Perez & Brady's

Principles and Practice of Radiation Oncology

EDITORS

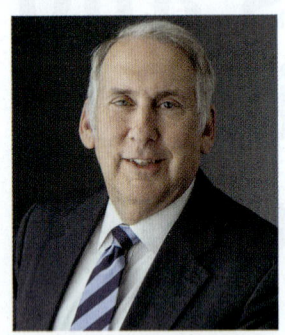

Edward C. Halperin, MD, MA

Chancellor for Health Affairs and Chief Executive Officer
New York Medical College
Professor of Radiation Oncology, Pediatrics, and History
Provost for Biomedical Affairs
Touro College and University
Valhalla, New York

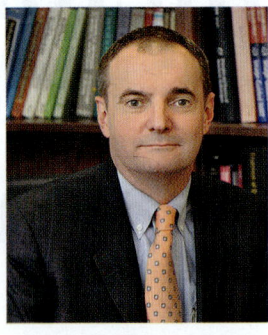

David E. Wazer, MD, FASTRO

Professor and Chairman
Radiation Oncologist-in-Chief
Department of Radiation Oncology
Tufts Medical Center
Tufts University School of Medicine
Boston, Massachusetts
Rhode Island Hospital
Alpert Medical School of Brown University
Providence, Rhode Island

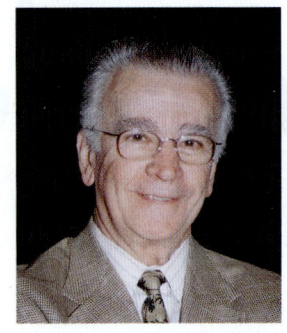

Carlos A. Perez, MD

Professor Emeritus
Department of Radiation Oncology
Mallinckrodt Institute of Radiology
Siteman Cancer Center
Washington University
St. Louis, Missouri

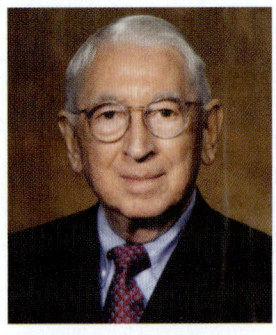

Luther W. Brady, MD

Distinguished University Professor
Hylda Cohn/American Cancer Society
Professor of Clinical Oncology
Professor, Department of Radiation Oncology
Drexel University College of Medicine
Philadelphia, Pennsylvania

Perez & Brady's

Principles and Practice of Radiation Oncology

Seventh Edition

Wolters Kluwer

Philadelphia • Baltimore • New York • London
Buenos Aires • Hong Kong • Sydney • Tokyo

Acquisitions Editor: Ryan Shaw
Editorial Coordinator: Lindsay Ries
Production Project Manager: Linda Van Pelt
Marketing Manager: Rachel Mante Leung
Designer: Teresa Mallon
Production Service: SPi Global

Library of Congress Cataloging-in-Publication Data
Names: Halperin, Edward C., editor. | Wazer, David E., editor. | Perez, Carlos A., 1934- editor. | Brady, Luther W., 1925- editor.
Title: Perez and Brady's principles and practice of radiation oncology / [edited by] Edward C. Halperin, David E. Wazer, Carlos A. Perez, Luther W. Brady.
Other titles: Principles and practice of radiation oncology
Description: Seventh edition. | Philadelphia : Wolters Kluwer, 2018. | Preceded by Perez and Brady's principles and practice of radiation oncology / editors, Edward C. Halperin ... [et al.]. 6th ed. c2013. | Includes bibliographical references and index.
Identifiers: LCCN 2018023918 | ISBN 9781496386793 (hardback)
Subjects: | MESH: Neoplasms—radiotherapy | Radiotherapy—methods | Radiometry
Classification: LCC RC271.R3 | NLM QZ 269 | DDC 616.99/40642—dc23 LC record available at https://lccn.loc.gov/2018023918

To our patients, who have taught us through both their courage and their suffering,

To our teachers, who inspired and mentored us with knowledge and wisdom,

To our trainees, who will make the cancer care of tomorrow better than today's,

To the universities where we work—institutions that are committed to generation, conservation, and dissemination of knowledge about the causes, prevention, and treatment of human disease and disability:

To our families, who unselfishly endorsed our work on this book.

Contributors

Todd Adams, MD
Radiation Oncologist
Department of Radiation Oncology
Virginia Commonwealth University
  Health
Assistant Professor
Department of Radiation Oncology
Massey Cancer Center
Virginia Commonwealth University
Richmond, Virginia

Anesa Ahamad, MD, FRCR
Associate Professor
Department of Radiation Oncology
Miller School of Medicine
University of Miami
Sylvester Comprehensive Cancer Center
University of Miami Health System
Miami, Florida

Mansoor M. Ahmed, PhD
Program Director
Radiation Research Program
Division of Cancer Treatment and
  Diagnosis
National Cancer Institute
National Institutes of Health
Bethesda, Maryland

Kaled M. Alektiar, MD
Radiation Oncologist
Department of Radiation Oncology
Memorial Sloan Kettering Cancer Center
New York, New York

Robert J. Amdur, MD
Department of Radiation Oncology
College of Medicine
University of Florida
Gainesville, Florida

Mark J. Amsbaugh, MD
Fellow
Radiation Oncology
The University of Texas MD Anderson
  Cancer Center
Houston, Texas

Douglas W. Arthur, MD
Chairman
Department of Radiation Oncology
Virginia Commonwealth University Health
Professor
Department of Radiation Oncology
Massey Cancer Center
Virginia Commonwealth University
Richmond, Virginia

Todd F. Atwood, PhD
Associate Professor
Department of Radiation Medicine and
  Applied Sciences
University of California, San Diego
La Jolla, California

Tracy A. Balboni, MD, MPH
Clinical Director
Supportive and Palliative Radiation
  Oncology
Women's Cancer Center
Department of Radiation Oncology
Dana-Farber/Brigham and Women's
  Cancer Center
Associate Professor
Department of Radiation Oncology
Harvard Medical School
Boston, Massachusetts

Elizabeth H. Baldini, MD, MPH
Associate Professor
Harvard Medical School
Radiation Oncology Director
Bone and Soft Tissue Sarcoma Program
Dana-Farber Cancer Institute and
  Brigham and Women's Hospital
Boston, Massachusetts

Michael Baumann, MD
Chief Physician
Department of Radiotherapy and
  Radiation Oncology
Faculty of Medicine and University
  Hospital Carl Gustav Carus
Technical University of Dresden
Dresden
Professor Dr. med.
Chairman and Scientific Director
German Cancer Research Center
Heidelberg, Germany

Jose G. Bazan, MD
Associate Professor
Department of Radiation Oncology
The James Cancer Hospital and Solove
  Research Institute
Associate Professor
Department of Radiation Oncology
The Ohio State University
Columbus, Ohio

Jennifer R. Bellon, MD
Associate Professor
Department of Radiation Oncology
Harvard Medical School
Director of Breast Radiation Oncology
Department of Radiation Oncology
Dana-Farber Cancer Institute and
  Brigham and Women's Hospital
Boston, Massachusetts

Stanley H. Benedict, PhD, FAAPM
*Professor and Vice Chair of Clinical
  Physics and Professor of Biomedical
  Engineering Graduate Group*
Department of Radiation Oncology
University of California at Davis Cancer
  Center
Sacramento, California

Ross Stuart Berkowitz, MD
Surgical Director
Department of Gynecologic Oncology
Dana-Farber/Brigham and Women's
  Cancer Center
Professor of Gynecology
Department of Obstetrics and Gynecology
Harvard Medical School
Boston, Massachusetts

Abigail T. Berman, MD, MSCE
Physician
Department of Radiation Oncology
Hospital of the University of
  Pennsylvania
Assistant Professor
Department of Radiation Oncology
University of Pennsylvania
Philadelphia, Pennsylvania

Eric J. Bernhard, PhD
Chief, Radiotherapy Development Branch
Radiation Research Program
Division of Cancer Treatment and
  Diagnosis
National Cancer Institute
National Institutes of Health
Bethesda, Maryland

Brian J. Boyce, MD
Assistant Professor
Department of Otolaryngology
University of Florida Health Shands
  Hospital
Associate Professor
Department of Otolaryngology
University of Florida
Gainesville, Florida

Luther W. Brady, MD
Distinguished University Professor
Hylda Cohn/American Cancer Society
Professor of Clinical Oncology
*Professor, Department of Radiation
  Oncology*
Drexel University College of Medicine
Philadelphia, Pennsylvania

Jeffrey D. Bradley, MD
*S. Lee Kling Endowed Professor of
  Radiation Oncology*
Department of Radiation Oncology
Washington University School of Medicine
St. Louis, Missouri

John C. Breneman, MD
*Charles M. Barrett Professor of
  Radiation Oncology and Adjunct
  Professor of Neurosurgery*
University of Cincinnati College of Medicine
Cincinnati Children's Hospital Medical
  Center
Cincinnati, Ohio

David J. Brenner, PhD, DSc
Professor
Center for Radiological Research
Department of Radiation Oncology
Columbia University Irving Medical Center
New York, New York

David M. Brizel, MD
*Leonard Prosnitz Professor of Radiation
    Oncology*
Professor, Head and Neck Surgery
*Co-Director, Head and Neck Cancer
    Program*
Duke Cancer Institute
Durham, North Carolina

Simon A. Brown, MD
Chief Resident and Instructor
Department of Radiation Medicine
Oregon Health & Science University
Portland, Oregon

Jeremy M. Brownstein, MD
Resident Physician
Department of Radiation Oncology
Duke University Medical Center
Durham, North Carolina

Thomas Buchholz, MD
Professor
Department of Radiation Oncology
Scripps Radiation Therapy Center
Medical Director
Department of Radiation Oncology
Scripps MD Anderson Cancer Center
San Diego, California

Jeffrey C. Buchsbaum, MD, PhD, AM
Medical Officer and Program Director
Radiation Research Program
Division of Cancer Treatment and
    Diagnosis
National Cancer Institute
National Institutes of Health
Bethesda, Maryland

Zachary Buchwald, MD, PhD
Resident
Department of Radiation Oncology
Emory University
Atlanta, Georgia

Jacek Capala, PhD, DSc
Program Director
Radiation Research Program
Division of Cancer Treatment and
    Diagnosis
National Cancer Institute
National Institutes of Health
Bethesda, Maryland

Dana L. Casey, MD
Radiation Oncology Resident
Department of Radiation Oncology
Memorial Sloan Kettering Cancer
    Center
New York, New York

Eric M. Chang, MD
Radiation Oncology Resident
Department of Radiation Oncology
David Geffen School of Medicine at
    University of California
Los Angeles, California

K. S. Clifford Chao, MD
Vice President
China Medical University
Superintendent
Cancer Center
China Medical University Hospital
Taichung, Taiwan

Yiyi Chen, PhD
Associate Professor in Biostatistics
OHSU-PSU School of Public Health,
    Knight Cancer Institute
Oregon Health & Science University
Portland, Oregon

Zhe (Jay) Chen, PhD
Smilow Chief Physicist
Department of Radiation Oncology
Yale New Haven Hospital
Professor
Department of Therapeutic Radiology
Yale University School of Medicine
New Haven, Connecticut

Skye Hung-Chun Cheng, MD
Chief
Department of Radiation Oncology
Koo Foundation Sun Yat-Sen Cancer
    Center
Taipei, Taiwan

Tsun-I Cheng, MD
Master Physician
Department of Internal Medicine
Koo Foundation Sun Yat-Sen Cancer Center
Taipei, Taiwan

Bhishamjit S. Chera
Associate Professor
Department of Radiation Oncology
University of North Carolina School of
    Medicine
UNC Hospitals
Chapel Hill, North Carolina

Indrin J. Chetty, PhD
Director of Medical Physics
Department of Radiation Oncology
Henry Ford Cancer Institute
Professor, Full-time Affiliate
Department of Radiation Oncology
Wayne State University Medical
    School
Detroit, Michigan

Arpit Chhabra, MD
Clinical Radiation Oncology Fellow
Department of Radiation Oncology
University of Maryland Medical
    Center
Baltimore, MD

Junzo P. Chino, MD
Associate Professor
Department of Radiation Oncology
Duke Cancer Center
Associate Professor
Department of Radiation Oncology
Duke University
Durham, North Carolina

Hak Choy, MD
Professor and Chairman
Department of Radiation Oncology
University of Texas Southwestern
    Medical Center
Dallas, Texas

Jared D. Christensen, MD
Associate Professor
Department of Radiation Oncology
Duke University School of Medicine
*Division Chief, Cardiothoracic
    Imaging*
*Director, Duke Lung Cancer Screening
    Program*
Department of Radiation Oncology
Duke University Medical Center
Durham, North Carolina

Hans T. Chung, MD, FRCPC
Assistant Professor
Department of Radiation
    Oncology
University of Toronto
Odette Cancer Centre
Sunnybrook Health Sciences
    Centre
Toronto, Ontario, Canada

Line Claude, MD
Chief
Department of Radiotherapy
Centre Leon Berard
Lyon, France

John J. Coen, MD
Radiation Oncologist
21st Century Oncology
Providence, Rhode Island

C. Norman Coleman, MD
Associate Director
Radiation Research Program
Division of Cancer Treatment and
    Diagnosis
National Cancer Institute
National Institutes of Health
Bethesda, Maryland

Stephanie E. Combs, MD, PhD
Professor and Chair
Department of Radiation Oncology
Technical University of Munich
Klinikum rechts der Isar Ismaninger
    Straße
München
Director
Institute of Innovative Radiotherapy
Oberschleißheim, Germany

Louis S. Constine, MD
Attending Physician
Department of Radiation Oncology and
    Pediatrics
Strong Memorial and Golisano Children's
    Hospitals
Professor
Department of Radiation Oncology and
    Pediatrics
University of Rochester
Rochester, New York

Stacy Lorine Cooper, MD
Assistant Professor of Oncology
Department of Medicine, Division of
    Oncology
Johns Hopkins School of Medicine
Baltimore, Maryland

Nils Cordes, MD
Professor
Department of Radiotherapy and
    Radiation Oncology
Faculty of Medicine
University Hospital Carl Gustav
    Carus
Technical University of Dresden
Professor
OncoRay—National Center for Radiation
    Research in Oncology
Technical University of Dresden
Dresden, Germany

Brian G. Czito, MD
Associate Professor
Department of Radiation
    Oncology
Duke University Medical Center
Durham, North Carolina

Roi Dagan, MD
Department of Radiation Oncology
College of Medicine
University of Florida
Gainesville, Florida

Rupak K. Das, PhD
Professor
Department of Human Oncology
University of Wisconsin
Madison, Wisconsin

Brittany A. Davidson, MD
Assistant Professor
Department of Obstetrics and
    Gynecology
Duke Cancer Center
Assistant Professor
Department of Obstetrics and
    Gynecology
Duke University School of Medicine
Durham, North Carolina

Roy H. Decker, MD, PhD
Professor
Department of Therapeutic Radiology
Yale University School of Medicine
New Haven, Connecticut

Phillip M. Devlin, MD, FACR, FASTRO, FFRRCSI (Hon)
Associate Professor
Department of Radiation Oncology
Harvard Medical School
Brigham and Women's Hospital
Boston, Massachusetts

Adam P. Dicker, MD, PhD
Enterprise Senior Vice President,
    Professor, and Chair
Director SKMC SI Program in Digital
    Health & Data Science
Department of Radiation Oncology
Sidney Kimmel Medical College &
    Cancer Center
Thomas Jefferson University
Philadelphia, Pennsylvania

Sarah S. Donaldson, MD
Catharine and Howard Avery Professor
Department of Radiation Oncology
Stanford University School of Medicine
Stanford, California

Anthony E. Dragun, MD
Chairman
Department of Radiation Oncology
MD Anderson Cancer Center at Cooper
    University Hospital
Camden, New Jersey

Dan G. Duda, DMD, PhD
Assistant Professor of Radiation
    Oncology
Edwin L. Steele Laboratory for Tumor
    Biology
Department of Radiation Oncology
Massachusetts General Hospital and
    Harvard Medical School
Boston, Massachusetts

Peter T. Dziegielewski, MD, FRCSC
Assistant Professor
Department of Otolaryngology
University of Florida
Chief of Head and Neck Surgical
    Oncology and Microvascular
    Reconstructive Surgery
Department of Otolaryngology
University of Florida Health
Gainesville, Florida

Tony Y. Eng, MD
Professor
Department of Radiation Oncology
Winship Cancer Institute of Emory
    University
Faculty
Department of Radiation Oncology
Emory University Hospital
Atlanta, Georgia

Natia Esiashvili, MD
Chief Quality Officer
Department of Radiation Oncology
Winship Cancer Institute
Associate Professor
Department of Radiation Oncology
Emory University
Atlanta, Georgia

Josh Evans, PhD, DABR
Assistant Professor
Department of Radiation Oncology
Virginia Commonwealth University
Richmond, Virginia

John C. Flickinger, MD
Professor of Radiation Oncology
University of Pittsburgh School of
    Medicine
Pittsburgh, Pennsylvania

Silvia C. Formenti, MD
Sandra and Edward Meyer Professor of
    Cancer Research
Chairman
Department of Radiation Oncology
Weill Cornell Medical College
Radiation Oncologist-in-Chief
Department of Radiation Oncology
New York Presbyterian Hospital
New York, New York

Steven J. Frank, MD
Associate Professor
Department of Radiation Oncology
The University of Texas MD Anderson
    Cancer Center
Houston, Texas

Clifton David Fuller, MD, PhD
Co-Medical Director
Program in Image-Guided Cancer Therapy
The University of Texas MD Anderson
    Cancer Center
Associate Professor
Department of Radiation Oncology
The University of Texas MD Anderson
    Cancer Center
Houston, Texas

Hiram A. Gay, MD
Radiation Oncologist
Department of Radiation Oncology
Barnes-Jewish Hospital
One Barnes-Jewish Hospital Plaza
Associate Professor
Department of Radiation Oncology
Washington University School of
    Medicine
St. Louis, Missouri

Jessica L. Geiger, MD
Clinical Assistant Professor
Medicine
Cleveland Clinic Lerner College of
    Medicine
Associate Staff
Hematology and Oncology
Taussig Cancer Institute
Cleveland Clinic
Cleveland, Ohio

Erin F. Gillespie, MD
Assistant Attending
Department of Radiation Oncology
Memorial Sloan Kettering Cancer Center
New York, New York

Daniel W. Golden, MD, MHPE
Assistant Professor
Department of Radiation and Cellular
    Oncology
University of Chicago
Chicago, Illinois

Daniel R. Gomez, MD
Associate Professor
Department of Radiation Oncology
The University of Texas MD Anderson
    Cancer Center
Houston, Texas

Vinai Gondi, MD
Co-Director
Brain and Spine Tumor Center
Northwestern Medicine Cancer Center
    Warrenville
Director of Research and Education
Northwestern Medicine Chicago Proton
    Center
Warrenville
Department of Radiation Oncology
Northwestern University Feinberg
    School of Medicine
Chicago, Illinois

Sharad Goyal, MD
Director
Department of Radiation Oncology
Professor and Chief
Department of Radiation Oncology
George Washington University Hospital
Washington, District of Columbia

Jimm Grimm, PhD, DABR
Senior Medical Physicist
Department of Radiation Oncology and
    Molecular Radiation Sciences
Johns Hopkins University
Baltimore, Maryland

Sean Grimm, MD
Health System Clinician
Department of Neurology
Chicago
Director of Medical Neuro-Oncology
Northwestern Medicine West Region
Warrenville, Illinois

Chandan Guha, MBBS, PhD
Director, Einstein Institute for Onco-Physics
Professor and Vice Chairman
Department of Radiation Oncology
Professor, Departments of Urology and
    Pathology
Montefiore Medical Center
Albert Einstein College of Medicine
Bronx, New York

Bruce G. Haffty, MD
Professor and Chairman
Department of Radiation Oncology
Rutgers Cancer Institute of New Jersey
New Brunswick, New Jersey

Edward C. Halperin, MD, MA
Chancellor for Health Affairs and Chief
    Executive Officer
New York Medical College
Professor of Radiation Oncology,
    Pediatrics, and History
Provost for Biomedical Affairs
Touro College and University
Valhalla, New York

Timothy P. Hanna, MD, MSc, FRCPC
Radiation Oncology Research Fellow
Collaboration for Cancer Outcomes
    Research and Evaluation
Liverpool Hospital
New South Wales, Australia

James E. Hansen, MD
Attending Physician
Department of Therapeutic Radiology
Smilow Cancer Hospital
Yale New Haven Health
Assistant Professor
Department of Therapeutic Radiology
Yale University School of Medicine
New Haven, Connecticut

Paul M. Harari, MD, FASTRO
Jack Fowler Professor and Chairman
Department of Human Oncology
University of Wisconsin School of
    Medicine and Public Health
Madison, Wisconsin

Alexander A. Harris, MD
Resident Physician
Department of Radiation Oncology
Stritch School of Medicine
Loyola University Chicago
Chicago, Illinois

William F. Hartsell, MD
Medical Director
CDH Proton Center, A ProCure Center
Warrenville, Illinois

Jaroslaw T. Hepel, MD, FACRO
Director of Radiosurgery
Department of Radiation Oncology
Lifespan Cancer Institute
Rhode Island Hospital
Associate Professor
Department of Radiation Oncology
Brown University
Providence, Rhode Island

James W. Hodge, PhD
*Deputy Chief, Laboratory of Tumor
    Immunology and Biology*
*Senior Investigator, Head, Recombinant
    Vaccine Group*
National Cancer Institute
National Institutes of Health
Bethesda, Maryland

David C. Hodgson, MD, MPH
Radiation Oncologist
Radiation Medicine Program
Princess Margaret Cancer Centre
Professor
Department of Radiation Oncology
University of Toronto
Faculty of Medicine
Toronto, Ontario, Canada

Henry T. Hoffman, MD
Department of Otolaryngology
University of Iowa
Iowa City, Iowa

Caroline Holloway, MD, FRCPC
Radiation Oncologist
Department of Radiation
    Oncology
BC Cancer—Victoria
Clinical Assistant Professor
Department of Radiation Oncology and
    Developmental Radiotherapeutics
University of British Columbia
Vancouver, British Columbia

Bradford S. Hoppe, MD, MPH
Associate Professor
Department of Radiation Oncology
University of Florida Health Proton
    Therapy Institute
Jacksonville
Associate Professor
Department of Radiation Oncology
University of Florida
Gainesville, Florida

Richard T. Hoppe, MD
Professor
Department of Radiation Oncology
Stanford Hospital and Clinics
*The Henry S. Kaplan-Harry Lebeson
    Professor in Cancer Biology*
Department of Radiation Oncology
Stanford University
Stanford, California

Andrew T. Huang, MD
President and CEO
Koo Foundation Sun Yat-Sen Cancer
    Center
Taipei, Taiwan
Professor of Medicine
Duke University
Durham, North Carolina

Jiayi Huang, MD
Assistant Professor
Department of Radiation Oncology
Washington University School of
    Medicine
Radiation Oncologist
Department of Radiation Oncology
Barnes-Jewish Hospital
St. Louis, Missouri

Paris-Ann Ingledew, MD
Radiation Oncologist
Department of Radiation Oncology
BC Cancer, Vancouver Cancer
    Center
Clinical Associate Professor
Division of Radiation Oncology and
    Radiotherapeutics
University of British Columbia
Vancouver, British Columbia

Jerry J. Jaboin, MD, PhD
Associate Professor and Vice Chair
Department of Radiation Medicine
Oregon Health & Science
    University
Portland, Orlando

Rakesh K. Jain, PhD
*A.W. Cook Professor of Tumor
    Biology*
*Director, Edwin L. Steele Laboratory for
    Tumor Biology*
Department of Radiation Oncology
Massachusetts General Hospital and
    Harvard Medical School
Boston, Massachusetts

**Peter A. S. Johnstone, MD, FACR,
FASTO**
Senior Member and Vice Chair
Departments of Radiation Oncology and
    Health Outcomes and Behavior
Moffitt Cancer Center and Research
    Institute
Professor
Department of Oncologic Science
University of South Florida
Tampa, Florida

John A. Kalapurakal, MD
Professor
Radiation Oncology
Northwestern University Feinberg
    School of Medicine
Chicago, Illinois

Tadashi Kamada, MD, PhD
Clinical Research Cluster
National Institute of Radiological
    Sciences
Inage-Ku, Chiba, Japan

Christopher J. Kandl, MD
Assistant Professor
Department of Otolaryngology Head and
    Neck Surgery
VCU Massey Cancer Center
Assistant Professor
Department of Otolaryngology Head and
    Neck Surgery
Virginia Commonwealth University
Richmond, Virginia

Josephine Kang, MD, PhD
Assistant Professor
Department of Radiation Oncology
Weill Cornell Medical Center
New York, New York

Brian D. Kavanagh, MD, MPH
Professor of Radiation Oncology
University of Colorado School of Medicine
Aurora, Colorado

Chris R. Kelsey, MD
Associate Professor
Department of Radiation Oncology
Duke University Medical Centre
Durham, North Carolina

Atif J. Khan, MD
Associate Attending
Department of Radiation Oncology
Memorial Sloan Kettering Cancer
    Center
New York, New York

Grace J. Kim, MD, PhD
Assistant Professor
Department of Radiation Oncology
Duke University
Durham, North Carolina

D. Nathan Kim, MD, PhD
Associate Professor
Department of Radiation Oncology
University of Texas Southwestern
    Medical Center
Dallas, Texas

Youn H. Kim, MD
Director/Professor
Dermatology-Cutaneous Lymphoma
Stanford Cancer Institute
Stanford
Director/Professor
Dermatology-Cutaneous Lymphoma
Stanford University
Palo Alto, California

**Timothy J. Kinsella, MD, MS, MA (ad
eundem), FASTRO**
Department of Radiation Oncology
Rhode Island Hospital
Research Scholar Professor
Department of Radiation Oncology
The Warner Alpert Medical School of
    Brown University
Providence, Rhode Island

John P. Kirkpatrick, MD, PhD
Clinical Director
Department of Radiation Oncology
Associate Professor
Department of Radiation Oncology and
  Neurosurgery
Duke University Medical Center
Durham, North Carolina

Jessica M. Kirwan, MA
Research Coordinator
Department of Radiation Oncology
University of Florida
Gainesville, Florida

Eric E. Klein, PhD
Professor
Department of Radiation Oncology
Brown University
Rhode Island Hospital
Providence, Rhode Island

Paul Patrick Koffer, MD
Resident
Department of Radiation Oncology
Tufts Medical Center
Boston, Massachusetts

**Andre A. Konski, MD, MBA, MA,
FACR, FASTRO**
Professor of Clinical Radiation Oncology
Department of Radiation Oncology
University of Pennsylvania
Perelman School of Medicine
Senior Fellow
Leonard Davis Institute of Health
  Economics
University of Pennsylvania
Medical Director
Department of Radiation Oncology
The Chester County Hospital
West Chester, Philadelphia

Mechthild Krause, MD
Director
OncoRay—National Center for Radiation
  Research in Oncology
Faculty of Medicine
Technical University of Dresden
Director
Department of Radiotherapy and
  Radiation Oncology
University Hospital Carl Gustav Carus
  Dresden
Dresden, Germany

Timothy J. Kruser, MD
Assistant Professor
Department of Radiation Oncology
Northwestern Memorial Hospital
Northwestern University Feinberg
  School of Medicine
Chicago, Illinois

Ina Kurth, PhD
Doctor Rerum Naturalium
Department of Radiooncology/
  Radiobiology
German Cancer Research Center
Heidelberg, Germany

Young Kwok, MD
Associate Professor
Department of Radiation Oncology
University of Maryland School of Medicine
Baltimore, Maryland

Corey J. Langer, MD
Professor
Director, Thoracic Oncology
University of Pennsylvania
Philadelphia, Pennsylvania

George E. Laramore, PhD, MD
*Peter Wootton Professor of Radiation
  Oncology*
Department of Radiation Oncology
University of Washington
Seattle, Washington

Larissa Lee, MD
*Director, Gynecologic Radiation
  Oncology*
Department of Radiation Oncology
Dana-Farber/Brigham and Women's
  Cancer Center
Assistant Professor
Department of Radiation Oncology
Harvard Medical School
Boston, Massachusetts

Nancy Y. Lee, MD
Radiation Oncologist
Memorial Sloan Kettering Cancer Center
New York, New York

Jonathan E. Leeman, MD
Instructor
Department of Radiation Oncology
Dana Farber Cancer Institute/Brigham
  and Women's Hospital
Longwood Radiation Oncology Center
Boston, Massachusetts

Zuofeng Li, DSc
Professor
Department of Radiation Oncology
University of Florida
Gainesville
Physics Director
UF Health Proton Therapy Institute
Jacksonville, Florida

Bruce Libby, PhD
Associate Professor
Department of Radiation Oncology
University of Virginia
Charlottesville, Virginia

Yolande Lievens, MD, PhD
*Head of Radiation Oncology
  Department*
Ghent University Hospital
Professor in Radiation Oncology
Ghent University
Ghent, Belgium

Annett Linge, MD
Clinician Scientist
Department of Radiotherapy and
  Radiation Oncology
University Hospital Carl Gustav Carus
German Cancer Consortium (DKTK)
German Cancer Research Center
  (DKFZ)
OncoRay
Dresden, Germany

Mirrorer Ming-Jiung Liu
Assistant Member
Department of Radiation Oncology
Koo-Foundation Sun Yat-Sen Cancer
  Center
Taipei, Taiwan

Benjamin H. Lok, MD
Staff Radiation Oncologist
Radiation Medicine Program
Princess Margaret Cancer Centre
Assistant Professor
Department of Radiation Oncology
University of Toronto
Faculty of Medicine
Toronto, Ontario, Canada

Laurel J. Lyckholm, MD
*Harvey M. Meyerhoff Professor of
  Bioethics and Medicine*
Clinical Professor of Internal Medicine
Section of Hematology, Oncology
  and Blood and Marrow
  Transplantation
*Faculty, Program in Bioethics and
  Humanities*
Carver College of Medicine
University of Iowa
Iowa City, Iowa

Roger M. Macklis, MD
Staff Physician
Department of Radiation Oncology
Taussig Cancer Institute
Cleveland Clinic
Professor of Medicine
Cleveland Clinic Lerner College of
  Medicine
Cleveland, Ohio

Anita Mahajan, MD
Professor
Department of Radiation Oncology
Mayo Clinic
Rochester, Minnesota

Brandon A. Mahal, MD
Physician
Department of Radiation Oncology
Brigham and Women's Hospital/
  Dana-Farber Cancer Institute
Physician
Department of Radiation Oncology
Harvard Medical School
Boston, Massachussets

Anthony A. Mancuso, MD
Professor and Chair
Department of Radiology
University of Florida Health Shands
  Hospital
Professor and Chair
Department of Radiology
University of Florida
Gainesville, Florida

Rafael R. Mañon, MD
Vice Chairman
Department of Radiation Oncology
Orlando Health
Orlando
Adjunct Faculty
Department of Radiation Oncology
University of Florida
Gainesville, Florida

David B. Mansur, MD
*Associate Professor and Vice Chair
  for Education*
Department of Radiation Oncology
Case Western Reserve University School
  of Medicine
*Director of Pediatric and Hematologic
  Radiation Oncology*
University Hospitals Seidman Cancer
  Center
Rainbow Babies and Children's
  Hospital
Cleveland, Ohio

Lawrence B. Marks, MD, FASTRO
Professor and Chair
Department of Radiation Oncology
University of North Carolina School of
  Medicine
North Carolina Cancer Hospital
Chapel Hill, North Carolina

John D. Martin, PhD
JSPS Postdoctoral Fellow
Department of Bioengineering
The University of Tokyo
Tokyo, Japan

Ursula A. Matulonis, MD
Chief, Division of Gynecologic Oncology
Department of Medical Oncology
Dana-Farber Cancer Institute
Professor of Medicine
Department of Medical Oncology
Harvard Medical School
Boston, Massachusetts

Joel L. Mayerson, MD
Professor
Orthopaedic Surgery
The Ohio State University School of
    Medicine
Director, Sarcoma Service
Orthopaedic Surgery
The Arthur G James Cancer Hospital
    at The Ohio State University Wexner
    Medical Center
Columbus, Ohio

Lukasz Mazur, PhD
Director of Healthcare Engineering
Department of Radiation Oncology
Assistant Professor
Department of Radiation Oncology,
    School of Medicine
School of Library and Information Science
University of North Carolina
Chapel Hill, North Carolina

William H. McBride, PhD, DSc
Distinguished Professor Emeritus
Department of Radiation Oncology
University of California at Los Angeles
Los Angeles, California

Minesh P. Mehta, MD, FASTRO
Deputy Director
Miami Cancer Institute
Chief of Radiation Oncology, and Professor
Florida International University
Miami, Florida

Loren K. Mell, MD
*Professor and Vice Chair, Clinical &
    Translational Research*
Department of Radiation Medicine and
    Applied Sciences
University of California San Diego
La Jolla, California

Nancy P. Mendenhall, MD, FASTRO
Professor and Associate Chair
Department of Radiation Oncology
University of Florida
Gainesville, Florida
Medical Director
University of Florida Health Proton
    Therapy Institute
Jacksonville, Florida

William M. Mendenhall, MD
Department of Radiation Oncology
University of Florida College of
    Medicine
Gainesville, Florida

Lucas C. Mendez, MD
Clinical Fellow
Department of Radiation Oncology
University of Toronto
Sunnybrook Odette Cancer Centre
Toronto, Ontario, Canada

Jeff M. Michalski, MD, MBA
*Vice Chair and Director of Clinical
    Programs*
Department of Radiation Oncology
Barnes-Jewish Hospital
*Carlos A. Perez Distinguished
    Professor*
Department of Radiation Oncology
Washington University School of
    Medicine
St. Louis, Missouri

Joseph Mikhael, MD, Med
Chief Medical Officer
Department of Hematology
International Myeloma Foundation
North Hollywood
Professor
Department of Hematology
City of Hope National Medical Centre
Duarte, California

Michael T. Milano, MD, PhD
Associate Professor
Department of Radiation Oncology
Strong Memorial Hospital
Associate Professor
Department of Radiation Oncology
University of Rochester
Rochester, New York

Eric D. Miller, PhD
Assistant Professor
Department of Radiation Oncology
Ohio State University Wexner Medical
    Center
Columbus, Ohio

Mark Mishra, MD
*Assistant Professor and Director of
    Clinical Research*
Department of Radiation Oncology
University of Maryland Medical Center
Baltimore, Maryland

**Gustavo S. Montana, MD, FACR,
FASTRO**
Emeritus Professor
Department of Radiation Oncology
Duke University Medical Center
Durham, North Carolina

Meena S. Moran, MD
*Director, Yale Radiation Breast
    Program*
Department of Therapeutic Radiology
Smilow Cancer Center
Professor
Department of Therapeutic
    Radiology
Yale University School of Medicine
New Haven, Connecticut

Gerard C. Morton, MB, MRCPI, FRCPC
Radiation Oncologist
Department of Radiation Oncology
Sunnybrook Health Sciences Centre—
    Odette Cancer Centre
Associate Professor
Department of Radiation Oncology
University of Toronto
Toronto, Ontario, Canada

Prithima Mosaly, PhD, MHA
Assistant Professor
Division of Healthcare Engineering
Department of Radiation Oncology
University of North Carolina School of
    Medicine
Chapel Hill, North Carolina

Benjamin Movsas, MD
Chair
Department of Radiation Oncology
Henry Ford Cancer Institute
Professor
Department of Radiation Oncology
Wayne State University
Detroit, Michigan

Yvonne Marie Mowery, MD, PhD
Butler Harris Assistant Professor
Department of Radiation Oncology
Duke Health
Department of Radiation Oncology
Duke University School of Medicine
Durham, North Carolina

Arno J. Mundt, MD
Professor and Chair
Department of Radiation Medicine and
    Applied Sciences
University of California San Diego
La Jolla, California

James D. Murphy, MD, MS
Associate Professor
Radiation Medicine and Applied
    Sciences
University of California San Diego
La Jolla, California

Sasa Mutic, PhD, FAAPM
*Vice Chair, Medical Physics and Clinical
    Strategy*
Director, Medical Physics Division
Professor of Radiation Oncology
Department of Radiation Oncology
Washington University School of Medicine
St. Louis, Missouri

Jeffrey N. Myers, MD, PhD, FACS
*Chair, Department of Head and Neck
    Surgery*
*Alando J. Ballantyne Distinguished
    Chair of Head and Neck Surgery*
University of Texas MD Anderson
    Cancer Center
Houston, Texas

**Subir Nag, MD, FACR, FACRO,
FASTRO, FABS**
Director
International Oncologic Health Center
Saratoga
Clinical Professor (Affiliated)
Department of Radiation Oncology
Stanford University School of Medicine
Stanford, California

Carsten Nieder, MD
Professor
Department of Clinical Medicine
The Arctic University of Norway
Troms
Consultant Oncologist
Department of Oncology and Palliative
    Medicine
Nerdland Hospital Trust
Bodes, Norway

William P. O'Meara, MD, MPH
Radiation Oncologist
Lahey Hospital & Medical Center
Peabody, Massachusetts

Sophie J. Otter, MBBChir, FRCR
Clinical Research Fellow
Department of Oncology
University of Surrey
Royal Surrey County Hospital
Guilford, United Kingdom

Laura Padilla, PhD, DABR
Assistant Professor
Department of Radiation Oncology
Virginia Commonwealth University
Richmond, Virginia

Manisha Palta, MD
Associate Professor
Department of Radiation Oncology
Duke University
Durham, North Carolina

Roy A. Patchell, MD
Chief of Neuro-Oncology
Capital Health
Hopewell, New Jersey

Arnold C. Paulino, MD
Professor
Department of Radiation Oncology
MD Anderson Cancer Center
Houston, Texas

Carlos A. Perez, MD
Professor Emeritus
Department of Radiation Oncology
Mallinckrodt Institute of Radiology
Siteman Cancer Center
Washington University
St. Louis, Missouri

Angelica Perez-Andujar, PhD, DABR
Assistant Professor
Radiation Oncology
University of California–San Francisco
San Francisco, California

Nikolai Podoltsev, MD
Attending Physician (Hematology)
Smilow Cancer Hospital—Yale New
    Haven Health
Assistant Professor of Medicine
Yale University School of Medicine
New Haven, Connecticut

Pascal Pommier, MD, PhD
Head of the Brachytherapy Unit
Department of Radiation Oncology
Centre Leon Bérard
Lyon, France

Pataje G. Prasanna, PhD
Program Director
Clinical Radiotherapy Development
    Branch
Radiation Research Program
Division of Cancer Treatment and
    Diagnosis
National Cancer Institute
National Institutes of Health
Bethesda, Maryland

Leonard R. Prosnitz, MD, FACR, FASTRO
Professor and Chair, Emeritus
Department of Radiation Oncology
Duke University Medical Center
Durham, North Carolina

James A. Purdy, PhD
Professor Emeritus
Department of Radiation Oncology
Washington University School of Medicine
St. Louis, Missouri

Ann C. Raldow, MD, MPH
Assistant Professor
Department of Radiation Oncology
David Geffen School of Medicine at
    University of California
Los Angeles, California

Avani Dholakia Rao, MD
Resident
Department of Radiation Oncology and
    Molecular Radiation Oncology
Johns Hopkins University School of Medicine
Baltimore, Maryland

William Regine, MD, FACR, FACRO
*Isadore & Fannie Schneider Foxman
    Chair*
Department of Radiation Oncology
University of Maryland Medical Center
Baltimore, Maryland

Ramesh Rengan, MD, PhD
Professor
Department of Radiation Oncology
University of Washington
Seattle, Washington

Mack Roach III, MD, FACR, FASTRO
Professor
Department of Radiation Oncology and
    Urology
Helen Diller Comprehensive Cancer
Mt. Zion Hospital
University of California, San Francisco
San Francisco, California

Kenneth B. Roberts, MD
Attending Physician
Department of Radiation Oncology
Yale New Haven Hospital
Professor
Department of Therapeutic Radiology
Yale University School of Medicine
New Haven, Connecticut

Clifford G. Robinson, MD
Associate Professor
Department of Radiation Oncology
Washington University School of
    Medicine
Radiation Oncologist
Department of Radiation Oncology
Barnes-Jewish Hospital
St. Louis, Missouri

Joseph K. Salama, MD
Associate Professor
Department of Radiation Oncology
Duke University
Durham, North Carolina

Nicholas J. Sanfilippo, MD
Assistant Professor
Department of Radiation Oncology
New York University School of
    Medicine
New York, New York

Rafael Santana-Davila, MD
Assistant Professor
Division of Medical Oncology
Department of Medicine
University of Washington/Seattle Cancer
    Care Alliance
Seattle, Washington

Dörthe Schaue, PhD
Associate Professor
Department of Radiation Oncology
University of California at Los Angeles
Los Angeles, California

Granger R. Scruggs, MD
*Texas Oncology—Department of
    Radiation Oncology*
Baylor University Medical
    Center—Dallas
Dallas, Texas

Stuart Evan Seropian, MD
Associate Professor of Medicine
Department of Hematology
Yale University
New Haven, Connecticut

Christiana M. Shaw, MD
Associate Professor
Department of Surgery
University of Florida
Associate Professor
Department of Surgery
UF Health Shands Hospital
Gainesville, Florida

Ron Y. Shiloh, MD
Attending Physician
Department of Radiation Oncology
Dana-Farber/Brigham and Women's
    Cancer Center
Instructor
Department of Radiation Oncology
Boston, Massachusetts

Shervin M. Shirvani, MD, MPH
Faculty Radiation Oncologist
Department of Radiation Oncology
Banner MD Anderson Cancer Center
Banner Boswell Medical Center
Sun City, Arizona
Adjunct Professor
Department of Radiation Oncology
The University of Texas MD Anderson
    Cancer Center
Houston, Texas

Daniel Robert Simpson, MD
Assistant Professor
Department of Radiation Medicine
University of California, San Diego
La Jolla, California

Tod W. Speer, MD
Radiation Oncologist
Department of Human Oncology
Radiation Oncology
University of Wisconsin School of
    Medicine and Public Health
Madison, Wisconsin

Michael L. Steinberg, MD
Professor and Chair
Department of Radiation Oncology
David Geffen School of Medicine at
    University of California
Los Angeles, California

Sarah Jo Stephens, MD
Resident
Department of Radiation Oncology
Duke University Medical Center
Durham, North Carolina

Alexandra J. Stewart, DM, MRCP, FRCR
Consultant Clinical Oncologist
St Luke's Cancer Centre
Royal Surrey County Hospital
Senior Lecturer
University of Surrey
Stag Hill, Guildford

Michael Story, PhD
*Professor, Vice Chair, and Chief, Division
    of Molecular Radiation Biology*
*David A. Pistenmaa, MD, PhD
    Distinguished Chair in Radiation
    Oncology*
Department of Radiation Oncology
UT Southwestern Medical Center
Dallas, Texas

Jeremy Sugarman, MD, MPH
Harvey M. Meyerhoff Professor of
  Bioethics and Medicine
Professor of Medicine
Professor of Health Policy and
  Management
Deputy Director for Medicine
Berman Institute of Bioethics
Johns Hopkins University
Baltimore, Maryland

Marie-Pierre Sunyach, MD
Department of Radiation therapy
Centre Leon Berard
Lyon, France

Ronan Tanguy, MD
Radiation Oncologist
Department of Radiation Therapy
Centre Leon Berard
Lyon, France

Roger E. Taylor, MA, FRCP, FRCR
Professor of Radiation Oncology
University of Wales
Swansea, Wales

Stephanie A. Terezakis, MD
Associate Professor
Department of Radiation Oncology and
  Molecular Radiation Sciences
Johns Hopkins School of Medicine
Baltimore, Maryland

Chris H. J. Terhaard, MD, PhD
Associate Professor
Radiation Oncologist
University Medical Center, Utrecht
Utrecht, The Netherlands

Bruce Thomadsen, PhD
Professor, Medical Physics
Departments of Medical Physics,
  Engineering Physics, Biomedical
  Engineering and Industrial and
  Systems Engineering
University of Wisconsin
Madison, Wisconsin

Charles R. Thomas Jr., MD
Service Chief
Department of Radiation Medicine
OHSU Health Care
Professor and Chair
Department of Radiation Medicine
Knight Cancer Institute
Oregon Health and Science University
Portland, Oregon

Wade L. Thorstad, MD
Chief, Head and Neck Service
Department of Radiation Oncology
Barnes-Jewish Hospital
Associate Professor
Department of Radiation Oncology
Washington University School of Medicine
St. Louis, Missouri

Robert D. Timmerman, MD
Professor of Radiation Oncology and
  Neurosurgery
Department of Radiation Oncology
University of Texas Southwestern
  Medical Center
Dallas, Texas

Filip T. Troicki, MD, MBA
Radiation Oncologist
Agnesian Cancer Center
SSM Health
Fond du Lac, Wisconsin

Pauline Truong, MDCM, FRCPC
Clinical Professor
Department of Radiation Oncology
University of British Columbia
Radiation Oncologist
Department of Radiation Oncology
British Columbia Cancer Agency
Victoria, British Columbia, Canada

Richard W. Tsang, MD
Radiation Oncologist
Radiation Medicine Program
Princess Margaret Cancer Centre
Professor
Department of Radiation Oncology
University of Toronto, Faculty of
  Medicine
Toronto, Ontario, Canada

Alfredo I. Urdaneta, MD
Radiation Oncologist
Department of Radiation Oncology
VCU Health
Assistant Professor
Department of Radiation Oncology
Massey Cancer Center
Virginia Commonwealth University
Richmond, Virginia

Brian A. Van Tine, MD, PhD
Associate Professor
Internal Medicine
Washington University
St. Louis, Missouri

Gregory M. M. Videtic, MD, CM,
FRCPC
Staff Physician
Department of Radiation Oncology
Taussig Cancer Institute
Cleveland Clinic
Associate Professor of Medicine
Cleveland Clinic Lerner College of
  Medicine
Cleveland, Ohio

Bhadrasain Vikram, MD, FACR
Chief, Clinical Radiation Oncology
  Branch
Radiation Research Program
Division of Cancer Treatment and
  Diagnosis
National Cancer Institute
National Institutes of Health
Bethesda, Maryland

Akila N. Viswanathan, MD, MPH
Executive Vice Chair
Department of Radiation Oncology and
  Molecular Radiation Sciences
Johns Hopkins Hospital
Professor
Department of Radiation Oncology and
  Molecular Radiation Sciences
Johns Hopkins University School of
  Medicine
Baltimore, Maryland

Michael A. Vogelbaum, MD, PhD
Associate Director of Neurosurgical
  Oncology
Brain Tumor and NeuroOncology
  Center
Cleveland Clinic
Professor of Neurosurgery
Department of Neurological Surgery
Cleveland Clinic Lerner College of
  Medicine of CWRU
Cleveland, Ohio

Gottfried von Keudell, MD, PhD
Assistant Attending
Department of Medicine/Lymphoma
  Service
Memorial Sloan Kettering Cancer
  Center
New York, New York

Zeljko Vujaskovic, MD, PhD
Professor
Department of Radiation Oncology
University of Maryland Medical
  System
Director, Division of Translational
  Radiation Science
Department of Radiation Oncology
University of Maryland School of
  Medicine
Baltimore, Maryland

Tony J. C. Wang, MD
Associate Attending
Department of Radiation Oncology
New York Presbyterian Hospital
Associate Professor
Department of Radiation Oncology
Columbia University
New York, New York

David E. Wazer, MD, FASTRO
Professor and Chairman
Radiation Oncologist-in-Chief
Department of Radiation Oncology
Tufts Medical Center
Tufts University School of
  Medicine
Boston, Massachusetts
Rhode Island Hospital
Alpert Medical School of Brown
  University
Providence, Rhode Island

Stephanie L. Wethington, MD, MSc
Assistant Professor
Department of Gynecology and
  Obstetrics
Johns Hopkins Hospital
Assistant Professor
Department of Gynecology and
  Obstetrics
Johns Hopkins University School of
  Medicine
Baltimore, Maryland

Christopher G. Willett, MD
Professor and Chair
Department of Radiation Oncology
Duke University Medical Center
Durham, North Carolina

Jeffrey F. Williamson, PhD, FAAPM,
FACR
Professor of Radiation Oncology
Department of Radiation Oncology
Virginia Commonwealth University
Richmond, Virginia

Lynn D. Wilson, MD, MPH
Attending Physician
Department of Radiation Oncology
Smilow Cancer Hospital
Yale-New Haven Health
Professor, Executive Vice Chairman
Director for Clinical Affairs
Department of Therapeutic
  Radiology
Yale School of Medicine
New Haven, Connecticut

Brian Winey, PhD
Medical Physicist
Department of Radiation Oncology
Physics Division
Massachusetts General Hospital
Assistant Professor
Department of Radiation Oncology
Harvard Medical School
Boston, Massachusetts

Matthew E. Witek, MD, MS
Assistant Professor
Department of Human Oncology
University of Wisconsin School of
    Medicine and Public Health
Madison, Wisconsin

H. Rodney Withers, AO, MD, DSc
Professor Emeritus (deceased)
Department of Radiation Oncology
University of California at Los Angeles
Los Angeles, California

Suzanne L. Wolden, MD, FACR
Member/Professor
Department of Radiation Oncology
Memorial Sloan Kettering Cancer Center
New York, New York

Serena Wong, MD
Associate Attending
Department of Medicine
Memorial Hospital for Cancer and Allied
    Diseases
New York, New York
Associate Clinical Member
Department of Medicine
Memorial Sloan Kettering Cancer Center
Middletown, New Jersey

Shiao Y. Woo, MD
Professor and Chairman
Radiation Oncology
University of Louisville
Louisville, Kentucky

Cheng-Shie Wuu, PhD
Director of Medical Physics
Department of Radiation Oncology
New York Presbyterian Hospital
Professor
Department of Radiation Oncology
Columbia University
New York, New York

Meng Xu-Welliver, MD, PhD
Assistant Professor
Department of Radiation
    Oncology
The Ohio State University Wexner
    Medical Center
Columbus, Ohio

**Theodore E. Yaeger, MD, FACRO,
FRSM**
*Associate Professor Radiation
    Oncology*
Wake Forest University School of
    Medicine
Winston-Salem, North Carolina

David S. Yoo, MD, PhD
Medical Instructor
Department of Radiation
    Oncology
Duke University Medical
    Center
Durham, North Carolina

Esther Yu, MD
*Clinical Assistant Professor of Radiation
    Oncology*
Department of Radiation Oncology
Warren Alpert Medical School of Brown
    University
Radiation Oncologist
Department of Radiation Oncology
Rhode Island Hospital
Providence, Rhode Island

Michael J. Zelefsky, MD
Professor of Radiation Oncology
Chief, Brachytherapy Service
Department of Radiation Oncology
Memorial Sloan Kettering Cancer
    Center
New York, New York

Jing Zeng, MD
Associate Professor
Department of Radiation Oncology
University of Washington
Seattle, Washington

Preface

The first edition of *Principles and Practice of Radiation Oncology* was published in 1987. This seventh edition is being published in 2018. After 31 years, approximately 11,000 pages of printed text, many tens of thousands of pages of typed and computer printed text, and an immeasurable number of meetings, phone calls, letters, e-mails, faxes, and text messages utilized to produce these seven volumes, many things have changed and others have stayed the same.

What has stayed the same? For 31 years, radiation therapy has remained a major component of the curative and palliative therapy of cancer and plays a major role in the management of many benign diseases. Patients with cancer are generally best managed by a combined modality approach that requires the participation of a well-informed, well-trained, and well-equipped radiation oncologist collaborating with a radiation oncology team. The radiation oncologist must be capable of taking a detailed medical history; performing a thorough and accurate physical examination of the patient; assessing and integrating the information from diagnostic imaging, from gross and microscopic pathology—incorporating a growing list of chemical and molecular markers that guide therapy and predict outcome—and from clinical chemistry; and formulating and implementing a treatment plan that is cognizant of the wishes of the patient and realistic in its goals. For this book, in particular, what has also stayed the same since 1987 is the vision and participation of Carlos A. Perez and Luther W. Brady, of Edward C. Halperin since 2004, and of David Wazer since 2008. We recognize that having such stability in the editorial team is exceptional in the history of textbook publishing and a blessing for the four of us. As we note below and in our acknowledgments, we remember and mourn those who contributed to previous editions of this book but are no longer with us: Ruth Aultman, Jonathan Pine, and Rupert Schmidt-Ullrich.

What has changed? There has been an explosion of knowledge concerning the molecular biology of cancer and tumor physiology. Concepts that were unknown in the 1980s are now considered fundamental building blocks of knowledge concerning cancer. As it concerns the technology of this specialty, when the first edition of this book was published, some radiation oncology residents were training, in part, on orthovoltage units; cobalt-60 machines remained in widespread use; simulation using diagnostic radiographs still vied with clinical setups of treatment fields using surface anatomy; and many radiation oncologists carried slide rules, protractors, right angle drafting triangles, and rulers to calculate and map radiation dose distributions. Now, elaborate linear accelerators with multileaf collimators, particle machines, intensity-modulated and/or image-guided radiation therapy, complex brachytherapy devices, dose painting, image fusion, metabolic imaging, and increasingly powerful computers that support the preceding list of technologies have become the norm in the developed world. (And, unfortunately, the paucity of even the most minimal radiation therapy services remains the norm in many parts of the economically less-developed world, and economic and racial disparities persist in cancer care and outcomes in the economically developed world....) In some diseases, the diagnostic and staging workup has changed profoundly in the past quarter of a century—for example, the role of staging laparotomy in Hodgkin disease. In other diseases, the role of radiotherapy in treatment has shifted dramatically, as demonstrated by the decline in the role or frequency of use of radiation therapy in the management of retinoblastoma and Wilms tumor, following balloon angioplasty and stenting for coronary artery disease, or for AIDS-associated malignancies, and the change in the use of radiation therapy for breast and prostate cancer.

The editors have striven to be cognizant of change by constantly adding and pruning chapters to document the current state of knowledge of cancer biology, medical radiation physics, dosimetry, cancer epidemiology, clinical radiation oncology, and radiation oncology economics, education, ethics, and policy. Particular attention in the fifth through seventh editions has been devoted to an attractive and useable design of the printed version of this book and the new electronic versions. We have taken care to have this book evolve with the times, and we have simultaneously striven to be true to the core mission of being "the book of record" for clinical care, providing the data that justify treatment recommendations as well as comprehensive illustrations and references in radiation oncology. We take this responsibility very seriously.

We have been gratified by the public reception of this book. Sales of the fifth edition rose dramatically compared to the fourth edition—an atypical pattern in the medical book business. It is, we like to believe, evidence that the pact wordlessly exchanged between the editors, the chapter authors, and our readers is being honored by all parties.

The editors sincerely hope that this seventh edition of *Principles and Practice of Radiation Oncology* will continue to advance understanding of the causes, prevention, and treatment of human cancer. We pray that this new edition will contribute to the cure of some malignancies, the amelioration of suffering for many patients and their families, the relief of pain, and the ultimate triumph of human knowledge over cancer.

Edward C. Halperin, MD, MA
David E. Wazer, MD, FASTRO
Carlos A. Perez, MD
Luther W. Brady, MD

In Memoriam

Luther W. Brady, MD (1925–2018)

The founding co-editor of this book, Luther W. Brady, died as the seventh edition of *Principles and Practice of Radiation Oncology* was being printed. As we note in the Acknowledgments section, this book has been through so many editions that we, as co-editors, have now sadly experienced the deaths of four of our collaborators: Ruth Aultman, Jonathan W. Pine, Jr., Rupert Schmidt-Ullrich, and now Luther W. Brady.

Raised in North Carolina, Luther Brady arrived at George Washington University (GWU) as, in his own words, a "wet-behind-the-ears 16-year-old" to encounter the professors, the packed lecture halls, and "the salacious lectures." He would go on to earn three degrees from GWU (AA in 1944, BA in 1946, MD in 1948) and serve on its board of trustees.

Writing 72 hours after his death, it is impossible for us to do justice to his life and career and meet the demands of publishing this book on time. This will be rectified in the lengthy tributes that will follow in the next few months.

Dr. Brady received post-graduate training in radiology and radiation oncology at the U.S. Naval Hospital in Bethesda, Jefferson Medical College, and the Hospital of the University of Pennsylvania. Except for a year at Harvard and a brief time at Columbia University, his entire academic career was in Philadelphia, first at the University of Pennsylvania and then at Hahnemann University Hospital and Drexel University School of Medicine. He was named professor in 1963; in 1970, he was appointed chair of the Department of Radiation Oncology and Nuclear Medicine. In 1975, he was named the Hylda Cohn/American Cancer Society Professor of Clinical Oncology. Hahnemann established the Luther W. Brady Pavilion in 1980.

He was president of the American College of Radiation Oncology, American Radium Society, American Society for Therapeutic Radiology and Oncology, American Board of Radiology, Intersociety Council for Radiation Oncology, Radiological Society of North America, Society of Chairmen of Academic Radiology Departments, and Society of Chairmen of Academic Radiation Oncology Departments. He was chair of the Radiation Therapy Oncology Group and of the radiation oncology committee for Accreditation Council for Graduate Medical Education.

Dr. Brady worked on behalf of the Philadelphia Museum of Art, chaired its executive committee, and was a member of the board of trustees. The museum established the Luther W. Brady Curatorship of Japanese Art. The Luther W. Brady Art Gallery at GWU was also created in his honor. He served on the board of directors of the Opera Company of Philadelphia, the Opera Company of New Mexico, the Santa Fe Opera Company, the Settlement Music School, and the Curtis Institute of Music.

In addition, Dr. Brady received multiple medals from universities and scholarly societies and honorary degrees, delivered many named lectures around the world, and was elected to honorary fellowships of many European scholarly societies.

His scholarly interests ranged from tumors of the eye and orbit to cancers of the breast, lung, and cervix to lymphoma. He had more than 600 publications to his name, was editor-in-chief of the *American Journal of Clinical Oncology,* and was a member of the editorial advisory boards of many other professional journals.

Dr. Brady was passionate about this book. He loved telling and retelling his "founding story" wherein, he claimed, he flipped a coin with Philip Rubin and thus decided who would become the founding editor of the *International Journal of Radiation • Oncology • Biology • Physics* and who would become the founding editor of this book. In the preparation of the fourth edition of this book, the representative of Lippincott Williams & Wilkins, J. Stuart Freeman, Jr., proposed the use of a specific thickness and type of paper for the pages. Dr. Brady strongly disagreed. One of us (ECH) gently suggested that after all, Mr. Freeman was in the publishing business and he probably knew what he was talking about when it came to paper. Mr. Freeman pressed his point. Dr. Brady responded in arched tones. "Don't tell me about paper, Stuart. I know paper. I am on the board of trustees of the Philadelphia Museum of Art and I know quality paper. I'll tell you the type of paper appropriate for our text and our illustrations."

Needless to say, when the dust settled, Dr. Brady got the kind of paper he wanted.

He was a gracious host and a cultured gentleman. We shall not see his like again.

May his memory be for a blessing.

Edward C. Halperin, MD, MA
David E. Wazer, MD, FASTRO
Carlos A. Perez, MD

July 16, 2018

Acknowledgments

We are grateful for the scholarly, meticulous, and thorough work of the contributors to this volume. Through seven editions, this book has become the "book of record" for the specialty of radiation oncology. It has achieved that distinction through the hard work of the individual chapter authors.

The staff of Wolters Kluwer have professionally seen this work through from planning to distribution. We are in their debt.

Our fellow faculty members, residents, and medical students have supported our work, providing consistent intellectual stimulation, valuable suggestions, and materials that have contributed to this book. We are grateful to the many librarians of our respective institutions who have come to our aid in finding the necessary books and articles to support the preparation of this book. Rupert K. Schmidt-Ullrich, MD, of the Medical College of Virginia/Virginia Commonwealth University, served as co-editor of the fourth edition. A consummate physician–scientist, a man who held himself and others to very high standards, and a valued colleague, his positive contributions live on. Ruth Aultman faithfully served as secretary to Dr. Halperin for 21 years and diligently worked on the fourth through sixth editions. She died in 2012 and was working on the manuscript for Chapter 1 until shortly before her death. Jonathan Pine served as our publisher's supervising editor for the fifth and sixth editions of this book. Jonathan was an endearing gentleman, kind, and possessed of gentle sense-of-humor. The four of us did not know of his long-standing diagnosis of lymphoma until what was perceived by us as his unexpected death in 2013. An obituary in *The Baltimore Sun* quoted one of Mr. Pine's friends, who calls him the "perfect gentleman. He had manners you don't see anymore, and he also had his first job. He was a rarity for this generation." Special recognition is due to Vilma Bordonaro, Mary Lou Chin, and Chris Trimble, who diligently worked on the preparation of materials for this volume. Our families have patiently endured the loss of time and attention to other matters that occurs as a result of the demands of a project of this magnitude. To them, especially, we express our gratitude and love.

Edward C. Halperin, MD, MA
David E. Wazer, MD, FASTRO
Carlos A. Perez, MD
Luther W. Brady, MD

Contents

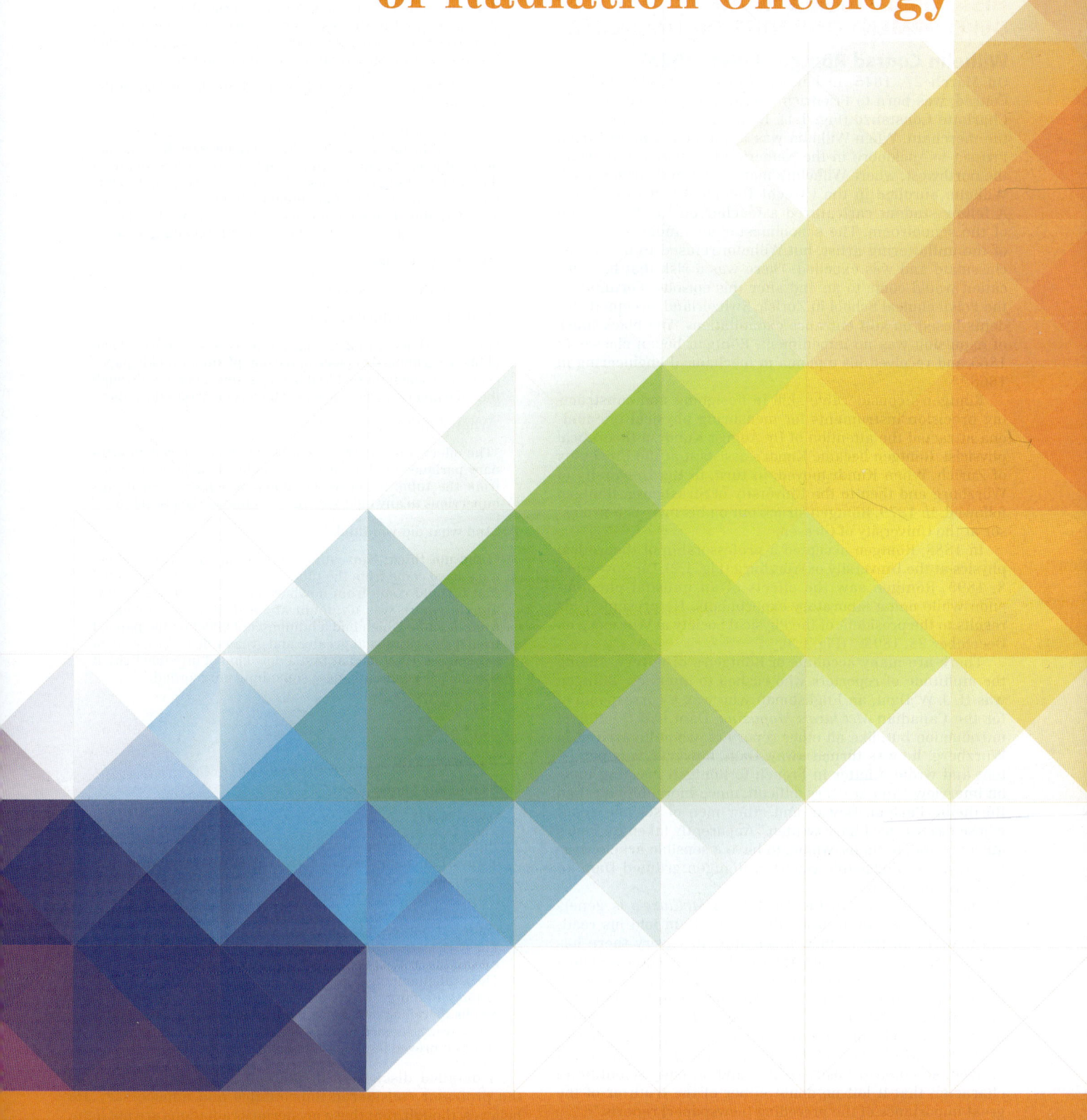

Overview and Basic Science of Radiation Oncology

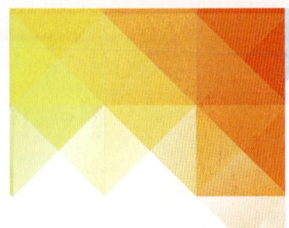

CHAPTER 1

The Discipline of Radiation Oncology

Edward C. Halperin

SKETCHES OF SOME IMPORTANT HISTORICAL FIGURES IN THE DEVELOPMENT OF RADIATION ONCOLOGY

Wilhelm Conrad Röntgen (1845–1923)

On March 27, 1845, in Lennep, Germany, a son, Wilhelm Conrad, was born to Friedrich Conrad Röntgen and his wife, Charlotte Constanze (Fig. 1.1). Röntgen's father was a textile merchant. When Wilhelm was 3, the family moved from Prussia to Apeldoorn in the Netherlands, about 100 miles to the northwest, where Wilhelm's maternal grandparents lived. Wilhelm enrolled in the Utrecht Technical School in 1862. A fellow student caricatured a teacher on the fire screen of the schoolroom. The schoolmaster demanded the name of the unflattering artist, but Wilhelm refused to betray his classmate and was expelled. There was a risk that his education would come to an end after this episode. Fortunately, the Polytechnical School in Zurich, Switzerland, accepted students based on stiff entrance examinations. The black mark of expulsion was no impediment. Röntgen began classes in 1865 and received his diploma in mechanical engineering in 1868.[1–3]

Röntgen's considerable skill in designing and constructing precision instruments for measuring physical phenomena attracted the attention of Dr. August Kundt, a theoretical physicist. Röntgen became Kundt's assistant at the University of Zurich. When Kundt moved, in turn, to the University of Würzburg and then to the University of Strasbourg, Röntgen followed. In 1879, Röntgen struck out on his own as a professor at the University of Giessen.

In 1888, Röntgen accepted a professorship of theoretical physics at the University of Würzburg (Fig. 1.2). On November 8, 1895, Röntgen saw the effects of an unusual phenomenon while doing laboratory experiments. He presented his results to the president of the Physical Society at Würzberg on December 28, 1895[2–5] (Fig. 1.3).

There are many accounts of Röntgen's discovery. Among the multitude of reporters who rushed to interview Röntgen was H. J. W. Dam, an Englishman who was a correspondent for the Canadian *McClure's Magazine*. Dam had a letter of introduction but, like all other reporters, when he arrived in Würzberg, he was turned away. Dam, however, was persistent and wrote a letter in French to Röntgen insisting upon an interview. "You are very difficult, much more difficult than Berthelot, Pasteur, Dewar, and other men of science about whose discoveries I have written." Apparently taken by Dam's audacity and, perhaps, willing to have a sensible article written by a knowledgeable reporter, Röntgen granted Dam an exclusive interview.

Dam's lead story in the April 1896 *McClure's* is generally regarded as an accurate depiction.[6] Dam told his readers that "in all the history of scientific discovery there has never been, perhaps, so general, rapid, and dramatic an effect wrought on the scientific centers of Europe as has followed, in the past four weeks, upon an announcement made to the Wurzburg Physio-Medical Society, at their December meeting, by Professor William Konrad Röntgen, professor of physics at the Royal University of Wurzberg.... Röntgen's own report arrived, so cool, so business-like, and so truly scientific in character, that it left no doubt either of the truth or of the great importance of the preceding [newspaper] reports."[6]

Dam, who was able to converse with Röntgen in English, French, and German, conducted an on-site interview in Röntgen's laboratories and had him describe the circumstances related to the discovery. Dam's charming description, excerpted here, gives an excellent insight into Röntgen the man and the nature of his scientific inquiry.

"Now, Professor," said I, "will you tell me the history of the discovery?"

"There is no history," he said. "I have been for a long time interested in the problems of the cathode rays from a vacuum tube as studied by Hertz and Lenard. I had followed theirs and other researches with great interest, and determined as soon as I had time to make some researches of my own. This time I found at the close of last October. I had been at work for some days when I discovered something new."

"What was the date?"

"The eighth of November."

"And what was the discovery?"

"I was working with a Crookes' tube covered with a shield of black cardboard. A piece of barium platinocyanoide paper lay on the bench there. I had been passing a current through the tube and I noticed a peculiar black line across the paper."

"What of that?"

"The effect was one which could only be produced, in ordinary parlance, by the passage of light. No light could come from the tube, because the shield which covered it was impervious to any light known, even that of the electric arc."

"And what did you think?"

"I did not think; I investigated. I assumed that the effect must have come from the tube, since its character indicated that it could come from nowhere else. I tested it. In a few minutes there was no doubt about it. Rays were coming from the tube which had a luminescent effect on the paper. I tried it successfully at greater and greater distances, even at two metres. It seemed at first a new kind of invisible light. It was clearly something new, something unrecorded."

"Is it light?"

"No."

"Is it electricity?"

"Not in any known form."

"What is it?"

"I don't know. Having discovered the existence of a new kind of rays, I of course began to investigate what they would do. It soon appeared from the tests that the rays had penetrative power to a degree hitherto unknown. They penetrated paper, wood and cloth with ease, and the thickness of the substance made no perceptible difference within reasonable limits. The rays passed through all the metals tested with the facility varying, roughly speaking, with the density of the metal. These phenomena I have discussed carefully in my report to the Würzburg Society and you will find all the technical results therein stated. Since the rays had this great penetrative power, it seemed natural that they should penetrate flesh, and so it proved in photographing the hand I showed you."

A detailed discussion of the characteristics of his rays the professor considered unprofitable and unnecessary. He believes, though, that these mysterious radiations are not light,

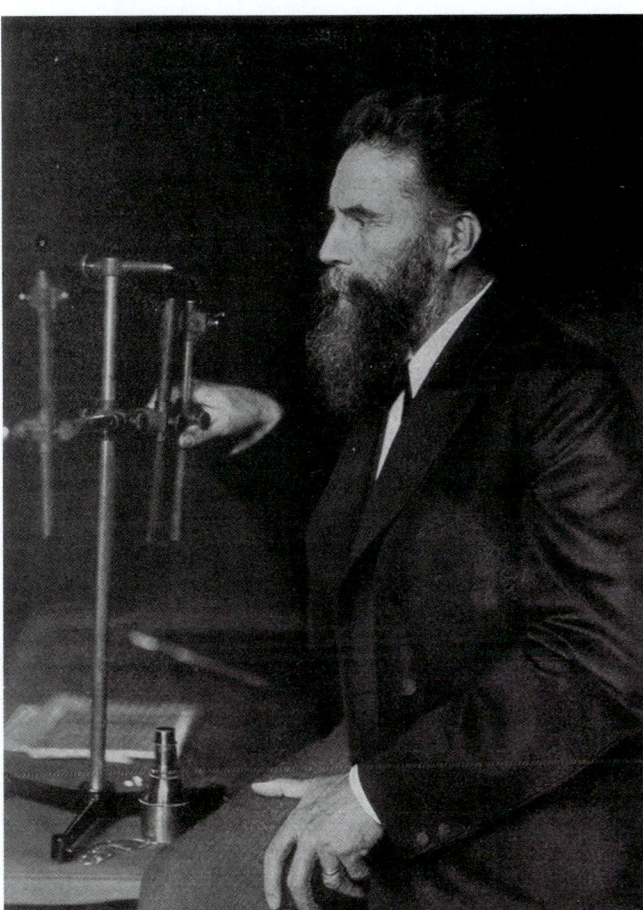

FIGURE 1.1. Wilhelm Conrad von Röntgen. He is shown in this photograph with physics instruments. (From Glasser O. *Wilhelm Conrad Röntgen and the early history of the Roentgen rays*. Springfield, IL: Charles C. Thomas, Publisher, Ltd., 1934, with permission.)

because their behavior is essentially different from that of light ways, even those light rays that are themselves invisible. The Röntgen rays cannot be reflected by reflecting surfaces, concentrated by lenses, or refracted or diffracted. They produce photographic action on a sensitive film, but their action is weak as yet, and herein lies the first important field of their development. The professor's exposures were comparatively long—an average of 15 minutes in easily penetrable media, and half an hour or more in photographing the bones of the

FIGURE 1.2. Photograph of the Physical Institute of the University of Würzburg from 1896. Professor Röntgen and his wife lived on the top floor. On the left side of the upper story can be seen the conservatory, of which Röntgen and his wife were particularly fond. (From Glasser O. *Dr. W.C. Röntgen*. Springfield: Charles C. Thomas, 1945, with permission.)

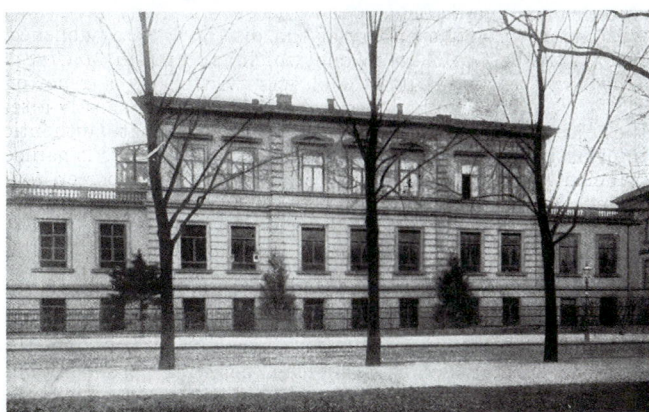

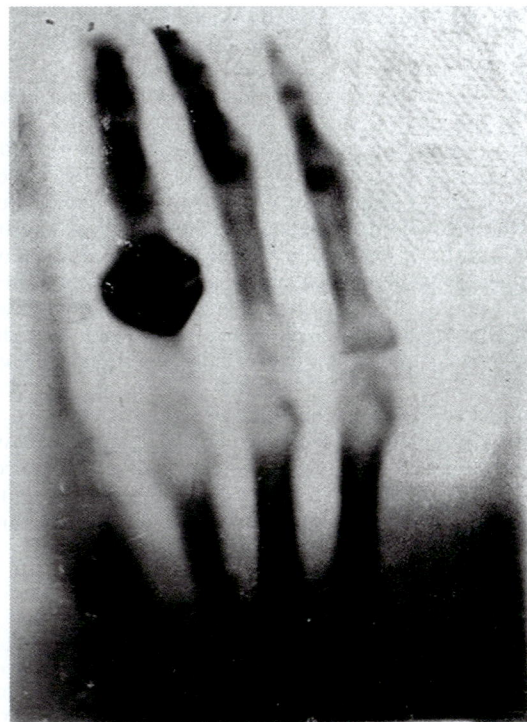

FIGURE 1.3. Röntgen made this image on December 22, 1895, and sent it to Vienna physicist F. Exner. (From Glasser O. *Dr. W.C. Röntgen*. Springfield: Charles C. Thomas, 1945, with permission.)

hand. Concerning vacuum tubes, he said that he preferred the Hittorf, because it had the most perfect vacuum, the highest degree of air exhaustion being the consummation most desirable. In answer to the question, "What of the future?" he said:

"I am not a prophet, and I am opposed to prophesying. I am pursuing my investigations, and as fast as my results are verified I shall make them public."

"Do you think the rays can be so modified as to photograph the organs of the human body?"

In answer he took up the photograph of the box of weights. "Here are already modifications," he said, indicating the various degrees of shadow produced by the aluminum, platinum, and brass weights, the brass hinges, and even the metallic stamped lettering on the cover of the box, which was faintly perceptible.

"But, Professor Neusser has already announced that the photographing of the various organs is possible."

"We shall see what we shall see," he said; "we have the start now; the developments will follow in time."

"You know the apparatus for introducing the electric light into the stomach?

"Yes."

"Do you think that this electric light will become a vacuum tube for photographing, from the stomach, any part of the abdomen or thorax?"

The idea of swallowing a Crookes tube, and sending a high frequency current down into one's stomach, seemed to him exceedingly funny. "When I have done it, I will tell you," he said, smiling, resolute in abiding by results.

"There is much to do, and I am busy, very busy," he said in conclusion. He extended his hand in farewell, his eye already wandering toward his work in the inside room. And his visitor promptly left him; the words, "I am busy," said in all sincerity, seeming to describe in a single phrase the essence of his character and the watchword of a very unusual man.[6]

Kaiser Wilhelm II invited Röntgen to the imperial court at Potsdam in January 1896, shortly after the scientist had mailed out reprints to prominent physicists. Röntgen demonstrated his findings and was decorated with the Prussian Order of the Crown, Second Class. On January 23, he gave a lecture to the Würzburg Physical-Medical Society and was startled and overwhelmed by the cheers of the audience. At the end of the talk, Röntgen invited Albert von Kölliker, one of Germany's most distinguished anatomists, to come to the podium and have his hand x-rayed. When the audience saw the bones of his hand, it erupted in thunderous applause. This was one of Röntgen's last formal lectures on x-rays. He became flustered before large groups and, when lecturing to small groups of students, was generally regarded as lusterless and dull.

Röntgen received the Nobel Prize in Physics in 1901 from the Swedish king. He thanked him but gave no speech. He willed the prize money to the University of Würzburg.[1] In the presentation speech, the president of the Royal Swedish Academy of Sciences, C. T. Odhner, commented on the enormous potential of Röntgen's discovery for diagnosis and therapy:

The Academy awarded the Nobel Prize in Physics to Wilhelm Conrad Röntgen, Professor in the University of Wurzburg, for the discovery with which his name is linked for all time: the discovery of the so-called Röntgen rays, or, as he himself called them, x-rays. These are, as we know, a new form of energy and have received the name "rays" on account of their property of propagating themselves in straight lines as light does. The actual constitution of this radiation of energy is still unknown. Several of its characteristic properties, however, have been discovered first by Röntgen himself and then by other physicists who have directed their research into this field. And there is no doubt that much success will be gained in physical science when this strange energy form is sufficiently investigated and its wide field has been thoroughly explored. Let us remind ourselves of one of the properties that has been found in Röntgen rays—the basis of the extensive use of x-rays in medical practice. Many bodies, just as they allow light to pass through them in varying degrees, behave likewise with x-rays but with the difference that some that are totally impenetrable to light can be penetrated easily by x-rays, whereas other bodies stop them. Thus, for example, metals are impenetrable to them; wood, leather, cardboard, and other materials are penetrable as are the muscular tissues of animal organisms. Now, when a foreign body impenetrable to x-rays (e.g., a bullet or a needle) has entered these tissues, its location can be determined by illuminating the appropriate part of the body with x-rays and taking a shadowgraph of it on a photographic plate, whereupon the impenetrable body is detected immediately. The importance of this for practical surgery and how many operations have been made possible and facilitated by it is well known to all. If we add that in many cases severe skin diseases (e.g., lupus) have been treated successfully with Röntgen rays, we can say at once that Röntgen's discovery already has brought so much benefit to mankind that to reward it with the Nobel Prize fulfills the intention of the testator to a very high degree.[7] (Figs. 1.4 and 1.5).

Antoine Henri Becquerel (1852–1908)

Antoine Henri Becquerel was born in Paris in 1852 into a family of scientists. His father was a professor of applied physics who had conducted research on solar radiation and phosphorescence. His grandfather was the inventor of an electrolytic method of extracting metals from ores.

Becquerel's early scientific work concerned the plane polarization of light, phosphorescence, terrestrial magnetism, and the absorption of light by crystals. Becquerel first heard of Röntgen's discovery in January 1896 at a meeting

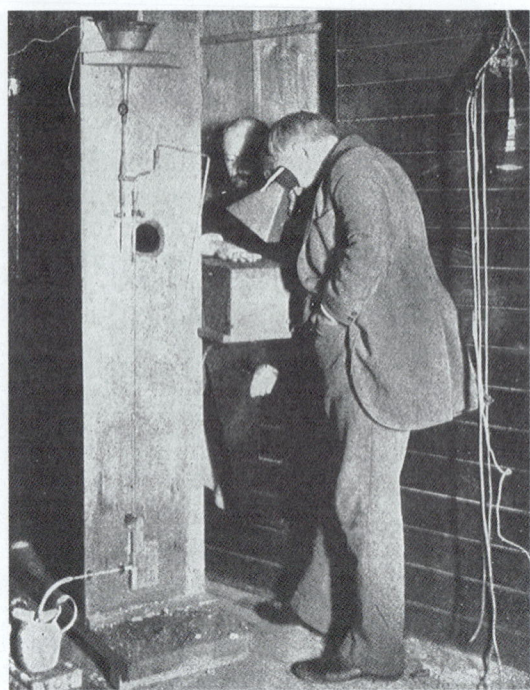

FIGURE 1.4. Thomas A. Edison experimenting with x-rays with, obviously, no radiation protection. (From Glasser O. *Dr. W.C. Röntgen*. Springfield: Charles C. Thomas, 1945, with permission.)

of the French Academy of Science. He wondered if there was a connection between phosphorescence and x-rays. He had inherited, from his father, a supply of uranium salts, which phosphoresced upon exposure to light.

Becquerel thought that the phosphorescent uranium salts might absorb sunlight and, in turn, re-emit the energy as x-rays. He placed crystals of the uranium salts on top of photographic plates wrapped in opaque black paper. After placing the experimental setup in the sun, he developed the plates and saw an outline of the crystals. When he placed coins and other metal objects between the crystals and the plates, he could produce outlines of the shapes of the metal objects. These initial experiments seemed to confirm his suspicions.

When he encountered several overcast days in February 1896, Becquerel put his uranium crystals and photographic plates in a drawer. On March 1, he opened the drawer and developed the plates. It is not clear why he did this. Nonetheless, he saw a clear image of the crystals on the plates. He had demonstrated that the uranium crystals were emitting x-rays on their own and had discovered spontaneous radioactivity.

Becquerel subsequently showed that the radioactive emissions from uranium could ionize gases and be deflected by electric or magnetic fields.[8–10]

Half of the 1903 Nobel Prize in Physics was awarded to Becquerel. The other half was given to Pierre and Marie Curie.[11]

Marie Sklodowska Curie (1867–1934) and Pierre Curie (1859–1906)

Marya Sklodowska was born in Warsaw on November 7, 1867. The youngest of four sisters and a brother, she lived under Russian rule in partitioned Poland. At 17, she left home to work as a governess to the daughters of the supervisor of a large sugar beet factory northeast of Warsaw in order to save enough money to attend university. In 1891, Sklodowska enrolled at the Faculte des Sciences at the Sorbonne in

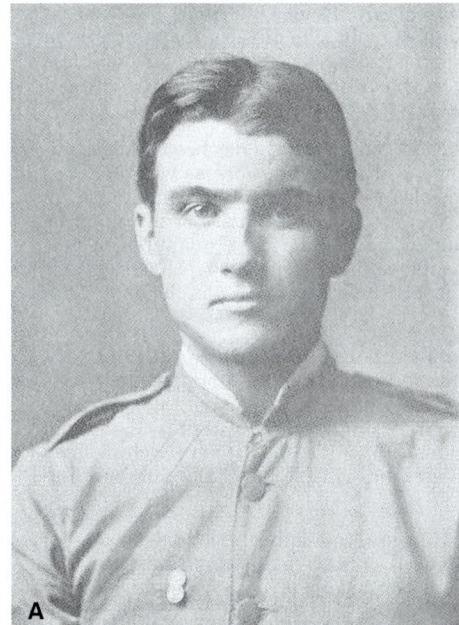

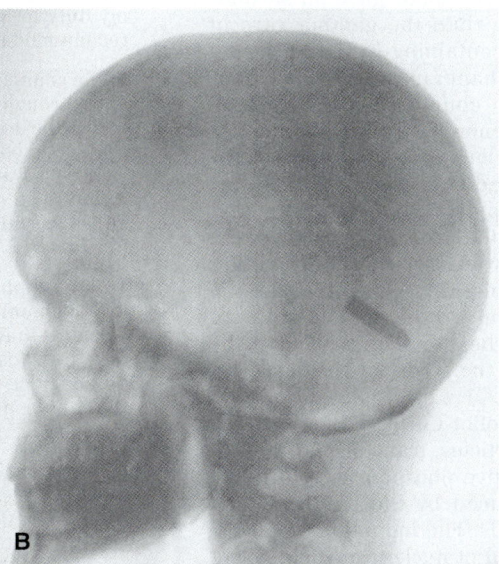

FIGURE 1.5. A and **B:** Private John Gretzer, Jr., Company D, First Nebraska Volunteers, U.S. Army injury, wounded above his left eye at long range in combat at Mariboa, Philippines. Five months after the injury, he returned to duty in the military mail service. Diagnostic x-ray units were utilized by the U.S. Army Medical Department in the 1898 war with Spain and the Philippine insurrection—within 4 years of the discovery of the x-ray. (From *The use of the Roentgen ray by the Medical Department of the United States Army in the war with Spain (1898)*. Washington, DC: Government Printing Office, 1900.)

Paris—one of just 23 women in a student body of about 1800. She completed degrees in mathematics and physics and in 1893 was hired by the Society for the Encouragement of National Industry to study the magnetic properties of steel. While in the process of securing additional laboratory space, she was introduced to Pierre Curie.

Curie was the son of a physician who had worked in the laboratory of Louis Pierre Gratiolet (1815–1865), who described the occipital visual pathways. Pierre Curie's doctoral thesis, "Magnetic Properties of Bodies at Diverse Temperatures," evaluated changes in magnetic properties of materials heated to high temperatures. He found that the magnetic properties of a substance change at a very specific temperature. This temperature is called the "Curie point" and is of great importance in studying plate tectonics, understanding extraterrestrial magnetic fields, and measuring the chemical contents of liquids. Curie also found that when crystals were pressed along their axis of symmetry, they produced an electric charge. This phenomenon is called "piezoelectricity," from the Greek word *piezin*, meaning "to squeeze," and is of importance in the operation of quartz watches, ink-jet printers, autofocus cameras, and medical ultrasound.

Marya Sklodowska (now using the French form of her first name, "Marie") and Pierre Curie wed on July 26, 1895.

For her doctoral thesis, Marie chose to investigate Becquerel's rays. She found that the intensity of the rays was affected neither by external conditions nor by any chemical process—they were an atomic property of the element. Marie observed that "it was obvious that a new science was in the course of development.... I coined the word *radioactivity*."[12]

After confirming Becquerel's observations, Marie and Pierre Curie in 1898 published a paper entitled "Sur une substance fortement nouvelle radio-active, continue dans la pechblende on a new, strongly radio-active substance contained in pitchblende." The new radioactive substance was called polonium (named in honor of Poland). In late 1898, while working on polonium, they noticed another substance, chemically akin to barium and more radioactive than polonium. Demarçay found specific spectral characteristics of this new element, which was called radium (from the Latin word for

"ray"). The Curies declined to patent their findings because, in Pierre's words, "it would be contrary to the scientific spirit." In 1903–1904, radium-226 began to be used in the treatment of patients with skin cancer and uterine cancer.[12] On June 25, 1903, Marie defended her thesis "Researches on Radioactive Substances" and became the first woman in France to receive a doctorate. Later that year, the Curies and Becquerel shared the Nobel Prize in Physics.

On April 19, 1905, Pierre Curie was killed while crossing the Rue Dauphine near the Seine—run down by a horse-drawn carriage carrying 13,000 pounds of military equipment. Marie returned to work and described the radioactive decay series of polonium. In 1911, she became the first person to win the Nobel Prize twice, this time in chemistry.

When France entered World War I, Marie Curie assembled hospital and mobile x-ray units for the care of the wounded. The mobile units were dubbed "petites Curies."[12] In March 1912, a glass tube containing 20 mg of radium was declared the international radium standard after comparison with a similar standard prepared in Vienna. The radioactivity unit was called Curie and defined as the emanation in equilibrium with 1 g of radium. In 1975, the International Commission on Radiation Units and Measurements replaced the Curie with the Becquerel (1 Curie = 3.7×10^{10} Bq). Marie Curie died on July 4, 1934, from the consequences of radiation exposure.

Irene (1897–1956) and Frederic Joliot-Curie (1900–1958)

In 1924, Marie Curie interviewed Frederic Joliot for a position in her laboratory. Joliot had a recommendation from the famed physicist Paul Langevin (1872–1946). Marie Curie's daughter Irene also worked in the laboratory. Romance blossomed and Frederic and Irene were married in 1926. The two worked together in the laboratory.[13] A reporter for *Time* magazine wrote:

> Husband and wife work like one person with two heads, four hands, 20 fingers. "We compare notes," says M. Joliot, "and exchange our thoughts so constantly that we honestly don't know which of us is the first to have an original idea. Don't you agree, ma chere?"[13]

Toward the end of 1931, the Joliot-Curies were studying the effects of alpha-particle irradiation of elements such as boron and beryllium. These metals gave off secondary radiations more penetrating than the gamma rays of radium. Interposing substances containing hydrogen in the beam, such as paraffin or cellophane, increased the intensity of secondary radiation. The couple considered these secondary radiations to be high-energy x-rays that knocked out protons from the atomic nucleus of hydrogenated substances. In England, James Chadwick conducted similar experiments with superior equipment. Remembering that Ernest Rutherford had predicted the probable existence of a nuclear chargeless particle, Chadwick correctly deduced that the secondary radiations were this chargeless particle, the neutron. Frederic Joliot-Curie admitted that he had not read Rutherford's Bakerian Lecture where he had predicted the existence of this particle and said the credit for the discovery ought go to Chadwick.

In 1934, Irene and Frederic Joliot-Curie, by bombarding aluminum targets with alpha particles, transformed a naturally stable element into radioactive phosphorus. Additional radioactive isotopes were produced by the irradiation of fluorine, sodium, and other metals. The induction of "artificial radioactivity" created the field of nuclear medicine—but Frederic always insisted that so-called artificial radioactivity was identical with natural radioactivity. In 1935, they learned that they had been awarded the Nobel Prize in Physics for their work. Husband and wife divided the Nobel Lecture between them Frederic predicted that researchers would find ways of exploiting progressive transmutations of elements by irradiation such that "veritable chemical chain reactions" would be produced—intimating the creation of self-sustaining nuclear fission chain reactions. In 1936, Irene Joliot-Curie was appointed by the Socialist President of France Léon Blum as undersecretary of state for scientific research.[12–14]

Frederic Joliot realized the possibility of atomic release of large amounts of energy and the potential of this for warfare. He pursued experiments designed to establish that a sustained chain reaction could be produced through nuclear fission leading to the production of vast amounts of energy.

Joliot may well have been the first to achieve a sustained nuclear chain reaction had not the German invasion of France and the capture of Paris intervened. Frederic Joliot-Curie and his scientific collaborators spirited their stock of heavy water and uranium out of France just ahead of the Germans. The Joliot-Curies hid their scientific papers on nuclear fission in a vault. Frederic joined the French Resistance, whereas Irene, her health in decline, moved to the French Alps with the couple's daughter. Eventually, mother and daughter crossed over to Switzerland in 1944. One wonders what would have been different in the history of science if the couple had taken the opportunity to escape to England in 1940 and continue their work. They would, perhaps, have played an even greater role in the development of atomic energy.[13]

The work of Joliot-Curie was invoked in the famous letter Albert Einstein signed sent to President Franklin D. Roosevelt on August 2, 1939. The letter, written by the Hungarian American physicist Leo Szilard, was designed to spur American action to assure that the United States would acquire nuclear weapons before Nazi Germany.

Einstein wrote:

Some recent work by E. Fermi and L. Szilard, which has been communicated to me in manuscript, leads me to expect that the element uranium may be turned into a new and important source of energy in the immediate future.

Certain aspects of the situation which has arisen seem to call for watchfulness and if necessary, quick action on the part of the Administration. I believe therefore that it is my duty to bring to your attention the following facts and recommendations.

In the course of the last four months it has been made probable through the work of Joliot in France as well as Fermi and Szilard in America—that it may be possible to set up a nuclear chain reaction in a large mass of uranium, by which vast amounts of power and large quantities of new radium-like elements would be generated. Now it appears almost certain that this could be achieved in the immediate future.

This new phenomenon would also lead to the construction of bombs, and it is conceivable—though much less certain—that extremely powerful bombs of this type may thus be constructed. A single bomb of this type, carried by boat and exploded in a port, might very well destroy the whole port together with some of the surrounding territory.

In view of this situation you may think it desirable to have some permanent contact maintained between the Administration and the group of physicists working on chain reactions in America.

I understand that Germany has actually stopped the sale of uranium from the Czechoslovakian mines which she has taken over. That she should have taken such early action might perhaps be understood on the ground that the son of the German Under-Secretary of State, von Weizsacker, is attached to the Kaiser-Wilhelm Institute in Berlin, where some of the American work on uranium is now being repeated.[13]

After the war, France created a civilian atomic energy authority. Frederic was appointed head of the Commisariate de l''Energie Atomique (CEA), the French Atomic Energy Commission. In 1946, he was promoted to Commandeur de la Legion d'Honneur and was awarded the Croix de Guerre for heroism during the Nazi occupation of France. A member of the French Communist Party, Joliot was dismissed as high commissioner for atomic energy in 1950 because of his political views.

Irene Joliot-Curie died of acute leukemia in 1956. Frederic Joliot-Curie died in 1958.[13,14]

James Ewing (1866–1943)

For much of the 20th century, if a person was selected by the editors of *Time* magazine to appear on the weekly newsmagazine's cover, it was a mark of distinction. Individuals on the cover of the magazine were "newsmakers": important, notable, and worthy of your attention. The January 12, 1931, issue of *Time* portrayed a dignified pathologist in a drawing. "Cancer Man Ewing": The "weapon" referred to dedicated cancer institutions. "He wants six $10,000,000 weapons" (Fig. 1.6).

James Ewing, born in Pittsburgh in 1866, was the son of Thomas Ewing who began his career as a teacher and undertook the study of law at age 36. He became a judge in the Court of Common Pleas in Pittsburgh, became an elder of the Presbyterian Church, and was viewed as a leading local citizen. Ewing's mother, Julia, graduated in the first class of Mt. Holyoke College and became a teacher.[15,16]

Ewing's personal life was marked by a series of illnesses and tragedies. He developed osteomyelitis of the femur when he was 14 and was bedridden for two years, his wife died after <3 years of marriage from toxemia of pregnancy, he suffered from tic douloureux and was operated on by Harvey Cushing, a urinary calculus developed later in life, and he ultimately died of bladder cancer. It was said of him that

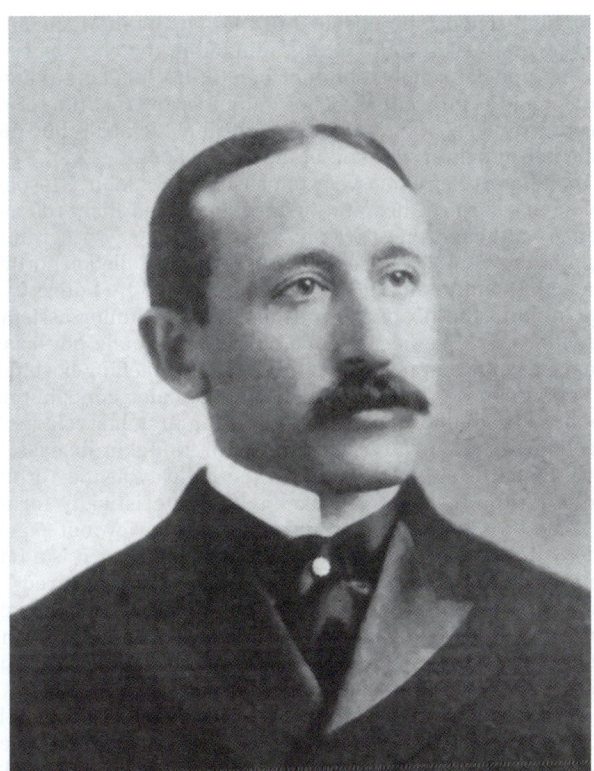

FIGURE 1.6. James Ewing was on the cover of *Time* on January 12, 1951.

adversity, suffering, disappointment, and sorrow left their mark on him not in the form of bitterness or disillusionment but in increasing sensibleness for the misfortune of others. "His sympathy and kindliness became almost legendary during his lifetime and the very legend of his benignity impressed itself on his character...That this benignity was not of the mere sentimental variety was shown by his intolerance of sham, hypocrisy, and mental laziness, which led him to be an unsparing critic."

Ewing received his undergraduate education at Amherst College and was in the first class of the College of Physicians and Surgeons of New York that graduated after the institution had become affiliated with Columbia University.[15,16]

In 1899, Ewing was appointed the first professor of pathology at Cornell Medical College and held that position for 33 years. Ewing began to focus his interest on cancer when Mrs. Collis P. Huntington (c1851–1924) established the C.P. Huntington Fund for Cancer Research in 1902. The thrice-married Mrs. Huntington was the heiress to a railway and industrial fortune and was said, by some, to be "the richest woman in America." Income from the fund was expended for cancer research at Cornell Medical College under Ewing's direction. Ewing's early studies focused on lymphosarcoma of dogs. (Many other US institutions benefited from the philanthropic support of C.P. Huntington and his wife including the Collis P. Huntington Memorial Hospital in Boston, the site of important early work in radiation therapy. After the closure of this hospital, some of its equipment was moved to the Massachusetts General Hospital.)

In 1919, after a decade of work, Ewing published the first of four editions of *Neoplastic Diseases*, the definitive reference of its time on tumor pathology. Unlike the multiauthored oncology books of today, including the one you are holding in your hands, *Neoplastic Diseases* was solely Ewing's work with >450 illustrations and 49 chapters (Box 1.1). He wrote in the preface to the first edition:

Box 1.1

A Definition of Cancer

For many years, it has been the habit of the author to ask medical students beginning a clinical elective on the radiation oncology service or new radiation oncology residents beginning their training, "How do you define the word cancer?" For someone beginning the study of cancer, this would seem to be the most fundamental question to answer at the outset. The question is most often met by a blank stare. Faced with the likelihood that, like these trainees, many of my readers have not grappled with this question, it seems worthy of some consideration in these pages.

James Ewing, who is profiled elsewhere in this chapter, spends many pages in the four editions of his definitive textbook, *Neoplastic Diseases*, trying to present a succinct definition. He settles on "a tumor is an autonomous new growth of tissue" while citing the attempts of others. He writes "Ziegler defined a tumor as a new growth of tissue which apparently originates and grows spontaneously, possesses an atypical structure, does not subserve the uses of the organism, and reaches no definite termination of its growth.... Adami accepts White's descriptive definition: 'A tumor proper is a mass of cells, tissues or organs resembling those normally present, but arranged atypically. It grows at the expense of the organism without at the same time subservient any useful function.'"[17]

The National Cancer Institute (NCI) Dictionary of Cancer Terms offers the following definition: Cancer is "a term for diseases in which abnormal cells divide without control and can invade nearby tissues. Cancer cells can also spread to other parts of the body through the blood and lymph systems."

If you were to line up a series of dictionaries and pathology textbooks on your desk, a turn each to the proffered definition of cancer, you will find phrases such as "an uncontrolled division of abnormal cells...," "a malignant tumor of potentially unlimited growth that expands locally by invasion and systemically by metastasis...," and "an abnormal growth of cells which tend to proliferate in an uncontrolled way and, in some cases, to metastasize (spread)."

No matter what definition what chooses, there will always be exceptions. The best is the enemy of good, as Voltaire reminded us, and the lack of a perfect definition should not dissuade us from finding a good, working, reasonable definition. Here is the one the author recommends:

Cancer is a heritable disease of abnormal cell proliferation. In their abnormal cell proliferation the cells do not respect the usual constraints of space and time. Cancer is characterized by invasion and metastases.

Let's unpack the definition and look at its components.

Heritable: cancerous behavior is passed from mother to daughter cells;

Abnormal cell proliferation: the fundamental disease-causing aspect of cancer is abnormal cell proliferation.

Cells do not respect the usual constraints of space and time: Normal cell growth is constrained. If you cut yourself then fibroblasts being to proliferation to heal the wound. They grow and grow and then a cellular switch turns the grown off (except in keloid formation). Similarly, in embryonic development our cells proliferate to grow organs, at some point, however, the growth stops. Cancer cells don't stop growing when they bump up against adjacent cells (contact inhibition) or according to some internal time clock. Their growth is not constrained.

Invasive: As Ewing wrote "growth is infiltrative, single cells or cell groups pushing their way through and destroying adjacent tissues";

Metastases: Cancers can send forth colonizing cells via the blood, lymph, cerebrospinal fluid, or in the pleural or peritoneal spaces which can establish themselves and grow.

Up to a very recent time it has been the prevailing impression that tumors fall into a limited number of grand classes in which the forms occurring in the several organs are so nearly related as to be virtually identical. Hence the practical physician or surgeon has been content without regard to the organ involved, and on this theory to treat the members of each class alike…I believe that this point of view has greatly retarded the progress of the knowledge of tumors, and it has been the writer's effort to combat such a conception, so far as present knowledge permits.[17]

In 1920, Ewing reported to the New York Pathological Society that he had observed a malignant tumor of the bone most frequently arising in teenagers and "composed of broad sheets of small polyhedral cells with pale cytoplasm, small hyperchromatic nuclei, well-defined cell borders, and complete absence of intercellular material." He considered the tumor to be an "endothelioma of bone" arising from blood vessels. In a second report, he called the tumor an "endothelial myeloma." Ewing commented on the tumor's marked radiosensitivity, its tendency to invade soft tissues, and its ability to metastasize to lymph nodes.[18,19]

Ewing was quick to recognize the potential of radiation therapy for cancer treatment. He called it "the first rational treatment of cancer ever devised."[20] Ewing revisited radiation therapy many times in his publications:

"From the most unexpected source, experimental physics, a new and powerful weapon has been brought into play."[21,22]

"Radiation therapy, by demanding a detailed knowledge of the symptoms, clinical course and pathology of tumors, has introduced a new era in the study of cancer."[21]

"Cancer research has entered a…fruitful era of therapeutics and more intelligent descriptive study…The developments of radiotherapy have opened a new biology of tumors, have stimulated new lines of research and suggested new concepts…many new facts and principles of tumor growth have been brought to light."[22,23]

Ewing conducted experimental work on cancer, vigorously worked to secure the funding for the establishment of New York's Memorial Hospital for Cancer and Allied Diseases (now called Memorial Sloan Kettering Cancer Center), investigated the role of radium in the treatment of cancer and worked to establish the production of radium in the United States, wrote four editions of the *Neoplastic Diseases*, and helped found the American Society for the Control of Cancer (now called the American Cancer Society) in 1913 and served on the organization's governing board for more than 30 years.[24]

Ewing viewed an organized war on cancer was a societal imperative and that success would be slow and incremental (Fig. 1.6):

It is a growing conviction that to know cancer in man, one must study the disease most carefully in the human subject. Personally, I do not look for any startling advances or sensational discoveries, since it is much more likely that a steady reduction in the mortality from cancer will come chiefly from a large number of separate factors, of which the most significant appear to be increased control of the conditions leading to cancer, more general recognition of the preliminary stages of the disease, early diagnosis, and treatment of the established disease. From the consideration of these various functions of the modern cancer research hospital, I think that it must be evident that such an institution not only can justify its existence, but fill a very urgent need without which progress of cancer research would be handicapped and much relief that might early be extended to cancer victims would be unavailable. Nor is there any doubt that the function of supporting such an institution is properly exercised by the State, which support should be continuous and liberal.[25]

At the age of 76, Ewing fractured his right femur. The fracture site showed metastatic bladder carcinoma. He died of bladder cancer in 1943.

M. Vera Peters (1911–1993)

Mildred Vera Peters (known throughout her career as Vera) was born and raised on a farm in Ontario, Canada, and received her elementary education in a one-room schoolhouse.

After high school, she enrolled in the Faculty of Medicine of the University of Toronto and graduated in the class of 1934. During medical school, she met her future husband. Peters' mother had been treated at the Radiotherapy Institute of the Toronto General Hospital by Dr. Gordon Richards but died while her daughter was still in medical school.

Dr. Peters, after a one-year internship at St. John's Hospital, a women's surgical hospital in Toronto, joined Richards as a trainee—although there was no formal residency program in radiotherapy. A 400-kV treatment unit was installed at Toronto General Hospital in 1937, the same year Dr. Peters was appointed to the hospital's full-time staff as junior assistant radiotherapist. She became one of the first female physicians to have a clinical appointment at a Toronto teaching hospital.

Peters can be justly credited for two major contributions to modern radiotherapy. We will consider, first, her role in the development of curative treatment for Hodgkin disease. In 1947, Richards stopped Peters in the hallway at the Toronto Radiotherapy Institute and in his characteristically formal way said, "Dr. Peters, how would you like to review out experience with Hodgkin's disease? All the textbooks say it is a fatal disease, but we seem to be seeing patients who are cured." In response, Peters carefully reviewed the Toronto clinical experience, working at night at home on records and files at her kitchen table while balancing her career, her marriage, and the care of her children[26].

Richards died in 1949 before Peters completed her study. By 1950, Peters published the first of a series of landmark papers in which she described a three-level staging system for Hodgkin disease and observed the prognostic importance of constitutional symptoms[26]. The current staging system of Hodgkin disease is based on the foundation laid by Peters. She also reported superior survival rates to those previously described and observed that irradiation of involved lymph nodes along with inclusion of adjacent nodal groups in the radiotherapy fields improved survival in early-stage disease. Peters also identified factors, which predicted findings in staging laparotomy and the value of lymphangiography. She persisted in reporting her findings and advocating for the curability of Hodgkin disease in spite of denigrating treatment by prominent male radiation oncologists.

Peters was also one of the pioneers in the development of techniques for the conservative management of early-stage breast cancer. She began to study a cohort of women who were treated with lumpectomy and radiation therapy in contrast to the prevailing wisdom favoring modified radical mastectomy. The patients Peters studied had received limited surgery and radiation either because of advanced age, poor general medical condition, the patients' refusal to accept their surgeon's advice to have radical surgery and, instead, insisting upon breast conservation, or the views of a limited number of surgeons favoring more conservative treatment. Peters observed that cancer-specific survival rates in these women seemed no different than those treated with radical surgery. In 1967, Peters published a paper in JAMA (*Journal of the American Medical Association*) titled "Wedge resection and irradiation: an effective treatment in early breast cancer."[27]. She also began giving lectures arguing that for stage I and early-stage II breast cancer patients, lumpectomy and radiotherapy were as effective as radical surgery. She continued to publish and lecture on the topic until her retirement in the mid-1970s. The rise of the women's movement and its associated contribution to the insistence of women to have a say in their treatment, and not be subservient to the dictates of a largely male-dominated medical profession, helped promote Peters' views. Large-scale randomized prospective clinical trials ultimately validated her initial observations.

Ernest Rutherford (1871–1937)

Many essential aspects of our understanding of atomic structure can be directly or indirectly attributed to the work of Ernest Rutherford. Rutherford's supervisor discovered the electron, Rutherford discovered the proton, and Rutherford predicted the existence of the neutron and his student discovered it. In the words of one of his biographers, the radiation oncologist Juan A. del Regato, "He became the outstanding atomic physicist of his time: amid a constellation of brilliant protagonists, he was second to none; in an era of rapidly developing, new revolutionary concepts, his own prevailed."[28]

Born in New Zealand, Ernest Rutherford received his BA and MS degrees at Canterbury College, Christchurch, New Zealand, received a scholarship to continue his studies at Cambridge University in England, and began work in the Cavendish Laboratories under the supervision of Professor Sir J. J. Thomson (1856–1940), discoverer of the electron and recipient of the 1906 Nobel Prize in Physics for his work on the conduction of electricity in gases. Within a few weeks of Rutherford's arrival in England, Röntgen's discovery of the x-ray became known. Thomson and Rutherford soon demonstrated the ability of x-rays to produce ionization in gases.

In 1898, Rutherford accepted the professorship of physics at Montreal's McGill University. It was at McGill that he identified and named alpha- and beta-radiation and also described the concept of radioactive half-life. In collaboration with the chemist Frederick Soddy (1877–1956), he developed a disintegration theory of radioactivity in which chemically different elements undergo a series of changes with decreasing radioactivity at each step. Most radioactive elements, they concluded, are the product of this successive decay[28].

In his 1904 Bakerian Lecture, he laid out a broad and prescient view of radioactivity. In 1907, Rutherford became professor of physics at Victorian University of Manchester, England. He demonstrated that alpha particles were helium atoms. The next year, he was awarded the Nobel Prize in Chemistry for "investigations into the disintegration of elements and the chemistry of radioactive substances."

Rutherford collaborated with Hans Wilhelm Geiger (1882–1945) and invented what is generally called the Geiger counter or scintillation counter to identify radioactivity. Working in Rutherford's laboratory, Geiger and Sir Ernest Marsden (1889–1970) observed that alpha particles that were streamed into a thin metal foil were sometimes scattered at very wide angles. Rutherford reasoned that this was the result of the alpha particles encountering an atomic particle of large size. The atom, he concluded, had a central, large, positively charged portion surrounded by negatively charged electrons.

After World War I ended, Rutherford returned to Cambridge University to succeed Thomson as professor and director of the Cavendish Laboratory. Rutherford proved that the hydrogen nucleus is present in other nuclei. He could show that hydrogen nuclei were produced as a product of the impact of alpha particles on nitrogen gas. The majority of air consists of nitrogen. When alpha particles passed through air scintillation, detectors showed the signatures of typical hydrogen nuclei as a product. When alphas were fired into pure nitrogen gas, the effect was larger. Rutherford determined that hydrogen could have come only from the nitrogen, and therefore nitrogen must contain hydrogen nuclei. One hydrogen nucleus was being knocked off by the impact of the alpha particle, producing oxygen-17. $^{14}N + \alpha \rightarrow {}^{17}O + p$.[86,88]

Insofar as the hydrogen nucleus is present in all other nuclei as an elementary particle, Rutherford decided to give the hydrogen nucleus a special name as a particle, since he suspected that hydrogen, the lightest element, contained only one of these particles. He named this new fundamental building block of the nucleus the *proton*, after the neuter singular of the Greek word for "first."

After the experiments of Walther Wilhelm Georg Franz Bothe (1891–1957) and Herbert Becker who, when they bombarded boron and beryllium with alpha particles, found that they produced a beam more penetrating than gamma rays, and the work of the Joliot-Curies (described in the section devoted to them), and Sir James Chadwick (1891–1974), the neutron was identified. Rutherford had predicted its existence in 1923. Chadwick was the 1935 Nobel Laureate in Physics. Bothe shared the 1954 Nobel Prize in Physics for his role in the description of wave–particle duality.[28]

THE ORIGINS OF CLINICAL RADIATION THERAPY

External beam radiation therapy (EBRT) quickly showed itself to be a useful form of cancer treatment. Only 8 years after Röntgen's discovery, Dr. Charles L. Leonard, in 1903, observed that:

> in spite of the most diligent study, there is nothing known of the etiology and histology of malignant disease that aids its treatment. Its development and fatal termination cannot be retarded, if the diseased tissue be permitted to remain in the body. Total extirpation by surgical intervention has been the only chance of cure.[29]

Leonard, however, discerned some promise in a new form of treatment"

> The results obtained by the use of the Röntgen rays seems to… have demonstrated their power to alter the character of malignant cells, to prevent their spread and development, and to produce retrograde changes that result in fatty and cystic degeneration or absorption, and often terminate in a restoration of the affected part to a nearly normal state…. The Röntgen treatment applied as a palliative in many hopeless, operatively impossible cases, has resulted frequently in cures that, if not permanent, have at least restored the patient to health and given months and even years of usefulness…. The results so far obtained are, therefore, very encouraging. An agent has been found which has a greater influence in retarding the growth of malignant tumors than any heretofore known. Many remarkable and apparently permanent cures have been obtained.[29]

Although it is controversial, most likely Leopold Freund was the first to report, in 1897, the use of ionizing radiation to "cure" a large nevus pigmentosus on the back of a young girl. Unfortunately, she later developed skin ulceration and scars.[30] Another pioneer in the therapeutic use of x-rays was Victor Despeignes who, in 1896, published on the treatment of a 52-year-old man who had an advanced stomach tumor (likely a lymphoma), with "considerable improvement in the condition of the patient."[31]

At the International Congress of Oncology in Paris in 1922, Coutard[32] and Hautant presented evidence that advanced laryngeal cancer could be cured without disastrous, treatment-induced sequelae. By 1934, Coutard[33] had developed a protracted, fractionated scheme that remains the basis for current radiation therapy, and, in 1933, Paterson[34] published results on the classification of tumors in relation to radiosensitivity.

The use of brachytherapy, starting with radium 226 (^{226}Ra) needles and tubes, is useful in the treatment of malignant tumors in many anatomic locations. Isotopes such as cesium, iridium 192 (^{192}Ir), iodine 125 (^{125}I), and palladium 103 (^{103}Pd) were generated from nuclear reactors, and the use of afterloading techniques, including remote afterloading devices and high–dose rate (HDR) brachytherapy, has contributed to this important treatment modality. With time, ionizing radiation became more precise; high-energy photons, electrons, protons, neutrons, and carbon ions became available for treatment; and treatment planning and delivery became more accurate and reproducible. Advances in computer and electronic technology fostered the development of more sophisticated treatment planning and delivery techniques, leading to the development and eventually broad implementation of three-dimensional conformal radiation therapy (3DCRT) and intensity-modulated radiation therapy (IMRT) (Box 1.2).

Box 1.2

A Call to Arms

An Institute on Cancer meeting was conducted at the University of Wisconsin in Madison in 1936. Among the prominent scientists in attendance were James Ewing, professor of oncology at Cornell University Medical College, after whom Ewing sarcoma is named; Gioacchino Failla, the famous radiation physicist of the Memorial Hospital for Cancer and Allied Diseases of New York; and Henri Coutard, pioneer radiation therapist of the Curie Institute of Paris. Glenn Frank, president of the University of Wisconsin, addressed the scientists on the first day of the meeting. Seventy-five years later, Frank's opening address remains a moving call to arms for basic science, translational, and clinical researchers, physicists, and clinicians.[35]

"Down the ages, cancer has been the most hideously persistent and the most persistently hideous enemy of mankind, the suffering it lays upon men intolerably horrible, its toll of life progressively devastating, its blows falling so often just when men have reached the years of ripest usefulness to family and state. But not all these tragic consequences together are the worse evil wrought by cancer. For every *body* that is *killed* by the *fact* of cancer, multiplied thousands of *minds* are *unnerved* by the *fear* of cancer. What cancer, as an unsolved mystery, does to the morale of millions who may never know its ravages is incalculable. This is an incidence of cancer that cannot be reached by the physician's medicaments, the surgeon's knife, or any organized advice against panic. Nothing but the actual conquest of cancer itself will remove this sword that today hangs over every head. I can remember, as a boy in rural Missouri, that death from cancer was rarely mentioned and then only with bated breath. I realize now that this reaction was born of a feeling of utter helplessness and awe in the presence of a mysterious enemy. That almost primitive reaction to cancer has happily vanished. We have not penetrated the mystery, but, thanks to you and your colleagues the world over, we have made notable rents in the veil surrounding the mystery. The world is determined to conquer this thing that steals upon men like a thief in the night and without warning strikes down the strong and weak alike. By one thing alone can this conquest come, and that is by the tireless, painstaking, and self-sacrificing genius of scientists who, like yourselves, go to their laboratory tables as to an altar and sink their lives in the great adventure of emancipating mankind from the fact and fear of this plague. Surely, if anywhere in the secular activities of men, there is a spark of divinity in lives so dedicated!"[35]

Box 1.3

The Etymology of *Radiate*

The defining verb of the discipline of radiation oncology, *radiate*, is derived from the Latin verb *radiatus*. *Radiatus* is the participial stem. Some dictionaries cite the origin of the word *radiate* as being from other tenses of the verb such as the present infinitive *radiarae* or the first-person singular present indicative *radio*. Radiate is defined as "to spread from the common center" or "to diverge or spread from the common point" or "to issue and raise." Radiate shares a common root and related meanings with other English words such as *ray*, *radius*, and *radial*. The verb *radiate* is more distantly related to other words. For example, if one proceeds along the ray from the political center to the extreme, then one is called *radical*.

The verb *irradiate* means "to direct rays upon" or "to cause rays to fall upon something." In Latin, the prefix *in* conveys the meaning of in, within, on, upon, or against. When the prefix *in* is used with the word that begins with the letter *r*, the letter *r* is substituted for the letter *n* in the prefix to assimilate the initial sound of the verb. Thus, the verb that indicates the placement of water within or on the ground changed from *inrigate* to *irrigate*. Similarly, *inradiate* was changed to *irradiate*.

An object may be said to radiate something or to emit a ray. For example, "The block of cobalt 60 radiates gamma rays." The verb that indicates directing rays on or into an object is *irradiate*. An example of proper usage would be "I recommend that we irradiate the tumor to a total dose of 45 Gy." Incorrect usage would be "I think the primary tumor should be radiated to a dose of 45 Gy."[37]

---

cost. In addition to curative efforts, radiation therapy plays a major role in cancer management in the effective palliation or prevention of symptoms of the disease: Pain can be alleviated, luminal patency can be restored, skeletal integrity can be preserved, and organ function can be re-established with minimal morbidity[36] (Box 1.2).

In 1962, Buschke defined a radiotherapist as a physician whose practice is limited to radiation therapy. He emphasized the active role of the radiation oncologist:

> While the patient is under our care we take full and exclusive responsibility, exactly as does the surgeon who takes care of a patient with cancer. This means that we examine the patient personally, review the microscopic material, perform examinations and take a biopsy if necessary. On the basis of this thorough clinical investigation we consider the plan of treatment and suggest it to the referring physician and to the patient. We reserve for ourselves the right to an independent opinion regarding diagnosis and advisable therapy and if necessary, the right of disagreement with the referring physician.... During the course of treatment, we ourselves direct any additional medication that may be necessary... and are ready to be called in an emergency at any time.[38]

To integrate the various disciplines and provide better care to patients, the radiation oncologist must cooperate closely with other specialists.[38,39]

A DEFINITION OF RADIATION ONCOLOGY

Radiation oncology is that discipline of human medicine concerned with the generation, conservation, and dissemination of knowledge concerning the causes, prevention, and treatment of cancer and other diseases involving special expertise in the therapeutic applications of ionizing radiation (Box 1.3). As a discipline that exists at the juncture of physics and biology, radiation oncology addresses the therapeutic uses of ionizing radiation alone or in combination with other treatment modalities such as biologic and immunologic and cellular therapies, surgery, drugs, oxygen, and heat. Furthermore, radiation oncology is concerned with the investigation of the fundamental principles of cancer biology, the biologic interaction of radiation with normal and malignant tissue, and the physical basis of therapeutic radiation. As a learned profession, radiation oncology is concerned with clinical care, scientific research, and the education of professionals within the discipline.

Radiation therapy is a clinical modality dealing with the use of ionizing radiations in the treatment of patients with malignant neoplasias (and occasionally benign diseases). The aim of radiation therapy is to deliver a precisely measured dose of irradiation to a defined tumor volume with as minimal damage as possible to surrounding healthy tissue, resulting in eradication of the tumor, a high quality of life, and prolongation of survival or palliation of symptoms at a reasonable

THE PLANNING AND CONDUCT OF A COURSE OF RADIATION THERAPY

When a physician proposes administering radiation therapy to a patient, six fundamental questions must be answered. Once these questions have been answered, an appropriate first step has been taken toward the development of a comprehensive justification and plan for the conduct of a course of radiation therapy. The six questions are:

1. What is the *indication* for radiation therapy?
2. What is the *goal* of radiation therapy?
3. What is the treatment *volume*?

4. What is the treatment *technique*?
5. What is the treatment *dose* and *fractionation*?
6. What is the radiation *tolerance* of surrounding normal tissues?

The *indication* for radiation therapy is that body of data that can be brought to bear showing that radiation therapy would be efficacious for the patient's condition. Such data might exist in the form of retrospective single-institution reviews of the specific malignancy, which provide evidence favoring the role of radiotherapy. Phase I and II studies demonstrating safety and possible efficacy could be invoked to justify a course of radiation therapy. For many physicians, the gold standard, however, is a prospective, randomized, phase III trial that demonstrates the value of radiation therapy. There remains a role for sound personal clinical experience. Although there is increasing reliance on published trials, and special deference is given to double-blind, prospective, randomized phase III trials, it is still appropriate for a physician to rely firmly on his or her clinical experience in the context of an intimate knowledge of the patient's problems. A sound scientific basis and an extensive knowledge of clinical research augment the essential nature of the physician–patient relationship, but they do not substitute for it.

Radiation therapy can be justified either because it improves local tumor control, ameliorates a specific symptom, improves the quality of life, or increases the probability of cure. Any data used to justify a course of radiation therapy must have a clearly defined endpoint, appropriate data analysis, and accepted statistical methodology. It is incumbent on the radiation oncologist to know how to critically evaluate the scientific literature and synthesize it in the best interest of the patient.

There are two possible *goals* of radiation therapy. *Curative* radiation therapy is used for the purpose of curing the patient where one is willing to engender a small risk of significant side effects in return for the possibility of cure. An example is the use of radiation therapy for the treatment of early-stage breast cancer. In return for a high probability of cure, one is willing to engender a very small risk of pneumonitis. *Palliative* radiation therapy is designed to ameliorate a specific symptom such as pain, obstruction, or bleeding. When palliative radiation therapy is used in the context of an incurable malignancy, one is not willing to engender a significant risk of side effects to achieve a palliative goal. Thus, if one wishes to relieve pain from lung cancer metastatic to a bone, one would pick a dose and technique of radiation therapy sufficient to relieve pain but not enough to run a risk of radiation osteonecrosis.

The questions of *indication* and *goal* are generic. They should be answered irrespective of the modality of therapy being used for the treatment of malignancy. It is reasonable to ask for indications and goal if one is planning on using chemotherapy, surgery, cellular therapy, immunotherapy, hyperthermia, biologic therapy, or radiation therapy.

Oncologists are often better at formulating indications for curative than for palliative therapy. It is not good palliative medicine to make the patient ill from therapy in order to make asymptomatic metastatic masses smaller. In palliative cancer treatment, one must treat the patient and his or her symptoms and not treat the mass devoid of its context.

The next three of the six major questions, *volume, dose,* and *technique,* are not generic—they are specific to the discipline of radiation oncology. First, the radiation oncologist must consider *volume* (Fig. 1.7). What is the appropriate volume of tissue that needs to be irradiated for the purpose of achieving the desired curative or palliative goal in the context of the justification? Does one need to treat strictly the visualized or palpable tumor mass? Is it also appropriate to treat the mass and surrounding lymphatic drainage? Does one have to worry about the routes of spread of microscopic

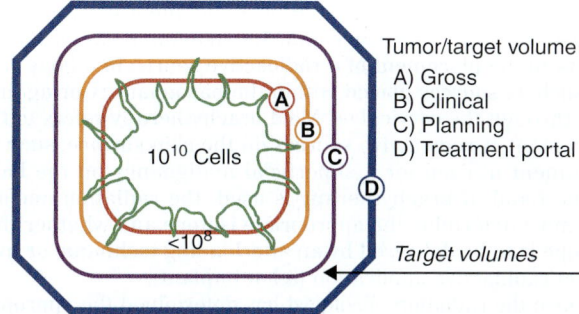

FIGURE 1.7. Schematic representation of "volumes" in radiation therapy. The treatment portal volume includes the tumor volume, potential areas of local and regional microscopic disease around the tumor, and a margin of surrounding normal tissue. (Modified from Perez CA, Purdy JA. Rationale for treatment planning in radiation therapy. In: Levitt SH, Khan FM, Potish RA, eds. *Levitt and Tapley's technological basis of radiation therapy: practical clinical applications.* 2nd ed. Philadelphia: Lea & Febiger, 1992. With permission.)

disease? All of these are crucial questions in formulating a plan for a course of radiation therapy. If radiation oncologists only needed to treat visible or palpable masses, then radiation oncology would be more of a physics exercise than the practice of human medicine. Understanding a cancer's routes of spread and the tolerance of organs surrounding the cancer requires honed clinical judgment.

An example of the problem of volume in the radiation therapy of cancer is medulloblastoma, a tumor that arises in the posterior fossa of the human brain. If, however, one treats with resection alone, patients almost uniformly relapse both locally and by leptomeningeal dissemination via the cerebrospinal fluid. Thus, the treatment volume for radiation therapy of medulloblastoma, in children >3 years old, is the area within the posterior fossa wherein the tumor arises and the entire craniospinal axis. Another example of the problem of treatment volume would be in head and neck cancer. Many of these tumors, by physical examination and by diagnostic imaging, appear to be localized at their site of origin. For many of these squamous cell cancers, there is, however, a high incidence of dissemination to the lymph nodes of the neck. Thus, the appropriate radiation therapy treatment volume would include both the primary tumor site and the neck.

The next question that the radiation oncologist must face is what is the appropriate *technique.*

Radiation oncologists, in general, have two techniques at their disposal. The first, *teletherapy,* has a similar etymology to telephone, telegraph, and telepathy. It refers to the projection of radiation through space. Teletherapy is administered with external beam sources such as a cobalt 60 (^{60}Co) machine or a linear accelerator. If one elects to treat a patient with teletherapy, one must derive appropriate external beam treatment plans. These plans include considerations such as whether the patient should be treated with photons, electrons, neutrons, carbon ions, or protons; with parallel-opposed fields, four fields, or multiple oblique fields; with IMRT; with or without respiratory gating; with or without compensators; and the like. There has been an explosion of interest in techniques of EBRT related to improvements in sophisticated diagnostic imaging and the rapidly increasing power of computers to allow manipulation of vast amounts of data.

Brachytherapy is the other important technique of radiation therapy. The word brachytherapy shares an etymology with words such as brachycephaly and brachydactyly. It refers to short or slow therapy (i.e., a radioactive implant). There are several broad categories of brachytherapy. These include *interstitial* brachytherapy, *intracavitary* brachytherapy, and *mold* therapy. Interstitial brachytherapy refers to the placement of radioactive sources directly into tissue. An example might be the implantation of the tumor bed for breast cancer or soft tissue sarcoma. Intracavitary radiotherapy refers to the placement of a radioactive source in a body cavity such as sources placed within the nasopharynx or against and through the cervical os. Mold brachytherapy refers to the placement of radioactive sources on the skin surface, such as treatment utilized for a superficial malignancy on the back of the hand. If brachytherapy is used, the radiation oncologist must determine the appropriate isotope and whether that isotope is to be delivered by an afterloading technique or by a direct radioactive application (a hot implant).

Once the radiation oncologist has determined the appropriate treatment volume and the treatment technique(s), he or she must determine the appropriate radiation *dose*. Radiation dose selection is a complex issue. One must determine the correct number of *fractions* of radiation per day, the correct dose per fraction, and the proposed total dose of irradiation. Furthermore, in certain situations, the dose rate (i.e., the number of cGy per minute) matters, such as in total-body irradiation (TBI) for bone marrow transplantation and in brachytherapy. Decisions concerning dose will, in part, be driven by decisions concerning treatment volume and technique. Paramount in the physician's mind will be the goal of treatment. The physician must determine what the correct dose is to achieve the proposed curative or palliative goal. In broad terms, the radiation oncologist must consider what is known about the dose–response relationship for tumor control in a particular clinical situation. This subject, addressed in detail elsewhere in this chapter, concerns the probability of tumor control within a radiation therapy field as a function of the dose administered.

Finally, the radiation oncologist must consider normal tissue *tolerance*. In general terms, the probability of acute and late ill effects of radiation is a function of dose. Ultimately, the prescription of a dose requires the radiation oncologist to engage in a balancing act between a sufficient dose of radiation to achieve the desired treatment goal and not giving so much dose as to engender an unacceptable risk of side effects.

The fundamental questions of radiation therapy are not for the physician alone. A patient has the right to be apprised of the physician's views on these questions, probability of tumor control (and cure, if possible), and sequelae. This information should be presented to the patient in an appropriate intellectual, social, and cultural context (i.e., in a manner in which the patient can understand), translated skillfully into the patient's preferred language if necessary, so that the patient becomes a full partner in his or her care. The signing of an informed consent document by the patient is the norm, but a signed document does not substitute for a proper doctor–patient conversation.

EXTERNAL BEAM RADIATION TREATMENT PLANNING

Treatment Volume

Tumor cell killing by ionizing radiation is an exponential function of dose (Box 1.4). The dose required for a certain level of tumor control probability (TCP, or local control) is proportional to the logarithm of the number of clonogenic cells in the tumor. Subclinical extensions of tumor (also called microscopic disease or disease below the level of ready clinical detection) should be controlled, in general, by a lower dose of radiation than is required for a palpable tumor mass. Microscopic tumor extensions may be less likely than bulky tumors to contain hypoxic cells. This also means that they may be more readily controlled by radiation.

Insofar as the dose tolerated by normal tissue is inversely related to the volume of normal tissue irradiated, delivering a uniform physical dose of radiation requires that one choose between the risks of marginal recurrence around small volumes of high dose, central recurrences in large volumes of low

---

Box 1.4

Logarithmic Cell Kill

Among the simplest exercises a radiation oncologist–in-training can undertake is the creation of a table of logarithmic cell kill. At first, such an exercise seems trivial. The effort expended on this somewhat tedious exercise will, however, be repaid many times over.

Let us assume that we have a tumor that follows a typical cell survival curve. These tumor cells have a 50% probability of cell survival after a radiation dose of 2 Gy. If we assume, for the purpose of this exercise, that there are no changes in the probability of cell kill wrought by changes in tumor oxygenation, pH, or other factors during the course of treatment; that there is no accelerated repopulation; and that only the simplest conditions apply (i.e., that there is 50% kill for each dose), then we can create a table showing the number of cells killed and the number of cells remaining after each dose (Table 1.7).

Let us assume that we begin with a relatively small tumor (i.e., a spherical tumor a bit more than 1 cm in diameter containing, say, 10^9 cells). At each dose of 2 Gy, 50% of the cells are killed. Thus, after the first dose, 500 million cells are killed and 500 million cells remain. At each successive dose, 50% of the cells are killed. Therefore, by the end of the course of radiation, very few cells are killed with each individual dose.

One can see, from going through the exercise, that even for a very small tumor, the number of initial cells is very large and the marginal killing of the absolute number of cells, with the last few doses, is small. It is not surprising, therefore, that for a tumor of average radiation sensitivity, quite a high dose of radiation is required.

Obviously, the exercise would change if we were to use a different radiation dose per fraction, producing a different probability of survival, or if the intrinsic radiosensitivity of the tumor cell line were different and the probability of survival were different.

Based on Suit HD. Radiation biology: a basis for radiotherapy. In Fletcher GH, ed. *Textbook of radiotherapy.* Philadelphia: Lea & Febiger, 1966.

---

dose, or excessive normal tissue damage and large volumes of high dose. We may conclude that different doses of radiation are required for a given probability of tumor control, depending on the type and initial number of clonogenic cells present.

A shrinking field technique is a rational approach to the problem of heterogeneous tumor distribution (Fig. 1.8). Withers and Taylor[40] have argued that "in the ideal case, the doses would be graded to provide a homogeneous TCP throughout the treatment volume rather than a homogeneous physical dose distribution." We are entering an era of "dose painting" where a heterogenous dose will be layered on a tumor as determined by sophisticated imaging tools.[41] The radiation oncologist delivers varying radiation doses to certain portions of the tumor (periphery vs. central portion or metabolically active vs. inactive on computed tomography [CT]/positron emission tomography [PET]) or may vary the dose in cases in which gross tumor has been surgically removed.

The International Commission on Radiation Units and Measurements (ICRU) Report 50 has recommended definitions of terms and concepts for radiation therapy treatment volumes and margins[42]:

- The gross tumor volume (GTV) denotes demonstrable tumor. It includes all known gross disease including abnormally enlarged regional lymph nodes. In the determination of GTV, it is important to use the appropriate imaging modality and physical examination to give the maximum dimension of what is considered potential gross disease.
- The clinical target volume (CTV) denotes the GTV and subclinical disease (i.e., volumes of tissue with suspected tumor).
- The planning target volume (PTV) denotes the CTV and includes margins for geometric uncertainties. One also should account for variation in treatment setup and other anatomic motion during treatment such as respiration.

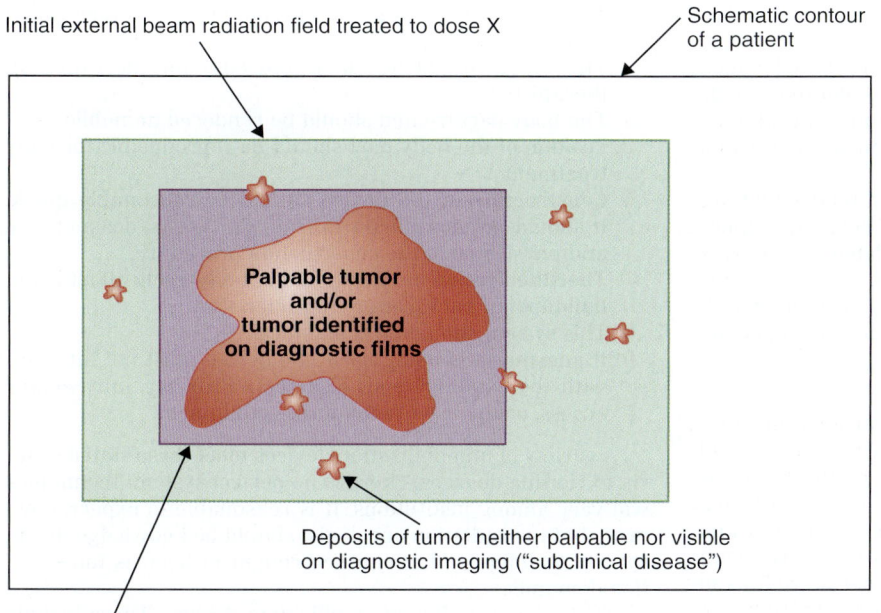

Initial external beam radiation field treated to dose X

Schematic contour of a patient

Palpable tumor and/or tumor identified on diagnostic films

Deposits of tumor neither palpable nor visible on diagnostic imaging ("subclinical disease")

"Conedown" or "boost" external beam radiation field treated to dose X + Y

FIGURE 1.8. Cell killing by ionizing radiation is an exponential function of dose. It follows that the dose required for a certain level of tumor control probability (TCP) is directly proportional to the logarithm of the number of clonogenic cells in the tumor deposit. It would be reasonable to expect that subclinical extensions of disease could be controlled by a lower dose of irradiation than what is required for a bulky palpable tumor mass. It has been argued by some researchers that microscopic tumor extensions are less likely to contain hypoxic foci that will minimize the requirement for reoxygenation for their control—but this is controversial. Insofar as the dose tolerated by a tissue is inversely related to the volume of tissue irradiated, delivering a uniform physical dose requires that one choose between the risk of marginal recurrences around small volumes of high dose, central occurrences in large volumes of low dose, or excessive normal tissue damage in large volumes of high dose. A reasonable approach is to use a shrinking-field technique in which one delivers an initial external beam field that is treated to dose X and then "cones down" to a smaller field to treat to dose X + Y. In the ideal case, doses are graded to provide a homogeneous TCP throughout the treatment volume rather than a homogeneous physical dose distribution. (Based on a concept articulated by Withers HR, Peters LJ. Biologic aspects of radiotherapy. In: Fletcher GH, ed. *Textbook of radiotherapy*. 3rd ed. Philadelphia: Lea & Febiger, 1980:142.)

Because the PTV does not account for treatment machine characteristics, the actual treated volume is that volume enclosed by an isodose surface that is selected and specified by the radiation oncologist as being appropriate to achieve the goal of treatment. It is impossible to design a radiation therapy treatment plan that limits the prescribed dose to the PTV only. Some tissues en route to the target or near the target also will be irradiated to the same dose as the target. The treated volume is, therefore, almost always larger than the PTV and usually has a somewhat simpler shape.

- The irradiated volume is that volume of tissue that receives a dose considered significant in relationship to tissue tolerance. This would include tissues in the exit region of unopposed photon, electron, or neutron beams or in the penumbra region of a beam.
- The planning organ at risk volume refers to the definition of margins around organs at risk (OARs) for injury by radiation. For example, one might define a 0.5-cm margin around the optic chiasm to avoid the risk of blindness.

Uncertainties

There are, inevitably, uncertainties in the planning and delivery of a course of radiation therapy. These were well characterized by the esteemed dosimetrist Gunilla Bentel[43,44] (1936–2000), to whom I am grateful for the following discussion (Box 1.5).

Uncertainties are divided into two general categories. First, there are uncertainties related to the delivery of dose. These include inhomogeneities in the beam, problems related to dose calculations, variables in the output of treatment machines, instability of the beam monitoring technique, and problems related to beam flatness. Spatial uncertainties in the delivery of radiation therapy may be divided into those related to mechanical inaccuracies in the equipment and those related to the patient.

Mechanical Uncertainties

- *Field-size settings.* There can be errors related either to mechanical dials or digital settings in which the field-size set on the machine is not precisely the same as that delivered.[290]

- *Rotational settings.* Mechanical or digital settings that display the degree of angulation of the gantry or the collimator may be in error.
- *Cross hairs.* Wires in the linear accelerator designed to show the central axis or the field edges may become displaced.
- *Isocenter.* Deviations in the position of the isocenter may occur as a result of sagging of the gantry head.
- *Light-beam congruence.* The light beam within the treatment machine may be in error. These misalignments may be caused by small shifts in the mirror or the light bulb.
- *Alignment systems.* The laser beam systems used for alignment may be in error.[386] They may not intersect exactly at the isocenter, they may not be perpendicular, and some systems may display relatively thick lines allowing for errors in judgment.

Box 1.5

Gunilla Bentel (1936–2000)

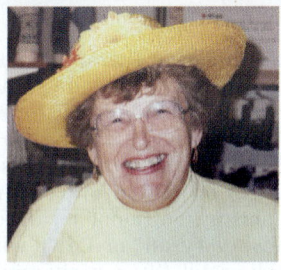

Gunilla Bentel was an international leader in the application of practical innovations to improve the accuracy of the planning and delivery of radiation therapy. Born in Sweden, Gunilla was formally trained as a nurse/radiation therapist, but spent most of her career functioning as a dosimetrist and physicist at Duke University in Durham North Carolina. She was a superb clinician who had a knack to develop practical solutions to real clinical problems. Her major contributions were in the areas of treatment planning, dose calculation, patient setup and immobilization, and she authored three textbooks on these topics (packed with helpful illustrations),which were the mainstay for students in our field for decades. She was active in the clinic, often working closely with her physician colleagues, assessing patients, and their technical challenges, together. She was a founding member of the American Association of Medical Dosimetrists (in 1975) and served as editor of the Medical Dosimetry journal. Through her books, her leadership, and other activities, Gunilla helped to improve the quality of care for patients around the world. Lawrence B. Marks MD, University of North Carolina—Chapel Hill.

- *Couch top.* There can be differences in sag between radiation treatment couches. In addition, there may be differences in sag between the simulator couch, the CT couch used for 3D or IMRT planning, and the accelerator couch. Sometimes, in the treatment room, a tennis racket–type insert is used. Over time, couch tops can become tilted from side to side or from end to end.
- *Beam-shaping blocks or collimators.* At institutions that are still using blocks rather than a multileaf collimator, there may be errors in constructing the blocks related to user error or because the cutting wire becomes too hot or is moved too fast around a corner when the Styrofoam mold is cut. If multileaf collimators are used, there may be errors in alignment.

Patient-Related Uncertainties

- *Target delineation.* No matter how sophisticated the computerized treatment planning system, it will be to no avail if the physician is uncertain about where the tumor is located. The inherent problems related to PET, MRI, CT, and our ability to make correlations between anatomic and functional imaging and the location of tumor may result in difficulty determining the extent of tumor as well as in transferring anatomic information from imaging studies to the 3D or IMRT treatment planning system.
- *Organ motion.* Organ motion can occur from respiration, heartbeat, or changes in the size or shape of an organ as a function of digestive or excretory function (i.e., changes in the size and position of the stomach, intestines, bladder, and rectum and, in the last case, its influence on prostate position)
- *Skin marks.* Skin marks can shift relative to deeper tissues. This can change as a result of alterations in patient weight, patient positioning, or the use of steroids during a course of radiation therapy. A particular problem is related to the width of set-up lines drawn by therapists on the patient's skin. The thickness of the point of the marking pen used can produce variation in the width of the lines drawn. When this is accompanied by variation in the position of the light fields in relationship to the lines, it can cause uncertainty in treatment delivery.
- *Repositioning.* Day-to-day problems in reproducing the position may occur.
- *Patient motion.* Some patients simply will not hold still during radiation therapy. Whether this is related to the patient being anxious, in pain, demented, or subject to a neurologic disorder, it can lead to uncertainties in radiation therapy treatment delivery.

Immobilization

The magnitude of uncertainties in radiation therapy treatment delivery varies. Furthermore, some uncertainties may be additive and some may cancel each other out. The net effect, on any given day, can be quite variable.

To irradiate a tumor while minimizing the radiation dose to uninvolved normal tissue, control of patient movement must be precise and absolute. Sophisticated tumor localization, 3D treatment planning, radiosurgery, and/or IMRT will be of no use if the patient is not holding still. Often, positioning and mobilization can be the weakest link in the chain of treatment planning.[45] Quality radiotherapy demands that a daily set-up accuracy of a few millimeters be ensured.

Mechanical immobilization of the awake radiotherapy patient is an adjunct to patient education and psychological preparation of the patient. Although not a substitute for education and psychological preparation, mechanical aids can greatly facilitate accurate treatment. The ideal mechanical aid for patient positioning will achieve the following goals[45]:

1. The patient must be comfortable and secure. There must be no danger of falling. The patient should not become claustrophobic.

2. The device must satisfy the radiotherapy treatment plan regarding patient position for correct geographic irradiation.
3. The setup should be quick and easy for the radiation therapist.
4. The body part treated should be rendered immobile.
5. Position of the body part should be reproducible for daily treatment.
6. Construction of the device should be reasonably quick. It should not be difficult to train therapists, dosimetrists, and physicians in the construction procedure.
7. The stabilization device should not adversely affect beam buildup and backscatter characteristics.
8. This system should be economical.
9. If anesthesia is being used, the device must not interfere with the establishment of a secure airway, intravenous access, or the use of monitoring equipment.

A variety of immobilization devices meet these stated criteria to varying degrees. There is no perfect system. Techniques will vary among institutions. It is reasonable to expect, however, that the radiation oncologist should be knowledgeable in several techniques that can be brought to bear as the situation demands.

There are a variety of stabilization devices. These include commercially available accessories such as plastic headholders and sponges; bite blocks; thermoplastics; plaster of Paris; vacuum-molded thermoplastics; polyurethane foams; vacuum bags; intrarectal balloons to stabilize the prostate and rectal wall during prostate radiotherapy, respiratory-gated radiotherapy, and therapy while breath holding to minimize respiratory excursion; and mechanical devices to compensate for patient movement by compensatory couch movement, collimator leaf movement, or robotic arms to move the linear accelerator.

Accuracy of external beam placement was typically assessed periodically with portal (localization) films. It is now more common to use online imaging verification (electronic portal imaging) devices or online CT, fluoroscopy, or ultrasound.[46,47] Portal localization errors may be systematic or occur at random. Online electronic portal imaging has been used to document inter- or intratreatment portal displacement.

Clinical evidence supports the benefit of stabilization devices in reducing patient motion. Marks et al.[48,49] demonstrated, by systematic use of verification films, a high frequency of localization errors in patients irradiated for head and neck cancer or malignant lymphomas. These errors were corrected with improved patient immobilization; with the use of a bite block in patients with head and neck tumors, localization errors were reduced from 16% to 1%[49] (Table 1.1). The use of 3DCRT and IMRT, as well as the emphasis on stereotactic body radiosur-

TABLE 1.1 THE IMPACT OF STABILIZATION DEVICES ON EXTERNAL BEAM SET-UP REPRODUCIBILITY

	Number of Position Adjustments per Number of Times Tested (%)	*P*
Hodgkin disease (*n* = 56)[a]		
Short cradle stabilization device	48/237 (20)	.009
Whole-torso cradle stabilization device	21/213 (10)	—
Head and neck cancer (*n* = 71)[b]		
Three casting strip stabilization device	55/307 (18)	.23
Customized mask device	40/291 (14)	—
Lung cancer (*n* = 60)[c]		
No stabilization device	17/119 (14)	.139
Cradle	14/171 (8)	—

[a]Bentel GC, Marks LB, Krishnamurthy R, et al. Comparison of two repositioning devices used during radiation therapy for Hodgkin's disease. *Int J Radiat Oncol Biol Phys* 1997;38(4):791–795.
[b]Bentel GC, Marks LB, Hendren K, et al. Comparison of two head and neck immobilization systems. *Int J Radiat Oncol Biol Phys* 1997;38(4):867–873.
[c]Bentel GC, Marks LB, Krishnamurthy R. Impact of cradle immobilization on setup reproducibility during external beam radiation therapy for lung cancer. *Int J Radiat Oncol Biol Phys* 1997;38(4):527–531.

gery, has led to several excellent contributions to the literature assessing the value of stabilization devices. Such devices are particularly important in the treatment of lung, liver, and paraspinal tumors. Often, these devices include a combination of a thermoplastic body cast, vacuum pillow, arm and leg support, wooden backing and/or sides, or a carbon plate. It has been demonstrated that such devices can achieve set-up errors and deviations in the 1- to 3-mm range.[50,51] Some institutions rely on vacuum-molded plastic shells. These devices, similarly, will achieve displacements on the order of 1 to 3 mm.[52]

In a randomized trial from the Karolinska University Hospital in Stockholm, Sweden, patients with head and neck cancer were randomly assigned to be stabilized with a thermoplastic head mask or a thermoplastic head and shoulder mask. Reproducibility was assessed by comparing port films in these three-dimensionally planned patients with simulator films. This was done twice during treatment and by comparing the actual treatment table positions weekly. Patient tolerance and skin reactions were also assessed. A total of 241 patients were evaluated. There were no statistically significant differences between the head mask stabilization device or the head and shoulder mask stabilization device in terms of reproducibility. It was of note, however, that patients with the thermoplastic mask extending over the head and shoulders experienced significantly more claustrophobic reactions and greater skin reactions. This study has been criticized for its reliance on thermoplastic devices rather than the vacuum-formed clear polyethylene masks.[53]

Because different stabilization devices are utilized in different clinical situations, there is no simple way to know which is the best stabilization device. An excellent comparative study done at the Northeast Proton Therapy Center analyzed the length for which there is a 95% probability that the total displacement will be smaller as a result of intrafractional patient motion. It is reasonable to expect that customized closely fitting molds should achieve intrafractional stabilization of 2 to 7 mm, with the best stabilization being obtained in precision treatment of the brain utilizing a rigid halo and bite block (Table 1.2).[54]

We may expect further benefits from research on stabilization. For example, air-filled rectal balloons have been shown to decrease prostate motion during prostate radiotherapy. The perturbation of the radiation dose near the air–tissue interface appears to produce some sparing of the rectal mucosa without incremental detriment to the dose to the prostate.[55] Active breathing control, gated radiotherapy, and compensatory motion of the treatment couch to account for patient motion are also all under active investigation.[56]

Respiratory-Dampened, Respiratory-Gated, and Respiration-Synchronized Radiotherapy

The movement associated with respiration affects the position of multiple organs. If the radiation oncologist wishes to administer highly conformal fractionated or single-fraction treatment(s)

TABLE 1.2 INTRAFRACTIONAL PATIENT MOTION AS A FUNCTION OF THE IMMOBILIZATION DEVICE[a]

Immobilization Device	Patient Motion
Alpha cradle	5.0 mm
Beanbag	6.8 mm
Head Aquaplast	3.6 mm
Duncan headrest	7.0 mm
Modified Gill-Thomas-Cosman frame	1.8 mm
Prone craniospinal head support	3.0 mm
Head Aquaplast with bite block	2.9 mm
Wing board	5.9 mm

[a]Based on an analysis of >10,000 fields, there is a 95% chance that the change in patient position between the initial patient setup and the position before the next treatment field setup will be less than the measurement shown.

Modified from Engelsman M, Rosenthal SJ, Michaud SL, et al. Intra and interfractional patient motion for a variety of immobilization devices. Med Phys 2005;32(11):3468–3474. Copyright © 2005 American Association of Physicists in Medicine. Reprinted by permission of John Wiley & Sons, Inc.

TABLE 1.3 AVERAGE DIAPHRAGM MOTION DURING ACTIVE BREATHING CONTROL (ABC) (MEAN, RANGE)[80,98,381]

By Fluoroscopy at Simulation	By Fluoroscopy During Treatment	Beam's Eye View During Treatment
1.4 mm (0–3.4 mm)	1.2 mm (0.4–2.5 mm)	0.5 mm (0–4.2 mm)

to tumors of the liver, lung, pancreas, kidney, retroperitoneum, thoracic wall, mediastinal region, and adjacent structures, it will be necessary to either account for respiration-induced movement by putting a larger margin around the tumor or use an intervention to reduce this movement (Table 1.3).

One method for limiting respiratory motion during radiotherapy is the *abdominal compression method*. This involves placing a plate or some other restrictive device above or around the abdomen and chest, sometimes in association with supplemental oxygen, in an effort to minimize the amount of diaphragmatic motion during radiotherapy.[57] This is also referred to as *respiratory-dampened radiotherapy*.[58] Many patients can be trained to modify their respiratory excursion by use of feedback by showing their respiration graphed on a video screen. Another technique involves general anesthesia and high-frequency jet ventilation to minimize diaphragm motion during liver radiosurgery.[59]

Respiratory-gated radiotherapy involves turning the beam on only during portions of the respiratory cycle. Some techniques call for the patient to hold his or her breath during the irradiation.[382]

DNA DAMAGE BY IONIZING RADIATION

The biologic effects of ionizing radiation are largely the result of DNA damage, which is caused directly by ionization within the DNA molecule or indirectly from the action of chemical radicals formed as a result of local ionizations in water. The general forms of DNA damage are base damage, DNA–protein cross-links, single-strand breaks, double-strand breaks, and complex combinations of all of these.[60]

Normal mammalian cells repair a significant proportion of radiation-induced DNA damage. Long-term biologic consequences are the result of those injuries, which are irreparable or misrepaired. The cell will attempt to repair DNA injury induced by radiation via several pathways. Key genes are involved in repair of double-strand DNA breaks.

There is some evidence that clustered local damage to DNA, such as a double-strand break accompanied by additional breaks, base damage, or DNA–protein cross-links, is especially difficult for cells to repair. Even lesions that are potentially repairable may be repaired incorrectly (misrepaired) if lesions are accumulating very rapidly because of HDR or dose rate radiation or if the cell enters M phase and attempts DNA synthesis while repair is in progress. Conversely, radiation, which is given at a low dose rate or is highly fractionated, provides an opportunity for repair of radiation-induced lesions and recovery from injury. DNA damage that is not repaired may cause cell death, prevent cell division, or permanently give rise to heritable lesions such as point mutations, small and large deletions and translocations of DNA sequences, and a wide variety of DNA aberrations[61–63].

RELEVANCE OF RADIOBIOLOGIC CONCEPTS IN CLINICAL RADIATION THERAPY

Radiation and Cancer Biology's Contributions to the Clinical Practice of Radiation Oncology

Generations of radiation oncologists have grappled with the question of radiation and cancer biology's contribution to the clinical practice of radiation oncology. The question was posed and addressed in two classic lectures: first by Stanford's Henry S. Kaplan[64] in his 1970 Failla Lecture to the Radiation Research Society and then by Harvard's Herman D. Suit[65,66] in his 1983 Failla Lecture. Treading on the ground prepared for us by Kaplan and Suit, we will reconsider the question in the context of the explosion of knowledge concerning the molecular and cellular basis of cancer.

One can look at the history of cancer biology's contribution to the clinical practice of radiation oncology in terms of two debates: *empiricism versus research-based radiation oncology* and *biology versus physics*.

Empiricism Versus Research-Based Radiation Oncology

Empiricism harkens to the views of David Hume (1711–1776) and other British philosophers of the 17th and 18th centuries and their distrust of the power of unaided reason. In the philosopher's view of empiricism, the best contact between one's understanding of knowledge and the world is not the point at which a mathematical proof crystallizes, but the point at which you see and touch a familiar object. Their paradigm was knowledge by sensory experience rather than by reason alone.[67–69]

Empirical radiation oncologists rely on accumulated clinical experience, also known as "what has worked in the past." They are suspicious of therapies based on theories and laboratory research and feel safest when treading the pathway of tested experience. One can find very strong signs of empiricism in the radiation oncology literature: case reports, single-institution retrospective clinical series, and a marked concern with retrospective clinical analyses of radiation therapy that mine clinical experience to aid the selection of radiation treatment volume, dose, and treatment techniques.

There can be no doubt that the development of radiation oncology has been extensively based on empiricism. We must note, however, that radiation biologists worked closely with the early radiation oncologists. It would be erroneous to suggest that the early history of radiation oncology was completely devoid of reliance on radiation biology.

The theme of hostility to empiricism and support for finding a firm basis for clinical radiation oncology in radiation and cancer biology research is easily identified in the development of the specialty. "Some people do the same thing wrong for 30 years and then call it accumulated clinical experience," said one critic; or it has been said, "If radiation oncologists were put in charge of the war against polio in 1945, they certainly would have perfected the iron lung by now."[70,71] Our growing knowledge of the genome, proteomics, secondary messengers, and solid tumor biology and the identification of new molecular targets for drugs, immunotherapies, cellular therapies, angiogenesis, oxygenation, and cell cycle control are changing the present and future of medicine. If clinical radiation oncologists have a future, these individuals say, then they must actively participate in the investigation of the molecular and cellular basis of cancer and in translational research.

Physics Versus Biology

One also may formulate the debate over the role of basic biology in clinical radiation oncology as a pull and tug between physics and biology. Medical radiation physics has dominated the thinking of clinical radiation oncologists. Among the major achievements of this discipline are the following:

- The identification and characterization of physical units of radiation dose
- Significant changes in photon and electron radiation therapy apparatus (initially, kilovoltage and later ^{60}Co, high-energy linear accelerators, the Gamma Knife [Elekta Corp., Stockholm, Sweden], and the CyberKnife [Accuray, Sunnyvale, CA])

- The development of 3D treatment planning for identification of tumor volume and characterization of irradiated normal tissue
- IMRT for improved conformality of treatment beams
- Particle therapy including neutrons, protons, pions, and stripped nuclei
- Improved stabilization devices to aid the reproducibility of treatment
- Advances in brachytherapy technology including new isotopes, the afterloading technique, and remote HDR machines
- The apparatus for intraoperative radiation therapy (IORT)
- Equipment for heat deposition in tumors leading to the clinical applications of hyperthermia

At present, a considerable effort in clinical radiation oncology is focused on the tools and techniques provided to the physician by the physicist. Radiation oncology meetings are dominated by discussions of proton therapy, IMRT, radiosurgery/conformal radiation, and innovations in equipment. Simply put, these techniques all offer better radiation dose distributions, which, one hopes, will lead to an increase in local control of tumors and a decrease in normal tissue toxicity. At present, a better dose distribution is the solution physics offers to the problems of oxygenation, monitoring of tumor blood flow, tumor pH, secondary messengers, tumor suppressor genes, oncogenes, the biology of metastasis, normal tissue radioprotectors, and tumor radiosensitizers. Could it be that "if all you have is a hammer, then everything looks like a nail"?

What has cancer biology ever done for the clinical radiation oncologist? It is, we think, a generally fair question, although it might be characterized as somewhat narcissistic, along the lines of "What have you done for me lately?"[65,70,72–74] Among the areas one should consider on the list of laboratory contributions to the clinic are the following:

- As early as 1906, Bergonie and Tribondeau[75] enunciated a series of famous laws of radiosensitivity. This was followed by the work of the French investigators Regaud and Ferroux,[76] who demonstrated that whereas a single dose of radiation to the testes always produced maximal damage to the scrotal skin, fractionated exposure spared the skin but destroyed spermatogenesis. They speculated that this same technique of fractionation might be differentially advantageous in the treatment of tumors. This led to Coutard's[32,33,77] studies that culminated in the fractionated EBRT techniques of today.
- The identification of the relationship between radiation dose and cell kill led to the characterization of the radiation cell survival curve. This contributed to our understanding of radiation therapy dose and fractionation and, consequently, contributed to our knowledge of radiation repair. This development placed our grasp of radiation fractionation on sound footing and led to investigations of alternative fractionation schemes. This has contributed to improved tumor control as well as limitation of normal tissue toxicity. Ultimately, the radiation cell survival curve also provided the underpinnings for our views of elements of the dose–response relationship for tumor control and normal tissue toxicity.
- In 1909, Schwarz[78,79] demonstrated that compression of the skin to diminish capillary blood flow reduces severity of cutaneous radiation reactions. This may have been the first demonstration of the "oxygen effect."[80] L. H. Gray[81] pointed out the relevance of the "oxygen effect" to radiation oncology by identifying the fact that human neoplasms contain a significant subpopulation of hypoxic cells.[82] A series of important developments has driven home the centrality of hypoxia to our understanding of radiation's effects on tumors. Clearly, histopathologic studies and invasive measurements of intratumoral partial oxygen pressure have shown that many human tumors contain regions with low oxygen tension.[83] We now believe that there are

at least two different mechanisms, called *diffusion-limited* and *perfusion-limited* hypoxia, behind this observation. Some have called these *permanent* and *transient* hypoxia.[84] Diffusion-limited hypoxia results from inadequate angiogenesis, whereas perfusion-limited hypoxia is associated with intermittent closure of tumor vessels, leading to acute hypoxic conditions for tumor cells downstream from the obstruction. In addition, we now understand how hypoxia activates genes and may produce tumor differentiation and increase a tumor's metastatic potential. Clinical studies have associated the prognostic value of hemoglobin level with tumor local control.[80,85] The characterization of the hypoxia problem has led to a variety of strategies to overcome it. One has been to have the patient breathe high–oxygen content gas mixtures or to irradiate patients in hyperbaric oxygen chambers. Another option involves the use of oxygen-mimetic chemicals. Other treatment strategies include blood transfusions or the specific use of hypoxic-specific cytotoxins such as mitomycin C.

- There has been considerable growth in our understanding of cell proliferation, the cell cycle, and cell repair mechanisms. We now understand that cells are more sensitive to radiation in M phase and more sensitive to hyperthermia in S-phase. Our understanding of the differential sensitivity

of cells to radiation during the cell cycle helps provide a rational basis for the use of radiation and chemotherapy.

- As an extension of the knowledge associated with the radiation cell survival curve, clinicians obviously need to have a good understanding of the radiation dose and response for both normal and malignant tissues. The development of research involving the lethal dose 50% (LD50), local control rates, and normal tissue toxicity in animal models has led to an improved understanding of the radiation dose–response relationship. Correlates of this understanding have included the use of the progressive shrinking-field technique, IORT, and brachytherapy as a "boost" and the use of increasingly conformal beams associated with our improved understanding of how radiation dose should be associated with tumor volume and dose painting. One expects, in the future, to see increasing work in intentional dose heterogeneity as a technique for improving local control.

In his 1983 Failla Lecture, Herman Suit[65] considered the evolution of the principles of clinical radiation therapy. He prepared a table in which he attempted to articulate the principles of radiation therapy invoked in the United States in 1956 and 1982. This is reproduced in the first two columns of Table 1.4. The author of this chapter has added a third column

TABLE 1.4 PRINCIPLES OF RADIATION ONCOLOGY DERIVED FROM THE INITIAL WORK OF SUIT

1956	1982	2013
1. Aim for uniform dose throughout the treatment volume. Treatment volume is constant for entire treatment (i.e., no shrinking field).	1. Use shrinking-field technique (i.e., a nonuniform dose distribution related to number of tumor cells).	1. Moderate, conform, and "paint" the external beam or brachytherapy dose distribution in accordance with the viable tumor cell distribution.
2. Initial large treatment volume is carried to tolerance.	2. Dose to the initial volume is usually less than tolerance. Only the final treatment volume is carried to tolerance dose level.	2. Dose to the initial volume is less than tolerance and may be moderated because of the specific host and treatment factors affecting tolerance.
3. No special emphasis to push dose to higher levels for larger tumors.	3. Dose aim is planned on the basis of tumor size or estimated tumor cell number. a. Maximum doses (with higher risk of morbidity) for large tumors. b. Modest well-tolerated dose levels for subclinical disease. c. For combination of radiation and surgery use less than radical dose level.	3. Dose aim is planned on the basis of tumor size, estimated tumor cell number, extent and completeness of surgical resection, biologic and genetic predictors of tumor aggressiveness, and response to induction chemotherapy. a. Maximum doses (with higher risk of morbidity) for large and more aggressive tumors. b. Modest well-tolerated dose levels for subclinical disease. c. For combinations of radiation and surgery, chemotherapy, and/or biologic therapy, one might use less than radical dose level in certain situations. d. For combinations of external beam radiation therapy and brachytherapy or radiation therapy and hyperthermia, the dose of each modality is modified as a function of the other modalities used.
4. Little priority given to planned combinations of radiation and surgery.	4. Major emphasis on planned combinations of radiation and surgery.	4. Major emphasis on planned combinations of radiation, surgery, chemotherapy, hormonal therapy, and biologic therapy.
5. Treatment fields are square or rectangular.	5. Secondary collimation is utilized on virtually all fields to reduce irradiation of tissues not suspected of involvement by tumor.	5. Multileaf collimators and intensity modulation are used on virtually all fields in an attempt to improve conformality of the radiation and reduce irradiation of tissue not suspected of being involved with tumor. Radiation dose distribution is based on sophisticated imaging technologies.
6. Radiation alone is the general rule.	6. Multidisciplinary approach accepted as most effective for most tumor problems.	6. The radiation oncologist is expected to be trained in and make use of pathology for tumor subtyping and grading; anatomic and molecular staging; diagnostic imaging; and the therapeutic role of chemotherapy, hormonal therapy, biologic therapy, and surgical therapy.
7. Results of treatment described almost exclusively in terms of absolute survival at a fixed period (e.g., 5 years).	7. Results analyzed on the basis of detailed assessment of causes of failure (e.g., local persistence or regrowth, local complication, marginal miss, regional spread, distant metastases, intercurrent disease).	7. The phase III randomized prospective trial is the gold standard for clinical decision-making. Decisions based on properly planned and conducted cancer trials concerning radiation therapy dose, volume, and technique are most appropriate. It is expected that evidence-based medicine will guide clinical decision-making. If such trials are not available or are inadequate, then phase II trials or retrospective reviews involving survival, local control, patterns of failure, and multivariate analysis of outcome are often useful. The future will depend on basic and translational research in cancer biology and medical physics being brought to the clinic.

identifying the appropriate principles for 2018. One can see, by scanning across the table, the significant changes that have taken place in our discipline. It is clear that the future holds a role both for empiricism and for research-based radiation oncology as well as a role for improvements in physics and biology. Through cooperation and constructive dialogue, all may contribute to the future of cancer care.

It is essential that radiation oncologists remaining current with scientific findings that will be critical in the development of improved therapeutic strategies. Approaches that alter the cell's surface membrane, receptors, secondary messengers, or nuclear contents may overcome cellular radiation resistance. By exploitation of cellular mechanisms related to apoptosis, it may be possible to kill cells with irradiation by inducing changes other than unrepaired DNA damage. With understanding of the tumor microenvironment and techniques such as complementary DNA (cDNA) microarrays, as well as an understanding of how growth factors may alter cellular processes, innovative bioinformatics and improved combined modality strategies may emerge. The ability to genetically sequence tumors will provide information beyond the era when biologic effects were attributed to a single gene. Better understanding of hypoxia may improve clinical outcome with antihypoxia strategies, including hypoxic cell radiosensitizers and hypoxic cytotoxic agents. Cyclins and growth factors may be useful as clinical radiation modifiers. Pharmacogenomics may inform how we prescribe drugs.

There is a critical need to balance the investment in technical aspects of radiation therapy with concepts and innovative approaches derived from better understanding of cancer biology. These scientific developments will greatly alter the way in which we practice our discipline.

EFFECTS OF IRRADIATION ON CELLS

The radiation-induced lesion most detrimental to cell survival involves damage to the DNA. This may result in either mitotic cell death or apoptosis. If the cell survives and repairs the damage, it may achieve a normal status. If there is misrepair, it may be associated with permanent mutations and induction of carcinogenesis. The physical interaction of ionizing radiation with the molecular infrastructure of the cell results in chemical reactions that occur within 10^{-18} to 10^{-3} seconds.[58] Absorption of the photon energy destabilizes the target molecule, resulting in molecular breaks or release of energetic electrons and secondary energy-attenuated photons, which may interact with other cellular molecules, leading to a chain reaction that produces a variety of short-lived ions and chemically unstable free radicals. The most common radicals are produced from the radiolysis of cellular water and include hydroxyl radicals ($\cdot$OH), hydrated electrons (e_{aq}), hydrogen atoms ($H\cdot$), and hydrogen peroxide (H_2O_2). Free radicals are extremely unstable and interact nearly instantaneously with neighboring molecules to produce chemically stable lesions. This process can be modified by free radical scavengers or by oxygen, which have opposing effects on the number of stable lesions and on the level of cellular radiosensitivity. However, if all factors remain constant, the permanent damage is linear with dose. Experiments in which the cell nucleus and the cytoplasm were selectively irradiated show that the dose required in the cytoplasm to kill a cell is larger than doses required in the nucleus.[231,232] It is generally accepted that most target molecules for radiation-induced cell killing are located in the nucleus and involve damage to the DNA.[233] However, other targets such as the cell membrane and the membrane of mitochondria have been proposed as the origin of apoptotic cascades that follow irradiation also contributing to cell death.

In many cells, radiation-induced lethality is not instantaneous because cells continue to function and even undergo several divisions before final mitotic death occurs. Noncycling lymphocytes, thymocytes, and hematopoietic cells were shown to undergo an interphase cell death without progressing through the mitotic phase of the cell cycle.[234,235] Two patterns of morphologic changes are associated with cell death in mammalian cells. Cell necrosis, which is degenerative, is the most usual type of cell damage. Necrotic cell death results from collapse of cellular metabolism and depletion of its adenosine triphosphate storage. The final events of necrosis involve membrane rupture, loss of lysosomal enzymes, degradation of nuclear chromatin, and karyolysis. The other process of radiation-induced cell death is apoptosis. Programmed cell death, or apoptosis, is a physiologic process that involves a series of characteristic, genetically controlled steps. These include chromatin condensation and segmentation, fragmentation of the nucleus into apoptotic bodies, cell shrinkage, and loss of cellular contact with neighboring cells.[64,236–238] Apoptosis culminates in the engulfment of the cell by neighboring cells, such as macrophages, without a concomitant inflammatory response.[239] Apoptosis occurs spontaneously in various solid tumors and contributes to the balance between tumor cell gain and cell loss.[240]

Within minutes after irradiation, signal transduction pathways mediated by protein kinase C and tyrosine kinase are stimulated.[86] Genes and enzymes involved in genetic control of radiation damage repair are activated, stress genes are induced, and growth factors and cytokines that modulate response of mammalian cells to ionizing radiation are activated.[116] Radiation-induced stimulation is probably critical to induction of many genes and proteins, including early response genes, which, in turn, activate other genes, including those for tumor necrosis factor, fibroblast growth factor, and transforming growth factor.[231] In addition, new proteins, such as tissue plasminogen activator, are synthesized.[241] This cascade of gene activation and transcription and protein synthesis is related to key cellular functions that the cell invokes in an attempt to survive a dose of radiation.[241]

Modifiers of Radiation Response

Several approaches have been used to enhance the therapeutic ratio in radiation therapy:

1. *Physical modifiers of low-LET radiations.* IMRT, three-dimensional treatment planning, improvements in anatomic and functional imaging, the increasing power of computer hardware and software, and treatment machine improvements have led to better photon, electron, and proton dose distributions; less side scatter; less differential absorption in the bone and normal tissues; and, with charged heavy particles, selective energy deposition at specific depths.[283]

2. *High-LET radiations.* The importance of tumor hypoxia and cells residing in relatively resistant phases of the mitotic cycle are factors that are less likely to cause unsatisfactory results with neutrons, pi mesons, and heavy ions than with standard radiation doses delivered with low-LET beams.[242]

3. *Hyperbaric oxygen or tourniquet techniques.* These techniques involve the use of increased oxygen tension to improve the effects of irradiation on the tumor or use of a tourniquet to produce severe hypoxia in the surrounding normal tissues so that higher irradiation doses can be delivered.[243] Theoretically, these approaches yield better tumor control without damaging normal tissues. Interest in the tourniquet technique waned years ago. Some investigators continue to evaluate hyperbaric oxygen. The logistics are formidable, and clinical trials have been inconclusive.[181,244–246]

4. *Hypoxic sensitizers.* Compounds with electron affinity, from the nitroimidazole group, theoretically produce free radicals in a manner similar to that of oxygen, selectively sensitizing hypoxic cells to radiation. Misonidazole (RO-07–0582) was evaluated in numerous clinical trials by the RTOG, with no evidence of clinical efficacy; however, in the Danish Head and Neck Cancer trial, there was

a highly significant survival benefit in the subgroup of patients with pharynx tumors.[247,248]

5. *Perfluorocarbons.* These agents are administered in emulsion (they are insoluble in water) in sufficient concentrations coupled with inhalation of 95% to 100% oxygen to enhance oxygen transport and release in the presence of low oxygen tension. Their potential application in the treatment of patients with cancer was evaluated.[249,250] Interest in the technique waned.

6. *Cytotoxic agents.* Actinomycin D, doxorubicin, 5-fluorouracil, cyclophosphamide, cisplatin, methotrexate, bleomycin, and others have been shown to interact with radiation in several forms to maximize tumor cell killing. In some instances, increased normal tissue reactions have been observed.[277]

7. *Epidermal growth factor receptor (EGFR).* EGFR, a member of the ErbB family of receptor tyrosine kinases, is activated in several epithelial cancers. Radiotherapy increases the expression of EGRF in cancer cells and blockade of EGFR signaling can sensitize cells to radiation. Cetuximab is a chimeric monoclonal antibody that targets EGFR. The drug appears to improve locoregional tumor control and survival in locally advanced squamous cell carcinoma of the head and neck.[234]

8. *Radioprotectors.* Sulfhydryl-containing compounds, such as cystine and cysteamine, have been used in animals to protect normal tissues against irradiation. Amifostine (WR-2721), a thiophosphate derivative of cysteamine, has been shown to selectively protect normal tissues, including the bone marrow, salivary glands, and intestinal mucosa, in animals, with little effect on tumor response to irradiation.[251] Amifostine undergoes dephosphorylation by cellular-bound alkaline phosphatase to an active metabolite, WR-1065. This alkaline phosphatase–dependent activation is thought to contribute to selective normal tissue protection because of a higher concentration of alkaline phosphatase in normal tissue. Cytoprotection is believed to be the result of the elimination of free radicals.[252] The compound was widely investigated in phase II and III clinical trials.[253] It is now approved by the U.S. Food and Drug Administration (FDA) and the European Medicines Agency for the reduction of xerostomia in patients with head and neck cancer undergoing radiotherapy.[212] A meta-analysis has shown that amifostine does not reduce overall or progression-free survival in patients treated with radiotherapy or chemoradiotherapy—arguing against amifostine protecting tumor tissue.[254]

9. *Hyperthermia.* Heat at temperatures of more than 42.5°C kills cells by itself or enhances the effects of irradiation and numerous cytotoxic agents. Heat selectively kills cells that are chronically hypoxic, acidotic, and nutritionally deficient—characteristics shared by tumor cells in comparison with the better-oxygenated and better-nourished normal cells. Furthermore, heat preferentially kills cells in the S-phase of the proliferative cycle, which are known to be relatively resistant to irradiation.[91,270,351]

RADIOSENSITIVITY AND RADIOCURABILITY

In 1906, Bergonie and Tribondeau[86] formulated a law relating radiosensitivity to reproductive capacity of cells, based on their experiments on rat testis in which they were able to destroy the germinal cells while the interstitial tissue and Sertoli syncytium remained unimpaired. They wrote that "X-rays are more effective on cells which have a greater reproductive activity; the effectiveness is greater on those cells which have a longer dividing future ahead.... From this law, it is easy to understand that roentgen radiation destroys tumors without destroying healthy tissues." Fletcher[87] felt that this observation, which was interpreted to indicate that radiosensitivity of tumors was linked to that of the mother organ,

did much harm to clinical radiation therapy, leading to the erroneous concept that undifferentiated tumors with mitotic activity were radiosensitive and that more differentiated tumors were radioresistant.

In 1914, Schwarz[78] introduced the concept of fractionation by postulating that it was inefficient to deliver the total radiation dose in one treatment because cells were in different states of radiosensitivity and because there was a better chance that multiple exposures could hit the cells in a radiosensitive phase (e.g., mitosis). Fractionation was assumed to create a favorable therapeutic ratio because the tolerance of normal tissues increased relative to that of tumors and because malignant cells had a greater reproductive capacity and were, therefore, more likely to be in a radiosensitive phase.

Based on these and other observations, the term *radiocurability* was coined. It refers to the eradication of tumor at the primary or regional site and reflects a direct effect of the irradiation producing logarithmic cell killing; this does not necessarily equate with the patient's cure from cancer (Table 1.5 and Box 1.5). In contrast, *radiosensitivity* is a measure of tumor–radiation response, thus describing the degree and speed of regression during and immediately after radiotherapy. However, for some malignant tumors, no significant correlation exists between the responsiveness of a tumor to irradiation and its radiocurability.

The response of human tumors to irradiation is a key issue for radiation oncologists and has been addressed by many leading radiobiologists.[88] At least four explanations have been considered that could alone or in combination account for the different radiosensitivities of tumors[89–91]:

1. *Hypoxia.* To explain the spectrum of clinical radioresponsiveness on this basis, it is likely that the less responsive tumors either have a high hypoxic fraction, have failed to reoxygenate during fractionated treatment, or both.[92]

TABLE 1.5 VARIOUS LEVELS OF IRRADIATION WILL YIELD DIFFERENT PROBABILITIES OF TUMOR CONTROL, DEPENDING ON THE SIZE OF THE LESION

Cumulative Dose (Gy)	Initial Cell Number	Probability of Survival	Remaining Cell Number
2	1,000,000,000	×0.5 =	500,000,000
4	500,000,000	×0.5 =	250,000,000
6	250,000,000	×0.5 =	125,000,000
8	125,000,000	×0.5 =	62,500,000
10	67,500,000	×0.5 =	31,250,000
12	33,750,000	×0.5 =	15,625,000
14	15,625,000	×0.5 =	7,812,500
16	7,823,500	×0.5 =	3,906,250
18	3,906,250	×0.5 =	1,953,125
20	1,953,125	×0.5 =	976,562
22	976,562	×0.5 =	488,281
24	488,281	×0.5 =	244,140
26	244,140	×0.5 =	122,070
28	122,070	×0.5 =	61,035
30	61,035	×0.5 =	30,517
32	30,517	×0.5 =	15,258
34	15,258	×0.5 =	7,629
36	7,629	×0.5 =	3,814
38	3,814	×0.5 =	1,907
40	1,907	×0.5 =	953
42	953	×0.5 =	476
44	476	×0.5 =	238
46	238	×0.5 =	119
48	119	×0.5 =	59
50	59	×0.5 =	29
52	29	×0.5 =	15
54	15	×0.5 =	7
56	7	×0.5 =	4
58	4	×0.5 =	2
60	2	×0.5 =	1
62	1	×0.5 =	<1

Direct oxygen electrode measurements have shown that cervical cancer, breast cancer, and squamous cell cancers are human tumors reported to have mean oxygen pressures below those of the surrounding tissue.[93–96] Despite a wide range of values, the oxygen pressure in tumors tends to decrease with increasing tumor size.[97] Although it is not possible to prove that hypoxia is unimportant in conventional radiation therapy, some doubts about its importance have been expressed based on the limited success of neutron therapy or hypoxic cell radiosensitizers.[98,99] Hypoxia can act as an important determinant of selecting for tumor cells of a more malignant phenotype that is likely to adversely affect treatment outcome.[94,98,100]

2. *Proportion of clonogenic cells.* Proliferating cells are more radiosensitive and have a greater turnover (cell loss) rate. Tumor regression during irradiation may be proportional to the total number of proliferating cells (growth fraction) or the proliferative rate, which may accelerate for certain tumor cells as a result of adaptive processes (accelerated repopulation) during fractionated irradiation.

3. *Inherent radiosensitivity of tumor cells.* Fertil and Malaise[101] and Deacon et al.[102] established a positive correlation between the steepness of the initial slope of the oxic cell survival curve for human tumor cells and their response to radiation. The magnitude of differences between cell lines at low doses is sufficient to explain the range of curability observed clinically. Steel and Peacock[103] analyzed human tumor radiosensitivity in light of existing concepts of cell killing based on the linear-quadratic (LQ) equation. However, despite encouraging correlations in some studies, these radiobiologic parameters have not been accepted for routine clinical use.

4. *Repair of radiation damage.* Repair of sublethal damage (SLD; split-dose effect) is observed in almost all tumor cell lines.[104–106,384] Potentially lethal damage (PLD) repair after a single dose varies considerably from one cell line to another and has been reported by Weichselbaum and Little[107] to correlate with clinical radiocurability, with less curable tumors showing the greatest degree of PLD recovery. These repair parameters have not been confirmed in larger clinical experiences to justify their use as predictors of radiotherapy outcomes (see later in this chapter).

Some investigators have reported a correlation between the clinical or pathologic response of a tumor after the completion of irradiation with ultimate probability of local tumor control.[108] For this analysis to be valid, it is necessary to compare patients with the same initial stage because, in general, more advanced lesions have a greater probability of tumor persistence at the completion of radiation therapy and local recurrence may be more frequent. Barkley and Fletcher[109] reported 82% tumor control in 88 patients with tumors of the oropharynx that had regressed completely at the end of therapy, in contrast to 41% in 237 patients with persistent tumor at completion of therapy. Sobel et al.[110] concluded that local tumor control in head and neck carcinomas could be predicted with the greatest accuracy and consistency 1 to 3 months after completion of radiotherapy. They noted that the prediction was 80% accurate in favorable tumors (T1 and T2) but decreased to 50% to 60% in more advanced primary lesions; complete tumor clearance was a more accurate predictor of tumor control. This was confirmed for the radiotherapeutic management of N2 (>3 cm) neck disease, where complete clinical resolution of tumor within 8 weeks of completion of irradiation correlated with a >90% freedom from neck failures.[111,112] Contemporary studies based on pathologic confirmation of complete tumor response or PET scan response show similar results.

Tumor Radiosensitivity and Predictive Assays

Since the inception of the use of ionizing radiation, many investigators have categorized the response of tumors according to their sensitivity to irradiation. Wetterer[113] in 1913 characterized tumor radiosensitivity based on histologic types, and Paterson[114] divided tumors into three groups: radiosensitive, intermediate, and radioresistant. The first category included germ cell tumors and reticuloses; the second included squamous cell and adenocarcinomas; and the third group included soft tissue and bone sarcomas and melanomas. However, depending on variation in proliferative rates and cell loss, endpoints for response assessment may vary substantially, as has been pointed out for malignant melanoma.[115] Attempts have been made to predict the response of tumors to radiation depending on several parameters, such as the assay proposed by Glucksmann[116] consisting of differential cell counts of mitotic, resting, and degenerating cells in biopsy samples from the growing edge of the tumor before and after initiation of radiotherapy. It is generally accepted that tumors contain mixed cell populations of stem cells with differing sensitivity to antineoplastic agents and that therapy can be selected for resistant cell populations or, in the case of certain cytotoxic agents, to induce cellular resistance.[117] Peters et al.[118,119] described a predictive assay to assess tumor response *in vitro* and the difficulties in predicting the probability of tumor control by irradiation in a given patient. Unfortunately, despite promising correlations between radiosensitivity *in vitro* and radioresponsiveness of normal tissues and tumors,[120,121] sufficiently powered predictive assays have not been identified. Given the inherent intertumor variability of predictive parameters, such as SF_2[122,123] or T_{POT},[124,125] and the genetic profile of tumor cells, a single predictive assay is unlikely to carry sufficient predictive power. The incorporation of multiple radiobiologic tumor cell parameters (e.g., markers for radiosensitivity and proliferation potential) into TCP (see later in this chapter) models appears more promising but awaits broader validation in clinical trials.[126]

Probability of Tumor Control

For many histologic types of cancer, higher radiation doses produce better tumor control. Numerous dose–response curves for a variety of tumors have been published. The first dose–response data were reported for skin cancer by Miescher[127] in 1934; 10 years later, Strandqvist[128] published a dose–response curve for skin cancer. The Strandqvist plots were refined by von Essen,[129] who demonstrated from a large skin carcinoma experience that the slopes for 97% tumor control and 3% skin necrosis differed and permitted, through appropriate fractionation schedules also considering the volume of disease, a dissociation of the two endpoints. As Fletcher[130] pointed out, meaningful dose–response curves can be generated only when a group of homogeneous tumors is given a range of radiation doses, indicating that tumor control is a probabilistic event. For every increment of radiation dose, a certain fraction of cells will be killed; therefore, the total number of surviving clonogenic cells will be proportional to the initial number present and the fraction killed with each dose.[104,105] Thus, various levels of irradiation will yield different probabilities of tumor control, depending on the extent of the lesion (number of clonogenic cells present). For subclinical disease in squamous cell carcinoma of the upper respiratory tract or for adenocarcinoma of the breast, doses of 45 to 50 Gy will result in disease control in more than 90% of patients.[130,131] Subclinical disease has been referred to as deposits of tumor cells that are too small to be detected clinically and even microscopically but, if left untreated, subsequently may evolve to clinically apparent tumor.[132,133] It must be emphasized that microscopic evidence of tumor, such as at the surgical margin, should not be regarded as subclinical disease; cell aggregates $\geq 10^5/cm^3$ are required for the pathologist to detect them. Therefore, these volumes must receive higher doses of irradiation, in the range of 60 to 65 Gy, in 6 to 7 weeks for epithelial tumors. This distinction of disease extent is re-emphasized by clinical results, demonstrating the need for irradiating patients with likely subclinical carcinoma to postoperative doses near 60 Gy.[134]

For clinically palpable head and neck tumors, doses of 65 (for T1) to 75 to 80 Gy or higher (for T4 tumors) are required at 2 Gy/day using five fractions weekly. This dose range and probability of tumor control have been documented for squamous cell carcinoma and adenocarcinoma.[87,130,131,135–138] Even with preoperative irradiation, the dose effect on probability of tumor control can be documented.

Baclesse[139] introduced the concept of different doses of irradiation for various portions of the tumor. The higher dose administered through small portals to residual disease is called a *boost*, which is delivered in an effort to achieve the same probability of tumor control as for subclinical aggregates.[130] One consequence of the concepts discussed earlier is use of portals that are progressively reduced in size. This *shrinking-field* technique administers higher radiation doses to the entire gross tumor where more clonogenic cells (including hypoxic cells) reside, relative to lower doses to tissues in the immediate proximity of the clinically apparent (gross) tumor. The tissues making up the "tumor margin" contain a lower number of tumor clonogens that are better oxygenated (see Fig. 1.8).

Normal Tissue Effects

A variety of normal tissue changes are induced by ionizing radiation, depending on the total dose, fractionation schedule (daily dose and overall treatment time), and volume treated.[307] These factors are closely interrelated (Fig. 1.9). Hermann Holthusen (1886–1971) created a diagram, which represented the hoped-for relationship between radiation dose and tumor control and radiation dose and normal tissue injury. First published by Holthusen in the 1930s, it has been reproduced innumerable times (Fig. 1.10). Holthusen "maintained that the margin of safety between effective tumor dose and safe tissue tolerance was dependant on volume of tissue irradiated and fractionation of the total dose… tolerance could be increased by fractionation."[140,141]

It has been postulated that for many normal tissues, the radiation dose necessary to produce a particular sequela increases as the irradiated fraction of volume of the organ decreases. This concept was demonstrated for skin by Paterson,[114] who plotted doses delivered with orthovoltage x-rays that would produce moist desquamation (Fig. 1.11). The same phenomenon later was reported for supervoltage irradiation of other organs[142] and for brachytherapy.

Higher tolerance doses (TDs) than initially reported have been observed for a variety of organs,[137,138,143–145] as a result of conform a-1 irradiation. This stresses the importance of updating tolerance information in light of more precise treatment planning and delivery of irradiation and more accurate evaluation and recording of sequelae. Examples are radiation

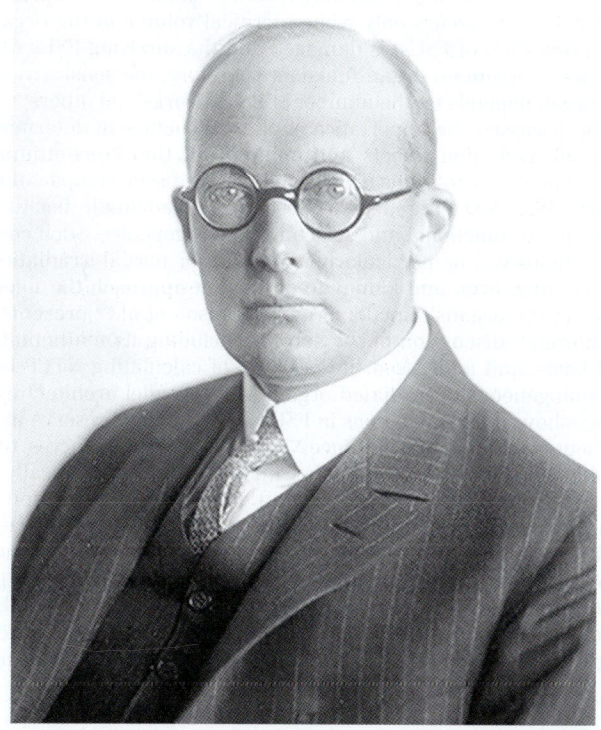

FIGURE 1.10. Hermann Holthusen (1886–1971) created these hypothetical curves for tumor control and normal tissue injury to demonstrate the dose–response of radiotherapy. One tries to shift the curves as far apart as possible.

dose escalation studies using conformal radiotherapy delivery techniques. A compilation from the literature of data on TDs for whole- or partial-organ irradiation was published by Emami et al.[146] The comprehensive update of this compilation, QUANTEC, is described in Chapter 14.

In studying late radiation effects, an organ can be considered to be made up of multiple functional subunits (FSUs) that are arranged serially or in parallel.[40,147] For serially structured organs, such as gastrointestinal tract or nervous tissue, damage to one portion of the organ may render the entire organ dysfunctional. In contrast, in organs with parallel structure, FSU damage

FIGURE 1.11. Graph showing the relationship between dose and size of area irradiated (healthy skin in an "average" site) to produce moist desquamation for various overall treatment times (daily irradiation at about 50 R/minute for each exposure with radiation of half-value layer 1.5 mm Cu). (From Paterson R. *The treatment of malignant disease by radium and x-rays*. Baltimore: Williams & Wilkins, 1949:39. With permission.)

FIGURE 1.9. Difference in cell survival curves for acute and late radiation effects with single or multifractionated doses of irradiation. (Reprinted from Fowler JF. Fractionation and therapeutic gain. In: Steel GG, Adams GE, Peckham MT, eds. *Biological basis of radiotherapy*. 2nd ed. Amsterdam: Elsevier Science, 1983: 181–194. Copyright © 1983 Elsevier. With permission.)

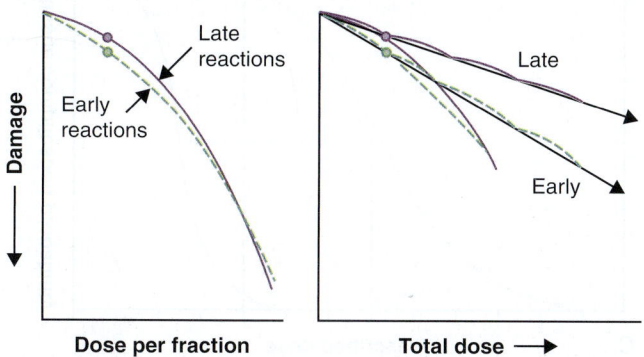

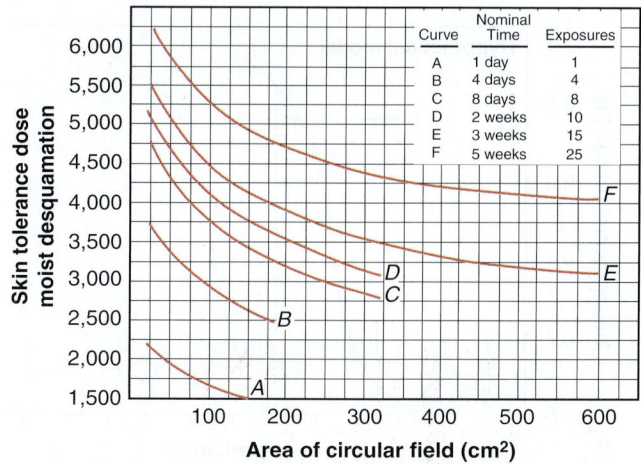

Curve	Nominal Time	Exposures
A	1 day	1
B	4 days	4
C	8 days	8
D	2 weeks	10
E	3 weeks	15
F	5 weeks	25

may not impair the entire organ function because the remaining FSUs operate independently from the damaged group, and clinical injury occurs only when a critical volume of the organ (or proportion of FSUs) is damaged and the surviving FSUs are unable to maintain organ function. Therefore, the sensitivity of an organ depends on the number of FSUs. Marks and others[148,149] have discussed the importance of organ structure in determining late radiation effects and pointed out that conventional dose–volume histograms (DVHs) and normal tissue complication probability (NTCP) models are frequently inadequate because they ignore functional and structural heterogeneities. Such considerations will be particularly important for partial irradiation of the lung, liver, and kidney to doses that approach the tolerance of the organs' functional units. Jackson et al.[150] presented a thorough discussion of the subject, including its mathematical basis, and addressed the problem of calculating NTCP for inhomogeneously irradiated organs with parallel architecture. They showed that variations in FSUs and functional reserve in a patient population may produce NTCP dose–response curves, the widths of which are comparable with those observed clinically.

Structural alterations without anatomic or functional impairment may be noted, whereas in other instances, substantial injuries with tissue destruction, severe dysfunction, or even death may occur. Normal tissues have a substantial capacity to recover from sublethal or PLD induced by radiation (at tolerable dose levels). Injury to normal tissues may be caused by the radiation effect on the microvasculature or the support tissues (stromal or parenchymal cells).[90]

Rubin et al.[151–153] indicated the usefulness of assigning a certain percentage of risk of complication, depending on the dose of the radiation. The minimal TD is defined as TD$_{5/5}$, which represents the dose of radiation that could cause no more than a 5% severe complication rate within 5 years after treatment. (Some authors use the equivalent terms "tissue tolerance dose," or TTD$_{5/5}$. Both the TD$_{5/5}$ and the TTD$_{5/5}$ are based on treatment at 2 Gy per fraction, five fractions per week.) Acceptable complication risk rate for severe injury of 5% in most curative clinical situations is generally viewed as acceptable. Moderate sequelae are noted in varying proportions (10% to 25% of patients), depending on the dose of irradiation given and the OARs.

Chronologically, the effects of irradiation are subdivided into acute (first 3 months) and late effects (more than 3 months after irradiation), according to the National Cancer Institute Common Toxicity Criteria. The gross manifestations depend on the kinetic properties of the cells (slow or rapid renewal) and the total radiation dose given.[310]

Early applications of time–dose considerations were applied by Baclesse[154,155] based on observations by Coutard[32,33,77] that various degrees of mucositis and moist desquamation were repaired by re-epithelialization of the mucosa and skin from the periphery of the irradiated field and from cells surviving in the center of the field. Protracted fractionation schedules for carcinoma of the breast with lower daily doses over 10 to 12 weeks were successful in avoiding acute moist desquamation,[155] but the higher radiation doses caused severe tissue damage in a large number of patients.[156]

No correlation has been established between the incidence and severity of acute reactions and the occurrence of late effects. Withers et al.[157] compiled data depicting isoeffect lines for acute or late effects in several organs. The slopes for late reactions were steeper than for acute effects, and there was a lack of correlation between the doses producing similar severities of acute or late effects.[158,159] This may result from the difference in the slopes of cell survival curves for acute or late-reacting tissues[70] (Figs. 1.12 and 1.13).

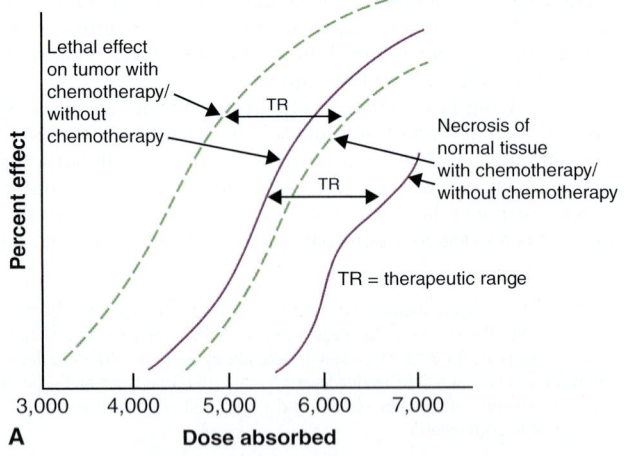

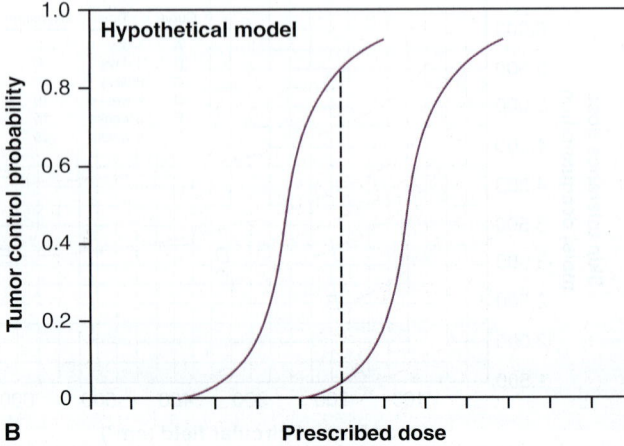

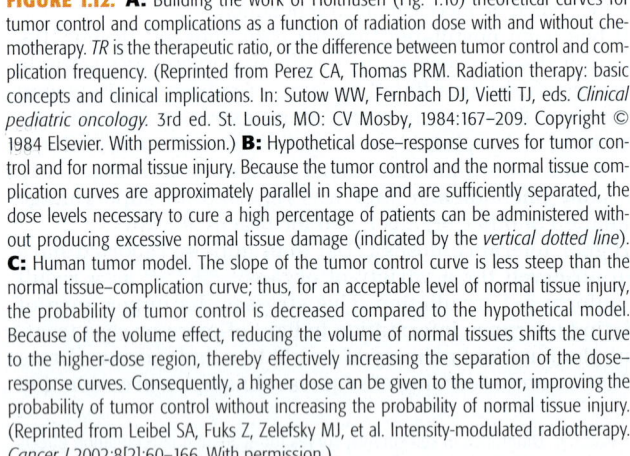

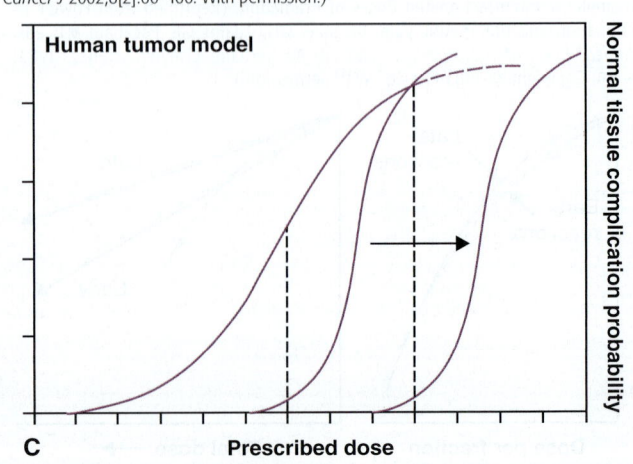

FIGURE 1.12. A: Building the work of Holthusen (Fig. 1.10) theoretical curves for tumor control and complications as a function of radiation dose with and without chemotherapy. *TR* is the therapeutic ratio, or the difference between tumor control and complication frequency. (Reprinted from Perez CA, Thomas PRM. Radiation therapy: basic concepts and clinical implications. In: Sutow WW, Fernbach DJ, Vietti TJ, eds. *Clinical pediatric oncology*. 3rd ed. St. Louis, MO: CV Mosby, 1984:167–209. Copyright © 1984 Elsevier. With permission.) **B:** Hypothetical dose–response curves for tumor control and for normal tissue injury. Because the tumor control and the normal tissue complication curves are approximately parallel in shape and are sufficiently separated, the dose levels necessary to cure a high percentage of patients can be administered without producing excessive normal tissue damage (indicated by the *vertical dotted line*). **C:** Human tumor model. The slope of the tumor control curve is less steep than the normal tissue–complication curve; thus, for an acceptable level of normal tissue injury, the probability of tumor control is decreased compared with the hypothetical model. Because of the volume effect, reducing the volume of normal tissues shifts the curve to the higher-dose region, thereby effectively increasing the separation of the dose–response curves. Consequently, a higher dose can be given to the tumor, improving the probability of tumor control without increasing the probability of normal tissue injury. (Reprinted from Leibel SA, Fuks Z, Zelefsky MJ, et al. Intensity-modulated radiotherapy. *Cancer J* 2002;8[2]:60–166. With permission.)

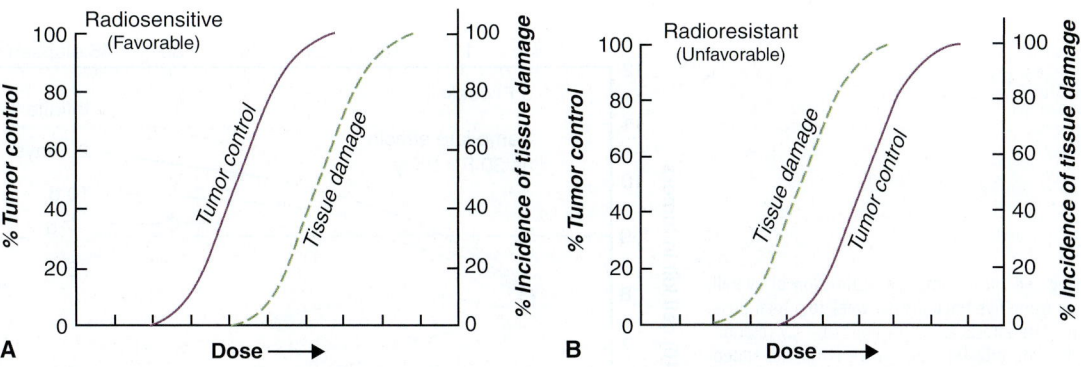

FIGURE 1.13. Different therapeutic ratios exist in different clinical circumstances depending on the radiosensitivity (dose–response curves) for the tumor versus critical normal tissue in the treatment field. **A:** Favorable. **B:** Unfavorable. (Reprinted from Rubin P. *Clinical oncology: a multidisciplinary approach for physicians and students.* 7th ed. Philadelphia: W. B. Saunders, 1993. Copyright © 1993 Elsevier. With permission.)

Combining irradiation with surgery or cytotoxic agents frequently modifies the tolerance of normal tissues to a given dose of irradiation, which may necessitate adjustments in treatment planning and dose prescription. The lack of correlation between acute and late-reacting tissues represents one rationale for combining radiotherapy with chemotherapy. As long as the enhanced acute toxicities of combined treatment can be managed, no significant increased damage in late-reacting tissues is expected.[159]

QUANTITATION OF TREATMENT TOXICITY

There is a critical need to accurately assess and record morbidity of treatment because this, in addition to therapeutic efficacy, is a crucial parameter in the evaluation of new regimens and in the selection of therapy for an individual patient. Multiple schemata have been developed, although a complete consensus has not been reached as to ideal grading scores. Toxicity grading systems for various organs were developed by RTOG and the European Organisation for Research and Treatment of Cancer (EORTC). Overgaard and Bartelink[34] stressed the importance of proper recording of morbidity in clinical radiation oncology, with quantification of the normal tissue effects and description of the treatment-related factors correlating with morbidity.

The evolution of radiation treatment planning and delivery, with innovative techniques (3DCRT, IMRT, image-guided radiation therapy, image-guided brachytherapy), particle therapy allowing for better definition of target and sensitive structure volumes and more precise quantitation of dose, has introduced more complexity into the evaluation of radiation effects on OARs. Journal articles and a book have been devoted to the "Quantitative Analysis of Normal Tissue Effects in the Clinic (QUANTEC)," which provided an updated review of knowledge in this area and practical guidance on toxicity risks and attempted to identify future research to elucidate radiation effects in normal tissues and organs. The QUANTEC program has continued its efforts and produced other publications. (See Chapter 14.)

Therapeutic Ratio (Gain)

The improved definitions of TCP and NTCP[160] imply that there is an optimal radiation dose that produces a maximum tumor control with a minimum (reasonably acceptable) frequency of complications, also called treatment sequelae. The farther the TCP and NTCP curves diverge, the more favorable is the therapeutic ratio (Fig. 1.14). The therapeutic ratio or therapeutic gain factor (TGF) of a given regimen could be expressed as a ratio:

$$TGF = \frac{\% \text{ tumor control with therapy A versus therapy B}}{\% \text{ complications with therapy A versus therapy B}}$$

FIGURE 1.14. Treatment outcomes. Uncomplicated curves (*dashed line*) are the desired results of treatment. This is illustrated as a function of the therapeutic ratio; that is, the greater the separation of the tumor control curve and the normal tissue–complication curve, the greater the number of uncomplicated cures that will result. The letters *A*, *B*, and *C* represent three different dose levels, which, if chosen, would lead to three different outcomes: *A* would result in few tumor cures but no complications; *C* would lead to complete cure in many cases, but virtually all patients would suffer complications. The optimal choice in this group of dose levels is *B*, which would result in the greatest number of cured patients without complications. (From Mendelsohn ML. The biology of dose-limiting tissues. In: *Time and dose relationships in radiation biology as applied to radiotherapy.* Brookhaven National Laboratory [BNL] Report 5023 [C-57]. Upton, NY: Brookhaven National Laboratory, 1969:154–173. Courtesy Brookhaven National Laboratory.)

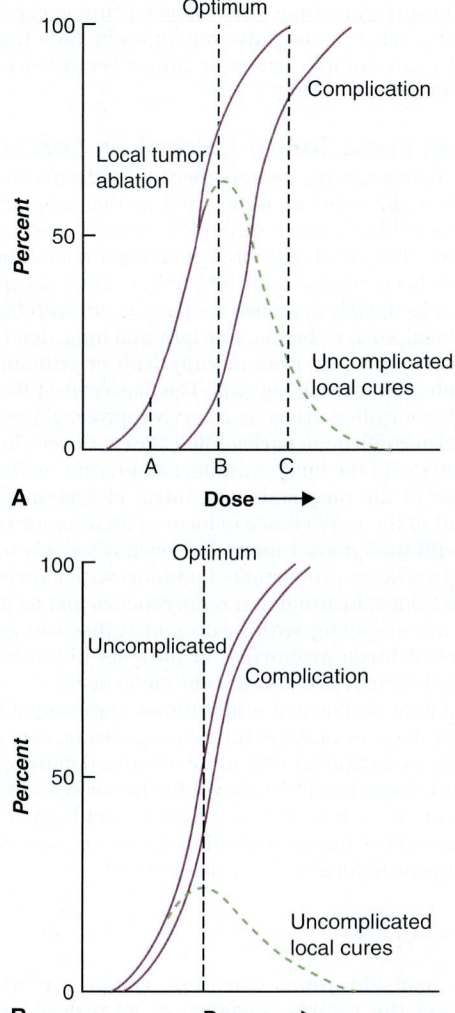

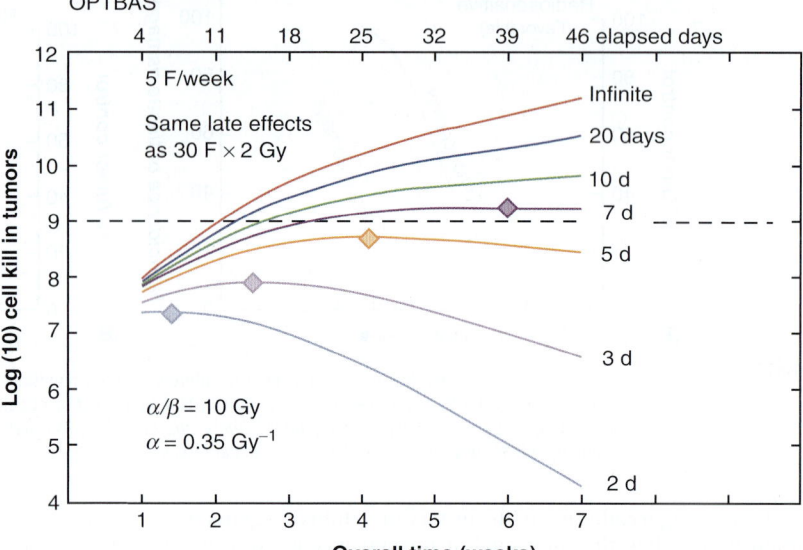

FIGURE 1.15. Log cell kill in tumors as a function of overall time, for schedules using five fractions per week to a total dose that gives the same late effects as 30 fractions of 2 Gy (assuming α/β = 3 Gy for late effects). Each curve is for the stated proliferation doubling time (average over the overall time). The diamond-shaped symbols show the maximum cell kill for that doubling time, at the optimum overall time for that number of fractions per week. If there is no diamond, the optimum overall time is longer than 7 weeks. The dotted line is drawn arbitrarily at 9 logs of cell kill. (Reprinted from Fowler JF. How worthwhile are short schedules in radiotherapy? A series of exploratory calculations. *Radiother Oncol* 1990;18[2]:165–181. Copyright © 1990 Elsevier Ireland Ltd. With permission.)

The higher the TGF, the more efficient a particular therapy. Such a quantitative expression could be used to compare different therapeutic strategies. Mendelsohn[161] expressed this concept in terms of "uncomplicated tumor ablation."

The selection of a dose must weigh the probability of major complications for any potential enhancement of tumor control. Models for decision-making, using Bayesian theory, incorporate values assigned to positive or negative outcomes.[161] Positive outcome is considered tumor cure without complication, whereas negative outcomes include tumor cure with significant complications or tumor recurrence with or without complications (Fig. 1.15).

Impact of Local Tumor Control on Survival

Systemic chemotherapy, immunotherapy, and molecularly targeted therapy have been emphasized as therapies that could improve survival of cancer through control of systemic metastatic disease. The effect of locoregional tumor control on patient survival has been emphasized repeatedly.[162] Clinical experiences and randomized trials demonstrate for cancers with high metastatic potential, such as breast, prostate, and lung, that improved locoregional control by radiotherapy with or without chemotherapy enhances overall survival. This has revived the interest in locoregional radiotherapy as a survival-prolonging treatment modality, also confirming earlier clinical experiences in patients with carcinoma of the lung, prostate, and uterine cervix.

Because of the emphasis on control of systemic disease, assessment of the importance of locoregional tumor control in patients with malignant tumors has been relatively underemphasized. In a large proportion of patients with cancer seen in the United States, locoregional recurrence is just as prevalent (69% of patients dying with locoregional disease) as distant metastases. A large proportion of patients (50%) have both locoregional recurrence and distant metastases.

Clinical data demonstrate that tumor persistence after initial therapy does, because of tumor progression, carry as poor a prognosis as treatment of a more advanced cancer. In addition, radiotherapy has been shown for tumor with high metastatic potential, such as breast, prostate, and lung, to prolong overall survival if higher radiation doses are delivered and achieve improved local control rates.[115,163,164]

DOSE–TIME FACTORS

Dose–time considerations constitute complex relationships that express the interdependence of total dose, time, and number of fractions in the production of a biologic effect within a given tissue volume. This phenomenon, from a radiobiologic viewpoint, is closely related to the four Rs of ionizing radiation:

1. *Repair* of sublethal and PLD
2. *Repopulation* of cells between fractions
3. *Redistribution* of cells throughout the cell cycle (partially, the result of radiation-induced synchrony secondary to transient arrest at cell cycle checkpoints and cell cycle–dependent cell killing)
4. *Reoxygenation* occurring during repeated radiation exposures

The advantages of dose fractionation include:

1. Reduction in the number of hypoxic cells occurs through cell killing and reoxygenation. There is increased oxygenation in the tumor after irradiation, whereas changes in normal tissue oxygen are slight or nonexistent.[165]
2. Reduction in the absolute number of clonogenic tumor cells by the preceding fractions with the killing of the better-oxygenated cells. Assuming a constant supply of oxygen, fewer cancer cells will have access to an increased amount of oxygen.
3. Blood vessels compressed by a growing cancer are decompressed secondary to tumor regression, thus permitting better oxygenation despite the constant diffusion distance of oxygen in tissue near 200 μm.
4. Fractionation exploits the difference in recovery rate between normal, acute, and late-reacting tissues and tumors. Radiation-induced redistribution of cells within the cell cycle tends to sensitize rapidly proliferating cells as they move into the more sensitive phases of the cell cycle.
5. The acute normal tissue toxicity of single radiation doses can be decreased with fractionation. Thus, patients' tolerance of radiotherapy will improve with fractionated irradiation.

In general, fractionated irradiation will spare acute reactions because of compensatory proliferation in the epithelium of the skin or the mucosa, acceleration of which can be measured experimentally 2 or 3 weeks after initiation of therapy, but most likely starts with initiation of irradiation.[166–169] However, a prolonged course of therapy with small daily fractions will decrease early acute reactions but not necessarily prevent serious late damage to normal tissues. This approach also promotes accelerated repopulation and permits the growth of rapidly proliferating tumors. A major research

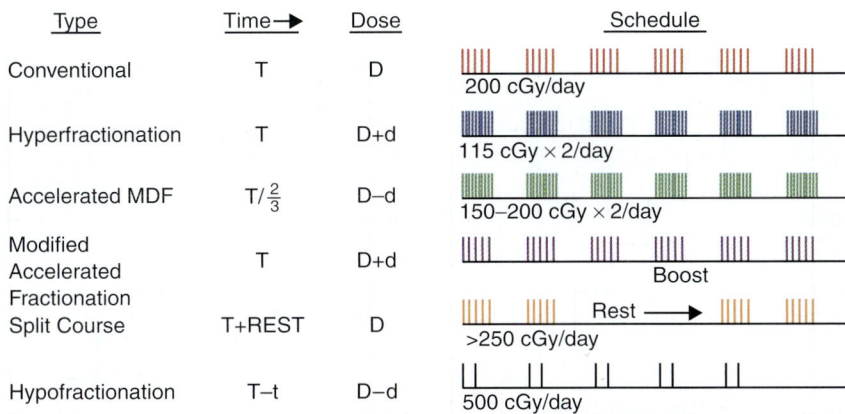

Type	Time→	Dose	Schedule

Conventional   T   D   200 cGy/day

Hyperfractionation   T   D+d   115 cGy × 2/day

Accelerated MDF   T/$\frac{2}{3}$ D−d   150–200 cGy × 2/day

Modified Accelerated Fractionation   T   D+d   Boost

Split Course   T+REST   D   Rest →   >250 cGy/day

Hypofractionation   T−t   D−d   500 cGy/day

FIGURE 1.16. Various types of fractionation used in radiation therapy.

effort in clinical radiobiology is and will be devoted to the optimization of dose–time fractionation schedules for various tumors that are individualized depending on cell kinetic characteristics, molecular biology, and clinical observations.[126,170,171] Fowler[71] published theoretic considerations based on a series of assumptions of the values used in the LQ equation with a time factor in which he attempted to predict the optimal dose fractionation schedules for tumors with various cell doubling times. He concluded that optimal overall times depend primarily on the doubling time of the tumor cells and intrinsic radiosensitivity, alpha (assumed to be proportional to α/β). Short overall treatment times are required for tumors with a low α/β ratio or fast proliferation. For median potential doubling times of 5 days and intermediate radiosensitivity, overall times of 2.5 to 4 weeks would be optimal. More slowly proliferating tumors, he argued, should be treated with longer overall times (Fig. 1.15). Clinical studies, however, support relatively short overall treatment times in several common solid malignancies, in contrast to Fawler's conclusions. *In vitro* techniques to assess tumor radiosensitivity in biopsy specimens ultimately may be helpful as predictive assays.

Altered Fractionation

Without a solid biologic basis and out of empiricism and convenience, the "standard fractionation" for radiation therapy has evolved into five fractions weekly. Other fractionation schedules have been proposed that deliver multiple fractions daily or six fractions weekly or use a hyperfractionation split-course regimen (Fig. 1.16). Based on the narrow window between improvements in tumor control and enhanced normal tissue toxicities,[55] any altered fractionation schedule is potentially harmful and must be approached with caution. However, the improved quality of clinical trials by national study groups and by individual institutions has generated a growing body of clinical outcome data that, together with improved biologic modeling, allows relatively accurate predictions of clinical outcomes based on relative biologic effectiveness (RBE) calculations[172] (Table 1.6).

Multiple daily fractions are likely to be more effective in rapidly growing tumors with a high growth fraction. Normal tissues behave as actively proliferating cells for expression of acute reactions but as slowly proliferating cells in the manifestation of late injury.[173,174] As suggested by several biologic studies,[175] clinical trial results conducted by EORTC and RTOG demonstrated that a minimum of 6 hours of interfraction interval should be allowed when multiple daily fractions are used to allow maximum repair of normal tissues. This is supported by reduced complication rates in patients irradiated for carcinoma of the lung and a highly uniform cohort of patients with tonsillar squamous cell carcinomas.[72,134]

Accelerated fractionation aims at shortening the overall treatment time. Schedules may use larger than standard size fractions five times weekly or more than five fractions per week of 2 Gy. In addition, multiple fractions of radiation may be given daily exclusively or in combination with standard fractions of 2 Gy. Some reduction in the total dose delivered may have to be used for fractions >2 Gy for normal tissue sparing. These schedules may be preferable with hypoxic cell sensitizers or other chemical modifiers of radiation response that require the presence of a high concentration of the compound in the tumor at the time of the radiation exposure.

With hyperfractionation, a larger number of smaller-than-conventional dose fractions are given daily; the total daily dose is usually 10% to 20% greater than with standard fractionation; the total period of time is minimally changed; and the total dose needs to be escalated to achieve tumor toxicity similar to that of standard fractionation. The aim of hyperfractionation is to achieve the same incidence of late effects on normal tissue as observed with a comparable conventional regimen while increasing the probability of tumor control through dose escalation.[176]

TABLE 1.6 COMPARISON OF VARIOUS FRACTIONATION SCHEDULES

	Conventional	Split-Course	Accelerated Fractionation	Hyperfractionation
Indication, in tumors, of growth rate	Average	Average or slow	Rapid	Slow (with large cell loss factors)
Normal tissue effects, acute	Standard	Standard or greater	Greater	Standard or greater
Normal tissue effects, late	Standard	Greater	Standard (if complete repair of sublethal damage occurs) or greater	Lower
Advantages	–	Shorter actual treatment time (fewer fractions)	Destroys more tumor cells; prevents tumor cell repopulation; less overall treatment time	Lower OER with small doses; spares late damage; allows reoxygenation; allows stem cell repopulation
Disadvantages	–	May permit tumor repopulation	–	More fractions

OER, oxygen enhancement ratio.

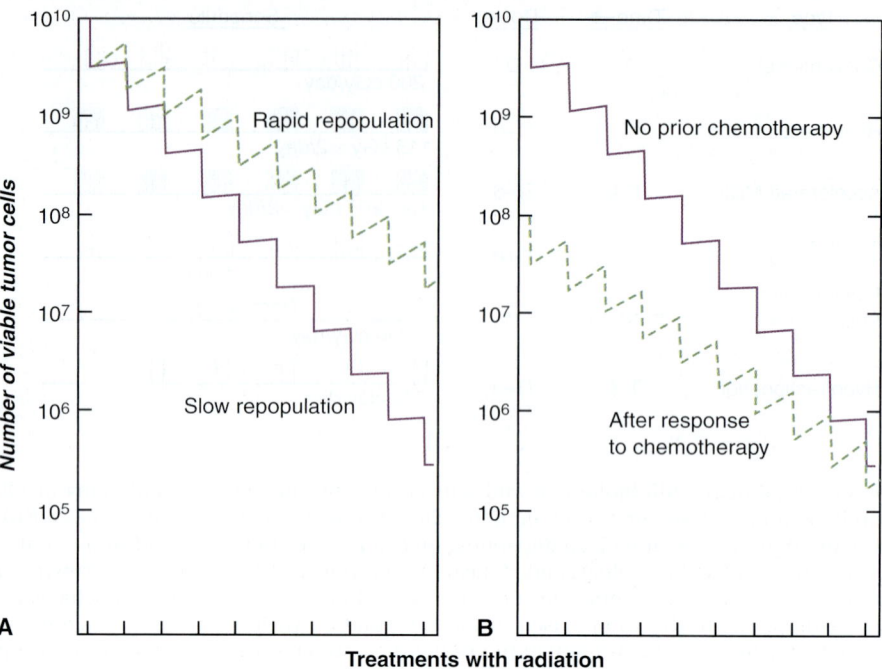

FIGURE 1.17. A: Schematic diagram indicating that cell survival during a course of fractionated irradiation depends not only on the proportion of cells killed with each dose (equal for the two curves shown) but also on the rate of proliferation of surviving cells between dose fractions, which differs for the two curves. **B:** Hypothetical diagram to illustrate the number of surviving cells in a tumor during treatment with irradiation alone (*solid line*) or during radiation therapy delivered to a tumor that has responded to chemotherapy (i.e., cell number reduced to 1% at start of irradiation) but where proliferation has been stimulated (*dashed line*). Note that cell survival is similar after fractionated irradiation, despite the initial response to drugs. (Reprinted from Tannock IF. Combined modality treatment with radiotherapy and chemotherapy. *Radiother Oncol* 1989;16[2]:83–101. Copyright © 1989 Elsevier Ireland Ltd. With permission.)

Accelerated Repopulation

Withers and Taylor[40] described experimental observations documenting accelerated repopulation of tumor cells during fractionated radiotherapy and provided convincing evidence that this phenomenon occurs in clinical situations (Figs. 1.17 and 1.18). Although Withers and Taylor's analyses suggested that accelerated repopulation occurs preferentially after the 4th week of radiotherapy, reanalysis of the same data by Bentzen[41] and Thames et al.[177] and independent derivations by Fowler[168] suggested that repopulation starts early during fractionated irradiation. The latter is supported by experimental data of Schmidt-Ullrich et al.,[169] showing that molecular processes of accelerated repopulation, mediated through radiation-induced receptor activation and cellular growth stimulation, occur after a single radiation exposure of 2 Gy. The effectiveness of a course of fractionated irradiation depends in part on the killing by individual fractions as well as on the rate of proliferation of surviving cells between irradiation fractions. Neoadjuvant chemotherapy also may lead to increased proliferation of surviving tumor cells after partial regression of the lesion, which could result in decreased cell killing by subsequent fractionated irradiation.

Isoeffect Graphs

To express an equal biologic effect produced by various fractionation schedules, isoeffect lines have been generated. Kronig and Friedrich[178] first published the observation that a specific physical dose of irradiation is less biologically effective if given in multiple fractions, which embodies the original concept of recovery between fractions. Later, MacComb and Quimby[179] and Reisner[180] established the rate of recovery in experimentally produced skin reactions in patients.

In 1944, Strandqvist[128] published a monograph describing the results of treatment of 280 patients with skin cancer (squamous cell and basal cell carcinoma); most tumors were treated within 14 and 29 days, and only one was treated within 45 days. An isoeffect line was drawn, with a slope of 0.22. He fitted the recovery factors of MacComb and Quimby and Reisner using an extrapolated value of 0.35 per day as the time for a single dose. He also produced a graph for various degrees of radiation reaction on the skin, ranging from erythema to necrosis (Fig. 1.19). It should be emphasized that in these curves, the vertical coordinate represents the total dose given, and the abscissa represents the total duration in days after the first irradiation. However, some authors have plotted similar graphs representing the number of fractions in the horizontal coordinate. It is critical to identify these two parameters because one could deliver 60 Gy in 6 weeks in 30 fractions given five times weekly or the same dose delivered in 18 fractions given three times weekly. The effects on normal tissues certainly would be different. von Essen,[181] using the Strandqvist data as well as his own, pointed out the importance of the volume irradiated when isoeffect parameters are studied and generated a 3D display of these data.

Dutreix et al.[182] published observations on the influence of fraction size in patients with cancer of the lung, on whom one of the supraclavicular areas received a single exposure and the other area received two exposures separated by 6 hours. They noticed that two fractions of 1 Gy produced the same skin reaction as one fraction of 2 Gy. As the fraction size increased,

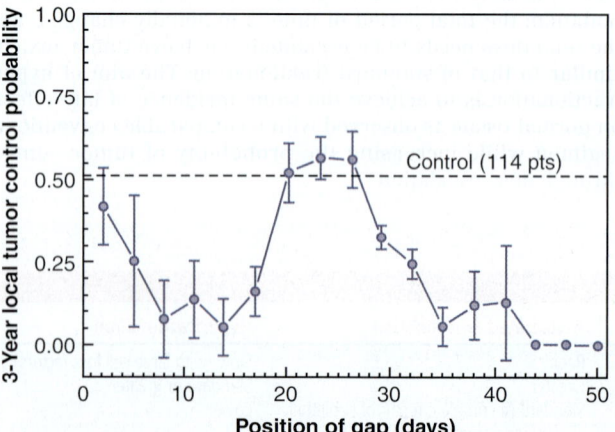

FIGURE 1.18. Dependence of tumor control probability (TCP) on the position of a single-treatment gap in 533 patients. Gap duration ranged from 3 to 20 days. Position of a gap is defined by its starting point. Each point shows the TCP averaged over 3 consecutive days (±SD). (Reprinted from Skladowski K, Law MG, Maciejewski B, et al. Planned and unplanned gaps in radiotherapy: the importance of gap position and gap duration. *Radiother Oncol* 1994;30[2]:109–120. Copyright © 1994 Elsevier Ireland Ltd. With permission.)

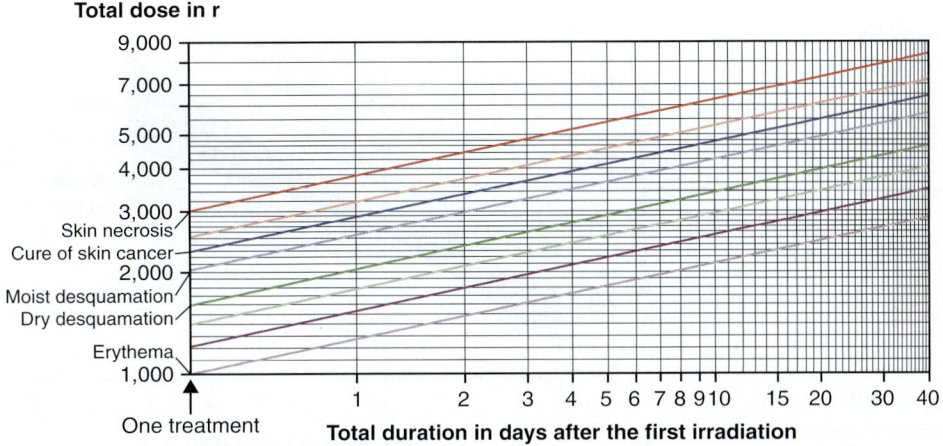

FIGURE 1.19. Strandqvist's curves on log paper. The slope of the curves (0.22) is the same for the tumoricidal dose for squamous cell carcinoma for various degrees of skin reactions. (From Strandqvist M. Sutdien uber die kumulative wirkung der rontgenstrahlen bie frakionierung. *Acta Radiol* [*Stockh*] 1944;55[Suppl]:1–300.)

however, it took a higher dose in the two-fraction schedule to produce the same reaction as with the single-fraction schedule. With mucositis of the faucial arch used as an endpoint, researchers at MD Anderson Cancer Center observed that 10 Gy per week given in five fractions of 2 Gy is equivalent to 11 Gy given in 10 fractions, twice a day, separated by 3 hours.[87]

The slopes for reactions for various normal tissues differ, as do slopes of tumor curability and normal tissue late effects. In general, the slope for tumor curability is less steep than that for normal tissue reactions. Isoeffect lines for various squamous cell carcinomas of the head and neck, different stages, have slopes varying from 0.33 to 0.38.[135,183] Furthermore, as stated earlier, tolerance of normal tissues is strongly related to the volume irradiated. Whereas 60 Gy could be given safely in 5 weeks for a small glottic tumor with a 5-cm by 4-cm portal, the same dose delivered in the same period for a supraglottic carcinoma, with a larger portal covering the entire larynx, would result in more severe acute and late sequelae[135] (Box 1.6).

Linear-Quadratic Equation (α/β Ratio)

Formulations based on dose survival models have been proposed to evaluate the biologic equivalence of various doses and fractionation schedules. These assumptions are based on an LQ survival curve represented by the equation:

$$\log_e S = \alpha D + \beta D^2,$$

in which α represents the *linear* (i.e., first-order dose-dependent) component of cell killing and β represents the *quadratic* (i.e., second-order dose-dependent) component of cell killing. Thus, β represents the more reparable (over a few hours) component of cell damage (Figs. 1.20–1.22). The dose at which the two components of cell killing are equal constitutes the α/β ratio.

In a study of 17 human tumor cell lines, Steel and Peacock[92] observed that the average surviving fraction at 2 Gy is 0.44 from the α component and 0.88 from the β component. The β effect at that dose level appears to be similar in radiosensitive and radioresistant tumors; thus, among radiosensitive tumors in which the survival from the α component is below 0.3, the β effect makes a very small contribution to overall radiosensitivity in the lower dose region. The overall effect of many small fractions is to amplify the dominance of the α component. The β effect is unimportant because repair will be almost complete. In the more radiocurable tumors, cell killing by the α component represents the predominant fraction of tumor cell killing.

The shape of the dose survival curve with photons differs for acutely and slowly responding normal tissues. This difference in shape is not observed with neutrons. The severity of

late effects changes more rapidly with a variation in the size of dose per fraction when a total dose is selected to yield equivalent acute effects. With a decreasing size of dose per fraction, the total dose required to achieve a certain isoeffect increases more for late-responding tissues than for acutely responding tissues. Thus, in hyperfractionated regimens, the tolerable dose would be increased more for late effects than for acute

Box 1.6

Nominal Standard Dose and Time–Dose Factor

The nominal standard dose (NSD) concept is of historic interest. For 20 years, NSD was used frequently to express equivalency of clinical doses of irradiation based on human skin tolerance and curability of squamous cell carcinoma. Cohen[378] pointed out that the regression coefficient for squamous cell carcinoma was different from that of normal skin (0.24). In 1969, Ellis[379] suggested that if one number could be used to represent the dose of irradiation that reached normal tissue tolerance, this would be advantageous in comparing different techniques. This figure should represent the normal connective tissue tolerance because this was, in his thinking, the limiting factor in most tumor therapies.

The unit for NSD expression was the *ret*. It could never be assumed that the NSD value represented a "single equivalent dose" because the isoeffect time calculated by Ellis used data from four to 30 fractions. Another flaw of the NSD calculation was that it did not allow for the effect of variations in volume treated or for interruptions of therapy (split-course therapy). Orton[380] estimated that NSD calculations were misused about 50% of the time by unaware clinicians comparing different radiation therapy regimens. The NSD formula did not predict isoeffect in pig skin irradiation with [184]Co using two to five fractions per week. Moreover, early reactions did not predict the magnitude of late damage when dose fractionation was altered from conventional daily schedules.

In 1973, Orton and Ellis[185] published a simplification of the NSD concept more applicable to clinical radiation therapy, stating that when a treatment did not result in normal connective tissue tolerance, treatment effectiveness should be described in terms of partial tolerance. Although there was no definite basis for the application of the time–dose factor (TDF) concept to clinical radiation therapy, equivalency of various dose schedules is sought constantly. For split-course regimens, the TDF values (in units of ret) were used by adding the TDF value for each of the partial tolerance factors corresponding to each component of the treatment and correcting for the decay of the first part of the treatment TDF.

In 1974, Orton[186] defined TDF values for continuous irradiation that could be used with temporary or permanent brachytherapy implants, using various isotopes. A standard radium therapy regimen of 60 Gy in 168 hours was used for comparison with other equivalent techniques. According to Ellis,[187] this was equivalent to 1,800 ret of fractionated external irradiation.

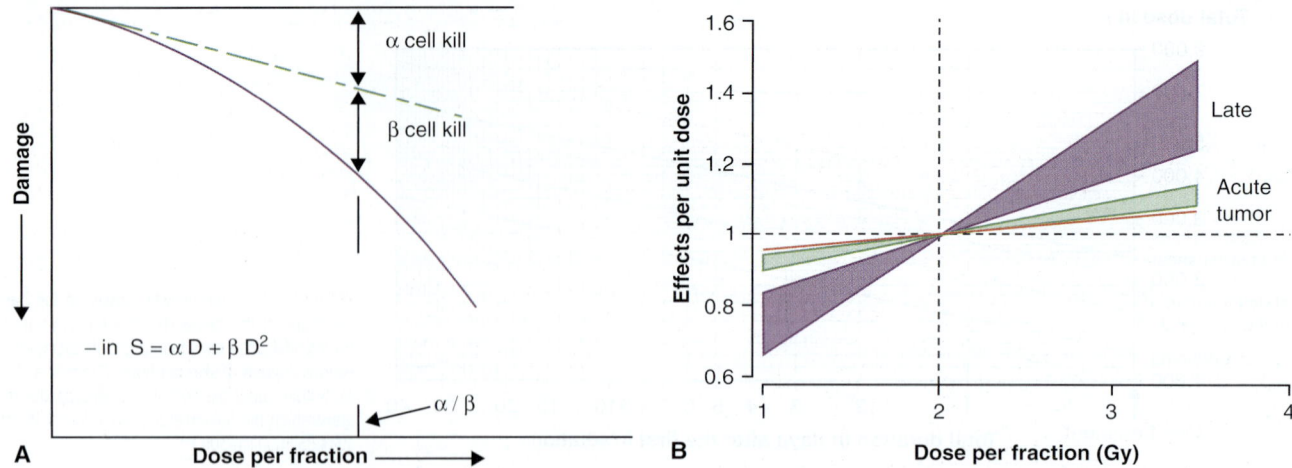

FIGURE 1.20. A: At a dose equal to the α/β ratio, the log cell kill because of the α-process (nonreparable) is equal to that because of the β-process (reparable injury); α/β is thus a measure of how soon the survival curve begins to bend over significantly. The α/β ratio for late effects on normal tissue generates a "curvier curve" than the α/β ratio for radiation's effects on acutely reacting normal tissue and tumor cells. Thus, the relative effect of dose per fraction is higher for late-responding tissue than for acutely responding tissues. In particular, for the central nervous system, high–dose-per-fraction radiation therapy is associated with an increased risk of late effects. An α/β ratio of 2 to 3 commonly is used in calculations of radiation effects on late-reacting tissue, whereas the ratio of 10 is used more commonly for acute-responding tissues or tumor. (Reprinted from Fowler JF. Fractionation and therapeutic gain. In: Steel GG, Adams GE, Peckham MT, eds. *Biological basis of radiotherapy.* 2nd ed. Amsterdam: Elsevier Science, 1983:181–194. Copyright © 1983 Elsevier. With permission.) **B:** A schematic representation of biologic data relating dose per fraction to effect on tumors, early-reacting, and late-reacting normal tissues. (Reprinted from Saunders MI. Programming of radiotherapy in the treatment of non-small-cell lung cancer—a way to advance cure. *Lancet Oncol* 2001;2[7]:401–408. Copyright © 2001 Elsevier. With permission.)

FIGURE 1.21. Hypothetical survival curves for the target cells for acute and late effects in normal tissues exposed to x-rays or neutrons. The α/β ratio in the equation for surviving fractions ($SF = e^{-\alpha D + \beta D_2}$) is higher for late effects than for acute effects in x-irradiated tissues, resulting in a greater rate of change in effect in late-responding tissues with change in dose. At dose A, survival of target cells is higher in late effects than in acute effect tissues, whereas at dose B, the reverse is true. Therefore, increasing the dose per fraction from A to B results in a relatively greater increase in late rather than acute injury. In the case of neutrons, the α/β ratio is low, with no detectable influence on the quadratic function ($e\beta D \pm D_2$) over the first two decades of reduction in cell survival, implying that accumulation of sublethal injury plays a negligible role in cell killing by doses of neutrons of clinical interest. At these doses, the relative biologic effectiveness is higher for late effects than it is for acute effects. (Reprinted from Fowler JF. Fractionation and therapeutic gain. In: Steel GG, Adams GE, Peckham MT, eds. *Biological basis of radiotherapy.* 2nd ed. Amsterdam: Elsevier Science, 1983:181–194. Copyright © 1983 Elsevier. With permission.)

effects. Conversely, if large doses per fraction are used, the total dose required to achieve isoeffects in late-responding tissues would be reduced more for late effects than for acute effects. In general, tumors and acutely reacting tissues have a high α/β ratio (8 to 15 Gy), whereas tissues involved in late effects have a low α/β ratio (1 to 5 Gy).

The values for α and β can be obtained from graphs in which the reciprocal of the total dose (Gy^{-1}) and the dose per

FIGURE 1.22. Values of α and β. If the reciprocal of total dose (for several multifraction schedules) is plotted against dose per fraction, a straight line will be obtained. The intercept of this line with the zero dose-per-fraction axis is proportional to α ($\alpha/\ln S$). The slope is proportional to β ($\beta/\ln S$). The α/β ratio is readily determined. For absolute values of α and β, clonogenic assay is necessary for the endpoint. (Reprinted from Fowler JF. Fractionation and therapeutic gain. In: Steel GG, Adams GE, Peckham MT, eds. *Biological basis of radiotherapy.* 2nd ed. Amsterdam: Elsevier Science, 1983:181–194. Copyright © 1983 Elsevier. With permission.)

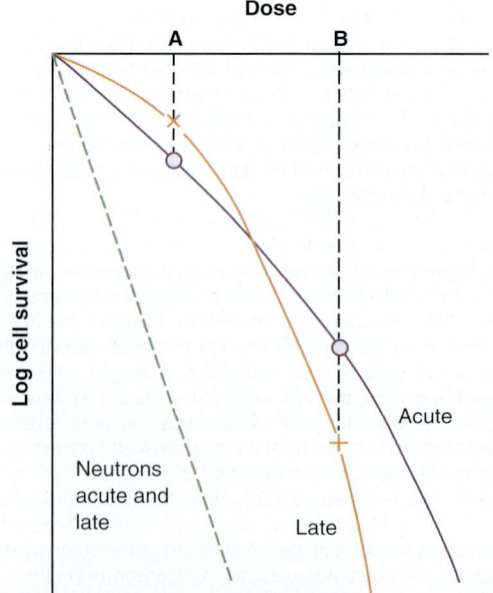

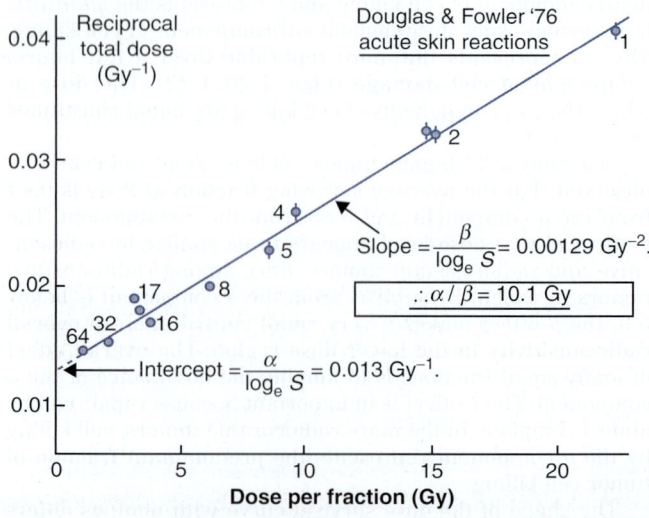

TABLE 1.7 RATIO OF LINEAR (α) TO QUADRATIC (β) TERMS FROM MULTIFRACTION EXPERIMENTS AND CLINICAL DATA

Tissue	α/β Ratio (Gy)	
	Experimental	Clinical
Early Reactions		
Skin/subcutaneous tissues	9–12	5–10
Jejunum	6–10	2.2–8
Colon	10–11	–
Testis	12–13	–
Callus	9–10	–
Late Reactions		
Spinal cord	1.0–4.9	3.3
Kidney	1.5–2.4	–
Lung	2.4–6.3	4.2–4.7
Bladder	3.1–7.0	3.4–4.5

Modified from Fowler JF. Fractionation and therapeutic gain. In: Steel GE, Adams GE, Peckham MT, eds. *Biological basis of radiotherapy.* 2nd ed. Amsterdam: Elsevier Science, 1983:181–194. Copyright © 1983 Elsevier. With permission.

fraction (Gy) are plotted (Table 1.7). A straight line is obtained. The intercept of this line with the zero dose-per-fraction axis is proportional to α and equal to $\alpha/\ln S$, wherein S is the natural logarithm of survival. The slope is proportional to β and equal to $\beta/\ln S$.

The algebraic functions to derive the straight line from the reciprocal total dose per fraction plot are as follows: Tumor cell survival following n fractions, each of dose d:

$$-\ln S = n(\alpha d + \beta d)^2$$
$$= \alpha nd + \beta nd^2$$
$$= nd(\alpha + \beta d)$$

Dividing both sides by total dose nd:

$$\frac{-\ln S}{nd} = \underset{\uparrow}{\alpha} + \underset{\uparrow}{\beta d}$$

Intercept Slope

Withers et al.[188] proposed a method for using these survival curve parameters for calculating the change in total dose necessary to achieve an equal response in tissue when the dose per fraction is varied, using the α/β ratios. This calculation accounts only for the effect of repair of cellular injury. The isoeffect curves vary for different tissues. A biologically equivalent dose (BED) can be obtained using this formula:

$$BED = \frac{\ln S}{\alpha}$$
$$BED = nd[1 + d/(\alpha/\beta)]$$

If one wishes to compare two treatment regimens, the following formula can be used:

$$\frac{Dr}{Dx} = \frac{\alpha/\beta + dx}{\alpha/\beta + dr}$$

in which Dr is the known total dose (reference dose), Dx is the new total dose (with different fractionation schedule), dr is the known fractionation (reference), and dx is the new fractionation schedule.

Let's consider an example of the use of this formula (with some reservations). Suppose 50 Gy in 25 fractions is delivered to yield a given biologic effect. If one assumes that the subcutaneous tissue is the limiting parameter (late reaction), it is desirable to know what the total dose to be administered will be using 4-Gy fractions. Assume α/β for late fibrosis equals 2 Gy.

Using the above formula:

$$Dx = \frac{Dr(\alpha/\beta + dr)}{\alpha/\beta + dx}$$

Thus,

$$Dx = 50\,Gy\left(\frac{5+2}{5+4}\right) = 39\,Gy$$

The basic LQ equation addresses the inactivation of a homogeneous population of cells. One should be wary, however, of accepting the basic equation as being complete. Because it is likely that accelerated repopulation of tumor clonogens occurs during the course of radiotherapy, and that cell cycle redistribution and reoxygenation also occur, we should consider how these factors can be accounted for in the formula.[89,189,190]

Repopulation may be accounted for, in broad approximation, by describing the number of clonogens (N) at time t as being related to the initial number of clonogens (No).

Then,

$$N = No^{e\lambda t}$$

The parameter λ determines the speed of cell repopulation and is given by

$$\lambda = \frac{\log e^2}{T\,pot} = \frac{0.693}{T\,pot}$$

where Tpot is the effective doubling time of cells in the tumor. If we ignore spontaneous cell loss, then Tpot is approximately the same as the measurable *in vitro* doubling time of tumor cells. Reported values of Tpot are 2 to 25 days with a median value of approximately 5 days. For late-responding tissues, Tpot is so large that λ is effectively zero.

Incorporating the allowance for tumor proliferation, with t representing time, the LQ equation becomes

$$BED = nd\left(1 + \frac{d}{\alpha/\beta}\right) - \frac{0.693t}{\alpha T pot}$$

Let's assume an α/β for an acutely reacting tissue, such as a tumor, of 10, and an α of 0.3 with a Tpot of 5. The BED of 70 Gy of 2 Gy/fraction, five fractions per week, in 46 days, is

$$BED = 70(1 + 0.2) = 84\,Gy_{10}.$$

Now let's add the correction for tumor repopulation during the course of treatment:

$$BED = 70\left(1 + \frac{2}{10}\right) - \frac{0.693}{0.3} \times \frac{46}{5}$$

$$BED = 84 - 21 = 63\,Gy_{10}$$

The decrease in clonogens by radiotherapy is attenuated, in part, by the repopulation of the surviving clonogens.

In the LQ equation, redistribution in the cell cycle and reoxygenation may be modeled by a single term called *resensitization.* Immediately after a dose of radiation, the average radiosensitivity of the cell population falls and then gradually returns to greater sensitivity. In contrast to tumor proliferation, resensitization probably increases as overall treatment time increases. Not enough is known about resensitization's clinical importance to make it useful to incorporate a numeric value for it in the LQ formula.

The LQ model can be used to construct a biologically oriented dose distribution algorithm for clinical radiation therapy.[94,191,192] A physical dose distribution can be translated to a BED using published biologic parameters. We are certainly not in a position to begin the routine use of this approach in clinical radiation therapy, although it may help clinicians to optimize treatment plans, and the technique may be used for outcome analysis in clinical research when the biologic parameters and the assumptions can be validated.

Brachytherapy and the Radiobiologic Dose Rate Effect

In 1901, Alexander Graham Bell suggested that cancer might be treated by directly implanting radioactive sources into a tumor. This form of radiotherapy is referred to as brachytherapy or endocurietherapy. The prefix brachy, from the Greek, means short, slow, or short range. The suffix therapy is derived from *therapeaia*, also Greek, meaning care or service to the sick. Some physicians use the alternative term endocurietherapy. The prefix endo, also from the Greek, means "within."

There are several ways we can describe the forms of brachytherapy. First, we can subdivide brachytherapy into a classification system based upon the physical placement of the radioactive sources. Thus, (1) interstitial brachytherapy is the placement of the radioactive sources directly into the tumor of tumor bed. Implanting radioactive seeds into the prostate would be an example of this form of treatment. (2) Intracavitary brachytherapy is the placement of the radioactive sources inside a body cavity and up against a tumor-bearing structure. The placement of tandem and ovoids for the treatment of carcinoma of the cervix or of a radioactive source-bearing catheter inside the nasopharynx are examples of this form of brachytherapy. Finally, (3) mold brachytherapy is the placement of radioactive sources upon the skin surface bearing a tumor. The use, for example, of radioactive sources embedded in a glove worn upon the hand for a period of time to treat a tumor of the dorsum of the hand, while preserving the function of the ligaments controlling the fingers, is an example of this form of treatment.

Another way we can subdivide the forms of brachytherapy is by duration of the treatment. A (1) temporary brachytherapy application resides in the tumor, body cavity, or adjacent to the tumor for a finite period of time before it is removed. Tandem and ovoid placement for carcinoma of the cervix is typically a temporary brachytherapy application. A (2) permanent brachytherapy application is placed permanently and, over time, the radioactive source decays. Injecting radioactive Au198 seeds into a bronchogenic carcinoma for palliation of bronchial obstruction by tumor is an example of a permanent implant.

Yet, a third way we can think about the forms of brachytherapy is by the speed with which the radiation is administered in cGy/minute. Three types are generally described. (1) Low–dose rate (LDR) brachytherapy typically administers its dose over a period of days. For example, administering 1,000 cGy/day to point A in a Cs 137 tandem and ovoid application would be a classic example of LDR brachytherapy. (2) High–dose rate (HDR) brachytherapy delivers the dose in a few minutes. The use of a robot referred to as a remote HDR remote afterloader to pump high-activity Ir-192 into and out of a series of Teflon catheters in the tumor bed for the postoperative treatment of a high-risk soft tissue sarcoma is an illustration of HDR brachytherapy. Finally, there is so-called (3) intermittent HDR brachytherapy or pulse–dose rate (PDR) brachytherapy. This usually refers to fractionating the HDR brachytherapy several times during the day, but the term is used by some physicians to refer to once per day or once every other day insertion of the HDR sources in the Teflon catheters. In either situation, a HDR remote afterloader machine is used.

When LDR brachytherapy is used for cancer treatment, we must give due consideration to its particular radiobiologic effects. We can think of LDR brachytherapy as the ultimate form of fractionation, being equivalent to an infinite number of small fractions with no interfraction intervals devoid of irradiation. What are the implications of this infinite fractionation on tumor cell killing and normal tissue tolerance?

The first point to consider is that much of the value of brachytherapy has less to do with biology than it has to do with physics. Brachytherapy is typically highly localized irradiation. The radiation beam in external beam radiotherapy comes "from the outside in" and passes through a block of normal tissue on its way to the tumor volume and, in the case of uncharged beams like photons and neutrons, passes through normal tissue on its way back out of the body after passing through the tumor. In contrast, the radiation beams in brachytherapy come "from the inside out" and are generally within or directly upon the tumor with the dose falling off rapidly as the square of the distance as one moves away from the radioactive source(s). Long before computer modeling of external beam irradiation and multileaf collimators for external beam treatment, brachytherapy was, to some extent, the first form of "dose painting" or "intensity-modulated radiation therapy." The ability to confine the radiation dose to a small area with brachytherapy, with the avoidance of exposing large areas of normal tissue, allows the treating clinician to safely give doses sometimes unimaginable with external beam treatment.

Perhaps, the ultimate clinical example of the volume effect of brachytherapy is the treatment of choroidal melanoma or retinoblastoma with a I-125 or Ir-192 or Co-60 or Ruthenium plaque sewn to the choroid and overlaying the tumor bed. In some cases, 40,000 to 70,000 cGy will be administered to a small area of the outer surface of the choroid with an acceptable long-term ill effects on normal tissue profile. This is only possible by the use of highly localized brachytherapy. This had led some wags to observe that "this isn't really radiotherapy as we know it. It is nuclear warfare."

It is also worth remembering that the dose in the tumor volume created by brachytherapy is often highly heterogenous. In the treatment of carcinoma of the cervix, for example, generations of radiation oncologists have prescribed and described the dose administered to "point A" and "point B," both located lateral to the cervix. Radiation dose, however, falls off as the square of the distance. Therefore, the dose at the surface of the tumor-containing cervix from a Cs137 tandem and ovoid application is much higher and more tumoricidal than the dose at point A.

The author has had the occasion to treat vaginal rhabdomyosarcoma in very young girls with intracavitary pulsed HDR brachytherapy and custom-built lead shields to both push uninvolved normal tissue away from the brachytherapy catheters and partially shield this tissue with lead. It is difficult to imagine achieving more exquisitely conformal radiation dose distributions by any means other than brachytherapy.

The second point to consider is the fundamental series of effects of LDR on cell death. We can think of the radiation damage to mammalian cells as divisible into (1) lethal, irreversible, and irreparable lethal damage; (2) PLD whose injurious effects can be either exacerbated or ameliorated by the postirradiation environmental conditions of the irradiated cells; and (3) SLD which, under normal circumstances, can be repaired unless additional SLD is heaped upon existing damage and converts it to lethal damage. Here's a simple way to think about SLD mathematically. Assume that A% of cells are killed by dose X of external beam irradiation. If you take dose X and split it into two equal fractions, then each fraction is X/2. Now, instead of giving all of the radiotherapy dose X at once, give X/2 today and the remaining X/2 tomorrow. What will happen? Instead of *A*% of cells dying as a result of radiation, A – B% will die. The improvement in the probability of cell survival, represented by B, is repaired SLD.

Let's turn our attention back to PLD. By definition, PLD is influenced by the conditions the cells find themselves in after being irradiated. Let's assume we do something to the cells, which prevents them from moving forward in the cell cycle. We might achieve this by lowering the ambient temperature or allowing the cells to be packed in closely so that density inhibition of growth occurs or by using a culture media, which starves the cells of nutrients. If we keep the cells from moving forward in the cell cycle, then we will inhibit the ability of radiation-induced DNA injury to manifest itself by causing cell death when the cells try to divide. Cell survival will rise compared to allowing the cells to vigorously march through the cell cycle into M phase. This diminution in cell mortality represents PLD.[394]

With LDR, several things happen simultaneously, which influence cell killing. The relative importance of these factors will vary based on the specifics of whether you are thinking about normal tissue tolerance to radiotherapy or the tumor type, the tumor's growth environment, and, for normal or tumor tissue, the dose rate. The factors are:

(a) Repair: As the dose rate slows, some cells will endeavor to repair the radiation injury as it occurs. The cell's ability to survive may gain the upper hand if the dose rate is low enough and the cell's intrinsic radiation repair functions can handle the injury as it occurs. Imagine you are sitting in a rowboat in the middle of a lake and the boat springs a pinhole-sized leak. If the rate of the water entering your boat is slow enough, you can bail the boat fast enough to get yourself back to shore. If the rate of the water entering the boat becomes too fast, you and your boat are going to find yourselves seated on the bottom of the lake. The hole in your boat is analogous to the rate of induction of radiation injury.

(b) Repopulation: Some cells will be killed by the radiation. For those that survive, they no longer have to compete with their adjacent newly dead neighbor for oxygen and other nutrients. They will start to grow faster and, to varying extents depending upon the type of tissue or tumor, repopulate the neighborhood with new cells.

(c) Reoxygenation: Oxygen is the most powerful radiosensitizer. To the extent that LDR kills cells, the "neighborhood effect" as described just above in (b) also applies to oxygen. The continuous reoxygenation will render the remaining cells, which have survived the initial onslaught or radiation more sensitive to subsequent radiation injury.[395]

(d) Reassortment: As a general principle, reassortment refers to the progression of cells through the cell cycle during the interval between split doses. To the extent that cells move into the more radiosensitive phases of the cell cycle, they are more likely to be killed by radiotherapy. To the extent that they move into less radiosensitive phases of the cell cycle, they are more likely to be spared. There is a paradoxical form of reassortment, which occurs in some cell lines during LDR. It is called the "inverse dose rate effect." When the inverse dose rate effect occurs, cells march through the cell cycle but become arrested in G2. G2 is a highly radiosensitive phase of the cell cycle, and the cells are more likely to be mowed down by radiation.[103]

Let's put all these factors together and think about what the net effect will be of LDR.

To the extent that cells repair SLD more effectively then the lower the dose rate, the better the cell survival. The magnitude of the effect will be dependent upon the efficacy and speed of SLD repair in an individual cell line.

To the extent that cells are redistributed into a more sensitive phase of the cell cycle, then the lower the dose rate, the worse the survival unless the dose rate is so low that the cells progress right on through into more resistant phases of the cell cycle. Then, their survival will rise.

To the extent that cells become better oxygenated as a result of LDR, then the worse the cell survival.

On net, from most mammalian cell lines, LDR produces a decrease in cell killing via a "flattening" of the cell survival curve and a "loss of the survival curve shoulder."

Brachytherapy is often a highly effective treatment for solid tumors as a result of its conformal dose distribution and radiobiologic effects on killing tumor cells and sparing normal tissue. Brachytherapy requires technical expertise, patience, access to a procedure room or operating room, and due attention to radiation safety and radiation protection. Catheters and seeds can be misplaced and there are risks of bleeding and infection. Practice makes perfect, and, unfortunately, many radiation therapy treatment centers do not do brachytherapy procedures frequently enough to develop local expertise and confidence with the techniques. It is not surprising that in the United States, inadequate brachytherapy experience is a common citation against radiation oncology residency programs. I am reminded of the words of wisdom of one of his beloved professors at the Massachusetts General Hospital in the early 1980s, Leonidas Harisiadis: "Brachytherapy is a highly effective form of treatment, but doing it can be a pain in the neck."

The radiation dose rate may significantly influence the biologic response, particularly for sparsely ionizing radiations such as x-rays and γ-rays. Three main biologic processes are involved in the dose rate effect (Figs. 1.23 and 1.24).[89,162]

With the advent of moderate– and high–dose rate remote control afterloading devices, increased emphasis has been placed on the biologic effects of dose rate. Many *in vitro* and *in vivo* experimental observations indicate variations in cell killing and repair of sublethal or PLD with varying dose rates. The so-called dose rate effect is most dramatic between 1 cGy/minute and 1 Gy/minute.[193] The biologic effect achieved by a

FIGURE 1.23. The dose rate effect as a result of repair of sublethal damage, redistribution in the cycle, and cell proliferation. The dose–response curve for acute exposures is characterized by a broad initial shoulder. As the dose rate is reduced, the survival curve becomes progressively shallower as more and more sublethal damage is repaired, but cells are "frozen" in their positions in the cycle and do not progress. As the dose rate is lowered further and for a limited range of dose rates, the survival curve steepens again because cells can progress through the cycle to pile up at a block in G2, a radiosensitive phase, but still cannot divide. A further lowering of dose rate allows cells to escape the G2 block and divide; cell proliferation then may occur during the protracted exposure, and survival curves become shallower as cell birth from mitosis offsets cell killing from the irradiation. (Based on the ideas of Dr. Joel Bedford, and from Hall EJ. *Radiobiology for the radiologist*. 4th ed. Philadelphia: J.B. Lippincott, 1994, with permission.)

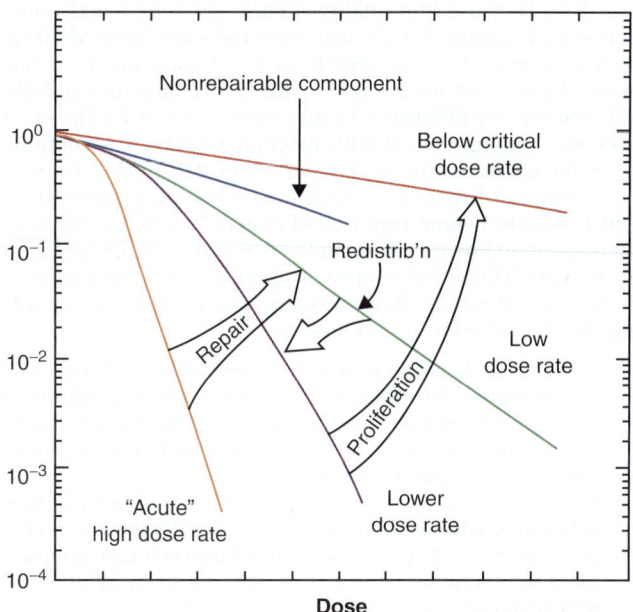

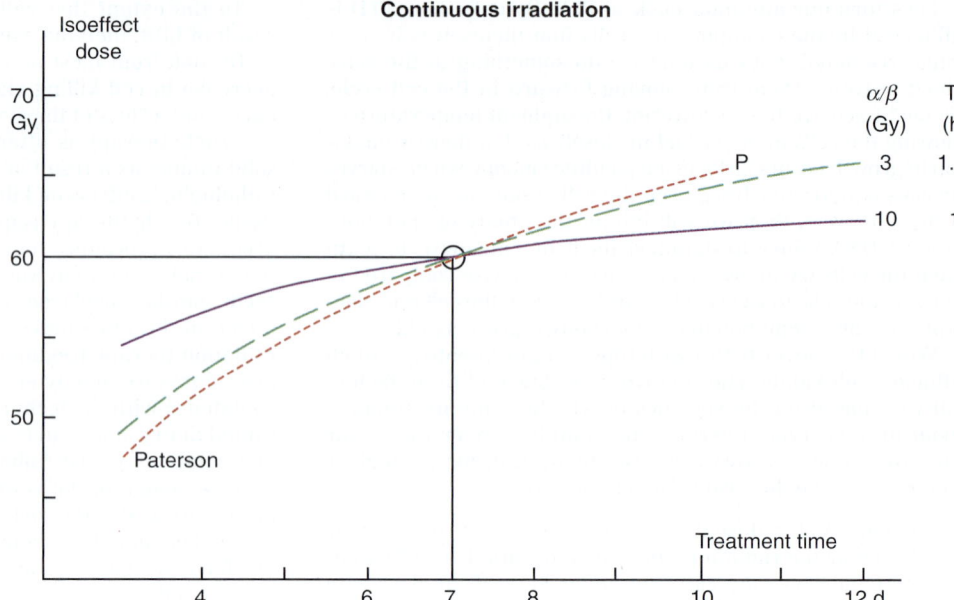

FIGURE 1.24. Low–dose rate irradiation. Isoeffect dose equivalent to 60 Gy in 7 days. Two sets of parameters have been considered for the computation, which would presumably correspond to skin and mucosa early reactions and to the effect on the epithelioma (α/β = 10 Gy, Tr = 1 hour) and to late reactions (α/β = 3 Gy, Tr = 1.5 hour). (Reprinted from Dutreix J. Expression of the dose rate effect in clinical curietherapy. *Radiother Oncol* 1989;15[1]:25–37. Copyright © 1989 Elsevier Ireland Ltd. With permission.)

given irradiation dose decreases as the dose rate diminishes, chiefly as a result of the increase in cell repair that occurs during continuous prolonged irradiation, because cell proliferation is virtually negligible in the range of treatment times used in LDR brachytherapy.[194]

In some experiments, a bending of the cell survival curve at very low dose rates has been noted, instead of the expected exponential result, possibly because of cell redistribution[388] or a decline in the repair capacity with large doses.[195] At a very low dose rate, because the cell killing is caused only by direct lethal events that are considered independent of the dose rate, cell repair is also negligible. The induction of sublethal injury is relatively slow compared with the rate of repair, and cell killing, by accumulation of sublethal injury, remains minimal. Variation of the isoeffect dose occurs mainly in the range of medium dose rates (1 to 10 Gy/hour), and it vanishes at very high dose rates because the cell repair is negligible during the short treatment time.[194]

The dose rate effect in clinical brachytherapy was described initially by Green and Paterson and reiterated by Ellis and Orton.[80,160,196–198] The historic isoeffect curve showed a significant increase in dose when time was increased from 2 to 7 days. However, the validity of Paterson's curve was questioned by Pierquin et al.,[199] who used the same dose of 70 Gy with treatment times ranging from 3 to 8 days for the treatment of head and neck tumors with Ir-192 implants and did not observe any difference in the control rate or incidence of necrosis. The agreement with Paterson's curve is acceptable when the α/β value equals 3 Gy and repair half-time (T$_r$) equals 1.5 hours, but the curve is shallower when α/β equals 10 Gy and T$_r$ equals 1 hour. One should expect Paterson's curve to correspond to late reactions and to overestimate the variation for early reactions and control of squamous cell carcinoma.

Several important concepts should be considered regarding the clinical relevance of dose rate[189,193,200]:

1. At ultra-high doses and instantaneous dose rates (i.e., 10 Gy pulsed in nanoseconds), the rapid deposition of energy consumes oxygen too quickly for diffusion to maintain an adequate level of oxygenation, and dose–response curves are characteristic of hypoxia.
2. Based on laboratory data, it may be possible to design schedules with a pulse width of several minutes and a pulse interval of about 1 hour to achieve cell killing equivalent to that obtained with a continuous 30 Gy in 60 hours (0.5 Gy/hour).

3. Using the LQ equation, it is possible to estimate the equivalency of HDR and LDR exposures with a variety of fractionation schedules (remembering that a lower number of fractions may result in enhanced late effects).

Special consideration should be given to the effect of HDR brachytherapy on normal tissues. The tumor dose must be decreased 30% to 50% in comparison with that delivered with conventional low dose rates.[201,202] (For further discussion, see Chapters 22 to 25.)

In the past, there was some interest in continuous LDR irradiation with external cobalt units.[203] Pierquin et al.[204] used a modified [185]Co unit with a small industrial source (activity 45 Ci). Radiation was delivered at 1 to 1.39 Gy/hour to administer daily tumor doses of 8 to 10 Gy in 7 to 8 hours. A minimum of five treatments was given per week, although occasionally weekends and holidays caused schedule modifications. Patients were given short rest periods every 1 or 2 hours. Tumor doses of approximately 63 Gy were delivered in 8 to 11 fractions, with the volume reduced to 8 by 10 cm after 45 Gy. Nineteen patients with advanced tumors of the mouth and pharynx were treated; 15 had no evidence of tumor 3 months after treatment. Only three patients developed recurrences. Of 19 patients, two developed moist desquamation and six developed dry desquamation; the others had only erythema. No significant late effects on the skin or the subcutaneous tissues were noted; 16/19 patients developed severe mucositis. Seven patients developed necrosis, six in large areas of the oral cavity and pharynx and, in several instances, at the tumor site.

The Target Theory of Radiobiology and How It Has Shaped Our Understanding of the Cell Survival Curve

We hold a dart in our hand and toss it at the dart board. What is our goal? To hit the target; to make a "bull's-eye." We go to a pistol range and, similarly, aim at the target. We try to "hit the target," whether it is a series of concentric circles or a paper outline of a man. A hunter stalks his or her prey in the woods with a rifle or a bow and arrow. They, similarly, want to cause a lethal injury and "bag the game."

A dart, a bullet, and an arrow are all physical modalities, not chemical, either used to inflict injury or death or show a person's ability to shoot straight and true. It is not much of a leap to envision how the early students of ionizing radiation's ability to kill cells envisioned that the physical modality of radiation would kill cells by hitting a target. Because many of these original investigators came from the world of physics, they sought to reduce the description of radiation's killing effect on viruses, bacteria, and cells to a series of mathematical equations, which described the cell survival curve. Furthermore, the empirical data, which were derived from radiation survival curves from the exposure of viruses and bacteria, could be fit to these equations.

The target theory is based on the concept that the biologic end product of cell death is related to the initial physical events, which occur upon irradiation. The fundamental principle of target theory is that inactivation of the target inside a cell or a bacteria or a virus results in its death.[200,238] The target is considered a unit of biologic function. The theory implies that the exact site where an ionizing event occurs, such as a double-strand DNA break, is the place where the primary ionizations responsible for that event occurred. Radiation-induced cell death can occur, in simplest terms, when there is a single hit of sufficient power to inactivate a single target and that target is sufficiently important that, when inactivated, the cell dies. This is called the single-hit/single-target model. One can also envision that some cells might not die unless multiple targets are inactivated. This is called the multiple-hit/multiple-target model. All manner of variations might be imagined such as a stubborn single target that required repetitive assaults to be inactivated (multiple hit/single target).[205,381,385]

With low–linear energy transfer (LET) radiation, ionizations occur in clusters and sporadically along the path traveled by the particle. The radiation survival of most bacteria and viruses is a constant exponential function of dose. To kill them, it would seem to require inactivation of at least one target per bacteria or virus. At this point, however, we need to rethink our metaphor of the dart, the bullet, or the arrow. Darts, bullets, or arrows are very consciously and with great intent aimed at a specific target. Radiation beams, however, while they are aimed at tumors, are not aimed at individual cells, and they certainly are not aimed with any knowledge of where, at any moment, the important target is located. The target, the DNA, is moving within the cell. This brings us to a crucial point: The deposition of ionizations from radiation and the production of radiochemical injury to the cell are random events. To better understand this concept, careful study of Figure 1.25 is recommended.[396,401]

Unlike the straight line survival curves of many bacteria and viruses, when you plot the cell survival curve of most mammalian cells on a semilog plot, you see a "shoulder" in the low-dose region indicative of a decreased efficiency of cell killing and then a straight or "exponential" component of the curve.

If we think about a strand of DNA as containing some regions that are essential to maintain the reproductive ability of the cell, then these regions are the specific targets for radiation damage. As we have pointed out, straight survival curves are usually found for the inactivation of bacteria and viruses and some very sensitive normal and malignant human cells, for the radiation response to low-LET radiation at very low dose rates and the response to high-LET radiation.

In Figure 1.25, we described how the dose D_0 is that dose of radiation, which gives an average of one hit per target and reduces the probability of cell survival from 1 to 0.37 or e−1. Using Poisson statistics, and understanding that the probability of the next hit occurring in any given cell is small, then the probability of a given cell surviving is the same as the probability that a cell suffers zero hits = $\exp(-D/D_0)$. (For a brief description of the Poisson distribution, see Box 1.7.) We could also look at the situation, mathematically, this way[396,398,399]:

If there is one target per cell, then the probability of that cell surviving (S) an average of one-hit per cell for a large number of cells is

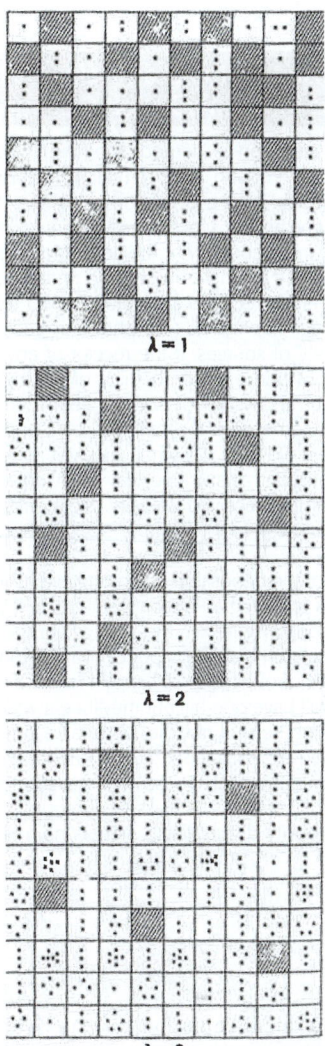

FIGURE 1.25. Let us assume that there are 100 equally sized tumor cells. Any individual cell will be killed if a crucial single target is hit at least once. This is a single-hit/single-target model. We fire a radiation beam capable of producing 100 lethal hits/ionizations at the 100 cells in the upper panel, and the deposition of ionizations occurs along the beam bath in clusters and randomly. Any individual cell's target is struck zero to four times with lethal ionizations. Any cell's target, which is struck at least once, is killed. Sixty-three cells die. Thirty-seven survive. The probability of any one cell surviving the onslaught is 37% which is e−1. In the next panel, in the middle, we fire a radiation beam capable of producing 200 lethal hits/ionizations at the same 100 cells. The targets of some cells are completely missed. Others are hit up to six times. Eight even cells die. Thirteen survive. Thirteen is 37% × 37% or e−2. In the lowest panel, we fire a radiation beam capable of producing 300 lethal hits/ionizations at the same 100 cells. How many cells survive? 37% × 37% × 37% or e−3 = 5 cells or 5% of the 100. It is the mathematical result of this random deposition of ionizing energy, which is part of target theory, helps us understand the derivation of the equations, which give mathematical representation to the cell survival curve, and helps define the concept of D_0. (Reproduced with permission from Withers HR, Peters LJ. Biologic aspects of radiotherapy. In: Fletcher GH. *Textbook of radiotherapy.* 3rd ed. Philadelphia: Lea and Febiger, 1980:103–180.)

$$P(1) = S = e^{-1}$$

If we gave a dose, which caused an average of two hits per cell, for a large number of cells, then the probability of any individual cell surviving is

$$P(2) = S = e^{-2}$$

If we gave a dose, which caused an average of X hits per cell, for a large number of cells, then the probability of any individual cell surviving is

Box 1.7

How the Poisson Distribution Helps Us Understand the Equations for the Radiation Cell Survival Curve

The Poisson distribution is named after the French mathematician Siméon Denis Poisson (1781–1840). A Poisson distribution expresses the probability of a given number of events occurring in a fixed interval of time and/or space if these events occur with a known average rate and independently of the time since the last event.

Let's think of some examples in order to understand this concept. Assume that a person receives an average of 50 text messages on their personal electronic device (cell phone or pad) every day from a very wide variety of sources. If the receipt of any particular email message does not affect the probability of getting the next email message, then some days the person will get 49 emails, some days they will get 51, some days they will get 100, and if enough time elapses then there will be a day when they get zero. While the average number of emails that arrive per day is 50, on any particular day the number of emails received will vary. Most days, the number of emails will cluster close to the number 50, but there will be a wide variation.

We can think of the deposition of ionizing events in cells and inactivating targets as following a Poisson distribution. If you look back at the panel at the top of Figure X-Y, the average number of hits per cells is 1, but the actual number of hits per cell varies from zero to four. If you plot the number of hits per cell, they'll follow a Poisson distribution. Most cells will have one hit, but they'll be a wide variation.

A Poisson distribution is not the same as a normal distribution (sometimes called a "bell-shaped curve") although, at first glance, they look somewhat similar. These two statistical concepts come from two different principles. A Poisson distribution is one example for discrete probability distribution, whereas normal belongs to the idea of a continuous probability distribution.

$$P(X) = S = e^{-X}$$

Because the typical radiation cell survival curve for normal and malignant mammalian cells has a "shoulder" and then an exponential component, it can be fit to a multitarget model. The initial slope of the curve, D_1, is the result of single-hit killing and has a slope, which represents the dose that is required to reduce the number of surviving cells from 100% to 37%. The final slope of the curve is the dose that is required to reduce survival from 0.1 to 0.037 or from 0.01 to 0.0037.

We can represent this "two-sloped" curve in the multitarget model by

$$P(X) = S = 1 - (1 - e^{-xD})^n$$

S is the probability of survival. D is the dose that causes a mean of hit per cell. X is the number of hits per cells. N is the number of targets that must be hit in an individual cell to cause cell death.

If we use the term D_0 for the slope of the exponential part of the curve, then

$$S = [1 - (1 - e^{-D/D_0})^n]^m$$

In this equation, S is the probability of survival, D is the dose of radiation administered, D_0 is the dose that causes a mean of one hit per cell, N is the heterodiploid number so that 1 is haploid, 2 is diploid, and 3 is triploid, and m is the number of targets that must be hit in an individual cell to cause cell death.

For a diploid cell with a average of one target per cell, the equation becomes

$$S = 1 - (1 - e^{-D/D_0})^2$$

Although there may or may not be discrete and identifiable target areas within DNA, the multitarget model does a pretty good job of predicting many cell survival curves, and the concepts of DQ, D_0, and n are understandable tools in describing radiation sensitivity.[396,400] There are radiation cell survival curves, which are not well represented by the target model, and the LQ theory was developed to be a more general concept (Fig. 1.25).

IMPORTANCE OF TREATMENT PLANNING IN RADIATION THERAPY

The predicted consequences of EBRT are based on the precision with which the dose and the irradiated volume are defined. An imprecise treatment system could lead to a high incidence of necrosis with, paradoxically, a low probability of tumor control (Fig. 1.26).[112] Decreasing irradiation doses to avoid complications will further reduce the probability of achieving tumor control if such action is based on the wrong assumption that the tumor control/complication ratio is related only to radiation dose levels. The ICRU recommends a ±5% accuracy for dose delivery computations.[42,206] However, every effort should be made to develop accurate dose calculation algorithms, including methods to correct for inhomogeneities in tissue density and the shape of the patient's body, and to develop practical treatment planning capabilities to obtain the highest possible dose optimization in the irradiated volume (tumor and normal tissues). There are benefits of reducing the treatment volume in an effort to deliver higher doses of irradiation. This may improve the quality of tumor control without excessively irradiating surrounding normal tissues, thereby decreasing treatment-related morbidity.

FIGURE 1.26. Frequency distribution of patients treated to different probabilities of complication. (From Orton CG. Other considerations in 3-dimensional treatment planning. In: Bagne F, ed. *Computerized treatment planning systems*. HHS Publication FDA 84–8223. Washington, DC: U.S. Government Printing Office, 1984:136–141.)

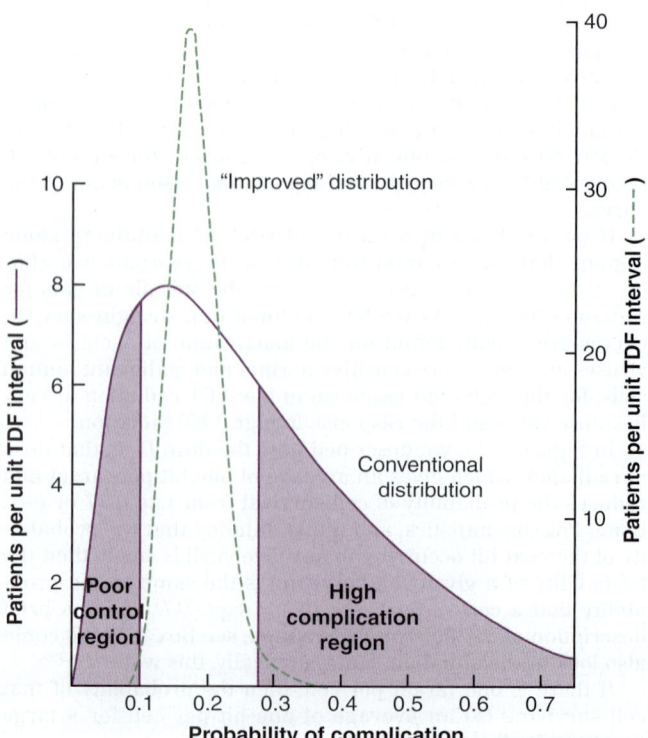

3-Dimensional treatment planning

Various steps can be taken to decrease toxicity in normal tissues, including precise treatment planning and irradiation techniques, selective decreased volume receiving higher doses dictated by estimated cell burden, and maneuvers to exclude sensitive organs from the irradiated volume. With the emphasis on organ preservation, treatment planning is critical to achieve maximum TCP and satisfactory cosmetic results.

Optimal dose distribution may be achieved by a combination of multiple stationary beams or by moving beam therapy, such as in arc or full rotational techniques or IMRT. In addition, the optimal dose distribution in many tumors requires access to more than one modality or beam energy particle type. A combination of external beams and intracavitary or interstitial therapy also may be required, depending on the location of the tumor.

Three-Dimensional Treatment Planning

Advances in computer technology have augmented accurate and timely computation, display of 3D radiation dose distributions, and DVHs.[207,208] These developments have stimulated sophisticated 3D treatment planning systems, which yield relevant information in evaluation of tumor extent, definition of target volume, delineation of normal tissues, virtual simulation of therapy, generation of digitally reconstructed radiographs, design of treatment portals including the use of multileaf collimators and aids (e.g., compensators, blocks), calculation of 3D dose distributions and dose optimization, and critical evaluation of the treatment plan.[209–211]

The potential benefits of 3D planning and delivery systems are great. It is, however, not clear which specific disease sites and treatment situations will be benefited by 3D planning.[212] With advanced computerized and display technologies, contiguous CT and/or MRI and/or PET slices are used to define anatomic structures and target volumes. External radiation beams of any possible orientation are simulated. A significant feature of these systems is the so-called beam's eye view, in which patient contours are viewed as if the observer's eye is placed at the source of radiation looking out along the axis of the radiation beam.[213] These systems allow simulation of the geometric setup; evaluation of the plan for dose optimization still is made on the merits of volumetric dose distributions.

Quantitative treatment planning evaluation is crucial in selection of the best portals and radiation beams to deliver an optimal dose to the tumor with relative sparing of normal tissues. The ICRU Report 50 and its supplement G2 define 3D volumes for the prescription and reporting of EBRT.[42] The GTV is defined as the gross demonstrable extent and location of malignant growth; the CTV allows a margin around the GTV for subclinical disease; the PTV allows margins on the CTV for variation in position, size, and shape so that the prescribed dose is received by the CTV; and the treated volume is that area receiving a dose considered appropriate to the purpose of treatment such as tumor eradication or palliation.

The DVH is useful as a means of dose display, particularly in assessing several treatment plan dose distributions.[214] A DVH provides a complete summary of the entire 3D dose matrix, showing the amount of target volume or critical structure receiving more than a specified dose level. Because a DVH does not provide spatial dose information, it cannot replace the other methods of dose display; it can only complement them.

Models for optimization of 3D dose distribution using biologic models of tumor and normal tissue responses correlated with physical radiation doses have been described. Mohan et al.,[172] in a theoretical analysis, concluded that for certain clinical situations, it is not sufficient to specify objectives of optimization purely on the basis of pattern of irradiation dose and that dose–volume effects and biologic indices also must be incorporated into the formulation.

Niemierko et al.[144] described a technique for optimization of 3D conformal radiation therapy plans with biologic models of tumor and normal tissue response to irradiation as well as with scores based on physical dose. Optimization programs attempted to minimize dose gradient across the target volume, match specified isodose contours to the target and critical organs, match specified dose–volume constraints, minimize integral dose to the entire volume of patient treated, minimize maximum dose to critical organs, and constrain dose to specified normal tissues below a TD level. The solutions were based on TCP, NTCP, various dose levels given to specified volumes of the patient, discrete or continuous values of beam parameters, number of beams, and logical combination of any constraints.

Intensity-Modulated Radiation Therapy

An increasingly popular approach to 3D treatment planning and conformal therapy optimizes the delivery of irradiation to irregularly shaped volumes through a process of complex inverse (or forward) treatment planning and dynamic delivery of irradiation that results in modulated fluence of photon or proton beam profiles and a more conformal dose to the target volume(s), with enhanced sparing of surrounding normal tissues.[185,215]

Treatment planning begins with the determination of the GTV and the CTV, which contains the GTV, and an estimate of where the tumor may spread. CT, MRI, and fluorodeoxyglucose positron emission tomography (FDG-PET) imaging along with image fusion have enhanced the possibilities for determining the target more accurately. The PTV accounts for inaccuracies in positioning patients and organ motion.

In "forward" planning, software calculates the dose distribution, displays it with a 3D anatomic model, and provides analytical and graphical metrics for assessing the adequacy of tumor treatment and normal tissue avoidance. The physician decides if the plan is acceptable. If not, an alteration is made in the beam arrangement, and the process is repeated.[271]

Computerized optimization techniques have led to "inverse" planning. Goals of an acceptable treatment plan are delineated, and the inverse planning algorithm searches through many thousands of possibilities to find a plan that best satisfies the goals. In IMRT, the beams are broken up into "beamlets" (on the order of 0.5 by 0.5 or 1 by 1 cm) that can each have a different intensity. IMRT may improve the ability to treat with a high radiation dose while minimizing dose to nearby critical structures.

There are a variety of forms in which IMRT can be administered:

1. A linear accelerator and multileaf collimation, with a variety of beam configurations at various angles, may be used; the MLC determines the portal shape of each of the portals. Photon-modulated fluency may be obtained (a step-and-shoot method). Analogous techniques may be used with protons.
2. Dynamic computer-controlled IMRT is delivered when the configuration of the beams outlined with the MLC is changing at the same time that the gantry or the accelerator is changing positions around the patient.
3. In helical TomoTherapy, the photon fan beam continually rotates around the patient as the couch transports the patient longitudinally through the ring gantry. The verification processes for helical TomoTherapy are enabled by the use of the ring gantry; the geometry of a CT scanner allows tomographic processes to be reliably performed. Dose reconstruction is a key process of tomography; the treatment detector sinogram computes the actual dose deposited in the patient. The length of the beam is 40 cm at the central axis and has a width that can vary between 0.5 and 5 cm. The lengths of the MLC in helical

tomography are temporally modulated or binary in the sense that they are rapidly driven either in or out by air system actuators rather than beam slowly pushed by motors driving lead screws as in the conventional MLC.

4. The robotic IMRT system consists of a miniaturized 6-MV photon linear accelerator mounted on a highly mobile arm and a set of ceiling-mounted x-ray cameras to provide near real-time information on patient position and target exposure during treatment.

The majority of the IMRT systems use 6-MV x-rays, but energies of 8 to 10 MV may be more desirable in some anatomic sites (to decrease skin and superficial subcutaneous tissue dose). Higher energies will increase neutron contamination of the therapeutic beam(s). The dose distribution and field-shaping parameters are based on inverse 3D planning using a specially defined minimal dose to target and dose constraints for surrounding normal tissues.[216-218] Inverse planning starts with an ideal dose distribution and finds through trial and error or multiple iterations (simulated annealing) the beam characteristics (fluence profiles) and then produces the best approximation to the ideal dose defined in a 3D array of dose voxels organized in a stack of two-dimensional (2D) arrays.[7,219]

A back-projection technique through careful choice of filters, beam placement, and shaping of the portals conforms the irradiation dose to the shape of the tumor, minimizing dose to critical adjacent structures. When this technique is used, it is critical to adhere to basic concepts of treatment planning and evaluation of the pathobiology of malignant disease. Well-designed treatment plans based on radiographic imaging (CT or MRI or PET), which in most instances demonstrates gross disease, are necessary to minimize the risk of missing or underirradiating adjacent microscopic or subclinical tumor.

Given the added time and labor involved in IMRT, numerous issues require study:

1. Can the tumor be localized with sufficient accuracy to take advantage of the improved dose localization?
2. Treatment plans that produce a rapid drop in dose between the edge of the tumor and the normal tissue require more exact patient positioning; otherwise, there is a high risk of underdosing the tumor or overdosing normal tissue.
3. Some IMRT plans treat the center of the tumor with a very high dose to achieve an acceptable dose at the edge. This may not be optimal.
4. Many IMRT techniques spread a low dose over a larger volume or normal tissue. This may increase the risk of secondary malignancies years later.

HEAVY PARTICLE BEAMS

One can imagine two possible mechanisms by which one could improve on therapeutic x-rays with an alternative particle. First, the alternative particle could have energy deposition characteristics that lead to a superior dose distribution. A beam, conceivably, could have more skin sparing than x-rays, better stopping characteristics, and/or less side scatter. This might allow a more conformal therapy. Second, the alternative particle could have advantageous radiobiologic properties. It might be more toxic than x-rays to hypoxic cells or cells in the late S-phase of the mitotic cell cycle. Such a particle would have, perhaps, a lower oxygen enhancement ratio (OER) and a higher RBE than x-rays. These two possible mechanisms of improving on x-rays are not mutually exclusive. A particle could have both superior physical dose distribution and radiobiologic properties.

The effort to identify improved alternatives to x-rays has focused on the group of particles called hadrons. These are particles constituted of strongly interacting particles called quarks and gluons. The hadrons include the mesons and the baryons. The latter include protons, neutrons, negative pions, and the nuclei of heavier atoms such as He^2 (helium), C^6 (carbon), O^8 (oxygen), Ne^{10} (neon), and Ar^{18} (argon). All of these forms of radiation are distinguished from x-rays and electrons by their greater masses. These alternative radiation modalities are relatively difficult to produce, are expensive, and are considerably more difficult to control.

Proton, heavy ion, and hadron beams have attracted radiation oncologists because they offer interesting and potentially beneficial dose distribution characteristics. Radiobiologically, their properties are not significantly different from x-rays. When a heavy particle beam traverses tissue, the dose is deposited in an approximately constant rate. The rate of energy loss (also called the "stopping power") of a heavy charged particle is proportional to the square of the particle charge and inversely proportional to the square of its velocity. As a proton or heavy ion slows down, its rate of energy loss increases and so does the ionization or absorbed dose to the tissue. Near the end of the proton's range, the deposition of energy rises very sharply before dropping to almost zero. This peaking of dose near the end of the particle range is called the Bragg peak. As a result of the Bragg peak effect and minimal scattering, the proton offers the potential advantage and the ability to concentrate dose inside and immediately adjacent to the tumor volume and minimize dose to surrounding normal tissues. There are multiple proton treatment facilities operational and under construction throughout the world.

For a thorough discussion of proton and neutron radiation, as well as a consideration of pi meson therapy and charged nuclei therapy such as helium ions and neon ions, the reader is referred to Chapters 19 and 20 of this volume.

BORON NEUTRON CAPTURE THERAPY

The fundamental concept of boron neutron capture therapy (BNCT) is the production of high–LET particles ($^7Li^{3+}$ and $^4He^{2+}$) when one "tags" or "labels" a tumor cell with a compound having a large cross-section capable of capturing a "slow" (thermal) neutron. After the compound captures the neutron, it goes into an excited state. The excited fission of the ^9B nucleus will release energy, which drives the heavy ion products over short distances comparable to the dimensions of one cell. A 0.48-MeV photon is also produced in 94% of the fission events. This is useful for monitoring the reaction but is of little consequence for cell killing.

The neutron has a mass of 0.782 MeV, more than that of the proton. Neutrons were identified in 1932 by Chadwick[120,384] at Cambridge University's Cavendish Laboratory. Subsequently, Fermi[220] discovered that neutrons react most efficiently with a number of elements after they are slowed by passage through a hydrogen-rich substance such as paraffin. Chadwick and Goldhaber,[120] Taylor and Goldhaber,[221] and Burcham and Goldhaber[222] showed that slow neutron bombardment of specific stable isotopes of boron, lithium, and nitrogen yields charged particle tracts in photographic plates. The tracts from boron's interaction with neutrons were short and straight and were consistent with the formation of two particles traveling in opposite trajectories. In photographic gelatin, their average travel distance was 7.6 μm. The boron neutron capture process is highly localized. In principle, one could kill a tumor cell containing boron while sparing an adjacent normal cell that does not contain boron. Box 1.8 provides a glossary of terms related to neutron capture therapy.

The complete chemical reaction is as follows:

$$^{10}B + {}^1n \rightarrow {}^7Li + {}^4He + \gamma + 2.4 \text{ MeV}.$$

The attraction of BNCT, for many clinicians, has been the notion of the "magic bullet." The idea that one could specifically label tumor cells with a compound with an enlarged

Box 1.8

A Glossary of Terms Pertinent to Neutron Capture Therapy

Epithermal neutrons: Energetic neutrons pass through an intermediate energy range on the way to becoming slow or thermal neutrons. This intermediate energy range is called epithermal.

Fast neutrons: Fast neutrons are highly energetic and travel quickly.

Moderation: Neutrons generated from the fission process or from particle bombardment of materials have significant energy. They lose that energy by colliding with atoms in their environment and create energetic recoil atoms. After a sufficient number of collisions, the neutrons lose essentially all of their energy and become thermal. This process of energy loss is called moderation. The material that provides the atoms the fast neutrons collide with is called a moderator. Water is the usual moderator.

Slow neutrons: Slow neutrons have little energy. They also are referred to as thermal neutrons because they have the same average kinetic energy as gas molecules in their environment.

Thermalize: Epithermal neutron beams, as they penetrate tissue, become additionally moderated. This is called becoming thermalized.

From Yanch JC, Shefer RE, Busse PM. Boron neutron capture therapy. In Fletcher GH, ed. *Science Med.* 1999; January/February:18–27.

cross-sectional area, not label surrounding normal tissue, and therefore deposit radiation only in the tumor is most attractive. Unfortunately, reality is far different from the ideal.

Fast neutrons differ from x-rays in the mode of their interaction with tissue. Whereas x-ray photons interact with the orbital electrons of atoms via the Compton or photoelectric process and set fast electrons in motion, neutrons interact with the nuclei of the atoms of the absorbing tissue. Neutrons put fast recoil protons, α-particles, and heavier nuclear fragments in motion. At energies above about 6 MeV, inelastic scattering by neutrons takes place.[99] A neutron may interact, for example, with a carbon or an oxygen nucleus to produce α-particles. These lead to nuclear fragments called spallation products. The LET is considerably higher for neutrons than for x-rays. Because the LET of neutron radiation is higher, the slope of the cell survival curve becomes steeper and the size of the initial shoulder gets smaller. This produces a beam with a lower OER than x-rays—neutrons are considerably more toxic to hypoxic cells than x-rays. Also, neutrons are more toxic to cells in phases of the cell cycle that are relatively radioresistant to x-rays. Thus, the RBE of neutrons is higher than x-rays.

In 1936, Locher[223] published a theoretical account of the possible biologic effects and therapeutic possibilities of boron neutron capture. In a prescient comment, he wrote:

The possibility of destroying or weakening cancerous cells, by the general or selective absorption of neutrons by themselves and particularly there is the possibility of introducing small quantities of neutron absorbers into the regions where it is desired to liberate ionizing energy. A simple illustration would be the injection of a soluble non-toxic compound of boron, lithium, or gold into a superficial cancer followed by bombardment with slow neutrons.

In 1950, Conger and Giles[224] from Oakridge National Laboratories reported that the trace amounts of boron normally present in lily bulbs were responsible for most of the radiation changes in the plants following exposure to slow neutrons. This demonstrated the biologic fact clearly and led William H. Sweet[225] and others to see if the normal brain could exclude enough boron and if tumor tissue could take up enough boron to produce an appropriate therapeutic ratio.

Sweet began work at the Brookhaven National Laboratory in New York with a 20-MW nuclear reactor in 1950.[226] He initially treated 10 glioblastoma multiforme patients who had undergone gross total resection of their tumors at the Massachusetts General Hospital in Boston. Sweet described the initial clinical work:

A portion of the shielding atop the reactor was removed to permit placing the lateral aspect of the patient's intact scalp and skull at the specially designed portal. To prevent scalp damage, we tied off the external carotid arteries and covered the entire scalp with tight elastic bandages in an attempt to prevent boron-containing blood from entering the scalp. These tactics, however, did not prevent the development of several large radiation erosions of the scalp. Five patients received a single radiation dose and the remaining 5 were given the treatment in 2 to 4 fractions. Although there were no life threatening complications of therapy, all of the patients died from 6 to 21 weeks after the first session of neutron capture therapy, which was usually the case in the 1950s for glioblastoma patients treated by any means. Postmortem studies done in 6 of the patients showed abundant viable tumor. Their painful scalp lesions together with the inadequacy of the radiation dose lead us to attempt to deliver the thermal neutron beam directly to the grossly normal but microscopically tumor-infiltrated brain. The Rockefeller Foundation made this approach possible with a $500,000 gift to the Massachusetts Institute of Technology [MIT] to provide additional features to a nuclear reactor that was then being constructed. Included was a surgical operating room immediately beneath the reactor core. This permitted us to turn down the scalp, bone, and dural flap used in the prior removal of gross tumor. At reopening the cerebrospinal fluid replacing tumor was also drained away to give maximally unimpeded access of the thermal neutrons through sterile air to the tumor-infiltrated brain.[225]

Sweet treated 18 patients at MIT. They died from 10 days to 11.5 months after radiation. In every patient, the cause of death was cerebral, and extensive irradiation necrosis of the brain was induced in nine cases. In two cases, only recurrent tumor was seen, and in one patient, there was extensive radiation necrosis and tumor.

Some of the initial work with BNCT was highly controversial and, decades later, led to investigations concerning the nature of informed consent for these human experiments. President William J. Clinton created, by executive order, a commission to study the ethics of cold war–era medical experimentation using radiation. One of the collateral effects of this commission's report was that Sweet and his colleagues were sued for malpractice 40 years after the BNCT experiments. Although the plaintiffs were awarded substantial damages at trial, the decision was eventually overturned on appeal.[227]

Lack of progress in BNCT may be attributed to two primary factors: inadequate tumor specificity of the boron compounds used to localize in the tumor and poor penetration into tissue of the thermal neutrons. In addition, the thermal and antithermal neutron beams produced by nuclear reactors have considerable contamination with γ-rays and fast neutrons. These can cause normal tissue damage even in the absence of boron concentration in tissues. In addition, there are a number of compounds in normal tissue that can interact with thermal neutrons and have capture events of their own, producing biologic damage even to non–boron-containing tissue.

The development of suitable boron-carrying agents remains a stumbling block to clinical programs. The ideal agent will be nontoxic, will have a high tumor-to-normal tissue ratio, and will have a high absolute boron concentration.

Investigations of improved ways of delivering thermal neutrons have centered on two areas: the use of nuclear reactors and useful alternatives to reactors.

The most intense way to generate a neutron beam is with a nuclear reactor. Despite the high neutron intensities available from these reactors, it is widely recognized that alternative neutron sources will be necessary for BNCT to be performed. First of all, there are few suitable nuclear reactors in operation. A patient would have to travel a long distance for treatment. Second, nuclear reactors, for political and social reasons, are not likely to be sited near major population centers in the future. A major reactor facility located far from a population center would have to be provided with its own clinical infrastructure, and it is not obvious that the target patient population would be large enough to support the operation of more than a few medical reactors. Therefore, some investigators have been pursuing nonreactive sources of thermal and epithermal neutrons with a sufficiently high flux to be used for BNCT.[225,228–230]

An alternative to the reactor would be a neutron source from radioactive decay such as californium-252 (^{252}Cf). However, production of a neutron beam with sufficient intensity for BNCT would require more than the entire present annual supply of ^{252}Cf. Another alternative source is a particle accelerator. Accelerator-based neutron beams are created when light ions such as protons or deuterons are accelerated in an electric field and are made to bombard target materials. Several accelerator techniques now exist that may be capable of producing intense beams for BNCT.

GENES AND THE BIOLOGY OF CANCER

The infectious nature of some cancers was demonstrated by Francis Peyton Rous (1879–1970) in a 1910 experiment showing that defined, submicroscopic, filterable agents (viruses) isolated from a chicken sarcoma could induce new sarcomas in healthy chickens. Rous and his work languished in obscurity before being rediscovered and recognized with the Nobel Prize in Physiology or Medicine in 1966 (Fig. 1.27).[84] In his Nobel Lecture, "The Challenge to Man of the Neoplastic Cell," Rous considered the possible existence of growth-promoting genes—what he called oncogens and what are now called oncogenes.

> Tumors destroy man in a unique and appalling way, as flesh of his own flesh which has somehow been rendered proliferative, rampant, predatory and ungovernable. They are the most concrete and formidable of human maladies, yet despite more than 70 years of experimental study they remain the least understood. This is the more remarkable because they can be evoked at will for scrutiny by any one

of a myriad chemical and physical means which are left behind as tumors grow. These had acted merely as initiation. Few situations are more exasperating to the inquirer than to watch a tiny nodule form on a rabbit's skin at a spot from which the chemical agent inducing it has long since been gone, and to follow the nodule as it grows, and only too often becomes a destructive epidermal cancer. What can be the why for these happenings?

> Every tumor is made up of cells that have been so singularly changed as to no longer obey the fundamental law whereby the cellular constituents of an organism exist in harmony and act together to maintain it. Instead the changed cells multiply at its expense and inflict damage that can be mortal. We term the lawless cells neoplastic because they form new tissue, and the growth itself is a neoplasm; but on looking into medical dictionaries, hoping for more information, we are told, in effect, that *neoplastic* means "of or pertaining to a neoplasm," and turning to *neoplasm* learn that it is "a growth which consists of neoplastic cells." Ignorance could scarcely be more stark.

> The chemical and physical initiators ordinarily are called *carcinogens*; but this is a misleading term because they not only induce the malignant epithelial growths known as carcinomas but also other neoplasms of widely various kinds. In this chapter the less often used term oncogenes will be used, meaning "thereby capable of producing a tumor." It hews precisely to the fact....

> What can be the nature of the generality of neoplastic changes, the reason for their persistence; for their irreversibility; and for the discontinuous, steplike alterations that they frequently undergo? A favorite explanation has been that oncogenes cause alterations in the genes of the body—somatic mutations as these are termed. But numerous facts, when taken together, decisively exclude this supposition.[84]

Rous, it turned out, was unequivocally wrong about oncogenes. Theodor Boveri[256] was right. In 1914, he used his studies of normal mitosis in sea urchins and worms as a platform for suggesting that cancer might be caused by the abnormal gain or loss of chromosomes and their function. In a 1929 English translation of his 1926 book, *The Origin of Malignant Tumors*, Boveri wrote:

> The unlimited tendency to rapid proliferation in malignant tumor cells [could result] from a permanent predominance of the chromosomes that promote division.... Another possibility [to explain cancer] is the presence of

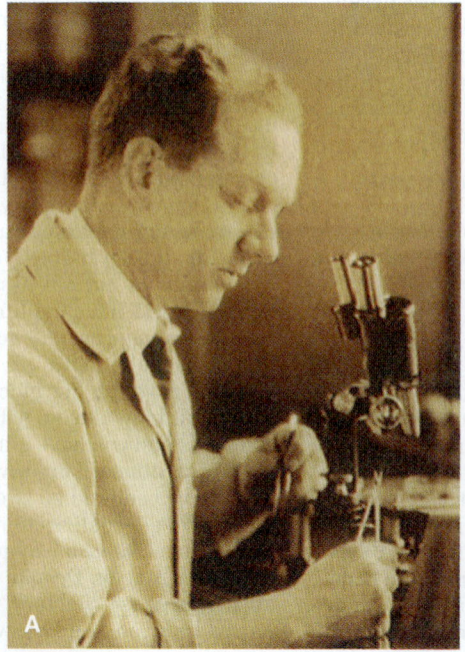
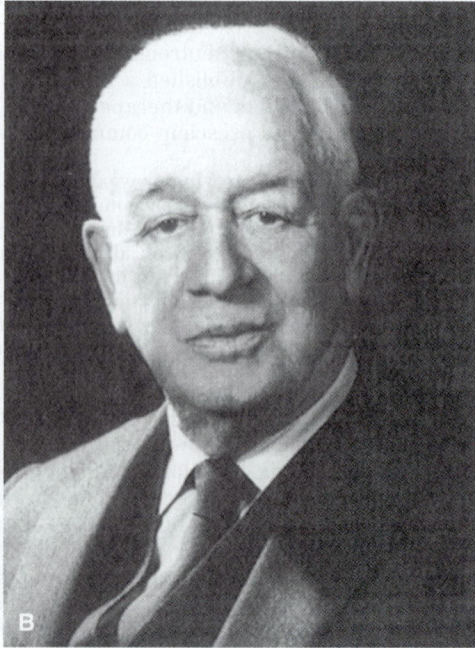

FIGURE 1.27. Peyton Rous won the Nobel Prize in 1966 for experiments he began in 1910. He demonstrated that a sarcoma could be transmitted from one chicken to another via a very small carcinogenic agent—a virus. **A:** Rous as a young investigator. **B:** At the time of the receipt of the Noble Prize. (Courtesy of Rockefeller Archives Center.)

definite chromosomes which inhibit division.... Cells of tumors with unlimited growth would arise if those "inhibiting chromosomes" were eliminated ... [since] each kind of chromosome is represented twice in the normal cell, the depression of only one of these two might pass unnoticed.[256]

Boveri predicted that the genetic abnormalities leading to the development of cancer are of two sorts: growth-promoting genes and growth-suppressing genes. If the growth-promoting genes are excessive in number or activity, they lead to cell proliferation. If, however, the growth-suppressing genes are defective in amount or activity, they fail to halt cell proliferation and lead to unbridled cell replication (Fig. 1.28). These growth-promoting genes are called *oncogenes*. The growth-suppressing genes are called *tumor suppressor genes*.

We may think of oncogenes and tumor suppressor genes as analogous to the accelerator pedal and the brake pedal of an automobile. The car can move forward when it is idling with the transmission in drive either by pushing on the accelerator pedal, by taking pressure off the brake pedal, or by doing both simultaneously. Similarly, cell growth and proliferation, leading to cancer, can occur either by the activity of the oncogenes or inactivity of the suppressor genes.

There are clearly a wide variety of physiologic conditions that call for the effective use of growth-promoting and growth-suppressing genes. There must be a mechanism to cause the fetus to grow and then, at the appropriate time, to restrain growth. There must be a way of causing fibroblasts to proliferate to heal a wound and then, at the appropriate time, halt the fibroblasts (except in the case of keloid formation). Uncontrolled cell growth, or cancer, may be thought of as a set of physiologic controls of cell growth gone awry.

Oncogenes

The experiments that initially identified oncogenes were based largely on transformed retroviruses in transplantable tumors in chickens, mice, and rats.[191] Oncogenes were described as the genetic material carried by RNA tumor viruses that resulted in rapid malignant transformation of target cells.[366,367] The name oncogene was given to virus-encoded single genes that alone or in combination with other genes induced a transformed phenotype in affected cells.[43,390,391]

The word oncogene derives from the Greek *onkos*, a "mass" or "tumor." Many oncogenes are those found in retroviruses. However, not all cellular genes capable of transforming cells have been identified within the genome of known retroviruses. It is accepted that an oncogene is a gene capable of contributing directly to the conversion of a normal cell to a tumorigenic one and that a proto-oncogene is a cellular gene convertible to an oncogene by various molecular mechanisms: sequence mutations, gene amplification, chromosomal translocation, viral transduction, and insertional mutagenesis. In general, these perturbations result in two net effects:

altered regulation or augmented expression of an oncogene through mutation or rearrangement of the nucleotide sequences that constitute signals for control of transcription, messenger RNA (mRNA) processing, and stability via insertion of a strong foreign promoter or by increased gene dosage and altered biochemical function or ectopic expression of a protein product as a result of a mutation or translocation within the protein-coding region of the oncogene. Proto-oncogene products are involved in the regulation of normal cellular growth and differentiation.

A large number of viral oncogenes have been identified. In addition, oncogenes have been identified that are not associated with RNA tumor viruses but are recognized either by their activity in transformation or by their association with chromosome translocations.[257] When DNA probing techniques were used, it was found that sequences homologous to the oncogene region of the virus were present in the DNA of all tissues of virus-free chickens. The normal cellular sequences are proto-oncogenes. The oncogene carried by a virus is referred to as *v-onc*, whereas the proto-oncogene is referred to as *c-onc*. In the normal cell, the expression of proto-oncogene is well controlled and appears to play a role in the growth and development of the organism. The function of some of these genes has been determined, whereas for others, a close association between cell proliferation and gene expression has been established.

Stimulation of a nonmalignant cell into a proliferative state often depends on an external signal, which is received by a receptor on the cell membrane and transferred through the membrane into the cytoplasm and ultimately to the nucleus where DNA synthesis is initiated. Proto-oncogenes have been found that function at each step of this pathway. The *erb*-B oncogene is homologous to the gene encoding for cell membrane receptor of epidermal growth factor (EGF). The interaction of EGF with this receptor reduces the proliferation of epidermal cells such as breast epithelium.

Strong evidence suggests that malignancy induction may be associated with genetic changes in the cell. Examples of this are the finding of specific chromosome abnormalities in malignant cells, association of tumor development with DNA-damaging agents such as ionizing irradiation and chemical carcinogens, and increasing incidence of cancer in hereditary diseases such as xeroderma pigmentosum. It is recognized that oncogenes are normal cellular genes that may contribute to the development of the malignant cell if their expression is altered through mutation, translocation, amplification, or some other mechanism. Evidence suggests that several genetic changes are needed to produce a cancer cell, and oncogene studies support this concept.

Chromosome translocations occur at a high frequency in some types of tumors, suggesting that they may play a role in their development. Examples of translocations are the t(9;22) Philadelphia chromosome in chronic myelogenous leukemia

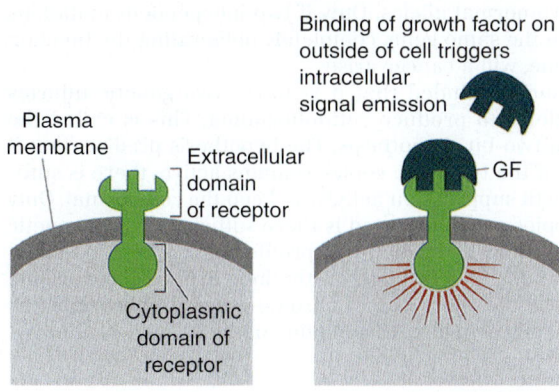

Binding of growth factor on outside of cell triggers intracellular signal emission

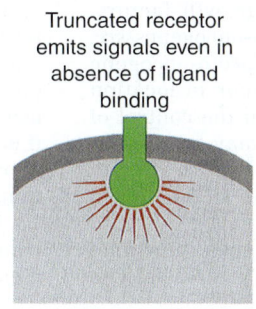

Truncated receptor emits signals even in absence of ligand binding

FIGURE 1.28. Oncogenes can act in multiple ways. One method is for a growth factor receptor, which ordinarily is only active when it binds to a ligand, to become active all the time even in the absence of a growth factor binding to it. This is called "being constitutively active" and is the result of an oncogenic mutation. (From Weinberg RA. *The biology of cancer*. New York: Garland Science, Taylor and Francis Group, 2007. Copyright © 2007 by Garland Science, Taylor & Francis Group, LLC. Used by permission of W. W. Norton & Company, Inc.)

(CML), the t(15;17) in promyelocytic leukemia, and several translocations involving chromosome 8 seen in lymphatic malignancies. Common sites of translocations in malignant cells are frequently near an oncogene. Those translocations such as the t(9;22) in CML can result in the formation of a new protein that is intimately involved in the tumorigenic transformation of the cell. In the CML example, the *ber*-gene is translocated next to the *abl*-oncogene, forming the new *bcr-abl* gene. The proteinaceous product of this newly formed gene is a hyperactive protein kinase that provides permanent growth signals to the cell.

Role of Proto-Oncogenes in Normal and Transformed Cells

Proto-oncogenes are genes with oncogenic potential, and because they are apparently present in all animals, some kind of activation of proto-oncogenes is likely to be associated with the initiation and progression of neoplasia. Activated oncogenes are detected in a large percentage of human tumors, suggesting a prominent role of these genes in their development; association between activated oncogenes and neoplastic diseases must have some kind of specificity for both the oncogene and the tumor.

Proto-oncogenes can be activated by genetic changes that affect either protein expression or structure. As succinctly stated by Weinberg:

The somatic mutations that caused proto-oncogene activation could be divided into two categories—those that caused changes in the structure of encoded proteins and those that led to elevated, deregulated expression of these proteins. Mutations affecting structure included the point mutations affecting ras proto-oncogenes and the chromosomal translocations that yielded hybrid genes such as bcr–abl. Elevated expression could be achieved in human tumors through gene amplification or chromosomal translocations, such as those that place the myc gene under the control of immunoglobulin enhancer sequences....

Gene amplification occurs through preferential replication of a segment (the amplicon) of chromosomal DNA. The result may be repeating end-to-end linear arrays of the segment, which appear as homogeneously staining regions (HSRs) of a chromosome when viewed under the light microscope. Alternatively, the region carrying the amplified segment may break away from the chromosome and can be seen as small, independently replicating, extra-chromosomal particles (double minutes). Gene amplification does not always result in overexpression of the gene....[382]

A variety of structural changes in proteins can also lead to oncogene activation. Examples include alterations in the structure of growth factor receptors (such as the EGF receptor) and translocations that fuse two distinct reading frames to yield a hybrid protein (such as Bcr-Abl). Both types of alterations deregulate the proteins, causing them to emit growth-promoting signals in a strong, unremitting fashion.[258]

Oncogene protein products can be grouped into several classes depending on their location and reactivity: nuclear, cytoplasmic, and membrane protein kinases; cytoplasmic guanosine triphosphate–binding proteins; growth factors; and others. The protein products of the proto-oncogenes *src*, *abl*, and *ras* are cytoplasmic in location. The proto-oncogene products of *myc*, *fos*, *ski*, and *myb* are nuclear in location and are believed to play an important role in the control of cell division. The expression of these genes may be responsible for the entry of the cell into DNA synthesis. Growth factors are proteins that act at the cell surface to stimulate cell growth.

Current evidence suggests that *ras* oncogenes contribute to both initiation and progression of human neoplasia. The incidence of proto-oncogene amplifications in biopsy specimens from tumors, although highly variable, is usually low. However, there may be a tendency toward association of amplification of specific proto-oncogenes and particular types of tumors. Amplifications of the c-*erb*-B-2/*neu* proto-oncogene (also referred to as *her*-2) may be involved in the etiology of human breast, salivary gland, and ovarian cancers and might serve as a useful prognostic marker for these malignancies.[327] The *erb*-B-2/*neu* locus is amplified in 30% of primary breast carcinomas and that amplification is associated with a worse prognosis.[183]

Amplification of another proto-oncogene, C-*myc*, occurs mainly in adenocarcinomas, squamous cell carcinomas, and sarcomas but not in hematologic malignancies, whereas N-*myc* amplification occurs most frequently in neuroblastomas and occasionally in retinoblastomas and a few small cell lung carcinomas.

Tumor Suppressor Genes

The concept that a gene product could inhibit or suppress proliferation of cells in a tumor was derived from experiments using somatic cell genetics.[259] Different chromosomes from normal human cells carry tumor suppression genes that are able to block tumor formation by the cancer cell. The cancer cells must sustain mutation in both alleles of these genes to develop the ability to produce tumors.[260,392,393]

These somatic cell genetic experiments relied on cell fusion. In the first type of experiment, a cancerous cell that was able to form a tumor in an animal was fused with a normal cell. The hybrid cell no longer produced tumors in animals. One could conclude that there was an element in the normal cell that was able to suppress the tumorigenic potential of the cancerous cell. It was found that, on occasion, one of the hybrid cell lines produced by fusion of cancerous and normal cells was tumorigenic. Why? These malignant cell lines were missing genetic material supplied by the normal parent cells. Further investigation identified the presence of tumor-suppressing genes from the normal parent. Eventually, several specific tumor suppressor genes were identified and named.[383,384]

The next important part of the story of tumor suppressor genes comes from studies of the ocular tumor of infancy—retinoblastoma. Retinoblastoma can be either unilateral and unifocal or bilateral and multifocal. The disease also can be heritable or nonheritable based on the presence of a positive family history. Alfred Knudson[261] noted that heritable retinoblastoma was more often bilateral and multifocal and occurred in younger children rather than nonheritable unilateral retinoblastoma, which occurred in older children (Figs. 1.29 and 1.30). Knudson postulated that there was a gene that renders children susceptible to retinoblastoma. Patients with early-onset bilateral, multifocal disease inherit one defective copy of this gene and one normal allele. With a very high frequency, mutations develop in the normal allele, and children develop the tumor. However, patients with nonheritable retinoblastoma inherit two normal alleles. Only if two independent mutations develop in the same gene, completely obliterating the function of that gene, will a cancer arise.

Knudson concluded that it requires two genetic injuries in two alleles to produce retinoblastoma. This is called the "Knudson two-hit" hypothesis. The hypothesis predicts that if only one of the two gene copies remains active, there is sufficient growth suppression activity to keep the cell normal. Only if both copies are inactivated is there sufficient loss of genetic activity to allow unbridled cell proliferation. The retinoblastoma gene, *Rb*, was isolated on the long arm of chromosome 13. Because the short arm of chromosomes is abbreviated as p and the long arm as q, the deletion of the *Rb* gene is abbreviated as 13q-.

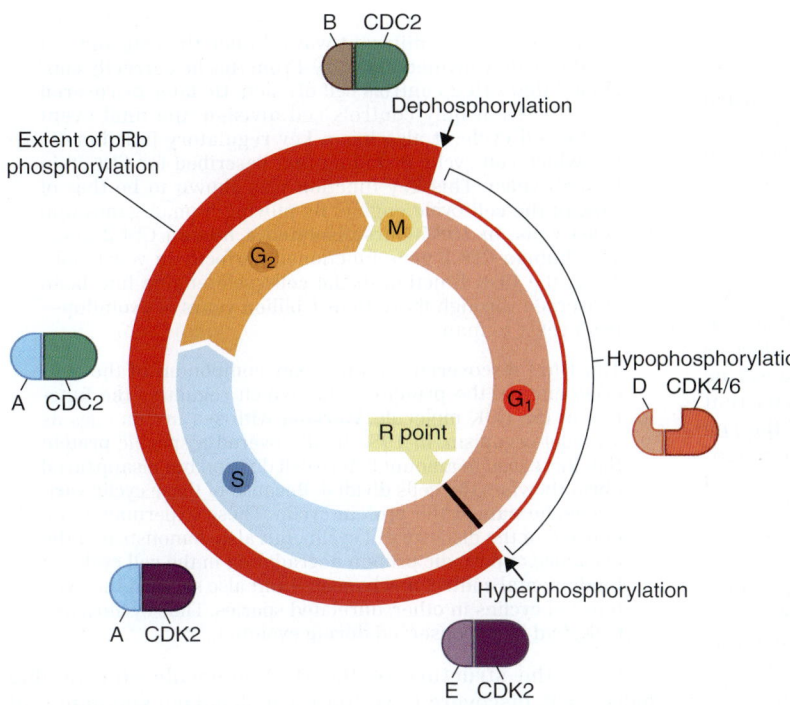

FIGURE 1.29. The phosphorylation of the retinoblastoma gene product protein, depicted as the red circle, helps to control the cell cycle. As the cell moves from M to G1, the protein is unphosphorylated; as the cell progresses through G1, the protein is hypophosphorylated; and after passing the R point (the restriction point), it is hyperphosphorylated. This process of phosphorylation is controlled by cyclins. (From Weinberg RA. *The biology of cancer*. New York: Garland Science, Taylor and Francis Group, 2007. Copyright © 2007 by Garland Science, Taylor & Francis Group, LLC. Used by permission of W. W. Norton & Company, Inc.)

How could one find tumor suppressor genes when their existence was most apparent by their absence? Robert Weinberg explains:

The dominantly acting oncogenes, in stark contrast, could be detected far more readily through their presence in a retrovirus genome, through the transfection-focus assay, or through their presence in a chromosomal segment that repeatedly undergoes gene amplification in a number of independently arising tumors....

A more general strategy was required that did not depend on the chance observation of interstitial chromosomal deletions or the presence of a known gene ... that, through good fortune, lay near a tumor suppressor gene on a chromosome. Both of these conditions greatly facilitated the isolation of the Rb gene. In general, however, the searches for most tumor suppressor genes were not favored by such strokes of good luck[258].

The tendency of tumor suppressor genes to undergo LOH (loss of heterozygosity) during tumor development provided cancer researchers with a novel genetic strategy for tracking them down. Because the chromosomal region flanking a tumor suppressor gene seemed to undergo LOH together with the tumor suppressor gene itself, one might be able to detect the existence of a still-uncloned tumor suppressor gene simply from the fact that an anonymous genetic marker lying nearby on the chromosome repeatedly undergoes LOH during the development of a specific type of human tumor.

The use of more powerful mapping techniques allowed geneticists to plant polymorphic markers more densely along the genetic maps of each chromosomal arm. Within a given chromosomal arm, some markers were found to undergo LOH far more frequently than others. Clearly, the closer these markers were to a sought-after tumor gene (i.e., the tighter the genetic linkage), the higher was the probability that such markers would undergo LOH together with the tumor suppressor gene. Conversely, markers located further away on a chromosomal arm were less likely to undergo LOH together with the tumor suppressor gene. Genetic analyses of DNAs prepared from various types of human tumors have revealed a large number of chromosomal regions that frequently suffer LOH. A subset of these regions have yielded

to the attacks of the gene cloners, resulting in the isolation of many tumor suppressor genes.[258]

A number of distinctions separate the oncogenes from the tumor suppressor genes. It is almost certain that, in most human cancers, there is a multistep pathway to tumor development, which involves the accumulation of mutations in a series of oncogenes and suppressor genes.[260]

Many tumor suppressor genes have been cloned. The suppressor p53 gene resides in 20 kilobase (kb) of DNA located in chromosome 17p13.1. The gene is a nuclear phosphoprotein composed of 393 amino acid residues in humans.[260] p53 mutations have been detected in a wide variety of malignant human tumors. The p53 gene encompasses 16 to 20 kb of DNA on the short arm of human chromosome 17. Loss of normal

FIGURE 1.30. Alfred Knudson (1922–2016) received a B.S. degree from California Institute of Technology (Caltech) in 1944, an M.D. from Columbia in 1947, and a Ph.D. from Caltech in 1956. He served in the Navy during World War II and the Army during the Korean war. In 1971 he published his "two hit" hypothesis for the etiology of some forms of cancer. We now know this to be the result of the disabling of a tumor suppressor gene.[397] (Photo courtesy of Fox Chase Cancer Center Archives, Philadelphia, PA.)

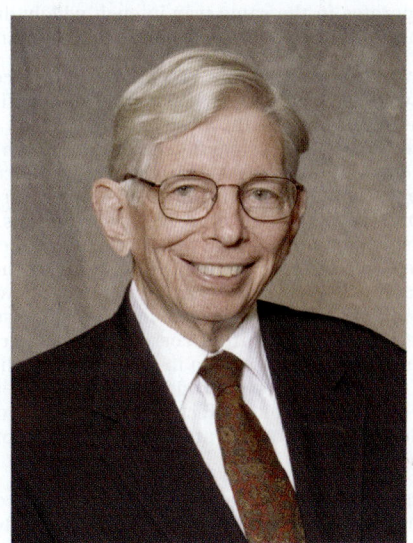

p53 function is associated with cell transformation *in vitro* and development of neoplasms *in vivo*. Abrogation of the normal p53 pathway is a common feature in human cancers, and it appears to be critical in the pathogenesis and progression of these tumors.[117] In some cases, candidate tumor suppressor genes have been identified based on an association between loss or inactivation and tumor development, the causal connection being only inferred.

Cell Cycle Control

The cell cycle, which consists of four phases (G1, S, G2, and M), regulates the duplication of genetic information and distribution of duplicated chromosomes to daughter cells. The phrases "cell cycle control" or "cell cycle clock" are used to describe the cell's molecular circuits operating in the nucleus that process and integrate afferent signals and decide if the cell will actively proliferate or remain quiescent. If the "go/no-go" decision is to "go" into proliferation, the circuitry is engaged to launch the biochemical changer necessary to allow the cell to double its contents and divide into two daughter cells. Key providers of the afferent information are tyrosine kinase receptors, G-protein–coupled receptors, transforming growth factor-*b* receptors, integrins, and the cell's nutritional status[258].

The Nobel Prize in Physiology or Medicine for 2001 was awarded to Leland H. Hartwell, R. Timothy Hunt, and Sir Paul M. Nurse for their discoveries regarding the control of the cell cycle. The Nobel presentation speech by Professor Anders Zetterberg succinctly describes the important controls of cell replication elucidated by these three scientists:

> Cell division is a fundamental process of life. All living organisms on earth are descended from an ancestral cell that appeared about 3 billion years ago, and which has undergone an unbroken series of cell divisions since then. Each human being also began life as one single cell—a cell that divided repeatedly to give rise to all one hundred thousand billion cells that we consist of.... Every second millions of cells divide in our body.

> The cycle of events that a cell completes from one division to the next is called the cell cycle. During the cell cycle the cell grows in size, duplicates its hereditary material—that is, it copies the DNA molecules in the chromosomes—and divides into two daughter cells.

> This year's Nobel Laureates have discovered the key regulators of the cell cycle—cyclin dependent kinase (CDK) and cyclin. Together these two components form an enzyme, in which CDK is comparable to a "molecular engine" that drives the cell through the cell cycle by altering the structure and function of other proteins in the cell. Cyclin is the main switch that turns the "CDK engine" on and off. This cell-cycle engine operates in the same way in such widely disparate organisms as yeast cells, plants, animals, and humans.

> How were the key regulators CDK and cyclin discovered? Lee Hartwell realized the great potential of genetic methods for cell-cycle studies. He chose baker's yeast as a model organism. In the microscope he could identify genetically altered cells—mutated cells—that stopped in the cell cycle when they were cultured at an elevated temperature. Using this method Hartwell discovered, in the early 1970s, dozens of genes specific to the cell-division cycle, which he named CDC genes. One of these genes, CDC28, controls the initiation of each cell cycle, the "start" function. Hartwell also formulated the concept of "checkpoints," which ensure that cell-cycle events occur in the correct order. Checkpoints are comparable to the program in a washing machine that checks if one step has been properly completed before the next can start. Checkpoint defects are considered to be one of the reasons behind the transformation of normal cells into cancer cells.

> Paul Nurse also used the genetic approach in his cell-cycle studies but in a different kind of yeast. In the late 1970s

> and early 1980s he discovered the gene CDC2, which could be mutated in two different ways. Either the cells did not divide, or they divided too early. From this he correctly concluded that CDC2 controls cell division. He later discovered that CDC2 not only controls cell division, the final event of the cell cycle; it also has a key regulatory function for the whole cell cycle, including that described for CDC28 in baker's yeast. This key function was shown to be that of CDK in the cell-cycle engine. By moving human genes into yeast cells, in 1987 Nurse isolated a human CDC2 gene. This human CDC2 gene functioned perfectly in yeast cells. Thus, the CDK function in the cell-cycle engine had been conserved through more than 1 billion years of evolution—from yeast to man.

> Tim Hunt discovered the other key component of the cell-cycle engine, the protein cyclin, which regulates the function of the CDK molecule. Working with sea urchin eggs as a model organism, in 1982 he discovered a specific protein that increased in amount before cell division but disappeared abruptly when the cells divided. Because of these cyclic variations, he named the protein cyclin. These experiments not only led to the discovery of cyclin, but also demonstrated the existence of periodic protein degradation in the cell cycle—a fundamental control mechanism. Hunt also showed the existence of cyclins in other, unrelated species. Thus cyclins, like CDK, had been conserved during evolution.[263]

Since the structure of the DNA molecule—the double helix—was discovered, we have a molecular explanation of how a gene can make a copy of itself. With the discoveries of CDK and cyclin, we are now beginning to understand, at the molecular level, how the cell can make a copy of itself.

To ensure that the daughter cells possess a full complement of genetic information, checkpoints exist to ensure fidelity of DNA duplication and accuracy of chromosome segregation.[48] Checkpoint pauses permit editing and repair of genetic information so that each daughter cell receives a full complement of genetic information identical to the parent cell. In some cells, there are checkpoints for initiation of mitosis. Mutation of the checkpoint genes allows the cell to enter mitosis after x-irradiation.[264] For example, the rad-9 gene is a G2/M checkpoint gene because it responds to two different types of signals.[265] Experimental observations suggest that the p53 gene, shown to be a transcriptional activator,[118] may be critical for G1 checkpoint control. p53 has been shown to induce transcription of p21, which in turn inhibits the association of CDK 4,6 with proliferating cell nuclear antigen and cyclin D. As a consequence, the retinoblastoma protein cannot be phosphorylated and stays in complex with the transcription factor E2 F, effectively blocking the transcription of cell cycle–promoting proteins and causing a cell cycle arrest.

Checkpoints are signal transduction systems that must receive a signal, amplify it, and transmit it to other components that regulate the cell cycle. Double-strand DNA breaks, unexcised ultraviolet light–induced dimers in DNA, and centromeres not engaged by the spindle are potential signals.[139,266] Checkpoints ensure the fidelity of genomic replication and segregation. Biologically significant levels of spontaneous damage require checkpoint control for cells to maintain a high fidelity of chromosome transmission. Therefore, restoration of compromised checkpoints could slow cancer cell evolution even in the absence of exogenous sources of DNA damage.[266] Many signal transduction systems, including checkpoint controls, exhibit adaptation; that is, in the presence of a constant stimulus, the response diminishes with time. As a consequence, the cell may proceed through the cell cycle, although the original perturbation has not been removed or cannot be repaired. Checkpoint activation may induce a variety of cell responses, including cell death. The checkpoint controlling entry into S-phase in mammalian cells includes p53. One function under the control of this pathway is apoptosis. Restoration of defective checkpoints could restore the apoptotic response of cancer cells and increase their sensitivity to DNA-damaging agents. It may be possible to achieve specificity for certain types of cancer cells because not all cells respond to the same apoptotic signals.[237,238,267,268]

Growth Factors and Signal Transduction

Transmission of biochemical signals to the cellular nucleus leads to altered expression of a wide variety of genes involved in microgenic and differentiation responses.[138] A number of growth factors exert their effects through receptors possessing intrinsic protein tyrosine kinase activity. On activation, these receptors phosphorylate both themselves and other intracellular proteins on the amino acid tyrosine. Among the receptors for growth factors are EGF, platelet-derived growth factor, insulin, nerve growth factor, and macrophage colony stimulatory factor. The mitogenic signaling pathway activated by protein tyrosine kinase receptors involves the activation of ras proteins. Ras undergoes conformational change and interacts with additional downstream targets. A protein kinase cascade is activated, which conveys the growth factor–initiated signal to the nucleus via the raf, mek, map kinase, and other proteins.

Telomeres

Human chromosomes are linear. At each end of the chromosome are structures known as telomeres, from the Greek *telo* for "end" and *mere* for "structure." Telomeres are composed of specialized DNA and DNA-binding proteins. As chromosomes are replicated, telomeres shorten each time during the process of cell division. Continued cycles of cell division result in shortened telomeres. The telomeres, for example, in the fibroblasts of older adults are shorter than those in children. Normal human cells senesce when the telomeres shorten to a critical length.

Stem cells and cancer cells must maintain their telomere lengths to prevent senescence. Two mechanisms of telomere maintenance have been identified: expression of the telomerase enzyme and the recombination of telomeres.

The telomere hypothesis states that critical telomere shortening prevents somatic cells from dividing. In contrast, the maintenance of telomere length allows cancer cells to continue to divide. An increasing body of experimental evidence supports the telomere hypothesis and its association with cancer.

The capacity of cells to respond to ionizing radiation is determined by multiple factors. There are a variety of syndromes associated with molecular defects that are characterized by clinical radiosensitivity. These include ataxia, telangiectasia, Nijmegen breakage syndrome, and ataxia telangiectasia–like disorder. These syndromes all have defective telomere maintenance in common. It has been hypothesized, therefore, that the radiosensitivity phenotype and the telomere dysfunction phenotype may be linked. A variety of experimental models suggest that telomere maintenance and radiosensitivity are associated, and this may offer the opportunity for a therapeutic target.

Apoptosis

Apoptosis or programmed cell death, a phenomenon distinct from necrosis, was described in 1972 by Kerr et al.[240] Apoptosis is programmed by specific signals in the cell that cause an endonuclease to cleave DNA at internucleosomal sites.

Apoptosis is detected by histologic evaluation of membrane blebbing and chromatin condensation, by flow cytometry using fluorescent nucleotides and terminal transferase to detect fragmented DNA, by detecting apoptotic cells that are usually very small with characteristic profiles of right-angle and forward light scattering, or by using DNA fluorochrome to detect a decrease in fluorescence as small DNA fragments diffuse from the cell that is undergoing apoptosis.[237,269,270] An early change in apoptosis, the flip-flop of the phospholipid phosphatidylserine (PS) from the inner to the outer leaflet of the bilayer membrane, also can be detected using a fluorescently labeled annexin V protein that has a high binding affinity to PS. Several oncogenes, cytokines, and growth factors have been reported to play a role in promoting or reducing radiation-induced apoptosis.[233]

Most radiation-induced cell lethality (loss of reproductive integrity) for dividing cells appears to be caused by mitotic-linked death resulting in loss of genetic information as cells with chromosomal aberrations divide. Apoptosis, frequently seen within 4 to 6 hours after irradiation, occurs spontaneously and is enhanced by radiation as observed *in vivo* in the intestinal crypt and salivary and lacrimal glands with nondividing cells and nondividing lymphocytes. Apoptotic cells are eliminated rapidly *in vivo*, making it difficult to quantify. In contrast, this cell death mechanism is easy to quantify *in vitro* because apoptotic cells persist in culture for many hours. However, cell division of nonapoptotic cells complicates quantification.[233] In cell lines susceptible to apoptosis, this process sometimes occurs early before cells enter mitosis or later after the cells divide. Late apoptosis may be associated with mitotically linked death and, in fact, may be triggered by chromosomal aberrations. Apoptosis may be quite important for clinically relevant doses of fractionated irradiation, even if it causes a relatively small reduction in clonogenic survival. However, this requires that cells be recruited into the apoptotic-susceptible fraction after each dose fraction.

It appears that with progression of certain tumors, spontaneous and therapy-related apoptosis occurs less frequently. The apoptotic response to irradiation can be modified by cytokines to protect normal tissues[170] or to induce tumor cell killing.[271-273] Tumor necrosis factor increases apoptosis after irradiation in some tumors while protecting the hematopoietic compartment, possibly by blocking apoptosis. Irradiation prevents extensive cellular proliferation by increasing differentiation in both tumors and normal tissues. Also, irradiation appears to increase the aging of normal cells. Another mechanism of reversible loss of proliferative capacity induced by irradiation is necrosis, which occurs with high doses of irradiation and is a major mechanism seen with large-dose fractions such as in stereotactic irradiation.

GRID Therapy, Bystander Effects, Abscopal Effects, REAP, and DAMP

Early in radiotherapy's history, some clinicians tried to improve normal tissue sparing, particularly the skin, by creating a shielding block which resembled a checkerboard. Imagine a checkerboard in which the black squares are lead and the white squares are open. This would permit radiation to travel through the open squares while the black squares would shield the patient, the patient's normal tissue, and the tumor from radiation. If a single-photon field was used to deliver the grid pattern of radiation, there would be a dose distribution of peaks and valleys across the normal tissue and the tumor because of penumbra and side scatter. A radiation dose, which is delivered to a continuous region, induces greater damage than the some dose fractionated in space. This concept is generally called GRID radiation therapy. It can now be performed with TomoTherapy, multileaf collimators, and/or a proton beam. In three dimensions, the GRID or "checkerboard" is probably better thought of as a honeycomb.

Spatially fractionated radiotherapy causes irradiated tumor cells to engage to cell-to-cell signaling. Neighboring unirradiated cancer cells are clearly affected. One observes cells undergoing a stress response, activation of repair enzymes, and antioxidant gene expression. It is as if the irradiated cells are sending a "Mayday...mayday...I am under attack" message to neighboring cells. Furthermore, in some experimental models, the irradiated cells provoke an immune response, which can kill irradiated and unirradiated cells. It appears that the radiation causes the emission of antigens and cell signals, which activate an immune reaction. The phenomena of the irradiated cells have an effect upon neighboring unirradiated calls is called "the bystander effect."[274]

The abscopal effect is a phenomenon where the localized treatment of a tumor causes not only a shrinking of the treated tumor but also a shrinking of tumors outside the scope of the localized treatment. Imagine, for example, an experimental mouse with a tumor implanted in the left thigh and a tumor of the same histology implanted in the right thigh. If a highly localized external radiation beam were directed against the tumor of the left thigh and it regressed and, in addition, the unirradiated tumor of the right thigh regressed, then the behavior of the tumor of the right thigh is called an abscopal effect. In a 1953 paper in the British Journal of Radiology, R.H. Mole proposed the term "abscopal" ("ab," away from; "scopus," target) to refer to radiation's effects "at a distance from the irradiated volume but within the same organism."[275]

A current active area of research addresses the idea that irradiation may augment the immunogenicity of tumors and accentuate the cytotoxic effects of radiotherapy both on the irradiated tumor and on distant tumors—a form of the abscopal effect. In combination with immunotherapeutic agents, an irradiated tumor might be able to act as an autologous *in situ* tumor vaccine. The mechanism of action might involved radiation-enhanced antigen presentation (REAP), damage-associated molecular patterns, or danger-associated molecular patterns (DAMP), by which host molecules initiate and perpetuate a noninfectious inflammatory response, immunomodulation of tumor cell surface molecules, and the modulation of cellular infiltrates in the tumor microenvironment.[276,277]

Stick the following references where they go, alphabetically, in the reference section of Chapter 1 but do not number them.

THE BIOLOGY OF METASTASIS

The prefix *meta* is of Greek origin and is defined as "after," "beyond," or "over." It is used to denote change or transformation. The word *stasis* means "stand" or "stationary." Thus, when the two words are combined to form *metastasis*, the new word is used to represent a change in location of a disease or its manifestations. It also means the transfer of a disease from one organ or body part to another organ or body part not directly connected. The oncologist uses the term *metastasis* to refer to the manifestation of malignancy that arises from the primary growth but is now in a secondary site.

It is clear that the pattern of metastatic spread of cancer is not random. The distribution of some secondary tumor deposits can be explained on mechanistic grounds (i.e., that the tumor cells are shed into the bloodstream and lodge in the first narrow capillary network that they encounter downstream). This would explain, for example, why the liver is the most common site for secondary tumors in patients with primary cancer within the catchment area of the hepatic portal vein, such as gastrointestinal malignancies. Similarly, the lung would be a favored site in patients with primary tumor spilling into the systemic veins. There can be no doubt that vascular drainage patterns influence the distribution of secondary tumor deposits from some types of primary cancer.

It is also clear, however, that the distribution of some metastatic tumors cannot be explained solely by patterns of encountering and lodging in the nearest narrow capillary bed. This is called "metastatic tropism": Carcinomas form detectable metastases in only a limited subset of possible distant organ sites. The seminal paper addressing the problem was metastatic tropism by Stephen Paget (Fig. 1.31). Paget was the fourth and youngest son of the famous British physician Sir James Paget. James Paget was one of the founders of modern pathology and is the nanesoke of Paget's disease. Stephen

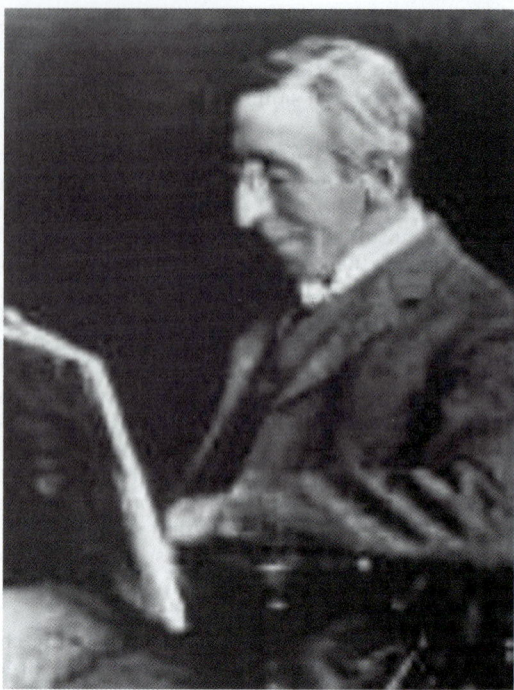

FIGURE 1.31. Stephen Paget (1855–1926). (Reprinted by permission from Nature: Fidler IJ. The pathogenesis of cancer metastasis: the 'seed and soil' hypothesis revisited. Nat Rev Cancer 2003;3[6]:453–458. Copyright © 2003 Springer Nature.)

Paget worked as an assistant surgeon at the West London and Metropolitan Hospitals in England. Later in life, he devoted himself to public health issues and became a highly regarded biographer and essayist.[278] Writing in the *Lancet* on March 23, 1889, on "The Distribution of Secondary Growth in Cancer of the Breast," Paget wondered:

> The question ought to be asked, and if possible answered: "What is it that decides what organs shall suffer in a case of disseminated cancer?" If the remote organs in such a case are all alike passive and, so to speak, helpless—all equally ready to receive and nourish any particle of the primary growth which may "slip through the lungs," and so be brought to them—then the distribution of cancer throughout the body must be a matter of chance. But if we can trace any sort of rule or sequence in the distribution of cancer, any relation between the character of the primary growth and the situation of the secondary growths derived from it, then the remote organs cannot be altogether passive or indifferent as regards embolism.... Every single cancer cell must be regarded as an organism, alive and capable of development. When a plant goes to seed, its seeds are carried in all directions; but they can only live and grow if they fall on congenial soil.[281]

Paget observed, in a large number of autopsies of women with breast cancer, that the lymph nodes, liver, lung, bone, and brain commonly were involved. However, he found that the kidney and spleen rarely were involved despite receiving a significant amount of blood flow. He was struck by the discrepancy between the relative blood supplies and the relative frequencies of metastatic tumors in various organs. From his data, Paget expounded his "seed and soil hypothesis." He argued that metastasis required both a willing seed (intrinsic cellular factors) and hospitable soil (host organ). There must be intrinsic cellular factors that lead to a satisfactory interaction between the tumor cell and the host organ resulting in successful metastasis. In contemporary terms, we understand this to mean that the tumor cell must have favorable adhesion molecules, and the host organ must be accepting receptors on its endothelial cells, which results in appropriate sites for the circulating tumor cells to bind, migrate into the organ, and subsequently grow, or, perhaps, that tumor cells promote upregulation of adhesion receptors in specific stromal cells.

As they grow, tumors almost certainly release large numbers of malignant cells into the blood and lymphatics continuously. It is clear, however, that the mere presence of tumor cells in the bloodstream does not always lead to the formation of distant metastases. A. J. Salisbury of the Brompton Hospital in London is credited as being one of the first to emphasize that the metastatic process is highly inefficient. The overwhelming majority of malignant cells released in the blood die.[282] They are battered in the circulation, assaulted by the immune system, and fail to reproduce. Irving Zeidman and Isaiah J. Fidler, at that time working at the University of Pennsylvania, injected mouse melanoma cells labeled with radioactive iodine into a peripheral vein of an experimental mouse. Within a few minutes, the melanoma cells had lodged in the nearest, narrowest capillary bed: the lungs. Most tumor cells died there. A day later, about 1% of the injected cells were still alive.[283,284]

The fact that only a small fraction of a tumor's cells can successfully form metastatic colonies implies that the survivors are, indeed, specially adapted cells. One might think of them in evolutionary terms. These successfully metastasizing cells must represent the survival of the fittest: the most hardy, most resilient, and most able to fend off the body's attempt to kill them. Isaiah J. Fidler performed an experiment with B16 melanoma cells in mice wherein he injected them into a peripheral vein, harvested the ones that grew in the lungs, grew the process in a tissue culture environment, and repeated the process over and over and showed that he could create increasingly efficient cancers, which became better and better of metastasizing to the lung. He shown that they truly were "the fittest" when he came to metastatic potential.

A long period of tumor growth leads to progressive changes in a tumor's structure, blood supply, oxygenation status, antigenic characteristics, doubling rate, growth properties, and metastatic potential. Several investigators have performed variations of the following experiment: Unselected tumor cell suspensions were divided into two parts. One part was injected intravenously into a group of mice. The other part was subdivided into separate cultures. From each culture, a single tumor cell was isolated and grown to produce a large number of different clones, that is, cells with identical genetic composition. Then, these clones were injected into groups of mice.[225,285]

If the metastatic potential of tumor cells was homogenous, then you would expect that the number and location of tumor colonies in injected mice would be similar in the mice receiving the unselected tumor cell suspensions and the mice receiving the cloned lines. If different cloned subpopulations gave rise to widely different numbers of colonies compared to the unclonced cells, it would indicate that the tumor was heterogenous—that the tumor contained cells with a variety of metastatic potential. The result was that there were widely different numbers of metastatic colonies. This implies the intrinsic heterogeneity of metastatic potential in a growing tumor.

As Stephen Paget suggested, there really a tendency for particular types of primary tumors to preferentially metastasize to particular organs. Can we show, experimentally, that this is true and that it really is not about "the nearest, narrowest capillary bed trapping the tumor cells"? Garth L. Nicholson and Isaiah J. Fidler took highly metastatic melanoma cells serially passed so that they were quite efficient at metastasizing to the lungs and injected some into the tail vein of mice where the first narrow capillary bed they would encounter was the lung and, in other animals, they injected the cells into the left ventricle, just beyond the lungs, where they would be more likely to be disseminated throughout the body. Initially, the animals who had cells injected into the tail vein had far more tumor cells in the lungs. One day after injection, there was no difference in the number of cells in the lungs irrespective of the site injection. After two weeks, the same number of lung tumors

were found for the two sites of injection. Tumor cells destined to form metastases in a particular organ appear capable of detaching from their first home and recirculating until they come to rest at their preferred site of ultimate metastases.[285]

Metastasis formation is an inefficient process. Fidler and colleagues[286] injected melanoma cells into the peripheral vein of a mouse whose DNA had been labeled with radioactive iodine. They found that, shortly after the injection, most of the injected cells rested in the lung (i.e., the nearest narrow capillary bed). Most of the tumor cells, however, went on to die in the lung. Only a few live cells continued to circulate. Within a day, only 1% of the injected cells were alive, and after 2 weeks, no known metastasis could be seen in the lungs. Only 0.1% of the cells originally injected were still alive.[286] Blood-borne metastasis must be a highly selective process. Only a very small proportion of malignant cells that enter into the bloodstream are able to survive and grow.

There are three major pathways of metastasis. They are:

- Across body cavities such as the peritoneal cavity or within the cerebrospinal fluid. This is the way, for example, that medulloblastoma disseminates via the leptomeninges or that ovarian tumors form on the peritoneal surface of the intestine.
- Via the lymphatic system. Axillary masses following breast cancer, which are easily palpable, would be a common example.
- Hematogenously, usually via veins rather than arteries. The spread of a limb sarcoma to the lungs would be an example (Fig. 1.32).

The molecular mechanism of tumor metastasis is a multistep process involving many tumor cells—host–cell interactions as well as cell–matrix associations.[312,338] This process is sometimes called the invasion–metastasis cascade. The crucial processes are as follows:

- Tumor cell adhesion to other tumor cells at the site of the primary malignancy, host cells, or components of the extracellular matrix
- Proteolysis of the extracellular matrix during invasion
- Tumor cell motility through the extracellular matrix to reach the vascular or lymphatic endothelium
- Intravasation into the lumina of blood vessels or lymphatics—this is facilitated by molecular changes that promote the ability of carcinoma cells to cross the pericytes and endothelial cell barriers
- Embolism into the lymphatic system and/or the blood circulation
- Tumor cell survival despite both the mechanical trauma endured by the cell in transit in the vascular system as well as the body's immunologic assault directed against the circulating tumor cell (insofar as most tumor cells have a diameter of 20 to 30 μm and capillaries have a diameter of approximately 8 μm; most tumor cells in circulation are probably quickly trapped in capillary beds)
- Adherence to the endothelium when the tumor cell comes to rest at the metastatic site in the secondary organ
- Dissolution of the cell–cell junction and the basement membrane of the blood vessel or lymphatic into the organ parenchyma
- Survival in the new host organ microenvironment and interaction with that new microenvironment in the host organ to permit growth of the tumor deposit
- Tumor cell proliferation in the new organ and angiogenesis to achieve metastatic colonization

Only if all of these steps can be negotiated successfully can the tumor cell ultimately "set up shop" as a metastatic focus. The fact that only a small fraction of tumor cells survive and successfully establish a metastasis would suggest that the

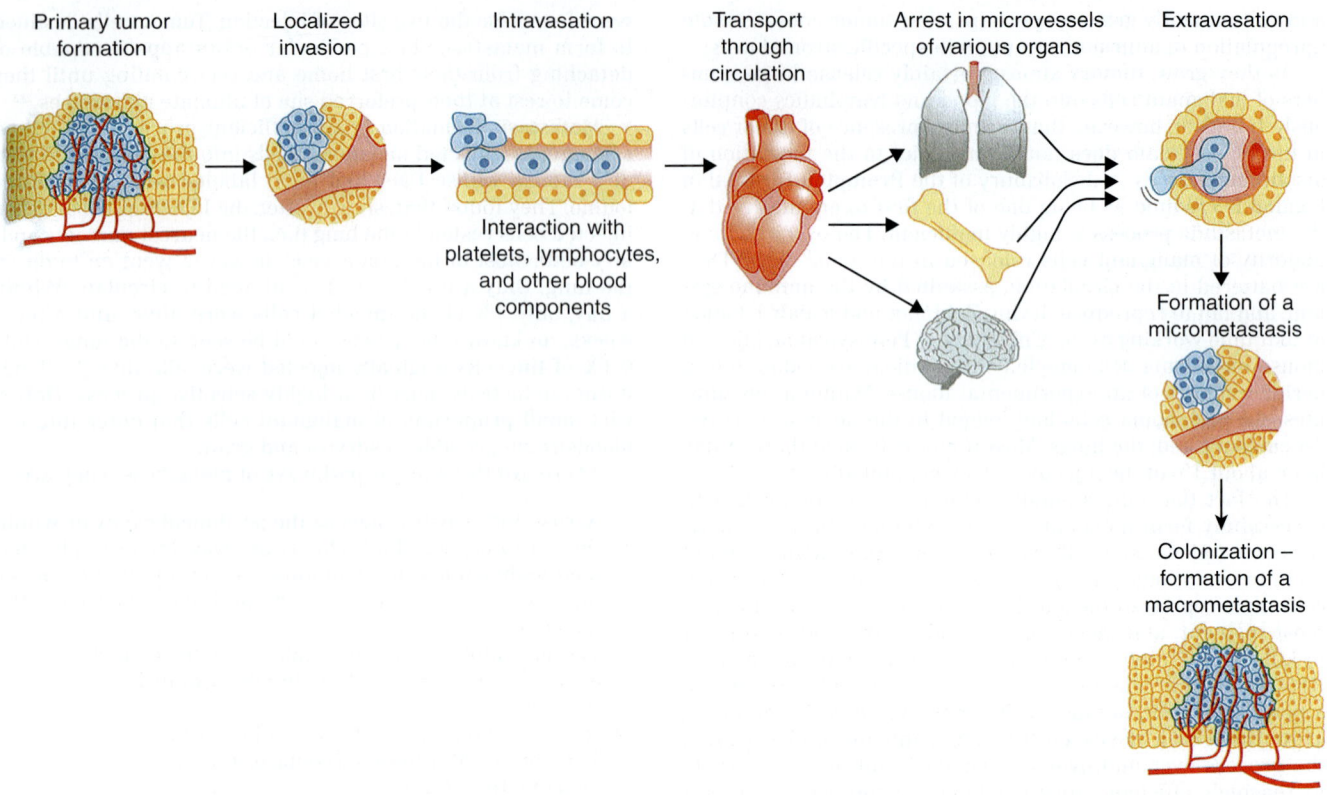

FIGURE 1.32. The development of metastasis is a multistep process that is highly inefficient. In order to form a metastasis, the tumor must breach the basement membrane and enter either a blood vessel or a lymphatic, travel through the bloodstream or the lymphatics and not be destroyed either by attack of the immune system or mechanical trauma, adhere to the endothelium at a distant anatomic site, invade the organ parenchyma, draw a blood supply into the metastatic deposit, and colonize the new organ. (From Weinberg RA. *The biology of cancer*. New York: Garland Science, Taylor and Francis Group, 2007. Copyright © 2007 by Garland Science, Taylor & Francis Group, LLC. Used by permission of W. W. Norton & Company, Inc.)

ultimately successful cells must be quite unusual. It would be reasonable to believe that they represent a subpopulation of tumor cells that are endowed with particular characteristics that make for successful metastasis. As the population of tumor cells evolves, it is likely that aggressive subpopulations, having diverse properties, will arise and that their frequency in the population increases under selective pressure of the host immune defenses. This will lead, ultimately, to the emergence of cells with enhanced malignancy.[287] Many people believe that tumor cells evolve via a Darwinian selection. Genetic variation continuously occurs in the tumor population and clones with a survival advantage become overrepresented. These cells have "metastasis virulence genes" enabling their spread. The successful metastatic cells will possess characteristics of neoplastic transformation—the ability to turn on an angiogenic switch, an invasive phenotype, and the capacity to evade the immune response—as well as favorable cell adhesion and motility characteristics.[258,288–290]

Metastatic progress involves not only the tumor's cells but also those cells' ability to recruit the aid of stromal cells. As tumors progress, the stroma becomes increasingly "reactive"—akin to the tissue of wound healing or chronic inflammation.

THE MOLECULAR BIOLOGY OF THE METASTATIC PHENOTYPE AND ANGIOGENESIS

Tumor progression is the acquisition of permanent, irreversible, qualitative changes in one or more characteristics of neoplasm that ultimately will lead to the tumor becoming more autonomous and malignant.[291] A genetic analysis of the stages

of tumor progression has led to the formulation of the multistep theory of tumorigenesis. The multistep theory involves activation of oncogenes, inactivation of tumor suppression genes, and identification of many tumor-associated molecules. The metastatic phenotype appears to require cells to have the additive effect of positive modulators (oncogenes) as well as the loss of negative effectors (tumor suppressor genes, invasion- and metastasis-suppressor genes). Thus, the molecular biology of a metastatic cell is clearly a multistep process of diversification and clonal selection for aggressive cells.

The mutated *ras* oncogene sequences, when transfected into mouse embryo–derived fibroblasts (NIH 3T3 cells), cause those transfected cells to produce numerous metastases. This finding has been confirmed in both fibroblasts and epithelial cells of human and rodent origin. A number of other metastasis-associated genes have been described. These include NM23-1 and stomelysm-3 (ST-3). NM23-1 has features similar to a transcription factor and may play a role not only in *c-myc* expression but also in the response of cells to transforming growth factor-β. ST-3 is a member of the matrix proteinase family.[292]

It would be far too simplistic to conclude that the metastatic phenotype arises only from genetic alterations associated with the acquisition of aggressive tumorigenicity. Cells clearly can be transformed by oncogene transfection, but not all cells acquire a metastatic phenotype after this oncogene transfection. Simply stated, we must bear in mind that there is separation between the genetic changes that drive tumorigenicity and the metastatic phenotype. Invasion and metastasis will require the activation of additional effector genes or loss of suppressor local inhibitors above those genetic changes required for uncontrolled growth alone.

The successful development of a metastatic focus requires new blood vessel growth. There are angiogenesis promoters and inhibitors that may be modified or removed during the tumor-induced angiogenic response. Tumor angiogenesis in the nascent metastasis is a tightly regulated process in a delicate balance between the pro- and antiangiogenic factors.[293]

Angiogenesis

The success of growth of a tumor is, in part, governed by a complex interplay between the tumor cells and the surrounding normal tissue. A dramatic example of this interplay is the process of tumor angiogenesis (also called tumor neovascularization).

The growth of the tumor depends on the tumor's access to nutrients and oxygen as well as its ability to eliminate metabolic waste and carbon dioxide. In very small tumors, these requirements are addressed by diffusion. As the tumor enlarges, however, diffusion is inadequate. The growing tumor requires direct access to the circulatory system.

Tumor access to the circulatory system is secured through angiogenesis, through which the tumor cells encourage the ingrowth of capillaries and larger vessels from the adjacent normal tissue. The tumor cells recruit these vessels through the release of angiogenic factors. These cause the proliferation of endothelial growth factor and, almost certainly, tissue growth factor-β. The generation of tumor vessels is the result of a delicate balance between angiogenesis-promoting factors and angiogenesis-inhibiting factors. These factors have now provided a growing body of therapeutic targets in the treatment of cancer.

Some authorities encourage us to think about the tumor as a structure composed of varied compartments including the actual clonogenic cells, a connective structure, and the blood vessels. Utilizing this way of thinking about tumors, we envision cancer treatment as striking at different components of the tumor (i.e., antiangiogenesis agents directed against the vasculature and anticlonogenic agents directed against proliferating cells). Experimental evidence suggests that, in certain tumor systems, the combination of radiation and antiangiogenic agents is a fruitful way of treating cancer. We may expect to see an increasing body of evidence for the use of combinations of radiation, chemotherapy, hormonal therapy, and antiangiogenesis agents in the coming years.

The hallmark of an invasive cancer is its ability to disrupt the epithelial basement membrane and the presence of cancer cells in the stromal compartment. It makes sense, therefore, that two broad classes of molecules have been implicated repeatedly in contributing to the metastatic ability: Cell–cell adhesion molecules and motility molecules play a crucial role in the development of metastatic potential.[294] The ability of tumor cells to adhere to other tumor cells, cells of the host, or components of the extracellular matrix affects multiple components of the metastatic cascade. These interactions depend on several classes of molecules expressed on the cell surface. Cadherins are calcium-dependent molecules that mediate homophilic cell–cell adherence. Integrins are heterodimeric transmemory proteins that are formed by the noncovalent association of α- and β-subunits. The binding of the extracellular matrix ligands to integrins is known to initiate similar transduction pathways. These pathways lead to cell proliferation, differentiation, migration, or cell death. Selectins act through a terminal calcium-dependent lexon domain. They are prominently involved in heterotypic cell–cell adhesion between blood cells and endothelial cells.[295]

Tumor adherence to the extracellular matrix and cell motility are the next crucial component of the metastatic cascade. Tumor cells are able to attach to a specific lipoprotein of the extracellular matrix such as fibronectin, collagen, and laminin. These adherences are formed either through integrin

---

Box 1.9

Antiangiogenesis Therapy of Cancer

Tumor vessels are fundamentally different from normal blood vessels insofar as they are usually irregular and disorganized. In vessels that are leaky, hemorrhagic, or torturous or in those containing poorly oxygenated blood that may flow backward and forward in the same vessel, tumor vasculature may provide an interesting therapeutic target. The general public and the scientific community have recently experienced a wave of considerable excitement associated with the possibility that antiangiogenesis agents may be employed clinically to disrupt tumor angiogenesis. This form of therapy may complement existing cancer treatments. Vascular endothelial growth factor (VEGF) is a key element in the stimulation of angiogenesis. VEGF binds to a receptor on endothelial cells (VEGFR), which stimulates tyrosine kinase activity, which in turn stimulates downstream signaling and activation of endothelial cells. The drugs in the therapeutic pipeline may be categorized as follows:

- Anti-VEGF agents: Some drugs prevent the binding of VEGF to its receptors. *Bevacizumab (Avastin)* is a monoclonal antibody that binds to VEGF, prevents it binding to VEGFR, and inhibits VEGFR activation. It is being utilized in the therapy of a variety of human malignancies.[262]
- Anti-VEGFR agents: Several receptors bind to VEGF: VEGFR1, VEGFR2, NRP-1, and NRP-2. VEGR2 is thought to mediate most of the angiogenic properties of VEGF and is expressed at high levels on the endothelial cells of tumor vasculature. Several monoclonal antibodies are under investigation in animal models to target the VEGF receptor.
- Receptor tyrosine kinase inhibitors: An antiangiogenesis strategy is to target the downstream activity of the binding of the VEGFR by inhibition of tyrosine kinase activity. The following drugs, now in human clinical trials, fall into this category: cediranib or recentin (AZD2171), pazopanib, BIBF 1120, sorafenib, and sunitinib (SU11248).

---

or nonintegrin cell surface receptors. CD44 is a crucial transmembrane glycoprotein with a large echo domain and a single cytoplasm domain. CD44 is involved in cell adhesion to hyaluronan[291] (Box 1.9).

The potentially metastatic cell must overcome a series of tissue barriers. These include the basement membrane and connective tissue. These must be traversed by the tumor cells during the metastatic process. Five classes of naturally occurring proteinases have been associated with aggressive tumor cells and implicated in metastases. These include members of the gene family of matrix metalloproteinases. These enzymes, each of which is secreted by a proenzyme that subsequently requires activation, may be divided into three general subclasses: interstitial collagenase, type 4 collagenase (gelatinases), and stromelysins. Once having dissolved barriers, active tumor cell motility is required for the penetration of the basement membrane and the interstitial stoma. Successful migration of metastatic cells requires transition of propulsive force from the extracellular matrix to the cytoskeleton. Tumor cells exhibit amoeboid movement, which is characterized by pseudopod extension. For the protrusion and retraction of pseudopods, the network of intracellular polymerized cross-linked filaments must be disassembled and then reassembled.[287]

MANAGEMENT OF THE PATIENT WITH CANCER

The optimal care of cancer patients is a multidisciplinary effort that may combine two or more disciplines: surgery, radiation therapy, and chemotherapy. Many professionals, including physicians, physicists, laboratory scientists, nurses, rehabilitation staff, sociologists, and social workers, are intimately involved. Pathologists, radiologists, clinical laboratory physicians, and immunologists are integral members of the team that renders the correct diagnosis. Biology, biochemistry, and pharmacology have contributed greatly to the advancement of methods used to evaluate and treat cancer patients (e.g., biomarkers, cell kinetic indicators, oncogenes).

The radiation oncologist, like any other physician, must assess all conditions relative to the patient and the tumor under consideration for treatment and systematically review the need for diagnostic and staging procedures as well as the best therapeutic strategy. This has been well illustrated in a series of "decision trees" designed by the Patterns of Care Study Group for radiation therapy.[296] In several instances, a clear relationship existed between compliance with guidelines for diagnostic or therapeutic procedures (best current management consensus) and therapy outcome, as defined by survival, recurrence patterns, or complications of treatment.

Emphasis on screening and early diagnosis of cancer, as well as improvements in therapeutic strategies, has had a significant positive impact on the survival of patients with cancer. In the United States, results of the Surveillance, Epidemiology, and End Results program have shown a small but steady improvement in survival for a variety of tumor sites. Relative survival of patients with cancer at various times after diagnosis has improved substantially since 1960.

Combination of Therapeutic Modalities

Irradiation and Surgery

The rationale for *preoperative radiation therapy* relates to its potential ability to eradicate subclinical or microscopic disease beyond the margins of the surgical resection, to diminish tumor implantation by decreasing the number of viable cells within the operative field, to sterilize lymph node metastases outside the operative field, to decrease the potential for dissemination of clonogenic tumor cells that might produce distant metastases, and to increase the possibility of resectability. The disadvantages of preoperative irradiation are that it may interfere with normal healing of the tissues affected by the radiation, it delays surgery, and it may disrupt surgical staging of the tumor and/or the expression of histologic or immunohistochemical prognostic factors.

The rationale for *postoperative irradiation* is based on the fact that it is possible to eliminate subclinical foci of tumor cells in the tumor bed (including lymph node metastases). By delivering higher doses to the volume of high-risk or known residual disease than can be achieved with preoperative irradiation, a greater tumor control may be obtained.

The potential disadvantages of postoperative irradiation are related to the delay in initiation of radiation therapy until wound healing is completed. Theoretic and experimental evidence suggests that the radiation effect may be impaired by vascular changes produced in the tumor bed by surgery (Fig. 1.33).

Irradiation and Chemotherapy

Tumor or *normal tissue enhancement* describes any increase in effect greater than that observed with either chemotherapy or irradiation alone.[297] Agents used in chemoirradiation include those with cytotoxic activity against the tumor, which may show additive, subadditive, or supra-additive effects, such as 5-fluorouracil or mitomycin C in anal carcinoma; agents with minimal or no significant activity against a specific tumor, which may, however, enhance the irradiation effect; radiation hypoxic cell cytotoxins or bioreductive agents; and radioprotectors.

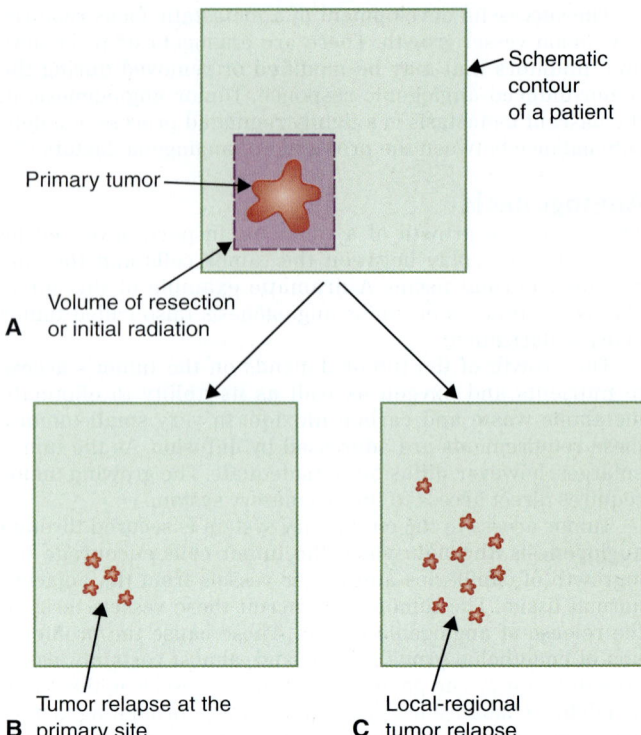

FIGURE 1.33. **A:** A pattern of failure analysis is useful to improve treatment of malignancies. **B:** If the tumor after surgery and/or radiotherapy tends to relapse at the primary site within the volume treated, it would suggest that the local therapy is insufficiently intense. **C:** If, however, there is a locoregional tumor relapse, it would suggest that the initial surgery or radiotherapy field size is insufficient to cover microscopic extension of disease that has the potential to be controlled. A pattern of failure as shown in panel **C** is not, by itself, sufficient to make the case for extended-field radiation. One must have a pattern of failure such as that which is seen in panel **C** and also be able to show that intervention with large field irradiation can alter that pattern in a favorable manner.

Chemotherapy alone or combined with irradiation may be used in several settings.[298] *Primary chemotherapy* is used as part of the primary lesion treatment (even if later followed by other local therapy) and when the primary tumor response to the initial treatment is the key identifier of systemic effects. *Adjuvant chemotherapy* is used as an adjunct to other local modalities as part of the initial curative treatment. The term *neoadjuvant chemotherapy* is used when this modality is used in the initial treatment of patients with localized tumors, before surgery or irradiation.

The effects of combined radiation therapy–chemotherapy can be independent, additive, or interactive. Chemotherapy and irradiation can be administered sequentially or concomitantly. Sequencing of treatment at the appropriate time is significantly related to the residual tumor cell burden at the point of introduction of each new treatment program.

Administration of chemotherapy before irradiation may produce cell killing and reduce the number of cells to be eliminated by the irradiation. Use of chemotherapy concurrently with radiation therapy has a strong rationale because it could interact with the local treatment (additive and even supra-additive action) and also could affect subclinical disease early in treatment. However, the combination of modalities may enhance normal tissue toxicity. When agents with added toxicity are used, lower tumor control may result because the added morbidity requires lowering the doses of the effective agents or prolonging overall irradiation treatment time. When fatal toxicity from chemotherapy occurs, it prevents some dying patients from demonstrating tumor response that could have been observed had they survived. Overall patient survival may be compromised as well.

Biologic Considerations in Combinations of Chemotherapy and Irradiation

Many experimental animal studies have shown therapeutic benefit from a combination of irradiation and drugs, but most are phenomenologic. Therapeutic benefit requires differential properties on tumor and normal tissues, which may be exploited for therapeutic gain. These include genetic instability of tumors compared with normal tissues, differences in cell proliferation (particularly cell repopulation during fractionated radiation therapy), and environmental factors such as hypoxia and acidity (which usually are confined to tumors). There are variations in sensitivity or resistance to irradiation or drugs. The mechanisms for resistance to these agents may be shared in some tumors and different in other tumors. Resistance to anticancer drugs may have implications for resistance to radiation therapy; many drug mechanisms for resistance are multifactorial, such as in cisplatin, in which this phenomenon may be the result of decreased drug uptake, increased repair of DNA, increased expression of sulfhydryl compounds such as glutathione and metallothionein, and increased expression of glutathione-*S*-transferase. Combined treatment with radiation and drugs might result in an improved therapeutic index if mechanisms of resistance are independent.[299]

Oxygen, pH, and nutrient supply can play an important role in the combined effects of chemotherapy and irradiation on tumor cells.[300] Hypoxic cells are less radiosensitive and chemosensitive to many drugs, and chronic hypoxia can alter cell cycle age distribution and proliferation rate—both important modifiers of cellular response to ionizing radiation and drugs. In addition, chronic hypoxia can affect cellular ability to repair radiation- and drug-induced DNA damage. Bioreductive drugs such as mitomycin C are activated to toxic species and affect solid animal tumors under hypoxic conditions. DNA repair, cell cycle age distribution, and the activity and stability of some chemotherapeutic drugs may be pH dependent; thus, this factor plays a role in the sensitivity of cells to irradiation and cytotoxic agents.

Hypoxic conditions, which commonly exist in tumors, may lead to amplification of genes. Under hypoxic conditions, hypoxia-inducible factor 1 (HIF-1) occur, levels rise, and functional HIF-1 transcription factor complexes induce angiogenesis, erythrocytopoiesis, glycolysis, and glucose transport into cells—all techniques to allow the cell to survive hypoxia. HIF-1 induces the genes encoding vascular endothelial growth factor (VEGF), platelet-derived growth factor, and transforming growth factor.[258] Some cytokines such as tumor necrosis factor-α or interleukin[235] and growth factors such as platelet-derived and fibroblast growth factors are seen in malignant and normal human cells after irradiation.[301] These cytokines and growth factors enhance the cytotoxic effects of irradiation and chemotherapy in tumor cells[302] or offer radioprotection in normal cells.[303]

Possible molecular or cellular mechanisms of interaction of chemotherapy and irradiation include:

1. Modification of the slope of the dose–response curves, such as has been shown with actinomycin D, cisplatin, doxorubicin, mitomycin C, 5-fluorouracil, and other agents.
2. Decreased accumulation or inhibition of repair of SLD, as induced by actinomycin D, cisplatin, bleomycin, hydroxyurea, and nitrosoureas.[304–307] Doxorubicin and other DNA intercalators decrease the shoulder widths but do not decrease the slope or suppress the repair of lethal damage in *in vitro* studies.[308]
3. Inhibition of repair of PLD, as has been shown with actinomycin D, doxorubicin, and cisplatin.[107,309]
4. Perturbation of cell kinetics, for example, after treatment with hydroxyurea, which kills cells in the S-phase, when cells may become partially synchronized and blocked at

the G1/S-phase of the cell cycle. If irradiation is delivered during this sensitive phase, as the cells subsequently emerge from the block, an enhanced cytotoxic effect may be expected.
5. Selective cytotoxicity and radiosensitization of hypoxic cells, which have been reported with mitomycin C and cisplatin.[310]
6. Inhibition of cell repopulation.
7. Decrease in tumor bulk leading to improved blood supply, reoxygenation, and cell cycle recruitment, resulting in increased radiosensitivity and chemosensitivity.

A possible danger in the administration of cytotoxic drugs before radiation therapy is accelerated cell proliferation or repopulation. Because some tumor regression is induced by the cytotoxic agent (drugs or irradiation), the distance between the tumor cells, and decreases in adjacent functional capillaries, this may induce tumor cell proliferation so that higher doses of irradiation would be required to produce a given tumor control. This may occur because, during radiation therapy, tumor cells surviving neoadjuvant chemotherapy may be stimulated to repopulate at a faster rate. Because of this effect, the initial advantage in cell killing by drugs is lost, and the survival curves for fractionated radiation therapy may come together or even cross over. Although this mechanism is hypothetical, it suggests caution in the use of induction chemotherapy and explains why an initial tumor response may not necessarily translate to a therapeutic advantage with combined modality treatment given in this fashion. For example, three courses of induction chemotherapy might reduce tumor cell numbers from 10^{10} to 10^8 (from 10 g to about 0.1 g), which is considered a complete clinical tumor regression. Even a pathologic complete response has limited long-term implications; a complete pathologic regression is consistent with the presence of about 10^6 tumor cells per gram, a substantial biologic cell burden (Fig. 1.34).

Integrated Multimodality Cancer Management and Organ Preservation

Combinations of two or all three of the classic modalities frequently are used to improve tumor control and patient survival. Steel and Peckham[311] postulated the biologic basis

FIGURE 1.34. Relationship between clinical remission and cure. A 10-g tumor containing 10^{10} cells is treated with three courses of chemotherapy, each of which kills 90% of the tumor cells present. After three courses, the number of viable tumor cells is <10^8 (<0.1 g) and the patient is judged to be in clinical and radiologic complete remission. Note that this is a small step toward tumor cure. Moreover, additional chemotherapy may not be helpful if drug-resistant cells have been selected after three courses of chemotherapy. (Reprinted from Tannock IF. Combined modality treatment with radiotherapy and chemotherapy. *Radiother Oncol* 1989;16[2]: 83–101. Copyright © 1989 Elsevier Ireland Ltd. With permission.)

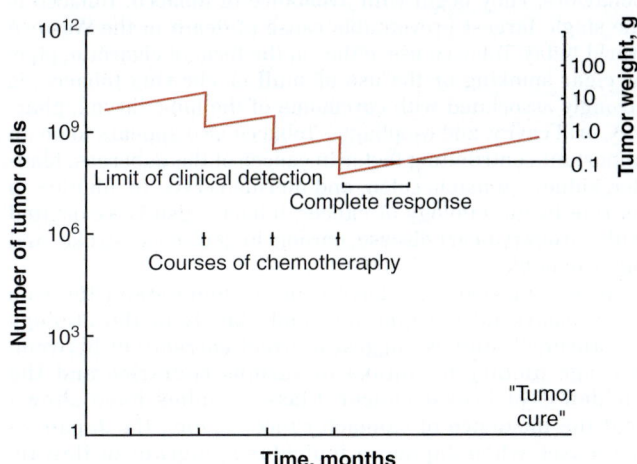

of cancer therapy as spatial cooperation, in which an agent is active against tumor cells spatially missed by another agent, addition of antitumor effects by two or more agents, and nonoverlapping toxicity and protection of normal tissues. Large primary tumors or metastatic lymph nodes must be removed surgically or treated with definitive radiation therapy. Regional microextensions are eliminated effectively by irradiation without the anatomic and at times physiologic deficit produced by equivalent medical surgery. Chemotherapy is applied mainly to control disseminated subclinical disease, although it also has an effect on some larger tumors.

Organ preservation is being vigorously promoted because it enhances the quality of life and psychoemotional feelings of patients with excellent tumor control and survival. In some types and stages of head and neck tumors, breast cancer, gastrointestinal malignancies, genitourinary tumors, soft tissue sarcomas, and pediatric tumors, studies have shown that less radical surgical procedures combined with chemotherapy and radiation therapy yield the same local tumor control at the primary site and survival as did radical procedures. Advances in reconstructive surgery have greatly improved our ability to repair defects of radical surgery.

CANCER PREVENTION

Cancer is a largely preventable disease. Epidemiologic studies have identified the causative agents for a significant proportion of adult cancers. Approximately 30% to 35% of cases of cancer in the United States are associated with tobacco use.[402] Another 30% to 35% of cases are associated with excessive dietary fat and obesity. Approximately 5% of cancer is related to alcohol use. Another 5% is associated with exposure to viral agents.[312] Among the other causative factors of cancer, each responsible for a small percentage of malignancies, are occupational exposures, a family history of cancer, environmental pollution, ionizing and ultraviolet irradiation, prescription drugs, and medical procedures (Table 1.6, Figs. 1.33–1.36).[280]

There are two general approaches to cancer prevention. They are referred to as *primary prevention strategies* and *secondary prevention strategies*. A primary preventive strategy may be invoked when there is an explicit and indisputable behavior that should be avoided or adopted because of its association with a predictable and certain reduction in cancer risk for an individual. A secondary prevention is distinguished from primary prevention in that it is an intervention focused on altering the natural history of a disease and thus avoiding disease-related adverse outcomes.[72] The most commonly used secondary prevention strategy is broad-based or targeted population screening.

The principal primary prevention strategies are directed against cancers that have been associated with certain behaviors. They begin with avoidance of tobacco. Tobacco is the single largest preventable cause of death in the Western world today. Tobacco use, either in the form of cigarette, pipe, or cigar smoking or the use of snuff or chewing tobacco, is strongly associated with carcinoma of the lung, larynx, pharynx, oral cavity, and esophagus. Tobacco also appears to be an important contributing factor in cancer of the pancreas, bladder, kidney, stomach, colon, and uterine cervix. In addition to its role in the etiology of cancer, tobacco also is associated with coronary heart disease, chronic lung disease, stroke, and other maladies.[388]

In recent years, we have come to understand the role of excessive fat consumption and obesity in the etiology of cancer.[387] Studies suggest a direct correlation between average dietary fat intake in various countries and the incidence of breast cancer. Classic studies have shown that the incidence of stomach cancer among the Japanese decreases when Japanese individuals migrate to Hawaii.

Second-generation Japanese residents of Hawaii have an incidence of stomach cancer equivalent to that of the White population.[313] Clearly, a more healthy diet could reduce the incidence of cancer.[297]

Excessive alcohol consumption also is associated with cancer. Alcohol consumption is particularly harmful among cigarette smokers. It appears that smoking acts as an initiator, producing injurious mutations, and alcohol acts as a promoter in cancer of the oral cavity, oropharynx, pharynx, larynx, and esophagus.

A variety of occupational exposures also are associated with specific cancers. These include cancer in asbestos miners and workers, various forms of cancer in workers in the chemical industry, cancers associated with pesticide exposure in agricultural workers, and radiation-associated cancers in uranium miners. An obvious preventive strategy is to minimize or eliminate such harmful exposures in the workplace.

In recent years, scientists have become increasingly aware of various genetic syndromes associated with the etiology of cancer. These include the multiple endocrine neoplasia syndromes and their association with medullary cancer of the thyroid, susceptibility genes that increase the risk of colon cancer, and the association of the BRCA1 and BRCA2 genes with carcinoma of the breast and ovary. For some of these genetic susceptibility traits, the best that the physician can offer is close follow-up. There are certain situations where the avoidance of a potentially lethal cancer may lead an individual to consider prophylactic surgery.

An exciting development in cancer prevention is the development of a vaccine capable of reducing, by about 70%, the incidence of human papillomavirus (HPV)-associated cervical cancer. The U.S. FDA approved this vaccine for clinical use in summer 2006. This vaccine, along with the use of routine Pap testing, has the potential to make invasive cervical cancer an exceedingly rare event.

Cancer screening is the most frequently considered secondary preventive strategy. A cancer screening procedure should lead to the early detection of an asymptomatic or unrecognized disease by the application of simple, inexpensive tests or examinations in a targeted population. For cancer screening to be appropriate and successful, several criteria should be met. These include the following:

1. The cancer for which one is screening should have a substantial morbidity and/or mortality rate that warrants the screening procedure.
2. The cancer for which one is screening should have a sufficiently high prevalence in a detectable, preclinical state to warrant screening.
3. Once the cancer is detected by a screening procedure, there should be an effective treatment related to early detection. This criterion is quite important because there is little value in screening for an untreatable malignancy.
4. The screening test should have a high sensitivity and specificity.
5. The screening test should be of low cost such that the expense of screening a large population would be more than offset by the reduced cost to society of treating early rather than advanced malignancy.
6. Individuals screened should suffer little inconvenience and discomfort.

There is no perfect screening test. Those tests currently used generally meet most, but not all, of the aforementioned criteria.[314,315]

There are several examples of currently used screening tests. For breast cancer, these include self-examination, examination by a trained health practitioner, and mammography, augmented, when appropriate, by ultrasound and MRI. The value of these tests in various populations of women is currently highly disputed. In screening for colorectal cancer, the tools available to the clinician include testing for fecal occult blood, sigmoidoscopy, colonoscopy, and barium enema studies and the developing field of virtual colonoscopy. There is a general consensus that screening for fecal occult blood and, in the appropriate aged population, screening colonoscopy are worthwhile. Among the most controversial areas for cancer screening is the role of screening in the detection of early prostate cancer. There was rapid general acceptance of the use of physical examination and prostate-specific antigen (PSA) testing to ascertain the presence of early prostate cancer. On further consideration, however, many investigators fear that we have, as a society, successfully identified large numbers of men who would never have been diagnosed with symptomatic prostate cancer in their remaining lifetime or required treatment. The appropriate role of screening for prostate cancer has generated as much controversy as the debate over mammography in breast cancer. A considerable amount of anxiety has been generated in asymptomatic men compulsively watching their PSA levels. The US oncology community has engaged in a very public debate over the recommendation of the U.S. Preventive Services Task Force ("USPSTF") to rescind a recommendation in favor of the widespread use of PSA for screening. The task force report in 2012 advised that healthy men should no longer receive the PSA blood test to screen for prostate cancer because the test does not save lives overall and often leads to more tests and treatments that needlessly cause pain, impotence, and incontinence in many.

The draft recommendation was based on the results of five clinical trials and had the potential to substantially change the care given to men aged 50 years and older. There are 44 million such men in the United States, and 33 million of them have already had a PSA test—sometimes without their knowledge—during routine physicals. As further evidence became available, the USPSTF revised its recommendations and, in 2018, recommended that men between 55 and 69 years discuss with the doctor the risks and benefits of PSA screening and make a decision based on personal values and risk factors. The USPTF does not recommend screening for men ≥70 years of age.[316]

It is likely that, in the future, efforts will be expended to identify that subset of men with biologic markers suggesting that they might benefit from PSA screening and, if diagnosed, treatment compared to those who are "best left alone."

Far less controversial, however, has been the use of the Pap test for early detection of carcinoma of the cervix. Where properly used, the test appears to have resulted in a decrease of mortality from this malignancy.

Cancer chemoprevention is defined as a pharmacologic intervention with specific nutrients or other chemicals intended to suppress or reverse carcinogenesis and to prevent the development of invasive cancer. Trials involving chemopreventive therapy require large numbers of individuals who are at high risk for malignancy because of family history, carcinogenic exposure, or the presence of a mutated gene. The ideal chemopreventive agent would have minimal side effects because it would be given to a considerable number of people, none of whom have cancer. Chemoprevention trials differ from other types of cancer prevention studies and from therapeutic studies in important ways. The participants are healthy volunteers, and one seeks to measure a reduction in morbidity and mortality in the long run. Chemoprevention trials are, by definition, large. There are strict enrollment criteria that reflect the group of interest. These studies are often long term and expensive. To date, the best-studied agents in human preventive trials are retinoids (the natural derivatives and synthetic analogs of vitamin A) and one member of the carotenoid class, β-carotene. A number of randomized cancer prevention trials involving carotenoids and retinoids have been completed. Some of these trials have reported chemopreventive effects for various retinoids and for β-carotene,

particularly in oral premalignancy. Other trials have been negative or even have suggested cancer promotional effects by β-carotene.[317]

CLINICAL TRIALS

These studies have been classified as phase I (toxicity), phase II (dose/efficacy), and phase III (efficacy and toxicity of a new drug compared with an established standard). Randomized phase III clinical trials and meta-analyses are the two most accepted sources of scientific information in evidence-based medicine. These randomized clinical studies, with sometimes complicated treatment schemas, large numbers of patients, defined endpoints, and rigorous statistical testing, which are increasingly required by the U.S. FDA to document the efficacy and safety of new drugs (and, I believe should add, should be required for medical devices), are logistically difficult and expensive to conduct. Cooperative clinical trial groups have been a major contributor, along with the participating institutions, investigators, and associated staff, to clinical investigation centered on the application of ionizing radiations, alone or combined with surgery or cytotoxic agents, hormones, and so forth, to improve the management of patients with cancer.

It is the responsibility of practicing radiation oncologists in academic and community centers to be active contributors, with both scientific input and encouragement of their patients to participate in many of these trials.

RADIATION-INDUCED SECOND PRIMARY MALIGNANT TUMORS

Patients cured of cancer have a significant probability of developing other cancers. Many publications document the frequency of second malignant neoplasms, associated with radiation therapy, in cancer survivors.[160] Several principles characterize radiation-induced cancers:

1. A wide variety of histologic types of cancers can be induced by radiation therapy. The current state of knowledge does not allow us to distinguish these tumors, morphologically, from "naturally" occurring cancers. In the future, it may be possible to identify specific genetic changes associated with radiation-induced malignancy. This future technology, termed *molecular forensics*, may, ultimately, affect our understanding of attributable risk of radiation-induced malignancies.[318,319]

2. The dose incidence curve for carcinogenesis generally rises more steeply with high-LET radiation doses than with low-LET doses, especially at low dose rates (Fig. 1.37).[96] In a liver cancer model in mice, neutron irradiation produces a greater incidence of hepatomas than gamma irradiation.[320] Low-LET radiation becomes less effective at carcinogenesis per cGy as the dose falls. High-LET radiation, however, does not.[321]

3. When one compares the frequency of second malignant neoplasms over time, it appears that orthovoltage radiation therapy is more likely to be carcinogenic than megavoltage therapy. This may be a dose-related phenomenon insofar as orthovoltage irradiation gives a higher dose to bone. It is also possible that the longer-term follow-up available for survivors of orthovoltage irradiation may, somewhat artifactually, lead to a higher reported incidence of tumors.[317,322,323]

4. The sensitivity of tissues to radiation-induced malignancies is not uniform. Current evidence indicates that the thyroid gland and the breast are sensitive to cancer induction at relatively low doses of radiation; lymphoid tissue, lung, and liver require moderate doses; and bone requires the highest dose. It also seems likely that the relationship

between dose and response may vary according to the type of induced tumor. One can estimate the cancer risk from radiation either per unit dose measured in Gy or per unit dose equivalent measured in sievert. When one measures in sieverts, a quality factor (Q) is used to take account of the varying biologic effectiveness of the different forms of radiation. For example, for a conventional γ-ray or x-ray, $Q = 1$. For neutron irradiation, $Q = 20$. A review of the available literature indicates that the lifetime cancer mortality risk for a working population of both sexes is 0.008 per Sv for high doses and 0.004 per Sv for low doses.[324] The cancer mortality risk for the general population after whole-body exposure is 0.0001 to 0.0004 per cGy per person.

5. One of the most puzzling aspects of radiation-induced cancer concerns the issue of the relation of low radiation dose to carcinogenesis. Most of the data we have concern relatively high doses. Much of the public debate, however, concerns exposure to relatively low doses. Because we have few exact data regarding low doses, extrapolation is, for the most part, used to predict risk at low doses. This can be a particularly vexing problem in litigation where a plaintiff sues for an alleged radiation-induced malignancy following relatively low-dose exposure to radiation.

6. Any assessment of the radiation dose–response curve for the production of second malignant neoplasms has to take into account the fact that neoplasms also can be induced by agents other than radiation. These include chemotherapy, environmental exposures, and hereditary disposition.

7. Because the risk of radiation-induced carcinogenesis is very small, a large denominator of irradiated patients followed for a long period with thorough follow-up would be necessary to calculate risk with any reliability.

8. Latent periods for the production of radiation-induced tumor vary according to the type of induced tumor. One type of latency is exemplified by the risk of leukemia in survivors of the atomic bomb. This consisted of an early pulse of increased risk followed by a gradual decline to baseline levels. The second pattern of occurrence, more typical of solid tumors, is an increase in the relative risk of second malignant neoplasms over many years that remains constant over time thereafter. It is important to remember, therefore, that the duration of follow-up for any study population is very likely to influence the frequency of tumors seen.

9. Age is a critical factor in determining radiation risk. In children, second cancers would be more likely to occur in tissues undergoing rapid proliferation such as the bone and thyroid tissue.

There are several classically cited episodes of human radiation carcinogenesis. These include:

1. Individuals who are treated with radiation for ankylosing spondylitis suffered from an increase in leukemia. Mortality from colon cancer, which is associated with spondylitis through a common association with ulcerative colitis, was increased in irradiated patients. Mortality for patients with cancers other than leukemia or colon cancer also rose.[325]

2. Diagnostic x-rays of the abdomen and pelvis taken of a pregnant woman to ascertain the size of the pelvic outlet before delivery are associated with an increased risk of malignancy in the offspring.

3. A large number of immigrants entered the State of Israel following its founding in 1948. X-ray epilation was used to treat tinea capitis. There was an increased incidence of brain and nervous system tumors (1.8 excess risk per 10,000 persons per year) in 10,834 children irradiated for tinea capitis compared with the same number of nonirradiated matched controls and 5,392 siblings. There were

12 malignant brain tumors in the irradiated patients versus five and one suspected in nonirradiated people. The average dose received was 4 Gy in 5 consecutive days. Irradiation doses of 1 to 2 Gy significantly increased the risk of neurologic tumors.[12]

4. The United States dropped atomic bombs on Hiroshima and Nagasaki in Japan in August 1945. Radiation-related risks among bomb survivors show that the incidence of leukemia rose. The increased risk appeared 1 to 3 years after the bombing and peaked at 6 to 7 years. In solid tumors, excess tumor risk was manifest only after exposed individuals reached the age at which the cancer was normally prone to develop.

5. Uranium miners suffered an increase of lung cancer as a result of inhalation of radon gas. Workers who painted luminous radium dials on watch faces developed bone sarcomas because of the habit of shaping the paintbrush in the mouth and ingesting bone-seeking radium.[326]

6. In the past, thorotrast was used as a contrast medium in diagnostic radiology. This material is a colloidal suspension of the α-emitter thorium dioxide. The compound was associated with the late development of angiosarcoma.

7. Canadian studies of women with tuberculosis who were fluoroscoped repeatedly for monitoring of an induced pneumothorax demonstrated an increased incidence of breast cancer.

8. The Chernobyl Nuclear Power Plant accident of April 26, 1986, is associated with an increased risk of thyroid cancer in Belarus and Ukraine.

An important review of radiation-induced sarcomas was published by Cahan et al.[327] in 1948. Cahan's criteria, which were used to define a radiation-induced sarcoma, have wide applicability and are used, by some investigators, as the standard for demonstration of any alleged radiation-induced malignancy. The Cahan criteria,[327] modified from his original definition, are:

a. A radiation-induced malignancy must have arisen in an irradiated field.

b. A sufficient latent period, preferably longer than 4 years, must have elapsed between the initial irradiation and the alleged induced malignancy.

c. The treated tumor must have been biopsied. The alleged induced tumor must have been biopsied. The two tumors must be of different histologies.

d. The tissue in which the alleged induced tumor arose must have been normal (i.e., metabolically and genetically normal) prior to radiation exposure.

QUALITY AND SAFETY

Quality and safety are important topics in radiotherapy. The issue of patient safety for radiation therapy and diagnostic imaging has been pulled to the forefront by press reports and associated congressional hearings. A number of misadministrations described in a series of *New York Times* articles triggered increased interest in improved patient safety in radiation oncology.[255,328] These articles have highlighted some of the risks inherent to advanced radiation therapy treatment planning and delivery systems and techniques. Many new patient safety initiatives, meetings, and other efforts have been organized to address the need to continue to enhance the safety of patients undergoing radiation therapy.

Safety and quality are different but related concepts. Safety generally relates to preventing errors that can have major therapeutic implications (e.g., treatment of the wrong patient, treatment with the wrong plan, incorrect placement of a block or wedge, failure to correctly transfer electronic data between the various computer systems). In contrast, quality often relates more to somewhat subjective issues such as ensuring that the defined volumes, doses, beams, and so forth are clinically appropriate and that the treatment is delivered as prescribed within acceptable clinical tolerance limits. To reconcile these concepts, in 2011, ASTRO sponsored the Intersociety Council to review and update previously published guidelines concerning the role of radiation oncology in integrated cancer management. In this updated document, entitled "Safety Is No Accident," every facet of patient evaluation, treatment planning, and treatment delivery was described with the specific goal of maximizing patient safety.[329] The process of care, the roles and responsibilities of staff, staff training and maintenance of competency, requirements for facilities and equipment, and the management of quality assurance (QA) were formally recognized as inextricably linked to the provision of safe, efficient, and effective radiation therapy. These ASTRO initiatives have involved cooperation with other organizations, including the American Association of Physicists in Medicine (AAPM), the American Brachytherapy Society, the American College of Radiology (ACR), the American College of Radiation Oncology, the American Board of Radiology, the American Society of Radiation Technologists, and the Society of Radiation Oncology Administrators.

Modern radiation therapy is complex and rapidly evolving. The safe delivery of radiation therapy requires the concerted and coordinated efforts of many individuals with varied responsibilities. Thus, all team members need to work together to create a *safe*, *high-quality*, and *efficient* clinical environment and workflow.

THE PROCESS OF CARE IN RADIATION ONCOLOGY

The "process of care" in radiation oncology refers to a conceptual framework for ensuring the appropriateness, quality, and safety of all patients treated with radiation for therapy. Each of the aspects of the process of care in radiation oncology requires knowledge and training in the natural history of cancer and certain benign diseases, radiobiology, medical physics, and radiation safety that can only be achieved by board certification in radiation oncology (or equivalent training) to synthesize and integrate the necessary knowledge base to safely and completely deliver care. This high level of training and board certification apply as a recommendation for all of the specialists on the radiation oncology team. The medical therapeutic application of ionizing radiation is irreversible, may cause significant morbidity, and is potentially lethal. Use of ionizing radiation in medical treatment, therefore, requires direct or personal physician management, as the leader of the clinical team, as well as input from various other essential coworkers.

The radiation oncology process of care can be separated into five categories:

- Patient evaluation
- Preparing for treatment
- Therapeutic simulation
- Treatment planning
- Pretreatment QA and plan verification
- Radiation treatment delivery
- Radiation treatment management
- Follow-up care management

A course of radiation therapy is composed of a series of distinct activities of varying complexity and is a function of the individual patient situation. All components of care involve intense cognitive medical evaluation, interpretation, management, and decision-making by the radiation oncologist and other members of the clinical team. Each time a procedure

is approved and reported, its level of effort/complexity should be appropriately documented in the patient record.

The clinical team, led by the radiation oncologist, provides the medical services associated with the process of care. Other team members involved in the patient's planning and treatment regimen include the medical physicist, dosimetrist, radiation therapist, and nursing staff. Many of the procedures within each phase of care will be carried to completion before the patient's care is taken to the next phase. Others will occur and recur during the course of treatment, and they are by necessity repeated during treatment because of patient tolerance, changes in tumor size, need for boost fields or port size changes, or protection of normal tissue, or as required by other clinical circumstances (i.e., certain procedures may need to occur multiple times during the treatment course). Each phase of care involves medical evaluation, interpretation, management, and decision-making by the radiation oncologist as well as other team members.

Patient Evaluation

Patient evaluation is a service provided by a physician at the request of another physician, the patient, or an appropriate source to either recommend care for a specific condition or problem or to determine whether to accept responsibility for ongoing management of the patient's entire care or for the care of a specific condition or problem. The physician as part of this process will review the pertinent radiologic and pathologic studies, the patient's complaints, and physical findings. This initial visit can also be used for patient counseling, coordinating care, and making recommendations about other aspects of oncologic management or staging.

Preparing for Treatment

The selection of a comfortable and appropriate patient position for treatment is an important part of the simulation processes. The selected position should consider the location of the target and anticipated orientation of the treatment beams. Appropriate immobilization devices provide comfort, support, and reproducibility. Immobilization of the patient in a comfortable position for treatment might involve the construction or selection of certain treatment devices for helping the patient remain in position during treatment. This step must consider the potential treatment planning considerations so that the treatment aids do not restrict the treatment techniques.

Simulation is the process of determining critical information about the patient's geometry, to permit safe and reproducible treatments on a megavoltage machine. Simulation for external beam radiation treatment is always image based. Simulation procedures have shifted away from the direct use of the treatment beam to using diagnostic x-rays, CT, or MRI. In general, this part of the overall process of care determines the relationship between the position of the target or targets and the surrounding critical structures. When a simulator of conventional design is used that mimics the geometry of the treatment unit or when direct simulation is performed on the treatment machine, this relationship is often determined indirectly through observation of skeletal anatomy that can act as a surrogate for the target position. Conventional simulators, like the CT simulator, can include the ability to produce volumetric data in addition to 2D images.

The preparation for external beam treatment can also depend on other imaging modalities that are directly or indirectly introduced in the simulation process. MRI, ultrasound, and/or PET is now available, and treatment planning systems that include image registration capabilities allow combining of information from other imaging modalities with the standard CT dataset obtained during simulation in appropriate situations. It is now possible to produce image datasets that quantify the motion of structures and targets because of respiration, cardiac motion, and physiologic changes in the body.

For most brachytherapy, treatment preparation is similar to the procedure described earlier for EBRT. The simulation process is also image based. Multiple imaging modalities may be important for some brachytherapy procedures, and these studies can be obtained as part of the preplanning imaging process. For clinical situations where therapy is delivered by unencapsulated radionuclides, a separate and distinct treatment planning process is necessary because of its multidisciplinary execution.[330]

Clinical treatment planning is a comprehensive, cognitive team effort performed under the direction of the radiation oncologist for each patient undergoing radiation treatment. The radiation oncologist is responsible for understanding the natural history of the patient's disease, knowing the extent of the disease relative to the adjacent normal anatomic structure, and integrating the patient's overall medical condition and associated comorbidities. A detailed understanding of the integration of chemotherapeutic and surgical treatment modalities with radiation therapy is also essential.

The skills of the trained and appropriately credentialed dosimetrist relate to the efficient and effective use of the complex treatment planning system hardware and software. This individual must also understand the clinical aspects of radiation oncology in order to interact with the radiation oncologist during the planning process. The role of the medical physicist is to guarantee proper functioning of the hardware and software used for the planning process, consult with the radiation oncologist and dosimetrist, check the accuracy of the selected treatment plan, and perform measurements and other checks aimed at ensuring accurate delivery of the plan.

For either EBRT or brachytherapy, treatment planning starts with a complete, formally documented, and approved directive. Details including total dose to all targets and OARs, fractionation, treatment modality, energy, time constraints, normal tissue constraints, and all other aspects of the radiation prescription in a written or electronic format must be provided by the radiation oncologist prior to the start of treatment planning. In some cases, this prescription can require modification based on the results of the treatment planning process.

Clinical treatment planning for either EBRT or brachytherapy is an important step in preparing for radiation oncology treatment. This planning includes the following components: determining the disease-bearing areas based on the imaging studies and pathology information, identifying the type (brachytherapy, photon beam, electric particle beam, other) and method of radiation treatment delivery, specifying areas to be treated, and specifying the dose and dose fractionation. In developing the clinical treatment plan, the radiation oncologist may use information obtained from the patient's clinical evaluation as well as any additional tests, studies, and procedures that are necessary to complete treatment planning. Studies ordered as part of clinical treatment planning may or may not be associated with studies necessary for staging the cancer and may be needed to obtain specific information to accomplish the clinical treatment plan. Review of imaging studies and laboratory tests must be performed to determine treatment volume and critical structures in close proximity to the treatment area.

At various steps in the treatment planning process, the radiation oncologist is presented with one or more treatment plans for review and selection. This process is often iterative and requires additional treatment planning. The radiation oncologist is responsible for selecting and formally approving the plan to be used for treatment.

The QA steps taken after completion of treatment planning and before the start of treatment are critical for guaranteeing patient safety. In the past, treatment verification consisted of field aperture imaging using radiographic film. These images are referred to as portal images or port films. With the introduction of IMRT, imaging of individual apertures is no longer practical. However, the traditional method of verifying the plan isocenter position using orthogonal imaging is often used for both 3DCRT and IMRT. For IMRT, this important QA technique is not considered to be sufficient to guarantee patient safety. In addition to this isocenter check procedure, for IMRT and other complex delivery techniques that use inverse treatment planning, patient-specific QA measurements are also required. In terms of clearly organizing the different steps in the process of care for radiation oncology, a blurring of the separation between the verification and treatment delivery occurs on the first day of treatment and whenever the treatment plan is changed.

Radiation Treatment Delivery

The physician is responsible for verification and documentation of the accuracy of treatment delivery as related to the initial treatment planning and set-up procedure. Image guidance (IGRT) may be performed to ensure accurate targeting of precise radiation beams. IGRT requires a target that is expected to move from day to day and can be reliably identified by the selected imaging modality. The physician is responsible for the supervision and review of these images and prescribing necessary positional shifts to ensure the therapy delivered conforms to the originally planned dosimetric constraints. Similarly, management of organ motion during treatment delivery is the responsibility of the treating physician.

Radiation Treatment Management

Radiation treatment management encompasses the radiation oncologist's overall management of the course of treatment and care for the patient as well as checks and approvals provided by other members of the radiation therapy team that are necessary at various points in the process. For the radiation oncologist, radiation treatment management requires and includes a minimum of one examination per week of the patient for medical evaluation and management. The professional services furnished during treatment management typically include:

- Review of portal images in a format appropriate to the technique of radiotherapy delivery
- Review of dosimetry, dose delivery, and treatment parameters
- Review of patient treatment setup
- Patient evaluation visit

Not all of these elements of treatment management are required for all patients for each week of management (except for the patient evaluation visit) because the clinical course of care may differ due to variation in treatment modality and individual patient requirements. Examinations and evaluations may be required more often than once weekly.

Follow-Up Care

Continued follow-up care of patients who have completed radiation therapy is necessary to manage acute and chronic morbidity resulting from treatment as well as to monitor the patient for tumor recurrence.

THE RADIATION ONCOLOGY TEAM

The radiation oncology team ensures every patient undergoing radiation treatment receives the appropriate level of medical, emotional, and psychological care before, during, and after treatment, through a collaborative multidisciplinary approach.

The radiation oncology team consists of but is not limited to radiation oncologists, physicists, dosimetrists, oncology nurses, and radiation therapists. The process of care in radiation oncology involves close collaboration of a team of qualified professionals. On-site or by consultation services can be provided by nonphysician providers, including nurse practitioners, clinical nurse specialists, advanced practice nurses and physician assistants, dentists, clinical social workers, psychologists/psychiatrists, nutritionists, speech pathologists, physical therapists, occupational therapists, genetic counselors, integrative medicine specialists, and pastoral care providers.

Board certification is the primary consideration for establishing proper qualifications and training for any professional working in radiation oncology. The relevant professional societies will establish the eligibility requirements to sit for a board exam. This may include education and training requirements such as a clinical residency. In addition, in some jurisdictions, professionals must meet additional requirements for obtaining appropriate licensure.

The applications, technologies, and methods of radiation oncology continue to expand and develop. Lifelong learning is vital to ensure incorporation of new knowledge into clinical practice. Therefore, each member of the interdisciplinary radiation oncology team should participate in available Continuing Education (CE) and Maintenance of Certification (MOC) programs. Each facility should have a policy regarding orientation, competency, credentialing, and periodic competency evaluations of all team members.

Staffing Requirements

Starting in 1986, the Intersociety Council for Radiation Oncology published a set of guidelines in a small pamphlet titled "Radiation Oncology in Integrated Cancer Management," often referred to as the "Blue Book."[331] This subsequently has been updated several times sought to improve it.[332] The document offers guidelines for staffing requirements and equipment utilization. The staffing needs of each facility are unique based on the patient mix and complexity of the services offered. The patient load, number of machines, and satellite clinics and affiliated treatment centers will influence the demand on management and clinical staff (Figs. 1.35 and 1.36). The minimum personnel requirements for a radiation oncology facility specify the need for one medical director (radiation oncologist), chief medical physicist, and department manager per program.[329]

FIGURE 1.35. Dose–response curves for incidence of tumors in relation to dose and dose rate of high–linear energy transfer (LET) and low-LET irradiation. (From Upton AC. Biological aspects of radiation carcinogenesis. In: Boice JD, Fraumeni JF, eds. *Radiation carcinogenesis: epidemiology and biological significance.* New York: Raven Press, 1984:9. With permission.)

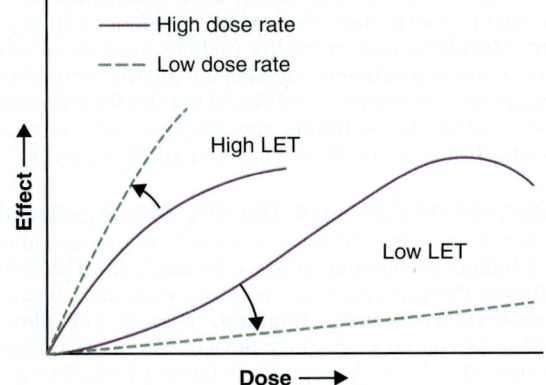

MANAGEMENT AND QUALITY ASSURANCE IN RADIATION ONCOLOGY

Quality assurance in radiation oncology is a set of processes and procedures designed to improve the practice of radiation therapy by confirming that radiation therapy will be or was administered appropriately and safely and documented properly. The overall goal of a QA process is the delivery of high-quality radiation oncology treatment to all patients.[272] Note that QA is an all-encompassing term that is often used to describe some or all of the different elements involved in quality management (QM) and a culture of safety. Cost and value are important in determining the quality of care.[268] To prove that technology adds value to patients, patients' reported outcome should be included.

A radiation oncology facility must satisfy numerous requirements[329]:

- A department must provide adequate clinic space, exam rooms and equipment, patient waiting and changing space, convenient patient parking, treatment rooms, simulation and imaging space, brachytherapy source preparation and storage space, dosimetry/treatment planning rooms, office space for professional staff, and medical physics laboratory and equipment storage space. The extent of facilities should be appropriate for the volume of patients seen and treated (Fig. 1.36).

FIGURE 1.36. The theoretical relation between the cost per patient and rate of use of a linear accelerator for cancer therapy. As the rate of use of a linear accelerator increases, the average cost (AC) of treatment per patient declines until all economies of scale have been achieved (*point B*). The average cost of a radiotherapy treatment will fall as long as any additional patients can be treated at a marginal cost (MC) lower than the AC. It is important to remember that point B represents only the minimized cost of operating the linear accelerator. If you add in costs such as the travel time for a patient to go a considerable distance to reach the linear accelerator, the lost time from work for the patient and anyone traveling with him or her, child care costs, and stress, then the total societal expenditure for a linear accelerator will not be minimized at point B. It will, instead, be reached at point A. We are, however, quite poor at accounting for costs such as travel, loss of work time, and stress, so it is difficult to determine point B and, in turn, the need for a new linear accelerator. If you wish to persuade a government regulatory agency to grant a certificate of need for a piece of radiotherapy equipment at a moderate distance from an existing facility, then you will have an economic incentive to inflate the importance of travel and inconvenience. In the United States, this behavior is increasing as institutions try to justify the need for linear accelerators, radiosurgery, and proton therapy units. The corporations that manufacture and market these units have a vested interest in contributing to this exaggeration of need. (Modified from Suit HD, Urie M. Proton beams in radiation therapy. *J Natl Cancer Inst* 1992;84[3]: 155–164. Reproduced by permission of Oxford University Press.)

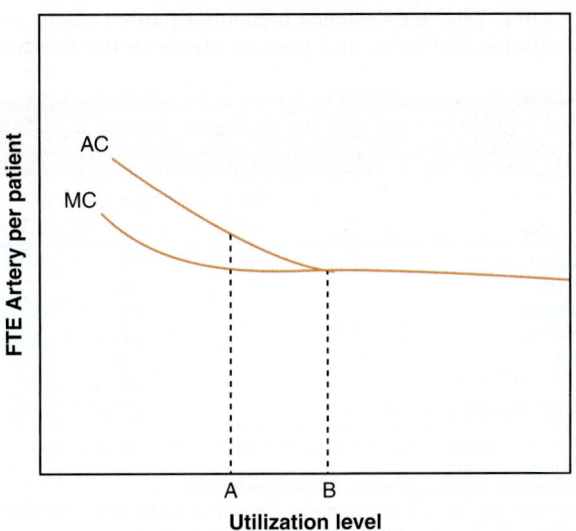

TABLE 1.8 ESTIMATED NEW CANCER CASES AND DEATHS, UNITED STATES, 2017

	Estimated New Cases	Estimated Deaths
All sites	1,688,780	600,920
Oral cavity and pharynx	49,670	9,700
Digestive system	310,440	157,700
Respiratory system	243,170	160,420
Bones and Joints	3,260	1,550
Soft tissue (including the heart)	12,390	4,990
Skin (excluding	95,360	13,590
Breast	255,180	41,070
Genital System	279,800	59,100
Urinary system	146,650	32,190
Eye and orbit	3,130	330
Brain and other nervous system	23,800	16,700
Endocrine system	59,250	3,010
Lymphoma	80,500	21,210
Myeloma	30,280	12,590
Leukemia	62,130	24,500
Other and unspecified primary sites	33,770	42,270

From Siegel RL, Muiller KD, Jemal A. Cancer Statistics, 2017. CA Cancer J Clin 2017;67(1):7–30. Copyright © 2017 American Cancer Society. Reprinted by permission of John Wiley & Sons, Inc.

- Treatment rooms must be carefully designed for radiation shielding, environmental conditions, adequate storage space for spare parts, testing and dosimetry equipment, and patient access and safety (Tables 1.8 and 1.9).
- There must be access to CT, MRI, and PET imaging for treatment planning.
- Rooms used for brachytherapy procedures require special attention to the specific radiation protection requirements associated with the particular brachytherapy modalities to be used. If the brachytherapy procedure load warrants it, a brachytherapy suite should be available, including patient waiting space, procedure rooms, recovery rooms, and brachytherapy source preparation and storage areas.
- Each department must have electronic access to the hospital or clinic information system for medical records and picture archiving and communication.

The following specific capabilities and methods for various aspects of the radiotherapy process are considered essential[329,333]:

- Calibration of treatment machines, CT and MRI scanners, treatment planning systems, and brachytherapy sources is to be carefully accomplished according to the appropriate protocols described by scientific/professional organizations.
- A safety program designed to monitor patient safety, avoid radiation incidents, and prevent errors in the treatment

process should be in place and subject to periodic review and update.
- A system for documenting radiotherapy treatment and other aspects of the patient's medical care should be rigorous and be subject to periodic review and update.
- High-quality and comprehensive treatment planning, using 3D computerized treatment planning for dose calculations, imaging, and other aspects of the planning process.
- A comprehensive QM program, including QA, quality control (QC), and other quality improvement tools.
- Radiation monitoring of simulators and treatment machines. A system to carefully control and monitor all radioactive sources in accordance with the requirements of regulatory agencies.
- A program for maintenance and repair of equipment.
- Staff training that is comprehensive, ongoing, and well documented.
- A well-developed process for continuous peer review. This should include a mechanism for peer review of the entire department and its procedures as well as for individual clinical care decisions.
- Access to medical oncology, surgical oncology, and other physician and nonphysician specialists involved in the multidisciplinary care and follow-up of the patient.
- Each department must implement careful and well-described policies and procedures for every aspect of patient care, for QA of the patient care process, for staff behavior, and for any issues that may impact the safety of patients and/or staff. Each specific treatment modality (e.g., IMRT, IGRT, stereotactic body radiation therapy [SBRT], etc.) should have detailed documentation of its treatment planning and delivery process including a description of the roles and responsibilities of each team member in that procedure, QA checklists, and a plan for continuous quality improvement and safety.

One of the most crucial activities in a quality radiation oncology department is the organized review and monitoring of all aspects of safety, errors, and outcome. Creating a "culture of safety" depends on guidance, direction, and financial support from the leadership of the institution and of the radiotherapy department, on individual effort by every member of the department, and on organized support for quality and safety at every level in the institution.

Each department should have a department-wide review committee that monitors specific quality metrics including near misses and errors in treatment, diagnosis, patient care, or other procedural problems that might lead to errors. This committee should organize the collection and analysis of such events, work to identify potential problems in devices or processes, and then try to mitigate these problems by modifying processes or adding new checks or actions to minimize the likelihood of further problems. Radiation oncology departments should hold regularly scheduled rounds to review patient morbidity and mortality, dose discrepancies, and any incident reports that involved an accident or injury to a patient. Morbidity and mortality include unusual or severe complications of treatment, unexpected deaths, or unplanned interruptions of treatment. Staff included should represent all the team members, including radiation oncologists, nurses, physicists, dosimetrists, therapists, and administrators.

Equipment and Device Quality Management
Radiation therapy is employed for treatment in a broad spectrum of human malignancy (Figs. 1.37 and 1.38). The delivery of radiation therapy relies on computer-controlled treatment machines, interconnected imaging, delivery and planning systems, and complex ancillary devices. Any new radiotherapy system should go through the following processes as it is prepared for clinical use:[330,334–336]

TABLE 1.9 STAFFING LEVELS FOR RADIATION ONCOLOGIST, MEDICAL PHYSICIST, DOSIMETRIST, AND RADIATION THERAPY TECHNOLOGIST

Clinical FTE[a]	Approximate Maximum # of Patients Treated per FTE per Year
Radiation oncologist	250
Physicist	250
Dosimetrist	250
Therapist	90
Nurse	250
Treatment machine	300[b]
Therapists/treatment machine	3.5[c]

[a]It is recommended that a minimum of two qualified individuals be present for any external beam patient treatment.
[b]Each treatment machine is assumed to be operational for 9 hours a day.
[c]The number of therapists per treatment machine is the ratio of the total number of therapists and the number of treatment delivery machines, not including the simulator.
FTE, full-time equivalent.

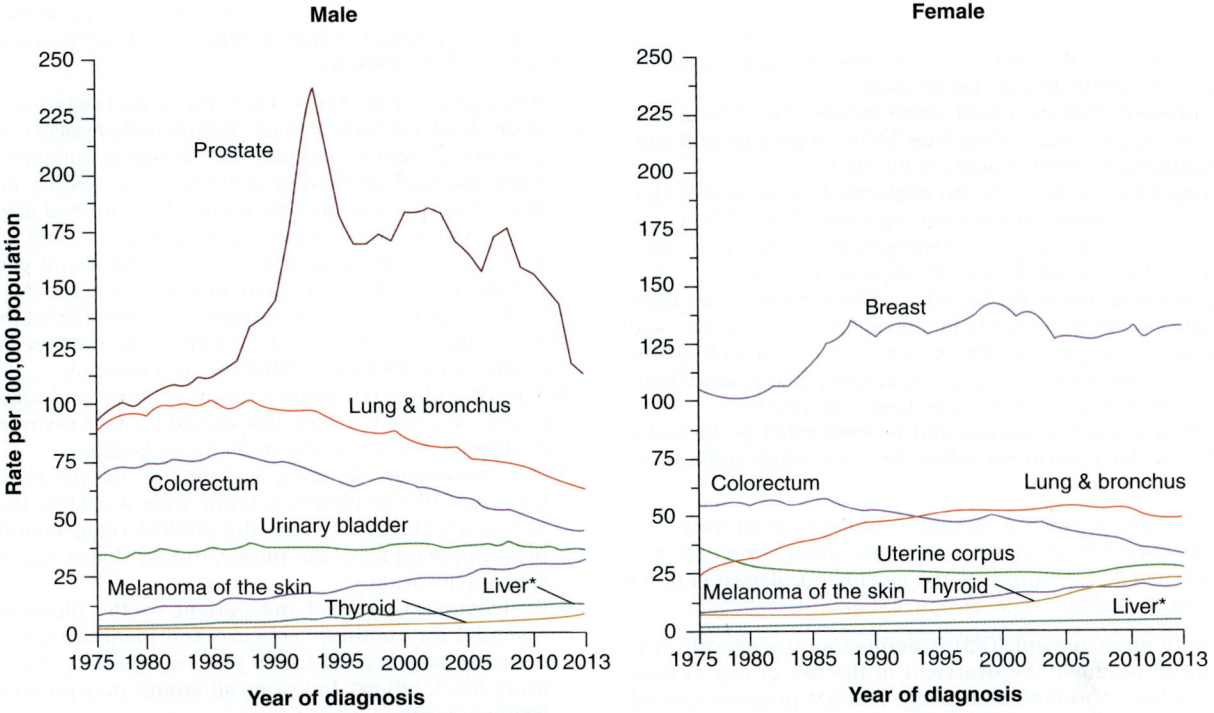

FIGURE 1.37. Trends in incidence rates for selected cancers by sex, United States, 1975–2013. Rates are age adjusted to the 2000 US standard population and adjusted for delays in reporting. (From Siegel RL, Miller KD, Jemal A. Cancer Statistics, 2017. *CA Cancer J Clin* 2017;67[1]:7–30. Copyright © 2017 American Cancer Society. Reprinted by permission of John Wiley & Sons, Inc.)

FIGURE 1.38. Ten leading cancer types for the estimated new cancer cases and deaths by sex, United States, 2017. Estimates are rounded to the nearest 10 and cases exclude basal cell and squamous cell skin cancers and *in situ* carcinoma except urinary bladder. (From Siegel RL, Miller KD, Jemal A. Cancer Statistics, 2017. *CA Cancer J Clin* 2017;67[1]:7–30. Copyright © 2017 American Cancer Society. Reprinted by permission of John Wiley & Sons, Inc.)

Estimated New Cases

Males			Females		
Prostate	161,360	19%	Breast	252,710	30%
Lung & bronchus	116,990	14%	Lung & bronchus	105,510	12%
Colon & rectum	71,420	9%	Colon & rectum	64,010	8%
Urinary bladder	60490	7%	Uterine corpus	61,380	7%
Melanoma of the skin	52,170	6%	Thyroid	42,470	5%
Kidney & renal pelvis	40,610	5%	Melanoma of the skin	34,940	4%
Non-Hodgkin lymphoma	40,080	5%	Non-Hodgkin lymphoma	32,160	4%
Leukemia	36,290	4%	Leukemia	25,840	3%
Oral cavity & pharynx	35,720	4%	Pancreas	25,700	3%
Liver & intrahepatic bile duct	29,200	3%	Kidney & renal pelvis	23,380	3%
All Sites	**836,150**	**100%**	**All Sites**	**852,630**	**100%**

Estimated Deaths

Males			Females		
Lung & bronchus	84,590	27%	Lung & bronchus	71,280	25%
Colon & rectum	27,150	9%	Breast	40,610	14%
Prostate	26,730	8%	Colon & rectum	23,110	8%
Pancreas	22,300	7%	Pancreas	20,790	7%
Liver & intrahepatic bile duct	19,610	6%	Ovary	14,080	5%
Leukemia	14,300	4%	Uterine corpus	10,920	4%
Esophagus	12,720	4%	Leukemia	10,200	4%
Urinary bladder	12,240	4%	Liver & intrahepatic bile duct	9,310	3%
Non-Hodgkin lymphoma	11,450	4%	Non-Hodgkin lymphoma	8,690	3%
Brain & other nervous system	9,620	3%	Brain & other nervous system	7,080	3%
All Sites	**318,420**	**100%**	**All Sites**	**282,500**	**100%**

- Each system should be carefully specified before acquisition, purchase, or development, including design, expectations, capabilities, tolerances, hazards, necessary training, usability, and technical specifications.
- To prevent data communication errors and clinical efficiency issues, each system must be interoperable and connectable with other systems in the clinic.
- Acceptance testing must be performed to document that the new system satisfies the specifications. Often, the acceptance criteria and/or testing methods should be documented as part of the specification for the system.
- Clinical commissioning includes all the activities that must be performed to understand, document, characterize, and prove that a given system is ready to be used clinically. Standard operating procedures, training, and hazard analysis should be part of the commissioning process.
- Each new system, device, and process must be formally released for clinical use after clinical commissioning has been completed.

Clinical use of a device, system, or process must involve the creation and application of a safety- and quality-oriented program designed to ensure that the machine or device is functioning in accordance with accepted standards[330,334-336]:

- Quality management (QM) is defined as the overall program to organize the oversight of the use of any system or process in radiation oncology. The QM program should include hazard analysis, QC, QA, training and documentation, and ongoing quality improvement efforts.
- Hazard analysis is the active evaluation of the potential for failures that will cause incorrect results or harm to the patient and should be performed for any new system.
- QC checks on the data that are input into a decision or process and is designed to prevent the propagation of error.
- QA is the typical shorthand term for the entire QM program and addresses quality checks that confirm that a given process is reasonable and generates appropriate results. QA checks, along with QC, are essential parts of the QM process for most devices and systems, as they can check the output of potentially very complicated decisions or actions performed by the system.
- Training of staff in goals, methods, results, operation, and evaluation of the quality of the output is important for the proper use of any system.

Patient-Related Quality Management

Within the complex and many-step process with which radiotherapy patients are treated, patient-specific issues must be carefully and comprehensively analyzed, documented, and verified. Each radiation oncology facility, regardless of its location or size, must appropriately manage and adhere to high-quality standards of practice for general medical issues,[337] including:

- Drug allergies
- Medication reconciliation
- Do-not-resuscitate codes
- Cleanliness and efforts to reduce infection
- Patient confidentiality and security of protected health information

Modern oncology patient care very often involves multiple modalities and requires the review and discussion of experts in various oncology-related disciplines. It is critical that the management of most cancer be addressed by the appropriate mix of disciplines. Regular presentation of these cases to a multidisciplinary tumor board is the standard of care and should be performed for most cancer cases to determine the appropriate combination (and coordination) of therapies for each individual case.

The details of the patient care process in radiation oncology vary from institution to institution. However, maintenance of the safety and quality of the radiotherapy process for most patients requires that a number of procedures be performed.[329] These include:

- A new patient conference that consists of a brief presentation of the details of each patient's history and physical examination, disease status, and plan for therapy to the other physicians and staff involved in patient care is used as an initial peer review for the basic treatment decisions and plan.
- The physician must obtain a clear, accurate, and detailed description of the patient's chief complaint and pertinent history in conjunction with an appropriate physical examination as part of the decision process for radiation therapy.
- Many patients who receive radiation therapy should receive a CT, PET/CT, or MRI-based simulation.
- After the physician defines target volumes and other normal tissues (contouring), this should be peer reviewed and confirmed before treatment planning begins.
- After treatment planning is complete, the physician and members of the planning team should review the plan and verify that it satisfies the clinical requirements and prescription(s) from the physician and that it can be carried out accurately.
- On-treatment visits of the patient by the physician are essential for continuity of care and monitoring of tumor response and normal tissue toxicity. Typically, this occurs every five fractions, but some situations may require more frequent visits.
- Patient chart rounds are an important peer review procedure used involving weekly review of all patients under treatment by the radiotherapy team, including physicians, therapists, nurses, dosimetrists, and physicists.
- Follow-up visits are a critical component of care for the radiotherapy patient. The frequency of follow-up visits will vary in accordance with the type of cancer, stage, degree of tumor response, normal tissue reactions, and other factors.
- Documentation is required of all the relevant details of patient care. Maintenance and continuous improvement of the quality and accessibility of the treatment record are essential.

The overall performance status of the patient prior to treatment should be recorded. Assessment of tumor response and normal tissue toxicity should occur both during and after treatment. Clinical assessment of patient response is a valuable independent check on the success of the overall QM system as unexpected outcomes may identify issues related to technique or equipment performance.

External Beam Quality Assurance

Nearly all external beam treatment requires the following steps, each of which must be carefully confirmed as part of the patient-specific QA process: determination of patient set-up position and immobilization; cross-sectional imaging (CT, PET/CT, or MRI simulation); creation of the anatomic model (contouring); specification of the treatment intent; creation of the planning directive and treatment prescription by the physician; computerized treatment planning and dose calculation; monitor unit calculation and/or IMRT leaf sequencing; plan and (electronic chart) preparation; plan evaluation; download to treatment management system (TMS); patient-specific QA as typically performed for IMRT, stereotactic radiosurgery (SRS), or SBRT; patient setup and delivery; plan verification checks; plan adaptation and modifications; chart checks; and more.[335,336,338,339]

Brachytherapy Quality Assurance

The QA process for brachytherapy is similar to that of external beam and involves several components that must be confirmed as part of the patient-specific QA management: treatment planning; treatment delivery systems; applicator commissioning and periodic checks; cross-sectional imaging (CT simulation); specification of the treatment intent, planning directive, and treatment prescription by the physician; plan preparation; plan evaluation; download to TMS; plan verification checks; plan modifications; and chart checks.[339-345]

LEGAL PRINCIPLES CONCERNING MALPRACTICE IN RADIATION ONCOLOGY

A plaintiff initiates a radiation oncology malpractice lawsuit by filing papers with the court claiming that he or she was harmed by the radiation oncologist and is entitled to legal redress. The claim of malpractice must be set out in the plaintiff's *prima facie* case. This will include a statement of the facts and legal theories that establish that the plaintiff believes he or she is legally entitled to enforceable claims against the physician.

There are four essential elements to a *prima facie* case of medical malpractice. They are the establishment of duty, breach, causation, and damages. To demonstrate medical malpractice, a plaintiff–patient must show that the radiation oncologist had a duty to provide nonnegligent care to the patient, that the provider breached that duty by providing negligent care, and that this breech caused the patient injury or damage.[261,295]

To establish a *duty*, the plaintiff must have facts that demonstrate a legal relationship between the radiation oncologist and the patient. It is a basic rule of Anglo American law that there is no duty to another person unless there is a legally recognized relationship with that person. The plaintiff–patient must demonstrate the existence of a physician–patient relationship.[346]

To establish a *breach*, the patient–plaintiff must demonstrate facts that illustrate the radiation oncologist breached the legal duties implied in the physician–patient relationship or duties that would be generally imposed on members of society. The plaintiff must establish that the appropriate standard of care was violated. Although, in theory, the establishment of the standard of care and the breach of that standard are legally separate, in reality, unless there is a factual question about what the radiation oncologist actually did, the proof of the standard of care also would demonstrate the defendant's breach. Most commonly, in law, the definition of *standard of care* is how similarly qualified radiation oncologists would have managed the patient's care under the same or similar circumstances. In most medical malpractice cases, both the standard of care and the breach are established through the testimony of expert witnesses.[347]

Negligence is defined as "the omission to do something which a reasonable man guided by those ordinary considerations which ordinarily regulate human affairs would do, or the doing of something which a reasonable and prudent man would not do." The person who brings a malpractice claim is asserting that he or she is owed some duty by the defendant physician and that the violation of that duty by the physician must have caused injury. The court will make a determination concerning the propriety or impropriety of the defendant physician's performance on the basis of "the reasonable man" had he or she been in the same situation as the individual being judged. Negligence may derive from the physician's lack of training or experience. It may also result from the physician's carelessness or inadvertence[348] (Box 1.10).

To understand the concept of an expert witness, we must consider the legal doctrines of the *school of practice*, the *locality rule*, and the concept of the *qualifications of an expert*.[376] The legal doctrine of the school of practice is designed to deal with the historic problem of the competing interests of physicians. Physicians generally do not want to testify against their

colleagues, but they often are tempted to try to run their competitors out of business. Allopathic physicians were happy to label homeopathic physicians as quacks, and many medical doctors would be happy to dispute the competence of a chiropractor. To deal with the problem, the courts use the legal doctrine of the *school of practice* in which they refuse to allow physician experts to question a different school based on philosophic or psychological beliefs.[346] The school of practice rule now generally is used to differentiate physicians in the self-designated specialties (we use the term *self-designated* because few state licensing boards recognize specialties or limit physicians' rights to practice the specialties in which they have been trained).

The *locality rule* refers to the concept that a physician's competence should be determined by comparison with other physicians in the community or in similar neighboring communities.[346] However, with the development of national standards for the practice of radiation oncology, there is no justification for rules that shelter substandard medical decision-making by using an excuse that it is the norm for a given community. A radiation oncologist, for example, could not be held at fault for failing to treat a patient with an unusual or exotic technology if that technology were not available in his or her local community. However, physicians are required to inform the patients of the limitations of the available facilities and recommend prompt transfer if indicated. Failure to refer patients when a provider lacks the experience to appropriately treat may create malpractice liability. Furthermore, if a radiation oncologist does not give a patient information

---

Box 1.10

The New York Times Investigates Radiation Therapy

Radiation therapy practice was severely shaken when *The New York Times* published an article on June 21, 2009, titled "At V.A. Hospital, a Rogue Cancer Unit" and a second article on January 23, 2010, titled "Radiation Offers New Cures, and Ways to Do Harm." Both articles were authored by Walt Bogdanich.[255,328]

The first article described allegations that the prostate brachytherapy program at the Philadelphia V.A. Medical Center was "a rogue cancer unit at the hospital, one that operated with virtually no outside scrutiny and botched 92 of 116 cancer treatments over a span of more than six years—and then kept quiet about it...." The article described allegations of repetitive misplacement of prostate brachytherapy seeds, the changing of treatment plans to cover up the alleged errors, lack of peer review and quality assurance procedures, and the development of severe complications in patients.

The second article focused on the death of a 43-year-old man who had been irradiated at St. Vincent's Hospital in Manhattan for a tongue carcinoma and a 32-year-old female breast cancer patient treated at the State University of New York Downstate Medical Center. In the former case, the multileaf collimator was left fully open during intensity-modulated radiation therapy. In the latter case, a wedge was left out of the linear accelerator. Both patients were significantly overdosed and the tongue cancer patient died of radiation injuries. Bogdanich explores the causes of the errors: possible software malfunctions, human error, and lack of quality assurance and safety check procedures. Furthermore, the reporter raised the serious question of whether or not governmental oversight was sufficient to ensure the safety of clinical radiation therapy.

The articles made the safety of radiation therapy a national concern and have produced considerable soul searching in the medical physics and clinical radiation therapy communities. Efforts are under way at many levels to understand what can go wrong in radiation therapy, what can be done to prevent these errors, how much can be done to engineer procedures to prevent machine and human error, and what types of oversight are necessary to minimize error. We must never forget the Hippocratic admonishment *primum non nocere*: "First do no harm."

about the potential result associated with not seeing a subspecialist able to use a specific technology, then the initial radiation oncologist may be held liable. Physicians must recognize when a particular medical problem is beyond their capacity for diagnosis or treatment. They are responsible for obtaining timely and adequate consultations when indicated and for referring the patient to an appropriate specialist or facility whenever the requirements for the appropriate or specialized care cannot be satisfied at the available facilities. The continued expansion of knowledge in radiation oncology and the increasingly specialized training of physicians make it essential that the radiation oncologist be able to recognize any limitations in his or her capabilities or ability to treat a given patient with what is perceived to be standard of care. Failure to obtain an appropriate consultation or make an appropriate referral may denote negligence.[192,349,350]

Qualified experts sometimes disagree as to the standard of care. When alternative schools of thought exist, the physician defendant is entitled to be judged by the tenants of the school he or she follows. In such states, this is called the *minority practice doctrine*. With this doctrine, also called the *respectable minority rule*, the physician may show that although the course of therapy followed was not the same as other practitioners would have followed, it was one that was accepted by a respectable minority group of practitioners.[351]

A problem that is increasingly facing physicians in the United States has been the pressure radiation oncologists face from their employers or from insurance companies to conform their proposed care to a predetermined regimen. Despite legislative initiatives to hold such organizations accountable, the radiation oncologist will, for the most part, carry a significant portion of the risk of liability in cases where the patient asserts that he or she was unable to obtain the most accurate and appropriate diagnostic and therapeutic measures. It is essential that the radiation oncologist come to his or her own conclusions about the standard of care irrespective of any pressures applied by an employer or an insurance company. In litigation, the radiation oncologist's best defense against a claim of malpractice is if he or she can demonstrate action only in the interest of the patient, regardless of any financial consideration or bureaucratic restraint imposed by an insurance company, an HMO, or any other financial consideration. If a conflict arises between the radiation oncologist's recommendations for the best course of treatment and the level of care authorized by his/her employer, or insurance company, or an HMO, the physician must give the best care to the patient even if it means he or she will not ultimately be compensated.[352]

Radiation oncologists will, on occasion, be called on to serve as expert witnesses in malpractice cases. Physicians, trained to give opinions, may find the give and take of the court room off-putting. For an expert witness, the foremost qualifications are effective presentation and teaching ability. The radiation oncologist, serving as an expert witness, must educate the attorneys, judge, and jury. Once there is a perception of understanding, the radiation oncologist may be able to convince the judge and jury that they can make an independent decision that his or her testimony is correct.

Both the plaintiff's attorney and the defense attorney will retain expert witnesses who will be persuaded to "take sides." The expert witness will be asked to swear, under oath, what influence the radiation dose, volume, or technique had on the risk of an ill effect of radiation therapy on normal tissue or alleged failure to control the tumor. This expert witness system troubles many physicians who feel that they can bring a dispassionate and scientific view to such cases and come to a reasonable conclusion about whether or not malpractice occurred outside the process of litigation.[352] Whatever the wishes of the physician, a trial is an adversarial process. The physician is best advised, therefore, to state his or her opinion

about the case frankly and not attempt to predict or handicap how a trial will turn out. The physician should do his or her best to provide an opinion and then step aside to let a system, in which he or she has little expertise, run its course in the hands of the attorneys and judge. Although often frustrating and distressing, the physicians will find themselves out of their league if they attempt to act as attorney or judge.

Each physician must make a determination as to whether he or she feels comfortable participating in the legal process as an expert witness. Some radiation oncologists accept employment as expert witnesses in both plaintiffs' actions and in defense. Some only choose to participate as expert witnesses for the defendant physicians or simply wash their hands of the matter and will have nothing to do with the process. The lure of money is strong and serving as an expert witness can be quite lucrative. Each physician must, however, determine for him- or herself whether the financial compensation for serving as an expert witness outweighs the considerable effort and troubling aspects of the process.

It is important that radiation oncologists understand that the concept in malpractice law of *res ipsa loquitur*,[346] roughly translated as "the thing speaks for itself," is used to deal with cases in which the actual negligent act may not be proved, but it is clear that the injury was caused by negligence. In law, this doctrine was first recognized in the case of a man who was injured when a barrel rolled out of a second-story window of a warehouse. The defense attorney argued that the plaintiff did not know what events preceded the barrel rolling out of the window, and, therefore, it could not be proven that an employee of the warehouse was negligent. The plaintiff, however, countered that barrels do not normally fall out of second-story warehouse windows. The simple fact that the barrel fell from the window and caused an injury "spoke for itself" and demonstrated that someone must have been negligent.

In medical malpractice law, *res ipsa loquitur* is used to shift the burden of proof to the defendant's position regarding causation. *Res ipsa loquitur* can be invoked if the patient suffers an injury that is not an expected complication of medical care, the injury does not normally occur unless someone has been negligent, and the defendant was responsible for the patient's well-being at the time of the injury. Examples in which this concept has been invoked include the dislocation of a patient's shoulder while aligning it for a chest x-ray, knocking out a patient's tooth while the patient was under anesthesia for a tonsillectomy, nerve injury because of a hypodermic injection, leaving a sponge in the abdomen during an operation, or fracturing a patient's jaw while extracting a tooth.[346]

An *intentional tort* is an action that can result in harm to the plaintiff. The classic intentional tort in medical malpractice law is forcing unwanted medical care on a patient. Even if care clearly would benefit a patient, if that care were refused and the radiation oncologist had no state mandate to force care on the patient, but did so anyway, the patient might sue for intentional tort. The most common intentional tort is *battery*. The legal standard for a battery is "an intentional unconsented touching."[347]

Battery is not the same, in law, as *assault*. Assault is the act of putting a person in fear of bodily harm. Most battery claims against physicians are based on real attacks. However, battery claims also can be created by the circumstances of the medical treatment. The legal standard of care is that male health care providers do not examine female patients without a female attendant present. Although the standard frequently is ignored, it should not be. An attorney representing a plaintiff–patient may attempt to demonstrate that allowing an unattended examination of a female patient by a male radiation oncologist is concrete evidence that, at the very least, the physician has very poor judgment.

Of particular concern to radiation oncologists, in the realm of malpractice, is the concept of *loss of chance*. This usually is evoked in circumstances where physicians failed to diagnose a terminal illness. The loss of chance stems from the failure to diagnose in time for the patient to have a chance of cure. Not all states recognize this standard. In those states that do, however, the patient must show that the loss of chance is statistically significant.[346]

It is generally viewed that any patient injured by exposure to a defective x-ray machine will be compensated as a matter of law.[348] If, however, the radiation oncologist did not know or could not have reasonably been expected to know that a machine was defective, he/she will generally not be held liable if they used the machine properly.[353] Radiation oncologists are bound by the usual standards of skill, knowledge, and appropriate diligence that apply to the specialists within the field.

If a patient is hypersensitive to radiation therapy, and in the absence of any reasonable way to predict this, the radiation oncologist will not be expected to predict or prevent it.[354-356] There is, however, the possibility that the plaintiff's attorney will invoke *res ipsa loquitur* in certain circumstances.[357] For example, in a patient who received radiation therapy for a benign condition and suffered a severe radiation cutaneous reaction that required bilateral amputation, the radiation oncologist was found to be negligent.[358] In the employment of diagnostic radiation, minimal exposure is involved, and it is not expected that a skin reaction will be produced. Thus, if a skin reaction does ensue, many courts would infer negligence.[359] If a part of the body is unintentionally irradiated and injured, liability will generally follow. For example, a patient who is undergoing radiation therapy to the head and neck was compensated when he suffered severe injury to the arms.[360] A patient given radiation therapy to the ear suffered reaction of the head, face, and neck. Liability was also imposed.[361] It is reasonable to expect that patients give informed consent for radiation therapy and will accept a certain risk of ill effects. This does not mean that the patient assumes a risk of negligent care.[362,363]

In a case where a patient with carcinoma of the rectum was given radiation therapy at a dose above that recognized as proper and suffered severe ill effects, the radiation oncologist offered a defense that such dosage had been given in accordance with the recommendation of a recently delivered scientific paper. The court rejected this claim. In the court's view, this was not a generally accepted course or program of therapy, and the patient's specific consent to the variance in therapy had not been obtained.[364]

One must be particularly cautious in dealing with a woman of childbearing age concerning the possibility of pregnancy before exposing her to radiation therapy. Because the fetus might be injured, producing birth defects or necessitating an abortion, the patient has a right to refuse or at least should be given the full chance of providing informed consent.[282]

One must also be wary of injury through other forms of negligence involving radiation therapy. Injuries of this type include allowing the patient to fall, unstrapped, off the couch of a treatment machine as it is being moved into the correct position, being struck by a fluoroscopic screen or other equipment from a treatment machine or a simulator, being shocked or burned, or being permitted to come in contact with high-tension electrical wires.

There are some data concerning the types of malpractice claims brought in radiation oncology. From 1975 through 1994, a total of 18,860 malpractice suits were brought in Cook County, Illinois, naming at least one codefendant physician; 8% named a radiation oncologist as one of the defendants. The number of suits directed against radiation oncologists fell sharply in Cook County after 1982. At that time, allegations that thyroid cancer in adults developed from tonsillar irradiation administered in childhood for benign disease halted when such suits proved unsuccessful. The most common complaints initiating radiation oncology suits in recent years relate to:

a. Alleged complications of radiation therapy
b. Alleged administration of radiation therapy for inappropriate indications
c. Alleged inappropriate withholding of radiation therapy[365]

An interesting survey of 107 radiation oncology lawsuits conducted by the Fletcher Society found that 59% of the plaintiff patients were female. The four most common organ sites involved in the suits were gynecologic (17%), breast (16%), head and neck (14%), and urologic (12%). The actuarial probability of a radiation oncologist remaining free of a lawsuit after 30 years in practice was 35%.[366]

From 1985 to 2007, I reviewed 20 cases of alleged malpractice involving radiation oncology in the capacity of an expert reviewer employed by an attorney—almost always for the defense. When there was sufficient information to determine intent of treatment, it was always curative rather than palliative. A few themes have emerged from an analysis of the primary complaints of the plaintiffs. In six of the 20 cases, the plaintiff alleged that a delay in diagnosis other than the radiation oncologist adversely affected the prognosis and/or increased the risk of adverse late effects of radiotherapy. In four of the 20 cases, the plaintiff alleged a breach of the standard of care caused radionecrosis, cognitive injury, or second malignant neoplasm induction. In two cases, the plaintiff alleged that the treating radiation oncologist should have obtained a second surgical pathology or cytology opinion and that failure to do so resulted in unnecessary ill effects of treatment.[367]

Marshall et al. reviewed 362 closed malpractice claims filed against radiation oncologists collected by a US liability trade association from 2003 to 2012. Of the 362 claims, 102 (28%) were paid, totaling $38 million or an average of $372,468/paid claim. The most common alleged error leading to a paid claim was improper performance of radiation therapy (18%). Examples include misplaced prostate brachytherapy seeds rectal toxicity, or forgetting a spinal cord block and causing radiation myelitis. Errors in diagnosis accounted for 12% of paid claims. Examples include failure to diagnose a new comer on a follow-up imaging study, stimulating a patient for prostate radiotherapy and not recognizing the presence of a colon cancer, or failure to diagnose appendicitis or an aortic aneurysm.

Death-related claims had a lower average payment and lower percentage of paid claims than claims for radiation injury. Why? It may be more difficult to blame a radiation oncologist for the death of a new comer patient than for radiation toxicity in a living patient.[368]

The National Association for Insurance Commissioners conducted an extensive study of medical liability claims and insurance indemnity. It was published yearly between 1977 and 1980. The final report was based on data collected from over 70,000 medical liability claims arising from over 62,000 alleged injuries or incidences that were closed with payments to the plaintiffs by insurers. These data show that 4% of paid claims were related to EBRT.[369]

Brachytherapy as the origin of a malpractice action poses particular problems for the radiation oncologist. Brachytherapy procedures are relatively rare. Therefore, expertise is often limited and the individual experience of the practicing radiation oncologist may be minimal. The existence of postimplant films, which document the location of the radioactive material, can be used to challenge the quality of the implant procedure. Brachytherapy complications can take years to occur and, because brachytherapy is often employed in treatment of carcinoma of the prostate, cervix, and uterus, the development of fistulas in long-term survivors can be the cause of a malpractice action.

Radiation oncologists conduct their practice with the assistance of others: physicists, dosimetrists, nurses, and therapists. It is necessary, therefore, for radiation oncologists to understand *vicarious liability*. In general, employers are responsible for the actions of their employees. This is called *respondent superior*—also called the master–servant relationship.[215] The fundamental issue that determines whether a person is legally treated as an employee is the extent to which the person hiring the worker may control the details of that work. Nurses, physician assistants, radiation therapists, and other physician extenders are professionals, but in most states in which they are licensed, they generally have a limited license. The extent to which they make medical decisions is determined by state law, but they usually must work under the supervision of a practicing physician. The physician's license, however, is unlimited. The physician, for example, may perform nursing tasks without violating nursing practice laws. Injury caused by extenders may, ultimately, lead to a malpractice claim against the physician. Physician liability for the actions of hospital employees is particularly problematic for radiation oncologists. Many radiation oncologists practice in hospital-based clinics. In general, the *doctrine of the borrowed-servant* or the *captain of the ship doctrine* states that all actions of hospital employees are attributable to the patient's attending physician. Under such a doctrine, the radiation oncologist may be found liable for the actions of a nurse, dosimetrist, or radiation therapist who the physician can neither hire, fire, nor otherwise directly control.[347]

When radiation oncologists are directors of clinical services, they also should be aware of the fact that they may be vicariously liable for the behavior of employees if they tolerate inappropriate activity or do not properly screen employees for dangerous tendencies. If, for example, a therapist has assaulted persons in the past and the radiation oncologist was negligent in discovering this, the radiation oncologist could be held liable under the theory of negligent hiring. The radiation oncologist also could be held liable for negligent retention if there were complaints about the behavior of the therapist and the physician failed to act on them.[346]

The captain of the ship doctrine means that physicians may have responsibility for the mistakes of their radiation therapists, dosimetrists, physicists, nurses, and fellow practicing physicians allegedly under their supervision or control. It is, therefore, incumbent upon the responsible radiation oncologist to take care in staff selection, training, and supervision. There is a risk in delegating such matters to an office manager. Ultimately, the physician must maintain an active role in ascertaining that he or she can fully trust the person selected to assist in all aspects of patient care. This means that the radiation oncologist must protect against allegations of sexual misconduct or abuse, alcohol or drug impairment, or mental illness potentially affecting patient care; because the physician is ultimately liable for the care given to a patient, the radiation oncologist must play an active role in ongoing training and professional development of his or her staff.

If an accident or allegation of misconduct occurs, the radiation oncologist must have a thorough, efficient, and adequate means of investigation of the matter and, if necessary, discipline or dismissal. Adequate employment records must be maintained.[352]

One of the most vexing problems now facing the practicing radiation oncologist is the matter of substance and alcohol abuse in the workplace and potential criminal records of employees. Some practices are instituting mandatory preemployment screening for alcohol and drug abuse and criminal background checks. These issues, however, are extremely complicated, and it is not yet clear which drugs should be tested for, when the testing should occur, who should be

evaluated for a potential criminal background, which positive criminal background checks merit a decision not to employ an individual or to dismiss the person, under what circumstances a person can be felt to have paid his or her debt to society in a way that allows the individual to practice in a health care environment, and to what extent a radiation oncologist can be held liable for failure to exercise due caution in this process. Obtaining sound advice from an expert in personnel relations and legal counsel is advisable.[365]

It is well recognized that no radiation oncologist can be available at all times and in all circumstances. A physician may arrange, during his or her absence for vacation or ill health, for practice coverage by another physician. When one radiation oncologist "covers" for another, there are risks to patient safety, and possible susceptibility to malpractice claims, if clinical care "falls through the cracks." To minimize the risk of malpractice claims, the following guidelines should be followed:

- When you are away from your practice, you should select a covering radiation oncologist who possesses knowledge and skill at least equal to yours.
- Inform and obtain consent from those patients who will be affected.
- Apprise your covering physician of any important clinical information pertaining to patients he or she will see in your absence.
- The covering physician is expected to do more than just "fill in." He or she must apply the same degree of medical skill and care as the regular radiation oncologist.
- When the regular radiation oncologist returns, he or she should receive a report of any noteworthy patient care events, laboratory tests or diagnostic imaging results that deserve follow-up, and any other "loose ends."[370]

It cannot be overemphasized that well-maintained medical records are crucial to a satisfactory legal defense in malpractice claims in radiation oncology. In law, the concept of *spoliation* refers to the destruction of evidence of significance or a meaningful alteration of a document. In medical malpractice cases, this would refer to the absence or disappearance of medical records. One radiation oncologist wisely counseled: Now and then look over an old chart, see if you can trace all of your steps in making decisions and executing treatments. Would this chart be sufficient to defend yourself against a malpractice claim?[366]

The Nature of Grievances, Malpractice Claims, and Insurance Disputes in Radiation Oncology

Dissatisfied patients might ignore their physician's advice or seek a new physician. Assertive patients may confront their physician. It is also commonplace for patients to discuss their complaints about physicians with friends and relatives.

In Anglo American law and custom, patients whose dissatisfaction prompts formal action have several options. These include bringing a malpractice claim and seeking redress in courts. Other options include filing a complaint with a government medical board; filing a complaint with the "patient relations office" of a hospital or group practice; directing a complaint to a hospital's chief of medical staff or credentials office; or submitting a grievance to the local, state, district, or national medical society. Why some dissatisfied patients do nothing and others take formal action is not well studied.[181] The general nature of patient grievances against physicians, however, has been evaluated by several authors.[371,372] Complaints fall into several broad categories:

- Alleged failure of physicians to fulfill the patient's expectations for examination and treatment (i.e., inadequate therapy, failure to obtain informed consent prior to a

procedure, inadequate physical examination, or lack of prompt attention following hospitalization)
- Alleged failure to make a prompt diagnosis
- Alleged rude or discourteous behavior
- Alleged unacceptable practice behavior, such as producing excessive pain or practicing outside an area of expertise
- Alleged inappropriate behavior related to billings and collections
- Alleged physician's use of alcohol or drugs
- Alleged sexual misconduct
- Alleged errors in prescribing
- Alleged insurance fraud

Formal complaints, including malpractice suits, represent only the tip of the iceberg of patient dissatisfaction. Patients far more often deal with their dissatisfaction by complaining to family and friends or switching doctors than by submitting a written complaint. A study by the Harvard Medical Practice Study Group, for example, found that <2% of patients who had adverse events because of medical malpractice ever filed malpractice claims.[373] Patients pursued medical malpractice claims for a variety of reasons. The four most common include an attempt to hold the offending caregiver accountable, to seek a more complete or satisfying explanation for the adverse event, to stop similar events from occurring to other patients, and to obtain financial compensation[368,372,373] (Boxes 1.11 and 1.12).

A disagreement between a patient and his or her radiation oncologist may cause the patient to have diminished trust in the physician, to be dissatisfied with the clinical results, to change physicians or health plans, to file a complaint, or to undertake litigation. For physicians, however, disagreements with patients may result in frustration, anger, a feeling of loss of control, and career dissatisfaction.

It is important to document your explanation of the risks and benefits of radiation therapy and to obtain the patient's written authorization to proceed, with a full understanding of those risks. In discussing any procedure or treatment with the patient or his or her guardian, the radiation oncologist should endeavor to explain all of the risks in sufficient detail to permit the patient to make a well-educated decision. Written informed consent should be obtained. But simply having the patient sign a standard form is not the end of the matter. The forms need to be easily understood and written in clear language. It is unwise for a physician to adopt standard printed forms without giving them proper scrutiny. Radiation oncologists must also be sure that the consent form is properly filled

out. If, for example, there are blanks for explanations of particular risks involved for the procedure, they should be properly filled in.[352]

It is essential that radiation oncologists use fundamental communication skills to avoid grievances and malpractice claims, understand the patient's worries and concerns, express empathy, actively discuss care options, negotiate differences of opinion, and allow time for adequate conversation. The challenge for radiation oncologists is to recognize patients' unfulfilled expectations and to engage patients in a discussion with the goal of identifying and avoiding dissatisfaction while building a trusting therapeutic relationship.[389]

Insurance disputes involving radiation oncology typically centered on one or more of the following questions: Is the recommended course of radiotherapy covered under the patient's insurance contract? Is the proposed treatment standard of care or experimental? Is the proposed course of treatment likely to be more beneficial than alternatives? What are the supporting references from the medical literature underpinning the doctor or the insurance company's decisions?

I was asked, between 1995 and 2007, to review 69 radiation oncology insurance disputes. Overwhelmingly, these disputes were about a radiation oncologist's desire to employ and bill for the use of an expensive technique of external become radiotherapy and the insurance company's response that the technology was not standard of care. Examples include Gamma Knife or Cyber Knife treatment of metastatic corner or proton therapy for prostate cancer or vestibular schwannian or IMRT for localized breast cancer.[367]

Box 1.12

The RAGE Campaign

In 1991, a group of women formed an organization in the United Kingdom called RAGE (Radiation in Action Group Exposure). Their campaign began when a patient developed serious brachial plexus damage following surgery and radiotherapy for breast cancer. The patient wrote a letter to several newspapers describing these events and criticizing the medical and legal processes. This produced an outpouring of concern from other patients who claimed to have suffered from the same side effects. RAGE called for significant changes in the use of radiotherapy for the treatment of breast cancer.[374] The group successfully applied to the legal aid board for funds to undertake research toward a group legal action and, in 1995, constituted a group of plaintiffs in a malpractice case. Publicity associated with the litigation prompted the Royal College of Radiology to establish a multidisciplinary working party that made recommendations to ensure that patients with symptoms that might be due to radiation-associated brachial plexus injury had access to a network of health care professionals and cancer centers with the necessary skills for diagnosis, functional assessment, and treatment. The case highlighted the risks of high-dose-per-fraction radiation therapy used in the 1970s and 1980s. When the case eventually came to judgment, Justice Ebsworth concluded that there was no negligence and costs were directed against the plaintiffs. The justice commented that "it was unfortunate that litigation in terms of medical negligence was felt to be the only mechanism available," particularly in view of the fact that the cost of litigation exceeded £4 million. The case is instructive on several grounds:

1. The ill effects of radiation therapy may take a long time to become manifest.
2. Communication with patients concerning the causes and treatment of an injury is crucial.
3. The cost of litigation is quite high, and one would certainly hope that in the future society can derive alternative mechanisms to costly malpractice actions to allow patients to understand how and why injuries occur.[280,374,375]

Box 1.11

Systematic Radiation Therapy Overdose and Underdose: Events in the United Kingdom

It was discovered in 1998 at Exeter that 207 patients were given a radiation dose >25% than that generally deemed appropriate for the treatment of breast cancer. Some patients had more marked radiation reactions than appropriate. When this became known, adverse publicity appeared in the press. At Stafford approximately 1,000 patients received approximately 25% underdosing over a 20-year period. An investigation concluded that in approximately 500 patients, there was a real possibility that underdosage may have affected the outcome of treatment and, in a small number of patients, produced a cancer recurrence higher rate than that expected.[279,280]

The causes of these two incidents were analyzed in great detail and may have been related to inadequate medical physics staffing. A Royal College of Radiologists survey showed that radiation oncologists in many UK radiotherapy departments were seeing ≥600 new patients per year as compared to the usual 250 to 300 patients seen in France, Germany, and the United States.

Health Insurance Portability and Accountability Act

Because the Health Insurance Portability and Accountability Act of 1996 (HIPAA) has come fully into effect, considerable changes have occurred in the area of health care fraud and abuse. HIPAA created new criminal offenses and brought civil remedies while strengthening existing ones. More important for the practicing radiation oncologist, however, HIPAA is part of a larger political initiative in which health care fraud and abuse became a top law enforcement priority. Large numbers of civil investigations have been brought regarding alleged abuses of Medicare and Medicaid. Many physicians and organizations have been excluded from federally funded health care programs, and there have been criminal convictions and collection of large amounts of money in criminal fines.

RISK MANAGEMENT IN RADIATION ONCOLOGY

In an era of increasing litigation and, unfortunately, a growth in adversarial situations between physicians and patients, it is critical for the radiation oncologist and staff to make every effort to decrease professional liability risks.

The origins of medical malpractice suits include[100]:

- Medical accidents that may not be adequately understood by the patient or explained by the treating physician.
- Less than successful or unexpected adverse results of treatment.
- Poor results from previous treatment elsewhere and ill-advised comments by other physicians or health care personnel.
- Rejection of a plan of therapy without appropriate documentation that the physician has advised the patient of the consequences of declining treatment. Some physicians document this discussion in the chart and send a certified letter advising the patient of the consequences of rejection of treatment.
- Complaint of experimentation when the patient has not been appropriately informed of the nature of the therapy to be administered.
- An angry patient who may find this a way to vent anger or frustration about any events surrounding treatment, including lack of communication, discourteous treatment by the physician or staff, or the amount of the medical bill.

The best prevention against a lawsuit is good rapport with the patient and relatives, effective communication and QA programs in all activities related to patient management, and clear and accurate documentation of all procedures, discussions, and events that take place before, during, and after treatment.

After appropriate clinical assessment, the histologic diagnosis of the patient must be confirmed at the treating institution; this often includes review of outside pathologic slides. Rationale of therapy and any changes in treatment plan should be duly explained and documented in the record. All procedures performed on the patient should be recorded in the chart, including details of daily treatments, such as use of special treatment aids (i.e., bight blocks, testicular shields, eye shields, immobilization devices), and any problems related to equipment operation. All treatment parameters and calculations should be accurately recorded and verified by a physicist or dosimetrist, in addition to the radiation oncologist. We should remember that, as professional liability attorneys say, "If it is not recorded on the chart, we may assume it never happened."

The physician and staff may help in their own professional liability defense in case a lawsuit occurs. It is extremely important for the physician to understand and, at an appropriate time, identify early warning signs of an impending malpractice suit. The physician should promptly contact his or her attorney, risk management office, and insurance carrier.

The physician should prepare an incident report in anticipation of potential litigation, describing the potential liability, including dates when

TABLE 1.10 POSSIBLE SPECIFIC SEQUELAE OF THERAPY DISCUSSED IN INFORMED CONSENT

Anatomic Site	Acute Sequelae	Late Sequelae
Brain	Earache, headache, dizziness, hair loss, erythema	Hearing loss Damage to middle or inner ear Pituitary gland dysfunction Cataract formation Brain necrosis
Head and neck	Odynophagia, dysphagia, hoarseness, xerostomia, dysgeusia, weight loss	Subcutaneous fibrosis, skin ulceration, necrosis Thyroid dysfunction Persistent hoarseness, dysphonia, xerostomia, dysgeusia Cartilage necrosis Osteoradionecrosis of mandible Delayed wound healing, fistulae Dental decay Damage to middle and inner ear Apical pulmonary fibrosis Rare: myelopathy
Lung and mediastinum or esophagus	Odynophagia, dysphagia, hoarseness, cough Pneumonitis Carditis	Progressive fibrosis of lung, dyspnea, chronic cough Esophageal stricture Rare: chronic pericarditis, myelopathy
Breast or chest wall	Odynophagia, dysphagia, hoarseness, cough Pneumonitis (asymptomatic) Carditis Cytopenia	Fibrosis, retraction of breast Lung fibrosis Arm edema Chronic endocarditis, myocardial infarction Rare: osteonecrosis of ribs
Abdomen or pelvis	Nausea, vomiting Abdominal pain, diarrhea Urinary frequency, dysuria, nocturia Cytopenia	Proctitis, sigmoiditis Rectal or sigmoid stricture Colonic perforation or obstruction Contracted bladder, urinary incontinence, hematuria (chronic cystitis) Vesicovaginal fistula Rectovaginal fistula Leg edema Scrotal edema, sexual impotency Vaginal retraction or scarring Sterilization Sexual impotence Damage to liver or kidneys
Extremities	Erythema, dry/moist desquamation	Subcutaneous fibrosis Ankylosis, edema Bone/soft-tissue necrosis

events took place and actors and witnesses to be identified by name, affiliation, and status. Incident reports are confidential information between the physician and the attorney, risk manager, or insurance carrier. The report should be prepared while the facts are still fresh so that documentation will be optimal.

Clear and well-kept records with notes documenting every discussion and procedure that is performed on the patient should help in case of a lawsuit. A full discussion with the patient and relatives regarding planned therapy, particularly side effects of irradiation, and a well-documented informed consent form are valuable in risk management.

Informed Consent

The need to obtain informed consent for treatment is based on the patient's right to self-determination and the fiduciary relationship between the patient and physician.[376] The law requires that the treating physician adequately apprise every patient of the nature of the disease requiring treatment, recommended course of therapy and details regarding it, alternative treatments available, benefits of recommended treatment, and all minor and major risks (acute and late effects) associated with the recommended therapy (Table 1.10). If the plan of therapy is modified, this should be discussed with the patient, and, if warranted, a second informed consent may be required. It is advisable to discuss the informed consent contents in the presence of a witness and have that person sign an informed consent form or the chart verifying that the information was discussed with the patient.

Informed consent is a process, not a form. A consent form documents and codifies the process but does not substitute for clear and appropriate provision of information to the patient with adequate time for questions, answers, and free discussion and exchange. Ultimately, the competent adult patient or a legal representative must agree to the treatment and give approval. For unemancipated minors or legally incompetent adults, informed consent must be signed by the parents, adult brothers or sisters, or a responsible near relative or legal guardian. For incompetent adults, spouses may be allowed by the state to sign. Emancipated minors may provide their own consent. It is extremely important for the radiation oncologist and the staff to spend as much time as is needed to ensure that the patient and, if necessary, relatives understand all aspects of the radiation therapy, particularly the specific description of the various potential deleterious effects of this modality.[221] Many physicians indicate which situations may require surgery to treat a complication and, specifically, when a gastrostomy, colostomy, ileal bladder, or other organ-substituting operation may be necessary to correct sequelae of therapy.

The radiation oncologist is always balancing a full disclosure of risks and options without overwhelming the patient with data and causing distress. It is reasonable to expect the patient to come away from a meeting with the treating radiation oncologist with a general realistic hope regarding the proposed course of treatment and honest understanding of the side effects and a sense of trust for the physician and the organization.[352] Good documentation is crucial and, if a malpractice action were to occur, liability may hinge on who said what to whom at what point of the treatment process. Absent or lost records will reflect extremely poorly on the radiation oncologist.[352]

It must be stressed that in dealing with children or mentally incompetent adults, a thorough discussion of the plan of therapy and sequelae should be held with the parents, relatives, or legal guardian of the patient. Also, they must sign the informed consent.

Although, in case of a lawsuit, having a properly executed informed consent form in the record is helpful, more important is the incontrovertible documentation in the chart of the pertinent discussion held with the patient. Table 1.10 describes many of the specific sequelae in several anatomic sites that should be included in the informed consent. Radiation oncologists also should be aware of court decisions that place a greater burden on the physician to disclose statistical life expectancy information to critically ill patients as part of the informed consent and as an affirmation of patient-centered decision-making (regarding treatment) in the context of a physician–patient relationship based on trust.[377]

SELECTED REFERENCES

A full list of references for this chapter is available online.

REFERENCES

1. Friedman M, Friedland GW. *Medicine's 10 greatest discoveries.* New Haven, CT: Yale University Press, 1998.
2. Glasser O. *Dr. W.C. Röntgen.* Springfield: Charles C. Thomas, 1945.
3. Glasser O. *Wilhelm Conrad Röntgen and the early history of the Roentgen rays.* Springfield: Charles C. Thomas, 1934.
4. Nitske WR. *The life of Wilhelm Conrad Röntgen: discoverer of the x ray.* Tucson, AZ: University of Arizona Press, 1971.
5. Roentgen WC. On a new kind of rays (preliminary communication). Translation of a paper read before the Physikalische-medicinischen Gesellschaft of Würzburg on December 28, 1985. *Br J Radiol* 1931;4:32.
6. Dam HJW. The new marvel in photography. *McClure's Magazine* 1896;6:403.
7. Odhner CT. *Award Ceremony Speech.* December 10, 1901. nobelprize.org. Accessed December 19, 2017.
8. Becquerel H. Sur les radiations invisibles emises par les sources d'uranium. *Cr Acad Sci Paris* 1896;122:689–694.
9. Becquerel H, Curie P. L'action physiologique des rayons du radium. *Cr Acad Sci Paris* 1901;132:1289–1291.
10. Nobel e-Museum. Available at: http://www.nobel.se.Nobel Prize. Henri Besquere-Biographical. Nobel Prize, org.
11. Del Regato JA. Marie Sklodowska Curie. *Int J Radiat Oncol Biol Phys* 1976;1:345–353.
12. Redniss L. *Radioactive: Marie & Pierre Curie. A tale of love and fallout.* New York: Harper Collins, 2011.
13. Del Regato JA. Jean Frederic Joliot. *Int J Radiat Oncol Biol Phys* 1980;6:621–640.
14. Kyle RA, Shampo MA. Irene Curie and her husband. Frederic Joliot. *JAMA* 1974;277:906.
15. Brand RA. *Biogrophicalsketch, James Stephen Ewing, M.D. (1884–1943). Clin Orth Relat Res* 2012;470:639–641.
16. Murphy JE. *James Ewing 1866–1945.* Washington, DC: National Academy of Science, 1951.
17. Ewing J. *Neoplastic diseases: a treatise on tumors.* 2nd ed. Philadelphia: W.B. Sauder Company, 1922.
18. Ewing J. Diffuse endothelium a of bone. *Proc New York Path Soc* 1921;21:17–24.
19. Ewing J. Further report on endothelial myeloma of bone. *Proc New York Path Soc* 1924;24:93–101.
20. Ewing J. An analysis of radiation therapy in cancer (The Mutter Lecture). *Trains Coll Phys Phila* 1922;44:190–235.
21. Ewing J. Early experiences in radiation therapy (The Janeway Lecture). *Am J Roentgenol* 1934;31:153–163.
22. Ewing J. Tissue reactions in radiation (The Caldwell Lecture, 1925). *Am J Roentgenol* 1926;15:93–115.
23. Ewing J. Radium therapy in cancer. *JAMA* 1917;68:1238–1247.
24. DeNyse A, Lawrence L. Behind the name. James Ewing: 'The chief' of cancer pathology. *HemOnc Today,* October 25, 2008, p. 39.
25. Del Regato JA. James Ewins. *Int J Radiat Oncol Biol Phys* 1977;2:185–198.
26. Cowan DH. Vera Peters and the curability of Hodgkin disease. *Curr Oncol* 2008;15:206–210.
27. Cowan DH. Vera Peter and the conservative management of early stage breast cancer. *Curr Oncol* 2010;17:30–54.
28. Del Regato JA. Ernest Rutherford. *Int J Radiat Oncol Biol Phys* 1979;5:539–582.
29. Leonard CL. The röntgen rays as a palliative in the treatment of cancer. *Am Med* 1903;6:854–855.
30. Freund L. Ein mit Roentgen-Strahlen behandelter Fall von neavus pigmentosus piliferu. *Wien Med Wochenschr* 1897;10:428–434.
31. Despeignes V. Observation concernant un cas de cancer l'estomac traite par les rayons Roentgen. *Lyon Med J* 1896;82:428–430.
32. Coutard H. Principles of x-ray therapy of malignant diseases. *Lancet* 1934;2:1–8.
33. Coutard H. Roentgentherapy of epitheliomas of the tonsillar region, hypopharynx and larynx from 1920 to 1926. *Am J Roentgenol* 1932;28:313–331.
34. Paterson R. Classification of tumors in relation to radiosensitivity. *BJR* 1933;218–233.
35. Kreyberg L, et al. *A symposium on cancer given at the Institute on Cancer conducted at the Medical School of the University of Wisconsin.* Madison, WI: University of Wisconsin Press, 1938.
36. Committee for Radiation Oncology Studies. *Criteria for radiation oncology in multidisciplinary cancer management: report to the director of the National Cancer Institute, National Institutes of Health.* Philadelphia: American College of Radiology, 1986.
37. Halperin EC. The right verb. *Int J Radiat Oncol Biol Phys* 1987;13:143.
38. Buschke F. What is a radiotherapist? [Editorial]. *Radiology* 1962;79:319–321.

39. Rosenthal RS. Malpractice: cause and its prevention. *Laryngoscope* 1978;88:1–11.

40. Withers HR, Taylor JM. Critical volume model. *Int J Radiat Oncol Biol Phys* 1992;25:151–152.

41. Bentzen SM. Dose-painting by numbers. Theranostic imaging for radiation oncology. *Lancet Oncol* 2005;6:112–117.

42. International Commission on Radiation Units and Measurements. *Prescribing, recording, and reporting photon beam therapy: ICRU report 50.* Bethesda, MD: International Commission of Radiation Units and Measurements, 1993.

43. Bentel GC. *Patient positioning and immobilization in radiation oncology.* New York: McGraw-Hill, 1999.

44. Bentel GC. *Radiation therapy planning.* 2nd ed. New York: McGraw-Hill, 1996.

45. Halperin EC, Constine LS, Kun LE, et al. Stabilization and immobilization devices. Chapter 22. In: Light KL, Halperin EC, eds. *Pediatric radiation oncology.* 7th ed. Philadelphia: Lippincott Williams & Wilkins, 2011:16.

46. Michalski JM, Wong JW, Gerber RL, et al. The use of on-line image verification to estimate the variation in radiation therapy dose delivery. *Int J Radiat Oncol Biol Phys* 1978;27:707–716.

47. Verhey LV, Goitein M, McNulty P, et al. Precise positioning of patients for radiation therapy. *Int J Radiat Oncol Biol Phys* 1982;8:289–294.

48. Marks JE, Haus AG. The effect of immobilization on localization errors in the radiotherapy of head and neck cancer. *Clin Radiol* 1976;27:175–177.

49. Marks JE, Haus AG, Sutton HG, et al. Localization error in the radiotherapy of Hodgkin's disease and malignant lymphoma with extended mantle fields. *Cancer* 1974;34:83–90.

50. Lovelock DM, Hua C, Wang P, et al. Accurate setup of paraspinal patients using a noninvasive patient immobilization cradle and portal imaging. *Med Phys* 2005;32:2606–2614.

51. Sause WT, Stewart JR, Plenk HP, et al. Late skin changes following twice-weekly electron beam radiation to post-mastectomy chest wall. *Int J Radiat Oncol Biol Phys* 1981;7:1541–1544.

52. Humphreys M, Guerrero Urbano MT, Mubata C, et al. Assessment of a customized immobilization system for head and neck IMRT using electronic portal imaging. *Radiother Oncol* 2005;77:39–44.

53. Roques T, Dagless M, Tames J. Randomized trial on two types of the thermoplastic masks for patient immobilization during radiation therapy for head-and-neck cancer: in regard to Sharp et al. *Int J Radiat Oncol Biol Phys* 2005;62:942.

54. Engelsman M, Rosenthal SJ, Michaud SL, et al. Intra and interfractional patient motion for a variety of immobilization devices. *Med Phys* 2005;32:3468–3474.

55. Suit HD. Impact of improved local control on survival in patients with soft tissues sarcoma. *Int J Radiat Oncol Biol Phys* 1986;12:699–700.

56. D'Souza WD, Naqvi SA, Yu CX. Real-time intra-fraction-motion tracking using the treatment couch: a feasibility study. *Phys Med Biol* 2005;50:4021–4033.

57. Benedict SH. Immobilization, localization, and repositioning methods in stereotactic body radiation therapy. In: Kavanagh BD, Timmerman RD, eds. *Stereotactic body radiation therapy.* Philadelphia: Lippincott Williams & Wilkins, 2005:51–56.

58. Timmerman RD, Kavangh BD. Stereotactic body radiation therapy. *Curr Probl Cancer* 2005;29:120–157.

59. Fritz P, Kraus HJ, Dolken W, et al. Technical note: gold marker implants and high-frequency jet ventilation for stereotactic, single-dose irradiation of liver tumors. *Technol Cancer Res Treat* 2006;5:9–14.

60. Upton AC. The biological effects of low-level ionizing radiation. *Scientific American* 1982;246:41–49.

61. Little JP. Cellular effectsof ionizing radiation. *N Engl J Med* 1968;278:269–376.

62. Little JP, Hahn GM, Frindel E, Tubiana N. Repair of potentially lethal damage in vitro and in vivo. *Radiology* 1973;106:689–694.

63. Little MP. Cancer after exposure to radiation in the course of treatment for benign and malignant disease. *Lancet Oncol* 2001;2:212–220.

64. Kaplan HS. Radiobiology's contribution to radiotherapy: promise or mirage? Failla Memorial Lecture. *Radiat Res* 1970;43:460–476.

65. Suit H. Radiation biology: the conceptual and practical impact on radiation therapy. *Radiat Res* 1983;94:10–40.

66. Suit HD. Radiation biology, a basis for radiotherapy. In: Fletcher GH, ed. *Textbook of radiotherapy.* 2nd ed. Philadelphia: Lee and Febiger, 1973:78.

67. Blackburn S. *Think: a compelling introduction to philosophy.* Oxford: Oxford University Press, 1999.

68. Nagel T. *What does it all mean? A very short introduction to philosophy.* New York: Oxford University Press, 1987.

69. Solomon RC, Higgins KM. *A passion for wisdom: a very brief history of philosophy.* New York: Oxford University Press, 1997.

70. Fowler JF. Fractionation and therapeutic gain. In: Steel GE, Adams GE, Peckham MT, eds. *Biological basis of radiotherapy.* Amsterdam: Elsevier Science, 1983:181–194.

71. Fowler JF. How worthwhile are short schedules in radiotherapy? A series of exploratory calculations. *Radiother Oncol* 1990;18:165–181.

72. Fowler JF. Late normal tissue complications: new insights. *Int J Radiat Oncol Biol Phys* 1995;33:759–760.

73. Suit HD. A personal philosophy of a radiation oncologist. *Radiother Oncol* 2011;100:10–14.

74. Ward JF. The yield of DNA double-strand breaks produced intracellularly by ionizing radiation: a review. *Int J Radiat Biol* 1990;57:1141.

75. Bergonie J, Tribondeau L. Interpretation of some results of radiotherapy and an attempt at determining a logical technique of treatment. *Radiat Res* 1959;11:587–588. [Translation of original article in *CR Acad Sci* 1906;143:983.]

76. Regaud C, Ferroux R. Disordance des effets de rayons X, d'une part dans le testicule, par le fractionnement de la dose. *Comptes Rendus Societe Biologique* 1927;97:431.

77. Coutard H. Cancer of the larynx: results of roentgen therapy after five and ten years of control. *Am J Roentgenol* 1938;40:509.

78. Schwarz G. Heilung teifliegender Karzinome durch Rontgen-bestrahlung von der Korperoberflache. *Munch Med Wochenschr* 1914;61:1733.

79. Schwarz G. Ueber desensibilisierung gegen Rontgen—und radiumstrahlen. *Munchener Med Wochenschr* 1909;24:1–2.

80. Overgaard J. *Sensitization of hypoxic tumour cells—clinical experience. Int J Radiat Biol* 1989;56(5):801–811.

81. Gray LH. Oxygenation in radiotherapy. I. radiobiological considerations. *Br J Radiol* 1957;30:403–406.

82. Thomlinson RH, Gray LH. The histological structure of some human lung cancers and the possible implications for radiotherapy. *Br J Cancer* 1955;9:539–549.

83. Brizel DM, Rosner GL, Harrelson J, et al. Pretreatment oxygenation profiles of human soft tissue sarcomas. *Int J Radiat Oncol Biol Phys* 1994;30(3):635–642.

84. nobelprize.org.peytonrous-biographical.nobelprize.org

85. Hirst DG. Anemia: a problem or an opportunity in radiotherapy. *Int J Radiat Oncol Biol Phys* 1986;12:2009–2017.

86. Bergonié J, Tribondeau L. Interprétation de quelques résultats de la radio-thérapie et essai de fixation d'une technique rationnelle. *Comptes-rendus des Seances de lAcadémie des Sciences* 1906;143:983–985.

87. Fletcher GH, ed. *Textbook of radiotherapy.* 3rd ed. Philadelphia: Lea & Febiger, 1980.

88. Regaud C, Ferroux R. Discordance des effects de rayons X, d'une part dans le testicule, par le fractionnement de la dose. *CR Soc Biol* 1927;97:431–434.

89. Hall EJ, Giaccia AJ. *Radiobiology for the radiologist.* 6th ed. Philadelphia: Lippincott Williams & Wilkins, 2006.

90. Travis EL. *Primer of medical radiobiology.* 2nd ed. Chicago, IL: Year Book Publishers, 1989.

91. Wile AG, Dahlman A, Burns RG, et al. Laser photoradiation therapy of cancer following hematoporphyrin sensitization. *Lasers Surg Med* 1982;2:163–168.

92. Steel GG, Peacock JH. Why are some human tumours more radiosensitive than others? *Radiother Oncol* 1989;15:63–72.

93. Höckel M, Knoop C, Schlenger K, et al. Intratumor pO2 predicts survival in advanced cancer of the uterine cervix. *Radiother Oncol* 1993;26:45–50.

94. Kaanders JH, Bussink J, van der Kogel AJ. Clinical studies of hypoxia modification in radiotherapy. *Semin Radiat Oncol* 2004;14:233–240.

95. Kagan AR. Malpractice in radiation oncology: redefining the role of the medical expert. *IJROBP* 2005;61:638–639.

96. Upton AC. Biological aspects of radiation carcinogenesis. In: Boice JD, Fraumeni JF, eds. *Radiation carcinogenesis: epidemiology and biological significance.* New York: Raven, 1984:9.

97. Vaupel P, Kelleher DK, Hockel M. Oxygen status of malignant tumors: pathogenesis of hypoxia and significance for tumor therapy. Treatment resistance of solid tumors: role of hypoxia and anemia. *Semin Oncol* 2001;28:29–35.

98. Denko NC, Giaccia AJ. Tumor hypoxia, the physiological link between Trousseau's syndrome (carcinoma-induced coagulopathy) and metastasis. *Cancer Res* 2001;61:795–798.

99. Duncan W. A clinical evaluation of fast neutron therapy. In: Steel GG, Adams GE, Peckham MJ, eds. *The biological basis of radiotherapy.* Amsterdam: Elsevier Science BV, 1983:277–286.

100. Kaanders JH, Wijffels KI, Marres HA, et al. Pimonidazole binding and tumor vascularity predict for treatment outcome in head and neck cancer. *Cancer Res* 2002;62:7066–7074.

101. Fertil B, Malaise EP. Inherent cellular radiosensitivity as a basic concept for human tumor radiotherapy. *Int J Radiat Oncol Biol Phys* 1981;7:621–629.

102. Deacon J, Peckham MJ, Steel GG. The radioresponsiveness of human tumours and the initial slope of the cell survival curve. *Radiother Oncol* 1984;2:317–323.

103. Steel GG, Peacock JH. Why are some human tumours more radiosensitive than others? *Radiother Oncol* 1989;15:63–72.

104. Elkind MM. DNA damage and cell killing: cause and effect. *Cancer* 1985;45:2123–2127.

105. Elkind MM, Sutton H. Radiation response of mammalian cells grown in culture. I. Repair of x-ray damage in surviving Chinese hamster cells. *Radiat Res* 1960;13:556–593.

106. Puck TT, Marcus PI. Actions of x-rays on mammalian cells. *J Exp Med* 1956;103:653–666.

107. Weichselbaum RR, Little JB. The differential response of human tumours to fractionated radiation may be due to a post-irradiation repair process. *Br J Cancer* 1982;46:532–537.

108. Suit HD, Westgate SJ. Impact of improved local tumor control on survival. *Int J Radiat Oncol Biol Phys* 1986;12:453–458.

109. Barkley HT, Fletcher GH. The significance of residual disease after external irradiation of squamous cell carcinoma of the oropharynx. *Radiology* 1977;124:493–495.

110. Sobel S, Rubin P, Keller B, et al. Tumor persistence as a predictor of outcome after radiation therapy of head and neck cancers. *Int J Radiat Oncol Biol Phys* 1976;1:873–880.

111. Northrop M, Fletcher GH, Jesse RH, et al. Evolution of neck disease in patients with primary squamous cell carcinoma of the oral tongue, floor of mouth, and palatine arch, and clinically positive neck nodes neither fixed nor bilateral. *Cancer* 1972;29:23–30.

112. Orton CG. Other considerations in 3-dimensional treatment planning. In: Bagne F, ed. *Computerized treatment planning systems.* HHS Publication FDA 84–8223. Washington, DC: U.S. Government Printing Office, 1984:136–141.

113. Wetterer J. *Handbuch der Rontgen Therapie.* Leipzig i:176, 1913–1914.

114. Paterson R. Studies in optimum dosage. *Br J Radiol* 1952;25:505–516.

115. Schmidt-Ullrich RK. Local tumor control and survival: clinical evidence and tumor biologic basis. *Surg Oncol Clin North Am* 2000;9:401–414.

116. Glucksmann A. Preliminary observations on the quantitative examination of human biopsy material taken from irradiated carcinomata. *Br J Radiol* 1941;14:187–198.

117. Calabresi P, Dexter DL, Heppner GA. Clinical and pharmacological implications of cancer cell differentiation and heterogeneity. *Biochem Pharmacol* 1979;28:1933–1941.

118. Peters LJ. Inherent radiosensitivity of tumor and normal tissue cells as a predictor of human tumor response. *Radiother Oncol* 1990;17:177–190.

119. Peters LJ, Brock WA, Chapman JD, et al. Predictive assays of tumor radiocurability. *Am J Clin Oncol* 1988;11:275–287.

120. Chadwick J, Goldhaber M. Disintegration by slow neutrons. *Nature* 1935;135:65.

121. Tucker SL, Geara FB, Peters LJ, et al. How much could the radiotherapy dose be altered for individual patients based on a predictive assay of normal-tissue radiosensitivity? *Radiother Oncol* 1996;38:103–113.

122. Bjork-Erikson T, West C, Karlsson E, et al. Tumor radiosensitivity (SF2) is a prognostic factor for local control in head and neck cancers. *Int J Radiat Oncol Biol Phys* 2000;46:13–19.

123. Mackay RI, Hendry JH. The modelled benefits of individualizing radiotherapy patients' dose using cellular radiosensitivity assays with inherent variability. *Radiother Oncol* 1999;50:67–75.

124. Roberts SA, Hendry JH. A realistic closed-form radiobiological model of clinical tumor-control data incorporating intertumor heterogeneity. *Int J Radiat Oncol Biol Phys* 1998;41:689–699.

125. Roberts SA, Hendry JH. Time factors in larynx tumor radiotherapy: lagtimes and intertumor heterogeneity in clinical datasets from four centers. *Int J Radiat Oncol Biol Phys* 1999;45:1247–1257.

126. Buffa FM, Davidson SE, Hunter RD, et al. Incorporating biologic measurements (SF(2), CFE) into a TCP model increases their prognostic significance: a study in cervical carcinoma treated with radiation therapy. *Int J Radiat Oncol Biol Phys* 2001;50:1113–1122.

127. Miescher G. Erfolge der karzinombehandlung an der Dermatologischen Klinik Zurich. Einzeitige Hochstdosis und Fraktionierte Behandlung. *Strahlentherapie* 1934;49:65–81.

128. Strandqvist M. Sutdien uber die kumulative wirkung der rontgenstrahlen bie frakionierung. *Acta Radiol (Stockh)* 1944;55(suppl):1–300.

129. Von Essen CF. A spatial model of time-dose-area relationships in radiation therapy. *Radiology* 1963;81:881–883.

130. Fletcher GH. Keynote address: the scientific basis of the present and future practice of clinical radiotherapy. *Int J Radiat Oncol Biol Phys* 1983;9:1073–1082.

131. Mendenhall WM, Million RR, Cassisi NJ. Elective neck irradiation in squamous cell carcinoma of the head and neck. *Head Neck Surg* 1980;3:15–20.

132. Parsons JT. Time-dose-volume relationships in radiation therapy. In: Million RR, Cassisi NJ, eds. *Management of head and neck cancer: a multidisciplinary approach*. Philadelphia: J.B. Lippincott, 1984:137–172.

133. Schneider JJ, Fletcher GH, Barkley HT Jr. Control by irradiation alone of nonfixed clinically positive lymph nodes from squamous cell carcinoma of the oral cavity, oropharynx, supraglottic larynx, and hypopharynx. *Am J Roentgenol Radium Ther Med* 1975;123:42–48.

134. Withers HR, Peters LJ, Taylor JM, et al. Late normal tissue sequelae from radiation therapy for carcinoma of the tonsil: patterns of fractionation study of radiobiology. *Int J Radiat Oncol Biol Phys* 1995;33:563–568.

135. Fletcher GH, Shukovsky LJ. The interplay of radiocurability and tolerance in the irradiation of human cancers. *J Radiol Electrol* 1975;56:383–400.

136. Shukovsky LJ. Dose, time, volume relationships in squamous cell carcinoma of the supraglottic larynx. *Am J Roentgenol* 1970;108:27–29.

137. Shukovsky LJ, Baeza MR, Fletcher GH. Results of irradiation of squamous cell carcinomas of the glossopalatine sulcus. *Radiology* 1976;120:405–408.

138. Shukovsky LJ, Fletcher GH. Time-dose and tumor volume relationships in the irradiation of squamous cell carcinoma of the tonsillar fossa. *Radiology* 1973;107:621–626.

139. Baclesse F. Clinical experience with ultrafractionated radiotherapy. *Progress in radiation therapy*. New York, NY: Grune Stratton, 1958:128–148.

140. Del Regato JA. Chapter 12. Herman Holthusen, (1886–1971). In: Del Regato JA, ed. *Radiological oncologists the unfolding of a medical specialty*. Reston VA: Radiology Centennial, Inc., 1985:109–118.

141. Holthusen H. Erfahrungen, über die vertraglichkeitsgrent Für Röntgenstrahlen und deren nutianwarendung. *Strahlentherapies* 1936;57:254-264.

142. Spanos WJ Jr, Shukovsky LJ, Fletcher GH. Time, dose, and tumor volume relationships in irradiation of squamous cell carcinomas of the base of the tongue. *Cancer* 1976;37:2591–2599.

143. Million RR. The larynx...so to speak: everything I wanted to know about laryngeal cancer I learned in the last 32 years. *Int J Radiat Oncol Biol Phys* 1992;23:691–704.

144. Niemierko A, Urie M, Goitein M. Optimization of 3D radiation therapy with both physical and biological end points and constraints. *Int J Radiat Oncol Biol Phys* 1992;23:99–108.

145. Ron E, Modan B, Boice JD, et al. Tumors of the brain and nervous system after radiotherapy in childhood. *N Engl J Med* 1988;319:1033–1039.

146. Emami B, Myerson RJ, Scott C, et al. Phase I/II study combination of radiotherapy and hyperthermia in patients with deep-seated malignant tumors: report of a pilot study by the Radiation Therapy Oncology Group. *Int J Radiat Oncol Biol Phys* 1991;20:73–79.

147. Schultheiss TE, Stephens LC, Ang KK, et al. Volume effects in rhesus monkey spinal cord. *Int J Radiat Oncol Biol Phys* 1994;29:67–72.

148. Marks LB, Yorke ED, Jackson A, et al. Use of normal tissue complication probability models in the clinic. *Int J Radiat Oncol Biol Phys* 2010;76:S10–S19.

149. Marks LB, Bentzen SM, Deasy JO, et al. Radiation dose-volume effects in the lung. *Int J Radiat Oncol Biol Phys* 2010;76:S70–S76.

150. Jackson A, Kutcher GJ, Yorke ED. Probability of radiation-induced complications for normal tissues with parallel architecture subject to non-uniform irradiation. *Med Phys* 1993;20:613–625.

151. Rubin P. The emergence of radiation oncology as a distinct medical specialty. *Int J Radiat Oncol Biol Phys* 1985;11:1247–1270.

152. Rubin P, Casarett GW. *Clinical radiation pathology*. vols. 1 and 2. Philadelphia: W.B. Saunders, 1968.

153. Rubin P, Cooper R, Phillips TL, eds. *Radiation biology and radiation pathology syllabus (Set RT 1: Radiation Oncology)*. Chicago, IL: American College of Radiology, 1975.

154. Baclesse F. Carcinoma of the larynx. *Br J Radiol* 1949;3:1–62.

155. Baclesse F. Roentgentherapy alone in the cancer of the breast. *Acta Unio Int Contra Cancrum* 1959;15:1023–1026.

156. Bush RS. The complete oncologist: the Buschke lecture. *Int J Radiat Oncol Biol Phys* 1982;8:1019–1027.

157. Withers HR, Thames HD, Peters LJ. Differences in fractionation response of acutely and late responding tissues. In: Karcher KH, Kogelnik HD, Reinartz G, eds. *Progress in radio-oncology II*. New York: Raven, 1982:287–296.

158. Thames HD, Withers HR, Mason KA, et al. Dose-survival characteristics of mouse jejunal crypt cells. *Int J Radiat Oncol Biol Phys* 1981;7:1591–1597.

159. Thames HD Jr, Withers HR, Peters LJ, et al. Changes in early and late radiation responses with altered dose fractionation: implications for dose-survival relationships. *Int J Radiat Oncol Biol Phys* 1982;8:219–226.

160. Nicholson G. Cancer metastasis. In: Friedberg EC, ed. *Cancer biology*. New York: W.H. Freeman and Company, 1986:138–148.

161. Mendelsohn ML. The biology of dose-limiting tissues. In: *Time and dose relationships in radiation biology as applied to radiotherapy*. Brookhaven National Laboratory (BNL) Report 5023 (C-57). Upton, NY: Brookhaven National Laboratory, 1969:154–173.

162. Hellman S. Roentgen Centennial Lecture: discovering the past, inventing the future. *Int J Radiat Oncol Biol Phys* 1996;35:15–20.

163. Coleman CN, Stevenson MA. The hallmark of modern radiation oncology. *Int J Radiat Oncol Biol Phys* 1994;30:1247–1249.

164. Hanks GE, Hanlon AL, Pinover WH, et al. Survival advantage for prostate cancer patients treated with high-dose three-dimensional conformal radiotherapy. *Cancer J Sci Am* 1999;5:152–158.

165. Cater DB, Silver IA. Quantitative measurements of oxygen tension in normal tissues and in the tumours of patients before and after radiotherapy. *Acta Radiol* 1960;53:233–256.

166. Bentzen SM. Potential clinical impact of normal-tissue intrinsic radiosensitivity testing. *Radiother Oncol* 1997;43:121–131.

167. Denekamp J. Changes in the rate of repopulation during multifraction irradiation of mouse skin. *Br J Radiol* 1973;46:381–387.

168. Fowler JF. Rapid repopulation in radiotherapy: a debate on mechanism. The phantom of tumor treatment—continually rapid proliferation unmasked. *Radiother Oncol* 1991;22:156–158.

169. Schmidt-Ullrich RK, Contessa JN, Dent P, et al. Molecular mechanisms of radiation-induced accelerated repopulation. *Radiat Oncol Invest* 1999;7:321–330.

170. Fuks Z, Alfieri A, Haimovitz-Friedman A, et al. Intravenous basic fibroblast growth factor protects the lung but not mediastinal organs against radiation-induced apoptosis. *Cancer J Sci Am* 1995;1:62–72.

171. Tubiana M, Richare JM, Malaise E. Kinetics of tumor growth and of cell proliferation in U.R.D.T. cancers: therapeutic implications. *Laryngoscope* 1975;85:1039–1052.

172. Mohan R, Wu Q, Niemierko A, et al. Optimization of IMRT plans based on biologically equivalent uniform dose. In: *Proceedings of Sixth International Conference on Dose, Time and Fractionation in Radiation Oncology. Biological and physical basis of IMRT and tomotherapy*. Madison, WI: Medical Physics Publishing, 2001.

173. Peschel RE, Fischer JJ. Multiple daily fractionation schedules. *Int J Radiat Oncol Biol Phys* 1982;8:1811–1812.

174. Withers HR, Thames HD Jr, Flow BL, et al. The relationship of acute to late skin injury in 2 and 5 fractions/week x-ray therapy. *Int J Radiat Oncol Biol Phys* 1978;4:595–601.

175. Fowler JF. The linear quadratic formula and progress in fractionated radiotherapy: a review. *Br J Radiol* 1989;62:679–694.

176. Withers HR, Peters LJ, Thames HD, et al. Hyperfractionation. *Int J Radiat Oncol Biol Phys* 1982;8:1807–1809.

177. Thames HD Jr., Withers HR, Peters LJ, et al. Changes in early and late radiation responses with altered dose fractionation: implications for dose-survival relationships. *Int J Radiat Oncol Biol Phys* 1982;8:219–226.

178. Kronig S, Friedrich W. *Physikalische und biologische Grundlagen der Strahlentherapie. Sonderbtrand der Strahlentherapie*. Berlin-Wien: Urban & Schwarzenberg, 1918.

179. MacComb WS, Quimby EH. The rate of recovery of human skin from the effects of hard or soft roentgen rays or gamma rays. *Radiology* 1936;27:196–207.

180. Reisner A. Hauterythem und rotgenstrahlung. *Ergeb Med Strahlenforsch* 1933;6:1.

181. Von Essen CF. A spatial model of time-dose-area relationships in radiation therapy. *Radiology* 1963;81:881–883.

182. Dutreix J, Wambersie A, Bounik C. Cellular recovery in human skin reactions: application to dose fraction number overall time relationship in radiotherapy. *Eur J Cancer* 1973;9:159–167.

183. Slamon DJ, Godolphin W, Jones LA, et al. Studies of the HER-2/neu proto-oncogene in human breast and ovarian cancer. *Science* 1989;244:707–712.

184. Chadwick J. The existence of a neutron. *Proc Roy Soc London* 1932;136:692–708.

185. Orton CG, Ellis F. A simplification in the use of the NSD concept in practical radiotherapy. *Br J Radiol* 1973;46:529–537.

186. Orton CG. Errors in applying the NSD concept. *Radiology* 1975;115:233–235.

187. Ellis F. Time, fractionation, and dose rate in radiotherapy. In: Vaeth JM, ed. *Frontiers of radiation therapy and oncology*. vol. 3. Basel, Switzerland: Karger, 1968:131–140.

188. Withers HR, Thames HD, Peters LJ. A new isoeffect curve for change in dose per fraction. *Radiother Oncol* 1983;1:187–191.

189. Brenner DJ, Dale R, Orton C, et al. Radiobiology of high dose-rate, low dose-rate, and pulsed-dose-rate brachytherapy. In: Joslin CAF, Flynn A, Hall EJ, eds. *Principles and practice of brachytherapy: using afterloading systems*. London: Arnold, 2001:189–204.

190. Yaes RJ. Linear-quadratic model isoeffect relations for proliferating tumor cells for treatment with multiple fractions per day. *Int J Radiat Oncol Biol Phys* 1989;17:901–905.

191. Land H, Parada LF, Weinberg RA. Cellular oncogenes and multistep carcinogenesis. *Science* 1983;222:771–778.

192. *Largess v. Tatem*, 291 A 2d 398, Vt 1972.

193. Hall EJ. Dose-rate considerations. In: Hilaris BS, Batata MA, eds. *Brachytherapy oncology—1983*. New York: Memorial Sloan-Kettering Cancer Center, 1983:33–39.

194. Dutreix J. Expression of the dose rate effect in clinical curietherapy. *Radiother Oncol* 1989;15:25–37.

195. Van Rongen E. Analysis of cell survival after multiple fractions and low dose-rate irradiation of two in vitro cultured rat tumor cell lines. *Radiat Res* 1985;104:28–46.

196. Ellis F. Time and dose relationships in radiation biology as applied to radiotherapy. Brookhaven National Laboratory. *BNL* 1969;50203(C-57):313.

197. Paterson R. *The treatment of malignant disease by radium and x-ray: being a practice of radiotherapy*. Baltimore, MD: Williams & Wilkins, 1949.378.

198. Paterson RP. The radical x-ray treatment of the carcinomata. *Br J Radiol* 1936;9:671–679.

199. Pierquin B, Chassagne D, Baillet F, et al. Clinical observations on the time factor in interstitial radiotherapy using Iridium 192. *Clin Radiol* 1973;24:506–509.

200. Orton CG. Time-dose factors (TDFs) in brachytherapy. *Br J Radiol* 1974;47:603–607.

201. Orton CG, Cohen L. A unified approach to dose-effect relationships in radiotherapy. I. Modified TDF and linear quadratic equations. *Int J Radiat Oncol Biol Phys* 1988;14:549–556.

202. Orton CG, Seyedsadr M, Somnay A. Comparison of high and low dose rate remote afterloading for cervix cancer and the importance of fractionation. *Int J Radiat Oncol Biol Phys* 1991;21:1425–1434.

203. Wilson JF. Low dose rate teletherapy: review of recent clinical study. In: *Proceedings of 2nd International Dose-Time Conference, University of Wisconsin, Madison, WI; September 12–14, 1984*.

204. Pierquin B, Baillet F, Brown CH. Low dose irradiation in advanced tumors of head and neck. *Acta Radiol* 1975;14:497–504.

205. Powers EL. Consideration of survival curves and target theory. *Phys Med Biol* 1962;7:3–28, 962.

206. *Prescribing, recording and reporting photon beam therapy (Supplement to ICRU report 50)*. Bethesda, MD: International Commission on Radiation Units and Measurements, 1999.

207. Goitein M. The comparison of treatment plans. *Semin Radiat Oncol* 1992;2:246–256.

208. Purdy JA. Photon dose calculations for three-dimensional radiation treatment planning. *Semin Radiat Oncol* 1992;2:235–245.

209. Goitein M, Abrams M. Multi-dimensional treatment planning. I. Delineation of anatomy. *Int J Radiat Oncol Biol Phys* 1983;9:777–787.

210. Perez CA, Michalski JM, Purdy JA, et al. Three-dimensional conformal therapy or standard irradiation in localized carcinoma of prostate: preliminary results of a nonrandomized comparison. *Int J Radiat Oncol Biol Phys* 2000;47:629–637.

211. Purdy JA, Wong JW, Harms WB, et al. Three dimensional radiation treatment planning system. In: *Proceedings of the 9th International Conference on the Use of Computers in Radiation Therapy*. North Holland, The Netherlands: Scheveningen, 1987.

212. Sharkey RM, Blumenthal RD, Hansen HJ, et al. Biological considerations for radioimmunotherapy. *Cancer Res* 1990;50(Suppl):964–969.

213. Purdy JA, Wong JW, Harms WB, et al. State of the art of high energy photon treatment planning. *Front Radiat Ther Oncol* 1987;21:4–24.

214. Chen GTY, Austin Seymour M, Castro JR, et al. Dose volume histograms in treatment planning evaluation of carcinoma of the pancreas. In: *International Conference on Computers in Radiation Therapy: proceedings of 8th International Conference*. Los Alamitos, CA: IEEE Computer Press, 1984.

215. Penagaricano JA, Papanikolaou N, Wu C, et al. An assessment of biologically-based optimization (BORT) in the IMRT era. *Med Dosim* 2005;30:12–19.

216. Brahme A. Optimized radiation therapy based on radiobiological objectives. *Semin Radiat Oncol* 1999;9:35–47.

217. Carol MP, Targovnik H. Importance of the user in creating optimized treatment plans with Peacock. *Med Phys* 1994;21:913.

218. Zelefsky MJ, Cowen D, Zuks Z, et al. Long term tolerance of high dose three-dimensional conformal radiotherapy in patients with localized prostate carcinoma. *Cancer* 1999;85:2460–2468.

219. Webb S. *The physics of three-dimensional radiation therapy: conformal radiotherapy, radiosurgery and treatment planning*. Bristol, England: Institute of Physics Publishing, 1993.

220. Fermi E. Artificial radioactivity produced by neutron bombardment. In: Holberg MA, ed. *Les Prix Nobel in 1939*. Stockholm: Norstedt and Söner, 1939.

221. Taylor JH, Goldhaber M. Detection of nuclear disintegration in a photographic emulsion. *Nature* 1935;135:34.

222. Burcham WE, Goldhaber M. The disintegration of nitrogen by slow neutrons. *Proc Cambridge Philos Soc* 1936;32:632–636.

223. Locher GL. Biologic effects and therapeutic possibilities of neutrons. *Am J Roentgenol* 1936;36:1.

224. Conger AD, Giles NH Jr. Cytogenic effect of slow neutrons. *Genetics* 1950;35:397–419.

225. Sweet WH. Early history of development of boron neutron capture therapy of tumors. *J Neuro Oncol* 1997;33:19–26.

226. Talmadge JE, Fidler IJ. Cancer metastasis is selective or random depending on the parent tumour population. *Nature* 1982; 297:593–594.

227. Halperin EC. Historical review: particle therapy for cancer. *Lancet Oncol* 2006;7:676–685.

228. Coderre JA, Morris GM. The radiation biology of boron neutron capture therapy. *Radiol Res* 1999;151:1–18.

229. Laramore GE. The use of neutrons in cancer therapy: a historical perspective through the modern era. *Semin Oncol* 1997;24:672–686.

230. Watson-Clarke RA, et al. Model studies directed toward the application of boron neutron capture theory of rheumatoid arthritis: boron delivery by liposomes to rat collagen-induced arthritis. *PNAS U S A* 1998;95:2531–2534.

231. Coleman CN. International Conference on Translational Research and Preclinical Strategies in Radio-Oncology (ICTR): conference summary. *Int J Radiat Oncol Biol Phys* 2001;49:301–309.

232. Munro TR. The relative radiosensitivity of the nucleus and the cytoplasm of the Chinese hamster fibroblast. *Radiat Res* 1990;42:451.

233. Dewey WC, Ling CC, Meyn RE. Radiation-induced apoptosis: relevance to radiotherapy. *Int J Radiat Oncol Biol Phys* 1995;33:781–796.

234. Allan DJ. Radiation-induced apoptosis: its role in a MADCaT (mitosis-apoptosis-differentiation-calcium toxicity) scheme of cytotoxicity mechanisms. *Int J Radiat Biol* 1992;62:145.

235. Woloschak GE, Liu GMC, Jones S, et al. Modulation of gene expression in Syrian hamster embryo cells following ionizing radiation. *Cancer Res* 1990;50:339–344.

236. Kaplan HS. Historic milestones in radiobiology and radiation therapy. *Semin Oncol* 1979;6(4):479–489.

237. Wyllie AH. Apoptosis. *Br J Cancer* 1993;67:205–208.

238. Wyllie AH. The biology of cell death in tumours. *Anti Cancer Res* 1985;5:131.

239. Martin GS. Normal cells and cancer cells. In: Bishop JM, Weinberg RA, eds. *Scientific American: molecular oncology*. New York: Scientific American, 1996:13–40.

240. Kerr JFR, Wyllie AH, Currie AR. Apoptosis: a basic biological phenomenon with wide-ranging implications in tissue kinetics. *Br J Cancer* 1972;26:239–257.

241. Fornace AJ Jr. Mammalian genes induced by radiation: activation of genes associated with growth control. *Annu Rev Genet* 1992;26:507–526.

242. Fowler JF. Rationale for high linear energy transfer radiotherapy. In: Steel GG, Adams GE, Peckham JM, eds. *The biological basis of radiotherapy*. Amsterdam: Elsevier Science, 1983:261–268.

243. Suit H, Lindberg R. Radiation therapy administered under conditions of tourniquet-induced local tissue hypoxia. *Am J Roentgenol* 1968;2:27–37.

244. Churchill DI. Oxygen effect on radiosensitivity. In: Proceedings of the conference on research of the radiotherapy of cancer. New York: American Cancer Society, 1961. Citing recent developments in radiotherapy. *N Engl J* 2017;377:1065–1075.

245. Dische S. Hyperbaric oxygen: the Medical Research Council trials and their clinical significance. *Br J Radiol* 1979;51:888–894.

246. Henk JM, Smith CW. Radiotherapy and hyperbaric oxygen in head and neck cancer. *Lancet* 1977;1:104–105.

247. Overgaard J, Hansen HS, Overgaard M, et al. A randomized double-blind phase III study of nimorazole as a hypoxic radiosensitizer of primary radiotherapy in supraglottic larynx and pharynx carcinoma. Results of the Danish head and neck cancer study (DAHANCA) protocol 5–85. *Radiother Oncol* 1998;46:135–146.

248. Overgaard J, Horsman MR. Modification of hypoxia-induced radio-resistance in tumors by the use of oxygen and sensitizers. *Semin Radiat Oncol* 1996;6:10–21.

249. Klein HG. Blood substitutes: how close to a solution? *Dev Biol (Basel)* 2005;120:45–52.

250. Rose C, Lustig R, McIntosh N, et al. A clinical trial of fluosol DA 20% in advanced squamous cell carcinoma of the head and neck. *Int J Radiat Oncol Biol Phys* 1988;12:1325–1327.

251. Utley JF, Seaver N, Newton GL, et al. Pharmacokinetics of WR-1065 in mouse tissues following treatment with WR-02721. *Int J Radiat Oncol Biol Phys* 1984;10:1525–1528.

252. Small W Jr, Winter K, Levenback C, et al. Extended-field irradiation and intracavitary brachytherapy combined with cisplatin and amifostine for cervical cancer with positive para-aortic or high common iliac lymph nodes. Results of arm II of radiation therapy oncology group (R TOG) 0116. *Int J Gynecol Cancer* 2011;21:1266–1275.

253. Brizel DM. Does amifostine have a role in chemoradiation treatment? *Lancet Oncol* 2003;4:378–81.

254. Bourhis J, Blanchard P, Maillard E, et al. Effect of amifostine on survival among patients treated with radiotherapy: a meta-analysis of individual patient data. *J Clin Oncol* 2011;29:2950–2957.

255. Bogdanich W. Radiation offers new cures, and ways to do harm. *New York Times*. Available at: http://www.nytimes.com/2010/01/24/health/24radiation.html. Accessed November 2, 2011.

256. Boveri T. *The origin of malignant tumors*. Baltimore, MD: Williams & Wilkins, 1929.

257. McShan DL, Fraass BA, Lichter AS. Full integration of the beam's eye view concept into computerized treatment planning. *Int J Radiat Oncol Biol Phys* 1990;18:1485–1494.

258. Weinberg RA. *The biology of cancer*. New York: Garland Science, Taylor and Francis Group, 2007.

259. Harris H, Miller OJ, Klein G, et al. Suppression of malignancy by cell fusion. *Nature* 1969;223:363.

260. Levine AJ. Tumor suppressor genes. In: Mendelsohn J, Howley PM, Israel MA, et al., eds. *The molecular basis of cancer*. Philadelphia: W.B. Saunders, 1995:86–104.

261. Knudson AG Jr. Mutation and cancer: statistical study of retinoblastoma. *Proc Natl Acad Sci U S A* 1971;68:820–823.

262. Goel S, Duda DG, Xu L, et al. Normalization of the vasculature for treatment of cancer and other diseases. *Physiol Rev* 2011;91:1071–1121.

263. Zeherberg A. *Award ceremony speech. The nobel prize in Physiology or Medicine 2001*. nobelprize.org. Accessed January 1, 2018.

264. Murakami MS, Strobel LMC, Vande Woude GF. Cell cycle regulation, oncogenes, and antineoplastic drugs. In: Mendelsohn J, Howley PM, Israel MA, et al., eds. *The molecular basis of cancer*. Philadelphia: W.B. Saunders, 1995:3–17.

265. Murray AW. Creative blocks: cell-cycle checkpoints and feedback controls. *Nature* 1992;359:599–604.

266. Hartwell LH, Kastan MB. Cell cycle control and cancer. *Science* 1994;266:1821–1828.

267. Rowley JD. Biological implications of consistent chromosome rearrangements in leukemia and lymphoma. *Cancer Res* 1984;44:3159–3168.

268. Williams GT, Smith CA. Molecular regulation of apoptosis: genetic controls of cell death. *Cell* 1993;74:777–779.

269. Chrest FJ, Buchholz MA, Kim YH, et al. Identification and quantitation of apoptotic cells following anti-CD3 activation of murine G0 T-cells. *Cytometry* 1993;14:883–890.

270. Wyllie AH, Kerr JFR, Currie AR. Cell death: the significance of apoptosis. *Int Rev Cytol* 1980;68:251–306.

271. Hallahan DE, Beckett MA, Kufe DW, et al. The interaction between recombinant human tumor necrosis factor and radiation in 13 human tumor cell lines. *Int J Radiat Oncol Biol Phys* 1990;19:69–74.

272. Hellman S, Weichselbaum RR. Radiation oncology. *JAMA* 1996;275:1852–1853.

273. Hellman S, Weichselbaum RR. Radiation oncology and the new biology. *Cancer J Sci Am* 1995;1:174–179.

274. Griffin RJ. *Biological response to spatially fractionated macro and microbeam radiotherapy. Defining shades of Gy: utilizing the biological consequences of radiation therapy in the development of new treatment approaches*. Shady Grove, MD: National Cancer Institute, September 11-12, 2017.

275. Mole, RH Whole body irradiation—radiobiology or medicine? *Br J Radiol* 1953;26:234–241.

276. Formenti S. *Can we modify radiation dose to the tumor or aspects of the tumor during the course of treatment without compromising control of tumor mass? Defining shades of Gy: utilizing the biological consequences of radiation therapy in the development of new treatment approaches*. Shady Grove, MD: National Cancer Institute, September 11–12, 2017.

277. Guha C. *Can we modify radiation dose to the tumor or aspects of the tumor during the course of treatment without compromising control of tumor mass? Defining shades of Gy: utilizing the biological consequences of radiation therapy in the development of new treatment approaches*. Shady Grove, MD: National Cancer Institute, September 11–12, 2017

278. Paget S. A centennial celebration of Dr. Stephen Paget's "Seed and Soil" hypothesis. *Cancer Metastasis Rev* 1989;8:93–97.

279. Ash DV. Breast radiation injury litigation and RAGE. *Clin Oncol (R Col Radiol)* 1999;11:138–139.

280. Kunkler I. Recommendations after the RAGE litigation. *Lancet* 1998;352:657.

281. Paget S. The distribution of secondary growths in cancer of the breast. *Lancet* 1889;1:571–573.

282. *Salinetro v. Nystrom*, 341 So 2d 1059, Fla, 1977.

283. Fidler IJ, Leidman I. Enhancement of experimental metoses by x-ray: a possible mechanism. *J Med* 1972;3:172-177.

284. Zeidman I, Fiedler IJ. Effect of irradiation on experimental metastases via lymph and blood streams. *J Med* 1970;1:9–14.

285. Fidler IJ, Nicholson GL. Organ selectivity for implantation survival and growth of B16 Melanoma variant tumor lines. *J Natl Cancer* 1976;57:1199–1202.

286. Fidler IJ, Hart IR. Biological diversity in metastatic neoplasms: origins and implications. *Science* 1982;217:998–1003.

287. Stracke M, Liotta L. *Molecular mechanisms of tumor cell metastasis. The molecular basis of cancer*. Philadelphia: W.B. Saunders, 1995:233–247.

288. Folkman J, Shing Y. Angiogenesis. *J Biol Chem* 1992;267:10931–10934.

289. Folkman J, Watson K, Ingber D, et al. Induction of angiogenesis during the transition from hyperplasia to neoplasia. *Nature* 1989;339:58.

290. Valastyan S, Weinberg RA. Tumor metastasis: molecular insights and evolving paradigms. *Cell* 2011;147:275–292.

291. Sneath RJ, Mangham DC. The normal structure and function of CD44 and its role in neoplasia. *Mol Pathol* 1998;51:191.

292. Stetler-Stevenson W, Kleiner D. Molecular biology of cancer: invasion and metastases. In: Devita V Jr, Hellman S, Rosenberg S, eds. *Cancer principles and practice of oncology*. 6th ed. Philadelphia: Lippincott Williams & Wilkins, 2001.

293. Li CY, Shan S, Huang Q, et al. Initial stages of tumor cell-induced angiogenesis: evaluation via skin window chambers in rodent models. *J Natl Cancer Inst* 2000;92(2):143–147.

294. Bracke, ME, van Roy FM, Mareel MM. The E-cadherin/catenin complex in invasion and metastasis. *Curr Top Microbiol Immunol* 1996;213(Pt 1):123.

295. Buck A. Adhesion mechanisms controlling cell-cell and cell-matrix interactions during the metastatic process. In: Mendelsohn J, Howley P, Israel M, eds. *The molecular basis of cancer*. Philadelphia: W.B. Saunders Company, 1995.

296. Hoppe RT, ed. *Patterns of care process study newsletter (Hodgkin's disease), 1990–1991*. Philadelphia: American College of Radiology, 1991.

297. Pawson T. The biochemical mechanisms of oncogene action. In: Bishop JM, Weinberg RA, eds. *Scientific American: molecular oncology*. New York: Scientific American, 1996.

298. Tannock IF. New perspectives in combined radiotherapy and chemotherapy treatment. *Lung Cancer* 1994;10(Suppl 1):29–51.

299. Tannock IF. Potential for therapeutic gain from combined-modality treatment. In: Meyer JL, Vaeth JM, eds. *Frontiers of radiation therapy and oncology. radiotherapy/chemotherapy interactions in cancer therapy*. vol. 26. Basel, Switzerland: Karger, 1992:1–15.

300. Durand RE. The influence of microenvironmental factors on the activity of radiation and drugs. *Int J Radiat Oncol Biol Phys* 1991;20:253–258.

301. Witte L, Fuks Z, Friedman-Himovitz A, et al. Effects of radiation on the release of growth factors from cultured bovine, porcine, and human endothelial cells. *Cancer Res* 1989;49:5066–5072.

302. Kwok TT, Sutherland RM. Enhancement of sensitivity of human squamous carcinoma cells to radiation by epidermal growth factor. *J Natl Cancer Inst* 1989;81:1020–1024.

303. Neta R, Oppenheim JJ, Douches SD. Interdependence of the radioprotective effects of human recombinant interleukin 1 alpha, tumor necrosis factor alpha, granulocyte colony stimulating factor, and murine recombinant granulocyte macrophage colony stimulating factor. *J Immunol* 1988;140:108–111.

304. Carde PL. Effects of cis-dichlorodiammineplatinum (II) and x-rays on mammalian cell survival. *Int J Radiat Oncol Biol Phys* 1981;7:929–933.

305. Kelland LR, Steel GG. Inhibition of recovery from damage induced by ionizing radiation in mammalian cells. *Radiother Oncol* 1988;13:285–299.

306. Saunders MI. Programming of radiotherapy in the treatment of non-small-cell lung cancer—a way to advance cure. *Lancet Oncol* 2001;2(7):401–408.

307. Siemann DW. Interactions between nitrosoureas and x-irradiation. In: Hill BT, Bellamy AS, eds. *Antitumor drug-radiation interactions*. Boca Raton, FL: CRC Press, 1990:141–151.

308. Donaldson SS, Moskowitz PS, Canty EL, et al. Combination radiation-adriamycin therapy: renoprival growth, functional and structural effects in the immature mouse. *Int J Radiat Oncol Biol Phys* 1980;6:851–859.

309. Dritschilo A, Piro AJ, Kelman AD. The effect of cisplatinum on the repair of radiation damage in plateau phase Chinese hamster (V-79) cells. *Int J Radiat Oncol Biol Phys* 1979;5:1345–1349.

310. Korbelik M, Skov KA. Inactivation of hypoxic cells by cisplatin and radiation at clinically relevant doses. *Radiat Res* 1989;119:145–156.

311. Steel GG, Peckham MJ. Exploitable mechanisms in combined radiotherapy-chemotherapy: the concept of additivity. *Int J Radiat Oncol Biol Phys* 1979;5:85–91.

312. Doll R, Peto R. *The causes of cancer: quantitative estimates of avoidable risks of cancer in the United States*. Oxford: Oxford University Press, 1981.

313. McLaughlin JR, Boyd NF. Epidemiology of cancer. In: Tannock IF, Hill RP, eds. *The basic science of oncology*. 3rd ed. New York: McGraw-Hill, 1998:6–25.

314. Costanza ME, Li FP, Finn LM, et al. Cancer prevention: strategies for practice. In: Lenhard RE Jr, Osteen RT, Gansler T, eds. *Clinical oncology*. Atlanta: American Cancer Society, 2001:75–122.

315. Rimer BK, Schildkraut J, Hiatt RA. Cancer screening. In: DeVita VT Jr, Hellman S, Rosenberg SA, eds. *Cancer principles and practice of oncology*. 6th ed. Philadelphia: Lippincott Williams & Wilkins, 2001:575–589.

316. US Preventive Services Task Force. Screening for prostate cancer: US Preventive Services Task Force Recommendation Statement. *JAMA* 2018;319:1901–1913.

317. Mayne ST, Lippman SM. Cancer prevention; diet and chemopreventive agents: retinoids, carotenoids, and micronutrients. In: DeVita VT Jr, Hellman S, Rosenberg SA, eds. *Cancer: principles and practice of oncology*. 6th ed. Philadelphia: Lippincott Williams & Wilkins, 2001:575–589.

318. Anonymous. Report on a workshop to examine methods to arrive at risk estimates for radiation-induced cancer in the human based on laboratory data. *Radiat Res* 1993;135:434–437.

319. Bogni A, Cheng C, Liu W, et al. Genome-wide approach to identify risk factors for therapy-related myeloid leukemia. *Leukemia* 2006;20:239–246.

320. Wiley AL Jr, Vogel HH Jr, Clifton KH. The effect of variations in LET and cell cycle on radiation hepatocarcinogenesis. *Radiat Res* 1973;54:284–293.

321. Kohn HI, Fry RJM. Radiation carcinogenesis. *N Engl J Med* 1984;310:504–511.

322. Haselow RE, Nesbit M, Dehner LP, et al. Second neoplasms following megavoltage radiation in a pediatric population. *Cancer* 1978;42:1185–1191.

323. Potish R, Dehner L, Haselow R, et al. The incidence of second neoplasms following megavoltage radiation for pediatric tumors. *Cancer* 1985;56:1534–1537.

324. Hall EJ, Wuu CS. Radiation-induced second cancers: the impact of 3D-CRT and IMRT. *Int J Radiat Oncol Biol Phys* 2003;56:83–88.

325. Darby SC, Dall R, Gill SK, et al. Long-term mortality after a single treatment course with x-rays in patients treated for ankylosing spondylitis. *Br J Cancer* 1987;55:179–190.

326. Fry SA. Studies of US radium dial workers: an epidemiological classic. *Radiat Res* 1998;150:521–529.

327. Cahan WG, Woodard HQ, Higinbotham ND, et al. Sarcoma arising in irradiated bone: report of eleven cases. *Cancer* 1948;1:3–29.

328. Bogdanich W, Rebelo K. A pinpoint beam strays invisibly, harming instead of healing. *New York Times*. Available at: http://www.nytimes.com/2010/12/29/health/29radiation.html. Accessed November 2, 2011.

329. Inter-Society Council for Radiation Oncology. *Safety is no accident*. Fairfax, VA: American Society for Radiation Oncology, May 2011.

330. *ACR-ASTRO practice guideline for the performance of therapy with unsealed radiopharmaceutical sources*. Available at: http://www.acr.org/SecondaryMainMenuCategories/quality_safety/guidelines/ro/unsealed_radiopharmaceuticals.aspx. Accessed November 2, 2011.

331. Inter-Society Council for Radiation Oncology. *Radiation oncology in integrated cancer management*. Philadelphia: American College of Radiation Oncology, December 1991.

332. Baltista JJ, Clark BG, Patterson MS, et al. Medical physics staffing for radiation oncology: a decade of experience in Ontario, Canada. *J Appl Clin Med Phys* 2012;13:93–110.

333. Kapur A, Potters L. Six sigma tools for a patient safety-oriented, quality checklist driven radiation medicine department. *Pract Radiat Oncol* 2012;2:86–96.

334. *ACR/ASTRO practice guideline for the performance of stereotactic radiosurgery. 2001. Revision approved May 2011.* Available at: http://www.acr.org/SecondaryMainMenuCategories/quality_safety/guidelines/ro/stereotactic_radiosurgery.aspx. Accessed November 2, 2011.

335. *ACR/ASTRO practice guideline for 3D external beam radiation planning and conformal therapy.* 2011. Revision approved May 2011. Available at: http://www.acr.org/SecondaryMainMenuCategories/quality_safety/guidelines/ro/3d_external_beam.aspx. Accessed November 2, 2011.

336. ACR/ASTRO practice guideline for the performance of total body irradiation (TBI). 2011 *Revision approved May 2011.* Available at: http://www.acr.org/SecondaryMainMenuCategories/quality_safety/guidelines/ro/total_body_irradiation.aspx. Accessed November 2, 2011.

337. Agarwal JP, Gupta T, Kalyani N, et al. Cetuximab with radiotherapy in patients with loco-regionally advanced squamous cell carcinoma of the head and neck unsuitable or ineligible for concurrent platinum-based chemo-radiotherapy: ready for routine clinical practice? *Indian J Cancer* 2011;48:148–153.

338. Hartford AC, Kavanagh B, Beyer DC, et al. ASTRO and ACR practice guideline for intensity modulated radiation therapy (IMRT). *Int J Radiat Oncol Biol Phys* 2009;73:9–14.

339. Nath R, Anderson LL, Meli JA, et al. Code of practice for brachytherapy physics: report of the AAPM Radiation Therapy Committee Task Group No. 56. *Med Phys* 1997;24:1557–1598.

340. Erickson BA, Demanes DJ, Ibbott GS, et al. American Society for Radiation Oncology (ASTRO) and American College of Radiology (ACR) practice guidelines for the performance of high-dose-rate (HDR) brachytherapy. *Int J Radiat Oncol Biol Phys* 2011;79:641–649.

341. Nath R, Bice WS, Butler WM, et al. AAPM recommendations on dose prescription and reporting methods for permanent interstitial brachytherapy for prostate cancer: report of Task Group 137. *Med Phys* 2009;36:5310–5322.

342. Thomadsen BR, Erickson BA, Eifel PJ, et al. ASTRO white paper: the status of high dose-rate brachytherapy practice guidance. *Practical Radiat Oncol* 2012. Available at: www.astro.org/uploadedFiles/content/clinical-practice/ASTRO%20HDR%20white%20paper%20v19b.pdf

343. Viswanathan AN, Beriwal S, Los Santos JD, et al. The American Brachytherapy Society treatment recommendations for locally advanced carcinoma of the cervix. Part II: high dose-rate brachytherapy. *Brachytherapy* 2012;11:47–52.

344. Viswanathan AN, Thomadsen BR; for the ABS Cervical Cancer Guidelines Writing Committee. The American Brachytherapy Society treatment recommendations for locally advanced carcinoma of the cervix. Part I: general principles. *Brachytherapy* 2012;11:33–46.

345. Yamada Y, Rogers L, Demanes J, et al. American Brachytherapy Society guidelines for high-dose-rate prostate brachytherapy. *Brachytherapy* 2012;11:20–32.

346. Richards EP, Rathbun KC. *Law and the physician: a practical guide.* Boston, MA: Little, Brown and Company, 1993.

347. Liang BA. *Health law and policy: a survival guide to medicolegal issues for practitioners.* Boston, MA: Butterworth Heinemann, 2000.

348. Blackman NS, Bailey CP. *Liability in medical practice: a reference for physicians.* Chur, Switzerland: Harwood Academic Publishers, 1990.

349. Anonymous. Duty to consult. *JAMA* 1973;226:111.

350. Anonymous. Duty to refer patient to medical specialist. *JAMA* 1968;204:281.

351. Prives C. Doing the right thing: feedback control and p53. *Curr Opin Cell Biol* 1993;5:214.

352. Horn C III, Caldwell DH Jr, Osborn DC. *Law for physicians: an overview of medical legal issues.* Chicago, IL: American Medical Association, 2002.

353. Anonymous. Radiation therapy. *JAMA* 1972;220:1807.

354. *Antowill v. Friedman N,* 188 NYS 777 NY, 1921.

355. *Runyan v. Goodrum,* 228 SW 397 Ark 1921.

356. *Wilkinson v. Harrington,* 243 A 2d, 745 RI, 1968.

357. *Costa v. Regents of the University of California,* 254 P 2d 85 Cal, 1953.

358. *Waddle v. Sutherland,* 126 SO 201 Miss, 1930.

359. Barnett GH. Evolution and organization of a regional Gamma Knife center. *Stereotactic Funct Neurosurg* 1996;66(Suppl 1):365–369.

360. *Martin v. Eschelman,* 33 SW 2d 827 Tex, 1930.

361. *Emrie v. Tice,* 258 P Td 332, Kans, 1953.

362. *Gross v. Robinson,* 218 SW 924, Mo, 1920.

363. *Holland v. Sisters of St. Joseph of Peace,* 552 P Td 208, Ore, 1974.

364. *Ahern v. Veterans' Administration,* 537 F 2d 1098, CCA 10 NM, 1976.

365. Berlin L. Malpractice issues in radiology: liability when covering for another radiation oncologist. *Am J Roent* 1999;172:1189–1192.

366. Sherman NE, Rich TA, Peters LJ. Professional liability in radiotherapy: experience of the Fletcher Society. *Int J Radiat Oncol Biol Phys* 1991;20:563–566.

367. Halperin, EC, Insurance and malpractice disputes in radiation oncology. *Am J Clin Oncol* 2009;32:452–435.

368. Marshall D, Tringalek, Connor M, Punglia R, Recht A, Hahangadi-Gluth J. Nature of medical malpractice claims against radiation oncologists. *Int J Radiat Oncol Biol Phys* 2017;98:21–30.

369. National Association for Insurance Commissioners. *NAIC malpractice claims, 1975–79: final compilation,* vol. 2, no. 2, Brookfield, WI, 1980.

370. *Bennett v. Los Angeles Tumor Institute,* 227 P 2d 473 Cal, 1951.

371. Halperin EC. Formal grievances directed against physicians. *Western Med J* 2000;173:235–238.

372. Vincent C, Young M, Phillips A. Why do people sue doctors? A study of patients and relative taking legal action. *Lancet* 1974;343:1609–1613.

373. Localio AR, Lawthers AG, Brennan TA, et al. Relation between malpractice claims and adverse events due to negligence: results of the Harvard Medical Practice study III. *N Engl J Med* 1991;325:245–251.

374. Dische S, Joslin CA, Miller S. The RAGE litigation. *Lancet* 1998;351:1967–1968.

375. Millington J. Breast radiation injury litigation and RAGE. *Clin Oncol (R Col Radiol)* 1999;11:137–138.

376. Reuter SR. An overview of informed consent for radiologists. *AJR Am J Roentgenol* 1987;148:219–227.

377. Annas GJ. Informed consent, cancer, and truth in prognosis. *N Engl J Med* 1994;330:223–225.

378. Cohen L. Clinical radiation dosage, Part II. Interrelation of time, area and therapeutic ratio. *Br J Radiol* 1949;22:706–713.

379. Ellis F. Time and dose relationships in radiation biology as applied to radiotherapy. Brookhaven National Laboratory. *BNL* 1969;50203(C-57):313.

380. Orton CG. Time-dose factors (TDFs) in brachytherapy. *Br J Radiol* 1974;47:603–607.

381. Atwood KC. Norman A on the interpretation of multi-hit survival curves. *Proc Natl Acad Sci U S A* 1949;35:696—709.

382. Dawson LA, Brock KK, Kazanjania S, et al. The reproducibility of organ position using active breathing control (ABC) during liver radiotherapy. *Int J Radiat Oncol Biol Phys* 2001;51:1410–1421.

383. Horsman MR. Realistic biological approaches for improving thermoradiotherapy. *Int J Hyperthermia* 2016;32(1):14–22.

384. Elkind MM, Sutton-Gilbert H, Moses VB, Alescio T, Swain RW. Radiosensitivity of mammalian cells grown in culture. Temperature dependence of the repair of X-ray damage in surviving cells (aerobic and hypoxic). *Radiat Res* 1965;25:359–376.

385. Namiya T. Discussions on target theory: past and present. *J Radiat Res* 2013;54:1161–1163.

386. Rabinowitz I, Broomberg J, Goitein M, et al. Accuracy of radiation field alignment in clinical practice. *Int J Radiat Oncol Biol Phys* 1985;11:1857–1867.

387. Risch HA, Jain M, Choi NW, et al. Dietary factors and the incidence of cancer of the stomach. *Am J Epidemiol* 1985;122:947–959.

388. Wynder EL, Graham EA. Tobacco smoking as a possible etiologic factor in bronchogenic carcinoma: a study of 684 proved cases. *JAMA* 1950;143:329–336.

389. Wallner K, Elliott K. Malpractice in radiation oncology: redefining the role of the medical expert in regard to Kagan. *Int J Radiat Oncol Biol Phys* 2005;62:1254–1255.

390. Varmus H, Weinberg RA. *Genes and the biology of cancer.* New York: Scientific American Library, 1993.

391. Varmus HE. The molecular genetics of cellular oncogenes. *Ann Rev Genet* 1984;18:553–612.

392. Weinberg RA. Tumor suppressor genes. *Science* 1991;254:1138–1146.

393. Weinberg RA, Hanahan D. The molecular pathogenesis of cancer. In: Bishop JM, Weinberg RA, eds. *Scientific American: molecular oncology.* New York: Scientific American, 1996.

394. Weichselbaum RR, Little JB. Radioresistance in some human tumor cells conferred in vitro by repair of potentially lethal x-ray damage. *Radiology* 1982;145:511–513.

395. Zeman EM, Brown JM. Aerobic radiosensitization by SR 4233 in rodent and human cell lines: mechanistic and therapeutic implications. *Int J Radiat Oncol Biol Phys* 1991;59:117–131.

396. Bacq ZM, Alexander P. *Fundamentals of radiobiology.* Completely revised second edition. New York: The MacMillan Company, Pergamon Press, 1961.

397. Chang K. Dr. Alfred G. Knudson, the 'Mendel of Cancer Genetics,' dies at 93. *NY Times* 2016.

398. Namiya T. Discussions on target theory: past and present. *J Radiol Res* 2013;54:1161–1163.

399. Suit HD. Radiation biology, a basis for radiotherapy. In Fletcher GH. *Textbook of radiotherapy.* Philadelphia, PA: Lea and Febiger, 1966:65–96.

400. Bodgi L, Canet A, Pujo-Menjouet L, et al. Mathematical models of radiation action on living cells: from the target theory to modern approaches. A historical and critical review. *J Theor Biol* 2016;364:93–101.

401. Withers HR, Peters LJ. Biologic aspects of radiotherapy. In: Fletcher GH. *Textbook of radiotherapy.* 3rd edition. Philadelphia: Lea and Febiger, 1980:103–180.

CHAPTER 2

Molecular Cancer and Radiation Biology

Michael Baumann, Ina Kurth, Nils Cordes, Mechthild Krause, and Annett Linge

During the last three decades, molecular cancer research has become a rapidly growing branch of the biomedical sciences. Many advances in our understanding of cancer are closely related to innovations in biotechnology—for example, gene editing techniques to modify the specific gene of interest, experimental maneuvers to manipulate temporal and spatial gene expression, the utilization of high-throughput methods to study the entire genome and proteome of cancer cells, and a vastly growing methodology to specifically interfere with signal transduction. Because of the rapidly expanding knowledge in molecular cancer and radiation biology, this chapter can only provide an introductory overview on selected topics.*Cell biology* approaches contribute to modern radiobiology and help to better understand effects of ionizing radiation on cells, tumors, and normal tissues. Knowledge in molecular cancer biology is important for clinical decision-making in oncology and the development of novel biology-driven strategies in the multidisciplinary clinical environment.[1-4] *Molecular pathology* of tumors increasingly supplements classic histopathology and immunohistochemistry, thereby providing the basis for improved treatment stratification in oncology.[5-7] *Molecular pathophysiology* describes mechanisms leading to a characteristic microenvironment of tumors or that eventually manifest radiation sequelae in normal tissues.[8] *Molecular imaging* has become important not only for staging but also for biologic characterization of tumors and for determination of target volumes in radiation oncology, including approaches such as dose painting.[9-12] *Molecular targeting* in radiotherapy may either increase the tumor response or protect normal tissues, thereby enhancing the therapeutic gain of the treatment.[13-17]Radiotherapy appears to be particularly promising to integrate molecular targeting approaches.[15,17] First, the radiobiologic mechanisms of the response of tumors and normal tissues to radiotherapy are well characterized, and the molecular pathways involved in these responses are increasingly known. Second, similar to conventional chemotherapeutic drugs, the novel drugs developed are not necessarily curative by themselves. In contrast, radiotherapy in itself is extremely efficient in eradicating cancer stem cells (CSCs), and recurrences often occur from only one or a few surviving CSCs.[18-20] Thus, even if novel drugs have the potential to kill only a limited number of CSCs, this might be sufficient to increase local control when combined with radiotherapy. The same argument applies when these drugs increase the radiosensitivity of tumor cells or when normal tissues are specifically protected. Third, in contrast to systemic chemotherapy, radiotherapy can be modulated in dose, time, and space. This allows individual tailoring of the effects of combined treatments in consideration of the spatial distribution of CSC burden as well as with consideration of normal tissues. Preclinical data and early clinical results corroborate these arguments[18,19,21-26] and support further translational research on biologically enhanced radiotherapy.

THE HALLMARKS OF CANCER

During carcinogenesis, neoplastic cells are gaining several biologic capabilities, which enable tumor growth and metastatic dissemination. Molecular biology of cancer can be summarized by a simplified concept based on a small number of underlying principles. In their seminal articles, Hanahan and Weinberg described these principles, which are being shared by most human tumor types, as the six core "*hallmarks of cancer,*" as well as "*emerging hallmarks*" and "*enabling characteristics*" facilitating tumor promotion.[27,28] These hallmarks are the consequence of specific genetic alterations or modifications in important oncogenes and tumor suppressor genes and are briefly outlined below.

Sustaining Proliferative Signaling

Mitogenic signals from growth factors, cytokines, extracellular matrix, and cell–cell adhesion molecules are transferred into the cell by different classes of transmembrane receptors.[27,28] Malignant cells acquire the capability to escape from the tightly regulated dependence on extracellular growth signals. The molecular mechanisms include overexpression of growth factors as well as growth factor receptors (autocrine and paracrine stimulation), receptor mutations leading to constitutive receptor activation without ligand binding, and molecular aberrations in the intracellular signal transduction pathways.[27,28]

Evading Growth Suppressors

Normal cell division is tightly regulated by stimulatory and inhibitory growth signals. Growth signaling involves interaction of diffusible growth factors or cytokines with transmembrane receptors, as well as regulation of growth by components of the extracellular matrix and by cell–cell interactions. Once a resting cell receives a sufficient growth stimulus, it enters the cell cycle by passing the restriction point and four distinct phases of cytokinesis and mitogenesis: gap-1 (G1), deoxyribonucleic acid (DNA) synthesis (S), gap-2 (G2), and mitosis (M).[29] The passage through the restriction point and the entry into S and M (G1/S and G2/M checkpoints) are governed by several proto-oncogenes and tumor suppressor genes such as *TP53* and *RB1* encoding for p53 and the retinoblastoma protein (pRb), respectively (Fig. 2.1).[27,28,30,31] Inactivation of tumor suppressor genes by genetic mutations or epigenetic mechanisms will ultimately lead to sustained cell proliferation.[27,32-34]

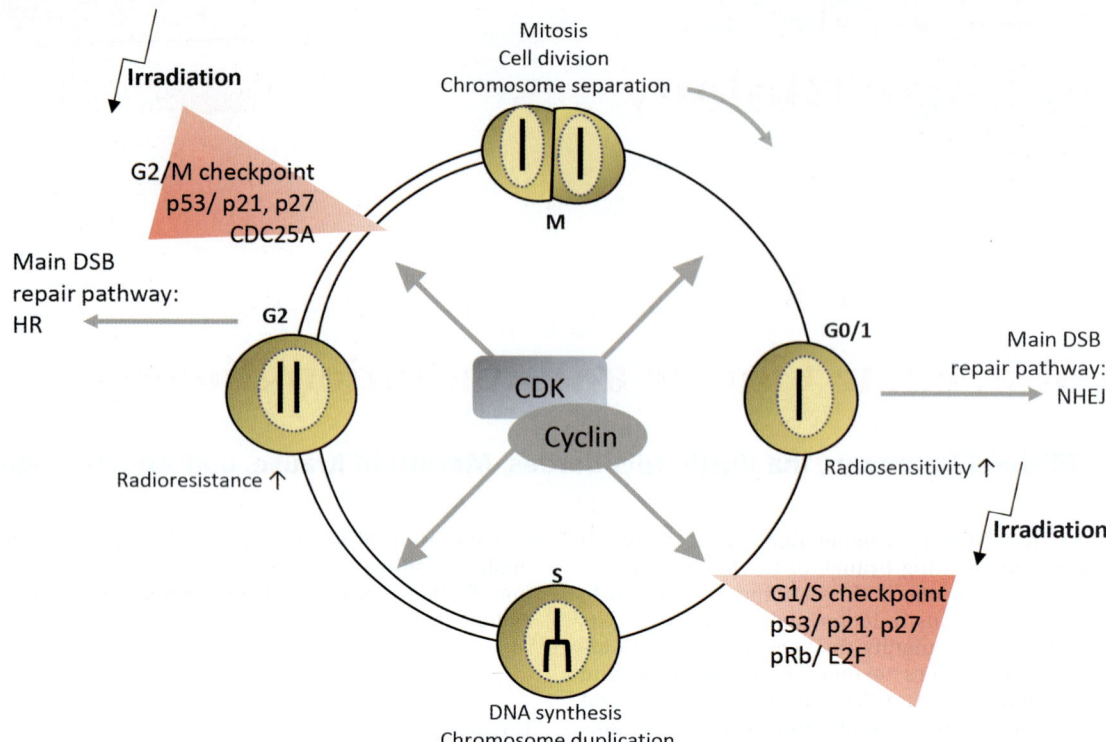

FIGURE 2.1. Cell cycle and checkpoints. The cell cycle is the backbone process that facilitates duplication of the DNA and cell division in order to generate two daughter cells. The distinct phases of the cell cycle are differently susceptible to irradiation damage. The highest radiation sensitivity is in early S and late G2/M phase. The cell cycle checkpoints in Gap 1 (G1) and Gap 2 phase ensure that the cell is ready for DNA synthesis (S-phase) or mitosis (M). If the DNA is damaged, the cell stops cycling and either the damage will get repaired and the cell continues with the cycle or the cell undergoes apoptosis and dies. Many types of cancer arise from mutations that lead to checkpoint misregulation or skipping of those. Cell cycle progression is governed by various cyclins and cyclin-dependent kinases (CDKs). Different cyclin–CDK complexes determine targeted downstream proteins that for example promote DNA replication and degrade S-phase inhibitors. NHEJ, nonhomologous end joining.

Activating Invasion and Metastasis

Locoregional and distant spread of tumor cells requires detachment from the primary tumor, invasion into surrounding tissues, intravasation into blood or lymphatic vessels, anoikis resistance, adhesion to endothelial cells at distant sites, extravasation, and eventually colonization in distant organs.[28,35] The acquired capability of cancer cells to grow invasively and to metastasize is associated with multiple genetic and biochemical alterations of the cell–cell and cell–matrix interactions.[27,28] Tissue invasion and metastasis require, at different steps, contrary capabilities—for example, detachment from the primary tumor versus adhesion at the metastatic site—suggesting that rapid adaptations, genetic instability, and clonal selection play an important role.[35] Also, the intratumoral microenvironment plays a key role; for example, hypoxia is described as one possible activator of metastasis.[36] In order to effectively metastasize, several critical steps are necessary, which involve epithelial to mesenchymal transition (EMT), extracellular matrix modulation, intravasation, circulation, extravasation, homing, forming the premetastatic niche for organotropic colonization and mesenchymal–epithelial transition (MET).[37,38]

Enabling Replicative Immortality

Loss of growth control and resistance to cell death are not sufficient for the development of macroscopic tumors. Normal cells have the capacity for a finite number of cell divisions, which results in a limited replicative potential. Thereafter, either cells stop proliferating and enter the process of senescence, which is a viable but nonproliferative state, or they die.[28,39] During tumorigenesis, some premalignant cells become immortal by circumventing senescence, that is, by acquiring a capability of limitless replicative potential.[27,28] Of importance, malignant tumors consist of heterogeneous populations differing in their replicative potential. Although most cancer cells have a limited replicative

potential, a small subpopulation (i.e., CSCs) have an infinite replicative capacity and the capability to reconstitute the tumor.[40] Thus, this subpopulation represents the target for curative cancer therapy, that is, all of these stem cells have to be inactivated by therapy or by host-related mechanisms to achieve cure.[18] It remains to be clarified whether CSCs represent distinct tumor cell subpopulations or whether they can switch between different stages in response to stress or environmental conditions.[41–43]

The molecular mechanisms underlying the escape from senescence and other modes of cell death include loss of tumor suppressor proteins such as p53 and pRB as well as telomere maintenance.[28] Telomeres are chromatin segments located at the ends of the chromosomes that protect these regions from recombination and degradation.[44] As telomeres are incompletely replicated, they become progressively shorter during cell divisions, subsequently resulting in loss of chromosomal protection, which in turn triggers senescence. Cancer cells generally have shorter telomeres than do normal cells but are able to perpetuate their replicative potential by expressing telomerase, a complex including DNA polymerase, which reconstitutes the telomeres.[44]

Inducing Angiogenesis

To grow beyond microscopically sized cell aggregates of around 1 mm, tumors depend on angiogenesis. Proliferating cells require appropriate oxygen and nutrient supply, which is physiologically limited to a distance of 100 to 200 μm from the next blood vessel. Therefore, malignant cells must induce and sustain their own vascular system to form tumors and metastases.[45] The process of the *angiogenic switch* during tumorigenesis (i.e., the transition from the avascular phase to the vascular stage) is governed by different molecular changes in tumor cells and in cells of the surrounding stroma.[27,28,46] The major event of the angiogenic switch is that proangiogenic factors—mostly growth factors such as vascular endothelial growth factors (VEGFs), fibroblast growth factors, and

TABLE 2.1 TYPES OF RADIATION-INDUCED CELL DEATH AND THEIR CHARACTERISTICS

Type of Cell Death	Important Morphologic Characteristics	Important Molecular Mechanisms
Mitotic catastrophe	During or after mitosis, missegregation of chromosomes, cell fusion, micronuclei, giant cell formation	Lethal chromosome damage, caspase independent
Apoptosis	Chromatin condensation, nuclear fragmentation, blebbing of cell membrane	Damage to DNA, and/or membranes, and/or alterations of intracellular signaling, caspase dependent (intrinsic pathway via caspase 9)
Senescence	Metabolically active but nondividing, functionally differentiated cells	Damage to DNA and/or alterations of intracellular signaling, generally p53-dependent terminal growth arrest, increased senescence-associated β galactosidase
Autophagy	Partial chromatin condensation, cell membrane blebbing, increased number of autophagic vesicles	Protein degradation characterized by double-membrane vesicles in the cytoplasm, possibly related to DNA protein kinase (DNA-PK) activity
Necroptosis	Early plasma membrane permeabilization, translucent cytosol, swollen mitochondria	Damage to DNA, and/or membranes, and/or alterations of intracellular signaling, caspase independent
Necrosis	Increased vacuolation, swelling of organelles and cells, rupture of cell membranes, formation of necrotic mass	Unregulated traumatic cell destruction; after irradiation as consequence of, for example, mitotic catastrophe or vascular damage

Adapted from Brown JM, Wouters BG. Apoptosis, p53, and tumor cell sensitivity to anticancer agents. *Cancer Res* 1999;59:1391–1399; Okada H, Mak TW. Pathways of apoptotic and non-apoptotic death in tumour cells. *Nat Rev Cancer* 2004;4(8):592–603.

platelet-derived growth factors (PDGFs)—outbalance anti-angiogenic factors, such as thrombospondin (*TSP-1*), *angiostatin*, and *endostatin*. Hypoxia promotes tumor angiogenesis via the hypoxia inducible factor 1, which transcriptionally regulates many angiogenic molecules.[47,48]

Resisting Cell Death

Under physiologic conditions, tissue homeostasis results from the balance of cell division and cell loss. This balance is disturbed in most tumors by an increased cell division rate due to the molecular mechanisms previously described and by a reduced rate of cell death, such as by apoptosis and senescence[27,28,49,50] (Table 2.1).

Deregulating Cellular Energetics and Metabolism

The sustained cell proliferation of cancer cells requires modifications and adjustments to their energy metabolism.[28] Under aerobic conditions, normal cells are processing glucose to pyruvate, and only under anaerobic conditions they are switching to glycolysis. Cancer cells were shown to favor glycolysis, also under aerobic conditions, and this has been termed "aerobic glycolysis" or Warburg effect.[28,51–53] Glutamine and lactate have also been shown to serve as metabolic fuel in cancer cells.[54–56] The deregulated cellular metabolism is an "emerging hallmark," because it is significantly independent from the main (initial) hallmarks.[28]

Evading Immune Destruction

During the development of cancer, antitumor responses are presenting a barrier that has to be overcome. The exact engagement of the immune system still remains to be determined and is therefore being referred to as an emerging hallmark.[28] It has been shown that many types of tumors utilize different strategies to evade immune destruction. Tumor cells change, for example, surface expression of antigens renders them invisible to cytotoxic T cells, or secrete immunity inhibitory proteins.[57]

Tumor-Promoting Inflammation

Immune cell infiltration can be seen in most neoplastic tissues, but to a varying extent.[58] Inflammation has been shown to be involved in a number of hallmark capabilities by supplying growth and survival factors, proangiogenic factors, and extracellular matrix–modifying enzymes.[28,59–61] Furthermore, inflammation can drive the progression of cancers from incipient neoplasias.[28,61] The release of reactive oxygen species (ROS) can also act mutagenic in surrounding cancer cells.[28,60] However, the immune system is also capable of evoking an antitumor response.[62]

Genome Instability and Mutation

Genomic alterations or modifications of neoplastic cells are largely necessary to acquire the hallmarks outlined above.

During tumor progression, mutations and epigenetic modifications but also nonmutational gene expression changes are leading to the accumulation of more favorable genotypes and clonal expansion of cells.[28] The identification of driver mutations leading to malignant progression is important also in terms of therapeutic targeting. For the detection of epigenomic changes, more comprehensive analyses such as histone modifications and DNA methylation are necessary.[28,63]

PRINCIPLES OF MOLECULAR CANCER BIOLOGY

Carcinogenesis describes the transformation of normal cells into cancer cells and the subsequent development of a tumor. This multistep process includes accumulating changes on the cellular, genetic, and epigenetic level and is also characterized by abnormal cellular proliferation. However, these changes can differ between tumor cells within the same tumor leading to intratumoral heterogeneity and also between patients causing intertumoral heterogeneity.

Genetic changes include point mutation, deletion, insertion, gene amplification, chromosomal instability, loss of heterozygosity, and translocation. Silencing of tumor suppressor genes by promoter hypermethylation, histone modifications, and microRNA (noncoding RNA) expression represents important epigenetic mechanisms of tumorigenesis.[32,34,64] Chemical agents, radiation, and errors during DNA replication and also infection with oncogenic viruses can contribute to the development of human cancer (e.g., human papillomaviruses [HPVs] in cervical or head and neck cancer, hepatitis B viruses in hepatocellular carcinoma, and human immunodeficiency viruses in Kaposi sarcoma).[65,66] The hostile micromilieu in solid tumors, particularly hypoxia, further promotes progressive genomic alterations and clonal selection.[67] Consequently, cells gain advantage in proliferation and survival, which eventually results in malignant transformation, a prerequisite for the development of cancer and metastatic spread.

Conceptually, two classes of cancer genes can be distinguished. First, *oncogenes* are activated in cancer cells by genetic alterations resulting in a gain of function. Mutations in proto-oncogenes acting in a dominant fashion (i.e., a genetic alteration in one of the alleles) are sufficient for gene activation. Typical oncogene functions are stimulation of cell proliferation (e.g., by activation of Ras) and increase in cell survival (e.g., by activation of PI3K/Akt signaling). Disorders in the second class of cancer genes, *tumor suppressor genes*, cause a loss of function. Mutations in one allele of a tumor suppressor gene are recessive because they can be functionally compensated by the second, nonmutated (wild-type) allele. Although some cancers can be attributed to single genetic alterations, most sporadic solid tumors exhibit a wide range of disorders in numerous cancer genes. Simplified mathematical modeling of the increasing incidence of common cancers as a function of age suggests that four to seven somatic gene alterations are required for carcinogenesis.[68,69] A typical example for multistep tumorigenesis is the adenoma–carcinoma sequence in colorectal cancer.[70]

Inherited cancer predisposition can be divided into the rare group of inherited cancer syndromes and familial cancers (strong predisposition) and the more frequent group of predisposition without evident family clustering (weak predisposition).[71] The first group includes syndromes caused by germ-line mutations affecting DNA repair, genomic stability, and cell cycle control, for example, *TP53* (Li-Fraumeni syndrome), nucleotide excision repair genes (xeroderma pigmentosum), *ATM* (ataxia telangiectasia), DNA mismatch repair genes (hereditary non-polyposis colorectal cancer), and *BRCA 1/2* (familial breast cancer). An example of a familial cancer syndrome related to oncogene activation is neurofibromatosis type I, in which the mutated *NF1* gene results in activation of the Ras oncogene.[71] Germline mutations causing inactivation of the cell–cell adhesion molecule E-cadherin can be found, for example, in familial diffuse gastric carcinoma.[72] A debate is ongoing on the question how close the risk of cancer depends on the number of normal stem cell divisions in contrast to the influence of environmental factors.[73,74] This issue is highly relevant for public health considerations as it points to the "bad luck" hypothesis versus a cancer risk importantly effected by external influences.

MOLECULAR RADIATION BIOLOGY

Biologic Consequences of Irradiation

The effects of ionizing radiation on cellular target molecules may lead to various functional consequences. These functional effects can be broadly categorized into cell death, repair, cell cycle effects, altered gene expression, modification of signal transduction, mutagenesis, and genomic instability (Fig. 2.2). These categories are not exclusive.

Cell Death

Among the functional consequences of ionizing radiation, cell death is the most important one for radiation oncology. Cells

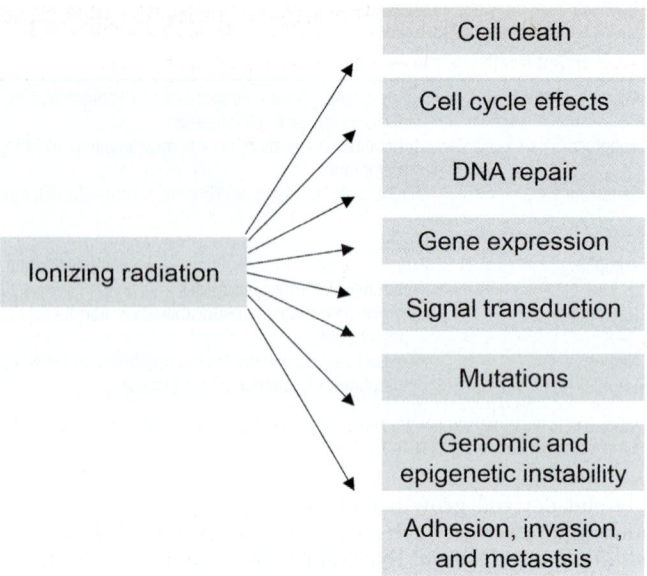

FIGURE 2.2. Illustration of cellular effects upon ionizing radiation.

can die in several ways[75]—by apoptosis, mitotic catastrophe, senescence, necrosis, necroptosis, and autophagy (Fig. 2.3; Table 2.1). Most important for the effect of radiotherapy of solid tumors is the *mitotic catastrophe*, which is caused by lethal chromosome damage.[76] After irradiation, cells can pass through one or few mitotic cycles before missegregation of chromosomes or cell fusion leads to the loss of their replicative potential (or clonogenicity). Often micronuclei, containing nonrepaired chromosome fragments, can be detected. Those micronuclei, and hence essential genetic information, will be lost during the following cell cycle, which results in cell death. Frequent multinucleate giant cells reflect a radiation-induced failure of cytoplasmatic separation on cell division.

Neoplastic hematopoietic or lymphatic cells often die from radiation-induced *apoptosis* via the intrinsic, caspase 9–dependent pathway. Two different forms of radiation-induced

FIGURE 2.3. Simplified illustration of cellular ROS effects. The generation of reactive oxygen species (ROS) causes DNA and non-DNA damage and results in different cellular effects.

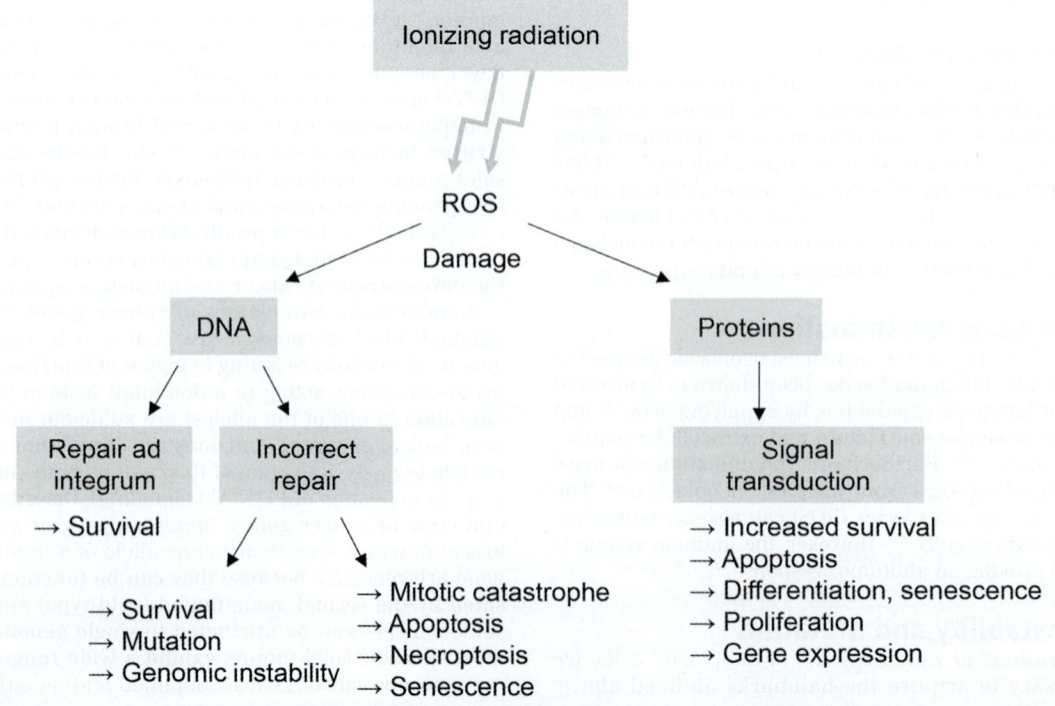

apoptosis can be distinguished—early or premitotic versus late or postmitotic apoptosis.[77] Early apoptosis is p53 dependent, occurs within few hours after irradiation before the cells enter mitosis, and is primarily a consequence of DNA damage. Early apoptosis represents a distinct mode of radiation-induced cell death. In contrast, secondary apoptosis occurs after mitosis and is one of several possible manifestations of radiation-induced lethal chromosome aberrations. In most cancers, particularly in solid tumors, apoptosis appears not to be the main mechanism of radiation-induced cell death.[78] No clear evidence exists that either apoptotic index or levels of p53, Bcl-2, or other Bcl-2 family members are predictive of the response of solid tumors to radiotherapy. For example, overexpression of Bcl-2 was shown to significantly decrease the apoptotic fraction in response to irradiation. However, this did not translate into a change of clonogenic cell survival after irradiation.[79]

Radiation-induced *senescence* plays an important role for development of normal tissue damage—for example, fibrosis[80]—but occurs also in response to nonlethal stress as in tumor cells.[81] Cells survive and are metabolically active but lose their replicative potential. *Necrosis* is an unregulated process of cell destruction by the release of intracellular components. This is usually the consequence of pathophysiologic conditions such as ischemia and inflammation.[75] It is well known that tumors often show massive necrosis after neoadjuvant radiotherapy or radiochemotherapy, which in some tumors correlates with improved prognosis.[82,83] It is likely that this radiation-induced necrosis is explained by several factors, including mitotic catastrophe of tumor cells and the effects of irradiation on tumor vessels leading to changes in the microenvironment, which consequently cause cell death.

Necroptosis, the prototype of regulated necrosis, is a caspase-independent form of programmed cell death and kills apoptosis-deficient cells. It is stimulated by death receptor ligands of the tumor necrosis factor receptor subfamily such as TNF-alpha (TNF-α), CD95 ligand, or tumor necrosis factor–related apoptosis-inducing ligand (TRAIL), but also by other receptors such as ectodermal dysplasia receptor.[84] Necroptosis can also be induced by other stress-inducing factors such as ionizing radiation, DNA-damaging agents, as well as ROS.[85] Recent experimental data show that knockout of necroptotic genes leads to significantly enhanced radiosensitivity and reduces tumor formation in mice.[86] Other reported forms of regulated necrosis are ferroptosis, oxytosis, ETosis, NETosis, cyclophilin D (CYPD)-mediated regulated necrosis, parthanatos, pyroptosis, and pyronecrosis.[85]

Autophagy is a form of nonapoptotic and nonnecrotic cell death that is related to lysosomal degradation of proteins and cell organelles that are then utilized for the production of new cells.[75] This mode of programmed cell death is triggered by growth factor withdrawal, differentiation, and developmental stimuli. Although the molecular regulation is not completely understood, data suggest that a high rate of autophagy contributes to radiation resistance and that autophagy is regulated through different hypoxia-dependent pathways, thereby facilitating survival during metabolic stress.[87,88]

Target Molecules of Radiation Damage

Radiation effects may occur as direct ionizations in an organic molecule or indirectly via free radical processes. As cells consist mostly of water, most ionizations produced by irradiation occur in water molecules. Within only 10^{-10} seconds, radiolysis of water leads, among other entities, to e^-aq, H·, and OH·. About 60% to 70% of cellular DNA damage produced by ionizing radiation is caused by OH·.[89] The radiation-induced ROS undergo further reactions—for example, production of H_2O_2 from two hydroxyl radicals. Aerobes have evolved antioxidant defenses to protect themselves against the oxygen-derived species generated *in vivo* or from external sources. These defenses include enzymes (such as superoxide dismutases, catalase, and glutathione peroxidase), low molecular mass agents (such as α-tocopherol and ascorbic acid), and proteins that bind metal ions in forms unable to catalyze the generation of free radicals. In contrast to those defensive mechanisms, the oxygen molecule has a high affinity to free radicals, which may give rise to further cascades of radical production and thereby to the fixation of free radical damage to important macromolecules of the cell (e.g., DNA). This is one explanation of the oxygen effect of radiation damage, that is, the fact that well-oxygenated cells are more radiosensitive than are hypoxic cells.[90,91]

By far the most important target for the biologic effects of ionizing radiation is the DNA (Fig. 2.3). This is obvious for the induction of mutations but has also been consistently demonstrated for the killing of cells in a number of different experiments. Irradiation of the cytoplasm of cells with short-range α-particles only leads to cell kill at very high doses, whereas 1,000-fold lower doses to the nucleus are sufficient to kill the cell.[92] Radioactive isotopes with short-range emission effectively kill cells when incorporated into the DNA but not when predominantly incorporated in cell membranes.[93] Modification of radiation-induced cell kill by different measures, including hypoxia, high–linear energy transfer radiation, or hyperthermia, is linked closely with a change in the induction and repair of DNA double-strand breaks (DSBs). Exposure of cells to about 1 Gy causes approximately 3,500 DNA injuries, 1,500 to 2,500 of which are damaged bases, 1,000 single-strand breaks (SSBs), 40 DSBs, and an estimated 100 to 200 local multiple-damaged sites, where one or several DSBs occur in close proximity to SSBs and base damage.[94] Most radiation-induced DNA damage is recognized and very efficiently repaired by the cell (*vide infra*). Importantly, it also has to be considered that different types of radiation treatment can cause different extent of damage to the DNA in a tumor cell. In contrast to photon therapy, particle therapy causes more severe DNA damage.[95]

Besides effects on DNA, ionizing radiation also evokes biologically important responses on proteins (e.g., transmembrane receptors) and on lipids (e.g., ceramides) (Fig. 2.3). Radiation-induced activation of receptors will be discussed later in this chapter. Ionizing irradiation induces rapid sphingomyelin hydrolysis by acid sphingomyelinase to generate ceramide, an inductor of apoptosis.[96]

Recognition of Radiation-Induced DNA Damage

DNA damage, in particular DSBs, is sensed by different proteins that trigger an ataxia telangiectasia–mutated (ATM)–dependent or, in some cases, ataxia telangiectasia and Rad3-related (ATR)–dependent signaling cascade (Fig. 2.4).[97] ATM activation requires the telomeric protein TRF2 and the MRN complex consisting of Rad50, meiotic recombination protein 11 (Mre11), Nijmegen breakage syndrome protein 1 (NBS1), mediator of DNA damage checkpoint protein-1 (MDC1), and 53BP1.[98] In addition to proper activation of downstream DNA repair proteins, histone H2AX molecules need to be phosphorylated in the vicinity of the DSB. All of these proteins assemble at the site of the breaks and presumably control the choice of one of several repair pathways. In addition to its role in repair, ATM is involved in the regulation of multiple cell cycle checkpoints (G1/S, S, G2/M) after DNA damage.[99] ATM, ATR, and DNA-dependent protein kinase catalytic subunit (DNA-PK$_{CS}$) phosphorylate p53 and a number of proteins involved in cell cycle delay, apoptosis, and induction of DNA repair. ATR appears to be important for sensing ultraviolet-related and other types of bulky lesions, as well as damage that induces a replication block, whereas ATM seems to be the sensor for DSB induced by ionizing radiation.[97] ATR may serve in some cases as a backup for ATM.

DNA Repair

Genome integrity is essential to the survival of cells and organisms. It is estimated that about 10^4 DNA lesions occur in a single human cell every day.[100] Most of the damage is caused by endogenous sources such as oxygen free radicals, replicative errors, and spontaneous deaminations. To cope with the plethora of permanent damage, a repair system was developed during evolution that also acts on external challenges such as radiation or chemical DNA damage. To enable repair of massive DNA damage, the cells stop proliferation. This may prevent replication or segregation of damaged genetic material. If repair is not possible, the cells either die or, in case of survival, may propagate mutated DNA (Fig. 2.4). When the DNA replication machinery meets damaged DNA, replication may continue despite the damage by translesion synthesis, which requires DNA polymerase with low fidelity. Different mechanisms are involved in DNA repair.[97,101]

Base Excision Repair

The mechanism of base excision repair (BER) is responsible for the repair of various kinds of base damage (abasic sites, oxidized bases, deaminated bases, and alkylated bases) and SSB. Base damages and SSB are the most frequent types of DNA damage after irradiation.[102,103] The major BER pathway is the short-patch pathway, which involves excision of only one base. The minor pathway—the long-patch repair—excises 2 to 10 nucleotides.

DSB Repair

Spontaneous DSBs either occur on topoisomerase failure during recombination and are forced by replication errors or are due to thermodynamic fluctuation. In germ cells, DSBs are produced during meiotic crossover in T- and B-lymphocytes

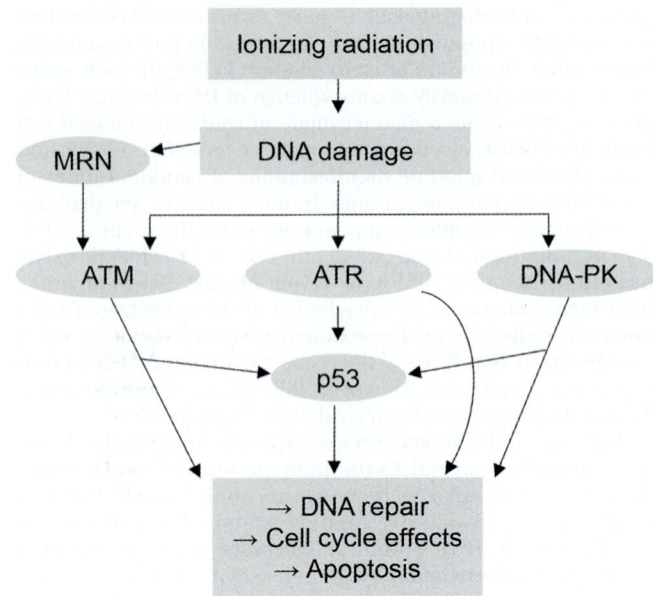

FIGURE 2.4. Simplified pathways of radiation-induced DNA damage recognition.

during a site-specific DNA recombination of variable diversity and joining genes (VDJ) on maturation of T-cell receptors and antibodies. Radiation-induced DSBs are, despite their relatively low induction frequency (40 per Gy per cell), biologically much more important than base damage and SSB. Two major pathways—homologous recombination (HR) and nonhomologous end joining (NHEJ)—have evolved to repair DSB (Fig. 2.5).[104,105] Whereas NHEJ occurs in all phases of the

FIGURE 2.5. Main DNA double-strand break damage repair mechanisms. The more error-prone nonhomologous end joining (NHEJ) is active throughout the whole cell cycle. For homologous recombination (HR), an identical DNA strand is necessary and used as template for precise repair.

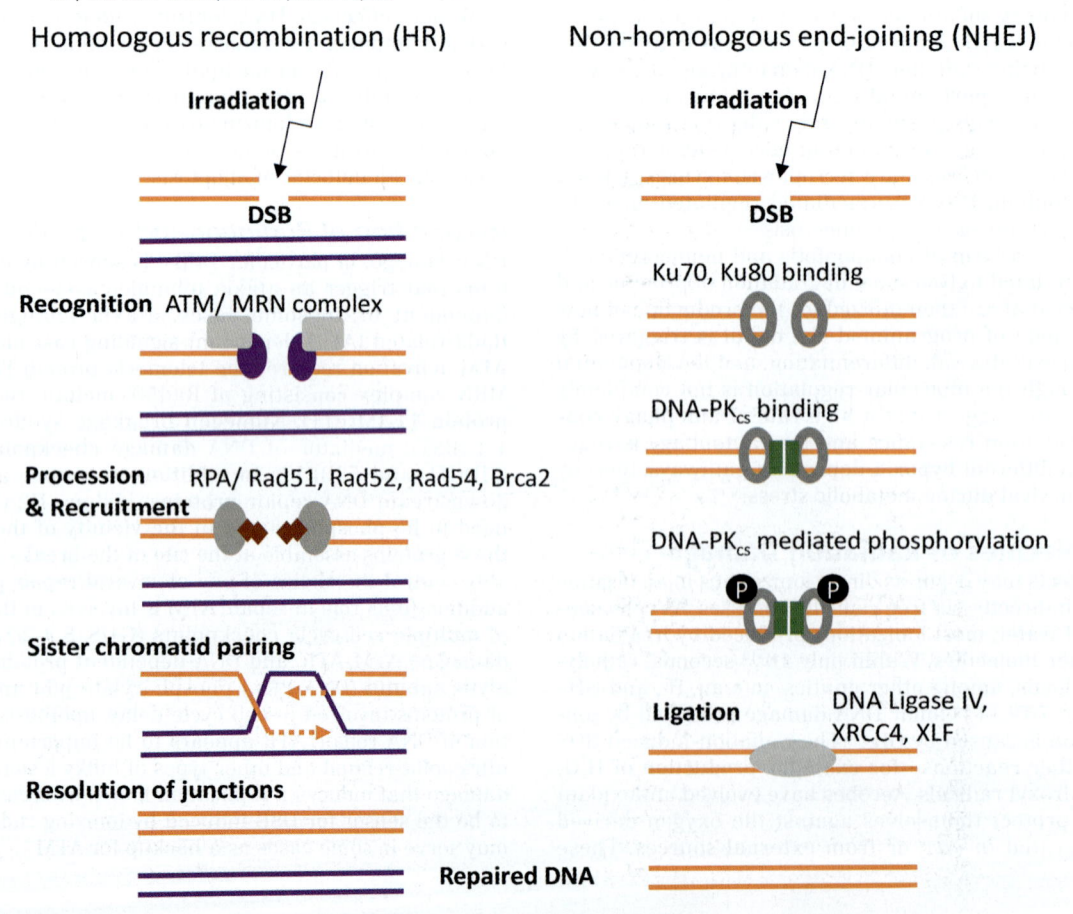

cell cycle, HR is particularly important in the S/G2 transition of the cell cycle.

HR is a slow, high-fidelity repair pathway. Regions of DNA homology—usually the sister chromatid—are used as the template. During HR, activated ATM recruits endonucleases that process broken ends, which ultimately creates single-stranded 3′ ends. For the processing, the MRN complex is required. In concert with BRCA1, BRCA2, and Rad51 paralogues (XRCC2, XRCC3, Rad51B, Rad51C, Rad51D, Rad52, Rad54), the Rad51 protein binds to single-stranded DNA with the aid of replication protein A and searches for a homologous sequence on the sister chromatid. On strand invasion, Rad51 enables the formation of a temporary triple helix. Once the complementary strands have paired, the 3′ end of the damaged DNA will be elongated by polymerases (not yet identified) beyond the position of the former DSB. When the 3′ single strand of the second end of the DSB also invades the structure, a quadruple helix is formed called a *Holliday junction*, which can be extended in both directions. After the gap has been safely bridged (usually about 50 base pairs will be copied), the Holliday junction is resolved, and the remaining nicks are sealed by a DNA ligase.[106,107]

NHEJ is a fast but error-prone, and thus potentially mutagenic, repair pathway that rejoins DNA ends, usually after removal of a limited number of base pairs. NHEJ is initiated by the Ku70/Ku80 heterodimer, which binds to DNA ends and recruits the DNA-PK$_{CS}$. DNA-PK$_{CS}$ can phosphorylate a variety of repair proteins such as Ku, x-ray cross-complementation protein 4 (XRCC-4), Artemis, p53, or replication protein A. However, only the autophosphorylation has been identified as being essential for repair. Artemis, in concert with DNA-PK$_{CS}$, trims the DSB ends for subsequent processing. After release of DNA-PK$_{CS}$ from the DNA, the end will be bridged by the complex of ligase IV/XRCC-4–/XRCC-4–like factor (XLF), which also performs the final ligation step. It has been observed that NHEJ can, to some extent, occur in the absence of several core proteins. This gave raise to the idea of a backup pathway that only operates when the DNA-PK–dependent NHEJ fails.[108] Besides the genuine repair proteins, the tumor suppressor p53 is involved in controlling the repair. P53 appears to suppress both HR and NHEJ in case an error-free repair is not possible and thereby reduces the mutagenic risk of error-prone repair.[109]

Despite our molecular knowledge about DSB repair, chromatin organization has also been shown to impact DSB induction and repair.[110-113] Chromatin is organized as euchromatin and heterochromatin, representing loose and condensed DNA areas, respectively. Whereas DSBs in euchromatin are easily accessible for repair proteins, DSBs in heterochromatic DNA regions need to be moved to less condensed areas for efficient repair.[111,113] Key molecules involved in these differential chromatin-dependent processes are ATM in association with heterochromatic marker proteins like KAP-1 and 53BP-1 and certain types of histones.[110,112]

Radiation-Induced Cell Cycle Delay

It has long been recognized that radiation-induced DNA damage is associated with delay in the cell cycle, which has been interpreted as allowing additional time for the cells to repair. Furthermore, DSBs can be found in all cell cycle phases, suggesting incomplete repair before entering the next phase. For example, tracking of radiation-induced γH2AX foci, representing DSBs, revealed transfer of DSBs induced in the G1 cell cycle phase to daughter cells.[114]

G1 Phase

The G1 cell cycle checkpoint prevents damaged DNA from being replicated and is the best understood checkpoint in mammalian cells.[115] Radiation-induced G1 phase cell cycle arrest is regulated by p53 (Fig. 2.1). Loss of p53 function, which is found in the majority of tumors, leads to a lack of G1-phase arrest. Instead, these cells exert a dose-dependent blockage in the G2 and M phases of the cell cycle. Central to the G1 checkpoint is the accumulation and activation of the p53 protein, which is controlled by the ATM and ATR kinases. These kinases, together with DNA-PK, are activated by and recruited to radiation-induced DNA lesions. Physiologically, p53 expression levels are low because of interaction with its negative regulator MDM2, which targets p53 for nuclear export and proteasome-mediated degradation in the cytoplasm.[116] Following radiation-induced DNA damage, ATM activates the downstream cell cycle checkpoint kinase Chk2 by phosphorylation, leading to p53 phosphorylation and finally resulting in p53 accumulation. Moreover, ATM exerts p53 stability and thereby prevents p53 nuclear export to the cytoplasm for degradation. P53 target genes include several genes that are involved in the DNA damage response (e.g., MDM2, GADD45a, p21^{Cip1}). Accumulation of the cyclin-dependent kinase inhibitor p21^{Cip1} blocks G1/S-phase progression by binding to the cyclinE/cdk2 complex, reducing cdk2 activity, which has an important function in phosphorylation of pRB. The retinoblastoma protein is an important regulator of cell cycling and cell differentiation.[117] Loss of pRB function is often found in malignant cells and leads to an uncontrolled G1/S transition, genomic instability, and loss of differentiation. Hypophosphorylated pRB binds to several proteins, including the E2F transcription factors and histone deacetylases.

S-Phase

After irradiation, the rate of DNA synthesis is decreased via ATM- and NBS1-dependent pathways.[118] Radiation-induced DNA damage activates ATM for Thr68 phosphorylation of Chk2.[119] Activated Chk2 targets CDC25A phosphatase for ubiquitination. As a result, Cdk2/cyclin E and Cdk2/cyclin A complexes remain inactive, which prevents completion of DNA synthesis and G2 entry. Alternatively, radiation-activated ATM phosphorylates several downstream substrates, including BRCA1, NBS1, and SMC1.[119,120] ATR phosphorylates the cell cycle checkpoint kinase Chk1. Subsequently, Chk1 phosphorylates CDC25A, which results in cytoplasmic sequestration and thereby in inhibition of S–G2 transition.[121]

G2 Phase

In contrast to the G1 checkpoint, all mammalian cells, normal or transformed, undergo cell cycle arrest in G2 after radiation-induced damage.[122] The G2 cell cycle checkpoint is the essential final determinant allowing cells to divide. The entry into mitosis is regulated by the activity of the cyclin-dependent kinase Cdk1[123] (Fig. 2.1). Phosphorylation of Cdk1 blocks cell cycling into G2. These phosphorylations are removed by the phosphatase CDC25C. After irradiation, ATR and ATM activate the downstream checkpoint kinases Chk1 and Chk2, which phosphorylate CDC25C.[124] This results in binding of 14-3-3 proteins. The CDC25C/14-3-3 protein complex is translocated into the cytoplasm for sequestration. As a consequence of this CDC25C degradation, Cdk1 remains phosphorylated, thereby preventing entry into mitosis. ATM appears to be more dominant at the early stage of G2/M checkpoint activation, whereas ATR seems to contribute mainly to sustained checkpoint events.[125]

Molecular Targets

Radiation Effects on Signal Transduction

Ionizing radiation affects intracellular signaling.[126] The general mechanisms of radiation-induced signal transduction activation involve the dose-dependent production of ROS and reactive nitrogen species (RNS), which stimulate, for example, cytoplasmic protein kinases, phosphatases, and cell membrane receptors or disturb, for example, lipid and protein metabolism.[127] Many signaling pathways are simultaneously activated in a dose- and cell-type–dependent manner, which may contribute to different radiation responses in different cell types. In addition, distinct radiation qualities such as photons or particles trigger different molecular signaling pathways.

Cooperative and mutual cross talk occurs between parallel and upstream and downstream signaling routes.[128] Examples of important intracellular signaling pathways and their modulation by ionizing radiation are discussed in the following paragraphs.

Receptor tyrosine kinases (RTKs) represent a group of oncogenic, transmembrane receptors consisting, if complete, of an extracellular ligand-binding domain, a transmembrane part, and an intracellular catalytic domain with tyrosine kinase activity.[129] On ligand binding and receptor homo-/heterodimerization, the protein kinase is subsequently activated, resulting in phosphorylation of tyrosine residues of the receptor itself (autophosphorylation) or target proteins. Depending on the cellular context, this triggers an intracellular signaling cascade that eventually leads to proliferation, survival, differentiation, and migration. Among the known human RTKs are the epidermal growth factor receptors (EGFRs), the platelet-derived growth factor receptors (PDGFRs), the vascular endothelial growth factor receptors (VEGFRs), the fibroblast growth factor receptors, the ephrin receptors, and tyrosine kinase receptor. This RTK signaling involves several distinct molecular pathways that are often deregulated in cancer cells. Prime examples of such deregulated pathways are the Ras–Raf–mitogen-activated protein kinase (MAPK) pathway, the phosphoinositide 3' kinase (PI3K)/Akt pathway, the Jak/Stat molecules, and protein kinase C. Cooperative and mutual cross talk between the different transduction pathways forms a complex signaling network.

The *EGFR family* consists of four distinct members (EGFR/ErbB-1, HER2/ErbB-2, HER3/ErbB-3, and HER4/ErbB-4) that are dimerized after ligand binding to the extracellular domain.[130,131] The receptor ligands, such as epidermal growth factor (EGF), tumor growth factor-α (TGF-α), and neuroregulin-1, as well as their cognate receptors, are abundantly expressed in a large variety of human cancers, including lung, breast, head and neck, and gliomas, and have been related to poor prognosis.

The EGFR is being activated through its natural ligands such as EGF, TGF-α, or amphiregulin and can be transactivated by cell adhesion molecules such as integrins or immunoglobulin-like receptors.[132] In addition, ionizing radiation is able to stimulate EGFR.[133] Radiation doses of 1 to 2 Gy activate the EGFR and its downstream signaling cascades with similar efficiency as physiologic EGF concentrations of 0.1 to 1 nM. Radiation-dependent production of ROS/RNS seems to play a critical role in EGFR activation and downstream signaling via MAPK.[127,134] It was shown that protein tyrosine phosphatases contain ROS-/RNS-sensitive cysteine residues at a site essential for phosphatase activity. Thus, the radiation-dependent activation of EGFR could be controlled by ROS-/RNS-regulated protein phosphatases. In addition, paracrine and autocrine activation of the EGFR can also result from radiation-induced release of TGF-α from irradiated cells or by release of growth factors stored in the extracellular matrix as result of activation of matrix-degrading proteases.[135–137]

EGFR signaling via Ras–Raf–MAPK after irradiation has been implicated in increased proliferation,[138] which corresponds to observations that EGFR overexpression is associated with repopulation during fractionated irradiation.[139–141] In addition, EGFR-dependent signaling via PI3K/Akt has been associated with increased cellular survival and cell cycle progression.[142,143]

After radiation-induced activation, the EGFR is internalized and may function as a nuclear transcription factor.[144] In addition, internalized EGFR can activate DNA-PK that is involved in cell cycle repair (see paragraph "DNA repair"). Pharmacologic inhibitors can block EGFR signaling at different levels and thereby influence several mechanisms of radioresistance, such as DNA repair, repopulation, antiapoptotic signaling, and tumor hypoxia.[24] The specific mutational status of the cells—for example, Ras mutations[136,145]—and the class of drugs[146,147] may modify effects of EGFR inhibition on radiation response. The concept of EGFR inhibition to improve outcome of radiotherapy has been proven in a phase III clinical trial.[23] However, considerable intertumoral heterogeneity has been observed, which is mechanistically only partly understood.[21]

RTK-Initiated Signal Transduction

Ras–Raf signaling

An important signal transduction route within EGFR signaling represents the Ras–Raf–MAPK pathway. The *Ras proteins* (H-Ras, K-Ras4A, K-Ras4B, and N-Ras) are GTPases and are attached in their active state (GTP bound) to the inner surface of the cell membrane. The Ras proto-oncogene, predominantly K-Ras, is mutated in about one-third of human cancers. Activating mutations are frequent in adenocarcinomas of the pancreas (up to 90%), the colorectum (about 50%), and the lung (about 30%).[148] The processing and membrane attachment of the functional Ras are governed by farnesyltransferases, which are the molecular target for specific pharmaceutical inhibitors of activated Ras.[149]

Activated Ras has an effect on various downstream molecules, including *PI3K*.[150] Signaling mediator molecules of PI3K include phosphoinositide-dependent kinase 1, Akt, protein kinase C, and subsequently the nuclear transcription factor NFκB. The cellular responses on activation of the PI3K pathway are cell-type specific and include changes in gene expression, cell cycle progression, survival, and apoptosis. The tumor suppressor protein *PTEN* negatively regulates the PI3K/Akt pathway. Akt overexpression or hyperactivity and PTEN mutations are found in numerous human malignancies.[151]

PDGF-Mediated Signaling

Radiation-induced autocrine and paracrine PDGF signaling plays an important role in fibroblast and endothelial cell activation and proliferation *in vitro*.[152] Combination of irradiation with PGDFR tyrosine kinase inhibitors resulted in decreased clonogenic survival of endothelial cells and fibroblasts *in vitro*.[152] PDGFR signaling may attenuate development of radiation-induced pulmonary fibrosis.[153]

VEGFR-Mediated Signaling

Transmembrane receptors for VEGF and related ligands include VEGFR-1 (Flt-1), VEGFR-2 (KDR/Flk-1), VEGFR-3 (Flt-4), neuropilin-1, and neuropilin-2.[154] On irradiation, VEGF is up-regulated via the EGFR/STAT signaling and released by tumor cells and exerts, via VEGFR/PI3K/Akt signaling, prosurvival stimuli on tumor and endothelial cells.[155] Up-regulated VEGFR expression has been found after ionizing irradiation.[156,157] Besides normalizing the tumor micromilieu,[158] inhibition of radiation-induced VEGF/VEGFR signaling represents the rationale for combining anti-VEGF strategies with radiotherapy. Besides, targeting immunomodulatory drugs to VEGF have recently been shown to reduce toxicity and increase local tumor control in the preclinical setting.[159]

Cytokine Receptors

A large number of growth-stimulating hormones, growth factors, and cytokines such as the interleukins, erythropoietin, and prolactin bind to the class of cytokine receptors that are structurally different from the previously described RTKs.[160] The intracellular signaling in response to cytokine receptor activation includes the *JAK* and *STAT* kinases. In addition to the cytokine receptors, also, many RTKs can activate the JAK/STAT pathway. In malignant cells, the autonomy of growth signaling can be associated with mutations in cytokine receptors (e.g., in the erythropoietin receptor) and constitutively up-regulated activity of the JAK/STAT pathway. Cancer cells can also evade drug-induced cell death by the secretion of cytokines leading to autocrine receptor stimulation.[161]

Wnt Signaling

Wnt proteins are diffusible growth factors that bind to specific surface receptors (Frizzled) and trigger distinct intracellular pathways leading to cell growth.[162] Wnt signaling involves the tumor suppressor protein adenomatous polyposis coli (APC) and regulates by phosphorylation the steady-state levels of cytosolic β-catenin. An increased level of β-catenin facilitates its transit into the nucleus, activation of transcription factors, and subsequently transcription of β-catenin target genes, including MYC, JUN, CCND1, and ALDH1A1.[163,164] The aberrant activation of Wnt signaling caused by mutations in the β-catenin and APC genes are typical findings in colon cancer and melanoma but also have been identified in a large variety of other human cancers. Wnt signaling has been shown to play an important role in tumorigenesis and in CSC self-renewal and differentiation and thus provides a promising target for anticancer treatment.[165,166]

Integrin-Mediated Signaling

Cross talk between tumor cells and tumor stroma emerges as an important determinant for tumor response to radiation and as a potential target for novel therapeutic combinations. Interactions between cells and ECM proteins are facilitated mainly by the integrin family of cell adhesion molecules.[167] Besides the influence of growth factors and cytokines, the cells' adhesion resistome adds further facets to the network of microenvironmental factors that modulate the cellular behavior on exposure to ionizing radiation.[168] Chemotherapeutic compounds, molecular-targeted compounds, and ionizing radiation showed less cytotoxic efficacy in cells adherent to ECM compared to cells growing in suspension or on plastic surfaces.[169] Resistance-promoting effects by integrin-mediated adhesion to ECM were found in cell lines from solid tumors of the lung,[170,171] breast,[172] liver,[173] colon,[174] pancreas,[169,175,176] ovary,[177] prostate,[178] brain,[179] and leukemia cells.[180] Certain integrins seem to communicate increased radiation and drug resistance, which is cooperatively influenced by RTKs like EGFR.[181,182] For example, $\alpha5\beta1$ integrin, the "classic" fibronectin receptor, acts as a major antagonist of cell death induced by doxorubicin or melphalan in multiple myeloma,[183] by paclitaxel in breast cancer or small cell and non–small cell lung cancer,[184,185] or by cisplatin or mitomycin C in non–small cell lung cancer.[184] Additional studies underscored the important role of $\beta1$ integrins in promoting resistance against ionizing radiation.[186,187] Further regulatory cytoplasmic cascades downstream of $\beta1$ integrins that exert survival advantage on treatment with genotoxic agents include regulation of the Akt1/FoxO cascade and the antiapoptotic Bcl-2–like proteins or Bcl-2/Bax.[180] In addition to regulating cell survival, cell–matrix interactions affect radiation-induced cell cycle arrest, that is, adhesion of cells to matrix proteins prolongs the G1 and G2 cell cycle blockage in parallel with enhanced activation of DNA repair pathways involving the checkpoint kinases Chk1, Chk2, and Cdk1, p53, and diverse cyclins.[184,188–190]

Following radiation exposure, the expression of several integrin subunits, including $\beta1$, $\beta3$, $\alpha5$, and αv, is up-regulated in human skin and lung fibroblasts,[169] endothelial cells, and keratinocytes,[191] as well as in tumor cells of the colon,[174] hematopoietic cells,[192] prostate,[193] lung,[194] brain,[195] and melanomas.[169] Generally, integrin-mediated adhesion to matrix proteins confers chemoresistance and radioresistance.[180,181,196,197]

Nonreceptor Kinases

Cytoplasmic, nonreceptor kinases are often activated in malignant disease. For example, the *Bcr/Abl* fusion protein kinase is a typical molecular finding in chronic myeloid leukemia and represents the molecular target for small molecule inhibitors such as imatinib.[198] This drug also inhibits KIT, a cytoplasmic tyrosine kinase, that has been shown to be activated by mutation in gastrointestinal stroma tumors, thus providing another molecular targeting approach.[199,200]

Transcription Factors

Transcription factors bind to the DNA and activate the expression of specific genes. Oncogenic transcription factors are overactive in most human cancers and contribute to the autonomy of growth signaling. Based on their mechanism of activation, three groups can be separated.[201] First are the *steroid receptors*, which are found in hormone-sensitive breast or prostate cancer. The second group of transcription factors resides in the nucleus, is governed by kinase signals, and consists of various members, including *myc*, *activator protein 1* (AP-1), and *E2F*. Myc transcription factors are induced in cancer by different mechanisms, including translocation and gene amplification. For example, c-myc is activated by the chromosomal translocation t(8;14), which results in a constitutive c-myc expression in 80% of Burkitt lymphomas. N-myc and L-myc amplifications are found in neuroblastoma and small cell lung cancer, respectively. AP-1, consisting of *JUN*, *FOS*, *ATF*, and *MAF*, can exhibit oncogenic or antioncogenic effects depending on the cellular context.[202] The third group of oncogenic transcription factors—the latent transcription factors—is activated by ligand–receptor interactions and includes the STATs (see previous discussion), the WNT–β-catenin pathway (see previous discussion), NFκB, and the stemness-related molecules Notch and Hedgehog. NFκB levels have been shown to be constitutively active in lymphomas, leukemias, and breast and colon cancer.[201]

Cancer Stem Cells

As described above, malignant tumors are composed of genetically and phenotypically heterogeneous cells in various differentiation states. Within this pool, CSCs are considered as the major cell population responsible for tumor initiation, growth, and relapse as well as for metastasis formation and therapy resistance.[203] Evidence shows that CSCs, which comprise a rather small fraction of the tumor mass, are often stunningly resistant to cytotoxic therapies as compared to the bulk tumor cells.[204] Therefore, the reduction of tumor mass is not an adequate measure of therapy success.[18] The identification of CSC populations within a tumor represents a promising strategy for prognosis, prediction, and also targeting of aggressive tumors (also see paragraph on "Molecular stratification in personalized radiotherapy"). However, identification and targeting of CSC is challenged by the high inter- and intratumoral diversity of different putative stem cell populations and CSC plasticity during cancer evolution and treatment. The CSC phenotype does not describe a static subpopulation but rather a highly dynamic intrinsic property of a tumor cell. This means that the CSC pool might be re-established by non-CSC tumor mass cells, and cancer therapy can only be effective when eradicating both tumor mass and CSC simultaneously.[205]

Targeting the signaling axes of CSC alone and in combination with cytotoxic drugs and/or radiotherapy is one approach. Those CSC signaling pathways often shared with normal stem cells include Notch, Hedgehog, and Wnt/β-catenin signaling.[206] Activated Wnt/β-catenin signaling, for instance, is one of the key pathways during embryonic development and is described for carcinogenesis, EMT, and radiation resistance. One target comprises the Wnt receptor Frizzled by blocking the association of Wnt with its receptor. First clinical studies with such an inhibitor ipafricept (FZD8-Fc, *OMP-54F28*) were just completed (clinicaltrials.gov, NCT01608867, NCT01345201). Another promising example for CSC signaling pathway targeting is the small molecule MK0752 that inhibits the Notch signaling pathway and is currently tested for treatment of advanced breast and pancreatic cancer (NCT00106145, NCT01098344). The combination of cytotoxic drugs with CSC inhibitors is tested for advanced stage small cell lung carcinoma and recurrent small cell lung carcinoma by using cisplatin and etoposide in combination with the Hedgehog inhibitor GDC-0449 (NCT00887159).

Metastatic spread is caused by disseminated tumor cells with CSC characteristics that leave the primary tumor and settle and grow at distant for them hostile places in the body. The transport phase of those cells, then called circulating tumor cells (CTCs), through the blood system represents another attractive diagnostic and therapeutic target. However, there is no standard definition of those CTC. To date, the magnetic bead–mediated CELLSEARCH system is the only FDA-approved method for the enrichment of epithelial cell adhesion molecule (EpCAM) expressing CTCs. Counts of EpCAM-positive cells show significant prognostic relevance for breast and prostate cancer patients.[207,208] Further biomarkers for the identification of CTCs are currently under investigation.

The CSC niche as a tumor-supporting microenvironment resembles another potential target for anti-CSC therapies. The niche maintains and sustains CSCs and orchestrates their fate decisions via extracellular matrix molecules (ECM), cell-to-cell contacts, pH value, vascularization, hypoxia, etc., that may induce for instance stem cell–related signaling cascades.[36] Thereby, the niche also provides a protective microenvironment for CSCs; for example, hypoxia can induce quiescence of the cells.[42] Thus, the cells escape chemotherapy, which mainly attacks rapidly proliferating cells. However, the ECM and their cognate receptors on the CSC surface represent potential drugable targets. The CSC metabolism, in parts intrinsically regulated also dependents on the microenvironment and the given nutrition supply, comprises a targetable CSC feature.

Epigenetics

Accumulating evidence suggests that a variety of epigenetic mechanisms contribute to tumor heterogeneity and to the initiation and maintenance of CSC traits. Per definition, epigenetics defines stable heritable changes in gene expression that are not caused by changes in the underlying DNA sequence.[34] Chromatin and histone modifications and DNA methylation are epigenetic key mechanisms that are influenced by cancer risk factors such as chronic inflammation, aging, and environmental changes. Replication of DNA methylation is highly error prone, and it is contemplated that not only genomic but also epigenetic instability drives tumorigenesis and heterogeneity.[63,209,210] Epigenetic alterations can silence or activate genes and thereby offer tumor cells two possible choices to rapidly evolve under therapy pressure, which can lead to therapy resistance and tumor relapse.[34] Epigenetic therapeutics can reverse those epigenetic changes and resensitize tumor cells. Epigenetic drugs such as enhancer of zeste homolog 2 (EZH2), isocitrate dehydrogenase (IDH), and bromodomain and extraterminal (BET) inhibitors are currently under investigation in clinical trials.[211] IDH1 mutations lead to DNA and histone hypermethylation. The IDH1 R132 mutation is of special interest as it may also serve as so-called neoantigen (*vide infra*). Peptide vaccines that capture this mutated region are currently under development and testing.[212] Epigenetic changes such as the IDH1 R132 mutation can directly affect tumor immune evasion because DNA hypermethylation and promoter methylation

can regulate the expression of cancer antigens and foster the evolvement of neoantigens. Therefore, epigenetic inhibitors also play an important role in immunotargeting.

Antitumor Immunity

Mutagenesis as well as genomic and epigenomic instability in the tumor can lead to the expression of tumor-specific mutant proteins (neoantigens) that are not present on normal cells.[213] Neoantigens are short peptides expressed on the tumor cell surface and thereby become recognizable to T cells as foreign antigen. Because of their tumor-selective expression, those neoantigens resemble attractive immune targets with minimal risk of autoimmunity and immunotolerance. Also, virus antigens expressed by tumors with a viral etiology (such as HPV-caused cancers of the cervix and the oropharynx) are representing an example of neoantigens. However, neoantigens arise in most cases from unique mutations, which complicates identification and needs individualized targeted immunotherapy. Current advancements in proteomics, genomics, and sequencing coupled with epitope prediction algorithms will speed up the future development of such therapy approaches. The development of immune checkpoint inhibitors targeting cytotoxic T-lymphocyte–associated protein 4 (CTL4) and programmed cell death protein 1 (PD1) was recently shown to provide clinical benefit in melanoma[214] and non–small cell lung cancer and is expected to be efficient in subsets of a wide variety of tumor entities.[215] Also, antibody-based therapies, including engineered bispecific T cells and chimeric antigen receptor (CAR) T cells, have been shown to be therapeutically active in several cancers, for example, leukemia.[216,217]

Human Papillomavirus

Oncogenic viruses such as the HPV are contributing to carcinogenesis and are driving malignant progression. Papillomaviruses are small, nonenveloped, double-stranded circular DNA viruses. To date, more than 200 HPV genotypes have been identified, including low-risk and high-risk subtypes.[218] Especially the high-risk subtypes HPV16 and HPV18 are known to cause a variety of carcinomas such as cervical cancer, oropharyngeal cancer, and anal cancer. In contrast to most viral infections, where virions are produced directly in the target cell, the syntheses of new HPV virions occur only after the target cell has undergone mitosis, followed by differentiation of one of its daughter cell.[219] HPV infects proliferating cells in the basal layer of stratified squamous epithelia following microtrauma and leads to the establishment of the HPV genome as extrachromosomal elements or episomes. Because these HPV genomes do not contain enzymes for viral replication, they depend on the DNA replication machinery of their host to mediate viral DNA synthesis.[220] Also after undergoing differentiation, virus-infected cells are remaining active in the cell cycle. In the suprabasal layers, some cells are still able to re-enter the S-phase in order to replicate HPV genomes and synthesize virions. When the epithelial cells are reaching the outer layer, the HPV virions are released.[219]

The proliferation of HPV-infected epithelial cells is independent from cellular differentiation. The HPV E7 oncoprotein binds to proteins of the Rb family and targets them for degradation. This leads consequently to the release and activation of the E2 transcription factors (E2F), which are driving the expression of S-phase genes and thereby initiating cell cycle progression.[221] The Rb-E2F protein normally acts via a negative feedback loop and inhibits gene transcription of CDKN2A, which encodes for p16. In contrast, the functional inactivation of the pRb pathway by the HPV E7 oncoprotein leads to loss of this negative feedback loop and thus to p16 overexpression[222] (Fig. 2.6).

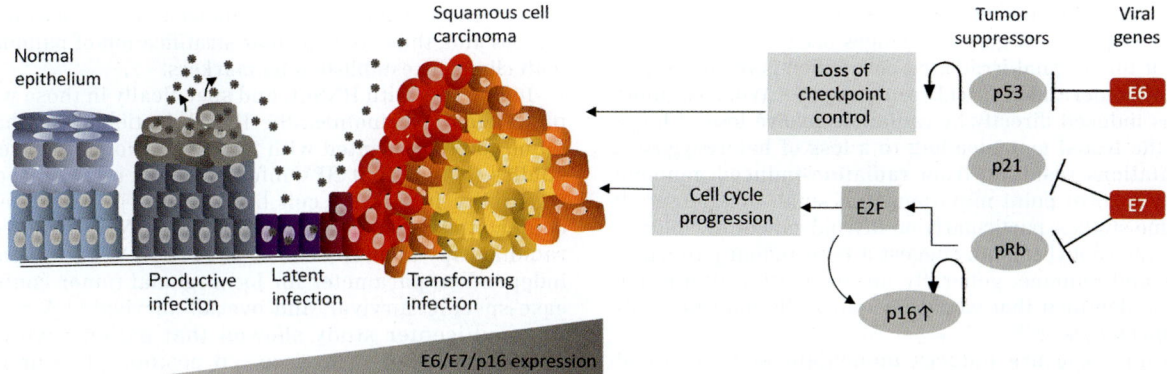

FIGURE 2.6. Human papillomavirus (HPV) infection and activation: Microtraumas allow the entrance of HPVs to the epithelial basal cell layer. This is followed by the coordinate expression of different viral genes. E6/E7 cause viral genome amplification and shedding of the newly produced viral particles. Persistent expression can lead to malignant dysplasia, once the HPV infection is established and evaded from immune recognition. Malignant transformation is characterized by loss of differentiation, high E6/E7 level, and no viral replication. The expression of the viral genes E6 and E7 inhibit the expression of the tumor suppressor genes p21, pRb, and p53, respectively. E6-triggered inhibition of the tumor suppressors p53 and p21 leads to loss of checkpoint control and with this to uncontrolled growth of squamous carcinoma cells. The E7 oncoprotein inactivates pRb, the effector protein of p16, via pRb/E2F degradation. This results in overexpression of p16 and cell cycle progression.

It is important to note that especially HPV E7 oncoprotein of high-risk HPV subtypes is binding strongly to the members of the Rb family. This efficient binding would then lead to the inhibition of cell growth and to apoptosis, via p53. To overcome this, the HPV oncoprotein E6 initiates ubiquitination and subsequent degradation of the p53 protein including disruption of the p53 pathway. The loss of the tumor suppressor gene p53 leads to defective control at the G1/S and G2/M checkpoints and subsequently to uncontrolled cell cycle progression.[223]

HPV-driven head and neck squamous cell carcinoma (HNSCC) are more radiosensitive than non–HPV-driven carcinoma, which is due to their cell cycle dysregulation (*vide supra*) including impaired DNA DSB repair capacity.[224]

Radiation-Induced Gene Expression

Radiation may significantly modify gene expression.[225] Many of the transcriptionally activated proteins have been shown to be centrally involved in the pathogenesis of radiation damage or to modulate the effect of radiation on tumor cells. Early responses may occur within hours after irradiation and involve mostly transcription factors such as the proto-oncogenes *JUN*, *FOS*, *JUNB*, and early growth response gene 1 (*EGR1*).[226] Sustained activation of early radiation response genes such as NFκB may contribute to late radiation damage.[227] Other examples of radiation-induced genes that may occur early and/or late after irradiation include TGF-β, TNF-α, bFGF, PDGF, and interleukin-1 (IL-1).[228]

Gene expression and DNA-binding activity of *NFκB* are induced soon after ionizing radiation.[229] NFκB is a sequence-specific DNA-binding protein complex that binds to DNA as a dimer. According to its multiple functions, NFκB can also be activated by a variety of agents, like membrane receptors such as TNFR or toll-like receptors and oxidative stress. Radiation-induced activation of NFκB is mediated by IKK.[230] This response does not depend on a nuclear signal, as it also occurs in enucleated cells.[231] However, it has been shown that ATM is required for chronic activation of the transcription factor NFκB.[232] NFκB acts in an antiapoptotic way and mediates radioresistance.[233]

Radiation exposure induces immediate and sustained *TGFβ1* gene expression, as well as activation of this cytokine.[234] On transcriptional activation, TGF-β is produced as an inactive latent form and secreted. Latent TGF-β is stored in the extracellular matrix and proteolytically activated in irradiated tissues.[235] Active TGF-β1 binds and activates the TGF-β1 type I receptor, resulting in TGF-β1–dependent gene expression, inducing, for example, p21, p27, collagen, and tissue inhibitors of metalloproteinase (TIMP).[15,236] This is most likely responsible for the cellular effects of TGF-β, such as modulation of proliferation, differentiation, and radiation sensitivity of fibroblasts, and for the biochemical events (e.g., collagen deposition, characteristic of radiation-induced fibrosis). In addition, TGF-β secreted by tumor cells on irradiation contributes to the development of radiation-induced fibrosis[237]. Intervention of TGF-β–mediated effects (e.g., by TGF-β1–neutralizing antibodies and superoxide dismutase) offers a promising strategy to prevent radiation-induced fibrosis. Moreover, a recent preclinical study showed that combined inhibition of TGF-β and PDGF with small molecules is a promising approach in diminishing radiation-induced lung toxicity.[238] Aside from fibrosis, TGF-β has been demonstrated to reduce latency, promote aggressive tumor growth, and increase estrogen receptor–negative breast cancers.[239] Moreover, the radiosensitivity of cancer cells can be enhanced by TGF-β–directed treatments.[240,241]

TNF-α belongs to the group of proinflammatory cytokines involved in radiation-induced normal tissue damage, such as pneumonitis and lung fibrosis. Immediately after irradiation, TNF-α is transcriptionally up-regulated and released by the bronchiolar epithelium. TNF-α enhances phagocytosis and cytotoxicity by neutrophilic granulocytes and modulates the expression of other cytokines such as IL-1 and IL-6.[242] Experimental data show that also tumor lines, particularly pediatric sarcomas, may produce large quantities of bioactive TNF-α after irradiation, which is of potential importance for tumor response and for normal tissue reactions after radiotherapy.[243]

Tracking of genetic changes during and after ionizing radiation will further elucidate the molecular and basic impact of how cancer and normal cells respond to radiation and may serve as predictors for therapy response.

Genome Instability and Mutation

Cells may survive radiation despite unrepaired or misrepaired DNA damage, that is, with mutations or chromosomal aberrations. These may remain silent or result in radiation-related secondary primary cancers or, as germline mutations, cause hereditary disease.[244–246] In addition to directly induced mutations, radiation may induce a heritable, genome-wide process of instability (i.e., genomic instability) that leads to an enhanced frequency of genetic changes occurring among the progeny of the original irradiated cell, which is transmissible over many generations of cell replication.[247] Whereas most mutations induced directly by radiation involve loss of large parts of the tested gene, leading to a loss of heterozygosity, most mutations resulting from radiation-induced genomic instability involve point mutations and small deletions.[247,248] While some studies, particularly on thyroid cancer in children after the Chernobyl fallout, suggest a nonrandom pattern of chromosomal damage, generally no fingerprint alterations have been identified that would unequivocally indicate radiation-induced cancer.[246]

Radiation exposure induces immediate and sustained *TGF-β1* gene expression, as well as activation of this cytokine.[234] On transcriptional activation, TGF-β is produced as an inactive latent form and secreted. Latent TGF-β is stored in the extracellular matrix and proteolytically activated in irradiated tissues.[235] Active TGF-β1 binds and activates the TGF-β1 type I receptor, resulting in TGF-β1–dependent gene expression, inducing, for example, p21, p27, collagen, and TIMP.[15,236] This is most likely responsible for the cellular effects of TGF-β, such as modulation of proliferation, differentiation, and radiation sensitivity of fibroblasts, and for the biochemical events (e.g., collagen deposition, characteristic of radiation-induced fibrosis). In addition, TGF-β secreted by tumor cells on irradiation might contribute to the development of radiation-induced fibrosis.[237] Intervention of TGF-β–mediated effects (e.g., by TGF-β1–neutralizing antibodies and superoxide dismutase) offers a promising strategy to prevent radiation-induced fibrosis. Aside from fibrosis, TGF-β has been demonstrated to reduce latency, promote aggressive tumor growth, and increase estrogen receptor–negative breast cancers.[239] Moreover, the radiosensitivity of cancer cells can be enhanced by TGF-β–directed treatments.

TNF-α belongs to the group of proinflammatory cytokines involved in radiation-induced normal tissue damage, such as pneumonitis and lung fibrosis. Immediately after irradiation, TNF-α is transcriptionally up-regulated and released by the bronchiolar epithelium. TNF-α enhances phagocytosis and cytotoxicity by neutrophilic granulocytes and modulates the expression of other cytokines such as IL-1 and IL-6.[242] Experimental data show that also tumor lines, particularly pediatric sarcomas, may produce large quantities of bioactive TNF-α after irradiation. This may be of potential importance for tumor response and for normal tissue reactions after radiotherapy.[243]

Induction of genes by ionizing radiation has been experimentally exploited for therapy. For example, the early-response gene *EGR1* was inserted upstream to TNF-α, which may act as a radiosensitizer. This provides a strategy for spatial and temporal control of the biologic effect by radiotherapy.[225,249]

Molecular Stratification Toward Personalized Radiotherapy

The treatment decision for patients with malignant tumors is clinically based on anatomical location and histopathologic features. To verify the anatomic extent of the disease, the TNM classification has been introduced, which considers the size of the primary tumor, the lymphatic spread (lymph node metastases), as well as distant metastases. The cell type and histopathologic features are being assessed based on the WHO classification. With recent advances in molecular pathology, implementation of DNA or RNA sequencing of cancer and normal tissue genomes, and biologic imaging techniques, a better understanding of the tumor and radiation biology is being gained and is leading toward molecular subclassification of tumors and, thus, to molecular stratification of patients along with clinically established biomarkers.

In patients with HNSCC and specifically in those with oropharyngeal carcinomas, the HPV infection status has been found to be associated with improved prognosis. Preclinical studies showed that HPV infection leads to increased radiosensitivity in HNSCC cell lines.[224,250] A prospective multicenter study including patients with HNSCC who received radiotherapy alone revealed that the HPV status is a strong independent parameter for locoregional tumor control, disease-specific survival, and overall survival.[251] A retrospective multicenter study showed that patients with locally advanced HNSCC who received postoperative or primary radiochemotherapy could be stratified according to their HPV status.[252,253] After postoperative radiochemotherapy, patients with HPV-positive HNSCC showed an excellent locoregional control of nearly 100%,[252] suggesting that these patients may benefit from de-escalation therapy, for example, by reducing the radiation dose. Such a de-escalation strategy is expected to reduce radiation-induced side effects while achieving an unchanged tumor control probability and is being currently tested in clinical trials. Patients with HPV-negative tumors could be further stratified by CSC marker expression as well as tumor hypoxia, which is in line with radiobiologic knowledge. Patients with HPV-negative, low hypoxic, and low CSC marker–expressing tumors also showed a superior locoregional control, whereas patients with hypoxic, CSC marker–overexpressing tumors showed a poor locoregional control and might benefit from intensified therapy regimens.[254] In contrast to the patients receiving postoperative radiochemotherapy, where only a few remaining tumor cells may have been left, the tumor volume is an important parameter for patients who are undergoing primary radiochemotherapy. The tumor volume is associated with the CSC number and is therefore important for local control. CSC marker expression reflecting CSC density varies widely between different tumors and can further enhance the powerful predictor tumor volume. Also, patients receiving primary radiochemotherapy could be stratified for their risk of locoregional failure based on their HPV status, tumor hypoxia, and CSC marker expression levels within the tumors.[253]

An important issue in research on biomarkers for radiotherapy is that parameters reflecting tumor response may change during treatment. For example, hypoxic tumors may reoxygenate during treatment, and it has been demonstrated that this is associated with improved local control compared to tumors with residual hypoxia.[255] Therefore, more extensive investigation into biomarker dynamics, by imaging, repeat tumor biopsies, or liquid biopsies, appears promising to improve their predictive value.

The identification of predictive biomarkers for the development of normal tissue toxicity in the individual patient is also a relevant issue in terms of personalized radiotherapy. It is well recognized that the degree of radiation-related toxicity varies between patients, which may be partly due to genotypic variation. The study of germ-line genotypic variations and the large clinical variability associated with the response to radiotherapy is also termed *radiogenomics*.[256] The overall aim of radiogenomics is to identify patients with common genetic variants who are very likely to develop normal tissue toxicity following radiotherapy. A recent meta-analysis of genome-wide association studies in prostate cancer identified two SNPs, which are associated with late toxicity following radiotherapy in patients with prostate cancer: rs17599026 on 5q31.2 with urinary frequency and rs7720298 on 5p15.2 with decreased urine stream.[257]

REFERENCES

1. Baumann M. Keynote comment: radiotherapy in the age of molecular oncology. *Lancet Oncol* 2006;7(10):786–787.

2. Okunieff P, Chen Y, Maguire DJ, et al. Molecular markers of radiation-related normal tissue toxicity. *Cancer Metastasis Rev* 2008;27(3):363–374.

3. Bentzen SM, Parliament M, Deasy JO, et al. Biomarkers and surrogate endpoints for normal-tissue effects of radiation therapy: the importance of dose-volume effects. *Int J Radiat Oncol Biol Phys* 2010;76(3 Suppl):S145–S150.

4. Baumann M, Krause M, Overgaard J, et al. Radiation oncology in the era of precision medicine. *Nat Rev Cancer* 2016;16(4):234–249.

5. Bentzen SM. Preventing or reducing late side effects of radiation therapy: radiobiology meets molecular pathology. *Nat Rev Cancer* 2006;6(9):702–713.

6. Grade M, Becker H, Ghadimi BM. The impact of molecular pathology in oncology: the clinician's perspective. *Cell Oncol* 2004;26(5–6):275–278.

7. Dietel M. Molecular pathology: a requirement for precision medicine in cancer. *Oncol Res Treat* 2016;39(12):804–810.

8. Vaupel P. Tumor microenvironmental physiology and its implications for radiation oncology. *Semin Radiat Oncol* 2004;14(3):198–206.

9. Bentzen SM, Gregoire V. Molecular imaging-based dose painting: a novel paradigm for radiation therapy prescription. *Semin Radiat Oncol* 2011;21(2):101–110.

10. Coleman CN. Linking radiation oncology and imaging through molecular biology (or now that therapy and diagnosis have separated, it's time to get together again!). *Radiology* 2003;228(1):29–35.

11. Bussink J, Kaanders JH, van der Graaf WT, et al. PET-CT for radiotherapy treatment planning and response monitoring in solid tumors. *Nat Rev Clin Oncol* 2011;8(4):233–242.

12. Ling CC, Humm J, Larson S, et al. Towards multidimensional radiotherapy (MD-CRT): biological imaging and biological conformality. *Int J Radiat Oncol Biol Phys* 2000;47(3):551–560.

13. Wilson GD, Bentzen SM, Harari PM. Biologic basis for combining drugs with radiation. *Semin Radiat Oncol* 2006;16(1):2–9.

14. Begg AC, Stewart FA, Vens C. Strategies to improve radiotherapy with targeted drugs. *Nat Rev Cancer* 2011;11(4):239–253.

15. Baumann M, Krause M, Zips D, et al. Molecular targeting in radiotherapy of lung cancer. *Lung Cancer* 2004;45(Suppl 2):S187–S197.

16. Rey S, Schito L, Koritzinsky M, et al. Molecular targeting of hypoxia in radiotherapy. *Adv Drug Deliv Rev* 2017;109:45–62.

17. Wahl DR, Lawrence TS. Integrating chemoradiation and molecularly targeted therapy. *Adv Drug Deliv Rev* 2017;109:74–83.

18. Baumann M, Krause M, Hill R. Exploring the role of cancer stem cells in radioresistance. *Nat Rev Cancer* 2008;8(7):545–554.

19. Baumann M, Krause M, Thames H, et al. Cancer stem cells and radiotherapy. *Int J Radiat Biol* 2009;85(5):391–402.

20. Kummermehr J, Trott K. Tumour stem cells. In: Potten C, ed. *Stem cells*. London, UK: Academic Press, 1997:363–400.

21. Ma BB, Bristow RG, Kim J, et al. Combined-modality treatment of solid tumors using radiotherapy and molecular targeted agents. *J Clin Oncol* 2003;21(14):2760–2776.

22. Bonner JA, Harari PM, Giralt J, et al. Radiotherapy plus cetuximab for squamous-cell carcinoma of the head and neck. *N Engl J Med* 2006;354(6):567–578.

23. Bonner JA, Harari PM, Giralt J, et al. Radiotherapy plus cetuximab for locoregionally advanced head and neck cancer: 5-year survival data from a phase 3 randomised trial, and relation between cetuximab-induced rash and survival. *Lancet Oncol* 2010;11(1):21–28.

24. Baumann M, Krause M, Dikomey E, et al. EGFR-targeted anti-cancer drugs in radiotherapy: preclinical evaluation of mechanisms. *Radiother Oncol* 2007;83(3):238–248.

25. Krause M, Gurtner K, Deuse Y, et al. Heterogeneity of tumour response to combined radiotherapy and EGFR inhibitors: differences between antibodies and TK inhibitors. *Int J Radiat Biol* 2009;85(11):943–954.

26. Sharma RA, Plummer R, Stock JK, et al. Clinical development of new drug-radiotherapy combinations. *Nat Rev Clin Oncol* 2016;13(10):627–642.

27. Hanahan D, Weinberg RA. The hallmarks of cancer. *Cell* 2000;100(1):57–70.

28. Hanahan D, Weinberg RA. Hallmarks of cancer: the next generation. *Cell* 2011;144(5):646–674.

29. Vermeulen K, Van Bockstaele DR, Berneman ZN. The cell cycle: a review of regulation, deregulation and therapeutic targets in cancer. *Cell Prolif* 2003;36(3):131–149.

30. Cowell JK. The nuclear oncoproteins: RB and p53. *Semin Cancer Biol* 1990;1(6):437–446.

31. Sager R. Tumor suppressor genes: the puzzle and the promise. *Science* 1989;246(4936):1406–1412.

32. Sharma S, Kelly TK, Jones PA. Epigenetics in cancer. *Carcinogenesis* 2010;31(1):27–36.

33. Feinberg AP, Koldobskiy MA, Gondor A. Epigenetic modulators, modifiers and mediators in cancer aetiology and progression. *Nat Rev Genet* 2016;17(5):284–299.

34. Jones PA, Issa JP, Baylin S. Targeting the cancer epigenome for therapy. *Nat Rev Genet* 2016;17(10):630–641.

35. Talmadge JE, Fidler IJ. AACR centennial series: the biology of cancer metastasis: historical perspective. *Cancer Res* 2010;70(14):5649–5669.

36. Peitzsch C, Perrin R, Hill RP, et al. Hypoxia as a biomarker for radioresistant cancer stem cells. *Int J Radiat Biol* 2014;90(8):636–652.

37. Gupta GP, Massague J. Cancer metastasis: building a framework. *Cell* 2006;127(4):679–695.

38. Nieto MA, Huang RY, Jackson RA, et al. Emt: 2016. *Cell* 2016;166(1):21–45.

39. Perez-Mancera PA, Young AR, Narita M. Inside and out: the activities of senescence in cancer. *Nat Rev Cancer* 2014;14(8):547–558.

40. Clarke MF, Dick JE, Dirks PB, et al. Cancer stem cells—perspectives on current status and future directions: AACR Workshop on cancer stem cells. *Cancer Res* 2006;66(19):9339–9344.

41. Marjanovic ND, Weinberg RA, Chaffer CL. Cell plasticity and heterogeneity in cancer. *Clin Chem* 2013;59(1):168–179.

42. Plaks V, Kong N, Werb Z. The cancer stem cell niche: how essential is the niche in regulating stemness of tumor cells? *Cell Stem Cell* 2015;16(3):225–238.

43. Chaffer CL, Brueckmann I, Scheel C, et al. Normal and neoplastic nonstem cells can spontaneously convert to a stem-like state. *Proc Natl Acad Sci U S A* 2011;108(19):7950–7955.

44. Blasco MA. Telomeres and human disease: ageing, cancer and beyond. *Nat Rev Genet* 2005;6(8):611–622.

45. Folkman J. Role of angiogenesis in tumor growth and metastasis. *Semin Oncol* 2002;29(6 Suppl 16):15–18.

46. Hanahan D, Folkman J. Patterns and emerging mechanisms of the angiogenic switch during tumorigenesis. *Cell* 1996;86(3):353–364.

47. Bergers G, Benjamin LE. Tumorigenesis and the angiogenic switch. *Nat Rev Cancer* 2003;3(6):401–410.

48. Liao D, Johnson RS. Hypoxia: a key regulator of angiogenesis in cancer. *Cancer Metastasis Rev* 2007;26(2):281–290.

49. Collado M, Serrano M. Senescence in tumours: evidence from mice and humans. *Nat Rev Cancer* 2010;10(1):51–57.

50. Kelly GL, Strasser A. The essential role of evasion from cell death in cancer. *Adv Cancer Res* 2011;111:39–96.

51. Warburg O. *The metabolism of tumours: investigations from the Kaiser Wilhelm Institute for Biology, Berlin-Dahlem*. London, UK: Arnold Constable, 1930.

52. Warburg O. On the origin of cancer cells. *Science* 1956;123(3191):309–314.

53. Warburg O. On respiratory impairment in cancer cells. *Science* 1956;124(3215):269–270.

54. Daye D, Wellen KE. Metabolic reprogramming in cancer: unraveling the role of glutamine in tumorigenesis. *Semin Cell Dev Biol* 2012;23(4):362–369.

55. Dhup S, Dadhich RK, Porporato PE, et al. Multiple biological activities of lactic acid in cancer: influences on tumor growth, angiogenesis and metastasis. *Curr Pharm Des* 2012;18(10):1319–1330.

56. Butler EB, Zhao Y, Munoz-Pinedo C, et al. Stalling the engine of resistance: targeting cancer metabolism to overcome therapeutic resistance. *Cancer Res* 2013;73(9):2709–2717.

57. Zindl CL, Chaplin DD. Immunology. Tumor immune evasion. *Science* 2010;328(5979):697–698.

58. Dvorak HF. Tumors: wounds that do not heal. Similarities between tumor stroma generation and wound healing. *N Engl J Med* 1986;315(26):1650–1659.

59. DeNardo DG, Andreu P, Coussens LM. Interactions between lymphocytes and myeloid cells regulate pro- versus anti-tumor immunity. *Cancer Metastasis Rev* 2010;29(2):309–316.

60. Grivennikov SI, Greten FR, Karin M. Immunity, inflammation, and cancer. *Cell* 2010;140(6):883–899.

61. Qian BZ, Pollard JW. Macrophage diversity enhances tumor progression and metastasis. *Cell* 2010;141(1):39–51.

62. Fridman WH, Pages F, Sautes-Fridman C, et al. The immune contexture in human tumours: impact on clinical outcome. *Nat Rev Cancer* 2012;12(4):298–306.

63. You JS, Jones PA. Cancer genetics and epigenetics: two sides of the same coin? *Cancer Cell* 2012;22(1):9–20.

64. Baylin SB, Ohm JE. Epigenetic gene silencing in cancer—a mechanism for early oncogenic pathway addiction? *Nat Rev Cancer* 2006;6(2):107–116.

65. zur Hausen H. Papillomaviruses causing cancer: evasion from host-cell control in early events in carcinogenesis. *J Natl Cancer Inst* 2000;92(9):690–698.

66. Haverkos HW. Viruses, chemicals and co-carcinogenesis. *Oncogene* 2004;23(38):6492–6499.

67. Vaupel P, Harrison L. Tumor hypoxia: causative factors, compensatory mechanisms, and cellular response. *Oncologist* 2004;9(Suppl 5):4–9.

68. Sarasin A. An overview of the mechanisms of mutagenesis and carcinogenesis. *Mutat Res* 2003;544(2–3):99–106.

69. Knudson AG. Two genetic hits (more or less) to cancer. *Nat Rev Cancer* 2001;1(2):157–162.

70. Fearon ER, Vogelstein B. A genetic model for colorectal tumorigenesis. *Cell* 1990;61(5):759–767.

71. Balmain A, Gray J, Ponder B. The genetics and genomics of cancer. *Nat Genet* 2003;33(Suppl):238–244.

72. Hazan RB, Qiao R, Keren R, et al. Cadherin switch in tumor progression. *Ann N Y Acad Sci* 2004;1014:155–163.

73. Tomasetti C, Li L, Vogelstein B. Stem cell divisions, somatic mutations, cancer etiology, and cancer prevention. *Science* 2017;355(6331):1330–1334.

74. Wu S, Powers S, Zhu W, et al. Substantial contribution of extrinsic risk factors to cancer development. *Nature* 2016;529(7584):43–47.

75. Okada H, Mak TW. Pathways of apoptotic and non-apoptotic death in tumour cells. *Nat Rev Cancer* 2004;4(8):592–603.

76. Eriksson D, Stigbrand T. Radiation-induced cell death mechanisms. *Tumour Biol* 2010;31(4):363–372.

77. Shinomiya N, Kuno Y, Yamamoto F, et al. Different mechanisms between premitotic apoptosis and postmitotic apoptosis in X-irradiated U937 cells. *Int J Radiat Oncol Biol Phys* 2000;47(3):767–777.

78. Brown JM, Attardi LD. The role of apoptosis in cancer development and treatment response. *Nat Rev Cancer* 2005;5(3):231–237.

79. Wouters BG, Denko NC, Giaccia AJ, et al. A p53 and apoptotic independent role for p21waf1 in tumour response to radiation therapy. *Oncogene* 1999;18(47):6540–6545.

80. Rodemann HP, Bamberg M. Cellular basis of radiation-induced fibrosis. *Radiother Oncol* 1995;35(2):83–90.

81. Ewald JA, Desotelle JA, Wilding G, et al. Therapy-induced senescence in cancer. *J Natl Cancer Inst* 2010;102(20):1536–1546.

82. Vecchio FM, Valentini V, Minsky BD, et al. The relationship of pathologic tumor regression grade (TRG) and outcomes after preoperative therapy in rectal cancer. *Int J Radiat Oncol Biol Phys* 2005;62(3):752–760.

83. Thomas M, Rube C, Semik M, et al. Impact of preoperative bimodality induction including twice-daily radiation on tumor regression and survival in stage III non-small-cell lung cancer. *J Clin Oncol* 1999;17(4):1185.

84. Fulda S. Therapeutic exploitation of necroptosis for cancer therapy. *Semin Cell Dev Biol* 2014;35:51–56.

85. Vanden Berghe T, Linkermann A, Jouan-Lanhouet S, et al. Regulated necrosis: the expanding network of non-apoptotic cell death pathways. *Nat Rev Mol Cell Biol* 2014;15(2):135–147.

86. Liu X, Zhou M, Mei L, et al. Key roles of necroptotic factors in promoting tumor growth. *Oncotarget* 2016;7(16):22219–22233.

87. Rouschop KM, Wouters BG. Regulation of autophagy through multiple independent hypoxic signaling pathways. *Curr Mol Med* 2009;9(4):417–424.

88. Vitale I, Manic G, De Maria R, et al. DNA Damage in Stem Cells. *Mol Cell* 2017;66(3):306–319.

89. Wallace SS. Enzymatic processing of radiation-induced free radical damage in DNA. *Radiat Res* 1998;150(5 Suppl):S60–S79.

90. Wright EA, Howard-Flanders P. The influence of oxygen on the radiosensitivity of mammalian tissues. *Acta Radiol* 1957;48(1):26–32.

91. Gray LH, Conger AD, Ebert M, et al. The concentration of oxygen dissolved in tissues at the time of irradiation as a factor in radiotherapy. *Br J Radiol* 1953;26(312):638–648.

92. Munro TR, Gilbert CW. The relation between tumour lethal doses and the radiosensitivity of tumour cells. *Br J Radiol* 1961;34:246–251.

93. Warters RL, Hofer KG, Harris CR, et al. Radionuclide toxicity in cultured mammalian cells: elucidation of the primary site of radiation damage. *Curr Top Radiat Res Q* 1978;12(1–4):389–407.

94. Ward JF. DNA damage produced by ionizing radiation in mammalian cells: identities, mechanisms of formation, and reparability. *Prog Nucleic Acid Res Mol Biol* 1988;35:95–125.

95. Allen C, Borak TB, Tsujii H, et al. Heavy charged particle radiobiology: using enhanced biological effectiveness and improved beam focusing to advance cancer therapy. *Mutat Res* 2011;711(1–2):150–157.

96. Kolesnick R, Fuks Z. Radiation and ceramide-induced apoptosis. *Oncogene* 2003;22(37):5897–5906.

97. Valerie K, Povirk LF. Regulation and mechanisms of mammalian double-strand break repair. *Oncogene* 2003;22(37):5792–5812.

98. Choudhury A, Cuddihy A, Bristow RG. Radiation and new molecular agents part I: targeting ATM-ATR checkpoints, DNA repair, and the proteasome. *Semin Radiat Oncol* 2006;16(1):51–58.

99. Khanna KK, Lavin MF, Jackson SP, et al. ATM, a central controller of cellular responses to DNA damage. *Cell Death Differ* 2001;8(11):1052–1065.

100. Lindahl T. Instability and decay of the primary structure of DNA. *Nature* 1993;362(6422):709–715.

101. Helleday T, Lo J, van Gent DC, et al. DNA double-strand break repair: from mechanistic understanding to cancer treatment. *DNA Repair* 2007;6(7):923–935.

102. Fortini P, Dogliotti E. Base damage and single-strand break repair: mechanisms and functional significance of short- and long-patch repair subpathways. *DNA Repair* 2007;6(4):398–409.

103. Wilson DM III, Bohr VA. The mechanics of base excision repair, and its relationship to aging and disease. *DNA Repair* 2007;6(4):544–559.

104. Mladenov E, Iliakis G. Induction and repair of DNA double strand breaks: the increasing spectrum of non-homologous end joining pathways. *Mutat Res* 2011;711(1–2):61–72.

105. Barker CA, Powell SN. Enhancing radiotherapy through a greater understanding of homologous recombination. *Semin Radiat Oncol* 2010;20(4):267–273, e263.

106. Wyatt HD, West SC. Holliday junction resolvases. *Cold Spring Harb Perspect Biol* 2014;6(9):a023192.

107. Li J, Xu X. DNA double-strand break repair: a tale of pathway choices. *Acta Biochim Biophys Sin (Shanghai)* 2016;48(7):641–646.

108. Iliakis G. Backup pathways of NHEJ in cells of higher eukaryotes: cell cycle dependence. *Radiother Oncol* 2009;92(3):310–315.

109. Willers H, McCarthy EE, Wu B, et al. Dissociation of p53-mediated suppression of homologous recombination from G1/S cell cycle checkpoint control. *Oncogene* 1999;19(5):632–639.

110. Storch K, Eke I, Borgmann K, et al. Three-dimensional cell growth confers radioresistance by chromatin density modification. *Cancer Res* 2010;70(10):3925–3934.

111. Jakob B, Splinter J, Conrad S, et al. DNA double-strand breaks in heterochromatin elicit fast repair protein recruitment, histone H2AX phosphorylation and relocation to euchromatin. *Nucleic Acids Res* 2011;39(15):6489–6499.

112. Goodarzi AA, Noon AT, Deckbar D, et al. ATM signaling facilitates repair of DNA double-strand breaks associated with heterochromatin. *Mol Cell* 2008;31(2):167–177.

113. Chiolo I, Minoda A, Colmenares SU, et al. Double-strand breaks in heterochromatin move outside of a dynamic HP1a domain to complete recombinational repair. *Cell* 2011;144(5):732–744.

114. Deckbar D, Jeggo PA, Lobrich M. Understanding the limitations of radiation-induced cell cycle checkpoints. *Crit Rev Biochem Mol Biol* 2011;46(4):271–283.

115. Bartek J, Lukas J. Mammalian G1- and S-phase checkpoints in response to DNA damage. *Curr Opin Cell Biol* 2001;13(6):738–747.

116. Alarcon-Vargas D, Ronai Z. p53-Mdm2—the affair that never ends. *Carcinogenesis* 2002;23(4):541–547.

117. Knudsen ES, Knudsen KE. Tailoring to RB: tumour suppressor status and therapeutic response. *Nat Rev Cancer* 2008;8(9):714–724.

118. Taylor AM, Groom A, Byrd PJ. Ataxia-telangiectasia-like disorder (ATLD)-its clinical presentation and molecular basis. *DNA Repair* 2004;3(8–9):1219–1225.

119. Falck J, Mailand N, Syljuasen RG, et al. The ATM-Chk2-Cdc25A checkpoint pathway guards against radioresistant DNA synthesis. *Nature* 2001;410(6830):842–847.

120. Kim ST, Xu B, Kastan MB. Involvement of the cohesin protein, Smc1, in Atm-dependent and independent responses to DNA damage. *Genes Dev* 2002;16(5):560–570.

121. Zhou XY, Wang X, Hu B, et al. An ATM-independent S-phase checkpoint response involves CHK1 pathway. *Cancer Res* 2002;62(6):1598–1603.

122. Denekamp J. Cell kinetics and radiation biology. *Int J Radiat Biol Relat Stud Phys Chem Med* 1986;49(2):357–380.

123. Nurse P. Universal control mechanism regulating onset of M-phase. *Nature* 1990;344(6266):503–508.

124. Peng CY, Graves PR, Thoma RS, et al. Mitotic and G2 checkpoint control: regulation of 14-3-3 protein binding by phosphorylation of Cdc25C on serine-216. *Science* 1997;277(5331):1501–1505.

125. Peng A, Chen PL. NFBD1/Mdc1 mediates ATR-dependent DNA damage response. *Cancer Res* 2005;65(4):1158–1163.

126. Schmidt-Ullrich RK, Dent P, Grant S, et al. Signal transduction and cellular radiation responses. *Radiat Res* 2000;153(3):245–257.

127. Mikkelsen RB, Wardman P. Biological chemistry of reactive oxygen and nitrogen and radiation-induced signal transduction mechanisms. *Oncogene* 2003;22(37):5734–5754.

128. Oda K, Matsuoka Y, Funahashi A, et al. A comprehensive pathway map of epidermal growth factor receptor signaling. *Mol Syst Biol* 2005;1:2005.0010.

129. Blume-Jensen P, Hunter T. Oncogenic kinase signalling. *Nature* 2001;411(6835):355–365.

130. Yarden Y, Sliwkowski MX. Untangling the ErbB signalling network. *Nat Rev Mol Cell Biol* 2001;2(2):127–137.

131. Hynes NE, Lane HA. ERBB receptors and cancer: the complexity of targeted inhibitors. *Nat Rev Cancer* 2005;5(5):341–354.

132. Morello V, Cabodi S, Sigismund S, et al. β1 integrin controls EGFR signaling and tumorigenic properties of lung cancer cells. *Oncogene* 2011;30(39):4087–4096.

133. Schmidt-Ullrich RK, Valerie K, Fogleman PB, et al. Radiation-induced autophosphorylation of epidermal growth factor receptor in human malignant mammary and squamous epithelial cells. *Radiat Res* 1996;145(1):81–85.

134. Leach JK, Black SM, Schmidt-Ullrich RK, et al. Activation of constitutive nitric-oxide synthase activity as an early signaling event induced by ionizing radiation. *J Biol Chem* 2002;277(18):15400–15406.

135. Barcellos-Hoff MH. Latency and activation in the control of TGF-beta. *J Mammary Gland Biol Neoplasia* 1996;1(4):353–363.

136. Toulany M, Dittmann K, Kruger M, et al. Radioresistance of K-Ras mutated human tumor cells is mediated through EGFR-dependent activation of PI3K-AKT pathway. *Radiother Oncol* 2005;76(2):143–150.

137. Dent P, Reardon DB, Park JS, et al. Radiation-induced release of transforming growth factor alpha activates the epidermal growth factor receptor and mitogen-activated protein kinase pathway in carcinoma cells, leading to increased proliferation and protection from radiation-induced cell death. *Mol Biol Cell* 1999;10(8):2493–2506.

138. Schmidt-Ullrich RK, Mikkelsen RB, Dent P, et al. Radiation-induced proliferation of the human A431 squamous carcinoma cells is dependent on EGFR tyrosine phosphorylation. *Oncogene* 1997;15(10):1191–1197.

139. Eriksen JG, Buffa FM, Alsner J, et al. Molecular profiles as predictive marker for the effect of overall treatment time of radiotherapy in supraglottic larynx squamous cell carcinomas. *Radiother Oncol* 2004;72(3):275–282.

140. Eriksen JG, Steiniche T, Askaa J, et al. The prognostic value of epidermal growth factor receptor is related to tumor differentiation and the overall treatment time of radiotherapy in squamous cell carcinomas of the head and neck. *Int J Radiat Oncol Biol Phys* 2004;58(2):561–566.

141. Bentzen SM, Atasoy BM, Daley FM, et al. Epidermal growth factor receptor expression in pretreatment biopsies from head and neck squamous cell carcinoma as a predictive factor for a benefit from accelerated radiation therapy in a randomized controlled trial. *J Clin Oncol* 2005;23(24):5560–5567.

142. Mendelsohn J, Baselga J. The EGF receptor family as targets for cancer therapy. *Oncogene* 2000;19(56):6550–6565.

143. Marmor MD, Skaria KB, Yarden Y. Signal transduction and oncogenesis by ErbB/HER receptors. *Int J Radiat Oncol Biol Phys* 2004;58(3):903–913.

144. Lin SY, Makino K, Xia W, et al. Nuclear localization of EGF receptor and its potential new role as a transcription factor. *Nat Cell Biol* 2001;3(9):802–808.

145. Toulany M, Dittmann K, Baumann M, et al. Radiosensitization of Ras-mutated human tumor cells in vitro by the specific EGF receptor antagonist BIBX1382BS. *Radiother Oncol* 2005;74(2):117–129.

146. Krause M, Schutze C, Petersen C, et al. Different classes of EGFR inhibitors may have different potential to improve local tumour control after fractionated irradiation: a study on C225 in FaDu hSCC. *Radiother Oncol* 2005;74(2):109–115.

147. Gurtner K, Deuse Y, Butof R, et al. Diverse effects of combined radiotherapy and EGFR inhibition with antibodies or TK inhibitors on local tumour control and correlation with EGFR gene expression. *Radiother Oncol* 2011;99(3):323–330.

148. Salomon DS, Brandt R, Ciardiello F, et al. Epidermal growth factor-related peptides and their receptors in human malignancies. *Crit Rev Oncol Hematol* 1995;19(3):183–232.

149. Brunner TB, Hahn SM, Gupta AK, et al. Farnesyltransferase inhibitors: an overview of the results of preclinical and clinical investigations. *Cancer Res* 2003;63(18):5656–5668.

150. Fresno JA, Casado E, de Castro J, et al. PI3K/Akt signalling pathway and cancer. *Cancer Treat Rev* 2004;30(2):193–204.

151. Sansal I, Sellers WR. The biology and clinical relevance of the PTEN tumor suppressor pathway. *J Clin Oncol Off J Am Soc Clin Oncol* 2004;22(14):2954–2963.

152. Li M, Ping G, Plathow C, et al. Small molecule receptor tyrosine kinase inhibitor of platelet-derived growth factor signaling (SU9518) modifies radiation response in fibroblasts and endothelial cells. *BMC Cancer* 2006;6:79.

153. Abdollahi A, Li M, Ping G, et al. Inhibition of platelet-derived growth factor signaling attenuates pulmonary fibrosis. *J Exp Med* 2005;201(6):925–935.

154. Cross MJ, Dixelius J, Matsumoto T, et al. VEGF-receptor signal transduction. *Trends Biochem Sci* 2003;28(9):488–494.

155. Wachsberger P, Burd R, Dicker AP. Tumor response to ionizing radiation combined with antiangiogenesis or vascular targeting agents: exploring mechanisms of interaction. *Clin Cancer Res* 2003;9(6):1957–1971.

156. Zips D, Eicheler W, Geyer P, et al. Enhanced susceptibility of irradiated tumor vessels to vascular endothelial growth factor receptor tyrosine kinase inhibition. *Cancer Res* 2005;65(12):5374–5379.

157. Kermani P, Leclerc G, Martel R, et al. Effect of ionizing radiation on thymidine uptake, differentiation, and VEGFR2 receptor expression in endothelial cells: the role of VEGF(165). *Int J Radiat Oncol Biol Phys* 2001;50(1):213–220.

158. Winkler F, Kozin SV, Tong RT, et al. Kinetics of vascular normalization by VEGFR2 blockade governs brain tumor response to radiation: role of oxygenation, angiopoietin-1, and matrix metalloproteinases. *Cancer Cell* 2004;6(6):553–563.

159. Schrand B, Verma B, Levay A, et al. Radiation-induced enhancement of antitumor T-cell immunity by VEGF-targeted 4-1BB costimulation. *Cancer Res* 2017;77(6):1310–1321.

160. Platanias LC. Mechanisms of type-I- and type-II-interferon-mediated signalling. *Nat Rev Immunol* 2005;5(5):375–386.

161. Jones VS, Huang RY, Chen LP, et al. Cytokines in cancer drug resistance: cues to new therapeutic strategies. *Biochim Biophys Acta* 2016;1865(2):255–265.

162. Karim R, Tse G, Putti T, et al. The significance of the Wnt pathway in the pathology of human cancers. *Pathology* 2004;36(2):120–128.

163. Peitzsch C, Cojoc M, Hein L, et al. An epigenetic reprogramming strategy to resensitize radioresistant prostate cancer cells. *Cancer Res* 2016;76(9):2637–2651.

164. de Sousa EMF, Vermeulen L. Wnt signaling in cancer stem cell biology. *Cancers (Basel)* 2016;8(7).

165. Wend P, Holland JD, Ziebold U, et al. Wnt signaling in stem and cancer stem cells. *Semin Cell Dev Biol* 2010;21(8):855–863.

166. Benoit YD, Guezguez B, Boyd AL, et al. Molecular pathways: epigenetic modulation of Wnt-glycogen synthase kinase-3 signaling to target human cancer stem cells. *Clin Cancer Res* 2014;20(21):5372–5378.

167. Hynes RO. Integrins: bidirectional, allosteric signaling machines. *Cell* 2002;110(6):673–687.

168. Dickreuter E, Cordes N. The cancer cell adhesion resistome: mechanisms, targeting and translational approaches. *Biol Chem* 2017;398(7):721–735.

169. Cordes N, Meineke V. Cell adhesion-mediated radioresistance (CAM-RR). Extracellular matrix-dependent improvement of cell survival in human tumor and normal cells in vitro. *Strahlenther Onkol* 2003;179(5):337–344.

170. Fridman R, Giaccone G, Kanemoto T, et al. Reconstituted basement membrane (matrigel) and laminin can enhance the tumorigenicity and the drug resistance of small cell lung cancer cell lines. *Proc Natl Acad Sci U S A* 1990;87(17):6698–6702.

171. Sethi T, Rintoul RC, Moore SM, et al. Extracellular matrix proteins protect small cell lung cancer cells against apoptosis: a mechanism for small cell lung cancer growth and drug resistance in vivo. *Nat Med* 1999;5(6):662–668.

172. Menendez JA, Vellon L, Mehmi I, et al. A novel CYR61-triggered 'CYR61-alphavbeta3 integrin loop' regulates breast cancer cell survival and chemosensitivity through activation of ERK1/ERK2 MAPK signaling pathway. *Oncogene* 2005;24(5):761–779.

173. Zhang H, Ozaki I, Mizuta T, et al. Beta 1-integrin protects hepatoma cells from chemotherapy induced apoptosis via a mitogen-activated protein kinase dependent pathway. *Cancer* 2002;95(4):896–906.

174. Hehlgans S, Haase M, Cordes N. Signalling via integrins: implications for cell survival and anticancer strategies. *Biochim Biophys Acta* 2007;1775(1):163–180.

175. Miyamoto H, Murakami T, Tsuchida K, et al. Tumor-stroma interaction of human pancreatic cancer: acquired resistance to anticancer drugs and proliferation regulation is dependent on extracellular matrix proteins. *Pancreas* 2004;28(1):38–44.

176. Cordes N, Frick S, Brunner TB, et al. Human pancreatic tumor cells are sensitized to ionizing radiation by knockdown of caveolin-1. *Oncogene* 2007;26(48):6851–6862.

177. Maubant S, Cruet-Hennequart S, Poulain L, et al. Altered adhesion properties and alphav integrin expression in a cisplatin-resistant human ovarian carcinoma cell line. *Int J Cancer* 2002;97(2):186–194.

178. Edlund M, Miyamoto T, Sikes RA, et al. Integrin expression and usage by prostate cancer cell lines on laminin substrata. *Cell Growth Differ* 2001;12(2):99–107.

179. Uhm JH, Dooley NP, Kyritsis AP, et al. Vitronectin, a glioma-derived extracellular matrix protein, protects tumor cells from apoptotic death. *Clin Cancer Res* 1999;5(6):1587–1594.

180. Damiano JS, Cress AE, Hazlehurst LA, et al. Cell adhesion mediated drug resistance (CAM-DR): role of integrins and resistance to apoptosis in human myeloma cell lines. *Blood* 1999;93(5):1658–1667.

181. Eke I, Cordes N. Dual targeting of EGFR and focal adhesion kinase in 3D grown HNSCC cell cultures. *Radiother Oncol* 2011;99(3):279–286.

182. Poschau M, Dickreuter E, Singh-Muller J, et al. EGFR and beta1-integrin targeting differentially affect colorectal carcinoma cell radiosensitivity and invasion. *Radiother Oncol* 2015;116(3):510–516.

183. Hazlehurst LA, Dalton WS. Mechanisms associated with cell adhesion mediated drug resistance (CAM-DR) in hematopoietic malignancies. *Cancer Metastasis Rev* 2001;20(1–2):43–50.

184. Cordes N, van Beuningen D. Arrest of human lung fibroblasts in G2 phase after irradiation is regulated by converging phosphatidylinositol-3 kinase and beta1-integrin signaling in vitro. *Int J Radiat Oncol Biol Phys* 2004;58(2):453–462.

185. Aoudjit F, Vuori K. Integrin signaling inhibits paclitaxel-induced apoptosis in breast cancer cells. *Oncogene* 2001;20(36):4995–5004.

186. Cordes N, Seidler J, Durzok R, et al. β1-integrin-mediated signaling essentially contributes to cell survival after radiation-induced genotoxic injury. *Oncogene* 2006;25(9):1378–1390.

187. Seidler J, Durzok R, Brakebusch C, et al. Interactions of the integrin subunit beta1A with protein kinase B/Akt, p130Cas and paxillin contribute to regulation of radiation survival. *Radiother Oncol* 2005;76(2):129–134.

188. Dimitrijevic-Bussod M, Balzaretti-Maggi VS, Gadbois DM. Extracellular matrix and radiation G1 cell cycle arrest in human fibroblasts. *Cancer Res* 1999;59(19):4843–4847.

189. Gadbois DM, Bradbury EM, Lehnert BE. Control of radiation-induced G1 arrest by cell-substratum interactions. *Cancer Res* 1997;57(6):1151–1156.

190. Kremer CL, Schmelz M, Cress AE. Integrin-dependent amplification of the G2 arrest induced by ionizing radiation. *Prostate* 2006;66(1):88–96.

191. Meineke V, Muller K, Ridi R, et al. Development and evaluation of a skin organ model for the analysis of radiation effects. *Strahlenther Onkol* 2004;180(2):102–108.

192. Dong L, Sun H, Liu W, et al. Effect of ligustrazine on expression of adherent molecule CD49d and cyclin D2 in hematopoietic cells in acute radiation injured mice. *J Tongji Med Univ* 1999;19(2):99–101.

193. Simon EL, Goel HL, Teider N, et al. High dose fractionated ionizing radiation inhibits prostate cancer cell adhesion and beta(1) integrin expression. *Prostate* 2005;64(1):83–91.

194. Cordes N, Blaese MA, Meineke V, et al. Ionizing radiation induces up-regulation of functional beta1-integrin in human lung tumour cell lines in vitro. *Int J Radiat Biol* 2002;78(5):347–357.

195. Cordes N, Hansmeier B, Beinke C, et al. Irradiation differentially affects substratum-dependent survival, adhesion, and invasion of glioblastoma cell lines. *Br J Cancer* 2003;89(11):2122–2132.

196. Monferran S, Skuli N, Delmas C, et al. Alphavbeta3 and alphavbeta5 integrins control glioma cell response to ionising radiation through ILK and RhoB. *Int J Cancer* 2008;123(2):357–364.

197. Eke I, Zscheppang K, Dickreuter E, et al. Simultaneous beta1 integrin-EGFR targeting and radiosensitization of human head and neck cancer. *J Natl Cancer Inst* 2015;107(2).

198. Kharas MG, Deane JA, Wong S, et al. Phosphoinositide 3-kinase signaling is essential for ABL oncogene-mediated transformation of B-lineage cells. *Blood* 2004;103(11):4268–4275.

199. Abbaspour Babaei M, Kamalidehghan B, Saleem M, et al. Receptor tyrosine kinase (c-Kit) inhibitors: a potential therapeutic target in cancer cells. *Drug Des Devel Ther* 2016;10:2443–2459.

200. Capdeville R, Buchdunger E, Zimmermann J, et al. Glivec (STI571, imatinib), a rationally developed, targeted anticancer drug. *Nat Rev Drug Discov* 2002;1(7):493–502.

201. Darnell JE, Jr. Transcription factors as targets for cancer therapy. *Nat Rev Cancer* 2002;2(10):740–749.

202. Eferl R, Wagner EF. AP-1: a double-edged sword in tumorigenesis. *Nat Rev Cancer* 2003;3(11):859–868.

203. Peitzsch C, Tyutyunnykova A, Pantel K, et al. Cancer stem cells: The root of tumor recurrence and metastases. *Semin Cancer Biol* 2017;44:10–24.

204. Kuhlmann JD, Hein L, Kurth I, et al. Targeting cancer stem cells: promises and challenges. *Anticancer Agents Med Chem* 2016;16(1):38–58.

205. Tang DG. Understanding cancer stem cell heterogeneity and plasticity. *Cell Res* 2012;22(3):457–472.

206. Takebe N, Miele L, Harris PJ, et al. Targeting Notch, Hedgehog, and Wnt pathways in cancer stem cells: clinical update. *Nat Rev Clin Oncol* 2015;12(8):445–464.

207. de Bono JS, Scher HI, Montgomery RB, et al. Circulating tumor cells predict survival benefit from treatment in metastatic castration-resistant prostate cancer. *Clin Cancer Res* 2008;14(19):6302–6309.

208. Pierga JY, Hajage D, Bachelot T, et al. High independent prognostic and predictive value of circulating tumor cells compared with serum tumor markers in a large prospective trial in first-line chemotherapy for metastatic breast cancer patients. *Ann Oncol* 2012;23(3):618–624.

209. Kendal WS, Frost P. Genomic instability, tumor heterogeneity and progression. *Adv Exp Med Biol* 1988;233:1–4.

210. Easwaran H, Johnstone SE, Van Neste L, et al. A DNA hypermethylation module for the stem/progenitor cell signature of cancer. *Genome Res* 2012;22(5):837–849.

211. Pfister SX, Ashworth A. Marked for death: targeting epigenetic changes in cancer. *Nat Rev Drug Discov* 2017;16(4):241–263.

212. Schumacher T, Bunse L, Pusch S, et al. A vaccine targeting mutant IDH1 induces antitumour immunity. *Nature* 2014;512(7514):324–327.

213. Yarchoan M, Johnson BA III, Lutz ER, et al. Targeting neoantigens to augment antitumour immunity. *Nat Rev Cancer* 2017;17(4):209–222.

214. Snyder A, Makarov V, Merghoub T, et al. Genetic basis for clinical response to CTLA-4 blockade in melanoma. *N Engl J Med* 2014;371(23):2189–2199.

215. Rizvi NA, Hellmann MD, Snyder A, et al. Cancer immunology. Mutational landscape determines sensitivity to PD-1 blockade in non-small cell lung cancer. *Science* 2015;348(6230):124–128.

216. Topp MS, Gokbuget N, Stein AS, et al. Safety and activity of blinatumomab for adult patients with relapsed or refractory B-precursor acute lymphoblastic leukaemia: a multicentre, single-arm, phase 2 study. *Lancet Oncol* 2015;16(1):57–66.

217. Porter DL, Levine BL, Kalos M, et al. Chimeric antigen receptor-modified T cells in chronic lymphoid leukemia. *N Engl J Med* 2011;365(8):725–733.

218. Conway MJ, Meyers C. Replication and assembly of human papillomaviruses. *J Dent Res* 2009;88(4):307–317.

219. Moody CA, Laimins LA. Human papillomavirus oncoproteins: pathways to transformation. *Nat Rev Cancer* 2010;10(8):550–560.

220. Cheng S, Schmidt-Grimminger DC, Murant T, et al. Differentiation-dependent up-regulation of the human papillomavirus E7 gene reactivates cellular DNA replication in suprabasal differentiated keratinocytes. *Genes Dev* 1995;9(19):2335–2349.

221. Khleif SN, DeGregori J, Yee CL, et al. Inhibition of cyclin D-CDK4/CDK6 activity is associated with an E2F-mediated induction of cyclin kinase inhibitor activity. *Proc Natl Acad Sci U S A* 1996;93(9):4350–4354.

222. Halperin CH, Gillison ML. Human papillomavirus in head and neck cancer: its role in pathogenesis and clinical implications. *Clin Cancer Res* 2009;15(22):6758–6762.

223. Nevins JR. The Rb/E2F pathway and cancer. *Hum Mol Genet* 2001;10(7):699–703.

224. Rieckmann T, Tribius S, Grob TJ, et al. HNSCC cell lines positive for HPV and p16 possess higher cellular radiosensitivity due to an impaired DSB repair capacity. *Radiother Oncol* 2013;107(2):242–246.

225. Kufe D, Weichselbaum R. Radiation therapy: activation for gene transcription and the development of genetic radiotherapy-therapeutic strategies in oncology. *Cancer Biol Ther* 2003;2(4):326–329.

226. Hallahan DE, Sukhatme VP, Sherman ML, et al. Protein kinase C mediates x-ray inducibility of nuclear signal transducers EGR1 and JUN. *Proc Natl Acad Sci U S A* 1991;88(6):2156–2160.

227. Haase MG, Klawitter A, Geyer P, et al. Sustained elevation of NF-kappaB DNA binding activity in radiation-induced lung damage in rats. *Int J Radiat Biol* 2003;79(11):863–877.

228. Barker HE, Paget JT, Khan AA, et al. The tumour microenvironment after radiotherapy: mechanisms of resistance and recurrence. *Nat Rev Cancer* 2015;15(7):409–425.

229. Brach MA, Hass R, Sherman ML, et al. Ionizing radiation induces expression and binding activity of the nuclear factor kappa B. *J Clin Invest* 1991;88(2):691–695.

230. Jung M, Kondratyev A, Lee SA, et al. ATM gene product phosphorylates I kappa B-alpha. *Cancer Res* 1997;57(1):24–27.

231. Devary Y, Rosette C, DiDonato JA, et al. NF-kappa B activation by ultraviolet light not dependent on a nuclear signal. *Science* 1993;261(5127):1442–1445.

232. Piret B, Schoonbroodt S, Piette J. The ATM protein is required for sustained activation of NF-kappaB following DNA damage. *Oncogene* 1999;18(13):2261–2271.

233. Ahmed KM, Li JJ. NF-kappa B-mediated adaptive resistance to ionizing radiation. *Free Radic Biol Med* 2008;44(1):1–13.

234. Hauer-Jensen M, Richter KK, Wang J, et al. Changes in transforming growth factor beta1 gene expression and immunoreactivity levels during development of chronic radiation enteropathy. *Radiat Res* 1998;150(6):673–680.

235. Barcellos-Hoff MH. Integrative radiation carcinogenesis: interactions between cell and tissue responses to DNA damage. *Semin Cancer Biol* 2005;15(2):138–148.

236. Martin M, Lefaix J, Delanian S. TGF-beta1 and radiation fibrosis: a master switch and a specific therapeutic target? *Int J Radiat Oncol Biol Phys* 2000;47(2):277–290.

237. Yarnold J, Brotons MC. Pathogenetic mechanisms in radiation fibrosis. *Radiother Oncol* 2010;97(1):149–161.

238. Dadrich M, Nicolay NH, Flechsig P, et al. Combined inhibition of TGFbeta and PDGF signaling attenuates radiation-induced pulmonary fibrosis. *Oncoimmunology* 2016;5(5):e1123366.

239. Minn AJ, Gupta GP, Siegel PM, et al. Genes that mediate breast cancer metastasis to lung. *Nature* 2005;436(7050):518–524.

240. Cook JA, Choudhuri R, Degraff W, et al. Halofuginone enhances the radiation sensitivity of human tumor cell lines. *Cancer Lett* 2010;289(1):119–126.

241. Bouquet F, Pal A, Pilones KA, et al. TGFbeta1 inhibition increases the radiosensitivity of breast cancer cells in vitro and promotes tumor control by radiation in vivo. *Clin Cancer Res* 2011;17(21):6754–6765.

242. Rube CE, Uthe D, Wilfert F, et al. The bronchiolar epithelium as a prominent source of pro-inflammatory cytokines after lung irradiation. *Int J Radiat Oncol Biol Phys* 2005;61(5):1482–1492.

243. Rube CE, van Valen F, Wilfert F, et al. Ewing's sarcoma and peripheral primitive neuroectodermal tumor cells produce large quantities of bioactive tumor necrosis factor-alpha (TNF-alpha) after radiation exposure. *Int J Radiat Oncol Biol Phys* 2003;56(5):1414–1425.

244. Allan JM, Travis LB. Mechanisms of therapy-related carcinogenesis. *Nat Rev Cancer* 2005;5(12):943–955.

245. Hall EJ. Intensity-modulated radiation therapy, protons, and the risk of second cancers. *Int J Radiat Oncol Biol Phys* 2006;65(1):1–7.

246. Trott KR, Rosemann M. Molecular mechanisms of radiation carcinogenesis and the linear, non-threshold dose response model of radiation risk estimation. *Radiat Environ Biophys* 2000;39(2):79–87.

247. Little JB. Induction of genetic instability by ionizing radiation. *C R Acad Sci III* 1999;322(2–3):127–134.

248. Trott KR, Teibe A. Lack of specificity of chromosome breaks resulting from radiation-induced genomic instability in Chinese hamster cells. *Radiat Environ Biophys* 1998;37(3):173–176.

249. Weichselbaum RR, Kufe DW, Hellman S, et al. Radiation-induced tumour necrosis factor-alpha expression: clinical application of transcriptional and physical targeting of gene therapy. *Lancet Oncol* 2002;3(11):665–671.

250. Mirghani H, Amen F, Tao Y, et al. Increased radiosensitivity of HPV-positive head and neck cancers: molecular basis and therapeutic perspectives. *Cancer Treat Rev* 2015;41(10):844–852.

251. Lassen P, Eriksen JG, Hamilton-Dutoit S, et al. Effect of HPV-associated p16INK4A expression on response to radiotherapy and survival in squamous cell carcinoma of the head and neck. *J Clin Oncol* 2009;27(12):1992–1998.

252. Lohaus F, Linge A, Tinhofer I, et al. HPV16 DNA status is a strong prognosticator of loco-regional control after postoperative radiochemotherapy of locally advanced oropharyngeal carcinoma: results from a multicentre explorative study of the German Cancer Consortium Radiation Oncology Group (DKTK-ROG). *Radiother Oncol* 2014;113(3):317–323.

253. Linge A, Lohaus F, Lock S, et al. HPV status, cancer stem cell marker expression, hypoxia gene signatures and tumour volume identify good prognosis subgroups in patients with HNSCC after primary radiochemotherapy: a multicentre retrospective study of the German Cancer Consortium Radiation Oncology Group (DKTK-ROG). *Radiother Oncol* 2016;121(3):364–373.

254. Linge A, Lock S, Gudziol V, et al. Low cancer stem cell marker expression and low hypoxia identify good prognosis subgroups in HPV(−) HNSCC after postoperative radiochemotherapy: a multicenter study of the DKTK-ROG. *Clin Cancer Res* 2016;22(11):2639–2649.

255. Zips D, Zophel K, Abolmaali N, et al. Exploratory prospective trial of hypoxia-specific PET imaging during radiochemotherapy in patients with locally advanced head-and-neck cancer. *Radiother Oncol* 2012;105(1):21–28.

256. Kerns SL, West CM, Andreassen CN, et al. Radiogenomics: the search for genetic predictors of radiotherapy response. *Future Oncol* 2014;10(15):2391–2406.

257. Kerns SL, Dorling L, Fachal L, et al. Meta-analysis of genome wide association studies identifies genetic markers of late toxicity following radiotherapy for prostate cancer. *EBioMedicine* 2016;10:150–163.

CHAPTER 3

Biologic Basis of Radiation Therapy*

William H. McBride, H. Rodney Withers, and Dörthe Schaue

INTRODUCTION

Clinically Relevant Physicochemical Events

Ionizing radiation (IR) interacts with biologic matter in many different ways, but in essence, high-energy photons produce electrons that directly ionize atoms and can break chemical bonds. Subsequently, free radical and other reactive species are generated whose actions can be heavily influenced by the intracellular milieu. For low linear energy transfer (LET) x- or γ-rays, there is about 1,000 ionization tracks per gray (Gy), and most of the free radicals, such as hydroxyls, singlet oxygen, superoxide, and hydrogen peroxide, come from ionization of water, a cell's major (about 90%) constituent. These oxygen-containing molecules are often collectively, although not totally accurately, referred to as reactive oxygen species (ROS) and have half-times generally of <1 ms. They cause oxidative damage by virtue of their unpaired valence shell electrons and are particularly relevant for low LET radiation (perhaps 70%). This indirect mechanism has numerous implications for the biologic effects of radiation therapy (RT) and is a major reason why biologic dose differs from physical dose. The type (quality) of radiation also determines the biologic effect. For all IRs, the density is especially high at the end of the electron tracks, but for high LET radiations, such as α-particles, ionization is dense all along and close to tracks, which number about 4 per Gy. As a result, more energy is deposited directly in biologic molecules, resulting in more direct than indirect damage.

The interaction between free radicals and the biologic microenvironment is complex but critical for the outcome of RT. Oxygen, and other electron affinic molecules,[1] participates in free radical cascadic reactions, but probably, its major effect is to "fix" chemical damage within biologic molecules, limiting their chemical repair. Oxygen is therefore a potent radiosensitizer, whereas hypoxia limits radiation damage and is a possible cause of failure of cancer RT. Considerable effort has gone into the search for oxygen-mimetic drugs that might penetrate tumor hypoxic regions and radiosensitize tumors. Some, such as the imidazoles, have been used successfully in the context of RT and for imaging hypoxia. Conversely, antioxidants such as glutathione, which is present in millimolar amounts in cells, protect cells by scavenging free radicals.

In general, IR is an oxidative stress forming numerous oxidative adducts, lowering antioxidant levels, and changing redox status. Numerous redox-sensing proteins are altered with biologic consequences. For example, Keap1 controls transcriptional activation of the nuclear factor (erythroid-derived)-like 2, also known as NFE2L2 or Nrf2. This pathway is highly dysregulated in several human cancers, most notably non–small cell lung cancer,[2] and strongly impacts cellular anabolic metabolism, tumor aggression, and response to IR.[3] Cell lineages also vary naturally in these pathways. For example, quiescent stem cells generally have high levels of free radical scavengers and antioxidants that confer relative radioresistance.[4]

The first wave of radiation-induced free radicals is amplified by further oxidative stress reactions that generate more ROS/RNS (reactive nitrogen species). One outcome is inflammation that plays a major role in physiologic and pathologic events, causing cell death, perpetuating damage, and producing even more ROS/RNS from biologic sources, most notably mitochondria, activated cation membrane channels, NADPH and other oxidases, and nitric oxide synthase induction. Radiation-induced inflammation in the form of skin burns was the earliest radiobiologic observation. Recently, interest has been revived in radiation-induced inflammation because of radiation-induced vascular changes, bystander effects, and immune cell infiltration into normal tissues and tumors. As early as 1916, roentgenologists were asking, "is the effect of radiation merely the result of the reaction between the rays and the cells they happen to hit, or do the rays in some way exert an indirect action over the entire organism." It was concluded that the systemic effects of radiation were important in RT and attributable in part to "radiovaccination," that is, systemic immune activation.[5] These concepts were swamped by mathematical models relating dose to direct target killing, only to be recently resurrected.[6]

DNA as a Biologic Target in RT

All cellular organelles are damaged by IR, but the biggest footprint relevant to RT is in DNA. Complex or clustered DNA double-strand breaks (DSBs), also referred to as multiply damaged sites, are most significant for radiation lethality and carcinogenesis, as opposed to "simple" DSBs and other forms of damage. These form in both cycling and noncycling cells as multiple lesions involving 15 to 20 base pairs clustered within about 1 helical turn of the DNA. They are a direct consequence of the characteristic and unique way that IR spatially deposits energy in dense "packets" and are the reason why IR is a powerful cytotoxic therapy. Low LET IR generates about 30% of DNA DSBs of this form, whereas for α-particles, it is >90%. By way of contrast, few complex lesions result from everyday, "natural" oxidative and chemical DNA damage. As many as 70,000 DNA lesions are produced per cell per day, mainly as single-strand break (SSB) and base damage that are readily repaired, although one study estimates that about 1% of such lesions are converted into DSBs as they encounter replicative DNA polymerase, forming 50 DSBs every cell cycle that may have larger consequences.[7]

---

*With the passing of H. Rodney Withers on February 25, 2015, the radiation oncology field lost its most pre-eminent clinically oriented thinker. The *in vivo* stem cell assays he developed over half a century ago were used by him and others to elucidate the biology behind many clinical radiation phenomena. The general principles he developed are forever enshrined in his 4Rs that fundamentally shaped the way we conceptualize fractionated radiation therapy for cancer treatment. The quantitation he developed spawned the phase III clinical trials on altered fractionation in the 1990s. However, perhaps more than anything else, his clarity of thought and attention to critical issues pertaining to the biologic effects of radiation delivery in the clinic remain his most brilliant contribution. Some of these concepts he expressed in earlier versions of this chapter. Here, we have tried to retain the flavor of many of his ideas. Their relevance is unchanged, and they form part of his lasting legacy.

Safeguarding the integrity of DNA is a biologic imperative that is achieved through highly efficient DNA repair mechanisms, each with a focus on a type of DNA lesion. The mechanisms are discussed in more detail in Chapter 2, but defective DNA repair mechanisms can account for many differences in the response to cancer RT. The two major DSB repair pathways are nonhomologous end joining (NHEJ), which is error prone, efficient, and not cell cycle phase specific, and homologous recombination (HR), which operates only in late S/G2 cell cycle phase, uses the sister chromatid as a template, and has slow kinetics. These have different functions and have been honed by evolution to deal with physiologic DSBs produced during meiosis (HR), DNA replication (HR), and the generation of specific immune receptors (NHEJ). The key proteins required for both NHEJ (Ku70, Ku80, DNA-PKcs, XRCC4, XLF, DNA ligase IV) and HR (Rad51, Rad52, Rad54, BRCA2, RPA) have been identified by a combination of genetic experiments and the use of fluorescent antibodies to examine the composition of IR-induced foci (IRIF) that form at sites of DSBs. The proteins MRE11, Rad50, and NBS1 act as a complex (MRSN) and participate in both HR and NHEJ. Simpler DNA SSBs and base damages formed by IR (1,000 per cell per Gy) are rapidly repaired largely by base excision repair (BER).

DNA repair mechanisms face considerable challenges partly because of diversity of the lesions. Complex DNA damage is especially difficult and slow to resolve, whereas repair in heterochromatin is slower than in euchromatin. Further, SSBs may be converted into DSBs at replication forks, making BER relevant to RT outcome in cycling cells. One consequence of this diversity is that the time taken for DNA repair varies substantially. "Fast" and "slow" components are a minimum consideration, with the latter having estimated half-lives of up to 4 hours and with "residual" unrepaired DNA damage often being most relevant to outcome. Estimates of "repair" rates within a tissue are therefore very uncertain. Note that when clinical fractionated treatments are discussed, the interfraction time interval left to allow "repair" really refers to tissue recovery rather than DNA repair *per se*.

The way cells respond to DNA damage is very important in RT. In general terms, DNA damage is recognized by "sensor" molecules that activate "transducer" protein kinase cascades to trigger downstream effectors of the DNA damage response (DDR). The protein mutated in ataxia telangiectasia (ATM) is one such sensor, whose loss results in extreme radiosensitivity and a complex human syndrome. Another sensor is ATR (ataxia telangiectasia and Rad3-related) that recognizes and repairs DNA replication complexes that have stalled at sites of DNA damage. IRIF form at DNA DSBs and signal the initiation of the DDR. IRIF are complex in composition and number depending on, for example, whether the DSB is in euchromatin or heterochromatin and the cell cycle phase irradiated.

In one early IRIF event, histone 2A subtype, H2AX, is phosphorylated by one of several phosphoinositol 3-kinase–related protein kinases (PIKKs), such as the ATM, DNA-PK, and ATR. The resulting gamma-H2AX molecules bind to DSB over several megabases along the flanking chromatin and can easily be detected using specific antibody. This highly sensitive assay has become the popular way to measure DSB formation and repair.[8] The histone provides interaction surfaces for IRIFs enrolling repair and checkpoint molecules to activate further kinase-dependent pathways leading to coherent downstream DDRs. The classic DDR pathway, which is a hallmark of radiation damage, is through ATM, which then phosphorylates various downstream substrates, including p53, the checkpoint kinase CHK2, p21, BRCA1, NBS1, and Bak and Bax to effect DNA repair, cell cycle progression, and cell death by apoptosis. Not surprisingly, defects in molecules in DDR and DNA repair, especially HR, are major causes of impaired IR-induced G_1-S, intra-S, and G_2-M cell cycle checkpoints, as well as radiosensitivity, genomic instability, increased mutational load, and

chromosomal abnormalities, and cancer predisposition, and are targets for therapeutic intervention.

The cell cycle phase restriction of HR repair to S and G2 has ramifications for cancer biology and treatment. Those chemotherapies that target proliferating cells will engage HR, which may be especially critical for chemo-RT combinations. Also, mutations in the BRCA1 or BRCA2 tumor suppressor genes compromise the ability of cells to perform HR and makes them especially sensitive to PARP-1 inhibitors, which block BER. This process, where a failure in either of two genes is not lethal but failure of both results in cell death, is known as synthetic lethality. DNA repair can therefore provide opportunities for therapeutic intervention, for example, targeting HR through iPARP or iATR with RT.[9]

Finally, DNA DSBs breaks may rejoin to form chromosome/chromatid aberrations, and their frequency can serve as an indicator of radiation dose received. Lesions take many forms, but deletions can result in acentric fragments (chromosome fragments lacking a centromere) and micronuclei or chromosomes that have difficulty migrating with the rest during anaphase and yet may persist through several divisions. The relevance of DNA fragments to cell signaling is discussed later. Exchanges can form symmetric translocation or inversions, or dicentrics or rings. The latter are generally lethal, whereas inversions are one of the mutational signatures of radiation-induced cancers.[10]

Radiation-Induced Cell Signaling

IR directly damages cellular structures other than DNA that rapidly trigger primary genetic programs (also known as immediate early response) in the absence of *de novo* protein synthesis. These evolve along with DDR pathways into more restricted secondary gene programs. The doses and times at which these different pathways "kick in" to trigger their downstream effects after RT are not well known, but they form an integral part of the overall response to IR.

Redox changes are one way primary programs can be generated, but are complex, for example, low ROS levels can activate molecular responses, whereas high levels can cause cell death. Redox changes can also activate transcriptional programs. In addition to Nrf2 mentioned earlier, NF-κB, AP-1, HIF-1α, PPARγ, p53, Sp1, c-abl, and STAT3 are redox sensitive, as are phosphatases that control activation of various pathways, for example, through epidermal growth factor receptor (EGFR).

One result of this signaling is the production of proinflammatory cytokines, such as members of the tumor necrosis factor (TNF) family (e.g., TNF-α, fasL, Trail), interleukin-1, type I interferons, etc. These can be induced through ROS/DDR p53–mediated pathways, or through activation of early growth response gene 1 (EGR1), or through pattern recognition receptors (PRRs)—a system for innate immune recognition of pathogen- and damage-associated molecular patterns (PAMPs and DAMPs).[11,12] RT releases numerous DAMPs to trigger PPR signaling, but the radiation-induced micronuclei and cytoplasmic DNA fragments, most likely left behind at mitosis, are of particular interest. The sensor is cyclic GMP-AMP (cGAMP) synthase (cGAS) that produces cGAMP upon activation and, with the adaptor molecule STING, triggers IRF3, STAT6, and NF-κB pathways to produce type 1 interferon, IL-6, and TNF family members, respectively. The cGAS-STING pathway also assists in the generation of tumor-specific CD8-mediated immunity. Interestingly, high single radiation doses, through nuclease controls, seem less effective than moderate fractionated doses at generating these responses.[13] Activation of this pathway is probably modified by proliferative status and/or mode of cell death and is likely to be more important days after exposure, whereas immediate early pathway responses are initiated within minutes to hours. The cGAS-STING pathway also responds to intracellular pathogens leading to potent immune activation, so it is not surprising that aberrant activation by self DNA can lead to autoimmune and inflammatory disease. Inflammation is therefore tightly integrated within responses to RT at multiple different levels. For example, TNF molecules may be on the cell surface or released, the latter contributing to mechanisms of IR-induced bystander effects; the former may be more involved in cell death, vascular responses, and proliferative responses to RT.[14] It is worth noting that some clinical symptoms are probably because of radiation-induced TNF-α and other proinflammatory cytokines rather than cell death, for example, nausea or vomiting within hours of RT involving the upper abdomen, acute erythema and edema associated with vascular leakage, fatigue in patients receiving RT to a large volume, and somnolence within a few hours of cranial irradiation. Radiation-induced proliferative responses such as gliosis or certain forms of fibrosis may also cause symptoms unrelated to cell depletion.

Cellular Damage Responses after Irradiation

The final cellular outcome of RT will depend in part upon how cells and tissues "perceive" damage through internal and external "sensors." Sensors in addition to those already mentioned include hypoxia, cytokines, cell–cell and cell–matrix interactions. Cancer-related mutations in DNA repair, cell cycle, and cell death pathway molecules and cell metabolism will inevitably alter the clinical response to RT. It is easy to see why "biologic dose" differs considerably from "physical dose."

A major and desired cellular outcome of RT is cell death. This can occur in several different ways that can change with dose[15] and can determine the outcome of RT.[16]

Mitotic death after irradiation was observed first in 1956 by Puck and Marcus,[17] who made the critical observation that "cells in which the ability to reproduce has been destroyed by doses below 800r can still multiply several times. At higher doses, even a single cell division is precluded." They were observing mitotic death, which is the most common form of cancer cell death caused by IR. So, mitotic death can be delayed at low dose, and the length of delay is inversely dose dependent. After around 8 Gy, the number of divisions and perhaps the persistence of damage may decrease, as may the number of mutations generated and the likelihood of radiation-induced genomic instability and cancer. The mode of death also may change.[15]

Mitotic death can be due to any of several molecular mechanisms, but in the M phase, chromothripsis can occur, which is a single catastrophic shattering event followed by the stitching of genomic fragments into derivative chromosomes that might generate numerous rearrangements, further genomic instability, fragmented genetic material, and cause cGAS-STING activation.

Apoptosis, by way of contrast, was first[18] seen as interphase death occurring within 4 to 6 hours of low dose IR in certain cell types, including many lymphocytes, and some cells in the endothelium, salivary gland, thyroid, intestinal crypt, and hair follicles. Radiation-induced apoptosis is often, although not always, "intrinsic" through the DDR involving p53 with Bax and Bak as primary downstream effectors.[19] Mitochondrial membranes are disrupted and factors released that activate a cascade of proteolytic caspases and an endonuclease that cleaves DNA between nucleosomes, producing DNA fragments that are multiples of a defined size. So, cells commit "suicide." Alternatively, TNF family members can trigger an "extrinsic" pathway through cell membrane receptors of the TNFR family that contain "death domains." This extrinsic TNFR-driven death pathway utilizes caspase-8 but overlaps mechanistically with the intrinsic mitochondrial factor pathway that activates caspase-9, and both converge on the same final executioner caspase-3–dependent pathway to complete apoptosis. Many cell types are protected against apoptosis. Only cells that have their internal molecular "rheostat" on a proapoptosis setting

are susceptible. For the intrinsic pathway, Bcl-2 and Bcl-XL are important antiapoptotic factors. The TNF pathway is also controlled. For example, mice lacking TNFR2, which counters the TNFR1 death pathway, are particularly sensitive to late effects of brain irradiation.[20] IR increases the frequency of apoptosis but does not change the rheostat settings, that is, it does not convert an inherently antiapoptotic phenotype into one that is proapoptotic. In clinical terms, tumors that have a high proportion of cells with a proapoptotic phenotype, such as lymphoma, tend to be radiosensitive. They respond rapidly to RT because of rapid cell loss. They may also regrow fast. The same general principles generally hold for normal tissues, where rapid apoptosis is often associated with proliferating sites.

Necrosis is a form of cell death most frequently seen in pathologic tissue injury settings. Cell membrane integrity is lost, cells swell, lysosomal enzymes are released, vasculature is damaged, and inflammatory responses are generated. It may be caused either directly by IR or indirectly by immune infiltrating cells that have infiltrated in response to radiation damage. Necrosis is often considered unregulated, but regulated forms exist, called necroptosis and pyroptosis, that differ primarily in their usage of proinflammatory cytokines, the former involving TNF-α and the latter IL-1β and IL-18.

Autophagy is another alternative death style that can follow IR. This is a primordial survival response in which cells internalize their cellular organelles within vacuoles and recycle them; it is most often seen in nutrient deprivation. Cells can be rescued from autophagy, although they die when the process is taken to excess. Again, death is delayed.

Senescence is another very delayed response of many proliferating cell types to IR that is relevant to many pathologic situations, including aging. It is akin to a permanent DDR with cell cycle arrest through activation of cell cycle checkpoint activators such as p21 and p16 and production of antiproliferative cytokines, such as IL-6 and transforming growth factor beta (TGF-β).[21] Cytoplasmic DNA and the cGAS pathway mentioned earlier may be essential.[22] Because senescence-associated cytokines drive collagen production, IR-induced senescence may be a reason for the fibrosis[23] that is so often seen as late damage in irradiated tissues. The relevance of senescence to "bystander" effects may be considerable because it is a long-lived secretory phenotype.

Mitotic death, apoptosis, necrosis, autophagy, and senescence may all remove damaged cells from the reproductive pool, decreasing the risk of radiocarcinogenesis, but the differences in timing may have additional consequences, apart from fibrosis and bystander effects. Some cells may resist death and checkpoint arrest and reenter the cell cycle precociously with persisting DNA damage or may reprogram into stem/progenitor cells.[24] The mechanisms of cell death are therefore likely critical to late as well as acute radiation effects, genomic instability, tissue regeneration, tumor regrowth, and antitumor immunity after RT.

TISSUE DAMAGE RESPONSES

Molecular and Cellular Aspects

Tissues can generally be classified as having either high or low turnover, that is, rate of cell loss and regeneration. This is important in RT because it determines the response to changes in the size of dose per fraction.

For example, the small intestine has the highest turnover rate in the body, with epithelial cells traveling from the crypt, up the villus, to be shed in about 5 days. Slow cycling columnar Lgr5+ stem cells intermingle with Paneth cells at the base of crypts to maintain the procession but easily apoptose after RT. Directly above, at position 4+ from the crypt base, is a population of some controversy.[25] It seems to contain radio-resistant stem cells that regenerate rapidly in response to IR but also are sufficiently plastic to replace the lost Lgr5+ stem cells at the base of the crypt.[26] In any event, the microcolony assay[27] showed that loss of >90% of surviving regenerating crypts at 3.5 days is lethal for mice. In contrast, in the colon, which is more radioresistant, radiation-induced apoptosis in Lgr5+ stem cells is not so marked and proliferative recovery is slower. These differences have been ascribed to less precocious entry of cells into the cell cycle in the colon compared with small intestine.[28]

In the thymus, about 98% of the cells generated die by apoptosis under normal conditions. Not surprisingly, IR causes a strong DDR and massive rapid, p53-dependent cell death in the thymic cortex. Similar responses are seen in most lymphoid tissues, in the small intestine, in hair follicles, and in the ependyma. In contrast, some normal tissues, in response to IR, up-regulate p53 without apoptosing, whereas others show neither radiation-induced p53 nor apoptosis, for example, liver, skeletal muscle, and brain.[19] The functional significance of apoptosis may depend upon the location and whether it is part of a natural process that removes excess proliferating cells or is more integral to lineage development. In humans, acute parotitis can develop within the first 24 hours in patients receiving head and neck RT, which is due to rapid death of serous cells.[29] Hence, xerostomia (dry mouth) occurs early, before acute mucositis.

A case has recently been made for a critical role of radiation-induced endothelial cell apoptosis through ceramide activation in both normal tissue and tumor responses.[30-32] The role of the vasculature in radiation responses is however a long-standing controversy best viewed in a wider context. There is little doubt that IR causes vascular damage, most obviously observed as microvascular "pruning," which may diminish a tissue's reserves following IR and possibly cause some hypoxia. An additional factor may be radiation-induced inflammation that activates vasculature to promote extravascular egress of neutrophils and other immune cells from the circulation and impacts endothelial cell viability and thrombus formation. RT can be thought of as generating a hub of oxidative stress reactions and danger signals leading to proinflammatory chemokines and cytokines, with consequential up-regulation of proteases, cell adhesion molecules, and extracellular matrix materials. The vasculature is part of this, but *in toto*, it is a regulated acute tissue reaction that has its evolutionary roots in fighting infection with cell death and inflammation and is normally resolved through tissue regeneration and remodeling. IR doses above approximately 6 to 7 Gy are especially proinflammatory[12] and are required for ceramide-mediated vascular responses.[30-32] Hypofractionation may favor these responses, although conventional fractions may also generate them over a longer time period.

Inflammation and danger signaling can extend the influence of RT outside the radiation field.[14,33] In addition to bystander effects, systemic tumor-specific immunity may be generated by RT promoting inflammatory microenvironments that are permissive for innate immune recognition. DAMPs and inflammatory cytokines further promote maturation of antigen-presenting dendritic cells to better stimulate adaptive immunity that may manifest systemically as "abscopal" distant antitumor responses that impact overall survival or assist in local tumor cure.[34] A key aspect of this response has come to the fore through the recent demonstration that many human tumors are immunogenic because of mutations caused by chemical or viral exposure that can be recognized as nonself by the adaptive immune system.[35] Defective DNA repair mechanisms increase the mutational load, as might RT.[10] It seems that dose, dose per fraction, and radiation quality are important to radiation-induced immunity as in other aspects of RT, with moderately hypofractionated SBRT perhaps showing some superiority.[13,36] In any event, these scenarios form the rationale behind combining immune checkpoint inhibitors

(ICIs) with RT, which is currently the subject of numerous clinical trials.[33] It should be noted that ICIs also disrupt normal tissue homeostasis and, although less toxic than conventional therapies, come with added risk of inflammation and autoimmunity that could exacerbate radiation toxicities.

In the longer term, a train of events is initiated after RT that may in fact not resolve the disturbance in tissue homeostasis, but perpetuate it. Dose-related oscillating waves of inflammatory responses and further DNA damage have been observed in preclinical models for months after tissue exposure that likely have clinical relevance. These waves presumably reflect continual failed attempts at tissue recovery and remodeling.[12,14] Late complications of RT therefore come to resemble chronic inflammation, which raises hope that better understanding may lead to some treatments for these debilitating diseases. The disturbances because of cancer itself, such as high local and systemic levels of TGF-β, may additionally critically impact outcome.

Kinetics of Normal Tissue Radiation Injury

As has been said, the rate of tissue turnover, that is, rate of cell loss and regeneration, is important in defining the response to RT, including changes in the size of dose per fraction. It has been known since the time of the Curies that it takes varying amounts of time for tissues to express radiation injury (*latency*), leading to use of the terms *acute*, *subacute*, and *late* effects. Note that these refer to symptoms not tissues *per se*, as any one tissue can express acute and late endpoints at different times. Acute and late effects appear largely independent of each other, although a severe acute radiation injury can lead to nonspecific late (consequential) changes, such as stenosis consequent to mucosal ulceration of the bowel, or fibrosis or necrosis of skin or oropharynx consequent to desquamation and acute ulceration.

Acute Responses

Acute responses to RT are defined as occurring during a standard 6- to 8-week course of RT and are seen in tissues that turn over rapidly (gastrointestinal, oropharyngeal and esophageal mucosa, bone marrow, skin). Such tissues are organized hierarchically, generally with a small number of relatively quiescent stem cells that proliferate slowly to produce highly proliferative progenitor cells that differentiate into mature, nonproliferative, functional cells. The functional population is little affected by RT, and the time it takes for an acute effect to become apparent (latency) is the time to the natural loss of functional cells without replacement. In contrast, IR generally depletes the more radiation-sensitive proliferating cell pool, often causing death by apoptosis. If depletion is sufficient, the functional pool is not replaced, and serious, even fatal, consequences may ensue.

The timing and extent of regeneration is classically assessed experimentally by giving two doses of IR and varying the time in between by days, weeks, or months. These assays have been invaluable guides for more modern studies into the *in vivo* effects of RT on stem/progenitor populations using biomarkers such as Lgr5. Remarkably, the depleted stem/progenitor pools are often dramatically expanded before functional recovery is initiated, although this varies with the tissue. A useful way to think of the impact of regeneration is that under normal steady-state circumstances, tissues have, by definition, a cell loss factor (φ) of 1. The only requirement for tissue growth is a decrease in (φ) to <1, as for embryos and fetuses, tissue regeneration, and malignancy. After IR exposure, some tissues (e.g., jejunal crypts) appear to reduce (φ) to zero and regenerate quickly; others (e.g., skin) may reduce it to about 0.5 and regenerate less quickly, continuously producing some functional cells; others such as seminiferous epithelium show little change in (φ) and mostly continue in steady state, producing sperm in numbers that are reduced for months or years in direct proportion to the extent of stem cell depletion.

It follows from the above that leukocyte and platelet numbers in blood drop quickly after bone marrow irradiation because they have a fast turnover rate, whereas anemia is not so obvious because red cells turn over slowly. In the testis, each spermatogenic stem cell produces more than 1,000 sperm through successive divisions of a small number of radiosensitive spermatogonia and spermatocytes—a process that in humans takes more than 60 days. So, sperm counts remain normal for several weeks after RT, falling steeply only when the progeny of the irradiated spermatogonia would normally have reached the seminal vesicles. In the small intestine, crypt stem/progenitor cells are lost within days of exposure, and the nonproliferative villus is unaffected initially but shortens as cells are shed into the lumen and not replaced. So, symptoms take about 2 weeks to appear in patients undergoing abdominal RT.

The *severity* of acute radiation injury increases with dose. Providing the reserve does not fall below a critical value, symptoms will be transient and recovery can be complete. Dose fractionation can lessen the severity of acute effects by allowing the stem/progenitor cell compartment to regenerate during the course of RT. The *latency* for acute injury, on the other hand, is relatively independent of dose because it is determined primarily by the physiologic turnover rate, that is, the kinetics of cell loss. Having said that, as dose increases, latency for an acute effect does decrease, but only by a few days, so the time, for example, to mucosal reactions seems fairly similar between individuals. For late effects, the inverse dose–time relationship is more marked.

Subacute Responses

Certain tissues may display subacute reactions several months after RT that are associated with cell loss and inflammation. Symptoms are often reversible, although in some instances, they may progress to severe damage and even death. Lhermitte syndrome after spinal cord irradiation is an example of a transient subacute reaction that is most likely because of diffuse demyelination and reversible by remyelination. Similarly, subacute pneumonitis can be seen by chest x-ray or CT scans 2 to 3 months after the start of lung RT with symptoms such as dyspnea, nonproductive cough, and poor lung function. The incidence depends on the dose and volume irradiated, as well as on smoking, and additional treatment. Loss of type I pneumocytes is associated with increased microvascular permeability, and host cell infiltrates, especially myeloid cells activated to secrete proinflammatory cytokines. It may resolve but can progress into chronic consolidated late pulmonary disease.

Late Responses

Late reactions to RT in normal tissues can be severe and with limited recovery. Because they occur after completion of treatment, dose adjustment is obviously not an option. Severity and latency are both dose dependent, with the latency increasing markedly with decreasing dose. This means that some late effects, such as atherosclerosis and heart disease, can occur decades after RT, which is becoming an increasing problem as patients survive longer. Late effects are generally considered to result from depletion of slowly proliferating "target" cells that are lost from the tissue at a slow rate or senesce after IR. However, chronic inflammation is also often present and is a hallmark that cannot be ignored. Pathologic findings are often variable and indicate more than one "target" mechanism. For instance, late demyelination after brain irradiation has often been ascribed to loss of oligodendrocytes, and subsequently of neurons, but proliferation and activation of astrocytes and microglial cells are common, as are vascular lesions with edema, hemorrhage, and inflammatory infiltrates. The

more chronic and debilitating nature of late reactions may be because of their relative inability to be readily repopulated from a stem cell pool, but regeneration may be additionally compromised by inflammation and fibrosis that is part of an ongoing alternative healing response for slow-responding tissues.

In late-responding tissues, proliferative cells may also be functional. When stimulated to proliferate, they may therefore also lose function, initiating a vicious "avalanche" effect. By the same token, late effects may be precipitously increased by insults such as surgery, chemotherapy, infection, or physical trauma. Depleted cellular reserves may also have an impact, as may expression of latent DNA damage. Latency decreases with dose as a result; however, late effects are complex and the critical cell type may change with time, making time–dose relationships and histopathology important when comparing responses.

An issue of growing clinical importance is the extent to which late radiation effects can be reversed. It has been shown recently that certain agents given after RT can modify injury in tissues. For example, captopril, an angiotensin-converting enzyme inhibitor, slows the development of radiation-induced nephritis and lung fibrosis in rats.[37] It is however clear that late effects are a reflection of dysregulated homeostasis that is in many cases linked to chronic inflammation. Reestablishing immune homeostasis may be required for full treatment.

Tolerance Doses and Functional Subunits

Generally accepted tissue tolerance doses exist and vary widely from tissue to tissue. Tolerance is determined by intrinsic radiosensitivity, capacity for regeneration, and many other factors. One factor is tissue organization. Tissues can be thought of as being composed of functional subunits (FSU), each FSU being defined as the tissue unit able to recover from one surviving clonogen. For example, epilation requires lower doses than desquamation, primarily because a smaller number of clonogenic cells are present in each hair FSU. Similarly, hair is depigmented by lower doses than epidermis because each hair follicle contains a smaller number of melanocytes, sometimes only one. In the kidney, each nephron is an FSU. If a tubule is completely de-epithelialized, it is lost permanently because it is not repopulated from adjacent nephrons. Therefore, the tolerance dose for the kidney is determined more by the number of tubule stem/progenitor cells per nephron than the number of nephrons. For example, if a kidney contained 10^{11} clonogenic tubule cells distributed as 10^4 cells in each of 10^7 nephrons, then most tubules should regenerate after a dose that reduced survival to 10^{-4}. From Poisson statistics, 37% of nephrons would be eliminated. If on the other hand, the 10^{11} clonogenic tubule cells were distributed as 10^7 in each of 10^4 nephrons, the dose required to eliminate 37% of the nephrons would have to reduce survival to 10^{-7}. In a multifractionated dose regimen with a logarithmic decline in cell number, a 7/4 (1.75) times higher dose would be needed. Tolerance doses can therefore vary greatly among tissues and organs even having the same intrinsic radiosensitivity. In mouse skin, the survival of about 10 out of approximately 10^6 basal stem/progenitor cells per cm^2 is required to prevent overt desquamation. Therefore, an FSU is about 1/10 cm^2.

Organs with more tubular architecture (e.g., salivary glands, pancreas, sweat glands, testis, mammary epithelium, spinal cord, nerve tracts, and central lung) may resemble the kidney in having better-defined FSUs organized "in series," whereas in dermis, mucosa, gut epithelium, and epidermis, FSUs may be considered to be organized "in parallel." The latter lack restricting physical barriers to cell migration, which may assist tissue regeneration. A tumor behaves as one FSU, as one surviving stem/progenitor cell can lead to recurrence, whereas a larger number of small metastatic deposits will be cured with lower radiation doses than a small number of larger metastases even if the total cell number is the same in the two cases. The FSU concept has some implications for "volume" effects.

Volume Effects

Traditionally, radiation oncologists reduce total dose when treating large volumes of normal tissue. In fact, the now widespread use of 1.8 rather than 2 Gy had its origin in a volume effect; the longer treatment duration enhanced mucosal tolerance in large head and neck treatment fields. A reduction in dose with increase in volume was generally recommended in the orthovoltage era, but this became less of an issue with the advent of skin-sparing megavoltage beams. In the modern era, dose–volume histograms (DVHs) are generated during intensity-modulated radiation therapy (IMRT) treatment planning. These are useful for avoiding excessive dosing to too high a volume for certain organs, but limited by the lack of spatial information and as a result do not predict toxicity very well.

In reality, the concept of decreasing dose with increasing treatment volume has little radiobiologic basis in cell kill, except in specific circumstances. For example, if FSUs are arranged in series, as in tubular structures, the loss of one FSU may result in injury regardless of the state of the other FSUs. The probability of injury increases with volume (number of FSUs exposed) (Fig. 3.1). Such a volume effect has been demonstrated clinically for small bowel obstruction and experimentally for myelitis.

The relationship between the number of FSUs irradiated (n) and the probability of a complication (P) can be quantified by:

$$P = 1 - (1 - p)^n,$$

where p is the probability of the loss of one FSU. This relationship is illustrated in Figure 3.2. When the average number of surviving cells per FSU is reduced to almost one, increasing the volume (number of FSUs exposed) reduces the dose necessary to produce a complication and increases the steepness of the dose–response curves.

FIGURE 3.1. Diagrammatic representation of the influence on the probability of a complication from increasing the treatment volume in a tissue where FSUs are arranged serially. The average survival of FSUs was 1 in 16, with sterilized FSUs being denoted by the *dark blue squares*. With the small volumes (A), the probability of myelitis was 6% (1/16), whereas it would approach 100% if 16 FSUs in one patient were exposed (E). The actual probabilities can be calculated using the equation in the text. (Reprinted from Withers HR, Taylor JM, Maciejewski B. Treatment volume and tissue tolerance. *Int J Radiat Oncol Biol Phys* 1988;14[4]:751–759. Copyright © 1988 Elsevier. With permission.)

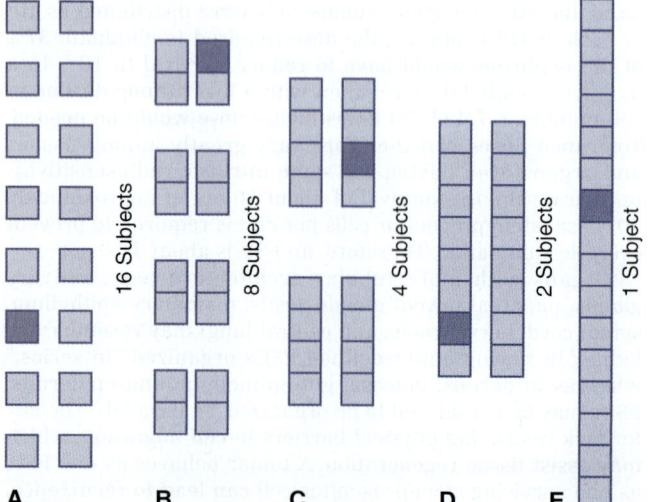

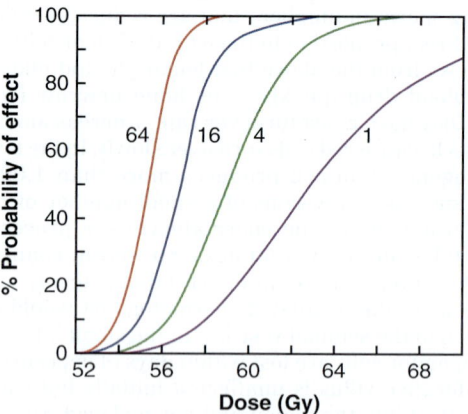

FIGURE 3.2. Curves illustrating how the probability of producing a complication increases with increase in the number of serially arranged FSUs included in the treatment volume. The curves were positioned by assuming that 58 Gy in 2-Gy fractions sterilized 10% of FSUs and that for a series of 2-Gy fractions, the effective D_0 for the target cells was 4 Gy. The curves are shifted to the left and are steeper with increase in number of FSUs exposed; however, this effect becomes less obvious once large numbers of subunits are involved. (Reprinted from Withers HR, Taylor JM, Maciejewski B. Treatment volume and tissue tolerance. *Int J Radiat Oncol Biol Phys* 1988;14[4]:751–759. Copyright © 1988 Elsevier. With permission.)

Spinal cord has been a favored model for volume effects. Experimental studies in spinal cord of rats have indicated a steep volume effect at <10 mm of length and an interesting "bath-and-shower" effect[38] for small fields with high tolerance for IR-induced paralysis. An additional modest "bath" dose (about 4 Gy) administered to 4-mm segments of the spinal cord surrounding a targeted "shower" 2 mm in size dramatically decreases the effective dose for 50% paralysis (ED_{50}) from 88 to 61 Gy. Proposed mechanisms are inhibition of angiogenesis or cell migration. Another recent study[39] showed IR-induced motor deficits in pigs to be independent of the irradiated volume in the lateral direction. This is of clinical relevance because it suggests that even partial spinal cord irradiation can have deleterious effects. However, in general, preclinical spinal cord dose–volume studies indicate that dose distribution may be more critical than the volume, suggesting that neither DVH analysis nor absolute volume constraints will be fully effective in predicting complications.

There is no evidence that direct cell kill after RT is affected by an increase in treatment volume. The radiosensitivity of skin epithelial clones is constant over a 5,000-fold range of treatment area. On the other hand, "volume effects," which are not related to cell death, can be seen when:

1. A small area of injury is tolerated better than a large area of the same severity. Pain, fluid leakage, and inflammation may be worse, and healing may be slower with more consequential contraction and scarring.
2. As volume increases, so does dose heterogeneity across the field. A tumor dose prescribed at the 80% level may be 25% higher dose at D_{max}, which could produce a marked increase in the incidence of complications, which would be further compounded for late effects by the "double trouble" of increased physical and biologic dose.[40] In addition, large fields may have large variations in contour that could cause a high dose region where tissue thickness is less than that measured at the midplane, as, for example, in the spinal cord at the thoracic inlet in thoracic irradiation and in tangential fields for treatment of the breast.
3. If organ "reserve" is obliterated as volume is increased (e.g., lung, salivary gland). This is not a true volume effect because sequelae are determined by the volume and functional status of the tissue *excluded* from the treatment volume, not the volume irradiated.

Regeneration (Repopulation)

As has been said, the latency and extent of regeneration after RT can be measured experimentally by a split-dose technique with two doses separated in time. The size of the second dose necessary for a constant level of effect (isoeffect) increases with time after the first dose because of regeneration/repopulation.

In acute-responding tissues, repopulation starts early because cell loss is rapid. In the irradiated jejunal mucosa, the lag time may be <24 hours. In the colon and stomach, it is slightly longer. In mouse renal tubules, there is no histologic evidence of cell depletion for many months after irradiation; there is a long lag period, and it takes more than 12 months to reconstitute a tubule.[41] The rate of repopulation has not been well quantified in tissues. In mice, some approximate doubling times for clonogenic cells are 8, 12, and 22 hours for jejunum, colon, and skin,[42] respectively.

In humans, tissue turnover kinetics are slower than in mice. Mucositis begins 14 to 21 days after the start of a regimen of 2 Gy given five times per week, but repopulation begins at about 10 to 12 days. The lag period may be shorter after high initial doses, but only by 1 or 2 days. Repopulation can increase the tolerance of the mucosa to a conventional regimen by an *average* of at least 1 Gy/day, which is equivalent to approximately a doubling of clonogenic cell numbers every 2 days, and it may be faster.[43] If daily irradiation is suspended (e.g., a 10- to 14-day break during an accelerated regimen), clonogenic cells may repopulate at two or three times this rate.[44] Figure 3.3 shows estimates for lengths of lag time and repopulation rates. The critical point is that there is a lag period followed by a phase of rapid exponential growth. In general, the lag period is shorter for chemotherapy, hyperthermia, and surgery because of more rapid cell loss.

The importance of repopulation is implicit in the history of RT. The current standard protracted overall treatment times confer a benefit by allowing regeneration of acute-responding tissues, which reduces toxicity. When attempts are made to accelerate therapy, acute responses become more severe and dose limiting.

Growth factors may shorten the apparent lag phase and accelerate recovery in irradiated tissues. Hematopoietic growth factors such as G-CSF, GM-CSF, erythropoietin, and IL-11 can accelerate proliferation of hematopoietic cells. In doing so, they minimize the danger of infection. In epithelial tissues, keratinocyte growth factor (KGF), which is specific for epithelial cells, has similar potential. It protects the oral mucosa, small intestine, lung, and hair follicles against chemo- or radiation injury in preclinical models.[45] In addition, mitigators of radiation damage have been developed[46–48] that can be given at least 24 hours after exposure.

"Remembered" Dose: Tolerance to Retreatment

According to conventional wisdom, heavily irradiated tissue cannot be retreated because of irreversible vascular damage. Although prior RT may decrease tissue tolerance, retreatment is often possible and may be better tolerated than expected. Factors that determine the limits include the tissue at risk, the amount of initial cell depletion, and the time elapsed since treatment and therefore the extent of regeneration. High prior doses, a short interval, and slow regeneration will reduce retreatment tolerance.

Data for experimental radiation myelitis in Figure 3.4 show the effect of size of a preceding dose on the dose required to produce a 50% incidence of myelitis. Recovery is complete after low doses but is progressively compromised as the initial dose approaches tissue tolerance.[50] It should be remembered that clinical "tolerance" doses for the spinal cord of 45 to 50 Gy in 1.8- to 2-Gy fractions are lower because the extent of injury tolerated is lower. The rate of recovery is not accurately known; however, in rats, at 100 days recovery is about 50% from what it would be at 200 days.[51] In monkeys, there was extensive recovery from 44 Gy in 2.2-Gy fractions by 2 years.[52]

FIGURE 3.3. Representation of the approximate kinetics of regeneration of irradiated normal tissues (*solid lines, solid symbols*) and tumors (*dashed lines, open symbols*). Curves are based on measurements or estimates of regeneration; symbols denote times at which an effect of regeneration has already appeared (*left-pointing arrow*) or has not yet appeared (*right-pointing arrow*). The logarithmic abscissa is for convenience of presentation only and has no biologic rationale. In general, the human data are displaced to the right of experimental animal data, reflecting a slower initiation of repopulation. Because human tissues proliferate more slowly than do their rodent counterparts, they were exposed to protracted dose regimens, and less-sensitive end points were used to detect onset of repopulation in humans. Numbers on the curve and symbols refer to different sources of data. These come from many sources. Further details are in the previous editions of this book.

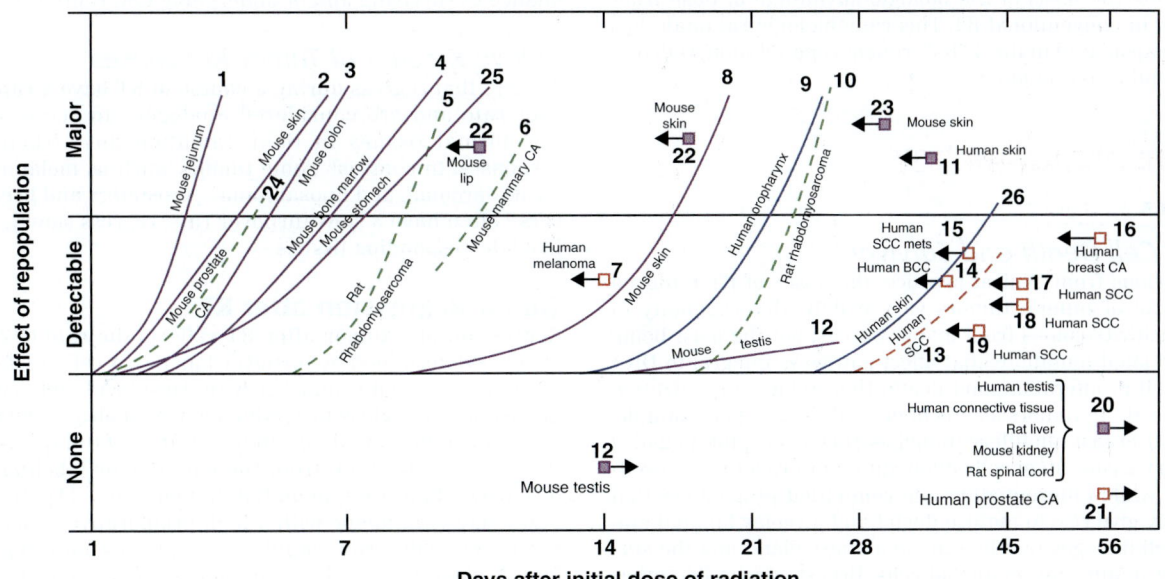

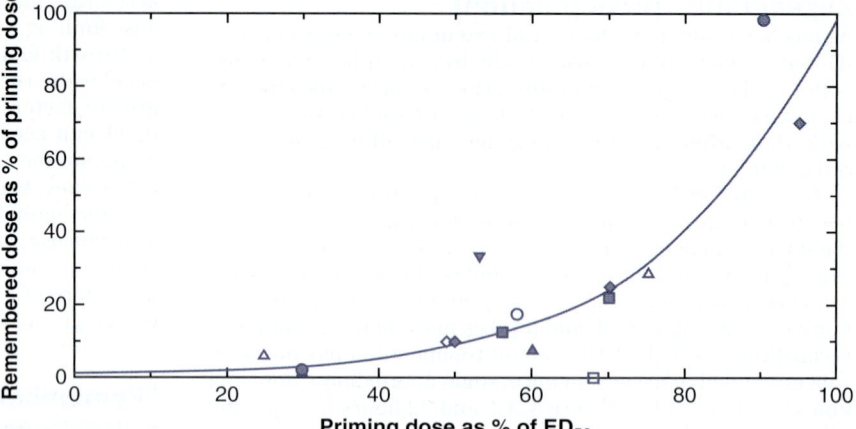

FIGURE 3.4. The dependence of remembered dose on size of priming dose (as a percentage of the ED_{50}) is shown for a variety of animal species at long periods (6 months to 2 years) after the initial radiation treatment: O, adult rhesus monkey; Δ, 12-week-old rat[49]; ◇, 1-day-old guinea pig; ●, young adult mouse; filled ▲, 8-week-old guinea pig; filled ▼, 8-week-old guinea pig; filled ■, 3-week-old weanling rat; ◆, young adult rat. (Reprinted from Mason KA, Withers HR, Chiang CS. Late effects of radiation on the lumbar spinal cord of guinea pigs: re-treatment tolerance. *Int J Radiat Oncol Biol Phys* 1993;26[4]:643–648. Copyright © 1993 Elsevier. With permission.)

Not all tissues or structures within tissues recover at an equal rate or extent after RT. Epithelial and hemopoietic tissues generally recover quickly and demonstrate a high tolerance to retreatment. However, the fibrovascular support structures in skin and mucosa and bone marrow respond more slowly. Kidney function shows poor retreatment tolerance in mice.[53] Retreatment tolerance is inversely related to the initial dose and decreases significantly with increasing interval between treatments, suggesting progression rather than recovery from the initial damage.

Because different tissues show different levels of tolerance to retreatment, caution should be exercised in the application of these concepts to the clinic. In addition, the experimental studies deal with well-defined end points within a limited time scale. If different end points in the same tissue are examined or the time is extended, the same guidelines may not apply. It should also be noted that if slowly proliferating cells involved in late responses are extensively or functionally inhibited, recovery may be permanently incomplete and the organ will be vulnerable to further injury, whether from radiation, trauma, cytotoxic drugs, or otherwise. For example, hyperthermia can precipitate myelitis in a patient who has had high but otherwise tolerable doses of x-irradiation, and trauma from dental intervention frequently precipitates mandibular necrosis.

Reproducible differences in tolerance of acute- and late-responding normal tissues, and between different types of tumors, to the same physical dose of IR are important because they define the basis of the biologic advantage of dose fractionation in conventional RT. This radiobiologic rationale has been encapsulated in the 4 "Rs" (repair, repopulation, redistribution, and reoxygenation).[49]

TUMOR RADIOBIOLOGY

Kinetics

Tumor Cell Death and Survival

As is obvious from clinical practice, the doses of RT required for control of human tumors vary widely. Heterogeneity in radiosensitivity comes from many sources, not the least being cancer-related mutations that affect pathways integral to DNA repair, cell proliferation, and death. Hierarchical organization is as relevant in tumors as it is in normal tissues. For example, in normal breast, undifferentiated estrogen receptor–negative mammary tissue, stem cells maintain themselves through self-renewal while differentiating into committed progenitors that ultimately give rise to mature ductal and alveolar luminal epithelial cell lineages that line the mammary gland and the surrounding mature myoepithelial cells. Breast cancer, like other

cancers, is a heterogeneous disease with subtypes that express luminal, mesenchymal or claudin-low, and basal-like phenotypes with distinct blocks imposed by BRCA1 loss and HER2 amplification. So most hierarchically organized tumors have more differentiated cells with limited proliferative potential and a cancer stem cell (CSC) compartment that maintains the tumor and contributes to RT resistance owing to its unique biologic properties. The importance of this concept is that tumor cure and regrowth are dependent on what may be a small minority of relatively quiescent cells that in several tumor types have been shown to be often very radioresistant and aggressive, which impacts how one thinks of the 4Rs related to cancer.[54] It also means that *in vitro* clonogenic assays are generally not good surrogates for *in vivo* radioresponse.

The mechanism of cell death may be important for radiocurability. The most radiocurable tumors have a tendency to apoptose, that is, lymphocytic > carcinomas > melanomas, sarcomas, astrocytomas. Importantly, the proportion of cells that undergo apoptosis tends to be regenerated between fractions.[55] In addition, genetic modification of cells to introduce a proapoptotic phenotype frequently, although not always, radiosensitizes.[56] Despite these findings, studies specifically designed to find relationships between molecular markers of apoptosis and radiocurability of human tumors have yielded mixed and sometimes contradictory results. This may be because the CSCs do not often express a proapoptotic phenotype. In contrast, cells that senesce or undergo autophagy or go through several mitotic divisions after RT may have a greater chance of surviving and of undergoing CSC reprogramming.

In Vivo Kinetics of Tumor Responses

Tumors that regress during a course of RT have a rapid turnover rate and are considered analogous to acute-responding normal tissues in their radiation dose–fractionation responses. In contrast, some tumors, such as melanoma, soft tissue sarcoma, and liposarcoma,[57] prostate,[58] and breast cancers[59] often have a slow turnover rate, regress slowly, and are like late-responding tissues.

Tumor Regression after RT

Regression of a tumor after RT reflects the *rate* of cell loss, which is determined by turnover kinetics. A cell loss factor (φ) of <1 is required for tumor growth. Most head and neck carcinomas have a φ close to 1, which is why their growth rate (on average, volume doubling times of about 60 days) is slower than one would think from their mitotic or labeling indices (LI), which indicate a potential doubling time (Tpot) of about 3 to 7 days. So, tumor with a high proliferative capacity does not necessarily grow rapidly, though they may regenerate fast. A classic example is the slow-growing basal cell skin carcinoma, in which numerous mitotic figures are commonly visible. They have a high φ owing to extensive apoptosis.[60] Tumor growth rate therefore does not equate with proliferation index, cell loss, or regrowth rate.

For standard RT, tumors with a high φ will regress rapidly during and after RT, regardless of pretreatment growth rate, and generally have a good prognosis. On the other hand, rapid regression would be expected if tumors have a high rate of cell production and high growth fraction, even if φ is low, but prognosis may be poor. Rapid regression is therefore not a universal prognostic indicator,[60] although it is usually a favorable prognostic sign.

Similar arguments can be applied to tumors that regress slowly, such as prostate carcinoma, some cases of nodular sclerosing Hodgkin disease, teratocarcinomas of testis, some soft tissue sarcomas, choroidal melanomas, meningiomas, pituitary adenomas, chordomas, or glomus tumors. Slow regression may reflect slow proliferation, low cell loss factor, or a high stroma content.

A practical implication of the complexity underlying tumor response to RT is that total dose should not be reduced just because a tumor regresses rapidly. In addition, tumors that are well-differentiated and grow slowly because of high cell loss factors may initiate an early repopulation response, and local control may be prejudiced by protraction of treatment time beyond normal, just as it is for fast-growing tumors.[61]

Potential Doubling Time

Repopulation with a decrease in φ occurs in all tumors and tissues as a homeostatic response to cell depletion. The potential regeneration rate of tumors after RT is better predicted by the pre-RT proliferative activity than by pre-RT tumor growth rate. The Tpot, which is the time required for clonogenic cells to double in number if the cell loss factor were zero, is a measure of this.[60] It can be estimated from the average duration of the S phase (Ts) and the fraction of cells in S phase, measured by LI:

$$\text{Tpot} = l\text{Ts/LI},$$

where l is a correction factor for the cell cycle distribution of the population.

Tpot is a logical predictor of the kinetics of a regenerative response, and attempts were made to use it clinically to predict which tumors would benefit from treatment acceleration aimed at minimizing repopulation. Early results indicated that it might be of some value, although later analyses indicated otherwise.[62] This may be because the cell cycle time in a tumor alters from before to during and after treatment.

Growth Fraction

The distinction between tumor and normal tissue is in a sense false, though convenient. In reality, perhaps 50% of cells in a tumor are host immune and stromal cells. The vasculature is obviously host derived. In addition, as in normal tissues, many cells in a tumor will be noncycling for a number of reasons; the most important are probably differentiation, hypoxia, and catabolic insufficiency. CSCs, for instance, are generally in a quiescent state. As a result, the *growth fraction*, which is simply the fraction of cycling cells in solid tumors, may be quite small (e.g., 20%). As tumors enlarge, they grow more slowly and the growth fraction may decrease even further (see control curve, Fig. 3.5). This changing growth rate can be approximated by a Gompertz equation. In contrast, after RT, the growth fraction may increase as CSCs are recruited to the proliferative pool and contribute to accelerated tumor regrowth, although other factors, such as hypoxia and necrosis, may be an influence. Of particular importance after RT may be an influx of tumor-associated macrophages that in many cases have been found to stimulate cell growth and metastasis.

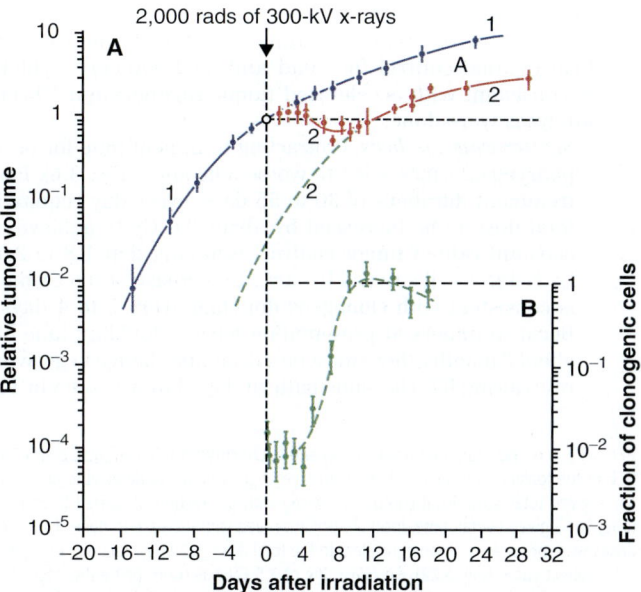

FIGURE 3.5. A: Growth curves for a rat rhabdomyosarcoma and its constituent clonogenic cells after a dose that reduced survival to 1%. The upper curve (*1*) shows unperturbed growth of tumors; the middle curve (*2*) shows regression and regrowth of tumors irradiated on day 0 with a dose that reduced cell survival to 1%; the lower curve **(B)** traces the repopulation of the tumor by surviving clonogens. Exponential regrowth of the surviving clonogenic cells occurs, whereas the gross tumor is regressing. (Reprinted from Hermens AF, Barendsen GW. Changes of cell proliferation characteristics in a rat rhabdomyosarcoma before and after x-irradiation. *Eur J Cancer* 1969;5[2]:173–189. Copyright © 1969 Elsevier. With permission.)

Regeneration in Experimental Tumors

Regeneration in tumors is similar to that found in normal tissues (liver, dermis) and largely involves rapid recruitment of resting, G0-phase cells. Hermens and Barendsen[63] showed a rapid exponential increase of surviving clonogenic tumor cells in a rat rhabdomyosarcoma several days after RT. Because only 1% of the initial clonogens survived, tumors did not visibly enlarge; rather, the tumor mass was still regressing when repopulation began (Fig. 3.5). This was later confirmed in other experiential tumors, and the same probably occurs during regression of clinical tumors. *In vitro* fractionated, daily irradiation can select for a small proportion of CSCs[64] and also promote reprogramming from more differentiated tumor cells.[65]

Regeneration in Human Tumors

Clonogen regeneration in human tumors can be assessed by the effect of increased treatment duration on the dose required for tumor control or the decrease in tumor control rate. Accelerated tumor regrowth occurs during standard RT for head and neck cancer[66,67] and is likely to occur in all but slow-growing tumor types with a low ϕ. The concept of accelerated repopulation in human tumors during and after a course of fractionated RT is supported by several observations.

1. *Time to Tumor Recurrence*
   If 10^4 head and neck cancer cells survived RT, they would have to undergo 15 doublings to present as a recurrence. Because most local recurrences are detectable within 12 months of RT, the *average* doubling time would have to be about 2 weeks, in contrast to about 2 months before RT, so the growth rate must accelerate following unsuccessful RT. Similar rapid regrowth was seen in pulmonary metastases after subcurative RT.[68]

2. *Split-Course Treatment*
   Split-course regimens for head and neck squamous cell carcinomas (SCCs) give lower local control rates than continuous regimens of the same total dose.

3. *Protracted Treatment*

Protraction of treatment time decreased the rate of locoregional control for head and neck cancer,[66] which is consistent with accelerated tumor regeneration. Three analyses were done:

a. *Scattergram analysis.* Protracting treatment time for oropharyngeal cancers led to worse outcome[66] (Fig. 3.6). For treatment durations of 30 to 55 days, every day required total dose to be increased by about 0.6 Gy to achieve a constant rate of tumor control. Assuming that 1.8 to 2.4 Gy reduces cell survival by 50%, an increase of 0.6 Gy/day is consistent with clonogens doubling every 3 to 4 days. Because tumors at presentation have a doubling time of about 2 months, there must be a dramatic change in growth rate during RT. The same pattern (Fig. 3.6) was seen in 11

other subsets of patients with oropharyngeal cancers and carcinomas of the supraglottic larynx[67] and for SCC of tonsil.[69] The latter is important because differences in overall treatment duration predominantly reflected institutional policy in this multicenter study. Because an increase in the tumor control dose 50 (TCD$_{50}$) was clearly noticed across all participating institutions with the extension of overall treatment time, any bias for worse tumors was unlikely.

b. *TCD$_{50}$ analysis.* Figure 3.7 presents TCD$_{50}$ values for SCC of head and neck calculated from the literature.[67] They are independent of treatment duration up to about 28 days, after which they increase rapidly (consistent with 0.6 Gy/day). The suggestion is that *on average*, head and neck SCCs exhibit a lag period of 3 to 4 weeks before beginning to repopulate, with an average doubling time of 3 to 4 days.

c. *Analysis of primary tumor control rate.* When a standard prescription (e.g., 50 Gy in 20 fractions in 4 weeks) is extended in time, the control rate decreases, commonly by 1% to 2% per day for head and neck and cervix cancer (Fig. 3.6B).

It should be noted that a lag period of up to 4 weeks and thereafter a 0.6 Gy/day increase in the "isocontrol" dose are *not* evidence that RT for head and neck cancer should be given in 4 weeks. Repopulation of mucosa begins at about 10 to 12 days and is more rapid than tumor. Thus, a therapeutic gain in mucosal tolerance relative to tumor control is still achieved by extending treatment beyond 4 weeks. Late-responding tissues, which do not benefit from repopulation, are unaffected by treatment prolongation, only by the size of dose per fraction and total dose. It follows that the overall therapeutic differential will be greatest if the tolerance dose for the critical late-responding tissue is delivered in the shortest overall time that is acceptable for acute responses, and without compromising the total dose delivered to the tumor, assuming the tumor has a high turnover rate.

4. *Accelerated Treatment*

If accelerated tumor growth contributes to treatment failure, it may be offset by accelerated RT. In nonrandomized studies, shortening the overall duration of treatment improved

FIGURE 3.6. A: Scattergram with TCD$_{50}$ and TCD$_{90}$ curves for 3-year local control of SCC of the tonsil (*1*, local control; *2*, recurrence; *3*, persistence of detectable disease). For a given total dose, local control decreased with protraction of overall treatment time. For a given overall time, local control improved with increase in dose. The total doses were normalized to be equivalent to the total dose in 2.5-Gy fractions using the LQ isoeffect curve (Fig. 3.22). An *α/β* value of 2.5 Gy was used, being the best estimate from these and other data. (Reprinted from Maciejewski B, Withers HR, Taylor JM, et al. Dose fractionation and regeneration in radiotherapy for cancer of the oral cavity and oropharynx: tumor dose-response and repopulation. *Int J Radiat Oncol Biol Phys* 1989;16[3]:831–843. Copyright © 1989 Elsevier. With permission.) **B:** Pelvic control as a function of treatment time for 621 patients treated with a total dose of 85 Gy. (Reprinted from Fyles A, Keane TJ, Barton M, et al. The effect of treatment duration in the local control of cervix cancer. *Radiother Oncol* 1992;25[4]:273–279. Copyright © 1992 Elsevier Ireland Ltd. With permission.)

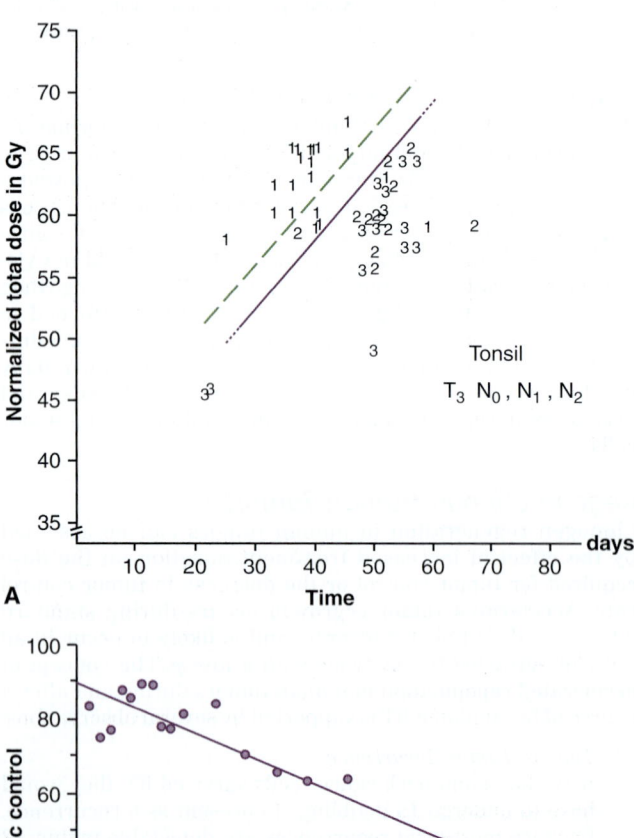

FIGURE 3.7. Estimated TCD$_{50}$ values as a function of treatment duration from published results of RT for squamous carcinomas of the head and neck excluding nasopharynx and true vocal cord. TCD$_{50}$ values are expressed as LQED$_{2Gy}$ (the equivalent dose given in 2-Gy fractions calculated using the LQ model). Total doses for an isoeffect increase steeply with protraction of treatment duration, implying accelerated repopulation by surviving tumor clonogens, consistent with the 3- to 4-day average doubling time calculated from scattergrams (Fig. 3.6A). The relatively constant TCD$_{50}$ value for treatments lasting up to 4 weeks is consistent with an average time of onset of accelerated growth at about 4 weeks. Growth of clonogens at the average preirradiation doubling rate of 2 month would have little detectable effect on TCD$_{50}$ values (about 2.5-Gy increase in 8 weeks). (From Withers HR, Taylor JM, Maciejewski B. The hazard of accelerated tumor clonogen repopulation during radiotherapy. *Acta Oncol* 1988;27[2]:131–146. Copyright © Acta Oncologica Foundation, reprinted by permission of Taylor & Francis Ltd, www.tandfonline.com on behalf of Acta Oncologica Foundation.)

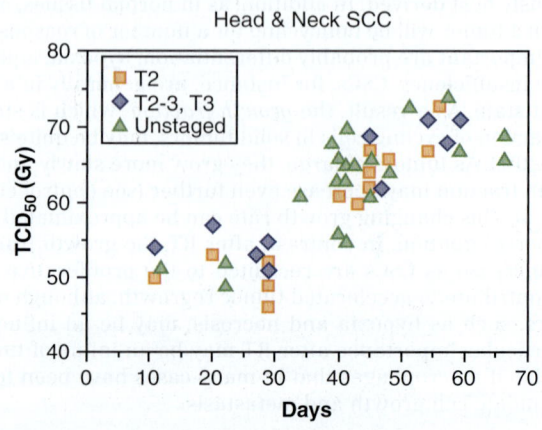

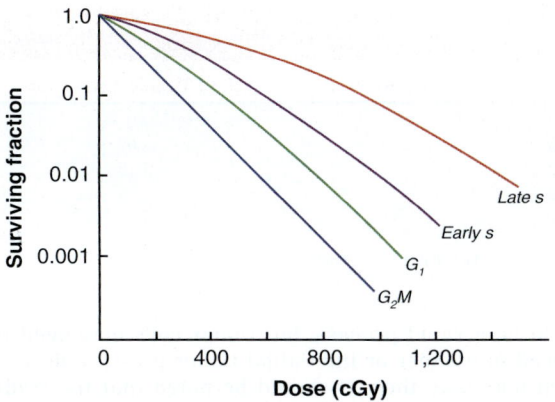

FIGURE 3.8. Radiation dose–survival curves for one line of mammalian cells (V-79 Chinese hamster) synchronized in four positions in the division cycle. Significant differences occur in the survival of cells at different ages, with the differences relative to absolute survival being greatest at lower doses. The survival ratio between late S and G_2M cells after 2 Gy is approximately 5. (From Withers HR, Peters LJ. Biological aspects of radiation therapy. In: Fletcher GH, ed. *Textbook of radiotherapy*. 3rd ed. Philadelphia: Lea & Febiger, 1980.)

the local control in inflammatory breast cancer,[70] melanoma metastases to the brain,[71] and head and neck cancer.[72] Randomized studies of accelerated treatment of head and neck cancer validated the benefit.[73] Exceptions may be cancer of the prostate, which has slow turnover rate, although hypofractionation with stereotactic body radiation therapy (SBRT) for prostate cancer has shown promise.[74] Dose-intensity studies suggest that chemotherapy also accelerates tumor regrowth.[75] As a result, two or three cycles of chemotherapy before the start of RT for head and neck cancer are rendered of little value because of accelerated regrowth.

Cell Cycle Redistribution after Radiation Therapy

Cells change in their radiosensitivity as they traverse the cell cycle[76] (Fig. 3.8). Irradiation will partially synchronize cells in relatively radioresistant cycle phases (e.g., S). When they resume cycling, they will move into more sensitive phases. If they were to be perfectly synchronized, this could be exploited by fractionation.[77] Unfortunately, synchronization is not perfect. Nevertheless, fractionation will still enhance the therapeutic ratio among tumor cells versus late-responding normal tissues by permitting redistribution. Radiosensitive cells in G2M will be eliminated by the first fraction and by the time the next fraction is given those originally in S phase will have moved into G2M, becoming more radiosensitive. This was the initial rationale for clinical trials of hyperfractionation, before intrinsic differences in response to low dose fractionation between late- and acute-responding tissues were appreciated.

The effect of cell cycle redistribution on tumor responses to multifraction RT is difficult to demonstrate. This may be because of intratumoral heterogeneity or because few cells are in radiosensitive G2/M phase. Also, CSCs are believed mainly to cycle slowly in niches, of which there are several, for example, glioma CSCs residing in both perivascular and hypoxic niches.[78,79] Most CSCs are negative for the proliferation marker Ki-67, but multiple fractions of IR may promote their recruitment from the niche and increase the proportion of cycling cells,[78,79] with a possible concomitant increase in radiosensitivity. Therefore, for CSCs, redistribution following RT may be tied to their mobilization into the cell cycle and thus regeneration.

The Oxygen Effect

In 1909, Schwarz reported that restricting the blood flow to a tissue decreased its radiation response, but it was not until 1952 that Read[80] showed that oxygen was a radiosensitizer. The relationship between oxygen tension and radiosensitivity varies, but about 3 to 10 mm Hg achieves a radiosensitivity halfway between that of hypoxic and euoxic (aerobic) cells (the k value[5]) (Fig. 3.9). Cells can survive at lower oxygen concentrations than this, so hypoxic radioresistant cells can retain viability. The inset in Figure 2.9 shows how survival curves are modified by oxygen concentration. The ratio of doses required to produce the same level of effect (e.g., cell survival) in hypoxic and euoxic conditions is the oxygen enhancement ratio (OER), which is between 2.5 and 3 for high doses of x- or γ-rays and slightly lower at low doses or low dose rates. This may be because at low doses, most damage comes from the densely ionizing component at the ends of electron tracks that are less affected by oxygen.

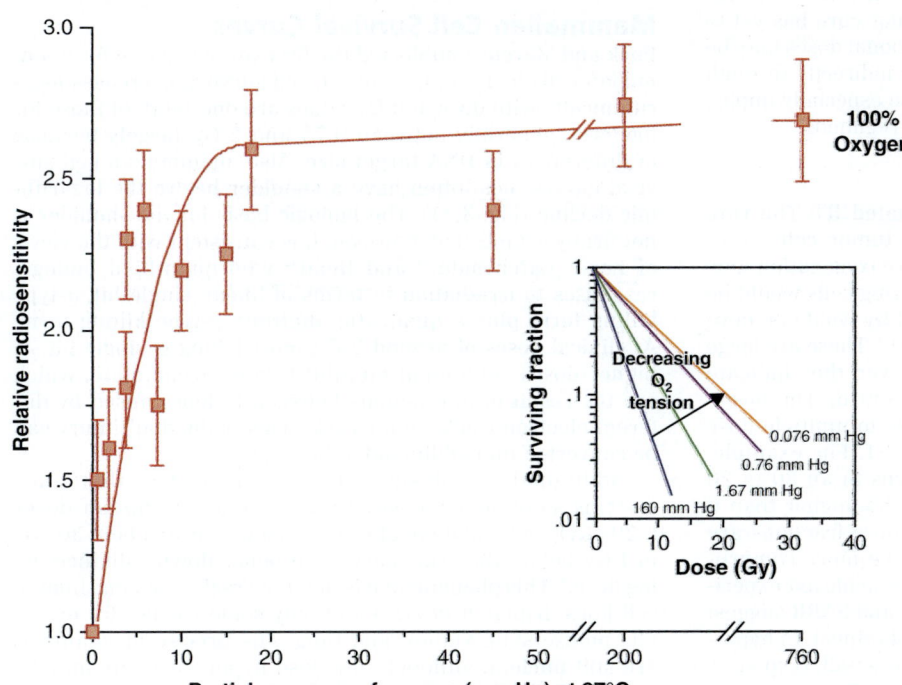

FIGURE 3.9. Curve relating cellular radiation sensitivity to partial pressure of oxygen at the time of irradiation. Data were obtained by scoring anaphase aberrations in Ehrlich ascites tumor cells, although similar curves have been obtained for killing of bacteria. About 50% of the total sensitization by oxygen is seen at a partial pressure of approximately 4 mm Hg at 37°C. The *inset* shows survival curves for different levels of oxygenation.

The electron affinity of oxygen is critical to radiosensitization. After this was realized, radiochemists developed electron-affinic drugs that could mimic the radiosensitizing effect of oxygen and that had more favorable properties, like being easier to administer, less rapidly metabolized, and able to diffuse further into hypoxic regions. The nitroimidazoles were most promising, for example, metronidazole, misonidazole, etanidazole, and nimorazole. Recently, other drugs have been developed, such as tirapazamine, that are selectively toxic to hypoxic cells and may radiosensitize.[81] Toxicity has somewhat limited the use of all of these drugs, but there is evidence of clinical efficacy.

Relevance of Hypoxia to Clinical Radiation Therapy

Tissue oxygenation is critically dependent on capillary blood flow, which is sluggish in solid tumors that develop hypoxic foci[82] because of poor blood supply, necrosis, shunts, or temporary occlusions. Temporary occlusion and blood shunting cause acute transient hypoxia that may be more important in RT than chronic hypoxia, which generally results from limited oxygen diffusion.[83] Chronic hypoxia may even radiosensitize as it decreases RAD51-mediated HR.[84]

Hypoxia has been linked with poor clinical outcome. Hyperbaric oxygen[85] or correction of anemia may help, although erythropoietin can support tumor CSC proliferation and survival, and so has the opposite effect.[86] Poor local control and survival rates have been correlated with hypoxia in head and neck and cervix cancer treated with RT.[82] However, outcome of surgical treatment alone in patients with uterine cervix cancers also correlated with hypoxia,[87] which can be explained by hypoxia selecting for more aggressive tumors.[88]

Despite the likely existence of hypoxic cells within many, if not all, solid human tumors, the importance of hypoxia as a predictor of individual response to RT has yet to be established, probably because the causes of tumor radioresistance are multifactorial and very complex. It is hard to routinely differentiate between acute and chronic hypoxia, and the status may change after RT as vascular damage preferentially eliminates acute hypoxia.[32,89] RT may also inhibit angiogenesis,[90] forcing the tumor to rely more on vascular supply through vasculogenesis. How common these radiation-induced alterations in the tumor microenvironment are in clinical reality, their intertumor variation, and their relationship to tumor cure has yet to be fully established, but higher than conventional doses may be required for vascular damage, directly[32] or indirectly through proinflammatory cytokines,[91] so they may be especially important in highly accelerated hypofractionated regimens.

Tumor Reoxygenation

Reoxygenation can occur during fractionated RT. The rate and extent seem variable, but if 30% of tumor cells were hypoxic and 70% euoxic and there was no reoxygenation during a course of conventional RT, most surviving cells would be hypoxic after the first few fractions and 70 Gy would be noncurative reducing survival to only about $<10^{-4}$. These are large assumptions and probably incorrect; however, they indicate the relevance of reoxygenation to tumor control. The possible effect of reoxygenation on the response to multiple dose fractions can be appreciated from Table 3.1. For example, the dose to a tumor that repeatedly returns to an 80 to 20 euoxic-to-hypoxic ratio would need to be 15% higher than if all tumor cells were euoxic. Where large dose fractions are given as a single exposure, outcome may be more compromised by hypoxia, but the high control rates achieved experimentally and clinically with brachytherapy and SABR suggest that reoxygenation is either adequate or not critical. In hyperfractionation, where the dose per fraction is small, responses will be little affected by 10% to 20% hypoxia. Reoxygenation

TABLE 3.1 RATIOS OF DOSE FOR ISOSURVIVAL EQUIVALENT TO THAT FROM 2 GY IN OXIC CONDITIONS[a]

Ratio of Euoxic to Hypoxic Cells	Dose Modification Factor
100/0	1.0
90/10	1.07
80/20	1.15
70/30	1.23
60/40	1.35

[a]Assuming a constant OER of 2.5 at all doses.

should be a rapid process, but tumor cells may need to be reduced in number or interstitial tumor pressure decreased, which may take time. It should be noted that free radicals generated during reoxygenation may be particularly toxic to cells, which may be why CSCs that resist considerable redox fluctuations can exist in a perivascular niche.[54] This could contribute to some of the vascular effects of RT mentioned above.

QUANTITATIVE RADIOBIOLOGY AND DOSE FRACTIONATION

Random Nature of Cell Killing

Our earliest understanding of dose–response relationships for irradiated cells came from studies with bacteria,[92] where survival decreases geometrically. In other words, the dose that reduces the survival rate to 50% will, when doubled, reduce it to 25%, and so forth, resulting in a straight line semilogarithmic plot, reflects random cell kill. Poisson statistics indicate that if 100 lethal lesions are distributed randomly throughout 100 equally radiation-sensitive cells (mean lethal dose = 1), 37 cells will be spared, 37 will have one lethal lesion, 18 will have two, etc. (Fig. 3.10), and all with >1 lesion will be dead. The 37% survival rate will recur for each additional mean lethal dose.

The mathematic bent of early radiation biologists, many of whom were also physicists, caused them to describe the slope of survival curves in terms of the mean lethal dose (D_{37} or D_0), which reduces survival by one natural logarithm (e^{-1}). D_{10}, which reduces it by one common logarithm ($\log_{10}$), is an easier term to think in with D_{10} about 2.3 times D_0.

Mammalian Cell Survival Curves

Puck and Marcus[17] published the first survival curve for mammalian cells in 1956. In general, cell survival decreases logarithmically with dose, but D_0 values are one-tenth of those for bacteria, generally between 0.75 and 2 Gy, largely because of differences in DNA target size. Also, mammalian cell survival curves most often have a shoulder before the logarithmic decline (Fig. 3.11). The biologic basis for the shoulder is not firmly established; however, it is consistent with the views of Lea,[93] Catcheside,[92] and Read[94] who quantified biologic responses to irradiation in terms of linear, single-hit, α-type killing term plus a quadratic, multihit, β-type killing term. At clinical doses of around 2 Gy, most killing is single hit. At higher doses, additional multihit lesions accumulate, which are the result of interactions between lesions caused by different electron tracks (intertrack). This "sublethal" injury can be converted into additional lethal injury.

Additional complexity comes from the fact that some systems show hypersensitivity to very low radiation doses (<20 cGy), and a plateau of radioresistance from about 30 cGy to 1 Gy, before the usual curve that bends down with increasing dose.[95] This phenomenon is not universal; only some human cell lines display it in vitro and only some tissues, for example, mouse skin, kidney, and lung. The precise mechanisms are still unclear, although low dose hypersensitivity may be due to a failure to activate G2-phase cell cycle checkpoints.[96]

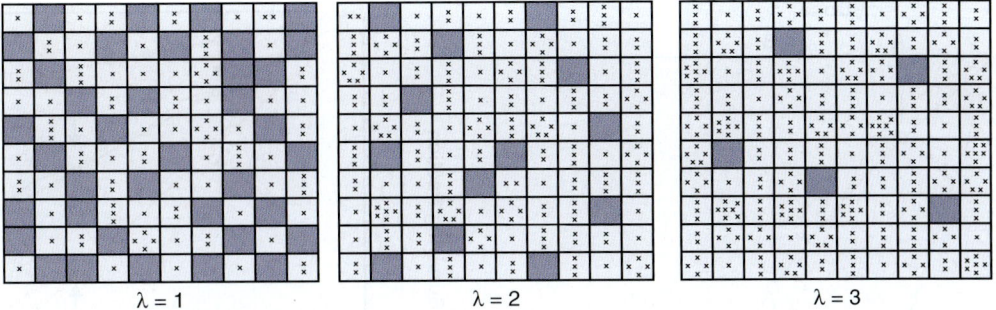

$\lambda = 1$ $\lambda = 2$ $\lambda = 3$

FIGURE 3.10. Random distribution in 100 equal-sized "targets" of 100, 200, or 300 "hits." The probability that any one of the 100 targets will not be struck when 100 hits are delivered randomly is e^{-1}, or 37%. The same probability of survival applies for each equal increment in the number of hits: 200 hits would result in a probability of survival of e^{-2}, or 0.37×0.37. Even after 300 hits are delivered, there is still a chance of $e^{-3} = 5\%$ that any one target will survive. This proportionate, or geometric, decrement in survival rate may be plotted as a *straight line* on semilogarithmic coordinates. (From Withers HR, Peters LJ. Biological aspects of radiation therapy. In: Fletcher GH, ed. *Textbook of radiotherapy.* 3rd ed. Philadelphia: Lea & Febiger, 1980.)

Obviously, many things can affect radioresponsiveness and therefore the dose–response curve. Mathematical models are derived to fit existing data, and their limitations must be considered when applying them in the clinic.

Linear Quadratic Formula

Assuming a linear dose coefficient (α) and a coefficient (β) for the square of the dose, the effect (E) is proportional

to $\alpha D + \beta D^2$, which can be used to fit a continuously bending curve to cell survival data.[97] The linear component (αD) is of major significance for conventionally fractionated RT (Fig. 3.12). Its importance was largely ignored in the 1960s

FIGURE 3.11. A TC survival curve for mammalian cells is characterized by a "shoulder" followed by a terminal exponential region, the slope of which is defined by a D_0 value (slope = $1/D_0$). The position of the curve on the radiation dose axis can be fixed by the intercepts of the terminal exponential region extrapolated back to the zero dose axis (n) or to the 100% survival level (D_q): n is termed the extrapolation number, and D_q the quasi-threshold dose. Although n and D_q are parameters that define the width of the shoulder on the survival curve, they do not indicate its shape, which is of prime importance in RT. The survival curve shoulder can be considered to consist of an initial exponential region (the slope of which is defined by $_1D_0$), followed by a downward-bending segment that merges asymptotically into the final exponential region of the survival curve. (From Withers HR, Peters LJ. Biological aspects of radiation therapy. In: Fletcher GH, ed. *Textbook of radiotherapy.* 3rd ed. Philadelphia: Lea & Febiger, 1980.)

FIGURE 3.12. Model dose–survival curves for mammalian cells showing that the experimentally determined curve for acute exposures (lowest curve) is the product of two mechanisms: single-hit injury described by an exponential curve ($e^{-\alpha d}$), and multihit, or cumulative, injury described by a continuously bending curve related by a coefficient, β, to the square of the dose. At doses of clinical relevance, cell death from the single-hit mechanism predominates. The rate at which the survival curve bends from an initial, essentially exponential region depends on the ratio (α/β) of the coefficients for single-hit and multihit killing: the lower the value, the sooner and more steeply the curve bends. The value of α/β is the dose at which single- and multihit mechanisms contribute equally to cell killing. In these curves, $\alpha/\beta = 10$ Gy, which is a value characteristic of acutely responding tissues. Target cells in late-responding normal tissues are characterized by low α/β values; hence, their survival curves are curvier. The flexure dose, D_f, is the dose at which deviation from the initial exponential part of the curve is difficult to detect and, for available biologic assay systems, is about one-tenth of α/β. When doses in a multifraction regimen are less than D_f, further dose fractionation does not produce detectable "sparing" (because cell killing is essentially all the result of single-hit events, the lesions potentially contributing to multievent killing being completely repaired during the fractionation intervals). The lower the α/β value, the lower the dose at which multihit mechanisms cause cell death, the lower the value of D_f, and the lower the dose per fraction below which a sparing effect of dose fractionation is lost. The curve for single-hit killing ($e^{-\alpha d}$) can be measured experimentally using very small dose fractions or a continuous low dose rate exposure; however, the curves for multihit killing ($e^{-\beta d^2}$) can be determined only indirectly from a knowledge of the other two curves.

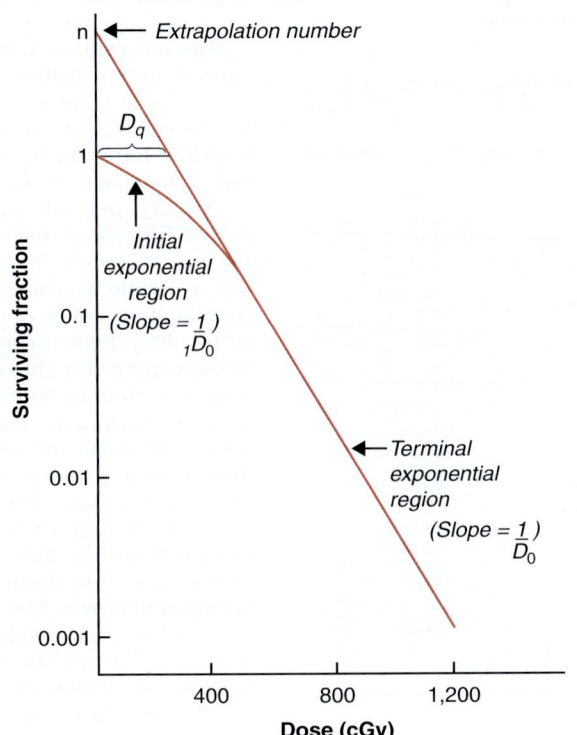

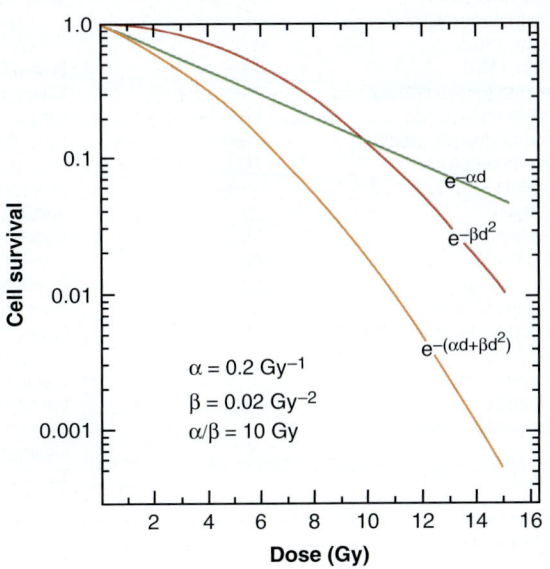

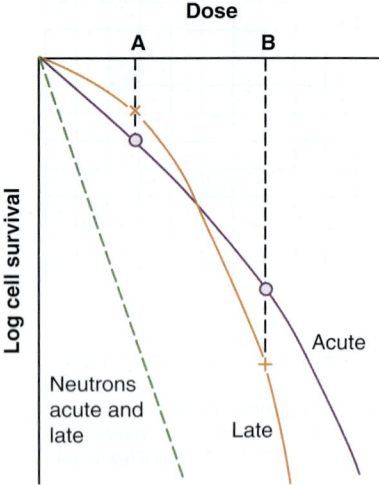

FIGURE 3.13. Hypothetical survival curves for the target cells for acute and late effects in normal tissues exposed to x-rays or neutrons. The α/β ratio is lower for late effects than for acute effects in x-irradiated tissues, resulting in a greater change in effect in late-responding tissues with change in dose. At dose A, survival of target cells is higher in late-effect than in acute-effect tissues; at dose B, the reverse is true. Increasing the dose per fraction from A to B results in a relatively greater increase in late than acute injury. For neutrons, the α/β ratio is high, with no detectable influence of the quadratic function (βd^2) over the first two decades of reduction in cell survival, implying that accumulation of sublethal injury plays a negligible role in cell killing by doses of neutrons of clinical interest.(Reprinted from Withers HR, Thames HD, Jr, Peters LJ. Biological bases for high RBE values for late effects of neutron irradiation. *Int J Radiat Oncol Biol Phys* 1982;8[12]:2071–2076. Copyright © 1982 Elsevier. With permission.)

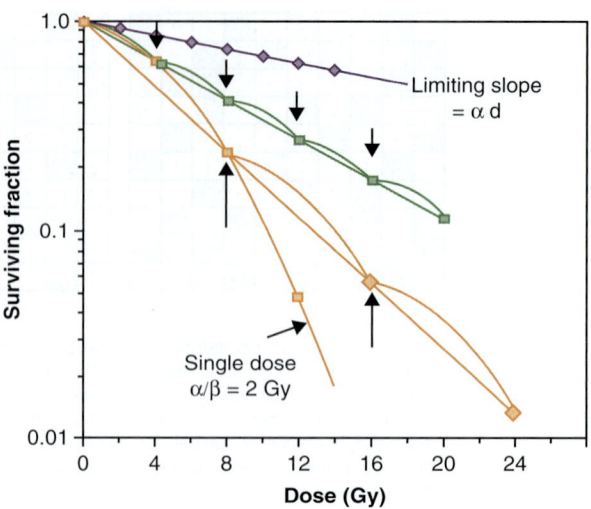

FIGURE 3.14. Multifraction dose–survival curves compared with a single-dose curve. Effective survival curves for multifraction regimens that produce an equal (proportionate) decrement in survival from each dose are linear, with shallower slopes than the single-dose curve at the same dose. Slopes of the multifraction curves become less steep with a decrease in fraction size until the dose per fraction is so low that multihit killing contributes negligibly and the slope is the limiting one determined by single-hit killing (and $_eD_0 = 1/\alpha$). The dose per fraction below which the effective survival curve becomes no shallower is a function of the curviness of the single dose–survival curve and is lower than the α/β value.

but was "rediscovered" in the early 1970s when Dutreix et al.[98] demonstrated that acute effects in human skin were not spared by decreasing fraction sizes below 3 Gy, that is, when the multihit component has become negligible and the effective survival curve is linear and has reached the slope of the α component in the single-dose curve. Now, it is accepted that single lethal hits are required for low dose rate brachytherapy or standard fractionated RT to eradicate cancer.[99]

$$\text{S.F. (survival fraction)} = e^{-(\alpha D + \beta D^2)}$$

The dose range over which the linear component dominates depends on the relative values of α and β. The α/β ratio

defines the dose at which cell killing by linear and quadratic components are equal. The higher the α/β ratio, the more linear and steeper is the dose–response curve and the less sensitive it is to dose fractionation. The lower the α/β coefficient, the "curvier" is the survival curve, bending down only after an initial linear region and allowing a marked sparing effect of dose fractionation (Figs. 3.13 and 3.14). The parameters can be estimated from multifraction data if the reciprocal of the total dose $1/nd$ is plotted against dose per fraction (d) (Fe plot).[100] The intercept on the ordinate is $\alpha/\log_e S$, and the slope is $\beta/\log_e S$. The ratio of the intercept to slope gives the α/β ratio. Fowler[101] also introduced the biologically effective dose (BED), which is the total dose multiplied by its relative effectiveness and changes linearly with a slope dependent on the α/β value of the tissue.

The α/β ratio is a measure of how sensitive different tissue responses are to changes in size of dose fraction. Importantly, it is not a measure of radiosensitivity *per se*. Late-responding, slow turnover tissues generally have a low α/β ratio and a large fractionation effect. Acute-responding, high turnover tissues generally have a large α/β ratio, as do many tumors, although melanoma, soft tissue sarcoma, liposarcoma, prostate, and breast tend to have low α/β ratios (Table 3.2). Variation observed within any one tumor type may indicate lineage differences. The linear quadratic (LQ) model is simple and useful in part because α/β ratios can be determined from *in vivo*

TABLE 3.2 α/β VALUES			
Early-Responding Tissues	**α/β (Gy)**	**Late-Responding Tissues**	**α/β (Gy)**
Skin (desquamation)	9.4–21.0	Spinal cord (paresis)	1.6–5
Skin–pig (desquamation)		—Cervical	2–3.4
—Time ≤16 d	8.7	—Lumbar	4–5
—Time >16 d	0.9	Brain (LD$_{50}$/10 mo)	2.1
Lip mucosa (desquamation)	7.9	Kidney (multiple endpoints)	0.4–5
Jejunal mucosa (clones)	7–13	Lung (pneumonitis)	1.6–4.5
Tongue mucosa (ulceration)	11.6	Lung (fibrosis)	2.3
Colonic mucosa (clones)	7–8.5	Heart failure	3.7
Hair follicles (epilation)		Liver (clones)	2.5
—Anagen	7.5	Bladder (frequency)	7.2
—Telogen	5.5	Bladder (contraction)	5.8–11.0
Testis (clones)	13.9	Bowel (stricture/perforation)	3.5–5
Spleen (clones)	8.9	Bowel (fistula/obstruction)	10.7
Bone marrow (clones)	9.0	Bowel (rectal stenosis, <5 d)	6.2
Melanocytes (depigmentation)	6.5	Bowel (rectal stenosis, >5 d)	1.1
Tumors (cure)		Dermal contraction	1.5–3.5
Experimental tumors	10–35	Dermal wound healing	2.5
Most human tumors	6–25	Eye cataracts	1.2
Human prostate cancer	1.5	Bone (human fracture)	2.2
		Cartilage and submucosa	1–4.9
		Total body irradiation (LD$_{50}$/1 y)	5.1

These values represent a synthesis from many sources. Individual values are means from one study. Where a range is given, it represents mean values from multiple studies.

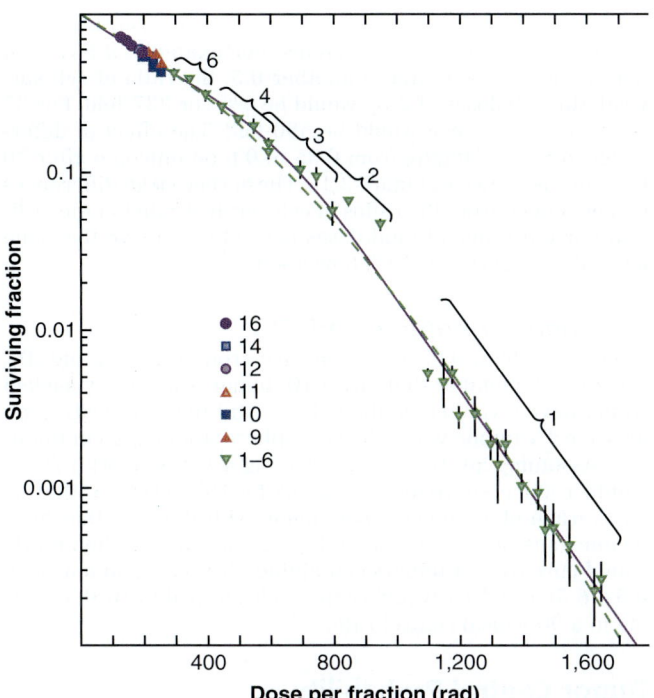

FIGURE 3.15. Effective single dose–survival curves for clonogenic cells of jejunal crypts fitted to multifraction data using LQ (*broken curves*) and TC (*solid lines*) models. Numbered brackets illustrate that the data were from experiments using that number of fractions. Mean survival curve parameters are as follows: for LQ model, n $\alpha = 0.23$ Gy, $\beta = 0.018$ Gy^{-2}; for TC model, $_1D_0 = 3.57$ Gy, $D_0 = 1.43$ Gy, $_nD_0 = 2.37$ Gy, and $n = 20.4$. (Reprinted from Thames HD, Jr, Withers R, Mason KA, et al. Dose-survival characteristics of mouse jejunal crypt cells. *Int J Radiat Oncol Biol Phys* 1981;7[11]:1591–1597. Copyright © 1981 Elsevier. With permission.)

multifraction experiments even though the absolute values of each coefficient are unknown.

Two-Component Model
Dose–survival curves can be well fitted by formulas other than the LQ formula. The two-component (TC) model combines a

single-hit component $e^{-D/_1D_0}$, where $_1D_0$ is the dose required to reduce survival to $0.37(e^{-1})$, with a multiple-hit $e^{-(1-e^{-D/_nD_0})n}$, where $_nD_0$ is the dose needed to reduce survival to e^{-1} in the final region of the curve and n is the extrapolation number (Fig. 3.11).

$$\text{S.F.} = e^{-D/D_1} \cdot (1 - [e^{-D_n/D_0}]^n)$$

Comparison of the Linear Quadratic and Two-Component Survival Models
Over a limited dose range (e.g., 2 to 8 Gy), relevant to most RT, both the TC and LQ models "fit" data similarly (Fig. 3.15). Outside this range, many experimental isoeffective curves are not very linear, and use of either model is unlikely to give realistic equivalent doses,[102] although there are other opinions.[103] The models differ significantly at predicting isoeffective doses at fractions of <2 Gy. The differences may appear small but are amplified if, for example, a dose of 1.15 Gy were to be repeated 70 times or more, as could happen in a hyperfractionated RT regimen (Fig. 3.16).

Multifraction Survival Curves
In 1959, Elkind and Sutton[77] showed recovery from sublethal damage (SLD) within a few hours, which can be estimated by split-dose experiments, that is, by increasing time between two dose fractions over a 24-hour period or by the increase in total dose necessary to achieve the same level of cell survival, or isoeffect (D2 to D1) (Fig. 3.17). If repair of SLD is complete, survivors of the first dose behave as though they had not been irradiated. So, if 2 Gy reduces survival to 50% (S.F.$_{2Gy}$ = 0.5), two doses of 2 Gy would reduce it to $(0.5)^2$ and n doses to $(0.5)^n$. Complete repair and no effect of redistribution, regeneration, or reoxygenation between doses are unlikely, but each dose fraction having an equal effect is a sufficient assumption for modeling purposes, and the multifraction dose–survival relationship gives a straight line when plotted on semilogarithmic coordinates (Fig. 3.18), extrapolating to 1 ($n = 1$) with a slope that is shallower the smaller the dose per fraction (Fig. 3.14). If the effects of the 4Rs were constant, the resulting survival curve would be linear and the slope would vary depending on the extent to which each phenomenon affected the response.

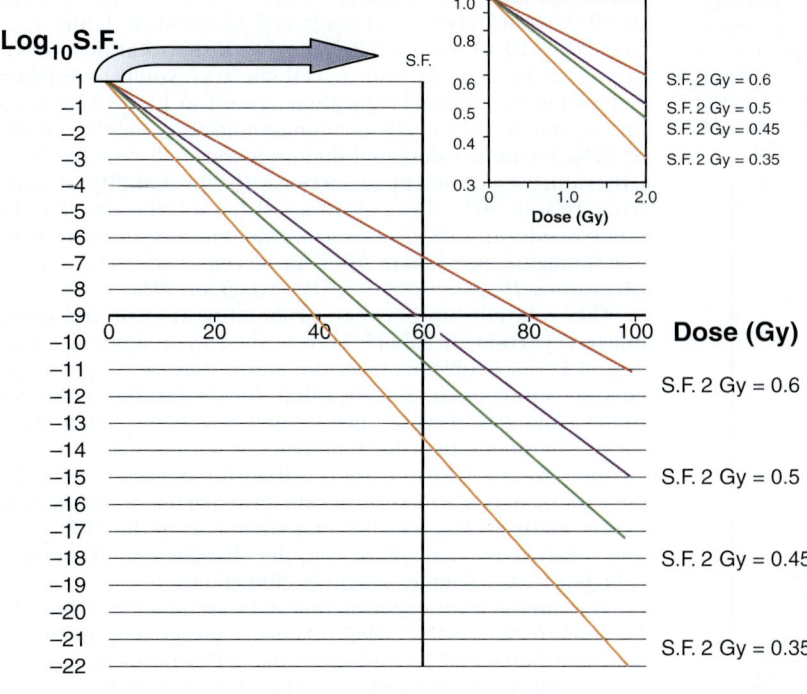

FIGURE 3.16. Effective multifraction dose–survival curves for cell populations, the survival of which from 2 Gy varies from 0.65 to 0.35. When survival from 2 Gy is 0.5, survival from 30 × 2 Gy is $(0.5)^{30}$ = approximately 10^{-9}. When this figure was constructed, this survival value was taken as an arbitrary standard against which the relative survival of other populations exposed to 30 × 2 Gy was plotted. The abscissa at the standard survival shows the total doses in 2-Gy fractions necessary to achieve that standard survival level in different cell populations. In all cases, an equal effect per dose fraction was assumed. The ratios of cell survival after a total dose of 60 Gy illustrate the exponential amplification of survival differences with increasing dose. Thus, dose fractionation can transform small differences in response at low doses (2 Gy) to large ultimate differences; measurements must be made accurately after a dose of 2 Gy to predict accurately the ultimate outcome of high dose multifraction irradiation. (Reprinted from Withers HR. Predicting late normal tissue responses. *Int J Radiat Oncol Biol Phys* 1986;12[4]:693–698. Copyright © 1986 Elsevier. With permission.)

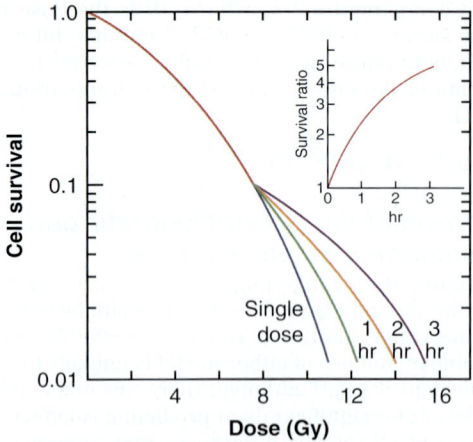

FIGURE 3.17. Recovery curves of the type first described by Elkind and Sutton.[77] The repair of sublethal injury begins immediately and can be measured in terms of survival ratio (*inset*) or the increment in dose to achieve isosurvival. (Reprinted by permission from Nature: Elkind MM, Sutton H. X-ray damage and recovery in mammalian cells in culture. *Nature* 1959;184:1293–1295. Copyright © 1959 Springer Nature.)

More likely, their influence varies with time. In some normal tissues (e.g., oropharyngeal mucosa), regeneration of surviving clonogenic cells late in a course of 1.8- to 2 Gy fractions may outstrip the cytocidal effect of treatment and the net survival curve will have a positive slope, as may happen to tumors on treatment. Despite these uncertainties, models of dose–response relationships can be useful.

The slope of a multifraction survival curve can be described by an "effective D_0" ($_{eff}D_0$, or $_eD_0$) that reduces survival to e^{-1}. If S.F.$_{2Gy}$ were 0.5, the corresponding $_eD_0$ value for a series of 2 Gy fractions would be 2.9 Gy (S.F. $= e^{-D/_{eff}D_0}$). If the S.F.$_{2Gy}$ values ranged from 0.45 to 0.67, the $_{eff}D_0$ values are from 2.5 to 5.0 Gy. In mice, S.F.$_{2Gy}$ values for jejunal crypt and spermatogenic stem cells are about 0.6 and for colonic cells about 0.65, giving $_{eff}D_0$ values for 2 Gy fractions of about 3.9 and 5.0 Gy, respectively. It can be calculated, in two ways, that 30 fractions of 2 Gy would reduce survival of jejunal crypt cells to 2×10^{-7}:

S.F. after 30×2 Gy $= $ (S.F.$_{2 Gy}$)^{30} $= (0.6)^{30} = 2 \times 10^{-7}$ or

S.F. after 60 Gy in 2-Gy fractions $= e^{-60/_{eff}D_0} = e^{-60/3.9} = 2 \times 10^{-7}$

FIGURE 3.18. Isoeffect curves in which the total dose necessary for a certain effect in various tissues is plotted as a function of dose per fraction (late effects, *solid lines*; acute effects, *broken lines*). Data were selected to exclude an influence on the total dose of regeneration during the multifraction experiments. The isodoses for late effects increase more rapidly with decrease in dose per fraction than is the case for acute effects. (From Withers HR. Biologic basis for altered fractionation schemes. *Cancer* 1985;55[9 Suppl]:2086–2095. Copyright © 1985 American Cancer Society. Reprinted by permission of John Wiley & Sons, Inc.)

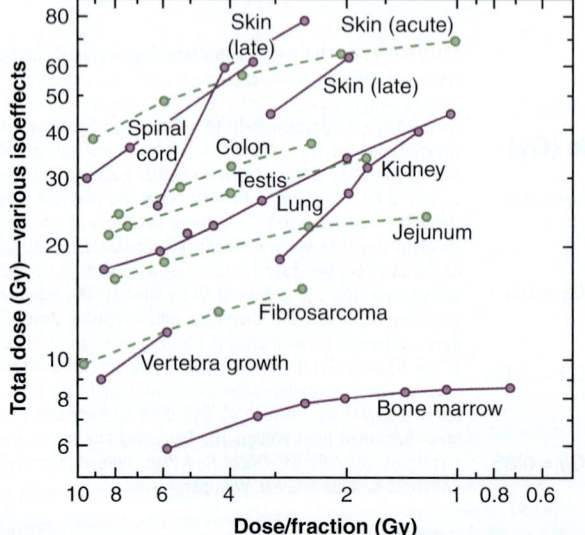

Small differences between cell types in intrinsic sensitivity amplify after many 2 Gy fractions. For example, if S.F.$_{2Gy}$ in one tissue were 0.6 and in another 0.5, the ratio of cell survival after 30 doses of 2 Gy would be $\left(\frac{0.6}{0.5}\right)^{30}$, or 237-fold. For 35 doses, the difference would be 590-fold. The effect of differences in S.F.$_{2Gy}$ ranging from 0.35 to 0.6 on outcome after 30 fractions is shown in Figure 3.16. These very large differences can be judged from the ratios of cell survival rate (on the ordinate) or the range of total doses needed to achieve the same level of cell survival (~10^{-9}) (abscissa).

Common Logarithms and $_eD_{10}$

If S.F.$_{2Gy}$ is about 0.5, $_{eff}D_0$ values are around 2.9 Gy, and $_eD_{10}$ is 6.7 Gy. Remember that about 10^9 tumor cells tightly packed would have a volume of about 1 cm^3 and that 10^{10} cells in an average T3 tumor would form a sphere about 2.2 cm diameter. Assuming an $_eD_{10}$ of 7 Gy, treating a T$_3$ tumor with 70 Gy would reduce surviving clonogens by 10^{-10} ($10^{-70/7}$), that is, on average of 1 clonogen per tumor, with the 37% that have 0 clonogens being eliminated. If $_eD_{10}$ were 6.5 Gy, then 65 Gy would cure 37% of tumors containing 10^{10} cells, and a dose of $(65 + 6.5) = 71.5$ Gy would reduce cell survival to 10^{-11}, resulting in a 90% local control rate.

Tumor Control Probability

Tumor Control Probability for Clinically Detectable Disease

The probability of tumor control increases as radiation dose increases, with success or failure depending on killing the last clonogen, so control is achieved abruptly. A plot of tumor control probability (TCP) versus dose therefore shows no response until a certain dose is reached, then a rapid increase to 100% following a Poisson distribution. If cell survival is reduced to an average of one clonogen per tumor, there would be, on average, 37% cured. The probability of tumor control with cell survival rate is given by:

$$P_{cure} = e^{-x} = e^{-(SF \cdot M)},$$

where x is the average number of surviving clonogens per tumor, which in turn is the product of S.F. (fraction of cells surviving) and M (initial cell number). For example, if a tumor contains 10^{10} clonogens, doses that reduce survival to 10^{-10} would give an average cell survival of 1 and P_{cure} to $e-(10^{10} \cdot 10^{-10}) = e^{-1} = 0.37$, or 37%. If the total dose were increased by two $_{eff}D_0$ values, cell survival would be further reduced by two natural logarithms, from 1 to $1 \times e^{-2}$, that is, to an average of 0.135 cells per tumor, and $P_{cure} = e^{-0.135} = 0.87$, or 87%. It can be calculated that an increase in dose by three $_{eff}D_0$ values is sufficient to increase the probability of cure from 10% to 90%. If $P_{cure} = 10\% = 0.1 = e^{-x}$, then $x = 2.3$. In other words, at 10% local control rate, there is an average of 2.3 clonogens per tumor. After an increase in dose by three $_{eff}D_0$ values, $P_{cure} = e^{-(2.3.e-3)} = e^{-(0.115)} = 0.89$, or 89%.

This relationship between probability of cure and dose, above a certain threshold, is described by a sigmoid curve (Fig. 3.19). It is obvious from the above that the slope of the curve is a function of the $_{eff}D_0$ values for the last few surviving tumor clonogens. It is steeper for neutrons or for single-dose x-ray treatments than for multifraction x-ray exposures and steeper (by the OER) for euoxic than for hypoxic cells. The dose that yields a 50% control rate for experimental studies is known as the TCD$_{50}$, which is in a steep part of the TCP curve and sensitive to small changes in the effectiveness of therapy. A higher rate is usually sought in clinical practice.

TCP curves from experimental data are steep but shallow for human tumors.[104–106] This reflects heterogeneity in tumor characteristics and RT prescriptions. RT is often individualized by physicians prescribing higher doses for larger tumors, which is not accounted for and flattens TCP curves. Even when variation has been minimized, TCP curves are fairly shallow, indicating a need for even better molecular profiling and examination of factors that impact their intrinsic radiosensitivity, redistribution, repopulation, and reoxygenation. The effect of constructing TCP curves for a series of tumors nonhomogeneous only in volume (T-stage) is illustrated in Figure 2.19. If tumors are stratified into three sizes varying in diameter by factors of 2, three distinct steep TCP curves would be obtained with a flatter overall TCP curve. It would not be appropriate to include a 64-fold volume range in a clinical TCP analysis, although the range in CSC numbers in human cancers of similar T-stage may be of this magnitude. The effect of CSC number would be further magnified by differences in repopulation kinetics during RT.

Normal tissue dose–response curves for the incidence of a certain complication are also sigmoid above a certain threshold, and probit analysis is used for estimating LD_{50} or ED_{50} values. Because normal tissues are more homogeneous than tumors, complication probability curves are steeper than those for tumor control, especially late effects.[107] The art of RT can be quantified in a risk–benefit analysis as a balance between the TCP and the probability of complications, NTCP (both represented by sigmoid curves illustrated in Fig. 3.20), with many factors involved. Different points illustrate this:

1. If there is to be a therapeutic gain, RT must be more effective against the tumor than normal tissues, that is, normal tissues must be preferentially spared.
2. In the steep midrange of TCP or NTCP, a small change in biologic effect can give a substantial change in clinical outcome. Conversely, if a change in RT produces a modest difference in TCP or NTCP, the change in biologic effectiveness may be small. It is better to quantify effectiveness as a change in dose to achieve a certain isoeffect, that is, the lateral shift of the TCP or NTCP curve. The ratio of isoeffect doses is the dose modification factor (DMF).
3. At incidences of less than about 10% and greater than about 85%, changes in biologically effectiveness may not

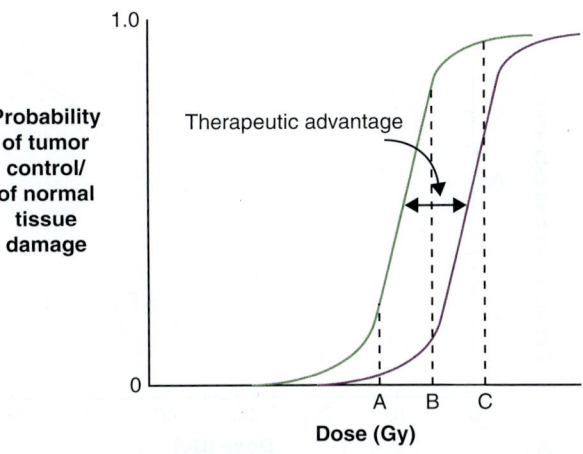

FIGURE 3.20. Theoretical curves showing the probability of tumor control and normal tissue complications. Both curves have a threshold and are log sigmoid in nature. The art of radiotherapy is to increase the distance between these two curves, that is, to derive a therapeutic benefit. If the normal tissue damage curve is to the left of that for TCP, tumor control is unlikely without unacceptable normal tissue complications.

be demonstrable or useful. For example, if the TCP is 90%, any gain to be had would be minor and may be of disadvantage if there was a risk of complications.

4. Because TCP and NTCP curves are generally close together, it is usually inappropriate to produce no complications (a.k.a. no pain, no gain). Within the treatment volume, a certain incidence of injury to normal tissues that is sufficient to be defined as a complication may be a prerequisite to good curative RT.
5. If the TCP is to the right of the NTCP curve, tumor control without a high incidence of complications is unlikely and other modalities should be considered. For example, a therapeutic gain might come from prior tumor excision or chemotherapy. However, 50% or even 90% debulking is of modest value. A 90% reduction in tumor volume may represent only a one-decade decrease in cell number, equivalent to about 6.5 to 7 Gy in 2 Gy fractions.
6. It defies scientific and ethic rationale to deny a patient the potential benefit from maximizing dose merely because TCP curves appear to be shallow in retrospective studies, as long as there is a finite chance of tumor control.

Tumor Control Probability for Subclinical Disease

The threshold–sigmoid TCP curve for clinically detectable tumors is not appropriate for subclinical metastases. If 10^n clonogens represent the upper limit of clinical undetectability of metastases, then patients who harbor subclinical metastases have a tumor burden of between 1 and 10^n cells. Given that micrometastases grow exponentially, it is reasonable (as a working hypothesis) to assume an even distribution of the logarithm of metastatic clonogens (between 1 and 10^n cells) within a series of patients.[108] If a reasonable value for n is 9, the assumption is that there will be the same number of patients with between 1 and 10 metastatic clonogens as between 10 and 10^2, and so forth, with 11% in each cohort. Although not completely accurate, this is a reasonable assumption, and TCP curves will generally exhibit no threshold and be shallow. The model in Figure 3.21A illustrates these concepts. Although the distribution could be modified by many factors, the analysis is generally consistent with results for RT of subclinical metastases (Fig. 3.21B) and suggests that relatively low doses could cure a percent of patients with micrometastatic disease.

FIGURE 3.19. Theoretic TCP curves for three sizes of spherical tumors (*solid lines*) and one that would result from a study incorporating into the dose–response analysis all three tumor sizes in equal proportions (*broken line*). They were calculated on the assumptions that the dose was given in 2-Gy fractions, that the $_eD_0$ value for 2 Gy/fraction was 3.5 Gy, and that a 1-cm diameter spherical tumor contained 10^7 clonogens. As tumor volume increases, so does the dose required for a certain probability of control. The cell number increases by 8 times and 64 times as the spherical tumor increases from 1-cm diameter to 2 and 4 cm, respectively. An exponential increase in clonogen number is related to a linear increase in dose for an isoeffect. Heterogeneity of even one factor, initial clonogen number, causes the TCP curve to be shallower (*broken line*). Retrospective clinical studies incorporate a large number of causes for heterogeneity of response.

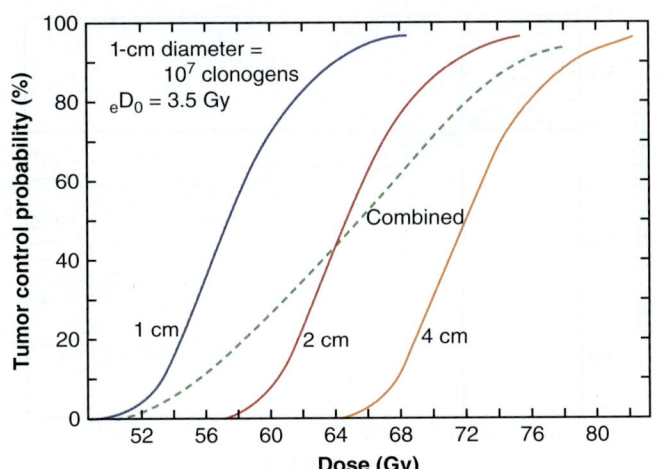

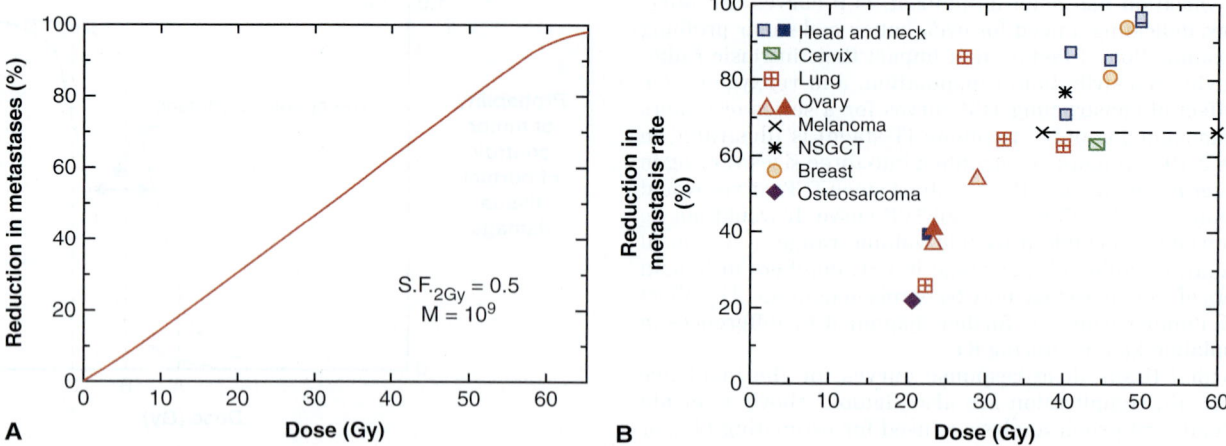

FIGURE 3.21. Percentage control rate as a function of dose for subclinical metastases. **A:** Modeling on the basis of a uniform distribution of the logarithm of numbers of metastatic tumor cells per patient ranging between 1 and 10^9. An S.F.$_{-2 Gy}$ value of 0.5 was used. The intercept of this theoretic curve is displaced slightly from zero because of the random statistical chance that any cell will survive any dose of radiation. In addition, at high doses, the probability of sterilizing all tumor cells approaches 100% asymptotically for the same reason. **B:** Percentage reductions in recurrence as a function of dose from reports in the literature for various tumor types. Solid symbols represent data from prospective randomized trials. Other data are retrospective comparisons between control rates with and without elective irradiation. (Reprinted from Withers HR, Peters LJ, Taylor JM. Dose-response relationship for radiation therapy of subclinical disease. *Int J Radiat Oncol Biol Phys* 1995;31[2]:353–359. Copyright © 1994 Elsevier. With permission.)

TIME–DOSE ISOEFFECT FORMULAS AND DOSE FRACTIONATION

History

Early isoeffect curves by Strandquist related the total dose required to produce certain skin reactions, or to achieve a certain TCP, to the treatment time over which the dose regimen was delivered.[109] Fowler and Stern[110] varied the number of fractions (N) and overall time (T) experimentally and showed that they were independent variables. Ellis[111] developed the nominal standard dose (NSD) formula to incorporate these two variables into an isoeffect curve that was used clinically for decades until the LQ model became popular, with or without modification for parameters related to the 4Rs.[112] In fact, there can be no single universally applicable isoeffect equation or curve because tissues (and tumors) differ greatly in characteristics that determine fractionation responses and kinetics that cannot be readily quantified.

Acute- Versus Late-Responding Tissues

The most clinically important biologic phenomenon influencing fractionated RT is differences between late- and early-responding tissues and tumors on changing the dose per fraction.[113] The exact reason is unknown but is entwined in differences in mechanisms of DNA repair and the mode of cell death that determine tissue turnover and recovery following RT. So, as the size of dose per fraction is reduced, the dose for an isoeffect increases more rapidly in late- than early-responding tissues, as is reflected in the slopes of isoeffect dose–survival and dose–function curves in Figures 3.18 and 3.22. Those in Figure 3.22 are constructed using the LQ formula to correct the total dose (normalized to 1) to that which would be given if the dose per fraction were a standard 2 Gy. Shown for comparison is a plot based on the NSD formula where the correction for time is ignored, that is, where $D = NSD \times N^{0.24}$.

Some specific clinical implications of the differences in fractionation responses between acute- and late-responding tissues are as follows:

1. For the same level of acute effects, large dose fractions are relatively more harmful to late-responding tissues than small dose fractions.[113]

2. Because of this therapeutic differential, the smallest practical dose per fraction should give the best therapeutic gain.[114] For example, for a hyperfractionated regimen, if two fractions of 1.15 Gy are isoeffective for 2 Gy in a late-responding tissue while 1.05 Gy is isoeffective for the tumor, the therapeutic gain would be $1.15/1.05 = 1.1$, increasing the biologically effective tumor dose by 10% with no increase in late complications, although acute-responding normal tissues will receive an increased biologic dose.

3. To maximize the potential therapeutic gain from hyperfractionation, repair of SLD in late-responding tissues must be complete, implying fractionation intervals of at

FIGURE 3.22. Isoeffect curves relating total dose to dose per fraction, with total dose being expressed as a ratio of that necessary in 2-Gy fractions (i.e., the LQED$_{2 Gy}$). α/β ratios (in Gy) are shown on the curves. Although the α/β ratios are not yet established accurately or even precisely for most normal tissues, especially late-responding ones (Table 2.2), the likely order of fractionation sensitivities is as shown. The *broken line* traces the change in dose, as it would have been predicted by a factor $N^{0.24}$ in the NSD formula. Phenomena other than repair of sublethal injury, specifically repopulation, are not accounted for by these curves. (From Withers HR. "Failla Memorial Lecture, Contrarian Concepts in the Progress of Radiotherapy." *Radiat Res* 1989;119:395–412. Reused with permission from Radiation Research. Copyright © 1989 Radiation Research Society.)

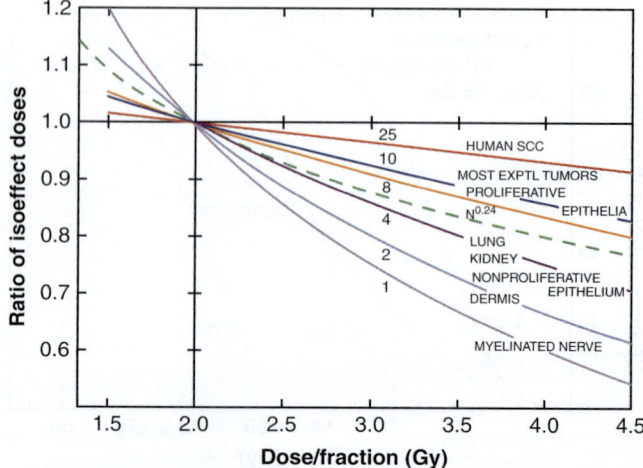

least 6 hours.[107,115] For the spinal cord, a longer interval may be prudent.[116]

4. The relative biologic efficiency (RBE) for high LET radiations is greater at low doses than high doses for late effects because the comparison is with x-rays that have a large sparing effect at low doses (Fig. 3.13).

Using the LQ Formula for Calculating Isoeffect Relationships

The LQ formula can be used to change the size of dose per fraction (within limits)[117,118]:

$$D_{new}/D_{ref} = (\alpha/\beta + d_{ref})/(\alpha/\beta = d_{new}),$$

where D_{new} is the new total dose for dose per fraction of d_{new}; D_{ref} is the previous total dose in fractions of d_{ref}; and α/β, in Gy, is for the tissue in question. For example, if d_{new} were 4 Gy and d_{ref} were 2 Gy, the ratio of total doses to achieve the same effects in a tissue with an α/β value of 2 Gy would be 0.66. For a tissue with an α/β value of 10 Gy, it would be 0.85. This calculation was used to derive the data in Figure 3.22.

The following caveats apply to this use of the LQ isoeffect formula:

1. The LQ response model does not apply equally at all dose levels. It fits well between about 1.5 to 8 Gy; however, its validity and precision above or below that range is in doubt.
2. Using uncertain values for α/β ratios affect late-responding tissues more and carry more risk. For tissues with α/β values of 10 Gy or more, isoeffect curves change little for different dose per fraction regimens, but this is not true for tissues with α/β values of around 2 Gy (Fig. 3.22).
3. The possible errors in dose corrections are greater at low doses per fraction. Using the isoeffect formula presented earlier, or the curves in Figure 3.22, compare the ratios of isoeffect doses for a tissue characterized by an α/β value of 2 Gy when the dose per fraction is changed from 2 to 1 Gy (a 33% increase) and from 2 to 3 Gy (a 20% decrease).
4. The basic LQ model has no time parameter. This is not so important for late-responding tissues that turnover slowly as it is for tumors and acute-responding tissues. Factors can be added to correct for incomplete repair, reoxygenation, and redistribution[112] and to the time to (kickoff time) and the extent of regeneration,[118] but the values are uncertain. The LQ formula should therefore be used cautiously.

Influence of Regeneration (Repopulation)

Normal Tissues

The influence of overall time on fractionated RT comes largely from differences in the time to (kickoff time) and extent of regeneration among various normal and neoplastic tissues (Fig. 3.3). As a result, simply adding a constant exponent for overall treatment time in an isoeffect formula without regard to tissue type is dangerous. For example, early regeneration in intestinal mucosa or bone marrow makes a major contribution to the net RT response if treatment is over several weeks, whereas it provides little or no benefit in spinal cord, kidney, or dermis.

Tumors

As with acute-responding normal tissues, tumors accelerate their growth in response to injury. Some clinical implications are:

1. Protracting treatment longer than necessary is likely a disadvantage, especially as it is difficult to predict the accelerated repopulation response of individual tumors. As an example, using 1.8 Gy rather than 2-Gy fractions given five times per week extends overall treatment time by about 10% and should be reserved for situations in which acute responses are likely to be limiting or where there may be substantial inhomogeneities in dose distribution that can lead to "double trouble," where the increase in physical dose has an added biologic component that will especially compromise late-responding tissues (Fig. 3.23).
2. If a treatment break is essential because of acute toxicity, it should be kept as short as tolerable.
3. Planned split-course therapy is inadvisable unless part of an accelerated protocol that ultimately shortens the overall treatment duration.
4. Breaks in therapy for nonmedical reasons (machine breakdown, holidays) may merit "catch-up" treatments, for example, by treating twice on some remaining days.
5. Obviously, rapidly growing tumors must be treated rapidly. Also, it is reasonable to accelerate treatment of tumors with a high proliferative index, regardless of their growth rate, because they are likely to reduce their rate of cell loss and regenerate earlier and faster during RT.

MODIFICATION OF DOSE FRACTIONATION PATTERNS

Standard RT regimens of about 2 Gy/day 5 days/week were developed empirically over decades and serve as a good overall regimen for dose fractionation. However, it should be obvious that it will not fit all clinical situations and that it is certainly inappropriate in some (e.g., obviously rapidly growing tumors).

FIGURE 3.23. Influence of dose heterogeneity on physical and biologic doses as a function of the isodose line chosen for defining the tumor dose and of α/β ratio of the tissue located at D_{max}. The divergence of biologic and physical doses reflects the change in biologic dose that results from change in dose per fraction that derives from the heterogeneity of dose distribution. The lower the α/β ratio, the greater the divergence between biologic and physical doses. This "double trouble" is not reflected in physics isodose distributions and not only may explain a spurious volume effect but also may contribute to low values of tolerance doses that have appeared in the literature from time to time.

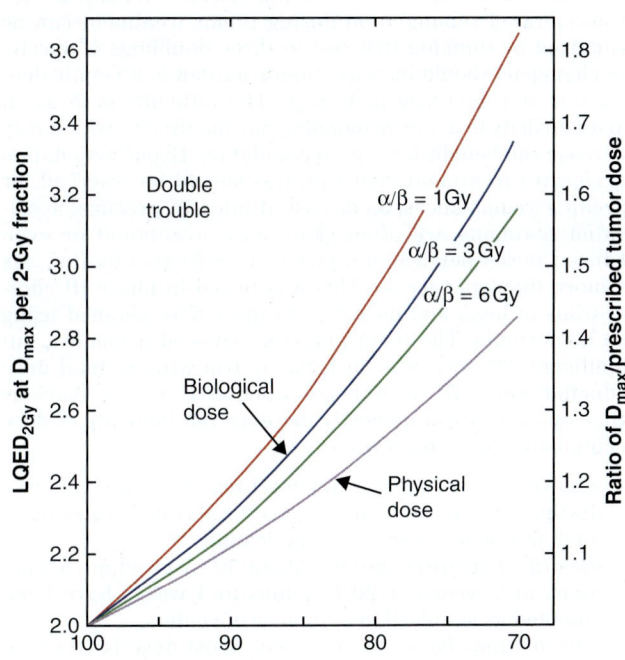

Some biologic factors relevant to modified dose fractionation are as follows:

1. Tissue-related factors have to be taken into account (Figs. 3.14, 3.18, and 3.22).
2. Acute-responding normal tissues have an enormous capacity for repopulation (Fig. 2.3).
3. Tumors can show accelerated repopulation (Figs. 3.5–3.7). There is probably great variability from tumor to tumor, but on average, the lag time is longer and its rate slower than for acute-responding normal tissues.
4. Cell cycle redistribution produces net sensitization in proliferative tissues but not in nonproliferative, late-responding tissues.
5. Hypoxia has less effect at low doses, and the kinetics of reoxygenation are probably rapid, so it may be a factor only for treatments employing single or a few large doses.
6. Slow-responding tissues "repair" better than acute-responding tissues.
7. Repopulation in normal tissues, and possibly in tumors, may be rapid during a treatment break.
8. The lag time to the onset of repopulation may be shortened to a limited extent by causing injury faster, for example, by increasing dose intensity or by concomitant chemotherapy.
9. Some tumors are similar to late-responding tissues in having a low α/β ratio and slow turnover.
10. True "stem" cells and CSCs are often relatively quiescent and have different characteristics from the bulk of the normal tissue and tumor. For example, long-term repopulating hematopoietic stem cells have a low α/β ratio[119] even though most bone marrow responses including lethality have a high α/β ratio. The target population for an endpoint therefore has to be carefully considered.

Accelerated Treatment

Accelerated treatment may be defined as a shortening of the overall treatment duration without a comparable reduction in total dose. However, in practice, for fraction sizes >2 Gy, lower doses are generally given (e.g., 50 to 55 Gy in 3 to 4 weeks), with an exception being continuous hyperfractionated accelerated radiotherapy (CHART) that gave 1.5 Gy three times per day, 7 days per week.[61,120] The essential aim is to minimize tumor regeneration during therapy. The importance of accelerated repopulation during tumor treatment can be visualized by thinking that two to three doublings of surviving clonogens should increase tumor burden to an equivalent of a one-step increase in T-stage. The difficulty is to avoid excess toxicity in acute-responding normal tissues, which may decrease the benefit from its repopulation. Hypofractionation accelerates treatment; however, this should be reserved for specific circumstances, as discussed later. In practice, accelerated regimens are often given as conventional or even reduced doses per fraction given more frequently (i.e., six or more times per week). This was tested in phase III clinical trials in head and neck SCC in the 1970s, planned using the LQ formula. The meta-analysis[73] showed a modest, but significant, 2% increases in local control without total dose reduction and 1.7% with dose reduction at 5 years. Various other approaches to modestly increase the intensity of dose accumulation have been tried.

1. *Continuous standard 2 Gy fractions per day:* A course lasting <2 weeks resulted in good local control rates but a high frequency of severe complications.[121]
2. *Relative hypofractionation:* About 50 Gy given in 15 fractions in 3 weeks or 20 fractions in 4 weeks have been adopted as standard in a number of centers.
3. *Concomitant boosting:* A second boost dose is given on several days to a reduced volume "concomitantly" with treatment of the initial larger volume, with an interfraction interval of at least 6 hours, and preferably during the later stages of treatment.[122] Concomitant boost with accelerated fractionation was part of a clinical trial that showed significantly improved locoregional control of head and neck cancer.[123]
4. *CHART:* With CHART, 51 to 54 Gy is given as 1.4- or 1.5-Gy fractions, three times daily at 6-hour intervals for 12 consecutive days.[61,124] In a large prospective, randomized CHART trial, tumor control rates were increased with acceptable acute morbidity. Some permanent sequelae (e.g., xerostomia, fibrosis) were reduced, although myelopathy was more likely when the spinal cord was treated three times per day.
5. *Split-course accelerated treatment:* Head and neck tumors were given about 38 Gy over about 10 days as 2 fractions of 1.6 Gy/day; after a break of 12 to 14 days, an additional 28 Gy (approximately) was delivered, with the total treatment lasting about 6 weeks. The results were better than in historic controls.[125,126]

Because accelerated tumor regrowth has its greatest effect late in a standard regimen, even a 1-week shortening could be advantageous (Figs. 3.5 and 3.6). However, excessive shortening to less than the lag time (e.g., to <3 to 4 weeks in head and neck cancer) is unlikely to improve tumor control rates, especially if the total dose is reduced to maintain acceptable acute toxicity.

Although modifying and individualizing fractionation patterns may improve the outcome for some patients, accelerated tumor growth, repopulation in acute-responding tissues, and differences in response between late-responding normal tissues and tumors have important implications for everyday conventional treatment. Consideration should be given to whether it is wise to complete RT on a Monday after a weekend break, start a course on a Friday, or to counter breaks in treatment (public holidays, patient demands, etc.) by delivering more than five fractions in at least one week of treatment b.i.d. Chemotherapy given before the start of RT may initiate accelerated repopulation and compromise local tumor control. It is best during or after RT when surviving tumor clonogens are actively proliferating.

Hyperfractionation

Hyperfractionation uses smaller-than-standard doses per fraction. It can be achieved without extending the overall treatment duration by treating once a day for 6 or 7 days per week but is usually given as 2 fractions per day, 5 days per week. It aims to increase the therapeutic differential between late-responding normal tissues and acute-responding tumors by exploiting differences in response to dose fractionation. It may also exploit cell cycle redistribution in the tumor and absent in late-responding normal tissues, and the OER being lower at low doses. When 2 fractions are given per day, the interfraction interval should preferably be not <6 hours, and longer if CNS tissue is involved. Hyperfractionation is unlikely to be advantageous for slowly proliferating tumors with a low α/β ratio.

Clinical evidence suggests that to stay within comparable toxicity constraints in fibrovascular tissues (late responding), one fraction of 2 Gy/day should be replaced with two fractions of about 1.2 Gy, whereas for acute-responding tissues and tumors, it is about 1.05 Gy, giving a therapeutic differential of 1.2/1.05 = 1.14, a 14% benefit. Hyperfractionation has improved tumor control rates but also increased acute toxicity. A meta-analysis of randomized trials treating mostly cancer of the oropharynx and larynx and comparing conventional RT with hyperfractionated RT with or without total dose reduction showed increased survival benefit of 8% at 5 years.[73]

Hypofractionation, SBRT, SRS, SABR

Classically trained radiation oncologists often fear giving high dose fractions because they have been associated with increased vascular injury, chronic inflammation, and severe late effects that can drastically affect quality and length of life of patients. However, these biologic disadvantages can sometimes be overcome. The advances in physics, particularly related to the use of IMRT, along with better imaging, and gating techniques to account for body motion, allow dose to be distributed to better avoid organs at risk and minimize tumor margins. Major issues remain as to what dose to give and how to fractionate.

From the radiobiologic perspective, if the fractionation response of the tumor is similar to that of late-responding normal tissues (low α/β ratio), there is little therapeutic advantage to be gained from conventional dose fractionation and, instead, moderate hypofractionation should be considered. Accelerated tumor repopulation would not be expected in tumors with low α/β ratios, so this is unlikely to be a factor. Acute toxicity may be increased, as might the risk of geographic miss and "cold spots," and tumor cure compromised by poor reoxygenation, but these may be countered by giving enough fractions. A recent SBRT analysis in low- and intermediate-risk prostate cancer (low α/β ratio), giving 36.25 Gy in 4 to 5 fractions, indicated PSA relapse-free survival rates comparable with other definitive treatments.[74] Fraction sizes of up to 8 Gy are convenient because they do not deviate much outside the limitations of the LQ model, but there are other reasons for thinking fractions around this size might be useful. Dose distributions optimized by IMRT mean less normal tissue receives high radiation doses, and although the integral body dose may be greater,[127] the rapid dose falloff outside the tumor may generate gradients of cytokines and chemokines that spatially organize infiltrating host immune cells. Such doses may also generate more "danger" signals for tumor immunity and abscopal effects, which could assist in combating micrometastatic disease. Preliminary data suggest that moderately high hypofractionated doses may be superior in this respect and in fact superior to even high single ablative doses.[36,128] The RT may cause more intratumoral vascular damage and prevent cells going through a single cycle and instead opt for a mode of rapid cell death. These factors will surely vary greatly with the tumor and are not easily investigated in the clinic, but they provide rationales for moderate hypofractionation under certain circumstances, especially in combination with ICIs.[33]

Single and high dose fractions, as used in stereotactic radiosurgery (SRS) or stereotactic ablative radiotherapy (SABR), are a separate consideration from moderately high doses used in hypofractionation. Leksell[129] introduced SRS in the late 1960s to treat inaccessible cerebral lesions and in particular small arteriovenous malformations with single-dose treatments, leading to development of the gamma knife. This was followed by the use of linear accelerators to give single dose SRS or stereotactic radiotherapy (SRT) in a small number of fractions. These approaches have proved clinically effective in treating a variety of benign and malignant brain diseases,[130] in particular well-defined metastatic masses. SRT has been extended to extracranial sites in the form of SBRT that may employ hypofractionation as above or SABR, which uses a small number of high dose fractions, such as three fractions of 15 to 20 Gy.[131,132] There is growing evidence that it dramatically improves outcome in medically inoperable early-stage non–small cell lung cancer patients[133] and may be of use against oligometastatic disease.[131,132] These findings, together with reports of excellent outcomes from high dose rate afterloading brachytherapy,[134] have prompted some re-evaluation of how traditional radiobiologic concepts apply to these new clinical procedures.[135]

SABR has a very different aim from conventional RT and aims at tumor ablation. Using the LQ formula, 3 × 20 Gy is equivalent to around 275 Gy in 2 Gy fractions to late-responding tissues with an α/β ratio of 3 Gy.[135] This extrapolation is probably not valid, but under any circumstances, the doses can be considered ablative. The normal tissue trade-off for SABR comes by minimizing the treatment volume and more consideration being given to tumor location. As discussed earlier, radiobiologic advantages of a high dose to a small volume may include allowing angiogenesis and stem cell migration from surrounding normal tissue to effect better normal tissue recovery and limit vascular damage and normal tissue hypoxia. As for location, SABR doses are moderated for tumors that are centrally located in the lung where serial structures are present. In the lung, loss of peripheral tissue function in small areas is not clinically important because there is ample residual lung function, which is not the case for all tissues and sites. Site and volume therefore appear to be the main SABR constraints, and provided they are adhered to, SABR appears to be well tolerated, with the caveat that there are not yet sufficient patients treated in this fashion to allow long-term effects to be properly assessed.

Low Dose Rate Continuous Irradiation

Low dose rate continuous irradiation, as in low dose brachytherapy, has the same biologic advantages as hyperfractionation. Additionally:

1. Proliferative cells may be delayed in their progression through the cell cycle,[136] in particular in late G2 phase. Such a skewed redistribution could self-sensitize proliferative tissues and tumors without affecting late-responding normal tissues.
2. The overall duration of therapy is shortened.
3. The high dose regions near the radioactive sources have a probability of being sterilized.
4. The volume of normal tissue receiving a high dose is minimized. Not only is the total dose beyond the treatment volume lower, the dose rate is as well, boosting further the sparing of late-responding tissues. This can be considered an inverse dose rate effect, that is, an inverse double-trouble effect or a double advantage.
5. Potential biologic disadvantages are the relatively rapid falloff in dose beyond the treatment volume and "cold spots" resulting from seed misplacement or movement. These could decrease the probability of tumor eradication if the tumor lay beyond the specified minimum tumor isodose (geographic miss).
6. Permanent implants of low dose rate radioisotopes with long half-lives (e.g., ^{125}I) may give late-responding normal tissues high doses, and if the total dose is delivered over a long time, the initial dose rate may have to be so low that CSCs "escape."

In contrast to low dose rate, the advantages of high dose rate brachytherapy come from improved logistics and staff protection and that some normal tissues can be tolerably displaced from the high dose field. Its biologic disadvantages may be loss of therapeutic differential between late-effect tissues and tumors endowed by the 4Rs.

Optimal Dose Rate

A change in dose rate, even 10 Gy/minute to 1 Gy/minute, can affect the response of tissues by allowing more SLD repair.[136] However, sparing of late-responding tissues is most pronounced with even lower dose rates, such as are characteristic of low dose rate brachytherapy, that is, between about 10 and 0.1 Gy/hour. In acute-responding tissues, and presumably also in a proportion of tumors, repopulation may be more important than repair at very low dose rates.

In late-responding tissues, such as rat spinal cord and lung,[137] a large dose rate effect is seen with change from

4 to 2 Gy/hour. If the 2 Gy per hour data are compared with multifraction data, the potential for substantial sparing with a further decrease in dose rate below 2 Gy/hour is indicated.[138] Such a large sparing effect of the reduced dose rate is to be expected in late-responding tissues.

Low Dose Rate Total Body Irradiation

Because proliferative bone marrow populations and leukemia cells are characterized by a high α/β ratio (Table 2.2), it is reasonable to prepare patients for bone marrow transplantation using either multiple small dose fractions or continuous low dose rate exposure. Between about 1 and 7 Gy/hour has been chosen for various continuous total body irradiation regimens, which is the dose where biologic effectiveness changes rapidly and even lower dose rates may provide better therapeutic differential.[139] Because the time to deliver the dose at such low dose rates is so long, many transplant centers give multifraction exposures. In general, low doses per fraction and low dose rates provide the best therapeutic differentials, provided the overall treatment duration is kept short in relation to the growth rate of the leukemic and normal stem cells.

Spatial Dose Considerations

Geographic Underdosage of Tumor

The impact of geographic underdosage (cold spots) of areas within tumor on the TCP depends on the number of CSCs in that area and the extent of the underdosage. This can be modeled under the assumption that cells and radiosensitivity are distributed uniformly. Each tumor can be regarded as being composed of a large number of "tumorlets," each receiving a specified, although variable, dose. The overall TCP can be estimated by summing the TCPs for all the tumorlets. As illustrated in Figure 3.24, the TCP decreases with the number of underdosed tumorlets (volume) and the larger the decrement in dose. (Note that physical dose inhomogeneities are amplified by "biologic" dose to an extent that will depend on the α/β ratio, that is, 2Gy + 2 Gy is not always 4 Gy, especially when the α/β is low.)

Figure 3.24 traces the decline in TCP as a function of volume and magnitude of tumor underdosage. The magnitude of the underdose is shown as multiples of D_{10}, the dose that would reduce the number of surviving clonogens to 10% of the initial number—about 7 Gy for a standard regimen of 2 Gy fractions. From Figure 3.24, it can be seen that a 7 Gy $(1 \times D_{10})$ underdosage to 10% of the tumor would reduce TCP from 90% to 83%, whereas a 14 Gy underdosage to only 5% of the tumor would reduce TCP from 90% to 55%; that is, the extent of underdosage is more important than the volume underdosed.

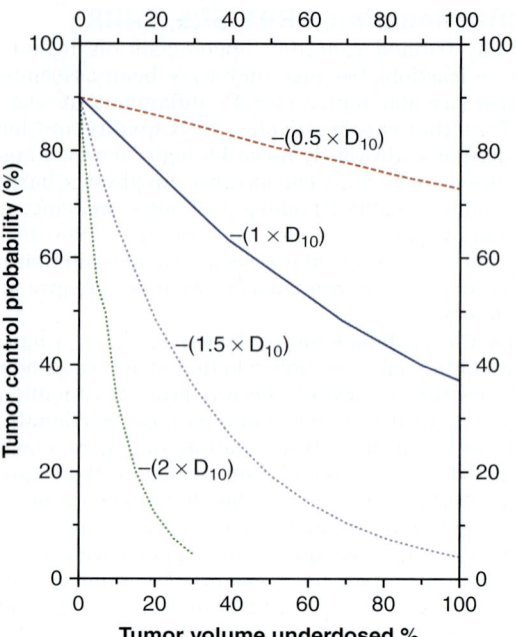

FIGURE 3.24. Effect of varying degrees of underdosage (in terms of D_{10} values) on TCP as a function of tumor volume underdosed. Note that the most important determinant is the magnitude of the underdosage.

Theoretical DVHs are presented in Figure 3.25. The smallest deviation from 100% dose to 100% tumor is outlined by a-e, showing 5% of the tumor being underdosed by about 5% $(0.5 \times D_{10})$. Underdosage by 10% $(1 \times D_{10})$, 15% $(1.5 \times D_{10})$, or 20% $(2 \times D_{10})$ in a 70-Gy regimen is shown by b-e, c-e, and d-e, respectively. The impact on TCP of the four levels of underdosage depicted by the DVHs in Figure 3.25 can be read from Figure 3.24. Assuming that 70 Gy in 2-Gy fractions yields a TCP of 90%, then the effect of underdosing 5% of the tumor by 5% $(0.5 \times D_{10})$, 10% $(1 \times D_{10})$, 15% $(1.5 \times D_{10})$, or 20% $(2 \times D_{10})$ would be a decline in TCP by 1%, 3.5%, 12.5%, and 35%, respectively (Fig. 3.24).

It is obvious that most of the DVH is irrelevant to TCP, but that small increments in the indentation along the x-axis in the upper right-hand corner may be critical, signifying that moderate to large reductions in dose to even small volumes are dangerous. The DVHs b-e, b-f, and b-g in Figure 3.25 illustrate a 10% underdosage to 5%, 10%, and 20% of the tumor, respectively. From Figure 3.24, it can be seen that this 10% underdosage would decrease the calculated TCP by 3.5%, 7%, and 14%, respectively, much less of a loss than associated with the smaller indentations along the x-axis.

FIGURE 3.25. Multiple theoretical DVH. By reference to Figure 3.24, the impact on TCP of indentations in the upper right corner of the DVH can be estimated (see text). The underdosage (a-e, b-e, c-e, d-e) is the most important determinant of TCP. The histogram h-j depicts a dangerous DVH for an organ with serially arranged FSUs such as spinal cord but benign for lung, liver, kidney, and so forth. Histogram k-m depicts danger for liver, lung, and kidney, although not for spinal cord.

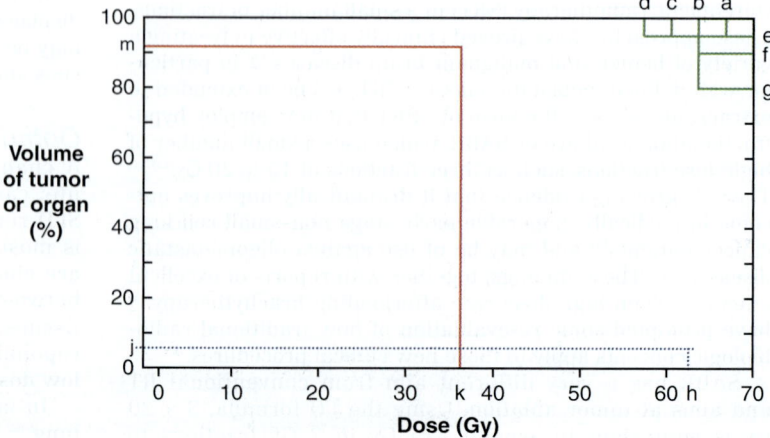

Again, the extent of underdosage is a more important determinant of TCP than the volume of tumor underdosed unlike overdosing.

Geographic Overdosage of Tumor

Small areas of elevated dose, or hot spots (e.g., in ≤30% of the tumor), produce a negligible change in overall TCP, especially if the TCP from the homogeneous dose is already high (Fig. 3.26). Obviously, the larger the volume of tumor included in the overdosed region, the greater the potential for an increase in TCP, especially if the TCP was low to begin with (lower curves, Fig. 3.26). In general, dose-painting subvolumes offer little advantage, whereas elevating the dose to the whole tumor could be of great value. For example, an escalation of dose to 30% of the tumor by $1 \times D_{10}$ could raise the TCP from 10% to nearly 18%, whereas the same increment to the whole tumor could raise the TCP from 10% to 80%.

A significant advantage would only derive from hot spot dose painting if the targeting was accurate and in areas of substantially and consistently greater radioresistance (e.g., a nidus of hypoxic cells, or a CSC niche) that would not be cured by a standard homogeneous dose. At present, there are no proven ways of localizing tumor foci that are consistently radioresistant. Thus, with current levels of understanding and technical expertise, the largest and most certain benefits are likely to be achieved if the dose to the whole tumor is escalated. This is illustrated by the increasing slope of the curves in Figure 3.26 as the volume receiving the higher dose approaches 100%.

Effective Uniform Dose

The effects of inhomogeneous dose distribution on TCP can be quantified by the equivalent uniform dose (EUD).[140] An EUD produces a constant probability of tumor control for different volumes of tumor under- or overdosed. In Figures 3.24 and 3.26, a horizontal line for any chosen TCP would join EUDs for various volumes exposed to doses differing by various multiples of D_{10}, the relevant EUD value being the homogeneous dose that produced that TCP.

FIGURE 3.26. Modeling of the effect on TCP of increasing dose to increasing proportions of the tumor. Small hot spots are not very useful, especially if TCP is already high. The closer to 100% the tumor being "overdosed," the steeper the TCP curve.

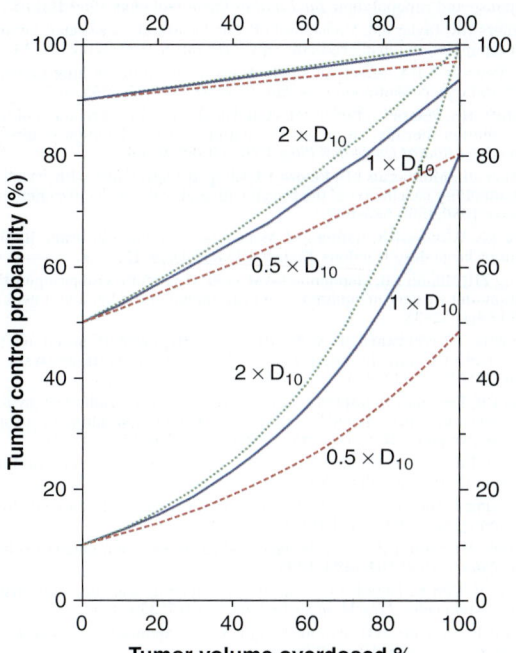

Dose–Volume Histograms for Normal Tissues

Obviously, heterogeneity in dose will also result in different levels of injury, with an outcome heavily dictated by the structure and function of the organ. Spinal cord, where FSUs are in series, can be injured by a high dose to even a small volume (Fig. 3.25, h-j) but not by a low dose to a large volume (k-m). However, a large dose to a small volume (h-i) is of little consequence if the tissue has a large "reserve" volume of FSUs. Conversely, a relatively low dose to a large volume (e.g., k-m), could be devastating if applied to lung, liver, or kidney. Thus, DVH configurations should be viewed against an understanding of the structure and physiology of the specific tissue.

QUALITY OF RADIATION

Linear Energy Transfer and Relative Biologic Efficiency

The rate at which a charged particle, such as an electron or proton, deposits its energy along its track is described as its LET; the heavier the particle, the higher its LET. Thus, electrons are predominantly low LET, protons slightly higher, neutrons even higher, and heavily charged particles the highest LET of clinically used radiations.

The rate of energy transfer increases as particles slow down, which means that LET is only an average value. As LET increases, so does its biologic efficiency, although the increase is most rapid and peaks around 100 to 150 kv/μm. This is thought to represent the sweet spot where individual ionization events are spaced exactly so that they are most likely to hit both strands of DNA. It then decreases per unit of measured physical dose with further increase in LET (an "overkill" phenomenon). As LET increases, OER decreases inversely with biologic effectiveness (i.e., oxygen is not needed as much to cause damage), and the impact of variations in cell cycle–related radiosensitivity become less.[141] At high LET, single-hit, nonrepairable cell killing increases relative to that from accumulation of SLD; thus, the survival curve for neutrons or heavily charged particles is essentially linear over at least the first decade of cell killing, and there is little sparing from dose fractionation.[142]

RBE is a ratio of doses from two beams to produce the same effect:

RBE = dose (standard beam)/dose (test beam)

Historically, RBE is used to compare high and low LET radiations; however, it has wider applicability for comparing the effectiveness of treatment approaches such as high and low dose rate x-irradiation. Initially, the standard photon beam was 250 kVp x-rays, but now, at least from the viewpoint of RT, it is ^{60}Co (250 kVp x-rays are about 15% more efficient than ^{60}Co in killing mammalian cells). It is not widely appreciated that even at relatively high dose rates, photon beam effectiveness varies with dose rate and is an important determinant of RBE. This can only be measured accurately if the same effect is achieved by both radiations. These uncertainties are magnified further when considering radiations that have a Bragg peak, where the RBE can vary markedly and rapidly over small tissue areas.

REFERENCES

1. Alper T, Howard-Flanders P. Role of oxygen in modifying the radiosensitivity of E. coli B. *Nature* 1956;178(4540):978–979.
2. DeNicola GM, Chen PH, Mullarky E, et al. NRF2 regulates serine biosynthesis in non-small cell lung cancer. *Nat Genet* 2015;47(12):1475–1481.
3. McDonald JT, Kim K, Norris AJ, et al. Ionizing radiation activates the Nrf2 antioxidant response. *Cancer Res* 2010;70(21):8886–8895.
4. Wu T, Harder BG, Wong PK, et al. Oxidative stress, mammospheres and Nrf2-new implication for breast cancer therapy? *Mol Carcinog* 2014.

5. Shohan J. Some theoretical considerations on the present status of roentgen therapy. *Boston Med Surg J* 1916;175:321–325.

6. Formenti SC, Demaria S. Combining radiotherapy and cancer immunotherapy: a paradigm shift. *J Natl Cancer Inst* 2013;105(4):256–265.

7. Vilenchik MM, Knudson AG. Endogenous DNA double-strand breaks: production, fidelity of repair, and induction of cancer. *Proc Natl Acad Sci U S A* 2003;100(22):12871–12876.

8. Banuelos CA, Banath JP, Kim JY, et al. gammaH2AX expression in tumors exposed to cisplatin and fractionated irradiation. *Clin Cancer Res* 2009;15(10):3344–3353.

9. Mahamud O, So J, Chua MLK, et al. Targeting DNA repair for precision radiotherapy: balancing the therapeutic ratio. *Curr Probl Cancer* 2017;41(4):265–272.

10. Behjati S, Gundem G, Wedge DC, et al. Mutational signatures of ionizing radiation in second malignancies. *Nat Commun* 2016;7:12605.

11. Ahmed MM. Regulation of radiation-induced apoptosis by early growth response-1 gene in solid tumors. *Curr Cancer Drug Targets* 2004;4(1):43–52.

12. Schaue D, McBride WH. Links between innate immunity and normal tissue radiobiology. *Radiat Res* 2010;173(4):406–417.

13. Vanpouille-Box C, Alard A, Aryankalayil MJ, et al. DNA exonuclease Trex1 regulates radiotherapy-induced tumour immunogenicity. *Nat Commun* 2017;8:15618.

14. McBride WH, Chiang CS, Olson JL, et al. A sense of danger from radiation. *Radiat Res* 2004;162(1):1–19.

15. Syljuasen RG, Hong JH, McBride WH. Apoptosis and delayed expression of c-jun and c-fos after gamma irradiation of Jurkat T cells. *Radiat Res* 1996;146(3):276–282.

16. Ratikan JA, Sayre JW, Schaue D. Chloroquine engages the immune system to eradicate irradiated breast tumors in mice. *Int J Radiat Oncol Biol Phys* 2013;87(4):761–768.

17. Puck TT, Marcus PI. Action of x-rays on mammalian cells. *J Exp Med* 1956;103(5):653–666.

18. Kerr JF, Wyllie AH, Currie AR. Apoptosis: a basic biological phenomenon with wide-ranging implications in tissue kinetics. *Br J Cancer* 1972;26(4):239–257.

19. Kemp CJ, Sun S, Gurley KE. p53 induction and apoptosis in response to radio- and chemotherapy in vivo is tumor-type-dependent. *Cancer Res* 2001;61(1):327–332.

20. Daigle JL, Hong JH, Chiang CS, et al. The role of tumor necrosis factor signaling pathways in the response of murine brain to irradiation. *Cancer Res* 2001;61(24):8859–8865.

21. Coppe JP, Rodier F, Patil CK, et al. Tumor suppressor and aging biomarker p16(INK4a) induces cellular senescence without the associated inflammatory secretory phenotype. *J Biol Chem* 2011;286(42):36396–36403.

22. Yang H, Wang H, Ren J, et al. cGAS is essential for cellular senescence. *Proc Natl Acad Sci U S A* 2017;114(23):E4612–E4620.

23. Bumann J, Santo-Holtje L, Loffler H, et al. Radiation-induced alterations of the proliferation dynamics of human skin fibroblasts after repeated irradiation in the subtherapeutic dose range. *Strahlenther Onkol* 1995;171(1):35–41.

24. Kyjacova L, Hubackova S, Krejcikova K, et al. Radiotherapy-induced plasticity of prostate cancer mobilizes stem-like non-adherent, Erk signaling-dependent cells. *Cell Death Differ* 2014.

25. Potten CS, Hendry JH. *Radiation and gut*. Amsterdam, The Netherlands: Elsevier Science, 1995.

26. Barker N, van Oudenaarden A, Clevers H. Identifying the stem cell of the intestinal crypt: strategies and pitfalls. *Cell Stem Cell* 2012;11(4):452–460.

27. Withers HR, Elkind MM. Radiosensitivity and fractionation response of crypt cells of mouse jejunum. *Radiat Res* 1969;38(3):598–613.

28. Hua G, Wang C, Pan Y, et al. Distinct Levels of Radioresistance in Lgr5+ Colonic Epithelial Stem Cells versus Lgr5+ Small Intestinal Stem Cells. *Cancer Res* 2017;77(8):2124–2133.

29. Stephens LC, Ang KK, Schultheiss TE, et al. Target cell and mode of radiation injury in rhesus salivary glands. *Radiother Oncol* 1986;7(2):165–174.

30. Kolesnick R, Fuks Z. Radiation and ceramide-induced apoptosis. *Oncogene* 2003;22(37):5897–5906.

31. Maj JG, Paris F, Haimovitz-Friedman A, et al. Microvascular function regulates intestinal crypt response to radiation. *Cancer Res* 2003;63(15):4338–4341.

32. Fuks Z, Kolesnick R. Engaging the vascular component of the tumor response. *Cancer Cell* 2005;8(2):89–91.

33. McBride WH, Ganapathy E, Lee MH, et al. A perspective on the impact of radiation therapy on the immune rheostat. *Br J Radiol* 2017:20170272.

34. Demaria S, Bhardwaj N, McBride WH, et al. Combining radiotherapy and immunotherapy: a revived partnership. *Int J Radiat Oncol Biol Phys* 2005;63(3):655–666.

35. Petljak M, Alexandrov LB. Understanding mutagenesis through delineation of mutational signatures in human cancer. *Carcinogenesis* 2016;37(6):531–540.

36. Schaue D, Ratikan JA, Iwamoto KS, et al. Maximizing tumor immunity with fractionated radiation. *Int J Radiat Oncol Biol Phys* 2012;83(4):1306–1310.

37. Moulder JE. 2013 Dade W. Moeller lecture: medical countermeasures against radiological terrorism. *Health Phys* 2014;107(2):164–171.

38. Philippens ME, Pop LA, Visser AG, et al. Bath and shower effect in spinal cord: the effect of time interval. *Int J Radiat Oncol Biol Phys* 2009;73(2):514–522.

39. Medin PM, Foster RD, van der Kogel AJ, et al. Spinal cord tolerance to single-session uniform irradiation in pigs: implications for a dose-volume effect. *Radiother Oncol* 2013;106:101–105.

40. Lee SP, Leu MY, Smathers JB, et al. Biologically effective dose distribution based on the linear quadratic model and its clinical relevance. *Int J Radiat Oncol Biol Phys* 1995;33(2):375–389.

41. Withers HR, Mason KA, Thames HD Jr. Late radiation response of kidney assayed by tubule-cell survival. *Br J Radiol* 1986;59(702):587–595.

42. Withers HR. Recovery and repopulation in vivo by mouse skin epithelial cells during fractionated irradiation. *Radiat Res* 1967;32(2):227–239.

43. Wang CC. Improved local control for advanced oropharyngeal carcinoma following twice daily radiation therapy. *Am J Clin Oncol* 1985;8(6):512–516.

44. Ang KK, Landuyt W, Xu FX, et al. The effect of small radiation doses per fraction on mouse lip mucosa assessed using the concept of partial tolerance. *Radiother Oncol* 1987;8(1):79–86.

45. Farrell CL, Bready JV, Rex KL, et al. Keratinocyte growth factor protects mice from chemotherapy and radiation-induced gastrointestinal injury and mortality. *Cancer Res* 1998;58(5):933–939.

46. Moulder JE, Cohen EP, Fish BL. Captopril and losartan for mitigation of renal injury caused by single-dose total-body irradiation. *Radiat Res* 2011;175(1):29–36.

47. Epperly MW, Francicola D, Shields D, et al. Screening of antimicrobial agents for in vitro radiation protection and mitigation capacity, including those used in supportive care regimens for bone marrow transplant recipients. *In Vivo* 2010;24(1):9–19.

48. Micewicz ED, Kim K, Iwamoto KS, et al. 4-(Nitrophenylsulfonyl)piperazines mitigate radiation damage to multiple tissues. *PLoS One* 2017;12(7):e0181577.

49. Withers HR. The 4Rs of radiotherapy. *Adv Radiation Biol* 1975;5:241–249.

50. Mason KA, Withers HR, Chiang CS. Late effects of radiation on the lumbar spinal cord of guinea pigs: re-treatment tolerance. *Int J Radiat Oncol Biol Phys* 1993;26(4):643–648.

51. Landuyt W, Fowler J, Ruifrok A, et al. Kinetics of repair in the spinal cord of the rat. *Radiother Oncol* 1997;45(1):55–62.

52. Ang KK, Jiang GL, Feng Y, et al. Extent and kinetics of recovery of occult spinal cord injury. *Int J Radiat Oncol Biol Phys* 2001;50(4):1013–1020.

53. Stewart FA, van der Kogel AJ. Retreatment tolerance of normal tissues. *Semin Radiat Oncol* 1994;4(2):103–111.

54. Pajonk F, Vlashi E, McBride WH. Radiation resistance of cancer stem cells: the 4 R's of radiobiology revisited. *Stem Cells* 2010;28(4):639–648.

55. Meyn RE, Stephens LC, Hunter NR, et al. Reemergence of apoptotic cells between fractionated doses in irradiated murine tumors. *Int J Radiat Oncol Biol Phys* 1994;30(3):619–624.

56. McBride WH, Dougherty GJ. Radiotherapy for genes that cause cancer. *Nat Med* 1995;1(11):1215–1217.

57. Thames HD, Bentzen SM, Turesson I, et al. Time-dose factors in radiotherapy: a review of the human data. *Radiother Oncol* 1990;19(3):219–235.

58. Brenner DJ, Hall EJ. Fractionation and protraction for radiotherapy of prostate carcinoma. *Int J Radiat Oncol Biol Phys* 1999;43(5):1095–1101.

59. Group ST, Bentzen SM, Agrawal RK, et al. The UK Standardisation of Breast Radiotherapy (START) Trial A of radiotherapy hypofractionation for treatment of early breast cancer: a randomised trial. *Lancet Oncol* 2008;9(4):331–341.

60. Steel GG. *Basic clinical radiobiology*. London, UK: Edward Arnold, 1993.

61. Dische S, Saunders MI. Continuous, hyperfractionated, accelerated radiotherapy (CHART): an interim report upon late morbidity. *Radiother Oncol* 1989;16(1):65–72.

62. Begg AC, Haustermans K, Hart AA, et al. The value of pretreatment cell kinetic parameters as predictors for radiotherapy outcome in head and neck cancer: a multicenter analysis. *Radiother Oncol* 1999;50(1):13–23.

63. Hermens AF, Barendsen GW. Changes of cell proliferation characteristics in a rat rhabdomyosarcoma before and after x-irradiation. *Eur J Cancer* 1969;5(2):173–189.

64. Phillips TM, McBride WH, Pajonk F. The response of CD24(-/low)/CD44+ breast cancer-initiating cells to radiation. *J Natl Cancer Inst* 2006;98(24):1777–1785.

65. Vlashi E, Pajonk F. Cancer stem cells, cancer cell plasticity and radiation therapy. *Semin Cancer Biol* 2014.

66. Maciejewski B, Withers HR, Taylor JM, et al. Dose fractionation and regeneration in radiotherapy for cancer of the oral cavity and oropharynx: tumor dose-response and repopulation. *Int J Radiat Oncol Biol Phys* 1989;16(3):831–843.

67. Withers HR, Taylor JM, Maciejewski B. The hazard of accelerated tumor clonogen repopulation during radiotherapy. *Acta Oncol* 1988;27(2):131–146.

68. van Peperzeel HA. Effects of single doses of radiation on lung metastases in man and experimental animals. *Eur J Cancer* 1972;8(6):665–675.

69. Withers HR, Peters LJ, Taylor JM, et al. Local control of carcinoma of the tonsil by radiation therapy: an analysis of patterns of fractionation in nine institutions. *Int J Radiat Oncol Biol Phys* 1995;33(3):549–562.

70. Barker JL, Montague ED, Peters LJ. Clinical experience with irradiation of inflammatory carcinoma of the breast with and without elective chemotherapy. *Cancer* 1980;45(4):625–629.

71. Choi KN, Withers HR, Rotman M. Metastatic melanoma in brain. Rapid treatment or large dose fractions. *Cancer* 1985;56(1):10–15.

72. Wang ZH, Million RR, Mendenhall WM, et al. Treatment with preoperative irradiation and surgery of squamous cell carcinoma of the head and neck. *Cancer* 1989;64(1):32–38.

73. Bourhis J, Overgaard J, Audry H, et al. Hyperfractionated or accelerated radiotherapy in head and neck cancer: a meta-analysis. *Lancet* 2006;368(9538):843–854.

74. King CR, Freeman D, Kaplan I, et al. Stereotactic body radiotherapy for localized prostate cancer: pooled analysis from a multi-institutional consortium of prospective phase II trials. *Radiother Oncol* 2013;109(2):217–221.

75. Kim JJ, Tannock IF. Repopulation of cancer cells during therapy: an important cause of treatment failure. *Nat Rev Cancer* 2005;5(7):516–525.

76. Terasima T, Tolmach LJ. Changes in x-ray sensitivity of HeLa cells during the division cycle. *Nature* 1961;190:1210–1211.

77. Elkind MM, Sutton H. X-ray damage and recovery in mammalian cells in culture. *Nature* 1959;184:1293–1295.

78. Vlashi E, Kim K, Lagadec C, et al. In vivo imaging, tracking, and targeting of cancer stem cells. *J Natl Cancer Inst* 2009;101(5):350–359.

79. Vlashi E, McBride WH, Pajonk F. Radiation responses of cancer stem cells. *J Cell Biochem* 2009;108(2):339–342.

80. Read J. Mode of addition of x-ray doses given with different oxygen concentrations. *Br J Radiol* 1952;25(294):336–338.

81. Brown JM, Giaccia AJ. Tumour hypoxia: the picture has changed in the 1990s. *Int J Radiat Biol* 1994;65(1):95–102.

82. Vaupel P, Schlenger KH, Hoeckel M, et al. Oxygenation of mammary tumors: from isotransplanted rodent tumors to primary malignancies in patients. *Adv Exp Med Biol* 1992;316:361–371.

83. Brown M. Henry S. Kaplan Distinguished Scientist Award Lecture 2007. The remarkable yin and yang of tumour hypoxia. *Int J Radiat Biol* 2010;86(11):907–917.

84. Chan N, Koritzinsky M, Zhao H, et al. Chronic hypoxia decreases synthesis of homologous recombination proteins to offset chemoresistance and radioresistance. *Cancer Res* 2008;68(2):605–614.

85. Henk JM, Kunkler PB, Smith CW. Radiotherapy and hyperbaric oxygen in head and neck cancer. Final report of first controlled clinical trial. *Lancet* 1977;2(8029):101–103.

86. Phillips TM, Kim K, Vlashi E, et al. Effects of recombinant erythropoietin on breast cancer-initiating cells. *Neoplasia* 2007;9(12):1122–1129.

87. Hockel M, Schlenger K, Hockel S, et al. Hypoxic cervical cancers with low apoptotic index are highly aggressive. *Cancer Res* 1999;59(18):4525–4528.

88. Graeber TG, Osmanian C, Jacks T, et al. Hypoxia-mediated selection of cells with diminished apoptotic potential in solid tumours. *Nature* 1996;379(6560):88–91.

89. Chen FH, Chiang CS, Wang CC, et al. Radiotherapy decreases vascular density and causes hypoxia with macrophage aggregation in TRAMP-C1 prostate tumors. *Clin Cancer Res* 2009;15(5):1721–1729.

90. Chen FH, Chiang CS, Wang CC, et al. Vasculatures in tumors growing from preirradiated tissues: formed by vasculogenesis and resistant to radiation and antiangiogenic therapy. *Int J Radiat Oncol Biol Phys* 2011;80(5):1512–1521.

91. van Horssen R, Ten Hagen TL, Eggermont AM. TNF-alpha in cancer treatment: molecular insights, antitumor effects, and clinical utility. *Oncologist* 2006;11(4):397–408.

92. Catcheside DG, Lea DE, Thoday JM. Types of chromosome structural change induced by the irradiation of Tradescantia microspores. *J Genet* 1946;47:113–136.

93. Lea DE. *Actions of radiations on living cells,1946.* Cambridge: Cambridge University Press, 1946.

94. Read J. The effect of ionizing radiations on the broad bean root—Part X. *Br J Radiol* 1952;25(291):154–160.

95. Joiner MC, Marples B, Johns H. The response of tissues to very low doses per fraction: a reflection of induced repair? *Recent Results Cancer Res* 1993;130:27–40.

96. Marples B, Lambin P, Skov KA, et al. Low dose hyper-radiosensitivity and increased radioresistance in mammalian cells. *Int J Radiat Biol* 1997;71(6):721–735.

97. Barendsen GW. Dose fractionation, dose rate and iso-effect relationships for normal tissue responses. *Int J Radiat Oncol Biol Phys* 1982;8(11):1981–1997.

98. Dutreix J, Wambersie A, Bounik C. Cellular recovery in human skin reactions: application to dose fraction number overall time relationship in radiotherapy. *Eur J Cancer* 1973;9:159–167.

99. Withers HR, Chen KY. Poor man's neutrons? *Br J Radiol* 1971;44(526):818.

100. Douglas BG, Fowler JF. Letter: fractionation schedules and a quadratic dose-effect relationship. *Br J Radiol* 1975;48(570):502–504.

101. Fowler JF. The linear-quadratic formula and progress in fractionated radiotherapy. *Br J Radiol* 1989;62(740):679–694.

102. McBride WH, Schaue D. Radiation Biology of SBRT: Is there a new biology involved? In: Pollock A, Ahmed MM, eds. *Hypofractionation. Scientific concepts and clinical experiences.* Ellicott City, MD: LumiText Publishing, 2011:3–18.

103. Brenner DJ. The linear-quadratic model is an appropriate methodology for determining isoeffective doses at large doses per fraction. *Semin Radiat Oncol* 2008;18(4):234–239.

104. Peters LJ, Fletcher GH. Causes of failure of radiotherapy in head and neck cancer. *Radiother Oncol* 1983;1(1):53–63.

105. Harwood AR, Beale FA, Cummings BJ, et al. Supraglottic laryngeal carcinoma: an analysis of dose-time-volume factors in 410 patients. *Int J Radiat Oncol Biol Phys* 1983;9(3):311–319.

106. Thames HD Jr, Peters LJ, Spanos W Jr, et al. Dose response of squamous cell carcinomas of the upper respiratory and digestive tracts. *Br J Cancer Suppl* 1980;4:35–38.

107. Thames HD, Peters LJ, Ang KK. Time-dose considerations for normal-tissue tolerance. *Front Radiat Ther Oncol* 1989;23:113–130.

108. McBride WH, Withers HR. Radiobiology of subclinical disease. *Front Radiat Ther Oncol* 1994;28:46–50.

109. Strandquist M. A study of the cumulative effects of fractionated x-ray treatment based on the experience at the radiumhemmet with the treatment of 280 cases of carcinoma of the skin and lip. *Acta Radiol* 1944;55 (Suppl):300–304.

110. Fowler JF, Stern BE. Dose-rate effects: some theoretical and practical considerations. *Br J Radiol* 1960;33:389–395.

111. Ellis F. Is NSD-TDF useful to radiotherapy? *Int J Radiat Oncol Biol Phys* 1985;11:1685–1697.

112. Brenner DJ, Hlatky LR, Hahnfeldt PJ, et al. A convenient extension of the linear-quadratic model to include redistribution and reoxygenation. *Int J Radiat Oncol Biol Phys* 1995;32:379–390.

113. Thames HD Jr, Withers HR, Peters LJ, et al. Changes in early and late radiation responses with altered dose fractionation: implications for dose-survival relationships. *Int J Radiat Oncol Biol Phys* 1982;8:219–226.

114. Horiot JC, Le Fur R, N'Guyen T, et al. Hyperfractionation versus conventional fractionation in oropharyngeal carcinoma: final analysis of a randomized trial of the EORTC cooperative group of radiotherapy. *Radiother Oncol* 1992;25:231–241.

115. Bentzen SM, Thames HD, Travis EL, et al. Direct estimation of latent time for radiation injury in late-responding normal tissues: gut, lung, and spinal cord. *Int J Radiat Biol* 1989;55:27–43.

116. Ang KK, Jiang GL, Guttenberger R, et al. Impact of spinal cord repair kinetics on the practice of altered fractionation schedules. *Radiother Oncol* 1992;25(4):287–294.

117. Withers HR, Thames HD Jr, Peters LJ. A new isoeffect curve for change in dose per fraction. *Radiother Oncol* 1983;1(2):187–191.

118. Fowler JF. Review: total doses in fractionated radiotherapy—implications of new radiobiological data. *Int J Radiat Biol Relat Stud Phys Chem Med* 1984;46(2):103–120.

119. Down JD, Boudewijn A, van Os R, et al. Variations in radiation sensitivity and repair among different hematopoietic stem cell subsets following fractionated irradiation. *Blood* 1995;86:122–127.

120. Saunders MI, Dische S, Grosch EJ, et al. Experience with CHART. *Int J Radiat Oncol Biol Phys* 1991;21:871–878.

121. Skladowski K, Maciejewski B, Golen M, et al. Randomized clinical trial on 7-day-continuous accelerated irradiation (CAIR) of head and neck cancer—report on 3-year tumour control and normal tissue toxicity. *Radiother Oncol* 2000;55(2):101–110.

122. Knee R, Fields RS, Peters LJ. Concomitant boost radiotherapy for advanced squamous cell carcinoma of the head and neck. *Radiother Oncol* 1985;4(1):1–7.

123. Fu KK, Pajak TF, Trotti A, et al. A Radiation Therapy Oncology Group (RTOG) phase III randomized study to compare hyperfractionation and two variants of accelerated fractionation to standard fractionation radiotherapy for head and neck squamous cell carcinomas: first report of RTOG 9003. *Int J Radiat Oncol Biol Phys* 2000;48(1):7–16.

124. Saunders MI, Dische S, Barrett A, et al. Randomised multicentre trials of CHART vs conventional radiotherapy in head and neck and non-small-cell lung cancer: an interim report. CHART Steering Committee. *Br J Cancer* 1996;73:1455–1462.

125. Wang CC. Accelerated hyperfractionation radiation therapy for carcinoma of the nasopharynx. Techniques and results. *Cancer* 1989;63(12):2461–2467.

126. Wang CC, Blitzer PH, Suit HD. Twice-a-day radiation therapy for cancer of the head and neck. *Cancer* 1985;55(9 Suppl):2100–2104.

127. Verellen D, Vanhavere F. Risk assessment of radiation-induced malignancies based on whole-body equivalent dose estimates for IMRT treatment in the head and neck region. *Radiother Oncol* 1999;53(3):199–203.

128. Dewan MZ, Galloway AE, Kawashima N, et al. Fractionated but not single-dose radiotherapy induces an immune-mediated abscopal effect when combined with anti-CTLA-4 antibody. *Clin Cancer Res* 2009;15(17):5379–5388.

129. Leksell L. Stereotactic radiosurgery. *J Neurol Neurosurg Psychiatry* 1983;46(9):797–803.

130. Hazard LJ, Jensen RL, Shrieve DC. Role of stereotactic radiosurgery in the treatment of brain metastases. *Am J Clin Oncol* 2005;28(4):403–410.

131. Iyengar P, Westover K, Timmerman RD. Stereotactic ablative radiotherapy (SABR) for non-small cell lung cancer. *Semin Respir Crit Care Med* 2013;34(6):845–854.

132. Desai NB, Laine AM, Timmerman RD. Stereotactic ablative body radiotherapy (SAbR) for oligometastatic cancer. *Br J Radiol* 2017;90(1070):20160500.

133. Fakiris AJ, McGarry RC, Yiannoutsos CT, et al. Stereotactic body radiation therapy for early-stage non-small-cell lung carcinoma: four-year results of a prospective phase II study. *Int J Radiat Oncol Biol Phys* 2009;75(3):677–682.

134. Martinez AA, Demanes J, Vargas C, et al. High-dose-rate prostate brachytherapy: an excellent accelerated-hypofractionated treatment for favorable prostate cancer. *Am J Clin Oncol* 2010;33(5):481–488.

135. Fowler JF, Tome WA, Fenwick JD, et al. A challenge to traditional radiation oncology. *Int J Radiat Oncol Biol Phys* 2004;60(4):1241–1256.

136. Hall EJ. Radiation dose-rate: a factor of importance in radiobiology and radiotherapy. *Br J Radiol* 1972;45(530):81–97.

137. Scalliet P, Landuyt W, van der Schueren E. Repair kinetics as a determining factor for late tolerance of central nervous system to low dose rate irradiation. *Radiother Oncol* 1989;14(4):345–353.

138. van der Kogel AJ. Radiation tolerance of the rat spinal cord: time-dose relationships. *Radiology* 1977;122(2):505–509.

139. Travis EL, Peters LJ, McNeill J, et al. Effect of dose-rate on total body irradiation: lethality and pathologic findings. *Radiother Oncol* 1985;4(4):341–351.

140. Niemierko A. Reporting and analyzing dose distributions: a concept of equivalent uniform dose. *Med Phys* 1997;24(1):103–110.

141. Broerse JJ, Barendsen GW, van Kersen GR. Survival of cultured human cells after irradiation with fast neutrons of different energies in hypoxic and oxygenated conditions. *Int J Radiat Biol Relat Stud Phys Chem Med* 1968;13(6):559–572.

142. Withers HR, Thames HD Jr, Peters LJ. Biological bases for high RBE values for late effects of neutron irradiation. *Int J Radiat Oncol Biol Phys* 1982;8:2071–2076.

143. Withers HR, Taylor JM, Maciejewski B. Treatment volume and tissue tolerance. *Int J Radiat Oncol Biol Phys* 1988;14(4):751–759.

144. Fyles A, Keane TJ, Barton M, et al. The effect of treatment duration in the local control of cervix cancer. *Radiother Oncol* 1992;25(4):273–279.

145. Thames HD Jr, Withers R, Mason KA, et al. Dose-survival characteristics of mouse jejunal crypt cells. *Int J Radiat Oncol Biol Phys* 1981;7(11):1591–1597.

146. Withers HR. Predicting late normal tissue responses. *Int J Radiat Oncol Biol Phys* 1986;12(4):693–698.

147. Withers HR. Biologic basis for altered fractionation schemes. *Cancer* 1985;55(9 Suppl):2086–2095.

148. Withers HR, Peters LJ, Taylor JM. Dose-response relationship for radiation therapy of subclinical disease. *Int J Radiat Oncol Biol Phys* 1995;31(2):353–359.

149. Withers HR. Failla memorial lecture. Contrarian concepts in the progress of radiotherapy. *Radiat Res* 1989;119(3):395–412.

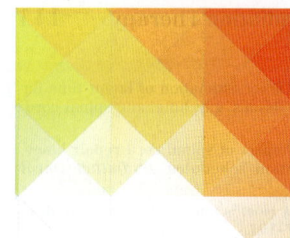

CHAPTER 4

Molecular Pathophysiology of Tumors

Rakesh K. Jain, John D. Martin, and Dan G. Duda

INTRODUCTION

A solid tumor is an organ-like structure containing neoplastic and stromal cells nourished by the tumor vasculature composed of endothelial cells (ECs), basement membrane, immune cells, and perivascular cells. All of these components are embedded in an extracellular matrix (ECM) (Fig. 4.1). The interactions between these cells, their surrounding matrix, and their local microenvironment influence the expression of various genes. The products encoded by these genes, in turn, control the pathophysiologic characteristics of the tumor. The tumor pathophysiology affects tumor growth, immune system evasion, invasion, and metastasis, as well as the response to radiation and other therapies. In this chapter, we will discuss various pathophysiologic parameters that characterize the vascular and extravascular compartments of a tumor as well as the molecular players involved in the formation and function of these compartments. Finally, we will point out some clinical implications of the findings and present a future perspective.

VASCULAR COMPARTMENT

Neoplastic cells, similar to normal cells, need oxygen and other nutrients for their survival and growth. Every reproductively intact normal cell in our body is located within 100 to 200 μm from a blood capillary so that it can receive adequate levels of oxygen and other nutrients by the process of diffusion. Likewise, cells undergoing neoplastic transformation depend on nearby capillaries for growth. These preneoplastic (i.e., dysplastic or hyperplastic) cells can grow as spherical or ellipsoidal cellular aggregates. However, once the size of the cellular aggregate reaches the diffusion limit for critical nutrients, the aggregate may become dormant. Indeed, human tumors may remain dormant for a number of years despite active cell proliferation because of a balance between proliferation and cell death. However, once they have access to new blood vessels, the tumor may grow and metastasize. What triggers the growth of new vessels? What molecular and cellular players are involved? How do these vessels compare with normal vessels with respect to their structure and function? How do they impact immunosuppression that allows tumors to evade the immune system?

Angiogenesis

The fact that the vascular system is associated with tumor growth in animals and humans has been known for more than a century.[1] Ide et al.[2] and Algire and Chalkley[3] provided powerful insight into the neovascularization of transplanted tumors using transparent window techniques (for reviews on this subject, see Refs.[4,5]). In 1968, Rijhsinghani et al.[6] and Ehrmann and Knoth[7] suggested the possibility that tumors produce an "angiogenic" substance. In 1971, Folkman[8,9] proposed the hypothesis that blocking angiogenesis should block tumor growth and metastasis. In 1978, Gullino[10] demonstrated that a tissue acquires angiogenic capacity during neoplastic transformation and proposed that antiangiogenesis approaches be used to prevent cancer. Both of these hypotheses have been validated in a number of preclinical studies.[11,12] A wide range of antiangiogenic strategies are currently being evaluated in the clinic to prevent or treat a large number of diseases, including cancer.[11] Most importantly, antiangiogenic strategies have yielded overall survival benefits in patients with advanced colorectal cancer, non–small cell lung cancer, renal cell cancer, cervical cancer, gastric cancer, hepatocellular carcinoma, and gastrointestinal stromal tumors and have shown increased response rates and progression-free survival benefits in advanced breast, medullary thyroid, and ovarian cancer, pancreatic neuroendocrine tumors (PNETs), and glioblastoma (reviewed in Refs.[13–16]). This has led so far to U.S. Food and Drug Administration (FDA) approval for 12 antiangiogenic drugs in the treatment of these diseases (Table 4.1).

The net balance between pro- and antiangiogenic factors governs both normal and pathologic angiogenic processes.[11] This balance is spatially and temporally regulated under physiologic conditions so that the "angiogenic switch" is "on" when needed (e.g., during embryonic development, wound healing, formation of corpus luteum) and "off" otherwise. During neoplastic transformation and tumor progression, this regulation is deranged, which results in ectopically formed blood vessels to support the growing mass.[11]

Cellular Mechanisms

Several cellular mechanisms have been described in the vascularization of tumors: (a) co-option, (b) intussusception, (c) sprouting (angiogenesis), (d) vasculogenesis from endothelial precursors, (e) cancer cell lining of vessels (vascular mimicry), or (f) transdifferentiation to the EC (Fig. 4.2).[11] Tumor cells can co-opt and grow around the existing vessels to form

FIGURE 4.1. Schematic representation of a solid tumor—an organ-like structure. The key components include cancer cells, host cells, and blood vasculature made of endothelial and perivascular cells—all embedded in a matrix bathed in interstitial fluid. The lymphatic vasculature, present in most normal tissues, is often lacking or is dysfunctional in solid tumors.

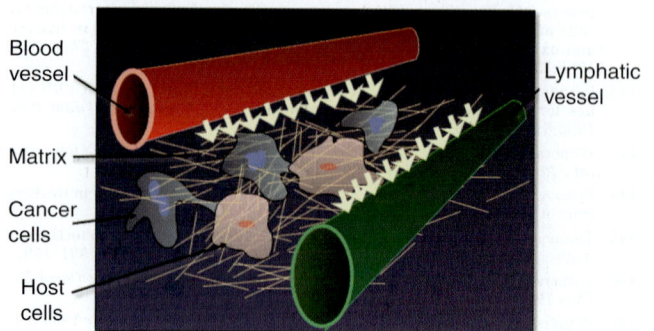

TABLE 4.1 FDA-APPROVED ANTIANGIOGENIC DRUGS

Drug	Approved Indication	Improvement in RR (%)	Improvement in PFS (mo)	Improvement in OS (mo)
Bevacizumab	Metastatic colorectal cancer (with chemotherapy)	10	4.4	4.7
		0	1.4	1.4
		7.8	2.8	2.5
		14.1	2.6	2.1
	Metastatic nonsquamous NSCLC (with chemotherapy)	20	1.7	2.0
		10.3–14.0	0.4–0.6	NS
	Metastatic breast cancer (with chemotherapy)	15.7	5.9	NS
		9–18	0.8–1.9	NS
		11.8–13.4	1.2–2.9	NS
		9.9	2.1	NS
	Metastatic RCC (with IFNa)	18	4.8	NS
		12.4	3.3	NS
Sunitinib	Metastatic RCC	35	6.0	4.6
	GIST	6.8	4.5	NS
	PNET	9.3	4.8	15
Sorafenib	Metastatic RCC	8	2.7	NS
	Unresectable HCC	1	NS	2.8
	Unresectable HCC	2	1.4	2.3
	Thyroid cancer	11.7	5.0	N/A
Pazopanib	Metastatic RCC	27	5.0	N/A
	Advanced soft tissue sarcoma	6.0	3.0	NS
Vandetanib	Advanced medullary thyroid cancer	43	6.2	N/A
Axitinib	Advanced RCC	10	2.0	N/A
Regorafenib	Chemorefractory metastatic colorectal cancer	0.6	0.2	1.4
Aflibercept	Chemorefractory metastatic colorectal cancer	8.7	2.2	1.4
Nintedanib	Metastatic nonsquamous NSCLC (with chemotherapy)	NS	0.8	NS
Lenvatinib	Thyroid cancer	63.3	14.7	N/A
Ramucirumab	Gastric or gastroesophageal junction cancer	26	N/A	1.4
	Platinum-based chemorefractory metastatic NSCLC (with chemotherapy)	9	1.5	1.4
	Chemorefractory metastatic colorectal cancer (with chemotherapy)	NS	1.2	1.6
Cabozantinib	Advanced RCC	14	4.7	4.3
	Thyroid cancer	28	7.2	5.5
	Unresectable HCC	5	1.1	2.2

GIST, gastrointestinal stromal tumor; HCC, hepatocellular carcinoma; NSCLC, non--small cell lung carcinoma; OS, overall survival; PFS, progression-free survival; PNET, primitive neuroectodermal tumor; RCC, renal cell carcinoma; RR, response rate.
Updated from Carmeliet P, Jain RK. Molecular mechanisms and clinical applications of angiogenesis. *Nature* 2011;473(7347):298–307.

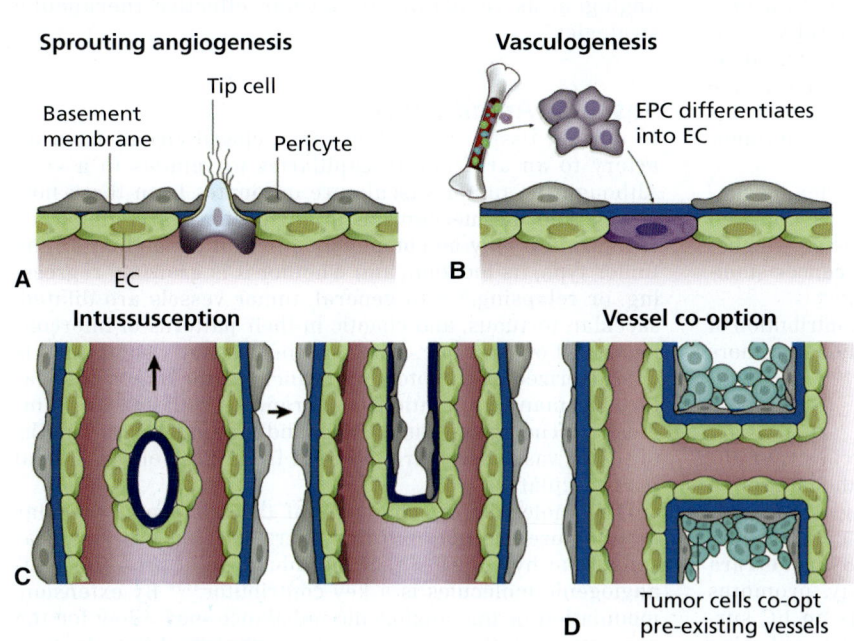
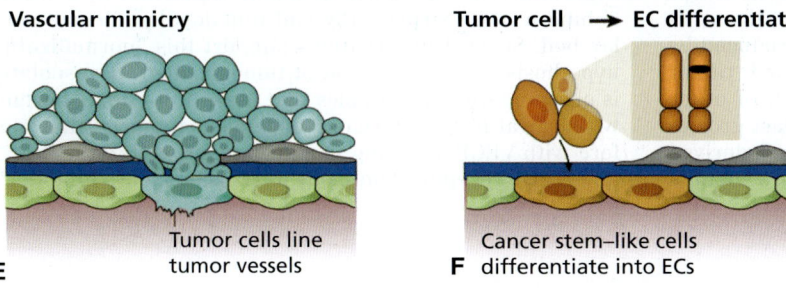

FIGURE 4.2. Modes of vessel formation in solid tumors. There are several known methods of blood vessel formation in normal tissues and tumors. **A–C:** Vessel formation can occur by sprouting angiogenesis **(A)**, by the recruitment of bone marrow–derived and/or vascular wall–resident endothelial progenitor cells (EPCs) that differentiate into ECs **(B)**, or by a process of vessel splitting known as intussusception **(C)**. **D–F:** Tumor cells can co-opt preexisting vessels **(D)**, or tumor vessels can be lined by cancer cells (vascular mimicry; **E**) or by ECs, with cytogenetic abnormalities in their chromosomes, derived from putative cancer stem cells **(F)**. Unlike normal tissues, which use sprouting angiogenesis, vasculogenesis, and intussusception **(A–C)**, tumors can use all six modes of vessel formation **(A–F)**. (Reprinted by permission from Nature: Carmeliet P, Jain RK. Molecular mechanisms and clinical applications of angiogenesis. *Nature* 2011;473[7347]:298–307. Copyright © 2011 Springer Nature.)

"perivascular" cuffs. However, as stated earlier, these cuffs cannot grow beyond the diffusion limit of critical nutrients, and they actually may cause the collapse of the vessels as a result of the growth pressure (referred to as "solid stress").[17-20] Alternatively, an existing vessel may enlarge in response to the growth factors released by tumors, and an interstitial tissue column may grow in the enlarged lumen and partition the lumen to form an expanded vascular network. This mode of microvascular growth termed intussusception occurs during tumor growth and wound healing.[21,22]

"Sprouting" angiogenesis is the most widely studied mechanism of vessel formation. During sprouting angiogenesis, the existing vessels become leaky in response to growth factors released by cancer or stromal cells; the basement membrane and the interstitial matrix dissolve; the pericytes dissociate from the vessel; ECs migrate and proliferate to form an array/sprout; a lumen is formed in the sprout (referred to as canalization); branches and loops are formed by confluence and anastomoses of sprouts to permit blood flow; and, finally, these immature vessels are invested with basement membrane and pericytes. During physiologic angiogenesis, these vessels differentiate into mature arterioles, capillaries, and venules, whereas in tumors, they may remain immature.[5,11,23]

During mammalian embryonic development, a primitive vascular plexus is formed from angioblasts or endothelial precursor cells (EPCs) by a process referred to as vasculogenesis. Distinct signals specify arterial or venous differentiation.[24] Several studies showed that circulating EPCs mobilized from the bone marrow or peripheral blood also can contribute to postnatal vasculogenesis in tumors and other tissues.[25] Although debated, the repair of healthy adult vessels or the expansion of pathologic vessels can be aided by the recruitment of bone marrow–derived cells (BMDCs) and/or EPCs to the vascular wall.[26] The progenitor cells then become incorporated into the endothelial lining in a process known as postnatal vasculogenesis. Collateral vessels, which bring bulk flow to ischemic tissues during revascularization, enlarge in size by distinct mechanisms, such as the attraction and activation of myeloid cells.[26,27] However, this process appears to be of rather limited importance in tumor neovascularization.[28-32]

Tissues can also become vascularized by other mechanisms, but the relevance of these processes is not well understood. For example, tumor cells can line vessels—a phenomenon known as vascular mimicry. Putative cancer stem-like cells can even generate tumor endothelium.[33-36]

The challenge now is to discern the relative contribution of each of these mechanisms of new vessel formation in tumors to optimize antiangiogenic treatment of cancer.[14,36,37]

Molecular Mechanisms

Various pro- and antiangiogenic molecules orchestrate different steps in vessel formation. Vascular endothelial growth factor (VEGF) is, perhaps, the most critical angiogenic molecule. Originally discovered in 1983 as the vascular permeability factor by Dvorak et al. and cloned in 1989 by Ferrara et al., VEGF increases vascular permeability, promotes migration and proliferation of ECs, serves as an EC survival factor, and is known to up-regulate leukocyte adhesion molecules on ECs.[38-40] During tumor progression, the variety and concentration of angiogenic molecules produced by a tumor can increase. Thus, if VEGF were blocked, tumor growth might continue as a result of the action of other angiogenic molecules, for example, basic fibroblast growth factor (bFGF), interleukin-8 (IL-8), and stromal cell–derived factor 1α (SDF1α).[37,41,42] Other positive regulators include

angiopoietins (Ang-1 and Ang-2) that are involved in blood vessel maturation[43], various proteases involved in extracellular matrix remodeling and growth factor release,[11,23] and organ-specific angiogenic stimulators such as endocrine gland VEGF[40] (Fig. 4.3).

Angiogenesis inhibitors include soluble receptors of various proangiogenic ligands as well as molecules that downregulate stimulator expression (e.g., interferons), interfere with stimulator release, or block binding of stimulators to their receptors (e.g., platelet factor 4). Thrombospondins are among the first and best characterized endogenous inhibitors that interfere with the growth, adhesion, migration, and survival of ECs. Other endogenous inhibitors include fragments of various plasma or matrix proteins, for example, angiostatin, fragment of plasminogen[44]; endostatin, fragment of collagen XVIII[45]; and tumstatin, fragment of collagen IV.[46]

The generation of pro- and antiangiogenic molecules can be triggered by injury, metabolic stress (e.g., low partial pressure of oxygen [Po_2], low pH, or hypoglycemia), mechanical stress (e.g., shear stress, solid stress), immune/inflammatory responses (e.g., immune/inflammatory cells that have infiltrated the tissue), and genetic mutations (e.g., activation of oncogenes or deletion of suppressor genes that control the production of angiogenesis regulators).[47-52] These molecules can emanate from cancer cells, ECs stromal cells, blood, and extracellular matrix[53-55] (Fig. 4.4). Because the host cells differ among organs, angiogenesis depends on host–tumor interactions.[54,56-60] Furthermore, because the tumor microenvironment is likely to change during tumor growth, regression, and relapse after treatment, profiles of pro- and antiangiogenic molecules are likely to change with time and space.[61-70] The challenge now is to develop a unified theoretic framework to describe the temporal and spatial profiles of this increasing number of angiogenesis regulators to develop effective therapeutic strategies.[37,71]

Vascular Architecture

In normal tissue, blood flows in a closed circuit from an artery to an arteriole to capillaries to venules to a vein. Although the tumor vasculature originates from these host vessels and the mechanisms of angiogenesis are similar, its organization may be completely different depending on the tumor type, its location, and whether it is growing, regressing, or relapsing.[72-74] In general, tumor vessels are dilated, saccular, tortuous, and chaotic in their patterns of interconnection. For example, whereas the normal vasculature is characterized by dichotomous branching, the tumor vasculature has many trifurcations and branches with uneven diameters.[75,76] The fractal dimensions and minimum path lengths of tumor vasculature are different from those of the normal host vasculature.[73,74,77]

The molecular mechanisms of this abnormal vascular architecture are not entirely understood, but it seems reasonable to hypothesize that an imbalance of pro- and antiangiogenic molecules is a key contributor.[11,78] By extension, modulation of this angiogenic imbalance may allow for the correction of the tumor vascular abnormalities, leaving behind a more structurally and functionally normal vascular bed. Several observations support this "normalization" hypothesis.[78] Normalization of tumor xenograft vasculature is observed during therapies that lower VEGF (e.g., hormone withdrawal from a hormone-dependent tumor),[79] that interfere with VEGF signaling (e.g., treatment with anti-VEGF or anti–VEGF receptor-2 antibody or tyrosine kinase inhibitor[80-85]

A Selection of tip cell

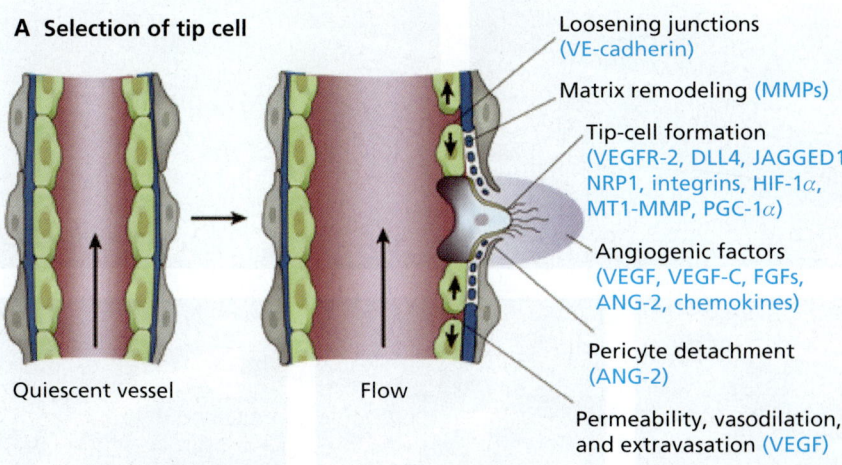

Quiescent vessel   Flow

Loosening junctions (VE-cadherin)

Matrix remodeling (MMPs)

Tip-cell formation (VEGFR-2, DLL4, JAGGED1, NRP1, integrins, HIF-1α, MT1-MMP, PGC-1α)

Angiogenic factors (VEGF, VEGF-C, FGFs, ANG-2, chemokines)

Pericyte detachment (ANG-2)

Permeability, vasodilation, and extravasation (VEGF)

B Stalk elongation and tip guidance

Lumen formation (VE-cadherin, CD34, sialomucins, VEGF)

Pericyte recruitment (PDGF-B, ANG-1, NOTCH, ephrin B2, FGF)

Tip-cell guidance and adhesion (semaphorins, ephrins, integrins)

Liberation of angiogenic factors from ECM (VEGF, FGFs)

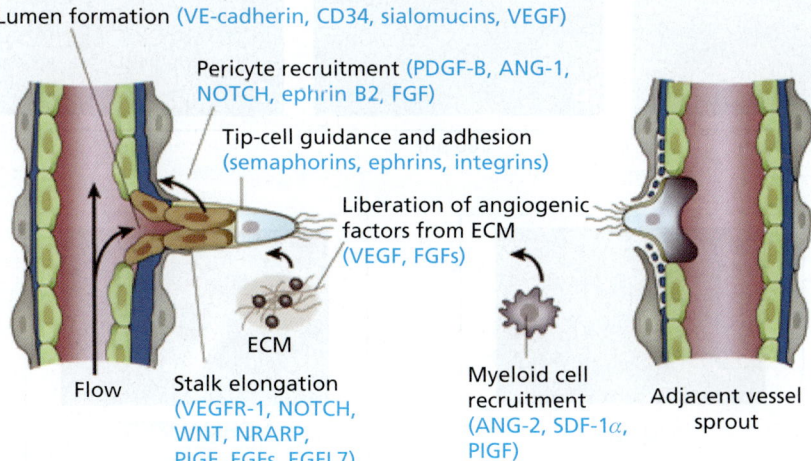

Flow

ECM

Stalk elongation (VEGFR-1, NOTCH, WNT, NRARP, PIGF, FGFs, EGFL7)

Myeloid cell recruitment (ANG-2, SDF-1α, PIGF)

Adjacent vessel sprout

C Quiescent phalanx resolution

Transendothelial lipid transport (VEGF-B)

Phalanx cell (PHD2, HIF-2α, VE-cadherin, TIE-2)

Vascular maintenance (VEGF, ANG-1, FGFs, NOTCH)

Barrier formation (VE-cadherin, ANG-1)

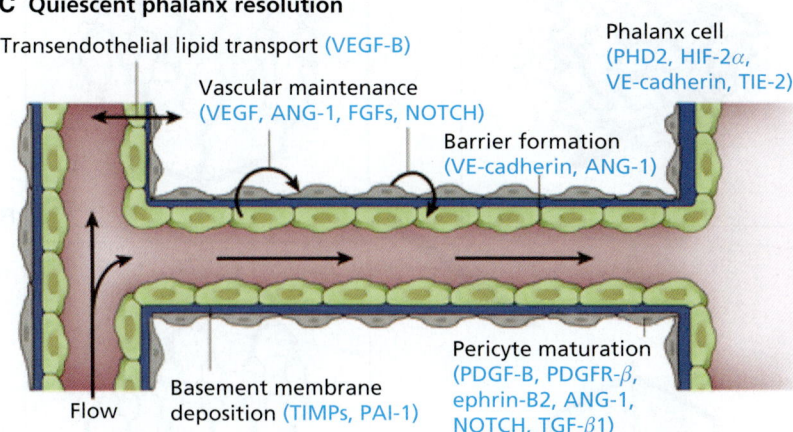

Flow

Basement membrane deposition (TIMPs, PAI-1)

Pericyte maturation (PDGF-B, PDGFR-β, ephrin-B2, ANG-1, NOTCH, TGF-β1)

FIGURE 4.3. Molecular basis of vessel branching. The consecutive steps of blood vessel branching are shown, with the key molecular players involved denoted in parentheses. **A:** After stimulation with angiogenic factors, the quiescent vessel dilates and an endothelial cell tip cell is selected (DLL4 and JAGGED1) to ensure branch formation. Tip cell formation requires degradation of the basement membrane, pericyte detachment, and loosening of EC junctions. Increased permeability permits extravasation of plasma proteins (such as fibrinogen and fibronectin) to deposit a provisional matrix layer and proteases remodel preexisting interstitial matrix, all enabling cell migration. For simplicity, only the basement membrane between ECs and pericytes is depicted, but in reality, both pericytes and ECs are embedded in this basement membrane. **B:** Tip cells navigate in response to guidance signals (such as semaphorins and ephrins) and adhere to the extracellular matrix (mediated by integrins) to migrate. Stalk cells behind the tip cell proliferate, elongate, and form a lumen, and sprouts fuse to establish a perfused neovessel. Proliferating stalk cells attract pericytes and deposit basement membranes to become stabilized. Recruited myeloid cells such as TAMs and Tie2-expressing monocytes (TEMs) can produce proangiogenic factors or proteolytically liberate angiogenic growth factors from the extracellular matrix. **C:** After fusion of neighboring branches, lumen formation allows perfusion of the neovessel, which resumes quiescence by promoting a phalanx phenotype, re-establishment of junctions, deposition of basement membrane, maturation of pericytes, and production of vascular maintenance signals. Other factors promote transendothelial lipid transport. (Reprinted by permission from Nature: Carmeliet P, Jain RK. Molecular mechanisms and clinical applications of angiogenesis. *Nature* 2011;473[7347]:298–307. Copyright © 2011 Springer Nature.)

(Fig. 4.5A–D), or that mimic an antiangiogenic cocktail (e.g., trastuzumab treatment of a HER2-overexpressing tumor)[65]. Emerging clinical data from cancer patients treated with bevacizumab, an anti–VEGF antibody, or pan-vascular endothelial growth factor receptor (VEGFR) tyrosine kinase inhibitors AZD2171 (cediranib) or sunitinib lend even more compelling support to this hypothesis.[14,36,61,62,64,66–68,70,78,86,87] More crucially, the

extent of vascular normalization directly correlates with the survival of patients with recurrent glioblastoma.[87] Moreover, the patients whose tumor blood flow increased most after cediranib treatment had the longest overall survival.[88,89]

Mechanical stress generated by proliferating and contracting cancer and stromal cells and transmitted by dense extracellular matrix also leads to compressed or totally collapsed vessels in

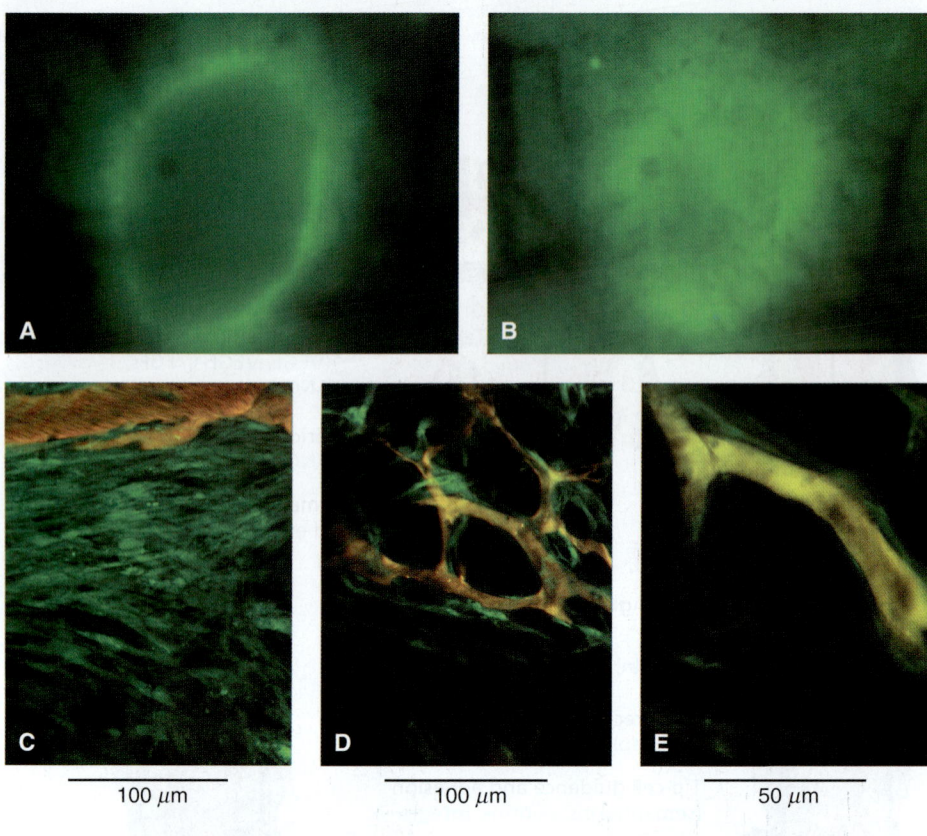

FIGURE 4.4. Tumor induction of host promoter activity in stromal cells. The expression of VEGF in host cells can be examined using transgenic mice expressing green fluorescent protein (GFP) under the control of the VEGF promoter. **A:** A murine mammary carcinoma xenograft shows host cell VEGF expression mainly at the periphery of the tumor after 1 week. **B:** After 2 weeks, the VEGF-expressing host cells have infiltrated the tumor. (Reprinted from Fukumura D, Xavier R, Sugiura T, et al. Tumor induction of VEGF promoter activity in stromal cells. *Cell* 1998;94[6]:715–725. Copyright © 2002 Cell Press. With permission.) **C:** A GFP-expressing layer of host cells can be seen at the tumor–host interface. **D** and **E:** The VEGF-expressing host cells colocalize with the angiogenic tumor vessels. (Reprinted by permission from Nature: Brown EB, Campbell RB, Tsuzuki Y, et al. In vivo measurement of gene expression, angiogenesis and physiological function in tumors using multiphoton laser scanning microscopy. *Nat Med* 2001;7[7]:864–868. Copyright © 2001 Springer Nature.)

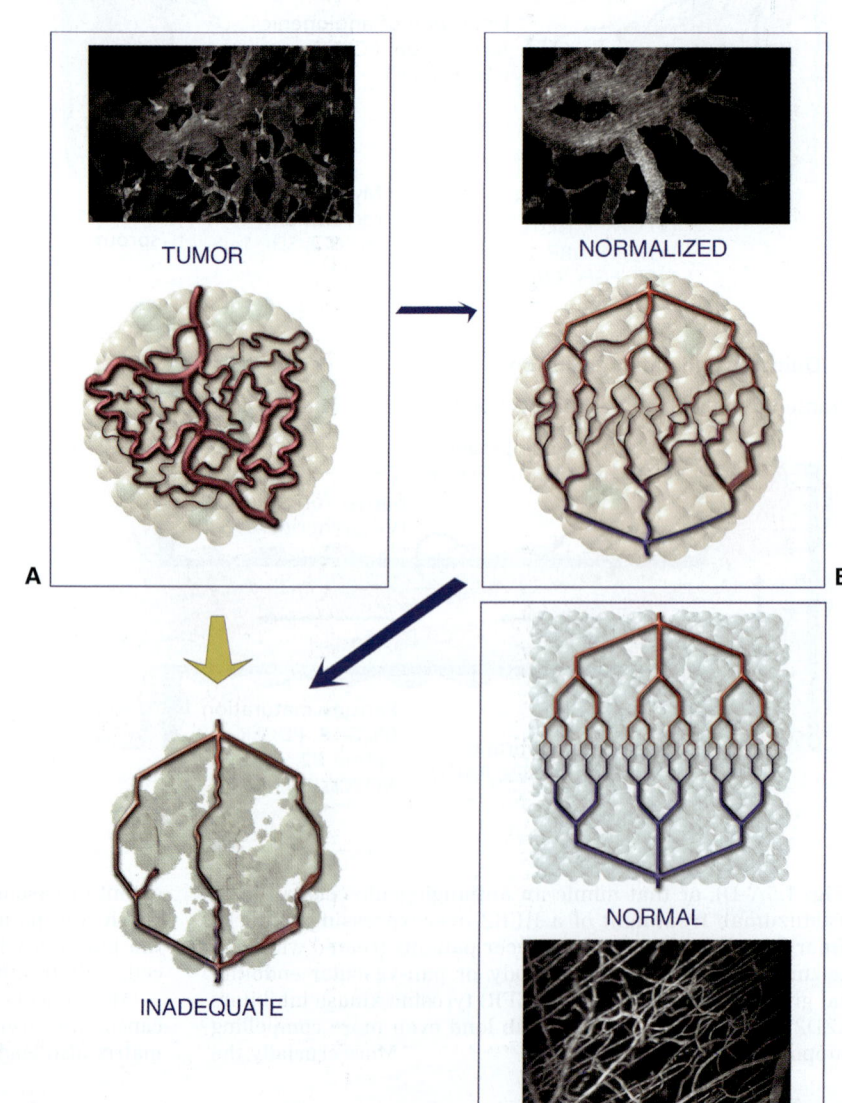

FIGURE 4.5. Normalization of tumor vasculature. **A:** Antiangiogenic therapies "normalize" the tumor vascular network. **B:** Tumor vessels are tortuous with increased vessel diameter, length, density, and permeability. **C:** Excessive pruning ultimately may reduce the vasculature to the point that it provides inadequate support for tumor growth. **D:** Normal vessels are well organized with even diameters. (Reprinted by permission from Jain RK. Normalizing tumor vasculature with anti-angiogenic therapy: a new paradigm for combination therapy. *Nat Med* 2001;7:987–989. Copyright © 2001 Nature; and Tong RT, Boucher Y, Kozin SV, et al. Vascular normalization by vascular endothelial growth factor receptor 2 blockade induces a pressure gradient across the vasculature and improves drug penetration in tumors. *Cancer Res* 2004;64[11]:3731–3736, with permission from AACR.)

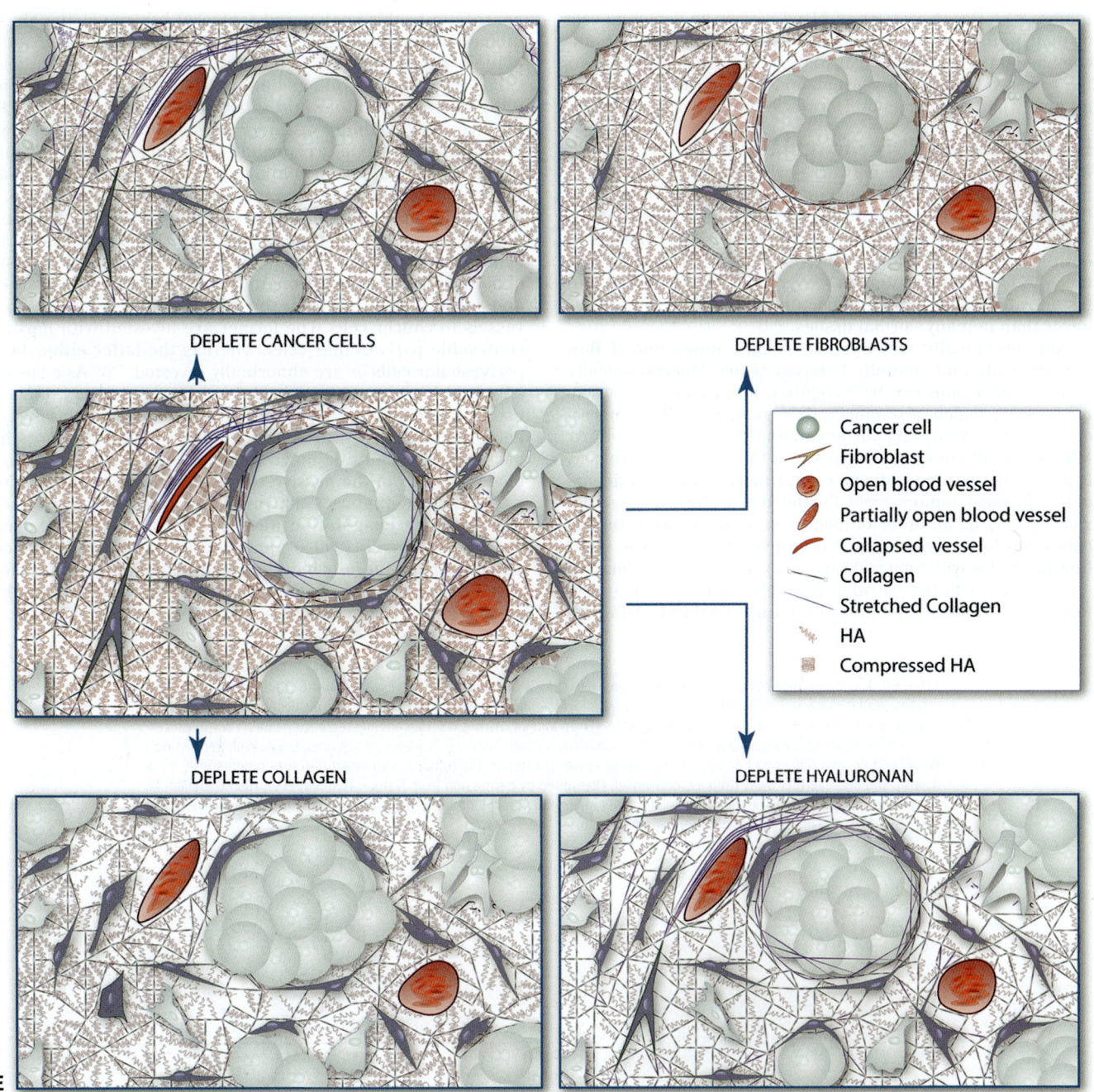

FIGURE 4.5. (*Continued*) **E:** Causes and remedies of vascular compression in tumors. *Middle panel*: In solid tumors, proliferating cancer cells and activated fibroblasts deform the interstitial matrix, resulting in stretched collagen fibers, compressed hyaluronan, and deformed cells—all storing solid stress, a type of mechanical force transmitted by solid tissue components. This stress compresses intratumor blood and lymphatic vessels. Potential strategies to alleviate solid stress and decompress vessels involve depleting these components. Depleting cancer cells (*top left*) or fibroblasts (*top right*) relaxes collagen fibers, hyaluronan, and the remaining cells, alleviating solid stress. Depleting collagen (*bottom left*) alleviates the stress that was held within these fibers while also relaxing stretched/activated fibroblasts and compressed cancer cells within nodules. Finally, depleting hyaluronan (*bottom right*) alleviates the stored compressive stress, allowing nearby components to decompress. Note that other stromal cells, such as pericytes, macrophages, and various immune cells that might also control production of collagen or hyaluronan, are not shown to simplify the schematic. Lymphatic vessels are also not shown for the same reason. (From Stylianopoulos T, Martin JD, Chauhan VP, et al: Causes, consequences, and remedies for growth-induced solid stress in murine and human tumors. *Proc Natl Acad Sci USA* 2012;109[38]: 15101–15108.)

tumors.[18,20,90] Decompression of blood vessels by depleting cells or matrix supports this mechanical hypothesis.[19,20,91–96] Thus, the combination of both molecular and mechanical factors renders the tumor vasculature abnormal, and both must be taken into account when designing novel strategies for cancer treatment.

Blood Flow and Microcirculation

Blood flow in a vascular network—whether normal or abnormal—is governed by arteriovenous pressure difference and flow resistance. The flow resistance is a function of the vascular architecture and the blood viscosity.[97] Abnormalities in both the vasculature and blood viscosity increase the resistance to blood flow in tumors.[75,76,98–100] As a result, overall perfusion rates (blood flow rate per unit volume) in tumors are lower than in many normal tissues.[101–103]

Macroscopically and microscopically, tumor blood flow is temporally and spatially heterogeneous. Macroscopically, four spatial regions can be recognized in a tumor: an avascular necrotic region, a seminecrotic region, a stabilized microcirculation region, and an advancing front[12,104] (Fig. 4.6A). Microscopically, in normal tissues, red blood cell (RBC) velocity is dependent on vessel diameter, but there is no such dependence in most tumors.[56,60,105] Furthermore, the average RBC velocity may be an order of magnitude lower in some tumors compared to the host tissue.[60] In a given tumor vessel, blood flow fluctuates with time and can even reverse its direction.[104–106]

In addition to the elevated geometric and viscous (rheologic) resistance, other molecular and mechanical factors contribute to this spatial and temporal heterogeneity. These include imbalance between pro- and antiangiogenic molecules,[105] solid stress generated by proliferating cancer cells,[18–20,96] vascular remodeling by intussusception, and coupling between luminal and interstitial fluid pressure (IFP) via hyperpermeability of tumor vessels.[73,107–109] As discussed later, this heterogeneity contributes to both acute and chronic hypoxia in tumors—a potential cause of resistance to radiation and other therapies and increased metastatic potential.

Considerable effort has gone into modulating tumor blood flow to improve cancer treatment. This has been difficult to achieve reproducibly because the tumor vasculature consists of both vessels co-opted from the preexisting host vasculature and vessels resulting from the angiogenic response of host vessels to cancer cells. The former are invested with normal contractile perivascular cells, whereas the latter either lack perivascular cells or are abnormally invested.[110–112] As a result, efforts to increase tumor blood flow and the delivery of cytotoxins, by pharmacologic or physical agents, have not always been successful.[97,113] In contrast, efforts to "starve" tumors by decreasing or shutting down tumor blood flow by "stealing" blood away from the passive component of the tumor vasculature by vasodilators[113] as well as by vascular targeting or intravascular coagulation have shown promise in experimental systems.[114] It also appears that judiciously applied antiangiogenic therapy may "normalize" the abnormal tumor vasculature, and the resulting "normalized" vessels might be more responsive to vasoactive agents[12,14,36,78,115] (Fig. 4.5A–D).

FIGURE 4.6. The tumor microenvironment is heterogeneous with proliferative, quiescent, and necrotic regions. **A:** These regions can be characterized in terms of various physiologic parameters. Decreasing magnitude of these parameters is indicated as + + +, + +, +, ±, and − in the adjoining table. (From Jain RK, Forbes NS. Can engineered bacteria help control cancer? *Proc Natl Acad Sci* USA 2001;98[26]:14748–14750, Copyright (c) 2001 National Academy of Sciences, U.S.A. With permission.) **B:** pH and Po₂ as a function of distance from a blood vessel in a tumor. The tumor environment becomes progressively more hypoxic and acidic farther away from a blood vessel. (Reprinted by permission from Nature: Helmlinger G, Yuan F, Dellian M, et al. Interstitial pH and pO₂ gradients in solid tumors in vivo: high-resolution measurements reveal a lack of correlation. *Nat Med* 1997;3[2]:177–182. Copyright © 1997 Springer Nature.)

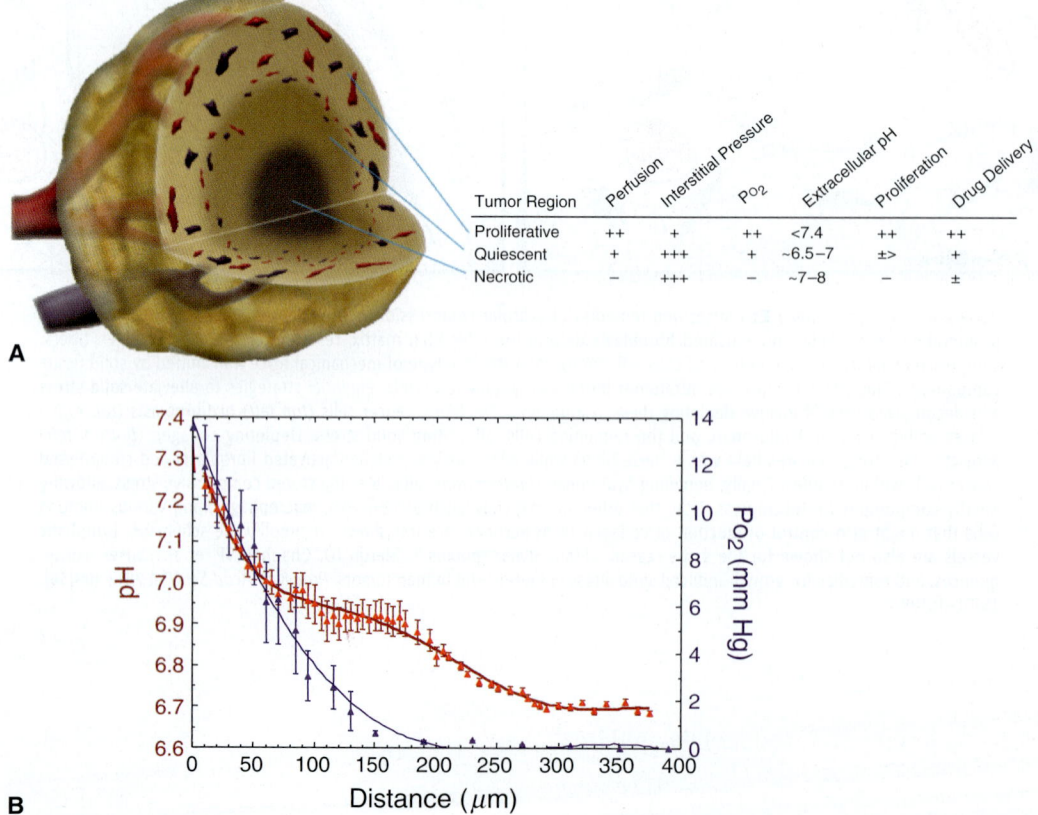

Tumor Region	Perfusion	Interstitial Pressure	Po₂	Extracellular pH	Proliferation	Drug Delivery
Proliferative	++	+	++	<7.4	++	++
Quiescent	+	+++	+	~6.5–7	±>	+
Necrotic	−	+++	−	~7–8	−	±

Vascular Permeability

Once a bloodborne molecule has reached an exchange vessel, its extravasation occurs by diffusion, convection, and, to some extent, presumably transcytosis.[116] The diffusive permeability of a molecule depends on the size, shape, charge, and flexibility of the molecule as well as the size, shape, charge, and dynamics of the transvascular transport pathway. In normal vessels, these pathways include diffusion through the EC membrane (for lipophilic solutes), trans-EC diffusion, interendothelial junctions (<7 nm), open or closed fenestrations (<10 nm), and transendothelial channels (including vesicles or vesicovacuolar organelles [VVOs]).[117] Some of these pathways may be lined with glycocalyx on ECs, thus effectively reducing the size of the pathway. A basement membrane may retard further the movement of molecules. Ultrastructural studies show widened interendothelial junctions; an increased number of fenestrations, vesicles, and VVOs in tumor vessels; and a lack of normal basement membrane and pericytes.[38,58,117-119]

In concert with these ultrastructural findings, both vascular permeability to solutes and water permeability (referred to as hydraulic conductivity) of tumors, in general, are significantly higher than that of various normal tissues.[60,100,120-123] Furthermore, unlike normal vessels, tumor vessels lack selectivity for the size of extravasating molecules.[124] However, positively charged molecules have a higher affinity for the negatively charged angiogenic tumor vessels.[125] Despite increased overall permeability, not all blood vessels of a tumor are leaky. Even the leaky vessels have a finite pore size that is tumor dependent, and ultrastructural studies show that the larger pore size in tumors represents wide interendothelial junctions.[58,119] Not only do the vascular permeability and pore size vary from one tumor to the next but also within the same tumor they vary both spatially and temporally as well as during tumor growth, regression, and relapse.[58,65,79]

The local microenvironment plays an important role in controlling vascular permeability. For example, a human glioma (HGL21) is fairly leaky when grown subcutaneously in immunodeficient mice, but it exhibits blood–brain barrier properties in the cranial window.[60] Such site-dependent differences for other tumors have been observed in other orthotopic sites.[56,59,126] One possible explanation is that the host–tumor interactions control the production and secretion of cytokines associated with permeability increase (e.g., VEGF) and decrease (e.g., Ang-1).[12,23,43,85,127] A better understanding of the molecular mechanisms of permeability regulation in tumors is likely to yield strategies for improved delivery of molecular medicine to tumors.[128]

Movement of Cells across Vessel Walls

Both cancer cells and immune cells frequently move across the walls of blood vessels—the former in the process of metastasis and the latter during immune response or cell-based immunotherapy. Both transendothelial and periendothelial pathways have been proposed as a route for intravasation and extravasation of cells. Very little is known about intravasation, except that a tumor may shed more than a million cells per gram per day and most of these are not clonogenic and that some may be shed as fragments along with stromal cells.[103,129-131] More is known about the molecular and cellular mechanisms of extravasation.[132-134] A cell within a blood vessel may continue to move with the flowing blood, collide with the vessel wall, adhere transiently or stably, and finally extravasate. These interactions are governed by both local hydrodynamic forces and adhesive forces. The former are determined by the vessel diameter and fluid velocity, and the latter by the expression, strength, and kinetics of binding between adhesion molecules and by the surface area of contact.[132,135-139] Deformability of cells affects both types of forces.[140]

Rolling of endogenous leukocytes is generally low in tumor vessels, whereas stable adhesion (≥30 seconds) is comparable between normal and tumor vessels.[141] However, both rolling and stable adhesion are nearly zero in angiogenic vessels induced in collagen gels by bFGF or VEGF, two of the most potent angiogenic factors. Whether the latter is due to a low flux of leukocytes into angiogenic vessels and/or down-regulation of adhesion molecules in these immature vessels is currently not known. Age may also play an important role in leukocyte–endothelial interactions.[142]

Further insight into the biology of cells that adhere to tumor vessels comes from studies on the localization of IL-2–activated natural killer (A-NK) cells in normal and tumor tissues in mice using positron emission tomography.[143,144] Immediately following systemic injection, these cells localized primarily in the lungs, whereas a nondetectable number of cells arrived in the tumor.[143] Increased rigidity caused by IL-2 activation may contribute to the mechanical entrapment of these cells in the lung microcirculation.[145,146] Constitutive expression of certain adhesion molecules in the lung vasculature also may facilitate their localization in the lungs.[132] One approach to reducing lung entrapment is to reduce the rigidity of these cells.[140,144] Alternatively, entrapment in lung vasculature can be circumvented by injecting A-NK cells directly into the blood supply of tumors. In this case, A-NK cells, both xenogeneic and syngeneic, adhered to some blood vessels in three different tumor models[144,147,148] via CD18 and very late antigen-4 (VLA-4) on the A-NK cells and intercellular adhesion molecule-1 (ICAM-1), vascular cell adhesion molecule-1 (VCAM-1), and E-selectin on the activated endothelium of angiogenic vessels.[39,149,150]

These molecules can be up-regulated by a number of cytokines, including tumor necrosis factor-α (TNF-α) and a protein of 90-kD molecular weight (p90); secreted by some neoplastic cells;[39,136] and down-regulated by others, for example, transforming growth factor-β (TGF-β) also, presumably, secreted by cancer cells.[57,151] Surprisingly, the proangiogenic VEGF also can up-regulate these molecules, whereas another proangiogenic molecule, bFGF, can down-regulate these molecules.[39,54,81,152] The challenge now is to decrease nonspecific entrapment of immune cells in normal vessels and to increase their delivery to tumor vessels to improve various cell-based therapies, including gene therapy. Judicious doses of anti-VEGF agents that "normalize" tumor vasculature can potentially realize this goal.[153,154] Moreover, more recent work implicates vascular normalization as a key contributor to antitumor immunity and showed that interferon-γ (IFN-γ)+ Th1 cells directly mediate vascular normalization.[155] Others showed that while decreased hypoxia secondary to vascular normalization promotes immunostimulatory macrophage programming, heightened IFN-γ levels might also induce the expression of programmed cell death ligand-1 (PD-L1) in tumor ECs and confer immunosuppressive properties to tumor blood vessels.[156] These recent findings highlight the intricate relationship between tumor blood vessels and effector immune cells.[157]

EXTRAVASCULAR COMPARTMENT

Composition and Origin

The extravascular compartment of a solid tumor consists of neoplastic cells (parenchyma) and host cells (e.g., inflammatory cells, fibroblasts) residing in an interstitial subcompartment bathed by the interstitial fluid (Fig. 4.1). Depending on the tumor type and its stage of differentiation, neoplastic cells may be dispersed in the matrix as individual cells (e.g., lymphomas, melanomas) or as clumps or nests (e.g., carcinomas). More than 80% of tumors are carcinomas arising from epithelial cells. The remaining 20% include sarcomas arising from mesenchymal cells (e.g., bone or muscle cells), lymphomas arising from lymphoid tissue, leukemias arising from hematopoietic cells, and hemangiomas arising from ECs. In a poorly differentiated carcinoma, the cancer cells may be loosely packed in clumps, whereas in a well-differentiated carcinoma, the cells may be connected with intercellular junctions and tightly packed in a nest enveloped by a basement membrane. With tumor progression, cancer cells may invade the basement membrane and spread to other regions.[38]

Unlike cancer cells, host cells must migrate into the tumor from normal tissue. Inflammatory cells may enter the tumor via blood vessels or may infiltrate from the adjacent tissue.[130] Other host cells, such as fibroblasts, may proliferate and migrate from the adjacent connective tissue[23,53,55,158,159] or from primary tumor to the metastatic site.[130] Increasingly, infiltrating host cells are being recognized as critical modulators of the tumorigenic process. For example, mesenchymal cells generically termed carcinoma-associated fibroblasts have been shown to promote tumor growth, metastasis, and angiogenesis, potentially through the secretion of SDF1α.[130,160–163] Furthermore, tumor-associated immune/inflammatory cells such as tumor-associated macrophages (TAMs), Tie2-expressing monocytes (TEMs), or Gr-1+ myeloid-derived suppressor cells (MDSCs) have been linked to both cancer immunosurveillance and suppression as well as to tumor promotion.[49,161,164–166] With the recent successes of immune therapy, a current challenge is promoting effector immune cell (e.g., T-lymphocyte) infiltration. Their limited infiltration can be attributed in part to the ECM providing a physical barrier[167] and to intratumoral hypoxia, which promotes an immunosuppressive phenotype of infiltrating cells.[168–171] The challenge now is to establish approaches for skewing immune cells (e.g., TAMs and T cells) toward a phenotype that promotes antitumor immune responses in cancer patients.[154,172,173]

The interstitial compartment of a tumor is bounded by the walls of the blood vessels on one side and by the membranes of cancer and stromal cells on the other. In normal tissues, the blood vessels are surrounded by a basement membrane, which is defective in tumors (see the Vascular Permeability section).[23,78] In addition, functional lymphatics may be confined to the tumor margin (see the Lymphatic Transport section).[174,175] Similar to normal tissues, the interstitial space of tumors is composed of a collagen and elastin fiber network that provides structural support to the tissue. Interdispersed in this cross-linked structure are the interstitial fluid and macromolecular constituents (polysaccharides hyaluronan and proteoglycans [PGs]), which form a hydrophilic gel.

Compared with our understanding of blood vessel formation, our understanding of stroma generation is minimal. Dvorak has proposed that the extravasated plasma protein fibrinogen, a key component of the tumor interstitial fluid (TIF), clots to form fibrin, which serves as a major component of the provisional stroma.[38] This provisional stroma eventually is replaced by more mature connective tissue stroma. The TIF also contains several proteins including fibronectin, vitronectin, osteopontin, thrombospondin, decorin, and tenascin. These proteins are present in both free and bound forms and contain the amino acid sequence Arg-Gly-Asp (RGD). The RGD sequence provides a binding site for adhesion that assists in the migration of various cells, including stromal cells. In addition to extravasating from the leaky tumor vessels, these proteins, along with collagen and various PGs, also are synthesized by the stromal cells, albeit in a form that is different from that in the plasma or normal tissues.[38] TIF also may contain various growth factors that facilitate stroma formation. For example, *in vitro* studies suggest that platelet-derived growth factor-β is involved in the recruitment of fibroblasts to tumors, and TGF-β controls the production of collagen and other matrix molecules in tumors.[23,176] With the increasing interest in using the fragments of matrix constituents for controlling angiogenesis, our understanding of the molecular and cellular mechanisms of stroma generation in tumors is likely to increase.[158]

Interstitial Transport

Once a molecule has extravasated, its movement through the interstitial space occurs by diffusion and convection.[117] Diffusion is proportional to the concentration gradient in the interstitium, and convection is proportional to the interstitial fluid velocity, which, in turn, is proportional to the pressure gradient in the interstitium. Just as the interstitial diffusion coefficient, D (cm²/s), relates the diffusive flux to the concentration gradient, the interstitial hydraulic conductivity, K (cm²/mm Hg·s), relates the interstitial velocity to the pressure gradient.[117] Values of these transport coefficients are governed by the structure and composition of the interstitial compartment as well as by the physicochemical properties of the solute molecule.[125,177–181]

The value of K (interstitial hydraulic conductivity) for a human colon carcinoma xenograft (LS174 T), measured using two different methods,[182,183] was found to be higher than that of a hepatoma,[181] which, in turn, was higher than that of the normal liver. Using fluorescence recovery after photobleaching, the diffusion coefficient (D) of various molecules in tumors was found to be about one-third that in water[184] and higher than the values in the host tissue.[178] Collagen content and structure have a significant effect on D in tumors.[180,182,185] This is surprising because hyaluronan and PGs, and not collagen, account for most of the resistance to transport in normal tissues. Because collagen is produced by the host-derived cells (e.g., fibroblasts), the penetrability of macromolecules into a tumor will depend on the host–tumor interaction. Thus, agents that interfere with collagen synthesis and/or organization (e.g., relaxin, bacterial collagenase, angiotensin system inhibitors) may increase interstitial transport in tumors.[177,186,187]

The time constant for a molecule with diffusion coefficient D to diffuse across a distance L is approximately $L^2/4D$. For diffusion of IgG (immunoglobulin G) in tumors, this time constant is on the order of 1 hour for a 100-μm distance, days for a 1-mm distance, and months for a 1-cm distance. So, for a 1-mm tumor, diffusional transport across the tumor would take days, and for a 1-cm tumor, it would take months. If the central vessels have collapsed completely as a result of cellular proliferation[18,19,19,96] and interstitial matrix rearrangement, the reduced delivery of macromolecules by blood flow would make diffusion the primary mechanism of delivery to this hypoxic center. Binding may further retard the transport in tumors.[184,188,189] The role of binding is illustrated clearly by comparing the rate of fluorescence recovery of a photobleached spot in tumor tissue injected with a nonspecific versus specific IgG. In addition to the heterogeneity of D in tumors, the most unexpected result of these photobleaching studies was the large extent (30% to 40%) of nonspecific binding.[184] These results collectively suggest that the interstitial compartment of a tumor can be a formidable barrier to the uniform delivery of therapeutic macromolecules (e.g., antibodies, genes using viruses, nanotherapeutics) in tumors, and strategies are needed to overcome this barrier.[91–94,116,125,186,187,190]

Lymphatic Transport

In most normal tissues, extravasated plasma and macromolecules are taken up by the lymphatics and returned to the central circulation. Although it is widely accepted that lymphatic vessels are present in the tumor margin and the peritumoral tissue, the hotly debated issue for nearly a century has been whether anatomically defined lymphatic vessels are present within solid tumors and, if so, whether they function.[175,191] Currently, available immunohistochemical markers stain for structures in some tumors that resemble lymphatic vessels. However, because many of these markers lack specificity,[174,175,192] it is not clear whether they stain functional lymphatic vessels, ECs from remnant lymphatic vessels, or some other structures or cell types (e.g., preferential fluid channels.[182]

It is likely that the stress induced by proliferating cancer cells compresses and impairs lymphatic vessels that are co-opted or formed in a tumor[18–20] and/or lymphatic valves are impaired by tumor growth.[193] The impaired lymphatic vessels, in turn, may contribute to the interstitial hypertension characteristic of animal and human tumors (see the Interstitial Hypertension section). In addition, invasion of the functional peritumoral lymphatics is considered to be a poor prognostic factor for a number of tumors, and lymphatic metastasis is a major cause of morbidity and mortality.

Our understanding of the mechanisms of lymphangiogenesis lags behind our understanding of the mechanisms of angiogenesis. However, considerable progress has recently been made toward identifying molecular players responsible for lymphangiogenesis. VEGF-C, acting through VEGFR-3, appears to play a central role in tumor-associated lymphangiogenesis. Several experimental[194–198] and clinical[199] studies have demonstrated a positive correlation between VEGF-C expression and peritumoral lymphatic vessel density, lymphatic metastasis, and, in some cases, poor clinical outcomes. Like in vascular angiogenesis, other positive and negative regulators, such as VEGF,[200,201] VEGF-D,[195] hepatocyte growth factor, platelet-derived growth factor-BB, and angiopoietins, are involved in lymphangiogenesis.[11,199] Furthermore, mechanisms analogous to co-option, intussusception, sprouting, and vasculogenesis may operate in lymphatic growth[11] (see the Angiogenesis: Cellular Mechanisms section). Similar to organ-specific angiogenic molecules (e.g., EG-VEGF)[40] and blood vascular EPCs,[25,202] there may be organ-specific lymphangiogenic molecules and lymphatic endothelial precursor cells that contribute to tumor-associated lymphangiogenesis.[203] Moreover, the proteolytic processing of lymphangiogenesis molecules, as well as the phenotype and function of the resulting lymphatics, may depend on the tumor type as well as on the host organ in which the tumor is growing.[23,81,174,199]

The precise roles for these lymphangiogenic molecules in the induction of lymphatic metastasis are imperfectly understood, even though phylogenetic tree analysis indicates that 35% of distant metastases arise from tumor-draining metastases.[204] Recent data demonstrate that tumor VEGF-C overexpression induces peritumoral lymphatic hyperplasia through activation of VEGFR-3. Consequently, lymph fluid volumetric flow increases.[194] This results in increased tumor cell delivery to lymph nodes and a higher rate of lymphatic metastasis[194] (Fig. 4.7). It remains unclear how VEGF-C overexpression impacts tumor cell entry into lymphatic vessels; however, an attractive hypothesis is that the increased lymphatic surface area simply increases the probability of tumor cell entry and dissemination. Alternatively, VEGF-C may stimulate the release of a chemotactic factor that recruits tumor cells into lymphatic vessels. Of potential clinical importance, VEGFR-3 blockade was shown to inhibit VEGF-C–induced lymphatic hyperplasia, tumor cell delivery to draining lymph nodes, and lymphatic metastasis when treatment was started at the time of tumor initiation. However, lymphatic metastases were not significantly reduced if VEGFR-3 blockade was started after

FIGURE 4.7. Schematic of lymphatics in low (*left*) versus high (*right*) VEGF-C–expressing tumors. VEGF-C secreted from tumor cells stimulates VEGFR-3 expressed in lymphatic ECs, inducing peritumor lymphatic hyperplasia (*top right*). An increase in lymphatic surface area may increase the opportunity for tumor cell entry into lymphatic vessels. Augmented lymph flow enhances tumor cell delivery to draining lymph nodes (*bottom right*). In the absence of VEGF-C overexpression, peritumor lymphatic hyperplasia is less pronounced and fewer tumor cells are delivered to draining lymph nodes (*left*). Anti–VEGF-C/anti–VEGFR-3 treatment inhibits VEGF-C–induced lymphatic hyperplasia and tumor cell delivery to draining lymph nodes (*bottom left*). (Reprinted from Hoshida T, Isaka N, Hagendoorn J, et al. Imaging steps of lymphatic metastasis reveals that vascular endothelial growth factor-C increases metastasis by increasing delivery of cancer cells to lymph nodes: therapeutic implications. *Cancer Res* 2006;66[16]:8065–8075. Copyright © 2006 American Association for Cancer Research. With permission from AACR.)

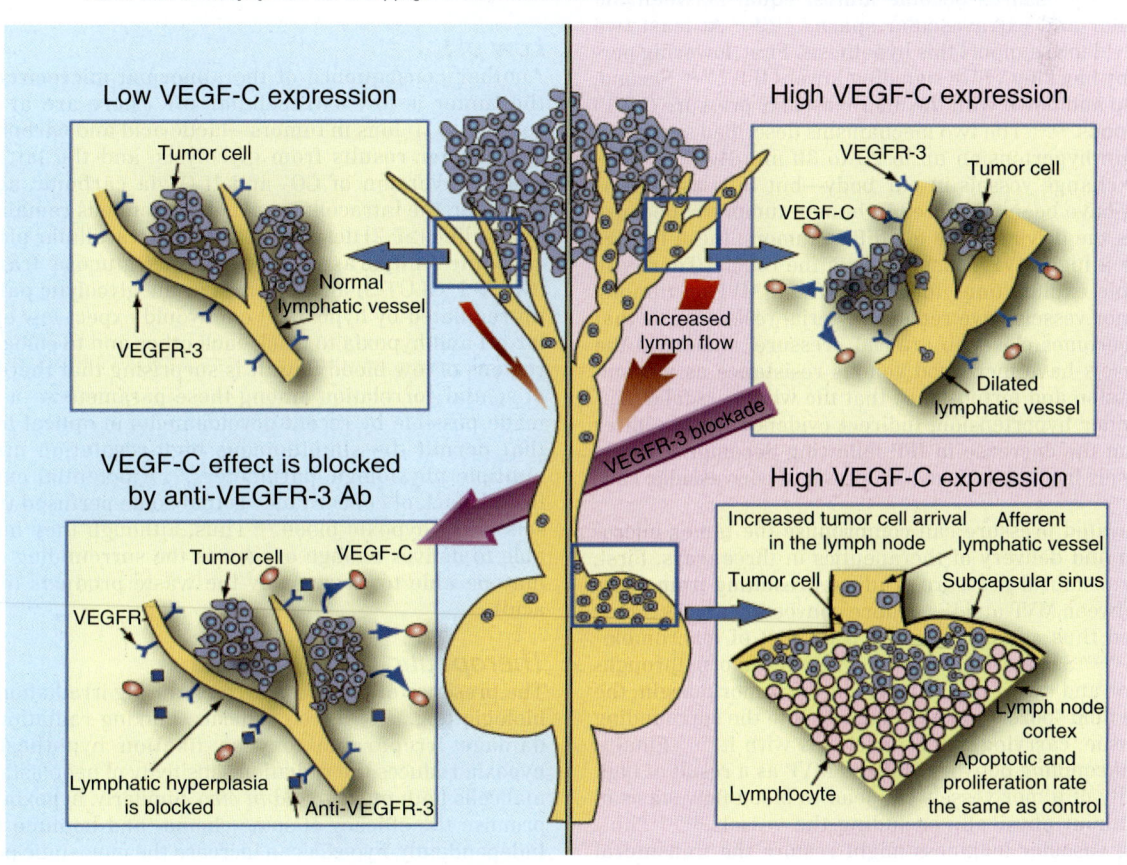

tumor cell seeding of draining lymph nodes.[194,205] These data suggest that anti–VEGFR-3 therapy may be effective in preventing, but not treating, lymphatic metastases—the more common clinical imperative—except in cases where a significant fraction of vascular ECs and/or cancer cells express VEGFR-3. The challenge now is to identify alternative strategies for treating lymphatic metastases, either through combination therapy (e.g., anti–VEGFR-2/anti–VEGFR-3) or modulation of other pathways.

Mechanical signals that trigger the lymphangiogenic switch are unknown. Because lymphatic vessels help maintain the balance of fluid in tissues, hydrostatic pressure is a likely trigger.[205,206] Whether the lymphatic hyperplasia seen in tumor margins is, in part, a response to the elevated hydrostatic pressure in tumors and whether the newly formed lymphatics remain open and relieve this pressure are open questions. Techniques such as microlymphangiography,[4,174,175,194,197,207,208] fluorescence photobleaching lymph flow quantitation,[191,194,207,209-211] and optical frequency domain imaging (OFDI)[212] will allow us to answer these important questions.

Interstitial Hypertension

Unlike normal tissues, where the IFP is around 0 mm Hg, both animal and human tumors exhibit interstitial hypertension.[64,66,68,117,175,183,213-224] The tumor IFP begins to increase as soon as the host vessels become leaky in response to angiogenic molecules such as VEGF.[225] Thus, IFP can be lowered by inhibiting the VEGF pathway using blocking antibodies.[64,66-68,83,226] The IFP increases with tumor size in some tumors[213,215,219] and remains independent of tumor size in others.[220]

Three mechanisms contribute to the interstitial hypertension in tumors. In normal tissues, lymphatics maintain fluid homeostasis; thus, the lack of functional lymphatics within tumors is a key contributor. Indeed, DiResta et al.[227] have shown that one could lower the IFP by placing "artificial lymphatics" in tumors. The second contributor is the leaky nature of tumor vessels. As a result, the hydrostatic and oncotic (colloid osmotic) pressures become almost equal between the intravascular and extravascular space.[77,83,214,228] At least two pieces of evidence support this hypothesis. First, lowering permeability by blocking VEGF signaling lowers IFP.[66,83,226] Second, IFP goes up and down with the microvascular pressure (MVP) within seconds.[229-231] The two mechanisms described so far can only explain hypertension up to 20 to 30 mm Hg—the MVP of most exchange vessels in our body—but IFPs as high as 94 mm Hg have been measured in human tumors.[223] Because the MVP is the driving force for IFP in tumors, these tumors must have a high MVP. Indeed, this is the case.[214] There are two possible explanations for the elevated MVP in tumors: (a) the tumor vessels have reduced arterial resistance so that the MVP becomes closer to arterial pressure, and/or (b) the tumor vessels have increased venous resistance as a result of compression and tortuosity so that the whole vascular network is under hypertension. Indirect evidence for the latter comes from the decrease in IFP following decompression of tumor vessels by drug-induced apoptosis of perivascular cancer cells.[19,96]

The elevated pressure can compromise the tumor microcirculation and delivery of therapeutics in three ways. First, reduced transmural pressure gradients resulting from equilibrium between MVP and IFP reduce convection across tumor vessels and thus compromise the transport of macromolecules.[77,83,97,214,230] Second, because IFP is nearly uniform throughout a tumor and drops precipitously in the tumor margin, the interstitial fluid "oozes" out of the tumor into the surrounding normal tissue, carrying macromolecules with it.[30,129] Finally, transmural coupling between IFP and MVP as a result of high permeability of tumor vessels can lead to blood flow stasis in tumors without physically occluding the vessels.[107-109] Thus, decreasing vascular leakiness might restore the transmural

pressure gradients and potentially resume/re-establish blood flow in the nonperfused regions of tumors.[154,232] Some direct and indirect antiangiogenic therapies may "normalize" the tumor vasculature through this mechanism[12,14,36,62,65,66,78,115,233] (Tables 4.2 and 4.3; Fig. 4.5).

Metabolic Environment

Hypoxia

A key function of the vasculature is to provide adequate levels of nutrients to the parenchymal cells and to remove waste products. Based on the anatomy of the capillary bed and a mathematical model of oxygen diffusion and consumption, the Nobel laureate August Krogh introduced the concept of a diffusion limit for oxygen of 100 to 200 μm nearly a century ago.[234] This unit of tissue—a single capillary surrounded by a 100- to 200-μm radius cylinder—is referred to as a Krogh cylinder in physiology. Nearly 50 years later, Thomlinson and Gray identified similar "cords" in human lung cancer and found necrotic cells beyond 180 μm away from blood vessels, presumably because of a lack of oxygen.[235] This is referred to as *chronic hypoxia* or *diffusion-limited hypoxia*. Although various hypoxia markers and microelectrodes have suggested these gradients, the first direct measurements of these perivascular Po2 gradients, as well as perivascular pH gradients, became possible only with the development of phosphorescence quenching microscopy[236,237] (Fig. 4.6B).

As discussed earlier, blood flow in tumor vessels is intermittent, and, thus, some regions of a tumor are periodically starved for oxygen. The resulting hypoxia is referred to as *acute hypoxia* or *perfusion-limited hypoxia*. A necessary consequence of intermittent blood flow is the resumption of blood flow after shutdown, and the resulting production of free radicals can lead to *ischemia–reperfusion injury* or *reoxygenation injury*; thus, applying additional selection pressure on cancer cells can cause them to become more locally aggressive, metastatic, and resistant to therapy.[238]

Low pH

Another consequence of the abnormal microcirculation of the tumor is low extracellular pH. There are at least two sources of H+ ions in tumors—lactic acid and carbonic acid.[239] The former results from glycolysis, and the latter results from conversion of CO_2 and H_2O via carbonic anhydrase. However, the intracellular pH of cancer cells remains neutral or alkaline (≥7.2) despite the acidic extracellular pH. Because carbonic anhydrase-9 and various glucose transporters (GLUT-1, GLUT-3) and enzymes in the glycolytic pathway are up-regulated by hypoxia,[238] one would expect low extracellular pH and hypoxia to track each other and to colocalize with regions of low blood flow. It is surprising that there is a lack of spatial correlation among these parameters—a discovery made possible by recent developments in optical techniques that permit the simultaneous high-resolution mapping of multiple physiologic parameters.[236] A potential explanation for this lack of concordance is that some perfused tumor vessels carry hypoxic blood.[236] Thus, although they may not be able to deliver enough oxygen to the surrounding cells, they may be able to carry away the waste products (e.g., lactic acid).

Therapeutic Consequences

The presence of molecular oxygen during irradiation can "fix" biologic (e.g., DNA) free radicals, making radiation-induced damage irreparable (oxygen fixation hypothesis). Thus, hypoxia reduces the radiation sensitivity of neoplastic and normal cells both *in vitro* and *in vivo*. Similarly, hypoxia can compromise the efficacy of some chemo- and immune therapies. Independently, hypoxia can increase the metastatic potential of

TABLE 4.2 STUDIES REPORTING ANTIANGIOGENIC THERAPY–INDUCED IMPROVEMENT IN TUMOR OXYGENATION

Antiangiogenic Therapy	Tumor Model	Effect on Oxygenation	Time Window of Improved Oxygenation
Antibody Therapy			
Bevacizumab	Melanoma, breast carcinoma, ovarian carcinoma	↑	2–4 d after start of therapy
Bevacizumab	GBM	↑	Up to 5 d
DC101	GBM	↑	2–8 days after start of therapy
Anti-PlGF Ab	Pancreatic carcinoma	No change	
TKI Therapy			
Sunitinib	Squamous carcinoma	↑	O_2 measured 4 d after start of therapy
Semaxanib	Melanoma	↑	O_2 measured 3 d after start of therapy
PI-103 (PI3 K inhibitor)	Fibrosarcoma, squamous carcinoma	↑	O_2 measured 10 d after start of therapy
Gefitinib (EGFR inhibitor)	Fibrosarcoma, squamous carcinoma	↑	O_2 measured 10 d after start of therapy
Erlotinib (EGFR inhibitor)	Squamous carcinoma, NSCLC	↑	O_2 measured 5 d after start of therapy
Endocrine Therapy			
Castration (androgen depletion)	Shionogi carcinoma	↑	O_2 measured 21 d after start of therapy
Metronomic Chemotherapy			
Low dose gemcitabine	Pancreatic carcinoma	↑	O_2 measured 28 d after start of therapy
Other Therapies			
FTIs (Ras inhibitors)	Prostate carcinoma, bladder carcinoma, glioma, fibrosarcoma, squamous carcinoma	↑	O_2 increased up to 7–10 d
Nelfinavir (AKT inhibitor)	Fibrosarcoma, squamous carcinoma	↑	O_2 measured 10 d after start of therapy
TNP-470	Breast carcinoma	↑	O_2 measured 9 d after start of therapy
Suramin	GBM	↑	O_2 measured 5–6 wk after start of therapy
Thalidomide	Liver carcinoma	↑	O_2 increased from day 2–4 after start of therapy
Thalidomide	Fibrosarcoma	↑	O_2 increased from day 2–3 after start of therapy
Genetic Models			
$VEGF^{-/-}$ (myeloid cells)	Lung carcinoma	↑	
$nNOS^{-/-}$ (tumor cells)	Glioblastoma	↑	
$\alpha_v\beta_3/\alpha_v\beta_5$ integrin–FAK–Rho knockdown (tumor cells)	Glioblastoma	↑	
SEMA3 A overexpression (transgene delivery)	Insulinoma	↑	O_2 increased after 4 wk
$Rgs5^{-/-}$ (stroma)	Insulinoma	↑	
$PHD2^{-/-}$ (stroma or EC specific)	Melanoma, pancreatic carcinoma	↑	
IFN-β overexpression (transgene delivery)	Glioblastoma, neuroblastoma	↑	

EC, endothelial cell; EGFR, epidermal growth factor receptor; FAK, focal adhesion kinase; FTI, farnesyl transferase inhibitor; GBM, glioblastoma multiforme; IFN, interferon; nNOS, neuronal nitric oxide synthase; NSCLC, non–small cell lung cancer; PHD, prolyl hydroxylase domain protein; PI3 K, phosphoinositide-3-kinase; PlGF, placental growth factor; TKI, tyrosine kinase inhibitor; VEGF, vascular endothelial growth factor. Reproduced with permission from Goel S, Duda DG, Xu L, et al. Normalization of the vasculature for treatment of cancer and other diseases. *Physiol Rev* 2011;91(3):1071–1121. Copyright © 2011 The American Physiological Society. All rights reserved.

TABLE 4.3 STUDIES REPORTING THE IMPACT OF ANTIANGIOGENIC/VASCULAR NORMALIZATION STRATEGIES UPON DELIVERY OF THERAPEUTIC COMPOUNDS/SYSTEMICALLY ADMINISTERED MOLECULES INTO TUMORS

Systemically Administered Molecule	Normalization Strategy	Tumor Model(s)	Effect on Delivery
Conventional Cytotoxics			
Irinotecan	A4.6.1	Colon carcinoma	↑
Topotecan, etoposide	Bevacizumab	Neuroblastoma	↑
Temozolomide	Sunitinib	Glioma	↑[a]
Cyclophosphamide, cisplatin	TNP-470	Lung carcinoma	↑
Temozolomide	TNP-470	Glioma	↓
Cyclophosphamide	Thalidomide	Liver carcinoma	↑
Doxorubicin	PDGF-D overexpression	Breast carcinoma	↑
Topotecan	IFN-β overexpression	Neuroblastoma	↑
Doxorubicin	Anti–TGF-β antibody or overexpression sTβrII	Breast carcinoma	↑
Nanoparticles			
Liposomal doxorubicin	Anti–TGF-β antibody or overexpression sTβrII	Breast carcinoma	↑
Antibodies			
Nonspecific IgG, anti–E-cadherin Ab	Axitinib	Lung carcinoma, pancreatic tumor	↑ (per vessel)
Viral Particles			
Oncolytic virus	Cilengitide	GBM	↑
Other Molecules			
BSA	DC101	Breast carcinoma, colon carcinoma	↑
FDG	Bevacizumab	Rectal carcinoma	↑ (per vessel)[b]

BSA, bovine serum albumin; FDG, fluorodeoxyglucose; GBM, glomerular basement membrane; IFN, interferon; PDGF, platelet-derived growth factor; TGF, transforming growth factor.
[a]Increased delivery of temozolomide noted with sunitinib 20 mg/kg but not at 60 mg/kg.
[b]Study performed in human subjects.
Reproduced with permission from Goel S, Duda DG, Xu L, et al. Normalization of the vasculature for treatment of cancer and other diseases. *Physiol Rev* 2011;91(3):1071–1121. Copyright © 2011 The American Physiological Society. All rights reserved.

cancer cells.[238] Therefore, for nearly half a century, considerable preclinical and clinical effort has been focused on alleviating hypoxia through a multitude of interventions such as improving tumor perfusion with mild hyperthermia or drugs, increasing oxygen content of the blood via hyperbaric oxygenation, and increasing hemoglobin/hematocrit by transfusion or exogenous erythropoietin. Unfortunately, the clinical outcomes have not met expectations. Although early studies suggested a marked benefit of transfusion in anemic cervical cancer patients undergoing definitive radiotherapy, careful analysis suggests that these studies are confounded by selection biases that preclude the conclusion that anemia correction by transfusion impacts outcome.[240,241] Furthermore, erythropoietin (or analog) treatment showed encouraging survival results in anemic cancer patients receiving nonplatinum chemotherapy and in anemic lung cancer patients receiving chemotherapy.[242,243] However, subsequent trials in anemic head and neck cancer patients and mainly nonanemic metastatic breast cancer patients actually suggested outcomes may be impaired by erythropoietic agents.[244,245] There are multiple possible reasons such interventions have yielded mixed results. These include the inability to increase tumor Po_2 as markedly as systemic Po_2,[246] the inability to increase Po_2 in all areas of a tumor to optimal levels because of abnormal vasculature,[77,115] and undesired "off-target" effects of interventions (e.g., immunosuppression with transfusion.[247–249] Furthermore, tumors may reoxygenate during radiation therapy with standard fractionation, potentially minimizing the impact of providing additional oxygen to the target tissue.

Similarly, low extracellular pH can adversely (or favorably) affect the uptake and cytotoxicity of some therapeutics. The pH gradient difference between tumor and normal tissue may offer a tumor-specific target for nanomedicines or weak acid chemotherapeutics for the treatment of cancer.[250,251] The development of specific drugs that exploit this pH difference and strategies to modulate pH in tumors has not yet reached the clinic but are anticipated.[238]

Two broad strategies targeting the unique tumor metabolic environment are emerging: (a) exploit hypoxia to activate drugs or attract tumoricidal anaerobic bacteria and (b) dissect hypoxia-induced pathways to identify novel targets for drug development. The first strategy has led to the development of drugs such as tirapazamine and to renewed interest in bacteriolytic therapy[252]; both approaches are in clinical trials, but promising data are yet to emerge.[253,254] The second strategy has revealed several molecular players in the physiologic and pathophysiologic response to hypoxia.[238,255,256] The balance between hypoxia-induced apoptosis/necrosis on one hand and the increased resistance to cell death mediated by various hypoxia-induced pathways on the other determines whether a tumor can survive and even grow under hypoxic conditions. Ultimately, hypoxia selects for tumor cells that are more malignant, more invasive, and genetically unstable, rendering them resistant to various therapies. Therefore, certain players in the hypoxia-induced pathways now are being targeted in the development of diagnostic and therapeutic agents. Hypoxia-induced pathways include genes involved in oxygen delivery, glycolysis and glucose uptake, pH control, stress response pathways, growth factor signaling, angiogenesis, transcription, apoptosis, growth inhibition, and invasion and metastasis (Fig. 4.3 and Box 4.1).[11,255]

Of the various molecular players involved in sensing and responding to hypoxia, hypoxia-inducible factor-1 a (HIF-1α) has received the most attention. This transcription factor is up-regulated in a number of human tumors.[255,264] Regulated by proline and asparagine hydroxylases, HIF-1α activates genes involved in an array of physiologic responses including angiogenesis, vasodilation, glycolysis, and RBC production by binding to the hypoxia-response element (HRE). Although HIF-1α is an attractive therapeutic target, its pleiotropic action may prove to be a major challenge for clinical exploitation. For example, teratomas arising from HIF-1α(−/−) embryonic cells grow more rapidly despite lower levels of VEGF and angiogenesis.[265] This counterintuitive finding may be a result of the ability of HIF-1α(−/−) cells to survive under hypoxic conditions, instead of undergoing apoptosis.[55] HIF-1α has also been shown to play an important role in determining tumor radioresponsiveness through the regulation of multiple, and sometimes opposing, processes.[266] Under some circumstances, HIF-1α inhibition *reduces* tumor cell radiosensitivity by protecting hypoxic cells from radiation-induced apoptosis and enhancing clonogenic survival potentially through reductions in adenosine triphosphate

---

Box 4.1

Hypoxia and Epigenetic Regulation of Angiogenesis

The prolyl hydroxylase domain (PHD) proteins PHD1–3 are oxygen-sensing enzymes that hydroxylate the HIF proteins HIF-1α and HIF-2α when sufficient oxygen is available. Once hydroxylated, HIFs are targeted for proteasomal degradation.[257] Under hypoxia, PHDs become inactive, and HIFs initiate broad transcriptional responses to increase the oxygen supply by angiogenesis, through the up-regulation of angiogenic factors such as VEGF.[258] HIFs are also activated in nonhypoxic conditions by oncogenes and growth factors, allowing tumor cells to stimulate angiogenesis before they become deprived of oxygen. In general, HIF-1α promotes vessel sprouting, whereas HIF-2α mediates vascular maintenance.[258] Reduced HIF-1α levels in mice impair embryonic vascular development, revascularization of ischemic tissues, and angiogenesis in injured tissues and tumors.[258] The use of HIF-1α inhibitors to block tumor or ocular angiogenesis has therefore received attention. Conversely, *Hif-1α* gene transfer in mice or activation of HIF-1α by pharmacologic blockade of PHDs promotes ischemic tissue revascularization.

HIF-1α also regulates tumor angiogenesis indirectly, by releasing chemoattractants such as SDF-1α to recruit proangiogenic BMDCs.[259] Gene silencing of Phd2 in mouse tumor cells enhances vessel growth by similar mechanisms. Hypoxia also regulates the polarization and proangiogenic activity of TAMs by means of HIF-1α and HIF-2α with different effects.[257] That hypoxia and inflammation are closely intertwined is illustrated by the finding that signaling by HIF-1α and nuclear factor-κB cross-activates each other. In certain cases, hypoxic up-regulation of VEGF occurs independently of HIF-1α and is mediated by the metabolic regulator peroxisome proliferator–activated receptor gamma coactivator (PGC)-1α in preparation for oxidative metabolism once the ischemic tissue is revascularized.[260] Because HIF signaling contributes to acquired resistance against anti–VEGF therapy, the combined blockade of VEGF and HIF-1α is being explored as a cancer treatment strategy.

There is increasing evidence for epigenetic control of angiogenesis, particularly by noncoding microRNAs (miRNAs),[261] which induce messenger RNA degradation or block translation. Because miRNAs target multiple genes, they are well positioned to regulate complex processes such as angiogenesis. ECs express several miRNAs that are induced by hypoxia or VEGF. Most of those stimulate angiogenesis by hijacking proangiogenic cascades while suppressing angiostatic pathways.[262] The expression of miR-126 is induced by the mechanosensitive transcription factor KLF2A and integrates the mechanosensory stimulus of blood flow to shape the vascular system.[263] EC-specific loss of DICER, an exonuclease involved in miRNA biogenesis, impairs pathologic angiogenesis. Angiogenic miRNAs seem to offer significant pro- or antiangiogenic potential.

Reprinted by permission from Nature: Carmeliet P, Jain RK. Molecular mechanisms and clinical applications of angiogenesis. *Nature* 2011;473(7347): 298–307. Copyright © 2011 Springer Nature.

---

metabolism, cellular proliferation, and p53 activation.[266] Furthermore, HIF-1α serves a key function in inflammatory cell energy metabolism, and its inhibition results in profound immunodeficiency.[267] Consequently, molecular therapies that target HIF-1α or HRE, as well as more selective therapies that target key downstream effectors of HIF-1α, are under intensive investigation for cancer detection and treatment.[238,255,268] Nonetheless, although oxygen and cancer drugs fail to reach tumor regions that are far from perfused vessels in adequate concentrations, this delivery limitation is more important for these strategies that depend on hypoxia or target hypoxia-induced pathways.

CLINICAL IMPLICATIONS

Two major problems currently plague the nonsurgical treatment of malignant solid tumors. First, physiologic barriers within tumors impede the delivery of therapeutics and oxygen (a key radiation sensitizer) at effective concentrations to all cancer cells.[36,78,269] Second, inherent or acquired resistance resulting from genetic and epigenetic mechanisms reduces the effectiveness of conventional as well as novel targeted therapies.[270,271] Can we take advantage of the unique pathophysiology of tumors to overcome these problems for better management of cancer? As discussed next, recent clinical data offer some hope.

Prognostic/Predictive Biomarker Implications

Multiple indices of tumor pathophysiology have been evaluated as potential predictors of treatment outcome including vessel density (reviewed in Refs.[37,272]), oxygen level (reviewed in Refs.[255,273]), interstitial pressure,[37,221,223,241] and blood or urine circulating molecules[68,86] (reviewed in Ref.[37]) Vessel density can be evaluated in biopsies and is measured either in "hot spots" (i.e., regions of most active angiogenesis) or in the tissue as a whole. The former presumably provides a measure of a tumor's aggressiveness, and the latter reflects the status of global oxygenation. Most studies to date show that poor outcome of radiation therapy correlates with high vessel density in "hot spots" and/or low overall microvessel density. There are, however, several studies showing a lack of correlation or an opposite correlation. This discrepancy may be the result of the morphometric techniques used or of differences in tumor types or treatment schedules.

The oxygen level in a tumor also has a potential prognostic value, and it can be directly measured with microelectrodes. Alternatively, immunohistochemical analysis of tumor tissue for endogenous or exogenous hypoxic markers (e.g., HIF-1α, glucose transporter-1, carbonic anhydrase-9, pimonidazole) can be used as a surrogate for tumor oxygenation status. However, immunohistochemical assessments of hypoxia do not necessarily correlate with oxygen status measured directly with microelectrodes.[274] A concerted effort is under way to assess hypoxia using novel, noninvasive imaging techniques.[256,275,276] Several studies have shown that tumor hypoxia is a predictor of a poor outcome of radiation therapy when used alone or in combination with other therapies. These findings are consistent with *in vitro* and *in vivo* preclinical studies showing the adverse effect of hypoxia on radiation responses.

Because the IFP is a reflection of the global physiology of tumors, a correlation between tumor IFP and the response to radiation therapy has been suggested. One cervical cancer study has shown that elevated tumor IFP can, indeed, independently predict a poor outcome of radiation therapy.[241] In breast cancer, IFP was not related to response to chemotherapy.[277] Further studies are needed to evaluate the prognostic significance of IFP in tumors. However, one potential application of the steep rise of pressure at the tumor periphery is improved localization of tumors before their removal.

Finally, circulating biomarkers may provide information about tumor pathophysiology and its changes after treatment. Of note, some of the emerging biomarkers—such as circulating collagen IV or soluble VEGFR-1—may represent biomarkers of vascular normalization and, if validated, could be useful in treatment decisions.[86,87,277,278]

Although each of these approaches has advantages, key disadvantages include their invasiveness and their potential for sampling error. With rapid developments in the field of noninvasive imaging, it is likely that the measurement of various physiologic and molecular parameters in tumors will become more refined and convenient for patients. Examples of such imaging approaches include blood oxygen level–dependent magnetic resonance imaging (BOLD MRI), electron paramagnetic resonance spectroscopy/imaging, and [18F]-misonidazole positron emission tomography (FMISO-PET).[275,276,279–281] The promise of such imaging approaches has just started to be realized. FMISO-PET has been evaluated in a substudy of patients with stage III or IV squamous cell carcinoma of the head and neck randomized to concurrent radiotherapy with either tirapazamine and cisplatin or infusional fluorouracil

and cisplatin. Pretreatment FMISO-PET–detected hypoxia was associated with a higher risk of locoregional recurrence among patients who did not receive the tirapazamine-containing regimen compared to patients who did receive tirapazamine.[281] This study suggests that FMISO-PET can provide clinically meaningful information about tumor physiology and simultaneously provides evidence that tirapazamine acts by specifically targeting hypoxic tumor cells. Furthermore, results from hypothesis-generating clinical trials involving noninvasive imaging approaches indicate that increased perfusion and oxygenation are potential predictive biomarkers of response to antiangiogenic therapy.[16,88,278,282–285] Such progress will continue, and physiologic/molecular profiles of patients' tumors will yield improved and better-tailored therapies for individual patients. Indeed, a current challenge is to verify increases in perfusion and oxygen as predictive biomarkers of response to antiangiogenic and solid stress–alleviating therapies.

Therapeutic Implications

Given the physiologic barriers to the delivery and effectiveness of various therapeutics, a strategy that is gaining increasing interest is destroying the tumor vasculature. This strategy has the advantage of targeting ECs that are easily accessible to a bloodborne drug and are presumably genetically stable. In addition, each EC supports multiple cancer cells, thus providing "therapeutic amplification." However, the inability to target *all* ECs in a tumor can reduce the effectiveness of antivascular therapy. Similarly, the dependence of ECs on multiple angiogenic molecules can limit the effectiveness of various antiangiogenic therapies when used alone.[36,78] Finally, destroying the stroma, including ECs, could promote disease progression.[286–289] These challenges may explain why currently available antiangiogenic agents, although demonstrating biologic activity, are usually unable to provide durable tumor control when used as monotherapy except in tumors that are highly VEGF-dependent (i.e., clear cell renal carcinoma, ovarian cancer, cervical cancer, and thyroid cancer) or highly vascularized (i.e., neuroendocrine cancers and hepatocellular carcinoma).[15] However, it should be noted that the anti–VEGFR-2 antibody ramucirumab led to an OS advantage of 1.4 months in advanced gastric or gastroesophageal junction (GEJ) adenocarcinomas. This may reflect the dependence of GEJ tumor vascularization or immunosuppression on VEGFR-2 signaling.

Although of limited utility when used alone especially in desmoplastic carcinomas with cancer cells clustered in nests surrounded by stroma, the judicious combination of antiangiogenic therapies with conventional cytotoxic therapies has led to improved tumor control in mice and lengthened survival in certain types of human tumors[14–16,251,290–293] (see Table 4.1). For example, in two human tumor xenograft models, a VEGFR-2–blocking antibody decreased the dose of fractionated radiation required to control 50% of tumors (TCD$_{50}$) by 11 to 27 Gy without modifying infield skin reactions.[251] Thus, to maximize clinical gains, these agents must be employed in combination with radiation and chemotherapy. The challenge now is to optimally combine these therapies in patients. Destruction of tumor vasculature by antiangiogenic agents would only antagonize chemo- and radiotherapy by compromising the delivery of therapeutics and oxygen, respectively.[289] However, judiciously applied antiangiogenic therapy can prune inefficient tumor vessels and render the remaining vasculature more efficient (Fig. 4.5A–D).[12,36,78,115,233] This "normalization" of tumor vasculature has been demonstrated in various preclinical models (reviewed in Refs.[36,78]) and in HER2-negative breast cancer, non–small cell lung cancer, rectal cancer, hepatocellular carcinoma, ovarian carcinoma, and glioblastoma patients[61,62,64,66,68,70,277,278] (Fig. 4.8).

To be effective, vascular "normalization" should result in improved delivery of cytotoxic chemotherapy and

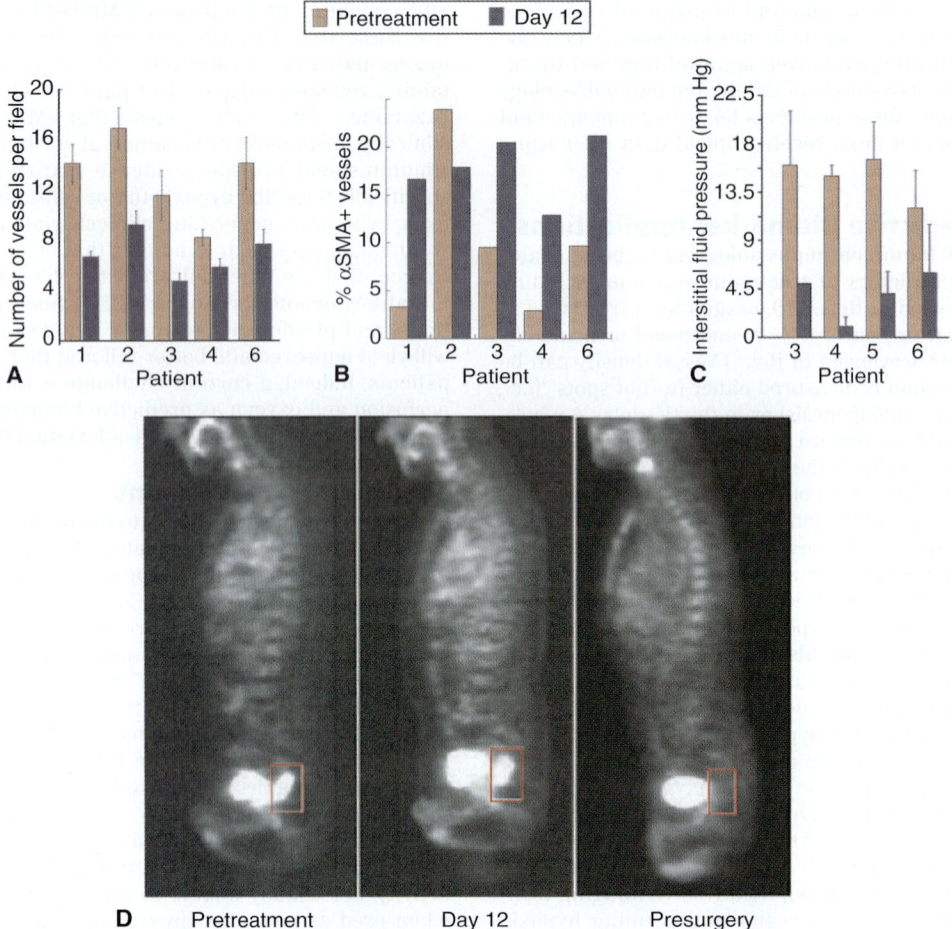

FIGURE 4.8. Vascular "normalization" in rectal cancer patients following treatment with the anti-VEGF antibody, bevacizumab. **A–C:** Tumor vessel normalization following a single injection of bevacizumab is suggested by the reduction of tumor microvessel density **(A)**, by the increase in fraction of tumor vessels with pericyte coverage **(B)**, and by the drop in IFP **(C)**. **D:** Positron emission tomography reveals no change in 18-fluorodeoxyglucose (FDG) uptake after a single dose of bevacizumab and complete resolution of FDG uptake following neoadjuvant chemoradiation (bevacizumab, 5-fluorouracil, pelvic external beam radiation therapy). The stability of FDG uptake following bevacizumab monotherapy, despite marked reductions in microvessel density, suggests the efficiency of residual tumor blood vessels after bevacizumab treatment is improved. (Reprinted by permission from Nature: Willett CG, Boucher Y, di Tomaso E, et al. Direct evidence that the VEGF-specific antibody bevacizumab has antivascular effects in human rectal cancer. *Nat Med* 2004;10[2]:145–147. Copyright © 2004 Springer Nature.)

radio- and immune-sensitizing oxygen, thereby improving tumor control. This principle has been rigorously tested in animal models[16,78,84,154,172,173,290,294–296] and investigated in large phase III trials and smaller hypothesis-driven trials. The lessons from these studies support the notion that optimally combining antiangiogenic therapies with radiation, chemotherapy, or immunotherapies will involve administering therapies in the window of maximized delivery of oxygen.[16] Furthermore, this window is dependent on the baseline vasculature, whether the vessels are fortified and whether vessel function is increased (Fig. 4.9A).[289]

In tumors that are hypovascular or hypoperfused, antiangiogenic treatments should be combined with solid stress–alleviating therapies to increase oxygenation (Fig. 4.5E).[297] Indeed, TGF-β1 inhibition with angiotensin system inhibitors increases perfusion and reduces hypoxia in hypovascular murine cancer models and has demonstrated promise in increasing resection rates induced by chemoradiation in neoadjuvant pancreatic ductal carcinoma patients (Fig. 4.9B).[91,298] These prospective studies are consistent with retrospective studies each surveying hundreds of patients with non–small cell lung cancer, pancreatic ductal adenocarcinoma, and renal cell carcinoma that show repurposing angiotensin system inhibitors from treating hypertension to reprogramming

the stroma of cancer might increase patient survival.[299–305] Furthermore, one retrospective study in hepatocellular carcinoma indicates that angiotensin system inhibitors and antiangiogenic agents in combination might increase survival.[304] Other strategies demonstrating potential in preclinical studies to decrease solid stress include vitamin D receptor agonism, antifibrotic medication losartan or tranilast, idiopathic pulmonary fibrosis medication pirfenidone, and diabetes medication metformin.[92–94,190] The current challenge is how to combine optimally antiangiogenic and solid stress–alleviating therapies particularly in tumors that are neither highly vascular nor highly desmoplastic.[297] Chemotherapy normalizes vessels when given metronomically, thereby complicating the task of optimizing treatment combinations.[306] Additionally, researchers must investigate how we can translate these lessons to treat patients with micrometastatic disease, which does not rely on sprouting angiogenesis.[307–309]

One emerging strategy to treat systemic disease could involve priming T cells with radiation locally administered to the tumor to promote immunogenicity of cancer cells and in turn immune response systemically against nonirradiated distant metastases.[310] This phenomenon, which is referred to as the "abscopal effect" of radiation, could potentially be used to increase the rate and duration of responses in patients treated

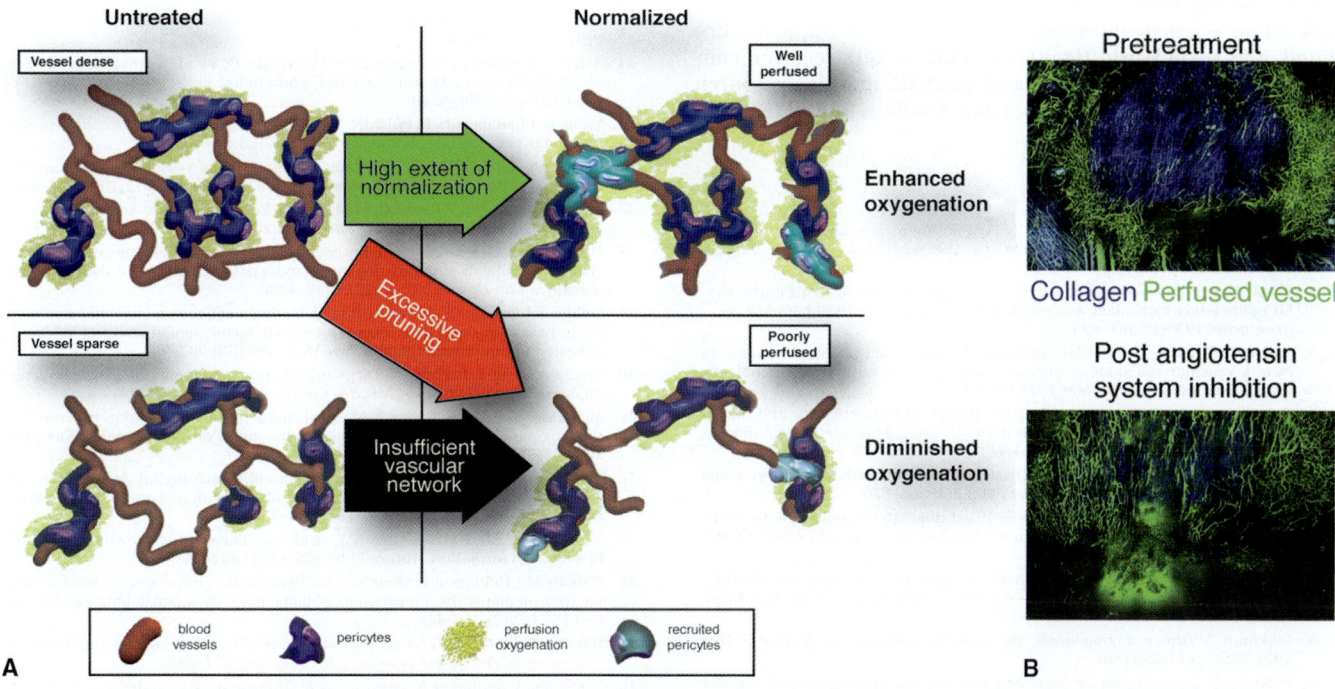

FIGURE 4.9. Vascular "normalization" in cancer patients. **A:** Preclinical and clinical studies support the hypothesis that the therapeutic effect of antiangiogenic therapies is best when vascular density is high and normalization fortifies rather than prunes vessels. The left quadrants depict tumor vessels (*red*) before antiangiogenic therapy. The right quadrants depict possible outcomes of antiangiogenic therapy. Tumors with low pretreatment vessel density do not respond to antiangiogenic therapy (*bottom left* to *right quadrant*), as the increase in vessel function from the recruitment of pericytes (teal) cannot overcome the paucity of vessels. In contrast, tumors with high baseline vascularity that recruit pericytes have better outcomes (*top left quadrant* to *top right quadrant*) than tumors with excessive pruning (*top left quadrant* to *bottom right quadrant*). (From Tolaney S, Duda DG, Boucher Y, et al. Role of vascular density and normalization in response to neoadjuvant bevacizumab and chemotherapy in breast cancer patients. *Proc Natl Acad Sci USA* 2015;112[46]:14325–14330.) **B:** Intravital microscopy images of a murine breast tumor before (*top panel*) and after (*bottom panel*) angiotensin system inhibition treatment to reduce solid stress. The treatment reduces the density of collagen fibers (*blue*) leading to a homogeneous distribution of perfused vessels (*green, bottom panel*). (Reprinted by permission from Nature: Chauhan VP, Martin JD, Liu H, et al. Angiotensin inhibition enhances drug delivery and potentiates chemotherapy by decompressing tumour blood vessels. *Nat Commun* 2013;4:2516. Copyright © 2013 Springer Nature.)

with immunotherapy.[311] To progress, tumors must successfully resist immune rejection, even though they are continuously producing neoantigens that T cells can recognize.[312] If cancer cells undergo immunogenic cell death, epitopes can be transferred from cancer cells to dendritic cells that are required to activate tumor-specific T cells.[313,314] Indeed, ionizing radiation and some chemotherapies induce immunogenic cell death.

Recent work focused on defining optimal dose and fractionation to schedule radiation with various immunotherapies.[315] Preclinical evidence indicates that fractionated rather single-dose radiotherapy might be required to induce an abscopal effect in combination with the immune checkpoint blocker anti–CTLA-4 antibody.[316,317] Furthermore, radiation doses above a certain level attenuate immunogenicity and thus should be avoided.[318] The attenuated immunogenicity is mediated by the DNA exonuclease Trex1, which could be a potential biomarker to determine the radiation dose and fractionation in combination with immunotherapy. These hypotheses have been generated in proof of principle clinical trials and require validation.[319,320]

In considering these disparate strategies together, several potentially synergistic combinations could be hypothesized to treat systemic disease. Antiangiogenic and solid stress–alleviating therapies could be administered in combination to alleviate hypoxia in tumors to potentiate subsequent fractionated, low dose radiotherapy. The resulting immunogenic cell death could lead to increased response through the abscopal effects when used in combination with immune therapy. One complementary pathway is TGF-β.[321] Inhibition of this pathway alleviates solid stress[91] and promotes radiotherapy-induced

antitumor immunity.[322] Future studies should uncover mechanisms through which these strategies complement each other toward developing more effective combination schedules.[16]

ACKNOWLEDGMENTS

This chapter is an update of Chapter 4 published in the sixth edition of *Principles and Practice of Radiation Oncology* and based on review articles by Carmeliet and Jain, *Nature*, 2011,[11] and Martin et al., *Cold Spring Harbor Perspectives in Medicine*, 2016,[289] and Chapter 8 of *Ableoff's Clinical Oncology* sixth edition forthcoming. The work summarized here was supported by continuous support from the National Cancer Institute since 1980 to R.K.J. R.K.J. is supported by grants from the National Cancer Institute (P01-CA080124, P50CA165962, R01-CA129371), the NCI Outstanding Investigator Award (R35-CA197743), the Lustgarten Foundation, and the National Foundation for Cancer Research. D.G.D. is supported through NIH grants R01-CA159258 and R21-CA139168 and Proton Beam/Federal Share Program, and the American Cancer Society grant 120733-RSG-11–073–01-TBG. J.D.M is supported by a Japan Society for the Promotion of Science Postdoctoral Fellowship P16731.

XTuit and Boards of Trustees of Tekla Healthcare Investors, Tekla Life Sciences Investors, Tekla Healthcare Opportunities Fund, and Tekla World Healthcare Fund. D.G.D. received consultant fees from Bayer Tilos and twoXAR, and has research grants from Bayer, Merrimack, Leap, Exelixis, and BMS.

REFERENCES

1. Goldmann E. The growth of malignant disease in man and the lower animals: with special reference to the vascular system. *Lancet* 1907;170(4392):1236–1240.

2. Ide A, Baker N, Warren S, et al. Vascularization of the Brown-Pearce rabbit epithelioma transplant as seen in the transplant ear chamber. *AJR Am J Roentgenol* 1939;42:891–899.

3. Algire G, Chalkley H. Vascular reactions of normal and malignant tissues *in vivo*. I. Vascular reactions of mice to wounds and to normal and neoplastic transplants. *J Natl Cancer Inst* 1945;6:73–85.

4. Fukumura D, Duda DG, Munn LL, et al. Tumor microvasculature and microenvironment: novel insights through intravital imaging in pre-clinical models. *Microcirculation* 2010;17(3):206–225.

5. Jain RK, Munn LL, Fukumura D. Dissecting tumour pathophysiology using intravital microscopy. *Nat Rev Cancer* 2002;2(4):266–276.

6. Rijhsinghani K, Greenblatt M, Shubik P. Vascular abnormalities induced by benzo [a] pyrene: an *in vivo* study in the hamster cheek pouch. *J Natl Cancer Inst* 1968;41(1):205–216.

7. Ehrmann RL, Knoth M. Choriocarcinoma: transfilter stimulation of vasoproliferation in the hamster cheek pouch—studied by light and electron microscopy. *J Natl Cancer Inst* 1968;41(6):1329–1341.

8. Folkman J. Tumor angiogenesis: therapeutic implications. *N Engl J Med* 1971;285(21):1182–1186.

9. Folkman J. Angiogenesis: an organizing principle for drug discovery? *Nat Rev Drug Discov* 2007;6(4):273–286.

10. Gullino PM. Angiogenesis and oncogenesis. *J Natl Cancer Inst* 1978;61(3):639–643.

11. Carmeliet P, Jain RK. Molecular mechanisms and clinical applications of angiogenesis. *Nature* 2011;473(7347):298–307.

12. Jain RK. Normalizing tumor vasculature with anti-angiogenic therapy: a new paradigm for combination therapy. *Nat Med* 2001;7(9):987–989.

13. Lu-Emerson C, Duda DG, Emblem KE, et al. Lessons from anti-vascular endothelial growth factor and anti-vascular endothelial growth factor receptor trials in patients with glioblastoma. *J Clin Oncol* 2015;33(10):1197–1213.

14. Jain RK, Duda DG, Clark JW, et al. Lessons from phase III clinical trials on anti-VEGF therapy for cancer. *Nat Clin Pract Oncol* 2006;3(1):24–40.

15. Jayson GC, Kerbel R, Ellis LM, et al. Antiangiogenic therapy in oncology: current status and future directions. *Lancet* 2016;388(10043):518–529.

16. Jain RK. Antiangiogenesis strategies revisited: from starving tumors to alleviating hypoxia. *Cancer Cell* 2014;26(5):605–622.

17. Jain RK, Martin JD, Stylianopoulos T. The role of mechanical forces in tumor growth and therapy. *Annu Rev Biomed Eng* 2014;16:321–346.

18. Helmlinger G, Netti PA, Lichtenbeld HC, et al. Solid stress inhibits the growth of multicellular tumor spheroids. *Nat Biotechnol* 1997;15(8):778–783.

19. Padera TP, Stoll BR, Tooredman JB, et al. Pathology: cancer cells compress intratumour vessels. *Nature* 2004;427(6976):695.

20. Stylianopoulos T, Martin JD, Chauhan VP, et al. Causes, consequences, and remedies for growth-induced solid stress in murine and human tumors. *Proc Natl Acad Sci U S A* 2012;109(38):15101–15108.

21. Patan S, Munn LL, Jain RK. Intussusceptive microvascular growth in a human colon adenocarcinoma xenograft: a novel mechanism of tumor angiogenesis. *Microvasc Res* 1996;51(2):260–272.

22. Patan S, Munn LL, Tanda S, et al. Vascular morphogenesis and remodeling in a model of tissue repair: blood vessel formation and growth in the ovarian pedicle after ovariectomy. *Circ Res* 2001;89(8):723–731.

23. Jain RK. Molecular regulation of vessel maturation. *Nat Med* 2003;9(6):685–693.

24. Swift MR, Weinstein BM. Arterial–venous specification during development. *Circ Res* 2009;104(5):576–588.

25. Rafii S, Lyden D, Benezra R, et al. Vascular and haematopoietic stem cells: novel targets for anti-angiogenesis therapy? *Nat Rev Cancer* 2002;2(11):826–835.

26. Jones R, Capen DE, Jacobson M, et al. VEGFR2+ PDGFRβ+ circulating precursor cells participate in capillary restoration after hyperoxia acute lung injury (HALI). *J Cell Mol Med* 2009;13(9b):3720–3729.

27. Schaper W. Collateral circulation: Past and present (INVITED EDITORIAL). *Basic Res Cardiol* 2008;104(1):5–21.

28. Duda DG, Cohen KS, Kozin SV, et al. Evidence for incorporation of bone marrow-derived endothelial cells into perfused blood vessels in tumors. *Blood* 2006;107(7):2774–2776.

29. Kozin SV, Kamoun WS, Huang Y, et al. Recruitment of myeloid but not endothelial precursor cells facilitates tumor regrowth after local irradiation. *Cancer Res* 2010;70(14):5679–5685.

30. Purhonen S, Palm J, Rossi D, et al. Bone marrow-derived circulating endothelial precursors do not contribute to vascular endothelium and are not needed for tumor growth. *Proc Natl Acad Sci* 2008;105(18):6620–6625.

31. Peters BA, Diaz LA, Polyak K, et al. Contribution of bone marrow–derived endothelial cells to human tumor vasculature. *Nat Med* 2005;11(3):261–262.

32. Kozin SV, Duda DG, Munn LL, et al. Is vasculogenesis crucial for the regrowth of irradiated tumours? *Nat Rev Cancer* 2011;11(7):532.

33. Ricci-Vitiani L, Pallini R, Biffoni M, et al. Tumour vascularization via endothelial differentiation of glioblastoma stem-like cells. *Nature* 2010;468(7325):824–828.

34. Soda Y, Marumoto T, Friedmann-Morvinski D, et al. Transdifferentiation of glioblastoma cells into vascular endothelial cells. *Proc Natl Acad Sci* 2011;108(11):4274–4280.

35. Wang R, Chadalavada K, Wilshire J, et al. Glioblastoma stem-like cells give rise to tumour endothelium. *Nature* 2010;468(7325):829–833.

36. Carmeliet P, Jain RK. Principles and mechanisms of vessel normalization for cancer and other angiogenic diseases. *Nat Rev Drug Discov* 2011;10(6):417–427.

37. Jain RK, Duda DG, Willett CG, et al. Biomarkers of response and resistance to antiangiogenic therapy. *Nat Rev Clin Oncol* 2009;6(6):327–338.

38. Dvorak HF. Vascular permeability factor/vascular endothelial growth factor: a critical cytokine in tumor angiogenesis and a potential target for diagnosis and therapy. *J Clin Oncol* 2002;20(21):4368–4380.

39. Melder RJ, Koenig GC, Witwer BP, et al. During angiogenesis, vascular endothelial growth factor and basic fibroblast growth factor regulate natural killer cell adhesion to tumor endothelium. *Nat Med* 1996;2(9):992–997.

40. Chung AS, Lee J, Ferrara N. Targeting the tumour vasculature: insights from physiological angiogenesis. *Nat Rev Cancer* 2010;10(7):505–514.

41. Mizukami Y, Jo W-S, Duerr E-M, et al. Induction of interleukin-8 preserves the angiogenic response in HIF-1α–deficient colon cancer cells. *Nat Med* 2005;11(9):992–997.

42. Yoshiji H, Harris SR, Thorgeirsson UP. Vascular endothelial growth factor is essential for initial but not continued *in vivo* growth of human breast carcinoma cells. *Cancer Res* 1997;57(18):3924–3928.

43. Yancopoulos GD, Davis S, Gale NW, et al. Vascular-specific growth factors and blood vessel formation. *Nature* 2000;407(6801):242–248.

44. O'Reilly MS, Holmgren L, Shing Y, et al. Angiostatin: a novel angiogenesis inhibitor that mediates the suppression of metastases by a Lewis lung carcinoma. *Cell* 1994;79(2):315–328.

45. O'Reilly MS, Boehm T, Shing Y, et al. Endostatin: an endogenous inhibitor of angiogenesis and tumor growth. *Cell* 1997;88(2):277–285.

46. Maeshima Y, Sudhakar A, Lively JC, et al. Tumstatin, an endothelial cell-specific inhibitor of protein synthesis. *Science* 2002;295(5552):140–143.

47. Fukumura D, Xu L, Chen Y, et al. Hypoxia and acidosis independently up-regulate vascular endothelial growth factor transcription in brain tumors *in vivo*. *Cancer Res* 2001;61(16):6020–6024.

48. Hanahan D, Weinberg RA. Hallmarks of cancer: the next generation. *Cell* 2011;144(5):646–674.

49. Huang Y, Snuderl M, Jain RK. Polarization of tumor-associated macrophages: a novel strategy for vascular normalization and antitumor immunity. *Cancer Cell* 2011;19(1):1–2.

50. Jain RK, Duda DG. Role of bone marrow-derived cells in tumor angiogenesis and treatment. *Cancer Cell* 2003;3(6):515–516.

51. Kerbel RS. Tumor angiogenesis. *N Engl J Med* 2008;358(19):2039–2049.

52. Xu L, Fukumura D, Jain RK. Acidic extracellular pH induces vascular endothelial growth factor (VEGF) in human glioblastoma cells via ERK1/2 MAPK signaling pathway: mechanism of low pH-induced VEGF. *J Biol Chem* 2002;277(13):11368–11374.

53. Fukumura D, Xavier R, Sugiura T, et al. Tumor induction of VEGF promoter activity in stromal cells. *Cell* 1998;94(6):715–725.

54. Tsuzuki Y, Fukumura D, Oosthuyse B, et al. Vascular endothelial growth factor (VEGF) modulation by targeting hypoxia-inducible factor-1alpha--> hypoxia response element--> VEGF cascade differentially regulates vascular response and growth rate in tumors. *Cancer Res* 2000;60(22):6248–6252.

55. Brown EB, Campbell RB, Tsuzuki Y, et al. *In vivo* measurement of gene expression, angiogenesis and physiological function in tumors using multiphoton laser scanning microscopy. *Nat Med* 2001;7(7):864–868.

56. Fukumura D, Yuan F, Monsky WL, et al. Effect of host microenvironment on the microcirculation of human colon adenocarcinoma. *Am J Pathol* 1997;151(3):679–688.

57. Gohongi T, Fukumura D, Boucher Y, et al. Tumor-host interactions in the gallbladder suppress distal angiogenesis and tumor growth: involvement of transforming growth factor beta1. *Nat Med* 1999;5(10):1203–1208.

58. Hobbs SK, Monsky WL, Yuan F, et al. Regulation of transport pathways in tumor vessels: role of tumor type and microenvironment. *Proc Natl Acad Sci U S A* 1998;95(8):4607–4612.

59. Monsky WL, Mouta Carreira C, Tsuzuki Y, et al. Role of host microenvironment in angiogenesis and microvascular functions in human breast cancer xenografts: mammary fat pad versus cranial tumors. *Clin Cancer Res* 2002;8(4):1008–1013.

60. Yuan F, Salehi HA, Boucher Y, et al. Vascular permeability and microcirculation of gliomas and mammary carcinomas transplanted in rat and mouse cranial windows. *Cancer Res* 1994;54(17):4564–4568.

61. Batchelor TT, Duda DG, di Tomaso E, et al. Phase II study of cediranib, an oral pan-vascular endothelial growth factor receptor tyrosine kinase inhibitor, in patients with recurrent glioblastoma. *J Clin Oncol* 2010;28(17):2817–2823.

62. Batchelor TT, Sorensen AG, di Tomaso E, et al. AZD2171, a pan-VEGF receptor tyrosine kinase inhibitor, normalizes tumor vasculature and alleviates edema in glioblastoma patients. *Cancer Cell* 2007;11(1):83–95.

63. Gerstner ER, Eichler AF, Plotkin SR, et al. Phase I trial with biomarker studies of vatalanib (PTK787) in patients with newly diagnosed glioblastoma treated with enzyme inducing anti-epileptic drugs and standard radiation and temozolomide. *J Neurooncol* 2011;103(2):325–332.

64. Horowitz NS, Penson RT, Duda DG, et al. Safety, efficacy, and biomarker exploration in a phase II study of bevacizumab, oxaliplatin, and gemcitabine in recurrent Müllerian carcinoma. *Clin Ovarian Cancer* 2011;4(1):26–33.

65. Izumi Y, Xu L, di Tomaso E, et al. Tumour biology: herceptin acts as an anti-angiogenic cocktail. *Nature* 2002;416(6878):279–280.

66. Willett CG, Boucher Y, di Tomaso E, et al. Direct evidence that the VEGF-specific antibody bevacizumab has antivascular effects in human rectal cancer. *Nat Med* 2004;10(2):145–147.

67. Willett CG, Boucher Y, Duda DG, et al. Surrogate markers for antiangiogenic therapy and dose-limiting toxicities for bevacizumab with radiation and chemotherapy: continued experience of a phase I trial in rectal cancer patients. *J Clin Oncol* 2005;23(31):8136–8139.

68. Willett CG, Duda DG, di Tomaso E, et al. Efficacy, safety, and biomarkers of neoadjuvant bevacizumab, radiation therapy, and fluorouracil in rectal cancer: a multidisciplinary phase II study. *J Clin Oncol* 2009;27(18):3020–3026.

69. Yoon SS, Duda DG, Karl DL, et al. Phase II study of neoadjuvant bevacizumab and radiotherapy for resectable soft tissue sarcomas. *Int J Radiat Oncol Biol Phys* 2011;81(4):1081–1090.

70. Zhu AX, Sahani DV, Duda DG, et al. Efficacy, safety, and potential biomarkers of sunitinib monotherapy in advanced hepatocellular carcinoma: a phase II study. *J Clin Oncol* 2009;27(18):3027–3035.

71. Zhu AX, Duda DG, Sahani DV, et al. HCC and angiogenesis: possible targets and future directions. *Nat Rev Clin Oncol* 2011;8(5):292–301.

72. Baish JW, Stylianopoulos T, Lanning RM, et al. Scaling rules for diffusive drug delivery in tumor and normal tissues. *Proc Natl Acad Sci U S A* 2011;108(5):1799–1803.

73. Baish JW, Jain RK. Fractals and cancer. *Cancer Res* 2000;60(14):3683–3688.

74. Gazit Y, Baish JW, Safabakhsh N, et al. Fractal characteristics of tumor vascular architecture during tumor growth and regression. *Microcirculation* 1997;4(4):395–402.

75. Less JR, Posner MC, Skalak TC, et al. Geometric resistance and microvascular network architecture of human colorectal carcinoma. *Microcirculation* 1997;4(1):25–33.

76. Less JR, Skalak TC, Sevick EM, et al. Microvascular architecture in a mammary carcinoma: branching patterns and vessel dimensions. *Cancer Res* 1991;51(1):265–273.

77. Jain RK, Tong RT, Munn LL. Effect of vascular normalization by antiangiogenic therapy on interstitial hypertension, peritumor edema, and lymphatic metastasis: insights from a mathematical model. *Cancer Res* 2007;67(6):2729–2735.

78. Goel S, Duda DG, Xu L, et al. Normalization of the vasculature for treatment of cancer and other diseases. *Physiol Rev* 2011;91(3):1071–1121.

79. Jain RK, Safabakhsh N, Sckell A, et al. Endothelial cell death, angiogenesis, and microvascular function after castration in an androgen-dependent tumor: role of vascular endothelial growth factor. *Proc Natl Acad Sci U S A* 1998;95(18):10820–10825.

80. Chae S-S, Kamoun WS, Farrar CT, et al. Angiopoietin-2 interferes with anti-VEGFR2–induced vessel normalization and survival benefit in mice bearing gliomas. *Clin Cancer Res* 2010;16(14):3618–3627.

81. Kadambi A, Mouta Carreira C, Yun CO, et al. Vascular endothelial growth factor (VEGF)-C differentially affects tumor vascular function and leukocyte recruitment: role of VEGF-receptor 2 and host VEGF-A. *Cancer Res* 2001;61(6):2404–2408.

82. Kamoun WS, Ley CD, Farrar CT, et al. Edema control by cediranib, a vascular endothelial growth factor receptor–targeted kinase inhibitor, prolongs survival despite persistent brain tumor growth in mice. *J Clin Oncol* 2009;27(15):2542–2552.

83. Tong RT, Boucher Y, Kozin SV, et al. Vascular normalization by vascular endothelial growth factor receptor 2 blockade induces a pressure gradient across the vasculature and improves drug penetration in tumors. *Cancer Res* 2004;64(11):3731–3736.

84. Winkler F, Kozin SV, Tong RT, et al. Kinetics of vascular normalization by VEGFR2 blockade governs brain tumor response to radiation: role of oxygenation, angiopoietin-1, and matrix metalloproteinases. *Cancer Cell* 2004;6(6):553–563.

85. Yuan F, Chen Y, Dellian M, et al. Time-dependent vascular regression and permeability changes in established human tumor xenografts induced by an antivascular endothelial growth factor/vascular permeability factor antibody. *Proc Natl Acad Sci U S A* 1996;93(25):14765–14770.

86. Duda DG, Willett CG, Ancukiewicz M, et al. Plasma soluble VEGFR-1 is a potential dual biomarker of response and toxicity for bevacizumab with chemoradiation in locally advanced rectal cancer. *Oncologist* 2010;15(6):577–583.

87. Sorensen AG, Batchelor TT, Zhang WT, et al. A "vascular normalization index" as potential mechanistic biomarker to predict survival after a single dose of cediranib in recurrent glioblastoma patients. *Cancer Res* 2009;69(13):5296–5300.

88. Sorensen AG, Emblem KE, Polaskova P, et al. Increased survival of glioblastoma patients who respond to antiangiogenic therapy with elevated blood perfusion. *Cancer Res* 2012;72(2):402–407.

89. Gerstner ER, Emblem KE, Chi AS, et al. Effects of cediranib, a VEGF signaling inhibitor, in combination with chemoradiation on tumor blood flow and survival in newly diagnosed glioblastoma. *J Clin Oncol* 2012;30:(suppl; abstr 2009).

90. Nia HT, Liu H, Seano G, et al. Solid stress and elastic energy as measures of tumour mechanopathology. *Nat Biomed Eng* 2016;1:0004.

91. Chauhan VP, Martin JD, Liu H, et al. Angiotensin inhibition enhances drug delivery and potentiates chemotherapy by decompressing tumour blood vessels. *Nat Commun* 2013;4:2516.

92. Incio J, Suboj P, Chin SM, et al. Metformin reduces desmoplasia in pancreatic cancer by reprogramming stellate cells and tumor-associated macrophages. *PLoS One* 2015;10(12):e0141392.

93. Papageorgis P, Polydorou C, Mpekris F, et al. Tranilast-induced stress alleviation in solid tumors improves the efficacy of chemo-and nanotherapeutics in a size-independent manner. *Sci Rep* 2017;7:4614.

94. Polydorou C, Mpekris F, Papageorgis P, et al. Pirfenidone normalizes the tumor microenvironment to improve chemotherapy. *Oncotarget* 2017;8(15):24506–24517.

95. Chauhan VP, Boucher Y, Ferrone CR, et al. Compression of pancreatic tumor blood vessels by hyaluronan is caused by solid stress and not interstitial fluid pressure. *Cancer Cell* 2014;26(1):14–15.

96. Griffon-Etienne G, Boucher Y, Brekken C, et al. Taxane-induced apoptosis decompresses blood vessels and lowers interstitial fluid pressure in solid tumors: clinical implications. *Cancer Res* 1999;59(15):3776–3782.

97. Jain RK. Determinants of tumor blood flow: a review. *Cancer Res* 1988;48(10):2641–2658.

98. Sevick EM, Jain RK. Geometric resistance to blood flow in solid tumors perfused ex vivo: effects of tumor size and perfusion pressure. *Cancer Res* 1989;49(13):3506–3512.

99. Sevick EM, Jain RK. Viscous resistance to blood flow in solid tumors: effect of hematocrit on intratumor blood viscosity. *Cancer Res* 1989;49(13):3513–3519.

100. Sevick EM, Jain RK. Measurement of capillary filtration coefficient in a solid tumor. *Cancer Res* 1991;51(4):1352–1355.

101. Jain RK, Shah SA, Finney PL. Continuous noninvasive monitoring of pH and temperature in rat Walker 256 carcinoma during normoglycemia and hyperglycemia. *J Natl Cancer Inst* 1984;73(2):429–436.

102. Vaupel P, Kallinowski F, Okunieff P. Blood flow, oxygen and nutrient supply, and metabolic microenvironment of human tumors: a review. *Cancer Res* 1989;49(23):6449–6465.

103. Butler TP, Grantham FH, Gullino PM. Bulk Transfer of Fluid in Interstitial Compartment of Mammary Tumors. *Cancer Res* 1975;35(11):3084–3088.

104. Endrich B, Reinhold HS, Gross JF, et al. Tissue perfusion inhomogeneity during early tumor growth in rats. *J Natl Cancer Inst* 1979;62(2):387–395.

105. Leunig M, Yuan F, Menger MD, et al. Angiogenesis, microvascular architecture, microhemodynamics, and interstitial fluid pressure during early growth of human adenocarcinoma LS174T in SCID mice. *Cancer Res* 1992;52(23):6553–6560.

106. Brizel DM, Klitzman B, Cook JM, et al. A comparison of tumor and normal tissue microvascular hematocrits and red cell fluxes in a rat window chamber model. *Int J Radiat Oncol Biol Phys* 1993;25(2):269–276.

107. Baish JW, Netti PA, Jain RK. Transmural coupling of fluid flow in microcirculatory network and interstitium in tumors. *Microvasc Res* 1997;53(2):128–141.

108. Mollica F, Jain RK, Netti PA. A model for temporal heterogeneities of tumor blood flow. *Microvasc Res* 2003;65(1):56–60.

109. Netti PA, Roberge S, Boucher Y, et al. Effect of transvascular fluid exchange on pressure-flow relationship in tumors: a proposed mechanism for tumor blood flow heterogeneity. *Microvasc Res* 1996;52(1):27–46.

110. Armulik A, Genové G, Betsholtz C. Pericytes: developmental, physiological, and pathological perspectives, problems, and promises. *Dev Cell* 2011;21(2):193–215.

111. Kashiwagi S, Izumi Y, Gohongi T, et al. NO mediates mural cell recruitment and vessel morphogenesis in murine melanomas and tissue-engineered blood vessels. *J Clin Invest* 2005;115(7):1816–1827.

112. Morikawa S, Baluk P, Kaidoh T, et al. Abnormalities in pericytes on blood vessels and endothelial sprouts in tumors. *Am J Pathol* 2002;160(3):985–1000.

113. Jain RK, Ward-Hartley KA. Tumor blood flow: characterization, modifications and role in hyperthermia. *IEEE Trans Sonics Ultrason* 1984;SU-31:504–526.

114. Heath VL, Bicknell R. Anticancer strategies involving the vasculature. *Nat Rev Clin Oncol* 2009;6(7):395–404.

115. Jain RK. Normalization of tumor vasculature: an emerging concept in antiangiogenic therapy. *Science* 2005;307(5706):58–62.

116. Jain RK, Stylianopoulos T. Delivering nanomedicine to solid tumors. *Nat Rev Clin Oncol* 2010;7(11):653–664.

117. Jain RK. Transport of molecules across tumor vasculature. *Cancer Metastasis Rev* 1987;6(4):559–593.

118. Baluk P, Morikawa S, Haskell A, et al. Abnormalities of basement membrane on blood vessels and endothelial sprouts in tumors. *Am J Pathol* 2003;163(5):1801–1815.

119. Hashizume H, Baluk P, Morikawa S, et al. Openings between defective endothelial cells explain tumor vessel leakiness. *Am J Pathol* 2000;156(4):1363–1380.

120. Endo M, Jain RK, Witwer B, et al. Water channel (aquaporin 1) expression and distribution in mammary carcinomas and glioblastomas. *Microvasc Res* 1999;58(2):89–98.

121. Gerlowski LE, Jain RK. Microvascular permeability of normal and neoplastic tissues. *Microvasc Res* 1986;31(3):288–305.

122. Lichtenbeld HC, Yuan F, Michel CC, et al. Perfusion of single tumor microvessels: application to vascular permeability measurement. *Microcirculation* 1996;3(4):349–357.

123. Yuan F, Leunig M, Berk DA, et al. Microvascular permeability of albumin, vascular surface area, and vascular volume measured in human adenocarcinoma LS174T using dorsal chamber in SCID mice. *Microvasc Res* 1993;45(3):269–289.

124. Yuan F, Dellian M, Fukumura D, et al. Vascular permeability in a human tumor xenograft: molecular size dependence and cutoff size. *Cancer Res* 1995;55(17):3752–3756.

125. Chauhan VP, Stylianopoulos T, Boucher Y, et al. Delivery of molecular and nanoscale medicine to tumors: transport barriers and strategies. *Annu Rev Chem Biomol Eng* 2011;2:281–298.

126. Tsuzuki Y, Mouta Carreira C, Bockhorn M, et al. Pancreas microenvironment promotes VEGF expression and tumor growth: novel window models for pancreatic tumor angiogenesis and microcirculation. *Lab Invest* 2001;81(10):1439–1451.

127. Monsky WL, Fukumura D, Gohongi T, et al. Augmentation of transvascular transport of macromolecules and nanoparticles in tumors using vascular endothelial growth factor. *Cancer Res* 1999;59(16):4129–4135.

128. Weis SM, Cheresh DA. Pathophysiological consequences of VEGF-induced vascular permeability. *Nature* 2005;437(7058):497–504.

129. Bockhorn M, Jain RK, Munn LL. Active versus passive mechanisms in metastasis: do cancer cells crawl into vessels, or are they pushed? *Lancet Oncol* 2007;8(5):444–448.

130. Duda DG, Duyverman AM, Kohno M, et al. Malignant cells facilitate lung metastasis by bringing their own soil. *Proc Natl Acad Sci* 2010;107(50):21677–21682.

131. Swartz MA, Kristensen CA, Melder RJ, et al. Cells shed from tumours show reduced clonogenicity, resistance to apoptosis, and *in vivo* tumorigenicity. *Br J Cancer* 1999;81(5):756–759.
132. Jain RK, Koenig GC, Dellian M, et al. Leukocyte-endothelial adhesion and angiogenesis in tumors. *Cancer Metastasis Rev* 1996;15(2):195–204.
133. Eichler AF, Chung E, Kodack DP, et al. The biology of brain metastases—translation to new therapies. *Nat Rev Clin Oncol* 2011;8(6):344–356.
134. Kienast Y, Von Baumgarten L, Fuhrmann M, et al. Real-time imaging reveals the single steps of brain metastasis formation. *Nat Med* 2010;16(1):116–122.
135. Hiratsuka S, Goel S, Kamoun WS, et al. Endothelial focal adhesion kinase mediates cancer cell homing to discrete regions of the lungs via E-selectin up-regulation. *Proc Natl Acad Sci* 2011;108(9):3725–3730.
136. Melder RJ, Munn LL, Yamada S, et al. Selectin- and integrin-mediated T-lymphocyte rolling and arrest on TNF-alpha-activated endothelium: augmentation by erythrocytes. *Biophys J* 1995;69(5):2131–2138.
137. Melder RJ, Yuan J, Munn LL, et al. Erythrocytes enhance lymphocyte rolling and arrest *in vivo*. *Microvasc Res* 2000;59(2):316–322.
138. Migliorini C, Qian Y, Chen H, et al. Red blood cells augment leukocyte rolling in a virtual blood vessel. *Biophys J* 2002;83(4):1834–1841.
139. Munn LL, Melder RJ, Jain RK. Role of erythrocytes in leukocyte-endothelial interactions: mathematical model and experimental validation. *Biophys J* 1996;71(1):466–478.
140. Melder RJ, Kristensen CA, Munn LL, et al. Modulation of A-NK cell rigidity: *in vitro* characterization and *in vivo* implications for cell delivery. *Biorheology* 2001;38(2–3):151–159.
141. Fukumura D, Salehi HA, Witwer B, et al. Tumor necrosis factor alpha-induced leukocyte adhesion in normal and tumor vessels: effect of tumor type, transplantation site, and host strain. *Cancer Res* 1995;55(21):4824–4829.
142. Yamada S, Mayadas TN, Yuan F, et al. Rolling in P-selectin-deficient mice is reduced but not eliminated in the dorsal skin. *Blood* 1995;86(9):3487–3492.
143. Melder RJ, Brownell AL, Shoup TM, et al. Imaging of activated natural killer cells in mice by positron emission tomography: preferential uptake in tumors. *Cancer Res* 1993;53(24):5867–5871.
144. Melder RJ, Jain RK. Reduction of rigidity in human activated natural killer cells by thioglycollate treatment. *J Immunol Methods* 1994;175(1):69–77.
145. Melder RJ, Jain RK. Kinetics of interleukin-2 induced changes in rigidity of human natural killer cells. *Cell Biophys* 1992;20(2–3):161–176.
146. Sasaki A, Jain RK, Maghazachi AA, et al. Low deformability of lymphokine-activated killer cells as a possible determinant of *in vivo* distribution. *Cancer Res* 1989;49(14):3742–3746.
147. Melder RJ, Salehi HA, Jain RK. Interaction of activated natural killer cells with normal and tumor vessels in cranial windows in mice. *Microvasc Res* 1995;50(1):35–44.
148. Sasaki A, Melder RJ, Whiteside TL, et al. Preferential localization of human adherent lymphokine-activated killer cells in tumor microcirculation. *J Natl Cancer Inst* 1991;83(6):433–437.
149. Munn LL, Koenig GC, Jain RK, et al. Kinetics of adhesion molecule expression and spatial organization using targeted sampling fluorometry. *Biotechniques* 1995;19(4):622–631.
150. Munn LL, Melder RJ, Jain RK. Analysis of cell flux in the parallel plate flow chamber: implications for cell capture studies. *Biophys J* 1994;67(2):889–895.
151. Gamble JR, Khew-Goodall Y, Vadas MA. Transforming growth factor-beta inhibits E-selectin expression on human endothelial cells. *J Immunol* 1993;150(10):4494–4503.
152. Detmar M, Brown LF, Schon MP, et al. Increased microvascular density and enhanced leukocyte rolling and adhesion in the skin of VEGF transgenic mice. *J Invest Dermatol* 1998;111(1):1–6.
153. Hamzah J, Jugold M, Kiessling F, et al. Vascular normalization in Rgs5-deficient tumours promotes immune destruction. *Nature* 2008;453(7193):410–414.
154. Huang Y, Yuan J, Righi E, et al. Vascular normalizing doses of antiangiogenic treatment reprogram the immunosuppressive tumor microenvironment and enhance immunotherapy. *Proc Natl Acad Sci U S A* 2012;109(43):17561–17566.
155. Tian L, Goldstein A, Wang H, et al. Mutual regulation of tumour vessel normalization and immunostimulatory reprogramming. *Nature* 2017;544(7649):250–254.
156. Schmittnaegel M, Rigamonti N, Kadioglu E, et al. Dual angiopoietin-2 and VEGFA inhibition elicits antitumor immunity that is enhanced by PD-1 checkpoint blockade. *Sci Transl Med* 2017;9(385):eaak9670.
157. De Palma M, Jain RK. CD4+ T cell activation and vascular normalization: Two sides of the same coin? *Immunity* 2017;46(5):773–775.
158. Kalluri R, Zeisberg M. Fibroblasts in cancer. *Nat Rev Cancer* 2006;6(5):392–401.
159. Qian B-Z, Pollard JW. Macrophage diversity enhances tumor progression and metastasis. *Cell* 2010;141(1):39–51.
160. Dawson MR, Chae S-S, Jain RK, et al. Direct evidence for lineage-dependent effects of bone marrow stromal cells on tumor progression. *Am J Cancer Res* 2011;1(2):144.
161. Hiratsuka S, Duda DG, Huang Y, et al. CXC receptor type 4 promotes metastasis by activating p38 mitogen-activated protein kinase in myeloid differentiation antigen (Gr-1)-positive cells. *Proc Natl Acad Sci* 2011;108(1):302–307.
162. Egeblad M, Nakasone ES, Werb Z. Tumors as organs: complex tissues that interface with the entire organism. *Dev Cell* 2010;18(6):884–901.
163. Orimo A, Weinberg RA. Stromal fibroblasts in cancer: a novel tumor-promoting cell type. *Cell Cycle* 2006;5(15):1597–1601.
164. De Visser KE, Eichten A, Coussens LM. Paradoxical roles of the immune system during cancer development. *Nat Rev Cancer* 2006;6(1):24–37.
165. Mazzieri R, Pucci F, Moi D, et al. Targeting the ANG2/TIE2 axis inhibits tumor growth and metastasis by impairing angiogenesis and disabling rebounds of proangiogenic myeloid cells. *Cancer Cell* 2011;19(4):512–526.
166. Rolny C, Mazzone M, Tugues S, et al. HRG inhibits tumor growth and metastasis by inducing macrophage polarization and vessel normalization through downregulation of PlGF. *Cancer Cell* 2011;19(1):31–44.
167. Salmon H, Franciszkiewicz K, Damotte D, et al. Matrix architecture defines the preferential localization and migration of T cells into the stroma of human lung tumors. *J Clin Invest* 2012;122(3):899.
168. Barsoum IB, Smallwood CA, Siemens DR, et al. A mechanism of hypoxia-mediated escape from adaptive immunity in cancer cells. *Cancer Res* 2013:canres. 0992.2013.
169. Calcinotto A, Filipazzi P, Grioni M, et al. Modulation of microenvironment acidity reverses anergy in human and murine tumor-infiltrating T lymphocytes. *Cancer Res* 2012;72(11):2746–2756.
170. Noman MZ, Desantis G, Janji B, et al. PD-L1 is a novel direct target of HIF-1α, and its blockade under hypoxia enhanced MDSC-mediated T cell activation. *J Exp Med* 2014;211(5):781–790.
171. Facciabene A, Peng X, Hagemann IS, et al. Tumour hypoxia promotes tolerance and angiogenesis via CCL28 and Treg cells. *Nature* 2011;475(7355):226–230.
172. Peterson TE, Kirkpatrick ND, Huang Y, et al. Dual inhibition of Ang-2 and VEGF receptors normalizes tumor vasculature and prolongs survival in glioblastoma by altering macrophages. *Proc Natl Acad Sci* 2016;113(16):4470–4475.
173. Kloepper J, Riedemann L, Amoozgar Z, et al. Ang-2/VEGF bispecific antibody reprograms macrophages and resident microglia to anti-tumor phenotype and prolongs glioblastoma survival. *Proc Natl Acad Sci* 2016;113(16):4476–4481.
174. Jain RK, Padera TP. Prevention and treatment of lymphatic metastasis by antilymphangiogenic therapy. *J Natl Cancer Inst* 2002;94(11):785–787.
175. Padera TP, Kadambi A, di Tomaso E, et al. Lymphatic metastasis in the absence of functional intratumor lymphatics. *Science* 2002;296(5574):1883–1886.
176. Elenbaas B, Weinberg RA. Heterotypic signaling between epithelial tumor cells and fibroblasts in carcinoma formation. *Exp Cell Res* 2001;264(1):169–184.
177. Brown E, McKee T, diTomaso E, et al. Dynamic imaging of collagen and its modulation in tumors *in vivo* using second-harmonic generation. *Nat Med* 2003;9(6):796–800.
178. Chary SR, Jain RK. Direct measurement of interstitial convection and diffusion of albumin in normal and neoplastic tissues by fluorescence photobleaching. *Proc Natl Acad Sci U S A* 1989;86(14):5385–5389.
179. Nugent LJ, Jain RK. Extravascular diffusion in normal and neoplastic tissues. *Cancer Res* 1984;44(1):238–244.
180. Pluen A, Boucher Y, Ramanujan S, et al. Role of tumor-host interactions in interstitial diffusion of macromolecules: cranial vs. subcutaneous tumors. *Proc Natl Acad Sci U S A* 2001;98(8):4628–4633.
181. Swabb EA, Wei J, Gullino PM. Diffusion and convection in normal and neoplastic tissues. *Cancer Res* 1974;34(10):2814–2822.
182. Boucher Y, Brekken C, Netti PA, et al. Intratumoral infusion of fluid: estimation of hydraulic conductivity and implications for the delivery of therapeutic agents. *Br J Cancer* 1998;78(11):1442–1448.
183. Znati CA, Rosenstein M, McKee TD, et al. Irradiation reduces interstitial fluid transport and increases the collagen content in tumors. *Clin Cancer Res* 2003;9(15):5508–5513.
184. Berk DA, Yuan F, Leunig M, et al. Direct *in vivo* measurement of targeted binding in a human tumor xenograft. *Proc Natl Acad Sci U S A* 1997;94(5):1785–1790.
185. Ramanujan S, Pluen A, McKee TD, et al. Diffusion and convection in collagen gels: implications for transport in the tumor interstitium. *Biophys J* 2002;83(3):1650–1660.
186. McKee TD, Grandi P, Mok W, et al. Degradation of fibrillar collagen in a human melanoma xenograft improves the efficacy of an oncolytic herpes simplex virus vector. *Cancer Res* 2006;66(5):2509–2513.
187. Diop-Frimpong B, Chauhan VP, Krane S, et al. Losartan inhibits collagen I synthesis and improves the distribution and efficacy of nanotherapeutics in tumors. *Proc Natl Acad Sci U S A* 2011;108(7):2909–2914.
188. Baxter LT, Jain RK. Transport of fluid and macromolecules in tumors. IV. A microscopic model of the perivascular distribution. *Microvasc Res* 1991;41(2):252–272.
189. Juweid M, Neumann R, Paik C, et al. Micropharmacology of monoclonal antibodies in solid tumors: direct experimental evidence for a binding site barrier. *Cancer Res* 1992;52(19):5144–5153.
190. Sherman MH, Yu RT, Engle DD, et al. Vitamin D receptor-mediated stromal reprogramming suppresses pancreatitis and enhances pancreatic cancer therapy. *Cell* 2014;159(1):80–93.
191. Leu AJ, Berk DA, Lymboussaki A, et al. Absence of functional lymphatics within a murine sarcoma: a molecular and functional evaluation. *Cancer Res* 2000;60(16):4324–4327.
192. Carreira CM, Nasser SM, di Tomaso E, et al. LYVE-1 is not restricted to the lymph vessels: Expression in normal liver blood sinusoids and down-regulation in human liver cancer and cirrhosis. *Cancer Res* 2001;61(22):8079–8084.
193. Isaka N, Padera TP, Hagendoorn J, et al. Peritumor lymphatics induced by vascular endothelial growth factor-C exhibit abnormal function. *Cancer Res* 2004;64(13):4400–4404.
194. Hoshida T, Isaka N, Hagendoorn J, et al. Imaging steps of lymphatic metastasis reveals that vascular endothelial growth factor-C increases metastasis by increasing delivery of cancer cells to lymph nodes: therapeutic implications. *Cancer Res* 2006;66(16):8065–8075.
195. Tammela T, Alitalo K. Lymphangiogenesis: Molecular mechanisms and future promise. *Cell* 2010;140(4):460–476.
196. Padera TP, Boucher Y, Jain RK. Correspondence re: S. Maula et al., Intratumoral Lymphatics Are Essential for the Metastatic Spread and Prognosis in Squamous Cell Carcinoma of the Head and Neck. Cancer Res., 63: 1920–1926, 2003. *Cancer Res* 2003;63(23):8555–8557.
197. Padera TP, Stoll BR, So PT, et al. Conventional and high-speed intravital multiphoton laser scanning microscopy of microvasculature, lymphatics, and leukocyte-endothelial interactions. *Mol Imaging* 2002;1(1):9–15.
198. Wong SY, Haack H, Crowley D, et al. Tumor-secreted vascular endothelial growth factor-C is necessary for prostate cancer lymphangiogenesis, but lymphangiogenesis is unnecessary for lymph node metastasis. *Cancer Res* 2005;65(21):9789–9798.

199. Norrmén C, Tammela T, Petrova TV, et al. Biological basis of therapeutic lymphangiogenesis. *Circulation* 2011;123(12):1335–1351.

200. Cursiefen C, Chen L, Borges LP, et al. VEGF-A stimulates lymphangiogenesis and hemangiogenesis in inflammatory neovascularization via macrophage recruitment. *J Clin Invest* 2004;113(7):1040–1050.

201. Nagy JA, Vasile E, Feng D, et al. Vascular permeability factor/vascular endothelial growth factor induces lymphangiogenesis as well as angiogenesis. *J Exp Med* 2002;196(11):1497–1506.

202. Lyden D, Hattori K, Dias S, et al. Impaired recruitment of bone-marrow–derived endothelial and hematopoietic precursor cells blocks tumor angiogenesis and growth. *Nat Med* 2001;7(11):1194–1201.

203. Religa P, Cao R, Bjorndahl M, et al. Presence of bone marrow–derived circulating progenitor endothelial cells in the newly formed lymphatic vessels. *Blood* 2005;106(13):4184–4190.

204. Naxerova K, Reiter JG, Brachtel E, et al. Origins of lymphatic and distant metastases in human colorectal cancer. *Science* 2017;357(6346):55–60.

205. Padera TP, Kuo AH, Hoshida T, et al. Differential response of primary tumor versus lymphatic metastasis to VEGFR-2 and VEGFR-3 kinase inhibitors cediranib and vandetanib. *Mol Cancer Ther* 2008;7(8):2272–2279.

206. Fukumura D, Jain RK. Tumor microenvironment abnormalities: causes, consequences, and strategies to normalize. *J Cell Biochem* 2007;101(4):937–949.

207. Hagendoorn J, Padera TP, Kashiwagi S, et al. Endothelial nitric oxide synthase regulates microlymphatic flow via collecting lymphatics. *Circ Res* 2004;95(2):204–209.

208. Jeltsch M, Kaipainen A, Joukov V, et al. Hyperplasia of lymphatic vessels in VEGF-C transgenic mice. *Science* 1997;276(5317):1423–1425.

209. Berk DA, Swartz MA, Leu AJ, et al. Transport in lymphatic capillaries. II. Microscopic velocity measurement with fluorescence photobleaching. *Am J Physiol* 1996;270(1 Pt 2):H330–H337.

210. Leu AJ, Berk DA, Yuan F, et al. Flow velocity in the superficial lymphatic network of the mouse tail. *Am J Physiol* 1994;267(4 Pt 2):H1507-1513.

211. Swartz MA, Berk DA, Jain RK. Transport in lymphatic capillaries. I. Macroscopic measurements using residence time distribution theory. *Am J Physiol Heart Circ Physiol* 1996;270(1):H324–H329.

212. Vakoc BJ, Lanning RM, Tyrrell JA, et al. Three-dimensional microscopy of the tumor microenvironment *in vivo* using optical frequency domain imaging. *Nat Med* 2009;15(10):1219–1223.

213. Boucher Y, Baxter LT, Jain RK. Interstitial pressure gradients in tissue-isolated and subcutaneous tumors: implications for therapy. *Cancer Res* 1990;50(15):4478–4484.

214. Boucher Y, Jain RK. Microvascular pressure is the principal driving force for interstitial hypertension in solid tumors: implications for vascular collapse. *Cancer Res* 1992;52(18):5110–5114.

215. Boucher Y, Kirkwood JM, Opacic D, et al. Interstitial hypertension in superficial metastatic melanomas in humans. *Cancer Res* 1991;51(24):6691–6694.

216. Boucher Y, Lee I, Jain RK. Lack of general correlation between interstitial fluid pressure and oxygen partial pressure in solid tumors. *Microvasc Res* 1995;50(2):175–182.

217. Boucher Y, Salehi H, Witwer B, et al. Interstitial fluid pressure in intracranial tumours in patients and in rodents. *Br J Cancer* 1997;75(6):829–836.

218. Curti BD, Urba WJ, Alvord WG, et al. Interstitial pressure of subcutaneous nodules in melanoma and lymphoma patients: changes during treatment. *Cancer Res* 1993;53(10):2204–2207.

219. Gutmann R, Leunig M, Feyh J, et al. Interstitial hypertension in head and neck tumors in patients: correlation with tumor size. *Cancer Res* 1992;52(7):1993–1995.

220. Less JR, Posner MC, Boucher Y, et al. Interstitial hypertension in human breast and colorectal tumors. *Cancer Res* 1992;52(22):6371–6374.

221. Milosevic M, Fyles A, Hedley D, et al. Interstitial fluid pressure predicts survival in patients with cervix cancer independent of clinical prognostic factors and tumor: Oxygen measurements. *Cancer Res* 2001;61(17):6400–6405.

222. Nathanson SD, Nelson L. Interstitial fluid pressure in breast-cancer, benign breast conditions, and breast parenchyma. *Ann Surg Oncol* 1994;1(4):333–338.

223. Roh HD, Boucher Y, Kalnicki S, et al. Interstitial hypertension in carcinoma of uterine cervix in patients: possible correlation with tumor oxygenation and radiation response. *Cancer Res* 1991;51(24):6695–6698.

224. Znati CA, Rosenstein M, Boucher Y, et al. Effect of radiation on interstitial fluid pressure and oxygenation in a human tumor xenograft. *Cancer Res* 1996;56(5):964–968.

225. Boucher Y, Leunig M, Jain RK. Tumor angiogenesis and interstitial hypertension. *Cancer Res* 1996;56(18):4264–4266.

226. Lee CG, Heijn M, di Tomaso E, et al. Anti-vascular endothelial growth factor treatment augments tumor radiation response under normoxic or hypoxic conditions. *Cancer Res* 2000;60(19):5565–5570.

227. DiResta GR, Lee J, Healey JH, et al. "Artificial lymphatic system": A new approach to reduce interstitial hypertension and increase blood flow, pH and pO(2) in solid tumors. *Ann Biomed Eng* 2000;28(5):543–555.

228. Stohrer M, Boucher Y, Stangassinger M, et al. Oncotic pressure in solid tumors is elevated. *Cancer Res* 2000;60(15):4251–4255.

229. Netti PA, Baxter LT, Boucher Y, et al. Time-dependent behavior of interstitial fluid pressure in solid tumors: implications for drug delivery. *Cancer Res* 1995;55(22):5451–5458.

230. Netti PA, Hamberg LM, Babich JW, et al. Enhancement of fluid filtration across tumor vessels: implication for delivery of macromolecules. *Proc Natl Acad Sci U S A* 1999;96(6):3137–3142.

231. Zlotecki RA, Boucher Y, Lee I, et al. Effect of angiotensin II induced hypertension on tumor blood flow and interstitial fluid pressure. *Cancer Res* 1993;53(11):2466–2468.

232. Chauhan VP, Stylianopoulos T, Martin JD, et al. Normalization of tumour blood vessels improves the delivery of nanomedicines in a size-dependent manner. *Nat Nanotechnol* 2012;7(6):383–388.

233. Jain RK. Taming vessels to treat cancer. *Sci Am* 2008;298(1):56–63.

234. Krogh A. *The anatomy and physiology of capillaries.* New York, NY: Yale University Press, 1922.

235. Thomlinson RH, Gray LH. The histological structure of some human lung cancers and the possible implications for radiotherapy. *Br J Cancer* 1955;9(4):539–549.

236. Helmlinger G, Yuan F, Dellian M, et al. Interstitial pH and pO2 gradients in solid tumors *in vivo*: high-resolution measurements reveal a lack of correlation. *Nat Med* 1997;3(2):177–182.

237. Torres Filho IP, Leunig M, Yuan F, et al. Noninvasive measurement of microvascular and interstitial oxygen profiles in a human tumor in SCID mice. *Proc Natl Acad Sci* 1994;91(6):2081–2085.

238. Pouysségur J, Dayan F, Mazure NM. Hypoxia signalling in cancer and approaches to enforce tumour regression. *Nature* 2006;441(7092):437–443.

239. Helmlinger G, Sckell A, Dellian M, et al. Acid production in glycolysis-impaired tumors provides new insights into tumor metabolism. *Clin Cancer Res* 2002;8(4):1284–1291.

240. Bush RS. The significance of anemia in clinical radiation therapy. *Int J Radiat Oncol Biol Phys* 1986;12(11):2047–2050.

241. Fyles A, Milosevic M, Hedley D, et al. Tumor hypoxia has independent predictor impact only in patients with node-negative cervix cancer. *J Clin Oncol* 2002;20(3):680–687.

242. Littlewood TJ. The impact of hemoglobin levels on treatment outcomes in patients with cancer. *Semin Oncol* 2001;28(2F):49–53.

243. Vansteenkiste J, Pirker R, Massuti B, et al. Double-blind, placebo-controlled, randomized phase III trial of darbepoetin alfa in lung cancer patients receiving chemotherapy. *J Natl Cancer Inst* 2002;94(16):1211–1220.

244. Henke M, Laszig R, Rübe C, et al. Erythropoietin to treat head and neck cancer patients with anaemia undergoing radiotherapy: randomised, double-blind, placebo-controlled trial. *Lancet* 2003;362(9392):1255–1260.

245. Leyland-Jones B, Semiglazov V, Pawlicki M, et al. Maintaining normal hemoglobin levels with epoetin alfa in mainly nonanemic patients with metastatic breast cancer receiving first-line chemotherapy: a survival study. *J Clin Oncol* 2005;23(25):5960–5972.

246. Sundfør K, Lyng H, Kongsgård U, et al. Polarographic Measurement of pO2 in Cervix Carcinoma. *Gynecol Oncol* 1997;64(2):230–236.

247. Dzik S, Mincheff M, Puppo F. Apoptosis, transforming growth factor-β, and the immunosuppressive effect of transfusion. *Transfusion* 2002;42(9):1221–1223.

248. Gharehbaghian A, Haque KM, Truman C, et al. Effect of autologous salvaged blood on postoperative natural killer cell precursor frequency. *Lancet* 2004;363(9414):1025–1030.

249. Santin AD, Bellone S, Palmieri M, et al. Effect of blood transfusion during radiotherapy on the immune function of patients with cancer of the uterine cervix: role of interleukin-10. *Int J Radiat Oncol Biol Phys* 2002;54(5):1345–1355.

250. Gerweck LE, Vijayappa S, Kozin S. Tumor pH controls the *in vivo* efficacy of weak acid and base chemotherapeutics. *Mol Cancer Ther* 2006;5(5):1275–1279.

251. Kozin SV, Boucher Y, Hicklin DJ, et al. Vascular endothelial growth factor receptor-2-blocking antibody potentiates radiation-induced long-term control of human tumor xenografts. *Cancer Res* 2001;61(1):39–44.

252. Jain RK, Forbes NS. Can engineered bacteria help control cancer? *Proc Natl Acad Sci U S A* 2001;98(26):14748–14750.

253. Hosseinidoust Z, Mostaghaci B, Yasa O, et al. Bioengineered and biohybrid bacteria-based systems for drug delivery. *Adv Drug Deliv Rev* 2016;106:27–44.

254. Rischin D, Peters LJ, O'Sullivan B, et al. Tirapazamine, cisplatin, and radiation versus cisplatin and radiation for advanced squamous cell carcinoma of the head and neck (TROG 02.02, HeadSTART): a phase III trial of the Trans-Tasman Radiation Oncology Group. *J Clin Oncol* 2010;28(18):2989–2995.

255. Semenza GL. Oxygen sensing, homeostasis, and disease. *N Engl J Med* 2011;365(6):537–547.

256. Mazzone M, Dettori D, Leite de Oliveira R, et al. Heterozygous deficiency of PHD2 restores tumor oxygenation and inhibits metastasis via endothelial normalization. *Cell* 2009;136(5):839–851.

257. Majmundar AJ, Wong WJ, Simon MC. Hypoxia-inducible factors and the response to hypoxic stress. *Mol Cell* 2010;40(2):294–309.

258. Fraisl P, Mazzone M, Schmidt T, et al. Regulation of angiogenesis by oxygen and metabolism. *Dev Cell* 2009;16(2):167–179.

259. Du R, Lu KV, Petritsch C, et al. HIF1α induces the recruitment of bone marrow-derived vascular modulatory cells to regulate tumor angiogenesis and invasion. *Cancer Cell* 2008;13(3):206–220.

260. Arany Z, Foo S-Y, Ma Y, et al. HIF-independent regulation of VEGF and angiogenesis by the transcriptional coactivator PGC-1α. *Nature* 2008;451(7181):1008–1012.

261. Buysschaert I, Schmidt T, Roncal C, et al. Genetics, epigenetics and pharmaco-(epi) genomics in angiogenesis. *J Cell Mol Med* 2008;12(6b):2533–2551.

262. Ohtani K, Dimmeler S. Control of cardiovascular differentiation by microRNAs. *Basic Res Cardiol* 2011;106(1):5–11.

263. Nicoli S, Standley C, Walker P, et al. MicroRNA-mediated integration of haemodynamics and Vegf signalling during angiogenesis. *Nature* 2010;464(7292):1196–1200.

264. Talks KL, Turley H, Gatter KC, et al. The expression and distribution of the hypoxia-inducible factors HIF-1α and HIF-2α in normal human tissues, cancers, and tumor-associated macrophages. *Am J Pathol* 2000;157(2):411–421.

265. Carmeliet P, Dor Y, Herbert JM, et al. Role of HIF-1alpha in hypoxia-mediated apoptosis, cell proliferation and tumour angiogenesis. *Nature* 1998;394(6692):485–490.

266. Moeller BJ, Dreher MR, Rabbani ZN, et al. Pleiotropic effects of HIF-1 blockade on tumor radiosensitivity. *Cancer Cell* 2005;8(2):99–110.

267. Cramer T, Yamanishi Y, Clausen BE, et al. HIF-1α is essential for myeloid cell-mediated inflammation. *Cell* 2003;112(5):645–657.

268. Melillo G. Inhibiting hypoxia-inducible factor 1 for cancer therapy. *Mol Cancer Res* 2006;4(9):601–605.

269. Duda DG, Jain RK, Willett CG. Antiangiogenics: the potential role of integrating this novel treatment modality with chemoradiation for solid cancers. *J Clin Oncol* 2007;25(26):4033–4042.

270. McCormick F. New-age drug meets resistance. *Nature* 2001;412(6844):281–282.

271. Kodack DP, Askoxylakis V, Ferraro GB, et al. The brain microenvironment mediates resistance in luminal breast cancer to PI3K inhibition through HER3 activation. *Sci Transl Med* 2017;9(391):eaal4682.

272. Sharma S, Sharma M, Sarkar C. Morphology of angiogenesis in human cancer: a conceptual overview, histoprognostic perspective and significance of neoangiogenesis. *Histopathology* 2005;46(5):481–489.

273. Varlotto J, Stevenson MA. Anemia, tumor hypoxemia, and the cancer patient. *Int J Radiat Oncol Biol Phys* 2005;63(1):25–36.

274. Nordsmark M, Loncaster J, Aquino-Parsons C, et al. Measurements of hypoxia using pimonidazole and polarographic oxygen-sensitive electrodes in human cervix carcinomas. *Radiother Oncol* 2003;67(1):35–44.

275. Serganova I, Humm J, Ling C, et al. Tumor hypoxia imaging. *Clin Cancer Res* 2006;12(18):5260–5264.

276. Sorensen AG, Batchelor TT, Wen PY, et al. Response criteria for glioma. *Nat Clin Pract Oncol* 2008;5(11):634–644.

277. Tolaney SM, Boucher Y, Duda DG, et al. Role of vascular density and normalization in response to neoadjuvant bevacizumab and chemotherapy in breast cancer patients. *Proc Natl Acad Sci* 2015;112(46):14325–14330.

278. Heist RS, Duda DG, Sahani DV, et al. Improved tumor vascularization after anti-VEGF therapy with carboplatin and nab-paclitaxel associates with survival in lung cancer. *Proc Natl Acad Sci* 2015;112(5):1547–1552.

279. Gallez B, Baudelet C, Jordan BF. Assessment of tumor oxygenation by electron paramagnetic resonance: principles and applications. *NMR Biomed* 2004;17(5):240–262.

280. Rajendran JG, Schwartz DL, O'Sullivan J, et al. Tumor hypoxia imaging with [F-18] fluoromisonidazole positron emission tomography in head and neck cancer. *Clin Cancer Res* 2006;12(18):5435–5441.

281. Rischin D, Hicks RJ, Fisher R, et al. Prognostic significance of [18F]-misonidazole positron emission tomography–detected tumor hypoxia in patients with advanced head and neck cancer randomly assigned to chemoradiation with or without tirapazamine: a substudy of Trans-Tasman Radiation Oncology Group Study 98.02. *J Clin Oncol* 2006;24(13):2098–2104.

282. Emblem KE, Mouridsen K, Bjornerud A, et al. Vessel architectural imaging identifies cancer patient responders to anti-angiogenic therapy. *Nat Med* 2013;19(9):1178–1183.

283. Batchelor TT, Gerstner ER, Emblem KE, et al. Improved tumor oxygenation and survival in glioblastoma patients who show increased blood perfusion after cediranib and chemoradiation. *Proc Natl Acad Sci* 2013;110(47):19059–19064.

284. Ueda S, Kuji I, Shigekawa T, et al. Optical imaging for monitoring tumor oxygenation response after initiation of single-agent bevacizumab followed by cytotoxic chemotherapy in breast cancer patients. *PLoS One* 2014;9(6):e98715.

285. Ueda S, Roblyer D, Cerussi A, et al. Baseline tumor oxygen saturation correlates with a pathologic complete response in breast cancer patients undergoing neoadjuvant chemotherapy. *Cancer Res* 2012;72(17):4318–4328.

286. Cooke VG, LeBleu VS, Keskin D, et al. Pericyte depletion results in hypoxia-associated epithelial-to-mesenchymal transition and metastasis mediated by met signaling pathway. *Cancer Cell* 2012;21(1):66–81.

287. Rhim AD, Oberstein PE, Thomas DH, et al. Stromal elements act to restrain, rather than support, pancreatic ductal adenocarcinoma. *Cancer Cell* 2014;25(6):735–747.

288. Lee JJ, Perera RM, Wang H, et al. Stromal response to Hedgehog signaling restrains pancreatic cancer progression. *Proc Natl Acad Sci U S A* 2014;111(30):E3091–E3100.

289. Martin JD, Fukumura D, Duda DG, et al. Reengineering the tumor microenvironment to alleviate hypoxia and overcome cancer heterogeneity. *Cold Spring Harb Perspect Med* 2016;6(12):a027094.

290. Ansiaux R, Baudelet C, Jordan BF, et al. Thalidomide radiosensitizes tumors through early changes in the tumor microenvironment. *Clin Cancer Res* 2005;11(2):743–750.

291. Browder T, Butterfield CE, Kräling BM, et al. Antiangiogenic scheduling of chemotherapy improves efficacy against experimental drug-resistant cancer. *Cancer Res* 2000;60(7):1878–1886.

292. Segers J, Di Fazio V, Ansiaux R, et al. Potentiation of cyclophosphamide chemotherapy using the anti-angiogenic drug thalidomide: importance of optimal scheduling to exploit the 'normalization' window of the tumor vasculature. *Cancer Lett* 2006;244(1):129–135.

293. Willett CG, Duda DG, Ancukiewicz M, et al. A safety and survival analysis of neoadjuvant bevacizumab with standard chemoradiation in a phase I/II study compared with standard chemoradiation in locally advanced rectal cancer. *Oncologist* 2010;15(8):845–851.

294. Huber PE, Bischof M, Jenne J, et al. Trimodal cancer treatment: beneficial effects of combined antiangiogenesis, radiation, and chemotherapy. *Cancer Res* 2005;65(9):3643–3655.

295. Salnikov AV, Roswall P, Sundberg C, et al. Inhibition of TGF-β modulates macrophages and vessel maturation in parallel to a lowering of interstitial fluid pressure in experimental carcinoma. *Lab Invest* 2005;85(4):512–521.

296. Wildiers H, Guetens G, De Boeck G, et al. Effect of antivascular endothelial growth factor treatment on the intratumoral uptake of CPT-11. *Br J Cancer* 2003;88(12):1979–1986.

297. Stylianopoulos T, Jain RK. Combining two strategies to improve perfusion and drug delivery in solid tumors. *Proc Natl Acad Sci U S A* 2013;110(46):18632–18637.

298. Murphy JE, Wo JY-L, Ferrone C, et al. *TGF-B1 inhibition with losartan in combination with FOLFIRINOX (F-NOX) in locally advanced pancreatic cancer (LAPC): Preliminary feasibility and R0 resection rates from a prospective phase II study. American Society of Clinical Oncology*; 2017.

299. Menter AR, Carroll N, Delate T, et al. Effect of angiotensin system inhibitors on survival in patients receiving chemotherapy for advanced non-small cell lung cancer. Paper presented at: 50th Annual Meeting of ASCO2014; Chicago, IL.

300. Keizman D, Huang P, Eisenberger MA, et al. Angiotensin system inhibitors and outcome of sunitinib treatment in patients with metastatic renal cell carcinoma: a retrospective examination. *Eur J Cancer* 2011;47(13):1955–1961.

301. Nakai Y, Isayama H, Ijichi H, et al. Inhibition of renin-angiotensin system affects prognosis of advanced pancreatic cancer receiving gemcitabine. *Br J Cancer* 2010;103(11):1644–1648.

302. Nakai Y, Isayama H, Sasaki T, et al. The inhibition of renin-angiotensin system in advanced pancreatic cancer: an exploratory analysis in 349 patients. *J Cancer Res Clin Oncol* 2015;141(5):933–939.

303. Wilop S, von Hobe S, Crysandt M, et al. Impact of angiotensin I converting enzyme inhibitors and angiotensin II type 1 receptor blockers on survival in patients with advanced non-small-cell lung cancer undergoing first-line platinum-based chemotherapy. *J Cancer Res Clin Oncol* 2009;135(10):1429–1435.

304. Pinter M, Weinmann A, Wörns M-A, et al. Use of inhibitors of the renin–angiotensin system is associated with longer survival in patients with hepatocellular carcinoma. *United European Gastroenterol J* 2017;5(7):987–996. doi:10.1177/2050640617695698.

305. Cerullo M, Gani F, Chen SY, et al. Impact of angiotensin receptor blocker use on overall survival among patients undergoing resection for pancreatic cancer. *World J Surg* 2017;41(9):2361–2370.

306. Mpekris F, Baish JW, Stylianopoulos T, et al. Role of vascular normalization in benefit from metronomic chemotherapy. *Proc Natl Acad Sci* 2017;114(8):1994–1999.

307. Jeong HS, Jones D, Liao S, et al. investigation of the lack of angiogenesis in the formation of lymph node metastases. *J Natl Cancer Inst* 2015;107(9):djv155.

308. Bridgeman VL, Vermeulen PB, Foo S, et al. Vessel co-option is common in human lung metastases and mediates resistance to anti-angiogenic therapy in preclinical lung metastasis models. *J Pathol* 2017;241(3):362–374.

309. Frentzas S, Simoneau E, Bridgeman VL, et al. Vessel co-option mediates resistance to anti-angiogenic therapy in liver metastases. *Nat Med* 2016;22(11):1294–1302.

310. Formenti SC, Demaria S. Systemic effects of local radiotherapy. *Lancet Oncol* 2009;10(7):718–726.

311. Formenti SC, Demaria S. Combining radiotherapy and cancer immunotherapy: a paradigm shift. *J Natl Cancer Inst* 2013;105(4):256–265.

312. Segal NH, Parsons DW, Peggs KS, et al. Epitope landscape in breast and colorectal cancer. *Cancer Res* 2008;68(3):889–892.

313. Schuler G, Steinman R. Dendritic cells as adjuvants for immune-mediated resistance to tumors. *J Exp Med* 1997;186(8):1183–1187.

314. Albert ML, Sauter B, Bhardwaj N. Dendritic cells acquire antigen from apoptotic cells and induce class I-restricted CTLs. *Nature* 1998;392(6671):86.

315. Vanpouille-Box C, Formenti SC, Demaria S. Towards precision radiotherapy for use with immune checkpoint blockers. *Clin Cancer Res* 2017:clincanres. 0037.2017.

316. Dewan MZ, Galloway AE, Kawashima N, et al. Fractionated but not single-dose radiotherapy induces an immune-mediated abscopal effect when combined with anti–CTLA-4 antibody. *Clin Cancer Res* 2009;15(17):5379–5388.

317. Demaria S, Kawashima N, Yang AM, et al. Immune-mediated inhibition of metastases after treatment with local radiation and CTLA-4 blockade in a mouse model of breast cancer. *Clin Cancer Res* 2005;11(2):728–734.

318. Vanpouille-Box C, Alard A, Aryankalayil MJ, et al. DNA exonuclease Trex1 regulates radiotherapy-induced tumour immunogenicity. *Nat Commun* 2017;8:15618.

319. Golden EB, Chhabra A, Chachoua A, et al. Local radiotherapy and granulocyte-macrophage colony-stimulating factor to generate abscopal responses in patients with metastatic solid tumours: a proof-of-principle trial. *Lancet Oncol* 2015;16(7):795–803.

320. Golden EB, Demaria S, Schiff PB, et al. An abscopal response to radiation and ipilimumab in a patient with metastatic non–small cell lung cancer. *Cancer Immunol Res* 2013;1(6):365–372.

321. Pinter M, Jain RK. Targeting the renin-angiotensin system to improve cancer treatment: implications for immunotherapy. *Sci Transl Med* 2017;9(410):eaan5616.

322. Vanpouille-Box C, Diamond JM, Pilones KA, et al. TGFβ is a master regulator of radiation therapy-induced antitumor immunity. *Cancer Res* 2015;75(11):2232–2242.

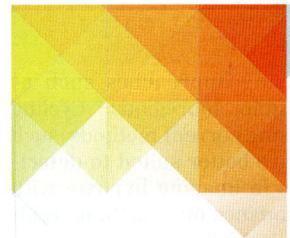

CHAPTER 5

SMART Radiotherapy

C. Norman Coleman, Pataje G. Prasanna, Jacek Capala, Mansoor M. Ahmed, Jeffrey C. Buchsbaum, Bhadrasain Vikram, and Eric J. Bernhard

INTRODUCTION

On being asked to write a second edition of this chapter, we realized that there may have been a few different conclusions drawn from the previous version. It might have been wildly successful, not very good requiring a remedial effort, or largely ignored. This is a serious science-based chapter, and to bring a new level of SMARTs to how a book chapter is viewed—of which our chapter is 4.7% of the total number of chapters—we have included a mini-survey for the reader in the conclusion. We are pleased to be among the first five chapters and to serve as the linker between biology and physics. As stated in the previous version, we anticipate that the radiation biology chapter will include molecular aspects of radiation therapy and the basic aspects of tumor microenvironment, the physics chapter will include essential aspects of particle therapy, and the clinical chapters will include molecular characterization of tumors, the use of molecular and functional imaging, and the current studies with molecular targeted agents for the various diseases.

The goal of this chapter is to take a broad view of what are likely to be some of the innovative concepts, now entering the practice of oncology, that are relevant to radiation therapy researchers and practitioners. A first major point is that perhaps now more than ever, radiation oncology needs to be at the center of the science of cancer care. Our clinical expertise transcends all diseases; our technology has impact in the most expensive, high-technology, upper-income-country care but can also reach people in dire need of cancer care in lower/middle-income countries. Although not always recognized as such, in the evolving era of "precision medicine," radiation is both "precision and accurate medicine" when one looks at radiation as a "drug." We can control the pharmacokinetics and pharmacodynamics of radiation by hitting specific physical targets and also by using doses and schedules that could be designed to activate molecular, cellular, and tissue pathways.[1] The term "focused biology" was coined 15 years ago,[2,3] and it is now increasingly relevant with image-guided radiation therapy, particle therapy, immune modulation, hypofractionation, and molecular targeted drug treatment.

Building from our definition of SMART radiotherapy from the previous edition, we will introduce new concepts *in italics*:

*S*cience-focused clinical care based on cancer, molecular, cellular, and tissue biology—*radiation as a drug, as part of combined modality therapy, and as an immune modulator*

*M*ultidimensional approach to all radiation issues facing society, including cancer treatment, prevention, and potential risk from radiation exposure—*normal tissue and biomarkers*

*A*ccess to care for all, including the underserved for whom radiation oncologists (often called clinical oncologists) are the primary oncology care provider—*progress in global health*

*R*esponsible implementation of technology so that we control our destiny based on data—*particles, systemic radionuclides, and nano-based treatments*

*T*raining and mentoring to ensure a broadly based, societal conscious next generation of clinicians, scientists, and educators—*radiation oncology as a key leader in cancer care*

By fortunate coincidence, our SMART components follow the same general organization as does this book. We start from the new biology, to the developing world, to physics and systemic radionuclides, and to education, training, and ethics.

SCIENCE-FOCUSED CLINICAL CARE BASED ON CANCER, MOLECULAR, CELLULAR, AND TISSUE BIOLOGY

Radiation as a Drug

A concept introduced in the previous edition of the chapter is radiation as a drug and immune modifier. Luo et al.[4] modified the "hallmarks of cancer" model of Hanahan and Weinberg[5] by targeting nononcogene addiction in addition to oncogene addiction. Logically, the biochemical and metabolic machinery of the cell carries out the functions of the genes be they normal or abnormal so that the target of cancer therapy can be to disrupt the turning on and off of genes directly and also to disrupt the metabolic and biochemical pathways that they activate. Nononcogene pathways include the stress responses: metabolic, proteotoxic, mitotic, oxidative, deoxyribonucleic acid (DNA) damage, and evading immune surveillance. Notably, all these pathways can be modulated by radiation.

The initial work by Tsai et al.[6] that showed what we now call "multifraction-adaptive (MF-adaptive)" responses used ribonucleic acid (RNA) microarrays to study the effects of 10 Gy as a single dose or as multifractionated radiation, 2 Gy × 5, in three tumor cell lines—breast, prostate, and brain—*in vitro* and *in vivo*. There is a substantially different gene expression pattern with fractionation compared to single dose, with immune response genes being a pathway significantly up-regulated with fractionation. Fractionated radiation made the cell lines somewhat more alike (one of the hypotheses tested), and there was substantial difference between tumors treated *in vivo* versus *in vitro*, which might reflect the effects of radiation as well as the presence of a variety of cell types within a tumor.

John-Aryankalayil et al.[7] studied the molecular changes in prostate cancer cells exposed to 10 Gy as a single dose (SD) or multiple fractions (MF) using 2 Gy × 5 (MF2) and 1 Gy × 10 (MF1). The gene profiles are markedly different between SD and MF, and MF1 induces more changes than does MF2. Summarizing substantial work in this regard[3,7–9] includes the following: (a) An inflection point occurs after six to seven 1 Gy doses with immune response genes being a major pathway so that this MF-adaptive response may be missed in schedules using only 3 to 5 fractions; (b) changes occur in micro ribonucleic acid (miRNA), metabolomics, and protein expression, which are now being correlated; (c) 0.5 Gy × 10 will induce changes so that many tissues know they've been hit; (d) similar changes are seen in endothelial cells, including immune response genes; and (e) as a proof-of-principle, drugs targeting the Akt–mTor pathway were effective after MF but not before, demonstrating that radiation could stimulate drug susceptibility. The above studies indicate potential unique use of the radiation in the "focused biology" concept for molecular targeted therapy and emphasize the importance of investigating the molecular phenotype in cells that survive radiation.

The Tumor Microenvironment

The efficacy of radiotherapy is in part determined by tumor microenvironmental factors, including, but not limited to, the extent of tumor oxygenation, the tumor pH, and the interaction of tumor cells with host stroma and with inflammatory cells. Tumors contain areas of poor vascular perfusion, low pH, and oxygen, which may provide regions in which both the delivery and activity of cytotoxic therapies is attenuated and in which cancer stem–like cells (CSCs) reside.[10,11] In addition, certain tumor environments may select for more aggressive or resistant tumor clonogens.[12] One factor that has received little clinical attention, but may provide an avenue for future advances, is the impact of mechanical force on transformation, progression, and treatment response of cancer cells.[13] Similarly, signaling originating from the interaction of stromal components with integrins on cancer cells can influence tumor survival and provide targets for intervention.[14,15]

The tumor microenvironment changes during radiotherapy.[16] Fractionated radiotherapy results in reoxygenation of the tumor due to elimination of well-oxygenated cells, thus increasing oxygen delivery to the previously hypoxic areas. Conversely, high-dose single fractions (over 13 Gy) have been shown to result in destruction of both tumor cells and vascular endothelium.[17] How and under what circumstances radiation-induced vascular injury impacts tumor responses continues to be a topic of investigation and is relevant to the current use of large fraction stereotactic radiosurgery or therapy.[18–21] Radiation also results in release of tumor antigens, and this release may be qualitatively and quantitatively modulated by fractionation schedules as discussed later.

Tumor Hypoxia

The longest-studied example of tumor microenvironment effects on cancer cell radiation survival is the impact of tumor oxygenation. Radiation under atmospheric oxygen conditions enhances killing by a factor of 2 to 3 compared to irradiation under anoxic conditions, which has been termed the oxygen enhancement ratio[22] (as reviewed by Horsman et al.[16]). In the clinical setting, hypoxia affects outcome after radiotherapy.[23,24] But hypoxia has also been shown to be a poor prognostic factor after chemotherapy[25] and surgery.[26,27] These findings were attributed to chronic hypoxia, and this has been studied under controlled oxygen concentrations *in vitro* or using electrodes or immunohistochemical staining to measure tissue oxygenation *in vivo*. Overcoming hypoxia by biochemical targeting of hypoxic regions in tumors has proven difficult to translate to the clinic.[28] Going forward, molecular targeting of hypoxic cells may prove more practicable and effective.[29] The approach of reducing tumor oxygen consumption may also be more effective than either targeting hypoxic cells or trying to increase tumor oxygen.[30] Recent advances in noninvasive tumor hypoxia imaging may also come into play in the future, allowing precise definition of hypoxic tumors and tumor subregions through imaging with positron emission tomography (PET),[31] magnetic resonance imaging (MRI),[32–34] or electron paramagnetic resonance oxygen imaging (recently reviewed in Colliez et al.[35]). The resolution of these imaging modalities will be critical.[36]

More recent studies have shown that acute fluctuations in tumor oxygenation ("transient" or "cycling" hypoxia) interspersed with periods of reoxygenation may be even more effective in promoting tumor survival and progression than chronic hypoxia.[37] A third type of hypoxia, termed "longitudinal hypoxia," has also been proposed, which occurs as a gradient along the length of tumor vessels.[38] Defining the relative contributions of these hypoxia mechanisms to radiobiologic responses is ongoing; however, it is likely that all could contribute to resistance. It is clear that cycling hypoxia may complicate efforts to identify and target radiobiologically important hypoxic regions within tumors using approaches such as radiation dose painting to hypoxic tumor subregions.[39] Cycling hypoxia is more difficult to image using current methods, such as nitroimidazole markers, which are better suited to detecting chronic hypoxia. Developments in imaging hypoxia with MRI and electron paramagnetic resonance may facilitate real-time detection of transient hypoxia in the future.

Hypoxic Cell Sensitizers and Cytotoxins

Targeting hypoxic cells should improve outcome in frequently hypoxic tumors. Nimorazole, a nitroimidazole hypoxic cell sensitizer has shown promising results when used with radiotherapy in patients with hypoxic tumors.[40,41] However, testing and adoption of this drug in countries other than Denmark have been limited. The alternative approach of using hypoxic cell cytotoxins has also been tested. Tirapazamine (TPZ, 3-amino-1,2,4-benzotriazine-1,4-dioxide) undergoes reduction under hypoxia to form a highly reactive radical that causes DNA damage leading to cell killing.[42] Under normoxic conditions, the reduction of nitroimidazoles and TPZ is reversed, thus providing the specificity for hypoxic tissues.[43,44] Despite promising early results, phase III testing of TPZ in combination with chemoradiotherapy failed to demonstrate improvement in failure-free survival, time to locoregional failure, or quality of life among patients with head and neck cancers.[45] However, patients in this trial were not selected for tumor hypoxia, and other treatment concerns were subsequently raised.[46] Development of new generation hypoxic cell cytotoxins with greater preclinical efficacy than TPZ is under way.[47] It will be crucial in future tests of hypoxia-targeting agents to select or stratify patients based on their tumor oxygenation status.[48]

The identification and selective treatment of hypoxic tumors may, in the future, enhance the results of radiotherapy. Novel imaging methods to identify hypoxia and new generation hypoxic cytotoxins and sensitizers will benefit this approach. In addition, hypoxia has been recently shown to impart susceptibility to DNA damage response inhibitors, as it down-regulates components of the homologous recombination (HR) DNA damage repair machinery.[49,50] Exploiting this finding in the context of radiotherapy with PARP or other HR inhibitors could prove effective for better elimination of otherwise resistant hypoxic tumor cells. The history and possible paths forward in exploiting hypoxia as a clinical target with a focus on lung cancer were recently reviewed.[51]

Tumor Angiogenesis and Antiangiogenic Approaches

Normal angiogenesis is a highly regulated process involving endothelial cells with differing functions (tip, stalk, and phalanx cells) under tight regulation of oxygen sensors (prolyl-hydroxylase-2 [PHD-2]), growth and maturation factors (vascular endothelial growth factor [VEGF], angiopoietins), and transmembrane receptors (Notch family) (reviewed in Carmeliet et al.[52]). Small changes or imbalance in the expression of these regulators can have a significant impact on vascular development and lead to the formation of abnormal tumor vessels that are inefficient in the transport of nutrients, oxygen, and metabolic wastes. Limited perfusion and convection also reduce the efficacy of chemotherapeutic delivery. Vascular endothelial cells, unlike tumor cells, are genetically stable and thus an attractive target. Antiangiogenic agents reduce or cut off tumor vascular flow by selective targeting of tumor vessel growth by blocking VEGF signaling. Targeting the tumor vasculature was originally proposed by Judah Folkman.[53] It is now clear, however, that this approach is complicated by the fact that development, structure, and the potential for recovery of tumor vasculature after treatment are influenced by bone marrow–derived progenitor cells in addition to the tumor and other stromal elements.[54] In addition, where tumor cell–derived vascular channeling (vasculogenic mimicry) plays a role in tumor circulation the effects of antiangiogenic strategies that target host vascular endothelial cells may not be as effective.[55]

VEGF can be induced in response to radiation, and inhibition of VEGF can increase tumor control after radiation in preclinical models.[56] VEGF receptor inhibition reduces endothelial cell proliferation *in vitro* after irradiation and also reduces microvessel density in irradiated tumors.[57] Clinical trials have suggested a potential benefit in combining radiation and antiangiogenic therapy in rectal cancer and sarcoma.[58,59] However, the toxicity of bevacizumab in combination with radiotherapy has been of concern in some tumors.[60]

Vascular normalization is a term coined to denote transient changes observed in tumor vessels after VEGF inhibition with a VEGF receptor-2 antibody.[60] Other antiangiogenic approaches have shown similar morphologic effects on tumor vasculature. Methylselenocysteine, which has antiangiogenic activity, has been shown to induce a more mature morphology in FaDu xenograft tumor vessels, accompanied by enhanced perfusion and a fourfold increase in doxorubicin delivery to treated tumors.[61] Normalization is characterized by a reduction in the chaotic branching and tortuosity of tumor vessels and is accompanied by a reduction in tumor hypoxia and enhanced radiosensitivity. The effects of vascular normalization may also involve reduction of tumor interstitial fluid pressure. High tumor interstitial fluid pressure has been shown to impact survival after irradiation and may also be influenced by the tumor stroma.[62] Tong et al.[63] have shown that blocking VEGF signaling results in decreased interstitial fluid pressure in tumor xenografts in mice. Although the normalization period offers an opportunity for improved response to radiation and chemotherapy, the period of normalization obtained with direct targeting of VEGF signaling in preclinical studies lasts less than a week, followed by vascular insufficiency. In addition, vascular normalization may not occur in all tumors and has not been observed in all studies (reviewed in Horsman and Siemann[64]). In the clinical setting, vascular normalization has been proposed as a predictive marker in patients undergoing cediranib (VEGF inhibitor) treatment for recurrent glioblastoma.[65] Elevated blood perfusion after cediranib treatment has recently been associated with increased survival in these patients.[66]

More durable normalization of tumor vasculature might be clinically achievable through growth factor or oncogenic signaling inhibition. Studies have shown changes in vascular morphology, function, and maturation accompanied by decreased tumor hypoxia after inhibition targeting epidermal growth factor (EGF) receptor, RAS, phosphoinositide (PI) 3-kinase, or AKT in human tumor xenografts and spontaneous mouse tumors that last up to 2 weeks.[67] Others have shown that blocking EGF signaling increased tumor uptake of cisplatin at the same time that enhanced vascular function and oxygenation were seen in tumor xenografts.[68] Signaling inhibition in these studies decreased, but did not eliminate, VEGF production by tumors, which might account for the effects seen and their duration.

Other approaches to altering tumor vasculature are being investigated. Inhibition of $\alpha(v)\beta(3)/\alpha(v)\beta(5)$ integrin has been reported to cause effects similar to signaling inhibition on tumor vascular morphology.[69] Using another approach, investigators showed that shutting off NOS1 production in U87 glioblastoma tumors restored a nitric oxide gradient around the tumor vessels. This was accompanied by a normalized phenotype with less tortuous and more abundant vessels that had increased perivascular cell coverage.[70] Hypoxia in these tumors was reduced and their response to radiation increased as measured by both relative tumor volume and survival endpoints. Modulation of host PHD-2 can affect tumor vascular structure and maturity.[71] Inhibitors of PHD-2, such as dimethyloxaloylglycine (DMOG), might be developed for clinical application. More recently, the interaction between T cells and tumor vasculature has been studied in the context of immunotherapy. Interferon-beta (INF-β) produced by T-helper type 1 cells has been shown to promote vascular normalization, which in turn facilitates T-effector functions.[72]

Inhibition of Vasculogenesis

Vasculogenesis, unlike angiogenesis, recruits cells from distant sites, including the bone marrow, to participate in the formation of new blood vessels (reviewed in Patenaude et al.[73]). The process is thought to be an important contributor to the tumor vasculature, although the precise contribution of the different recruited cell types is still a matter of debate.[54] The CD11b-positive, matrix metalloproteinase-9 (MMP-9) expressing myeloid cells appear to be central to this process.[74] A neutralizing antibody to CD11b inhibited the recruitment of myeloid cells to tumors and prolonged radiation-induced regrowth delay. Additionally, mice with reduced CD11b expression showed enhanced xenograft radiosensitivity.[75] Stromal derived factor-1 (SDF-1) and the chemokine receptor CXCR4 also contribute to recruitment of endothelial cell precursors and could be targeted. Inhibition of the CXCR4/ SDF-1 interaction reduced bone marrow–derived progenitor cell recruitment into irradiated glioblastoma orthotopic xenografts and slowed tumor regrowth.[76] An inhibitor of CXCR4 activation by SDF1, AMD3100 (plerixafor), is in clinical use for stem cell mobilization and could be quickly adopted for this purpose. This drug has been shown to have promising effects in chemoradiotherapy for cervical cancer.[77]

Antivascular Therapy

Selectively destroying tumor vasculature with vascular disrupting agents (VDAs) is an approach that seeks to kill tumors by shutting off their blood supplies (reviewed in McKeage and Baguley[78]). This approach, however, acts primarily on the tumor core and does not eradicate host vessels that border the tumor and are in proximity of normal host vasculature. Tumor cells at the host–tumor interface can remain viable after this treatment to repopulate the tumor. Furthermore, vascular disruption could generate areas of hypoxia that still contain viable tumor cells, thereby selecting for more resistant clones.[12] Combining VDA treatment with a cytotoxic modality could overcome this problem. The effects of VDAs both alone and in combination with antiangiogenics, chemotherapy, radiation, or other modalities have been examined in a number of preclinical studies (reviewed by Horsman and Siemann[64]). VDAs are currently in phase II to III clinical trials alone or in combination with cytotoxic chemotherapies.[79]

Tumor Stroma and Extracellular Matrix

The tumor stromal compartment, including the extracellular matrix, host fibroblasts, and immune cells, is known to contribute to tumor progression and survival.[80,81] In certain tumors, like pancreatic cancers, activation of quiescent stromal cells, known as stellate cells, to myofibroblast-like cells involved in extracellular matrix production contributes significantly to tumor progression.[82] Activated fibroblasts deposit collagens, leading to changes in stromal rigidity. Stromal rigidity can impact both transformation and progression.[83] This mechanism of stromal-induced tumor promotion includes intercellular signaling initiation via integrins to prosurvival pathways, including PI3-kinase.[84]

There are multiple points at which stromal changes can be inhibited, including inhibition of fibroblast or stellate cell activation by angiotensin-converting enzyme (ACE) inhibitors or other antifibrogenic compounds such as halofuginone.[85] This class of agents can also protect from normal tissue fibrosis and inhibit tumor growth factor-β (TGF-β).[86,87] Signaling by the cytokine TGF-β strongly promotes fibrosis, both in response to tumor growth and in normal tissues in response to treatment with radiation. Direct inhibition of TGF-β in tumors can interrupt or mitigate desmoplasia and reduce tumor growth.[88] Angiotensin-II (Ang II) can promote stellate cell growth under pathologic conditions, and ACE inhibitors act in part through blocking Ang II.[89] Angiotensin-(1-7), an endogenous 7 amino acid peptide antagonist of Ang II, has been shown to reduce TGF-β expression, block proliferation of cancer-associated fibroblasts, and inhibit tumor growth.[90] Inhibition of hedgehog pathway signaling is another approach that has been tested in pancreatic cancer mouse models,[91] but there is controversy surrounding the role of hedgehog signaling in pancreatic and other cancers.[92]

Integrin binding and signaling have been identified as a potential target for cancer treatment, as these receptors are involved in tumor growth and angiogenesis (reviewed in Desgrosellier and Cheresh[93]) as well as therapy resistance.[94] Cilengitide is a pentapeptide mimic of the RGD binding site that blocks $\alpha(v)\beta3$ and $\alpha(v)\beta(5)$ integrin binding to extracellular matrix components.[95] In addition to its antiangiogenic activity, it inhibits focal adhesion kinase signaling.[96] Cilengitide is well tolerated and has some antitumor activity as a single agent.[97] It has been shown to be active in combination with radiation in several, but not in all reports.[98-100] However, questions remain about potential normal tissue toxicity in combined modality treatment because integrin signaling is required for normal cell function and survival.[98] A phase III trial of cilengitide with temozolomide radiotherapy for GBM saw no unanticipated toxicities but failed to meet its endpoints.[101] There are currently (2017) no open trials of this agent listed in Clinicaltrials. gov, but integrin targeting remains an active area of research.

Targeting Stem Cells

The CSCs model is currently used to as a framework for understanding cancer proliferation, growth, and treatment resistance (reviewed in Bednar and Simeone[102]). CSCs are thought to be a subset of cells at the peak of a developmental chain within a tumor with the capacity for unlimited self-renewal and lineage plasticity.[103] These cells give rise to more differentiated daughter cells with less replicative and tumorigenic potential that make up the bulk of the tumor cell population. The CSC may be more quiescent than the general population of cells in a tumor and relatively resistant to cytotoxic therapy.[104,105] Some studies have identified perivascular niches for these cells[106,107] and the conditions that promote their colonization and survival,[10] but the identification of both the stem cells and their niches in a disorganized and dynamic tumor environment remains challenging.[108] The perivascular niche and, in particular, the endothelial cells may both aid in tissue repair and promote tumor growth by secreting "angiocrine factors."[109] Targeting these factors could be an approach to cancer treatment. Disruption of the perivascular niche with VDAs or antiangiogenics might also reduce CSC numbers. The potential for CSCs as targets and potential biomarkers for radiotherapy has recently been reviewed by Krause et al.[110]

Recent work indicates a novel potential target within the tumor stroma, fibroblast activation protein, which has the potential to enhance innate antitumor immune responses. In a transgenic mouse model, the elimination (through genetic manipulation) of fibroblasts and pericytes expressing fibroblast activation protein enhanced antitumor immune responses. Activation of tumor-infiltrating T cells and the resulting increase in interferon-γ and tumor necrosis factor-α (TNF-α) promoted the antitumor immune response in a transgenic mouse model.[111] A possible pharmacologic approach to elimination of these activated fibroblasts is by inhibition of the matrix enzyme lysyl oxidase-like-2 (LOXL-2). Inhibition of this enzyme using a monoclonal antibody decreased desmoplasia

and both primary and metastatic tumor growth[112]; small molecule inhibitors of this enzyme also exist. Targeting lysyl oxidase (LOX), which has been shown to promote tumor growth in orthotopic and spontaneous mouse tumor models, might also be a means of inhibiting tumor growth.[84]

Summary of Microenvironment

It is not possible to predict exactly how radiotherapy will evolve in its utilization of knowledge regarding the tumor microenvironment and host–tumor interactions. What appears clear is that increasing emphasis will be placed on these factors. Targeting changes specific to the microenvironment has the advantage of being largely tumor specific and potentially less toxic than cytocidal therapies. Future developments may allow for hypoxic tumor region dose painting. Alternatively, hypoxia-targeting drugs may finally reach clinical maturity. Inhibition of hypoxia in tumors may also arise from strategies that revert tumor vasculature to a more normal morphology and function. This strategy has the added advantage of reducing hypoxia selection for aggressive tumor clones and enhancing chemotherapy delivery. The impact of the immune response on tumors and in turn the effects of different radiotherapeutic interventions on immunity are now being exploited with the explosion of trials combining checkpoint inhibitors and radiation (see the next section). Findings relating to the impact of host stromal elements on tumor cell radiation survival through direct intercellular signaling, autocrine stimulation, or mechanical force may also soon reveal new targets and interventions applicable to radiotherapy.

In addition to the host and tumor microenvironment, external environmental factors may also play a role in response to therapy. These have yet to be fully evaluated or exploited. Temperature (hyperthermia) is well known to impact radiation response,[113-115] but its evaluation and clinical application, at least in the United States, has lagged. Conversely, preclinical studies have shown that lower ambient temperatures can induce resistance to cytotoxic therapies[116] and influence both tumor growth and immune responses.[117] The impact of time of day of treatment and the role of circadian clock proteins is another understudied area that could be exploited.[118] Preclinical work points to the possibility that the clock proteins influence tumor radiosensitivity.[119] There are indications from clinical studies that both toxicity and treatment failure could be impacted by the time of irradiation, but the data are not yet conclusive.[120] At a minimum, the further study of these factors could inform preclinical study conditions and perhaps enhance translation and reproducibility of results.

Combining agents that alter the tumor environment with radiotherapy requires strong preclinical data demonstrating at least additive effect and acceptable toxicities. Careful preclinical testing, including normal tissue response evaluation, may avoid subsequent problems in many instances. Having markers and imaging that detect the targets of interventions, such as hypoxia, cancer-associated fibroblasts, or immune-infiltrating cells, and that can be used to assess intervention-mediated changes in the environment will be critical to fully exploiting this approach. Recent developments in the analysis of circulating tumor cells and cell-free DNA may revolutionize treatment monitoring as discussed later in this chapter.

Immunomodulating Events in Response to Ionizing Radiation

The surge in interest in immunotherapy for cancer offers an opportunity for radiation oncology and radiation biology to play central roles in the development and delivery of this aspect of precision medicine. The tumor microenvironment harbors clones that can escape from immune editing and surveillance processes. These processes are regulated by several cytokines and checkpoint proteins. Ionizing radiation (RT) causes changes in the tumor microenvironment that can lead to intratumoral as well as distal immune modulation (the so-called abscopal effect). Tumor-associated antigens (TAAs) are released by irradiated dying cancer cells triggering danger signals such as heat shock protein (Hsp), HMGB1, and calreticulin ("eat-me" signal for phagocytes). These TAAs and cell debris are taken up by phagocytes such as macrophages, neutrophils, and dendritic cells for antigen processing and presentation. At the same time, RT can induce increased expression of tumor antigens and MHC class I molecules on tumor cells. Consequently, activated antigen-presenting cells (APCs) migrate to the draining lymph node, further mature upon encountering T helper cells, and release interferons (IFNs) and IL-12/18 to stimulate Th₁ responses that support the differentiation and proliferation of antigen-specific CTLs. Activated antigen-specific CTLs traffic systemically from the draining lymph node to infiltrate and lyse cells in primary as well as distal tumors. Concomitantly, tumor irradiation can also recruit immunosuppressive cells into the tumor microenvironment and induce expression of certain negative stimulatory molecules on T cells and tumor cells (CTLA-4, PD-1, PDL1) that can curtail the activation of T cells leading to an immunosuppressive environment. Other immunosuppressive function of radiation can occur through induction IL-10 and TGF-β (Fig. 5.1).[121–123] These immunomodulating events can also impact tumor growth at a distance from the irradiated tumor site, the "abscopal effect," that is mostly immune, and in certain instances, it can be non–immune mediated through ceramide signaling.

Harnessing Radiation Modulation of the Immune Response

Several factors can influence the ability of radiation to enhance immunotherapy, including (a) the dose of radiation per fraction and the number of fractions and (b) the volume of the irradiated tumor tissue and target location. However, the impact of these variables is not well understood. Historical evidence and recent literature point out that radiation doses at opposite ends of the dose spectrum induce robust immune activation.[124,125] For the sake of clarity, this section divides three dose ranges, low-dose RT (0.1 to 1 Gy), high-dose RT including ablation (8 Gy and above), and clinically relevant dose (1.8 to 2.2 Gy), to define immune modulation events and how these events can be harnessed with cancer immunotherapy.

Low-Dose Radiation

At low doses of radiation from 0.1 to 1 Gy, immune activation is achieved by increased Th1 response that attract naïve T cells and promote its differentiation and activation.[126] Because the D_{10} for CD4+/CD8+ lymphocytes ranges from 3.32 to 3.84 Gy,[127,128] low-dose chronic and acute irradiation stimulate enhanced immune function leading to in situ vaccination, trafficking, infiltration, and killing. Low-dose radiation at 0.5 Gy is associated with greatest number of infiltrating T cells with a decline at >1 Gy, and this was accompanied with redirecting macrophage differentiation from a "tumor-promoting/immunosuppressive state" to one that enables cytotoxic T lymphocytes

FIGURE 5.1. A schematic view of radiotherapy-induced immune modulations. #1, Tumor-associated antigens are released by irradiated dying cancer cells. TAAs and cell debris are engulfed in the tumor microenvironment by phagocytes such as macrophages, neutrophils, and dendritic cells for antigen processing and presentation. #2, Radiotherapy-induced cell death releases danger signals, including HSP, HMGB1, and calreticulin ("eat-me" signal for phagocytes). #3, Radiotherapy induces increased expression of tumor antigens and MHC class I molecules on tumor cells. #4, Radiotherapy-induced T-cell activation increases expression of negative stimulatory molecules such as CTLA-4. #5, Certain radiation doses may increase tumor production/secretion of immunosuppressive cytokines such as IL-10 and TGF-β. #6, Activated APCs migrate to the draining lymph node, further mature upon encountering TH cells, and release IFNs and IL-12/18 to stimulate TH1 responses that support the differentiation and proliferation of antigen-specific CTLs. Activated antigen-specific CTLs traffic systematically from the draining lymph node to infiltrate and lyse primary and distal tumors. RT, radiotherapy. (Reprinted from Ahmed MM, Hodge JW, Guha C, et al. Harnessing the potential of radiation-induced immune modulation for cancer therapy. *Cancer Immunol Res* 2013;1[5]:280–284. Copyright © 2013 American Association for Cancer Research. With permission from AACR.)

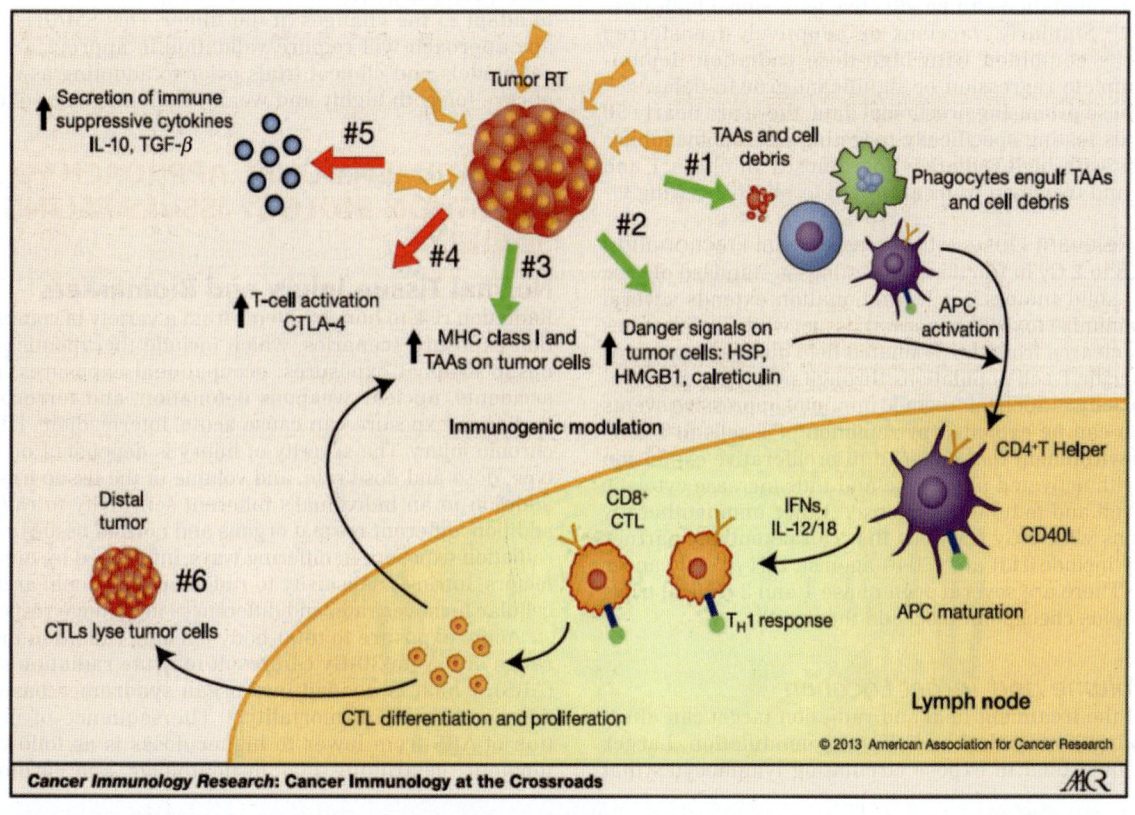

Cancer Immunology Research: Cancer Immunology at the Crossroads

to infiltrate tumors and kill cancer cells.[129] Moreover, low-dose RT causes an increase in homing of activated T cells[129] in tumor milieu unlocking the barriers of cancer immunotherapy. Furthermore, tumor cells when irradiated with 1 Gy fractions can robustly activate immune gene program[130] that can be conducive for trafficking and homing of T cells that is similar to antimicrobial/inflammatory response. All these immune modulation conditions can be harnessed with drugs that augment dendritic cell maturation such as TLR or CD40 agonist or IFN-β to further intensify antitumor immunity effects.[125] Kinetics of immune gene activation in tumor cells treated with 1 Gy multifraction demonstrates that the opportunistic widow (inflection point) to exploit the maximal immune function for adjuvant immunotherapy is around 6 to 10 Gy total dose.[130] Cancer vaccines and adoptive T-cell therapy could boost radiation-induced in situ vaccination.[125] Furthermore, agonistic antibodies directed against costimulatory/coinhibitory molecules on T cells can synergize an increase in T-cell function.[125] Even though there are many preclinical studies to support the above low-dose RT combinations with immunotherapy, there is currently only one clinical trial that is opened by NCI CTEP utilizing 0.5 Gy bid fractions with dual checkpoint inhibitor in NSCLC and metastatic colorectal cancer (NCT02888743).

High-Dose Radiation

With radiation doses of 8 Gy and above in single or multiple fractions, TAAs initiate DAMPs to release IFNs to help mature T-cell differentiation and activation leading to immunogenic cell death and antitumor immunity with a potential to significantly increase the incidence of distal (so-called abscopal) effects.[131] These events lead to T-cell priming, trafficking, infiltration, *in situ* vaccination, and immunogenic killing.[125] The immune modulation events by high-dose RT can be exploited to enhance immunotherapeutic efficacy by activating T cells using antibodies targeted against coinhibitory T-cell receptors/ligands such as PD-1/PD-L1 and TIM-3 and TGF-β and LAG-3 blockers.[125] In several preclinical tumor models, efficacy of immune checkpoint-targeted therapies improved when combined with high-dose radiation.[132] Significant downregulation of PDL-1 was observed in tumor cells treated with single fraction of 10 Gy but not with multifraction, and hence, anti-PDL1 combination can be effective with single high-dose treatment.[130] Similarly, vaccines or adoptively transferred CD8+ T cells combined with high-dose radiation demonstrated complete regression or significant growth delay.[133,134] Based on these promising preclinical data, there are nearly 50 clinical trials testing specifically targeting checkpoint inhibitor proteins with high radiation dose, mostly in phase 1 and 2 settings, and two open trials are there in phase 3 setting.[135]

Clinically Relevant Dose with Conventional Fractionation

Doses at 1.8 to 2 Gy in fractionated settings is standard of care for several solid tumors. Such fractionation extends several weeks to minimize toxicity to normal tissue, while lymphocytes are rapidly cleared from the irradiated field diminishing tumor antigen-specific T-cell populations through persistent site-specific cytotoxicity.[136] Such tolerogenic immunosuppressive events of radiation can be exploited by repletion of T cells in T-cell–deficient environment that can lead to proliferative expansion of T cells with activated phenotype and thus increase cytolytic activity to self and to tumor antigens.[136] Other immunotherapy combinations with 2 Gy fractions that can potentially partner for synergy include TLR and CD40 agonist, IFN-β, and cancer vaccines.[125] There are several open phase 1 and 2 clinical trials with EBRT plus checkpoint blockade therapy.[135]

Tumor Volume and Target Location

The size of the treatment field and radiation target can affect the exploiting potential of radioimmunomodulation. Larger treatment field tend to expose circulating lymphocytes that can impact proliferating T cells and T-cell priming in draining lymph nodes. This is similar to protracted RT regimens that are lymphotoxic, which may lead to T-cell clearance and lymphopenia.[137,138] To protect lymphocytes and T cells and reduce lymphopenia, one can adopt strategies such as reducing the treatment field size, shortening beam-on treatment times, hypofractionation,[135] and lattice radiotherapy.[139,140]

Another important facet to consider when it comes to combining RT with immunotherapy is the site of radiation. As abscopal responses have been observed during irradiation of bone metastasis, there are reports to demonstrate that such abscopal events can result more from irradiation of visceral metastases.[141] This is supported by a recently failed phase 3 trial when single fraction of 8 Gy with anti-CTLA-4 to osseous metastasis.[142]

SMART Radiotherapy in Context of Immune Modulation and Immunotherapy

Current evidence indicates that either low-dose radiation or high-dose ablative radiotherapy can elicit immune stimulation more robustly than standard clinical regimens of fractionated radiotherapy. This is an area that requires further study and experimental validation. Based on the results to date, a potentially effective smart radiotherapy schema to boost immune response might be a preboost high-dose or ablative dose with single or less than three fractions directed toward partial treatment volume to trigger in situ vaccination, T-cell priming, trafficking, infiltration, and immunogenic killing. This would be followed by low-dose radiotherapy with 0.5 to 1 Gy fraction directed toward gross tumor volume to increase Th1-type response and facilitate the homing of activated T cells. At this time, dual checkpoint blockade immunotherapy can be effective in differentiation and proliferation of CTLs and to reactivate T-effector cells. Perhaps the most important point is that radiotherapy will best be used as a "drug," which may mean varying the dose, fractionation, and target during a course of treatment to achieve the desired effect. The "one-size-fits-all" thinking is not an appropriate approach as it could lead to a lack of success by virtue of the wrong choice and not allow for the thoughtful development of the field. Biomarkers of response including circulating molecules or cells, imaging, and tumor sampling may be critical along the course of treatment to adapt to the changes in the tumor. This SMART radiotherapy approach will require validation in appropriate preclinical models and clinical trials prior to adopting as a standard of care for both highly and weakly immunogenic solid tumors.

MULTIDIMENSIONAL APPROACH TO ALL RADIATION BIOLOGY ISSUES FACING SOCIETY

Normal Tissue Injury and Biomarkers

Radiation risk to humans stems from a variety of complex radiation exposure scenarios, which include therapeutic and diagnostic medical exposures, occupational exposures, radiation accidents, nuclear weapons detonation, and terrorist events. Radiation exposure can cause acute, intermediate, late, and/or chronic injury. The severity of injury is dependent on radiation type, dose and dose rate, and volume of the tissue irradiated in addition to an individual's inherent sensitivity to radiation. In addition, different normal organs and normal tissues respond to radiation exposure in differing ways, influenced by, among other factors, intrinsic sensitivity to radiation, functional architecture, cellular turnover rate, and differences in damage response.

Acute exposure to total-body ionizing radiation in the dose range of 0.5- to 30-Gy can result in acute radiation syndrome (ARS), which is divided into organ syndromes based on the dose and cause of mortality.[143] The sequence of manifestation of ARS from lower to higher doses is as follows: hematopoietic, gastrointestinal, dermatologic, and cardiovascular and neurologic. However, syndromes overlap. For example, damage to the gastrointestinal or dermatologic systems can impact the outcome of hematologic syndrome at sublethal doses. Bioindicators or biomarkers of radiation exposure, even in the lower dose range, can reflect a response by multiple organs, all of which sense and respond to the radiation.[144]

At radiation doses below 0.5-Gy, acute effects are not observed but the probability of late effects such as cancer and hereditary effects begin to occur.[145] The possibility of exposure of a large number of people to radiation following a nuclear incident has raised the public's concerns about the increase in the chances of developing radiation-induced cancers.[146] However, public perception and "fear of radiation" appear to be well beyond the actual risk. This fear was elevated as a consequence of the Fukushima disaster, despite the lack of evidence for acute radiologic injury in the general population.[147] Quantifying the risk associated with low-level radiation exposures is problematic and uncertain because of the unresolved shape of the dose–response curve for radiation-induced cancer in the low-dose region.[148] For the purposes of radiation protection, it is assumed that there is a linear relationship between exposure and future cancer risk. A linear no-threshold (LNT) model is used to assess risk at doses below 100 mSv, recognizing that epidemiologic information in this dose region cannot unambiguously support or refute the model assumptions.[149] However, recent data from the Radiation Effects Research Foundation (RERF, Japan) seem to be more in line with a linear relationship between radiation dose and cancer risk.[150] Evidence is also now emerging on the possibility of additional late developing effects on health following somewhat higher doses, such as cardiovascular[151] and respiratory disease,[152] premature senescence,[153] and damage to endothelial cells.[154]

A multidimensional approach is necessary to address the complexity of the radiobiologic issues facing society. Various agencies of the U.S. government have been conducting studies on radiation-induced normal tissue injury and developing medical countermeasures (MCMs) to mitigate a multitude of risks to individuals or populations associated with radiation exposures, addressing different dose ranges relevant to an agency's mission. Successful development of risk mitigation strategies requires a multidimensional approach with mechanistic scientific underpinnings to address the complex biologic variables. A summary of ongoing research efforts among various government agencies related to radiation-induced normal tissue injury is summarized in Figure 5.2.

The Department of Energy (DoE) under the Biological Systems Sciences Division studies radiation-related health risks from exposures to low levels of radiation. Exposures to low doses can occur in a number of scenarios including (a) around nuclear power plants, (b) during isolation of materials for nuclear weapons and nuclear power production and waste cleanup, (c) medical diagnostic exposures, (d) radiation terrorism incidents, etc. The DoE's low-dose program (now closed) focused on cellular and molecular responses to doses relevant to workplace exposure limits, radioadaptive responses, genetics of interindividual variation, low-dose and dose-rate effects, effects on immune system, and epigenetic regulations.

FIGURE 5.2. U.S. government research efforts among various government agencies related to radiation-induced normal tissue injury. AFRRI, Armed Forces Radiobiology Research Institute; ARS, acute radiation syndrome; BARDA, Biomedical Advanced Research and Development Authority; CMCRC, Center for Medical Countermeasures against Radiation Consortium; CNS, central nervous system; DEARE, Delayed Effects of Acute Radiation Exposure; DoD, Department of Defense; DoE, Department of Energy; GCR, galactic cosmic rays; HRP, Human Research Program; HZE, High (H) Atomic number (Z) and Energy (E); NASA, National Aeronautics and Space Administration; NCI, National Cancer Institute; NIAID, National Institute of Allergy and Infectious Diseases; NSBRI, National Space Biomedical Research Institute; NSRL, National Space Radiation Laboratory; RNCP, Radiation and Nuclear Countermeasures Program; SMART, **S**ocietal focused, **M**olecularly aware, **A**ltruistic, **R**esearch supportive, and wary of **T**echnological solutions to biologic problems; TRI, Translational Research Institute (also known as The Translational Research Institute for Space Health [TRISH]).

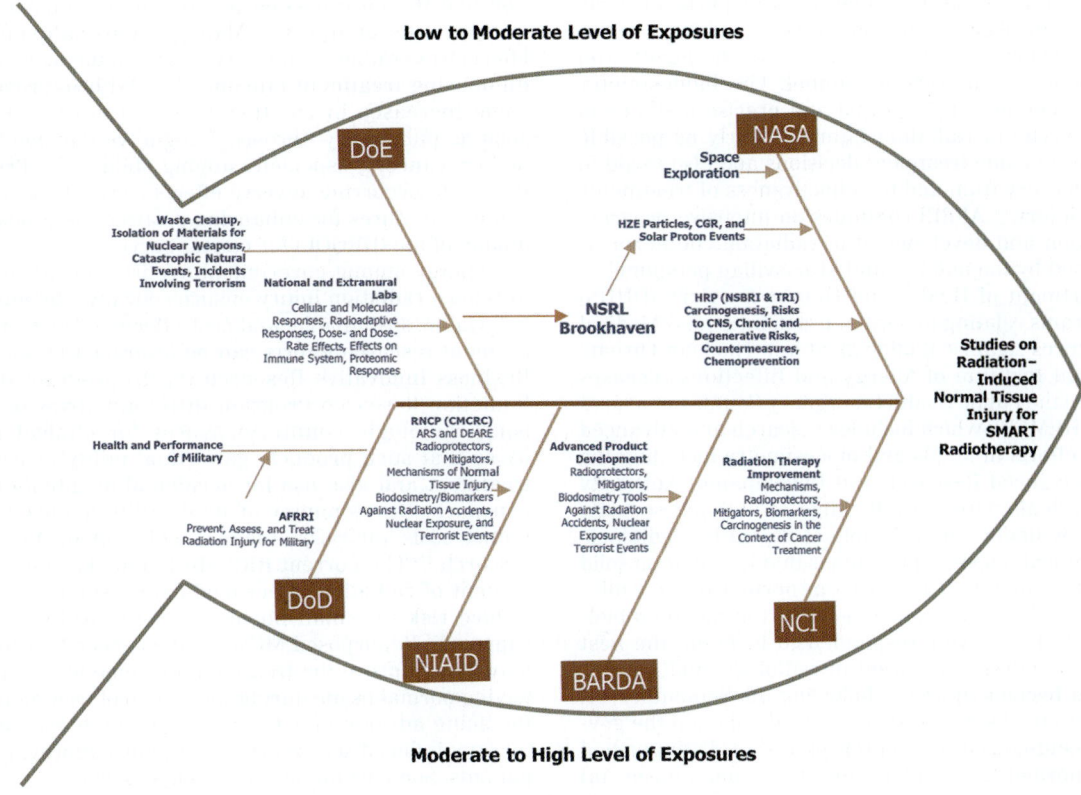

NASA's interest in radiation research focuses on space exploration including earth orbits and more recently potential manned missions to Mars and beyond. The duration of Mars mission necessitates understanding immediate health risks in the space radiation environment and long-term postmission quality of life. The Human Research Program (HRP) was developed to refocus the space program in early 2004. NASA identified major risk categories attributable to space radiation including carcinogenesis,[155] risks to central nervous system (CNS),[156] and chronic and degenerative tissue risks.[157] High charge and energy ion components of galactic cosmic radiation (CGR) can cause genetic mutations,[158] inflammation, and CNS structural damage and dysfunction.[159] The HRP is focused on understanding the possibility of reducing these health risks by developing countermeasures for acute exposures of greater than one Gy associated with large solar particle events, and mitigators for lower-level exposures, particularly iron ions that will be encountered in the Mars mission. NASA's National Space Biomedical Research Institute (NSBRI) conducts integrated biomedical research to support long-term human presence during exploration of space and also on the enhancement of life on earth by applying these advances. The NASA Translational Research Institute was founded in 2016 to work in partnership with the HRP to translate cutting-edge terrestrial research into applications for space flight focusing on human risk mitigation strategies for exploratory missions. Teaming up with Department of Energy's Office of Science, NASA has established National Space Radiation Laboratory (NSRL) at the Brookhaven National Laboratory. NSRL makes use of the Brookhaven ion beam facilities to enhance understanding of the link between radiation and cellular damage and also seeks approaches to limit the damage to the healthy tissues by cosmic radiation in a simulated space radiation environment. NSRL uses beams of heavy ions extracted from Brookhaven's booster accelerator to simulate cosmic rays found in space environment. NSRL has a beam line dedicated to radiobiology research. These studies are also relevant in particle therapy research for cancer treatment.

The Armed Forces Radiobiology Research Institute (AFRRI), within the Department of Defense (DoD), conducts basic and applied research to identify and perform early development of measures to prevent, assess, and treat radiation injury in order to preserve and protect the health and performance of U.S. military personnel. The biodosimetry program has been developing rapid and precise methods to assess the severity of radiation injury as early as possible after the event to guide treatment decisions and also to aid in monitoring recovery from and the effectiveness of treatments for radiation injury.[160] AFRRI continues an intensive program on identification and development of radiation countermeasures to be used by the military and also civilian personnel.

The Department of Health and Human Services (DHHS) has two programs relating to normal tissue injury: (a) Medical Countermeasures Against Radiological and Nuclear Threats at the National Institute of Allergy and Infectious Diseases (NIAID) and (b) the Public Health Emergency Countermeasures Enterprise (PHEMCE), which includes research and advanced development efforts in MCMs and biodosimetry including the Biomedical Advanced Research and Development Authority (BARDA) that deals with the full range of national security threats.[161] A key underlying principle of the entire radiologic or nuclear medical response program is that it is built on solid scientific underpinnings.[161] Research in normal tissue radiation biology received a substantial boost as the radiation biology community proactively responded to bringing the best science to help address the threat of radiologic and nuclear terrorism that became apparent following the September 11, 2001, terrorist attacks. Scientists from academia and the government conceptualized a research plan that distinguished modifiers of normal tissue injury into three time phases: (a)

protectors that are administered before radiation, (b) mitigators that are used following radiation exposure but before the damage has been fully manifest, and (c) treatment that is given for established radiation injury.[162] Some agents may function in more than one role. The radiologic or nuclear incident research plan includes the broad categories of (a) MCMs, which are drugs or biologics developed as radiation mitigators, (b) biomarkers that can quantify an individual's radiation dose as a guide to treatment, and (c) agents that serve to reduce the exposure to internalized radionuclides by blocking uptake or enhancing excretion. The medical consequences of interest are those that result from a total-body exposure (or significant partial-body exposure) of a dose that can produce ARS.[144] A radiologic or nuclear incident will be a "no-notice" event, and for a large-scale nuclear incident, the requirement for an MCM is that it should be effective if started up to 24 hours after radiation.[163,164] A longer window of opportunity would be better given the chaos of the situation and that is part of the MCM development effort. What is not often appreciated is the concept of latency between exposure and clinical manifestation of radiation injury. To that end, there are two terms used to convey the concept: ARS and Delayed Effects of Acute Radiation Exposure (DEARE). The development of next generation of MCMs will exploit the evolving understandings on mechanisms by which radiation induces injury in normal tissue and its manifestation over time, from acute to DEARE to long-term late effects. The challenges to employing radioprotectors to reduce normal tissue injury during the course of radiotherapy are different. Here, a major concern is the protection of the tumor itself, which would result in a compromised therapeutic benefit.

NCI's Radiation Research Program (RRP) has been supporting studies of normal tissue injury in the context of radiation therapy for several decades. In the clinical context, a radioprotective drug might allow dose escalation to the tumor, leading to a better tumor control or to same local control with less toxicity. Although many novel approaches of dose delivery to the tumor volume significantly reduce collateral normal tissue injury and improve the therapeutic ratio, location of the tumor within an organ of inherent sensitivity to radiation and the dose needed to cure the tumor can still result in normal tissue injury.[162] Many patients still suffer adverse effects from radiotherapy, largely due to the biologic variables influencing treatment outcome.[165,166] With improved survival come increases in treatment-related adverse late effects, such as pulmonary fibrosis,[167] cognitive damage,[168] and secondary cancers, especially among children.[169] Prevention of these late-occurring adverse effects warrants development of countermeasures for enhancing posttreatment health-related quality of life (HRQOL) for cancer survivors.

Synergy among government agencies in supporting drugs to reduce radiation injury ensures our investments are rational, viable, sustainable, and cost-effective. Academic and government research efforts can be leveraged by the NCI Small Business Innovative Research (SBIR) program through the Radiation Research Program (RRP) initiatives to test promising radiologic countermeasures for clinical applicability so that such products gain "dual utility"—use in cancer treatment and also use for accidental or intentional civilian exposure. Development of dual-utility agents will greatly reduce costs and risks of failure while enhancing the value of research.[170] The current RRP-SBIR effort for advanced development of radiation-effect modulators serves as a model to reduce risk for small businesses by providing government support.[171] Repurposed MCMs in the cancer treatment setting may help improve the treatment outcome by specifically protecting normal tissue during the course of treatment, reducing the acute adverse effects or mitigating late effects including therapy-induced secondary cancers thus improving HRQOL of patients. Some examples are discussed below.

Among patients undergoing radiation treatment for head and neck cancers, oral mucositis is a frequent and potentially serious symptomatic toxicity. Currently available treatment options could be augmented by innovative compounds that target underlying biologic pathways associated with mucositis.[172] Colby Pharmaceutical (Menlo Park, CA) via a fast-track contract from the NCI's SBIR Development Center is formulating MnSOD as a mouthwash to prevent or reduce the severity of mucositis.[170] Similarly, radiation-induced lung damage is an intermediate to late-occurring side effect of radiotherapy in some patients after thoracic irradiation. Fibrogenesis, excessive extracellular matrix and collagen deposition, and TGF-β are involved in the development and expression of lung and other forms of tissue fibrosis.[167] Humanetics Corp (Minneapolis, MN) is developing BIO300, a patented nanoparticle formulation of genistein as a postirradiation treatment option to prevent radiation-induced pulmonary injury.[170] BIO300 was originally developed as a medical radiation countermeasure with funding from US Department of Defense and BARDA. Radiation exposure is a core component in the treatment of brain tumors; however, many patients experience neurocognitive dysfunction, which is a late-occurring side effect. Chrysalis Biotherapeutics (Galveston, TX; formerly RADIX Therapeutics) proposed to accelerate the development of TP508 (Chrysalin) by repurposing it for mitigating the radiation effects on brain tissue.[170]

A nuclear accident or terrorist incident could potentially expose a large number of people to low to moderate doses of ionizing radiation and increase their lifetime cancer risk. There is an urgent need to develop low or nontoxic mitigators for this purpose. Current status, issues, and challenges regarding development of mitigators against radiation-induced cancers has recently been published.[173] These challenges include the long latency between exposure and cancer manifestation, limitations of animal models, potential side effects of the mitigator itself, potential need for long-term use, the complexity of human trials to demonstrate its effectiveness, and statistical power constraints for measuring health risks (and reduction of health risks after mitigation) following relatively low radiation doses (<0.75 Gy). Nevertheless, progress in the understanding of the molecular mechanisms resulting in radiation injury, along with parallel progress in dose assessment technologies, make this an opportune, if not critical, time to invest in research strategies that result in the development of agents to lower the risk of radiation-induced cancers for populations that survive a significant radiation exposure incident. Such mitigators will also be of immense value to counter late effects including secondary cancers after radiation therapy among cancer survivors.

Products that target the tumor promotion stage of a multistep carcinogenesis model, which involves initiation, promotion, and progression,[174] have largely come from the field of chemoprevention. Modifiers of radiation-induced transformation reported *in vitro* systems include the following classes of compounds: (a) vitamins (or vitamin-like compounds), their precursors (e.g., vitamin A, its precursor carotene and other carotenoids), and derivatives (e.g., retinoids), (b) protease inhibitors (e.g., the soybean-derived protease inhibitor, Bowman-Birk inhibitor), (c) hormones (e.g., glucocorticoid hormones, testosterone, dihydrotestosterone), (d) modifiers of arachidonic acid metabolism (eicosanoids), (e) inhibitors of protein kinase C, and (f) antioxidants, including numerous products that scavenge free radicals.[173] Many cancer-preventive products recognized by Division of Cancer Prevention (DCP, National Cancer Institute) also may be useful as mitigators of carcinogenesis after exposures to carcinogens implying their potential to intervene in radiation-induced carcinogenesis at the promotion stage as exemplified by a Curcumin study in which dietary administration significantly reduced the incidence of mammary tumors in rats.[175]

However, testing MCM drugs for use after radiation accidents for effectiveness as well as mitigators to counter radiation-induced cancers are challenging. The Food and Drug Administration's Animal Rule provides a regulatory framework for obtaining regulatory approval for MCMs. Neupogen (filgrastim), a granulocyte colony–stimulating factor (G-CSF) and Neulasta has been approved by the FDA to counter radiation-induced neutropenia in the event of a radiation emergency. Regulatory challenges regarding mitigators have been even a greater challenge, given the uncertain relationship between low-dose exposures and late effects, lack of suitable models, and early predictive biomarkers.[173]

Biomarkers

Clinical Application of Circulating Cell-Free DNA and Circulating Tumor Cell DNA to the Assessment of Tumor Response and Evolution Under Treatment

One of the limiting factors slowing the integration of molecular therapies in the context of radiotherapy has been the lack of radiation biomarkers to monitor and predict clinical responses of both tumor and normal tissues. For monitoring tumor responses, the capacity to rapidly analyze cell free and circulating tumor DNA (ctDNA) promises to overcome this limitation. Analysis of free circulating DNA in plasma by droplet digital PCR (ddPCR) can reveal the presence of cancer in as little as 3 days compared to 4 weeks to obtain the results of next generation sequencing (NGS). In ddPCR, the purified plasma DNA is emulsified with oil into thousands of droplets containing at most one target DNA molecule that is PCR amplified and fluorescently labeled and then read in an automated droplet flow cytometer. Each droplet is individually scored based on fluorescent intensity for the mutant or wild-type allele of a target locus.[176] The high sensitivity and specificity of this technology has been demonstrated in a prospective study of non–small cell cancer.[177] The limitations of this test are that it is useful only when the tumor sheds DNA into the bloodstream, it detects only known genotypes, and it cannot detect rearrangements and is difficult to multiplex.

NGS can detect a broad range of targetable genomic alterations with 100% specificity. The sensitivity of this technique is equivalent to that of ddPCR.[178] When assessing for the presence of a driver or resistance-associated mutation, this technique applied to circulating DNA could avoid biopsy when results are positive, but sensitivity limitations mean that it cannot rule out mutation with a negative result. Circulating tumor DNA (ctDNA) analysis can also be used to monitor the evolution of a tumor under treatment. Novel methods are being developed to use circulating tumor DNA analysis as a longitudinal diagnostic tool for patients with localized and metastatic cancers.[179-181] The mutation levels in patient plasma samples reflect the clonal hierarchy inferred from sequencing of tumor biopsies. Serial changes in circulating levels of subclone-specific mutations correlate with different treatment responses between metastatic sites. Comparison of biopsy and plasma samples in individual patients with metastatic breast cancer demonstrates that circulating tumor DNA provides a dynamic sampling of somatic alterations that reflect the size and activity of distinct tumor subclones. Analysis of ctDNA also mirrors the clonal hierarchy determined by multiregional tumor sequencing and tracks the variability of treatment responses by different metastases.

The identification of actionable somatic mutations or alterations that are known to confer resistance to specific therapies and their relative circulating levels in pretreatment plasma samples could inform an individualized choice of targeted treatments and represent a breakthrough for precision radiotherapy and cancer treatment in general.

The NGS-based approach of using Cancer Personalized Profiling by Deep Sequencing (CAPP-Seq) for analysis of ctDNA enhances both the sensitivity and specificity of ctDNA detection and mutation analysis.[182] This method uses labeled DNA oligonucleotides (selector) that target known DNA sequences mutated in the cancer of interest. The selector is applied to tumor or circulating DNA to identify, by hybrid affinity capture, a patient's cancer-specific genetic aberrations (including driver mutations and rearrangements) and then used to quantitate their presence and change over time in circulating DNA. When combined with integrated digital error suppression (iDES), which eliminates most technical artifacts observed in cell-free DNA (cfDNA) sequencing data,[183] CAPP-Seq can achieve the same sensitivity as the digital drop PCR (ddPCR) technique. CAPP-Seq can achieve the equivalent or better sensitivity to digital PCR techniques (down to 4 in 10^5 cfDNA molecules) but can test a much wider number of sites on the genome.

These new minimally invasive genomic analysis techniques can monitor response and minimal residual disease and give advanced warning of recurrence allowing for early changes in therapy. They may in the future be adapted to early detection, allowing for early-stage radiotherapy treatment of currently intractable diseases such as pancreatic and CNS malignancies. An example of this is the demonstration of the sensitivity of ctDNA in cases of new melanoma brain metastases.[184]

Biomarkers to Predict Normal Tissue Responses

The application of predictive biomarkers of radiation injury is another rapidly evolving area of research, with potential to integrate with SMART radiotherapy by (a) predicting individual differences in radiation sensitivity,[185] (b) predicting severity of normal tissue injury among patients,[186] and (c) assessing and monitoring tumor response to radiation therapy.[187] A biomarker-based test that can predict the risks of developing severe radiotherapy-related complications not only will allow the delivery of alternative treatment modalities and the use of mitigators and protectors but also may allow dose escalation to the tumor in less sensitive patients. This might improve the overall therapeutic benefit and improve outcomes among all cohorts of patients. A variety of radiation biomarkers have already been explored or are currently under development at different technology readiness levels in the context of their potential application for individual dose assessment in accidental exposures to radiation or malevolent use of radiation.[188] However, discovery, development, and validation of predictive biomarkers of radiation hypersensitivity are as challenging, if not more challenging, than radiation-effect modulators. This is due to the low prevalence of normal tissue complications in the clinic, a need for long-term studies for predicting late effects (e.g., radiation-induced cognitive damage),[168] and complexity related to the combination of chemotherapy with radiation as standard of care for most tumors.

Mitigating the risk of radiation-induced cancers will require the use of three categories of biomarkers: (a) radiation dose assessment biomarkers (biodosimeters), (b) genomic health predictors, and (c) cancer surveillance biomarkers.[173] Diagnostic biomarkers for determining radiation dose of individuals following accidental exposures or therapeutic exposures may also be useful in assigning risk to the exposed population for developing delayed health risks including cancer. This would help identify "at-risk" individuals who may benefit from mitigators of late and/or enhanced cancer screening. In this context, well-established/validated cytogenetic assays, such as cytokinesis-block micronucleus assay[189] performed using peripheral blood lymphocytes for assessing "total genomic health risk,"[190] will be useful. There is also a need for using an enhanced cancer surveillance program for selected high-risk radiation-exposed cohort, especially following a radiologic mass casualty. The Early Detection Research Network of Division of Cancer Prevention at NCI, a consortium of laboratories, is focused on identifying, testing, and validating methods to noninvasively and accurately detect cancers at their earliest stages. Biomarker-based treatment decisions may eventually drive personalized medicine. Issues related to designing clinical trials with biomarkers have been discussed elsewhere.[191]

Several biomarker technologies are currently under development across government agencies, which have been reviewed.[188] The biomarker development and MCM development efforts complement one another. Commercial development and use of radiation risk mitigators will benefit from predictive biomarkers for radiation dose and genomic health concurrently, and these would help in the understanding of the impact of nutrition, repurposed drugs, or other interventions.

In summary, Figure 5.2 provides a glimpse of ongoing multidimensional efforts in radiobiology related to radiation-induced normal tissue injury at various government agencies. These efforts over the past decades has significantly advanced our understanding of mechanisms of radiation injury to normal tissue and its manifestation in different cell renewal and organ systems, allowing discovery and development of next-generation radiation countermeasures and biomarkers with foundational mechanistic radiobiology, which could be used to enhance SMART radiotherapy.

ACCESS TO CARE FOR ALL, INCLUDING THE UNDERSERVED FOR WHOM RADIATION ONCOLOGISTS (OFTEN CALLED CLINICAL ONCOLOGISTS) ARE THE PRIMARY ONCOLOGY CARE PROVIDER

At the time of writing this chapter, there is a major debate as to the future of health care in the United States. The Affordable Care Act (ACA) versus the American Health Care Act (AHCA) (so-called Obamacare vs. Trumpcare) issue is not likely to be resolved by the completion date of this chapter. Even more relevant is that entering this debate with the hope of a logical, scientific, and data-based outcome would not be SMART. As controversial as health care access and equity are for resource-rich countries, it is many times more dismal and complex for underserved people globally. This issue is covered in detail elsewhere in this book in the chapter "Radiation Oncology in the Developing World" by Timothy Hanna and Norman Coleman.

RESPONSIBLE IMPLEMENTATION OF TECHNOLOGY SO THAT WE CONTROL OUR DESTINY BASED ON DATA, … PARTICLES AS A SOCIETAL ISSUE AND SCIENCE

SMART Particles

Particle therapy is in many ways a paradox in terms of SMART. It is both very SMART, and it is not SMART at all. It has the most complex infrastructure of the external beam modalities in terms of physics support and costs. As such, it is relatively uncommon in most countries and is often considered the most specialized form of radiation. It has been touted as having fewer side effects and is often considered the first choice when treating pediatric tumors.[192] It also may be the most problematic on multiple levels. It is, in some sectors, the most promoted form of radiation therapy, and yet it is the most immature form of radiotherapy.[193]

Particle therapy can be divided into two major categories: protons and the so-called heavy ions, which include, typically, helium, carbon, and oxygen among others (although these are often termed "light ions" in the physics literature because of their position on the periodic table). Unlike photons that are generated from electrons hitting a target or from radioactive decay from isotopes such as cobalt-60, particles must be accelerated to near the range of the speed of light to do their work. To achieve this, large machines employing large magnetic fields are used to accelerate particles. Typical devices to do this include cyclotrons, synchrotrons, and other devices—areas of discussion in other chapters so we are only mentioning them here. This section applies to both of these subgroups unless otherwise stated explicitly.

To explore the concept of SMART particles, a number of interrelated domains that will likely change simultaneously will be presented in this section. Although not exhaustive of all the possible changes to this type of radiation therapy, they are meant to be broadly reflective of the overall trends to be seen in particle therapy. What they have in common is that they are likely to reflect decreasing cost of the devices and a crucial, newfound willingness to treat particles as imperfect and in need of rigorous study. These changes are all based on financial change and increasing translational knowledge.

Hopefully, the field will conduct and complete prospective randomized trials to better define and develop where particle therapy has clear advantages and where is not only "less good" but perhaps "uniquely bad." This is something we have needed in the field for a long time—with published articles at one point actually debating if trials were needed, in this case to evaluate protons, because of the fact that protons superiority was supposedly obvious and not up for debate.[194] Many things have conspired to make that supposedly obvious truth less obvious in the current space of using physical dose to prescribe dose in the case of proton therapy. We really don't know if they have unique problems long term based on their biology to normal tissue.[195] We do think they are likely better if used carefully by those with experience, but with RBEs of higher than 1.1, how will doses that are 75 to 100 Gy equivalent affect normal tissues over time[196]? Conversely, if used poorly, they are at best likely to be far worse in that it is far easier to dosimetrically miss a tumor with particles. Plans with photons and standard planning target volumes (PTVs) are generally more robust making widespread use of particles, without widespread expertise in the subtleties of their use, a somewhat risky prospect moving forward for the field unless methods can be developed to make their use more robust and to contain the complexity in manageable planning interfaces.

Trials and the development of new tools are needed to address these issues and will generate a host of data to be incorporated prospectively into the field. Honest evaluation of planning skill and time spent in planning with outcome will need to be performed. The risks particle therapy presents to the field because of biologically incomplete planning will be one of the forces that may drive the inclusion of artificial intelligence into the planning process—as a means of giving patients more expertise wherever they are treated. The very earliest vestiges of this exist in the literature of autocontouring and expert training. In time, proper particle therapy will demand they be used as the number of users increases but patients who benefit remains about the same. Beam selection will need to optimize (a) not only Bragg peak location (b) but also all areas of high linear energy transfer (LET) dose deposition such as the penumbra of each field, perhaps of each spot, (c) inherent geometric motion statistics for site in three and four dimensions, and (d) specific tissue data based on voxel-by-voxel beam data and situational awareness of other medical issues such as oxygenation of tissue, concurrent agent concentration, and prior tissue injury status.[196,197]

These changes due in the domain of particle therapy are a component of the parallel SMART radiation therapy concept of radiation as drug. It just becomes more unique to each particle because particles are biologically different. Each particle will finally be seen and considered as a different drug. Trials will be designed in this way. What we have done to date—allowing a mixture of photon and proton patients and looking at the results only after the fact—will no longer be a viable trial design. Trials will need to be powered for each "drug" used. What each particle does to DNA and even the normal components of cells like the membranes, organelles, and proteins are vastly different and may yield opportunities for therapeutic index gain. Each particle will be thought of as a new agent rather than just radiation therapy.[198] As such, agent mixes and even new agents designed to work specifically with our newly appreciated war chest of radiation "drugs" will allow further optimization of treatment and perhaps even cost savings. It might turn out that mixtures of particles of different types in specific sequences in time and space will be far superior than any monotherapy of particle or photon in use today.

These new data are likely to shed light on the reality of particle therapy and allow it to reach the level of promise many have envisioned for it from the beginning. To do this, the resulting new set of biologic data will be the basis of a major, global change in radiation oncology driven by particle therapy but affecting all modalities: biologic treatment planning. The software methodologies discussed above will collapse to classical photons as the control state much like classical mechanics is the default state of special relativity when one's velocity is far slower than the speed of light.[199] Plans for patients will move from physical energy dose prescription to this integrative form of a biologic dose prescription and organ at risk (OAR) risk tolerance mapping model. Computer models incorporation libraries of biologic data will be invoked to do this work. Imaging-based biomarkers will be used in real time to monitor biologic response to fit the models to actual host response. This new paradigm could be called adaptive biologic treatment planning.[200] It will be very labor intensive to build the models in ways that allow for real-time adjustment via the incorporation of biomarker data, but once built, what we do now with physical dose will seem extremely crude in comparison. This is perhaps the most real form of SMART radiation therapy that is to come in the future. It will involve and allow for the use of all sorts of new agents and combinations of agents and the idea that radiation is very much biologically driven by the point in space and time it is being used rather and "a Gy is a Gy" will be the new paradigm.

Inexorably linked in time with more trials being performed will be a combination of decreasing cost of the devices, increasing availability of computing resources that can scale to these issues affordably, increasing numbers of particle treatment machines, more narrowly defined uses for radiation in general based on concurrent research expanding our biologic understanding, and likely decreased reimbursement. This is a metastable situation at best on several levels. The most profound level of which is the reality that everyone who wants one of these centers might not be able to support it with sufficient patient numbers where it is indicated to keep staff expert and bills paid. Financial uncertainty in radiation oncology is increasing, and these centers are likely to be the most uncertain financial component of any given center unless they are run with a "break-even at best" long-term business plan somehow supported by institutional commitment to the science involved despite risk of losses, the rare disease capacity, or development support.[201]

SMART Use of Visible Light and Related Technologies

Photodynamic therapy (PDT), where light is used to interact with chemical agents to deliver energy to tissue is currently in the midst of a large number of prospective trials as sponsored by several program project grants from the NCI and other support mechanisms. Areas of interest involve tumors of many regions, both from a definitive perspective in a postoperative setting and in a preventative setting. Additionally, some studies are evaluating the interplay between the immune system and PDT usage.[202-204] PDT is under intense investigation and its use may become more widespread if these trials define areas of significant therapeutic benefit. This active milieu of trials will be the contemporaneous environment of PDT for the reader of this text during the active period of this edition.

Much of the work described in the last edition[205] has progressed in terms of both molecular mechanistic understanding of how PDT therapy works and of new light plus photo agents that expand the use of the technology spatially.[206] These data will likely both inform the use of rationalized drug combinations with PDT, including checkpoint inhibitors,[203,207,208] and expand the spatial and temporal use of the methodology to new clinical indications.

Beyond this natural evolution of PDT, there have been exciting, promising developments in the dimension of creating agents that interact with traditional ionizing radiation much like light does in PDT to make the range of action not just millimeters as in the case of light but centimeters.[209,210] This area may allow yet another way to use ionizing radiation with chemotherapy but with the agents being inert until radiated, that is, to be triggered with the radiation therapy like a mousetrap. This will move the scope of radiation therapy into a more diverse set of clinical situations as it opens up the ability to spatially constrain side effects further. Obviously, care will be needed to optimize this approach given the fact that radiation entry and exit doses may limit the ability to prevent damage to normal tissue in, at a minimum, entry dose regions. One could envision a mixture of old and new radiation modalities being used to harness these new agents' potentials.

The implications here are broad for radiation therapy departments globally. Orthovoltage optimization may become useful in this context again as could the use of heavy ions at low dose. If the agents can be designed to require a dosimetric threshold for action of say 0.25 Gy, one can imagine simple plans being very much able to address this with three-dimensional conformal radiotherapy at relative low doses, opening up the possibility of being able to avoid treating to normal tissue tolerance in the future routinely. This would better enable retreatment and would likely lower costs to society overall. Given radiation's unique capacity to be spatially delivered, this approach has promise. The biodistribution of these agents, like any chemical, will impact the success of these methods radically.

Combinatory Therapies

Systemic administration of therapeutic agents (TA) for cancer treatment is a common practice. However, their presence in normal tissue is generally not favorable as it could lead to adverse toxicities. The undue toxicity might be avoided if the TA remained encapsulated or inactive until exposed to an extremal stimulus within well-defiled volume. In addition, the time of activation could be adjusted so that concentration of the TA in the target volume reaches levels necessary for an effective treatment. The key criteria toward achieving effective and safe treatment include minimal invasiveness of the external stimuli and quantitative control of localized TA release or activation. Remote triggering mechanisms may include photodynamic, photothermal, photo-triggered chemotherapeutic release, ultrasound, electrothermal, magnetothermal, x-ray, particle beam, and radiofrequency. Examples of three combinatory strategies using nanoparticles are presented in Figure 5.3.

Use of radiation or ultrasound to activate or release TA has been an active research front in many academic centers with fruitful results. Thermal release of drugs from liposomes has been in clinical practice for years. An example is ThermoDox (Cesion Corporation; http://celsion.com/thermodox/), which uses LTSL (lysolipid thermally sensitive liposome) technology to encapsulate doxorubicin, a proven and commonly used cancer drug. The heat-sensitive liposome rapidly changes structure when heated to 40°C to 45°C, creating openings in the liposome that release doxorubicin directly into and around the targeted tumor. Other "smart" systems that might

FIGURE 5.3. Examples of three combinatory strategies using nanoparticles. The top two panels utilize radiation to trigger liposomes and PDT. The lower panel uses nanoparticles to internalize drugs/molecules that enhance effects of x-rays. Nano-RDE, nano-encased radiation dose.

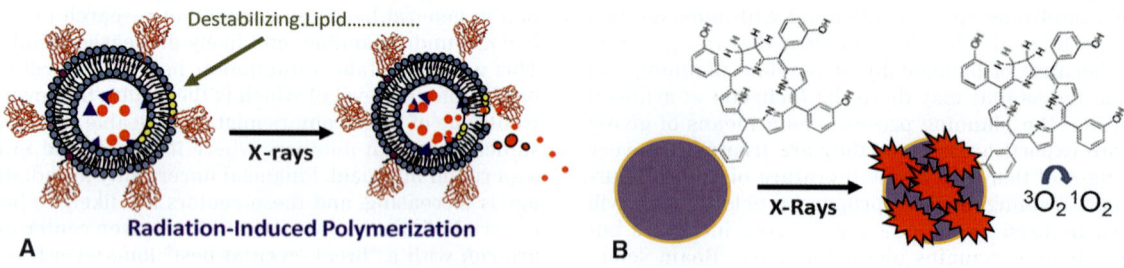

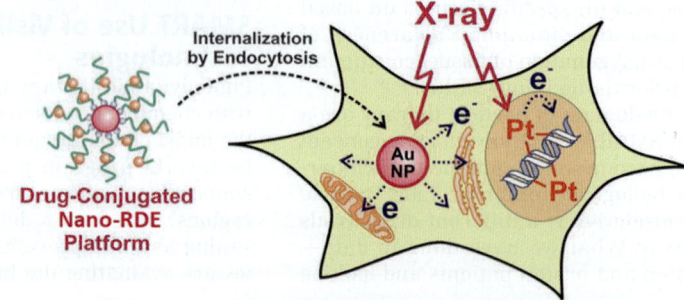

release drugs or induce a toxic effect in response to an externally controlled stimulus promise unique clinical benefits over conventional systems that release their cargo passively or are activated internally. In combination with RT, x-rays might be used to stimulate local release of encapsulated drugs in tumor volume or the combination of x-rays with nanoscintillators producing light used in PDT would allow its extension to deep-seated tumors.

Nanotechnology

Multifunctional nanoparticles allow simultaneous targeted delivery of diagnostic and TA to the tumor tissue giving rise to a new, fast-growing field of theragnostics that combines the modalities of diagnosis and therapy.[211]

Gold Nanoparticles

Over the last two decades, radiation dose enhancement by high atomic number elements such as iodine has been explored for cancer radiotherapy.[212] As a small molecule radiation dose enhancer (smRDE), iododeoxyuridine (IUdR) has been used because of its facile incorporation into cellular DNA.[212,213] The subsequent external irradiation of high-energy photons on the IUdR-containing target cells can trigger the secondary emission of photoelectric radiation (i.e., Auger/secondary electron emission or x-ray fluorescence).[214] The resulting triggered emission from smRDE can cleave the nuclear DNA double strands that can induce the radiosensitized cell death.[215] In this smRDE-mediated radiotherapy, several advantages have been demonstrated. The triggered emission from smRDEs generally decays in several millimeters, which is a typical length scale of a cell so that the resulting cytotoxicity is highly dependent on the cellular location of smRDEs. Therefore, only the smRDEs located inside the target cells can deliver high toxicity upon radiation, but their off-target toxicity can be reduced by virtue of their being outside of the cells.[216]

Although such smRDEs can improve the radiotherapeutic efficacy with reduced side effects, safe and effective delivery of smRDE to target tissue remains one of the major drawbacks to clinical applications.[216] As iodine-attached tumor-targeting antibodies were used to improve their biodistribution, their targeting and therapeutic efficacies were not satisfied because of the rapid dehalogenation mechanism in DNA as well as the heterogeneity and limited expression of target receptors on cancer cells.[217] Furthermore, the prolonged treatments with high dosages of iodine compounds should be avoided because of their toxic side effects to the host organs.

These limitations might be circumvented by development of a nano-encased RDE (nano-RDE) platform, based on functionalizable polymer-modified nanoparticles. Nano-RDE platforms can demonstrate several advantages: First, the biodistribution of nano-RDE can be highly improved by the "enhanced permeation and retention" effect in solid tumor tissue that allows for the selective accumulation of nano-RDE at diseased sites (passive targeting).[218,219] Second, high amount of nano-RDE can be readily internalized in target cells by endocytic pathways, which are known as a completely different cellular internalization mechanism from that of small molecules.[220] In addition, the subsequent acidic endosomal environments can be used as a trigger for the pH-sensitive release of additional chemotherapeutic agents.[221]

In conventional chemotherapy, the rapid developments of multidrug-resistant characteristics in cancer cells cause a critical problem in clinical cancer treatments.[222] As such, it is obvious that a combinational therapy is more effective than a single modality treatment. To this end, anticancer drug-conjugated nano-RDE would be "smart-combined modality therapy" as a multimodal delivery platform for *both* radio- and chemotherapy.

Gold nanoparticles have been tested for improvement of both chemotherapy[223] and radiotherapy.[224] The TNFα-PEG-colloidal gold nanoparticle, CYT-6091 (CytImmune,

Gaithersburg, MD), has been shown to selectively traffic to tumor tissue. This agent was evaluated in a phase I trial and shown to selectively deliver TNF-α to tumors with reduced toxicity compared to recombinant human TNF-α alone.[225]

In addition to its properties as a nanocarrier, colloidal gold, being a high-Z element, may also increase the radiation dose delivered specifically to the target cells. In this system, gold nanoparticles (AuNPs) are used as inorganic nano-RDEs for radiotherapy as well as a delivery platform for chemotherapeutic agents. Because of the K-edge of gold at 80.7 keV, x-ray radiation with the energy level of Au K-edge can trigger the secondary emission of photoelectric radiation from AuNPs.[226,227] The resulting radiation can induce the degradation of target molecules by ionization and can interact with surrounding water molecules to produce reactive oxygen species that can damage the target molecules.[228] As such, AuNP-sensitized degradations of plasmid DNA[229] and human proteins[230] upon x-ray radiation have been demonstrated in *in vitro* model systems. Additionally, when AuNP-containing tumor cells were irradiated, increased apoptotic cell death was detected because of the continuous stress on cytosolic organelles.[231] Furthermore, enhanced *in vivo* efficacy of AuNPs upon radiotherapy was also observed in human cancer-bearing mouse models.[224] However, these AuNPs have shown very poor pharmacokinetic results due in part to their limited surface functionality as a bare colloidal particle.

Recently, AuNPs have been used in a wide range of biologic applications because of their biocompatibility and well-known surface chemistry. Using the known reactions, AuNPs can be readily modified with thiol-end–capped polymers[232] that can significantly alter the pharmacokinetics.[233,234] This functional polymer can be prepared by reversible addition–fragmentation chain transfer (RAFT) radical polymerization, which allows for copolymerization of a wide range of monomers.[235]

As the gold K-edge is at 80.7 keV and the enhancement is optimal in the photoelectric-dominated x-ray spectrum, irradiation conditions could be optimized by using monoenergetic x-rays. However, a significant enhancement of the treatment efficacy might also be obtained in standard megavoltage x-ray beams.[236] To track biodistribution of gold nanoparticles, these can be easily activated with thermal neutrons prior to administration to emit 411 keV gamma rays, which can be detected by SPECT.

Liposomes

Another alternative approach would be using radiation as a trigger releasing or activating drugs delivered to the tumor prior to irradiation. One option could provide radiosensitive liposomes. Liposomes have been explored as viable carriers for targeting, imaging, and delivery of payload of drugs for decades.[237] To date, various triggering modalities such as local hyperthermia and pH-triggered, tissue-associated enzyme, and light-triggered drug release have been developed.[238] Among these, electromagnetic radiation-triggered release of liposomal drugs appears a promising approach and includes strategically designed phospholipid molecules to initiate a light-induced trigger. These liposomes are based on the principle of photopolymerization of lipids,[239] photosensitization by membrane-anchored hydrophobic probes,[240,241] and/or photoisomerization[242] of photoreactive lipids. However, none of the formulations developed so far have been successful for *in vivo* applications presumably because of the lack of adequate photon energy produced by the radiation source(s) and/or inability of radiation to penetrate into biologic tissues.

Radiation-Activated Photodynamic Therapy

PDT is increasingly being recognized as an attractive and useful tool in the treatment of many diverse human diseases, including macular degeneration, several dermatologic disorders, and oncology.[243] PDT utilizes photosensitizers that can be preferentially localized in malignant tissues. The interaction of the photosensitizer and light results in the generation of cytotoxic species, including singlet oxygen ($^1O_2$), free radicals, and peroxides, that attack key structural entities within the targeted cells. Those very toxic species are characterized by a short lifetime (<0.04 μs) and a short radius of action. Therefore, the damaged area is essentially confined to tissue that both contains the photosensitizer and is exposed to light.

Relative to current treatments, such as surgery, radiation therapy, and chemotherapy, PDT is also comparatively noninvasive, can be more accurately targeted, and is not subject to the total-dose limitations associated with radiotherapy; in addition, the healing process typically results in little or no scarring.[244] Despite these advantages, PDT has not yet gained general clinical acceptance. The photosensitizers that have been approved for routine PDT treatment absorb light in the visible spectral regions below 700 nm, thus preventing access to deeper residing tumors. As a result, even with the advent of more sophisticated light delivery systems, the clinical application of PDT is limited to superficial solid tumors, endoscopically accessible regions, or skin lesions. The development of photosensitizers with absorbance in the near-infrared region, which would help overcome the limitation on the penetration depth, is an active area of research. There is also still need for isomerically pure photosensitizers. Improving the efficiency of singlet oxygen production in the tissue microenvironment would permit reduction of the concentration of the photosensitizer necessary to treat the tumor. Finally, it would be helpful to develop better molecular targeting in order to improve the selectivity of the photosensitizers for the diseased tissue.

The combination of radiotherapy with PDT, exploiting the tissue penetration of ionizing x-ray radiation and the cell-level targeting of PDT, might provide a novel approach to overcome the problems with penetration depth and might help with the delivery and targeting of photosensitizing agents. It has been already observed that under certain conditions, some photosensitizers act as radiosensitizers. The combination of Photofrin, an FDA-approved photosensitizer, with radiation therapy led to significant enhancements in cytotoxic and apoptotic death of cancer cells.[245,246] However, the molecular mechanism for this effect is still unknown.

More recently, there has been interest in developing a nanoparticle-based photosensitizer delivery system for a combination of PDT with radiation therapy. Chen and Zhang[247] proposed using scintillating nanoparticles conjugated to photosensitizers; in response to irradiation with deeply penetrating x-rays, these nanoscintillators would produce light capable of activating the attached photosensitizers, thereby producing toxic amounts of free radicals in any desired location of the body. These nanoparticles would overcome the limitations imposed on current PDT and expand its application to deeply located tumors. In addition, it might be possible to conjugate molecules for receptor-mediated internalization to the nanoparticles as well, ensuring delivery to the intracellular space; perhaps, delivery could even be targeted to vulnerable subcellular structures.

Several doped nanoparticles ($LaF_3:Ce^{3+}$, $LuF_3:Ce^{3+}$, $CaF_2:Mn^{2+}$, $CaF_2:Eu^{2+}$, $BaFBr:Eu^{2+}$) and semiconductor nanoparticles (ZnO, ZnS, and TiO_2) are potential light sources for use in a nanoparticle-PDT system. The emission spectra of these nanoparticles can be matched perfectly to the absorption spectra of Photofrin, fullerenes, and TiO_2 nanoparticles. For example, $BaFBr:Eu^{2+}:Mn^{2+}$ nanoparticles excited by x-ray have three emission bands, one peaking at approximately 400, 500, and 640 nm, respectively. The emission spectrum of these nanoparticles is well matched to the absorption spectrum of hematoporphyrin. Another example is the x-ray luminescence spectrum of $LaF_3:Ce^{3+}$ nanoparticles with maximum emission at 350 nm, tailing to 500 nm. This emission spectrum matches the absorption spectra of most photosensitizers as well. The rationale for this approach is to combine the effects of PDT and radiation therapy while reducing toxicity.

Boron Neutron Capture Therapy

Another example of combinatory treatment that in theory provides a way to selectively destroy malignant cells and spare normal cells is boron neutron capture therapy (BNCT). It is based on the nuclear capture that occurs when a stable isotope of boron, ^{10}B, is irradiated with low-energy thermal neutrons leading to fission reactions producing high LET alpha particles (^4He) and recoiling lithium-7 (^7Li) nuclei. Because the high LET particles have limited path lengths in tissue (5 to 9 μm), the destructive effects of these high-energy particles is limited to boron-containing cells. When a sufficient amount of ^{10}B accumulates in the tumor and enough thermal neutrons are absorbed by them to sustain lethal damage from the $^{10}B(n, \alpha)^7Li$ capture reaction, tumor cells dispersed in normal tissue can be selectively destroyed.

The development of BNCT began approximately 60 years ago. Since then, many research groups worldwide and 15 different neutron facilities using nuclear research reactors have been involved in development of BNCT. Only two boron delivery agents, the polyhedral boron anion, sodium mercaptoundecahydro-*closo*-dodecaborate ($Na_2B_{12}H_{11}SH$), known as sodium borocaptate (BSH), and the boron-containing amino acid (L)-4-dihydroxy-borylphenyalanine known as boronophenylalanine (BPA) have been used in humans.[248] Clinical trials of BNCT have been focused primarily on high-grade gliomas[249,250] and head and neck cancers.[251] The lack of success of these trials could be attributed to slow progress in the development of compounds that would deliver adequate amounts of boron specifically to tumor cells and to the use of expensive and often obsolete nuclear reactors at physics laboratories apart from medical centers as the neutron sources. A positive development is the application of accelerator-based neutron sources, such as the one commercially available from Sumitomo Heavy Industries.[252] The new accelerator-based neutron sources will be more compact and their operation will be much less expensive than nuclear reactors. They might be located at a radiation department of any hospital, facilitating interactions with other departments, and particularly radiology that would improve diagnosis and treatment planning.

Development of new boron delivery agents characterized by low systemic toxicity and rapid clearance from blood and normal tissues, combined with high tumor uptake (at least $\sim$20 μg ^{10}B/g tumor) and persistence in tumor during the BNCT procedure, is crucial for the success of future clinical trials. Special attention should be paid to targeting the CSCs known for efficient exocytosis that might be responsible for the failure of the clinical trials using BPA to deliver boron to cancer cells.[253] Promising new boron delivery agents based on peptides, purines, pyrimidines, porphyrin derivatives, thymidines, nucleosides, and nucleotides are being developed. In addition, monoclonal antibodies (MAb), liposomes, and nanoparticles are used to design high molecular weight BNCT agents.[254,255]

Targeted Radionuclide Therapy

Systemic targeted radionuclide therapy (TRT) is an evolving and promising modality of cancer treatment. It provides a unique means to efficiently eradicate disseminated tumors cells and small metastases before they are detectable by currently available methods. In combination with external RT, TRT might be used as a boost to deliver additional radiation dose specifically to the tumor.

The key characteristic of systemic targeted radiotherapy is its specificity. Using tumor-homing characteristics of a radioactive compound or conjugating therapeutic radionuclei with a tumor-targeting molecule (antibody, antibody fragment, or peptide), it can deliver higher amounts of a radionuclide to cancer cells than to normal tissue. A number of antigens and receptors present on the tumor cell surface including CD20, CD45, PSMA, mucin 1 (MUC1), HER2, EGFR, tumor necrosis factor, as well as VEGF and avb3 abundant on the vascular endothelial cells within newly developed blood vessels have been advocated as potential targets for radioimmunotherapy (RIT) in patients.[256]

The targeting pharmaceuticals are radiolabeled with various radionuclides to deliver radiation directly to the target. In contrast to biologic targeted therapy, TRT does not require detailed knowledge of cancer phenotype signaling pathways. Rather than disrupting cancer-associated signaling, TRT directly kills tumor cells by radiation-induced DNA damage. Although DNA damage-induced tumor cell killing is also the mechanism used by chemotherapy, TRT is far less toxic because the radiation is delivered predominantly to cells that express a TAA. The fundamental and distinguishing aspect of TRT relative to other cancer therapeutics is the ability to select the radionuclide and, in particular, the type of radiation emissions that are delivered. The majority of TRT applications have used beta-particle emitting radionuclides such as ^{131}I, ^{90}Y, and ^{177}Lu. Beta-particle path length in tissue ranges from 0.8 to 5 mm; the energy deposited per distance traveled is approximately 0.2 keV/μm and has been characterized as low LET.

Medullary thyroid cancer treatment with targeted radionuclides illustrates the potential of molecular radiotherapy in a situation where few other treatment options exist. Treatment of indolent non-Hodgkin lymphoma (NHL) provides another example. There are two FDA-approved antibody-based molecular radiotherapeutics, Bexxar and Zevalin, for this disease. Both ^{131}I-tositumomab (Bexxar) and ^{90}Y-ibritumomab tiuxetan (Zevalin) are radiolabeled antibodies; they target different regions (epitopes) on the B-cell–associated CD20 antigen.

A lower molecular weight class of molecular radiotherapeutics, radiolabeled peptides (peptides are typically made up of less than 50 amino acids), has been the focus of European investigators. These peptides can achieve binding affinities in the low nanomolar range and have been found to be nonimmunogenic. One of the first of these, ^{111}In-DTPA-octreotide (Octreoscan) was approved by the FDA in 1994 for imaging/detection of neuroendocrine tumors with somatostatin receptors based on trials conducted exclusively outside the United States (in Europe). Although not as successful as the radiolabeled antibodies against lymphoma, radiopeptides have nevertheless demonstrated efficacy in patients with late-stage, refractory neuroendocrine tumors.[257] Such tumors are substantially more radioresistant than lymphomas. These agents clear the circulation rapidly, reducing the bone marrow–absorbed dose and allowing greater administered activities and increased tumor-absorbed doses. The amount that can be administered in a single injection has been limited by renal toxicity.[257] Several interventions have been adopted to reduce uptake by the kidneys, the most prevalent one involves infusion of cationic amino acids. Over 400 patients with neuroendocrine tumors have been treated with radiolabeled peptides and overall response rates between 60% and 75% have been reported; only a small percentage of these, however, have been complete responses.[257] As in NHL, new promising peptide-based RPTs continue to be developed and comparative trials will be needed to determine how these will be used with current treatment against neuroendocrine tumors.

Metaiodobenzylguanidine (MIBG) is an aralkylguanidine analog of catecholamine precursors, structurally similar to norepinephrine that concentrates within secretory granules of catecholamine-producing cells. It has been labeled with ^{123}I for diagnostic imaging and with ^{131}I for therapy of neuroblastoma, pheochromocytoma, and, to a lesser extent, other neuroendocrine tumors.[258] Neuroblastoma constitutes approximately 8% to 10% of pediatric cancers at an annual incidence of 8 to 10 cases per million children. Approximately 600 new cases are seen in the United States each year. Once metastasized, the 5-year survival rate is only 30% to 40%. In these trials, ^{131}I-MIBG has demonstrated highly specific uptake and prolonged intracellular retention in tumor and not in normal organs. ^{131}I-MIBG has also been investigated in pheochromocytoma in adults.[259] In neuroblastoma treatment ^{131}I-MIBG has been investigated in progressive or recurrent neuroblastoma after conventional therapy or in combination with myeloablative therapy; it has also been applied prior to surgery in inoperable stage III and IV disease. In a very difficult to successfully treat patient population, a 40% to 60% rate of objective responses has been observed, including some complete responses. These responses are typically observed at doses that lead to high-grade hematologic toxicity.

The application of TRT for the treatment of solid tumors has been less successful than in patients with malignant lymphoma. There are several problems that should be addressed to improve its efficacy.[260] First, the cells in bulky solid tumors are generally less radiosensitive. Secondly, the delivery of therapeutic radionuclide to solid tumors might be less effective because of limited vascularization, elevated intratumoral hydrostatic pressure, and heterogeneous uptake of the radionuclide. Nevertheless, a recently completed global phase III clinical trial (ALSYMPCA) with radium-223 chloride (Xofigo) in patients with castration-resistant prostate cancer and bone metastases showed that these limitations can be successfully circumvented and nuclear medicine may become an effective treatment modality for disseminated solid tumors as well.[261,262]

The success of ALSYMPCA leads to an increased interest in using alpha-particle–emitting radionuclides for TRT. Aside from the ability to target cells from within, targeted delivery of alpha-emitters provides the additional fundamental advantage of a more potent, cytotoxic type of radiation. Alpha particles are helium nuclei that deposit DNA damaging energy along their track that is 100 to 1,000 times greater than that of beta particles; the damage caused by alpha particles is predominately double-stranded DNA breaks severe enough to make the DNA repair mechanism ineffective. Therefore, a small number of tracks through a cell nucleus can sterilize a cell and alpha-particle radiation is not susceptible to resistance as seen with external radiotherapy (e.g., in hypoxic tissue). Animal and cell culture studies have shown that relative biologic effectiveness (RBE) of alpha particles is in the range of 3 to 7. Although one might expect that this high potency against targeted cells would also be accompanied by high toxicity to normal bystander cells, the short 50 to 100 μm range of alpha particles limits the amount of damage that is incurred by normal tissue.

In addition, the Big Pharma companies that have developed antibodies for targeted cancer therapies are interested in extending their application for delivery of therapeutic loads to the cancer cells. One example is Roche, which has recently introduced to the clinical practice trastuzumab emtansine (trade name Kadcyla), an antibody–drug conjugate consisting of the monoclonal antibody trastuzumab (Herceptin) linked to the cytotoxic agent DM1, and, in collaboration with AREVA Med, is currently developing ^{212}Pb-trastuzumab. The positive results of phase 1 clinical trials of this radioconjugate have been recently reported in the American Journal of Clinical Oncology.[263]

There are two different approaches that have been introduced into clinical practice including the use of direct conjugation of radioisotope tagged to mAb or pretargeting of the tumor. In the first case, the patient receives a diagnostic dose of an antibody labeled with radionuclide compatible with appropriate imaging modality (SPECT or PET). If the conjugate is stable and there is sufficient localization of an antibody at the site of disease, the patient can be injected with a therapeutic dose capable of inducing cytoreductive and potentially curative effects. This approach, however, has some limitations. First, radiation dose delivered to solid tumors might be insufficient because of poor penetration of the large-size radioimmunoconjugate. Moreover, rather long serum half-life of mAbs together with long decay time of the radioisotope increases the radiation exposure to normal organs and can contribute to bone marrow toxicity.

In a pretargeting approach, the radionuclide is administrated separately from the antibody vehicle. There are two strategies; one involves the administration of radioactive biotin for selective localization on antibody–streptavidin conjugates. This approach takes advantage of the rapid pharmacokinetics of the small biotin molecule and the high affinity of avidin–biotin binding.[264] Alternatively, chelators of radioactive metals and multispecific antibodies that are capable to simultaneously bind to a TAA and a metal chelator could be used.[265]

The advance in imaging and radiation transport will allow new approaches to radionuclide therapy treatment planning. By administration of the dosimetric (trace-labeled) dose and determination of the patient's residence time (a measure of how long the radionuclide is retained in the body), the therapeutic dose can be precisely adjusted to maximize the therapeutic effect and minimize toxicity. The paradigm of a targeted drug with a patient-specific dose may become more routine as targeted therapies are further developed along with better assays to directly measure drug levels. For the present, whole-body dosimetry is routinely applied for RIT but in the near future, the patient-specific maximally tolerated therapeutic radiation dose will be used to maximize efficacy while minimizing organ and bone marrow toxicity.[266] The ability to access the radiation dose delivered to the tumor by TRT will enable its combination with external RT.

TRAINING AND MENTORING TO ENSURE A BROADLY BASED, SOCIETAL CONSCIOUS NEXT GENERATION OF CLINICIANS, SCIENTISTS, AND EDUCATORS

Contemplating the future requires careful scrutiny of the present and how we got here. That things that were "obvious truths"—more dose is better and protons must outperform photons—have had successes but also failures. Changing paradigms requires a willingness to look beyond conventional wisdom and embrace rather than fear change.

A number of prospective, randomized trials during the latter part of the 20 century showed that adding certain drugs to RT prolonged patients' survival (TMZ in GBM, cisplatin in H&N, cisplatin in cervix, cisplatin/etoposide in NSCLC, cetuximab in H&N, ADT in prostate). For the most part, however, our understanding of why those drugs were successful whereas many others have failed remains poor. This has hampered industry investment. Exploiting for therapeutic gains, our growing knowledge about radiation response and (from initiatives such as TCGA) the vulnerabilities of specific subtypes of cancers is a high priority for the field.

Exploiting physics and engineering technology for escalating radiation dose to tumors for prolonging survival has unfortunately not been very successful so far (GBM, lung, prostate) and in some instances even counterproductive. One exception is tumor-treating fields wherein the application of low-energy electrical fields to the brain in conjunction with radiochemotherapy prolonged the survival of patients with GBM. The mechanism of action however remains poorly understood. Another bright spot is Radium 223 that prolonged the survival of patients with metastatic CRPC.[262,267] That has ignited interest in an area that had been ignored by radiation oncologists, namely, targeted radionuclide therapy (TRT). The knowledge gained from the human genome project, TCGA, etc., has led to the development of numerous molecularly "targeted" agents that can localize to the tumor or its microenvironment. Their ability to eradicate the tumor is limited however by the fact that (a) not all tumor cells may express the target and (b) tumor cells may develop secondary resistance. Adding a radioactive "payload" to such a drug may prevent the cell from developing secondary resistance. Furthermore, using beta particles of the appropriate energy may help kill even neighboring cancer cells that did not express the target.

Physics and engineering developments have had some success in decreasing adverse events (AEs). It must be pointed out however that these relatively expensive technologies (such as protons, SRT, and IMRT) in the United States have often been deployed in situations where no RT (or even no treatment at all) is a viable or even preferred alternative; examples include low-risk prostate cancer and breast cancer ductal carcinoma in situ (DCIS). Decreasing AEs is a laudable objective, but it must always be simultaneously demonstrated that it did not compromise tumor control. In that context, preliminary data showing decreased AEs should be supplemented by robust data showing at least noninferiority with regard to tumor control. Unfortunately, most studies reported to date fall short in that respect. Those concerns include worse tumor control after IMRT in H&N cancer, worse brainstem toxicity after proton RT for postfossa tumors, and worse intracranial tumor control after SRT for brain metastases.

Drug companies routinely sponsor prospective, randomized trials for demonstrating the superiority of their products, but the device industry in general and the RO industry in particular do so rarely because they are usually not required to by the U.S. FDA. Why the latter has this double standard is beyond the scope of this discussion, but there is no reason why radiation oncologists, just like medical oncologists, should not demand robust evidence before paying millions, sometimes hundreds of millions, of dollars for what the manufacturer is trying to sell.

CONCLUSIONS

That there is so much new material to discuss in this second edition of this chapter is encouraging. There are improvements in the use of the existing technology including amalgamation of imaging and therapy to better hit the desired anatomic targets. Particle therapy is understood to be much more than better dose distribution. Indeed, it is time to begin to think of radiation in terms of the biologic changes it produces and future inverse planning will include biologic events rather than just physical dose. The era of precision medicine has already changed how cancer is diagnosed and classified and elucidated the remarkable heterogeneity in the cancer cells before and during treatment that makes drug targeting ever more challenging and exciting. Perhaps the focal stress response induced by radiation and/or the other new technologies described in this chapter can help homogenize and/or modify the cancer phenotype and make it susceptible to drug treatment or immunotherapy.

The introduction indicated that we would engage the readers in a SMART experiment. We would be interested in knowing how many people read this chapter, if there were any suggestions of what to include and if this would be useful as a journal publication in concert with this book that would ensure both broader and timely dissemination of this information as it is rapidly changing. Please send comments to ccoleman@mail.nih.gov and bernhardej@mail.nih.gov with the subject line SMART Rad (or something close to that).

To be a SMART radiation oncology health care provider requires the interest, ability, and dedication to stay current in one's own field but also to remain aware of the rapid advances in cancer biology. Advances in imaging, machine learning, and computer-driven planning and treatment delivery may actually free us up to spend more time with patients and in creative activities. Knowing the limit of one's toolkit provides incentive to reach into new domains and take on new challenges. Radiation oncology lives day-to-day at the interface of cancer biology, innovative technology, imaging, economics, long-term outcomes from many cured patients, societal fears of radiation, and an opportunity to bring care to the millions of underserved people. Be **S**ocietal focused, **M**olecularly aware, **A**ltruistic, **R**esearch supportive, and wary of **T**echnological solutions to biologic problems: Be *SMART*.

REFERENCES

1. Coleman CN. The radiation stress response: of the people, by the people and for the people. *Radiat Res* 2017;187(2):129–146.

2. Coleman CN. Linking radiation oncology and imaging through molecular biology (or now that therapy and diagnosis have separated, it's time to get together again!). *Radiology* 2003;228(1):29–35.

3. Makinde AY, John-Aryankalayil M, Palayoor ST, et al. Radiation survivors: understanding and exploiting the phenotype following fractionated radiation therapy. *Mol Cancer Res* 2013;11(1):5–12.

4. Luo J, Solimini NL, Elledge SJ. Principles of cancer therapy: oncogene and non-oncogene addiction. *Cell* 2009;136(5):823–837.

5. Hanahan D, Weinberg RA. The hallmarks of cancer. *Cell* 2000;100(1):57–70.

6. Tsai MH, Cook JA, Chandramouli GV, et al. Gene expression profiling of breast, prostate, and glioma cells following single versus fractionated doses of radiation. *Cancer Res* 2007;67(8):3845–3852.

7. John-Aryankalayil M, Palayoor ST, Cerna D, et al. Fractionated radiation therapy can induce a molecular profile for therapeutic targeting. *Radiat Res* 2010;174(4):446–458.

8. Palayoor ST, John-Aryankalayil M, Makinde AY, et al. Differential expression of stress and immune response pathway transcripts and miRNAs in normal human endothelial cells subjected to fractionated or single-dose radiation. *Mol Cancer Res* 2014;12(7):1002–1015.

9. Simone CB, 2nd, John-Aryankalayil M, Palayoor ST, et al. mRNA expression profiles for prostate cancer following fractionated irradiation are influenced by p53 status. *Transl Oncol* 2013;6(5):573–585.

10. Mohyeldin A, Garzon-Muvdi T, Quinones-Hinojosa A. Oxygen in stem cell biology: a critical component of the stem cell niche. *Cell Stem Cell* 2010;7(2):150–161.

11. Tredan O, Galmarini CM, Patel K, et al. Drug resistance and the solid tumor microenvironment. *J Natl Cancer Inst* 2007;99(19):1441–1454.

12. Graeber TG, Osmanian C, Jacks T, et al. Hypoxia-mediated selection of cells with diminished apoptotic potential in solid tumours. *Nature* 1996;379(6560):88–91.

13. Lin CH, Pelissier FA, Zhang H, et al. Microenvironment rigidity modulates responses to the HER2 receptor tyrosine kinase inhibitor lapatinib via YAP and TAZ transcription factors. *Mol Biol Cell* 2015;26(22):3946–3953.

14. Dickreuter E, Eke I, Krause M, et al. Targeting of beta1 integrins impairs DNA repair for radiosensitization of head and neck cancer cells. *Oncogene* 2016;35(11):1353–1362.

15. Nam JM, Chung Y, Hsu HC, et al. Beta1 integrin targeting to enhance radiation therapy. *Int J Radiat Biol* 2009;85(11):923–928.

16. Horsman M, Wouters B, Joiner M, et al. The oxygen effect and fractionated radiotherapy. In: Kogel Jvd, ed. *Basic clinical radiobiology*. London, UK: Hodder Arnold; 2009:207–216.

17. Garcia-Barros M, Paris F, Cordon-Cardo C, et al. Tumor response to radiotherapy regulated by endothelial cell apoptosis. *Science* 2003;300(5622):1155–1159.

18. Budach W, Taghian A, Freeman J, et al. Impact of stromal sensitivity on radiation response of tumors. *J Natl Cancer Inst* 1993;85(12):988–993.

19. Garcia-Barros M, Thin TH, Maj J, et al. Impact of stromal sensitivity on radiation response of tumors implanted in SCID hosts revisited. *Cancer Res* 2010;70(20):8179–8186.

20. Gerweck LE, Vijayappa S, Kurimasa A, et al. Tumor cell radiosensitivity is a major determinant of tumor response to radiation. *Cancer Res* 2006;66(17):8352–8355.

21. Ogawa K, Boucher Y, Kashiwagi S, et al. Influence of tumor cell and stroma sensitivity on tumor response to radiation. *Cancer Res* 2007;67(9):4016–4021.

22. Gray LH, Conger AD, Ebert M, et al. The concentration of oxygen dissolved in tissues at the time of irradiation as a factor in radiotherapy. *Br J Radiol* 1953;26(312):638–648.

23. Brizel DM, Dodge RK, Clough RW, et al. Oxygenation of head and neck cancer: changes during radiotherapy and impact on treatment outcome. *Radiother Oncol* 1999;53(2):113–117.

24. Nordsmark M, Bentzen SM, Rudat V, et al. Prognostic value of tumor oxygenation in 397 head and neck tumors after primary radiation therapy. An international multi-center study. *Radiother Oncol* 2005;77(1):18–24.

25. Kovacic P, Osuna JA Jr. Mechanisms of anti-cancer agents: emphasis on oxidative stress and electron transfer. *Curr Pharm Des* 2000;6(3):277–309.

26. Brizel DM, Scully SP, Harrelson JM, et al. Tumor oxygenation predicts for the likelihood of distant metastases in human soft tissue sarcoma. *Cancer Res* 1996;56(5):941–943.

27. Hockel M, Schlenger K, Aral B, et al. Association between tumor hypoxia and malignant progression in advanced cancer of the uterine cervix. *Cancer Res* 1996;56(19):4509–4515.

28. Horsman MR, Overgaard J. The impact of hypoxia and its modification of the outcome of radiotherapy. *J Radiat Res* 2016;57(Suppl 1):i90–i98.

29. Rey S, Schito L, Koritzinsky M, et al. Molecular targeting of hypoxia in radiotherapy. *Adv Drug Deliv Rev* 2017;109:45–62.

30. Gallez B, Neveu MA, Danhier P, et al. Manipulation of tumor oxygenation and radiosensitivity through modification of cell respiration. A critical review of approaches and imaging biomarkers for therapeutic guidance. *Biochim Biophys Acta* 2017;1858:700–711.

31. Mahy P, Geets X, Lonneux M, et al. Determination of tumour hypoxia with [18F]EF3 in patients with head and neck tumours: a phase I study to assess the tracer pharmacokinetics, biodistribution and metabolism. *Eur J Nucl Med Mol Imaging* 2008;35(7):1282–1289.

32. Yasui H, Matsumoto S, Devasahayam N, et al. Low-field magnetic resonance imaging to visualize chronic and cycling hypoxia in tumor-bearing mice. *Cancer Res* 2010;70(16):6427–6436.

33. Wong KH, Panek R, Bhide SA, et al. The emerging potential of magnetic resonance imaging in personalizing radiotherapy for head and neck cancer: an oncologist's perspective. *Br J Radiol* 2017;90(1071):20160768.

34. Panek R, Welsh L, Baker LCJ, et al. Noninvasive imaging of cycling hypoxia in head and neck cancer using intrinsic susceptibility MRI. *Clin Cancer Res* 2017;23:4233–4241.

35. Colliez F, Gallez B, Jordan BF. Assessing tumor oxygenation for predicting outcome in radiation oncology: a review of studies correlating tumor hypoxic status and outcome in the preclinical and clinical settings. *Front Oncol* 2017;7:10.

36. Grimes DR, Warren DR, Warren S. Hypoxia imaging and radiotherapy: bridging the resolution gap. *Br J Radiol* 2017;90:20160939.

37. Michiels C, Tellier C, Feron O. Cycling hypoxia: a key feature of the tumor microenvironment. *Biochim Biophys Acta* 2016;1866(1):76–86.

38. Koch CJ, Jenkins WT, Jenkins KW, et al. Mechanisms of blood flow and hypoxia production in rat 9L-epigastric tumors. *Tumor Microenviron Ther* 2013;1:1–13.

39. Lin Z, Mechalakos J, Nehmeh S, et al. The influence of changes in tumor hypoxia on dose-painting treatment plans based on 18F-FMISO positron emission tomography. *Int J Radiat Oncol Biol Phys* 2008;70(4):1219–1228.

40. Overgaard J, Eriksen JG, Nordsmark M, et al. Plasma osteopontin, hypoxia, and response to the hypoxia sensitiser nimorazole in radiotherapy of head and neck cancer: results from the DAHANCA 5 randomised double-blind placebo-controlled trial. *Lancet Oncol* 2005;6(10):757–764.

41. Overgaard J, Hansen HS, Overgaard M, et al. A randomized double-blind phase III study of nimorazole as a hypoxic radiosensitizer of primary radiotherapy in supraglottic larynx and pharynx carcinoma. Results of the Danish Head and Neck Cancer Study (DAHANCA) Protocol 5-85. *Radiother Oncol* 1998;46(2):135–146.

42. Brown JM. Therapeutic targets in radiotherapy. *Int J Radiat Oncol Biol Phys* 2001;49(2):319–326.

43. Lloyd RV, Duling DR, Rumyantseva GV, et al. Microsomal reduction of 3-amino-1,2,4-benzotriazine 1,4-dioxide to a free radical. *Mol Pharmacol* 1991;40(3):440–445.

44. Wang J, Biedermann KA, Brown JM. Repair of DNA and chromosome breaks in cells exposed to SR 4233 under hypoxia or to ionizing radiation. *Cancer Res* 1992;52(16):4473–4477.

45. Rischin D, Peters LJ, O'Sullivan B, et al. Tirapazamine, cisplatin, and radiation versus cisplatin and radiation for advanced squamous cell carcinoma of the head and neck (TROG 02.02, HeadSTART): a phase III trial of the Trans-Tasman Radiation Oncology Group. *J Clin Oncol* 2010;28(18):2989–2995.

46. Peters LJ, O'Sullivan B, Giralt J, et al. Critical impact of radiotherapy protocol compliance and quality in the treatment of advanced head and neck cancer: results from TROG 02.02. *J Clin Oncol* 2010;28(18):2996–3001.

47. Hicks KO, Siim BG, Jaiswal JK, et al. Pharmacokinetic/pharmacodynamic modeling identifies SN30000 and SN29751 as tirapazamine analogues with improved tissue penetration and hypoxic cell killing in tumors. *Clin Cancer Res* 2010;16(20):4946–4957.

48. Hill RP, Bristow RG, Fyles A, et al. Hypoxia and predicting radiation response. *Semin Radiat Oncol* 2015;25(4):260–272.

49. Chan N, Pires IM, Bencokova Z, et al. Contextual synthetic lethality of cancer cell kill based on the tumor microenvironment. *Cancer Res* 2010;70(20):8045–8054.

50. Pires IM, Olcina MM, Anbalagan S, et al. Targeting radiation-resistant hypoxic tumour cells through ATR inhibition. *Br J Cancer* 2012;107(2):291–299.

51. Salem A, Asselin M-C, Reyman B, et al. Targeting hypoxia to improve non-small cell lung cancer outcome. *J Natl Cancer Inst* 2018;110. doi:10.1093/jnci/djx160.

52. Carmeliet P, De Smet F, Loges S, et al. Branching morphogenesis and antiangiogenesis candidates: tip cells lead the way. *Nat Rev Clin Oncol* 2009;6(6):315–326.

53. Folkman J. Tumor angiogenesis: therapeutic implications. *N Engl J Med* 1971;285(21):1182–1186.

54. Ahn GO, Brown JM. Role of endothelial progenitors and other bone marrow-derived cells in the development of the tumor vasculature. *Angiogenesis* 2009;12(2):159–164.

55. Hendrix MJ, Seftor EA, Seftor RE, et al. Tumor cell vascular mimicry: novel targeting opportunity in melanoma. *Pharmacol Ther* 2016;159:83–92.

56. Gorski DH, Beckett MA, Jaskowiak NT, et al. Blockage of the vascular endothelial growth factor stress response increases the antitumor effects of ionizing radiation. *Cancer Res* 1999;59(14):3374–3378.

57. Hess C, Vuong V, Hegyi I, et al. Effect of VEGF receptor inhibitor PTK787/ZK222584 [correction of ZK222548] combined with ionizing radiation on endothelial cells and tumour growth. *Br J Cancer* 2001;85(12):2010–2016.

58. Crane CH, Eng C, Feig BW, et al. Phase II trial of neoadjuvant bevacizumab, capecitabine, and radiotherapy for locally advanced rectal cancer. *Int J Radiat Oncol Biol Phys* 2010;76(3):824–830.

59. Yoon SS, Duda DG, Karl DL, et al. Phase II study of neoadjuvant bevacizumab and radiotherapy for resectable soft tissue sarcomas. *Int J Radiat Oncol Biol Phys* 2011;81:1081–1090.

60. Spigel D, Hainsworth J, Yardley D, et al. Tracheoesophageal fistula formation in patients with lung cancer treated with chemoradiation and bevacizumab. *J Clin Oncol* 2010;28:43–48.

61. Bhattacharya A, Seshadri M, Oven SD, et al. Tumor vascular maturation and improved drug delivery induced by methylselenocysteine leads to therapeutic synergy with anticancer drugs. *Clin Cancer Res* 2008;14(12):3926–3932.

62. Rofstad EK. Orthotopic human melanoma xenograft model systems for studies of tumour angiogenesis, pathophysiology, treatment sensitivity and metastatic pattern. *Br J Cancer* 1994;70(5):804–812.

63. Tong RT, Boucher Y, Kozin SV, et al. Vascular normalization by vascular endothelial growth factor receptor 2 blockade induces a pressure gradient across the vasculature and improves drug penetration in tumors. *Cancer Res* 2004;64(11):3731–3736.

64. Horsman MR, Siemann DW. Pathophysiologic effects of vascular-targeting agents and the implications for combination with conventional therapies. *Cancer Res* 2006;66(24):11520–11539.

65. Sorensen AG, Batchelor TT, Zhang WT, et al. A "vascular normalization index" as potential mechanistic biomarker to predict survival after a single dose of cediranib in recurrent glioblastoma patients. *Cancer Res* 2009;69(13):5296–5300.

66. Batchelor TT, Gerstner ER, Emblem KE, et al. Improved tumor oxygenation and survival in glioblastoma patients who show increased blood perfusion after cediranib and chemoradiation. *Proc Natl Acad Sci U S A* 2013;110(47):19059–19064.

67. Qayum N, Muschel RJ, Im JH, et al. Tumor vascular changes mediated by inhibition of oncogenic signaling. *Cancer Res* 2009;69(15):6347–6354.

68. Cerniglia GJ, Pore N, Tsai JH, et al. Epidermal growth factor receptor inhibition modulates the microenvironment by vascular normalization to improve chemotherapy and radiotherapy efficacy. *PLoS One* 2009;4(8):e6539.

69. Alghisi GC, Ponsonnet L, Ruegg C. The integrin antagonist cilengitide activates alphaVbeta3, disrupts VE-cadherin localization at cell junctions and enhances permeability in endothelial cells [Electronic Resource]. *PLoS One* 2009;4(2):e4449.

70. Kashiwagi S, Tsukada K, Xu L, et al. Perivascular nitric oxide gradients normalize tumor vasculature. *Nat Med* 2008;14(3):255–257.

71. Mazzone M, Dettori D, Leite de Oliveira R, et al. Heterozygous deficiency of PHD2 restores tumor oxygenation and inhibits metastasis via endothelial normalization. *Cell* 2009;136(5):839–851.

72. Tian L, Goldstein A, Wang H, et al. Mutual regulation of tumour vessel normalization and immunostimulatory reprogramming. *Nature* 2017;544(7649):250–254.

73. Patenaude A, Parker J, Karsan A. Involvement of endothelial progenitor cells in tumor vascularization. *Microvasc Res* 2010;79(3):217–223.

74. Ahn GO, Brown JM. Matrix metalloproteinase-9 is required for tumor vasculogenesis but not for angiogenesis: role of bone marrow-derived myelomonocytic cells. *Cancer Cell* 2008;13(3):193–205.

75. Ahn GO, Tseng D, Liao CH, et al. Inhibition of Mac-1 (CD11b/CD18) enhances tumor response to radiation by reducing myeloid cell recruitment. *Proc Natl Acad Sci U S A* 2010;107(18):8363–8368.

76. Kioi M, Vogel H, Schultz G, et al. Inhibition of vasculogenesis, but not angiogenesis, prevents the recurrence of glioblastoma after irradiation in mice. *J Clin Investig* 2010;120(3):694–705.

77. Chaudary N, Pintilie M, Jelveh S, et al. Plerixafor improves primary tumor response and reduces metastases in cervical cancer treated with radio-chemotherapy. *Clin Cancer Res* 2017;23(5):1242–1249.

78. McKeage MJ, Baguley BC. Disrupting established tumor blood vessels: an emerging therapeutic strategy for cancer. *Cancer* 2010;116(8):1859–1871.

79. Chase DM, Chaplin DJ, Monk BJ. The development and use of vascular targeted therapy in ovarian cancer. *Gynecol Oncol* 2017;145(2):393–406.

80. Josson S, Sharp S, Sung SY, et al. Tumor-stromal interactions influence radiation sensitivity in epithelial- versus mesenchymal-like prostate cancer cells. *J Oncol* 2010;2010. pii: 232831.

81. Tsai KK, Stuart J, Chuang YY, et al. Low-dose radiation-induced senescent stromal fibroblasts render nearby breast cancer cells radioresistant. *Radiat Res* 2009;172(3):306–313.

82. Korc M. Pancreatic cancer-associated stroma production. *Am J Surg* 2007;194(4 Suppl):S84–S86.

83. Butcher DT, Alliston T, Weaver VM. A tense situation: forcing tumour progression. *Nat Rev Cancer* 2009;9(2):108–122.

84. Levental KR, Yu H, Kass L, et al. Matrix crosslinking forces tumor progression by enhancing integrin signaling. *Cell* 2009;139(5):891–906.

85. Spector IH, Honig H, Kawada N, et al. Inhibition of pancreatic stellate cell activation by halofuginone prevents pancreatic xenograft tumor development. *Pancreas* 2010;39(7):1008–1015.

86. Chen Y, Liu W, Wang P, et al. Halofuginone inhibits radiotherapy-induced epithelial-mesenchymal transition in lung cancer. *Oncotarget* 2016;7(44):71341–71352.

87. Lin R, Yi S, Gong L, et al. Inhibition of TGF-beta signaling with halofuginone can enhance the antitumor effect of irradiation in Lewis lung cancer. *Onco Targets Ther* 2015;8:3549–3559.

88. Medicherla S, Li L, Ma JY, et al. Antitumor activity of TGF-beta inhibitor is dependent on the microenvironment. *Anticancer Res* 2007;27(6B):4149–4157.

89. Shimizu K. Mechanisms of pancreatic fibrosis and applications to the treatment of chronic pancreatitis. *J Gastroenterol* 2008;43(11):823–832.

90. Cook KL, Metheny-Barlow LJ, Tallant EA, et al. Angiotensin-(1-7) reduces fibrosis in orthotopic breast tumors. *Cancer Res* 2010;70(21):8319–8328.

91. Olive KP, Jacobetz MA, Davidson CJ, et al. Inhibition of Hedgehog signaling enhances delivery of chemotherapy in a mouse model of pancreatic cancer [see comment]. *Science* 2009;324(5933):1457–1461.

92. Rhim AD, Oberstein PE, Thomas DH, et al. Stromal elements act to restrain, rather than support, pancreatic ductal adenocarcinoma. *Cancer Cell* 2014;25(6):735–747.

93. Desgrosellier JS, Cheresh DA. Integrins in cancer: biological implications and therapeutic opportunities. *Nat Rev Cancer* 2010;10(1):9–22.

94. Eke I, Cordes N. Focal adhesion signaling and therapy resistance in cancer. *Semin Cancer Biol* 2015;31:65–75.

95. Dechantsreiter MA, Planker E, Matha B, et al. N-methylated cyclic RGD peptides as highly active and selective alpha(V)beta(3) integrin antagonists. *J Med Chem* 1999;42(16):3033–3040.

96. Oliveira-Ferrer L, Hauschild J, Fiedler W, et al. Cilengitide induces cellular detachment and apoptosis in endothelial and glioma cells mediated by inhibition of FAK/src/AKT pathway. *J Exp Clin Cancer Res* 2008;27:86.

97. Reardon DA, Fink KL, Mikkelsen T, et al. Randomized phase II study of cilengitide, an integrin-targeting arginine-glycine-aspartic acid peptide, in recurrent glioblastoma multiforme. *J Clin Oncol* 2008;26(34):5610–5617.

98. Albert JM, Cao C, Geng L, et al. Integrin alpha v beta 3 antagonist Cilengitide enhances efficacy of radiotherapy in endothelial cell and non-small-cell lung cancer models. *Int J Radiat Oncol Biol Phys* 2006;65(5):1536–1543.

99. Burke PA, DeNardo SJ, Miers LA, et al. Cilengitide targeting of alpha(v)beta(3) integrin receptor synergizes with radioimmunotherapy to increase efficacy and apoptosis in breast cancer xenografts. *Cancer Res* 2002;62(15):4263–4272.

100. Mikkelsen T, Brodie C, Finniss S, et al. Radiation sensitization of glioblastoma by cilengitide has unanticipated schedule-dependency. *Int J Cancer* 2009;124(11):2719–2727.

101. Stupp R, Hegi ME, Gorlia T, et al. Cilengitide combined with standard treatment for patients with newly diagnosed glioblastoma with methylated MGMT promoter (CENTRIC EORTC 26071-22072 study): a multicentre, randomised, open-label, phase 3 trial. *Lancet Oncol* 2014;15(10):1100–1108.

102. Bednar F, Simeone DM. Pancreatic cancer stem cell biology and its therapeutic implications. *J Gastroenterol* 2011;46(12):1345–1352. doi:10.1007/s00535-011-0494-7.

103. Ge Y, Gomez NC, Adam RC, et al. Stem cell lineage infidelity drives wound repair and cancer. *Cell* 2017;169(4):636.e614–650.e614.

104. Meacham CE, Morrison SJ. Tumour heterogeneity and cancer cell plasticity. *Nature* 2013;501(7467):328–337.

105. Shibue T, Weinberg RA. EMT, CSCs, and drug resistance: the mechanistic link and clinical implications. *Nat Rev Clin Oncol* 2017;14(10):611–629.

106. Sharma A, Shiras A. Cancer stem cell-vascular endothelial cell interactions in glioblastoma. *Biochem Biophys Res Commun* 2016;473(3):688–692.

107. Borovski T, De Sousa EMF, Vermeulen L, et al. Cancer stem cell niche: the place to be. *Cancer Res* 2011;71(3):634–639.

108. LaBarge MA. The difficulty of targeting cancer stem cell niches. *Clin Cancer Res* 2010;16(12):3121–3129.

109. Butler JM, Kobayashi H, Rafii S. Instructive role of the vascular niche in promoting tumour growth and tissue repair by angiocrine factors. *Nat Rev Cancer* 2010;10(2):138–146.

110. Krause M, Yaromina A, Eicheler W, et al. Cancer stem cells: targets and potential biomarkers for radiotherapy. *Clin Cancer Res* 2011;17(23):7224–7229.

111. Kraman M, Bambrough PJ, Arnold JN, et al. Suppression of antitumor immunity by stromal cells expressing fibroblast activation protein-alpha. *Science* 2010;330(6005):827–830.

112. Barry-Hamilton V, Spangler R, Marshall D, et al. Allosteric inhibition of lysyl oxidase-like-2 impedes the development of a pathologic microenvironment. *Nat Med* 2010;16(9):1009–1017.

113. Datta NR, Puric E, Klingbiel D, et al. Hyperthermia and radiation therapy in locoregional recurrent breast cancers: a systematic review and meta-analysis. *Int J Radiat Oncol Biol Phys* 2016;94(5):1073–1087.

114. Datta NR, Rogers S, Klingbiel D, et al. Hyperthermia and radiotherapy with or without chemotherapy in locally advanced cervical cancer: a systematic review with conventional and network meta-analyses. *Int J Hyperthermia* 2016;32(7):809–821.

115. Datta NR, Rogers S, Ordonez SG, et al. Hyperthermia and radiotherapy in the management of head and neck cancers: a systematic review and meta-analysis. *Int J Hyperthermia* 2016;32(1):31–40.

116. Eng JW, Reed CB, Kokolus KM, et al. Housing temperature-induced stress drives therapeutic resistance in murine tumour models through beta2-adrenergic receptor activation. *Nat Commun* 2015;6:6426.

117. Kokolus KM, Capitano ML, Lee CT, et al. Baseline tumor growth and immune control in laboratory mice are significantly influenced by subthermoneutral housing temperature. *Proc Natl Acad Sci U S A* 2013;110(50):20176–20181.

118. Rich TA, Shelton CH, 3rd, Kirichenko A, et al. Chronomodulated chemotherapy and irradiation: an idea whose time has come? *Chronobiol Int* 2002;19(1):191–205.

119. Zhanfeng N, Yanhui L, Zhou F, et al. Circadian genes Per1 and Per2 increase radiosensitivity of glioma in vivo. *Oncotarget* 2015;6(12):9951–9958.

120. Chan S, Rowbottom L, McDonald R, et al. Does the time of radiotherapy affect treatment outcomes? A review of the literature. *Clin Oncol (R Coll Radiol)* 2017;29(4):231–238.

121. Ahmed MM, Hodge JW, Guha C, et al. Harnessing the potential of radiation-induced immune modulation for cancer therapy. *Cancer Immunol Res* 2013;1(5):280–284.

122. Wattenberg MM, Fahim A, Ahmed MM, et al. Unlocking the combination: potentiation of radiation-induced antitumor responses with immunotherapy. *Radiat Res* 2014;182(2):126–138.

123. Ahmed MM, Guha C, Hodge JW, et al. Immunobiology of radiotherapy: new paradigms. *Radiat Res* 2014;182(2):123–125.

124. Rubner Y, Wunderlich R, Ruhle PF, et al. How does ionizing irradiation contribute to the induction of anti-tumor immunity? *Front Oncol* 2012;2:75.

125. Herrera FG, Bourhis J, Coukos G. Radiotherapy combination opportunities leveraging immunity for the next oncology practice. *CA Cancer J Clin* 2017;67(1):65–85.

126. Farooque A, Mathur R, Verma A, et al. Low-dose radiation therapy of cancer: role of immune enhancement. *Expert Rev Anticancer Ther* 2011;11(5):791–802.

127. Anderson RE, Warner NL. Ionizing radiation and the immune response. *Adv Immunol* 1976;24:215–335.

128. Nakamura N, Kusunoki Y, Akiyama M. Radiosensitivity of CD4 or CD8 positive human T-lymphocytes by an in vitro colony formation assay. *Radiat Res* 1990;123(2):224–227.

129. Klug F, Prakash H, Huber PE, et al. Low-dose irradiation programs macrophage differentiation to an iNOS(+)/M1 phenotype that orchestrates effective T cell immunotherapy. *Cancer Cell* 2013;24(5):589–602.

130. Aryankalayil MJ, Makinde AY, Gameiro SR, et al. Defining molecular signature of pro-immunogenic radiotherapy targets in human prostate cancer cells. *Radiat Res* 2014;182(2):139–148.

131. Popp I, Grosu AL, Niedermann G, et al. Immune modulation by hypofractionated stereotactic radiation therapy: Therapeutic implications. *Radiother Oncol* 2016;120(2):185–194.

132. Ngwa W, Ouyang Z. Following the preclinical data: leveraging the abscopal effect more efficaciously. *Front Oncol* 2017;7:66.

133. Chakraborty M, Abrams SI, Camphausen K, et al. Irradiation of tumor cells up-regulates Fas and enhances CTL lytic activity and CTL adoptive immunotherapy. *J Immunol* 2003;170(12):6338–6347.

134. Chakraborty M, Abrams SI, Coleman CN, et al. External beam radiation of tumors alters phenotype of tumor cells to render them susceptible to vaccine-mediated T-cell killing. *Cancer Res* 2004;64(12):4328–4337.

135. Kang J, Demaria S, Formenti S. Current clinical trials testing the combination of immunotherapy with radiotherapy. *J Immunother Cancer* 2016;4:51.

136. Kaur P, Asea A. Radiation-induced effects and the immune system in cancer. *Front Oncol* 2012;2:191.

137. Yovino S, Kleinberg L, Grossman SA, et al. The etiology of treatment-related lymphopenia in patients with malignant gliomas: modeling radiation dose to circulating lymphocytes explains clinical observations and suggests methods of modifying the impact of radiation on immune cells. *Cancer Invest* 2013;31(2):140–144.

138. Chadha AS, Liu G, Chen HC, et al. Does unintentional splenic radiation predict outcomes after pancreatic cancer radiation therapy? *Int J Radiat Oncol Biol Phys* 2017;97(2):323–332.

139. Kanagavelu S, Gupta S, Wu X, et al. In vivo effects of lattice radiation therapy on local and distant lung cancer: potential role of immunomodulation. *Radiat Res* 2014;182(2):149–162.

140. Blanco Suarez JM, Amendola BE, Perez N, et al. The use of lattice radiation therapy (LRT) in the treatment of bulky tumors: a case report of a large metastatic mixed Mullerian ovarian tumor. *Cureus* 2015;7(11):e389.

141. Abuodeh Y, Venkat P, Kim S. Systematic review of case reports on the abscopal effect. *Curr Probl Cancer* 2016;40(1):25–37.

142. Kwon ED, Drake CG, Scher HI, et al. Ipilimumab versus placebo after radiotherapy in patients with metastatic castration-resistant prostate cancer that had progressed after docetaxel chemotherapy (CA184-043): a multicentre, randomised, double-blind, phase 3 trial. *Lancet Oncol* 2014;15(7):700–712.

143. Anno GH, Baum SJ, Withers HR, et al. Symptomatology of acute radiation effects in humans after exposure to doses of 0.5-30 Gy. *Health Phys* 1989;56(6):821–838.

144. DiCarlo AL, Maher C, Hick JL, et al. Radiation injury after a nuclear detonation: medical consequences and the need for scarce resources allocation. *Disaster Med Public Health Prep* 2011;5(Suppl 1):S32–44.

145. Mullenders L, Atkinson M, Paretzke H, et al. Assessing cancer risks of low-dose radiation. *Nat Rev Cancer* 2009;9(8):596–604.

146. Knebel AR, Coleman CN, Cliffer KD, et al. Allocation of scarce resources after a nuclear detonation: setting the context. *Disaster Med Public Health Prep* 2011;5(Suppl 1):S20–S31.

147. Brumfiel G. Fukushima: fallout of fear. *Nature* 2013;493(7432):290–293.

148. Paunesku T, Haley B, Brooks A, et al. Biological basis of radiation protection needs rejuvenation. *Int J Radiat Biol* 2017:1–8.

149. Protection ICoR. The 2007 Recommendations of the International Commission on Radiological Protection. *Ann ICRP* 2007;37(2–4):1–332.

150. Ozasa K, Shimizu Y, Suyama A, et al. Studies of the mortality of atomic bomb survivors, Report 14, 1950–2003: an overview of cancer and noncancer diseases. *Radiat Res* 2012;177(3):229–243.

151. Little MP, Tawn EJ, Tzoulaki I, et al. A systematic review of epidemiological associations between low and moderate doses of ionizing radiation and late cardiovascular effects, and their possible mechanisms. *Radiat Res* 2008;169(1):99–109.

152. Marks LB, Bentzen SM, Deasy JO, et al. Radiation dose-volume effects in the lung. *Int J Radiat Oncol Biol Phys* 2010;76(3 Suppl):S70–S76.

153. Meng A, Wang Y, Brown SA, et al. Ionizing radiation and busulfan inhibit murine bone marrow cell hematopoietic function via apoptosis-dependent and -independent mechanisms. *Exp Hematol* 2003;31(12):1348–1356.

154. Paris F, Fuks Z, Kang A, et al. Endothelial apoptosis as the primary lesion initiating intestinal radiation damage in mice. *Science* 2001;293(5528):293–297.

155. Cucinotta FA, Durante M. Cancer risk from exposure to galactic cosmic rays: implications for space exploration by human beings. *Lancet Oncol* 2006;7(5):431–435.

156. Parihar VK, Allen B, Tran KK, et al. What happens to your brain on the way to Mars. *Sci Adv* 2015;1(4):e1400256.

157. Chancellor JC, Scott GB, Sutton JP. Space radiation: the number one risk to astronaut health beyond low earth orbit. *Life (Basel)* 2014;4(3):491–510.

158. Barcellos-Hoff MH, Blakely EA, Burma S, et al. Concepts and challenges in cancer risk prediction for the space radiation environment. *Life Sci Space Res (Amst)* 2015;6:92–103.

159. Cucinotta FA, Alp M, Rowedder B, et al. Safe days in space with acceptable uncertainty from space radiation exposure. *Life Sci Space Res (Amst)* 2015;5:31–38.

160. Blakely WF, Salter CA, Prasanna PG. Early-response biological dosimetry—recommended countermeasure enhancements for mass-casualty radiological incidents and terrorism. *Health Phys* 2005;89(5):494–504.

161. Coleman CN, Sullivan JM, Bader JL, et al. Public health and medical preparedness for a nuclear detonation: the nuclear incident medical enterprise. *Health Phys* 2015;108(2):149–160.

162. Stone HB, Moulder JE, Coleman CN, et al. Models for evaluating agents intended for the prophylaxis, mitigation and treatment of radiation injuries. Report of an NCI Workshop, December 3-4, 2003. *Radiat Res* 2004;162(6):711–728.

163. Homer MJ, Raulli R, DiCarlo-Cohen AL, et al. United States Department of Health and Human Services Biodosimetry and Radiological/Nuclear Medical Countermeasure Programs. *Radiat Prot Dosimetry* 2016;171(1):85–98.

164. Grace MB, Cliffer KD, Moyer BR, et al. The U.S. government's medical countermeasure portfolio management for nuclear and radiological emergencies: synergy from interagency cooperation. *Health Phys* 2011;101(3):238–247.

165. Prasanna PG, Stone HB, Wong RS, et al. Normal tissue protection for improving radiotherapy: where are the gaps? *Transl Cancer Res* 2012;1(1):35–48.

166. Citrin D, Cotrim AP, Hyodo F, et al. Radioprotectors and mitigators of radiation-induced normal tissue injury. *Oncologist* 2010;15(4):360–371.

167. Citrin D, Prasanna PGS, Walker AJ. Radiation-induced fibrosis: mechanisms and opportunities to mitigate. Report of an NCI Workshop, September 19, 2016. *Radiat Res* 2017;188(1):1–20.

168. Prasanna PG, Ahmed MM, Stone HB, et al. Radiation-induced brain damage, impact of Michael Robbins' work and the need for predictive biomarkers. *Int J Radiat Biol* 2014;90(9):742–752.

169. Hall EJ, Wuu CS. Radiation-induced second cancers: the impact of 3D-CRT and IMRT. *Int J Radiat Oncol Biol Phys* 2003;56(1):83–88.

170. Prasanna PG, Narayanan D, Hallett K, et al. Radioprotectors and radiomitigators for improving radiation therapy: the Small Business Innovation Research (SBIR) gateway for accelerating clinical translation. *Radiat Res* 2015;184(3):235–248.

171. Coleman CN, Hrdina C, Casagrande R, et al. User-managed inventory: an approach to forward-deployment of urgently needed medical countermeasures for mass-casualty and terrorism incidents. *Disaster Med Public Health Prep* 2012;6(4):408–414.

172. Yuan A, Sonis S. Emerging therapies for the prevention and treatment of oral mucositis. *Expert Opin Emerg Drugs* 2014;19(3):343–351.

173. Yoo SS, Jorgensen TJ, Kennedy AR, et al. Mitigating the risk of radiation-induced cancers: limitations and paradigms in drug development. *J Radiol Prot* 2014;34(2):R25–R52.

174. Vogelstein B, Papadopoulos N, Velculescu VE, et al. Cancer genome landscapes. *Science* 2013;339(6127):1546–1558.

175. Inano H, Onoda M, Inafuku N, et al. Chemoprevention by curcumin during the promotion stage of tumorigenesis of mammary gland in rats irradiated with gamma-rays. *Carcinogenesis* 1999;20(6):1011–1018.

176. Oxnard GR, Paweletz CP, Kuang Y, et al. Noninvasive detection of response and resistance in EGFR-mutant lung cancer using quantitative next-generation genotyping of cell-free plasma DNA. *Clin Cancer Res* 2014;20(6):1698–1705.

177. Sacher AG, Paweletz C, Dahlberg SE, et al. Prospective validation of rapid plasma genotyping for the detection of EGFR and KRAS mutations in advanced lung cancer. *JAMA Oncol* 2016;2(8):1014–1022.

178. Paweletz CP, Sacher AG, Raymond CK, et al. Bias-corrected targeted next-generation sequencing for rapid, multiplexed detection of actionable alterations in cell-free DNA from advanced lung cancer patients. *Clin Cancer Res* 2016;22(4):915–922.

179. Murtaza M, Dawson SJ, Pogrebniak K, et al. Multifocal clonal evolution characterized using circulating tumour DNA in a case of metastatic breast cancer. *Nat Commun* 2015;6:8760.

180. Murtaza M, Dawson SJ, Tsui DW, et al. Non-invasive analysis of acquired resistance to cancer therapy by sequencing of plasma DNA. *Nature* 2013;497(7447):108–112.

181. Perdigones N, Murtaza M. Capturing tumor heterogeneity and clonal evolution in solid cancers using circulating tumor DNA analysis. *Pharmacol Ther* 2017;174:22–26.

182. Newman AM, Bratman SV, To J, et al. An ultrasensitive method for quantitating circulating tumor DNA with broad patient coverage. *Nat Med* 2014;20(5):548–554.

183. Newman AM, Lovejoy AF, Klass DM, et al. Integrated digital error suppression for improved detection of circulating tumor DNA. *Nat Biotechnol* 2016;34(5):547–555.

184. Chang GA, Tadepalli JS, Shao Y, et al. Sensitivity of plasma BRAFmutant and NRASmutant cell-free DNA assays to detect metastatic melanoma in patients with low RECIST scores and non-RECIST disease progression. *Mol Oncol* 2016;10(1):157–165.

185. Beaton LA, Marro L, Samiee S, et al. Investigating chromosome damage using fluorescent in situ hybridization to identify biomarkers of radiosensitivity in prostate cancer patients. *Int J Radiat Biol* 2013;89(12):1087–1093.

186. Chua ML, Rothkamm K. Biomarkers of radiation exposure: can they predict normal tissue radiosensitivity? *Clin Oncol (R Coll Radiol)* 2013;25(10):610–616.

187. Torres-Roca JF. A molecular assay of tumor radiosensitivity: a roadmap towards biology-based personalized radiation therapy. *Per Med* 2012;9(5):547–557.

188. Sullivan JM, Prasanna PG, Grace MB, et al. Assessment of biodosimetry methods for a mass-casualty radiological incident: medical response and management considerations. *Health Phys* 2013;105(6):540–554.

189. Fenech M. Cytokinesis-block micronucleus cytome assay. *Nat Protoc* 2007;2(5):1084–1104.

190. Bauer DC, Gaff C, Dinger ME, et al. Genomics and personalised whole-of-life healthcare. *Trends Mol Med* 2014;20(9):479–486.

191. Freidlin B, McShane LM, Korn EL. Randomized clinical trials with biomarkers: design issues. *J Natl Cancer Inst* 2010;102(3):152–160.

192. Conroy R, Gomes L, Owen C, et al. Clinical equipoise: protons and the child with craniopharyngioma. *J Med Imaging Radiat Oncol* 2015;59(3):379–385.

193. Cheng CW, Das IJ, Srivastava SP, et al. Dosimetric comparison between proton and photon beams in the moving gap region in cranio-spinal irradiation (CSI). *Acta Oncol* 2013;52(3):553–560.

194. Suit H, Kooy H, Trofimov A, et al. Should positive phase III clinical trial data be required before proton beam therapy is more widely adopted? No. *Radiother Oncol* 2008;86(2):148–153.

195. Buchsbaum JC, McDonald MW, Johnstone PA, et al. Range modulation in proton therapy planning: a simple method for mitigating effects of increased relative biological effectiveness at the end-of-range of clinical proton beams. *Radiat Oncol* 2014;9:2.

196. Kralik SF, Ho CY, Finke W, et al. Radiation necrosis in pediatric patients with brain tumors treated with proton radiotherapy. *AJNR Am J Neuroradiol* 2015;36(8):1572–1578.

197. Buchsbaum JC. Are treatment toxicity issues in particle therapy a clarion call for biologic treatment planning overall? *Int J Radiat Oncol Biol Phys* 2017;97(5):1085–1086.

198. Suit H, DeLaney T, Goldberg S, et al. Proton vs carbon ion beams in the definitive radiation treatment of cancer patients. *Radiother Oncol* 2010;95(1):3–22.

199. Renn J. The relativity revolution from the perspective of historical epistemology. *Isis* 2004;95(4):640–648.

200. Bradley JD, Perez CA, Dehdashti F, et al. Implementing biologic target volumes in radiation treatment planning for non-small cell lung cancer. *J Nucl Med* 2004;45(Suppl 1):96S–101S.

201. Johnstone PA, Kerstiens J. Doing poorly by doing good: the bottom line of proton therapy for children. *J Am Coll Radiol* 2014;11(10):995–997.

202. Tanaka N, Ohata C, Ishii N, et al. Comparative study for the effect of photodynamic therapy, imiquimod immunotherapy and combination of both therapies on 40 lesions of actinic keratosis in Japanese patients. *J Dermatol* 2013;40(12):962–967.

203. He C, Duan X, Guo N, et al. Core-shell nanoscale coordination polymers combine chemotherapy and photodynamic therapy to potentiate checkpoint blockade cancer immunotherapy. *Nat Commun* 2016;7:12499.

204. Korbelik M, Naraparaju VR, Yamamoto N. Macrophage-directed immunotherapy as adjuvant to photodynamic therapy of cancer. *Br J Cancer* 1997;75(2):202–207.

205. Hahn SM, Fraker DL, Mick R, et al. A phase II trial of intraperitoneal photodynamic therapy for patients with peritoneal carcinomatosis and sarcomatosis. *Clin Cancer Res* 2006;12(8):2517–2525.

206. Wang L, Meng D, Hao Y, et al. Gold nanostars mediated combined photothermal and photodynamic therapy and X-ray imaging for cancer theranostic applications. *J Biomater Appl* 2015;30(5):547–557.

207. Lu K, He C, Guo N, et al. Chlorin-based nanoscale metal-organic framework systemically rejects colorectal cancers via synergistic photodynamic therapy and checkpoint blockade immunotherapy. *J Am Chem Soc* 2016;138(38):12502–12510.

208. Xu J, Xu L, Wang C, et al. Near-infrared-triggered photodynamic therapy with multitasking upconversion nanoparticles in combination with checkpoint blockade for immunotherapy of colorectal cancer. *ACS Nano* 2017;11(5):4463–4474.

209. Chen MH, Jenh YJ, Wu SK, et al. Non-invasive photodynamic therapy in brain cancer by use of Tb3+-doped LaF3 nanoparticles in combination with photosensitizer through x-ray irradiation: a proof-of-concept study. *Nanoscale Res Lett* 2017;12(1):62.

210. Tang Y, Hu J, Elmenoufy AH, et al. Highly efficient FRET system capable of deep photodynamic therapy established on x-ray excited mesoporous LaF3:Tb scintillating nanoparticles. *ACS Appl Mater Interfaces* 2015;7(22):12261–12269.

211. Kelkar SS, Reineke TM. Theranostics: combining imaging and therapy. *Bioconjug Chem* 2011;22(10):1879–1903.

212. Laster BH, Thomlinson WC, Fairchild RG. Photon activation of iododeoxyuridine: biological efficacy of Auger electrons. *Radiat Res* 1993;133(2):219–224.

213. O'Donoghue JA, Wheldon TE. Targeted radiotherapy using Auger electron emitters. *Phys Med Biol* 1996;41(10):1973–1992.

214. Karnas SJ, Yu E, McGarry RC, et al. Optimal photon energies for IUdR K-edge radiosensitization with filtered x-ray and radioisotope sources. *Phys Med Biol* 1999;44(10):2537–2549.

215. Kassis AI, Walicka MA. Double-strand break yield following ^{125}I decay effects of DNA conformation. *Acta Oncol* 2000;39(6):721–726.

216. Hofer KG. Biophysical aspects of Auger processes. *Acta Oncol* 2000;39(6):651–657.

217. Milenic DE, Brady ED, Brechbiel MW. Antibody-targeted radiation cancer therapy. *Nat Rev Drug Discov* 2004;3(6):488–499.

218. Ferrari M. Cancer nanotechnology: opportunities and challenges. *Nat Rev Cancer* 2005;5(3):161–171.

219. Peer D, Karp JM, Hong S, et al. Nanocarriers as an emerging platform for cancer therapy. *Nat Nanotechnol* 2007;2(12):751–760.

220. Savic R, Luo L, Eisenberg A, et al. Micellar nanocontainers distribute to defined cytoplasmic organelles. *Science* 2003;300(5619):615–618.

221. Maxfield FR, McGraw TE. Endocytic recycling. *Nat Rev Mol Cell Biol* 2004;5(2):121–132.

222. Gottesman MM, Pastan I, Ambudkar SV. P-glycoprotein and multidrug resistance. *Curr Opin Genet Dev* 1996;6(5):610–617.

223. Paciotti GF, Myer L, Weinreich D, et al. Colloidal gold: a novel nanoparticle vector for tumor directed drug delivery. *Drug Deliv* 2004;11(3):169–183.

224. Hainfeld JF, Slatkin DN, Smilowitz HM. The use of gold nanoparticles to enhance radiotherapy in mice. *Phys Med Biol* 2004;49(18):N309–315.

225. Libutti SK, Paciotti GF, Byrnes AA, et al. Phase I and pharmacokinetic studies of CYT-6091, a novel PEGylated colloidal gold-rhTNF nanomedicine. *Clin Cancer Res* 2010;16(24):6139–6149.

226. Cho SH. Estimation of tumour dose enhancement due to gold nanoparticles during typical radiation treatments: a preliminary Monte Carlo study. *Phys Med Biol* 2005;50(15):N163–N173.

227. Carter JD, Cheng NN, Qu Y, et al. Nanoscale energy deposition by X-ray absorbing nanostructures. *J Phys Chem B* 2007;111(40):11622–11625.

228. Boudaiffa B, Cloutier P, Hunting D, et al. Resonant formation of DNA strand breaks by low-energy (3 to 20 eV) electrons. *Science* 2000;287(5458):1658–1660.

229. Brun E, Sanche L, Sicard-Roselli C. Parameters governing gold nanoparticle X-ray radiosensitization of DNA in solution. *Colloid Surf B Biointerfaces* 2009;72(1):128–134.

230. Brun E, Duchambon P, Blouquit Y, Gold nanoparticles enhance the X-ray-induced degradation of human centrin 2 protein. *Radiat Phys Chem* 2009;78(3):177–183.

231. Chang M-Y, Shiau A-L, Chen Y-H, et al. Increased apoptotic potential and dose-enhancing effect of gold nanoparticles in combination with single-dose clinical electron beams on tumor-bearing mice. *Cancer Sci* 2008;99(7):1479–1484.

232. Boyer C, Whittaker MR, Luzon M, et al. Design and synthesis of dual thermoresponsive and antifouling hybrid polymer/gold nanoparticles. *Macromolecules* 2009;42(18):6917–6926. doi:10.1021/ma9013127.

233. Harris JM, Chess RB. Effect of pegylation on pharmaceuticals. *Nat Rev Drug Discov* 2003;2(3):214–221.

234. Duncan R. Polymer conjugates as anticancer nanomedicines. *Nat Rev Cancer* 2006;6(9):688–701.

235. Chiefari J, Chong YK, Ercole F, et al. Living free-radical polymerization by reversible addition? Fragmentation chain transfer: the RAFT process. *Macromolecules* 1998;31(16):5559–5562.

236. Berbeco RI, Ngwa W, Makrigiorgos GM. Localized dose enhancement to tumor blood vessel endothelial cells via megavoltage X-rays and targeted gold nanoparticles: new potential for external beam radiotherapy. *Int J Radiat Oncol Biol Phys* 2011;81(1):270–276.

237. Abu Lila AS, Ishida T. Liposomal delivery systems: design optimization and current applications. *Biol Pharm Bull* 2017;40(1):1–10.

238. Lee Y, Thompson DH. Stimuli-responsive liposomes for drug delivery. *Wiley Interdiscip Rev Nanomed Nanobiotechnol* 2017;9(5). doi:10.1002/wnan.1450.

239. Regen SL, Singh A, Oehme G, et al. Polymerized phosphatidyl choline vesicles. Stabilized and controllable time-release carriers. *Biochem Biophys Res Commun* 1981;101(1):131–136.

240. Lavi A, Weitman H, Holmes RT, et al. The depth of porphyrin in a membrane and the membrane's physical properties affect the photosensitizing efficiency. *Biophys J* 2002;82(4):2101–2110.

241. Chandra B, Mallik S, Srivastava DK. Design of photocleavable lipids and their application in liposomal "uncorking". *Chem Commun (Camb)* 2005;(24):3021–3023.

242. Morgan CG, Bisby RH, Johnson SA, et al. Fast solute release from photosensitive liposomes: an alternative to 'caged' reagents for use in biological systems. *FEBS Lett* 1995;375(1–2):113–116.

243. Palumbo G. Photodynamic therapy and cancer: a brief sightseeing tour. *Expert Opin Drug Deliv* 2007;4(2):131–148.

244. Brown SB, Brown EA, Walker I. The present and future role of photodynamic therapy in cancer treatment. *Lancet Oncol* 2004;5(8):497–508.

245. Schaffer M, Ertl-Wagner B, Schaffer PM, et al. The application of Photofrin II (R) as a sensitizing agent for ionizing radiation—a new approach in tumor therapy? *Curr Med Chem* 2005;12(10):1209–1215.

246. Kulka U, Schaffer M, Siefert A, et al. Photofrin as a radiosensitizer in an in vitro cell survival assay. *Biochem Biophys Res Commun* 2003;311(1):98–103.

247. Chen W, Zhang J. Using nanoparticles to enable simultaneous radiation and photodynamic therapies for cancer treatment. *J Nanosci Nanotechnol* 2006;6(4):1159–1166.

248. Soloway AH, Tjarks W, Barnum BA, et al. The chemistry of neutron capture therapy. *Chem Rev* 1998;98(4):1515–1562.

249. Chanana AD, Capala J, Chadha M, et al. Boron neutron capture therapy for glioblastoma multiforme: interim results from the phase I/II dose-escalation studies. *Neurosurgery* 1999;44(6):1182–1192; discussion 1192–1183.

250. Capala J, Stenstam BH, Skold K, et al. Boron neutron capture therapy for glioblastoma multiforme: clinical studies in Sweden. *J Neurooncol* 2003;62(1–2):135–144.

251. Kankaanranta L, Seppala T, Koivunoro H, et al. Boron neutron capture therapy in the treatment of locally recurred head-and-neck cancer: final analysis of a phase I/II trial. *Int J Radiat Oncol Biol Phys* 2012;82(1):e67–e75.

252. Tanaka H, Sakurai Y, Suzuki M, et al. Experimental verification of beam characteristics for cyclotron-based epithermal neutron source (C-BENS). *Appl Radiat Isot* 2011;69(12):1642–1645.

253. Sun T, Zhou Y, Xie X, et al. Selective uptake of boronophenylalanine by glioma stem/progenitor cells. *Appl Radiat Isot* 2012;70(8):1512–1518.

254. Capala J, Barth RF, Bendayan M, et al. Boronated epidermal growth factor as a potential targeting agent for boron neutron capture therapy of brain tumors. *Bioconjug Chem* 1996;7(1):7–15.

255. Carlsson J, Kullberg EB, Capala J, et al. Ligand liposomes and boron neutron capture therapy. *J Neurooncol* 2003;62(1–2):47–59.

256. Steiner M, Neri D. Antibody-radionuclide conjugates for cancer therapy: historical considerations and new trends. *Clin Cancer Res* 2011;17(20):6406–6416.

257. Weiner RE, Thakur ML. Radiolabeled peptides in oncology: role in diagnosis and treatment. *BioDrugs* 2005;19(3):145–163.

258. Pasieka JL, McEwan AJ, Rorstad O. The palliative role of 131I-MIBG and 111In-octreotide therapy in patients with metastatic progressive neuroendocrine neoplasms. *Surgery* 2004;136(6):1218–1226.

259. Pashankar FD, O'Dorisio MS, Menda Y. MIBG and somatostatin receptor analogs in children: current concepts on diagnostic and therapeutic use. *J Nucl Med* 2005;46(Suppl 1):55s–61s.

260. Oyen WJ, Bodei L, Giammarile F, et al. Targeted therapy in nuclear medicine—current status and future prospects. *Ann Oncol* 2007;18(11):1782–1792.

261. Parker C, Nilsson S, Heinrich D, et al. Alpha emitter radium-223 and survival in metastatic prostate cancer. *N Engl J Med* 2013;369(3):213–223.

262. Parker C, Zhan L, Cislo P, et al. Effect of radium-223 dichloride (Ra-223) on hospitalisation: an analysis from the phase 3 randomised Alpharadin in Symptomatic Prostate Cancer Patients (ALSYMPCA) trial. *Eur J Cancer* 2017;71:1–6.

263. Meredith RF, Torgue JJ, Rozgaja TA, et al. Safety and outcome measures of first-in-human intraperitoneal alpha radioimmunotherapy with 212Pb-TCMC-Trastuzumab. *Am J Clin Oncol* 2016. [Epub ahead of print.]

264. Zhang M, Zhang Z, Garmestani K, et al. Pretarget radiotherapy with an anti-CD25 antibody-streptavidin fusion protein was effective in therapy of leukemia/lymphoma xenografts. *Proc Natl Acad Sci U S A* 2003;100(4):1891–1895.

265. Karacay H, Sharkey RM, McBride WJ, et al. Pretargeting for cancer radioimmunotherapy with bispecific antibodies: role of the bispecific antibody's valency for the tumor target antigen. *Bioconjug Chem* 2002;13(5):1054–1070.

266. He B, Wahl RL, Du Y, et al. Comparison of residence time estimation methods for radioimmunotherapy dosimetry and treatment planning—Monte Carlo simulation studies. *IEEE Trans Med Imaging* 2008;27(4):521–530.

267. Croke J, Leung E, Segal R, et al. Clinical benefits of alpharadin in castrate-chemotherapy-resistant prostate cancer: case report and literature review. *BMJ Case Rep* 2012;2012. doi:10.1136/bcr-2012-006540.

PART B
Medical Radiation Physics

CHAPTER 6

Principles of Radiation Physics and Dosimetry

James A. Purdy and Sasa Mutic

A solid foundation in the principles of radiation physics, dosimetry, and treatment planning is essential for the practice of modern-day radiation oncology. This chapter discusses the basic concepts in radiation physics, radiation therapy treatment machines, and the dosimetry parameters used for photon external beam treatment planning and dose/monitor unit calculations methods. As this textbook is aimed at practicing radiation oncologists and physician residents, these topics are not treated in the detail required for medical physicists. More details on these topics can be found in the medical physics textbooks listed in the references.[1-3]

ATOMIC AND NUCLEAR STRUCTURE

The *atom* may be thought of as consisting of a centrally located core, the *nucleus*, surrounded by small orbiting particles called *electrons*. The overall dimension of an atom is about 10^{-10} m, and the nucleus is about 10^{-14} m. An electron has a rest mass (m_e) of 9.109×10^{-31} kg and has a negative electrical charge equal to 1.602×10^{-19} Coulomb (C). Most of the mass of the atom is contained in the nucleus, making it extremely dense (10^{15} kg/m^3). The nucleus is composed of two kinds of particles—*protons* and *neutrons*, known collectively as *nucleons*. A proton has a rest mass (m_p) of 1.673×10^{-27} kg and has a positive electrical charge equal in magnitude to the charge of the electron (1.602×10^{-19} C). Collectively, the protons constitute the electrical charge of the nucleus. A neutron is slightly more massive than a proton ($m_n = 1.675 \times 10^{-27}$ kg) and has no electrical charge.

Units used to describe atomic processes include the *atomic mass unit (amu)* for mass, *nanometer (nm)* for distance, *electron volt (eV)* for energy, and *electronic charge (e)* for electrical charge. The amu is defined as 1/12 the mass of the neutral carbon-12 atom. Thus, 1 amu = 1.660×10^{-27} kg. In terms of amu, a proton's rest mass is equal to 1.00727 amu, a neutron's rest mass is equal to 1.00866 amu, and an electron's rest mass is equal to 0.000548 amu. The electron volt (eV) is defined as the kinetic energy acquired by an electron accelerated through a potential difference (voltage) of 1 volt (V). One electron volt is equal to 1.6×10^{-19} joule (J) of energy. One writes 1,000 electron volts (keV) as 10^3 eV, and 1 million electron volts (MeV) as 10^6 eV. The nanometer is defined as equal to 10^{-9} m, and the electronic unit of charge is defined as equal to 1.602×10^{-19} C.

The planetary model of the atom is attributed to Niels Bohr, who in 1913 theorized that the hydrogen atom consisted of an electron orbiting around a nucleus of equal and opposite charge. He extended his theory to multielectron atoms, requiring the electrons surrounding a nucleus to be arranged in distinct, concentric shells or energy levels as shown in Figure 6.1. Energy is released when an electron moves to an orbit closer to the nucleus, and energy is required to move an electron into a higher orbit. Historically, the shells are labeled, from innermost outward, by the letters *K*, *L*, *M*, and so forth. There are a maximum number of electrons that can be accommodated in each shell: 2 in the first shell, 8 in the second, 18 in the third, and so on. The maximum number of electrons allowed in each shell is given by $2n^2$, where *n* is an integer specific to each shell and is called the *principal quantum number*. Other properties of the electron also have discrete values specified by quantum numbers. These include the electron's angular momentum as it orbits the nucleus, denoted by quantum number *l* ($l = 0, 1,...,$ $n - 1$); its spin about its axis, denoted by *s* ($s = \pm 1/2$); and its magnetic moment, denoted by m_l ($m_l = 0, \pm 1,..., \pm l$). Thus, each electron in an atom has an associated set of quantum numbers (n, l, s, m_l). This is the basis of the *Pauli exclusion principle*, which states that no two electrons can have the same set of quantum numbers within a particular atom.

Modern physics has replaced the simplistic orbiting electron model of Bohr with a complex quantum mechanical model of diffuse electron clouds that represent probability functions of the electron's position. However, for an understanding of radiologic physics, the simple Bohr model of a nucleus composed of protons and neutrons and surrounded by orbiting electrons in distinct orbits (energy levels) is sufficient.

The atom of an *element* is specified by its *atomic number*, denoted by the symbol *Z*, and its *mass number*, denoted by the symbol *A*. The atomic number is equal to the number of protons in the nucleus, and the mass number is equal to the number of nucleons (protons and neutrons) in the nucleus. Hence, *A* minus *Z* is equal to the number of neutrons, denoted by the symbol *N*, within the nucleus. In addition, each element has an associated chemical symbol (e.g., Co for cobalt). When these definitions are used, the standard notation to specify an atom is $^A_Z X$, as illustrated by $^{60}_{70} Co$, which is a radioactive isotope of the element cobalt that has an atomic number of 27 (i.e., 27 protons) and a mass number of 60 (i.e., 60 nucleons, or 27 protons and 33 neutrons).

Isotopes of an element (e.g., $^{58}_{27} Co$, $^{59}_{27} Co$, and $^{60}_{27} Co$) have the same atomic number but different numbers of neutrons and therefore different mass numbers. Isotopes have the same chemical properties but have different physical properties. Atoms such as $^{60}_{27} Co$ and $^{60}_{28} Ni$, which have the same mass number but different numbers of protons and neutrons, are called *isobars*. Atoms such as $^{57}_{27} Co$ and $^{56}_{26} Fe$, which have the same number of neutrons but different atomic and mass numbers, are called *isotones*.

Every atom has a characteristic atomic mass A_m (sometimes referred to as atomic weight). The *gram-atomic mass* of an isotope is the amount of isotope in grams that is numerically equaled to the isotope's atomic mass. For example,

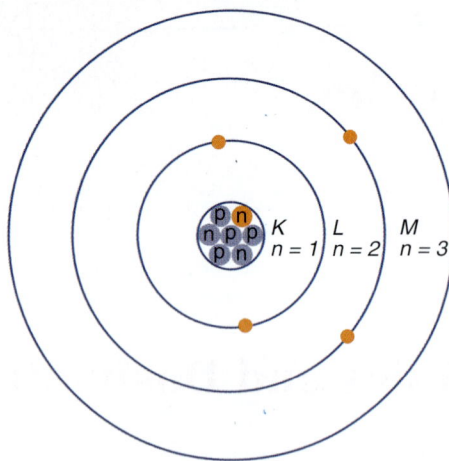

FIGURE 6.1. Schematic drawing of the Bohr model of the atom. The nucleus contains protons (p) and neutrons (n). Electrons revolve around the nucleus in specific orbits having discrete energy levels. By convention, the orbits (energy levels) are assigned either quantum numbers ($n = 1, 2, 3, \ldots$) or letters ($K, L, M, \ldots$).

1 g-atomic mass of carbon-12 is 12 g. One gram-atomic mass contains 6.0228×10^{23} atoms, a constant that is called *Avogadro number* (N_A). Useful parameters that can be calculated using Avogadro number are as follows:

Number of atoms/gram $= N_A / A_m$
Number of electrons/gram $= (N_A Z)/A_m$
Number of grams/atom $= A_m / N_A$

The closer the electrons are to the nucleus, the more tightly bound they are to the nucleus. This results from the attraction between the negatively charged electrons and the positively charged nucleus and is referred to as the *Coulomb* or *electrostatic force*. To move an electron from an inner shell to an outer shell (*excitation*) or to remove it completely from the atom (*ionization*), energy must be supplied. The energy required to remove an electron completely from an atom is called the *binding energy* for the electron. Binding energies are considered negative because energy must be supplied to remove the electron from its orbit. Atomic shells often are described in terms of binding energy, as shown in Figure 6.2 for the tungsten atom. The binding energies for the $K, L,$ and M shells are $-69,500, -11,000,$ and $-2,500$ eV, respectively. The electrons in the outermost shells are called *valence electrons* and have a binding energy of only a few electron volts because they are very loosely bound. These electrons determine the atom's chemical properties.

FIGURE 6.2. Schematic drawing of tungsten atom showing electron configuration and energy levels. (From Johns HE, Cunningham JR. *The physics of radiology.* 4th ed. Springfield, IL: Charles C Thomas, 1983:19. Courtesy of Charles C Thomas Publisher, Ltd., Springfield, Illinois.)

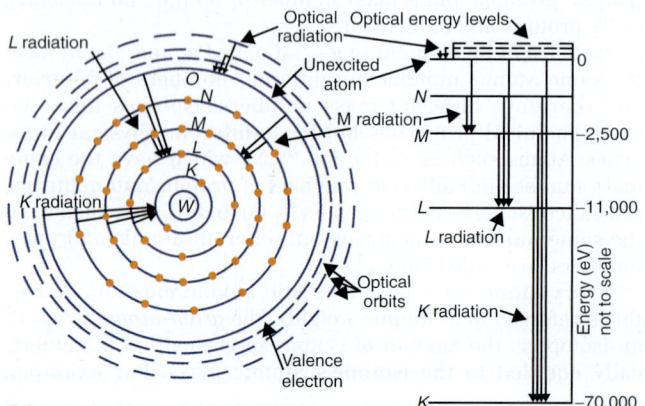

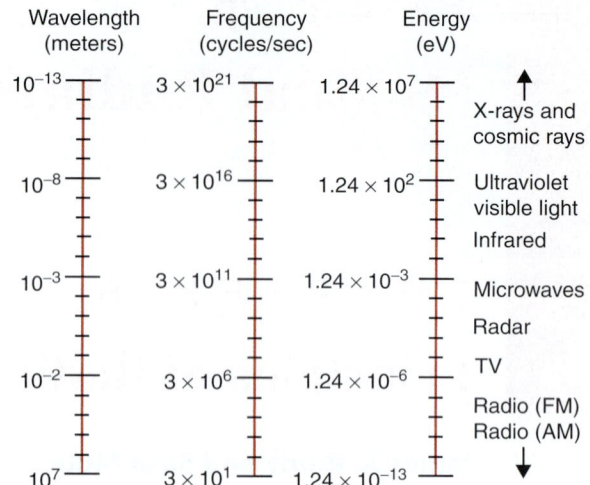

FIGURE 6.3. Electromagnetic spectrum extending over several orders of magnitude, with values of wavelength and frequency, and identifying values in some of the more common regions of the spectrum.

ELECTROMAGNETIC RADIATION

Electromagnetic radiation can be represented by a varying electric and magnetic field that is conveniently described using a sine-wave model. The sine wave is characterized by two parameters: the *frequency*, represented by the Greek letter v, and the *wavelength*, represented by the Greek letter λ. The wavelength is the distance from one crest of the sine wave to another; the frequency is the number of complete cycles or oscillations per second and is measured in *hertz* (Hz). The product of the frequency and wavelength is the speed with which the wave is propagated, which in a vacuum is the speed of light ($c = 3 \times 10^8$ m/s).

Electromagnetic radiation wavelengths extend from approximately 10^7 to 10^{-13} m. The frequencies associated with these radiations are approximately 10^1 to 10^{21} Hz. The electromagnetic spectrum shown in Figure 6.3 includes the radio and television bands; radar and microwaves; the infrared, visible, and ultraviolet regions; and x-rays and cosmic rays.

Quantum physics allows electromagnetic radiation to be represented as waves and also as particles, called *photons*. This is referred to as the *wave–particle duality of nature*. The photon energy is directly proportional to the classic wave frequency and is related to it through a constant of proportionality known as *Planck constant* (h), which has a numerical value of 6.625×10^{-34} J-sec. The relationship between energy, E, and frequency, v, is given by the following equation:

$$E = hv$$

The relationship between photon energy and photon wavelength is given by the following equation:

$$E = hc/\lambda$$

in which c is the speed of light in a vacuum. These relationships show that as the wavelength becomes shorter or the frequency becomes larger, the energy of the photon becomes greater.

X-RAYS

Wilhelm Conrad Röentgen discovered *x-rays* on November 8, 1895.[4] He observed that a paper screen coated with fluorescent material glowed when placed in the vicinity of a tube of gas at low pressure through which electricity was being passed. We now know that the x-rays were produced where the electron beam struck the anode. Energetic electrons that impinge on matter interact with either the orbital electrons or the nuclei of target atoms. The kinetic energy of the electrons

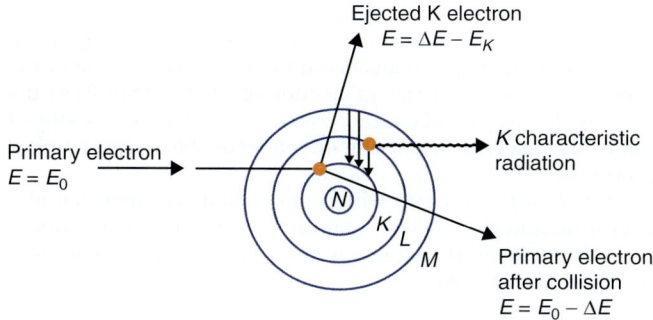

FIGURE 6.4. Schematic diagram illustrating characteristic x-ray production.

then is converted into thermal energy or electromagnetic energy (in the form of x-rays).

The impinging electron's kinetic energy is converted into thermal energy through interaction with an outer-shell electron of a target atom, which raises it to a higher energy level (referred to as *excitation*). The excited electron then returns to the normal energy level with the emission of low-energy electromagnetic radiation (*infrared*).

If the impinging electron's kinetic energy is high enough, the interaction can free an orbital electron (referred to as *ionization*), which then can result in the production of electromagnetic radiation (*characteristic x-rays*) when an outer orbital electron moves to the electron vacancy produced via ionization (Figure 6.4). The characteristic x-ray energy is equal to the difference in the binding energies of the two orbital electrons involved. Occasionally, this excess energy is transferred directly to another orbital electron, causing it to be emitted from the atom. Such electrons are called *Auger electrons*.

The impinging electron also can lose its kinetic energy via a process called *bremsstrahlung* (braking radiation), which occurs when the incident electron interacts with the electric field of the nucleus (rather than the orbiting electrons) and is deflected and loses energy. This loss of energy reappears in the form of an x-ray photon. The impinging electron can lose any amount of its kinetic energy in the bremsstrahlung process. Thus, the x-radiation produced via the bremsstrahlung process is characterized by having a continuous range of energy values, unlike characteristic x-rays, which have only discrete energy values. A bremsstrahlung spectrum (i.e., a graph of x-ray intensity vs. energy) is shown in Figure 6.5. Superimposed on the continuous bremsstrahlung x-ray spectrum are the characteristic x-rays. The maximum energy of a bremsstrahlung x-ray is numerically equal to the maximum energy of the incident electrons.

FIGURE 6.5. A bremsstrahlung x-ray spectrum calculated for a thick tungsten target extending from zero to the maximum energy of the electron. The *dotted lines* are for no filtration, and the solid curves are for a filtration of 1-mm aluminum. Note the superimposed characteristic x-ray emission spectrum. (From Johns HE, Cunningham JR. *The physics of radiology.* 4th ed. Springfield, IL: Charles C Thomas, 1983:271. Courtesy of Charles C Thomas Publisher, Ltd., Springfield, Illinois.)

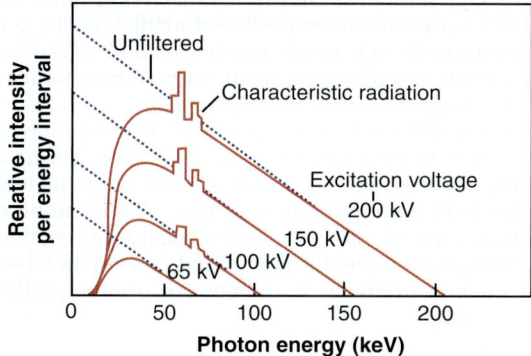

The direction of emission of the bremsstrahlung x-ray depends on the energy of the incident electron, with higher-energy electrons producing more-forward-directed x-rays.

RADIOACTIVITY

In 1896, Henri Becquerel conducted experiments in which he wrapped a photographic plate in black paper to keep out the light and then placed pieces of various elements against the wrapped plate.[5] He discovered that the mineral pitchblende emitted x-rays. Other elements—such as thorium, actinium, and two new elements (polonium and radium) discovered by Pierre and Marie Curie[6]—also emitted x-rays. Further experiments showed that the radioactive elements emitted three types of radiation: α-*particles*, having a positive electrical charge; β-*particles*, having a negative charge; and high-energy γ-*rays*, having no charge at all. We now know that an α-particle is a helium nucleus, β-particles are electrons, and γ-rays are electromagnetic radiation that is similar to x-rays except that they originate from within the nucleus of the atom.

Many other elementary particles have since been discovered and are important topics of current physics research, but they are not germane to our discussion of radiation oncology physics. Properties of the particles relevant to radiation therapy are listed in Table 6.1.

The radioactive decay processes are related to the forces involved. Huge electrostatic (Coulomb) forces of repulsion exist between the positively charged and closely spaced protons in a nucleus. However, a nuclear force of attraction (called the *strong nuclear force*) exists among the neutrons and protons, binding them together to form the nucleus. The strong nuclear force is much more complicated than the *electrostatic (Coulomb) force* and is still not completely understood. However, it is known that the strong nuclear force between nucleons depends on the distance between them and is effective only over a very short distance, whereas the electrostatic force decreases with the square of the distance. The strong nuclear force easily overcomes the repelling electrostatic force as long as the protons are very close together. However, for a large nucleus, the strong nuclear force binding the nucleons together may be weaker on opposite sides of the nucleus than the repelling electrostatic force. Therefore, a large nucleus is not as stable as a smaller nucleus.

Because neutrons interact through the attractive strong nuclear force and not the repelling electrostatic force, they can be considered stabilizing particles for the nucleus. For example, in light nuclei, only an equal number of neutrons and protons are required, but in heavier nuclei, the number of neutrons must be about 1.5 times greater than the number of protons to counteract the repelling electrostatic forces of the protons. A nuclide having too many more protons than neutrons is said to have an unfavorable N-to-Z ratio and thus undergoes *radioactive decay* to reach a stable configuration.

TABLE 6.1 PARTICLES OF INTEREST IN RADIATION THERAPY

Particle	Symbol	Charge	Mass
Photon	$h\nu$, γ	0	0
Electron	e, e$^-$, β^-	−1	0.000549 amu
Positron	e$^+$, β^+	+1	0.000549 amu
Proton	p, $^1_1$H	+1	1.007277 amu
Neutron	n, $^1_0$n	0	1.008665 amu
Alpha particle	α, $^4_2$He^{++}	+2	4.002604 amu
Neutrino	ν	0	$<1/2{,}000\, m_0$
Pi mesons	π^+, π^-	+1, −1	$273\, m_0$
	π°	0	$264\, m_0$
Mu mesons	μ^+, μ^-	+1, −1	$207\, m_0$
K mesons	K$^+$, K$^-$	+1, −1	$967\, m_0$
	K^0	0	$973\, m_0$

1 amu = 1.66043×10^{-27} kg. m_0, rest mass of an electron, 9.1091×10^{-31} kg.

The *decay constant* of a radioactive nucleus is defined as the fraction of the total number of atoms that decay per unit of time and is denoted by the symbol λ. The decay process can be represented mathematically. If N_0 radioactive nuclei are initially present in a particular sample, the number of radioactive nuclei, N, remaining at a particular time, t, is given by the following equation:

$$N = N_0 e^{-\lambda t}$$

Activity, which describes the radioactivity of a sample and is denoted by the symbol A, is defined as the total number of disintegrations per unit of time interval and is given by the following relationship:

$$A = \frac{\Delta N}{\Delta t} = -\lambda N$$

This decay-constant equation can be expressed in terms of activity:

$$A = A_0 e^{-\lambda t}$$

where A is the activity at time t and A_0 is the initial activity. The *curie* (Ci), a unit of activity, is equal to 3.7×10^{10} disintegrations per second, the approximate number of decays per second by 1 g of ^{226}Ra. The *becquerel* (Bq), the special name in the International System of Units (SI) for the measure of activity, is equal to one disintegration per second (Table 6.2).

The *half-life* of a radioactive nuclide is the time required for the number of atoms in a particular sample to decrease by one-half. The half-life, $T_{1/2}$, is related to the decay constant by the following equation:

$$T_{1/2} = \frac{0.693}{\lambda}$$

The *average life*, T_a, of a radioactive nuclide is related to the decay constant and the half-life by the following equation:

$$T_a = \frac{1}{\lambda} = 1.44\, T_{1/2}$$

The average life represents the time period that a hypothetical source would need—if it retained its original activity for that time period and then suddenly decayed to zero activity—to produce the same number of disintegrations as produced over an infinite time period by the source if it decayed exponentially.

Gamma decay occurs when a nucleus undergoes a transition from a higher to a lower energy level. In this process, a high-energy photon, called a γ-ray, is emitted. These γ-rays are identical to the x-rays emitted by excited atoms, except that γ-rays originate from within the nucleus and x-rays originate from outside the nucleus. Half-lives for γ decay are usually very short, typically 10^{-15} second.

Closely related to γ decay is the process called *internal conversion*. Instead of emitting a γ-ray, the excess energy from the excited nucleus is transferred to an electron in one of the inner atomic shells, causing ejection of the electron from the atom with emission of characteristic x-rays. The probability of internal conversion occurring increases as the atomic number increases.

In β *decay*, a neutron within the nucleus is converted into a proton, and an electron and an *antineutrino* are emitted, or a proton is converted into a neutron, and a *positron* and a *neutrino* are emitted:

$$\beta^- \text{ decay: } n \rightarrow p + \beta^- + \bar{v}$$
$$\beta^+ \text{ decay: } p \rightarrow n + \beta^+ + v$$

The positron was discovered in cosmic ray experiments in 1932. It is a positively charged particle with the same mass and spin as the electron and is considered the antiparticle of the electron. The neutrino and its antiparticle, the *antineutrino*, are massless particles (or at least have only a very small mass) having no charge that carry opposite spins and account for the conservation of energy and continuous energy spectrum observed for β decay. Particle–antiparticle pairs interact by annihilating each other, converting all their mass into electromagnetic energy (two γ-ray photons, each of 0.51 MeV). In β decay, the emitted particles may vary in the kinetic energy they possess, which is rarely >3 MeV. Half-lives for β decay are long compared with γ decay half-lives, varying from seconds to years. The forces responsible for the β decay processes are weak compared with both the *strong nuclear force* and the *electrostatic force* among the nucleons. Accordingly, the force responsible for β decay is referred to as the *weak nuclear force*.

Electron capture is an alternative to *positron decay*. In this process, an electron, usually in the K shell, is captured within the nucleus and combined with a proton to create a neutron. Electron capture most often is followed by γ decay to release any excess nuclear energy.

Alpha decay occurs in nuclides with atomic number >82 and where the ratio of neutrons to protons is low, thus resulting in the repulsive Coulomb force of the protons overcoming the attractive strong nuclear force. The emitted α-particle is a helium nucleus (two protons and two neutrons). The kinetic energy for a particular α decay is monoenergetic (i.e., the transition may be to an excited energy state with subsequent γ emission) and often 4 to 5 MeV. Half-lives range from 10^{-3} to 10^{10} years. The radioactive decay of radium to radon is an example of α decay, where the Q term represents the total energy release in the transition (called *transition energy*). For example,

$$^{226}_{88}\text{Ra} \rightarrow\, ^{222}_{86}\text{Rn} + ^4_2\alpha + \gamma + Q$$

The most recent version of the periodic table of the elements shows a grouping of 118 elements (elements 117 and 118 have not yet been observed but are included to show their expected positions). Only the first 92 occur naturally; the remaining ones have been produced artificially. In general, the elements with high atomic number tend to be radioactive; in fact, all but one of the elements with atomic number >82 (lead) are radioactive; only Bi is stable.

The naturally occurring radioactive elements have been grouped into three radioactive series called the *uranium series*, the *actinium series*, and the *thorium series*, all of which terminate with a stable isotope of lead. The uranium series provides an example of radioactive nuclides undergoing successive transformations through α and β decay in which the parent nuclide produces a radioactive product called the *daughter nuclide*.

TABLE 6.2 INTERNATIONAL SYSTEM OF UNITS (SI UNITS) FOR RADIATION THERAPY

Quantity	SI Unit (Special Name)	Non-SI Unit	Conversion Factor
Exposure	C kg^{-1}	roentgen (R)	1 C kg^{-1} $\approx$ 3,876 R
Absorbed dose, kerma	J kg^{-1} (gray [Gy])	rad	1 Gy = 100 rad
Dose equivalent	J kg^{-1} (sievert [Sv])	rem	1 Sv = 100 rem
Activity	s^{-1} (becquerel [Bq])	curie	1 Bq = 2.7 $\times$ 10^{-11} Ci

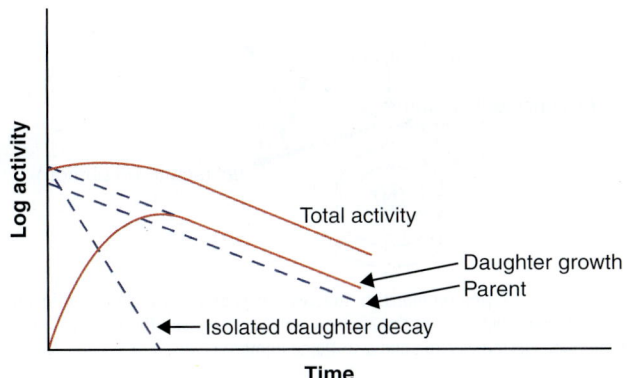

FIGURE 6.6. Transient equilibrium. Shown is a semilog plot of activity versus time for parent and daughter radionuclides illustrating conditions of transient equilibrium that may be achieved when the parent nuclide's half-life is not much greater than the half-life of the daughter nuclide. Once equilibrium is established, the daughter activity exceeds the parent activity, and both decay with the half-life of the parent.

When the half-life of the parent nuclide is longer than the half-life of the daughter nuclide, an equilibrium condition exists. When this occurs, the ratio of the activity of the daughter nuclide to the activity of the parent nuclide becomes constant, and the apparent decay rate of the daughter nuclide is controlled by the parent nuclide's decay rate. Two types of radioactive equilibrium conditions are defined: *transient equilibrium* and *secular equilibrium*. Transient equilibrium is established when the parent nuclide's half-life is not much greater than the daughter nuclide's half-life (Figure 6.6). In secular equilibrium, the half-life of the parent nuclide is much greater than that of the daughter nuclide (Figure 6.7). The two types of equilibrium are described mathematically by the following equations, in which A_P and A_D represent the activity of the parent and daughter nuclides, respectively:

$$\text{Transient equilibrium:} \quad \frac{A_D}{A_P} = \frac{\lambda_D}{\lambda_D - \lambda_P}$$

$$\text{Secular equilibrium:} \quad A_D = A_P$$

FIGURE 6.7. Secular equilibrium. Shown is a semilog plot of activity versus time for parent and daughter radionuclides illustrating conditions of secular equilibrium that may be achieved when the parent nuclide's half-life is much greater than the half-life of the daughter nuclide. Once secular equilibrium is established, activities of both parent and daughter are equal.

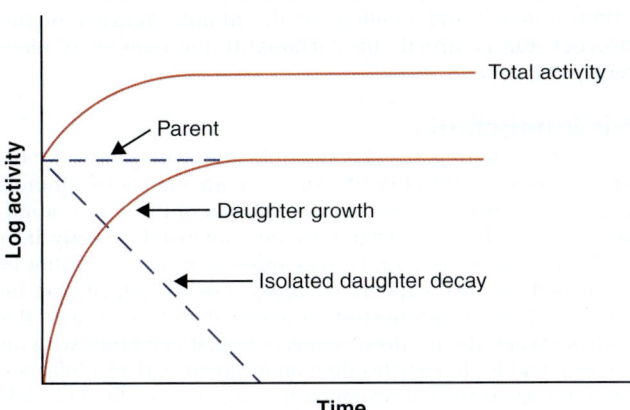

INTERACTION OF PHOTONS WITH MATTER

As stated previously, x-rays and γ-rays may be considered as bundles of energy called *photons*. If an x-ray photon enters a thin layer of matter, it is possible that it will pass through without interaction, or it may interact (usually with the atomic electrons, but sometimes with the atomic nuclei) in one of five different ways (*coherent scattering, photoelectric effect, Compton scattering, pair production,* and *photodisintegration*). The probability that a photon will interact when it traverses through a given thickness of material is the product of the individual interaction probabilities for each of these processes. The attenuation process can be described mathematically by the following equation:

$$N = N_0 e^{-\mu x}$$

where N_0 is the number of photons in the beam impinging on an absorber of thickness x, e is the base of the natural logarithms, and μ is the linear attenuation coefficient. The quantity μ is actually the sum of the individual attenuation coefficients for the five processes. Its numerical value depends on the energy of the photon and the type of attenuating material.

There are a variety of tabulated attenuation coefficients, including the *linear attenuation coefficient* (μ), the *mass attenuation coefficient* (μ/ρ), the *mass energy-transfer coefficient* (μ_{tr}/ρ), and the *mass energy-absorption coefficient* (μ_{en}/ρ). Each type of coefficient is intended for use in the solution of different types of attenuation or energy-absorption problems; division by ρ, the physical density of the medium, makes the coefficient medium independent. Figure 6.8 shows the mass attenuation coefficient for lead and water as a function of incident photon energy. The discontinuities where the attenuation coefficient suddenly increases are called *absorption edges* and occur at photon energies just equal to the binding energy of a specific electron shell.

The thickness of material that reduces the number of photons transmitted to one-half the incident number is termed the *half-value layer* (HVL). The HVL is related to the linear attenuation coefficient by the following equation:

$$\text{HVL} = \frac{0.693}{\mu}$$

This parameter is used to describe the *quality* or *penetrability* of the radiation and is discussed later in this chapter.

FIGURE 6.8. Mass attenuation coefficient for lead and water. Note sharp discontinuities, which are called *absorption edges*. (From Johns HE, Cunningham JR. *The physics of radiology*. 4th ed. Springfield, IL: Charles C Thomas, 1983:147. Courtesy of Charles C Thomas Publisher, Ltd., Springfield, Illinois.)

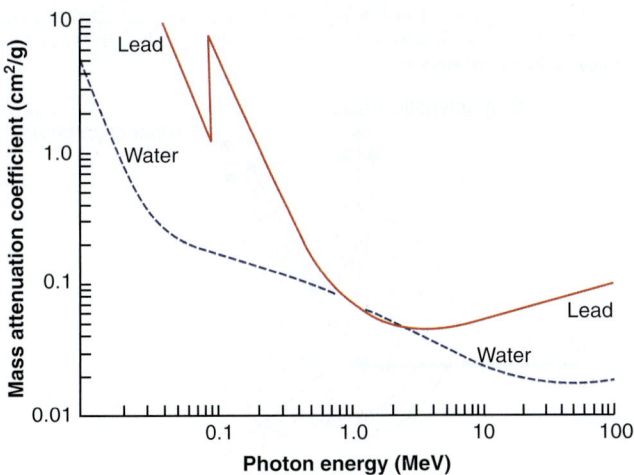

Coherent or Classical Scattering

If the photon energy is low enough that the quantum effects of the interaction are unimportant and the bound electron(s) can be regarded as essentially "free," the interaction corresponds to the "classical scattering" situation (called *coherent scattering*), in which the incident electrical field accelerates one or more orbital electrons and causes them to radiate. There are two types of coherent scattering: *Thomson scattering*, in which a single orbital electron is involved, and *Rayleigh scattering*, in which the orbital electrons act as a single group. In coherent scattering, no energy is transferred; only the direction of the incident photon is changed. The coherent mass attenuation coefficient is denoted by σ_{coh}/ρ.

Photoelectric Effect

In the *photoelectric effect*, the total energy of the photon is transferred to an orbital electron, usually close to the nucleus, and the photon disappears. The electron then is ejected from the atom with an energy equal to the energy of the photon minus the binding energy of the electron (Fig. 6.9). The direction in which the electron is emitted depends on the energy of the incident photon. For the low-energy photons (e.g., 50 keV), the photoelectron is ejected at a large angle with respect to the incoming photon's direction, increasing in the forward direction as the photon's energy increases. After ejection of the electron, the neutral atom becomes a positively charged ion with a vacancy in an inner shell that must be filled. The atom returns to a stable condition by filling the vacancy with a nearby, less tightly bound electron farther out from the nucleus, and characteristic x-rays or an Auger electron is emitted.

The probability that a given photon will interact by means of the photoelectric process (denoted by τ/ρ) is a function of both the photon's energy and the atomic number of the target atom. For the process to occur, the incident photon must have energy greater than the binding energy of the involved orbital electron. In general, the probability per electron that a photon will undergo a photoelectric interaction is inversely proportional to the third power of the photon's energy and directly proportional to the third power of the atomic number of the target atom.

Compton Scattering

In *Compton scattering*, the incident photon interacts with a loosely bound orbital electron in which part of the photon's energy is transferred to the electron as kinetic energy and the remaining energy is carried away by another photon

FIGURE 6.9. Photoelectric effect. In this type of photon interaction, the incident photon disappears, and an electron is ejected with kinetic energy equal to the incident photon's energy minus the binding energy of the electron. Characteristic x-rays and Auger electrons are emitted as the atom's electrons cascade to fill the vacancy created by the ejected electron.

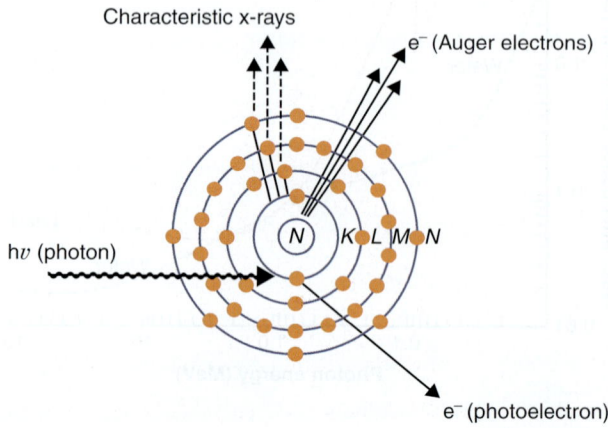

Characteristic x-rays

e⁻ (Auger electrons)

hv (photon)

N   K L M N

e⁻ (photoelectron)

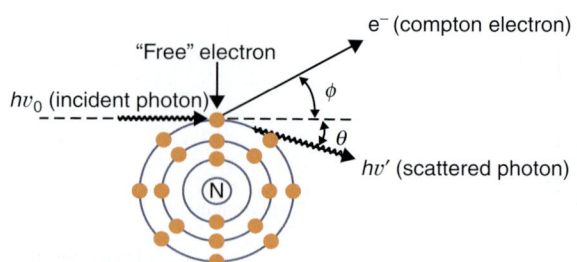

FIGURE 6.10. Compton effect. In this type of photon interaction, the incident photon interacts with one of the atom's outer electrons, and the energy is shared between the ejected electron and a scattered photon.

(Fig. 6.10). The binding energy of the electron is insignificant compared with the incident photon's energy and thus can be ignored. The energy of the Compton-scattered photon is equal to the difference between the energy of the incident photon and the energy transferred to the electron. If the incoming photon's energy is low (e.g., 100 keV), very little energy is transferred to the electron. As the photon's energy increases, a greater proportion of the energy is transferred to the electron, so the scattered photon necessarily retains a smaller proportion of the incident energy. The photon may be scattered at any angle with respect to the direction of the incident photon, but the Compton electron is confined to angles between 0 and 90 degrees with respect to the direction of the incident photon. If the incoming photon's energy is low, the distribution of the scattered photons is isotropic (equal in all directions). The scatter angles decrease for photons and electrons as the incident photon's energy increases (e.g., at megavoltage photon energies, both are scattered predominantly in the forward direction).

As a result of conservation of energy and momentum, the energies of the incident photon, hv_0; the scattered photon, hv'; and the scattered electron, E, are given by the following relationships:

$$E = hv_0 \frac{\alpha(1 - \cos \theta)}{1 + \alpha(1 - \cos \theta)}$$

$$hv' = hv_0 \frac{1}{1 + \alpha(1 - \cos \theta)}$$

$$\cot(\varphi) = (1 + \alpha) \tan(\theta/2)$$

where $\alpha = hv_0/m_0c^2$, and m_0c^2 is the rest energy of the electron (0.511 MeV). If hv_0 is expressed in MeV, then $\alpha = hv_0/0.511$.

The probability that a photon will interact with a target atom via the Compton process (σ_c/ρ) depends on the energy of the incoming photon, generally decreasing as the energy of the photon is increased. The probability of a Compton interaction is nearly independent of the atomic number of the absorber and is directly proportional to the number of electrons per gram.

Pair Production

Pair production (Fig. 6.11) is possible only with photons having energies >1.02 MeV. When such an energetic photon approaches closely enough to the nucleus of the target atom, the incident photon energy may be converted directly into an electron–positron pair. Energy possessed by the photon in excess of 1.02 MeV appears as kinetic energy, which may be distributed in any proportion between the electron and the positron. When the positron comes to rest, it combines with an electron, and both particles then undergo mutual annihilation, with the appearance of two photons with energy of 0.511 MeV traveling in opposite directions. The probability of pair production (π/ρ) occurring increases rapidly with incident photon

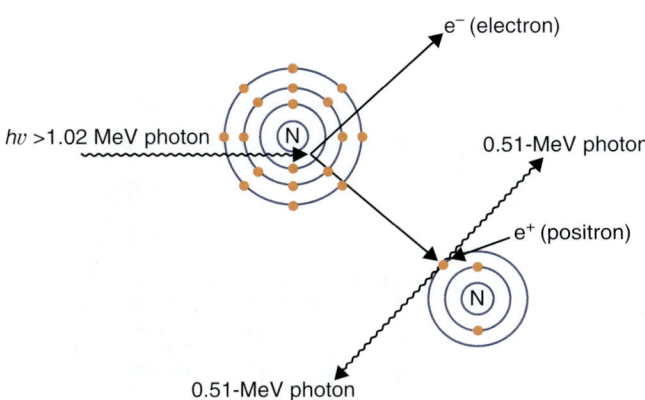

e⁻ (electron)

hv >1.02 MeV photon

0.51-MeV photon

e⁺ (positron)

0.51-MeV photon

FIGURE 6.11. Pair production. In this type of photon interaction, the incident photon interacts with the electromagnetic field of the nucleus. The incident photon disappears, and two energetic electrons (a positron and a negatron) are produced. Two annihilation photons of energy 0.511 MeV then are produced when the positron interacts with its antiparticle, another electron.

energy above the 1.02-MeV threshold and is proportional to Z^2 per atom, Z per electron, and approximately Z per gram.

Photodisintegration

In *photodisintegration*, a high-energy photon interacts with the nucleus of an atom, totally disrupting the nucleus, with the emission of one or more nucleons. It typically occurs at photon energies much higher than those encountered in radiation therapy. However, it is important to account for this in designing shielding around high-energy accelerators, as this interaction is a source of low-energy neutrons.

Relative Importance of Interaction Processes

Figure 6.12 illustrates the relative importance of the photoelectric, Compton, and pair-production processes—the three principal modes of interactions pertinent to radiation therapy—as a function of energy and atomic number of the absorber. For example, for an absorber with an atomic number approximately equal to that of tissue ($Z = 7$) and for monoenergetic photons, the photoelectric effect is the dominant interaction below about 30 keV. Above 30 keV, the Compton effect becomes dominant and remains so until approximately 24 MeV, at which point pair production becomes the dominant interaction. The total mass attenuation coefficient accounting

FIGURE 6.12. Relative importance of the three principal modes of interaction as a function of photon energy and atomic number of absorber. (Reprinted from Hendee WR, Ritenour ER. *Medical imaging physics*. 3rd ed. St. Louis: Mosby-Year Book, 1992. Copyright © 1992 Elsevier. With permission.)

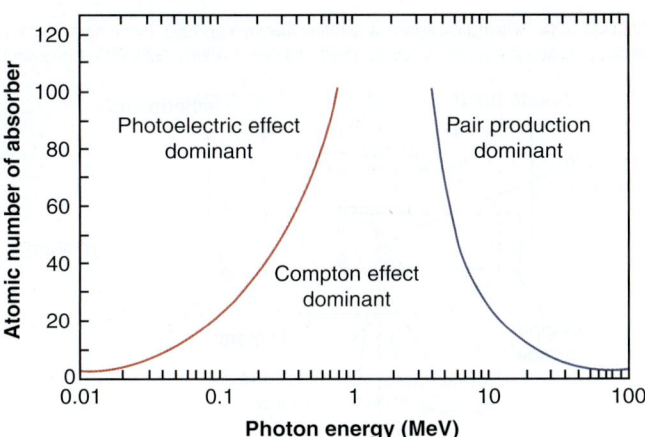

for all the photon interactions discussed is given by the sum of the individual coefficients:

$$\mu_{en}/\rho = \sigma_{coh}/\rho + \tau/\rho + \sigma_c/\rho + \pi/\rho$$

INTERACTION OF PARTICLES WITH MATTER

Electrons

An electron loses its kinetic energy when traversing matter via interactions that can be either *elastic*, in which no kinetic energy is lost, or *inelastic*, in which some portion of the kinetic energy is changed into some other form of energy. The term *linear energy transfer (LET)* is used to describe how much energy an ionizing particle transfers to the material traversed per unit distance. Elastic collisions occur with either atomic electrons or with atomic nuclei and are characterized by a change in direction of the incident electron with no loss of kinetic energy. Inelastic collisions can occur with atomic electrons, resulting in *ionizations* and *excitations* of atoms, or inelastic collisions with atomic nuclei, which result in the production of bremsstrahlung x-rays (*radiative losses*). In the case of ionization, it is possible for the ejected electron to acquire enough kinetic energy to cause additional ionizations of its own. These electrons are called *secondary electrons* or *δ rays*, and they can go on to produce additional ionizations and excitations. The typical energy loss in tissue for a therapeutic electron beam, averaged over its entire range, is about 2 MeV/cm in water.

The complete description of the energy and depth of penetration of the moving electrons at any point in the medium is complicated by the fact that the electrons are very much lighter than the atomic nuclei. As a result, the electron can lose a very large fraction of its energy in a single process and thus can be deflected by very large angles. This means that even if the electron beam is monoenergetic when first impinging on a medium, there will be a large variation among all the moving electrons as to where in the medium each will stop. This is referred to as *range straggling*.

Protons and Heavier Ions

Protons traverse relatively straight paths through matter, slowing down continuously by interactions with atomic electrons and with atomic nuclei. This results in depth–dose characteristics that show an approximately constant absorbed dose value over most of the beam range until near the end of the proton's range, where a very sharp increase in dose occurs (called the *Bragg peak*), as shown in Figure 6.13. Dose at the peak is approximately four times the dose at the surface, and the distal width of the peak is on the order of 1 cm, depending on beam energy and beam energy spread. Depth–dose characteristics customized for individual patients can be generated by superposition of multiple proton beams having different energies. This technique creates a *spread-out Bragg peak (SOBP)* that covers the target volume and decreases sharply to zero dose a few millimeters beyond the target. Protons are somewhat more effective biologically than photons, that is, a lower dose is required to cause the same biological effect. This concept of *relative biological effectiveness (RBE)* of protons is defined as the dose of a reference radiation (typically ⁶⁰Co) divided by the proton dose to achieve the same biological effect. Paganetti et al.[7] has shown that proton RBE varies (≅10%) along the Bragg peak, particularly at the distal end where LET is high. Current clinical practice and ICRU recommendations[8] advocate that an overall RBE factor of 1.1 be applied.

Heavier ions, such as carbon, are also being used in modern radiation therapy at a few medical heavy-ion facilities in Europe and Asia.[9-11] Because of the greater mass of carbon ions, multiple scattering and range straggling are much less

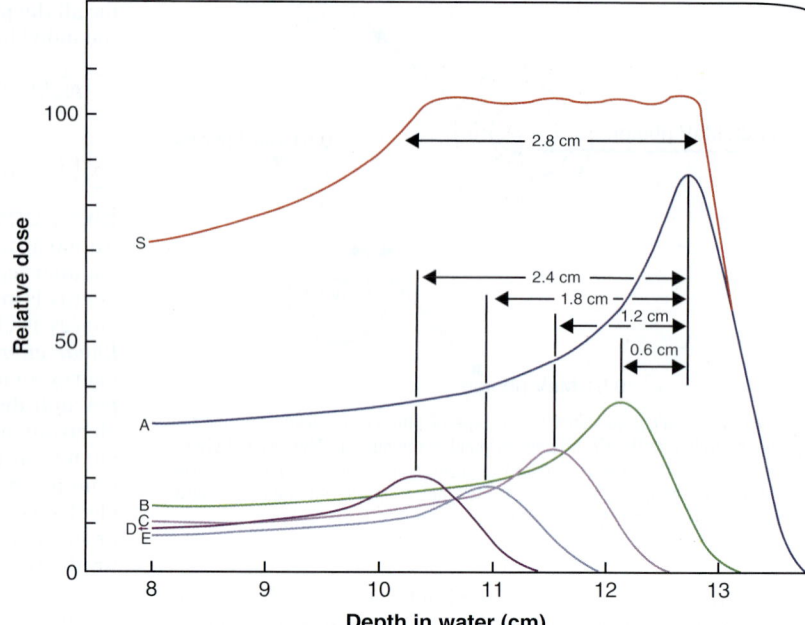

FIGURE 6.13. Drawing illustrating the way in which the Bragg peak for a proton beam can be spread out. Curve A is the depth–dose distribution for the primary beam of 160-MeV protons at the Harvard cyclotron. Beams of lower intensity and shorter range, as illustrated by curves B to E, can be added to give a composite curve, S, which results in a uniform dose of >2.8 cm. (From Hall EJ. *Radiobiology for the radiologist.* 4th ed. Philadelphia: JB Lippincott, 1994. With permission.

than protons, resulting in a sharper lateral and longitudinal edge. Also, because the LET in the peak of a carbon beam is larger than that of proton beams, the RBE is far greater for carbon ions.

Neutrons

Neutrons, like photons, are uncharged and thus are an indirectly ionizing radiation, which are exponentially attenuated by matter. The interactions are through processes that are primarily nuclear. They include elastic scattering with nuclei that make up the body's tissues (hydrogen, oxygen, carbon, nitrogen, etc.). Neutron interactions result in recoil protons and charged nuclear fragments that have relatively low energy. The RBEs of these resultant particles are not fully known, thereby complicating the understanding of the relationship between clinical response and absorbed dose.

RADIATION THERAPY TREATMENT MACHINES

Kilovoltage Units

Before 1951, most radiation treatment units were kilovoltage x-ray machines capable of producing photon beams having only limited penetrability. Today, this type of machine is still used in some clinics for the treatment of skin cancer. In these machines, the electrons are accelerated by an electric field produced from a high voltage generated in a transformer that is applied directly between the filament (cathode) and the x-ray target (anode). A schematic diagram of a radiation therapy x-ray tube is shown in Figure 6.14. The potential difference (kVp) is variable on these machines, and metal filters can be added to absorb the lower-energy photons preferentially, changing the penetrability of the beam. The combination of variable kVp and different filtration provides the capability of generating multiple x-ray beams. The degree of penetrability is used to categorize the units as *contact*, *superficial*, and *orthovoltage* (deep-therapy) x-ray machines. A more detailed review of these type of treatment machine is provided by Biggs et al.[12]

Contact Units

A contact x-ray machine typically operates at potentials of 40 to 50 kVp and at a tube current of 2 to 5 milliamperes (mA).

Attached cones are used for a source–skin distance (SSD) of typically 2 cm or less. Filters of 0.5- to 1.0-mm aluminum are used to give a typical HVL of 0.6-mm aluminum. The x-ray tube is rod shaped with an extremely thin mica–beryllium window, having an inherent filtration of 0.03-mm-aluminum equivalence, and the radiation is emitted axially. The primary radiation therapy application of a contact x-ray unit is for endocavitary irradiation of selected small rectal carcinomas.[13]

Superficial Units

A superficial unit is an x-ray machine that operates at potentials of 50 to 150 kVp and 5 to 10 mA. Added thickness of filtration (1-mm Al to 1-mm Al + 0.25-mm Cu) produces HVLs of 1.0 to 8.0 mm of aluminum. Attached cones typically are used; lead masks are used to define irregular fields. The SSD is typically 15 or 20 cm. These machines are used primarily to treat skin lesions.

Orthovoltage (Deep-Therapy) Units

Orthovoltage x-ray machines operate at potentials between 150 and 500 kV, with most operating between 200 and 300 kV, and with tube currents of 10 to 20 mA. HVLs of 1 to 4 mm of copper are common with the use of added filters, such as the *Thoraeus filter*, a combination of thin sheets of tin, copper, and aluminum arranged so that the highest–atomic number sheet is always closest to the x-ray target, ensuring

FIGURE 6.14. Schematic diagram of radiation therapy x-ray tube. (From Khan FM. *The physics of radiation therapy*. 2nd ed. Baltimore: Williams & Wilkins, 1994. With permission.)

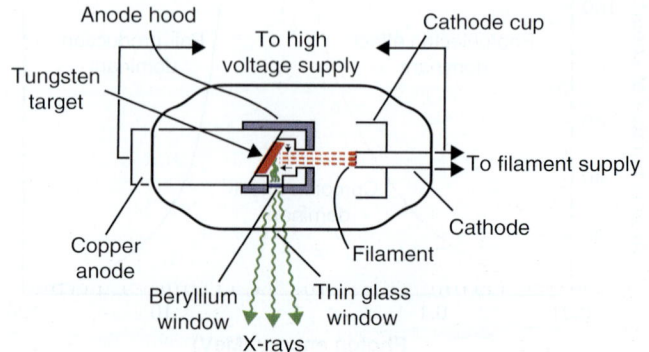

that the higher-energy characteristic x-rays are absorbed by the lower-Z metal. Treatment fields usually are defined using detachable cones. The SSD is typically 50 cm. Very few of these types of machines are still in clinical use.

Supervoltage and Megavoltage Photon and Electron Beam Treatment Units

X-ray treatment machines operated in the range of 500 to 1,000 kV were designated as *supervoltage therapy* machines.[14] The *resonant transformer x-ray machine* is an example of this type of kilovoltage machine. X-ray treatment machines that can produce beams 1 MV or greater have been designated as *megavoltage therapy* machines. One of the first megavoltage machines was the *Van de Graaff generator*, which operated at 1 to 2 MV. Another early type of megavoltage machine was the *betatron*, first developed in 1941 by Kerst.[15] Betatrons used in radiation oncology produced x-ray beams with energies of >40 MV. All of these early machines are now obsolete and no longer in clinical use. Details on the history and development of these early accelerators used in radiation therapy can be found in the textbook by Karzmark et al.[16]

Cobalt-60 Teletherapy

The first *cobalt-60* (^{60}Co) *teletherapy* machine was loaded with its ^{60}Co source in August 1951 in the Saskatoon Cancer Clinic, Saskatoon, Canada, and the first patient was treated on November 8 of that year.[17,18] A very readable history of the development of the first cobalt-60 teletherapy machine in the United States is provided by Almond.[19] A technical review of ^{60}Co teletherapy machines is provided by Glasgow.[20] The advantages of a ^{60}Co teletherapy machine are its relative constancy of beam output, predictability of decay because of a well-defined half-life, and lack of day-to-day small-output fluctuations typically found in electrical machines. Disadvantages include the need for source replacement approximately every 4 to 5 years, poor field flatness for large fields and large penumbra, and lower depth dose compared with high-energy photons generated by medical linear accelerators and discussed later. Isocentric units with source-to-axis distance (SAD) of 80 or 100 cm were designed with maximum field sizes of 40 × 40 cm at the machine isocenter for the 100-cm SAD machine. Source activities vary from about 5,000 to 13,000 Ci in 1.5- to 2.0-cm-diameter sources and yield exposure rates from 150 to 250 R/min at 1 m. The radiation consists of 1.17- and 1.33-MeV γ-rays having a $d_{1/2}$ in tissue (the depth at which the dose has been reduced to 50% of the maximum dose value) of about 10 cm.

Cobalt teletherapy machines became a mainstay for radiation therapy for nearly three decades but are rarely used in US clinics today. Cobalt-based teletherapy machines do remain a valuable radiotherapy solution in developing countries, though there are several active programs to provide economical solutions which do not rely on radioactive materials.

Two exceptions for use of cobalt in modern radiotherapy machines are the Elekta Gamma Knife (Elekta AB, Stockholm, Sweden) stereotactic radiosurgery machines and the magnetic resonance (MR) guided radiotherapy machine by ViewRay (ViewRay Inc., Oakwood Village, OH).[21] Both of these technologies offer state-of-the-art radiotherapy solutions based on cobalt.

Gamma Knife

Elekta *Gamma Knife* is a dedicated stereotactic radiosurgical device that was developed in 1968 by Dr. Lars Leksell,[22] a Swedish neurosurgeon. This machine initially made it possible to deliver a single, large dose of highly conformal radiation (γ-rays) precisely to a number of intracranial sites using multiple fixed ^{60}Co sources aimed at a center point. As the field of cranial stereotactic radiosurgery evolved, Gamma

Knife started offering solutions for fractionated treatments, named *stereotactic radiotherapy*. In stereotactic radiotherapy patients are treated with several fractions of highly conformal doses without use of ring frames and relying on thermoplastic masks for immobilization. The Gamma Knife traditionally consisted of three basic components—a spherical source housing/gantry, four collimator helmets, and a couch with electronic controls. The source housing (models U, B, and C) contains 201 ^{60}Co sources distributed in a quasihemispherical arrangement. The γ-rays from each source converge to the *unit center point* (UCP), which is 40 cm away from each source. The UCP is analogous to the isocenter of a teletherapy machine and is the location where the target volume must be positioned during a treatment. This is accomplished by the three-axis coordinate system on the Leksell stereotactic frame. Each source has an activity of approximately 30 Ci when newly installed, and the 201 sources combined provide a dose rate of approximately 300 cGy/min at the UCP. Along the path to the UCP, the radiation beam from each source is collimated twice—once by a primary collimator and then by one of four secondary collimator helmets. For each helmet, 201 tungsten collimators define specified circular apertures (4, 8, 14, or 18 mm projected at the UCP). To conform the radiation dose to the shape of the target in the patent, various combinations of aperture diameters, aperture blocking (*plugging*), irradiation times, and head positions are used. A specific combination of these four parameters defines what is referred to as a *shot* in Gamma Knife terminology. Hundreds of thousands of patients have been treated using this type of treatment machine.

In 2006, Elekta introduced the Gamma Knife Perfexion, which was a major change in design from the previous models, with several advanced features, including an enlarged internal patient cavity for extended access to peripheral cranial anatomy. Unlike the earlier models, the Perfexion moves the entire patient on the couch to each stereotactic x, y, and z coordinate. The collimation was also placed within the source housing part of to the machine gantry, eliminating the external helmets. The sources are arranged radially and divided into eight moving sectors with 24 sources each. Each sector is independently selectable, thereby providing various sector combinations for aperture (collimation) size or blocking at each shot position during treatment. With the introduction of its associated Extend System accessory, the Perfexion has an increased reach to allow treatments to the upper cervical spine.

In 2015, Elekta introduced the Gamma Knife Icon (Fig. 6.15), which added image-guided radiation therapy (IGRT) imaging capability. The Icon enables cone beam computed tomography (CBCT)-based patient localization capability and intrafraction patient monitoring with infrared camera. CBCT isocenter is placed away from the cobalt sources isocenter, but the two isocenters are linked in software and hardware and the Icon provides workflows for patient localization, treatment evaluation, and adjustments when need. In this sense the Icon offers modern IGRT capabilities in combination with cobalt radiotherapy.

Image-Guided Cobalt (ViewRay)

A concept of combining a linac-based radiation therapy treatment machine with a magnetic resonance imaging (MRI) scanner originated in 1990s, and several research groups worked on development of such system. ViewRay system (Fig. 6.16) was a parallel commercial effort, which concentrated on combining a 0.35-T split bore MRI, which straddles a radiotherapy gantry housing three cobalt heads spaced 120 degrees apart. Each head contains a nominally 15,000 Ci cobalt source mated to a multileaf collimator (MLC). The three sources contributed to the combined initial dose rate of approximately 600 cGy/min. The MRI scanner and radiotherapy gantry

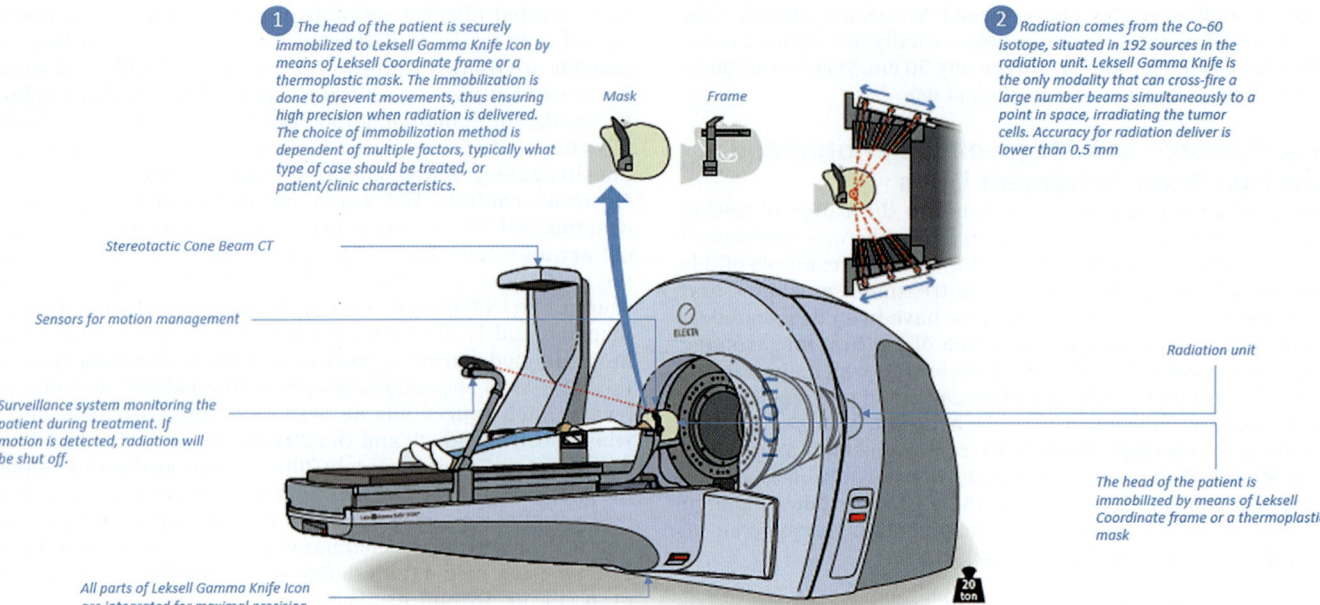

① *The head of the patient is securely immobilized by Leksell Gamma Knife Icon by means of Leksell Coordinate frame or a thermoplastic mask. The immobilization is done to prevent movements, thus ensuring high precision when radiation is delivered. The choice of immobilization method is dependent of multiple factors, typically what type of case should be treated, or patient/clinic characteristics.*

② *Radiation comes from the Co-60 isotope, situated in 192 sources in the radiation unit. Leksell Gamma Knife is the only modality that can cross-fire a large number beams simultaneously to a point in space, irradiating the tumor cells. Accuracy for radiation deliver is lower than 0.5 mm*

Mask Frame

Stereotactic Cone Beam CT

Sensors for motion management

Surveillance system monitoring the patient during treatment. If motion is detected, radiation will be shut off.

Radiation unit

The head of the patient is immobilized by means of Leksell Coordinate frame or a thermoplastic mask

All parts of Leksell Gamma Knife Icon are integrated for maximal precision

FIGURE 6.15. Elekta Gamma Knife (Elekta AB, Stockholm, Sweden) is a dedicated stereotactic radiosurgical device first developed in 1968 by Dr. Lars Leksell, a Swedish neurosurgeon, to provide highly accurate radiation ablative treatment of intracranial targets. Shown is the latest model, the Gamma Knife Icon, which now includes an integrated immobilization system and an integrated stereotactic cone beam CT system.

shared a common isocenter enabling MR-based treatment localization as well as intrafractional treatment monitoring with MRI. The first MR-guided radiotherapy treatment occurred at Washington University in St. Louis on January 15, 2014. The clinical system relied exclusively on Monte Carlo–based dose calculation and intensity-modulated radiation therapy (IMRT), 2D, and 3D treatment capabilities. While the ViewRay system relied on cobalt sources, which inherently have large penumbra than do linac-based systems, the doubly focused MLCs offered better collimation than did the contemporary linear accelerators resulting in equivalent treatment dose distributions between the two technologies.[23,24] The initial ViewRay system also enabled practical online adaptive radiotherapy where patients could be imaged, new plan generated, patient specific QA performed, and treatment delivered all

FIGURE 6.16. ViewRay system combines a 0.35 T split bore MRI, which straddles a radiotherapy gantry housing three cobalt heads spaced 120 degrees apart. The MRI scanner and radiotherapy gantry shared a common isocenter enabling MR-based treatment localization as well as intrafractional treatment monitoring with MRI.

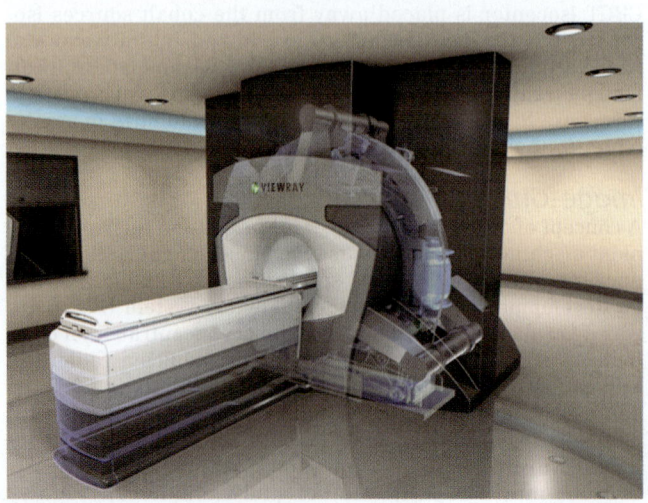

within the time compatible with conventional radiotherapy treatment times.[25,26] This really also marked the initiation of the first practical online adaptive radiotherapy program, and Washington University treated the first online MR-guided adaptive radiotherapy treatment on September 8, 2014. This program quickly grew with several hundred adaptive treatments administered within the first 2 years of operation. The third key distinguishing functionality that the ViewRay system offered was intrafractional anatomy tracking and treatment control (gating). In this application, the ViewRay systems enabled acquisition of four sagittal orientated single image frames per second. On each of the acquired images, the system automatically contoured the tracked anatomy (target or organ at risk), determined if the object was within the treatment bounds or not, and gated the treatment off when necessary. This functionality enabled treatment gating based on the actual anatomy rather than on surrogates. With the MR guidance, online adaptive radiotherapy, and MR-based gating, the ViewRay system offered state-of-the-art radiotherapy in combination with cobalt teletherapy. While this technology was adopted by several institutions around the world, ViewRay introduced a linac-based version of their system in 2016, which initiated the end of MR-guided cobalt-based machines.

Linear Accelerators

The first microwave electron linear accelerator (8 MV) for medical use became operational in 1953 at the Radiation Research Center of the Medical Research Council at Hammersmith Hospital in London.[27] The design for an isocentric gantry mount for the accelerator first was conceived by P. Howard-Flanders.[28] Shortly thereafter, Ginzton et al.[29] at Stanford University developed a 6-MV isocentric medical linear accelerator (*linac*). The history of the development of this first medical linear accelerator in the United States is provided by Jacobs.[30] Since then, there have been continued advances in accelerator design and construction, and today, medical linear accelerators account for most of the operational megavoltage treatment units in clinical use.[16,31]

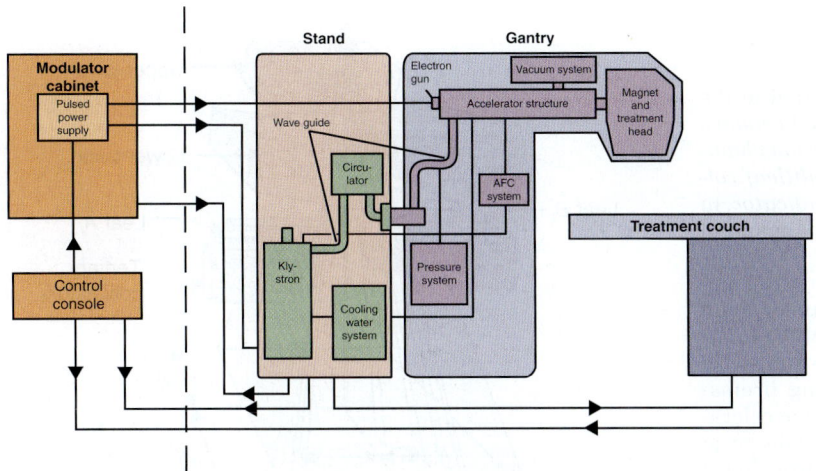

FIGURE 6.17. Schematic block diagram showing major components of a high-energy bent-beam medical linear accelerator. (Courtesy of Varian, Palo Alto, CA.)

Figure 6.17 is a block diagram of a high-energy, bent-beam medical linear accelerator showing the major components. The linac uses electromagnetic waves of frequencies in the *S-band* microwave region (2,856 megahertz [MHz]) to generate an electric field. The microwave radiation is propagated through a device called an *accelerator structure*, and the electrons injected into the structure are accelerated by the electric field in a straight line. The accelerator structure consists of a stack of cylindrical metal cavities having an axial hole through which the accelerated electrons pass. The accelerator structure's electric field produced by the microwaves can be either a *traveling wave* or *standing wave* design. In a traveling wave design, the electrons travel with the electric field as the field propagates through the structure with time, somewhat in the manner of a surfboarder riding the crest of an ocean wave. In a standing wave accelerator, the reflected microwave power is used to produce a standing wave electric field. In that case, the microwave power is coupled into the accelerator structure by side-coupling cavities rather than through the accelerator structure's axial cavity apertures.

The accelerator structure in low-energy (4 to 6 MV) linacs most often is mounted vertically in the treatment head

collinear along with the components associated with producing, controlling, and monitoring the x-ray beam (Fig. 6.18, left). High-energy (15 to 18 MV) linacs use a horizontally mounted accelerator structure with a beam-bending magnet system (Fig. 6.18, right). Accelerator structure technology now makes possible multiple high–dose rate photon beams of widely separated energies.

Other important components of a linac are the modulator, microwave power sources, electron gun, and the beam-handling components. The *modulator* is the source of pulsed direct current (DC) power, which is needed for the production of *microwave power*. Pulsed DC power is also supplied to the *electron gun* (a hot-wire filament that serves as the source of the accelerated electrons). The electrons are bunched before acceleration by a device called a *buncher*. The electron beam thus consists of pulses of bunched electrons in the form of a narrow pencil beam. The *magnetron* is a device that serves both as the source of the microwaves and as a power amplifier. The *klystron* is a device used to amplify the microwave power that is generated from a separate microwave source *(RF driver)*. The microwave power coming from the magnetron or klystron is transported to the accelerator

FIGURE 6.18. Schematic cutaway diagram of treatment heads for low-energy, straight-beam (*left*) and high-energy, bent-beam (*right*) medical linear accelerators. (Courtesy of Varian, Palo Alto, CA.)

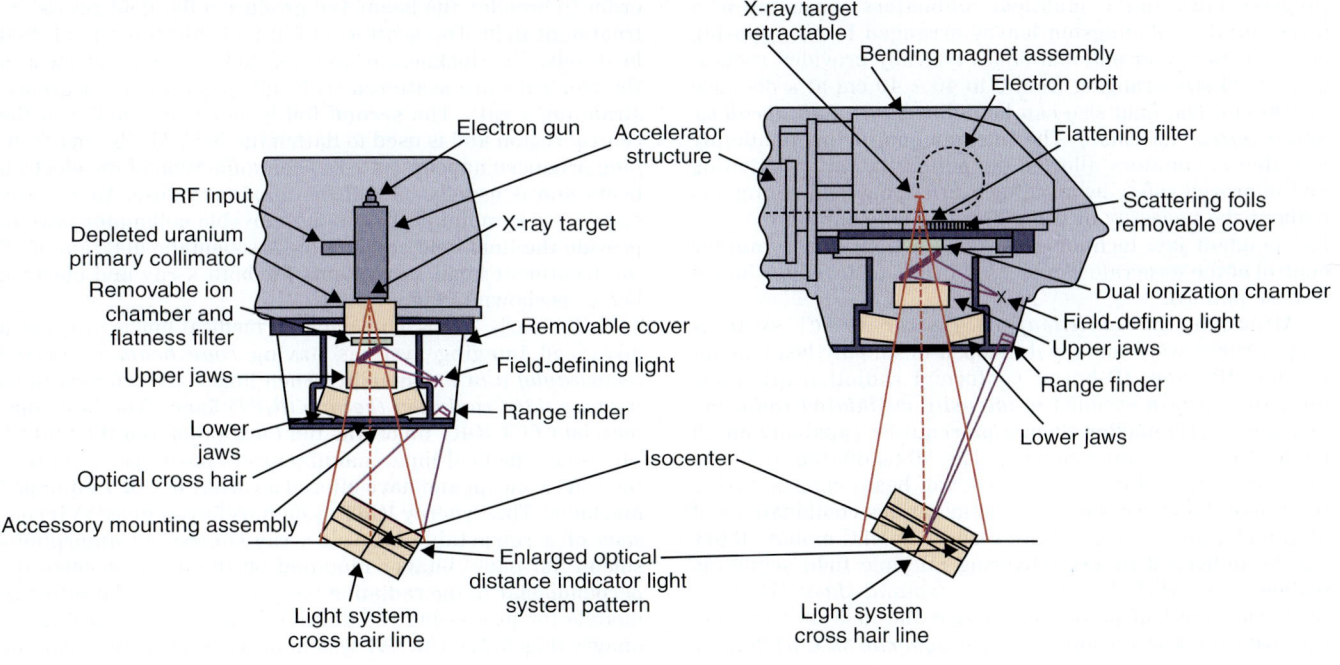

structure by a metallic pipe called a *waveguide*. A device called the *circulator* is used to isolate the klystron/magnetron from the reflected microwave power.

Other important components in a linac are located in the treatment head. These include the *x-ray target, fixed primary collimator, scattering foils, flattening filter, monitor ion chamber, movable secondary collimator jaws and/or mulitleaf collimator, light field localizer*, and *optical distance indicator*. In addition, the treatment head contains a significant amount of shielding material to minimize leakage radiation.

At the exit window of the accelerator structure, the high-energy electrons emerge in the form of a pencil beam of about 2 to 3 mm in diameter. In a low-energy (4 to 6 MeV) linac, the accelerated electrons proceed in a straight line and strike an x-ray target when in photon mode, producing bremsstrahlung x-rays. In high-energy linacs, because the accelerator structure is much longer and is placed horizontally or at some angle with respect to the horizontal, the electrons must be bent through a suitable angle, usually 90 or 270 degrees between the accelerator structure and the target. This is enabled by the beam transport system, which consists of an *achromatic focusing and bending magnet*, as well as *steering* and *focusing coils*.

The *primary collimator* is a fixed collimator located just below the x-ray target and is used to collimate the x-ray beam in the direction of the patient treatment and reduces the leakage radiation from the x-ray source. The angular distribution of the bremsstrahlung x-rays produced by megavoltage electrons incident on a target is forward peaked. To make the x-ray beam intensity uniform across the field, a conical metal *flattening filter* is inserted in the beam. Filters are constructed of lead, tungsten, uranium, steel, and aluminum (or some combination of these), depending on x-ray energy. The flattened x-ray beam then passes through a *monitor ionization chamber*. In most cases, this system consists of several transmission-type parallel-plate ionization chambers, which cover the entire beam. These ion chambers are used to monitor the field symmetry, dose rate, and integrated dose per monitor unit. In 2010s, several linacs offering flattening filter-free beams were commercially introduced. Some of these systems provided only flattening filter-free beams, whereas some provided dual capability with and without flattening filters.

After passing through the monitor chamber, the beam can be further collimated by continuously and independently movable x-ray collimators consisting of two pairs of lead or tungsten jaws and/or mulitleaf collimators consisting of a large number of tungsten leaves arranged in an opposing configuration. Conventional linacs typically provided rectangular field sizes ranging from 0 to 40 × 40 cm at a distance of 100 cm. The field size can be defined by a *light localizer* and a *mirror assembly*. The introduction of independently movable collimators allowed simplified patient positioning and improved safety by avoiding overlapping field abutments without the necessity of using heavy beam-splitting blocks.[32] Independent jaw technology in conjunction with computer control of the dose rate can be used to create a wedge-shaped isodose pattern.[33]

Although the *multileaf collimator* (*MLC*) systems (Fig. 6.19)[34,35] were initially developed to simplify beam shaping for 2D- and 3D-based conformal radiotherapy, their ultimate purpose excelled in *intensity-modulated radiation therapy* (*IMRT*) making them a prerequisite capability on all modern radiotherapy machines. The MLCs offered ability to electronically and dynamically control beam shapes during treatment. IMRT can be delivered in various combinations of MLC and gantry motions. With respect to MLC motion, IMRT can be delivered by (a) delivering multiple field segments (called *segmental MLC* [*SMLC*] or *step-and-shoot IMRT*) or (b) having the leaf pairs move across the field at a varying rate with the x-ray beam on (called *dynamic MLC* [*DMLC*] or

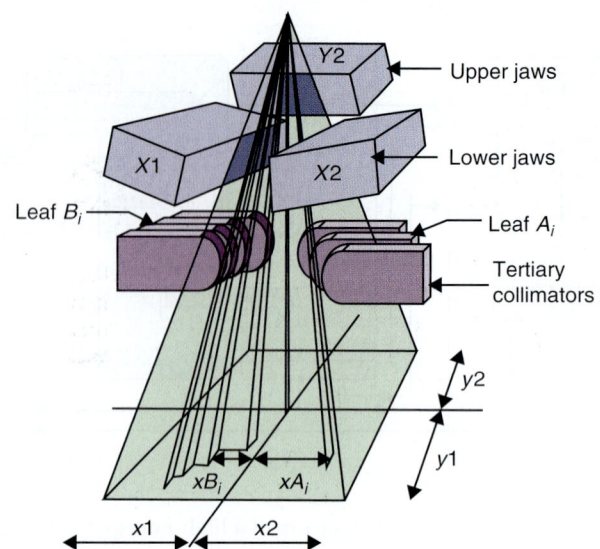

FIGURE 6.19. Schematic illustrating the geometry of a multileaf collimator for Varian linear accelerators. The *x*-direction is the field width across each leaf pair, and the *y*-direction is the field length. (Courtesy of Varian, Palo Alto, CA.)

sliding window IMRT)[36] With respect to gantry motion, the VMAT capability involves continuous gantry motion during delivery of typically coplanar beams,[37–39] while 4Pi delivery involves complex combinations of gantry and couch rotations enabling highly conformal dose distributions with noncoplanar delivery.[40] Initial designs of MLCs relied on in-line opposing pairs of MLC leafs. Alternate MLCs arrangements have been a long-standing topic of interest and double focused and/or multilayer MLCs eventually became available. The double focused MLCs offer improved penumbra compared to inline MLCs by being able to match the leaf edge with the beam divergence across all field sizes. The inline MLCs require a compromise of the beam penumbra as a function of the MLC position. The multilayer MLCs offer greater flexibility in field shape resolution, reduced leakage, greater speed, and simplification of operation.

In the electron mode, the accelerator's beam current is reduced 1,000-fold and the x-ray target is retracted. An *electron-scattering foil* is moved into place on the beam centerline so that the accelerated pencil electron beam strikes it in order to broaden the beam and produce a flat field across the treatment field. The scattering foil typically consists of dual lead foils. The thickness of the first foil ensures that most of the electrons are scattered with only a minimum of bremsstrahlung x-rays. The second foil is generally thicker in the central region and is used to flatten the field. The bremsstrahlung produced appears as x-ray contamination of the electron beam and is usually <5% of the maximum dose. An *electron applicator* is mounted below the movable collimator jaws to provide the final field collimation. A schematic diagram of all the treatment head subsystems for both x-ray and electron beams is shown in Figure 6.20.

In the early 2000s, conventional medical linacs integrated advanced imaging systems having *cone beam computed tomography* (*CBCT*) capability. Such linacs are referred to as *image-guided radiation therapy* (*IGRT*) linacs. The first commercial CBCT IGRT linac was the *Elekta Synergy* (Elekta).[41,42] The other medical linac manufacturers have also embraced the IGRT concept and have offered a variety of CBCT-equipped machines. The Synergy IGRT system (referred to as XVI) consists of a retractable kilovolt x-ray source, an amorphous silicon flat-panel imager mounted on the linear accelerator perpendicular to the radiation beam direction, and a software module for processing the data and tools for registering the images (Fig. 6.21). The XVI system provides for planar, motion,

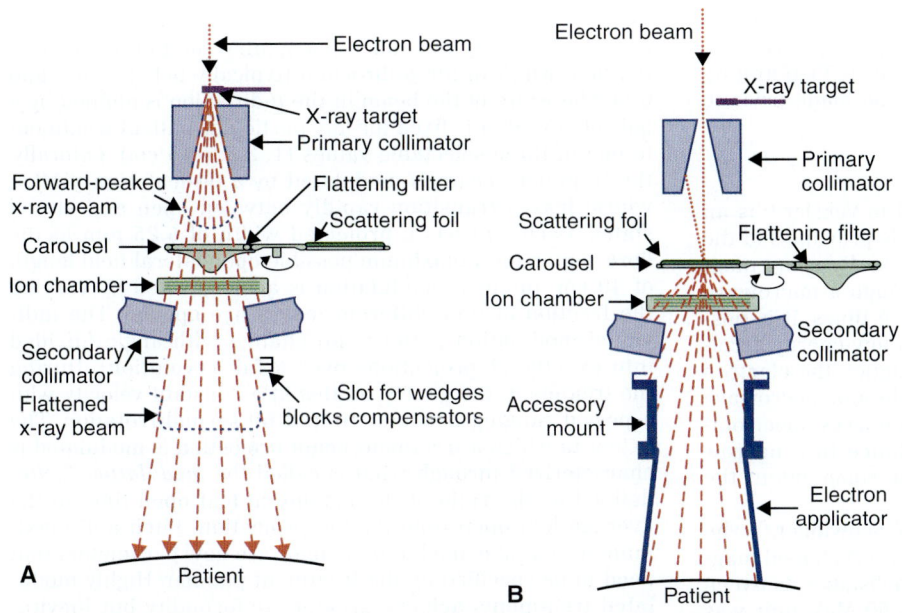

FIGURE 6.20. Schematic diagram of beam subsystems for x-ray beam **(A)** and electron beam therapy **(B)**. (From Karzmark CJ, Morton RJ. *A primer on theory and operation of linear accelerators in radiation therapy*. Rockville, MD: Department of Health and Human Services, Public Health Service, Food and Drug Administration, Bureau of Radiological Health, 1997.)

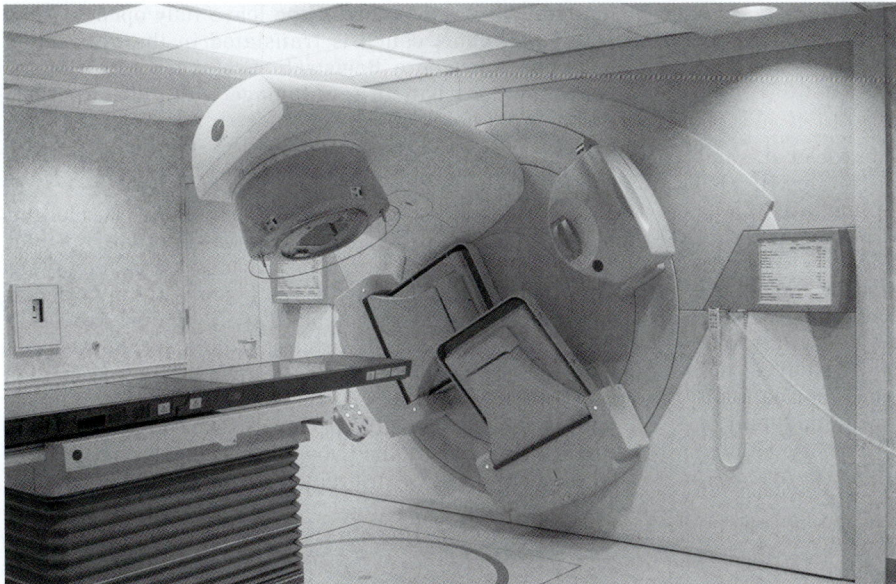

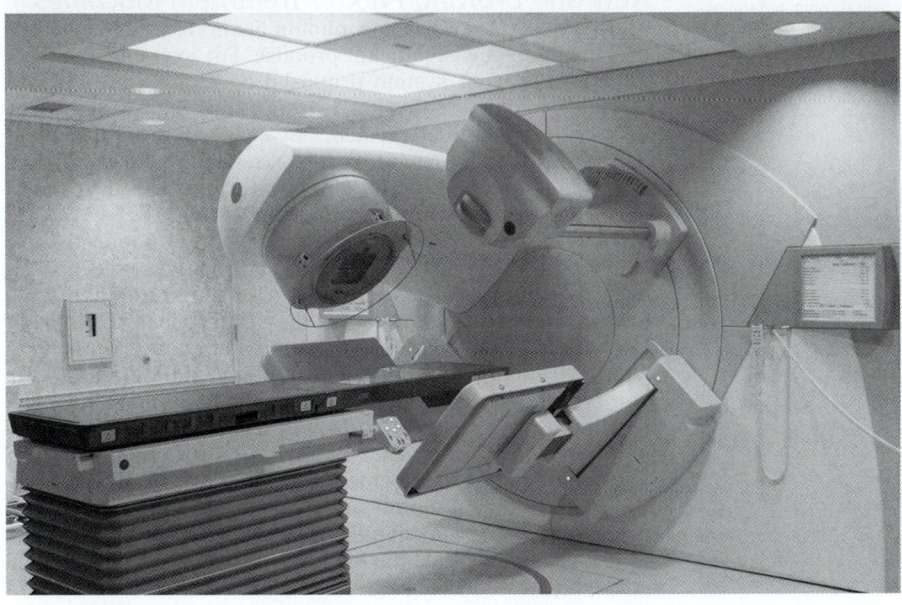

FIGURE 6.21. Elekta Synergy installed at the University of California, Davis. The unit consists of a conventional multimodality medical linac with a retractable kilovolt x-ray source, an amorphous silicon flat-panel imager mounted on the linear accelerator perpendicular to the radiation beam direction, and a software module (referred to as the XVI system). **Top:** The x-ray source, with the amorphous silicon flat panels retracted. **Bottom:** With the panels extended.

and volumetric imaging capabilities. Registration software is provided to compare the daily patient setup image with the stored prescription computed tomography (CT)–planning image, after which table adjustments can be made prior to treating the patient.

Microtrons

The microtron, whose concept is credited to Veksler,[43] is an electron accelerator that combines the basic principles of the electron linear accelerator and the cyclotron. By using magnets to recirculate the electron beam through a microwave accelerator cavity (or cavities) one or more times, it is possible to achieve a high beam energy with a low-energy accelerating section. After each orbit in the magnet, the electron bunch must arrive in phase with the accelerator microwave field. Thus, the magnet system acts as an energy spectrometer, limiting the electron energy acceptance to a narrow energy width and consequently limiting to some extent the beam current.

This concept was developed further by Schwinger,[44] who proposed the *racetrack microtron*. It uses two D-shaped magnet pole pieces that are separated by a fixed distance, between which is a linac accelerator structure. A 50-MeV unit was developed for radiation therapy applications by the Swedish firm Scanditronics (Uppsala, Sweden) and was one of the first modern IMRT delivery systems described in the literature.[45] Only two of this type of microtron were installed in the United States, and both have been replaced.

Tomotherapy

Helical tomotherapy was first proposed by Mackie et al.[46] and became commercially available as the TomoTherapy HI-ART system (Accuray, Madison, WI).[47] A short, in-line, 6-MV linac (Siemens Oncology Systems, Concord, CA) rotated on a ring gantry at a source–axis distance of 85 cm. Figure 6.22 shows the unit installed at the University of California, Davis. The IMRT treatment is delivered while the patient-support couch is translated in the *y*-direction (toward the gantry) through the gantry bore in the same way as a helical CT study is conducted. Thus, in the patient's reference frame, the treatment beam is angled inward along a helix, with the midpoint of the fan beam passing through the center of the bore. Similar

to helical CT, the treatment beam *pitch* is defined as the distance traveled by the couch per gantry rotation divided by the field width in the *y*-direction (typically between 0.2 and 0.5). The width of the beam in the *y*-direction is defined by a pair of jaws that is fixed for any particular patient treatment to one of three selectable values (1, 2.5, or 5 cm). Laterally, the treatment beam is modulated by a 64-leaf binary MLC, whose leaves transition rapidly between open and closed states. Each leaf has a projected width of 6.25 mm at the bore center, for a maximum possible open lateral field length of 40 cm. Intensity modulation is accomplished by varying the fraction of time different leaves are opened. The individual modulation pattern can change with angle (divided into exactly 51 projections over a full revolution). During the treatment, the gantry rotates at a constant velocity with a period ranging between 10 and 60 seconds/rotation. The extent to which a treatment beam projection is modulated is characterized through what is called the *modulation factor*, defined as the ratio of the maximum leaf open time to the average leaf open time for the projection. Pitch and maximum permissible modulation factor are new parameters that need to be specified by the treatment planner. Highly modulated treatments achieve greater conformality but inevitably take longer to deliver. A helical MVCT image is acquired using the onboard xenon CT detector system and the 6-MV linac (detuned to 3.6 MV) with the leave fully opened when the patient-support couch is translated in the *y*-direction through the gantry bore. Registration software is provided to compare the daily patient setup image with the stored prescription CT planning image.

CyberKnife

The use of a small X-band (~10,000 MHz) linear accelerator mounted on an industrial robotic arm was first developed for radiosurgery.[48,49] The robotic arm provides the capability for aiming a narrowly collimated x-ray beam with any orientation relative to the target volume. The system uses two ceiling-mounted diagnostic x-ray sources and amorphous silicon image detectors mounted flush to the floor. The treatment is specified by the trajectory of the robot and by the number of monitor units delivered at each robotic orientation. During the patient's treatment, the CyberKnife system correlates live radiographic images with preoperative CT or MRI scans in real time to determine patient and tumor position repeatedly over the course of treatment.

New and Evolving Photon Treatment Machines

There are several other new photon beam treatment machine designs that show significant promise. For example, the four-dimensional IGRT system proposed by Kamino et al. has a unique, gimbaled x-ray head design that allows the linear accelerator head to be pivoted.[50] By easily allowing noncoplanar beams without couch rotations, new degrees of freedom are made available for IMRT optimization, and even more conformal dose distributions may be possible.

In May 2017, Varian Medical Systems announced their Halcyon machine (Figure 6.23), which was specifically designed to address challenges of deploying radiotherapy in low resource settings. Some of the specific features include lower power consumption, simpler installation process, easier serviceability, greatly simplified operation, and specific aim for higher throughput than conventional machines. The machine is also designed to benefit from a 100% IGRT treatment approach where all treatments require imaging guidance and imaging dose is included in the treatment dose. The Halcyon also has a double-layer MLC, which in early studies has shown to provide significant dosimetric advantages. It is worth noting that all of the features, which make this machine advantageous in emerging markets also, make it attractive in

FIGURE 6.22. TomoTherapy HI-ART system installed at the University of California, Davis. A short, in-line 6-MV linac rotates on a ring gantry. Intensity-modulated radiation therapy treatment is delivered while the patient-support couch is translated through the gantry bore in the same way as a helical computed tomography study is conducted. The width of the beam in the patient-translated direction is defined by a pair of jaws that is fixed for any particular patient treatment, and laterally, the treatment beam is modulated by a 64-leaf binary multileaf collimator.

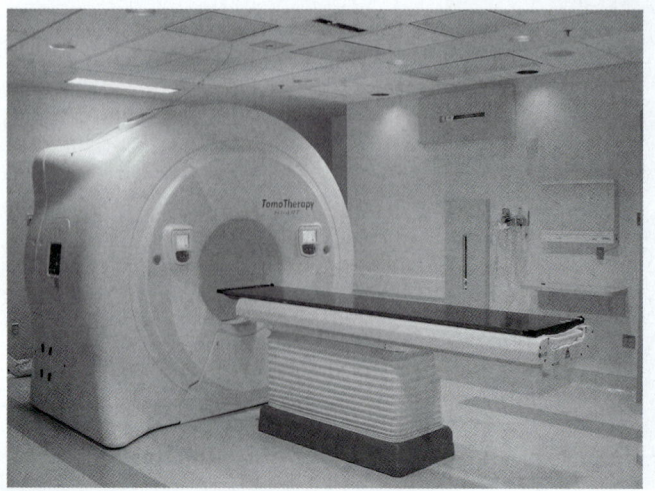

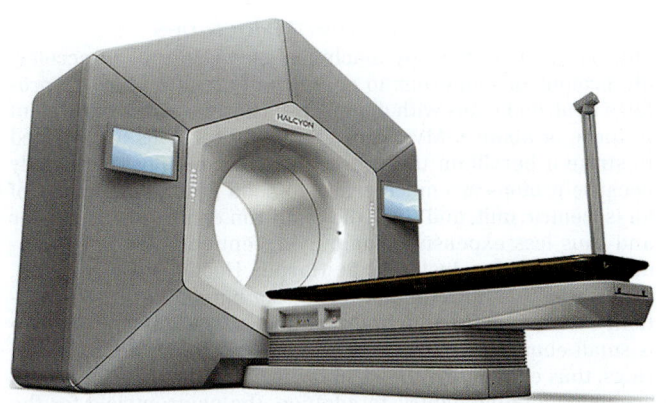

FIGURE 6.23. Varian Medical Systems' Halcyon introduced in 2017, which is specifically designed to provide highly efficient IGRT treatments. Note that the system does not offer electron beam treatment capability and has an "O" shape design, as opposed to the conventional "C" shape design used for other Varian and Elekta medical linacs.

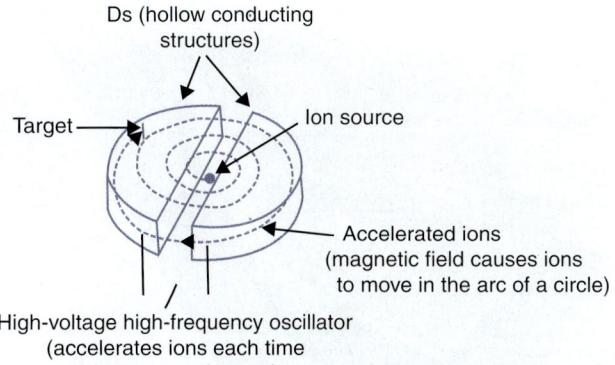

FIGURE 6.24. Schematic drawing showing principles of cyclotron operation. This machine is used for accelerating positive ions and is used clinically to produce proton and neutron beams. Metal half-disks (Ds) have an evacuated center through which the protons can travel. The protons are accelerated by an oscillating electric field operating between the half-disks. A magnetic field perpendicular to the plane of the half-disks confines the charged particles in the half-disks.

developed settings. As such, it is expected that this machine will play a role in a variety of settings and may have a significant impact on global access to radiotherapy. The machine does not offer electron beam treatment capability. Another noteworthy point is that the system has an "O" shape design, as opposed to the conventional "C" shape design for Varian, Elekta, Siemens, etc., machines. This design joins a host of other advanced machines with "O" shape (Tomotherapy, ViewRay, Elekta Unity) and potentially signals that this may become a more prevalent approach to radiotherapy patient treatments.

Several investigators have also pointed out the utility of very high-energy (VHE) electron beams (150 to 250 MeV).[51,52] Such high-energy beams are not yet available, and so only beam simulation software has been used to demonstrate the use of multi-VHE beams from opposed directions and the ability to modulated VHE beam intensity.[51,52] Such machines are clearly some time away, but these early studies show promise.

Proton, Light-Ion, and Neutron Beam Treatment Units

The first use of proton beams for radiation therapy is credited to Wilson,[53] who in 1946 pointed out the superior depth–dose characteristics provided by protons. Details on the history and development of proton beam radiation therapy (PBRT) machines are provided by Breuer and Smith[54] and Delaney and Kooy.[55] PBRT is seeing increasing interest worldwide because its depth–dose characteristics show advantages over those of photon beams.[56]

In most existing or proposed proton and light-ion particle treatment facilities, either a *cyclotron* or a *synchrotron* is used to accelerate proton beams to sufficient energy (200 to 250 MeV) and beam intensity.

Cyclotron

The cyclotron (Fig. 6.24) was invented by Ernest Lawrence of the University of California in 1929. It accelerates charged particles such as protons, deuterons, and light ions using a high-frequency, alternating voltage (potential difference) applied across two conducting D-shaped evacuated half-cylinders (Ds). A fixed magnetic field, perpendicular to the top of the two Ds, forces the charged particles to travel in a circular path. The charged particles accelerate only when passing through the gap between the two Ds. The beam spirals out to the edge of the container as the particle speed increases. At this point, the particle speed approaches the speed of light. Proton beam energies of 200 to 250 MeV are

considered adequate for most radiation therapy applications. Beam intensity from the accelerator must be adequate to overcome losses in the beam delivery system and provide tolerable treatment times.

Synchrocyclotron and Synchrotron

A *synchrocyclotron* varies either the magnetic field or the frequency of the applied electric field; a *synchrotron* varies both. By increasing these parameters appropriately as the particles gain energy, one can hold their path constant as they are accelerated. This allows the vacuum container for the particles to be a large, thin torus. In reality, it is easier to use some straight sections and some bent sections using multiple bend magnets, thus creating the shape of a rounded-corner polygon. The proton beam facility at Loma Linda University Medical Center (Loma Linda, CA) is an example of this type of accelerator.[57]

The synchrotron has the advantage of simple energy variability, whereas the cyclotron produces continuous beams with a fixed energy and higher beam intensity, making their design somewhat simpler. Beam-spreading mechanisms obtain suitable field sizes for radiation therapy by passive modulation (scattering foil) systems or by dynamic pencil-beam spot-scanning systems,[57] which allow dose conformation not only at the distal edge of the tumor but also at the proximal edge. Hall[58] pointed out that there is significant neutron leakage radiation for proton treatment machines that use a scattering foil and recommended moving to the pencil-beam scanning systems.

Size and Scope of Proton and Heavy-Ion Treatment Machines

The initial clinical proton systems involved either utilization of research system or commercial systems, which relied on multiroom solutions. Although the research systems enabled patient treatments, they did not allow broad scale deployment of this technology. The commercial multiroom solutions enabled broader deployment of this technology, but the significant initial cost and the size of the operation limited deployment of this type of technology. Single-gantry proton systems reduced the overall cost of proton facility and offered a scale that was easier to deploy. The first single room proton solutions included the MEVION S250 Proton Therapy System (Mevion Medical Systems, Littleton, MA) shown in Figure 6.25 and IBA Proteus One (IBA, Louvain-La-Neuve, Belgium). The first Proteus One treatment occurred at Willis-Knighton

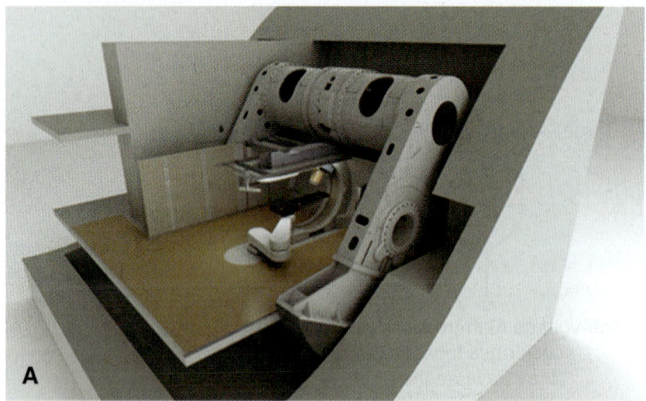

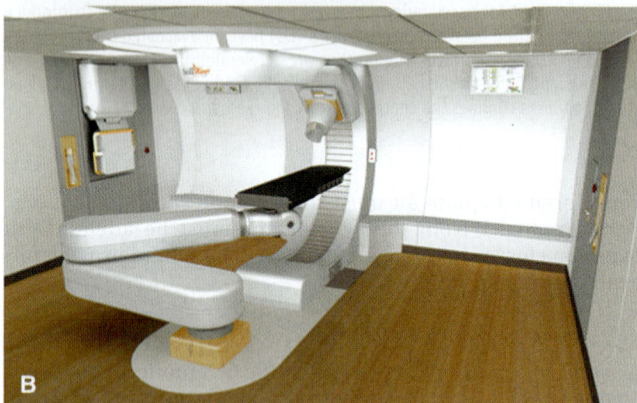

FIGURE 6.25. Rendering of next-generation proton therapy system (MEVION S250 Proton Therapy System, Mevion Medical Systems, Littleton, MA; formerly Still River Systems). **A:** Outer gantry holds the proton accelerator in the center, pointing directly to the isocenter. Accelerator is a 250-MeV cyclotron specifically designed (uses superconducting magnets) for proton therapy (with intensity-modulated proton therapy capabilities, high dose rate, high reliability, and easy maintenance). **B:** Treatment room depicting inner gantry and six-degree-of-freedom robotic couch.

Cancer Center in Shreveport, Louisiana, in September 2014, and the first Mevion S250 treatment occurred at Washington University in St. Louis, Missouri, in December 2014. This system uses a superconducting synchrocyclotron that is gantry mounted and incorporates image guidance and robotic patient positioning. The first unit was installed at Washington University (St. Louis, MO) in late 2011.

Several heavy-ion (carbon ion) radiation therapy facilities are now available in several centers in Asia and Europe,[9–11,56,59] and the first such facility in the United States will likely start construction in the next few years. Heavy-ion radiation therapy requires beams at much higher energies than proton therapy. For example, a proton beam of 150 MeV can penetrate 16 cm in water. To achieve the same penetration with carbon ions, energy of 3,000 MeV or 250 MeV/nucleon is needed. Synchrotrons are the only available sources for such high-energy ion beams, and they are large, complex machines requiring large facilities and similarly large capital expenditures.

Interest in heavy-ion radiation therapy is due primarily to its combination of two important physical advantages: (a) its depth–dose characteristics and (b) high LET in the Bragg peak region of the beam. For its depth characteristics, the ratio of the Bragg peak dose to the entrance region dose is even larger than for protons. In addition, there is a large increase in the radiation LET in the Bragg peak region of the beam. The combination of these two characteristics results in a potentially unique advantage of providing a high LET region that can be closely conformed to the target volume.

Neutron Therapy Treatment Machines

Modern neutron therapy machines use cyclotrons to accelerate protons or deuterons to energies of about 50 MeV to produce neutron beams with depth–dose characteristics equivalent to those of about 6-MV x-rays. The p,Be (protons accelerated to strike a beryllium target) reaction is used most commonly because protons are much easier to bend around the gantry of an isocentric unit, and thus, the cyclotron can be much smaller and thus less expensive. The only exception is the superconducting cyclotron installed at Harper Hospital (Detroit, MI), which uses the d,Be (deuterions strike beryllium target) reaction.[60] With superconducting technology, the entire cyclotron is small enough to be rotated around the patient on isocentric rings, thus eliminating the need for bending the deuteron beam around a rotating gantry. In addition, the neutron yield for the d,Be reaction is about five times that for the p,Be reaction. More details on the history and development of neutron beam therapy machines are provided in the review by Maughan and Yudelev.[61]

SIMULATORS

Conventional Simulator

Details on the development of the *radiation therapy simulator* and the selection, acceptance testing, and quality assurance of conventional radiation therapy simulators are provided in the review article by Van Dyk and Munro.[62] The conventional simulator mimics the functions and allowed motions of a therapy unit and uses a diagnostic x-ray tube to simulate the radiation properties of the treatment beam (Fig. 6.26). A simulator allows the beam direction and the treatment fields to be determined to encompass the projection of the target volume. Radiographic visualization of internal structures in relation to external landmarks allows special shielding devices (Cerrobend blocks) to be constructed to help minimize the dose to normal critical structures. Gantry arms are rigid enough to

FIGURE 6.26. The basic components and motions of a radiation therapy simulator. *A:* Gantry rotation. *B:* Source–axis distance. *C:* Collimator rotation. *D:* Image intensifier (lateral). *E:* Image intensifier (longitudinal). *F:* Image intensifier (radial). *G:* Patient table (vertical). *H:* Patient table (longitudinal). *I:* Patient table (lateral). *J:* Patient table rotation about isocenter. *K:* Patient table rotation about pedestal. *L:* Film cassette. *M:* Image intensifier. Motions not shown include field-size delineation, radiation beam diaphragms, and source–tray distance. (From Van Dyk J, Mah K. Simulators and CT scanners. In: Williams JR, Thwaites DI, eds. *Radiotherapy physics*. New York: Oxford Medical Publications, 1993:118. Reproduced by permission of Oxford University Press.)

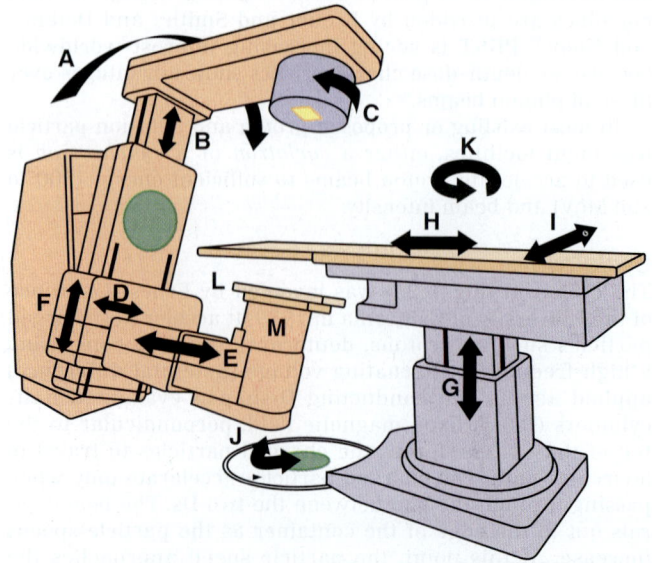

support heavy shielding blocks and simulated electron cones. Couch widths are similar to therapy-unit couch widths, and operating consoles feature digital displays of parameters and programmable settings for SAD, gantry angles, and field sizes. Older models of conventional simulators were equipped with an x-ray fluoroscopy system consisting of an image intensifier and video camera system to expedite field setup and beam angulations. Modern simulator design has replaced the image intensifier with amorphous silicon technology. The new imagers produce high spatial- and contrast-resolution images that approach film quality, facilitating the concept of filmless radiation oncology departments, and provide CBCT capability. Although this feature allows volumetric imaging on a conventional simulator, they have been virtually completely replaced with CT simulators.

CT Simulators

In the 1980s and early 1990s, research led to the integration of a diagnostic CT scanner with what was essentially a three-dimensional (3D) treatment-planning system, which led to the concept of *virtual simulation*.[63–65] Such a system is now referred to as a *CT simulator* and consists of a CT scanner, a flat-tabletop patient position–alignment system, including an orthogonal laser system, and a digital interface (DICOM) to a planning system that is equipped with virtual simulation software (Fig. 6.27). Modern CT simulation systems incorporate large-bore CT scanners especially designed for radiation oncology, with multislice capability, high-quality laser patient positioning/marking systems, and sophisticated virtual simulation software features. Conventional diagnostic CT scanners are typically equipped with 70-cm-diameter bore, whereas large-bore scanners have openings 80 to 90 cm in diameter. While the CT scanners used for CT simulation tend to be specifically designed for radiation oncology, there has been a steady adoption of technology developed for diagnostic purposes to CT simulators. Most of this technology concentrates on ever-evolving image reconstruction improvements as well as improvements in image acquisition technology. For example, iterative image reconstruction techniques and dual kV acquisition have found application in radiotherapy. Details of the virtual simulation process are discussed in some detail in Chapter 9. More details on CT simulation can be found in the review article by Van Dyk and Taylor[66] and articles by Mutic et al.[67,68]

New and Evolving Simulation Machines

Positron emission tomography (PET)/CT simulators and MR simulators have been available for radiotherapy purposes for a while. The adoption of this technology has been relatively modest and is somewhat limited by reimbursement practices and generally good access to these modalities through diagnostic radiology departments. Recent developments in radiotherapy treatment planning based on functional imaging and monitoring of response to therapy may increase the presence of MR- and PET-based simulators. However, this will likely need to be facilitated by clinical evidence, which would result in modifications of reimbursement practices to allow broader use of multimodality scanners in radiotherapy departments.

QUALITY OF RADIATION

The penetrability of an x-ray beam, referred to as the *quality* of the beam, is completely specified by its spectral distribution curve (i.e., the relative intensities of photons of various energies), which is the result of fluctuations of tube potential, the bremsstrahlung radiation process, characteristic radiation, and multiple interactions of the incident electrons and the x-ray target. The distribution of the photon energies, including the peak photon energy, in the continuous spectrum is governed solely by the x-ray tube potential. However, the energy of the characteristic photons increases with increasing atomic number of the target element. All other factors being equal, the radiation intensity is proportional to the atomic number of the target element.

Spectral distribution of an x-ray beam can be modified by placing absorbing materials of various thicknesses (i.e., filters) in the beam. In general, a filter removes relatively more low-energy photons than high-energy photons, although photons of all energies are removed to some extent. For radiation in the orthovoltage region (except for the absorption edge effect), the lower the energy of the photons, the larger is the total mass attenuation coefficient and therefore the greater is the likelihood that the photon will be absorbed. Thus, the beam emerges from the filter with a larger percentage of high-energy photons than it had on entering the filter. The beam has a greater penetration power and is said to have been "*hardened*" by the filter. The quality of an x-ray beam improves with increasing tube

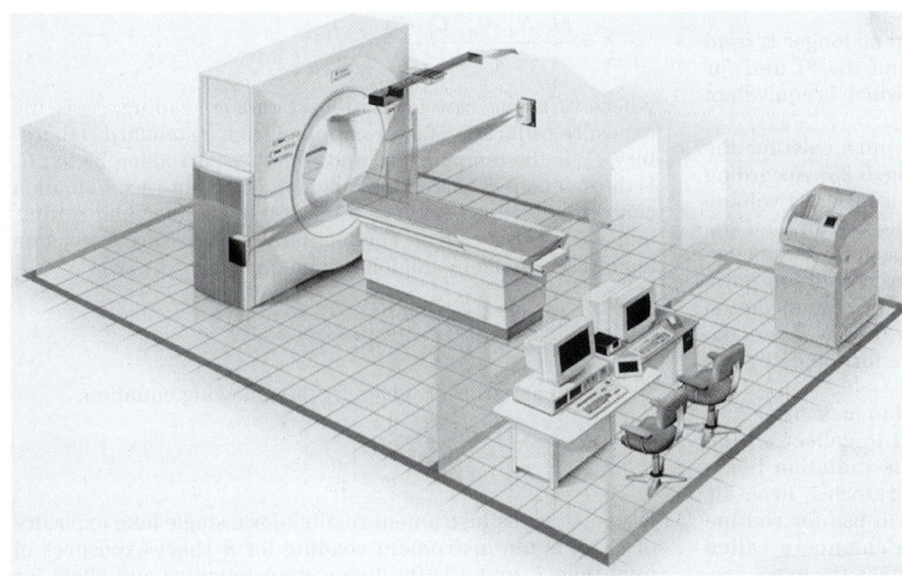

FIGURE 6.27. Typical computed tomography simulation suite showing the scanner, flat tabletop, orthogonal laser system, virtual simulation workstation, and hardcopy output device.

potential and with increasing thickness and atomic number of the filter.

A specification of beam quality-based entirely on a spectral distribution is too cumbersome for radiation therapy. The usual method of specifying beam quality in superficial and orthovoltage therapy is to list the HVL and the accelerating potential. For megavoltage beams, only the maximum energy of the electrons striking the x-ray target typically is used. The *homogeneity coefficient* denotes how homogeneous an x-ray beam is with respect to its photon energies. It is defined as the ratio of the first HVL to the second HVL. As the filtration is increased, the exposure rate decreases; therefore, there is a practical limit of filter thickness in orthovoltage therapy with a given combination of kilovolts, milliamperes, and treatment distance. In certain situations, it is convenient to express the quality of the x-ray beam in terms of an "equivalent energy," which can be derived from knowledge of the HVL. The type of x-ray beam that is used in radiation therapy is always heterogeneous; however, the x-ray beam can be considered to have an *equivalent energy* of a monoenergetic x-ray beam that has a HVL equal to the measured HVL of the heterogeneous beam.

RADIATION EXPOSURE

In 1928 at the Second International Congress of Radiology, the ionization of air, called *exposure*, was adopted as the measurable effect of radiation of a photon beam.[69] As the beam passes through a material, it creates ion pairs via the ionization process. In air, these ion pairs have some mobility and can be collected by applying an electric field across the air. The number of ion pairs collected is a measure of the quantity of radiation passing through the air.

The *roentgen* (R), the unit for exposure, also was defined at the 1928 Congress. The definition has been modified slightly by subsequent congresses, but the basic concept remains the same. The roentgen is that amount of x- or γ-radiation that causes the associated corpuscular emission per 0.001293 g of air to produce, in air, ions carrying one electrostatic unit of charge of either sign. The value 0.001293 g is the mass of 1 cm³ of air at 0°C and 760 mm Hg pressure; "associated corpuscular emission" refers to the Compton and pair-production electrons set in motion by the interactions between the incident photons and the air molecules. By conversion of units, the roentgen can be expressed as follows:

$$1\,\text{R} = 2.58 \times 10^{-4}\ \text{C/kg of air}$$

With the advent of SI units, the roentgen no longer is used as a special name for a radiation unit, and the SI unit for exposure is Coulombs per kilogram (C/kg), which is equivalent to approximately 3,876 R (Table 6.2).

The condition of electronic equilibrium must exist for the definition of the roentgen to be satisfied (Fig. 6.28). According to the definition, the electrons produced in a specified volume must spend all of their energies by ionization in air, and the total charge must be measured. However, because some electrons produced inside the specified volume create ion pairs outside the volume and some electrons produced outside the volume contribute ionization inside the specified volume, the gain and loss of ion pairs must be the same for the definition of the roentgen to be satisfied.

The free-air ionization chamber is used to measure exposure directly in roentgens.[1] It is designed to collect all the ions produced in a defined volume by the radiation beam and is used primarily by standards laboratories. Free-air chambers are bulky and too complicated to use for routine measurements. Instead, small ionization chambers called *thimble chambers* are typically used to measure exposure. The chamber gives a measure of the ionization produced,

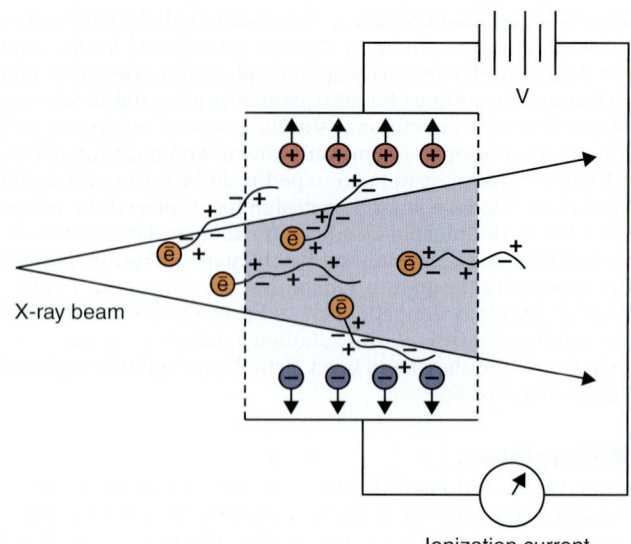

FIGURE 6.28. Schematic illustrating electronic equilibrium. (From Khan FM. *The physics of radiation therapy*. 2nd ed. Baltimore: Williams & Wilkins, 1994. With permission.)

which then is converted to exposure in roentgens by use of an *exposure calibration factor*, N_x, traceable to the National Institute of Standards and Technology (Gaithersburg, MD). Thimble chambers are designed for use at specific energies; the thickness of the chamber wall is equal to the maximum electron range (electronic equilibrium established). If they are used at higher energies, at which the electron range is greater, an added wall thickness or *buildup cap* must be used.

To determine the exposure rate from an x-ray or γ-ray machine, an exposure-calibrated thimble chamber (with appropriate wall thickness) and connected to an *electrometer* is placed at beam center, in air, at right angles to the beam's central axis and at the point where the exposure rate is to be specified. The field size for which the exposure rate is to be measured is set, and the radiation machine is turned on for a specified time, T, to achieve a reading, M, on the connected electrometer. The reading is corrected for *temperature and atmospheric pressure*, *timer error*, *stem effect*, and *ion-recombination effects*. The therapy machine exposure rate, $\dot{X}$, is given in roentgens per minute by the following equation:

$$\dot{X} = \frac{M \cdot N_x \cdot C_{tp} \cdot C_{st} \cdot C_s}{T + \alpha}$$

where M is the raw ionization chamber reading, N_x is the exposure calibration factor obtained from a standards laboratory, C_{tp} is the temperature and pressure correction factor, C_{st} is the stem effect correction factor, C_s is the ion-recombination correction factor, T is timer (minutes) or monitor unit setting, and α is the timer error. The temperature-pressure correction factor C_{tp} is given by the following equation:

$$C_{tp} = \left(\frac{t + 273.16}{295.16}\right)\left(\frac{760}{p}\right)$$

The timer error α is given by the following equation:

$$\frac{M_1}{T + \alpha} = \frac{M_2}{T + n\alpha}$$

where M_1 is the instrument reading for a single long exposure of T, M_2 is the instrument reading for n short exposures of total time T, and α is the timer error (monitor end effect for linacs) for a single exposure.[70]

Beyond 3 MeV, the roentgen cannot be measured accurately, and thus calibrations of radiation therapy machines at these higher energies are performed using an exposure-calibrated ionization chamber such as a Bragg–Gray cavity, and the ionization readings are converted to absorbed dose as discussed in the following section.

ABSORBED DOSE

In 1953 the International Commission on Radiological Units and Measurements introduced the concept of *absorbed dose* and defined its unit, the *rad*.[69] Before its definition can be presented, the reader must understand the concept of dose absorption. As a beam of radiation passes through an absorbing medium, it interacts with it in a two-stage process. The first step occurs when energy carried by the photons—the indirectly ionizing particles—is transformed into kinetic energy of high-speed electrons; the second step occurs as these electrons—the directly ionizing particles—are slowed down and deposit their energy in the medium.

Kerma, an acronym for "kinetic energy released in the medium," represents the transfer of energy from the photons to the directly ionizing particles (step 1). The subsequent transfer of energy from the directly ionizing particles to the medium (step 2) is represented by the absorbed dose and is defined in terms of the energy deposited by the radiation beam as it passes through the medium. The relationship between kerma and absorbed dose is illustrated in Figure 6.29.

The *rad* represents the absorption of 0.01 J/kg of the absorbing material (1 rad = 0.01 J/kg). The rad now has been replaced with the SI unit for absorbed dose (1 J/kg) given the

special name of *gray* (*Gy*) (Table 6.2). By conversion of units, the gray can be expressed as follows:

$$1 \text{ Gy} = 1 \text{ J/kg} = 100 \text{ cGy} = 100 \text{ rad}$$

Determination of Absorbed Dose

It is difficult to measure absorbed dose directly, but two direct methods—*calorimetry* and *Fricke dosimetry*—are available in some laboratories. Neither method is particularly practical nor widely used, and the reader is referred to the literature for more details.[71] Instead, a simpler, indirect method using an exposure-calibrated ionization chamber is used to determine absorbed dose.

Absorbed Dose Calculation from Exposure Measurement

For photon energies of ^{60}Co and lower, an ionization chamber having an exposure calibration factor assigned by an appropriate national calibration facility (e.g., a dosimetry calibration laboratory accredited by the National Institute of Standards and Technology or the American Association of Physicists in Medicine [AAPM; College Park, MD]) can be used to measure exposure in air as described in the section "Radiation Exposure." Absorbed dose then can be calculated from the exposure as explained here. The energy deposited in a fixed mass of air from a known exposure can be calculated because it is known that an exposure of 1 R creates a finite number of ion pairs per unit mass of air (i.e., 1.61×10^{15} ion pairs per kilogram of air) and that the mean energy required to create an ion pair in air (denoted by W) is equal to 33.97 eV per ion pair. When these values are used, the relationship between the exposure, X, and the dose to air, D_{air}, is given by the following expression:

$$D_{air}(\text{rad}) = 0.876 \left(\frac{rad}{R} \right) \cdot X(R)$$

The *dose in free space*, D_{fs}, is defined as the dose at the center of a small mass of phantom-like material just large enough to provide electronic equilibrium (Fig. 6.30) and can be derived from D_{air} using the ratio of the mass energy-absorption coefficients (u_{en}/ρ) and an attenuation correction factor, A_{eq}, that accounts for the photon attenuation in the small mass of phantom-like material:

$$D_{fs} = \left[0.876 \frac{\mu_{en}\rho_{med}}{\mu_{en}\rho_{air}} \right] \cdot X \cdot A_{eq}$$

The term in brackets is called the *f-factor* or the *roentgen-to-rad conversion factor* and is represented as f_{med}, giving the dose in free space as follows:

$$D_{fs} = f_{med} \cdot X \cdot A_{eq}$$

Values of f_{med} are shown in Figure 6.31 over the energy range commonly used in radiation therapy. Notice that the

FIGURE 6.29. Graphs showing schematic relationship of kerma and absorbed dose. (From Johns HE, Cunningham JR. *The physics of radiology*. 4th ed. Springfield, IL: Charles C Thomas, 1983:222. Courtesy of Charles C Thomas Publisher, Ltd., Springfield, Illinois.)

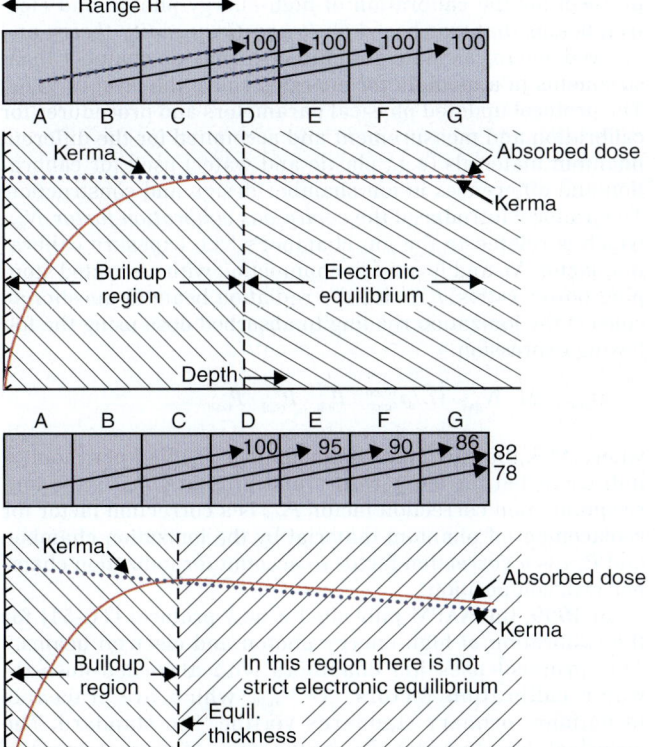

FIGURE 6.30. Schematic illustrating ionization measurement in air to determine dose in free space. (From Khan FM. *The physics of radiation therapy*. 2nd ed. Baltimore: Williams & Wilkins, 1994. With permission.)

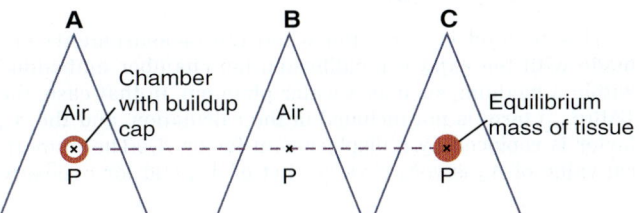

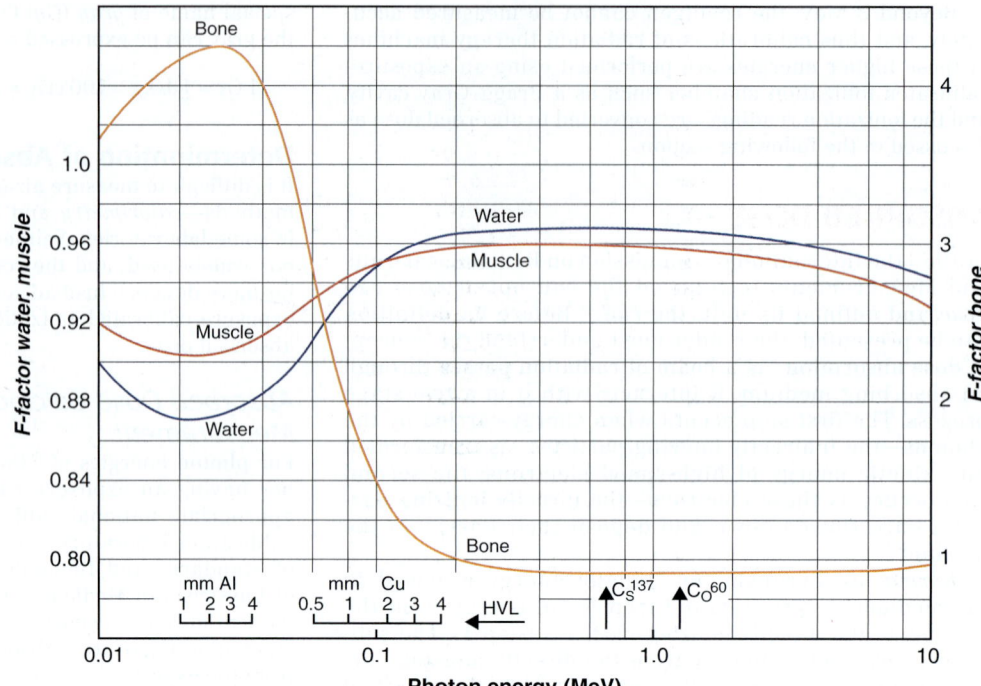

FIGURE 6.31. The roentgen-to-rad conversion factor for bone, muscle, and water as a function of photon energy. (From Johns HE, Cunningham JR. *The physics of radiology.* 4th ed. Springfield, IL: Charles C Thomas, 1983:287. Courtesy of Charles C Thomas Publisher, Ltd., Springfield, Illinois.)

f-factor is a function of the medium and the energy of the photon beam. Typical values of A_{eq} are 0.989 and 1.00 for ^{60}Co and 250-kV energies, respectively.

An in-air calibration procedure is performed as follows. The calibrated ion chamber (with wall thick enough to ensure electronic equilibrium) is placed in air with its sensitive volume on the central axis of the beam and its stem at right angles to the beam direction. The center of the chamber most often is placed at a distance from the source (or target) equal to the nominal SSD of the machine plus the buildup depth. A standard field size is set, usually 10 × 10 cm, using either movable collimators or the standard treatment applicator. An exposure is made for a known time or number of monitor units. The ionization chamber reading is converted to units of Gy/min at the depth of the maximum dose within a phantom, d_{med}, using the following equation:

$$\dot{D}_{med} = \frac{M \cdot N_x \cdot C_{tp} \cdot C_{st} \cdot C_s \cdot A_{eq} \cdot f_{med} \cdot TAR(d_{max})}{T + \alpha}$$

where M, N_x, C_{tp}, C_{st}, C_s, A_{eq}, f_{med}, T, and α are used as defined earlier. The term $TAR(d_{max})$ represents the tissue-air ratio at the depth of maximum dose (i.e., the *backscatter* or *peakscatter factor*) and converts the dose in free space to the dose in a phantom at the depth of maximum dose. This parameter is discussed in more detail later. The preceding equation can be rewritten as follows:

$$\dot{D}_{med} = \dot{X} \cdot f_{med} \cdot A_{eq} \cdot TAR(d_{max})$$

and

$$\dot{D}_{med} = \dot{D}_{fs} \cdot TAR(d_{max})$$

This method is also valid when the measurements are made with the exposure-calibrated ion chamber embedded within a medium, such as a water phantom. In that case, the $TAR(d_{max})$ term is not included in the calculation, and the A_{eq} factor is replaced by a displacement factor, A_m. The numerical value of A_m is very close to that of A_{eq}, and for exposure measurements made within a water phantom, the dose rate is given by the following expression:

$$\dot{D}_{med} = \dot{X} \cdot f_{med} \cdot A_m$$

Absorbed Dose Calculation from Bragg–Gray Cavity Ionization Measurement

For energies above the level of ^{60}Co, exposure calibration factors are not available from the standards laboratories because of measurement limitations. In 1983, the AAPM introduced a protocol for the calibration of high-energy photon and electron beams that was based on *Bragg–Gray cavity theory* and allowed one to calculate dose directly from ion chamber measurements in a medium for energies above the level of ^{60}Co.[72] The protocol updated physical parameters and procedures for calibration and measurement and accounted for the different phantom materials (e.g., plastic and water) used for calibration and differences in ion chamber design and construction. The protocol introduced the *cavity-gas calibration factor*, N_{gas}, which is related to the ion chamber's ^{60}Co exposure calibration factor, N_x, and is used in conjunction with restricted stopping-power ratios, $\bar{L}/\rho$, for the radiation beam in question to convert the ionization reading to absorbed dose using the following expression:

$$D_{med} = M \cdot N_{gas} \cdot (\bar{L}/\rho)_{gas}^{med} \cdot P_{ion} \cdot P_{repl} \cdot P_{wall}$$

where M is the raw ionization chamber reading per monitor unit corrected for temperature and pressure, P_{ion} is the ion-recombination correction factor, P_{repl} is a correction factor for replacement of phantom material by the ionization chamber, and P_{wall} is a correction factor to account for ionization chamber wall composition.

In 1999, the AAPM published a new protocol (TG-51) for the calibration of high-energy photon and electron beams.[73] This protocol uses ion chambers with absorbed-dose-to-water calibration factors, $N^{Co-60}_{D,W}$, which are traceable to national primary standards via the ^{60}Co standard. The absorbed dose to water D_W^Q at the point of measurement of the ion chamber placed under reference conditions is given by the following equation:

$$D_W^Q = M \cdot k_Q \cdot N_{D,W}^{Co\text{-}60}$$

where Q is the beam quality of the clinical beam, M is the fully corrected ion chamber reading, and k_Q is the *quality conversion factor* that converts the calibration factor for a ^{60}Co beam to that for a beam of quality Q. The protocol is designed to be a simplification of the AAPM's TG-21 protocol in the sense that large tables of stopping-power ratios and mass energy-absorption coefficients are no longer needed, and the user does not need to calculate any theoretical dosimetry factors.[74-76]

Other Dosimetry Methods

Thermoluminescent Dosimetry

Certain crystalline materials exhibit a phenomenon known as *thermoluminescence*. When a crystal capable of thermoluminescence is irradiated, a small portion of the energy absorbed is stored in the structure of the crystal lattice. If the material is heated, the energy is released in the form of visible light. Several thermoluminescent phosphors are available, but lithium fluoride, with an effective atomic number of 8.2, is the most commonly used.

The physical theory of thermoluminescent dosimetry can be explained as follows. In the individual atom, electrons occupy discrete energy levels. However, in the crystal lattice, the electronic energy levels are perturbed by mutual interactions between atoms, giving rise to energy bands, so-called *allowed energy bands* and *forbidden energy bands*. Impurities in the crystal create energy traps in the forbidden bands, allowing metastable states to exist; for example, when the phosphor is irradiated, some of the electrons in the valence band (ground state) receive sufficient energy to be raised to the conduction band. If there is an instantaneous emission of light, the phenomenon is called *fluorescence*. If an electron in the trap requires energy to get out of the trap and return to the valence band, the emission of light is called *phosphorescence*. If the emission of light is slow at room temperature but can be sped up with heating, the process is called *thermoluminescence*.

Thermoluminescent dosimeters must be calibrated before they can be used for measuring an unknown dose. Because the response of the thermoluminescent material is affected by its radiation and thermal histories, the material must be annealed to remove residual effects. The standard preirradiation annealing procedure for lithium fluoride is 1 hour of heating at 400°C and 24 hours at 80°C. More details can be found in the review article by DeWerd et al.[77]

Film Dosimetry

When an x-ray film is exposed to ionizing radiation, the exposed silver bromide crystals form a latent image. In the film development process, the affected crystals cause a darkening of the film, and the unaffected crystals leave the film clear. The degree of blackening of the film is proportional to the energy absorbed and is measured by determining the optical density with a densitometer. The optical density is defined as follows:

$$OD = \log(I_0/I_T)$$

where I_0 is the amount of light detected without the film in place and I_T is the amount of light detected with the film in place. For radiation dosimetry, the net optical density is obtained by subtracting the densitometric reading for the base fog (clear portion of the film) from the measured optical density. Most films are exposed to yield an optical density between 1.3 and 1.7 for optimal viewing.

A plot of net optical density as a function of radiation exposure or dose is called the *sensitometric curve* or the *Hunter–Driffield (H-D) curve*. If the curve is nonlinear, appropriate corrections must be applied to convert net optical density to absorbed dose.

The use of film is a relatively straightforward method of dosimetry for electron beams, but it must be done with extreme care in photon dosimetry. The problem is that the photoelectric effect depends on Z^3 ($Z_{silver} = 47$), and the film emulsion strongly absorbs radiation below 100 kV. A concise review of radiographic film dosimetry can be found in the article by Das.[78]

Radiochromic Film Dosimetry

Radiochromic film consists of a thin (7 to 23 mm), radiosensitive, colorless leuco dye bonded to a 100-mm-thick Mylar base. Radiochromic films are colorless before irradiation and turn deep blue when irradiated without physical, chemical, or thermal processing. The film is approximately tissue equivalent, integrates simultaneously at all measurement points, and has a high spatial resolution (>1,200 lines/mm). It shows a stable, reproducible response if protected from ultraviolet light, unstable temperatures, and humidity. Because radiochromic dye is an aromatic hydrocarbon, like plastic scintillators, it has an energy response superior to that of diodes and comparable with thermoluminescent dosimetry. Interest in radiochromic film as a quantitative dosimeter has been stimulated by the appearance of a fourfold-more-sensitive film (model MD-55), which extends its response down to the 5-Gy level. More details on radiochromic film dosimetry are given in the article by Soares et al.[79]

Diode Dosimetry

Semiconductor diodes offer many advantages for clinical dosimetry, including high sensitivity, real-time read-out, robustness, and independence of air pressure. Most semiconductor diodes are made from silicon, which is either *n* type (silicon doped with group V material, such as phosphorus) or *p* type (silicon doped with group III material, such as boron). To form a diode detector, a *p-n* junction must be created.

The physical theory of semiconductor dosimetry can be explained as follows. During irradiation, electron–hole pairs are created both within and outside the depletion region in the body of the diode detector. The charge carriers are swept across the depletion region and collected rapidly under the action of the electric field that exists across it. In this way, a current is generated, flowing in the reverse direction to normal diode current flow, which can be measured and related to absorbed dose.

Dosimetry diodes are operated without an external reverse bias voltage and connected via cable to a simple electrometer. Details on their use for *in vivo* dosimetry are provided in AAPM Report 87.[80] Calibration of diodes typically is performed by comparison of readings against an ion chamber in a standard setup to establish a diode calibration factor for absorbed dose to water and the establishment of a series of correction factors to account for calibration differences when measurements are performed under various experimental conditions. Typical concerns are energy dependence, temperature sensitivity, directional dependence, and radiation damage. Each radiation therapy center should establish the responses of their diodes under the various conditions encountered and monitor them as the cumulative dose to the diodes increases. Frequency of checks should be adjusted according to the frequency of use of the diodes and the variability encountered. More details on diode dosimetry are given in the article by Zhu and Saini.[81]

Metal Oxide Semiconductor-Field Effect Transistor Dosimetry

Metal oxide semiconductor-field effect transistors represent another example of a semiconductor dosimeter. Originally developed for space dosimetry, the operation is based on the buildup of charge in the silicon oxide transistor gate created by ionizing radiation. The reader is referred to the article by Cygler and Scalchi[82] for more details on this type of dosimeter.

Polymer-Gel Dosimetry

Gel dosimetry is based on quantifying the effects of radiation-induced chemical changes occurring within some volume of material filled with an aqueous gel matrix. The degree of chemical change in the gel is related to dose. The dose-dependent changes are determined by imaging techniques, including MRI, CT, and optical CT. Hence, gel dosimetry has the potential to provide full 3D dosimetry throughout the volume of the irradiated gel dosimeter.

For example, one form of this method exploits the radiation-induced free-radical chain polymerization of acrylic monomers dispersed in an aqueous gel. When irradiated, discrete, microscopic regions of cross-linked polymer are formed, the concentration of which is proportional to radiation dose. The water proton nuclear MR relaxation rates in the gel are strongly affected by local changes in the polymer molecular structure and dynamics; thus, the distribution of radiation dose may be visualized and quantified with high resolution using MRI. Because the polymer microparticles scatter light, the dose distribution also can also be visualized in the transparent gel as a dose-dependent 3D optical turbidity and read by optical CT.

Unfortunately, gel dosimetry, while having the potential for tissue-equivalent 3D dosimetry for a almost three decades, has not come into common clinical use, as it has proven too difficult to use in the clinic setting.[83] Research continues in gel dosimetry, as there is clearly a need for a robust 3D high-resolution dosimetry system.[83,84] Recent publications indicate that these research efforts may result in viable clinical and commercial solutions.[85]

DOSIMETRY PARAMETERS

Percentage Depth Dose

Percentage depth dose (PDD) can be understood by reference to Figure 6.32. It is the ratio, expressed as a percentage, of the absorbed dose on the central axis at depth d to the absorbed dose at the reference point d_0. PDD is given by

$$\text{PDD}(d, d_0, S, f, E) = \frac{D_d}{D_{d0}} \times 100$$

FIGURE 6.32. Schematic drawing illustrating definition of percentage depth dose, where d is any depth and d_0 is the reference depth, usually $d_{\max}$.

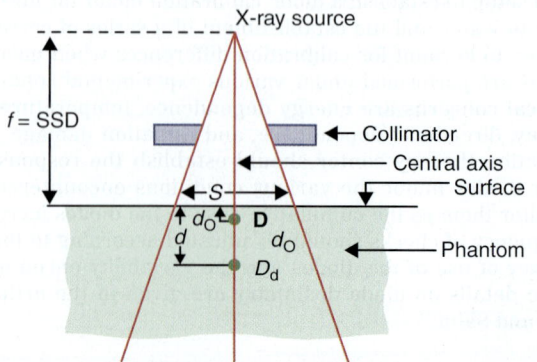

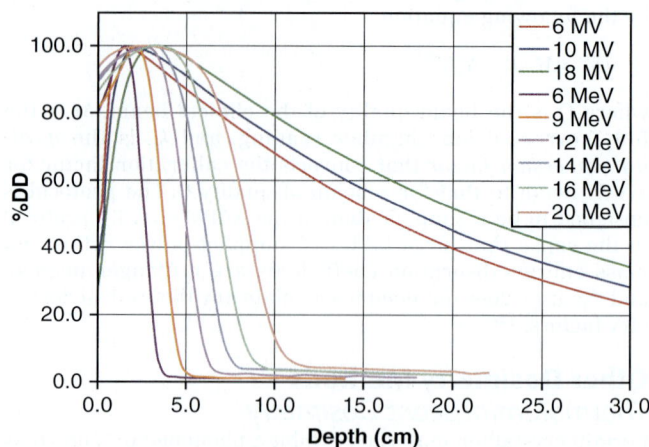

Photon and electron beam %DDs

FIGURE 6.33. Examples of central axis percentage depth dose (DD) for megavoltage x-ray beams ranging from ^{60}Co to 18-MV x-rays and 6- to 20-MeV electron beams.

The functional symbols have been inserted in the expression to make it clear that the PDD is affected by a number of parameters, including d, d_0, field dimension S, source-to-surface distance f, and radiation beam energy (or quality) E. S refers to the side length of a square beam at a specified reference depth. Nonsquare beams may be designated by their equivalent square. Field shape and added beam collimation also can affect the central axis depth–dose distribution. Photon-beam PDD increases with increasing energy, SSD, and field size. Figure 6.33 shows that the depth of the 50th percentile increases from approximately 14 cm for 4-MV x-rays to nearly 23 cm for 25-MV x-rays. The depth of maximum dose varies from about 1 cm for 4-MV x-rays to >3.5 cm for 25-MV x-rays.

The PDD for one SSD is related to the PDD at a second SSD by the following equation:

$$\text{PDD}(d, S, f_2) = \text{PDD}(d, S, f_1)\left(\frac{f_1 + d}{f_2 d} \cdot \frac{f_2 + d_{\max}}{f_1 + d_{\max}}\right)^2$$

The term in the brackets is called the *Mayneord F-factor*.[86]

Tissue–Air Ratio

The tissue–air ratio (TAR) is defined as the ratio of the absorbed dose D_d at a given point in the phantom by the absorbed dose in free space, D_{fs}, that would be measured at the same point but in the absence of the phantom, if all other conditions of the irradiation (e.g., collimator, distance from the source) are equal (Fig. 6.34). The TAR is expressed as follows:

$$\text{TAR}(d, S_d, E) = \frac{D_d}{D_{fs}}$$

FIGURE 6.34. Schematic drawing illustrating the definition of tissue-air ratio, where d is the thickness of overlying material.

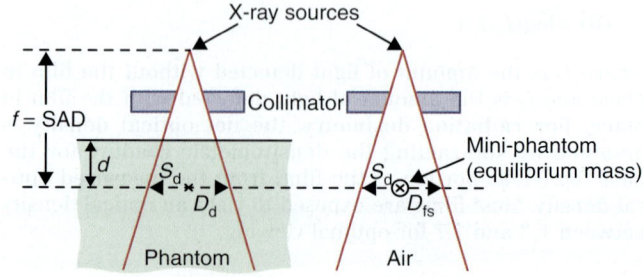

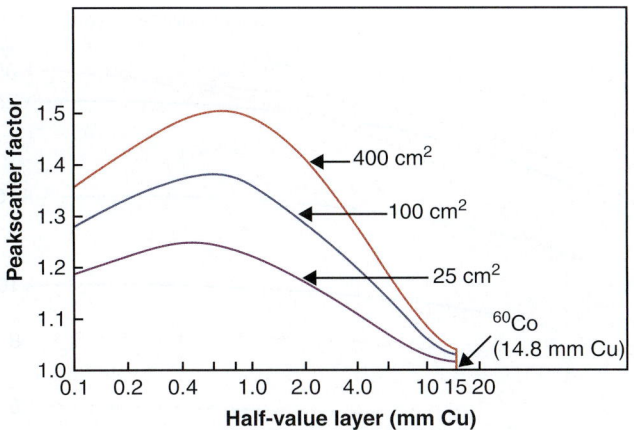

FIGURE 6.35. Variation of peakscatter factor with beam quality (half-value layer). (From Johns HE, Cunningham JR. *The physics of radiology*. 4th ed. Springfield, IL: Charles C Thomas, 1983:248. Courtesy of Charles C Thomas Publisher, Ltd., Springfield, Illinois.)

where d is depth, E is radiation beam energy, and S_d is the beam dimension measured at depth d. TAR depends on depth, field size, and beam quality, but for all practical purposes, it is independent of the distance from the source.

The TAR at the depth of maximum dose is called the *peakscatter factor*. It is perhaps better known as the backscatter factor, but because of the finite depth d_0, this tends to be misleading. Figure 6.35 shows the peakscatter factors for various field sizes and beam qualities.

Tissue–Phantom Ratio and Tissue–Maximum Ratio

The concepts of tissue–phantom ratio (TPR) and tissue–maximum ratio (TMR) were proposed for high-energy radiation as alternatives to TAR in response to arguments raised against the use of in-air measurement for a photon beam with a maximum energy >3 MeV.[87,88] As originally defined, TPR is given by the ratio of two doses:

$$TPR(d, d_r, S_d, E) = \frac{D_d}{D_{d_r}}$$

where D_{d_r} is the dose at a specified point on the central axis in a phantom with a fixed reference depth, d_r, of tissue-equivalent material overlying the point; D_d is the dose in the phantom at the same spatial point as before but with an arbitrary depth, d, of overlying material; and S_d is the beam width at the level of measurement (Fig. 6.36). In each instance, underlying material is sufficient to provide for full backscatter. There is no general agreement about the magnitude of

FIGURE 6.36. Schematic drawing illustrating the definition of tissue–phantom ratio and tissue–maximum ratio, where d is the thickness of overlying material and d_r is the reference thickness.

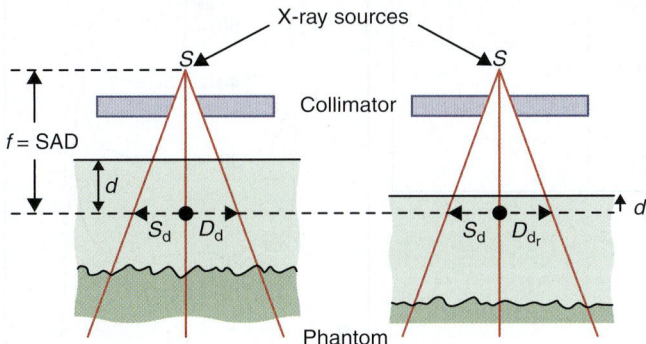

the reference depth to be used for this quantity, particularly for high energies. The TPR is intended to be analogous to the TAR but has an advantage because the reference dose, D_{d_r}, is directly measurable over the entire range of x-rays and γ-rays in use, eliminating problems in obtaining a value for the dose in free space when the depth for electronic buildup is great.

The original TMR definition is similar to the definition of TPR, except that the reference depth, d_r, is the depth of maximum dose. However, the depth of maximum dose for megavoltage x-ray beams varies significantly with field size and also is a function of SSD. Thus, the definition of TMR creates a measurement problem because a variable d_r is required and the TMR depends on SSD. A modification by Khan et al.[89] proposed that the reference depth, d_r, must be equal to or greater than the largest depth of maximum dose.

Purdy[90] reported on the relationships between the central axis PDD and the TPR, TMR, and TAR. This work suggested that the degree to which the TPR and TMR are independent of distance from the radiation source depends largely on the linac's collimator/flattening filter scatter component of the beam.

Scatter–Air Ratio and Scatter–Maximum Ratio

The scatter–air ratio (SAR) can be thought of as the scatter component of the TAR.[91] It is defined as follows:

$$SAR(d, S_d, E) = TAR(d, S_d, E) = TAR(d, 0, E)$$

SAR is the difference between the TAR for a field of finite area and the TAR for a zero-area field size. The zero-area TAR is a mathematical abstraction obtained by extrapolation of the TAR values measured for finite field sizes.

Similarly, the scatter–maximum ratio (SMR), the scatter component of the TMR, is defined as follows:

$$SMR(d, S_d, E) = TMR(d, S_d, E) \cdot \frac{S_p(S_d, E)}{S_p(S_0, E)} - TMR(d, 0, E)$$

where S_p is a phantom scatter correction factor, which takes into account changes in scatter radiation originating in the phantom at the reference depth as the field size is changed.[89]

Output Factor

The output factor for a given field size is defined as the ratio of the dose rate at the depth of maximum dose for a given field size to that for the reference field size (usually 10×10 cm) at its d_{max}. The output factor varies with field size (Fig. 6.37) as a result of two distinct phenomena. As the collimator jaws are opened, the primary dose, D_p, at d_{max} on the central ray per monitor unit increases as a result of a larger number of primary x-ray photons scattered out of the flattening filter. In addition, the scatter dose, $D_s(d_{max}, r)$, at the measurement point per unit D_p increases as the scattering volume irradiated by primary photons increases with increasing collimated field size. These two components can vary independently of one another if nonstandard treatment distances or extensive secondary blocking is used.

Khan et al.[89] described a method for separating the overall output factor, $S_{c,p}$, into two components. One is the collimator scatter factor, $S_c(r_c)$, which is a function only of the collimator opening, r_c, projected to isocenter. The other is the phantom scatter factor, $S_p(r)$, which is a function only of the cross-sectional area or effective field size, r, irradiated at the treatment distance. They demonstrate that

$$S_{c,p}(r) = S_c(r_c) \cdot S_p(r)$$

In practice, the total and collimator scatter factors both are measured and the phantom scatter factor is calculated using the relationship listed previously. $S_c(r_c)$ is measured in air using an ion chamber fitted with an equilibrium-thickness buildup

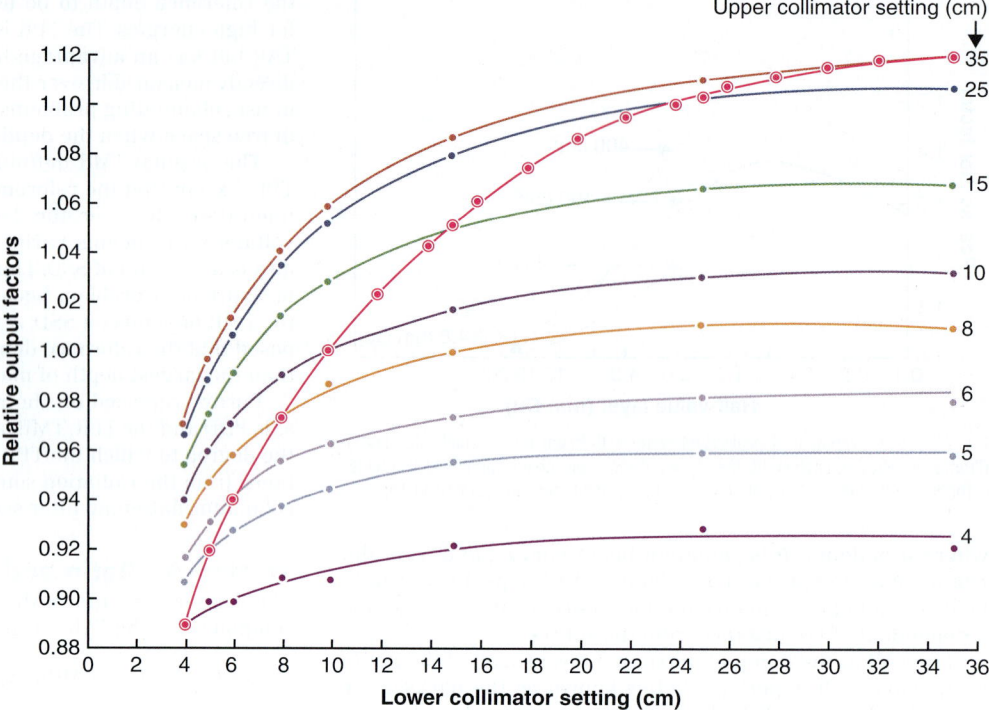

FIGURE 6.37. Example of output factor as a function of lower and upper collimator settings for a medical linear accelerator 18-MV x-ray beam.

cap and given by the ratio of the reading for the given collimator opening to the reading for a reference field (typically 10 × 10 cm) collimator opening. The overall output factor is measured in-phantom using the standard treatment distance and is given by the reading relative to that for a 10 × 10 cm field size. By carefully extrapolating this measured ratio to zero-field size, one obtains the zero-field-size phantom scatter factor, $S_p(0)$. If a small-ion chamber is positioned axially in the beam, it is possible to measure $S_{c,p}$ for field sizes as small as 1 × 1 cm. Because of the loss of lateral secondary electron equilibrium encountered near the edges of high-energy photon beams, S_p deviates significantly from unity. Consistent separation of primary and scatter dose components significantly improves the accuracy of dose predictions for irregular field calculations, especially near block edges and the resultant dose falloff resulting from lateral electron disequilibrium, and under blocks, overcoming many of the dose-modeling problems presented by use of extensive customized blocking.

Isodose Curves

An isodose curve represents points of equal dose. A set of these curves, normally given in 10% increments normalized to the dose at the reference depth, can be plotted on a chart (i.e., isodose chart) to give a visual representation of the dose distribution in a single plane (Fig. 6.38). Beam parameters, such as source size, flattening filter, field size, and SSD, play important roles in the shape of the isodose curve.

Dose Profiles

A dose profile is a representation of the dose in an irradiated volume as a function of spatial position along a single line. Dose profiles are particularly well suited to the description of field flatness and penumbra. The data most often are given as ratios of doses normalized to the dose on the central axis (Fig. 6.39). The profiles, called *off-axis factors* or *off-center ratios*, may be measured in air (i.e., with only a buildup cap)

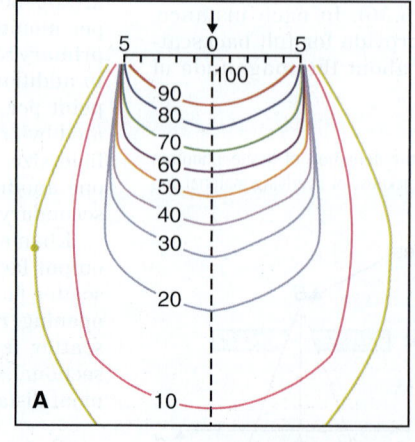

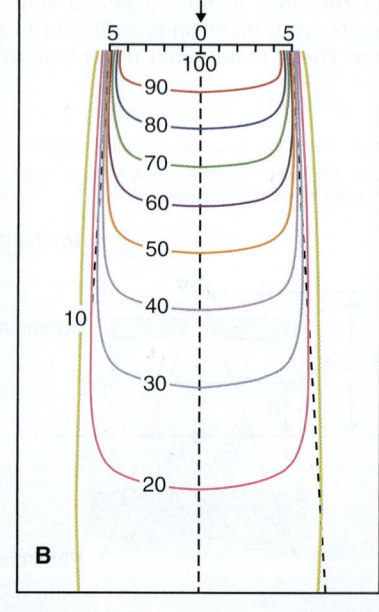

FIGURE 6.38. Isodose distributions for different quality radiations. **A:** 200 kVp, source–skin distance (SSD) = 50 cm, half-value layer (HVL) = 1 mm Cu, field size = 10 × 10 cm. **B:** ^{60}Co, SSD = 80 cm, field size = 10 × 10 cm.

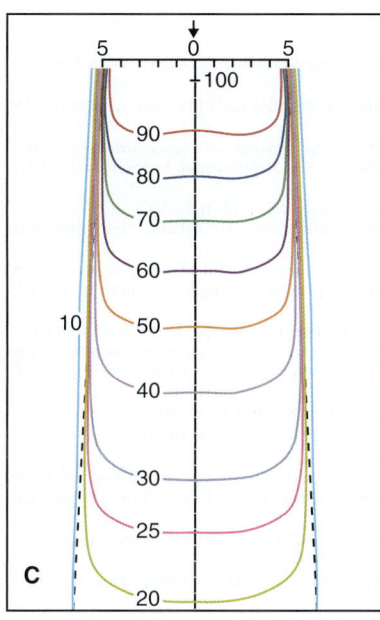

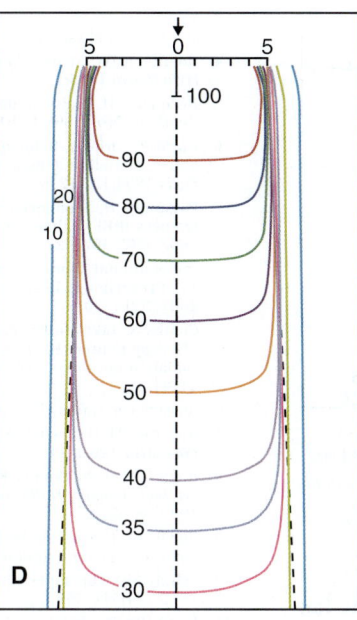

FIGURE 6.38. (*Continued*) **C:** 4-MV x-rays, SSD = 100 cm, field size = 10 × 10 cm. **D:** 10-MV x-rays, SSD = 100 cm, field size = 10 × 10 cm. (From Khan FM. *The physics of radiation therapy*. 2nd ed. Baltimore: Williams & Wilkins, 1994. With permission.)

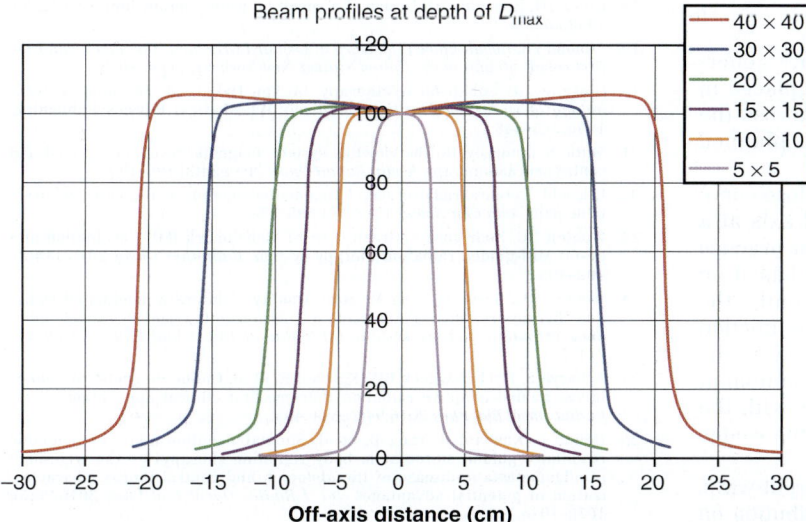

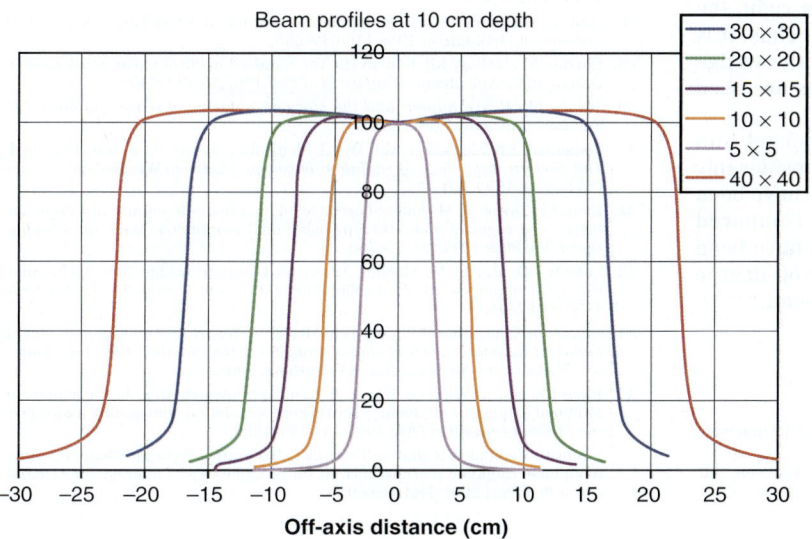

FIGURE 6.39. Example of dose profiles for an 18-MV linear accelerator x-ray beam measured at depths of 3 and 10 cm.

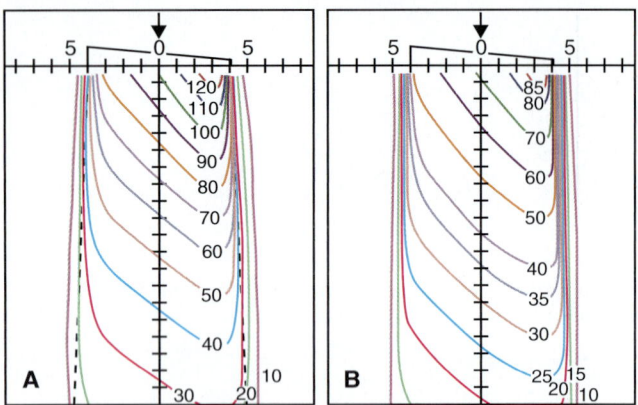

FIGURE 6.40. Isodose curves for a wedge filter. **A:** Normalized to D_{max}. **B:** Normalized to D_{max} without the wedge. ^{60}Co, wedge angle = 45 deg, field size = 8 × 10 cm, source–skin distance = 80 cm. (From Khan FM. *The physics of radiation therapy*. 2nd ed. Baltimore: Williams & Wilkins, 1994. With permission.)

or in a phantom at selected depths. The in-air off-axis factor gives only the variation in primary beam intensity; the in-phantom off-center ratio shows the added effect of phantom scatter.

Wedge Filter

Wedge filters, first introduced by Ellis and Miller,[92] generally are constructed of brass, steel, or lead. When placed in the beam they progressively decrease intensity across the field, causing the isodose distribution to have a planned asymmetry.

The wedge angle is defined as the angle the isodose curve subtends with a line perpendicular to the central axis at a specific depth and for a specified field size. Current practice is to use a depth of 10 cm. Past definitions were based on the 50th-percentile isodose curve and, more recently, the 80th-percentile isodose curve. The wedge angle is a function of field size and depth. The wedge factor is defined as the ratio of the dose measured in a tissue-equivalent phantom at the depth of maximum buildup on the central axis with the wedge in place to the dose at the same point with the wedge removed.

Wedge isodose curves can be normalized in different ways, as shown in Figure 6.40. The wedged isodose distribution on the left side of the figure has been normalized to 100% at d_{max} on the central axis with the wedge in place; on the right, the normalization is done without the wedge in place. Thus, it is imperative that the normalization and the use of the wedge factor should be clearly understood before wedges are used clinically.

Beam hardening occurs when a wedge is inserted into the radiation beam. The PDD, therefore, can be considerably increased at depth. Differences in PDD of nearly 7% have been reported for a 4-MV x-ray, 60-deg wedge field, compared with the open field at a depth of 12 cm, and there have been reports of as much as a 3% difference between the 60-degree wedge field and the open field for a 25-MV x-ray beam.[93,94]

REFERENCES

1. Khan FM. *The physics of radiation therapy*. 4th ed. Philadelphia, PA: Lippincott Williams & Wilkins, 2010.
2. Van Dyk J, ed. *The modern technology of radiation oncology*. Madison, WI: Medical Physics Publishing, 1999.
3. Van Dyk J, ed. *The modern technology of radiation oncology*. Vol. 2. Madison, WI: Medical Physics Publishing, 2005.
4. Roentgen WC. A new kind of rays [in German]. *Sitzungber Phys Med Ges (Wurzburg)* 1895;137.
5. Becquerel H. Emission de radiations nouvilles par l'uranium métallique. *C R Acad Sci Paris* 1896;122:1086.
6. Curie P, Curie M, Belmont MG. Sur une nouvelle substance fortement radio-active, contenue dans la pechblende. *C R Hebdomadaires Séances Acad Sci Paris* 1898;127:1215.
7. Paganetti H, Niemierko A, Ancukiewicz M, et al. Relative biological effectiveness (RBE) values for proton beam therapy. *Int J Radiat Oncol Biol Phys* 2002;53(2):407–421.
8. International Commission on Radiation Units and Measurements. Report 78: Prescribing, Recording, and reporting proton beam therapy. *J ICRU* 2007;7(2):1–201.
9. Combs S, Jäkel O, Haberer T, et al. Particle therapy at the Heidelberg Ion Therapy Center (HIT)–Integrated research-driven university hospital-based radiation oncology service in Heidelberg, Germany. *Radiother Oncol* 2010;95:41–44.
10. Rossi S. The status of CNAO. *Eur Phys J Plus* 2011;126:1–39.
11. Benedikt M, Wrulich A. Medaustron–project overview and status. *Eur Phys J Plus* 2011;126:1–11.
12. Biggs P, Ma C-M, Doppke K, et al. Kilovoltage x-rays. In: Van Dyk J, ed. *The modern technology of radiation oncology*. Madison, WI: Medical Physics Publishing, 1999:287–312.
13. Purdy JA, Prasad SC, Walz BJ, et al. Radiation protection considerations for endocavitary. *Int J Radiat Oncol Biol Phys* 1985;11:2177–2181.
14. Schulz MD. The supervoltage story. *Am J Roentgenol Radium Ther Nucl Med* 1975;124:541–559.
15. Kerst DW. The betatron. *Radiology* 1943;40:120–127.
16. Karzmark CJ, Nunan CS, Tanabe E. *Medical electron accelerators*. New York: McGraw-Hill, 1993.
17. Johns HE, Bates IM, Watson TA. 1000 curie cobalt units for radiation therapy. I. The Saskatchewan cobalt-60 unit. *Br J Radiol* 1952;25:296.
18. Green DT, Errington RF. Design of a cobalt 60 beam therapy unit. *Br J Radiol* 1952;25:309.
19. Almond PR. *Cobalt blues (The story of Leonard Grimmett, the man behind the first cobalt-60 unit in the United States)*. New York: Springer, 2013.
20. Glasgow GP. Cobalt-60 teletherapy. In: Van Dyk J, ed. *The modern technology of radiation oncology*. Madison, WI: Medical Physics Publishing, 1999:313–348.
21. Mutic S, Dempsey JF. The ViewRay system: magnetic resonance-guided and controlled radiotherapy. *Semin Radiat Oncol* 2014;24(3):196–199.
22. Leksell L. Cerebral radiosurgery: I. Gammathalamotomy in two cases of intractable pain. *Acta Chir Scand* 1968;134:585–595.
23. Wooten HO, Rodriguez V, Green O, et al. Benchmark IMRT evaluation of a Co-60 MRI-guided radiation therapy system. *Radiother Oncol* 2015;114(3):402–405.
24. Wooten HO, Green O, Yang M, et al. Quality of intensity modulated radiation therapy treatment plans using a ^{60}Co magnetic resonance image guidance radiation therapy system. *Int J Radiat Oncol Biol Phys* 2015;92(4):771–778.
25. Acharya S, Fischer-Valuck BW, Kashani R, et al. Online magnetic resonance image guided adaptive radiation therapy: first clinical applications. *Int J Radiat Oncol Biol Phys* 2016;94(2):394–403.
26. Henke L, Kashani R, Yang D, et al. Simulated online adaptive magnetic resonance-guided stereotactic body radiation therapy for the treatment of oligometastatic disease of the abdomen and central thorax: characterization of potential advantages. *Int J Radiat Oncol Biol Phys* 2016;96(5):1078–1086.
27. Miller CW. Traveling-wave linear accelerator for x-ray therapy. *Nature* 1953;171:297–298.
28. Howard-Flanders P. The development of the linear accelerator as a clinical instrument. *Acta Radiol* 1954;116:649–655.
29. Ginzton EL, Mallory KB, Kaplan HS. The Stanford medical linear accelerator. I. Design and development. *Stanford Med Bull* 1957;15:123–140.
30. Jacobs CD. *Henry Kaplan and the story of hodgkin's disease*. Stanford, CA: Stanford University Press, 2010.
31. Podgorsak EB, Metcalfe P, Van Dyk J. Medical accelerators. In: Van Dyk J, ed. *The modern technology of radiation oncology*. Madison, WI: Medical Physics Publishing, 1999:349–435.
32. Klein EE, Taylor M, Michaletz-Lorenz M, et al. A mono-isocentric technique for breast and regional nodal therapy using dual asymmetric jaws. *Int J Radiat Oncol Biol Phys* 1994;28:753–760.
33. Leavitt DD, Martin M, Moeller JH, et al. Dynamic wedge field techniques through computer-controlled collimator motion and dose delivery. *Med Phys* 1990;17:87–91.
34. American Association of Physicists in Medicine. *Report 72: basic applications of multileaf collimators: report of task group 50 of the radiation therapy committee*. Madison, WI: Medical Physics Publishing, 2001.
35. Klein EE, Harms WB, Low DA, et al. Clinical implementation of a commercial multileaf collimator: dosimetry, networking, simulation, and quality assurance. *Int J Radiat Oncol Biol Phys* 1995;33:1195–1208.
36. Intensity Modulated Radiation Therapy Collaborative Working Group. Intensity modulated radiation therapy: current status and issues of interest. *Int J Radiat Oncol Biol Phys* 2001;51(4):880–914.

37. Yu CX. Intensity modulated arc therapy with dynamic multileaf collimation: an alternative to tomotherapy. *Phys Med Biol* 1995;40(9):1435–1449.

38. Yu CX, Tang G. Intensity-modulated arc therapy: principles, technologies and clinical implementation. *Phys Med Biol* 2011;56(5):R31–R54.

39. Otto K. Volumetric modulated arc therapy: IMRT in a single gantry arc. *Med Phys* 2008;35(1):310–317.

40. Dong P, Lee P, Ruan D, et al. 4π non-coplanar liver SBRT: a novel delivery technique. *Int J Radiat Oncol Biol Phys* 2013;85(5):1360–1366.

41. Jaffray DA, Drake DG, Moreau M, et al. A radiographic and tomographic imaging system integrated into a medical linear accelerator for localization of bone and soft-tissue targets. *Int J Radiat Oncol Biol Phys* 1999;45:773–789.

42. Jaffray DA, Siewerdsen JH, Wong JW, et al. Flat-panel cone-beam computed tomography for image-guided radiation therapy. *Int J Radiat Oncol Biol Phys* 2002;53(5):1337–1349.

43. Veksler VJ. A new method for acceleration of relativistic particles [in Russian]. *Dokl Akad Nauk SSSR* 1944;43:329.

44. Schwinger J. On the classical radiation of accelerated electrons. *Phys Rev* 1949;75:1912–1925.

45. Brahme A. Design principles and clinical possibilities with a new generation of radiation therapy equipment. *Acta Oncol* 1987;26:403–412.

46. Mackie TR, Holmes T, Swerdloff S, et al. Tomotherapy: a new concept for the delivery of dynamic conformal radiotherapy. *Med Phys* 1993;20(6):1709–1719.

47. Jeraj R, Mackie TR, Balog J, et al. Radiation characteristics of helical tomotherapy. *Med Phys* 2004;31(2):396–404.

48. Adler JR, Chang SD, Murphy MJ, et al. The CyberKnife: a frameless robotic system for radiosurgery. *Stereotact Funct Neurosurg* 1997;69:124–128.

49. Adler JR, Murphy MJ, Chang SD, et al. Image-guided robotic radiosurgery. *Neurosurgery* 1999;44:1299–1307.

50. Kamino Y, Takayama K, Kokubo M, et al. Development of a four-dimensional image-guided radiotherapy system with a gimbaled x-ray head. *Int J Radiat Oncol Biol Phys* 2006;66(1):271–278.

51. DesRosiers C, Moskvin V, Bielajew AF, et al. 150–250 MeV electron beams in radiation therapy. *Phys Med Biol* 2000;45:1781–1805.

52. Fuchs T, Szymanowski H, Oelfke U, et al. Treatment planning for laser-accelerated very-high energy electrons. *Phys Med Biol* 2009;54:3315–3328.

53. Wilson RW. Radiological use of fast protons. *Radiology* 1946;47:487–491.

54. Breuer H, Smith BJ. *Proton therapy and radiosurgery*. Berlin, Germany: Springer-Verlag, 2000.

55. Delaney TF, Kooy HM. *Proton and charged particle radiotherapy*. Philadelphia, PA: Lippincott Williams & Wilkins, 2008.

56. Schulz-Ertner D, Jakel O, Schlegel W. Radiation therapy with charged particles. *Semin Radiat Oncol* 2006;16(4):249–259.

57. Coutrakon G, Bauman M, Lesyna D, et al. A prototype beam delivery system for the proton medical accelerator at Loma Linda. *Med Phys* 1991;18(6):1093–1099.

58. Hall EJ. Intensity-modulated radiation therapy, protons, and the risk of second cancer. *Int J Radiat Oncol Biol Phys* 2006;65(1):1–7.

59. Henning W, Shank C, eds. *Accelerators for America's future*. Washington, DC: U.S. Department of Energy, 2010:25.

60. Maughan RL, Powers WE. A superconducting cyclotron for neutron radiation therapy. *Med Phys* 1994;21(6):779–785.

61. Maughan RL, Yudelev M. Neutron therapy. In: Van Dyk J, ed. *The modern technology of radiation oncology*. Madison, WI: Medical Physics Publishing, 1999:871–917.

62. Van Dyk J, Munro PN. Simulators. In: Van Dyk J, ed. *The modern technology of radiation oncology*. Madison, WI: Medical Physics Publishing, 1999:95–129.

63. Nishidai T, Nagata Y, Takahashi M, et al. CT simulator: A new 3-D planning and simulation system for radiotherapy. I. Description of system. *Int J Radiat Oncol Biol Phys* 1990;18:499–504.

64. Perez CA, Purdy JA, Harms WB, et al. Design of a fully integrated three-dimensional computed tomography simulator and preliminary clinical evaluation. *Int J Radiat Oncol Biol Phys* 1994;30(4):887–897.

65. Sherouse GW, Bourland JD, Reynolds K, et al. Virtual simulation in the clinical setting: some practical considerations. *Int J Radiat Oncol Biol Phys* 1990;19(4):1059–1065.

66. Van Dyk J, Taylor JS. CT simulators. In: Van Dyk J, ed. *The modern technology of radiation oncology*. Madison, WI: Medical Physics Publishing, 1999:131–168.

67. Mutic S, Palta JR, Butker EK, et al. Quality assurance for computed-tomography simulators and the computed-tomography-simulation process: Report of the AAPM Radiation Therapy Committee Task Group No. 66. *Med Phys* 2003;30(10):2762–2792.

68. Mutic S, Purdy JA, Michalski JM, et al. The simulation process in the determination and definition of the treatment volume and treatment planning. In: Levitt SH, Purdy JA, Perez CA, et al., eds. *Technical basis of radiation therapy*. Berlin, Germany: Springer, 2006:107–133.

69. Almond P. A historical perspective: a brief history of dosimetry, calibration protocols, and the need for accuracy. In: Rogers DWO, Cygler JE, eds. *Clinical dosimetry measurements in radiotherapy*. Madison, WI: Medical Physics Publishing, 2009:1×27.

70. Orton CG, Seibert JB. The measurement of teletherapy unit timer errors. *Phys Med Biol* 1972;17:198.

71. Kron T. Dose measuring tools. In: Van Dyk J, ed. *The modern technology of radiation oncology*. Madison, WI: Medical Physics Publishing, 1999:753–821.

72. American Association of Physicists in Medicine, Task Group 21, Radiation Therapy Committee. A protocol for the determination of absorbed dose from high-energy photon and electron beams. *Med Phys* 1983;10:741–771.

73. Almond PR, Biggs PJ, Coursey BM, et al. AAPM's TG-51 protocol for clinical reference dosimetry of high-energy photon and electron beams. *Med Phys* 1999;26:1847–1870.

74. Huq MS, Andreo P. Reference dosimetry in clinical high-energy photon beams: comparison of the AAPM TG-51 and AAPM TG-21 dosimetry protocols. *Med Phys* 2001;28(1):46–54.

75. Huq MS, Andreo P, Song H. Comparison of the IAEA TRS-398 and AAPM TG-51 absorbed dose to water protocols in the dosimetry of high-energy photon and electron beams. *Phys Med Biol* 2001;46(11):2985–3006.

76. Huq MS, Song H. Reference dosimetry in clinical high-energy electron beams: comparison of the AAPM TG-51 and AAPM TG-21 dosimetry protocols. *Med Phys* 2001;28(10):2077–2087.

77. DeWerd LA, Bartol LJ, Davis SD. Thermoluminescent dosimetry. In: Rogers DWO, Cygler JE, eds. *Clinical dosimetry measurements in radiotherapy*. Madison, WI: Medical Physics Publishing, 2009:815–840.

78. Das IJ. Radiographic film. In: Rogers DWO, Cygler JE, eds. *Clinical dosimetry measurements in radiotherapy*. Madison, WI: Medical Physics Publishing, 2009:865–890.

79. Soares CG, Trichter S, Devic S. Radiochromic film. In: Rogers DWO, Cygler JE, eds. *Clinical dosimetry measurements in radiotherapy*. Madison, WI: Medical Physics Publishing, 2009:759–813.

80. American Association of Physicists in Medicine. *Report 87. Diode in vivo dosimetry for patients receiving external beam radiation therapy: report of task group 62 of the radiation therapy committee*. Madison, WI: Medical Physics Publishing, 2005.

81. Zhu TC, Saini AS. Diode dosimetry for megavoltage electron and photon beams. In: Rogers DWO, Cygler JE, eds. *Clinical dosimetry measurements in radiotherapy*. Madison, WI: Medical Physics Publishing, 2009:913–939.

82. Cygler JE, Scalchi P. MOSFET dosimetry in radiotherapy. In: Rogers DWO, Cygler JE, eds. *Clinical dosimetry measurements in radiotherapy*. Madison, WI: Medical Physics Publishing, 2009:941–977.

83. Baldock C, De Deene Y, Doran S, et al. Polymer gel dosimetry. *Phys Med Biol* 2010;(55):R1–R51.

84. Schreiner LJ, Olding T. Gel dosimetry. In: Rogers DWO, Cygler JE, eds. *Clinical dosimetry measurements in radiotherapy*. Madison, WI: Medical Physics Publishing, 2009:979–1025.

85. Rankine LJ, Mein S, Cai B, et al. Three-Dimensional dosimetric validation of a magnetic resonance guided intensity modulated radiation therapy system. *Int J Radiat Oncol Biol Phys* 2017;97(5):1095–1104.

86. Burns JE. Conversion of depth doses from one FSD to another. *Br J Radiol* 1958;31:643.

87. Holt JD, Laughlin JS, Moroney JP. The extension of the concept of tissue-air (TAR) to high energy x-ray beams. *Radiology* 1970;96:437–446.

88. Karzmark CJ, Deubert A, Loevinger R. Tissue-phantom ratios—an aid to treatment planning. *Br J Radiol* 1965;38:158–159.

89. Khan FM, Sewchand W, Lee J, et al. Revision of tissue-maximum ratio and scatter-maximum ratio concepts for cobalt 60 and higher energy x-ray beams. *Med Phys* 1980;7:230–237.

90. Purdy JA. Relationship between tissue-phantom ratio and percentage depth dose. *Med Phys* 1977;4:66.

91. Cunningham JR. Scatter-air ratios. *Phys Med Biol* 1972;17:42–51.

92. Ellis F, Miller H. The use of wedge filters in deep x-ray therapy. *Br J Radiol* 1944;17:90.

93. Abrath FG, Purdy JA. Wedge design and dosimetry for 25-MV x rays. *Radiology* 1980;136:757–762.

94. Sewchand W, Khan FM, Williamson J. Variations in depth-dose data between open and wedge fields for 4-MV x rays. *Radiology* 1978;127:789–792.

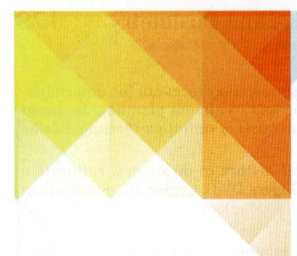

CHAPTER 7

Photon External-Beam Dosimetry and Treatment Planning

James A. Purdy and Sasa Mutic

INTRODUCTION

When planning the treatment of a patient with cancer, the radiation oncologist is faced with the problem of prescribing a treatment regimen with a radiation dose that is large enough to potentially cure or control the disease but does not cause serious normal tissue complications. This task is a difficult one because tumor control and normal tissue effect responses for most disease sites are typically steep functions of radiation dose; that is, a small change in the dose delivered (±5%) can result in a dramatic change in the local response of the tissue (±20%).[1–3] Moreover, the prescribed curative doses are often, by necessity, very close to the doses tolerated by the normal tissues. Thus, for optimum treatment, the radiation dose must be planned and delivered with a high degree of precision.

One can readily compute the dose distribution resulting from photons, electrons, protons, or a mixture of these radiation beams impinging on a regularly shaped, flat-surface, homogeneous unit-density phantom. However, the patient presents a much more complicated situation because of irregularly shaped topography and having tissues of varying densities and atomic composition (called *heterogeneities*). In addition, beam modifiers, such as wedges, compensating filters, or bolus, are sometimes inserted into the radiation beam, further complicating the calculation of the absorbed dose.

In this chapter, several aspects of photon external-beam treatment planning and dosimetry are reviewed, including methods used for dose/monitor unit (MU) calculations, correction for the effects of the patient's irregular surface and internal heterogeneities on the calculated photon dose distribution, isodose distributions for combined fields, field junctions, field shaping and design of treatment aids, and related clinical dosimetry issues.

DOSE CALCULATION METHODS

For purposes of discussion, it is convenient to characterize photon beam dose calculation methods as either *correction based* or *model based*.[4] In the former method, the dose at a given point is calculated using measured central-axis data, for example, percent depth dose (PDD), tissue–air ratios (TARs), tissue-maximum ratios (TMRs), tissue–phantom ratios (TPRs), and off-axis ratios (OARs). These quantities are measured under reference conditions (i.e., in a homogeneous water phantom with a flat surface normal to the incident radiation beam at a standard distance from the x-ray source). Hence, specific correction factors (CFs) are used in planning the treatment of real patients to account for varying patient surfaces, tissue heterogeneities, irregular field shapes, and any beam modifiers used.

In the model-based algorithms, the dose distribution is computed in a phantom or patient from more of a first-principles approach accounting for lateral transport of radiation, beam energy, geometry, beam modifiers, patient surface topography, and electron density distribution rather than correcting parameterized dose distributions measured in a water phantom. These models utilize convolution energy deposition kernels that describe the distribution of dose about a single primary photon interaction site and provide much more

accurate results even for complex heterogeneous geometries. Both methods are discussed in the following sections, and more details on model-based photon dose calculation algorithms can be found in the references listed.[4,5] It should be noted that with the evolution of advanced computing methods, modern treatment planning systems generally do not rely on correction methods and are included here for historic reference rather than for practical treatment planning purposes. The correction-based models remain relevant for purposes of manual dose calculations and secondary/independent dose verification applications. However, many of the modern-day independent dose calculation programs include more sophisticated dose calculation algorithms.

Correction-Based Dose Calculation Methods

Using the notation of Khan et al.,[6] the dose at a point (D_P) at a depth d of overlying tissue on the central ray for an irregularly shaped field is given by:

$$D_P = D_{\text{ref}} \cdot S_c\left(r_c\right) \cdot S_p\left(r_d\right) \cdot \text{TF} \cdot \text{WF} \left(\frac{\text{SCD}}{\text{SAD}}\right)^2 \cdot \text{TMR}\left(d, r_d\right)$$

where S_c denotes the *collimator scatter factor;* S_p the *phantom scatter factor;* and TMR the *tissue-maximum ratio.* TF and WF denote the tray and wedge factors, respectively, and are defined as the ratio of the central ray dose with the tray or wedge filter in place relative to the dose in the open-beam geometry. The collimated field size is denoted by r_c and is usually described as the square field size equivalent to the rectangular collimator opening projected to isocenter. The effective field size is denoted by r_d and is specified to the iso-center distance (SAD). The inverse-square law factor accounts for the difference in distances from the source to point of dose calculation relative to the source to calibration point distance (SCD). Note that when isocentric calibration is used, this factor is unity. Also, note that collimator-defined field size is used for lookup of the collimator scatter factor, S_c, whereas effective field size projected to isocenter is used for lookup of the TMR value and the phantom scatter factor, S_p. By separately accounting for the effect of collimator opening on the primary dose component and the influence of cross-sectional area of tissue irradiated, most of the difficulties in accurately calculating a dose in the presence of extensive blocking are overcome. Details on determining the effective field size for an irregularly shaped field, taking into account both the primary and scatter dose components, will be discussed in a later section.

Correction for Varying Patient Topography (Air Gaps)

In the previous equation, it is assumed that the beam is normally incident on a unit-density uniform phantom. The following CF methods can be applied to the equation to account for the nonnormal beam incidence caused by the patient's varying surface.[7]

Air Gap CF: Ratio of Tissue–Air Ratio Method
In the ratio of TAR or TPR method, the surface (along a ray line) directly above point A (source-to-skin distance [SSD] = S′)

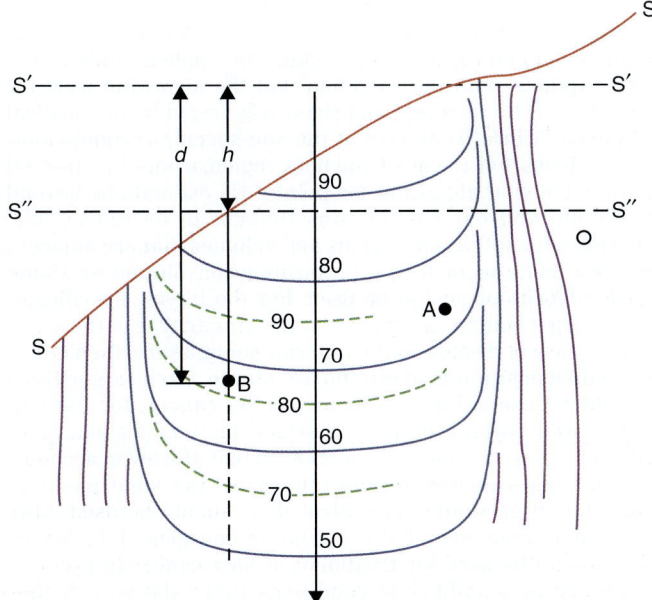

FIGURE 7.1. Schematic drawing illustrating tissue–air ratio and effective source-to-skin distance (SSD) methods for the correction of isodose curves under a sloping surface (*solid lines* for SSD = S'; *dashed lines* for SSD = S"). (From International Commission of Radiation Units and Measurements. Report 24: Determination of absorbed dose in a patient irradiated by beams of × or gamma rays in radiotherapy procedures. Washington, DC: International Commission of Radiation Units and Measurements, 1976. Reproduced by permission of International Commission on Radiation Units and Measurements.)

is unaltered, so the primary component to the dose distribution at this point is unchanged (and the scatter component is also assumed to be unaltered) (see Fig. 7.1). Thus, the dose at point A can be considered as unaltered by patient shape. However, for point B, where there are considerable variations in the patient's topography, both the primary and scatter components of the radiation beam are altered. The CF may be determined using two TARs or TPRs as follows:

$$CF = \frac{T(d-h, s_d)}{T(d, s_d)}$$

where h = air gap.

Air Gap CF: Effective Source–Skin Ratio Method
In the effective SSD method, the isodose chart to be used is placed on the patient's contour representation, positioning the central axis at the distance for which the curve was measured (Fig. 7.1). It then is shifted down along the ray line for the length of the air gap, h, resulting in SSD = S". The PDD value at point B is read and modified by an inverse-square calculation to account for the effective change in the peak dose. The CF can be expressed as follows:

$$CF = \frac{P(d-h, d_0, S, f, E)}{P(d, d_0, S, f, E)} \cdot \left(\frac{f+d_0}{f+h+d_0}\right)^2$$

Correction for Tissue Heterogeneities
The following CF methods can be used to account for the tissue heterogeneities found within the patient.

Tissue Heterogeneities CF: Ratio of Tissue–Air Ratio Method
The ratio of TAR (RTAR) method of correction for inhomogeneities is given by

$$CF = \frac{T(d_{eff}, S_d)}{T(d, S_d)}$$

where the numerator is the TAR for the equivalent water thickness, d_{eff}, and the denominator is the TAR for the actual thickness, d, of tissue between the point of calculation and the surface along a ray passing through the point. S_d is the dimension of the beam cross section at the depth of calculation. The RTAR method accounts for the field size and depth of calculation. It does not account for the position of the point of calculation with respect to the heterogeneity. It also does not take into account the shape of the inhomogeneity; instead, it assumes that it extends the full width of the beam and has a constant thickness (i.e., referred to as *slab geometry*).

Tissue Heterogeneities CF: Power Law TAR Method
The *power law TAR method* was proposed by Batho[8] and generalized by Young and Gaylord.[9] This method, sometimes called the *Batho method*, attempts to account for the nature of the inhomogeneity and its position relative to the point of calculation. However, it does not account for the extent or shape of the inhomogeneity. The CF for the point P is given by

$$CF = \left(\frac{T(d_2, S_d)}{T(d_1, S_d)}\right)^{\rho_2 - 1}$$

where d_1 and d_2 refer to the distances from point P to the near and far side of the non–water-equivalent material, respectively; S_d is the beam dimension at the depth of P; and ρ_2 is the relative electron density of the inhomogeneity with respect to water.

Sontag and Cunningham[10] derived a more general form of this CF, which can be applied to a case in which the effective atomic number of the inhomogeneity is different from that of water and the point of interest lies within the inhomogeneity. The CF in this situation is given by

$$CF = \frac{T(d_2, S_d)^{(\rho_b - 1)}}{T(d_1, S_d)^{(\rho_b - \rho_a)}} \times \frac{(\mu_{en}/\rho)_a}{(\mu_{en}/\rho)_b}$$

where ρ_a is the density of the material in which point P lies at a depth d below the surface and ρ_b is the density of an overlying material of thickness $(d_2 - d_1)$; $(\mu_{en}/\rho)_a$ and $(\mu_{en}/\rho)_b$ are the mass energy absorption coefficients for the medium a and b.

Model-Based Dose Calculation Methods
Advanced three-dimensional dose calculation algorithms, such as the convolution/superposition algorithm and Monte Carlo, have for many years now been the standard of practice.[4,5,11–13] These models provide accurate results even for complex heterogeneous geometries.

Convolution/Superposition Dose Calculation Algorithm
The convolution/superposition dose calculation algorithm is based on the following equation[4]:

$$D(\vec{r}) = \iiint T_E(\vec{s}) h(E, \vec{r} - \vec{s}) d^3 s \, dE$$

where D represents the dose at some point, $T_E(\vec{s})$ represents the total energy released by primary photon interactions per unit mass (or TERMA), and $h(E, \vec{r} - \vec{s})$ is the *point spread function* (also called *dose spread array, differential pencil beam,* and *energy deposition kernel*). The point spread function represents the fraction of the energy deposited (per unit volume) at a point that is subsequently transported to the calculation point. Hence, the dose at a point is computed by integrating over all space the dose contributions from photons and electrons that are produced at all other points in the phantom or patient.

Ahnesjö et al.[14] showed that the point spread function, $h(E, \vec{r} - \vec{s})$, changes only slightly as a function of energy and, thus, can be replaced by $h(\vec{r} - \vec{s})$ (defined as the average point spread function weighted by the spectral components of the beam), reducing the basic convolution four-dimensional integral to a three-dimensional integral overall space. Point spread functions for monoenergetic photons are generally precomputed using Monte Carlo methods.[14] The energy dependence of the TERMA, $T_E(\vec{s})$, can be expressed by applying the inverse-square law and exponential attenuation to the photon fluence at the surface of the phantom or patient.

The three-dimensional integral is typically evaluated in a two-step process. The first step takes into account the properties of the accelerator (including the finite source size, primary collimator, flattening filter, collimator jaws, multileaf collimators, and any beam-modifying devices used for the treatment, such as wedges, alloy blocks, and compensating filters) to compute the energy fluence at the phantom or patient surface. The second step of the calculation takes into account the inverse-square law and exponential attenuation to this incident fluence to determine the TERMA, $T_E(\vec{s})$, at each point within the phantom or patient and convolve the result with the point spread function, $h(\vec{r} - \vec{s})$.

The convolution equation is strictly valid only for homogeneous media (i.e., $h(\vec{s})$ must be spatially invariant). To account for the effects of tissue heterogeneities, all physical distances in the convolution integral are replaced with radiologic distances, that is, the physical distance multiplied by the average density along the line in question.[11,14] Hence, the convolution/superposition algorithm accounts for the effects of heterogeneities anywhere in the vicinity of the calculation point in three dimensions. In contrast, most CF-based dose calculation techniques require only a simple one-dimensional evaluation of radiologic path length and can thus account for the effects of only those tissue heterogeneities that lie along a ray connecting the radiation source to the calculation point.

Several investigators have tested the convolution/superposition algorithm against measurements and Monte Carlo–generated data for complex phantom geometries including both homogeneous and heterogeneous phantoms and found that the convolution/superposition model gave accurate results, even in parts of the buildup region and penumbra.[15,16]

Monte Carlo Method

Monte Carlo is, in principle, the only method capable of computing the dose distribution accurately for all situations encountered in radiation therapy, including being able to accurately predict the dose near interfaces of materials with very dissimilar atomic numbers, such as near metal prostheses, or different densities such as tumors in lung tissue.[17] The Monte Carlo method uses the known cross sections for electron and photon interactions in matter and follows individual photons and the associated electrons set in motion through the entire heterogeneous phantom or patient. By calculating the trajectories and interactions of a very large number of photons and electrons, one can accurately model the dose distribution. Recently, several Monte Carlo codes have been developed for radiotherapy treatment planning,[13,18] many of which have been implemented commercially. The reader is referred to the American Association of Physicists in Medicine (AAPM) Task Group (TG) 105 Report, which summarizes commercial use of Monte Carlo for radiation therapy treatment planning.[12] The reader is also referred to the review article by Siebers et al. for even more details on Monte Carlo calculation for external-beam radiation therapy.[17] More recently, Monte Carlo dose calculations have been extended to account for magnetic field effects on deposition of radiation dose for MR-guided treatment machines.[19–21]

Dose Calculation Algorithms and Tissue Heterogeneities

In 2004, the AAPM published Report 85 (Task Group 65) on tissue inhomogeneity corrections for megavoltage photon beams.[22] The task group recommended an accuracy goal for tissue heterogeneity corrections of 2% in order to achieve an overall 3% accuracy in dose delivery. The AAPM report recommended heterogeneity corrections be applied to plans and prescriptions, with the condition that the algorithm used for calculations be reviewed and rigorously tested by the medical physicist. A brief summary of the site-specific recommendations follows. For the head and neck region, a one-dimensional path correction algorithm for point-dose estimations beyond mandible and ear cavities was thought to be reasonable. However, for soft tissue regions and volumes that are adjacent to these heterogeneities, superposition/convolution or Monte Carlo algorithms should be used. For the larynx, specifically, if the target volume is adjacent to the air cavity or if there is a severe case of disease in the anterior commissure, then either the superposition/convolution or Monte Carlo algorithms should be used. For treatment of lung cancer, for interest points well beyond the lung interface, one-dimensional path corrections were thought to be reasonable. However, accounting for doses at tumor–lung interfaces, the superposition/convolution or Monte Carlo algorithms should be used. Also, the report recommended that photon energies of 12 MV or less should be used for treatment of lung cancer in order to minimize nonequilibrium conditions that exist with higher energies. For breast cancer treatment (particularly if the dose of interest of the target volume is considered to be chest wall), it is recommended that calculations be performed with superposition/convolution or Monte Carlo. However, for simple intact breast planning, one-dimensional algorithms were adequate. For the upper gastrointestinal tract, one-dimensional corrections were adequate. However, one should be leery if barium contrast is used as it can erroneously impact the dose calculation because of its high Z. In terms of the pelvis and prostate, one-dimensional corrections were quite reasonable except in the presence of high-Z implanted hip prostheses. (Note that the dosimetric considerations for patients with hip prostheses undergoing pelvic irradiation are discussed in a later section). The study by Frank et al.[23] provides a clear method for safely transitioning clinical use from one based on planning that assumes a homogeneous unit-density patient to one using a heterogeneous patient model.

The Radiological Physics Center published the results of a study comparing measured results of irradiated lung phantoms having various geometries with dose calculations for similar conditions using commercial treatment planning systems. They found significant differences if algorithms less sophisticated than the superposition-/convolution-type algorithms were used.[24]

MONITOR UNIT CALCULATION METHODS

MU calculations refer to determining the linac MU setting per field to deliver the prescribed dose taking into account the tumor depth, treatment distance, multileaf collimator setting or secondary blocking configuration, and primary collimator opening. This is accomplished by using the various dosimetric quantities described in the preceding chapter to relate the dose corresponding to an arbitrary set of treatment parameters to the reference calibration geometry where the output of the machine is specified in terms of cGy/MU. The reference source to calibration point distance, field size, and depth of output specification are denoted by the symbols SCD, r_{cal}, and d_{cal}, respectively. For a fixed SSD calibration geometry:

$$SCD = SAD\ (source - axis\ distance) + d_{max}$$
$$r_{cal} = 10\ cm \times 10\ cm$$
$$d_{cal} = d_{max}$$

Normal incidence and open-beam geometry (i.e., absence of trays or any beam-modifying filters) are specified.

For treatment machines calibrated isocentrically, the point of MU specification is located at distance SAD rather than at distance SAD + d_{max} as stated previously. For isocentric calibration, SCD = SAD.

The linac is calibrated by adjusting the sensitivity of its internal monitor transmission ion chamber so that 1 MU equals 1 cGy for the reference calibration geometry condition. Several reports providing more details on MU calculations and their verification are listed in the references.[25-27]

MU Calculation for Fixed Fields

When the patient is to be treated isocentrically, the point of dose prescription is located at the isocenter regardless of the target depth. Using the notation of Khan et al.,[6] the MU needed to deliver a prescribed tumor dose to isocenter (TD$_{iso}$) for a depth d of overlying tissue on the central ray is given by

$$MU = \frac{TD_{iso}}{TMR(d,r_d) \cdot S_c(r_c) \cdot S_p(r_d) \cdot TF \cdot WF\left(\frac{SCD}{SAD}\right)^2}$$

where TF and WF denote the tray and wedge factors, respectively. They are defined as the ratio of the central ray dose with the tray or wedge filter in place relative to the dose in the open-beam geometry. The collimated field size is denoted by r_c and is usually described as the square field size equivalent to the rectangular collimator opening projected to isocenter. The effective field size is denoted by r_d and is always specified to the isocenter distance (SAD). The inverse-square law factor accounts for the difference in distances from the source to point of dose prescription relative to the point of MU specification. When isocentric calibration is used, this factor is unity. Note that collimator-defined field size is used for lookup of the collimator scatter factor, S_c, whereas effective field size projected to isocenter is used for lookup of TMR and the phantom scatter factor, S_p. By separately accounting for the effect of collimator opening on the primary dose component and the influence of cross-sectional area of tissue irradiated, most of the difficulties in accurately delivering a dose in the presence of extensive blocking are overcome.

When a fixed distance between the target and entry skin surface (SSD) is used to treat the patient, a dose calculation formalism based on PDD is used rather than one based on isocentric dose ratios. When a dose TD is to be delivered to depth d, MUs are given by:

$$MU = \frac{TD \cdot 100}{PDD(SSD,d,r) \cdot S_c(r_c) \cdot S_p(r) \cdot TF \cdot WF\left(\frac{SCD}{SSD+d_{max}}\right)^2}$$

The field size (or its equivalent square) on the skin surface at central axis is denoted by r and is used for lookup of both PDD and S_p. The collimated field size r_c at the isocenter must be used for lookup of S_c. When an extended treatment distance is used, the collimated field size at isocenter differs significantly from that at the skin surface of the patient. Note that PDD is a function of SSD, depth, and effective field size. Collimator scatter factors measured at SAD are valid over a wide range of extended treatment distances.[6]

When this dose calculation formalism for highly extended treatment distances such as encountered in administering total-body irradiation is used, care must be taken to verify the validity of inverse-square law at these distances. It is recommended that such setups always be verified by ion chamber measurement at the extended distance. Because of the large scatter contribution to effective primary dose originating from the flattening filter and other components in the treatment head, the virtual source of radiation may be as much as 2 cm proximal to the target of the accelerator.

The TAR system of dose calculation is a widely used alternative to the Khan formalism. It is simply an extension of the familiar TAR and backscatter factor concepts, as used in ^{60}Co and orthovoltage dosimetry, to the megavoltage photon energy range. The needed dosimetry parameters are determined from ion chamber measurements (both in-phantom and in-air) like those performed for ^{60}Co, but now using a much larger buildup cap (radius thickness = d_{max}). Thus, the megavoltage peak scatter factor, PSF(r), for an effective field size r is simply the ratio of the two ion chamber readings as shown here.

$$PSF(r) = \frac{\text{ionization at depth } d_{max} \text{ in phantom}}{\text{ionization with buildup cap in air at same point in space}}$$

And the megavoltage beam dose rate (Gy/MU) in free space, $\dot{D}_{fs}$, is given by

$$\dot{D}_{fs}(SAD+d_{max},r_c) = \frac{\dot{D}(SSD,r_c,d_{max})}{PSF(r_c)}$$

where the numerator is the measured d_{max} dose at distance SSD = SAD + d_{max} and collimator setting r_c. Implementation of this system requires a table of $\dot{D}_{fs}$ (SAD + d_{max}, r_c) values for each collimator opening and a table of PSF versus effective field size. Then, dose at d_{max} per MU for any distance, effective field size, and collimator opening can be calculated easily.

When the patient is to be treated isocentrically, the MU needed to deliver a prescribed isocenter dose (ID) to a depth d on the central axis is given by:

$$MU = \frac{ID}{TAR(d,r_d) \cdot \dot{D}_{fs}(SAD+d_{max},r_c) \cdot TF \cdot WF\left(\frac{SCD}{SAD}\right)^2}$$

If the treatment is fixed SSD, the MU needed to deliver a prescribed dose (TD) to a depth d on the central ray is given by:

$$MU = \frac{TD \times 100}{PDD(d,r) \cdot \dot{D}_{fs}(SAD+d_{max},r_c) \cdot PSF(r) \cdot TF \cdot WF\left(\frac{SCD}{SSD+d_{max}}\right)^2}$$

All MU calculation formalisms require some means of estimating the square field size, r, that is equivalent, in terms of scattering characteristics, to an arbitrary rectangular field of width a and length b. Perhaps the most widely used rectangular equivalency principle is the "A/P" rule. It states that a square and a rectangle are equivalent if they have the same area/perimeter ratio; that is:

$$r = \frac{2(a \times b)}{(a+b)}$$

Another widely used approach to reducing rectangular estimates of effective field size to square field sizes is the equivalent square table published in the *British Journal of Radiology*.[28] Estimating the effective field size equivalent to an irregular field is best handled via irregular-field calculations as discussed later in this chapter.[29,30]

MU Calculations for Asymmetric X-Ray Collimators

Asymmetric x-ray collimators (also referred to as independent jaws) allow independent movement of an individual jaw and may be available for one jaw pair or both pairs. Because MU calculations and treatment planning methods generally rely on symmetric jaw data, the dosimetric effects for asymmetric jaws must be fully documented before being implemented in the clinic. Several investigators have examined the effects of asymmetric jaws on PDD, collimator scatter, and iso-dose distributions.[31,32] MU calculations for asymmetric jaws are only slightly more complex than for symmetric jaws.[25] Typically, one simply applies an *off-axis ratio (OAR)* or *off-center ratio (OCR)* CF that depends only on the distance from the machine's central axis to the center of the independently collimated open field.[33,34] PDD is only minimally affected, but isodose curve shape can be altered and must be investigated for the particular treatment unit. Calculations for asymmetric wedge fields follow similar procedures by simply incorporating a wedge OAR or OCR.[32,35]

MU Calculations for Multileaf Collimator

Multileaf collimators (MLCs) have nearly completely replaced conventional alloy field shaping for photon beams in most clinics around the world. Several investigators have examined the effects of the Varian MLC design (tertiary system) on PDD, collimator scatter, and isodose distributions.[36] The effects due to field area shaped by this type of MLC on PDD and beam output parameters are similar to those resulting from Cerrobend field shaping. Thus, the dose/MU calculation methods discussed previously apply by simply using the equivalent area defined by the MLC. The collimator scatter factor and the dose in free space are determined using the x-ray collimator jaw settings, with an off-axis factor applied for any asymmetric jaw settings.

It should be noted, however, that for MLC systems that replace one of the collimating jaws, the MLC field shape can be a determining factor in selecting the appropriate output factor.[37] For example, in the case of the Elekta linacs (Elekta AB, Crawley, United Kingdom), in which the lower jaws are replaced by the MLC system, the calculation takes into consideration the collective blocked area that is created by both the MLC leaves and the lower backup diaphragms.[38] For an MLC system that replaces the upper jaw (e.g., Siemens linac, Siemens Medical Solutions USA, Inc., Malvern, PA), Das et al.[39] describe a method that relies on the blocked area for determining all the calculation parameters (mainly output, PDD, and scatter factor).

Hence, because of MLC design differences and the fact that vendors are continuing to modify/improve MLC designs, the authors caution that when a new linac is installed, the impact of the MLC on the institution's MU calculation procedure should be fully documented before clinical use. The reader is also encouraged to review the AAPM Task Group 50 Report, which provides more detail on various MLC types and discusses quality assurance (QA) and MU calculations.[40]

MU Calculations for Irregular Fields

For large, irregularly shaped fields and at points off the central axis, it is necessary to take account of the off-axis change in intensity (relative to the central axis) of the beam, the variation of the SSD within the field of treatment, the influence of the primary collimator on the output factor, and the scatter contribution to the dose. Changes in the beam quality as a function of position in the radiation field also should be considered.[41,42]

The general method used for irregular-field calculations consists of summation at each point of interest of the primary and scatter irradiation, with allowance for the off-axis change in intensity (off-axis factor) and SSD.[29,30] The MUs required to deliver a specified tumor dose at an arbitrary point in an irregular field (Fig. 7.2) can be calculated as follows:

$$MU = \frac{TD}{[TAR(d,0) + \overline{SAR}(d)] \cdot \dot{D}_{fs}(SSD + d_{max}, r_c) \cdot TF \cdot OAF \left(\frac{SSD + d_{max}}{SSD + g + d}\right)^2}$$

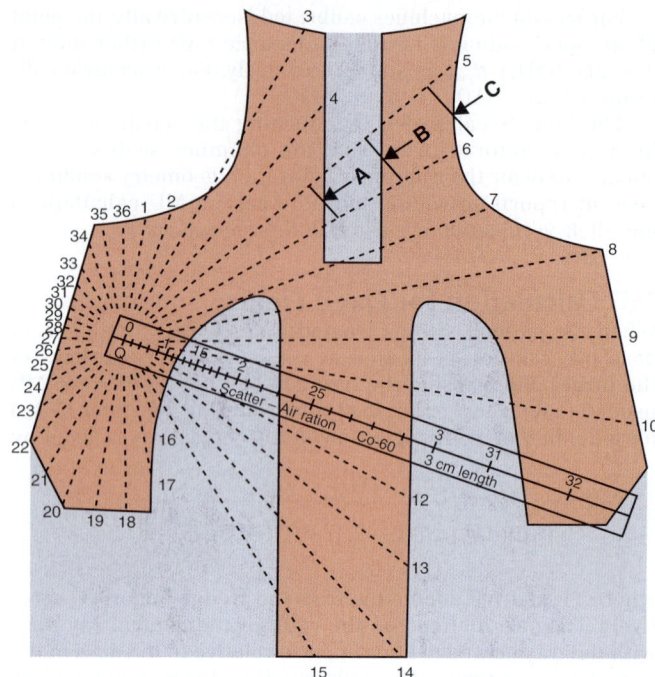

FIGURE 7.2. Outline of mantle field illustrating method of determining scatter-to-air ratio, used for irregular-field dose calculations. (From Cundiff JH, Cunningham JR, Golden R, et al. A method for the calculation of dose in the radiation treatment of Hodgkin's disease. *Am J Roentgenol* 1973;117:30–34. Reprinted with permission from the American Journal of Roentgenology.)

where the parameters used are

TAR $(d,0)$ = zero-field size TAR at depth d
SAR (d) = average SAR for point in question at depth d determined using the Clarkson technique
D_{fs} = Gy/MU in a small mass of tissue, in-air, on the central axis at normal SSD + d_{max} for the collimated field size
SSD = nominal SSD for treatment constraints
d_{max} = depth of dose maximum
TF = blocking tray attenuation factor
g = vertical distance between skin surface over point in question and nominal
SSD = (bean vertical)
d = vertical depth, skin surface to point in question
OAF = in-air off-axis factor

Computer implementations vary but typically include using the expanded field size at a depth for the SAR calculation, determining the off-axis factor using the distance from the central axis to the slant projection of the point of calculation to the SSD plane along a ray from the source and determining the zero-area TAR using the slant depth along a ray going from the source to the point of calculation. It is generally accepted that the off-axis factor should be multiplied by the sum of the zero-area TAR and the SAR as originally proposed.

Beam quality is a function of position in the field for beams generated by linear accelerators.[41,42] The TAR$_0$ may be expressed as a function of position in the beam so that changes in beam quality can be incorporated into calculations, and it can be related to the half-value layer (HVL) of water by the following equation:

$$TAR(d,0,r) = e\left[\frac{-0.693(d - d_{max})}{HVL(r)}\right]$$

where d is the depth of the point of reference, d_{max} is the depth of maximum dose, r is the radial distance from the central axis of the beam to the point of calculation, *e* is the base of the natural logarithm, and HVL*(r)* is the beam quality expressed as the HVL measured in water.

MU Calculations for Rotation Therapy

The classic method for MU calculations for rotation therapy is given by the following equation:

$$MU = \frac{ID}{TAR_{avg} \cdot \dot{D}_{fs} \left(\frac{SCD}{SAD}\right)^2}$$

and the MU per degree setting is given by

$$MU/deg = \frac{monitor\ unit\ setting}{degrees\ of\ rotation}$$

where the symbols have the previous meaning and TAR_{avg} is an average TAR (averaged over radii [depth in the patient] at selected angular intervals, such as 10 or 20 degrees).

Most recently, manufacturers of linacs and their associated planning systems have introduced features that provide rotational intensity-modulated radiation therapy (IMRT) capability[43,44] (e.g., Elekta VMAT[45] and Varian RapidArc[46]). The linac-based rotational IMRT concept was first proposed by Yu[47,48] and called *intensity-modulated arc therapy (IMAT)*, but planning software was not commercially available at that time. Rotational IMRT approaches on conventional linacs may provide even more conformal dose distributions delivered in a shorter treatment time, compared with *SMLC-IMRT (step and shoot)* or *DMLC-IMRT (dynamic)* approaches that use only a limited number of gantry directions. In addition, plan optimization is simpler because it eliminates the planner's iterative choices of beam number and direction. MU calculations for this more complex form of rotational therapy are generated via advanced treatment planning systems having this capability. All are techniques in which the MLC shape changes during a rotation therapy, and depending on the specific linac, other parameters, such as dose rate, may also change. This advanced type of treatment delivery is currently predominantly checked via phantom measurements rather than manual calculations prior to the patient's treatment. Secondary computer programs can also be used to perform independent dose calculations and MU as well as 3D dose calculations.

It is apparent that the simple MU manual calculation methods described here are no longer adequate for the complex technologies in use today. Modern computer plans utilize dose weight points of interest, which classical MU calculation methods may not address; in addition, geometries that include the presence of heterogeneities, added tertiary devices such as MLCs and asymmetric jaws, and beam intensity modulation can all be problematic for manual check calculations. For example, when the dose weight point is within a small volume of mass surrounded by low-density tissue (e.g., a coin lesion in lung) or one that is at the border of a chest wall and lung (as in a postmastectomy patient), MU calculations cannot easily be confirmed by simple hand-calculated MU methods, and one must rely on the planning system for calculations such as these, emphasizing the importance of fully testing such system prior to clinical use. Dedicated commercial software for MU verification is widely available; for example, RadCalc (LifeLine Software Inc, Austin, TX)[49,50] offers a variety of independent MU beam on time calculations, including that for the Gamma Knife (software developed at Washington University and licensed to RadCal).[51] Obviously, such systems must be validated by the physics user prior to clinical use.

CLINICAL PHOTON BEAM DOSIMETRY

Percent Depth Dose and Single-Field Isodose Charts

The central-axis PDD expresses the penetrability of a radiation beam. Table 7.1 summarizes beam characteristics for x-ray and γ-ray beams typically used in radiation therapy and lists the depth at which the dose is maximum (100%) and the 10-cm depth PDD value. Representative PDD curves are shown in Figure 7.3 for conventional SSDs. As a rule of thumb, an 18-MV, 6-MV, and ^{60}Co photon beam loses approximately 2%, 3.5%, and 4.5% per centimeter, respectively, beyond the depth of maximum dose, d_{max} (values are for a 10- × 10-cm field, 100-cm SSD). There is no agreement as to what is the single optimal x-ray beam energy; instead, institutional bias or radiation oncologist training typically influences its selection, and it is usually treatment site specific. As pointed out in Chapter 6, most modern linacs are multimodality and provide a range of photon and electron beam energies ranging from 4 to 25 MV, with 6-, 10-, and 15-MV x-ray beams becoming the most common. It should be noted that in the case of IMRT, the impact of energy on the quality of the delivered radiation dose distribution is less compared to 2D and 3DCRT treatments and that all recent developments in radiotherapy use lower-energy beams exclusively (e.g., CyberKnife, TomoTherapy, ViewRay, Halcyon).[52] The choice of high-energy beams in the era of predominantly IMRT delivery likely has much larger effect on operational efficiency and facility design than on the quality of delivered radiation. Selection of treatment machines with the highest energy of 10 MV or less results in simplification of radiotherapy treatment rooms, typically allowing elimination of the maze and use of thinner and faster room entry doors. These shielding gains come from the elimination of shielding requirements for secondary neutron radiation.

TABLE 7.1 BEAM CHARACTERISTICS FOR PHOTON BEAM ENERGIES OF INTEREST IN RADIATION THERAPY

200 kVp, 2-mm Cu HVL, SSD = 50 cm
- Depth of maximum dose = surface
- Rapid falloff with depth due to (a) low energy and (b) short SSD
- Sharp beam edge due to small focal spot
- Significant dose outside beam boundaries due to Compton scattered radiation at low energies

[60]CO, SSD = 80 cm
- Depth of maximum dose = 0.5 cm
- Increased penetration (10 cm PDD = 55%)
- Beam edge not as well defined—penumbra due to source size
- Dose outside beam low because most scattering is in forward direction
- Isodose curvature increases as the field size increases

4-MV x-ray, SSD = 80 cm
- Depth of maximum dose = 1–1.2 cm
- Penetration slightly greater than cobalt (10 cm PDD = 61%)
- Penumbra smaller
- "Horns" (beam intensity off-axis) due to flattening filter design ≈14%

6-MV x-ray, SSD = 100 cm
- Depth of maximum dose = 1.5 cm
- Slightly more penetration than ^{60}Co and 4 MV (10 cm PDD = 67%)
- Small penumbra
- Horns (beam intensity off-axis) due to flattening filter design ≈9%

15- to 18-MV x-ray, SSD = 100 cm
- Depth of maximum dose = 3–3.5 cm
- Much greater penetration (10 cm PDD = 80%)
- Small penumbra
- Horns (beam intensity off-axis) due to flattening filter design ≈5%
- Exit dose often higher than entrance dose

HVL, half-value layer; PDD, percentage depth dose; SSD, source-to-skin distance.

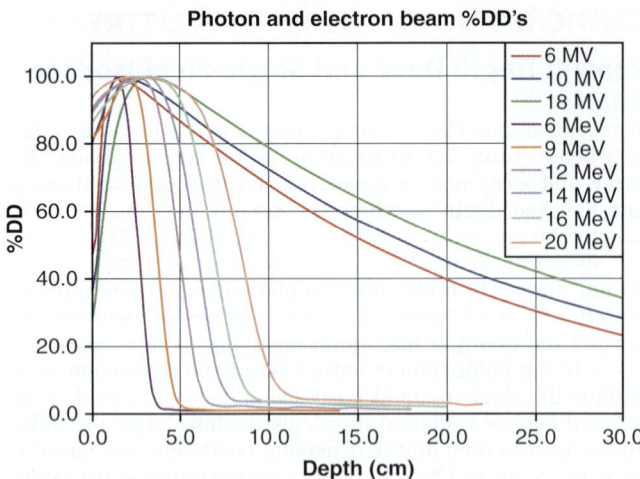

FIGURE 7.3. Typical photon and electron beam central-axis percentage depth-dose (DD) curves for a 10- × 10-cm beam for megavoltage beams ranging from ⁶⁰Co to 18-MV x-rays and 6- to 20-MeV electron beams.

Isodose charts provide much more information about the radiation beam characteristics than do central-axis PDD data alone. However, even isodose charts are limited in that they represent the dose distribution in only one plane (typically the one containing the beam's central axis) and are usually available only for square or rectangular fields. Isodose charts are usually measured in a water phantom with the radiation beam directed perpendicular to the phantom's flat surface. Isodose curves show the relative uniformity of the beams across the field at various depths and also provide a graphical depiction of the width of the beam's penumbra region. ⁶⁰Co teletherapy units exhibit a relatively large penumbra, and their isodose distributions are more rounded than those from linac x-ray beams. This is due to the relatively large source size (typically 1 to 2 cm in diameter vs. only a few millimeters for linacs). Linac beam penumbra width does increase slightly as a function of energy and if unfocused MLC leaves are used but is still much less than that for ⁶⁰Co units. The beam penumbra can be improved if focused MLCs are used. For example, the ViewRay's ⁶⁰Co could produce treatment plans equivalent in quality to that of modern linacs. This equivalence between ⁶⁰Co and linac plans was achieved through combining ⁶⁰Co with doubly focused MLCs on ViewRay.[53] This ability to improve the IMRT plan quality through MLC design will undoubtedly lead to further refinements in approaches to MLC design. ViewRay's double-layer doubly focused and Varian Halcyon's dual-layer MLCs are early indication of this possibility. In addition to the smaller penumbra, linac x-ray isodose distributions have relatively flat isodose curves at depth. However, at shallow depths, particularly at d_{max}, linac x-ray beams typically exhibit an increase in beam intensity away from the central axis; this beam characteristic is referred to as the dose profile *horns* and depends on flattening filter design. In general, each treatment unit has unique radiation beam characteristics, and thus, isodose distributions must be measured, or at least verified, for each specific treatment unit. Excellent dosimetric reproducibility between modern treatment machines has been observed, and there is now a trend toward verification of the expected beam dosimetry rather than attempting to fully characterize dosimetry for each machine.[54]

Another important point to understand is how the radiation field size is defined. The radiation field size dimensions refer to the distance perpendicular to the beam's direction of incidence that corresponds to the 50% isodose at the beam's edge. It is defined at the skin surface for SSD treatments, and at the SAD for isocentric treatments.

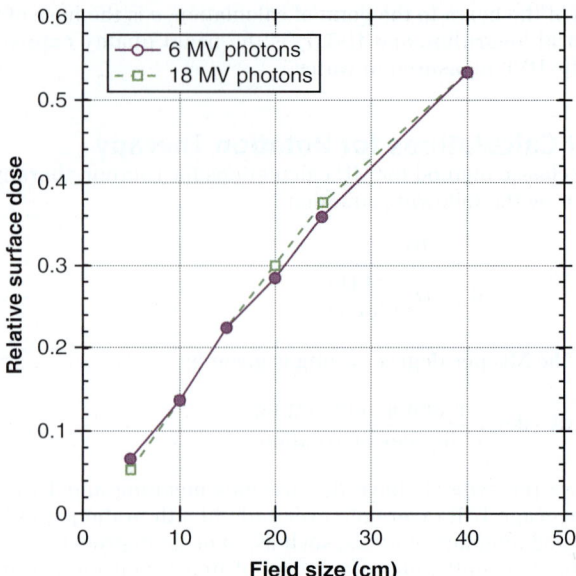

FIGURE 7.4. Relative surface dose versus field size with blocking tray in place for 6- and 18-MV photons. (Reprinted from Klein EE, Purdy JA. Entrance and exit dose regions for Clinac-2100 C. *Int J Radiat Oncol Biol Phys* 1993;27[2]:429–435. Copyright © 1993 Elsevier. With permission.)

Depth-Dose Buildup Region

When a photon beam strikes the tissue surface, electrons are set in motion, causing the dose to increase with depth until the maximum dose is achieved at depth d_{max}. As the energy of the photon beam increases, the thickness of the buildup region is increased. The subcutaneous tissue-sparing effects of higher-energy x-rays, combined with their great penetrability, make them well suited for treating deep lesions. In general, the dose to the surface and in the buildup region for megavoltage photon beams generally increases with increasing field size and with the insertion of blocking trays made of plastic or other type of material in the beam (Fig. 7.4). The blocking trays should be at least 20 cm above the skin surface because skin doses are significantly increased for lesser distances. Copper, lead, or lead glass filters beneath the blocking tray can be used to remove the undesired lower-energy electrons that contribute to skin dose, but this is nowadays rarely done routinely in the clinic.[55,56]

As the angle of the incident radiation beam becomes more oblique, the surface dose increases, and d_{max} moves toward the surface (Fig. 7.5). This is primarily due to more secondary electrons' contribution from the media below the surface along the oblique path of the beam.[57]

FIGURE 7.5. The variation of surface dose and depth of maximum dose as a function of the angle of incidence of the x-ray beam with the surface (4 MV, 10 × 10 cm).

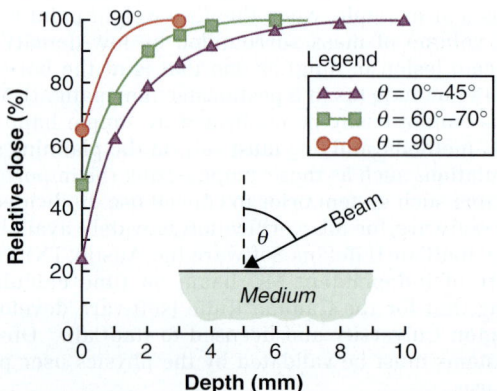

Depth-Dose/Exit Dose Region

The skin and superficial tissue on the side of the patient from which the beam exits receive a reduced dose if there is insufficient backscatter material present. The amount of dose reduction is a function of x-ray beam energy, field size, and the thickness of tissue that the beam has penetrated reaching the exit surface. For a 6-MV beam, a 15% reduction in dose with little dependency on field size has been reported,[55] and for 18-MV beams, an 11% reduction in exit dose was measured.[58] In general, the addition of a thickness of tissue-equivalent material on the exit side equivalent in thickness to approximately two-thirds of the d_{max} depth is sufficient to provide full dose to the build-down region on the exit side. Figure 7.6 shows the effects of various backscattering media when placed directly behind the exit surface.

FIGURE 7.6. Enhancement of exit dose for **(A)** 6-MV and **(B)** 18-MV photons for a 15 × 15 cm field at 100-cm source-to-axis distance versus backscatter depth for various backscattering materials. (Reprinted from Klein EE, Purdy JA. Entrance and exit dose regions for Clinac-2100 C. *Int J Radiat Oncol Biol Phys* 1993;27[2]:429–435. Copyright © 1993 Elsevier. With permission.)

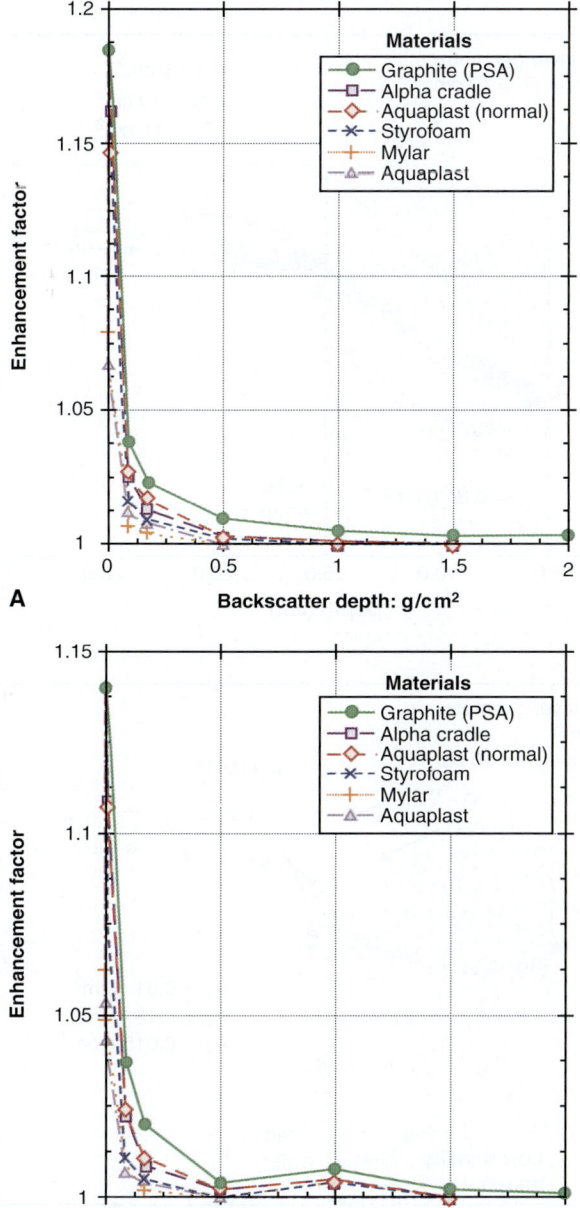

Tissue Heterogeneities and Tissue Interface Dosimetry

The presence of tissue heterogeneities, such as air cavities, lungs, bony structures, and prostheses, can greatly impact the calculated dose distribution. The change in dose is due to the perturbation of the transport of primary and scattered photons and that of the secondary electrons set in motion from photon interactions. Depending on the energy of the photon beam and the shape, size, and constituents of the inhomogeneities, the resultant change in dose can be large.

Perturbation of photon transport is more noticeable for lower-energy beams. There is usually an increase in transmission, and therefore dose, when the beam traverses a low-density inhomogeneity. The reverse applies when the inhomogeneity has a density higher than that of water. However, the change in dose is complicated by the concomitant decrease or increase in the scatter dose. For a modest lung thickness of 10 cm, there will be about a 15% increase in the dose to the lung for a ^{60}Co or 6-MV x-ray beam, but only about 5% for an 18-MV x-ray beam.[59]

When there is a net imbalance of electrons leaving and entering the region near an inhomogeneity (interfaces of different media), the condition of electron equilibrium is disrupted. The dose distribution in the patient in such transition zones depends on radiation field size (scatter influence), distance between interfaces (e.g., air cavities), differences between physical densities and atomic number of the interfacing media, and the size and shape of the different media. Because electrons have finite travel, the resultant change in dose is usually local to the vicinity of the inhomogeneity but may be quite large. The effects are more noticeable for the higher photon energy beams because of the increased energy and range of the scattered electrons. Near the edge of the lungs and air cavities, the reduction in dose can be larger than 15%.[60]

For inhomogeneities with density larger than water, there will be an increase in dose locally due to the generation of more electrons. However, most dense inhomogeneities have atomic numbers higher than that of water so that the resultant dose perturbation is further compounded by the perturbation of the multiple Coulomb scattering of the electrons. Near the interface between a bony structure and water-like tissue, large hot and cold dose spots can be present. Several benchmark measurements have been reported for various geometries simulating clinical situations and are discussed briefly in the following sections.

Air Cavities

Air cavities that appear in various locations of the body, most particularly in the head and neck region, pose a problem because of loss of equilibrium at the air–tissue boundaries internal to the patient. Epp et al.[61] reported that for cobalt beams, a reduction in dose of approximately 12% was found for a typical larynx air cavity, which recovered within 5 mm in the new buildup region. The loss was due to a lack of forward scattered electrons. Epp et al.[62] reported that for a 10-MV x-ray beam, a 14.5% loss was measured at the distal interface of the air cavity with a buildup curve that plateaued within 20 mm of the interface. Klein et al.[63] measured distributions about air cavities for 4-MV and 15-MV x-ray beams in both the distal and proximal regions. The combined dose distribution in a parallel-opposed fashion showed a 10% loss at the interfaces for both beam energies.

Lung Tissue

Although the problem of reestablishing equilibrium for lung interfaces is not as severe as with air cavities, a transition zone region at the lung–tissue interface still exists over the range of typical clinical photon beam energies. Rice et al. measured responses within various simulated lung media for 4- and 15-MV x-rays using a parallel-plate ion chamber and a phantom constructed of solid water and simulated lung material (average lung material density, $\rho = 0.31$ g/cm^3; some additional measurements made with materials having densities of 0.015 and 0.18 g/cm^3).[64] Figure 7.7 shows the results in terms of measured CFs for the 15-MV beam. A considerable buildup curve was observed (10% change in CF) for small fields (5 × 5 cm^2) for the 15-MV beam, which began in the distal region of the lung and plateaued about 5 cm beyond the simulated lung interface.

Bone–Soft Tissue Interfaces

Das et al.[65] measured dose perturbation factors (DPFs) proximal and distal for simulated bone–tissue interface regions using a parallel-plate chamber for both 6- and 24-MV x-ray beams. They reported DPFs of 1.1 for the 6-MV beam and 1.07 for the 24-MV beam at the proximal interface. At the distal interface, a DPF of 1.07 was measured for the 24-MV

beam, whereas the 6-MV beam exhibited a DPF of 0.95, resulting in a new buildup region in soft tissue. Note that both buildup and build-down regions dissipate within a few millimeters from the interfaces and the perturbations are independent of thickness and lateral extent of the bone or radiation field size.

Metal Prostheses

Das and associates measured DPFs following a 10.5-mm-thick stainless steel layer simulating a hip prosthesis geometry.[65] They reported a DPF of 1.19 for 24-MV photons, but only 1.03 for 6-MV photons; on the proximal side, they reported a DPF of 1.30 due to the backscattered electrons that was independent of energy, field size, or lateral extent of the steel. These interface effects dissipated within a few millimeters in polystyrene. Other reports dealing with dosimetry perturbations due to metal objects are included in the references.[66,67]

Niroomand-Rad et al. reported on dose perturbation effects at the tissue–titanium alloy implant interfaces in patients with

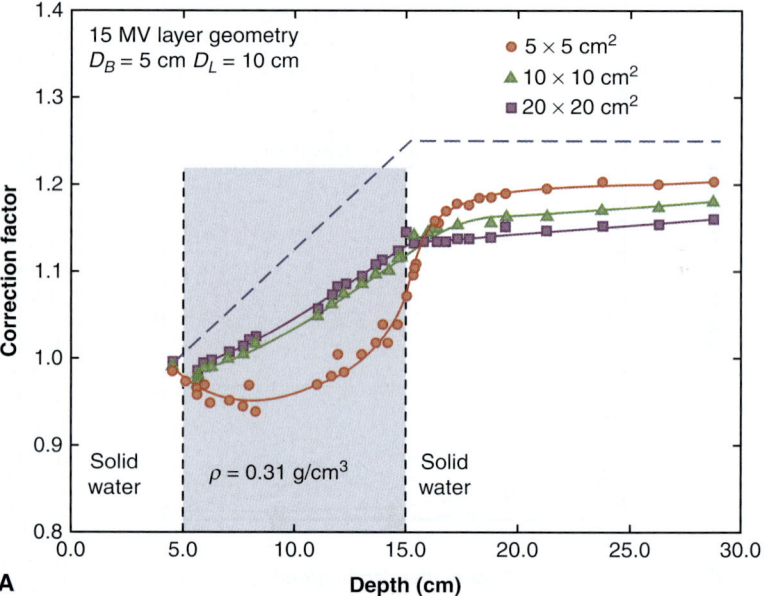

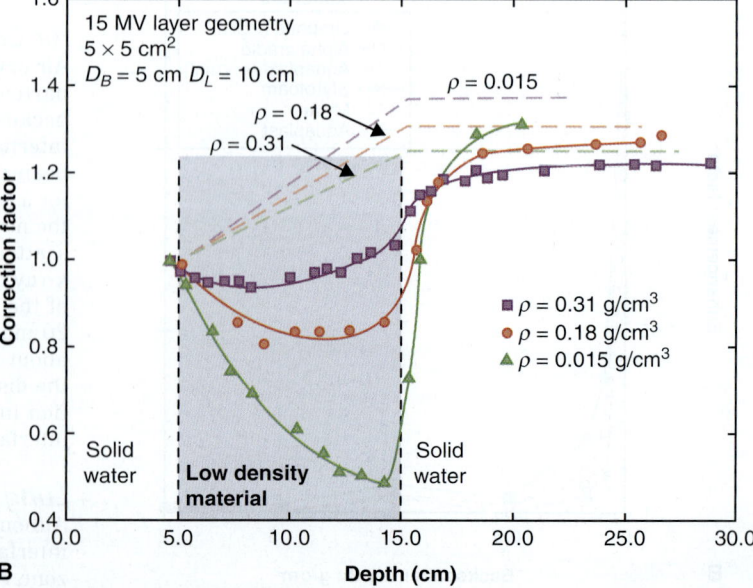

FIGURE 7.7. A: Dose correction factors as a function of depth for a transition zone geometry that simulates a lung–tissue interface for three different field sizes and a lung thickness of 10 cm for 15-MV x-rays. The modification to the primary dose only on the central axis (shown by the *dashed curve*) is independent of field size. **B:** Dose correction factors as a function of depth for a transition zone geometry that simulates a lung–tissue interface for three different densities, a 5- × 5-cm field and a lung thickness of 10 cm for 15-MV x-rays. The modification to the primary dose only on the central axis is shown by the *dashed curve*. (Reprinted from Rice RK, Mijnheer BJ, Chin LM. Benchmark measurements for lung dose corrections for x-ray beams. *Int J Radiat Oncol Biol Phys* 1988;15[2]:399–409. Copyright © 1988 Elsevier. With permission.)

head and neck cancer treated with 6- and 10-MV photon beams.[68] They found at the upper surface (toward the source) of the tissue–dental implant interface DPFs of 1.22 and 1.20 for the 6- and 10-MV photon beams, respectively. At the lower interface, dose reduction was approximately −13.5% and −9.5% for the 6- and 10-MV beams, respectively.

The most complete information currently available on hip prosthesis dosimetry is found in AAPM Report 81 (TG 63).[69] The report provides the current state of scientific understanding and clinical dosimetry in use for patients with high-Z hip prostheses undergoing radiation therapy. Beam arrangements that avoid the prosthesis should always be a first consideration. If this cannot be done, valuable information is available in Report 81, including values for different prostheses' electron density, approximate attenuation of the beam passing through the prosthesis, and possible dose increase to the hip bone. It should also be noted that some of the data provided and recommendations are also applicable to patients having other implanted high-Z prosthetic devices such as pins and humeral head replacements.

Silicone–Soft Tissue Interfaces

Klein and Kuske reported on interface perturbations with silicone breast prostheses.[70] Such prostheses have a density similar to breast tissue but have a different atomic number. They observed a 6% enhancement at the proximal interface and a 9% loss at the distal interface.

Wedge Filter Dosimetry

When a wedge filter is inserted into the beam, the dose distribution is angled at some specified depth to some desired angle relative to the incident beam direction over the entire transverse dimension of the radiation beam (Fig. 7.8). For cobalt units, the depth of the 50% isodose usually is selected for specification of the wedge angle, whereas for high-energy linacs, higher-percentile isodose curves, such as the 80% curve, or the isodose curves at a specific depth (10 cm) are used to define the wedge angle.

Linacs are typically equipped with multiple wedges that may be used with an allowed range of field sizes. Although linac wedges can be designed for any desired *wedge angle*, 15-, 30-, 45-, and 60-degree wedges are the most common.

Some linacs (Elekta AB, Sweden) feature a single wedge, referred to as a *universal wedge*, located in the treatment head, and the desired wedged dose distribution is obtained by the proper combination of wedged and unwedged

treatment. A simple approximate model for combining open and wedged fields was first proposed by Tatcher,[71] in which the effective wedge angle θ_E, resulting by the addition of a wedged and unwedged beam, is equal to the nominal wedge angle θ_W for the wedged beam, weighted by the fraction of wedged field B:

$$B = \theta_E / \theta_W$$

The Philips Medical Systems Division[72] proposed a slightly different method as follows:

$$B = \tan(\theta_E) / \tan(\theta_W)$$

Petti and Siddon[73] investigated both methods and showed that these are approximations to an exact theoretical solution, which is given by

$$B = f / ([\tan(\theta_W) / \tan(\theta_E)] + f - 1)$$

Most importantly, their investigations showed that Tatcher's approximation is good only for values of $\theta_W < 45$ degrees and thus is inadequate for accelerators such as Elekta, which use a 60-degree motorized universal wedge. They did show that for the field sizes studied (up to 20 × 20 cm), the Philips relationship was valid to within 3 degrees.

The wedged isodose curves can be normalized in two different ways. In some older systems, the wedge dose distributions have the wedge factor (i.e., the ratio of the measured central-axis dose rate with and without the wedge in place) incorporated into the wedged isodose distribution. More commonly, the wedge isodose curves are normalized to 100% at d_{max}, and a separate *wedge factor* is used to calculate the actual treatment MUs or time. McCullough et al.[74] noted that wedge factors measured at d_{max} usually are accurate to within 2% for depths up to 10 cm but, at greater depths, can be inaccurate to 5% or more. The inclusion (or noninclusion) of the wedge factor is an extremely important point to understand because serious error in dose delivered to the patient can occur if used improperly.

Sewchand et al.[75] and Abrath and Purdy[76] pointed out that beam hardening results when a wedge is inserted into the radiation beam. The PDD, therefore, can be considerably increased at depth. Differences reported were nearly 7% for a 4-MV 60-degree wedge field PDD from the open field PDDs at 12-cm depth, and a 3% difference in depth-dose values between the wedge field and the open field for a 60-degree wedge using 25-MV x-rays was reported.

Modern computer-controlled medical linacs now have software features that allow the user to create a wedge-shaped dose distribution by moving one collimator jaw across the field in conjunction with adjustment of the dose rate over the course of the daily single-field treatment.[77] This technology provides superior dose distributions and eliminates the previously mentioned beam-hardening problem seen in physical wedges. This feature can deliver a greater number of wedge angles, and over larger field sizes, including asymmetric field sizes (30 cm in the wedge direction, with 20 cm toward the wedge "heel" and 10 cm toward the wedge "toe"). The increased number of angles enhances planning options but also complicates commissioning and QA.[78]

When the patient's treatment is planned, wedged fields are commonly arranged such that the angle between the beams, the *hinge angle* (θ), is related to the wedge angle (φ) by the following relationship (Fig. 7.9):

$$\theta = 90 \text{ degrees} - \phi / 2$$

For example, as shown in Figure 7.10, 45-degree wedge fields orthogonal to one another yield a uniform dose distribution.

FIGURE 7.8. Isodose distributions for a 6-MV x-ray beam with an 8- × 8-cm field size. **A:** Open field. **B:** Field with a 45-degree wedge. (From Khan FM. *The physics of radiation therapy.* 2nd ed. Baltimore: Williams & Wilkins; 1994. With permission.)

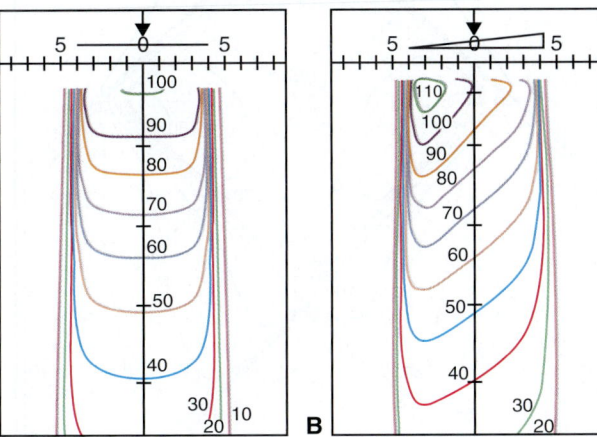

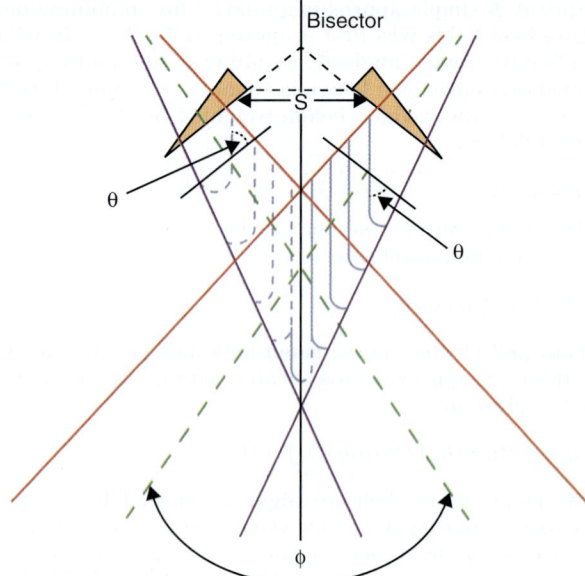

FIGURE 7.9. Parameters of the wedge beams: ϕ is the wedge angle, θ is the hinge angle, and S is separation. Isodose curves for each wedge field are parallel to the bisector. (From Khan FM. *The physics of radiation therapy*. 2nd ed. Baltimore: Williams & Wilkins; 1994. With permission.)

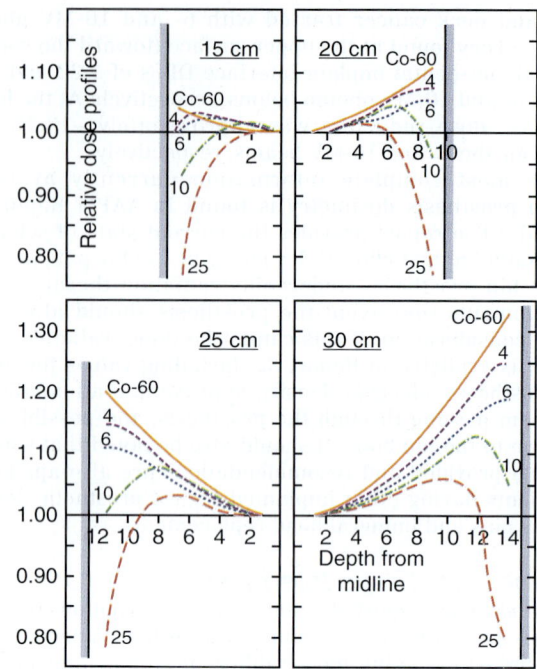

FIGURE 7.11. Relative central-axis dose profiles as a function of x-ray energy (^{60}Co or 4, 6, 10, and 25 MV) and patient thickness (15, 20, 25, and 30 cm). The parallel-opposed beams are equally weighted, and the profiles are normalized to unity at midline. Because of symmetry, only half of each profile is shown.

TREATMENT PLANNING: COMBINATION OF TREATMENT FIELDS

Parallel-Opposed Fields

When only two unmodified x-ray beams are used in radiation therapy, they usually are parallel-opposed beams (i.e., directed toward each other from opposite sides of the anatomic site with the central axes coinciding). Figure 7.11 presents the normalized relative axis dose profiles from parallel-opposed photon beams for a 10- × 10-cm field at an SSD of 100 cm and for patient diameters of 15 to 30 cm in 5-cm increments. The weight of a beam denotes a numeric value assigned to the beam at some normalization point. For SSD beams, the weight specifies the relative dose assigned to the beam at d_{max}, and for isocentric beams, at isocenter. The

beams shown are weighted 1 to 1 (i.e., assigned equal value 100% at d_{max}), and the dose profiles have been normalized to the cumulative midline PDD.

The maximum patient diameter easily treated with parallel-opposed beams for a midplane tumor requiring 50 Gy or less with low-energy megavoltage beams is approximately 18 cm. For "thicker" patients, higher x-ray energies produce improved dose profiles with less dose variation along the central axis without resorting to more complex multibeam arrangements.

For some treatment sites, the underdosing achieved near the skin surface with very–high-energy, parallel-opposed

FIGURE 7.10. Isodose distribution for two angled beams. **A:** Without wedges. **B:** With wedges. Both: 4 MV; field size, 10 × 10 cm; source-to-skin distance, 100 cm; wedge angle, 45 degrees. (From Khan FM. *The physics of radiation therapy*. 2nd ed. Baltimore: Williams & Wilkins; 1994. With permission.)

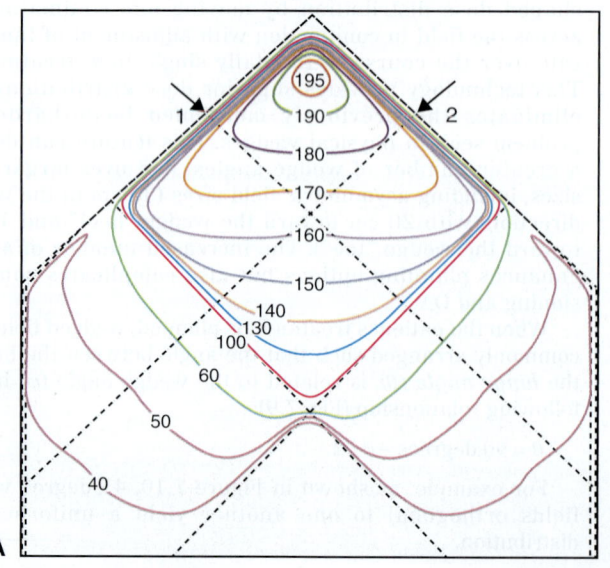

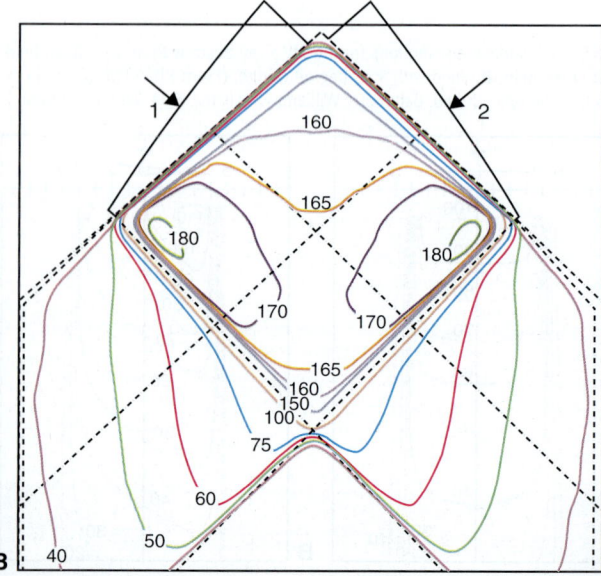

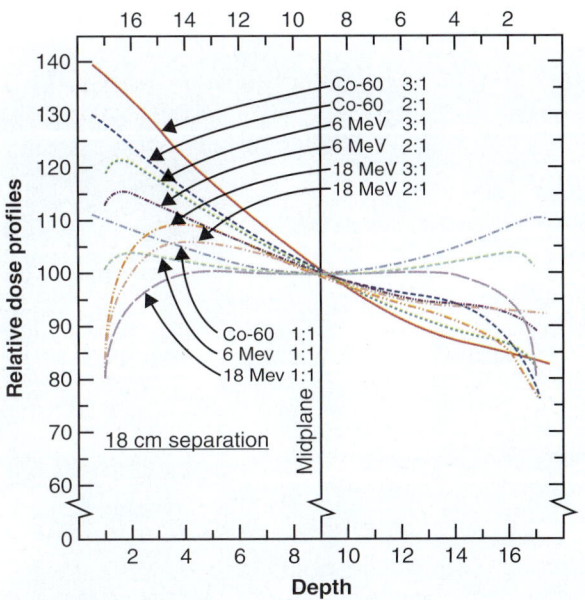

FIGURE 7.12. Dose profiles achieved with unequal weightings of parallel-opposed photon beams; profiles are normalized to unity at midline.

x-ray beams is a highly advantageous feature; but in others, it may be desirable to achieve a higher dose nearer to the skin. With very–high-energy x-ray beams traversing small anatomic thicknesses, the exit dose can exceed the entry dose, and the exact dose distribution in the regions beneath the entry and exit surfaces from parallel-opposed high-energy x-ray beams must be carefully evaluated to consider properly the contribution from both entrance and exit components.

Unequal beam weightings are advantageous if the target volume is not midline. Figure 7.12 shows normalized central-axis dose profiles for other weightings, such as 2 to 1 and 3 to 1. The greater the unequal weighting, the greater will be the shift of the higher-dose region toward one surface and away from midline. Although in some anatomic sites unequal

weighting may be advantageous, special attention must be directed to the anatomic structures in the high-dose volume.

Multiple-Beam Arrangements

Figure 7.13 shows three commonly used coaxial three-field beam arrangements. A direct anterior field with two anterior oblique fields can be used to generate a high-dose region where the three fields overlap, whereas a low-dose region exists beyond this intersection point. For example, if this arrangement is used for treating the mediastinum, the spinal cord might be included in the anterior beam but spared by the anterior oblique beams. Moving the anterior oblique fields laterally to form a parallel-opposed pair yields a rectangular isodose region with a more uniform dose gradient; however, the magnitude of the dose gradient is determined by the relative weighting of the beams and the thickness of tissue traversed. An anterior field with two symmetrically placed posterior oblique beams yields elongated isodose curves. The degree of elongation is determined by the relative thickness of tissue each beam traverses to the point of intersection and by the relative weights of the beams. Three-field arrangements are often useful for treating tumors lateral to the midline of a patient.

Three-field nonaxial (noncoplanar) arrangements are readily achieved with linacs by rotating the table and gantry. A common technique for treating pituitary tumors uses two lateral fields and a vertex field with the beam entering through the top of the head. Astrocytomas often are treated with parallel-opposed lateral fields and a frontal field entering through the forehead. A 90-degree couch rotation is used with the gantry rotated laterally for the vertex or frontal fields. The lateral fields are also rotated by collimator to ensure the "heels" of the wedges are in the plane of the vertex/frontal field trajectory.

Four-field techniques typically are used in such sites as the abdomen or the pelvis. In most instances, the arrangements consist of pairs of parallel-opposed fields, with a common intersecting point, which yield a "boxlike" isodose distribution. Figure 7.14 compares the dose distributions achieved with a four-field "box technique" for 6- and 18-MV x-ray beams. The

FIGURE 7.13. Three-field coaxial beam arrangements: dose distribution for two different beam arrangements using 6-MV x-ray beams, 8- × 10-cm field size, 100-cm source-to-skin distance. Isodose curves have been renormalized to show the 100% line almost encompassing the target volume. **A:** Anterior field with two anterior oblique fields at 40 degrees off the midline, all equally weighted. **B:** Anterior field with a weight of 0.8 with two equally weighted (1) posterior oblique fields separated by 120 degrees.

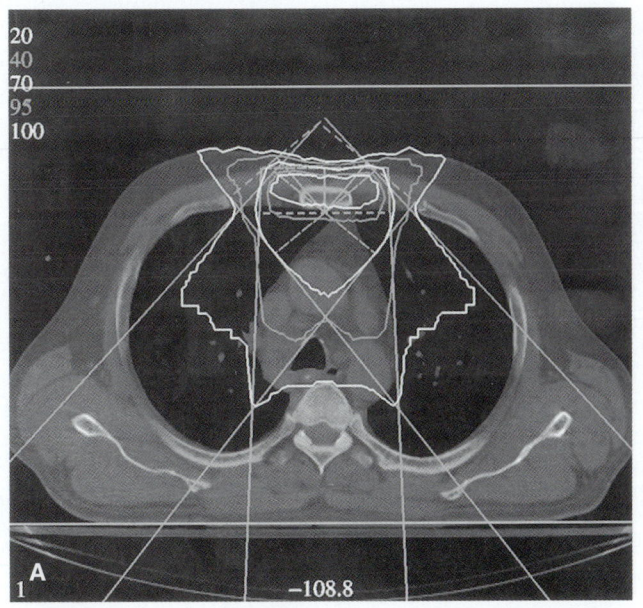

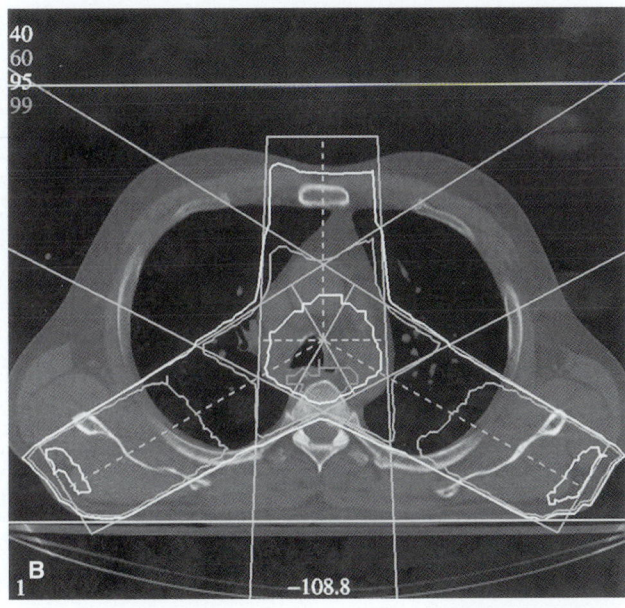

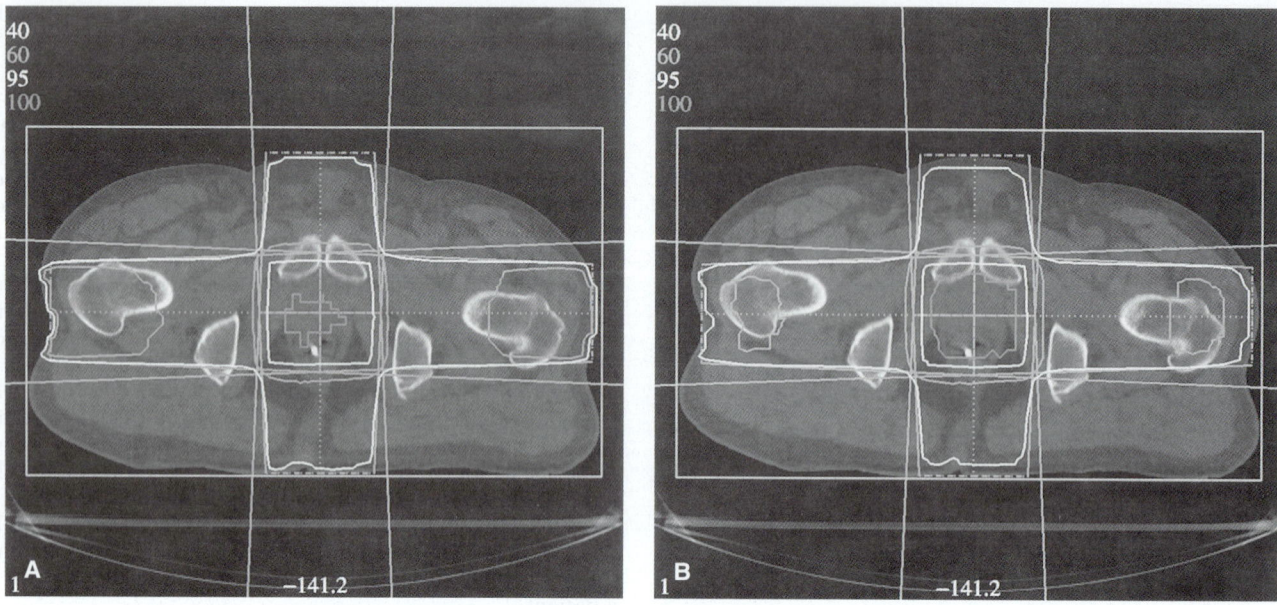

FIGURE 7.14. Four-field "box technique" coaxial beam arrangements (equal beam weightings). **A:** 6-MV x-ray beams. **B:** 18-MV x-ray beams. Note the improved dose distribution with the higher-energy beam technique (more uniform dose in the target region and lower doses near the femoral head region of the lateral fields) as a result of the increased percentage depth for 18-MV x-rays.

central dose distribution is similar for all beam energies, but the greater penetrability of the higher-energy beams yields a lower dose to the region outside the box. Variations in the dose gradient are achieved by differential weighting of each pair of beams. Figure 7.15 shows other possible four-beam arrangements. Angulation of the beams yields a diamond-shaped dose distribution. A butterfly-shaped distribution is achieved if each pair of beams has a point of intersection lying on a common line but separated by a few centimeters.

Treatments involving more than four gantry angles, historically required with orthovoltage x-ray units to treat deep, midline lesions, were originally rarely used with high-energy megavoltage therapy units. However, with the broad introduction of *three-dimensional conformal radiation therapy*

(3DCRT) and *IMRT*, there has been an increase in multibeam treatments such as the 3DCRT six-field technique commonly used for the treatment of prostate carcinoma[79] and the nine-field technique commonly used for head and neck cancer IMRT treatments.[80] More recently, these multibeam arrangements are further refined by adding segments of field with the same beam angle either to improve dose homogeneity or to intentionally generate an inhomogeneous dose distribution (e.g., the simultaneous integrated boost technique).[81]

Rotation Therapy

Rotational (or *arc*) *therapy* techniques, in which the treatment is delivered while the gantry (and thus the radiation beam) rotates around the patient, can be thought of as an infinite

FIGURE 7.15. Four-field "oblique technique" coaxial beam arrangements (6-MV x-rays, equal beam weightings). **A:** With common isocenter resulting in a diamond-shaped dose distribution. **B:** Each beam pair intersecting at two different points on a common line resulting in a butterfly-shaped isodose distribution.

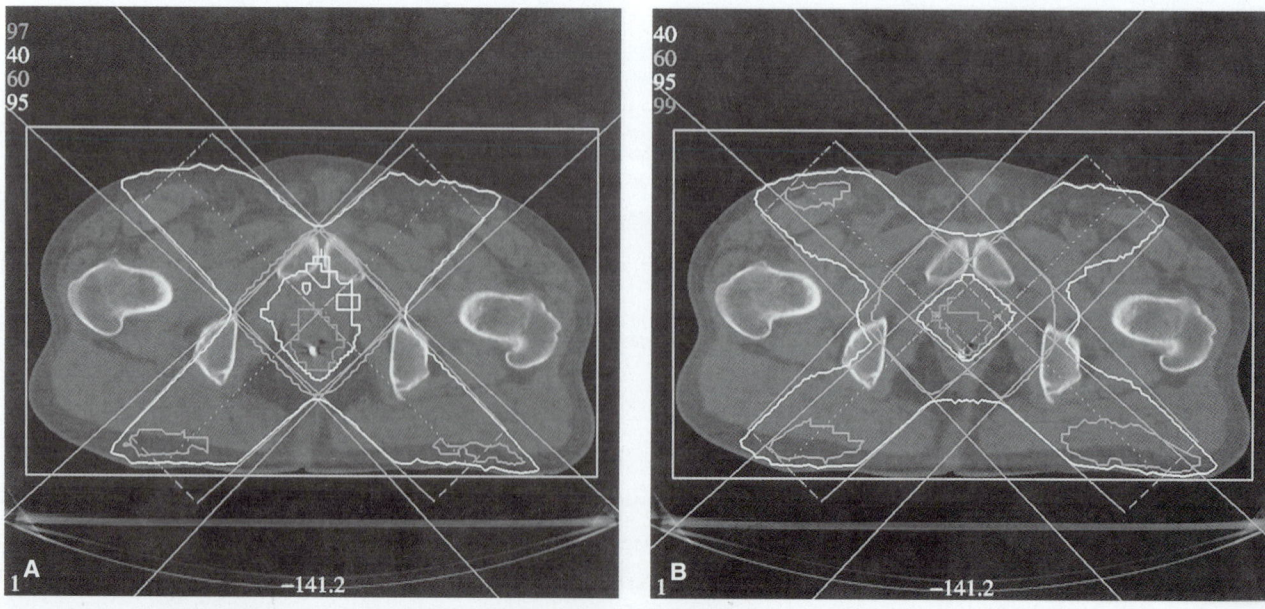

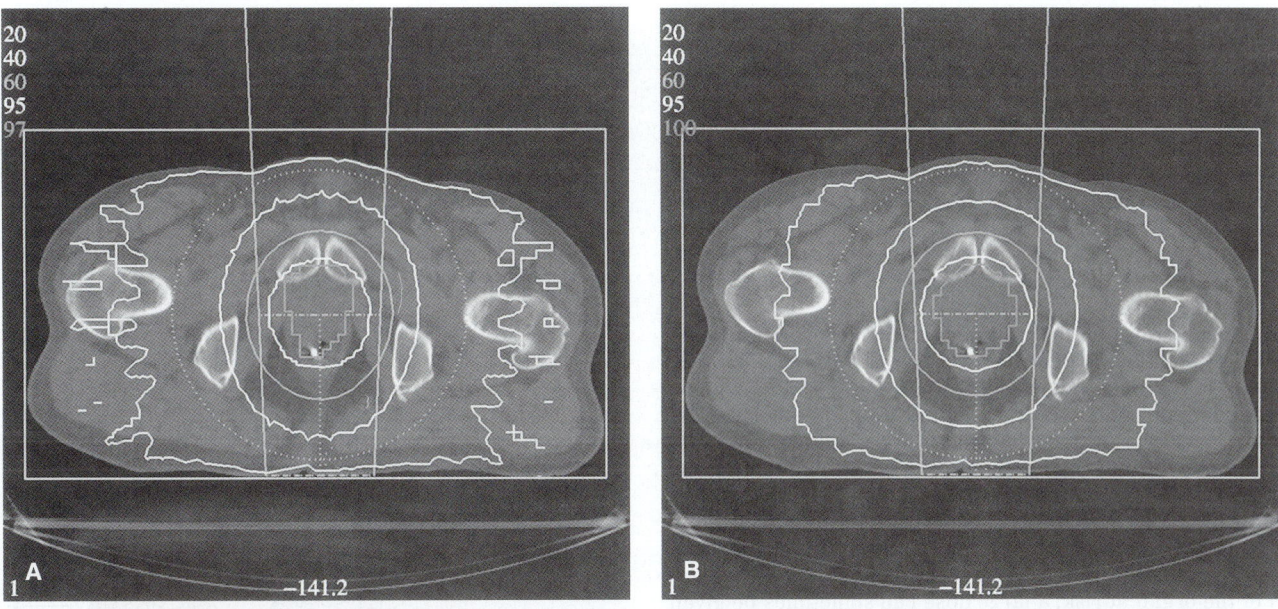

FIGURE 7.16. A 360-degree rotational therapy technique. **A:** 6-MV x-ray beams. **B:** 18-MV x-ray beams. Note that there is little difference in the dose distribution when using a higher-energy beam as a result of the offsetting effects of increased percentage depth versus higher exit dose.

extension of the multiple-field techniques already described. This technique is most useful when applied to small, symmetric, deep-seated tumors and usually is limited to field sizes less than approximately 10 cm in width for the treatment of centrally located lesions (i.e., there is approximately an equal amount of tissue in all directions around the lesion).

Dose distributions generated by rotational techniques are not very sensitive to the energy of the photon beam. Figure 7.16 illustrates this fact, showing the dose distribution achieved using a 6-MV x-ray beam and also the distribution using an 18-MV x-ray beam. There is a little less elongation in the direction of the shorter dimension of the patient's anatomy for the 18-MV beam, and the dose distribution in the periphery is slightly lower.

In arc therapy techniques, one or more sectors of a 360-degree rotation are skipped to reduce the dose to critical normal structures. When a sector is skipped, the high-dose region is shifted away from the skipped region. Therefore, the isocenter must be moved toward the skipped sector; this technique is referred to as *past-pointing*, as illustrated in Figure 7.17.

The prostate, bladder, cervix, and pituitary are clinical sites that have been treated, either initially or for boost doses, with rotational or arc therapy techniques. Although the dose distributions achieved by rotation or arc therapy yield high target-volume doses, these techniques normally result in a greater volume of normal tissue being irradiated (albeit at low doses) than fixed, multiple-field techniques.

FIGURE 7.17. Arc therapy technique for 6-MV x-rays. **A:** 240-degree arc. Note that when a sector of the full 360-degree rotation is skipped, the high-dose isodose curves are shifted away from the skipped sector. **B:** 240-degree arc, but patient positioned so that isocenter is 2 cm lower toward the skipped sector (this technique is called *past-pointing*). Note high-dose isodose curves now encompass the target volume.

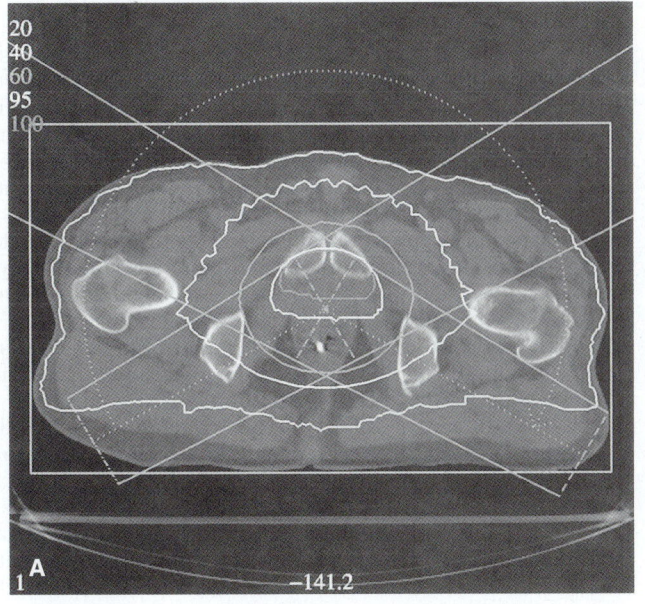
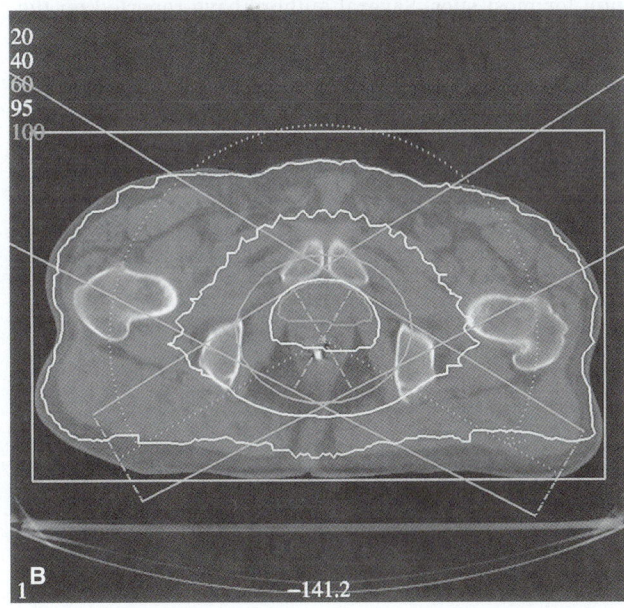

As previously indicated, modern-day rotational therapy is now delivered by a variety of techniques (e.g., TomoTherapy, RapidArc, VMAT). Recent developments also include rotational therapy with *flattening filter free (FFF)* beams.[82] The FFF feature allows dose rates up to 2,400 MUs per minute, thus greatly improving efficiency in dose delivery, which is particularly important for patients receiving treatments where very high daily doses are delivered, such as stereotactic body radiation therapy (SBRT).[83]

FIELD SHAPING

A major constraint in the treatment of cancer using radiation is the limitation in the dose that can be delivered to the tumor because of the dose tolerance of the tissue (critical organs) surrounding or near the target volume. Shielding normal tissue and critical organs has allowed the radiation oncologist to increase the dose to the tumor volume while maintaining the dose to critical organs below some tolerance level. The frequently used tolerance doses for these organs are not absolute and depend on a number of clinical and treatment factors. Depending on the predominantly serial or parallel organization of the organ at risk, a large dose can sometimes be given to fractional volumes of organs with a parallel structure (liver, kidneys, lungs).[84,85] Shielding is usually accomplished using collimator jaws (with the asymmetric feature) and multileaf collimators, in which the beam aperture (field shape) is customized for individual patients. Use of low–melting-point alloy blocks is rapidly being replaced with the MLC technology.

MLC and Associated Dosimetry

Asymmetric Collimator Jaws

Field shaping and abutted field radiation therapy techniques have been made even more versatile with the asymmetric jaw feature found on modern-day linacs. This feature allows each set of jaws to open and close independently of each other (Fig. 7.18). The collimator jaw provides greater attenuation than the MLC leaf or alloy block, thus providing an advantage (which is readily apparent on portal films) in reducing the dose to blocked regions.

Depth-dose characteristics for asymmetric fields are similar to those of symmetric fields as long as the degree of asymmetry is not too extreme. Clinical sites where asymmetric jaws are typically used include breast (Fig. 7.19), head and neck, craniospinal, and prostate. In addition, the use of asymmetric jaws as beam splitters, for field reductions, and with MLCs is helpful for most sites. Several authors have reported on the

FIGURE 7.18. Independent or asymmetric collimators. **A:** Conventional symmetric pairs of collimators. **B:** Asymmetric collimators in which collimator jaws are allowed to move independently of each other.

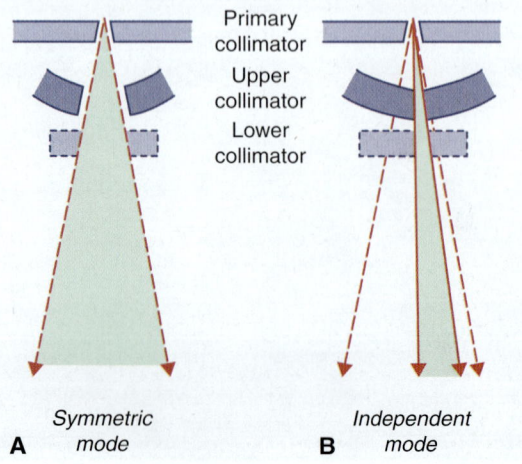

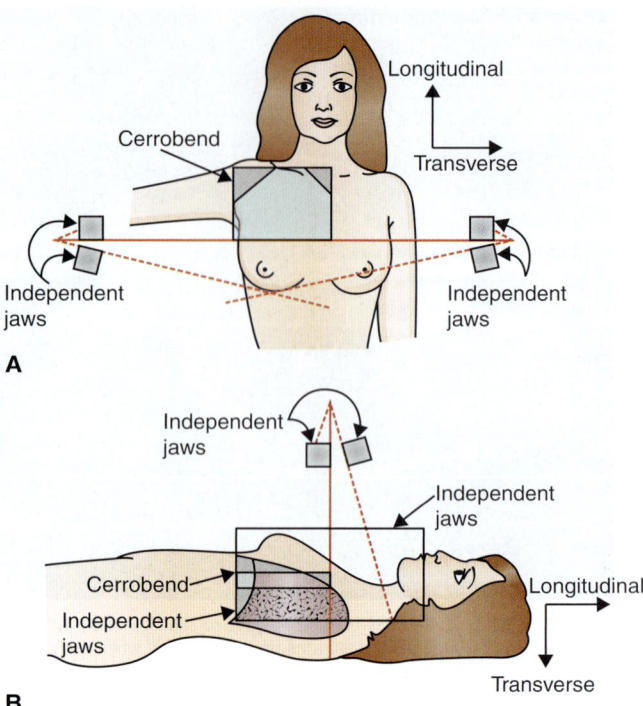

FIGURE 7.19. A and **B:** Treatment technique for breast cancer using independent collimators. (Reprinted from Klein EE, Taylor M, Michaletz-Lorenz M, et al. A mono isocentric technique for breast and regional nodal therapy using dual asymmetric jaws. *Int J Radiat Oncol Biol Phys* 1994;28[3]:753–760. Copyright © 1994 Elsevier. With permission.)

use of asymmetric jaws to match supraclavicular and tangential fields for breast irradiation.[86–88] Such technology allows a single setup point for all of the treatment fields, including the posterior axillary field. The Y-jaws can beam split the caudal and cephalic regions for the supraclavicular and tangential beams, respectively, and the X-jaws are used to shield the ipsilateral lung and contralateral breast. Hence, a common match plane with one common isocenter can be used for all portals, eliminating the need to move the patient between portals, thus reducing overall patient setup time by almost a factor of two. In addition, the increased attenuation by the jaws reduces the dose to the contralateral breast and lung.[89] A technique for matching lateral head and neck fields and the supraclavicular field using asymmetric jaws was described by Sohn et al.[90]

Multileaf Collimation

Multileaf collimation, first introduced in Japan in the 1960s,[91] has now gained widespread acceptance and has replaced alloy blocking as the standard of practice for field shaping in modern radiation therapy clinics. The different manufacturers' MLC systems vary with respect to MLC location, leaf design, and field size coverage. The leaves are typically carried on two opposed carriages that transport the leaves in unison. The leaves have individual controls that are computer assigned and positioned. Initially, most commercial MLC systems were designed to serve as a block replacement but now provide for dynamic IMRT delivery as well.

Elekta first introduced its MLC system in the late 1980s.[92] Their current MLC system replaces the upper photon collimator jaws, and therefore, the maximum field size can open to a full 40 × 40 cm. The MLC system is augmented by parallel diaphragms, which increase the leaf's attenuation by an additional two HVLs.

The Varian MLC system is considered a tertiary system placed below the photon collimator jaws. The latest Varian MLC (non-SRS) is a 120-leaf (60 on each side) system, in which the middle 20 cm consists of 0.5-cm-wide leaves, whereas the outer 20-cm leaves still project to 1.0-cm widths. This set of leaves projects to 16.0 cm in length at isocenter, and the leaf span range (maximum–minimum positions on the same carriage) is limited to 14.5 cm. The leaves move perpendicular to the beam's central axis. The distance from the x-ray target to the bottom of the leaves (on the central axis) is 54.0 cm. The leaves fan away from the central axis so that their sides are divergent with the beam's fan lines. The leaves are interdigitated by a tongue-and-groove design. In May of 2017, Varian introduced the Halcyon machine, which does not have movable jaws and only has a double-layer MLCs with the two layers being offset by half of a leaf width and with each leaf being 1 cm wide. This "stacked and staggered" MLC design aims to provide optimized modulation and reduce interleaf leakage. The Halcyon also support 4 gantry rotations per minute (as opposed to 1 rotation per minute for conventional C shape linear accelerators), and the MLC have 5 cm/s speed to support this faster gantry rotation. The MLCs are also designed to have full overtravel and cover the full span of the field.

For the single-layer Varian MLC system, leaf transmission values of 1.5% to 2.0% for a 6-MV beam and 1.5% to 5% for an 18-MV beam have been reported.[36,93] These values are lower than those found for alloy blocks (3.5%) but higher than those for collimator jaw transmission (that being <1.0%). Transmission through abutted (closed) leaf pairs was as high as 28% for 18-MV photons on the central axis. The abutment transmission decreased as a function of off-axis distance to as low as 12%. The data for the double-layer MLC are not available as of this writing, but the MLC is specifically designed to reduce leaf transmission, and it is expected that this will translate into clinical benefits.

Figure 7.20 shows a comparison of MLCs and alloy blocks regarding penumbra. The discrete steps of the MLC systems introduce undulations in the isodose lines. This effect causes an apparent increase in penumbra with wave patterns after the undulations. Single, focused MLC systems have a slightly larger penumbra than do alloy shields and have an even larger difference in comparison with collimator jaws. Boyer et al. found the penumbra (80% to 20% isodose lines) generated by leaf ends to be wider than those generated by upper collimator jaws by 1.0 to 1.5 mm, and 1.0 to 2.5 mm compared with the lower jaws, depending on energy and field size.[94] Powlis and associates compared multileaf collimation and alloy field shaping and found few differences.[95] LoSasso and Kutcher found similar results and concluded that geometric accuracy is even improved with MLCs.[96] ViewRay recently introduced a

double-layer, doubly focused MLC and the design was reviewed by Li et al.[97] However, as of the writing of this chapter, there are no publications characterizing the performance of this MLC. The recently introduced Varian's MLC is also double layered with specially designed leaf tips to improve some of the above described shortcomings of the conventional MLCs.

The penumbras measured for the leaf sides are comparable with those found for upper jaws because of their divergent nature. The penumbra increase and stair-stepping effect are most prominent at d_{max}. The effects diminish at depth because of the influence of scattered electrons and photons as the scatter-to-primary ratio increases with depth. Adding an opposed beam leads to further smoothing of the undulations and penumbra differences become less significant. For multibeam arrangements, the differences in dose distribution between MLC and alloy shields are negligible.

The main limitation in optimizing the MLC leaf settings to conform to the shaped field is the discrete leaf steps. Most field shapes require only minor adjustment of collimator angle to achieve minimal discrepancy between the desired and resultant field shape. The criteria for optimizing the MLC leaf settings are governed by placing the most leaf ends tangent to the field and also maintaining the same internal area as originally prescribed. MLC shaping systems typically provide an option to place the leaf ends entirely outside the field (exterior), entirely within the field (interior), or crossing the field at midleaf (leaf-center insertion). The last is the most widely used criterion because the desired field area is more closely maintained. However, this choice leads to regions in which some treatment areas are shielded and some normal tissues are irradiated. Zhu et al. reported on a variable insertion technique in which leaves are placed only far enough into the field to cause the 50% isodose contour to undulate outside and up to the desired contour.[98] LoSasso et al. reported on a method in which each leaf is inserted such that the treatment area covered by the leaf equals the normal tissue area that is not spared.[99] Brahme also demonstrated optimal choices for choosing a collimator angle to optimize leaf direction, depending on whether the field shape is convex or concave.[100] Du et al. reported on a method that defines optimal leaf positioning in combination with optimal collimator angulation.[101] Typically, the optimal direction for the leaf motion is along the narrower axis. For a simple ellipse, the optimal leaf direction is parallel to the short axis. Reports on the effects of tissue heterogeneities on penumbra and resultant field definition indicate that the penumbra in lung increases (especially for 18-MV photons), whereas in bone, it decreases for both alloy blocks and MLCs.[36]

As indicated previously, because MLC systems are still evolving, a careful evaluation of the effect of MLCs on MU calculations must be performed before clinical use. Extensive testing over the clinical range of field sizes and shapes should be undertaken before the MLC system is used clinically.

Low-Melting Alloy Blocks

Although alloy blocks are rapidly disappearing from clinical use, a short section is included in this chapter for completeness. The Lipowitz metal (Cerrobend) shielding block system was introduced by Powers et al.[102] Lipowitz metal consists of 13.3% tin, 50% bismuth, 26.7% lead, and 10% cadmium. The physical density at 20°C is 9.4 g/cm³, compared with 11.3 g/cm³ for lead. The block fabrication procedure is illustrated in Figure 7.21, and more details on using this form of field shaping can be found in the review article by Leavitt and Gibbs.[103]

Specific doses to critical organs may be limited by using either a full-thickness block, usually five HVLs (3.125% transmission) or six HVLs (1.562% transmission), or a partial transmission shield, such as a single HVL (50% transmission) of shielding material. The actual dose delivered under the shielded area is usually greater than these stated transmission levels because of scatter radiation beneath the blocks

FIGURE 7.20. Comparison of beam's-eye view isodose curves at 10-cm depth for multileaf collimator (*solid line*) and Cerrobend-shaped (*dashed line*) beam apertures for 18-MV photons. (Reprinted from Klein EE, Harms WB, Low DA, et al. Clinical implementation of a commercial multileaf collimator: dosimetry, networking, simulation, and quality assurance. *Int J Radiat Oncol Biol Phys* 1995;33[5]:1195–1208. Copyright © 1995 Elsevier. With permission.)

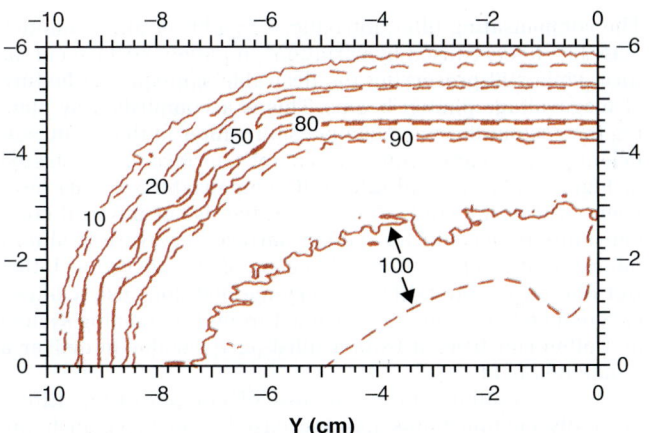

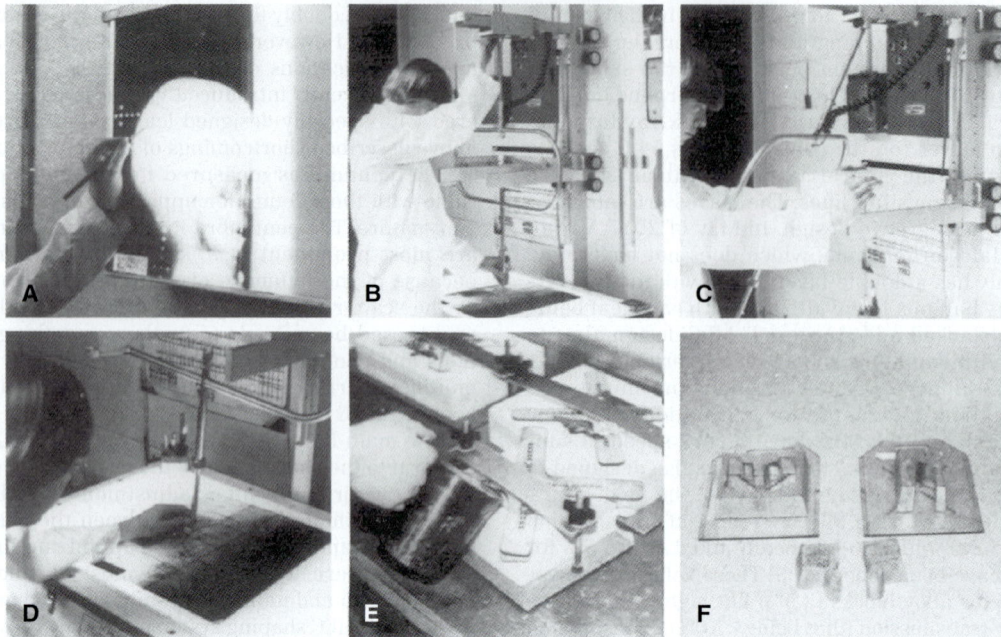

FIGURE 7.21. Composite photographs illustrating the low–melting-point alloy shielding block design and fabrication process. **A:** Physician defining the treatment volume on the x-ray simulator radiograph. **B:** Physics technician adjusting the source-to-skin distance and skin-to-film distance of a hot-wire cutter to emulate simulator geometry. **C:** Proper-thickness foam block aligned to the central axis of the cutter. **D:** Foam mold cut with hot-wire cutter. **E:** Foam pieces aligned and held in place using a special clamping device. Molten alloy is poured into the mold and allowed to harden. **F:** Examples of typical shielding blocks cast using this system. (From Purdy JA. Secondary field shaping. In: Wright AE, Boyer AL, eds. *Advances in radiation therapy treatment planning*. New York: American Institute of Physics, 1983:456–476. Copyright © 1983 by American Association of Physicists in Medicine. Reprinted by permission.)

from adjacent unshielded portions of the field. The scatter component of the dose increases with depth as more radiation scatters into the shielded volume beneath the block. Thus, the dose to the blocked area is a function of block material, thickness (and width), field size, and energy. Figure 7.22 shows the attenuation of Lipowitz metal of x-rays produced at 2, 4, 10,

FIGURE 7.22. Attenuation in Lipowitz metal of x-rays produced at 2, 4, 10, and 18 MV and γ-rays from ^{60}Co. (From Huen A, Findley DO, Skov DD. Attenuation in Lipowitz's metal of x-rays produced at 2, 4, 10, and 18 MV and gamma rays from cobalt-60. *Med Phys* 1979;6[2]:147–148. Copyright © 1979 American Association of Physicists in Medicine. Reprinted by permission of John Wiley & Sons, Inc.)

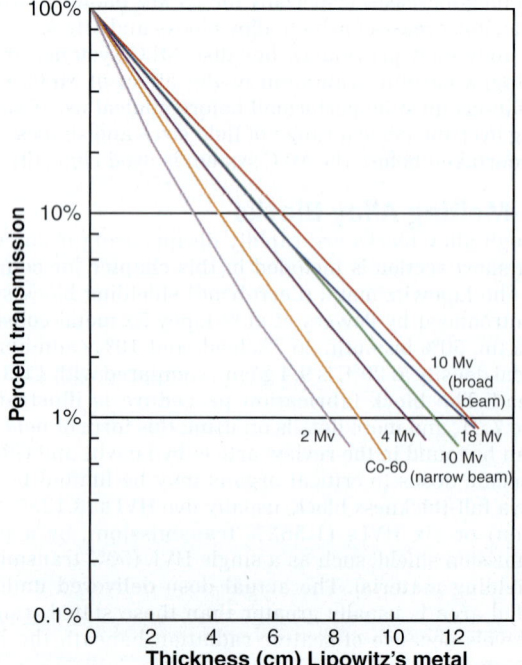

and 18 MeV and ^{60}Co γ-rays.[104] Alloy blocks made from the standard thickness (7.6 cm) of foam molds reduce the primary beam intensity to 5% of its unattenuated value. Increasing the block thickness usually is not worthwhile because it makes the block heavier, whereas the scatter radiation contributes an equal or greater share of the dose under the blocks.

Because of the advent of multileaf collimation, metal blocks for photon beams are rarely used, as multileaf collimation afforded there to be no room for entry between treatment fields. In addition, the construction of blocks was time consuming and expensive. Also, the materials themselves, as they were heated, gave off potentially toxic air, particularly because of the lead and cadmium. The one advantage of blocks is that they provide smooth boundaries by having a continuous shape around the field and incur no field size limitation. However, the weight of the blocks can be excessive, sometimes up to 15 pounds, leading to the potential for injury to therapists and patients should they be mishandled.

COMPENSATING FILTERS

The compensating filter, introduced by Ellis et al.,[105] counteracts the effects caused by variations in patient surface curvature while still preserving the desirable skin-sparing feature of megavoltage photon beams. This is accomplished by placing the custom-designed compensating filter in the beam, sufficiently "upstream" from the patient's surface, as illustrated in Figure 7.23. Several different compensator systems have been used in the clinic.[106] However, the use of physical compensators to account for patient surface curvature is almost nonexistent in clinics today because of the advent of IMRT. But one particular IMRT delivery method does use a physical compensator, which is designed from the planning system and often constructed from a third-party vendor to deliver a modulated field.[107]

One exception where the use of compensating filters or really custom bolus has increased is in electron beam applications.[108] The decimal company (Sanford, FL) offers a

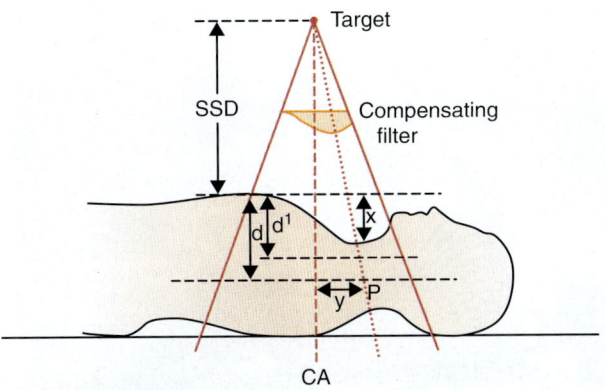

FIGURE 7.23. Schematic illustrating typical geometry used in the design of a compensator filter to account for patient's irregularly shaped surface. SSD, source-to-skin distance; CA, central axis.

product BolusECT, which enables creation of custom three-dimensional bolus to improve conformality of electron beams at depth. These devices offer a simple and relatively inexpensive method to significantly improve electron beam dosimetry. The main shortcoming is the delay involved in ordering and shipping the devices, but overall, this approach appears to be clinically manageable.

BOLUS

Tissue-equivalent material placed directly on the patient's skin surface to reduce the skin sparing of megavoltage photon beams is referred to as *bolus*. A tissue-equivalent bolus should have electron density, physical density, and atomic number similar to those of tissue or water and be pliable so that it conforms to the skin surface contour. Inexpensive, nearly tissue-equivalent materials used as a bolus in radiation therapy include slabs of paraffin wax, rice bags filled with soda, gauze coated with petrolatum, and synthetic-based substances, such as Superflab or Super Stuff.[109]

Thin slabs of bolus that follow the surface contour increase the dose to the skin beneath the bolus with a maximum reduction when the bolus thickness is approximately equal to the d_{max} depth for the photon beam. In addition, adding bolus to fill a tissue deficit may smooth an irregular surface. A bolus also can be shaped to alter the dose distribution as well, but normally, wedges are used to alter the dose distribution for megavoltage photon beams to retain skin sparing.

PATIENT POSITIONING, REGISTRATION, AND IMMOBILIZATION

Ensuring accurate daily positioning of the patient in the treatment position and reduction of patient movement during treatment is essential to deliver the prescribed dose and achieve the planned dose distribution. The reproducibility achievable in the daily positioning of a patient for treatment depends on several factors other than the anatomic site under treatment, including the patient's age, general health, and weight. In general, obese patients and small children are the most difficult to position.

The fields to be treated typically are delineated in the computed tomography (CT) simulation process using either visible skin markings or skin markings visible only under an ultraviolet light. In some instances, external tattoos are applied. These markings are used in positioning a patient on the treatment machine using the machine's field localization light and distance indicator and the laser alignment lights mounted in the treatment room that project transverse, coronal, and sagittal light lines (or dots) on the patient's skin surface.

It is vital that the rigidity of the mask maintain consistency over the course of treatment. In the last 10 years, the normal method of aligning the patient for treatment relied on the marks on a patient before placing a mask on. Therefore, the systems that interface with the immobilization systems and the treatment couch need to also be rigid and registered. As of now, patients are set up to treatment coordinates once they are fit onto the mobilization systems.

Numerous patient restraint and repositioning devices have been designed and used in treating specific anatomic sites. For example, the disposable foam plastic head holder provides stability for the head when the patient is in the supine position. If the patient is treated in the prone position, a face-down stabilizer can be used. This device has a foam rubber lining covered by disposable paper with an opening provided for the patient's eyes, nose, and mouth. It allows comfort and stability as well as air access for the patient during treatment in the prone position.

A vacuum-form body immobilization system is commercially available. This system consists of a vacuum pump and an outer rubber bag filled with plastic minispheres. The rubber bag containing the minispheres is positioned to support the patient's treatment position. A vacuum is then applied, causing the minispheres to come together to form a firm, solid support molded to the patient's shape. The bite block (Fig. 7.24) is another device used as an aid in patient

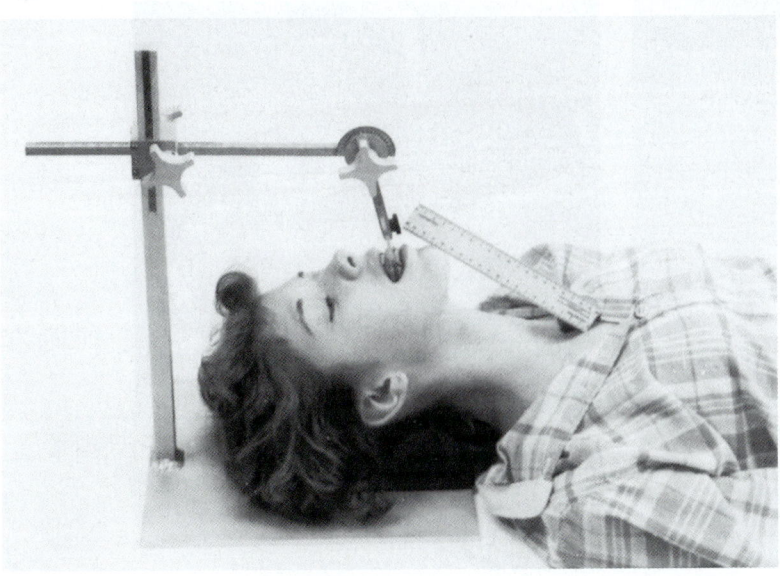

FIGURE 7.24. Example of a bite-block registration and immobilization system used in treatment of head and neck cancer. (Courtesy of Radiation Products Design, Inc.)

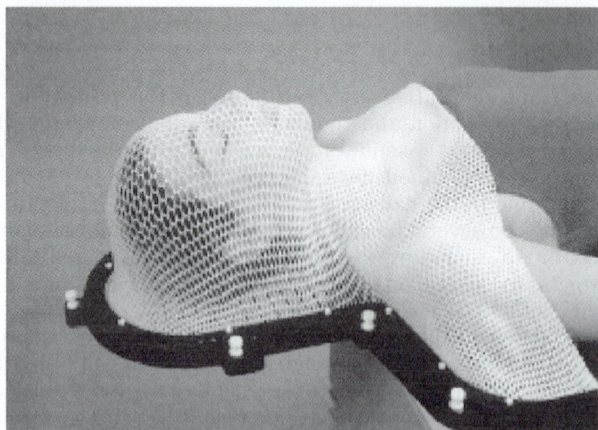
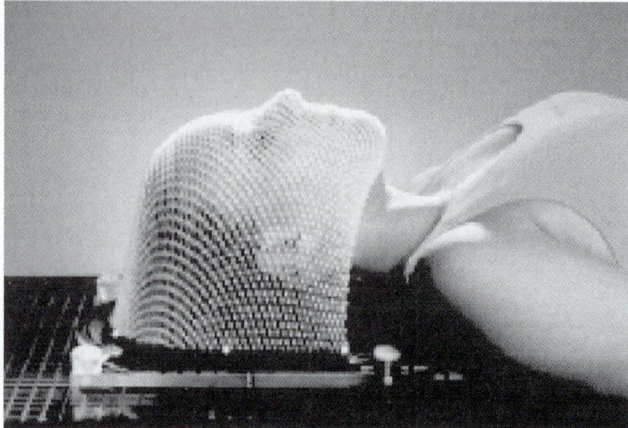

FIGURE 7.25. Example of a registration and immobilization system (thermal plastic mask) used in treatment of head and neck cancer.

repositioning in the treatment of head and neck cancer. With this device, the patient, in the treatment position, bites into a specially prepared dental impression material layered on a fork that is attached to a supporting device. When the material hardens, the impression of the teeth is recorded. The bite-block fork is connected to a support arm, which is attached to the treatment couch, and may be used either with or without scales for registration.

Thermal plastic masks are widely used in the United States (Fig. 7.25). A plastic sheet is placed in warm water or an oven and, once soft, draped over the site. As the plastic sheet cools, it hardens and forms a permanent mask.[110] The use of thermal plastic masks allows treatments with few skin marks made on the patient because most of the reference lines can be placed on the mask. Treatments can be given through the mask; however, there is some minimal loss of skin sparing. When skin sparing is critical, the mask may be cut out to match the treatment portal, although some of the structural rigidity is lost. One of the concerns with use of plastic masks is that they sometimes shrink a bit. This shrinkage can cause changes in patient positioning or can introduce discomfort. A problem with discomfort is that patients often overcorrect their position to avoid pain caused because of poorly fitting immobilization. As a general rule, comfortable patients are easier to reproduce the daily setup and they tend to be less movable during an individual fraction. Therefore, it is important to monitor masks for shrinkage and to follow manufacturer instructions for making masks. These instructions often have procedures designed to minimize shrinkage.

Custom molds constructed from polyurethane formed to patient contours have gained widespread use as aids in immobilization and repositioning (Fig. 7.26). The constituent chemicals for the polyurethane foam are mixed in liquid form and allowed to expand and harden around the patient while the patient is in the treatment position. These molds are used for treatment of Hodgkin disease with the mantle irradiation technique, in patients with cancer of the thorax or prostate, and for extremity repositioning/immobilization. Johnson et al.[111] reported on the effect on surface dose caused by the mold for ^{60}Co, 6- and 18-MV photon beams. Also, when concerned about surface dose effects caused by immobilization devices, one should not neglect understanding the effects also caused by carbon fiber couch inserts.[112]

A bite-block system or a thermal plastic face mask system is commonly used to immobilize patients with head and neck tumors. Patients immobilized with the bite-block system

FIGURE 7.26. Examples of registration and immobilization systems (foam mold) used in treatment of the thorax. **A:** Mold is registered to table and the patient is registered to the mold by fiducial markings. **B:** Mold with cutout area to allow clear access to the treatment area and built-in handgrip.

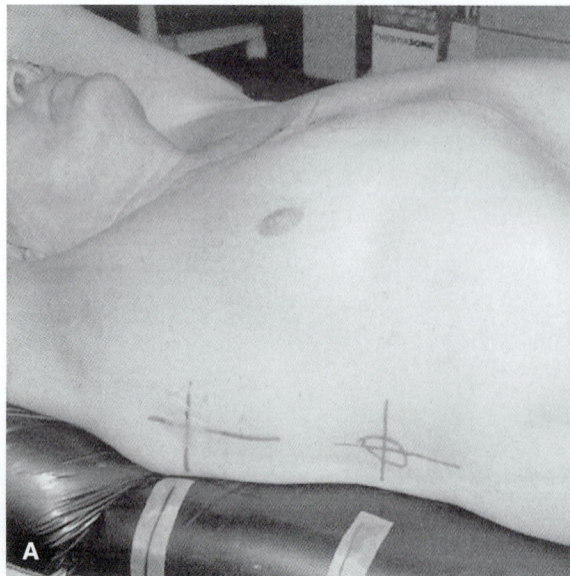
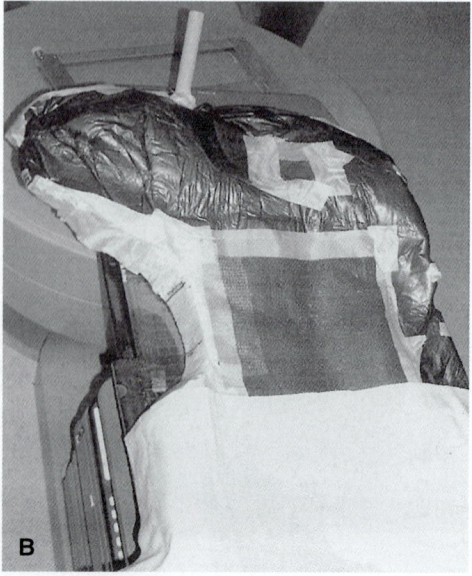

typically require a larger number of adjustments than when more effective systems like the thermal face mask are used. Also, patients may prefer the face mask because most of the reference marks are on the mask rather than on the skin. However, the final assessment of accuracy and reproducibility of the daily treatment is obtained by radiographic imaging of the area treated because there is the possibility of patient movement within the mask, especially if significant tumor shrinkage or weight loss has taken place.

SEPARATION OF ADJACENT X-RAY FIELDS

Field Junctions

Different techniques for matching adjacent fields are illustrated in Figure 7.27. A commonly used gap calculation method for adjacent radiation fields is illustrated in Figure 7.28A. The separation between adjacent field edges necessary to produce junction doses similar to central-axis doses follows from the similar triangles formed by the half-field length and SSD in each field. The field edge is defined by the dose at the edge that is 50% of the dose at $d_{\max}$. For two contiguous fields of lengths L_1 and L_2, the separation, S, of these two fields at the skin surface can be calculated using the following expression:

$$S = \tfrac{1}{2} L_1 \left(\frac{d}{\text{SSD}} \right) + \tfrac{1}{2} L_2 \left(\frac{d}{\text{SSD}} \right)$$

A slight modification of this formula is needed when sloping surfaces are involved, as shown in Figure 7.28B.[113] Typically, the skin gap location is moved a number of times to reduce the hot and cold spots that arise with this technique. Figure 7.29 illustrates the dose distribution for three different field separations.[114]

Beam divergence may be eliminated by using a "beam splitter," created using a five- or six-HVL block over one-half of the treatment field. The central axes of the adjacent fields, where there is no divergence, are then matched. As previously discussed, this is a useful method on linacs with the asymmetric jaws feature. Match-line wedges or penumbra generators that generate a broad penumbra for linac beams have been reported but have not found widespread use.[115] Here, the intent is to broaden the narrow penumbra of the linacs so that it is not so difficult to match the 50% isodose levels. The resulting dose distributions are similar to those obtained with a moving gap technique. Finally, there are several reports of edge-matching techniques based on the mathematical relationships between adjacent beams and the allowed angles of the gantry, collimators, and couch.[116]

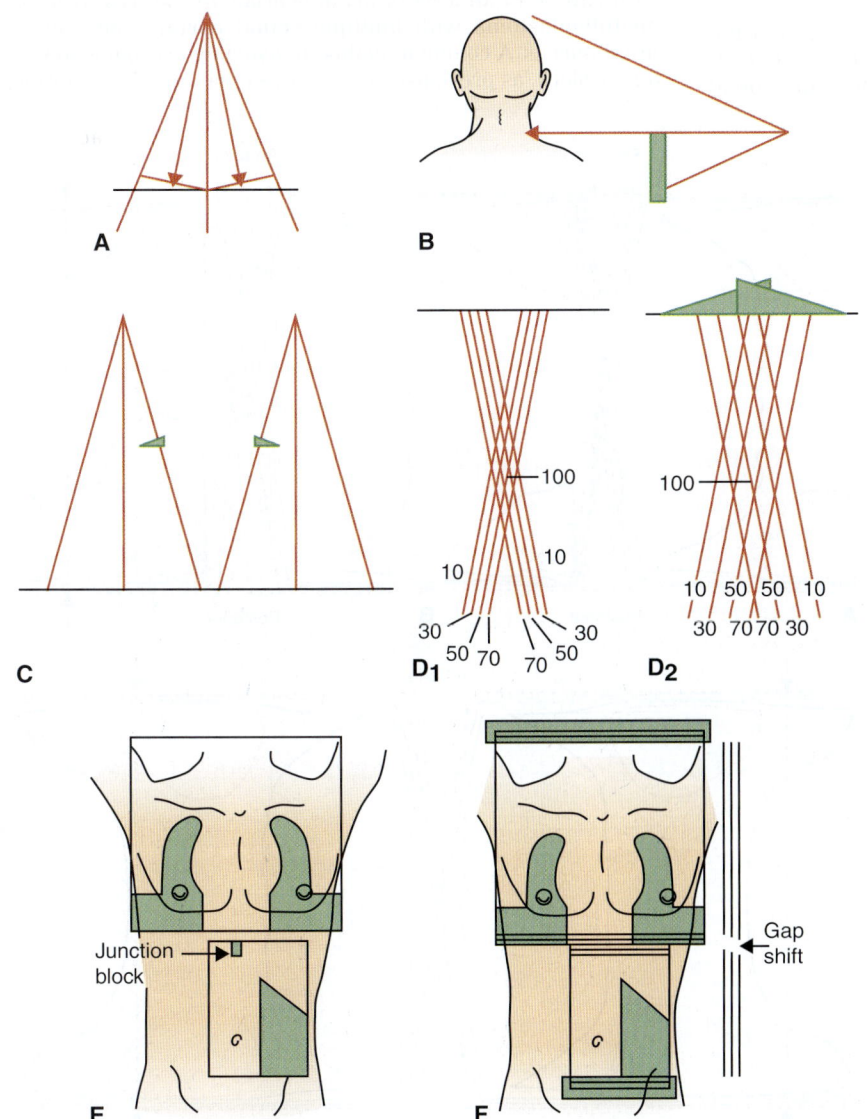

FIGURE 7.27. Different techniques for matching adjacent fields. **A:** Beam's central rays are angled slightly away from one another so that the diverging beams are parallel. **B:** Half-beam block to eliminate divergence. **C:** Penumbra generators (small wedges) to increase width of penumbra, as illustrated in **D₁** and **D₂**. **E:** Junction block over spinal cord. **F:** Moving gap technique. (Reprinted from Bentel GC, ed. *Radiation therapy planning.* 2nd ed. New York: McGraw-Hill, 1996:141. Copyright © 1996 McGraw-Hill Education. All rights reserved.)

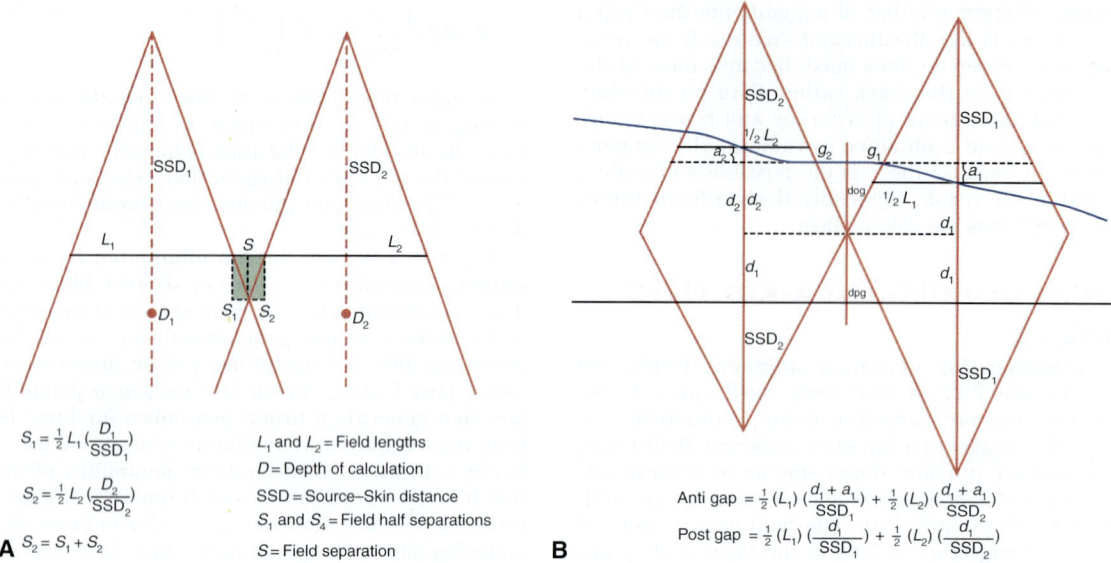

$$S_1 = \tfrac{1}{2} L_1 \left(\frac{D_1}{SSD_1}\right)$$

$$S_2 = \tfrac{1}{2} L_2 \left(\frac{D_2}{SSD_2}\right)$$

A $S_2 = S_1 + S_2$

L_1 and L_2 = Field lengths
D = Depth of calculation
SSD = Source–Skin distance
S_1 and S_4 = Field half separations
S = Field separation

$$\text{Anti gap} = \tfrac{1}{2}(L_1)\left(\frac{d_1 + a_1}{SSD_1}\right) + \tfrac{1}{2}(L_2)\left(\frac{d_1 + a_1}{SSD_2}\right)$$

$$\text{Post gap} = \tfrac{1}{2}(L_1)\left(\frac{d_1}{SSD_1}\right) + \tfrac{1}{2}(L_2)\left(\frac{d_1}{SSD_2}\right)$$

FIGURE 7.28. A: Standard formula for calculating the gap at the skin surface for a given depth using similar triangles. **B:** Modified formula for calculating the gap for matching four fields on a sloping surface. (Reprinted from Keys RA, Grigsby PW. Gapping fields on sloping surfaces. *Int J Radiat Oncol Biol Phys* 1990;18[5]:1183–1190. Copyright © 1990 Elsevier. With permission.)

Orthogonal Field Junctions

Figure 7.30 illustrates the geometry of matching abutting orthogonal photon beams. Such techniques are necessary, particularly in the head and neck region where the spinal cord can be in an area of beam overlap, in the treatment of medulloblastoma with multiple spinal portals and lateral brain portals. A common method of avoiding overlap is to use a half-block, as previously discussed, so that abutting anterior

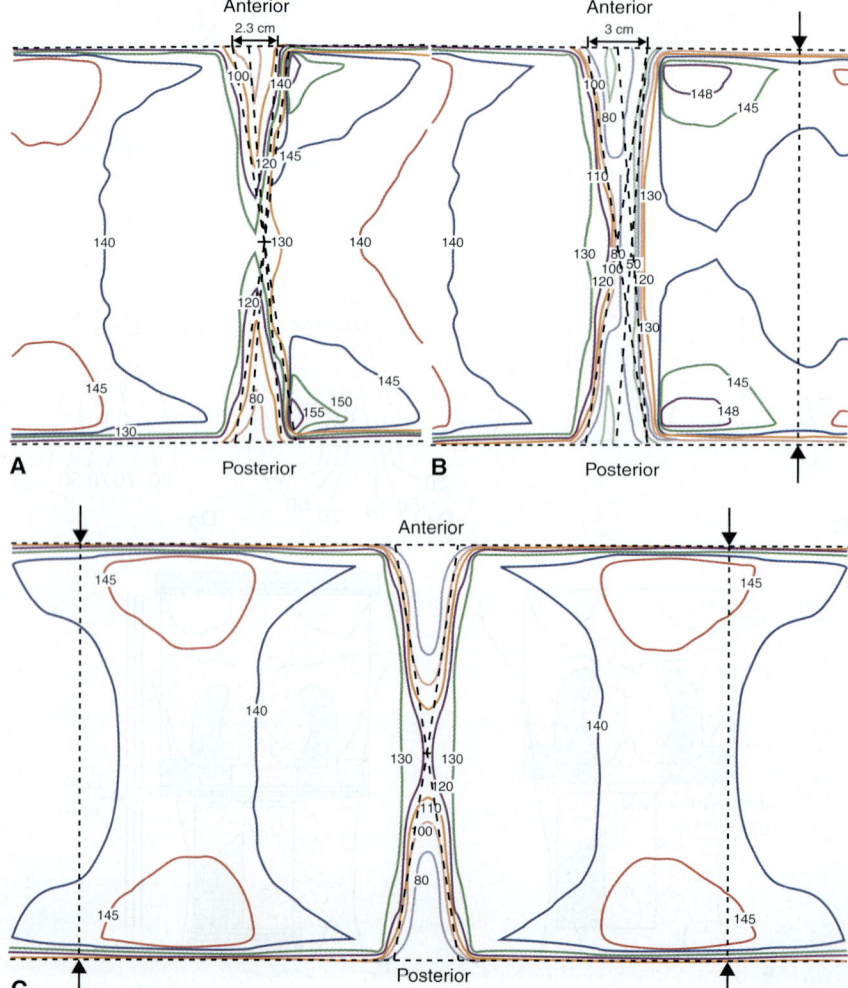

FIGURE 7.29. Dose distribution for geometric separation of fields with all four beams intersecting at midpoint. Adjacent field sizes: 30 × 30 cm and 15 × 15 cm; source-to-skin distance (SSD), 100 cm; anteroposterior thickness, 20 cm; 4-MV x-ray beams. **A:** Field separation at surface is 2.3 cm. A three-field overlap exists in this case because the fields have different sizes but the same SSD. **B:** The adjacent field separation increased to eliminate three-field overlap on the surface. **C:** Field separation adjusted to 2.7 cm to eliminate three-field overlap at the cord at 15 cm depth from anterior. (From Khan FM. *The physics of radiation therapy*. 2nd ed. Baltimore: Williams & Wilkins; 1994. With permission.)

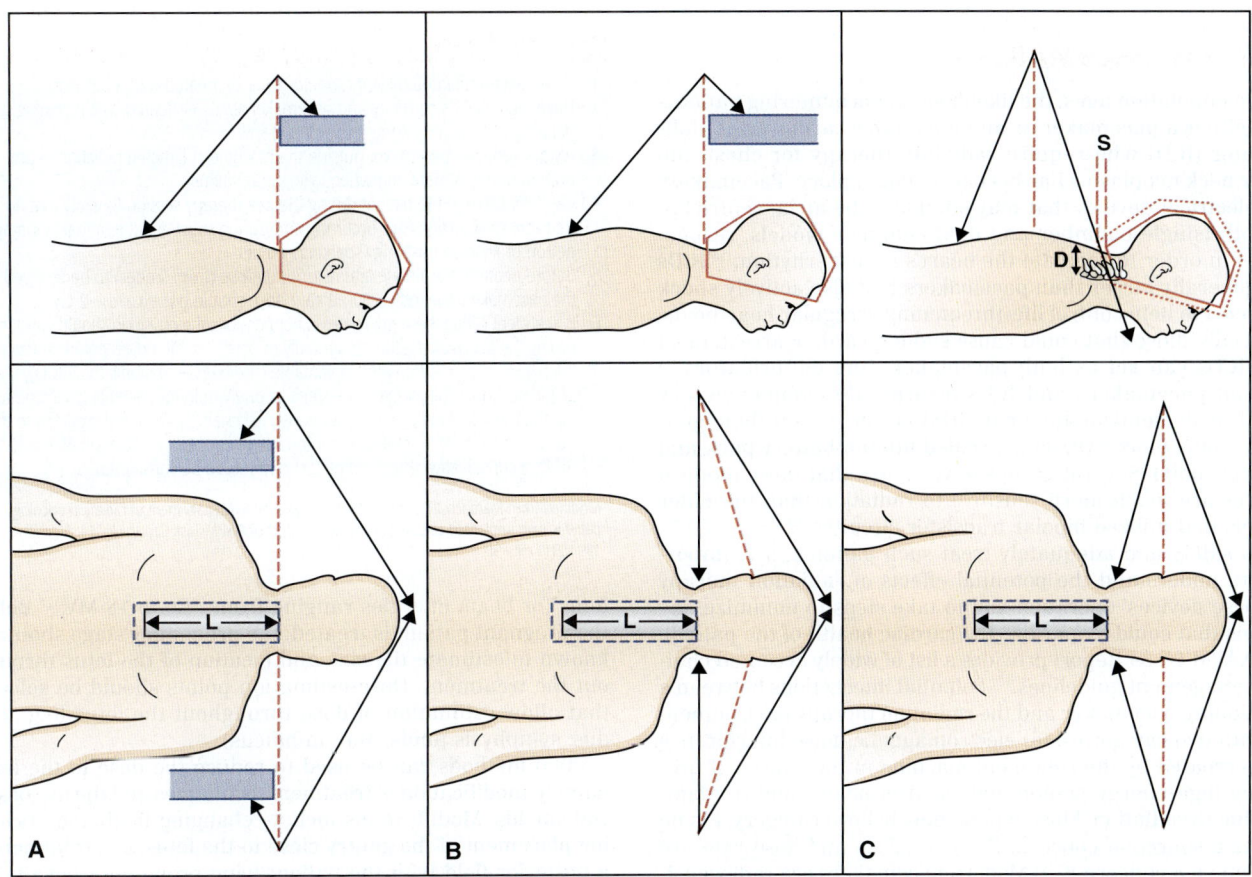

FIGURE 7.30. Some solutions for the problem of overlap for orthogonal fields. **A:** A beam splitter, a shield that blocks half of the field, is used on the lateral and posterior fields and on the spinal cord portal to match the nondivergent edges of the beams. **B:** The divergence in the lateral beams may also be removed by angling the lateral beams so that their caudal edges match. Because most therapy units cannot be angled like this, the couch is rotated through small angles in opposite directions to achieve the same effect. **C:** A gap technique allows the posterior and lateral field to be matched at depth using a gap *S* on the skin surface. The *dashed lines* indicate projected field edges at depth *D*, where the orthogonal fields meet. (Reprinted from Williamson TJ. A technique for matching orthogonal megavoltage fields. *Int J Radiat Oncol Biol Phys* 1979;5[1]:111–116. Copyright © 1979 Elsevier. With permission.)

and lateral field edges are perpendicular to the gantry axis. In head and neck cancer, a notch in the posterior corner of the lateral oral cavity portal is commonly used to ensure overlap avoidance of the spinal cord when midline cord blocks cannot be used on anteroposterior portals irradiating the lower neck and matched to the oral cavity portals. Other techniques rotate the couch about a vertical axis to compensate for the divergence of the lateral field.[117] The angle of rotation is given by

$$\tan \theta^{-1} = \left(\frac{\frac{1}{2} \text{field width}}{\text{SAD}} \right)$$

Another technique is to leave a gap, *S*, on the anterior neck surface between the posterior field of length *L* and lateral field edges.[118] *S* can be calculated using the following formula where d is the depth of the spine beneath the posterior field:

$$S = \frac{1}{2}(L)\left(\frac{d}{\text{SAD}} \right)$$

The potential for the occurrence of radiation myelopathy resulting from a potentially excessive dose from misaligned overlapping fields is always a concern when central nervous system tumors are treated. Craniospinal irradiation is well established as a standard method of treating suprasellar dysgerminoma, pineal tumors, medulloblastomas, and other tumors involving the central nervous system. Uniform

treatment of the entire craniospinal target volume is possible using separate parallel-opposed lateral cranial portals rotated so that their inferior borders match with the superior border of the spinal portal, which is treated with either one or two fields, depending on the length of the spine to be treated.[119] Two junctional moves are typically made at one-third and two-thirds of the total dose. The spinal field central axis is shifted away from the brain by 0.5 cm and the field size length reduced by 0.5 cm with corresponding increases in the length of the cranial field, so that a match exists between the inferior border of the brain portal and the superior border of the spine portal. To achieve the match, a collimator rotation for the whole-brain portals must be done for an angle given by the following relationship:

$$\tan \theta^{-1} = \left(\frac{\frac{1}{2} \text{spinal field length}}{\text{SAD}} \right)$$

In addition, in order to eliminate the divergence between the cranial portal and spinal portal, the table is rotated through a floor angle given by the following relationship:

$$\tan \alpha^{-1} = \left(\frac{\frac{1}{2} \text{cranial field length}}{\text{SAD}} \right)$$

RADIATION THERAPY PATIENTS WITH CARDIAC PACEMAKERS

As the population ages, the likelihood of encountering patients with either a pacemaker or an implantable cardioverter–defibrillator (ICD) who require radiation therapy for chest and lower neck neoplasms has become commonplace. Pacemakers are electrical devices that may stimulate the atria, ventricles, or both (single-chamber and dual-chamber models, respectively) in order to regulate the heart's natural rhythm.[120] ICDs are generally larger than pacemakers and also actively shock the heart to help control life-threatening, irregular heartbeats, especially those that could cause sudden cardiac arrest; most new ICDs can act as both pacemakers and defibrillators.[121] Modern pacemakers and ICDs incorporate complementary metal oxide semiconductor (CMOS) circuitry into their generator units (encompassing a sealed lithium battery pack and circuitry only). Several groups have shown that these modern devices are much more sensitive to radiation than the older models that utilized bipolar transistor circuitry.[122–124]

To safely and adequately treat such patients, it is important to understand the potential effects of radiation therapy on these devices' operation and to take steps to minimize any actions that could jeopardize the cardiac health of the patient. The AAPM TG 34 Report provides a list of widely accepted clinical management guidelines.[125] Potential interactions between a functioning pacemaker and the radiation therapy environment fall into two categories: (a) electromagnetic noise interference (EMI) created by the treatment machine in the course of producing high-energy photon and electron beams and (b) damage due to radiation. Most experts now believe category 1 is no longer a source of concern. However, dose and dose rate are very much a concern.[122,124] Modern pacemakers are radiosensitive and have a significant probability of failing catastrophically at radiation doses well below normal tissue tolerance and, therefore, should never be irradiated by the direct beam. Also, several authors have shown that recommended maximum doses obtained from manufacturers have not proven to be reliable and vary greatly among manufacturers.[126] A recent review by Hudson et al. provides the latest information and points out that radiation-induced device malfunctions are rare, and death associated with that malfunction is even more uncommon.[126] However, they conclude that the adequacy of published guidelines is not supported by hard data. They recommend that it is important to consider all aspects of radiation therapy treatment, not just accumulated dose. These include the effect of backscatter, dose rate, fractionation, and potential EMI with new technologies such as IMRT and respiratory gating. They recommend that each radiation oncology department employ their own policy for the management of patients with pacemakers and ICDs, potentially based on an updated standard national or international guideline similar to that released by the AAPM in 1994 (Table 7.2).

FETAL DOSE

Radiation therapy is standard treatment for several malignancies (e.g., Hodgkin lymphoma, breast cancer) in which the population of women is often of child-bearing age. The issues are complex, and the patient along with the radiation oncologist must evaluate treatment risk to the fetus in such cases. Radiation effects to the fetus are not fully understood and cannot be comfortably predicted for each individual case. If the decision is to irradiate, the dose levels outside the treatment fields should be quantified, and every effort should be made to lower the dose to the fetus. This may require changes in irradiation technique (i.e., modified mantle fields), elimination of double-exposure portal images, and the addition of special patient shields. The AAPM TG 36 Report provides data and techniques to estimate and reduce radiation dose to the

TABLE 7.2 MANAGEMENT GUIDELINES FOR RADIATION THERAPY PATIENTS WITH CARDIAC PACEMAKERS

1. Pacemaker-implanted patients should never be treated with a betatron.
2. Have the patient's coronary and pacemaker status evaluated by a cardiologist before and soon after completion of therapy.
3. Always keep the pacemaker outside the machine-collimated radiation beam, both during treatment and when taking portal films.
4. Carefully observe the patient during the first therapy session to verify that no transient malfunctions are occurring and during subsequent treatments if magnetron or klystron misfiring (sparking) occurs.
5. Before treatment, estimate and record the dose (from scatter) to be received by the pacemaker. The total accumulated dose should not exceed ~2 Gy.
6. If treatment within these guidelines is not possible, the physician should consider having the pacemaker either temporarily or permanently moved before irradiation.
7. If a patient has an automatic implantable cardioverter–defibrillator (AICD), the physicist should follow the same steps as one would for pacemakers in contacting the manufacturer and simultaneously ascertaining the dose expected to the AICD. If there is no manufacturer information concerning radiation effects to the AICD, a conservative threshold of 100 cGy should be considered.

Modified from Marbach JR, Sontag MR, Van Dyk J, et al. Management of radiation oncology patients with implanted cardiac pacemakers: report of AAPM Task Group No. 34. *Med Phys* 1994;21(1):85–90.

fetus for beam energies ranging from ^{60}Co to 18 MV.[127] Before the pregnant patient is treated, the pregnancy stage should be known to estimate the size and location of the fetus throughout the treatment. Dose-estimation points should be selected that allow estimation of dose throughout the fetus (e.g., fundus, symphysis pubis, and umbilicus).

Two methods can be used to reduce the dose to the fetus, namely, modification of treatment techniques and the use of special shields. Modifications include changing field angle (avoiding placement of the gantry close to the fetus, i.e., treatment of a posterior field with the patient lying prone on a false tabletop), reducing field size, choosing a different radiation energy (avoiding ^{60}Co because of high leakage or energies of >10 MV because of neutrons), and using tertiary collimation to define the field edge nearest to the fetus. When shields are designed, the shielding device must allow for treatment fields above the diaphragm and on the lower extremities. Safety to the patient and personnel is a primary consideration in shield design. As part of the management of a pregnant patient, the treatment planning tasks listed in Table 7.3 should be performed to ensure that the dose to the fetus is kept to a minimum.[127]

It should be noted that the aforementioned AAPM TG Report was based on treatment machines that predated modern MLCs. One study showed that the use of tertiary MLC systems such as those found on Varian linacs actually reduced fetal dose during

TABLE 7.3 TREATMENT PLANNING TASKS TO ENSURE THAT DOSE TO THE FETUS IS KEPT TO A MINIMUM

1. Complete all planning as though the patient were not pregnant.
2. Consider modifications of the plan that would minimize the fetal dose (e.g., changing field size and angle, using a different energy).
3. Estimate dose to fetus without shielding using a phantom or data from the AAPM report.[120]
4. Design and construct special shielding if necessary; four or five HVLs of lead usually suffice.
5. Measure dose to fetus in a phantom during simulated treatment with shielding in place.
6. Document the treatment plan and discuss the treatment with all personnel involved with the treatment.
7. Check all aspects of safety, including the load-bearing limits of the couch and support and movement of the shields, to ensure that there will be no injury to the patient or to personnel. The setup of each field should be photographed for documentation.
8. Monitor fetal size and location throughout the course of therapy and update estimates of fetal dose if necessary.
9. Document the completion of treatment by estimating the total dose to the fetus because of the radiation therapy.

Modified from Stovall M, Blackwell CR, Cundiff J, et al. Fetal dose from radiotherapy with photon beams: report of AAPM Radiation Therapy Committee Task Group No. 36. *Med Phys* 1995;22(1):63–82.

irradiation of a pregnant patient.[128] The leaf and carriage system provided some absorption, and if the MLC leaves were oriented in direction along the plane of concern, such as typically when a patient with Hodgkin disease is treated (i.e., leaves oriented along the length of the table), the reduction difference when compared to having no MLCs was on the order of 2.5 to 3.

GONADAL DOSE

Many of the reports used to estimate peripheral dose and fetal dose apply to dose estimations to both testes and ovaries.[129,130] Simultaneously, there have been studies to determine the genetically significant dose (GSD) as it applies to peripheral radiotherapy dosage to ovaries and testes. Niroomand-Rad and Cumberlin[131] combined measured data and GSD data to determine the GSD for particular treatment techniques that deliver peripheral dose to ovaries and testes. They summarized that GSDs from conventional therapies are minimal. However, there are circumstances, such as treatment of seminoma, when it is necessary to use a testicular shield to surround the testes to reduce head scatter and leakage, and some internal scatter.[132]

REFERENCES

1. Fischer JJ, Moulder JE. The steepness of the dose-response curve in radiation therapy. *Radiology* 1975;117:179–184.
2. Herring DF. The consequences of dose response curves for tumor control and normal tissue injury on the precision necessary in patient management. *Laryngoscope* 1975;85:119–125.
3. Stewart J, Jackson A. The steepness of the dose response curve for both tumor cure and normal tissue injury. *Laryngoscope* 1975;85:1107–1111.
4. Mackie RT, Liu HH, McCullough EC. Treatment planning algorithms: model-based photon dose calculations. In: Khan FM, ed. *Treatment planning in radiation oncology.* 2nd ed. Philadelphia: Lippincott Williams & Wilkins, 2007:63–77.
5. Ahnesjö A, Aspradakis MM. Dose calculations for external photon beams in radiotherapy. *Phys Med Biol* 1999;44:R99–R155.
6. Khan FM, Sewchand W, Lee J, et al. Revision of tissue-maximum ratio and scatter-maximum ratio concepts for cobalt 60 and higher energy x-ray beams. *Med Phys* 1980;7:230–237.
7. International Commission on Radiation Units and Measurements. *ICRU report 24: determination of absorbed dose in a patient irradiated by beams of X or gamma rays in radiotherapy procedures.* Washington, DC: International Commission on Radiation Units and Measurements, 1976.
8. Batho HF. Lung corrections in Cobalt 60 beam therapy. *J Can Assoc Radiol* 1964;15:79–83.
9. Young MEJ, Gaylord JD. Experimental tests of corrections for tissue inhomogeneities in radiotherapy. *Br J Radiol* 1970;43:349–355.
10. Sontag MR, Cunningham JR. Corrections to absorbed dose calculations for tissue inhomogeneities. *Med Phys* 1977;4:431–436.
11. Mackie TR, Scrimger JW, Battista JJ. A convolution method of calculating dose for 15-MV x-rays. *Med Phys* 1985;12:188–196.
12. Chetty IJ, Curran B, Cygler JE, et al. Report of the AAPM Task Group No. 105: issues associated with clinical implementation of Monte Carlo-based photon and electron external beam treatment planning. *Med Phys* 2007;34(12):4818–4853.
13. Verhaegen F, Seuntjens J. Monte Carlo modelling of external radiotherapy photon beams (topical review). *Phys Med Biol* 2003;48(21):R107–R164.
14. Ahnesjö A, Andreo P, Brahme A. Calculation and application of point spread functions for treatment planning with high energy photon beams. *Acta Oncol* 1987;26:49–56.
15. Lydon JM. Photon dose calculations in homogeneous media for a treatment planning system using a collapsed cone superposition convolution algorithm. *Phys Med Biol* 1998;43:1813–1822.
16. Ahnesjö A. Collapsed cone convolution of radiant energy for photon dose calculation in heterogeneous media. *Med Phys* 1989;16:577–592.
17. Siebers JV, Keall PJ, Kawrakow I. Monte Carlo dose calculations for external beam radiation therapy. In: Dyk JV, ed. *The modern technology of radiation oncology—a compendium for medical physicists and radiation oncologists.* vol. 2. Madison, WI: Medical Physics Publishing, 2005:91–130.
18. Cygler JE, Daskalov GM, Chan GH, et al. Evaluation of the first commercial Monte Carlo dose calculation engine for electron beam treatment planning. *Med Phys* 2004;31(1):142–153.
19. Malkov VN, Rogers DW. Charged particle transport in magnetic fields in EGSnrc. *Med Phys* 2016;43:4447–4458.
20. Ahmad SB, Sarfehnia A, Paudel MR, et al. Evaluation of a commercial MRI linac based Monte Carlo dose calculation algorithm with GEANT4. *Med Phys* 2016;43:894–907.
21. Wang Y, Mazur T, Park J, et al. Development of a fast Monte Carlo dose calculation system for online adaptive radiation therapy quality assurance. *Phys Med Biol* 2017;62(12):4970–4990.
22. American Association of Physicists in Medicine. *Report 85: tissue inhomogeneity corrections for megavoltage photon beams: report of Task Group 65 of the Radiation Therapy Committee.* Madison, WI: Medical Physics Publishing, 2004.
23. Frank SJ, Forster KM, Stevens CW, et al. Treatment planning for lung cancer: traditional homogeneous point-dose prescription compared with heterogeneity-corrected dose-volume prescription. *Int J Radiat Oncol Biol Phys* 2003;56(5):1308–1318.
24. Davidson SE, Popple RA, Ibbott GS, et al. Heterogeneity dose calculation accuracy in IMRT: study of the commercial treatment planning systems using an anthropomorphic thorax phantom. *Med Phys* 2008;35:5434–5439.
25. Gibbons JP, ed. *Monitor unit calculations for external photon and electron beams.* Madison, WI: Advanced Medical Publishing, 2000.
26. Georg D, Huekelom S, Venselaar J. Formalisms for MU calculations, ESTRO booklet 3 versus NCS report 12. *Radiother Oncol* 2001;60(3):319–328.
27. Stern RL, Heaton R, Fraser MW, et al. Verification of monitor unit calculations for non-IMRT clinical radiotherapy: report of AAPM Task Group 114. *Med Phys* 2011;38(1):504–530.
28. Central axis depth dose data for use in radiotherapy. *Br J Radiol* 1996;25(Suppl).
29. Cundiff JH, Cunningham JR, Golden R, et al. A method for the calculation of dose in the radiation treatment of Hodgkin's disease. *Am J Roentgenol* 1973;117:30–44.
30. Cunningham JR. Scatter-air ratios. *Phys Med Biol* 1972;17:42–51.
31. Chui C, Mohan R, Fontanela D. Dose computation for asymmetric fields defined by independent jaws. *Med Phys* 1986;15:92.
32. Rosenberg I, Chu JC, Saxena V. Calculation of monitor units for a linear accelerator with asymmetric jaws. *Med Phys* 1995;22:55–61.
33. Slessinger ED, Gerber RG, Harms WB, et al. Independent collimator dosimetry for a dual photon energy linear accelerator. *Int J Radiat Oncol Biol Phys* 1993;27(3):681–687.
34. Palta JR, Ayyangar KM, Suntharalingam N. Dosimetric characteristics of a 6 MV photon beam from a linear accelerator with asymmetric collimator jaws. *Int J Radiat Oncol Biol Phys* 1988;14:383–387.
35. Khan F. Dosimetry of wedged fields with asymmetric collimation. *Med Phys* 1993;20:1447.
36. Klein EE, Harms WB, Low DA, et al. Clinical implementation of a commercial multileaf collimator: dosimetry, networking, simulation, and quality assurance. *Int J Radiat Oncol Biol Phys* 1995;33:1195–1208.
37. Palta JR, Yeung DK, Frouhar V. Dosimetric considerations for a multileaf collimator system. *Med Phys* 1996;23(7):1219–1224.
38. Jordan TJ, Williams PC. The design and performance characteristics of a multileaf collimator. *Phys Med Biol* 1994;39:231–251.
39. Das IJ, Desobry GE, McNeeley SW, et al. Beam characteristics of a retrofitted double-focused multileaf collimator. Med Phys 1998;25(9):1676–1684.
40. Boyer A, Biggs P, Galvin J, et al. *AAPM report 72: basic applications of multileaf collimators, report of Task Group 50. Published for the American Association of Physicists in Medicine.* Madison, WI: Medical Physics Publishing, 2001.
41. Hanson WF, Berkley LW. Calculative technique to correct for the change in linear accelerator beam energy at off-axis points. *Med Phys* 1980;7(2):147–150.
42. Hanson WF, Berkley LW. Off-axis beam quality change in linear accelerator x-ray beams. *Med Phys* 1980;7(2):145–146.
43. Otto K. Volumetric modulated arc therapy: IMRT in a single gantry arc. *Med Phys* 2008;35(1):310–317.
44. Bedford JL, Warrington AP. Commissioning of volumetric modulated arc therapy (VMAT). *Int J Radiat Oncol Biol Phys* 2009;73(2):537–545.
45. Rao M, Yang W, Chen F, et al. Comparison of Elekta VMAT with helical tomotherapy and fixed field IMRT: plan quality, delivery efficiency and accuracy. *Med Phys* 2010;37(3):1350–1359.
46. Ling CC, Zhang P, Archambault Y, et al. Commissioning and quality assurance of RapidArc radiotherapy delivery system. *Int J Radiat Oncol Biol Phys* 2008;72(2):575–581.
47. Yu CX. Intensity modulated arc therapy with dynamic multileaf collimation: an alternative to tomotherapy. *Phys Med Biol* 1995;40(9):1435–1449.
48. Yu CX, Tang G. Intensity-modulated arc therapy: principles, technologies and clinical implementation. *Phys Med Biol* 2011;56(5):R31–R54.
49. Kung JH, Chen GTY, Kuchnir FK. A monitor unit verification calculation in intensity modulated radiotherapy as a dosimetry quality assurance. *Med Phys* 2000;27(10):2226–2230.
50. Yang Y, Xing L, Li JG, et al. Independent dosimetric calculation with inclusion of head scatter and MLC transmission for IMRT. *Med Phys* 2003;30(11):2937–2947.
51. Purdy JA. Buildup/surface dose and exit dose measurements for 6-MV linear accelerator. *Med Phys* 1986;13:259.
52. Mamalui-Hunter M, Yaddanapudi S, Zhao T, et al. Patient-specific independent 3D GammaPlan quality assurance for Gamma Knife Perfexion radiosurgery. *J Appl Clin Med Phys* 2013;14(1):3949.
53. Followill DS, Nüsslin F, Orton CG. IMRT should not be administered at photon energies greater than 10 MV. *Med Phys* 2007;34:1877–1879.
54. Wooten HO, Green O, Yang M, et al. Quality of intensity modulated radiation therapy treatment plans using a ^{60}Co magnetic resonance image guidance radiation therapy system. *Int J Radiat Oncol Biol Phys* 2015;92(4):771–778.
55. Glide-Hurst C, Bellon M, Foster R, et al. Commissioning of the Varian TrueBeam linear accelerator: a multi-institutional study. *Med Phys* 2013;40(3):031719-1-031719-15.
56. Rustgi SN, Rodgers JE. Improvement in the buildup characteristics of a 10-MV photon beam with electron filters. *Phys Med Biol* 1985;30:587.
57. Gerbi BJ, Meigooni A, Khan FM. Dose buildup for obliquely incident photon beams. *Med Phys* 1987;14:393–399.
58. Klein EE, Purdy JA. Entrance and exit dose regions for Clinac-2100 C. *Int J Radiat Oncol Biol Phys* 1993;27:429–435.
59. Cunningham JR. Tissue inhomogeneity corrections in photon-beam treatment planning. In: Orton CG, ed. *Progress in medical physics.* vol. 1. New York, NY: Plenum Press, 1982:103–131.
60. Kornelsen RO, Young MEJ. Changes in the dose-profile of a 10 MV x-ray beam within and beyond low density material. *Med Phys* 1982;9:114–116.

61. Epp ER, Lougheed MN, McKay JW. Ionization build-up in upper respiratory air passages during teletherapy units with cobalt-60 irradiation. *Br J Radiol* 1958;31:361.
62. Epp ER, Boyer AL, Doppke KP. Underdosing of lesions resulting from lack of electronic equilibrium in upper respiratory air cavities irradiated by 10 MV x-ray beams. *Int J Radiat Oncol Biol Phys* 1977;2:613.
63. Klein EE, Chin LM, Rice RK, et al. The influence of air cavities on interface doses for photon beams (abstract). *Int J Radiat Oncol Biol Phys* 1993;27:419.
64. Rice RK, Mijnheer BJ, Chin LM. Benchmark measurements for lung dose corrections for x-ray beams. *Int J Radiat Oncol Biol Phys* 1988;15:399–409.
65. Das IJ, Kase KR, Meigooni AS, et al. Validity of transition-zone dosimetry at high atomic number interfaces in megavoltage photon beams. *Med Phys* 1990;17(1):10–16.
66. Sibata CH, Mota HC, Hoggins PD, et al. Influence of hip prostheses on high energy photon dose distribution. *Int J Radiat Oncol Biol Phys* 1990;18:455–461.
67. Thatcher M. Perturbation of Cobalt 60 radiation doses by metal objects implanted during oral and maxillofacial surgery. *J Oral Maxillofac Surg* 1984;42:108–110.
68. Niroomand-Rad A, Razavi R, Thobejane S, et al. Radiation dose perturbation at tissue-titanium dental interfaces in head and neck cancer patients. *Int J Radiat Oncol Biol Phys* 1996;34(2):475–480.
69. Reft C, Alecu R, Das IJ, et al. Dosimetric considerations for patients with HIP prostheses undergoing pelvic irradiation. Report of the AAPM Radiation Therapy Committee Task Group 63. *Med Phys* 2003;30(6):1162–1182.
70. Klein EE, Kuske RR. Changes in photon dosimetry due to breast prosthesis. *Int J Radiat Oncol Biol Phys* 1993;25(3):541–549.
71. Tatcher M. A method for varying effective angle of wedge filters. *Radiology* 1970;97:132.
72. Philips Medical Systems Division. *Product data 764*. Eindhoven, The Netherlands: Philips Medical Systems Division, 1983.
73. Petti PL, Siddon RL. Effective wedge angles with a universal wedge. *Phys Med Biol* 1985;30(9):985–991.
74. McCullough EC, Gortney J, Blackwell CR. A depth dependence determination of the wedge transmission factor for 4–10 MV photon beams. *Med Phys* 1988;15:621–623.
75. Sewchand W, Khan FM, Williamson J. Variations in depth-dose data between open and wedge fields for 4-MV x rays. *Radiology* 1978;127:789–792.
76. Abrath FG, Purdy JA. Wedge design and dosimetry for 25-MV x rays. *Radiology* 1980;136:757–762.
77. Leavitt DD, Martin M, Moeller JH, et al. Dynamic wedge field techniques through computer-controlled collimator motion and dose delivery. *Med Phys* 1990;17:87–91.
78. Klein EE, Low DA, Meigooni AS, et al. Dosimetry and clinical implementation of dynamic wedge. *Int J Radiat Oncol Biol Phys* 1995;31:583–592.
79. Akazawa PF, Roach MI, Pickett B, et al. Three dimensional comparison of blocked arcs vs four and six field conformal treatment of the prostate. *Radiother Oncol* 1996;41:83–88.
80. Wu Q, Manning M, Schmidt-Ullrich R, et al. The potential for sparing of parotids and escalation of biologically effective dose with intensity-modulated radiation treatments of head and neck cancers: a treatment design study. *Int J Radiat Oncol Biol Phys* 2000;46(1):195–205.
81. Wu Q, Mohan R, Morris M, et al. Simultaneous integrated boost intensity-modulated radiotherapy for locally advanced head-and-neck squamous cell carcinomas. I: dosimetric results. *Int J Radiat Oncol Biol Phys* 2003;56(2):573–585.
82. Verbakel WF, Senan S, Cuijpers JP, et al. Rapid delivery of stereotactic radiotherapy for peripheral lung tumors using volumetric intensity-modulated arcs. *Radiother Oncol* 2009;93(1):122–124.
83. Xiao Y, Kry SF, Popple R, et al. Flattening filter-free accelerators: a report from the AAPM Therapy Emerging Technology Assessment Work Group. *J Appl Clin Med Phys* 2015;16(3):12-29.
84. Emami B, Lyman J, Brown A, et al. Tolerance of normal tissue to therapeutic irradiation. *Int J Radiat Oncol Biol Phys* 1991;21:109–122.
85. Marks LB, Ten Haken RK, Martel MK. Guest editor's introduction to QUANTEC: a user's guide. *Int J Radiat Oncol Biol Phys* 2010;76(3, Suppl 1):S1–S2.
86. Rosenow UF, Valentine ES, Davis LW. A technique for treating local breast cancer using a single set-up point and asymmetric collimation. *Int J Radiat Oncol Biol Phys* 1990;19:183–188.
87. Marshall M. Three-field isocentric breast irradiation using asymmetric jaws and a tilt board. *Radiother Oncol* 1993;28:228–232.
88. Klein EE, Taylor M, Michaletz-Lorenz M, et al. A mono-isocentric technique for breast and regional nodal therapy using dual asymmetric jaws. *Int J Radiat Oncol Biol Phys* 1994;28:753–760.
89. Foo ML, McCullough EC, Foote RL, et al. Doses to radiation sensitive organs and structures located outside the radiotherapeutic target volume for four treatment situations. *Int J Radiat Oncol Biol Phys* 1993;27:403.
90. Sohn JW, Suh JH, Pohar S. A method for delivering accurate and uniform radiation dosages to the head and neck with asymmetric collimators and a single isocenter. *Int J Radiat Oncol Biol Phys* 1995;32:809–814.
91. Takahaski S. Conformation radiotherapy-rotation techniques as applied to radiography and radiotherapy of cancer. *Acta Radiol Suppl* 1965;242:1–142.
92. Hounsell AR, Sharrock PJ, Moore CJ, et al. Computer-assisted generation of multileaf collimator settings for conformation therapy. *Br J Radiol* 1992;65:321–326.
93. Galvin JM, Smith AR, Lally B. Characterization of a multileaf collimator system. *Int J Radiat Oncol Biol Phys* 1993;25:181–192.
94. Boyer AL, Ochran TG, Nyerick CE, et al. Clinical dosimetry for implementation of a multileaf collimator. *Med Phys* 1992;19(5):1255–1261.
95. Powlis WD, Smith AR, Cheng E, et al. Initiation of multileaf collimator conformal radiation therapy. *Int J Radiat Oncol Biol Phys* 1993;25:171–179.
96. LoSasso T, Kutcher GJ. Multi-leaf collimation vs. Cerrobend blocks: analysis of geometric accuracy. *Int J Radiat Oncol Biol Phys* 1995;32:499–506.
97. Li H, Mutic S, Low D, et al. A novel doubly-focused multileaf collimator design for MR-guided radiation therapy. *Med Phys* 2016;43(6):3853.
98. Zhu Y, Boyer AL, Desorby GE. Dose distributions of x-ray fields as shaped with multileaf collimators. *Phys Med Biol* 1992;37:163–173.
99. LoSasso T, Chui CS, Kutcher GJ. The use of a multi-leaf collimator for conformal radiotherapy of carcinomas of the prostate and nasopharynx. *Int J Radiat Oncol Biol Phys* 1993;25:161–170.
100. Brahme A. Optimization of stationary and moving beam radiation therapy techniques. *Radiother Oncol* 1988;12:129–140.
101. Du MN, Yu CX, Symons M, et al. A multi-leaf collimator prescription preparation system for conventional radiotherapy. *Int J Radiat Oncol Biol Phys* 1995;32:513–520.
102. Powers WE, Kinzie JJ, Demidecki AJ, et al. A new system of field shaping for external-beam radiation therapy. *Radiology* 1973;108:407–411.
103. Leavitt DD, Gibbs FA Jr. Field shaping. In: Purdy JA, ed. *Advances in radiation oncology physics: dosimetry, treatment planning, and brachytherapy*. New York, NY: American Institute of Physics, 1992:500–523.
104. Huen A, Findley DO, Skov DD. Attenuation in Lipowitz's metal of x-rays produced at 2, 4, 10, and 18 MV and gamma rays from cobalt-60. *Med Phys* 1979;6:147–148.
105. Ellis F, Hall EJ, Oliver R. A compensator for variations in tissue thickness for high energy beams. *Br J Radiol* 1959;32:421–422.
106. Reinstein LE. New approaches to tissue compensation in radiation oncology. In: Purdy JA, ed. *Advances in radiation oncology physics: dosimetry, treatment planning, and brachytherapy*. New York, NY: American Institute of Physics, 1992:535–572.
107. Chang SX, Cullip TJ, Deschesne KM, et al. Compensators: an alternative IMRT delivery technique. *J Appl Clin Med Phys* 2004;5(3):15–36.
108. Kudchadker RJ, Antolak JA, Morrison WH, et al. Utilization of custom electron bolus in head and neck radiotherapy. *J Appl Clin Med Phys* 2003;4(4):321–333.
109. Humphries SM, Boyd K, Cornish P, et al. Comparison of super stuff and paraffin wax bolus in radiation therapy of irregular surfaces. *Med Dosim* 1996;21(3):155–157.
110. Gerber RL, Marks JE, Purdy JA. The use of thermal plastics for immobilization of patients during radiotherapy. *Int J Radiat Oncol Biol Phys* 1982;8:1461.
111. Johnson MW, Griggs MA, Sharma SC. A comparison of surface doses for two immobilizing systems. *Med Dosim* 1995;20(3):191–194.
112. Higgins DM, Whitehurst P, Morgan AM. The effect of carbon fiber couch inserts on surface dose with beam size variation. *Med Dosim* 2001;26(3):251–254.
113. Keys R, Grigsby PW. Gapping fields on sloping surfaces. *Int J Radiat Oncol Biol Phys* 1990;18:1183–1190.
114. Johnson JM, Khan FM. Dosimetric effects of abutting extended source to surface distance electron fields with photon fields in the treatment of head and neck cancers. *Int J Radiat Oncol Biol Phys* 1994;28:741–747.
115. Fraass BA, Tepper JE, Glatstein E, et al. Clinical use of a match line wedge for adjacent megavoltage radiation field matching. *Int J Radiat Oncol Biol Phys* 1983;9:209–216.
116. Christopherson D, Courlas GJ, Jette D. Field matching in radiotherapy. *Med Phys* 1984;3:369.
117. Siddon RL, Tonnesen GL, Svensson GK. Three-field techniques for breast treatment using a rotatable half-beam block. *Int J Radiat Oncol Biol Phys* 1981;7:1473–1477.
118. Williamson TJ. A technique for matching orthogonal megavoltage fields. *Int J Radiat Oncol Biol Phys* 1979;5:111.
119. Lim MLF. A study of four methods of junction change in the treatment of medulloblastoma. *Am Assoc Med Dosim J* 1985;10:17–24.
120. National Heart, Lung, and Blood Institute (NHLBI). *What is a pacemaker?*, 2011. Available at: http://www.nhlbi.nih.gov/health/dci/Diseases/pace/pace_whatis.html
121. National Heart, Lung, and Blood Institute (NHLBI). *What is an implantable cardioverter defibrillator?* 2011. Available at: http://www.nhlbi.nih.gov/health/dci/Diseases/icd/icd_whatis.html
122. Hurkmans CW, Scheepers E, Springorum BGF, et al. Influence of radiotherapy on the latest generation of implantable cardioverter-defibrillators. *Int J Radiat Oncol Biol Phys* 2005;63(1):282.
123. Solan AN, Solan MJ, Bednarz G, et al. Treatment of patients with cardiac pacemakers and implantable cardioverter-defibrillators during radiotherapy. *Int J Radiat Oncol Biol Phys* 2004;59(3):897–904.
124. Sundar S, Symonds RP, Deehan C. Radiotherapy to patients with artificial cardiac pacemakers. *Cancer Treat Rev* 2005;31(6):474–486.
125. Marbach JR, Sontag MR, Van Dyk J, et al. Management of radiation oncology patients with implanted cardiac pacemakers: report of AAPM Task Group No. 34. *Med Phys* 1994;21(1):85–90.
126. Hudson F, Coulshed D, D'Souza E, et al. Effect of radiation therapy on the latest generation of pacemakers and implantable cardioverter defibrillators: a systematic review. *J Med Imaging Radiat Oncol* 2010;54(1):53–61.
127. Stovall M, Blackwell CR, Cundiff J, et al. Fetal dose from radiotherapy with photon beams: report of AAPM Radiation Therapy Committee Task Group No. 36. *Med Phys* 1995;22:63–82.
128. Mutic S, Klein EE. A reduction in the AAPM TG-36 reported peripheral dose distributions with tertiary multileaf collimation. *Int J Radiat Oncol Biol Phys* 1999;44(4):947–953.
129. Francois P, Beurtheret C, Dutreix A. Calculation of the dose delivered to organs outside the radiation beams. *Med Phys* 1988;15(6):879–883.
130. van der Giessen PH. A simple and generally applicable method to estimate the peripheral dose in radiation teletherapy with high energy x-rays or gamma radiation. *Int J Radiat Oncol Biol Phys* 1996;35(5):1059–1068.
131. Niroomand-Rad A, Cumberlin RL. Measured dose to ovaries and testes from Hodgkin's fields and determination of genetically significant dose. *Int J Radiat Oncol Biol Phys* 1993;25(4):745–751.
132. Fraass BA, Kinsella TJ, Harrington ES, et al. Peripheral dose to the testes: the design and clinical use of a practical and effective gonadal shield. *Int J Radiat Oncol Biol Phys* 1985;11(3):609–616.

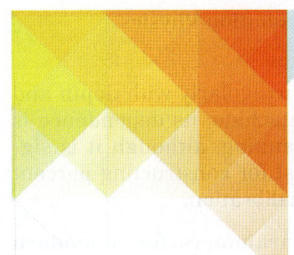

CHAPTER 8

Electron Beam Therapy Dosimetry, Treatment Planning, and Techniques

Angelica Perez-Andujar and Eric E. Klein

INTRODUCTION

Megavoltage-photon–based radiation therapy treatment of shallow tumor volumes is complicated by the buildup and radiation transport properties of photon beams. These beams are capable of treating both shallow and deep tumors; however, when treating shallow tumors, the radiation beams transit through the entire patient, exposing distal normal tissues. Megavoltage electron beams have the property of a finite range and therefore do not deliver significant radiation doses to distal depths. Electron beam therapy is therefore suitable for shallow tumors (<5 cm deep), such as head and neck cancers, skin cancers, chest wall irradiation for breast cancer, and boost dose to nodes. Electrons typically provide dose uniformity in these target volumes, with minimal dose to distal organs. In fact, G.H. Fletcher[1] had gone as far as saying, "There is no alternative treatment to electron-beam therapy." Even the strongest proponents of photon or proton therapy acknowledge that electron therapy is necessary to complete any radiotherapy program.

In 1976, Tapley[2] published one of the earlier comprehensive treatises on electron radiation therapy, in which she states, "There is no practical way for every radiation therapy department, in either hospitals or private offices, to be equipped with all modalities of irradiation beams. Ideally, electron beams should be available for those clinical situations where electrons are indispensable or very clearly superior." Electrons are now used at most radiation therapy centers. It still might be advantageous to refer patients to regional centers for special treatment techniques utilizing electrons.

Since the late 1970s, there have been three developments in electron beam radiation therapy technology that have improved significantly our ability to deliver electron therapy. First, the advent of computed tomography (CT)-based treatment planning allowed for coverage of the planning target volume (PTV) by the therapeutic dose and the dose to normal tissues and structures to be more accurately assessed. Use of CT provides a physical description of the anatomy, which is required for accurate dose calculations.[3,4] Second, the development of the electron pencil beam algorithms (PBAs) and their implementation into treatment planning systems in the early 1980s provided a mechanism for accurately calculating dose.[5,6] More recently, the use of Monte Carlo calculations has moved development to commercial platforms.[7] They have demonstrated high degrees of accuracy, especially with the presence of inhomogeneities. Third, manufacturers have refined the quality of their electron beams (i.e., depth dose, off-axis uniformity, and penumbral width) by providing dual-scattering foil systems and electron applicators. Klein et al.[8] describe dosimetric improvement with the most recent Varian electron beam delivery system. Presently, the differences in the electron beam dose characteristics of various radiation therapy machines from different vendors are minimal. Kashani et al.[9] described electron beam characteristics of a new configured beam line for the Varian TrueBeam machine.

Electron beam therapy is advantageous because it delivers a reasonably uniform dose from the surface to a specific depth, after which dose falls off rapidly, eventually to a near-zero value. The depth of treatment is controlled by selecting the appropriate energy and, when necessary, the bolus thickness. Using electron beams with energies up to 20 MeV allows disease within approximately 6 cm of the surface to be treated effectively, sparing distal normal tissues.

Electron beam therapy is useful in treating cancer of the skin and lips, upper respiratory and digestive tract, head and neck,[10,11] breast, and a variety of other sites.[2,12,13] Treatment sites of the skin include the eyelids, nose, ear,[14] scalp,[2,15] and more widely spread diseases of the limbs (e.g., melanoma and lymphoma)[16] or total skin (e.g., mycosis fungoides).[17,18] Treatment sites of the upper respiratory and digestive tract include the floor of mouth, soft palate, retromolar trigone, and salivary glands.[10,19] Treatments of the breast include chest wall irradiation following mastectomy[2,20,21]; nodal irradiation, often internal mammary chain (IMC) and occasionally axillary; and boost to the surgical bed following mastectomy or lumpectomy.[22] Current techniques of using tangential photon adjunct fields abutting supraclavicular and posterior axillary fields are difficult enough without the addition of treating a separate medial breast internal mammary field with a mixture of photon and electrons. Other sites of electron beam therapy include the retina,[23] orbit,[24] paraspinal muscles,[3,25] pancreas and other abdominal structures (intraoperative therapy),[26] vulva,[27] and cervix (intracavitary irradiation).[28]

The purpose of this chapter is to discuss the treatment and treatment planning techniques necessary to deliver the most effective electron beam therapy. This requires a basic knowledge of dose distribution in water, dose in the heterogeneous patient, treatment planning tools and principles, and special techniques using electron beams.

DOSE DISTRIBUTION IN WATER

To appreciate the clinical use of electron beams, their dose distributions in water must be understood. Understanding the properties of depth dose, off-axis ratios (OARs), and two-dimensional (2-D) isodose contour plots will clarify the concept of dose distribution in water. As well, an understanding of the dependence of the dose distribution on incident energy, field size, and source-to-surface distance (SSD) is required. It is assumed that the dose distribution for a specified energy, field size, and SSD is machine dependent. Applicator design may have a minor influence on dose distributions.

Depth Dose

This section discusses percentage of dose (values are normalized to 100% at the depth of dose maximum, R_{100}) versus depth in water. Central-axis depth dose implies that the electron field is symmetric about the central axis, and the focus initially will be on square fields. Electron depth dose varies with field size; however, once the field reaches a certain size, side-scatter equilibrium is achieved, and further increasing the size has an insignificant effect on depth dose.[29,30] In the energy range of up to 20 MeV, a 10 by 10 cm^2 field size typically will achieve side-scatter equilibrium on central axis. The

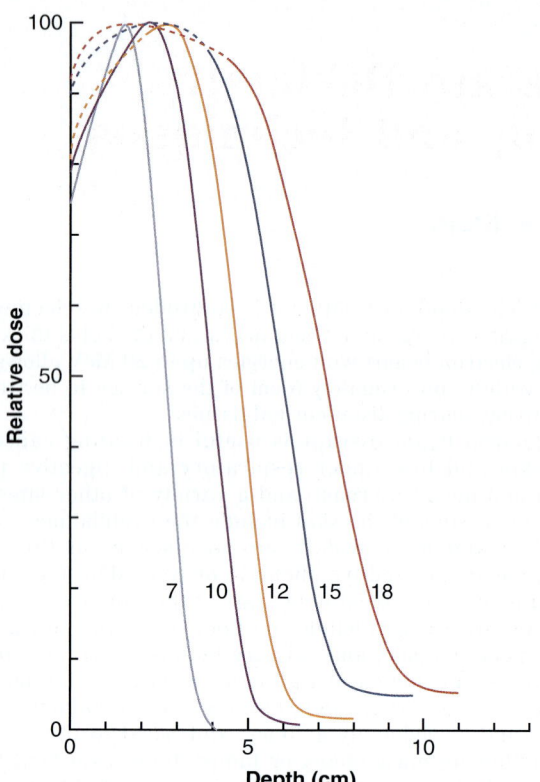

FIGURE 8.1. Energy dependence of depth dose. Plot of relative dose (%) versus depth for a 10 by 10 cm² field size for 7- to 18-MeV beams on a Siemens Mevatron 77 radiation therapy unit (source-to-surface distance, or SSD = 100 cm). (From Meyer JA, Palta JR, Hogstrom KR. Demonstration of relatively new electron dosimetry measurement techniques on the Mevatron 80. *Med Phys* 1984;11[5]:670–677. Copyright © 1984 American Association of Physicists in Medicine. Reprinted by permission of John Wiley & Sons, Inc.)

5. The R_{100} depth (d_{max}) can vary irregularly with depth and model of electron treatment machine; its dependence is insignificant for treatment planning, although it is significant to the medical physicist for constructing percent depth-dose data and in beam calibration.

Table 8.1 gives dosimetric parameters for a modern (Trilogy, Varian) linear accelerator.

Depth dose has a significant dependence on field size, which varies with incident electron energy. The primary reason for the field-size dependence is loss of side-scatter equilibrium, which has been discussed in detail by Hogstrom[29] and Khan et al.[30] Figure 8.2, which shows the field-size dependence of percentage depth dose at 9 and 20 MeV, clearly illustrates that it is a greater issue at higher energies. Loss of side-scatter equilibrium, which begins first at the deeper depths, results in R_{90} shifting toward the surface as field size decreases. As the field size gets even smaller, the maximum dose decreases; and when it is normalized to 100%, the relative dose at the surface, D_s, increases. In addition, the effects on the distal portion of the depth-dose curve are greater. The most clinically significant effect is the decrease in R_{90} with decreasing field size, which can require a greater energy than initially proposed for treatment using very small fields (<5 cm).

Depth-dose variations with SSD are usually minimal. Differences in the depth dose resulting from inverse square effect are small because electrons do not penetrate that deep (≤6 cm in the therapeutic region) and because the significant growth of penumbra width with SSD restricts the SSD in clinical practice to typically 115 cm or less. The primary effect of inverse square is that R_{90} penetrates a few millimeters deeper at extended SSD at the higher energies, as illustrated in Figure 8.3. In relatively few cases (e.g., when the electron beam has a large component of collimator-scattered electrons), the variation in depth dose with SSD can become more significant. In such cases, the collimator-scattered electrons are scattered out of the beam, resulting in a depth dose with a lower D_s and greater R_{90}.[31]

For rectangular fields, Hogstrom[32] derived and others have confirmed[31,33] that percentage of depth dose can be calculated by taking the geometric mean of the percentage of depth doses for a square field of length dimension (L) and one of width dimension (W). That is:

$$\%D(d; LxW) = \sqrt{\%D(d; LxL) \cdot \%D(d; WxW)} \qquad (1)$$

If the square field percentage of depth-dose curves do not have a common R_{100}, then the result of Eq. (1) must be normalized such that its maximum equals 100%. This method is referred to as the square-root method.

In some instances (e.g., intraoperative, intraoral, or intravaginal cones), circular fields are used. In such cases, it is necessary to measure dose distributions independent of those determined for square or rectangular fields.

Usually, a collimating insert is placed inside an electron applicator to form an irregular-shaped field, occasionally blocking the central axis. In this instance, central-axis depth dose makes little sense, and the term *central-field depth dose* should be used, provided that the field has an axis of

energy dependence of depth dose is illustrated in Figure 8.1, where central-axis depth dose is plotted for a 10 by 10 cm² field for energies in the range of 7 to 18 MeV. The family of curves illustrates how the dosimetric characteristics vary with the incident electron energy:

1. Surface dose (D_s) increases from approximately 75% to 95% as energy increases. The slow increase in dose from the surface to the depth of maximum dose (R_{100}) occurs as a result of electrons undergoing multiple Coulomb scattering in water.[29]
2. Depth of distal 90% (R_{90}), often the therapeutic prescription depth, increases as energy increases. A physician may also prescribe to the 80% or 100% depth.
3. The practical range (R_p) (maximum penetration) of the electrons increases as energy increases.
4. X-ray dose attributable to bremsstrahlung that lies beyond the electron dose component is characterized by its value (D_x) and is taken from the PDD curve 10 cm beyond the practical range (R_p). D_x increases as energy increases. Machines are designed to provide Rx values to be <5%.

TABLE 8.1	VARIAN TRILOGY MEASURED ELECTRON DEPTHS (R_p, R_{50}) AND CALCULATED ENERGIES (E_p, E_0)					
Nominal Energy	Measured E_o (MeV)	Measured E_p (MeV)	R_{90}: Depth of 90% (cm)	R_{50}: Depth of 50% (cm)	R_p (cm)	Dx (%)
6	5.55	6.08	1.53	2.38	2.95	0.1
9	8.41	8.84	2.69	3.61	4.33	0.3
12	11.77	12.23	3.85	5.05	6.02	0.9
16	15.63	16.02	5.10	6.71	7.900	1.6
20	19.62	20.78	6.14	8.42	10.25	2.1

E_o: Average energy at the surface, where $E_0 = 2.33 \times R_{50}$.
E_p: Most probable electron energy at the surface, where $E_p = C_1 + C_2 R_p = C_3 R_p^2$ and where C1, C2, and C3 are constants, with C1 = 0.22 MeV, C2 = 1.98 MeV cm¹, and C3 = 0.01025 MeV cm².

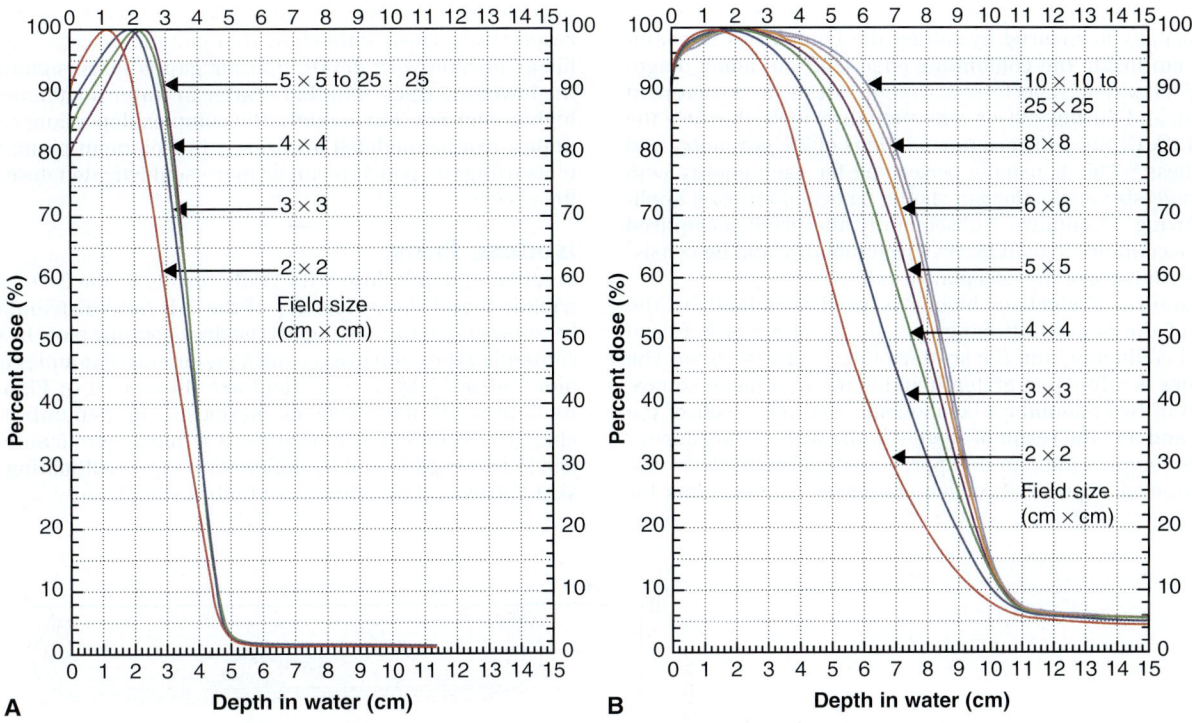

FIGURE 8.2. Field-size dependence of depth dose. Plot of percent dose versus depth for field sizes from 2 by 2 to 25 by 25 cm² for 9-MeV **(A)** and 20-MeV **(B)** beams on a Varian Clinac 2100C radiation therapy unit (source-to-surface distance, or SSD = 100 cm). (Courtesy of Varian, Palo Alto, CA.)

symmetry. In cases where the insert is irregular, the depth dose can be approximated using a rectangular-shaped field that approximates the irregular-shaped field.[34] In highly irregular-shaped fields, the dose distribution should be calculated using an appropriate dose algorithm in a three-dimensional (3-D) treatment planning system. For very small fields, irregular or otherwise, it is highly recommended that PPD measurements be performed to properly determine prescriptive choices (i.e., R_{90}).

Off-Axis Dose

Dose profiles in the dimensions perpendicular to the central axis can be described by OARs. The OAR is defined as the ratio of dose at an off-axis position to that on the central axis at the same depth. The OARs measured in water are used to assess off-axis beam quality, which is characterized by flatness and symmetry in the uniform portion of the beam and by its falloff in the region of the penumbra (e.g., 90% to 10%, or 80% to 20%).

Manufacturers should be able to provide electron beams with a symmetry specification of 2% for opposing points in the beam and a flatness specification of ±3% of the *central-axis value* along the major axes (±4% along diagonals). The American Association of Physicists in Medicine (AAPM) Task Group 25 recommended that flatness and symmetry should be evaluated along major axes (lines containing central axis and perpendicular to the collimator edges) and along diagonal axes.[30] Task Group 25 also recommended that flatness and symmetry be evaluated at depths near the surface and therapeutic depth. Practically, this is performed at R_{100}.

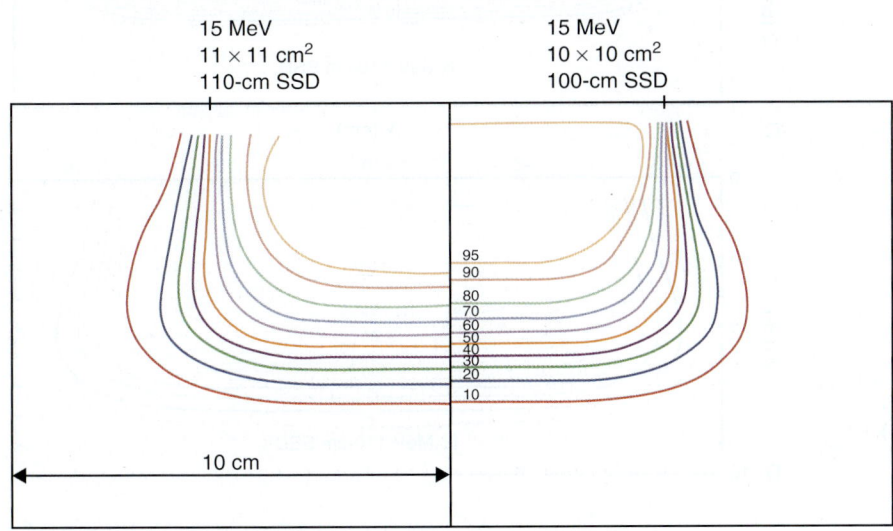

15 MeV
11 × 11 cm²
110-cm SSD

15 MeV
10 × 10 cm²
100-cm SSD

95
90
80
70
60
50
40
30
20
10

10 cm

FIGURE 8.3. Source-to-surface distance (SSD) dependence of depth dose. Comparison of isodose plots for 15-MeV beam, 10 by 10 cm² at 100-cm SSD with 11 by 11 cm² field at 110-cm SSD. (From Hogstrom KR. Clinical electron-beam dosimetry: basic dosimetry data. In: Purdy JA, ed. *Advances in radiation oncology physics: dosimetry, treatment planning, and brachytherapy. Woodbury*: American Institute of Physics, 1992:390–429. Copyright © 1992 by American Association of Physicists in Medicine. Reprinted by permission.)

Flatness and symmetry are evaluated inside the penumbra, which usually is ensured by setting the boundaries of evaluation 2 cm inside the collimating edge ($2\sqrt{2}$ cm along diagonals). When physicist perform acceptance-tests for a treatment machine, and during subsequent annual reviews, they use the AAPM Task Group 142 recommendations of 2% symmetry and 5% flatness.[35] This is usually performed for each energy with an average-size applicator but should be tested for each applicator during acceptance. Subsequently, the profiles acquired during acceptance should be reviewed monthly and be consistent to within 1% of the acceptance values.[35,36]

Penumbra of electron beams is predetermined by the design of the beam flattening system, the air gap between the final collimator, and the scatter of electrons in water. The penumbra is a function of depth and is the root mean square addition of two penumbral components: one the result of the air gap and one the result of scatter in the water.[6] This dependence is complex but can be appreciated qualitatively by the illustration in Figure 8.4, which compares isodose plots for normal (100 cm) and extended (110 cm) SSD at 6 and 16 MeV, respectively. These data show that penumbra grows in a nonlinear fashion with depth, that air gap is more significant at the lower energies, and that scatter in water dominates at the higher energies. Fortunately, the complex dependence of penumbra can be modeled accurately in treatment planning systems using the pencil beam or more sophisticated dose algorithms.[29,32,34,37]

Isodose Plots

Combining depth dose with OARs results in the 3-D dose distribution, and the properties of the 3-D dose distribution can be appreciated by viewing 2-D isodose contour plots in a plane containing the central axis and a major axis. Examples of these plots for a 15 by 15 cm² field are illustrated in Figure 8.5. As field width decreases or increases, the penumbra shape changes insignificantly because it is most significantly influenced by air gaps and by collimation type. Collimating on the skin, for example, reduces penumbra significantly.

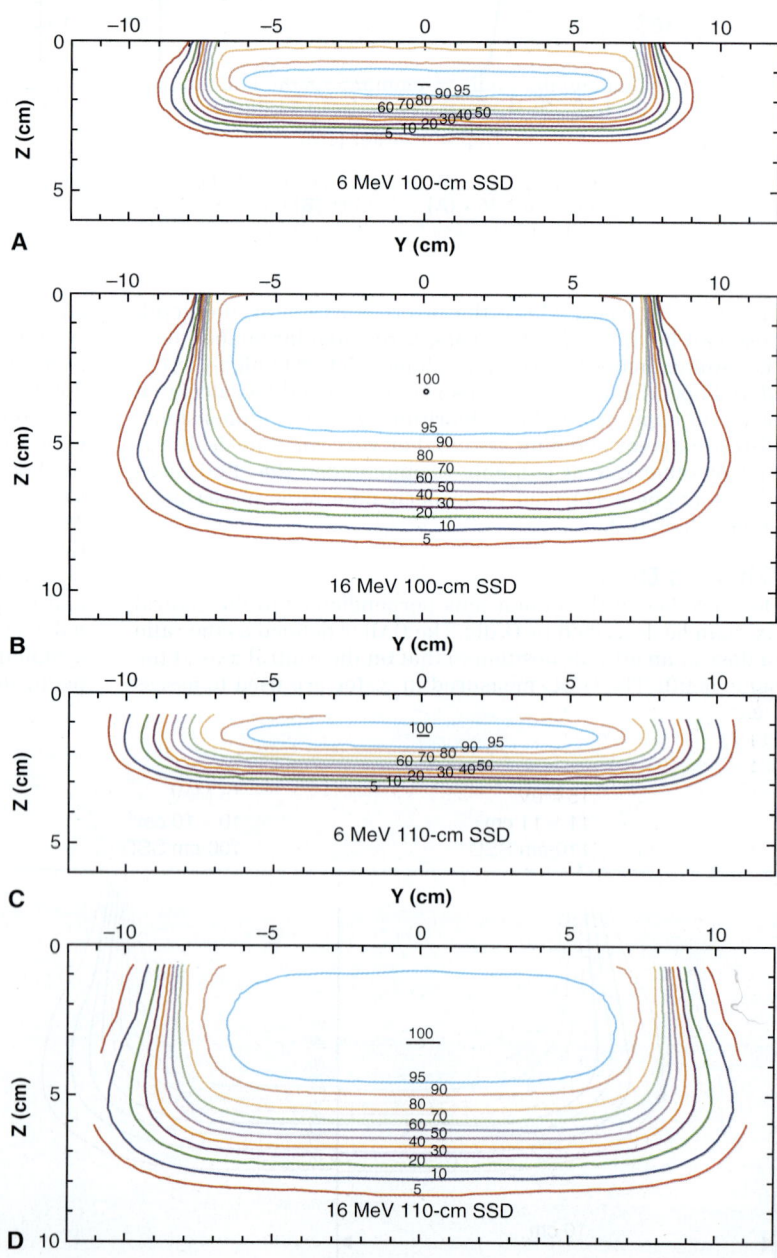

FIGURE 8.4. Variation of dose distribution with energy and SSD. Isodose plots (5% to 100%) in water for open 15 by 15 cm² applicator and for 6 MeV, 100-cm SSD **(A)**; 16 MeV, 100-cm SSD **(B)**; 6 MeV, 110-cm SSD **(C)**; and 16 MeV, 110-cm SSD **(D)** (Varian Clinac 2100C). (Courtesy of Varian, Palo Alto, CA.)

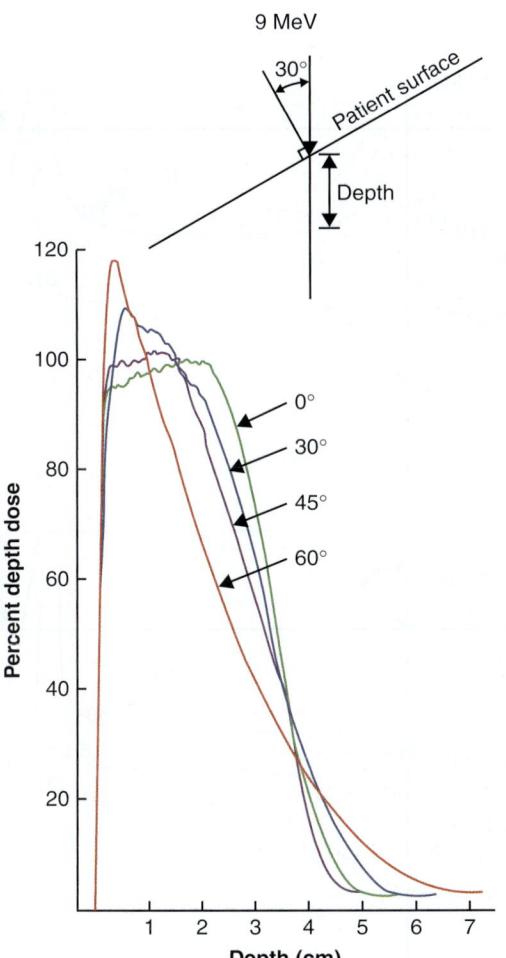

FIGURE 8.5. Effect of angle of incidence on depth dose. Dose versus depth for a 9-MeV beam incident on water angled 0 degrees to 60 degrees from the normal. (From Ekstrand KE, Dixon RL. The problem of obliquely incident beams in electron-beam treatment planning. *Med Phys* 1982;9[2]:276–278. Copyright © 1982 American Association of Physicists in Medicine. Reprinted by permission of John Wiley & Sons, Inc.)

Data required for isodose contours are acquired for an inclusive spread of field sizes at each energy. Two-dimensional isodose contour plots and data are useful for manual treatment planning, input data required by dose algorithms, verification of dose calculated by a treatment planning system, and quality assurance standards.[29,30,38]

DOSE IN THE HETEROGENEOUS PATIENT

For most clinical circumstances, the ideal irradiation condition is for the electron beam to be incidentally normal to a flat surface with underlying homogeneous soft tissues. The dose distribution for this condition, similar to that for a water phantom described previously, contains a reasonably uniform dose inside the penumbra from the surface to R_{90}, and it has the sharpest possible falloff laterally and with depth. As the angle of incidence deviates from normal, as the surface becomes irregular, and as internal heterogeneous tissues (e.g., air, lung, and bone) become present, the qualities of the dose distribution degrade.[39] Internal heterogeneities can change the depth of beam penetration as a result of differences in the rate of energy loss, which can result in PTV underdose and critical structure overdose. Both irregular surfaces and internal heterogeneities create

changes in side-scatter equilibrium, producing volumes of increased dose (hot spots) and decreased dose (cold spots), potentially leading to an increased dose to critical structures and decreased dose to the PTV.[3,39] These perturbations can be reduced or eliminated by modifying the treatment technique.

Irregular Surfaces

Two geometries that illustrate the effects on the dose distribution caused by an irregular patient surface are the sloped skin surface and the stepped skin surface. Figure 8.5 illustrates changes in the depth-dose curve as a result of nonnormal incidence of an electron beam onto a flat surface. Compared with normal incidence, the nonnormal incident electron beam, central-axis, depth-dose curve shows the following: (a) an increased surface dose, (b) an increased maximum dose, (c) a decreased penetration of the therapeutic dose (R_{90}), and (d) an increased range of penetration.[30,40] These changes can be clinically significant, particularly at angles of incidence >30 degrees from the normal. Such conditions can occur when irradiating curved patient surfaces with large fields (e.g., chest wall, limbs, neck, and scalp). In addition, it should be appreciated that the depth of R_{90} is specified along the central axis of the beam; and if the depth is taken perpendicular to the surface, then the depth is further reduced (approximately) by a factor cos (φ), where φ is the deviation of the incident angle from the normal.

Any time a sharp gradient (stepped surface) occurs on the patient's surface, side-scatter equilibrium will be lost, resulting in a cold spot beneath the proximal surface and a hot spot beneath the distal surface.[32,39,41,42] This can occur as a result of a sharp bolus edge, surgical defects, or within normal anatomy. For example, in the use of a uniform-thickness bolus that partially covers a field, a 90-degree step can result in hot or cold spots as great as 20%, as illustrated in Figure 8.6. In such a case, the bolus should be tapered as much as possible. The results of a 45-degree tapered bolus in Figure 8.6 show a reduction in the hot spot but more significantly an increased coverage of the 90% isodose contour. The nose is a protrusion that creates a cold spot, often the location of the tumor.[5,33,39] The ear canal (Fig. 8.7) and surgical voids, which are characterized by a depression in the patient's surface, can result in hot spots in excess of 50%, depending on void dimension and beam energy.[43,44] Such depressions normally should be filled with some type of bolus material. Normal anatomy contains many irregular surface depressions and protrusions (e.g., the ear canal and the nose, respectively) and should be accounted for by accurate treatment planning.

Air Cavities

The influence of an internal air cavity is illustrated in Figure 8.8, which compares isodose contours beneath an air cavity to those without the air cavity. Results show that (a) the isodose contours in the shadow of air are shifted distally, (b) the dose beneath the air cavity increases as a result of loss of side-scatter equilibrium, and (c) the influence of the air increases laterally with depth. Internal air cavities of clinical interest primarily occur in treatment of the head and neck (e.g., nasal passages, ethmoid sinuses, maxillary sinuses, larynx, and mastoids).[32,39]

Another significant effect is the reduction in dose in unit density tissue lateral to an air cavity. Electrons scattering from the unit density tissue into the air are not replaced because air is unable to scatter an equal amount back into the unit density tissue. Frequently, nose tumors can spread into the septum, in which case bolus should be used to eliminate or reduce underdosing.

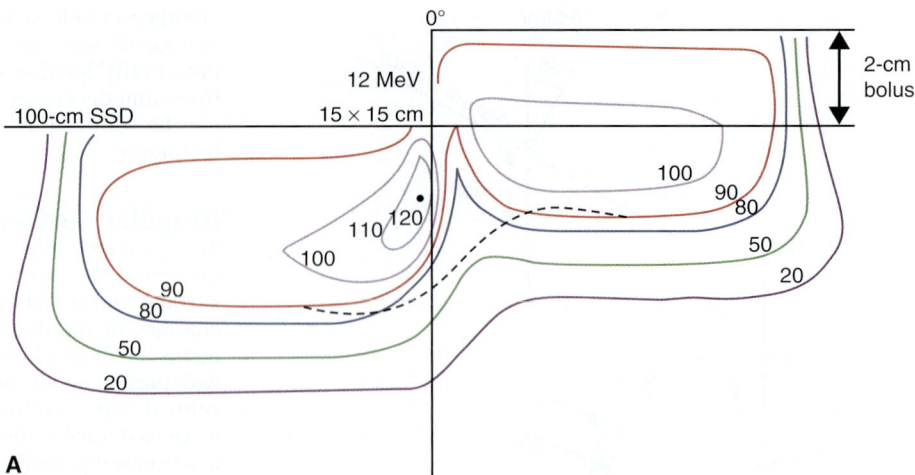

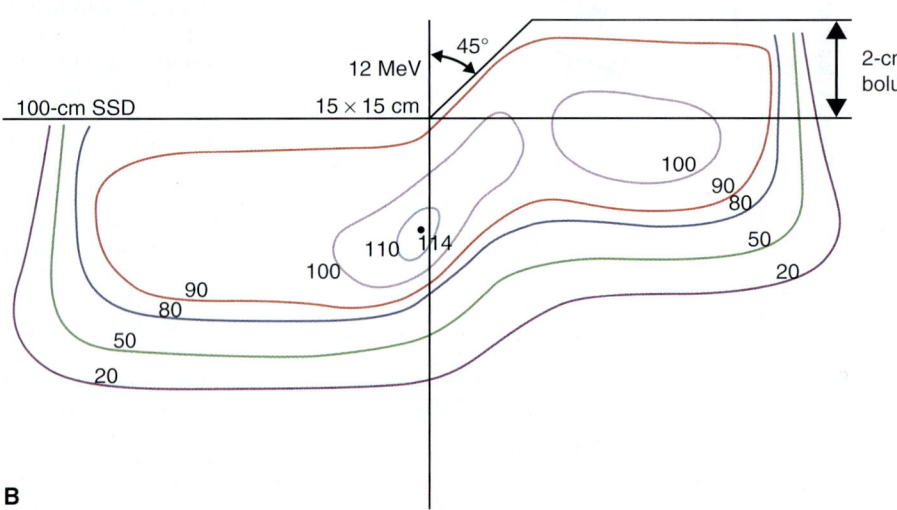

FIGURE 8.6. Effect of irregular patient surface on dose distribution. Plot of isodose contours for a 12-MeV, 15 by 15 cm² beam incident on water at 100-cm source-to-surface distance (SSD) having a stepped surface resulting from a 2-cm slab of bolus **(A)** and a beveled edge (45 degree) on the stepped surface **(B)**. The *dashed line* in the top figure shows the location of the 90% isodose contour in the bottom one. (From Hogstrom KR. Treatment planning in electron-beam therapy. In: Vaeth JM, Meyer JL, eds. *Frontiers of radiation therapy and oncology vol. 25: the role of high energy electrons in the treatment of cancer.* Basel: S. Karger AG, 1991:30–52. Copyright © 1991 Karger Publishers, Basel, Switzerland. Reprinted by permission.)

FIGURE 8.7. Impact of irregular surface anatomy on dose distribution. A 15-MeV electron beam irradiates the left side of a patient treated for dermal squamous carcinoma with perineural invasion. A beeswax bolus protects the posterior cranial fossa and the maxillary sinus. Isodose contours, expressed as a percentage of given dose, show how the ear canal results in an unacceptable hot spot of 160% to the middle ear **(A)** and how filling the ear canal with bolus (saline solution) eliminates that hot spot **(B)**. The residual hot spot of 125% is a result of the external ear. (Reprinted from Morrison WH, Wong PF, Starkschall G, et al. Water bolus for electron irradiation of the ear canal. *Int J Radiat Oncol Biol Phys* 1995;33[2]:479–483. Copyright © 1995 Elsevier. With permission.)

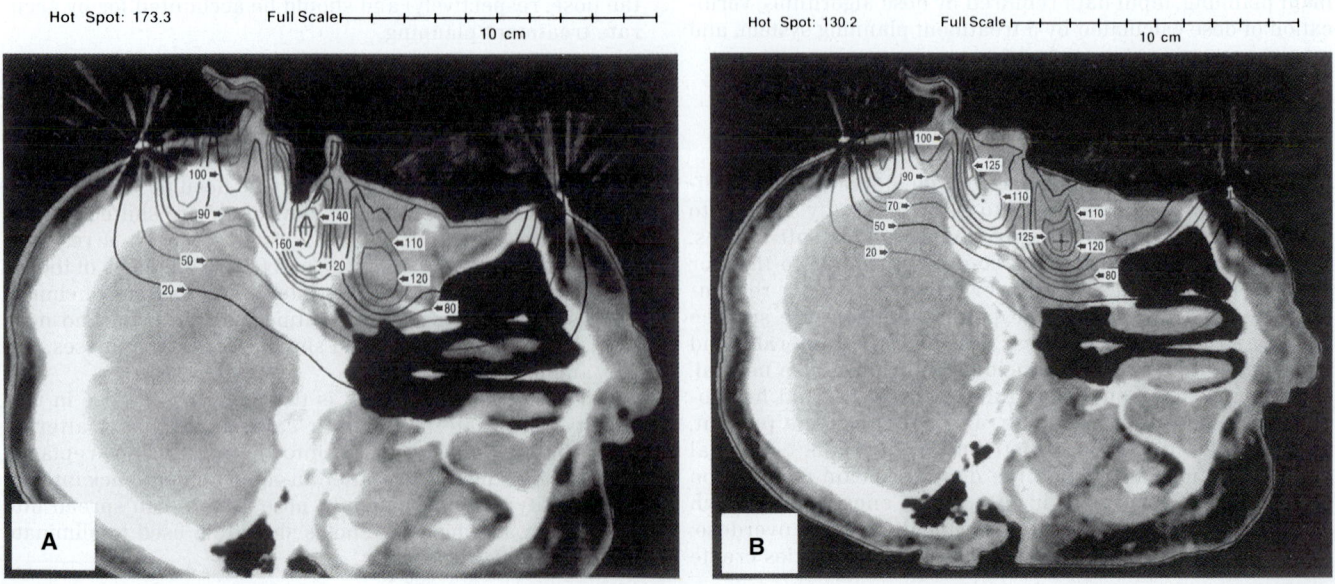

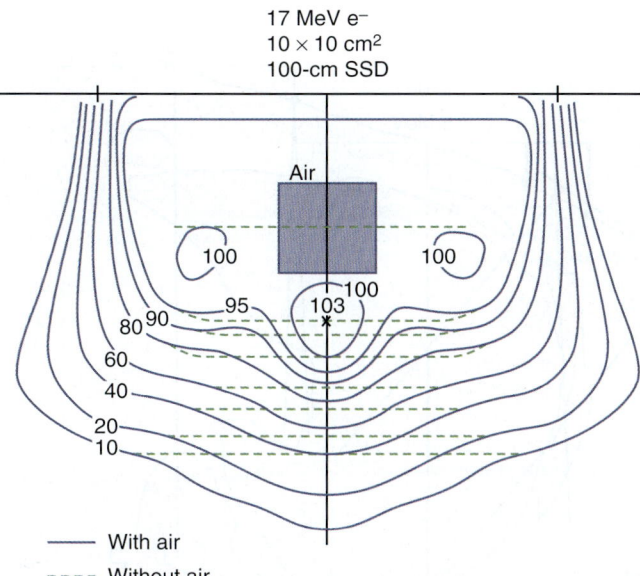

17 MeV e⁻
10 × 10 cm²
100-cm SSD

FIGURE 8.8. Effect of internal air cavity on underlying dose distribution. Dose calculated by the pencil beam algorithm (PBA) for a 2 by 2 cm² cylinder of air located 2 cm below the surface in water is compared to that in its absence. (From Hogstrom KR. Dosimetry of electron heterogeneities. In: Wright AE, Boyer AL, eds. *Advances in radiation therapy treatment planning*. New York: American Institute of Physics, 1983:223–243, with permission. Copyright © 1983 by American Association of Physicists in Medicine. Reprinted by permission.)

Lung

In lung, electrons can penetrate three to four times farther than in unit density tissue. This is demonstrated in Figure 8.9, where isodose contours from a typical electron chest wall treatment are compared with those in which the lung is assumed unit density. Assuming a given dose of 50 Gy, the 40% isodose contour corresponds to 20 Gy, approximately the threshold for pneumonitis, if significant lung volume is irradiated. Ignoring the low density of lung would grossly underestimate the volume of lung receiving more than 20 Gy.[32]

This effect increases with energy. For example, increasing the beam energy from 9 to 12 MeV results in an additional 1.5 cm of penetration in water-like tissue (electrons lose energy at a rate of ~2 MeV per centimeter in water), and this corresponds to as much as 6.0 cm in lung (assuming a lung physical density of 25%). Consider the patient whose chest wall thickness requires an energy of 10 MeV for treatment and that 12 MeV must be selected. This results in as much as 4 cm in depth of needless irradiation in lung, unless 1 cm of bolus is used to effectively lower the energy incident on the patient to 10 MeV.

Care must be taken when irradiating targets where the lung is immediately distal, such as with entire chest wall post-mastectomy irradiation.

Bone

Interactions of electrons with bone are complex and interesting. The influence of bone is illustrated in Figure 8.10, which compares isodose contours beneath the hard bone to those without the bone. The results show that:

1. The isodose contours in the shadow of the bone are shifted proximally,
2. Dose outside (inside) the bone–water interface increases (decreases) by approximately 5% as a result of loss of side-scatter equilibrium, and
3. The lateral dimension of the region having its dose perturbed by the bone increases with depth.

Living bones are not uniformly dense throughout their cross-section, and in most cases, their edges are not parallel to the incident beam. Both differences decrease the influence of bone in generating inhomogeneity in the patient's dose distribution. Dense bones that significantly affect the dose distribution include the mandible, bones of the skull (e.g., frontal bone and zygoma in orbit treatment or temporal bone in treatment of parotid), clavicles, and vertebral processes (e.g., craniospinal irradiation).

One might ask, "What is the clinical significance of the increase in dose in or around bone because of increased scatter?" The maximum dose increase expected as a result of backscattered electrons is 5%, and the maximum dose increase expected inside bone and in adjacent exit tissues is approximately 7%.[45] These increases represent maximum dose estimates because actual bones are not as dense through and through as are the bone substitute in which these data were taken. These estimates of the increased dose are not expected to be clinically significant. In fact, untoward effects in or around bone that can be attributed to dosimetry have not been observed in patients treated with electron beam therapy.

DOSE PRESCRIPTION AND CALCULATION OF MONITOR UNITS

Dose Prescription

It is recommended that dose be prescribed to given dose or 90% of given dose. Intermediate or lower prescription (95%, 85%, 80%) can be prescribed if the energy (typically stepped in 3- to 4-MeV increments) choices are too coarse to maintain a single baseline prescription recipe. Given dose is defined as the maximum central-axis dose in a water phantom at the SSD of the patient for the energy, applicator, and field size identical to that used for patient treatment. If the field shape is irregular, then the field size is taken to be a rectangular field representative of the irregular field shape. The most representative rectangular field is not well defined; however, Hogstrom et al.[37] have provided one methodology for determining its estimate.

It is recommended that the dose is prescribed to given dose or a percentage of it and not to a point in the patient. It is quite possible that a dose prescription point in the patient could be in a region of increased or decreased dose because of tissue heterogeneity or irregular surface, which could result in PTV underdose or overdose, respectively.

Calculation of Monitor Units

Monitor units can be determined by

$$MU = \frac{D_{\text{prescribed}} / \%D}{O(E, C, LxW, SSD)}, \qquad (2)$$

where $D_{\text{prescribed}}$ is the prescribed dose, $\%D$ is the percentage of given dose to which dose is prescribed (e.g., 90%), and $O(E, C, LxW, SSD)$ is the output (dose per monitor unit) for a beam of energy E, applicator C, field size LxW, and SSD. To use this methodology, the medical physicist must measure dose output as a function of square field size and SSD for each energy–applicator combination at the time of commissioning the accelerator. Output for rectangular fields can be determined using the square-root method of Mills et al.[14,46] and Shiu et al.[31]:

$$O(E, C, LxW, SSD) = [O(E, C, LxL, SSD) \cdot O(E, C, WxW, SSD)]^{1/2}. \qquad (3)$$

Output for rectangular fields also can be determined using an equivalent square method[30,33,47,48]; however, Biggs et al.[47] recommend limiting this method to an aspect ratio (L:W)

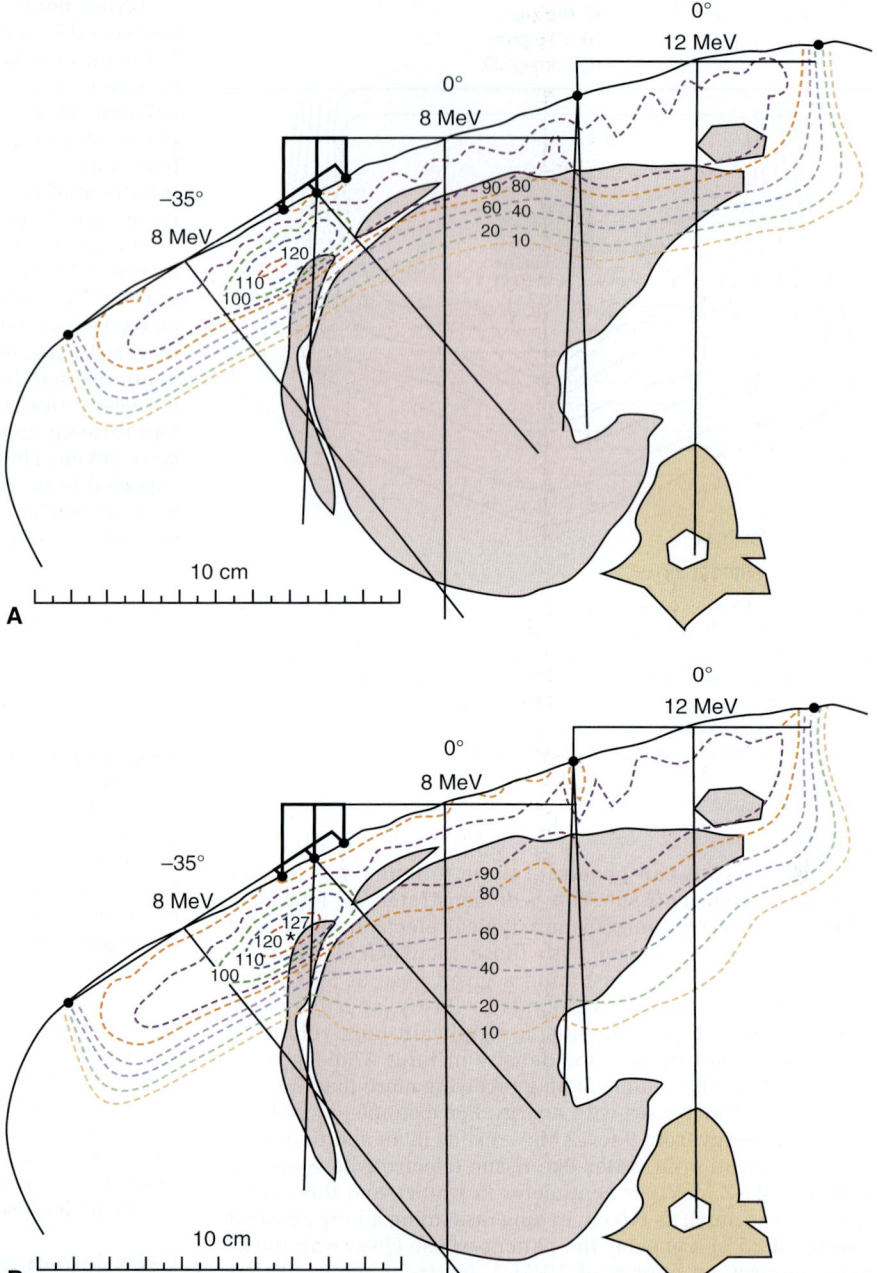

FIGURE 8.9. Effect of lung on dose distribution underlying chest wall. Comparison of dose calculated by the pencil beam algorithm (PBA) for 8-MeV chest wall irradiation, assuming patient's water **(A)** and heterogeneous anatomy **(B)** based on computed tomography data.

of 2:1. The square-root method is not limited to the aspect ratio, and Shiu et al.[31] have shown it to be more accurate. Figure 8.11 illustrates beam output data at 9 MeV for four common applicators used on the Varian Clinac 2100C (Varian Medical Systems, Palo Alto, CA) at 100 cm SSD.

Output at extended SSD can be determined by either the air-gap method or the effective-source method.[30] The effective-source method is covered in detail by Khan.[48] The air-gap method has a sounder physical basis. Although both methods give similar answers, only the air-gap method will be covered here.[33] Output at extended SSD is given by the product of output at the nominal SSD (SSD_0), the air-gap factor (fair), and an inverse square term,

$$O(E, C, LxW, SSD) = O(E, C, LxW, SSD_0) f_{air}(E, LxW, SSD)$$

$$\times \left(\frac{SSD_o + R_{100}}{SSD + R_{100}} \right) \quad (4)$$

f_{air} is determined by measuring dose output for square fields at the extended SSD and then solving equation 4. For rectangular fields, the air-gap factor is determined using the square-root method[31]:

$$f_{air}(E, LxW, SSD) = \sqrt{f_{air}(E, LxL, SSD) \cdot f_{air}(E, WxW, SSD)} \quad (5)$$

As f_{air} is assumed independent of applicator, the dose output needs to be measured only for the smallest applicator that contains the square field size. Figure 8.12 plots the square field air-gap factors for the 9-MeV beam of the Varian Clinac 2100C for SSD from 100 to 120 cm. For a more detailed explanation of dose output and sample calculations of monitor units for electron beams, refer to Hogstrom et al.[34] Another practical option is to fix incremented SSDs to be used clinically (i.e., 100, 105, 110, 115 cm) and establish tabular outputs for each energy–applicator SSD combination.

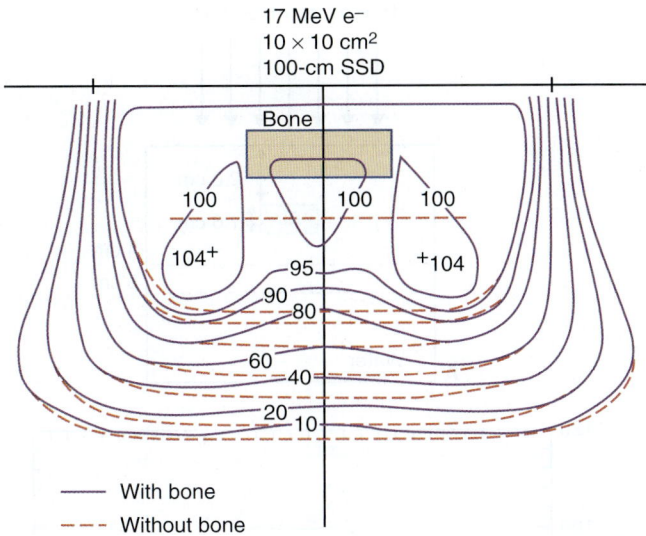

17 MeV e⁻
10 × 10 cm²
100-cm SSD

—— With bone
- - - Without bone

FIGURE 8.10. Effect of hard bone on underlying dose distribution. Dose calculated by the pencil beam algorithm (PBA) for a 3 by 1 cm² cylinder of hard bone substitute located 1 cm below the surface in water is compared to that in its absence. (From Hogstrom KR. Dosimetry of electron heterogeneities. In: Wright AE, Boyer AL, eds. *Advances in radiation therapy treatment planning.* New York: American Institute of Physics, 1983:223–243, with permission. Copyright © 1983 by American Association of Physicists in Medicine. Reprinted by permission.)

CALCULATION OF DOSE IN PATIENT

Standards for Patient Dose Calculations

Sound treatment planning decisions require accurate dose calculation in the patient. Therefore, the following recommendations are made for electron beam treatment planning. First, dose should be calculated in the full three dimensions to allow for evaluation of dose homogeneity in the PTV, coverage of the PTV by the 90% isodose contour, and dose to critical structures. Second, the dose algorithm should account for patient heterogeneity. Failure to properly account for patient heterogeneity can result in failure to appreciate dose heterogeneity, PTV underdose, or normal-tissue overdose.[5,39,49] Third, the dose algorithm should be accurate; and for those conditions for which this is not the case, physicians and physicists should discuss the proper interpretation of the dose calculations.

To expand on the final recommendation, a dose algorithm must meet certain criteria to be most effective in the clinic.[50]

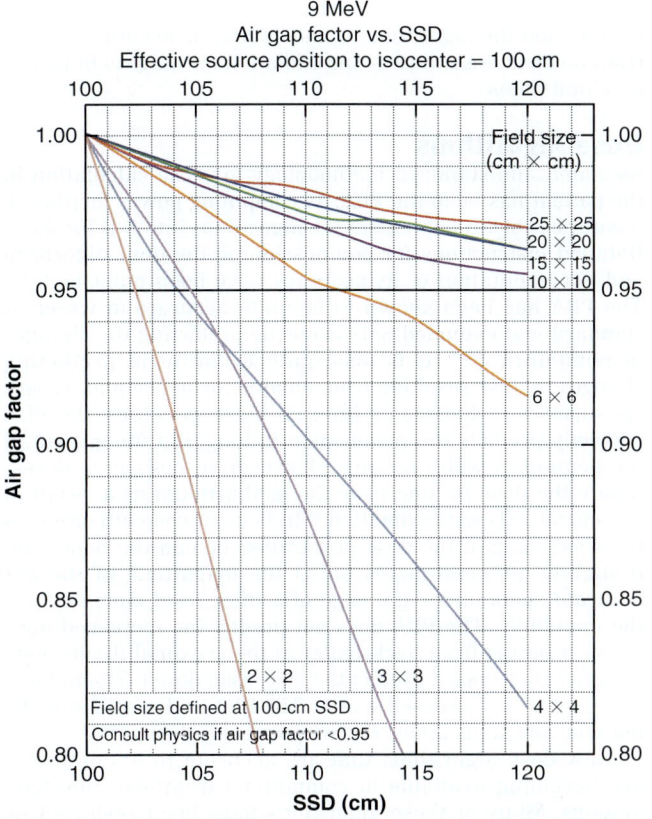

9 MeV
Air gap factor vs. SSD
Effective source position to isocenter = 100 cm

Field size defined at 100-cm SSD
Consult physics if air gap factor <0.95

FIGURE 8.12. Dependence of air-gap factors on source-to-surface distance (SSD) and field size. Plot of f_{air} versus SSD for field sizes ranging from 2 by 2 to 25 by 25 cm² and for the 9-MeV beam (Varian Clinac 2100C).(Courtesy of Varian, Palo Alto, CA.)

First, it should be accurate to within 4% in regions of low dose gradients or within 2 mm in regions of high dose gradient (e.g., penumbra or depth-dose falloff region).[38,51] Second, the dose algorithm should be commissioned easily by a qualified medical physicist. Third, the accuracy of the dose algorithm should be well documented. Since 1981, the PBA has best this requirement. Presently, several new, more accurate algorithms, both analytical- and Monte Carlo–based, are being implemented into commercial treatment planning systems and will replace or supplement the PBA in due time.[52] Regardless

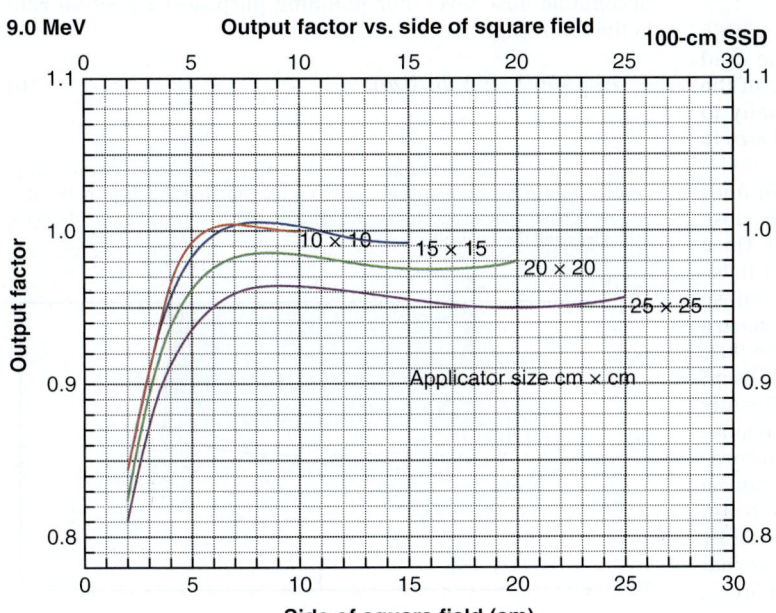

9.0 MeV   Output factor vs. side of square field   100-cm SSD

Applicator size cm × cm

FIGURE 8.11. Field-size dependence of output (dose/monitor unit). Plot of output factor (cGy/MU) versus side of square field from 2 by 2 cm² to the open applicator for four applicators and for the 9-MeV beam of a Varian Clinac 2100C. (Courtesy of Varian, Palo Alto, CA.)

of the algorithm, it is the medical physicist's responsibility to commission the algorithm, to understand its accuracy, and to train medical dosimetrists and radiation oncologists in its use and limitations.

Dose Algorithms

As stated, the standard methodology for dose calculation in the patient has been the PBA. As computing power increased, it was possible to implement the algorithms into 3-D format.[53] Detailed instructions for commissioning the dose algorithm and documentation of its accuracy have been published.[5,6,50] The PBA has been shown to be quite accurate in water at standard and extended SSD, correctly predicting the changes in penumbra.[29,32,34] It is also quite accurate in predicting changes in dose resulting from oblique incidence and irregular surfaces.[5,50] Regarding internal heterogeneities, the PBA correctly predicts the penetration in lung and the growth of the penumbra width in lung[50]; however, it tends to underestimate the dose in lung near the mediastinum as a result of its central-axis approximation.[50] In bone, it correctly predicts the shortening of the dose penetration behind the bone, and it slightly underestimates (<5%) the magnitude of the *hot* and *cold* spots under the edge of a thick hard bone such as the mandible.[5] The PBA does not predict the increased dose (<5%) resulting from backscatter at the proximal tissue–bone interface, nor does it predict the increased dose (>7%) in bone resulting from increased scatter. The PBA underestimates the hot and cold spots under the air–tissue interfaces.[5,50]

New dose algorithms that are accurate to 4% or better are becoming available in commercial treatment planning systems. Many of these algorithms have been reviewed by Hogstrom and Steadham.[50] One of these is the pencil beam redefinition algorithm (PBRA), whose commissioning is similar to that of the conventional PBA, although its accuracy is significantly improved.[54–56] Figure 8.13 illustrates the improvement of the PBRA.

Many of the newer algorithms are based on Monte Carlo methods, which allow them to be quite accurate.[57–61] Cygler et al.[52] published a report on the first commercial system using Monte Carlo–based electron calculations, demonstrating excellent results. Ding et al.[62] demonstrated outstanding results for a macro–Monte Carlo algorithm, along with a companion report showing superior results for Monte Carlo compared with PBA.[63]

TREATMENT PLANNING PRINCIPLES, TOOLS, AND METHODS

Electron therapy is usually restricted to a PTV that is within 6 cm distal from the patient's surface. Electrons may be used alone or in conjunction with photon beams. In the case of the former, the objective of the treatment planner is usually to select the appropriate beam direction, energy, and field size to provide as uniform a dose as possible to the PTV while delivering minimal dose to normal tissue and structures. To optimize dose homogeneity, the beam direction should be as close to normal incidence to the patient surface as practical. Once beam direction is specified, the selection of energy and field-size specification follows. Figure 8.14 compares the isodose contours in water with the beam edges and R_{90}. Electrons are unique in that the uniform region of dose lies inside the 90% isodose contour. Dose outside the 90% isodose contour falls off rapidly. However, the patient anatomy can differ significantly from water so that effects resulting from patient heterogeneity make the resulting treatment plan unacceptable, according to the original prescription. In addition, the PTV can be at a variable depth beneath the surface so that a single beam energy is inadequate. The treatment plan can be improved by utilization of special treatment aids such as skin or internal collimation, bolus, field abutment, or other special techniques.

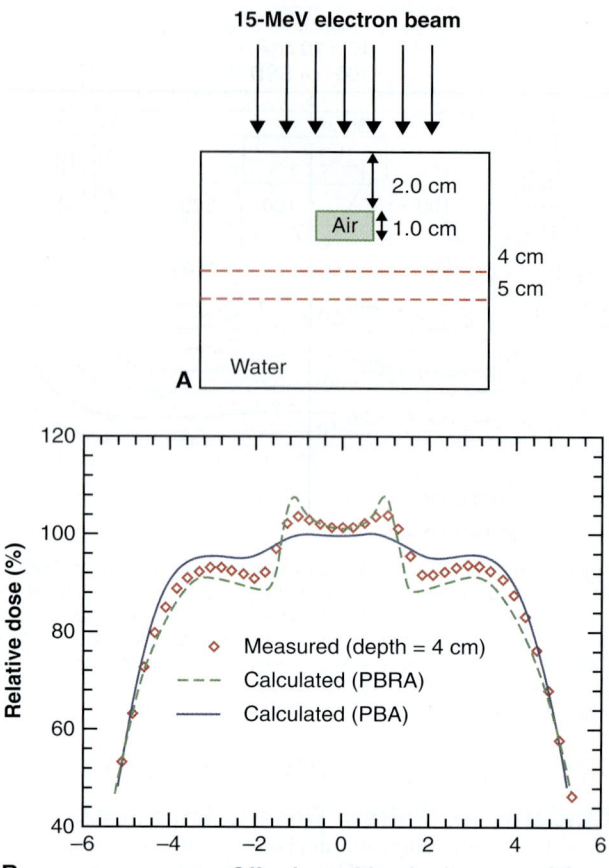

FIGURE 8.13. Evaluation of accuracy of dose algorithms below air cavity. **A:** Dose is measured distal to an internal air cavity. **B:** Measured dose profile at a depth of 4 cm is compared to that calculated by the pencil beam algorithm and the pencil beam redefinition algorithm. PBA, pencil beam algorithm; PRBA, pencil beam redefinition algorithm. (From Shiu AS, Hogstrom KR. Pencil-beam redefinition algorithm for electron dose distributions. *Med Phys* 1991;18[1]:7–18, with permission. Copyright © 1991 American Association of Physicists in Medicine. Reprinted by permission of John Wiley & Sons, Inc.)

Selection of Energy

The energy of the incident electron beam should be selected so that the distal surface of the 90% (of given dose) dose surface encompasses the PTV and that critical structures lie beyond the maximum penetration of the electrons or at an acceptable dose level. For planning purposes, a general rule is the following:

$$E_{p,0}(MeV) \sim 3.3 \cdot R_{90}(cm), \tag{6}$$

FIGURE 8.14. Plot of isodose curves for a 15-MeV, 10 by 10 cm² electron beam in water (source-to-surface distance, or SSD = 100 cm). Note the shape of the 90% isodose contour with respect to the shaded area, which is framed by the diverging field edges and the R_{90} depth.

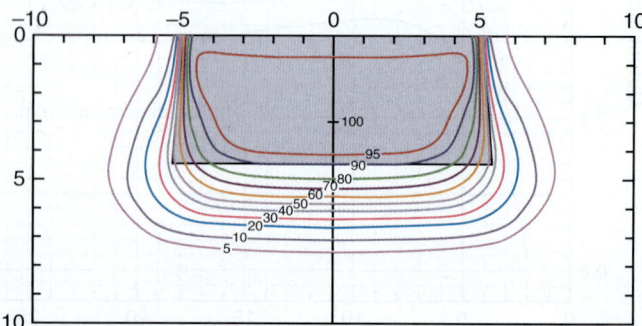

where $E_{p,0}$ is the most probable incident electron energy in MeV. The energy should be selected such that R_{90} just exceeds the maximum depth of the PTV. This approximation is true in water for field sizes large enough to have side-scatter equilibrium on the central axis. For small field sizes that do not have side-scatter equilibrium, R_{90} will be less; thus, a higher energy might be required. As well, heterogeneous tissue (e.g., bone or air) can affect the penetration, requiring greater or lesser energy, respectively.

Similarly, for planning purposes, a general rule is the following:

$$E_{p,0}(MeV) = 2 \cdot R_p(cm), \qquad (7)$$

where R_p is the practical range in centimeters of the electron beam.[32] The treatment planner can select an energy such that R_p is less than the minimal depth of a critical structure. This approximation has no field-size limitation; however, as before, heterogeneous tissue (e.g., bone, lung, or air) can affect the penetration, allowing greater or lesser energy.

As an example of how to use these general rules, consider treating the posterior cervical nodes of the neck with electrons to spare the spinal cord because its dose is already near tolerance. If the maximum depth of the nodes is 3 cm and the minimum depth of the spinal cord is 6 cm, then Eqs. (6) and (7) indicate that the minimum energy to cover the PTV is 9.9 MeV, and the maximum energy that protects the spinal cord is 12 MeV, respectively. Hence, beam energies in the range of 10 to 12 MeV are acceptable. In all cases, the energy of the beam should be confirmed by performing a 3-D dose calculation for the planned treatment using a CT representation of the patient. Bolus may be strategically used to tune the beam penetration either globally or in discrete areas and ideally should be placed at the time of the CT.

Design of Electron Collimation

Electron collimation consists of multiple collimating components; however, the electron field shape usually is defined by an applicator's collimating insert and/or skin collimation. Custom electron collimators are constructed from lead or low–melting-point lead alloy (Lipowitz metal). The lead thickness in millimeters required to stop the primary electrons equals one-half the incident of most probable energy of the electron beam in MeV.[29,30] To account for small variations in thickness resulting from the lead-sheet manufacturing process, a 1-mm surplus can be added. That is:

$$t_{pb}(mm) = 0.5 \cdot E_{p,0}(MeV) + 1 \qquad (8)$$

For example, an 18-MeV beam requires 10 mm of lead. Lipowitz metal is comprised mostly of lead along with bismuth that has a density of 20% less lead; therefore, its thickness should be increased by 20%. For example, an 18-MeV beam requires 12 mm of Lipowitz metal. Lipowitz metal collimating inserts usually are fabricated at a constant thickness—namely, that sufficient for the greatest energy on the treatment machine. For a machine whose maximum energy is 20 MeV, the Lipowitz metal thickness should be at least 13 mm.

Skin Collimation

The closer the field-defining collimator is to the patient, the sharper the beam's penumbra; hence, skin collimation provides the sharpest possible penumbra. Because of the significant effort often required to fabricate skin collimation, its use is restricted to applications for which it has the greatest benefit, for example, (a) small-field (<4 cm) treatments providing maximal protection to adjacent critical structures, (b) sharpening penumbra (c) reducing penumbra when treating at an extended air gap, (d) reducing penumbra in electron arc

therapy, and (e) where patient motion may be an issue. Proper use of skin collimation requires that it be in contact with the skin surface and that it extend sufficiently inwardly and outwardly to intercept the penumbra from upstream collimation.

Skin collimation absorption can be accomplished using lead sheets and normally is taken to be the minimum thickness necessary to shield the maximum. The maximum possible dose beneath the skin collimation occurs at the skin surface with no air gap between the two.[30,33] The transmitted dose, which is the result of bremsstrahlung photons from the incident beam and those generated by electrons stopping in the lead, is slightly greater than that with no lead present. It is recommended that a table of measured dose under the lead, as a function of lead thickness, is available for each beam energy.[29] As the air gap between the lead and the patient increases, the transmitted dose to the patient decreases. These values can be measured at the time of beam commissioning. If not, and for cases where precise determination of dose beneath a block is critical, *in vivo* dosimetry (e.g., thermoluminescent dosimetry) should be used.

In designing the shape of the aperture of a collimating insert, due consideration is made for the penumbra. Typically, there is approximately a 1-cm margin between the projected edge of the collimator and outer boundary of target volume when both are projected to the isocenter. This margin varies with energy, depth, and air gap; and it only can be appreciated by utilization of isodose curves (Figs. 8.4 and 8.14). Again, the adequacy of the margin between the aperture and PTV should be confirmed by performing 3-D dose calculations using CT images.

The utility of skin collimation for small-field treatments is illustrated in Figure 8.15. A 6-MeV, 3 by 3 cm² field with a 10-cm air gap (collimator to surface) is essentially all penumbra, resulting in an unsatisfactory dose distribution. However,

FIGURE 8.15. Impact of skin collimation for small electron fields. Isodose plots are compared for results of a computer simulation of a 6-MeV electron beam in water for a 3 by 3 cm² field formed by an applicator insert 10 cm above the patient **(A)** and a 3 by 3 cm² field formed by collimation at the surface with a 6 by 6 cm² applicator insert 10 cm above the patient **(B)**. (From Hogstrom KR. Clinical electron-beam dosimetry: basic dosimetry data. In: Purdy JA, ed. Advances in radiation oncology physics: dosimetry, treatment planning, and brachytherapy. Woodbury: American Institute of Physics, 1992:390–429. Copyright © 1992 by American Association of Physicists in Medicine. Reprinted by permission.)

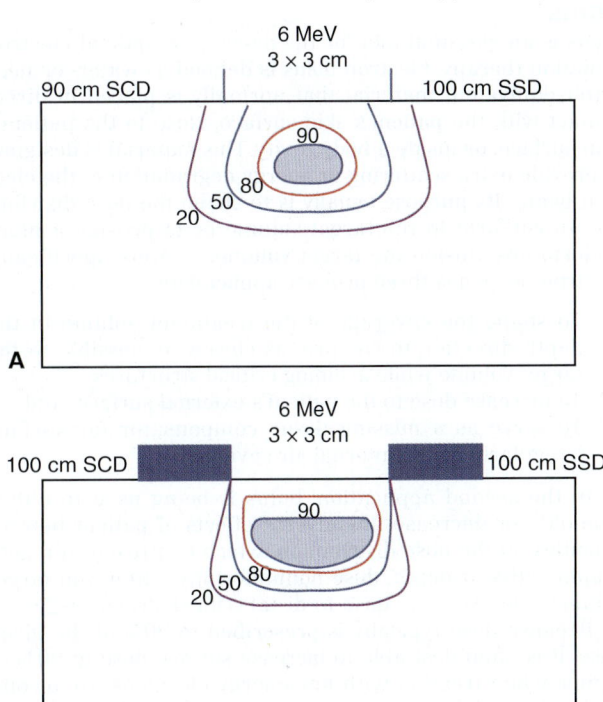

by opening the collimator to 6 by 6 cm² and then forming the 3 by 3 cm² field using skin collimation, the dose distribution becomes clinically satisfactory. This application is used for treatment of the eyelid, nose, and other small target volumes.

In the presence of skin collimation, the depth dose is approximated by that for the field size on the skin surface (i.e., that defined by the skin collimator). In contrast, the dose output is approximated by that for the field-size incident on the skin collimation (i.e., that defined by the applicator cutout). For the example in Figure 8.15, the depth dose is taken to be that of the 3 by 3 cm² field; the dose output is taken to be that of the 6 by 6 cm² field. This simple approximation slightly overestimates dose output, if the depths of maximum dose for the two field sizes differ. In such a case, the output of the larger field is multiplied by the depth-dose factor of the larger field at the depth of maximum dose of the smaller field.[34]

Multileaf Collimation

The use of existing photon multileaf collimators (MLCs) to modulate electron beams has been shown to be somewhat feasible, although a report by Klein et al.[64] showed that an SSD of 70 cm was necessary to provide clinical acceptable fields using the photon MLC. This is because of the dispersion of the electrons in air. They performed a feasibility study of using existing photon MLC to modulate electron beams, which was shown to be somewhat feasible. An important aspect from that work demonstrated that when using existing photon MLC to produce narrow electron beam segments, the large generated penumbra could be an advantage in terms of beam matching.

The other possibility is not to use the existing photon MLC but rather to have a tertiary electron MLC system that is closer to the patient, thereby narrowing the penumbra that is produced when the MLC is far from the patient. Lee et al.[65] found that replacing air with helium in the treatment head made a significant impact in predicted dose distributions. Karlsson et al.[66] demonstrated that penumbra, effective-source position, field shape, and matching could be optimized by replacing air with helium in the treatment head below the MLC leaves and by shifting the position of the scattering foils, monitor chamber, and MLC position.

Bolus

Bolus is an essential tool for the delivery of optimal electron radiation therapy. Electron bolus is defined as water- or near water-equivalent material that normally is placed in direct contact with the patient's skin surface, close to the patient's skin surface, or inside a body cavity. This material is designed to provide extra scattering or energy degradation of the electron beam. Its purpose usually is to shape the dose distribution to conform to the target volume or to provide a more uniform dose inside the target volume.[29,32] More specifically, electron bolus has three primary applications:

1. To shape the coverage of the treatment volume in the depth direction to conform as closely as possible to the target volume while avoiding critical structures,
2. To increase dose to the patient's external surface, and
3. To serve as a missing tissue compensator for surface irregularities and internal air cavities.

In the second application, bolus is being used to either eliminate or decrease the adverse effects of patient heterogeneities on the dose distribution, which can result in a geographic miss at depth, dose nonuniformity within the target volume, and excessive dose-to-critical structures.[29,32]

Because dose typically is prescribed to 90% of the given dose, it is often desirable to increase surface dose to 90% or higher when treating with low-energy electrons. To accomplish this, a higher energy beam is selected and a uniformly thick bolus is placed on or near the skin surface. The surface

TABLE 8.2 VALUES OF SURFACE DOSE AND THERAPEUTIC DEPTH FOR VARIOUS ENERGY–BOLUS COMBINATIONS						
Superflab Thickness (cm)	**0.0**	**0.3**	**0.5**	**1.0**	**1.5**	**2.0**
Energy: 6 MeV						
D_s (%)	72	79	83	93	100	–
R_{90} (cm)	2.0	1.7	1.5	1.0	0.5	–
Energy: 9 MeV						
D_s (%)	78	83	85	89	95	99
R_{90} (cm)	3.0	2.7	2.5	2.0	1.5	1.0
Energy: 12 MeV						
D_s (%)	83	88	89	91	94	96
R_{90} (cm)	4.0	3.7	3.5	3.0	2.5	2.0
Energy: 16 MeV						
D_s (%)	87	92	93	96	97	98
R_{90} (cm)	5.0	4.7	4.5	4.0	3.5	3.0
Energy: 20 MeV						
D_s (%)	91	96	97	98	99	100
R_{90} (cm)	6.1	5.8	5.6	5.1	4.6	4.1

dose of the higher energy electron beam is greater, and the bolus places the skin at a deeper depth, further increasing the surface dose. The energy–bolus thickness combination is selected to place R_{90} at the prescription depth while increasing the surface dose (D_s) to near 90%. To assist in usage of this technique, a table that allows selection of the optimal energy–bolus thickness combination is recommended. Table 8.2 illustrates a sample for the five electron beam energies of a typical radiation therapy machine.

Two bolus methods are used for this function. One places flexible sheet material (e.g., Superflab) directly on the skin surface. Materials are approximately water equivalent and come in thickness increments of 0.3 to 4 cm. It is particularly useful for chest wall irradiation, for both fixed beam and arced-beam therapies. In some treatments, the bolus is used for only a portion of the field, in which case care must be taken to ensure that the edge of the bolus is tapered to reduce the magnitude of the hot or cold spot created by the surface irregularity (such as is seen in Fig. 8.6).[29,32]

For highly irregular or sensitive skin surfaces, which often are encountered in head and neck or postsurgical irradiations, it is advantageous to have a rigid bolus sheet (often referred to as a scatter plate because it not only degrades the energy of the electron beam but also scatters the beam) close to but not necessarily in direct contact with the patient.[32] For such cases, standard thicknesses of polymethylmethacrylate (PMMA) (0.125 to 0.25 inches) are placed perpendicular to the beam. To restore a sharp penumbra, skin collimation usually is recommended with use of the scatter-plate bolus method. Rules for using skin collimation with the bolus have been discussed by Hogstrom.[32] It is important that the bolus be in contact or close to the patient because too large of an air gap can create an exceedingly large penumbra.

Bolus is considered part of the beam; however, it also can be considered part of the patient, effectively shortening the SSD. For uniform bolus thickness (t), it is recommended to adjust the dose output for inverse square.[34] That is:

$$O_{bolus} = O \cdot \left[\frac{SSD + t + R_{100}}{SSD + R_{100}} \right]^2 \qquad (9)$$

A more sophisticated use of bolus is to design custom bolus for the purpose of electron conformal therapy. In this application, the bolus usually is designed to conform the 90% isodose line to the PTV while minimizing dose to nearby critical structures and maintaining dose uniformity as much as possible within the 90% dose contour. Proper design of custom bolus requires use of a 3-D treatment planning system[67] that utilizes bolus design operators[68] and a 3-D PBA.[53] The methodology of bolus design to optimize target coverage and critical structure

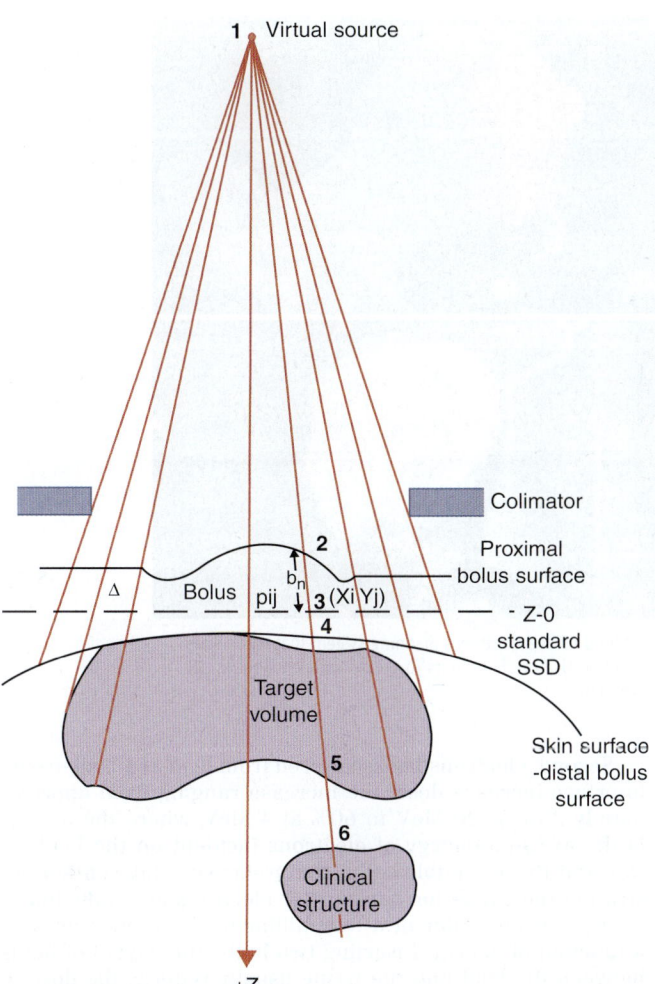

FIGURE 8.16. Schematic representation of the patient contour, target volume, and compensating bolus designed to optimize the coverage of the target while minimizing the dose to the underlying critical structure. (From Low DA, Starkschall G, Bujnowski SW, et al. Electron bolus design for radiation therapy treatment planning: bolus design algorithms. *Med Phys* 1992;19[1]:115–124. Copyright © 1992 American Association of Physicists in Medicine. Reprinted by permission of John Wiley & Sons, Inc.)

searing is seen in Figure 8.16. Perkins et al.[20] showed the use of custom bolus for chest wall irradiation in the cases of highly distorted anatomy and of a chest wall recurrence (Fig. 8.17), and Kudchadker et al.[69] have demonstrated its use in head and neck treatment. And Low et al.[25] have shown its utilization for sparing spinal cord, lung, and kidney in treatment of the paraspinal muscles.

It is recommended that the intent of bolus be verified by measurement or calculation. Bolus used to increase skin dose can be verified by performing *in vivo* dosimetry measurements (e.g., using thermoluminescent dosimetry). Complex bolus shapes, as used to remove surface irregularities or for electron conformal therapy, can be verified by CT scanning the patient with the bolus in place.[20,25] The dose distribution then can be recalculated using the electron dose algorithm in a treatment planning system.

This method of electron conformal therapy may be facilitated by a commercial vendor that can create the custom bolus from treatment plan machinist coordinates.[70]

Along these lines, customization could also be achieved with the use of a 3-D printer.[71–73] In this process, a customized bolus is made using the patient's CT with a commercial treatment planning system. Figure 8.18 shows an example of such process. The bolus' structure is sent to a 3-D modeling software that will convert the file to the appropriate language (standard tessellation language), which will be used by the 3-D printer to manufacture the bolus.[71]

The dimensions of the bolus are dependent on the type of 3-D printer available, which will also determine the composition of bolus material. There are printers that could print using only one material, whereas there are others that can print multiple materials at once [71]. Mainly, the materials used are some type of variation of acrylonitrile butadiene styrene (ABS) and polylactic acid (PLA). It is important to clearly characterize the material's electron density in order to calculate the correct dose that will be delivered to the patient. In addition, the 3-D printed bolus might have air bubbles, which will affect the dose distribution. It is recommended, as for any type of bolus, to perform the necessary measurement to characterize the 3-D printed bolus as well as to develop the necessary quality assurance procedures before using the bolus for any patient.

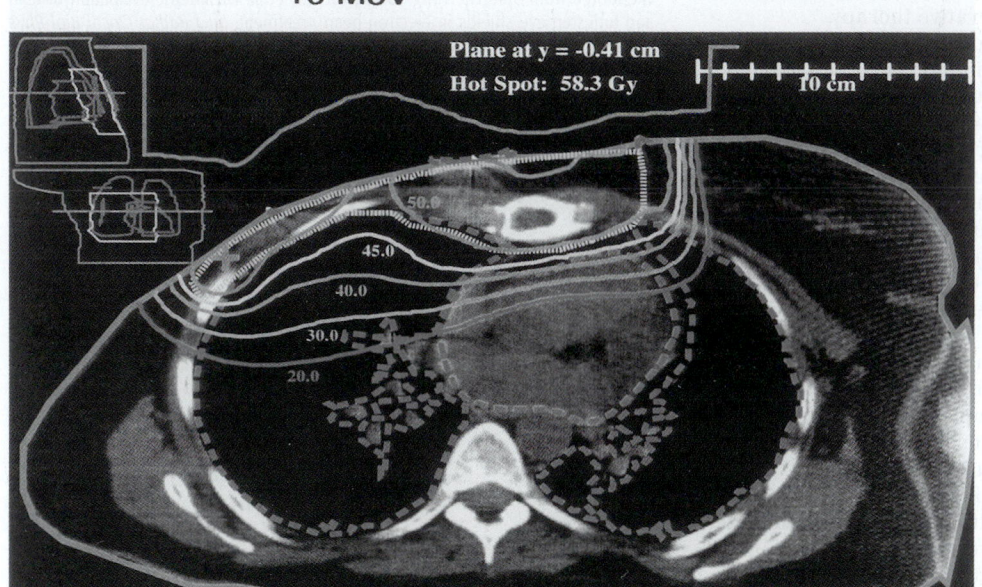

FIGURE 8.17. Conformal electron therapy using variable thickness bolus. Bolus is used to shape the 90% isodose surface (45 Gy) to the distal surface of the chest wall in treating a chest wall occurrence, optimally sparing lung. (Reprinted from Perkins GH, McNeese MD, Antolak JA, et al. A custom three-dimensional electron bolus technique for optimization of postmastectomy irradiation. *Int J Radiat Oncol Biol Phys* 2001;51[4]:1142–1151. Copyright © 2001 Elsevier. With permission.)

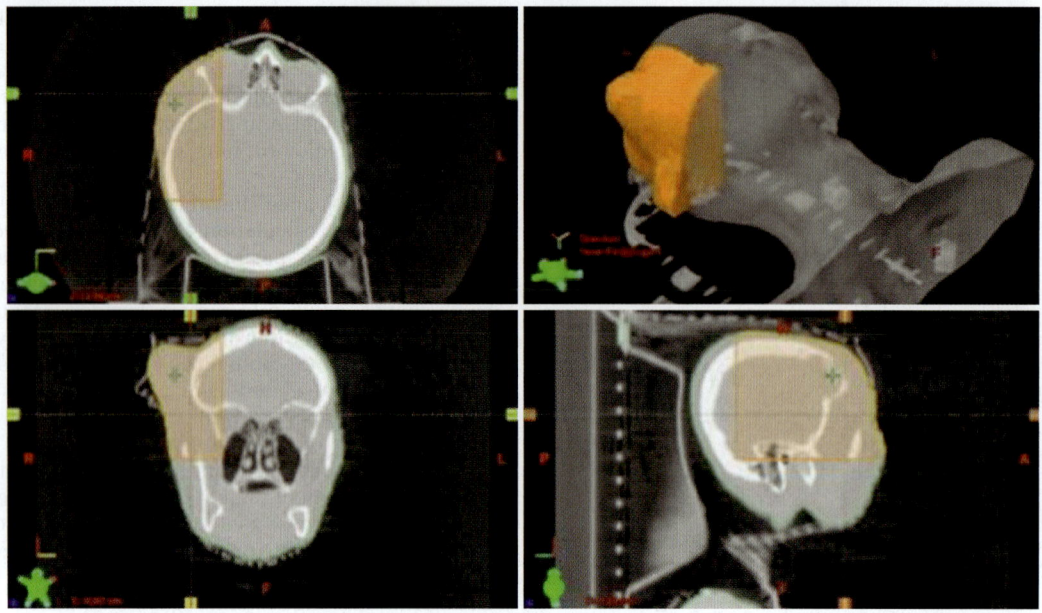

FIGURE 8.18. Example of a bolus structure (shown in orange) defined on the treatment planning system that was subsequently made by a 3-D printer. (From Burleson S, Baker J, Hsia AT, et al. Use of 3D printers to create a patient-specific 3D bolus for external beam therapy. *J Appl Clin Med Phys* 2015;16[3]:166–178.)

Two of the main limitation of using 3-D printed bolus routinely for radiotherapy is the availability of a 3-D printer and the time that it takes to print a complete bolus. Although 3-D printers should become more affordable as these are gaining popularity in radiotherapy. The printing time could also vary widely among printers. The time that it takes to print a bolus is highly dependent on the type of printer's filament and, of course, on the dimensions and complexity of the bolus. Printing could take from 4 to 24 hours.[71,72] This time could be doubled if by any chance there is any failure in the printing process.

Internal Shielding

Internal shields stops electrons that enter the body before they reach critical structures and deposit any significant dose. Examples of clinical utilization of internal shielding are intraoral blocks protecting salivary glands during head and neck treatments[2]; eye blocks protecting the lens in irradiation of the eyelid,[74] orbit, or retina; and sheets of lead used to protect internal structures during intraoperative therapy.

There are two important concepts to remember in the use of internal shielding. First, the collimator must be sufficiently thick to stop the energy of the electrons in the beam at depth. Electron beam energy is reduced by 2 MeV per centimeter in unit density tissue; hence, the energy of a 12-MeV beam at a depth of 2 cm is 8 MeV. The thickness of lead required to stop 8-MeV electrons is 4 mm (8 MeV to 0.5 mm/MeV).

One application where ensuring that collimation is sufficiently thick that has been sometimes overlooked is the use of internal eye shields. Shiu et al.[74] showed that x-ray eye shields constructed of plastic-coated lead and designed to shield the eyes from kilovoltage x-rays did not stop 6-MeV electrons, resulting in penetration of approximately 50% of the given dose. However, electron eye shields constructed of enamel-coated tungsten can stop electrons with energies as great as 9 MeV (Fig. 8.19). By using higher-density tungsten (ρ = 19.3 g/cm³) instead of lead (ρ = 11.5 g/cm³), the eye shields remain sufficiently thin to fit under the eyelid. If only x-ray eye shields are available, bolus should be placed on top of the eye and eye shield to ensure that the electron energy is reduced sufficiently so that electrons do not penetrate the eye shield.

Second, electrons backscattered from lead at a lead–tissue interface increase dose, the increase ranging from approximately 20% at 20 MeV to 60% at 4 MeV, where the energy is the average energy of electrons incident on the lead.[30,75] Das and Bushe[76] published a comprehensive dataset demonstrating the range for backscatter electrons as a function of energy, on the order of a few millimeters, and increases as a function of energy. Inserting two half-value layers of bolus between the lead and the tissue usually reduces the dose to upstream tissue to a clinically acceptable value. The thickness of one half-value layer ranges from approximately 1 cm at 10 MeV to 0.5 cm at 3 MeV.[30,77] Intraoral lead stents are routinely coated with acrylic,[28] and a material such as den-

FIGURE 8.19. Electron eye shields. The dose distribution under tungsten electron eye shields demonstrates its ability to stop 9-MeV electrons. The dose distribution under a lead x-ray eye shield shows its inability to stop 6-MeV electrons. (Reprinted from Shiu AS, Tung SS, Gastorf RJ, et al. Dosimetric evaluation of lead and tungsten eye shields in electron-beam treatment. *Int J Radiat Oncol Biol Phys* 1996;35[3]:599–604. Copyright © 1996 Elsevier. With permission.)

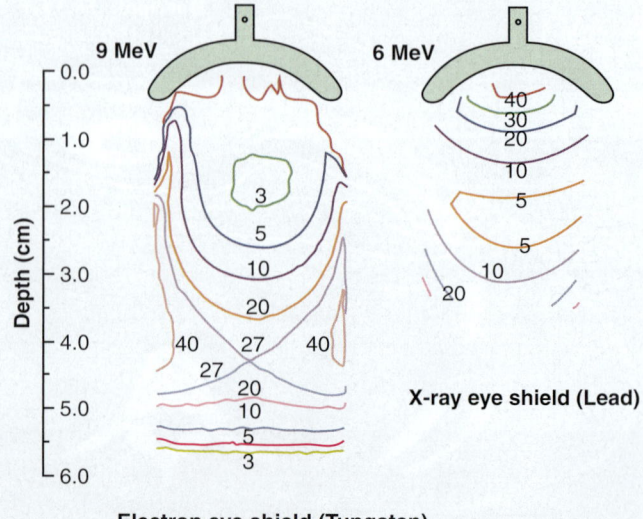

tal wax can be applied easily to lead sheets placed between the mucosa and gums. Eye shields, however, only have clearance for 1 to 2 mm of coating; hence, backscatter dose to the eyelids is an important consideration in treatment management.[77] When determining lead thickness for an internal shielding at a particular depth, one must first determine the energy of the electron beam at that location. The energy of the electron beam on the surface is $E_{o,p}$ typically close to the nominal stated energy. As electrons lose energy by 2 MeV per centimeter, one can determine the remaining energy of any depth. For example, 12 MeV beams at surface would be approximately 6 MeV after 3 cm.

Field Abutment

The purpose of field abutment is to enlarge the radiation area by using parallel matched beams or to change the beam energy or modality. In either case, beam uniformity requires that three criteria be met. First, the beams must abut along the entire border.[29,30,32,78] If the edges of the two beams coincide exactly (Fig. 8.20A), then the two beams will be equivalent to a single beam and optimal uniformity will be achieved. If the central axes of the two beams are parallel (Fig. 8.20B), then the diverging beam edges will overlap, creating a cold spot upstream and a hot spot downstream of the region of intersection. This is least significant for narrow fields, as encountered in irradiation of the cervical nodes of the neck or abutting the internal mammary and medial chest wall fields. If the central axes are converging (Fig. 8.20C), then there is an even greater amount of overlap. This is the case for abutting lateral and medial chest wall fields. In such cases, feathering the beam edge ±1 cm can reduce the dose heterogeneity. This is illustrated in Figure 8.21 for a standard postmastectomy chest wall irradiation using electrons.

The second criterion is that the beam penumbra must be matched. This is the case for the two spinal fields referred to earlier; however, it is not the case in general, particularly in abutting electron to photon fields. In such cases, either one or both of the field edges must be feathered. Third, it is

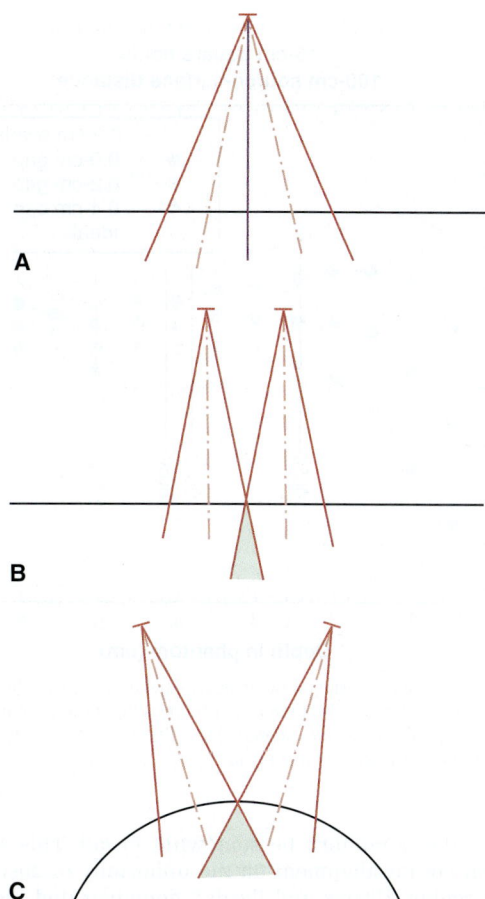

FIGURE 8.20. Comparison of abutment geometries. **A:** Common edge is created by having diverging central axes. **B:** Parallel central axes result in overlapping edges. **C:** Converging central axes result in the greatest overlap. (From Svensson H, Almond P, Brahme A, et al. ICRU Report 35. *Radiation dosimetry: electron beams with energies between 1 and 50 MeV.* Bethesda, MD: International Commission on Radiation Units and Measurement, 1984. Reproduced by permission of International Commission on Radiation Units and Measurements.)

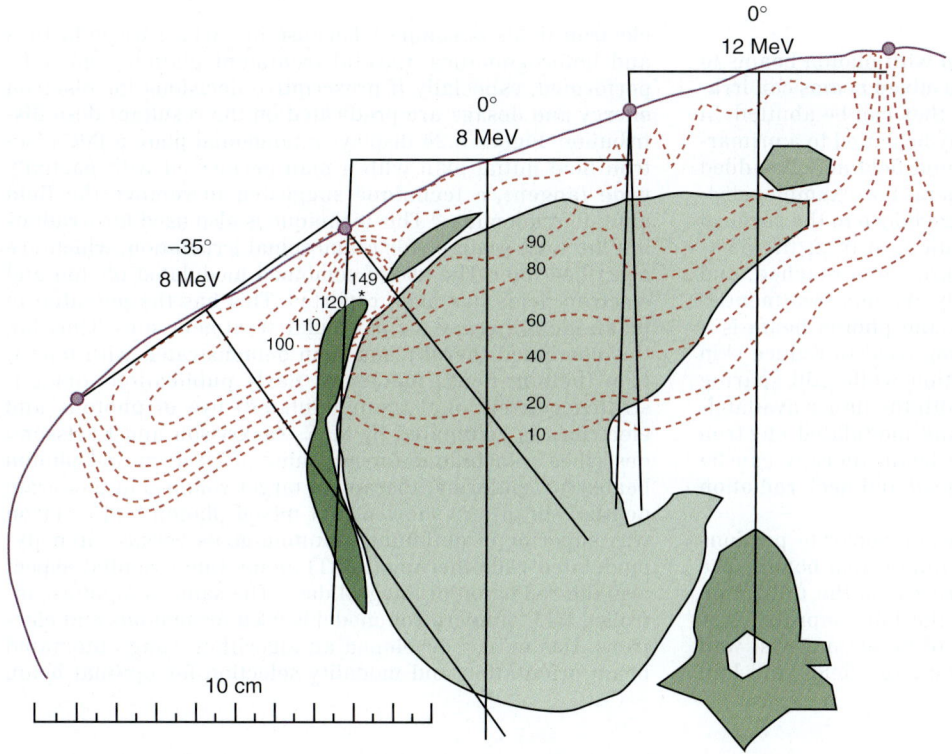

FIGURE 8.21. Clinical example of abutting electron fields in chest wall treatment. Dose homogeneity is acceptable at the border of internal mammary chain (IMC) and medial chest wall fields because central axes are parallel and field widths are small. Dose homogeneity is unacceptable at the border of medial and lateral chest wall fields because central axes are converging (Fig. 8.10B). Dose homogeneity is improved at border of medial and lateral chest wall fields by delivering equal doses with the match line being moved 1 cm twice during treatment.

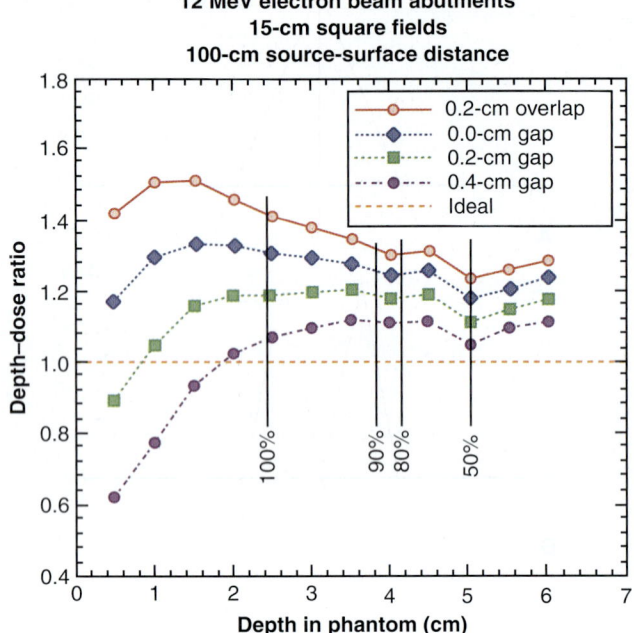

FIGURE 8.22. Graph depicting dose homogeneity for abutted 12-MeV electron fields for a series of gaps. (Reprinted from Harms WB, Purdy JA. Abutment of high energy electron fields. *Int J Radiat Oncol Biol Phys* 1991;20[4]:853–858. Copyright © 1991 Elsevier. With permission.)

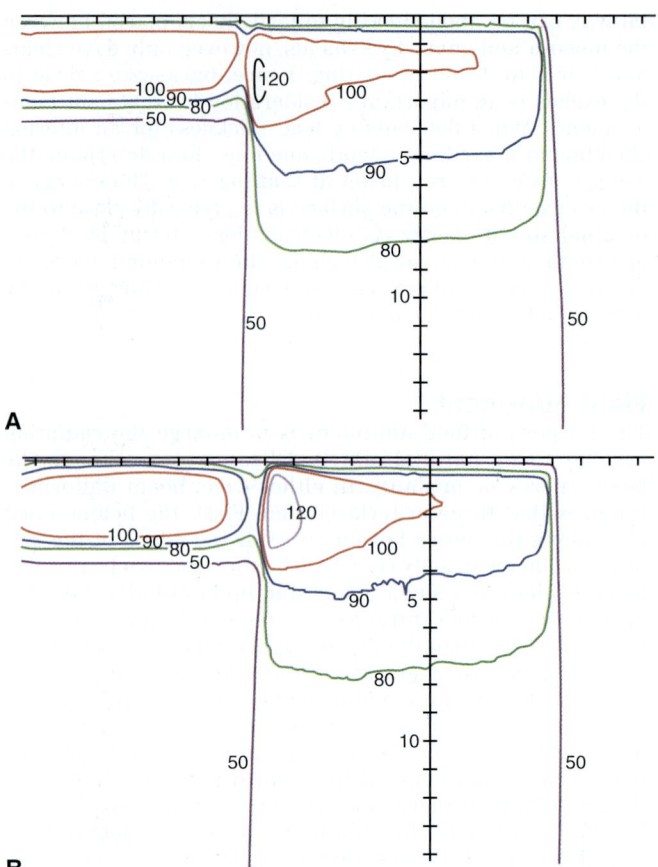

FIGURE 8.23. Isodose curves in a plane perpendicular to the junction line between abutting photon and electron fields. 9-MeV electron beam; field size equals 10 by 10 cm²; 6-MV photon beam; source-to-surface distance (SSD) equals 100 cm. **A:** Electron beam at standard SSD of 100 cm. **B:** Electron beam at extended SSD of 120 cm. (Reprinted from Johnson JM, Khan FM. Dosimetric effects of abutting extended source to surface distance electron fields with photon fields in the treatment of head and neck cancers. *Int J Radiat Oncol Biol Phys* 1994;28[3]:741–747. Copyright © 1994 Elsevier. With permission.)

best that the penumbra be somewhat broad. This reduces the impact of misalignment on the uniformity of dose in the abutted region. Harms and Purdy[49] demonstrated the influence of SSD energy and match bolus on match-line dosimetry. Figure 8.22 displays dose homogeneity for abutted 12-MeV fields depending on gap. In addition, the matching of electron and photo fields is a planning challenge, as two differing penumbra are abutted. Johnson and Khan[79] performed a study of matched electron–photon fields as a function of energy and SSD. Figure 8.23 demonstrates match-line profiles for a typical head and neck field match.

Mixed Beam Therapy

Electron beams frequently are mixed with photon beams to create an appropriate treatment. The mixed beams can irradiate a common volume of tissue, or they can be abutted. In the former case, an electron field may be added to a primarily photon beam treatment, or a photon field may be added to a primarily electron beam treatment. For example, electron boosts are used to deliver localized dose to the surgical site following photon breast irradiation, to treat the postcervical nodes once spinal cord tolerance is reached, and to reduce spinal cord dose (e.g., in lymphoma treatment).[80] In some head and neck treatments, the photon beam is a surrogate to the electron beam, being used to reduce skin dose and to increase dose penetration while still sparing the contralateral salivary gland.[2,10] With the future availability of intensity-modulated photon and modulated electron therapy, the effectiveness of mixed beam therapy can be expected to increase in breast and head and neck radiation therapy.

Abutted mixed beams are used when separate portions of the anatomy can benefit from two individual beams. The most common application of this process is the utilization of electron fields for irradiation of the IMC, supraclavicular, or axillary lymph nodes as part of breast or chest wall irradiation.[2] Matching of tangential photon fields and IMC

electron fields is complex because of surface irregularities and heterogeneities. Careful treatment planning must be performed, especially if prescriptive decisions for electron energy and dosage are predicated on the resultant dose distribution. Figure 8.24 displays a tangential photon IMC electron field initial plan with a plan performed with partially wide tangent, a technique suggested to remove the field abutment dilemma.[81] This technique is also used for irradiating the total scalp or for craniospinal irradiation, which are described later. The use of combined modulated photon and electron fields has been reported. This has the potential to be an ideal therapy for particular treatment sites. Thus far, this combined therapy has been demonstrated with microtron (helium head) machines. Early publications demonstrated conventional (nonmodulated) use of photons and electrons as collimated by MLC. Zackrisson and Karlsson[82] described a technique for matching of electron and photon beams for conformal therapy of target volumes at moderate depths. Mu et al.[83] showed that mixed photon and electron was superior in obtaining planning goals versus intensity-modulated radiotherapy (IMRT) alone. One essential aspect was the reduction of integral dose. The same computer-controlled MLC of microtron model is used for photons and electrons. Das et al.[84] developed an algorithm using automated beam orientation and modality selection for optimal beam

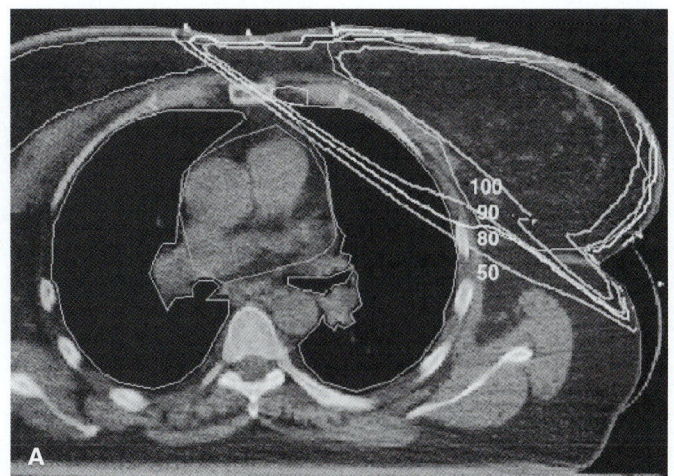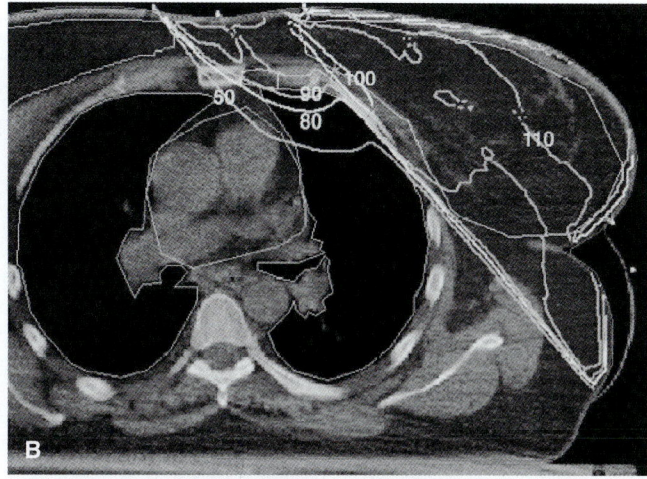

FIGURE 8.24. Dose distribution with partially wide tangentials (PWTs) versus photon/electron (P/E) illustrating difference in position of hot spots. Left lung, heart, internal mammary chain, left breast or chest, and right breast were outlined. The 50%, 80%, 90%, 100%, 110%, and 120% isodose lines are displayed. **A:** Dose distribution with intact breast and PWT. **B:** Dose distribution with intact breast and P/E. (Reprinted from Severin D, Connors S, Thompson H, et al. Breast radiotherapy with inclusion of internal mammary nodes: a comparison of techniques with three-dimensional planning. *Int J Radiat Oncol Biol Phys* 2003;55[3]:633–644. Copyright © 2003 Elsevier. With permission.)

arrangement selection in IMRT of mixed photon and electron beams. Finally, Ma et al.[85] performed a comparative study on tangential photon beams, IMRT, and modulated electron radiotherapy (MERT) for breast cancer treatment.

SPECIALIZED ELECTRON TECHNIQUES

Although electron beam therapy is used less frequently than is photon beam therapy, it remains an essential modality. To fully use electron beam therapy, there must be access to comprehensive electron treatment and treatment planning techniques. This includes specialized electron techniques, which, in the present context, are defined as those that are seldom required and that use a complex treatment geometry, special treatment delivery hardware, or special treatment planning software. It is not recommended that all radiation therapy facilities offer all techniques. However, radiation oncologists should be aware of these techniques and should be able to refer patients to a regional center for those that are impractical in smaller settings. This recommendation is based on the significant time, resources, and costs of implementing, maintaining, and providing some of the more complex special electron procedures. The American College of Medical Physics (absorbed into the AAPM) has reviewed the manpower effort and cost associated with several special procedures, which include electron arc therapy, intraoperative electron therapy, and total skin electron irradiation.[86]

Four types of special techniques are discussed here. First, the treatment of internal tissues is exemplified by intraoperative radiation therapy and intracavitary radiation therapy. Second, the utilization of abutted electron and photon fields is exemplified by craniospinal and total-scalp treatment techniques. Third, the treatment of superficial tissues for a cylindric geometry is exemplified by the total-limb and total skin treatment techniques. Fourth, an alternative to fixed beam therapy of the chest wall is exemplified by arc therapy.

Intracavitary Irradiation

Applicators of appropriate design can be used for intracavitary electron irradiation, which delivers an improved dose

distribution over that traditionally delivered using orthovoltage x-rays. Intracavitary irradiation most frequently is used to boost the primary site while sparing nearby normal tissues. Intracavitary irradiation has been a choice for intraoral, transvaginal, and intraoperative treatments. Wang[19] showed the benefit of intraoral cones for boosting the oral lesions of the floor of the mouth, soft palate, tongue, and retromolar trigone while sparing mandible, teeth, gum, and salivary glands. McGinnis et al.[28] reported using a transvaginal applicator to boost carcinoma of the cervix with electrons, reducing bulk tumor to subsequently allow intracavitary brachytherapy. Intraoperative radiation therapy can be used in many sites[13]; however, it is used primarily for abdominal sites. Merrick et al.[26] reviewed the experience in the United States of using intraoperative radiotherapy for treatment of pancreatic, biliary, and gastric carcinomas.

The criteria for intracavitary electron irradiation are similar regardless of site. A treatment applicator is necessary so that healthy tissue can be restrained from intercepting electrons irradiating the tumor. The applicator wall must be sufficiently thick to stop electrons from escaping to outside tissue while being thin enough not to interfere with tumor access. Guidelines for accomplishing this for intraoperative applicators have been discussed by Hogstrom et al.[87] Another issue is how to ensure accurate alignment while maintaining patient safety with an applicator. Appropriate cone positioning requires having a method for looking down the cone to view the tumor. Proper alignment of the applicator after inserting it into the patient requires methods for docking it to the machine. For soft docking, the applicator is not physically attached to the machine[87,88] (Fig. 8.25). For hard docking, the applicator is physically attached to the machine, and there are methods for its breaking away under stress.[28,89]

Treatment planning for intracavitary cones typically is done manually because it is not possible to CT scan the patient in the treatment position or under operating room conditions. The electron energy and cone size are selected to match measured isodose distributions to the dimensions of the clinical target volume. Examples of dose distributions

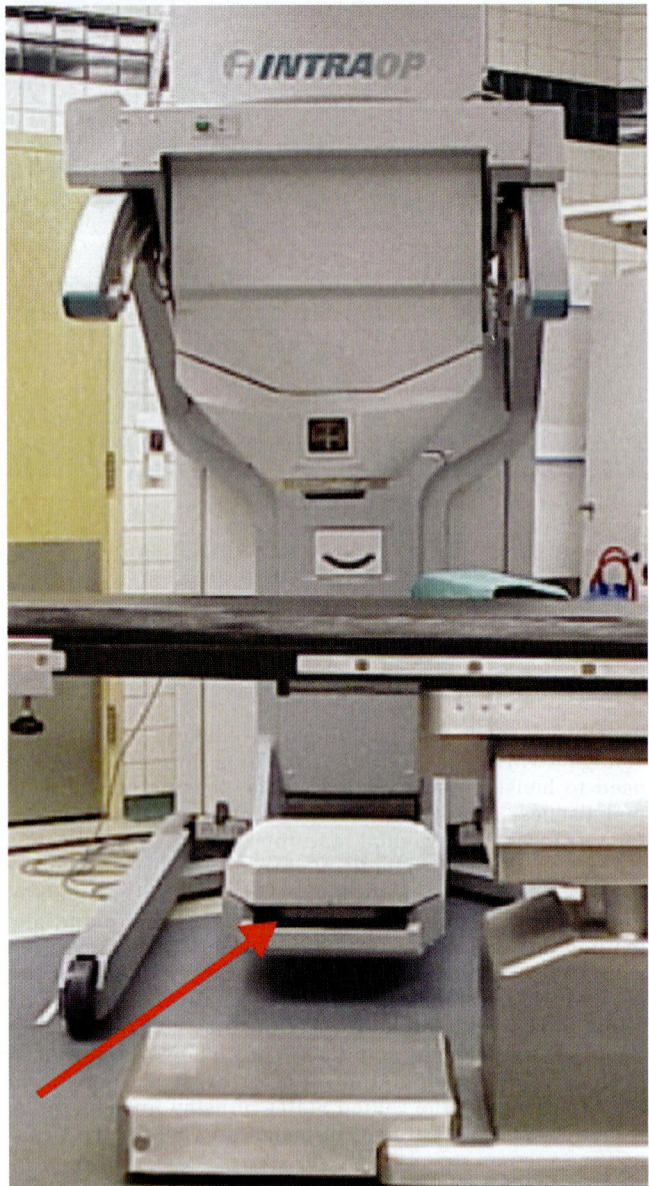

FIGURE 8.25. Intraoperative electron radiation therapy accelerator. View of the Mobetron self-shielded mobile intraoperative radiation therapy unit by IntraOp Medical Corporation. (From Beddar AS, Biggs PJ, Chang S, et al. Intraoperative radiation therapy using mobile electron linear accelerators. AAPM Radiation Therapy Committee Task Group No. 72, Report No. 92, 2006. Copyright © 2006 The Authors.)

for intraoperative applicators are shown in Figure 8.26.[90] These examples show two characteristics of such applicators. First, for the larger diameter applicators, scattering off the wall of the applicator can lead to hot spots near the applicator's periphery. Second, ends of the applicator often are beveled to make it easy to establish contact when the anatomic plane is not perpendicular to the direction of approach (i.e., the central axis of the beam). Note how the depth of the 90% isodose contour beneath the surface decreases from 3.6 cm at 0 degree incidence to 3.0 cm at 30 degrees incidence, as a result of the effects described earlier.

Total-Scalp Irradiation

Total-scalp irradiation is sometimes necessary in the management of malignancies (e.g., cutaneous lymphoma, melanoma, and angiosarcoma) that present with widespread involvement of the scalp and forehead.[2,15] Electron beam therapy is a practical means of achieving the therapeutic goal of delivering a uniform dose to the scalp with minimal dose to underlying brain. For many years, total-scalp irradiation was achieved by patching multiple electron fields.[2,91] Although effective, the treatment was tedious as a result of the large number of fields, their requirement for skin collimation, and the need to move the abutment border to improve dose homogeneity.[91] Akazawa[92] from the University of California–San Francisco reported a simpler technique that abuts lateral electron fields to parallel-opposed photon fields, the latter of which treats the rind of the scalp while avoiding brain tissue. Tung et al.[15] modified the abutment scheme to account for beam divergence and demonstrated improved dose uniformity by comparing 3-D dose calculations with in vivo dose measurements. Figure 8.27 illustrates the abutment scheme. The outer edge of the electron field overlaps the inner edge of the 6-MV x-ray field by 3 mm to account for the divergence of the contralateral 6-MV x-ray field. Because the electron and x-ray penumbras are not matched, their common border is moved 1 cm toward beam center halfway through treatment to improve dose homogeneity. Figure 8.28 shows the dose distribution in a transverse CT plane, which illustrates the dose homogeneity achieved in the region of abutment and the sparing of brain tissue. Initially, the common border is set at approximately 0.5 cm inside the inner table of the skull. Moving the common border farther toward the inner table of the skull reduces brain irradiation at the expense of the x-ray beam being replaced by an electron beam that would begin to graze the skull. As discussed earlier, grazing radiation penetrates less deeply, possibly underdosing the scalp in this region. Also noticeable in Figure 8.28 is a 6-mm thick wax bolus, which increases surface dose for both the electron and x-ray fields. Although this technique is straightforward to plan and implement, concern of hot spots along to the midline superior brain tissue along the plane is a concern.

Walker et al.[93] described a six-field electron beam technique for treatment of mycosis fungoides of the scalp. This technique of overlapping beams was verified with thermoluminescent dosimetry measurements. The dose prescriptions were 20 and 30 Gy for the two patients in this study. Yaparpalvi et al.[94] developed a technique for scalp irradiation that used a single posterior-superior field with concentric circles that varied in electron energy. This interesting technique was not confirmed with anthropomorphic phantom dosimetry studies. Peters[95] described use of an electron reflector to improve dose uniformity to the scalp during total skin electron therapy.

Total-Limb Irradiation

It may be advantageous to irradiate the superficial anatomy of a limb for management of cancer (e.g., melanoma, lymphoma, Kaposi sarcoma). If the depth beneath the surface is 2 cm or less, electrons offer a uniform dose while sparing deep tissues and structures. This technique has been described by Wooden et al.[16] for the treatment of the lower calf of a patient with Kaposi sarcoma. Illustrated in Figure 8.29, six equally spaced 5-MeV electron beams are used to irradiate a 9-cm diameter cylinder. Each beam is sufficiently wide so that the entire circle falls within the uniform portion of each beam. Tangential radiation to the surface of the cylinder delivers a greater dose as a result of oblique incidence, which is partially offset by the inverse square effect. Additionally, the tangential radiation penetrates less deeply. The utilization of six or more beams begins to simulate 360-degree arc therapy (which is not feasible because of collisions). The resulting dose distribution illustrates three interesting characteristics. First, the average

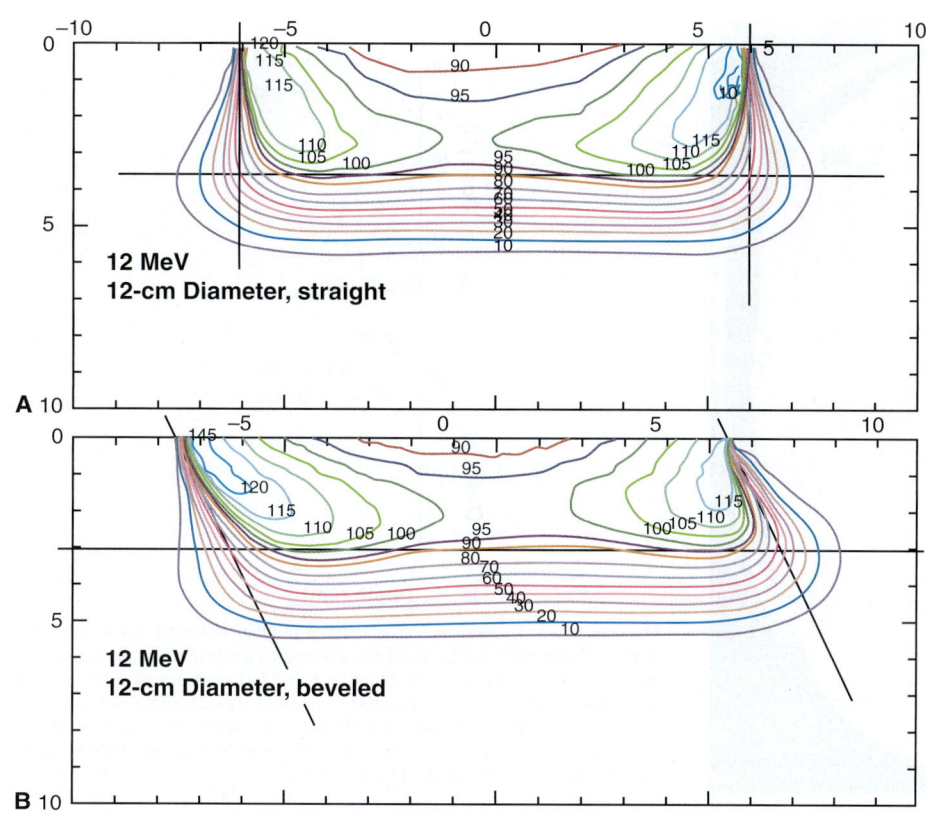

FIGURE 8.26. Isodose plots illustrating typical intraoperative dose distributions at 12 MeV. **A:** 12-cm diameter cone, normal incidence. **B:** 30-degree beveled, 12-cm diameter cone. Note the decreased depth of the 90% dose beneath the surface for the beam 30 degrees from normal incidence relative to that for normal incidence. (Reprinted from Nyerick CE, Ochran TG, Boyer AL, et al. Dosimetry characteristics of metallic cones for intraoperative radiation therapy. *Int J Radiat Oncol Biol Phys* 1991;21[2]:501–510. Copyright © 1991 Elsevier. With permission.)

maximum dose along each radius is approximately 2.5 times the given dose of each of the six fields. Second, 90% of the average maximum dose penetrates 8 to 10 mm, reduced from the value of 15 mm for a single beam incident normally on a flat surface (Fig. 8.30). Third, the surface dose has increased to 90% or greater of average maximum dose compared with approximately 70% of the given dose for a single beam incident normally on a flat surface. This is the result of the self-bolusing effect of tangential electron radiation.

The dosimetric characteristics should be carefully evaluated using one's treatment planning system.

Total-Skin Irradiation

Total-skin electron irradiation is a modality designed for management of diseases that require irradiation of the entire skin surface or a significant portion of it. The technique is used most frequently for treatment of mycosis fungoides, whose management is reviewed by Hoppe,[17] and Kaposi sarcoma.

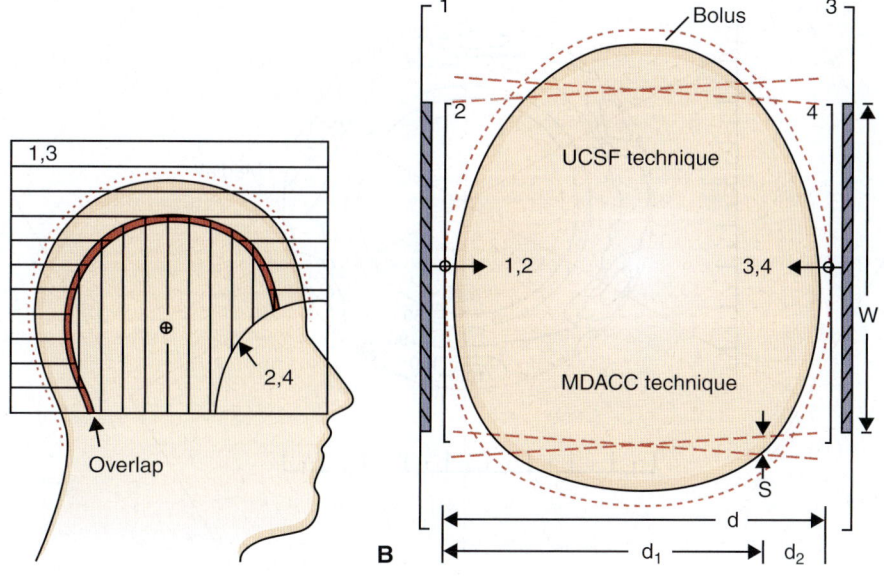

FIGURE 8.27. Abutment scheme for total-scalp irradiation (x-ray fields, 1, 3; electron fields, 2, 4). **A:** The electron field edge, placed just inside the skull, overlaps the edge of the ipsilateral x-ray field by approximately 3 mm to account for divergence of the edge of the contralateral x-ray field. Halfway through treatment, the field edges are moved 1 cm to improve dose homogeneity in the region of abutment. **B:** The need for the 3-mm overlap (MD Anderson Cancer Center [MDACC] technique) is better appreciated viewing the divergent edges of all fields in a transverse plane. (Reprinted from Tung SS, Shiu AS, Starkschall G, et al. Dosimetric evaluation of total scalp irradiation using a lateral electron-photon technique. *Int J Radiat Oncol Biol Phys* 1993;27[1]:153–160. Copyright © 1993 Elsevier. With permission.)

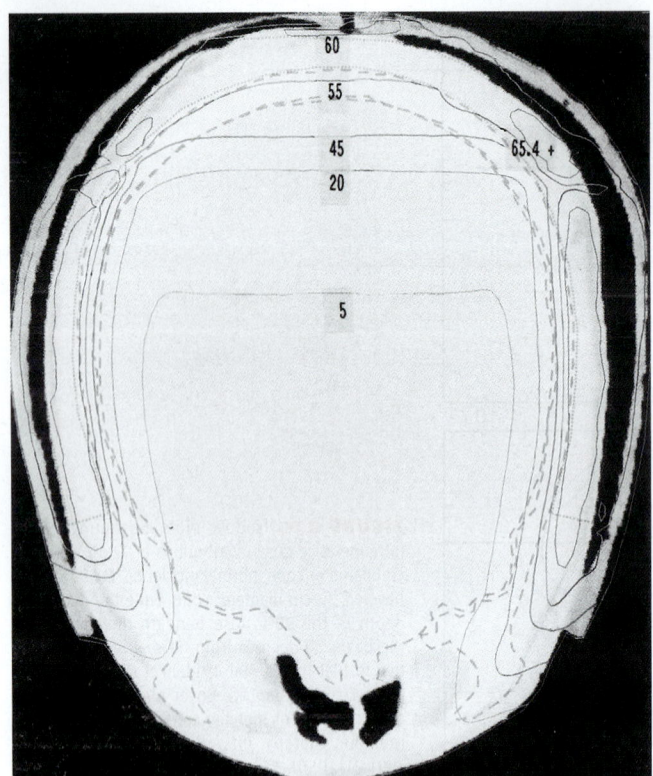

FIGURE 8.28. Dose distribution in a transverse computed tomography plane, illustrating the homogeneity of dose in the abutment region and the degree of brain sparing with this technique. Isodose values in *gray*. (Reprinted from Tung SS, Shiu AS, Starkschall G, et al. Dosimetric evaluation of total scalp irradiation using a lateral electron-photon technique. *Int J Radiat Oncol Biol Phys* 1993;27[1]:153–160. Copyright © 1993 Elsevier. With permission.)

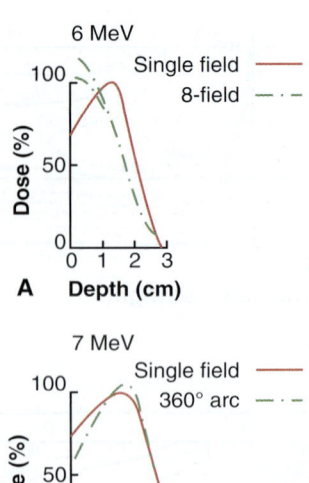

FIGURE 8.30. Treating circular anatomy with multiple beams spaced over 360 degrees. Depth dose along a radial axis depends on the field width. **A:** Depth dose for a broad, 6-MeV beam, resulting from an 8-field technique around a 20-cm diameter water cylinder, is governed by grazing radiation, typical of total skin and total-limb irradiation. **B:** Depth dose for a narrow, 7-MeV beam, resulting from rotating around a 20-cm diameter water cylinder, is governed by focusing of the radiation toward isocenter, typical of arc electron therapy.

Multiple techniques for total skin electron therapy have been reviewed in AAPM Report No. 23.[18] The underlying principles of the various techniques are similar, which are exemplified by the modified Stanford technique, illustrated in Figure 8.31. First, the treatment requires a broad beam from right to left, which can be achieved by a combination

FIGURE 8.29. Dose distribution for total-limb irradiation. Six equally spaced 17-cm wide, 5-MeV electron beams are used to irradiate a 9-cm diameter cylinder. 100% equals 2.55 times the given dose from a single field. (Reprinted from Wooden KK, Hogstrom KR, Blum P, et al. Whole-limb irradiation of the lower calf using a six-field electron technique. *Med Dosim* 1996;21[4]:211–218. Copyright © 1996 Elsevier. With permission.)

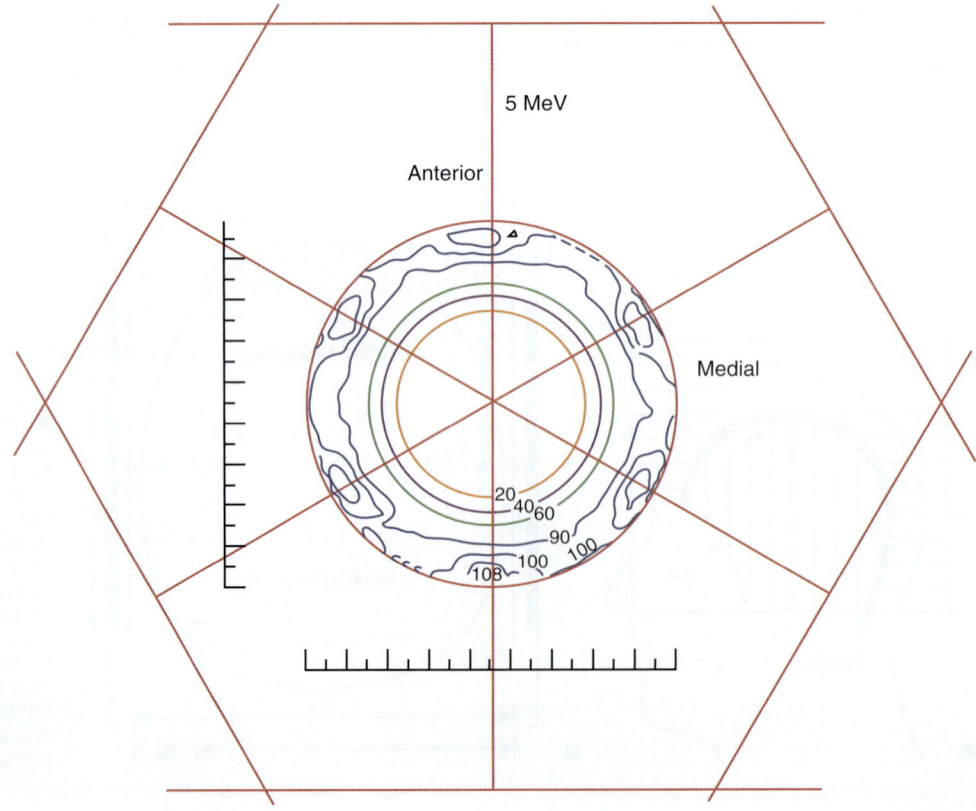

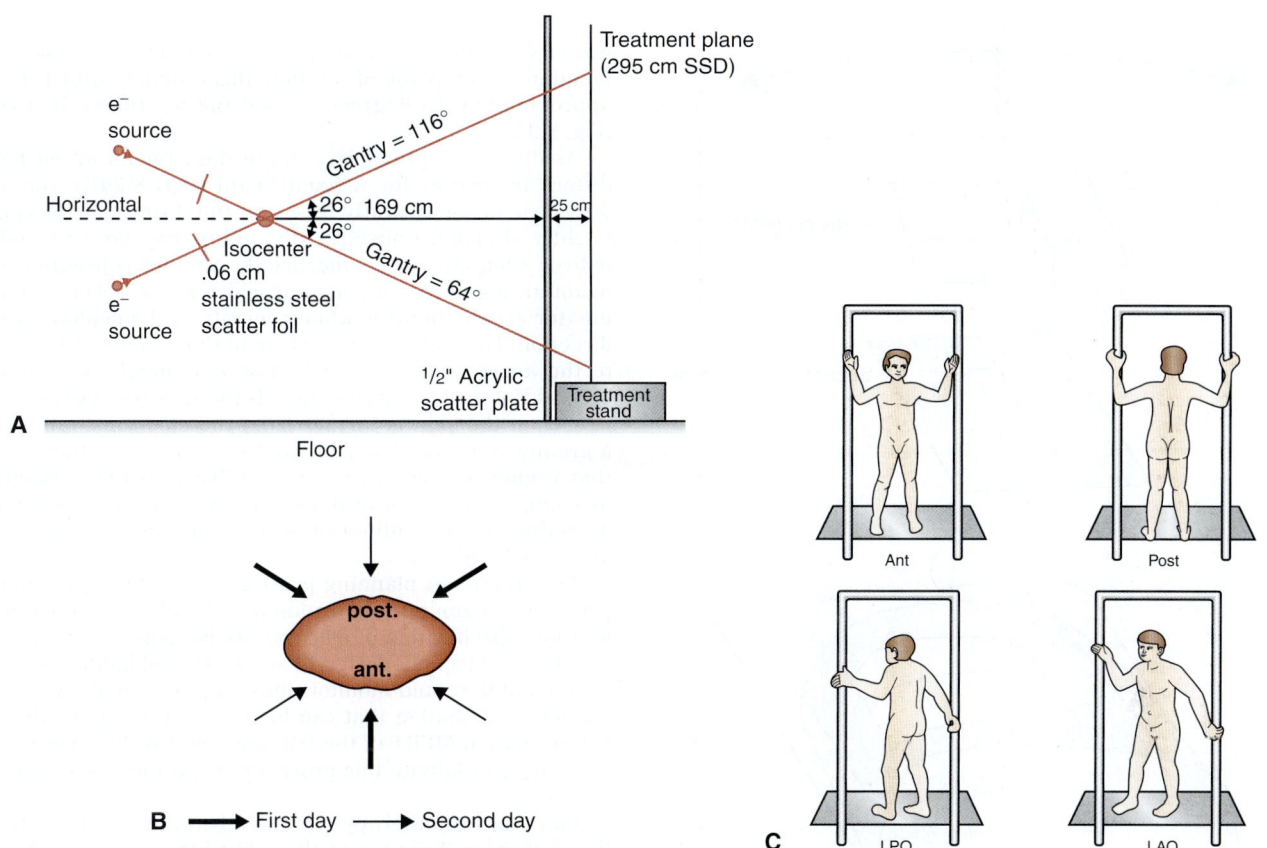

FIGURE 8.31. Schematic of modified Stanford technique for total skin irradiation. Side view of setup shows the relative position of patient plane, scatter plate, isocenter, and gantry angles **(A)**. Six beam directions **(B)** are achieved by placing the patient in six patient positions **(C)**. (From Almond PR. Total skin electron irradiation technique and dosimetry. In: Kereiakes JG, Elson HR, Born CG, eds. *Radiation oncology physics 1986.* New York: American Institute of Physics, 1987:296–332; and Karzmark CJ, Anderson J, Fessenden P, et al. *AAPM Report No. 23, total skin electron therapy: technique and dosimetry.* New York: American Institute of Physics, 1987. Reprinted by permission of American Association of Physicists in Medicine.)

of treating the patient at an extended SSD (300 to 400 cm). The beam is made uniform from head to foot by abutting two fields at the 50% OAR (Fig. 8.31A). (Note that the 50% OAR lies outside the edge of the light field; thus, when properly abutted, there is a gap between the edges of the respective light fields.) By aiming the beams up and down, the largest bremsstrahlung contribution (central axis) misses the patient. The dose is made uniform around the circumference of the patient by irradiating from six different directions (Fig. 8.31B). Similar to total-limb irradiation, tangential radiation results in a higher surface dose and a less penetrating dose. Placed upstream of the patient is a plastic screen that serves as both an energy degrader and a scatterer. Dose homogeneity depends on patient position, and reproducing the positions of the Stanford technique (Fig. 8.31C) is important. Despite efforts to create a homogeneous dose, there always will be areas that are underdosed (e.g., top of scalp, sole of feet, perineum, and under the breast or under the panniculus of obese individuals). These areas and sometimes tumorous lesions require separate treatment and boosting, respectively. In contrast, fingers, feet, and toes typically receive excess dose and are shielded for a portion of the treatment. *In vivo* measurement of patient dose on an individual basis is important when making decisions on prescriptions for supplemental treatments.

Implementation of this technique is complex. It requires an external patient stand with a plastic diffuser, special

dosimetry equipment for quality assurance and calibration, special shields for selected parts of the patient, and access to *in vivo* dosimetry.[96] It is also necessary for the radiation therapy accelerator to have a high dose rate mode and interlocks for electron energy, gantry angle, and x-ray jaws. Implementation of this technique has been estimated at 105 hours.[86] An institution must have a warranted patient population requiring this technique.

Electron Arc Therapy

Electron arc therapy is a useful technique for treating postmastectomy chest wall(s).[21] It is used in lieu of parallel-opposed tangential photon irradiation. It is more useful in "barrel-chested" women, where tangential beams can irradiate too much lung. It is also difficult to achieve homogeneous dose in the region where the medial tangential beam used for the chest wall abuts the anterior beam used for the IMC. In such cases, treating both areas with only opposed tangent photon beams irradiates too much lung. In such cases, electron arc therapy is a viable option. This can be particularly important in patients with bilateral disease.

The treatment geometry and dosimetry for arc therapy are unique. There are three levels of collimation in electron arc therapy: the primary x-ray collimators, a shaped secondary Cerrobend insert, and skin collimation (Fig. 8.32). The secondary collimator typically projects a 5- to 6-cm beam width at isocenter. There is typically a large air gap between the

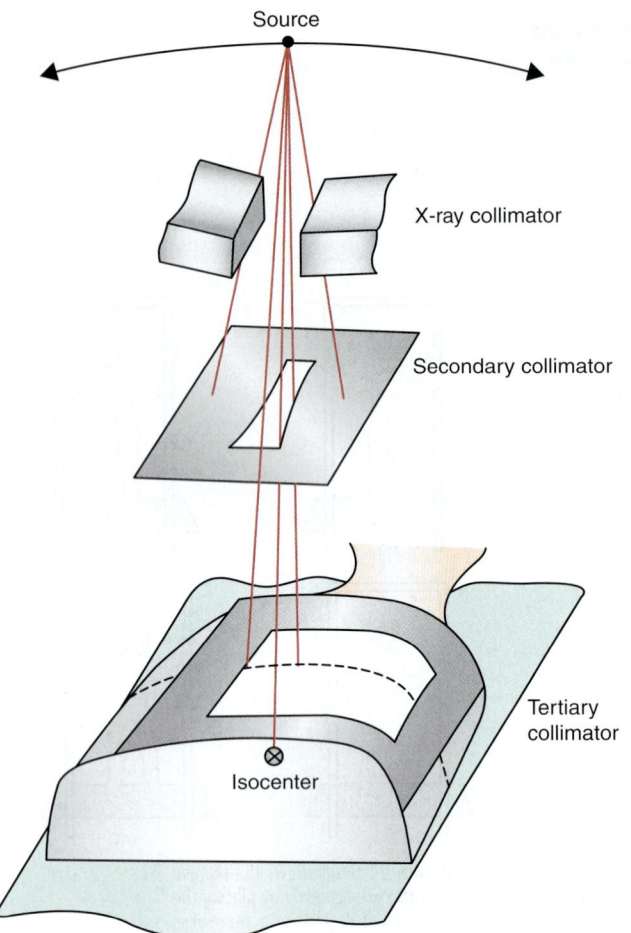

FIGURE 8.32. Schematic of treatment geometry for electron arc therapy. Skin collimation is required because of the large air gap between secondary collimator and patient, which is needed to allow rotation of the gantry around the patient.

secondary collimating insert and the patient, resulting in a large penumbra; also in addition, the finite width of the field results in a broad edge at the end of the arc. The sharpness of the penumbra is restored utilizing skin collimation. This

requires that the edge of the field of the secondary collimator extends well beyond the edge of the field defined by skin collimation. In the plane of rotation, this is achieved by rotating approximately 15 degrees beyond the treatment field edge (Fig. 8.33).

As discussed previously, depth dose for an arced beam differs from that for a fixed beam (Fig. 8.24B); the surface dose is significantly less, and the dose falloff becomes slightly sharper. Consequently, bolus may be required to deliver adequate dose superficially. Another consequence of beam arcing is that a constant width of the secondary collimator results in dose inhomogeneity in the cephalocaudal direction. The radius of curvature of the patient with respect to the accelerator isocentric axis is typically less superiorly, as the neck is approached. If the radius of curvature is less, then the skin is farther from the electron source (i.e., a greater SSD). Contrary to fixed beam therapy, the dose to that region increases rather than decreases as a result of focusing of the electron fluence toward isocenter. However, by reducing the collimator width, the dose can be made more uniform.

The treatment planning process for arc therapy requires patient CT scanning, delineation of PTV, selection of isocenter location, specification of electron arc boundaries, energy and slab bolus selection, design of secondary collimator, and calculation of dose and monitor units. Figure 8.34 shows a typical dose distribution that can be achieved using arc therapy for irradiation MERT of the IMC and chest wall. Physics commissioning to initiate this procedure is on the order of 4 to 6 weeks.

Electron radiotherapy has not advanced beyond conventional therapy because of the labor-intensive (cutouts and bolus) tasks to shape and modulate beams, limited conformity in the depth direction, limited lateral conformity, no inverse planning, and no dynamic beam delivery. If these were overcome via an automated method, the conformation of dose distributions to shallow tumors might greatly improve—hence the advent of MERT. There is a definitive niche for MERT to complement a photon IMRT program. MERT will be able to achieve lateral dose conformity by intensity modulation (such as photon IMRT) and dose conformity along the depth direction using energy modulation (unique to electron beams). In addition, MERT may increase dose uniformity in the target both laterally and along the depth direction, reduce high or

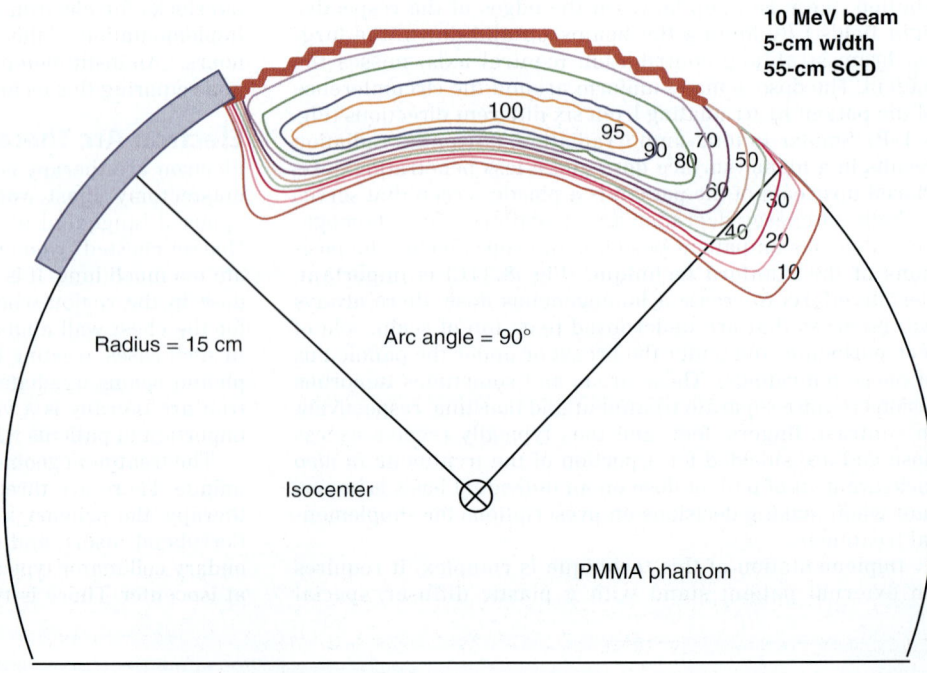

FIGURE 8.33. Comparison of dose distribution with and without skin collimation. The uncollimated edge has a slow dose falloff that is useful for abutting to other arced fields. The skin collimation restores the beam edge but requires rotating the beam 15 degrees beyond the edge of the skin collimator.

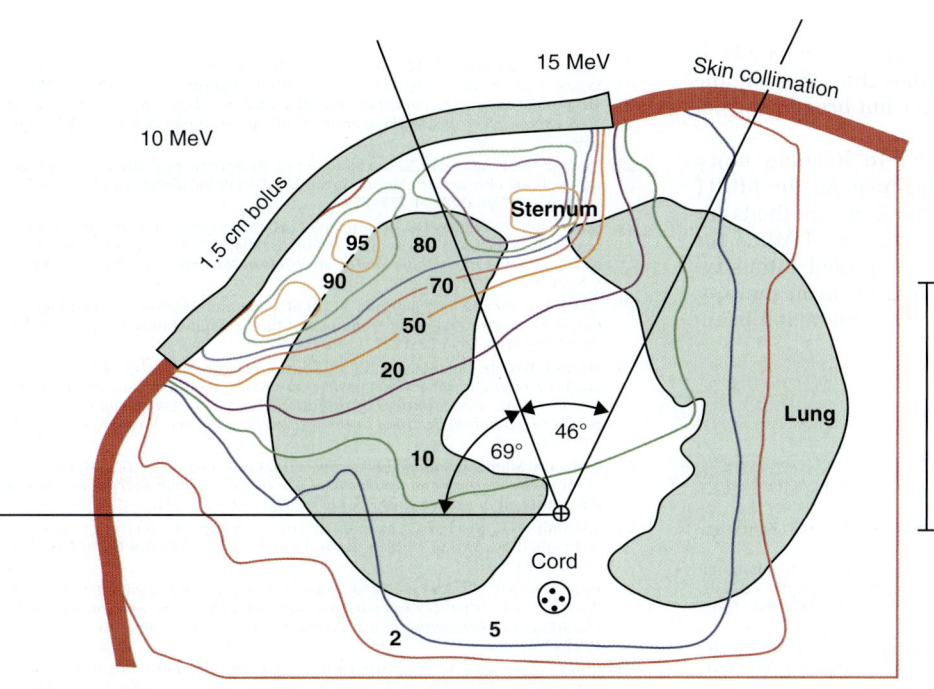

FIGURE 8.34. Typical dose distribution achieved by arc electron therapy. Note the different energies used for the internal mammary chain (IMC) and chest wall fields, the exact abutment of the IMC and chest wall fields, the rotation 15 degrees beyond the skin edges of the skin collimator, and the use of bolus to increase the surface dose. (From Hogstrom KR, Kurup RG, Shiu AS, et al. A two-dimensional pencil-beam algorithm for calculation of arc electron dose distributions. *Phys Med Biol* 1989;34[3]:315–341. doi:10.1088/0031-9155/34/3/005. © Institute of Physics and Engineering in Medicine. Reproduced by permission of IOP Publishing. All rights reserved.)

moderate concomitant dose to distal organs (e.g., lung, heart, and contralateral breast for breast treatments), and improve skin coverage or sparing when combined with photon IMRT.[88,97]

Disease sites such as postmastectomy chest wall, and mycosis fungoides or any cutaneous manifestation of lymphoma of the scalp, and so forth are likely best suited for modulated electrons, either with or without photons, or perhaps a combination of both. However, the inherent collimation systems in modern accelerators were optimized for megavoltage photons and are not conducive to electron beam delivery (in lieu of extended applicators), nor do commercial treatment planning systems model electrons collimated without applicators.

As an example of targeted sites that would be improved with MERT, treatment to the chest wall stands out. Current techniques of using tangential photon adjunct fields abutting supraclavicular and posterior axillary fields are difficult enough without the addition of treating a separate medial breast internal mammary field with a mixture of photon and electrons. Although there has been extensive work to optimize these techniques,[98] there are shortcomings because of match-line problems and delivery of unacceptable doses to volumes of heart, lung, and contralateral breast. Clinical side effects include edema, fibrosis, heart disease, and pneumonitis. Delivery by tangential photon beams to the chest wall is also not ideal because of the heterogeneous dose delivered in the secondary electron buildup region of the breast. Bolus may be used; however, this unfortunately reduces skin sparing. Electron arc therapy was developed in the 1980s to address the limitations of tangential photon beam treatments,[99] although it was extremely time consuming to implement. Use of MERT will phase out electrons arcs.

Many centers have used photon IMRT to improve dose conformity; however, the fundamental limitations because of megavoltage photon beams, such as excess distal dose and the buildup dose, are still challenges. MERT has been proposed as an alternative, particularly for postmastectomy patients.[8,62] The principal advantage is the rapid distal dose falloff. In principle, electron beams are well suited for these shallow targets, as they will spare distal regions, such as lung and heart.

Optimization is another important aspect for a MERT program. Many people have come up with inverse planning techniques for photons and even more recently for electrons. Al-Yahya et al.[100] came up with a method of optimizing electron beam planning for a few leaf-electron collimator (FLEC). Planning was performed via Monte Carlo calculations and optimization using simulated annealing—a powerful mathematical tool that is the basis for inverse planning. The FLEC system consists of four motor-driven trimmer bars at the end of an applicator that creates rectangular shapes. The report claims potential treatment times of 15 minutes or less. Very comprehensive work by Lee et al.[65] described a Monte Carlo optimization scheme for modulated electron beam radiotherapy based on a stop-and-shoot technique. One of the most challenging things in both calculating and optimizing is the leaf scatter, where distributions could vary up to 20% depending on leaf positions. Lee et al.[65] performed MLC planning accomplished by calculating composite distributions for electron beamlets as collimated by tertiary electron MLC. Scatter and leakage contributions were included in the final dose calculation. An inverse planning dose optimization engine designed weights for each beamlet. The particle generation and absorption within the MLC leaves created demanding calculations but were necessary for accurate organ-at-risk calculations. Therefore, modeling of leaf scatter and transmissions is vital for accurate dose calculations. It is key that a multiple source model be developed. Publications describing the use of photon MLCs to modulate electrons have promoted an effective method to reform conformal electron therapy.[101–103]

Summary

Electron beam therapy remains an important modality to the practice of radiation therapy. As discussed earlier, its effective use requires knowledge of the unique properties of electron beam dose distributions, the impact of the patient on the dose distribution, and the basic principles for good practice. It requires access to and the proper use of comprehensive treatment planning and delivery tools. It also requires access to special techniques that offer unique treatment solutions for a limited number but broad range of patient conditions.

Electron therapy can be expected to become more sophisticated in the future as the enthusiasm for MERT grows. Advances in electron dose calculations, methods for electron beam optimization, and availability of MLCs for electrons will enable the practice of combined intensity-modulated photon and energy-modulated electron therapy. This will advance both electron conformal and mixed beam therapy.

REFERENCES

1. Fletcher GH. Introduction. In: Tapley N, ed. *Clinical applications of the electron beam*. New York: John Wiley and Sons, 1976:1.
2. Tapley ND, ed. *Clinical applications of the electron beam*. New York: John Wiley and Sons, 1976.
3. Hogstrom KR, Fields RS. Use of CT in electron beam treatment planning: current and future development. In: Ling CC, Rogers CC, Morton RJ, eds. *Computed tomography in radiation therapy*. New York: Raven Press, 1983:241–252.
4. Hogstrom KR. Implementation of CT treatment planning. In: Wright AE, Boyer AL, eds. *Advances in radiation therapy treatment planning*. New York: American Institute of Physics, 1983:268–281.
5. Hogstrom KR, Mills MD, Meyer JA, et al. Dosimetric evaluation of a pencil-beam algorithm for electrons employing a two-dimensional heterogeneity correction. *Int J Radiat Oncol Biol Phys* 1984;10:561–569.
6. Hogstrom KR. Evaluation of electron pencil beam dose calculations. In: Kereiakes JG, Elson HR, Born CG, eds. *Radiation oncology physics 1986*. New York: American Institute of Physics, 1987:532–557.
7. Popple RA, Weinber R, Antolak JA, et al. Comprehensive evaluation of a commercial macro Monte Carlo electron dose calculation implementation using a standard verification data set. *Med Phys* 2006;33(6):1540–1551.
8. Klein EE, Low DA, Purdy JA. Dosimetric changes with the new scattering foil applicator system on a C12100 C. *Int J Radiat Oncol Biol Phys* 1995;32:483–490.
9. Kashani R, Santanam L, Moore K, et al. Electron beam dosimetric characteristics for the Varian TrueBeam [abstract]. *Med Phys* 2011;38:3662.
10. Fields RS, Hogstrom KR. Optimization of electron-photon mixed beam planning. In: *Proceedings of the Eighth International Conference on the Use of Computers in Radiation Therapy*. Silver Spring, MD: IEEE Computer Society Press, 1984:248–254.
11. Million RR, Parson JT, Bova FJ, et al. Electron beam: the management of head and neck cancer. In: Vaeth JM, Meyer JL, eds. *Frontiers of radiation therapy and oncology vol. 25: the role of high energy electrons in the treatment of cancer*. Basel: S. Karger AG, 1991:107–127.
12. Kun LE. Electron beam therapy in children. In: Vaeth JM, Meyer JL, eds. *Frontiers of radiation therapy and oncology vol. 25: the role of high energy electrons in the treatment of cancer*. Basel: S. Karger AG, 1991:201–206.
13. Vaeth JM, Meyer JL, eds. *Frontiers of radiation therapy and oncology vol. 25: the role of high energy electrons in the treatment of cancer*. Basel: S. Karger AG, 1991.
14. Mills MD, Hogstrom KR, Fields RS. Determination of electron beam output factors for a 20-MeV linear accelerator. *Med Phys* 1985;12:473–476.
15. Tung SS, Shiu AS, Starkschall G, et al. Dosimetric evaluation of total scalp irradiation using a lateral electron-photon technique. *Int J Radiat Oncol Biol Phys* 1993;27:153–160.
16. Wooden KK, Hogstrom KR, Blum P, et al. Whole-limb irradiation of the lower calf using a six-field electron technique. *Med Dosim* 1996;21:211–218.
17. Hoppe RT. Total skin electron beam therapy in the management of mycosis fungoides. In: Vaeth JM, Meyer JL, eds. *Frontiers of radiation therapy and oncology vol. 25: the role of high energy electrons in the treatment of cancer*. Basel: S. Karger AG, 1991:80–89.
18. Karzmark CJ, Anderson J, Fessenden P, et al. *AAPM Report No. 23, total skin electron therapy: technique and dosimetry*. New York: American Institute of Physics, 1987.
19. Wang CC. Intraoral cone for carcinoma of the oral cavity. In: Vaeth JM, Meyer JL, eds. *Frontiers of radiation therapy and oncology vol. 25: the role of high energy electrons in the treatment of cancer*. Basel: S. Karger AG, 1991:128–131.
20. Perkins GH, McNeese MD, Antolak JA, et al. A custom three-dimensional electron bolus technique for optimization of postmastectomy irradiation. *Int J Radiat Oncol Biol Phys* 2001;51:1142–1151.
21. Stewart JR, Leavitt DD, Prows J. Electron arc therapy of the chest wall for breast cancer: rationale, dosimetry, and clinical aspects. In: Vaeth JM, Meyer JL, eds. *Frontiers of radiation therapy and oncology vol 25: the role of high energy electrons in the treatment of cancer*. Basel: S. Karger AG, 1991:134–150.
22. Recht A, Triedman SA, Harris JR. The "boost" in the treatment of early-stage breast cancer: electrons versus interstitial implants. In: Vaeth JM, Meyer JL, eds. *Frontiers of radiation therapy and oncology vol. 25: the role of high energy electrons in the treatment of cancer*. Basel: S. Karger AG, 1991:169–179.
23. Kirsner SM, Hogstrom KR, Kurup RG, et al. Dosimetric evaluation in heterogeneous tissue of anterior electron beam irradiation for treatment of retinoblastoma. *Med Phys* 1987;14:772–779.
24. Donaldson SS, Findley DO. Treatment of orbital lymphoid tumors with electron beams. In: Vaeth JM, Meyer JL, eds. *Frontiers of radiation therapy and oncology vol. 25: the role of high energy electrons in the treatment of cancer*. Basel: S. Karger AG, 1991:187–200.
25. Low DA, Starkschall G, Sherman NE, et al. Computer-aided design and fabrication of an electron bolus for treatment of the paraspinal muscles. *Int J Radiat Oncol Biol Phys* 1995;33:1127–1138.
26. Merrick HW III, Dobelbower RR Jr, Konski AA. Intraoperative radiation therapy for pancreatic, biliary and gastric carcinoma: the US experience. In: Vaeth JM, Meyer JL, eds. *Frontiers of radiation therapy and oncology vol. 25: the role of high energy electrons in the treatment of cancer*. Basel: S. Karger AG, 1991:246–257.
27. Perez CA. Management of vulvar cancer. In: Vaeth JM, Meyer JL, eds. *Frontiers of radiation therapy and oncology vol. 25: the role of high energy electrons in the treatment of cancer*. Basel: S. Karger AG, 1991:183–186.
28. McGinnis WL, Bischof CJ, Latourette HB. Transvaginal cone electron beam technique for a Varian 18 MeV linear accelerator. *Int J Radiat Oncol Biol Phys* 1979;5:123–125.
29. Hogstrom KR. Clinical electron beam dosimetry: basic dosimetry data. In: Purdy JA, ed. *Advances in radiation oncology physics: dosimetry, treatment planning, and brachytherapy*. Woodbury, NY: American Institute of Physics, 1991:390–429.
30. Khan FM, Doppke KP, Hogstrom KR, et al. Clinical electron-beam dosimetry: report of AAPM Radiation Therapy Committee Task Group No. 25. *Med Phys* 1991;18:73–109.
31. Shiu AS, Tung SS, Nyerick CE, et al. Comprehensive analysis of electron beam central axis dose for a radiation therapy linear accelerator. *Med Phys* 1994;21:559–566.
32. Hogstrom KR. Treatment planning in electron beam therapy. In: Vaeth JM, Meyer JL, eds. *Frontiers of radiation therapy and oncology vol. 25: the role of high energy electrons in the treatment of cancer*. Basel: S. Karger AG, 1991:30–52.
33. Meyer JA, Palta JR, Hogstrom KR. Demonstration of relatively new electron dosimetry measurement techniques on the Mevatron 80. *Med Phys* 1984;11:670–677.
34. Hogstrom, KR, Steadham RE, Wong PF, et al. Monitor unit calculations for electron beams. In: Gibbons JP, ed. *Monitor unit calculations for external photon and electron beams*. Madison, WI: Advanced Medical Publishing, 2000:113–126.
35. Klein EE, Hanley J, Bayouth J, et al. Task Group 142 report: quality assurance of medical accelerators. *Med Phys* 2009;36(9):4197–4212.
36. Kutcher GJ, Coia L, Gillin M, et al. Comprehensive QA for radiation oncology: report of AAPM Radiation Therapy Committee Task Group 40. *Med Phys* 1994;21(4):581–618.
37. Hogstrom KR, Horton JL, Kutcher GJ, et al. *ACMP Task Group Report: survey of physics resources for radiation oncology special procedures*. Reston, VA: American College of Medical Physics, 1998.
38. Fraass B, Doppke K, Hunt M, et al. American Association of Physicists in Medicine Radiation Therapy Committee Task Group 53: quality assurance for clinical radiotherapy treatment planning [review]. *Med Phys* 1998;25(10):1773–1829.
39. Hogstrom KR. Dosimetry of electron heterogeneities. In: Wright AE, Boyer AL, eds. *Advances in radiation therapy treatment planning*. New York: American Institute of Physics, 1983:223–243.
40. Ekstrand KE, Dixon RL. The problem of obliquely incident beams in electron-beam treatment planning. *Med Phys* 1982;9:276–278.
41. Boyd RA, Hogstrom KR, Antolak JA, et al. A measured data set for evaluating electron-beam dose algorithms. *Med Phys* 2001;28:950–958.
42. Shiu AS, Tung S, Hogstrom KR, et al. Verification data for electron beam dose algorithms. *Med Phys* 1992;19:623–636.
43. Morrison WH, Wong PF, Starkschall G, et al. Water bolus for electron irradiation of the ear canal. *Int J Radiat Oncol Biol Phys* 1995;33:479–483.
44. Perry DJ, Holt JG. A model for calculating the effects of small inhomogeneities on electron beam dose distributions. *Med Phys* 1980;7:207–215.
45. Shiu AS, Hogstrom KR. Dose in bone and tissue near bone-tissue interface from electron beam. *Int J Radiat Oncol Biol Phys* 1991;21:695–702.
46. Mills MD, Hogstrom KR, Almond PR. Prediction of electron beam output factors. *Med Phys* 1982;9:60–68.
47. Biggs PJ, Boyer AL, Doppke KP. Electron dosimetry of irregular fields on Clinac-18. *Int J Radiat Oncol Biol Phys* 1979;5:433–440.
48. Khan FM. *The physics of radiation therapy*. 4th ed. Baltimore, MD: Lippincott Williams & Wilkins, 2009.
49. Harms WB, Purdy JA. Abutment of high energy electron fields. *Int J Radiat Oncol Biol Phys* 1991;20(4):853–858.
50. Hogstrom KR, Steadham RE. Electron beam dose computation. In: Palta JR, Mackie TR, eds. *Teletherapy: present and future*. Madison, WI: Advanced Medical Publishing, 1996:137–174.

51. Craig T, Brochu D, Van Dyk J. A quality assurance phantom for three-dimensional radiation treatment planning. *Int J Radiat Oncol Biol Phys* 1999;44(4):955–966.

52. Cygler JE, Daskalov GM, Chan GH, et al. Evaluation of the first commercial Monte Carlo dose calculation engine for electron beam treatment planning. *Med Phys* 2004;31(1):142–153.

53. Starkschall G, Shiu AS, Bujnowski SW, et al. Effect of dimensionality of heterogeneity corrections on the implementation of a three-dimensional electron pencil-beam algorithm. *Phys Med Biol* 1991;36:207–227.

54. Boyd RA, Hogstrom KR, Rosen II. Effect of using an initial polyenergetic spectrum with the pencil-beam redefinition algorithm for electron-dose calculations in water. *Med Phys* 1998;25:2176–2185.

55. Boyd RA, Hogstrom KR, Starkschall G. Electron pencil-beam redefinition algorithm dose calculations in the presence of heterogeneities. *Med Phys* 2001;28:2096–2104.

56. Shiu AS, Hogstrom KR. Pencil-beam redefinition algorithm for electron dose distributions. *Med Phys* 1991;18:7–18.

57. Faddegon B, Balogh J, Mackenzie R, et al. Clinical considerations of Monte Carlo for electron radiotherapy treatment planning. *Radiat Phys Chem* 1998;53:217–227.

58. Jiang SB, Kapur A, Ma CM. Electron beam modeling and commissioning for Monte Carlo treatment planning. *Med Phys* 2000;27(1):180–191.

59. Ma CM, Mok E, Kapur A, et al. Clinical implementation of a Monte Carlo treatment planning system. *Med Phys* 1999;26(10):2133–2143.

60. Neuenschwander H, Born EJ. A macro Monte-Carlo method for electron-beam dose calculations. *Phys Med Biol* 1992;37(1):107–125.

61. Neuenschwander H, Mackie TR, Reckwerdt PJ. MMC—a high-performance Monte Carlo code for electron beam treatment planning. *Phys Med Biol* 1995;40(I):543–574.

62. Ding GX, Duggan DM, Coffey CW, et al. First macro Monte Carlo based commercial dose calculation module for electron beam treatment planning—new issues for clinical consideration. *Phys Med Biol* 2006;51(11):2781–2799.

63. Ding GX, Cygler JE, Yu CW, et al. A comparison of electron beam dose calculation accuracy between treatment planning systems using either a pencil beam or a Monte Carlo algorithm. *Int J Radiat Oncol Biol Phys* 2005;63(2):622–633.

64. Klein EE, Li Z, Low DA. A feasibility study of multileaf collimated electrons with a scattering foil based accelerator. *Radiother Oncol* 1996;41:189–196.

65. Lee MC, Jiang SB, Ma CM. Monte Carlo and experimental investigations of multileaf collimated electron beams for modulated electron radiation therapy. *Med Phys* 2000;27(12):2708–2718.

66. Karlsson MG, Karlsson M, Ma CM. Treatment head design for multileaf collimated high-energy electrons. *Med Phys* 1999;26(10):2161–2167.

67. Starkschall G, Antolak JA, Hogstrom KR. Electron beam bolus for 3-D conformal radiation therapy. In: Purdy JA, Emami B, eds. *3-D radiation treatment planning and conformal therapy, proceedings of an international symposium.* Madison, WI: Medical Physics Publishing, 1995:265–282.

68. Low DA, Starkschall G, Bujnowski SW, et al. Electron bolus design for radiation therapy treatment planning: bolus design algorithms. *Med Phys* 1992;19:115–124.

69. Kudchadker RJ, Hogstrom KR, Garden AS, et al. Electron conformal radiation therapy using bolus and intensity modulation. *Int J Radiat Oncol Biol Phys* 2002;53:1023–1037.

70. Zeidan OA, Chauhan BD, Estabrook WW, et al. Image-guided bolus electron conformal therapy—a case study. *J Appl Clin Med Phys* 2010;12(1):3311.

71. Burleson S, Baker J, Hsia AT, Xu Z. Use of 3D printers to create a patient-specific 3D bolus for external beam therapy. *J Appl Clin Med Phys* 2015;16(3):166.

72. Canters RA, Lips IM, Wendling M, et al. Clinical implementation of 3D printing in the construction of patient specific bolus for electron beam radiotherapy for non-melanoma skin cancer. *Radiother Oncol* 2016;121:148.

73. Su S, Moran K, Robar JL. Design and production of 3D printed bolus for electron radiation therapy. *J Appl Clin Med Phys* 2014;15(4):194

74. Shiu AS, Tung SS, Gastorf RJ, et al. Dosimetric evaluation of lead and tungsten eye shields in electron beam treatment. *Int J Radiat Oncol Biol Phys* 1996;35:599–604.

75. Klevenhagen SC, Lambert GD, Arbabi A. Backscattering in electron beam therapy for energies between 3 and 35 MeV. *Phys Med Biol* 1982;27:363–373.

76. Das IJ, Bushe HS. Backscattering and transmission through a high Z interface as a measure of electron beam energy. *Med Phys* 1994;21(2):315–319.

77. Lambert GD, Klevenhagen SC. Penetration of backscattered electrons in polystyrene for energies between 1 and 25 MeV. *Phys Med Biol* 1982;27:721–725.

78. ICRU Report 35. *Radiation dosimetry: electron beams with energies between 1 and 50 MeV.* Bethesda, MD: International Commission on Radiation Units and Measurement, 1984.

79. Johnson JM, Khan FM. Dosimetric effects of abutting extended source to surface distance electron fields with photon fields in the treatment of head and neck cancers. *Int J Radiat Oncol Biol Phys* 1994;28(3):741–747.

80. Mills MD, Fuller LM, Zagars GK, et al. Spinal cord dose reduction using an anterior 13 MeV electron field situated between a split anterior ⁶⁰Co supraclavicular field. *Int J Radiat Oncol Biol Phys* 1987;13:1571–1575.

81. Severin D, Connors S, Thompson H, et al. Breast radiotherapy with inclusion of internal mammary nodes: a comparison of techniques with three-dimensional planning. *Int J Radiat Oncol Biol Phys* 2003;55(3):633–644.

82. Zackrisson B, Karlsson M. Matching of electron beams for conformal therapy of target volumes at moderate depths. *Radiother Oncol* 1996;39(3):261–270.

83. Mu X, Olofsson L, Karlsson M, et al. Can photon IMRT be improved by combination with mixed electron and photon techniques? *Acta Oncol* 2004;43(8):727–735.

84. Das SK, Bell M, Marks LB, et al. A preliminary study of the role of modulated electron beams in intensity modulated radiotherapy, using automated beam orientation and modality selection. *Int J Radiat Oncol Biol Phys* 2004;59(2):602–617.

85. Ma CM, Ding M, Li JS, et al. A comparative dosimetric study on tangential photon beams, intensity-modulated radiation therapy (IMRT) and modulated electron radiotherapy (MERT) for breast cancer treatment. *Phys Med Biol* 2003;48(7):909–924.

86. Mills MD. Analysis and practical use: the Abt Study of Medical Physicist Work Values for Radiation Oncology Physics Services—round II. *J Am Coll Radiol* 2005;2(9):782–789.

87. Hogstrom KR, Boyer AL, Shiu AS, et al. Design of metallic electron beam cones for an intraoperative therapy linear accelerator. *Int J Radiat Oncol Biol Phys* 1990;18:1223–1232.

88. Beddar AS, Biggs PJ, Chang S, et al. Intraoperative radiation therapy using mobile electron linear accelerators: report of AAPM Radiation Therapy Committee Task Group No. 72, Report No. 92. *Med Phys* 2006;33(5):1476–1489.

89. Biggs PJ, Wang CC. Breakaway safety feature for an intra-oral cone system. *Int J Radiat Oncol Biol Phys* 1984;10:1117–1119.

90. Nyerick CE, Ochran TG, Boyer AL, et al. Dosimetry characteristics of metallic cones for intraoperative radiation therapy. *Int J Radiat Oncol Biol Phys* 1991;21:501–510.

91. Able CM, Mills MD, McNeese MD, et al. Evaluation of a total scalp electron irradiation technique. *Int J Radiat Oncol Biol Phys* 1991;21:1063–1072.

92. Akazawa C. Treatment of the scalp using photon and electron beams. *Med Dosim* 1989;14:129–131.

93. Walker C, Wadd NJ, Lucraft HH. Novel solutions to the problems encountered in electron irradiation to the surface of the head. *Br J Radiol* 1999;72(860):787–791.

94. Yaparpalvi R, Fontenla DP, Beitler JJ. Improved dose homogeneity in scalp irradiation using a single set-up point and different energy electron beams. *Br J Radiol* 2002;75(896):670–677.

95. Peters VG. Use of an electron reflector to improve dose uniformity at the vertex during total skin electron therapy. *Int J Radiat Oncol Biol Phys* 2000;46(4):1065–1069.

96. Almond PR. Total skin electron irradiation technique and dosimetry. In: Kereiakes JG, Elson HR, Born CG, eds. *Radiation oncology physics 1986.* New York: American Institute of Physics, 1987:296–332.

97. Alexander A, Soisson E, Hijal T, et al. Comparison of modulated electron radiotherapy to conventional electron boost irradiation and volumetric modulated photon arc therapy for treatment of tumour bed boost in breast cancer. *Radiother Oncol* 2011;100(2):253–258.

98. Jin JY, Klein EE, Kong FM, et al. An improved internal mammary irradiation technique in radiation treatment of locally advanced breast cancers. *J Appl Clin Med Phys* 2005;6(1):84–93.

99. Gaffney DK, Leavitt DD, Tsodikov A, et al. Electron arc irradiation of the postmastectomy chest wall with CT treatment planning: 20-year experience. *Int J Radiat Oncol Biol Phys* 2001;51:994–1001.

100. Al-Yahya K, Hristov D, Verhaegen F, et al. Monte Carlo based modulated electron beam treatment planning using a few-leaf electron collimator—feasibility study. *Phys Med Biol* 2005;50(5):847–857.

101. Klein EE, Vicic M, Ma CM, et al. Validation of calculations for electrons modulated with conventional photon multileaf collimators. *Phys Med Biol* 2008;53(5):1183–1208.

102. Klein EE, Mamalui-Hunter M, Low DA. Delivery of modulated electron beams with conventional photon multi-leaf collimators. *Phys Med Biol* 2009;54(2):327–339.

103. Surucu M, Klein EE, Mamalui-Hunter M, et al. Planning tools for modulated electron radiotherapy. *Med Phys* 2010;37(5):2215–2224.

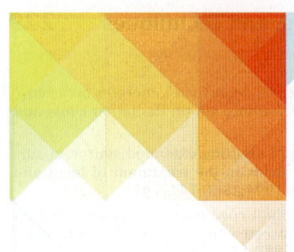

CHAPTER 9

Conformal Radiation Therapy Physics, Treatment Planning, and Clinical Aspects

James A. Purdy and Sasa Mutic

INTRODUCTION

Modern anatomic imaging technologies, such as x-ray computed tomography (CT) and magnetic resonance imaging (MRI), provide a fully three-dimensional model of the cancer patient's anatomy, which is often complemented with functional imaging, such as positron emission tomography (PET) or magnetic resonance spectroscopy (MRS). Such advanced imaging allows the radiation oncologist to more accurately identify tumor volumes and their relationship with other critical normal organs. Powerful x-ray CT simulation and three-dimensional treatment planning systems (3DTPS) have been commercially available since the early 1990s, and three-dimensional conformal radiation therapy (3DCRT) has been the standard of practice for many years.[1–3] In addition, advances in radiation treatment delivery technology continue to evolve, as evident by developments in MRI-LINAC technology by Elekta (Stockholm, Sweden) and ViewRay (Oakwood Village, OH) as well as developments in proton beam delivery. Although these machines have different goals and features and it is beyond the scope of this text to provide an in-depth analysis of these technologies, some of the topics that are relevant in the designs of these technologies include improving imaging localization and intrafractional patient monitoring, increasing delivery efficiency, improving quality of delivered dose distributions, reducing cost of the equipment and of operation, improving clinical outcomes, simplifying use, and improving global access to modern day radiotherapy.

3DCRT treatment plans generally use an increased number of radiation beams that are shaped to conform to the target volume. To improve the conformality of the dose distribution, conventional beam modifiers (e.g., wedges, partial transmission blocks, and/or compensating filters) are sometimes used.

This *forward planning* approach used for 3DCRT (Fig. 9.1) is rapidly giving way to an *inverse planning* approach used for *intensity-modulated radiation therapy* (IMRT) (Fig. 9.2), which can achieve even greater conformity by optimally modulating the individual beamlets that make up the radiation beams.[4,5] IMRT dose distributions can be created to conform much more closely to the target volume, particularly for those volumes having complex/concave shapes, and also shaped to avoid critical normal tissues in the irradiated volume. This increased conformality results in IMRT treatments being much more sensitive to geometric uncertainties than the two-dimensional or forward-planned 3DCRT approaches and has spurred the development of treatment machines integrated with advanced volumetric imaging capabilities.[2,3,6,7,8] This has pushed the frontiers in conformal radiation therapy (CRT) practice from IMRT to what is now referred to *image-guided radiation therapy* (IGRT).[2,3,9] Of course, the concept of image guidance is not revolutionary and really should be viewed as an evolutionary component in the development of CRT. In the past, many systems and/or processes have been developed to help better localize the patient for treatment (and hence conform the dose), including dedicated x-ray simulators, megavoltage radiographic port films, electronic portal imaging devices (EPIDs), implanted radiopaque markers, ultrasound imaging systems, optical surface tracking systems, etc.[10,11] Even the early isocentric cobalt-60 teletherapy machines in the 1960s came equipped with a kilovolt x-ray tube attached to the beam stop.

This chapter will review the critical components that make up the CRT planning and delivery process, focusing mainly on the forward-planned 3DCRT process. However, it should be understood that most of the concepts and tasks discussed apply equally well to IMRT and IGRT, particularly with regard to target volume definition, plan evaluation, and many aspects of clinical quality assurance (QA). The reader should also

FIGURE 9.1. Three-dimensional conformal radiation therapy (3DCRT), considered a "forward planning" CRT approach that uses an increased number of radiation beams that are shaped to conform to the target volume. To improve the conformality of the dose distribution, beam modifiers (e.g., wedges, partial transmission blocks, and/or compensating filters) are sometimes used. Shown is a prostate seven-field coplanar beam arrangement.

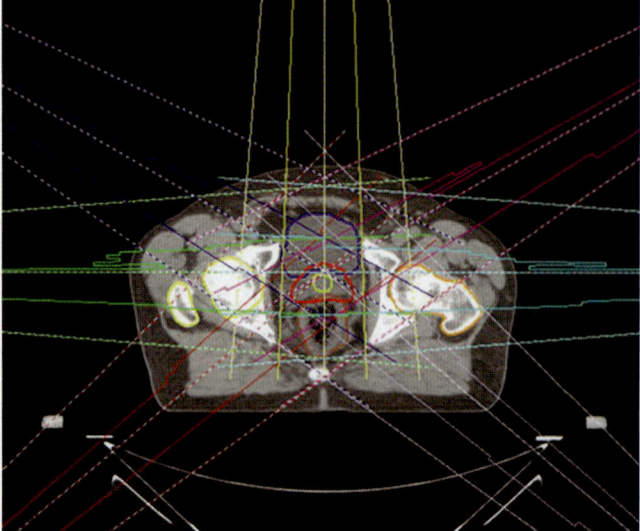

FIGURE 9.2. Intensity-modulated radiation therapy (IMRT) is considered an "inverse planning" conformal radiation therapy approach that can achieve even greater conformity than three-dimensional conformal radiation therapy by optimally modulating the individual beamlets that make up the radiation beams. IMRT dose distributions can be created to conform much more closely to the target volume, particularly for those volumes having complex/concave shapes, and also shaped to avoid critical normal tissues in the irradiated volume.

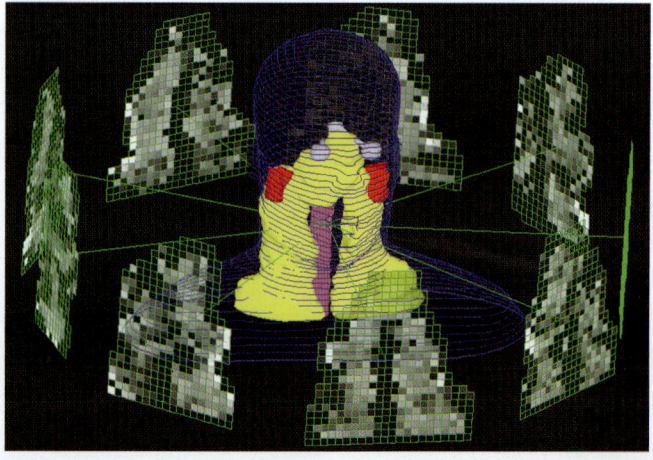

understand that the use of the terms two-dimensional (*2-D*), three-dimensional (*3-D*), and even four-dimensional (*4-D*)[12] as descriptors for the CRT planning and delivery process refers to a process and the various tools used and not merely to beam arrangements. For example, 3-D treatment planning certainly does not require the use of "noncoplanar" beams—a common misconception—but does require the ability to plan and visualize volumetric dose distributions for such beam arrangements. Even today, newer tools are being developed that allow 4-D, image-based CRT planning, that is, target-volume segmentation and dose calculation in the presence of moving organs and target volumes. Hence, the reader will be able to appreciate the CRT approach much more fully if it is viewed as a constantly evolving planning and treatment delivery workflow process using ever-advancing computer software and technology.

HISTORICAL DEVELOPMENT OF CONFORMAL RADIATION THERAPY AND 3-D TREATMENT PLANNING SYSTEMS

Conformational treatment methods were pioneered in the 1950s and 1960s by several groups, including Takahashi[13] in Japan; Proimos,[14] Trump, and Wright et al.[15] in the United States; and Green et al.[16] in Great Britain. Work continued into the 1970s, when several groups actually implemented computer-controlled radiation therapy, including a project of the Joint Center for Radiation Therapy in Boston led by Bjarngard and Kijewski[17] and the Tracking Cobalt Project led by Davy et al.[18] at the Royal Free Hospital in London.

Sterling et al.[19,20] are credited with the first 3-D approach to treatment planning (dose calculation and display). They demonstrated a technique by which a computer-generated film loop gave the illusion of a 3-D view of the patient's relevant anatomic features and the calculated isodose distribution (2-D color washes) throughout a treatment volume. However, this effort did not result in a practical 3DTPS and was viewed as simply a demonstration project. The Rhode Island Hospital/Brown University group made the first real step in implementing a clinically usable 3DTPS based on a new type of display, called beam's-eye view (BEV), which simulated the treatment planner's viewing point from the perspective of the radiation source looking out along the axis of the radiation beam, similar to that obtained when viewing a simulation radiograph.[21,22]

The advent of CT spurred further development of 3-D planning systems. In 1983, Goitein and coworkers[23,24] reported on their system, which took advantage of CT and increased minicomputer capabilities. The system produced high-quality color BEV displays and could display radiographic images computed from the digital CT data; such computed radiographs are now called digitally reconstructed radiographs (DRRs). By the latter half of the 1980s, several other academic groups had developed 3-D planning systems having powerful new features.[25–28]

In the 1990s, the commercial availability of 3DTPS led to widespread adoption of 3-D planning and CRT as the standard of practice. One of the keys to this development was a series of research contracts funded by the National Cancer Institute (NCI) in the 1980s and 1990s to evaluate the potential of 3-D planning and to make recommendations to the NCI for future research in this area.[29] Each of the research contracts funded a collaborative working group (CWG). The participating institutions in each CWG are shown in Table 9.1. Their charge was to evaluate various aspects of this new planning process and develop new software tools needed. The CWGs were composed of physicists, clinicians, and computer scientists. Many important developments and/or refinements in 3-D planning came from these NCI research CWGs, particularly planning evaluation software tools such as *dose–volume histograms* (DVHs),[30,31] *electronic view box*,[32] and biologic effect models such as *tumor control probability* (TCP)

TABLE 9.1 NATIONAL CANCER INSTITUTE RESEARCH CONTRACTS IN SUPPORT OF THREE-DIMENSIONAL RADIATION THERAPY TREATMENT PLANNING

Evaluation of Treatment Planning for Heavy Particles (1982–1986)
Lawrence Berkeley Laboratory and University of California
Massachusetts General Hospital, Harvard University
MD Anderson Cancer Center, University of Texas
University of Pennsylvania School of Medicine and Fox Chase Cancer Center

Evaluation of Treatment Planning for External Beam Photons (1984–1987)
Massachusetts General Hospital, Harvard University
Memorial Sloan Kettering Cancer Center
University of Pennsylvania School of Medicine and Fox Chase Cancer Center
Washington University in St. Louis

Evaluation of Treatment Planning for External Beam Electrons (1986–1989)
MD Anderson Cancer Center, University of Texas
University of Michigan
Washington University in St. Louis

Development of Radiation Therapy Treatment Planning Software Tools (1989–1994)
University of North Carolina
University of Washington
Washington University in St. Louis

and *normal tissue complication probability* (NTCP) models.[33] Even IMRT has benefited from the CWG approach, as a consensus statement was developed in 2001 that helped clarify many issues and pointed to important research areas regarding that form of CRT.[34]

VOLUME SPECIFICATION FOR CONFORMAL RADIATION THERAPY

The International Commission on Radiation Units and Measurements (ICRU) first addressed the issue of consistent volume and dose specification in radiation therapy with the publication of ICRU Report 29 in 1978.[35] That report defined the *target volume* as *the volume containing those tissues that are to be irradiated to a specified absorbed dose according to a specified time–dose pattern* (Fig. 9.3A). It is interesting to note that this report (even though published in the 2-D era) attempted to address spatial uncertainties by pointing out that the size and shape of a target volume may change during the course of a treatment and that one should take into account the following parameters when describing the target volume:

1. Expected movements (e.g., caused by breathing) of those tissues that contain the target volume relative to anatomic reference points (e.g., skin markings, suprasternal notch)

FIGURE 9.3. A: Schematic illustration of the boundaries of the volumes defined by International Commission on Radiation Units and Measures (ICRU) Report 29: target volume, treatment volume, and irradiated volume. **B:** Boundaries of the volumes defined by ICRU Report 50: gross tumor volume (GTV), clinical target volume (CTV), planning target volume (PTV), treated volume, and irradiated volume. **C:** Boundaries of the volumes defined by ICRU Report 62: GTV, CTV, internal target volume (ITV), PTV, treated volume, and irradiated volume.

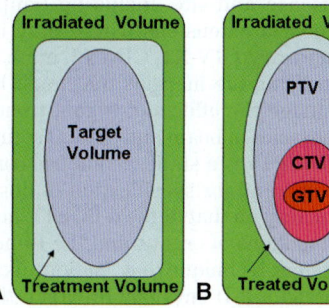
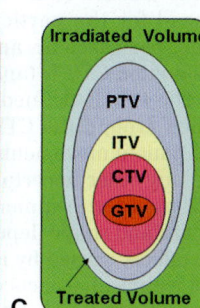

Section I

2. Expected variation in shape and size of the target volume during a course of treatment (e.g., urinary bladder, stomach)
3. Inaccuracies or variations in treatment setup during the course of treatment

However, the report did not address the issues of coordinate systems (e.g., patient vs. treatment machine), and no attempt was made to define and explicitly separate the margins for the different types of uncertainties.

In addition to the target volume, ICRU Report 29 defined two other volumes: (a) the *treatment volume* and (b) the *irradiated volume*. These volumes were not based on anatomy, but instead were based on the dose distribution. The treatment volume was defined as *the volume enclosed by the isodose surface representing the minimal target dose*, and the irradiated volume was defined as *the volume that receives a dose considered significant in relation to normal tissue tolerance* (e.g., 50% isodose surface).

Report 29 defined *organs at risk* (OARs) as *especially radiosensitive organs in or near the target volume whose presence influences treatment planning and/or prescribed dose*. The report also recognized the importance of tissues outside the target area that received a dose higher than 100% of the specified target dose. This was defined as a *hot spot* and was considered clinically meaningful only if the corresponding isodose curve enclosed an area of at least 2 cm^2 in a section.

In retrospect, ICRU Report 29 recommendations were well suited for the technology of the 1970s and 1980s, that is, using a conventional simulator to generate a planning radiograph for designing beam portals based on bony and soft tissue landmarks for standardized beam arrangement techniques applied to whole classes of comparable patients. Several generations of radiation oncologists were trained using this nomenclature and method, and the ICRU recommendation for reporting dose and volumes helped advance radiation oncology.

In 1993, the ICRU updated its recommendations for specifying dose/volume in Report 50, which was well suited for conformal therapy.[36] The target volume definition was separated into three distinct volumes: (a) visible tumor, that is, *gross tumor volume* (GTV); (b) a volume to account for uncertainties in microscopic tumor spread, that is, *clinical target volume* (CTV); and (c) a volume to account for geometric and other uncertainties, that is, *planning target volume* (PTV), as illustrated in Figure 9.3B.

The GTV and CTV are anatomic–clinical concepts that should be defined before a choice of treatment modality and technique is made. Labels or subscripts with the GTV nomenclature can be used to distinguish between primary disease and other areas of macroscopic tumor involvement such as involved lymph nodes that are visible on imaging studies (e.g., GTV$_{primary}$ and GTV$_{nodal}$, or GTV-T and GTV-N). Similarly, the GTV together with this surrounding volume of local subclinical involvement that defines the CTV can be denoted as CTV-T. Note that even if the GTV has been removed by radical surgery, the volume can be designated as CTV-T. In specifying the CTV, the physician must consider not only microextensions of the disease near the GTV but also the natural avenues of spread for the particular disease and site, including lymph node, perivascular, and perineural extensions. These may be designated CTV-N (and, if necessary, CTV-N1, CTV-N2, etc.).

The *PTV* is defined by specifying the margins that must be added around the CTV to manage the effects of organ, tumor and patient movements, inaccuracies in beam and patient setup, and any other uncertainties. The PTV is a static, geometric concept used for treatment planning and for specification of dose. Its size and shape depend primarily on that of the GTV/CTV and the effects caused by internal motions of organs and the tumor and technical aspects of treatment technique (e.g., patient fixation). The PTV can be considered a 3-D envelope in which the tumor and any microscopic extensions reside and move. Once

the PTV is defined, appropriate beam sizes to account for penumbra and beam arrangements must be selected to ensure the desired dose coverage of the PTV. Note that multiple PTVs may be defined for a patient's radiation therapy treatment. For example, it is common practice to plan a higher dose to the PTV enclosing the GTV and a lower dose to the PTV containing the CTV. Such planning volumes are typically subscripted using the dose level prescribed; for example, PTVs for 66 Gy and 54 Gy can be represented as PTV$_6$ and PTV$_{54}$, respectively.

ICRU Report 50 essentially retained the definition of the two dose volumes defined in ICRU Report 29, changing the treatment volume name to *treated volume* and refining the definition as *the volume enclosed by an isodose surface, selected and specified by the radiation oncologist as being appropriate to achieve the purpose of treatment* (e.g., tumor eradication, palliation), and the irradiated volume as that *tissue volume that receives a dose that is considered significant in relation to normal tissue tolerance*.

Report 50 refined the definition of organs at risk as *normal tissues whose radiation sensitivity may significantly influence treatment planning and/or prescribed dose*. The report did state that any possible movement of the organ at risk during treatment, as well as uncertainties in the setup during the whole treatment course, must be considered, but did not provide a method to do so.

The hot spot definition was modified to be *a volume outside the PTV that received a dose larger than 100% of the specified PTV dose*. This was considered clinically meaningful only if the minimum diameter exceeded 15 mm (note: previously, it had been 2 cm^2). However, if the hot spot occurs in a small organ, such as the optic nerve, a dimension smaller than the recommended 15 mm should be considered.

As previously stated, Report 50 was well suited to conformal therapy, and it stimulated broad interest in the radiation oncology community. However, irradiation techniques continued to evolve (e.g., IMRT, IGRT), and advances in imaging procedures (e.g., PET, MRI) provided even more information on functionality, the location; shape, and limits of tumor/target volumes; and organs at risk. In response to these developments, the ICRU in 1999 published Report 62,[37] which expanded on some of the definitions and concepts of Report 50 and took into account the consequences of the technical and clinical progress referred to previously. However, it should be clearly understood that Report 62 is intended to complement the recommendations contained in Report 50 and not to replace it.

ICRU Report 62 refined the definition of PTV by introducing the concept of an *internal margin* to take into account variations in size, shape, and position of the CTV in reference to the patient's coordinate system using anatomic reference points, as well as the concept of a *set-up margin* to take into account all uncertainties in patient beam positioning in reference to the treatment machine coordinate system. Identification of these two types of margins is needed, as they compensate for different types of uncertainties and refer to different coordinate systems. Internal margin uncertainties are due to physiologic variations (e.g., filling of the rectum, movements because of respiration) and are difficult or almost impossible to control from a practical viewpoint. Set-up margin uncertainties are related largely to technical factors that can be dealt with by more accurate setup and immobilization of the patient and improved mechanical stability of the machine. However, exactly how these margins should be combined is still not clear. This point will be discussed further in a later section, but for now, it is necessary to understand that the selection of an overall margin and delineation of the border of the PTV typically involve a compromise that requires the experience and the judgment of the radiation oncologist and the treatment planning team.

ICRU Report 62 defines the volume formed by the CTV and the internal margin as the *internal target volume* (ITV) (Fig. 9.3C). The ITV represents the movements of the CTV

TABLE 9.2 SUMMARY OF THE INTERNATIONAL COMMISSION ON RADIATION UNITS AND MEASUREMENTS (ICRU) NOMENCLATURE FOR VOLUMES (1970S TO PRESENT)

ICRU Report 29: 1970s–1993	ICRU Report 50: 1993–Present	ICRU Report 62: 1999–Present	ICRU Report 83: 2010–Present
Target volume	GTV CTV PTV	GTV CTV ITV PTV	GTV CTV ITV PTV
Treatment volume Irradiated volume Organ at risk	Treated volume Irradiated volume Organ at risk	Treated volume Irradiated volume Organ at risk PRV	Treated volume Irradiated volume Organ at risk PRV RVR
Hot spot (area outside target that receives dose >100% of specified target dose; at least 2 cm² in a section)	Hot spot (volume outside PTV that receives dose >100% of specified PTV dose; >15 mm diameter)	Hot spot (volume outside PTV that receives dose >100% of specified PTV dose; 15 mm diameter)	High dose to RVR
Dose heterogeneity (no value given)	Dose heterogeneity (+7% to −5% of prescribed dose)	Dose heterogeneity (+7% to −5% of prescribed dose)	Not specified

CTV, clinical target volume; GTV, gross tumor volume; ITV, internal target volume; PRV, planning risk volume; PTV, planning target volume; RVR, remaining volume at risk.

referenced to the patient coordinate system and is specified in relation to internal and external reference points, which preferably should be rigidly related to each other through bony structures. In cases not involving significant internal organ motion, the radiation oncologist can simply ignore having to explicitly define the ITV and use only the GTV, CTV, and PTV concepts. However, in cases involving significant motion, such as often is the case with lung cancer, the ITV concept has proven useful and should be used.[38]

ICRU Report 62 refined the definition of the two dose volumes defined ICRU Report 50 as follows:

The treated volume is the tissue volume that (according to the approved treatment plan) is planned to receive at least a dose selected and specified by radiation oncology team as being appropriate to achieve the purpose of the treatment, e.g., tumor eradication or palliation, within the bounds of acceptable complications.

The irradiated volume is the *tissue volume that receives a dose that is considered significant in relation to normal tissue tolerance.*

Report 62 refined the definition of organs at risk as *normal tissues (e.g., spinal cord) whose radiation sensitivity may significantly influence treatment planning and/or prescribed dose.* The report also included a discussion regarding a system of classifying organs at risk as "serial," "parallel," or "serial–parallel." Report 62 also addressed what was perhaps the most criticized limitation of Report 50, which was that it did not provide a method to account for organ-at-risk movements and changes in shape and/or size, as well as set-up uncertainties. To account for such spatial uncertainties, Report 62 introduced the concept of the *planning organ at risk volume* (PRV), in which a margin is added around the organ at risk to compensate for that organ's geometric uncertainties. The PRV margin around the organ at risk is analogous to the PTV margin around the CTV. The introduction of the PRV concept is timely, as its use is even more important for those conformal therapy cases involving IMRT because of the increased sensitivity of this type treatment to geometric uncertainties. For example, it is common practice to add a 0.5-cm rind around the spinal cord contour. Note that the PTV and the PRV may overlap, and often do so, which implies searching for a compromise in weighting the importance of each in the planning process. A summary of the ICRU volume nomenclature recommendations per report is presented in Table 9.2.

CONFORMAL RADIATION THERAPY PLANNING PROCESS

As previously stated, CRT treatment planning and delivery is best considered as a process and the tools used. This process is summarized in Table 9.3 and includes (a) establishing the

patient's treatment position, constructing a patient repositioning immobilization device when needed, and obtaining a volumetric image data set of the patient in treatment position; (b) contouring target volume(s) and organs at risk using the volumetric planning image data set; (c) specifying a prescription

TABLE 9.3 CONFORMAL RADIATION THERAPY PROCESS

1. Patient treatment position, immobilization, and planning imaging
   a. Position patient in proposed treatment position.
   b. Fabricate immobilization devices.
   c. Place radiopaque markers, and mark repositioning lines on patient and immobilization devices.
   d. Obtain topograms to check patient alignment.
   e. Perform volumetric computed tomography (CT) scan of patient in treatment position.
   f. Make illustrative photographs to assist in repositioning the patient at the treatment couch.
   g. Transfer CT images to three-dimensional treatment planning system (3DTPS).
   h. Perform imaging studies (e.g., MRI, PET/CT, etc.) as requested by treating physician, and transfer image data to 3DTPS.
2. Delineation of tumor/target volumes and organs at risk
   a. Physician contours target volume(s).
   b. Physician or dosimetrist contours organs at risk.
3. Dose prescription
   a. Physician provides prescription dose for planning target volume (PTV) and dose–volume constraints for organs at risk.
   b. Forward planning (three-dimensional conformal radiation therapy)
      i. Set up initial beam configuration and design field shapes; wedges/bolus/ no beam modifiers; beam weights.
      ii. Compute 3-D dose matrix.
      iii. Compute treatment machine monitor units.
   c. Inverse planning (intensity-modulated radiation therapy [IMRT])
      i. Set up initial beam configuration.
      ii. Enter desired dose–volume constraints for PTV(s) and all regions of interest.
      iii. Initiate treatment planning system optimization process, which generates beam fluences, resulting dose distribution, monitor units, and leaf motion files.
4. Plan evaluation and improvement
   a. Evaluate plan (dose–volume histograms, planar isodose display, 3-D isodose display) and modify until plan is found to be acceptable by treating physician.
   b. Transfer patient's plan to patient's chart (electronic medical record) and treatment machine verify and record (V&R) system.
5. Plan implementation and treatment verification
   a. Physicist performs second check of treatment plan and transfer of data to V&R system.
   b. For IMRT plans, perform phantom dosimetric verification.
   c. Verify patient position and isocenter placement on treatment machine using orthogonal portal electronic portal imaging devices (EPIDs) vs. digitally reconstructed radiograph (DRRs) or using onboard CT vs. planning CT.
   d. For 3DCRT, check field shapes by comparing treatment field DRRs with treatment beam EPIDs.
   e. Capture treatment machine settings in V&R system.
   f. Check first-day treatment with diode measurements.
   g. Perform periodic imaging verification checks during treatment (e.g., orthogonal EPIDs/DRRs or beam EPIDs/DRRs, cone-beam CT/planning CT).

dose for the PTV and dose–volume constraints for any OARs; (d1) for 3DCRT forward planning, determining beam orientation and designing beam apertures and computing a 3-D dose distribution according to the dose prescription; (d2) for IMRT inverse planning, setting up initial beam orientations and entering optimization parameters (i.e., dose–volume constraints for PTV[s] and all regions of interest) and initiating the TPS optimization process, which generates beam fluences, resulting dose distribution, monitor units (MUs), and leaf motion files; (e) evaluating the treatment plan and, if needed, modifying the plan (e.g., beam orientations, apertures, beam weights, etc.) until an acceptable plan is approved by the radiation oncologist; and (f) implementing the approved plan on the treatment machine and verifying the patient's treatment using appropriate QA procedures throughout the treatment. All of these tasks make up the CRT process and are discussed in the ensuing sections.

Patient Treatment Position and Immobilization and Planning of Imaging

In the initial part of the CRT process (preplanning), the proposed treatment position of the patient is determined, and the immobilization device to be used during simulation/treatment is selected. It should be clearly understood that repositioning patients and accounting for internal organ movement for fractionated radiation therapy in order to accurately reproduce the planned dose distribution remain difficult technical aspects of the CRT process. Errors may occur if patients are inadequately immobilized, with resultant treatment fields inaccurately aligned from treatment to treatment (interfraction). In addition, patients and/or their tumor volume may also move during treatment (intrafraction) because of either inadequate immobilization or physiologic activity. Accounting for all of the uncertainties in the CRT planning and delivery process remains a challenge for radiation oncology, and research and development is ongoing.

Determining the treatment position of the patient and constructing the immobilization device are typically done in a dedicated radiation therapy CT simulator facility. A radiation therapy CT simulator consists of a diagnostic-quality CT scanner, laser patient positioning/marking system, virtual simulation 3-D treatment planning software, as well as various digital display systems for viewing the DRRs.[39,40] The CT scanner is used to acquire a volumetric planning CT scan of a patient in treatment position. The use of intravenous or other contrast to help delineate target volumes needs to be considered during simulation in some cases. CT topograms should be generated first and reviewed prior to acquiring the planning scan to ensure that patient alignment is correct, with adjustments to be made if needed. Radiopaque markers can be placed on the patient's skin and the immobilization device to serve as fiducial marks to assist in any coordinate transformation needed as a result of 3-D planning and eventual plan implementation. An example of a typical immobilization repositioning system used for patients undergoing radiation therapy for head and neck (H&N) cancer is shown in Figure 9.4. PET-CT simulators[41] are also used in a number of departments. Trend for replacement of CT simulators with PET-CT simulators was especially active in the 2000s. More recently, there is a trend for use of MR simulators in RT- and MR-only–based simulation, and treatment planning has been an active topic of research and development.[42,43]

Planning CT scan protocols are tumor site dependent and typically range from 2 to 5 mm in slice thickness and 50 to 200 slices. In general, a 3-mm slice thickness provides adequate-quality DRR. In some sites, such as those of H&N cancer, slice thicknesses of 1 mm are often needed for delineation of very small volumes, such as the optic chiasm and the optic

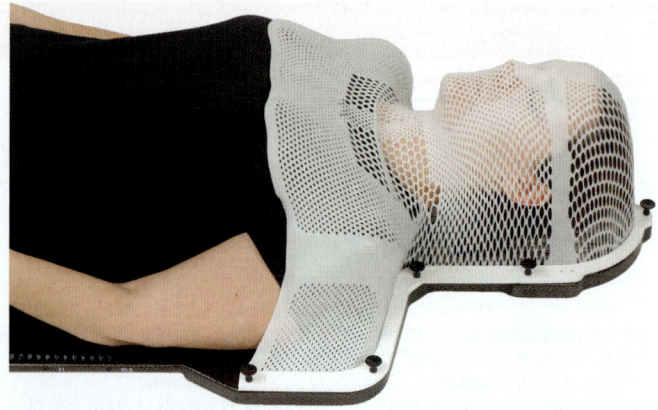

FIGURE 9.4. Example of immobilization repositioning system used for patients undergoing radiation therapy for head and neck cancer. It should be clearly understood that being able to accurately reposition the patient and account for internal organ movement in order to accurately deliver the planned dose distribution is one of the most important steps in the conformal therapy process. (Courtesy of CIVCO Radiotherapy.)

nerves. The same holds true for optimal reconstruction of the position of any implanted markers used, such as in prostate cancer radiation therapy.

The planning CT data set is typically transferred to a 3DTPS via a computer network. The planning CT data set provides an accurate geometric model of the patient, as well as the electron density information needed for the calculation of the 3-D dose distribution that takes into account tissue heterogeneities.

Delineation of Tumor/Target Volumes and Organs at Risk

Delineation of tumor/target volume and organs at risk contours using the volumetric CT data set is typically performed by the radiation oncologist and the medical dosimetrist working as a team. The CT data are displayed at the 3DTPS workstation (Fig. 9.5), and contours are drawn manually by the radiation oncologist/dosimetrist, most often using a computer mouse or stylus on a slice-by-slice basis. Some OARs with distinct boundaries (e.g., skin, lung) can be contoured automatically, with only minor editing required; others (e.g., brachial plexus) require the hands-on effort of the radiation oncologist.[44] With modern 3DTPS image segmentation software, contouring generally takes 0.5 to 1 hour, depending on the disease site. However, for some complex sites, such as H&N cancer, where many OARs and complex tumor/target volumes are the norm, this task can take several hours.

CT is still the principal source of imaging data used for defining the GTV for most sites, but this imaging modality presents several potential pitfalls. First, when contouring the GTV, it is essential that the appropriate CT window and level settings be used in order to determine the maximum dimension of what is considered potential gross disease (Fig. 9.6). Second, for those treatment sites in which there is considerable organ motion, such as for tumors in the thorax, CT images do not correctly represent either the time-averaged position of the tumor or its shape, and hence newer 4-D CT technology must be used.[45–47] This can be understood by appreciating the fact that CT simulators rely almost exclusively on the use of fast spiral CT technology and thus acquire data essentially in limited width slices and combine them to construct a 3-D matrix. This has the effect of capturing the tumor cross-sectional images at particular positions in the breathing cycle. If the tumor motion is significant, different, and possibly noncontiguous, transverse sections of the tumor could be imaged at different points of the breathing cycle, leading

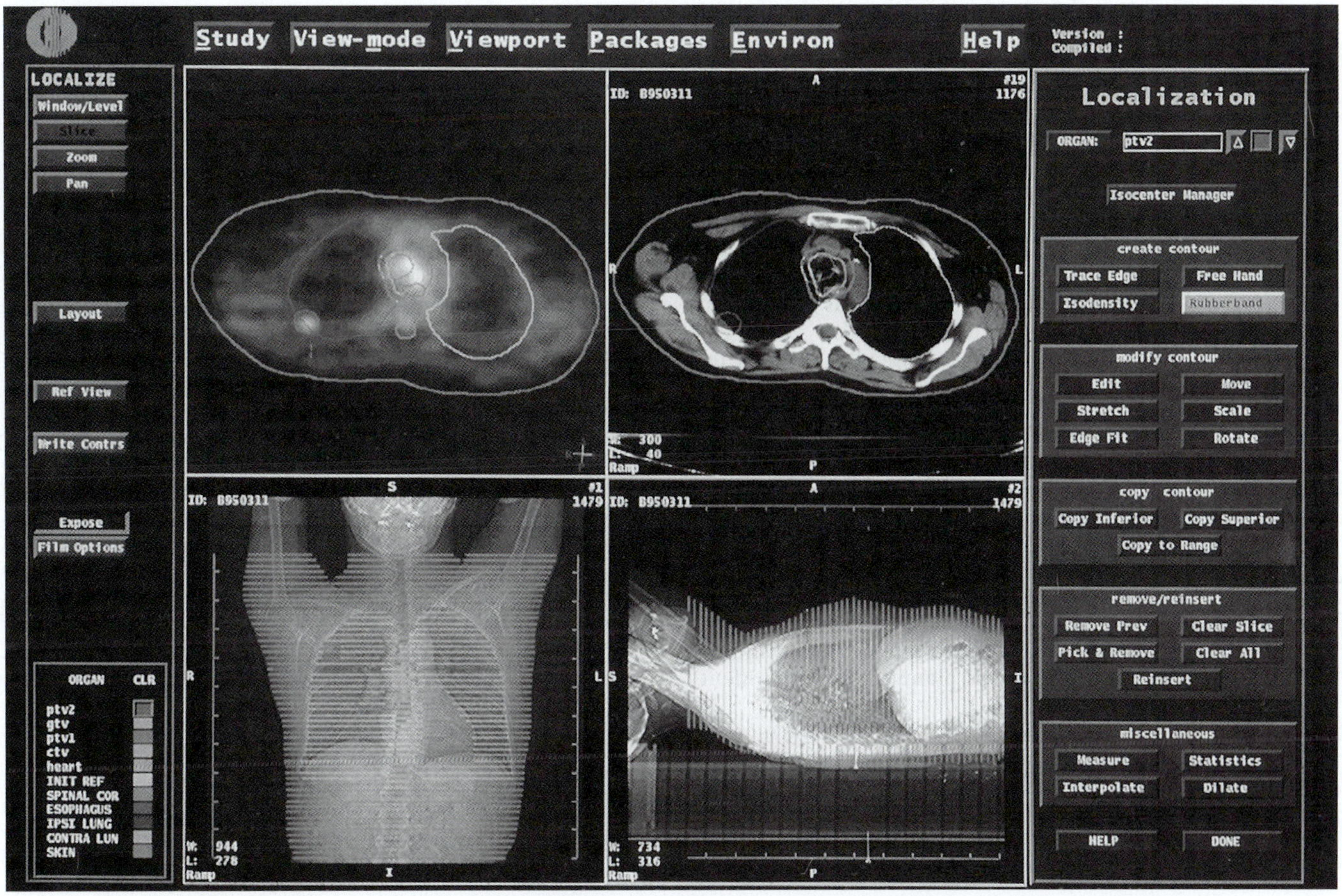

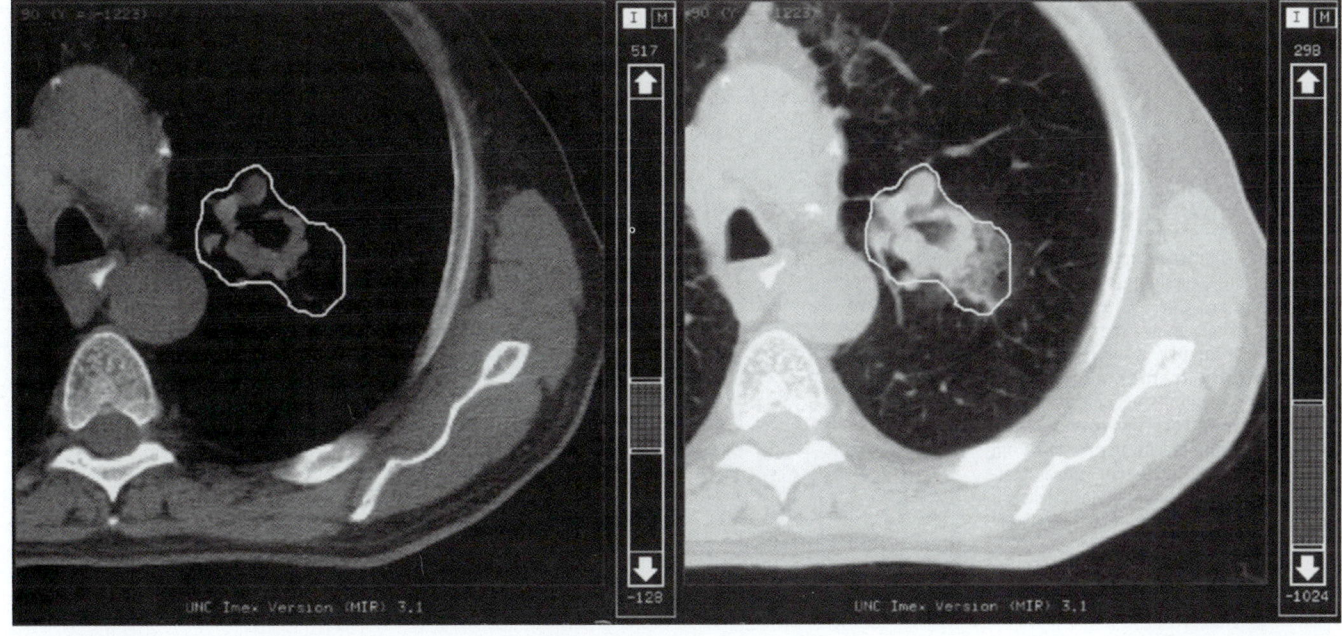

FIGURE 9.5. Advanced image segmentation software provides tools for radiation oncologists and treatment planners to determine critical structures and tumor and target volumes for three-dimensional planning. Computed tomography (CT) data are displayed, and contours are drawn by the treatment planner/radiation oncologist around the tumor, target, and normal tissues on a slice-by-slice basis, as seen in **upper right panel**. At the same time, planar images from both anterior–posterior and lateral projections are displayed in **bottom right** and **left panels**. **Upper left panel** shows positron emission tomography scan data with overlying contours after image registration with the CT data.

FIGURE 9.6. Computed tomography (CT) slice for patient with lung cancer showing that the appropriate CT window and level settings **(right frame)** must be used to determine the maximum dimensions of the gross tumor volume (GTV). Note that a much smaller GTV would have been contoured with the settings used in the left frame. (Reprinted from Purdy JA. Advances in three-dimensional treatment planning and conformal dose delivery. *Semin Oncol* 1997;24[6]:655–671. Copyright © 1997 Elsevier. With permission.)

to volume uncertainties. The interpolation process in spiral CT technology adds further to the uncertainty. As a result, the 3-D reconstruction of the GTV from temporally variant 2-D images often results in a poor representation of the tumor and its motion. Currently, 4-D CT technology has become the standard for CT simulators, making it possible to capture images in each phase of the respiratory cycle.[48,49] In addition, other technologies and methodologies to explicitly help manage the movements induced by the respiratory motion (to the order of <5 mm during treatment preparation and delivery) continue to be developed, including respiratory-gated techniques, respiration-synchronized techniques, breath hold techniques, and forced shallow-breathing methods.[50]

Delineating the CTV is even more difficult and must be done by the radiation oncologist based on clinical experience (and/or the use of published CTV atlases for certain clinical sites) because current imaging techniques cannot be used to directly detect subclinical tumor involvement. This field has seen a virtual explosion in the use of multimodality imaging over the last decade, and radiation oncologists have developed considerable imaging expertise in order to accurately define GTVs and be able to define nonimaged CTVs. However, the need for a higher level of image-based cross-sectional anatomy training in this field is well recognized.[51] The AAPM Task Group 132 addresses integration of multimodality imaging in the treatment planning and treatment processes.[52]

The PTV margin is specified by the radiation oncologist, often in consultation with the radiation oncology physicist and/or dosimetrist. In most occasions, it is based on published clinical experience that is not calculated based on measurements performed by the department for a particular treatment machine/technique and team. Van Herk and colleagues

reported extensively on the influence of systematic and random errors/variations on the required margins to account for set-up error and organ motion and developed margin recipes for calculating individualized (for a department, machine, and team) margins as given by the following equation[53,54]:

$$PTV \text{ margin} = 2.5\Sigma + 0.7\sigma$$

where Σ is the standard deviation of the systematic errors and σ is the standard deviation of the random errors.

When defining the PTV, the radiation oncologist should account for the asymmetric nature of positional uncertainties (Fig. 9.7). For example, it is recognized that prostate organ motion and daily set-up errors may be anisotropic (side-to-side or rotational shifts of the position of the patients are likely to have a different result compared to movement in the anterior–posterior direction). Thus, the PTV margin around a CTV generally should not be uniform.

Typically, when the beam portal is defined, additional margin beyond the PTV is required to obtain dose coverage because of beam penumbra and treatment technique. This emphasizes that treatment portal margins in relation to the PTV must be set according to the dosimetric characteristics of the beams being used. Often, a 5-mm margin (portal edge to PTV) is a good starting point, which can be increased if needed, but one must be knowledgeable about the characteristics of the actual beams used to make this starting-point determination. An additional point to understand is that in the case of coplanar treatment techniques, the margins required across the plane of treatment and the margins orthogonal (say superior–inferior) to this plane will be different. To clarify this point, consider a pelvic four-field axial technique as an example. Portions of the lateral aspects of

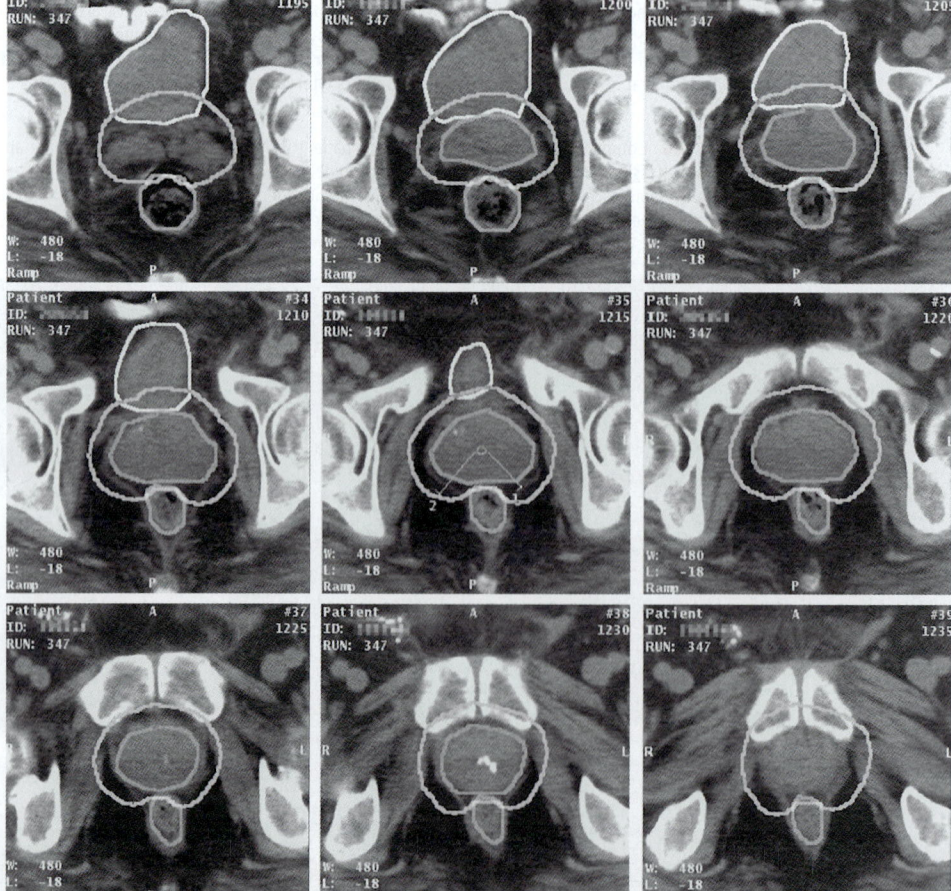

FIGURE 9.7. Computed tomography images of patient with prostate cancer showing the contour outlines for the gross tumor volume (GTV), planning target volume (PTV), bladder, and rectum. The physician made the decision that no additional margin around the prostate for the clinical target volume (CTV) was required (i.e., CTV = GTV). Note that a nonuniform margin around the GTV/CTV was used to define the PTV in the region of the rectum **(middle frame)**. Also, note the additional PTV contours needed to cap the GTV/CTV **(upper left** and **lower right frames)**. (Reprinted by permission from Springer: Purdy JA. Three-dimensional treatment planning and conformal dose delivery: a physicist's perspective. In: Mittal BB, Purdy JA, Ang KK, eds. *Advances in radiation therapy.* Boston: Kluwer Academic Publishers, 1998:1–33. Copyright © 1998 Springer Science+Business Media New York.)

the PTV that are in the low dose regions (near the penumbra) of the anterior–posterior and posterior–anterior fields will be in the high dose regions (well away from the beam penumbra) of the lateral fields. However, the superior and inferior aspects of the PTV will always be in the same low dose regions of all four fields, so there will be no dose filling from any of the fields. Thus, a larger portal margin in the inferior–superior dimension is needed to ensure that the prescription isodose resulting from all beams contains the PTV, whereas the lateral and anterior–posterior portal margins for each field may be reduced due to the other beams filling in the dose. The same holds true for the portals of the boost fields used in the so-called integrated boost technique, in which the beams used for treating the large volume fill up the dose in the buildup region of the boost volume. Last, the size of the margins will also be affected by the relative beam weighting. Hence, making hard rules about margin sizes is impossible and requires some planning iteration to find the right mix of beam margins.

When a PTV overlaps with a contoured normal structure, it is important to be explicit as to which volume the overlapping voxels are assigned for optimization purposes and for DVH calculations. Planning systems should allow the overlapping voxels to be included in both volumes for plan evaluation and reporting purposes. This ensures that the clinician is aware of the potential for the high dose region to include part of the normal structure as well as the PTV when reviewing the DVHs.

In addition, most 3DTPS cannot accurately account for a PTV contour that extends outside the skin surface, resulting in a DVH that does not reflect clinical reality because of the lack of dose generated in air and in the buildup region just below the skin. In those cases, the best solution is to delineate the PTV 3 to 5 mm below the skin surface. This will also help reduce acute skin reactions by preventing the optimization process from increasing the skin dose to excessive levels. In all cases, however, the treating physician should be aware of this approximation when setting or approving actual field margins.

All of the issues discussed in this section point out the fact that the PTV/PRV concept is a useful tool that simplifies accounting for geometric uncertainties. However, its use does give rise to several dilemmas. Particularly important is the loss of actual tumor and normal organ volume information reported for researchers developing TCP and NTCP models. Although it does not appear possible to totally eliminate the PTV concept at this time, it does appear possible to use smaller margins for some sites if more frequent imaging or other technical innovation is used to reduce geometric uncertainties. For example, for prostate cancer, the use of daily imaging and other technologies to relocate the target volume in reference to the machine isocenter does allow for a smaller margin for the PTV.[11,55] However, one must still be prudent in the amount of margin reduction for the prostate PTV when using these technologies. The different methods include various trade-offs ranging from treatment machine control, which is not dependent on the patient, to systems that are completely dependent on the patient. Again, regardless of which technique is used to reduce the overall PTV margin, one must be prudent in deciding the amount of margin reduction. Data do exist for support of margin reduction, but one must be systematical in approaching such reductions and ensure that there are no adverse effects on expected patient outcomes.[56]

Dose Prescription

Dose prescription is the responsibility of the radiation oncologist, generally using institutional protocols based on evidence published in the literature combined with institutional experience. Typically, the CRT prescription is specified as a dose at

or near the center of the PTV or (particularly for IMRT) as a dose covering a certain percentage of the PTV—for example, $D_{95\%}$, a dose that covers 95% of the PTV. Because the resulting dose distribution can be quite different depending on the dose prescription methodology, it is imperative that publications provide a clear and unambiguous description of the dose specification for the radiation treatment results being reported. The ICRU recently updated their recommendations for dose specification, and these will be discussed in a later section.[57]

Conformal Planning

For 3DCRT planning, beams can be arranged and beam apertures shaped with MLC leaves or shielding blocks to help conform the prescribed dose to the PTV and avoid OARs using BEV displays. This "forward planning" approach to CRT has now been supplemented—but not replaced—by an "inverse planning" approach as used for IMRT, which can achieve even greater conformity and OAR dose avoidance.

Forward Planning: 3DCRT

Design of the beam arrangement is the next step in the planning process for 3DCRT. The ability to orient beams in 3-D allows one to develop treatment plans that use noncoplanar beams. However, when noncoplanar beam arrangements are used, care must be taken to avoid the selection of gantry and couch angles that results in table/gantry collisions or a conflict with other treatment room restrictions. The *BEV* and the *DRR display*,[24,58] as shown in Figure 9.8, allows the planner to easily view the target volume and the organs at risk so that shielding blocks or MLC apertures can be drawn using a computer mouse or, as available with most current 3DTPS software versions, automatically generated with a chosen margin around the selected volume. DRRs also provide planar reference images that can be used in facilitating the plan implementation and treatment verification phases of CRT.

Inverse Planning: IMRT

The major differences between 3DCRT forward planning and IMRT inverse planning are the use of a computer optimization program that requires a formal description of the requirements using a mathematical *objective function* and constraints that are used by the program to find the solution. For example, after the design of the initial beam geometry, the physician/treatment planner puts into the TPS the desired dose–volume constraints for the PTVs and all OARs. The TPS optimization algorithm then divides each beam into many small *beamlets* (i.e., pencil beams that together make up the IMRT beam) and then iteratively alters the beamlet intensities until the 3-D dose distribution best conforms to the *a priori* specified dose–volume objectives. After the optimal beam intensities and resulting dose distribution have been determined, the TPS then calculates the MLC leaf sequence motions that will achieve this dose distribution and the dose recalculated. Typically, there may be some differences in the optimized dose distribution and the final dose distribution that is delivered with the computer-controlled MLC system, but this difference is usually acceptable.

Noncoplanar Multibeam Delivery

Sheng and colleagues recently investigated benefits of increasing the number of beams in noncoplanar delivery and showed that significant normal tissue sparing and dose conformality gains can be achieved when 14 to 22 beams are used for delivery.[59] In this approach, an optimization algorithm, in addition to conventional fluence optimization, also optimizes noncoplanar beam orientations considering a patient-specific deliverable beam geometry solution space, parameterized with patient and linear accelerator gantry orientations. This

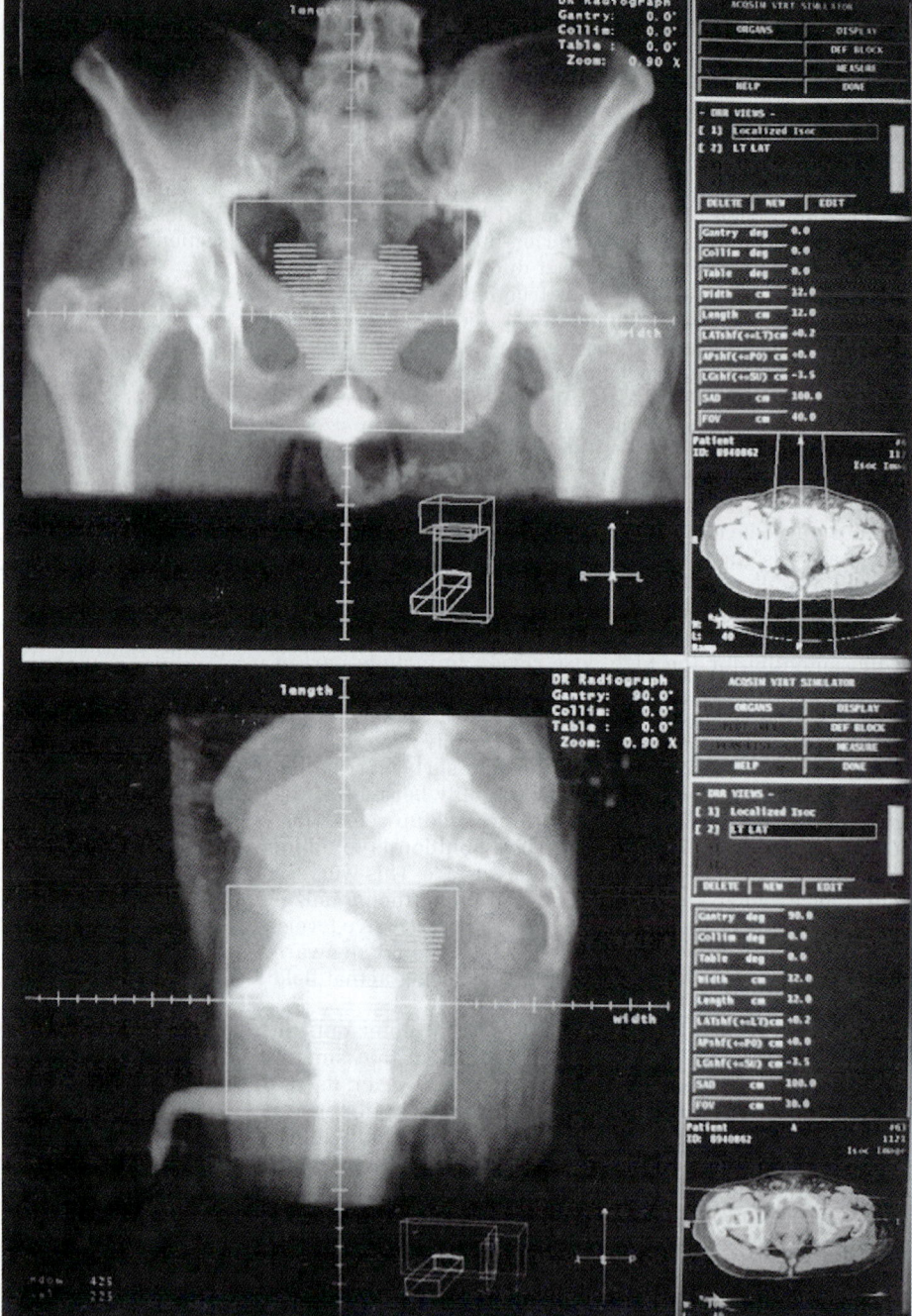

FIGURE 9.8. Beam's-eye–view (BEV) and digitally reconstructed radiograph (DRR) display of three-dimensional radiation therapy treatment planning for a prostate cancer patient. BEV display is useful in identifying best gantry, collimator, and couch angles at which to irradiate the target and avoid irradiating adjacent normal structures by interactively moving patient and treatment beam. Critical structures and target volumes are outlined on the patient's serial computed tomography sections. Contours are seen in perspective, as though the observer's eye is at the radiation source looking out along the axis of the radiation beam. The beam shape is defined by multileaf collimator (MLC). (Reprinted from Purdy JA. Advances in three-dimensional treatment planning and conformal dose delivery. *Semin Oncol* 1997;24[6]:655–671. Copyright © 1997 Elsevier. With permission.)

delivery technique, dubbed 4π, has been extended to other disease sites and has shown that research can lead to additional improvements in radiotherapy photon dose distributions.[60,61]

Dose Distribution Calculation

A rectilinear coordinate system affixed to the patient 3-D CT image set is typically used for calculating the dose distribution. This "patient or CT system" coordinate system typically has its x-axis along the horizontal axis of the transverse CT images, the y-axis along the vertical axis, and the z-axis along the couch motion. Contour points are specified as a sequence of points having x-, y-, and z-coordinates in this system. The center of each voxel in the 3-D CT image matrix is computed relative to the same coordinate system and is used to look up the relative electron density values that are related to the CT numbers (see later discussion). The selection of grid spacing for the 3-D dose matrix is an important consideration

regarding dose computational accuracy, calculation speed, and computer hardware requirements. Drzymala et al.[31] pointed out that a 2% dose accuracy or 2-mm isodose positional accuracy can generally be achieved with a grid spacing of 5 mm. However, in regions of high dose gradients, a finer grid is typically needed, which creates larger computer files and increases the 3DTPS memory and mass storage requirements. With modern computing capabilities, these issues are not a practical limitation, and high-resolution dose computations are achievable that can lead to dosimetric benefits.[62]

The reader should also understand that CT numbers are not used directly in photon dose calculations. Instead, the CT numbers are correlated with the electron density of the corresponding tissues at each voxel relative to the electron density of water.[63] This is because Compton scattering is the dominant mode of interaction for the type of photon beam used in radiation therapy (cobalt 60 through 25-MV x-rays), and the absorption and scattering of photons in tissue depend primarily on the electron density of the tissue. Errors in CT numbers can result in inaccurate dose calculations. Generally, however, errors of 10% or less in electron density (CT numbers) will not result in significant errors in the dose distribution.[63] A recent development has been direct electron density imaging[64]; full clinical impact of this technology remains to be investigated.

Details on specific dose calculation algorithms are discussed in a separate chapter, and so only issues pertinent to the CRT planning process are discussed in this section. In the past, dose calculation algorithms were traditionally based on parameterizing dose distributions measured in water phantoms under standard conditions and applying correction factors to the beam representations for the nonuniform surface contour of the patient or the obliquity of the beam, tissue heterogeneities, and beam modifiers such as blocks, wedges, and compensator. However, more advanced models, such as the superposition/convolution method, have been developed for CRT planning[63] and are now the standard of practice today for CRT planning. The study by Frank et al.[65] provides a clear method for safely transitioning from a clinical experience based on planning assuming a homogeneous unit density patient to a heterogeneous patient model.

Plan Evaluation and Improvement

The 3DCRT plan evaluation/improvement process involves an iterative, interactive approach. Typically, the initial beam arrangement has been selected based primarily on clinical experience using BEV displays. The generated dose distribution is reviewed by the planner/physician, and the beam arrangement is then modified based on the review of DVHs (Fig. 9.9) and multilevel 2-D displays showing isodose lines superimposed on CT images (Fig. 9.10); sometimes, the display is in the form of a *color wash*, that is, a spectrum of colors superimposed on the anatomic information. Historically, the planned dose distribution approved by the radiation oncologist is most often one in which a uniform dose is delivered to the target volume (e.g., +7% and −5% of the prescribed dose) with doses to critical structures held below tolerance levels,[66–69] as well as within the constraints for the absolute maximum dose, median dose, or a volume (e.g., V_{20Gy}) that has been specified by the radiation oncologist. With IMRT and SBRT approaches, there is an increased acceptance of larger-dose heterogeneities, whereas the approach to other evaluation parameters remains unchanged.

Over the recent years, the plan creation and evaluation process has significantly evolved adding several new options and tools to the process. The calculation of Pareto surfaces in multicriteria optimization (MCO) based IMRT treatment planning involves creation of several treatment plan options where each plan offers a combination of different dose volume trade-offs.[70] Pareto optimal plans offer a plan bundle where each plan favors an organ at risk or a combination of organs at risk at an expense of some other organ or organs. In other words, radiotherapy treatment planning is all about trade-offs between doses delivered to target volumes and various organs at risk. These trade-offs involve physicians making decisions on dose sacrifices and sparing, which critical organs to give less dose at expense of some other organs getting more dose or they involve compromises in the balance of dose delivery between targets and organs at risk. In MCO, a set of plans optimized for unique combinations of dose trade-offs is combined with tools to offer a physician an efficient way to navigate through these trade-offs or plan options and to select a plan offering the trade-offs favored by that physician. This approach has been shown to have quantifiable dosimetric advantages.[71] Both RaySearch (Garden City, NY) and Varian (Palo Alto, CA) offer MCO approaches. The advantages of this technique include the flexibility offered to physicians in guiding the treatment delivery; however, there can be inconsistencies in physician selection process, which can increase the variability of clinical practices.

In knowledge-based planning (KBP), treatment plans of previously treated patients are used to create models of achievable dose distributions for future plans.[72,73] The historical plans constitute a training data set, and machine learning–like approaches are used to create DVH range predictions unique to a patient's specific organ geometry (Fig. 9.11). In the KBP approach, a DVH or 3-D dose prediction can be created

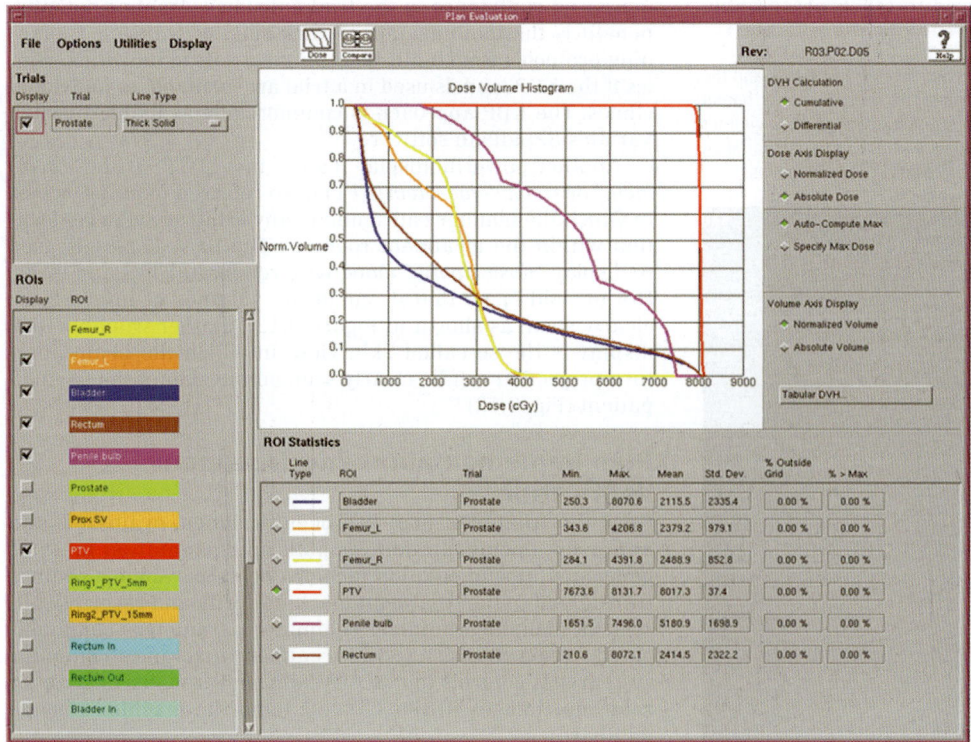

FIGURE 9.9. Example of a treatment planning system display (Pinnacle; Philips Medical Systems, Highland Heights, OH), showing the cumulative dose–volume histograms for a typical prostate cancer patient's plan: the prostate PTV (*red*) and multiple OARs (penile bulb, *magenta*; right femur, *yellow*; left femur, *orange*; rectum, *brown*; bladder, *blue*); also shown are associated dose statistics for the various defined volumes.

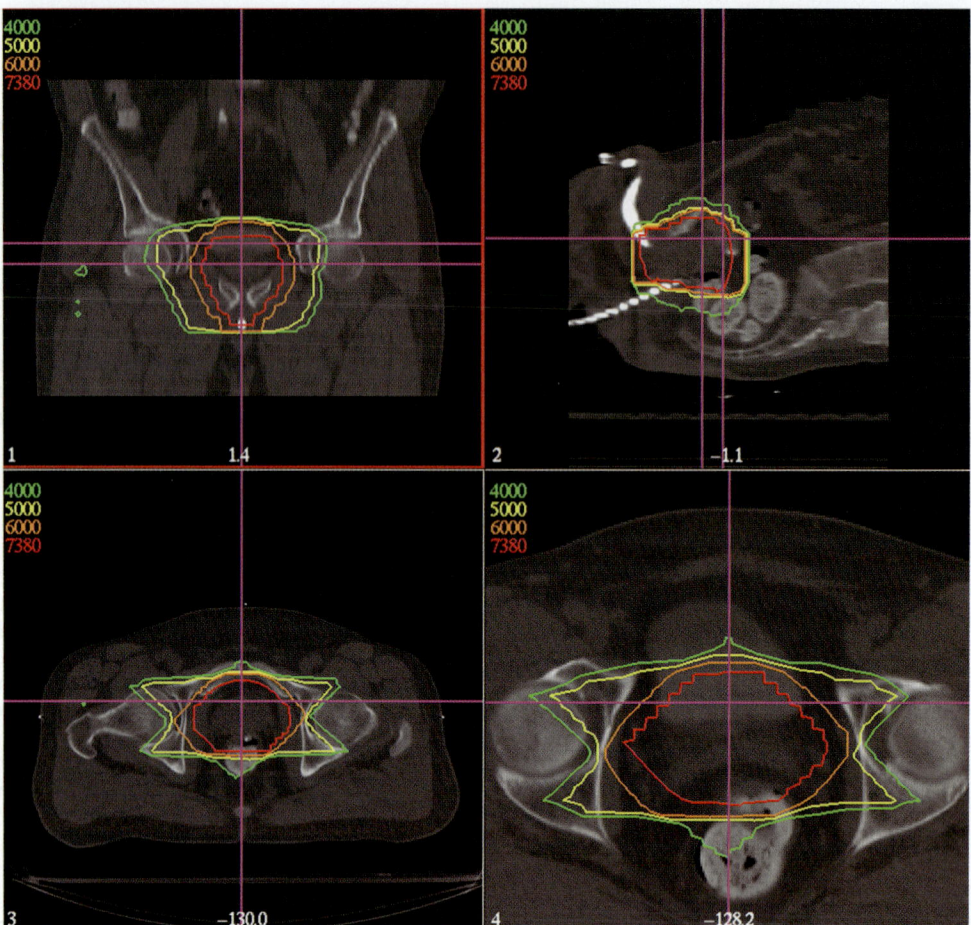

FIGURE 9.10. Dose distribution displays for a patient with prostate cancer showing coronal, sagittal, and two axial computed tomography (CT) sections with superimposed color-coded isodose lines (73.8, 60, 50, and 40 Gy). *Vertical* and *horizontal lines* displayed on each CT section indicate the positions of each section. Evaluating volumetric three-dimensional dose distributions using only this type of two-dimensional display is difficult and time-consuming.

as soon as there are contours of the patient geometry and the prescription.[74] The proposed solution is driven by the prior treatment planning practices and results in a single-treatment plan rather than multiple plan options as in the MCO. In this approach, treatment models can be created at one institution or globally and transferred to other, presumably

FIGURE 9.11. Colored range is the DVH prediction range for two OARS, and the *dotted lines* are treatment planning objectives, which are set at the lower bound of these predictions and are automatically passed to the optimization engine for treatment planning purposes. The use of lower bound setting in the optimization ensures that the system is driven in the direction of optimal dose distributions.

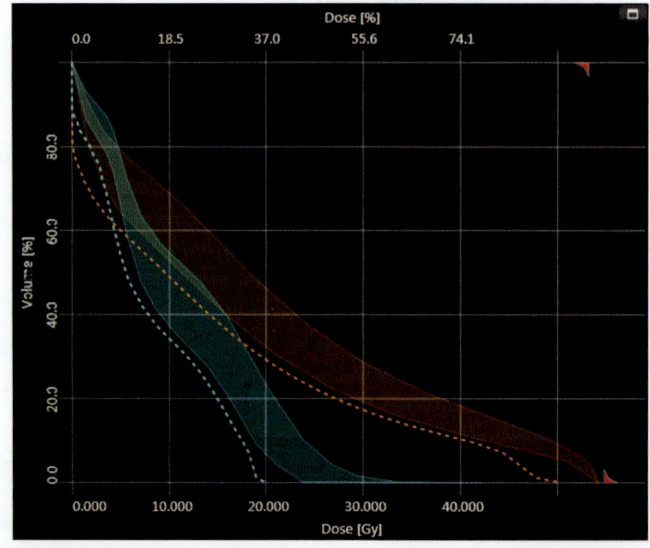

less experienced, institutions[72,73] as well as used to standardize treatment planning quality in multi-institutional trials.[75,76] The ability to standardize plan quality in multi-institutional trials minimizes a significant source of historical variability and shortcoming in these trials, which should translate in increased confidence in the trial outcomes. Another potential benefit is the minimization of variability of transfer of planning protocols from multi-institutional trials to individual clinics if the KBP models used in a trial are available to individual clinics. The KBP approach is commercially available through Varian's RapidPlan software.

Another powerful display feature in a 3DTPS is the "*room-view*" or *room's-eye–view* (*REV*) (also referred to as 3-D view), in which the planner can simulate any arbitrary viewing location within the treatment room.[27,77] The REV display is used to display "*dose clouds*" along with rendered PTVs and OARs. Hot or cold spots that occur in the volumes of interest are clearly seen, as shown in Figure 9.12. Another valuable REV display is the so-called Skin View, in which the beam aperture projection can be clearly seen on the skin of the (virtual) patient (Fig. 9.13).

Plan Implementation and Treatment Verification

Once the treatment plan has been designed, evaluated, and approved, documentation for plan implementation must be generated. Documentation includes beam parameter settings transferred to the treatment machine verify and record (V&R) system, including multileaf collimator parameters communicated over a network to the treatment machine's computer system that controls the MLC system, and transfer of setup or reference images (DRRs, CTs, etc.) and the machine's image database.

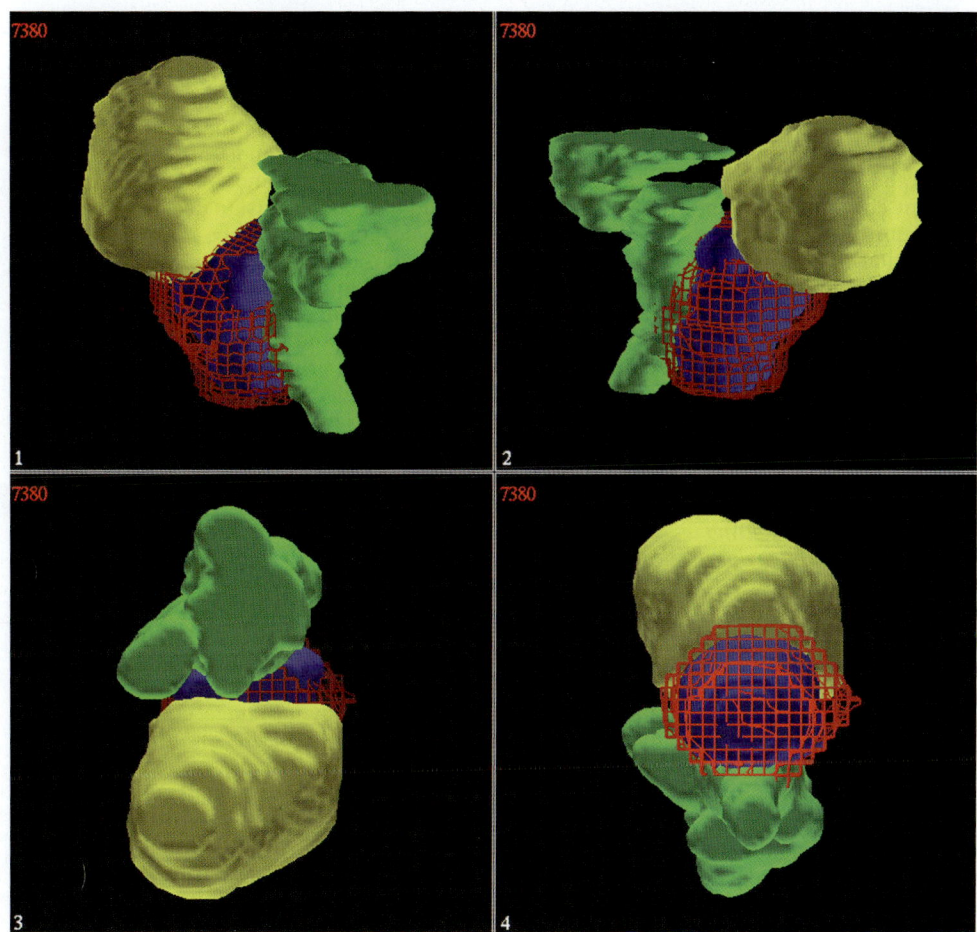

FIGURE 9.12. Room's-eye–view (REV) three-dimensional (3-D) isodose surface display with real-time interactivity is a valuable tool for evaluation of 3-D dose distributions in terms of adequate coverage of target volumes and sparing of critical structures. The REV display enables radiation oncologists to view target volume or normal tissue volume with superimposed isodose surfaces or "dose clouds" from any arbitrary viewing angle. Shown is a four-panel REV display of the 73.8-Gy isodose volume, the prostate planning target volume (PTV), bladder, and rectum of a patient with prostate cancer treated with a six-field technique. The location of the PTV region not covered by the specified dose level is easily discernible using the REV display.

Validation of patient position and treatment setup may involve acquiring images of all individual treatment beams. However, with IMRT, SBRT, TomoTherapy, ViewRay, etc., these processes are not practical and are generally not done. Instead, orthogonal radiographs, CBCTs, and other images of the patient (rather than of treatment beams) are now the preferred method to ensure correct isocenter positioning. When available, the optical distance indicator is also useful

FIGURE 9.13. Room's-eye–view (REV) display showing simulated skin surface for a breast cancer patient undergoing radiation therapy using tangential, supraclavicular, and internal mammary fields. Beam aperture projection can be clearly seen on the skin of the (virtual) patient.

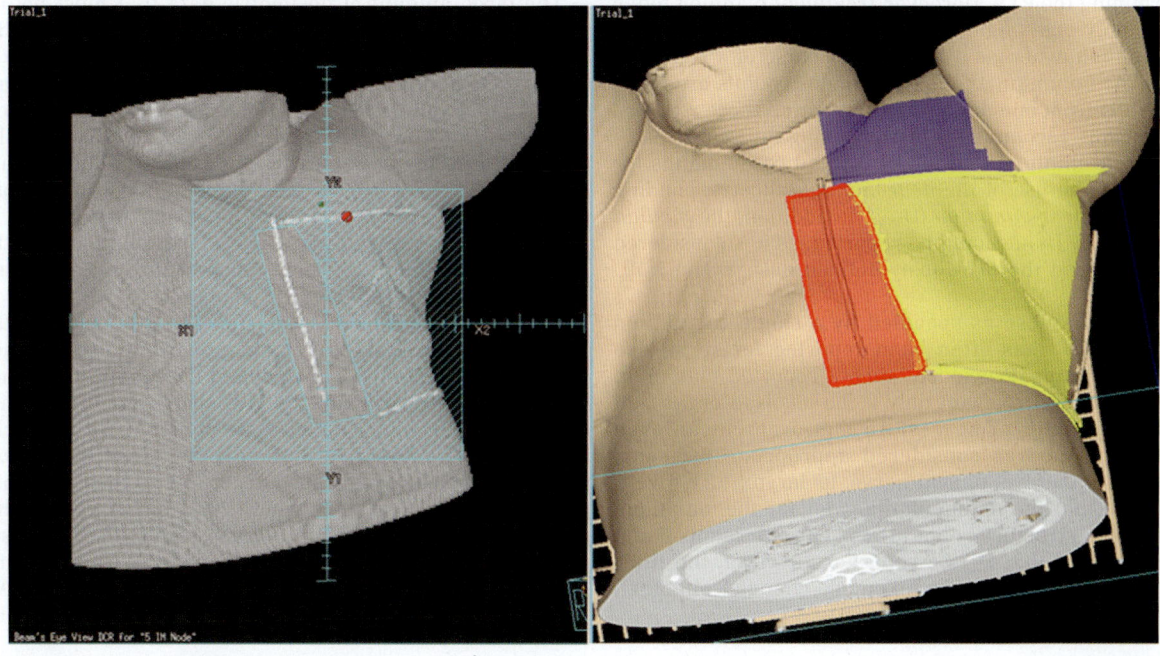

in assessing the correctness of the setup of a particular beam. Documentation provides the depth of isocenter below the skin surface on the central ray of the beam, which can then be compared with the isocenter depth measured on the simulator or treatment machine after the beam is set up using the couch and gantry positions specified by the treatment plan.

QA checks used to confirm the validity and accuracy of the CRT plan typically include an independent check of the plan and MU calculation by a physicist; radiation therapists also evaluate the integrity of the plan information that is passed to them for treatment (i.e., therapist new start check). Most importantly, careful scrutiny must be given to the input of data into the V&R system to assure that it is correct. These checks are discussed in more detail in a separate section. Additional information on standards for CRT plan verification can be obtained from the most current AAPM Task Group reports, ACR, and ASTRO practice accreditation guidelines.

Dose Reporting and Dose Prescription

ICRU Reports 50 and 62 define a series of doses, including the minimum, maximum, mean dose, and *ICRU reference dose* (defined at the *ICRU reference point*), for reporting dose relevant to CRT. The *ICRU reference point* for a particular treatment plan should be chosen based on the following criteria: It should be (a) clinically relevant and defined in an unambiguous way, (b) located where the dose can be accurately determined, and (c) located in a region where there are no steep dose gradients. In general, this point should be in the central part of the PTV. In cases in which the treatment beams intersect at a given point, it is recommended that the intersection point be chosen as the ICRU reference point.

ICRU Report 83[57] updates the previous ICRU recommendation on CRT dose reporting and recommends moving from single spatial point reporting (i.e., the ICRU reference point dose, minimum and maximum dose) to dose–volume reporting. This is justified based on the availability of more accurate dose calculation algorithms and the advances and ubiquity of modern-day anatomic/functional imaging.

It also should be understood that in the past, *minimum dose* and *maximum dose* referred to point doses in the dose calculation grid assigned to a single voxel. It is now acknowledged that the minimum dose may not be accurately determined because it is often located in a high-gradient region at the edge of the PTV, making it highly sensitive to the resolution of the calculation and the accuracy of delineating the CTV and determining the PTV. Moreover, treatment planning today represents only one single representation of the calculated dose distribution, whereas over the full course of a radiation treatment, the minimum and maximum dose points are likely to shift slightly from one day to another. For all those reasons, ICRU Report 83[57] recommends discontinuing the use of maximum dose and minimum dose and instead recommends for dose reporting the use of the *near-maximum* (corresponding to $D_{2\%}$) and the *near-minimum* ($D_{98\%}$). In addition, the *median dose*, specified by $D_{50\%}$, should be reported, as it is considered to best correspond the previously defined dose at the ICRU reference point.

The maximum dose as specified by a single calculation point (D_{max} or $D_{0\%}$) has often been reported for serial-like organs or structures. Previously, such a reported maximum dose was considered relevant only if the involved organ had a minimum diameter of at least 15 mm, whereas an even smaller dimension was considered appropriate for some organs, such as the eye, optical nerve, or larynx.[36] The ICRU acknowledged that the minimum diameter for the maximum dose region in a structure is not always easy to establish and hence recommend that $D_{2\%}$ be reported. However, the ICRU pointed out that care should be taken in a change from maximum dose to the near-maximum dose, $D_{2\%}$.

As stated previously, with regard to dose homogeneity, ICRU Report 50 recommends that the dose coverage of the PTV be kept within specific limits, namely, +7% and −5% of the prescribed dose.[36] However, this level of dose homogeneity might not be achieved in all cases (particularly for current IMRT techniques), and ICRU Report 50 explicitly states that if this degree of homogeneity cannot be achieved, it is the responsibility of the radiation oncologist to decide whether the dose heterogeneity is acceptable. Similarly, a slight underdose to the PTV might be required (particularly if in close proximity to an OAR) or result for lung tumors surrounded by low-density lung tissue as a result of electronic disequilibrium.

Note that ICRU Reports 50 and 62 do not make strict recommendations regarding dose prescription; instead, the ICRU states "the radiation oncologist should have the freedom to prescribe the parameters in his/her own way, mainly using what is current practice to produce an expected clinical outcome of the treatment."[36] For dose reporting, however, it is recommended to also state the prescribed dose if the actual prescription was not done accordingly.

It is now recognized that there is a large variability among institutional results in IMRT planning and reporting.[78,79] Studies strongly support the ICRU Report 83 recommendation to move away from single-spatial-point prescription/reporting to dose–volume prescription/reporting. In addition, ASTRO has gone even further and recommends that specific details of the inverse treatment planning and image-guided treatment processes be recorded using (a) an *IMRT treatment planning directive*, (b) a *treatment goal summary*, (c) an *image guidance summary*, and (d) a *motion management summary*.[80] Das et al.[81] recently evaluated compliance with ICRU-83 prescribing guidelines and found that the overwhelming majority of patient treatments in the surveyed institutions do not comply with these guidelines. The KBP planning approach and automatic DVH analysis are both aimed in reducing these variabilities. More extensive and standardized methods and supporting software for treatment prescribing currently do not exist. Just as the tools have emerged for more consistent plan creation and evaluation, it is critical that a process be developed, which will improve the standardization and quantification of radiation therapy prescribing. It would be very beneficial if the prescription parameters (treatment planning goals) and the evaluation metrics overlap.

Dose–Volume Histograms

The large amount of dosimetric data that must be analyzed when a CRT plan is evaluated has prompted the development of methods of condensing and presenting the data in more easily understandable formats. One such data reduction tool is the *dose–volume histogram*.[30,31] Two types of DVHs, *differential* and *cumulative*, are available in CRT planning, with the latter now universally used in plan evaluation for assessing PTV(s) coverage and dose to OARs, as displayed in Figure 9.14. However, it must be clearly understood that the DVH does not provide any spatial information and thus can only complement and not replace spatial dose distribution display tools such as isodose displays.

The *differential DVH (dDVH)*, as shown in Figure 9.14A, is essentially a plot of the frequency distribution of the individual dose distribution elements (called dose voxels) obtained from the dose grid. Typically, the grid size is small enough so that the dose can be assumed to be constant within each voxel. The volume's dose distribution is then divided into *dose bins*, and the voxels are grouped according to their dose bin value without regard to their spatial location. A plot of the number of voxels in each bin (*y*-axis) versus the bin dose range (*x*-axis) is by definition a differential DVH. The size of the dose bin used determines the height of each bin of the dDVH. For example, if the bin widths were increased, the heights of the

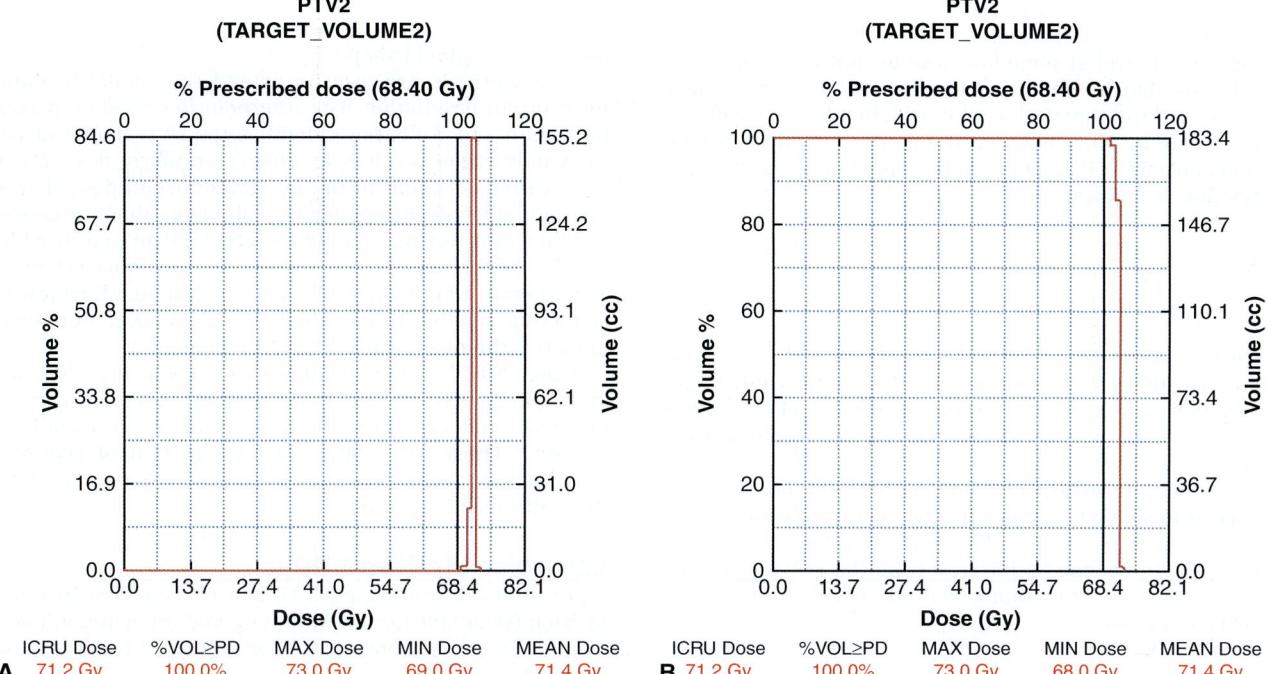

FIGURE 9.14. A: The differential dose–volume histogram (dDVH) for a specified target volume (PTV2)—the volume is subdivided into individual elements (called voxels) and tagged according to dose received as determined from the three dimensional dose grid. Voxels are then grouped according to each specified dose bin value without regard to their spatial location. A plot of the number of voxels in each bin (*y*-axis) versus the bin dose range (*x*-axis) is by definition a dDVH. **B:** The corresponding cumulative DVH (cDVH) is generated by summing for each dose bin all of the voxels of the PTV2 dDVH to the right of each dose bin; the *y*-axis gives the volume, or percentage of volume, that receives a dose equal to or greater than the indicated dose on the *x*-axis.

histogram bins would increase because more voxels would fall into any given bin. Thus, it should be clearly understood that the detailed shape of a differential DVH depends on the dose bin size used, even though the underlying dose–volume data are the same.

A *cumulative DVH* (*cDVH*), as shown in Figure 9.14B, is a plot in which each bin represents the volume, or percentage of volume (*y*-axis), that receives a dose equal to or greater than the indicated dose on the *x*-axis. The cDVH is generated by summing all of the voxels of the corresponding dDVH to the right of each dose. The volume value for the first bin (dose origin) is the full volume of the structure because the total volume receives at least zero dose and the volume for the last bin is that which receives the maximum dose. Note that in the literature, the "c" in the cDVH is generally dropped, leaving just DVH.

Explicit values of dose–volume parameters can be extracted from the DVH data and are called dose–volume statistics or simply *dose statistics*. Examples for target volumes include maximum dose, minimum dose, mean dose, and percentage volume receiving greater than or equal to the prescription dose; for OARs, they typically include maximum point dose, mean dose, and percentage volume receiving greater than or equal to an established tolerance dose. As previously stated, ICRU Report 83[57] recommends replacing the *minimum dose* and *maximum dose* point doses with *near-maximum* (corresponding to $D_{2\%}$) and *near-minimum* ($D_{98\%}$).[57]

There is an ever-increasing reliance on DVH-based evaluation of treatment plans. Because the majority of planning objectives in clinical trials and QUANTEC recommendations are based on dose–volume tolerances of individual organs, it is natural to extend plan evaluation with a primary focus on DVH or derived metric (e.g., R_{50}) evaluation. There are now also several commercial and homegrown software packages for automatic extraction and evaluation of these parameters

with easy to assess indicators for which parameters meet the planning goals and which ones fail. Although the automatic evaluation is fundamentally more efficient, its main advantage is reduced likelihood for error and greater efficiency in the evaluation process. Also, the transfer and implementation of multi-institutional plan evaluation parameters are easier and more systematic to implement with automated dose–volume metric evaluation. It should be reemphasized that DVH review is not a substitute for reviewing the actual isodose distributions and plans are best evaluated in combination of all these review parameters.

Biologic Models for Dose–Volume Response

Evaluation of the quality of a treatment plan (i.e., is plan A better than plan B?) is difficult and at best a qualitative procedure. For example, it is not clear what degree of dose uniformity within the PTV is optimum, as dose levels can now be significantly escalated using CRT techniques, nor is it always clear which plan is best if the two DVHs for a specific OAR cross each other (i.e., difficulty in weighting importance of dose vs. volume).

Researchers have developed biophysical models that attempt to translate the dose–volume information into estimates of biologic response—*tumor control probability* (*TCP*) and *normal tissue complication probability* (*NTCP*) models.[68,69,82] Most authors agree that the TCP and NTCP models developed thus far are not accurate enough such that the absolute values can be used to predict clinical outcome; however, they are used to compare rival plans and as such help to rank plan quality. In any case, such biologic indices should be used clinically only when their utility has been firmly established for well-defined clinical conditions. ICRU Report 83 is clear in stating that if biologically based metrics are to be reported, the assumptions used in the models, their parameters, and the model itself must be unambiguously specified.[57]

Tumor Control Probability

TCP plotted as a function of dose has a classic sigmoid shape, having zero control at some low dose to control at some high dose. Rather than attempt to review in detail the various models, here I discuss some relevant issues. Readers are referred to the article by Moiseenko et al. for more details.[83] Simple phenomenologic TCP models can be represented by the logistic function as follows:

$$TCP = \cfrac{1}{1+\left(\cfrac{D_{50\%}}{D}\right)^{4\gamma_{50\%}}}$$

where $D_{50\%}$ is the dose at which the TCP is 50%, $\gamma_{50\%}$ is the slope of the dose–response curve at 50% tumor control, and D is the dose administered.[84] Note that the use of the logistic function assumes an approximate uniform cell response and a uniform dose distribution.

For a nonuniform dose distribution, the total tumor volume is reduced to smaller volumes having "uniform" doses within each subvolume element v_i. The TCP value for each volume element, TCP(v, D), can be inferred from the TCP for uniform irradiation of the entire tumor volume, TCP(1, D), using the following equation:

$$TCP(v, D) = TCP(1, D)^v$$

Thus, the TCP for the tumor receiving an inhomogeneous dose is given by the product of the individual volume element TCPs as follows:

$$TCP = \prod_{i=1}^{N} TCP(v_i, D_i)$$

Here, TCP(v_i, D_i) is the TCP for the ith volume element receiving dose D_i, and N is the total number of tumor volume elements. Recall that the validity of this equation is highly dependent on the validity of the assumptions that the individual tumor volume elements are uniformly distributed throughout the tumor volume and are equally radiosensitive.

Normal Tissue Complication Probability

There are mainly two different approaches used in radiation therapy in modeling NTCP: the *empiric model* introduced by Lyman and Wolbarst[85,86] and *functional models* that introduced concepts of *serial* and *parallel* tissue organization and *functional subunits (FSUs)*.[84,87–89]

The *Lyman NTCP model* can be expressed in terms of an error function of dose (D) and volume (v) as follows:

$$NTCP(D, v) = \frac{1}{\sqrt{2\pi}} \int_{-\infty}^{1} \exp\left(-t^2/2\right) dt,$$

where

$$t = \left[D - D_{50}(v)\right] / \left[m \cdot D_{50}(v)\right],$$

with v equal to the partial volume (V/V_{ref}) and the tolerance dose volume dependence given by the following power–law relationship:

$$D_{50}(v) = D_{50}(1) \cdot v^{-n}$$

$D_{50}(1)$ is the tolerance dose for 50% complications for uniform whole-organ irradiation, and $D_{50}(v)$ is the 50% tolerance dose for uniform partial-organ irradiation to the fractional volume v. The arbitrary variables m and n are found by fitting tolerance doses for uniform whole- and uniform partial-organ irradiation, where m characterizes the gradient (slope) of the dose–response function at D_{50} and n characterizes the effect of volume. When n is near unity, the volume effect is large;

conversely, when n is near zero, the volume effect is small. When NTCP is plotted against dose, the NTCP equation demonstrates a sigmoid shape.

Two methods are used to extend this model to nonuniform organ irradiation. The *interpolation method*, proposed by Lyman and Wolbarst,[86] modifies the DVH to one in which the whole organ receives an effective uniform dose, D_{eff}, that is less than or equal to the maximum organ dose. The second method, called the effective volume method, proposed by Kutcher and Burman,[90] modifies the DVH to one in which a fraction of the organ, v_{eff}, receives the maximum organ dose. The Lyman model coupled with the Kutcher-Burman DVH reduction scheme (now called the Lyman-Kutcher-Burman model) is the most widely used NTCP model.[82]

Other NTCP models include two developed by Niemierko and Goitein—the *critical element model*, used for serial-like organs,[91] and the *critical volume model*, for parallel-like organs.[92] These are similar in form to that of Lyman and Wolbarst[85] but include additional terms to better account for the radiosensitivity of the FSUs.

Equivalent Uniform Dose

Equivalent uniform dose (EUD) is a concept first introduced by Niemierko[93] for use in evaluating and reporting inhomogeneous dose distributions and later redefined by the following equation[94]:

$$EUD = \left(\sum_i v_i D_i^\alpha\right)^{1/\alpha}$$

where v_i is the volume of the dose–volume bin with a dose D_i and the exponent α is a complication-specific parameter.

The EUD concept assumes that any two dose distributions are equivalent if they cause the same radiobiologic effect and appears well suited for use in evaluating competing conformal plans. However, McGary et al. pointed out that there are conditions in which EUD is not adequate as a single parameter to report or analyze inhomogeneous dose distributions—for example, when the minimum dose is significantly lower than the mean dose.[95–97]

MANAGEMENT OF CONFORMAL RADIATION THERAPY DATA

To accurately perform the steps involved in CRT, several forms of patient imaging and other data must be acquired, displayed, manipulated, and stored. Typically, patient image data acquired from several imaging subsystems must be communicated to a TPS to permit these images to be used for treatment planning. Several software components also must be integrated so that the output of one processing step can be made available for use as input to the next step. Daily IGRT imaging is also putting large demands on data storage, and the need for more robust image processing tools is evident. These issues in data management in CRT are complex and continue to be somewhat problematic, although some progress is being made through the Integrating the Healthcare Enterprise in Radiation Oncology effort initiated by ASTRO.[98]

This issue is just part of larger informatics issues facing radiation oncology. There is an explosion in the types and volume of data that must be made available for scientific query. Difficulty in accessing the data in practical ways has become a critical limitation to investigators in the field and to its advancement. Unfortunately, the commercially available radiation oncology information systems are not yet adequate to meet this challenge. The great volume and diversity of the data have rendered their storage, management, and processing extremely problematic, resulting in situations in which important data and information are inefficiently disseminated and sometimes lost. In the busy clinic, failure to manage critical information may compromise patient safety. Here, a major issue is the lack of integration of the radiation oncology electronic medical record (EMR), based on systems such as Elekta-Impac MOSAIQ (Sunnyvale, CA) or Varian ARIA, with the electronic hospital record (EHR), based on systems such as those provided by Epic (Verona, WI). In most cases, we must resort to hybrid charting systems (ad hoc combinations of EMR, EHR, and paper charting), which entails risks and gives rise to a dangerous situation. Immediate and focused efforts in achieving these integrations and improving the radiation oncology informatics infrastructure are urgently needed.

QUALITY ASSURANCE FOR CONFORMAL RADIATION THERAPY

It is most important to realize that a QA program for CRT is an interdisciplinary effort involving radiation oncologists, radiation physicists, dosimetrists, radiation therapists, clinical engineers, and information technology specialists and that the efforts of each group often overlap substantially. To be effective, it is also essential to have the full support of the department chair and hospital administration.

Although in general, radiation therapy has a long, successful history of QA, most authors have come to realize that the current approach (which relies heavily on prescriptive QA tests, tolerances, and frequencies as provided by consensus expert groups from national/international professional/scientific organizations) is likely inadequate by itself for more advanced modalities such as CRT.[99–101]

For example, today's imaged-guided CRT planning and delivery processes have become much more complex and much less intuitive. These complexities, coupled with the inadequate informatics infrastructure and outdated national QA guidelines, have created enormous QA challenges. Communication among members of the planning team, including physician, resident, simulation therapist, dosimetrist, physicist, and treating therapist, is often rushed, cryptic, and complicated by the lack of integration of the radiation oncology EMR (e.g., Elekta-Impac MOSAIQ) with the hospital's EHR (e.g., Epic software). In fact, in most cases, one must resort to a hybrid charting system (ad hoc combinations of EMR, EHR, and paper charts), which is a dangerous situation. In addition, multiple imaging modalities are often used to define target volumes, all complicating the processing of the information. CRT plan data, transferred over a network to the V&R system and computer-controlled LINAC systems, carry complex specifications for treatment, including positioning of MLC leaves, sometimes variable dose rates, collimator rotation, gantry angles, and, in some instances, a moving treatment table or gantry or both. In some cases, different vendor software systems are used, and interoperability is not always robust. This continuing increasing complexity of devices and systems is clearly problematic for a totally prescriptive QA approach, and it results in increased time demands on staff and groups where there are already shortages. A series of *New York Times* articles[100] brought needed attention to this issue and spurred national organizations to work to improve the current QA situation.[102,103]

Although it is believed that the prescriptive QA approach is valid and valuable for much of the CRT technology and procedures currently in place, new and different approaches need to be developed in parallel.[104,105] These must be risk/evidence based and process oriented rather than device and procedure oriented; they likely need to be multidisciplinary in nature, resource and risk optimized, and flexible enough to cope with current and anticipated changes in technology.[106] Such process-oriented QA includes risk-based analysis, process mapping, application of failure modes and effects analysis (FMEA), and fault tree analysis (FTA), including analyses of human actions and responses.[107]

In support of this direction, the AAPM recently published recommendations of Task Group 100 on the application of risk analysis methods to radiation therapy quality management.[108] This report provides a mechanism for individual facilities to create custom QA protocols based on their individual situation and risk profile. This task group also calls on the future AAPM task groups to embrace the same methodology. The significance of the TG-100 is the departure of more or less purely prescriptive QA guidelines to the provision of a tool set for individual clinics to establish their own QA methods. Advantages of this approach, as described above, include the ability to create custom QA protocols considering the unique needs and circumstances of the particular institution. Shortcomings include the time required to create these QA protocols and potential absence of local expertise that can objectively assess individual facility needs. However, both of these are likely transient limitations as efficiency and proficiency in this process will be developed over time. Another great advantage of this approach is the evaluation of new processes and establishment of QA methods and QA tool development based on that analysis. For example, Noel et al.[109] analyzed QA processes and tools needed for implementation of online adaptive radiotherapy, and Acharya et al.[110] subsequently relied on that analysis for clinical implementation of an actual online adaptive radiotherapy program. The TG-100 report is poised to make a major impact on QA practices in radiotherapy and our future practices should proceed with that in mind.

That said, radiation oncology departments must do all that they can now to ensure that processes for safe planning and delivery of CRT are in place and appropriately resourced. Table 9.4 provides a list of guiding principles to help a department prioritize QA efforts for improving patient safety and quality for CRT. This list is a compilation of pertinent key recommendations made by several national and international groups.[99,102,111–115]

Quality Assurance: Treatment Planning System

The complexity of 3DTPS continues to increase to better facilitate the accurate delivery of CRT. In a number of instances, the TPS is an integral component of the treatment machine. Hence, this results in having more than one planning system in the department, thus increasing QA complexity. Rigorous acceptance and commissioning of the TPS are essential to ensure it is functioning accurately before it is used clinically; in this respect, it is no different than other medical devices. AAPM recently published Medical Physics Practice Guideline 5.a on commissioning and QA of treatment planning systems.[116] There has also been activity in automating QA of treatment planning systems, and the automation in this area should offer improvements in consistency and efficiency as well as reduction in errors.[117] More details on acceptance, commissioning, and periodic QA tests are available elsewhere.[118–125]

The accuracy of dose calculations must be examined thoroughly during the 3DTPS commissioning process. Periodic checks of calculations versus measured dose are also essential because of possible data corruptions in the TPS itself and to how well treatment machine parameters such as flatness and symmetry are maintained. It should be appreciated that the 3DTPS can never be fully tested, nor can the manufacturer assure the user that the system is "bug-free." Rather, the system should be tested over a range of parameters that are typical of those used in the clinic. For example, tests should include (a) consistency of input/output data; (b)

TABLE 9.4 GUIDING PRINCIPLES FOR CONFORMAL RADIATION THERAPY QUALITY ASSURANCE PROGRAM

1. Establish a safety-conscious culture within the department and ensure that the processes for safe delivery of conformal radiation therapy (CRT) are in place and appropriately resourced. To that end, perform the following:
   a. Establish a formal covenant and commitment to safety. The radiation therapy team should work under a radiation safety covenant, and each member of the team should pledge a commitment to protect the safety of each and every patient.
   b. Make sure it is clear that each member of the treatment team has the right and the responsibility to declare a "time-out" if he or she has concerns or questions about the plan or course of treatment for a patient.
   c. Make sure that the quality assurance (QA) program is properly resourced.
2. Seek practice accreditation by the appropriate national body, for example, the American College of Radiology (ACR)/American Society for Radiation Oncology (ASTRO).
3. Participate in external dosimetric audits such as provided by the Radiological Physics Center (RPC) annual External Reference Dosimetry Audit.
4. Expand the use of checklists in CRT treatment planning and treatment delivery.
5. Implement a formal policy that ensures that CRT policy and procedures (P&Ps), including checklists, are in place and are regularly updated and reviewed on an annual basis (require documentation that this is actually done).
6. Conduct periodic reviews of staffing levels to ensure that the staffing and skills mix are appropriate for the numbers of patients treated and the complexity of treatments delivered.
7. Implement a Clinical Operations Committee (COC), with supervisor representatives from each group, to address any problematic issues in the clinic and to help ensure that good communication exists among all groups involved in the CRT treatment process.
8. Conduct town hall meetings (with QA program being a major focus) with department faculty/staff at least quarterly to help ensure good communication exists among all groups involved in the treatment process.
9. Maintain training records for all staff involved in radiation therapy. They should be detailed and specific to particular procedures, that is, an internal form of CRT credentialing.
10. Maintain funding to support training and continuing education, particularly when new CRT techniques are introduced.
11. Introduction of new CRT techniques always needs to be carefully planned with a thorough risk assessment, review of staffing levels and skills required, and development of pertinent P&Ps. All staff involved in the process should undergo specific training in the new treatment technique or process prior to clinical use.
12. Working environment, particularly in two areas—treatment machine console and treatment planning—needs to be conducive to safety and designed such that it ensures that staff can work without inappropriate interruptions.
13. Prescriptive QA program should be in place but continually evaluated to ensure that each specific test adds value and that those that do not add the required value are eliminated.
14. Perform systematic risk analysis and improvement using industrial engineering–based tools such as process mapping, failure modes and effects analysis (FMEA), and fault tree analysis (FTA) for all advanced treatment modalities.
15. Implement a treatment table registration system (CT simulator and treatment machines) so that all patient/immobilization device positions on the table can be registered.
16. Use treatment planning/delivery systems tolerance tables for specific procedures, and monitor set-up variability (i.e., any therapist overrides of treatment couch, gantry, collimator position, etc., settings in order to treat patient).
17. Perform on-treatment verification imaging as needed, but be mindful of imaging dose, and look for ways to become more efficient.
18. Perform *in vivo* dosimetry (e.g., diode checks) at the beginning of treatment for all 3DCRT patients when physically possible.
19. Conduct weekly peer review chart rounds (review prescription, verification images, dose distribution, and other pertinent documentation, e.g., signed consent, pathology, etc.).
20. Conduct weekly peer review planning conference to review CRT plans. Review of GTV, CTV, and PTV contours, DRRs, and dose distributions helps to develop a consistent approach in implementing ICRU 50/62/83 methodology.
21. Implement a treatment planning workflow monitoring software system.
22. Implement a software system for reporting and analyzing errors and near misses, with feedback to the staff at town hall meetings.
23. Strive to have the right balance between accountability and openness in the department's incident reporting culture.
24. Department should strongly endorse a national/international incident reporting system for radiotherapy incidents.

monitor unit calculations, (c) relative dose distributions, (d) graphical data, including BEV and field aperture display, and (e) plan evaluation tools such as DVHs and DRRs. The test procedures and results should be fully documented, as they will provide the baseline data to which the periodic QA tests can be compared.

It has been a practice to validate IMRT treatments with patient-specific dose measurements. However, for online adaptive radiotherapy, it is not practical to perform a phantom-based measurement, and an alternative approach to validation of dose calculation accuracy is needed.[110] The prevailing method for assurance of online adaptive treatment is to perform a secondary independent dose calculation combined with a rules engine to verify integrity of the treatment plan. As online adaptive radiotherapy becomes more mainstream practice, it is expected that the patient-specific measurement-based QA will diminish in prevalence.

Quality Assurance: Patient Positioning and Immobilization and Imaging Data Acquisition

CT, MRI, PET, and ultrasound imaging are used, depending on disease site, for acquiring imaging data to determine patient external contours and target and organs-at-risk volumes. Hence, there are a number of additional QA demands placed on imaging units that are specific to CRT treatment planning.[40] Because the patient needs to be repositioned reproducibly on the treatment machine, special patient positioning immobilization devices are needed. Such devices should be constructed so that they can be attached in a similar manner to the treatment machine couch and the CT, MR, or PET imaging system couches used in obtaining the planning imaging data. These devices should not only attach and lock to all couches, but they also should do so in a configurable manner to allow indexing of the devices to the treatment couch for daily reproducibility.

In some instances, the composition of these devices is also important; for example, low–atomic number materials are necessary for CT scanners, whereas carbon fiber devices are not compatible with MRI. In addition, patient motion can distort MRI and CT images, which can lead to inaccuracies in organ delineation and plan calculation. Large-bore CT simulators often offer extended or extrapolated field of view option.[126] With this option, the native image field of view can be extended by reconstructing the image in the portion of the CT scanner bore opening where partial data collection occurred. Depending on the scanner model and image reconstruction software age, there can be spatial and quantitative CT distortions in those areas of images, which ultimately can translate to treatment planning errors.

Geometric accuracy of all imaging modalities used for planning must be checked. This can be accomplished by imaging suitably designed phantoms on the various machines and comparing the results with the known values. Special care should be given to MRI units, which may suffer from appreciable spatial distortions. If a PET-CT is used, special attention should be paid to the physical alignment of the table couch and both imaging rings. If images from CT, MR, and/or PET are registered and fused, a QA program must be implemented to ensure that the inherent algorithm used and departmental procedures are able to produce accurate composite images for planning.[127,128] Finally, for CT, it is necessary to obtain or confirm the relationship between CT number and electron density.

The transfer of image data routinely occurs directly via a computer network but should be checked on a regular basis. Vigilance is also necessary to eliminate any systematic errors; for example, an error in the specification of a scan diameter can lead to geometric distortions of the image.

Quality Assurance: Volume(s) Delineation

Target volume delineation is viewed by many experts in the field as being the weakest link in the entire CRT workflow chain. A high variation continues to be seen in all studies evaluating consistency of delineation of target volumes and organs at risk among physicians.[129-134] This can be explained by a lack of generally accepted guidelines for volume delineation and also, most likely, insufficient training of radiation oncology residents in modern cross-sectional imaging. It is clear that errors/inconsistencies in volume delineation can seriously undermine the goals of CRT. One approach toward solving this difficult issue is to adopt guidelines and consensus volumes based on the delineation performed by a number of experts in the field.[133,135] Both the Radiation Therapy Oncology Group and the European Society of Therapeutic Radiation Oncology have placed high priority on this approach and now offer more online guidelines for several sites. Standardization in naming convention of targets and organs at risk[136] should be a component of the effort to improve organ delineation process. To this end, the AAPM has formed the TG 263 on standardizing nomenclature in radiation therapy, and it is expected that the results of this work will lead to significant improvements in standardization in this area.

It is also possible to improperly define an OAR because of faulty or incomplete CT procedures. For example, the base of the brain may be better defined on the CT slice if sagittal reconstructions are also available while contouring. In addition, if contrast is used, density overrides may be needed before treatment planning is performed to avoid the erroneous effects of the high-Z media. Related to this is the situation that occurs when high-Z materials like hip prostheses are found within the patient and density overrides are required to account for artifacts. Because of likelihood and significance of contouring errors in radiotherapy, there is an ever-increasing emphasis on peer review of contoured volumes. In certain situations (e.g., solo practices, online adaptive radiotherapy), it may not be practical to perform peer review or independent review of contoured organs. It is expected that automatic contour checking will play a role in the future of radiotherapy.[137-139]

Quality Assurance: Designing Beams

MLC leaf settings or block apertures and beam orientation displays must be confirmed prior to clinical use and checked after any software modification. In addition, it is possible to define beam orientations that are physically impossible to set up, and this process requires use of clinical judgment by the dosimetrist generating the treatment plan. Thus, the ability to physically set up a particular beam orientation must be reviewed and verified, particularly for beam orientations involving couch rotation. In such cases, tests might have to be performed to verify clearance between the treatment machine gantry and the patient or the gantry and the treatment couch before finalizing the treatment plan. This is especially true for SBRT treatments and will likely be the case for 4π treatments.

Quality Assurance: Treatment Plan Review

All CRT treatment plans should be reviewed, signed, and dated by the treatment planner. The treating physician should of course also review, approve, and sign the treatment plan. Because most of the clinics are paperless today, various combinations of treatment planning systems, V&R systems, and EMR pose unique challenges as to where to approve plans and how to document plan reviews by treatment planner, medical physicist, and radiation oncologist. Each clinic should develop a process where there is a traceability of these approvals and it is transparent as to who was involved in the planning and plan review processes. In addition, all plans should be independently checked prior to initiation of radiation therapy by a physicist who was not involved directly in the production of the plan. The independent plan check should assure that set-up instructions have been properly recorded—for example, field size, gantry angle, and so on. In addition, beam normalization points (normally at isocenter) can be problematic if near nontissue medium or under or near an MLC leaf edge and hence should be moved to a more suitable location. The number of MUs to realize the dose prescription is typically obtained directly from the 3DTPS. These values must be independently checked either by hand calculations or, more typically, independent computer calculations. An action level should be established based upon the accuracy of the computer algorithm and independent dose calculation procedure. Obviously, any MU check system must be tested prior to clinical use and following any change or software upgrade. The American Association of Physicists in Medicine Task Group 114 report provides valuable information on the verification of MU calculations for non-IMRT radiotherapy treatments.[140]

Note that IMRT plans require additional checks, including review of optimization parameters, minimum gap size, minimum MU/segment, and maximum doses in and outside of the target. In addition, in the United States, the patient's plan must undergo phantom measurement checks on the intended treatment machine to verify both point dose and spatial dose distribution agreement.

AAPM plan checks are becoming largely automated through homegrown[141,142] and commercial solutions. These software packages range from basic secondary dose calculation to more sophisticated rules engine and industrial methods-driven software. The AAPM's Task Group 275 on Strategies for Effective Physics Plan and Chart Review in Radiation Therapy is in part charged with developing recommendations for software vendors for development of patient plan checking software. Although, in the past, most could afford the time needed to perform plan checks manually, the online adaptive radiotherapy process does not afford that time. In the age of adaptive radiotherapy, automated plan checks are becoming the necessity, and that will undoubtedly change the field's overall approach to plan checks moving systematically away from manual work and toward computer-assisted checks.

Quality Assurance: Planning Conference

One of the most important components of a CRT QA program is the establishment of a weekly planning QA conference that is attended by radiation oncologists, medical physicists, radiation therapists, and dosimetrists. This is in addition to the normal new-patient chart rounds conference, at which the patient's pertinent medical history, physical, pathology, and diagnostic imaging findings along with the tumor staging and proposed plan of treatment, including the prescription, are presented by the attending radiation oncologists or residents. In a planning QA conference, the group can review the CRT plans using a high-resolution, large-screen video projector connected to the 3DTP network. GTV, CTV, and PTV contours, DRRs, and dose distributions can all be reviewed very efficiently. This type of planning conference helps the staff to develop a very consistent approach in implementing ICRU 50/62/83 methodology for specifying volumes and provides a very effective peer review mechanism for a CRT clinical program.

Quality Assurance: Plan Implementation and Treatment Verification

If a clinic is in the initial phases of implementing CRT techniques or if experienced users implement new CRT modalities using nonconventional beam orientations, a verification simulation procedure is recommended to confirm the correctness of the beam orientations. It is important to check that all treatment plan parameters are properly implemented. This can be best accomplished by having the treatment planning team available (or on call) during this procedure so that any detected ambiguities or problems can be addressed immediately. When a beam orientation cannot be simulated, EPIDs can be used to obtain orthogonal images for comparison with similar DRRs to ensure correct isocenter positioning. Today, even more advanced onboard imaging and other data localization systems (i.e., ultrasound, video surfacing, static kilovolt imaging, kilovolt cone-beam CT, megavolt helical CT, megavolt cone-beam CT, and MRI) are available.[11,55] Clearly written policy and procedures (P&Ps) should be in place with regard to (a) localization procedures, (b) therapist instructions and tolerance criteria to move (or not move) a patient, (c) whether post imaging is required when a move is made, (d) subsequent reviews by physicians, and (e) the process for peer review of verification images. Special care should be taken to ensure that all beam-modifying devices are correctly positioned. Although errors in MLC settings or block fabrication/mounting should be observed when reviewing the portal images, wedge or compensator misalignment is much more problematic and may only be revealed by careful observation during patient setup.

When available, the optical distance indicator is also useful in assessing the correctness of the setup of a particular beam. Documentation provides a depth of isocenter below the skin surface on the central ray of the beam, which can then be compared with the isocenter depth measured on the simulator or treatment machine after the beam is set up using the couch and gantry positions specified by the treatment plan.

A V&R system should be used to assure that the same parameters (within tolerance limits) are used each day. Such systems are valuable for the verification and recording of at least the following parameters: (a) monitor units, (b) energy, (c) mode, (d) collimator settings (including independent jaws and multileaf collimator), (e) collimator angle, (f) gantry angle, (g) table position, and (h) wedge number and orientation. However, V&R systems must be used with care because they can give the user a false sense of security. For example, if a set-up error is made on the first day and the machine geometry parameters are captured, the system will faithfully verify this erroneous setting from day to day. To reduce the chance of this occurring, the patient should be carefully set up according to the treatment plan (best if there is a direct electronic transfer of plan parameters to the V&R system), and a robust P&P for approval of patient treatment position should be in place; upon approval, the parameters are captured with the V&R system. As vendor implementation of Digital Imaging and Communications in Medicine data exchange has matured significantly, the direct transfer of data from the TPS to the V&R system has undoubtedly reduced such errors; however, a careful check of patient position is still recommended.

Thermoluminescent dosimeters (TLDs), diodes, optically stimulated luminescence dosimeters (OSLs), and MOSFET detectors are often used for *in vivo* dosimetry. Diodes or MOSFETS are most used for dose checks at the beginning of treatment for non-IMRT patients. TLDs or OSLs are typically used for checking multiple dose locations for unusual treatment conditions or for critical structures in or near the treatment volume. Recently, exit portal dosimetry using EPIDs has been used to provide full-field information, even for IMRT fields.[143,144] Transmission detectors are also playing an increasing role in patient treatment verification. In transmission dosimetry, a large-area detector is mounted on the exit surface of the gantry head, and it compares radiation (fluence and shape) exiting the LINAC with the expectations from the treatment planning system.[145] There has also been a push to use machine log files for daily analysis of patient treatments.[146-148] It is difficult to determine which one of these methods is most effective as they all have some unique benefits and a combination of techniques may be needed for in-depth defense. To the extent that some of these processes (e.g., log file analysis) are passive and run in background, they are easy and inexpensive to perform and almost offer free information for prevention of patient treatment errors.

Summary

We strongly believe that the use of 3-D treatment planning and CRT has had (and will continue to have) a major impact on the practice of radiation therapy. Phase I/II and III CRT dose escalation studies in several disease sites have been conducted (or are underway) by the Radiation Therapy Oncology Group under cooperative agreement with the NCI.[149] In addition, there are many other individual institutional studies that have shown the benefits of 3-D planning and conformal therapy, particularly for prostate cancer, head and neck cancer, and lung cancer, as documented in the literature.[150] Patients identified to benefit most from 3-D planning and CRT are those with tumors in sites with complex anatomy, irregularly shaped tumor volumes, tumors adjacent to radiation-sensitive normal structures, and undergoing small-volume or high dose treatments. However, as with any major technical advance in radiation oncology, CRT use must be supported with enhanced quality assurance from all members of the treatment team.

REFERENCES

1. Purdy JA. 3-D radiation treatment planning: a new era. In: Meyer JL, Purdy JA, eds. *3-D conformal radiotherapy: a new era in the irradiation of cancer.* Basel, Switzerland: Karger, 1996:1–16.

2. Purdy JA. From new frontiers to new standards of practice: advances in radiotherapy planning and delivery. In: Meyer JL, ed. *IMRT, IGRT, SBRT.* Basel, Switzerland: Karger, 2007:18–39.

3. Purdy JA. Advances in the planning and delivery of radiotherapy: new expectations, new standards of care. In: Meyer JL, ed. *IMRT, IGRT, SBRT.* 2nd ed. Basel, Switzerland: Karger, 2011:1–28.

4. Purdy JA. Intensity-modulated radiation therapy. *Int J Radiat Oncol Biol Phys* 1996;35(4):845–846.

5. Webb S. *Intensity-modulated radiation therapy.* Bristol, UK: Institute of Physics Publishing, 2000.

6. Jaffray DA, Drake DG, Moreau M, et al. A radiographic and tomographic imaging system integrated into a medical linear accelerator for localization of bone and soft-tissue targets. *Int J Radiat Oncol Biol Phys* 1999;45:773–789.

7. Jaffray DA, Siewerdsen JH, Wong JW, et al. Flat-panel cone-beam computed tomography for image-guided radiation therapy. *Int J Radiat Oncol Biol Phys* 2002;53(5):1337–1349.

8. Mutic S, Dempsey JF. The ViewRay system: magnetic resonance-guided and controlled radiotherapy. *Semin Radiat Oncol* 2014;24(3):196–199.

9. Bortfeld T, Schmidt-Ullrich R, De Neve W, et al. *Image-guided IMRT.* Berlin, Germany: Springer, 2006.

10. Ling CC, York E, Fuks Z. From IMRT to IGRT: frontierland or neverland? *Radiother Oncol* 2006;78:119–122.

11. Dawson LA, Balter JM. Interventions to reduce organ motion effects in radiation delivery. *Semin Radiat Oncol* 2004;14(1):76–80.

12. Keall PJ. 4-Dimensional computed tomography imaging and treatment planning. *Semin Radiat Oncol* 2004;14(1):81–90.

13. Takahaski S. Conformation radiotherapy-rotation techniques as applied to radiography and radiotherapy of cancer. *Acta Radiol Suppl* 1965;242:1–142.

14. Proimos BS. Synchronous field shaping in rotational megavoltage therapy. *Radiology* 1960;74:753–757.

15. Trump JG, Wright KA, Smedal MI, et al. Synchronous field shaping and protection in 2-million-volt rotational therapy. *Radiology* 1961;76:275–283.

16. Green A, Jennings WA, Christie HM. Rotational roentgen therapy in the horizontal plane. *Acta Radiol* 1960;31:275–320.

17. Bjarngard BE, Kijewski PK. Computer-controlled radiation therapy. In: *Proceedings 2nd Annual Symposium on Computer Applications in Medical Care.* Long Beach, CA, 1978.

18. Davy TJ, Brace J. Dynamic 3-D treatment using a computer-controlled cobalt unit. *Br J Radiol* 1979;53:612–616.

19. Sterling TD, Knowlton KC, Weinkam JJ, et al. Dynamic display of radiotherapy plans using computer-produced films. *Radiology* 1973;107:689–691.

20. Sterling TD, Perry H, Katz L. Automation of radiation treatment planning. V. Calculation and visualization of the total treatment volume. *Br J Radiol* 1965;38:906–913.

21. McShan DL, Silverman A, Lanza D, et al. A computerized three-dimensional treatment planning system utilizing interactive color graphics. *Br J Radiol* 1979;52:478–481.

22. Reinstein LE, McShan D, Webber BM, et al. A computer-assisted three-dimensional treatment planning system. *Radiology* 1978;127:259–264.

23. Goitein M, Abrams M. Multi-dimensional treatment planning: I. Delineation of anatomy. *Int J Radiat Oncol Biol Phys* 1983;9:777–787.

24. Goitein M, Abrams M, Rowell D, et al. Multi-dimensional treatment planning: II. Beam's eye view, back projection, and projection through CT sections. *Int J Radiat Oncol Biol Phys* 1983;9:789–797.

25. Fraass BA, McShan DL. 3-D treatment planning. I. Overview of a clinical planning system. In: *Proceedings of the 9th International Conference on the Use of Computers in Radiation Therapy*. Scheveningen, The Netherlands, 1987.
26. Mohan R, Barest G, Brewster LJ, et al. A comprehensive three-dimensional radiation treatment planning system. *Int J Radiat Oncol Biol Phys* 1988;15:481–495.
27. Purdy JA, Wong JW, Harms WB, et al. Three dimensional radiation treatment planning system. In: *Proceedings of the 9th International Conference on the Use of Computers in Radiation Therapy*. Scheveningen, The Netherlands, 1987.
28. Sherouse GW, Mosher CE, Novins K, et al. Virtual simulation: concept and implementation, in the use of computers in radiation therapy. In: *Proceedings of the 9th International Conference on the Use of Computers in Radiation Therapy*. Scheveningen, The Netherlands, 1987.
29. Smith AF, Purdy JA. Editors' note. *Int J Radiat Oncol Biol Phys* 1991;21(1):1.
30. Drzymala RE, Holman MD, Yan D, et al. Integrated software tools for the evaluation of radiotherapy treatment plans. *Int J Radiat Oncol Biol Phys* 1994;30(4):909–919.
31. Drzymala RE, Mohan R, Brewster L, et al. Dose–volume histograms. *Int J Radiat Oncol Biol Phys* 1991;21(1):71–78.
32. Bosch WR, Low DA, Gerber RL, et al. The electronic viewbox: a software tool for radiation therapy treatment verification. *Int J Radiat Oncol Biol Phys* 1995;31(1):135–142.
33. Goitein M. The probability of controlling an inhomogeneously irradiated tumor. In: Goitein M, Lyman J, Maor M, et al., eds. *Report of the working groups on the evaluation of treatment planning for particle beam radiotherapy*. Bethesda, MD: National Cancer Institute, 1987.
34. IMRT Collaborative Working Group. Intensity modulated radiation therapy: current status and issues of interest. *Int J Radiat Oncol Biol Phys* 2001;51(4):880–914.
35. International Commission on Radiation Units and Measurements. *Report 29: dose Specification for reporting external beam therapy with photons and electrons*. Washington, DC: International Commission on Radiation Units and Measurements, 1978.
36. International Commission on Radiation Units and Measurements. *Report 50: prescribing, recording, and reporting photon beam therapy*. Bethesda, MD: International Commission on Radiation Units and Measurements, 1993.
37. International Commission on Radiation Units and Measurements. *Report 62: prescribing, recording, and reporting photon beam therapy (Supplement to ICRU Report 50)*. Bethesda, MD: International Commission on Radiation Units and Measurements, 1999.
38. Jin J-Y, Ajlouni M, Chen Q, et al. A technique of using gated-CT images to determine internal target volume (ITV) for fractionated stereotactic lung radiotherapy. *Radiother Oncol* 2006;78(2):177–184.
39. Perez CA, Purdy JA, Harms WB, et al. Design of a fully integrated three-dimensional computed tomography simulator and preliminary clinical evaluation. *Int J Radiat Oncol Biol Phys* 1994;30(4):887–897.
40. Mutic S, Palta JR, Butker EK, et al. Quality assurance for computed-tomography simulators and the computed-tomography-simulation process: report of the AAPM Radiation Therapy Committee Task Group No. 66. *Med Phys* 2003;30(10):2762–2792.
41. Mutic S. Patient positioning, immobilization devices, and fiducial markers in PET/CT scanner based RT simulation. *Semin Ultrasound CT MR* 2010;31(6):462–467.
42. Paulson ES, Erickson B, Schultz C, et al. Comprehensive MRI simulation methodology using a dedicated MRI scanner in radiation oncology for external beam radiation treatment planning. *Med Phys* 2015;42(1):28–39.
43. Tyagi N, Fontenla S, Zhang J, et al. Dosimetric and workflow evaluation of first commercial synthetic CT software for clinical use in pelvis. *Phys Med Biol* 2017;62(8):2961–2975.
44. Hall WH, Guiou M, Lee NY, et al. Development and validation of a standardized method for contouring the brachial plexus: preliminary dosimetric analysis among patients treated with IMRT for head-and-neck cancer. *Int J Radiat Oncol Biol Phys.* 2008;72(5):1362–1367.
45. Caldwell CB, Mah K, Skinner M, et al. Can PET provide the 3D extent of tumor motion for individualized internal target volumes? A phantom study of the limitations of CT and the promise of PET. *Int J Radiat Oncol Biol Phys* 2003;55(5):1381–1393.
46. Chen GTY, Kung JH, Beaudette KP. Artifacts in computed tomography scanning of moving objects. *Semin Radiat Oncol* 2004;14(1):19–26.
47. Rietzel E, Chen GT, Choi NC, et al. Four-dimensional image-based treatment planning: target volume segmentation and dose calculation in the presence of respiratory motion. *Int J Radiat Oncol Biol Phys* 2005;61(5):1535–1550.
48. Rietzel E, Pan T, Chen GT. Four-dimensional computed tomography: image formation and clinical protocol. *Med Phys* 2005;32(4):874–889.
49. Qi XS, White J, Rabinovitch R, et al. Respiratory organ motion and dosimetric impact on breast and nodal irradiation. *Int J Radiat Oncol Biol Phys* 2010;78(2):609–617.
50. Bortfeld T, Jiang S, Rietzel E. Effects of motion on the total dose distribution. *Semin Radiat Oncol* 2004;14(1):41–51.
51. Chino JP, Lee WR, Madden R, et al. Teaching the anatomy of oncology: evaluating the impact of a dedicated oncoanatomy course. *Int J Radiat Oncol Biol Phys* 2011;79(3):853–859.
52. Brock K, Mutic S, McNutt T, et al. Use of image registration and fusion algorithms and techniques in radiotherapy: report of the AAPM Radiation Therapy Committee Task Group No. 132. *Med Phys* 2017;44(7):e43–e76. doi: 10.1002/mp.12256.
53. van Herk M. Errors and margins in radiotherapy. *Semin Radiat Oncol* 2004;14(1):52–64.
54. van Herk M, Remeijer P, Lebesque JV. Inclusion of geometric uncertainties in treatment plan evaluations. *Int J Radiat Oncol Biol Phys* 2002;52(5):1407–1422.
55. Keall P. Locating and targeting moving tumors with radiation beams. In: Meyer JL, ed. *IMRT, IGRT, SBRT*, 2nd ed. Basel, Switzerland: Karger, 2011:118–131.
56. Chen AM, Farwell DG, Luu Q, et al. Evaluation of the planning target volume in the treatment of head and neck cancer with intensity-modulated radiotherapy: what is the appropriate expansion margin in the setting of daily image guidance? *Int J Radiat Oncol Biol Phys* 2011;81(4):943–949.
57. International Commission on Radiation Units and Measurements. Report 83: prescribing, recording, and reporting photon-beam intensity-modulated radiation therapy (IMRT). *J ICRU* 2010;10(1):1–106.
58. Sherouse GW, Novins K, Chaney EL. Computation of digitally reconstructed radiographs for use in radiotherapy treatment design. *Int J Radiat Oncol Biol Phys* 1990;18(3):651–658.
59. Dong P, Lee P, Ruan D, et al. 4π non-coplanar liver SBRT: a novel delivery technique. *Int J Radiat Oncol Biol Phys* 2013;85(5):1360–1366.
60. Dong P, Lee P, Ruan D, et al. 4π noncoplanar stereotactic body radiation therapy for centrally located or larger lung tumors. *Int J Radiat Oncol Biol Phys* 2013;86(3):407–413.
61. Rwigema JC, Nguyen D, Heron DE, et al. 4π noncoplanar stereotactic body radiation therapy for head-and-neck cancer: potential to improve tumor control and late toxicity. *Int J Radiat Oncol Biol Phys* 2015;91(2):401–409.
62. Ong CL, Cuijpers JP, Senan S, et al. Impact of the calculation resolution of AAA for small fields and RapidArc treatment plans. *Med Phys* 2011;38(8):4471–4479.
63. Mackie RT, Liu HH, McCullough EC. Treatment planning algorithms: model-based photon dose calculations. In: Khan FM, ed. *Treatment planning in radiation oncology*. 2nd ed. Philadelphia, PA: Lippincott Williams & Wilkins, 2007:63–77.
64. Zhao T, Mistry N, Raupach R, et al. Evaluation of the use of direct electron density CT images in radiation therapy (abstract). *Med Phys* 2016;43(6):3876.
65. Frank SJ, Forster KM, Stevens CW, et al. Treatment planning for lung cancer: traditional homogeneous point-dose prescription compared with heterogeneity-corrected dose-volume prescription. *Int J Radiat Oncol Biol Phys* 2003;56(5):1308–1318.
66. Emami B, Lyman J, Brown A, et al. Tolerance of normal tissue to therapeutic irradiation. *Int J Radiat Oncol Biol Phys* 1991;21:109–122.
67. Milano MT, Constine LS, Okunieff P. Normal tissue tolerance dose metrics for radiation therapy of major organs. *Semin Radiat Oncol* 2007;17(2):131.
68. Marks LB, Ten Haken RK, Martel MK. Guest Editor's introduction to QUANTEC: a users guide. *Int J Radiat Oncol Biol Phys* 2010;76(3 Suppl):S1–S2.
69. Marks LB, Yorke ED, Jackson A, et al. Use of normal tissue complication probability models in the clinic. *Int J Radiat Oncol Biol Phys* 2010;76(3 Suppl):S10–S19.
70. Monz M, Küfer KH, Bortfeld TR, et al. Pareto navigation: algorithmic foundation of interactive multi-criteria IMRT planning. *Phys Med Biol* 2008;53(4):985–998.
71. Kamran SC, Mueller BS, Paetzold P, et al. Multi-criteria optimization achieves superior normal tissue sparing in a planning study of intensity-modulated radiation therapy for RTOG 1308-eligible non-small cell lung cancer patients. *Radiother Oncol* 2016;118(3):515–520.
72. Good D, Lo J, Lee WR, et al. A knowledge-based approach to improving and homogenizing intensity modulated radiation therapy planning quality among treatment centers: an example application to prostate cancer planning. *Int J Radiat Oncol Biol Phys* 2013;87(1):176–181.
73. Moore KL, Brame RS, Low DA, et al. Experience-based quality control of clinical intensity-modulated radiotherapy planning. *Int J Radiat Oncol Biol Phys* 2011;81(2):545–551.
74. Shiraishi S, Moore KL. Knowledge-based prediction of three-dimensional dose distributions for external beam radiotherapy. *Med Phys* 2016;43(1):378.
75. Giaddui T, Chen W, Yu J, et al. Establishing the feasibility of the dosimetric compliance criteria of RTOG 1308: phase III randomized trial comparing overall survival after photon versus proton radiochemotherapy for inoperable stage II-IIIB NSCLC. *Radiat Oncol* 2016;11:66.
76. Moore KL, Schmidt R, Moiseenko V, et al. Quantifying unnecessary normal tissue complication risks due to suboptimal planning: a secondary study of RTOG 0126. *Int J Radiat Oncol Biol Phys* 2015;92(2):228–235.
77. Purdy JA, Harms WB, Matthews JW, et al. Advances in 3-dimensional radiation treatment planning systems: room-view display with real time interactivity. *Int J Radiat Oncol Biol Phys* 1993;27(4):933–944.
78. Das IJ, Chang C-W, Chopra KL, et al. Intensity-modulated radiation therapy dose prescription, recording, and delivery: patterns of variability among institutions and treatment planning systems. *J Natl Cancer Inst* 2008;100(5):300–307.
79. Willins J, Kachnic L. Clinically relevant standards for intensity-modulated radiation therapy dose prescription. *J Natl Cancer Inst* 2008;100(5):288–290.
80. Holmes T, Das R, Low D, et al. American Society for Radiation Oncology recommendations for documenting intensity-modulated radiation therapy treatments. *Int J Radiat Oncol Biol Phys* 2009;74(5):1311–1318.
81. Das IJ, Andersen A, Chen ZJ, et al. State of dose prescription and compliance to international standard (ICRU-83) in intensity modulated radiation therapy among academic institutions. *Pract Radiat Oncol* 2017;7(2):e145–e155.
82. Bentzen SM, Constine LS, Deasy JO, et al. Quantitative Analyses of Normal Tissue Effects in the Clinic (QUANTEC): an introduction to the scientific issues. *Int J Radiat Oncol Biol Phys* 2010;76(3 Suppl):S3–S9.
83. Moiseenko V, Deasy JO, Van Dyk J. Radiobiological modeling for treatment planning. In: Van Dyk J, ed. *The modern technology of radiation oncology*, Vol. 2. Madison, WI: Medical Physics Publishing, 2005:185–220.
84. Schultheiss TE, Orton CG, Peck RA. Models in radiotherapy: volume effects. *Med Phys* 1983;10:410–415.
85. Lyman JT, Wolbarst AB. Optimization of radiation therapy. III. A method of assessing complication probabilities from dose-volume histograms. *Int J Radiat Oncol Biol Phys* 1987;13:103–109.
86. Lyman JT, Wolbarst AB. Optimization of radiation therapy. IV. A dose-volume histogram reduction algorithm. *Int J Radiat Oncol Biol Phys* 1989;17(2):433–436.
87. Källman P, Lind BK, Brahme A. An algorithm for maximizing the probability of complication free tumor control in radiation therapy. *Int J Radiat Oncol Biol Phys* 1992;37:871–890.
88. Olsen DR, Kambestad BK, Kristoffersen DT. Calculation of radiation induced complication probabilities for brain, liver and kidney, and the use of a reliability model to estimate critical volume fractions. *Br J Radiol* 1994;67:1218–1225.

89. Withers HR, Taylor JMG, Maciejewski B. Treatment volume and tissue tolerance. *Int J Radiat Oncol Biol Phys* 1988;14:751–759.

90. Kutcher G, Berman C. Calculation of complication probability factors for nonuniform tissue irradiation: the effective volume method. *Int J Radiat Oncol Biol Phys* 1989;16:1623–1630.

91. Niemierko A, Goitein M. Calculation of normal tissue complication probability and dose-volume histogram reduction schemes for tissues with a critical element architecture. *Radiother Oncol* 1991;20:166–176.

92. Niemierko A, Goitein M. Modeling of normal tissue response to radiation: the critical volume module. *Int J Radiat Oncol Biol Phys* 1993;25:135–145.

93. Niemierko A. Reporting and analyzing dose distributions: a concept of equivalent uniform dose. *Med Phys* 1997;24(1):103–110.

94. Niemierko A. A generalized concept of equivalent uniform dose (EUD) [Abstract]. *Med Phys* 1999;26:1100.

95. McGary JE, Grant W, Woo SY, et al. Comment on "Reporting and analyzing dose distributions: a concept of equivalent uniform dose" [Med. Phys. 24, 103–109 (1997)]. *Med Phys* 1997;24(8):1323–1324.

96. McGary JE, Grant W, Woo SY. Applying the equivalent uniform dose formulation based on the linear-quadratic model to inhomogeneous tumor dose distributions: caution for analyzing and reporting. *J Appl Clin Med Phys* 2000;1(4):126–137.

97. Niemierko A. Response to Comment on "Reporting and analyzing dose distributions: a concept of equivalent uniform dose" [*Med. Phys.* 24, 1323–1324 (1997)]. *Med Phys* 1997;24(8):1325–1327.

98. Abdel-Wahab M, Rengan R, Curran B, et al. Integrating the healthcare enterprise in radiation oncology plug and play—the future of radiation oncology? *Int J Radiat Oncol Biol Phys* 2010;76(2):333–336.

99. Kutcher GJ, Coia L, Gillin M, et al. Comprehensive QA for radiation oncology: report of AAPM Radiation Therapy Committee Task Group 40. *Med Phys* 1994;21(4):581–618.

100. Bogdanovitch W. Radiation offers new cures, and ways to do harm. *New York Times* January 24, 2010. Available at: http://www.nytimes.com/2010/01/24/health/24radiation.html

101. Williamson JF, Dunscombe PB, Sharpe MB, et al. Quality assurance needs for modern image-based radiotherapy: recommendations from 2007 interorganizational symposium on "Quality Assurance of Radiation Therapy: Challenges of Advanced Technology". *Int J Radiat Oncol Biol Phys* 2008;71(1 Suppl):S2–S12.

102. Klein EE, Hanley J, Bayouth J, et al. Task Group 142 report: quality assurance of medical accelerators. *Med Phys* 2009;36(9):4197–4212.

103. ASTRO. Press release: ASTRO reaffirms commitment to quality, issues progress report on patient safety plan, 2011. Available at: http://www.astro.org/News-and-Media/News-Releases/2011/Target-Safely,-a-six-point-patient-protection-plan-developed-in-January-2010,-to-improve-the-safety-and-quality-of-radiation.aspx

104. Pawlicki T, Mundt AJ. Quality in radiation oncology. *Med Phys* 2007;34(5):1529–1534.

105. Ford EC, Gaudette R, Myers L, et al. Evaluation of safety in a radiation oncology setting using failure mode and effects analysis. *Int J Radiat Oncol Biol Phys* 2009;74(3):852–858.

106. Pawlicki T, Dunscombe PB, Mundt AJ, et al., eds. *Quality and safety in radiotherapy.* New York, NY: Taylor & Francis, 2011.

107. Rath F. Tools for developing a quality management program: proactive tools (process mapping, value stream mapping, fault tree analysis, and failure mode and effects analysis). *Int J Radiat Oncol Biol Phys* 2008;71(1 Suppl):S187–S190.

108. Huq MS, Fraass BA, Dunscombe PB, et al. The report of Task Group 100 of the AAPM: application of risk analysis methods to radiation therapy quality management. *Med Phys* 2016;43(7):4209–4262.

109. Noel CE, Santanam L, Parikh PJ, et al. Process-based quality management for clinical implementation of adaptive radiotherapy. *Med Phys* 2014;41(8):081717.

110. Acharya S, Fischer-Valuck BW, Kashani R, et al. Online Magnetic Resonance Image Guided Adaptive Radiation Therapy: First Clinical Applications. *Int J Radiat Oncol Biol Phys* 2016;94(2):394–403.

111. American College of Radiology. *Practice guidelines and technical standards.* Reston, VA: American College of Radiology, 2010.

112. International Atomic Energy Agency. *Safety Report Series No. 17: Lessons learned from accidental exposures in radiotherapy.* Vienna, Austria: International Atomic Energy Agency, 2000.

113. International Atomic Energy Agency. *Comprehensive audits of radiotherapy practices: a tool for quality improvement.* Vienna, Austria: International Atomic Energy Agency, 2007.

114. Royal College of Radiologists, Society and College of Radiographers, Institute of Physics and Engineering in Medicine, National Patient Safety Agency, British Institute of Radiology. *Towards safer radiotherapy.* London, UK: Royal College of Radiologists, 2008.

115. Hendee WR, Herman MG. Improving patient safety in radiation oncology. *Med Phys* 2011;38(1):78–82.

116. Smilowitz JB, Das IJ, Feygelman V, et al. AAPM Medical Physics Practice Guideline 5.a.: Commissioning and QA of Treatment Planning Dose Calculations—Megavoltage Photon and Electron Beams. *J Appl Clin Med Phys* 2016;17(1):6166.

117. Wexler A, Gu B, Goddu S, et al. FMEA of manual and automated methods for commissioning a radiotherapy treatment planning system. *Med Phys* 2017;44(9):4415–4425. doi: 10.1002/mp.12278.

118. Fraass B, Doppke K, Hunt M, et al. AAPM Radiation Therapy Committee Task Group 53: quality assurance for clinical radiotherapy treatment planning. *Med Phys* 1998;25:1773–1829.

119. Jacky J, White CP. Testing a 3-D radiation therapy planning program. *Int J Radiat Oncol Biol Phys* 1990;18:253–261.

120. Van Dyk J, Barnett RB, Cygler JE, et al. Commissioning and quality assurance of treatment planning computers. *Int J Radiat Oncol Biol Phys* 1993;26(2):261–273.

121. Van Dyk J. Quality assurance of radiation therapy planning systems: current status and remaining challenges. *Int J Radiat Oncol Biol Phys* 2008;71 (1 Suppl):S23–S27.

122. International Atomic Energy Agency. *Commissioning and quality assurance of computerized planning systems for radiation treatment of cancer.* Vienna, Austria: International Atomic Energy Agency, 2004.

123. Ezzell GA, Burmeister JW, Dogan N, et al. IMRT commissioning: multiple institution planning and dosimetry comparisons, a report from AAPM Task Group 119. *Med Phys* 2009;36(11):5359–5373.

124. Bruinvis IAD, Keus RB, Lenglet WJM, et al. Quality assurance of 3-D treatment planning systems for external photon and electron beams: report 15 of The Netherlands Commission on Radiation Dosimetry. Delft, The Netherlands; 2005.

125. Mijnheer B, Olszewska A, Fiorino C, et al. Quality assurance of treatment planning systems: practical examples of non-IMRT photon beams. ESTRO Booklet No. 7. Brussels, 2004.

126. Mutic S. Use of imaging systems for patient modeling: commissioning and use of conventional CT. In: Curran BH, Chetty IJ, Balter JM, eds. *Integrating new technologies into the clinic: Monte Carlo and image guided radiation therapy.* Maryland: American Association of Physicists in Medicine, 2006:1–31.

127. Lavely WC, Scarfone C, Cevikalp H, et al. Phantom validation of coregistration of PET and CT for image-guided radiotherapy. *Med Phys* 2004;31(5):1083–1092.

128. Mutic S, Dempsey JF, Bosch WR, et al. Multimodality image registration quality assurance for conformal three-dimensional treatment planning. *Int J Radiat Oncol Biol Phys* 2001;51(1):244–260.

129. Gregoire V, Coche E, Cosnard G, et al. Selection and delineation of lymph node target volumes in head and neck conformal radiotherapy. Proposal for standardizing terminology and procedure based on the surgical experience. *Radiother Oncol* 2000;56(2):135–150.

130. Gregoire V, Levendag P, Ang KK, et al. CT-based delineation of lymph node levels and related CTVs in the node-negative neck: DAHANCA, EORTC, GORTEC, NCIC, RTOG consensus guidelines. *Radiother Oncol* 2003;69(3):227–236.

131. Matzinger O, Gerber E, Bernstein Z, et al. EORTC-ROG expert opinion: radiotherapy volume and treatment guidelines for neoadjuvant radiation of adenocarcinomas of the gastroesophageal junction and the stomach. *Radiother Oncol* 2009;92:164–175.

132. Poortmans PMP, Ataman F, Bernard Davis J, et al. Guidelines for target volume definition in post-operative radiotherapy for prostate cancer, on behalf of the EORTC Radiation Oncology Group. *Radiother Oncol* 2007;82:121–127.

133. Symon Z, Tsvang L, Wygoda M, et al. An interobserver study of prostatic fossa clinical target volume delineation in clinical practice: are regions of recurrence adequately targeted? *Am J Clin Oncol* 2011;34(2):145–149.

134. van Mourik AM, Elkhuizen PHM, Minkema D, et al. Multiinstitutional study on target volume delineation variation in breast radiotherapy in the presence of guidelines. *Radiother Oncol* 2010;94(3):286–291.

135. Miralbell R, Vees H, Lozano J, et al. Endorectal MRI assessment of local relapse after surgery for prostate cancer: a model to define treatment field guidelines for adjuvant radiotherapy in patients at high risk for local failure. *Int J Radiat Oncol Biol Phys* 2007;67(2):356–361.

136. Santanam L, Hurkmans C, Mutic S, et al. Standardizing naming conventions in radiation oncology. *Int J Radiat Oncol Biol Phys* 2012;83(4):1344–1349.

137. Altman MB, Kavanaugh JA, Wooten HO, et al. A framework for automated contour quality assurance in radiation therapy including adaptive techniques. *Phys Med Biol* 2015;60(13):5199–5209.

138. Chen HC, Tan J, Dolly S, et al. Automated contouring error detection based on supervised geometric attribute distribution models for radiation therapy: a general strategy. *Med Phys* 2015;42(2):1048–1059.

139. Olsen LA, Robinson CG, He GR, et al. Automated radiation therapy treatment plan workflow using a commercial application programming interface. *Pract Radiat Oncol* 2014;4(6):358–367.

140. Stern RL, Heaton R, Fraser MW, et al. Verification of monitor unit calculations for non-IMRT clinical radiotherapy: report of AAPM Task Group 114. *Med Phys* 2011;38(1):504–530.

141. Yang D, Wu Y, Brame RS, et al. Technical note: electronic chart checks in a paperless radiation therapy clinic. *Med Phys* 2012;39(8):4726–4732.

142. Li HH, Wu Y, Yang D, et al. Software tool for physics chart checks. *Pract Radiat Oncol* 2014;4(6):e217–e225. doi: 10.1016/j.prro.2014.03.001.

143. Kruse JJ. On the insensitivity of single field planar dosimetry to IMRT inaccuracies. *Med Phys* 2010;37(6):2516–2524.

144. Mans A, Wendling M, McDermott LN, et al. Catching errors with in vivo EPID dosimetry. *Med Phys* 2010;37(6):2638–2644.

145. Prabhakar R. Real-time dosimetry in external beam radiation therapy. *World J Radiol* 2013;5(10):352–355.

146. Rangaraj D, Zhu M, Yang D, et al. Catching errors with patient-specific pretreatment machine log file analysis. *Pract Radiat Oncol* 2013;3(2):80–90.

147. Sun B, Rangaraj D, Palanisswamy G, et al. Initial experience with TrueBeam trajectory log files for radiation therapy delivery verification. *Pract Radiat Oncol* 2013;3(4):e199–e208.

148. Yang D, Wooten HO, Green O, et al. A software tool to automatically assure and report daily treatment deliveries by a Cobalt-60 radiation therapy device. *J Appl Clin Med Phys* 2016;17(3):6001.

149. RTOG. Image-Guided Radiation Therapy Committee. *Int J Radiat Oncol Biol Phys* 2001;51(3 Suppl 2):60.

150. Meyer JL, ed. *IMRT, IGRT, SBRT.* 2nd ed. Basel, Switzerland: Karger; 2011.

CHAPTER 10

Physics and Dosimetry of Proton Therapy

Brian Winey

PHYSICS OF PROTON

As protons travel through media, protons interact with the media through electromagnetic interactions, nuclear interactions, and Coulomb scattering.[1,2] The electromagnetic interactions between the proton and the media can be described according to the stopping power equation, known as the Bethe equation:

$$\frac{S_{el}}{\rho} = -\frac{1}{\rho}\frac{dE}{dx} = \frac{4\pi r_e^2 m_e c^2}{\beta^2}\frac{1}{u}\frac{Z}{A}z^2 L(\beta)$$

where r_e is the electron radius, $m_e c^2$ is the electron rest energy, u is the atomic mass unit, β is the particle velocity, Z is the atomic number of the medium, A is the relative atomic mass of the medium, and z is the charge number of the particle ($p = 1$, $C = 6$).

The term $L(\beta)$ can be expanded as:

$$L(\beta) = L_0(\beta) + zL_1(\beta) + z^2 L_2(\beta)$$

where the individual terms are as follows:

$$L_0(\beta) = \frac{1}{2}\ln\left(\frac{2m_e c^2 \beta^2 W_m}{1-\beta^2}\right) - \beta^2 - \ln(I) - \frac{C}{Z} - \frac{\delta}{2}$$

$$L_1(\beta) = g_1 \beta^{-2g2}$$

$$z^2 L_2(\beta) = -\left(\frac{z a}{\beta}\right)^2 \sum_{n=1}^{\infty}\frac{1}{\left[n\left(n^2+\left(\frac{z a}{\beta}\right)^2\right)\right]}$$

where W_m is the largest possible energy loss in a single collision with a free electron, C/Z is the shell correction to account for the bound state of K and L shell electrons, and $\delta/2$ is the Fermi density effect correction. The second factor, L_1, is known as the Barkas correction factor and is an empirical fit with variable g dependent upon the medium. The final term can be approximated in the limit of the particle traveling faster than the atomic electron as the Bloch approximation:

$$z^2 L_2(\beta) = -\left(\frac{z a}{\beta}\right)^2\left[1.20-\left(\frac{z a}{\beta}\right)^2\left(1.04-0.85\left(\frac{z a}{\beta}\right)^2+0.343\left(\frac{z a}{\beta}\right)^4\right)\right]$$

which now gives the Bethe-Bloch equation that describes the proton stopping power in a medium:

$$\frac{S_{el}}{\rho} = -\frac{1}{\rho}\frac{dE}{dx} = \frac{4\pi r_e^2 m_e c^2}{\beta^2}\frac{1}{u}\frac{Z}{A}z^2$$
$$\left[\frac{1}{2}\ln\left(\frac{2m_e c^2 \beta^2 W_m}{1-\beta^2}\right)-\beta^2-\ln(I)-\frac{C}{Z}-\frac{\delta}{2}+L_1(\beta)+z^2 L_2(\beta)\right]$$

In general, the electromagnetic interactions increase as the proton velocity (energy) decreases (Fig. 10.1).

In addition to the electromagnetic interactions, the nuclear interactions are comprised of both elastic and nonelastic interactions with the majority of dose deposited by the nonelastic interactions that result in secondary nuclear particles, primarily protons along with gamma radiation. The nonelastic nuclear interactions are mostly independent of particle velocity until the particle slows to a resonance velocity, which results in an increase in the nuclear interaction cross section, similarly to the electromagnetic interactions. Combined, the nuclear and electromagnetic interactions give rise to the famous Bragg curve of particle therapy (Fig. 10.2). The relationship between proton energy and proton range[3] is detailed in Figure 10.3. Typical clinical proton therapy centers provide proton energies from about 70 MeV to 235 or 250 MeV.

Because particles traveling through media is a stochastic process, the particles can lose energy at different rates. The energy straggling of the protons broadens the Bragg peak as the particles travel deeper into the media and the spectrum of energies in the beam increases in width. The clinical result is the broadening of the distal penumbra of the particle beam particularly evident when treating deep targets (Fig. 10.2).

As the particles travel through the medium, the particles undergo Coulomb scattering events with the nuclei. Because of the elastic nature, little energy is lost in the Coulomb scattering events, but the effect is most pronounced in the shape of the beam as it progresses through the medium. Multiple Coulomb scattering (MCS) affects the beam output for small fields, dose coverage of targets, dose homogeneity, range straggling, and increased lateral penumbra (Fig. 10.4). In fact, for small proton beams (diameter < 1 cm for ranges > 10 cm), the MCS events can result in a loss of the Bragg peak along the central axis and inside the treatment target (Fig. 10.4).

FIGURE 10.1. The energy loss (dE/dx) as a function of proton kinetic energy for protons traveling through water. Most importantly, the energy loss increases rapidly as the proton slows in the medium. This rapid energy loss gives rise to the Bragg peak.

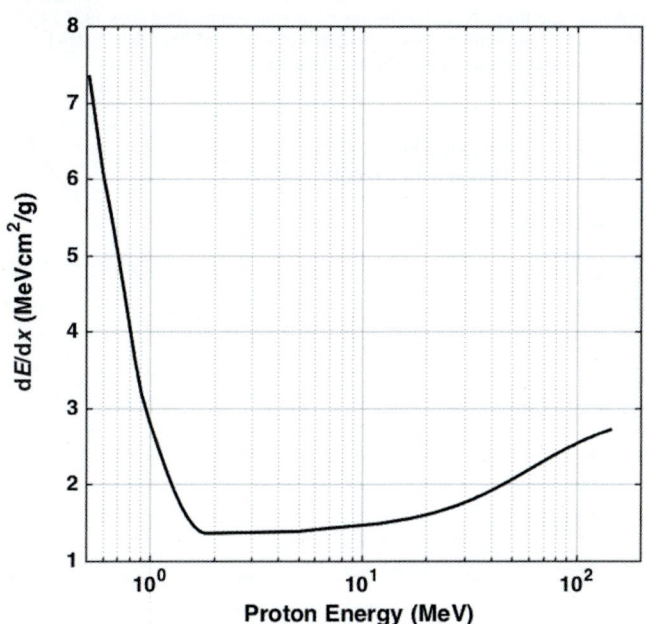

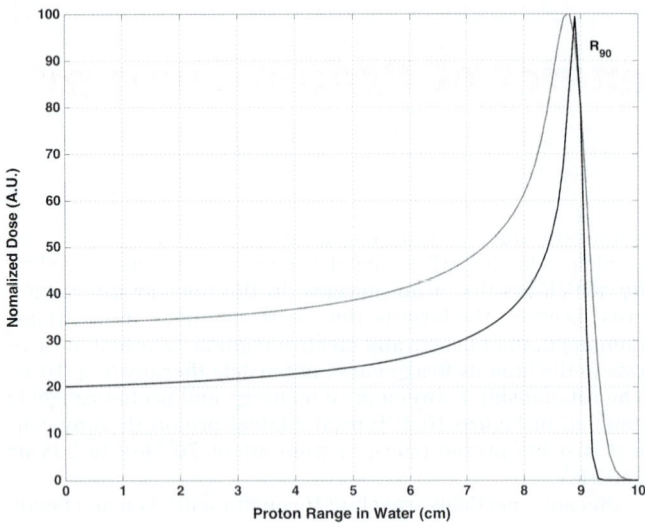

FIGURE 10.2. The proton energy deposited into the medium (water) as a function of proton range. The *dotted line* represents the effects of proton energy straggling as the protons stochastically interact with the medium. The R_{90} range is labeled.

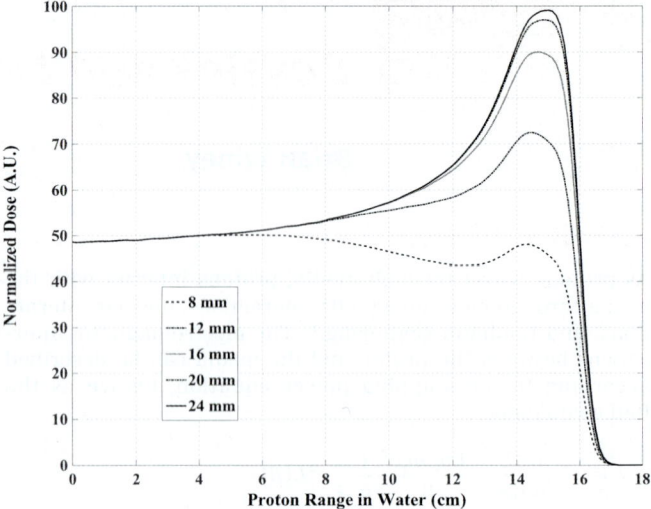

FIGURE 10.4. A central axis depth dose curve for a Bragg peak with a range of 15.5 versus field size. All fields are given for a range of 15.5 cm, and the field size decreases from 24 to 8 mm. Similar effects can be observed with single pencil beams. As the field size increases, the lateral scatter of neighboring pencil beams provides lateral equilibrium along the central axis and restores the Bragg peak.

DOSIMETRY

Absolute dosimetry in proton therapy is typically performed using Faraday cups or calorimetry, with Faradays cups being more common[2]. Aside from absolute dosimetry, most clinical proton therapy centers rely upon ionization chambers to perform beam calibrations. In many ways, proton beam dosimetry is similar to photon therapy. Dosimetry must be traceable to a primary standard radiation source (e.g., NIST in the United States), where radiation dose is typically defined in a free air ionization chamber with a cobalt source. Institutions can rely on Accredited Dosimetry Calibration Laboratories to supply an absolute calibration factor for ionization chambers. Current protocols utilize dose to water calculations and correct for the proton beam quality relative to Cobalt.

FIGURE 10.3. The relationship of proton energy and range (R_{90}) in water. The graph is a commonly cited fit[3] to empirical data that are not displayed. Typical clinical proton therapy accelerators provide proton energies from about 70 MeV (R_{90} = 4 cm) to 235 MeV (R_{90} = 35 cm). (From Bortfeld, T. An analytical approximation of the Bragg curve for therapeutic proton beams. *Med Phys* 1997;24[12]: 2024–2033. Copyright © 1997 American Association of Physicists in Medicine. Reprinted by permission of John Wiley & Sons, Inc.)

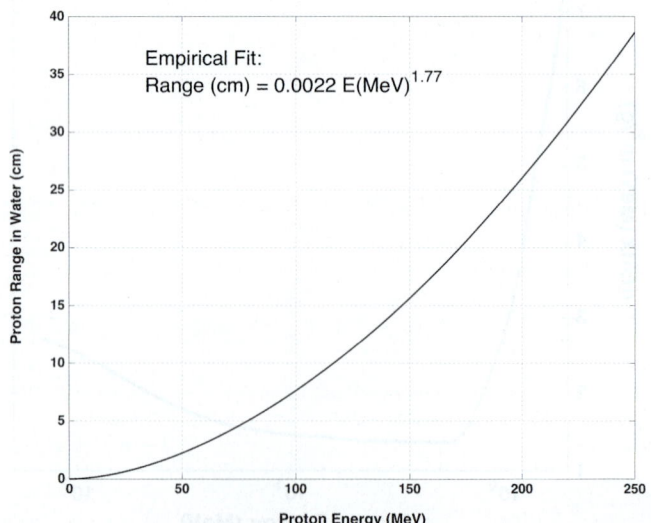

According to TRS-398 and ICRU Report 78,[1] a calibrated ionization chamber can be used to perform calibration of a proton beam according to the following equation:

$$D_{w,Q_p} = M_{Q_p} N_{D,w,Q_{p0}} k_{Q_p,Q_{p0}}$$

where the measurement, M, is corrected for pressure, temperature, polarization, and recombination. The k_q factor is a function of residual range (R_{res}) of the proton beam, which is correlated with the spectrum of proton energies at the point of measurements.

Of particular note in scanned beam proton therapy, instantaneous dose rates in the volume of the ionization chamber can be significantly higher than most proton beams and recombination can become a problem. Some proton therapy accelerators can deliver lower beam currents, or an institution can purchase ionization chambers designed for scanned proton beams. A proton beam calibration measurement will be performed in an irradiated volume large enough to reduce the effects of scattering and volume averaging in the volume of the ionization chamber. Typically, an ionization chamber will be placed in the center of a field size of 10 cm × 10 cm and a modulation width of at least 10 cm (R_{res} = 5 cm).

Although the physical dose of protons is measured and recorded similarly to photon therapy beams, the biologic dosimetry is different. The historical and still common practice is to apply a relative biologic effectiveness (RBE) correction factor of 1.1 to the physical dose in order to correct for the increased clinical effectiveness of the proton physical dose delivered to the patient relative to a photon treatment of the same physical dose.[4] Proton beam radiation therapy is typically quoted in Gy RBE such that the physical dose is multiplied by the RBE correction factor:

$$D_{Gy,RBE} = 1.1 \times D_{Gy}$$

The RBE factor of 1.1 is not constant for all cell types, clinical end points, or locations along the proton dose curve. There are more recent studies analyzing the effects of variable RBE or measuring cell- and end point–specific RBE values. There remains uncertainty regarding the most accurate RBE factor for proton beam therapy, but there is little clinical evidence that the current practice requires immediate remedy.

UNCERTAINTIES

Physical dose and particle interactions have long been described in the literature, and the fundamental physics is generally well understood. There remains some uncertainty in the cross-section interactions between protons and nuclei (I) in the above equations, but commissioning measurements of clinical systems can greatly reduce the uncertainties of the underlying physics.

Uncertainties in proton therapy delivery remain and affect the accuracy of the proton beam delivery to the intended target. Because of the sharpness of the Bragg peak, uncertainties that affect the proton range can result in large underdosing in the target when the Bragg peak stops prematurely or overdosing of the surrounding tissues when the Bragg peak travels farther than intended into the patient.

There are generally two classes of uncertainties that affect the range of the proton Bragg peak in the patient: systematic and random. Uncertainties in both categories can be mitigated with various methods during pretreatment imaging, treatment planning, and treatment room imaging. A summary of both categories of uncertainties can be found in Table 10.1. The important note is the larger dosimetric effect of systematic versus random uncertainties in the proton beam delivery. It is also important to note that many of the uncertainties are present in photon or electron beam therapy, but the Bragg peak in proton therapy can create unique dosimetric uncertainties.

Many of the uncertainties have both systematic and random contributions because of the differences of calibration and delivery or treatment planning system calculation versus delivery. For example, anatomy might not be accurately captured in the computed tomography (CT) in the case of a filled sinus cavity, which can become a systematic range error for the treatment of a nasopharyngeal lesion if the sinus were to drain prior to the first treatment. Other anatomic changes such as motion can be random.

To mitigate the dosimetric effects of the listed uncertainties, or increase the robustness of the treatment plan, there are multiple methods that can be employed. One of the simplest and most robust methods is to utilize more than one treatment beam. The use of multiple beams can spread the uncertainty of a single beam direction and reduce the magnitude of a dose uncertainty to a single location. Depending upon the time scale of the random uncertainties, multiple beams can also reduce the magnitude of the random uncertainty simply by the increased time of delivery.

Although the Bragg peak reduces both the entrance and exit dose compared to photon beams to greatly reduce the integral dose to organs outside of the target, the use of multiple beams can increase the integral dose. It is a clinical decision whether the increase of robustness using multiple beams is worth the increased integral dose. In some treatment sites, the increased integral dose can be deposited in the surrounding tissues that have a low risk of toxicities. In other sites, the risk of toxicities is greater and the clinical decision leads to the use of a single treatment beam.

A second method to increase robustness of the treatment delivery is to use margins, similar to photon therapy. Specific to proton therapy is the distal edge of the target, and distal margins are often determined separately from the lateral margins in a beam angle geometry. In addition to margins, the distal edge of a treatment beam can be "smeared," which decreases the distal conformality in the lateral direction of the beam such that tissue motion or patient setup uncertainties have a reduced effect on the target dose.

A third method that can be used in more recent treatment planning systems is a "robust optimization" technique. The basic premise of a robust optimizer is to include random and systematic uncertainties in the dose optimization in addition to the more common dose objectives and constraints for the targets and organs. Generally, more robust plans result in less sharp dose gradients in close proximity to avoidance regions such that the effect of range or dose uncertainties will be reduced.

TREATMENT PLANNING

Although the Bragg peak is commonly known, it is less known how the Bragg peak is optimized for the treatment of a target volume. There are essential two methods for proton therapy delivery: scattered and scanned. Scattered therapy was the dominant solution for more than 50 years of treatment but is fading as most proton therapy centers purchase scanning systems.

Scattered Beams

Briefly, scattered systems use scatters composed of various plastic and metals to increase the diameter of the proton beam within a specified flatness and symmetry. A proton beam exits the accelerator with a sigma on the scale of millimeters or 1 to 2 cm, depending upon the system and energy selection method. A typical ocular line requires very little scattering, but targets larger than an ocular target require larger beam diameters. Common double-scattering systems that use multiple scattering elements can achieve flat proton beams up to a clinically flat 25 cm diameter. Once the beam is scattered to the appropriately specified diameter, apertures are used to laterally shape the proton beam to the shape of the target volume.

In addition to the lateral shape of the proton beam, the size of the beam along the beam axis is variable and specified by the modulation of the Bragg peak. There are multiple methods of modulation, which essentially modulate the energy of the proton beam to change the range of the protons in the patient. The summation of the multiple energy proton beams results in a spread out Bragg peak (SOBP) that provides a flat dose distribution inside the target volume (Fig. 10.5). The modulation of the proton beam energy can occur at the accelerator, in the energy selection system, with a modulation wheel, or generally with any technique that adds material in the beam path. One of the more common modulation methods uses a modulation wheel that is composed of a wheel with increasing steps of material thickness. The wheel rotates through the beam path

TABLE 10.1 A BRIEF AND NONEXHAUSTIVE LIST OF UNCERTAINTIES THAT AFFECT THE DOSIMETRIC DELIVERY OF PROTONS. THE MAGNITUDE OF THE UNCERTAINTIES IS NOT LISTED.	
Systematic	**Random**
CT stopping power calibration	CT noise
Beam energy/range calibration	Beam energy tuning
Ion chamber calibration	Spot position and weight
Immobilization densities	Patient positioning
Implanted device densities/artifacts	Anatomic motion
Anatomic changes	Anatomic changes
Heterogeneities *in silico*	Heterogeneities *in vivo*

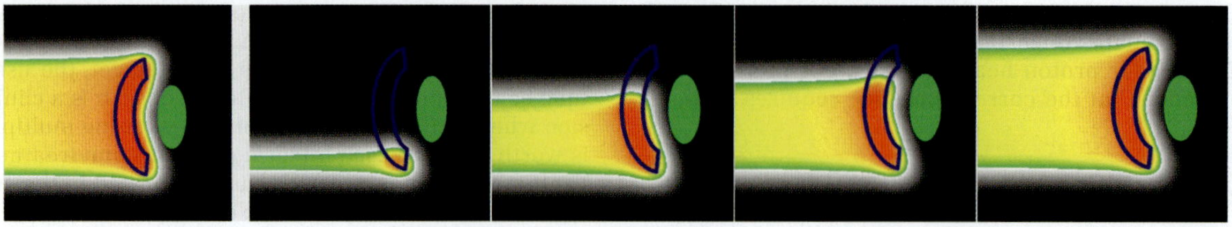

FIGURE 10.5. A comparison of the dose delivered by a scattered beam (*left*) and a scanned beam at different times in the field delivery beginning with the first pencil beam and scanned across the blue target volume.

and essentially sweeps the proton Bragg peak through the treatment volume multiple (hundreds) times each second.

Scanned Beams

Although scattered beams spread the beam laterally, shaped by an aperture, to deliver a uniform dose to the specific target volume, scanned beams sweep a single proton pencil beam (Fig. 10.5) laterally to deposit dose to a volume of tissue, either continuously or spot scanning. In most scattered beam deliveries, the entire target receives a uniform dose, and the beam continues to deliver a uniform dose to the entire target until the time that the prescription dose is delivered. In a scanning system, a small portion of the target is irradiated with a single Bragg peak pencil beam until the prescribed dose of that pencil beam is delivered and then the pencil beam is scanned to the next location. The pencil beam is scanned over the entire volume, using energy changes when necessary to modulate the depth of the pencil beam, until the prescribed dose pattern is delivered (Fig. 10.5).

Although a scanned beam delivery does not require apertures to provide lateral conformality to the target volume, apertures can provide additional conformality for shallow targets and larger spot sizes. The target depth when the apertures no longer provide a clinical advantage depends upon the spot size of the delivery system.

In addition to reducing the need for physical hardware, scanning systems can provide multiple dosimetric benefits over scattered beams. The primary benefits include the following:

1. Reduced proximal dose in the entrance region
2. Greater proximal conformality because of nonuniform modulation
3. Ability to deliver nonuniform doses to the target (intensity modulation)
4. Greater conformality and organ sparing for complex-shaped targets
5. Gradient match lines for large targets, particularly craniospinal irradiation (CSI) treatments

Scanned beam dosimetry can be less robust to motion and other uncertainties listed above, but the robustness of the scanned beam delivery can be improved using robust optimization, margins, rescanning, rapid scanning, and variable spot sizes.

With greater effort toward the deployment of scanned beam systems, the challenges of robustness are being overcome and the utility of scattered beams is diminishing.

Site-Specific Proton Treatment Planning

The earliest proton therapy treatments were delivered to cranial (pituitary) and ocular targets. Currently, ocular proton therapy is the most common proton therapy site by patient numbers worldwide.[5] The primary reasons for the popularity of ocular treatment popularity are the target location, low proton energy, and small treatment fields. When proton

therapy began in the physics accelerator laboratories, there were many accelerators capable of reaching 70 MeV and the beam delivery required little scattering to achieve the lateral field sizes needed for the ocular targets.

Brain

Cranial targets were the first recorded treatments with proton and ion beams.[6-11] The treatments were straightforward with opposed lateral beams targeting the sella for pituitary therapies. With the advent of 3D imaging, more diagnoses in the brain are currently treated, including both conventional and stereotactic radiosurgery fractionation techniques.

When considering a treatment plan for a cranial target, protons can reduce the normal brain integral dose and dose to sensitive structures such as the optic apparatus and the brainstem. The clinical significance of the dose reduction to normal brain is not discussed here. Cranial targets present an excellent proton therapy site because of the ability to use multiple beam entrance angles to increase the dose conformality, reduce the uncertainties from any single beam, and increase the overall robustness of the proton delivery. Typical treatment plans are displayed in Figures 10.6.

Base of Skull

From a treatment planning perspective, base of skull targets such as chordomas can be treated with protons to reduce integral dose to the brain and spare many organs in close proximity to the target volume, particularly the brainstem. Prior to the clinical deployment of scanned beams, the treatment of concave base of skull targets with scattered beams required the use of matched beams inside the target volume. Scanned beam treatment plans can now provide more robust treatments with gradient match lines and increase the dose sparing of organs in close proximity to the targets. Similar to cranial targets, the base of skull lesions can be treated with multiple beam entrance angles, including superior oblique beams to increase the dose conformality, treatment robustness, and normal tissue sparing (Fig. 10.7).

Head and Neck

The treatment of head and neck lesions can provide some challenges to treatment planning and delivery, irrespective of the method of proton delivery. Large anatomic variations because of sinus filling, tumor shrinkage, and patient weigh loss can greatly affect the accuracy of the proton treatment. The treatment planning advantages for head and neck targets are typically the sparing of normal tissues to reduce acute and chronic toxicities.

Typical treatment plans for targets in the nasal region employ two or more treatment fields, but the possible beam angles are often reduced because of the location of the target with respect to the eyes and optic nerves. Beam angles for lesions around the oral cavity and inferior have greater flexibility than nasal targets. Additionally, simultaneous boost volumes can also be treated easily with scanned proton beams. Tumor shrinkage or sinus filling/draining can also

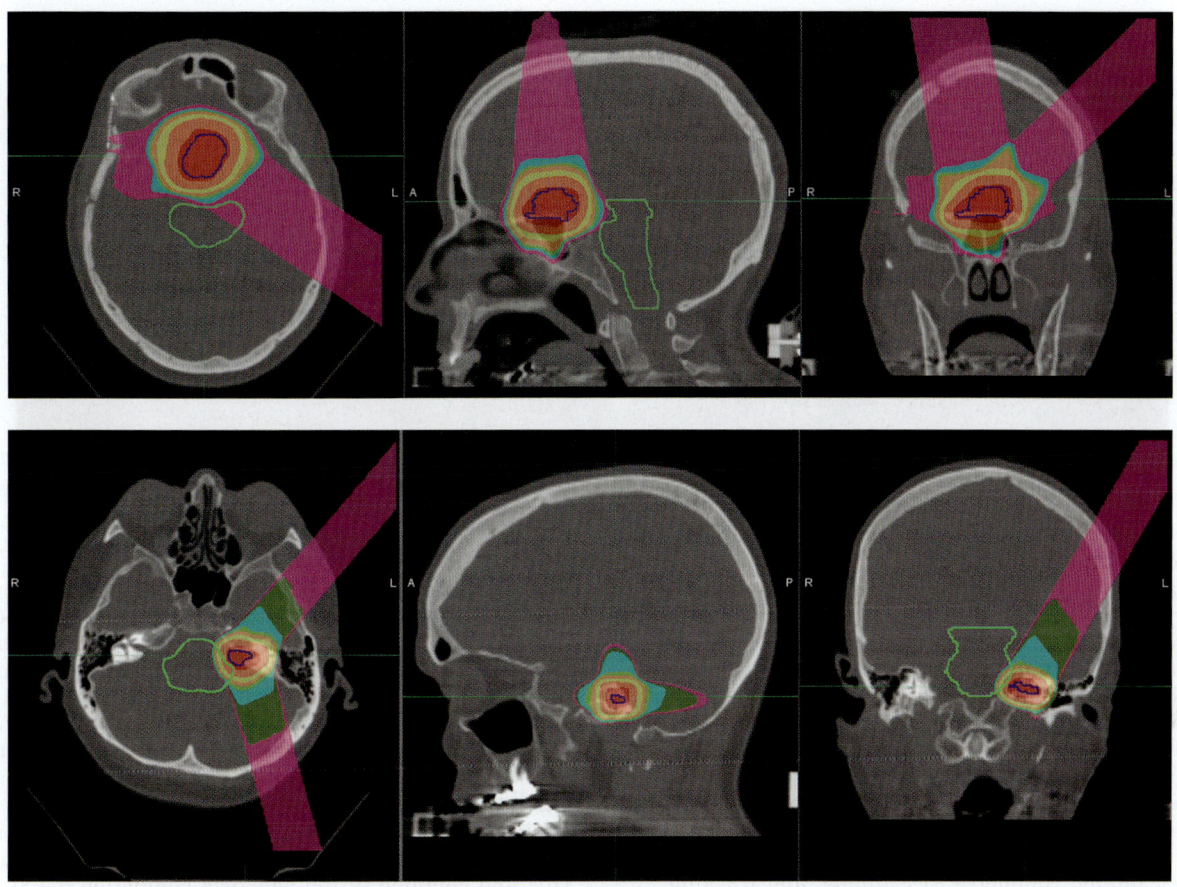

FIGURE 10.6. An example of cranial target treatment plans for a meningioma **(top)** and an acoustic schwannoma **(bottom)**. The beam angles can be visualized by the low dose.

increase the uncertainty of proton treatment. Adaptive proton therapy will greatly benefit targets in the nasal and oral cavities and neck locations.

Breast

Recently, breast proton therapy has become an option for breast radiation therapy.[12,13] The typical treatment employs a single *en face* proton beam. Breathing motion is mostly oriented along the beam angle such that the motion has little effect on the treatment delivery. With the use of proton therapy, nodal target volumes can be included in a single scanned beam so long as the total target volume fits in the maximum field size of the treatment delivery system. Additionally, simultaneous boost volumes can also be treated easily with scanned proton beams (Fig. 10.8).

Compared to photon therapy, protons do not have a buildup region because protons are directly ionizing radiation. The increased surface dose can be reduced in the optimization process of a scanned beam plan. Additionally, range uncertainties at the distal edge of the treatment volume in the region of the chest wall and lung interface should be accounted in the plan optimization.

FIGURE 10.7. A representative treatment plan for a base of skull lesion utilizing beam angles in the axial plane as well as superior oblique beams.

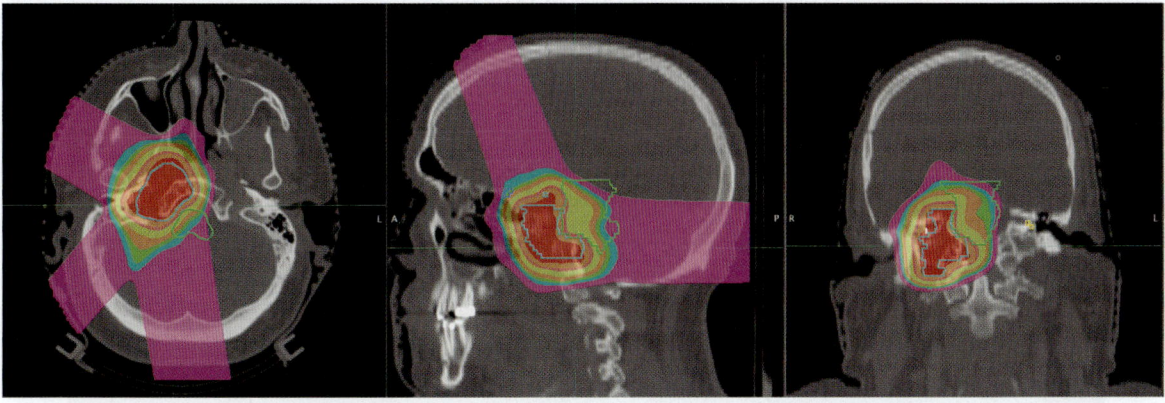

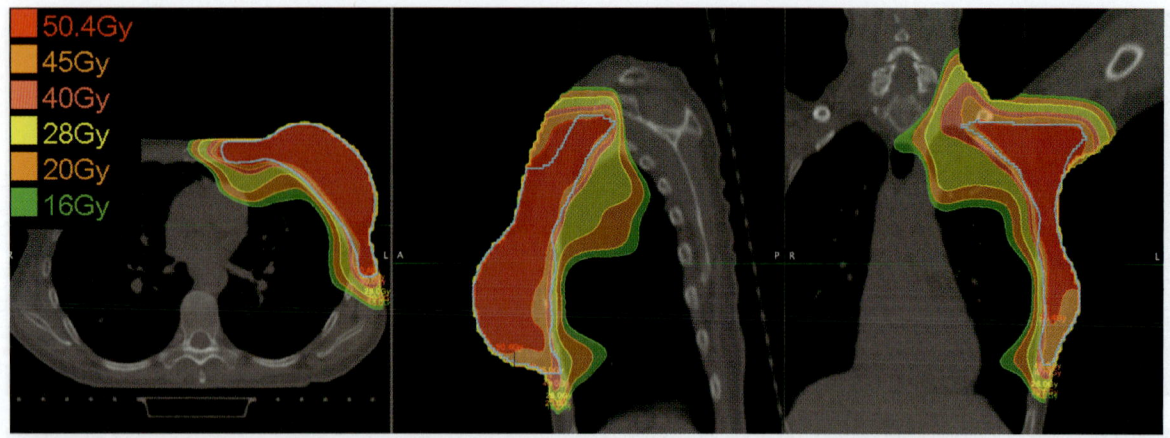

FIGURE 10.8. An example of a scanned beam breast treatment plan with nodal volumes. The treatment uses a single *en face* proton beam from the anterior oblique direction.

Thoracic and Abdominal

All thoracic lesions require extensive quality assurance (QA) to determine the optimal method of addressing the tissue heterogeneities in the region of the target volume. Range uncertainties in lung tissue can greatly increase the amount of healthy lung irradiated. Additionally, shrinkage of thoracic lesions must be assessed during the course of treatment to reduce the risk of errantly irradiating healthy tissues.

The motion of thoracic and abdominal lesions has long been studied in the context of proton therapy.[2,14–22] Methods to provide robust treatment plans include density overrides inside the ITV, use of 4D CT for optimization, gating, layer rescanning, volumetric rescanning, and tracking.[2,14–22] Although there is not yet a consensus regarding the optimal method for treating lesions with large amplitudes of motion (>1 to 2 cm), it is necessary for any institution to perform a complete analysis of their treatment protocols because the dosimetry is dependent on spot size, scanning speed, dose rate, time for energy (layer) changes, and fractionation scheme.

Generally, as the spot size becomes smaller and the fraction number decreases, the effects of the interplay between the breathing motion and the treatment delivery increase the risk of dosimetric errors. Combinations of the previously mentioned motion management techniques can be deployed to reduce the magnitude of the interplay effects. Briefly, rescanning can effectively increase the number of "fractions" by scanning the same target volume or layer multiple times similar to repeating the same field over multiple fractions.

Sarcomas

Sarcomas can be located in various regions of the body. Some locations, such as the sacral, pelvic, and vertebral locations, can be treated with protons to avoid dose delivery to radiosensitive organs. Typical beam arrangements for sarcomas located along the vertebral column use a single or a couple posterior or posterior oblique beams to provide maximal sparing of organs located anterior to the treated volume.

Pediatric

Pediatric treatments can cover many of the aforementioned treatment sites in the brain and other body sites. More specific and common in the pediatric population is CSI. Proton therapy is commonly used for CSI treatment delivery because of the zero dose exposure in the organs anterior to the vertebral column and whole brain. The long-term secondary cancer risk is much lower for protons, especially for soft tissues of the abdomen and thoracic region. Because the in-field doses are similar for both photon and proton pediatric treatments, the secondary risk is assumed to be similar, that is, secondary meningiomas following brain irradiation.

In the past, proton CSI treatments with scattered fields required three levels to reduce the risk of dosimetric hot and cold spots at the match lines. Each level required 4 to 5 treatment fields, each with custom apertures and range compensators. The total of 12 to 15 fields and custom hardware can be challenging for treatment planning and delivery workflows. Scanned beams greatly simplified the CSI treatment because of the ability to easily delivery gradient match lines instead of feathering with three levels (Fig. 10.9).[23,24]

FIGURE 10.9. An example of a scanned beam CSI treatment. The plan uses gradient match lines.

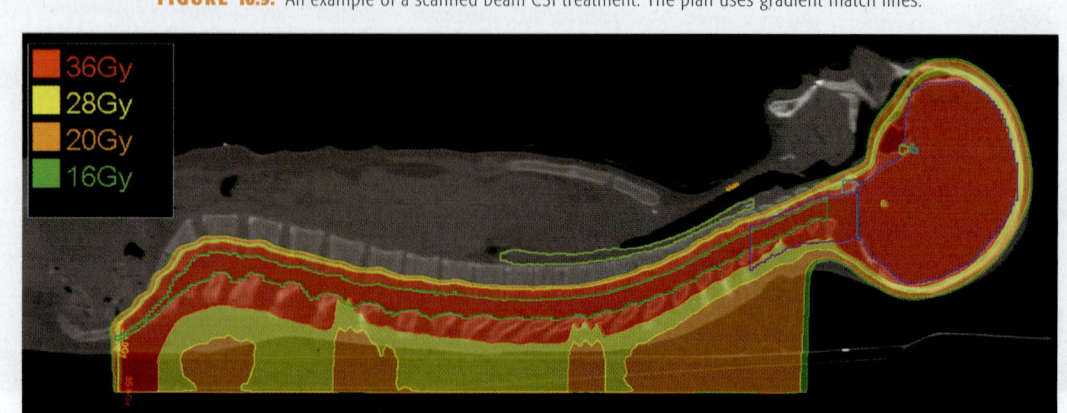

QUALITY ASSURANCE

There are several distinct challenges for quality assurance in a proton therapy clinic.[25] First, there are very few national or international protocols specific for proton therapy quality assurance. The ICRU Report 78[1] specifies the calibration procedure and recommends other QA measurements. The AAPM is currently developing several proton-specific protocols, but photon protocols are typically referenced until the proton-specific documents are published. Although the imaging and mechanical systems should operate with similar specifications, the dose delivery systems and dose measurements are lacking in photon protocols. To supplement the photon documents, previously published single-institution studies are often used.[2,26–39]

Second, there are three common treatment planning system (TPS) dose verification methods. Photon TPS dose verification is typically performed with a secondary dose calculation in an independent software application that is independently commissioned. Monte Carlo dose calculations might be the most similar independent check in proton therapy, and several institutions have deployed such software for dose checks.[37,40–44] Other institutions measure every field prior to delivery.[26,32] The third option is an analytic model based on empirical data.[34]

Third, the proton therapy user base is much more diverse than the photon radiotherapy clinic. There are currently multiple proton therapy vendors with multiple beam delivery and verification systems. Each system can have different beam parameters, hardware, and software, in addition to the aforementioned scattered and scanning delivery techniques. Such diversity of systems can make consensus protocols difficult to design and requires extensive expertise at each center or appropriate credentialing processes.

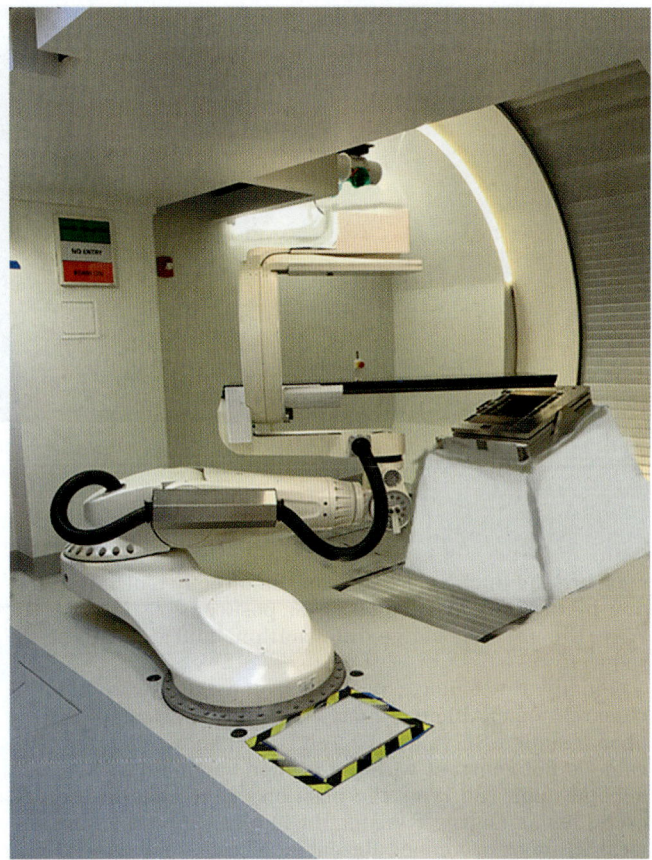

FIGURE 10.10. Example of a novel CBCT design such that the imaging ring is attached to the patient positioner.

DEVELOPMENTS

Image guidance in proton therapy is beginning to incorporate volumetric imaging solutions. The Paul Scherrer Institute in Switzerland was one of the first centers to install an in-room CT device. Other centers in Trento (Italy), Dresden (Germany), and the Mayo Clinic (Rochester, MN) have also installed in-room CT devices. The advantage is high-quality imaging and the option for 4D imaging. A diagnostic CT cannot, however, perform imaging at isocenter and always requires transferring the patient from an imaging position, up to several meters from isocenter, to the treatment position.

Other institutions have deployed cone beam computed tomography (CBCT) as a volumetric imaging solution. Recent advances in CBCT image quality improvement have allowed for better soft tissue visualization and HU accuracy for dose calculations.[45–53] Some proton vendors have deployed CBCT using the proton gantry as the mechanical rotation mount, and others have deployed C-arm or couch-mounted 0-ring systems (Fig. 10.10).

Simultaneously with the deployment of in-room volumetric imaging, there are multiple institutions attempting to integrate the 3D imaging into adaptive workflows.[45–48,50–52] Previously, adaptive proton therapy required separate imaging sessions with external imaging systems such as a CT or MR. In-room options can provide more streamlined workflows for adaptations based upon CT information. At this time, there are no in-room MR deployments at proton therapy centers, but there are multiple feasibility studies.[54,55]

More than photon therapy, proton therapy greatly benefits from adaptive workflows when the patient has anatomic variations or the target has motion because of breathing or bowel movements. Even in other target locations, online adaptive proton therapy might reduce the need for some margin expansions.

In addition to adaptive methods, robust planning methods can reduce the need for some margins and increase the certainty of the dosimetry calculated in the treatment planning system being delivered to the patient. The basic premise of robust optimization in the treatment planning system is to incorporate any random range uncertainties as variables in the cost function that controls the optimizer.[24,56–58] In other words, the optimizer not only considers the dose to the target or organs at risk (OAR) but also considers the risk of overdosing the OAR or underdosing the target in the presence of range uncertainties. The cost function penalizes plans that have higher risk of dose uncertainty and essentially reduces the presence of high-dose gradients in the optimized plan. More robust plans may have higher OAR doses, but the certainty of the delivery is much higher if the model accurately captures the uncertainties of the treatment workflow.

Although patient setup, anatomic, and dosimetric uncertainties have been addressed by the previous developments, range uncertainties remain in the delivery of proton therapy. There are multiple methods being explored to measure the *in vivo* range of the proton beam during or post treatment. A simultaneous measurement of the range can be accomplished using implanted devices for lesions located in close proximity to the rectal or vaginal cavity.[59–61] Other methods

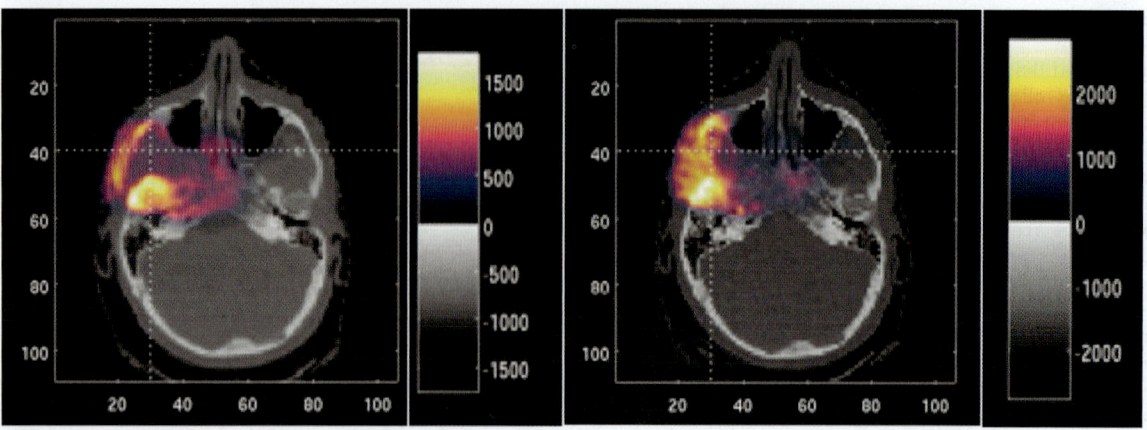

FIGURE 10.11. A sample of a PET signal following a proton beam irradiation as simulated in Monte Carlo **(left)** and measured **(right)**.

measure the nuclear products of the directly ionizing radiation by the prompt gammas[62–65] or positrons[66–72] (Fig. 10.11). With the *in vivo* range information, margins might be reduced.

Finally, the biologic dose of proton therapy remains a research topic. Although most clinical dose calculations rely upon a static RBE value of 1.1, it is well known that the RBE value is not constant within a treated volume. The RBE can depend upon cell type, the position of the cells in the cell cycle, linear energy transfer (LET) of the protons, and the local tissue environment. Recent studies continue to evaluate the RBE[73–79] and the local (micro) dosimetry through biologic Monte Carlo simulations.[80–82]

CONCLUSIONS

The physics of proton therapy are generally well understood, and the physical dose distributions greatly reduce the integral dose to healthy tissues as well as organs in close proximity to the targeted volume. There are many topics for further discovery including the integration of 3D imaging, adaptive workflows, range measurements, and biologic modeling, and more discoveries will increase the therapeutic ratio of proton therapy.

REFERENCES

1. *Prescribing, recording and reporting proton-beam therapy.* Oxford, UK: Oxford University Press, 2007.
2. American Association of Physicists in Medicine Summer School; Das IJ, Paganetti H. *Principles and practice of proton beam therapy: American Association of Physicists in Medicine 2015 Summer School proceedings* (Chapter 3: Proton Beam Interactions: Basic), Colorado College, Colorado Springs, Colorado, June 14–18, 2015.
3. Bortfeld T. An analytical approximation of the Bragg curve for therapeutic proton beams. *Med Phys* 1997;24:2024–2033.
4. Paganetti H, et al. Relative biological effectiveness (RBE) values for proton beam therapy. *Int J Radiat Oncol Biol Phys* 2002;53:407–421.
5. PTCOG. PTCOG Patient Statistics. (PTCOG). Available at: https://www.ptcog.ch/index.php/ptcog-patient-statistics
6. Kjellberg RN, Koehler AM, Preston WM, et al. Stereotaxic instrument for use with the Bragg peak of a proton beam. *Confin Neurol* 1962;22:183–189.
7. Kjellberg RN, Sweet WH, Preston WM, et al. The Bragg peak of a proton beam in intracranial therapy of tumors. *Trans Am Neurol Assoc* 1962;87:216–218.
8. Larsson B, et al. The high-energy proton beam as a neurosurgical tool. *Nature* 1958;182:1222–1223.
9. Lawrence JH. Proton irradiation of the pituitary. *Cancer* 1957;10:795–798.
10. Leksell L. The stereotaxic method and radiosurgery of the brain. *Acta Chir Scand* 1951;102:316–319.
11. Leksell L, et al. Lesions in the depth of the brain produced by a beam of high energy protons. *Acta Radiol* 1960;54:251–264.
12. MacDonald SM. Proton Therapy for Breast Cancer: Getting to the Heart of the Matter. *Int J Radiat Oncol Biol Phys* 2016;95:46–48.
13. MacDonald SM, et al. Proton therapy for breast cancer after mastectomy: early outcomes of a prospective clinical trial. *Int J Radiat Oncol Biol Phys* 2013;86:484–490.
14. Knopf A, Mori S. *Principles and practice of proton beam therapy,* (Chapter 25: Motion Management), 2015.
15. Bush DA, et al. Hypofractionated proton beam radiotherapy for stage I lung cancer. *Chest* 2004;126:1198–1203.
16. Chang JY, et al. Consensus Statement on Proton Therapy in Early-Stage and Locally Advanced Non-Small Cell Lung Cancer. *Int J Radiat Oncol Biol Phys* 2016;95:505–516.
17. Dowdell S, Grassberger C, Paganetti H. Four-dimensional Monte Carlo simulations demonstrating how the extent of intensity-modulation impacts motion effects in proton therapy lung treatments. *Med Phys* 2013;40:121713.
18. Dowdell S, Grassberger C, Sharp GC, et al. Interplay effects in proton scanning for lung: a 4D Monte Carlo study assessing the impact of tumor and beam delivery parameters. *Phys Med Biol* 2013;58:4137–4156.
19. Dueck J, et al. Robustness of the Voluntary Breath-Hold Approach for the Treatment of Peripheral Lung Tumors Using Hypofractionated Pencil Beam Scanning Proton Therapy. *Int J Radiat Oncol Biol Phys* 2016;95:534–541.
20. Gomez DR, et al. Phase 1 study of dose escalation in hypofractionated proton beam therapy for non-small cell lung cancer. *Int J Radiat Oncol Biol Phys* 2013;86:665–670.
21. Grassberger C, et al. Quantification of proton dose calculation accuracy in the lung. *Int J Radiat Oncol Biol Phys* 2014;89:424–430.
22. Grassberger C, et al. Motion interplay as a function of patient parameters and spot size in spot scanning proton therapy for lung cancer. *Int J Radiat Oncol Biol Phys* 2013;86:380–386.
23. Farace P, et al. Supine craniospinal irradiation in pediatric patients by proton pencil beam scanning. *Radiother Oncol* 2017;123:112–118.
24. Lin H, et al. Supine craniospinal irradiation using a proton pencil beam scanning technique without match line changes for field junctions. *Int J Radiat Oncol Biol Phys* 2014;90:71–78.
25. Dicker AP, Williams TR, Ford E. *Quality and safety in radiation oncology: implementing tools and best practices for patients, providers, and payers.* New York: Demos Medical Publishing, 2017.
26. Arjomandy B, Sahoo N, Ding X, et al. Use of a two-dimensional ionization chamber array for proton therapy beam quality assurance. *Med Phys* 2008;35:3889–3894.
27. Bednarz B, Daartz J, Paganetti H. Dosimetric accuracy of planning and delivering small proton therapy fields. *Phys Med Biol* 2010;55:7425–7438.
28. Clasie B, et al. Golden beam data for proton pencil-beam scanning. *Phys Med Biol* 2012;57:1147–1158.
29. Daartz J, Engelsman M, Paganetti H, et al. Field size dependence of the output factor in passively scattered proton therapy: influence of range, modulation, air gap, and machine settings. *Med Phys* 2009;36:3205–3210.
30. Engelsman M, Lu HM, Herrup D, et al. Commissioning a passive-scattering proton therapy nozzle for accurate SOBP delivery. *Med Phys* 2009;36:2172–2180.
31. Fontenot JD, et al. Determination of output factors for small proton therapy fields. *Med Phys* 2007;34:489–498.

32. Gillin MT, et al. Commissioning of the discrete spot scanning proton beam delivery system at the University of Texas M.D. Anderson Cancer Center, Proton Therapy Center, Houston. *Med Phys* 2010;37:154–163.

33. Koch N, Newhauser W. Virtual commissioning of a treatment planning system for proton therapy of ocular cancers. *Radiat Prot Dosimetry* 2005;115:159–163.

34. Kooy HM, Schaefer M, Rosenthal S, et al. Monitor unit calculations for range-modulated spread-out Bragg peak fields. *Phys Med Biol* 2003;48:2797–2808.

35. Lorin S, et al. Reference dosimetry in a scanned pulsed proton beam using ionisation chambers and a Faraday cup. *Phys Med Biol* 2008;53:3519–3529.

36. Meier G, Besson R, Nanz A, et al. Independent dose calculations for commissioning, quality assurance and dose reconstruction of PBS proton therapy. *Phys Med Biol* 2015;60:2819–2836.

37. Pedroni E, et al. Experimental characterization and physical modelling of the dose distribution of scanned proton pencil beams. *Phys Med Biol* 2005;50:541–561.

38. Slopsema RL, et al. Development of a golden beam data set for the commissioning of a proton double-scattering system in a pencil-beam dose calculation algorithm. *Med Phys* 2014;41:091710.

39. Zhu XR, et al. Commissioning dose computation models for spot scanning proton beams in water for a commercially available treatment planning system. *Med Phys* 2013;40:041723.

40. Koch N, et al. Monte Carlo calculations and measurements of absorbed dose per monitor unit for the treatment of uveal melanoma with proton therapy. *Phys Med Biol* 2008;53:1581–1594.

41. Paganetti H, Jiang H, Lee SY, et al. Accurate Monte Carlo simulations for nozzle design, commissioning and quality assurance for a proton radiation therapy facility. *Med Phys* 2004;31:2107–2118.

42. Schuemann J, Dowdell S, Grassberger C, et al. Site-specific range uncertainties caused by dose calculation algorithms for proton therapy. *Phys Med Biol* 2014;59:4007–4031.

43. Paganetti H. Monte Carlo simulations will change the way we treat patients with proton beams today. *Br J Radiol* 2014;87:20140293.

44. Testa M, et al. Experimental validation of the TOPAS Monte Carlo system for passive scattering proton therapy. *Med Phys* 2013;40:121719.

45. Kim J, Park YK, Sharp G, et al. Water equivalent path length calculations using scatter-corrected head and neck CBCT images to evaluate patients for adaptive proton therapy. *Phys Med Biol* 2017;62:59–72.

46. Kurz C, et al. Comparing cone-beam CT intensity correction methods for dose recalculation in adaptive intensity-modulated photon and proton therapy for head and neck cancer. *Acta Oncol* 2015;54:1651–1657.

47. Kurz C, et al. Investigating deformable image registration and scatter correction for CBCT-based dose calculation in adaptive IMPT. *Med Phys* 2016;43:5635.

48. Kurz C, et al. Feasibility of automated proton therapy plan adaptation for head and neck tumors using cone beam CT images. *Radiat Oncol* 2016;11:64.

49. Landry G, et al. Phantom based evaluation of CT to CBCT image registration for proton therapy dose recalculation. *Phys Med Biol* 2015;60:595–613.

50. Landry G, et al. Investigating CT to CBCT image registration for head and neck proton therapy as a tool for daily dose recalculation. *Med Phys* 2015;42:1354–1366.

51. Park YK, Sharp GC, Phillips J, et al. Proton dose calculation on scatter-corrected CBCT image: feasibility study for adaptive proton therapy. *Med Phys* 2015;42:4449–4459.

52. Veiga C, et al. First Clinical Investigation of Cone Beam Computed Tomography and Deformable Registration for Adaptive Proton Therapy for Lung Cancer. *Int J Radiat Oncol Biol Phys* 2016;95:549–559.

53. Wang P, et al. Quantitative assessment of anatomical change using a virtual proton depth radiograph for adaptive head and neck proton therapy. *J Appl Clin Med Phys* 2016;17:427–440.

54. Hartman J, et al. Dosimetric feasibility of intensity modulated proton therapy in a transverse magnetic field of 1.5 T. *Phys Med Biol* 2015;60:5955–5969.

55. Raaymakers BW, Raaijmakers AJ, Lagendijk JJ. Feasibility of MRI guided proton therapy: magnetic field dose effects. *Phys Med Biol* 2008;53:5615–5622.

56. Depauw N, et al. A novel approach to postmastectomy radiation therapy using scanned proton beams. *Int J Radiat Oncol Biol Phys* 2015;91:427–434.

57. Unkelbach J, Bortfeld T, Martin BC, et al. Reducing the sensitivity of IMPT treatment plans to setup errors and range uncertainties via probabilistic treatment planning. *Med Phys* 2009;36:149–163.

58. Unkelbach J, Chan TC, Bortfeld T. Accounting for range uncertainties in the optimization of intensity modulated proton therapy. *Phys Med Biol* 2007;52:2755–2773.

59. Gottschalk B, et al. Water equivalent path length measurement in proton radiotherapy using time resolved diode dosimetry. *Med Phys* 2011;38:2282–2288.

60. Hoesl M, et al. Clinical commissioning of an in vivo range verification system for prostate cancer treatment with anterior and anterior oblique proton beams. *Phys Med Biol* 2016;61:3049–3062.

61. Testa M, et al. Proton radiography and proton computed tomography based on time-resolved dose measurements. *Phys Med Biol* 2013;58:8215–8233.

62. Verburg JM, Riley K, Bortfeld T, et al. Energy- and time-resolved detection of prompt gamma-rays for proton range verification. *Phys Med Biol* 2013;58:L37–L49.

63. Verburg JM, Seco J. Proton range verification through prompt gamma-ray spectroscopy. *Phys Med Biol* 2014;59:7089–7106.

64. Verburg JM, Shih HA, Seco J. Simulation of prompt gamma-ray emission during proton radiotherapy. *Phys Med Biol* 2012;57:5459–5472.

65. Verburg JM, Testa M, Seco J. Range verification of passively scattered proton beams using prompt gamma-ray detection. *Phys Med Biol* 2015;60:1019–1029.

66. Knopf AC, et al. Accuracy of proton beam range verification using post-treatment positron emission tomography/computed tomography as function of treatment site. *Int J Radiat Oncol Biol Phys* 2011;79:297–304.

67. Min CH, et al. A Recommendation on How to Analyze In-Room PET for In Vivo Proton Range Verification Using a Distal PET Surface Method. *Technol Cancer Res Treat* 2015;14:320–325.

68. Min CH, et al. Clinical application of in-room positron emission tomography for in vivo treatment monitoring in proton radiation therapy. *Int J Radiat Oncol Biol Phys* 2013;86:183–189.

69. Parodi K, Bortfeld T, Haberer T. Comparison between in-beam and offline positron emission tomography imaging of proton and carbon ion therapeutic irradiation at synchrotron- and cyclotron-based facilities. *Int J Radiat Oncol Biol Phys* 2008;71:945–956.

70. Parodi K, et al. Patient study of in vivo verification of beam delivery and range, using positron emission tomography and computed tomography imaging after proton therapy. *Int J Radiat Oncol Biol Phys* 2007;68:920–934.

71. Zhu X, El Fakhri G. Proton therapy verification with PET imaging. *Theranostics* 2013;3:731–740.

72. Zhu X, et al. Monitoring proton radiation therapy with in-room PET imaging. *Phys Med Biol* 2011;56:4041–4057.

73. Carabe A, Espana S, Grassberger C, et al. Clinical consequences of relative biological effectiveness variations in proton radiotherapy of the prostate, brain and liver. *Phys Med Biol* 2013;58:2103–2117.

74. Giantsoudi D, et al. Linear energy transfer-guided optimization in intensity modulated proton therapy: feasibility study and clinical potential. *Int J Radiat Oncol Biol Phys* 2013;87:216–222.

75. Giantsoudi D, et al. Incidence of CNS Injury for a Cohort of 111 Patients Treated With Proton Therapy for Medulloblastoma: LET and RBE Associations for Areas of Injury. *Int J Radiat Oncol Biol Phys* 2016;95:287–296.

76. Paganetti H. Relative biological effectiveness (RBE) values for proton beam therapy. Variations as a function of biological endpoint, dose, and linear energy transfer. *Phys Med Biol* 2014;59:R419–R472.

77. Paganetti H. Significance and implementation of RBE variations in proton beam therapy. *Technol Cancer Res Treat* 2003;2:413–426.

78. Wouters BG, et al. Radiobiological intercomparison of the 160 MeV and 230 MeV proton therapy beams at the Harvard Cyclotron Laboratory and at Massachusetts General Hospital. *Radiat Res* 2015;183:174–187.

79. Zeng C, et al. Maximizing the biological effect of proton dose delivered with scanned beams via inhomogeneous daily dose distributions. *Med Phys* 2013;40:051708.

80. McNamara A, et al. Validation of the radiobiology toolkit TOPAS-nBio in simple DNA geometries. *Phys Med* 2017;33:207–215.

81. Polster L, et al. Extension of TOPAS for the simulation of proton radiation effects considering molecular and cellular endpoints. *Phys Med Biol* 2015;60:5053–5070.

82. Underwood TS, et al. Comparing stochastic proton interactions simulated using TOPAS-nBio to experimental data from fluorescent nuclear track detectors. *Phys Med Biol* 2017;62:3237–3249.

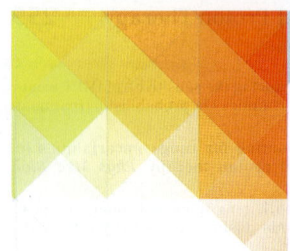

CHAPTER 11

Intensity-Modulated Radiation Treatment Techniques and Clinical Applications

Tony J. C. Wang, Cheng-Shie Wuu, and K. S. Clifford Chao

INTRODUCTION

The previous edition of this chapter included literature reports through 2013. For the past 10 years, intensity-modulated radiation therapy (IMRT) has become the *de facto* standard practice for many tumors. IMRT's coming of age is described in thorough terms in the 2010 International Commission on Radiation Units (ICRU) report (hereafter ICRU 83), which spans 106 pages with over 350 references.[1] Readers new to the field will find this report an excellent synthetic introduction to IMRT and other techniques; experienced physicians should also note that it contains new reporting guidelines for clinical treatments.

The use of ionizing radiation for treatment of cancer has more than a century of history; for a wonderfully concise review, see Bernier et al.[2] An enduring clinical problem has been to achieve high doses of irradiation at the tumor site without causing extremely toxic or even fatal consequences in normal tissues in the path of the treatment beam. Developments in technology allowed true three-dimensional (3D) tailoring of radiation fluence with equipment and a planning time scale feasible for clinical application. Since its introduction into clinical use,[3–5] IMRT has generated widespread utilization. IMRT optimally assigns nonuniform intensities (i.e., weights) to tiny subdivisions of beams, which have been called rays or "beamlets." The ability to optimally manipulate the intensities of individual rays within each beam permits greatly increased control over the radiation fluence, enabling custom design of optimum dose distributions. These improved dose distributions potentially may lead to improved tumor control and reduced normal tissue toxicity. For example, tumors of the head and neck often require concave-shaped treatment volumes to spare closely adjacent sensitive critical structures (e.g., brainstem, spinal cord). Such fluence distributions are easily done with IMRT but may be difficult or impossible by other techniques, including three-dimensional conformal radiation therapy (3DCRT). This is illustrated in Figure 11.1, which is taken from ICRU 83.

IMRT requires designing the intensities of tens of thousands of rays (beamlets) that make up an intensity-modulated treatment plan. This task requires the use of specialized computer-aided optimization methods. Optimal beamlet intensities are determined using a systematic iterative process, which a computer sequentially generates intensity-modulated plans one by one, evaluates each of them according to user-selected criteria ("desired objectives"), and makes changes in the ray intensities based on the desired objectives. The quality of an intensity-modulated treatment plan produced in this manner depends on a variety of factors. These include the parameters used by the optimization process to evaluate and compare competing treatment plans; the mathematics and algorithms of optimization; the number, orientation, and energy of radiation beams; margins assigned to the planning target volume (PTV) and to normal structures; dose calculation algorithms; and so on.

Both ICRU 83 report and the ASTRO report[6] have some important conceptual changes in plan evaluation and dose reporting. The previous ICRU reports for photon therapy (No. 50 in 1993 and its supplement, No. 62 in 1999) defined a reference point within the treatment volume, one that was easily located with anatomic landmarks and where dosage could be accurately measured. The prescription dose was something of an ideal to be sought. With IMRT, treatment *volumes* are more relevant, and doses are given and bounds set within those volumes. The prescription dose itself is taken to be the final result of treatment planning by the physicists and radiation oncologists. With literally thousands of degrees of freedom available to the planner, the dosage to a single point is not adequate to describe or evaluate a plan.

ICRU 83 report and the ASTRO report cite the increase in the clinical impact and use of IMRT in the recent past: "In a survey performed in 2003 in the USA, among 168 radiation oncologists randomly selected, one-third was using IMRT. In 2005, a similar survey showed that more than two-thirds of radiation oncologists were using some form of IMRT, mainly for increased normal-tissue sparing or target-dose escalation."[1,7,8] Another noteworthy metric is the number of research reports in the peer-reviewed literature concerning IMRT. A scan of the Web of Science database showed full papers with IMRT in the title as numbering <50 per year through 2001. It reached 100 in 2005, and it plateaued at about 140 for the years 2009 to 2011 and continues to increase incrementally.

IMRT RATIONALE

IMRT is a form of 3DCRT in which a *computer-aided iterative optimization process is used to determine customized nonuniform fluence distributions to attain certain specified dosimetric and clinical objectives*. IMRT is intimately tied to 3D imaging. As ICRU 83 states: "Three-dimensional CRT, in general, and IMRT, in particular, increase the need for accurate anatomic delineation. This requires an adequate specification of the tumor location and a thorough knowledge of the processes of likely infiltration and spread."[1]

IMRT has many advantages. It can be used to produce dose distributions that are far more conformal than those possible with standard 3DCRT. Dose distributions within the PTV can be more homogeneous and a sharper falloff dose at the PTV boundary can be achieved. With respect to dose homogeneity, the IMRT plan always should produce more homogeneous dose distribution (dose conformality) than a plan made with uniform beams. A sharper falloff dose at the PTV boundary, in turn, means that the volume of normal tissues exposed to high doses may be reduced significantly. These factors may allow escalation of tumor dose, reduction of normal tissue dose, or both, leading to improved outcomes, including reducing morbidity. IMRT has the potential to be more efficient with treatment planning and delivery than standard 3DCRT. The treatment design process is relatively insensitive to the choice of planning parameters, such as beam direction.[9–11] There are no secondary field-shaping devices other than the computer-controlled multileaf collimator (MLC). Furthermore, large fields and boosts can be integrated into a single treatment plan, and electrons can be dispensed with, permitting the use of the same integrated boost plan for the entire course of treatment.[12,13] An integrated boost treatment may offer an additional radiobiologic advantage[14] in terms of lower dose per fraction to normal tissues while delivering higher dose per

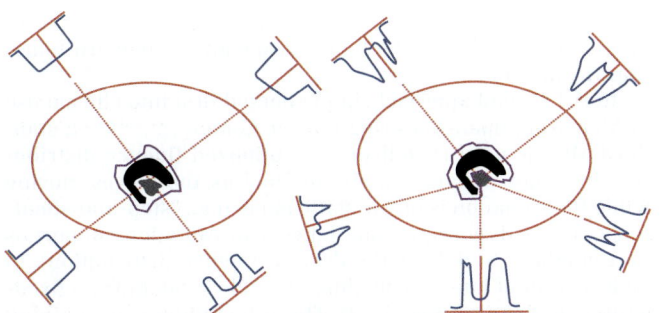

FIGURE 11.1. Comparison of conformal radiation therapy (CRT) (*left*) and intensity-modulated radiation therapy (IMRT) (*right*). The ability for CRT to alter isodose lines was limited to shaping of field boundaries with multileaf collimators (MLCs) or blocks, the use of wedges or compensators for missing tissues, and the use of central blocks for shielding critical structures. The IMRT beams can have highly nonuniform beam intensities (fluences) and are capable of producing a more concave-shaped absorbed dose distribution. With neither conformal therapy nor IMRT can the planning organ at risk volume (PRV) always be completely avoided, but with IMRT the concave isodose curve that includes the planning target volume (PTV) better avoids the PRV. The black region indicates the PTV, the gray region indicates a PRV, and the line surrounding the PTV is a typical isodose contour. (From International Commission of Radiation Units and Measurements. ICRU Report 83: prescribing, recording, and reporting photon-beam intensity-modulated radiation therapy [IMRT]. *J ICRU* 2010;10[1]:1–106. Reproduced by permission of International Commission on Radiation Units and Measurements.)

fraction to the target volume. Higher dose per fraction also reduces the number of fractions and hence lowers the cost and burden to the patient for a treatment course. IMRT also offers the potential of adaptive therapy—revision of the treatment plan according to imaging of tumor reduction and organ movement during the course of radiation therapy. Mechalakos et al. presented a case study where weekly cone beam computed tomography (CBCT) was used to track treatment of a recurrent neck mass from a nasopharyngeal cancer.[15]

IMRT Limitations and Risks

We should recognize that IMRT has limitations. There are many dose distributions (or dose–volume combinations) that are simply not physically or technically achievable. Furthermore, our knowledge about what is clinically optimal and achievable and how best to define clinical and dosimetric objectives of IMRT is often limited. Moreover, the best solution may elude us because of the limitations of the mathematical formalism used or because of the practical limits of computer speed and the time required for finding it.

Uncertainties of various types (e.g., those related to daily or interfraction patient positioning; displacement and distortions of internal anatomy; intrafraction motion; and changes in physical and radiobiologic characteristics of tumors and normal tissues during the course of treatment) may limit the applicability and efficacy of IMRT. Dosimetry characteristics of a delivery device, such as radiation scattering and transmission through the MLC leaves, introduce limitations in the accuracy and deliverability of IMRT fluence distributions. In addition, the limited spatial and temporal coverage and overall accuracy of current IMRT dosimetric verification systems diminish the confidence in the delivered dose. Furthermore, dose calculation models are limited in their accuracy, especially for the small, complex fields. It is quite conceivable that inaccuracies in dose calculations may yield a solution different from the one derived if dose calculations were accurate. However, an important factor that may limit IMRT is the inadequacy of imaging technology to define the true extent of the tumor, its extensions, and radiobiologic characteristics as well as geometric, dose–response, and functional characteristics of normal tissues.

We should be aware of the potential risks of IMRT. The effect of large fraction doses used in integral boost IMRT on

tissues embedded within the gross tumor volume (GTV) is uncertain and may present an increased risk of injury.[16] There also may be an increased risk that improper use of spatial margins, coupled with the high degree of conformality with IMRT, may lead to geographic misses of the disease and recurrences, especially for disease sites where positioning and motion uncertainties play a large role or where there are significant changes in anatomy and radiobiology during the course of radiotherapy. This uncertainty has been decreased with newer image guidance technology. Similarly, high doses in close proximity to normal critical structures may pose a greater risk of normal tissue injury. In addition, although IMRT can spare specific tissues compared to conventional radiation therapy, the use of many more beams and irradiation angles resulting in a higher integral dose exposure.

IMRT: An Unconventional Paradigm

The application, process, and dose distributions of IMRT are different from those of conventional two-dimensional (2D) CRT or 3DCRT. This means the conventional methods of specification and fractionation of treatments, evaluation of treatment plans, and reporting of results are limited and new methods are required.

The traditional 3DCRT process involves "forward planning," in which beam parameters (directions, apertures and their margins, beam weights, beam modifiers) are specified and dose distributions are computed. The treatment plan is evaluated by a human being, and if necessary, beam parameters are modified to achieve an acceptable dose distribution. In IMRT, an inverse process ("inverse planning") is used in which the desired dosimetric and clinical objectives are stated mathematically (in the form of an "objective function").[10,17–19] The term *inverse planning* should not be confused with the mathematical operation of matrix inversion. In the present context, the word *inverse* is used to distinguish it from forward planning for conventional 3DCRT. As ICRU 83 concisely notes:

> The word "inverse" is used in reference to the established body of mathematical inverse problem-solving techniques, which start at the final or desired result and works backwards to establish the best way to achieve it. So-called inverse treatment planning starts by describing a goal, i.e., a series of descriptors characterizing the desired absorbed dose distribution within the tumor, with additional descriptors designed to spare normal tissues.

The inverse planning process works iteratively to determine beam shapes and fluence patterns to achieve an optimal or acceptable absorbed dose distribution. The IMRT optimization software iteratively adjusts beam parameters with the aim of obtaining the best possible approximation of the desired dose distribution. In each optimization iteration, the optimization software computes the value of the objective function (i.e., the IMRT plan score) to judge the overall quality of each of a large number of plans to choose the optimum one. However, it must be kept in mind that limitations of planning time may preclude full exploration of all the degrees of freedom (there can be many thousands), so whether the optimization is done by a variant of gradient or stochastic methods, the computed solution may not be the true global one. Importantly, the final review by the radiation oncologist of any plan is required.

IMRT is the most conformal and efficient technique when all target volumes (gross disease, subclinical extensions, and electively treated nodes) are treated simultaneously using different fraction sizes. Such a treatment strategy has been called the simultaneous integrated boost (SIB).[16,20] This is in contrast to conventional radiation therapy in which the same fraction size (typically 1.8 or 2 Gy) is used for all target volumes with successive reductions in field sizes to protect critical normal structures and to limit the dose to electively treated and subclinical disease regions.

Alternative IMRT Approaches

During the past 20 years, a variety of techniques have been explored for designing and delivering optimized IMRT.[3–5,9,16,18,21–43] Many of these are implemented in commercial IMRT systems. The most significant differences among the various approaches are in terms of the mechanisms they use for the delivery of nonuniform fluences. Although the merits of each often are speculated, the superiority of any of the approaches is difficult to assess because there have been no systematic comparisons of clinical treatment plans.

Of the various approaches proposed, two dominant but significantly different techniques have emerged. Mackie et al.[30] proposed an approach called *tomotherapy* in which intensity-modulated photon therapy is delivered using a rotating slit beam. A temporally modulated slit MLC is used to rapidly move leaves in or out of the slit. Like a computed tomography (CT) unit, the radiation source and the collimator continuously revolve around the patient. The patient is translated either stepwise between successive rotations (serial tomotherapy) or continuously during rotation (helical tomotherapy). For helical tomotherapy, the system looks like a conventional CT scanner and includes a megavoltage portal detector to provide for the tomographic reconstruction of the delivered dose distribution.

A commercial slit collimator (called *MIMiC*) of the type proposed by Mackie et al.[30] was designed and built by the NOMOS Corporation (North American Scientific, Chatsworth, CA), and it was incorporated into the company's serial tomotherapy system, known as Peacock, for planning and rotational delivery of intensity-modulated treatments.[3,25] Figure 11.2 shows an original "binary" collimator built by NOMOS and as mounted on a LINAC. The figure also shows a modern tomotherapy machine.

In the second approach, implemented first into clinical use at Memorial Sloan-Kettering Cancer Center,[4,5,18,32,33,40,44] a standard MLC is used to deliver the optimized fluence distribution in either dynamic mode (defined as the leaves moving while the radiation is on) or static mode (i.e., "step-and-shoot" mode, defined as sequential delivery of radiation subportals that combine to deliver the desired fluence distribution), to deliver a set of intensity-modulated fields incident from fixed-gantry angles (see Fig. 11.3). These techniques are gaining wide acceptance rapidly. Every major commercial treatment planning system manufacturer has implemented one or both of these.

A third approach, called *intensity-modulated arc therapy* or IMAT, developed by Yu,[43] uses a combination of dynamic multileaf collimation and arc therapy. The method is similar to the step and shoot in that each field is subdivided into subfields of uniform intensity, which are superimposed to produce the desired intensity modulation. However, the MLC moves dynamically to shape each subfield while the gantry is rotating and the beam is on all the time. Multiple superimposing arcs are delivered with the leaves moving to new positions at a regular angular interval, for example, 5 degrees. Each arc is programmed to deliver one subfield at each gantry angle. A new arc is started to deliver the next subfield and so on until all the arcs and their associated subfields have been all delivered. A typical treatment takes three to five arcs, and

FIGURE 11.2. Commercial serial tomotherapy delivery hardware mounted on a conventional linear accelerator. **A:** View looking into the collimator toward the radiation source. A leaf pattern is shown that highlights the system's capability for delivering complex fluence patterns. **B:** The multileaf collimator mounted to a conventional linear accelerator. **C:** Modern tomotherapy TomoHD machine. (**C**, Courtesy of Accuray Incorporated, Sunnyvale, CA)

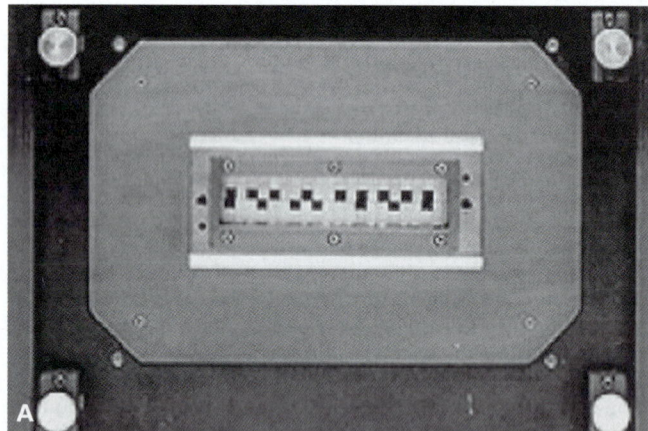

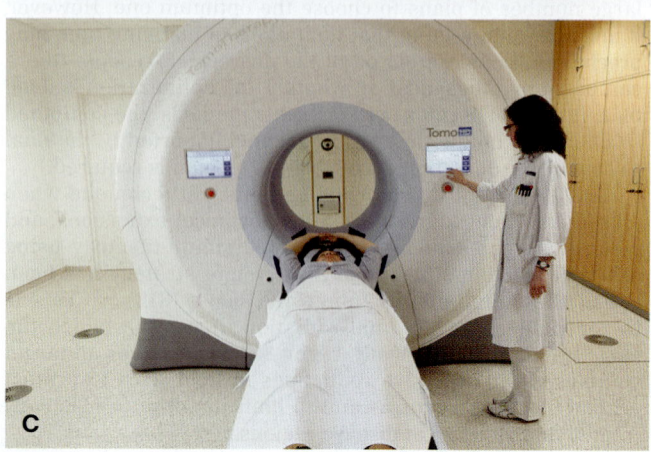

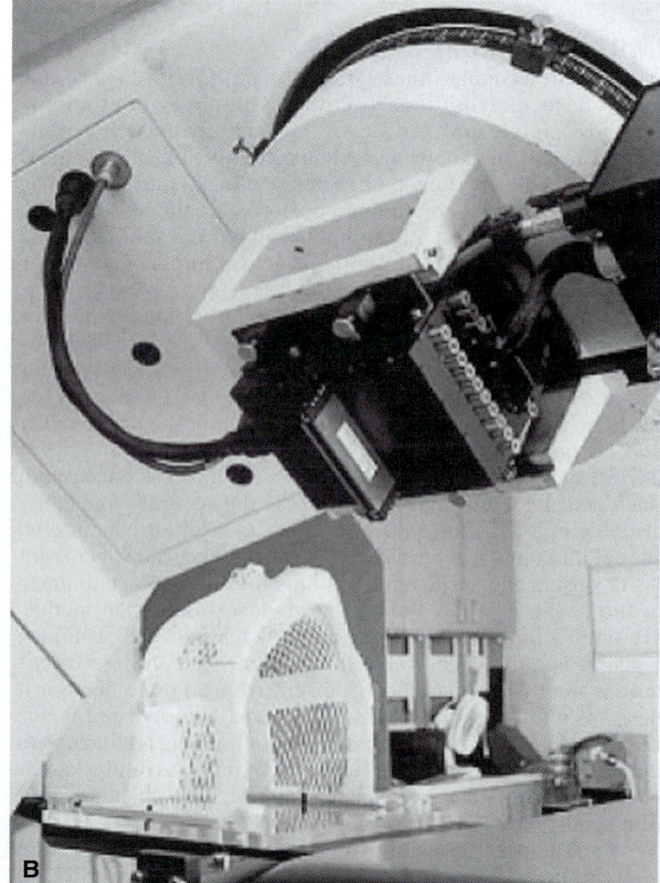

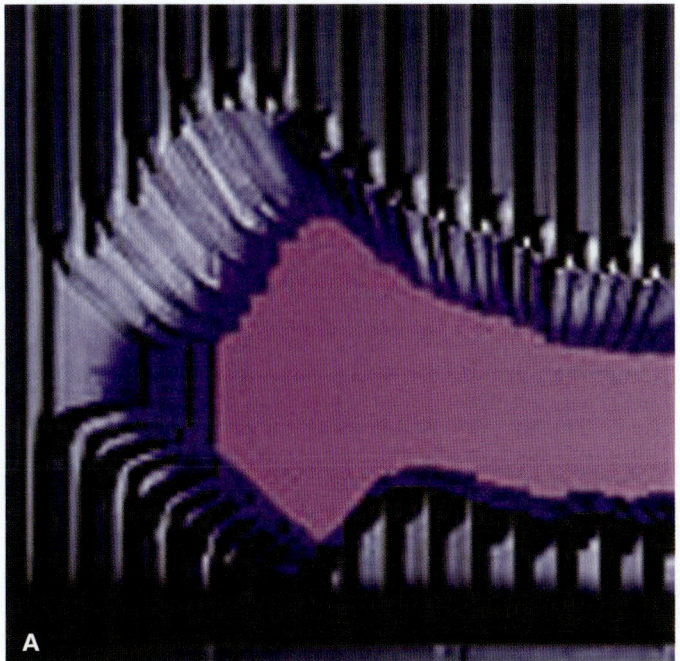

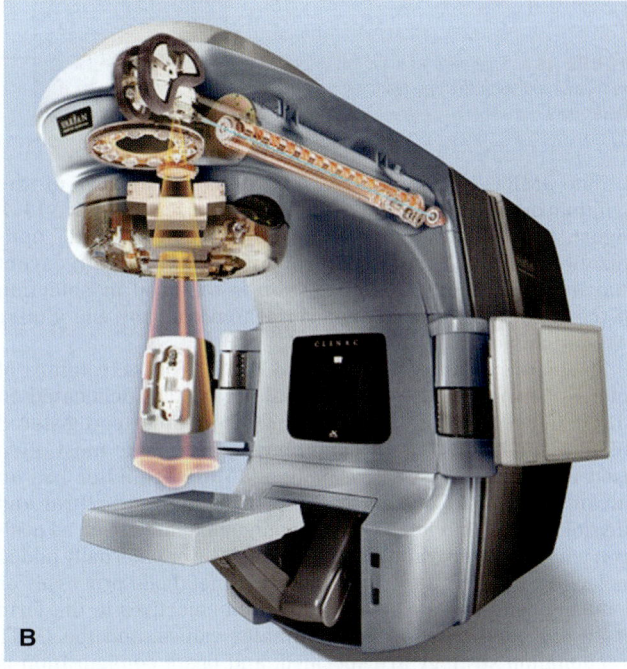

FIGURE 11.3. A: A typical multileaf collimator used for delivery of intensity-modulated radiation therapy looking toward the radiation source. In the dynamic mode, the leaves move back and forth or sweep across the field continuously to form the sequence of required field shapes while the beam is on. In the static or step-and-shoot mode, the beam is turned off when the leaves move to form the required field shapes. **B:** Cutaway diagram of LINAC head, Varian Clinac. (Courtesy of Varian, Palo Alto, CA.)

the operational complexity is comparable to conventional arc therapy.[45] It has the theoretical advantage of increased flexibility in delivering highly conformal plans by using a large number of beam directions. The IMAT delivery technique was never widely utilized partly because of the necessity of treating several arcs to deliver a single IMAT treatment field. In the late 2000s, both Varian and Elekta introduced variable dose rate rotational delivery options into their linear accelerators. The delivery of a rotational cone beam with variable shape and intensity is commonly called volumetric-modulated arc therapy (VMAT). In a VMAT treatment, in order to create a satisfactory dose plan with a single arc, it is necessary to optimize the field shapes and beam intensities from a large number of gantry angles. However, the field shapes are restricted by the constraints placed on MLC leave motions. The MLC leaves must be able to move to their new positions within the time required for the gantry to rotate between consecutive gantry positions. Unfortunately, the larger the sampled gantry angles, the more difficult it is for the TPS to optimize the MLC leave motion constraints. A novel plan optimization for a VMAT delivery was first proposed by Otto.[46] Other optimization algorithms have since been developed.[47,48] The biggest advantage of a VMAT delivery is in its delivery efficiency. Several investigators have reported significant reductions in treatment times and possible MUs over conventional IMRT.[49–51] One major benefit of VMAT compared with tomotherapy is the possibility of delivering this treatment on conventional linear accelerators, which are configured to have this capability. Currently, there are several VMAT systems available under various names (RapidArc, Varian; SmartArc, Phillips; and Elekta VMAT, Elekta). Arc therapy is discussed in a recent review of various intensity-modulated techniques.[52]

IMRT techniques have led to improved conformal dose delivery methods. However, IMRT tends to have higher monitor units (MU) compared to 3DCRT technique. This contributes to higher leakage from the gantry head and consequently increased dose to normal tissues and whole body in general.[53]

This undesirable dose is likely to result in higher second tumor induction rate.[54] It is, therefore, desirable to reduce the unnecessary scatter from the gantry head and shorten the treatment time for IMRT delivery. The removal of the flattening filter has been a logical choice to reduce the scatter.[55] The development of IMRT eliminates the need for a flattening filter in modern linear accelerator (LINAC) systems. In recent years, the application of the flattening filter-free (FFF) photon beam has been studied extensively.[56–61] Forward peaked dose profile is the major characteristic of the FFF beam.[62–65] Compared with the flattened beam, the FFF beam also has increased dose rate,[57,58] reduced dose to organ at risk (OAR),[66,67] reduced neutron contamination for high-energy beams (>15 MV),[68] and reduced uncertainty in dose calculation.[57] Thus, clinical application of the FFF beam would lead to reduced treatment time and secondary cancer risk induced by radiation.[58,59]

In addition to these approaches, the University of Michigan has used the so-called multisegment approach in which each of a number of beams is divided into multiple segments.[69] One segment for each beam frames the entire target, whereas the others spare one or more normal structures. Each segment is uniform in intensity. The weights of segments of all beams are optimized to produce the desired treatment plan. The treatments are delivered as a sequence of multiple uniform field segments. A similar approach previously was proposed by Mohan et al.[70] In almost all of these significantly different treatment delivery approaches, the underlying principles of optimization are similar, although the specifics may be quite different.

THE IMRT PROCESS OVERVIEW

As mentioned previously, there are significant differences in 3DCRT and IMRT concepts and processes. Yet, there are also many similarities. In particular, IMRT relies on many of the same imaging, dose calculations, plan evaluation, quality assurance (QA), and delivery tools as 3DCRT.

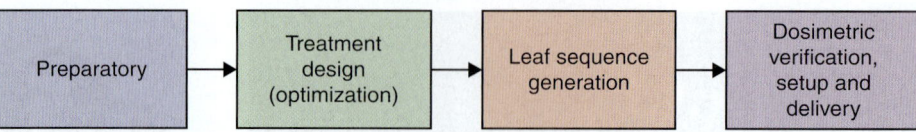

FIGURE 11.4. Overview of a typical intensity-modulated radiation therapy planning and delivery process.

The IMRT planning, QA, and delivery phases of the dynamic or static MLC process are summarized in Figure 11.4. Figure 11.5 shows the steps in each phase of the IMRT optimization process. The tomotherapy process is similar, except that the fixed beam angle selection is replaced by selection of the slice thickness and, for serial tomotherapy, the gantry rotation angles.

In the preparatory phase of the IMRT process, volumes of interest (such as tumors and normal organs) are delineated on 3D CT images,[71] often with assistance from other coregistered imaging modalities. The second imaging technique most often used is magnetic resonance imaging (MRI); the latter has an advantage over CT in that it can provide both structural and physiologic information.[72] Other imaging modalities such as positron emission tomography (PET) use intrinsic or externally added molecular markers to visualize specific metabolic processes or cellular phenotypes.[73-77] Also, the desired objectives in the form of an objective function, its parameter values, and the IMRT fractionation strategy are specified, and beam configuration is defined. Typically, the objective function[78] assigns a weighted "cost" to the square of the difference between the desired 3D fluence distribution and that calculated at a given iteration. The software attempts to minimize the costs—maximizing dosage to the tumor volume and minimizing exposure of normal tissues.

In the treatment plan optimization phase, an iterative process is used to adjust and set the intensities of rays of each beam (or portion of the arc) so that the resulting intensity distributions yield the best approximation of the desired objectives. The IMRT plan then is evaluated to ensure that the trade-offs

FIGURE 11.5. Comparison between traditional (*left*) and intensity-modulated radiation therapy (IMRT) (*right*) optimization processes. (From International Commission of Radiation Units and Measurements. ICRU Report 83: prescribing, recording, and reporting photon-beam intensity-modulated radiation therapy [IMRT]. *J ICRU* 2010;10[1]:1–106. Reproduced by permission of International Commission on Radiation Units and Measurements.)

made by the optimization system are acceptable. If further improvement is deemed necessary and possible, the objective function parameters are modified, and the optimization process is repeated until a satisfactory treatment plan is achieved.

In the leaf sequence generation phase, the intensity distributions are converted into sequences of leaf positions. It is conceivable that certain dose distributions cannot be delivered as a result of the leakage characteristics of the delivery devices. Therefore, in most treatment planning systems, the leaf sequences are used in a reverse process to calculate the dose distributions they are expected to deliver. These dose distributions, called the *deliverable dose distributions*, are evaluated for clinical adequacy. If necessary, objective function parameters are further adjusted to produce an intensity distribution that leads to a deliverable dose distribution that meets the desired objectives. This is the practice in most systems. However, in some systems, the leaf sequence generation process is incorporated into the IMRT plan optimization loop so that the optimized and deliverable dose distributions are identical. More details on this are given later in this chapter.

The leaf sequences then are transmitted to the treatment machine and used to verify that the dose distribution that will be delivered to the patient is correct and accurate. The patient then is set up in the usual fashion and treated. In general, the entire treatment is delivered remotely without the need to re-enter the treatment room in between fields.

PREPARATORY AND IMRT PLANNING PHASES

This section discusses each of the steps of the preparatory and IMRT plan design phases. For reasons of clarity, the order in which these steps are discussed is not the same as the order in which they occur as shown in Figure 11.5. Figure 11.6 sketches the QA process.

Imaging and Volumes of Interest

ICRU 83 presents updated definitions for the assorted volumes that will form the skeleton of the treatment plan.[1] Conceptually, the volumes contain three types of tissue: (a) malignant/benign lesion, (b) otherwise normal tissue near the tumor that is already or likely to be infiltrated by microscopic disease, and (c) more distant normal tissue and organs. The quoted definitions that follow are from ICRU 83.

- *Gross tumor volume (GTV)*: "The GTV is the gross demonstrable extent and location of the tumor. The GTV may consist of a primary tumor (primary tumor GTV or GTV-T), metastatic regional node(s) (nodal GTV or GTV-N), or distant metastasis (metastatic GTV or GTV-M)."[1] They note that in some cases, it may not be possible to differentiate expanding primary lesions from nearby metastatic disease. The GTV for IMRT is always defined from anatomic images, usually CT with or without MRI, and increasingly supplemented by PET.

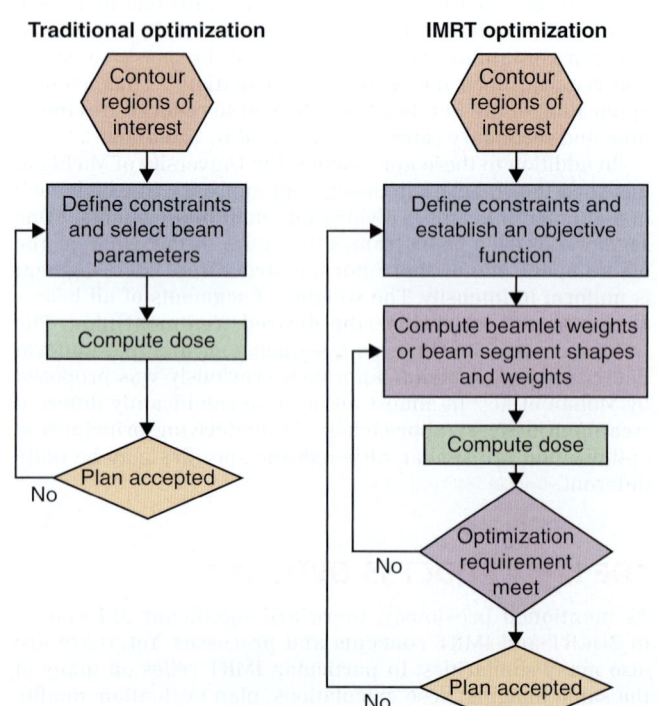

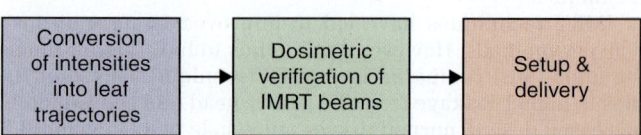

FIGURE 11.6. Intensity-modulated radiation therapy (IMRT) process: quality assurance (QA) and delivery phase.

- *Clinical target volume (CTV)*: "The CTV is a volume of tissue that contains a demonstrable GTV and/or subclinical malignant disease with a certain probability of occurrence considered relevant for therapy. There is no general consensus on what probability is considered relevant for therapy, but typically, a probability of occult disease higher than from 5% to 10% is assumed to require treatment."[1] The volumes outside the GTV encompassed by the CTV will depend a great deal on the particular tumor (e.g., with high or low propensity for lymph node extension). In the past, the CTV was effectively the GTV (including affected nodes) plus a 1- to 2-cm margin. The current definition stresses more the physiologic criteria based on the specifics of disease spread for each tumor. Gregoire et al.[79] have compiled studies on CTV margins into a book. In postoperative situations, following an R0 or R1 resection, there is no gross tumor, so only the CTV need be defined. Readers are strongly encouraged to consult ICRU 83 for details.
- *Planning target volume (PTV)*: "The PTV is a geometrical concept introduced for treatment planning and evaluation. It is the recommended tool to shape absorbed dose distributions to ensure that the prescribed absorbed dose will actually be delivered to all parts of the CTV with a clinically acceptable probability, despite geometrical uncertainties such as organ motion and setup variations."[1]
- *Organ at risk (OAR)*: "The OAR or critical normal structures are tissues that if irradiated could suffer significant morbidity and thus might influence the treatment planning and/or the absorbed dose prescription. In principle, all nontarget tissues could be OARs. However, normal tissues considered as OARs typically depend on the location of the CTV and/or the prescribed absorbed dose."[1] All normal tissue exposed to radiation during treatment is at risk, but the OAR is generally taken to be rather more specific—structures in the immediate vicinity of the PTV, sparing of which may demand specific recontouring of the CTV or PTV. Historically, OARs have been loosely grouped into "serial" or "parallel" organs or a combination of the two, following the work of Withers et al. using the concept of functional subunits in each organ.[80,81] Serial organs, such as the spinal cord, can suffer unacceptable damage if only a small portion is irradiated, whereas parallel organs, such as the liver, can suffer loss of a portion without total loss of function.
- *Planning organ at risk volume (PRV)*: "As is the case with the PTV, uncertainties and variations in the position of the OAR during treatment must be considered to avoid serious complications. For this reason, margins have to be added to the OARs to compensate for these uncertainties and variations, using similar principles as for the PTV. This leads, in analogy with the PTV, to the concept of PRV."[1] As with the OAR itself, margins in the PRV will be affected by the serial or parallel attributes of the adjacent tissues.
- *Remaining volume at risk (RVR)*: "The RVR is operationally defined by the difference between the volume enclosed by the external contour of the patient and that of the CTVs and OARs on the slices that have been imaged."[1] Definition of an RVR and its inclusion in the treatment plan (at least in the form of dose constraints) is essential in IMRT. Without such limits, the optimization software could craft excellent dose distributions for the CTV and OAR but cause toxic irradiation levels in otherwise uncontoured tissues.
- *Treated volume (TV)*: "The TV is the volume of tissue enclosed within a specific isodose envelope, with the absorbed dose specified by the radiation oncology team as appropriate to achieve tumor eradication or palliation, within the bounds of acceptable complications."[1] The TV is what is physically deliverable given limitations of beam collimation and homogeneity and, more importantly, the risks of treatment-associated morbidity acceptable to the

oncologist and the patient. ICRU 83 proposes that, in conformity with its proposal for proton therapy, the TV be defined as the dosage received by 98% of the PTV. This serves as a measure of the minimum absorbed dose and is also referred to as $D_{\text{near minimum}}$. In an analogous manner, a $D_{\text{near maximum}}$ is defined as $D_{2\%}$, the dose received by 2% of the PTV receiving the highest fluence. Readers are referred to Section 3 of ICRU 83.

It should be noted that the GTV, CTV, and OAR represent volumes based on anatomic and physiologic judgments on the location of malignant growths or normal tissues in danger from metastatic spread and/or treatment-induced toxicity. These are independent of the particular irradiation protocol employed (i.e., 3DCRT, IMRT, or particle beams). The PTV, PRV, and TV are intimately tied to the specific radiation therapy used.

Beam Configurations
Systems Using Fixed Intensity-Modulated Fields
The beam configuration can have a significant impact on the quality of an optimized IMRT plan. It may be argued that, because of the greater control over dose distributions afforded by optimized intensity modulation, the fine-tuning of beam angles may not be as important for IMRT as it is for standard radiotherapy. However, optimization of beam angles may find paths least obstructed by critical normal tissues, thus facilitating the achievement of desired distribution with a minimum of compromise.

Beam angle optimization, however, is not a trivial problem. There have been some attempts to solve this problem,[82-84] and advances in mathematical operations research applied to the problem have been reviewed recently.[85] To appreciate the magnitude of the problem, consider the following example. If the angle range is divided into 5-degree steps, nearly 60,000 combinations would need to be tested for three beams, nearly 14 million combinations for five beams, nearly 1.5 billion combinations for seven beams, and so on. Considering the magnitude of the search space, none of the optimization methods is likely to be able to demonstrate a significant improvement in treatment plans, let alone find a truly optimum combination when the number of beams is five or more. Furthermore, the beam angle optimization problem is known to have multiple minima,[86] which means that fast gradient-based optimization techniques may fail. Stochastic methods,[87,88] in principle, should avoid the local minimum problem but may present excessive computing time demands. These should prove less of a problem in the near future, especially with the use of dedicated parallel processors, which can drastically reduce computation time. For a review, see Pratx and Xing.[89]

Another question that may be asked is how many beams are optimal. In principle, a larger number of beams would provide a larger number of parameters to adjust and therefore a greater opportunity to achieve desired dose distributions. (Thus, in theory, a rotational beam would be the ultimate.) However, for fixed beam IMRT, it may be desirable to minimize the number of beams to reduce the time and effort required for planning, QA, dosimetric verification, and delivery of treatments. Fewer intensity-modulated beams would be needed if beam angles were optimized than if the beams were placed at equiangular steps. Calculations by Webb[10] indicate that seven or nine fields give adequate conformal dose distributions for both serial tomography and fixed-gantry IMRT. Consideration of technical feasibility of the plan is very important.

Figure 11.7 compares prostate treatment plans employing different numbers of fields using 3DCRT, serial tomography, and step-and-shoot IMRT. Consistent with published experience, the plan quality improves, but the incremental improvement diminishes with increasing number of beams. Optimum nonuniform placement of beams can further improve dose distribution. Figure 11.8A and B shows a head and neck IMRT

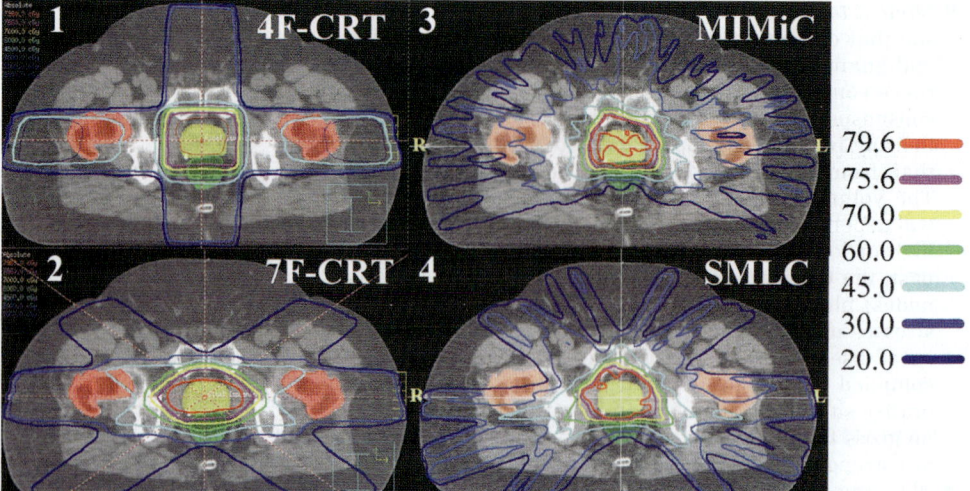

FIGURE 11.7. Typical isodose distributions for treating prostate cancer from (*1*) a four-field three-dimensional conformal radiation therapy (3DCRT) plan; (*2*) a seven-field 3DCRT plan; (*3*) an intensity-modulated radiation therapy (IMRT) plan delivered by serial tomotherapy using MIMiC (NOMOS Corp, Sewickley, PA); and (*4*) a 10-field step-and-shoot segmental multileaf collimator (SMLC) plan. (Reprinted from Clifford Chao KS, Apisarnthanarax S, Ozyigit G. *Practical essentials of IMRT.* 2nd ed. Philadelphia: Lippincott Williams & Wilkins, 2005. With permission.)

case for two different beam angles. The patient, treated with the beam configuration shown in Figure 11.8A, developed significant mucositis at the early phase of treatment. This was consistent with the "horn" in dose distribution shown by the arrow. Revising the beam angle arrangement as shown in Figure 11.8C led to improved dose distribution, shown in Figure 11.8D.

In general, it is most advantageous to place beams so that they are maximally avoiding each other and the opposing beams with the stipulation that directions that overlap significant obstructions, such as heavily attenuating bars in the treatment couch, be avoided. For simplicity, beams often are constrained to lie in the same transverse plane. However, non-coplanar beams will provide an additional degree of freedom and potentially an additional gain in the quality of treatments

but at the expense of setup variability. It should be noted that the beam configurations used for 3DCRT may not be optimal for IMRT.[90]

Although reducing the number of beams is a desirable goal for IMRT delivered with several fixed-gantry angles and dynamic MLC, it should not be the overriding consideration. IMRT can be planned and delivered automatically in times not significantly different from the times for much simpler conventional treatments. Therefore, the delivery times for 6 to 20 beams may be quite acceptable.

Systems Using Rotating Arc Approach

Tomotherapy delivery has substantial differences from fixed-portal IMRT. Mackie[91] has published a historical review of tomotherapy, intertwined as it is with his career. The linear

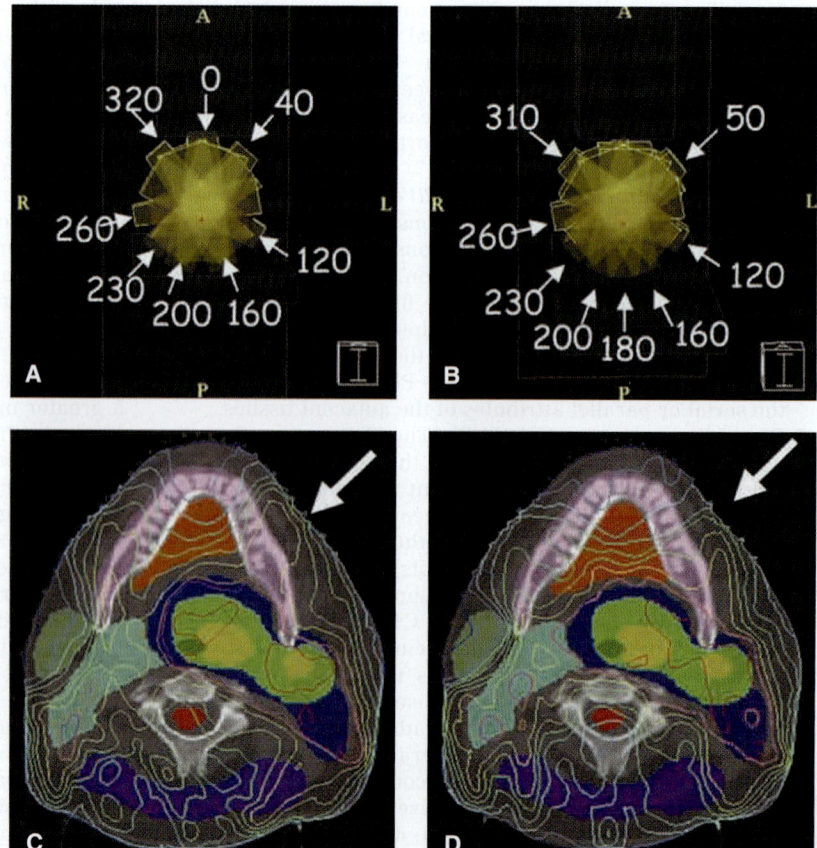

FIGURE 11.8. A patient with carcinoma of the base of the tongue was treated with intensity-modulated radiation therapy. **A** and **B** depict the beam angle arrangement and the resulting isodose distribution. *Arrow* on **(C)** indicated a "horn" of high dose to the left oral tongue and buccal mucosa. Rearrangement of anterior beam placement as shown in **(B)** led to improvement of dose distribution to the normal mucosa of the left anterior oral cavity **(D)**.

accelerator rotates during delivery, and the beams are modulated during rotation. Typically, the modulation is subdivided into small gantry angle ranges (e.g., 5 degrees), and the beam is independently modulated at each gantry angle. Each leaf is used to deliver a single rotating pencil. The pencil-beam modulation is conducted for each leaf by opening that leaf for a fraction of the gantry range consistent with the fractional fluence to be delivered from that gantry angle. For example, for a 5-degree-angle-range bin, if a leaf is to deliver 50% fluence, the leaf will be open for 2.5 degrees over the 5-degree range. Because of geometric constraints of modulating the radiation fan beams, only one or two thin planes can be treated with each rotation. The Peacock system,[3] for instance, uses two banks of opposing leaves projecting to 1.7 or 3.4 cm, depending on user-selected mechanical stops. This delivers modulated beams to two abutting, independently modulated planes. The helical tomotherapy unit uses a single leaf bank with a backup collimator that allows the radiation field width to be continuously adjusted. Narrower leaf widths provide higher spatial resolution for modulation but require more treatment arcs and consequently more delivery time. The current TomoHD MLC uses tungsten leaves 10 cm thick (in beam direction) and with a width of 0.625 cm. Leaves are driven pneumatically and switch in 20 msec.

In a VMAT treatment, the gantry rotates continuously, with MLC leaves, gantry rotation speed, and dose rates varying throughout the arc. VMAT is similar to tomotherapy in that the LINAC source rotates through a 360-degree arc around the patient. The most important difference between the two methods arise from the slice-by-slice delivery of tomotherapy versus the single arc volumetric delivery of VMAT. The difficulty with the optimization of VMAT field shaping throughout the arc is that the MLC leaf position changes between consecutive gantry positions must be restricted. The novel optimization for VMAT proposed by Otto employed a technique called progressive sampling to alleviate this problem.[46] In this approach, the arc is subdivided into a small number of gantry angle samples (e.g., 6), whose beam shapes and/or intensities are varied during the first iteration of the optimization. There are little if any restrictions on MLC leaf position for these fields, because the initial samples are spaced far apart. After several iterations, a new arc sample is added with a field shape interpolated between the first two samples, and optimization continues. After more iterations, another new arc sample is added in the fashion midway between samples 2 and 3. This process continues until desired gantry sampling is met. By starting with a small number of samples and gradually introducing new samples, a high-quality plan can be achieved in a short period of time. Also, a sufficient number of samples ensure the preservation of dose modeling accuracy.

Aperture Margins

IMRT has the inherent capacity to reduce margins attributable to the beam penumbra. When a photon beam traverses the body, it is scattered, depositing dose not only along the path of each ray of the beam but also at points away from it. The electrons knocked out by the incident photons travel laterally to points in the neighborhood of each ray, depositing dose along the way. Near the middle of a uniform beam, outgoing electrons are offset by incoming electrons and equilibrium exists. However, at and just inside the boundaries of the beam, there are no incoming electrons to balance electrons flowing out of the beam. Therefore, a "lateral electronic disequilibrium" exists that leads to a dose deficit inside the boundaries of beams. For lower-energy beams and at large depths, scattered photons significantly contribute to this effect also. The conventional approach to overcome this deficiency is to add a margin for the "beam penumbra" to the PTV so that the tumor dose is maintained at the required level.

For IMRT plans, there is another method to counterbalance the dose deficit. The intensity of rays just inside the beam boundary may be increased. Because some of the increased energy must also flow out, a very large increase would be required if the margin for the penumbra were set to zero or to a very small value. Therefore, an increase in boundary fluence alone is not enough. A combination of an increased fluence and the addition of a margin, albeit a much smaller one, is a better solution. This reduction in margin can be exploited quite usefully to reduce the volume of normal tissues exposed to high doses of radiation with a corresponding reduction in toxicity and a further potential for dose escalation.

The beam boundary–sharpening and margin reduction feature of IMRT can be taken advantage of only if the dose computation method is able to adequately take into account the lateral transport of radiation[92] and if the intensity matrix grid size is sufficiently small. Initially, dose distribution for a given configuration of beams is computed by taking lateral transport into consideration. In each optimization iteration, the intensity distribution first is designed ignoring lateral transport. At the end of the iteration, the dose distribution is recalculated, thereby incorporating the effects of field-shaping devices on lateral transport and revealing the resulting deviations from the anticipated dose distribution. In the next iteration, ray intensities are adjusted further to rectify the deviations, and so on.[44] Carrasco et al.[92] compared several dose computation algorithms in lung phantoms.

A schematic example shown in Figure 11.9 illustrates the issues involved. Figure 11.9A shows a normal organ overlapping the target volume. The target volume is being irradiated by two parallel-opposed beams. It is desired that the dose to the region of overlap be 60% of the target dose. If more dose is delivered, damage to the normal organ may result; but lower than the desired dose may cause local failure. If the role of lateral transport in optimization is ignored, the intensity resulting from the optimization process is essentially a step function, as shown in Figure 11.9B (solid curve). The corresponding dose distribution (the dotted curve) shows a dose deficit inside the high-dose target volume as well as the outside edge of the region of overlap and an excess of dose in the region of overlap adjacent to the high-dose volume. If lateral transport is incorporated by adjusting fluence, the fluence and dose patterns shown in Figure 11.9C result. Fluence is increased at both boundaries. It also is increased in the high-dose side of the interface with the overlap region and decreased on the lower-dose side. The dose is now much closer to the desired dose. Comparing Figure 11.9B and C, it also appears that a modest increase in fluence just inside the boundary does not lead to a perceptible increase in dose outside the beam boundary. This is presumably the result of the fact that the excess dose flowing out of the target periphery is deposited in a much larger volume of tissue. A reduction of margins attributable to penumbra by as much as 8 mm has been found to be feasible for prostate treatments.[44]

IMRT Fractionation

In principle, conventional fractionation strategies can be used to design IMRT plans as well. For example, in a strategy similar to the conventional 1.8-Gy to 2-Gy/fx schedule, a major portion of the dose could be delivered in the initial phase using uniform fields designed with standard 3D conformal methods followed by an IMRT boost. Alternatively, separate IMRT plans could be designed for both the initial large-field treatment and the boost treatment. It may be intuitively obvious that, if a large portion of the dose already has been delivered using large fields, it may be very difficult, if not impossible, to achieve a high level of dose conformation with the remaining fractions in the IMRT boost phase.[16] As indicated earlier in this chapter, IMRT may be most conformal if all target volumes (gross disease, subclinical extensions, and electively

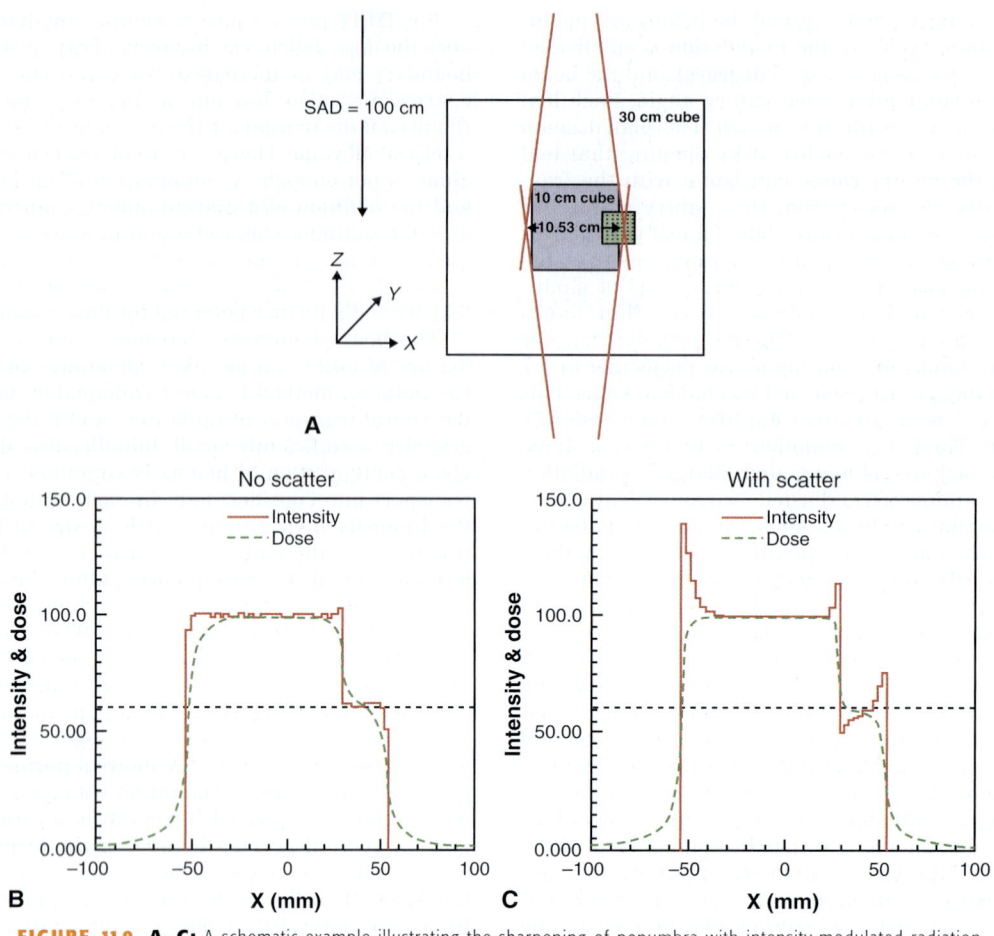

FIGURE 11.9. A–C: A schematic example illustrating the sharpening of penumbra with intensity-modulated radiation therapy.

treated nodes) are treated simultaneously using different fraction sizes.[15] Such a treatment strategy has been called the SIB.[12,13,16,20] Mackie et al.[30] had also indicated the possibilities for irradiation boost in their first paper on serial tomography. The SIB IMRT strategy not only produces superior dose distributions but also is an easier, more efficient, and perhaps less error-prone way of planning and delivering IMRT because it involves the use of the same plan for the entire course of treatment. Furthermore, in many cases, there is no need for electron fields, and the nodal volumes can be included in the IMRT fields; thus, the perennial problem of field matching[93] encountered in the treatment of many sites is thereby avoided.

Because each of the target regions receives different doses per fraction in the SIB IMRT strategy, prescribed nominal (physical) dose and dose per fraction must be adjusted appropriately. The adjusted nominal dose and fraction size for each target region depend on the number of IMRT fractions. The fraction sizes may be estimated using an isoeffect relationship based on the linear-quadratic model and the values of its parameters (such as α/β ratios, tumor doubling time).

The effect of the modified fractionation on acute and late toxicity of normal tissues both outside and within the volumes to be treated also should be considered. Because of the improved conformality of IMRT plans, dose to normal tissues outside the target volume is typically lower than for conventional treatment plans. In addition, if the number of fractions is greater than the number of fractions used to deliver large fields in conventional therapy, the dose per fraction to normal tissues is lower. Therefore, the biologically effective dose would be lower still. However, normal tissues embedded within or adjacent to the target volumes would receive high doses per fraction and may be at higher risk. Isoeffect formulae for

normal tissues also may be derived to estimate the effect of a particular fractionation strategy (see ICRU 83, pp. 36–38). These formalisms would need to incorporate regeneration and change in sensitivity over the treatment course.

The values of parameters for the computation of altered fractionation may, in theory, be obtained from published studies. Studies by Maciejewski et al.[94] and Withers et al.[95–97] for example, have yielded important information for estimating tumor parameters for head and neck carcinoma. In general, the data available are limited. Furthermore, there is considerable uncertainty in the data, and there are concerns about the validity of numerous assumptions in the linear-quadratic model and the isoeffect formalism, especially with regard to normal tissues. (For an early review of the linear-quadratic model, see Fowler.)[98] Much of the accumulated data on normal tissue complications comes from clinical experience in the era of wide-field radiation therapy, so the dosage limits reported from such studies may not be immediately applicable to IMRT. Nevertheless, various investigators have carried out the necessary calculations and adopted SIB IMRT fractionation strategies. Continued investigations and clinical trials are needed to develop more reliable time–dose fractionation models, to produce better estimates of their parameters, and to evaluate alternate SIB IMRT fractionation strategies for all sites.[14] The following are some examples of IMRT fractionation strategies that have been used for IMRT of head and neck cancers.

In the Radiation Therapy Oncology Group H-0022 protocol for early-stage oropharyngeal cancer, 30 daily fractions (5 per week × 6 weeks) are used to simultaneously deliver 66 Gy (2.2 Gy per fraction) to the PTV, 60 Gy (2 Gy per fraction) to the high-risk subclinical disease ("levels II to IV bilaterally, Ib ipsilaterally, and level V and retropharyngeal nodes if the jugular nodes were involved"), and 54 Gy (1.8 Gy per fraction) to subclinical disease. These are biologically equivalent to 70, 60, and 50 Gy, respectively, if given in 2 Gy per fraction. For normal structures, brainstem, spinal cord, and mandible are maintained below 54, 45, and 70 Gy, respectively. The mean dose to the parotid glands is maintained below 26 Gy, and/or 50% of one of the parotids is maintained below 30 Gy and/or at least 20 mL of the combined volume of both parotids is constrained to receive no more than 20 Gy. Sixty-nine patients were accrued at 14 institutions. Treatment-associated xerostomia improved following therapy, in contrast to regular radiation therapy. High locoregional control was achieved with stringent adherence to protocol guidelines.[99]

The SIB strategy at Virginia Commonwealth University involves a dose escalation protocol in which primary nominal dose levels of 68.1, 70.8, and 73.8 Gy, given in 30 fractions (biologically equivalent to 74, 79, and 85 Gy, respectively, if given in 2 Gy per fraction), are used.[100] Simultaneously, the subclinical disease and electively treated nodes were prescribed 60 and 54 Gy, respectively (biologically equivalent to 60 and 50 Gy, respectively, if given in 2 Gy fractions). Spinal cord and brainstem are maintained below 45 and 55 Gy, respectively, and an attempt is made to allow no more than 50% of at least one parotid to receive higher than 26 Gy.

At the Mallinckrodt Institute of Radiology, the SIB strategy for definitive IMRT prescribes 70 Gy in 35 fractions in 2 Gy per fraction to the volume of gross disease with margins. The adjacent soft tissue and nodal volumes at high risk were treated to 63 Gy in 1.8 Gy per fraction and simultaneously 56 Gy in 1.6 Gy per fraction to the elective nodal regions. This regimen has been shown to be well tolerated when combined with concurrent chemotherapy.[101]

The normal tissue constraints for head and neck sites based on the most recent NRG and RTOG protocols (0912, HN001, HN002, HN003) are optic nerve and chiasm <54 Gy; eyes <45 Gy; brainstem <50 to 54 Gy to any 0.03 cc volume; brain <60 Gy to any 0.03 cc volume; spinal cord <45 to 50 Gy to any 0.03 cc volume; ipsilateral cochlea <50 Gy; parotid glands mean dose <26 Gy and at least 20 cc volume <20 Gy; submandibular glands mean <39 Gy; mandible <60 Gy; cervical esophagus mean <34 Gy; and pharynx mean <40 to 45 Gy (for details, see www.nrgoncology.org). Other workers[102–104] have determined dose levels to the pharyngeal constrictors above which severe dysphagia will occur: V (65 Gy) >30%, V (55 Gy) >80%, and a mean dose >60 Gy were predictive of feeding tube dependence.

Optimization of Intensity Maps

The optimization of ray intensities may be carried out using one of several mathematical formalisms and algorithms, also termed *optimization engines*.[85] Each method has its strengths and weaknesses. The choice depends in part on the nature of the objective function and in part on individual preference. Although the details are complex, the basic principles are not difficult to comprehend. Each ray of each beam is traced from the source of radiation through the patient. Only the rays that pass through the target volume need to be traced (plus through a small margin assigned to ensure that the lateral loss of scattered radiation does not compromise the treatment). Others are set to a weight of zero.

The patient's 3D image is divided into voxels. The dose at every voxel in the patient is calculated for an initial set of ray weights. The resulting dose distribution is used to compute the "score" of the treatment plan (i.e., the value of the objective function that mathematically states the clinical objectives of the intended treatment).

The ray-tracing process identifies the tumor and normal tissue voxels that lie along the path of the ray. The effect of a small change in a ray weight on the score then is calculated. If the increase in ray weight would result in favorable

consequences for the patient, the weight is increased, and vice versa. Mathematically speaking, the ray weight is changed by an amount proportional to the gradient of the score with respect to the ray weight. Realizing that the improvement in the plan at each point comes from rays from many beams and that each ray affects many points, only a small change in ray weight may be permitted at a time. This process is repeated for each ray. At the end of each complete cycle (an iteration), a small improvement in the treatment plan results. The new pattern of ray intensities then is used to calculate a new dose distribution and the new score of the plan, which then is used as the basis of further improvement in the next iteration. The iterative process continues until no further improvement takes place, the optimization process is assumed to have converged, and the optimum plan is assumed to have been achieved.

Many current optimization systems use variations of gradient techniques to optimize IMRT plans. These calculations are prodigious given the thousands of free parameters in variation—it was only with the advent of powerful and affordable computers that such calculations could become clinically realistic. Direct aperture optimization has been proposed as an alternative that reduces the parameter space and eliminates nonphysical dose distributions at the start; for a review, see Broderick.[105] The use of gradient techniques assumes that there is a single extremum (a minimum or a maximum, depending on the form of the objective function). This is indeed the case for objective functions based on variance of dose and when only ray weights are optimized. For other cases, it would be necessary to determine whether multiple extrema exist and whether such multiple extrema have an impact on the quality of the solution found. Multiple extrema have been found to exist when beam directions are optimized or when dose–response-based objective functions are used to optimize weights of uniform beams.[70,86,87] One can expect that multiple minima also exist when dose–response-based objective functions are used to optimize IMRT plans. Using simple schematic examples, it also has been shown that multiple minima exist when dose–volume-based objectives are used.[106] Although this may be the case in theory, the existence of multiple minima has not been found to be a serious impediment in dose–volume-based or dose–response-based optimization using gradient techniques. In fact, in a study of dose–volume-based IMRT optimization, Wu and Mohan[107] found that, starting from vastly different initial intensities, the solutions converged to nearly the same plans. The reasons for this have been speculated but not conclusively proven and need to be investigated further.

If multiple minima are discovered to be a factor, then some form of stochastic optimization technique may need to be considered. At the simplest, one may use a random search technique in conjunction with one of the gradient techniques. A more sophisticated stochastic technique is "simulated annealing" or its variation, the "fast simulated annealing."[9,41,70,87] These techniques allow the optimization process to escape from the local minima traps. Other forms of stochastic approaches, such as "genetic algorithms," also have been proposed.[108] In principle, the simulated annealing technique and other stochastic approaches can find the global minimum, but, practically, there is no guarantee that the absolute optimum has been found, only that the best among the solutions examined has been found. (This, of course, is true for gradient techniques as well.) Stochastic techniques tend to be extremely slow and should be used in routine work only if it is established that they are necessary. Nevertheless, some commercial systems have implemented the simulated annealing approach for IMRT optimization.[3] Also, as noted earlier, rapid advances in parallel processing using off-the-shelf components can dramatically reduce computation times.[89] In 2005, Xu and Mueller[109] reported an order of magnitude decrease in the time to process a CT image on a PC when equipped with a dedicated graphics board.

OBJECTIVE FUNCTIONS

Dose-Based Objective Functions

A simple example of an objective function is the criteria stated in terms of the sum of the squares of the differences of desired dose and computed dose at each point within each of the volumes of interest. That is,

$$S = \sum_i (D_{T,0} - D_{T,i})^2 + \sum_n \sum_j p_n \times H(D_{n,0} - D_{n,j}) \times (D_{n,0} - D_{n,j})^2 \quad (1)$$

This type of objective function is called the *quadratic* or *variance* objective function. The optimization process attempts to minimize the treatment plan score S. $D_{T,0}$ in expression Eq. (1) is the desired dose to the target volume, and $D_{n,0}$ is the tolerance dose of the nth normal structure. $D_{T,i}$ is the computed dose at the ith voxel of the target, and $D_{n,j}$ is the computed dose at the jth voxel of the nth normal structure. For normal organs, the function $H(D_{n,j} - D_{n,0})$ is a Heaviside step function defined as follows:

$$H(D_{n,j} - D_{n,0}) = 0 \quad \text{for} \quad D_{n,j} \leq D_{n,0} \quad \text{and}$$
$$= 1 \quad \text{for} \quad D_{n,j} > D_{n,0} \quad (2)$$

In other words, so long as the dose in a normal tissue voxel does not exceed the tolerance limit, the voxel does not contribute to the score function. The quantity p_n is the "relative penalty" for exceeding the tolerance dose.

Dose–Volume-Based Objective Functions

Purely dose-based criteria, such as the one previously described, are not sufficient. In general, the response of the tumor and normal tissues is a function of not only radiation dose but also (to varying degrees depending on the tissue type) the volume subjected to each level of dose. Currently, dose–volume-based objective functions are the most widely used clinically. Dose–volume-based objective functions are expressed in terms of the limits on the volumes of each structure that may be allowed to receive a certain dose or higher. ICRU 83 sets its IMRT reporting guidelines in terms of dose–volume criteria, and dose–volume histograms (DVHs) are a mandatory part of treatment planning.

A practical scheme to incorporate dose–volume-based objectives has been suggested by Bortfeld et al.[110] It is explained in Figure 11.10 using a simple schematic example of one organ at risk. The dose–volume constraint is specified as $V(>D_1) < V_1$. In other words, the volume receiving dose greater than D_1 should be less than V_1. To implement such a constraint into the objective function, we seek another dose value D_2 so that in the current DVHs $V(D_2) = V_1$. The objective function component for this OAR then may be written as:

$$p_n \cdot \sum_i H(D_2 - D_j) \cdot H(D_j - D_1) \cdot (D_j - D_1)^2 \quad (3)$$

That is, only the points with dose values between D_1 and D_2 contribute to the score. Therefore, they are the only ones penalized.

For the target volumes, two types of dose–volume criteria may be specified to limit both the hot and cold spots. For instance, for the desired target dose of 80 Gy, we may specify $V (>85 \text{ Gy}) \leq 5\%$ and $V (>79 \text{ Gy}) \geq 95\%$. In other words, the volume of the target receiving dose >85 Gy should be no more than 5%, and the volume of target receiving 79 Gy or higher should be at least 95%. Dose-based criteria can be considered as a subset of the dose–volume criteria in which the volume is set to an extreme value (0% or 100%, as appropriate). Dose–volume criteria provide more flexibility for the optimization process and greater control over dose distributions. The reason is that dose-based optimization penalizes all the points above the dose limit, whereas the dose–volume-based optimization penalizes only the subset of points within the lower end of range of dose values above the dose limit. For the example of Figure 11.10A, the dose–volume-based optimization process attempts to bring only the points between D_1 and D_2 into compliance with the constraint. In contrast, the dose-based optimization process attempts to constrain all of the points above D_1. Furthermore, dose–volume criteria are highly "degenerate" functions of dose distributions (i.e., there is a very large number of dose distributions that correspond to the same dose–volume constraint). Therefore, the optimization system has a large solution space to choose from, making it easier to find a better solution.

Limitations of Dose–Volume-Based Objective Functions

Dose–volume-based criteria have been demonstrated to have limitations. To illustrate one such limitation, consider the example in Figure 11.10B of a normal structure for which a constraint has been specified that no more than 25% of the volume is to receive 50 Gy or higher. All three DVHs shown meet this criteria. However, the DVH represented by the solid curve clearly causes the least damage. One can argue that we can overcome this limitation by specifying multiple dose–volume constraints or even the entire DVH. However, as illustrated in Figure 11.10C, this would be too limiting. Multiple DVHs could lead to an equivalent injury to a particular organ,

FIGURE 11.10. A: Incorporation of dose–volume constraints in intensity-modulated radiation therapy optimization. (Adapted from Wu Q, Mohan R. Multiple local minima in IMRT optimization based on dose-volume criteria. *Med Phys* 2002;29[7]:1514–1527. Copyright © 2002 American Association of Physicists in Medicine. Reprinted by permission of John Wiley & Sons, Inc.) **B** and **C:** Limitations of dose–volume-based criteria (see text).

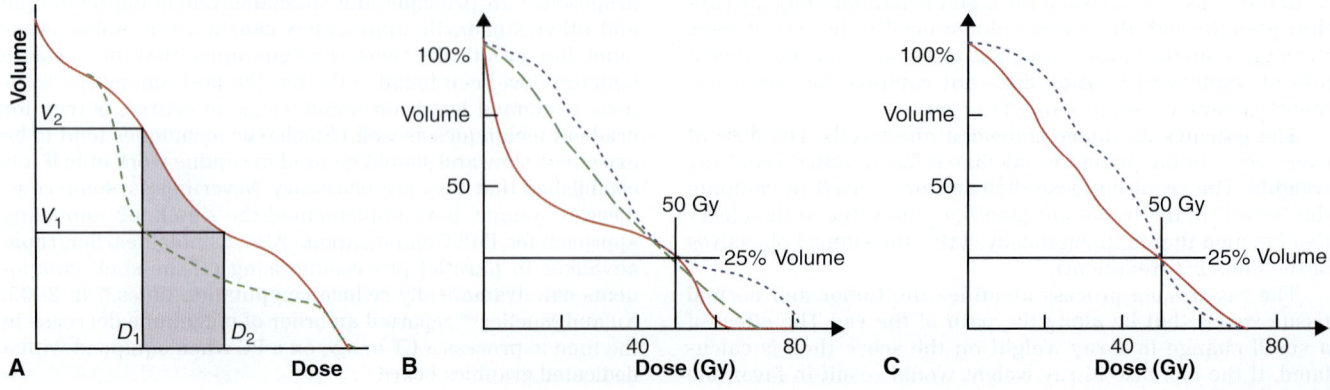

but each DVH may produce a different effect on other organs and the tumor. When this happens, DVHs usually cross each other, as shown in Figure 11.10C. Only one of them is optimum so far as the tumor and other organs are concerned.

To overcome the limitations of dose–volume-based criteria, they may be supplemented with biologic (or dose–response-based) criteria, for instance, in terms of such indices as tumor control probability (TCP), normal tissue complication probabilities (NTCPs), and equivalent uniform dose (EUD).[92] Dose–response-based objective functions are the subject of ongoing investigations.[44,111] The ICRU currently includes NTCP and EUD projections in its level 3 reporting (i.e., still investigative). The report (see p. 51) notes that most of the tissue tolerance data go back to the period before 3D imaging, but they do cite newer prospective studies involving 3DCRT or IMRT.[112,113]

Objective Function Parameters

The desired IMRT dose distributions are specified in terms of parameters of the objective function. In Eq. (1), for instance, the parameters of the objective function are the desired dose limits $D_{T,0}$ and $D_{n,0}$ for target and normal structures, respectively, and the relative importance (or penalty) factors p_n for deviating from desired dose limits. Most often, the objective functions are specified in terms of one or more "soft" dose–volume constraints for each volume of interest, one for each constraint. That is, if the computed dose deviates from the desired value, the plan is not rejected, but it is assessed a penalty. The optimization software computes a "subscore" corresponding to each constraint. The subscore value depends on the deviation of dose distribution from the desired dose distributions and the penalty factor. The overall score of an IMRT plan is an accumulation of subscores of individual volumes of interest. The IMRT optimization system uses the IMRT plan score to arrive at the optimum plan according to the specified objective function. The optimized solution involves trade-offs that balance specified normal tissue objectives against each other and against tumor objectives. An IMRT treatment planning system should provide parameters that allow the treatment planner to adjust the trade-off for each critical structure in a straightforward manner. An example of this is shown in Figure 11.11, where a head and neck target volume nearly abuts the parotid gland.[114] Two of six plans are shown—plans C and F use parameters that emphasize parotid gland sparing and tumor coverage, respectively. This is an excellent example of the flexibility of moving the steep dose gradient in and out of the target volume.

The plan considered to be the best by the computer may not be judged the best (or even good enough) by the treatment planner. Parameters are adjusted by trial and error to obtain a satisfactory plan. A confounding factor is that a change in a parameter of one volume of interest affects not only its own subscore and DVH but also the subscores and DVHs of other structures in a complicated manner. For a complex IMRT problem, in which there may be several dozen parameters, their adjustment is an extremely difficult task. The trial-and-error approach used currently is time consuming and leads to suboptimal results. Future research based on artificial intelligence techniques may provide a systematic means of determining optimum parameter values.

Treatment Plan Evaluation

IMRT dose distributions tend to be highly conformal but complex and unconventional. Traditional methods of evaluation and reporting may be too limited for such dose distributions. In principle, the target dose distributions for IMRT should be more homogeneous than for 3DCRT. In practice, the opposite is the case, due in part to the competing demands of sparing of normal tissues and in part to the inadequacy of objective functions. Dose distributions in normal structures as well are, in general, more nonuniform than for 3DCRT.

In the current practice of radiation therapy, treatment plans are evaluated using dose and dose–volume parameters including such quantities as dose to a point in the volume of interest, minimum dose, maximum dose, minimum dose to a specified fractional volume, or the volume of the structure receiving a specified dose or higher. MUs are set to deliver the prescribed dose to a specified point or to an isodose line (or surface) just enclosing the target volume. For some sites and techniques (e.g., stereotactic radiosurgery of brain tumors), an index of conformality (the ratio of volume occupied by the prescription isodose surface and the volume of the target) is used for plan evaluation. Cumulative dose and dose–volume data are reported as a part of the patient's chart and used for correlation with outcome.

Because of the unconventional nature of IMRT dose distributions, especially the high degree of dose heterogeneity and fluctuations in dose as a function of position in volumes of interest, indices such as dose to a point, minimum dose, or maximum dose may not correlate well with dose response. Instead, dose to a specified fractional volume is more appropriate, and this is the approach taken by ICRU 83. ICRU reporting now specifies a $D_{98\%}$ or $D_{near\ minimum}$ (dose to at least 98% of the PTV) and a corresponding $D_{2\%}$ (dose received by the most heavily irradiated 2% of the PTV).[1]

Limitations of dose and dose–volume plan evaluation parameters have been articulated in the literature.[115] These limitations become more significant for the complex dose distributions of IMRT. It has been argued that biophysical dose–response indices, which summarize complex dose distributions using a single clinically relevant index in each volume of interest, may be more appropriate. Currently, indices such

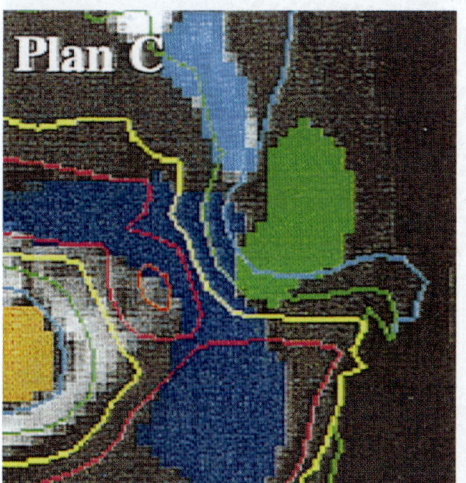

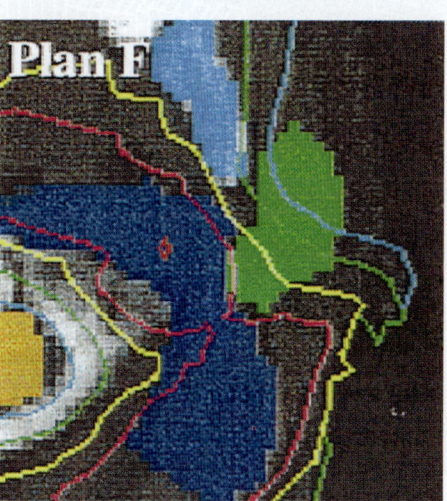

FIGURE 11.11. Effect of adjusting dose prescription parameters on the resulting treatment plan. The parotid gland and target are shown in *green* and *blue*, respectively. *Plan C* emphasizes parotid sparing, and *plan F* emphasizes tumor coverage. (Interested readers should view the full set of six plans as presented in the original paper. From Chao KS, Low DA, Perez CA, et al. Intensity-modulated radiation therapy in head and neck cancers: the Mallinckrodt experience. *Int J Cancer* 2000;90[2]:92–103.)

as TCP, NTCPs, and biologically EUD often are computed and recorded but rarely are used for routine plan evaluation. This is because of the unreliability of published dose–response data and weaknesses of models to compute these indices. This is, in turn, the result of the various sources of uncertainty both in the quantification of response and in doses delivered to the structures. Levegrun et al.[116] analyzed data from patients with prostate cancer treated at Memorial Sloan-Kettering Cancer Center and concluded that the biopsy-based response did not correlate with minimum tumor dose, EUD, or TCP. Instead, they found the mean dose to be a very good predictor of response. They attributed this observation to large treatment margins for PTV, substantial target motion, and relatively homogeneous dose distributions. As functional imaging (e.g., PET and nanoparticle optical probes) becomes more widespread, treatment will become more adaptive, with planning readjusted to reflect tumor regression or persistence. Recently, Moeller et al.[77] reported a prospective study using 18-fluorodeoxyglucose (FDG)-PET to assess tumor response in head and neck cancers. PET was seen to be superior to CT in the subset of patients with high-risk disease.

GENERATION OF LEAF SEQUENCES

Fixed Intensity-Modulated Fields

For the IMRT mode using multiple fixed fields, the plan optimization process produces nonuniform intensity distributions (see Fig. 11.12) for each set of fields. In principle, such intensity distributions can be delivered using custom-fabricated compensators made of lead alloys to attenuate the appropriate amount of radiation along each ray of the beam. Such devices would have to be produced using computerized milling machines. In addition, to use them it would be necessary for the operator (radiation therapist) to enter the treatment room to insert the device for each field. This process would be highly labor intensive and impractical considering that a large number of beams often may be needed for optimum intensity-modulated treatments.

The most efficient means of delivering fixed-field IMRT is the standard MLC in dynamic mode using such methods as the "sliding-window" technique or the step-and-shoot technique. In either case, leaf position sequences as a function of MUs need to be generated. The MLC leaves are made of approximately 5- or 6-cm-thick tungsten and are typically 0.5 or 1 cm wide (projected to isocenter). MLCs with leaves of a width as

small as 1 mm have been introduced. Smaller leaf width may be of greater value for IMRT than for standard 3DCRT. For the former, the leaf width affects the dose delivered to the entire slice, whereas for the latter, it affects only the shape of the boundary. A smaller leaf width undoubtedly would produce more conformal dose distributions, but the electromechanical complexity and cost of the device would increase. Because of the smearing caused by finite-sized radiation sources, lateral secondary electron transport, and the use of multiple fields, and because of motion and positioning uncertainties, an acceptable leaf width may not need to be very small. The minimum desirable leaf width would depend on numerous factors including shapes and locations of volumes of interest, dose gradients desired, and number and orientations of beams. Although the issue of leaf width has been debated for quite some time, there are no definitive studies to guide the choice of the most suitable width.

MLCs transmit only 0.5% to 2% of incident radiation (except through small interleaf gaps and the rounded ends of some MLCs). However, as discussed later in this chapter, because intensity-modulated treatments require a substantially larger number of MUs than do the conventional uniform field treatments, the cumulative effective transmission may be considerably larger.

Leaf Sequence Generation: Sliding-Window Technique

In the sliding-window method, the gap formed by each pair of opposing leaves is swept across the target volume under computer control while the radiation is on. The gap opening and its speed are optimally adjusted. Because the dose rate of the treatment machine might fluctuate slightly, the motion is indexed to MUs rather than time. The basic principle is that as the gap slides across a point, the radiation received by the point is proportional to the number of MUs delivered during the time the tip of the leading leaf goes past the point and exposes it until the tip of the trailing leaf moves in to block it again. (The point also receives additional radiation transmitted through or scattered from the leaves, which must be accounted for. See later discussion in this chapter.) The setting of the gap opening and its speed for each pair at any instant are determined by a technique first introduced by Convery and Rosenbloom[117] and refined and studied further by Bortfeld et al.,[24] Spirou and Chui,[36,37] Stein et al.,[38] Svensson et al.,[118] and others.[40,119] Knowledge of the maximum leaf speed

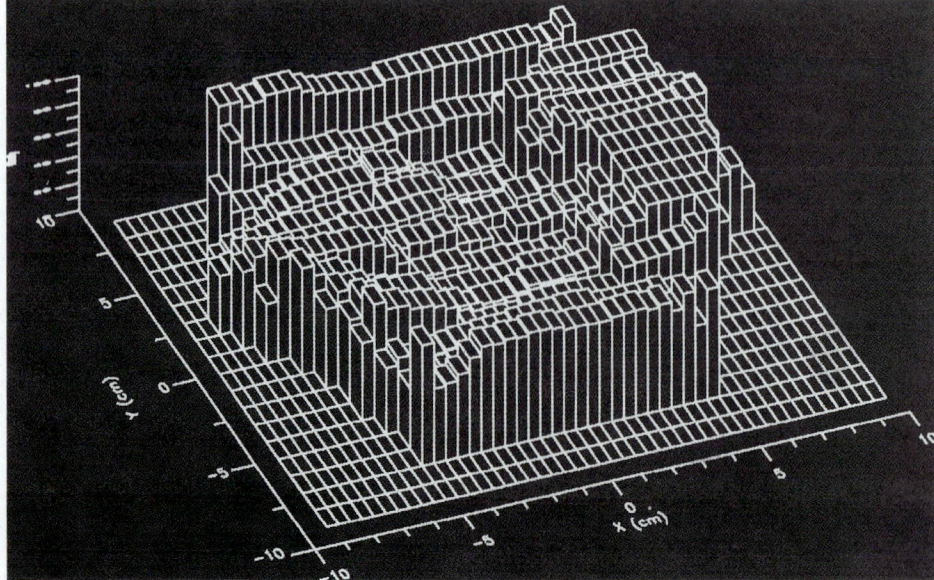

FIGURE 11.12. Intensity profile of the left lateral beam of an intensity-modulated radiation therapy plan designed for the treatment of the cervix. Intensity distribution in a plane through the isocenter and normal to the direction of the beam is plotted. The grid size along the *y*-axis is 1 cm, corresponding to the width of multileaf collimator leaves. Each intensity curve along the *x*-axis corresponds to one pair of opposing leaves.

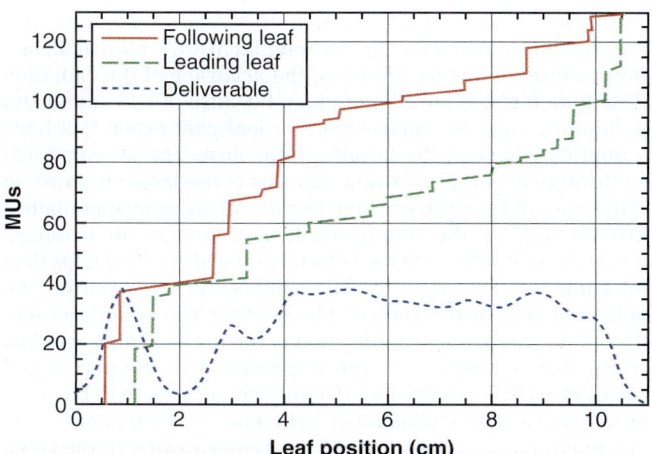

FIGURE 11.13. A typical trajectory of one of the pairs of leaves used to deliver intensity-modulated beam profiles of the type shown in Figure 11.12. Intensity-modulated radiation therapy optimization based on deliverable dose distributions using the sliding-window technique. Positions of the leading and following leaves are plotted as a function of monitor units (MUs). The gap formed by the pair of leaves moves from left to right. Its width and speed are adjusted by the computer to allow a predetermined amount of radiation to reach each point within the field. Note that the fluence is the differences in MUs for the left leaf and the right leaf.

is taken advantage of to maximize the gap between the opposing pair of leaves and, therefore, to minimize the treatment time. The number of leaves participating in the delivery of a beam depends on the projected size of the target volume. The data describing leaf trajectories, produced by the leaf sequence generation process, are in the form of a table of positions of leaves versus the corresponding MUs (depicted graphically in Fig. 11.13).

Leaf Sequence Generation: Step-and-Shoot and Multisegment Techniques

With the step-and-shoot technique (as well as for multisegment technique), the fixed-gantry radiation beam is composed of multiple static MLC segments, with each segment having its own aperture shape and weight or monitor (MU) settings. The leaf sequence generation algorithms take the optimized intensity pattern as the input and decompose it into multiple segments, each to be shaped as an aperture formed by the MLC. Fluence intensity throughout each MLC segment is relatively uniform. The summation of all static segments yields the required intensity-modulated dose distributions. Ideally, the segments are sorted to minimize the MLC leaf travel time between the segments. Note that such sorting is neither necessary nor possible for the sliding-window technique.

The first step of the leaf sequence generation process is the discretization of the continuous intensity distribution into a limited number of intensity levels. These intensity levels then are converted into leaf sequences using one of several methods described in the literature. Bortfeld et al.,[24] for example, have proposed a method in which each row of intensity is handled separately, similar to the sliding-window algorithm. The advantage is that the total number of MUs is small but at the cost of possibly large numbers of segments. Xia and Verhey[120] proposed the so-called areal algorithm. Instead of dividing the intensities into levels of equal steps, they divided them into levels in powers of 2 to reduce the number of steps and to gain efficiency. Wu et al.[111] proposed a technique called the *K-means clustering* in which the intensity levels are grouped together based on their values and the user-specified error tolerance levels. The intensity levels are not equally spaced and can be arbitrary.

Unlike the sliding-window algorithm, the maximum leaf speed is not important for the step-and-shoot and multisegment techniques. Similarly, although the number of segments

is not an issue for the sliding-window techniques, it could affect the step-and-shoot delivery efficiency significantly. For the former, the only penalty of the large number of segments is the size of computer storage, whereas for the latter, it leads to inefficiency because the beam is off during the transition between the segments. Furthermore, for some linear accelerators, there is an overhead time associated with each segment.

Que[121] compared several step-and-shoot algorithms and found that the algorithm used by Xia and Verhey[120] frequently, but not always, produces the least number of segments. Other investigators have reported methods to minimize the number of segments as well. The algorithm of Dai and Zhu[122] checks numerous candidates for each segment, and the candidate that would result in a residual intensity matrix with the least complexity is selected. If more than one candidate exists with the same complexity, the one with the largest size is chosen. Langer et al.[123] reported a technique based on the integer programming that can minimize the number of segments under the constraints that the MUs do not exceed a certain limit. It was found that the technique produces considerably fewer segments than the algorithms of Bortfeld et al.[9,110] and Xia and Verhey[120] for the same or fewer MUs.

Monitor Units of IMRT Beams

Based on methods similar to those previously described, software systems have been developed to convert intensity distributions to leaf trajectories. The input to this software is the intensity distribution for each field in terms of MUs or, to be more precise, "effective" MUs. Effective MUs are fractions of MUs transmitted through the intensity modulation or compensation device. The intensity distribution-to-leaf trajectory conversion software not only produces trajectories but also computes actual MU settings for each beam as a natural by-product of the conversion process. Trajectories of leaves and the MUs for each beam are transmitted to the computer-controlled radiation treatment machine for dosimetric verification and the delivery of treatment.

It is important to note that the relationship between the prescribed dose and MUs required for delivering each of the intensity-modulated beams is highly complex and not obvious. There is no practical way to calculate MUs by hand as is done for traditional treatments as an independent check of the predicted MU values. To ensure patient safety and to satisfy the requirements of the independent check, some systems have implemented independent software for a second MU calculation. Others have adopted the policy to measure the dose or dose distribution for each of the beams before the first treatment.

Impact of MLC Characteristics

ICRU 83 notes that the tolerances for MLC operation must be more stringent than even those required for beam blockage in 3DCRT. This stems from the steep dose gradients made possible by and employed with IMRT. Slippage of leaf position would cause a cumulative degradation of the dose distribution actually delivered. Leakage through closed leaves may also pose a problem for which consideration in planning must be taken.[124] Adjustments to leaf trajectories are required to account for the various effects associated with MLC characteristics, including the rounded leaf tips, tongue-and-groove leaf design, interleaf and intraleaf transmission, leaf scatter, and collimator scatter upstream from the MLC. The accuracy of dose delivered and the agreement between calculated and measured dose distributions depend on the adequate accounting of these effects. Approximate empirical corrections are applied for these effects by algorithms and software that convert optimized intensity distributions into leaf trajectories.

MLCs have an interlocking tongue-and-groove leaf design to minimize interleaf leakage. However, there is a difference in interleaf leakage and leakage through the leaves.

This difference can become significant for beams that require a large number of MUs and in portions of the beams that receive large fractions of their dose through leakage. Currently, this effect is ignored, although the use of Monte Carlo techniques to account for it is being investigated.[125,126]

In addition, there are circumstances during creation of intensity profiles when a thin strip of the irradiated medium is shielded by the tongue of one leaf pair or the groove of the adjacent leaf pair rather than being completely exposed or completely blocked. Van Santvoort and Heijmen[39] have demonstrated that this leads to an underdosage in the thin strip. They, and subsequently Webb et al.,[42] also showed that this effect could be removed by the use of leaf motion-synchronizing techniques. However, such techniques result in an increase in the number of MUs. Furthermore, this effect is not considered to be of significant clinical consequence because of the smearing caused by multiple fields and the positioning and motion uncertainties. Using different collimator angles for each field can reduce this effect further.

Depending on the complexity (the frequency and amplitudes of peaks and valleys) of the intensity pattern, points within the field aperture may receive a substantial portion of the dose as a result of radiation transmitted through or scattered from the leaves when the points are in the shadow of the leaves. Points outside the leaf aperture receive their entire dose through these "indirect" sources. The complexity of intensity distributions produced by the IMRT optimization process depends on a combination of several clinical factors including the shapes, sizes, and relative locations of tumor and normal tissues; required tumor dose; dose homogeneity; and dose–volume limits of normal tissues. Intensity distributions for head and neck cases, for example, tend to be considerably more complex than for prostate cases. For beams with highly complex intensity patterns, the average window width to deliver the treatment tends to be small, and for the same dose received by the tumor, the treatment time (i.e., the number of MUs) is long. Consequently, the contribution of radiation transmitted through and scattered from the leaves may form a significant fraction of the total dose delivered. Because these contributions are accounted for approximately, the uncertainty in dose delivered is increased. In addition, the differences between interleaf and intraleaf transmissions may no longer be negligible. Another consequence of complex intensity patterns is that the lower limit of the deliverable intensity is high.

The deliverable dose distributions may be significantly different from the original optimized ones. There are different ways to overcome the difficulties resulting from the differences in desired and deliverable dose distributions. For example, if the deliverable dose to a particular normal structure is higher than the original optimized dose, the planner could modify the objective function to demand an appropriately lower dose. Alternatively, the optimization loop could include a pass-through leaf sequence generation and calculation of deliverable dose distributions. The optimizer then adjusts ray weights based on deliverable dose distributions rather than the idealized ones. This scheme has been investigated by Siebers et al.[127]

QA FOR INTENSITY-MODULATED TREATMENTS

A number of QA steps unique to IMRT are needed to ensure the accuracy and safety of treatments. These include QA of the MLC in dynamic mode, dosimetric verification for each dynamic beam as well as for the composite treatment plans, portal imaging, treatment verification, *in vivo* dosimetry, and reduction in uncertainty associated with daily positioning and internal organ motion during irradiation. In recognition of the special demands of IMRT, the American Association of Physicists in Medicine (AAPM) commissioned Task Force 142[128]

to replace the earlier Task Group 40[129] and recommend new QA guidelines. When using conventional 3DCRT, MLC leaf position calibration errors influence the accuracy of the radiation distribution at the portal boundary. Because of PTV and beam penumbra margins, small errors in leaf calibration will have a minimal effect on the target volume dose. The accepted leaf calibration accuracy is 2 mm, but this is too large[1] because in IMRT the MLCs are used to generate inhomogeneous fluence distributions. In the sliding-window technique, for instance, this is done by adjusting the velocity and width of leaf gaps during radiation delivery. If the MLC calibration is inaccurate, the delivered dose distribution will be in error. The error is a function of the ratio of leaf calibration error to the sliding-window width. For example, a 1-mm imprecision in the gap would result in a 10% error in dose if a uniform field were to be delivered using a sliding window of 1 cm. For step-and-shoot delivery, magnitudes of dose errors are greater (owing to the steep dose gradients near the MLC leaf edges), but they are confined to the subfield edges. Thus, it is essential to verify the IMRT absorbed dose calculation algorithm against measurements for the IMRT accelerator in question using a suitable small-field detector.[130] In addition, it is absolutely essential for leaf-positioning accuracy to be verified. The AAPM TG-142 protocol recommends that a leaf should be positioned with an accuracy of 1.0 mm and the physicists must ensure through routine QA procedures that such precise positioning is achieved and maintained. It is interesting that integral dose error is similar for both the step-and-shoot and sliding-window techniques, but the distribution of the error is different.

Because MLC leaf calibration and the accuracy of MLC operations influence the delivered dose distribution, new, more rigorous MLC QA procedures have been developed. Chui et al.,[131] LoSasso and Chui,[132] and Ling et al.,[5] among others, have developed QA procedures specifically for MLCs used in dynamic mode. Periodic QA checks must ensure that the leaves of the MLC do indeed move to their designated positions at the specified values of MUs. Moreover, to ensure safe and accurate delivery of treatments with an MLC, the manufacturers must include redundant and independent sensors for the leaves of the MLC. Furthermore, in the event of treatment field interruption and resumption, there should be no perceptible change in dose delivered.

Another aspect of QA important for IMRT is the daily positioning uncertainty and motion during irradiation. IMRT is a highly conformal and highly precise form of radiotherapy frequently used to escalate dose. Dose distributions may have steep dose gradients between the target and the neighboring normal structures. Furthermore, margins may be much smaller than in conventional treatments. Patient positioning and immobilization requirements are more stringent than ever to ensure that the target volumes are covered adequately and the normal tissues are spared adequately. In fact, special immobilization devices and techniques are being developed to reproducibly and accurately position the target volume and normal anatomy. Many of these devices already are available commercially (e.g., rectal inserts to improve positioning for prostate IMRT).

Similarly, motion during treatment, mainly as a consequence of respiration, also can be a serious problem for IMRT of sites in the thorax and abdomen. Because IMRT is delivered dynamically, the moving target volume may move in and out of the instantaneous field of radiation. Some portions of the target volume may get more than the planned dose, whereas others may get less. A way to minimize effects of respiratory motion would be to use "gated treatments" in which radiation and leaf motion are turned on only during a specific, reproducible portion of the respiratory cycle or in an interval during which the patient's breath is voluntarily, or involuntarily, held.[133] New methodologies, typically employing CT imaging, are being used to synchronize patient breathing motion with the irradiation beam.[134–136]

DOSIMETRIC VERIFICATION OF INTENSITY-MODULATED TREATMENTS

To implement a new treatment technology into routine clinical use, there are usually three distinct but closely related phases. *Acceptance tests*: This is the initial set of tests that ensures the hardware and software meet the factory- or customer-provided specifications. Usually, but not always, the written specifications contain the necessary instructions or guidelines for these tests (in order to avoid legal ambiguity in the measurements). It is also a good opportunity for the users to establish some performance baselines, especially for the hardware purchased. *Commissioning tests*: The IMRT commissioning is a process to implement IMRT treatments using the customer's hardware and beam data. Various groups have studied the general guidelines for commissioning a treatment planning system, and the AAPM issued a new report on IMRT commissioning in 2009.[137] The process usually starts with collection of essential beam data for beam modeling. The parameters of the dose calculation algorithm are then tuned to provide the best performance for the user's beam. Additional tests should be performed to evaluate the limitations of the treatment planning system and a solution or a work-around should be found if the problem is clearly identified. Then IMRT phantom measurements should be performed to test the accuracy of the delivery system and data connectivity. If the accuracy is judged to be acceptable, the system can be released to the clinic after the necessary user training and procedural implementations. It is recommended that a small (interdisciplinary) focus group should be assigned to lead the IMRT implementation in the clinic. The "train-the-trainer" approach has proven to be effective in translating new technology into routine clinical practice. *Ongoing QA*: After the system is released to the clinic, it is important to establish a routine QA program. The performance of various steps involved in performing IMRT treatments needs to be tracked so that the quality of the treatments can be maintained. The ongoing QA program can be separated into patient-specific QA and equipment QA, which will be described in more detail in the following section.

Patient- and Equipment-Specific QA

Because of the complexity of irregular field shapes, small-field dosimetry, and time-dependent deliverable leaf sequences, it is recommended by the AAPM and ASTRO that patient-specific QA should be performed as a part of the IMRT management process and a requirement for billing for IMRT services. Figure 11.14 shows the general categories of patient- and equipment-specific QA, which are detailed in the following.

Patient setup, although not specific to IMRT dosimetry, is considered a key step in ensuring accurate IMRT treatments. A variety of image-guided localization techniques have been proposed for use with IMRT treatments, from simple orthogonal portal films to the beam's eye view portal film with IMRT intensity pattern overlays,[138] imaging of implanted fiducials,[139,140] daily ultrasound-guided localization,[141–143] conventional CT, megavoltage CT, cone beam CT, orthogonal kV images, and to the most integrated tomotherapy solutions.[144] Emerging technologies also allow the acquisition of MR images. These images, when approved by the radiation oncologist, assure that the subsequent treatment is properly administered to the designated clinical volumes. The detailed discussion of these specific image-guided procedures is out of the scope of this chapter, but QA in patient positioning remains an important issue for IMRT. A somewhat related problem of organ motion because of breathing has been discussed earlier. Several recent studies have examined the use of cone beam CT for patient setup or respiratory gating.[145–148] The implementation of patient-specific QA depends highly on each institution. For example, dosimetric measurements

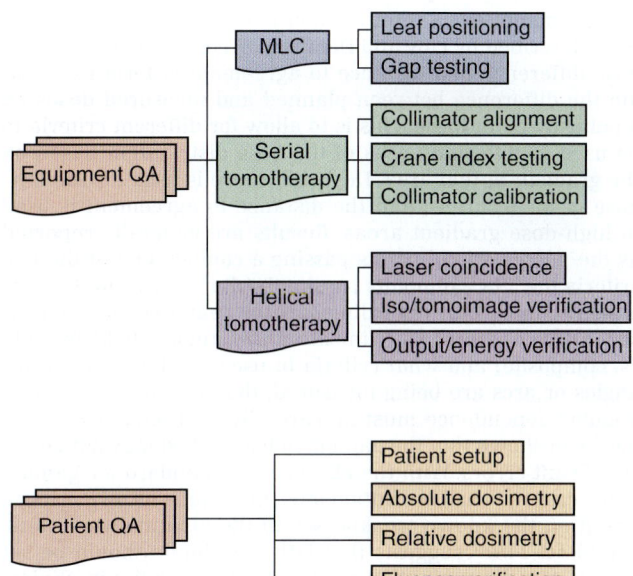

FIGURE 11.14. Overview of intensity-modulated radiation therapy quality assurance (QA) includes patient-specific and equipment-specific procedures. MLC, multileaf collimator.

of MU settings can be verified for each beam individually (usually in a flat [slab] phantom geometry) or for the composite treatment plan (usually in a specially designed phantom, but it is also possible to use the simple slab phantom setup). Unlike single-beam verification in which the single-beam dose distribution can be significantly different from the original patient plan, the advantage of measuring the composite treatment plan in a phantom (regardless of the shape of the phantom) is that the composite dose distribution or the dose "pattern" generated in a phantom is usually similar to those in the original patient plan. This can be useful in selecting the measurement points or in visualizing potential dose errors. Absolute dosimetry is usually referred to as "MU verification" for IMRT. The traditional manual process for MU verification is virtually impossible to perform because of the large number of fields involved and the irregular shape and size of the treatment segments. Attempts have been made to verify MU settings in an IMRT plan using alternative calculation methods.[149] However, these alternative calculation methods cannot predict the uncertainties during the actual delivery at the treatment machines and are also subject to limitations and approximations in their dose calculation models. The most reliable and practical technique currently for IMRT MU verification is still the ion chamber-based point dose measurement in a phantom. Absolute dose measurement in a phantom is usually performed through a process called the *hybrid phantom plan*. In this plan, all beam angles and deliverable intensity patterns for a patient plan are transferred to the phantom, and doses in the phantom are computed for QA. The basic assumption in this process is that if the dose calculated in the phantom agrees with the measurement in the phantom, then the dose delivered to the patient agrees with the dose calculated in the patient. Originally, IMRT QA involved the use of an ion chamber to verify absolute dose and film to verify the relative 2D dose distribution. Subsequently, detector arrays and the necessary software became widely adopted tool for this verification.[149–151] For film dosimetry, it is important to convert film density into relative dose using a film calibration process. Because of the additional dimensionality, it becomes difficult to define good numerical criteria for evaluating relative 2D/3D measurements. Various numerical indicators (such as the distance to agreement, and gamma, or normalized agreement test) were proposed. In particular, the

most common evaluation method is the gamma index originally described by Low and Dempsey.[152] This method uses both
dose difference and distance to agreement criteria to evaluate the difference between planned and measured doses on
a point-by-point basis. This is to allow for different criteria to
be used in different areas of the dose distribution based on
the gradient in that area. Dose difference is used for the low-
dose gradient areas, and the distance to agreement is used
in high-dose gradient areas. Results are generally reported
as the percentage of points passing a combination of the two
criteria (i.e., 98% of points passing 3%/3 mm criterion). There
is some controversy regarding how the beams should be measured (fixed-gantry vs. clinical gantry angles, field by field
vs. composite) and what criteria to use.[153,154] If clinical gantry
angles or arcs are being measured, the measurement device
angular dependence must be carefully characterized.[155–158] It
has been shown that the gamma index method may not detect
significant errors. With the absence of a standard for gamma
index criteria, each institution must determine its own criteria
based on the known weaknesses in the institution's system.
AAPM TG-119[137] suggests that IMRT QA limits should be set
based on a determination of statistical variability in clinical
practice. Special attention should be paid to the low-dose
regions near critical structures in the original patient plan.
Attention should also be paid to the systematic shifts of isodose lines, which may reveal if the isocenter or any reference
setup point may be off. It would be useful if the relative dose
distribution can be normalized to the absolute dose measurement point, which converts the relative dose measurement
into absolute dose distributions.

Figure 11.14 also illustrates equipment-specific QA procedures. In general, IMRT QA is a subset of general equipment
QA processes. The technology of IMRT and techniques for QA
are also evolving. It is strongly suggested that users of IMRT
should attempt to attend national meetings and technology
conferences or training courses so that their knowledge about
the use of IMRT can be updated regularly.

IMRT has been variously termed as *opaque, unintuitive,*
and *nontransparent,* partly because it is delivered using
dynamic techniques. Many are skeptical about whether
the dose distribution displayed on an IMRT plan is, in fact,
delivered. Furthermore, because of the complexity of computations involved, there is no practical way to verify the MU
settings by hand calculations, as is done for conventional
treatments. Moreover, because of the inherent nonuniformity
of IMRT fields, it is important to know the dose accurately at
every point within the beam. One way to check if the intended
dose would be delivered to the patient at the time of the treatment is to conduct dosimetric verification measurements.

Two broad categories of IMRT treatment plan verification approaches have been developed for MLC-based IMRT.
First, the dose distribution from radiation fields is independently measured and evaluated. This often is accomplished
by using a flat homogeneous water-equivalent phantom and
irradiating each field independently. The dose distributions
measured with a film or 2D detector array are compared
against calculations conducted by the treatment planning
system under the same geometric conditions. The process
is explained in Figure 11.15. For calculation of dose distributions, each field is transferred to a treatment plan with a
flat homogeneous phantom. A typical example for a sliding-
window intensity-modulated beam dosimetric verification is
shown in Figure 11.16. This technique has the advantage that
discrepancies between the planned and delivered dose can be
attributed to individual radiation portals. However, the total
integrated dose distribution is not checked.

The second method uses a phantom irradiated by all beam
portals, allowing the evaluation of the total dose distribution delivered.[159,160] Typically, ionization chambers and radiographic film are the dosimeters used for these measurements.
Although ionization chambers can be benchmark-quality
dosimeters, they suffer from volume averaging and are inefficient for measuring multiple points. Because of the complexity
of the dose distributions being measured, a 2D dosimeter is
required for thorough evaluations of nonuniform dose distribution. Quantitative radiographic film measurements require
careful dose calibrations using independently measured sensitometric curves. The film optical densities are measured
and converted to absolute dose using film calibration data
and compared with the predictions of the treatment planning
system.[40]

In vivo dosimetry commonly is used to verify the dose
delivered by conformal therapy radiation fields. The complex
fluence distribution of IMRT fields makes quantitative use of
in vivo dosimetry, specifically the use of skin surface–mounted
dosimeters, difficult.

Film, thermoluminescent dosimeters, and diodes may not
be sufficiently accurate; are laborious to use; and, in the case
of thermoluminescent dosimeters and diodes, are incapable of
providing detailed information. In the long run, the most efficient way to verify fixed intensity-modulated fields is expected
to be with real-time 2D or 3D dosimetry systems using appropriately calibrated electronic portal imaging devices (EPIDs).
A general review of EPIDs was published in 2008.[161] Such
devices could be used for dosimetric verification of IMRT
beams before treatment delivery and for exit dosimetry using
transmitted portal dose images (PDIs). For EPIDs to be used
for pretreatment dosimetric verification and exit dosimetry,

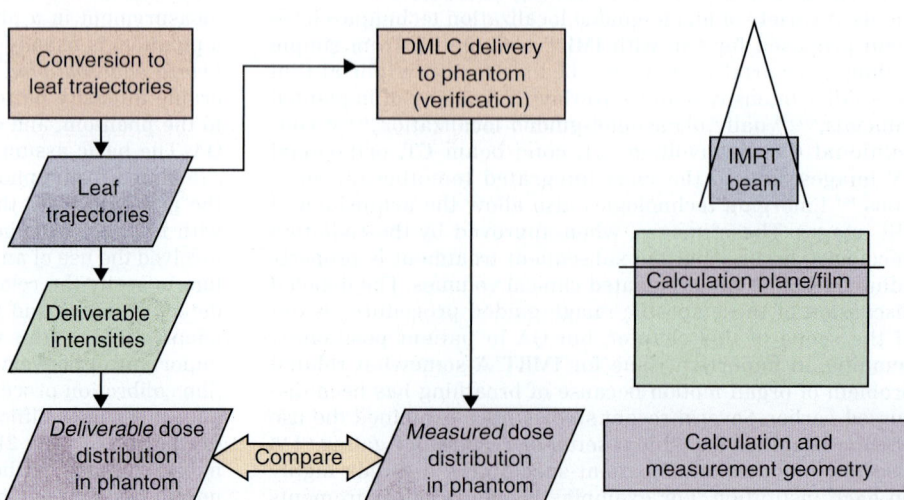

FIGURE 11.15. Diagram illustrating dosimetric verification of individual intensity-modulated
radiation therapy fields. DMLC, dynamic multileaf
collimator; IMRT, intensity-modulated radiation
therapy.

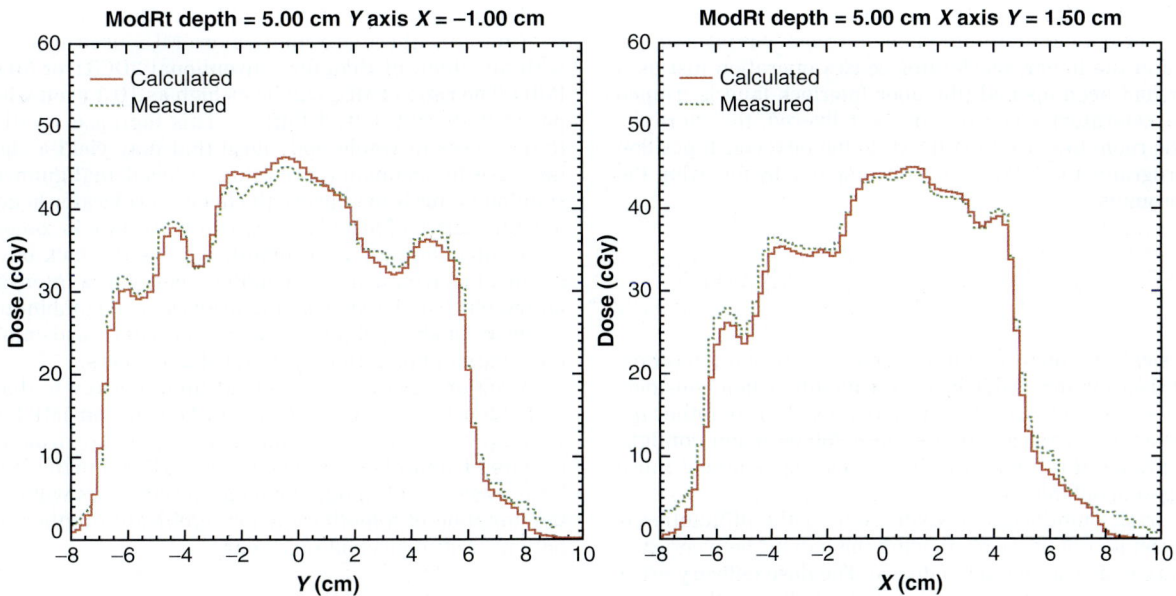

FIGURE 11.16. Dosimetric verification example comparing measured and calculated dose profiles of a right lateral field generated with sliding-window technique for the intensity-modulated radiation therapy of gynecologic cancer.

they must operate in the integration mode to capture the transmitted radiation over the entire exposure of each beam. The result is a PDI that can be compared with an intensity-modulated digitally reconstructed PDI. For pretreatment dosimetric verification of a given beam, a PDI may be created using a 3D treatment planning system to compute dose deposited in the EPID detector.[162–165] For exit dosimetry, the PDI may be calculated using the 3D CT image of the patient.[166,167] In either case, for accurate dosimetric verification, the effect of scattered radiation and the variation in response of the detector with energy must be included. The former effect can be taken into account with dose-spread kernel superposition methods, but both can be accounted for using Monte Carlo techniques. 3D *in vivo* dose verification for IMRT and VMAT using a-Si EPIDs has also been developed recently. The EPID-based 3D dose distribution can be reconstructed using either a back-projection algorithm[168,169] or a model-based forward-calculation algorithm.[170,171]

TREATMENT SETUP AND DELIVERY

Fixed-Gantry Intensity-Modulated Fields

Similar to conventional radiotherapy, for IMRT techniques using fixed intensity-modulated fields, it is necessary to verify the patient alignment using portal images with beams used for actual treatment or other image guidance technology before the delivery of the first treatment and then periodically thereafter. However, no beam apertures are required for IMRT. Therefore, special fields for portal imaging with apertures are created in which the shape of each aperture is defined by the terminal positions of the leading leaf tips and the starting positions of the trailing leaf tips.

Intensity-modulated treatments may be delivered remotely or automatically under computer control. The treatment machine computer may automatically set up the various components of the machine and switch on the radiation beam. For the sliding-window technique, the leaves move during radiation in the sequence specified in the leaf motion dataset. In the step-and-shoot mode, the radiation pauses while the leaves move. At the completion of the first field, the computer sets the machine for the next field and again goes through its leaf motion sequence and irradiation. This process is repeated until all fields have delivered. The treatment times may vary

somewhat and depend on the number of fields involved and the complexity of the fluence distribution. Current time estimates range from 5 to 20 minutes, excluding patient setup.[4,5,40]

SETUP AND IMRT DELIVERY WITH SERIAL TOMOTHERAPY

Current delivery of serial tomotherapy is concisely described in a review.[172] A new-generation serial treatment machine with multiple photon heads as well as an electron source has been described by Achterberg and Müller.[173] Because there are no specific beam directions or portals associated with serial tomotherapy beam delivery, the treatment QA concentrates on patient positioning and immobilization. The add-on multileaf collimator (MIMiC) is relatively heavy and its removal is time consuming, so portal films often are acquired with the MIMiC in place. This limits the portal fields to a roughly 3.4- × 20-cm² field size. Therefore, the imaging of useful, immobile, bony anatomic landmarks is critical for each port film, meaning that the selection of the portal film locations is critical to the accurate determination of patient-treated indices, but the digitally reconstructed radiograph that is used to compare against the portal film must be simulated at the same relative couch position as the portal film is acquired. Typically, anterior–posterior and lateral films are acquired, and if the target is longer than 10 cm and is in a location where patient structures are flexible (e.g., in the neck), portal films may be required at multiple couch positions to ensure the patient is in the correct orientation throughout the length of treatment.

Treatments are conducted by placing the patient on the couch and aligning the patient to the linear accelerator in the standard fashion. Once the patient is aligned (to a point analogous to isocenter for conventional treatments), the couch translation device (called *CRANE*) coordinates are set to zero, and the couch is moved to the location of the first index. This position is determined by the treatment planning system. The gantry is rotated to the starting arc position, and the patient treatment plan is loaded onto the MIMiC control computer. The linear accelerator is operated in normal arc mode, and the MIMiC control computer determines if the treatment can proceed. If the gantry speed is within acceptable limits, the MLC leaves are opened in their programmed sequence. The MIMiC communicates with the linear accelerator using the conventional door interlock. If the MIMiC control computer determines the treatment should not continue, the door interlock circuit is interrupted, and the linear accelerator ceases operation just as if the door had been opened (the door interlock fault is tripped on the accelerator). Once the arc is delivered, the therapist enters the room to move the CRANE to the next couch position and reprograms the MIMiC control computer by following the screen prompts.

TOMOTHERAPY VERSUS FIXED-GANTRY IMRT

The physical and operational differences between tomotherapy and fixed-gantry IMRT lead to trade-offs when considering each system. The rotational beams used in tomotherapy could be a significant advantage until robust beam configuration optimization tools are developed, particularly those involving noncoplanar beams.

For serial tomotherapy delivery, one of the difficulties is the requirement of precisely moving the patient between successive arc deliveries (couch indexes). The dose delivery error made for an incorrect junction move is similar to the errors in abutting conventional fields. Studies have shown that the maximum dose error is 25% mm^{-1} in the abutment region for errors in couch index movement or intrajunction patient motion.[174] When conventional fields are abutted, feathering often is used to reduce the risk of systematic dose errors. A similar technique has been suggested for distributing the abutment regions for serial tomotherapy[175] by creating multiple treatment plans with modified target volumes to force a redistribution of indexes.

Even when perfectly abutted, there are dose heterogeneities within the abutment region caused by the divergent radiation fields, especially when arcs of <360 degrees are used. Low et al.[174] studied the abutment region dose distributions for arcs ranging from 180 to 340 degrees and determined that the tumor doses can have significant cold spots when short arcs are used. These become more severe when the longer leaf setting (1.7 cm) is used. The accuracy of the treatment planning system in predicting these heterogeneities was not evaluated, but the system tends to underestimate the severity of the heterogeneities. Although the divergence in the radiation beams is still present in helical tomotherapy, the helical path of the field edge distributes the diverging distribution such that dose errors caused by inaccuracies in couch motion, or by patient movement, are significantly smaller than with serial tomotherapy.

One of the advantages of fixed-gantry IMRT is the availability of noncoplanar directions. The commercial hardware device used to precisely move the couch between successive indexes also is produced in a model that attaches directly to the couch, allowing for couch rotations. Although limited noncoplanar dose delivery is possible when using serial tomotherapy, especially when treating the brain, this has not been widely adopted.

Gating for serial tomotherapy is impractical because of the use of conventional linear accelerators and the lack of shared information between the MLC and the linear accelerator control computers. Breath hold techniques are also impractical because of the relatively long time to rotate the linear accelerator gantry. Because of the potentially large abutment region dosimetry errors, it is important to consider the immobilization accuracy of targets and critical structures when selecting targets for serial tomotherapy. Gating for helical tomotherapy is possible by pausing the radiation beam and the couch motion when the gating circuitry dictates that no treatment should be delivered. However, there will be a delay in restarting the treatment after the gating signal has been restarted while waiting for the gantry to return to its position when the gating signal was interrupted.

Because the dose is delivered over many indexes or gantry rotations, there are many more MUs used when treating with tomotherapy than for conventional 3DCRT or MLC-based IMRT. The ratio of MUs can be as high as 10:1 even when compared with MLC-based IMRT.[176] This increase in MUs leads to increases in whole-body dose that may yield a significant increase in secondary radiation-induced malignancies. The solution to this is to improve the linear accelerator head shielding, the source of most of the whole-body dose in tomotherapy.

Another limitation of tomotherapy is the lack of electron beams. Electron beams (including energy and intensity-modulated electron beams), by themselves or in combination with intensity-modulated photon beams, currently are employed in the treatment of both breast and skin cancers.

A major advantage of helical tomotherapy is that it is a dedicated IMRT device. However, MLC-based IMRT is likely to compete as a delivery mode resulting in part from the limitations of tomotherapy discussed earlier. Furthermore, the large base of MLC-mounted linear accelerators will mean that the adoption of tomotherapy for significant numbers of IMRT patient treatments will take years.

SPECIAL REQUIREMENTS OF FACILITY DESIGN FOR IMRT

The room-shielding design characteristics for IMRT delivery are different than those for conventional radiotherapy. Shielding requirements are determined separately for primary and scattered radiation barriers and for tomotherapy and MLC-based IMRT. For MLC-based IMRT, the total integrated radiation fluence remains similar to that used in conformal therapy, so no change in primary barrier thicknesses is expected. However, the increase in MUs of about a factor of 3 is expected to increase the required secondary shielding barrier attenuation, at least until the linear accelerator manufacturers improve the head leakage characteristics. For serial tomotherapy without a beam stopper, the same primary barrier is struck for each couch index, indicating that an increase in primary barrier thickness may be required. However, the use of a rotating beam, and the relatively small angle subtended by the MIMiC, reduces effective use factor to the point that it almost exactly cancels the number of times the beam strikes the primary barrier. Increases in secondary shielding, however, may be greater than for IMRT because the total number of MUs is significantly greater.

CLINICAL EXPERIENCE WITH IMRT

IMRT of Head and Neck Cancer

The first report of the application of IMRT to head and neck neoplasms was from Baylor College. Kuppersmith et al.[177] reported a decrease in dose to the parotid glands to <30 Gy in 28 patients treated with IMRT using serial tomotherapy. They also found the incidence of acute toxicity to be drastically lower than with conventional radiation therapy. Later, Butler et al.[178] implemented the "simultaneous modulated accelerated radiation therapy"[179] technique, an equivalent of the SIB technique, and found that 19 out of 20 patients treated had complete response with acceptable toxicity. Low et al.[180] described the application of the serial tomotherapy technique and QA practices for head and neck treatments at Washington University in St. Louis. Preliminary results of the use of these techniques for 17 patients were reported by Chao et al.[101] and showed that the tumor control is promising with no severe adverse acute side effects. A subsequent prospective clinical study conducted by Chao et al.[181] also showed that the sparing of parotid glands translated into objective and subjective improvement of both xerostomia and quality of life scores in patients with head and neck cancers treated with IMRT.

In another study, Chao et al.[182] also reported the dosimetric advantage of IMRT treatment in patients with oropharyngeal carcinoma (260 with primary tumors in the tonsil and 170 with primary tumors at the base of the tongue). No adverse impact on local tumor control or disease-free survival (DFS) was seen, but there was a significant reduction of late salivary toxicity. Fixed-field IMRT and serial tomography gave superior GTV coverage and lower parotid doses compared to conventional RT in nasopharyngeal cancer.[183] Groups at Memorial Sloan-Kettering[184] and UCSF[185] found similar results for nasopharyngeal patients. IMRT likewise showed promise for oral and oropharyngeal cancer[186] and in dose escalation studies of head and neck squamous cell carcinoma.[13,100] Examples of target delineation for nasopharyngeal and hypopharyngeal cancer are shown in Figures 11.17 and 11.18, respectively.

Since the early part of the past decade, IMRT usage in head and neck cancers has become the standard of care. The Web of Science database records 2,087 papers with "head and neck" and "IMRT" in the title from 2002 through 2016. Of these, 1,044 appeared in or after 2012. Review articles pertaining to head and neck cancers include the following: Lee and Terezakis[187] in 2008 and Maingon et al.[188] in 2010. Lu and Yao[189] found improved quality of life and survival benefit in IMRT treatment of nasopharyngeal cancer. Reviews focused on quality of life issues include Scott-Brown et al.[190] and Tribius and Bergelt[191]; swallowing issues are reviewed by Roe et al.[192] Early work by Chao et al.[181,182] showed significant reduction in salivary gland toxicity in the IMRT-treated patients. Nutting et al.[193] reported the results from a head-to-head phase III trial of IMRT versus conventional radiation therapy in patients with pharyngeal squamous cell carcinoma (T1–T4, N0–N3, M0). The IMRT arm showed significantly less grade 2 (or worse) xerostomia compared to radiation therapy: at 12 months, 74% for radiation therapy versus 38% for IMRT, and at 24 months, 83% for radiation therapy versus 29% for IMRT. At 24 months, no significant differences were seen in other toxicities or in local tumor control or overall survival.

This raises a question—given the increased complexity and cost in equipment and physician/physicist/staff time for IMRT compared to conventional radiation therapy, is the improvement in quality of life alone worth the cost? This was the *raison d'être* for the study by Tribius and Bergelt.[191] and the answer is obviously yes for the patient. More to the point, what possibilities are there for improvement of outcome in survival and locoregional control? IMRT by itself is still radiation therapy—the photon sources do not have the coherence of an optical laser, so there are beam-edge effects and also beam scattering from the MLC leaves and within the patient's body as the depth increases. This puts limits on the dose gradients that can actually be achieved, and if OAR sparing is to occur, it will mean less homogeneous doses to the GTV. There are several ways to approach this problem:

1. Better imaging during a course of treatment. Changes in tumor size and/or location during treatment will require imaging to adjust the IMRT plan and possibly adaptive radiation therapy. Various promising imaging modalities useful for radiation oncology were reviewed by Apisarnthanarax and Chao[74]; more recently Moeller et al.[77] reported on a prospective trial using FDG-PET and CT imaging in head and neck cancer. Cone beam CT has also been reviewed recently.[194]

2. Accelerated fractionation. One makes use of the radiobiologic advantages of IMRT to perform dose escalation to tumor while constraining the dose to critical normal tissue.[14] Ling et al.[195] have discussed the effects of dose rate in terms of the widely used linear-quadratic model. Chakraborty et al.[196,197] observed 95% DFS in 20 patients with squamous cell carcinomas at various head and neck sites, but the SIB group treated at a higher dose did have more acute toxicities.

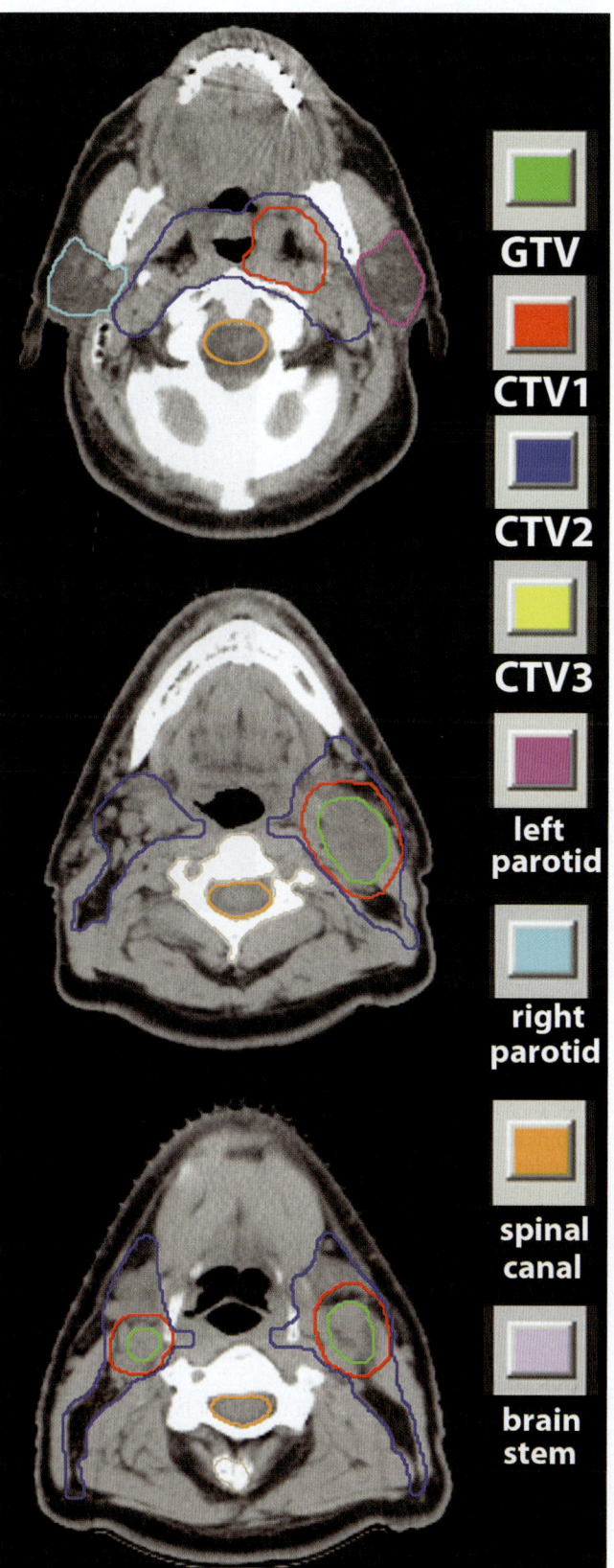

FIGURE 11.17. Intensity-modulated radiation therapy (IMRT) target delineation for stage T2N2 nasopharyngeal cancer. Three axial slices are shown. CTV, clinical tumor volume; GTV, gross tumor volume.

3. Combined modality treatment. Combined chemotherapy and radiation treatment is the current approach for locally advanced head and neck squamous cell carcinoma.[198] Chemoradiation for locally advanced head and

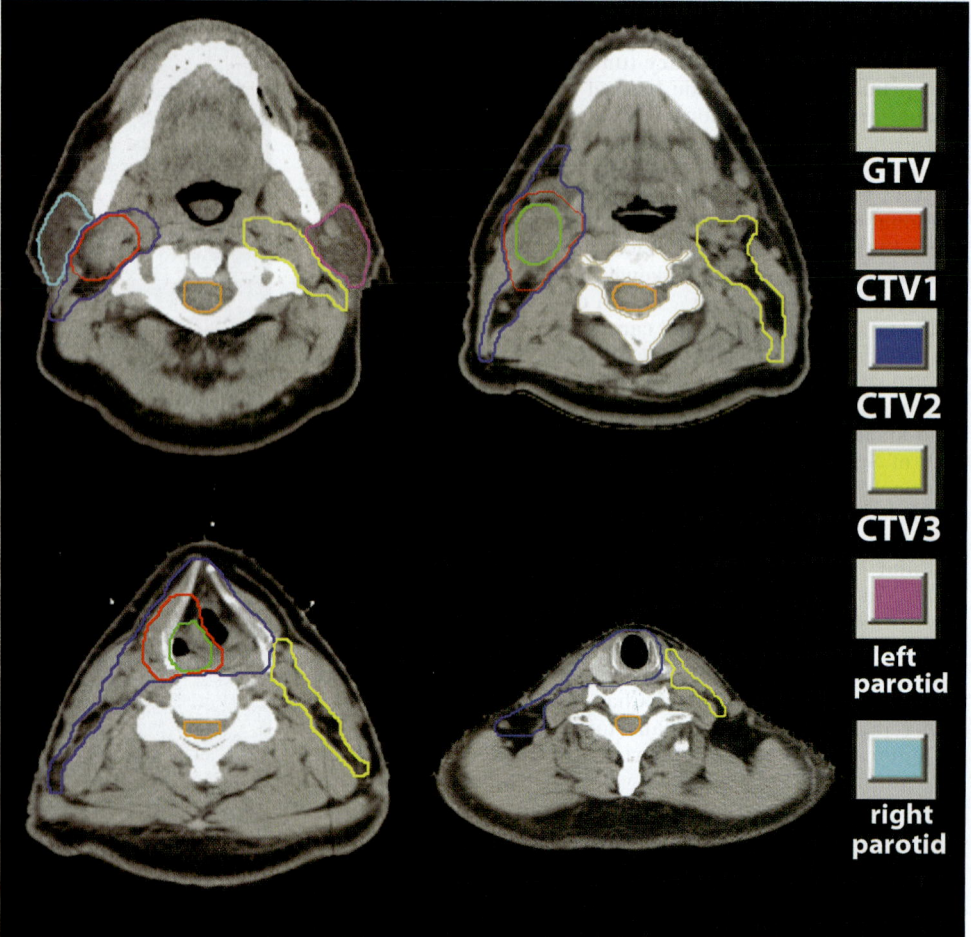

FIGURE 11.18. Intensity-modulated radiation therapy (IMRT) target delineation for stage T2N1 hypopharyngeal cancer. Four axial slices are shown; the spinal canal is contoured in orange. CTV, clinical tumor volume; GTV, gross tumor volume.

neck disease has also been reviewed by Seiwert et al.[199] Similar themes were expressed in the 2008 Southwest Oncology Group report.[200] Riesterer et al. discuss the last decade of work on chemosensitization with molecular signaling agents followed by radiation.[201]

New technologies, in particular beams of charged heavy ions (protons or carbon), show promise because of their highly depth-dependent energy deposition profile (the spread-out Bragg peak). Thariat et al. recently published a concise review of these and other techniques as applied to head and neck cancers.[202] Heavy ion beam therapy is very costly and available only at a few centers, so in the immediate future, it will likely be limited to those cases such as malignancies close to the eyes or optic chiasm where photon beams cause unacceptable vision loss.

IMRT of Prostate Cancer

The prostate was one of the first targets of IMRT in the work of Ling et al. at Memorial Sloan-Kettering.[4,5] Studies involving hundreds of patients followed: in 2000, Zelefsky et al.[203] demonstrated superior target coverage with IMRT compared to conventional RT and 3DCRT; in 2002, they reported a larger study showing the feasibility of high-dose IMRT with reduced acute toxicities.[204]

A total of 772 patients were treated: 698 to 81.0 Gy and 74 to 86.4 Gy. Acute grade 2 rectal toxicity was seen in 35 (4.5%), but none at grade 3 or above. Acute grade 2 urinary symptoms developed in 217 patients (28%), but only 1 patient with grade 3 problems. Late rectal bleeding (grade 2) was experienced by 11 patients (1.5%). PSA relapse-free survival rates (3-year actuarial) were 92%, 86%, and 81% for the favorable, intermediate, and high-risk groups, respectively.

This early work was extended by other workers,[205,206] and the field has been extensively reviewed.[207–209]

Combined radiation and hormonal therapy is used for patients at higher risk. For a review, see Sanfilippo et al.,[210] who reported on a phase I/II trial in 22 patients with locally advanced hormone-ablated disease (T1–T3). Paclitaxel was given biweekly, with four-field 3DCRT starting at 63 Gy and escalating to 66.6, 70.2, and 73.8 Gy. Acute toxicities included diarrhea (mostly grade 1 and 2, but with grade 3 in four patients); at 38 months, 21 (95%) were alive. But 6 of 22 (27%) had developed relapsed disease. Tucker et al.[211,212] analyzed Radiation Therapy Oncology Group (RTOG) 9406 data to obtain Lyman NTCP parameters and the linear-quadratic α/β ratio for late rectal toxicity in prostate-irradiated patients.

The treatment of prostate cancer has been greatly impacted by advances in magnetic resonance, both standard MRI and magnetic resonance spectroscopic imaging (MRSI). This growing field has been extensively reviewed; for two recent articles, see Sciarra et al.[213] and Mazaheri et al.[174,214] Magnetic resonance can often "see" details of the prostate tumor that are not observable on a CT scan. MRI can be used for much more precise tumor target delineation for IMRT than would otherwise be possible, and this has had significant clinical impact.

IMRT of Intracranial Malignancies

With FDG-PET and/or MRI, tumors within the brain can be visualized more clearly than on CT. Given the desire to avoid extensive neurologic damage, IMRT is expected to offer some advantages in sparing normal tissues and possibly improving the often bleak prognosis of central nervous system cancer patients. For example, Gutierrez et al.[215] reported a planning study with tomotherapy to provide an integrated boost to whole-brain irradiation in an effort to spare the hippocampus. This has also been replicated in RTOG and ongoing NRG Oncology trials.

Iuchi et al.[216] from Japan published a retrospective report on 25 patients with malignant astrocytomas (World Health Organization grade III and IV) treated with IMRT using a hypofractionated regimen of 48 to 68 Gy in eight fractions. Thirteen patients were treated to 68 Gy and 12 patients received doses of 48 to 65 Gy. The IMRT group was compared to 60 patients treated with conventional techniques to doses of 40 to 60 Gy using 2 Gy daily fractions. The 2-year overall survival was significantly improved ($P = .043$) in patients treated with hypofractionated IMRT (55.6%) compared to those patients treated with conventional techniques (19.4%).

Huang et al.[217] reported on 15 patients with pediatric medulloblastoma treated with conventional craniospinal radiotherapy followed by a boost to the posterior fossa using IMRT. IMRT delivered lower doses of radiation to the auditory apparatus while maintaining full doses to the desired target volume. Their findings suggested that, despite receiving higher doses of cisplatin and despite receiving radiotherapy before cisplatin therapy, IMRT can significantly decrease the rate of hearing loss in children treated for medulloblastoma.

Glioblastoma multiforme (GBM) has a very poor outcome, with a median survival of 12 to 16 months following resection.[218] Floyd et al.[219] used hypofractionated IMRT tomotherapy to treat 20 patients with primary disease. Fifty Gy in 10 daily fractions was given with 30 Gy (10 fx) to surrounding edema. Time to disease progression was 7 months, so no gain in survival was seen, but the treatment time was reduced from 6 to 2 weeks. Stupp et al.[220] studied outcomes in GBM patients after resection who were treated with RT with or without adjuvant temozolomide: the chemoradiation group had a median survival of 14.6 months compared to 12.1 months with RT alone. A review of temozolomide therapy for brain tumors was recently done by Koukourakis et al.[221] Amelio et al.[222] recently reviewed the use of IMRT, including hypofractionation, in the treatment of glioblastoma and in particular for elderly patients. They concluded that there is clinical advantage with IMRT because higher doses can be given in shorter times without increasing toxicity.

IMRT of Breast Cancer

Radiation therapy for breast cancer poses challenges, in particular large differences in tissue thickness in the radiation field and the close proximity of the lung apex and the heart, coupled with target motion during the breathing cycle. Taylor et al.[223] reviewed excess mortality because of cardiac damage in patients treated from 1950 through 1990, when cardiac doses of up to 14 to 17 Gy were given. In addition, part of the radiation field contains the skin boundary between tissue and air. Because air scatters much less of the x-ray fluence, there can be significant dose inhomogeneities and overdosing of the skin ("skin flash"). Commercial systems are available that can autocontour the volume of breast tissue within conventionally designed tangential photon portals and then use an inverse planning algorithm to optimize dose homogeneity within these tangential portals. However, most commercial inverse planning systems could not handle the "skin flash" appropriately. The traditional IMRT technique to overcome target motion uncertainty (such as breathing) is to expand the PTV and optimize the dose coverage to the entire PTV. However, this strategy may not work because a portion of the PTV will be expanded into the air, which does not have the necessary mass to absorb the dose. Some treatment planning systems ignore the regions outside the skin contour entirely. Therefore, it may be necessary to add "virtual" tissues in the PTV for the inverse planning system. Sometimes, it may require users to manually open certain IMRT segments to take care of the skin flash effect.

Nevertheless, there has been interest in using IMRT for left-sided breast cancers in order to spare myocardium from the high-dose region of the radiotherapy fields. The Guerrero

Urbano and Nutting IMRT review includes a concise summary of early work through about 2002.[224] No robust data regarding clinical outcomes after IMRT for breast cancer exist; however, a variety of dosimetric studies[225-231] have suggested reductions in lung and myocardium doses when IMRT is compared to conventional radiotherapeutic techniques. Hurkmans et al.[232] used an NTCP model to estimate the NTCP for cardiac and lung complications because of radiotherapy and found that IMRT did decrease the NTCP for late cardiac toxicity compared to more conventional radiotherapy techniques but had a minimal effect on the NTCP for radiation pneumonitis. A potential drawback is a larger volume of normal tissue in the thorax receiving lower radiation dose levels.

Hong et al.[227] reported a dosimetric study of IMRT in 10 cases of intact breast cancer showing significant reduction of dose to the coronary arteries, ipsilateral lung, and surrounding soft tissues. It simultaneously improved dose homogeneity throughout the target volume. Li et al.[228] described a combined electron and IMRT technique for breast cancer treatment, which led to improvement over the conventional treatment technique using tangential fields with reduced dose to the ipsilateral lung and the heart. Other studies[226,231] also confirmed that IMRT reduces the high-dose volume in tangential breast irradiation significantly and enables more complete cardiac sparing without compromising PTV coverage in some patients. Furthermore, IMRT creates a possibility to improve field matching in case of multiple field irradiations of the breast and lymph nodes.[231,233,234] In addition, IMRT for tangential breast radiation therapy was found to be an effective and efficient method to achieve uniform dose throughout the breast. Preliminary findings showed minimal or no acute skin reactions with different breast sizes in 32 patients with early-stage breast cancer.[233] Taylor et al.[235] reviewed results of RT of breast cancer patients in 2006 and found that use of more modern planning had significantly reduced mean heart doses to 2.3 Gy but that a small part of the heart still received more than 20 Gy in left-sided irradiation.

IMRT of Gynecologic Cancer

In regard to the targeting of pelvic lymphatics with IMRT, Taylor et al.[236] mapped the pelvic lymphatics of 20 patients using MRI with the administration of iron oxide particles and found that a modified CTV margin of 7 mm around the iliac vessels resulted in adequate coverage of the pelvic lymphatics.

Ahamad et al.[237] analyzed the normal tissue-sparing effects of IMRT in the treatment of the pelvis after hysterectomy in patients with gynecologic cancers and found that although more small bowel, bladder, and rectum could be spared with IMRT compared to conventional radiotherapeutic techniques, these benefits rapidly diminished with even small expansions of the target volumes. D'Souza et al.[238] used the same dataset of patients as Ahamad et al.[237] and found that IMRT may allow higher doses of radiation (54 Gy) to be delivered safely to the node-bearing regions of the pelvis and the vaginal apex compared to conventional techniques that administer 50.4 Gy. Gielda et al.[179] reported on a small study of gynecologic cancer patients ineligible for brachytherapy who were treated with tomotherapy in an attempt to reduce toxicity to bowel and femoral heads.

Salama et al.[239] reported on 13 patients treated with extended field pelvic and para-aortic radiotherapy using IMRT and found that two patients experienced grade 3 or higher toxicity. Both of these patients received concurrent cisplatin-based chemotherapy.

Portelance et al.[240] described dosimetric comparison between 3DCRT and IMRT for 10 patients with cervical cancer. They demonstrated that, with similar target coverage, normal tissue sparing was superior with IMRT. Mundt et al.[241] reported the clinical experience of 40 patients with gynecologic malignancy who underwent IMRT to the pelvis. Compared with 35 historic control patients who were treated with conventional techniques, patients treated with IMRT experienced fewer acute gastrointestinal (GI) symptoms than those treated with conventional whole-pelvic radiotherapy. The ability of IMRT to deliver local control while reducing grade ≥2 bowel toxicity was shown in a recent report by Portelance et al.[242] from the multi-institutional RTOG 0418 cervical cancer trial. Ring et al.[243] did a study on 36 patients with FIGO (International Federation of Gynecology and Obstetrics) stage IB2 to IIIB cervical cancer. They were treated with extended field radiation therapy with concurrent cisplatin to target suspicious pelvic or para-aortic lymph nodes or excessive local pelvic tumor burden. At 32 months, 24 patients were disease-free and an additional 8 were still alive but with disease.

IMRT of Gastrointestinal Cancer

Pancreatic cancer remains a disease with a poor prognosis. In 1995, Lillemoe[244] reviewed then-current disease management. By this time, mortality from surgical resection had been reduced to 2% or 3%, but the weighted average 5-year overall survival was still only about 22%. In 2011, Showalter et al.[245] reanalyzed the data from RTOG 9704 on the results of surgical resection and adjuvant chemoradiation. Interpolating their Figure 11.2, one can estimate 5-year overall survival as about 28% for node negative and 19% for one to three positive nodes—not significantly different in 15 years.

Crane et al.[246] attempted a dose escalation study with RT and gemcitabine in unresectable pancreatic cancer patients but had to discontinue due to dose-limiting toxicity.

Ben-Josef et al.[247] reported on 15 patients with pancreatic cancer treated with concurrent capecitabine and IMRT (45 to 55 Gy) and reported that only one patient had grade 3 GI toxicity, specifically GI ulceration, which responded to medical management.

Brown et al.[248] performed a dosimetric analysis of 15 patients with pancreatic cancer and compared 3DCRT, IMRT with sequential boost, and IMRT with integrated boost and found that IMRT with integrated boost allowed dose escalation up to 64.8 Gy to the primary tumor. More recently, Yovino et al.[249] reported that IMRT produced a statistically significant reduction in upper and lower GI toxicity compared to 3DCRT in chemoradiation treatment following RTOG 9704 guidelines.

IMRT for GI cancers (including pancreas) was recently reviewed by Bockbrader and Kim[250] from the radiobiologic and dosimetric as well as clinical outcomes viewpoint. Meyer et al.[251] gave the rationale for IMRT with PET/CT in anorectal cancers as to reduce radiation-associated morbidity. They also present some clinical data.

Guerrero Urbano et al.[252] performed a dosimetric evaluation in five patients with locally advanced rectal cancer and found that IMRT with SIB theoretically reduced the radiation dose to the small bowel compared to 3D conformal techniques. Milano et al.[253] reported on 17 patients with squamous cell carcinomas of the anal canal treated with IMRT with whole-pelvic radiation doses of 45 Gy followed by boost to the anal canal. Thirteen patients received concurrent 5-fluorouracil and mitomycin C chemotherapy. Treatment was well tolerated with no grade 3 or higher nonhematologic toxicity and no required treatment breaks from skin or GI toxicity. However, one patient receiving mitomycin C chemotherapy did experience grade 4 hematologic toxicity. Three patients who did not achieve a complete response required abdominoperineal resection and colostomy. With a mean follow-up of 20.3 months, there were no other local failures.

Milano et al.[254] also reported on seven patients with gastric cancer treated with IMRT to a dose of 50.4 Gy. No patient experienced grade 3 toxicity. The treated IMRT plans were compared to conventional anterior–posterior/posterior–anterior and three-field plans, and the IMRT plans were found to provide better coverage of the target volumes compared to conventional techniques, with better sparing of the liver and kidneys.

RTOG0529 reported in their dose-painted IMRT technique that dose–volume normal tissue design is somewhat predictive for acute and late GI toxicity for anal carcinoma chemoradiotherapy.[255]

IMRT of Lung Cancer

Because of concerns regarding respiratory motion in radiation therapy of lung cancer, the use of IMRT requires some method to account for tumor and organ motion during treatment planning and delivery; these techniques include both respiratory gating[134] and four-dimensional CT planning.[256] Starkschall et al.[257] recently reported direct 4D CT measurements of interfraction GTV movement during free breathing and concluded that breath hold gating provides reproducible tumor localization. With cone beam CT or orthovoltage x-ray, the appropriate margins are 0.3 cm for implanted fiducials and 0.8 cm for bony landmarks.

The poor local tumor control rates of conventional radiation therapy doses in the treatment of lung cancer[258] have led to much interest in using IMRT to allow for dose escalation to improve local control. Holloway et al.[259] reported the initial results of five patients with unresectable stage II and III non–small cell carcinoma treated on a phase I dose escalation trial using induction chemotherapy followed by IMRT to a dose of 84 Gy (2.4 Gy daily fractions). PET/CT was used to define target volumes. One patient developed lethal radiation pneumonitis and the trial was halted. Murshed et al.[260] performed a dosimetric analysis of 41 patients initially treated with 3DCRT to a dose of 63 Gy. IMRT plans were generated using these patients' initial planning CT scans, and IMRT was found to decrease the volume of lung irradiated to both 10 and 20 Gy. Target coverage was improved with IMRT, and the volumes of heart and esophagus irradiation were also reduced. Figures 11.19 and 11.20 illustrate MLC portals and IMRT treatment plans for lung cancer.

Grills et al.[261] performed a dosimetric comparison of four radiotherapy techniques in 18 patients with stages I to IIB lung cancer comparing IMRT, optimized multiple-beam 3DCRT, two- to three-beam 3DCRT, and traditional wide-field radiotherapy with elective nodal irradiation. This study found that IMRT and optimized 3DCRT resulted in similar doses of radiotherapy to normal tissues in node-negative patients; however, in node-positive patients, IMRT resulted in a 15% decrease in the volume of lung treated to 20 Gy (V_{20} GY) and a 30% decrease in the NTCP for radiation pneumonitis. In 2010, Liao et al.[262] reported the outcomes of 409 non–small cell lung carcinoma patients treated at MD Anderson. Three hundred and eighteen patients received CT/3DCRT and 91 received 4D CT/IMRT to a median dose of 63 Gy. The mean lung dose was slightly higher for the IMRT group (24.9 Gy compared to 22.1), but the mean and 95% confidence interval range was lower for IMRT (34.4% ± 1.2% vs. 37.0% ± 1.1%). When corrected for factors such as smoking status, histology, and nodal status, the hazard ratio for IMRT to 3DCRT was significantly less than one, as was that for toxicity (grade 3 pneumonitis), whereas distant metastases were similar. Therefore, IMRT gave similar or better results in terms of survival and local control while reducing treatment toxicity. Vogelius et al.[263,264] pose a cautionary warning—their dosimetric modeling showed that when RT is used in combination with chemotherapy, the larger volume exposed to lower radiation doses in IMRT could pose problems with pneumonitis as compared to 3DCRT or proton therapy.

IMRT Experience with Other Cancer Sites

Complementing strong evidence supporting the use of IMRT in head and neck and prostate cancer, a number of studies report the feasibility and outcomes of IMRT in other cancers;

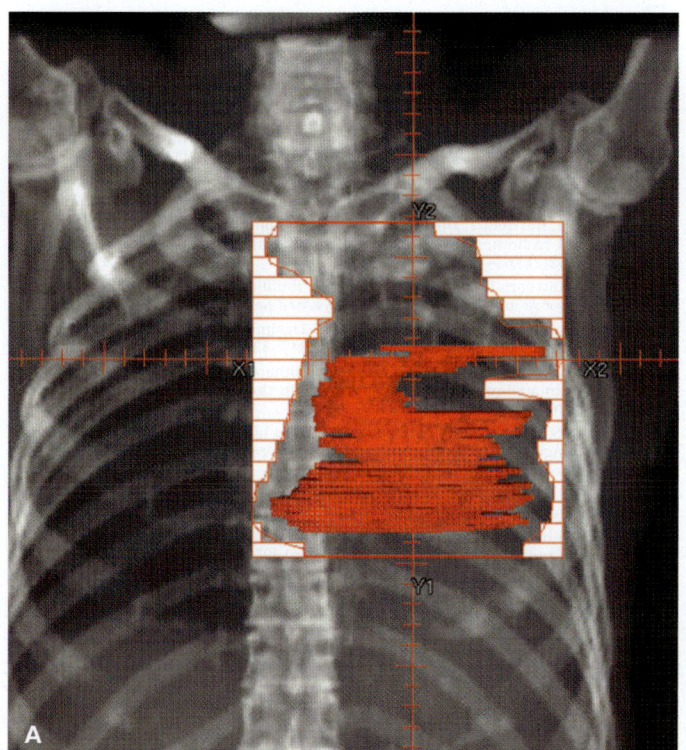

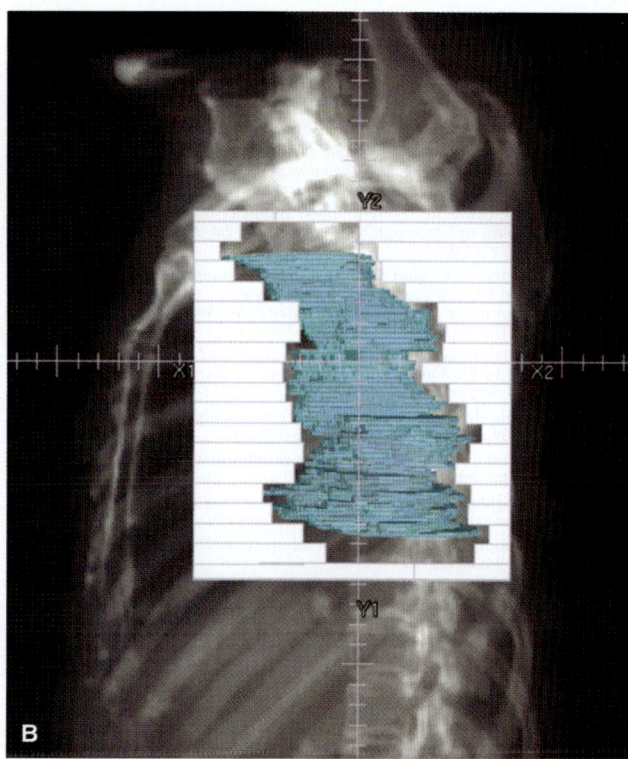

FIGURE 11.19. Illustration of anterior–posterior **(A)** and oblique **(B)** multileaf collimator configuration.

many of these reports are theoretical dosimetric studies. Theoretically, improved dosimetry alone probably does not serve as sufficient justification for the routine use of IMRT in these cases, and in the absence of robust clinical data regarding actual treatment outcomes, IMRT in these settings should be considered investigational.

In closing, IMRT results in improved radiation dose distributions in a variety of cancers. In some cases, the superior dosimetry of IMRT has resulted in improved clinical outcomes for patients; however, the scientific evidence documenting these clinical improvements lags far behind the data documenting

improved dosimetry. Many patients present with disease for which the likelihood of cure is remote, but for whom reduction of tumor burden with fewer debilitating toxicities will be an attractive option. Reduction in treatment morbidity is an immediately realizable benefit of IMRT. Improvement of survival will require better ability to image the biologic activity of malignancies, and this is an area of very active research. It is incumbent on radiation oncologists to continue to document improved clinical outcomes with IMRT in the peer-reviewed literature if we wish to justify the use of this expensive technology to our communities in an era of skyrocketing medical costs.

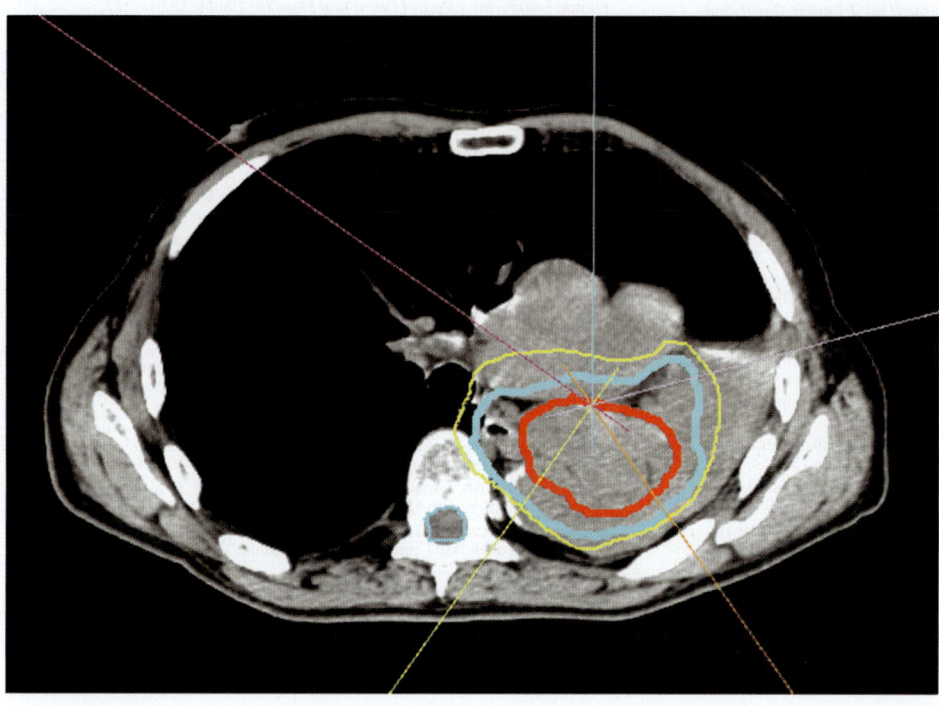

FIGURE 11.20. Intensity-modulated radiation therapy (IMRT) plan for locally advanced non–small cell lung cancer. Inner red line is the gross tumor volume (GTV); clinical tumor volume (CTV) is shown as a light blue aqua contour, which includes nodal regions to left of the GTV. The outermost yellow contour is the 60-Gy iso-dose line.

REFERENCES

1. ICRU. ICRU report 83: prescribing, recording, and reporting photon-beam intensity-modulated radiation therapy (IMRT). *J ICRU* 2010;10(1):1–106.
2. Bernier J, Hall EJ, Giaccia A. Timeline—radiation oncology: a century of achievements. *Nat Rev Cancer* 2004;4(9):737–747.
3. Carol MP. Peacock (TM)—a system for planning and rotational delivery of intensity-modulated fields. *Int J Imaging Syst Technol* 1995;6(1):56–61.
4. Ling CC, Burman C, Chui CS, et al. Conformal radiation treatment of prostate cancer using inversely-planned intensity-modulated photon beams produced with dynamic multileaf collimation. *Int J Radiat Oncol Biol Phys* 1996;35(4):721–730.
5. Ling CC, Burman C, Chui CS, et al. Implementation of photon IMRT with dynamic leaf MLC for the treatment of prostate cancer. In: Sternick ES, ed. *The theory and practice of intensity-modulated radiation therapy*. Pittsburgh, PA: NOMOS, 1997:219–228.
6. Holmes T, Das R, Low D, et al. American Society of Radiation Oncology recommendations for documenting intensity-modulated radiation therapy treatments. *Int J Radiat Oncol Biol Phys* 2009;74(5):1311–1318.
7. Mell LK, Mehrotra AK, Mundt AJ. Intensity-modulated radiation therapy use in the U.S., 2004. *Cancer* 2005;104(6):1296–1303.
8. Mell LK, Roeske JC, Mundt AJ. A survey of intensity-modulated radiation therapy use in the United States. *Cancer* 2003;98(1):204–211.
9. Bortfeld T, Schlegel W. Optimization of beam orientations in radiation therapy: some theoretical considerations. *Phys Med Biol* 1993;38(2):291–304.
10. Webb S. Optimizing the planning of intensity-modulated radiotherapy. *Phys Med Biol* 1994;39(12):2229–2246.
11. Sodertrom S, Brahme A. Optimization of the dose delivery in a few field techniques using radiobiological objective functions. *Med Phys* 1993;20(4):1201–1210.
12. Bai YR, Wu GH, Guo WJ, et al. Intensity modulated radiation therapy and chemotherapy for locally advanced pancreatic cancer: results of feasibility study. *World J Gastroenterol* 2003;9(11):2561–2564.
13. Lauve A, Morris M, Schmidt-Ullrich R, et al. Simultaneous integrated boost intensity-modulated radiotherapy for locally advanced head-and-neck squamous cell carcinomas: II–clinical results. *Int J Radiat Oncol Biol Phys* 2004;60(2):374–387.
14. Orlandi E, Palazzi M, Pignoli E, et al. Radiobiological basis and clinical results of the simultaneous integrated boost (SIB) in intensity modulated radiotherapy (IMRT) for head and neck cancer: a review. *Crit Rev Oncol Hematol* 2010;73(2):111–125.
15. Mechalakos J, Lee N, Hunt M, et al. The effect of significant tumor reduction on the dose distribution in intensity modulated radiation therapy for head-and-neck cancer: a case study. *Med Dosim* 2009;34(3):250–255.
16. Mohan R, Wu Q, Manning M, et al. Radiobiological considerations in the design of fractionation strategies for intensity-modulated radiation therapy of head and neck cancers. *Int J Radiat Oncol Biol Phys* 2000;46(3):619–630.
17. Preiser K, Bortfeld T, Hartwig K, et al. Inverse radiotherapy planning for intensity-modulated photon fields. *Radiologe* 1998;38(3):228–234.
18. Wang XH, Mohan R, Jackson A, et al. Optimization of intensity-modulated 3D conformal treatment plans based on biological indexes. *Radiother Oncol* 1995;37(2):140–152.
19. Mackie TR, Holmes TW, Reckwerdt PJ, et al. Tomotherapy–optimized planning and delivery of radiation-therapy. *Int J Imaging Syst Technol* 1995;6(1):43–55.
20. Allison RR, Gay HA, Mota HC, et al. Image-guided radiation therapy: current and future directions. *Future Oncol (London, England)* 2006;2(4):477–492.
21. Barth NH. An inverse problem in radiation therapy. *Int J Radiat Oncol Biol Phys* 1990;18(2):425–431.
22. Bortfeld T, Burkelbach J, Boesecke R, et al. Methods of image reconstruction from projections applied to conformation radiotherapy. *Phys Med Biol* 1990;35(10):1423–1434.
23. Bortfeld T, Burkelbach J, Boesecke R, et al. Three-dimensional solution of the inverse problem in conformation radiotherapy. In: Breit A, ed. *Advanced radiation therapy: tumor response monitoring and treatment planning*. Berlin, Germany: Springer Verlag, 1992:503–508.
24. Bortfeld TR, Kahler DL, Waldron TJ, et al. X-ray field compensation with multileaf collimators. *Int J Radiat Oncol Biol Phys* 1994;28(3):723–730.
25. Carol M, Grant WH III, Pavord D, et al. Initial clinical experience with the Peacock intensity modulation of a 3-D conformal radiation therapy system. *Stereotact Funct Neurosurg* 1996;66(1-3):30–34.
26. Chen Z, Wang X, Bortfeld T, et al. The influence of scatter on the design of optimized intensity modulations. *Med Phys* 1995;22(11 Pt 1):1727–1733.
27. Chui CS, LoSasso T, Spirou S. Dose calculation for photon beams with intensity modulation generated by dynamic jaw or multileaf collimations. *Med Phys* 1994;21(8):1237–1244.
28. Holmes T, Mackie TR. A filtered backprojection dose calculation method for inverse treatment planning. *Med Phys* 1994;21(2):303–313.
29. Kallman P, Lind B, Eklof A, et al. Shaping of arbitrary dose distributions by dynamic multileaf collimation. *Phys Med Biol* 1988;33(11):1291–1300.
30. Mackie TR, Holmes T, Swerdloff S, et al. Tomotherapy: a new concept for the delivery of dynamic conformal radiotherapy. *Med Phys* 1993;20(6):1709–1719.
31. Mohan R, Leibel SA. Intensity modulation of the radiation beam. In: DeVita VT, Hellman S, Rosenberg SA, eds. *Cancer: principles and practice of oncology*. Philadelphia: Lippincott-Raven, 1997:3093–3106.
32. Mohan R, Ling CC, Stein J, et al. The number of beams in intensity-modulated treatments: in response to Drs. Soderstrom and Brahme. *Int J Radiat Oncol Biol Phys* 1996;34(3):758–759.
33. Mohan R, Wang X, Jackson A, et al. The potential and limitations of the inverse radiotherapy technique. *Radiother Oncol* 1994;32(3):232–248.
34. Soderstrom S, Brahme A. Selection of suitable beam orientations in radiation therapy using entropy and Fourier transform measures. *Phys Med Biol* 1992;37(4):911–924.
35. Soderstrom S, Brahme A. Optimization of the dos delivery in a few field techniques using radiobiological objective functions. *Med Phys* 1993;20(4):1201–1210.
36. Spirou SV, Chui CS. Generation of arbitrary intensity profiles by dynamic jaws or multileaf collimators. *Med Phys* 1994;21(7):1031–1041.
37. Spirou SV, Chui CS. Generation of arbitrary intensity profiles by combining the scanning beam with dynamic multileaf collimation. *Med Phys* 1996;23(1):1–8.
38. Stein J, Bortfeld T, Dorschel B, et al. Dynamic X-ray compensation for conformal radiotherapy by means of multi-leaf collimation. *Radiother Oncol* 1994;32(2):163–173.
39. van Santvoort JP, Heijmen BJ. Dynamic multileaf collimation without 'tongue-and-groove' underdosage effects. *Phys Med Biol* 1996;41(10):2091–2105.
40. Wang X, Spirou S, LoSasso T, et al. Dosimetric verification of intensity-modulated fields. *Med Phys* 1996;23(3):317–327.
41. Webb S. Optimization of conformal radiotherapy dose distributions by simulated annealing: 2. Inclusion of scatter in the 2D technique. *Phys Med Biol* 1991;36(9):1227–1237.
42. Webb S, Bortfeld T, Stein J, et al. The effect of stair-step leaf transmission on the 'tongue-and-groove problem' in dynamic radiotherapy with a multileaf collimator. *Phys Med Biol* 1997;42(3):595–602.
43. Yu CX. Intensity-modulated arc therapy with dynamic multileaf collimation: an alternative to tomotherapy. *Phys Med Biol* 1995;40(9):1435–1449.
44. Mohan R, Wu Q, Wang X, et al. Intensity modulation optimization, lateral transport of radiation, and margins. *Med Phys* 1996;23(12):2011–2021.
45. Yu CX. Intensity modulated arc therapy: a new method for delivering conformal radiation therapy. In: Sternick ES, ed. *The theory and practice of intensity modulated radiotherapy*. Madison, WI: Advanced Medical Publishing, 1997:107–120.
46. Otto K. Volumetric modulated arc therapy: IMRT in a single gantry arc. *Med Phys* 2008;35(1):310–317.
47. Bedford JI. Treatment planning for volumetric modulated arc therapy. *Med Phys* 2009;36(11):5128–5138.
48. Yu CX, Tang G. Intensity modulated arc therapy: principles, technologies and clinical implementation. *Phys Med Biol* 2011;56(5):R31–R54.
49. Rao M, Yang W, Chen F, et al. Comparison of elekta vmat with helical tomotherapy and fixed field IMRT: plan quality, delivery efficiency and accuracy. *Med Phys* 2010;37(3):1350–1359.
50. Rao M, Cao D, Chen F, et al. Comparison of anatomy-based, fluence-based and aperture-based treatment planning approaches for vmat. *Phys Med Biol* 2010;55(21):6475–6490.
51. Matuszak MM, Yan D, Grills I, et al. Clinical applications of volumetric modulated arc therapy. *Int J Radiat Oncol Biol Phys* 2010;77(2):608–616.
52. Jin JY, Wen N, Ren L, et al. Advances in treatment techniques arc-based and other intensity modulated therapies. *Cancer J* 2011;17(3):166–176.
53. Followill D, Geis P, Boyer A. Estimates of whole-body dose equivalent produced by beam intensity modulated conformal therapy. *Int J Radiat Oncol Biol Phys* 1997;38(3):667–672.
54. Diallo I, Haddy N, Adjadj E, et al. Frequency distribution of second solid cancer locations in relation to the irradiated volume among 115 patients treated for childhood cancer. *Int J Radiat Oncol Biol Phys* 2009;74(3):876–883.
55. Yan Y, Yadav P, Bassetti M, et al. Dosimetric differences in flattened and flattening filter free beam treatment plans. *J Med Phys* 2016;41(2):92–99.
56. Cashmore J, Ramtohul M, Ford D. Lowering whole-body radiation doses in pediatric intensity-modulated radiotherapy through the use of unflattened photon beams. *Int J Radiat Oncol Biol Phys* 2011;80(4):1220–1227.
57. Georg D, Knöös T, McClean B. Current status and future perspective of flattening filter free photon beams. *Med Phys* 2011;38(3):1280–1293.
58. Reggiori G, Mancosu P, Castiglioni S, et al. Can volumetric modulated arc therapy with flattening filter free beams play a role in stereotactic body radiotherapy for liver lesions? A volume-based analysis. *Med Phys* 2012;39(2):1112–1118.
59. Kry SF, Vassiliev ON, Mohan R. Out-of-field photon dose following removal of the flattening filter from a medical accelerator. *Phys Med Biol* 2010;55(8):2155–2166.
60. Kragl G, Baier F, Lutz S, et al. Flattening filter free beams in SBRT and IMRT: dosimetric assessment of peripheral doses. *Z Med Phys* 2011;21(2):91–101.
61. Wang Y, Khan MK, Ting JY, et al. Surface dose investigation of the flattening filter-free photon beams. *Int J Radiat Oncol Biol Phys* 2012;83(2):e281–e285.
62. Vassiliev ON, Titt U, Pönisch F, et al. Dosimetric properties of photon beams from a flattening filter free clinical accelerator. *Phys Med Biol* 2006;51(7):1907–1917.
63. Pönisch F, Titt U, Vassiliev ON, et al. Properties of unflattened photon beams shaped by a multileaf collimator. *Med Phys* 2006;33(6):1738–1746.
64. Kragl G, Albrich D, Georg D. Radiation therapy with unflattened photon beams: dosimetric accuracy of advanced dose calculation algorithms. *Radiother Oncol* 2011;100(3):417–423.
65. Hrbacek J, Lang S, Klöck S. Commissioning of photon beams of a flattening filter-free linear accelerator and the accuracy of beam modeling using an anisotropic analytical algorithm. *Int J Radiat Oncol Biol Phys* 2011;80(4):1228–1237.
66. Titt U, Vassiliev ON, Pönisch F, et al. A flattening filter free photon treatment concept evaluation with Monte Carlo. *Med Phys* 2006;33(6):1595–1602.
67. Ghahremani S, Chavez R, Li Y, et al. SU-E-T-435: flattening filter free beams for head and neck IMRT and VMAT optimization. *Med Phys* 2015;42(6):3434.
68. Kry SF, Titt U, Pönisch F, et al. Reduced neutron production through use of a flattening-filter-free accelerator. *Int J Radiat Oncol Biol Phys* 2007;68(4):1260–1264.
69. Fraass BA, Kessler ML, McShan DL, et al. Optimization and clinical use of multisegment intensity-modulated radiation therapy for high-dose conformal therapy. *Semin Radiat Oncol* 1999;9(1):60–77.

70. Mohan R, Mageras GS, Baldwin B, et al. Clinically relevant optimization of 3-D conformal treatments. *Med Phys* 1992;19(4):933–944.

71. Kak AC, Slaney M. *Principles of computerized tomographic imaging.* New York: IEEE Press, 1988.

72. Bradbury M, Hricak H. Molecular MR imaging in oncology. *Magn Reson Imaging Clin N Am* 2005;13:225–240.

73. Gregoire V, Haustermans K, Lee JJ. Molecular image-guided radiotherapy with positron emission tomography. In: Joiner MC, van der Kogal A, eds. *Basic clinical radiobiology.* London, UK: Hodder Arnold, 2009:271–286.

74. Apisarnthanarax S, Chao KSC. Current imaging paradigms in radiation oncology. *Radiat Res* 2005;163(1):1–25.

75. Frank SJ, Chao KSC, Schwartz DL, et al. Technology insight: PET and PET/CT in head and neck tumor staging and radiation therapy planning. *Nat Clin Pract Oncol* 2005;2(10):526–533.

76. Cheebsumon P, Yaqub M, van Velden FHP, et al. Impact of (18)F FDG PET imaging parameters on automatic tumour delineation: need for improved tumour delineation methodology. *Eur J Nucl Med Mol Imaging* 2011;38(12):2136–2144.

77. Moeller BJ, Rana V, Cannon BA, et al. Prospective risk-adjusted (18)F fluorodeoxyglucose positron emission tomography and computed tomography assessment of radiation response in head and neck cancer. *J Clin Oncol* 2009;27(15):2509–2515.

78. Spirou SV, Chui CS. A gradient inverse planning algorithm with dose-volume constraints. *Med Phys* 1998;25(3):321–333.

79. Gregoire VP, Scallkiet P, Ang KK. *Clinical target volumes in conformal and intensity modulated radiation therapy. A clinical guide to cancer treatment.* Berlin, Germany: Springer Verlag, 2003.

80. Withers HR, Taylor JMG, Maciejewski B. Treatment volume and tissue tolerance. *Int J Radiat Oncol Biol Phys* 1988;14(4):751–759.

81. Withers HR, Thames HD. Dose fractionation and volume effects in normal-tissues and tumors. *Am J Clin Oncol* 1988;11(3):313–329.

82. Pugachev AB, Boyer AL, Xing L. Beam orientation optimization in intensity-modulated radiation treatment planning. *Med Phys* 2000;27(6):1238–1245.

83. Stein J, Mohan R, Wang XH, et al. Number and orientations of beams in intensity-modulated radiation treatments. *Med Phys* 1997;24(2):149–160.

84. Webb S. The physical basis of IMRT and inverse planning. *Br J Radiol* 2003;76(910):678–689.

85. Ehrgott M, Guler C, Hamacher HW, et al. Mathematical optimization in intensity modulated radiation therapy. *Ann Oper Res* 2010;175(1):309–365.

86. Deasy JO. Multiple local minima in radiotherapy optimization problems with dose-volume constraints. *Med Phys* 1997;24(7):1157–1161.

87. Mageras GS, Mohan R. Application of fast simulated annealing to optimization of conformal radiation treatments. *Med Phys* 1993;20(3):639–647.

88. Webb S. Optimization by simulated annealing of 3-dimensional, conformal treatment planning for radiation-fields defined by a multileaf collimator. 2. Inclusion of 2-dimensional modulation of the x-ray-intensity. *Phys Med Biol* 1992;37(8):1689–1704.

89. Pratx G, Xing L. GPU computing in medical physics: a review. *Med Phys* 2011;38(5):2685–2697.

90. Mohan R, Bortfeld T. The potential and limitations of IMRT: a physicist's point of view. In: Bortfeld T, Schmidt-Ullrigh R, De Neve W, et al., eds. *Image-guided IMRT.* Heidelberg, Germany: Springer, 2006:11–18.

91. Mackie TR. History of tomotherapy. *Phys Med Biol* 2006;51(13):R427–R453.

92. Carrasco P, Jornet N, Duch MA, et al. Comparison of dose calculation algorithms in phantoms with lung equivalent heterogeneities under conditions of lateral electronic disequilibrium. *Med Phys* 2004;31(10):2899–2911.

93. Li JG, Xing L, Boyer AL, et al. Matching photon and electron fields with dynamic intensity modulation. *Med Phys* 1999;26(11):2379–2384.

94. Maciejewski B, Withers HR, Taylor JM, et al. Dose fractionation and regeneration in radiotherapy for cancer of the oral cavity and oropharynx: tumor dose-response and repopulation. *Int J Radiat Oncol Biol Phys* 1989;16(3):831–843.

95. Withers HR, Peters LJ, Taylor JM, et al. Late normal tissue sequelae from radiation therapy for carcinoma of the tonsil: patterns of fractionation study of radiobiology. *Int J Radiat Oncol Biol Phys* 1995;33(3):563–568.

96. Withers HR, Peters LJ, Taylor JM, et al. Local control of carcinoma of the tonsil by radiation therapy: an analysis of patterns of fractionation in nine institutions. *Int J Radiat Oncol Biol Phys* 1995;33(3):549–562.

97. Withers HR, Taylor JM, Maciejewski B. The hazard of accelerated tumor clonogen repopulation during radiotherapy. *Acta Oncol* 1988;27(2):131–146.

98. Fowler JF. The linear-quadratic formula and progress in fractionated radiotherapy. *Br J Radiol* 1989;62(740):679–694.

99. Eisbruch A, Harris J, Garden AS, et al. Multi-institutional trial of accelerated hypofractionated intensity-modulated radiation therapy for early-stage oropharyngeal cancer (RTOG 00–22). *Int J Radiat Oncol Biol Phys* 2010;76(5):1333–1338.

100. Wu Q, Mohan R, Morris M, et al. Simultaneous integrated boost intensity-modulated radiotherapy for locally advanced head-and-neck squamous cell carcinomas. I: dosimetric results. *Int J Radiat Oncol Biol Phys* 2003;56(2):573–585.

101. Chao KS, Ozyigit G, Tran BN, et al. Patterns of failure in patients receiving definitive and postoperative IMRT for head-and-neck cancer. *Int J Radiat Oncol Biol Phys* 2003;55(2):312–321.

102. Li BQ, Li D, Lau DH, et al. Clinical-dosimetric analysis of measures of dysphagia including gastrostomy-tube dependence among head and neck cancer patients treated definitively by intensity-modulated radiotherapy with concurrent chemotherapy. *Radiat Oncol* 2009;4:52–61.

103. Schwartz DL, Hutcheson K, Barringer D, et al. Candidate dosimetric predictors of long-term swallowing dysfunction after oropharyngeal intensity-modulated radiotherapy. *Int J Radiat Oncol Biol Phys* 2010;78(5):1356–1365.

104. Gokhale AS, McLaughlin BT, Flickinger JC, et al. Clinical and dosimetric factors associated with a prolonged feeding tube requirement in patients treated with chemoradiotherapy (CRT) for head and neck cancers. *Ann Oncol* 2010;21(1):145–151.

105. Broderick M, Leech M, Coffey M. Direct aperture optimization as a means of reducing the complexity of intensity modulated radiation therapy plans. *Radiat Oncol* 2009;4.

106. Dogan N, Leybovich LB, King S, et al. Improvement of treatment plans developed with intensity-modulated radiation therapy for concave-shaped head and neck tumors. *Radiology* 2002;223(1):57–64.

107. Wu Q, Mohan R. Multiple local minima in IMRT optimization based on dose-volume criteria. *Med Phys* 2002;29(7):1514–1527.

108. Ezzell GA. Genetic and geometric optimization of three-dimensional radiation therapy treatment planning. *Med Phys* 1996;23(3):293–305.

109. Xu F, Mueller K. Accelerating popular tomographic reconstruction algorithms on commodity PC graphics hardware. *IEEE Trans Nucl Sci* 2005;52(3):654–663.

110. Bortfeld T, Schlegel W, Dykstra C, et al. Physical vs. biological objectives for treatment plan optimization. *Radiother Oncol* 1996;40(2):185–187.

111. Wu Y, Yan D, Sharpe MB, et al. Implementing multiple static field delivery for intensity modulated beams. *Med Phys* 2001;28(11):2188–2197.

112. Adkison JB, Khuntia D, Bentzen SM, et al. Dose escalated, hypofractionated radiotherapy using helical tomotherapy for inoperable non-small cell lung cancer: preliminary results of a risk-stratified phase I dose escalation study. *Technol Cancer Res Treat* 2008;7(6):441–447.

113. De Ruysscher D, Wanders R, van Haren E, et al. HI-CHART: a phase I/II study on the feasibility of high-dose continuous hyperfractionated accelerated radiotherapy in patients with inoperable non-small-cell lung cancer. *Int J Radiat Oncol Biol Phys* 2008;71(1):132–138.

114. Chao KS, Low DA, Perez CA, et al. Intensity-modulated radiation therapy in head and neck cancers: the Mallinckrodt experience. *Int J Cancer* 2000;90(2):92–103.

115. Goitein M. The comparison of treatment plans. *Semin Radiat Oncol* 1992;2(4):246–256.

116. Levegrun S, Jackson A, Zelefsky MJ, et al. Analysis of biopsy outcome after three-dimensional conformal radiation therapy of prostate cancer using dose-distribution variables and tumor control probability models. *Int J Radiat Oncol Biol Phys* 2000;47(5):1245–1260.

117. Convery DJ, Rosenbloom ME. The generation of intensity-modulated fields for conformal radiotherapy by dynamic collimation. *Phys Med Biol* 1992;37(6):1359–1374.

118. Svensson R, Kallman P, Brahme A. An analytical solution for the dynamic control of multileaf collimators. *Phys Med Biol* 1994;39(1):37–61.

119. Mohan R, Arnfield M, Tong S, et al. The impact of fluctuations in intensity patterns on the number of monitor units and the quality and accuracy of intensity modulated radiotherapy. *Med Phys* 2000;27(6):1226–1237.

120. Xia P, Verhey LJ. Multileaf collimator leaf sequencing algorithm for intensity modulated beams with multiple static segments. *Med Phys* 1998;25(8):1424–1434.

121. Que W. Comparison of algorithms for multileaf collimator field segmentation. *Med Phys* 1999;26(11):2390–2396.

122. Dai J, Zhu Y. Minimizing the number of segments in a delivery sequence for intensity-modulated radiation therapy with a multileaf collimator. *Med Phys* 2001;28(10):2113–2120.

123. Langer M, Thai V, Papiez L. Improved leaf sequencing reduces segments or monitor units needed to deliver IMRT using multileaf collimators. *Med Phys* 2001;28(12):2450–2458.

124. Hardcastle N, Metcalfe P, Ceylan A, et al. Multileaf collimator end leaf leakage: implications for wide-field IMRT. *Phys Med Biol* 2007;52(21):N493–N504.

125. Kim JO, Siebers JV, Keall PJ, et al. A Monte Carlo study of radiation transport through multileaf collimators. *Med Phys* 2001;28(12):2497–2506.

126. Siebers JV, Keall PJ, Kim JO, et al. A method for photon beam Monte Carlo multileaf collimator particle transport. *Phys Med Biol* 2002;47(17):3225–3249.

127. Siebers JV, Lauterbach M, Keall PJ, et al. Incorporating multi-leaf collimator leaf sequencing into iterative IMRT optimization. *Med Phys* 2002;29(6):952–959.

128. Klein EE, Hanley J, Bayouth J, et al. Task Group 142 report: quality assurance of medical accelerators. *Med Phys* 2009;36(9):4197–4212.

129. Kutcher GJ, Coia L, Gillin M, et al. Comprehensive QA for radiation oncology: report of AAPM Radiation Therapy Committee Task Group 40. *Med Phys* 1994;21(4):581–618.

130. Martens C, De Wagter C, De Neve W. The value of the PinPoint ion chamber for characterization of small field segments used in intensity-modulated radiotherapy. *Phys Med Biol* 2000;45(9):2519–2530.

131. Chui CS, Spirou S, LoSasso T. Testing of dynamic multileaf collimation. *Med Phys* 1996;23(5):635–641.

132. LoSasso T, Chui CS, Ling CC. Comprehensive quality assurance for the delivery of intensity modulated radiotherapy with a multileaf collimator used in the dynamic mode. *Med Phys* 2001;28(11):2209–2219.

133. Kubo HD, Hill BC. Respiration gated radiotherapy treatment: a technical study. *Phys Med Biol* 1996;41(1):83–91.

134. Keall P, Vedam S, George R, et al. The clinical implementation of respiratory-gated intensity-modulated radiotherapy. *Med Dosim* 2006;31(2):152–162.

135. Chang J, Mageras GS, Yorke E, et al. Observation of interfractional variations in lung tumor position using respiratory gated and ungated megavoltage cone-beam computed tomography. *Int J Radiat Oncol Biol Phys* 2007;67(5):1548–1558.

136. Mageras GS, Yorke E, Rosenzweig K, et al. Fluoroscopic evaluation of diaphragmatic motion reduction with a respiratory gated radiotherapy system. *J Appl Clin Med Phys* 2001;2(4):191–200.

137. Ezzell GA, Burmeister JW, Dogan N, et al. IMRT commissioning: multiple institution planning and dosimetry comparisons, a report from AAPM Task Group 119. *Med Phys* 2009;36(11):5359–5373.

138. Low DA, Parikh P, Dempsey JF, et al. Ionization chamber volume averaging effects in dynamic intensity modulated radiation therapy beams. *Med Phys* 2003;30(7):1706–1711.

139. Kitamura K, Shirato H, Shimizu S, et al. Registration accuracy and possible migration of internal fiducial gold marker implanted in prostate and liver treated with real-time tumor-tracking radiation therapy (RTRT). Radiother Oncol 2002;62(3):275–281.

140. Murphy MJ. Fiducial-based targeting accuracy for external-beam radiotherapy. Med Phys 2002;29(3):334–344.

141. Lattanzi J, McNeeley S, Hanlon A, et al. Ultrasound-based stereotactic guidance of precision conformal external beam radiation therapy in clinically localized prostate cancer. Urology 2000;55(1):73–78.

142. Morr J, DiPetrillo T, Tsai JS, et al. Implementation and utility of a daily ultrasound-based localization system with intensity-modulated radiotherapy for prostate cancer. Int J Radiat Oncol Biol Phys 2002;53(5):1124–1129.

143. Serago CF, Chungbin SJ, Buskirk SJ, et al. Initial experience with ultrasound localization for positioning prostate cancer patients for external beam radiotherapy. Int J Radiat Oncol Biol Phys 2002;53(5):1130–1138.

144. Mackie TR, Kapatoes J, Ruchala K, et al. Image guidance for precise conformal radiotherapy. Int J Radiat Oncol Biol Phys 2003;56(1):89–105.

145. Li H, Zhu XR, Zhang L, et al. Comparison of 2D radiographic images and 3D cone beam computed tomography for positioning head-and-neck radiotherapy patients. Int J Radiat Oncol Biol Phys 2008;71(3):916–925.

146. Lu J, Guerrero TM, Munro P, et al. Four-dimensional cone beam CT with adaptive gantry rotation and adaptive data sampling. Med Phys 2007;34(9):3520–3529.

147. Perks JR, Lehmann J, Chen AM, et al. Comparison of peripheral dose from image-guided radiation therapy (IGRT) using kV cone beam CT to intensity-modulated radiation therapy (IMRT). Radiother Oncol 2008;89(3):304–310.

148. Sillanpaa J, Chang J, Mageras G, et al. Developments in megavoltage cone beam CT with an amorphous silicon EPID: reduction of exposure and synchronization with respiratory gating. Med Phys 2005;32(3):819–829.

149. Xing L, Chen Y, Luxton G, et al. Monitor unit calculation for an intensity modulated photon field by a simple scatter-summation algorithm. Phys Med Biol 2000;45(3):N1–N7.

150. Jursinic PA, Nelms BE. A 2-D diode array and analysis software for verification of intensity modulated radiation therapy delivery. Med Phys 2003;30(5):870–879.

151. Kung JH, Chen GT, Kuchnir FK. A monitor unit verification calculation in intensity modulated radiotherapy as a dosimetry quality assurance. Med Phys 2000;27(10):2226–2230.

152. Low DA, Dempsey JF. Evaluation of the gamma dose distribution comparison method. Med Phys 2003;30(9):2455–2464.

153. Nelms BE, Zhen H, Tomee WA. Per-beam, planar IMRT QA passing rates do not predict clinically relevant dose errors. Med Phys 2011;38(2):1037–1044.

154. Nelms BE, Chan MF, Jarry G, et al. Evaluating IMRT and VMAT dose accuracy: practical examples of failure to detect systematic errors when applying a commonly used metric and action levels. Med Phys 2013;40(11):111722.

155. Boggula R, Birkner M, Lohr F, et al. Evaluation of a 2D detector array for patient-specific VMAT QA with different setups. Phys Med Biol 2011;56(22):7163–7177.

156. O'Daniel J, Das S, Wu QJ, et al. Volumetric-modulated arc therapy: effective and efficient end-to-end patient-specific quality assurance. Int J Radiat Oncol Biol Phys 2012;82(5):1567–1574.

157. Zhu J, Chen L, Jin G, et al. A comparison of VMAT dosimetric verifications between fixed and rotating gantry positions. Phys Med Biol 2013;58(5):1315–1322.

158. Jin H, Keeling VP, Johnson DA, et al. Interplay effect of angular dependence and calibration field size of MapCHECK2 on Rapid Arc quality assurance. J Appl Clin Med Phys 2014;15(3):4638.

159. Low DA. Quality assurance of intensity-modulated radiotherapy. Semin Radiat Oncol 2002;12(3):219–228.

160. Verhey LJ. Issues in optimization for planning of intensity-modulated radiation therapy. Semin Radiat Oncol 2002;12(3):210–218.

161. van Etmpt W, McDermott L, Nijsten S, et al. A literature review of electronic portal imaging for radiotherapy dosimetry. Radiother Oncol 2008;88(3):289–309.

162. Siebers JV, Kim JO, Ko L, et al. Monte Carlo computation of dosimetric amorphous silicon electronic portal images. Med Phys 2004;31(7):2135–2146.

163. Van Esch A, Depuydt T, Huyskens DP. The use of an aSi-based EPID for routine absolute dosimetric pre-treatment verification of dynamic IMRT fields. Radiother Oncol 2004;71(2):223–234.

164. Parent L, Seco J, Evans PM, et al. Monte Carlo modelling of a-Si EPID response: the effect of spectral variations with field size and position. Med Phys 2006;33(12):4527–4540.

165. Varian-Medical-Systems. Eclipse Algorithms Reference Guide. Vol. B500298R01A. Finland, 2006;7-1-7-28.

166. Berry SL, Sheu RD, Polvorosa CS, et al. Implementation of EPID transit dosimetry based on a through-air dosimetry algorithm. Med Phys 2012;39(1):87–98.

167. Berry SL, Polvorosa, CS, Cheng S, et al. Initial clinical experience performing patient treatment verification with an electronic portal imaging device transit dosimeter. Int J Radiat Oncol Biol Phys 2014;88(1):204–209.

168. Wendling M, McDermott LN, Mans A, et al. A simple backprojection algorithm for 3D in vivo EPID dosimetry of IMRT treatments. Med Phys 2009;36(7):3310–3321.

169. Mans A, Remeijer P, Olaciregui-Ruiz I, et al. 3D dosimetric verification of volumetric-modulated arc therapy by portal dosimetry. Radiother Oncol 2010;94(2):181–187.

170. Van Uytven E, Van Beek T, McCowan PM, et al. Validation of a method for in vivo 3D dose reconstruction for IMRT and VMAT treatments using on-treatment EPID images and a model-based forward-calculation algorithm. Med Phys 2015;42(12):6945–6954.

171. McCowan PM, Van Uytven E, Van Beek T, et al. An in vivo dose verification method for SBRT-VMAT delivery using the EPID. Med Phys 2015;42(12):6955–6963.

172. Bailat CJ, Baechler S, Moeckli R, et al. The concept and challenges of TomoTherapy accelerators. Rep Prog Phys 2011;74(8).

173. Achterberg N, Müller RG. Multibeam tomotherapy: a new treatment unit devised for multileaf collimation, intensity-modulated radiation therapy. Med Phys 2007;34(10):3926–3942.

174. Low DA, Mutic S, Dempsey JF, et al. Abutment region dosimetry for serial tomotherapy. Int J Radiat Oncol Biol Phys 1999;45(1):193–203.

175. Dogan N, Leybovich LB, Sethi A, et al. Improvement of dose distributions in abutment regions of intensity modulated radiation therapy and electron fields. Med Phys 2002;29(1):38–44.

176. Mutic S, Low DA, Klein EE, et al. Room shielding for intensity-modulated radiation therapy treatment facilities. Int J Radiat Oncol Biol Phys 2001;50(1):239–246.

177. Kuppersmith RB, Greco SC, Teh BS, et al. Intensity-modulated radiotherapy: first results with this new technology on neoplasms of the head and neck. Ear Nose Throat J 1999;78(4):238, 241–236, 248 passim.

178. Butler EB, Teh BS, Grant WH III, et al. Smart (simultaneous modulated accelerated radiation therapy) boost: a new accelerated fractionation schedule for the treatment of head and neck cancer with intensity modulated radiotherapy. Int J Radiat Oncol Biol Phys 1999;45(1):21–32.

179. Gielda BT, Shah AP, Marsh JC, et al. Helical tomotherapy delivery of an IMRT boost in lieu of interstitial brachytherapy in the setting of gynecologic malignancy: feasibility and dosimetric comparison. Med Dosim 2011;36(2):206–212.

180. Low DA, Chao KS, Mutic S, et al. Quality assurance of serial tomotherapy for head and neck patient treatments. Int J Radiat Oncol Biol Phys 1998;42(3):681–692.

181. Chao KS, Deasy JO, Markman J, et al. A prospective study of salivary function sparing in patients with head-and-neck cancers receiving intensity-modulated or three-dimensional radiation therapy: initial results. Int J Radiat Oncol Biol Phys 2001;49(4):907–916.

182. Chao KS, Majhail N, Huang CJ, et al. Intensity-modulated radiation therapy reduces late salivary toxicity without compromising tumor control in patients with oropharyngeal carcinoma: a comparison with conventional techniques. Radiother Oncol 2001;61(3):275–280.

183. Cheng JC, Chao KS, Low D. Comparison of intensity modulated radiation therapy (IMRT) treatment techniques for nasopharyngeal carcinoma. Int J Cancer 2001;96(2):126–131.

184. Hunt MA, Zelefsky MJ, Wolden S, et al. Treatment planning and delivery of intensity-modulated radiation therapy for primary nasopharynx cancer. Int J Radiat Oncol Biol Phys 2001;49(3):623–632.

185. Lee N, Xia P, Quivey JM, et al. Intensity-modulated radiotherapy in the treatment of nasopharyngeal carcinoma: an update of the UCSF experience. Int J Radiat Oncol Biol Phys 2002;53(1):12–22.

186. Claus F, Duthoy W, Boterberg T, et al. Intensity modulated radiation therapy for oropharyngeal and oral cavity tumors: clinical use and experience. Oral Oncol 2002;38(6):597–604.

187. Lee NY, Terezakis SA. Intensity-modulated radiation therapy. J Surg Oncol 2008;97(8):691–696.

188. Maingon P, Marchesi V, Crehange G. Intensity modulated radiation therapy. Bull Cancer 2010;97(7):759–768.

189. Lu HM, Yao M. The current status of intensity-modulated radiation therapy in the treatment of nasopharyngeal carcinoma. Cancer Treat Rev 2008;34(1):27–36.

190. Scott-Brown M, Miah A, Harrington K, et al. Evidence-based review: quality of life following head and neck intensity-modulated radiotherapy. Radiother Oncol 2010;97(2):249–257.

191. Tribius S, Bergelt C. Intensity-modulated radiotherapy versus conventional and 3D conformal radiotherapy in patients with head and neck cancer: is there a worthwhile quality of life gain? Cancer Treat Rev 2011;37(7):511–519.

192. Roe JWG, Carding PN, Dwivedi RC, et al. Swallowing outcomes following intensity modulated radiation therapy (IMRT) for head & neck cancer—a systematic review. Oral Oncol 2010;46(10):727–733.

193. Nutting CM, Morden JP, Harrington KJ, et al. Parotid-sparing intensity modulated versus conventional radiotherapy in head and neck cancer (PARSPORT): a phase 3 multicentre randomised controlled trial. Lancet Oncol 2011;12(2):127–136.

194. Boda-Heggemann J, Lohr F, Wenz F, et al. kV cone-beam CT-based IGRT: a clinical review. Strahlenther Onkol 2011;187(5):284–291.

195. Ling CC, Gerweck LE, Zaider M, et al. Dose-rate effects in external beam radiotherapy redux. Radiother Oncol 2010;95(3):261–268.

196. Chakraborty S, Ghoshal S, Patil VM, et al. Preliminary results of SIB-IMRT in head and neck cancers: report from a regional cancer center in northern India. J Cancer Res Ther 2009;5(3):165–172.

197. Chakraborty S, Ghoshal S, Patil V, et al. Acute toxicities experienced during simultaneous integrated boost intensity-modulated radiotherapy in head and neck cancers—experience from a North Indian regional cancer centre. Clin Oncol 2009;21(9):676–686.

198. Wirth LJ, Posner MR. Recent advances in combined modality therapy for locally advanced head and neck cancer. Curr Cancer Drug Targets 2007;7(7):674–680.

199. Seiwert TY, Salama JK, Vokes EE. The chemoradiation paradigm in head and neck cancer. Nat Clin Pract Oncol 2007;4(3):156–171.

200. Okunieff P, Kachnic LA, Constine LS, et al. Report from the Radiation Therapy Committee of the Southwest Oncology Group (SWOG): Research Objectives Workshop 2008. Clin Cancer Res 2009;15(18):5663–5670.

201. Riesterer O, Milas L, Ang KK. Combining molecular therapeutics with radiotherapy for head and neck cancer. J Surg Oncol 2008;97(8):708–711.

202. Thariat J, Bolle S, Demizu Y, et al. New techniques in radiation therapy for head and neck cancer: IMRT, CyberKnife, protons, and carbon ions. Improved effectiveness and safety? Impact on survival? Anticancer Drugs 2011;22(7):596–606.

203. Zelefsky MJ, Fuks Z, Happersett L, et al. Clinical experience with intensity modulated radiation therapy (IMRT) in prostate cancer. Radiother Oncol 2000;55(3):241–249.

204. Zelefsky MJ, Fuks Z, Hunt M, et al. High-dose intensity modulated radiation therapy for prostate cancer: early toxicity and biochemical outcome in 772 patients. Int J Radiat Oncol Biol Phys 2002;53(5):1111–1116.

205. Pollack A, Hanlon AL, Horwitz EM, et al. Dosimetry and preliminary acute toxicity in the first 100 men treated for prostate cancer on a randomized hypofractionation dose escalation trial. Int J Radiat Oncol Biol Phys 2006;64(2):518–526.

206. Kupelian PA, Thakkar VV, Khuntia D, et al. Hypofractionated intensity-modulated radiotherapy (70 gy at 2.5 Gy per fraction) for localized prostate cancer: long-term outcomes. *Int J Radiat Oncol Biol Phys* 2005;63(5):1463–1468.
207. Guckenberger M, Flentje M. Intensity-modulated radiotherapy (IMRT) of localized prostate cancer—a review and future perspectives. *Strahlenther Onkol* 2007;183(2):57–62.
208. Hatano K, Araki H, Sakai M, et al. Current status of intensity-modulated radiation therapy (IMRT). *Int J Clin Oncol* 2007;12(6):408–415.
209. Shridhar R, Bolton S, Joiner MC, et al. Dose escalation using a hypofractionated, intensity-modulated radiation therapy boost for localized prostate cancer: preliminary results addressing concerns of high or low alpha/beta ratio. *Clin Genitourin Cancer* 2009;7(3):E52–E57.
210. Sanfilippo N, Hardee ME, Wallach J. Review of chemoradiotherapy for high-risk prostate cancer. *Rev Recent Clin Trials* 2011;6(1):64–68.
211. Tucker SL, Jin HK, Wei XO, et al. Impact of toxicity grade and scoring system on the relationship between mean lung dose and risk of radiation pneumonitis in a large cohort of patients with non-small cell lung cancer. *Int J Radiat Oncol Biol Phys* 2010;77(3):691–698.
212. Tucker SL, Thames HD, Michalski JM, et al. Estimation of alpha/beta for late rectal toxicity based on RTOG 94-06. *Int J Radiat Oncol Biol Phys* 2011;81(2):600–605.
213. Sciarra A, Barentsz J, Bjartell A, et al. Advances in magnetic resonance imaging: how they are changing the management of prostate cancer. *Eur Urol* 2011;59(6):962–977.
214. Mazaheri Y, Shukla-Dave A, Muellner A, et al. MRI of the prostate: clinical relevance and emerging applications. *J Magn Reson Imaging* 2011;33(2):258–274.
215. Gutierrez AN, Westerly DC, Tome WA, et al. Whole brain radiotherapy with hippocampal avoidance and simultaneously integrated brain metastases boost: a planning study. *Int J Radiat Oncol Biol Phys* 2007;69(2):589–597.
216. Iuchi T, Hatano K, Narita Y, et al. Hypofractionated high-dose irradiation for the treatment of malignant astrocytomas using simultaneous integrated boost technique by IMRT. *Int J Radiat Oncol Biol Phys* 2006;64(5):1317–1324.
217. Huang E, Teh BS, Strother DR, et al. Intensity-modulated radiation therapy for pediatric medulloblastoma: early report on the reduction of ototoxicity. *Int J Radiat Oncol Biol Phys* 2002;52(3):599–605.
218. Simpson JR, Horton J, Scott C, et al. Influence of location and extent of surgical resection on survival of patients with glioblastoma-multiforme—results of 3 consecutive Radiation-Therapy Oncology Group (RTOG) clinical-trials. *Int J Radiat Oncol Biol Phys* 1993;26(2):239–244.
219. Floyd NS, Woo SY, Teh BS, et al. Hypofractionated intensity-modulated radiotherapy for primary glioblastoma multiforme. *Int J Radiat Oncol Biol Phys* 2004;58(3):721–726.
220. Stupp R, Mason WP, van den Bent MJ, et al. Radiotherapy plus concomitant and adjuvant temozolomide for glioblastoma. *N Engl J Med* 2005;352(10):987–996.
221. Koukourakis GV, Kouloulias V, Zacharias G, et al. Temozolomide with radiation therapy in high grade brain gliomas: pharmaceuticals considerations and efficacy; a review article. *Molecules* 2009;14(4):1561–1577.
222. Amelio D, Lorentini S, Schwarz M, et al. Intensity-modulated radiation therapy in newly diagnosed glioblastoma: a systematic review on clinical and technical issues. *Radiother Oncol* 2010;97(3):361–369.
223. Taylor CW, Nisbet A, McGale P, et al. Cardiac exposures in breast cancer radiotherapy: 1950s-1990s. *Int J Radiat Oncol Biol Phys* 2007;69(5):1484–1495.
224. Urbano MTG, Nutting CM. Clinical use of intensity-modulated radiotherapy: part II. *Br J Radiol* 2004;77(915):177–182.
225. Cho BC, Schwarz M, Mijnheer BJ, et al. Simplified intensity-modulated radiotherapy using pre-defined segments to reduce cardiac complications in left-sided breast cancer. *Radiother Oncol* 2004;70(3):231–241.
226. Evans PM, Donovan EM, Partridge M, et al. The delivery of intensity modulated radiotherapy to the breast using multiple static fields. *Radiother Oncol* 2000;57(1):79–89.
227. Hong L, Hunt M, Chui C, et al. Intensity-modulated tangential beam irradiation of the intact breast. *Int J Radiat Oncol Biol Phys* 1999;44(5):1155–1164.
228. Li JG, Williams SS, Goffinet DR, et al. Breast-conserving radiation therapy using combined electron and intensity-modulated radiotherapy technique. *Radiother Oncol* 2000;56(1):65–71.
229. Remouchamps VM, Vicini FA, Sharpe MB, et al. Significant reductions in heart and lung doses using deep inspiration breath hold with active breathing control and intensity-modulated radiation therapy for patients treated with locoregional breast irradiation. *Int J Radiat Oncol Biol Phys* 2003;55(2):392–406.
230. Thilmann C, Sroka-Perez G, Krempien R, et al. Inversely planned intensity modulated radiotherapy of the breast including the internal mammary chain: a plan comparison study. *Technol Cancer Res Treat* 2004;3(1):69–75.
231. van Asselen B, Raaijmakers CP, Hofman P, et al. An improved breast irradiation technique using three-dimensional geometrical information and intensity modulation. *Radiother Oncol* 2001;58(3):341–347.
232. Hurkmans CW, Cho BC, Damen E, et al. Reduction of cardiac and lung complication probabilities after breast irradiation using conformal radiotherapy with or without intensity modulation. *Radiother Oncol* 2002;62(2):163–171.
233. Kestin LL, Sharpe MB, Frazier RC, et al. Intensity modulation to improve dose uniformity with tangential breast radiotherapy: initial clinical experience. *Int J Radiat Oncol Biol Phys* 2000;48(5):1559–1568.
234. Landau D, Adams EJ, Webb S, et al. Cardiac avoidance in breast radiotherapy: a comparison of simple shielding techniques with intensity-modulated radiotherapy. *Radiother Oncol* 2001;60(3):247–255.
235. Taylor CW, Povall JM, McGale P, et al. Cardiac dose from tangential breast cancer radiotherapy in the year 2006. *Int J Radiat Oncol Biol Phys* 2008;72(2):501–507.
236. Taylor A, Rockall AG, Reznek RH, et al. Mapping pelvic lymph nodes: guidelines for delineation in intensity-modulated radiotherapy. *Int J Radiat Oncol Biol Phys* 2005;63(5):1604–1612.
237. Ahamad A, D'Souza W, Salehpour M, et al. Intensity-modulated radiation therapy after hysterectomy: comparison with conventional treatment and sensitivity of the normal-tissue-sparing effect to margin size. *Int J Radiat Oncol Biol Phys* 2005;62(4):1117–1124.
238. D'Souza WD, Ahamad AA, Iyer RB, et al. Feasibility of dose escalation using intensity-modulated radiotherapy in posthysterectomy cervical carcinoma. *Int J Radiat Oncol Biol Phys* 2005;61(4):1062–1070.
239. Salama JK, Mundt AJ, Roeske J, et al. Preliminary outcome and toxicity report of extended-field, intensity-modulated radiation therapy for gynecologic malignancies. *Int J Radiat Oncol Biol Phys* 2006;65(4):1170–1176.
240. Portelance L, Chao KS, Grigsby PW, et al. Intensity-modulated radiation therapy (IMRT) reduces small bowel, rectum, and bladder doses in patients with cervical cancer receiving pelvic and para-aortic irradiation. *Int J Radiat Oncol Biol Phys* 2001;51(1):261–266.
241. Mundt AJ, Lujan AE, Rotmensch J, et al. Intensity-modulated whole pelvic radiotherapy in women with gynecologic malignancies. *Int J Radiat Oncol Biol Phys* 2002;52(5):1330–1337.
242. Portelance L, Moughan J, Jhingran A, et al. A phase II multi-institutional study of postoperative pelvic intensity modulated radiation therapy (IMRT) with weekly cisplatin in patients with cervical carcinoma: two year efficacy results of the RTOG 0418. *Int J Radiat Oncol Biol Phys* 2011;81(2):S3–(abstr).
243. Ring KL, Young JL, Dunlap NE, et al. Extended-field radiation therapy with whole pelvis radiotherapy and cisplatin chemosensitization in the treatment of IB2-IIIB cervical carcinoma: a retrospective review. *Am J Obstet Gynecol* 2009;201(1):6.
244. Lillemoe KD. Current management of pancreatic-carcinoma. *Ann Surg* 1995;221(2):133–148.
245. Showalter TN, Winter KA, Berger AC, et al. The influence of total nodes examined, number of positive nodes, and lymph node ratio on survival after surgical resection and adjuvant chemoradiation for pancreatic cancer: a secondary analysis of RTOG 9704. *Int J Radiat Oncol Biol Phys* 2011;81(5):1328–1335.
246. Crane CH, Antolak JA, Rosen II, et al. Phase I study of concomitant gemcitabine and IMRT for patients with unresectable adenocarcinoma of the pancreatic head. *Int J Gastrointest Cancer* 2001;30(3):123–132.
247. Ben-Josef E, Shields AF, Vaishampayan U, et al. Intensity-modulated radiotherapy (IMRT) and concurrent capecitabine for pancreatic cancer. *Int J Radiat Oncol Biol Phys* 2004;59(2):454–459.
248. Brown MW, Ning H, Arora B, et al. A dosimetric analysis of dose escalation using two intensity-modulated radiation therapy techniques in locally advanced pancreatic carcinoma. *Int J Radiat Oncol Biol Phys* 2006;65(1):274–283.
249. Yovino S, Poppe M, Jabbour S, et al. Intensity-modulated radiation therapy significantly improves acute gastrointestinal toxicity in pancreatic and ampullary cancers. *Int J Radiat Oncol Biol Phys* 2011;79(1):158–162.
250. Bockbrader M, Kim E. Role of intensity-modulated radiation therapy in gastrointestinal cancer. *Expert Rev Anticancer Ther* 2009;9(5):637–647.
251. Meyer JJ, Willett CG, Czito BG. Emerging role of intensity-modulated radiation therapy in anorectal cancer. *Expert Rev Anticancer Ther* 2008;8(4):585–593.
252. Guerrero Urbano MT, Henrys AJ, Adams EJ, et al. Intensity-modulated radiotherapy in patients with locally advanced rectal cancer reduces volume of bowel treated to high dose levels. *Int J Radiat Oncol Biol Phys* 2006;65(3):907–916.
253. Milano MT, Jani AB, Farrey KJ, et al. Intensity-modulated radiation therapy (IMRT) in the treatment of anal cancer: toxicity and clinical outcome. *Int J Radiat Oncol Biol Phys* 2005;63(2):354–361.
254. Milano MT, Garofalo MC, Chmura SJ, et al. Intensity-modulated radiation therapy in the treatment of gastric cancer: early clinical outcome and dosimetric comparison with conventional techniques. *Br J Radiol* 2006;79(942):497–503.
255. Olsen JR, Moughan J, Myerson R, et al. Predictors of radiation therapy-related gastrointestinal toxicity from anal cancer dose-painted intensity modulated radiation therapy: secondary analysis of NRG Oncology RTOG 0529. *Int J Radiat Oncol Biol Phys* 2017;98(2):400–408.
256. Alasti H, Cho YB, Vandermeer AD, et al. A novel four-dimensional radiotherapy method for lung cancer: imaging, treatment planning and delivery. *Phys Med Biol* 2006;51(12):3251–3267.
257. Starkschall G, Balter P, Britton K, et al. Interfractional reproducibility of lung tumor location using various methods of respiratory motion mitigation. *Int J Radiat Oncol Biol Phys* 2011;79(2):596–601.
258. Byhardt RW, Scott C, Sause WT, et al. Response, toxicity, failure patterns, and survival in five Radiation Therapy Oncology Group (RTOG) trials of sequential and/or concurrent chemotherapy and radiotherapy for locally advanced non-small-cell carcinoma of the lung. *Int J Radiat Oncol Biol Phys* 1998;42(3):469–478.
259. Holloway CL, Robinson D, Murray B, et al. Results of a phase I study to dose escalate using intensity modulated radiotherapy guided by combined PET/CT imaging with induction chemotherapy for patients with non-small cell lung cancer. *Radiother Oncol* 2004;73(3):285–287.
260. Murshed H, Liu HH, Liao Z, et al. Dose and volume reduction for normal lung using intensity-modulated radiotherapy for advanced-stage non-small-cell lung cancer. *Int J Radiat Oncol Biol Phys* 2004;58(4):1258–1267.
261. Grills IS, Yan D, Martinez AA, et al. Potential for reduced toxicity and dose escalation in the treatment of inoperable non-small-cell lung cancer: a comparison of intensity-modulated radiation therapy (IMRT), 3D conformal radiation, and elective nodal irradiation. *Int J Radiat Oncol Biol Phys* 2003;57(3):875–890.
262. Liao ZX, Komaki RR, Thames HD Jr, et al. Influence of technologic advances on outcomes in patients with unresectable, locally advanced non-small-cell lung cancer receiving concomitant chemoradiotherapy. *Int J Radiat Oncol Biol Phys* 2010;76(3):775–781.
263. Vogelius IR, Westerly DC, Aznar MC, et al. Estimated radiation pneumonitis risk after photon versus proton therapy alone or combined with chemotherapy for lung cancer. *Acta Oncol* 2011;50(6):772–776.
264. Vogelius IS, Westerly DC, Cannon GM, et al. Intensity-modulated radiotherapy might increase pneumonitis risk relative to three-dimensional conformal radiotherapy in patients receiving combined chemotherapy and radiotherapy: a modeling study of dose dumping. *Int J Radiat Oncol Biol Phys* 2011;80(3):893–899.

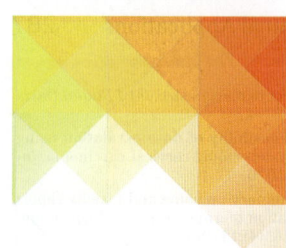

CHAPTER 12

Image-Guided Radiation Therapy

Daniel Robert Simpson, Loren K. Mell, Arno J. Mundt, and Todd F. Atwood

INTRODUCTION

Over the past few decades, the field of radiation oncology has seen rapid and extensive technologic advancements that have completely transformed radiation therapy planning and delivery. Undoubtedly, this transformation would not have been possible without the introduction of image-guided radiotherapy (IGRT). Although there are various definitions of IGRT, for the discussion herein, the term broadly refers to applications that incorporate imaging into radiation therapy planning and delivery with the overarching goal of improving treatment accuracy. Thus, this chapter will discuss a wide range of imaging modalities, old and new, and their applications in radiation therapy.

Why is IGRT Necessary?

As clinical radiation therapy devices continue to evolve with improving capabilities for precision treatment delivery, so increases the need for improved treatment accuracy. Modern treatment techniques such as intensity-modulated radiation therapy (IMRT), stereotactic radiosurgery (SRS), and stereotactic body radiation therapy (SBRT) are able to conform radiation dose to a much greater degree than conventional techniques. These technologies create highly conformal dose gradients that allow for potential dose reduction to surrounding normal organs at risk (OAR), but in turn, there is increased risk of missing the target. Although this presents opportunity for mitigation of radiation-related toxicity, this also increases the likelihood of subtherapeutic tumor dose delivery, which can have catastrophic clinical consequences. In addition, practitioners of radiation oncology still face the common challenges inherent to radiation therapy caused by tumor heterogeneity, anatomic variation, physiologic motion, and patient positioning error. IGRT applications designed to address these issues can be classified into two categories: image-guided *tissue delineation* and *in-room imaging*.

Tissue delineation refers to identification and definition of tumor or normal tissue during the treatment planning process. In modern radiation therapy practices, 3-D planning is standard and tissue volumes are delineated using computed tomography (CT) images. Although CT imaging provides adequate information for treatment planning in many cases, there are limitations in soft tissue definition and identification of physiologic subregions within tumors and normal tissues. The first part of this chapter will focus on applications of IGRT designed to improve tissue delineation through integration of advanced functional and biologic imaging modalities. In-room setup before and during radiation delivery introduces further potential uncertainty in target positioning. This uncertainty stems from various factors including human error, weight loss, tumor regression, and physiologic changes. These factors can cause drastic changes in target and normal tissue positioning over seconds to weeks and are often difficult to identify at the outset of treatment planning. The second part of this chapter will discuss various in-room IGRT modalities used to address these hurdles.

IMAGE-GUIDED TARGET/TISSUE DELINEATION

Positron Emission Tomography

Positron emission tomography (PET) has dramatically changed the way oncologists stage and treat cancer. PET scanning involves the systemic administration of a tracer labeled with a radioactive isotope, which emits positrons as it decays. PET scanners are able to detect the interaction of positrons in tissues and thus detect regions of increased radiotracer accumulation. Radiation therapy planning systems are equipped with rigid image registration software that can readily fuse PET images to planning CT images for purposes of target delineation. In addition, commercial software systems that incorporate deformable image registration can aid delineation by accommodating changes in patient anatomy and positioning between scans and segmenting target volumes based on quantitative methods (Fig. 12.1).[1,2]

FIGURE 12.1. Reductions in contour variability are observed with automatic contouring. Physician manual contours shown in *blue*, automatic contours modified by physicians shown in *purple*, and manual contours using Simultaneous Truth and Performance Level Estimation (STAPLE) algorithm shown in *brown*. (Reprinted from Stapleford LJ, Lawson JD, Perkins C, et al. Evaluation of automatic atlas-based lymph node segmentation for head-and-neck cancer. *Int J Radiat Oncol Biol Phys* 2010;77[3]:959–966. Copyright © 2010 Elsevier. With permission.)

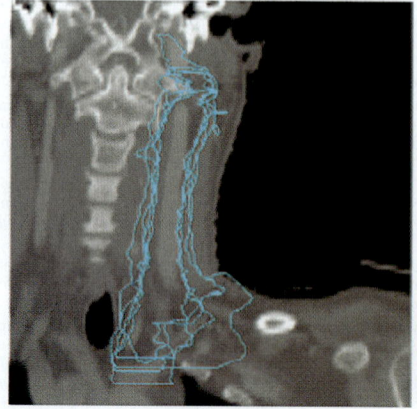
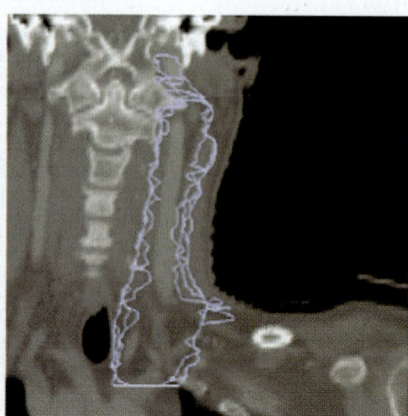
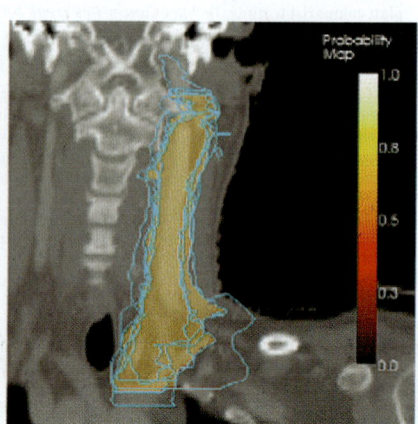

¹⁸F-Fluorodeoxyglucose-Positron Emission Tomography

The most widely used tracer is F18-fluorodeoxyglucose (¹⁸F-FDG), which is taken into cells and trapped intracellularly. ¹⁸F decays to ¹⁸O, and the molecule enters the glycolytic pathway, but the metabolism of ¹⁸F-FDG is slow relative to normal glucose, accounting for the high relative accumulation in metabolically active cells, including inflammatory tissue, neurons, brown fat, bone marrow, gastrointestinal (GI) epithelium, and tumors.[3] Studies in many different types of cancer have found that ¹⁸F-FDG-PET improves staging,[4–8] thus improving risk-adapted management. In addition, multiple studies have shown correlation with ¹⁸F-FDG uptake values and cancer prognosis,[9–11] making PET a desirable potential imaging biomarker for use in patient-directed treatment paradigms.

Multiple studies have evaluated the utility of ¹⁸F-FDG-PET in radiotherapy planning for lung cancer.[12–17] Many of these studies have shown that incorporation of ¹⁸F-FDG-PET imaging leads to significant alterations in treatment volumes in non–small cell lung cancer (NSCLC)[15–18] and mesothelioma.[19] PET aids in detection of occult nodal involvement and improves distinction of tumor from atelectasis compared to CT alone (Fig. 12.2).[16,20] Vanuytsel et al.[15] found that ¹⁸F-FDG-PET-CT altered treatment volumes in over 60% of lymph node–positive patients staged by mediastinoscopy. The results of the Radiation Therapy Oncology Group's (RTOG) study RTOG-0515, a phase II trial with 52 NSCLC patients, demonstrated that ¹⁸F-FDG-PET–guided treatment planning led to altered nodal volumes in 51% of patients and in general led to smaller tumor gross tumor volumes (GTV) and mean lung dose. Although there is controversy regarding the optimal method of PET-guided target volume delineation, the use of PET does appear to reduce interobserver variation in target definitions.[12] Although early studies[18] reported on the use of standardized uptake values (SUV) for tumor demarcation, recent studies in both phantoms and patients indicate that gradient-based methods may be a more accurate and consistent technique for target volume contouring.[2,21]

Several studies have shown that ¹⁸F-FDG-PET has similar utility for target definition in head and neck cancer (HNC).[17,22–26,26a,26b] Paulino et al.[27] compared CT and ¹⁸F-FDG-PET–guided IMRT planning in HNC patients and found that CT-based plans were suboptimal in covering the PET-delineated GTV in 25% of patients. In a prospective analysis of 20 patients, Schwartz et al.[23] found that IMRT plans could be optimized with ¹⁸F-FDG-PET-CT to improve parotid and laryngeal sparing and allow dose escalation up to 81 Gy. A study from Memorial Sloan Kettering Cancer Center found significant differences in magnetic resonance imaging (MRI) and PET-delineated target volumes drawn, thus indicating that various modalities provide important and complementary information for accurate target delineation.[24] GTVs delineated by using ¹⁸F-FDG-PET appear to be significantly smaller than those delineated on CT alone.[24–26] Some concerns exist regarding the technical aspects of PET-guided radiation therapy in HNC, including difficulties in establishing optimal image registration[28] and large variability in target definition.[29] Recent studies indicate that automated techniques to guide delineation in HNC can improve consistency.[1,30,31] Leclerc et al.[32] tested a gradient-based ¹⁸F-FDG-PET segmentation method in HNC patients in a prospective multicentric study. They found that this method consistently decreased the size of target volumes with resultant reduction in dose to the parotid glands and oral cavity. Importantly, they saw comparable clinical outcomes in terms of survival and no marginal tumor recurrences with a minimum follow-up of 2 years. Nonetheless, target delineation is still highly dependent on both segmentation and reconstruction methods, emphasizing the importance of clarifying and standardizing methodologies across institutions.[33,34]

¹⁸F-FDG-PET–guided target delineation has also been evaluated in GI malignancies including both esophageal[8,35–40] and rectal[41–45] cancer. Hong et al.[37] studied 25 esophageal cancer patients undergoing ¹⁸F FDG PET-CT for radiotherapy planning; PET influenced target delineation in 21 patients (84%), with changes classified as major in 9 (34%). However, Muijs et al.[8] reviewed 30 studies spanning 1,222 patients and found no conclusive evidence supporting the necessity of PET for radiation therapy planning. It is clear that PET is helpful in determining lymph node status and detecting occult metastases, but whether it is superior to other modalities for GTV delineation remains unclear. If used to delineate GTV, a threshold of 2.5 for either absolute SUV or SUV relative to liver uptake has been proposed.[40] As for rectal cancer, Braendengen et al.[41] compared GTV delineation with MRI versus ¹⁸F-FDG-PET-CT in 77 patients. The results of this study indicate that PET-guided volumes tend to be smaller than MRI volumes, but PET guidance also often complements data from MRI. Dynamic ¹⁸F-FDG-PET-CT may also play a role in the future.[43]

FIGURE 12.2. ¹⁸F-FDG-positron emission tomography/computed tomography (PET-CT) scan in a patient with a right middle lobe lung carcinoma. On CT (*left*), the limits of the tumor are obscured by postobstructive pneumonia and atelectasis. On the fused scan (*right*), the tumor is intensely FDG-avid and more easily differentiated. (Reprinted from Spratt DE, Diaz R, McElmurray J, et al. Impact of FDG PE T/CT on delineation of the gross tumor volume for radiation planning in non-small-cell lung cancer. *Clin Nucl Med* 2010;35[4]:237–243. With permission.)

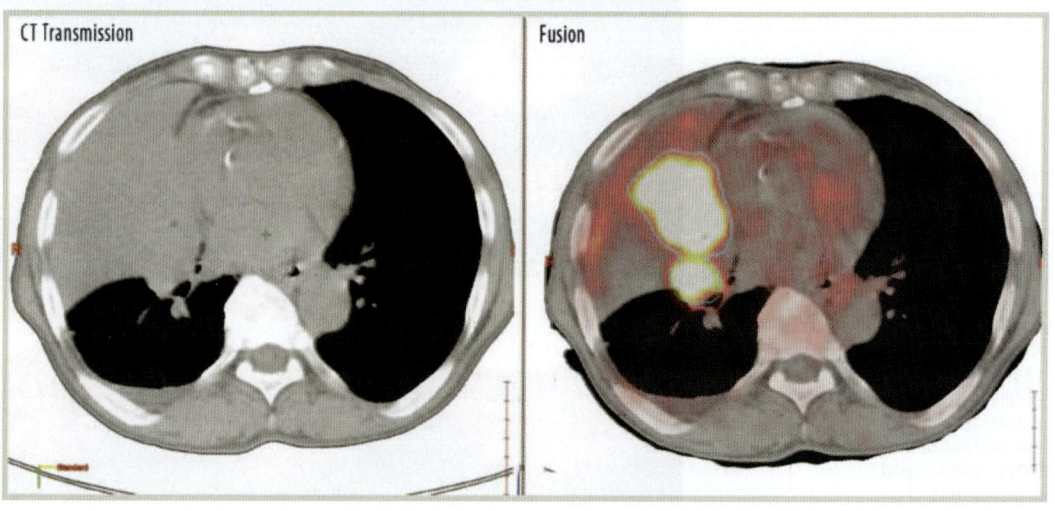

Investigators at Washington University have carried out extensive research in ^{18}F-FDG-PET for cervical cancer.[46–48] They have shown that PET-guided target delineation for cervical cancer patients with involved para-aortic lymph nodes can facilitate safe dose escalation to 60 Gy when used in conjunction with IMRT.[49] Serial changes in cervical tumor volume during brachytherapy[50] and external beam RT[51] have been documented, but the optimal treatment approach for metabolically unresponsive tumors is yet to be determined. Lin et al.[52] reported that ^{18}F-FDG-PET–based brachytherapy planning significantly optimized GTV coverage without increasing bladder or rectal dose. Liang et al.[53] found that ^{18}F-FDG-PET–guided bone marrow–sparing IMRT for pelvic malignancies was feasible and reduced dose to active bone marrow. Related work by Rose et al.[46] has indicated that dose to metabolically active bone marrow subregions identified by ^{18}F-FDG-PET is a significant predictor of hematologic toxicity. Recently, Mell et al.[47] showed that reducing dose specifically to PET-identified active pelvic bone marrow mitigates hematologic toxicity in gynecologic cancer patients undergoing chemoradiotherapy, potentially permitting delivery of more intensive chemotherapy regimens.

The utility of ^{18}F-FDG-PET–guided radiation therapy in other disease sites is less clear. Although ^{18}F-FDG-PET can aid in contouring lumpectomy cavities in breast cancer[48] that involved nodal radiation therapy for lymphoma[54,55] and GTV delineation for pancreatic cancer,[56] the results from studies in sarcoma, central nervous system (CNS) tumors, and prostate cancer show ^{18}F-FDG-PET to be less helpful.[57,58] The data for ^{18}F-FDG-PET guidance in pediatrics are limited. Kornerup et al.[59] analyzed the utility of PET-CT simulation in pediatric patients with primary cancers in various sites. They compared target volumes contoured with and without ^{18}F-FDG-PET and used normal tissue complication probability (NTCP) modeling to estimate the effect of PET-guided treatment planning. Although their results indicated an impact for some individual patients, overall they found no consistent impact in target volume or NTCP across the cohort.

Non–[18]F-FDG-Positron Emission Tomography

In addition to ^{18}F-FDG, many other radiotracers have been studied, including ^{18}F-thymidine (FLT), ^{18}F-misonidazole (^{18}F-MISO), ^{18}F-azomycin arabinoside ([18]FAZA), ^{18}F-choline, ^{11}C-choline, ^{11}C-methionine (^{11}C-MET), ^{11}C-acetate, and [60]Cu(II)-diacetyl-bis(N[4]-methylosemicarbazone) ([60]Cu-ATSM). [15]O and [13]N—labeled H_2O, CO_2, O_2, or NH_3—molecules have also been used to measure blood flow, apoptosis, or hypoxia with PET.[60–62] New tracers are continually being developed and tested. For further discussion of novel molecular imaging applications, refer to several reviews.[60–64] Because of low physiologic uptake in brain tissue, ^{11}C-MET is a potentially useful radiotracer for image-guided planning of brain tumors. Grosu et al.[65] analyzed the use of ^{11}C-MET in patients with glioblastoma multiforme (GBM) and found that ^{11}C-MET uptake extended (up to 4.5 cm) beyond the tumor identified by MRI in nearly 75% of patients. ^{11}C-MET has also been shown to improve GTV delineation for skull base meningiomas.[66] A limitation of ^{11}C-MET PET, however, is the short half-life of [11]C (20 minutes). ^{18}F-ET leads to different GTV compared to MRI alone[67] but appears to be comparable to ^{11}C-MET (Fig. 12.3),[68] with the advantage of a longer isotope half-life. Milker-Zabel

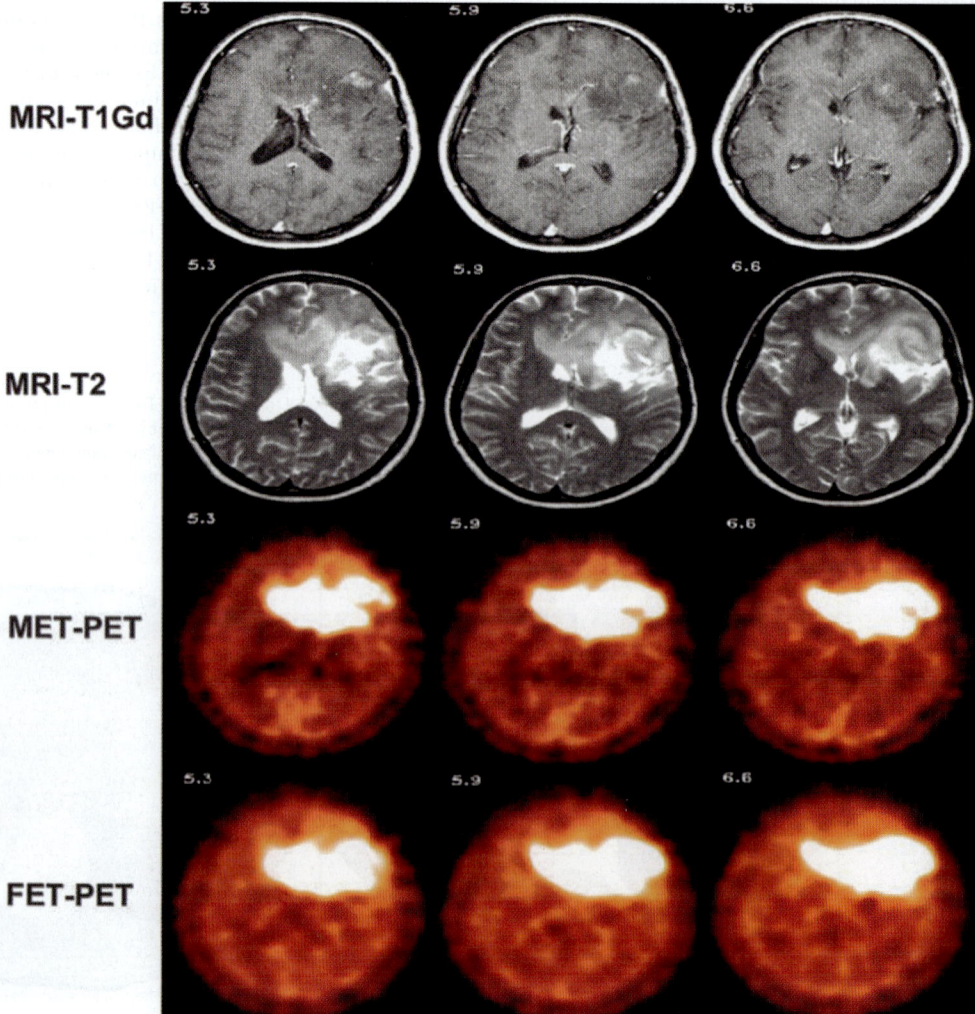

FIGURE 12.3. Comparison of magnetic resonance imaging, ^{11}C-methionine (^{11}C-MET) positron emission tomography (PET), and ^{18}F-fluoroethyl-L-tyrosine (^{18}F-ET) PET for a patient with grade III astrocytoma. (Reprinted from Grosu AL, Astner ST, Riedel E, et al. An interindividual comparison of O-(2-[^{18}F]fluoroethyl)-L-tyrosine (FET)- and L-[methyl-^{11}C]methionine (MET)-PET in patients with brain gliomas and metastases. *Int J Radiat Oncol Biol Phys* 2011;81[4]:1049–1058. Copyright © 2011 Elsevier. With permission.)

MRI-T1Gd

MRI-T2

MET-PET

FET-PET

et al.[69] evaluated [68]Ga-(0)-D-Phe (1)-Tyr (221)-octreotide (^{68}Ga-DOTATOC) PET in meningioma patients and demonstrated that ^{68}Ga-DOTATOC PET significantly influenced target delineation in the majority of cases. Gehler et al.[70] found similar results, with ^{68}Ga-DOTATOC PET-CT changing target volumes in 17 of 26 patients.

Several investigators have explored PET-guided RT using ^{18}F-MISO[71,72] and ^{18}F-AZA.[73] The Trans-Tasman Radiation Oncology Group correlated hypoxia identified on ^{18}F-MISO PET with outcomes in 45 stage III or IV HNC patients undergoing chemoradiation therapy, with or without the hypoxic cytotoxin tirapazamine.[72] Baseline hypoxia and residual hypoxia (detected on ^{18}F-MISO PET scans at week 4 or 5 of treatment) were correlated with higher rates of locoregional failure. [60]Cu-ATSM has attracted attention for hypoxia imaging because of its potential biokinetic advantages and better resolution. [60]Cu-ATSM PET-guided hypoxia imaging has been investigated in HNC and cervical cancer.[74,75] In a pilot study in 14 cervical cancer patients, [60]Cu-ATSM appeared to provide good prognostic discrimination; 5 of 5 patients with hypoxic tumors developed recurrence versus 3 of 9 with normoxic tumors.[75]

[11]C-choline and ^{18}F-choline have both been studied in prostate cancer,[76,77] but their utility for routine clinical care is unclear. SUV values from ^{11}C-choline PET appear to correlate well with histopathologic specimens as a threshold for contouring dominant intraprostatic lesions.[76] ^{18}F-FLT PET can be potentially useful in certain cancers, such as esophageal cancer, where its positive predictive value for involved nodes may be higher than for ^{18}F-FDG-PET.[39] In a study of five NSCLC patients undergoing serial baseline and on-treatment ^{18}F-FLT PET, reductions in ^{18}F-FLT uptake within both tumor and bone marrow were observed.[78] However, ^{18}F-FLT PET guidance appears to provide less benefit for tumor and nodal delineation in rectal cancer and HNC.[79,80] Arens et al.[81] tested the use of an ^{18}F-FLT PET–based adaptive segmentation method in HNC. They demonstrated robustness and reproducibility with this method as well as clinical prognostic value associated with serial ^{18}F-FLT PET parameters. Novel PET agents have also been used for normal tissue sparing. Investigators at the University of Melbourne[82] conducted a prospective clinical trial using 4-D ^{68}Ga-labeled macroaggregated albumin PET for functionally adapted lung sparing in 20 patients with NSCLC. Their results showed a significant reduction in functional mean lung dose with this method (Fig. 12.4).

MRI

MRI-guided RT planning has well-established utility, particularly for CNS, HNC, and pelvic malignancies.[83–91] Some radiation departments have even transitioned to using MR simulators, and MRI-only planning approaches are becoming more widely available (Fig. 12.5).[92] In addition to standard MRI modalities, functional MRI (fMRI) techniques have been used to enhance radiation planning. For example, fMRI has been used to reduce radiation dose to a normal functioning brain during planning for CNS tumors.[93–97] Aoyama et al.[96] evaluated the use of magnetoencephalography and anisotropic diffusion-weighted MRI for CNS targets including arteriovenous malformation (AVM). In 15 patients, target volumes were modified with significant reduction in the volume of sensitive regions receiving more than 15 Gy. Fast imaging employing steady-state acquisition can facilitate visualization of the trigeminal nerve during radiosurgery planning.[98,99] The ^{1}H MR spectroscopy (MRS) has also been used to guide planning in gliomas.[100,101] Underdosing of volumes delineated using ^{1}H MRS metabolically active areas has been associated with worse outcomes in GBM.[101]

In patients with prostate cancer, van Lin et al.[102] have reported the feasibility of escalating doses to 90 Gy to dominant intraprostatic lesions identified by ^{1}H MRS. MR lymphography with intravenous ferumoxtran-10 has also been used to identify pathologic nodal involvement in prostate cancer (Fig. 12.6).[103,104] In a study of 47 patients treated with salvage RT for rising postprostatectomy prostate-specific antigen (PSA), 79% were found to have at least one aberrant positive lymph node, including 10 of 18 (61%) with a PSA <1.0 ng/mL. MR lymphography may therefore be useful in helping to define nodal boost volumes in prostate cancer. Dynamic contrast-enhanced (DCE) MRI has been investigated for RT planning in a variety of tumors including HNC, lung, rectal, and cervical cancers.[105–108] Mayr et al.[108] studied 102 cervical cancer patients treated with DCE MRI. Patients with a low total volume of tumor voxels with low DCE signal had significantly worse tumor control and disease-specific survival. Carmona et al.[109] used an MRI technique called iterative decomposition of water and fat with echo asymmetry and least squares estimation (IDEAL) to study fractional changes in fat content of pelvic bone marrow during pelvic chemoradiation therapy (Fig. 12.7). Conversion of the bone marrow from low fat, high cellularity to high fat, low cellularity during RT is readily observed, enabling noninvasive quantitative methods to analyze the impact of local changes in radiation dose.

FIGURE 12.4. Axial slices from 4-D ^{68}Ga-labeled macroaggregated albumin positron emission tomography in a patient with severe emphysema. Dose color wash shown for a conventional intensity-modulated radiation therapy plan optimized to anatomic lung **(A)** and a functionally adapted plan optimized to the "highly perfused" (HP) lung volume **(B)**. (Reprinted from Siva S, Thomas R, Callahan J, et al. High-resolution pulmonary ventilation and perfusion PET/CT allows for functionally adapted intensity modulated radiotherapy in lung cancer. *Radiother Oncol* 2015;115[2]:157–162. Copyright © 2015 Elsevier Ireland Ltd. With permission.)

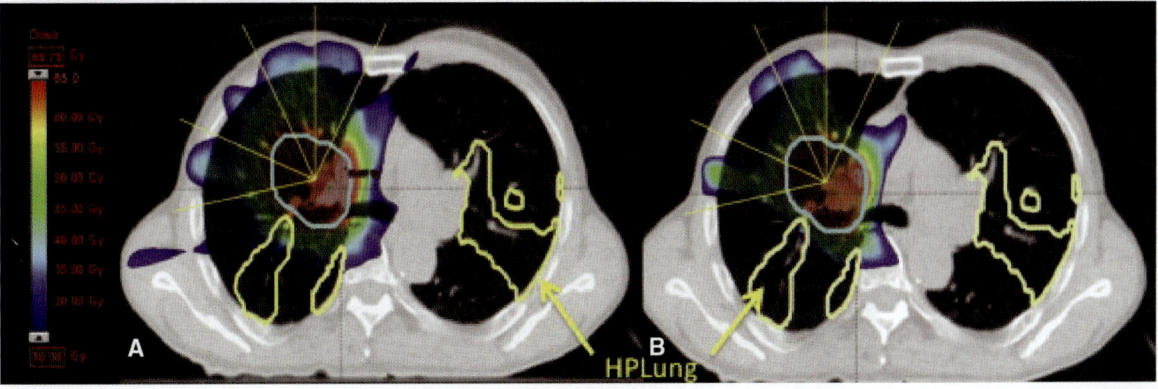

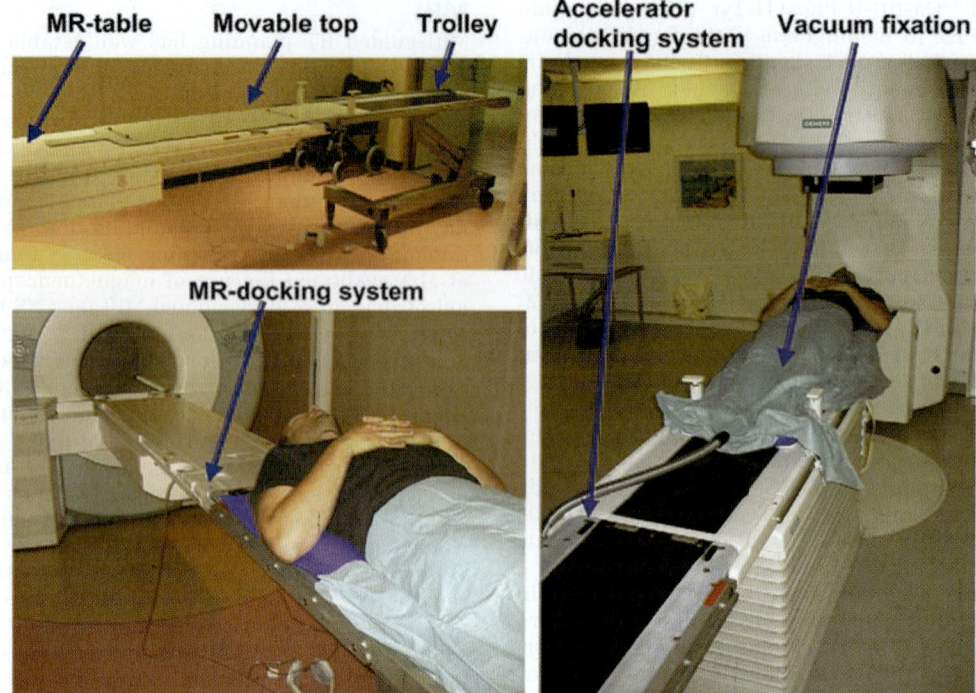

FIGURE 12.5. Integration of magnetic resonance imaging (MRI) and radiotherapy, with trolley solution and specialized docking device for smooth transfer between MR and linear accelerator. (Reprinted from Karlsson M, Karlsson MG, Nyholm T, et al. Dedicated magnetic resonance imaging in the radiotherapy clinic. *Int J Radiat Oncol Biol Phys* 2009;74[2]:644–651. Copyright © 2009 Elsevier. With permission.)

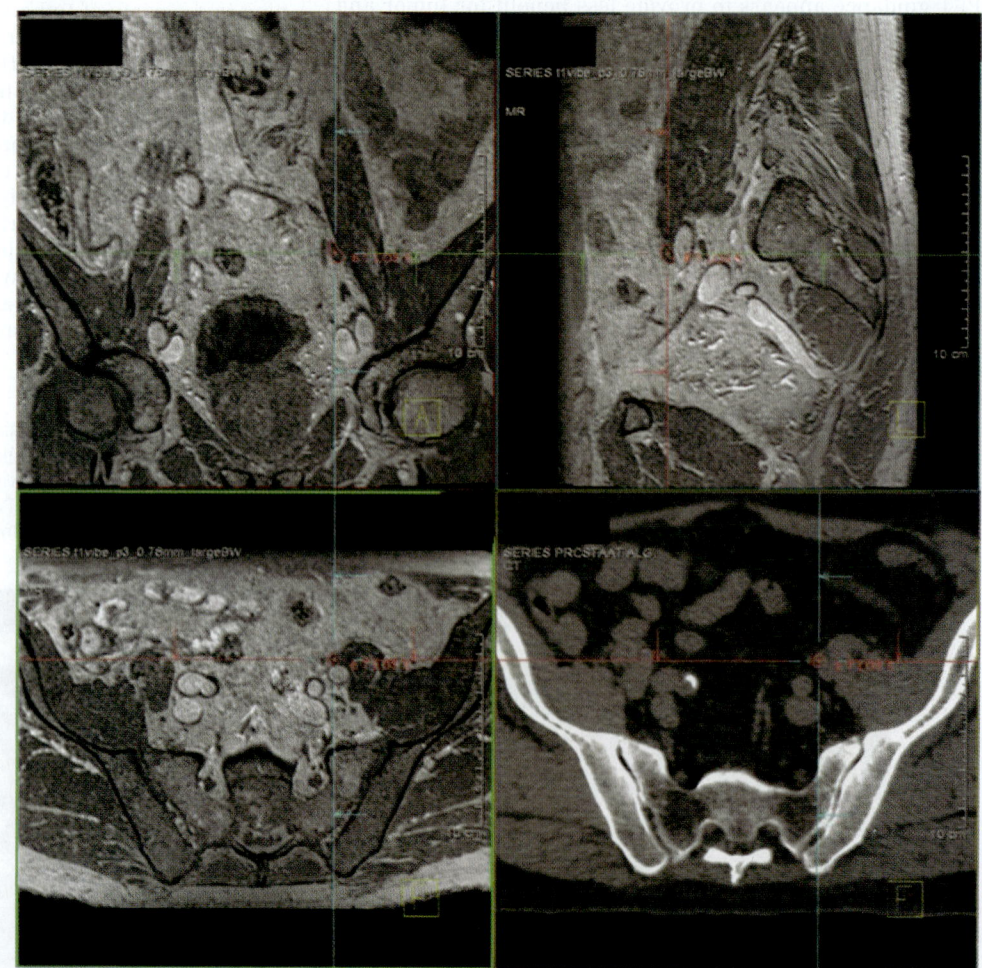

FIGURE 12.6. Fusion of magnetic resonance (MR) lymphography (*upper right* and *left* and *lower left*) and computed tomography (CT) (*lower right*). With the help of MR lymphography, the node identified on CT is identified as pathologic. (Reprinted from Meijer HJ, Debats OA, Kunze-Busch M, et al. Magnetic resonance lymphography-guided selective high-dose lymph node irradiation in prostate cancer. *Int J Radiat Oncol Biol Phys* 2012;82[1]:175–183. Copyright © 2012 Elsevier. With permission.)

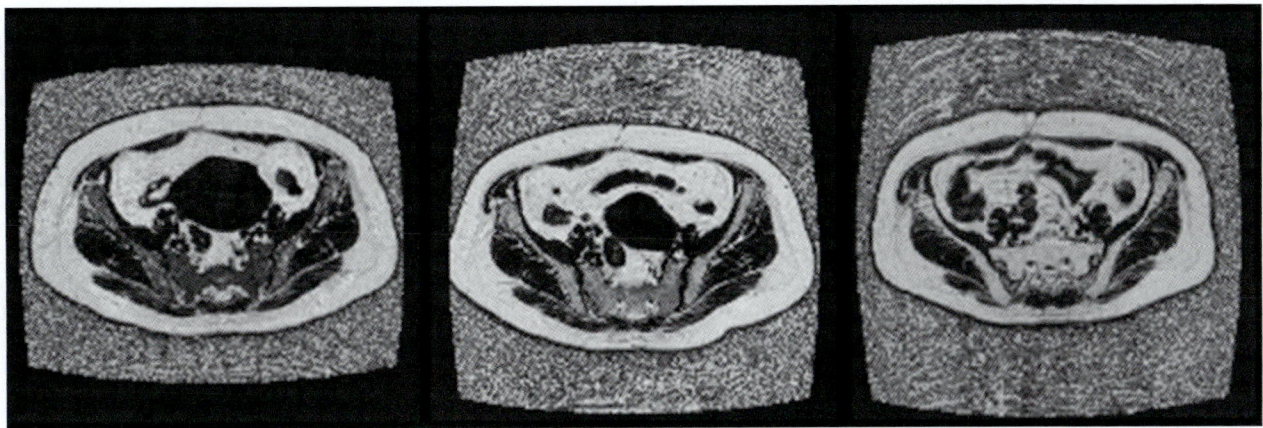

FIGURE 12.7. Axial iterative decomposition of water and fat with echo asymmetry and least squares estimation (IDEAL) magnetic resonance imaging scans of the pelvis in a gynecologic cancer patient undergoing chemoradiotherapy. Scans were acquired at baseline (*left*), midtreatment (*middle*), and posttreatment (*right*) and show a steady increase in fraction of fat relative to water within the pelvic bones, indicated by conversion to progressively higher signal.

SPECT

Single-photon emission computed tomography (SPECT) is a well-established functional imaging technique, with a wide range of potential tracers. In addition to being relatively cost-effective compared to PET, SPECT has some dosimetric advantages. Although PET can provide more accurate quantitative information regarding *in vivo* radiation dose distribution,[63] SPECT tracers typically have longer half-lives and release less energy, leading to favorable dosimetry and utility for studying slower biologic processes.[63] Nonetheless, SPECT-guided treatment appears to be less widely adopted in radiation oncology.[110]

Several studies have demonstrated utility of ^{111}In-capromab pendetide radioimmunoscintigraphy (RIS) guidance for both external beam RT[111–113] and brachytherapy[114,115] for prostate cancer. Jani et al.[116] found that RIS guidance led to alteration of RT volumes and decision-making in a significant proportion of patients undergoing post-prostatectomy salvage RT. Of 54 evaluable patients, 18.5% had treatment plans altered by RIS, including 4 patients who were not offered RT based on the RIS findings. In a multivariate analysis of 107 patients (53 planned with RIS), RIS was associated with an improved 3-year biochemical failure-free survival (bFFS).[112] A similar analysis of 82 patients undergoing RIS for salvage therapy, however, did not reveal a clear benefit of RIS.[116] Ellis et al.[114] treated 80 low–intermediate-risk prostate cancer patients with RIS-assisted brachytherapy. Regions of the prostate showing increased RIS uptake were prescribed 150% of the standard dose. The overall 4-year bFFS was 97.4%.

Other applications of SPECT-guided treatment planning have been studied, including [123]IMT (^{123}I-alpha-methyl-L-tyrosine) SPECT for gliomas[117–119] and meta-[123]iodo-benzylguanidine scans for neuroblastoma.[120] Krengli et al.[119] studied 21 patients with high-grade gliomas using fused ^{99m}Tc-MIBI SPECT and MRI. Similar to findings of Grosu et al.,[118] target volumes were significantly augmented by SPECT, with an average increase of 33% over MRI alone, particularly in resected cases.

SPECT has also been used to guide normal tissue avoidance. In patients with NSCLC, Christian et al.[121] used ^{99m}Tc SPECT to identify functional lung to avoid using inverse RT planning and showed the V20 of functioning lung could be reduced without compromising target coverage. Roeske et al.[122] used ^{99m}Tc SPECT to identify active bone marrow subregions to reduce hematologic toxicity in patients receiving pelvic chemoradiation therapy.

Four-Dimensional Imaging and Motion Management

Respiratory-induced organ motion is a significant problem in radiation therapy. Tumors located in the thorax and upper abdomen can move in large amounts during normal respiration. If ignored, respiratory motion can result in substantial imaging artifacts on the treatment planning images, which can lead to inaccurate target delineation and/or unnecessarily large target volumes.[123,124] Several motion management strategies currently exist: free breathing (target compensates for the full range of tumor motion), abdominal compression (device limits diaphragm expansion and tumor motion), respiratory gating (select portions of the respiratory cycle are utilized for treatment), and real-time tumor tracking (radiation beam follows the moving target).[125] Although all of these techniques have their advantages and disadvantages, choosing the optimal technique for an individual institution depends on the clinical needs and staff expertise.

Respiratory Gating

Respiratory gating refers to the process of limiting the radiation beam to select portions of the respiratory cycle, thus treating the tumor at a specific position. Respiratory gating has two main approaches: internal (utilizing internal surrogates for tumor motion) and external (utilizing an external device to monitor respiration as a surrogate for tumor motion).[126–128] The external approach is far more prevalent in radiation oncology today, where respiration information is determined from markers on the patient's abdomen, a compression belt, or spirometer signals.

The Real-time Position Management (RPM) system (Varian Medical Systems, Palo Alto, CA) is a popular example of an external respiratory gating system. This system consists of a lightweight plastic block containing multiple passive reflective markers, which is monitored by a charge-coupled device video camera mounted in the treatment room. When the block is placed on the patient's abdomen, the system can be used to generate a respiratory waveform surrogate for tumor motion during both simulation and treatment.

External surrogates, such as the RPM system, are advantageous because they are noninvasive, easy to use, and well-tolerated by patients and don't require additional imaging radiation dose. However, because only an external respiratory signal is acquired, the correlation between tumor motion and patient respiration must be closely monitored throughout treatment. Other systems, such as the ExacTrac X-Ray Monitoring System (BrainLAB, Westchester, IL), combine x-ray imaging of internal anatomy with an external respiratory signal.[129] This technique allows the correlation between tumor position and patient respiration to be continuously updated at a reasonable frequency, keeping patient x-ray exposure in mind.

Regardless of the gating system, patient respiration is typically divided into ten discrete time points per period. These time points, typically referred to as phases, are used to assess tumor motion and determine a gating strategy. An example of a respiration period is illustrated in Figure 12.8 (top), where the 0% phase corresponds to maximum inspiration and the 50% phase corresponds to maximum expiration. On average, most patients spend more time in expiration than they do in inspiration, which creates a beneficial scenario for respiratory gating around expiration (Fig. 12.8, middle). More specifically, if no respiration is occurring, no respiration-induced tumor motion

is occurring, providing a large window to treat the tumor with limited motion. On the other hand, if a patient is a candidate for deep inspiration breath hold (DIBH), they can be asked to hold their breath for an extended amount of time, creating a large window to treat the tumor with little motion (Fig. 12.8, bottom). Both of these respiratory gating strategies are contingent on the ability to generate the necessary four-dimensional treatment planning images during simulation.

Four-Dimensional Imaging

Four-dimensional (4-D) imaging combines three-dimensional (3-D) spatial information with the time-dependent motion resulting from respiration. Although 4-D MRI[130] and PET[131] techniques currently exist, 4-D CT is currently the most prevalent imaging technique utilized in radiation oncology.[132,133]

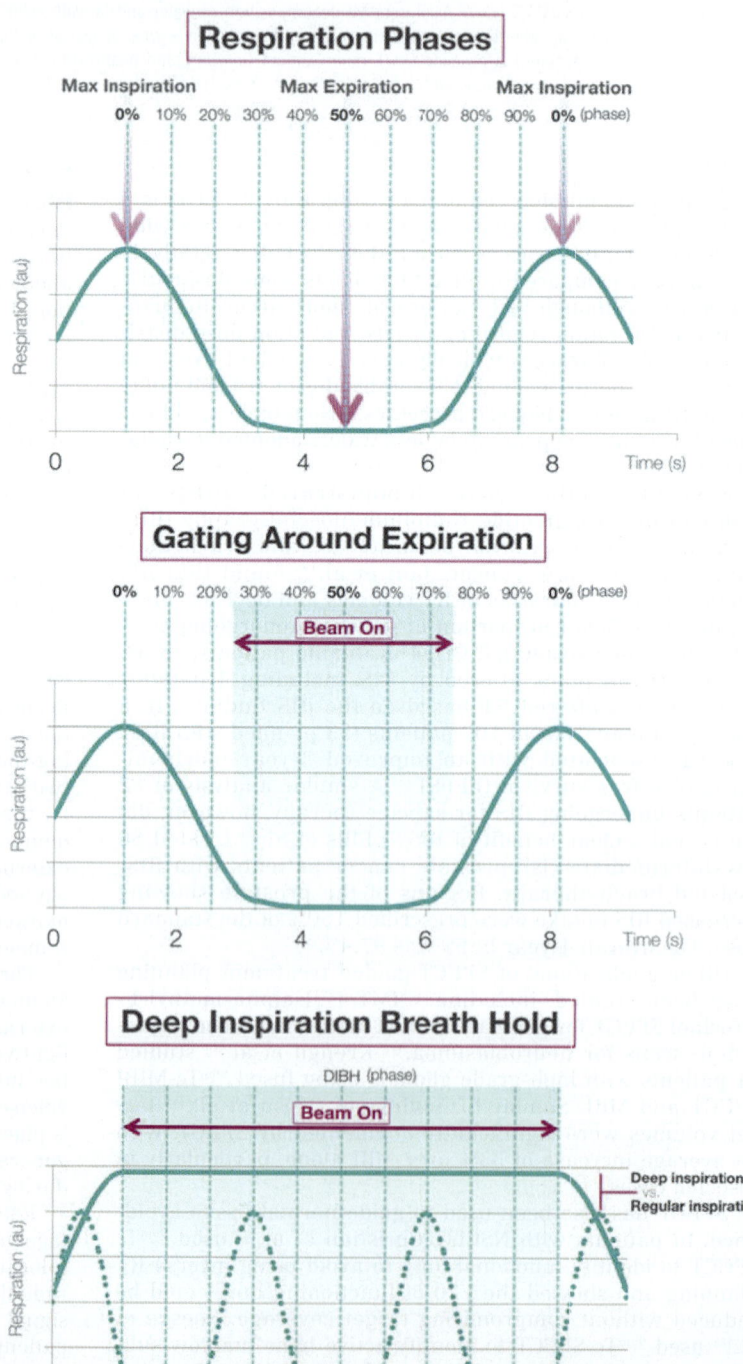

FIGURE 12.8. Top: A sample period of patient respiration, with ten phases labeled (0% to 90% phases). **Middle:** An illustration of respiratory gating around expiration (30% to 70% phases). **Bottom:** An illustration of deep inspiration breath hold gating.

Motion artifacts can occur in free-breathing CT scans for a variety of reasons. If the scan speed is slower than the tumor motion speed, the image of the tumor is blurred. If the scan speed is faster than the tumor motion speed, the tumor image represents an arbitrary phase of respiration. If the scan speed is comparable to the tumor motion speed, the tumor image is distorted (shape and/or position). All of these scenarios present significant challenges for motion management and treatment planning.[123,124,134]

Four-dimensional CT provides a solution to these imaging problems by correlating the CT data acquisition with patient respiration. By associating each position of interest along the patient's superior–inferior axis with the corresponding breathing phase, multiple 3-D datasets can be generated (typically ten) that represent the patient's anatomy throughout respiration. During the CT scan, real-time breathing phase information can be obtained through a variety of methods: RPM system, surface imaging, pressure belts, or spirometry. After completion of the scan, images are sorted using the corresponding breathing phase or amplitude signals. However, this additional information comes at a cost. By acquiring redundant information to generate multiple phase images, the patient is exposed to more radiation dose. Figure 12.9 illustrates the motion of a simulated lung tumor (top) and the corresponding CT slices (bottom) during the various phases of respiration.

Four-Dimensional Target Delineation

Creating an internal target volume (ITV) or an internal gross tumor volume (IGTV) for a moving lung tumor can be done in multiple ways.[135–140] Simplistic techniques such as "slow" CT scanning or forced shallow breathing have shown to be beneficial when compared to free-breathing CT-derived ITV techniques alone.[136] However, more sophisticated techniques, utilizing 4-D CT imaging, are preferred for target delineation.

Four-dimensional CT-based target delineation techniques for lung tumors are most commonly broken up into two approaches: maximum intensity projection (MIP)-based or individual phase-based.[138–140] The MIP-based technique is popular because of its simplicity. By creating a single 3-D image that represents the maximum intensity of all phases of interest,

FIGURE 12.9. **Top:** Motion of a simulated lung tumor (magenta circle) during the various phases of respiration. In the 50% phase (max expiration), the tumor is in the most superior position. In the 30% and 70% phases, the tumor is pushed slightly inferior as the lungs expand, but the majority of the tumor is in the corresponding slice as the 50% phase (*blue shading*). In the 0% phase (max inspiration), the tumor is pushed greatly inferior, leaving only a small cross-section of the tumor in the corresponding slice. **Bottom:** Computed tomography (CT) slices of the above scenario, illustrating the changing tumor cross-section with respiration.

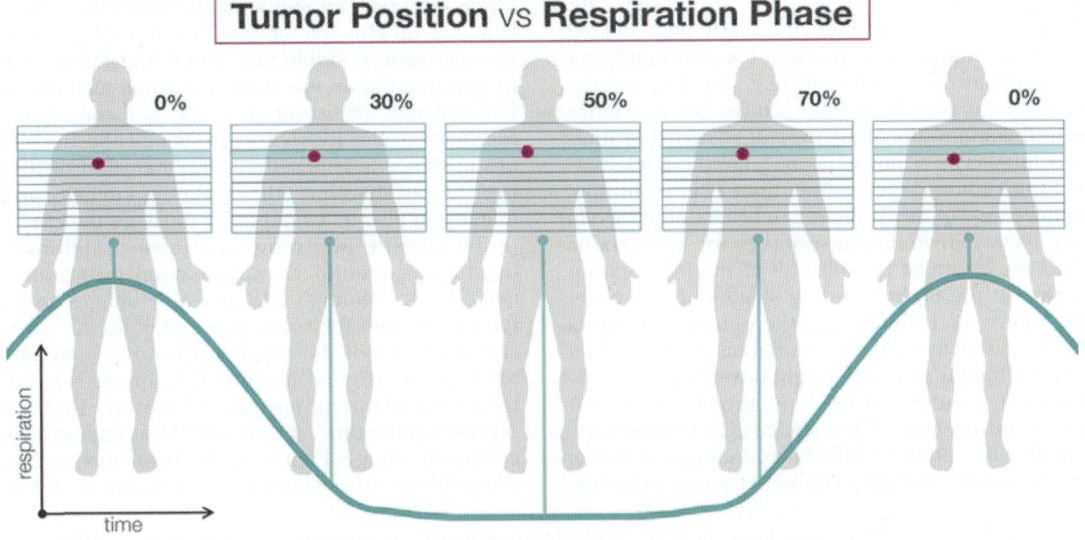

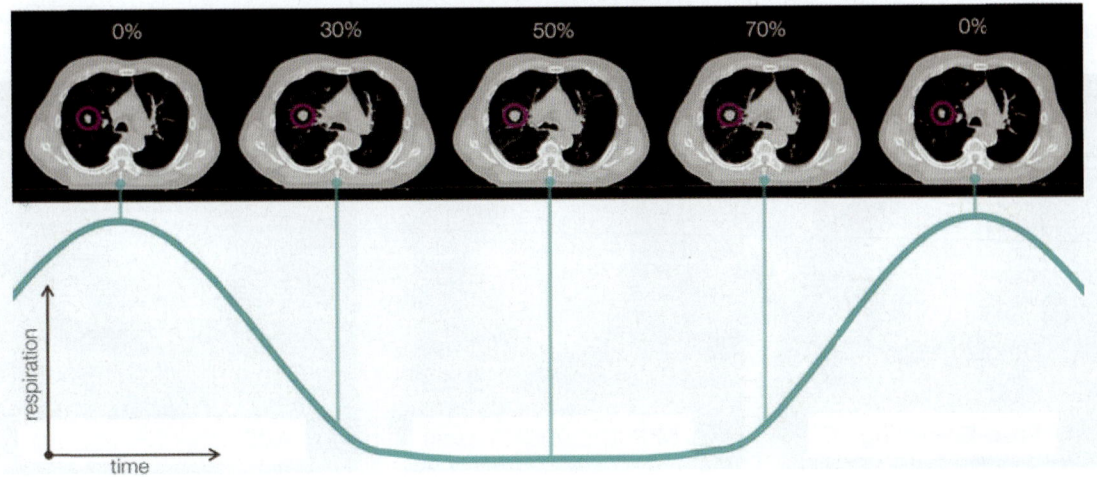

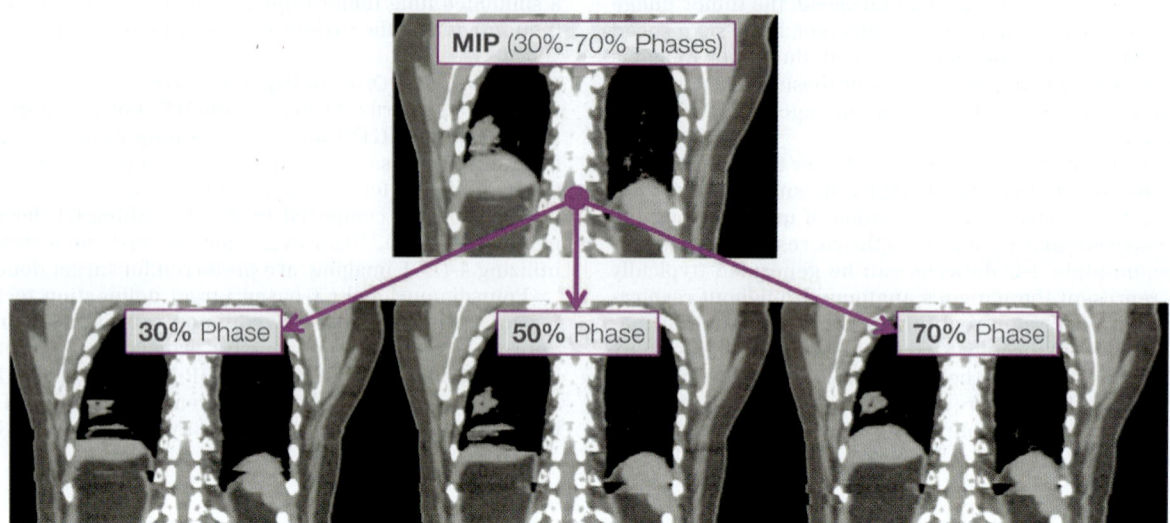

FIGURE 12.10. **Top:** A maximum intensity projection (MIP) image of a right lower lobe lung lesion around expiration (30% to 70% phases), which appears to illustrate a large lesion abutting the diaphragm. **Bottom:** The 30%, 50%, and 70% phase images (*left to right*) used to create the MIP image. All of these individual phase images contain significant motion artifacts that could lead to overestimating the size of the lung tumor in the MIP image.

the target can be visualized in all positions simultaneously. This allows for easy target delineation, if the MIP was created from accurate phase images and the target is not abutting a structure with a similar electron density (e.g., the diaphragm). However, as treatment planning systems have become more sophisticated and computationally powerful, visualizing multiple 3-D phase images as a movie has become the gold standard for 4-D lung tumor target delineation. This technique allows for the full range of tumor motion to be evaluated while also inspecting each individual phase image for artifacts or distortions. This method also provides all of the information necessary to choose the optimal gating strategy for a given set of images. Figure 12.10 illustrates the potential dangers of using a MIP-based alone, without examining the individual phase images for a lung tumor in the right lower lobe.

For moving tumors outside of the lung, target delineation can be more difficult because of the similarities between the tumor electron density and that of the surrounding soft tissue. In these cases, the use of surrogates can be extremely valuable.

When available, implanted metal fiducials, stents, and surgical clips are all effective options for quantifying target motion. If the surrogate is stable (i.e., is not migrating) and is located in or near the tumor, the aforementioned techniques can be used to determine the extent of motion and choose the optimal gating strategy. For liver cancers specifically, the electron density of the tumor is generally lower than that of the surrounding liver tissue. Therefore, the minimum intensity projection (MIN) image can also be valuable for deriving the ITV.

Treatment planning and dose calculation for moving tumors should be approached differently than target delineation. Although MIP and MIN images both provide useful information for contouring, they do not provide an accurate depiction of the tumor for dose calculation. Instead, the average intensity projection (AVG) image is recommended for treatment planning because of the fact that it more closely represents the time-averaged patient anatomy than any other composite image. Figure 12.11 illustrates an image comparison between a free-breathing CT image, a MIP image, and an

FIGURE 12.11. A comparison of a free-breathing computed tomography (CT) image, a maximum intensity projection (MIP) image, and an average intensity projection (AVG) image (*left to right*) for a lung tumor. The free-breathing image provides a snapshot of the tumor in an arbitrary phase. The MIP image illustrates the position of the tumor in all 10 phases. The AVG image illustrates the time-averaged position of the tumor.

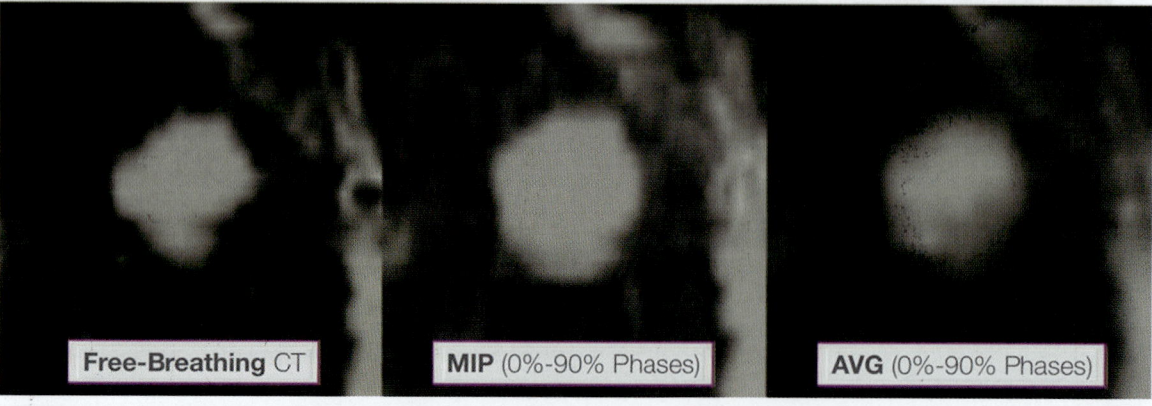

AVG image for a lung tumor. As the field of radiation oncology continues to evolve, and the computational resources for commercial RT products continue to increase, the field will move toward 4-D planning as the gold standard (i.e., calculating dose on each individual phase image and accumulating the dose).[141,142]

IN-ROOM IMAGING

Ultrasound

Ultrasound (US) remains a clinically available IGRT modality in modern radiation oncology; however, the technique is typically confined to prostate cancer.[142,143] US systems work by first transmitting high-frequency sound waves into the body from a probe and then waiting for the sound waves to reflect back to the probe from a tissue boundary. This information can then be used by the US system to calculate the distances from the probe and the tissue or organ (boundary) of interest. Furthermore, anatomical images can be generated by sweeping the probe across an entire region of interest. Readers interested in a more in-depth description of US technology are referred elsewhere.[144]

IGRT using US requires a system to map the US image coordinate system to the linear accelerator coordinate system and subsequently the simulation images. This is typically done in one of two ways: tracking the position of the stereotactic arm holding the probe or tracking the position of the probe itself via infrared imaging. An example of tracking the position of the stereotactic arm is the B-mode acquisition and targeting (BAT) transabdominal system (NOMOS, North American Scientific, Chatsworth, CA). In this system, the stereotactic arm is attached to the linear accelerator gantry, providing information on the probe location. An example of tracking the location of the probe itself is the SonArray system (Varian Medical Systems, Palo Alto, CA). In this system, an optical guidance platform provides real-time feedback of the US probe position in the treatment room. Using either of these techniques, the target location can be determined in the treatment room prior to treatment, and the necessary shifts can be calculated to move the target into the correct position for treatment.

Very little information has been published regarding the use of US IGRT for nonprostate patients. Most notably are studies to confirm bladder volume and position in gynecologic patients[145] and evaluate intracavitary brachytherapy treatment planning for perforations.[146,147] However, there is an extensive amount of research regarding the use of US IGRT for prostate cancer. Numerous studies have been published comparing US-based patient set-up methods versus conventional set-up methods (i.e., utilizing external skin markers),[148–152] and several studies have been published comparing US-based patient set-up versus implanted fiducial markers.[152–154]

As newer IGRT approaches continue to develop, the role of US-based IGRT is likely to continue to decrease.[143] However, US will likely always have a role in prostate cancer care because of the fact that it offers an IGRT solution that does not require additional ionizing radiation.

Video and Surface Imaging

Video and surface imaging techniques for radiation therapy were first introduced over 30 years ago. Early versions of this technology were based on the ability of closed circuit cameras to compare an image of the patient's setup to a stored reference image[155] or for image subtraction techniques to automatically determine differences in patient set-up images.[156,157]

An example of a modern surface imaging technology is the AlignRT system (Vision RT Ltd., London, UK). This system is designed to aid in initial patient setup as well as patient position monitoring. Through the use of three 3-D stereo camera units mounted to the ceiling of the treatment vault, the patient surface can be constantly monitored and compared to the ideal position (determined from the treatment planning CT) with submillimeter accuracy. This system can also be incorporated into the linear accelerator management system to automatically trigger the beam to turn off when a patient is out of position.

Although this technology has been used for many IGRT applications, one of its most popular applications involved breast cancer. AlignRT has been used to assess interfraction variation for whole breast radiotherapy,[158,159] as well as to examine positioning accuracy for left-sided breast DIBH techniques.[160,161] In addition to breast, the AlignRT system has also shown value when used for intracranial SRS cases with minimal immobilization. Cerviño et al. have shown that an open-mask approach (i.e., leaving the face exposed) provides enough surface area to accurately detect head motion in real time.[162,163] Figure 12.12 illustrates the use of AlignRT for an intracranial SRS case.

As surface and video imaging technologies continue to evolve, the uses for these IGRT techniques are expected to expand. Building on the success of frameless radiosurgery, other novel uses for this nonionizing IGRT technique will likely appear in the future.

Planar Imaging

Megavoltage (MV) and kilovoltage (kV) planar imaging techniques are the most common in-room IGRT approaches used in radiation therapy today. These systems have proven valuable for nearly all disease sites and are incorporated into a variety of linear accelerator-based treatment systems.[143,164] As the field of radiation oncology has evolved, so has the quality and performance of these planar imaging systems, making them a staple in modern radiation oncology.

Electronic Portal Imaging Devices

Electronic portal imaging devices (EPIDs) utilize the therapeutic beam (MV) to generate an image on a movable flat-panel detector. These devices have entirely replaced portal films in most cases, by providing higher-quality 2-D digital images of the treatment field with the patient in the treatment position. Although EPID design has gone through numerous iterations, most commercial systems today consist of amorphous silicon (aSi) detectors. These systems work by first converting the x-rays to visible light using a scintillator and then converting the visible light to electrons using a photodiode array. In the last step, the electrons activate pixels in a layer of aSi to generate an image. For a more comprehensive overview of EPID technology and development, readers are referred elsewhere.[165,166]

EPID-based planar imaging is often used for patient setup when the size and shape of the treatment field need to be verified in reference to the patient anatomy (i.e., 3-D conformal techniques). Although different energy beams are available for treatment and imaging, EPID-based imaging is limited by the lack of contrast available for the Compton interactions that dominate the 2.5- to 18-MV therapeutic energy range. Because of this, EPIDs are most beneficial when the region of interest contains boney anatomy or implanted fiducial markers.[167–170] However, as more sophisticated IGRT techniques become commonplace, the use of EPID-based imaging is decreasing for complex IMRT/VMAT treatments.

kV Imaging Devices

Utilizing the therapeutic treatment (MV) beam for IGRT has two main limitations: increased patient dose and decreased image quality. Because of this, kV-based imaging systems have become the standard for modern IGRT. Diagnostic kV imaging systems are incorporated into treatment delivery systems in

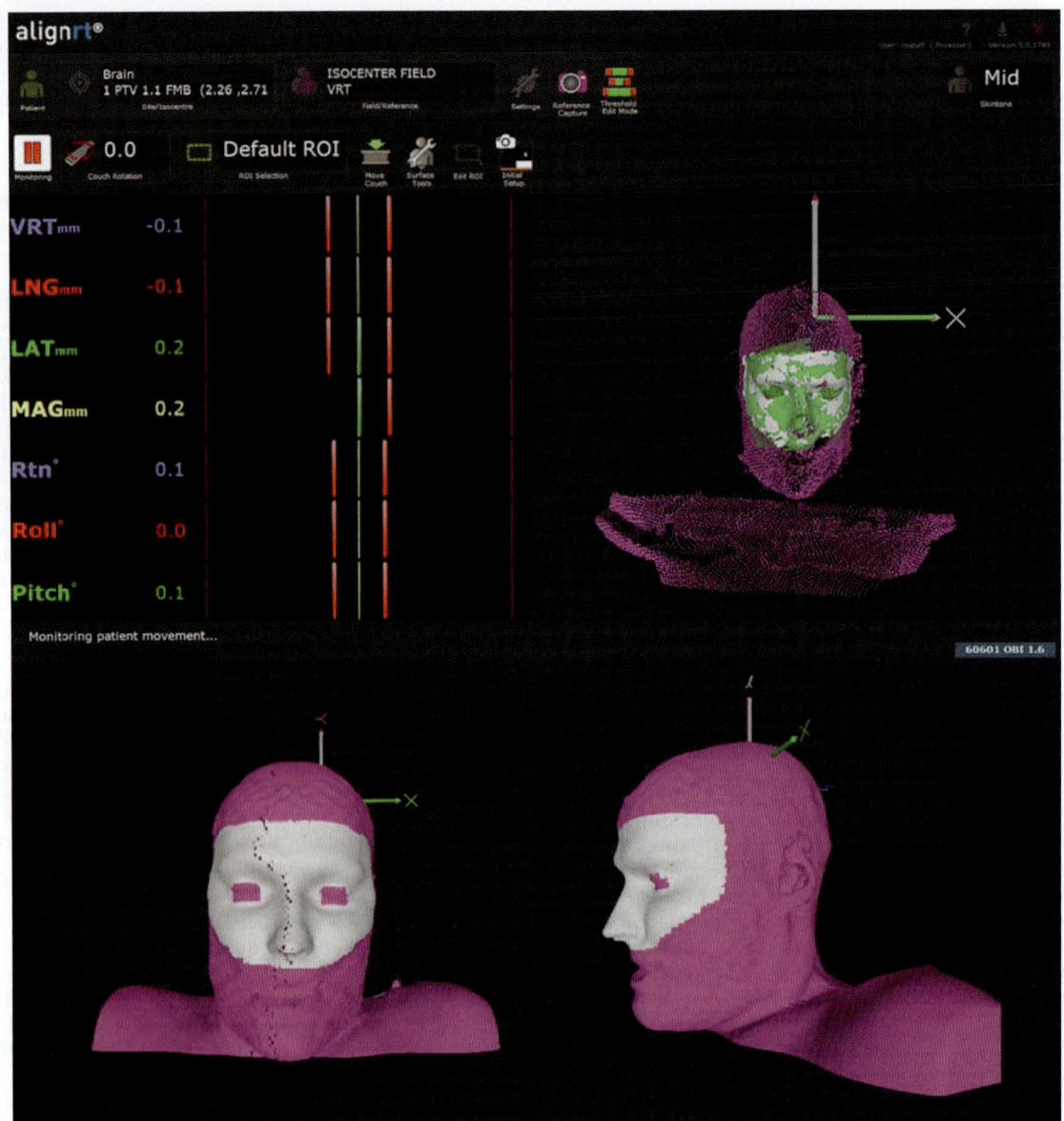

FIGURE 12.12. The use of AlignRT during an intracranial stereotactic radiosurgery case. **Top:** AlignRT monitoring the alignment of a patient's surface (face in an open mask), with deviations from the intended position listed in a column on the *left*. **Bottom:** The chosen surface to monitor (*white*), selected from the simulation computed tomography body contour (*pink*).

a variety of ways, but regardless of the implementation, all are designed to provide high-quality 2-D pretreatment digital images of the patient anatomy.

The On-Board Imager (OBI) system (Varian Medical Systems, Palo Alto, CA) is a popular example of a linear accelerator equipped with gantry-mounted kV imaging. This system incorporates a retractable diagnostic quality kV imaging tube and a movable flat-panel aSi detector perpendicular to the treatment beam (i.e., offset by 90 degrees). The OBI system allows high-quality and low-dose images to be compared to digitally reconstructed radiographs (DRRs) of the patient anatomy for orthogonal pairs of images, taken at any angle. Fox et al. presented a comprehensive overview of the OBI software and hardware implementation and performance.[171] An example of the Varian gantry–mounted OBI system is illustrated in Figure 12.13.

Although gantry-mounted kV imaging systems are the most popular design, other implementations also exist. CyberKnife (Accuray Inc, Sunnyvale, CA) consists of a linear accelerator attached to a robotic manipulator with 6 degrees of freedom.

In this system, diagnostic x-ray tubes are mounted to the ceiling and nearly orthogonal aSi flat-panel detectors are mounted to the floor. The Novalis system (BrainLAB Inc, Westchester, IL) is a more conventional gantry-mounted linear accelerator design, but the diagnostic x-ray tubes are mounted on the floor of the treatment room, and the nearly orthogonal flat-panel detectors are located on the ceiling. In both systems, images are automatically compared with DRRs from the treatment planning CT to verify and adjust patient alignment.[172–174]

Volumetric Imaging

Cone-beam computed tomography (CBCT) systems (both MV and kV) offer the natural progression from planar 2-D IGRT to volumetric 3-D IGRT. Over the past several years, CBCT systems have quickly become the standard of care for a variety of disease sites and have been incorporated into numerous linear accelerator-based treatment systems.[144,164] As IGRT continues to progress, the use of CBCT will most likely continue to play an integral role.

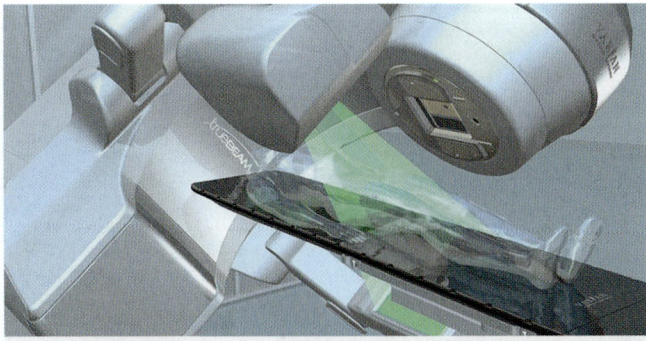

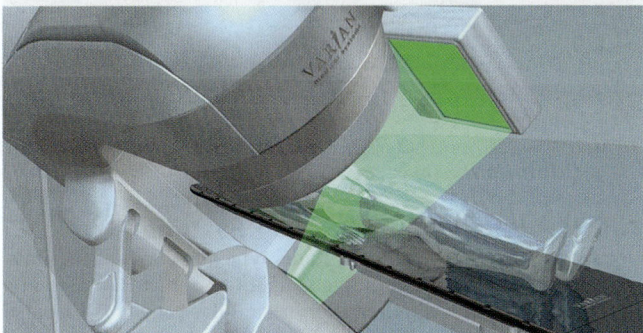

FIGURE 12.13. An illustration of the gantry-mounted Varian On-Board Imager system. Planar kilovoltage images (*green* overlay) are being taken at two orthogonal positions (*top and bottom*). (Courtesy of Varian, Palo Alto, CA.)

MV CBCT

MV CBCT systems utilize the treatment beam and the EPID to generate a 3-D image that is comparable to the treatment planning CT. MV CBCT images are created by collecting a series of 2-D projections, followed by reconstruction of the 3-D dataset in a process similar to that of conventional CT imaging. MV CBCT has the same limitations as that of MV planar imaging. When compared to kV techniques, MV CBCT is associated with a higher patient dose and lower contrast. An example of a MV CBCT is illustrated in Figure 12.14.

Multiple studies have evaluated the usefulness of MV CBCT, with the largest number of publications coming from UCSF utilizing a Primus linear accelerator (Siemens Oncology Systems, Concord, CA).[175–178] Although many of these studies illustrate the utility of MV CBCT imaging for a variety of cancers, most vendors have moved away from this technology because of the aforementioned downsides. One unique exception is the

Halcyon system (Varian Medical Systems, Palo Alto, CA), which offers integrated MV planar and CBCT imaging, with the imaging dose accounted for in the treatment planning system. Although kV imaging is available for Halcyon systems, MV imaging–only systems are available at a lower price point.

kV CBCT

Most large linear accelerator manufacturers currently offer gantry-mounted kV CBCT systems. For example, the previously discussed Varian OBI system, consisting of a diagnostic x-ray tube mounted across from a flat-panel aSi detector, is also capable of generating high-quality kV CBCT images. The OBI system, along with the Elekta Synergy system (Elekta Oncology Systems, Norcross, GA), acquires kV projections through a full 360-degree gantry rotation or smaller 180-degree rotation, which are then reconstructed into a 3-D dataset.[179] An example of a kV CBCT is illustrated in Figure 12.15.

Similar to MV CBCT imaging, multiple studies have evaluated the utility of kV CBCT imaging systems.[179–182,182a] However, unlike MV CBCT imaging, kV CBCT imaging has become the standard of care for modern IGRT. Higher-contrast high-quality kV CBCT images allow users to identify important anatomy for a variety of cancers throughout the body, creating the best 3-D–3-D registration possible with the treatment planning CT. As kV CBCT techniques continue to evolve, image quality will continue to improve as advances such as 4-D CBCT will become the norm.

MRI

As discussed earlier, MRI provides superior soft tissue visualization compared to other CT and other clinically available in-room imaging modalities. Until recently, there have been technical barriers making it difficult to combine MRI with clinical radiation therapy devices. However, there are now clinically available hybrid machines capable of real-time MR imaging during radiotherapy. One of the first of these devices of its kind developed by ViewRay Inc. (Oakwood Village, OH) utilizes a 0.35-T MR, 3-KCi cobalt sources, and three double-focused MLCs (Fig. 12.16). This system was developed using cobalt sources rather than a linear accelerator to overcome some of the technical issues that arise due to electron interactions with high-strength magnetic fields.[183]

Chen et al.[184,185] recently reported on their initial clinical experience in the use of MR-guided radiotherapy. Using an integrated MR–cobalt system, they treated 31 patients with newly diagnosed or recurrent HNC with MRI-guided IMRT (Fig. 12.17). The results were promising with excellent rates of locoregional control in both newly treated and recurrent patients as well as modest rates of toxicity consistent with previously published literature. Of note, the authors commented

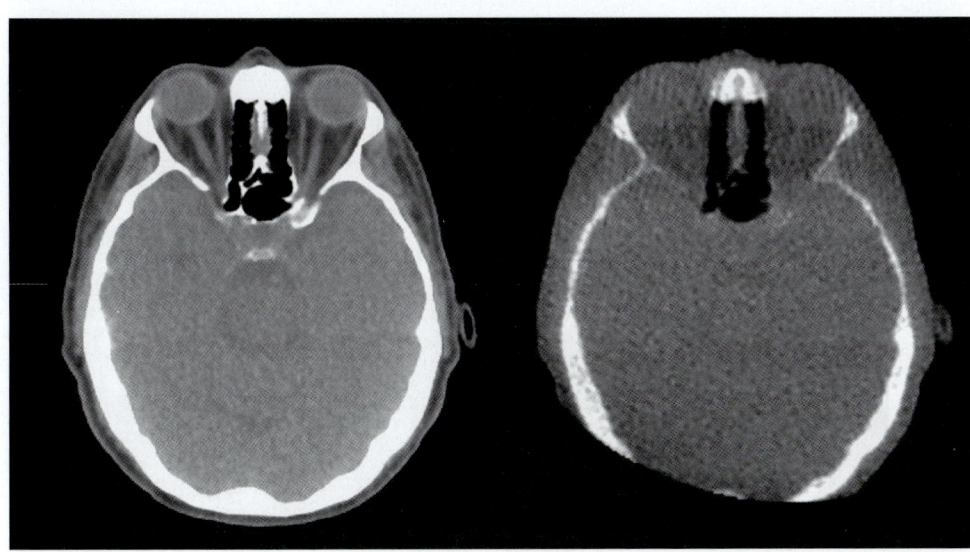

FIGURE 12.14. Comparison of a megavoltage cone-beam computed tomography (*right*) with the treatment planning computed tomography (*left*). The axial slice shown includes the brain, skull, and optic structures.

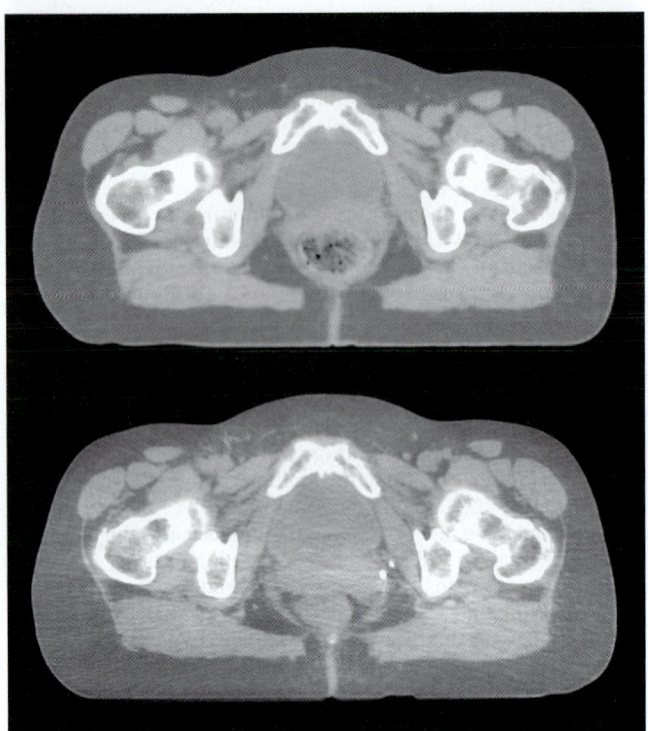

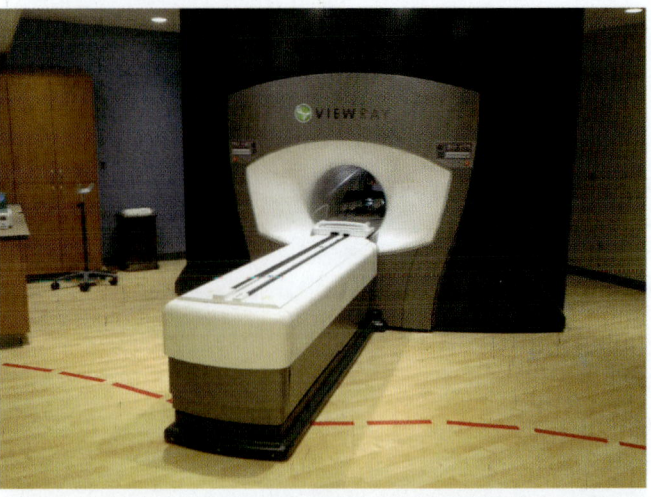

FIGURE 12.16. ViewRay cobalt-magnetic resonance imaging system. (Courtesy of Viewray, Oakwood Village, OH.)

FIGURE 12.15. Comparison of a kilovoltage cone-beam computed tomography (*bottom*) with the treatment planning computed tomography (*top*). The axial slice shown includes the femoral heads, bladder, rectum, etc.

that only a small subset of these patients were treated with adaptive replanning, and they felt that expanded use of this approach would be feasible and provide potential to improve the therapeutic ratio.

In an attempt to overcome some of the technical limitations of cobalt therapy, several centers worldwide have begun development of MR-LINAC prototypes. Investigators at the University of Utrecht and Cross Cancer Institute in Alberta are pioneers in this area and have been working for over a decade to development hybrid MR-LINAC prototypes.[186,187] There are now multiple other MR-LINAC systems currently under development, but to date these have not been employed in routine clinical use.

Radiofrequency Localization Systems

Electromagnetic localization systems typically consist of a magnetic dipole source and multiple sensors to detect the magnetic field created by the dipole. When a radiofrequency (RF) pulse excites the dipole, a magnetic field is created. When the RF signal is removed, it results in an oscillating magnetic dipole. The dipole sources in clinical RF localization systems are typically referred to as transponders, where each transponder is approximately the size of a gold fiducial. These transponders are implanted directly into the tissue of interest. Electromagnetic localization systems have several benefits. The transponders can be implanted directly into the target area, no ionizing radiation is used, and the system provides real-time positional feedback. The Calypso system (Varian Medical Systems, Palo Alto, CA) is an example of a commercially available RF localization system.[188]

Although most of the research published with RF localization systems is focused on prostate cancer localization and continuous monitoring during treatment,[189–193] other treatment sites such as pancreatic cancer have also shown potential.[193a] As a whole, RF localization systems such as Calypso are a valuable IGRT tool for performing real-time monitoring of target position for sites in which intrafraction motion is a concern.

FIGURE 12.17. Axial and coronal magnetic resonance images (MRI) from an MRI-guided intensity-modulated radiation therapy plan in a patient with locoregionally advanced head and neck cancer. The gross tumor volume (**A**), planning tumor volume (PTV) receiving 70 Gy (PTV70) (**B** and **C**; *red line*), PTV59.4 (**B** and **C**; *blue line*), PTV54 (**B** and **C**; *purple line*), and parotid gland (**C**; *green line*) are shown. The *arrow* demonstrates sparing of the contralateral parotid gland. (Reprinted by permission from Springer: Chen AM, Hsu S, Lamb J, et al. MRI-guided radiotherapy for head and neck cancer: initial clinical experience. *Clin Transl Oncol* 2018;20[2]:160–168. Copyright © 2017 Federación de Sociedades Españolas de Oncología [FESEO].)

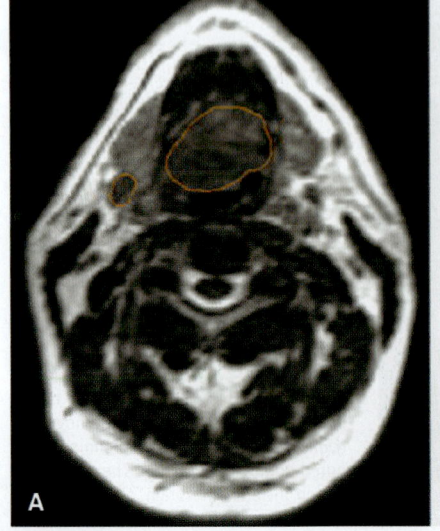

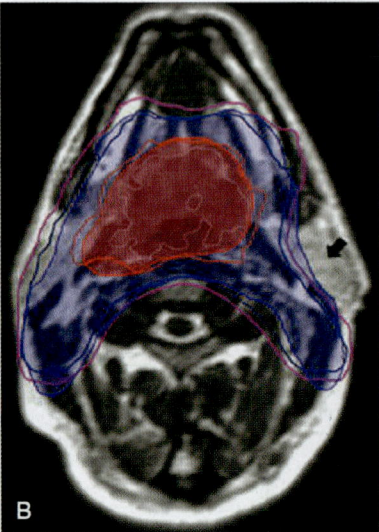

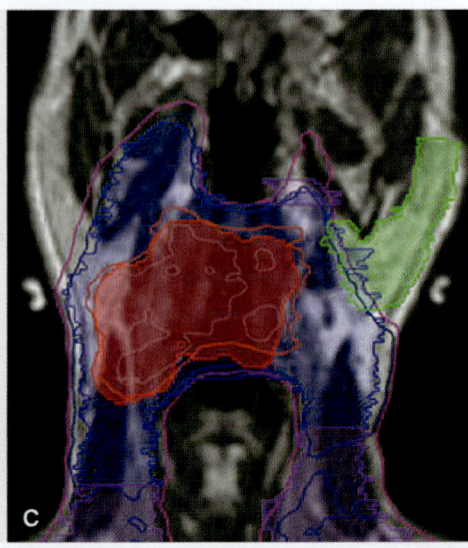

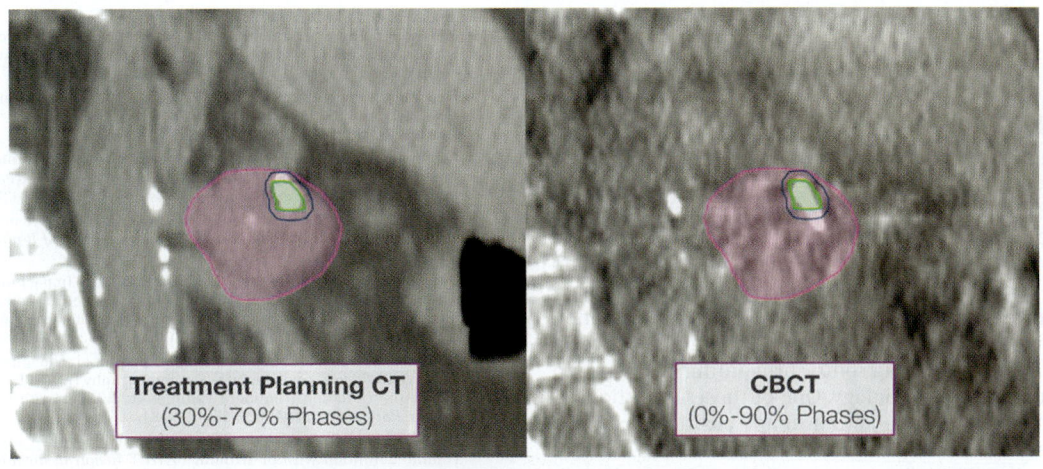

FIGURE 12.18. A comparison of the treatment planning computed tomography (CT) (*left*) created from the phases around expiration (30% to 70%) and a cone-beam CT (*right*) created from all 10 respiratory phases (0% to 90%). In both cases, the *pink* contour represents the planning target volume, and the *green and blue* contours represent the fiducial and a 1-mm margin, respectively.

Four-Dimensional Imaging and Motion Management

Regardless of the respiratory-induced motion management strategy utilized for target delineation and treatment planning, effective in-room imaging is a necessity to ensure proper treatment delivery. For free breathing, abdominal compression, respiratory gating, and real-time tumor tracking techniques, in-room imaging must be used to verify that that the treatment planning conditions are appropriately replicated.

2-D, CBCT, and Fluoroscopic Imaging

Two-dimensional and 3-D (CBCT) imaging have well-defined roles in patient setup and treatment verification. However, in 4-D motion management cases (e.g., gating around expiration or DIBH), the use of these technologies becomes more complex and crucial. Although orthogonal kV images are the standard for initial patient alignment, little attention is paid to the breathing phase at this stage of the patient set-up process. This is not the case for CBCT imaging, which has proven to be valuable for tumor and soft tissue alignment in both gated and nongated treatments. In nongated cases, the 3-D–3-D matching process is relatively straightforward. However, the lack of

commonplace 4-D CBCT imaging creates a significant 3-D–3-D registration problem for gated cases. For example, when gating around expiration, the treatment planning CT is generated from the phases around expiration only (i.e., 30% to 70%), but most in-room CBCT systems only have the capability to generate images from all respiratory phases (i.e., 0% to 90%). When substantial motion is present, this results in the target or surrogate appearing larger or elongated in the CBCT image. Figure 12.18 illustrates a common registration issue where the CBCT image of an implanted fiducial appears much larger than the contour from the treatment planning CT. This is the result of the CBCT image including the phases around inspiration, where the fiducial is pushed inferiorly. As 4-D CBCT systems become more commonplace, the problems associated with motion-induced blurring will become less prohibitive.

Fluoroscopic imaging is a unique and beneficial tool for gated treatment verification. Unlike static kV imaging, this technique provides a "live" look at the target anatomy and/or surrogate throughout the patient's respiratory cycle. This allows the position of the target to be compared to an aperture representing the correct breathing phase (e.g., around expiration or DIBH), allowing the position of the target and the gating window to be determined simultaneously. The diagrams in Figure 12.19

FIGURE 12.19. Simulated fluoroscopic images (anterior–posterior) of a lung tumor (*purple circle*) in the correct phase (*left side*—within the internal target volume [ITV] aperture) and in the incorrect phase (*right side*—outside of the ITV aperture).

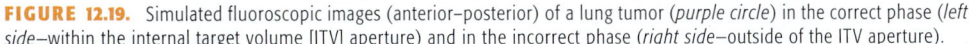
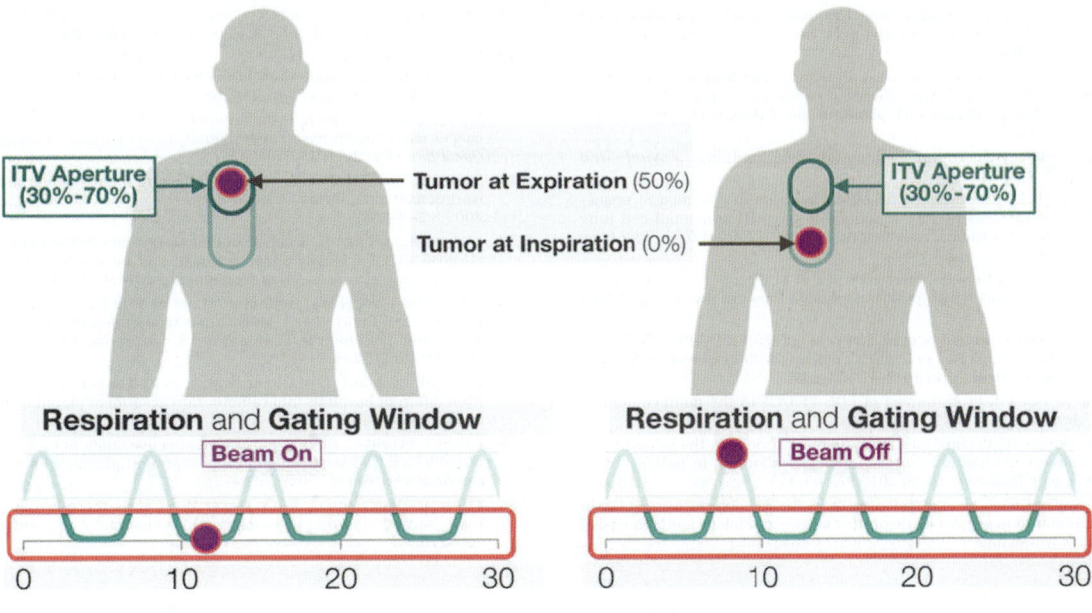

illustrate how fluoroscopic imaging can be used to determine that the target is in the correct location for a gated treatment delivery.

Tumor Tracking

Tumor tracking is a sophisticated motion management strategy that provides a technologically intense alternative to respiratory gating, DIBH, or abdominal compression. Instead of limiting target motion or treating at specific phases of respiration, tumor tracking utilizes real-time tumor localization to continually reposition the treatment beam, thus decreasing residual target motion and increasing delivery efficiency. However, this ideal motion management strategy has several technical hurdles that are currently preventing widespread clinical adoption of this technology. One of these limitations is treatment planning. All of the actual tumor positions, relative to the surrounding tissues, cannot be known at the time of treatment planning. Therefore, treatment planning for tumor tracking is typically done on an average patient geometry or 4-D simulation data, and an adaptive scheme is applied throughout the treatment course. Although some specialized commercial systems are already available, more LINAC-based systems are currently investigating ways to obtain real-time 3-D tumor position information and to decrease system latency.

CONCLUSIONS

IGRT has become ubiquitous in radiation oncology clinics, and new applications are constantly being developed to improve treatment accuracy with the ultimate goal of improving clinical outcomes. Although numerous studies have shown dosimetric benefits with implementation of IGRT, only a handful have tested the use of IGRT in a prospective fashion and reported clinical outcomes. Additional research is still needed to test the clinical impact and safety of various IGRT applications. Furthermore, the question of cost-effectiveness of routine use of IGRT needs to be addressed. There are numerous ongoing trials analyzing the utility of image-guided radiation therapy in a variety of cancer types.[194] The results of these studies should help to guide clinical decision-making in radiation oncology in regard to IGRT implementation and provide further hypotheses for incorporation of novel imaging modalities into prospective clinical trial design.

REFERENCES

1. Stapleford LJ, Lawson JD, Perkins C, et al. Evaluation of automatic atlas-based lymph node segmentation for head-and-neck cancer. *Int J Radiat Oncol Biol Phys* 2010;77:959–966.
2. Werner-Wasik M, Nelson AD, Choi W, et al. What is the best way to contour lung tumors on PET scans? Multiobserver validation of a gradient-based method using a NSCLC digital PET phantom. *Int J Radiat Oncol Biol Phys* 2012;82(3):1164–1171.
3. Plathow C, Weber WA. Tumor cell metabolism imaging. *J Nucl Med* 2008;49(Suppl 2):43S–63S.
4. MacManus MP, Hicks RJ, Matthews JP, et al. High rate of detection of unsuspected distant metastases by PET in apparent stage III non-small-cell lung cancer: implications for radical radiation therapy. *Int J Radiat Oncol Biol Phys* 2001;50:287–293.
5. Pieterman RM, van Putten JW, Meuzelaar JJ, et al. Preoperative staging of non-small-cell lung cancer with positron-emission tomography. *N Engl J Med* 2000;343:254–261.
6. Haerle SK, Schmid DT, Ahmad N, et al. The value of (18)F-FDG PET/CT for the detection of distant metastases in high-risk patients with head and neck squamous cell carcinoma. *Oral Oncol* 2011;47:653–659.
7. Baba S, Abe K, Isoda T, et al. Impact of FDG-PET/CT in the management of lymphoma. *Ann Nucl Med* 2011;25:701–716.
8. Muijs CT, Beukema JC, Pruim J, et al. A systematic review on the role of FDG-PET/CT in tumour delineation and radiotherapy planning in patients with esophageal cancer. *Radiother Oncol* 2010;97:165–171.
9. Schoder H, Noy A, Gonen M, et al. Intensity of 18-fluorodeoxyglucose uptake in positron emission tomography distinguishes between indolent and aggressive non-Hodgkin's lymphoma. *J Clin Oncol* 2005;23:4643–4651.
10. Suzuki A, Xiao L, Hayashi Y, et al. Prognostic significance of baseline positron emission tomography and importance of clinical complete response in patients with esophageal or gastroesophageal junction cancer treated with definitive chemoradiotherapy. *Cancer* 2011;117:4823–4833.
11. Schwarz JK, Siegel BA, Dehdashti F, et al. Metabolic response on posttherapy FDG-PET predicts patterns of failure after radiotherapy for cervical cancer. *Int J Radiat Oncol Biol Phys* 2012;83(1):185–190.
12. Ashamalla H, Rafla S, Parikh K, et al. The contribution of integrated PET/CT to the evolving definition of treatment volumes in radiation treatment planning in lung cancer. *Int J Radiat Oncol Biol Phys* 2005;63:1016–1023.
13. Bradley J, Thorstad WL, Mutic S, et al. Impact of FDG-PET on radiation therapy volume delineation in non-small-cell lung cancer. *Int J Radiat Oncol Biol Phys* 2004;59:78–86.
14. Deniaud-Alexandre E, Touboul E, Lerouge D, et al. Impact of computed tomography and 18F-deoxyglucose coincidence detection emission tomography image fusion for optimization of conformal radiotherapy in non-small-cell lung cancer. *Int J Radiat Oncol Biol Phys* 2005;63:1432–1441.
15. Vanuytsel LJ, Vansteenkiste JF, Stroobants SG, et al. The impact of (18)F-fluoro-2-deoxy-D-glucose positron emission tomography (FDG-PET) lymph node staging on the radiation treatment volumes in patients with non-small cell lung cancer. *Radiother Oncol* 2000;55:317–324.
16. Bradley J, Bae K, Choi N, et al. A phase II comparative study of gross tumor volume definition with or without PET/CT fusion in dosimetric planning for non-small-cell lung cancer (NSCLC): primary analysis of Radiation Therapy Oncology Group (RTOG) 0515. *Int J Radiat Oncol Biol Phys* 2012;82:435.e1–441.e1.
17. Grosu AL, Piert M, Weber WA, et al. Positron emission tomography for radiation treatment planning. *Strahlenther Onkol* 2005;181:483–499.
18. Yu J, Li X, Xing L, et al. Comparison of tumor volumes as determined by pathologic examination and FDG-PET/CT images of non-small-cell lung cancer: a pilot study. *Int J Radiat Oncol Biol Phys* 2009;75:1468–1474.
19. Pehlivan B, Topkan E, Onal C, et al. Comparison of CT and integrated PET-CT based radiation therapy planning in patients with malignant pleural mesothelioma. *Radiat Oncol* 2009;4:35.
20. Spratt DE, Diaz R, McElmurray J, et al. Impact of FDG PET/CT on delineation of the gross tumor volume for radiation planning in non-small-cell lung cancer. *Clin Nucl Med* 2010;35:237–243.
21. Wanet M, Lee JA, Weynand B, et al. Gradient-based delineation of the primary GTV on FDG-PET in non-small cell lung cancer: a comparison with threshold-based approaches, CT and surgical specimens. *Radiother Oncol* 2011;98:117–125.
22. Arens AI, Troost EG, Schinagl D, et al. FDG-PET/CT in radiation treatment planning of head and neck squamous cell carcinoma. *Q J Nucl Med Mol Imaging* 2011;55:521–528.
23. Schwartz DL, Ford EC, Rajendran J, et al. FDG-PET/CT-guided intensity modulated head and neck radiotherapy: a pilot investigation. *Head Neck* 2005;27:478–487.
24. Thiagarajan A, Caria N, Schöder H, et al. Target volume delineation in oropharyngeal cancer: impact of PET, MRI, and physical examination. *Int J Radiat Oncol Biol Phys* 2012;83(1):220–227.
25. Delouya G, Igidbashian L, Houle A, et al. ¹⁸F-FDG-PET imaging in radiotherapy tumor volume delineation in treatment of head and neck cancer. *Radiother Oncol* 2011;101:362–368.
26. Guido A, Fuccio L, Rombi B, et al. Combined 18F-FDG-PET/CT imaging in radiotherapy target delineation for head-and-neck cancer. *Int J Radiat Oncol Biol Phys* 2009;73:759–763.
26a. MacManus M, Nestle U, Rosenzweig KE, et al. Use of PET and PET/CT for radiation therapy planning: IAEA expert report 2006–2007. *Radiother Oncol* 2009;91:85–94.
26b. Schwartz DL, Ford E, Rajendran J, et al. FDG-PET/CT imaging for preradiotherapy staging of head-and-neck squamous cell carcinoma. *Int J Radiat Oncol Biol Phys* 2005;61:129–136.
27. Paulino AC, Koshy M, Howell R, et al. Comparison of CT- and FDG-PET-defined gross tumor volume in intensity-modulated radiotherapy for head-and-neck cancer. *Int J Radiat Oncol Biol Phys* 2005;61:1385–1392.
28. Gregoire V, Daisne JF, Geets X. Comparison of CT- and FDG-PET-defined GT: in regard to Paulino et al. *Int J Radiat Oncol Biol Phys* 2005;63:308–309.
29. Breen SL, Publicover J, De Silva S, et al. Intraobserver and interobserver variability in GTV delineation on FDG-PET-CT images of head and neck cancers. *Int J Radiat Oncol Biol Phys* 2007;68:763–770.
30. Yu H, Caldwell C, Mah K, et al. Automated radiation targeting in head-and-neck cancer using region-based texture analysis of PET and CT images. *Int J Radiat Oncol Biol Phys* 2009;75:618–625.
31. Simon E, Fox TH, Lee D, et al. PET lesion segmentation using automated iso-intensity contouring in head and neck cancer. *Technol Cancer Res Treat* 2009;8:249–255.
32. Leclerc M, Lartigau E, Lacornerie T, et al. Primary tumor delineation based on (18)FDG PET for locally advanced head and neck cancer treated by chemoradiotherapy. *Eur J Nucl Med Mol Imaging* 2014;41(5):915–924.
33. Schinagl DA, Vogel WV, Hoffmann AL, et al. Comparison of five segmentation tools for 18F-fluoro-deoxy-glucose-positron emission tomography-based target volume definition in head and neck cancer. *Int J Radiat Oncol Biol Phys* 2007;69:1282–1289.
34. Ollers M, Bosmans G, van Baardwijk A, et al. The integration of PET-CT scans from different hospitals into radiotherapy treatment planning. *Radiother Oncol* 2008;87:142–146.
35. Leong T, Everitt C, Yuen K, et al. A prospective study to evaluate the impact of FDG-PET on CT-based radiotherapy treatment planning for oesophageal cancer. *Radiother Oncol* 2006;78:254–261.
36. Vrieze O, Haustermans K, De Wever W, et al. Is there a role for FDG-PET in radiotherapy planning in esophageal carcinoma? *Radiother Oncol* 2004;73:269–275.

37. Hong TS, Killoran JH, Mamede M, et al. Impact of manual and automated inter-pretation of fused PET/CT data on esophageal target definitions in radiation planning. *Int J Radiat Oncol Biol Phys* 2008;72:1612–1628.

38. Vesprini D, Ung Y, Dinniwell R, et al. Improving observer variability in target delineation for gastro-oesophageal cancer—the role of (18F)fluoro-2-deoxy-D-glucose positron emission tomography/computed tomography. *Clin Oncol (R Coll Radiol)* 2008;20:631–638.

39. Han D, Yu J, Yu Y, et al. Comparison of (18)F-fluorothymidine and (18) F-fluorodeoxyglucose PET/CT in delineating gross tumor volume by optimal threshold in patients with squamous cell carcinoma of thoracic esophagus. *Int J Radiat Oncol Biol Phys* 2010;76:1235–1241.

40. Vali FS, Nagda S, Hall W, et al. Comparison of standardized uptake value-based positron emission tomography and computed tomography target volumes in esophageal cancer patients undergoing radiotherapy. *Int J Radiat Oncol Biol Phys* 2010;78:1057–1063.

41. Braendengen M, Hansson K, Radu C, et al. Delineation of gross tumor volume (GTV) for radiation treatment planning of locally advanced rectal cancer using information from MRI or FDG-PET/CT: a prospective study. *Int J Radiat Oncol Biol Phys* 2011;81:e439–e445.

42. Buijsen J, van den Bogaard J, Janssen MH, et al. FDG-PET provides the best correlation with the tumor specimen compared to MRI and CT in rectal cancer. *Radiother Oncol* 2011;98:270–276.

43. Janssen MH, Aerts HJ, Ollers MC, et al. Tumor delineation based on time-activ-ity curve differences assessed with dynamic fluorodeoxyglucose positron emis-sion tomography-computed tomography in rectal cancer patients. *Int J Radiat Oncol Biol Phys* 2009;73:456–465.

44. Krengli M, Cannillo B, Turri L, et al. Target volume delineation for preoperative radiotherapy of rectal cancer: inter-observer variability and potential impact of FDG-PET/CT imaging. *Technol Cancer Res Treat* 2010;9:393–398.

45. Patel DA, Chang ST, Goodman KA, et al. Impact of integrated PET/CT on vari-ability of target volume delineation in rectal cancer. *Technol Cancer Res Treat* 2007;6:31–36.

46. Rose BS, Liang Y, Lau SK, et al. Correlation between radiation dose to (18) F-FDG-PET defined active bone marrow subregions and acute hematologic toxicity in cervical cancer patients treated with chemoradiotherapy. *Int J Radiat Oncol Biol Phys* 2012;83(4):1185–1191.

47. Mell LK, Sirák I, Wei L, et al. Bone marrow-sparing intensity modulated radia-tion therapy with concurrent cisplatin for stage IB-IVA cervical cancer: an International Multicenter Phase II Clinical Trial (INTERTECC-2). *Int J Radiat Oncol Biol Phys* 2017;97(3):536–545.

48. Ford EC, Lavely WC, Frassica DA, et al. Comparison of FDG-PET/CT and CT for delineation of lumpectomy cavity for partial breast irradiation. *Int J Radiat Oncol Biol Phys* 2008;71:595–602.

49. Esthappan J, Chaudhari S, Santanam L, et al. Prospective clinical trial of positron emission tomography/computed tomography image-guided intensity-modulated radiation therapy for cervical carcinoma with positive para-aortic lymph nodes. *Int J Radiat Oncol Biol Phys* 2008;72:1134–1139.

50. Lin LL, Mutic S, Malyapa RS, et al. Sequential FDG-PET brachytherapy treat-ment planning in carcinoma of the cervix. *Int J Radiat Oncol Biol Phys* 2005;63:1494–1501.

51. Schwarz JK, Lin LL, Siegel BA, et al. 18-F-fluorodeoxyglucose-positron emis-sion tomography evaluation of early metabolic response during radiation therapy for cervical cancer. *Int J Radiat Oncol Biol Phys* 2008;72:1502–1507.

52. Lin LL, Mutic S, Low DA, et al. Adaptive brachytherapy treatment planning for cervical cancer using FDG-PET. *Int J Radiat Oncol Biol Phys* 2007;67:91–96.

53. Liang Y, Bydder M, Yashar CM, et al. Prospective study of functional bone marrow-sparing intensity modulated radiation therapy with concur-rent chemotherapy for pelvic malignancies. *Int J Radiat Oncol Biol Phys* 2013;85(2):406–414.

54. Girinsky T, Ghalibafian M, Bonniaud G, et al. Is FDG-PET scan in patients with early stage Hodgkin lymphoma of any value in the implementation of the involved-node radiotherapy concept and dose painting? *Radiother Oncol* 2007;85:178–186.

55. Hutchings M, Loft A, Hansen M, et al. Clinical impact of FDG-PET/CT in the planning of radiotherapy for early-stage Hodgkin lymphoma. *Eur J Haematol* 2007;78:206–212.

56. Topkan E, Yavuz AA, Aydin M, et al. Comparison of CT and PET-CT based plan-ning of radiation therapy in locally advanced pancreatic carcinoma. *J Exp Clin Cancer Res* 2008;27:41.

57. Karam I, Devic S, Hickeson M, et al. PET/CT for radiotherapy treatment planning in patients with soft tissue sarcomas. *Int J Radiat Oncol Biol Phys* 2009;75:817–821.

58. Douglas JG, Stelzer KJ, Mankoff DA, et al. [F-18]-fluorodeoxyglucose positron emission tomography for targeting radiation dose escalation for patients with glioblastoma multiforme: clinical outcomes and patterns of failure. *Int J Radiat Oncol Biol Phys* 2006;64:886–891.

59. Kornerup JS, Brodin NP, Bjork-Eriksson T, et al. PET/CT-guided treatment plan-ning for paediatric cancer patients: a simulation study of proton and conven-tional photon therapy. *Br J Radiol* 2015;88:1047.

60. Schöder H, Ong SC. Fundamentals of molecular imaging: rationale and applica-tions with relevance for radiation oncology. *Semin Nucl Med* 2008;38:119–128.

61. Blankenberg FG. The state of the art of molecular imaging: in vivo detection of apoptosis. *J Nucl Med* 2008;49(Suppl):81–95.

62. Krohn KA, Link JM, Mason RP. Molecular imaging of hypoxia. *J Nucl Med* 2008;49(Suppl):129–148.

63. Bading JR, Shields AF. Imaging of cell proliferation: status and prospects. *J Nucl Med* 2008;49(Suppl):64–80.

64. Wahl RL, Herman JM, Ford E. The promise and pitfalls of positron emission tomography and single-photon emission computed tomography molecular imaging-guided radiation therapy. *Semin Radiat Oncol* 2011;21:88–100.

65. Grosu AL, Weber WA, Riedel E, et al. L-(methyl-11C) methionine positron emis-sion tomography for target delineation in resected high-grade gliomas before radiotherapy. *Int J Radiat Oncol Biol Phys* 2005;63:64–74.

66. Astner ST, Dobrei-Ciuchendea M, Essler M, et al. Effect of 11C-methionine-positron emission tomography on gross tumor volume delineation in stereo-tactic radiotherapy of skull base meningiomas. *Int J Radiat Oncol Biol Phys* 2008;72:1161–1167.

67. Niyazi M, Geisler J, Siefert A, et al. FET-PET for malignant glioma treatment planning. *Radiother Oncol* 2011;99:44–48.

68. Grosu AL, Astner ST, Riedel E, et al. An interindividual comparison of O-(2-[18F]fluoroethyl)-L-tyrosine (FET)- and L-[methyl-11C]methionine (MET)-PET in patients with brain gliomas and metastases. *Int J Radiat Oncol Biol Phys* 2011;81:1049–1058.

69. Milker-Zabel S, Zabel-du Bois A, Henze M, et al. Improved target volume defi-nition for fractionated stereotactic radiotherapy in patients with intracranial meningiomas by correlation of CT, MRI, and [68Ga]-DOTATOC-PET. *Int J Radiat Oncol Biol Phys* 2006;65:222–227.

70. Gehler B, Paulsen F, Oksüz MO, et al. [68Ga]-DOTATOC-PET/CT for meningioma IMRT treatment planning. *Radiat Oncol* 2009;4:56.

71. Rasey JS, Koh WJ, Evans ML, et al. Quantifying regional hypoxia in human tumors with positron emission tomography of [18F]fluoromiso-nidazole: a pretherapy study of 37 patients. *Int J Radiat Oncol Biol Phys* 1996;36:417–428.

72. Rischin D, Hicks RJ, Fisher R, et al. Prognostic significance of [18F]-misonidazole positron emission tomography-detected tumor hypoxia in patients with advanced head and neck cancer randomly assigned to chemoradiation with or without tirapazamine: a substudy of Trans-Tasman Radiation Oncology Group Study 98.02. *J Clin Oncol* 2006;24:2098–2104.

73. Grosu AL, Souvatzoglou M, Röper B, et al. Hypoxia imaging with FAZA-PET and theoretical considerations with regard to dose painting for individualization of radiotherapy in patients with head and neck cancer. *Int J Radiat Oncol Biol Phys* 2007;69:541–551.

74. Chao KS, Bosch WR, Mutic S, et al. A novel approach to overcome hypoxic tumor resistance: Cu-ATSM-guided intensity-modulated radiation therapy. *Int J Radiat Oncol Biol Phys* 2001;49:1171–1182.

75. Dehdashti F, Grigsby PW, Mintun MA, et al. Assessing tumor hypoxia in cer-vical cancer by positron emission tomography with 60Cu-ATSM: relationship to therapeutic response-a preliminary report. *Int J Radiat Oncol Biol Phys* 2003;55:1233–1238.

76. Chang JH, Joon DL, Lee ST, et al. Histopathological correlation of (11)C-choline PET scans for target volume definition in radical prostate radiotherapy. *Radiother Oncol* 2011;99:187–192.

77. Wang H, Vees H, Miralbell R, et al. 18F-fluorocholine PET-guided target volume delineation techniques for partial prostate re-irradiation in local recurrent prostate cancer. *Radiother Oncol* 2009;93:220–225.

78. Everitt S, Hicks RJ, Ball D, et al. Imaging cellular proliferation during chemo-radiotherapy: a pilot study of serial 18F-FLT positron emission tomography/computed tomography imaging for non-small-cell lung cancer. *Int J Radiat Oncol Biol Phys* 2009;75:1098–1104.

79. Muijs CT, Beukema JC, Widder J, et al. 18F-FLT-PET for detection of rectal can-cer. *Radiother Oncol* 2011;98:357–359.

80. Troost EG, Vogel WV, Merkx MA, et al. 18F-FLT PET does not discriminate between reactive and metastatic lymph nodes in primary head and neck can-cer patients. *J Nucl Med* 2007;48:726–735.

81. Arens AI, Troost EG, Hoeben BA, et al. Semiautomatic methods for segmenta-tion of the proliferative tumour volume on sequential FLT PET/CT images in head and neck carcinomas and their relation to clinical outcome. *Eur J Nucl Med Mol Imaging* 2014;41(5):915–924.

82. Siva S, Thomas R, Callahan J, et al. High-resolution pulmonary ventilation and perfusion PET/CT allows for functionally adapted intensity modulated radio-therapy in lung cancer. *Radiother Oncol* 2015;115(2):157–162.

83. Aoyama H, Shirato H, Nishioka T, et al. Magnetic resonance imaging system for three-dimensional conformal radiotherapy and its impact on gross tumor volume delineation of central nervous system tumors. *Int J Radiat Oncol Biol Phys* 2001;50:821–827.

84. Stall B, Zach L, Ning H, et al. Comparison of T2 and FLAIR imaging for target delineation in high grade gliomas. *Radiat Oncol* 2010;5:5.

85. Emami B, Sethi A, Petruzzelli GJ. Influence of MRI on target volume delineation and IMRT planning in nasopharyngeal carcinoma. *Int J Radiat Oncol Biol Phys* 2003;57:481–488.

86. Gardner M, Halimi P, Valinta D, et al. Use of single MRI and 18F-FDG PET-CT scans in both diagnosis and radiotherapy treatment planning in patients with head and neck cancer: advantage on target volume and critical organ delinea-tion. *Head Neck* 2009;31:461–467.

87. Buyyounouski MK, Horwitz EM, Price RA, et al. Intensity-modulated radio-therapy with MRI simulation to reduce doses received by erectile tissue during prostate cancer treatment. *Int J Radiat Oncol Biol Phys* 2004;58:743–749.

88. Parker CC, Damyanovich A, Haycocks T, et al. Magnetic resonance imaging in the radiation treatment planning of localized prostate cancer using intra-prostatic fiducial markers for computed tomography co-registration. *Radiother Oncol* 2003;66:217–224.

89. Usmani N, Sloboda R, Kamal W, et al. Can images obtained with high field strength magnetic resonance imaging reduce contouring variability of the prostate? *Int J Radiat Oncol Biol Phys* 2011;80:728–734.

90. Yeung AR, Vargas CE, Falchook A, et al. Dose-volume differences for com-puted tomography and magnetic resonance imaging segmentation and planning for proton prostate cancer therapy. *Int J Radiat Oncol Biol Phys* 2008;72:1426–1433.

91. Viswanathan AN, Dimopoulos J, Kirisits C, et al. Computed tomography versus magnetic resonance imaging-based contouring in cervical cancer

brachytherapy: results of a prospective trial and preliminary guidelines for standardized contours. *Int J Radiat Oncol Biol Phys* 2007;68:491–498.

92. Karlsson M, Karlsson MG, Nyholm T, et al. Dedicated magnetic resonance imaging in the radiotherapy clinic. *Int J Radiat Oncol Biol Phys* 2009;74:644–651.

93. Hamilton RJ, Sweeney PJ, Pelizzari CA, et al. Functional imaging in treatment planning of brain lesions. *Int J Radiat Oncol Biol Phys* 1997;37:181–188.

94. Liu WC, Schulder M, Narra V, et al. Functional magnetic resonance imaging aided radiation treatment planning. *Med Phys* 2000;27:1563–1572.

95. Schad LR, Bock M, Baudendistel K, et al. Improved target volume definition in radiosurgery of arteriovenous malformations by stereotactic correlation of MRA, MRI, blood bolus tagging, and functional MRI. *Eur Radiol* 1996;6:38–45.

96. Aoyama H, Kamada K, Shirato H, et al. Integration of functional brain information into stereotactic irradiation treatment planning using magnetoencephalography and magnetic resonance axonography. *Int J Radiat Oncol Biol Phys* 2004;58:1177–1183.

97. Chang J, Narayana A. Functional MRI for radiotherapy of gliomas. *Technol Cancer Res Treat* 2010;9:347–358.

98. Wang TJ, Brisman R, Lu ZF, et al. Image registration strategy of T(1)-weighted and FIESTA MRI sequences in trigeminal neuralgia gamma knife radiosurgery. *Stereotact Funct Neurosurg* 2010;88:239–245.

99. Chávez GD, De Salles AA, Solberg TD, et al. Three-dimensional fast imaging employing steady-state acquisition magnetic resonance imaging for stereotactic radiosurgery of trigeminal neuralgia. *Neurosurgery* 2005;56:E628.

100. Pirzkall A, Li X, Oh J, et al. 3D MRSI for resected high-grade gliomas before RT: tumor extent according to metabolic activity in relation to MRI. *Int J Radiat Oncol Biol Phys* 2004;59:126–137.

101. Chan AA, Lau A, Pirzkall A, et al. Proton magnetic resonance spectroscopy imaging in the evaluation of patients undergoing gamma knife surgery for Grade IV glioma. *J Neurosurg* 2004;101:467–475.

102. van Lin EN, Futterer JJ, Heijmink SW, et al. IMRT boost dose planning on dominant intraprostatic lesions: gold marker-based three-dimensional fusion of CT with dynamic contrast-enhanced and 1H-spectroscopic MRI. *Int J Radiat Oncol Biol Phys* 2006;65:291–303.

103. Meijer HJ, van Lin EN, Debats OA, et al. High occurrence of aberrant lymph node spread on magnetic resonance lymphography in prostate cancer patients with a biochemical recurrence after radical prostatectomy. *Int J Radiat Oncol Biol Phys* 2012;82(4):1405–1410.

104. Meijer HJ, Debats OA, Kunze-Busch M, et al. Magnetic resonance lymphography-guided selective high-dose lymph node irradiation in prostate cancer. *Int J Radiat Oncol Biol Phys* 2012;82:175–183.

105. Craciunescu OI, Yoo DS, Cleland E, et al. Dynamic contrast-enhanced MRI in head-and-neck cancer: the impact of region of interest selection on the intra- and interpatient variability of pharmacokinetic parameters. *Int J Radiat Oncol Biol Phys* 2012;82:e345–e350.

106. Lazanyi KS, Abramyuk A, Wolf G, et al. Usefulness of dynamic contrast enhanced computed tomography in patients with non-small-cell lung cancer scheduled for radiation therapy. *Lung Cancer* 2010;70:280–285.

107. Kierkels RG, Backes WH, Janssen MH, et al. Comparison between perfusion computed tomography and dynamic contrast-enhanced magnetic resonance imaging in rectal cancer. *Int J Radiat Oncol Biol Phys* 2010;77:400–408.

108. Mayr NA, Huang Z, Wang JZ, et al. Characterizing tumor heterogeneity with functional imaging and quantifying high-risk tumor volume for early prediction of treatment outcome: cervical cancer as a model. *Int J Radiat Oncol Biol Phys* 2012;83(3):972–979.

109. Carmona R, Pritz J, Bydder M, et al. Fat composition changes in bone marrow during chemotherapy and radiation therapy. *Int J Radiat Oncol Biol Phys* 2014;90:155–163.

110. Simpson DR, Lawson JD, Nath SK, et al. Utilization of advanced imaging technologies for target delineation in radiation oncology. *J Am Coll Radiol* 2009;6:876–883.

111. Ganswindt U, Paulsen F, Corvin S, et al. Intensity modulated radiotherapy for high risk prostate cancer based on sentinel node SPECT imaging for target volume definition. *BMC Cancer* 2005;5:91.

112. Jani AB, Blend MJ, Hamilton R, et al. Influence of radioimmunoscintigraphy on postprostatectomy radiotherapy treatment decision making. *J Nucl Med* 2004;45:571–578.

113. Jani AB, Blend MJ, Hamilton R, et al. Radioimmunoscintigraphy for post-prostatectomy radiotherapy: analysis of toxicity and biochemical control. *J Nucl Med* 2004;45:1315–1322.

114. Ellis RJ, Vertocnik A, Kim E, et al. Four-year biochemical outcome after radioimmunoguided transperineal brachytherapy for patients with prostate adenocarcinoma. *Int J Radiat Oncol Biol Phys* 2003;57:362–370.

115. Ellis RJ, Sodee DB, Spirnak JP, et al. Feasibility and acute toxicities of radioimmunoguided prostate brachytherapy. *Int J Radiat Oncol Biol Phys* 2000;48:683–687.

116. Liauw SL, Weichselbaum RR, Zagaja GP, et al. Salvage radiotherapy after postprostatectomy biochemical failure: does pretreatment radioimmunoscintigraphy help select patients with locally confined disease? *Int J Radiat Oncol Biol Phys* 2008;71:1316–1321.

117. Grosu AL, Weber W, Feldmann HJ, et al. First experience with I-123-alpha-methyl-tyrosine SPECT in the 3-D radiation treatment planning of brain gliomas. *Int J Radiat Oncol Biol Phys* 2000;47:517–526.

118. Grosu AL, Feldmann H, Dick S, et al. Implications of IMT-SPECT for postoperative radiotherapy planning in patients with gliomas. *Int J Radiat Oncol Biol Phys* 2002;54:842–854.

119. Krengli M, Loi G, Sacchetti G, et al. Delineation of target volume for radiotherapy of high-grade gliomas by 99m Tc-MIBI SPECT and MRI fusion. *Strahlenther Onkol* 2007;183:689–694.

120. Fenig E, Mishaeli M, Yerushalmi R, et al. Treatment of neuroblastoma using the fused imaging guided radiotherapy (FIGURA) system. *Clin Nucl Med* 2006;31:256–258.

121. Christian JA, Partridge M, Nioutsikou E, et al. The incorporation of SPECT functional lung imaging into inverse radiotherapy planning for non-small cell lung cancer. *Radiother Oncol* 2005;77:271–277.

122. Roeske JC, Lujan A, Reba RC, et al. Incorporation of SPECT bone marrow imaging into intensity modulated whole-pelvic radiation therapy treatment planning for gynecologic malignancies. *Radiother Oncol* 2005; 77:11–17.

123. Kitamura K, Shirato H, Shinohara N, et al. Reduction in acute morbidity using hypofractionated intensity-modulated radiation therapy assisted with a fluoroscopic real-time tumor-tracking system for prostate cancer: preliminary results of a phase I/II study. *Cancer J* 2003;9:268–276.

124. Seppenwoolde Y, Shirato H, Kitamura K, et al. Precise and real-time measurement of 3D tumor motion in lung due to breathing and heartbeat, measured during radiotherapy. *Int J Radiat Oncol Biol Phys* 2002;53:822–834.

125. Keall PJ, Mageras GS, Balter JM, et al. The management of respiratory motion in radiation oncology report of AAPM Task Group 76. *Med Phys* 2006;33:3874–3900.

126. Li R, Lewis JH, Cervino LI, et al. A feasibility study of markerless fluoroscopic gating for lung cancer radiotherapy using 4DCT templates. *Phys Med Biol* 2009;54:N489–N500.

127. Lin T, Li R, Tang X, et al. Markerless gating for lung cancer radiotherapy based on machine learning techniques. *Phys Med Biol* 2009;54:1555–1563.

128. Zhang T, Keller H, O'Brien MJ, et al. Application of the spirometer in respiratory gated radiotherapy. *Med Phys* 2003;30:3165–3171.

129. Chang Z, Liu T, Cai J, et al. Evaluation of integrated respiratory gating systems on a Novalis Tx system. *J Appl Clin Med Phys* 2011;12:3495.

130. Shimizu S, Shirato H, Aoyama H, et al. High-speed magnetic resonance imaging for four-dimensional treatment planning of conformal radiotherapy of moving body tumors. *Int J Radiat Oncol Biol Phys* 2000;48:471–474.

131. Nath SK, Sandhu AP, Kim D, et al. Locoregional and distant failure following image-guided stereotactic body radiation for early-stage primary lung cancer. *Radiother Oncol* 2011;99:12–17.

132. Vedam SS, Keall PJ, Kini VR, et al. Acquiring a four-dimensional computed tomography dataset using an external respiratory signal. *Phys Med Biol* 2003;48:45–62.

133. Pan T, Lee TY, Rietzel E, et al. 4D-CT imaging of a volume influenced by respiratory motion on multi-slice CT. *Med Phys* 2004;31:333–340.

134. Chen GT, Kung JH, Beaudette KP. Artifacts in computed tomography scanning of moving objects. *Semin Radiat Oncol* 2004;14:19–26.

135. ICRU Report 62. *Prescribing, recording, and reporting photon beam therapy (supplement to ICRU Report 50)*. Washington, DC: ICRU, 1999.

136. Lagerwaard FJ, Van Sornsen de Koste JR, Nijssen-Visser MR, et al. Multiple "slow" CT scans for incorporating lung tumor mobility in radiotherapy planning. *Int J Radiat Oncol Biol Phys* 2001;51:932–937.

137. Wong JW, Sharpe MB, Jaffray DA, et al. The use of active breathing control (ABC) to reduce margin for breathing motion. *Int J Radiat Oncol Biol Phys* 1999;44:911–919.

138. Rietzel E, Liu AK, Doppke KP, et al. Design of 4D treatment planning target volumes. *Int J Radiat Oncol Biol Phys* 2006;66:287–295.

139. Underberg RW, Lagerwaard FJ, Slotman BJ, et al. Use of maximum intensity projections (MIP) for target volume generation in 4DCT scans for lung cancer. *Int J Radiat Oncol Biol Phys* 2005;63:253–260.

140. Muirhead R, McNee SG, Featherstone C, et al. Use of maximum intensity projections (MIPs) for target outlining in 4DCT radiotherapy planning. *J Thorac Oncol* 2008;3:1433–1438.

141. Starkschall G, Britton K, McAleer MF, et al. Potential dosimetric benefits of four-dimensional radiation treatment planning. *Int J Radiat Oncol Biol Phys* 2009;73:1560–1565

142. Mexner V, Wolthaus JWH, van Herk M, et al. Effects of respiration-induced density variations on dose distributions in radiotherapy of lung cancer. *Int J Radiat Oncol Biol Phys* 2009;74:1266–1275.

143. Simpson DR, Lawson JD, Nath SK, et al. A survey of image-guided radiation therapy use in the United States. *Cancer* 2010;116:3953–3960.

144. Hangiandreou NJ. B-mode US: basic concepts and new technology. *Radiographics* 2003;23:1019–1033.

145. Serago CF, Chungbin SJ, Buskirk SJ, et al. Initial experience with ultrasound localization for positioning prostate cancer patients for external beam radiotherapy. *Int J Radiat Oncol Biol Phys* 2002;53:1130–1138.

146. Trichter F, Ennis RD. Prostate localization using transabdominal ultrasound imaging. *Int J Radiat Oncol Biol Phys* 2003;56:1225–1233.

147. Fuss M, Cavanaugh SX, Fuss C, et al. Daily stereotactic ultrasound prostate targeting: inter-user variability. *Technol Cancer Res Treat* 2003;2:161–170.

148. Little DJ, Dong L, Levy LB, et al. Use of portal images and BAT ultrasonography to measure setup error and organ motion for prostate IMRT: implications for treatment margins. *Int J Radiat Oncol Biol Phys* 2003;56: 1218–1224.

149. Dobler B, Mai S, Ross C, et al. Evaluation of possible prostate displacement induced by pressure applied during transabdominal ultrasound image acquisition. *Strahlenther Onkol* 2006;182:240–246.

150. Artignan X, Smitsmans MH, Lebesque JV, et al. Online ultrasound image guidance for radiotherapy of prostate cancer: impact of image acquisition on prostate displacement. *Int J Radiat Oncol Biol Phys* 2004;59:595–601.

151. Fung AYC, Enke CA, Ayyangar KM, et al. Prostate motion and isocenter adjustment from ultrasound-based localization during delivery of radiation therapy. *Int J Radiat Oncol Biol Phys* 2005;61:984–992.

152. Langen KM, Pouliot J, Anezinos C, et al. Evaluation of ultrasound-based pros-tate localization for image-guided radiotherapy. *Int J Radiat Oncol Biol Phys* 2003;57:635–644.

153. Van den Heuvel F, Powell T, Seppi E, et al. Independent verification of ultra-sound based image-guided radiation treatment, using electronic portal imag-ing and implanted gold markers. *Med Phys* 2003;30:2878–2887.

154. Scarbrough TJ, Golden NM, Ting JY, et al. Comparison of ultrasound and implanted seed marker prostate localization methods: implications for image-guided radiotherapy. *Int J Radiat Oncol Biol Phys* 2006;65:378–387.

155. Connor W, Boone M, Veomett R, et al. Patient repositioning and motion detection using a video cancellation system. *Int J Radiat Oncol Biol Phys* 1975;1:147–153.

156. Milliken BD, Rubin SJ, Hamilton RJ, et al. Performance of a video-image-subtraction-based patients positioning system. *Int J Radiat Oncol Biol Phys* 1997;38:855–866.

157. Johnson S, Milliken BD, Hadley SW, et al. Initial clinical experience with a video-based patient positioning system. *Int J Radiat Oncol Biol Phys* 1999;45:205–213.

158. Padilla L, Kang H, Washington M, et al. Assessment of interfractional varia-tion of the breast surface following conventional patient positioning for whole-breast radiotherapy. *J Appl Clin Med Phys* 2014;15:4921.

159. Shah AP, Dvorak T, Curry MS, et al. Clinical evaluation of interfractional varia-tions for whole breast radiotherapy using 3-dimensional surface imaging. *Pract Radiat Oncol* 2013;3:16–25.

160. Tanguturi SK, Lyatskaya Y, Chen Y, et al. Prospective assessment of deep inspi-ration breath-hold using 3-dimensional surface tracking for irradiation of left-sided breast cancer. *Pract Radiat Oncol* 2015;5:358–365.

161. Tang X, Cullip T, Dooley J, et al. Dosimetric effect due to the motion during deep inspiration breath hold for left-sided breast cancer radiotherapy. *J Appl Clin Med Phys* 2015;16:5358.

162. Cerviño LI, Pawlicki T, Lawson JD, et al. Frame-less and mask-less cranial ste-reotactic radiosurgery: a feasibility study. *Phys Med Biol* 2010;55:1863–1873.

163. Cerviño LI, Detorie N, Taylor M, et al. Initial clinical experience with a fra-meless and maskless stereotactic radiosurgery treatment. *Pract Radiat Oncol* 2012;2:54–62.

164. Nabavizadeh N, Elliott DA, Chen Y, et al. Image Guided Radiation Therapy (IGRT) practice patterns and IGRT's impact on workflow and treatment planning: results from a National Survey of American Society for Radiation Oncology Members. *Int J Radiat Oncol Biol Phys* 2016;94(4):850–857.

165. Antonuk L. Electronic portal imaging devices: a review and historical perspective of contemporary technologies and research. *Phys Med Biol* 2002;47:R31–R65.

166. Boyer AL, Antonuk L, Fenster A, et al. A review of electronic portal imaging devices (EPIDs). *Med Phys* 1992;19:1–16.

167. Vigneault E, Pouliot J, Laverdiere J, et al. Electronic portal imaging device detection of radiopaque markers for the evaluation of prostate position during megavoltage radiation: a clinical study. *Int J Radiat Oncol Biol Phys* 1997;37:205–212.

168. Welsh JS, Berta C, Borzillary S, et al. Fiducial markers implanted during pros-tate brachytherapy for guiding conformal external beam radiation therapy. *Technol Cancer Res Treat* 2004;3:359–364.

169. Pouliot J, Aubin M, Langen KM, et al. (Non)-migration of radiopaque markers used for on-line localization of the prostate with an electronic portal imaging device. *Int J Radiat Oncol Biol Phys* 2003;56:862–866.

170. Chung PWM, Haycocks T, Brown T, et al. On-line aSi portal imaging of implanted fiducial markers for the reduction of interfraction error during conformal radiotherapy of prostate carcinoma. *Int J Radiat Oncol Biol Phys* 2004;60:329–334.

171. Fox T, Huntzinger C, Johnstone P, et al. Performance evaluation of an auto-mated image registration algorithm using an integrated kilovoltage imaging and guidance system. *J Appl Clin Med Phys* 2006;7:97–104.

172. Adler JR, Murphy MJ, Chang SD, et al. Image guided robotic radiosurgery. *Neurosurgery* 1999;44:1299–1306.

173. Yan H, Yin FF, Kim JH. A phantom study on the positioning accuracy of the Novalis Body system. *Med Phys* 2003;30:2052–2060.

174. Rahimian J, Chen JC, Rao AA, et al. Geometrical accuracy of the Novalis stereotactic radiosurgery system for trigeminal neuralgia. *J Neurosurg* 2004;101:351–355.

175. Jaffray DA. Emergent technologies for 3-dimensional image-guided radiation delivery. *Semin Radiat Oncol* 2005;15:208–216.

176. Ford EC, Chang J, Mueller K, et al. Cone-beam CT with megavoltage beams and an amorphous silicon electronic portal imaging device: poten-tial for verification of radiotherapy of lung cancer. *Med Phys* 2002;29:2913–2934.

177. Sidhu K, Ford EC, Spirou S, et al. Optimization of conformal thoracic radio-therapy using cone-beam CT imaging for treatment verification. *Int J Radiat Oncol Biol Phys* 2003;55:757–767.

178. Pouliot J, Bani-Hashemi A, Chen J, et al. Low-dose megavoltage cone-beam CT for radiation therapy. *Int J Radiat Oncol Biol Phys* 2005;552–650.

179. Sykes JR, Amer A, Czjka J, et al. A feasibility study for image guided radio-therapy using low dose, high speed, cone beam x-ray volumetric imaging. *Radiother Oncol* 2005;77:45–52.

180. Thilmann C, Nill S, Tucking T, et al. Correction of patient positioning errors based on in-line cone beam CTs: clinical implementation and first experiences. *Radiat Oncol* 2006;1:16–21.

181. Oldham M, Letourneau D, Watt L, et al. Cone-beam-CT guided radiation ther-apy: a model for on-line application. *Radiother Oncol* 2005;75:271–278.

182. Letourneau D, Martinez AA, Lockman D, et al. Assessment of residual error for online cone-beam XT-guided treatment of prostate cancer patients. *Int J Radiat Oncol Biol Phys* 2005;62:1239–1246.

182a. McBain CA, Henry AM, Sykes J, et al. X-ray volumetric imaging in image-guided radiotherapy: the new standard in on-treatment imaging. *Int J Radiat Oncol Biol Phys* 2006;64:625–634.

183. Kron T, Eyles D, John SL, et al. Magnetic resonance imaging for adaptive cobalt tomotherapy: a proposal. *J Med Phys* 2006;31:242–254.

184. Chen AM, Hsu S, Lamb J, et al. MRI-guided radiotherapy for head and neck can-cer: initial clinical experience. *Clin Transl Oncol* 2018;20:160–168. doi:10.1007/s12094-017-1704-4.

185. Chen AM, Cao M, Hsu S, et al. Magnetic resonance imaging guided reirradia-tion of recurrent and second primary head and neck cancer. *Adv Radiat Oncol* 2017;2:167–175.

186. Lagendijk JJ, Raaymakers BW, Raaijmakers AJ, et al. MRI/Linac integration. *Radiother Oncol* 2008;86:25–29.

187. Raaymakers BW, de Boer JC, Knox C, et al. Integrated MV portal imaging with a 1.5 T MRI Linac. *Phys Med Biol* 2011;56:N207–N214.

188. Litzenberg DW. Electromagnetic tracking. In: Mundt AJ, Roeske JC, eds. *Image-guided radiation therapy: a clinical perspective*. Shelton, CT: People's Medical Publishing House-USA, 2011:143–155.

189. Kupelian P, Willoughby T, Mahadevan A, et al. Multi-institutional clinical expe-rience with the Calypso System in localization and continuous, real-time moni-toring of the prostate gland during external radiotherapy. *Int J Radiat Oncol Biol Phys* 2007;67:1088–1098.

190. Rajendran RR, Palastaras JP, Mick R, et al. Daily isocenter correction with electromagnetic-based localization improves target coverage and rectal sparing during prostate radiotherapy. *Int J Radiat Oncol Biol Phys* 2010;76:1092–1099.

191. Su Z, Zhang L, Murphy M, et al. Analysis of prostate patient setup and track-ing data: potential intervention strategies. *Int J Radiat Oncol Biol Phys* 2011;81:880–887.

192. King BL, Butler WM, Merrick GS, et al. Electromagnetic transponders indicate prostate size increase followed by decrease during the course of external beam radiation therapy. *Int J Radiat Oncol Biol Phys* 2011;79:1350–1357.

193. Tanyi JA, He T, Summers PA, et al. Assessment of planning target vol-ume margins for intensity-modulated radiotherapy of the prostate gland: role of daily inter- and intrafraction motion. *Int J Radiat Oncol Biol Phys* 2010;78:1579–1585.

193a. Shinohara ET, Kassaee A, Mitra N, et al. Feasibility of electromagnetic tran-sponder use to monitor inter- and intrafractional motion in locally advanced pancreatic cancer patients. *Int J Radiat Oncol Biol Phys* 2012;83:566–573.

194. https://clinicaltrials.gov/

Techniques, Modalities, and Modifiers in Radiation Oncology

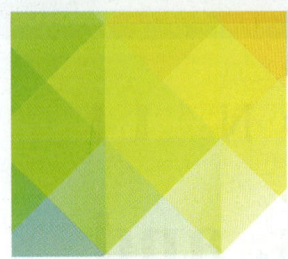

CHAPTER 13

Altered Fractionation Schedules

Anthony E. Dragun

INTRODUCTION

Conventionally fractionated radiotherapy (CFRT) is typically defined as the delivery of doses of 1.8 to 2 Gy, once daily, 5 days/week. This chapter discusses the history of and rationale and evidence for altered radiotherapy fractionation schedules for some of the most common cancers seen in clinical practice. The first section addresses background radiobiology. The second section reports outcomes of clinical studies of hyperfractionated radiotherapy (HyperRT), as well as new results of hypofractionated radiotherapy (HypoRT) for prostate and breast cancer, which have been added to this edition. The purpose of this chapter is to explore the experience of altered fractionation in cases where the traditional target and delivery technique remains (e.g., tangential whole-breast radiotherapy portals), but the dose per fraction is changed. Altered radiation schedules using special treatment procedures such as stereotactic radiosurgery (SRS) or stereotactic body radiotherapy techniques (SBRT), partial breast irradiation, or brachytherapy are discussed in dedicated chapters elsewhere in this book.

BACKGROUND RADIOBIOLOGY

The most important consideration of altered fractionation is the sensitivity of late effects to changes in dose per fraction.[1] Alternatively, acute reactions are more dependent on changes in total dose.

The traditional understanding of early and late reactions is couched in terms of target cell killing. This description is better characterized for acute effects, where direct connections can be made between cell loss and measurable injury, than with late effects, where that association is less well understood[2] (see also Chapter 3 of this book). Nonetheless, the conventional understanding of the potential risks and benefits of altered fractionation is framed within this target cell concept.

Time–Dose Parameters

The time–dose parameters that determine normal tissue tolerance are total dose, dose per fraction, fraction frequency, and duration of treatment. Fraction size and frequency determine rate of dose accumulation, sometimes referred to as the *weekly dose rate*. The intensity of acute reactions in tissues that are organized into stem cell, maturation, and functional compartments (e.g., epithelium, bone marrow) reflects the balance between cell killing by irradiation and the rate of regeneration of surviving stem cells, driven primarily by the weekly dose rate. After an acute reaction has peaked (e.g., moist desquamation of the skin), further stem cell killing cannot produce an increase in *intensity* of the acute reaction but manifests as a delay in healing, which may ultimately result in a *consequential* late injury.[3]

Late reactions differ in that they are thought to occur in tissues characterized by slow cellular turnover, such as mature connective tissues and the parenchymal cells of various organs. Because cellular depletion in such tissues does not manifest until well after the completion of the course of radiation, weekly dose rate would be of minor significance in determining the severity of late reactions. Therefore, late reactions would depend more on size of dose per fraction, and interfraction interval.

The understanding of late effects, however, does not lend itself well to simplification. For example, we have already mentioned evidence that the frequency of some late reactions correlates with the weekly dose rate and intensity of acute reactions (consequential late effects).[4-6] Moreover, there is evidence that late effects can be modified by pharmacologic intervention. For example, amifostine administration protects lung tissue and the esophageal mucosa in the treatment of lung cancer,[7] and other agents have been shown to affect the development of radiation-induced nephritis (captopril) and breast fibrosis (pentoxifylline and vitamin E).[8]

Size of Dose per Fraction and Length of Interfraction Interval

The influence of fraction size on radiation therapy outcome is manifest through the slope of fractionated dose response curves, and this is a reflection of cellular *repair capacity*. In Chapter 3 of this book, Figure 3.18 shows that changes in isoeffect doses for late effects with changing dose per fraction (solid curves) are steeper than for acute effects (dashed curves).[9] Therefore, for tumors with fraction sensitivity similar to acutely responding normal tissues, a gain in therapeutic ratio can be realized by significantly reducing the fraction sizes and escalating the total dose (hyperfractionation). It is convenient to mathematically estimate fractionation sensitivity, and this is most easily done using the linear quadratic (LQ) model. Assuming that the target cell hypothesis is correct and that the LQ model correctly describes the target cell survival curves, the ratio α/β of the LQ model becomes a quantitative measure of sensitivity to changes in fraction size[9]: low ratios signify high fractionation sensitivity, and high ratios signify low fractionation sensitivity. The implication is that the tolerance dose for late effects can be increased more by the use of smaller fraction sizes than the tolerance dose for tumors and acute effects (hyperfractionation). The α/β ratios for some animal normal tissues are set out in Chapter 3 and clinical data in human tissues and tumors in Table 13.1.

In general, the estimated values of α/β for early and late reactions in human normal tissues are consistent with results from experimental animals. With regard to tumors, squamous cell carcinomas of the head and neck, cervix, and skin and non–small cell lung cancers (NSCLCs) are characterized by high α/β ratios, in agreement with rodent models. However, data from melanomas and sarcomas suggest somewhat lower α/β ratios for these tumor types. The α/β ratio for breast adenocarcinomas may be lower than those for other carcinomas listed in Table 13.1.[42] The situation is different with prostate tumors, which contain unusually small fractions of cycling cells.[43] Prostate tumors might not respond to changes in fractionation in the same way as do other cancers,[44,45] and respond to changes in fractionation more like a late-responding normal tissue.[36,46–48] There is evidence both from animal[44,49–54] and from human[5,55–57] studies that for late rectal sequelae a value of α/β of >4 Gy is higher than for most other late sequelae. And so, if the α/β value for prostate cancer (range: 1 to 3) is indeed less than that for this adjacent late-responding normal tissue, then hypofractionation would be expected to yield increased tumor control for a given level of late complications or decreased late complications for a given level of tumor control.

TABLE 13.1 ESTIMATES OF α/β FOR HUMAN TISSUES AND TUMORS

Tissue/Tumor	Reference	Estimate/Bound of α/β in Gy (95% CI)
Acutely Responding		
Skin		
Desquamation (time $\leq$ 29 d)	Turesson and Thames[6]	11.2 (8.5–17.6)
Erythema	Turesson and Thames[6]	8.8 (6.9–11.6)
	Bentzen et al.[10]	12.3 (2–23)
Mucous membrane–ulcer	Rezvani et al.[11]	15 (0–45.2)
Lung–acute	Cox[12]	>8.8
Late Responding		
Supraglottic larynx–late sequelae	Maciejewski et al.[13]	3.8 (0.8–14)
Larynx–cartilage necrosis	Henk and James[14]	~3.4
	Horiot et al.[15]	$\leq$4.4
	Fletcher et al.[16]	
	Stell and Morrison[17]	$\leq$4.2
Larynx–pharynx	Taylor et al.[18]	7.8 (3–∞)
	Rezvani et al.[11]	3.5 (1.1–5.9)
Oropharynx–late sequelae	Horiot et al.[15]	~4.5
Skin		
Subcutaneous fibrosis	Bentzen et al.[10]	1.9 (0.8–3)
Telangiectasia	Turesson and Thames[6]	3.9 (2.7–4.8)
	Bentzen et al.[10]	3.7 (0.2–4.7)
	Bentzen and Overgaard[19]	2.8 (0–8.1)
Mucosal ulceration (consequential effects)	Withers et al.[20]	21.3 (5.2–∞)
Shoulder–impaired movement	Bentzen et al.[21]	3.5 (0.7–6.2)
Rib–fracture	Overgaard[22]	1.8–2.8
Bone–exposure/necrosis	Withers et al.[20]	0.8 (0–2.4)
Lung		
Pneumonitis	Cox[23]	$\leq$3.8
Computed tomography density	van Dyk et al.[24]	3.3 (0.5–6.5)
Spinal cord–myelopathy	Dische et al.[25]	$\leq$3.3
Brachial plexus–plexopathy	Powell et al.[26]	$\leq$5.3
Bowel–stricture/perforation	Bennett[27], Edsmyr et al.[28]	$2.2 \leq \alpha/\beta \leq 8$
Tumors		
Tonsil	Withers et al.[20]	14.7 (4.4–∞)
Vocal cord	Harrison et al.[29]	>9.9
Larynx	Rezvani et al.[30]	T2[a]: 18 (0–42), T3[a]: 13 (3–23)
Oral cavity/oropharynx	Maciejewski et al.[31]	~25
	Byhardt et al.[32]	>6.5
	Cox et al.[23]	~10.3
	Handa et al.[33]	>7
Lung–non-small cell carcinomas	Cox et al.[23]	50–90
Cervix	Watson et al.[34]	>13.9
Skin	Trott et al.[35]	8.5 (4.5–11.3)
Prostate	Brenner et al.[36]	1.2 (0.03–4.1)
	Brenner and Hall[37]	1.5 (0.8–2.2)
	Fowler et al.[38]	1.5 (1.3–1.8)
	King and Fowler[39]	1.8–2.8
Melanoma	Bentzen et al.[40]	0.6 (0–2.5)[b]
Liposarcoma	Thames and Suit[41]	0.4 (0–5.4)[b]

CI, confidence interval.
[a]American Joint Committee on Cancer staging system.
[b]Lower confidence limit is negative but is listed as 0 because a negative α/β has no biologic meaning.

Repair Kinetics

During altered fractionation schedules, the time interval between the dose fractions becomes crucial for allowing adequate repair of normal tissue. If doses are too closely spaced, injury will accumulate between dose fractions, and successive doses will become increasingly more damaging. This concept is described as *repair kinetics,* which is quantified by the half-time for repair. Of tissue models in which repair kinetics

have been studied, half-times for repair tend to be longest (1 to several hours) in the skin, kidney, and spinal cord, shortest (~1/2 hour) in the jejunal mucosa, and intermediate in the lung and colon.[2,58–67] The exact values vary according to the experimental protocol, and considerable overlap exists in the confidence limits of repair half-time. The important point is to ensure an adequate interfraction interval during hyperfractionation.

Repair kinetics is of particular importance in determining the response of the spinal cord to fractionation schedules of more than one daily fraction. In rats, experimental data showed that repair is best described by a biexponential function in which the slower component has a half-time of 3.8 hours.[68] This would imply that any fractionation schedule using more than one fraction per day is associated with some degree of incomplete repair in the spinal cord. A clinical report of radiation myelopathy occurring in four patients whose spinal cords received 45 to 48 Gy in 28 fractions of 1.5 Gy three times a day with a 6-hour interval over 9 consecutive days supports this observation.[69,70] Two reports from the Radiation Therapy Oncology Group (RTOG)[71,72] showed an increased rate of other late complications in patients treated with HyperRT when the mean interval was <4.5 hours.

Bentzen et al.[73] analyzed late complications in the Continuous, Hyperfractionated, Accelerated Radiation Therapy (CHART) randomized trial, estimated repair half-times, were 4.9 hours (95% CI, 3.2 to 6.4) for laryngeal edema, 3.8 hours (95% CI, 2.5 to 4.6) for skin telangiectasia, and 4.4 hours (95% CI, 3.8 to 4.9) for subcutaneous fibrosis. These results are consistent with observations from two other randomized altered fractionation trials: European Organization for Research and Treatment of Cancer (EORTC) 22791 and EORTC 22851.[74,75] For clinical practice, it is crucial to be mindful of compounding effect of incomplete repair, and a minimum 6-hour interval between dose fractions is typically advised.[76]

Overall Time

The cure rates of some cancers (particularly squamous cell carcinomas) are highly dependent on overall treatment time. Decrease in tumor control with longer treatment times is thought to be due to accelerated repopulation of tumor cells.[77] After a variable lag period, surviving tumor clonogens regenerate rapidly during fractionated radiation therapy to the extent that each additional day of treatment requires approximately 0.6 Gy, to offset potential regeneration, again. This hypothesis suggests a clonogenic cell doubling time of 3.5 to 5 days.[78–80]

Conversely, reduction of the overall treatment time may increase the probability of local tumor control. Molecular marker profiles (TP53, E-cadherin, Ki 67, and EGFR) may aid in the selection of patients likely to benefit from reduction in overall treatment time.[81]

Isoeffect Formulas

The commensurate adjustment of total dose to account for the effect of changes in dose fractionation in the production of a desired is approximated by isoeffect formulas. The first clinical isoeffect curve was produced by Strandqvist.[82] This was followed by other studies,[83–86] culminating in the nominal standard dose formula of Ellis[87]: $D = N^{0.24} \times T^{0.11}$, where D is the dose, N is the number of dose fractions, and T is the overall time. None of these explicitly included dose per fraction.

In the early 1980s, it was recognized that isoeffect doses for various late effects in normal tissues are more sensitive to changes in dose per fraction than are corresponding doses for acute effects. With the widespread use of the LQ model to quantify the fractionation sensitivity, the following model has gained in popularity: $D_1 = D_2(\alpha/\beta + d_2)/(\alpha/\beta + d_1)$, where D_2 is the reference total dose given in fractions of size d_2, and it is desired to calculate the total dose D_1 in fractions of size d_1 that would be isoeffective. This basic formula assumes complete repair between dose fractions, and no time factor is incorporated in it (see Chapter 3 for a detailed discussion). Whereas the LQ-based isoeffect model is remarkably consistent for a wide range of clinical applications, it is limited by at least two factors. First, there is the lack of precision of estimates of α/β. In both animal and human studies, estimates of α/β show large confidence intervals (Table 13.1). Second, as discussed earlier, the severity of complications can be modulated by various agents, including growth factors, radioprotectors, and pharmacologic agents. In the end, the isoeffect formula is neither perfect nor sufficiently reliable to substitute for sound judgment, and each new fractionation schedule must be tested clinically to establish its safety and efficacy.

Rationale for Hyperfractionated Radiotherapy

Hyperfractionation employs small-dose fractions to allow higher total doses to be delivered within the tolerance of late-responding normal tissues, thus enabling a higher biologically effective dose to the tumor. For this rationale to hold, the α/β ratio for both tumor cells and acute responding tissues must be greater than that for the dose-limiting normal tissue. Other rationales for HyperRT include radiosensitization through cell cycle redistribution and lesser dependence on oxygen effect.[88]

HyperRT has been tested in more than 20 randomized trials, and these are summarized in the data presented in Table 13.2. Regimens are classified as either hyperfractionated or accelerated. In hyperfractionation, the total dose and number of fractions are increased whereas the size of dose per fraction is reduced, and overall time is relatively unchanged. In accelerated fractionation, overall time is significantly reduced.

Rationale for Accelerated Fractionation

The rationale for accelerated fractionation is that reduction in overall treatment time decreases the opportunity for tumor cell regeneration, thereby increasing the probability of tumor control for a given total dose. Because overall treatment time has little influence on the probability of late normal tissue injury, a therapeutic gain should be realized, provided the interval between dose fractions is sufficient for complete repair to take place.

Strategies to accelerate radiation can be divided into two categories: (a) *pure accelerated fractionation* regimens, with reduced overall treatment time without concurrent changes in the fraction size or total dose (Table 13.3), and (b) *hybrid accelerated fractionation*, with reduced overall treatment time in conjunction with changes in other parameter(s), such as the fraction size, total dose, and time distribution (Table 13.4). The categories are further described as follows (Figs. 13.1–13.3):

Type A: There is drastic reduction of the overall time, with substantial decrease in the total dose.
Type B: Duration of treatment is more modestly reduced, with total dose kept in the same range, and there is a break in treatment.
Type C: Duration of treatment is more modestly reduced, with total dose kept in the same range, with a concomitant boost phase.

CLINICAL STUDIES

This section summarizes the results of hyperfractionated (HF) radiotherapy trials and accelerated fractionation (AF) radiotherapy trials. A new subsection summarizes results of pure hypofractionated radiotherapy (fraction size of >2 Gy). There is also a summary of combined altered fractionation with concurrent chemotherapy, critical fractionation issues to consider when intensity-modulated radiotherapy (IMRT) is used, common clinically practiced fractionation schedules, and future directions in combining molecular targeting with altered fractionation.

Results of HyperRT Trials

The key findings of HyperRT include the following:

- HF offers better locoregional control than standard fractionation when radiotherapy alone is used in the treatment of locally advanced head and neck carcinoma. This was also associated with an improvement in survival in three trials.[78]
- Reducing the fraction size from 2 Gy to 1.1 to 1.2 Gy permits a 7% to 17% total radiation dose escalation without increase in late complications. This supports the existence of differential fractionation sensitivity (variable α/β ratios) between human late-responding normal tissues and head and neck carcinomas.

Altered fractionation radiotherapy improves survival in patients with head and neck squamous cell carcinoma (HNSCC).[120] Comparison of the different types of altered radiotherapy suggests that hyperfractionation provides the greatest benefit. An individual patient data meta-analysis was conducted to see the effect of altered fractionation radiotherapy. It revealed a significant absolute survival benefit of 3.4% at 5 years with altered fractionation radiotherapy (hazard ratio [HR], 0.92; 95% confidence interval [CI], 0.86 to 0.97; $P = .003$) among 6,515 patients with nonmetastatic HNSCCs in 15 randomized trials comparing conventional radiotherapy with altered fractionation. The survival benefit at 5 years with HyperRT was 8%, with accelerated radiotherapy was 2% (without total dose reduction), and was 1.7% (with total dose reduction; $P = .02$). Locoregional control was better with altered fractionation (6.4% at 5 years; $P < .0001$), with particularly effect improved local control and less benefit for nodal control. The benefit was significantly higher in the youngest patients, <50 years old.

Table 13.2 summarizes reported prospective, randomized trials addressing hyperfractionation for the treatment of patients with head and neck, bladder, lung, and brainstem tumors; whole-brain radiotherapy for pediatric acute lymphoblastic leukemia; whole-brain radiotherapy for brain metastases or prophylactic whole-brain radiotherapy; and rhabdomyosarcoma. The most striking results are from trials in HNSCC, for which HyperRT was accompanied by an increase in dose.

Head and Neck

In all four head and neck trials,[75,89-92] HyperRT allowed a higher total dose to be delivered, which produced improved locoregional control by 8% to 20%. In three of these trials, HyperRT improved overall survival by 10% to 19%. In all four studies, HyperRT produced more severe acute mucositis but no increase in late morbidity. A Brazilian group[89] tested HyperRT of 70.4 Gy at 1.1 Gy twice daily and showed improved local response by 20% and 3.5-year overall survival from 8% to 27%. The EORTC tested 80.5 Gy HyperRT at 1.15 Gy/fraction twice per day for 7 weeks.[75] The 10-Gy increase in dose improved locoregional control from 38% to 56% and overall survival.[78,90] The Princess Margaret Hospital (Toronto, Canada) tested 58 Gy at 1.45 Gy twice per day over 4 weeks versus 51 Gy at 2.55 Gy/fraction once daily (a standard fractionation at that institute).[91] The 7-Gy increase in dose improved locoregional control from 37% to 45% and improved 5-year overall survival from 30% to 40%.

TABLE 13.2 DATA OF PHASE III CLINICAL TRIALS ADDRESSING HYPERFRACTIONATION

Tumor Site and Type	Number of Patients	Dose/ Fx (Gy)	Fx/ Day	Total Dose (Gy)	Overall Time (wk)	Tumor Response	Side Effects	Reference
Head and Neck Carcinomas								
Oropharynx, stage III–IV	98	1.1 2.0	2 1	70.4 66.0	6.5 6.5	Tumor response: 84% vs. 64% (P = .02) 3.5-y OS: 27% vs. 8% (P = .03)	Earlier onset of acute reactions with HF Late complications: no details	Pinto et al.[89]
Oropharynx, T2–T3, N0–N1	356	1.15 2.0	2 1	80.5 70.0	7.0 7.0	5-y LRC: 59% vs. 40% (P = .02) Improved local control of T3 tumors.	More acute mucositis with HF No difference in late complication rate	Horiot et al.[75] Horiot[90]
Various sites, T3–T4, N0, or any T, N+	331	1.45 2.55	2 1	58.0 51.0	4.0 4.0	5-y LRC: 45% vs. 37% (P = .01) 5-y OS: 40% vs. 30% (P = .01)	More acute mucositis with HF 5-y grade 3–4 late toxicity: 8% vs. 14% (P = .31)	Cummings et al.[91]
Various sites, stage III–IV, stage II of tongue base, hypopharynx	1,0+73	1.2 1.8 1.6 2.0	2 1–2 2 1	81.6 72.0 67.2 70.0	6.0 7.0 6.0 7.0	LRC: higher with HF and CB (P = .045 and .05) DFS: trend in favor of HF and CB (P = .067 and .054) but no difference in OS	More acute mucositis with all altered fractionations No difference in late complication rate	Fu et al.[92]
Bladder Cancer (TCC)								
T2–T4	168	1.0 2.0	3 1	84.0 64.0	8.0 8.0	Survival: higher with HF with an RH of 1.52 (95% CI, 1.10–2.09) OS benefit persists at 10 y	Trend for increase in bowel injury requiring surgical treatment	Naslund et al.[93]
Non–Small Cell Lung Cancer								
Stage II–III (surgically unresectable)	458	1.2 2.0	2 1	69.6 60.0	5.8 6.0	No significant difference in median or 5-y survival (induction chemotherapy arm yielded better OS)	Late toxicity not presented in detail	Sause et al.[94]
Stage III (RTOG 9410); arm A, neoadjuvant chemotherapy; arms B and C, concurrent chemotherapy	610	A: 2.0 B: 2.0 C: 1.2	1 1 2	60.0 60 69.6	6.0 6.0 5.8	No significant difference in median survival between arms B and C; improved 5-y survival for concurrent chemotherapy	Acute grade 3–5 nonhematologic toxic effects were higher with concurrent than sequential therapy, but late toxic effects were similar	Curran et al.[95]
Brainstem Tumors								
Age, 3–21 y	130	1.17 1.80	2 1	70.2 54.0	6.0 6.0	No significant difference in time to disease progression and overall survival	Morbidity similar in both arms	Mandell et al.[96]
Cranial Radiation for Treatment of High-Risk Acute Lymphoblastic Leukemia								
Children treated on two consecutive protocols for high-risk ALL	369	0.9 1.8	2 1	18.0 18.0	2.0 2.0	8-y EFS 72% ± 3% vs. 80% ± 3% (P = .06), OS 78% ± 3% vs. 85% ± 3% (P = .06); CNS HF may compromise antileukemic efficacy	Provides no benefit in terms of cognitive late effects No difference in intelligence, academic achievement, visuospatial reasoning, or verbal learning. Children on HF arm exhibited a modest advantage for visual memory (P ≤ .05).	Weber et al.[97] LeClerc et al.[98]
Children with Rhabdomyosarcoma								
Children enrolled into the Intergroup RMS Study IV with group III RMS	490	1.1 1.8	2 1	59.4 50.4	5.5 5.5	No difference in 5-y FFS or OS between HF and SF	Analysis by intention to treat; high noncompliance analysis by actual treatment also shows no difference; higher acute toxicity with HF	Donaldson et al.[99]
Unresected Brain Metastases (Hyperfractionation vs. Accelerated Hypofractionation)								
RTOG 9104; patients with measurable brain metastasis and KPS at least 70; AHF vs. AF	429	1.6 3.0	2 1	54.4 30.0	3.5 2.0	No difference in 1-y OS: 19% in AF vs. 16% in AHF	Grade III or IV toxicity was equivalent in both arms.	Murray et al.[100]
Prophylactic Cranial Irradiation for Limited-Stage Small Cell Lung Cancer in Complete Remission After Chemotherapy and Thoracic Radiotherapy								
Standard or higher total dose using either conventional or accelerated hyperfractionated radiotherapy	720	2.5 2.0 1.5	1 1 2	25 36.0 36	2.0 3.5 3	No difference in incidence of brain metastases; significant increase in mortality after higher-dose PCI	Slightly higher acute toxicity in the higher-dose arm but greater serious adverse events in the standard-dose group	Le Péchoux et al.[101]

The outcome data given x% vs. y% imply that x is the experimental-arm result. AF, accelerated fractionation; AHF, accelerated hyperfractionation; ALL, acute lymphoblastic leukemia; CI, confidence interval; CNS, central nervous system; DFS, disease-free survival; EFS, event-free survival; FFS, failure-free survival; Fx, fraction(s); Gy, gray; HF, hyperfractionation; KPS, Karnofsky performance score; LC, local control; LRC, locoregional control; MST, median survival time; N+, nodal stage; NSCLC, non–small cell lung cancer; OS, overall survival; PCI, prophylactic cranial irradiation; RMS, rhabdomyosarcoma; SF, standard fractionation; T, tumor stage; TCC, transitional cell carcinoma; wk, week.

TABLE 13.3 DATA OF PHASE III CLINICAL TRIALS ADDRESSING PURE ACCELERATED FRACTIONATION

Tumor Site and Type	Number of Patients	Dose/ Fx (Gy)	Fx/Day (Ti, h)	Total Dose (Gy)	Overall Time (wk)	Tumor Response	Side Effects	Reference
Inoperable non–small cell lung cancer	204	2.0 2.0	2 1	60 ± Carbo 60 ± Carbo	3.0 6.0	No significant difference in median survival time and 2-y OS	Esophageal toxicity significantly greater in AF	Ball et al.[102]
Various head and neck carcinomas, stage III–IV	82	2.0 2.0	2 (≥6) 1	66.0 66.0	3.4 6.8	CR: 35% vs. 29% (P = .18) No difference in 3-y relapse-free survival	Grade 3–4 reactions: 27 vs. 8 (P = .00005) Grade 4 late toxicity: 8 vs. 2 (P = .10)	Jackson et al.[103]
Various head and neck carcinomas, T2–T4, N0–N1	100	1.8–2.0 1.8–2.0	1 1	~70.0 ~70.0	5.0 7.0	3-y LC: 82% vs. 37% (P ≤ .0001) and 3-y OS: 78% vs. 32% (P ≤ .0001)	Severe mucositis: 62% vs. 26% Late complications: 10% vs. 0%	Skladowski et al.[104]
Various head and neck carcinomas, all stages	1,485	2.0 2.0	1 1	~66.0 ~66.0	6.0 7.0	5-y LRC: 66% vs. 57% (P = .01). 5-y DFS: 72% vs. 65% (P = .04); no difference in OS	More acute mucositis with AF No difference in late complication rate	Overgaard et al.[105]
Larynx carcinomas, T1–T3, N0	395	2.0 2.0	1–2 (≥6) 1	66.0 66.0	5.5 6.5	LRC: higher with AF (P = .03).	More acute reactions with AF; no difference in late complications except for telangiectasia	Hliniak et al.[106]
Nasopharynx cancer	416	1.8–1.9 1.8–1.9 2.0	1 1 1	74–76 74–76 +Cis/5-FU 70–76	6.0 6.0 7.0	LR 16.7% vs. 13.6% vs. 27.3% (P ≤ .05) 5-y OS 53.6% vs. 57.6% vs. 43.8% (P ≤ .05) Acceleration had a similar improvement as concurrent chemotherapy	Acute reactions higher with acceleration	Wang et al.[107]

The outcome data given as x% vs. y% imply that x is the experimental-arm result. AF, accelerated fractionation; Carbo, carboplatin; Cis, cisplatin; CR, complete response; DFS, disease-free survival; Fx, fraction(s); 5-FU, 5-flourouracil; Gy, gray; hr, hours; LC, local control; LR, local recurrence; LRC, locoregional control; OS, overall survival; Ti, interfraction interval time; wk, week.

TABLE 13.4 DATA OF PHASE III CLINICAL TRIALS ADDRESSING HYBRID ACCELERATED FRACTIONATION

Tumor Site and Type	Number of Patients	Dose/Fx (Gy)	Fx/Day (Ti, h)	Total Dose (Gy)	Overall Time (wk)	Tumor Response	Side Effects	Reference
Accelerated Fractionation with Total Dose Reduction (Type A)								
Various head and neck carcinomas, mainly stage II–IV	918	1.5 2.0	3 (6) 1	54.0 66.0	2.0 6.5	No difference in LRC, disease-free interval, and OS	More acute mucositis but less epidermis, telangiectasia, mucosal ulceration, and edema with AF	Dische et al.[108]
Various head and neck carcinomas, stage III–IV	350	1.8 2.0	2 (≥6) 1	59.4 70.0	3.5 7.0	5-y LRC: 52% vs. 47% (P = .30) 5-y DFS: 41% vs. 35% (P = .32) 5-y DSS: 46% vs. 40% (P = .40)	More severe acute mucositis (P = .00008) but reduced incidence of grade ≥ 2 late soft tissue effects (P ≤ .05) with AF (except for mucosal late effect)	Poulsen et al.[109]
All sites of head and neck carcinomas; oropharynx 75%; T4 70%	268	2.0 2.0	2 1	~63.0 70.0	3.3 7.0	2-y LRC: 58% vs. 34% (P ≤ 0.01) No difference in OS	Grade 3–4 mucositis: 83% vs. 28% (P ≤ .01) Similar late toxicity	Bourhis et al.[110]
Postoperative head and neck	70	1.4 2.0	3 (6) 1	46.2 60.0	2.0 6.0	3-y LRC: 88% ± 4% vs. 57% ± 9% (p = .01) OS: 60% ± 10% vs. 46% ± 9% (p = .29)	More rapid and more severe mucositis; fibrosis and edema more frequent after accelerated	Awwad et al.[111]
RTOG 9104; patients with measurable brain metastasis and KPS at least 70; AHF vs. AF	429	3.0 1.6	1 2	30.0 54.4	2.0 3.5	No difference in 1-y OS: 19% in AF vs. 16% in AHF	Grade III or IV toxicity was equivalent in both arms.	Murray et al.[100]
Locally advanced non–small cell lung cancer	563	1.5 2.0 split course	3 (6) 1	54.0 60.0	2.0 6.0	2-y OS: 29% vs. 20% (P = .008) Lower risk of local progression (P = .033)	No difference in short- or long-term morbidity	Saunders et al.[112]

TABLE 13.4 DATA OF PHASE III CLINICAL TRIALS ADDRESSING HYBRID ACCELERATED FRACTIONATION (*Continued*)

Tumor Site and Type	Number of Patients	Dose/Fx (Gy)	Fx/Day (Ti, h)	Total Dose (Gy)	Overall Time (wk)	Tumor Response	Side Effects	Reference
Stage IIIA and B non–small cell lung cancer	141	1.5 2.0	3 1	57.6 60.0	2.5 6.5	Trend suggesting a survival advantage in MS 20.3 vs. 14.9 mo (*P* = .28); 2-y OS 44% vs. 34%, 3-y OS 24% vs. 14%	Study included induction CT closed prematurely because concurrent CRT now seems more effective; 388 patients were needed.	Belani et al.[113]
Locally advanced non–small cell lung cancer CHARTWEL (CHART weekend less)	406	1.5 2.0	3 (6) 1	60.0 60.0	2.5 6.0	No difference in 2, 3, and 5 y (31%, 22%, and 11%) vs. CF (32%, 18%, and 7%; HR, 0.92; 95% CI, 0.75–1.13, *P* = .43)	Acute dysphagia and radiologic pneumonitis were more pronounced after CHARTWEL.	Baumann et al.[114]

Split-Course (Type B) and Concomitant Boost (Type C) Accelerated Fractionation

Tumor Site and Type	Number of Patients	Dose/Fx (Gy)	Fx/Day (Ti, h)	Total Dose (Gy)	Overall Time (wk)	Tumor Response	Side Effects	Reference
Various head and neck carcinomas, T2–T4, N0–N1	500	1.6 2.0 split course	3 1	72.0 70.0	5.0 7.0	5-y LRC: 59% vs. 46% (*P* = .02) Trend for higher 5-y DFS (*P* = .08) but no difference in OS (*P* = .96)	More severe acute mucositis and higher incidence of severe late morbidity (*P* ≤ .001) with AF	Horiot et al.[74]
Various head and neck carcinomas, stage III–IV, stage II of tongue base, hypopharynx	1,073	1.8[a] 1.20 1.60 split course 2.0	1–2 2 2 1	72.0 81.6 67.2 70.0	6.0 7.0 6.0 7.0	LRC: higher with CB and HF (*P* = .05 and .045) DFS: strong trend in favor of CB and HF (*P* = .054 and .067) but no difference in OS	More acute mucositis with all altered fractionations No difference in late complication rate	Fu et al.[92]
Unresectable epidermoid tumors of oropharynx	192	2.0 1.6 split course 2[b]	1 2 1	66–70 64–67.2 66–70	6.5–7 5.5 6.5–7	Concurrent chemotherapy almost doubled the 5-y overall survival, relapse-free survival, and locoregional control rates but did not reach statistical significance.	SF had less severe mucositis than AFS or SF chemo; concurrent chemotherapy showed slightly more subcutaneous and mucosal G3+ late side effects.	Fallai et al.[116]
T2–T3, N0–N1 bladder tumors	229	1.8 (a.m.), 2 (p.m.) split course 2.0	2 1	60.8 64.0	5.0 6.5	No difference in 3- or 5-y DFS and OS 5-y OS 37% vs. 40%	More acute bowel reactions with AF	Horwich et al.[117]
Various head and neck carcinomas, high-risk surgical–pathologic features	151	1.8 1.8	1–2 1	63.0 63.0	5.0 7.0	A trend for higher LRC (*P* = .11) and OS (*P* = .08) with CB. Cumulative time was a significant prognostic factor for LRC (*P* = .005) and OS (*P* = .03).	More acute mucositis with CB No difference in late complication rate	Ang et al.[115]
High-risk features (pT4, + margins, pN > 1, perineural/lymphovascular invasion, extracapsular extension, subglottic extension) after surgery	226		1–2 1	64.0 60.0	5.0 6.0	No difference in OS and LRC but trend for improved LRC among patients who had delayed RT	More acute mucositis with CB	Sanguineti et al.[118]

Accelerated Hyperfractionation

Tumor Site and Type	Number of Patients	Dose/Fx (Gy)	Fx/Day (Ti, h)	Total Dose (Gy)	Overall Time (wk)	Tumor Response	Side Effects	Reference
Glioblastoma multiforme	231	1.6 1.8	2 1	70.4 ± DMFO 59.4 ± DMFO	4.4 6.5	No difference in PFS (*P* = .32) and OS (*P* = .48)	Cerebral necrosis was not observed; morbidity more common in the DFMO arms	Prados et al.[119]

The outcome data given as *x*% vs. *y*% imply that *x* is the experimental-arm result. There are three types of hybrid accelerated: accelerated with dose reduction (A), accelerated with split course (B), and accelerated with concomitant boost (C). AF, accelerated fractionation; AFS, accelerated hyperfractionated split course; AHF, accelerated hyperfractionated; CB, concomitant boost; CHART, continuous, hyperfractionated, accelerated radiotherapy; CI, confidence interval; CRT, concurrent chemoradiation; CT, chemoradiation; DFS, disease-free survival; DMFO, difluoromethylornithine; DSS, disease-specific survival; EFS, event-free survival; Fx, fraction(s); Gy, gray; HF, hyperfractionation; hr, hours; KPS, Karnofsky performance score; LRC, locoregional control; MS, median survival; OS, overall survival; PFS, progression-free survival; RTOG, Radiation Therapy Oncology Group; SF, standard fractionation; SF chemo, standard fraction plus concomitant chemotherapy; Ti, interfraction interval time; wk, week.
[a]Boost dose given in 1.5-Gy fractions.
[b]Third arm with concurrent chemotherapy.

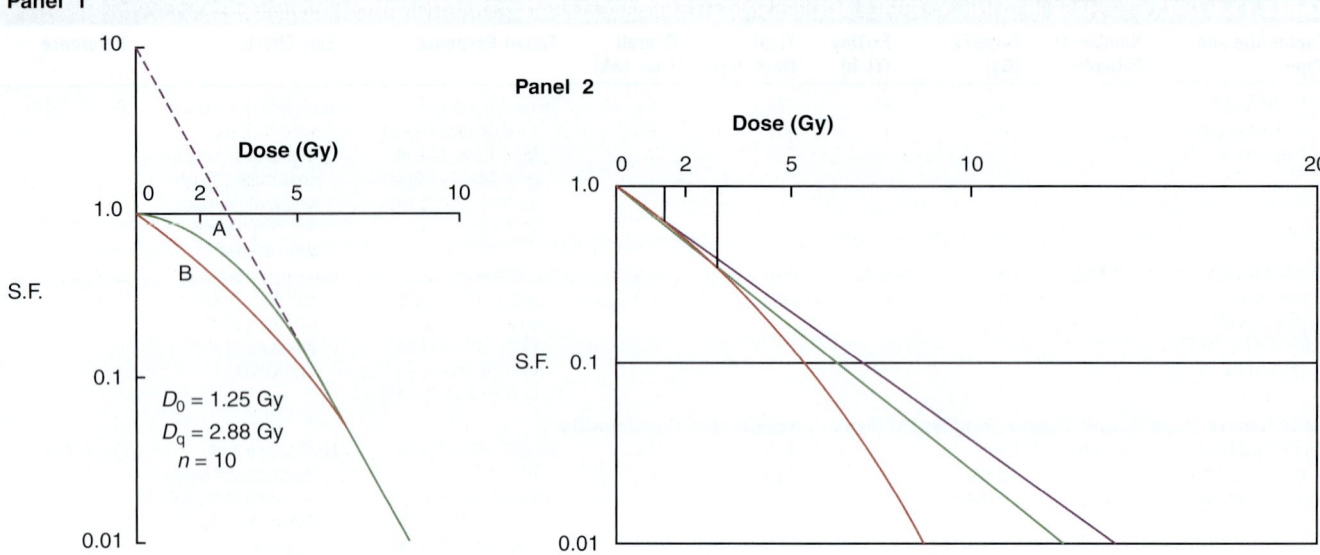

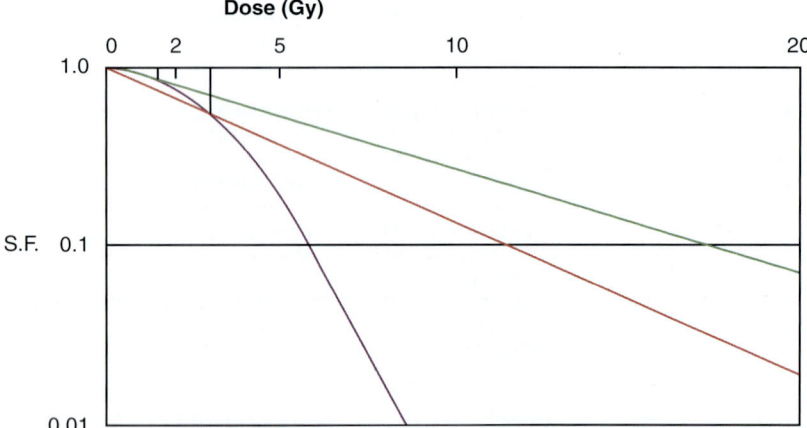

FIGURE 13.1. The importance of survival curve shoulder *shape* rather than width for the response to fractionated irradiation. *Panel 1:* Two survival curves with the same D_o, D_q, and n but with different initial slopes and shoulder curvatures. In terms of the linear quadratic model of cell survival, the α/β ratio is lower for curve A than for curve B. *Panels 2 and 3:* Effect of change in fraction size on the dose required for a given effect. *Panel 2:* When the shoulder has a steep initial slope and little curvature (high α/β), a change in dose per fraction from 3 to 1.5 Gy would only slightly increase the total dose needed to produce a given survival fraction. *Panel 3:* When the shoulder has a shallow initial slope and marked curvature (low α/β), a much greater increase in total dose is necessary to produce a given survival fraction when the same change in dose per fraction is made. (From Peters LJ, Brock WA, Travis EL. Radiation biology at clinically relevant fractions. In: DeVita V, Hellman S, Rosenberg SA, eds. *Important advances in oncology.* Philadelphia: JB Lippincott, 1991:65–83. With permission.)

The RTOG 9003 trial[92] tested 81.6 Gy at 1.2 Gy/fraction HyperRT twice per day over 6 weeks versus 70 Gy at 2 Gy/fraction versus two accelerated regimens (a continuous and a split-course accelerated regimen), as shown in Tables 13.2 and 13.4. HyperRT improved locoregional control from 46% to 54.4% (similar to the improvement by AF with the concomitant boost arm of the trial). This trial gives strong evidence that total dose and treatment duration are important to outcome. Locoregional control was significantly improved by an increase of the total dose without changing overall time using HyperRT or by accelerated overall treatment time without changing total dose using concomitant boost fractionation.

Meta-analysis of HyperRT and accelerated radiotherapy in unresected locally advanced squamous cell carcinoma of the head and neck showed a substantial prolongation of median survival (14.2 months; $P < .001$) for HyperRT compared to CFRT.[121] Of the four hyperfractionation trials,[75,90,122] one from Barcelona[122] has been criticized for questionable quality.[123] All

four trials showed a statistically significant survival benefit. Studies testing HyperRT without dose escalation did not show a survival advantage.[124,125] Overall, HyperRT is a useful tool to enable dose escalation without an increase of severe late toxicity.

Bladder Cancer

In the study by Edsmyr et al.,[28] T2–T4 bladder tumors were randomized to either three 1-Gy daily fractions 4 hours apart with interfraction intervals to 84 Gy or a single daily fraction of 2 Gy to total dose of 64 Gy, both given in a split course over 8 weeks. Cystoscopic complete response rate increased from 36% to 65% with HyperRT ($P < .001$), and the 5-year survival rate also significantly increased. However, severe late complications were higher in the hyperfractionated arm, indicating that the dose chosen might not be equivalent for late normal tissue injury. An updated analysis revealed that the survival benefit persisted for 10 years, but there was a

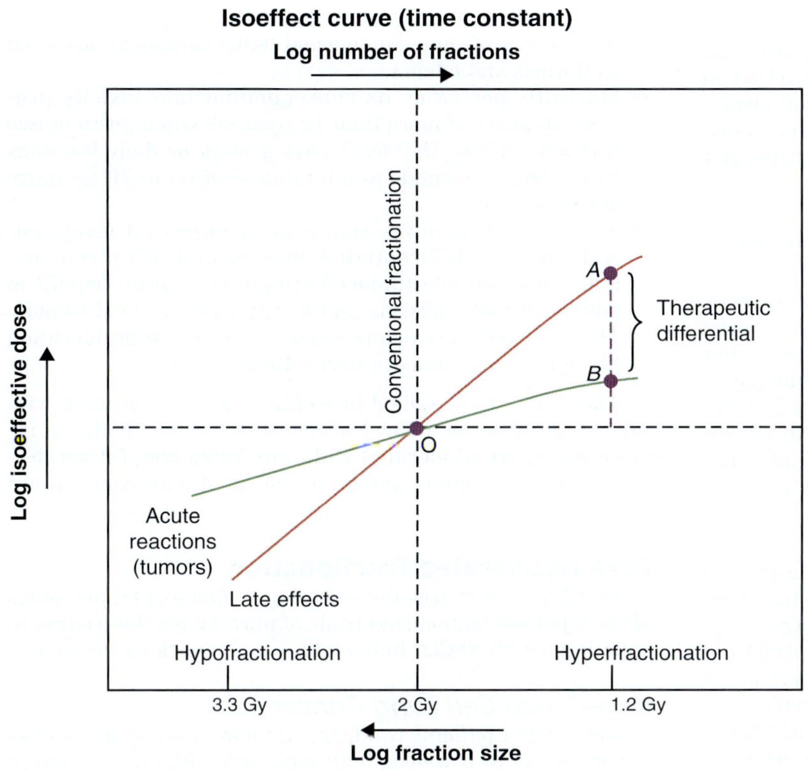

Isoeffect curve (time constant)

Log number of fractions

Log isoeffective dose

Conventional fractionation

A

Therapeutic differential

B

O

Acute reactions (tumors)

Late effects

Hypofractionation

Hyperfractionation

3.3 Gy   2 Gy   1.2 Gy

Log fraction size

FIGURE 13.2. Effect of change in size of dose fraction (with overall time held constant) on the total dose necessary to produce a given level of acute and late effects. The curves are normalized to the "conventional" 2 Gy/fraction. Changes in fraction size have a relatively greater effect on the isoeffective doses for late reactions than for acute reactions and for the response of tumors with high α/β ratios. Consequently, by reducing the dose per fraction—for example, from 2 to 1.2 Gy—the total dose for equivalent late effects can be increased from O to A, which is greater than the increase (O to B) required to achieve an equivalent tumor response. The increment in dose from B to A represents the therapeutic differential achieved by hyperfractionation.

trend for higher bowel complications requiring surgery in the HyperRT group.[93]

Non–Small Cell Lung Cancer

The joint Intergroup trial[94] of the RTOG, the Eastern Cooperative Oncology Group (ECOG), and the Southwest Oncology Group compared induction chemotherapy (cisplatin and vinblastine) plus 60 Gy in 2-Gy fractions or HyperRT (69.6 Gy in 1.2-Gy fractions) with CFRT (60 Gy in 2-Gy fractions). Though considered slightly more effective, HyperRT did not significantly improve survival over CFRT.

Two concurrent regimens with standard or HyperRT were tested as part of three arms of RTOG 9410, a phase III trial.

Six hundred ten patients had either neoadjuvant cisplatin and vinblastine or the same chemotherapy concurrent with 60-Gy standard fractionation versus concurrent cisplatin and etoposide with HyperRT (69.6 Gy delivered as 1.2-Gy twice-daily fractions). Median survival times were 14.6, 17.0, and 15.6 months, respectively. Five-year survival was statistically significantly higher for patients treated with the concurrent regimen with once-daily radiotherapy (TRT) compared with the sequential treatment (5-year survival: sequential, arm 1, 10% [20 patients], 95% CI = 7% to 15%; concurrent, arm 2, 16% [31 patients], 95% CI, 11% to 22%, P = .046; concurrent, arm 3, 13% [22 patients], 95% CI, 9% to 18%). Late toxic effects were similar.[95]

Comparison of conventional and four prototypes of accelerated fractionation schedules

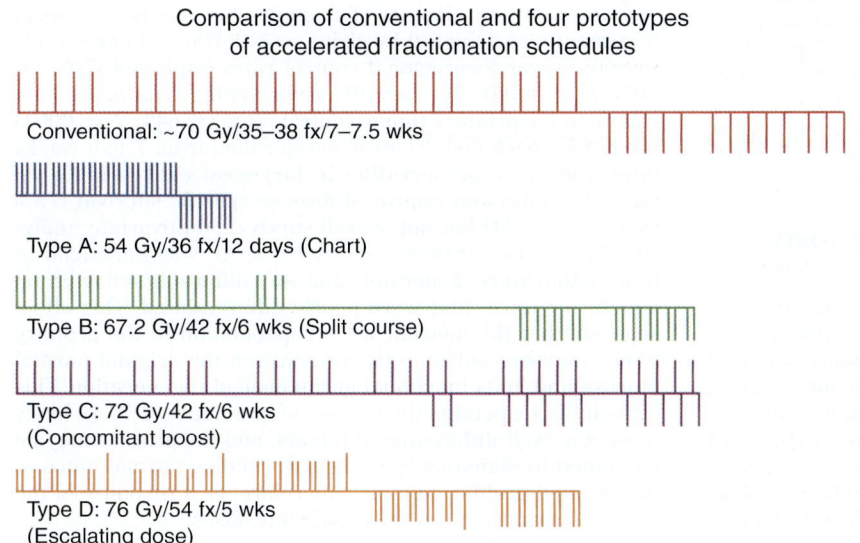

Conventional: ~70 Gy/35–38 fx/7–7.5 wks

Type A: 54 Gy/36 fx/12 days (Chart)

Type B: 67.2 Gy/42 fx/6 wks (Split course)

Type C: 72 Gy/42 fx/6 wks (Concomitant boost)

Type D: 76 Gy/54 fx/5 wks (Escalating dose)

FIGURE 13.3. Conventional and accelerated fractionation schedules. For each regimen, the large-field treatment is depicted by the bars above the horizontal line and the boost-field irradiation by the bars below the line. The dotted bars represent treatment omitted in the lower ranges of total dose. fx, fraction.

Childhood Brainstem Tumor

The trial of the Pediatric Oncology Group[96] compared the efficacy of 70.2 Gy given as 1.17 Gy/fraction versus 54 Gy in 1.8-Gy fractions, both in combination with 100 mg/m² cisplatin. This study showed no difference in the median time to disease progression, median time to death, or survival rates at 1 and 2 years, with no significant difference in toxicity.

Cranial Radiation Therapy for High-Risk Acute Lymphoblastic Leukemia

To test whether HyperRT could reduce incidence and severity of late toxicities associated with 18-Gy prophylactic cranial radiotherapy, 369 children on two consecutive Dana-Farber Cancer Institute Consortium protocols were randomized to 18 Gy delivered in ten 1.8-Gy fractions once daily over 2 weeks versus 18 Gy delivered in twenty 0.9-Gy fractions. No benefit was seen in terms of cognitive late effects, and the results suggested that HF may compromise antileukemic efficacy.[97,98]

Group III Rhabdomyosarcoma

A total of 490 children with group III rhabdomyosarcoma (RMS) were randomized to HyperRT (59.4 Gy in fifty-four 1.1-Gy twice-daily fractions) versus CFRT to 50.4 Gy in the Intergroup RMS Study IV. This trial showed that HyperRT did not improve local/regional control, failure-free survival, or overall survival compared with CFRT and that HyperRT actually produced more acute toxicity.[99] Unlike studies in HNSCC showing positive results with dose-escalated HyperRT, an escalation of dose by 9.5 Gy did not improve outcome for RMS.

Unresected Brain Metastasis

RTOG 9104 compared 1-year survival and acute toxicity rates between an accelerated HyperRT (1.6 Gy twice a day) to a total dose of 54.4 Gy and an accelerated hypofractionated (HypoRT) arm of 30 Gy in 10 daily fractions in patients with unresected brain metastasis. Of 429 analyzable patients, the median survival time was 4.5 months in both arms. The 1-year survival rate was 19% in the HypoRT arm versus 16% in the HyperRT arm. Grade III or IV toxicity was equivalent in both arms. In spite of an escalated dose, HyperRT was of no benefit.[100]

Prophylactic Cranial Irradiation for Limited-Stage Small Cell Lung Cancer

To test whether higher-dose prophylactic cranial irradiation (PCI) would reduce brain metastases, 720 patients with limited-stage small cell lung cancer (SCLC) who were in complete remission after chemotherapy and thoracic radiotherapy were randomized to standard 25 Gy in 10 daily versus 36 Gy either as 18 daily 2-Gy fractions or accelerated HyperRT as 24 twice-daily 1.5-Gy fractions in 16 days. There was no significant difference in the 2-year incidence of brain metastases and a lower overall survival in the higher-dose group. PCI at 25 Gy was recommended as the standard of care in limited-stage SCLC.[101]

Results of Accelerated Radiotherapy Trials

Key findings of accelerated regimens include the following:

- Modest acceleration by 1 week by delivering six fractions of 2 Gy/week or a concomitant boost regimen without dose reduction or treatment break yields superior locoregional control of head and neck carcinomas without increase in late toxicity but without clear impact on survival. Acceleration by more than 3 weeks with a 10% total dose reduction (<6 to 7 Gy) also improves the locoregional control without demonstrable increase in late complications. However, a further 5% to 8% total dose reduction

abrogates the gain in tumor control but appears to reduce the severity of some late normal tissue complications, such as fibrosis and edema.
- Mucositis per se or its consequential late toxicity prevents delivery of more than 12 Gy/week when given in two fractions of 2 Gy/day for 5 days a week or daily fractions throughout weekends to a total dose of 66 to 70 Gy (pure acceleration).
- Acceleration achieves significantly improved local control for well-differentiated tumors and advanced primary mucosal site tumors but may be of little benefit to advanced nodal disease and poorly differentiated tumors. This supports the existence of the accelerated proliferation phenomenon in mucosa-derived tumor cells.

The trials are classified into either pure accelerated, with same total dose, or hybrid accelerated, of which there are three types: (a) accelerated with dose reduction, (b) accelerated with split course, and (c) accelerated with concomitant boost.

Pure Accelerated Fractionation

Table 13.3 summarizes the radiation regimens and outcomes of six reported randomized trials of pure AF for the treatment of patients with NSCLC lung and head and neck carcinoma.

Non–Small Cell Lung Cancer

A study of 204 patients randomized them to 60 Gy in 3 weeks versus 60 Gy in 6 weeks, both with and without concurrent carboplatin.[102] The results showed no survival advantage with either acceleration or concurrent carboplatin. The study showed that 60 Gy in 3 weeks induced a significantly greater esophagitis than did 60 Gy in 6 weeks.

Head and Neck Cancer

The first two HNSCC studies shown in Table 13.3[103,104] induced unacceptable toxicity, leading to early termination, and these two fractionations have been abandoned. However, two of the other three trials showed positive results,[105,107] whereas one[106] showed no benefit and similar late toxicity.

The Polish Cooperative Group compared 66 Gy given in 33 fractions over 38 days (two fractions every Thursday) as compared with a conventional regimen of 66 Gy given in 33 fractions over 45 days. In the study, 395 patients with T1–T3, N0, M0 glottic, and supraglottic laryngeal cancer were randomized. There was no difference in terms of locoregional control (P = .37).[106]

The Danish trial, one of the largest trials of altered fractionation,[105] accrued 1,485 patients with larynx, oropharynx, and oral cavity carcinomas of all stages. Six versus 7 weeks of treatment was achieved by giving a sixth fraction each week. Overall 5-year locoregional control rates improved (70% vs. 60%; P = .0005). The benefit of shortening treatment time was seen for primary tumor control (76% vs. 64%; P = .0001) but not for neck node control. Acceleration from 7 to 6 weeks improved voice preservation in laryngeal cancer (80% vs. 68%; P = .007) and improved disease-specific survival (73% vs. 66%; P = .01) but not overall survival. Multivariate analysis of 754 larynx cancers showed that AF was beneficial in tumors that were moderately and well differentiated, with no benefit for those that were poorly differentiated. This effect suggests that the mechanism of repopulation in the primary tumor may be similar to the response in the original normal mucosa and in its functional mechanism of regeneration. This capacity to respond to the trauma of irradiation is more likely to exist in well-differentiated tumors, and the process may be facilitated by signaling from the surrounding normal mucosa. Accelerated proliferation may, therefore, be a response of the primary tumor and not the nodal metastases.[126]

Nasopharynx

Pure acceleration for nasopharynx cancer was tested in Guangxi, China. In the study, 416 patients were randomized to three arms: all had 7,400 to 7,600 cGy given as accelerated six fractions per week with or without concurrent cisplatin and 5-fluorouacil versus the conventional five 2-Gy fractions per week. The local recurrence rates were 16.7% in the accelerated group, 13.6% in the accelerated-concurrent group, and 27.3% in the CFRT group ($P < .05$). The 5-year survival rates were 53.6%, 57.6%, and 43.8% ($P < .05$), respectively. The interesting finding was that acceleration had a similar effect as concurrent chemotherapy with acceleration for nasopharynx cancer.[107]

Hybrid Accelerated Fractionation

Table 13.4 summarizes the details of regimens and outcomes of reported prospective, randomized trials addressing the role of types A to C hybrid accelerated fractionation (Fig. 13.4).

Type A

Accelerated fractionation regimens (with dose reduction) were addressed in trials shown in Table 13.4, including a trial in HNSCC (definitive and postoperative), brain metastases, and NSCLC. It includes trials by the British Medical Research Council (MRC), the Trans-Tasman Radiation Oncology Group (TROG), the French Radiotherapy Oncology Group for Head and Neck Cancer (GORTEC), and the ECOG.

Head and Neck

As shown in Table 13.4, two trials for HNSCC—the MRC CHART[126] and TROG regimens[109]—did not yield improvement in locoregional control and disease-free and overall survival rates. In contrast, the GORTEC regimen[110] for locally advanced head and neck carcinoma, with a 3.5-week acceleration and only 7-Gy (10%) dose reduction, significantly improved the locoregional control, with no gain in the overall survival rate.

Based on the potential for accelerated proliferation after surgery, Awwad et al.[111] in Cairo explored acceleration in postoperative radiotherapy of locally advanced HNSCC. Seventy patients with T2/N1–N2 or T3–T4/any N squamous cell carcinoma of the oral cavity, larynx, and hypopharynx were randomized to accelerated HyperRT of 46.2 Gy in 12 days versus CFRT (60 Gy per 6 weeks). The 3-year locoregional control rate was better with accelerated treatment (88% ± 4%) versus CFRT (57% ± 9%; $P = .01$), with no difference in survival (60% ± 10% vs. 46% ± 9%; $P = .29$). As expected, acute mucositis was more severe in the accelerated group, and fibrosis and edema also tended to be more frequent; this finding contrasts with the results in two postoperative studies of type C (concomitant boost) described later and in Table 13.4.[115,118]

Non–Small Cell Lung Cancer

One randomized, controlled trial showed that CHART improves survival over standard radiotherapy of 60 Gy in 30 fractions in patients with locally advanced, unresectable stage III NSCLC. This MRC trial[112] showed that CHART with a 4-week acceleration and 6-Gy (10%) dose reduction decreased the risk for local progression and improved the overall survival significantly without increasing short- and long-term morbidity. These patients are now routinely given concurrent chemotherapy. However, in some countries, selected patients who are not fit for chemotherapy or patients who prefer radiotherapy only may be considered for CHART. The ECOG tested accelerated radiotherapy after induction chemotherapy (two cycles of carboplatin plus paclitaxel) in stage IIIA and B NSCLC. Acceleration was achieved with 57.6 Gy (1.5 Gy three times a day for 2.5 weeks) versus CFRT (64 Gy in 2 Gy/day). Of 141 patients enrolled, 83% were randomly assigned—60 accelerated and 59 conventional. The median survival was 20.3 and 14.9, respectively ($P = .28$). With the acceptance that concurrent chemoradiation is more effective than sequential treatment, this trial closed early.[113]

Further acceleration to 2.5 weeks was tested in a trial of CHARTWEL (CHART weekend less), in which 406 patients with NSCLC were randomized to receive three-dimensional planned radiotherapy to 60 Gy/40 fractions/2.5 weeks (CHARTWEL) or 66 Gy/33 fractions/6.5 weeks (conventional fractionation [CF]). Overall survival (OS; primary endpoint) at 2, 3, and 5 years was not significantly different after CHARTWEL (31%, 22%, and 11%) versus CF (32%, 18%, and 7%; HR, 0.92; 95% CI, 0.75 to 1.13, $P = .43$). Local tumor control rates and distant metastases did not significantly differ.[114]

Split-Course Accelerated Fractionation Regimen (Type B)

Split-course accelerated regimens (type B) are also shown in Table 13.4. This was addressed by EORTC[74] and RTOG,[92] by a study from Florence, Italy,[116] of patients with locally advanced head and neck carcinomas, and by the Royal Marsden NHS Trust, Institute of Cancer Research, London, for bladder cancer.[117] The EORTC regimen consisted of 28.8 Gy over 7 days, followed by a 2-week break, then 43.2 Gy over 11 days to a cumulative dose of 72 Gy in 45 fractions over 5 weeks. Although the 2-week acceleration improved locoregional control, it produced twice as many grade 3 to 4 acute morbidities, more late toxicity ($P < .001$), seven cases of permanent peripheral neuropathy, and two cases of myelopathy. This regimen has been abandoned.

The RTOG split regimen was comparable to that of the Massachusetts General Hospital study[127]: two fractions of 1.6 Gy/day to a total dose of 67.2 Gy in 6 weeks, including a 2-week break in treatment after 38.4 Gy, with the standard 70 Gy in 7 weeks. This 1-week acceleration with a 3.8-Gy (5%) dose reduction increased acute mucositis without improving the locoregional control rate, with the concomitant boost and hyperfractionation arm being superior. Fallai et al.[116] reported an Italian multicenter randomized trial that treated 192 patients with advanced carcinoma of the oropharynx with CFRT (arm A: 66 to 70 Gy in 33 to 35 fractions for 5 days

FIGURE 13.4. Zone of therapeutic gain in squamous cell carcinomas (SCCs) of the head and neck for different accelerated fractionation schedules. Type A is 54 Gy in 36 fractions over 12 days, type B is 67.2 Gy in 42 fractions over 42 days, and type C is 72 Gy in 42 fractions over 40 days. For explanation, see text. (From Peters LJ, Brock WA, Travis EL. Radiation biology at clinically relevant fractions. In: DeVita V, Hellman S, Rosenberg SA, eds. *Important advances in oncology*. Philadelphia: JB Lippincott, 1991:65–83. With permission.)

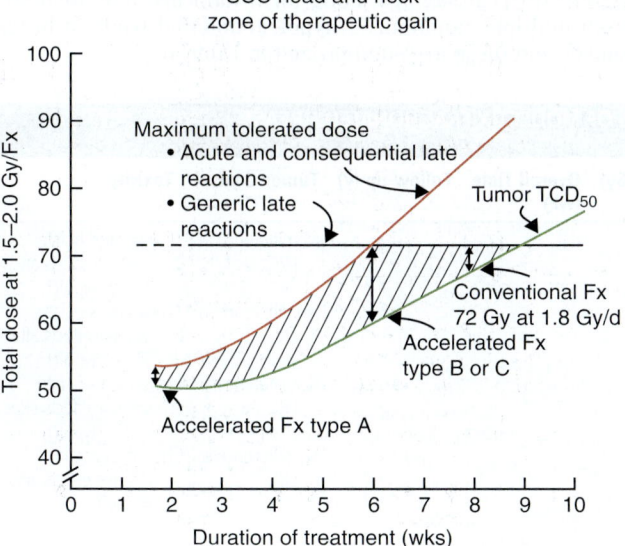

SCC head and neck zone of therapeutic gain

a week over 6.5 to 7 weeks) versus accelerated split-course radiotherapy (arm B: 64 to 67.2 Gy in two fractions of 1.6 Gy for 5 days a week with 2-week split at 38.4 Gy) versus concomitant chemoradiation (arm C: same radiotherapy as arm A plus concomitant carboplatin and 5-fluorouracil). Although the results did not reach statistical significance, chemoradiation almost doubled the 5-year overall survival (21%, 21%, and 40% for arms A, B, and C, respectively) and relapse-free survival (15%, 17%, and 36% for arms A, B, and C, respectively). There was a slight trend toward better 5-year locoregional control ($P = .07$) for the combined arm: patients without locoregional relapse in arm C, 21%, 18%, and 48% for arms A, B, and C, respectively. The occurrence of persistent G3 xerostomia was comparable in the three treatment arms.

The Royal Marsden study in London evaluated the efficacy and toxicity of an accelerated regimen to treat T2 or T3, N0 or N1 muscle-invasive bladder cancer. The 229 patients were randomized into two groups and given 60.8 Gy in 32 fractions over 5 weeks with a 1-week treatment gap after the first 12 fractions versus 64 Gy in 32 fractions over 6.5 weeks. Acceleration was achieved by two fractions per day of 1.8 and 2.0 Gy. RTOG grade 2 or 3 bowel toxicity in the accelerated arm was 44% versus 26% in the CFRT arm (P trend = .001), with no difference in acute grade 2 or 3 bladder toxicity or late RTOG grade 2 toxicity equivalent. There was no significant difference in disease-free survival and overall survival at 3 and 5 years.[117]

Concomitant Boost Accelerated Fractionation Regimen (Type C)

Concomitant boost acceleration (type C) was also addressed by the RTOG[92]; this regimen was designed at the MD Anderson Cancer Center[128] and delivers 54 Gy of wide-field irradiation in 1.8-Gy fractions over 6 weeks and 18 Gy of boost dose given in 1.5-Gy fractions as second daily fractions during the last 2.5 weeks. This regimen was found to improve the locoregional control rate, with a strong trend for a higher disease-free survival rate and with more severe mucositis but no detectable increase in late complications.

Concomitant boost-type fractionation was also tested for postoperative radiation therapy in two phase III trials.[118,128] Ang et al.[129] randomized patients with high-risk pathologic features to 63 Gy given in 35 fractions over either 5 weeks (daily fractions for 3 weeks and then two fractions per day for 2 weeks) or 7 weeks. This study showed that the cumulative time of the combined treatment was a significant determinant of locoregional control and overall survival. Concomitant boost partially offsets the detrimental effect of a delay in initiating radiation therapy beyond 6 weeks after surgery without inducing a detectable increase in late complications. These findings were confirmed by Sanguineti et al.[118] in Genoa, Italy, who randomized patients from four institutions with one

or more high-risk features after surgery to CFRT (60 Gy in 6 weeks) versus 64 Gy in 5 weeks with twice-daily treatment in the first and last weeks of treatment. Once again, there was no difference in outcome between the two arms; however, there was a trend for improved locoregional control for patients who had a delay in starting radiotherapy and who were treated with acceleration compared with those with a delay who were treated with CFRT (HR, 0.5; 95% CI, 0.2 to 1.1). Acceleration does not seem worthwhile postoperatively for carcinoma of the head and neck, although it might be an option for patients who delay starting radiotherapy.

A phase III trial in patients with glioblastoma multiforme (GBM) assessed the role of a combined accelerated, hyperfractionated regimen with a 2-week reduction of therapy duration and a dose increment of 11 Gy (18%).[119] This radiation regimen, with or without difluoromethylornithine, was found to yield no better progression-free and overall survival rates.

Pure Hypofractionated Radiotherapy (HypoRT) for Breast Cancer

Elective mastectomy rates among breast conservation candidates are consistently highest among underserved patients with limited access to radiotherapy services.[130,131] For such a common disease, the commitment to daily CFRT has significant barriers, mainly related to the inconvenience of a 3- to 7-week regimen and the cost of treatment—both direct health care expenditures and opportunity costs to the patient and society due to time away from home and work.[132] Hypofractionated radiotherapy (HypoRT) for breast cancer has therefore been seen as a logical solution to these disparities, but has a long and controversial history dating back to the 1960s.[87,133–135] Early understandings of radiobiology (inadequate reductions of total dose to compensate for increased fraction size) along with limitations in technology (high skin doses, gross off-axis inhomogeneities) contributed to poor outcomes in the mid-to-late twentieth century.[136] Fortunately, perseverance to better understand the biologic dose–response of breast cancer and normal tissue as well as the desire to improve access and cost of adjuvant radiotherapy led to a modern renaissance of HypoRT in the late 1990s.

Modest HypoRT

Although 2.0-Gy fraction size has been considered standard since the beginning of the breast conservation era, modest, daily hypofractionation with fractional doses between 2.5 and 3.3 Gy has been common practice in countries with centralized healthcare systems such as the United Kingdom and Canada, where reduction in total treatment time represents significant cost savings. Long-term data are now available from multiple randomized hypofractionated trials in breast cancer and these are summarized in Table 13.5.

TABLE 13.5 RECENTLY PUBLISHED PROSPECTIVE, RANDOMIZED TRIALS OF MODESTLY FRACTIONATED BREAST HYPOFRACTIONATED RADIOTHERAPY

Study	Enrollment	Number of Patients	Dose/Fx (Gy)	Total Dose (Gy)	Overall Time (wk)	Follow-up (y)	Tumor Control	Toxicity
RMH Trial[137]	Post-BCS for early breast cancer (pT1-3a, pN0-1, M0)	1,410	3.3	42.9	5	9.7	No difference in LRC	Lower rates of late adverse effects after 39-Gy HypoRT
			3	39	5			
			2	50	5			
START A Trial[138]	Post-BCS or mastectomy for early breast cancer (pT1-3a, pN0-1, M0)	2,236	3.2	41.6	5	9.3	No difference in LRC	Lower rates of late adverse effects after 39-Gy HypoRT
			3	39	5			
			2	50	5			
START B Trial[138]	Post-BCS or mastectomy for early breast cancer (pT1-3a, pN0-1, M0)	2,215	2.67	40	3	9.9	No difference in LRC	Lower rates of late adverse effects after 40-Gy HypoRT
			2	50	5			
Canadian Trial[139]	Post-BCS for early breast cancer (pT1-2, pN0, M0)	1,234	2.67	42.5	3	10	No difference in LRC	No difference in adverse effects after HypoRT
			2	50	5			

BCS, breast-conserving surgery; HypoRT, hypofractionated radiotherapy; LRC, locoregional control; RMH, Royal Marsden Hospital.

Phase III trials from the United Kingdom began with the Royal Marsden Hospital (RMH) study and progressed to include the two multi-institutional Standardisation of Breast Radiotherapy Trials (START A and B). All of these studies used 50 Gy in 25 fractions as the standard arm and tested multiple iterations of modest hypofractionation schemes over 3 to 5 weeks in an endeavor to determine the most appropriate biologically equivalent dose for both efficacy and toxicity. The RMH study accrued 1,410 patients from 1986 to 1998 and used an every-other-day schedule to test two HypoRT regimens (39.0 or 42.9 Gy in 13 fractions).[137] In this study, all patients had undergone BCS and nearly 75% of patients were prescribed an additional tumor bed boost. At 10 years follow-up, there were no differences in local control among the treatment arms. The 39-Gy HypoRT arm of the RMH study exhibited cosmetic outcome that was equivalent to CFRT, and so it was chosen as the "standard-experimental" arm of the START A Trial.

START A (1999 to 2002) tested two dose levels of a 13-fraction schedule, again every other day, against the sCFRT with the aim of measuring the sensitivity of normal and malignant tissues to fraction size.[138] Two thousand two hundred thirty-six women with early breast cancer (pT1-3a, pN0-1, M0) were randomized to receive after primary surgery (85% BCS) standard 50 Gy in 25 fractions versus 41.6 Gy or 39 Gy in 13 fractions of 3.2 Gy or 3.0 Gy over the same 5 weeks. Over 60% of patients who had BCS as primary surgery received an additional tumor bed boost. After a median follow-up of 9.3 years, the rate of locoregional tumor relapse was at 7.2% after 50 Gy, 6.3% after 41.6 Gy, and 8.8% after 39 Gy. There was a lower rate of late adverse effects after 39 Gy than with 50 Gy in terms of breast induration, telangiectasia, and edema. The START B Trial (1999–2001) ran concurrently with START A and randomized 2,215 women with pT1-3a, pN0-1, M0 breast cancer to 50 Gy in 25 fractions over 5 weeks versus 40 Gy in 15 fractions of 2.67 Gy, (this time once daily) over 3 weeks.[138] A total of 92% of patients had undergone BCS of which 43% received an additional tumor bed boost. After a median follow-up of 9.9 years, treatment with daily HypoRT 40 Gy in 15 fractions produced the same rates of locoregional tumor relapse as that with 50 Gy in 25 fractions (4.3% vs. 5.5%). The rates of late adverse effects (breast shrinkage, telangiectasia, and edema) were lower after 40-Gy than after 50-Gy treatment by photographic and patient self-assessments.

Similar to START B, a Canadian study in 1,234 stage I, postmenopausal women tested daily HypoRT (42.5 Gy in 16 fractions, 3 weeks) versus CFRT (50.0 Gy in 25 fractions, 5 weeks). All patients in this study underwent BCS with clear resection margins and none received an additional boost.[139] At 10 years, the risk of local recurrence was similar: 6.7% with standard fractionation versus 6.2% with hypofractionated regimen and the rate of women with a good or excellent cosmetic outcome was also similar. A meta-analysis of nearly 8,200 patients included in the four abovementioned trials as well as nine additional published studies showed that for early breast cancer, there are no significant differences in local failure, regional failure, or survival in patients treated with HypoRT versus CFRT.[140] In addition, HypoRT is associated with significantly less acute toxicity while providing equivalent late cosmetic outcomes.

There are differing opinions as to whether routine use of HypoRT should be restricted to patients that represent the majority of subjects enrolled in these clinical trials (postmenopausal, stage I, post-BCS) or whether they should be considered studies of biologic equivalence to be reasonably extrapolated to underrepresented subgroups. The American Society for Radiation Oncology therefore developed an evidence-based guideline to provide direction for clinical practice.[141] The panel considered the data sufficient to support the use of hypofractionated whole-breast irradiation for patients with early-stage breast cancer who were of age 50 years or older, had disease stage pT1-2, pN0, and did not receive chemotherapy. However, it remains highly unlikely that separate clinical trials on the scale and scope of those described above will ever be practical or feasible for patients with earlier (DCIS) or more advanced disease. In the United Kingdom, where the published experience of HypoRT remains the longest and broadest, the view is that modest HypoRT should be available to any identifiable subset of subclinical breast cancers.[136] The National Institute for Health and Clinical Excellence (NICE) in the United Kingdom has adopted a much more broad view of modest HypoRT and endorses it as standard of care for the majority of patients (either BCS or postmastectomy) with early breast cancer.[142] Although NICE acknowledges that the use of HypoRT in the treatment of DCIS is a matter of debate, it seems paradoxical to insist on CFRT for this more favorable subset of breast cancers. It is likely that in the coming years, multi-institutional collaboration and registry studies will continue to shed light on the efficacy of HypoRT for the treatment of subsets of patients not fitting the mold of those in the original clinical trials.

Large-Fraction HypoRT

The accumulation of sufficient modest HypoRT experience has allowed investigators to further push the limits of hypofractionation in order to eliminate the requirement of daily therapy. Large-fraction HypoRT, which delivers approximately 30 to 33 Gy in 5 to 6 Gy/fraction, once or twice weekly, was initially tested in small, institutional nonrandomized studies in Europe and the United Kingdom. First employed only for elderly patients, early studies have shown toxicity, cosmesis, and outcomes comparable to CFRT regimens.[143–148] A summary of studies that used once-weekly hypofractionated breast irradiation (WHBI) published in the modern era is listed in Table 13.6.

TABLE 13.6 RECENTLY PUBLISHED TRIALS OF LARGE-FRACTION BREAST HYPOFRACTIONATED RADIOTHERAPY

Study	Enrollment	Number of Patients	Dose/Fx (Gy)	Total Dose (Gy)	Overall Time (wk)	Follow-up (y)	Tumor Control	Cosmesis (% G/E)
French Prospective Single-Arm Trial[143]	Elderly (T1–T3, N0–N1, M0)	150	6.5	32.5	5	5	97.7%	NR
French Retrospective Study[144]	Elderly (T1–T3, N0, M0)	367	6.5	32.5	5	7.8	95%	88%
			2	50	5			
Italian Retrospective Study[145]	Elderly (T1–T3, N0–N2, M0)	298	6.5	32.5	5	4	98%	86%
			6	30	5			
UK Prospective Single-Arm Trial[146]	Postmenopausal (T1, N0, M0)	30	6	30	2.5	3	100%	77%
UK FAST Prospective Randomized Trial[147]	Postmenopausal (T1, N0, M0)	915	6	30	5	3	99%	83%–90%[a]
			5.7	28.5	5			
			2	50	5			
US Prospective Double Cohort Trial[148]	Pre- or postmenopausal (Tis-2, N0–N1, M0)	158	6	30	5	3.5	98%	82%
			5.7	28.5	5			

G/E: good–excellent; HypoRT: hypofractionated radiotherapy; NR: breast-conserving surgery; NR: not reported.
[a]Reported as "significant photographic change," cosmetic outcome was statistically significantly better in the 28.5-Gy HypoRT arm.

The first prospective phase III randomized study of large-fraction HypoRT against CFRT is the UK FAST trial.[147] This trial (n = 915) tested 50 Gy in 25 fractions of CFRT against two different regimens of HypoRT delivered in a five-fraction schedule over 5 weeks (30 Gy or 28.5 Gy/fraction). The two experimental arms represented the most commonly used regimen to date (30 Gy per 5 fractions) and a dose-reduced regimen (28.5 Gy per 5 fractions) based on radiobiologic estimations derived from the outcomes of the UK START trials. The first published report of this trial, which was open to node-negative postmenopausal women, showed an overall rate of grade 2 or higher skin toxicity of 23.9%, with a lower rate found in both experimental arms (14.4% and 10.4%) versus those treated with CFRT (46.4%).[147] At 3 years' follow-up, there were only 5 local recurrences, 3 in the CFRT arm and 2 in the HypoRT arms. The rate of significant photographic cosmetic change was slightly higher (17.3%) for patients treated with 30 Gy compared to 28.5 Gy or CFRT (11.1% and 9.5%, respectively). A phase II trial from the United States, which had a broader eligibility criteria and used the same large-fraction HypoRT dosing schemes, showed similar results for both toxicity and local control.[148]

Longer-term follow-up from these studies will ultimately provide clarity before large HypoRT regimens can be considered for routine use outside of a clinical trial. In the meantime, the investigators in the United Kingdom have proceeded with the FAST-Forward study aims to further reduce treatment times.[149] Patients on this trial are randomized to modest HypoRT (40 Gy in 15 fractions, 3 weeks) versus one of two large-fraction HypoRT arms (27 or 26 Gy, 5 fractions, 1 week). Fortunately, this study includes patients outside of traditionally targeted low-risk (i.e., postmenopausal, node-negative, no chemotherapy) populations. This will prove vital to facilitate reasonable extrapolation of alternative fractionation so as to improve access to care among women with breast cancer.

Concerns Related to Dosimetry and Organs at Risk

Despite the level of evidence described above, widespread, wholesale changes in practice patterns away from CFRT have been slow, especially in the United States.[150] The reasons for this are multifactorial and include health care physician reimbursement economics as well as a general risk aversion based on historical reports. Given the superb and predictable outcomes achieved with CFRT, physicians in practice must balance the improved convenience of HypoRT versus the more rigorous attention to dosimetric criteria in order to deliver it safely. In terms of dose heterogeneity within the breast, "hot spots" in a dose plan that receives a higher dose per fraction

carry more significance and will ultimately be penalized more severely.[136] Therefore, it is generally advised that distributions within the breast are kept within 95% to 107% of the reference isodose, where the risk of additional adverse effects is predicted to be clinically insignificant.

As with any breast radiotherapy plan, it is also vital to limit the exposure of the underlying heart and lung tissue using customized physical dose sculpting and shielding. Lung volumes exposed in modern, CT-based tangential field arrangements are minimal, but doses to lung tissue exceed tolerance no matter which fractionation scheme is employed. One prospective, randomized study of CFRT versus HypoRT used spirometry, plethysmography, and hemoglobin-corrected diffusing capacity at baseline and post treatment.[151] Investigators found that although mild lung restriction could be detected within 3 years of treatment completion, there were no differences between the two fractionation regimens. In terms of cardiac risk, the priority is to protect the heart from exposure using custom blocking or respiratory management techniques. Radiation exposure to the heart in the modern era therefore is less from direct irradiation and more from low-dose internal scatter. Because it is widely accepted that there is no "safe" heart dose, and because the most robust risk models are based on "mean heart dose,"[152] it is unclear if or how altered fractionation might confer an additional risk. In a large prospective registry of over 5,000 women treated with CFRT or HypoRT for left-sided breast cancer, there were no differences in 15-year cardiac mortality (4.2% vs. 4.8%).[153] Future studies may shed light on risks associated with changes in dose per fraction when it comes to specific cardiac substructures.

Pure HypoRT for Prostate Cancer

Similar to breast cancer, hypofractionation schedules are particularly attractive because of the sheer impact of cost and convenience benefits for the treatment of the most common cancer seen in men. Moreover, prostate cancers are slow proliferating with estimated α/β ratios of 1 to 3 Gy—even lower than those for breast cancer.[36,46] Early results for HypoRT for prostate cancer are somewhat mixed, as they differ in structure (superiority vs. noninferiority hypotheses) and inconsistencies regarding conventional doses delivered in the standard arm. As of now, there is no clear consensus to replace conventional fractionation with a new "gold standard"; however, the most recent data offers more favorable evidence for the present use and future growth of HypoRT as a very valid option for many prostate cancer patients. A summary of the largest, most modern randomized trials of HFRT in prostate cancer is shown in Table 13.7.

TABLE 13.7 RECENTLY PUBLISHED PROSPECTIVE, RANDOMIZED TRIALS OF PROSTATE HYPOFRACTIONATED RADIOTHERAPY

Study	Enrollment	Number of Patients	CFRT Arm	HypoRT Arm	Follow-up Time (y)	Tumor Control	Toxicity
Fox Chase Cancer Center[154]	Low–high risk	303	76 Gy/38 Fx	70.2 Gy/26 Fx	5y	No significant differences, HypoRT not superior	No significant differences. Late GU toxicity higher for men with preexisting urinary symptoms
MDACC[155]	Intermediate risk	203	75.6 Gy/42 Fx	72 Gy/30 Fx	6y	No significant differences, HypoRT not superior	No significant differences. Suggestion of higher late GI toxicity for HypoRT
HYPRO[156,157]	Intermediate–high risk	820	78 Gy/39 Fx	64.6 Gy/19 Fx	5y	No significant differences, HypoRT not superior	Cumulative ≥ grade 3 late GU toxicity for HypoRT
NRG 0415[158]	Low risk	1092	73.8 Gy/41 Fx	70 Gy/28 Fx	5.5y	No significant differences, HypoRT not inferior	Increased late grade 2–3 GI and GU toxicity for HypoRT
CHHiP[159]	Low–intermediate risk	3216	74 Gy/37 Fx	60 Gy/20 Fx or 57 Gy/19 Fx	5y	60 Gy/20 Fx HypoRT not inferior	No significant differences. Suggestion of higher acute toxicity for HypoRT and higher late toxicity for standard RT
PROFIT[160]	Intermediate risk	1206	78 Gy/39 Fx	60 Gy/20 Fx	6y	No significant differences, HypoRT not inferior	No significant differences in ≥ grade 3 late GI or GU toxicity

Early trials of HypoRT for prostate cancer were conducted before dose escalation benefits were fully understood. For instance in 2005, a Canadian study of 936 low-risk patients could not exclude the possibility that HFRT might be inferior to the standard regimen.[161] However, the two arms (66 Gy in 33 fractions versus 52.5 Gy in 20 fractions) were both less biologically effective than what we consider standard today. Recently there have emerged smaller, randomized studies from two highly regarded US cancer centers that employed more modern radiotherapy doses and techniques. The Fox Chase Cancer Center tested 76 Gy in 38 fractions versus 70.2 Gy in 26 fractions in 303 patients, whereas investigators at the MD Anderson Cancer Center tested 75.6 Gy in 42 fractions versus 72 Gy in 30 fractions. Both centers employed IMRT, and both found the efficacy and toxicity of HFRT schedules to be comparable to conventional treatment.[154,155]

In the last few years, there has been a rising tide of data from larger, cooperative group organizations from all over the world. The first of these reports came from the European HYPRO study involving 820 intermediate- to high-risk patients.[156,157] This randomized phase 3 trial treated patients to 78 Gy in 39 fractions or 64.6 Gy in 19 fractions (every other day) and hypothesized that HypoRT would increase 5-year relapse-free survival by 10% over CFRT (80% vs. 70%). After a median follow-up of 5 years, the actual RFS for patients treated with HypoRT versus CFRT was 80.5% versus 77.1% ($P = .36$). What was statistically significant, however, was grade 3 late GU toxicity in the HypoRT arm ($P = .021$).

In contrast to the HYPRO study, three larger cooperative group endeavors were structured as noninferiority trials. The NRG Oncology group in the United States randomized 1,092 low-risk patients to 73.8 Gy in 41 fractions versus 70 Gy in 28 fractions.[158] This study found that the hazard ratio for DFS was 0.85 (95% CI, 0.64 to 1.14), consistent with its predefined noninferiority benchmark of <1.52 ($P < .001$). Late grade 2 to 3 GI and GU toxicities were higher for patients treated with HypoRT in this study, which employed both 3D conformal radiation therapy and IMRT techniques. The Conventional or Hypofractionated High-Dose Intensity-Modulated Radiotherapy in Prostate Cancer (CHHiP) trial in the United Kingdom randomized 3,216 patients to receive either CFRT (74 Gy in 37 fractions) or HFRT in one of two regimens (57 Gy or 60 Gy in 3 Gy/fraction).[159] This study featured a more heterogeneous enrollment, with 12% of patients having high-risk disease. At a median follow-up of over 5 years, failure-free rates were 88.3% for CFRT, 85.9% for 57 Gy HypoRT, and 90.6% for 60 Gy HypoRT. The 60-Gy experimental arm was judged to be noninferior to CFRT; however, noninferiority could not be established for the 57-Gy schedule. Patterns of toxicity were different with higher acute symptoms seen in HypoRT and higher late reactions noted after CFRT, but these differences were not statistically significant. Finally, the international PROFIT trial compared 78 Gy in 39 fractions to 60 Gy in 30 fractions for 1,206 patients with intermediate-risk disease.[160] This noninferiority study allowed either 3D conformal radiation therapy or IMRT but mandated strict, centrally reviewed radiation quality control. At 5 years, the study found no difference in biochemical failure or grade 3 or higher late GI or GU toxicity.

These studies have contributed greatly to our understanding of the efficacy of altered fractionation in the treatment of prostate cancer and provided cautionary tales along the way. Although the optimal fractionation regimen has yet to be revealed, enough evidence exists for clinicians to discuss HypoRT as an alternative to standard fractionation with a wide variety of patients. As with breast cancer, the cost and convenience drivers for patients must be accompanied by an even greater attention to quality of radiation dosimetry and technique on the part of the treating physician who offers HypoRT.

The Combination of Altered Fractionation with Concurrent Chemotherapy

In a meta-analysis conducted at the Institut Gustave Roussy (Villejuif, France), an absolute benefit of 3% (from 36% to 39%; HR, 0.92; 95% CI, 0.87 to 0.97; $P = .004$) was observed at 5 years in favor of the altered fractionation regimens.[162] In light of the data in support of the superiority of altered fractionation to standard radiotherapy alone and findings of improved local control and survival with the addition of concurrent chemotherapy to radiotherapy in several randomized studies[163–165] and two recent meta-analyses,[166,167] at least 11 studies reported on investigation of addition of chemotherapy to altered fractionation (Table 13.8). These studies did not explore chemotherapy results with varying fractionation regimens, except for one study,[146,174] which tested the addition of chemotherapy to radiation in patients with unresectable squamous cell HNSCC by adding chemotherapy to either standard fractionation or a complicated prolonged split-course regimen.

Key Findings of Combined Altered Fractionation with Concurrent Chemotherapy

Although the magnitude of its effect was less marked for survival indices than for locoregional control, the addition of chemotherapy to altered fractionation regimens results in a clear improvement compared with hyperfractionated or accelerated regimens alone; however, the effect on late toxicity of normal tissues is not fully known.

In nasopharynx cancer, the benefit of concurrent chemotherapy is similar to that of acceleration without chemotherapy. The potential biologic interactions between chemotherapy and radiotherapy by the addition of radiation can be summarized as follows[147]:

1. Shift of cell survival curves toward higher cell-killing levels and lower cell-surviving fractions for a given dose of irradiation
2. Cooperation to prevent the emergence of resistant clones
3. A decrease in tumor mass and reoxygenation
4. Specific toxicity for hypoxic cells
5. Selective toxicity depending on cell cycle phase
6. Cytokinetic cooperation
7. Inhibition of DNA repair
8. Increased apoptosis

Table 13.8 summarizes the results of randomized studies investigating the efficacy of concurrent chemotherapy regimens with altered fractionation.

Acceleration Versus Chemoradiation or with Chemotherapy

An Austrian three-arm trial tested the addition of mitomycin C (MMC) on day 5 of treatment to the Vienna variation of continuous, hyperfractionated, accelerated radiotherapy (V-CHART): 55.3 Gy in 17 days. The three arms were 70 Gy of conventional fractionation alone versus V-CHART and versus V-CHART with concurrent MMC on day 5 (V-CHART plus MMC).[148] Two hundred thirty-nine patients were randomized. Locoregional tumor control was 31% after conventional fractionation, 32% after V-CHART, and 48% after V-CHART plus MMC, respectively ($P < .05$). Overall, crude survival was 24% after conventional fractionation, 31% after V-CHART, and 41% after V-CHART plus MMC, respectively ($P < .05$). Therefore, reducing the treatment time from 7 weeks to 17 consecutive days and dose of radiotherapy from 70 to 55.3 Gy produced identical results, whereas the addition of MMC on day 5 to the accelerated fractionated treatment produced a significant improvement in local tumor control and survival. This supports an argument for adding chemotherapy to AF.

TABLE 13.8 PHASE III TRIALS ADDRESSING CONCURRENT CHEMOTHERAPY AND ALTERED FRACTIONATION IN PATIENTS WITH HEAD AND NECK CANCER

Reference	Tumor Site and Stage	Number of Patients	Therapy Regimen	Tumor Response	Complications
Accelerated Fractionation Plus Chemotherapy					
Dobrowsky and Naude[168]	Various sites T1–T4, N0–N3	239	V-CHART: 55.3 Gy/17 d (2.5 Gy on d 1, then 1.65 Gy, b.i.d., on d 2–17) V-CHART + MMC: 20 mg/m² on d 5 CF: 70 Gy/7 wk	V-CHART + MMC yielded higher LRC ($P < .05$) and survival ($P \leq .03$) than V-CHART and CF	V-CHART induced more mucositis than CF but not intensified by MMC Late toxicity not reported
Staar et al.[169]	Stage III–IV unresectable oropharynx and hypopharynx	240	69.9 Gy/5.5 wk + carboplatin (70 mg/m²/d) and 5-FU (600 mg/m²/d) for 5 d ×2 69.9 Gy/5.5 wk (1.8 Gy every day for 3.5 wk, then b.i.d., 1.8 Gy + 1.5 Gy, for 2 wk)	2-y OS: 48% vs. 39% ($P = .11$) 2-y LRC 51% vs. 45% ($P = .14$) Patients receiving G-CSF had worse LRC ($P = .007$)	Grade 3–4 mucositis: 68% vs. 52% ($P = .01$) Grade 3–4 vomiting: 8.2% vs. 1.6% ($P = .02$) Late swallowing problems and feeding tube dependency: 51% vs. 25% ($P = .02$)
Bourhis et al.[110]	Various sites Advanced inoperable	109	62–64 Gy/5 wk + Cis (100 mg/m² on d 1, 16, 32) and 5-FU (1 g/m²/d on d 1–5, 31–35) 62–64 Gy/3 wk	Not reported yet	Early cessation because of higher treatment-related deaths in the combined arm
Wang et al.[107]	Nasopharynx cancer	416	74–76 Gy in 6 wk (6 fractions/wk) + Cis/5-FU 74–76 Gy in 6 wk (6 fractions/wk) 70–76 Gy in 7 wk	LRC 13.6% vs. 16.7% vs. 27.3% ($P < .05$), 5-y OS 57.6% vs. 53.6% vs. 43.8% ($P < .05$); acceleration had a similar improvement as concurrent chemotherapy.	Acute reactions higher with acceleration
Alternating Chemoradiation Versus Partly Accelerated Radiotherapy in Locally Advanced Squamous Cell Carcinoma of the Head and Neck					
Corvo et al.[170]	Unfavorable stage II or stage III–IV	136	1 wk Cis (20 mg/m²/d + 5-FU 200 mg/m²)/d for 5 d alternated with three 2-wk courses of 20 Gy 2 Gy/d, 5 d/wk (60 Gy) vs. 75 Gy/40 CB in 6 wk	3-y OS: 37% vs. 29%; 3-y PFS: 35% vs. 27% 3-y LRC: 32% vs. 27%	Acute skin and late mucosal and skin toxicities significantly less with chemoradiation, but radiotherapy dose was 15 Gy or less
Split-Course Accelerated Fractionation Plus Chemotherapy					
Denham et al.[4]	Various sites T2–T4, N0–N3	122	RT: 70 Gy/47 d in 1.25 Gy b.i.d. (7–10/d break after 40 Gy) + Cis and 5-FU wk 1 and 6 RT alone: 75 Gy/42 d in 1.25 Gy, b.i.d.	3-y LRC: 70% vs. 44% ($P = .01$) 3-y RFS: 61% vs. 41% ($P = .07$) 3-y OS: 55% vs. 34% ($P = .07$)	Similar mucositis; increased internal feeding and sepsis Similar late complications
Byhardt et al.[32]	Various sites, stage III–IV	270	70.2 Gy/51 d plus Cis, 5-FU, and leucovorin 70.2 Gy/51 d (23.4 Gy in 1.8-Gy fractions, b.i.d., for 3 cycles with 10-d break)	3-y LRC: 36% vs. 17%, ($P < .004$) 3-y OS: 48% vs. 24% ($P < .0003$)	Grade 3–4 acute mucositis: 38% vs. 16% ($P < .001$) Serious late side effects: 10% vs. 6.4% (NS)
Chemoradiation with Split-Course Prolonged Radiotherapy					
Adelstein et al.[171]	Stage III or IV unresectable disease	295	30 Gy at 2 Gy/d with concurrent 5-FU and Cis wk 1–3, 5-wk break with chemotherapy followed by 30–40 Gy/wk 8–11 vs. 70 Gy at 2 Gy/d plus Cis on d 1, 22, and 43 vs. (3) 70 Gy at 2 Gy/d alone	3-y projected OS: 27% vs. 37% vs. 23%. Median survival: 13.8 vs. 19.1 vs. 12.6 mo; no difference between arms 1 and 3 3-y DSS 41% vs. 51% vs. 33%; arm 2 was better ($P = .01$)	Grade 3 or worse toxicity: 77% vs. 89% vs. 52% ($P < .001$)
Hyperfractionation Plus Chemotherapy					
Denham et al.[172]	Various sites, stage III–IV	130	77 Gy/7 wk + Cis (6 mg/m²/d) 77 Gy/7 wk (1.1 Gy, b.i.d.)	5-y LRPFS: 50% vs. 36% ($P = .04$) 5-y PFS: 46% vs. 25% ($P = .007$) 5-y DMFS: 86% vs. 57% ($P = .001$) 5-y OS: 46% vs. 25% ($P = .008$)	No significant difference in acute morbidity (except for leucopenia, $P = .006$) or late toxicity
Hugeunin et al.[173]	Squamous cell carcinomas of the head and neck	224	74.4 Gy; 1.2 Gy b.i.d. + Cis 20 mg/m² (on 5 d wk 1 and 5) 74.4 Gy; 1.2 Gy b.i.d.	Failure-free rate at 2.5 y was 45% and 33%; LRC was significantly improved, log-rank test ($P < .039$).	Late toxicity was comparable.
Hyperfractionated Accelerated Chemoradiation with Concurrent Chemotherapy Versus Dose-Escalated Hyperfractionated Accelerated Radiation Therapy Alone in Locally Advanced Head and Neck Cancer					
Budach et al.[121]	Various sites, stage III–IV	384	70.6 Gy in 6 wk (30 Gy, 2 Gy/d + 40.6 at 1.4 Gy b.i.d.) + 5-FU (600 mg/m²) + mitomycin (10 mg/m²) 77.6 Gy (14 Gy at 2 Gy/d + 1.4 Gy b.i.d.): dose-escalated radiotherapy	5-y LRC 49.9% vs. 37.4% ($P = .001$) 5-y OS: 28.6% vs. 23.7% ($P = .023$)	Maximum acute mucositis, moist desquamation, and erythema were higher in dose-escalated radiotherapy; no differences in late reactions.

5-FU, 5-flourouracil; b.i.d., twice-a-day irradiation; CB, concomitant boost; CF, conventional fractionation; Cis, cisplatin; DMFS, distant metastasis–free survival; DSS, disease-specific survival; G-CSF, granulocyte colony–stimulating factor; LC, local control; LRC, locoregional control; LRPFS, locoregional progression-free survival; MMC, mitomycin C; NS, not significant; OS, overall survival; PFS, progression-free survival; RFS, relapse-free survival; V-CHART, Vienna variation of continuous hyperfractionated accelerated radiotherapy.

A German Cooperative Group compared a concomitant boost radiation regimen with or without carboplatin and 5-fluorouracil.[149] The addition of chemotherapy produced a trend for better locoregional control and survival rates, but it induced a significantly higher incidence of chronic dysphagia, resulting in feeding tube dependence (51% vs. 25%). A secondary randomization to receive or not receive granulocyte colony–stimulating factor to reduce mucositis produced the startling finding that *the administration of granulocyte colony–stimulating factor significantly reduced the probability of locoregional control in both treatment arms.*

The French Cooperative Group GORTEC tested the combination of 62 to 64 Gy given in 5 weeks with cisplatin and 5-fluorouracil but terminated the trial prematurely because of unacceptable toxicity.[89] The nasopharynx trial from China gave a very interesting finding that accelerated radiotherapy provides the same benefit as adding concurrent chemotherapy; this was discussed earlier in the section on accelerated radiotherapy.[56]

Alternating chemoradiotherapy was studied in Italy by Corvo et al.[170] and compared with high-dose accelerated radiotherapy. The 136 patients with unfavorable stage II or stage III to IV head and neck carcinoma were randomized to alternating cisplatin and 5-fluorouracil with three 2-week courses of radiotherapy (20 Gy at 2 Gy/day: 60 Gy vs. 75 Gy at 40 fractions in 6 weeks) using a concomitant boost technique. At 60 months, there were no differences in overall survival, progression-free survival, or locoregional control.

Split-course altered fractionation with or without concurrent chemotherapy was tested in two trials. Both added cisplatin and 5-fluorouracil to split-course AF schedules (70 Gy in 42 to 51 days).[143,151] Both showed that a chemotherapy regimen improved locoregional control versus altered fractionation alone. However, a split-course accelerated regimen is now known to be no more effective than standard fractionation. The locoregional control improved, with an 18% to 26% increase in late effects. The larger trial showed improved overall survival.

Adelstein et al.[171] reported on the Head and Neck Intergroup's trial to test the addition of chemotherapy to radiation in patients with unresectable squamous cell HNSCC by adding chemotherapy to either standard fractionation or a prolonged split-course regimen. The 295 patients were randomized into three arms: 70 Gy at 2 Gy/day (radiation [RT] only) versus the same radiation therapy with concurrent bolus cisplatin (RT + chemotherapy [C]) versus a third arm: split-course radiotherapy with chemotherapy during the break in radiotherapy (split RT + C) from week 9. They did not meet the accrual goal. Grade 3 or worse toxicity occurred in 52% of patients in the RT-only arm, 89% in the RT + C arm ($P < .0001$), and 77% in the split RT + C arm ($P < .001$). The 3-year projected overall survival for patients in the RT-only arm was 23%, compared with 37% for the RT + C arm ($P = .014$) and 27% for the split RT + C arm ($P = $ not significant). The addition of concurrent high-dose, single-agent cisplatin to conventional radiation significantly improves survival and increases toxicity; however, multiagent chemotherapy did not offset the loss of efficacy resulting from prolongation by split-course radiation.

Concurrent Chemotherapy in Addition to Hyperfractionated Radiotherapy

A randomized trial by Jeremic et al.[175] tested the addition of low-dose daily cisplatin to 77 Gy at 1.1 Gy/fraction twice daily over 7 weeks. Daily cisplatin improved the results of HF radiation, with better locoregional progression-free survival (50% vs. 36%; $P = .04$), 5-year progression-free survival (46% vs. 25%; $P = .007$), 5-year distant metastases–free survival (86% vs. 57%; $P = .001$), and 5-year overall survival (46% vs. 25%; $P = .008$). This was a true therapeutic gain because there was no difference in late side effects.

A study conducted in Zurich reported similar results.[173] The 224 patients with squamous cell carcinomas were randomized to two cycles of concurrent cisplatin 20 mg/m² on 5 days of weeks 1 and 5 with HF radiotherapy (median dose, 74.4 Gy; 1.2 Gy twice daily) versus the same radiotherapy. Locoregional control and distant disease–free survival were significantly improved with cisplatin (log-rank test; $P = .039$ and .011, respectively) with no difference in overall survival and similar late toxicity. The therapeutic index of HyperRT was improved by concomitant cisplatin.

A third trial, reported by the German Cancer Society with an even greater number of patients, confirmed this outcome, using a nonplatinum regimen with HyperRT-accelerated radiation versus dose-escalated HyperRT-accelerated radiation.[176] The 84 patients with stage III (6%) and IV (94%) oropharyngeal (59.4%), hypopharyngeal (32.3%), and oral cavity (8.3%) cancer were randomized to concurrent chemotherapy and accelerated radiation therapy to 70.6 Gy in 6 weeks versus accelerated radiation therapy alone to 77.6 Gy. Chemotherapy was 5-fluoroucil (600 mg/m², 120-hour continuous infusion) days 1 through 5 and mitomycin (10 mg/m²) on days 5 and 36. At 5 years, the locoregional control was 49.9% versus 37.4% ($P = .001$), and overall survival was 28.6% versus and 23.7% ($P = .023$), respectively. Progression-free and metastases-free rates were 29.3% and 51.9% versus 26.6% and 54.7%, respectively ($P = .009$ and .575, respectively). There were no differences in late reactions. They concluded that concurrent chemotherapy with accelerated HyperRT to 70.6 Gy is superior to dose-escalated HyperRT to 77.6 Gy, with less acute reactions and equivalent late reactions, indicating an improvement of the therapeutic ratio.[176]

Results of Radiation Therapy Oncology Group Trial of Concurrent Chemotherapy to Select Fractionation Schedules

The RTOG conducted a randomized trial to determine whether accelerated fractionation improves the outcome of concurrent cisplatin chemotherapy (i.e., whether the benefit of altered fractionation remains true in the setting of concurrent chemotherapy).[177] Acceleration of radiotherapy did not improve outcome in the setting of concurrent cisplatin chemotherapy. Seven hundred forty-three patients with stage III or IV squamous cell carcinoma of the oral cavity, oropharynx, hypopharynx, or larynx were randomized into two arms: *standard radiation* (70 Gy in 35 fractions once daily over 7 weeks [SFX]) with three cycles of concurrent cisplatin (100 mg/m² given every 3 weeks during radiotherapy) versus accelerated *fractionation with concomitant boost* 72 Gy in 42 fractions in 6.5 weeks (AFX-C) with *two cycles* of the same chemotherapy. Seven hundred twenty-one cases were analyzable (360 for AFX-C; 361 for SFX). Two arms were balanced by site, stage, performance status, and age. At analysis, 418 patients were alive with median follow-up of 4.8 (0.3 to 6.5) years. First analysis of this trial showed that, when combined with concurrent cisplatin, AFX-C did not improve outcome or increase late toxicity. No differences were observed in OS (5 years: 59% vs. 56%; HR, 0.90; CI = 0.72 to 1.13; $P = .18$), disease-free survival (45% vs. 44%; $p = .42$), locoregional failure (31% vs. 28%; $P = .76$), or metastasis (18% vs. 22%; $P = .06$). There were also no differences in the overall grade 3 to 4 acute mucositis (33% vs. 40%) and worst grade 3 to 4 late toxicity (26% vs. 21%). Feeding tube rates were 22% and 25% pretreatment, 67% and 69% at therapy end, and 28 and 29% at 1 year, respectively, but declined later to 5% to 15%. When analyzed for the effect of radiotherapy duration and cisplatin dose, they both affected survival significantly. Cisplatin improved OS more by reducing locoregional progression, but it also increased toxicity. The effect of AFX-C approximated the third cisplatin dose, suggesting that cisplatin acted, in part, by inhibiting clonogen repopulation.

This finding suggests that for patients undergoing standard fractionation and who are unable to have their full planned concurrent chemotherapy, acceleration of the remaining course of radiotherapy may be of benefit. This may be achieved by treating two fractions per day on one of their treatment days each week.

As a continuous variable, each day of radiotherapy delay in RTOG 0129 was associated with compromised OS, progression-free survival, and locoregional progression by 5%, 4%, and 4% (P = .001, .006, and .02), respectively.[178]

Critical Fractionation Issues to Consider When Intensity-Modulated Radiation Treatment Is Used

There is great diversity in IMRT fractionation. A survey of international practice of IMRT fractionation showed that among 14 international centers, 12 different dose fractionations were practiced: conventional daily 2 Gy/fraction was used in 3 of 14 centers with concurrent chemotherapy, whereas 11 of 14 centers used altered fractionation, including a 6-fractions/week Danish Head and Neck Cancer Group regimen in 3 centers, $\leq$2.2 Gy/fraction in 3 centers, dose-escalated hypofractionation ($\geq$2.3 Gy/fraction) in 4 centers, hyperfractionation in 1 center, continuous acceleration in 1 center, and concomitant boost in 1 center. Reasons for fractionation practice included (a) dose escalation, (b) total irradiated volume, (c) number of target volumes, (d) synchronous systemic treatment, (e) shorter overall treatment time, (f) resources availability, (g) longer time on treatment couch, (h) variable gross tumor volume margins, (i) confidence in treatment setup, (j) late tissue toxicity, and (k) use of lower neck anterior fields.[179]

The new era of high-precision radiation therapy brings two major advantages: improved coverage of tumor volumes by the prescribed dose without the use of multiple matched fields and increased sparing of normal tissues, such as parotid gland, spinal cord, brainstem, brain, and optic using IMRT. However, there are two important fractionation issues to be considered:

- If a single plan is used, all targets are treated in the same overall number of fractions. This may result in treating secondary targets to a lower dose per fraction. This has to be corrected by alteration of the total dose to the secondary targets to avoid the potentially serious disadvantage of delivering a lower biologically effective dose.
- IMRT may allow an increased dose to be delivered if the dose-limiting toxicity can be spared by organ avoidance. This may be delivered as additional fractions with prolongation of the duration of treatment or by giving more than one fraction per day. Alternatively, the dose per fraction may be increased and the total escalated dose delivered in the same or shortened treatment time.

Potential Delivery of Lower Biologically Effective Dose to Targets and Lower Probability of Cure

Classic non-IMRT techniques for HNSCC deliver doses at a fixed dose per fraction to all targets. A large initial field delivers an initial dose to the entire volume, and the field is reduced sequentially to boost additional regions to a higher dose (shrinking-field technique). For example, a classic head and neck three-field plan uses opposed lateral photon fields and abutting electron fields to deliver 50 Gy at 2 Gy/fraction to gross disease at the primary site and nodes, elective

nodal regions, and regions around the tumor that may contain microscopic tumor cells. Smaller fields are then used to deliver an additional 16 to 20 Gy in 8 to 10 fractions to boost the gross tumor and nodal disease to 66 to 70 Gy, depending on the size of the gross tumor. A posterior electron field may be added to bring the dose adjacent to the gross nodal tumor to 56 to 60 Gy. This type of fractionation is used especially with concurrent chemotherapy. This contrasts with IMRT, with which the dose prescribed to various portions of the treatment volume is delivered simultaneously. Each fraction delivers a specific constant dose per fraction throughout the treatment to each target. All targets are treated in the same number of fractions. For example, 70 Gy in 35 fractions prescribed to the gross tumor will deliver 2 Gy/fraction to this volume. The 56 and 50 Gy prescribed to secondary target volumes will also be delivered in 35 fractions in 7 weeks using IMRT at a 1.6 and 1.43 dose per fraction over 7 weeks, respectively. The biologically effective dose to 56 and 50 Gy in 35 fractions in 7 weeks is lower using IMRT because of the effect of the smaller dose per fraction and longer treatment time. This must be compensated for by increasing the total dose to the elective and intermediate dose targets, as suggested in Table 13.9.

TABLE 13.9 COMMONLY USED FRACTIONATION REGIMENS FOR HEAD AND NECK CANCER

Dose/Fractionation	GTVs (Gy)	Intermediate-Risk Target Volume (Gy)	Low-Risk Target Volume Suspicious of Microscopic Disease (Gy)
United States: IMRT[a]			
70/33 Fx; s.i.d. with chemotherapy	70 Gy	60–63	57–60
Concomitant Boost			
72 Gy/42 Fx b.i.d. for 10–12 d	72	57–63	54
66/30 Fx s.i.d. Without chemotherapy postoperative	66	60	54
60–66/30 FX s.i.d.	66	56–57	54
Canada (PMH): IMRT[a]			
70 Gy/35 Fx s.i.d.	70	63	56
60 Gy/25 Fx T2, N0 larynx small, T1–T2 oropharynx	60	56	50
64 Gy/40 Fx; b.i.d. T3, T4 with low-volume nodal disease Postoperative boost	64	56	46
66 Gy/33 Fx; s.i.d.	66	60	56
60 Gy/30 Fx; s.i.d. 51 Gy/20 Fx T1a, N0, M0 glottic cancer	60	60	54
Manchester (United Kingdom; Christie Hospital)			
50–52.5/16 Fx for small volume (5–6 cm) larynx			
55 Gy in 20 Fx for modest volumes up to 10 cm long			
Postoperative 50 Gy/20 Fx with chemotherapy			
50–52.5 Gy/20 Fx without chemotherapy			
Denmark			
70 Gy/35 Fx; 6 Fx/wk			

The biologically isoeffective dose for tumor control to targets in the third and fourth columns with IMRT takes into consideration the effect of reduced dose per fraction and the effect of prolonged overall treatment time. b.i.d., twice a day; Fx, fraction; Gy, gray; GTVs, gross tumor volumes; IMRT, intensity-modulated radiotherapy; N, nodal stage; PMH, Princess Margaret Hospital; s.i.d., once per day; T, tumor stage; wk, week.
[a]Single-phase treatment schedule.

Prospect for Improving the Therapeutic Ratio by Dose Escalations to Targets without Increased Dose to Normal Tissues

The experience and conclusions of altered fractionation studies are based entirely on results of traditional radiotherapy techniques and conventional conformal techniques. These techniques deliver the boost dose to a much larger volume of tissue of normal tissues, which inevitably receive the full boost dose. However, IMRT delivers much reduced doses to normal structures with potential for less toxicity. For example, IMRT produced significant reduction in incidence and severity of xerostomia with parotid-sparing head and neck.[180–182] However, a further advantage of IMRT may be its potential for dose escalation. Preclinical comparative dosimetry studies suggested that dose escalation may be feasible using simultaneous boosts to tumor subvolumes.[183] Further work is ongoing to explore whether the boost volume may be localized using metabolic or hypoxic imaging.[184]

Common Standard Clinical Practice

An analysis by the Meta-Analysis of Chemotherapy on Head and Neck Cancer Collaborative Group revealed that concurrent chemoradiation yielded a larger survival benefit than that achieved with altered fractionation regimens.[167] This benefit is seen predominantly in more locally advanced (i.e., stage IV) HNSCC, and concurrent chemoradiation is often recommended for patients with large T3 or T4 tumors or with N2–N3 nodes usually given with standard fractionation.

Because accelerated regimens seem to preferentially benefit local control at the primary site and not nodal control, it is reasonable to choose altered fractionation for patients with T2, exophytic T3, or N0–N1 disease who are not routinely given chemotherapy and those with more advanced locoregional tumor who are unfit to receive chemotherapy.[185]

In much of the United States and Europe, standard fractionation remains 2 Gy/day. However, there is considerable variation in common practice, and despite the results of randomized studies, institutions tend to adhere to dose fractionation schedules with which they are experienced. Examples of commonly used schedules in Manchester (United Kingdom), Canada, Denmark, and the United States are shown in Table 13.9.

FUTURE DIRECTIONS: COMBINING THE GAINS OF MOLECULAR IMAGING AND MOLECULAR TARGETING WITH ALTERED FRACTIONATION

Up to the present day, the choice of fractionation scheme for a particular cancer has been based largely on mathematical estimations based on tissue models and clinical experience. Our understanding of the effects of radiation on crucial cellular processes and DNA repair mechanisms is largely based on conventional fractionation. There may be significant differences in gene expression response patterns resulting from the various forms of altered fractionation. Further investigation into these differences may reveal targetable pathways to enhance tumor response to fractionated radiotherapy. Molecular profiling of tumors in preclinical studies has revealed an array of targetable molecules (such as NF-κB and STAT1), the presence of which varies with dose and fractionation.[186] Advances in the understanding of molecular biology, immunotherapy, and genomics have opened exciting

possibilities and broadened our ability to identify subgroups of tumors that will best respond to—as well as patients who will best tolerate—altered fractionation.

ACKNOWLEDGMENT

I gratefully acknowledge the work of Anesa W. Ahmad, M.D., whose previous work on this chapter served as a framework for this updated version.

REFERENCES

1. Marks LB, Yorke ED, Jackson A, et al. Use of normal tissue complication probability models in the clinic. *Int J Radiat Oncol Biol Phys* 2010;76(3 Suppl):S10–S19.
2. Thames HD, Hendry JH. *Fractionation in radiotherapy*. London, UK: Taylor & Francis, 1987.
3. Peters LJ, Ang KK, Thames HD Jr. Accelerated fractionation in the radiation treatment of head and neck cancer. A critical comparison of different strategies. *Acta Oncol* 1988;27(2):185–194.
4. Denham JW, Hauer-Jensen M, Kron T, et al. Treatment-time-dependence models of early and delayed radiation injury in rat small intestine. *Int J Radiat Oncol Biol Phys* 2000;48(3):871–887.
5. Jereczek-Fossa BA, Jassem J, Badzio A. Relationship between acute and late normal tissue injury after postoperative radiotherapy in endometrial cancer. *Int J Radiat Oncol Biol Phys* 2002;52(2):476–482.
6. Turesson I, Thames HD. Repair capacity and kinetics of human skin during fractionated radiotherapy: erythema, desquamation, and telangiectasia after 3 and 5 year's follow–up. *Radiother Oncol* 1989;15(2):169–188.
7. Tannehill SP, Mehta MP, Larson M, et al. Effect of amifostine on toxicities associated with sequential chemotherapy and radiation therapy for unresectable non–small-cell lung cancer: results of a phase II trial. *J Clin Oncol* 1997;15(8):2850–2857.
8. Jacobson G, Bhatia S, Smith BJ, et al. Randomized trial of pentoxifylline and vitamin E vs standard follow-up after breast irradiation to prevent fibrosis, evaluated by tissue compliance meter. *Int J Radiat Oncol Biol Phys* 2013;85(3):604–608.
9. Thames HD Jr, Withers HR, Peters LJ, et al. Changes in early and late radiation responses with altered dose fractionation: implications for dose–survival relationships. *Int J Radiat Oncol Biol Phys* 1982;8(2):219–226.
10. Bentzen SM, Christensen JJ, Overgaard J, et al. Some methodological problems in estimating radiobiological parameters from clinical data. Alpha/beta ratios and electron RBE for cutaneous reactions in patients treated with postmastectomy radiotherapy. *Acta Oncol* 1988;27(2):105–116.
11. Rezvani M, Alcock CJ, Fowler JF, et al. Normal tissue reactions in the British Institute of Radiology Study of 3 fractions per week versus 5 fractions per week in the treatment of carcinoma of the laryngo-pharynx by radiotherapy. *Br J Radiol* 1991;64(768):1122–1133.
12. Cox JD. Fractionation: a paradigm for clinical research in radiation oncology. *Int J Radiat Oncol Biol Phys* 1987;13(9):1271–1281.
13. Maciejewski B, Taylor JM, Withers HR. Alpha/beta value and the importance of size of dose per fraction for late complications in the supraglottic larynx. *Radiother Oncol* 1986;7(4):323–326.
14. Henk JM, James KW. Comparative trial of large and small fractions in the radiotherapy of head and neck cancer. *Clin Radiol* 1978;29(6):611–616.
15. Horiot JC, Fletcher GH, Ballantyne AJ, et al. Analysis of failures in early vocal-cord cancer. *Radiology* 1972;103(3):663–665.
16. Fletcher GH, Barkley HT Jr, Shukovsky LJ. Present status of the time factor in clinical radiotherapy. II. The nominal standard dose formula. *J Radiol Electrol Med Nucl* 1974;55(11):748–751.
17. Stell PM, Morrison MD. Radiation necrosis of the larynx. Etiology and management. *Arch Otolaryngol* 1973;98(2):111–113.
18. Taylor JM, Mendenhall WM, Lavey RS. Dose, time, and fraction size issues for late effects in head and neck cancers. *Int J Radiat Oncol Biol Phys* 1992;22(1):3–11.
19. Bentzen SM, Overgaard M. Relationship between early and late normal-tissue injury after postmastectomy radiotherapy. *Radiother Oncol* 1991;20(3):159–165.
20. Withers HR, Peters LJ, Taylor JM, et al. Local control of carcinoma of the tonsil by radiation therapy: an analysis of patterns of fractionation in nine institutions. *Int J Radiat Oncol Biol Phys* 1995;33(3):549–562.
21. Bentzen SM, Overgaard M, Thames HD. Fractionation sensitivity of a functional endpoint: impaired shoulder movement after post-mastectomy radiotherapy. *Int J Radiat Oncol Biol Phys* 1989;17(3):531–537.
22. Overgaard M. Spontaneous radiation-induced rib fractures in breast cancer patients treated with postmastectomy irradiation. A clinical radiobiological analysis of the influence of fraction size and dose–response relationships on late bone damage. *Acta Oncol* 1988;27(2):117–122.
23. Cox JD, Byhardt RW, Komaki R, et al. Reduced fractionation and the potential of hypoxic cell sensitizers in irradiation of malignant epithelial tumors. *Int J Radiat Oncol Biol Phys* 1980;6(1):37–40.
24. Van Dyk J, Mah K, Keane TJ. Radiation-induced lung damage: dose-time-fractionation considerations. *Radiother Oncol* 1989;14(1):55–69.
25. Dische S, Martin WM, Anderson P. Radiation myelopathy in patients treated for carcinoma of bronchus using a six fraction regime of radiotherapy. *Br J Radiol* 1981;54(637):29–35.

Section II

26. Powell S, Cooke J, Parsons C. Radiation-induced brachial plexus injury: follow-up of two different fractionation schedules. *Radiother Oncol* 1990;18(3):213–320.

27. Bennett MR. The treatment of stage III squamous carcinoma of the cervix in air and hyperbaric oxygen. *Br J Radiol* 1978;51:68.

28. Edsmyr F, Andersson L, Esposti PL, et al. Irradiation therapy with multiple small fractions per day in urinary bladder cancer. *Radiother Oncol* 1985;4(3):197–203.

29. Harrison D, Crennan E, Cruickshank D, et al. Hypofractionation reduces the therapeutic ratio in early glottic carcinoma. *Int J Radiat Oncol Biol Phys* 1988;15(2):365–372.

30. Rezvani M, Fowler JF, Hopewell JW et al. Present status of the time factor in clinical radiotherapy. II. Present status of the time factor in clinical radiotherapy. II. The nominal standard dose formula, Present status of the time factor in clinical radiotherapy. II. The nominal standard dose formula. Sensitivity of human squamous cell carcinoma of the larynx to fractionated radiotherapy. *Br J Radiol* 1993;66(783):245–255.

31. Maciejewski B, Withers HR, Taylor JM, et al. Dose fractionation and regeneration in radiotherapy for cancer of the oral cavity and oropharynx: tumor dose–response and repopulation. *Int J Radiat Oncol Biol Phys* 1989;16(3):831–843.

32. Byhardt RW, Greenberg M, Cox JD. Local control of squamous carcinoma of oral cavity and oropharynx with 3 vs 5 treatment fractions per week. *Int J Radiat Oncol Biol Phys* 1977;2(5–6):415–420.

33. Handa K, Edoliya TN, Pandey RP, et al. A radiotherapeutic clinical trial of twice per week vs. five times per week in oral cancer. *Strahlentherapie* 1980;156(9):626–631.

34. Watson ER, Halnan KE, Dische S, et al. Hyperbaric oxygen and radiotherapy: a Medical Research Council trial in carcinoma of the cervix. *Br J Radiol* 1978;51(611):879–887.

35. Trott KR, Maciejewski B, Preuss-Bayer G, et al. Dose–response curve and split-dose recovery in human skin cancer. *Radiother Oncol* 1984;2(2):123–129.

36. Brenner DJ, Martinez AA, Edmundson GK, et al. Direct evidence that prostate tumors show high sensitivity to fractionation (low alpha/beta ratio), similar to late-responding normal tissue. *Int J Radiat Oncol Biol Phys* 2002;52(1):6–13.

37. Brenner DJ, Hall EJ. Fractionation and protraction for radiotherapy of prostate carcinoma. *Int J Radiat Oncol Biol Phys* 1999;43(5):1095–1101.

38. Fowler J, Chappell R, Ritter M. Is alpha/beta for prostate tumors really low? *Int J Radiat Oncol Biol Phys* 2001;50(4):1021–1031.

39. King CR, Fowler JF. A simple analytic derivation suggests that prostate cancer alpha/beta ratio is low. *Int J Radiat Oncol Biol Phys* 2001;51(1):213–214.

40. Bentzen SM, Thames HD, Overgaard M. Latent-time estimation for late cutaneous and subcutaneous radiation reactions in a single-follow-up clinical study. *Radiother Oncol* 1989;15(3):267–274.

41. Thames HD, Suit HD. Tumor radioresponsiveness versus fractionation sensitivity. *Int J Radiat Oncol Biol Phys* 1986;12(4):687–691.

42. Notter G, Turesson I. Multiple small fractions per day versus conventional fractionation. Comparison of normal tissue reactions and effect on breast carcinoma. *Radiother Oncol* 1984;1(4):299–308.

43. Haustermans KM, Hofland I, Van Poppel H, et al. Cell kinetic measurements in prostate cancer. *Int J Radiat Oncol Biol Phys* 1997;37(5):1067–1070.

44. Brenner D, Armour E, Corry P, et al. Sublethal damage repair times for a late-responding tissue relevant to brachytherapy (and external-beam radiotherapy): implications for new brachytherapy protocols. *Int J Radiat Oncol Biol Phys* 1998;41(1):135–138.

45. Duchesne GM, Peters LJ. What is the alpha/beta ratio for prostate cancer? Rationale for hypofractionated high-dose-rate brachytherapy. *Int J Radiat Oncol Biol Phys* 1999;44(4):747–748.

46. Brenner DJ. Toward optimal external-beam fractionation for prostate cancer. *Int J Radiat Oncol Biol Phys* 2000;48(2):315–316.

47. Lindsay PE, Moiseenko VV, Van Dyk J, et al. The influence of brachytherapy dose heterogeneity on estimates of alpha/beta for prostate cancer. *Phys Med Biol* 2003;48(4):507–522.

48. Logue JP, Cowan RA, Hendry JH. Hypofractionation for prostate cancer. *Int J Radiat Oncol Biol Phys* 2001;49(5):1522–1523.

49. Martinez AA, Demanes J, Vargas C, et al. High-dose-rate prostate brachytherapy: an excellent accelerated–hypofractionated treatment for favorable prostate cancer. *Am J Clin Oncol* 2010;33(5):481–488.

50. Dewit L, Oussoren Y, Bartelink H, et al. The effect of cis-diamminedichloroplatinum(II) on radiation damage in mouse rectum after fractionated irradiation. *Radiother Oncol* 1989;16(2):121–128.

51. Dubray BM, Thames HD. Chronic radiation damage in the rat rectum: an analysis of the influences of fractionation, time and volume. *Radiother Oncol* 1994;33(1):41–47.

52. Gasinska A, Dubray B, Hill SA, et al. Early and late injuries in mouse rectum after fractionated x-ray and neutron irradiation. *Radiother Oncol* 1993;26(3):244–253.

53. Terry NH, Denekamp J. RBE values and repair characteristics for colo-rectal injury after caesium 137 gamma-ray and neutron irradiation. II. Fractionation up to ten doses. *Br J Radiol* 1984;57(679):617–629.

54. van der Kogel AJ, Jarrett KA, Paciotti MA, et al. Radiation tolerance of the rat rectum to fractionated x-rays and pi-mesons. *Radiother Oncol* 1988;12(3):225–232.

55. Brenner DJ. Fractionation and late rectal toxicity. *Int J Radiat Oncol Biol Phys* 2004;60(4):1013–1015.

56. Dorr W, Hendry JH. Consequential late effects in normal tissues. *Radiother Oncol* 2001;61(3):223–231.

57. Wang CJ, Leung SW, Chen HC, et al. The correlation of acute toxicity and late rectal injury in radiotherapy for cervical carcinoma: evidence suggestive of consequential late effect (CQLE). *Int J Radiat Oncol Biol Phys* 1998;40(1):85–91.

58. Ang KK, Thames HD Jr, van der Kogel AJ, et al. Is the rate of repair of radiation-induced sublethal damage in rat spinal cord dependent on the size of dose per fraction? *Int J Radiat Oncol Biol Phys* 1987;13(4):557–562.

59. Ang KK, Xu FX, Landuyt W, et al. The kinetics and capacity of repair of sublethal damage in mouse lip mucosa during fractionated irradiations. *Int J Radiat Oncol Biol Phys* 1985;11(11):1977–1983.

60. Down JD, Easton DF, Steel GG. Repair in the mouse lung during low dose–rate irradiation. *Radiother Oncol* 1986;6(1):29–42.

61. Fowler JF, Whitsed CA, Joiner MC. Repair kinetics in mouse lung: a fast component at 1.1 Gy per fraction. *Int J Radiat Biol* 1989;56(3):335–353.

62. Henkelman RM, Lam GK, Kornelsen RO, et al. Explanation of dose-rate and split-dose effects on mouse foot reactions using the same time factor. *Radiat Res* 1980;84(2):276–289.

63. Huczkowski J, Trott KR. Jejunal crypt stem-cell survival after fractionated gamma-irradiation performed at different dose rates. *Int J Radiat Biol Relat Stud Phys Chem Med* 1987;51(1):131–137.

64. Travis EL, Thames HD, Watkins TL, et al. The kinetics of repair in mouse lung after fractionated irradiation. *Int J Radiat Biol Relat Stud Phys Chem Med* 1987;52(6):903–919.

65. Vegesna V, Withers HR, Thames HD Jr, et al. Multifraction radiation response of mouse lung. *Int J Radiat Biol Relat Stud Phys Chem Med* 1985;47(4):413–422.

66. Rojas A, Joiner M, Ninis J. Rate of repair of radiation injury (kidney). *Gray Lab Annu Rep* 1986:42–43.

67. Thames HD, Withers HR, Peters LJ. Tissue repair capacity and repair kinetics deduced from multi-fractionated or continuous irradiation regimens with incomplete repair. *Br J Cancer* 1984;49(Suppl VI):263–269.

68. Ang KK, Jiang GL, Guttenberger R, et al. Impact of spinal cord repair kinetics on the practice of altered fractionation schedules. *Radiother Oncol* 1992;25(4):287–294.

69. Saunders MI, Dische S, Grosch EJ, et al. Experience with CHART. *Int J Radiat Oncol Biol Phys* 1991;21(3):871–878.

70. Guttenberger R, Thames HD, Ang KK. Is the experience with CHART compatible with experimental data? A new model of repair kinetics and computer simulations. *Radiother Oncol* 1992;25(4):280–286.

71. Cox JD, Pajak TF, Marcial VA, et al. ASTRO plenary: interfraction interval is a major determinant of late effects, with hyperfractionated radiation therapy of carcinomas of upper respiratory and digestive tracts: results from Radiation Therapy Oncology Group protocol 8313. *Int J Radiat Oncol Biol Phys* 1991;20(6):1191–1195.

72. Marcial VA, Pajak TF, Chang C, et al. Hyperfractionated photon radiation therapy in the treatment of advanced squamous cell carcinoma of the oral cavity, pharynx, larynx, and sinuses, using radiation therapy as the only planned modality: (preliminary report) by the Radiation Therapy Oncology Group (RTOG). *Int J Radiat Oncol Biol Phys* 1987;13(1):41–47.

73. Bentzen SM, Saunders MI, Dische S. Repair halftimes estimated from observations of treatment-related morbidity after CHART or conventional radiotherapy in head and neck cancer. *Radiother Oncol* 1999;53(3):219–226.

74. Horiot JC, Bontemps P, van den Bogaert W, et al. Accelerated fractionation (AF) compared to conventional fractionation (CF) improves loco-regional control in the radiotherapy of advanced head and neck cancers: results of the EORTC 22851 randomized trial. *Radiother Oncol* 1997;44(2):111–121.

75. Horiot JC, Le Fur R, N'Guyen T, et al. Hyperfractionation versus conventional fractionation in oropharyngeal carcinoma: final analysis of a randomized trial of the EORTC cooperative group of radiotherapy. *Radiother Oncol* 1992;25(4):231–241.

76. Thames HD, Peters LJ, Ang KK. Time-dose considerations for normal-tissue tolerance. *Front Radiat Ther Oncol* 1989;23:113–130.

77. Withers HR, Taylor JM, Maciejewski B. The hazard of accelerated tumor clonogen repopulation during radiotherapy. *Acta Oncol* 1988;27(2):131–146.

78. Bentzen SM, Thames HD. Clinical evidence for tumor clonogen regeneration: interpretations of the data. *Radiother Oncol* 1991;22(3):161–166.

79. Dubben HH. Local control, TCD50 and dose–time prescription habits in radiotherapy of head and neck tumours. *Radiother Oncol* 1994;32(3):197–200.

80. Thames HD, Bentzen SM. Time factor for tonsillar carcinoma. *Int J Radiat Oncol Biol Phys* 1995;33(3):755–758.

81. Eriksen JG, Buffa FM, Alsner J, et al. Molecular profiles as predictive marker for the effect of overall treatment time of radiotherapy in supraglottic larynx squamous cell carcinomas. *Radiother Oncol* 2004;72(3):275–282.

82. Strandqvist M. Studien uber die kumulative wirkung der rontgenstrahlen bei fraktionierung. *Acta Radiol* 1944;55(Suppl):1.

83. Cohen L. Clinical radiation dosage. *Br J Radiol* 1949;22(255):160–163.

84. Cohen L. Clinical radiation dosage; inter–relation of time, area and therapeutic ratio. *Br J Radiol* 1949;22(264):706–713.

85. Cohen L. Estimation of biological dosage factors in clinical radiotherapy. *Br J Cancer* 1951;5(2):180–194.

86. Fowler JF, Stern BE. Fractionation and dose-rate. II. Dose–time relationships in radiotherapy and the validity of cell survival curve models. *Br J Radiol* 1963;36:163–173.

87. Ellis F. Nominal standard dose and the ret. *Br J Radiol* 1971;44(518):101–108.

88. Palcic B, Skarsgard LD. Reduced oxygen enhancement ratio at low doses of ionizing radiation. *Radiat Res* 1984;100(2):328–339.

89. Pinto LH, Canary PC, Araujo CM, et al. Prospective randomized trial comparing hyperfractionated versus conventional radiotherapy in stages III and IV oropharyngeal carcinoma. *Int J Radiat Oncol Biol Phys* 1991;21(3):557–562.

90. Horiot JC. Controlled clinical trials of hyperfractionated and accelerated radiotherapy in otorhinolaryngologic cancers [in French]. *Bull Acad Natl Med* 1998;182(6):1247–1260.

91. Cummings B, O'Sullivan B, Keane T. 5-year results of a 4 week/twice daily radiation schedule: the Toronto Trial. *Radiother Oncol* 2000;56:S8.

92. Fu KK, Pajak TF, Trotti A, et al. A Radiation Therapy Oncology Group (RTOG) phase III randomized study to compare hyperfractionation and two variants of accelerated fractionation to standard fractionation radiotherapy for head and neck squamous cell carcinomas: first report of RTOG 9003. *Int J Radiat Oncol Biol Phys* 2000;48(1):7–16.

93. Naslund I, Nilsson B, Littbrand B. Hyperfractionated radiotherapy of bladder cancer. A ten-year follow-up of a randomized clinical trial. *Acta Oncol* 1994;33(4):397–402.

94. Sause W, Kolesar P, Taylor SI, et al. Final results of phase III trial in regionally advanced unresectable non–small cell lung cancer: Radiation Therapy Oncology Group, Eastern Cooperative Oncology Group, and Southwest Oncology Group. *Chest* 2000;117(2):358–364.

95. Curran WJ Jr, Paulus R, Langer CJ, et al. Sequential vs. concurrent chemoradiation for stage III non–small cell lung cancer: randomized phase III trial RTOG 9410. *J Natl Cancer Inst* 2011;103(19):1452–1460.

96. Mandell LR, Kadota R, Freeman C, et al. There is no role for hyperfractionated radiotherapy in the management of children with newly diagnosed diffuse intrinsic brainstem tumors: results of a Pediatric Oncology Group phase III trial comparing conventional vs. hyperfractionated radiotherapy. *Int J Radiat Oncol Biol Phys* 1999;43(5):959–964.

97. Waber DP, Silverman LB, Catania L, et al. Outcomes of a randomized trial of hyperfractionated cranial radiation therapy for treatment of high-risk acute lymphoblastic leukemia: therapeutic efficacy and neurotoxicity. *J Clin Oncol* 2004;22(13):2701–2707.

98. LeClerc JM, Billett AL, Gelber RD, et al. Treatment of childhood acute lymphoblastic leukemia: results of Dana-Farber ALL Consortium Protocol 87–01. *J Clin Oncol* 2002;20(1):237–246.

99. Donaldson SS, Meza J, Breneman JC, et al. Results from the IRS-IV randomized trial of hyperfractionated radiotherapy in children with rhabdomyosarcoma—a report from the IRSG. *Int J Radiat Oncol Biol Phys* 2001;51(3):718–728.

100. Murray KJ, Scott C, Greenberg HM, et al. A randomized phase III study of accelerated hyperfractionation versus standard in patients with unresected brain metastases: a report of the Radiation Therapy Oncology Group (RTOG) 9104. *Int J Radiat Oncol Biol Phys* 1997;39(3):571–574.

101. Le Pechoux C, Dunant A, Senan S, et al. Standard-dose versus higher-dose prophylactic cranial irradiation (PCI) in patients with limited-stage small-cell lung cancer in complete remission after chemotherapy and thoracic radiotherapy (PCI 99–01, EORTC 22003–08004, RTOG 0212, and IFCT 99–01): a randomised clinical trial. *Lancet Oncol* 2009;10(5):467–474.

102. Ball D, Bishop J, Smith J, et al. A randomised phase III study of accelerated or standard fraction radiotherapy with or without concurrent carboplatin in inoperable non–small cell lung cancer: final report of an Australian multi-centre trial. *Radiother Oncol* 1999;52(2):129–136.

103. Jackson SM, Weir LM, Hay JH, et al. A randomised trial of accelerated versus conventional radiotherapy in head and neck cancer. *Radiother Oncol* 1997;43(1):39–46.

104. Skladowski K, Maciejewski B, Golen M, et al. Randomized clinical trial on 7-day-continuous accelerated irradiation (CAIR) of head and neck cancer—report on 3-year tumour control and normal tissue toxicity. *Radiother Oncol* 2000;55(2):101–110.

105. Overgaard J, Hansen HS, Grau C. The DAHANCA 6 and 7 trial: a randomized multicenter study of 5 versus 6 fractions per week of conventional radiotherapy of squamous cell carcinoma (SCC) of the head and neck. *Radiother Oncol* 2000;56:S4.

106. Hliniak A, Gwiazdowska B, Szutkowski Z. Radiotherapy of the laryngeal cancer: the estimation of the therapeutic gain and the enhancement of toxicity by the one–week shortening of the treatment time. Results of the randomized phase III multicenter trial. *Radiother Oncol* 2000;56:S5.

107. Wang RS, Liu WQ, Li J, et al. Accelerated fractionated radiotherapy with concurrent chemotherapy in advanced nasopharyngeal carcinoma [in Chinese]. *Ai Zheng* 2003;22(9):982–984.

108. Dische S, Saunders M, Barrett A, et al. A randomised multicentre trial of CHART versus conventional radiotherapy in head and neck cancer. *Radiother Oncol* 1997;44(2):123–136.

109. Poulsen MG, Denham JW, Peters LJ, et al. A randomised trial of accelerated and conventional radiotherapy for stage III and IV squamous carcinoma of the head and neck: a Trans-Tasman Radiation Oncology Group Study. *Radiother Oncol* 2001;60(2):113–122.

110. Bourhis J, Lapeyre M, Tortochaux J, et al. Preliminary results of the GORTEC 96–01 randomized trial, comparing very accelerated radiotherapy versus concomitant radio-chemotherapy for locally inoperable HNSCC. *Int J Radiat Oncol Biol Phys* 2001;51(3, Suppl 1):39.

111. Awwad HK, Lotayef M, Shouman T, et al. Accelerated hyperfractionation (AHF) compared to conventional fractionation (CF) in the postoperative radiotherapy of locally advanced head and neck cancer: influence of proliferation. *Br J Cancer* 2002;86(4):517–523.

112. Saunders M, Dische S, Barrett A, et al. Continuous, hyperfractionated, accelerated radiotherapy (CHART) versus conventional radiotherapy in non–small cell lung cancer: mature data from the randomised multicentre trial. CHART Steering committee. *Radiother Oncol* 1999;52(2):137–148.

113. Belani CP, Wang W, Johnson DH, et al. Phase III study of the Eastern Cooperative Oncology Group (ECOG 2597): induction chemotherapy followed by either standard thoracic radiotherapy or hyperfractionated accelerated radiotherapy for patients with unresectable stage IIIA and B non–small-cell lung cancer. *J Clin Oncol* 2005;23(16):3760–3767.

114. Baumann M, Herrmann T, Koch R, et al. Final results of the randomized phase III CHARTWEL-trial (ARO 97–1) comparing hyperfractionated-accelerated versus conventionally fractionated radiotherapy in non–small cell lung cancer (NSCLC). *Radiother Oncol* 2011;100(1):76–85.

115. Ang KK, Trotti A, Brown BW, et al. Randomized trial addressing risk features and time factors of surgery plus radiotherapy in advanced head-and-neck cancer. *Int J Radiat Oncol Biol Phys* 2001;51(3):571–578.

116. Fallai C, Bolner A, Signor M, et al. Long-term results of conventional radiotherapy versus accelerated hyperfractionated radiotherapy versus concomitant radiotherapy and chemotherapy in locoregionally advanced carcinoma of the oropharynx. *Tumori* 2006;92(1):41–54.

117. Horwich A, Dearnaley D, Huddart R, et al. A randomised trial of accelerated radiotherapy for localised invasive bladder cancer. *Radiother Oncol* 2005;75(1):34–43.

118. Sanguineti G, Richetti A, Bignardi M, et al. Accelerated versus conventional fractionated postoperative radiotherapy for advanced head and neck cancer: results of a multicenter Phase III study. *Int J Radiat Oncol Biol Phys* 2005;61(3):762–771.

119. Prados MD, Wara WM, Sneed PK, et al. Phase III trial of accelerated hyperfractionation with or without difluoromethylornithine (DFMO) versus standard fractionated radiotherapy with or without DFMO for newly diagnosed patients with glioblastoma multiforme. *Int J Radiat Oncol Biol Phys* 2001;49(1):71–77.

120. Baujat B, Bourhis J, Blanchard P, et al. Hyperfractionated or accelerated radiotherapy for head and neck cancer. *Cochrane Database Syst Rev* 2010;(12):CD002026.

121. Budach W, Hehr T, Budach V, et al. A meta-analysis of hyperfractionated and accelerated radiotherapy and combined chemotherapy and radiotherapy regimens in unresected locally advanced squamous cell carcinoma of the head and neck. *BMC Cancer* 2006;6:28.

122. Sanchiz F, Milla A, Torner J, et al. Single fraction per day versus two fractions per day versus radiochemotherapy in the treatment of head and neck cancer. *Int J Radiat Oncol Biol Phys* 1990;19(6):1347–1350.

123. Bourhis J, Lapeyre M, Tortochaux J, et al. Very accelerated versus conventional radiotherapy in HNSCC: results of the GORTEC 94–02 randomized trial. *Int J Radiat Oncol Biol Phys* 2000;51(Suppl 1):39.

124. Beck-Bornholdt HP, Dubben HH, Liertz-Petersen C, et al. Hyperfractionation: where do we stand? *Radiother Oncol* 1997;43(1):1–21.

125. Willers H, Liertz-Petersen C, Dubben HH, et al. Outcome of hyperfractionated radiation therapy in randomized clinical trials. *Int J Radiat Oncol Biol Phys* 1998;40(1):257–259.

126. Overgaard J, Hansen HS, Specht L, et al. Five compared with six fractions per week of conventional radiotherapy of squamous-cell carcinoma of head and neck: DAHANCA 6 and 7 randomised controlled trial. *Lancet* 2003;362(9388):933–940.

127. Wang CC. Local control of oropharyngeal carcinoma after two accelerated hyperfractionation radiation therapy schemes. *Int J Radiat Oncol Biol Phys* 1988;14(6):1143–1146.

128. Ang KK, Berkey BA, Tu X, et al. Impact of epidermal growth factor receptor expression on survival and pattern of relapse in patients with advanced head and neck carcinoma. *Cancer Res* 2002;62(24):7350–7356.

129. Ang KK, Landuyt W, Xu FX, et al. The effect of small radiation doses per fraction on mouse lip mucosa assessed using the concept of partial tolerance. *Radiother Oncol* 1987;8(1):79–86.

130. Dragun AE, Huang B, Tucker TC, et al. Disparities in the application of adjuvant radiotherapy after breast-conserving surgery for early stage breast cancer: impact on overall survival. *Cancer* 2011;117(12):2590–2598.

131. Dragun AE, Huang B, Tucker TC, et al. Increasing mastectomy rates among all age groups for early stage breast cancer: a 10-year study of surgical choice. *Breast J* 2012;18(4):318–325.

132. Barry PN, Dragun AE. Once-weekly hypofractionated breast irradiation: fool's gold or diamond in the rough? *J Comp Eff Res* 2015;4(2):147–156.

133. Cox JD. Large-dose fractionation (hypofractionation). *Cancer* 1985;55(9 Suppl):2105–2111.

134. Peters LJ, Withers HR. Morbidity from large dose fractions in radiotherapy. *Br J Radiol* 1980;53(626):170–171.

135. Collins CD, Lloyd-Davies RW, Swan AV. Radical external beam radiotherapy for localised carcinoma of the prostate using a hypofractionation technique. *Clin Oncol* 1991;3(3):127–132.

136. Yarnold J, Bentzen SM, Coles C, et al. Hypofractionated whole-breast radiotherapy for women with early breast cancer: myths and realities. *Int J Radiat Oncol Biol Phys* 2011;79(1):1–9.

137. Owen JR, Ashton A, Bliss JM, et al. Effect of radiotherapy fraction size on tumour control in patients with early-stage breast cancer after local tumour excision: long-term results of a randomised trial. *Lancet Oncol* 2006;7(6):467–471.

138. Haviland JS, Owen JR, Dewar JA, et al. The UK Standardisation of Breast Radiotherapy (START) trials of radiotherapy hypofractionation for treatment of early breast cancer: 10-year follow-up results of two randomised controlled trials. *Lancet Oncol* 2013;14(11):1086–1094.

139. Whelan TJ, Pignol JP, Levine MN, et al. Long–term results of hypofractionated radiation therapy for breast cancer. *N Engl J Med* 2010;362(6):513–520.

140. Valle LF, Agarwal S, Bickel KE, et al. Hypofractionated whole breast radiotherapy in breast conservation for early-stage breast cancer: a systematic review and meta-analysis of randomized trials. *Breast Cancer Res Treat* 2017;162(3):409–417.

141. Smith BD, Bentzen SM, Correa CR, et al. Fractionation for whole breast irradiation: an American Society for Radiation Oncology (ASTRO) evidence-based guideline. *Int J Radiat Oncol Biol Phys* 2011;81(1):59–68.

142. Harnett A. Fewer fractions of adjuvant external beam radiotherapy for early breast cancer are safe and effective and can now be the standard of care. Why the UK's NICE accepts fewer fractions as the standard of care for adjuvant radiotherapy in early breast cancer. *Breast* 2010;19(3):159–162.

143. Ortholan C, Hannoun-Lévi JM, Ferrero JM, et al. Long-term results of adjuvant hypofractionated radiotherapy for breast cancer in elderly patients. *Int J Radiat Oncol Biol Phys* 2005;62(2):479–485.

144. Kirova YM, Campana F, Savignoni A, et al. Breast-conserving treatment in the elderly: long-term results of adjuvant hypofractionated and normofractionated radiotherapy. *Int J Radiat Oncol Biol Phys* 2009;75(1):76–81.

145. Rovea P, Fozza A, Franco P, et al. Once-weekly hypofractionated whole-breast radiotherapy after breast-conserving surgery in older patients: a potential alternative treatment schedule to daily 3-week hypofractionation. *Clin Breast Cancer* 2015;15(4):270–276.

146. Martin S, Mannino M, Rostom A, et al. Acute toxicity and 2-year adverse effects of 30 Gy in five fractions over 15 days to whole-breast after local excision of early breast cancer. *Clin Oncol* 2008;20:502–505.

147. Agrawal RK, Alhasso A, Berrett-Lee PJ, et al. First results of the randomised UK FAST Trial of radiotherapy hypofractionation for treatment of early breast cancer (CRUKE/04/015). *Radiother Oncol* 2011;100(1):93–100.

148. Dragun AE, Ajkay NJ, Riley EC, et al. First Results of a Phase 2 Trial of Once-Weekly Hypofractionated Breast Irradiation (WHBI) for Early-Stage Breast Cancer. *Int J Radiat Oncol Biol Phys* 2016;96(2):S7.

149. Brunt AM, Wheatley D, Yarnold J, et al. Acute skin toxicity associated with a 1-week schedule of whole breast radiotherapy compared with a standard 3-week regimen delivered in the UK FAST-Forward Trial. *Radiother Oncol* 2016;120(1):114–118.

150. Bekelman JE, Sylwestrzak G, Barron J, et al. Uptake and costs of hypofractionated vs conventional whole breast irradiation after breast conserving surgery in the United States, 2008–2013. *JAMA* 2014;312(23):2542–2550.

151. Verbanck S, Hanon S, Schuermans D, et al. Mild lung restriction in breast cancer patients after hypofractionated and conventional radiation therapy: a 3-year follow-up. *Int J Radiat Oncol Biol Phys* 2016;95(3):937–945.

152. Darby SC, Ewertz M, McGale P, et al. Risk of ischemic heart disease in women after radiotherapy for breast cancer. *N Engl J Med* 2013;368(11):987–998.

153. Chan EK, Woods R, Virani S, et al. Long-term mortality from cardiac causes after adjuvant hypofractionated vs. conventional radiotherapy for localized left-sided breast cancer. *Radiother Oncol* 2015;114(1):73–78.

154. Pollack A, Walker G, Horwitz EM, et al. Randomized trial of hypofractionated external-beam radiotherapy for prostate cancer. *J Clin Oncol* 2013;31(31):3860–3868.

155. Hoffman KE, Voong KR, Pugh TJ, et al. Risk of late toxicity in men receiving dose-escalated hypofractionated intensity modulated prostate radiation therapy: results from a randomized trial. *Int J Radiat Oncol Biol Phys* 2014;88(5):1074–1084.

156. Aluwini S, Pos F, Schimmel E, et al. Hypofractionated versus conventionally fractionated radiotherapy for patients with prostate cancer (HYPRO): late toxicity results from a randomised, non-inferiority, phase 3 trial. *Lancet Oncol* 2016;17(4):464–474.

157. Incrocci L, Wortel RC, Alemayehu WG, et al. Hypofractionated versus conventionally fractionated radiotherapy for patients with localised prostate cancer (HYPRO): final efficacy results from a randomised, multicentre, open-label, phase 3 trial. *Lancet Oncol* 2016;17(8):1061–1069.

158. Lee WR, Dignam JJ, Amin MB, et al. Randomized phase III noninferiority study comparing two radiotherapy fractionation schedules in patients with low-risk prostate cancer. *J Clin Oncol* 2016;34(20):2325–2332.

159. Dearnaley D, Syndikus I, Mossop H, et al. Conventional versus hypofractionated high-dose intensity-modulated radiotherapy for prostate cancer: 5-year outcomes of the randomised, non-inferiority, phase 3 CHHiP trial. *Lancet Oncol* 2016;17(8):1047–1060.

160. Catton CN, Lukka H, Gu CS, et al. Randomized trial of a hypofractionated radiation regimen for the treatment of localized prostate cancer. *J Clin Oncol* 2017:JCO2016717397.

161. Lukka H, Hayter C, Julian JA, et al. Randomized trial comparing two fractionation schedules for patients with localized prostate cancer. *J Clin Oncol* 2005;23(25):6132–6138.

162. Bourhis J, Audry H, Overgaard J, et al. Meta-analysis of conventional versus altered fractionated radiotherapy in head and neck squamous cell carcinoma (HNSCC): final analysis. *Int J Radiat Oncol Biol Phys* 2004;60(1, Suppl):S190–S191.

163. Calais G, Alfonsi M, Bardet E, et al. Randomized trial of radiation therapy versus concomitant chemotherapy and radiation therapy for advanced-stage oropharynx carcinoma. *J Natl Cancer Inst* 1999;91(24):2081–2086.

164. Merlano M, Benasso M, Corvo R, et al. Five-year update of a randomized trial of alternating radiotherapy and chemotherapy compared with radiotherapy alone in treatment of unresectable squamous cell carcinoma of the head and neck. *J Natl Cancer Inst* 1996;88(9):583–589.

165. Wendt TG, Grabenbauer GG, Rodel CM, et al. Simultaneous radiochemotherapy versus radiotherapy alone in advanced head and neck cancer: a randomized multicenter study. *J Clin Oncol* 1998;16(4):1318–1324.

166. El-Sayed S, Nelson N. Adjuvant and adjunctive chemotherapy in the management of squamous cell carcinoma of the head and neck region. A meta-analysis of prospective and randomized trials. *J Clin Oncol* 1996;14(3):838–847.

167. Pignon JP, Bourhis J, Domenge C, et al. Chemotherapy added to locoregional treatment for head and neck squamous-cell carcinoma: three meta-analyses of updated individual data. MACH-NC Collaborative Group. Meta-Analysis of Chemotherapy on Head and Neck Cancer. *Lancet* 2000;355(9208):949–955.

168. Dobrowsky W, Naude J. Continuous hyperfractionated accelerated radiotherapy with/without mitomycin C in head and neck cancers. *Radiother Oncol* 2000;57(2):119–124.

169. Staar S, Rudat V, Stuetzer H, et al. Intensified hyperfractionated accelerated radiotherapy limits the additional benefit of simultaneous chemotherapy—results of a multicentric randomized German trial in advanced head-and-neck cancer. *Int J Radiat Oncol Biol Phys* 2001;50(5):1161–1171.

170. Corvo R, Benasso M, Sanguineti GL, et al. Alternating chemoradiotherapy versus partly accelerated radiotherapy in locally advanced squamous cell carcinoma of the head and neck: results from a phase III randomized trial. *Cancer* 2001;92(11):2856–2867.

171. Adelstein DJ, Li Y, Adams GL, et al. An intergroup phase III comparison of standard radiation therapy and two schedules of concurrent chemoradiotherapy in patients with unresectable squamous cell head and neck cancer. *J Clin Oncol* 2003;21(1):92–98.

172. Denham JW, Hauer-Jensen M, Peters LJ. Is it time for a new formalism to categorize normal tissue radiation injury? *Int J Radiat Oncol Biol Phys* 2001;50(5):1105–1106.

173. Huguenin P, Beer KT, Allal A, et al. Concomitant cisplatin significantly improves locoregional control in advanced head and neck cancers treated with hyperfractionated radiotherapy. *J Clin Oncol* 2004;22(23):4665–4673.

174. Akimoto T, Muramatsu H, Takahashi M, et al. Rectal bleeding after hypofractionated radiotherapy for prostate cancer: correlation between clinical and dosimetric parameters and the incidence of grade 2 or worse rectal bleeding. *Int J Radiat Oncol Biol Phys* 2004;60(4):1033–1039.

175. Jeremic B, Shibamoto Y, Milicic B, et al. Hyperfractionated radiation therapy with or without concurrent low-dose daily cisplatin in locally advanced squamous cell carcinoma of the head and neck: a prospective randomized trial. *J Clin Oncol* 2000;18(7):1458–1464.

176. Budach V, Stuschke M, Budach W, et al. Hyperfractionated accelerated chemoradiation with concurrent fluorouracil–mitomycin is more effective than dose-escalated hyperfractionated accelerated radiation therapy alone in locally advanced head and neck cancer: final results of the radiotherapy cooperative clinical trials group of the German Cancer Society 95–06 prospective randomized trial. *J Clin Oncol* 2005;23(6):1125–1135.

177. Ang K, Pajak TF, Wheeler R, et al. A phase III trial to test accelerated versus standard fractionation in combination with concurrent cisplatin for head and neck carcinomas (RTOG 0129): report of efficacy and toxicity. *Int J Radiat Oncol Biol Phys* 2010;77(1):1–2.

178. Ang K, Zhang Q, Wheeler R, et al. A phase III trial (RTOG 0129) of two radiation–cisplatin regimens for head and neck carcinomas (HNC): impact of radiation and cisplatin intensity on outcome. *J Clin Oncol* 2010;28(15, Suppl):5507.

179. Ho KF, Fowler JF, Sykes AJ, et al. IMRT dose fractionation for head and neck cancer: variation in current approaches will make standardisation difficult. *Acta Oncol* 2009;48(3):431–439.

180. Lin A, Kim HM, Terrell JE, et al. Quality of life after parotid-sparing IMRT for head-and-neck cancer: a prospective longitudinal study. *Int J Radiat Oncol Biol Phys* 2003;57(1):61–70.

181. Munter MW, Thilmann C, Hof H, et al. Stereotactic intensity modulated radiation therapy and inverse treatment planning for tumors of the head and neck region: clinical implementation of the step and shoot approach and first clinical results. *Radiother Oncol* 2003;66(3):313–321.

182. Parliament MB, Scrimger RA, Anderson SG, et al. Preservation of oral health–related quality of life and salivary flow rates after inverse-planned intensity-modulated radiotherapy (IMRT) for head-and-neck cancer. *Int J Radiat Oncol Biol Phys* 2004;58(3):663–673.

183. Mohan R, Wu Q, Manning M, et al. Radiobiological considerations in the design of fractionation strategies for intensity-modulated radiation therapy of head and neck cancers. *Int J Radiat Oncol Biol Phys* 2000;46(3):619–630.

184. Chao KS, Bosch WR, Mutic SL, et al. A novel approach to overcome hypoxic tumor resistance: Cu-ATSM–guided intensity-modulated radiation therapy. *Int J Radiat Oncol Biol Phys* 2001;49(4):1171–1182.

185. Nguyen LN, Ang KK. Radiotherapy for cancer of the head and neck: altered fractionation regimens. *Lancet Oncol* 2002;3(11):693–701.

186. Makinde AY, Eke I, Aryankalayil MJ, et al. Exploiting gene expression kinetics in conventional radiotherapy, hyperfractionation, and hypofractionation for targeted therapy. *Semin Radiat Oncol* 2016;26(4):254–260.

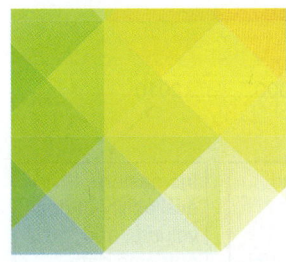

CHAPTER 14

Late Effects and QUANTEC

John P. Kirkpatrick, Michael T. Milano, Jimm Grimm, Louis S. Constine, Zeljko Vujaskovic, and Lawrence B. Marks

INTRODUCTION

Modern cancer therapy is largely predicated on the safe intensification of radiation, chemotherapy, and biologic and, now, immunologic adjuvants. This has resulted in a markedly increased survivorship, which now exceeds 64% overall, and for some malignancies, such as breast and prostate cancer, is much higher. Malignancies resistant to therapy may demand an aggressive treatment approach that often resides at the limit of, or even exceeds, normal tissue tolerance to some "acceptable" degree. Clearly, the potential to ameliorate or prevent such normal tissue damage, or to manage and rehabilitate affected patients, requires an understanding of tissue tolerance to therapy. Because "late effects" manifest months or years after cessation of treatment, therapeutic decisions intended to obviate such effects can be based only on the probability, not the certainty, that such effects will develop. In making such decisions, the balance between efficacy and potential for toxicity should be considered, as well as the influence of host, disease, and treatment-related risk factors.

Historically, radiation therapy fields and doses were selected empirically, based largely on physicians' clinical experience and judgment. They understood that these empiric guidelines were imprecise and did not completely reflect the underlying anatomy, physiology, molecular biology, and dose distributions. The introduction of three-dimensional (3D) treatment planning offered the promise of quantitative correlates of doses/volumes with clinical outcomes. This promise was partly delivered. When 3D dosimetric information became widely available, guidelines were needed to help physicians predict the relative safety of proposed treatment plans, although only limited data were available.

In 1991, investigators pooled their clinical experience, judgment, and information regarding partial organ tolerance doses and produced the "Emami paper."[1] As discussed later, this paper clearly stated the uncertainties and limitations in its recommendations, and it is rightly admired for addressing a critical clinical need. Over the past two decades, numerous studies have reported associations between dosimetric parameters and normal tissue outcomes. In 2007, a joint task force of physicists and physicians was formed, with the support of the American Society for Therapeutic Radiology and Oncology (ASTRO) and the American Association of Physicists in Medicine (AAPM), to summarize the available data in a format useful to clinicians and to update/refine the estimates provided by Emami et al.

The resulting QUANTEC reviews[2] (*qu*antitative *a*nalysis of *n*ormal *t*issue *e*ffects in the *c*linic), published in a special issue of the *International Journal of Radiation Oncology, Biology and Physics* in March 2010, are summarized in this chapter.

HISTORICAL BACKGROUND

The relationship between dose–volume parameters and outcome has been the focus of numerous investigators for decades. A brief summary of historical landmarks is

provided to follow, along with our opinion regarding the key contributions and shortcomings of these reviews (Fig. 14.1 and Table 14.1).

THE INCORPORATION OF 3D DOSE–VOLUME INFORMATION INTO CLINICAL GUIDELINES

The pre-Emami reports[3] were novel in that there were typically no good tools available (to either the authors or clinicians) to accurately quantify the fraction of various organs that were being irradiated. Thus, the dose/volume/outcome information presented consisted largely of estimates based on expert opinion. Similarly, clinicians needed to estimate the partial volumes of different organs that were being irradiated in their patients in order to apply the provided information.

In the late 1980s and early 1990s, 3D planning systems were providing clinicians with a plethora of information. However, systematic dose/volume/outcome data to guide clinical decisions based on this information were limited. There was an urgent need for clinicians to have some guidance in making clinical dose–volume decisions. The report by Emami et al.[1] met this critical need. This report was, and remains, a landmark summary of decades worth of data for a wide variety of organs, supplemented with expert opinion where data were lacking. This article remains a required reading for all trainees in our field.

During the 1990s and 2000s, a large number of studies related dose–volume data to clinical outcomes. The QUANTEC review was an attempt to refine the guidelines based on the available 3D dose/volume/outcome data.

DOSE–VOLUME HISTOGRAMS AND ASSOCIATED FIGURES OF MERIT

Three-dimensional dose–volume data can be difficult for clinicians to readily digest. Visualizing isodose distributions is challenging, and comparing competing distributions is almost impossible. Therefore, dose–volume histograms (DVHs; essentially two-dimensional [2D] representations of the 3D data) were embraced as a rapid way to summarize the dose distribution. Note that DVHs discard information regarding the spatial character of dose as well as (usually) variations in fraction size. However, DVHs can also be challenging for clinicians to consider and compare. Therefore, it has become attractive to extract "figures of merit" from the DVH, such as the V_x (the percent of an organ receiving $\geq x$ Gy). Thus, DVHs and their associated figures of merit are necessary tools to enable clinicians to readily apply 3D information clinically. They are excellent tools but obviously have their shortcomings.

MODEL-BASED ESTIMATES OF OUTCOMES

The Emami et al. report systematically used the same DVH-based construct across many organs, for example, the $TD_{5/5}$ and $TD_{50/5}$ for the uniform irradiation of one-third, two-thirds,

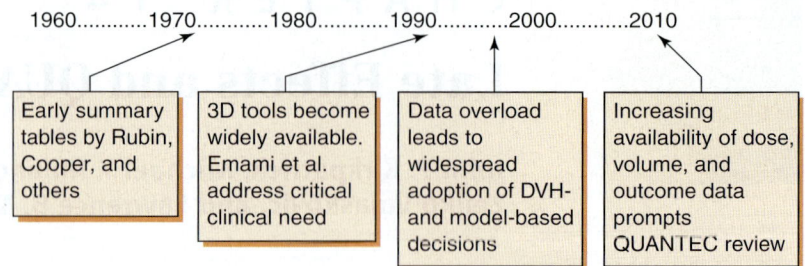

FIGURE 14.1. Key events in the development of dose–volume and normal tissue toxicity relationships in radiation oncology.

and the whole volume of an organ. This uniform approach enabled the application of "single unifying models" of dose/volume/outcome across organs. For example, the dose/volume/outcome estimates from Emami et al. were used by Burman et al.,[4] Kutcher et al.,[5] and Lyman et al.[6] to generate a set of organ-specific model parameters. Such a uniform approach is attractive to modelers and busy clinicians.

During the last two decades, many clinical dose/volume/outcome reports computed parameters for these "unifying models" (e.g., Ten Haken et al.).[7–9] Other investigators have suggested alternative models that appeared to be better suited to specific organs (*vide infra*).

The dose/volume/outcome data available for the QUANTEC review were not of a uniform format. Outcomes across organs were correlated with a diverse array of dose–volume metrics (e.g., threshold volumes [V_x], threshold doses [D_x], mean doses). Therefore, the QUANTEC review included model-based parameters for just a few organs, and not always in a systematic fashion.

MAJOR DIFFERENCES BETWEEN THE QUANTEC AND EMAMI REVIEWS

Emami et al.[1] provided information for 26 organs, judged necessary to support protocols for "three-dimensional treatment planning for high-energy photons (RFP #NCI-CM-36716-21)." Conversely, the QUANTEC review was focused on organs for which the steering committee thought that there were meaningful dose/volume/outcome data (Table 14.2).

Emami et al. addressed a wide variety of clinical outcomes and thus provided the reader with a set of dose–volume parameters for *essentially* all clinical situations. Conversely, the QUANTEC review was focused on end points where there were dose/volume/outcome data. In this regard, the Emami tables are more complete. For example, consider the QUANTEC summary for the small bowel. A volume restriction is provided for the end point of acute grade ≥3 toxicity. No guidance is provided for late small bowel injury, as the authors did not believe that there was meaningful dose/volume/outcome data for late injury. This is a shortcoming of the QUANTEC review as it is not "complete." When evaluating a proposed 3D treatment plan, one obviously must consider both acute and late injury.

Emami et al. presented information in a systematic/uniform manner, facilitating interorgan comparisons and model-based parameter estimates. The QUANTEC review presented dose/volume/outcome data in the diverse manner in which they were available in the literature.

MOLECULAR MECHANISMS OF LATE RADIATION DAMAGE

The design of optimal radiation treatment plans and identification of therapeutic strategies to prevent radiation-induced damage would benefit from an understanding of the underlying late effects from ionizing radiation. Both of these issues are further complicated by the variability in sensitivity to radiation observed across disease types and between patients, as well as the current absence of identifiable factors that predict a propensity for radiation-induced toxicity.[10–13]

An early theory for describing the development of acute and late side effects after radiation exposure was based on the target cell hypothesis. This hypothesis is focused on radiation as a direct cause of cell killing in tissues and organs, thus depleting crucial cell populations and resulting in functional deficiency. Radiation is thought to cause irreversible damage to predominantly rapidly proliferating cell populations. These damaged cells in turn lose their ability to replicate and induce a regenerative response. The latent period between radiation exposure and repopulation appears to depend on both tissue turnover time and radiation dose. Both parenchymal cell loss and vascular endothelium damage occur; vascular hyperpermeability and venous exudation follow and have been theorized to contribute to clinically devastating toxicities, such as radiation myelopathy. Although the target cell hypothesis may explain some of the mechanisms by which acute side effects occur, it does not appear to fully explain the development late side effects. Recent research has shown a complex interaction between multiple cell types, leading to persistent overexpression of reactive oxygen species (ROS), activation of signaling pathways, and production of proinflammatory and profibrotic cytokines.

Although the initial damage done to the DNA, proteins, and membrane lipids of cells by exposure to ionizing radiation is well known, the mechanisms behind the sustained changes in gene expression and signaling pathways that contribute to latent and permanent tissue injury are less clear. This section will focus on the established mechanisms of radiation-induced tissue injury and identify areas in which further efforts are needed to determine the mechanisms driving tissue injury and prognostic markers for the development of radiation injury.

TABLE 14.1 HISTORICAL OVERVIEW OF SUMMARIES OF DOSE/VOLUME/OUTCOME INFORMATION		
Report	**Key Contributions**	**Key Shortcomings**
Rubin, 1975[3]	Introduced the concept of TD$_{5/5}$ and TD$_{50/5}$	Minimal dose–volume data
Emami, 1991[1]	Concise summary addressing most clinically meaningful end points in a uniform manner	Dose–volume relationship based on limited data and, thus, much expert opinion
	Based on available data and expert opinion	
QUANTEC, 2010[2]	Driven largely by the available 3D dose/volume/outcome data.	Because dose/volume/outcome data on all meaningful clinical outcomes are *not* available, the summary is not able to guide all clinical practice.
	Systematic review addressing many challenges such as organ delineation and confounding factors such as chemotherapy	

TABLE 14.2 COMPARISON OF THE CHARACTER/CONTENT OF EMAMI ET AL. AND QUANTEC

Characteristic	Emami et al.[1]	QUANTEC[2]
Number of organs	26	16
3D data available	Minimal	More/moderate (18-y interval)
Format dose–volume limits	Uniform $TD_{5/5}$ and $TD_{50/5}$ for one-third, two-thirds, whole organ	Nonuniform
End points	Specific, complete	Specific, incomplete
Expert opinion	Dominant	Much less
Impact of chemotherapy	Not explicitly discussed	Addressed individually for each organ

Early Cellular Effects of Radiation

Exposure to ionizing radiation causes direct DNA damage through linear energy transfer as well as indirect damage by radiolytic cleavage of water, yielding hydroxyl radicals capable of abstracting hydrogen from the backbone of DNA to cause double-stranded breaks.[14,15] This damage to genomic DNA causes cell death by apoptosis or mitotic catastrophe. Although the ability of hydroxyl radicals to cause DNA damage is significant, the initial increase in hydroxyl radical and other ROS attributable to radiation exposure is negligible compared to the baseline presence of ROS in the cell.[15] Within a few hours of radiation exposure, however, the cell responds by increasing ROS production, creating a cellular environment capable of exacerbating the initial injury by causing oxidative damage to proteins and lipids.[16] This is thought to occur via ROS-mediated activation of mitochondria-dependent and mitochondria-independent metabolic enzymes, including nitric oxide synthases (NOSs) and oxidoreductase enzymes.

Sources of Reactive Oxygen Species

NADPH Oxidases

Nicotinamide adenine dinucleotide phosphate (NADPH) oxidases are a family of broadly distributed oxidoreductase enzymes. Membrane-associated NADPH oxidases are the primary source of ROS in nonphagocytic cells.[17] Under normal conditions, NADPH oxidase–derived superoxide anion is a mediator of maintenance and smooth muscle tone of the vasculature.[18] When these enzymes are induced to begin pathologic overproduction of ROS, however, they can contribute to the development of oxidative stress, resulting in cell damage and disruption of signaling pathways.[19] Nox4, a hydrogen peroxide–producing isoform, is of particular interest, as overproduction of hydrogen peroxide by Nox4 has been shown to be a necessary element of transforming growth factor-β1 (TGF-β1)–mediated cell death.[20]

Mitochondria

Under normal conditions, electrons from the electron transport chain can leak into the mitochondrial matrix and react with oxygen to form superoxide anion.[21] Following radiation, Leach et al.[22] observed that mitochondria in squamous carcinoma cells undergo a permeability transition, causing release of high levels of ROS into the cytoplasm. They further showed that inhibition of this transition not only attenuates the increase in cytoplasmic free radicals but also prevents radiation-induced activation of mitogen-activated protein (MAP) kinase, suggesting a causal link between mitochondrial ROS/reactive nitrogen species (RNS) generation and a large group of signal transduction pathways. The role of mitochondrial-generated ROS/RNS in radiation injury is further supported by the radioprotective effect of Mn porphyrin superoxide dismutase (SOD) mimetics, which accumulate preferentially within the mitochondria.[23]

Augmentation of Reactive Oxygen Species from Other Sources

Superoxide anion from any source can react with nitric oxide to form peroxynitrite (ONOO–), itself a powerful oxidizing species capable of reacting with other molecules and cellular elements to perpetuate free radical overproduction and cause oxidative damage to the cell.[24]

Free Radicals and the Tissue Response to Radiation

When the increase in ROS production exceeds the antioxidant capacity of the cell, the intracellular environment becomes strongly oxidizing. This change results in altered gene expression as a part of the response to oxidative damage to genomic DNA, modification of redox-sensitive protein activity, and membrane lipid oxidation.[25] All of these insults can affect the structure, function, and signaling capacity of the cell. Of particular importance to the radiation response is the persistent upregulation of transcription factors, including hypoxia-inducible factor-1α (HIF-1α) and nuclear factor κB (NFκB), and cytokines, including TGF-β, which contributes to the development of radiation-induced tissue injury.[16,26] These molecules all contribute to the vascular changes, inflammation, and cell death observed in response to radiation, but their roles in complex signaling pathways suggest that early changes in the activity of these molecules may also contribute to the disease process of latent injury. The role of ROS in radiation-induced tissue injury has been confirmed by the finding that SOD overexpression and the use of SOD mimetics can mitigate tissue injury following ionizing radiation exposure.[11,23,27–30]

The Role of Inflammation in the Response to Radiation

Although the manifestations of radiation injury can be divided into early and late effects, irradiated tissues show a dynamic population of different inflammatory cell types throughout the "latency" period, suggesting that, on a cellular level, radiation injury is an ongoing disease process.[31] Localization of inflammatory cells is mediated by vascular adhesion markers, and preferentially blocking intercellular adhesion molecule-1 (ICAM-1) does indeed reduce the inflammatory response to radiation in the lungs of C57BL/6 mice.[32,33] The resulting reduction in inflammation was, however, not sufficient to suppress development of latent pulmonary damage, suggesting that there are other mechanisms at work during this latent period that contribute to disease processes.[32] With the changing inflammatory cell populations come changes in cytokine activity, specifically interleukins, tumor necrosis factor-α (TNF-α), TGF-β, monocyte chemoattractant protein-1 (MCP-1), and keratinocyte chemoattractant (KC).[31,34,35] Expression of interleukin-1 (IL-1) messenger RNA (mRNA), together with a two-part upregulation of TGF-β expression, is known to coincide with the development of fibrosis in C57BL/6J mice, suggesting that the inflammatory response does indeed contribute to the development of latent tissue injury.[36] This idea is further supported by the finding that early inhibition of TGF-β reduces radiation-induced pulmonary fibrosis and improves lung function.[37–39] Further studies indicate that administration of exogenous SOD following thoracic radiation reduced the early upregulation of IL-1, TNF-α, and TGF-β and extended postradiation survival.[40] The apparent link between ROS, inflammatory signaling, and latent injury development suggests that early changes in ROS production do affect delayed tissue damage through ongoing perturbations of signaling pathways.

Radiation-Induced Vascular Changes

Exposure to ionizing radiation causes damage to endothelial cells and vascular structural elements, causing increased vascular permeability.[41] This vascular dysfunction results in edema as well as decreased perfusion, which can lead to development of hypoxic regions within the affected tissues.[42] Hypoxia exacerbates the initial injury by increasing recruitment of inflammatory cells that, in the process of undergoing the respiratory burst, produce ROS and increase tissue hypoxia by consuming the available oxygen.[43] Hypoxia also results in activation of HIFs. HIF-1α is an ROS-stabilized transcription factor that, under hypoxic conditions, forms a heterodimer with HIF-1β. This heterodimer is translocated to the nucleus where it binds the hypoxia response element (HRE), inducing transcription of genes involved in migration proliferation, apoptosis, and angiogenesis.[44] This element of the hypoxia response contributes to endothelial cell damage, increasing vascular permeability and, as a result, leakage of fibrin into the extracellular matrix.

Vascular endothelial growth factor (VEGF) is an HIF-mediated growth factor. Under hypoxic conditions, VEGF expression is increased, resulting in aberrant vascular network formation, which leads to irregular perfusion.[45] The resulting cycles of hypoperfusion and reperfusion contribute to oxidative stress, further damaging tissue.[38]

Macrophage accumulation further contributes to the self-perpetuating nature of radiation-induced tissue injury. Accumulation of macrophages is known to occur in areas of low perfusion and inadequate supply of oxygen and is observed in tissues following radiation exposure.[46,47] When activated, these cells produce HIF-1α in order to initiate angiogenesis to correct low perfusion.[47] This response on the part of macrophages increases the level of oxidative stress, continuing the spread of damage through inappropriate continuation of wound healing mechanisms.

Possible Metabolic Changes

Carbonic anhydrase-9 (CA-9) is commonly used as a hypoxia marker because CA-9 transcription is dependent on HIF-1α. Because carbonic anhydrases act to catalyze the conversion of metabolically produced carbon dioxide to bicarbonate,[48] this increase in CA-9 suggests that cells may also be undergoing a metabolic shift in response to their hypoxic environments. The observed changes in mitochondrial activity would support altered metabolism in postradiation cells, but further work is necessary to determine the nature of such a change.

Implications

Exposure to ionizing radiation disrupts DNA, causing cell death, but it also causes increased production of ROS in viable cells. The oxidizing environment that results from ROS production exceeding the antioxidant capacity of the cell causes further damage by disrupting cell function and signaling pathways. This disturbance results in changes in vascular integrity, an ongoing inflammatory response, and aberrant angiogenesis. Because overproduction of ROS is self-perpetuating, these effects are amplified, increasing the area and severity of damage.

Though many of the mechanisms through which ROS production affects the development of late radiation effects remain unclear, it is likely that these early changes initiate disease processes that progress over time to cause the observed late injury.

SUMMARY BY ORGAN SYSTEM

To provide a consistent summary of the extensive information in the individual organ reviews, the following outline is utilized:

1. Clinical Significance
2. End points
3. Challenges Defining Volumes
4. Dose/Volume/Toxicity Data
5. Factors Affecting Risk
6. Mathematic/Biologic Models
7. Special Situations
8. Recommended Dose–Volume Limits
9. Future Studies
10. Toxicity Scoring Criteria

Note that the brief summaries for each review do not substitute for reading and understanding the original papers and, as necessary, the underlying literature. In addition, the dose–volume limits described in the QUANTEC reviews are intended to supplement, not supplant, clinical judgment.

CENTRAL NERVOUS SYSTEM

Brain

Clinical Significance

The acute and late effects of radiotherapy on the brain are common and represent a significant source of morbidity.[49] In particular, patients with tumor-related neurocognitive dysfunction may exhibit exacerbated deficits after radiotherapy. In addition, the radiation fields used to treat the upper aerodigestive tract (e.g., sinuses and pharynx) often include a portion of the brain.

End Points

The acute side effects of radiation therapy (RT) to the brain include nausea, vomiting, and headache; seizures, visual disturbances, and vertigo are less common.[49] These symptoms are typically transient and generally respond well to medication. The end points for assessing long-term radiation-induced complications are typically radiation necrosis or asymptomatic radiologic changes as seen on serial magnetic resonance imaging (MRI) scans.[49] Other measures have included steroid usage, preservation of performance status, and neurocognitive function.[50-52]

Challenges Defining Volumes

Contouring the entire brain is straightforward, and with appropriate immobilization, there is little intra- or interfraction motion. However, delineation of subregions (e.g., the border between the brainstem and thalamus) and functional segments (e.g., Broca area) of the brain is challenging, and the utility of defining such areas has not yet been proven.[49]

Dose/Volume/Toxicity Data

For fractionated radiotherapy to the brain, the relationship between dose and radiation necrosis for partial brain irradiation is shown in Figure 14.2 for various fractionation schemes.[53-60] Lawrence et al. compared different fractionation schemes by calculating the biologically effective dose (BED),[61] with an α/β ratio of 3 Gy.[49] For standard fractionation, a dose–response relationship appears to exist, such that an incidence of side effects of 5% and 10% occurs at a BED of 120 Gy$_3$ (range, 100 to 140) and 150 Gy$_3$ (range, 140 to 170), respectively (corresponding to 72 Gy [range 60 to 84] and 90 Gy [range, 84 to 102] in 2-Gy fractions). For twice-daily fractionation, a steep increase in toxicity is apparent when the BED exceeds 80 Gy. For daily large-fraction sizes (>2.5 Gy), the incidence and severity of toxicity are unpredictable. Lawrence et al. caution against overinterpreting this analysis given the heterogeneity of the data pool (i.e., different target volumes, end points, sample sizes, and brain regions).

In children, whole-brain radiotherapy appears associated with neurocognitive decline. With central nervous system prophylaxis for acute lymphoblastic leukemia, the addition of 24-Gy radiation to the whole brain (to a chemotherapy regimen) is associated with a median 13-point intelligence

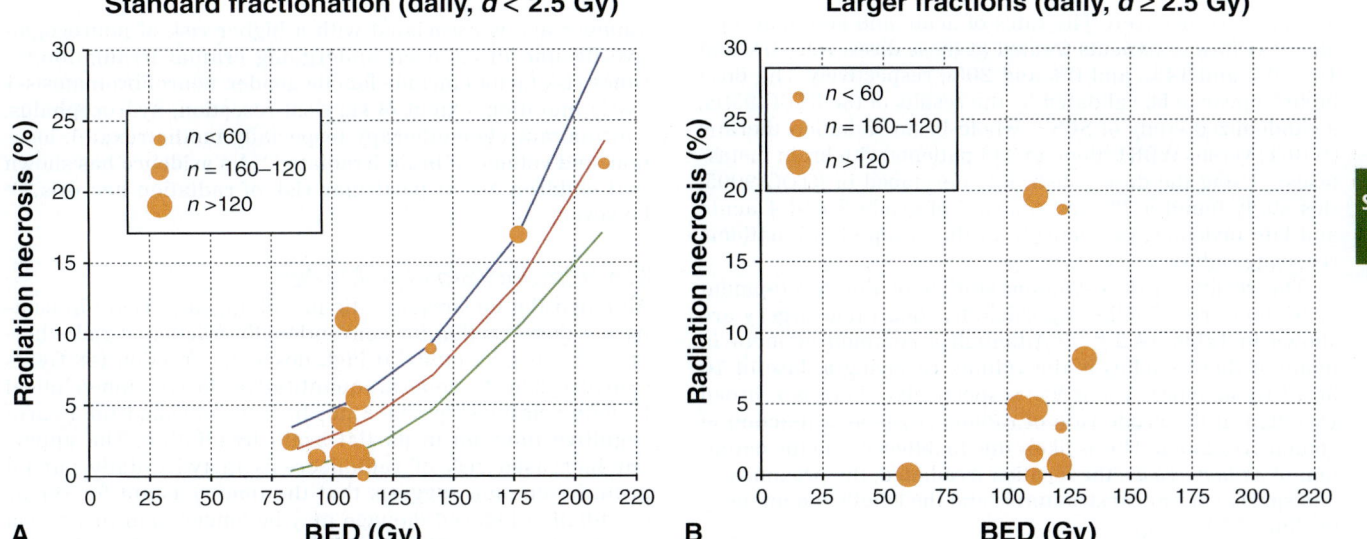

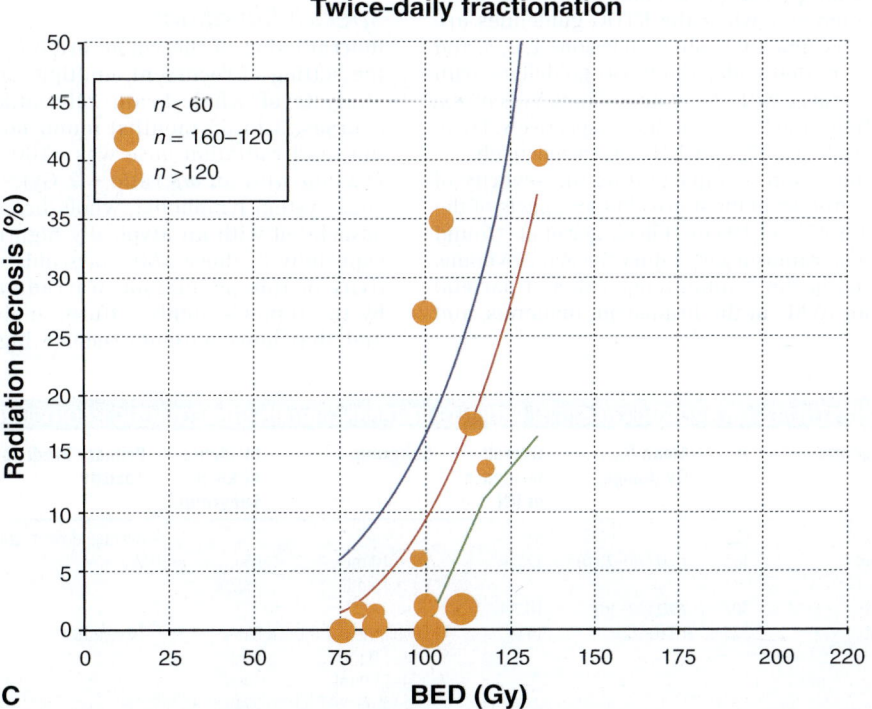

FIGURE 14.2. Incidence of radiation necrosis in brain irradiation from selected studies. Biologic effective dose (BED) calculated from the linear-quadratic model with $\alpha/\beta = 3$ Gy; n = patient numbers as shown. *Solid line* represents least-squares best fit of data to probit model; *dotted lines* represent 95% confidence limits. **A:** Once-daily fractions <2.5 Gy. **B:** Once-daily fractions ≥2.5 Gy (data too scattered to allow plotting of "best fit" line). **C:** Twice-daily radiotherapy. (Reprinted from Lawrence YR, Li XA, el Naqa I, et al. Radiation dose-volume effects in the brain. *Int J Radiat Oncol Biol Phys* 2010;76[3 Suppl]:S20–S27. Copyright © 2010 Elsevier. With permission.)

quotient reduction at 5 years after radiotherapy, as well as poorer academic performance and greater psychological distress.[62] Reported toxicities have been lower when 14 to 18 Gy was used.[63–65] In medulloblastoma, the post-RT intelligence quotients were 10 to 15 points higher for a total whole-brain dose of 23.4 versus 36 Gy.[66,67] In adults, the neurocognitive effects of whole-brain irradiation are less clear. The RTOG 0933 phase II study of hippocampal sparing (which required that 100% dose and maximum dose not exceed 10 and 17 Gy, respectively) analyzed 113 patients with brain metastases. With hippocampal sparing, memory preservation at 4 and 6 months was significantly better than that in historical controls.[68]

In stereotactic radiosurgery (SRS) of brain lesions, normal tissue toxicity appears to be a function of dose, volume, and location in the brain. The Radiation Therapy Oncology Group (RTOG) conducted a dose escalation study (RTOG 9005) of radiosurgery to recurrent brain metastases and primary tumors in patients who previously received whole or partial brain irradiation.[69] The goal of this study was to determine the maximal tolerated dose as a function of maximum diameter of the lesion. Unacceptable toxicity was defined as acute irreversible severe neurologic symptoms, requiring inpatient or outpatient medications, any life-threatening neurologic toxicity, or death. This study found a maximum tolerated prescription dose to the tumor margin of ≥24, 18, and 15 Gy for tumors with a maximal diameter of ≤2.0, 2.1 to 3.0, and 3.1 to 4.0 cm, respectively. The rates of acute and late unacceptable toxicities in patients treated at these doses were 0% and 10%, 0% and 14%, and 0% and 20%, respectively. The dose limits appear to be validated by the results of the RTOG 9508, a randomized study of SRS + whole-brain radiation therapy (WBRT) versus WBRT alone in 333 patients with brain metastases.[50] Using the dose constraints developed in RTOG 9005, this study found a 3% and 6% rate of grade 3 and 4 acute and late toxicities, respectively, in the group of 167 patients receiving radiosurgery.

The results of dose–volume studies of the development of "radionecrosis" following single-fraction radiosurgery are shown in Table 14.3.[49,70–79] Although a common element in many of these studies is the volume receiving a dose of 10 or 12 Gy or more (V_{10} or V_{12}, respectively), there is a broad variation in the crude rate of radionecrosis as a function of volume irradiated. This is likely due to difference in the definition of *radionecrosis*, the location irradiated, the proximity to and sparing of critical structures, and the length and intensity of clinical follow-up.

These results suggest that the rate of complications increases rapidly as the V_{12} increases beyond 5 to 10 cm³. Note, however, that V_{12} will far exceed these limits for lesions 2 cm or greater in mean diameter when the RTOG guidelines are utilized. For example, assume that spherical lesions 1, 2, 3, and 4 cm in diameter are treated under the RTOG guidelines with single-fraction radiosurgery with the plans yielding V_{12}'s of six, five, four, and three times the lesion volume, respectively. Then, the calculated V_{12}'s are 3, 21, 57, and 101 cm³, respectively.

The location of the lesion is important as the severity of expressed damage is greater in the more eloquent parts of the brain. For example, for a V_{12} of 10 cm³, Flickinger et al.[72] found a <5% symptomatic postradiosurgery injury for arteriovenous malformations (AVMs) in the frontal, temporal, and parietal lobes versus >20% for AVMs in the brainstem, thalamus, and basal ganglia.

Factors Affecting Risk

Younger age is associated with a higher risk of neurocognitive decline in children undergoing cranial irradiation.[80,81] Other risk factors include female gender, neurofibromatosis-1 (NF1) mutation, extent of surgical resection, hydrocephalus, concomitant chemotherapy (especially methotrexate), location, and volume of brain irradiated.[82] No evidence has shown that children are at particular risk of radiation necrosis,[83,84] however.

Mathematic/Biologic Models

Although the linear-quadratic model appears useful in comparing dose/fraction for conventionally fractionated radiotherapy schemes, its utility at high doses per fraction (≥8 Gy) is controversial. In general, quantitative dose/volume/clinical toxicity relationships have not been established for neurocognitive function in partial brain irradiation. The apparent increased risk of radionecrosis in twice-daily partial brain irradiation suggests that the time constant for repair of radiation-induced damage may be longer than the typical interfraction interval, but this has not been modeled for this specific system.

Special Situations

Reirradiation of the whole brain is frequently performed in the setting of recurrent, multiple brain metastases. A meta-analysis of whole-brain reirradiation (interval between courses, 3 to 55 months) found no cases of necrosis when the total radiation dose was <100 Gy (normalized to 2 Gy/fraction with an α/β ratio = 2 Gy).[85] In primary central nervous system lymphoma, whole-brain radiotherapy has been associated with an atypically high risk of cognitive decline, especially in those >60 years old.[86,87] The heightened sensitivity of this population to irradiation might be explained by the tumor's highly diffuse, angiocentric growth pattern and that most patients receive high-dose methotrexate, a

TABLE 14.3 SELECTED STUDIES OF RADIONECROSIS IN PATIENTS RECEIVING BRAIN STEREOTACTIC RADIOSURGERY

Reference	Diagnosis	n	Mean D_{min}, Gy (Range)	Overall Incidence of RN	Subgroup	Incidence of RN in Subgroup	Primary Predictor of Toxicity	Other Risk Factors
Lax and Karlsson[70]	AVM	823	?	5%			Average dose in 20 cm³	
Voges et al.[71]	Mixed	133	15.0 (7.0–25.0)	12.8%	V_{10} < 10 mL V_{10} > 10 mL	0% 23.7%	V_{10}	Location
Flickinger et al.[72]	AVM	307	20.9 (12–30)	10.7%			V_{12}	Location
Miyawaki et al.[73]	AVM	73	16 (0–22)	14%	Tx volume: <1 mL 1–3.9 mL 4–13.9 mL >14 mL	0% 15% 14% 27%	Tx volume	Dose, prior brain insult
Chin et al.[74]	Mixed	243	20 (10–30)	7%			V_{10}	Repeated radiosurgery, glioma
Nakamura et al.[75]	Mixed	749	18 (16–19)[a]	?	Rx volume: 0.05–0.66 mL 0.67–3 mL 3.1–8.6 mL 8.7–95.1 mL	0% 3% 7% 9%	Rx volume	
Barker et al.[76]	AVM	1,250	10.5 (4–65)	4.1%			Dose and volume combined	Age, location
Friedman et al.[77]	AVM	269	?	4.7%			V_{12}	
Varlotto et al.[78]	Brain metastases	137	16 (12–25)	11.4%	Tx volume: <2 mL >2 mL	3.7% 16%	Volume	
Korytko et al.[79]	Tumor	129	17.3 (11–25)	30%	V_{12}: 0–5 mL 5–10 mL 10–15 mL >15 mL	23% 20% 54% 57%	V_{12}	Location, previous WBRT, male

[a]Range refers to 25th to 75th quartile.

?, not specified in study; AVM, arteriovenous malformation; RN, radionecrosis; Rx, prescription; Tx, treatment; V_{10}, volume receiving 10 Gy; V_{12}, volume receiving 12 Gy; WBRT, whole-brain radiotherapy.

Adapted from Lawrence YR, Li XA, el Naqa I, et al. Radiation dose-volume effects in the brain. *Int J Radiat Oncol Biol Phys* 2010;76(3 Suppl):S20–S27. Copyright © 2010 Elsevier. With permission.

potent neurotoxin. As a result, up-front full-dose RT is now often avoided in elderly patients with this disease. A lower radiation dose of 23.4 Gy delivered in 1.8-Gy daily fractions appears to be associated with minimal cognitive toxicity, even in older patients.[88]

Recommended Dose–Volume Limit[49]

For partial brain irradiation at a conventional dose per fraction, there is a predicted 5% and 10% risk of symptomatic radiation necrosis at a BED of 120 Gy_3 (range, 100 to 140) and 150 Gy_3 (range, 140 to 170), respectively, which corresponds to 72 Gy (range 60 to 84 Gy) and 90 Gy (range 84 to 102 Gy) for 2-Gy daily fractions. This is a less conservative estimate than the 5% risk of radionecrosis for one-third of the brain irradiated to 60 Gy in the Emami paper.[1] The authors stress that for most cancers, there is no clinical indication for partial brain dose above 60 Gy and that, in some scenarios, an incidence of 1% to 5% radiation necrosis at 5 years would be unacceptably high. The brain appears especially sensitive to fraction sizes >2 Gy and, surprisingly, twice-daily irradiation.

For radiosurgery, the available data suggest that it is prudent to minimize the volume of normal brain receiving >12 Gy in a single fraction and to consider both target diameter and anatomic location when prescribing dose. However, the QUANTEC authors admit that "the substantial variation between the reported treatment parameters and outcomes from different centers has prevented [more] precise toxicity risk predictions."

Future Studies

Key questions that would benefit from systematic study include the following:

1. What is the dose/volume/location/clinical toxicity relationship for brain metastases and other common lesions treated with single-fraction SRS?
2. What is the rate of local and distant failure for the aforementioned sets of patients as a function of prescribed dose?
3. How does the gross tumor volume (GTV) to planning target volume (PTV) expansion influence the incidence of normal tissue toxicity and failure rates in single-fraction SRS?
4. How is the incidence of normal tissue toxicity affected by previous large-field irradiation to the brain, particularly the combination of WBRT and SRS in the treatment of brain metastases?
5. How do systemic treatments affect the incidence of normal tissue toxicity?
6. What is the time interval for repair of radiation-induced damage in the brain?

Toxicity Scoring Criteria

Studies of brain radiotherapy should report detailed dosimetric and outcome data, including neurocognitive and neurologic dysfunction (e.g., per the Common Terminology Criteria for Adverse Events, version 4.0 [CTCAE v. 4.088]), the prescription dose, dose/fraction, target volume, V_{12}, anatomic location treated, and clinical outcome data (e.g., adverse events, patterns of failure).

Optic Apparatus

Clinical Significance

The optic nerves and chiasm frequently receive a substantial dose during therapeutic irradiation of the brain, base of the skull, and head and neck targets, and the optic apparatus is frequently the dose-limiting structure in these cases. While rare, damage to the optic apparatus can produce devastating and, at present, irreversible visual deficits.[89]

End Points

The primary end point for radiation-induced optic neuropathy (RION) is visual impairment, defined by visual acuity and the size/extent of visual fields.[90] Of course, damage to the lens (development of cataracts), retina (retinitis), and lacrimal apparatus and trigeminal nerve (dry eye syndrome) can also produce impaired vision.[91] Although toxicity may be objectively scored using CTCAE version 4[92] and late effects of normal tissues and subjective, objective, medical management, and analytical (LENT–SOMA) evaluation of injury criteria,[93,94] it is important to obtain a comprehensive ophthalmologic examination of patients with suspected RION.

Challenges Defining Volumes

The optic nerve originates roughly at the posterior center of the globe and is bracketed by the rectus muscles as it tracks posteriorly through the orbit to pass through the optic notch, just medially to the anterior clinoid process. The optic nerves join and decussate to form the optic chiasm, an X-shaped structure that sits just superiorly to the sella turcica with the center immediately anterior to the pituitary stalk.[95] The optic nerves and chiasm are thin (<5 mm diameter), and visualization is best performed using thin-cut (≤3 mm) T1- or T2-weighted MRI. Contouring the optic nerves/chiasm is challenging, and it is important to ensure that these structures are drawn in continuity (i.e., there is no gap in the contours). Appropriate contouring of these structures is facilitated by visualizing this region in multiple planes and using fused imaging modalities (e.g., utilizing the magnetic resonance images in the axial and coronal planes to track the optic nerves/chiasm and sagittal computed tomography [CT] views to see the sella turcica).

Dose/Volume/Toxicity Data

The data for the incidence of RION with conventional fractionation for selected studies[96–103] are summarized in Figure 14.3. The risk of RION appears to rise steeply past 60 Gy. None of the patients in the study by Parsons et al.[96] with a maximum point dose (D_{max}) to the optic nerves/chiasm <59 Gy developed RION. In the study by Martel et al.,[97] the average maximum chiasm and nerve dose was 53.7 Gy (range 28 to 70 Gy) and 56.8 Gy (range 0 to 80.5 Gy) for patients without RION. The optic nerves had received a D_{max} of 64 Gy with 25% of the volume receiving >60 Gy for patients with moderate to severe complications. Jiang et al.[98] reported no incidence of ipsilateral RION for a dose <56 Gy and a <5% incidence at 10 years for a dose <60 Gy at approximately 2.5 Gy/fraction.

The risk of RION appears to be related to the fraction size. Parsons et al.[96] reported 15-year actuarial rates of RION for total doses of 60 to <70 Gy of 50% versus 11% at ≥1.9 versus <1.9 Gy dose/fraction, respectively. No patients treated twice daily with 1.2 Gy/fraction developed RION. At total doses of 70 to 83 Gy, the incidence was 33% versus 11% for ≥1.9 versus <1.9 Gy/fraction and 12% for 1.2 Gy twice-daily fractions. Bhandare et al.[104] noted reductions in RION rates for twice- versus once-daily treatment.

Results from proton treatments appear consistent with those utilizing photons.[103,105–107] Note that the proton doses are reported as cobalt gray equivalent (CGE), reflecting their greater biologic effect, and that photons were often used in combination with protons. Most proton series have reported a very low incidence of RION, and in the few cases of reported RION, a threshold dose in the range of 55 to 60 CGE has been observed, consistent with the photon experience. As with photons, many patients exceeding this threshold did not develop RION. Wenkel et al.,[107] Noel et al.,[105] Weber et al.,[103] and Nishimura et al.[106] used a D_{max} constraint to the optic structures of 54, 55, 56, and 60 CGE, respectively.

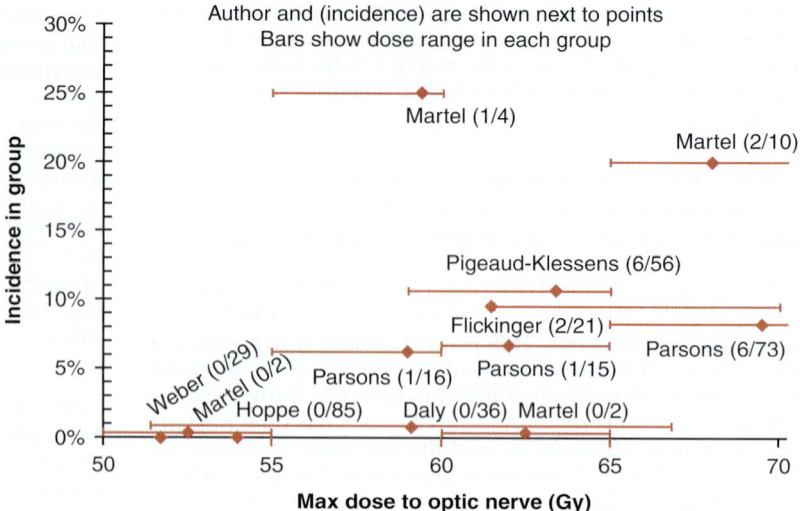

FIGURE 14.3. Incidence of radiation-induced optic neuropathy (RION) in selected studies.[96-103] Points offset from 0% to 1% were shifted to clearly show range bars. The single patients in the studies by Parsons et al.[96] and Martel et al.[97] with events in the 55 to 60 Gy range were treated to 59 Gy and 59.5 Gy, respectively. (Reprinted from Mayo C, Martel MK, Marks LB, et al. Radiation dose-volume effects of optic nerves and chiasm. *Int J Radiat Oncol Biol Phys* 2010;76[3 Suppl]:S28–S35. Copyright © 2010 Elsevier. With permission.)

Because of the small size of the optic nerves/chiasm and steep dose gradients in radiosurgery, most studies of RION involving SRS use the D_{max} to the optic nerves/chiasm as the critical dose metric.[89] As shown in Table 14.2, single-fraction SRS studies describe a range of threshold D_{max} for RION. In analyzing their early experience with radiosurgery, Tishler et al.[108] reported RION at D_{max} as low as 9.7 Gy and recommended 8 Gy as the dose limit for the optic nerves/chiasm in SRS. Stafford et al.[109] found RION in 4 of 215 patients receiving a median D_{max} of 10 Gy. The D_{max} in the patients ranged from 0.4 to 16 Gy, and 3 of the 4 had received previous external beam radiotherapy to this area. They estimated a 1.7%, 1.8%, 0%, and 6.9% incidence of RION for D_{max} of <8, 8 to 10, 10 to 12, and >12 Gy, respectively.

Pollock et al.[110] observed no cases of RION in 62 patients with nonfunctioning pituitary adenomas receiving a median D_{max} of 9.5 ± 1.7 Gy to the optic apparatus during single-fraction SRS, using a 12-Gy D_{max} as the dose constraint for the optic apparatus. From a study of 50 patients with benign base of the skull tumors treated with single-fraction SRS and a median follow-up of 40 months, Leber et al.[111] estimated a 0%, 27%, and 78% risk of RION for D_{max} of <10, 10 to <15, and ≥15 Gy, respectively. No data for dose–volume and RION were available for hypofractionated stereotactic radiotherapy (HFSRT) (4 to 8 Gy/fraction).[89]

Factors Affecting Risk

There appears to be an increased risk of RION with increasing age.[96] Parsons et al.[96] reported that none of the 38 patients in the 20- to 50-year-old range developed RION, even though the reported optic nerve doses were >60 Gy for 58% and >70 Gy for 26%. In contrast, for patients with doses >60 Gy, the incidence was 26% and 56% for the 50- to 70- versus >70-year-old age groups. RION in children is poorly characterized, but treatment of the developing optic apparatus should be approached cautiously. Reports on the effect of other factors such as adjuvant chemotherapy, diabetes mellitus, and hypertension have been inconsistent. Minimal data are available on reirradiation of the optic apparatus and the effect of the interval between courses on RION. Flickinger et al.[112] found that one of 10 patients undergoing reirradiation of the optic apparatus developed RION—the affected received an initial 40 Gy and, after a 7.5-year interval, an additional 46 Gy, both at 2 Gy/fraction.

Mathematic/Biologic Models

The original Lyman-Kutcher-Burman normal tissue complication probability (NTCP) volumetric modeling[4] estimated

TD_{50} = 65 Gy, n = 0.25, and m = 0.14. The dose–response data from Jiang et al.[98] (1.5 to 2.2 Gy/fraction) suggest $TD_{50} \approx$ 72 to 75 Gy. Martel et al.[97] and Brizel et al.[113] estimated TD_{50} at 72 and 70 Gy, respectively. Extrapolation of the Parsons dose–response data[96] suggests that TD_{50} exceeds 70 Gy.

Special Situations

There is a suggestion that RION may occur at lower doses in patients with pituitary tumors, as complications at doses as low as 46 Gy at 1.8 Gy/fraction have been reported.[101,114,115] Mackley et al.[101] and van den Bergh et al.[114] constrained the optic structure D_{max} to 46 and 45 Gy, respectively. The RION latency also appeared shorter in patients with pituitary tumors. The average latency was 10.5 and 31 months (range 5 to 168 months) in patients with pituitary targets and nonpituitary targets, respectively.[101,115] The apparent increased sensitivity in these patients might be related to tumor-associated compression and/or postsurgical trauma of these nerves.

Recommended Dose–Volume Limits

The estimate by Emami et al.[1] of a 5% risk of blindness within 5 years of treatment for a dose of 50 Gy appears inaccurate. The QUANTEC review[89] suggests that the incidence of RION was unusual (<2%) for D_{max} < 55 Gy, particularly for fraction sizes <2 Gy. The risk increases (3% to 7%) in the region of 55 to 60 Gy and becomes more substantial (>7% to 20%) for doses >60 Gy when dose per fraction of 1.8 to 2.0 Gy is used. The patients with RION treated in the 55 to 60 Gy range were typically treated to doses in the very high end of that range (i.e., 59 Gy). For particles, most investigators found that the incidence of RION was low for a D_{max} < 54 CGE. One exception to this range was for pituitary tumors, in which investigators used a constraint of D_{max} < 46 to 48 Gy for 1.8 Gy/fraction.

The aforementioned studies suggest that the incidence of RION in single-fraction radiosurgery is rare for D_{max} < 8 Gy, increases in the range of 8 to 12 Gy D_{max}, and becomes >10% when D_{max} exceeds 12 Gy. Though the QUANTEC paper presents isoeffect curves for RION over a range of 2 to 12 Gy/fraction using various radiobiologic models, the authors emphasize that there are no data in the hypofractionated range and caution that the curves should not be used to predict toxicity in this regimen.

Future Studies

In addition to reporting detailed dose–volume data for patients with and without RION receiving radiation to the optic apparatus, investigators must consistently, completely, and accurately contour the optic apparatus.

Toxicity Scoring Criteria

Visual deficits should be scored using the CTCAE v. 4.0.[37]

Brainstem

Clinical Significance

As with the optic apparatus, irradiation of the brain, base of the skull, and the neck can deliver a significant dose to the brainstem, which is frequently the dose-limiting structure.

End Points

Radiation-induced damage to the brainstem may be manifest as specific cranial neuropathies; focal motor, sensory, or balance deficits; or mild to life-threatening global dysfunction. This is reflected in the CTCAE,[92] which scores brainstem-related toxicity on the basis of symptoms. The study of radiation-induced brainstem injury is challenging because (a) the reported incidence of injury is low, (b) survival time is short for many patients, (c) formal grading of brainstem effects is subjective and is often characterized categorically (i.e., "yes–no") for cranial neuropathy, and (d) for patients with intracranial tumors, it is often difficult to distinguish between side effects and disease progression.[116]

Challenges Defining Volumes

Contouring the brainstem on axial MRI is usually straightforward, although it requires special attention to the superior extent and interfaces at the cerebral and cerebellar peduncles where the borders are indistinct. Coronal and sagittal views, in addition to axial images, are frequently helpful in visualizing the brainstem and its interfaces. The adult brainstem volume is on the order of 35 ± 8 mL.[117]

Dose/Volume/Toxicity Data

Studies of potential radiation-induced brainstem toxicity in conventionally fractionated partial brain, base-of-skull, or neck irradiation variably report crude radiographic and functional toxicities over typically short follow-up periods.[100,103,105–107,118–127] Reported toxicities attributable to radiation of the brainstem and dose constraints are presented in Table 14.4. Uy et al.[127] reported brainstem necrosis in one of 40 adult meningioma patients treated with intensity-modulated radiation therapy (IMRT). For this patient, the D_{max} was 55.6 Gy, and the absolute volume of brainstem that exceeded 54 Gy was 4.7 mL. Jian et al.[122] noted a grade 1 neurologic

deficit in three of 48 patients with nasopharyngeal cancer treated with 1.2 Gy twice-daily photons to 74.4 Gy and concomitant chemotherapy.

In the largest study, Debus et al.[118,119] reported on 367 patients with base-of-skull tumors with a combination of conformal photon and proton radiation therapy. Nineteen late brainstem-related toxicities were observed, including three deaths. On univariate analysis, significant predictors of toxicity were $D_{max} > 64$ CGE, V_{50} CGE > 5.9 mL, V_{55} CGE > 2.7 mL, V_{60} CGE > 0.9 mL, two or more skull-based surgeries, diabetes, and high blood pressure. On multivariate analysis only $V_{60} > 0.9$ mL, two or more skull-based surgeries, and diabetes were predictive. In a study of 46 patients with recurrent base-of-skull meningiomas, treated to a median brainstem D_{max} of 58.0 CGE, Wenkel et al.[107] found that one patient developed brainstem injury at a dose that exceeded an unspecified constraint value by 10%. Two others with neurologic toxicities had brainstem doses that exceeded the constraints as shown in Table 14.4.

In pediatric patients with brainstem glioma (treated with opposed lateral fields that encompassed the majority of the brainstem), no toxicity was reported at doses of 54 to 60 Gy at 2 Gy/fraction, 75.6 Gy at 1.26 Gy twice daily,[120] or 78 Gy at 1 Gy twice daily.[124] The primary limitation of these studies was the short median survival, <12 months. Of 32 patients treated to 72 Gy twice daily in combination with recombinant β-interferon, there was at least one treatment-related death.[125]

Most pediatric protocols for central nervous system tumors recommend doses >54 Gy, and separate brainstem dose constraints are often absent. Merchant et al. studied 68 patients with infratentorial ependymoma treated with surgery and conformal RT (54 to 59.4 Gy).[123] In patients with full recovery, a considerable portion of the brainstem received over 60 Gy ($V_{60} = 7.8 \pm 1.4$ mL). There was no difference in brainstem recovery based on absolute or percent volume of the brainstem that received more than 54 Gy. Differences in these values for patients without full recovery were not statistically significant. One patient died with autopsy-confirmed residual tumor and focal areas of brainstem necrosis. The mean brainstem dose was 59 Gy, and he also exhibited severe perioperative morbidity after two surgeries.

A limited number of studies report brainstem toxicity in single-fraction SRS or HFSRT.[128–132] A broad range of prescription isodose levels and dose metrics are reported, making it difficult to develop a predictive dose–volume model for

TABLE 14.4 SELECTED STUDIES OF RADIATION-INDUCED BRAINSTEM TOXICITY WITH CONVENTIONAL FRACTIONATION OR HYPERFRACTIONATION

Reference	Patients/Disease	Modality	Dose Constraint	Radiation-Induced Brainstem Toxicity
Jian et al.[122]	48 Adults/nasopharyngeal cavity	Photons	$V_{65} < 3$ mL, $V_{60} < 5$ mL	3 grade 1 neurologic toxicities
Hoppe et al.[121]	85 Adults/nasal cavity and/or paranasal sinus	Photons	$D_{max} < 50$ Gy	
Daly et al.[100]	36 Adults/nasal cavity and/or paranasal sinus cavity	Photons	$D_{1\%} < 54$ Gy	
Schoenfeld et al.[126]	100 Adults/pharynx or larynx	Photons	$V_{55} < 0.1$ mL	
Uy et al.[127]	40 Adults/intracranial meningioma	Photons	Unknown	1 BS necrosis @ D_{max} 55.6 Gy, V_{54} 4.7 mL
Merchant et al.[123]	68 Children/infratentorial ependymoma	Photons	No separate brainstem constraint	1 BS necrosis @ D_{mean} 59 Gy
Freeman et al.[120]	136 Children/brainstem glioma	Photons	Prescribed 54–60 Gy at 2 Gy once daily or 75.6 Gy at 1.26 Gy twice daily	None reported
Packer et al.[124,125]	98 Children/brainstem glioma	Photons	Prescribed 72 or 78 Gy total @ 1 Gy twice daily	One treatment-related death at 72 Gy total @ 1 Gy twice daily and concurrent β-IFN
Weber et al.[103]	29 Adults/chordoma, chondrosarcoma	Protons	Surface ≤ 63 CGE Center ≤ 54 CGE	None reported
Nishimura et al.[106]	14 Adults/olfactory neuroblastoma	Protons	Surface ≤ 64 CGE Center < 53 CGE	None reported
Noel et al.[105]	45 Adults/BOS tumors	Photons + protons	Surface ≤ 63 CGE Center ≤ 54 CGE	
DeBus et al.[118,119]	367 Adults/BOS tumors	Photons + protons	Surface ≤ 64 CGE Center ≤ 53 CGE	19 BS toxicities, including 3 deaths
Wenkel et al.[107]	46 Adults/BOS meningiomas	Photons + protons	Surface ≤ 64 CGE Center ≤ 53 CGE	1 BS injury, 2 neurologic toxicities

β-IFN, recombinant β-interferon; BOS, base of skull; BS, brainstem; CGE, cobalt gray equivalent.

brainstem toxicity.[116] In the study with the largest number of patients, Foote et al.[128] analyzed the outcome in 149 vestibular schwannoma patients treated with SRS between 1988 and 1998; 41 were treated before 1994, when radiosurgery was primarily based on CT imaging, and 108 after 1994, when planning was MRI based. Large single-fraction doses (10 to 22.5 Gy) were used. Their analysis revealed a "learning curve," with a 5% and 2% actuarial 2-year rate of facial and trigeminal neuropathies, respectively, for patients treated after 1994 compared with 29% for both neuropathies for the earlier patients. This study found a significant difference, with a 2-year actuarial rate of facial and trigeminal neuropathies of 29% and 7% for patients treated before and after 1994, respectively. The authors ascribe this difference to the use of MRI rather than CT-based imaging and lower prescription doses in the latter years. A univariate analysis showed an incidence of cranial nerve neuropathy of 2% for <12.5 Gy versus 24% for >12.5 Gy ($P < .0003$). On multivariate analysis, the prescription dose >12.5 Gy, prior surgery, and treatment prior to 1994 were significant variables.

Mathematic/Biologic Models

The Emami review estimates a 5-year, 5% rate of complications, defined in that study as "necrosis/infarct," at 50, 53, and 60 Gy delivered to the whole, two-thirds of, and one-third of the brainstem, respectively.[1] The corresponding Lyman-Kutcher-Berman (LKB) parameters for calculation of the NTCP were $n = 0.16$, $m = 0.14$, and a tolerance dose for 50% probability of these complications (TD_{50}) equal to 65 Gy.[26] These estimates and model parameters appear overly conservative. For example, the LKB model estimates a 12% risk of severe complications for 54 Gy to the whole brainstem or a 3% risk of complications when the proton dose constraints (Table 14.4) are utilized. The clinical data would suggest that a larger TD_{50}, smaller m, or larger m values might produce more reasonable estimates of toxicity. For example, an LKB model with a larger TD_{50} (72 Gy) or smaller m (0.1) would reduce the predicted risks to <5% or <1%, respectively. However, there are insufficient existing dose/volume/complication data to generate a more accurate model estimate at this time.

Recommended Dose–Volume Limits

The QUANTEC study concludes that the entire brainstem may be treated to 54 Gy using conventional fractionation with limited risk of severe or permanent neurologic effects.[116,123] Although the precise dose–volume relationship is unclear, partial volumes of the brainstem (1 to 10 mL) may be irradiated to a maximum dose of 59 Gy for dose fractions ≤2 Gy. The risk appears to increase markedly at doses >64 Gy. In radiosurgery, it appears that a maximum brainstem dose of 12.5 to 13 Gy is associated with a low (<5%) risk of cranial neuropathy in patients with vestibular schwannomas treated with single-fraction SRS. The risk appears to increase rapidly when the marginal prescription dose is >15 Gy or when the target volume exceeds 4 mL.[116,128,133] However, doses of 15 to 20 Gy have been used to treat brainstem metastases with a low reported rate of complications, potentially because of the limited survival time for these patients.[130,134]

Future Studies

Uniform, complete reporting of patient-specific dose/volume/outcome data for patients with and without complications are required.

Toxicity Scoring Criteria

Patients should undergo a complete history and physical examination at regular intervals with particular attention to the neurologic exam. Toxicity should be scored and reported using the CTCAE v. 4.0.[92]

Auditory Apparatus

Clinical Significance

Radiation therapy to brain tumors and head and neck cancers may damage the cochlea and/or acoustic nerve, leading to sensorineural hearing loss (SNHL) and compromised quality of life.[135]

End Points

SNHL following conventionally fractionated radiotherapy is typically measured by a decrease in the bone conduction threshold (BCT) at 0.5 to 4 kHz,[135] the primary range for human speech, using pure-tone audiometry (PTA). Although the technique is well established and standardized, a broad range of specific audiometric parameters are used to characterize SNHL, including the frequency (range) used for testing, the threshold chosen for a clinically significant change in the BCT (10 to 20 dB), and the control/standard used for comparison. In stereotactic radiosurgery, SRS, or HFSRT, hearing status is more commonly evaluated using the Gardner-Robertson scale, which is based on both PTA and speech discrimination. Hearing loss after SRS/HFSRT may be characterized by changes in Gardner-Robertson hearing grade or retention of serviceable hearing (i.e., functional hearing with the aid of a hearing aid) or any measurable hearing. In addition, the length of follow-up will influence reported hearing loss, as deficits may develop more rapidly following single-fraction SRS than HFSRT, and hearing loss increases over time in both situations.

Challenges Defining Volumes

Contouring of the acoustic nerve and brainstem is best accomplished on high-resolution, contrast-enhanced T1-weighted and fast imaging with steady-state precession MRI. The cochlea and associated bony anatomy are better delineated on fine-cut (≤1 mm slice thickness) CT scans. Both the acoustic nerve and cochlea are small structures, and the dose gradient at the latter structure is often quite steep. Moreover, the acoustic nerve anatomy is distorted by the tumor, significantly increasing its apparent diameter. Thus, the dose to these structures is typically characterized by an average or maximum dose, rather than a dose–volume distribution. In many studies, the primary dose metric was the dose to the acoustic neuroma, rather than the normal tissue structures per se, which is not unreasonable as the dose to the tumor appears to be correlated with the dose received by the acoustic nerve.[45]

Dose/Volume/Toxicity Data

SNHL at key frequencies following radiotherapy for head and neck cancer with conventionally fractionated radiotherapy[135–142] is summarized in Figure 14.4. Pan et al.[136] prospectively studied the BCT in 31 patients after unilateral RT with standard fractionation using changes seen in the contralateral ear as standard (0.25 to 8 kHz). Changes in BCT > 10 dB were rarely observed unless the corresponding difference in mean cochlear dose was >45 Gy. The dose to the contralateral cochlea ranged from 0.5 to 31.3 Gy (mean, 4.2 Gy). Honore et al.[141] retrospectively estimated mean cochlear doses in 20 patients treated with radiation therapy for head and neck cancer.[143–145] A dose–response relationship was observed at 4 kHz, but not at other frequencies.

Chen et al.[137] retrospectively studied 22 patients treated with RT for nasopharyngeal cancer (with fraction sizes from 1.6 to 2.3 Gy and concurrent/adjuvant chemotherapy) and studied BCT 12 to 79 months post RT. A significant increase in hearing loss (change in BCT of >20 dB at one frequency or >10 dB at two consecutive frequencies) was observed for all frequencies (0.5 to 4 kHz) when the mean dose received by the cochlea exceeded 48 Gy. Van der Putten et al.[142] retrospectively evaluated changes in BCT after head and neck radiotherapy in 21 patients with unilateral parotid tumors (fraction sizes

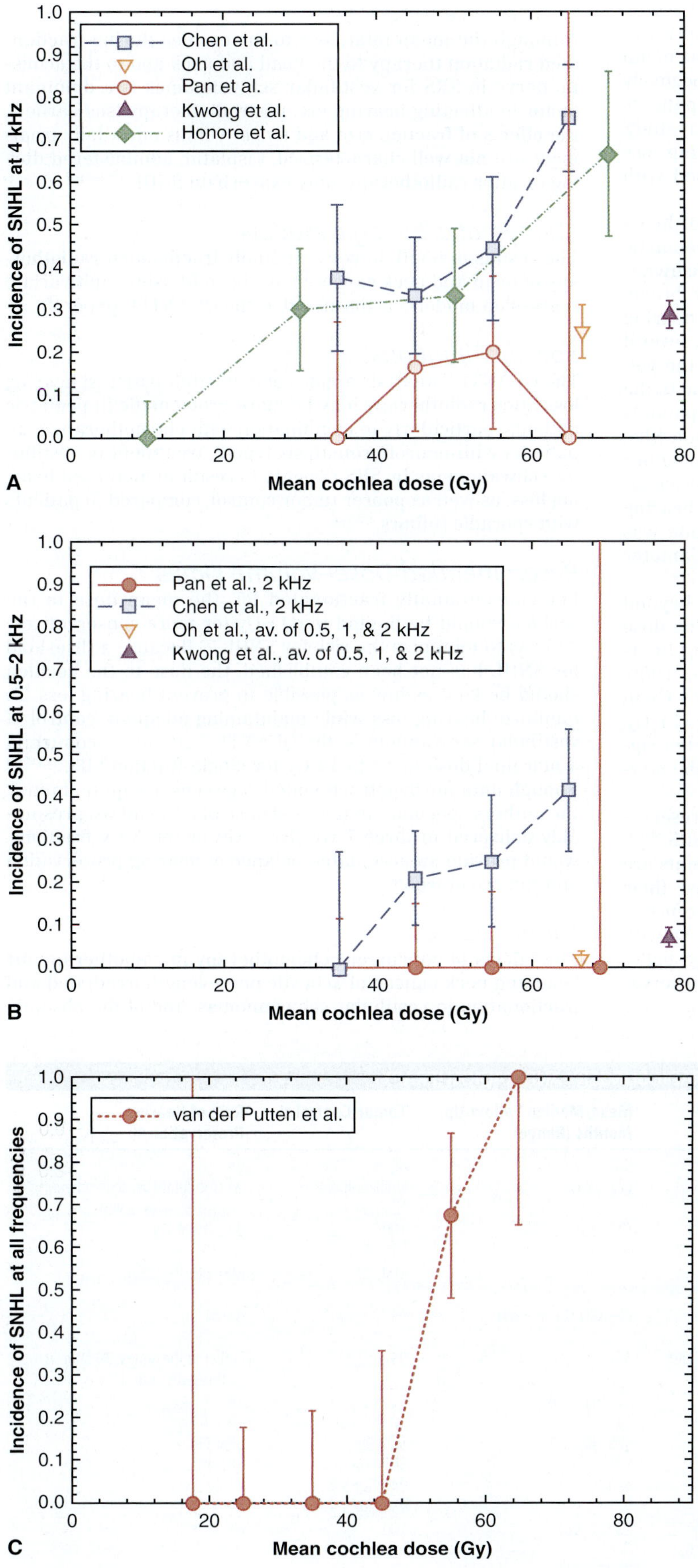

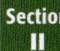

FIGURE 14.4. Mean dose response for sensorineural hearing loss (SNHL) at **(A)** 4 kHz,[136,138,140–142] **(B)** 0.5 to 2 kHz,[136,138,140–142] and **(C)** all frequencies[142] (0.25 to 12 kHz). (Reprinted from Bhandare N, Jackson A, Eisbruch A, et al. Radiation therapy and hearing loss. *Int J Radiat Oncol Biol Phys* 2010;76[3 Suppl]:S50–S57. Copyright © 2010 Elsevier. With permission.)

1.8 to 3.0 Gy). Using the contralateral ear as a control, SNHL, defined as a >15 dB difference in BCT at three or more frequencies between 0.25 and 12 kHz, was seen when mean doses received by the cochlea were >50 Gy. Oh[140] prospectively studied changes in BCT (0.25 to 4 kHz) post RT in 25 patients with nasopharyngeal cancer (fraction size 2 Gy). In that study, inner ear doses were high (63 to 70 Gy), and hearing loss (a >15 dB decrease in BCT from baseline) correlated with total dose received by the inner ear.

Table 14.5 summarizes the reported incidence of hearing loss for single-fraction SRS and fractionated stereotactic radiotherapy (FSRT) in the treatment of vestibular schwannomas.[143,144,146-155] The range of hearing loss reported is broad, in part because of the variation in the definition of hearing preservation and the length of follow-up. Nonetheless, several studies suggest that there is a relationship between the volume/length of acoustic nerve irradiated and/or the dose to the nerve and cochlea with hearing loss. In a study of 82 patients treated to a marginal dose of 12 Gy in single-fraction SRS, Massager et al.[156] found that increased intracanalicular tumor volume (<100 vs. ≥100 mm³) and volume-averaged intracanalicular dose were significant predictors of increased hearing loss. Pollock et al.[157] reported that hearing preservation was more likely when tumors <3 cm versus >3 cm in diameter were treated with single-fraction SRS.

Niranjan et al.[158] found that the dose extending beyond the intracanalicular tumor volume and the prescription dose were the most important factors adversely affecting hearing. In that study, serviceable hearing was preserved in 100% of patients treated with a marginal tumor dose of ≤14 Gy in single-fraction SRS versus 20% in those receiving >14 Gy. Similarly, Kondziolka et al. and Lunsford et al. reported significantly improved hearing preservation rates when the marginal dose was reduced from 16–20 to 12–14 Gy.[150,151]

Several studies suggest that the rate of hearing preservation is improved with FSRT versus single-fraction SRS.[143-145] However, there is an issue of selection bias in that patients are frequently selected for fractionated treatment because their hearing is good. Meijer et al.[154] found no significant difference in hearing preservation in acoustic neuroma patients treated with four to five fractions of 5 Gy HFSRT versus 10 to 12.5 Gy single-fraction SRS (61% vs. 75%), though trigeminal nerve preservation was significantly higher with HFSRT (98% vs. 92%).

Factors Affecting Risk

Although the mean total dose to the cochlea during fractionated radiation therapy to the head and neck and to the acoustic nerve in SRS for vestibular schwannomas is a dominant factor in affecting hearing loss postradiotherapy (see earlier), the effects of fraction size and twice- versus once-daily treatment are not well characterized. Cisplatin, administered during or after radiotherapy, may exacerbate SNHL.[137,159,160]

Mathematic/Biologic Models

The results of SNHL in conventionally fractionated radiotherapy of head and neck cancers have been fit using multivariate regression models, as discussed in the QUANTEC paper.[135]

Special Situations

The QUANTEC analysis applies only to adult patients; hearing loss after radiotherapy may be more problematic in pediatric patients, particularly in combination with chemotherapy.[161] In patients with neurofibromatosis type 2, treatment of vestibular schwannomas by SRS appears to result in increased hearing loss, as well as poorer tumor control, compared to patients with sporadic tumors.[162-164]

Recommended Dose–Volume Limits

For conventionally fractionated RT, the mean dose to the cochlea should be limited to ≤45 Gy (or more conservatively ≤35 Gy) to minimize the risk for SNHL.[135] Because a threshold for SNHL has not been established, the dose to the cochlea should be kept as low as possible to prevent hearing loss. To minimize hearing loss while maintaining adequate control of vestibular schwannomas, the QUANTEC authors recommend a marginal dose of 12 to 14 Gy for single-fraction SRS.[128,135,165] Though data for hypofractionated regimens are quite limited, the authors speculate that a total dose of 21 to 30 Gy, presumably delivered in three 7-Gy, five 5-Gy, or ten 3-Gy fractions, would provide an acceptable balance of hearing preservation and tumor control.[135]

Future Studies

The effects of concurrent chemotherapy in radiotherapy for head and neck cancer, of acoustic nerve length irradiated and fractionation in vestibular schwannomas, and of the absolute

TABLE 14.5 HEARING PRESERVATION IN STEREOTACTIC RADIOSURGERY AND RADIOTHERAPY

Reference	Technique: Number of Patients	Treatment Dose, Gy	Mean/Median Follow-Up, Months (Range)	Tumor Control,%	Rate of Hearing Preservation,%
Hirsch and Noren[146]	SRS: 126	18–25	56	86	26
Noren et al.[147]	SRS: 254 (NF2: 61)	18–20 / 10–15	(12–204)	Unilateral: 94 / NF2: 84	22 (moderate vs. severe hearing loss: 55% vs. 23%)
Foote et al.[148]	SRS: 36	16–20	(2.5–36)	100	42 ± 17 at 2 y
Flickinger et al.[149]	SRS: 273 (CT vs. MRI planned: 118 vs. 155)	12–20		CT: 44 / MRI: 32	CT: 39 / MRI: 68
Kondziolka et al.[150]	SRS: 162	12–20 Mean: 16.6	(6–102) (60% > 60)	94	47–51
Lunsford et al.[151]	SRS: 402	Earlier in the series: 17 later in the series: 12–14	36	93	Earlier in the series: 39 later in the series: 68
Flickinger et al.[152]	SRS: 190	11–18 Median: 13	30 (max: 80)	91 at 5 y	74
Andrews et al.[143]	SRS: 64 (NF2: 5) FSRT: 46 (NF2: 10)	SRS: 12 FSRT: 50 (2 Gy/fx)	SRS: 30 ± 17 SRT: 30 ± 24	SRS: 98 SRT: 97	SRS: 33 SRT: 81
Combs et al.[144]	FSRT: 106	57.6 Gy (1.8 Gy/fx)	49 (3–172)	94% @ 3 y 93% @ 5 y	94 @ 5 y
Williams[153]	HFSRT: 125	Tumors < 3 cm: 25/5 fxs Tumors ≥3 cm: 30/10 fxs	22 (12–68)	100	64
Meijer et al.[154]	SRS: 12 HFSRT: 25	SRS: 10–12 HFSRT: 20–25	25 (12–61)	–	91

CT, computed tomography; FSRT, fractionated stereotactic radiotherapy; fx, fraction; HFSRT, hypofractionated stereotactic radiotherapy; MRI, magnetic resonance imaging; NF2, neurofibromatosis type 2; SRS, stereotactic radiosurgery.

dose to the cochlea in all settings would benefit from prospective, multi-institutional studies.

Toxicity Scoring Criteria

An audiometric evaluation should be performed for both ears immediately before radiotherapy and biannually thereafter. The QUANTEC authors recommend that a "clinically significant hearing loss" should be defined as an increase in the threshold of 10 dB in postradiotherapy BCT or a decline of 10% in a speech discrimination evaluation.[135]

Spinal Cord
Clinical Significance

Although the spinal cord proper is from the base of the skull through the top of the lumbar spine, individual nerves continue down the spinal canal to the level of the pelvis. Thus, portions of the spinal cord and canal are often included in radiotherapy fields during treatment of malignancies involving the neck, thorax, abdomen, and pelvis.[166] In addition, metastatic disease to the bony spine is encountered in approximately 40% of all cancer patients,[167] and this disease is often treated with radiotherapy. Though rare, radiation-induced spinal cord injury (i.e., myelopathy) can be severe, resulting in pain, paresthesias, sensory deficits, paralysis, Brown-Séquard syndrome, and bowel/bladder incontinence.[168]

End Points

Myelopathy is defined as a grade 2 or higher myelitis, per CTCAE v. 4.0.[92] Under this definition, asymptomatic changes in the cord detected radiographically and mild signs/symptoms, such as the Babinski sign or Lhermitte syndrome, would not be classified as myelopathy. Consequently, a diagnosis of myelopathy is based on the appearance of signs/symptoms of sensory or motor deficits, loss of function, or pain, now frequently confirmed by MRI. Radiation myelopathy rarely occurs <6 months after completion of radiotherapy and, in most cases, appears within 3 years.[169]

Challenges Defining Volumes

In conventional external beam RT, the field generally encompasses the entire circumference of the cord, vertebral body, and spinal nerve roots, and precise organ definition is not critical apart from correctly identifying the level of the involved cord. Delineation of the cord in radiosurgery is unsettled, with various studies contouring the critical organ in the axial plane as the spinal cord, the spinal cord expanded 2 to 3 mm, the thecal sac and its contents, or the entire spinal canal.[170] As the volume receiving a high dose often extends superiorly and inferiorly to the target, several studies expand the critical organ volume above and below the target volume. For example, RTOG protocol 0631, a study of image-guided radiosurgery of spine metastases, defines the cord as the unexpanded cord itself visualized in MRI and extends the volume of the partial spinal cord 5 to 6 mm above and below the target volume.

Dose/Volume/Toxicity Data

Schultheiss[166,171] compiled and analyzed published reports of radiation myelopathy in 335 and 1,946 patients receiving radiotherapy to the full circumference, previously unirradiated cervical[169,172–175] and thoracic[176–187] spines, respectively (Fig. 14.5A and B). Although a small number of these patients received relatively high doses per fraction, none were treated using stereotactic techniques to exclude a portion of the

Cervical spine

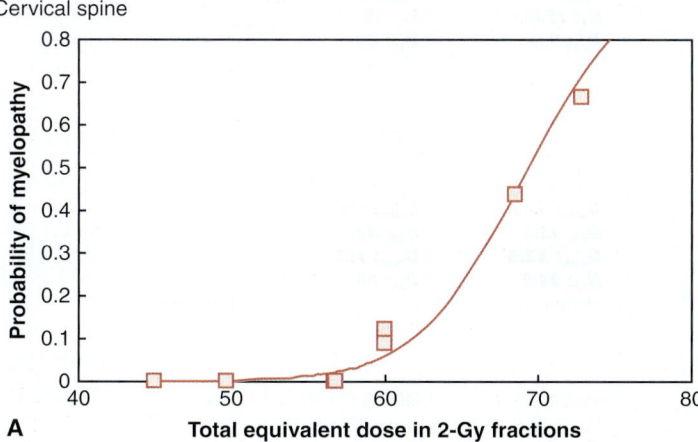

A

Thoracic spine

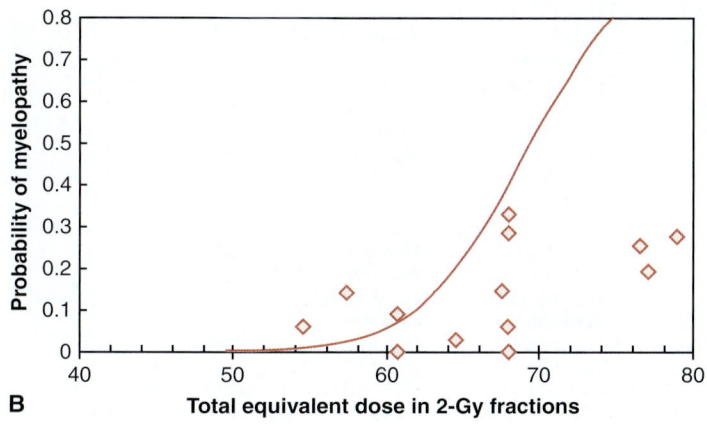

B

FIGURE 14.5. Incidence of transverse myelopathy from selected studies. **A:** Cervical cord: data for selected studies[169,172–175] shown by □ with probability of myelopathy corrected for estimated survival and *solid line* fit to these data by the method of Schultheiss. **B:** Thoracic cord: data for selected studies[176–187] shown by ◊ with probability of myelopathy corrected for estimated survival. *Solid line* is the best fit to the cervical cord data, as thoracic cord data were insufficient to permit an adequate fit. (Adapted from Schultheiss TE. The radiation dose-response of the human spinal cord. *Int J Radiat Oncol Biol Phys* 2008;71[5]:1455–1459. Copyright © 2008 Elsevier. With permission.)

circumference of the cord. Note that the dose to the cord is the prescribed dose reported in those studies; typically, dosimetric data were not available to calculate the true cord dose. As discussed later, the rate of myelopathy appears very low below total doses of 50 Gy for conventional radiation delivered at 2 Gy per fraction.

Published reports of radiation myelopathy from radiosurgery to the spine are summarized in Table 14.6.[188,190-196] Of the exactly 1,400 cases of spinal radiosurgery presented in the published literature, there are only 12 reported instances of radiation-induced myelopathy, equaling a crude rate of 0.8%. Because the survival is generally short for most of these patients, this may be an underestimate of the true rate of injury. Given the small number of reported cases of myelopathy, as well as the variation in published dosimetric parameters, it is not feasible to construct a quantitative model for the risk of myelopathy as a function of cord dose in spinal radiosurgery. In fact, most of the cases of myelopathy involved cord doses well within the range of doses *not* associated with myelopathy, as discussed later.

Factors Affecting Risk

Animal studies suggest that the immature cord is somewhat more susceptible to radiation-induced complications and the time to manifestation of damage is shorter.[197-200] Though the literature on radiation-induced myelopathy in children is

TABLE 14.6 TRANSVERSE MYELOPATHY IN STEREOTACTIC RADIOSURGERY (SRS) OF THE SPINE

Reference	Cases of Myelopathy/ Total Patients	Total Dose (Gy)	Dose/Fraction (Gy)	Dose to Cord (Gy)	BED to Cord (Gy$_3$)	Proportion of Patients Previously Irradiated to Involved Segment of Spine
Gibbs et al.[188]	6/1,075	12.5–25	5–25	D_{max}: 3–28	Range: 24–121 Gy$_3$	>55%
		25	**12.5**	**D_{max}: 26.2**	**D_{max}: 141**	
		20	**12.5**	**D_{max}: 29.9**	**D_{max}: 81**	
		21	**10.5**	**D_{max}: 19.2**	**D_{max}: 46**	
		24	**8**	**D_{max}: 13.9**	**D_{max}: 129**	
		20	**10**	**D_{max}: 10**	**D_{max}: 33**	
		20	**20**	**D_{max}: 8.5**	**D_{max}: 43**	
Ryu et al.[189]	1/86	<10–18	<10–18	*Mean ± SD* D_{max}: 12.2 ± 2.5 D_{10}: 8.6 ± 2.1 *Maximum* D_{max}: 19.2 D_{10}:13	*Mean ± SD* D_{max}: 62 ± 4.6 D_{10}: 33 ± 3.6 *Maximum* D_{max}: 142 D_{10}: 69	0%
		18	18	*Mean ± SD* D_{max}: 13.8 ± 2.2 D_{10}: 9.8 ± 1.5	*Mean ± SD* D_{max}: 77 ± 3.8 D_{10}: 42 ± 2.3	
		16	**16**	**D_{max}: 14.8** **D_1: 13.0** **D_{10}: 9.6**	**D_{max}: 88** **D_1: 69** **D_{10}: 40**	
Gwak et al.[190]	2/9	21–44	3–5	*Median* D_{max}: 32.9 D_{25}: 11.0 *Range* D_{max}: 11–37 D_{25}: 1.2–24	*Median* D_{max}: 106 D_{25}: 21 *Range* D_{max}: 19–172 D_{25}: 1–88	33%
		30	**10**	**D_{max}: 35.2** **D_{25}: 15.5**	**D_{max}:172** **D_{25}: 42**	
		33	**11**	**D_{max}: 32.9** **D_{25}: 24.0**	**D_{max}: 153** **D_{25}: 88**	
Benzil et al.[191]	3/31	Median: 10 **100** **12** **20**	Median: 5 **50** **12** **5**	Median: 6.0	Median: 12	Unknown
Sahgal et al.[192]	0/38	24	8	*Median* $D_{0.1 mL}$: 10.5 $D_{1 mL}$: 7.4	*Median* $D_{0.1 mL}$: 23 $D_{1 mL}$: 14	62%
Sahgal et al.[193]	0/16	21	7	*Median* D_{max}: 20.9 $D_{1 mL}$: 13.8 *Range* D_{max}: 4.3–23 $D_{1 mL}$: 2.8–19	*Median* $D_{1 mL}$: 22 *Range* $D_{1 mL}$: 6–54	6%
Chang et al.[194]	0/63	30 pts: 30 Gy 33 pts: 27 Gy	30 pts: 6 Gy 33 pts: 9 Gy	30 pts: <10 33 pts: <9	30 pts: <16.7 33 pts: <18	56%
Gerszten et al.[195]	0/50	19	19	*Mean* D_{max}: 10 *Range* D_{max}: 6.5–13	*Mean* D_{max}: 21 *Range* D_{max}: 11–32	96%
Nelson et al.[196]	0/32	Median: 18	Median: 7	*Mean ± SD* D_{max}: 14.4 ± 2.3 D_{10}: 11.5 ± 2.1 *Maximum* D_{max}: 19.2 D_{10}: 15.2	*Mean ± SD* D_{max}: 46.0 ± 13.2 D_{10}: 31.2 ± 8.1 *Maximum* D_{max}: 78.3 D_{10}: 46.5	58%

sparse, care should be exercised in irradiating a child's spine because of the increased sensitivity of the developing central nervous system and bone to ionizing radiation.[201] There are a handful of reports of myelopathy at relatively low radiation doses to the spine postchemotherapy.[202-205] Many chemotherapeutic agents are directly neurotoxic[206] and should be used with caution during irradiation of the central nervous system.[207]

Mathematic/Biologic Models

Schultheiss[171] calculated the risk of myelopathy as a function of dose using a probability distribution model, using the data for cervical and thoracic spinal cord myelopathy adjusted for estimated overall survival. A good fit to the combined cervical and thoracic cord data was not possible, and separate analyses were performed. For the cervical cord data, D_{50} = 69.4 Gy and α/β ratio = 0.87 Gy provided a reasonable fit of the data, as shown in Figure 14.5. The 95% confidence interval was 66.4 to 72.6 Gy for D_{50} and 0.54 to 1.19 Gy for α/β ratio. At 2 Gy per fraction, the calculated probability of myelopathy is 0.03% at a total dose of 45 Gy and 0.2% at 50 Gy. Because of the dispersion of the thoracic data, it was not possible to obtain a good fit to those data. As shown in Figure 14.5B, the data points for the thoracic cord generally lie to the right of the dose–response curve generated from the cervical cord. This suggests that the thoracic cord may be less radiation sensitive than the cervical cord.

At the high doses per fraction encountered in radiosurgery, the applicability of the linear-quadratic model is controversial, and the biologically equivalent doses presented in Table 14.6 should be used solely for making rough comparisons of the different dose regimens. In particular, data obtained at a low dose per fraction should not be extrapolated to regimens employing doses of 10 Gy or more per fraction.[166,208] Applying the Schultheiss model[171] to spinal radiosurgery appears to overestimate the risk of myelopathy. For example, using the α/β ratio of 0.87 Gy, the model yields an estimated risk of myelopathy of 0.8%, 13.6%, 50%, and 73% for 12, 13, 13.7, and 14 Gy, respectively, delivered in a single fraction.

In contrast, Ryu et al.[189] found only one case of myelopathy in 86 patients treated with single-fraction spine radiosurgery at a mean cord D_{max} of 12.2 Gy (±2.5 Gy standard deviation) and no cases in the subset of 39 lesions prescribed 18 Gy and treated to a mean cord D_{max} of 13.8 Gy. Note that the Medin et al.[209] study of single-fraction irradiation of the swine spinal cord shows a steep dose–response curve with a median effective D_{max} of 20 Gy.

Special Situations

The need to reirradiate previously treated cord is often encountered in the setting of recurrent spine metastases following spinal irradiation or new spine lesions within, for example, a previously treated lung, pancreas, or esophageal field. In evaluating reirradiation of the spinal cord, the dose regimen for each course, the volume and region (re)irradiated, and the time interval between the courses of radiation therapy must be considered.[210] Animal studies support a time-dependent model of repair for radiation damage to the spinal cord.[197,211-215] For example, Ang et al.[197] treated the thoracic and cervical spines of rhesus monkeys to 44 Gy and then reirradiated these animals with an additional 57 Gy at 1 to 2 years or 66 Gy at 2 to 3 years, yielding aggregate doses of 101 and 110 Gy, respectively. Of 45 animals evaluated, 4 developed myelopathy by the end of the observation period. The reirradiation tolerance model developed from these and similar data[211] estimates a recovery of 34 Gy (76%), 38 Gy (85%), and 45 Gy (101%) at 1, 2, and 3 years, respectively. Under conservative assumptions, an overall recovery of 26 Gy (61%) was calculated.

Table 14.7 summarizes published reports involving reirradiation of the spinal cord in humans using both conventional and full circumference external beam radiotherapy.[210,216-228] For purposes of comparing different regimens, an α/β ratio of 3 Gy was used to calculate the biologically equivalent dose in Gy$_3$. In all of these studies, the median interval between courses was at least 6 months, and only a small number of cases were treated at intervals <6 months. Note that few cases of myelopathy are reported despite large cumulative doses,

TABLE 14.7 TRANSVERSE MYELOPATHY IN REIRRADIATION OF THE SPINE							
Reference	Cases of Myelopathy/ Total Patients	Median F/U (Months)	BED, Initial Course (Gy$_3$) Median (Range)	BED, Reirradiation (Gy$_3$) Median (Range)	Interval Between Courses (Months) Median (Range)	Total BED (Gy$_3$) Median (Range)	2-Gy Dose Equivalent, α/β = 3 Gy Median (Range)
Wright et al.[216]	0/37	8	60 (10–101)	16 (5–50)	19 (2–125)	79 (21–117)	47 (13–70)
Langendijk et al.[217]	0/34	–	–	–	–	<100	<60
Nieder et al.[210,218,219]	0/15	30	70 (34–83)	50 (38–83)	30 (6–96)	115 (91–166)	69 (54–100)
Schiff et al.[220]	4/54 4	4[a]	60 All 60	37 73[b] (29–115)	10 (1–51) 9 (5–21)	97 133 (109–175)	58 80 (65–105)
Ryu et al.[221]	0/1	60	75	72	144	147	88
Kuo et al.[222]	0/1	8	75	42	37	117	70
Bauman et al.[223]	0/2	>3–9	(40–56)	(18–35)	(8–20)	(58–91)	(35–57)
Sminia et al.[224]	0/8	–	56 (29–78)	42 (36–83)	30 (4–152)	106 (65–159)	64 (39–96)
Magrini et al.[225]	0/5	168	47 (32–47)	55 (33–67)	24 (12–36)	94 (80–113)	57 (48–68)
Rades et al.[226]	0/62	12	29 (29–47)	29 (29–47)	6 (2–40)	69 (59–77)	41 (35–46)
Jackson and Ball[227]	0/6	15	All 73	36 (32–39)	15	106 (103–109)	63 (62–65)
Wong et al.[228]	11/–[c]	11	72 (28–96)	42 (14–86)	11 (2–71)	115 (100–138)	69 (60–83)

[a]Overall survival.
[b]One patient received two courses of reirradiation; another received three courses.
[c]Total number of patients not reported.
After Kirkpatrick JP, van der Kogel AJ, Schultheiss TE. Radiation dose-volume effects in the spinal cord. *Int J Radiat Oncol Biol Phys* 2010;76(3 Suppl):S42–S49. Copyright © 2010 Elsevier. With permission.

with essentially no cases of myelopathy observed for cumulative doses <60 Gy in 2 Gy equivalent doses. These observations are consistent with the predictions of postradiotherapy repair observed in the animal models.

As discussed earlier, radiosurgery at a high dose per fraction is increasingly employed in the treatment of spinal lesions. Though reports of toxicity are rare, the follow-up time is short and patient numbers small. Prudence should be observed when prescribing the dose and every reasonable effort made to limit the dose to the cord by immobilization, image guidance, and attention to patient comfort. Estimates of toxicity based on conventional fractionation should not be applied to such treatments without further careful study.

Recommended Dose–Volume Limits

With conventional fractionation of 2 Gy/d including the full cord cross-section, total doses of 50 Gy, 60 Gy, and approximately 69 Gy are associated with a 0.2%, 6%, and 50% rate of myelopathy. The level of acceptable risk will depend on the clinical scenario; that is, a 5% risk of myelopathy may be acceptable in treatment of a primary spinal cord tumor but not in irradiation of a lung lesion. For reirradiation of the full cord cross-section at 2 Gy per daily fraction after prior conventionally fractionated treatment, cord tolerance appears to increase at least 25% 6 months after the initial course of RT. In spine radiosurgery, a maximum cord dose of 13 Gy in a single fraction or 20 Gy in three fractions appears associated with a <1% risk of myelopathy. In comparison, Sahgal et al.[229] recommend a *de novo* single-fraction maximum point dose to the thecal sac of 10 Gy to avoid myelopathy entirely, and RTOG protocol 0631 specifies a cord D_{10} and $D_{0.35\,mL}$ of 10 Gy and D_{max} of 14 Gy for the involved spine.

Future Studies

A model of dose/volume/outcome for spinal cord toxicity will require that more extensive and detailed data be collected over many years, including data on entire cohorts of patients treated with radiotherapy and radiosurgery, not just those with myelopathy. Extensive dosimetric parameters should be collected, specifically D_{max}, D_1, D_{10}, D_{50}, $D_{0.1\,mL}$, $D_{0.35\,mL}$, and $D_{1\,mL}$, and the volume of the involved segment of the spinal cord, as well as the prescribed total dose, dose per fraction, involved spinal level(s), portion of the vertebral body irradiated, irradiation technique, and patient characteristics/demographics. In addition, preclinical studies identifying the fundamental mechanisms of radiation-induced toxicity would be valuable.

Toxicity Scoring Criteria

Toxicity should be scored and reported using CTCAE v. 4.0.[92]

NECK

Larynx and Pharynx

Clinical Significance

Radiation therapy is often utilized as the primary treatment of early-stage laryngeal cancers in an effort to preserve speech and swallowing. However, radiation-induced progressive edema and associated fibrosis can lead to long-term problems with phonation and swallowing.[230] Irradiation of the pharynx and larynx, particularly in combination with concurrent chemotherapy, can produce severe dysphagia, compromising nutrition, protection of the airway, and quality of life.

End Points

The critical larynx-specific end points examined were laryngeal edema and vocal function.[231] Dysphagia, resulting from laryngeal and/or pharyngeal dysfunction, may be assessed by instrument-based swallowing studies,[232] by observer-based criteria (e.g., CTCAE v. 4.0[92]), or by patient-reported quality of life questionnaires.

Challenges Defining Volumes

Phonation and swallowing are complex processes involving multiple anatomic structures in close proximity to one another. The relative importance of various normal tissue structures affecting vocal function and swallowing is controversial. In studying vocal dysfunction, doses to the epiglottis, base of tongue, lateral pharyngeal walls, preepiglottic space, aryepiglottic folds, false vocal cords, upper esophageal sphincter, and cricoid cartilage have been considered.[231,233,234] Radiation-induced dysphagia has been correlated with the dose to the pharyngeal constrictor muscles and specific points in the supraglottic and glottic larynx.[233,235–238] Precise identification of these structures for treatment planning requires a high-resolution, contrast-enhanced CT scan.

Dose/Volume/Toxicity Data

On multivariate analysis, Sanguineti et al.[234] found that the mean laryngeal dose or percentage of volume receiving >50 Gy and neck stage were the only independent predictors of grade 2 or greater laryngeal edema. Vocal function is usually well preserved after radiotherapy for stage T1 laryngeal cancer[231] (typically 60 to 66 Gy). Less information is available regarding voice quality after treatment of more locally advanced laryngeal cancers. However, Dornfeld et al.[233] found a strong correlation between speech quality and the doses delivered to the aryepiglottic folds, preepiglottic space, false vocal cords, and lateral pharyngeal walls at the level of the false vocal cords. In particular, a steep decrease in vocal function was observed when the dose to these structures exceeded 66 Gy.

In a prospective study using intensity-modulated radiotherapy to reduce dysphagia in patients undergoing chemoradiation, Feng et al.[236] observed a strong correlation between the mean doses and the dysphagia end points (Fig. 14.6). Aspiration was observed when the mean dose to the pharyngeal constrictors was >60 Gy and the dose–volume threshold for the pharyngeal constrictor volume receiving ≥40, ≥50, ≥60, and ≥65 Gy was 90%, 80%, 70%, and >50%, respectively. For aspiration to occur, the glottic/supraglottic larynx dose–volume threshold was >50% of volume receiving ≥50 Gy. In a retrospective study of conventional radiotherapy, Jensen et al.[237] found that doses <60 Gy to the supraglottic area, larynx, and upper esophageal sphincter were associated with a low risk of aspiration. Dornfeld et al.[233] found that swallowing difficulties increased progressively with radiation doses >50 Gy to the aryepiglottic folds, false vocal cords, and lateral pharyngeal walls near the false cord.

Levendag et al.[238] reported that a median dose of 50 Gy to the superior and middle pharyngeal constrictor muscles predicted a 20% probability of dysphagia and that this increased significantly beyond a mean dose of 55 Gy. The V_{60-65} and mean inferior pharyngeal constrictors were most predictive of gastrostomy tube dependence in one study,[239] whereas V_{50}[240] and mean dose[240,241] of the middle pharyngeal constrictors were most predictive of dysphagia in other studies. In an analysis of 96 patients from Dana-Farber, the inferior pharyngeal constrictor V_{50} and larynx V_{50} were significantly associated with aspiration and stricture risk.[242] MDACC recommends a V_{55} < 80% and V_{65} < 30% for superior pharyngeal constrictors,[243] whereas UAB recommends V_{60} < 12% to the inferior pharyngeal constrictors, V_{65} < 75% to the middle pharyngeal constrictors, and V_{65} < 33% to the superior pharyngeal constrictors.[244]

Factors Affecting Risk

The addition of concurrent chemotherapy to high-dose RT appears to at least double the risk of laryngeal edema and

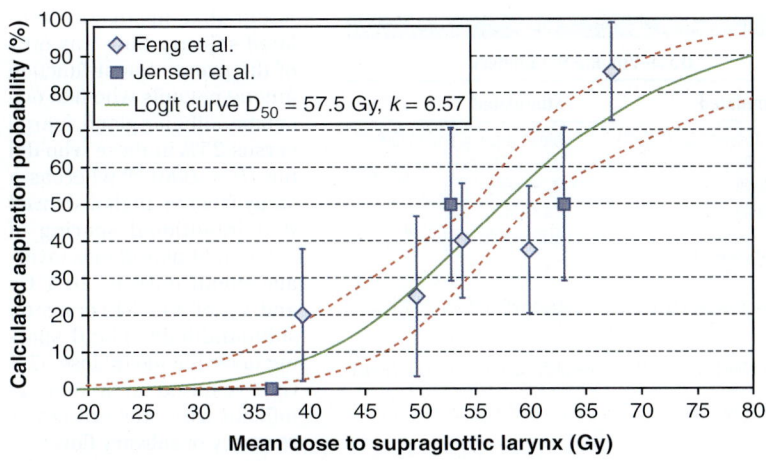

FIGURE 14.6. Probability of aspiration (proxy for dysphagia) versus larynx dose for selected studies.[236,237] *Solid line* fit of logit model to combined data; *dotted lines* represent 68% confidence area. (Reprinted from Rancati T, Schwarz M, Allen AM, et al. Radiation dose-volume effects in the larynx and pharynx. *Int J Radiat Oncol Biol Phys* 2010; 76[3 Suppl]:S64–S69. Copyright © 2010 Elsevier. With permission.[69])

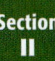

dysfunction.[231] Severe laryngeal dysfunction secondary to tumor will often persist following radiotherapy, and a laryngectomy may be preferred to chemoradiation in this setting.

Mathematic/Biologic Models

Rancati et al.[245] fit dose–volume data for grade 2 to 3 laryngeal edema using the Lyman-Kutcher-Burman model and the logit model with the DVH reduced to the equivalent uniform dose (EUD). Both models fit the clinical data well. The best fit parameters for the Lyman-Kutcher-Burman model were $n = 0.45 \pm 0.28$, $m = 0.16 \pm 0.05$, and $TD_{50} = 46.3 \pm 1.8$ Gy. Based on these findings, the investigators suggested an EUD of <30 to 35 Gy to reduce the risk of grade 2 to 3 laryngeal edema. The Feng et al. study[236] suggests that a 50% NTCP is observed at mean doses of 50 to 60 Gy to the pharyngeal constrictors and the larynx (Fig. 14.6).

Special Situations

Pretherapy vocal and swallowing function should be considered when assessing the functional response to radiation therapy of the larynx and pharynx.[246]

Recommended Dose–Volume Limits

To minimize the risk of laryngeal edema, the QUANTEC authors recommend limiting the mean noninvolved larynx dose to 40 to 45 Gy and the maximal dose to <63 to 66 Gy, if possible, according to the tumor extent.[231] Minimizing the volume of the pharyngeal constrictors and larynx receiving >60 Gy and reducing, when possible, the volume receiving >50 Gy is associated with reduced dysphagia/aspiration.[231] Of course, the impact of any such dose reduction on tumor control must be considered, given the uncertainties in target delineation.

Future Studies and Toxicity Scoring Criteria

Prospective studies that include pretherapy assessments of vocal and swallowing function should be conducted to correlate observer-rated scores such as the CTCAE v. 4.0 system,[92] patient-reported quality scores, and objective swallowing.[231] Such studies should focus on patients receiving concurrent chemoradiation, as this population is at the greatest risk of laryngeal/pharyngeal toxicity. Although CTCAE-based scoring is simple and widely utilized, objective measurement by a speech pathologist is often necessary to quantify swallowing dysfunction following radiotherapy.

Salivary Glands

Clinical Significance

In radiotherapy of head and neck tumors, the parotid, submandibular, and minor salivary glands often receive substantial doses of radiation. Reduced salivary production is a common toxicity and adversely affects the patient's quality of life. Inadequate salivary function leads to multiple problems, including poor dental hygiene, a propensity to oral infections, sleep disturbances, pain, and difficulty chewing and swallowing.[247] The majority of stimulated salivary production comes from the parotid glands, whereas resting (unstimulated) salivary production is due primarily to the submandibular, sublingual, and numerous small oral salivary glands.[248]

End Points

Xerostomia (dry mouth secondary to inadequate saliva production) can be assessed based on the patient's symptoms (altered taste or sensation of dryness) and/or quantitative saliva production.

Challenges Defining Volumes

Parotid and submandibular salivary glands can be adequately delineated on contrast-enhanced CT scans. However, during irradiation, parotid glands typically shrink during RT, potentially resulting in decreased gland sparing. For example, Robar et al.[249] found that while the medial position of the parotid gland was stable over a course of radiation therapy, the lateral borders shrank approximately 1 mm/wk, yielding total displacements of 4 to 6 mm.

Dose/Volume/Toxicity Data

A variety of dose–volume parameters have been correlated with salivary end points, including subjective xerostomia and objective stimulated/unstimulated salivary flow. In particular, mean parotid gland dose[249–252] appears associated with whole-mouth or individual gland salivary production. Table 14.8 summarizes the reported dose–volume predictors for salivary flow, the incidence of complications, and salivary function recovery. Minimal reduction in flow is observed at mean doses <10 to 15 Gy, decreases gradually over the range of 20 to 40 Gy, and is markedly reduced above 40 Gy.[250,254] The risk of xerostomia is reduced when at least one parotid gland or submandibular gland is spared.[255] In the study by Portaluri et al.,[256] patients receiving <30 Gy to the contralateral parotid reported either no or mild subjective xerostomia.

Some recovery of salivary function occurs over time, with the dose required to obtain an equivalent reduction in salivary flow increasing at longer follow-up times (Fig. 14.7).[252,255,257–260] The whole-mouth or ipsilateral salivary measurement-based tissue dose required for a 50% response (TD$_{50}$) tends to be lower than the scintigraphy-based TD$_{50}$, yielding a higher TD$_{50}$ compared with those derived from salivary flow data. The wide variation in the reported TD$_{50}$ values may be the result of several factors, including variations in dose distributions, salivary measurement methods, segmentation, and inherent tissue sensitivity.

Section II

TABLE 14.8 DOSIMETRIC PREDICTORS OF XEROSTOMIA

Reference	Patients (n)/ Follow-Up	Total Prescribed Target Dose (Gy)[a]	Dose–Volume Parameters	
			Unstimulated	Stimulated
Eisbruch et al.[253]	88/1–12 mo	58–72	Mean dose ≤ 22–25 Gy[b] $V_{15} < 66\%$ $V_{30} < 43\%$ $V_{45} < 26\%$	Mean dose ≤ 25–26 Gy[c] $V_{15} < 67\%$ $V_{30} < 45\%$ $V_{45} < 24\%$
Maes et al.[252]	39/1–4 mo	66–70	–	Mean dose ≤ 20 Gy[d]
Blanco et al.[250]	55/6 mo 29/12 mo	50–71	Mean dose < 25.8 Gy	–
Li et al.[251]	142/1–24 mo	60–75	Mean dose < 25–30 Gy	Mean dose < 25–30 Gy

[a]Treated at 1.5 to 2.0 Gy per fraction.
[b]24 Gy at 1 and 3 months, 22 Gy at 6 months, and 25 Gy at 12 months; threshold dose defined as mean dose above which saliva production appeared to abruptly approach zero.
[c]26 Gy at 1, 3, and 6 months, 25 Gy at 12 months; threshold dose defined as mean dose above which saliva production appeared to abruptly approach zero.
[d]Corresponds to probability of 70% that loss of salivary excretion fraction was <50%.
V_x, percentage of gland volume receiving >x Gy.

Factors Affecting Risk

Patient factors (e.g., gender and age) and the use of chemotherapy have typically not correlated with xerostomia risk. However, pretreatment salivary function and medications affecting salivary function can influence the risk of xerostomia.[247]

Mathematic/Biologic Models

As noted earlier, there is a wide variation in the observed dose/volume/toxicity relationship, depending on the patient population, treatment technique, and end point selected. Thus, models predicting the risk of xerostomia as a function of dose–volume parameters have yielded a broad range of parameters.[247,250,254,259,262,263] Because the glands seem to respond independently to irradiation, the function of the parotid glands should be modeled separately. NTCP modeling of 178 patients treated with IMRT showed that baseline salivary function and mean contralateral parotid gland dose were predictors for xerostomia and that mean contralateral submandibular gland dose, mean sublingual dose, and mean dose to minor salivary glands in the soft palate were predictive for sticky saliva.[264,265]

Attempts to predict the effect of fraction size on toxicity using the linear-quadratic model have returned low to high α/β ratios, perhaps because the different end points examined represent acute versus late effects.[247]

Special Situations

Submandibular gland sparing appears to reduce the risk of both stimulated and unstimulated xerostomia.[255] A Finnish study found that mean unstimulated salivary flow was 60% of the pretreatment function among patients who had one submandibular gland spared versus 25% in those who did not (P = .006),[266] whereas a study from Shanghai showed that intentional sparing of submandibular glands (average mean dose of 20.4 Gy and V_{30} of 14.7%) versus no submandibular gland sparing (average mean dose 57.4 Gy), resulted in a nonsignificant trend toward better recovery of salivary flow.[267]

The mean dose to the oral cavity (which contains minor salivary glands) has also been found to be an independent risk factor in some studies[261,268] but not others,[269] probably because of differences in technique. Although quantitative data are admittedly sparse, amifostine has been shown to increase the functional tolerance of the parotid and submandibular glands to therapeutic radiation.[270] Much of the existing data is derived from patients with oropharyngeal cancers being treated to ≈70 Gy. With the increasing incidence of HPV-associated oropharynx cancers, which appear to be more sensitive to therapy, lower doses of radiation (e.g., 60 Gy) are sometimes being used. Because the dosimetric parameters such as mean dose and V_x are likely surrogates for more complex 3D dose/volume distributions within the glands, the appropriate dose/volume constraints in the setting of a prescribed dose of 70 Gy may or may not be appropriate in the setting of a prescribed dose of 60 Gy.[271]

Recommended Dose–Volume Limits

Severe xerostomia (long-term salivary function <25% of baseline) can usually be avoided if at least one parotid gland receives a mean dose of less than about 20 Gy or if both glands receive a mean dose of less than approximately 25 Gy.[272,273] In patients with head and neck cancer treated with IMRT, the mean dose to each parotid gland should be kept as low as possible, taking into account the desired target coverage. Similarly, keeping the dose to the submandibular glands to modest levels (<35 Gy) may reduce the severity of xerostomia.[247]

Future Studies

Key questions on radiation-induced salivary gland dysfunction and xerostomia include the following:

1. Does partially sparing the submandibular glands or salivary minor glands have a positive impact on quality of life (QOL)?
2. Is the (arbitrary) 25% salivary threshold the best quantitative measure with respect to QOL?
3. Should parotid gland shrinkage during RT explicitly be accounted for in functional predictions?
4. How should submandibular sparing be incorporated into predictive salivary function models?
5. How does oral cavity sparing quantitatively affect xerostomia?
6. Does the radioprotector amifostine provide a clinically significant benefit for whole-mouth salivary function?
7. How does the use of lower tumor target doses (as are being increasingly suggested in patients with HPV-associated cancers) impact the dose/volume limits?

Toxicity Scoring Criteria

The QUANTEC authors recommend that an observer-based system (e.g., CTCAE v. 4.0) be supplemented by a validated quality of life instrument (e.g., the xerostomia questionnaire[261]) and/or quantitative salivary measurements.

FIGURE 14.7. Mean percentage of reduction in stimulated salivary flow rate versus mean parotid gland dose for selected studies[252,255,257–261] using different follow-up durations. Nominal follow-up intervals of 1, 6, and 12 months represent ranges of 1 to 1.5, 6 to 7, and 12 months, respectively. *Lines* represent least-squares fit of data for each nominal follow-up interval. (Reprinted from Deasy JO, Moiseenko V, Marks LB, et al. Radiotherapy dose-volume effects on salivary gland function. *Int J Radiat Oncol Biol Phys* 2010;76[3 Suppl]:S58–S63. Copyright © 2010 Elsevier. With permission.)

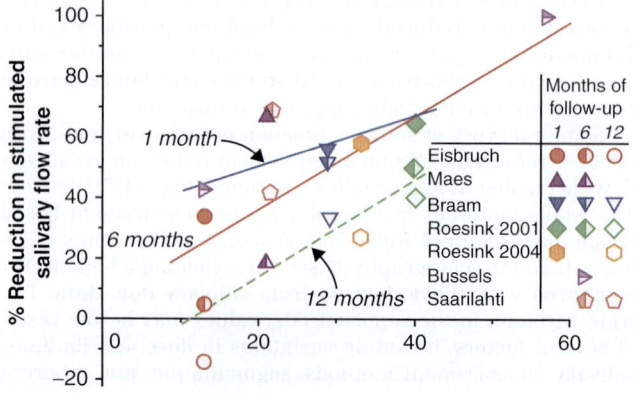

CHEST

Lung

Clinical Significance

The lung's primary function is the exchange of oxygen for carbon dioxide. Radiation-associated lung injury is one of the most common side effects seen in clinical oncology, and its risk limits the dose of radiation that can be used for treatment of thoracic tumors.

End Points

Radiation damage to the lung can result in symptomatic pneumonitis and fibrosis. Symptomatic radiation pneumonitis is characterized by dyspnea, cough, and occasionally a low-grade fever, typically occurring several weeks to months after radiation. Long-term lung fibrosis can lead to respiratory insufficiency. It is often challenging to distinguish radiation-related pulmonary symptoms from comorbid illnesses (e.g., exacerbation of chronic obstructive pulmonary disease, infection, cardiac events).[274] Objective reductions in the lungs' ability to move and exchange gas can be measured by formal pulmonary function tests (PFTs). The various end points shown in Table 14.9 are arbitrarily segregated by their manifestation (clinical vs. subclinical) and whether they reflect regional or global lung function.

Challenges Defining Volumes

Because the lungs move and their volume changes with respiration, there are inherent inaccuracies when defining the lung volume. As the mass of the lung is relatively constant during respiration and its density must decline with increased lung volumes, one could consider using dose–mass histograms

TABLE 14.9 END POINTS FOR RADIATION-INDUCED LUNG INJURY

| Manifestation | Geographic Distribution | |
	Regional	Global
Clinical	Symptomatic bronchial stenosis	Respiratory symptoms (dyspnea, cough)
Subclinical	Radiologic abnormalities (computed tomography, perfusion/ventilation scans)	Pulmonary function tests, exercise testing results

rather than DVHs. To our knowledge, this approach has not been widely applied. Because of this variation in volumes with respiration, it is very likely that the dose/volume/outcome data are dependent on the type (if any) of respiratory control. The vast majority of dose/volume/outcome data are derived from free-breathing scans/treatment. These may not apply to patients being treated under, for example, breath hold techniques. Further, there are uncertainties in defining the lung borders in the vicinity of the central airways. Variable inclusion of the conducting airways in the "defined lung" can influence interpatient/institutional comparisons.

Dose/Volume/Toxicity Data

Several parameters have been shown to be associated with the risk of radiation pneumonitis, including V_5 to V_{70}, mean lung dose (MLD), and model-based parameters.[9,275] These dosimetric parameters are mutually correlated, accounting for the fact that in most studies examining a range of V_x's, many appear statistically significant.[276–291] Figure 14.8 summarizes the studies discussed here.

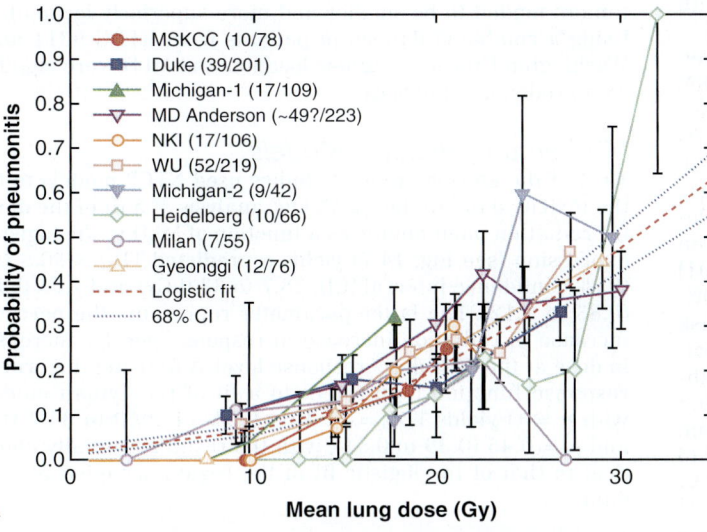

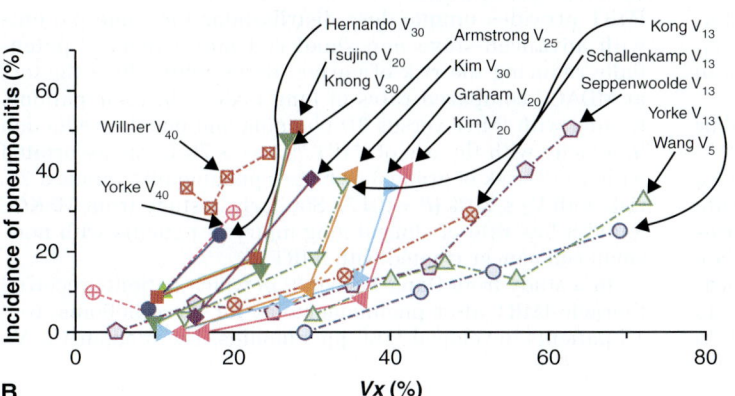

FIGURE 14.8. The rate of radiation pneumonitis after fractionated partial lung radiotherapy as a function of **(A)** mean lung dose (MLD) and **(B)** lung volume receiving x Gy (V_x). **A:** MLD: Confidence intervals (*bars*) represent ± 1 standard deviation. Results from Memorial Sloan-Kettering Cancer Center (MSKCC),[290] Radiation Therapy Oncology Group (RTOG) grade 3 or higher pulmonary toxicity at 6 months; Duke,[279] Common Terminology Criteria for Adverse Events (CTCAE) grade 1 or higher at 6 months; Michigan,[292] Southwest Oncology Group (SWOG) grade 2 or higher at 6 months; M.D. Anderson Cancer Center,[287] CTCAE grade 3 or higher, 1 year actuarial—includes concurrent chemotherapy patients; Netherlands Cancer Institute (NKI),[293] SWOG grade 2 or higher at 6 months; Washington University (WU),[280] SWOG grade 2 or higher; Michigan,[294] SWOG grade 1 or higher; Heidelberg,[295] RTOG acute grade 1 or higher; Milan,[296] SWOG grade 2 or higher, no time limit, patients without chronic obstructive pulmonary disease, includes induction chemotherapy patients; Gyeonggi,[281] RTOG grade 3 or higher at 6 months, includes concurrent chemotherapy patients. Dashed line is best fit of these data fit to the logistic expression of the form $[f/(1 + f)]$, where $f = \exp(b0 + b1 * MLD)$. Best fit values (95% confidence intervals) are b0 = −3.87 (−3.33, −4.49) and b1 = 0.126 (0.100, 0.153), corresponding to TD$_{50}$ = 30.75 (28.7, 33.9) Gy and γ_{50} = 0.969 (0.833, 1.122), where γ_{50} represents the increase in response (measured as percentage) per 1% increase in dose around the 50% dose–response level. **B:** V_x: Data from Yorke,[290] Willner,[288] Hernando,[279] Tsujino,[298] Kong,[292] Armstrong,[299] Kim,[281] Graham,[275] Seppenwoolde,[285] Wang,[287] and Schallenkamp.[284] Some of the above data were modified or derived from the original publications, as described in Marks et al.[100] (Reprinted from Marks LB, Bentzen SM, Deasy JO, et al. Radiation dose-volume effects in the lung. *Int J Radiat Oncol Biol Phys* 2010;76[3 Suppl]:S70–S76. Copyright © 2010 Elsevier. With permission.)

A NTCP analysis from the Netherlands, in collaboration with the University of Michigan, suggests that using the MLD (linear function) is more predictive than using V_x (step function).[285] However, V_{13} tended to be more predictive in situations where the MLD exceeded 20 Gy or V_{13} exceeded 50%. The TD_{50} values in this study were an MLD of 30.8 Gy, $V_{13} > 77\%$, and $V_{20} > 65\%$, similar to the MLD of 31.8 Gy reported in an earlier multi-institutional study.[282] From a study at the Memorial Sloan-Kettering Cancer Center (MSKCC),[291] a MLD of approximately 26 Gy, V_{13} of >80% to the ipsilateral lung, or V_{40} of >32% to the lower lung results in a 50% risk of developing late complications. A MLD of approximately 12 Gy or a V_{13} of >40% to the ipsilateral lung results in a 5% late complication risk. A V_{13} of 36% to the lower lung, 42% to the total lung, or 62% to the ipsilateral lung results in a 20% risk of developing late grade 3 or higher complications.

Another study from MSKCC of patients treated with radiation alone reported a significantly increased risk of grade 3 or higher pulmonary toxicity, 38% for $V_{25} > 30\%$ versus 4% for $V_{25} < 30\%$ ($P = .04$).[276] In subsequent studies from this same group, significant variables for predicting grade 3 or higher pulmonary toxicity include MLD, the range of V_5 to V_{40} of total lung, V_5 to V_{40} of ipsilateral lung, and V_5 to V_{50} of lower lung.[290,291] The range of V_5 to V_{20} ipsilateral lung was most predictive.

Washington University was another of the early investigators to show that the risk of pneumonitis significantly correlates with the V_{20}; the 2-year incidence of grade 2 or higher radiation pneumonitis was 36%, 13%, 7%, and 0% with a V_{20} of >40%, 32% to 40%, 22% to 31%, and <22% ($P = .0013$), respectively.[275] In another study by Washington University, radiation pneumonitis was significantly correlated with V_5 to V_{80}, with peak significance in the V_5 to V_{15} and V_{70} to V_{75} ranges; radiation pneumonitis was also significantly correlated with the dose delivered to 5% to 100% of the lung (D_5 to D_{100}), with peak significance in the D_{30} to D_{40} and V_{90} to V_{95} ranges.[280]

A study from Duke, in which 18% of patients received concurrent chemoradiotherapy, found that a V_{30} of >18% versus <18% was associated with a risk of grade 1 or higher radiation pneumonitis of 24 versus 6% ($P = .0003$).[279] MLDs of <10, 10 to 20, 21 to 30, and >30 Gy were associated with risks of 10%, 16%, 27%, and 44%, respectively. A Japanese study of patients treated with platinum-based chemoradiotherapy found a 6-month risk of grade 2 or higher radiation pneumonitis to be 85%, 51%, 18.3%, and 8.7% ($P < .0001$) with a V_{20} of ≥31%, 26% to 30%, 21% to 25%, and ≤20%, respectively.[298] In a University of Michigan study, a 10% risk for grade 2 or higher pneumonitis and fibrosis was associated with a V_{20} of >30% and an MLD of >20 Gy. These thresholds provided a positive predictive value of 50% to 71% and a negative predictive value of 85% to 89%.[292] In a study from M.D. Anderson Cancer Center (MDACC), the MLD and V_5 to V_{65} were highly correlated with risk of pneumonitis, and V_5 was the most significant factor in a multivariate analysis.[287] For a $V_5 \le 42\%$ versus >42%, the risk of grade 3 or higher pneumonitis at 1 year was 3% versus 38% ($P = .001$). In a Mayo Clinic study, V_{10} to V_{13} was most predictive of radiation pneumonitis; a $V_{10} = 32\%$ to 43%, $V_{13} = 29\%$ to 39%, $V_{15} = 27\%$ to 34%, and $V_{20} = 21\%$ to 31% resulted in a 10% to 20% risk of pneumonitis.

Several dose escalation studies have used V_{20}, V_{eff}, and/or NTCP to stratify the risk of toxicity as a function of dose.[301-304] In the RTOG 9311 dose escalation study,[301] patients with a V_{20} of <25% experienced a 7% to 16% 18-month actuarial rate of grade 3 or higher late lung toxicity with prescribed doses of 70.9 to 90.3 Gy; the absolute risk of grade 2 or higher late lung toxicity was 30% to 45%, with one fatal lung complication at the 90.3 Gy dose level. Patients with a V_{20} of 25% to 36% treated to doses of 70.9 to 77.4 Gy experienced 15%

grade 3 or higher late toxicity at 18 months and a 40% to 60% risk of grade 2 or higher late lung toxicity. D_{15} was the most predictive variable for radiation pneumonitis.[277]

Factors Affecting Risk

Recent meta-analyses have shown that patient-related adverse risk factors for radiation pneumonitis among NSCLC[305-307] and breast cancer[308] patients include older age,[305,306] history of chronic lung disease, or diabetes.[307] Smoking was an adverse risk factor in one meta-analysis,[307] whereas not being an active or prior smoker[305] was an adverse risk factor in another, a discrepancy that is attributed to the complexity of the relationship between smoking, chronic lung disease, and pneumonitis.[307] Chemotherapy concurrent with radiation therapy,[307] particularly carboplatin/paclitaxel chemotherapy,[306] has been reported to increase the pneumonitis risk.

The effect of dose to regions of the lung was investigated in a Dutch study,[293] dividing the lung into central and peripheral, ipsilateral and contralateral, caudal and cranial, and anterior and posterior subvolumes. The mean regional doses to the posterior, caudal, ipsilateral, central, and peripheral lung subvolumes were significantly correlated with the incidence of steroid-requiring radiation pneumonitis. In a similar study from MSKCC, the risk of radiation pneumonitis was better correlated with the radiation dose to the inferior, as opposed to the superior, aspect of the lung.[291]

Tumor location within the chest may also be a factor affecting risk of pneumonitis. In the study from Washington University,[280] inferior tumor location was the most significant predictor of radiation pneumonitis. Tumor location was not a strong correlate with radiation pneumonitis in RTOG 9311, perhaps attributable, in part, to differences in treatment (with RTOG 9311 treating smaller volumes to higher doses) and differences in tumor size and location (the RTOG 9311 tumors tended to be smaller and more superiorly located).[277] Using a combined dataset of patients from RTOG 9311 and Washington University, tumor location and MLD were significant predictors of toxicity.

Mathematic/Biologic Models

Most of the aforementioned studies used NTCP models to fit the toxicity data. In the QUANTEC analysis,[300] a fit of the data for radiation pneumonitis as a function of MLD to the logistic expression (see Fig. 14.7) yields a predicted $TD_{50} = 30.8$ Gy (95% confidence interval [CI], 28.7 to 33.9 Gy) and $\gamma_{50} = 0.97$ (0.83 to 1.12). The latter parameter represents the percent increase in radiation increase in response per 1% increase in dose at the 50% dose–response level. A fit using the probit response function (equivalent to a fit of the Lyman model with $n = 1$) yields $TD_{50} = 31.4$ Gy (95% CI, 29.0 to 34.7 Gy) and $m = 0.45$ (0.39 to 0.51), with the result essentially identical to that of the logistic fit in the region occupied by the data.

Special Situations

IMRT provides unique dose distributions for some patients with advanced-stage non–small cell lung cancer,[309] potentially reducing the risk of normal tissue injury. Investigators at MDACC compared rates of lung toxicity in their patients treated with IMRT versus 3D planning and noted a reduction in toxicity with the use of IMRT.[310] A $V_5 > 70\%$ was associated with a 21% risk of grade 3 or higher pneumonitis versus a 2% risk with $V_5 \le 70\%$ ($P = .017$). Similarly, a study from MSKCC found a low rate of clinical lung injury in patients with non–small cell cancer treated with IMRT.[311]

In a study from Dana-Farber,[312] in which patients received thoracic IMRT after pneumonectomy for mesothelioma, 6 of 13 patients developed fatal pneumonitis. The median V_{20}, V_5, and MLD for patients who developed pneumonitis was 17.6%, 98.6%, and 15.2 Gy, respectively, versus 10.9%, 90%, and 12.9 Gy for those who did not develop pneumonitis. Although these differences were not significant, the severity of the toxicities suggests caution in treating patients to large volumes after a pneumonectomy. In a study from Duke,[313] 1 of 13 patients treated with IMRT for mesothelioma died from pneumonitis, and two others developed symptomatic pneumonitis. The median V_{20}, V_5, and MLD for patients developing pneumonitis were 2.3%, 92%, and 7.9 Gy, respectively, versus 0.2%, 66%, and 7.5 Gy for those who did not develop pneumonitis and 6.9%, 92%, and 11.4 Gy for the patient who developed fatal pneumonitis. In a study of mesothelioma patients treated at MDACC,[314] 6 of 63 died from pulmonary-related causes (including two patients with fatal pneumonitis). The V_{20} was significant on univariate and multivariate analyses ($P = .017$), with $V_{20} > 7\%$ corresponding to a 42-fold increase in the risk of pulmonary death.

Stereotactic body radiotherapy (SBRT) generally involves a few large fractions (e.g., three 18-Gy or five 10-Gy fractions) given over 5 to 20 days.[315–317] Typically, the high-dose volumes in SBRT are small and dose gradients steep, minimizing dose to surrounding critical structures. However, because multiple beams are used, large volumes of lung receive low to medium doses.[317] Consequently, the dose–volume characteristics of lung SBRT are quite different from those of conventional RT and deserve special consideration. Radiation pneumonitis is relatively uncommon after SBRT, usually <10%[316,318,319] but as high as 25% in one study.[320] Bronchial injury/stenosis, an unusual complication with conventional dose fractionation,[321] has been associated with SBRT to perihilar/central tumors.[316]

A recent review from Zhao et al.[322] suggests that the risk of RT-associated lung injury was <10% to 15% after lung SBRT with a MLD of the combined lungs <8 Gy, and the percent of total lung volume receiving more than 20 Gy (V_{20}) <10% to 15%. Patients with interstitial lung disease appear to be especially susceptible to severe radiation-associated lung toxicity.

Recommended Dose–Volume Limits

Individual studies note a dose–response relationship for radiation pneumonitis based on a variety of metrics. However, the QUANTEC analysis[300] of the pooled data shows that there is no specific threshold for pneumonitis, with risks increasing gradually as dose increases. Because many dose–volume parameters of the lung (i.e., V_5 through V_{30}, MLD) are correlated with each other, there likely is not an "optimal" parameter. For patients with non–small cell lung cancer, it is prudent to limit the V_{20} to <30% to 35%, and the MLD to <20 to 23 Gy, in order to reduce the risk of pneumonitis to <20%. In patients irradiated after pneumonectomy for mesothelioma, it is prudent to limit the V_5 to below 60%, V_{20} to <4% to 10%, and the MLD to <8 Gy.

Future Studies

Radiation-induced pneumonitis appears more commonly in patients with lower versus upper lobe tumors and may be better correlated with radiation doses to the lower versus upper lung. The cause of this correlation is presently unknown and requires further investigation, though it may be related to heart irradiation. Additional work is needed to better understand the impact of clinical factors (e.g., preradiotherapy functional status, tobacco use) and systemic agents (e.g., chemotherapy) on the risk of lung injury. Studies aimed at determining and exploiting the ability of biomarkers such as TGF-β (measured before and/or during lung radiotherapy) on radiation pneumonitis would be valuable.

Toxicity Scoring Criteria

The LENT–SOMA system should be used for scoring toxicity as it explicitly captures symptomatic, functional, and radiographic end points. A global score can be generated, but the granular data should be recorded and maintained.

Heart

Clinical Significance

The heart is a muscular organ typically located in the left hemithorax, which, via continuous rhythmic contraction, pumps blood throughout the blood vessels. The functional and structural complexity of the heart places it at risk for a spectrum of radiation and chemotherapy injuries that can manifest months to years following therapy.[323]

End Points

All components of the heart and pericardium are susceptible to radiation damage. Radiation-induced cardiac injury includes pericarditis, congestive heart failure, restrictive cardiomyopathy, valvular insufficiency and stenosis, coronary artery disease, ischemia, and infarction.

Challenges Defining Volumes

The substructures of the heart, as well as the intersection/border of the heart, great vessels, liver, diaphragm, and stomach, can be challenging to delineate on CT imaging. The heart moves during the respiratory and cardiac cycles, with different regions moving to different degrees. The uncertainties that accompany these anatomic/physiologic realities must be considered when contouring targets and normal tissue structures and when interpreting DVHs.

Dose/Volume/Toxicity Data

Multiple studies show an increased risk of cardiac morbidity following left-sided versus right-sided thoracic radiation in patients undergoing treatment for breast cancer. It is generally recognized that reducing the dose prescribed to the mediastinum and reducing the volume of heart in the radiation field reduce the risk of late toxicity.[324–326] Recent studies from Duke demonstrated that an increased percentage of the left ventricle irradiated correlates with a greater risk of cardiac perfusion defects.[327–329] Even over the range of low-dose exposure (~8 to 20 Gy) to small volumes of the cardiac apex, an increased risk of heart disease has been reported.[330]

A study from Stockholm used NTCP modeling to predict the risk of late heart toxicity in women treated for breast cancer.[331] The models predicted a TD_{50} of 52 Gy for dose to the myocardium. A 5% risk of excess cardiac mortality at 15 years was associated with a myocardial dose of approximately 30 Gy, $V_{33} > 60\%$, $V_{38} > 33\%$, or $V_{42} > 20\%$. Calculations using the whole-heart volume (as opposed to myocardium) yielded equivalent results.

The same group from Stockholm used a similar analysis to assess cardiac risk in Hodgkin disease patients.[332] Patients were stratified based on a $V_{38} > 35\%$ versus <35%. The excess mortality risk at 15 years was 7.9% and 4.7%, respectively. The TD_{50} was calculated to be 70 Gy. Heart doses of 42 and 53 Gy resulted in a 5% and 10% risk of cardiac complications, respectively. The corresponding values in the breast cancer patients were 37 and 44 Gy, respectively (lower threshold doses and steeper gradient). The differences in complication probabilities and TD_{50} between the breast cancer and Hodgkin disease cohorts (Fig. 14.9) suggest that radiation exposure to different portions of the heart results in differences in cardiac risk, though there may be other confounding variables (i.e., patient age at treatment, overlapping breast cancer, cardiac disease risk factors, etc.).

Section II

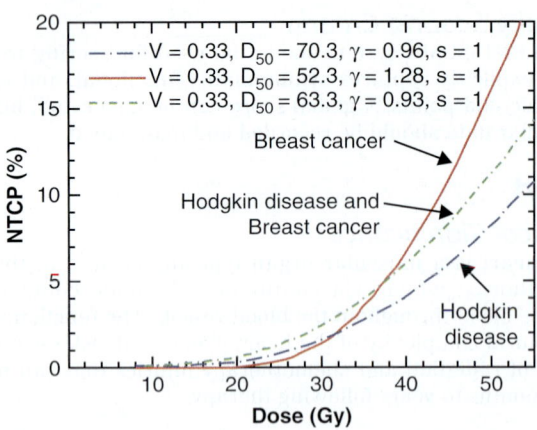

FIGURE 14.9. Dose–response curves for long-term cardiac mortality in patients with Hodgkin disease (HD) and breast cancer treated with thoracic radiotherapy. NTCP = normal tissue complication probability, defined in that study as the excessive risk of ischemic heart disease. *Curves were obtained by fitting data from breast cancer trials, a cohort of patients with Hodgkin disease, and the combined dataset. Plotted curves correspond to uniform irradiation of one-third of the heart volume.* (Reprinted from Eriksson F, Gagliardi G, Liedberg A, et al. Long-term cardiac mortality following radiation therapy for Hodgkin's disease: analysis with the relative seriality model. *Radiother Oncol* 2000;55[2]:153–162. Copyright © 2000 Elsevier Science Ireland Ltd. With permission.)

A study from MDACC described the risk of pericardial effusions in patients treated for esophageal cancer.[333] A mean dose >26 Gy and relative volumes of the pericardium treated at doses >3 to 50 Gy (V_3 to V_{50}) showed the greatest risk, with the association strongest at V_{30}. For $V_{30} < 46\%$ versus >46%, the rate of pericardial effusion was 73% versus 13% ($P = .001$) 18 months postradiation. For a mean pericardium dose <26 versus >26 Gy, the rate of pericardial effusion was 73% versus 13% ($P = .001$). A study from the University of Michigan[334] also demonstrated that a mean dose >27 Gy and a maximum dose of 47 Gy correlated with risk of pericardial effusion. However, only patients treated with 3.5-Gy fractions developed pericardial effusions.

The incidence of valvular disease has been related to mediastinal radiation doses >30 Gy and younger age at irradiation.[335] Subclinical valvular disease has been detected at 2 to 20+ years postradiation, but it appears to take much longer for clinical symptoms to become apparent (median interval 22 years from radiation to symptoms). For patients treated for Hodgkin lymphoma more than 10 years prior with radiation, aortic disease, usually consisting of mixed stenosis and regurgitation, is more common than mitral and right-sided valvular disease.[335,336]

Factors Affecting Risk and Special Situations

Anthracycline chemotherapy can exacerbate radiation-elated cardiac toxicity. In Hodgkin disease patients, radiation exposure, in conjunction with anthracyclines, may impair ejection fraction and increase risk of myocardial infarction, congestive heart failure, and valvular disorders. A Dutch study[337] of 1,474 Hodgkin lymphoma survivors showed that risks of myocardial infarction and congestive heart failure were significantly increased, with standard incidence ratios of 3.6 and 4.9, respectively, for these survivors versus the general population. Mediastinal radiation alone increases the risks of myocardial infarction, angina pectoris, congestive heart failure, and valvular disorders (two- to sevenfold). The addition of anthracyclines further elevated the risks of congestive heart failure and valvular disorders, with hazard ratios of 2.81 and 2.10, respectively. The 25-year cumulative incidence of congestive heart failure following combined radiation and anthracycline chemotherapy was 7.9%.

Other risk factors for cardiac disease, particularly coronary artery disease, also must be considered. For example, a University of Rochester study[338] assessed the risk of coronary artery disease in survivors of Hodgkin lymphoma and also the prevalence of cardiac risk factors. The relative risk of cardiac death was 3.1 for males versus 1.8 for females. Other risk factors were more common than in the general population; among patients with Hodgkin lymphoma experiencing morbid cardiac events, 72% smoked, 72% were male, 78% had hypercholesterolemia, 61% were obese, 28% had a positive family history, 33% had hypertension, and 6% had diabetes.

Evolving data from patients irradiated for breast or lung cancer suggest that RT-associated cardiac injury may occur earlier than previously believed (i.e., within a few years of RT).[339–342] For example, in patients with non–small cell lung cancer prescribed to receive >70 Gy, the mean heart dose and preexisting cardiac disease have been implicated as predictors for cardiac injury[342]; the 2-year competing risk–adjusted cardiac event rates for patients with heart mean doses <10 Gy, 10 to 20 Gy, or ≥20 Gy were 4%, 7%, and 21%, respectively.

Mathematic/Biologic Models

There are no well-accepted models for cardiac toxicities. Nevertheless, several authors have computed model parameters for various cardiac end points, as summarized in the QUANTEC review.[323]

Recommended Dose–Volume Limits

A heart V_{30} to V_{40} of approximately 30% to 35% is associated with an approximately 5% excess risk of cardiac death at approximately 15 years. A heart V_{30} of >45% and a mean cardiac dose of >26 Gy are associated with a higher risk of pericarditis. In patients with breast and lung cancer, it is recommended that the irradiated heart volume be minimized as much as possible without compromising target coverage. In patients with lymphoma, the whole heart should be limited to 30 Gy if treated with radiation alone and to 15 Gy for patients also receiving anthracycline chemotherapy. Although there is no direct evidence that eliminating traditional cardiac risk factors alters the natural history of radiation-associated cardiac disease, it seems prudent to minimize such factors.[323,343,344]

Future Studies

Issues that would benefit from further systematic study are the effects of radiation on specific subvolumes of the heart, the impact of modern radiotherapy techniques on cardiac toxicity, the relationship between heart irradiation and baseline cardiovascular risk factors on the development of cardiac disease, the effect of hypofractionation encountered in thoracic SBRT, and the global physiologic effects of thoracic radiotherapy (e.g., interactions between simultaneous heart and lung irradiation).[323]

Toxicity Scoring Criteria

The QUANTEC authors recommend that the LENT–SOMA system[94,345] be considered to describe cardiac toxicity, as it explicitly includes clinical, radiologic, and functional assessments of cardiac dysfunction.

Esophagus

Clinical Significance

Acute esophagitis is very common and often severe in patients receiving radiation for intrathoracic malignancies (e.g., primary lung cancer and esophageal cancer). Patients with severe esophagitis may require a feeding tube and/or treatment interruptions.

End Points

Because most patients with thoracic cancers have a poor prognosis, acute toxicity may be considered more clinically relevant than late injury. Late esophageal complications include dysphagia, stricture, dysmotility, odynophagia, and rarely necrosis or fistula.

Challenges Defining Volumes

The esophagus can be challenging to visualize on axial imaging, and the use of dilute oral contrast can assist in its identification. Also, the esophagus often has folds such that its external contour as seen on an axial image may not accurately represent its true circumference. Indeed, in CT imaging, the circumference of the esophagus appears highly variable on different axial levels, when in fact the esophagus has a relatively uniform circumference. One study has suggested that the dosimetric parameters that apply this prior anatomic knowledge are better predictors of acute and late esophageal injury than are traditional dosimetric parameters.[346]

Dose/Volume/Toxicity Data

A variety of dose–volume parameters have been associated with the incidence of esophagitis.[333,347-384] Although a continuous dose–response curve for acute esophagitis is observed based on a range of dosimetric parameters, as shown in Figure 14.10, there is no consensus as to the optimal dosimetric predictors of esophageal injury.

In a series from Washington University, grade 3 to 5 esophageal toxicity (acute and late) was associated with a maximal dose (D_{max}) of >58 Gy, a mean dose of >34 Gy, and the administration of concurrent chemotherapy.[353] The V_{55} was not significant. A study from China reported that maximal dose >60 Gy, as well as the use of concurrent chemotherapy, was a significant factor for esophageal toxicity (acute and late).[352] In a study from Duke, V_{50}, the surface dose receiving ≥50 Gy (S_{50}), the length of esophagus receiving >50 to 60 Gy, and a circumferential D_{max} > 80 Gy were significant predictors of late esophageal toxicity.[351] A V_{50} > 32% or an S_{50} > 32% resulted in crude rates of approximately 30% late esophageal toxicity versus 7% below these thresholds. With >3.2 cm of the esophagus receiving >50 Gy, late toxicity occurred in approximately 30%, versus 4% in those with <3.2 cm receiving >50 Gy (P = .008).

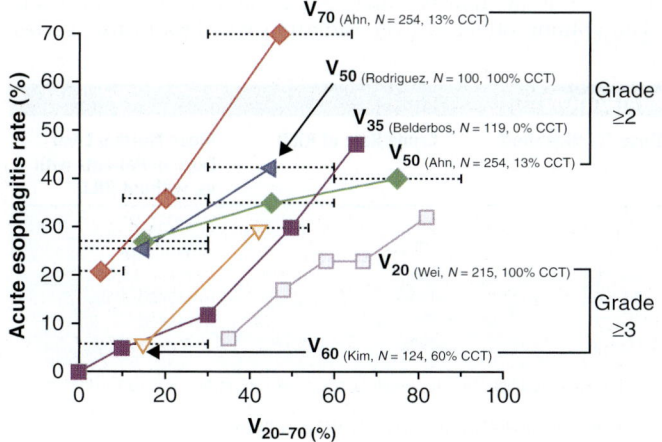

FIGURE 14.10. Incidence of acute esophagitis according to V_x (volume receiving more than x Gy) for selected studies. *X*-axis values estimated from range of doses reported. Datasets annotated as follows: V_{dose} (investigator, number of patients, percentage with concurrent chemotherapy [CCT]). (Reprinted from Werner-Wasik M, Yorke E, Deasy J, et al. Radiation Dose-Volume Effects in the Esophagus. *Int J Radiat Oncol Biol Phys* 2010;76[3]:S86–S93. Copyright © 2010 Elsevier. With permission.)

In another study from Duke, grade 1 or higher late toxicity was correlated with several dose parameters: the entire circumference receiving ≥50 Gy and ≥55 Gy; 75% of the circumference receiving ≥70 Gy; and maximal percentage of circumference receiving ≥60 to 80 Gy.[347] The rate of grade 1 or higher late toxicity was approximately 5% in patients with a V_{50} to V_{70} of 0% to 30% versus approximately 25% in those with a V_{70} of 31% to 64% and approximately 10% in those with a V_{50} > 60% (nonsignificant). Acute esophageal toxicity was the greatest predictor of late toxicity. In two studies, most of the patients who developed late grade 3 or higher toxicity had developed acute grade 3 or higher toxicity, though roughly 25% to 40% of patients who developed grade 3 or higher late toxicity had only grade 0 to 2 acute esophageal toxicity.[352,353]

A 2013 meta-analysis (published after QUANTEC) of 1,082 NSCLC patients treated with chemoradiation analyzed esophageal V_5 to V_{70} parameters (in 5 Gy increments); all significant predictors of grade ≥2 esophagitis and on multivariate analyses V_{60} proved to be the most significant predictor of grade ≥2 to 3 esophagitis (PMID 24035329). Recursive partitioning identified 3 risk groups: low (29% and 4% risk of grade ≥2 and ≥3 esophagitis with V_{60} < 0.07%), intermediate (41% and 10% risk of grade ≥2 and ≥3 esophagitis with V_{60} 0.07% to 17%), and high (59% and 22% risk of grade ≥2 and ≥3 esophagitis with V_{60} ≥ 17%).

Factors Affecting Risk

Greater rates of acute esophagitis have been observed with more aggressive radiotherapy regimens (e.g., hyperfractionation, concurrent boost), the addition of concurrent chemotherapy, increasing age, and several other clinical factors (e.g., preexisting dysphagia, increasing nodal stage). The incidence of grade 3 or higher acute esophagitis is approximately 1% for patients treated with once-daily radiotherapy alone versus as high as 49% with concurrent gemcitabine. Several studies have assessed the putative radioprotector amifostine. Three single-institution phase III studies suggested a benefit for amifostine in reducing the rate of grade 2 or higher esophagitis, but this result was not confirmed in a large cooperative group phase III randomized trial (RTOG trial 9801).[355-358]

Mathematic/Biologic Models

Using data on grade 2 or higher acute esophagitis, two studies obtained relatively consistent estimates of Lyman-Kutcher-Burman model parameters, including TD_{50} of 47 to 51 Gy.[7,348] Note that these parameters differ significantly from those derived from the Emami data,[4] which examined a more clinically severe end point (stricture and perforation).

Special Situations

Esophageal toxicity data for hypofractionated treatments in SBRT to central thoracic lesions are quite limited,[359] and long-term data in this and other altered fractionation settings (e.g., accelerated fraction and concomitant boosts) have not been comprehensively reported.[360]

Recommended Dose–Volume Limits

Given the available data, there are no strict dose–volume limits for the esophagus. Several parameters are associated with the risk of adverse events, and clinicians can apply these data as seems reasonable for the clinical situation. Unfortunately, the anatomic reality for many patients with locally advanced non–small cell lung cancer is that the PTV (and certainly the GTV) is often immediately adjacent to the esophagus, and thus, it is not possible to limit the doses as desired without compromising target coverage. The ongoing phase III intergroup trial, RTOG 0617, has recommended (but has not mandated) that the mean dose to the esophagus be kept to <34 Gy.

Future Studies

IMRT may provide increased flexibility in sparing the esophagus during lung irradiation,[385] and outcome as function of dose–volume should be systematically studied for this treatment technique. As in other organ systems, detailed outcome and dosimetric data should be reported, based on clearly defined methods of contouring the target and organs at risk.

Toxicity Scoring Criteria

Esophageal toxicities should be scored using the CTCAE v. 4.0.[37]

ABDOMEN/PELVIS

Liver

Clinical Significance

The liver is a vital organ, involved in the metabolism of ingested nutrients, detoxification, protein synthesis, bile production, glycogen storage, and red blood cell decomposition. The liver may be incidentally irradiated during radiation therapy of abdominal or thoracic tumors and will be irradiated in patients undergoing partial hepatic radiation for liver metastases or hepatocellular carcinoma. There is no effective treatment to reverse the process of radiation-induced liver disease (RILD); therefore, prophylaxis and prevention are best. Anticoagulants, paracentesis, and diuretics can be used to mitigate symptoms, whereas liver transplantation is required for frank radiation hepatopathy.

End Points

RILD generally presents as vague to intense right upper abdominal pain followed by abdominal swelling because of hepatomegaly and ascites, resulting in weight gain. Anicteric ascites often develops 2 to 4 months after irradiation; chemoradiation-induced liver disease may occur more rapidly (e.g., 1 to 4 weeks post radiation therapy in a bone marrow transplantation setting). Other sequelae of RILD include elevation of liver enzymes, jaundice, asterixis (tremor), encephalopathy, or coma.

The basic pathophysiologic sequelae of classic RILD is central vein thrombosis at the lobular level, which results in retrograde congestion leading to hemorrhage and secondary alterations in surrounding hepatocytes. This often occurs between 2 weeks and 3 months after therapy. Severe acute hepatic changes often progress to fibrosis or cirrhosis and liver failure.

Nonclassic RILD implies dramatic elevations of liver transaminases (greater than five times the upper limit) or decline in liver function in the absence of classic RILD. The underlying pathology of nonclassic RILD is unclear.[361]

Challenges Defining Volumes

The liver is readily identified on CT and MRI. For radiation planning, it must be recognized that the liver moves with the respiratory cycle.[361]

Dose/Volume/Toxicity Data

The liver parenchyma is composed of innumerable, redundant, parallel functional subunits, which allows the liver to potentially tolerate focal injury without clinical sequelae if adequate normal liver parenchyma can be spared.

In a study of 79 patients treated with liver radiotherapy at the University of Michigan, 9 of 33 patients who received whole-liver radiotherapy developed late radiation toxicity versus none of 46 who underwent partial liver radiation.[362] Several studies have explored partial liver radiation in more detail, many of which used mean liver dose as a dose–volume metric (Table 14.10). In a series from Taipei, patients with irradiated hepatocellular carcinoma who developed late liver toxicity had received a mean hepatic dose of 25 Gy (vs. 20 Gy in patients without toxicity, $P = .02$).[371] In a Korean study of 105 patients with hepatocellular carcinoma, the mean dose and V_{20} to V_{40} parameters to total liver and normal liver (total liver minus GTV) were investigated.[370] The total liver V_{30} was the only significant parameter ($P < .001$). Grade 2 or higher liver toxicity was observed in only 2.4% of patients with a total liver V_{30} of approximately 60% and 55% of patients with a total liver V_{30} of >60% ($P < .001$).

Factors Affecting Risk and Mathematic/Biologic Models

A wide variety of agents have been reported to elevate liver enzymes: nitrosoureas (BCNU), methotrexate, and some combinations of chemotherapy agents such as cyclophosphamide, doxorubicin, vincristine, and prednisone (CHOP) and proMace-MOPP (prednisone, methotrexate, doxorubicin, cyclophosphamide, etoposide, and MOPP). In bone marrow transplantation, preparatory regimens can be toxic.

As described earlier, the dose to partial liver volumes can impact the risk of RILD. Several studies have used NTCP modeling to help predict risks. In a study from University of Michigan, no late liver toxicity was observed with a mean liver dose <31 Gy, with NTCP models being optimized with a TD_{50} of 43 Gy and TD_5 of 31 Gy for whole-liver radiation; the risk of complications was strongly dependent on volume of liver irradiated.[363] Other risk factors for late toxicity included primary hepatobiliary carcinoma (as opposed to metastatic disease), use of bromodeoxyuridine chemotherapy (as opposed to fluorodeoxyuridine), and male gender. The NTCP models predict a TD_5 in excess of 80 Gy if less than one-third of the liver is irradiated. With irradiation of two-thirds of the liver, the TD_5 is on the order of 50 Gy and TD_{50} on the order of 60 Gy.

In the series of hepatocellular carcinoma patients from Taipei (discussed earlier),[371] the TD_{50} for whole-liver, two-thirds liver, and one-third liver radiation was modeled to be approximately 43, 50, and 67 Gy, respectively. The TD_5 for whole-liver, two-thirds liver, and one-third liver radiation was modeled to be approximately 25, 28, and 38 Gy, respectively. The volume effect of liver radiation was less in this series.

TABLE 14.10 RADIATION-INDUCED LIVER DISEASE IN PARTIAL LIVER IRRADIATION					
Reference	n/% C-P A	Diagnosis	Dose Fractionation	Crude Rate of RILD	Mean Normal Liver Dose in Patients with vs. without RILD
Michigan[363,364]	203/100%	PLC + LMC	1.5 Gy bid	9%	37 vs. 31.3 Gy
Taipei[365]	89/76%	HCC	1.8–3 Gy qd	19%	23 vs. 19 Gy
Shanghai[366,367]	109/85%	PLC	4–6 Gy qd	16%	24.9 vs. 19.9 Gy
Guangdong[368]	94/46%	HCC	4–8 Gy qd	17%	Not stated
S. Korea (Seong et al.)[369]	158/74%	HCC	1.8 Gy qd	7%	Not stated
S. Korea (Kim et al.)[370]	105/81%	HCC	2.0 Gy qd	12%	25.4 vs. 19.1 Gy

% C-P A, percent of patients with baseline Child-Pugh A score (in all studies, patients were either A or B); bid, twice-daily treatment; HCC, hepatocellular carcinoma; LMC, metastatic disease to the liver; PLC, primary liver cancer; qd, once-daily treatment; RILD, radiation-induced liver disease.
After Pan CC, Kavanagh BD, Dawson LA, et al. Radiation-associated liver injury. *Int J Radiat Oncol Biol Phys* 2010;76(3 Suppl):S94–S100. Copyright © 2010 Elsevier. With permission.

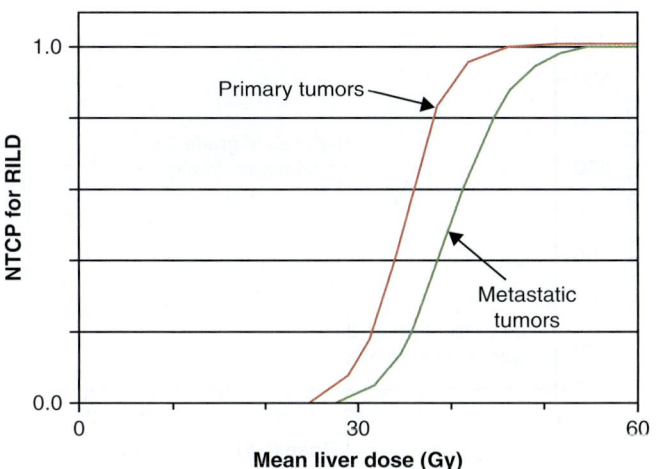

FIGURE 14.11. Mean liver dose, corrected with linear-quadratic modeling for 2-Gy fractions versus Lyman normal tissue complication probability (NTCP) of classic radiation-induced liver disease (RILD) for primary and metastatic liver cancer. (Reprinted from Pan CC, Kavanagh BD, Dawson LA, et al. Radiation-associated liver injury. *Int J Radiat Oncol Biol Phys* 2010;76[3 Suppl]:S94–S100. Copyright © 2010 Elsevier. With permission.)

In another study from the same group, the mean liver dose and hepatitis B virus positivity were significant predictors of radiation toxicity; with NTCP modeling, the TD_{50} was approximately 50 Gy.[365]

The data from Asia differs from that in the West, perhaps reflecting differences in the treated malignancy (mostly metastases in the West vs. primary liver cancer in Asia, which often occurs in the setting of liver cirrhosis), as shown in Figure 14.11. In addition, radiation fractionation, concurrent therapies delivered with radiation, and the fact that the majority of patients with hepatocellular carcinoma from Asia have hepatitis B viral infections may impact liver tolerance.[361] Poor preexisting liver function is also predictive of poorer tolerance to radiation.[361]

Special Situations

The hypofractionated delivery of radiation, using novel techniques such as SBRT and/or image-guided radiation therapy (IGRT), for primary and metastatic liver lesions presents a unique situation in which small volumes of normal liver receive very high doses of radiation per fraction. In a collaborative phase I study, the University of Colorado and Indiana University enrolled 18 patients with one to three liver metastases treated with three fractions of SBRT.[372] No patients developed grade 2 or higher toxicity. Late radiographic changes of well-circumscribed hypodense lesions were commonly seen, corresponding to the 30-Gy dose distribution. In a follow-up analysis, including an additional 18 patients treated in a phase II study of three fractions of 20 Gy, one patient developed subcutaneous tissue breakdown; no radiation-related liver toxicity occurred.[373] In a subsequent study, in which ≥700 mL of normal liver was required to receive <15 Gy in three fractions, no patient experienced RILD.[374]

Princess Margaret Hospital treated 41 patients with primary hepatocellular or intrahepatic biliary cancer in a phase I study of 24 to 60 Gy in six fractions.[375] Using normal tissue complication modeling, patients were stratified into three different dose escalation groups, based on the effective liver volume to be irradiated. Acute (<3 months) elevation of liver enzymes occurred in 24%, acute grade 3 nausea occurred in 7%, and acute transient biliary obstruction occurred in 5% of patients. In contrast, among 68 patients with liver metastases treated similarly with SBRT, two patients (3%) developed grade 3 liver enzyme changes, but no RILD or other grade 3 or higher liver toxicity was reported.[376]

Recommended Dose–Volume Limits

For patients with liver metastases undergoing partial volume liver radiation, the risk of radiation-induced liver toxicity appears to be more dependent upon the volume of liver irradiated. Partial volumes of liver can tolerate relatively high doses. Liver tolerances, however, are lower for patients with primary liver cancer (who are more apt to have underlying liver disease). For whole-liver radiation, doses ≤28 to 30 Gy in 2-Gy fractions (28 Gy for liver metastases and 30 Gy for primary liver cancer) and ≤21 Gy in 3-Gy fractions are recommended. For partial liver radiation, treated with standard fractionation, the mean dose to normal liver (liver minus GTV) is suggested to be <30 Gy for liver metastases and <28 Gy for primary liver cancer.

Future Studies

Studies that better correlate dose–volume parameters with long-term clinical/objective outcomes are needed. The impact of treatment-related (including fractional dose and systemic therapies) and host-related variables should be better defined.

Toxicity Scoring Criteria

The CTCAE v. 3.0 grades hepatobiliary toxicity according to clinical criteria of jaundice, asterixis, and encephalopathy or coma for grades 2, 3, and 4, respectively. The much more commonly occurring alteration in liver enzymes, in the absence of symptomatic manifestations, is classified under the CTCAE metabolic/laboratory category of elevations of alanine aminotransferase (ALT) and aspartate aminotransferase (AST). The use of CTCAE criteria for elevations of AST and ALT and other metabolic effects is advisable to promote consistency of reporting.

Small Bowel/Stomach

Clinical Significance

The stomach and small bowel aid in the digestion and absorption of food and nutrients. Symptoms from radiation-related late toxicities include dyspepsia, gastric ulceration, diarrhea, bowel obstruction, and ulceration, fistula, or perforation.[377]

End Points

Nausea and vomiting can occur immediately or within hours after RT to the stomach or small bowel. The radiosensitivity of the gastric mucosa is reflected in the early depression of hydrochloric acid and pepsin secretion after modest radiation doses of 15 to 20 Gy. Although some recovery of cellular structure occurs, suppression can continue for 6 months to many years after irradiation. Usually, at total doses at or above 50 Gy, cellular and functional recovery is never complete. Ulcers are the most common complication of gastric irradiation and present clinically with dyspepsia, significant pain, and sometimes hemorrhage. An ulcer in this anatomic setting can lead to hemorrhage and perforation, which, although rare, can be fatal. Ulcerations have been described as typically antral, perhaps because of placement of radiation therapy fields, and develop as early as 2 to 12 months after treatment. Pyloric obstruction may be a late development because of fibrosis after ulcer healing.

The early onset of malabsorption of fat and hypermotility after modest doses of radiation illustrates the radiosensitivity of the small intestine. Usually, recovery at dose levels below 40 to 45 Gy occurs, although some persistence of small bowel dysfunction and mesenteric cramping may be noted. Surgical intervention and adhesions can precipitate a more serious course of events. Higher doses result in diarrhea, malabsorption of fat, and leakage of albumin into the bowel. If an obliterative arteritis develops, the risk of infarction and perforation remains despite recovery. The underlying lesion is one of ulceration and segmental enteritis that can lead to stenosis of the bowel lumen, with varying degrees of obstruction during the chronic period.

Challenges Defining Volumes

The stomach and small bowel are well visualized, particularly with the use of intravenous contrast and/or oral contrast. The stomach and small bowel position can be variable, and it is therefore recommended that patients avoid large meals or carbonated beverages prior to simulation and treatment.

Dose/Volume/Toxicity Data

Because the stomach and small bowel are mobile and distensible, determining accurate dose–volume (or dose–surface) constraints is challenging. A 2013 systematic review of women undergoing extended field radiation suggested a point dose maximum of 55 Gy to small bowel would yield a 10% toxicity risk within 5 years.[386] In a study of women undergoing posthysterectomy IMRT, the V_{40}/small bowel volume ratio (optimal threshold of 28%) and maximal dose (optimal threshold of 55.9 Gy) were significant prognostic factors for chronic grade 1 to 2 toxicity.[387]

Late radiation-induced stomach injury has been reported to occur with increasing frequency with increasing doses. In a study from Walter Reed, the rates of gastric ulceration were 4% and 16% after treatment of <50 versus >50 Gy, respectively. Similarly, the rates of perforation were 2% and 14% in the same dose cohorts, respectively. Overall, the dose of approximately 50 Gy to the stomach is associated with about a 2% to 6% incidence of severe late injury. The volume effect for late stomach injury is not well defined. For late small bowel toxicity, doses of approximately 50 Gy are associated with obstruction/perforation rates that are approximately 2% to 9%. There is a paucity of good quantitative data on dose–volume metrics that predict for gastric or bowel late toxicity. Nevertheless, there are data that demonstrate a volume effect. The risk of bowel obstruction among patients with rectal cancer whose fields extended to L1 or L2 was 30% versus 9% in those treated with pelvis-only fields.[378] The University of Michigan investigated gastric and duodenal bleeding after radiation of patients with liver tumors.[379] Normal tissue complication modeling was consistent with a dose threshold (~60 Gy) for bleeding without a large volume effect.

Two studies of locally advanced pancreatic cancer patients correlated small bowel toxicity risks with dose–volume metrics. After concurrent gemcitabine and radiotherapy, duodenal $V_{35} > 20\%$ was associated with a 41% risk of grade ≥3 small bowel toxicity (acute or late) versus 0% for a $V_{35} < 20\%$.[388] In another study, $V_{55} \geq 1$ mL versus <1 mL was significantly correlated with grade ≥2 toxicity (47% vs. 9%, $P = .0003$).[389] Among patients treated with neoadjuvant radiation for rectal cancer, a 10% risk of grade ≥3 small bowel toxicity was correlated with a $V_{15} < 275$ cm³ for contoured bowel loops and <830 cm³ for the peritoneal space.[390]

Factors Affecting Risk

Factors affecting risk of late toxicity include total dose (with doses in excess of 40 to 50 Gy increasing the risk of late complications), fractional dose, prior abdominal surgery (which increases the risk of bowel obstruction), and concurrent chemotherapy use. In the European Organisation for Research and Treatment of Cancer (EORTC) Hodgkin lymphoma study, the rate of complications was 3% without prior abdominal surgery versus 12% with prior abdominal surgery.[380]

Mathematic/Biologic Models

The University of Michigan analyzed gastric bleeding among patients treated with radiation for liver tumors.[379] Variables significantly impacting bleeding risk included NTCP, mean dose to stomach, and presence of cirrhosis. Data from William

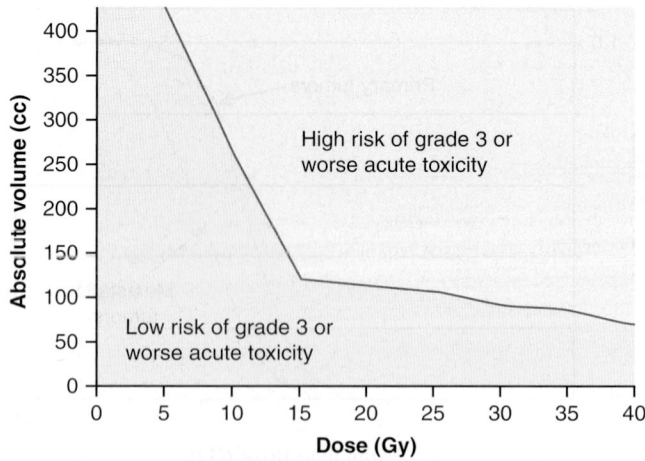

FIGURE 14.12. Graphic representation of the Baglan–Robertson[381,382] threshold model for acute small bowel toxicity. "Low risk" implies <10% and "high risk" >40% grade 3 toxicity. Absolute volume is based on contouring individual bowel loops, not the entire peritoneal space. (Reprinted from Kavanagh BD, Pan CC, Dawson LA, et al. Radiation dose-volume effects in the stomach and small bowel. *Int J Radiat Oncol Biol Phys* 2010;76[3 Suppl]:S101–S107. Copyright © 2010 Elsevier. With permission.)

Beaumont Hospital has suggested that the volume of bowel exposed to radiation doses of >5 to 40 Gy correlates with risk of acute grade 3 toxicity; their studies[381,382] and others have shown small bowel V_{15} to be highly significant ($P < .0001$).[383] The model results are graphically depicted in Figure 14.12. Using NTCP modeling for patients undergoing preoperative radiation for rectal cancer, IMRT has been shown to reduce the anticipated rate of grade 2 or higher diarrhea from 40% to 27% (with further reductions if IGRT is also used).[377]

Special Situations

High-grade small bowel mucositis, ulceration, and perforation, as well as acute gastroparesis, have been reported in patients undergoing hypofractionated SBRT for pancreatic malignancies,[384] though the reported rate of such grade 3 to 4 toxicities (albeit in a patient population with poor survival) has been relatively low in US studies.[391–393] Among patients undergoing three- to five-fraction SBRT for liver metastases, bowel toxicity has been reported to occur with maximal doses to the bowel of >30 Gy.[361]

Recommended Dose–Volume Limits

Using the entire potential small bowel space, it is suggested that the small bowel exposed to V_{45} to V_{50} should be <195 mL to reduce acute toxicity (not discussed earlier)[377,394]; while using the visualized loops of bowel, it is recommended that the V_{15} should be <120 mL.[377,381] Although these dose constraints were derived from acute toxicity data, they do provide guidelines that should help minimize risk of late toxicity as well. For the stomach, it is recommended to maintain the dose to the whole stomach to <45 Gy; a maximum point dose might be an important predictor of toxicity, but more data are needed to confirm this hypothesis.

Future Studies

More detailed dose–volume effects for late bowel toxicity are needed, particularly for altered fractionation (i.e., SBRT). As many gastrointestinal cancers are treated with chemotherapy, data on the impact of chemotherapy on acute and late stomach and bowel toxicity are needed.

Toxicity Scoring Criteria

The CTCAE v. 4.0 is used to grade gastric and small bowel toxicity.[92]

Kidneys

Clinical Significance

The kidney functions to remove wastes; regulate electrolytes; produce erythropoietin, which stimulates red blood cell production; and modulate blood pressure through the renin–angiotensin pathway as well as through fluid/electrolyte balance. Radiation nephropathy is an uncommonly reported toxicity, not because kidneys are radioresistant, but because clinicians carefully respect renal tolerance doses.

End Points

Five distinct clinical syndromes may overlap in symptoms, signs, and time sequence: acute radiation nephropathy, chronic radiation nephropathy, benign hypertension, malignant hypertension, and hyperreninemic hypertension secondary to a scarred encapsulated kidney (Goldblatt kidney). The signs (i.e., decreased glomerular filtration rate) and symptoms of radiation nephropathy are not distinguishable from other causes of renal damage, and these should be excluded. Acute (within 6 months) radiation-induced kidney injury is generally subclinical. Urinary findings consist of microscopic hematuria, proteinuria, and urinary casts. Blood alterations in β_2-microglobulin correlate linearly with both inulin and creatinine clearance and with later elevations of blood urea nitrogen (BUN). There is a 6- to 12-month latency period before the clinical expression of acute radiation nephropathy. In this subacute phase, the signs and symptoms include dyspnea, headaches, ankle edema, lassitude, anemia, hypertension, albuminuria, papilledema, elevated blood urea, and urinary abnormalities (granular and hyalin casts, red blood cells). Death may occur from chronic uremia or left ventricular failure, pulmonary edema, pleural effusion, and hepatic congestion. Chronic radiation nephropathy and hypertension do not develop until after 12 to 18 months. When chronic nephropathy is severe, death may result.

Challenges Defining Volumes

The kidneys are readily defined on contrast and noncontrast CT imaging. Ideally, the "functional" kidney parenchyma as opposed to the collecting system should be contoured.

Dose/Volume/Toxicity Data

Several studies have investigated whole-kidney dose tolerance, either after whole-abdominal radiation or total-body irradiation (TBI) (generally delivered with lower fractional doses). Renal toxicity can occur after bilateral kidney doses ≥10 Gy, and the risk is quite high (50% to 80%) after 20 Gy. Thus, the kidneys have a relatively low threshold for damage. The dose–volume effect on the kidneys has been long recognized, even prior to the planning CT era, because kidneys are well visualized on plain simulation films. From these studies, when greater than half of the kidney receives doses >20 to 30 Gy, or greater than one-third receives >30 to 40 Gy, patients are at increased risk of developing renal atrophy, decreased kidney function, and hypertension.[1,297,395,396]

There is little published on dose–volume parameters to predict late renal toxicity, in part because clinicians make an effort to minimize the volume of kidney exceeding the accepted tolerance dose. Low doses, 10 to 15 Gy, to large volumes of kidney increase the risk of nephrotoxicity,[78,397,398] whereas smaller volumes of kidney with doses exceeding approximately 20 to 25 Gy can result in late renal toxicity.[78,397,399,400] In a series from Heidelberg, normal tissue complication modeling was used to estimate the risk of late complications.[399] A median dose of approximately 17.5 to 21.5 Gy and 22 to 26 Gy corresponded to a 5% and 50% late complication risk (anemia, azotemia, hypertension, and edema), respectively. In another German study, reduced kidney function, as measured by scintigraphy changes, was analyzed as a function of

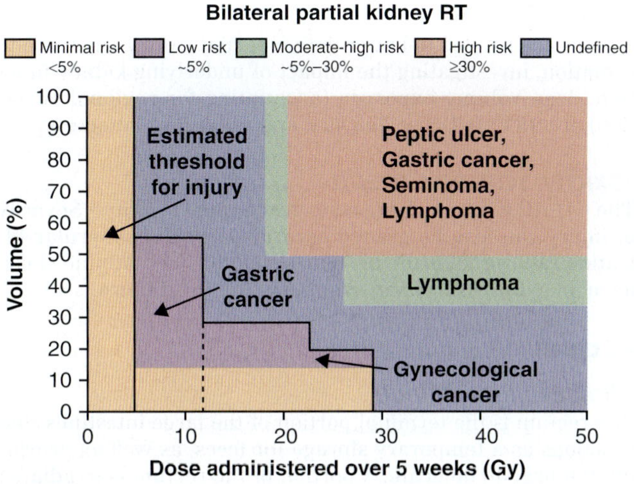

Bilateral partial kidney RT

| Minimal risk <5% | Low risk ~5% | Moderate-high risk ~5%–30% | High risk ≥30% | Undefined |

FIGURE 14.13. Schematic diagram of bilateral kidney dose–volume histogram from selected studies, represented as regions associated with minimal (<5%), low (~5%), moderate to high (~5% to 30%), high (>30%), or undefined estimated risk of toxicity. Clinical situation that yielded risk estimates for each region is also indicated. Actual risks are patient and plan specific and are associated with substantial uncertainty. (Adapted from Dawson LA, Kavanagh BD, Paulino AC, et al. Radiation-associated kidney injury. *Int J Radiat Oncol Biol Phys* 2010;76[3 Suppl]:S108–S115. Copyright © 2010 Elsevier. With permission.)

dose and volume.[397] After irradiation of 10% to 30%, 30% to 60%, and 60% to 100% of the kidney volume to 20 Gy, the incidence of reduced activity was <10%, approximately 40%, and >70%, respectively. After irradiation of 10% to 30%, 30% to 60%, and 60% to 100% of the kidney volume to 30 Gy, the incidence of reduced activity was approximately 35%, >90%, and >98%, respectively. In a Dutch study of patients with gastric cancer (treated with concurrent radiation and cisplatin or capecitabine), the left kidney V_{20} of ≥64% and mean left kidney dose of ≥30 Gy were associated with a significant decrease in left kidney function as compared to the right.[400]

Recognizing the limitations described earlier, the QUANTEC study summarized the toxicity data for bilateral kidney irradiation in Figure 14.13.

Factors Affecting Risk

A variety of agents have been implicated as toxic or as radiosensitizers (i.e., retinoic acid, cisplatin, BCNU, actinomycin D), administered either singly or in combination chemotherapy. Of note, angiotensin-converting enzyme (ACE) inhibitors and angiotensin II receptor blockers have been shown to delay the progression of radiation injury in the experimental setting.[401] TBI dose rates (≤6 cGy/min vs. ≥10 cGy/min) have been shown to significantly impact risk of renal toxicity.[402] Patient-related factors may include underlying renal insufficiency, diabetes, hypertension, liver disease, heart disease, and smoking.[403]

Special Situations

Several reports have described the use of SBRT in the treatment of medically unresectable kidney cancer and/or in patients with only one functioning kidney. With limited follow-up, SBRT with high dose (≥10 Gy) has been reportedly well tolerated.[403]

Recommended Dose–Volume Limits[403]

For whole (bilateral) kidney radiation, doses <10 Gy delivered over five to six fractions (at a <6 cGy/min dose rate) and <15 to 18 Gy for radiation delivered over ≥5 weeks are recommended. For partial kidney radiation, the volume of kidneys receiving >20 Gy predicts risk of renal toxicity. The recommendation for partial kidney radiation is to maximally spare the kidneys and maintain a mean dose of <18 Gy to both kidneys, or maintain a V_6 < 30% if one kidney cannot be adequately spared.

Future Studies

Studies are needed to better define partial kidney tolerance to radiation, investigating the impact of underlying kidney function, dose–volume exposure (accounting for regional variation), fractionated dose delivery, and radiation protectors.

Toxicity Scoring Criteria

The CTCAE v. 4.0 can be used to grade renal toxicity.[92] Severity of injury can also be graded according to the glomerular filtration rate, serial urine protein, serum BUN, creatinine clearance, blood pressure, and symptoms of renal failure.

Rectum

Clinical Significance

The rectum is the terminal portion of the large intestines that functions as a temporary storage for feces, as well as providing the urge to defecate. A portion of the rectum is irradiated in patients undergoing radiation for prostate cancer, gynecologic cancers, and other pelvic tumors (such as sarcomas).

End Points

Acute rectal toxicity includes diarrhea or loose stools, tenesmus, proctitis, and rectal urgency and/or frequency. The most common late radiation-related rectal complication is bleeding. Rectal ulceration and fistula are much less common. Other late injuries include stricture and decreased rectal compliance, which can result in frequent small stool and/or tenesmus. The anus is also at risk of late complications including stricture and laxity, leading to fecal incontinence.

Challenges Defining Volumes

The rectum extends from the rectosigmoid junction to the anus, with the inferior extent variably defined as the level of the anal verge the ischial tuberosities or 2 cm below the ischial tuberosities, or above the anus (the most inferior 3 cm of the intestines). The rectum should be segmented from above the anal verge to the turn into the sigmoid colon, though the superior and inferior borders of the rectum are not always easy to define on CT imaging, and definition of the cranial and caudal extents is variable.[404] The rectum is mobile and distensible, and therefore, its position and volume can vary between and during radiation fractions.

The percentage of rectum or rectal wall receiving a given dose can be somewhat subjective (i.e., based on how much of the rectum is segmented); using the absolute volume of rectum[405] or rectal wall is less subjective, though defining the rectal wall is not standardized. William Beaumont Hospital demonstrated that the rectal volume as well as rectal wall V_{50} to V_{70} values predict late toxicity, with the rectal wall being more predictive of grade 2 to 3 late effects; acute toxicity is also predictive of late toxicity.[406] MDACC has also shown the rectal wall to be better predictive of late rectal bleeding.[407]

Review of Dose/Volume/Toxicity Data

Abundant dosimetric data have shown a correlation of risk with rectal volume and surface/rectal wall doses among patients undergoing radiation for prostate cancer. Figure 14.14 summarizes many of the studies discussed here.

MSKCC has shown a significant difference in the DVHs between patients who developed rectal bleeding versus those who did not after conformal radiation for prostate cancer.[408] The percent rectum exposed to 62% and 102% of the prescription dose (70.2 or 75.6 Gy) was significant; the rectal wall being encompassed by the 50% isodose line, higher maximal dose to the rectum, and smaller rectal volume were also significantly adverse risk factors.[408,417] In a recent study of 1,571 patients treated at MSKCC, the use of IMRT and the lack of acute rectal toxicity predicted for lower risk of late rectal toxicity.[418]

In a randomized trial of 70 versus 78 Gy from MDACC in the treatment of early- to intermediate-risk early-stage prostate cancer, the risk of grade 2 or higher late rectal complications was significantly greater with a rectal $V_{70} \geq 25\%$ versus $V_{70} < 25\%$ (46 vs. 16%, $P = .001$).[419] A retrospective analysis from MDACC showed that the risk is a continuous function of dose and volume, with suggested cutoff points for lowering the complication risk: $V_{60} \leq 41\%$, $V_{70} \leq 26\%$, $V_{76} \leq 16\%$ or 3.8 mL, and $V_{78} \leq 5\%$ or 1.4 mL.[409] At 6 years, the risk of grade 2 or higher late rectal complications was 54% for patients with a rectal $V_{70} \geq 26\%$ versus 13% for a $V_{70} < 26\%$.

Among patients treated in the Dutch randomized trial of 68 versus 78 Gy for prostate cancer,[420] the mean anal dose (as well as V_5 to V_{60}) significantly predicted the rate of grade 2 or higher gastrointestinal toxicity (at 4 years, 16% vs. 31% for a mean dose of <19 vs. >52 Gy).[421] The mean dose (as well as V_5 to V_{70}) also predicted the risk for use of incontinence pads (at 5 years, <5% vs. >20% for a mean dose <28 vs. >46 Gy). The anorectal V_{65} (as well as V_{55} to V_{60}) was significantly predictive of rectal bleeding (4-year risk <1% and >10% for a $V_{65} < 23\%$ vs. >29%).[421] Several other studies have shown that the volume of rectum receiving >50 to 70 Gy has been shown to significantly correlate with late rectal toxicity.[410,411,422,423] From a 1998 Dutch study, recommendations for the volume of rectal wall (vs.

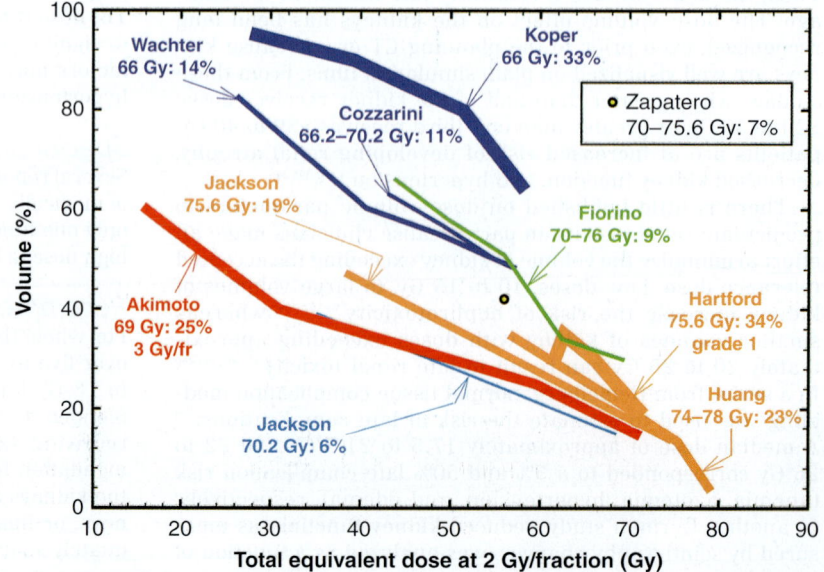

FIGURE 14.14. Dose–volume histogram thresholds for grade 2 or higher rectal toxicity from selected studies.[408–416] *Thicker lines* indicate higher rates of overall toxicity (percentages are indicated on the figure along with the physical prescription dose). Threshold doses are expressed as the total equivalent dose delivered in 2-Gy fractions, adjusted using the linear-quadratic model with $\alpha/\beta = 3$ Gy. The associated equivalent prescription doses are coded by color spectrum from lowest (*blue*) to highest (*red*). Volumes shown in the graph are based on the full length of the anatomic rectum. Note that these curves converge in the high-dose range, implying that doses in this range are more consistently associated with rectal toxicity. (Reprinted from Michalski JM, Gay H, Jackson A, et al. Radiation dose-volume effects in radiation-induced rectal injury. *Int J Radiat Oncol Biol Phys* 2010;76[3 Suppl]:S123–S129. Copyright © 2010 Elsevier. With permission.)

rectal volume) exceeding 65, 70, and 75 Gy are <40%, <30%, and <5%, respectively.[424] Data from the Cleveland Clinic[405] and William Beaumont Hospital[406] showed a significantly increased risk of grade 2 or higher rectal toxicity with rectal or rectal wall V_{70} to V_{78} of ≥15 versus <15 mL (~20% to >30% vs. ~5% to 10%).[406] V_{75} was the only dosimetric measure significantly associated with late rectal toxicity in a phase I/II RTOG 9406 study of 1,009 prostate cancer patients.[425] In an analysis of 748 patients randomized to the 79.2-Gy arm of the RTOG 0126 protocol, rectal V_{70} ≥ 15% was associated with grade 2+ rectal toxicity (P = .034 on multivariate analysis). At 3-years, V_{70} ≥ 15% was associated with an approximately 24% risk of late gastrointestinal toxicity versus 12% for V_{70} < 15%.[426] In a study of 1,285 prostate cancer patients who received proton therapy, the rectal (P = .010) and rectal wall (P = .0017) V_{75} were significant for risk of rectal bleeding on multivariate analysis.[427]

Women undergoing radiation for gynecologic malignancies are also susceptible to rectal toxicity. From historical data, the incidence of severe proctitis in patients with cancer of the cervix is dependent on the prescribed point A dose, with a <4% incidence with doses of <80 Gy, a 7% to 8% incidence after 80 to 95 Gy, and a 13% incidence for doses of ≥95 Gy.[428,429] With modern radiation delivery, particularly with IMRT planning, the rate of severe gastrointestinal toxicity is low. In a University of Chicago series of 183 patients treated with conventional radiation and brachytherapy, 9% developed grade 1 to 2 rectal toxicity and 7% developed grade 3 toxicity; a history of diabetes, point A dose, and the pelvic external beam radiotherapy dose were most significantly correlated with rectal toxicity. Among patients experiencing diarrhea or loose stools after pelvic radiotherapy, rectal toxicity becomes difficult to differentiate from small bowel toxicity. In another report from the University of Chicago, of 50 women treated with pelvic IMRT for gynecologic malignancies, acute gastrointestinal toxicity was correlated with small bowel dose (see above), but not rectum receiving 25% to 110% of the prescription.[251] However, the rectum was constrained to receive <40 Gy to >40% with a maximum dose of 49 Gy.

Factors Affecting Risk

Several patient-related variables, such as history of diabetes and/or vascular disease, inflammatory disease, and age, may impact the risk of late toxicity.[420,430,431] Prior abdominal surgery is also relevant.[432] From 1,010 prostate cancer patients enrolled in the RTOG 9406, cardiovascular disease was significantly (P = .015) associated with a higher rate of late rectal toxicity, whereas diabetes, hypertension, rectal volume, rectal length, neoadjuvant hormone therapy, and prescribed dose per fraction (1.8 vs. 2 Gy) were not significant factors.

Mathematic/Biologic Models

Rectal toxicity has been modeled using the Lyman-Kutcher-Burman NTCP model, mostly from patients treated with 3D conformal radiation. Most data are suggestive of a small volume effect, meaning that small volumes receiving high dose are most predictive for late effects.[404] The TD_{50} of grade 2 or higher late rectal toxicity is estimated to be around 77 to 79 Gy (with 95% CIs of ~74 to 82 Gy).[404] From the largest study to date of 1,010 patients enrolled in the RTOG 9406, the TD_{50} was 79 Gy; the fit based on dose-wall histogram data was not significantly different. EUD has also been modeled as a predictor of late rectal toxicity.[433]

Special Situations

SBRT for prostate cancer is under investigation. In one study, 67 patients were treated with 7.25 Gy × 5, in which rectal DVH goals were $V_{18.1\%}$ < 50%, $V_{29\%}$ < 20%, $V_{32.6\%}$ < 10%, and $V_{36.3\%}$ < 5%.[434] Grade 3, 2, and 1 rectal toxicities were seen in 0%, 2%, and 12.5% of patients, respectively. Persistent rectal bleeding was not observed. In another study, after SBRT (9.5 Gy

× 4), acute grade 1 to 2 and 3 rectal toxicity occurred in 33% and 0% of patients, respectively, and late grade 1 to 2 and 3 acute genitourinary toxicity occurred in 8% and 0%, respectively.[435] For patients treated with permanent interstitial brachytherapy[436,437] or afterloaded high-dose rate brachytherapy[438] for prostate cancer (either as monotherapy or as a boost), the dose–volume exposure of rectum has been correlated with late rectal toxicity. Combined external beam radiation and brachytherapy may lower the threshold for rectal toxicity after prostate brachytherapy.[439]

Recommended Dose–Volume Limits

For patients undergoing radiation therapy in which the rectum is irradiated, it is recommended to limit the rectal V_{50}, V_{60}, V_{65}, V_{70}, and V_{75} to <50%, 35%, 25%, 20%, and 15%, respectively. Although the data supporting these dose constraints primarily are from prostate cancer patients treated with conventional radiotherapy, studies of patients undergoing IMRT for prostate cancer suggest similar dose constraints.[440]

Future Studies

Future studies should be directed at achieving accurate dose–volume distributions for the rectum, which is a mobile, distensible structure, and correlating these dosimetric characteristics with toxicity. More robust data are needed for hypofractionated radiation delivery to the rectum, as with SBRT or HDR brachytherapy, as well as with low-dose brachytherapy and combined modality approaches.

Toxicity Scoring Criteria

The CTCAE v. 4.0[92] or RTOG scoring criteria can be used to grade rectal toxicity.

Urinary Bladder

Clinical Significance

The bladder is a highly distensible organ that collects urine. Symptoms from late radiation-related toxicities include increased urinary frequency, hematuria, and dysuria. Necrosis, contracted bladder, and hemorrhage are less common, severe effects. Perhaps, late bladder toxicity is underreported due to its long latency as well as toxicity being attributed to more common causes.

End Points

Bladder injury can be broadly classified as focal damage (e.g., bleeding) or more global injury (e.g., reduced bladder capacity with secondary urinary frequency). Acute side effects from incidental bladder irradiation are common and include urinary frequency, urgency, and dysuria (symptoms that may also reflect acute urethral toxicity). Late effects attributable to global injury include dysuria, frequency, urgency, contracture, spasm, reduced flow, and incontinence. In contrast, late effects arising from focal injury include hematuria, fistula, obstruction, ulceration, and necrosis.

Challenges Defining Volumes

The bladder is a mobile and distensible structure, depending upon the volume of urine within the bladder. Postvoid residuals may vary due to variable emptying and constant filling. In contouring the bladder, either the volume of the bladder and contents or the bladder wall alone can be segmented (with the latter more representative of a surface).

Dose/Volume/Toxicity Data

Because the bladder is mobile and distensible, determining accurate dose–volume (or dose-surface) constraints is challenging. Detailed dose–volume (or dose-surface) constraints have not been published, in part because of the complexities of assigning dose–volume or dose-surface metrics to a mobile, distensible structure. Whole-bladder tolerances have been mostly studied in patients with urinary bladder cancer, whereas partial bladder tolerances have been mostly studied in patients with genitourinary (mostly prostate) and gynecologic cancers.[441]

For whole-bladder irradiation, doses in excess of 60 Gy, particularly with fraction sizes >2 Gy and/or accelerated radiation regimens, result in a significant risk of grade 3 or higher late toxicity. Risks are lower when the whole bladder receives 45 to 55 Gy followed by a boost to >60 Gy to a portion of the bladder, though toxicity risk has not been correlated to dose–volume metrics. With prostate cancer treated to high doses (≥72 Gy), the inferior portion of the bladder (e.g., trigone area) also receives ≥70 Gy. This tends to be well tolerated with respect to bladder toxicity. Arguably, the urinary toxicity that does develop after radiation is due in part to the prostatic urethra receiving suprathreshold doses.

Mean bladder dose and area under the DVH were significant predictors of grade ≥2 genitourinary toxicity in a study of 503 prostate cancer patients.[442] In a study of 296 prostate cancer patients (in whom the bladder was contoured as whole organ, after drainage and infusion of 120 mL of saline), no bladder dose–volume relationships were associated with the risk of grade ≥2 genitourinary toxicity.[440]

Factors Affecting Risk
Prior pelvic surgery can result in increased risk of bladder toxicity as a direct result of bladder or urethral trauma and/or denervation of the bladder, which can cause urinary hesitancy or retention, resulting in overflow incontinence.[441] Patients receiving anticoagulants may be at greater risk of hematuria. Cytoxan, independently or with radiation, can cause chronic hemorrhagic cystitis, incontinence, contractions, and vesicoureteral reflux. Radiation-sensitizing chemotherapy may increase risk of acute and late bladder toxicity, though data supporting this are lacking.

Mathematic/Biologic Models
Quantitative mathematic modeling of bladder toxicity is lacking.

Special Situations
SBRT for prostate cancer is an emerging investigative approach. In one study, after SBRT (7.25 Gy × 5), grade 1 to 2 genitourinary toxicity occurred in 28%, and grade 3 toxicity was reported in 3% of patients (two patients required cystoscopies and dilation procedures for dysuria).[434] Urinary incontinence, complete obstruction, or persistent hematuria was not observed. In another study, after SBRT (9.5 Gy × 4), acute grade 1 to 2 and 3 acute genitourinary toxicity occurred in 71% and 0% of patients, respectively, and grade 1 to 2 and 3 late acute genitourinary toxicity occurred in 11% and 5%, respectively; grade 3 toxicity included temporary urinary catheterization and intermittent self-catheterization.[435]

Recommended Dose–Volume Limits
For whole-bladder radiation, the reported risks of grade 3 or higher toxicity in doses of 50 to 60 Gy range from ≤5% to 40%. This variation is likely attributable to the challenges of correlating toxicity with dose delivered to a mobile structure, which is even more problematic when correlating partial volume exposures to toxicity. With the caveat of these issues, bladder constraints of approximately 15%, 25%, 35%, and 50% receiving ≥80, ≥75, ≥70, and ≥65 Gy, respectively, as recommended in the RTOG 0415 study of prostate cancer, are suggested. The protocol advises an empty bladder at the time of simulation and treatment; the bladder is segmented from the base to the dome.

Future Studies
Studies that incorporate the changing size and shape of the bladder may provide a better understanding of the dose–volume tolerance of the bladder. Incorporating day-to-day variation with adaptive planning DVHs and/or use of deformable modeling would be informative. More detailed studies are needed to assess regional variation in radiation susceptibility (i.e., trigone vs. dome).

Toxicity Scoring Criteria
The CTCAE v. 4.0 or RTOG scoring criteria can be used to grade genitourinary toxicity.

Penile Bulb
Clinical Significance
Radiation dose to the penile bulb can affect erectile function, as a direct result either of damage to this structure or of damage to surrounding structures, whose radiation-induced damage is correlated with the dose exposure of the penile bulb. The most common scenario in which the penile bulb is irradiated is in the treatment of prostate cancer. IMRT is often used to minimize the dose to the penile bulb.[443,444]

End Points
Erectile dysfunction reported by the patient can be the result of treatment or other confounding factors including age, medications (particularly hormonal therapy), or comorbid conditions (e.g., diabetes, peripheral vascular disease, hypertension). Objective diagnostic tests can be performed to help establish the etiology of erectile dysfunction; these include nocturnal penile tumescence, somatosensory-evoked potentials, bulbocavernosus reflex latency, penile electromyography, color duplex Doppler ultrasound, dynamic infusion cavernosometry, and pharmacologic testing.

Challenges Defining Volumes
The anatomy of the pelvic floor is challenging to visualize on CT or MRI, and hence, definition of the penile bulb is somewhat subjective. The QUANTEC authors recommend defining the penile bulb as the most proximal portion of the penis sitting immediately caudal to the prostate.[445]

Dose/Volume/Toxicity Data
Several studies have investigated dose–volume parameters to predict risk of erectile dysfunction. In several studies, no correlation was discerned for penile bulb dose and erectile function.[443,446,447] In one study, attempts were made to reduce the dose to the penile bulb (mean dose of 25 Gy), and thus, few patients received high dose to the penile bulb.[443] In another study of 70 patients, no correlation was found for mean dose or maximal dose to the penile bulb, penile crura, or superior most 1 cm of the penile crura; DVHs were also compared and found to be similar.[447]

In a small (21 patients), early study from University of California, San Francisco, patients receiving a D_{70} of <40%, 40% to 70%, and >70% to the penile bulb had a 0%, 80%, and 100% risk, respectively, of experiencing radiation-induced impotence.[448] In a study (29 patients) from Thomas Jefferson University, several dose–volume metrics were analyzed; a D_{30} > 67 Gy, D_{45} > 63 Gy, D_{60} > 42 Gy, and D_{75} > 20 Gy to the proximal penis were correlated with increased erectile dysfunction as well as decreased ejaculatory function.[449] In a study from Royal Marsden Hospital, a D_{90} > 50 Gy to the penile bulb was associated with significantly worse erectile function, whereas D_{15}, D_{30}, and D_{50} showed a similar (albeit not significant) trend toward increased doses in impotent versus intermediately potent versus potent patients.[450] The largest study (158 patients) to date to investigate penile bulb dose is an analysis of the RTOG 9406 dose escalation study.[451] A median dose of ≥52.5 Gy was associated with a greater risk of impotence (50% vs. 25% at 5 years).

Factors Affecting Risk

The etiology of erectile dysfunction following radiation is likely multifactorial. In additional to radiation effects, pre-treatment erectile function, diabetes, smoking history, and a history of hypertension have been implicated as important factors affecting risk, though the data to date have been somewhat conflicting.[450]

Special Situations

Hormonal therapy, which is commonly used in patients with early-stage intermediate- to high-risk prostate cancer or advanced-stage prostate cancer, in and of itself can result in erectile dysfunction. However, the interaction (if any) of hormonal therapy and dose–volume delivery to the penile bulb is not well established.[445] Proton therapy is a well-established treatment approach for prostate cancer and is becoming more widely utilized as more proton centers are developed. Although proton therapy can reportedly lower penile bulb dose, the impact on erectile dysfunction is unknown.[452] Proton therapy may reduce postradiation testosterone suppression.[453] Interstitial brachytherapy (either with high-dose rate sources using afterloaded catheters or with permanent low-dose rate seeds) is a standard radiation modality as well. Data correlating erectile function with penile bulb dose from brachytherapy are sparse. In one study, there was no correlation between the penile bulb dose and postbrachytherapy erectile dysfunction.[454] SBRT for prostate cancer is an emerging investigative approach. The impact of hypofractionated SBRT on erectile dysfunction or the dose–volume parameters predictive of risk after prostate SBRT are not well studied. In one small study of 32 patients, penile bulb dose did not correlate with erectile dysfunction.[455]

Recommended Dose–Volume Limits

Based on published data for photon external beam radiation, the QUANTEC authors recommend keeping the mean dose to 95% of the penile bulb below 50 Gy and limiting D_{70} and D_{90} to 70 and 50 Gy, respectively.[445]

Future Studies

Studies should be directed at better anatomic definition of the putative anatomic sites impacted by erectile dysfunction and rigorous prospective correlation of dose–volume parameters with erectile dysfunction.

Toxicity Scoring Criteria

Pre- and posttreatment assessment of erectile dysfunction should be performed using the International Index of Erectile Function Scale.[445]

COMPOSITE SUMMARY OF DOSE/VOLUME/OUTCOME DATA

Table 14.11 summarizes the dose/volume/outcome findings in the QUANTEC reviews. Note that clinicians must understand the clinical situations from which the QUANTEC recommendations were derived, and there is no substitute for reading the original QUANTEC papers. At the same time, clinical judgment as applied to a specific patient is essential. In addition to the QUANTEC papers, the Emami paper continues to play an important role in estimating normal tissue toxicity during radiotherapy. Finally, as more comprehensive dose/volume/outcome data are developed—particularly in combination with emerging and evolving chemotherapy regimens—the

radiation oncologist will need to continually and critically keep abreast of the clinical literature on normal tissue toxicity. There is an ongoing effort to perform a similar dose–volume outcome summary for organs that are of particular interest for pediatric patients (PENTEC), but no information is available from that initiative.

CLINICAL APPLICATION, LIMITATIONS, AND IMPLICATIONS OF QUANTEC

Implications for Understanding the Underlying Mechanisms of Radiation-Induced Normal Tissue Injury

The consistent structure of the Emami dose–volume limits, and the application of that information to predictive models, may be taken to imply a uniform mechanism of radiation-induced injury. The diversity of the structure of the information obtained in the QUANTEC review suggests a more diverse mechanism of radiation-induced injury. An interorgan comparison of dose–response functions from the QUANTEC review is interesting (Fig. 14.15) and may have implications for our understanding of radiation-induced normal tissue injury.

1. There are marked variations in the dose–response curves for different organs, suggesting that there are different mechanisms for radiation-induced injury in different organs and/or that the end points selected for the different organs reflect a varied type of injury.
2. Organs that are classically considered structured in series (e.g., spinal cord, optic nerve, and small bowel, analogous to electrical circuits in series) have steep dose–response curves at doses beyond an apparent critical threshold. This is expected based on our understanding of the structure/anatomy of the series of organs: damage to a functional subunit can render the entire structure dysfunctional.
3. Several neural structures exhibit a similar threshold dose for injury: ≈55 to 60 Gy (corresponding to a BED of ≈100 for an α/β ratio of 3 Gy) for the brain, brainstem, optic nerve, and spinal cord. This suggests that there may be a common mechanism of injury in these structures. Because all of these organs are dependent on the vasculature, it is tempting to implicate vascular injury as the common target for these organs.
4. Organs that are classically considered structured in parallel (e.g., lung, liver, parotid, and kidney, analogous to electrical circuits) experience injury at far lower doses and have more gradual dose–response curves compared to series organs. The presence of injury at lower doses suggests that a different mechanism of injury is occurring in these organs as compared to series organs. It appears that these organs each have critical components that are more sensitive to the radiation than are the critical components within the neuronal tissues. It is thus tempting to conclude that subunits such as hepatocytes, nephrons, and alveoli are relatively radiation sensitive.
5. During heterogeneous organ irradiation, the predictive value of mean organ dose in some parallel-structured organs is interesting but counterintuitive. Consider the lung. Relatively uniform fractionated whole-lung doses as high as 15 to 23 Gy have a very low risk of symptomatic pneumonitis. Thus, the lung's "functional subunit" must generally be able to tolerate these doses. However, heterogeneous lung irradiation to a MLD of ≈15 to 23 Gy is associated with a 10% to 25% risk of symptomatic pneumonitis. Thus, during heterogeneous lung irradiation, it is likely that the mean dose is merely a surrogate for the percent of lung exposed to various other doses of radiation. The same may be true in other parallel organs as well.

TABLE 14.11 QUANTEC SUMMARY: CLINICAL DOSE/VOLUME/OUTCOME DATA

Organ	Volume Segmented	Irradiation Type (Partial Organ Unless Otherwise Stated)[a]	End Point	Dose (Gy), or Dose–Volume Parameters[a]		Rate (%)	Notes on Dose–Volume Parameters
Brain	Whole organ	3DCRT	Symptomatic necrosis	D_{max}	<60	<3	Data at 72 and 90 Gy extrapolated from BED models
	Whole organ	3DCRT	Symptomatic necrosis	D_{max}	72	5	
	Whole organ	3DCRT	Symptomatic necrosis	D_{max}	90	10	
	Whole organ	SRS (single fraction)	Symptomatic necrosis	V_{12}	<5–10 mL	<20	Rapid rise when V_{12} > 5–10 mL
Brainstem	Whole organ	Whole organ	Permanent cranial neuropathy or necrosis	D_{max}	<54	<5	
	Whole organ	3DCRT	Permanent cranial neuropathy or necrosis	$D_{1-10\ mL}$	≤59	<5	
	Whole organ	3DCRT	Permanent cranial neuropathy or necrosis	D_{max}	<64	<5	Point dose << 1 mL
	Whole organ	SRS (single fraction)	Permanent cranial neuropathy or necrosis	D_{max}	<12.5	<5	For patients with acoustic tumors
Optic nerve/ chiasm	Whole organ	3DCRT	Optic neuropathy	D_{max}	<55	<3	Given the small size, 3DCRT often covers the whole circumference of the organ[b]
	Whole organ	3DCRT	Optic neuropathy	D_{max}	55–60	3–7	
	Whole organ	3DCRT	Optic neuropathy	D_{max}	>60	>7–20	
	Whole organ	SRS (single fraction)	Optic neuropathy	D_{max}	<12	<10	
Spinal cord	Partial organ	3DCRT	Myelopathy	D_{max}	50	0.2	Including full cord cross-section
	Partial organ	3DCRT	Myelopathy	D_{max}	60	6	
	Partial organ	3DCRT	Myelopathy	D_{max}	69	50	
	Partial organ	SRS (single fraction)	Myelopathy	D_{max}	13	1	Partial cord cross-section irradiated
	Partial organ	SRS (hypofraction)	Myelopathy	D_{max}	20	1	3 fractions, partial cord cross-section irradiated
Cochlea	Whole organ	3DCRT	Sensory neural hearing loss	Mean dose	≤45	<30%	Mean dose to cochlea, hearing at 4 kHz
	Whole organ	SRS (single fraction)	Sensory neural hearing loss	Prescription dose	≤14	<25%	Serviceable hearing
Parotid	Bilateral whole parotid glands	3DCRT	Long-term parotid salivary function reduced to <25% of pre-RT level	Mean dose	<25	<20%	For combined parotid glands[c]
	Unilateral whole parotid gland	3DCRT	Long-term parotid salivary function reduced to <25% of pre-RT level	Mean dose	<20	<20%	For single parotid gland At least one parotid gland spared to <20 Gy[c]
	Bilateral whole parotid glands	3DCRT	Long-term parotid salivary function reduced to <25% of pre-RT level	Mean dose	<39	<50%	For combined parotid glands[c]
Pharynx	Pharyngeal constrictors	Whole organ	Symptomatic dysphagia and aspiration	Mean dose	<50	<20	Based on Section B4 of paper
Larynx	Whole organ	3DCRT	Vocal dysfunction	D_{max}	<66	<20	With chemotherapy
	Whole organ	3DCRT	Aspiration	Mean dose	<50	<30	With chemotherapy
	Whole organ	3DCRT	Edema	Mean dose	<44	<20	Without chemotherapy, based on single study in patients without larynx cancer[a]
	Whole organ	3DCRT	Edema	V_{50}	<27%	<20	
Lung	Whole organ	3DCRT	Symptomatic pneumonitis	V_{20}	≤30%	<20	For combined lung. Gradual dose response
	Whole organ	3DCRT	Symptomatic pneumonitis	Mean dose	7	5	Excludes purposeful whole-lung irradiation
	Whole organ	3DCRT	Symptomatic pneumonitis	Mean dose	13	10	
	Whole organ	3DCRT	Symptomatic pneumonitis	Mean dose	20	20	
	Whole organ	3DCRT	Symptomatic pneumonitis	Mean dose	24	30	
	Whole organ	3DCRT	Symptomatic pneumonitis	Mean dose	27	40	
Esophagus	Whole organ	3DCRT	Grade 3 or higher acute esophagitis	Mean dose	<34	5–20	Based on RTOG and several studies
	Whole organ	3DCRT	Grade 2 or higher acute esophagitis	V_{35}	<50%	<30	A variety of alternate threshold doses have been implicated. Appears to be a dose–volume response
	Whole organ	3DCRT	Grade 2 or higher acute esophagitis	V_{50}	<40%	<30	
	Whole organ	3DCRT	Grade 2 or higher acute esophagitis	V_{70}	<20%	<30	
Heart	Pericardium	3DCRT	Pericarditis	Mean dose	<26	<15	Based on single study
	Pericardium	3DCRT	Pericarditis	V_{30}	<46%	<15	
	Whole organ	3DCRT	Long-term cardiac mortality	V_{25}	<10%	<1	Overly safe risk estimates based on model predictions
Liver	Whole liver–GTV	3DCRT or whole organ	Classic RILD	Mean dose	<30–32	<5	Excluding patients with preexisting liver disease or hepatocellular carcinoma, as tolerance doses are lower in these patients
	Whole liver–GTV	3DCRT	Classic RILD	Mean dose	<42	<50	

TABLE 14.11 QUANTEC SUMMARY: CLINICAL DOSE/VOLUME/OUTCOME DATA (*Continued*)

Organ	Volume Segmented	Irradiation Type (Partial Organ Unless Otherwise Stated)[a]	End Point	Dose (Gy), or Dose–Volume Parameters[a]		Rate (%)	Notes on Dose–Volume Parameters
	Whole liver–GTV	3DCRT or whole organ	Classic RILD	Mean dose	<28	<5	In patients with Child-Pugh A preexisting liver disease or hepatocellular carcinoma, excluding hepatitis B reactivation as an end point
	Whole liver–GTV	3DCRT	Classic RILD	Mean dose	<36	<50	
	Whole liver–GTV	SBRT (hypofraction)	Classic RILD	Mean dose	<13	<5	3 fractions, for primary liver cancer
					<18	<5	6 fractions, for primary liver cancer
	Whole liver–GTV	SBRT (hypofraction)	Classic RILD	Mean dose	<15	<5	3 fractions, for liver metastases
					<20	<5	6 fractions, for liver metastases
	>700 mL of normal liver	SBRT (hypofraction)	Classic RILD		<15	<5	Critical volume based, in 3–5 fractions
Kidney	Bilateral whole kidney[d]	Bilateral whole organ or 3DCRT	Clinically relevant renal dysfunction	Mean dose	<15–18	<5	
	Bilateral whole kidney[d]	Bilateral whole organ	Clinically relevant renal dysfunction	Mean dose	<28	<50	
	Bilateral whole kidney	3DCRT	Clinically relevant renal dysfunction	V_{12}	<55%	<5	For combined kidney
				V_{20}	<32%		
				V_{23}	<30%		
				V_{28}	<20%		
Stomach	Whole organ	Whole organ	Ulceration	D_{max}	<45	<7	
Small bowel	Individual small bowel loops	3DCRT	Grade 3 or higher acute toxicity[e]	V_{15}	<120 mL	<10	Volume based on segmentation of the individual loops of bowel, not the entire potential space within the peritoneal cavity
	Entire potential space within peritoneal cavity	3DCRT	Grade 3 or higher acute toxicity[e]	V_{45}	<195 mL	<10	Volume based on the entire potential space within the peritoneal cavity
Rectum	Whole organ	3DCRT	Grade 2 or higher late rectal toxicity	V_{50}	<50%	<15	Prostate cancer treatment
			Grade 3 or higher late rectal toxicity			<10	
	Whole organ	3DCRT	Grade 2 or higher late rectal toxicity	V_{60}	<35%	<15	
			Grade 3 or higher late rectal toxicity			<10	
	Whole organ	3DCRT	Grade 2 or higher late rectal toxicity	V_{65}	<25%	<15	
			Grade 3 or higher late rectal toxicity			<10	
	Whole organ	3DCRT	Grade 2 or higher late rectal toxicity	V_{70}	<20%	<15	
			Grade 3 or higher late rectal toxicity			<10	
	Whole organ	3DCRT	Grade 2 or higher late rectal toxicity	V_{75}	<15%	<15	
			Grade 3 or higher late rectal toxicity			<10	
Bladder	Whole organ	3DCRT	Grade 3 or higher late RTOG	D_{max}	<65	<6	Bladder cancer treatment Variations in bladder size/shape/location during RT hamper ability to generate accurate data
	Whole organ	3DCRT	Grade 3 or higher late RTOG	V_{65}	≤50%		Prostate cancer treatment Based on current RTOG 0415 recommendation
				V_{70}	≤35%		
				V_{75}	≤25%		
				V_{80}	≤15%		
Penile bulb	Whole organ	3DCRT	Severe erectile dysfunction	Mean dose to 95% of gland	<50	<35	
	Whole organ	3DCRT	Severe erectile dysfunction	D_{90}	<50	<35	
	Whole organ	3DCRT	Severe erectile dysfunction	$D_{60–70}$	<70	<55	

Clinically, these data should be applied with caution. Clinicians are strongly advised to use the individual QUANTEC articles to check the applicability of these limits to the clinical situation at hand. These end points largely do not reflect modern IMRT.

[a] All at standard fractionation (i.e., 1.8–2.0 Gy per daily fraction) unless otherwise noted.
[b] For optic nerve, the cases of neuropathy in the 55–60 Gy range received ~59 Gy (see optic nerve paper for details). Excludes patients with pituitary tumors where the tolerance may be reduced.
[c] Severe xerostomia is related to additional factors including the doses to the submandibular glands.
[d] Nontraumatic brain injury.
[e] With combined chemotherapy.
3DCRT, three-dimensional conformal radiotherapy; D_x, minimum dose received by the "hottest" x% (or x mL) of the organ; RILD, radiation-induced liver disease (characterized by anicteric hepatomegaly and ascites, typically occurring between 2 weeks and 3 months after therapy; classic RILD also involves elevated alkaline phosphatase, more than twice the upper limit of normal or baseline value); RTOG, Radiation Therapy Oncology Group; SBRT, stereotactic body radiotherapy; SRS, stereotactic radiosurgery.
Adapted from Marks LB, Yorke ED, Jackson A, et al. Use of normal tissue complication probability models in the clinic. *Int J Radiat Oncol Biol Phys* 2010;76(3 Suppl):S10–S19. Copyright © 2010 Elsevier. With permission.

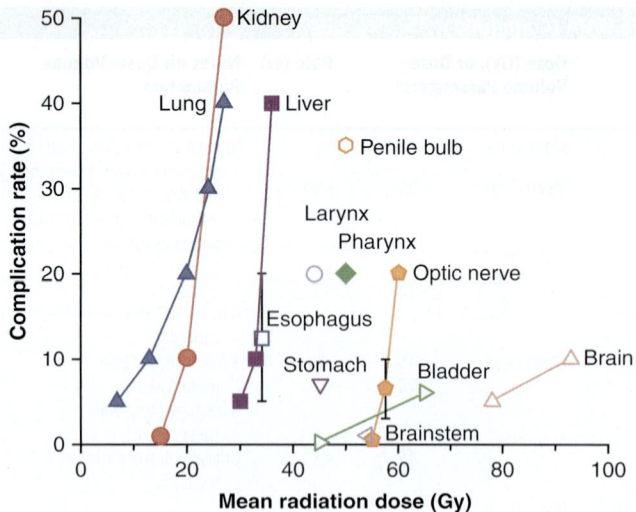

FIGURE 14.15. Composite diagram of normal tissue complication rates versus mean radiation dose.

NEXT STEPS: HYTEC (HIGH DOSE PER FRACTION, HYPOFRACTIONATED TREATMENT EFFECTS IN THE CLINIC)

A similar methodology to QUANTEC is now being applied to SBRT, in a multidisciplinary effort termed HyTEC: High Dose per Fraction, Hypofractionated Treatment Effects in the Clinic,[457,458] addressing hypofractionated treatments versus the predominantly conventionally fractionated regimens in QUANTEC. In addition, whereas QUANTEC focused primarily on normal tissue tolerance, HyTEC will also address tumor

control. This collaboration of physicians, physicists, radiobiologists, and biomathematicians is officially organized as the SBRT Working Group (WGSBRT) within the American Association of Physicists in Medicine (AAPM). The working group received the following charge from AAPM:

The radiobiology of hypofractionated treatments may differ considerably from that of standard fractionated treatments, in regards to repair, reoxygenation, dose-rate effects, volume effects, fraction size effects, etc. The working group will generate reports, including but not limited to, critically surveying the published data regarding: 1. Tumor response: review of the effect of hypofractionation on local control. 2. Normal tissue response: review of the effect of hypofractionation on normal tissue tolerances. 3. Radiobiology of hypofractionated treatments. 4. Clinical rationales for the diverse prescription schemes in current use (e.g., 20Gy x 3 fractions vs 24Gy x 1 fraction). 5. Standards for reporting outcome, including end points, defining/contouring of target and normal structures, dose definitions.

These studies are well underway, and peer-reviewed publication is expected in late 2017. In an independent effort outside of HyTEC (which includes only existing peer-reviewed data), a series of articles[459,460] presented hypofractionated dose–response models for 10 critical structures: optic pathway, cochlea, oral mucosa, aorta/major vessels, esophagus, chest wall, bronchi, small bowel, and spinal cord.

In the Emami paper,[1] all dose tolerance limits were specified in terms of TD 5/5 and TD 50/5, the dose at which a complication rate of 5% and 50%, respectively, was expected 5 years post radiotherapy. This standardized definition was important for establishing the concept of dose tolerance limits and normal tissue injury. Today, however, we recognize that the rate of normal tissue complications encountered in practice is much lower, typically well under 10% for serious adverse events. In addition, using the profile likelihood[461] or

FIGURE 14.16. Construction of the DVH Risk Map for maximum point dose of aorta/major vessels in 1 to 5 fractions. **A:** The portion of the DVH Risk Map corresponding to aorta/major vessel maximum point dose; datapoints in this figure are only from the newer dataset.[463] **B:** The dose–response model. The red squares represent the D_{max} doses corresponding to the grade 3 to 5 complications, whereas the *green* and *blue dots* correspond to the noncomplications. All published dose tolerance limits are shown as *blue diamonds*, and a selected subset is circled and labeled to show a high-risk (*solid red line*) and low-risk trend (*dashed green line*). The tabular portion of the figure shows the numerical values of each selected dose tolerance limit, as well as the corresponding risk estimate from the logistic model. Because the median number of fractions was 5, the model was constructed in terms of 5-fraction equivalent dose with the linear-quadratic model and $\alpha/\beta = 3$ Gy and converted back to effective dose in 1 to 5 fractions for the 5 rows in the table. No risk estimates were provided for 1 and 2 fractions because that data were too sparse. In light of the extremely low-risk values for the low-risk trend line (all less than half a percent), an alternate low-risk trend line was selected in Figure 14.17, which is closer to 1% to 2% risk.

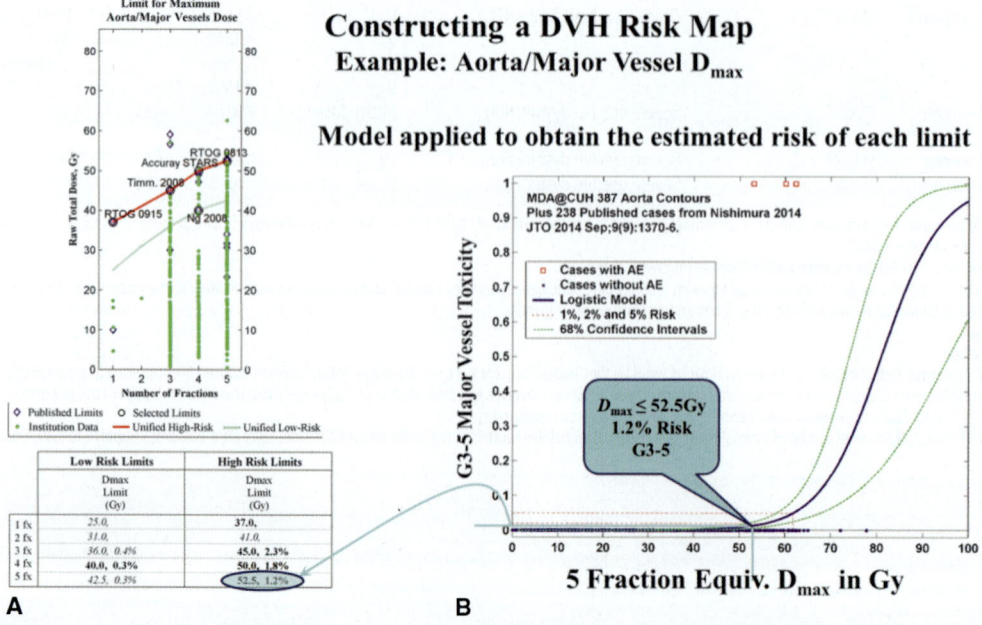

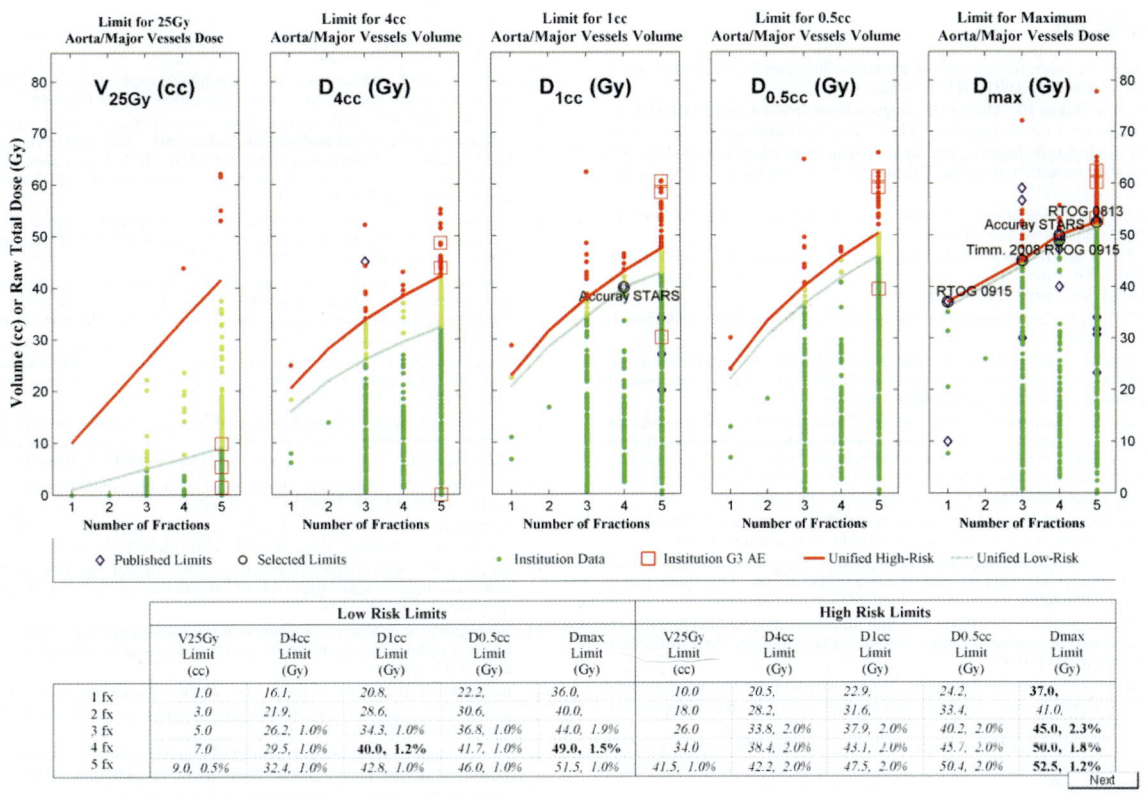

	Low Risk Limits					High Risk Limits				
	V25Gy Limit (cc)	D4cc Limit (Gy)	D1cc Limit (Gy)	D0.5cc Limit (Gy)	Dmax Limit (Gy)	V25Gy Limit (cc)	D4cc Limit (Gy)	D1cc Limit (Gy)	D0.5cc Limit (Gy)	Dmax Limit (Gy)
1 fx	1.0	16.1.	20.8.	22.2.	36.0.	10.0	20.5.	22.9.	24.2.	**37.0,**
2 fx	3.0	21.9.	28.6.	30.6.	40.0.	18.0	28.2.	31.6.	33.4.	41.0.
3 fx	5.0	26.2. 1.0%	34.3. 1.0%	36.8. 1.0%	44.0. 1.9%	26.0	33.8. 2.0%	37.9. 2.0%	40.2. 2.0%	**45.0, 2.3%**
4 fx	7.0	29.5. 1.0%	40.0. 1.2%	41.7. 1.0%	49.0. 1.5%	34.0	38.4. 2.0%	43.1. 2.0%	45.7. 2.0%	**50.0, 1.8%**
5 fx	9.0 0.5%	32.4. 1.0%	42.8. 1.0%	46.0. 1.0%	51.5. 1.0%	41.5. 1.0%	42.2. 2.0%	47.5. 2.0%	50.4. 2.0%	**52.5, 1.2%**

Next

FIGURE 14.17. DVH Risk Map for aorta/major vessels in 1 to 5 fractions, including dose–volume data from 625 aorta or other major vessel contours, combined from both datasets.[463,464] From left to right, the 5 panels present data for V_{25Gy}, D_{4cc}, D_{1cc}, $D_{0.05cc}$, and D_{max}. All other annotations are the same style as described in the legend of Figure 14.16. In comparison to the Emami TD 5/5 and TD 50/5, these low-risk levels are about 1%, and the high-risk levels are about 2%, reflecting the evolution over the past 25 years, from the notions of 5% and 50% risk toward lower levels of around 1% to 2% risk encountered in today's clinical practice. Caution must be advised as these data are from only two institutions, and the outcomes may depend strongly on the exact treatment techniques employed; the goal of HyTEC is to generalize results such as these by combining many such datasets and to determine insights into the factors affecting outcomes by detailed comparisons of the studies.

bootstrap methods,[462] it was apparent that the lack of clinical data at doses producing a 50% complication resulted in broad confidence intervals at these high-dose/high-risk levels. In contrast, the confidence in the models was reasonably good at the low complication rates encountered in clinical practice. Specific details regarding the models for each of the 10 critical structures are presented, although the focus is on simplicity and clinical utility, as in the Emami study and QUANTEC.

As an example of this approach, Figures 14.16 and 14.17 present the results for radiation-induced damage to the aorta/major vessels. Nishimura et al.[464] provided full DVH data for the entire portion of 238 aorta or major vessel contours that received 25 Gy or higher dose. Among the 133 patients whose lung tumor was treated with SBRT in 5 fractions, 3 developed late grade 3 to 5 toxicity in the pulmonary artery. These data were combined with major vessel contours from 387 additional patients who were treated with CyberKnife at the M.D. Anderson Cancer Center at Cooper University Hospital.[463] Logistic dose–response models were generated from the aggregate dataset, and all information was organized into a DVH Risk Map[460] as shown in Figures 14.16 and 14.17. The actual dose–volume major vessel data points planned for each patient are shown as the green dots in these figures, and the dose–volume points corresponding to the grade 3 to 5 complications are shown as the red squares. These are overlaid onto the published dose tolerance limits (blue diamonds), also including a selected representative low-risk and high-risk subset of those, denoted as the black circles with text descriptions. A high-risk trend line is depicted as the red solid line and the low-risk trend line as the dashed green line; these selections were somewhat arbitrary but now using the clinical datasets, the estimated risk level for each selected limit is interpolated from the dose–response model, as illustrated in Figure 14.16. The upshot is that, although the dose tolerance limits were extracted from a variety of publications, each with its own unique characteristics, the estimated risk levels are all from the aggregate data of these two institutions. Clinical application must carefully consider the relevance of the particular treatment techniques of those two manuscripts as compared to an institution's own patient population. The goal of the HyTEC effort is to combine all appropriate published datasets to more fully characterize the general principles for broad classes of patients while identifying the unique aspects of each dataset to determine factors that affect outcomes.

CONCLUSIONS

The QUANTEC effort is one further step in our field's decades-long effort to better quantify the relationship between dose–volume parameters and clinical outcomes. As the scope of the QUANTEC review was largely limited to organ systems with meaningful dose/volume/outcome data, the review, by itself, is an incomplete tool to guide clinical care. Consistent and clear reporting of dose/volume/outcome data[465] will enable further refinements in clinical guidelines and will hopefully improve patient care.

ACKNOWLEDGMENTS

Supported in part by grants from the National Institutes of Health CA69579 (L.B.M.) and the Lance Armstrong Foundation (L.B.M.). Parts of this chapter were adapted from Rubin et al., *ALERT: Adverse Late Effects of Radiation Therapy.*

REFERENCES

1. Emami B, et al. Tolerance of normal tissue to therapeutic irradiation. *Int J Radiat Oncol Biol Phys* 1991;21(1):109–122.
2. Marks LB, Ten Haken RK, Martel MK. Guest editors introduction to QUANTEC: a users guide. *Int J Radiat Oncol Biol Phys* 2010;76(3 Suppl):S1–S2.
3. Rubin P, Cooper RA, Phillips TL. *Radiation biology and radiation pathology syllabus. Set RT1: radiation oncology.* Chicago, IL: American College of Radiology, 1975:2–7.
4. Burman C, et al. Fitting of normal tissue tolerance data to an analytic function. *Int J Radiat Oncol Biol Phys* 1991;21(1):123–135.
5. Kutcher GJ, et al. Histogram reduction method for calculating complication probabilities for three-dimensional treatment planning evaluations. *Int J Radiat Oncol Biol Phys* 1991;21(1):137–146.
6. Lyman JT. Complication probability as assessed from dose-volume histograms. *Radiat Res Suppl* 1985;8:S13–S19.
7. Chapet O, et al. Normal tissue complication probability modeling for acute esophagitis in patients treated with conformal radiation therapy for non-small cell lung cancer. *Radiother Oncol* 2005;77(2):176–181.
8. Ten Haken RK, Lawrence TS, Dawson LA. Prediction of radiation-induced liver disease by Lyman normal-tissue complication probability model in three-dimensional conformal radiation therapy for primary liver carcinoma: in regards to Xu et al. (Int J Radiat Oncol Biol Phys 2006;65:189–195). *Int J Radiat Oncol Biol Phys* 2006;66(4):1272; author reply 1272–1273.
9. Ten Haken RK, et al. Use of Veff and iso-NTCP in the implementation of dose escalation protocols. *Int J Radiat Oncol Biol Phys* 1993;27(3):689–695.
10. Azria D, et al. Single nucleotide polymorphisms, apoptosis, and the development of severe late adverse effects after radiotherapy. *Clin Cancer Res* 2008;14(19):6284–6288.
11. Gauter-Fleckenstein B, et al. Early and late administration of MnTE-2-PyP5+ in mitigation and treatment of radiation-induced lung damage. *Free Radic Biol Med* 2010;48(8):1034–1043.
12. Kelsey CR, et al. A polymorphism within the promoter of the TGFbeta1 gene is associated with radiation sensitivity using an objective radiologic endpoint. *Int J Radiat Oncol Biol Phys* 2012;82(2):e247–e255.
13. Kong FM, et al. The use of blood biomarkers to predict radiation lung toxicity: a potential strategy to individualize thoracic radiation therapy. *Cancer Control* 2008;15(2):140–150.
14. Hoglund E, et al. DNA damage induced by radiation of different linear energy transfer: initial fragmentation. *Int J Radiat Biol* 2000;76(4):539–547.
15. Ward JF. The complexity of DNA damage: relevance to biological consequences. *Int J Radiat Biol* 1994;66(5):427–432.
16. Robbins ME, Zhao W. Chronic oxidative stress and radiation-induced late normal tissue injury: a review. *Int J Radiat Biol* 2004;80(4):251–259.
17. von Lohneysen K, et al. Structural insights into Nox4 and Nox2: motifs involved in function and cellular localization. *Mol Cell Biol* 2010;30(4):961–975.
18. Bengtsson SH, et al. Novel isoforms of NADPH oxidase in vascular physiology and pathophysiology. *Clin Exp Pharmacol Physiol* 2003;30(11):849–854.
19. Collins-Underwood JR, et al. NADPH oxidase mediates radiation-induced oxidative stress in rat brain microvascular endothelial cells. *Free Radic Biol Med* 2008;45(6):929–938.
20. Carnesecchi S, et al. A key role for NOX4 in epithelial cell death during development of lung fibrosis. *Antioxid Redox Signal* 2011;15(3):607–619.
21. Kim GJ, Chandrasekaran K, Morgan WF. Mitochondrial dysfunction, persistently elevated levels of reactive oxygen species and radiation-induced genomic instability: a review. *Mutagenesis* 2006;21(6):361–367.
22. Leach JK, et al. Ionizing radiation-induced, mitochondria-dependent generation of reactive oxygen/nitrogen. *Cancer Res* 2001;61(10):3894–3901.
23. Spasojevic I, et al. Mn porphyrin-based superoxide dismutase (SOD) mimic, MnIIITE-2-PyP5+, targets mouse heart mitochondria. *Free Radic Biol Med* 2007;42(8):1193–1200.
24. Cernanec JM, et al. Influence of oxygen tension on interleukin 1-induced peroxynitrite formation and matrix turnover in articular cartilage. *J Rheumatol* 2007;34(2):401–407.
25. Mikkelsen RB, Wardman P. Biological chemistry of reactive oxygen and nitrogen and radiation-induced signal transduction mechanisms. *Oncogene* 2003;22(37):5734–5754.
26. Zhao W, Diz DI, Robbins ME. Oxidative damage pathways in relation to normal tissue injury. *Br J Radiol* 2007;80(Spec No 1):S23–S31.
27. Epperly MW, et al. Radioprotection of lung and esophagus by overexpression of the human manganese superoxide dismutase transgene. *Mil Med* 2002;167(2 Suppl):71–73.
28. Gauter-Fleckenstein B, et al. Comparison of two Mn porphyrin-based mimics of superoxide dismutase in pulmonary radioprotection. *Free Radic Biol Med* 2008;44(6):982–989.
29. Rabbani ZN, et al. Overexpression of extracellular superoxide dismutase reduces acute radiation induced lung toxicity. *BMC Cancer* 2005;5:59.
30. Vujaskovic Z, et al. A small molecular weight catalytic metalloporphyrin antioxidant with superoxide dismutase (SOD) mimetic properties protects lungs from radiation-induced injury. *Free Radic Biol Med* 2002;33(6):857–863.
31. Rubin P, et al. A perpetual cascade of cytokines postirradiation leads to pulmonary fibrosis. *Int J Radiat Oncol Biol Phys* 1995;33(1):99–109.
32. Hallahan DE, Geng L, Shyr Y. Effects of intercellular adhesion molecule 1 (ICAM-1) null mutation on radiation-induced pulmonary fibrosis and respiratory insufficiency in mice. *J Natl Cancer Inst* 2002;94(10):733–741.
33. Hallahan DE, Virudachalam S. Intercellular adhesion molecule 1 knockout abrogates radiation induced pulmonary inflammation. *Proc Natl Acad Sci U S A* 1997;94(12):6432–6437.
34. Herskind C, Bamberg M, Rodemann HP. The role of cytokines in the development of normal-tissue reactions after radiotherapy. *Strahlenther Onkol* 1998;174(Suppl 3):12–15.
35. Rube CE, et al. Irradiation induces a biphasic expression of pro-inflammatory cytokines in the lung. *Strahlenther Onkol* 2004;180(7):442–448.
36. Epperly MW, et al. Manganese [correction of magnesium] superoxide dismutase (MnSOD) plasmid/liposome pulmonary radioprotective gene therapy: modulation of irradiation-induced mRNA for IL-I, TNF-alpha, and TGF-beta correlates with delay of organizing alveolitis/fibrosis. *Biol Blood Marrow Transplant* 1999;5(4):204–214.
37. Anscher MS, et al. Small molecular inhibitor of transforming growth factor-beta protects against development of radiation-induced lung injury. *Int J Radiat Oncol Biol Phys* 2008;71(3):829–837.
38. Nishioka A, et al. Histopathologic amelioration of fibroproliferative change in rat irradiated lung using soluble transforming growth factor-beta (TGF-beta) receptor mediated by adenoviral vector. *Int J Radiat Oncol Biol Phys* 2004;58(4):1235–1241.
39. Xavier S, et al. Amelioration of radiation-induced fibrosis: inhibition of transforming growth factor-beta signaling by halofuginone. *J Biol Chem* 2004;279(15):15167–15176.
40. Epperly MW, et al. Intratracheal injection of adenovirus containing the human MnSOD transgene protects athymic nude mice from radiation-induced organizing alveolitis. *Int J Radiat Oncol Biol Phys* 1999;43(1):169–181.
41. Evans ML, et al. Changes in vascular permeability following thorax irradiation in the rat. *Radiat Res* 1986;107(2):262–271.
42. Vujaskovic Z, et al. Radiation-induced hypoxia may perpetuate late normal tissue injury. *Int J Radiat Oncol Biol Phys* 2001;50(4):851–855.
43. Rabbani ZN, et al. Hypoxia inducible factor 1alpha signaling in fractionated radiation-induced lung injury: role of oxidative stress and tissue hypoxia. *Radiat Res* 2010;173(2):165–174.
44. Brahimi-Horn C, Mazure N, Pouyssegur J. Signalling via the hypoxia-inducible factor-1alpha requires multiple posttranslational modifications. *Cell Signal* 2005;17(1):1–9.
45. Bartholdi D, Rubin BP, Schwab ME. VEGF mRNA induction correlates with changes in the vascular architecture upon spinal cord damage in the rat. *Eur J Neurosci* 1997;9(12):2549–2560.
46. Fleckenstein K, et al. Temporal onset of hypoxia and oxidative stress after pulmonary irradiation. *Int J Radiat Oncol Biol Phys* 2007;68(1):196–204.
47. Lewis JS, et al. Macrophage responses to hypoxia: relevance to disease mechanisms. *J Leukoc Biol* 1999;66(6):889–900.
48. Olive PL, et al. Carbonic anhydrase 9 as an endogenous marker for hypoxic cells in cervical cancer. *Cancer Res* 2001;61(24):8924–8929.
49. Lawrence YR, et al. Radiation dose-volume effects in the brain. *Int J Radiat Oncol Biol Phys* 2010;76(3 Suppl):S20–S27.
50. Andrews DW, et al. Whole brain radiation therapy with or without stereotactic radiosurgery boost for patients with one to three brain metastases: phase III results of the RTOG 9508 randomised trial. *Lancet* 2004;363(9422):1665–1672.
51. Aoyama H, et al. Neurocognitive function of patients with brain metastasis who received either whole brain radiotherapy plus stereotactic radiosurgery or radiosurgery alone. *Int J Radiat Oncol Biol Phys* 2007;68(5):1388–1395.
52. Chang EL, et al. Neurocognition in patients with brain metastases treated with radiosurgery or radiosurgery plus whole-brain irradiation: a randomised controlled trial. *Lancet Oncol* 2009;10(11):1037–1044.
53. Lee AW, et al. Effect of time, dose, and fractionation on temporal lobe necrosis following radiotherapy for nasopharyngeal carcinoma. *Int J Radiat Oncol Biol Phys* 1998;40(1):35–42.
54. Lee AW, et al. Factors affecting risk of symptomatic temporal lobe necrosis: significance of fractional dose and treatment time. *Int J Radiat Oncol Biol Phys* 2002;53(1):75–85.
55. Corn BW, et al. White matter changes are correlated significantly with radiation dose. Observations from a randomized dose-escalation trial for malignant glioma (Radiation Therapy Oncology Group 83-02). *Cancer* 1994;74(10):2828–2835.
56. Ruben JD, et al. Cerebral radiation necrosis: incidence, outcomes, and risk factors with emphasis on radiation parameters and chemotherapy. *Int J Radiat Oncol Biol Phys* 2006;65(2):499–508.
57. Shaw E, et al. Prospective randomized trial of low- versus high-dose radiation therapy in adults with supratentorial low-grade glioma: initial report of a North Central Cancer Treatment Group/Radiation Therapy Oncology Group/Eastern Cooperative Oncology Group study. *J Clin Oncol* 2002;20(9):2267–2276.
58. Murray KJ, et al. A randomized phase III study of accelerated hyperfractionation versus standard in patients with unresected brain metastases: a report of the Radiation Therapy Oncology Group (RTOG) 9104. *Int J Radiat Oncol Biol Phys* 1997;39(3):571–574.
59. Sause WT, et al. Phase I/II trial of accelerated fractionation in brain metastases RTOG 85-28. *Int J Radiat Oncol Biol Phys* 1993;26(4):653–657.
60. Jen YM, et al. Different risks of symptomatic brain necrosis in NPC patients treated with different altered fractionated radiotherapy techniques. *Int J Radiat Oncol Biol Phys* 2001;51(2):344–348.
61. Fowler JF. The linear-quadratic formula and progress in fractionated radiotherapy. *Br J Radiol* 1989;62(740):679–694.
62. Hill JM, et al. A comparative study of the long term psychosocial functioning of childhood acute lymphoblastic leukemia survivors treated with intrathecal methotrexate with or without cranial radiation. *Cancer* 1998;82(1):208–218.
63. Smibert E, et al. Risk factors for intellectual and educational sequelae of cranial irradiation in childhood acute lymphoblastic leukaemia. *Br J Cancer* 1996;73(6):825–830.
64. Moore IM, et al. Cognitive function in children with leukemia. Effect of radiation dose and time since irradiation. *Cancer* 1991;68(9):1913–1917.

65. Waber DP, et al. Neuropsychological outcomes from a randomized trial of triple intrathecal chemotherapy compared with 18 Gy cranial radiation as CNS treatment in acute lymphoblastic leukemia: findings from Dana-Farber Cancer Institute ALL Consortium Protocol 95-01. *J Clin Oncol* 2007;25(31):4914–4921.
66. Mulhern RK, Fairclough D, Ochs J. A prospective comparison of neuropsychologic performance of children surviving leukemia who received 18-Gy, 24-Gy, or no cranial irradiation. *J Clin Oncol* 1991;9(8):1348–1356.
67. Mulhern RK, et al. Neuropsychologic functioning of survivors of childhood medulloblastoma randomized to receive conventional or reduced-dose craniospinal irradiation: a Pediatric Oncology Group study. *J Clin Oncol* 1998;16(5):1723–1728.
68. Gondi V, et al. Preservation of memory with conformal avoidance of the hippocampal neural stem-cell compartment during whole-brain radiotherapy for brain metastases (RTOG 0933): a phase II multi-institutional trial. *J Clin Oncol* 2014;32(34):3810–3816.
69. Shaw E, et al. Single dose radiosurgical treatment of recurrent previously irradiated primary brain tumors and brain metastases: final report of RTOG protocol 90-05. *Int J Radiat Oncol Biol Phys* 2000;47(2):291–298.
70. Lax I, Karlsson B. Prediction of complications in gamma knife radiosurgery of arteriovenous malformation. *Acta Oncol* 1996;35(1):49–55.
71. Voges J, et al. Risk analysis of linear accelerator radiosurgery. *Int J Radiat Oncol Biol Phys* 1996;36(5):1055–1063.
72. Flickinger JC, et al. Complications from arteriovenous malformation radiosurgery: multivariate analysis and risk modeling. *Int J Radiat Oncol Biol Phys* 1997;38(3):485–490.
73. Miyawaki L, et al. Five year results of LINAC radiosurgery for arteriovenous malformations: outcome for large AVMS. *Int J Radiat Oncol Biol Phys* 1999;44(5):1089–1106.
74. Chin LS, Ma L, DiBiase S. Radiation necrosis following gamma knife surgery: a case-controlled comparison of treatment parameters and long-term clinical follow up. *J Neurosurg* 2001;94(6):899–904.
75. Nakamura JL, et al. Dose conformity of gamma knife radiosurgery and risk factors for complications. *Int J Radiat Oncol Biol Phys* 2001;51(5):1313–1319.
76. Barker FG II, et al. Dose-volume prediction of radiation-related complications after proton beam radiosurgery for cerebral arteriovenous malformations. *J Neurosurg* 2003;99(2):254–263.
77. Friedman WA, et al. Analysis of factors predictive of success or complications in arteriovenous malformation radiosurgery. *Neurosurgery* 2003;52(2):296–307; discussion 307–308.
78. Varlotto JM, et al. Analysis of tumor control and toxicity in patients who have survived at least one year after radiosurgery for brain metastases. *Int J Radiat Oncol Biol Phys* 2003;57(2):452–464.
79. Korytko T, et al. 12 Gy gamma knife radiosurgical volume is a predictor for radiation necrosis in non-AVM intracranial tumors. *Int J Radiat Oncol Biol Phys* 2006;64(2):419–424.
80. Bleyer WA, et al. Influence of age, sex, and concurrent intrathecal methotrexate therapy on intellectual function after cranial irradiation during childhood: a report from the Children's Cancer Study Group. *Pediatr Hematol Oncol* 1990;7(4):329–338.
81. Jannoun L, Bloom HJ. Long-term psychological effects in children treated for intracranial tumors. *Int J Radiat Oncol Biol Phys* 1990;18(4):747–753.
82. Duffner PK. Long-term effects of radiation therapy on cognitive and endocrine function in children with leukemia and brain tumors. *Neurologist* 2004;10(6):293–310.
83. Tanaka T, et al. [The comparison between adult and pediatric AVMs treated by gamma knife radiosurgery]. *No Shinkei Geka* 1995;23(9):773–777.
84. Smyth MD, et al. Stereotactic radiosurgery for pediatric intracranial arteriovenous malformations: the University of California at San Francisco experience. *J Neurosurg* 2002;97(1):48–55.
85. Mayer R, Sminia P. Reirradiation tolerance of the human brain. *Int J Radiat Oncol Biol Phys* 2008;70(5):1350–1360.
86. Omuro AM, et al. Delayed neurotoxicity in primary central nervous system lymphoma. *Arch Neurol* 2005;62(10):1595–1600.
87. Schlegel U, et al. Neurologic sequelae of treatment of primary CNS lymphomas. *J Neurooncol* 1999;43(3):277–286.
88. Shah GD, et al. Combined immunochemotherapy with reduced whole-brain radiotherapy for newly diagnosed primary CNS lymphoma. *J Clin Oncol* 2007;25(30):4730–4735.
89. Mayo C, et al. Radiation dose-volume effects of optic nerves and chiasm. *Int J Radiat Oncol Biol Phys* 2010;76(3 Suppl):S28–S35.
90. Danesh-Meyer HV. Radiation-induced optic neuropathy. *J Clin Neurosci* 2008;15(2):95–100.
91. Gordon KB, Char DH, Sagerman RH. Late effects of radiation on the eye and ocular adnexa. *Int J Radiat Oncol Biol Phys* 1995;31(5):1123–1139.
92. Program, C.T.E. *Common Terminology Criteria for Adverse Events (CTCAE) Version 4.0*. Available at: http://evs.nci.nih.gov/ftp1/CTCAE. Accessed January 16, 2011.
93. Pavy JJ, et al. EORTC Late Effects Working Group. Late Effects toxicity scoring: the SOMA scale. *Int J Radiat Oncol Biol Phys* 1995;31(5):1043–1047.
94. Rubin P, et al. RTOG Late Effects Working Group. Overview. Late Effects of Normal Tissues (LENT) scoring system. *Int J Radiat Oncol Biol Phys* 1995;31(5):1041–1042.
95. Celesia GG, DeMarco PJ Jr. Anatomy and physiology of the visual system. *J Clin Neurophysiol* 1994;11(5):482–492.
96. Parsons JT, et al. Radiation optic neuropathy after megavoltage external-beam irradiation: analysis of time-dose factors. *Int J Radiat Oncol Biol Phys* 1994;30(4):755–763.
97. Martel MK, et al. Dose-volume complication analysis for visual pathway structures of patients with advanced paranasal sinus tumors. *Int J Radiat Oncol Biol Phys* 1997;38(2):273–284.
98. Jiang GL, et al. Radiation-induced injury to the visual pathway. *Radiother Oncol* 1994;30(1):17–25.
99. Flickinger JC, et al. Megavoltage external beam irradiation of craniopharyngiomas: analysis of tumor control and morbidity. *Int J Radiat Oncol Biol Phys* 1990;19(1):117–122.
100. Daly ME, et al. Intensity-modulated radiation therapy for malignancies of the nasal cavity and paranasal sinuses. *Int J Radiat Oncol Biol Phys* 2007;67(1):151–157.
101. Mackley HB, et al. Intensity-modulated radiotherapy for pituitary adenomas: the preliminary report of the Cleveland Clinic experience. *Int J Radiat Oncol Biol Phys* 2007;67(1):232–239.
102. Pigeaud-Klessens ML, Kralendonk JH. Radiation retino- and opticopathy. A prospective study. *Doc Ophthalmol* 1992;79(3):285–291.
103. Weber DC, et al. Results of spot-scanning proton radiation therapy for chordoma and chondrosarcoma of the skull base: the Paul Scherrer Institut experience. *Int J Radiat Oncol Biol Phys* 2005;63(2):401–409.
104. Bhandare N, et al. Does altered fractionation influence the risk of radiation-induced optic neuropathy? *Int J Radiat Oncol Biol Phys* 2005;62(4): 1070–1077.
105. Noel G, et al. Combination of photon and proton radiation therapy for chordomas and chondrosarcomas of the skull base: the Centre de Protontherapie D'Orsay experience. *Int J Radiat Oncol Biol Phys* 2001;51(2):392–398.
106. Nishimura H, et al. Proton-beam therapy for olfactory neuroblastoma. *Int J Radiat Oncol Biol Phys* 2007;68(3):758–762.
107. Wenkel E, et al. Benign meningioma: partially resected, biopsied, and recurrent intracranial tumors treated with combined proton and photon radiotherapy. *Int J Radiat Oncol Biol Phys* 2000;48(5):1363–1370.
108. Tishler RB, et al. Tolerance of cranial nerves of the cavernous sinus to radiosurgery. *Int J Radiat Oncol Biol Phys* 1993;27(2):215–221.
109. Stafford SL, et al. A study on the radiation tolerance of the optic nerves and chiasm after stereotactic radiosurgery. *Int J Radiat Oncol Biol Phys* 2003;55(5):1177–1181.
110. Pollock BE, et al. Gamma knife radiosurgery for patients with nonfunctioning pituitary adenomas: results from a 15-year experience. *Int J Radiat Oncol Biol Phys* 2008;70(5):1325–1329.
111. Leber KA, Bergloff J, Pendl G. Dose–response tolerance of the visual pathways and cranial nerves of the cavernous sinus to stereotactic radiosurgery. *J Neurosurg* 1998;88(1):43–50.
112. Flickinger JC, Deutsch M, Lunsford LD. Repeat megavoltage irradiation of pituitary and suprasellar tumors. *Int J Radiat Oncol Biol Phys* 1989;17(1):171–175.
113. Brizel DM, et al. Conformal radiation therapy treatment planning reduces the dose to the optic structures for patients with tumors of the paranasal sinuses. *Radiother Oncol* 1999;51(3):215–218.
114. van den Bergh AC, et al. Radiation optic neuropathy after external beam radiation therapy for acromegaly. *Radiother Oncol* 2003;68(2):95–100.
115. Aristizabal S, Caldwell WL, Avila J. The relationship of time-dose fractionation factors to complications in the treatment of pituitary tumors by irradiation. *Int J Radiat Oncol Biol Phys* 1977;2(7–8):667–673.
116. Mayo C, Yorke E, Merchant TE. Radiation associated brainstem injury. *Int J Radiat Oncol Biol Phys* 2010;76(3 Suppl):S36–S41.
117. Luft AR, et al. Patterns of age-related shrinkage in cerebellum and brainstem observed in vivo using three-dimensional MRI volumetry. *Cereb Cortex* 1999;9(7):712–721.
118. Debus J, et al. Brainstem tolerance to conformal radiotherapy of skull base tumors. *Int J Radiat Oncol Biol Phys* 1997;39(5):967–975.
119. Debus J, et al. Dose-volume tolerance of the brainstem after high-dose radiotherapy. *Front Radiat Ther Oncol* 1999;33:305–314.
120. Freeman CR, et al. Final results of a study of escalating doses of hyperfractionated radiotherapy in brain stem tumors in children: a Pediatric Oncology Group study. *Int J Radiat Oncol Biol Phys* 1993;27(2):197–206.
121. Hoppe BS, et al. Treatment of nasal cavity and paranasal sinus cancer with modern radiotherapy techniques in the postoperative setting–the MSKCC experience. *Int J Radiat Oncol Biol Phys* 2007;67(3):691–702.
122. Jian JJ, et al. Improvement of local control of T3 and T4 nasopharyngeal carcinoma by hyperfractionated radiotherapy and concomitant chemotherapy. *Int J Radiat Oncol Biol Phys* 2002;53(2):344–352.
123. Merchant TE, et al. Factors associated with neurological recovery of brainstem function following postoperative conformal radiation therapy for infratentorial ependymoma. *Int J Radiat Oncol Biol Phys* 2010;76(2):496–503.
124. Packer RJ, et al. Outcome of children with brain stem gliomas after treatment with 7800 cGy of hyperfractionated radiotherapy. A Childrens Cancer Group Phase I/II Trial. *Cancer* 1994;74(6):1827–1834.
125. Packer RJ, et al. Treatment of children with newly diagnosed brain stem gliomas with intravenous recombinant beta-interferon and hyperfractionated radiation therapy: a childrens cancer group phase I/II study. *Cancer* 1996;77(10):2150–2156.
126. Schoenfeld GO, et al. Patterns of failure and toxicity after intensity-modulated radiotherapy for head and neck cancer. *Int J Radiat Oncol Biol Phys* 2008;71(2):377–385.
127. Uy NW, et al. Intensity-modulated radiation therapy (IMRT) for meningioma. *Int J Radiat Oncol Biol Phys* 2002;53(5):1265–1270.
128. Foote KD, et al. Analysis of risk factors associated with radiosurgery for vestibular schwannoma. *J Neurosurg* 2001;95(3):440–449.
129. Fuentes S, et al. Brainstem metastases: management using gamma knife radiosurgery. *Neurosurgery* 2006;58(1):37–42; discussion 37–42.
130. Kased N, et al. Gamma knife radiosurgery for brainstem metastases: the UCSF experience. *J Neurooncol* 2008;86(2):195–205.
131. Maruyama K, et al. Stereotactic radiosurgery for brainstem arteriovenous malformations: factors affecting outcome. *J Neurosurg* 2004;100(3):407–413.
132. Pollock BE, Gorman DA, Brown PD. Radiosurgery for arteriovenous malformations of the basal ganglia, thalamus, and brainstem. *J Neurosurg* 2004;100(2):210–214.
133. Spiegelmann R, et al. Linear accelerator radiosurgery for vestibular schwannoma. *J Neurosurg* 2001;94(1):7–13.

134. Lorenzoni JG, et al. Brain stem metastases treated with radiosurgery: prognostic factors of survival and life expectancy estimation. *Surg Neurol* 2009;71(2):188–195; discussion 195, 195–196.
135. Bhandare N, et al. Radiation therapy and hearing loss. *Int J Radiat Oncol Biol Phys* 2010;76(3 Suppl):S50–S57.
136. Pan CC, et al. Prospective study of inner ear radiation dose and hearing loss in head-and-neck cancer patients. *Int J Radiat Oncol Biol Phys* 2005;61(5):1393–1402.
137. Chen WC, et al. Sensorineural hearing loss in combined modality treatment of nasopharyngeal carcinoma. *Cancer* 2006;106(4):820–829.
138. Kwong DL, et al. Sensorineural hearing loss in patients treated for nasopharyngeal carcinoma: a prospective study of the effect of radiation and cisplatin treatment. *Int J Radiat Oncol Biol Phys* 1996;36(2):281–289.
139. Ho WK, et al. Long-term sensorineural hearing deficit following radiotherapy in patients suffering from nasopharyngeal carcinoma: a prospective study. *Head Neck* 1999;21(6):547–553.
140. Oh YT, et al. Sensory neural hearing loss after concurrent cisplatin and radiation therapy for nasopharyngeal carcinoma. *Radiother Oncol* 2004;72(1):79–82.
141. Honore HB, et al. Sensori-neural hearing loss after radiotherapy for nasopharyngeal carcinoma: individualized risk estimation. *Radiother Oncol* 2002;65(1):9–16.
142. van der Putten L, et al. Permanent unilateral hearing loss after radiotherapy for parotid gland tumors. *Head Neck* 2006;28(10):902–908.
143. Andrews DW, et al. Stereotactic radiosurgery and fractionated stereotactic radiotherapy for the treatment of acoustic schwannomas: comparative observations of 125 patients treated at one institution. *Int J Radiat Oncol Biol Phys* 2001;50(5):1265–1278.
144. Combs SE, et al. Management of acoustic neuromas with fractionated stereotactic radiotherapy (FSRT): long-term results in 106 patients treated in a single institution. *Int J Radiat Oncol Biol Phys* 2005;63(1):75–81.
145. Williams JA. Fractionated radiotherapy for acoustic neuromas. In *Congress of Neurological Surgeons: 50th Annual Meeting*. San Antonio, TX. 2000.
146. Hirsch A, Noren G. Audiological findings after stereotactic radiosurgery in acoustic neurinomas. *Acta Otolaryngol* 1988;106(3–4):244–251.
147. Noren G, et al. Gamma knife surgery in acoustic tumours. *Acta Neurochir Suppl (Wien)* 1993;58:104–107.
148. Foote RL, et al. Stereotactic radiosurgery using the gamma knife for acoustic neuromas. *Int J Radiat Oncol Biol Phys* 1995;32(4):1153–1160.
149. Flickinger JC, et al. Evolution in technique for vestibular schwannoma radiosurgery and effect on outcome. *Int J Radiat Oncol Biol Phys* 1996;36(2):275–280.
150. Kondziolka D, et al. Long-term outcomes after radiosurgery for acoustic neuromas. *N Engl J Med* 1998;339(20):1426–1433.
151. Lunsford LD, Kondziolka D, Pollock BE. Acoustic neuroma management: evolution and revolution. In: Kondziolka D, ed. *Radiosurgery*. Basel, Switzerland: Karger, 1998:1–7.
152. Flickinger JC, et al. Results of acoustic neuroma radiosurgery: an analysis of 5 years' experience using current methods. *J Neurosurg* 2001;94(1):1–6.
153. Williams JA. Fractionated stereotactic radiotherapy for acoustic neuromas. *Int J Radiat Oncol Biol Phys* 2002;54(2):500–504.
154. Meijer OW, et al. Single-fraction vs. fractionated linac-based stereotactic radiosurgery for vestibular schwannoma: a single-institution study. *Int J Radiat Oncol Biol Phys* 2003;56(5):1390–1396.
155. Flickinger JC, Kondziolka D, Lunsford LD. Dose and diameter relationships for facial, trigeminal, and acoustic neuropathies following acoustic neuroma radiosurgery. *Radiother Oncol* 1996;41(3):215–219.
156. Massager N, et al. Role of intracanalicular volumetric and dosimetric parameters on hearing preservation after vestibular schwannoma radiosurgery. *Int J Radiat Oncol Biol Phys* 2006;64(5):1331–1340.
157. Pollock BE, et al. Outcome analysis of acoustic neuroma management: a comparison of microsurgery and stereotactic radiosurgery. *Neurosurgery* 1995;36(1):215–224; discussion 224–229.
158. Niranjan A, et al. Dose reduction improves hearing preservation rates after intracanalicular acoustic tumor radiosurgery. *Neurosurgery* 1999;45(4): 753–762; discussion 762–765.
159. Bhandare N, et al. Ototoxicity after radiotherapy for head and neck tumors. *Int J Radiat Oncol Biol Phys* 2007;67(2):469–479.
160. Low WK, et al. Sensorineural hearing loss after radiotherapy and chemoradiotherapy: a single, blinded, randomized study. *J Clin Oncol* 2006;24(12):1904–1909.
161. Hua C, et al. Hearing loss after radiotherapy for pediatric brain tumors: effect of cochlear dose. *Int J Radiat Oncol Biol Phys* 2008;72(3):892–899.
162. Mathieu D, et al. Stereotactic radiosurgery for vestibular schwannomas in patients with neurofibromatosis type 2: an analysis of tumor control, complications, and hearing preservation rates. *Neurosurgery* 2007;60(3):460–468; discussion 468–470.
163. Phi JH, et al. Radiosurgical treatment of vestibular schwannomas in patients with neurofibromatosis type 2: tumor control and hearing preservation. *Cancer* 2009;115(2):390–398.
164. Rowe J, Radatz M, Kemeny A. Radiosurgery for type II neurofibromatosis. *Prog Neurol Surg* 2008;21:176–182.
165. Flickinger JC, et al. Acoustic neuroma radiosurgery with marginal tumor doses of 12 to 13 Gy. *Int J Radiat Oncol Biol Phys* 2004;60(1):225–230.
166. Kirkpatrick JP, van der Kogel AJ, Schultheiss TE. Radiation dose-volume effects in the spinal cord. *Int J Radiat Oncol Biol Phys* 2010;76(3 Suppl):S42–S49.
167. Klimo P Jr, et al. A meta-analysis of surgery versus conventional radiotherapy for the treatment of metastatic spinal epidural disease. *Neuro Oncol* 2005;7(1):64–76.
168. Schultheiss TE, et al. Radiation response of the central nervous system. *Int J Radiat Oncol Biol Phys* 1995;31(5):1093–1112.
169. Abbatucci JS, et al. Radiation myelopathy of the cervical spinal cord: time, dose and volume factors. *Int J Radiat Oncol Biol Phys* 1978;4(3–4):239–248.
170. Sahgal A, Larson DA, Chang EL. Stereotactic body radiosurgery for spinal metastases: a critical review. *Int J Radiat Oncol Biol Phys* 2008;71(3): 652–665.
171. Schultheiss TE. The radiation dose–response of the human spinal cord. *Int J Radiat Oncol Biol Phys* 2008;71(5):1455–1459.
172. Atkins HL, Tretter P. Time-dose considerations in radiation myelopathy. *Acta Radiol Ther Phys Biol* 1966;5:79–94.
173. Jeremic B, Djuric L, Mijatovic L. Incidence of radiation myelitis of the cervical spinal cord at doses of 5500 cGy or greater. *Cancer* 1991;68(10):2138–2141.
174. Marcus RB Jr, Million RR. The incidence of myelitis after irradiation of the cervical spinal cord. *Int J Radiat Oncol Biol Phys* 1990;19(1):3–8.
175. McCunniff AJ, Liang MJ. Radiation tolerance of the cervical spinal cord. *Int J Radiat Oncol Biol Phys* 1989;16(3):675–678.
176. Abramson N, Cavanaugh PJ. Short-course radiation therapy in carcinoma of the lung. A second look. *Radiology* 1973;108(3):685–687.
177. Choi NC, et al. Basis for new strategies in postoperative radiotherapy of bronchogenic carcinoma. *Int J Radiat Oncol Biol Phys* 1980;6(1):31–35.
178. Dische S, Warburton MF, Saunders MI. Radiation myelitis and survival in the radiotherapy of lung cancer. *Int J Radiat Oncol Biol Phys* 1988;15(1): 75–81.
179. Eichhorn HJ, Lessel A, Rotte KH. Einfluss verschiedener Bestrahlungsrhythmen auf Tumor- und Normalgewebe in vivo [Influence of various irradiation rhythms on neoplastic and normal tissue in vivo]. *Strahlentherapie* 1972;143(6):614–629.
180. Fitzgerald RH Jr, Marks RD Jr, Wallace KM. Chronic radiation myelitis. *Radiology* 1982;144(3):609–612.
181. Guthrie RT, Ptacek JJ, Hass AC. Comparative analysis of two regimens of split course radiation in carcinoma of the lung. *Am J Roentgenol Radium Ther Nucl Med* 1973;117(3):605–608.
182. Hatlevoll R, Host H, Kaalhus O. Myelopathy following radiotherapy of bronchial carcinoma with large single fractions: a retrospective study. *Int J Radiat Oncol Biol Phys* 1983;9(1):41–44.
183. Hazra TA, et al. Survival in carcinoma of the lung after a split course of radiotherapy. *Br J Radiol* 1974;47(560):464–466.
184. Macbeth FR, et al. Randomized trial of palliative two-fraction versus more intensive 13-fraction radiotherapy for patients with inoperable non-small cell lung cancer and good performance status. Medical Research Council Lung Cancer Working Party. *Clin Oncol (R Coll Radiol)* 1996;8(3):167–175.
185. Macbeth FR, et al. Radiation myelopathy: estimates of risk in 1048 patients in three randomized trials of palliative radiotherapy for non-small cell lung cancer. The Medical Research Council Lung Cancer Working Party. *Clin Oncol (R Coll Radiol)* 1996;8(3):176–181.
186. Madden FJ, et al. Split course radiation in inoperable carcinoma of the bronchus. *Eur J Cancer* 1979;15(9):1175–1177.
187. Scruggs H, et al. The results of split-course radiation therapy in cancer of the lung. *Am J Roentgenol Radium Ther Nucl Med* 1974;121(4):754–760.
188. Gibbs IC, et al. Delayed radiation-induced myelopathy after spinal radiosurgery. *Neurosurgery* 2009;64(2 Suppl):A67–A72.
189. Ryu S, et al. Partial volume tolerance of the spinal cord and complications of single-dose radiosurgery. *Cancer* 2007;109(3):628–636.
190. Gwak HS, et al. Hypofractionated stereotactic radiation therapy for skull base and upper cervical chordoma and chondrosarcoma: preliminary results. *Stereotact Funct Neurosurg* 2005;83(5–6):233–243.
191. Benzil DL, et al. Safety and efficacy of stereotactic radiosurgery for tumors of the spine. *J Neurosurg* 2004;101(Suppl 3):413–418.
192. Sahgal A, et al. Proximity of spinous/paraspinous radiosurgery metastatic targets to the spinal cord versus risk of local failure. *Int J Radiat Oncol Biol Phys* 2007;69:S243.
193. Sahgal A, et al. Image-guided robotic stereotactic body radiotherapy for benign spinal tumors: the University of California San Francisco preliminary experience. *Technol Cancer Res Treat* 2007;6(6):595–604.
194. Chang EL, et al. Phase I/II study of stereotactic body radiotherapy for spinal metastasis and its pattern of failure. *J Neurosurg Spine* 2007;7(2):151–160.
195. Gerszten PC, et al. Single-fraction radiosurgery for the treatment of spinal breast metastases. *Cancer* 2005;104(10):2244–2254.
196. Nelson JW, et al. Stereotactic body radiotherapy for lesions of the spine and paraspinal regions. *Int J Radiat Oncol Biol Phys* 2009;73(5):1369–1375.
197. Ang KK, et al. The tolerance of primate spinal cord to re-irradiation. *Int J Radiat Oncol Biol Phys* 1993;25(3):459–464.
198. Ruifrok AC, Kleiboer BJ, van der Kogel AJ. Fractionation sensitivity of the rat cervical spinal cord during radiation retreatment. *Radiother Oncol* 1992;25(4):295–300.
199. Ruifrok AC, Kleiboer BJ, van der Kogel AJ. Radiation tolerance and fractionation sensitivity of the developing rat cervical spinal cord. *Int J Radiat Oncol Biol Phys* 1992;24(3):505–510.
200. Ruifrok AC, Stephens LC, van der Kogel AJ. Radiation response of the rat cervical spinal cord after irradiation at different ages: tolerance, latency and pathology. *Int J Radiat Oncol Biol Phys* 1994;29(1):73–79.
201. Friedman DL, Constine LS. Late effects of cancer treatment. In: Halperin EC, et al., eds. *Pediatric radiation oncology*. Philadelphia, PA: Lippincott Williams & Wilkins, 2011:353–396.
202. Bloss JD, et al. Radiation myelitis: a complication of concurrent cisplatin and 5-fluorouracil chemotherapy with extended field radiotherapy for carcinoma of the uterine cervix. *Gynecol Oncol* 1991;43(3):305–308.
203. Chao MW, et al. Radiation myelopathy following transplantation and radiotherapy for non-Hodgkin's lymphoma. *Int J Radiat Oncol Biol Phys* 1998;41(5):1057–1061.
204. Ruckdeschel JC, et al. Sequential radiotherapy and adriamycin in the management of bronchogenic carcinoma: the question of additive toxicity. *Int J Radiat Oncol Biol Phys* 1979;5(8):1323–1328.

205. Seddon BM, et al. Fatal radiation myelopathy after high-dose busulfan and melphalan chemotherapy and radiotherapy for Ewing's sarcoma: a review of the literature and implications for practice. *Clin Oncol (R Coll Radiol)* 2005;17(5):385–390.

206. Lee YY, Nauert C, Glass JP. Treatment-related white matter changes in cancer patients. *Cancer* 1986;57(8):1473–1482.

207. Schultheiss TE, et al. Effect of latency on calculated complication rates. *Int J Radiat Oncol Biol Phys* 1986;12(10):1861–1865.

208. Kirkpatrick JP, Meyer JJ, Marks LB. The linear-quadratic model is inappropriate to model high dose per fraction effects in radiosurgery. *Semin Radiat Oncol* 2008;18(4):240–243.

209. Medin PM, et al. Spinal cord tolerance to single-fraction partial-volume irradiation: a swine model. *Int J Radiat Oncol Biol Phys* 2011;79(1):226–232.

210. Nieder C, et al. Proposal of human spinal cord reirradiation dose based on collection of data from 40 patients. *Int J Radiat Oncol Biol Phys* 2005;61(3):851–855.

211. Ang KK, et al. Extent and kinetics of recovery of occult spinal cord injury. *Int J Radiat Oncol Biol Phys* 2001;50(4):1013–1020.

212. Ang KK, van der Kogel AJ, van der Schueren E. The effect of small radiation doses on the rat spinal cord: the concept of partial tolerance. *Int J Radiat Oncol Biol Phys* 1983;9(10):1487–1491.

213. Knowles JF. The radiosensitivity of the guinea-pig spinal cord to X-rays: the effect of retreatment at one year and the effect of age at the time of irradiation. *Int J Radiat Biol Relat Stud Phys Chem Med* 1983;44(5):433–442.

214. Ruifrok AC, Kleiboer BJ, van der Kogel AJ. Repair kinetics of radiation damage in the developing rat cervical spinal cord. *Int J Radiat Biol* 1993;63(4):501–508.

215. Wong CS, Hao Y. Long-term recovery kinetics of radiation damage in rat spinal cord. *Int J Radiat Oncol Biol Phys* 1997;37(1):171–179.

216. Wright JL, et al. Clinical outcomes after reirradiation of paraspinal tumors. *Am J Clin Oncol* 2006;29(5):495–502.

217. Langendijk JA, et al. A phase II study of primary reirradiation in squamous cell carcinoma of head and neck. *Radiother Oncol* 2006;78(3):306–312.

218. Grosu AL, et al. Retreatment of the spinal cord with palliative radiotherapy. *Int J Radiat Oncol Biol Phys* 2002;52(5):1288–1292.

219. Nieder C, et al. Update of human spinal cord reirradiation tolerance based on additional data from 38 patients. *Int J Radiat Oncol Biol Phys* 2006;66(5):1446–1449.

220. Schiff D, Shaw EG, Cascino TL. Outcome after spinal reirradiation for malignant epidural spinal cord compression. *Ann Neurol* 1995;37(5):583–589.

221. Ryu S, et al. 'Full dose' reirradiation of human cervical spinal cord. *Am J Clin Oncol* 2000;23(1):29–31.

222. Kuo JV, et al. Intensity-modulated radiation therapy for the spine at the University of California, Irvine. *Med Dosim* 2002;27(2):137–145.

223. Bauman GS, et al. Reirradiation of primary CNS tumors. *Int J Radiat Oncol Biol Phys* 1996;36(2):433–441.

224. Sminia P, et al. Re-irradiation of the human spinal cord. *Strahlenther Onkol* 2002;178(8):453–456.

225. Magrini SM, et al. Neurological damage in patients irradiated twice on the spinal cord: a morphologic and electrophysiological study. *Radiother Oncol* 1990;17(3):209–218.

226. Rades D, et al. Spinal reirradiation after short-course RT for metastatic spinal cord compression. *Int J Radiat Oncol Biol Phys* 2005;63(3):872–875.

227. Jackson MA, Ball DL. Palliative retreatment of locally-recurrent lung cancer after radical radiotherapy. *Med J Aust* 1987;147(8):391–394.

228. Wong CS, et al. Radiation myelopathy following single courses of radiotherapy and retreatment. *Int J Radiat Oncol Biol Phys* 1994;30(3):575–581.

229. Sahgal A, et al. Spinal cord tolerance for stereotactic body radiotherapy. *Int J Radiat Oncol Biol Phys* 2010;77(2):548–553.

230. Fung K, et al. Effects of head and neck radiation therapy on vocal function. *J Otolaryngol* 2001;30(3):133–139.

231. Rancati T, et al. Radiation dose-volume effects in the larynx and pharynx. *Int J Radiat Oncol Biol Phys* 2010;76(3 Suppl):S64–S69.

232. Kendall KA, et al. Timing of swallowing events after single-modality treatment of head and neck carcinomas with radiotherapy. *Ann Otol Rhinol Laryngol* 2000;109(8 Pt 1):767–775.

233. Dornfeld K, et al. Radiation doses to structures within and adjacent to the larynx are correlated with long-term diet- and speech-related quality of life. *Int J Radiat Oncol Biol Phys* 2007;68(3):750–757.

234. Sanguineti G, et al. Dosimetric predictors of laryngeal edema. *Int J Radiat Oncol Biol Phys* 2007;68(3):741–749.

235. Eisbruch A, et al. Dysphagia and aspiration after chemoradiotherapy for head-and-neck cancer: which anatomic structures are affected and can they be spared by IMRT? *Int J Radiat Oncol Biol Phys* 2004;60(5):1425–1439.

236. Feng FY, et al. Intensity-modulated radiotherapy of head and neck cancer aiming to reduce dysphagia: early dose-effect relationships for the swallowing structures. *Int J Radiat Oncol Biol Phys* 2007;68(5):1289–1298.

237. Jensen K, Lambertsen K, Grau C. Late swallowing dysfunction and dysphagia after radiotherapy for pharynx cancer: frequency, intensity and correlation with dose and volume parameters. *Radiother Oncol* 2007;85(1):74–82.

238. Levendag PC, et al. Dysphagia disorders in patients with cancer of the oropharynx are significantly affected by the radiation therapy dose to the superior and middle constrictor muscle: a dose-effect relationship. *Radiother Oncol* 2007;85(1):64–73.

239. Li B, et al. Clinical-dosimetric analysis of measures of dysphagia including gastrostomy-tube dependence among head and neck cancer patients treated definitively by intensity-modulated radiotherapy with concurrent chemotherapy. *Radiat Oncol* 2009;4:52.

240. Deantonio L, et al. Dysphagia after definitive radiotherapy for head and neck cancer. Correlation of dose-volume parameters of the pharyngeal constrictor muscles. *Strahlenther Onkol* 2013;189(3):230–236.

241. Dirix P, et al. Dysphagia after chemoradiotherapy for head-and-neck squamous cell carcinoma: dose-effect relationships for the swallowing structures. *Int J Radiat Oncol Biol Phys* 2009;75(2):385–392.

242. Caglar HB, et al. Dose to larynx predicts for swallowing complications after intensity-modulated radiotherapy. *Int J Radiat Oncol Biol Phys* 2008;72(4):1110–1118.

243. Schwartz DL. et al. Candidate dosimetric predictors of long-term swallowing dysfunction after oropharyngeal intensity-modulated radiotherapy. *Int J Radiat Oncol Biol Phys* 2010;78(5):1356–1365

244. Caudell JJ, et al. Dosimetric factors associated with long-term dysphagia after definitive radiotherapy for squamous cell carcinoma of the head and neck. *Int J Radiat Oncol Biol Phys* 2010;76(2):403–409.

245. Rancati T, Fiorino C, Sanguineti G. NTCP modeling of subacute/late laryngeal edema scored by fiberoptic examination. *Int J Radiat Oncol Biol Phys* 2009;75(3):915–923.

246. Langerman A, et al. Aspiration in chemoradiated patients with head and neck cancer. *Arch Otolaryngol Head Neck Surg* 2007;133(12):1289–1295.

247. Deasy JO, et al. Radiotherapy dose-volume effects on salivary gland function. *Int J Radiat Oncol Biol Phys* 2010;76(3 Suppl):S58–S63.

248. Dawes C, Wood CM. The contribution of oral minor mucous gland secretions to the volume of whole saliva in man. *Arch Oral Biol* 1973;18(3):337–342.

249. Robar JL, et al. Spatial and dosimetric variability of organs at risk in head-and-neck intensity-modulated radiotherapy. *Int J Radiat Oncol Biol Phys* 2007;68(4):1121–1130.

250. Blanco AI, et al. Dose-volume modeling of salivary function in patients with head-and-neck cancer receiving radiotherapy. *Int J Radiat Oncol Biol Phys* 2005;62(4):1055–1069.

251. Li Y, et al. The impact of dose on parotid salivary recovery in head and neck cancer patients treated with radiation therapy. *Int J Radiat Oncol Biol Phys* 2007;67(3):660–669.

252. Maes A, et al. Preservation of parotid function with uncomplicated conformal radiotherapy. *Radiother Oncol* 2002;63(2):203–211.

253. Eisbruch A, et al. Dose, volume, and function relationships in parotid salivary glands following conformal and intensity-modulated irradiation of head and neck cancer. *Int J Radiat Oncol Biol Phys* 1999;45(3):577–587.

254. Chao KS, et al. A prospective study of salivary function sparing in patients with head-and-neck cancers receiving intensity-modulated or three-dimensional radiation therapy: initial results. *Int J Radiat Oncol Biol Phys* 2001;49(4):907–916.

255. Saarilahti K, et al. Intensity modulated radiotherapy for head and neck cancer: evidence for preserved salivary gland function. *Radiother Oncol* 2005;74(3):251–258.

256. Portaluri M, et al. Three-dimensional conformal radiotherapy for locally advanced (stage II and worse) head-and-neck cancer: dosimetric and clinical evaluation. *Int J Radiat Oncol Biol Phys* 2006;66(4):1036–1043.

257. Braam PM, et al. Quality of life and salivary output in patients with head-and-neck cancer five years after radiotherapy. *Radiat Oncol* 2007;2:3.

258. Bussels B, et al. Dose–response relationships within the parotid gland after radiotherapy for head and neck cancer. *Radiother Oncol* 2004;73(3):297–306.

259. Roesink JM, et al. Quantitative dose-volume response analysis of changes in parotid gland function after radiotherapy in the head-and-neck region. *Int J Radiat Oncol Biol Phys* 2001;51(4):938–946.

260. Roesink JM, et al. Scintigraphic assessment of early and late parotid gland function after radiotherapy for head-and-neck cancer: a prospective study of dose-volume response relationships. *Int J Radiat Oncol Biol Phys* 2004;58(5):1451–1460.

261. Eisbruch A, et al. Xerostomia and its predictors following parotid-sparing irradiation of head-and-neck cancer. *Int J Radiat Oncol Biol Phys* 2001;50(3):695–704.

262. Buus S, et al. Individual radiation response of parotid glands investigated by dynamic 11C-methionine PET. *Radiother Oncol* 2006;78(3):262–269.

263. Deasy JO, Chao KS, Markman J. Uncertainties in model-based outcome predictions for treatment planning. *Int J Radiat Oncol Biol Phys* 2001;51(5):1389–1399.

264. Beetz I, et al. Development of NTCP models for head and neck cancer patients treated with three-dimensional conformal radiotherapy for xerostomia and sticky saliva: the role of dosimetric and clinical factors. *Radiother Oncol* 2012;105(1):86–93.

265. Beetz I, et al. NTCP models for patient-rated xerostomia and sticky saliva after treatment with intensity modulated radiotherapy for head and neck cancer: the role of dosimetric and clinical factors. *Radiother Oncol* 2012;105(1):101–106.

266. Saarilahti K, et al. Sparing of the submandibular glands by intensity modulated radiotherapy in the treatment of head and neck cancer. *Radiother Oncol* 2006;78(3):270–275.

267. Wang ZH, et al. Impact of salivary gland dosimetry on post-IMRT recovery of saliva output and xerostomia grade for head-and-neck cancer patients treated with or without contralateral submandibular gland sparing: a longitudinal study. *Int J Radiat Oncol Biol Phys* 2011;81(5):1479–1487.

268. Little M, et al. Reducing xerostomia after chemo-IMRT for head-and-neck cancer: beyond sparing the parotid glands. *Int J Radiat Oncol Biol Phys* 2012;83(3):1007–1014.

269. Jellema AP, et al. Does radiation dose to the salivary glands and oral cavity predict patient-rated xerostomia and sticky saliva in head and neck cancer patients treated with curative radiotherapy? *Radiother Oncol* 2005;77(2):164–171.

270. Munter MW, et al. Changes in salivary gland function after radiotherapy of head and neck tumors measured by quantitative pertechnetate scintigraphy: comparison of intensity-modulated radiotherapy and conventional radiation therapy with and without amifostine. *Int J Radiat Oncol Biol Phys* 2007;67(3):651–659.

271. Chera BS, et al. Dosimetric predictors of patient reported xerostomia and dysphagia with deintensified chemoradiotherapy for HPV-associated oropharyngeal squamous cell carcinoma. *Int J Radiat Oncol Biol Phys* 2017;98(5):1022–1027.

272. Moiseenko V, et al. Treatment planning constraints to avoid xerostomia in head-and-neck radiotherapy: an independent test of QUANTEC criteria using a prospectively collected dataset. *Int J Radiat Oncol Biol Phys* 2012;82(3):1108–1114.
273. Tribius S, et al. Xerostomia after radiotherapy. What matters—mean total dose or dose to each parotid gland? *Strahlenther Onkol* 2013;189(3):216–222.
274. Kocak Z, et al. Challenges in defining radiation pneumonitis in patients with lung cancer. *Int J Radiat Oncol Biol Phys* 2005;62(3):635–638.
275. Graham MV, et al. Clinical dose-volume histogram analysis for pneumonitis after 3D treatment for non-small cell lung cancer (NSCLC). *Int J Radiat Oncol Biol Phys* 1999;45(2):323–329.
276. Armstrong J, et al. Promising survival with three-dimensional conformal radiation therapy for non-small cell lung cancer. *Radiother Oncol* 1997;44(1):17–22.
277. Bradley JD, et al. A nomogram to predict radiation pneumonitis, derived from a combined analysis of RTOG 9311 and institutional data. *Int J Radiat Oncol Biol Phys* 2007;69(4):985–992.
278. Fay M, et al. Dose-volume histogram analysis as predictor of radiation pneumonitis in primary lung cancer patients treated with radiotherapy. *Int J Radiat Oncol Biol Phys* 2005;61(5):1355–1363.
279. Hernando ML, et al. Radiation-induced pulmonary toxicity: a dose-volume histogram analysis in 201 patients with lung cancer. *Int J Radiat Oncol Biol Phys* 2001;51(3):650–659.
280. Hope AJ, et al. Modeling radiation pneumonitis risk with clinical, dosimetric, and spatial parameters. *Int J Radiat Oncol Biol Phys* 2006;65(1):112–124.
281. Kim TH, et al. Dose-volumetric parameters for predicting severe radiation pneumonitis after three-dimensional conformal radiation therapy for lung cancer. *Radiology* 2005;235(1):208–215.
282. Kwa SL, et al. Radiation pneumonitis as a function of mean lung dose: an analysis of pooled data of 540 patients. *Int J Radiat Oncol Biol Phys* 1998;42(1):1–9.
283. Piotrowski T, Matecka-Nowak M, Milecki P. Prediction of radiation pneumonitis: dose-volume histogram analysis in 62 patients with non-small cell lung cancer after three-dimensional conformal radiotherapy. *Neoplasma* 2005;52(1):56–62.
284. Schallenkamp JM, et al. Incidence of radiation pneumonitis after thoracic irradiation: dose-volume correlates. *Int J Radiat Oncol Biol Phys* 2007;67(2):410–416.
285. Seppenwoolde Y, et al. Comparing different NTCP models that predict the incidence of radiation pneumonitis. Normal tissue complication probability. *Int J Radiat Oncol Biol Phys* 2003;55(3):724–735.
286. Tsujino K, et al. Radiation pneumonitis following concurrent accelerated hyperfractionated radiotherapy and chemotherapy for limited-stage small-cell lung cancer: dose-volume histogram analysis and comparison with conventional chemoradiation. *Int J Radiat Oncol Biol Phys* 2006;64(4):1100–1105.
287. Wang S, et al. Analysis of clinical and dosimetric factors associated with treatment-related pneumonitis (TRP) in patients with non-small-cell lung cancer (NSCLC) treated with concurrent chemotherapy and three-dimensional conformal radiotherapy (3D-CRT). *Int J Radiat Oncol Biol Phys* 2006;66(5):1399–1407.
288. Willner J, et al. A little to a lot or a lot to a little? An analysis of pneumonitis risk from dose-volume histogram parameters of the lung in patients with lung cancer treated with 3-D conformal radiotherapy. *Strahlenther Onkol* 2003;179(8):548–556.
289. Yom SS, et al. Initial evaluation of treatment-related pneumonitis in advanced-stage non-small-cell lung cancer patients treated with concurrent chemotherapy and intensity-modulated radiotherapy. *Int J Radiat Oncol Biol Phys* 2007;68(1):94–102.
290. Yorke ED, et al. Correlation of dosimetric factors and radiation pneumonitis for non-small-cell lung cancer patients in a recently completed dose escalation study. *Int J Radiat Oncol Biol Phys* 2005;63(3):672–682.
291. Yorke ED, et al. Dose-volume factors contributing to the incidence of radiation pneumonitis in non-small-cell lung cancer patients treated with three-dimensional conformal radiation therapy. *Int J Radiat Oncol Biol Phys* 2002;54(2):329–339.
292. Kong FM, et al. Final toxicity results of a radiation-dose escalation study in patients with non-small-cell lung cancer (NSCLC): predictors for radiation pneumonitis and fibrosis. *Int J Radiat Oncol Biol Phys* 2006;65(4):1075–1086.
293. Seppenwoolde Y, et al. Regional differences in lung radiosensitivity after radiotherapy for non-small-cell lung cancer. *Int J Radiat Oncol Biol Phys* 2004;60(3):748–758.
294. Martel MK, et al. Dose-volume histogram and 3-D treatment planning evaluation of patients with pneumonitis. *Int J Radiat Oncol Biol Phys* 1994;28(3):575–581.
295. Oetzel D, et al. Estimation of pneumonitis risk in three-dimensional treatment planning using dose-volume histogram analysis. *Int J Radiat Oncol Biol Phys* 1995;33(2):455–460.
296. Rancati T, et al. Factors predicting radiation pneumonitis in lung cancer patients: a retrospective study. *Radiother Oncol* 2003;67(3):275–283.
297. Dewit L, et al. Compensatory renal response after unilateral partial and whole volume high-dose irradiation of the human kidney. *Eur J Cancer* 1993;29A(16):2239–2243.
298. Tsujino K, et al. Predictive value of dose-volume histogram parameters for predicting radiation pneumonitis after concurrent chemoradiation for lung cancer. *Int J Radiat Oncol Biol Phys* 2003;55(1):110–115.
299. Armstrong JG, et al. Strategy for dose escalation using 3-dimensional conformal radiation therapy for lung cancer. *Ann Oncol* 1995;6(7):693–697.
300. Marks LB, et al. Radiation dose-volume effects in the lung. *Int J Radiat Oncol Biol Phys* 2010;76(3 Suppl):S70–S76.
301. Bradley J, et al. Toxicity and outcome results of RTOG 9311: a phase I-II dose-escalation study using three-dimensional conformal radiotherapy in patients with inoperable non-small-cell lung carcinoma. *Int J Radiat Oncol Biol Phys* 2005;61(2):318–328.
302. Hayman JA, et al. Dose escalation in non-small-cell lung cancer using three-dimensional conformal radiation therapy: update of a phase I trial. *J Clin Oncol* 2001;19(1):127–136.
303. Narayan S, et al. Results following treatment to doses of 92.4 or 102.9 Gy on a phase I dose escalation study for non-small cell lung cancer. *Lung Cancer* 2004;44(1):79–88.
304. Rosenzweig KE, et al. Final report of the 70.2-Gy and 75.6-Gy dose levels of a phase I dose escalation study using three-dimensional conformal radiotherapy in the treatment of inoperable non-small cell lung cancer. *Cancer J* 2000;6(2):82–87.
305. Vogelius IR, Bentzen SM. A literature-based meta-analysis of clinical risk factors for development of radiation induced pneumonitis. *Acta Oncol* 2012;51(8):975–983.
306. Palma DA, et al. Predicting radiation pneumonitis after chemoradiation therapy for lung cancer: an international individual patient data meta-analysis. *Int J Radiat Oncol Biol Phys* 2013;85(2):444–450.
307. Zhang XJ, et al. Prediction of radiation pneumonitis in lung cancer patients: a systematic review. *J Cancer Res Clin Oncol* 2012;138(12):2103–2116.
308. Gokula K, et al. Meta-analysis of incidence of early lung toxicity in 3-dimensional conformal irradiation of breast carcinomas. *Radiat Oncol* 2013;8:268.
309. Murshed H, et al. Dose and volume reduction for normal lung using intensity-modulated radiotherapy for advanced-stage non-small-cell lung cancer. *Int J Radiat Oncol Biol Phys* 2004;58(4):1258–1267.
310. Liao ZX, et al. Influence of technologic advances on outcomes in patients with unresectable, locally advanced non-small-cell lung cancer receiving concomitant chemoradiotherapy. *Int J Radiat Oncol Biol Phys* 2010;76(3):775–781.
311. Sura S, et al. Intensity-modulated radiation therapy (IMRT) for inoperable non-small cell lung cancer: the Memorial Sloan-Kettering Cancer Center (MSKCC) experience. *Radiother Oncol* 2008;87(1):17–23.
312. Allen AM, et al. Fatal pneumonitis associated with intensity-modulated radiation therapy for mesothelioma. *Int J Radiat Oncol Biol Phys* 2006;65(3):640–645.
313. Miles EF, et al. Intensity-modulated radiotherapy for resected mesothelioma: the Duke experience. *Int J Radiat Oncol Biol Phys* 2008;71(4):1143–1150.
314. Rice DC, et al. Dose-dependent pulmonary toxicity after postoperative intensity-modulated radiotherapy for malignant pleural mesothelioma. *Int J Radiat Oncol Biol Phys* 2007;69(2):350–357.
315. Heinzerling JH, Kavanagh B, Timmerman RD. Stereotactic ablative radiation therapy for primary lung tumors. *Cancer J* 2011;17(1):28–32.
316. Timmerman R, et al. Accreditation and quality assurance for Radiation Therapy Oncology Group: multicenter clinical trials using stereotactic body radiation therapy in lung cancer. *Acta Oncol* 2006;45(7):779–786.
317. Timmerman RD, Park C, Kavanagh BD. The North American experience with stereotactic body radiation therapy in non-small cell lung cancer. *J Thorac Oncol* 2007;2(7 Suppl 3):S101–S112.
318. Hara R, et al. Serum levels of KL-6 for predicting the occurrence of radiation pneumonitis after stereotactic radiotherapy for lung tumors. *Chest* 2004;125(1):340–344.
319. Timmerman R, et al. Extracranial stereotactic radioablation: results of a phase I study in medically inoperable stage I non-small cell lung cancer. *Chest* 2003;124(5):1946–1955.
320. Yamashita H, et al. Exceptionally high incidence of symptomatic grade 2–5 radiation pneumonitis after stereotactic radiation therapy for lung tumors. *Radiat Oncol* 2007;2:21.
321. Miller KL, et al. Bronchial stenosis: an underreported complication of high-dose external beam radiotherapy for lung cancer? *Int J Radiat Oncol Biol Phys* 2005;61(1):64–69.
322. Zhao J, et al. Simple factors associated with radiation-induced lung toxicity after stereotactic body radiation therapy of the thorax: A pooled analysis of 88 studies. *Int J Radiat Oncol Biol Phys* 2016;95(5):1357–1366.
323. Gagliardi G, et al. Radiation dose-volume effects in the heart. *Int J Radiat Oncol Biol Phys* 2010;76(3 Suppl):S77–S85.
324. Adams MJ, et al. Radiation-associated cardiovascular disease. *Crit Rev Oncol Hematol* 2003;45(1):55–75.
325. Gagliardi G, Lax I, Rutqvist LE. Partial irradiation of the heart. *Semin Radiat Oncol* 2001;11(3):224–233.
326. Hancock SL, Tucker MA, Hoppe RT. Factors affecting late mortality from heart disease after treatment of Hodgkin's disease. *JAMA* 1993;270(16): 1949–1955.
327. Das SK, et al. Predicting radiotherapy-induced cardiac perfusion defects. *Med Phys* 2005;32(1):19–27.
328. Evans ES, et al. Impact of patient-specific factors, irradiated left ventricular volume, and treatment set-up errors on the development of myocardial perfusion defects after radiation therapy for left-sided breast cancer. *Int J Radiat Oncol Biol Phys* 2006;66(4):1125–1134.
329. Marks LB, et al. The incidence and functional consequences of RT-associated cardiac perfusion defects. *Int J Radiat Oncol Biol Phys* 2005;63(1):214–223.
330. Carr ZA, et al. Coronary heart disease after radiotherapy for peptic ulcer disease. *Int J Radiat Oncol Biol Phys* 2005;61(3):842–850.
331. Gagliardi G, et al. Long-term cardiac mortality after radiotherapy of breast cancer–application of the relative seriality model. *Br J Radiol* 1996;69(825):839–846.
332. Eriksson F, et al. Long-term cardiac mortality following radiation therapy for Hodgkin's disease: analysis with the relative seriality model. *Radiother Oncol* 2000;55(2):153–162.
333. Wei X, et al. Risk factors for pericardial effusion in inoperable esophageal cancer patients treated with definitive chemoradiation therapy. *Int J Radiat Oncol Biol Phys* 2008;70(3):707–714.
334. Martel MK, et al. Fraction size and dose parameters related to the incidence of pericardial effusions. *Int J Radiat Oncol Biol Phys* 1998;40(1):155–161.
335. Heidenreich PA, et al. Asymptomatic cardiac disease following mediastinal irradiation. *J Am Coll Cardiol* 2003;42(4):743–749.
336. Hull MC, et al. Valvular dysfunction and carotid, subclavian, and coronary artery disease in survivors of Hodgkin lymphoma treated with radiation therapy. *JAMA* 2003;290(21):2831–2837.

337. Aleman BM, et al. Late cardiotoxicity after treatment for Hodgkin lymphoma. *Blood* 2007;109(5):1878–1886.

338. King V, et al. Symptomatic coronary artery disease after mantle irradiation for Hodgkin's disease. *Int J Radiat Oncol Biol Phys* 1996;36(4):881–889.

339. Darby SC, et al. Risk of ischemic heart disease in women after radiotherapy for breast cancer. *N Engl J Med* 2013;368(11):987–998.

340. Dess RT, et al. Cardiac events after radiation therapy: combined analysis of prospective multicenter trials for locally advanced non-small-cell lung cancer. *J Clin Oncol* 2017;35(13):1395–1402.

341. Wang K, et al. Cardiac toxicity after radiotherapy for stage iii non-small-cell lung cancer: pooled analysis of dose-escalation trials delivering 70 to 90 Gy. *J Clin Oncol* 2017;35(13):1387–1394.

342. Chun SG, et al. Impact of intensity-modulated radiation therapy technique for locally advanced non-small-cell lung cancer: a secondary analysis of the NRG oncology RTOG 0617 randomized clinical trial. *J Clin Oncol* 2017;35(1):56–62.

343. Jones LW, et al. Early breast cancer therapy and cardiovascular injury. *J Am Coll Cardiol* 2007;50(15):1435–1441.

344. Mosca L, et al. Evidence-based guidelines for cardiovascular disease prevention in women: 2007 update. *J Am Coll Cardiol* 2007;49(11):1230–1250.

345. Rubin P, et al.; EORTC Late Effects Working Group. Overview of late effects normal tissues (LENT) scoring system. *Radiother Oncol* 1995;35(1):9–10.

346. Kahn D, et al. "Anatomically-correct" dosimetric parameters may be better predictors for esophageal toxicity than are traditional CT-based metrics. *Int J Radiat Oncol Biol Phys* 2005;62(3):645–651.

347. Ahn SJ, et al. Dosimetric and clinical predictors for radiation-induced esophageal injury. *Int J Radiat Oncol Biol Phys* 2005;61(2):335–347.

348. Belderbos J, et al. Acute esophageal toxicity in non-small cell lung cancer patients after high dose conformal radiotherapy. *Radiother Oncol* 2005;75(2):157–164.

349. Bradley J, et al. Dosimetric correlates for acute esophagitis in patients treated with radiotherapy for lung carcinoma. *Int J Radiat Oncol Biol Phys* 2004;58(4):1106–1113.

350. Kim TH, et al. Dose-volumetric parameters of acute esophageal toxicity in patients with lung cancer treated with three-dimensional conformal radiotherapy. *Int J Radiat Oncol Biol Phys* 2005;62(4):995–1002.

351. Maguire PD, et al. Clinical and dosimetric predictors of radiation-induced esophageal toxicity. *Int J Radiat Oncol Biol Phys* 1999;45(1):97–103.

352. Qiao WB, et al. Clinical and dosimetric factors of radiation-induced esophageal injury: radiation-induced esophageal toxicity. *World J Gastroenterol* 2005;11(17):2626–2629.

353. Singh AK, Lockett MA, Bradley JD. Predictors of radiation-induced esophageal toxicity in patients with non-small-cell lung cancer treated with three-dimensional conformal radiotherapy. *Int J Radiat Oncol Biol Phys* 2003;55(2):337–341.

354. Werner-Wasik M, et al. Predictors of severe esophagitis include use of concurrent chemotherapy, but not the length of irradiated esophagus: a multivariate analysis of patients with lung cancer treated with nonoperative therapy. *Int J Radiat Oncol Biol Phys* 2000;48(3):689–696.

355. Antonadou D, et al. Randomized phase III trial of radiation treatment +/– amifostine in patients with advanced-stage lung cancer. *Int J Radiat Oncol Biol Phys* 2001;51(4):915–922.

356. Komaki R, et al. Effects of amifostine on acute toxicity from concurrent chemotherapy and radiotherapy for inoperable non-small-cell lung cancer: report of a randomized comparative trial. *Int J Radiat Oncol Biol Phys* 2004;58(5):1369–1377.

357. Leong SS, et al. Randomized double-blind trial of combined modality treatment with or without amifostine in unresectable stage III non-small-cell lung cancer. *J Clin Oncol* 2003;21(9):1767–1774.

358. Movsas B, et al. Randomized trial of amifostine in locally advanced non-small-cell lung cancer patients receiving chemotherapy and hyperfractionated radiation: radiation therapy oncology group trial 98-01. *J Clin Oncol* 2005;23(10):2145–2154.

359. Onimaru R, et al. Tolerance of organs at risk in small-volume, hypofractionated, image-guided radiotherapy for primary and metastatic lung cancers. *Int J Radiat Oncol Biol Phys* 2003;56(1):126–135.

360. Werner-Wasik M, et al. Radiation dose-volume effects in the esophagus. *Int J Radiat Oncol Biol Phys* 2010;76(3 Suppl):S86–S93.

361. Pan CC, et al. Radiation-associated liver injury. *Int J Radiat Oncol Biol Phys* 2010;76(3 Suppl):S94–S100.

362. Lawrence TS, et al. The use of 3-D dose volume analysis to predict radiation hepatitis. *Int J Radiat Oncol Biol Phys* 1992;23(4):781–788.

363. Dawson LA, et al. Analysis of radiation-induced liver disease using the Lyman NTCP model. *Int J Radiat Oncol Biol Phys* 2002;53(4):810–821.

364. Jackson A, et al. Analysis of clinical complication data for radiation hepatitis using a parallel architecture model. *Int J Radiat Oncol Biol Phys* 1995;31(4):883–891.

365. Cheng JC, et al. Biologic susceptibility of hepatocellular carcinoma patients treated with radiotherapy to radiation-induced liver disease. *Int J Radiat Oncol Biol Phys* 2004;60(5):1502–1509.

366. Liang SX, et al. Radiation-induced liver disease in three-dimensional conformal radiation therapy for primary liver carcinoma: the risk factors and hepatic radiation tolerance. *Int J Radiat Oncol Biol Phys* 2006;65(2):426–434.

367. Xu ZY, et al. Prediction of radiation-induced liver disease by Lyman normal-tissue complication probability model in three-dimensional conformal radiation therapy for primary liver carcinoma. *Int J Radiat Oncol Biol Phys* 2006;65(1):189–195.

368. Wu DH, Liu L, Chen LH. Therapeutic effects and prognostic factors in three-dimensional conformal radiotherapy combined with transcatheter arterial chemoembolization for hepatocellular carcinoma. *World J Gastroenterol* 2004;10(15):2184–2189.

369. Seong J, et al. Clinical results and prognostic factors in radiotherapy for unresectable hepatocellular carcinoma: a retrospective study of 158 patients. *Int J Radiat Oncol Biol Phys* 2003;55(2):329–336.

370. Kim TH, et al. Dose-volumetric parameters predicting radiation-induced hepatic toxicity in unresectable hepatocellular carcinoma patients treated with three-dimensional conformal radiotherapy. *Int J Radiat Oncol Biol Phys* 2007;67(1):225–231.

371. Cheng JC, et al. Radiation-induced liver disease after three-dimensional conformal radiotherapy for patients with hepatocellular carcinoma: dosimetric analysis and implication. *Int J Radiat Oncol Biol Phys* 2002;54(1):156–162.

372. Schefter TE, et al. A phase I trial of stereotactic body radiation therapy (SBRT) for liver metastases. *Int J Radiat Oncol Biol Phys* 2005;62(5):1371–1378.

373. Kavanagh BD, et al. Interim analysis of a prospective phase I/II trial of SBRT for liver metastases. *Acta Oncol* 2006;45(7).848–855.

374. Rusthoven KE, et al. Multi-institutional phase I/II trial of stereotactic body radiation therapy for liver metastases. *J Clin Oncol* 2009;27(10):1572–1578.

375. Tse RV, et al. Phase I study of individualized stereotactic body radiotherapy for hepatocellular carcinoma and intrahepatic cholangiocarcinoma. *J Clin Oncol* 2008;26(4):657–664.

376. Lee MT, et al. Phase I study of individualized stereotactic body radiotherapy of liver metastases. *J Clin Oncol* 2009;27(10):1585–1591.

377. Kavanagh BD, et al. Radiation dose-volume effects in the stomach and small bowel. *Int J Radiat Oncol Biol Phys* 2010;76(3 Suppl):S101–S107.

378. Mak AC, et al. Late complications of postoperative radiation therapy for cancer of the rectum and rectosigmoid. *Int J Radiat Oncol Biol Phys* 1994;28(3):597–603.

379. Pan CC, Dawson LA, McGinn CJ. Analysis of radiation-induced gastric and duodenal bleeds using the Lyman-Kutcher-Burman model. *Int J Radiat Oncol Biol Phys* 2003;57:S217.

380. Cosset JM, et al. Late radiation injuries of the gastrointestinal tract in the H2 and H5 EORTC Hodgkin's disease trials: emphasis on the role of exploratory laparotomy and fractionation. *Radiother Oncol* 1988;13(1):61–68.

381. Baglan KL, et al. The dose-volume relationship of acute small bowel toxicity from concurrent 5-FU-based chemotherapy and radiation therapy for rectal cancer. *Int J Radiat Oncol Biol Phys* 2002;52(1):176–183.

382. Robertson JM, et al. The dose-volume relationship of small bowel irradiation and acute grade 3 diarrhea during chemoradiotherapy for rectal cancer. *Int J Radiat Oncol Biol Phys* 2008;70(2):413–418.

383. Engels B, et al. Preoperative helical tomotherapy and megavoltage computed tomography for rectal cancer: impact on the irradiated volume of small bowel. *Int J Radiat Oncol Biol Phys* 2009;74(5):1476–1480.

384. Hoyer M, et al. Phase-II study on stereotactic radiotherapy of locally advanced pancreatic carcinoma. *Radiother Oncol* 2005;76(1):48–53.

385. Kelsey CR, et al. Phase 1 dose escalation study of accelerated radiation therapy with concurrent chemotherapy for locally advanced lung cancer. *Int J Radiat Oncol Biol Phys* 2015;93(5):997–1004.

386. Stanic S, et al. Tolerance of the small bowel to therapeutic irradiation: a focus on late toxicity in patients receiving para-aortic nodal irradiation for gynecologic malignancies. *Int J Gynecol Cancer* 2013;23(4):592–597.

387. Chen Z, et al. Dose-volume histogram predictors of chronic gastrointestinal complications after radical hysterectomy and postoperative intensity modulated radiotherapy for early-stage cervical cancer. *BMC Cancer* 2014;14:789.

388. Huang J, et al. Dose-volume analysis of predictors for gastrointestinal toxicity after concurrent full-dose gemcitabine and radiotherapy for locally advanced pancreatic adenocarcinoma. *Int J Radiat Oncol Biol Phys* 2012;83(4):1120–1125.

389. Kelly P, et al. Duodenal toxicity after fractionated chemoradiation for unresectable pancreatic cancer. *Int J Radiat Oncol Biol Phys* 2013;85(3):e143–e149.

390. Banerjee R, et al. Small bowel dose parameters predicting grade ≥ 3 acute toxicity in rectal cancer patients treated with neoadjuvant chemoradiation: an independent validation study comparing peritoneal space versus small bowel loop contouring techniques. *Int J Radiat Oncol Biol Phys* 2013;85(5):1225–1231.

391. Chang DT, et al. Stereotactic radiotherapy for unresectable adenocarcinoma of the pancreas. *Cancer* 2009;115(3):665–672.

392. Mahadevan A, et al. Induction gemcitabine and stereotactic body radiotherapy for locally advanced nonmetastatic pancreas cancer. *Int J Radiat Oncol Biol Phys* 2011;81(4):e615–e622.

393. Rwigema JC, et al. Stereotactic body radiotherapy in the treatment of advanced adenocarcinoma of the pancreas. *Am J Clin Oncol* 2011;34(1):63–69.

394. Roeske JC, et al. A dosimetric analysis of acute gastrointestinal toxicity in women receiving intensity-modulated whole-pelvic radiation therapy. *Radiother Oncol* 2003;69(2):201–207.

395. Kim TH, Somerville PJ, Freeman CR. Unilateral radiation nephropathy–the long-term significance. *Int J Radiat Oncol Biol Phys* 1984;10(11):2053–2059.

396. Willett CG, et al. Renal complications secondary to radiation treatment of upper abdominal malignancies. *Int J Radiat Oncol Biol Phys* 1986;12(9):1601–1604.

397. Köst S, et al. Effect of dose and dose-distribution in damage to the kidney following abdominal radiotherapy. *Int J Radiat Biol* 2002;78(8):695–702.

398. Welz S, et al. Renal toxicity of adjuvant chemoradiotherapy with cisplatin in gastric cancer. *Int J Radiat Oncol Biol Phys* 2007;69(5):1429–1435.

399. Flentje M, et al. Renal tolerance to nonhomogenous irradiation: comparison of observed effects to predictions of normal tissue complication probability from different biophysical models. *Int J Radiat Oncol Biol Phys* 1993;27(1):25–30.

400. Jansen EPM, et al. Prospective study on late renal toxicity following postoperative chemoradiotherapy in gastric cancer. *Int J Radiat Oncol Biol Phys* 2007;67(3):781–785.

401. Moulder JE, Fish BL. Influence of nephrotoxic drugs on the late renal toxicity associated with bone marrow transplant conditioning regimens. *Int J Radiat Oncol Biol Phys* 1991;20(2):333–337.

402. Cheng JC, Schultheiss TE, Wong JY. Impact of drug therapy, radiation dose, and dose rate on renal toxicity following bone marrow transplantation. *Int J Radiat Oncol Biol Phys* 2008;71(5):1436–1443.

403. Dawson LA, et al. Radiation-associated kidney injury. *Int J Radiat Oncol Biol Phys* 2010;76(3 Suppl):S108–S115.

404. Michalski JM, et al. Radiation dose-volume effects in radiation-induced rectal injury. *Int J Radiat Oncol Biol Phys* 2010;76(3 Suppl):S123–S129.

405. Kupelian PA, et al. Dose/volume relationship of late rectal bleeding after external beam radiotherapy for localized prostate cancer: absolute or relative rectal volume? *Cancer J* 2002;8(1):62–66.

406. Vargas C, et al. Dose-volume analysis of predictors for chronic rectal toxicity after treatment of prostate cancer with adaptive image-guided radiotherapy. *Int J Radiat Oncol Biol Phys* 2005;62(5):1297–1308.

407. Tucker SL, et al. Comparison of rectal dose-wall histogram versus dose-volume histogram for modeling the incidence of late rectal bleeding after radiotherapy. *Int J Radiat Oncol Biol Phys* 2004;60(5):1589–1601.

408. Jackson A, et al. Late rectal bleeding after conformal radiotherapy of prostate cancer. II. Volume effects and dose-volume histograms. *Int J Radiat Oncol Biol Phys* 2001;49(3):685–698.

409. Huang EH, et al. Late rectal toxicity: dose-volume effects of conformal radiotherapy for prostate cancer. *Int J Radiat Oncol Biol Phys* 2002;54(5):1314–1321.

410. Wachter S, et al. Rectal sequelae after conformal radiotherapy of prostate cancer: dose-volume histograms as predictive factors. *Radiother Oncol* 2001;59(1):65–70.

411. Cozzarini C, et al. Significant correlation between rectal DVH and late bleeding in patients treated after radical prostatectomy with conformal or conventional radiotherapy (66.6–70.2 Gy). *Int J Radiat Oncol Biol Phys* 2003;55(3):688–694.

412. Akimoto T, et al. Rectal bleeding after hypofractionated radiotherapy for prostate cancer: correlation between clinical and dosimetric parameters and the incidence of grade 2 or worse rectal bleeding. *Int J Radiat Oncol Biol Phys* 2004;60(4):1033–1039.

413. Fiorino C, et al. Clinical and dosimetric predictors of late rectal syndrome after 3D-CRT for localized prostate cancer: preliminary results of a multicenter prospective study. *Int J Radiat Oncol Biol Phys* 2008;70(4):1130–1137.

414. Hartford AC, et al. Conformal irradiation of the prostate: estimating long-term rectal bleeding risk using dose-volume histograms. *Int J Radiat Oncol Biol Phys* 1996;36(3):721–730.

415. Koper PC, et al. Impact of volume and location of irradiated rectum wall on rectal blood loss after radiotherapy of prostate cancer. *Int J Radiat Oncol Biol Phys* 2004;58(4):1072–1082.

416. Zapatero A, et al. Impact of mean rectal dose on late rectal bleeding after conformal radiotherapy for prostate cancer: dose-volume effect. *Int J Radiat Oncol Biol Phys* 2004;59(5):1343–1351.

417. Skwarchuk MW, et al. Late rectal toxicity after conformal radiotherapy of prostate cancer (I): multivariate analysis and dose–response. *Int J Radiat Oncol Biol Phys* 2000;47(1):103–113.

418. Zelefsky MJ, et al. Incidence of late rectal and urinary toxicities after three-dimensional conformal radiotherapy and intensity-modulated radiotherapy for localized prostate cancer. *Int J Radiat Oncol Biol Phys* 2008;70(4):1124–1129.

419. Pollack A, et al. Prostate cancer radiation dose response: results of the M. D. Anderson phase III randomized trial. *Int J Radiat Oncol Biol Phys* 2002;53(5):1097–1105.

420. Peeters ST, et al. Acute and late complications after radiotherapy for prostate cancer: results of a multicenter randomized trial comparing 68 Gy to 78 Gy. *Int J Radiat Oncol Biol Phys* 2005;61(4):1019–1034.

421. Peeters ST, et al. Localized volume effects for late rectal and anal toxicity after radiotherapy for prostate cancer. *Int J Radiat Oncol Biol Phys* 2006;64(4):1151–1161.

422. Fiorino C, et al. Rectal dose-volume constraints in high-dose radiotherapy of localized prostate cancer. *Int J Radiat Oncol Biol Phys* 2003;57(4):953–962.

423. Fiorino C, et al. Relationships between DVHs and late rectal bleeding after radiotherapy for prostate cancer: analysis of a large group of patients pooled from three institutions. *Radiother Oncol* 2002;64(1):1–12.

424. Boersma LJ, et al. Estimation of the incidence of late bladder and rectum complications after high-dose (70–78 GY) conformal radiotherapy for prostate cancer, using dose-volume histograms. *Int J Radiat Oncol Biol Phys* 1998;41(1):83–92.

425. Tucker SL, et al. Do intermediate radiation doses contribute to late rectal toxicity? An analysis of data from Radiation Therapy Oncology Group protocol 94-06. *Int J Radiat Oncol Biol Phys* 2012;84(2):390–395.

426. Michalski JM, et al. Preliminary toxicity analysis of 3-dimensional conformal radiation therapy versus intensity modulated radiation therapy on the high-dose arm of the Radiation Therapy Oncology Group 0126 prostate cancer trial. *Int J Radiat Oncol Biol Phys* 2013;87(5):932–993.

427. Colaco RJ, et al. Rectal toxicity after proton therapy for prostate cancer: an analysis of outcomes of prospective studies conducted at the university of Florida Proton Therapy Institute. *Int J Radiat Oncol Biol Phys* 2015;91(1):172–181.

428. Perez CA, et al. Impact of dose in outcome of irradiation alone in carcinoma of the uterine cervix: analysis of two different methods. *Int J Radiat Oncol Biol Phys* 1991;21(4):885–898.

429. Pourquier H, Dubois JB, Delard R. Cancer of the uterine cervix: dosimetric guidelines for prevention of late rectal and rectosigmoid complications as a result of radiotherapeutic treatment. *Int J Radiat Oncol Biol Phys* 1982;8(11):1887–1895.

430. Eifel PJ, et al. Time course and incidence of late complications in patients treated with radiation therapy for FIGO stage IB carcinoma of the uterine cervix. *Int J Radiat Oncol Biol Phys* 1995;32(5):1289–1300.

431. Schultheiss TE, et al. Late GI and GU complications in the treatment of prostate cancer. *Int J Radiat Oncol Biol Phys* 1997;37(1):3–11.

432. Peeters ST, et al. Rectal bleeding, fecal incontinence, and high stool frequency after conformal radiotherapy for prostate cancer: normal tissue complication probability modeling. *Int J Radiat Oncol Biol Phys* 2006;66(1):11–19.

433. Fleming C, et al. A method for the prediction of late organ-at-risk toxicity after radiotherapy of the prostate using equivalent uniform dose. *Int J Radiat Oncol Biol Phys* 2011;80(2):608–613.

434. King CR, et al. Long-term outcomes from a prospective trial of stereotactic body radiotherapy for low-risk prostate cancer. *Int J Radiat Oncol Biol Phys* 2012;82(2):877–882.

435. Jabbari S, et al. Stereotactic body radiotherapy as monotherapy or post-external beam radiotherapy boost for prostate cancer: technique, early toxicity, and PSA response. *Int J Radiat Oncol Biol Phys* 2012;82(1):228–234.

436. Aoki M, et al. Evaluation of rectal bleeding factors associated with prostate brachytherapy. *Jpn J Radiol* 2009;27(10):444–449.

437. Keyes M, et al. Rectal toxicity and rectal dosimetry in low-dose-rate iodine-125 permanent prostate implants: a long-term study in 1006 patients. *Brachytherapy* 2012;11(3):199–208.

438. Konishi K, et al. Correlation between dosimetric parameters and late rectal and urinary toxicities in patients treated with high-dose-rate brachytherapy used as monotherapy for prostate cancer. *Int J Radiat Oncol Biol Phys* 2009;75(4):1003–1007.

439. Kalakota K, et al. Late rectal toxicity after prostate brachytherapy: influence of supplemental external beam radiation on dose-volume histogram analysis. *Brachytherapy* 2010;9(2):131–136.

440. Pederson AW, et al. Late toxicity after intensity-modulated radiation therapy for localized prostate cancer: an exploration of dose-volume histogram parameters to limit genitourinary and gastrointestinal toxicity. *Int J Radiat Oncol Biol Phys* 2012;82(1):235–241.

441. Viswanathan AN, et al. Radiation dose-volume effects of the urinary bladder. *Int J Radiat Oncol Biol Phys* 2010;76(3 Suppl):S116–S122.

442. Ahmed AA, et al. A novel method for predicting late genitourinary toxicity after prostate radiation therapy and the need for age-based risk-adapted dose constraints. *Int J Radiat Oncol Biol Phys* 2013;86(4):709–715.

443. Brown MW, et al. An analysis of erectile function after intensity modulated radiation therapy for localized prostate carcinoma. *Prostate Cancer Prostatic Dis* 2007;10(2):189–193.

444. Kao J, et al. Sparing of the penile bulb and proximal penile structures with intensity-modulated radiation therapy for prostate cancer. *Br J Radiol* 2004;77(914):129–136.

445. Roach M III, et al. Radiation dose-volume effects and the penile bulb. *Int J Radiat Oncol Biol Phys* 2010;76(3 Suppl):S130–S134.

446. Selek U, et al. Erectile dysfunction and radiation dose to penile base structures: a lack of correlation. *Int J Radiat Oncol Biol Phys* 2004;59(4):1039–1046.

447. van der Wielen GJ, et al. Dose-volume parameters of the corpora cavernosa do not correlate with erectile dysfunction after external beam radiotherapy for prostate cancer: results from a dose-escalation trial. *Int J Radiat Oncol Biol Phys* 2008;71(3):795–800.

448. Fisch BM, et al. Dose of radiation received by the bulb of the penis correlates with risk of impotence after three-dimensional conformal radiotherapy for prostate cancer. *Urology* 2001;57(5):955–959.

449. Wernicke AG, et al. Radiation dose delivered to the proximal penis as a predictor of the risk of erectile dysfunction after three-dimensional conformal radiotherapy for localized prostate cancer. *Int J Radiat Oncol Biol Phys* 2004;60(5):1357–1363.

450. Mangar SA, et al. Evaluating the relationship between erectile dysfunction and dose received by the penile bulb: using data from a randomised controlled trial of conformal radiotherapy in prostate cancer (MRC RT01, ISRCTN47772397). *Radiother Oncol* 2006;80(3):355–362.

451. Roach M, et al. Penile bulb dose and impotence after three-dimensional conformal radiotherapy for prostate cancer on RTOG 9406: findings from a prospective, multi-institutional, phase I/II dose-escalation study. *Int J Radiat Oncol Biol Phys* 2004;60(5):1351–1356.

452. Schwarz M, et al. Helical tomotherapy and intensity modulated proton therapy in the treatment of early stage prostate cancer: a treatment planning comparison. *Radiother Oncol* 2011;98(1):74–80.

453. Nichols RC Jr, et al. Proton radiotherapy for prostate cancer is not associated with post-treatment testosterone suppression. *Int J Radiat Oncol Biol Phys* 2012;82(3):1222–1226.

454. Solan AN, et al. There is no correlation between erectile dysfunction and dose to penile bulb and neurovascular bundles following real-time low-dose-rate prostate brachytherapy. *Int J Radiat Oncol Biol Phys* 2009;73(5):1468–1474.

455. Wiegner EA, King CR. Sexual function after stereotactic body radiotherapy for prostate cancer: results of a prospective clinical trial. *Int J Radiat Oncol Biol Phys* 2010;78(2):442–448.

456. Marks LB, et al. Use of normal tissue complication probability models in the clinic. *Int J Radiat Oncol Biol Phys* 2010;76(3 Suppl):S10–S19.

457. Marks L et al. Doses, modeling and outcomes of hypofractionated treatments-results of the WGSBRT. *ASTRO*, Oct 2015.

458. Grimm J, et al. Joint symposium of AAPM and ASTRO: normal tissue dose-volume effects of HN and liver/GI SBRT. *AAPM*, July 2017.

459. Grimm J. Dose tolerance for stereotactic body radiation therapy. *Semin Radiat Oncol* 2016;26(2):87–88.

460. Asbell SO, et al. Introduction and clinical overview of the DVH risk map. *Semin Radiat Oncol* 2016;26(2):89–96.

461. Levegrün S, et al. Fitting tumor control probability models to biopsy outcome after three-dimensional conformal radiation therapy of prostate cancer: pitfalls in deducing radiobiologic parameters for tumors from clinical data. *Int J Radiat Oncol Biol Phys* 2001;51(4):1064–1080.

462. Iwi G, et al. Bootstrap resampling: a powerful method of assessing confidence intervals for doses from experimental data. *Phys Med Biol* 1999;44:N55–N62.

463. Xue J, et al. Validity of current stereotactic body radiation therapy dose constraints for aorta and major vessels. *Semin Radiat Oncol* 2016;26(2):135–139.

464. Nishimura S, et al. Toxicities of organs at risk in the mediastinal and hilar regions following stereotactic body radiotherapy for centrally located lung tumors. *J Thorac Oncol* 2014;9(9):1370–1376.

465. Deasy JO, et al. Improving normal tissue complication probability models: the need to adopt a "data-pooling" culture. *Int J Radiat Oncol Biol Phys* 2010;76(3 Suppl):S151–S154.

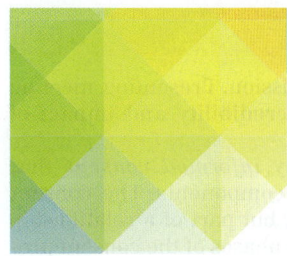

CHAPTER 15

Methodology of Clinical Trials

Abigail T. Berman, Erin F. Gillespie, Clifton David Fuller, Yiyi Chen, and Charles R. Thomas Jr.

In this chapter, we discuss the design, conduct, and analysis of oncology clinical trials, along the way pointing out particular areas of interest to radiation oncology and reviewing some recent ideas in clinical trials and related research studies. This chapter provides only a brief and essentially nontechnical sketch of the main concepts and current research areas, and we refer the reader to comprehensive texts on clinical trial conduct in oncology for further details. Excellent recent texts, the *Handbook of Statistics in Clinical Oncology*,[1] *Clinical Trials in Oncology*,[2] and *Oncology Clinical Trials: Successful Design, Conduct and Analysis*,[3] provide the fundamentals, as well as up-to-date discussion of new challenges and active research in statistical methods for oncology clinical trials.

Clinical trials enable physicians to advance medical care in a safe, scientific, and ethical manner. Formally defined, clinical trials are a set of procedures in medical research conducted to allow safety and efficacy data to be collected for health interventions.[4] A more detailed definition for our purposes would describe a clinical trial as a prospective study that includes an active intervention, carried out in a well-defined patient cohort and producing interpretable information about the action of the intervention.[5] Although in some ways similar to a well-designed laboratory experiment, the involvement of living human subjects demands adherence to strict ethical principles while also adding to the complexity of interpretation of the results. The last 60 years has witnessed an unprecedented appreciation of the importance of clinical trials and a consequent surge in the number of clinical trials performed. In the field of radiation oncology alone, according to a PubMed search, 376 clinical trials were published in 2010, of which 65 were phase III trials.

Over the course of less than a century, the evidence upon which medicine is practiced has evolved from being entirely empirical to a highly regulated scientific process based upon vigorously designed clinical trials tightly overseen by numerous scientific and governmental agencies. Cardinal chapters in the history of clinical trial design and implementation include:

- 1747—James Lind's work on the effect of citrus fruits in the prevention of scurvy among sailors in the Royal Navy
- 1863—Austin Flint's use of a placebo group for comparison with an experimental treatment in the treatment of rheumatic fever
- 1947—Nuremburg Codex, a result of the appreciation that much of the medical experimentation performed by physicians in Nazi Germany was both ethically wrong and scientifically uninterpretable
- 1948—The first double-blind trial, performed by the British Medical Research Council, to assess the value of streptomycin in the treatment of tuberculosis
- 1964—Declaration of Helsinki, ethical guidelines for the performance of clinical trials developed by the World Medical Association and frequently updated since
- 2000—Creation of ClinicalTrials.gov Web site, a registry of clinical trials under the auspices of the National Institute of Health (NIH)

The performance of high-quality cancer clinical trials involves the cooperation of multiple bodies, so-called stakeholders, including cancer patients and their families, physicians (who accrue the patients), their operating environment (academic institution or practice), the research team (who run the trial on a day-to-day basis), sponsors (who oversee and fund the trial), independent monitors (to ensure the correct performance of the research team), government regulatory agencies, contract research organizations (CROs, who may carry out specific aspect of the trial such as auditing), and medical insurance companies. Modern clinical trials may often require involvement of translational scientists, clinical psychologists, and experts in quality of life, cost-effectiveness, and other disciplines. The complexity of clinical trials adds to the regulatory work involved; for instance, a multi-institutional federally sponsored clinical trial protocol will require the approval of at least three different research ethics oversight committees (Institutional Review Boards or IRBs): within the group coordinating the trial, at each institution that opens the trial to accrue patients, and at the sponsor.

Although many phase I and phase II trials are carried out by investigators within a single institution, many larger phase II and most phase III trials are generally multi-institutional. Thus, clinical trial investigator networks have emerged as essential players in the performance of large phase II and III clinical trials. The U.S. National Cancer Institute–sponsored cancer cooperative group program is an example,[6] as are similar groups such as the European Organisation for Research and Treatment of Cancer (EORTC). One cooperative group, the Radiation Therapy Oncology Group (RTOG), founded by Simon Kramer in 1968, is dedicated to trials involving radiation therapy, has activated 460 protocols, and has accrued approximately 90,000 patients to its trials. Early studies sought to answer questions regarding radiation dose and fractionation. As cancer therapy became multimodal, the group addressed questions relating to combining systemic chemotherapy with radiation therapy. The majority of recent trials seek to combine targeted agents with contemporary radiation therapy techniques.[6]

Clinical trials are extremely expensive to perform, with costs continuing to rise as a result of both increased regulatory oversight and greater trial complexity. For instance, it has been estimated that implementation of the European Union's Clinical Trials Directive (laws and regulations relating to implementation of good clinical practice [GCP] in the conduct of clinical trials) led to a doubling of the cost of running noncommercial cancer trials in the United Kingdom.[7] Large phase III trials can cost in excess of $100 million, and as a result, clinical trials are frequently financed by the pharmaceutical industry. An unfortunate consequence is that clinical trials are rarely performed on established "generic drugs" where there is little commercial interest in establishing new indications. Conversely, the performance of rigorous clinical trials contributes significantly to the costs involved in the development of new pharmaceutical agents, which are subsequently reflected in the commercial pricing of the product.

RESPONSIBILITIES OF THE PRINCIPAL INVESTIGATOR

Although much progress has been made over the past several decades since the Tuskegee Study and other shoddy research debacles came to widespread public attention, there persists an inconsistency in the conduct of rigorous research, both preclinical and clinical, to the extent that it is becoming well known that a significant portion of research results are not readily reproducible.[8] The radiation oncology research community is not immune to this quandary and must be committed to improving the research climate on multiple levels.

High-quality research involving human subjects demands accountability on multiple levels, starting foremost with the *responsibilities* of the principal investigator (PI). Although we recommend that prospective PIs proactively enroll in courses that have been developed by one's IRB, we will briefly summarize some of the essential elements.

All clinical trials must be based on testable objectives that are based upon a sound hypothesis. There should be appropriate end points that can actually measure whether the objectives have been met (or not). The eligibility, trial design, and statistical power (including estimate of the effect size, accrual, specimen availability, imaging interpretation, etc.) must be defined up-front. Bioassays and imaging should be performed by qualified personnel who do not have any knowledge of the outcome for patients enrolled onto the study. The study data must be maintained in a secure database at a recognized institution (not at the PIs' private home server).

The PI is responsible for making sure that research is conducted in a manner that is consistent with the guidelines of the International Council for Harmonisation of Technical Requirements for Pharmaceuticals for Human Use (ICH) by using accepted best practices, also known as good clinical practice (GCP). To participate in the conduct of clinical trials, the PI will need to review and sign the investigator statement (form FDA 1572), which basically is a voluntary commitment to follow the IRB-approved protocol and related requirements, including all applicable federal, state, and institutional regulations. The PI is responsible for controlling all investigational devices and/or agents for a protocol. For the radiation oncologist, this requires a cadre that may include—nurse, research associate, protocol coordinator, regulatory and budget coordinator, medical physicists, dosimetrists, lead radiation therapists, and other oncology coinvestigators. Finally, the PI must be committed to protecting the rights, safety, benevolence, and overall welfare of patients who are evaluated and eventually enrolled onto the trial.

There are core *qualifications* of the PI. Primarily, the PI should possess the necessary qualifications with respect to educational training and experience to make sure that research, including a clinical trial, can be conducted properly and ethically. The PI should be cognizant of the essentials of GCP and be committed with complying. Although intuitive to most readers, it is necessary to reiterate that the PI should be familiar with the use of investigational treatment approaches, including devices and/or agents. The PI should have a serious time commitment to successful execution of the trial. This commitment includes reading and approving the protocol as well as being involved in a rational plan to identify and enroll patients, proactively addressing barriers to the conduct of increasingly common ancillary or translational research components of trials such as procurement of blood, tissue, and/or novel imaging tests. The PI should have an assessment plan to make sure that the end points are set up to measure the objectives of the trial, especially the primary objective. The PI needs to have a team and the necessary resources to conduct the trial; if not, then it is not ethical to open a trial regardless of the scientific enthusiasm or merit. The PI needs to understand that certain tasks are delegated to qualified members of the research team. There should be an expectation that routine auditing, and expectation by sponsoring organizations as well as government and institutional regulatory bodies, is normal. Finally, it is critical that the PI is committed to evaluating the results and dissemination to the scientific community via a peer-reviewed manuscript submission. Presenting meeting abstracts alone undermines the credibility and impact of cancer research.

All patients must submit truly *informed consent* that includes both verbal and written components. The consent *process* is not purely transactional, but part of a relationship between the patient and the PI. The phases of the consent process include: (a) prestudy review and approval by the IRB; (b) during the recruitment of subjects with a number of caveats that the patient must understand, primarily that any conflict of interest (COI) on the part of the PI is proactively disclosed and that subjects can withdraw from the study at any time without prejudice; (c) prior to beginning the trial, a signed copy of the consent must be given to the patient (or qualified surrogate such as a parent in the case of a pediatric radiation oncology trial) and also remain on file in the official medical record as well as the protocol office; and (d) during the trial, any revised consent form must have IRB approval, and new information that can impact the outcome for patients must be proactively shared.

Earlier, we mentioned the concept of GCP. The essential values of GCP are listed below[9]:

- Comply with ethical principles.
- Minimize risk to human subjects.
- Maintain dignity, welfare, and human rights.
- Accurate investigational study product information.
- Rigorous peer-reviewed protocol.
- IRB review and approval of protocol.
- Bioethics review (either separate or in concert with IRB approval).
- PI must be qualified.
- Research team must be qualified to carry out delegated responsibilities.
- Enrolled patients must sign uncoerced and voluntary informed consent (written and verbal).
- Data generated must be accurate and verifiable.
- Study records must be kept confidential in a secure environment and readily made available to auditing and/or regulatory authorities.
- Investigational produce functionality and manufacturing standard should be verifiable.
- Quality assurance (QA) and quality control must be in place.

Essential Questions for the PI to Consider (adapted with permission from Lillian Siu, MD and Patricia LoRusso, DO)

1. It is absolutely critical that the PI be clear on why it is of value to perform the trial and what the rationale is. The scientific insights, including the robustness of the preclinical and other published data, must be understood. Is there a gap in theranostic efficacy?

2. If the trial is positive, will a meaningful vertical impact and penetration in the field result? Some trials may prove a proof of concept and others may have a clinical impact. In the latter case, is the PI testing a low-risk strategy in incremental steps such that a new standard of care may result? In radiation, this might be the addition of Manuka honey to prevent radiation-induced oral mucositis. Or, is a higher-risk strategy being tested, which may involve a significant step forward. An example of this would be the addition of pembrolizumab to chemoradiation for locally advanced lung cancer, which is currently a trial concept being developed by the NRG.

3. Where does the trial concept lay within the innovation spectrum? If a low-risk question, will the field really care about the results and is the research question worth the investment in resources (i.e., time, money, and patients)? If a high-risk question, will the feasibility and dissemination be limited to a few very specialized centers?

4. Does the study have a primary clinical end point and what are the pros/cons of candidate end points? It is important to have an idea as to how quick one can determine an early end point (i.e., response rate), reliability (i.e., overall survival), clinical significance, and impact of subsequent factors on the end point (i.e., PFS vs. overall survival). Because no end point will be perfect to show an increase in the therapeutic ratio, the PI should have a rational justification for choosing it.

5. The study must be feasible with respect to scientific, pragmatic, financial, and ethical boundaries.

6. Are you able to assemble the nonphysician investigative team, beginning with an experienced biostatistician? Other component personnel include imaging and basic science investigators, research nurses, study coordinator, pharmacist, regulatory affairs, and IRB.

7. The PI must have dedicated (protected) time to remain engaged in the study.

8. Barriers always exist. It is important that the PI learn, early on, which barriers are permanent versus temporary, which require a doable work-around versus a fatal flaw. A mentor who is committed to helping navigate the oncopolitical landscape is valued.

9. It should be clear who and what are competing in this research space. Is a more capable investigator at another institution actually more capable of executing your original idea? Are your colleagues as enthusiastic about your concept as you are? Is there a competing institutional and/or multi-institution trial that will limit patients? If so, is this a temporary concern?

10. The PI needs to discern if they are ready to start working on the protocol immediately or perhaps at a time in the future. Time management is paramount.

OVERVIEW OF ETHICAL CONSIDERATIONS

Medical ethics are based upon the principles of autonomy (the patient's right to refuse or choose their treatment), beneficence (a practitioner should act in the best interest of the patient), nonmaleficence (first, do no harm), justice (fairness and equality), dignity, and honesty. Without due diligence, physicians may infringe upon these principles when encouraging patient participation in clinical trials. Are the physicians confident that the proposed treatment is beneficial and not harmful? Are the potential subjects fully aware of the implications of participation? Do all segments of the population have equivalent chance to participate and receive potentially better treatment? Despite the universal acceptance of these principles, there have been numerous examples of grossly unethical research being performed in the Western world within living memory. Documents seeking to address these issues include the Nuremberg Code, the Declaration of Helsinki, and the Belmont Report. Emanuel has listed seven requirements that provide a systematic and coherent framework for determining whether clinical research is ethical.[10]

Ethical principles themselves, and the creation of guidelines, are insufficient to ensure the ethical conduct of medical research. Physicians within Nazi Germany performed atrocities despite the existence of German guidelines published in 1931,[11] reflecting the need for legislation. The International Council for Harmonisation of Technical Requirements for Pharmaceuticals for Human Use (ICH) brought together the regulatory authorities of Europe, Japan, and the United States and experts from the pharmaceutical industry to regulate scientific and technical aspects of pharmaceutical product registration. The ICH guidelines are legally binding in many countries (although not in the United States) and are updated every few years, reflecting the increasing sophistication of the field. An example of a recent addition is the introduction of data and safety monitoring committees (DSMCs), an independent group of experts who monitor patient safety and treatment efficacy data while a clinical trial is ongoing. Another recent advance is the requirement for the registration of clinical trials, at sites such as *ClinicalTrials.gov*. Such registration both improves transparency concerning what clinical trials have been or are being performed and empowers patients to find relevant clinical trials.

OVERVIEW OF TRADITIONAL CLINICAL TRIAL DEVELOPMENT

Traditionally, a new anticancer agent is tested in a three-step process, starting with a small dose-finding trial (phase I), followed by a pilot efficacy trial (phase II), and culminating with a large comparative randomized (phase III) trial. Although this development paradigm was created and established in the era of cytotoxic chemotherapies, it continues to be used today in the era of often less toxic (and possibly not dose dependent) targeted therapies, with some adaptations and innovations that we will discuss later. Here, we review the traditional paradigm without technical details, which can be found in many excellent sources for clinical trial design and conduct.[2,5]

Phase II

The primary purpose of the phase II trial is to determine the response rate of the treatment, seeking early evidence of clinical activity. An important secondary purpose is to gather more robust adverse event (AE) information at the established dose. The primary efficacy end point of the phase II trial has traditionally been tumor response, but duration of response, progression-free survival (PFS), and site-specific activity such as locoregional control are all relevant and increasingly used. Measures of patient survival are usually secondary end points in phase II trials, because of the limited sample size and follow-up duration of these trials. In general, phase II trials usually are not designed to provide definitive evidence that the test treatment is superior to current options. In fact, phase II trials have traditionally been single-arm studies comparing against a benchmark historical response rate. Reliance on this nonconcurrent external control rate can be problematic.[12–14] Furthermore, patient selection factors can influence the results, for example, overall response rates in a single-institution phase II trials can be significantly higher than in multicenter studies or subsequent phase III controlled trials.[15] Randomized phase II trials have historically had a role in multiarm trials aimed at selecting the best treatment(s) to take forward for further testing[16] and have more recently become favored as a means of providing more reliable pilot efficacy data.[17] However, the preferred approach is changing as described later.

Phase III

Phase III trials are randomized comparisons between a new treatment regimen that has already shown promise in phase I/II trials and the current best standard of care (i.e., the control). Randomization offers a critical advantage over nonrandomized studies. Specifically, randomization balances the distribution of prognostic factors between treatment arms and assures that treatment is assigned independent of these factors, thereby minimizing or eliminating these effects when comparing outcomes by treatment. When randomization is combined with treatment blinding of patients, researchers, or both, then even subjective outcomes can be assessed with minimal bias. Also, in multicenter studies, randomization can balance any systematic bias of the treating physicians or institutions.

Phase III trials can address one of several types of primary questions. For example, a study can be designed to determine if standard treatment is better than the best supportive care. More often, phase III studies are designed to compare a new treatment with the current standard treatment. Phase III studies can also compare two or three different regimens with each other, as well as with standard treatment. Finally, a trial may be designed to demonstrate that a given treatment option is not worse than another by more than a tolerable margin. These "equivalence" trials, more accurately referred to as noninferiority trials, play an important role in the development of less invasive or less burdensome treatment regimens.

The primary end point of a phase III trial is most typically overall survival (time to death from any cause), but other important clinical end points such as disease-free survival (DFS) are increasingly justified. Because these trials aim to definitively demonstrate benefit with respect to these end points, the number of participants and follow-up period required for the phase III trial is much longer than in phase II trials. Important secondary end points can include locoregional control and other site-specific failure end points, AE profiles, and quality of life measures.

Phase IV

Phase IV trial is also known as postmarketing surveillance trial. Phase IV trials involve the safety surveillance of a drug after it receives regulatory approval for standard use. The safety surveillance is designed to detect any rare or long-term adverse effects over a much larger patient population and longer time period than was possible during the phase I to III clinical trials.

Phase 0 or Window Studies

The goal of phase 0 trials is to evaluate the pharmacodynamics (PD) and/or pharmacokinetics (PK) of an antitumor modality prior to traditional phase 1 studies (see Fig. 15.1 from Murgo et al.[18]).

PD is considered to represent "what the modality does to the body," whereas PK measures "what the body does to the modality," be it radiation and/or a systemic agent.[19] PD parameters may include nadir hematologic counts, nonhematologic toxicity, molecular correlates, and/or imaging end points. PK parameters such as C_{max}, AUC (area under the curve drug exposure), half-life, and clearance all help to quantitate absorption, distribution, metabolism, and/or excretion of an agent. This can impact the bioavailability of an agent that is intended to sensitize radiation. Phase 0 studies can help to refine a target or biomarker assay for drug impact in human samples by incorporating methods developed and validated in representative preclinical models.

Therapeutic clinical trials in radiation oncology typically involve the introduction of new technologies (e.g., the use of stereotactic body radiation for a new indication) or more frequently the novel combination of radiation therapy with a systemic agent. There are unique challenges—biologic and clinical—that characterize clinical trials in radiation oncology compared to those not involving radiation.

Response rate is frequently used in early-phase medical oncology trials to indicate activity; however, because radiation therapy itself is highly effective at shrinking tumors, this end point is not useful in radiation trials. A more appropriate "activity" end point for radiation trials may be PFS, but this itself is often difficult to objectively assess. Modern imaging end points (such as FDG uptake) show promise as early readouts of activity, but still require vigorous validation for individual disease sites. Furthermore, efficacy and toxicity end points in radiation trials are dependent on multiple biologic factors including size of the target, proximity of tumor to sensitive normal tissues, accuracy of target volume definition, degree of patient immobilization, dose of radiation, and fractionation scheme. Consequently, quality assurance measures are an essential feature of radiation trials, especially in the multi-institutional setting.[20] Inadequate QA and lack of consistency in radiation delivery have led to the conclusions obtained from large expensive clinical trials being questioned.[21-27] As a recent example in the RTOG trial 9704, which evaluated postoperative adjuvant chemoradiation treatment of pancreatic cancer, subtle protocol violations in target definition influenced both toxicity and survival.[28]

In medical oncology trials, AEs typically occur during or within days of completing treatment. In contrast, toxicity following radiation therapy follows a biphasic course, early (within 3 months of starting treatment) and late (months to years later). Late toxicity is typically irreversible and hence important in determining the tolerability of an experimental treatment. Although utilizing long-term toxicity as the primary end point in clinical trials is not practical, it is nonetheless imperative to collect and report robust information on long-term outcomes from radiation therapy trials. In fact, even in phase I radiation therapy trials, the follow-up period can be significantly longer than for those evaluating chemotherapy. A recent approach to dose escalation in phase I trials that considers late toxicities when deciding whether to advance to the next dosing level is discussed later.[29]

A further difference relates to the population studied. In medical oncology early-phase trials, participants have often received several lines of treatment and lack further therapeutic options. In contrast, patients on phase I radiation trials typically receive full-dose radiation treatment and subjects may be treatment naïve. Furthermore, phase I trials in medical oncology are frequently "first-in-human" experience for the agent; toxicity is unpredictable and PK studies are essential. Conversely, most multimodality phase I trials in radiation oncology involve systemic agents that have already been through extensive clinical testing; systemic toxicity is known and PK studies are unnecessary. The purpose of the trial is to define the extent of local toxicity within the radiation field; consequently, radiation oncology phase I trials are organ specific. A recent study demonstrated that in reality, radiation phase I trials rarely utilize "first-in-human" agents, are associated with qualitatively predictable toxicity, and are comparatively safe.[30]

STATISTICAL ISSUES IN CLINICAL TRIAL DESIGN

Patient Population Definition and Stratification

A key issue in a clinical trial is a well-defined patient population to which the potential therapy applies. This is typically defined in terms of traditional disease characteristics reflecting putative prognosis, such as stage or its components. Increasingly, tumor pathology or marker features may be included. In any case, these must be unambiguously defined. Because factors defining eligibility are often critically related to prognosis, any randomized comparative study may use a stratified randomization approach in order to ensure equal representation of prognostic risk among treatment arms. Stratification factors need to be limited to a reasonable number, because the total number of strata equals the product of the number of categories for each. For example, in a recently completed RTOG for prostate cancer, stratification factors consisted of two levels of PSA (<4 vs. 4 to 20), three cell differentiation categories (well, moderate, poor), and nodal status (N0 vs. NX). The possible combinations of these variables create $2 \times 3 \times 2 = 12$ strata within which treatments are to be balanced in allocation.

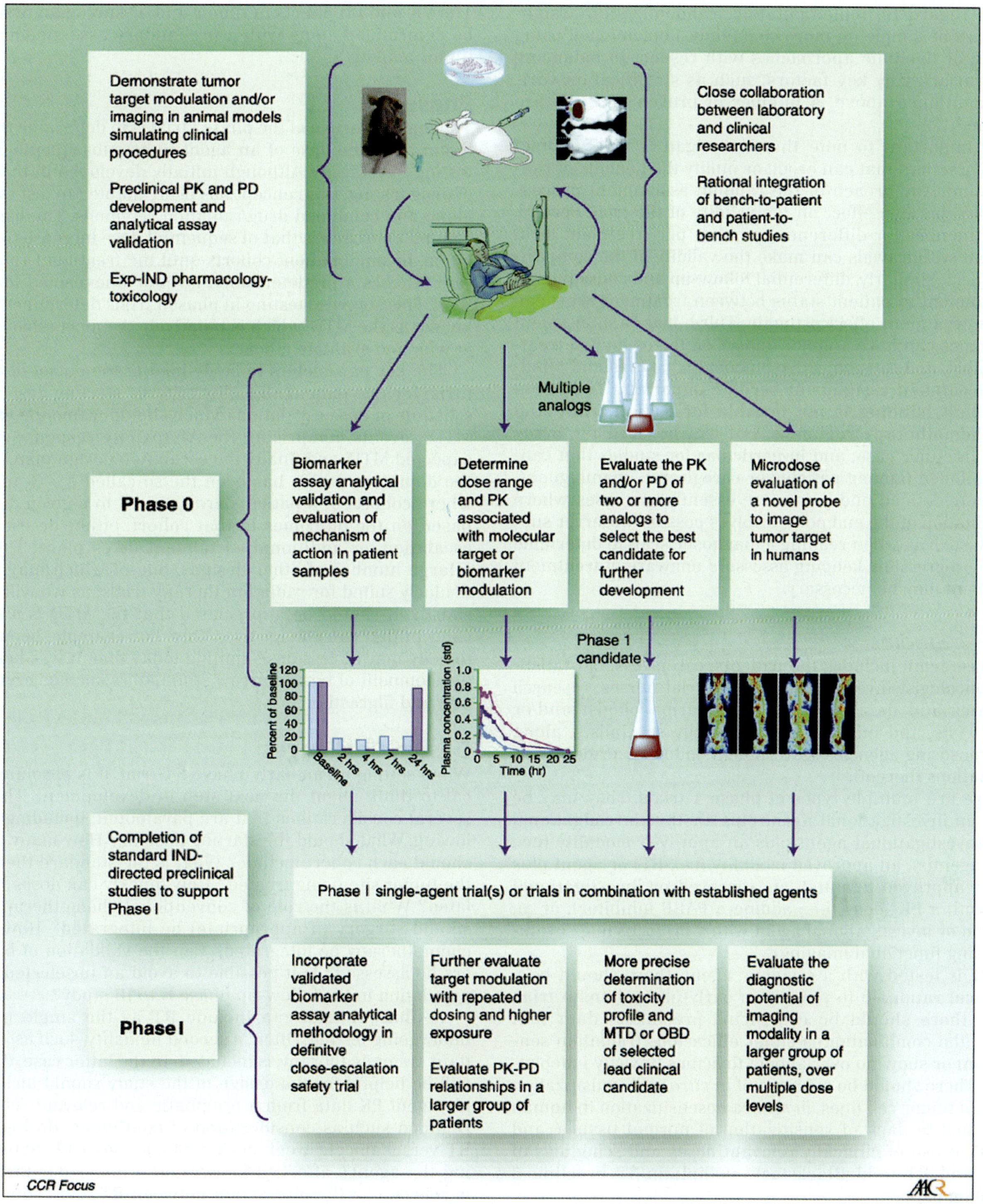

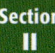

Demonstrate tumor target modulation and/or imaging in animal models simulating clinical procedures
Preclinical PK and PD development and analytical assay validation
Exp-IND pharmacology-toxicology
Close collaboration between laboratory and clinical researchers
Rational integration of bench-to-patient and patient-to-bench studies
Multiple analogs
Phase 0
Biomarker assay analytical validation and evaluation of mechanism of action in patient samples
Determine dose range and PK associated with molecular target or biomarker modulation
Evaluate the PK and/or PD of two or more analogs to select the best candidate for further development
Microdose evaluation of a novel probe to image tumor target in humans
Phase 1 candidate
Percent of baseline
Baseline
2 hrs
4 hrs
7 hrs
24 hrs
Plasma concentration (std)
Time (hr)
Completion of standard IND-directed preclinical studies to support Phase I
Phase I single-agent trial(s) or trials in combination with established agents
Phase I
Incorporate validated biomarker assay analytical methodology in definitve close-escalation safety trial
Further evaluate target modulation with repeated dosing and higher exposure
Evaluate PK-PD relationships in a larger group of patients
More precise determination of toxicity profile and MTD or OBD of selected lead clinical candidate
Evaluate the diagnostic potential of imaging modality in a larger group of patients, over multiple dose levels
CCR Focus

FIGURE 15.1. Preclinical, phase 0, and phase 1 clinical trial development. (From Murgo AJ, Kummar S, Rubinstein L, et al. Designing phase 0 cancer clinical trials. *Clin Cancer Res* 2008;14:3675–3682.)

Randomization

Randomization is used differently in different phases of development, but serves a similar purpose, which is to render treatment groups similar with respect to factors other than treatment that can influence outcomes. In phase I trials, there typically are not comparative groups, although there are situations where parallel cohorts of patients are being evaluated, and thus randomization into cohorts assures that these groups can be compared later for response biomarkers or other factors of interest. In phase II trials, randomization has been used in two similar but distinct ways. First, so-called selection designs have been used to help decide which of several potential candidate treatments to take forward to further definitive testing.[16] In these trials, interest is not in statistically significant differences between treatments but rather the ability to nominally rank candidates in terms of best potential efficacy. It can be shown that this approach has high probability of identifying the most likely superior arm but at the cost of false-positive findings, particularly if misused.[31] A second and more recent role of randomization in phase II trials is to provide evidence, albeit at a less stringent criteria, that a test treatment is indeed promising.[17] In phase III, randomization is critical for definitive unbiased evaluation.

With regard to implementation, randomization assignments can be simple or, more commonly, implemented using blocking or dynamic approaches with respect to balancing treatment arms by key factors, such as stratification variables mentioned above. A number of proven methods are available.[5]

It is important to note that investigators must protect against practices that can erode or nullify the benefits of randomization. Any breach of the random assignment process has an irreparable effect on the validity of the trial. Second, a large number (or differential number per treatment arm) of patient withdrawals can make the validity of the comparison suspect. Similarly, differential follow-up and consequently ascertainment of patient status between treatment arms can bias the treatment effect estimate. Third, bias in assessment of outcomes can have a major impact on the estimated treatment effect, and thus objective outcome measures and blinding of treatment assignment become important. Treatment assignment blinding is not feasible for radiotherapy and most chemotherapy regimens, but can be used for many agents. In either case, and in particular for studies that cannot be blinded (among patients or caregivers), unambiguous, objectively defined end points are essential. In cases where determination of the end point involves possible observer subjectivity, such as when reading a diagnostic scan to determine disease progression, keeping assessors unaware of treatment assignment may be necessary.

Phase 1 Studies

The phase team includes the patients, caregivers, biostatisticians, oncologist investigators, clinical trial nurses, research associates and data coordinators, pharmacologist and/or pharmacists, and imaging and pathology specialists, along with sponsoring agencies (government, industry, academic, or combinations thereof).

There are multiple types of phase 1 trials. They may be testing an investigational agent plus another investigational agent, investigational agent plus an approved modality (i.e., RT) or agent(s), an approved modality (i.e., RT) or agent plus another approved agent(s), an approved or investigational agent with a PK focus (i.e., adding a PARP inhibitor), or an approved or investigational agent with a PD focus (e.g., evaluation using functional imaging).

If RT is tested with a systemic agent, there should be a preclinical rationale to pursue an early-phase human trial. Ideally, there should be convincing preclinical data that indicate the combination is either efficacious (radiation sensitization) or show no overlapping toxicities (toxicity independence). There should be evidence of *in vitro* radiosensitization in human tumor cell lines, *in vivo* radiosensitization in human tumor models, lack of sensitization of normal tissues, and preclinical use of clinically relevant doses and schedules of agents and RT (add Blackstock oxaliplatin/RT preclinical scheduling paper).

The primary objective is to determine the maximum tolerated dose (MTD) based on scientifically defined dose-limiting toxicities (DLTs). The MTD found in phase I stage is often used as the recommended phase II dose(s) (RP2D). DLT is often defined as a toxicity that is considered serious, typically based on standard criteria CTCAE (most recent version). The DLT must be defined in advance prior to beginning the trial, is protocol-specific, and is usually based, in the case of a systemic agent, on toxicity seen in the first cycle. The MTD is a dose level that yields reasonable rate of DLTs in targeting patient populations. It is a dose that is believed to be efficacious and adequately safe. A dose higher than the MTD is unacceptable. The secondary objectives of phase I studies are to define toxicity profile of new therapy(s) or schedule of an existing modality, such as radiotherapy, under evaluation.

The PK and PD effects in tumor and/or surrogate tissues can be determined along with a preliminary assessment of antitumor activity.

Phase I

The main objective of the phase I trial is to determine the maximum tolerable dose of an agent to be subsequently used in testing for efficacy. Although initially developed in the setting of drug testing, this concept has been adapted to test radiation alone and combined drug/radiation regimens. The basic conceptual approach is that of sequential dose increases, or escalation, in small patient cohorts until the treatment-related AE rate reaches a predetermined level or unexpected toxicity is seen. This stepwise testing in phase I trials determines what is known as the MTD, which is putatively the most effective level at which to evaluate efficacy.

The key parameters to be defined at the outset of a phase I trial include patient eligibility criteria, starting dose and the schedule of dose escalation (which should frame the expected MTD), events comprising the AE/toxicity response and the expected MTD, and finally the escalation design plan.[32] By far, the dominant design has been the so-called 3 + 3 approach, where cohorts of 3 patients are exposed to a given dose, and based on the outcomes in that cohort, either de-escalation, escalation, or additional enrollment takes place. There are a large number of other designs, one of which may be particularly suited for radiation therapy trials, as we will discuss shortly. It should be appreciated that the MTD is a relative concept that can change over time. For example, hematologic toxicity may be less dose limiting today than it was before the development of bone marrow stimulators such as erythropoietin and filgrastim.

Design Challenges

When setting up an early-phase RT trial, it is absolutely critical to think about the next step in development. There are several considerations that are paramount, including the following: What should the starting dose be? How many patients should each cohort include? What is the standard therapy for the tumor site being treated? How quickly can doses be escalated? What is the role of conventional chemotherapy? How should surgery (if appropriate) be integrated? How should chemotherapy be integrated? Can the validation of biomarkers be assessed? Is it possible to avoid an unselected subject population in the follow-up phase II to III study?

A phase 1 trial can include RT as the single modality undergoing testing. Often, a second modality, such as concomitant systemic therapy, is included. In the latter case, data that will be helpful for the design of the study should include single-agent PK data from a pragmatic and relevant scheduling regimen such as consideration of continuous dosing during RT versus once-a-week dosing. Single-agent PD data including the agent's affect (if known) on a molecular target that is relevant to the interaction between RT and radiation are necessary as are safety data.

Dose escalation guidelines have been developed and refined in order to effectively identify the RPTD. Basic principles of dose escalation include starting with a safe starting dose, minimizing the number of patients treated at subtoxic (and thus maybe subtherapeutic) doses, escalating dose rapidly in the absence of toxicity, and escalating dose slowly in the presence of toxicity.

The Fibonacci sequence typically includes three patients per cohort until the DLT is reached; then, additional three patients are accrued at the dose level. Some of the accelerated titration designs attempt to minimize patients within the early dose levels. Typically, a single patient is enrolled at each cohort until ≥grade 2 toxicity, and then the number of patients accrued at the dose level increased to 3 (or perhaps a total

Phase I Trial Design: Standard 3 + 3 Design

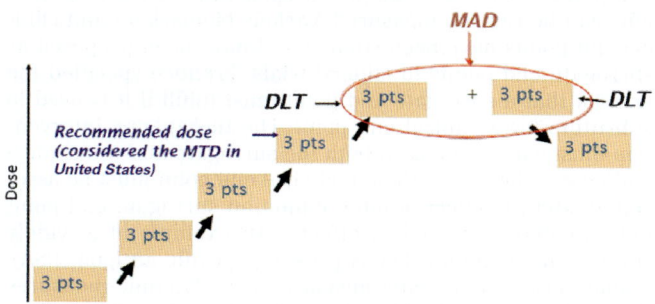

FIGURE 15.2. Example of standard 3 + 3 phase I design.

of 6 if that turns out to the MTD). Standard dose escalation rules are acceptable especially if multiple agents are being used (including conventional chemotherapy). The *Maximum Administered Dose* (MAD) and *Maximum Tolerated Dose* (MTD) can be confusing, and these phrases vary with country. More importantly, the RP2D is often one dose level below that which the DLT occurred in a prespecified proportion of patients (e.g., ≥33%) (Fig. 15.2)

It is recommended to consider using a toxicity assessment in association with clinical or biologic end points. With targeted small molecular agents, it may be necessary to define the optimal biologic dose (OBD) as opposed to MTD. The OBD is the *dose associated with a prespecified desired effect on a biomarker. For example, it may be the* modality dose at which ≥20% of patients have inhibition of a key target in tumor/surrogate tissues. It may also be the modality dose at which ≥20% of patients achieve a prespecified immunologic parameter. Caution is advised because the biologic end point is often considered a surrogate for therapeutic effect, and this may not be completely understood during the early drug development period.

Patient selection is important in early-phase study design. For example, the tumor site(s) to be studied needs to be defined because this will impact the assessment of toxicity. Not all normal tissue is equal (as discussed in more detail in Chapter 14). The selection of tumor site may also be impacted by the agent being used in combination with RT, such as the choice to study the epidermal growth factor receptor monoclonal antibody, cetuximab, with radiotherapy in the head and neck setting. Also, are the patients being enrolled onto a phase 1 study going to receive curative or palliative radiotherapy? This will affect total radiation dose and fractionation utilized. This will affect the patient population and perhaps the ability to tolerate combined modality therapy. In general, phase I data are generated from studies that are cancer specific and/or site specific.

Starting dose and schedules of the modality under investigation will need to be defined. If the goal is radiosensitization, then delivery of the agent during as many fractions of radiation is desirable. Timing may be critical. A typical approach especially in the curative setting is to start with a standard radiation dose; however, escalation (or even de-escalation) of the radiation dose may be desirable in certain clinical situations.

A limited dose escalation design is more commonly being used. DLTs may include, though not limited to, the following: grade IV hematologic toxicity, grade III nonhematologic toxicity with exceptions for grade III GI (nausea and emesis) in the setting of upper abdominal RT, unscheduled breaks during the RT course, inability to administer systemic agent, and/or surgical morbidity for trials where the dose escalation component occurs in the preoperative setting.

As stated earlier, not all normal tissues are equal. A parallel track dose escalation design may allow one to test the combination of one (or more) agent(s) plus different doses of RT for different anatomical disease sites. After the RP2D of the dual-targeted agents is identified and thereafter fixed, then the RT dose is escalated.

Lead-in administration of a novel agent, prior to piggybacking onto a standard combined modality backbone, may allow for independent assessment of toxicity as well as evaluation of a biomarker with respect to proof of principal preliminary exploration of possible mechanisms of target inhibition (see Fig. 15.3).

In addition, this approach may be particularly helpful in selecting patients for phase II studies. Furthermore, an expanded cohort at final dose may allow for a more precise evaluation of biomarker.

Phase I Trial of Protease Inhibitor, Nelfinavir, With Concurrent Chemoradiotherapy For Stage IIIA/IIIB Inoperable NSCLC

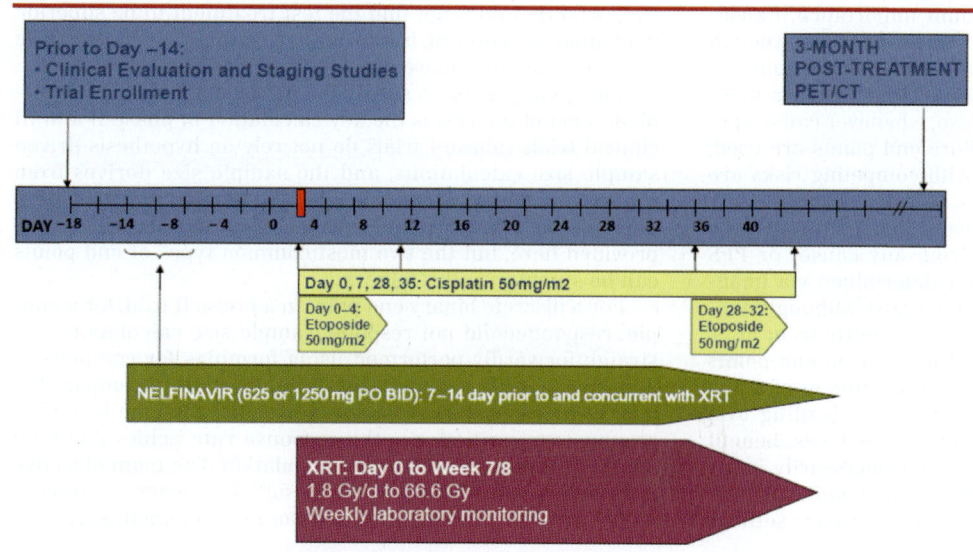

FIGURE 15.3. Example of lead-in administration of a novel agent, which may allow for independent assessment of toxicity as well as evaluation of a biomarker. (Courtesy of Ramesh Rengan.)

End Points

In clinical trials, end points must be unambiguously defined, be assessable and reproducible, and reflect the action of the intervention. Typically, there is a single primary end point in a clinical trial, but there may be numerous secondary end points.

Traditionally in phase II cancer trials, treatment activity has been defined in terms of reduction in tumor burden. The most recent criteria for measuring activity are known as the Response Evaluation Criteria in Solid Tumors, or RECIST.[33] The criteria require the identification of target and nontarget lesions at baseline and their largest single dimensions. Categories of response are then defined, for example, complete response (CR, disappearance of all target and nontarget lesions and no new lesions), partial response (PR, 30% or greater decrease in the sum of the longest diameter of all target lesions, no progression of nontarget lesions, and no new lesions), and progressive disease (PD, 20% or greater increase in target lesions, progression of nontarget lesions, or the occurrence of new lesions). A patient not satisfying either response or progression criteria is classified as having a stable disease (SD). Those achieving either a CR or PR are typically defined as objective responders, and the proportion of patients responding is then the primary end point of interest. Although widely used, there has long been concern that response defined this way is an inadequate substitute for more clinically relevant and objective end points such as survival time. In one study, <25% of agents that produced tumor response were eventually found to extend survival in comparative trials,[34] whereas another suggested that tumor response is a reasonable surrogate for survival extension.[35] Additional problems with the use of response rates in phase II trials include subjectivity and lack of reproducible assessments.[36]

As mentioned earlier, response is not as frequently used when radiation therapy is the test question, and in any case, other discrete binary end points can readily be used. For example, the proportion free of a given event (i.e., proportion alive, proportion recurrence-free, etc.) at a fixed time landmark, such as 2 years, is a common and straightforward end point.

A more informative end point that is used in many phase II and most phase III trials is the elapsed time from trial entry until occurrence of some event. The most straightforward of these is overall survival time, or time to death from any cause. This simple end point does not depend on adjudication of cause of death and its attendant complexities and naturally corrects for both favorable and unfavorable consequences of treatment. Although it can be verified or even ascertained from public records because of its simplicity, active follow-up per protocol remains of paramount importance. Cause-specific survival end points may also be considered, although as mentioned, assigning cause of death is not simple, and one must account for "other cause" of deaths and whether these have any relationship to treatment. Also, whenever cause-specific deaths or other site-specific failure end points are used, methods for appropriately dealing with competing risks are required.[37,38]

Other commonly used time-to-event end points include DFS (time to recurrence or death from any cause) or PFS (time to disease progression, possibly determined via imaging or other assessments at regular intervals), although definitions of these are not standardized (e.g., see Hudis et al.[39]), and the specific failure events comprising a given end points should be carefully specified. The main advantage of using DFS or PFS is the more rapid rate of events, leading to a smaller required sample size. In many cancer types, benefit with respect to these end points does not necessarily imply subsequent lengthened survival, although they may still represent clinical benefit for patients. For other disease settings

(e.g., adjuvant therapy in colon cancer), DFS is a reliable and well-accepted primary end point that is strongly correlated with survival.[40] This raises the topic of so-called surrogate end points, which are end points upon which treatment benefits can be reliably measured. Various biomarkers and clinical end points have been studied and have been proposed as surrogate end points in clinical trials. Prentice specified the criteria that a surrogate end point must fulfill if it is used to substitute for a clinical end point: The therapeutic intervention must exert benefit on both the surrogate and the clinical end points; the surrogate and clinical end point must be associated; and the effect of intervention on surrogate end point must mediate the clinical effect.[41] An example of a widely studied surrogate marker is prostate-specific antigen (PSA), applied either as a static measure or as dynamic measures (PSA velocity; PSA doubling time; time to PSA nadir, particularly useful after radiation therapy of the intact prostate), to assess time to biochemical failure in patients with nonmetastatic adenocarcinoma of the prostate.[42,43] This continues to be a developing area, and there remain many caveats and cautions regarding surrogate end points in clinical trials.[44]

Statistical Power and Sample Size

The overarching design consideration in clinical trials is to obtain sufficient information about an intervention so that a reliable decision can be made regarding its further development or use. In the classical (e.g., frequentist) statistical hypothesis testing paradigm, one sets up a null hypothesis of no treatment effect and an alternative hypothesis (which one hopes to validate) indicating a treatment effect. The type II or β error equals the probability that a statistical test fails to produce a decision in favor of a treatment effect when in fact the treatment is superior in the population. The complement of this probability $(1 - \beta)$ is referred to as *statistical power* and equals the probability of correctly deciding in favor of a treatment benefit. Statistical power depends on the other principal parameters considered when planning the trial, specifically the probability of incorrectly finding in favor of a difference when none exists (type I or alpha error, usually set to 0.05 or 0.01 by convention), the *a priori* specification of a treatment effect that is considered both realistic and clinically material, and of course the sample size. It is imperative that trials be designed to achieve adequate statistical power; typically, 0.80 to 0.90 is desirable, so as not to obtain equivocal findings concerning the potential worth of new treatments under consideration. Studies with low statistical power can cause delay or even abandonment of the development of promising treatments, and waste valuable resources, not least of which is the participation and goodwill of patients.[45] In contrast, a "negative" trial that does not find the test treatment to be superior, if adequately powered, is informative, in that resources can be directed into other more promising alternatives.

Thus, sample size to satisfy the power desired for the specified effect of interest is the key calculation in phase II and III clinical trials (phase I trials do not rely on hypothesis-driven sample size calculations, and the sample size derives from the specific design used). The specific sample size calculation depends on the end point, and technical details will not be provided here, but the two most common types of end points can be summarized as follows.

For a discrete binary end point in a phase II trial, for example, responded/did not respond, sample size calculations are straightforwardly performed using formulas for comparison of proportions. In a single-arm study, one aims to compare the observed response rate for the new agent to some historical response proportion, p_0—the response rate achievable with standard therapy in the target population. The main objective is to determine whether there is sufficient evidence to conclude that the response rate for the new regimen is greater than p_0. We designate p_A a response rate, which, if true, would be clinically material. We test the null hypothesis H_0: $p = p_0$ against the alternative hypothesis H_0: $p = p_A$. The values of p_0 and p_A (and more importantly the difference), along with the sample size, will determine the power of the study. Note that to detect a small improvement (say, ≤10%) requires a large sample size. For example, to detect an improvement from a historical value of 20% to 30% with 85% power, over 120 subjects are required. Also, the value for both p_0 and p_A must be realistic; it is of little value to design and carry out a study to detect an effect size $p_A - p_0$ that is unlikely to be realized, simply because it is compatible with the number of patients that can be recruited.

For two-arm randomized phase II trials with discrete end points, the above is simply redefined in terms of two-sample comparisons of proportions, and the sample size is consequently much larger. Finally, if the end point is a fixed time landmark such as proportion event-free or alive at one year, then the estimates of the proportions may be derived from survival analysis methods to appropriately account for losses to follow-up.

In many randomized phase II and nearly all phase III trials, the time from randomization until occurrence of the event is of principal interest, rather than the event status at some fixed time landmark. In larger phase II trial and phase III trials, recruitment may take place over a lengthy interval, and each patient will have a different follow-up duration, and the use of follow-up time per patient is more efficient than waiting until all patients have reached some fixed time. The treatment effect measure is then specified in terms of failure *hazards*, which can be thought of as failure rates per unit of time. Hypotheses are thus usually formulated in terms of the hazard ratio (HR) as H_0: $\lambda_A/\lambda_B = HR = 1.0$ where λ_A and λ_B are the hazards for treatments A and B versus alternative H_A: $HR < 1.0$, for some value of the HR that represents a clinically important difference in outcomes. Under the assumption that this ratio is relatively constant over time, a given HR can be converted to an absolute difference between groups in proportions remaining event-free at a specific follow-up time. For example, a new/standard HR equals to 0.75, or a 25% reduction in failure rate in the experimental group relative to the standard group may translate into an absolute difference in the proportion of patients remaining free of the event between groups of 4.6% at 5 years, if the standard group 5-year survival percentage is 80%.

From the specification of difference of interest or effect size, then the sample size in terms of number of *events* required to detect this difference with desired statistical power and significance level is determined. Depending on the anticipated accrual rate and the prognosis (e.g., rapidity of failure events) in the control treatment group, the number of *patients* required can then be approximated. The number of events required depends strongly on the HR, becoming dramatically larger as the HR approaches 1.0. The number of patients required and total duration of the trial depend on the rate of patient accrual and the failure rate in the control group, both of which contribute to the determination of how rapidly the requisite events will be observed. The accrual rate is typically estimated from previous experience and may also involve querying investigators to project the accrual rate per unit of time. Similarly, the failure rate for patients under standard therapy is derived from available data. The final computations are straightforward but generally require computer programs,[46] but, under certain assumptions, can be approximated.[47] Sample size methods have been extended to take into account other factors that will influence power, such as patients withdrawing from treatment (dropout), switching from the assigned treatment to the other group (crossover), or deviating from protocol treatment (noncompliance).[48-50]

Interim Analysis and Stopping Rules

Primarily for ethical considerations but also to make best use of resources, interim analysis plans are used in all phases of clinical trials. These plans provide for early decision-making in a trial regarding continuation, disclosure of findings, or modification of the trial while preserving integrity of the study with respect to power and type I error control described earlier. These methods are needed because with repeated hypothesis tests, the probability of at least one test resulting in an erroneous rejection of the null hypothesis increases.

Phase I trials have stopping rules that are integral to the design, in that termination of enrollment to a given dose is based on observed cumulative AE rates at a given time. We refer to a review of the designs for more details.[1]

Phase II trials more formally incorporate stopping rules, usually restricted to "futility stopping", or discontinuation when results do not appear promising. For trials with discrete end points such as tumor response, this is accomplished through multistage study designs, whereby a cohort of patients is enrolled and assessed for response, and if a specific minimum response proportion is observed, the trial continues to full accrual; otherwise, it discontinues enrollment. The most commonly used designs are those proposed by Simon,[51] although there are other similar approaches. In trials with time-to-event end point, futility rules similar to those for phase III trials (discussed next) can be used to discontinue after a period of follow-up if results appear unpromising. Early stopping of single-arm phase II trials for extraordinary efficacy is unusual but certainly not prohibited.

Phase III trials use repeated testing strategies derived from an area of statistics known as group sequential methods. Briefly, the primary hypothesis is evaluated at predefined increments (typically 3 to 5 looks) of the total information (usually in the form of failure events) needed for definitive analysis. The individual tests are designed to (a) protect against spurious early stopping because of the unstable nature of "early" results and (b) correct for the effect of repeated testing on type I error, which can also lead to spurious declaration of treatment effects that may not be reliable. Commonly used approaches include the Haybittle-Peto approach, for which each test through the penultimate look requires a constant highly significant result, such as $P < .0001$, in order to stop,[52,53] and the O'Brien-Fleming approach and its subsequent approaches,[54] in which the required significance level decreases over the looks, becoming less extreme as more information accumulates. There are many variations and extensions of the latter approach, with different properties and advantages in special circumstances. In addition to efficacy monitoring rules, phase III trials increasingly also incorporate formal futility-stopping rules, although methods such as conditional power calculations have been available and used for some time.[55,56] Futility-stopping rules similarly involve setting a boundary such that when the test statistic falls beyond it, then one considers stopping because the new treatment will not ultimately prevail. Stopping for futility is a complex decision requiring careful consideration,[57] and methods continue to be studied and developed.[58,59]

Definitive Analysis and Secondary Analyses

When the trial reaches maturity either as planned or earlier as a result of the monitoring plan, then definitive analysis takes place. Prior to this, it is not conventional or recommended to disclose any results from the trial,[60] and this policy is adhered to in NCI Cooperative Group trials.

A critical aspect of clinical trial analysis is the definition of the analyzed cohort. The concept of analysis by *intention to treat* is often cited, but the definition of this term can sometimes be unclear, so it is best to explicitly describe which patients are included.[61] In the strictest sense, the intention-to-treat cohort includes all patients randomized, regardless of eligibility, adherence to assigned treatment, or any other post-randomization deviations from protocol. However, it is often the case that patients found ineligible for the trial after randomization because of having been incorrectly staged or for other reasons are excluded from the primary analysis, and this practice (used with caution) is sometimes advocated, as it allows for evaluation of the therapy in the population for whom it was intended.[2] A rarely acceptable practice involves exclusion of patients who did not or could not comply with assigned therapy regimens or received nonprotocol therapy or other postrandomization conditions. Such exclusions can easily lead to biased comparisons, and in general, any post hoc analysis of treatment benefit by dose received is fraught with interpretational difficulties and should be avoided in primary analysis.[62]

The primary analysis methods follow naturally from a well-written protocol (see below) and thus should be straightforward. Given that major journals increasingly require that study protocols be provided at the time of publication, and that regulatory agencies and public sponsors do likewise, it behooves the trialist to outline the analysis plan in the protocol and then carry it out at study conclusion. This does not suggest that additional analyses cannot be carried out, but having a framework for the planned analysis adds credibility to the findings.

Secondary prognostic factor analysis using statistical models or other techniques often follows primary analysis of phase III trials. Of particular interest is whether there are particularly responsive or nonresponsive subsets of patients, in an attempt to render the findings more relevant to practice. The modeling process, which entails deciding which factors to include, determining the correct way to represent a given factor (i.e., in categories, on a continuous scale, etc.), consideration of interrelationships (e.g., interactions) among factors, and many other issues, can be complex, and it should be recognized that these analyses will be largely viewed as exploratory. Although possibly worth exploring, true differential effects of treatment by other factors usually require a large sample size, unless the effects are very large.[63] A comprehensive review of current modeling methods applied to oncology data is provided by Schmoor et al.[63]

PRACTICAL ISSUES IN THE DESIGN, CONDUCT, AND REPORTING OF CLINICAL TRIALS

Protocol Document and Study Conduct

The goal of a clinical trial is to answer a well-formulated question that will change clinical practice. To achieve that, the investigators must know the current state of knowledge on the studied disease, clearly describe the eligibility criteria of the studied population, understand the number of patients who will be eligible in their institution/cooperative group, choose simple and achievable end points, establish statistical assumptions based on thorough review of preexisting data, and collaborate with a biostatistician to decide on study design, sample size, and power.

The clinical trial protocol document must contain the title, investigators and sponsor's name, phase (I, II, or III), protocol synopsis, background knowledge, study design and schema, objectives, methodology, subject selection criteria, registration procedures, treatment plan, dosing modifications, AE reporting, data and safety monitoring plan, study calendar, outcome measures, data reporting, statistical considerations, and the informed consent.[64]

Choosing the right study end points is crucial, as it needs to reflect the primary goal of the trial. Any number of end points may be of suitable scientific and clinical value, but if there is interest in regulatory approval, then obviously the end point must reflect the requirements of those parties involved. Overall survival largely remains the "gold standard" for a registration trial designed to gain marketing approval. However, survival length may be affected by effective salvage therapies or by patient's "crossing over" to the other study arm. End points such as DFS and PFS have been used for either expedited drug approval or regular approval, depending on the disease site.[65] If end points subject to assessment bias are to be used (e.g., PFS or tumor response), then appropriate bias reduction measures are needed. One approach to circumvent this problem is an independent review panel (e.g., radiologists reviewing baseline and follow-up images to quantify tumor responses and note the moment of tumor progression), consisting of experts not associated with the trial and unaware of the arm to which the patient was enrolled. One must also consider validity of modern end points even under unbiased review. For example, the phenomena of pseudoprogression and pseudoresponse have made imaging-based end points, including overall radiographic response and PFS, problematic.[66]

Successful completion of a clinical trial requires constant attention to its practical aspects. Sufficient personnel are necessary in order to assure the smooth running of the study and safety of the participating subjects. Clinical research nurses, clinical research associates, data managers, and investigational pharmacists are crucial components of the research team.[67] Of particular importance are careful and immediate recording and attribution of all AEs. Severe AEs have to be reported promptly to appropriate regulatory agencies (IRB in the institution where the study is open, FDA, and others) and to the study sponsor. Because most protocols have amendments added during their lifetime and new toxicities are reported from other studies, the research protocol commonly evolves over several successive versions. As a result, new versions of consent forms must be created as well, and IRB approval may again be required. It is imperative that patients enrolled to the study sign the most current version of the consent form. All the prescribed follow-up tests (imaging, blood work, etc.) have to be scheduled ahead of time and coincide with the study calendar. Departures from any of the procedures are scored as protocol deviations during periodic audits and will impact adversely on the study's validity. Additionally, designated independent medical monitors are assigned to high-risk trials (such as most single-institution investigator-initiated trials) to continuously review any reported events, which are later evaluated periodically by the institutional data safety monitoring committee.

Data and Safety Monitoring Committees

The decision to alter clinical trial in progress, including discontinuation of accrual and/or treatment, depending on its current state, and early release of findings is typically vested in an independent DSMC. In addition to evaluating according to the monitoring rules described earlier, the DSMC considers the information available from the trial as well as external information that bear on treatment for the disease under study. Specifically, it should be noted that the early stopping rules described above are meant to serve as guidelines, and there may at any decision point be additional considerations that must be taken into account.[68] The policies and procedures for U.S. National Cancer Institute–sponsored Cooperative Group trials provide a good overview of DSMC structure and function.[69]

Trial Reporting

Once the study is completed and the data are fully analyzed, its results should be reported promptly. Publication of the results of the trial in a scientific journal represents culmination of the investigators' efforts and allows wide distribution of the findings. However, lack of precise requirements of reporting may lead to inaccurate or biased result presentation. The CONSORT (Consolidated Standards of Reporting Trials) statement is used worldwide to improve the quality of reporting of randomized controlled trials.[70] It provides a 25-item checklist of all required elements and a flow diagram to assure that all patients enrolled are accounted for. Many journals require the authors to follow the CONSORT guidelines, because "diligent adherence by authors to the checklist items facilitates clarity, completeness, and transparency of reporting."[70] The ICMJE (International Committee of Medical Journal Editors) similarly publishes guidelines on uniform requirements for manuscripts submitted to biomedical journals.[71] There have also been calls for improvements in reporting of phase I and II trials.[72,73] In addition to quality with respect to content, a full disclosure of the financial COI by the investigators to the readers is necessary as well. Redundant publications (repeating the same results in several journals) are discouraged and there is an obligation to publish negative studies. Study of the publication rate of cancer cooperative group trials regardless of findings shows there is room for improvement with respect to responsible approach to clinical trial conduct.[74]

In the United States, reporting requirements are currently trending toward an expansion to more "open access" sources, based on mandates arising from recently enacted legislation. ClinicalTrials.gov is the largest clinical trial database in the world, run by the National Library of Medicine in the National Institutes of Health. Initially including information only on NIH-sponsored studies, NILM now also contains studies sponsored by the pharmaceutical companies and demands "basic results" information not later than one year after the study's primary completion date (ClinicalTrials.gov). The requirements for results reporting were prompted by removal of several drugs from the market because of earlier unrealized toxicity, knowledge about which was obscured by lack of publication or other public documentation.

RECENT APPROACHES TO CLINICAL TRIAL DESIGN

An Alternative Phase I Trial Design for Radiation Oncology Trials

As mentioned earlier, phase I trials in radiation therapy present a unique challenge in that toxicities may occur long after treatment and need to be incorporated into dose evaluation. The traditional stepwise designs do not accommodate this, and thus an extension of the Continual Reassessment Method[75] that incorporates the time-to-event (i.e., time to toxicity) information for each patient was developed.[76] Designated the TITE-CRM approach, a dose–response model is first posited that identifies the starting dose and range to be considered, along with a time frame for events occurring anywhere up to T time units from administration of therapy. Rather than waiting for each cohort of patients to be followed for this length of time, however, one can enter new patients at, say, half-month intervals. As in the original CRM, the first patient is assigned to a dose level based on prior information or, as in the modified CRM, to the lowest candidate dose. At the time the next patient(s) is (are) to be enrolled, the observed toxicities and follow-up times of patients already entered are used to form an updated estimate of the β parameter that defines the dose–response curve and the dose level for the next patient(s) selected according to the usual CRM or modified CRM criteria. In simulation studies, the TITE-CRM produced results comparable to its CRM counterpart while significantly reducing the average duration of the trial. However, the TITE-CRM method was associated with slightly more toxicities, particularly in

situations where events tend to occur near the end of the observation period, because escalation to the next dose may have already occurred before toxicities were observed.[76] Another problematic issue is rapid accrual, where premature escalation of dose may be indicated. A recent review and suggested modifications may make this approach even more suitable for radiation oncology trials.[77]

Alternative Phase II Trial Designs

As indicated earlier, the value of traditional single-arm phase II trials has been called into question in terms of providing a reliable basis for further pursuit of promising treatments. The currently favored design is a randomized phase II trial with a standard of care comparison group.[13,17,78] This approach and the goal of accelerating development have led to consideration enhancements to the phase II design, including adaptive randomization, where one favors enrollment to the arm(s) that seem to be prevailing while reducing probability of enrollment on other arms and even dropping some treatment arms. This is an idea with a long history,[79] but recent innovations in computing and Bayesian methods, as well as a newfound interest in accelerated development, have brought it to wider use in some settings.[80] In some instances, it may offer advantages but must be weighed against simpler approaches with similar or even greater efficiency.[81]

Changes in therapeutic approaches also suggest design changes. Because primarily cytostatic agents (i.e., most biologic drugs) are not expected to necessarily result in tumor response in the traditional sense, there is a need to consider alternative phase II designs based on end points other than response rates. For trials enrolling patients who have failed prior therapy, Mick et al.[82] propose a method that uses each patient as his/her own control, comparing the time to progression (possibly censored) under the new agent with the time to progression under prior therapy. Rosner et al.[83] propose a randomized discontinuation design to evaluate cytostatic drugs in which all patients are initially treated with the experimental agent. After a specified interval, responders remain on drug and those who progress discontinue, whereas those patients with SD are randomized to either continued active treatment or placebo. This randomized comparison allows one to assess whether the drug is truly slowing the rate of growth of the tumor, as opposed to the investigators having simply selected patients with slow-growing tumors. Because the patients with SD form a more homogeneous subgroup, this design also requires a smaller sample size than would a trial that randomized all patients at entry. It is important to note that the purpose of this design is to determine whether the drug is active in an explanatory sense. Whether the percentage of patients exhibiting SD is high or low has bearing on the efficiency of the approach, because in the latter case the total sample size required may be quite large and any demonstration of activity in the randomized component would only be relevant to a small subset of the population. Korn et al.[84] point out other caveats with this design. For example, patients may find it unattractive to potentially discontinue a treatment that they perceive to be helping their disease.

Using Biomarkers as Inclusion Criteria

It is increasingly understood that the response of tumors to targeted agents is highly dependent on their molecular subtype. Consequently, trials increasingly screen for molecular characteristics of tumors to use as eligibility criteria or, at a minimum, stratification factors. For example, recent and currently accruing RTOG brain tumor trials require MGMT status, whereas the head and neck cancer trials are now requiring HPV status to be determined at entry. When studies enroll sufficient numbers of patients, then treatment by marker synergisms, referred to statistically as interaction effects, can be investigated. Robust evaluation of true differential benefit according to markers requires that treatments be randomized, and so randomized phase II and phase III trials are ideal setting for developing tailored treatments.

In many instances, potentially responsive subsets of patients may be small and may also be identified after trials have initiated enrollment. For instance, ALK inhibitors are highly effective, but only in the 3% to 5% of lung cancers that have *ALK* gene rearrangements. It may simply not be feasible to perform separate phase III trials for each lung cancer subtype. One possible alternative is "adaptive randomized" trial designs in which the data gathered as the trial progresses are used to change some aspect of the trial as it progresses. Some recent examples are the Biomarker-Integrated Approaches of Targeted Therapy for Lung Cancer Elimination (BATTLE) trial in lung cancer[85] and the I-SPY trials in breast cancer.[86] However, there are limitations and challenges to these complex trial designs. For example, in order to be able to acquire information rapidly enough to undertake weighted randomization favoring more promising arms or eliminate nonresponsive arms, surrogate end points such as "disease control rate at 8 weeks" must be used. It is not clear such short-term end points are relevant to radiation oncology where local control is very frequently achieved.

A number of recent papers in the clinical literature have provided excellent reviews of the opportunities and challenges involved in incorporating modern molecular medicine into clinical trial design.[87,88]

MOVING BEYOND CLINICAL TRIALS

Comparative Effectiveness Research

The randomized phase III clinical trial is considered the most robust method of comparing the efficacy of a new treatment with the standard of care. Grading systems for evaluating clinical evidence universally place "randomized controlled trials" above observational trials.[89] More recently, this hierarchical approach to scientific evidence has been attacked by[20] criticisms including the high fiscal cost of clinical trials, the length of time that it takes to obtain a conclusion (by which time the results are frequently no longer relevant because the standard of care has changed), and the large number of trials with negative results.

A specific criticism relates to clinical protocols that typically allow enrollment of only the fittest patients that lack comorbidities and have good performance status, criteria that subsequently limit the generalizability of the results. Studies have indeed shown that, for example, older patients are excluded unnecessarily out of concern for potential AEs.[90-92] There have indeed long been calls for simpler and more inclusive eligibility criteria.[93]

In some sense, the desire to reduce exclusivity and broaden trial enrollment to more closely match the population is antithetical to "personalized medicine" and more focused trials as mentioned above. However, there are some ways in which the two concepts can possibly work in concert. Larger trials that can robustly support subset analysis according to biologic, clinical, and health history/behavior factors can at once be more inclusive and address questions about particularly responsive subgroups.

Another response to the criticism of phase III trials has been a reappreciation of the importance of population-based retrospective studies as a way to appreciate a treatment's effectiveness in the "real world." Even more useful are well-designed prospective cohort studies, such as the Cancer of the Prostate Strategic Urologic Research Endeavor (CaPSURE) study in prostate cancer, which will provide information both on factors driving treatment choice and the effects of specific intervention strategies for which randomized trial evidence is currently lacking.[94] Another key strategy is conducting trials in parallel with concurrent registries of patients treated according to physician and patient choice and/or common convention, such as the Trial Assigning IndividuaLized Options for Treatment (**Rx**) (TAILORx) trial.[95] In this trial, 7,000 women with breast cancer are screened using a molecular profiling tool, and for those with profiles in the range where the utility of the tool is uncertain, randomization between "hormonal therapy alone" and "hormonal therapy plus chemotherapy" is performed. Patients obtaining scores below or above this range are registered in order to accurately record treatment choices and ensure that good follow-up data are obtained. This trial will both serve to determine the utility of the profiling tool in the uncertain range and provide high-quality data on the validity of treatment decisions based upon it.

Meta-analysis

A formal quantitative means of combining evidence from multiple clinical trials is by meta-analysis, a widely used analytic tool in many areas of social and medical science. Meta-analysis refers to a process whereby data from independent studies are combined to form a quantitative summary estimate of a given effect. Meta-analyses are considered by some to be a level I evidence source along with large randomized clinical trials. A meta-analysis combines results of several studies, all of which ask a similar research question, but may be individually too small to have enough statistical power to definitively answer the question. Performing a systematic analysis of data from all identified randomized trials can define a modest but real advantage associated with a new therapeutic approach. The goals of combined modality phase I studies are similar to single-agent studies. However, the design and application often differ. The primary end point is usually an assessment of toxicity and to identify a RP2D. The investigation of biomarkers can also occur, although some investigators have tended to attach this end point as part of a phase 0 trial design.

Toxicity assessment is typically during the entire radiation course and some defined period of time afterward, for example, 30 to 60 days. It is frankly impractical to wait an extended period of time for late and/or chronic RT toxicity to be assessed. The TITE-CRM Bayesian methodology may allow for more prompt dose escalation and continuous inclusion of new toxicity data from prior patients enrolled onto the trial.[29,96]

TIME-TO-EVENT CONTINUAL REASSESSMENT METHOD (TITE-CRM)

The TITE-CRM was initially described by Cheung and Chappell[76] where the time to toxicity was incorporated for each patient. This allows both acute and late toxicities to be accounted for, all while patient enrollment continues. Studies have shown that the TITE-CRM design is usually more efficient, treating more patients closer to the MTD and shorter trial durations.

Statistically, the TITE-CRM design assumes that the hazard of developing toxicity is constant over time. In radiotherapy, that is often not the case. For example, pneumonitis is a subacute toxicity after thoracic radiotherapy that occurs 1 to 6 months after the end of radiotherapy, but not before or after. Therefore, assuming a constant risk for pneumonitis after time is inaccurate.

In radiotherapy, where late toxicity is a major concern, the TITE-CRM has multiple advantages. Normolle et al. performed a Monte Carlo simulation and found that, compared with a traditional 3 + 3 design, it can produce more accurate estimates of the MTD and not expose patients to significant excess risk.[29]

One concern in chemoradiotherapy trials is that with fast patient accrual and late toxicities, the TITE-CRM could lead

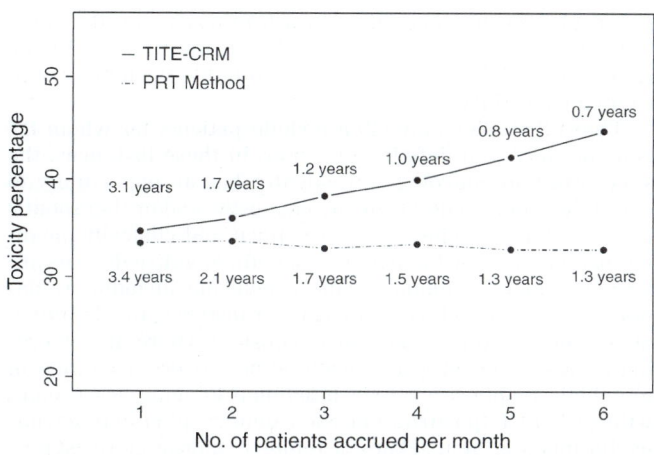

FIGURE 15.4. Comparison of toxicities seen using both methods with different accrual rates. (From Bekele BN, Ji Y, Shen Y, Thall PF. Monitoring late-onset toxicities in phase I trials using predicted risks. *Biostatistics* 2008;9[3]:442–457. Reproduced by permission of Oxford University Press.)

to overdose. Polley et al.[77] have proposed a modification to the TITE-CRM using accrual suspension. Bekele et al. proposed yet another variation on the TITE-CRM using time to toxicity. In this model, if the anticipated risk to patients while conducting a trial becomes too high, but then normalizes, the trial is restarted. The authors propose that this affords greater safety than the classic TITE-CRM, although the trial may take longer (Fig. 15.4).[97]

A radiotherapy-specific model-based method has also been developed. Mehta et al.[98] reported on an alternative Bayesian methodology, which determines the probability of pneumonitis as a function of mean normalized lung dose, and the dose per fraction is escalated accordingly.

Despite the advantages of CRM design, Rogatko et al.[99] have shown that only 1.6% of 1,235 phase I cancer trials published between 1991 and 2006 used Bayesian designs. Le Tourneau et al.[100] found that only 3.3% of 181 evaluable phase I trials performed in 2007 to 2008 used CRM design (5 modified CRM, 1 TITE CRM).

Multiple CMT studies have used the TITE-CRM design. For example, in pancreatic cancer, TITE-CRM has been used in a phase I/II to dose escalate the radiotherapy dose with fixed-dose gemcitabine.[101] It has been used to dose escalate both oxaliplatin and gemcitabine with fixed-dose radiotherapy.[102] And, lastly, it has been used to escalate cisplatin with fixed-dose gemcitabine and radiotherapy.[103]

Lawrence et al.[104] published on the early-stage development of radiosensitizers. They advocated for the use of the TITE-CRM design in its ability to enroll new patients while simultaneously monitoring for the development of late toxicity and incorporating that data into the model. They specifically note that intrapatient dose escalation is likely not appropriate in trials that use radiotherapy because of the cumulative nature of radiation toxicity. Likewise, TITE-CRM has been used to dose escalate radiotherapy when combined with radioprotectants, for example, in liver radiation and concurrent amifostine.[105]

Accordingly, there is an urgent need for predictive biomarkers of normal tissue toxicity. Finding such biomarkers is an area of fruitful research. One example that appears promising in the cardio-oncology arena is troponin and/or N-terminal pro–B-type natriuretic peptide (NT-proBNP) blood levels along with strain analysis of 2-D speckle-tracking echocardiography.[106–109]

Pitfalls

Chronic and cumulative toxicities usually cannot be assessed and may be missed, because most patients do not stay on trial beyond 2 cycles if systemic agent is being added onto

an RT backbone. Furthermore, uncommon toxicities will be missed, because few patients are enrolled onto early-phase trial. Finally, the variations in target delineation by different investigators have the potential to inadvertently impact the toxicity profile. The use of anatomic atlases may help mitigate this critical variable. Chronic and cumulative toxicities usually cannot be assessed and may be missed, because most patients have been lost to follow up.

History of Phase 1 RT–Drug Trials

Over the past 3 decades, most of these clinical trials ($N = 162$ phase 1 only, $N = 66$ phase 1 to 2) have utilized a rule-based design for dose escalation, usually a 3 + 3.[110] RT has only been tested for dose escalation approximately one-eighth of the time (27 trials) when combined with a drug. In these trials, RT was the only modality being tested for dose escalation two-thirds of the time. Only a single anatomical site has been usually studied (98%), with head and neck (20%), lung (18%), brain (11%), and pancreas (10%) being the most common. Over 90% of published studies did report grade 3 to 4 AE, with two-fifths (42%) comprising hematologic AEs and 50% nonhematologic (with plurality being mucositis). The mean number of events described as DLT per number of grade 3 to 4 AE was reported to be 4, and the description of the DLT period (mean of 69 days) was only described in only nearly two-thirds (62%) of the studies. This published benchmark although helpful cannot account for the much larger number of trials that were never written up in full manuscript form. With the increasing cadre of radiation oncologist learning how to design prospective clinical trials as part of dedicated career development course, including the ASCO (American Society of Clinical Oncology)/AACR (American Association for Cancer Research) Methods in Clinical Cancer Research Vail Workshop, the ECCO (European CanCer Organisation) Methods in Clinical Cancer Research Zeist (formerly Flims) Workshop, and other smaller courses developed exclusively to training radiation oncologist, this future may be brighter.

Phase 2 Trials

The decision to proceed with a combined modality phase II study is dependent upon the safety and early efficacy results from the phase I trial. A major goal of a combined modality study is *efficacy* or clinical activity, as defined as increasing the therapeutic window (or therapeutic ratio).[111,112] These trials can screen out suboptimal treatments and identify promising strategies worthy of further validation in a more definitive or confirmatory trial setting. Phase 2 trials can also provide a more extended safety profile than may have been possible in the phase 1 trial.

Design

When designing phase 2 trials involving RT, there are a number of challenges, some of which are unique to the modality and others are compounded by combined modality therapeutic designs. These include the fact that (a) many phase II studies are of unselected patient populations, (b) they are often introduced in the curative setting (i.e., plus/minus boost for ductal carcinoma *in situ*) such that the interval for observation may be extended (i.e., years), (c) recent data on RT/immunotherapy are promising for some metastatic scenarios resulting in both a redefinition of the classic mantra of spatial cooperation between modalities and considering whether RT may be a vaccine or primer for novel immunotherapy agents such as checkpoint inhibitors, (d) combination with classic cytotoxic-based chemotherapy, (e) difficulty in assessing late effects, and (f) the low prioritization from the drug development industry. As a consequence of this latter reality, there is a prolong delay (median 6 years, interquartile range 5 to 8 years) between the opening of the phase I trial without RT

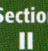

and the opening of the phase I with RT.[113] In addition, the median lag time P between the *published* phase I trial without RT and the *opening* phase I with RT was 3 years (interquartile range of 1 to 6 years).

An important consideration is to be cost-efficient in the design of the trial, as the PI should seek to minimize the number of patients exposed to an ineffective treatment by enrolling as few patients as "necessary" to show benefit or failure.

One of the most important design decisions is to determine if a single-arm study will suffice or whether a multiarm trial is preferable. The latter may be required if the historical data for comparison are lacking or considered generally weak. Single-arm studies may include a two-stage design with early stopping rules for futility or lack of response. The most common single-arm trial designs are the Simon two-stage,[51] the balanced design,[114] Gehan two-stage,[115] and the Fleming two-stage.[116] These are considered frequentist approaches (as opposed to Bayesian designs). A multiarm phase 2 trial may include a (a) phase 2 selection design (prioritization) or (b) phase 2 design with a reference control am (control). The former involves parallel single-arm studies that do not directly compare the arms to each other. They compare each to the "null rate." The Simon "pick-the-winner" design is an example.[16] This approach is useful when there are more than one candidate new drugs, new schedules, new doses, or even combinations of different drugs, schedules, and doses to be evaluated. It is not powered to directly compare the treatment efficacies, and hence, the number of patients needed to complete the study is smaller. On the other hand, a randomized phase 2 design with a reference control arm directly compares the new treatment with the control treatment. The randomization is effective to remove potential bias that is often unavoidable in single-arm trials where treatment effect of the new treatment (represented by efficacy end points, e.g., local control, response rate, colostomy-free survival, nodal failure, etc.) is indirectly compared with the historical controls. The comparison is indirect in that the point estimate from historical controls is often treated as the null hypothesis in the single-arm trials. Therefore, the uncertainty associated with the estimate is neglected in the testing. As a consequence, the single-arm trials often require one-third or smaller a sample size compared to randomized two-arm trials with the same hypothesis to be tested. As a trade-off, the findings in the single-arm trial are often much unreliable compared with randomized trials.[117]

Phase 2 studies may often include patients for whom RT is a standard and definitive therapy. In these instances, the savvy radiation oncology investigator has an opportunity to carefully define goals, strategic diagnostic, and/or therapeutic interventions, to achieve a well-defined and clinically meaningful end point for the patient's benefit. Adaptive designs are becoming more common in cancer medicine, including radiation oncology–based trials (Bhatt). For instance, the definition of response rate is important to consider. There are emerging data to suggest that a well-defined, *a priori* change in metabolic response rate via functional imaging assessment with FDG-PET (positron emission tomography) may harbor useful imaging biomarkers of tumor response or resistance much earlier than classic pure anatomic imaging using conventional CT scanning.[118–120] Adaptive trials will need to incorporate serial data inputs, including though not limited to imaging, -omic (genomic and proteomic), and anatomic changes during treatment in order to enhance response and get ahead of the tendency of tumors to develop radioresistant phenotypes (Fig. 15.5).

In order to exploit the promise of precision medicine, alternative phase 2 designs have emerged in the form of umbrella and basket trials.[121] The umbrella trial is set up to test one type of cancer (i.e., lung), which may harbor multiple mutations, some of which may be actionable with various therapeutic interventions. The basket trial can include patients with multiple anatomic types of cancer though each tumor must harbor a common genetic mutation for which the same candidate therapy is tested.

End Points

Response rates alone may be challenging for selecting efficacious regimens, because of several factors including (a) delayed time to response with RT, (b) residual unevaluable masses versus scarring or fibrosis, (c) progressive disease outside of the RT field, and/or (d) underlying high local response rates to RT.

Response rate is commonly measured by the RECIST and sometimes the PRECIST (Positron Emission Tomography

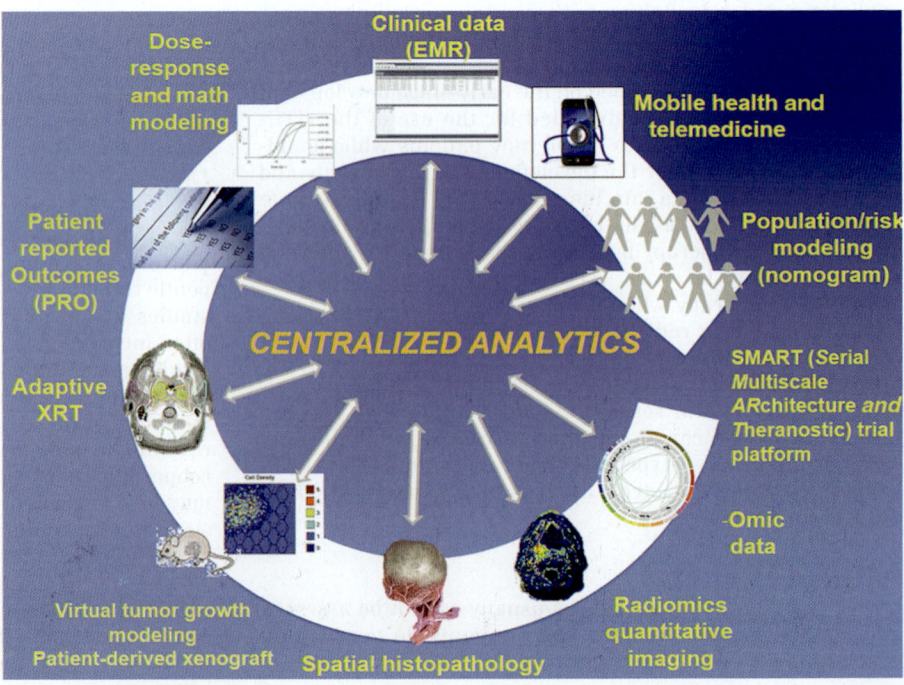

FIGURE 15.5. Centralized analytics allows for phenotyping using all patient and tumor-specific data.

Response Criteria in Solid Tumors) criteria. A CR plus a PR is added together to determine the overall objective response rate. If patients whose best response is SD or no change, that may also be important because many of the targeted agents (sometimes called cytostatic agents) inactivate a driver tumor target though no objective shrinkage of tumor may be noted by conventional imaging.

Efficacy end points commonly used include (a) CR rate, (b) pathologic CR rate based on examination of tissue, (c) undetectable blood biomarkers such as circulating tumor DNA and/or circulating tumor cells, (d) local or locoregional control rates, (e) time to progression, (f) survival, and/or (g) a decrease in toxicity. In the instance of the latter end point of decreased toxicity, RTOG 0529 is a good example of a clinical trial that was primarily designed to show that the way that RT was delivered (i.e., IMRT) may yield a preferable therapeutic window compared to historical experience for invasive anal cancer.[122,123] The end point selected will depend upon the tumor and the current standard therapy.

Robust documentation of both acute and late toxicities is essential. In particular, collection of late toxicity data will be helpful as the phase III study is designed. This should involve provider assessment via the usual tools such as the next-generation CTC profile, as well as validated patient-related outcome (PRO) tools. There are emerging data that the concordance of AE documentation between patients and providers on cancer cooperative group setting could even improve overall survival.[174]

Summary

Phase II trials are designed to generate a signal of antitumor activity and to inform the phase III decision. The ideal phase II trial uses a good PK/PD drug against a validated disease target and shows convincing antitumor activity. Results of phase II trials must be interpreted cautiously, in the context of the availability of other therapies. It does, however, estimate clinical activity and provide further safety information, which is important in the "go/no-go" decision for a phase III trial. A phase II randomized trial is still considered exploratory and does not obviate the need for a larger more definitive phase III trial. Adaptive designs can be very efficient for selection, but require more maintenance.

Phase 3 Trials

These trials usually involve two or more arms, including one that is considered a standard of care. The goal is to show superiority of a new therapeutic approach, such as the addition of postoperative (adjuvant) chemoradiotherapy for resected gastric cancer[125] or perhaps to demonstrate noninferiority, the latter which can lead to a more cost-effective treatment approach, such as hypofractionated radiotherapy for breast cancer.[126] The essential components to consider for phase III trials are study design, randomization approach, blinding strategy, and monitoring of end points. The CONSORT 2010 checklist (www.consort-statement.org) summarizes information that must be considered when analyzing phase III trial reports.[127]

Design

The design is randomized in most phase III trials, and the patients enrolled should all have the disease to be studied as well as comparable pretreatment characteristics. A *parallel* design involves randomization to a standard (or control) intervention versus an experimental (new) intervention. The experimental intervention may include ≥1 arm, such that the variable between the experimental arms may be the number of radiation fractions and/or fraction size, with a theoretically equal BED. *Factorial* designs, such as utilized in the ACT II anal cancer trial, allow for more multiple intervention vari-

ables to be compared to a single gold standard or control.[128] Crossover designs allow for patients randomized to arm A to undergo crossover therapy to arm B after the efficacy end point of arm A has been measured. This occurs when the efficacy end point is PFS.[129]

Randomization

This is a process that provides each patient an equal chance of being assigned to an intervention arm or a control arm, unless it has been predetermined that an unequal randomization allocation (i.e., 2:1) is warranted to enhance accrual. Ideally, the patient and the PI should not influence or be aware of which arm the former will be randomized to prior the decision has been made to provide informed consent to participate in the study. This requires equipoise on the part of the investigator, an area of active controversy among the radiation oncology community when deciding how to study new and expensive technology, such as particle therapy. *The following section on Statistical Issues will provide a more in-depth discussion on randomization and blinding considerations in clinical trials.*

Superiority, Noninferiority, and Equivalence Designs

A superiority design is fairly common and seeks to show that a new radiation approach (i.e., higher dose of radiotherapy) is superior to that standard of care, such as was tested in RTOG-0123.[130]

A noninferiority design is often used to show that a less aggressive (or potentially toxic) approach (i.e., lower dose of radiotherapy or less intense systemic therapy) is not worse to a clinically meaningful degree compared to the standard intervention. The difference or delta (Δ) in the *a priori* defined end point should only be slightly worse (or inferior) to the standard. Confidence intervals estimate the difference in outcome between the control and experimental arms as an approach to confirm the hypothesis. Sample sizes of noninferiority trials are often bigger than superiority trials.[131] Several studies have been *a priori* designed and reported on for localized prostate cancer,[132] resectable rectal cancer,[133] and brain metastases.[134] Some trials combine noninferiority and superiority testing into one study. This is because the noninferiority and superiority can both be evaluated at 0.05 significance level without a need to adjust for multiple testing because of the closed testing principle.[131] Two things need to be paid attention to when conducting such combination testings: (a) the study needs to be powered for noninferiority and (b) the noninferiority needs to be tested before testing for the superiority.

An equivalence design seeks to show that the control and the experimental arm(s) are equal with respect to the primary outcome. Equivalence can be defined as the treatment effect residing between −delta (−Δ) and delta (Δ) (two-sided problem). This design *is not* the same as a noninferiority design. RTOG 9704 was a phase III trial that sought to show that by excluding mitomycin C (an antitumor antibiotic with a well-known profile of significant hematologic and renal toxicity) from a backbone of fluorinated pyrimidine chemotherapy (5-fluorouracil) and external beam radiotherapy for anal canal cancer, the therapeutic outcomes would remain equal, whereas the therapeutic ratio would be increased by lessening the toxicity.[135] This study showed that the doublet, including mitomycin C, was actually superior. It is problematic to routinely relay on null hypothesis testing of equality if statistical significance of the *a priori* differences is not met.

Quality Assurance/Contouring

In the era of highly conformal radiation treatment, safe and effective treatment planning depends increasingly on precisely identifying tumor and normal tissues through contour delineation, with evidence from clinical trials emerging that correlates poor contouring with inferior outcomes. In head and neck cancer, both TROG 02.02 and RTOG 0129 found a 20% decrease in overall survival for patients with radiation protocol violations.[136,137] Similar trends have been identified in pancreatic cancer and Hodgkin lymphoma.[28,138] Although multiple aspects of the radiation planning process can lead to protocol violations,[139,140] between 13% and 83% of protocol violations have been attributed to contouring.[28,136,138,141] In response, an increasing emphasis is being placed on trial QA programs that actively perform contour evaluation and train providers.

First, development of a visual atlas for anorectal cancer was shown to reduce contour variation[142] and improve predicted toxicity[143] among providers that intended to enroll patients on a SWOG-sponsored study (SWOG S0713). This atlas was initially developed for RTOG 0529 in response to the observation from the first five cases submitted with coverage of the mesorectum and elective nodes.[122] Visual atlases have been duplicated in contouring studies performed outside of the clinical trial setting for disease sites that have a well-defined high-risk clinical target volume such as prostate fossa[144] and nasopharyngeal cancer.[144] However, RTOG 1106 recently reported that development of a visual atlas for lung cancer, which relies primarily on identification of gross tumor, did not reduce variation in contours submitted through its trial QA credentialing process.[145]

Given the limitations of a visual atlas, disease sites such as lung cancer have been moving toward prospective centralized contour review prior to patient treatment. However, the administrative burden and potential for treatment delays warrant consideration by the QA committee when determining feasibility of their contouring QA program. Multiple trials show that radiation protocol deviations are more frequent among low-accruing treatment centers,[136–139,146] so perhaps a risk-stratified approach should be considered. It is important to keep in mind that the more strict the trial QA, the less generalizable the results may be to routine practice. Instead, development of robust resources and training processes that could be implemented and easy to use in routine practice would be ideal.

STATISTICAL ISSUES IN TRADITIONAL CLINICAL TRIAL DESIGN

Patient Population and Subject Eligibility

Defining patient population is an essential step in the design of clinical trial. The inclusion and exclusion criteria of subject should be carefully defined and specified for any clinical trial before study initiation. Several aspects need to be considered when defining the subject eligibility of enrollment to specific trials: (a) generalizability, (b) feasibility, (c) competing risks, (d) projected AEs, and (e) homogeneity. The patient inclusion and exclusion criteria of a trial should be the result of a nice balancing of all the above five aspects.

Generalizability and Feasibility

To begin with, investigators should first think about the targeting patient population to which the new treatment will be adopted. Ideally, a phase III clinical trial should relax the exclusion criteria as much as possible to mirror the target patient population. Less restricted eligibility criteria will make the findings in the trial more generalizable to the targeting population. In addition, relatively relaxed inclusion criteria are likely to lead to quicker accrual and make the study treatment more available to a broader patient population who may benefit from it.

Adverse Events, Competing Risks, and Homogeneity

Although inclusive eligibility criteria will boost the generalizability and feasibility, it can be risky and harmful to include subjects who should be excluded. For instance, if subjects with HIV/AIDs are suspected to have exceptional high risk of experiencing treatment-related toxicity in a pancreatic cancer trial, they should better be excluded. Otherwise, not only the subgroup of patients are exposed to high risk of toxicity, including them may put the whole trial to the risk of closure for excessive toxicity. Even if the trial continued as planned, these subjects are likely to add complexity to the efficacy and toxicity analysis of the trial.

Another thing to keep in mind is the competing risk. For example, if a trial is to evaluate the response rate after six cycles of radiation therapy, then including subjects with high risk of dying before completing the six cycles is undesired. In this example, the competing risk is death of cancer or other disease before treatment completion or before the primary end point becomes available.

The last thing to aware is the homogeneity of subjects as defined in the eligibility criteria. Exclusive eligibility criteria often help to pick more homogeneous subjects, which could add power in detecting a true treatment effect if the certain type of subjects as defined in the eligibility criteria has a good response to the treatment. However, as we discussed previously, findings of a trial with exclusive eligibility criteria lack generalizability, and exclusive eligibility criteria may also jeopardize the speed of accrual. Therefore, it is typically acceptable to have more exclusive eligibility criteria in phase I and phase II trials, but the criteria should be relaxed to be more inclusive in phase III trials. A relatively heterogeneous patient population in a phase III trial will also allow the detection of efficacy difference in subgroups of subjects, which is an added bonus of having inclusive eligibility criteria in a clinical trial with relatively large sample size.

Historically, there are not much guidelines to follow for determining the inclusion and exclusion criteria of a clinical trial. Starting August 2016, ASCO and Friends of Cancer Research (Friends) had a joint effort to form four working groups to develop consensus recommendations on clinical trial eligibility criteria that are both scientifically and clinically appropriate.

Randomization

Randomization is an effective way to assign patients to treatment groups without systematic imbalances in important factors and patient characteristics. A well-designed and implemented randomized trial is often viewed as the "gold standard" for evaluating an experimental treatment when compared with either placebo or standard treatment.

In this section, we introduce a few randomization schemes that are most well-known or widely used for implementing random treatment assignments.

Simple Randomization

Considering a randomized controlled study where subjects are to be 1:1 assigned to either an experimental treatment or a control group, the simple randomization is no different from flipping a fair coin and assigning subjects to the experimental group if "head" and to the control group if "tail." Although, in theory, the assignment can be quite balanced in treatment assignment and in patient characteristics between groups on average; very few trials choose to use simple randomization in practice. This is because reasonable balance can only be achieved using simple randomization if the sample size is large. However, large clinical trials often are multisite and have interim analyses. A multisite trial typically requires stratified randomization by site, and interim analyses require balance in assignment be achieved with relatively smaller sample size.

Permuted Block Randomization

One easy way to address the unbalanced group size at interim analysis or at other time points during the trial is to use permuted block randomization (PBR), which imposes a balance restriction by blocks. The size of the block can be a prefixed or be selected at random. If we again consider a 1:1 randomized controlled trial, implementing PBR with block size of 4 will ensure balance in group size for every four subjects. That means for every four subjects, two must be assigned to the experimental group (E) and two must be assigned to the control group (C). We can easily permute the potential sequences for assignment of two treatments for block size of 4: EECC, CCEE, CECE, ECEC, CEEC, and ECCE. The same can be done essentially for any block size. Common choices of the block size are 2, 4, 6, and 8. We may randomly pick one of the generated sequences for any block if using PBR with fixed block size. For using PBR with random block size, one additional random pick needs to be made before starting any block: Randomly pick the block size for the coming block from all available choices, say 2, 4, or 6. Once the size of coming block is determined, we can use the same procedure as PBR to implement the randomization.

We discourage using a block size of 2 for PBR with fixed block size because that adds too much restriction on randomization. We also discourage using a block size of 8 or more for any PBR as the imbalance can still be substantial with larger block sizes. A well-known and criticized drawback of PBR with fixed block size is that it may hinder blinding. With relatively small block size, there is a good chance for physicians or researchers to figure out who are assigned to which treatment although they should be blinded of such assignment. Therefore, we suggest using PBR with random block size over PBR with fixed block size whenever appropriate and necessary.

Stratified Randomization and Covariate-Adaptive Randomization

Achieving balance in the number of subjects assigned to each arm throughout the duration of the trial is often not sufficient for most randomized clinical trials in oncology. It is also important to ensure balancing on known covariates that may affect outcomes. If the covariates to be balanced are all categorical variables and the number of covariates is less than 3, stratified randomization is often appropriate for achieving balance in covariates. The idea of stratified randomization is simple: We first create different strata based on the covariates to be stratified and then conduct PRB or simple randomization within each stratum. The number of strata is jointly determined by the number of stratifying covariates and the levels of each covariate. For k stratifying covariates with levels of each covariate denoted by $l_1, l_2, ..., l_k$, the number of strata is $l_1 \times l_2 \times \cdots \times l_k$. For example, if a randomized trial has two stratifying covariates, site (three participating sites) and type of cancer (breast and prostate cancer), then the number of strata is 6. The number of strata increases quickly with more stratifying covariates. Once the number of subjects in each stratum becomes too small, there is an increased chance of imbalanced assignment within each stratum, which influences the balance of the whole trial. Therefore, when the number of stratifying factors exceeds 3, or if one or more continuous covariates are to be balanced, we suggest using covariate-adaptive randomization, also called minimization. The covariate-adaptive randomization assigns treatment to a new subject for minimizing the covariate imbalances within treatment groups. There are multiple ways of doing so, such as Zelen's rule, the Pocock-Simon procedure, and Wei's marginal urn design.[147]

Response-Adaptive Randomization

Most adaptive clinical trials that use Bayesian design adopt response-adaptive randomization, which has a changing probability of assigning a new patient to treatments based on the observed data from previously treated patients in the trial. The response-adaptive randomization allows more subjects be assigned to the more promising treatment arm and thus is viewed as a more ethical design. The response-adaptive randomization is preferred for many trials, but not all, because it typically requires an added complexity in designing, implementing, and analyzing the trial and often has slightly reduced power in detecting treatment difference for a fixed sample size.

Statistical Power and Sample Size

All clinical trials require the computation and justification of sample size, because the number of subjects evaluated in the trial is a key factor that determines the quality of scientific findings in the study. A clinical trial with too small a sample size fails to yield meaningful scientific results, whereas a trial with too large a sample size will waste resources in finding a result and may expose more subjects than necessary to inferior treatment.

We need to know the design of a clinical trial and the variable type of the primary end point before doing sample size computation. In general, if a hypothesis testing is going to be conducted, we should specify the desired power, the null and the alternative hypothesis, the statistical test procedure to be conducted, and the type I error rate. The type I error is the probability of rejecting the null hypothesis when the null hypothesis is true. In other words, it is the chance of claiming a new drug is effective although it actually is not. As type I error can be a very serious error for all clinical trials, it is typically controlled at a low rate (α) of 0.05 or less. Another error we take into consideration when computing sample size is the type II error, the probability of not rejecting the null hypothesis when the alternative hypothesis is true. It can be viewed as the chance of incorrectly determining a therapy is not effective although it actually is. Although type II error is also critical, it is often not as serious error as the type I error. Therefore, it is acceptable for a trial to have 20% or less type II error rate (β). The power is simply $1 - \beta$. Therefore, clinical trials are typically designed to have 80% or more power.

For some early-phase pilot studies, the major goal may not be to determine whether a treatment is effective or not but to gain preliminary information on the level of effectiveness for planning future studies. For such a trial, it makes sense to plan the sample size based on the precision of a confidence interval. The precision of an estimate is directly based on the width of a confidence limit. The smaller the width, the narrower is the confidence interval, and the better precision is the estimate. For example, if we want to gain preliminary information on the 6-month objective response rate for a new radiation therapy in a single-arm phase II pilot trial, and we believe a 95% confidence limit ±0.15 is narrow enough no matter what the estimated response rate locates, we can then propose a sample size of 47 evaluable subjects to ensure the computed width of confidence interval is within 0.3.

Figure 15.6 shows the relationship between width of confidence limit, sample size, and the estimated proportion computed using Clopper-Pearson exact method (produced by Power Analysis and Sample size Software, 2017, NCSS, LLC, Kaysville, Utah, USA, http://ucss.com/software/pass). We can tell the width of confidence limit monotonically gets smaller as the sample size increases, and the width of confidence is also influenced by the point estimate of the response rate. The width is always the widest at point estimate of 0.5 and gets narrower as the point estimate moves away from 0.5 in either direction.

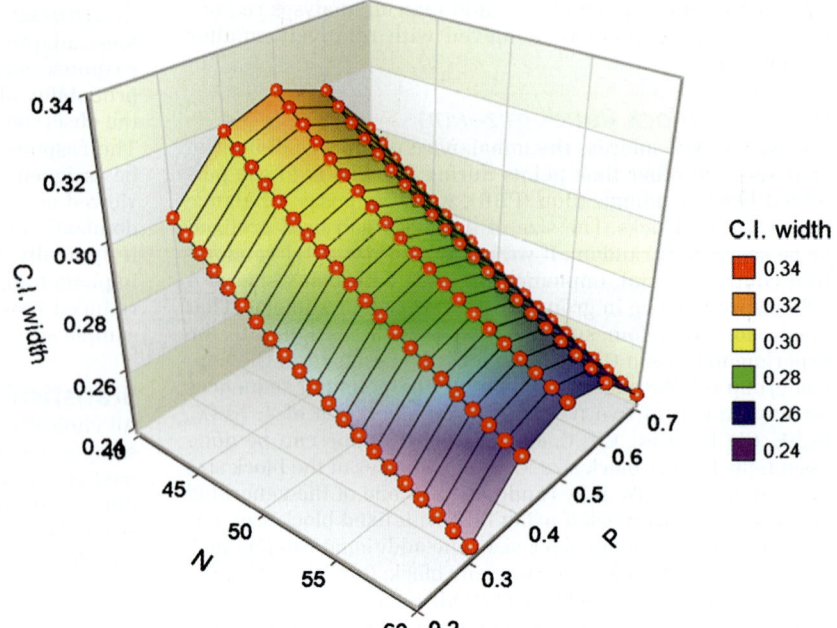

FIGURE 15.6. Relationship between width of confidence limit, sample size, and the estimated proportion.

We should keep in mind that the proposed sample size of enrollment in a clinical trial typically is larger than the computed sample size, because it is likely for patients to either drop off or become invaluable after enrollment. The proposed sample size should be inflated accordingly to make sure the final evaluable sample size has adequate power.

Although most trials require a predetermined fixed sample size at the design stage, some allows flexible total sample size depending on the findings during the trial. For example, the well-known 3 + 3 design, continual reassessment design, and Simon's two-stage design all allow flexible total sample size. Any clinical trials with interim looks and associated stopping rules allow flexible total sample size. However, the procedures of determining the sample size based on findings in the trial and the potential range of the trial need to be specified clearly in the protocol at the design stage.

Interim Analysis and Stopping Rules

Most phase III clinical trials and some phase II trials are designed to have interim analyses that allow the trial to be stopped early based on the findings in the interim analysis. A major purpose of a stopping rule is to protect patients from unsafe and/or ineffective drug. Many trials with interim analysis only allow early stopping because of evidence of futility or excessive toxicity. For example, the famous Simon's two-stage design only stops the trial for futility. In the design, n_1 subjects are enrolled to stage 1. If only r_1 or fewer subjects had successes, the trial will be stopped early. Otherwise, it will continue to enroll another n_2 subject. The final analysis is based on all $n_1 + n_2$ subjects. In general, the decision on whether to stop early for futility is predetermined based on the conditional power, the conditional probability of having statistically significant result if the trial continues to the end given the accumulated data in the interim analysis.[148] If such a probability is very low, lower than a preset threshold, then the trial may be terminated early because of futility.

Many other trials with interim looks allow early stopping for clear evidence in efficacy of the treatment. For such trials, it is extremely important to make sure the overall type I error rate is not inflated by the interim looks. For example, the well-known Pocock group sequential design[149] and the O'Brien-Fleming group sequential design proposed stopping boundaries for interim looks with appropriate α spending functions.[54] The Pocock design makes the interim looks equally spaced and requires the same level of evidence (i.e., using the same z, the boundary of rejection for the test statistic) for early and late interim looks. These requirements can be too restricted. Therefore, O'Brien and Fleming proposed a group sequential design that makes it harder to stop in early interim looks by letting the boundaries of early stopping decrease with the number of looks being conducted before the interim look.

Many other sequential or group sequential designs have been proposed and implemented. The key requirements for such trials are as follows: (a) the end point for interim analysis is relatively quick to evaluate. It is not desirable to use an end point that requires longtime follow-up (e.g., 10-year overall survival), because the trial will be halted for each interim look. (b) The number of interim looks, when to take the looks, and under which condition the trial will be stopped early should all be clearly specified in the protocol before the initiation of the trial. (c) An appropriate spending function is used to control for the overall type I error rate.

In general, unplanned interim looks are not allowed for any clinical trials. The exception is that when the unplanned interim look is proposed by data safety monitoring board for protecting patients. In such situation, stopping boundaries can be constructed and modified for the added looks.[150]

Many sequential and group sequential clinical trials are designed using Bayesian methods. Unlike the frequentist methods that completely rely on the data in the current trial to make inferences and decisions, Bayesian methods incorporate outside information (e.g., published similar studies, pilot data, expert's opinion, etc.) into the procedure. A Bayesian method typically starts with specifying a prior distribution for the parameters of interest and updates the distributions using data from the trial. The updated distribution is called the posterior distribution, and the updates can be applied as many times as necessary in theory. The stopping rule of a Bayesian group sequential design is based on the posterior probability of efficacy or futility, which is computed combing the prior and the current data of the trial.

SURVIVAL ANALYSIS AND CATEGORICAL DATA ANALYSIS

Many oncology clinical trials include overall survival or time to PFS as primary or secondary end points. Such end points are called time-to-event end points, and statistical analysis for time-to-event end points is called survival analysis. Patients are followed sufficiently long so that a subset of subjects will experience the event of interest during the trial. The event of interest is death for overall survival and is progression or death for time to PFS.

Without loss of generalizability, we use overall survival as the event of interest from now on. The method is exactly the same for all other time-to-event end points.

The survival end point is actually a combination of two measures: (a) a binary variable indicating whether the subject died by the end of the study or at the last follow-up of the subject and (b) a continuous variable measuring time from a common starting point (e.g., the initiation of a treatment or at the time of randomization) to death if the subject has died. For those subjects who are still alive by their last follow-up time, the component of the survival time is not known and is thus treated as missing. Noticed that the information is only partially missing for these subjects because we do know they were still alive by the time of their last follow-up. A special terminology is used in survival analysis for such partial missingness—censored.

For most survival data, the first step is to use Kaplan-Meier estimate to describe the distribution of survival time.[151] The Kaplan-Meier method utilizes the information of all subjects, including those who had observed death and those who censored, to describe the cumulative survival over time, which is the product of survival ratio of the number of subject still alive to those who are at risk.

Let us illustrate the computation and the plot of Kaplan-Meier curve using a simple example.

Suppose that we have 20 patients randomized to 2 arms. The observed survival time for subjects in each arm is as follows:

A: 8+, 11+, 16+, 18+, 23, 24, 26, 28, 30, 31.
B: 9, 13, 13, 14, 14, 16, 19+, 22+, 23+, 29+.

The unit was in month, and "+" indicates a censored observation.

Figure 15.7 shows the plot of the Kaplan-Meier curve.

Using arm A as example, we show step by step how the Kaplan-Meier curve was determined. Before plotting, the data should be sorted from low to high, regardless of whether the subject is censored or not. The Kaplan-Meier plot is a step function with steps formulated at one of more observed death. Starting at baseline, all 10 patients are alive, so the initial ratio of subject still alive to those who are at risk is 1 (=10/10). This is also the cumulative survival at baseline. At 8 months, one subject had censored, so the ratio of subject still alive to those at risk remains the same 1 (=9/9). As the baseline cumulative survival is 1, the cumulative survival at 8 months is still 1 (=1*1). Afterward, 3 more subjects are censored, which did not change the ratio, whereas the number of subjects at risk dropped to 6. The fifth subject died at 23 months. This makes the ratio dropped to 0.83 (=5/6). The cumulative survival at 23 months is still 0.83, because the cumulative survival at 18 months (the previous time point) is 1; thus, 0.83*1 = 0.83. The ratio was further dropped to 0.8 (=4/5) at 24th month, making the cumulative survival to be 0.664 (=0.8*0.83). The seventh subject died at month 26, with the computed ratio being 0.75 (=3/4) and the cumulative survival being 0.498 (=0.75*0.664). The ratio for the last subject at 31 months was 0 (=0/1), making the cumulative survival to become 0 as well. For a Kaplan-Meier plot, the cumulative survival is always 0 if the last subject is an observed death, as shown in the plot for arm A. Otherwise, if the last subject is censored, the Kaplan-Meier plot is flat with a positive cumulative survival, as seen in the plot for arm B.

The Kaplan-Meier plot can be used to compute the median survival time, a common statistic of interest showing the estimated time that half of the patients will have died. Again, using the arm A plot as example, the median survival is month 26, when the cumulative survival first fell under 0.5. The median survival time is often reported with a confidence interval because this is an estimate. We omit the computation of the confidence interval here because of limited space. The median survival time and its associated confidence interval typically can be computed by almost all software for survival analysis.

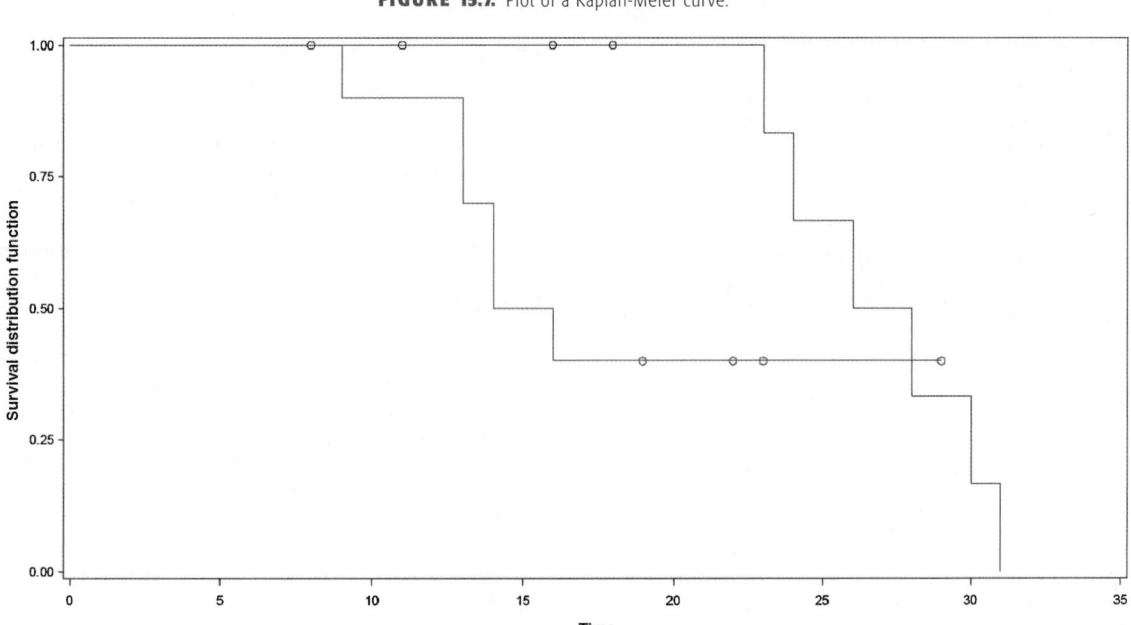

FIGURE 15.7. Plot of a Kaplan-Meier curve.

STRATA: —— treatment=A   ○ ○ ○ Censored treatment=A   —— treatment=B   ○ ○ ○ Censored treatment=B

However, sometimes, the median survival is not estimable. This is because the Kaplan-Meier curve never fell below 0.5 for the study or for the particular arm under evaluation.

As the observed survival data rely a lot on the length of follow-up, it is important for any clinical trial with survival analysis to report the follow-up time.

The Kaplan-Meier plot is often accompanied by a log-rank test, a nonparametric test for comparing the survival distribution in two treatment groups. A significant log-rank test suggests the survival distribution in the Kaplan-Meier plot differs significantly for the two treatment arms.

The log-rank test only compares the survival distribution of the two arms without considering and controlling the effect of other influential factors, potential confounder, and effect modifiers. In order to control for those covariates, a Cox regression model is typically used to estimate the HR of the two treatments. In survival analysis, the hazard rate is the instantaneous risk of death at a given time and can be thought of loosely as the probability of death at time t given that the patient is alive just before time (t^2). The Cox regression model is also called proportional hazards model because it assumes the HR for two specified strata are constant over time.

Another type of end points often seen in oncology clinical trial is the categorical end points, such as tumor response. The first thing to describe for categorical end points is the response rate and the associated confidence interval in each arm if this is a randomized trial. Pearson's chi-square test is the most often used test to evaluate the difference in response rate for two treatments without controlling for other factors. When the sample size is small, P values from Fisher's exact test are often reported instead. Logistic regression model is the most common choice for comparing treatment effects using statistical modeling. It provides estimation to the odds ratio of treatment after controlling for important covariates other than the treatment.

In addition to traditional statistical modeling, machine learning methods can also be used to analyze survival end point and categorical end points.

PRACTICAL ISSUES IN THE DESIGN, EXECUTION, AND REPORTING OF CLINICAL TRIALS

The Institutional Review Board

Several different groups share responsibility for the monitoring and oversight of ethical and safety issues in clinical trials. According to U.S. Federal Regulations, the role of the IRB is primarily to ensure that "risks to subjects are minimized" and "risks to subjects are reasonable in relation to anticipated benefits."[90] This involves review of the study protocol, informed consent document, background information, and proposed research plan.

Data and Safety Monitoring Committees

Once trials are initiated, ongoing monitoring of accumulating data regarding safety, effectiveness, and trial conduct is required. In the late 1960s, federal agencies (such as the National Institutes of Health and the Department of Veterans Affairs in the United States) began to mandate an *external* review by a DSMC, because investigators may not be fully objective in their interim data analysis. Meanwhile, industry-sponsored trials have been slower to incorporate this practice.[81] However, not all trials warrant the cost of a DSMC, including trials of short duration or those that have end points such as relief of symptoms (rather than survival or severe toxicity). For this reason, the IRB review serves to inquire about the safety monitoring plan and can request establishment of a DMSC, if warranted because of perceived potential risk to patients.

Conflict of Interest

Industry sponsorship of clinical trials in oncology has increased over the past 2 decades. Compared to the pharmaceutical industry, radiation oncology is limited to a small number of equipment vendors. Nonetheless, one study found that among clinical trials led by radiation oncologists and reporting conflicts of interest, over half of COI was related to industry sponsorship.[152] A literature review of COI in radiation therapy trials for breast cancer from 2004 to 2014 found that 13% of studies reported funding from profit organizations, whereas an additional 49% of trials were supported by not-for-profit organizations.[153] They found that funded trials and those with a positive conclusion were more likely to be published in journals with a higher impact factor, but the presence of COI did not influence study conclusions. In a randomized survey of internal medicine physicians, the perceived impact of trial results from industry-sponsored studies was lower than that from NIH-sponsored studies.[154] Nonetheless, any financial support should be reported given the potential for conflicts of interest to arise.

Role of Cooperative Groups

Clinical trials are truly only ethical if the foreseeable risks outweigh the benefits. It is considered unethical to launch a trial if it is unlikely to enroll enough patients to ensure statistically significant results. This has led to the initiation of trials by multicenter cooperative groups, such as the European Organisation for Research and Treatment of Cancer (EORTC), and more recently the combination of the National Surgical Adjuvant Breast and Bowel Project (NSABP), Radiation Therapy Oncology Group (RTOG), and Gynecologic Oncology Group (GOG) into the NRG. Meanwhile, the Human Health Division of the International Atomic Energy Agency (IAEA) supports coordinated research activities (CRAs) between their member states, which aims to support well-designed trials that maximize impact.[155] Important randomized trials have been conducted under the auspices of the IAEA including the evaluation of the safety and efficacy of hypofractionated radiation in elderly patients with GBM[156] and brachytherapy boost in nasopharyngeal cancer.[157] One ongoing IAEA trial randomizes patients to SBRT versus transarterial chemoembolization (TACE) for hepatocellular carcinoma, with practical components of trial design that include training on treatment techniques and use of novel QA phantoms in credentialing processes.[89]

Register on ClinicalTrials.gov

Maintained by the National Institutes of Health, ClinicalTrials.gov serves to inform researchers, physicians, and patients of ongoing and completed clinical trials both in the United States and around the world. The Web site was created as part of the Food and Drug Administration Modernization Act of 1997, which mandated that both federally and privately funded trials conducted under investigational new drug applications be registered in a publicly accessible platform. Although requirements for registration were expanded in 2007, still many clinical trials do not require registration, though it is strongly encouraged to improve transparency. As of April 2017, ClinicalTrials.gov reported 41,919 registered trials, of which 56% represented exclusively non-US trials from 197 countries. The trial sponsor or PI is responsible for registering trials at ClinicalTrials.gov at study initiation, as well as providing timely updates and submitting summary results.

Consolidated Standards of Reporting Trials (CONSORT)

By the early 1990s, medical journal editors and clinical trialists identified a need for a scale to assess the quality of

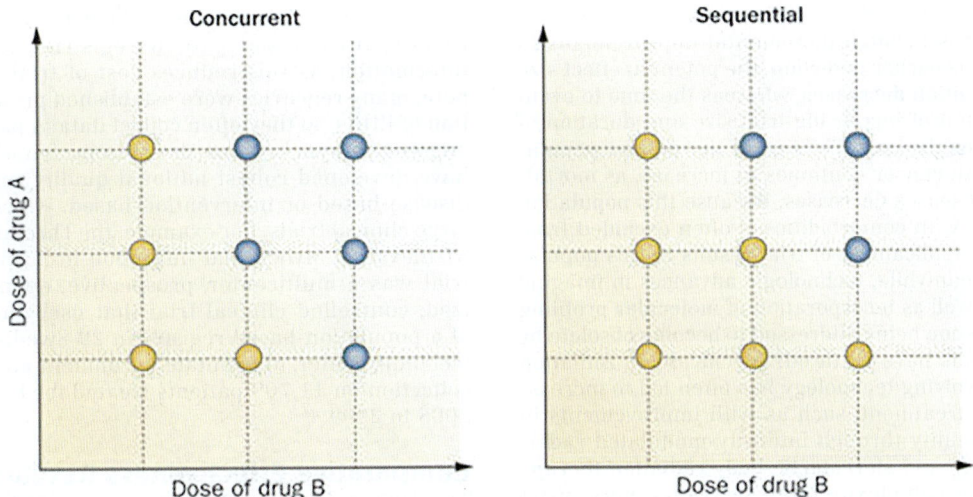

FIGURE 15.8. Different schedules of two drugs given concurrently or sequentially. (Reprinted by permission from Nature: Berry DA. Adaptive clinical trials in oncology. *Nat Rev Clin Oncol* 2011;9[4]:199–207. Copyright © 2011 Springer Nature.)

randomized controlled trials. Groups of these experts meeting separately in Canada and the United States created the SORT and Asilomar reports, respectively, which merged in 1996 into a single, coherent, evidence-based recommendation known as the CONSORT Statement (http://www. consort-statement.org/). Most notably, this guideline statement includes both a checklist and flow diagram (Figure: http://www.consort-statement.org/consort-statement/flow-diagram) to enable readers to understand a trial's design, conduct, and analysis and to encourage adherence and transparency by authors.[158]

NOVEL APPROACHES TO CLINICAL TRIAL DESIGN

Seamless Phase I to II Trial

As have been discussed thus far, typically, phase I trials evaluate toxicity and phase II efficacy. However, seamless phase I/II trials—or trials that achieve the goals of both phases I and II in one umbrella protocol—have been developed to address both of these questions.[22] In these two-stage designs, information from the initial phase I study is incorporated into the phase II study. Different variations on this have been developed. Figure 15.8 from the manuscript by Berry et al.[159] shows the concept behind a seamless phase I/II trial using two drugs, A and B, given either concurrently or sequentially in one of the 10 dose combinations indicated by the yellow dots.

This adaptive randomization takes into account the toxicity and efficacy of these combinations.

Another Bayesian adaptive phase I to II clinical trial has been designed for evaluating efficacy and toxicity with delayed outcomes,[160] which, as previously discussed, is crucial in radiotherapy trials. This approach evaluates both efficacy and toxicity as binary outcomes, both as time-to-event models. The authors' simulations showed that this method significantly reduces the study duration.

Pan et al.[161] propose a phase I/II seamless dose escalation/ expansion with adaptive randomization scheme (SEARS). There are three critical components to this model: First, it applies the modified toxicity probability interval (mTPI) method as a way of monitoring toxicity. Then, in the phase II portion, it adaptively randomizes, based on efficacy, patients to any doses showing promising efficacy and safety. Posterior probabilities are calculated using both the phase I and II information (Fig. 15.9 from Pan et al.[161]).

REDEFINING THE APPROACH TO CLINICAL TRIALS

The randomized phase III clinical trial is considered the most robust method of comparing the efficacy of a new treatment with the standard of care. Grading systems for evaluating clinical evidence universally place RCTs above observational trials. However, multiple features of modern medicine

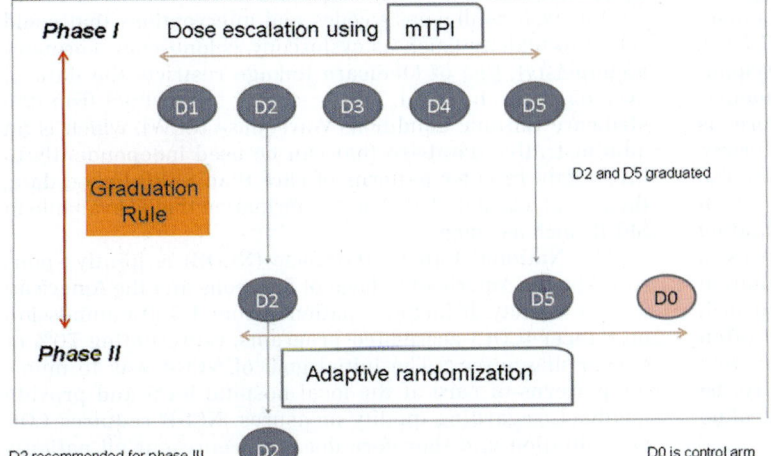

FIGURE 15.9. Phase I/II SEARS. (Reprinted by permission from Pan H, Xie F, Liu P, et al. A phase I/II seamless dose escalation/ expansion with adaptive randomization scheme (SEARS). *Clin Trials* 2014;11[1]:49–59. Copyright © 2014 SAGE Publications.)

challenge the feasibility of this traditional approach. First, as medicine progresses through incremental improvements in treatment as well as earlier detection, the potential effect size of the next intervention decreases, whereas the time to event increases. The result of increasing trial size and duration of follow-up increases the cost. The age of the patient population diagnosed with cancer continues to increase, as mortality from cardiac diseases decreases. Because this population of elderly patients with comorbidities is often excluded from clinical trials, the applicability of trial results to this population is difficult. Meanwhile, technologic advances in imaging and treatment as well as incorporation of molecular profiling can cause the question being addressed to become obsolete by the time trial results have matured. Specifically in radiation therapy, rapidly evolving technology has often led to increasing complexity of treatment, such as with improvements in treatment conformality through intensity-modulated radiation therapy (IMRT) and stereotactic body radiation therapy (SBRT). Increasing complexity often warrants more strict QA mechanisms to ensure that the intervention is applied appropriately in order to adequately test its utility, thereby reducing the ability to generalize the results to routine clinical practice.

Pragmatic Clinical Trials

The concept of pragmatic clinical trials arose out of the concern that clinical trials were being optimized to determine efficacy while potentially overestimating benefit and underestimating harm when applied to the general population.[162] Pragmatic trials thus focus on applicability of a new intervention to general practice, whereas explanatory trials aim to address questions of biologic mechanism. In 2009, a tool called the PRagmatic-Explanatory Continuum Indicator Summary (PRECIS) was published to provide clinical trialists with a guide to understanding how different components of design would impact the applicability, or pragmatism, of the trial.[163] An updated version (PRECIS-2) was published in 2013 in which 9 domains get scored on a Likert-type scale (1 = most explanatory, 5 = most pragmatic).[164] The primary goal of PRECIS-2 is to match the trial design to the intended application of trial results.

Meanwhile, CONSORT published an "extension for pragmatic trials" that specifies that trial publications include all the information on the context of their conducted trial so that future readers can judge applicability of the results to their own clinical context, where they may be considering implementing the intervention tested in that randomized trial.[165] So although PRECIS-2 encourages appropriate trial design, CONSORT ensures trial results and information are reported adequately for health system decision-makers to determine applicability of trial results to their clinical setting.

A study design often employed in pragmatic trials is cluster randomization. This allows the intervention to be implemented at the group level rather than the individual level, which affords more opportunity for training of interdisciplinary teams of professionals and assurance that implementation is appropriate for the clinical context. Furthermore, as a result, all patients within a center are treated uniformly, which improves efficiency and reduces the risk of errors. The comparator arm, meanwhile, is generally usual care, which is not always the case on explanatory trials. By facilitating training, cluster designs also help to address differences in provider experience, which have been shown in radiation oncology to influence outcomes and must be considered such as to avoid confounding. Although pragmatic trials often include providers with a representative mix of experience levels to increase generalizability, trial quality must always be closely monitored. A pragmatic trial conducted poorly is of no use for decision support.

Pragmatic trials rely more heavily on electronic health records (EHRs) and patient registries to collect patient information, as this reduces cost of trial coordinators. Of note, many registries were established prior to implementation of EHRs, so they often collect data in parallel, with work ongoing to synchronize the system. Some health systems have developed robust national quality registries that are disease-based or intervention-based, which has facilitated large clinical trials. For example, the Thrombus Aspiration in ST-Elevation Myocardial Infarction in Scandinavia (TASTE) trial was a multicenter, prospective, open-label, randomized, controlled clinical trial that used the infrastructure of a population-based registry in 29 Swedish centers and 1 Icelandic center, to facilitate enrollment and long-term data collection on 11,709 patients treated for heart attacks from 2008 to 2009.[166]

Comparative Effectiveness Research

The 1999 Institute of Medicine's report "To Err Is Human" called attention to serious concerns about patient safety in the United States. The Agency for Healthcare Research and Quality (AHRQ) was established to address these concerns by focusing on the safety and quality improvement in health care delivery. The AHRQ defines comparative effectiveness research (CER) as that which is "designed to inform healthcare decisions by providing evidence on the effectiveness, benefits, and harms of different treatment options."[87] Then, in 2010, an independent nonprofit, nongovernmental organization called the Patient-Centered Outcomes Research Institute (PCORI) was authorized by Congress to further address the need for information to guide better-informed health decisions by patients, providers, and policy makers. PCORI is the single largest public funder of CER in the United States, supporting primarily large pragmatic studies and large-scale observational studies.[88]

Over the past few decades, government agencies, professional societies, and private corporations have established patient registries that collect standardized data from patients diagnosed and treated in a variety of settings, in order to provide data regarding patterns of care and patient outcomes.

The Surveillance, Epidemiology, and End Results (SEER) Program of the National Cancer Institute was established in 1974 to provide cancer statistics in order to reduce the burden of cancer.[86] SEER is a population-based registry representing 17 regions and 28% of the US population. It is therefore a useful epidemiologic tool for calculating incidence (new cases per population), prevalence (existing cases per population), and mortality (deaths per population) for different cancers, and it documents tumor-specific information. SEER, a clinical database, is often linked to the Medicare claims data, in order to provide more detailed indirect information regarding treatment of cancer (including number of fractions of radiation) as well as diagnosis codes and interventions that could relate to toxicity (such as cystoscopy, colonoscopy, coronary angioplasty). Use of Medicare linkage restricts the data to over 65 years, however. This is similar but distinct from the Medicare Chronic Conditions Warehouse (CCW), which is an administrative database that can be used independently to investigate broader patterns of care than SEER-linked data, though it lacks detailed cancer information that is available in SEER, such as stage.

The National Cancer Database (NCDB) is jointly sponsored by the American College of Surgeons and the American Cancer Society. It includes patients from 1,500 Commission on Cancer (COC)-accredited programs, representing 70% of cancer diagnoses.[85] The initial goal of NCDB was to monitor patterns of care at the local hospital level and provide feedback regarding quality measures. NCDB requires COC accreditation and therefore does not represent all patients in a population. It is therefore technically not a population-based database and thus not appropriate for incidence/prevalence but can be used to assess outcomes after diagnosis. NCDB includes details of margin status, radiation dose, and technique, which are not captured in the SEER database. Although NCDB enables important patterns of care studies, it lacks robust outcome data, including cancer-specific survival, and recently has been used extensively to assess efficacy of radiation treatment with overall survival as the primary end point, which has significant limitations. Because of the observational nature of this registry, confounders exist in treatment selection (including patient performance status), which can bias the perceived efficacy of the treatment. In a retrospective database, one can never fully control for this selection bias and therefore should interpret overall survival results with extreme caution.

A major limitation of SEER, NCDB, and CCW, however, is the lack of patient-reported outcomes. The CaPSURE represents a prostate-specific registry that was initiated in 1995 to enable prospective cohort studies in men with prostate cancer that focused on incorporating patient-reported outcomes.[167] Approximately 40 urology practices, primarily community-based, enroll patients in a database that tracks over 1,000 clinical and patient-reported variables. Though this is not a population-based sample, it provides much richer clinical detail than SEER. Given the long natural history of prostate cancer, CaPSURE is regarded as a cost-effective alternative to randomized trials that reflects "real world" practice and has resulted in nearly 200 peer-reviewed publications.

Newer registries are being developed to address the limitations of current databases and therefore include a robust interface for data collection that facilitates prospective clinical trials (such as the Swedish TASTE trial) and incorporation of radiation-specific information (including that captured in Digital Imaging and Communications in Medicine (DICOM) files). Cancer Learning Intelligence Network for Quality (CancerLinQ) is a national initiative sponsored by the American Society for Clinical Oncology (ASCO) that involves a cloud-based platform that communicates nightly with the EHR at each individual practice to collect, deidentify, and update patient information, which serves as both a database to evaluate quality metrics and also real-time decision support tool that recommends guideline-concordant therapies.[168] As of October 2016, CancerLinQ had registered over 1 million patients treated at 70 clinics by 1,500 oncologists, and shortly thereafter, the American Society for Radiation Oncology (ASTRO) announced partnership to incorporate critical radiation-specific data into the database.[84] Developing a DICOM-based registry for radiation oncology requires first standardizing naming conventions to enable harmonization of the digital information. This process is in progress in the United States, with AAPM Task Group 263 defining the naming convention and the Radiation Oncology Institute developing the National Radiation Oncology Registry and piloting it in prostate cancer at 30 centers. Meanwhile, Sweden has successfully implemented the naming convention and is collecting RT data in DICOM files through their Medical Information Quality Archive at the majority of their radiation centers.[169]

Meta-analysis

A formal quantitative means of combining evidence from multiple clinical trials is by meta-analysis—a widely used analytic tool in many areas of social and medical science. Meta-analysis refers to a process whereby data from independent studies are combined to form a quantitative summary estimate of a given effect.

Meta-analyses are considered by some to be a source of level I evidence along with large randomized clinical trials. A meta-analysis combines results of several studies, all of which ask a similar research question but may be individually too small to have enough statistical power to definitively answer the question. Performing a systematic analysis of data from all identified randomized trials can define a modest yet real advantage associated with a therapeutic approach, such as overall survival associated with radiation in breast cancer[170] and concurrent chemotherapy with radiation in head-and-neck cancer.[171] To address the likelihood of publication bias (i.e., a greater representation of trials with positive results appearing in the literature), a meta-analysis should include unpublished studies as well, though assessing quality is critical given the lack of peer review.

Meta-analyses can be performed with or without access to the raw data, though the methods employed are critical to ensuring quality results. Cochrane is an independent, non-profit, nongovernmental organization consisting of a group of more than 37,000 volunteers in more than 130 countries that aims to improve access to high-quality reviews that guide decision-making.[82] Researchers interested in undertaking meta-analyses are encouraged to contact the Cochrane Methods Groups, which provide access to methodologists that can assist with responsible conduct of meta-analyses (http://methods.cochrane.org/methods-groups).

Clinical trials in radiation therapy often restrict access to raw patient data, including detailed treatment planning information in DICOM files, much of which is not reported or even investigated in the primary publication. For example, multiple trials have reported the presence of a major protocol deviation predicting inferior overall survival.[146] Even determining the reason for the deviation can be difficult to find, because the process has been retrospectively defined until only recently. Access to the original images, treatment plans, and setup images could elucidate important information regarding details in QA that could better explain the differences in patient outcomes. An ideal system would promote the public availability of trial data to facilitate further research, with a currently available resource including figshare (https://figshare.com/).

NEXT-GENERATION RADIATION ONCOLOGY TRIALS

Next-generation trials will need to include iterative, adaptive designs that are not *a priori* committed to studying uniform fraction intervals (i.e., q daily, Monday to Friday, *or* qod, Mon, Wed, Fri), but are based on the constant incorporation of serial imaging and liquid biopsies, which can serve as surrogates of early response and/or resistance for most or a small component of the tumor. All patients will have omic information available, and all patients will likely have their tumors growing in an avatar to generate patient-derived xenografts (PDX). There is increased evidence that immunotherapy radiation may enhance the therapeutic capacity of immunotherapy, as shown in Fig. 15.10.

Furthermore, the emerging field of radiomics[172] and mathematical modeling,[173] an outgrowth of evolutionary biology, will provide personalized radiotherapy prescriptions that may change multiple times during a course of treatment.[174-176]

Although the patient and providers may not know the length and schedule of the prescription at the time of the initial consultation, positive results will demand that trials incorporate disruptive algorithms in order to test promising and disruptive treatment paradigms. Figure 15.11 provides a snapshot of the next-generation clinical trial approach for radiation-based cancer research.

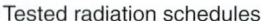

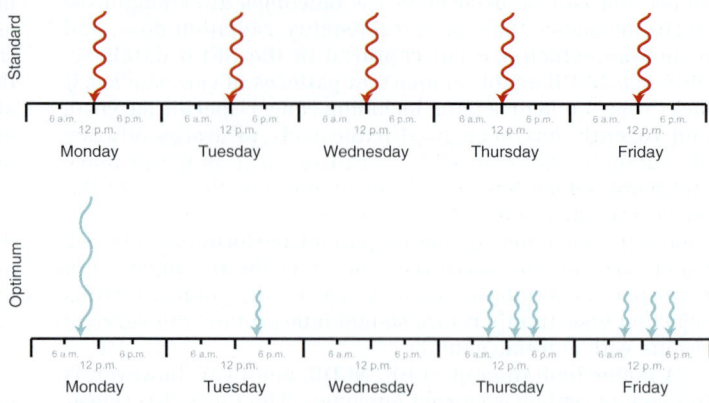

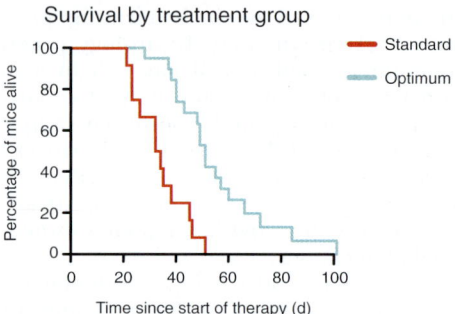

FIGURE 15.10. Testing of two radiation schedules in a mouse model. (Adapted from Leder K, Pitter K, LaPlant Q, et al. Mathematical modeling of PDGF-driven glioblastoma reveals optimized radiation dosing schedules. *Cell* 2014;156[3]:603–616. Copyright © 2014 Elsevier. With permission.)

FIGURE 15.11. The varied considerations of the interplay of a heterogeneous population of cancer cells. (Reprinted from Michor F, Beal K. Improving Cancer Treatment via Mathematical Modeling: Surmounting the Challenges is Worth the Effort. *Cell* 2015;163[5]:1059–1063. Copyright © 2015 Elsevier. With permission.)

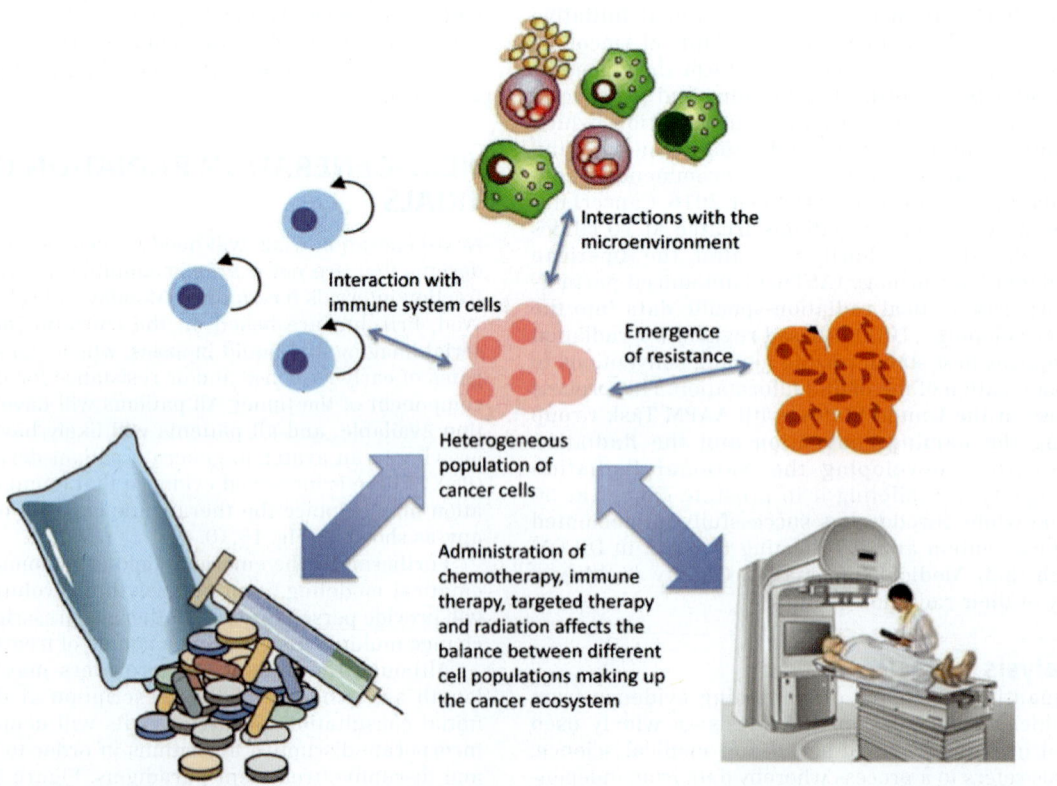

ACKNOWLEDGMENTS

Some content was modified from previous editions of this chapter. The current authors gratefully acknowledge the previous editions' authors' contributions.

Jan Bussink
Richard Chappell
Chaitanya Divgi
Joe Gray
Stephen Hahn
Kevin Harrington
Reshma Jagsi
Patricia LoRusso
Joseph Rajendran
Ramesh Rengan
Yu Shyr
Bridgett Sparkman
Lillian Siu
Miguel Villalona-Calero
James Welsh
Kristina H. Young
Chelsea Davis

REFERENCES

1. Crowley J, Ankerst D. *Handbook of statistics in clinical oncology*. New York, NY: Chapman Hall/CRC, 2006.
2. Green S, Benedetti J, Smith A, et al. *Clinical trials in oncology*. Boca Raton, FL: Chapman Hall/CRC Interdisciplinary Statistics, 2012.
3. Kelly K, Halabi S. *Oncology clinical trials: successful design, conduct and analysis*. New York, NY: Demos Medical Publishing, 2009.
4. Unknown. Wikipedia. Available at http://en.wikipedia.org/wiki/Clinical_trial2011.
5. Piantadosi S. *Clinical trials: a methodologic perspective*. New York, NY: John Wiley & Sons, 2005.
6. Available at http://www.cancer.gov/cancertopics/factsheet/NCI/clinical-trials-cooperative-group.
7. Hearn J, Sullivan R. The impact of the 'Clinical Trials' directive on the cost and conduct of non-commercial cancer trials in the UK. *Eur J Cancer* 2007;43:8–13.
8. Begley CG, Ellis LM. Drug development: raise standards for preclinical cancer research. *Nature* 2012;483:531–533.
9. Fromell GJ. Good clinical practice standards: what they are and some tools to support them. *Hum Gene Ther* 2008;19:431–440.
10. Emanuel EJ, Wendler D, Grady C. What makes clinical research ethical? *JAMA* 2000;283:2701–2711.
11. Wendler D, Zalta EN. *The ethics of clinical research*. Oxford: Oxford University Press, 2009.
12. Ratain MJ, Sargent DJ. Optimising the design of phase II oncology trials: the importance of randomisation. *Eur J Cancer* 2009;45:275–280.
13. Mandrekar SJ, Sargent DJ. Randomized phase II trials: time for a new era in clinical trial design. *J Thorac Oncol* 2010;5:932–934.
14. Tang H, Foster NR, Grothey A, et al. Comparison of error rates in single-arm versus randomized phase II cancer clinical trials. *J Clin Oncol* 2010;28:1936–1941.
15. Leventhal BG. An overview of clinical trials in oncology. *Semin Oncol* 1988;15:414–422.
16. Simon R, Wittes RE, Ellenberg SS. Randomized phase II clinical trials. *Cancer Treat Rep* 1985;69:1375–1381.
17. Rubinstein LV, Korn EL, Freidlin B, J. Design issues of randomized phase II trials and a proposal for phase II screening trials. *J Clin Oncol* 2005;23:7199–7206.
18. Murgo AJ, Kummar S, Rubinstein L, et al. Designing phase 0 cancer clinical trials. *Clin Cancer Res* 2008;14:3675–3682.
19. Bates SE. The language of pharmacodynamics. *Clin Cancer Res* 2014;20(10):2524. doi:10.1158/1078-0432.CCR-14-0739.
20. Vogelbaum MA. The future of clinical research beyond phase III trials. *Clin Neurosurg* 2009;56:37–39.
21. FitzGerald TJ, Urie M, Ulin K. Processes for quality improvements in radiation oncology clinical trials. *Int J Radiat Oncol Biol Phys* 2008;71:S76–S79.
22. Justin EB, Joachim Y. Quality of radiotherapy reporting in randomized controlled trials of Hodgkin's lymphoma and non-Hodgkin's lymphoma: review. *Int J Radiat Oncol Biol Phys* 2009;73:492–498.
23. Morris SL, Beasley M, Leslie M. Chemotherapy for pancreatic cancer. *N Engl J Med* 2004;350:2713–2715. author reply 2713–2715.
24. Bydder S, Spry N. Chemotherapy for pancreatic cancer. *N Engl J Med* 2004;350:2713–2715. author reply 2713–2715.
25. Crane CH, Ben-Josef E, Small W Jr. Chemotherapy for pancreatic cancer. *N Engl J Med* 2004;350:2713–2715. author reply 27132715.
26. Rischin D, Peters L, Fisher R. Tirapazamine, cisplatin, and radiation versus fluorouracil, cisplatin, and radiation in patients with locally advanced head and neck cancer: a randomized phase II trial of the Trans-Tasman Radiation Oncology Group (TROG 98. 02). *J Clin Oncol* 2005;23:79–87.
27. Weiner MA, Leventhal B, Brecher ML, et al. Randomized study of intensive MOPP-ABVD with or without low-dose total-nodal radiation therapy in the treatment of stages IIB, IIIA2, IIIB, and s disease in pediatric patients: a Pediatric Oncology Group study. *J Clin Oncol* 1997;15:2769–2779.
28. Abrams RA, Winter KA, Regine WF, et al. Failure to adhere to protocol specified radiation therapy guidelines was associated with decreased survival in RTOG 9704 – a phase III trial of adjuvant chemotherapy and chemoradiotherapy for patients with resected adenocarcinoma of the pancreas. *Int J Radiat Oncol Biol Phys* 2012;82:809–816.
29. Normolle D, Lawrence T. Designing dose-escalation trials with late-onset toxicities using the time-to-event continual reassessment method. *J Clin Oncol* 2006;24:4426–4433.
30. Glass C, Den R, Dicker AP, et al. *Toxicity of phase I radiation oncology trials: worldwide experience, abstract #1605. American Society for Therapeutic Radiation Oncology (ASTRO) 52nd Annual Meeting*, October 31–November 4, 2010, San Diego, CA.
31. Liu PY, LeBlanc M, Desai M. False positive rates of randomized phase II designs. *Control Clin Trials* 1999;20:343–352.
32. Piantadosi S. Principles of clinical trial design. *Semin Oncol* 1988;15:423–433.
33. Therasse P, Arbuck SG, Eisenhauer EA, et al. New guidelines to evaluate the response to treatment in solid tumors. European Organization for Research and Treatment of Institute of the United States of Canada. *J Natl Cancer Inst* 2000;92:205–216.
34. Chen TT, Chute JP, Feigal E. A model to select chemotherapy regimens for phase III trials for extensive-stage small-cell lung cancer. *J Natl Cancer Inst* 2000;92:1601–1607.
35. Buyse M, Thirion P, Carlson RW. Relation between tumour response to first-line chemotherapy and survival in advanced colorectal cancer: a meta-analysis. Meta-Analysis Group in Cancer. *Lancet* 2000;356:373–378.
36. Moertel CG. Improving the efficiency of clinical trials: a medical perspective. *Stat Med* 1984;3:455–468.
37. Gaynor JJ, Feuer EJ, Tan CC. On the use of cause-specific failure and conditional failure probabilities: examples from clinical oncology data. *J Am Stat Assoc* 1993;88:400–409.
38. Dignam JJ, Kocherginsky MN. Choice and interpretation of statistical tests used when competing risks are present. *J Clin Oncol* 2008;26:4027–4034.
39. Hudis CA, Barlow WE, Costantino JP. Proposal for standardized definitions for efficacy end points in adjuvant breast cancer trials: the STEEP system. *J Clin Oncol* 2007;25:2127–2132.
40. Sargent DJ, Wieand HS, Haller DG. Disease-free survival versus overall survival as a primary end point for adjuvant colon cancer studies: individual patient data from 20,898 patients on 18 randomized trials. *J Clin Oncol* 2005;23:8664–8670.
41. Prentice RL. Surrogate endpoints in clinical trials: definition and operational criteria. *Stat Med* 1989;8:431–440.
42. Buyyounouski MK, Hanlon AL, Horwitz EM. Interval to biochemical failure highly prognostic for distant metastasis and prostate cancer-specific mortality after radiotherapy. *Int J Radiat Oncol Biol Phys* 2008;70:59–66.
43. Denham JW, Steigler A, Wilcox C. Time to biochemical failure and prostate-specific antigen doubling time as surrogates for prostate cancer-specific mortality: evidence from the TROG 96. 01 randomised controlled trial. *Lancet Oncol* 2008;9:1058–1068.
44. Schatzkin A, Gail M. The promise and peril of surrogate end points in cancer research. *Nat Rev Cancer* 2002;2:19–27.
45. Halpern SD, Karlawish JH, Berlin JA. The continuing unethical conduct of underpowered clinical trials. *JAMA* 2002;288:358–362.
46. Shuster J. *Power and sample size for phase III clinical trials of survival. Handbook of Statistics in Clinical Oncology*. New York, NY: Chapman Hall–CRC, 2006:207–226.
47. Freedman LS. Tables of the number of patients required in clinical trials using the logrank test. *Stat Med* 1982;1:121–129.
48. Ahn S, Anderson SJ. Sample size determination in complex clinical trials comparing more than two groups for survival endpoints. *Stat Med* 1998;17:2525–2534.
49. Lachin JM, Foulkes MA. Evaluation of sample size and power for analyses of survival with allowance for nonuniform patient entry, losses to follow-up, noncompliance, and stratification. *Biometrics* 1986;42:507–519.
50. Shih JH. Sample size calculation for complex clinical trials with survival endpoints. *Control Clin Trials* 1995;16:395–407.
51. Simon R. Optimal two-stage designs for phase II clinical trials. *Control Clin Trials* 1989;10:1–10.
52. Haybittle JL. Repeated assessment of results in clinical trials of cancer treatment. *Br J Radiol* 1971;44:793–797.
53. Peto R, Pike MC, Armitage P, et al. Design and analysis of randomized clinical trials requiring prolonged observation of each patient. II analysis and examples. *Br J Cancer* 1977;35:1–39.
54. Fleming TR, Harrington DP, O'Brien PC. Designs for group sequential tests. *Control Clin Trials* 1984;5:348–361.
55. Halperin M, Lan KK, Ware JH. An aid to data monitoring in long-term clinical trials. *Control Clin Trials* 1982;3:311–323.
56. Lan KK, The B, Wittes J. Value: a tool for monitoring data. *Biometrics* 1988;44:579–585.

Section II

57. Dignam JJ, Bryant J, Wieand HS. Early stopping of a clinical trial when there is evidence of no treatment benefit: protocol B-14 of the National Surgical Adjuvant Breast and Bowel Project. *Control Clin Trials* 1998;19:575–588.

58. Freidlin B, Korn EL, Gray R. A general inefficacy interim monitoring rule for randomized clinical trials. *Clin Trials* 2010;7:197–208.

59. Freidlin B, Korn EL. A comment on futility monitoring. *Control Clin Trials* 2002;23:355–366.

60. Fleming TR, Sharples K, McCall J. Maintaining confidentiality of interim data to enhance trial integrity and credibility. *Clin Trials* 2008;5:157–167.

61. Gail MH. Eligibility exclusions, losses to follow-up, removal of randomized patients, and uncounted events in cancer clinical trials. *Cancer Treat Rep* 1985;69:1107–1113.

62. Redmond C, Fisher B, Wieand HS. The methodologic dilemma in retrospectively correlating the amount of chemotherapy received in adjuvant therapy protocols with disease-free survival. *Cancer Treat Rep* 1983;67:519–526.

63. Schmoor C, Sauerbrei W, Schumacher M. Sample size considerations for the evaluation of prognostic factors in survival analysis. *Stat Med* 2000;19:441–452.

64. Grant N, Sacatos M, Kelly K, et al. The trials and tribulations of writing an investigator initiated clinical study. In: Kelly WK, Halabi S, eds. *Oncology clinical trials successful design conduct and analysis.* New York, NY: Demos Medical, 2009:119–130.

65. U.S. Food and Drug Administration. Guidance for Industry: Clinical Trial Endpoints for the Approval of Cancer Drugs and Biologics, 2011.

66. Brandsma D, Stalpers L, Taal W. Clinical features, mechanisms, and management of pseudoprogression in malignant gliomas. *Lancet Oncol* 2008;9:453–461.

67. De Pourcq F. Defining the roles and responsibilities of study personnel. In: Kelly K, Halabi S, eds. *Oncology clinical conduct and analysis.* New York, NY: Demos Medical, 2009:321–326.

68. Lan KK, Lachin JM, Bautista O. Over-ruling a group sequential boundary-a stopping rule versus a guideline. *Stat Med* 2003;22:3347–3355.

69. Smith MA, Ungerleider RS, Korn EL. Role of independent data-monitoring committees in randomized clinical trials sponsored by the National Cancer Institute. *J Clin Oncol* 1997;15:2736–2743.

70. Schulz KF, Altman DG, Moher D; CONSORT Group. CONSORT 2010 statement: updated guidelines for reporting parallel group randomised trials. *PLoS Med* 2010;7:e1000251.

71. International Committee of Medical Journal Editors (ICMJE). Uniform Requirements for Manuscripts Submitted to Biomedical Journals: writing and editing for biomedical publication. *Haematologica* 2004;89(3):264.

72. Mariani L, Marubini E. Content and quality of currently published phase II cancer trials. *J Clin Oncol* 2000;18:429–436.

73. Zohar S, Lian Q, Levy V. Quality assessment of phase I dose-finding cancer trials: proposal of a checklist. *Clin Trials* 2008;5:478–485.

74. Krzyzanowska MK, Pintilie M, Tannock IF. Factors associated with failure to publish large randomized trials presented at an oncology meeting. *JAMA* 2003;290:495–501.

75. O'Quigley J, Pepe M, Fisher L. Continual reassessment method: a practical design for phase 1 clinical trials in cancer. *Biometrics* 1990;46:33–48.

76. Cheung YK, Chappell R. Sequential designs for phase I clinical trials with late-onset toxicities. *Biometrics* 2000;56:1177–1182.

77. Polley MY. Practical modifications to the time-to-event continual reassessment method for phase I cancer trials with fast patient accrual and late-onset toxicities. *Stat Med* 2011;30:2130–2143.

78. Cannistra SA Phase II trials in journal of clinical oncology. *J Clin Oncol* 2009;27:3073–3076.

79. Zelen M. Play the winner rule and the controlled clinical trial. *J Am Stat Assoc* 1969;64:131–146.

80. Biswas S, Liu DD, Lee JJ, et al. Bayesian clinical trials at the University of Anderson Cancer Center. *Clin Trials* 2009;6:205–216.

81. Korn EL, Freidlin B. Outcome-adaptive randomization: is it useful? *J Clin Oncol* 2011;29:771–776.

82. Mick R, Crowley JJ, Carroll RJ. Phase II clinical trial design for noncytotoxic anticancer agents for which time to disease progression is the primary endpoint. *Control Clin Trials* 2000;21:343–359.

83. Rosner GL, Stadler W, Ratain MJ Randomized discontinuation design: application to cytostatic antineoplastic agents. *J Clin Oncol* 2002;20:4478–4484.

84. Korn EL, Arbuck SG, Pluda JM. Clinical trial designs for cytostatic agents: are new approaches needed? *J Clin Oncol* 2001;19:265–272.

85. Kim ES, Herbst RS, Wistuba II. Battle trial: the personalizing therapy for lung cancer. *Cancer Discov* 2011;1:44–53.

86. Barker AD, Sigman CC, Kelloff GJ. I-SPY an adaptive breast cancer trial design in the setting of neoadjuvant chemotherapy. *Clin Pharmacol Ther* 2009;86:97–100.

87. Freidlin B, McShane LM, Korn EL. Randomized clinical trials with biomarkers: design issues. *J Natl Cancer Inst* 2010;102:152–160.

88. Simon R. The use of genomics in clinical trial design. *Clin Cancer Res* 2008;14:5984–5993.

89. Harbour R, Miller J. A new system for grading recommendations in evidence based guidelines. *BMJ* 2001;323:334–336.

90. Hutchins LF, Unger JM, Crowley JJ. Underrepresentation of patients 65 years of age or older in cancer-treatment trials. *N Engl J Med* 1999;341:2061–2067.

91. Kumar A, Soares HP, Balducci L. Treatment tolerance and efficacy in geriatric oncology: a systematic review of phase III randomized trials conducted by five National Cancer Institute-sponsored cooperative groups. *J Clin Oncol* 2007;25:1272–1276.

92. Lewis JH, Kilgore ML, Goldman DP. Participation of patients 65 years of age or older in cancer clinical trials. *J Clin Oncol* 2003;21:1383–1389.

93. George SL. Reducing patient eligibility criteria in cancer clinical trials. *J Clin Oncol* 1996;14:1364–1370.

94. Lubeck DP, Litwin MS, Henning JM, et al. The CaPSURE database: a methodology for clinical practice and research in prostate cancer. CaPSURE Research Panel. Cancer of the Prostate Strategic Urologic Research Endeavor. *Urology* 1996; 48:773–777.

95. Sparano JA. TAILORx: trial assigning individualized options for treatment (Rx). *Clin Breast Cancer* 2006;7:347–350.

96. Pijls-Johannesma M, van Mastrigt G, Hahn SM, et al. A systematic methodology review of phase I radiation dose escalation trials. *Radiother Oncol* 2010;95:135–141.

97. Bekele BN, Ji Y, Shen Y, et al. Monitoring late-onset toxicities in phase I trials using predicted risks. *Biostatistics* 2008;9:442–457.

98. Mehta M, Scrimger R, Mackie R, et al. A new approach to dose escalation in non-small-cell lung cancer. *Int J Radiat Oncol Biol Phys* 2001;49:23–33.

99. Rogatko A, Schoeneck D, Jonas W, et al. Translation of innovative designs into phase I trials. *J Clin Oncol* 2007;25:4982–4986.

100. Le Tourneau C, Lee JJ, Siu LL. Dose escalation methods in phase I cancer clinical trials. *J Natl Cancer Inst* 2009;101:708–720.

101. Ben-Josef E, Schipper M, Francis IR, et al. A phase I/II trial of intensity modulated radiation (IMRT) dose escalation with concurrent fixed-dose rate gemcitabine (FDR-G) in patients with unresectable pancreatic cancer. *Int J Radiat Oncol Biol Phys* 2012;84:1166–1171.

102. Desai SP, Ben-Josef E, Normolle DP, et al. Phase I study of oxaliplatin, full-dose gemcitabine, and concurrent radiation therapy in pancreatic cancer. *J Clin Oncol* 2007;25:4587–4592.

103. Muler JH, McGinn CJ, Normolle D, et al. Phase I trial using a time-to-event continual reassessment strategy for dose escalation of cisplatin combined with gemcitabine and radiation therapy in pancreatic cancer. *J Clin Oncol* 2004;22:238–243.

104. Lawrence YR, Vikram B, Dignam JJ, et al. NCI-RTOG translational program strategic guidelines for the early-stage development of radiosensitizers. *J Natl Cancer Inst* 2013;105:11–24.

105. Feng M, Smith DE, Normolle DP, et al. A phase I clinical and pharmacology study using amifostine as a radioprotector in dose-escalated whole liver radiation therapy. *Int J Radiat Oncol Biol Phys* 2012;83:1441–1447.

106. Bellinger AM, Arteaga CL, Force T, et al. Cardio-oncology: how new targeted cancer therapies and precision medicine can inform cardiovascular discovery. *Circulation* 2015;132:2248–2258.

107. Witteles RM. biomarkers as predictors of cardiac toxicity from targeted cancer therapies. *J Card Fail* 2016;22:459–464.

108. Jacob L, Uvarova M, Boulet S, et al. Evaluation of a multi-arm multi-stage Bayesian design for phase II drug selection trials—an example in hemato-oncology. *BMC Med Res Methodol* 2016;16:67.

109. Henri C, Heinonen T, Tardif JC. The role of biomarkers in decreasing risk of cardiac toxicity after cancer therapy. *Biomark Cancer* 2016;8:39–45.

110. Rivoirard R, Vallard A, Langrand-Escure J, et al. Thirty years of phase I radio-chemotherapy trials: latest development. *Eur J Cancer* 2016;58:1–7.

111. Higgins GS, O'Cathail SM, Muschel RJ, et al. Drug radiotherapy combinations: review of previous failures and reasons for future optimism. *Cancer Treat Rev* 2015;41:105–113.

112. Sharma RA, Plummer R, Stock JK, et al. Clinical development of new drug-radiotherapy combinations. *Nat Rev Clin Oncol* 2016;13:627–642.

113. Blumenfeld P, Pfeffer RM, Symon Z, et al. The lag time in initiating clinical testing of new drugs in combination with radiation therapy, a significant barrier to progress? *Br J Cancer* 2014;111:1305–1309.

114. Ye F, Shyr Y. Balanced two-stage designs for phase II clinical trials. *Clin Trials* 2007;4:514–524.

115. Gehan EA. The determination of the number of patients required in a preliminary and a follow-up trial of a new chemotherapeutic agent. *J Chronic Dis* 1961;13:346–353.

116. Fleming TR. One-sample multiple testing procedure for phase II clinical trials. *Biometrics* 1982;38:143–151.

117. Chen Y, Chen Z, Mori M. A new statistical decision rule for single-arm phase II oncology trials. *Stat Methods Med Res* 2016;25:118–132.

118. Ohri N, Piperdi B, Garg MK, et al. Pre-treatment FDG-PET predicts the site of in-field progression following concurrent chemoradiotherapy for stage III non-small cell lung cancer. *Lung Cancer* 2015;87:23–27.

119. Goodman KA, Niedzwiecki D, Hall N, et al. Initial results of CALGB 80803 (Alliance): a randomized phase II trial of PET scan-directed combined modality therapy for esophageal cancer. *J Clin Oncol* 2017;35(suppl 4S; abstract 1):1–1.

120. Kong FM, Ten Haken RK, Schipper M, et al. Effect of midtreatment PET/CT-adapted radiation therapy with concurrent chemotherapy in patients with locally advanced non-small-cell lung cancer: a phase 2 clinical trial. *JAMA Oncol* 2017;3:1358–1365.

121. West HJ. Novel precision medicine trial designs: umbrellas and baskets. *JAMA Oncol* 2017;3:423.

122. Kachnic LA, Winter K, Myerson RJ, et al. RTOG 0529: a phase 2 evaluation of dose-painted intensity modulated radiation therapy in combination with 5-flurorouracil and mitomycin-C for the reduction of acute morbidity in carcinoma of the anal canal. *Int J Radiat Oncol Biol Phys* 2013;86:27–33.

123. Herman JM, Thomas CR Jr. RTOG 0529: intensity modulated radiation therapy and anal cancer, a step in the right direction? *Int J Radiat Oncol Biol Phys* 2013;86:8–10.

124. Basch E, Deal AM, Dueck AC, et al. Overall survival results of a trial assessing patient-reported outcomes for symptom monitoring during routine cancer treatment. *JAMA* 2017;318:197–198.

125. MacDonald WC, Owen DA. Gastric carcinoma after surgical treatment of peptic ulcer: an analysis of morphologic features and a comparison with cancer in the nonoperated stomach. *Cancer* 2001;91:1732–1738.

126. Whelan TJ, Pignol JP, Levine MN, et al. Long-term results of hypofractionated radiation therapy for breast cancer. *N Engl J Med* 2010;362:513–520.

127. Moher D, Hopewell S, Schulz KF, et al. CONSORT 2010 explanation and elaboration: updated guidelines for reporting parallel group randomised trials. *BMJ* 2010;340:c869.

128. James RD, Glynne-Jones R, Meadows HM, et al. Mitomycin or cisplatin chemoradiation with or without maintenance chemotherapy for treatment of squamous-cell carcinoma of the anus (ACT II): a randomised, phase 3, open-label, 2 × 2 factorial trial. *Lancet Oncol* 2013;14:516–524.

129. Hendlisz A, Van den Eynde M, Peeters M, et al. Phase III trial comparing protracted intravenous fluorouracil infusion alone or with yttrium-90 resin microspheres radioembolization for liver-limited metastatic colorectal cancer refractory to standard chemotherapy. *J Clin Oncol* 2010;28:3687–3694.

130. Minsky BD, Pajak TF, Ginsberg RJ, et al. INT 0123 (Radiation Therapy Oncology Group 94-05) phase III trial of combined-modality therapy for esophageal cancer: high-dose versus standard-dose radiation therapy. *J Clin Oncol* 2002;20:1167–1174.

131. Lesaffre E. Superiority, equivalence, and non-inferiority trials. *Bull NYU Hosp Jt Dis* 2008;66:150–154.

132. Dearnaley D, Syndikus I, Mossop H, et al. Conventional versus hypofractionated high-dose intensity-modulated radiotherapy for prostate cancer: 5-year outcomes of the randomised, non-inferiority, phase 3 CHHiP trial. *Lancet Oncol* 2016;17:1047–1060.

133. Erlandsson J, Holm T, Pettersson D, et al. Optimal fractionation of preoperative radiotherapy and timing to surgery for rectal cancer (Stockholm III): a multicentre, randomised, non-blinded, phase 3, non-inferiority trial. *Lancet Oncol* 2017;18:336–346.

134. Mulvenna P, Nankivell M, Barton R, et al. Dexamethasone and supportive care with or without whole brain radiotherapy in treating patients with non-small cell lung cancer with brain metastases unsuitable for resection or stereotactic radiotherapy (QUARTZ): results from a phase 3, non-inferiority, randomised trial. *Lancet* 2016;388:2004–2014.

135. Flam M, John M, Pajak TF, et al. Role of mitomycin in combination with fluorouracil and radiotherapy, and of salvage chemoradiation in the definitive nonsurgical treatment of epidermoid carcinoma of the anal canal: results of a phase III randomized intergroup study. *J Clin Oncol* 1996;14:2527–2539.

136. Peters LJ, O'Sullivan B, Giralt J, et al. Critical impact of radiotherapy protocol compliance and quality in the treatment of advanced head and neck cancer: results from TROG 02.02. *J Clin Oncol* 2010;28:2996–3001.

137. Wuthrick EJ, Zhang Q, Machtay M, et al. Institutional clinical trial accrual volume and survival of patients with head and neck cancer. *J Clin Oncol* 2015;33:156–164.

138. Duhmke E, Franklin J, Pfreundschuh M, et al. Low-dose radiation is sufficient for the noninvolved extended-field treatment in favorable early-stage Hodgkin's disease: long-term results of a randomized trial of radiotherapy alone. *J Clin Oncol* 2001;19:2905–2914.

139. Fairchild A, Straube W, Laurie F, et al. Does quality of radiation therapy predict outcomes of multicenter cooperative group trials? A literature review. *Int J Radiat Oncol Biol Phys* 2013;87:246–260.

140. Ohri N, Shen X, Dicker AP, et al. Radiotherapy protocol deviations and clinical outcomes: a meta-analysis of cooperative group clinical trials. *J Natl Cancer Inst* 2013;105:387–393.

141. Eisbruch A, Harris J, Garden AS, et al. Multi-institutional trial of accelerated hypofractionated intensity-modulated radiation therapy for early-stage oropharyngeal cancer (RTOG 00-22). *Int J Radiat Oncol Biol Phys* 2010;76:1333–1338.

142. Fuller CD, Nijkamp J, Duppen JC, et al. Prospective randomized double-blind pilot study of site-specific consensus atlas implementation for rectal cancer target volume delineation in the cooperative group setting. *Int J Radiat Oncol Biol Phys* 2011;79:481–489.

143. Mavroidis P, Giantsoudis D, Awan MJ, et al. Consequences of anorectal cancer atlas implementation in the cooperative group setting: radiobiologic analysis of a prospective randomized in silico target delineation study. *Radiother Oncol* 2014;112:418–424.

144. Gillespie EF, Panjwani N, Golden DW, et al. Multi-institutional randomized trial testing the utility of an interactive three-dimensional contouring atlas among radiation oncology residents. *Int J Radiat Oncol Biol Phys* 2017;98:547–554.

145. Cui Y, Chen W, Kong FM, et al. Contouring variations and the role of atlas in non-small cell lung cancer radiation therapy: analysis of a multi-institutional preclinical trial planning study. *Pract Radiat Oncol* 2015;5:e67–e75.

146. Weber DC, Tomsej M, Melidis C, et al. QA makes a clinical trial stronger: evidence-based medicine in radiation therapy. *Radiother Oncol* 2012;105:4–8.

147. Lachin JM, Rosenberger WF. *Randomization in clinical trials: theory and practice*. 2nd ed. New York, NY: John Wiley & Sons, 2015.

148. Proschan MA, Lan F, Wittes JT. *Statistical monitoring of clinical trials: a uniform approach*. New York, NY: Springer, 2006.

149. Pocock SJ. Group sequential methods in the design and analysis of clinical trials. *Biometrika* 1977;64:191–199.

150. Lan K, DeMets D. Discrete sequential boundaries for clinical trials. *Biometrika* 1983;70:659–663.

151. Kaplan EL, Meier P. Nonparametric estimation from incomplete observations. *J Am Stat Assoc* 1958;53:457–481.

152. Jagsi R, Sheets N, Jankovic A, et al. Frequency, nature, effects, and correlates of conflicts of interest in published clinical cancer research. *Cancer* 2009;115:2783–2791.

153. Leite ETT, Moraes FY, Marta GN, et al. Trial sponsorship and self-reported conflicts of interest in breast cancer radiation therapy: an analysis of prospective clinical trials. *Breast* 2017;33:29–33.

154. Kesselheim AS, Robertson CT, Myers JA, et al. A randomized study of how physicians interpret research funding disclosures. *N Engl J Med* 2012;367:1119–1127.

155. Abdel-Wahab M, Zubizarreta E, Polo A, et al. Improving quality and access to radiation therapy—an IAEA perspective. *Semin Radiat Oncol* 2017;27:109–117.

156. Roa W, Kepka L, Kumar N, et al. International atomic energy agency randomized phase III study of radiation therapy in elderly and/or frail patients with newly diagnosed glioblastoma multiforme. *J Clin Oncol* 2015;33:4145–4150.

157. Rosenblatt E, Abdel-Wahab M, El-Gantiry M, et al. Brachytherapy boost in locoregionally advanced nasopharyngeal carcinoma: a prospective randomized trial of the International Atomic Energy Agency. *Radiat Oncol* 2014;9:67.

158. Schulz KF, Altman DG, Moher D. CONSORT statement: updated guidelines for reporting parallel group randomised trials. *BMJ* 2010;340:c332.

159. Berry DA. Adaptive trial design. *Clin Adv Hematol Oncol* 2007;5:522–524.

160. Koopmeiners JS, Modiano J. A Bayesian adaptive Phase I–II clinical trial for evaluating efficacy and toxicity with delayed outcomes. *Clin Trials* 2014;11(1):38–48. doi:10.1177/1740774513500589.

161. Pan H, Xie F, Liu P, et al. A phase I/II seamless dose escalation/expansion with adaptive randomization scheme (SEARS). *Clin Trials* 2014;11(1):49–59.

162. Ford I, Norrie J. Pragmatic trials. *N Engl J Med* 2016;375:454–463.

163. Thorpe KE, Zwarenstein M, Oxman AD, et al. A pragmatic-explanatory continuum indicator summary (PRECIS): a tool to help trial designers. *J Clin Epidemiol* 2009;62:464–475.

164. Loudon K, Treweek S, Sullivan F, et al. The PRECIS-2 tool: designing trials that are fit for purpose. *BMJ* 2015;350:h2147.

165. Zwarenstein M, Treweek S, Gagnier JJ, et al. Improving the reporting of pragmatic trials: an extension of the CONSORT statement. *BMJ* 2008;337:a2390.

166. Frobert O, Lagerqvist B, Olivecrona GK, et al. Thrombus aspiration during ST-segment elevation myocardial infarction. *N Engl J Med* 2013;369:1587–1597.

167. Porten SP, Cooperberg MR, Konety BR, et al. The example of CaPSURE: lessons learned from a national disease registry. *World J Urol* 2011;29:265–271.

168. Miller RS. CancerLinQ update. *J Oncol Pract* 2016;12:835–837.

169. Nyholm T, Olsson C, Agrup M, et al. A national approach for automated collection of standardized and population-based radiation therapy data in Sweden. *Radiother Oncol* 2016;119:344–350.

170. Early Breast Cancer Trialists' Collaborative Group; Darby S, McGale P, et al. Effect of radiotherapy after breast-conserving surgery on 10-year recurrence and 15-year breast cancer death: meta-analysis of individual patient data for 10,801 women in 17 randomised trials. *Lancet* 2011;378:1707–1716.

171. Pignon JP, le Maitre A, Maillard E, et al.; MACH-NC Collaborative Group. Meta-analysis of chemotherapy in head and neck cancer (MACH-NC): an update on 93 randomised trials and 17,346 patients. *Radiother Oncol* 2009;92:4–14.

172. Aerts HJ. The potential of radiomic-based phenotyping in precision medicine: a review. *JAMA Oncol* 2016;2:1636–1642.

173. Dolgin E. The mathematician versus the malignancy. *Nat Med* 2014;20:460–463.

174. Leder K, Pitter K, LaPlant Q, et al. Mathematical modeling of PDGF-driven glioblastoma reveals optimized radiation dosing schedules. *Cell* 2014;156:603–616.

175. Grassberger C, Scott JG, Paganetti H. Biomathematical optimization of radiation therapy in the era of targeted agents. *Int J Radiat Oncol Biol Phys* 2017;97:13–17.

176. Michor F, Beal K. Improving cancer treatment via mathematical modeling: surmounting the challenges is worth the effort. *Cell* 2015;163:1059–1063.

177. Takenaga K. Modification of the metastatic potential of tumor cells by drugs. *Cancer Metastasis Rev* 1986;5(2):67–75.

Section II

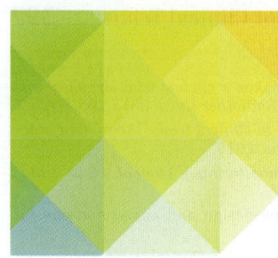

CHAPTER 16

Stem Cell Transplantation and Total-Body Irradiation

Sarah Jo Stephens, Kenneth B. Roberts, Zhe (Jay) Chen, Stuart Evan Seropian, and Chris R. Kelsey

INTRODUCTION

Historically, total-body irradiation (TBI) was used without stem cell support for palliation of radiation-sensitive diseases such as chronic lymphocytic leukemia and follicular lymphoma. Currently, TBI is primarily performed in the context of hematopoietic transplantation for its cytotoxic and immunologic effects. The patient's hematopoietic system is reconstituted after high-dose chemotherapy, with or without TBI, from either the patient's own stem cells (autologous) or stem cells from a donor (allogeneic). In the case of donor stem cells from an identical twin, the term syngeneic transplantation is appropriate. This chapter will also briefly address hemibody irradiation (HBI), which is occasionally utilized for palliation of diffuse metastatic disease. Stem cell support is not required in this setting.

RATIONALE FOR STEM CELL TRANSPLANTATION

Hematopoietic stem cell transplantation (SCT), while utilized in a variety of settings, is primarily pursued for patients with high-risk or relapsed/refractory hematologic malignancies to decrease the risk of disease recurrence. Multipotent stem cells have the capacity to differentiate into all blood cell lineages and can be obtained from several sources including bone marrow, peripheral blood, and umbilical cord blood. Stem cells can be harvested directly from the marrow or through apheresis of the peripheral blood following administration of granulocyte colony-stimulating factor (G-CSF). The conditioning regimen for hematopoietic SCT has several important functions and depends on the type of transplant—autologous (auto-SCT) or allogeneic (allo-SCT). For the former, the sole purpose of the conditioning regimen is cytotoxicity. For allogeneic transplants, the conditioning regimen also facilitates immunosuppression, so the host does not reject the donor stem cells, and to create space in the bone marrow for the graft. Conditioning regimens can consist of chemotherapy alone or a combination of chemotherapy and TBI.

Autologous Transplantation

Autologous transplantation relies upon higher doses of chemotherapy to overcome the resistance of malignant cells with subsequent reinfusion of stem cells to reconstitute the hematopoietic system. The most common indications for auto-SCT are multiple myeloma, relapsed diffuse large B-cell lymphoma, and relapsed Hodgkin lymphoma. Peripheral blood stem cells are the graft product of choice for auto-SCT and are associated with improvements in rates of engraftment, quality of life, and reduced cost when compared with cells derived from bone marrow.[1,2] Patients undergoing auto-SCT must be reasonably fit to tolerate high-dose chemotherapy/TBI. With modern supportive care and increasing experience with this procedure, the risk of mortality from auto-SCT is quite low (~1%).[3]

The timing of auto-SCT depends on the underlying disease. For most patients with relapsed aggressive lymphomas, auto-SCT is preceded by a salvage chemotherapy regimen. If the patient has chemotherapy-sensitive disease, ideally demonstrated by achievement of a negative positron emission tomography/computed tomography (PET-CT) scan, then the patient proceeds with high-dose chemotherapy and auto-SCT. The high-dose chemotherapy regimen is based on the underlying disease. For example, in the setting of relapsed Hodgkin lymphoma, BEAM (carmustine, etoposide, cytarabine, melphalan) or CBV (cyclophosphamide, carmustine, and etoposide) is often utilized. High-dose melphalan is the most common conditioning regimen for multiple myeloma.

When adjunctive radiotherapy is indicated, the optimal timing is not well characterized. Historically, radiotherapy has been given after auto-SCT, but there is increasing experience of giving it before. Some concern exists for radiation therapy (RT) to the chest prior to auto-SCT having an undue risk of pneumonitis, as initially reported by a Toronto group.[4] Other investigators, such as from Memorial Sloan Kettering Cancer Center, dispute this and prefer to give RT prior to high-dose therapy and transplant.[5]

Allogeneic Transplantation

As opposed to auto-SCT, which relies completely on cytotoxicity from high-dose chemotherapy/TBI to eradicate persistent tumor clones, allo-SCT relies in part on an immunologic graft-versus-tumor effect to eradicate malignant cells. The most common indication for allo-SCT is high-risk and relapsed acute leukemia, particularly acute myelogenous leukemia (AML) and acute lymphocytic leukemia (ALL). Allo-SCT may be preceded by full-dose (myeloablative) conditioning designed to have maximal antitumor effect and also to condition the patient for the infusion of the donor cells as an immunologic therapy. Increasingly, allo-SCT is preceded by a nonmyeloablative or reduced intensity conditioning program. In this latter situation, the major antitumor effect is postulated to derive from the infused donor stem cells, and the intensity of the condition regimen is modified to allow the procedure in patient populations previously ineligible because of age or medical condition. Nonmyeloablative allogeneic transplants are associated with lower treatment-related morbidity compared with myeloablative allogeneic transplants.[6,7] Most transplant centers utilize peripheral blood progenitor cells, as opposed to bone marrow, for allo-SCT.

Thus, allo-SCT is largely an immunologic therapy. Allogeneic hematopoietic cells must be matched with the recipient for the majority of the major histocompatibility antigens to avoid rejection and minimize graft versus host disease (GVHD). Differences in minor human leukocyte antigens (HLA) facilitate the graft-versus-tumor effect that enhances transplantation efficacy. Early studies demonstrated improved leukemia control with allogeneic bone marrow cells as compared to syngeneic (identical twin) donor cells.[8] Further evidence for graft-versus-tumor effect derives from the efficacy of donor lymphocyte infusions after relapse of leukemia following allo-SCT.[9,10]

Despite HLA matching, allo-SCT is limited by GVHD. GVHD results from the release of inflammatory cytokines as a result of activation of mature donor T cells that recognize recipient HLA alloantigens, presented as peptide molecules by antigen-presenting cells (APCs). Normally, mature T cells express "tolerance" to these peptides derived from self-proteins because of thymic depletion or peripheral suppression of autoreactive T cells.[11] However, in the setting of allo-SCT, despite HLA matching, a repertoire of peptides displayed on recipient cells can be recognized as minor histocompatibility antigens by donor T cells because of polymorphisms in genes outside of the HLA system.[12] The activation of donor T cells after contact with specialized APCs leads to differentiation to effector cells that produce cytokines such as interferon gamma (IFN-γ) and tumor necrosis factor (TNF) as well as mediate cytotoxicity against normal recipient organs. Acute GVHD includes clinical damage to the skin, GI tract, and liver, but other organs can also be involved. GVHD may evolve, or develop de novo, later after transplantation with distinct clinical features resembling sporadic autoimmune diseases (termed chronic GVHD). Common presentations include sicca syndrome, sclerotic or lichenoid skin disease, and immune hepatitis. Fasciitis/myositis and bronchiolitis obliterans syndrome (BOS) are less common presentations, which may cause significant morbidity.

Despite the prophylactic use of immunosuppressive agents such as cyclosporine, tacrolimus, methotrexate, sirolimus, and mycophenolate mofetil, HLA-matched sibling hematopoietic transplants result in some degree of GVHD in approximately 60% of patients.[13,14] Increased immunosuppression may ameliorate symptoms from GVHD but may also abrogate the graft-versus-tumor effect and place patients at higher risk for posttransplant infections.[15] Acute GVHD can be effectively prevented by T-cell depletion of the donor cells prior to stem cell infusion, but this may also lead to an increased risk for infections as well as the concern that the desirable graft-versus-tumor effects will be diminished or lost. Nevertheless, there has been clinical success with T-cell–depleted allo-SCT in reducing GVHD. Such techniques require more intensive immunosuppression to prevent graft rejection and therefore often employ TBI in the conditioning regimens.[16,17]

Myeloablative Allogeneic Stem Cell Transplantation

TBI has been a central part of allo-SCT for leukemias since the pioneering work of Thomas and associates beginning in the late 1950s. Historically, a single dose of 10 Gy utilizing a low dose rate (~10 cGy/min) was used. The premise that TBI had to be given as a single fraction was challenged in the late 1970s when Peters et al. demonstrated the marked sensitivity of most normal tissues to altered fractionation and dose rate with minimal effects on bone marrow progenitors and leukemic cells.[18,19] It was concluded that with the same total dose, an improved therapeutic ratio would be expected from a reduction in the dose rate of single-fraction TBI or by TBI fractionation. Calculations of various fractionation schemes and dose rates have been published based on the linear quadratic model.[20–22] O'Donoghue et al. calculated that for very low dose rate single-fraction TBI to be equivalent radiobiologically to the more common fractionated TBI schedules, an unreasonable radiation time of 20 to 24 hours would be necessary.[22] With concepts of both radiobiology and practicality in mind, a large variety of fractionated TBI schedules have been used. After a generation of clinical investigation, no one regimen is clearly superior to another. Currently, most myeloablative TBI programs use a twice or three times a day fractionation scheme over 3 to 5 days to deliver a total dose of 12 to 15 Gy.

Nonmyeloablative or Reduced Intensity Allogeneic Stem Cell Transplantation

In the past decade, growing recognition of the immunotherapeutic potential of allografts has led to a reconsideration of the need for high-dose myeloablative conditioning regimens traditionally administered prior to transplantation.

Pioneering work of Storb et al. and others in canine models established that highly immunosuppressive, but nonmyeloablative, regimens could establish stable mixed hematopoietic chimerism in major histocompatibility complex–matched littermates using one-sixth of the usual ablative dose of TBI in combination with postgrafting immunosuppressive drugs.[23,24] Subsequently, numerous clinical trials have established that a spectrum of subablative conditioning regimens of varying intensity may allow engraftment of donor cells with reduction in transplant-related toxicity, permitting transplantation of patients traditionally excluded from allo-SCT because of age or medical comorbidities.[25,26] The primary purpose of a nonmyeloablative preparatory regimen is to suppress the patient's immune system sufficiently to allow the engraftment of donor cells with minimal host toxicity. The graft-versus-tumor effect is relied upon to eradicate tumor cells.

Common to these regimens is sufficient immunosuppression to overcome host resistance to engraftment using either antimetabolites such as fludarabine, TBI, or both, in combination with other agents. Other factors, such as patient age, HLA disparity with the donor, tumor burden, and prior therapy may also affect the degree of engraftment. A series from the Seattle transplant group, for example, demonstrated that a single 2-Gy fraction of TBI, in combination with postgrafting cyclosporine and mycophenolate, is sufficient to achieve a high rate of donor engraftment in patients with a prior history of auto-SCT, but additional immunosuppression in the form of fludarabine is necessary to assure engraftment in less heavily pretreated patients or patients receiving unrelated donor grafts.[27]

Reduced intensity transplants now account for roughly 25% of all allo-SCTs. Efficacy is difficult to evaluate in the absence of randomized trials, but reduced intensity conditioning regimens have allowed for an expanded use of transplants in high-risk populations. As an example, elderly patients with acute leukemias in first remission have long-term survival rates over 40% with reduced intensity transplants, which would be considered a remarkable achievement compared to historical experience in which very few patients would be expected to survive.[28] Toxicity is significantly lower than traditional myeloablative transplants. The Seattle group has reported a 1-year non–relapse-related mortality of allo-SCT of 30% for ablative regimens compared to 16% for reduced intensity conditioning regimens ($P = .04$).[29] The toxicity of a single-fraction 2-Gy TBI, for example, should be minimal. Most transplant centers delivering this dose of TBI would dispense with the complexities of lung blocks as well as compensating filters for dose homogeneity.

PURPOSES OF CONDITIONING

The purpose of high-dose chemotherapy, with or without TBI, prior to auto-SCT is simply to give a higher intensity of treatment to overcome intrinsic tumor resistance, thereby decreasing the risk of a relapse. The purpose of conditioning in the setting of allo-SCT is more complex and serves three key functions: (a) to provide sufficient immunosuppression in the recipient to prevent rejection of the graft, (b) to create space in the bone marrow for donor stem cells, and (c) to provide further cytoreduction to achieve a minimal residual disease state prior to transplant. Myeloablative regimens address all three whereas reduced-intensity regimens provide immunosuppression and create space for the donor stem cells but with variable, and lesser degrees of, further cytoreduction.

The choice of conditioning regimen prior to transplantation depends upon a variety of factors that include the type of transplant (allogeneic vs. autologous), conditioning intensity (myeloablative vs. nonmyeloablative), disease type (AML vs. ALL), expected patient tolerance, and disease status.

TBI-Based Conditioning Regimens

There is wide variability between centers in regard to the techniques utilized for TBI including total dose, fractionation scheme, dose rate, lung shielding, and patient positioning (see below for further discussion). Some aspects have been formally evaluated with randomized studies, whereas many others have not.

In regard to total dose, two randomized trials have compared 12 Gy versus 15.75 Gy in patients with AML and chronic myelogenous leukemia (CML). In the AML study, patients randomized to the higher-dose arm were noted to have improved relapse-free survival (RFS) (P = .06) but at the cost of increased transplant-related mortality (P = .04) and moderate to severe GVHD (P = .02).[30] There was no difference in overall survival (OS). In the CML series, a disease that is rarely transplanted anymore given the efficacy of tyrosine kinase inhibitors, the investigators also noted improvement in RFS (P = .008) with a nonsignificant trend toward increased transplant-related mortality (P = .13) and moderate to severe GVHD (P = .15) in patients receiving the 15.75-Gy regimen.[31] As OS was not improved in either study, more moderate total doses seem preferable.

Several studies have evaluated single-fraction compared with multifraction regimens. Deeg et al. evaluated 75 patients with acute nonlymphoblastic leukemia in first remission. The first 22 patients enrolled on the study received 9.2 Gy in a single fraction at 4 to 6 cGy/min utilizing opposed cobalt sources. The remaining patients were randomized to either 10 Gy in a single fraction or 12 Gy in 6 fractions. Survival was improved in the patients receiving either 9.2 Gy in a single fraction or 12 Gy in 6 fractions compared to 10 Gy in a single fraction (P = .04). There was an increase in early toxicity, particularly veno-occlusive disease or sinusoidal obstructive syndrome (VOD/SOS), in patients receiving 10 Gy in a single fraction. Pneumonitis appeared more common in single fraction (both 10 Gy and 9.2 Gy) compared to the fractionated regimen.[32] Girinsky et al. randomized 160 patients to either 10-Gy single-fraction (12.5 cGy/min instantaneous dose rate, 4.5 cGy/min average dose rate) or hyperfractionated TBI to 14.85 Gy in 11 fractions (25 cGy/min instantaneous dose rate). They noted no difference in OS or cause-specific survival. There was an increase in incidence of VOD/SOS in patients who received single-fraction TBI (P = .044).[33] In a study from the Hôspital Tenon in Paris, 157 patients were randomized to single-fraction TBI with variable dose rate (6 vs. 15 cGy/min) or fractionated TBI with variable dose rate (3 vs. 6 cGy/min). No significant differences were noted between the single-fraction and fractionated TBI schedules, or by dose rate.[34] The preponderance of data favors a fractionated regimen using a low dose rate approach.

The choice of chemotherapy agents used in conjunction with TBI depends on the underlying disease. For AML, and in many other settings, high-dose cyclophosphamide is utilized given its effectiveness in both immunosuppression and cytotoxicity. A typical dose is 120 mg/kg over 2 days. In other settings, agents such as etoposide, melphalan, and fludarabine are combined with TBI. Reduced intensity or nonmyeloablative transplant regimens using low-dose TBI are often combined with fludarabine.[35]

Chemotherapy and TBI are given sequentially rather than concurrently to avoid any potential increase in normal tissue toxicity. Whether chemotherapy should be given before or after TBI is unclear. One study of 1,769 patients undergoing myeloablative allo-SCT for acute leukemia did not show any differences in outcomes with cyclophosphamide given before or after TBI.[36] Typically, TBI over 3 to 5 days is best delivered during the regular work week, when the full technical support staff is available. TBI may be better tolerated if given first when the patient is less fatigued and not experiencing the side effects of chemotherapy. The risk of nosocomial infections may be marginally lower when the patient travels to the radiotherapy department before becoming neutropenic later in the conditioning course. Alternatively, TBI at the end of the preparative regimen allows the stem cell transplant to proceed immediately thereafter. Unlike chemotherapy, there is no washout period needed for TBI, theoretically decreasing the time the patient spends neutropenic prior to engraftment.

Chemotherapy-Alone Conditioning Regimens

Although the evolution of TBI has led to significant reduction in toxicities, the initial concern about the risk of fatal radiation pneumonitis led to the development of non-TBI regimens. For example, Santos at Johns Hopkins and other groups began administering busulfan in place of radiotherapy.[37] These approaches were initially developed for use in the auto-SCT setting but have been expanded for use in the allo-SCT, as well. The hope was that these regimens would result in less toxicity compared to TBI-containing regimens. In addition, conditioning with chemotherapy alone can be used in practice settings where TBI is unavailable. Combinations have been developed based on biologic activity of a particular drug, drug tolerability, and nonoverlapping drug toxicities. The most commonly used ablative regimens to condition patients with AML are the combination of busulfan and cyclophosphamide (BuCy) or busulfan and fludarabine.[38,39] A regimen utilizing carmustine, etoposide, cytosine arabinoside, and melphalan (BEAM) or carmustine, etoposide, and cyclophosphamide is commonly used to treat patients with non-Hodgkin and Hodgkin lymphoma.[40] Single-agent high-dose melphalan is also used frequently prior to auto-SCT for treatment of multiple myeloma. For patients with aplastic anemia, the combination of cyclophosphamide and antithymocyte globulin is often used for immunosuppression while avoiding excessive myelotoxicity.[41] There is interfacility variation in dosing and drug delivery schedules making it somewhat difficult to make direct comparisons between these regimens.

Most of the initial trials using BuCy used high-dose oral busulfan, which has highly variable pharmacokinetics, poor gastrointestinal tolerability, high rates of VOD/SOS, and increased frequency of seizures.[42] An intravenous formulation of busulfan has been developed, which is much better tolerated, has more predictable pharmacokinetics, and has been associated with less toxicity.[43] Some chemotherapy agents are associated with pulmonary toxicity, which may be a significant issue in patients with a prior history of chest radiotherapy.[44,45]

TBI-Based Versus Chemotherapy-Alone Conditioning Regimens

Randomized studies comparing chemotherapy-alone conditioning regimens to TBI-based regimens are few, often enrolled multiple leukemia subtypes, included a variety of patients (e.g., first complete remission, relapse, etc.), and used antiquated TBI and chemotherapy platforms. These limitations make it difficult to reach firm conclusions.

A French randomized trial compared BuCy to TBI-Cy before allo-SCT for adult AML in first remission.[46] TBI-Cy was superior for disease-free survival (DFS) (P < .01), leukemia relapse (P < .04), and transplant mortality (P < .06). Long-term follow-up also demonstrated worse OS and leukemia-free survival (LFS) in the patients receiving BuCy compared to TBI-Cy, felt to be the result of higher transplant-related mortality and relapse rates.[47]

Bunin et al. published a randomized series of patients with ALL treated with either etoposide–cyclophosphamide–TBI or etoposide–BuCy. The authors found an improvement in event-free survival (P = .03) for patients in the TBI arm.[48]

A randomized study from the Southwest Oncology Group (SWOG 8612) compared fractionated TBI plus etoposide versus high-dose BuCy in patients who had failed prior conventional therapy for ALL, AML, or CML. Patients were stratified as "good risk" (second complete remission for acute leukemia or accelerated phase CML) or "poor risk" (more advanced stages of leukemia). There was no difference noted in OS or DFS between the two treatment groups.[49]

Ringdén et al. of the Nordic Bone Marrow Transplantation Group compared BuCy to TBI-Cy in patients with AML, CML, and ALL. Patients treated with BuCy had higher rates of VOD/SOS ($P = .009$), hemorrhagic cystitis ($P = .003$), transplant-related mortality in those with advanced disease ($P = .002$), seizures ($P = .03$), high-grade chronic GVHD ($P = .04$), and death associated with GVHD ($P = .003$). There were similar rates of acute GVHD between the two groups. RFS was similar upon analysis of all patients, but in the subgroup of adult patients ($P = .05$) and advanced disease ($P = .005$), TBI-containing regimen appeared superior.[50] Long-term follow-up of this study demonstrated a 7-year relapse rate of 29% in both groups. In patients with advanced disease, there was a significant increase in transplant-related mortality in patients who received BuCy ($P = .004$). There was no difference in LFS in patients with early disease, but there was an improvement in LFS in patients with advanced disease receiving TBI ($P < .01$).[51]

A randomized trial from the French Society of Bone Marrow Graft (SFGM), which also evaluated the impact of single fraction versus fractionated TBI, showed no difference in overall 5-year survival or DFS for patients with CML treated with BuCy versus TBI-Cy.[52] Similarly, the study by Clift et al. showed no significant difference for 3 year OS, relapse, event-free survival, or speed of engraftment for BuCy versus TBI-Cy for CML.[53]

Socié et al. published long-term follow-up of 4 randomized controlled trials. For patients with AML, there was a strong trend toward improved survival ($P = .068$) and DFS ($P = .051$) with TBI-Cy.[54] A meta-analysis by Hartman et al. evaluated 5 prospective randomized control trials with 652 patients treated from 1966 to 1996 and showed trends not reaching statistical significance in favor of TBI for both OS and DFS.[55] Another meta-analysis by Shi-Xia et al. evaluated 18 trials with a total of 3,172 patients. For patients with ALL or AML, TBI-Cy was associated with lower rates of leukemia relapse, lower transplant-related mortality, and higher rates of DFS. However, for patients with CML, the TBI-Cy regimen was associated with higher rates of leukemia relapse, lower transplant-related mortality, and similar DFS. The risk for cataracts ($P = .01$), pneumonitis, and growth/developmental problems ($P = .008$) was higher with a TBI-containing regimen. Alternatively, the risk of VOD/SOS ($P < .00001$), hemorrhagic cystitis, and transplant-related mortality appeared higher for patients treated with BuCy.[56]

Given the conflicting randomized studies, a number of retrospective series, most using registry data, have evaluated TBI-based versus chemotherapy-alone conditioning regimens in AML. The majority of retrospective analyses demonstrate equivalent outcomes when comparing oral busulfan-containing regimens compared to TBI-Cy.[57–60] A single-institution retrospective series from Duke showed superior LFS and OS in patients with AML treated with TBI-Cy compared to BuCy, at the expense of increased pulmonary toxicity.[61] Intravenous busulfan has the added advantage of better tolerability and pharmacokinetics. The data are inconsistent whether intravenous busulfan with cyclophosphamide is more effective than TBI-Cy regimens.[57,62,63]

To summarize, limited randomized data, with obvious limitations, have not demonstrated any difference in outcomes with TBI and non–TBI-based regimens for CML. For ALL, TBI appears to be an important component of the conditioning regimen. For AML, the available randomized studies and meta-analyses favor TBI-Cy, though this is controversial given negative findings from nonrandomized registry studies (Table 16.1).

TABLE 16.1 CONDITIONING REGIMENS FOR AML				
Study	**N**	**Conditioning Regimen**	**Leukemia-Free Survival**	**Comments**
Randomized Trials				
Blaise et al.[47]	101	TBI–Cy	55%	PO busulfan
		BuCy	35% ($P = .02$)	
SWOG 8612[49]	122	TBI-etoposide	NS ($P = .69$)[a]	PO busulfan
		BuCy		
Ringdén et al.[51]	69	TBI–Cy	56%	PO busulfan
		BuCy	59% ($P = .7$)	Increased incidence of VOD/SOS, hemorrhagic cystitis, chronic GVHD, and obstructive bronchiolitis with BuCy. Cataracts more frequent with TBI/Cy[a]
Meta-Analysis				
Socié et al.[54]	172	TBI–Cy	57%	PO busulfan
		BuCy	47% ($P = .051$)	
Shi-Xia et al.[56]	1,289	TBI–Cy	OR 1.49 (1.01, 2.20) in favor of TBI	PO busulfan
		BuCy		Higher rates of cataracts, interstitial pneumonitis, and developmental problems for patients receiving TBI–Cy. Higher rates of VOD/SOS and hemorrhagic cystitis in patients receiving BuCy
Registry Studies				
Nagler et al.[57]	1,659	TBI–Cy	64%	Intravenous busulfan
		BuCy	61% ($P = .27$)	Lower incidence of acute GVHD (grades 2–4) and chronic GVHD in IV BuCy group
Copelan et al.[62]	1,230	TBI–Cy	RR 0.70 (0.55, 0.88)	Examined both IV and PO busulfan formulations
		BuCy	($P = .003$) in favor of IV busulfan	No statistically significant difference between oral busulfan and TBI-based regimens
Litzow et al.[59]	581	TBI–Cy	58%	PO busulfan
		BuCy	54% ($P = .438$)	Higher rates of VOD/SOS with busulfan-based regimen
Ringdén et al.[60]	824	TBI–Cy	66%	PO busulfan
		BuCy	64% (NS)	Higher rates of VOD/SOS and hemorrhagic cystitis with busulfan-based regimen
Institutional Series				
Stephens et al.[61]	206	Cy-TBI	43%	PO busulfan
		BuCy	30% ($P = .12$)	LFS improved with Cy-TBI on multivariate analysis. Higher rates of pulmonary toxicity in TBI-based regimen

ALL, acute lymphocytic leukemia; AML, acute myelogenous leukemia; Bu, busulfan; CML, chronic myelogenous leukemia; Cy, cyclophosphamide; DFS, disease-free survival; LFS, leukemia-free survival; TBI, total-body irradiation.
[a]Included data from patients with ALL/CML.

The side effect profile of different conditioning regimens is also an important consideration. Although there can be significant overlap in treatment-related toxicities between chemotherapy and TBI-based conditioning regimens, such as fatigue and nausea, some toxicities are more common with one modality versus another. Although both chemotherapy and TBI can cause lung toxicity, TBI-based regimens appear to be associated with a higher risk of pneumonitis and other lung complications.[46,50,54,55] Prior thoracic radiotherapy may increase the risk of fatal pneumonitis. One study demonstrated a 32% risk of fatal pneumonitis after TBI in patients with prior chest radiation doses above 20 Gy.[64] Avoiding TBI may be prudent in such patients. One contemporary series of allo-SCT documented a 33% risk of severe pulmonary toxicity after TBI-based conditioning, with the number of prior chemotherapy regimens being the only independent risk factor for lung toxicity.[65] Cataracts and endocrine deficiencies are also more common with TBI.

In contrast, hepatic VOD/SOS[66] and hemorrhagic cystitis are more common with BuCy.[55,67] The Nordic Bone Marrow Transplantation showed a VOD/SOS incidence of 12% in patients treated with busulfan compared to 1% for the TBI-treated patients ($P = .009$). Hemorrhagic cystitis risk was 24% for busulfan-based therapy versus 8% for TBI ($P = .002$).[50] Oral busulfan-conditioning regimens also have an appreciable risk for seizures.[68]

A relative advantage in using TBI for SCT is that the dose delivery throughout the body is highly controllable. In contrast to chemotherapy, dose distribution is independent of such factors as blood supply, and there are no concerns about agent activation, metabolism, excretion, or dose modifications based on liver or kidney function. TBI may also reach chemotherapy sanctuary sites, which is of particular concern in patients at risk for testicular or CNS involvement.

GRAFT FAILURE

Failure to engraft is a potential life-threatening complication of allo-SCT. Historically, approximately 6% of patients fail to engraft with myeloablative conditioning.[69] Given the expanded use of alternative donor transplants and nonmyeloablative regimens, more recent estimates of failure to engraft are between 12% and 15%.[70-72] Not surprisingly, graft failure is associated with worse outcomes.[73] For those patients who fail to engraft, salvage allo-SCT with a TBI-based regimen is possible. Several small, single-institution studies have described using a nonablative regimen in this setting,[74-76] although use of a second myeloablative regimen has also been described.[77] Second myeloablative transplants are generally associated with increased risk of severe toxicity. Reduced intensity regimens can be used to escalate host immunosuppression and increase the probability of successful engraftment.[78]

TOTAL-BODY IRRADIATION—RADIOBIOLOGY

Radiobiologic Effects on the Normal Hematopoietic System

Successful hematopoietic stem cell engraftment requires (a) eradication of the recipient bone marrow, (b) immunosuppression to prevent rejection of donor stem cells in the case of an allo-SCT, and (c) relative sparing of the recipient's bone marrow stromal cells. The use of the classic radiobiologic parameter D_0 gives a rough indication of the radiosensitivity of various cell populations. The reported D_0 values of bone marrow stem cells usually range from 0.5 to 1.4 Gy, indicating intrinsic radiosensitivity.[79,80] Although conventional wisdom assumes that recipient marrow cells must be removed to leave space for donor cells in the stem cell microenvironment to favor competitive repopulation, this concept has been

challenged. In fact, mixed bone marrow chimerism resulting from less cytotoxic, nonmyeloablative transplantation may be acceptable or even desirable.

Immunosuppression in the setting of allo-SCT is necessary to avoid rejection of donor stem cells. TBI is a very efficient immunosuppressant. In animal work by Storb and colleagues, equivalent doses of fractionated TBI were significantly less effective than single-dose TBI to condition dog leukocyte antigen (DLA)-identical littermate dogs before bone marrow transplantation.[24,81] The investigators concluded that significant repair of DNA damage by lymphoid cells occurs during interfraction intervals. In a murine model, Salamon et al. looked at 3 TBI schemas from schedules that had been developed for human TBI therapy (8.5-Gy single-fraction TBI, 2 Gy × 6 fractions of TBI, and 1.2 Gy × 12 fractions of hyperfractionated TBI).[82] In terms of the immunosuppressive effects, the results favored single-fraction TBI. A marked initial shoulder on the dose survival curve has been reported for T-lymphocyte precursors[83] and for a human lymphoblastoid cell line.[84] The immunosuppressive effects of TBI show marked fractionation sensitivity, leading one to conclude fractionated TBI might be associated with more graft rejections than the same dose delivered in a single fraction.

If bone marrow stromal cells and their progenitors (colony-forming unit fibroblasts) are damaged, delayed engraftment or even graft failure may follow.[85] Progenitors of human bone marrow stromal cells have been found to have a D_0 of 1.46 Gy.[86] They are also sensitive to dose rate effects and fractionation. Thus, fractionated TBI spares bone marrow stromal cells and their progenitors better than does single-fraction TBI.[87]

Radiobiologic Effects on Leukemia

In the setting of SCT, TBI achieves significant leukemia cell killing in conjunction with chemotherapy and the subsequent graft-versus-tumor effect, leading to eradication of malignant clones in a significant portion of cases. Most D_0 values for both animal and human leukemia cell lines range from 0.8 to 1.5 Gy,[88-91] although extreme values range from 0.3 to >5 Gy. Leukemic cell lines frequently show a minimal initial shoulder in radiation cell survival curves, leading to the hypothesis that fractionation (or reduced dose rate exposure) should have only a minor effect on cell survival. Split-dose radiation experiments lend further support to this hypothesis. Greater repair capacity is seen with more differentiated leukemias or lymphocytes (e.g., B- or T-cell phenotypes).

TOTAL-BODY IRRADIATION—TECHNIQUES AND DOSIMETRY

Basic Requirements

Historically, radiation oncologists have aimed to deliver a relatively homogenous dose of TBI throughout the whole body given the concern that leukemias are systemically distributed. Because microscopic disease burden during remission may not be uniform throughout the body, the importance of homogeneous dose delivery is unclear. Some TBI programs use photon energies above 20 MV, which may theoretically deliver higher marrow doses because of increased pair production and higher bone absorption.[92] Many correct for skin-sparing effects of megavoltage irradiation with the use of beam spoilers, although this is probably not necessary for low-energy photons in the absence of leukemia cutis or a tropism for skin involvement such as in monocytic leukemias. Where there is concern for a higher burden of disease, boost radiation fields may be added to TBI. Augmented doses of radiation may be delivered to the brain in the setting of CNS involvement or to the testes in males with ALL, for example.

To ensure the planned dose distribution is accurately delivered, all TBI techniques must undergo a rigorous and comprehensive dosimetric characterization. Because of large variations in body geometry and tissue density between patients, it is recommended that dose homogeneity remain within a specified window of ±10% of the prescribed dose, though ±5% is typically attainable. For TBI and HBI, there is evidence that a 5% change in lung dose could result in 20% change in the incidence of radiation pneumonitis, a complication that is sometimes fatal.[93,94] Therefore, the basic dosimetry of TBI (and HBI) techniques should be performed as precise as readily achievable. Accurate dosimetry coupled with an effective quality assurance program, including adjustments to dose delivery after *in vivo* measurements on the first day of treatment, will ensure not only safe delivery of TBI treatments but also accurate dosimetry data for meaningful dose–response analysis. Once a patient begins a course of TBI, within a comprehensive conditioning program, the timing of successive fractions becomes critical to the outcome of the procedure. It is imperative to have a backup TBI system either within the same institution or in a nearby radiation therapy department when establishing a TBI program. When the primary system is down, a fully commissioned backup TBI system can be utilized to complete the remaining treatments.

Total-Body Irradiation Techniques

Many TBI techniques have been described, and improvements in both the irradiation technique and physical dosimetry continue.[95–98] Much of the early clinical experience with TBI was obtained at centers with facilities designed specifically for large-field irradiation.[99] Although a few dedicated systems still exist, current TBI procedures are largely performed with techniques established on linear accelerators that are also used for conventional radiotherapy. Common to these TBI techniques is the use of radiation fields that are larger than the maximum field size (~40 by 40 cm) available at standard source-to-surface distance (SSD) by treating TBI patients at extended SSDs of 200 to 600 cm. For treatment rooms large enough to accommodate an SSD of 5 m or more, a single square field at maximum collimator opening is usually sufficient to completely encompass patients of typical height placed along the diagonal of the field (Fig. 16.1A–E). At shorter SSDs, multiple

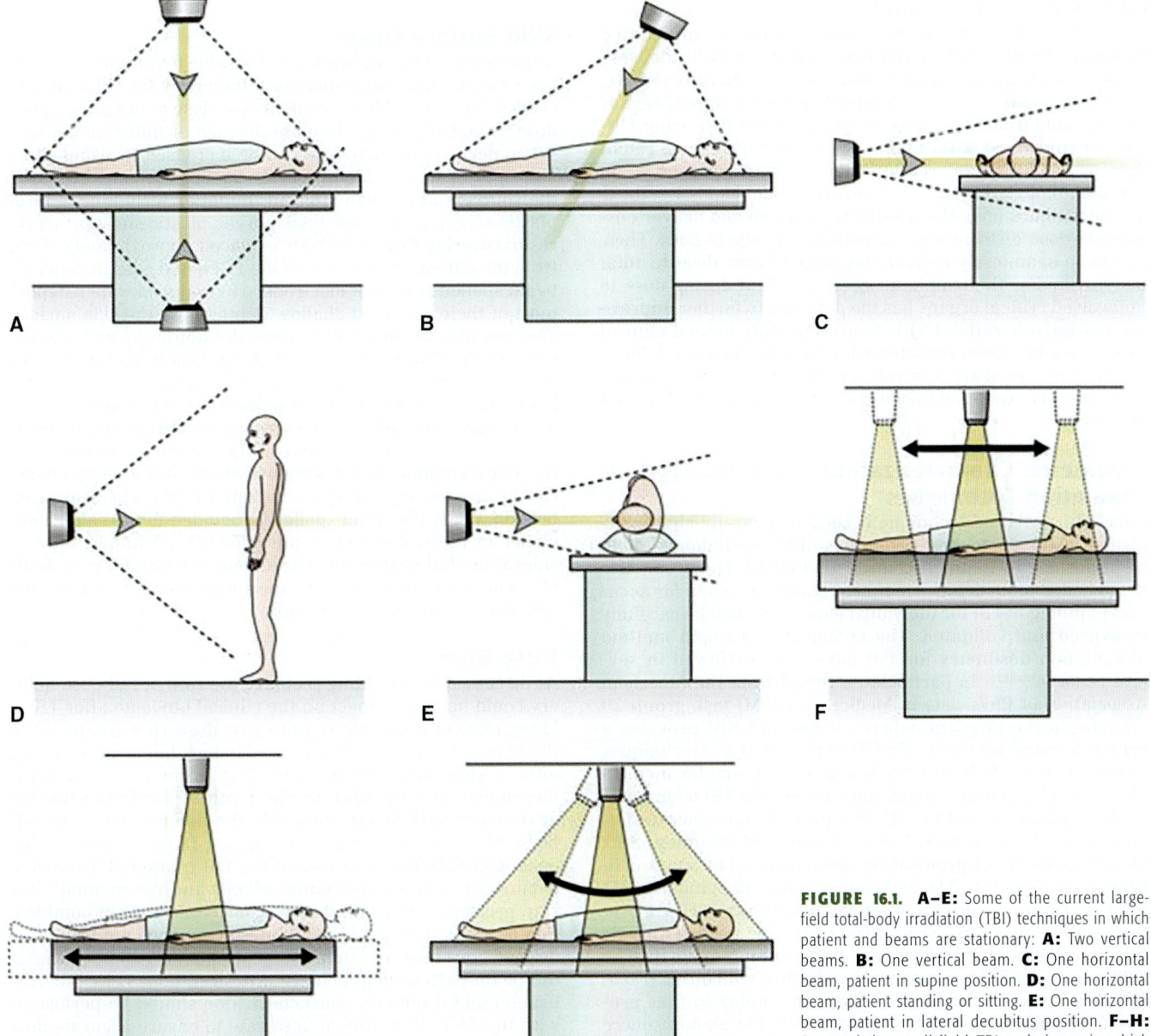

FIGURE 16.1. **A–E:** Some of the current large-field total-body irradiation (TBI) techniques in which patient and beams are stationary: **A:** Two vertical beams. **B:** One vertical beam. **C:** One horizontal beam, patient in supine position. **D:** One horizontal beam, patient standing or sitting. **E:** One horizontal beam, patient in lateral decubitus position. **F–H:** Some of the small-field TBI techniques in which patient or beam moves. **F:** Source scans horizontally. **G:** Patient moves horizontally. **H:** Sweeping beam.

abutting fields may be necessary, and irradiation of the whole body can be achieved by translating the radiation field[100] or the patient[101] or by sweeping the radiation field over a stationary patient (Fig. 16.1F–H).[102] For these irradiation techniques, patients are typically treated with two parallel-opposed fields. When a single radiation source is used, this can be accomplished by rotating the patient 180 degrees along the patient's longitudinal axis between the two fields. In a dedicated system with two radiation sources mounted opposite to each other, the treatment can be accomplished by irradiating the two fields simultaneously without changing the patient's position. Various patient positions, ranging from sitting, standing upright, to lying horizontally in a supine or lateral decubitus positions, have been used (Fig. 16.1A–H).

The technique using a single large field encompassing the entire patient at extended SSD is by far the simplest and the most prevalent TBI technique used today. The treatment is typically delivered with a horizontal field directed toward the primary shielding wall. It eliminates the dosimetry complications occurring in the junctions of multiple abutting fields. It also alleviates the concern that cells circulating through the body may potentially receive a reduced dose when abutting fields are delivered sequentially.

Recently, with the introduction of intensity-modulated radiation therapy (IMRT) and other advanced IMRT delivery systems, such as volumetric modulated arc therapy (VMAT) on conventional linear accelerators and spiral TomoTherapy on dedicated treatment units, the possibility of delivering TBI-type treatments at SSDs similar to that of conventional radiotherapy has been explored by several research groups.[96–98] In addition to obviating the need for using extended SSDs, these new techniques open the possibility to design and deliver customized dose distributions throughout the whole body. Their ability to seamlessly deliver integrated boost dose to total marrow and/or the lymphatic system while reducing dose to uninvolved critical organs has the potential to further improve the therapeutic ratio of TBI. At present, only limited clinical experience has been reported with these techniques.[103] More carefully designed and controlled clinical testing of these new techniques is needed to fully establish their clinical utility and efficacy.

Dosimetric Characterization of Total-Body Irradiation Techniques

Once an irradiation technique is chosen, a careful characterization of the dosimetric properties of the technique should be performed by a qualified medical physicist. The dosimetric data needed to model the treatment planning system for accurate planning of TBI for individual patients should be carefully measured and validated. The technical issues and method of radiation dosimetry for TBI have been reviewed in several reports.[99,104,105] In particular, a report from the American Association of Physicists in Medicine (AAPM) task group 29 (TG-29) on the physical aspects of TBI and HBI provides a comprehensive discussion on dosimetry issues and techniques specific to large-field TBI.[99] It is a good resource for medical physicists charged to commission a large-field TBI technique.

Since publication of the TG-29 report, the reference dosimetry protocol for external beams at standard treatment SSD, known as the TG-21 protocol, has been updated by a new calibration protocol (TG-51). For photon beams at standard SSD, the TG-51 protocol produces similar results as the TG-21 protocol. However, the TG-51 protocol cannot be applied directly for large fields at extended SSD as encountered in TBI. The calibration of a TBI beam can be established with direct traceability to TG-51 by using an approach similar to that proposed by Curran et al.[106] In this approach, the photon source of the TBI beam is first calibrated under the TG-51 reference condition at standard SSD. The dose per unit beam-on time at a reference point of the TBI beam under TBI treatment conditions is then related to the dose per unit beam-on time of the same photon source at the TG-51 reference point by a correction factor that accounts for the TBI setup geometry and scattering conditions. This correction factor, as well as the relative dose factors that characterize the spatial distribution of the TBI beam, such as the percent depth dose (PDD) or tissue maximum ratio (TMR) along the central axis, can be measured directly under the TBI treatment conditions using a phantom with size similar to that of a typical patient. In-phantom off-axis beam profiles at various depths, especially along the diagonal near the corners of the field, should also be measured at TBI treatment distances to evaluate the dose variation across the radiation beam. Independent verification of the TBI calibration should be performed after the initial commissioning. The modeling of the treatment planning system should also be verified on an anthropomorphic phantom.[107–109] A thermoluminescent dosimeter calibrated on an independent linear accelerator can be used to verify TBI calibration and doses at other points of interest. Ion chamber and film may be used to assess dose distributions.[110]

Skin Surface Dose

Although skin sparing is often a desirable feature of megavoltage irradiation in conventional radiotherapy, for TBI, it may be desirable to have skin surface receive close to full prescription dose as leukemia may circulate through or infiltrate the skin. When needed, the skin dose can be increased by using either bolus placed on the skin or a beam spoiler positioned between the source and the patient.[111] In the latter technique, a large plastic screen (e.g., 2-cm-thick acrylic plastic sheet or acrylic resin) covering the whole body is placed approximately 10 cm from the patient. As photons of the TBI beam pass through the beam spoiler, scattered electrons are produced, which deposit most of their energy at shallow depths near the skin surface. The use of a beam spoiler alters the depth-dose characteristics of the TBI beam in the buildup region. The magnitude of this modifying effect depends on the photon energy of the beam, the composition and thickness of the scatter screen, and the distance between the screen and the patient. It should be carefully evaluated as part of the commissioning task for the TBI technique. The dosimetric effect of the beam spoiler can be treated separately or included in the TBI beam calibration. When the beam spoiler is included in the calibration, choice of the calibration depth becomes an important consideration. Calibration measurements performed at a depth of 5 cm or greater decrease the influence of beam spoiler-generated electrons significantly.

Dose Rate

As discussed in preceding sections, the rate of TBI dose delivery could have an impact on the clinical outcome after TBI.[112] Many clinical protocols require low dose rate treatment at the rate of 0.05 to 0.20 Gy/min.[99] Modern linear accelerators offer a wide range of dose rates (e.g., from 1 to 6 Gy/min in increments of 1 Gy/min), to the depth of maximum buildup at standard SSD. At extended SSD, the nominal dose rate will be smaller because of inverse-square falloff of photon fluence with SSD. The dose rate at the TBI treatment distance is dependent on the combination of SSD and the nominal dose rate programmed at the LINAC console. If a given combination of SSD and nominal LINAC dose rate does not produce a desired dose rate, a custom-made attenuator can be placed in the beam path to help achieve a desired dose rate. TBI calibration and dosimetry characterization should be performed with the desired treatment dose rate to ensure accurate dose delivery.[99]

Patient Positioning

As treatment times may last up to 30 or 40 minutes for each fraction of a TBI protocol (even longer for single-fraction protocols), patients must be placed in a comfortable and reproducible position. When a pair of parallel-opposed fields is used, irradiation along the anteroposterior/posteroanterior (AP/PA) direction is advantageous as the body thickness in the AP/PA direction is usually smaller than in the lateral direction, which results in better dose uniformity along the beam path for a given photon energy. As depicted in Figure 16.1A and B, this may be accomplished with the patient lying in the supine/prone position under a vertical beam arrangement or with the patient lying on the side in a lateral decubitus position when a horizontally directed beam is used (Figs. 16.1E and 16.2A and B). Irradiation with the patient lying supine using a horizontally directed beam (Figs. 16.1C and 16.2C) is also a reasonable technique, especially for patients with small lateral separations, such as pediatric patients, or when a higher-energy photon beam is employed. Because of clinical problems associated with patient fatigue and orthostatic hypotension, special patient stands are used in some institutions to facilitate upright patient positioning (Fig. 16.1D).

Treatment Planning

The calculation of radiation beam-on time for a prescribed TBI dose is often performed with a specialized in-house program or by manual computation. This is because most commercial treatment planning systems are designed and commissioned using standard datasets for conventional radiotherapy, which do not automatically apply to a TBI configuration. Some newer versions of commercial treatment planning systems can be adapted for isodose planning of TBI at extended SSDs by using depth dose, beam profiles, and other parameters measured directly under TBI conditions. For example, a special TBI beam model was successfully commissioned on the Theraplan Plus 3D system and used in routine TBI treatment planning at Yale. Others have commissioned and evaluated an extended SSD photon model on the Pinnacle[3] planning system for TBI.[113] Newer techniques for total marrow and/or lymphatic irradiation using TomoTherapy or VMAT at standard treatment distances can take advantage of the beam models already commissioned in an existing treatment planning system, although the dosimetric accuracy must undergo a careful validation for irradiating large and complex target volumes demanded by TBI and total marrow irradiation (TMI).

In addition to TBI beam characteristics, an accurate description of patient geometry is needed for patient-specific treatment planning. The external body contour of a TBI patient in treatment position can be reconstructed from the measurements of body thickness at representative anatomic points judiciously distributed over the patient's body. A CT scan of the entire body provides the best description of patient geometry and is required for IMRT-based TBI/TMI techniques. For extended SSD, TBI techniques using two parallel-opposed beams, dose variation over the patient's body arises primarily from (a) photon attenuation along the beam path, (b) the changing body contour across the patient, and (c) variations in tissue density.

The dose variation caused by photon attenuation along the beam path is dependent upon both the beam energy and the body thickness. It decreases with decreasing body thickness and increasing photon energy. Because the body is typically thinner in AP direction, treating patients using an AP/PA technique with higher photon energy will improve the dose uniformity along the beam path. Using lateral-opposed beams will usually result in greater dose variation compared to AP/PA treatments, especially for adult patients. The dose variation caused by changing body contour may be reduced by using missing-tissue compensators or tissue-equivalent bolus material placed directly on the patient. The ability to compute isodose distribution across the body is highly desirable for compensator design. Missing-tissue compensator for TBI is typically constructed to even out the variation of body thickness along the head to toe direction. Such a one-dimensional compensator can be constructed manually using multiple thin copper (or material) plates. As the compensator is usually mounted at the head of the linear accelerator, small variations in the placement of compensating plates will be magnified at extended SSD distance. Care must be exercised in constructing these compensators. For example, when compensating plates are used for the head and neck region, mounting the compensator too far inferiorly could result in a lower dose to the shoulders. In addition, careful alignment of the patient to the planned position becomes important to achieve the desired missing-tissue compensation.

Dose variation caused by tissue heterogeneity in the thoracic region requires special attention because the lungs are a critical dose-limiting structure in TBI. Without compensation for air density, particularly for AP/PA treatments, dose inhomogeneity can exceed the prescribed dose by 10% to 24%, depending on the energy of beams used.[99] In order to reduce lung toxicity, correction for lung air density should be taken into account. Further, many institutions attenuate the dose to the lungs using lung shielding. This can take many forms including customized lung blocks (typically in the setting of AP/PA fields; Fig. 16.2B and E) or attenuation using brass compensators (typically in the setting of lateral fields; Fig. 16.2D) The use of lung blocks increases the complexity of the TBI procedure, and accurate repositioning of lung blocks can be a challenge for fractionated treatments. Several techniques have been reported to increase the repositioning accuracy of lung blocks.[114-116] At Yale, individualized thin lung blocks (with ~85% photon transmission) are mounted close to the patient on an acrylic resin tray using a hook and loop fastener system that allows easy repositioning of lung blocks for each fraction (Fig. 16.2B). Verification of correct lung block positioning is carried out by using customized online electronic portal imaging. For the lateral technique, the arms can be used, in addition to shielding using brass compensators, to decrease dose to the lungs (Fig. 16.2C). For pediatric patients, the arm may not be large enough laterally to cover the entire lung.

Dose Description and Reporting

Because there is no standard treatment technique for TBI, significant differences in dose distributions can exist with different treatment methods. Two institutions can prescribe the same dose at some selected prescription point, but dose to other points could vary considerably if different treatment techniques are used. Without supplemental information on the dose distribution, it would be difficult to assess the clinical effectiveness of different TBI programs based on the reported prescription dose alone. To facilitate treatment comparison among institutions, various methods for prescribing the dose for TBI treatments have been reported.[117,118] One method uses a single-point prescription dose supplemented with the specified limits of highest and lowest dose levels acceptable for any point within the body. In addition, dose limits are also set for certain tissues, such as the lungs. An example of such a TBI prescription is given in AAPM TG-29, which uses the midpoint at the level of the umbilicus as the prescription point. A prescription would read as follows: "The dose to the midpoint at the level of the umbilicus is 14 Gy to be delivered in 8 fractions with 2 fractions on each day separated by at least 6 hours. All points in the body should receive doses within the limits of −5% and +10% of prescription dose. The dose to lung should be no more than 85% of the prescription dose." When reporting results from a TBI-based conditioning regimen, ideally, the actual values of the corresponding dose descriptors

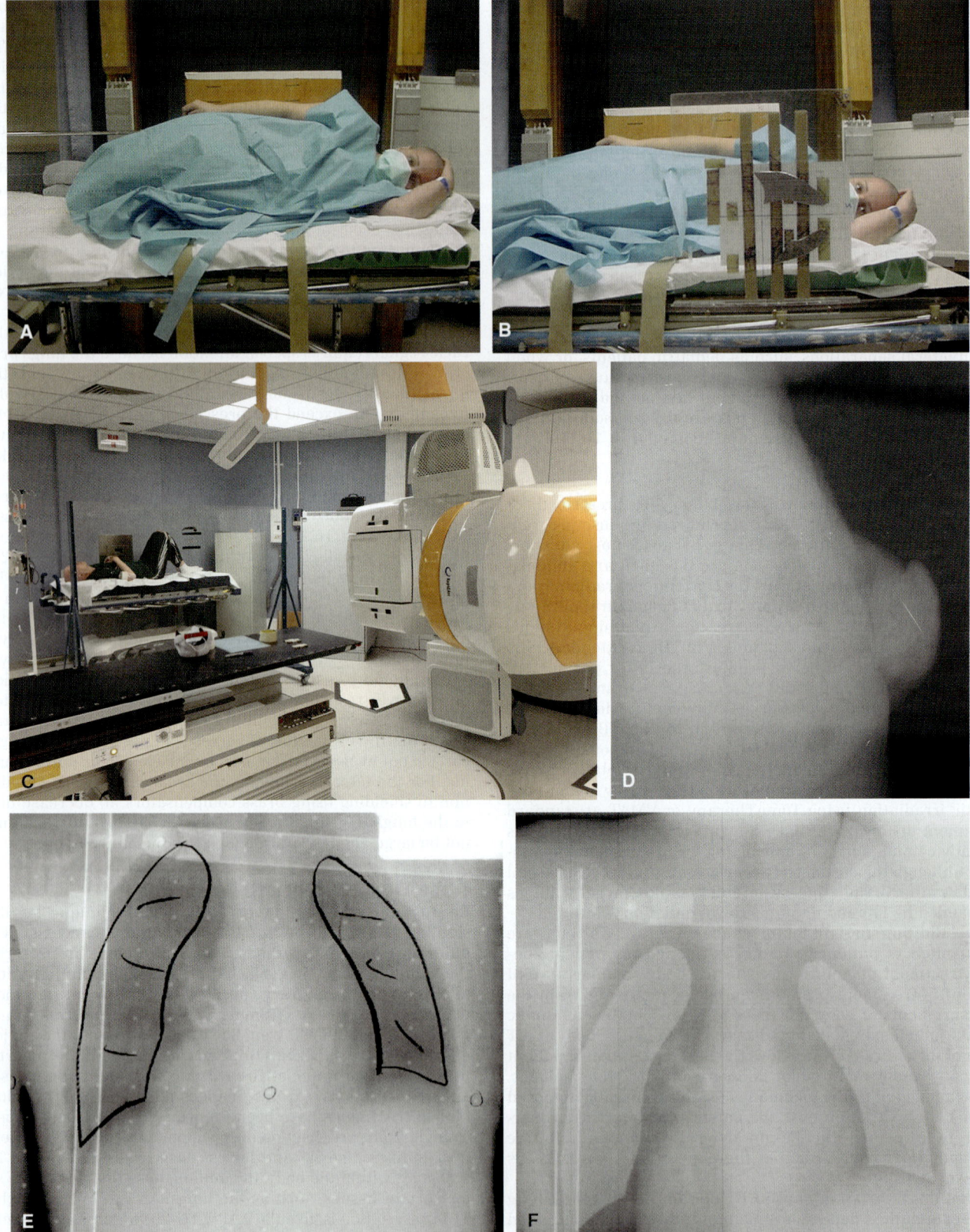

FIGURE 16.2. A: Patient in decubitus position for total-body irradiation (TBI), anterior beam. **B:** Thin lung blocks placed close to the thorax using a Velcro–plexiglass system to reposition blocks with each fraction. **C:** Patient in supine position for TBI using lateral fields. **D:** A megavoltage port film confirming position of brass compensators to attenuate the dose to the lungs when lateral fields are utilized. **E:** A megavoltage simulation film taken in decubitus position. **F:** Treatment portal imaging taken in decubitus position.

would be provided. When CT-based TBI treatment planning is available, dose–volume histogram of the target volume and critical organs should be reported.

Quality Assurance

To improve dosimetric accuracy and consistency, periodic assessment of TBI calibration and beam characteristics should be performed as part of an ongoing quality assurance program. Each patient's treatment plan, including the design of customized tissue compensators when used, should be checked by an independent physicist. In addition, *in vivo* dosimetry verification of the treatment plan should be performed during the first fraction for all TBI patients. Changes in patient body shape (e.g., due to weight loss between the time of simulation and treatment delivery) and positioning can alter the dose distribution. Adjustment of radiation beam-on time and tissue compensators may be needed for subsequent treatments based on the *in vivo* verification (assuming the accuracy and confidence of *in vivo* measurement have already been established). Thermoluminescent dosimeters and diode detectors are typical choices for *in vivo* monitoring of doses delivered to patients.[110,119] These detectors should be calibrated in the TBI beam under the treatment condition prior to commencing patient treatment. A diode dosimetry system with multiple diode detectors is especially convenient for these types of measurements because they allow simultaneous measurement of doses at multiple anatomic sites in nearly real time.

Lung (and Other Organ) Dose Attenuation

Many transplant centers use lung blocks or lung shielding during TBI in order to correct for the dosimetric effects of lung density or to specifically reduce the dose to lung tissue, thereby reducing the risk for pneumonitis. This is particularly important in patients who have baseline lung dysfunction.[120] Lung shielding will reduce the risk of pneumonitis, all other factors being equal.[121] Overcompensation, however, risks an increase in leukemia recurrence. A study from the Institut Gustave Roussy delivering 10 Gy as a single fraction of TBI over four hours showed a higher incidence of relapse in patients whose lung dose was reduced to 6 Gy with lung blocks compared with 8 Gy.[122]

There are many techniques to attenuate the dose to the lungs. The technique at Yale utilizes 1/8-inch lead filters that attenuate the dose by 10% to 15%, in essence a slight overcorrection for the dosimetric effects of pulmonary air density[123] (Fig. 16.2E and F). At Duke University, where lateral TBI fields are utilized, the dose to the lungs is attenuated to 8 to 10 Gy, based on baseline lung function and other clinical factors, using brass compensators (Fig. 16.2D). The Memorial Sloan Kettering Cancer Center (MSKCC) group utilizes lung shielding with the use of electron boosts to the chest wall under the blocks.[124] There are considerable dosimetric challenges with this technique: electron treatments are planned in a supine position yet delivered standing; overlap issues of photon and electron fields; surface contour variability, especially from breast tissue in women; and delivering unwanted radiation dose to some limited volume of the lungs. The Institut Gustave Roussy has reported no clinical benefit to electron boosts to the chest wall under such lung blocks.[125] The Johns Hopkins group has reported using thick (7 HVL) blocks for just 1 fraction of their TBI course over several days.[126] The Seattle group uses 1 or 2 HVL blocks for half of the TBI fractions without a chest wall boost. Other transplant groups such as the University of Minnesota have reported using partial transmission blocks to the liver and kidneys to reduce the risk of hepatic VOD/SOS or nephropathy.[127,128]

When TBI is used for nonneoplastic diseases (e.g., aplastic anemia), where the main objective is immunosuppression, one may also consider shielding radiosensitive structures such as the gonads or eyes (i.e., the lens).[129]

Boosting of Selected Organs with TBI

A relative advantage of TBI is the treatment of chemotherapy sanctuary sites. This is particularly important when treating diseases with a propensity to involve the CNS or testes. Theoretically, regions of the body where there is a higher burden of disease at the time of transplant may be boosted with additional radiation to supplement TBI. In selected patients with acute lymphoblastic leukemia, CNS-preventative therapy may include cranial irradiation. When such patients are determined at diagnosis to be best managed with an allo-SCT, it is reasonable to defer prophylactic cranial irradiation until the time of TBI. Augmented doses of radiation may be delivered to the CNS bringing the cumulative cranial dose to approximately 18 Gy (a current standard in children and many adults with ALL). Higher total doses to the brain and perhaps the spine can be considered in patients being managed with overt CNS leukemia. Boost doses to the brain using lateral fields may be given in 1.8- to 2.0-Gy fractions. Caution is necessary for additional CNS boost treatments when patients have received prior cranial irradiation because of toxicity concerns. Similarly, the testes in males with ALL may be boosted to a cumulative dose of approximately 16 to 18 Gy. The scrotum may be treated with en face electrons of appropriate energy or a single superior/anterior/oblique photon field. Because the incremental toxicity of such testicular irradiation is low regardless of fraction size, and the fact that some programs have not observed testicular relapses after TBI, dose prescriptions for testicular boosting vary from 0 to 4 Gy.

TOTAL-BODY IRRADIATION—ACUTE AND LATE TOXICITIES

Side effects from TBI used with SCT have complex interactions with cytotoxic drugs and posttransplant immunosuppressive agents. In addition, GVHD has its own unique toxicities, which have complex interactions with the conditioning regimen. Infectious complications are also prevalent after transplant. Isolating which toxicities are strictly related to TBI is not always straightforward.

Low-Dose TBI (Nonmyeloablative Regimens)

With TBI-based nonmyeloablative regimens, 2 Gy in a single fraction being commonly employed, the chief side effect after treatment is nausea and vomiting, which can be ameliorated using prophylactic antiemetics. The primary long-term risk is cataract development, which can be corrected surgically. The risk of injury to other normal organs with a single 2-Gy fraction is very low.

Full-Dose TBI (Myeloablative Regimens)

Acute Toxicity

Nausea, vomiting, and diarrhea are the most common early side effects when a single fraction of 8- to 10-Gy TBI is given. Xerostomia, headaches, fevers, and hypertension were historically reported in roughly half of patients receiving single-fraction TBI.[130] The use of fractionated TBI reduces the incidence, as well as the severity of these and other side effects. Moreover, fever and hypertension are rarely seen with fractionated TBI.[131,132] Patients can also develop a transient xerostomia, reduction in tear formation, and mucositis within 10 days. Reversible alopecia develops at approximately 2 weeks in all patients.[19] Parotiditis, which usually occurs after the first day of irradiation and subsides within 24 to 48 hours, is unique to TBI and is very common with single-fraction RT but occurs in <10% of cases with fractionated regimens.[131]

Nausea may be controlled with the use of serotonin receptor-3 antagonists, as shown in several small randomized trials.[133,134] Mucositis resulting from both radiation and chemotherapy may be ameliorated by good dental hygiene[135] along with a variety of topical agents. Adjunctive agents that have been studied include topical chlorhexidine digluconate,[136,137] calcium phosphate slurry,[138] sucralfate,[139] and clarithromycin.[140] Amifostine was studied in one trial of allo-SCT showing a reduction in duration of mucositis with fewer severe infections but no effect on hepatic toxicity, renal toxicity, or hematopoietic engraftment.[141] Recombinant human keratinocyte growth factor was found to reduce mucositis after TBI and intensive chemotherapy resulting in reduced narcotic and parenteral nutrition usage in one auto-SCT study.[142] Despite such supportive care, parenteral nutrition and narcotics are often necessary.

Late Toxicity

Lung

Interstitial pneumonitis is the major dose-limiting toxicity for TBI. The lung-sparing effect for fractionation has been shown to be important down to approximately 1 Gy.[143] This dose roughly corresponds to the lowest fraction size in some hyperfractionated TBI schedules. The marked lung-sparing effect of fractionation, or of a decrease in dose rate, has been confirmed by the work of Penney and colleagues showing a progressive sparing of the lung with increased fractionation for both early pneumonitis and late fibrosis.[144] The rate of lung repair between fractions was reviewed by Travis et al., indicating the presence of two significantly different repair rates corresponding to a fast repair half-time of 0.40 hours and a slow repair half-time of 4.01 hours.[145] The slow repair component needs to be kept in mind when designing TBI schedules that include 2 or 3 fractions per day.

Reduction in the risk of pneumonitis by fractionation is supported by the previously described randomized clinical trial comparing single-fraction TBI (9.2 or 10 Gy) with fractionated TBI (12 Gy in 6 fractions over 3 days) for patients with AML in first remission. This study demonstrated a significant improvement in event-free survival with fractionation, primarily due to a reduction in early mortality. Interstitial pneumonitis was decreased from 26% to 15% with fractionation.[32] Other studies have confirmed that fractionated TBI regimens markedly reduce the incidence of interstitial pneumonitis to <20% without increasing the rate of tumor recurrence.[124,132,146] Within a range of conventional fraction sizes of 1.5 to 2 Gy given once or twice daily, no significant increase in the incidence of interstitial pneumonitis is noted up to total doses as high as 15 Gy.[30,31,146] Nevertheless, total dose delivered to the lung is a key determinant of pneumonitis risk.[93,147]

Another radiobiologic approach to reduce the incidence of interstitial pneumonitis is to lower the radiation dose rate. Within the context of fractionated TBI schemes, instantaneous dose rates of 5 to 20 cGy/min have been generally employed and are often determined by the available output of linear accelerators at extended treatment distances. It is unclear whether or not higher instantaneous dose rates are detrimental despite theoretical concerns in this regard. One small study that compared dose rates of 7.5 cGy/min versus 15 cGy/min in context of a TBI prescription of 12 Gy in 6 fractions reported a pneumonitis risk of 13% versus 43%, respectively, although there were many confounding covariates.[148] Other studies have not shown dose rate to be an important predictor of pneumonitis from fractionated TBI, but rather total dose to the lung is the more critical determinant.[121]

Pneumonitis in the transplant setting has a multifactorial etiology, reflecting not only the effects of radiation but also the effects of chemotherapy,[149] performance status,[150] GVHD, lung injury from tumor, baseline lung function, opportunistic infections, patient age, and other risk factors.[121,147,151] Many chemotherapy drugs are known to injure the lung. GVHD may cause lung injury directly and the drugs used to control GVHD may also cause pulmonary toxicity.[152] T-cell–depleted transplants tend to have lower risk for pneumonitis.[153]

Lens

The lens of the eye is one of the most radiation-sensitive structures in the body. Schenken and Hagemann derived an alpha/beta ratio of 1.2 Gy (0.6 to 2.1), suggesting a high fractionation and/or dose rate sensitivity for cataract induction.[154] In the Seattle experience, >75% of patients developed cataracts 5 years or more after single-fraction TBI.[155] The risk is markedly reduced with fractionation. Ozsahin et al. calculated a difference in the 5-year estimated cataract incidence between single-fraction TBI (39%) and fractionated TBI (13%) while also showing a beneficial effect of lower dose rate.[156] Tichelli et al. reported that the probability of requiring cataract surgery was 85% after single-fraction TBI and 20% after fractionated TBI.[157] This has been confirmed in the Seattle long-term analysis showing the risk of cataracts to be 85%, 50%, 34%, and 19% after 10-Gy single-fraction TBI, >12-Gy fractionated TBI, 12-Gy fractionated TBI, and no TBI, respectively.[158] Steroid therapy is an independent risk factor for cataract formation after bone marrow transplantation, even in the absence of TBI. Lens shielding during TBI is not recommended because of the risk of retro-ocular relapse of leukemia but is a consideration in aplastic anemia and other nonneoplastic diseases managed with SCT.

Growth and Gonadal and Endocrine Effects

Almost all children who undergo bone marrow transplantation with TBI experience decreased growth velocity, which is less with fractionated than single-dose TBI.[159,160] Growth hormone deficiency may be detected in 34% of adults who received TBI in their childhood. Other endocrine effects in this setting include Leydig cell dysfunction in 23% and primary hypothyroidism in 34%.[161] High-dose TBI produces primary gonadal failure in almost all patients, but recovery may occur in females.[160] In children, puberty is usually delayed but can be induced by appropriate hormone replacement.[162,163] Thyroid dysfunction is reported in as many as 43% of patients after TBI.[159,164] Subclinical hypothyroidism is the most common picture, with raised thyroid-stimulating hormone and normal thyroxine levels. The incidence of thyroid dysfunction is lower when hyperfractionated TBI is used.[165]

Liver

Hepatic veno-occlusive disease (VOD) has been renamed sinusoidal obstructive syndrome (SOS) given the recognition that this clinical problem, principally seen in myeloablative transplants, is an endothelial injury to hepatic sinusoids and this hepatocyte injury and hepatic thrombosis are secondary late-stage effects.[166–168] This syndrome accounting for significant morbidity and mortality in high-dose transplant regimens is characterized by hepatic enlargement, ascites, jaundice, encephalopathy, and weight gain in 10% to 40% of patients.[131,169] This disease, which needs to be distinguished from cholestatic drug injury and acute GVHD, is best diagnosed by transvenous hepatic biopsy where an elevated hepatic venous pressure gradient is documented along with characteristic histology showing hepatic sinusoidal and central vein fibrosis and accompanying hepatocyte necrosis. The etiology of VOD/SOS is thought to be related to acrolein, a cyclophosphamide metabolite also implicated in causing hemorrhagic cystitis, which acts as an endothelial toxin. Other toxic agents give rise to this disease, but in the transplant setting, TBI, busulfan, cytosine arabinoside, and preexisting or concomitant liver disease are risk factors, possibly due to depletion of intracellular glutathione levels or matrix metalloproteinase activity. Radiobiologically, hepatocytes respond to dose fractionation (or dose rate) in a manner similar to late-responding tissues with large variations in the isoeffect dose when fraction size (or dose rate) is modified.[170,171] An alpha/beta ratio of 1 to 2 Gy has been estimated.[172]

The incidence of VOD/SOS has been minimized by fractionating TBI and keeping total doses below 13.2 Gy. The Seattle group has reported considerably more VOD/SOS after 10-Gy single-fraction TBI than after 12-Gy fractionated TBI in a randomized trial.[32] A nonrandomized retrospective study found that fractionated TBI resulted in less VOD/SOS disease but with borderline significance.[173] Barrett showed a decrease in the incidence of VOD/SOS with a lower dose rate.[174] Others have shown that modifications of chemotherapy dosing and scheduling based on individual pharmacodynamics may also lower the risk.[50,168] Other prevention strategies for VOD/SOS include the administration of low molecular weight heparins and ursodiol as part of the pretransplant supportive care regimen.[168] In one well-designed clinical trial, ursodiol prevented cholestatic liver injury and GVHD, but had no effect on VOD/SOS.[175] Treatment is mainly supportive care, but there is some limited evidence that defibrotide, a single-stranded polydeoxyribonucleotide drug with antithrombotic and anti-ischemic properties, may be helpful.[176]

Kidney

Renal toxicity has been underreported as a major late complication of SCT. A report by Tarbell et al. in 1988 showed a 35% rate of renal dysfunction in ALL patients receiving transplants.[177] More contemporary reports place this risk at 17%, influenced by the use of TBI, cyclosporine for immunosuppression, and presence of significant GVHD.[178] Alpha/beta ratio calculations for kidney in a variety of animal and human models have consistently shown relatively low values indicative of fractionation and dose rate radiosensitivity.[179–181] A protracted value of the half-time for repair ($t\frac{1}{2}$) for late damage of 2.10 hours (1.90 to 2.34) was found by VonRongen.[182] Because transplant patients also receive various nephrotoxic drugs (etoposide, teniposide, amphotericin B, aminoglycoside antibiotics) before, during, and after intensive cytoreductive therapy, the contribution of TBI to renal dysfunction is not clearly established.[183] GVHD also has complex interactions with TBI in affecting the risk of transplant-related nephritis.[184] Helenglass reported a trial comparing cyclophosphamide-TBI with melphalan-TBI. The benefit obtained from melphalan in reducing the relapse rate was offset by its nephrotoxic effect.[185] Other studies suggest that use of TBI and chronic GVHD are risk factors for posttransplant chronic kidney disease.[178,186] Some transplant programs have used partial transmission blocks over the kidneys or limiting the total dose, suggesting that kidney doses over 12 Gy are associated with increased risks of nephropathy.[128] This is not done at our institutions.

Secondary Cancers

The risk for development of a second tumor 15 years after intensive chemoradiation and SCT is estimated to be 13% to 20%.[163,187–190] The risk for a secondary malignancy is approximately 4 times higher than the general population.[191] Increasing TBI doses has been associated with increased risk of solid cancers in one study[187] but has not been observed in others.[192] The largest series of secondary malignancy from combined registries of the International Bone and Marrow Transplant Research Centers and the Fred Hutchinson Cancer Research Center has observed 189 solid cancers among 28,874 transplant patients, more than 6,000 of whom had survived >5 years.[192] Two-thirds of this cohort received radiotherapy as part of their conditioning and was a major determinant for a secondary cancer along with chronic immunosuppression. Common posttransplant nonsquamous cell cancers include melanoma, cervical or uterine cancer, thyroid cancer, breast cancer, and gliomas.[191] Patients < 30 years of age at the time of treatment have an approximately 9-fold increased risk for nonsquamous cell cancers over those who did not receive radiotherapy. Myelodysplastic syndrome and AML are the most common secondary tumors in patients treated for lymphoid malignancies. Patients who are older, who experienced acute GVHD, who were treated with antithymocyte globulin or anti-CD3 antibodies, or who receive TBI are at greatest risk.[189,190] Some lymphoproliferative disorders that occur after allo-SCT are associated with Epstein-Barr virus and may be successfully managed with anti–B-cell antibodies,[193,194] adoptive immunotherapy,[195–197] or donor lymphocyte transfusions.[196] Chronic GVHD and male age increase the risk for squamous cell cancers. Other studies have documented an increased risk for skin cancers and oral cavity cancers, the latter related to chronic lichenoid oral lesions and the historical use of azathioprine for GVHD immunosuppression.[198]

HEMIBODY IRRADIATION

HBI has been used for many years to palliate widely metastatic solid tumors, often very late in the course of the disease.[199–201] As the field of medical oncology has developed a larger array of systemic therapies for disseminated cancers, this form of radiotherapy has been less frequently employed.

Applications

Patients with osseous metastases tend to have multiple sites of disease, often with multiple painful areas that can be challenging to treat with conventional RT. The pain relief produced by single-fraction HBI for skeletal metastases is prompt, with nearly 50% of all responding patients doing so within 48 hours and 80% within 1 week after treatment.[202,203] More than 70% of treated patients experience pain relief as documented in a number of studies including various RTOG trials from the 1980s.[202,204–207] The duration of pain relief persists for at least 50% of the patient's remaining life.[199,202] The most effective HBI doses found by the RTOG were 6 Gy for upper HBI and 8 Gy for lower and middle HBI. Doses beyond these levels do not appear to increase pain relief, duration of pain relief, or rapidity of response.[202]

When treatment of the other half of the body is also indicated, it is advisable to wait 6 to 8 weeks to allow sufficient recovery of blood cells and irradiated marrow.[199] Planned sequential upper and lower HBI 6 to 8 weeks apart has been used to treat multiple myeloma, malignant lymphoma, and other widely disseminated tumors.[199,208–212] HBI appears to be capable of delaying the progression of existing asymptomatic metastasis and the clinical development of new metastases,[204,208,209,213] which eliminates or reduces the need for patients to spend a substantial portion of their remaining lives commuting to treatment centers. At least for multiple myeloma, however, a randomized trial did not support routine use of hemibody radiotherapy.[212] In this trial, patients were initially treated with chemotherapy. Eligible patients were then randomized to 1 year of vincristine, melphalan, cyclophosphamide, and prednisone (VMCP) versus sequential HBI with vincristine and prednisone (VP). RFS and OS were better with VMCP than with HBI ($P = .04$ and $P = .018$, respectively).

Technique

The physical considerations for HBI are similar to those for TBI. The field size required for HBI is much smaller than that for TBI, and HBI can often be delivered on a conventional linear accelerator, albeit using extended distances. By convention, subtotal-body irradiation is usually divided into upper HBI, lower HBI, and middle HBI.[202,214] An arbitrary line at the bottom of L4 is commonly used to separate upper and lower HBI,[214] although this may be modified based on individual circumstances. Treatment is delivered using AP/PA parallel-opposed fields. The patient is positioned with a vertical beam allowing coverage of the hemibody, and the treatment table is lowered to the appropriate level or to the floor. Shielding of previously irradiated areas or other body regions to reduce toxicity, such as the salivary glands and the lungs, may be employed. The dose is prescribed to the midplane of the patient at the central axis of the beam.

Complications

In general, HBI is well tolerated. The most common side effects associated with single-dose HBI are nausea and vomiting, mainly when the abdomen is included within the fields. These occur shortly after radiation administration and last a few hours.[199,202,203] Premedication with steroids and antiemetics is highly recommended. As these patients are frequently anorexic or cachectic from their underlying illness, dehydration and need for intravenous fluids are common with HBI, and hospitalization for supportive care may be desirable.[214] A series from the University of Maryland examined single-fraction HBI with escalating doses of 4 to 10 Gy, split-course HBI with two 4-Gy fractions separated by 2 weeks, and daily fractionated HBI with 15 Gy given in 5 fractions. Fractionated HBI was found to be more acutely tolerable, similar to the experience with TBI.[215] Diarrhea occurs commonly when a significant volume of the intestines are irradiated and may last for several days. The severity of this side effect can be reduced by limiting the dose to the abdomen to 6 Gy.[202] The risk of pneumonitis is very low if the single-fraction dose to the whole lungs is limited to 7 Gy (uncorrected for air density). If 8 Gy is delivered to the upper body, partial transmission lung blocks to limit the lung dose at 6 to 7 Gy is recommended. Hematologic recovery usually occurs in 4 to 6 weeks.

REFERENCES

1. Vellenga E, van Agthoven M, Croockewit AJ, et al. Autologous peripheral blood stem cell transplantation in patients with relapsed lymphoma results in accelerated haematopoietic reconstitution, improved quality of life and cost reduction compared with bone marrow transplantation: the Hovon 22 study. *Br J Haematol* 2001;114(2):319–326.
2. Vose JM, Sharp G, Chan WC, et al. Autologous transplantation for aggressive non-Hodgkin's lymphoma: results of a randomized trial evaluating graft source and minimal residual disease. *J Clin Oncol* 2002;20(9):2344–2352.
3. Gertz MA, Ansell SM, Dingli D, et al. Autologous stem cell transplant in 716 patients with multiple myeloma: low treatment-related mortality, feasibility of outpatient transplant, and effect of a multidisciplinary quality initiative. *Mayo Clin Proc* 2008;83(10):1131–1138.
4. Tsang RW, Gospodarowicz MK, Sutcliffe SB, et al. Thoracic radiation therapy before autologous bone marrow transplantation in relapsed or refractory Hodgkin's disease. PMH Lymphoma Group, and the Toronto Autologous BMT Group. *Eur J Cancer* 1999;35(1):73–78.
5. Yahalom J, Rimner A, Tsang R. Salvage therapy for relapsed and refractory Hodgkin lymphoma. In: Specht L, Yahalom J, eds. *Radiotherapy for Hodgkin lymphoma*. Berlin Heidelberg: Springer; 2011:31–44.
6. Baron F, Maris MB, Sandmaier BM, et al. Graft-versus-tumor effects after allogeneic hematopoietic cell transplantation with nonmyeloablative conditioning. *J Clin Oncol* 2005;23(9):1993–2003.
7. Dean RM, Bishop MR. Allogeneic hematopoietic stem cell transplantation for lymphoma. *Clin Lymphoma* 2004;4(4):238–249.
8. Gale RP, Horowitz MM, Ash RC, et al. Identical-twin bone marrow transplants for leukemia. *Ann Intern Med* 1994;120(8):646–652.
9. Kolb HJ, Schmid C, Barrett AJ, et al. Graft-versus-leukemia reactions in allogeneic chimeras. *Blood* 2004;103(3):767–776.
10. Depil S, Deconinck E, Milpied N, et al. Donor lymphocyte infusion to treat relapse after allogeneic bone marrow transplantation for myelodysplastic syndrome. *Bone Marrow Transplant* 2004;33(5):531–534.
11. Goodnow CC, Sprent J, Fazekas de St Groth B, et al. Cellular and genetic mechanisms of self tolerance and autoimmunity. *Nature* 2005;435(7042):590–597.
12. Chao NJ. Minors come of age: minor histocompatibility antigens and graft-versus-host disease. *Biol Blood Marrow Transplant* 2004;10(4):215–223.
13. Chao NJ, Chen BJ. Prophylaxis and treatment of acute graft-versus-host disease. *Semin Hematol* 2006;43(1):32–41.
14. Storb R, Deeg HJ, Whitehead J, et al. Methotrexate and cyclosporine compared with cyclosporine alone for prophylaxis of acute graft versus host disease after marrow transplantation for leukemia. *N Engl J Med* 1986;314(12):729–735.
15. Brown JM. Exogenous administration of immunomodulatory therapies in hematopoietic cell transplantation: an infectious diseases perspective. *Curr Opin Infect Dis* 2005;18(4):352–358.
16. Papadopoulos EB, Carabasi MH, Castro-Malaspina H, et al. T-cell-depleted allogeneic bone marrow transplantation as postremission therapy for acute myelogenous leukemia: freedom from relapse in the absence of graft-versus-host disease. *Blood* 1998;91(3):1083–1090.
17. Jakubowski AA, Small TN, Young JW, et al. T cell depleted stem-cell transplantation for adults with hematologic malignancies: sustained engraftment of HLA-matched related donor grafts without the use of antithymocyte globulin. *Blood* 2007;110(13):4552–4559.
18. Peters L. Total Body Irradiation Conference: discussion: the radiobiological bases of TBI. *Int J Radiat Oncol Biol Phys* 1980;6(6):785–787.
19. Thomas E, Storb R, Clift RA, et al. Bone-marrow transplantation (first of two parts). *N Engl J Med* 1975;292(16):832–843.
20. Barendsen GW. Dose fractionation, dose rate and iso-effect relationships for normal tissue responses. *Int J Radiat Oncol Biol Phys* 1982;8(11):1981–1997.
21. Dale RG. The application of the linear-quadratic model to fractionated radiotherapy when there is incomplete normal tissue recovery between fractions, and possible implications for treatments involving multiple fractions per day. *Br J Radiol* 1986;59(705):919–927.
22. O'Donoghue JA. Fractionated versus low dose-rate total body irradiation. Radiobiological considerations in the selection of regimes. *Radiother Oncol* 1986;7(3):241–247.
23. Storb R, Yu C, Wagner JL, et al. Stable mixed hematopoietic chimerism in DLA-identical littermate dogs given sublethal total body irradiation before and pharmacological immunosuppression after marrow transplantation. *Blood* 1997;89(8):3048–3054.
24. Storb R, Raff RF, Appelbaum FR, et al. Fractionated versus single-dose total body irradiation at low and high dose rates to condition canine littermates for DLA-identical marrow grafts. *Blood* 1994;83(11):3384–3389.
25. McSweeney PA, Niederwieser D, Shizuru JA, et al. Hematopoietic cell transplantation in older patients with hematologic malignancies: replacing high-dose cytotoxic therapy with graft-versus-tumor effects. *Blood* 2001;97(11):3390–3400.
26. Slavin S, Nagler A, Naparstek E, et al. Nonmyeloablative stem cell transplantation and cell therapy as an alternative to conventional bone marrow transplantation with lethal cytoreduction for the treatment of malignant and nonmalignant hematologic diseases. *Blood* 1998;91(3):756–763.
27. Nakamae H, Storer BE, Storb R, et al. Low-dose total body irradiation and fludarabine conditioning for HLA class I-mismatched donor stem cell transplantation and immunologic recovery in patients with hematologic malignancies: a multicenter trial. *Biol Blood Marrow Transplant* 2010;16(3):384–394.
28. Niederwieser D, Gentilini C, Hegenbart U, et al. Allogeneic hematopoietic cell transplantation (HCT) following reduced-intensity conditioning in patients with acute leukemias. *Crit Rev Oncol Hematol* 2005;56(2):275–281.
29. Diaconescu R, Flowers CR, Storer B, et al. Morbidity and mortality with nonmyeloablative compared with myeloablative conditioning before hematopoietic cell transplantation from HLA-matched related donors. *Blood* 2004;104(5):1550–1558.
30. Clift RA, Buckner CD, Appelbaum FR, et al. Allogeneic marrow transplantation in patients with acute myeloid leukemia in first remission: a randomized trial of two irradiation regimens. *Blood* 1990;76(9):1867–1871.
31. Clift RA, Buckner CD, Appelbaum FR, et al. Allogeneic marrow transplantation in patients with chronic myeloid leukemia in the chronic phase: a randomized trial of two irradiation regimens. *Blood* 1991;77(8):1660–1665.
32. Deeg HJ, Sullivan KM, Buckner CD, et al. Marrow transplantation for acute nonlymphoblastic leukemia in first remission: toxicity and long-term follow-up of patients conditioned with single dose or fractionated total body irradiation. *Bone Marrow Transplant* 1986;1(2):151–157.
33. Girinsky T, Benhamou E, Bourhis JH, et al. Prospective randomized comparison of single-dose versus hyperfractionated total-body irradiation in patients with hematologic malignancies. *J Clin Oncol* 2000;18(5):981–986.
34. Ozsahin M, Pene F, Touboul E, et al. Total-body irradiation before bone marrow transplantation. Results of two randomized instantaneous dose rates in 157 patients. *Cancer* 1992;69(11):2853–2865.
35. Miller KB, Roberts TF, Chan G, et al. A novel reduced intensity regimen for allogeneic hematopoietic stem cell transplantation associated with a reduced incidence of graft-versus-host disease. *Bone Marrow Transplant* 2004;33(9):881–889.
36. Holter-Chakrabarty JL, Pierson N, Zhang MJ, et al. The Sequence of Cyclophosphamide and Myeloablative Total Body Irradiation in Hematopoietic Cell Transplantation for Patients with Acute Leukemia. *Biol Blood Marrow Transplant* 2015;21(7):1251–1257.
37. Santos GW. The development of busulfan/cyclophosphamide preparative regimens. *Semin Oncol* 1993;20(4 Suppl 4):12–16; quiz 17.
38. Tutschka PJ, Copelan EA, Klein JP. Bone marrow transplantation for leukemia following a new busulfan and cyclophosphamide regimen. *Blood* 1987;70(5):1382–1388.
39. O'Donnell MR, Long GD, Parker PM, et al. Busulfan/cyclophosphamide as conditioning regimen for allogeneic bone marrow transplantation for myelodysplasia. *J Clin Oncol* 1995;13(12):2973–2979.
40. Gaspard MH, Maraninchi D, Stoppa AM, et al. Intensive chemotherapy with high doses of BCNU, etoposide, cytosine arabinoside, and melphalan (BEAM) followed by autologous bone marrow transplantation: toxicity and antitumor activity in 26 patients with poor-risk malignancies. *Cancer Chemother Pharmacol* 1988;22(3):256–262.
41. Storb R, Leisenring W, Anasetti C, et al. Long-term follow-up of allogeneic marrow transplants in patients with aplastic anemia conditioned by cyclophosphamide combined with antithymocyte globulin. *Blood* 1997;89(10):3890–3891.
42. Slattery JT, Clift RA, Buckner CD, et al. Marrow transplantation for chronic myeloid leukemia: the influence of plasma busulfan levels on the outcome of transplantation. *Blood* 1997;89(8):3055–3060.

43. Schuler US, Renner UD, Kroschinsky F, et al. Intravenous busulphan for conditioning before autologous or allogeneic human blood stem cell transplantation. *Br J Haematol* 2001;114(4):944–950.

44. Peters WP, Shpall EJ, Jones RB, et al. High-dose combination alkylating agents with bone marrow support as initial treatment for metastatic breast cancer. *J Clin Oncol* 1988;6(9):1368–1376.

45. Valteau D, Hartmann O, Benhamou E, et al. Nonbacterial nonfungal interstitial pneumonitis following autologous bone marrow transplantation in children treated with high-dose chemotherapy without total-body irradiation. *Transplantation* 1988;45(4):737–740.

46. Blaise D, Maraninchi D, Archimbaud E, et al. Allogeneic bone marrow transplantation for acute myeloid leukemia in first remission: a randomized trial of a busulfan Cytoxan versus Cytoxan-total body irradiation as preparative regimen: a report from the Group d'Etudes de la Greffe de Moelle Osseuse. *Blood* 1992;79(10):2578–2582.

47. Blaise D, Maraninchi D, Michallet M, et al. Long-term follow-up of a randomized trial comparing the combination of cyclophosphamide with total body irradiation or busulfan as conditioning regimen for patients receiving HLA-identical marrow grafts for acute myeloblastic leukemia in first complete remission. *Blood* 2001;97(11):3669–3671.

48. Bunin N, Aplenc R, Kamani N, et al. Randomized trial of busulfan vs total body irradiation containing conditioning regimens for children with acute lymphoblastic leukemia: a Pediatric Blood and Marrow Transplant Consortium study. *Bone Marrow Transplant* 2003;32(6):543–548.

49. Blume KG, Kopecky KJ, Henslee-Downey JP, et al. A prospective randomized comparison of total body irradiation-etoposide versus busulfan-cyclophosphamide as preparatory regimens for bone marrow transplantation in patients with leukemia who were not in first remission: a Southwest Oncology Group study. *Blood* 1993;81(8):2187–2193.

50. Ringden O, Ruutu T, Remberger M, et al. A randomized trial comparing busulfan with total body irradiation as conditioning in allogeneic marrow transplant recipients with leukemia: a report from the Nordic Bone Marrow Transplantation Group. *Blood* 1994;83(9):2723–2730.

51. Ringden O, Remberger M, Ruutu T, et al. Increased risk of chronic graft-versus-host disease, obstructive bronchiolitis, and alopecia with busulfan versus total body irradiation: long-term results of a randomized trial in allogeneic marrow recipients with leukemia. Nordic Bone Marrow Transplantation Group. *Blood* 1999;93(7):2196–2201.

52. Devergie A, Blaise D, Attal M, et al. Allogeneic bone marrow transplantation for chronic myeloid leukemia in first chronic phase: a randomized trial of busulfan-cytoxan versus cytoxan-total body irradiation as preparative regimen: a report from the French Society of Bone Marrow Graft (SFGM). *Blood* 1995;85(8):2263–2268.

53. Clift RA, Buckner CD, Thomas ED, et al. Marrow transplantation for chronic myeloid leukemia: a randomized study comparing cyclophosphamide and total body irradiation with busulfan and cyclophosphamide. *Blood* 1994;84(6):2036–2043.

54. Socie G, Clift RA, Blaise D, et al. Busulfan plus cyclophosphamide compared with total-body irradiation plus cyclophosphamide before marrow transplantation for myeloid leukemia: long-term follow-up of 4 randomized studies. *Blood* 2001;98(13):3569–3574.

55. Hartman AR, Williams SF, Dillon JJ. Survival, disease-free survival and adverse effects of conditioning for allogeneic bone marrow transplantation with busulfan/cyclophosphamide vs total body irradiation: a meta-analysis. *Bone Marrow Transplant* 1998;22(5):439–443.

56. Shi-Xia X, Xian-Hua T, Hai-Qin X, et al. Total body irradiation plus cyclophosphamide versus busulphan with cyclophosphamide as conditioning regimen for patients with leukemia undergoing allogeneic stem cell transplantation: a meta-analysis. *Leuk Lymphoma* 2010;51(1):50–60.

57. Nagler A, Rocha V, Labopin M, et al. Allogeneic hematopoietic stem-cell transplantation for acute myeloid leukemia in remission: comparison of intravenous busulfan plus cyclophosphamide (Cy) versus total-body irradiation plus Cy as conditioning regimen—a report from the acute leukemia working party of the European group for blood and marrow transplantation. *J Clin Oncol* 2013;31(28):3549–3556.

58. Uberti JP, Agovi MA, Tarima S, et al. Comparative analysis of BU and CY versus CY and TBI in full intensity unrelated marrow donor transplantation for AML, CML and myelodysplasia. *Bone Marrow Transplant* 2011;46(1):34–43.

59. Litzow MR, Perez WS, Klein JP, et al. Comparison of outcome following allogeneic bone marrow transplantation with cyclophosphamide-total body irradiation versus busulphan-cyclophosphamide conditioning regimens for acute myelogenous leukaemia in first remission. *Br J Haematol* 2002;119(4):1115–1124.

60. Ringden O, Labopin M, Tura S, et al. A comparison of busulphan versus total body irradiation combined with cyclophosphamide as conditioning for autograft or allograft bone marrow transplantation in patients with acute leukaemia. Acute Leukaemia Working Party of the European Group for Blood and Marrow Transplantation (EBMT). *Br J Haematol* 1996;93(3):637–645.

61. Stephens SJ, Thomas S, Rizzieri DA, et al. Myeloablative conditioning with total body irradiation for AML: balancing survival and pulmonary toxicity. *Adv Radiat Oncol* 2016;1(4):272–280.

62. Copelan EA, Hamilton BK, Avalos B, et al. Better leukemia-free and overall survival in AML in first remission following cyclophosphamide in combination with busulfan compared with TBI. *Blood* 2013;122(24):3863–3870.

63. Bredeson C, LeRademacher J, Kato K, et al. Prospective cohort study comparing intravenous busulfan to total body irradiation in hematopoietic cell transplantation. *Blood* 2013;122(24):3871–3878.

64. Van der Jagt RH, Appelbaum FR, Petersen FB, et al. Busulfan and cyclophosphamide as a preparative regimen for bone marrow transplantation in patients with prior chest radiotherapy. *Bone Marrow Transplant* 1991;8(3):211–215.

65. Kelsey CR, Horwitz ME, Chino JP, et al. Severe pulmonary toxicity after myeloablative conditioning using total body irradiation: an assessment of risk factors. *Int J Radiat Oncol Biol Phys* 2011;81(3):812–818.

66. Rozman C, Carreras E, Qian C, et al. Risk factors for hepatic veno-occlusive disease following HLA-identical sibling bone marrow transplants for leukemia. *Bone Marrow Transplant* 1996;17(1):75–80.

67. Nevill TJ, Barnett MJ, Klingemann HG, et al. Regimen-related toxicity of a busulfan-cyclophosphamide conditioning regimen in 70 patients undergoing allogeneic bone marrow transplantation. *J Clin Oncol* 1991;9(7):1224–1232.

68. De La Camara R, Tomas JF, Figuera A, et al. High dose busulfan and seizures. *Bone Marrow Transplant* 1991;7(5):363–364.

69. Kernan NA, Bartsch G, Ash RC, et al. Analysis of 462 transplantations from unrelated donors facilitated by the National Marrow Donor Program. *N Engl J Med* 1993;328(9):593–602.

70. Niederwieser D, Maris M, Shizuru JA, et al. Low-dose total body irradiation (TBI) and fludarabine followed by hematopoietic cell transplantation (HCT) from HLA-matched or mismatched unrelated donors and postgrafting immunosuppression with cyclosporine and mycophenolate mofetil (MMF) can induce durable complete chimerism and sustained remissions in patients with hematological diseases. *Blood* 2003;101(4):1620–1629.

71. Laport GG, Sandmaier BM, Storer BE, et al. Reduced-intensity conditioning followed by allogeneic hematopoietic cell transplantation for adult patients with myelodysplastic syndrome and myeloproliferative disorders. *Biol Blood Marrow Transplant* 2008;14(2):246–255.

72. Maris MB, Niederwieser D, Sandmaier BM, et al. HLA-matched unrelated donor hematopoietic cell transplantation after nonmyeloablative conditioning for patients with hematologic malignancies. *Blood* 2003;102(6):2021–2030.

73. Rondon G, Saliba RM, Khouri I, et al. Long-term follow-up of patients who experienced graft failure postallogeneic progenitor cell transplantation. Results of a single institution analysis. *Biol Blood Marrow Transplant* 2008;14(8):859–866.

74. Byrne BJ, Horwitz M, Long GD, et al. Outcomes of a second non-myeloablative allogeneic stem cell transplantation following graft rejection. *Bone Marrow Transplant* 2008;41(1):39–43.

75. Heinzelmann F, Lang PJ, Ottinger H, et al. Immunosuppressive total lymphoid irradiation-based reconditioning regimens enable engraftment after graft rejection or graft failure in patients treated with allogeneic hematopoietic stem cell transplantation. *Int J Radiat Oncol Biol Phys* 2008;70(2):523–528.

76. Gyurkocza B, Cao TM, Storb RF, et al. Salvage allogeneic hematopoietic cell transplantation with fludarabine and low-dose total body irradiation after rejection of first allografts. *Biol Blood Marrow Transplant* 2009;15(10):1314–1322.

77. Radich JP, Sanders JE, Buckner CD, et al. Second allogeneic marrow transplantation for patients with recurrent leukemia after initial transplant with total-body irradiation-containing regimens. *J Clin Oncol* 1993;11(2):304–313.

78. Baron F, Storb R, Storer BE, et al. Factors associated with outcomes in allogeneic hematopoietic cell transplantation with nonmyeloablative conditioning after failed myeloablative hematopoietic cell transplantation. *J Clin Oncol* 2006;24(25):4150–4157.

79. Hendry JH. The cellular basis of long-term marrow injury after irradiation. *Radiother Oncol* 1985;3(4):331–338.

80. Uckun FM, Song CW. Radiobiological features of human pluripotent bone marrow progenitor cells (CFU-GEMM). *Int J Radiat Oncol Biol Phys* 1989;17(5):1021–1025.

81. Storb R, Raff RF, Appelbaum FR, et al. Comparison of fractionated to single-dose total body irradiation in conditioning canine littermates for DLA-identical marrow grafts. *Blood* 1989;74(3):1139–1143.

82. Salomon O, Lapidot T, Terenzi A, et al. Induction of donor-type chimerism in murine recipients of bone marrow allografts by different radiation regimens currently used in treatment of leukemia patients. *Blood* 1990;76(9):1872–1878.

83. Triebel F, Gluckman JC, Chapuis F, et al. T-lymphocyte progenitors in man: phenotypic characterization of blood and bone marrow T-colony forming cells. *Immunology* 1985;54(2):241–247.

84. Rigaud O, Papadopoulo D, Moustacchi E. Decreased deletion mutation in radio-adapted human lymphoblasts. *Radiat Res* 1993;133(1):94–101.

85. Gallini R, Hendry JH, Molineux G, et al. The effect of low dose rate on recovery of hemopoietic and stromal progenitor cells in gamma-irradiated mouse bone marrow. *Radiat Res* 1988;115(3):481–487.

86. FitzGerald TJ, Santucci MA, Harigaya K, et al. Radiosensitivity of permanent human bone marrow stromal cell lines: effect of dose rate. *Int J Radiat Oncol Biol Phys* 1988;15(5):1153–1159.

87. Cosset JM, Socie G, Dubray B, et al. Single dose versus fractionated total body irradiation before bone marrow transplantation: radiobiological and clinical considerations. *Int J Radiat Oncol Biol Phys* 1994;30(2):477–492.

88. Cosset JM, Socie G, Girinsky T, et al. Radiobiological and Clinical Bases for Total Body Irradiation in the Leukemias and Lymphomas. *Semin Radiat Oncol* 1995;5(4):301–315.

89. O'Donoghue JA, Wheldon TE, Gregor A. The implications of in-vitro radiation-survival curves for the optimal scheduling of total-body irradiation with bone marrow rescue in the treatment of leukaemia. *Br J Radiol* 1987;60(711):279–283.

90. Song CW, Kim TH, Khan FM, et al. Radiobiological basis of total body irradiation with different dose rate and fractionation: repair capacity of hemopoietic cells. *Int J Radiat Oncol Biol Phys* 1981;7(12):1695–1701.

91. Weichselbaum RR, Greenberger JS, Schmidt A, et al. In vitro radiosensitivity of human leukemia cell lines. *Radiology* 1981;139(2):485–487.

92. Bradley J, Reft C, Goldman S, et al. High-energy total body irradiation as preparation for bone marrow transplantation in leukemia patients: treatment technique and related complications. *Int J Radiat Oncol Biol Phys* 1998;40(2):391–396.

93. Keane TJ, Van Dyk J, Rider WD. Idiopathic interstitial pneumonia following bone marrow transplantation: the relationship with total body irradiation. *Int J Radiat Oncol Biol Phys* 1981;7(10):1365–1370.

94. Van Dyk J, Keane TJ, Kan S, et al. Radiation pneumonitis following large single dose irradiation: a re-evaluation based on absolute dose to lung. *Int J Radiat Oncol Biol Phys* 1981;7(4):461–467.
95. Leer JW, Broerse JJ, De Vroome H, et al. Techniques applied for total body irradiation. *Radiother Oncol* 1990;18(Suppl 1):10–15.
96. Schultheiss TE, Wong J, Liu A, et al. Image-guided total marrow and total lymphatic irradiation using helical tomotherapy. *Int J Radiat Oncol Biol Phys* 2007;67(4):1259–1267.
97. Aydogan B, Yeginer M, Kavak GO, et al. Total marrow irradiation with RapidArc volumetric arc therapy. *Int J Radiat Oncol Biol Phys* 2011;81(2):592–599.
98. Yeginer M, Roeske JC, Radosevich JA, et al. Linear accelerator-based intensity-modulated total marrow irradiation technique for treatment of hematologic malignancies: a dosimetric feasibility study. *Int J Radiat Oncol Biol Phys* 2011;79(4):1256–1265.
99. Van Dyk J, Glavin JM, Glasgow GP. *The physical aspects of total and half body photon irradiation: a report of Task Group 29 Radiation Therapy Committee*. American Association of Physicists in Medicine, 1986.
100. Cunningham JR, Wright DJ. A simple facility for wholebody irradiation. *Radiology* 1962;78:941–949.
101. Quast U. Physical treatment planning of total-body irradiation: patient translation and beam-zone method. *Med Phys* 1985;12(5):567–574.
102. Pla M, Chenery SG, Podgorsak EB. Total body irradiation with a sweeping beam. *Int J Radiat Oncol Biol Phys* 1983;9(1):83–89.
103. Wong JYC, Rosenthal J, Liu A, et al. Image-guided total-marrow irradiation using helical tomotherapy in patients with multiple myeloma and acute leukemia undergoing hematopoietic cell transplantation. *Int J Radiat Oncol Biol Phys* 2009;73(1):273–279.
104. Van Dyk J. Dosimetry for total body irradiation. *Radiother Oncol* 1987;9(2):107–118.
105. Briot E, Dutreix A, Bridier A. Dosimetry for total body irradiation. *Radiother Oncol* 1990;18(Suppl 1):16–29.
106. Curran WJ Jr, Galvin JM, D'Angio GJ. A simple dose calculation method for total body photon irradiation. *Int J Radiat Oncol Biol Phys* 1989;17(1): 219–224.
107. Kirby TH, Hanson WF, Cates DA. Verification of total body photon irradiation dosimetry techniques. *Med Phys* 1988;15(3):364–369.
108. Scarpati D, Mancini G, Corvo R, et al. Tissue air ratio in total body irradiation. An in vivo evaluation. *Acta Oncol* 1989;28(2):283–285.
109. Syh HW, Chu WK, Kumar PP, et al. Estimation of the mean effective organ doses for total body irradiation from Rando phantom measurements. *Med Dosim* 1992;17(2):103–106.
110. Sanchez-Doblado F, Terron JA, Sanchez-Nieto B, et al. Verification of an on line in vivo semiconductor dosimetry system for TBI with two TLD procedures. *Radiother Oncol* 1995;34(1):73–77.
111. Shank B. Techniques of magna-field irradiation. *Int J Radiat Oncol Biol Phys* 1983;9(12):1925–1931.
112. Appelbaum FR. The influence of total dose, fractionation, dose rate, and distribution of total body irradiation on bone marrow transplantation. *Semin Oncol* 1993;20(4 Suppl 4):3–10; quiz 11.
113. Lavallee MC, Gingras L, Chretien M, et al. Commissioning and evaluation of an extended SSD photon model for PINNACLE3: an application to total body irradiation. *Med Phys* 2009;36(8):3844–3855.
114. Breneman JC, Elson HR, Little R, et al. A technique for delivery of total body irradiation for bone marrow transplantation in adults and adolescents. *Int J Radiat Oncol Biol Phys* 1990;18(5):1233–1236.
115. Miralbell R, Rouzaud M, Grob E, et al. Can a total body irradiation technique be fast and reproducible? *Int J Radiat Oncol Biol Phys* 1994;29(5): 1167–1173.
116. Niroomand-Rad A. Physical aspects of total body irradiation of bone marrow transplant patients using 18 MV x rays. *Int J Radiat Oncol Biol Phys* 1991;20(3):605–611.
117. Galvin JM. Calculation and prescription of dose for total body irradiation. *Int J Radiat Oncol Biol Phys* 1983;9(12):1919–1924.
118. Kim TH, Khan FM, Galvin JM. Total Body Irradiation Conference: a report of the work party: comparison of total body irradiation techniques for bone marrow transplantation. *Int J Radiat Oncol Biol Phys* 1980;6(6):779–784.
119. Svahn-Tapper G, Nilsson P, Jonsson C, et al. Calculation and measurements of absorbed dose in total body irradiation. *Acta Oncol* 1990;29(5):627–633.
120. Singh AK, Karimpour SE, Savani BN, et al. Pretransplant pulmonary function tests predict risk of mortality following fractionated total body irradiation and allogeneic peripheral blood stem cell transplant. *Int J Radiat Oncol Biol Phys* 2006;66(2):520–527.
121. Sampath S, Schultheiss TE, Wong J. Dose response and factors related to interstitial pneumonitis after bone marrow transplant. *Int J Radiat Oncol Biol Phys* 2005;63(3):876–884.
122. Girinsky T, Socie G, Ammarguellat H, et al. Consequences of two different doses to the lungs during a single dose of total body irradiation: results of a randomized study on 85 patients. *Int J Radiat Oncol Biol Phys* 1994;30(4): 821–824.
123. Dutreix J, Janoray P, Bridier A, et al. Biologic and anatomic problems of lung shielding in whole-body irradiation. *J Natl Cancer Inst* 1986;76(6): 1333–1335.
124. Shank B, Hopfan S, Kim JH, et al. Hyperfractionated total body irradiation for bone marrow transplantation: I. Early results in leukemia patients. *Int J Radiat Oncol Biol Phys* 1981;7(8):1109–1115.
125. Cosset JM, Baume D, Pico JL, et al. Single dose versus hyperfractionated total body irradiation before allogeneic bone marrow transplantation: a non-randomized comparative study of 54 patients at the Institut Gustave-Roussy. *Radiother Oncol* 1989;15(2):151–160.
126. Pino y Torres JL, Bross DS, Lam WC, et al. Risk factors in interstitial pneumonitis following allogenic bone marrow transplantation. *Int J Radiat Oncol Biol Phys* 1982;8(8):1301–1307.
127. Lawton CA, Barber-Derus S, Murray KJ, et al. Technical modifications in hyperfractionated total body irradiation for T-lymphocyte deplete bone marrow transplant. *Int J Radiat Oncol Biol Phys* 1989;17(2):319–322.
128. Lawton CA, Cohen EP, Murray KJ, et al. Long-term results of selective renal shielding in patients undergoing total body irradiation in preparation for bone marrow transplantation. *Bone Marrow Transplant* 1997;20(12):1069–1074.
129. Shank B, Brochstein JA, Castro-Malaspina H, et al. Immunosuppression prior to marrow transplantation for sensitized aplastic anemia patients: comparison of TLI with TBI. *Int J Radiat Oncol Biol Phys* 1988;14(6):1133–1141.
130. Chaillet MP, Cosset JM, Socie G, et al. Prospective study of the clinical symptoms of therapeutic whole body irradiation. *Health Phys* 1993;64(4):370–374.
131. Buchali A, Feyer P, Groll J, et al. Immediate toxicity during fractionated total body irradiation as conditioning for bone marrow transplantation. *Radiother Oncol* 2000;54(2):157–162.
132. Thomas ED, Clift RA, Hersman J, et al. Marrow transplantation for acute nonlymphoblastic leukemic in first remission using fractionated or single-dose irradiation. *Int J Radiat Oncol Biol Phys* 1982;8(5):817–821.
133. Tiley C, Powles R, Catalano J, et al. Results of a double blind placebo controlled study of ondansetron as an antiemetic during total body irradiation in patients undergoing bone marrow transplantation. *Leuk Lymphoma* 1992;7(4):317–321.
134. Spitzer TR, Bryson JC, Cirenza E, et al. Randomized double-blind, placebo-controlled evaluation of oral ondansetron in the prevention of nausea and vomiting associated with fractionated total-body irradiation. *J Clin Oncol* 1994;12(11):2432–2438.
135. Borowski B, Benhamou E, Pico JL, et al. Prevention of oral mucositis in patients treated with high-dose chemotherapy and bone marrow transplantation: a randomised controlled trial comparing two protocols of dental care. *Eur J Cancer B Oral Oncol* 1994;30B(2):93–97.
136. Ferretti GA, Ash RC, Brown AT, et al. Chlorhexidine for prophylaxis against oral infections and associated complications in patients receiving bone marrow transplants. *J Am Dent Assoc* 1987;114(4):461–467.
137. Ferretti GA, Ash RC, Brown AT, et al. Control of oral mucositis and candidiasis in marrow transplantation: a prospective, double-blind trial of chlorhexidine digluconate oral rinse. *Bone Marrow Transplant* 1988;3(5):483–493.
138. Papas AS, Clark RE, Martuscelli G, et al. A prospective, randomized trial for the prevention of mucositis in patients undergoing hematopoietic stem cell transplantation. *Bone Marrow Transplant* 2003;31(8):705–712.
139. Castagna L, Benhamou E, Pedraza E, et al. Prevention of mucositis in bone marrow transplantation: a double blind randomised controlled trial of sucralfate. *Ann Oncol* 2001;12(7):953–955.
140. Yuen KY, Woo PC, Tai JW, et al. Effects of clarithromycin on oral mucositis in bone marrow transplant recipients. *Haematologica* 2001;86(5):554–555.
141. Hwang WY, Koh LP, Ng HJ, et al. A randomized trial of amifostine as a cytoprotectant for patients receiving myeloablative therapy for allogeneic hematopoietic stem cell transplantation. *Bone Marrow Transplant* 2004;34(1):51–56.
142. Spielberger R, Stiff P, Bensinger W, et al. Palifermin for oral mucositis after intensive therapy for hematologic cancers. *N Engl J Med* 2004;351(25):2590–2598.
143. Parkins CS, Fowler JF, Maughan RL, et al. Repair in mouse lung for up to 20 fractions of X rays or neutrons. *Br J Radiol* 1985;58(687):225–241.
144. Penney DP, Siemann DW, Rubin P, et al. Morphological correlates of fractionated radiation of the mouse lung: early and late effects. *Int J Radiat Oncol Biol Phys* 1994;29(4):789–804.
145. Travis EL. The sequence of histological changes in mouse lungs after single doses of x-rays. *Int J Radiat Oncol Biol Phys* 1980;6(3):345–347.
146. Phillips GL, Herzig RH, Lazarus HM, et al. Treatment of resistant malignant lymphoma with cyclophosphamide, total body irradiation, and transplantation of cryopreserved autologous marrow. *N Engl J Med* 1984;310(24):1557–1561.
147. Weiner RS, Bortin MM, Gale RP. Interstitial pneumonitis after bone marrow transplantation. Assessment of risk factors. *Ann Intern Med* 1986;104(2):168–175.
148. Carruthers SA, Wallington MM. Total body irradiation and pneumonitis risk: a review of outcomes. *Br J Cancer* 2004;90(11):2080–2084.
149. Kelsey CR, Horwitz ME, Chino JP, et al. Severe pulmonary toxicity after myeloablative conditioning using total body irradiation: an assessment of risk factors. *Int J Radiat Oncol Biol Phys* 2011;81(3):812–818.
150. Kelsey CR, Scott JM, Lane A, et al. Cardiopulmonary exercise testing prior to myeloablative allo-SCT: a feasibility study. *Bone Marrow Transplant* 2014;49(10):1330–1336.
151. Ho VT, Weller E, Lee SJ, et al. Prognostic factors for early severe pulmonary complications after hematopoietic stem cell transplantation. *Biol Blood Marrow Transplant* 2001;7(4):223–229.
152. Weiner RS, Bortin MM, Gale RP, et al. Interstitial pneumonitis after bone marrow transplantation. Assessment of risk factors. *Ann Intern Med* 1986;104(2):168–175.
153. Huisman C, van der Straaten HM, Canninga-van Dijk MR, et al. Pulmonary complications after T-cell-depleted allogeneic stem cell transplantation: low incidence and strong association with acute graft-versus-host disease. *Bone Marrow Transplant* 2006;38(8):561–566.
154. Schenken LL, Hagemann RF. Time/dose relationships in experimental radiation cataractogenesis. *Radiology* 1975;117(1):193–198.
155. Deeg HJ. Acute and delayed toxicities of total body irradiation. Seattle Marrow Transplant Team. *Int J Radiat Oncol Biol Phys* 1983;9(12):1933–1939.
156. Ozsahin M, Belkacemi Y, Pene F, et al. Total-body irradiation and cataract incidence: a randomized comparison of two instantaneous dose rates. *Int J Radiat Oncol Biol Phys* 1994;28(2):343–347.
157. Tichelli A, Gratwohl A, Egger T, et al. Cataract formation after bone marrow transplantation. *Ann Intern Med* 1993;119(12):1175–1180.

158. Benyunes MC, Sullivan KM, Deeg HJ, et al. Cataracts after bone marrow transplantation: long-term follow-up of adults treated with fractionated total body irradiation. *Int J Radiat Oncol Biol Phys* 1995;32(3):661–670.

159. Keilholz U, Korbling M, Fehrentz D, et al. Long-term endocrine toxicity of myeloablative treatment followed by autologous bone marrow/blood derived stem cell transplantation in patients with malignant lymphohematopoietic disorders. *Cancer* 1989;64(3):641–645.

160. Sanders JE, Buckner CD, Leonard JM, et al. Late effects on gonadal function of cyclophosphamide, total-body irradiation, and marrow transplantation. *Transplantation* 1983;36(3):252–255.

161. Felicetti F, Manicone R, Corrias A, et al. Endocrine late effects after total body irradiation in patients who received hematopoietic cell transplantation during childhood: a retrospective study from a single institution. *J Cancer Res Clin Oncol* 2011;137(9):1343–1348.

162. Barrett AJ. Bone marrow transplantation. *Cancer Treat Rev* 1987;14(3–4):203–213.

163. Deeg HJ. Delayed complications and long-term effects after bone marrow transplantation. *Hematol Oncol Clin North Am* 1990;4(3):641–657.

164. Sklar CA, Kim TH, Ramsay NK. Thyroid dysfunction among long-term survivors of bone marrow transplantation. *Am J Med* 1982;73(5):688–694.

165. Boulad F, Bromley M, Black P, et al. Thyroid dysfunction following bone marrow transplantation using hyperfractionated radiation. *Bone Marrow Transplant* 1995;15(1):71–76.

166. DeLeve LD, Shulman HM, McDonald GB. Toxic injury to hepatic sinusoids: sinusoidal obstruction syndrome (veno-occlusive disease). *Semin Liver Dis* 2002;22(1):27–42.

167. Shulman HM, Fisher LB, Schoch HG, et al. Veno-occlusive disease of the liver after marrow transplantation: histological correlates of clinical signs and symptoms. *Hepatology* 1994;19(5):1171–1181.

168. Wingard JR, Nichols WG, McDonald GB. Supportive care. *Hematology Am Soc Hematol Educ Program* 2004:372–389.

169. McDonald GB, Sharma P, Matthews DE, et al. The clinical course of 53 patients with venocclusive disease of the liver after marrow transplantation. *Transplantation* 1985;39(6):603–608.

170. Fisher DR, Hendry JH, Scott D. Long-term repair in vivo of colony-forming ability and chromosomal injury in X-irradiated mouse hepatocytes. *Radiat Res* 1988;113(1):40–50.

171. Thames HD Jr, Hendry JH. *Fractionation in radiotherapy*. London, England: Taylor and Francis, 1987.

172. Fisher DR, Hendry JH. Dose fractionation and hepatocyte clonogens: alpha/beta congruent to 1–2 Gy, and beta decreases with increasing delay before assay. *Radiat Res* 1988;113(1):51–57.

173. Baume D, Cosset JM, Pico JL, et al. Veno-occlusive disease of the liver after bone marrow graft. Possible value of fractionation of whole body irradiation. *Presse Med* 1987;16(35):1759.

174. Barrett A. Total body irradiation (TBI) before bone marrow transplantation in leukaemia: a co-operative study from the European Group for Bone Marrow Transplantation. *Br J Radiol* 1982;55(656):562–567.

175. Ruutu T, Eriksson B, Remes K, et al. Ursodeoxycholic acid for the prevention of hepatic complications in allogeneic stem cell transplantation. *Blood* 2002;100(6):1977–1983.

176. Richardson PG, Murakami C, Jin Z, et al. Multi-institutional use of defibrotide in 88 patients after stem cell transplantation with severe veno-occlusive disease and multisystem organ failure: response without significant toxicity in a high-risk population and factors predictive of outcome. *Blood* 2002;100(13):4337–4343.

177. Tarbell NJ, Guinan EC, Niemeyer C, et al. Late onset of renal dysfunction in survivors of bone marrow transplantation. *Int J Radiat Oncol Biol Phys* 1988;15(1):99–104.

178. Ellis MJ, Parikh CR, Inrig JK, et al. Chronic kidney disease after hematopoietic cell transplantation: a systematic review. *Am J Transplant* 2008;8(11):2378–2390.

179. Jen YM, Hendry JH. Dose-fractionation sensitivity of mouse kidney clonogens measured using different interfraction intervals and postirradiation assay times. *Radiother Oncol* 1993;26(2):117–124.

180. Jordan SW, Anderson RE, Lane RG, et al. Fraction size, dose and time dependence of X ray induced late renal injury. *Int J Radiat Oncol Biol Phys* 1985;11(6):1095–1101.

181. Williams MV, Denekamp J. Radiation induced renal damage in mice: influence of fraction size. *Int J Radiat Oncol Biol Phys* 1984;10(6):885–893.

182. van Rongen E, Kuijpers WC, Madhuizen HT. Fractionation effects and repair kinetics in rat kidney. *Int J Radiat Oncol Biol Phys* 1990;18(5):1093–1106.

183. Guinan EC, Tarbell NJ, Niemeyer CM, et al. Intravascular hemolysis and renal insufficiency after bone marrow transplantation. *Blood* 1988;72(2):451–455.

184. Miralbell R, Bieri S, Mermillod B, et al. Renal toxicity after allogeneic bone marrow transplantation: the combined effects of total-body irradiation and graft-versus-host disease. *J Clin Oncol* 1996;14(2):579–585.

185. Helenglass G, Powles RL, McElwain TJ, et al. Melphalan and total body irradiation (TBI) versus cyclophosphamide and TBI as conditioning for allogeneic matched sibling bone marrow transplants for acute myeloblastic leukaemia in first remission. *Bone Marrow Transplant* 1988;3(1):21–29.

186. Abboud I, Porcher R, Robin M, et al. Chronic kidney dysfunction in patients alive without relapse 2 years after allogeneic hematopoietic stem cell transplantation. *Biol Blood Marrow Transplant* 2009;15(10):1251–1257.

187. Curtis RE, Rowlings PA, Deeg HJ, et al. Solid cancers after bone marrow transplantation. *N Engl J Med* 1997;336(13):897–904.

188. Darrington DL, Vose JM, Anderson JR, et al. Incidence and characterization of secondary myelodysplastic syndrome and acute myelogenous leukemia following high-dose chemoradiotherapy and autologous stem-cell transplantation for lymphoid malignancies. *J Clin Oncol* 1994;12(12):2527–2534.

189. Lowsky R, Lipton J, Fyles G, et al. Secondary malignancies after bone marrow transplantation in adults. *J Clin Oncol* 1994;12(10):2187–2192.

190. Witherspoon RP, Fisher LD, Schoch G, et al. Secondary cancers after bone marrow transplantation for leukemia or aplastic anemia. *N Engl J Med* 1989;321(12):784–789.

191. Kolb HJ, Socie G, Duell T, et al. Malignant neoplasms in long-term survivors of bone marrow transplantation. Late Effects Working Party of the European Cooperative Group for Blood and Marrow Transplantation and the European Late Effect Project Group. *Ann Intern Med* 1999;131(10):738–744.

192. Rizzo JD, Curtis RE, Socie G, et al. Solid cancers after allogeneic hematopoietic cell transplantation. *Blood* 2009;113(5):1175–1183.

193. Benkerrou M, Jais JP, Leblond V, et al. Anti-B-cell monoclonal antibody treatment of severe posttransplant B-lymphoproliferative disorder: prognostic factors and long-term outcome. *Blood* 1998;92(9):3137–3147.

194. Kuehnle I, Huls MH, Liu Z, et al. CD20 monoclonal antibody (rituximab) for therapy of Epstein-Barr virus lymphoma after hemopoietic stem-cell transplantation. *Blood* 2000;95(4):1502–1505.

195. O'Reilly RJ, Small TN, Papadopoulos E, et al. Biology and adoptive cell therapy of Epstein-Barr virus-associated lymphoproliferative disorders in recipients of marrow allografts. *Immunol Rev* 1997;157:195–216.

196. Papadopoulos EB, Ladanyi M, Emanuel D, et al. Infusions of donor leukocytes to treat Epstein-Barr virus-associated lymphoproliferative disorders after allogeneic bone marrow transplantation. *N Engl J Med* 1994;330(17):1185–1191.

197. Barker JN, Doubrovina E, Sauter C, et al. Successful treatment of EBV-associated posttransplantation lymphoma after cord blood transplantation using third-party EBV-specific cytotoxic T lymphocytes. *Blood* 2010;116(23):5045–5049.

198. Curtis RE, Metayer C, Rizzo JD, et al. Impact of chronic GVHD therapy on the development of squamous-cell cancers after hematopoietic stem-cell transplantation: an international case-control study. *Blood* 2005;105(10):3802–3811.

199. Fitzpatrick PJ, Rider WD. Half body radiotherapy. *Int J Radiat Oncol Biol Phys* 1976;1(3–4):197–207.

200. Saenger EL, Silberstein EB, Aron B, et al. Whole body and partial body radiotherapy of advanced cancer. *Am J Roentgenol Radium Ther Nucl Med* 1973;117(3):670–685.

201. Tobias JS, Richards JD, Blackman GM, et al. Hemibody irradiation in multiple myeloma. *Radiother Oncol* 1985;3(1):11–16.

202. Salazar OM, Rubin P, Hendrickson FR, et al. Single-dose half-body irradiation for palliation of multiple bone metastases from solid tumors. Final Radiation Therapy Oncology Group report. *Cancer* 1986;58(1):29–36.

203. Salazar OM, Rubin P, Keller B, et al. Systemic (half-body) radiation therapy: response and toxicity. *Int J Radiat Oncol Biol Phys* 1978;4(11–12):937–950.

204. Poulter CA, Cosmatos D, Rubin P, et al. A report of RTOG 8206: a phase III study of whether the addition of single dose hemibody irradiation to standard fractionated local field irradiation is more effective than local field irradiation alone in the treatment of symptomatic osseous metastases. *Int J Radiat Oncol Biol Phys* 1992;23(1):207–214.

205. Qasim MM. Half body irradiation (HBI) in metastatic carcinomas. *Clin Radiol* 1981;32(2):215–219.

206. Rowland CG, Bullimore JA, Smith PJ, et al. Half-body irradiation in the treatment of metastatic prostatic carcinoma. *Br J Urol* 1981;53(6):628–629.

207. Wilkins MF, Keen CW. Hemi-body radiotherapy in the management of metastatic carcinoma. *Clin Radiol* 1987;38(3):267–268.

208. Lombardi F, Rottoli L, Gianni C, et al. Advanced neuroblastoma: results of two treatment programs including sequential hemibody irradiation. *Int J Radiat Oncol Biol Phys* 1989;17(3):485–491.

209. MacLennan I, Selim HM, Rubin P. Sequential hemibody radiotherapy in poor prognosis localized adenocarcinoma of the prostate gland: a preliminary study of the RTOG. *Int J Radiat Oncol Biol Phys* 1989;16(1):215–218.

210. McSweeney EN, Tobias JS, Blackman G, et al. Double hemibody irradiation (DHBI) in the management of relapsed and primary chemoresistant multiple myeloma. *Clin Oncol (R Coll Radiol)* 1993;5(6):378–383.

211. Rubin P, Heilmann HP. International Clinical Trials in Radiation Oncology. Large field trials. *Int J Radiat Oncol Biol Phys* 1988;14(Suppl 1):S65–S76.

212. Salmon SE, Tesh D, Crowley J, et al. Chemotherapy is superior to sequential hemibody irradiation for remission consolidation in multiple myeloma: a Southwest Oncology Group study. *J Clin Oncol* 1990;8(9):1575–1584.

213. Hazra TA, Giri S. Prophylactic pelvic girdle irradiation in the treatment of prostatic carcinoma. *Int J Radiat Oncol Biol Phys* 1981;7(6):817–819.

214. Rubin P, Salazar O, Zagars G, et al. Systemic hemibody irradiation for overt and occult metastases. *Cancer* 1985;55(9 Suppl):2210–2221.

215. Salazar OM, DaMotta NW, Bridgman SM, et al. Fractionated half-body irradiation for pain palliation in widely metastatic cancers: comparison with single dose. *Int J Radiat Oncol Biol Phys* 1996;36(1):49–60.

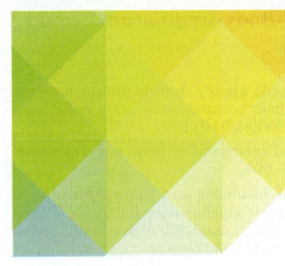

CHAPTER 17

Stereotactic Radiosurgery

John C. Flickinger

INTRODUCTION

Stereotactic radiosurgery (SRS) and stereotactic radiotherapy (SRT) are techniques to administer precisely directed, high-dose irradiation that tightly conforms to an intracranial target to create a desired radiobiologic response while minimizing radiation dose to surrounding normal tissue. These techniques exploit the fact that the radiation tolerance of normal tissue is volume dependent. Compared to conventional radiotherapy with standard 1- to 2-cm treatment margins allowing for patient movement and setup error, stereotactic techniques reduce complication risks for any radiation dose delivered by minimizing or eliminating normal tissue treatment margins. The term radiosurgery is used when all of the irradiation is done in 1 to 5 sessions or fractions, whereas the term stereotactic radiotherapy (SRT) is appropriate when 6 or more radiation fractions are administered. Table 17.1 lists the key requirements for successful stereotactic irradiation. Advances in imaging, computers, and treatment planning in the last two decades have led to the development of a variety of different stereotactic radiosurgery/radiotherapy techniques and their wider applications. Successful clinical experience with intracranial radiosurgery for a variety of applications has lead to a reexamination of radiobiology and exploration of both fractionated approaches and extracranial applications. Margin reduction with radiosurgery and fractionated stereotactic irradiation techniques makes target definition accuracy more critical. Drawing contours from different imaging techniques or by different physicians are approaches to reduce target definition error (Fig. 17.1).

TERMINOLOGY

Stereotactic refers to using a precise three-dimensional mapping technique to guide a procedure. The terminology used in stereotactic irradiation can be confusing. The term radiosurgery or stereotactic radiosurgery (SRS) is best used for stereotactically guided conformal irradiation of a defined target volume in a single session but may be also used for 2 to 5 sessions, although fractionated stereotactic radiosurgery (FSR)

is a clearer description for that use. Radiosurgery or SRS can be delivered with Gamma Knife, modified LINAC radiosurgery systems (including CyberKnife and image-guided radiotherapy systems), TomoTherapy, or proton beam systems. The terms stereotactic radiation therapy (SRT), stereotactic body radiotherapy (SBRT), and stereotactic ablative radiotherapy (SABR) can be used to refer to stereotactically guided delivery of highly conformal radiation to a defined target volume in 6 or more fractions, typically using noninvasive positioning techniques, although they are often used with treatment courses with 2 to 5 fractions as well. While SRT could potentially refer to precision image-guided radiotherapy used with the same doses and schedules used for conventional radiotherapy, SABR is normally reserved for high, ablative doses of radiation usually with hypofractionated schedules. Adding specific references to intensity-modulated radiation therapy (IMRT) to the nomenclature can further complicate or confuse the terminology. Any radiation treatment plan that uses individual treatment beams that irradiate only part of the target at a time is IMRT. Strictly speaking, multiple-isocenter radiosurgery (of a single target volume) meets the criteria for IMRT or stereotactic IMRT (SIMRT), although the term SIMRT is usually only used when multileaf collimators are employed. The terminology is useful to distinguish when the same linear accelerator is equipped to treat with either fixed circular collimators for radiosurgery (SRS or SRT mode) or to deliver IMRT using multileaf collimators (SIMRT mode).

RADIOBIOLOGIC CONSIDERATIONS

Prior to the introduction of radiosurgery, essentially all clinical irradiation was administered with radiation dose fractions between 1.2 and 3 Gy for intracranial targets. Extracranial targets were usually treated with 1.2- to 4-Gy fractions with 6- to 8-Gy fractions used occasionally for treatment of bone metastases or malignant melanoma. Before the rapid adaption of radiosurgery into the clinic in the late 1980s, most radiation oncologists and radiation biologists believed that fractionating radiation treatment lessens the relative risk of injury to normal tissue compared to tumor in essentially all circumstances. Radiobiologic analysis of a limited number of malignant tumors in cell culture and clinical experience with conventionally fractionated radiotherapy of fast-growing malignant tumors established this radiobiologic dogma. Increasing the fractionation of radiotherapy for slow-growing benign tumors may not necessarily improve the balance between tumor control and radiation complication. Slow-growing benign tumors are difficult to study in either cell culture or animal models, so the effect of fractionation has not been well delineated. Stereotactic radiosurgery allowed clinicians to administer high single doses of radiation to intracranial targets with relative safety, thereby leading to a new appreciation of the underlying radiobiology. Laboratory studies suggest that the radiation response for the high-dose single fractions used in radiosurgery is predominantly related to the supporting endothelial cells.[1] Pathology studies of benign and malignant tumors treated by radiosurgery also support a vascular response dominated by the response of endothelial cells.[1,2]

TABLE 17.1 KEY REQUIREMENTS FOR OPTIMAL STEREOTACTIC IRRADIATION	
Requirement	**Rationale**
Small target/treatment volume	Reducing the volume of normal and target tissue irradiated to high doses improves tolerance
Sharply defined target	Sharply defined targets can be treated with little or no extra margin of surrounding normal tissue and/or without unintentional underdosage of the target (marginal miss)
Accurate radiation delivery	No margin of normal tissue needed for set-up error and/or reduced chance of underdosing target
High conformality	Reduces the treatment volume to match the target volume
Sensitive structures excluded from target	Dose-limiting structures (optic chiasm, spinal cord, etc.) should be able to be defined and excluded from the target volume to limit the risk of radiation injury

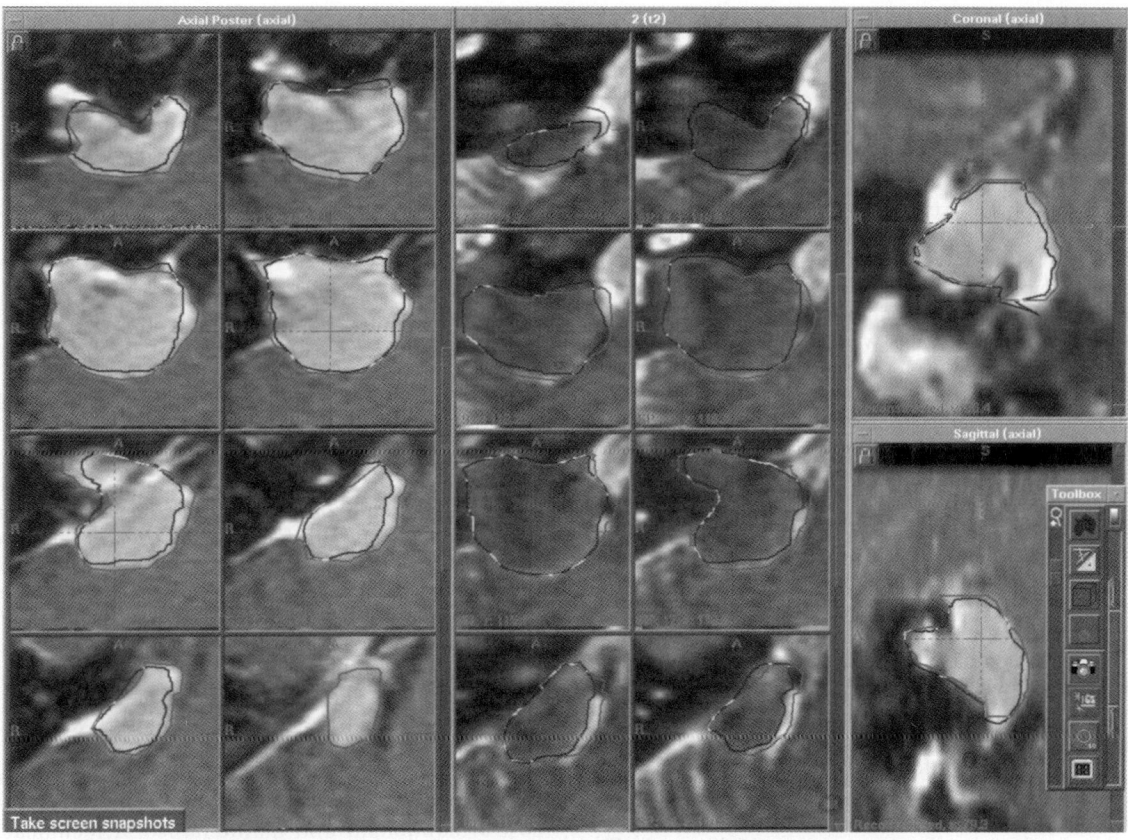

FIGURE 17.1. Comparisons of acoustic schwannoma contours drawn from T1-contrast MR images (eight axial images on the left side with coronal and sagittal images on the right side) with contours drawn from T2 MR images (the darker eight axial images in the center). T1 contours can sometimes slightly overestimate extension into the internal auditory canal and unnecessarily include adjacent blood vessels.

Analysis of clinical data from radiosurgery to delineate dose–response relationships and define radiobiologic parameters is fraught with difficulties. Typical radiosurgery treatment plans use inhomogeneous dose distributions with the prescription isodose covering anywhere from 90% to 100% of the target volume. The absolute minimum dose to the target typically is 5% to 30% lower than the prescription dose. Contours of the same tumor/target volume or critical structures may vary slightly from one clinician to another. Using the linear-quadratic formula to extrapolate from experience with conventional radiotherapy experience with low-dose fractions to high-dose single fractions for radiosurgery appears problematic. Using single-fraction radiosurgery dose–response curves for arteriovenous malformation (AVM) obliteration, radiation injury to brain parenchyma and cranial nerves to calculate α/β ratios yields values of negative 30 to negative 60 rather than 2 to 3 as expected from conventional fractionated radiotherapy data.[3,4] Comparing dose–responses for fractionated stereotactic radiotherapy to radiosurgery is hampered by limited data with dose–response curves that have insufficient slopes for accurate comparison.

There are several reasons that radiosurgery/SABR might potentially be better than conventional radiotherapy for combined treatment with immune modulation. The immune responses from cells within the additional margin of normal tissue irradiated around the tumor with conventional radiotherapy could potentially be dampened within that margin but should be less affected with SRS/SABR. Also, the higher proportion of tumor cells killed with ablative doses of radiation used in SRS/SABR should expose more tumor antigens to stimulate immune responses both against the irradiated

tumor and also possibly against more distant nonirradiated tumor (referred to as the abscopal response). Dewan et al.[5] looked at three schedules of ablative radiotherapy (20 Gy × 1, 8 Gy × 3, or 6 Gy × 5 fractions in consecutive days) delivered to one out of a pair of identical implanted mouse tumors in combination with immunotherapy using a 9H10 monoclonal antibody against CTLA-4. The immunotherapy alone had no effect on either tumor, whereas radiotherapy alone caused growth delay in only irradiated tumor. The combination of immunotherapy with either 3- or 5-fraction radiotherapy increased tumor response at the irradiated site ($P < .0001$) and, unlike the mice treated to 20 Gy in 1 fraction, inhibited growth of unirradiated tumor (which correlated with CD8+ T cells showing tumor-specific IFN-γ production). Marconi et al.[6] performed a meta-analysis of abscopal effects in preclinical animal models that correlated abscopal tumor responses with increasing biologic effective dose (BED) assuming an α/β ratio of 10 for the tumors. Abscopal effects were detected in 50% occurred with BED (10) doses of 60 Gy (such as with 10 Gy × 3 fractions).

RADIOSURGICAL TECHNIQUES

Radiosurgery was originally envisioned to treat intracranial lesions by delivering a high dose of ionizing radiation in a single treatment session using multiple beams precisely collimated to a target inside the cranium. Advances in both imaging and computer technologies resulted in wider applications of radiosurgery. There are now a variety of different radiosurgery and stereotactic radiotherapy techniques available for intracranial and extracranial use.

Gamma Knife Radiosurgery

After Leksell's initial experiences with stereotactic treatment using orthovoltage radiotherapy in 1951 and proton beam irradiation in 1957, Leksell and Larson created the first prototype of the Gamma Knife in 1967. The Gamma Knife uses a relatively hemispherical array of multiple fixed Co-60 beams (201 in most models) that are sharply collimated to create small relatively spherical treatment volumes of varied diameter with sharp dose falloff. The earlier model originally was referred to as the U (for university) style and contained cobalt sources arranged in hemispherical array including sources at the pole of the hemisphere. These units present challenging loading and reloading issues with the cobalt-60 sources, particularly with radiation protection. To eliminate this problem, the B-unit (named after Bergen, Norway, the first site) was redesigned so that sources were arranged in an annular section of a hemisphere, similar to the northern hemisphere with the Arctic Circle excluded. In 1999, the Model C version of the Gamma Knife was introduced with the option to use robotic positioning to set treatment coordinates. This expedited execution of multiple-isocenter treatment plans. Manual positioning was still needed for some targets away from the center of the head. The Model 4-C introduced in 2005 was equipped with enhancements designed to improve workflow, increase accuracy, and provide integrated imaging capabilities. The Perfexion model introduced in 2006 uses a larger patient aperture and internally mounted secondary collimators that can be blocked or treated with different diameters of 4, 8, or 16 mm for any of eight different sectors around the circumference of the unit. Because of the larger patient aperture, the Perfexion unit is able to treat all intracranial and even C1-2 level spine targets quickly and efficiently with robotic positioning. The latest version, the ICON unit, is similar to a Perfexion but equipped with a cone-beam CT scan for use with a frameless thermoplastic mask system with infrared patient position monitoring to facilitate FSR. Figure 17.2 shows the infrared monitor tracking of patient movement within an ICON unit during treatment. Clinical experience with the ICON unit has found that despite the relatively tight thermoplastic immobilization mask used, patient motion exceeding 1.0- or 1.5-mm total deviation (requiring repeat cone-beam CT for realignment) tends to occur more frequently with treatments over 30 minutes and in patients who fall asleep during treatment. Patients requiring longer treatments or sedation are more easily treated with stereotactic frame-based techniques with this unit. In addition to reducing patient motion, another advantage of radiosurgery using a magnetic resonance (MR)-compatible stereotactic frame is the elimination of any error (though usually small) from MR to CT image coregistration.

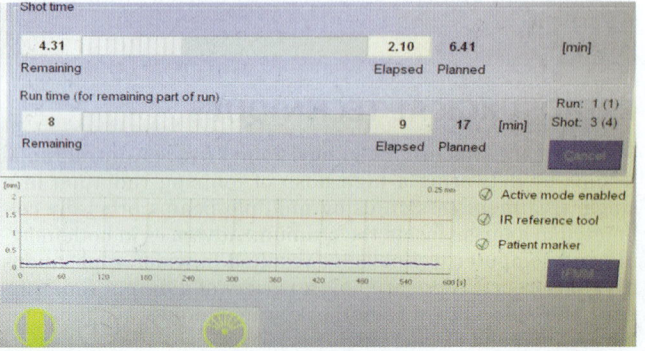

FIGURE 17.2. Infrared motion tracking on an ICON model Gamma Knife displaying real-time maximum combined position deviation within a thermoplastic immobilization mask during radiosurgery.

Rotating Gamma System

A radiosurgery device called the rotating gamma system (RGS) was developed in China. The RGS (OUR International Inc., Shenzhen, China) employs thirty cobalt-60 radiation sources in a revolving hemispherical shell. The secondary collimator is a coaxial hemispheric shell with six groups of five different collimators to produce spherical treatment volumes of different diameter. The experience with this system is somewhat limited.

Proton Radiosurgery

The chief advantage of charged proton radiosurgery is that the beams stop at a depth related to the beam's energy. Electron beams also use charged particles but lack the sharp beam edge of the proton beam. The lack of an exit dose and the sharp beam profile of protons allow target irradiation with lower integral doses than are delivered with photon (LINAC x-ray or cobalt-60 gamma) irradiation. An unmodified proton beam irradiation deposits increased energy in the last couple millimeters of the path length. This area of increased ionization, where cell killing is even higher because of an increased radiobiologic effect, is termed the Bragg peak or Bragg-Gray peak. To allow homogeneous irradiation of targets greater than a millimeter or two, the Bragg peak is normally modulated or spread out throughout the target, essentially eliminating its effect. The first treatment of a malignant tumor by irradiation with a proton beam Bragg peak was carried out in 1957 followed by functional neurosurgery done for advanced Parkinson disease in 1958. Presently, proton beam irradiation is available at a limited number of centers because of high cost of equipment and maintenance. If technical improvements and increased competition lead to continued cost reductions, proton beam irradiation will become increasingly used because of its dosimetric advantages

LINAC Radiosurgery

The pioneering work of many researchers in the 1980s led to the gradual modifications of linear accelerators (LINACs) designed for conventional radiotherapy to be used for radiosurgery. LINAC technologies were modified by incorporating improved guiding (stereotactic) devices and methods to measure and improve accuracy of various components. Unmodified LINACs for conventional radiotherapy tend to deviate from isocenter alignment at different gantry angles. Most early LINAC-based radiosurgery techniques used multiple radiation arcs with circular secondary collimators to create spherical dose distributions for stereotactically defined 3-D targets. Improved hardware and advanced dose planning software have been developed to enhance conformity. These include beam shaping with micromultileaf collimators and intensity modulation with inverse treatment planning algorithms. Many LINAC-based systems are commercially available. Most are modifications of standard linear accelerators equipped with more precise treatment couches (some capable of alignment with three degrees of rotation) and highly stable treatment isocenters, usually with cone-beam CT scans for targeting and often with patient monitoring system. The CyberKnife combines a miniaturized LINAC mounted on an industrial robot with a system for orthogonal x-ray target tracking and beam realignment. This system utilizes a 6-MeV LINAC with different-sized circular collimators attached to a six-axis robotic manipulator. Stereotactic frames are not normally used for targeting. CyberKnife plans use multiple fixed beam positions and multiple isocenters. Before the radiation is delivered from any beam position, the target position is tracked using an integrated x-ray image processing system (IPS), consisting of two orthogonal diagnostic x-ray cameras and an optical tracking system. During treatment, the IPS acquires x-ray images of the patient's body multiple times throughout the treatment, while stealth tracking software compares the actual images with the target images to correct alignment of the beam. The tracking interval is set by the user with many CyberKnife centers usually using 1-minute intervals. There are some other LINAC radiosurgery systems that have capability for intratreatment patient movement monitoring and correction and others that do not. Respiratory gating/tracking is necessary for optimal treatment (with minimum treatment volumes) of SBRT targets that move with respiration.

The combination of diagnostic 3-D imaging with highly conformal treatment delivery in a single unit to maintain accuracy is the basis of various treatment techniques and processes collectively known as image-guided radiation therapy (IGRT). Most IGRT techniques add CT imaging capability to a LINAC radiotherapy unit equipped for stereotactic and IMRT use. Because any patient movement between image acquisition and treatment delivery (or during treatment delivery) can introduce error, these IGRT systems utilize noninvasive immobilization devices and patient position tracking systems. Several manufacturers currently offer IGRT using LINAC technology capable of delivering stereotactic radiosurgery and radiotherapy. Equipping LINAC units with image guidance from the addition of positron emission tomography (PET) scanning and MR imaging are other possible developments.

TomoTherapy

TomoTherapy, literally "slice" therapy, is a new form of radiotherapy that modifies the design of a diagnostic CT (computerized tomography) scan into a treatment delivery machine, thereby combining the precision of CT imaging with the radiation treatment. This is done by adding a LINAC megavoltage treatment beam to the rotating x-ray source and moving table design of a diagnostic CT unit, which normally uses only a kilovoltage diagnostic x-ray beam. Unlike traditional radiation therapy systems with a slow-moving external gantry designed for positioning individual beams onto the tumor from a few different directions, TomoTherapy rapidly rotates the beam around the patient (and inside the housing of the unit), thus allowing the beam to enter the patient from many different angles in succession. Beam intensity modulation (IMRT) is possible through the use of a multileaf collimator system. The inclusion of CT imaging technology within the TomoTherapy unit allows precise localization of the target before and during treatment.

NORMAL TISSUE TOLERANCE IN SRS AND SRT

Radiosensitivity

Estimating the risks of a proposed treatment plan with various doses is an essential part of treatment planning and dose prescription for SRS and SRT. The ability of normal tissue to tolerate radiation without injury depends on the radiation dose administered, the volume of tissue irradiated, the sensitivity of the tissue affected, history of any prior radiation treatment to the region, as well as any individual variation in radiation sensitivity between different people. At present, with the exception of patients with known increased radiation sensitivity, such as those with ataxia–telangiectasia, there is usually no information routinely available to modify treatment plans for individual differences in radiosensitivity. Prior fractionated radiotherapy appears to have limited effects on the risks of developing postradiosurgery parenchymal edema and neurologic sequelae after radiosurgery but has been observed to effect optic nerve tolerance.

Location Effects

Analysis of postradiosurgery injury reactions in AVM patients revealed no difference in the likelihood of postradiosurgery injury imaging changes (increased signal developing in

TABLE 17.2 PREDICTED RISKS OF DEVELOPING ANY SYMPTOMATIC (AND PERMANENT) NEUROLOGIC SEQUELAE AFTER AVM RADIOSURGERY ACCORDING TO 12-GY VOLUME AND LOCATION FROM 755 PATIENTS WITH 2-YEAR MINIMUM FOLLOW-UP

12-Gy Volume	Brainstem	Thalamus	Other
0.1 cm³	11% (8%)	5% (3%)	1% (0.3%)
10 cm³	28% (15%)	15% (7%)	4% (1%)
20 cm³	55% (30%)	37% (15%)	10% (2%)
30 cm³	79% (50%)	64% (28%)	27% (5%)
40 cm³	92% (69%)	84% (48%)	53% (12%)

From Kano H, Flickinger JC, Tonetti D, et al. Estimating the risks of adverse radiation effects after Gamma Knife radiosurgery for arteriovenous malformations. *Stroke* 2017;48(1):84–90.

surrounding brain on long relaxation time or T2 images) in different regions of the brain.[6,7] Dramatic differences were seen in the rates of developing persistent neurologic sequelae after AVM radiosurgery between the brainstem, thalamus, and other regions of the brain as shown in Table 17.2.

Radiosurgery Dose Escalation Studies

The RTOG Radiosurgery Dose-Escalation Study (95-05) established tolerance doses for radiosurgery of recurrent brain metastases and high-grade gliomas not involving the brainstem.[8] They administered radiosurgery to 156 patients with brain metastases or primary brain tumors that recurred or progressed after conventional radiotherapy following a dose escalation protocol. Starting with initial doses of 18, 15, and 12 Gy for diameters <20, 21 to 30, and 31 to 40 mm, respectively, they escalated prescription doses in 3-Gy intervals until irreversible toxicity was seen in over 20% of patients within 3 months. The exception was with tumors <20 mm in diameter where dose-limiting toxicity was not reached and investigators were reluctant to escalate above 24 to 27 Gy. The recommended tolerance doses from that protocol were 24, 18, and 15 Gy for diameters of <20 mm, 21 to 30, and 31 to 40 mm, respectively. The data with longer follow-up beyond 3 months to assess late toxicity were fitted to individual logistic dose–response curves in Figure 17.3. These tolerance doses have been widely used as dose guidelines for single-fraction radiosurgery of malignant tumors, often with interpolation for tumors close to 20 and 30 mm in diameter (e.g., 20 Gy for 18- to 22-mm diameter and 16.5 Gy for 28- to 32-mm diameter treatment volumes).

Murai et al.[9] performed a limited dose escalation study of CyberKnife radiosurgery of 48 brain metastases 2.5 to 4 cm in average diameter with 18 to 30 Gy in 3 fractions and

FIGURE 17.3. Phase 1 RTOG dose escalation data for radiosurgery of recurrent brain metastases and glioblastoma fit to logistic dose–response curves. The numbers at each data point indicate the number of patients in each dose/diameter group. (From Dewan MZ, Galloway AE, Kawashima N, et al. Fractionated but not single-dose radiotherapy induces an immune-mediated abscopal effect when combined with anti-CTLA-4 antibody. *Clin Cancer Res* 2009;15[17]:5379–5388.)

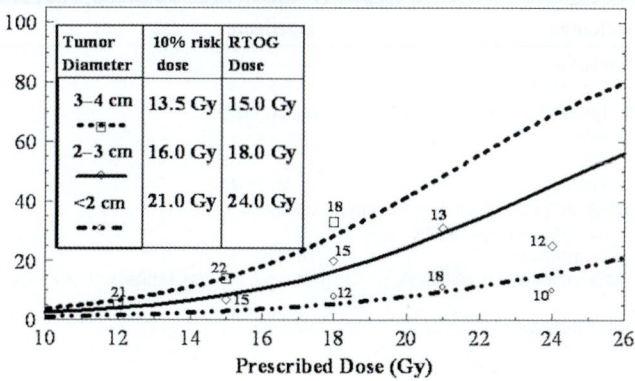

% Developing Late Neurological Sequelae

Tumor Diameter	10% risk dose	RTOG Dose
3–4 cm	13.5 Gy	15.0 Gy
2–3 cm	16.0 Gy	18.0 Gy
<2 cm	21.0 Gy	24.0 Gy

13 metastases >4-cm diameter with 21 to 35 Gy in 5 fractions. They reported grade 2 brain necrosis developing in 1/19 patients at the penultimate level of either 22 to 27 Gy/3 fractions or for >4 cm 25 to 31 Gy/5 fractions and 3/23 patients (two grade 2 and one grade 3) at the highest level of 27 to 30 Gy/3 fractions or for >4 cm 31 to 35 Gy/5 fractions.

Schwer et al.[10] performed a 3-fraction SRS dose escalation study from 18 to 36 Gy in 15 patients with recurrent gliomas treated in combination with gefitinib. With a median treatment volume of 41 cm[3] (8 to 151 cm[3]), three patients were treated at the 18, 24, and 30 Gy levels and 16 at 36 Gy. They failed to identify any radiation-related toxicity.

Clarke et al.[11] reported a dose escalation study of 3 fractions of radiosurgery delivered with 10 mg/kg bevacizumab q2 weeks to doses of 27, 30, and 33 Gy in groups of 3, 5, and 7 patients, respectively, with recurrent glioblastoma and anaplastic astrocytoma after prior conventional chemoradiotherapy. They identified no cases of clearly symptomatic radionecrosis, but one patient in the 33-Gy level exhibited cognitive deterioration and grade 3 fatigue, which they counted as treatment-related toxicity. Three patients underwent subsequent resections for presumed local progression with viable tumor and substantial radiation necrosis found in each, one of which had necrosis in >90% of the specimen.

Pollom et al.[12] also reported a somewhat unenlightening dose escalation trial of 5-fraction radiosurgery to doses of 25, 30, 35, and 40 Gy delivered with a 5-mm margin along with concurrent and adjuvant temozolomide in 30 patients with newly diagnosed supratentorial glioblastoma. Six patients were entered at each of the 4 lower-dose levels and 12 at the highest level of 40 Gy. With a median follow-up of 13.5 months (0.4 to 62.4 months) and 10.4 months for quality of life (QOL) assessment, 8/30 showed evidence of adverse radiation effects (ARE), which were symptomatic in 6 of those patients, but no dose/volume breakdown of the toxicity was reported nor was a maximum tolerated radiation dose. The 12-month ARE rate was 38% with 4/5 survivors with >2 years of health-related QOL follow-up developing ARE. Survival and tumor control seemed similar to that expected with standard chemoradiotherapy. ARE did not significantly affect health-related QOL, possibly because all patients developing ARE were treated with bevacizumab.

Optic Nerve Tolerance for Radiosurgery

The first analysis of optic nerve tolerance to radiosurgery, a combined Harvard/University of Pittsburgh study of patients with cavernous sinus meningiomas, craniopharyngioma, and pituitary adenomas, recommended 8 Gy as a safe maximum dose limit for the optic nerves/chiasm, although most centers now use 10 Gy.[13] The lowest optic chiasm dose at which optic neuropathy developed in that study was reported as being 9.7 Gy. Optic nerve/chiasm doses were estimated from isodose distributions overlaid on CT images, unlike the present day

when the entire optic system is usually outlined on detailed MR images and maximum doses are assessed from dose–volume histograms. It is highly likely that the true maximum doses to the optic system were higher and lay in portions of the nerve that were poorly visualized.

Stafford et al.[14] reported a later analysis of four cases of optic neuropathy occurring out of 215 Mayo clinic radiosurgery patients with a median dose of 10 Gy to the optic chiasm. One case developed after an optic nerve/chiasm dose of 12.8 Gy with radiosurgery alone, at which the risk level appeared to be approximately 3%. The other cases developed in patients with prior fractionated radiotherapy (7 Gy after 58.8 Gy, 9 Gy after 45 Gy and two procedures delivering 9, and later 12 Gy to the optic system after 50.4 Gy).

Leber et al.[15] analyzed optic nerve injury risks in 50 patients with 24- to 60-month follow-up (median 40 months) who underwent Gamma Knife radiosurgery for benign skull base tumors. Their risks of optic neuropathy were 0% with <10 Gy, 27% with 10 to 15 Gy, and 78% with >15 Gy. They found no cavernous sinus nerve injury with doses of 5 to 30 Gy.

Hiniker et al.[16] found <1% risk of optic neuropathy with 12 Gy in 1 fraction, 19.5 Gy in 3 fractions, and 25 Gy among 262 patients with perioptic tumors treated with SRS.

What is not clear at this point is what doses of repeat radiation can be delivered for 1%, 5%, and 10% risks of injury to the optic system nerves and chiasm to 6 months or more after they have received standard tolerance doses of 10, 18, or 25 Gy in 1, 3, or 5 fractions, respectively.

Tolerance of Other Cranial Nerves

From clinical experience with fractionated conventional radiosurgery and radiosurgery, it appears that special sensory nerves (optic and auditory) are the most radiosensitive, followed by somatic sensory nerves (trigeminal) and finally the motor nerves (cranial nerves II, IV, VI, VII, and IX to XII). After acoustic schwannoma radiosurgery to doses of 12 to 13 Gy, FSR to 18 Gy in 3 fractions, or SRT to 45 to 50 Gy in 25 to 28 fractions, decreased hearing develops in 30% to 50% of patients, facial numbness in 2% to 3%, and facial weakness in 0.5% or less. Single-fraction radiosurgery with present techniques for meningiomas involving the cavernous sinus is associated with a risk of trigeminal neuropathy of approximately 3% of patients with radiation injuries to cranial nerves III, IV, or VI more uncommon.[17–21] The risk of injury correlates with the length of nerve irradiated.[22]

CLINICAL USES OF SRS AND SRT

Table 17.3 lists the most commonly used indications for radiosurgery with representative references. Except for functional radiosurgery, there are varied levels of experience with SRT for each of these indications.

TABLE 17.3 COMMON INDICATIONS FOR RADIOSURGERY OR HYPOFRACTIONATED STEREOTACTIC RADIOTHERAPY

Indication	Experience	Value	References
Functional a. Trigeminal neuralgia b. Unilateral tremor	a. Extensive b. Moderate	1. Less numbness than rhizotomy 2. In poor candidates for deep brain stimulation	a. [18–22] b. [23–26]
Vascular a. AVM b. Cavernous	a. Extensive b. Moderate	a. High b. Controversial	a. [4,27–29] b. [30–32]
Benign tumors: schwannoma, pituitary adenoma meningioma, etc.	Extensive	High tumor control, acceptable morbidity for selected small tumors	[11–13,33–64]
Brain metastases	Extensive	Control rates ≥ surgery for small mets	[65,66]
Primary malignant brain tumors	Extensive for GBM. Limited with other uses	Initial SRS appears ineffective for GBM. Helpful for recurrent tumors, possibly initial pilocytic, neurocytoma	[67–75]
Spinal metastases	Moderate	High for recurrent tumors. No phase 3 comparison with conventional XRT for initial treatment	[16,17]

Functional Radiosurgery

The most widely used functional application for radiosurgery is in the management of typical trigeminal neuralgia refractory to medical therapy.[23–27] Atypical or constant pain does not respond. Other alternatives for managing typical trigeminal neuralgia are medication, open surgery with microvascular decompression, and rhizotomy procedures using glycerol injection, balloon compression, or radiofrequency injury to the nerve. Typically 4-mm collimators are used for radiosurgery to a maximum dose of 80 to 90 Gy. Response rates reach approximately 85%, typically 1 week to 4 months after the procedure, but can develop as late as 6 months afterward. Approximately 50% of typical trigeminal neuralgia patients remain pain-free and off medication 5 years following radiosurgery. A typical radiosurgery plan for trigeminal neuralgia is shown in Figure 17.4. Kotecha et al.[25] analyzed the dose response for trigeminal neuralgia in 352, 85, and 433 patients undergoing SRS with maximum doses of ≤82, 83 to 86, and ≥90 Gy. They found 4-year pain responses of 79%, 82%, and 92% and 4-year rates of BNI class 3 to 4 numbness developing in 25%, 49%, and 40% of patients at maximum doses of <82, 73 to 86, and >90 Gy, respectively. The numbness in nine patients (1%) was classified as anesthesia dolorosa, all of whom with maximum doses ≤86 Gy.

Recent studies have suggested that radiosurgery within 3 years of onset of trigeminal neuralgia lead to better long-term pain control and that selective dose reduction to 70 to 75 Gy may reduce risks of radiation-induced trigeminal neuropathy in patients with larger treatment volumes resulting from having thicker trigeminal nerves.[26,27]

A small destructive lesion in the ventralis intermedius nucleus of the thalamus can be created either invasively with a needle equipped with a radiofrequency generator or noninvasively with radiosurgery using 4-mm diameter collimators and a maximum dose of 130 Gy to alleviate medically refractory unilateral tremor in patients with essential tremor and/or Parkinson disease.[28–31] Nondestructive management through insertion of a deep brain stimulator is preferred in most patients, but not all patients are acceptable candidates

and radiosurgery appears more cost-effective.[31] Although targeting the globus pallidus for bradykinesia, rigidity, and dyskinesia from Parkinson's has been successful with deep brain stimulation, limited early radiosurgical pallidotomy has not achieved established success.[32,33] There is limited experience with bilateral radiosurgical capsulotomy (targeting the anterior limb of the internal capsule) for managing severe, refractory obsessive–compulsive disorder, including a small randomized controlled study that was retracted after it was found that only 2/8 patients responded to radiosurgery (vs. 3/8 as originally thought) compared to 0/8 without radiosurgery.[34] Radiosurgery to hypothalamic hamartomas may help control refractory gelastic seizures.[35] The use of radiosurgery as an alternative to extensive surgery in medically refractory mesial temporal lobe epilepsy shows promise and continues to be investigated.[36] Improvements in functional imaging such as MR tractography should eventually lead to improvements in functional neurosurgical interventions including radiosurgery. Another recent development is the substitution of focused ultrasound as a substitute for radiation to create focal areas of necrosis.[65]

Vascular Malformations

Untreated intracranial AVMs have a bleeding risk of approximately 2% to 3% per year or higher if prior bleeds have occurred.[66–68] This results in an average of 1% of untreated AVM patients dying per year from hemorrhage. Management options include observation, surgical resection, embolization, and radiosurgery. The ARUBA trial for AVMs with no prior bleeds compared observation to treatment intervention with institutional choices of embolization, resection, and/or radiosurgery.[69] Because the initial morbidity from intervention by surgery, embolization, and/or radiosurgery was compared to the relatively low annual bleeding risk of unruptured AVM with observation, the ARUBA trial identified observation as the best management option for their relatively short 33-month mean follow-up period. Although this trial could be used to justify observation for older patients with low-risk AVMs, the relatively short follow-up ARUBA trial was inadequate to see the long-term benefits from definitive management of AVM with surgery or radiosurgery in younger patients.

After 3 to 5 years, radiosurgery can dramatically reduce the risk of hemorrhage. Radiosurgery obliterates the AVM nidus in approximately 75% of patients within 3 years of the procedure.[3,70,71] Individual obliteration rates vary from 50% to 88% depending upon marginal dose administered as shown in the dose–response curve illustrated in Figure 17.5. Although AVM obliteration rates appear to be optimized

FIGURE 17.4. Typical radiosurgery plan for right trigeminal neuralgia. The right trigeminal nerve is outlined in white. The 30% and 50% isodose volumes from treating a single isocenter with 4-mm diameter collimators with a gamma unit are shown. A maximum dose of 80 Gy will deliver 40 Gy to the 50% isodose value and 16 Gy to the 20% volume.

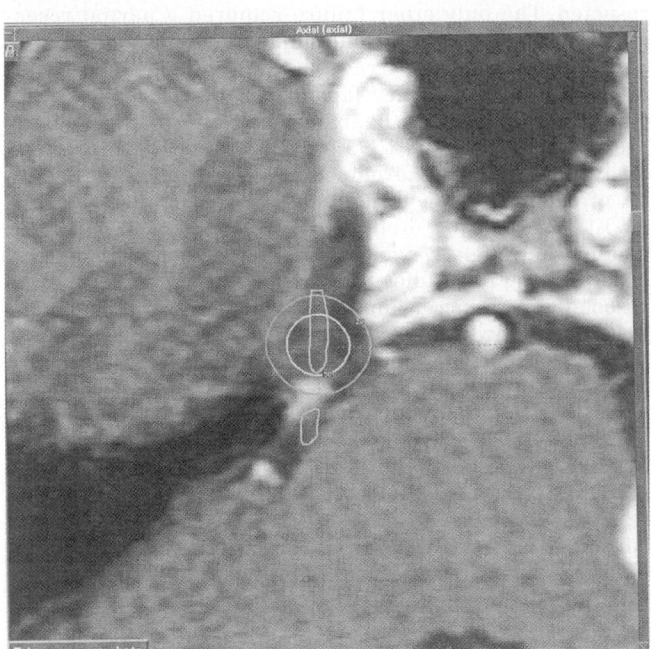

FIGURE 17.5. Dose response for obliteration of AVM after radiosurgery from 297 patients treated at the University of Pittsburgh without embolization. (Reprinted by permission from Flickinger JC, Kondziolka D, Lunsford LD. Radiobiological analysis of tissue responses following radiosurgery. *Technol Cancer Res Treat* 2003;2[2]:87–92. Copyright © 2003 SAGE Publications.[72])

% with Overall Angiographic or MR Obliteration

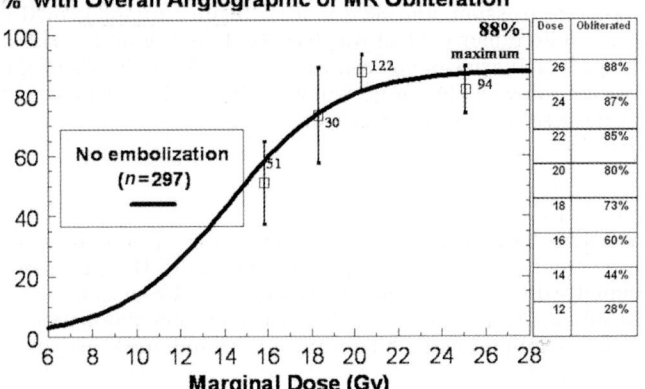

Dose	Obliterated
26	88%
24	87%
22	85%
20	80%
18	73%
16	60%
14	44%
12	28%

with marginal doses of approximately 23 Gy, lower doses are selected for most patients to minimize complications. The risk of neurologic sequelae from radiosurgery averages approximately 3% but varies with treatment volume, dose, and location (Fig. 17.2). The risk of hemorrhage while waiting for complete obliteration to develop seems unaltered.[66] All of these risks and benefits of radiosurgery need to be considered together to optimize management of individual AVM patients.

When an AVM nidus fails to completely obliterate by 3 years after radiosurgery, irradiation can be repeated with acceptable morbidity.[73,74] Although some residual radiation injury effect would be expected within the previously irradiated unobliterated AVM nidus vasculature, re-treatment appears to require similar, if not higher doses to achieve similar rates of complete obliteration as initial radiosurgery.[73,74]

Management of large AVMs is presently difficult because radiosurgery may be associated with high complication risks and low obliteration rates. Recent improvements in embolization with liquid glue or onyx polymer can sometimes help reduce the target volume but add to the total risks of the overall management.[75] Another promising approach is staged radiosurgery, in which large AVMs are treated in two or three sections separated by 4- to 6-month intervals to reduce acute toxicity. Whether there is any benefit to fractionating stereotactic irradiation of AVMs is presently unclear.[76]

Cavernous malformations do not show detectable flow on angiography but nevertheless are vascular lesions with annual hemorrhage risks of 0.5% per year with no prior bleed, 4.5% with one prior hemorrhage, and approximately 32% per year after a history of two or more hemorrhages.[77-81] Lower pressures in these lesions lead to smaller bleeds than are typically seen with AVM. Repeated bleeds from brainstem cavernous malformations can cause considerable neurologic morbidity. Symptomatic surgically accessible lesions should be resected. Radiosurgery of brainstem cavernous malformations with a history of two or more prior hemorrhages appears to reduce the risk of subsequent bleeds to approximately 1% per year with acceptable morbidity.[82-88]

Benign Tumors

Most small benign intracranial tumors are well managed with radiosurgery, FSR, or SRT. Radiosurgery control rates are high with radiosurgery with single-fraction prescription doses on the order of 12 to 14 Gy or their equivalent with hypofractionation.[17-21,37-62,89-98] Kondziolka et al. evaluated long-term tumor control in 285 consecutive patients who underwent radiosurgery for benign intracranial tumors between 1987 and 1992 with a median follow-up period of 10 years.[17] This included 157 patients with vestibular schwannomas, 10 with other cranial nerve schwannomas, 85 with meningiomas, 28 with pituitary adenomas, and 5 with craniopharyngiomas. 44% had prior surgical resection and 5% had prior fractionated radiotherapy. They found that 95% of the 285 patients had imaging-defined local tumor control (63% had tumor regression, and 32% had no further tumor growth). The crude tumor control was 95% (271/285 patients) with a 15-year actuarial tumor control rate of 93.7%. In 5% of the patients, delayed tumor growth was identified. Resection was performed after radiosurgery in 13 patients (5%) for tumor growth.

Vestibular Schwannomas

Vestibular schwannomas, also known as acoustic neuromas, are benign tumors arising from Schwann cells. They are associated with loss of genetic information on chromosome 22.[93] Vestibular schwannomas either occur on one side as spontaneous mutations or bilaterally as the hallmark of type 2

neurofibromatosis (NF-2). Vestibular schwannomas usually arise within the internal auditory canal and later extend intracranially into the cerebellar–pontine angle. Because these tumors lack the ability to invade bone, the portion of tumor outside the canal in the cerebellar–pontine angle eventually grows into a globular extension that is larger than the intracanalicular portion (Fig. 17.1). The differential diagnosis of a cerebellar–pontine angle tumor includes vestibular schwannoma (90%), meningioma (close to 10%), cholesteatomas, facial or trigeminal schwannoma, and rare primary or metastatic malignant tumors. Cerebellar–pontine angle meningiomas (which can be managed similarly to vestibular schwannomas) also may involve the internal auditory canal, but usually be distinguished by a broad, flat, dural attachment that is lacking in vestibular schwannomas.

Observation and surgical resection were essentially the only management strategies offered to acoustic schwannoma patients until favorable experiences with Gamma Knife radiosurgery were reported in the 1980s. Observation may be appropriate in selected NF-2 patients and some elderly patients with small, minimally symptomatic vestibular schwannomas, but early intervention appears to be the best strategy for long-term hearing preservation for most patients.[94,95] Surgery appears to be the best initial strategy in patients with vestibular schwannomas large enough to cause symptomatic brainstem compression with obstructive hydrocephalus. For small to medium vestibular schwannomas, tumor control rates with radiosurgery or SRT are comparable to surgical resection.[37-58,94-98]

Early radiosurgery series including patients treated during the 1980s with higher doses (14 to 18 Gy) and less conformal treatment plans had higher rates of postradiosurgery cranial neuropathies (15% to 20% trigeminal and/or facial and 67% with a drop in their Gardner-Robertson hearing level).[98] This prompted some groups to pursue SRT for vestibular schwannomas, whereas others pursued radiosurgery with refined techniques and lower doses. Both approaches lead to improved results.[37-55,94-98] The University of Pittsburgh reported on 313 previously untreated unilateral acoustic schwannoma patients that underwent Gamma Knife radiosurgery doses of 12 to 13 Gy between February 1991 and February 2001.[38] Median follow-up was 24 months and maximum follow-up 115 months, and 36 patients had >60 months of follow-up. The actuarial clinical tumor control rate, free of surgical intervention, was 98.6% at 7 years. One patient's growing tumor was subsequently completely resected. The only other failure required a partial resection because of an enlarging adjacent subarachnoid cyst, despite control of the irradiated tumor. The 7-year actuarial rates for unchanged facial strength, unchanged facial sensation, unchanged hearing level, and useful hearing preservation were 100%, 95.6%, 70.3%, and 78.6%, respectively. Eight patients developed new trigeminal neuropathy, six of whom developed numbness (7-year actuarial rate = 2.5%), whereas the other two developed new typical trigeminal neuralgia (7-year actuarial rate = 1.9%). The risk of developing postradiosurgery trigeminal neuropathy was associated with increasing tumor volume ($P = .038$). Similar results with low-dose radiosurgery of vestibular schwannomas were reported by Iwai et al.[41], Paek et al.,[44] Muacevic et al.,[42] and Rowe et al.[46]

Various fractionation schemes (18 Gy/3, 20 Gy/4 to 5, 25 Gy/5, 45 to 50 Gy/25, and 54 Gy/30) have been used with vestibular schwannoma with minor differences in results. After accounting for length and quality of follow-up treatment, results seem similar to radiosurgery with 12 to 13 Gy, but an advantage for fractionation can't be excluded entirely.[43] UCLA reported unusually good hearing preservation (93%) for their experience with 50 unilateral acoustic schwannoma patients irradiated to 54 Gy in 30 fractions to a 90% isodose treatment volume including a 1- to 3-mm margin around gross tumor.[56] All tumors were controlled with a median follow-up of 36 months (range: 6 to 74 months). They defined useful hearing preservation as the ability to talk on the telephone with the affected ear. New facial numbness developed in one patient (2%) and facial weakness also in one patient (2%) after radiotherapy.

Andrews et al. analyzed the Jefferson vestibular schwannoma experience, comparing 69 radiosurgery patients to 50 SRT patients who received 50 Gy/25 fractions.[50] Their first 25 vestibular schwannoma patients were treated using a linear accelerator, whereas later radiosurgery patients were treated with Gamma Knife radiosurgery. The authors reported similar facial and trigeminal neuropathy rates for the radiosurgery and fractionated radiotherapy groups, but the rate of hearing loss was significantly higher in their radiosurgery group. There were only a small number of patients with serviceable (useful) hearing in each group prior to irradiation (12 in the radiosurgery and 21 in the FSRT groups), and follow-up was limited. Meijer et al., from Amsterdam, also reported a single-institution comparison of radiosurgery (LINAC to 10 or 12.5 Gy) and SRT (20 Gy/4 to 5 fractions) for vestibular schwannoma.[49] They selected 49 edentulous patients (mean age = 63 years) for radiosurgery and 80 patients (mean age = 43 years) with intact dentition for SRT. They found a higher rate of trigeminal neuropathy following radiosurgery (8%) than SRT. (2%) at 5 years (*P* = .048), but similar hearing loss with radiosurgery (25%) than SRT (39% FSRT, *P* > 0.05), similar, but higher than usual rates of new facial neuropathy (7% radiosurgery vs. 3% FSRT, *P* > 0.05) and similar 5-year actuarial tumor control rates (100% with radiosurgery vs. 94% with SRT). Combs et al.[53] compared the results of vestibular schwannoma management with single-fraction radiosurgery to a median dose of 13 Gy in 169 patients to FSRT at 1.8 Gy/fraction to a median dose of 57.6 Gy in 291 patients with a median follow-up of 67 months. Local control rates were similar at 95% and 94% at 5 and 10 years. Useful hearing preservation rates were also similar at 84% and 86% in the SRS and FSRT groups, as was trigeminal and facial neuropathy were similar at approximately 1% for both. Akpinar et al.[58] reported the results of hearing preservation after single-fraction radiosurgery with a median dose of 12.5 Gy (11 to 13 Gy) to a median volume of 0.72 cm³ (0.11 to 12.8 cm³) in 88 University of Pittsburgh patients with vestibular schwannomas with no subjective hearing loss at the time of diagnosis with 75 months of median follow-up. For the 57 patients who underwent SRS ≤2 years from diagnosis, the serviceable hearing (class 1 to 2) and normal hearing preservation rates (class 1) at 5 years after SRS were 88% and 77%, whereas those for the 31 patients who underwent late SRS (>2 years after diagnosis) were 55% and 33%, respectively (*P* = 0.006 and *P* < .001).

Nonacoustic Schwannomas

Schwannomas may occasionally involve other cranial nerves, particularly V, VII, and XI-XII in the jugular foramen. Tumor control rates are similar, but postradiosurgery neuropathies seem less common as somatic sensory and particularly motor nerves seem less sensitive to radiation injury than special sensory nerves like VIII.[59–63] Kano et al.[63] reported on 92 jugular foramen schwannomas managed at multiple institutions with a median single-fraction dose of 12.5 Gy (10 to 18 Gy) to volumes of 0.8 to 22.6 cm³ (median = 4.1 cm³). Tumor control rates at 5 and 10 years were 87% and 82%. Preexisting cranial neuropathies improved in 32% and 37% of patients. Because spinal schwannomas involving motor nerves are difficult to completely resect without causing motor deficits, they are often managed with radiosurgery. Shin et al.[64] reported one of

the larger series of neurogenic spinal nerve root tumors (47 schwannomas, 7 neurofibromas, and 4 malignant peripheral nerve sheath tumors managed with radiosurgery). Local control for the schwannomas was 86%.

Meningiomas

Radiosurgery and SRS are both excellent management options for most small benign meningiomas with infield tumor control rates well above 90%, as has been seen with most other benign tumors.[17,89] Marginal recurrences rates as high as 25% may develop because of the tight margins used for radiosurgery or SRT treatment volumes limited to small recurrences or residual tumor after resection of large parasagittal meningiomas.[17,89,99–101] Marginal recurrences are far less of a problem with unresected (and usually unbiopsied) meningiomas. A University of Pittsburgh study[89] analyzed 219 imaging diagnosed (unbiopsied) meningiomas managed with single-fraction Gamma Knife radiosurgery to a prescription dose of 8.9 to 20 Gy (14 Gy median) and treatment volumes of 0.47 to 56.5 mL (median 5.0 mL) with 2 to 164 months of follow-up (median 29 months). Tumors progressed in 7 patients, two of which proved to be different tumors (metastatic nasopharyngeal adenoid cystic carcinoma and chondrosarcoma). Another patient with locally control of the lesion developed a subsequent brain metastasis, changing the diagnosis of the first lesion to the same. The actuarial tumor control rate was 93.2% at both 5 and 10 years. The actuarial rate of identifying a diagnosis other than meningioma was at both 5 and 10 years. No pretreatment variables, including dose, correlated with tumor control in univariate or multivariate analysis. The actuarial rate for developing any postradiosurgical injury reaction was 8.8% at 5 and 10 years. The risk of postradiosurgery sequelae was lower (5.3%) after 1991 (with stereotactic MRI and lower doses; *P* = .0104).

Atypical and malignant (anaplastic) meningiomas have higher rates of local and marginal recurrence after therapeutic intervention. Complete surgical resection is advocated whenever possible followed by a full course of conventional radiotherapy with at least 1-cm margins around the tumor volume. Radiosurgery has been recommended to improve local control of unresectable tumor.[101–104] Malik et al. reported 5-year actuarial control rates of 87% for typical meningiomas, 49% for atypical, and 0% for malignant meningioma in the Sheffield Gamma Knife experience.[101] Harris et al. reported on the Pittsburgh Gamma Knife experience in 12 malignant and 18 atypical meningiomas.[103] Their 5-year local tumor control was 72% for malignant and 83% for atypical meningiomas; however, 10-year actuarial survival rates were only 59% and 0%, respectively. Katz et al. could not substantiate that either accelerated fractionated radiotherapy or a radiosurgery boost improved tumor control or survival in their analysis of 27 atypical and 9 malignant meningioma patients managed at the University of Florida.[104]

One controversy in radiosurgical management of meningiomas is whether an additional dural margin or dural tail needs to be routinely included in the treatment volume. Dibiase et al.[105] analyzed a series of 162 benign meningioma patients treated to a median single fraction of 14 Gy and found improved tumor control with treatment of the dural tail (96% vs. 78%). Most centers do not follow this policy and other authors[106] have argued against this policy with WHO grade 1 meningiomas. Outlining the tumor target volume with T2 imaging sometimes discloses gross tumor extension into what otherwise appears to be normal dura adjacent to the tumor. Any WHO grade 2 or 3 meningioma should be treated with a 1-cm margin of additional normal dura whenever possible.

Pituitary Adenoma

Management of pituitary adenomas requires a multidisciplinary approach to properly select which patients are suitable for different approaches with medical therapy, surgery, fractionated radiotherapy and radiosurgery, or combinations of these. Most patient with visual compromise, particularly with a hemianopsia or greater, will do better with initial surgical decompression. Prolactinomas are usually initially managed with medical therapy.[90] Most other small pituitary adenomas, where the target volume can be separated from the optic nerves, are reasonable candidates for radiosurgery.[17,90–92]

Sheehan et al.[92] performed a review of 35 peer-reviewed reports of radiosurgery for pituitary adenoma, which included 1,621 patients. Most studies reported a >90% control of tumor size (range: 68% to 100%). His weighted average tumor control rate for all published series (encompassing 1,283 patients) was 96%. In eight published series with mean or median patient follow-up periods of 4 or more years, tumor growth control rates varied from 83% to 100%.

Twenty-two series results published radiosurgery results for 314 Cushing disease patients. The mean radiosurgical prescription (margin) doses for these series varied from 15 to 32 Gy. In those series with at least ten patients and a median follow-up of 2 years, endocrinologic remission rates range from 17% to 83%. Many of the patients in older series were treated in the pre-CT and MRI era of radiosurgery sometimes as often as four times before their Cushing disease went into remission. Mehta et al.[93] reported a multi-institutional experience with SRS to a mean single-fraction dose of 23.7 Gy in 278 Cushing disease patients with a mean follow-up of 5.6 years (0.5 to 20.5 years). Cumulative initial control of hypercortisolism was 80% at 10 years with a mean time to cortisol normalization of 14.5 months. Recurrences after initial cortisol normalization developed in 18% of patients, which made the overall rate of durable hormonal control to 64% at 10 years and 68% among patients who received SRS as a primary treatment. AREs included hypopituitarism (25%) and cranial neuropathy (3%). Development of visual deficits correlated with tumors involving the suprasellar cistern ($P = .01$), whereas both visual ($P < .0001$) and nonvisual cranial neuropathies ($P = .02$) were related to prior pituitary irradiation. The North American Gamma Knife Consortium series[94] of 512 nonfunctioning pituitary adenoma patients reported 5- and 10-year tumor control rates of 91% and 85% with a mean dose of 16 Gy (range: 5 to 35 Gy) to a mean volume of 3.33 Gy (range: 0.08 to 33 cm³). Higher tumor control rates were found in tumors <5 cm³ and those without suprasellar extension. Tumor control rates in patients receiving <12 Gy, 12 to 20 Gy, and >20 Gy were 73.5%, 95.5%, and 92%. New or progressive cranial neuropathies developed in 9% of patients (including 6.6% optic). Decreasing age, increasing volume, history of prior radiation therapy, and history of prior pituitary axis deficiency correlated with new or worsening cranial neuropathy.

Malignant Tumors

Management of brain metastases with radiosurgery is discussed elsewhere in this book. The most important controversies in brain metastasis radiosurgery involve the management of larger brain metastases. For brain metastasis radiosurgery, both local tumor recurrence rates and complication rates increase with increasing tumor target volume, particularly for tumors >3 cm in diameter. Strategies to improve the radiosurgical management of brain metastases include switching from single fraction to different forms of fractionated SRS or SRT and also combining radiosurgery with surgical resection.

Two different overall types of fractionation strategies have been used. One strategy is to fractionate the radiation treatment for a single treatment plan over a short time period, usually within 1 to 2 weeks to limit tumor repopulation. The other approach is a two-staged adaptive radiosurgery with the fractions separated by approximately 1 month. This allows tumor to shrink before the second fraction is delivered and so requires reimaging with a second treatment plan. Cho et al.,[107] for example, compared the outcome of treating 81 small brain metastases with a median volume of 1.0 cm³ (range: 0.12 to 4.4 cm³), with single-fraction radiosurgery to a median dose of 22 Gy to that with 38 larger brain metastases with a median volume of 17.6 cm³ (range 12.8 to 23.7 cm³) treated with 3 to 5 fractions to a median dose of 35 Gy. Tumor control rates at 1 year for single versus 3 to 5 fractions were similar at 89.7% versus 87% as were radiation necrosis rates at 12.3% versus 15.8%, respectively. The second strategy for radiosurgery of large brain metastases is a two-staged adaptive radiosurgery with time in between to allow for tumor shrinkage. Angelov et al.,[108] for example, treated 63 brain metastases with a median volume of 10.5 cm³ in 54 patients with a median initial dose of 15 Gy (12 to 18 Gy) and to a median second dose of 15 Gy (range 12 to 15 Gy) to a median volume of 7.0 cm³(1.0 to 29.7 cm³) and a median of 34 days later. Tumor control was 88% at 6 months and only 11% adverse radiation effects.

The other approach for dealing with large brain metastases is combining surgical resection with radiosurgery to the tumor bed. Patel et al.[109] compared the results of surgical resection of brain metastases with radiosurgery delivered either preoperatively to a median dose of 14.5 Gy with no margin in 66 patients or postoperatively with 2-mm margin in 114 patients. Although no significant differences were found in overall survival ($P = .1$), local recurrence ($P = .24$), or distant brain recurrence ($P = .75$), patients undergoing postop SRS developed significantly more leptomeningeal disease (16.6% vs. 3.2%) and symptomatic radiation injury (16.4% vs. 4.9%) at 2 years despite a higher proportion of breast cancer with similar median gross tumor volumes (9.2 vs. 8.3 cm³) and a higher proportion of breast cancer cases in the preoperative group (27.2% vs. 10.5%). Atalar et al.[110] had previously reported higher risks of leptomeningeal seeding with postop SRS for brain metastases from breast cancer (24% vs. 9% at 1 year) than other primaries.

Brain Metastases

Brain metastases are the most common and best studied of the indications for radiosurgery.[103] Early clinical investigations found impressive tumor control with radiosurgery for brain metastases that progressed after prior whole-brain radiotherapy (WBXRT). RTOG's phase I dose escalation trial in recurrent brain tumors to some degree standardized dose prescription for brain metastasis radiosurgery.[72] Because of the success of radiosurgery in controlling brain metastases after WBXRT and the high rate of eventual local tumor progression in brain metastases after conventional WBXRT, radiosurgery has been increasingly used in initial management of brain metastases.[72] RTOG's subsequent phase III randomized trial, RTOG 95-08, established that radiosurgery immediately following standard WBXRT (37.5 Gy in 15 fractions) improves local control and quality of life for patients with one to three brain metastases while also improving overall survival for patients with solitary metastasis, all compared to patients initially managed with only WBXRT.[36]

Although RTOG 95-08 established radiosurgery's role after WBXRT in managing one to three brain metastases, questions remained about managing brain metastases with radiosurgery alone and preserving full-dose WBXRT as an option for later managing cases with subsequent progression. Aoyama published the outcome of a prospective randomized controlled trial to evaluate whether initial WBXRT provides better outcomes when added to stereotactic radiosurgery (SRS) compared to using SRS alone.[1] Aoyama's 11 hospital study randomized 132 patients with one to four brain metastases <3 cm in diameter to radiosurgery either with or without initial WBXRT. They found that the median survival time and the 1-year actuarial survival rates were not significantly different with or without WBXRT.[35] The 1-year brain tumor "recurrence rate" (corresponding to the development of additional brain metastases) was higher in the SRS-alone group compared to the patient group who received both WBRT and SRS. Earlier retrospective studies had similar observations. The most common primary site in these studies was the lung. Separate analyses of brain metastases radiosurgery of different histologies with and without whole-brain radiosurgery found that WBXRT reduced subsequent development of brain metastases in lung cancer patients but not in patients with melanoma or renal cell carcinoma. Administering initial WBXRT and waiting a month before radiosurgery for subsequent tumor shrinkage are a reasonable strategy to limit radiation injury reactions and/or improve tumor control for brain metastases >3 cm in diameter and for brainstem metastases >2 cm in diameter.

There is no clear limit to how many metastases and what total volume of metastases can or should be treated by radiosurgery. RTOG 9508 was limited to 1 to 3 metastases, whereas Aoyama's trial and a smaller University of Pittsburgh trial included patients with up to four brain metastases.[104] Bhatnagar et al.[111] analyzed 205 patients who underwent radiosurgery for 4 to 18 brain metastases (median = 5). They reported a median survival of 8 months after radiosurgery and found that survival correlated with the total volume of metastases, age, and RTOG-RPA class, but not the total number of brain metastases. Presently, many centers use WBXRT alone to initially manage patients with five or more metastases and subsequently consider radiosurgery for patients who are unable to be withdrawn from steroid medication and for patients whose brain metastases progress after WBXRT.

Radiosurgery has also largely supplanted WBXRT for postoperative radiotherapy following initial resection of brain metastases. Luther et al.[112] reported the outcome for 120 brain metastasis patients undergoing tumor resection bed radiosurgery. Although overall tumor control was satisfactory at 85.8%, the 2-year local control for target volumes ≥8 cm³ was only 65% (compared to 86%) for <8 cm³. Soltys et al.[113] recommended adding a 2-mm margin to the postoperative cavity radiosurgery treatment volume. In their experience, it improved local control from 70% ($n = 79$) to 100% ($n = 10$), though not significantly ($P = 0.15$). Minnetti et al.[114] reported on 101 solitary brain metastases >3-cm diameter resections managed with postoperative SRS to 27 Gy in 3 fractions with a 2-mm margin added to resection cavity volumes of 12.6 to 35.7 cm³. The 1- and 2-year rates of local control rates were 93% and 84%, whereas those for radiation necrosis (developing in 9 patients) were 7% and 16%.

Patel et al.[115] compared the results of surgical resection of brain metastases with radiosurgery delivered either preoperatively to a median dose of 14.5 Gy with no margin in 66 patients or postoperatively with 2-mm margin in 114 patients. Although no significant differences were found in overall survival ($P = 0.1$), local recurrence ($P = .24$), or distant brain recurrence ($P = .75$), patients undergoing postop SRS developed significantly more leptomeningeal disease (16.6% vs. 3.2%) and symptomatic radiation injury (16.4% vs. 4.9%) at

2 years despite a higher proportion of breast cancer similar median gross tumor volumes (9.2 vs. 8.3 cm³) and a higher proportion of breast cancer cases in the preoperative group (27.2% vs. 10.5%). Atalar et al.[116] had previously reported higher risks of leptomeningeal seeding with postop SRS for brain metastases from breast cancer (24% vs. 9% at 1 year) than other primaries.

Glioblastomas

During the late 1980s and 1990s, many centers that had been using brachytherapy for recurrent high-grade gliomas and as boosts after conventional radiotherapy switched to radiosurgery.[69,106] Although retrospective series appeared to show that initial brachytherapy or radiosurgery boosts after conventional radiotherapy improved survival of glioblastoma patients, prospective randomized trials of both modalities used prior to conventional radiotherapy of glioblastoma patients were negative[69,106]. Radiosurgery appears to be a reasonable option for small well-circumscribed high-grade gliomas that recur after prior conventional large-field radiotherapy and chemotherapy. Clark et al.[117] reported dose-escalated radiosurgery delivered with 10 mg/kg bevacizumab q2 weeks to 27, 30, and 33 Gy for recurrent glioblastoma and anaplastic astrocytoma in 3, 5, and 7 patients with no cases of clearly symptomatic radionecrosis but with one patient in the 33-Gy level exhibiting cognitive deterioration and grade 3 fatigue. Three patients underwent subsequent resections for presumed local progression with viable tumor and substantial radiation necrosis found in each, one of which with necrosis in >90% of the specimen.

Summary

Stereotactic radiosurgery and radiotherapy techniques have become a dominant way of managing a large number of benign and malignant tumors and other conditions in the brain and central nervous system. The safety and effectiveness of these techniques continue to improve along with technical improvements in radiation targeting and delivery as well as improvements in our understanding of radiobiologic responses.

REFERENCES

1. Garcia-Barros M, Paris F, Cordon-Cardo C, et al. Tumor response to radiotherapy regulated by endothelial cell apoptosis. *Science* 2003;300(5622): 1155–1159.
2. Szeifert GT, Massager N, DeVriendt D, et al. Observations of intracranial neoplasms treated with gamma knife radiosurgery. *J Neurosurg* 2002;97: 623–626.
3. Flickinger JF, Kondziolka D, Maitz AH, et al. An analysis of the dose-response for arteriovenous malformation radiosurgery and other factors affecting obliteration. *Radiother Oncol* 2002;63:347–354.
4. Flickinger JC, Kondziolka D, Pollock BE, et al. Complications from arteriovenous malformation radiosurgery: multivariate analysis and risk modeling. *Int J Radiat Oncol Biol Phys* 1997;38:485–490.
5. Dewan MZ, Galloway AE, Kawashima N, et al. Fractionated but not single-dose radiotherapy induces an immune-mediated abscopal effect when combined with anti-CTLA-4 antibody. *Clin Cancer Res* 2009;15(17):5379–5388.
6. Marconi R, Strolin S, Bossi G, et al. A meta-analysis of the abscopal effect in preclinical models: is the biologically effective dose a relevant physical trigger? *PLoS One* 2017;12(2):e0171559.
7. Flickinger JC, Kondziolka D, Lunsford LD, et al. Development of a model to predict permanent symptomatic postradiosurgery injury for arteriovenous malformation patients. Arteriovenous Malformation Radiosurgery Study Group. *Int J Radiat Oncol Biol Phys* 2000;46(5):1143–1148.
8. Shaw E, Scott C, Souhami L, et al. Single dose radiosurgical treatment of recurrent previously irradiated primary brain tumors and brain metastases: final report of RTOG protocol 90-05. *Int J Radiat Oncol Biol Phys* 2000;47(2):291–298.
9. Murai T, Ogino H, Manabe Y, et al. Fractionated stereotactic radiotherapy using CyberKnife for the treatment of large brain metastases: a dose escalation study. *Clin Oncol (R Coll Radiol)* 2014;26(3):151–158.

10. Schwer AL, Damek DM, Kavanagh BD, et al. A phase I dose-escalation study of fractionated stereotactic radiosurgery in combination with gefitinib in patients with recurrent malignant gliomas. *Int J Radiat Oncol Biol Phys* 2008;70(4):993–1001.

11. Clarke J, Neil E, Terziev R, et al. Multicenter, Phase 1, Dose escalation study of hypofractionated stereotactic radiation therapy with bevacizumab for recurrent glioblastoma and anaplastic astrocytoma. *Int J Radiat Oncol Biol Phys* 2017;99(4):797–804. doi: 10.1016/j.ijrobp.2017.06.2466.

12. Pollom EL, Fujimoto D, Wynne J, et al. Phase 1/2 trial of 5-fraction stereotactic radiosurgery with 5-mm margins with concurrent and adjuvant temozolomide in newly diagnosed supratentorial glioblastoma: health-related quality of life results. *Int J Radiat Oncol Biol Phys* 2017;98(1):123–130. doi: 10.1016/j.ijrobp.2017.01.242.

13. Tishler RB, Loeffler JS, Lunsford LD, et al. Tolerance of cranial nerves of the cavernous sinus to radiosurgery. *Int J Radiat Oncol Biol Phys* 1993;27:215–221.

14. Stafford SL, Pollock BE, Leavitt JA, et al. A study on the radiation tolerance of the optic nerves and chiasm after stereotactic radiosurgery. *Int J Radiat Oncol Biol Phys* 2003;55(5):1177–1181.

15. Leber KA, Bergloff J, Pendl G. Dose-response tolerance of the visual pathways and cranial nerves of the cavernous sinus to stereotactic radiosurgery. *J Neurosurg* 1998;88(1):43–50.

16. Hiniker SM, Modlin LA, Choi CY, et al. Dose-response modeling of the visual pathway tolerance to single-fraction and hypofractionated stereotactic radiosurgery. *Semin Radiat Oncol* 2016;26(2):97–104. doi: 10.1016/j.semradonc.2015.11.008.

17. Kondziolka D, Nathoo N, Flickinger JC, et al. Long-term results after radiosurgery for benign intracranial tumors. *Neurosurgery* 2003;53(4):815–821; discussion 821–822.

18. Lee JY, Niranjan A, McInerney J, et al. Stereotactic radiosurgery providing long-term tumor control of cavernous sinus meningiomas. *J Neurosurg* 2002;97(1):65–72.

19. Pollock BE, Stafford SL. Results of stereotactic radiosurgery for patients with imaging defined cavernous sinus meningiomas. *Int J Radiat Oncol Biol Phys* 2005;62(5):1427–1431.

20. Nicolato A, Foroni R, Alessandrini F, et al. The role of Gamma Knife radiosurgery in the management of cavernous sinus meningiomas. *Int J Radiat Oncol Biol Phys* 2002;53(4):992–1000.

21. Morita A, Coffey RJ, Foote RL, et al. Risk of injury to cranial nerves after gamma knife radiosurgery for skull base meningiomas: experience in 88 patients. *J Neurosurg* 1999;90(1):42–49.

22. Flickinger JC, Pollock BE, Kondziolka D, et al. Does increased nerve length within the treatment volume improve trigeminal neuralgia radiosurgery? A prospective double-blind, randomized study. *Int J Radiat Oncol Biol Phys* 2001;51(2):449–454.

23. Tempel ZJ, Chivukula S, Monaco EA III, et al. The results of a third Gamma Knife procedure for recurrent trigeminal neuralgia. *J Neurosurg* 2015;122(1):169–179.

24. Regis J, Metellus P, Hayashi M, et al. Prospective controlled trial of gamma knife surgery for essential trigeminal neuralgia. *J Neurosurg* 2006;104(6):913–924.

25. Kotecha R, Kotecha R, Modugula S, et al. Trigeminal neuralgia treated with stereotactic radiosurgery: the effect of dose escalation on pain control and treatment outcomes. *Int J Radiat Oncol Biol Phys* 2016;96(1):142–148. doi: 10.1016/j.ijrobp.2016.04.013.

26. Mousavi SH, Niranjan A, Huang MJ, et al. Early radiosurgery provides superior pain relief for trigeminal neuralgia patients. *Neurology* 2015;85(24):2159–2165.

27. Mousavi SH, Niranjan A, Akpinar B, et al. A proposed plan for personalized radiosurgery in patients with trigeminal neuralgia. *J Neurosurg* 2017;128(2):452–459.

28. Niranjan A, Jawahar A, Kondziolka D, et al. A comparison of surgical approaches for the management of tremor: radiofrequency thalamotomy, gamma knife thalamotomy and thalamic stimulation. *Stereotact Funct Neurosurg* 1999;72(2–4):178–184.

29. Niranjan A, Raju SS, Kooshkabadi A, et al. Stereotactic radiosurgery for essential tremor: retrospective analysis of a 19-year experience. *Mov Disord* 2017;32(5):769–777.

30. Raju SS, Niranjan A, Monaco Iii EA, et al. Stereotactic radiosurgery for intractable tremor-dominant parkinson disease: a retrospective analysis. *Stereotact Funct Neurosurg* 2017;95(5):291–297.

31. McClelland S III, Jaboin JJ. Treatment of the ventral intermediate nucleus for medically refractory tremor: a cost-analysis of stereotactic radiosurgery versus deep brain stimulation. *Radiother Oncol* 2017;125(1):136–139.

32. Elaimy AL, Arthurs BJ, Lamoreaux WT, et al. Gamma knife radiosurgery for movement disorders: a concise review of the literature. *World J Surg Oncol* 2010;8:61.

33. Andrade P, Carrillo-Ruiz JD, Jiménez F. A systematic review of the efficacy of globus pallidus stimulation in the treatment of Parkinson's disease. *J Clin Neurosci* 2009;16(7):877–881. doi: 10.1016/j.jocn.2008.11.006.

34. Lopes AC, Greenberg BD, Canteras MM, et al. Gamma ventral capsulotomy for obsessive-compulsive disorder: a randomized clinical trial. *JAMA Psychiatry* 2014;71(9):1066–1076. doi: 10.1001/jamapsychiatry.2014.1193. Retraction in: *JAMA Psychiatry* 2015;72(12):1258.

35. Régis J, Lagmari M, Carron R, et al. Safety and efficacy of Gamma Knife radiosurgery in hypothalamic hamartomas with severe epilepsies: a prospective trial in 48 patients and review of the literature. *Epilepsia* 2017;58(Suppl 2):60–71. doi: 10.1111/epi.13754.

36. 38. McGonigal A, Sahgal A, De Salles A, et al. Radiosurgery for epilepsy: systematic review and International Stereotactic Radiosurgery Society (ISRS) practice guideline. *Epilepsy Res* 2017;137:123–131. doi: 10.1016/j.eplepsyres.2017.08.016.

37. Pollock BE, Lunsford LD, Kondziolka D, et al. Outcome analysis of acoustic neuroma management: a comparison of microsurgery and stereotactic radiosurgery. *Neurosurgery* 1995;36(1):215–225.

38. Flickinger JC, Kondziolka D, Niranjan A, et al. Acoustic neuroma radiosurgery with marginal tumor doses of 12 to 13 Gy. *Int J Radiat Oncol Biol Phys* 2004;60(1):225–230.

39. Foote KD, Friedman WA, Buatti JM, et al. Analysis of risk factors associated with radiosurgery for vestibular schwannoma. *J Neurosurg* 2001;95(3):440–449.

40. Inoue HK. Low-dose radiosurgery for large vestibular schwannomas: long-term results of functional preservation. *J Neurosurg* 2005;102(Suppl):111–113.

41. Iwai Y, Yamanaka K, Shiotani M, et al. Radiosurgery for acoustic neuromas: results of low-dose treatment. *Neurosurgery* 2003;53(2):282–287; discussion 287–288.

42. Muacevic A, Jess-Hempen A, Tonn JC, et al. Results of outpatient gamma knife radiosurgery for primary therapy of acoustic neuromas. *Acta Neurochir Suppl* 2004;91:75–78.

43. Flickinger JC, Kondziolka D, Lunsford L. Fractionation of radiation treatment in acoustics. Rationale and evidence in comparison to radiosurgery. *Neurochirurgie* 2004;50(2–3 Pt 2):421–426.

44. Paek SH, Chung HT, Jeong SS, et al. Hearing preservation after gamma knife stereotactic radiosurgery of vestibular schwannoma. *Cancer* 2005;104(3):580–590.

45. Regis J, Pellet W, Delsanti C, et al. Functional outcome after gamma knife surgery or microsurgery for vestibular schwannomas. *J Neurosurg* 2002;97(5):1091–1100.

46. Rowe JG, Radatz MW, Walton L, et al. Gamma knife stereotactic radiosurgery for unilateral acoustic neuromas. *J Neurol Neurosurg Psychiatry* 2003;74(11):1536–1542.

47. Weber DC, Chan AW, Bussiere MR, et al. Proton beam radiosurgery for vestibular schwannoma: tumor control and cranial nerve toxicity. *Neurosurgery* 2003;53(3):577–586.

48. Wowra B, Muacevic A, Jess-Hempen A, et al. Outpatient gamma knife surgery for vestibular schwannoma: definition of the therapeutic profile based on a 10-year experience. *J Neurosurg* 2005;102(Suppl):114–118.

49. Meijer OW, Vandertop WP, Baayen JC, et al. Single-fraction vs. fractionated linac-based stereotactic radiosurgery for vestibular schwannoma: a single-institution study. *Int J Radiat Oncol Biol Phys* 2003;56(5):1390–1396.

50. Andrews DW, Suarez O, Goldman HW, et al. Stereotactic radiosurgery and fractionated stereotactic radiotherapy for the treatment of acoustic schwannomas: comparative observations of 125 patients treated at one institution. *Int J Radiat Oncol Biol Phys* 2001;50(5):1265–1278.

51. Bush DA, McAllister CJ, Loredo LN, et al. Fractionated proton beam radiotherapy for acoustic neuroma. *Neurosurgery* 2002;50(2):270–273.

52. Chang SD, Gibbs IC, Sakamoto GT, et al. Staged stereotactic irradiation for acoustic neuroma. *Neurosurgery* 2005;56(6):1254–1261; discussion 1261–1263.

53. Combs SE, Engelhard C, Kopp C, et al. Long-term outcome after highly advanced single-dose or fractionated radiotherapy in patients with vestibular schwannomas—pooled results from 3 large German centers. *Radiother Oncol* 2015;114(3):378–383. doi: 10.1016/j.radonc.2015.01.011.

54. Lederman G, Lowry J, Wertheim S, et al. Acoustic neuroma: potential benefits of fractionated stereotactic radiosurgery. *Stereotact Funct Neurosurg* 1997;69(1–4 Pt 2):175–182.

55. Lin VY, Stewart C, Grebenyuk J, et al. Unilateral acoustic neuromas: long-term hearing results in patients managed with fractionated stereotactic radiotherapy, hearing preservation surgery, and expectantly. *Laryngoscope* 2005;115(2):292–296.

56. Selch MT, Pedroso A, Lee SP, et al. Stereotactic radiotherapy for the treatment of acoustic neuromas. *J Neurosurg* 2004;101(Suppl 3):362–372.

57. Williams JA. Fractionated stereotactic radiotherapy for acoustic neuromas. *Int J Radiat Oncol Biol Phys* 2002;54(2):500–504.

58. Akpinar B, Mousavi SH, McDowell MM, et al. Early radiosurgery improves hearing preservation in vestibular schwannoma patients with normal hearing at the time of diagnosis. *Int J Radiat Oncol Biol Phys* 2016;95(2):729–734.

59. Mabanta SR, Buatti JM, Friedman WA, et al. Linear accelerator radiosurgery for nonacoustic schwannomas. *Int J Radiat Oncol Biol Phys* 1999;43(3):545–548.

60. Pan L, Wang EM, Zhang N, et al. Long-term results of Leksell gamma knife surgery for trigeminal schwannomas. *J Neurosurg* 2005;102(Suppl):220–224.

61. Pollock BE, Kondziolka D, Flickinger JC, et al. Preservation of cranial nerve function after radiosurgery for nonacoustic schwannomas. *Neurosurgery* 1993;33(4):597–601.

62. Zabel A, Debus J, Thilmann C, et al. Management of benign cranial nonacoustic schwannomas by fractionated stereotactic radiotherapy. *Int J Cancer* 2001;96(6):356–362.

63. Kano H, Meola A, Yang HC, et al. Stereotactic radiosurgery for jugular foramen schwannomas: an international multicenter study. *J Neurosurg* 2017:1–9. doi: 10.3171/2017.5.JNS162894.

64. Shin DW, Sohn MJ, Kim HS, et al. Clinical analysis of spinal stereotactic radiosurgery in the treatment of neurogenic tumors. *J Neurosurg Spine* 2015;23(4):429–437.

65. Bond AE, Shah BB, Huss DS, et al. Safety and efficacy of focused ultrasound thalamotomy for patients with medication-refractory, tremor-dominant parkinson disease: a randomized clinical trial. *JAMA Neurol* 2017;74(12):1412–1418. doi: 10.1001/jamaneurol.2017.3098.

66. Pollock BE, Flickinger JC, Lunsford LD, et al. Factors that predict the bleeding risk of cerebral arteriovenous malformations. *Stroke* 1996;27(1):1–6.

67. Stapf C, Mast H, Sciacca RR, et al. Predictors of hemorrhage in patients with untreated brain arteriovenous malformation. *Neurology* 2006;66(9): 1350–1355.

68. Ondra SL, Troupp H, George ED, et al. The natural history of symptomatic arteriovenous malformations of the brain: a 24-year follow-up assessment. *J Neurosurg* 1990;73:387–391.

69. Mohr JP, Parides MK, Stapf C, et al. international ARUBA investigators. Medical management with or without interventional therapy for unruptured brain arteriovenous malformations (ARUBA): a multicentre, non-blinded, randomised trial. *Lancet* 2014;383(9917):614–621. doi: 10.1016/S0140-6736(13)62302-8.

70. Maruyama K, Kawahara N, Shin M, et al. The risk of hemorrhage after radiosurgery for cerebral arteriovenous malformations. *N Engl J Med* 2005;352(2):146–153.

71. Karlsson B, Lindquist C, Steiner L. Prediction of obliteration after gamma knife surgery for cerebral arteriovenous malformations. *Neurosurgery* 1997;40(3):425–430.

72. Flickinger JC, Kondziolka D, Lunsford LD. Radiobiological analysis of tissue responses following radiosurgery. *Technol Cancer Res Treat* 2003;2(2): 87–92.

73. Maesawa S, Flickinger JC, Kondziolka D, et al. Repeated radiosurgery for incompletely obliterated arteriovenous malformations. *J Neurosurg* 2000;92(6):961–970.

74. Kano H, Kondziolka D, Flickinger JC, et al. Stereotactic radiosurgery for arteriovenous malformations, Part 3: outcome predictors and risks after repeat radiosurgery. *J Neurosurg* 2012;116:21–32.

75. Florio F, Lauriola W, Nardella M, et al. Endovascular treatment of intracranial arterio-venous malformations with Onyx embolization: preliminary experience. *Radiol Med* 2003;106(5–6):512–520.

76. Kano H, Kondziolka D, Flickinger JC, et al. Stereotactic radiosurgery for arteriovenous malformations, Part 6: multistaged volumetric management of large arteriovenous malformations. *J Neurosurg* 2012;116:54–65.

77. Kupersmith MJ, Kalish H, Epstein F, et al. Natural history of brainstem cavernous malformations. *Neurosurgery* 2001;48(1):47–53.

78. Kim DS, Park YG, Choi JU, et al. An analysis of the natural history of cavernous malformations. *Surg Neurol* 1997;48(1):9–17.

79. Kondziolka D, Lunsford LD, Flickinger JC, et al. Reduction of hemorrhage risk after stereotactic radiosurgery for cavernous malformations. *J Neurosurg* 1995;83(5):825–831.

80. Kondziolka D, Lunsford LD, Kestle JR. The natural history of cerebral cavernous malformations. *J Neurosurg* 1995;83(5):820–824.

81. Aiba T, Tanaka R, Koike T, et al. Natural history of intracranial cavernous malformations. *J Neurosurg* 1995;83(1):56–59.

82. Monaco EA, Khan AA, Niranjan A, et al. Stereotactic radiosurgery for the treatment of symptomatic brainstem cavernous malformations. *Neurosurg Focus* 2010;29(3):E11. doi: 10.3171/2010.

83. Pollock BE, Garces YI, Stafford SL, et al. Stereotactic radiosurgery for cavernous malformations. *J Neurosurg* 2000;93(6):987–991.

84. Huang YC, Tseng CK, Chang CN, et al. LINAC radiosurgery for intracranial cavernous malformation: 10-year experience. *Clin Neurol Neurosurg* 2006;108(8):750–756.

85. Liu KD, Chung WY, Wu HM, et al. Gamma knife surgery for cavernous hemangiomas: an analysis of 125 patients. *J Neurosurg* 2005;102(Suppl.): 81–86.

86. Liscak R, Vladyka V, Simonova G, et al. Gamma knife surgery of brain cavernous hemangiomas. *J Neurosurg* 2005;102(Suppl):207–213.

87. Hasegawa T, McInerney J, Kondziolka D, et al. Long-term results after stereotactic radiosurgery for patients with cavernous malformations. *Neurosurgery* 2002;50(6):1190–1197; discussion 1197–1198.

88. Kim MS, Pyo SY, Jeong YG, et al. Gamma knife surgery for intracranial cavernous hemangioma. *J Neurosurg* 2005;102(Suppl.):102–106.

89. Flickinger JC, Kondziolka D, Maitz AH, et al. Gamma knife radiosurgery of imaging-diagnosed intracranial meningioma. *Int J Radiat Oncol Biol Phys* 2003;56(3):801–806.

90. Pouratian N, Sheehan J, Jagannathan J, et al. Gamma knife radiosurgery for medically and surgically refractory prolactinomas. *Neurosurgery* 2006;59(2):255–266.

91. Mingione V, Yen CP, Vance ML, et al. Gamma surgery in the treatment of nonsecretory pituitary macroadenoma. *J Neurosurg* 2006;104(6):876–883.

92. Sheehan JP, Niranjan A, Sheehan JM, et al. Stereotactic radiosurgery for pituitary adenomas: an intermediate review of its safety, efficacy, and role in the neurosurgical treatment armamentarium. *J Neurosurg* 2005;102(4): 678–691.

93. Mehta GU, Ding D, Patibandla MR, et al. Stereotactic radiosurgery for cushing disease: results of an international, multicenter study. *J Clin Endocrinol Metab* 2017;102(11):4284–4291.

94. Sheehan JP, Starke RM, Mathieu D, et al. Gamma Knife radiosurgery for the management of nonfunctioning pituitary adenomas: a multicenter study. *J Neurosurg* 2013;119(2):446–456. doi: 10.3171/2013.3.JNS12766.

95. Narod SA, Parry DM, Parboosingh J, et al. Neurofibromatosis type 2 appears to be a genetically homogeneous disease. *Am J Hum Genet* 1992;51(3):486–496.

96. Shirato H, Sakamoto T, Sawamura Y, et al. Comparison between observation policy and fractionated stereotactic radiotherapy (SRT) as an initial management for vestibular schwannoma. *Int J Radiat Oncol Biol Phys* 1999;44:545–550.

97. Sakamoto T, Shirato H, Takeichi N, et al. Annual rate of hearing loss falls after fractionated stereotactic irradiation for vestibular schwannoma. *Radiother Oncol* 2001;60(1):45–48.

98. Kondziolka D, Lunsford LD, McLaughlin MR, et al. Long-term outcomes after radiosurgery for acoustic neuromas. *N Engl J Med* 1998;339:1426–1433.

99. Kondziolka D, Flickinger JC, Perez B. Judicious resection and/or radiosurgery for parasagittal meningiomas: outcomes from a multicenter review. Gamma Knife Meningioma Study Group. *Neurosurgery* 1998;43(3):405–413.

100. Kondziolka D, Levy EI, Niranjan A, et al. Long term outcomes after meningioma radiosurgery: physician and patient perspectives. *J Neurosurg* 1999;91(1):44–50.

101. Malik I, Rowe JG, Walton L, et al. The use of stereotactic radiosurgery in the management of meningiomas. *Br J Neurosurg* 2005;19(1):13–20.

102. Modha A, Gutin PH. Diagnosis and treatment of atypical and anaplastic meningiomas: a review. *Neurosurgery* 2005;57(3):538–550; discussion 538–550.

103. Harris AE, Lee JY, Omalu B, et al. The effect of radiosurgery during management of aggressive meningiomas. *Surg Neurol* 2003;60(4):298–305.

104. Katz TS, Amdur RJ, Yachnis AT, et al. Pushing the limits of radiotherapy for atypical and malignant meningioma. *Am J Clin Oncol* 2005;28(1): 70–74.

105. DiBiase SJ, Kwok Y, Yovino S, et al. Factors predicting local tumor control after gamma knife stereotactic radiosurgery for benign intracranial meningiomas. *Int J Radiat Oncol Biol Phys* 2004;60(5):1515–1519.

106. Bulthuis VJ, Hanssens PE, Lie ST, et al. Gamma Knife radiosurgery for intracranial meningiomas: do we need to treat the dural tail? A single-center retrospective analysis and an overview of the literature. *Surg Neurol Int* 2014;5(Suppl 8):S391–S395. doi: 10.4103/2152-7806.140192. eCollection 2014.

107. Cho YH, Lee JM, Lee D, et al. Experiences on two different stereotactic radiosurgery modalities of Gamma Knife and Cyberknife in treating brain metastases. *Acta Neurochir (Wien)* 2015;157(11):2003–2009; discussion 2009. doi: 10.1007/s00701-015-2585-3.

108. Angelov L, Mohammadi AM, Bennett EE, et al. Impact of 2-staged stereotactic radiosurgery for treatment of brain metastases ≥2 cm. *J Neurosurg* 2017:1–17. doi: 10.3171/2017.3.JNS162532.

109. Patel KR, Burri SH, Asher AL, et al. Comparing preoperative with postoperative stereotactic radiosurgery for resectable brain metastases: a multi-institutional analysis. *Neurosurgery* 2016;79(2):279–285.

110. Atalar B, Modlin LA, Choi CY, et al. Risk of leptomeningeal disease in patients treated with stereotactic radiosurgery targeting the postoperative resection cavity for brain metastases. *Int J Radiat Oncol Biol Phys* 2013;87(4):713–718. doi: 10.1016/j.ijrobp.2013.07.034.

111. Bhatnagar AK, Flickinger JC, Kondziolka D, et al. Stereotactic radiosurgery for four or more intracranial metastases. *Int J Radiat Oncol Biol Phys* 2006;64(3):898–903.

112. Luther N, Kondziolka D, Kano H, et al. Predicting tumor control after resection bed radiosurgery of brain metastases. *Neurosurgery* 2013;73(6):1001–1006; discussion 1006.

113. Soltys SG, Adler JR, Lipani JD, et al. Stereotactic radiosurgery of the postoperative resection cavity for brain metastases. *Int J Radiat Oncol Biol Phys* 2008;70(1):187–193.

114. Minniti G, Esposito V, Clarke E, et al. Multidose stereotactic radiosurgery (9 Gy × 3) of the postoperative resection cavity for treatment of large brain metastases. *Int J Radiat Oncol Biol Phys* 2013;86(4):623–629. doi:10.1016/j.ijrobp.2013.03.037.

115. Patel KR, Burri SH, Asher AL, et al. Comparing preoperative with postoperative stereotactic radiosurgery for resectable brain metastases: a multi-institutional analysis. *Neurosurgery* 2016;79(2):279–285.

116. Atalar B, Modlin LA, Choi CY, et al. Risk of leptomeningeal disease in patients treated with stereotactic radiosurgery targeting the postoperative resection cavity for brain metastases. *Int J Radiat Oncol Biol Phys* 2013;87(4): 713–718.

117. Clarke J, Neil E, Terziev R, et al. Multicenter, Phase 1, Dose Escalation Study of Hypofractionated Stereotactic Radiation Therapy With Bevacizumab for Recurrent Glioblastoma and Anaplastic Astrocytoma. *Int J Radiat Oncol Biol Phys* 2017;99(4):797–804.

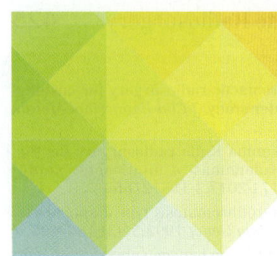

CHAPTER 18

Stereotactic Irradiation of Tumors Outside the Central Nervous System

Brian D. Kavanagh, Jeffrey D. Bradley, and Robert D. Timmerman

INTRODUCTION

Departing from the established traditions of conventionally fractionated external beam radiotherapy, in the late 1980s and early 1990s, investigators in the United States, Sweden, and Japan began to explore the use of extremely brief hypofractionated radiation treatment regimens for the spine, lung, liver, and selected other malignant extracranial tumors.[1-3] In essence, these clinical researchers were modifying techniques proven clinically valuable in the context of cranial and spine stereotactic radiosurgery in an effort to exploit the efficiency and biologic potency of high–dose per fraction irradiation.[4] This idea was soon appreciated for its clinical promise by other researchers in numerous countries across the world.

Pioneers in the field initially used customized ancillary equipment constructed in their own institutions to immobilize patients and to adapt ordinary linear accelerators for the task of precise internal tumor targeting. Now, however, the administration of high-dose, tightly focused external-beam radiation therapy is greatly facilitated by a wide assortment of commercially available systems that immobilize patients, address the problem of respiratory motion during treatment, and ensure accurate treatment with the use of image guidance. The newest generation of linear accelerators from several manufacturers is either exclusively dedicated to cranial or extracranial stereotactic radiotherapy or is equipped with a built-in package of features that provide an easy means of administering this type of treatment.

Stereotactic body radiation therapy (SBRT) is the term applied in the United States by the American Society of Therapeutic Radiology and Oncology (ASTRO) for the management and delivery of image-guided high-dose radiation therapy with tumor-ablative intent within a course of treatment that does not exceed 5 fractions.[5] Other descriptive terms have been occasionally applied to describe what is officially called SBRT, including the acronym SABR, an abbreviation for *stereotactic ablative radiotherapy*.[6]

BIOLOGIC AND ONCOLOGIC RATIONALE FOR SBRT

The appeal of SBRT is based on the nonlinear relation between radiation dose and cytotoxic effect, whereby one or a few large individual doses of radiation therapy may have substantially more cell-killing effect than the same dose of radiation given in smaller individual doses. Traditionally, the expected relation between radiation dose and tumor cell kill has been commonly estimated by the well-known linear-quadratic (LQ) model of radiation dose response, often relied on for the purpose of comparing the biologic potency of different schedules of conventionally fractionated radiation therapy. In the range of dose per fraction used in SBRT, however, there has been an emerging appreciation that the LQ model overestimates the potency of fraction sizes on the order of 8 to 10 Gy or higher.

A variety of alternative mathematical models have been proposed to account for the observed inaccuracy of the LQ model for doses in this range. For example, Guerrero and Li[7] have proposed a modification of Curtis's[8] lethal-potentially lethal model that accounts for ongoing repair processes occurring during the time of an individual radiation treatment, thus predicting lower cytotoxicity from high doses administered over time intervals resembling typical clinical treatment times. Experimental data modeling cranial radiosurgery offer support for this concept.[9] Alternatively, Park et al.[10] have offered the universal survival curve formalism, which combines the LQ model for doses in the range used in conventional fractionation with a multitarget model for doses in the range used for SBRT. This piecewise function effectively achieves the same key mathematical result as other departures from the LQ model applied to SBRT, namely, a more linear slope in the relation between dose and log cell kill in the high-dose region.

In the special case of prostate cancer, the rationale for evaluating SBRT for prostate cancer has also included an additional LQ model-based hypothesis. Retrospective outcomes comparisons that involve a variety of doses and schedules of treatments had suggested that if the LQ model was applicable, the α/β ratio for prostate cancer might be very low, likely in the range of 1.5 to 3.0 Gy.[11,12] If this estimate of α/β ratio for prostate cancer were correct, then higher doses per fraction should provide a more favorable therapeutic ratio than a conventionally fractionated regimen. Accumulating evidence from randomized clinical trials comparing conventional daily fractions of 2 Gy with hypofractionated regimens using fractions sized on the order of 2.5 to 3 Gy/d offer conflicting evidence in this regard, raising some questions about the initial parameter estimates.[13-15] Clinical reports involving SBRT for prostate cancer have involved doses that are higher than 3 Gy and are discussed later in the chapter.

None of the aforementioned models of high–dose per fraction tumor cell–killing effects explicitly incorporate a mechanism of tumor cell kill that might be of equal or greater importance than tumor DNA damage-based injury, namely, the antiangiogenic effect of endothelial cell apoptosis occurring above an apparent threshold dose on the order of 8 to 10 Gy. First observed preclinically and reported by Garcia-Barros et al.,[16] clinical evidence indirectly supporting the importance of this mechanism includes measures of an increase in serum markers of apoptosis post-SBRT.[17] Challenging the importance of this mechanism, however, is the work of Kirsch and colleagues, who used a genetically engineered mouse model to evaluate the influence of endothelial cell apoptosis in a mouse sarcoma model,[18,19] observing minimal impact on tumor radiosensitivity from the degree of endothelial apoptosis achieved. The impact of high–dose per fraction radiotherapy upon immune responses is a topic of current high interest. One early preclinical study demonstrated that a single dose of 20 Gy, unlike a fractionated regimen of lower dose per fraction, can trigger a strong T-cell response that enhances the cytotoxic effect in a preclinical melanoma model.[20]

Beyond its uses as primary therapy for selected early-stage cancers, SBRT can also be used as a noninvasive and efficient means of eradicating discrete tumors in the setting of oligometastatic disease. As articulated by Hellman and Weichselbaum,[21] the spectrum theory or theory of oligometastases proposes that there is a subgroup of patients with metastatic disease that is intermediate between completely absent and widely metastatic. For such patients, the entire systemic disease burden is contained within the finite number of individual sites of gross disease recognized by the relevant imaging studies. This condition would reflect an intermediate point in the natural history of that individual's cancer; therefore, these patients might be cured if their limited numbers of metastatic sites are eradicated. There have been numerous reports of patients enjoying a high rate of 3- to 5-year survival following various forms of aggressive local treatment (e.g., surgical resection, radiofrequency ablation, cryotherapy) for limited metastases in the liver or lung from an assortment of solid tumor types.[22] SBRT is a valid, noninvasive substitute for other local modalities if it can provide similar efficacy and the same or less toxicity. Among the many examples of studies lending indirect support to the theory of oligometastases and the potential value of SBRT in this setting would be the report by Stinauer et al.[23] involving patients treated with SBRT for metastases from melanoma or renal cell carcinoma, where there was significantly longer survival for patients with oligometastatic disease, there defined as three or fewer sites, than for patients with more extensive disease.

The indications for SBRT in the setting of metastatic disease might be alternatively couched in terms of a patterns-of-failure model. Rusthoven et al.[24] reviewed a large series of patients who received chemotherapy for metastatic non–small cell lung cancer and observed, not surprisingly, that patients are most likely to suffer tumor recurrence in sites initially involved prior to chemotherapy. The hypothesis that eradicating all known sites of non–small cell lung cancer present in patients with limited metastatic disease can extend disease-free survival was tested in a clinical trial by Gomez et al.[25] After appropriate induction systemic therapy (at least four cycles of platinum doublet therapy or at least 3 months of erlotinib/crizotinib for patients with EGFR mutations/ALK fusions, respectively), patients were randomized to either local consolidative therapy (LCT) or systemic therapy alone. LCT could be radiotherapy, chemoradiotherapy, or surgical resection. The study was closed early on advice from the data safety monitoring committee because of significant efficacy benefit observed in the LCT arm. At a median follow-up time of over 16 months, the median progression-free survival time in the LCT arm was 14.4 months, compared to 3.9 months in the no-LCT arm (hazard ratio = 0.36, P = .013).

Numerous studies of similar structure to the Gomez trial have been launched. For example, Palma and colleagues have conducted a multicenter randomized phase II trial to assess the impact of a comprehensive oligometastatic SBRT treatment program on overall survival and quality of life in patients with up to five metastatic cancer lesions, compared to patients who receive standard of care treatment alone.[26] Patients are stratified by the number of metastases (1 to 3 vs. 4 to 5) and then randomized between Arm 1: current standard of care treatment, and Arm 2: standard of care treatment + SBRT to all sites of known disease. Patients will be randomized in a 1:2 ratio to Arm 1:Arm 2, respectively. Salam and Milano have provided a thorough review of the use of ablative-intent radiotherapy for extracranial oligometastases.[27]

Especially intriguing is the possibility that stereotactic irradiation can initiate immunologic responses that can trigger an abscopal responsive to novel agents such as ipilimumab, as described in a number of case reports.[28,29] Additional indirect evidence for a favorable relationship between the use of radiotherapy and another immunotherapeutic agent, pembrolizumab, has emerged from a secondary single institutional analysis of the KEYNOTE-001 trial.[30] Among 98 patients who were enrolled and received their first cycle of pembrolizumab, 42 (43%) had previously received any radiotherapy for the treatment of NSCLC before the first cycle of pembrolizumab. Overall survival with pembrolizumab was significantly longer in patients who previously received any radiotherapy than

in patients without previous radiotherapy (P = .026; median overall survival 10.7 months [95% CI 6.5–18.9] vs. 5.3 months [2.7–7.7]) and for patients who previously received extracranial radiotherapy compared with those without previous extracranial radiotherapy (P = .034; median overall survival 11.6 months [95% CI 6.5–20.5] vs. 5.3 months [3.0–8.5]). The optimal timing of immunotherapeutic agent and dose prescription for radiotherapy given in combination is a topic of active investigation at numerous centers.

STEREOTACTIC BODY RADIATION THERAPY GUIDELINES, PHYSICS OVERVIEW, AND SAFETY CONSIDERATIONS

ASTRO and the American College of Radiology (ACR) have published guidelines that characterize the personnel qualifications and responsibilities, documentation, quality control, and clinical operations recommended for the safe and proper administration of SBRT and follow-up care for patients treated.[5] The ASTRO-ACR guidelines advise that the following components should be in place within and institution's SBRT program:

1. Qualified personnel:
   a. Board-certified radiation oncologist
   b. Qualified medical physicist
   c. Licensed radiation therapist
   d. Other support staff as indicated (dosimetrists, oncology nurses, and so forth)
2. Ongoing machine quality assurance program
3. Documentation in accordance with the *ACR Practice Guideline for Communication: Radiation Oncology*
4. Quality control of treatment accessories
5. Quality control of planning and treatment images
6. Quality control of treatment planning system
7. Simulation and treatment systems that account for systematic and random errors associated with setup and target motion in a manner that is based on actual measurement of organ motion and setup uncertainty.

The American Association of Physicist in Medicine Task Group 101 (TG101) moved forward from the ASTRO-ACR guidelines to generate a report that considers additional important nuances in the planning and treatment delivery of SBRT.[31] Included within the TG101 report are discussions of potential imaging artifacts and their impact on treatment planning, the challenges of small-field dosimetry, and the importance of using an acceptable dose calculation algorithm, among other issues.

Proper patient repositioning, target localization, and management of breathing-related motion are essential for SBRT. A variety of patient immobilization devices are available, including several types of body frames with external fiducial markers. So-called frameless systems incorporate ultrasound, kilovolt-range imaging, or near real-time computed tomography (CT) scanning to verify the location of internal targets relative to the beams to be used. Because SBRT treatment sessions are lengthier than conventional external-beam treatments, patient comfort is an important issue.

Breathing-related motion control devices and systems fall into three general categories: (a) dampening, (b) gating, and (c) tracking or "chasing." Respiratory dampening techniques include systems of abdominal compression intended to diminish one of the largest contributors to breathing-related motion, namely, diaphragmatic excursion, by obliging the inspiratory–expiratory lung motion pattern to involve more intracostal expansion and shallower breathing overall. Also included in this category are the systems employing breath-holding maneuvers to stabilize the tumor in a reproducible stage of the respiratory cycle (e.g., deep inspiration). Gating systems for SBRT, as for any radiotherapy application, follow the respiratory cycle using a surrogate indicator for respiratory motion, for example, chest wall motion, and employ an electronic beam activation trigger allowing irradiation to occur only during a specified range of expected tumor locations. Tracking or "chasing" systems move the radiation beam or patient to follow the movement of the tumor.

Regardless of the system employed, the procedure of treatment planning must include the same consideration for respiratory motion management to be used during treatment. Despite available motion control equipment, some positional uncertainty will remain. The planning target volume (PTV) margins used to account for this residual motion of the gross tumor volume (GTV) will typically range from 3 to 5 mm.

The word *stereotactic* has heretofore usually implied that some sort of external reference markers indexed to internal structures facilitate internal target relocalization, but the definition has expanded to include systems of image-guided radiation therapy (IGRT) that relate the position of internal targets to a three-dimensional coordinate geometry registered to the treatment machine without the use of external markers on the patient. SBRT always involves some form of IGRT to guide for treatment delivery.

Most reports describing SBRT published to date have employed high-energy photons (x-rays) as the source of therapeutic radiation, although other particles can also be used. There is no absolute standard for the combination of beam or arc angles ideal for any given clinical situation, and each case can present unique challenges. In general to achieve a tightly focused high-dose distribution within the PTV and rapid dose falloff outside the PTV, a combination of multiple (often 10 or more) noncoplanar beams or multiple arcs are required. Intensity modulation across the individual beams or arc segments can be incorporated within SBRT.

As part of ASTRO's Target Safely campaign, the Multidisciplinary Quality Assurance Subcommittee of the Clinical Affairs and Quality Committee of ASTRO commissioned a white paper on the topic of cranial radiosurgery and SBRT titled "Quality and Safety Considerations in Stereotactic Radiosurgery and Stereotactic Body Radiation Therapy."[32] Of particular importance within the white paper are sections emphasizing the importance of creating a proactive culture of safety with procedural checkpoints and error analysis mechanisms.

CLINICAL EXPERIENCE WITH STEREOTACTIC BODY RADIATION THERAPY IN SELECTED SITES

Liver

The two major reasons for considering SBRT for hepatocellular cancer (HCC) is that underlying severe liver disease often renders patients medically inoperable and that other nonsurgical therapies have generally achieved at best rather modest success in that setting. The natural history of untreated HCC has been reported to involve a median survival in the range of 3 to 8 months,[33-35] and so a safe and effective therapy is needed in this setting.

The earliest observations following SBRT for HCC were reported by a group at Karolinska Hospital,[2] and more recent formal prospective studies have followed. The Princess Margaret Hospital group utilized a 6-fraction regimen in a prospective phase I study in patients with HCC (*n* = 31) or intrahepatic cholangiocarcinoma (*n* = 10).[36] Prescription doses were selected according to a normal tissue complication probability (NTCP) model based on conventionally fractionated radiotherapy to the liver. The median dose to the tumor was 36 Gy (range, 24 to 54 Gy). The NTCP model overestimated the chance of radiation-induced liver disease, and it is

possible that the dose could have been escalated to a higher level in most cases. Nevertheless, in this group of heavily pretreated patients (over 60% had had at least one prior therapy for HCC), a remarkable median survival of 12 months was observed.

Méndez Romero et al.[37] at Erasmus University Medical Center treated eight patients with 11 separate lesions of HCC in 3 to 5 fractions to a dose of 25.0 to 37.5 Gy. A 1-year survival of 75% was observed. Choi et al.[38] at the Catholic University of Korea treated 23 patients with 32 individual lesions in a 3-fraction regimen to a median dose of 36 Gy (range, 30 to 39 Gy). No patient experienced severe toxicity, although follow-up was limited (median 11 months). Interestingly, in a subsequent analysis of predictors for decline in liver function after SBRT, on multivariate analysis the only predictor for a decrease in Child-Pugh classification (CPC) from baseline level was the volume of normal liver receiving 18 Gy or more (V18). The rate of negative impact on CPC rose sharply when the V18 exceeded 800 cc.[39] This latter observation favors a model of SBRT effect on normal liver in line with a critical volume model, whereby it is important to preserve a certain minimum level of function by sparing an adequate volume of normal liver from receiving a dose above a certain threshold.

The group from the Korea Institute of Radiological and Medical Sciences treated a prospectively registered cohort of 38 patients with inoperable HCC with SBRT, all of whom had failed prior transarterial chemoembolization.[40] The median tumor volume was 40.5 cc (range, 11 to 464). The SBRT dose was 33 to 57 Gy in 3 or 4 fractions. Minimal grade 3 toxicity (<3%) was observed, and the 2-year overall survival was 61%.

Cardenes et al.[41] from Indiana University and the University of Colorado reported a multi-institutional phase I dose escalation study of SBRT given in 3 fractions for HCC. Eligibility requirements were CPC-A or -B, medical or technical inoperability, and three or fewer lesions of cumulative tumor diameter 6 cm or less. The study enrolled 17 patients with 25 individual lesions. Dose was escalated from 36 to 48 Gy (16 Gy per fraction) in CPC-A patients without dose-limiting toxicity (DLT); however, two patients with CPC-B status at baseline developed grade 3 hepatic toxicity at the 42 Gy (14 Gy per fraction) dose level. Consequently, the dose for CPC-B patients was reduced to 40 Gy in 5 fractions. There were no local failures within the treated volume, and six patients proceeded to liver transplantation. The 2-year overall survival for the entire group was 60%.

The Indiana University group has separately reported their single institution experience involving a total of 60 patients: 34 CPC-A, 25 CPC-B, and 1 CPC-C.[42] The median number of fractions, dose per fraction, and total dose, was 3, 14, and 44 Gy, respectively, for those with CPC-A cirrhosis and 5, 8, and 40 Gy, respectively, for those with CPC-B. With a median follow-up time of 27 months, the 2-year local control rate was 90%. Two-year overall survival was 67%. SBRT served as a bridge to liver transplant for 23 patients who underwent transplant at a median time of 7 months following SBRT. A progression in CPC was observed in 20% of patients within 3 months of treatment.

Numerous other series have been reported in the last several years. Among the larger is the experience of Bibault et al., who treated 75 patients with 96 liver-confined HCC with SBRT.[43] There were 67 patients with Child-Turcotte-Pugh (CTP) Class A and eight patients with CTP Class B. Treatment was administered in three sessions. A total dose of 40 to 45 Gy to the 80% isodose line was delivered. The local control rate was 89.8% at 1 and 2 years. Overall survival was 78.5% and 50.4% at 1 and 2 years, respectively. Toxicity mainly consisted of grade 1 and grade 2 events. Higher alpha-fetoprotein (aFP) levels were associated with less favorable local control, and a higher dose was associated with better local control. A Child-Pugh score higher than 5 was associated with worse overall survival.

A provocative analysis has been reported by Su et al.[44] A propensity matching technique was used to pair 82 patients who received SBRT with a group of 35 patients who underwent liver resection. Before propensity score matching, the 1-, 3-, and 5-year OS was 96.3%, 81.8%, and 70.0% in the SBRT group and 93.9%, 83.1%, and 64.4% in the resection group, respectively (P = NS). After propensity score matching, 33 paired patients were selected from the SBRT and resection groups. The 1-, 3-, and 5-year OS was 100%, 91.8%, and 74.3% in the SABR group and 96.7%, 89.3%, and 69.2% in the resection group, respectively (P = NS). There was a similarity of hepatotoxicity between the 2 groups. The SBRT group experienced more acute nausea but suffered lower rates of complications such as hepatic hemorrhage, hepatic pain, and weight loss.

Outcomes following SBRT for liver metastases have also been reported by numerous groups[45–53] and are summarized in Table 18.1. Regimens of 1 to 5 fractions have been employed, and total doses up to 60 Gy to the PTV have been administered. Taken together, the results show good survival outcomes achieved in heavily pretreated individuals and a trend toward improved local control with increasing dose.

Chang et al.[54] reported a pooled analysis from three institutions with the use of liver SBRT for liver metastases from colorectal primary cancers. The combined experience from Stanford, Princess Margaret Hospital, and the University of Colorado included 65 patients with a total of 102 individual liver metastases from colorectal cancer treated. More than half of the patients had had at least one prior systemic therapy regimen, and over 40% of the patients had had two or more prior systemic regimens. The analysis indicated that to achieve durable local control of treated lesion, a 3-fraction total dose on the order of 48 Gy is needed. Sustained local control after SBRT was closely associated with improved survival on multivariate analysis (P = .06).

Technical issues and posttreatment imaging follow-up considerations unique to liver SBRT have been included in these reports and in review papers.[55,56] Briefly, target delineation and image guidance can be difficult, because liver metastases are not well visualized on CT scans or in-room volumetric imaging used for IGRT. In many centers, radiopaque fiducial markers are place in or near the metastases to facilitate IGRT. In all centers, the PTV is an expansion of the GTV in consideration of the setup and intrafraction motion to be expected with the particular setup and delivery system employed. Typically, the margin used to expand a GTV into a PTV is on the order of 5 mm axially and 5 to 10 mm craniocaudally.

The Colorado group first applied the critical volume approach to normal liver dose constraints in their initial phase I study[57] and subsequent phase II study. Noted above in relation to the observations of the Catholic University of Korea in their treatment of primary liver tumors, the critical volume model liver SBRT is an adaptation of the early work of Yeas and Kalend.[58] Applicable for organs of radiobiologically parallel structure, the crux of this application is to work backward, in a sense, from an estimate of how much volume of the organ is essential and must be protected from functional ablation. The estimate for liver that at least 700 cm^3 should receive <15 Gy during a 3-fraction SBRT course was derived from a combination of prior reports of outcomes after partial hepatectomy documenting approximate minimum volumes required and estimates of the effects of that dose of radiation extrapolated from prior reports of conventionally fractionated treatment.

One feature of the normal tissue effect of liver SBRT consistently observed within the first few months after SBRT is a zone of hypodensity observed on follow-up CT scans corresponding to the volume that received approximately 30 Gy.[57] This phenomenon, first described by Herfarth et al.[59] following single-dose liver SBRT, is likely related to local veno-occlusive effects.[60] There is no known clinical consequence associated with the finding per se, but it can cloud the assessment of tumor response within the first few months after liver SBRT.

CASE STUDY

Liver Stereotactic Body Radiation Therapy

A 45-year-old female had been diagnosed with stage IV breast cancer 2 years previously. Biopsy-proven liver metastases were present at the time of diagnosis. Numerous systemic agents had been given, most recently gemcitabine and trastuzumab. Although all other measurable or assessable sites of disease were stable or regressing, a mass in the liver had progressed from 2.5-by-2.9 cm to 6.0-by-4.2 cm within the past 3 months. Because the patient was tolerating the regimen well and apparently having a response in most sites, she was offered SBRT in an effort to eradicate tumor in the liver.

The lesion diameter (>6 cm) rendered the patient ineligible for an ongoing phase II trial of SBRT for liver metastases, and the dose given was lower than the protocol doses (Fig. 18.1). The 53 cm^3 GTV was expanded by 5 mm radially and 10 mm in the superior–inferior direction to generate the PTV. The dose distribution shown was administered in 3 fractions within 1 week using multiple

TABLE 18.1 STEREOTACTIC BODY RADIATION THERAPY FOR LIVER METASTASES			
Institution	Patients/ Lesions	SBRT Dose and Fractionation	Results
Heidelberg[45]	37/60	11–21 Gy × 1	18-month LC: Low dose (<16): 0% High dose (>16): 81%
Würzburg[46]	39/51	7 Gy × 4 10 Gy × 3 12.5 Gy × 3 26 Gy × 1	2-year LC: Low dose (28–30): 58% High dose (others): 82%
Aarhus-Copenhagen[47]	44/not stated	10 Gy × 3	2-year LC: 79% All pts CRC 3 ulcers with intestinal dose >30 Gy
Erasmus[48]	17/34	10 Gy × 3 12.5 Gy × 3	54% 15 pts CRC; 1 late portal hypertension in multiply treated patient
Colorado/multi-institutional[49]	47/63	12–20 Gy × 3	2-year LC: ≤3 cm: 100% >3 cm: 75%
Princess Margaret Hospital[50]	68/141	Variable, NTCP based Median 7 Gy × 6	1-year LC: 71% Better for higher dose, smaller volume
Stanford[51]	19/35	18–30 Gy × 1	1-year LC: 77% Combined with 7 patients with primarily liver cancer; maximum tolerated dose not reached
University of Texas–Southwestern[52]	26/35	6–12 Gy × 5	2-year LC 56%, 89%, 100% for total dose 30, 50, 60 Gy, respectively
Humanitas Clinical and Research Center[53]	42/52	Mean dose 75 Gy in 3 fractions	2-year LC 91%, 2-year OS 65%

CRC, colorectal cancer; LC, local control; NTCP, normal tissue complication probability; OS, overall survival; PTV, planning target volume.

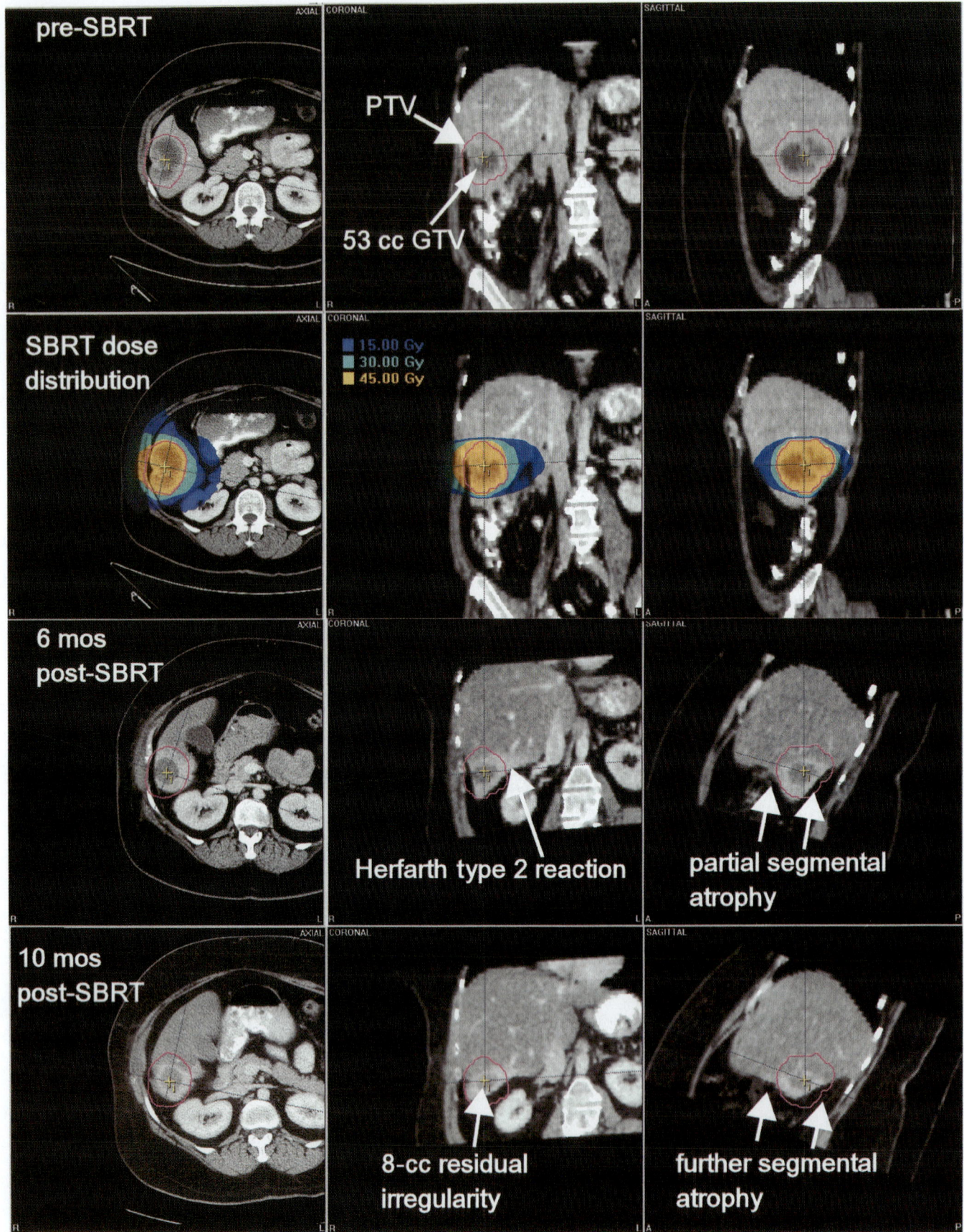

FIGURE 18.1. Example of liver stereotactic body radiation therapy (SBRT). **Top panel:** Pre-SBRT planning computed tomography images with *thin arrow* pointing to the gross tumor volume (GTV) and *wide arrow* showing the planning target volume (PTV), which is outlined. **Second panel:** SBRT composite dose distribution. **Third panel:** Images obtained 6 months post-SBRT illustrating a Herfarth type 2 reaction in adjacent parenchyma and partial segmental atrophy. **Bottom panel:** Shows images 10 months post-SBRT, indicating continued tumor regression as the ablated liver volume continues to recede.

dynamic conformal arcs and a controlled breath-holding device. The nominal prescription dose was 45 Gy. The maximum point dose was 59 Gy, and the equivalent uniform dose was 54 Gy. The volume of normal liver receiving <15 Gy was 1,800 cm³. The portion of the right kidney receiving above 15 Gy was 13%. Follow-up scans at 6 and 10 months show a Herfarth type 2 reaction with hyperdensity in the treated normal liver.[59] There is also volume loss in the nearby normal liver parenchyma surrounding the lesion, a phenomenon that has also been described.[60] The lesion remained controlled for the duration of the patient's life; she eventually died of complications related to central nervous system metastases.

Lung

Medically inoperable early-stage lung cancer has historically provided a substantial management challenge. Conventionally fractionated radiotherapy has yielded generally unsatisfactory outcomes with high rates of local failure and 3-year survivals in the range of approximately 30%. For this reason, medically inoperable early-stage lung cancer was the first clinical indication for which SBRT was studied in prospective clinical trials. Following the early exploratory studies of lung SBRT for stage I non–small cell lung cancer at the Karolinska Hospital in Stockholm[61] and National Medical Defense Hospital in Saitama,[3] numerous formal prospective studies of SBRT for medically inoperable non–small cell lung cancer have been now been reported. Table 18.2 lists the major prospective studies (N = 50 or more) with a minimum median follow-up of 24 months at the time of reporting, along with local control and overall survival at 3 years.[62-65] The consistent observation is that 3-year survival on the order of 50% to 60% has been achieved. A randomized clinical trial comparing SBRT (66 Gy in 3 fractions) to conventionally fractionated radiotherapy (70 Gy in 35 fractions) in this setting revealed equivalent overall survival despite slightly worse prognostic features in the SBRT arm. Patients who received SBRT also had lower rates of pulmonary toxicity and better self-reported quality of life.[66]

One important observation from the Indiana University studies was that although the treatment was generally well tolerated, tumor location near large airways in the vicinity of the pulmonary hilum (called the zone of the proximal bronchial tree) was associated with a markedly higher risk of toxicity. For this reason, in the Radiation Therapy Oncology Group's (RTOG) study RTOG-0236 of SBRT for medically inoperable non–small cell lung cancer, patients with tumors located in the zone of the proximal bronchial tree were excluded.[64] The RTOG launched a separate dose escalation study (ROTG-0813) in which tumors near the proximal bronchial tree were treated to doses in the range of 50 to 60 Gy in 5 fractions.[67] Protocol specified DLT rate were low, though some late toxicity outside those definitions occurred. The American Society for Radiation Oncology (ASTRO) has issued a guideline on SBRT for early-stage lung cancer that addresses key questions of patient selection and dose regimen for peripheral and central tumors.[68]

Although many retrospective studies of lung SBRT contain a mixture of both primary and metastatic lesions, a few prospective studies exclusively focused on SBRT for lung metastases have been reported. In the University of Colorado phase I SBRT trial for lung metastases,[69] eligible patients had one to three pulmonary metastases from a solid tumor, cumulative tumor diameter <7 cm, and adequate pulmonary function (forced expiratory volume in the first second of expiration [FEV_1] >1.0 L). The PTV was typically constructed from the GTV by adding a 5-mm radial and 10-mm craniocaudal margin. The first cohort received 48 Gy to the PTV in 3 fractions. The SBRT dose was escalated in subsequent cohorts up to a preselected maximum of 60 Gy in 3 fractions. The percentage of normal lung receiving more than 15 Gy (V15) was restricted to <35%. DLT included acute grade 3 lung or esophageal toxicity or any acute grade 4 toxicity. No patient experienced a DLT, and the SBRT dose was escalated to 60 Gy in 3 fractions without reaching a maximum tolerated dose. No consistent significant effects on pulmonary functions tests were noted.

The phase II study of SBRT for lung metastases the Colorado study group included 38 patients with 63 lesions.[70] Most had received at least one prior systemic regimen for metastatic disease, and approximately one-third had received two or more prior regimens. The incidence of any grade 3 toxicity was 8% (3/38), and no grade 4 toxicity was seen. Symptomatic pneumonitis occurred in one patient (2.6%). For 50 lesions assessable for local control, the median follow-up was 15.4 months. The median GTV was 4.2 cc. The actuarial 2-year local control was 96%. Median overall survival was 19 months.

CASE STUDY

Lung Stereotactic Body Radiation Therapy

A 74-year-old female had undergone wedge resection for a pT1N0M0 non–small cell cancer of the right lung 7 years previously. She had a right pneumonectomy 3 years later as salvage treatment for a locoregional recurrence. She was later observed to have developed a left lung nodule on a surveillance chest x-ray, and needle biopsy proved it to be a non–small cell lung cancer, presumed to be a second primary. Staging studies revealed no other sites of disease. She was given systemic therapy and enjoyed a transient minor response and then regrowth of the lesion (Fig. 18.2).

The patient used supplemental oxygen, 2 L/min at bedtime and occasionally during the day. She was offered SBRT as potentially curative therapy for a new T1N0M0 lung cancer. The 4 cm³ GTV was expanded by 5 mm radially and 10 mm in the superior–inferior direction to generate the 29 cm³ PTV. The dose distribution shown was administered in 3 fractions within 1 week using multiple dynamic conformal arcs. The patient did not comfortably tolerate a breath-holding technique because of her supplemental oxygen requirements; therefore, an abdominal compression technique was used during simulation and treatment. The nominal prescription dose was 60 Gy. The maximum point dose was 79 Gy, and the equivalent uniform dose was 72 Gy. The portion of normal lung receiving <15 Gy was 12.7%. The lesion remained controlled for the duration of the patient's life; she died of unrelated causes more than 2 years after SBRT.

Spine

The earliest investigation into what would now be termed spine SBRT was that of Hamilton et al.,[1,71] who used a rigid immobilization with a device surgically attached to the spinal column. Conservative doses in the range of 8 to 10 Gy were given in 1 fraction to nine patients with recurrent lesions in the spine following prior conventional radiotherapy. Spinal cord doses were very low using this technique (0.5 to 3.2 Gy).

TABLE 18.2 MAJOR PROSPECTIVE STUDIES OF STEREOTACTIC BODY RADIATION THERAPY FOR MEDICALLY INOPERABLE NON–SMALL CELL LUNG CANCER

Institution	Number of Patients	SBRT Dose and Fractionation	3-Year Results
Indiana University[62]	70	60–66 Gy/3 fractions	LC 88%, OS 43%
Nordic Group[63]	57	45 Gy/3 fractions	LC 92%, OS 60%
RTOG[64]	55	54 Gy/3 fractions	LC 98%, OS 56%
University of Torino[65]	62	45 Gy/3 fractions	LC 88%, OS 57%

LC, local control; OS, overall survival; RTOG, Radiation Therapy Oncology Group.

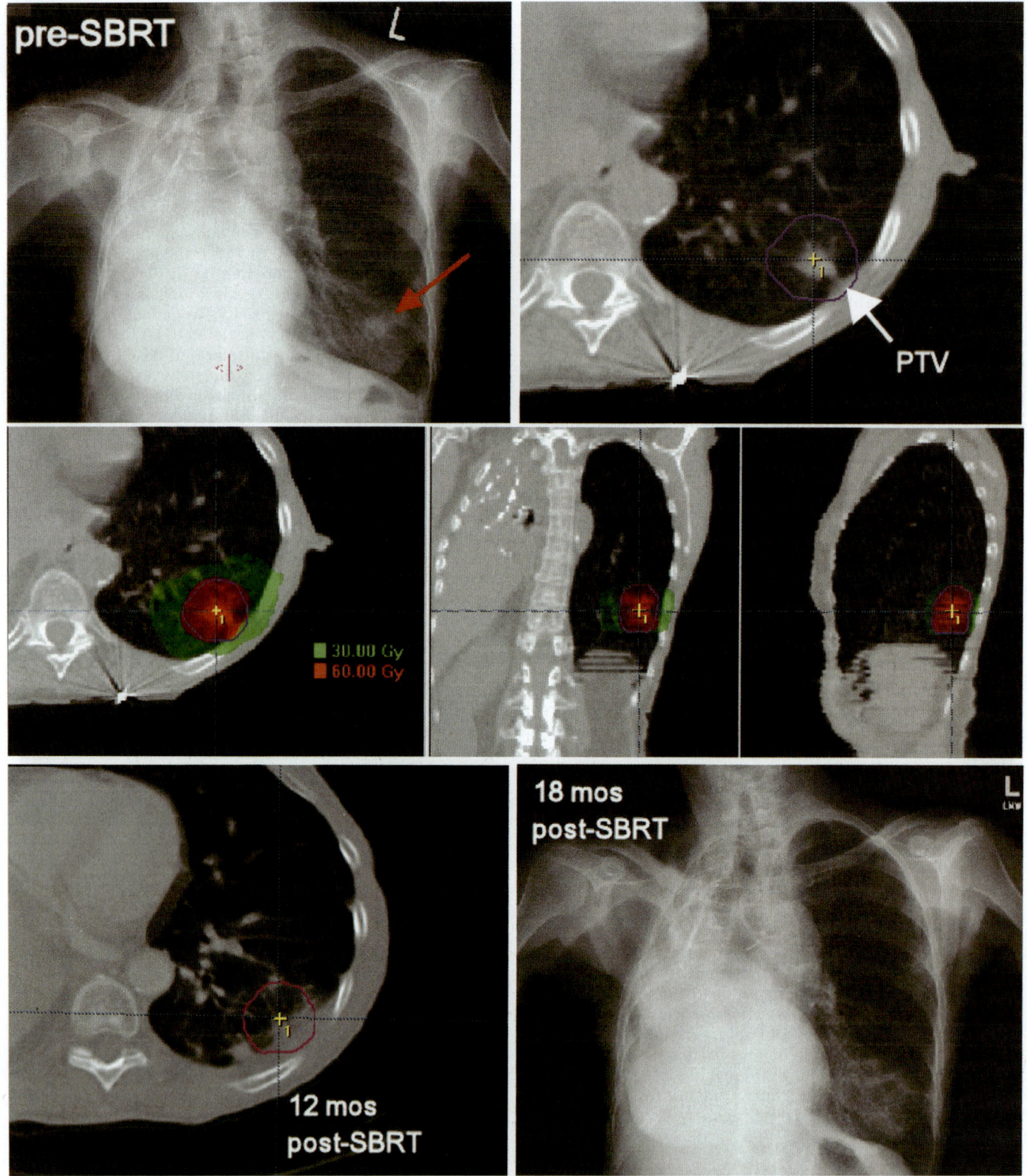

FIGURE 18.2. Example of lung stereotactic body radiation therapy (SBRT). **Top panel:** Pre-SBRT chest x-ray showing the left lung nodule (*red arrow*) and axial planning computed tomography (CT) image with *white arrow* pointing to the planning target volume (PTV), which is outlined. **Middle panel:** SBRT composite dose distribution shown in axial, coronal, and sagittal perspectives. **Bottom panel:** Follow-up CT scan axial image obtained 12 months post-SBRT illustrating stable patchy fibrosis in the high-dose region (*left*) and chest x-ray obtained 12 months post-SBRT, indicating minimal residual haziness in the region treated.

Limited follow-up suggested a favorable clinical effect in some patients, and no complications were observed. More recently, less invasive techniques have been investigated.

Ryu et al.[72] at the Henry Ford Hospital initially studied the treatment of spine metastases with initial fractionated radiotherapy followed by a spinal radiosurgery boost (6 to 8 Gy), observing prompt relief of pain in nearly all 10 treated patients. In a subsequent study of single-fraction spinal radiosurgery alone (10 to 16 Gy), this group observed complete or partial pain relief in 85% of the 49 patients treated.[73] Perhaps even more importantly, pain relief was rapid after SBRT, sometimes within hours of treatment.

Chang et al.[74,75] at the M.D. Anderson Cancer Center performed a prospective phase I dose escalation study in treating spinal metastases and later updated their institutional experience. The equipment used included a "CT on rails" that allowed for imaging immediately to guide patient repositioning. Sixty-three cancer patients underwent near-simultaneous CT-guided SBRT. Spinal magnetic resonance imaging was conducted at baseline and at each follow-up visit. The median tumor volume of 74 spinal metastatic lesions was 37.4 cc. Approximately half the patients received 30 Gy in 5 fractions, and the other half received 27 Gy in 3 fractions. A conservative constraint of 9 to 10 Gy maximum dose to the spinal cord was applied. No neuropathy or myelopathy was observed during a median follow-up period of nearly 2 years. The actuarial 1-year tumor progression-free rate was 84%. The investigators noted two characteristic patterns of failure: (a) recurrence in the bone adjacent to the site of previous treatment and (b) recurrence in the epidural space adjacent to the spinal cord. A low rate of any grade 3 toxicity was observed.

Similar observations of good tumor control and minimal toxicity have been reported from other centers.[76-81] For example, Gerszten et al.[78] of the University of Pittsburgh analyzed a cohort of 500 cases of spinal metastases. The maximum intratumoral dose ranged from 12.5 to 25 Gy (mean, 20). Tumor volume ranged from 0.20 to 264 mL (mean, 46). Durable pain reduction was achieved in 86% of patients, and durable tumor control was demonstrated for approximately 90% of the lesions treated. The vast majority of patients with a progressive neurologic deficit before treatment experienced at least some clinical improvement.

Regarding normal tissue toxicities, the Memorial Sloan-Kettering Cancer Center group reported that post-SBRT vertebral fracture is common when there is metastatic lytic disease involving more than 40% of the vertebral body and location at or below T10.[81] The MD Anderson Cancer Center group also analyzed the risk of fracture after spine SBRT and noted that fractures were more common among patients of age over 55 years, those with a pre-existing fracture, and pain at the time of treatment,[82] suggesting that patients at very high risk might appropriately be considered for prophylactic vertebral stabilization or augmentation procedures. Fortunately, spinal cord toxicity has only rarely been observed after SBRT. Case-control comparisons offer some suggestions of parameters that might elevate the risk, but the paucity of events evaluable make it difficult to draw firm conclusions.[83,84] Constraints used to guide spine SBRT have included maximum point dose to the cord in the range of 10 to 14 Gy and limiting the volume of adjacent spinal cord receiving more than 10 Gy in a single fraction to 10% or less.

The International Spine Radiosurgery Consortium group has published guidelines to inform target definition and response assessment after spine SBRT.[85] The SPIne response assessment in Neuro-Oncology (SPINO) Group has likewise issued guidance on response assessment.[86]

Prostate Cancer

The first publication on SBRT for prostate cancer was the work of Madsen et al.,[80,87] who recently updated their observations. In a prospective trial, 40 patients with low-risk cancer (Gleason score ≤6 and prostate-specific antigen [PSA] ≤10 ng/mL) were treated to a dose of 33.5 Gy in 5 daily fractions The median age was 69 years (range, 50 to 82), and the median follow-up period was 5 years. The overall 5-year Phoenix definition (nadir plus 2 ng/mL) biochemical relapse-free survival (bRFS) rate was 93%. No patients died of prostate cancer. Late grade 3 genitourinary toxicity was rare, occurring in only one patient, and no late grade 3 or higher gastrointestinal was observed.[88]

The groups at Winthrop University and the University of California–San Francisco have also reported trials of SBRT for early-stage prostate cancer.[89,90] Using doses of 35 to 38 Gy in 4 or 5 fractions, both groups reported similarly low rates of grade 3 or higher toxicity of any kind (<1% in aggregate between the studies) after a median follow-up of 1 year. King et al.[91] from Stanford University reported a prospective trial in which 67 patients with clinically localized low-risk prostate cancer were treated with SBRT to a dose of 36.25 Gy, administered in 5 fractions. The 4-year bRFS was 94%, and no grade 3 or higher rectal toxicity was observed. There were only two cases (3%) of grade 3 or higher bladder toxicity, both of which were believed to have been caused or exacerbated by procedures performed for dysuria (cystoscopies or dilatation).

The combined observations from multiple prospective trials at eight institutions were pooled and reported.[92] SBRT to a median dose of 36.35 Gy in 4 to 5 fractions was given to 1,100 patients with clinically localized prostate cancer. Most patients were low-risk, though nearly 40% had intermediate-risk or high-risk disease. A minority (14%) received a short course of androgen deprivation therapy. The 5-year bRFS rate was 93% for all patients; 95%, 83%, and 78% for GS ≤6, 7 and ≥8, respectively (P = .001), and 95%, 84%, and 81% for low-, intermediate- and high-risk patients, respectively (P < .001). For 135 patients with a minimum of 5 years follow-up, the 5-year bRFS rate for low- and intermediate-risk patients was 99% and 93%, respectively. A parallel quality of life analysis in the same group of patients indicated a transient decline in the urinary and bowel domains within the first 3 months after SBRT, which typically returned to baseline status or better within 6 months and remained so beyond 5 years.[93] Sexual quality of life decline was predominantly observed within the first 9 months

Boike et al.[94] from the University of Texas–Southwestern have completed a dose escalation for prostate SBRT, aiming for a more aggressive regimen potentially suitable for patients with intermediate- or high-risk disease. At the highest dose level, 6.6% of patients treated (6 of 91) developed high-grade rectal toxicity, 5 of whom required colostomy.[95] Grade 3+ delayed rectal toxicity was correlated with volume of rectal wall receiving 50 Gy >3 cm³ (P < .0001) and treatment of >35% circumference of rectal wall to 39 Gy (P = .003). Grade 2+ acute rectal toxicity was significantly correlated with treatment of >50% circumference of rectal wall to 24 Gy (P = .010). The anticipated incorporation of hydrogel spacers inserted between the rectum and prostate is expected to reduce bowel toxicity after prostate SBRT and allow the evaluation of dose escalation in high-risk patients in the future.[96]

Pancreas Cancer

The role of conventionally fractionated radiotherapy in combination with chemotherapy for locally advanced pancreas cancer remains unresolved. An effect on overall survival is not seen consistently, though there is likely at least a moderate benefit in terms of achieving treatment-free intervals in this challenging clinical scenario.[97,98] SBRT would be an appealing alternative if equivalent or better survival could be achieved with lower rates of toxicity related to the reduction of the volume of normal tissue exposed to a high dose of radiation.

SBRT regimens for pancreas cancer have included treatments given in 1 to 5 fractions. The relation of risk of toxicity to the volume of normal tissue receiving a high dose is illustrated by the Danish cooperative group study. Here, a dose of 45 Gy in 3 fractions to a volume that included generous margins around the GTV, such that the median volume receiving more than 30 Gy, was 136 cc.[99] The toxicity from this high-volume treatment was unacceptably high.

More recent studies have incorporated tighter planning margins around the primary tumor and achieved reduction in toxicity and improvement in survival. The Stanford experience included 55 patients treated with a single 25 Gy fraction to the GTV plus 3-mm margin, with gemcitabine (GEM) given for 1 cycle prior to and 4 to 6 cycles after SBRT.[100] A median survival of 13 months was observed. The San Bartolo Hospital group gave 30 Gy in 3 fractions to a similar target volume, again with GEM given before and after SBRT, and observed an 11-month median survival.[101] The Beth Israel Deaconess group used a dose of 24 to 36 Gy in 3 fractions, with the GEM given after SBRT for 6 cycles, and observed a 14-month median survival.[102] The incidence of grade 3 or higher SBRT-related toxicity was very low for each study. In the San Bartolo Hospital and Beth Israel Deaconess studies, the rates of grade 3 or higher nonhematologic toxicity were 0% and 14%, respectively.

The Stanford group analyzed potential dosimetric factors that predicted for a risk of duodenal toxicity after single-fraction SBRT for pancreatic cancer.[103] Among 73 patients evaluable, 6 patients experienced grade 2 toxicity and 6 experienced grade 3 or 4 toxicity. Numerous interrelated metrics proved to be able to distinguish groups of lower versus higher risk of toxicity. For example, the volume of duodenum receiving a dose of 15 Gy or higher (V15) was significant: for V15 ≥ 9.1 cc, the rate of toxicity was 52%, whereas for V15 < 9.1 cc, the rate was 11% (P = .002).

In a more recent phase 2 multi-institutional study, 49 patients with locally advanced pancreas cancer received up to 3 doses of gemcitabine (1,000 mg/m^2) followed by a 1-week break and then SBRT (33.0 gray [Gy] in 5 fractions).[104] After SBRT, patients continued to receive gemcitabine until disease progression or toxicity. The median overall survival was 13.9 months (95% confidence interval, 10.2 to 16.7 months). Freedom from local disease progression at 1 year was 78%. Rates of acute and late (primary endpoint) grade ≥2 gastritis, fistula, enteritis, or ulcer toxicities were 2% and 11%, respectively. QLQ-C30 global quality of life scores remained stable from baseline to after SBRT (67 at baseline, median change of 0 at both follow-ups; P > .05 for both). Patients reported a significant improvement in pancreatic pain (P = .001) 4 weeks after SBRT on the QLQ-PAN26 questionnaire. The median plasma carbohydrate antigen 19-9 (CA 19-9) level was reduced after SBRT (median time after SBRT, 4.2 weeks; 220 vs. 62 U/mL [P < .001]). Freedom from local disease progression at 1 year was 78%.

CONCLUSIONS

SBRT has emerged as a versatile strategy with a wide range of applications for many different types and stages of cancer. As with any form of radiation therapy, careful attention to matters of patient selection and technical quality assurance is essential for the effective and safe implementation of SBRT. Future advances will refine our understanding of the biologic mechanisms and optimal integration and sequencing of SBRT with other anticancer therapies.

REFERENCES

1. Hamilton AJ, Lulu BA, Fosmire H, et al. Preliminary clinical experience with linear accelerator-based spinal stereotactic radiosurgery. *Neurosurgery* 1995;36:311–319.
2. Blomgren H, Lax I, Naslund I, et al. Stereotactic high dose fraction radiation therapy of extracranial tumors using an accelerator. Clinical experience of the first thirty-one patients. *Acta Oncol* 1995;34:861–870.
3. Uematsu M, Shioda A, Tahara K, et al. Focal, high dose, and fractionated modified stereotactic radiation therapy for lung carcinoma patients: a preliminary experience. *Cancer* 1998;82:1062–1070.
4. Kavanagh BD, Timmerman RD. Stereotactic radiosurgery and stereotactic body radiation therapy: an overview of technical considerations and clinical applications. *Hematol Oncol Clin North Am* 2006;20:87–95.
5. Potters L, Kavanagh B, Galvin JM, et al. American Society for Therapeutic Radiology and Oncology (ASTRO) and American College of Radiology (ACR) practice guideline for the performance of stereotactic body radiation therapy. *Int J Radiat Oncol Biol Phys* 2010;76(2):326–332.
6. Loo BW, Chang JY, Dawson LA, et al. Stereotactic ablative radiotherapy: what's in a name? *Pract Radiat Oncol* 2011;1:38–39.
7. Guerrero M, Li X. Extending the linear–quadratic model for large fraction doses pertinent to stereotactic radiotherapy. *Phys Med Biol* 2004;49:4825–4835.
8. Curtis SB. Lethal and potentially lethal lesions induced by radiation—a unified repair model. *Radiat Res* 1986;106:252–270.
9. Benedict SH, Lin PS, Zwicker RD, et al. The biological effectiveness of intermittent irradiation as a function of overall treatment time: development of correction factors for LINAC-based stereotactic radiotherapy. *Int J Radiat Oncol Biol Phys* 1997;37:765–769.
10. Park C, Papiez L, Zhang S, et al. Universal survival curve and single fraction equivalent dose: useful tools in understanding potency of ablative radiotherapy. *Int J Radiat Oncol Biol Phys* 2008;70:847–852.
11. Brenner DJ, Hall EJ. Fractionation and protraction for radiotherapy of prostate carcinoma. *Int J Radiat Oncol Biol Phys* 1999;43:1095–1101.
12. Williams SG, Taylor JM, Liu N, et al. Use of individual fraction size data from 3756 patients to directly determine the alpha/beta ratio of prostate cancer. *Int J Radiat Oncol Biol Phys* 2007;68:24–33.
13. Lee WR, Dignam JJ, Amin MB, et al, Seaward SA. Randomized phase III noninferiority study comparing two radiotherapy fractionation schedules in patients with low-risk prostate cancer. *J Clin Oncol* 2016;34(20):2325–2332.
14. Pollack A, Walker G, Horwitz EM, et al. Randomized trial of hypofractionated external-beam radiotherapy for prostate cancer. *J Clin Oncol* 2013;31(31):3860–3868.
15. Arcangeli S, Strigari L, Gomellini S, et al. Updated results and patterns of failure in a randomized hypofractionation trial for high-risk prostate cancer. *Int J Radiat Oncol Biol Phys* 2012;84:1172–1178.
16. Garcia-Barros M, Paris F, Cordon-Cardo C, et al. Tumor response to radiotherapy regulated by endothelial cell apoptosis. *Science* 2003;300(5622):1155–1159.
17. Zhang L, Kavanagh B, Thorburn A, et al. Preclinical and clinical estimates of a cancer's basal apoptotic rate predict for the amount of apoptosis induced by subsequent pro-apoptotic stimuli. *Clin Cancer Res* 2010;16:4478–4489.
18. Moding EJ, Lee CL, Castle KD et al. Atm deletion with dual recombinase technology preferentially radiosensitizes tumor endothelium. *J Clin Invest* 2014;124:3325–3338.
19. Moding EJ, Castle KD, Perez BA et al. Tumor cells, but not endothelial cells, mediate eradication of primary sarcomas by stereotactic body radiation therapy. *Sci Transl Med* 2015;7:278ra34.
20. Lee Y, Auh SL, Wang Y, et al. Therapeutic effects of ablative radiation on local tumor require CD8+ T cells: changing strategies for cancer treatment. *Blood* 2009;114:589–595.
21. Hellman S, Weichselbaum RR. Oligometastases. *J Clin Oncol* 1995;13:8–10.
22. Timmerman RD, Bizekis CS, Pass HI, et al. Local surgical, ablative, and radiation treatment of metastases. *CA Cancer J Clin* 2009;59:145–170.
23. Stinauer MA, Kavanagh BD, Schefter TE, et al. Stereotactic body radiation therapy for melanoma and renal cell carcinoma: impact of single fraction equivalent dose on local control. *Radiat Oncol* 2011;6(1):34.
24. Rusthoven K, Hammerman SF, Kavanagh BD, et al. Is there a role for consolidative stereotactic body radiation therapy following first-line systemic therapy for metastatic lung cancer? A patterns-of-failure analysis. *Acta Oncol* 2009;48:578–583.
25. Gomez DR, Blumenschein GR, Lee JJ, et al. Local consolidative therapy versus maintenance therapy or observation for patients with oligometastatic non-small-cell lung cancer without progression after first-line systemic therapy: a multicentre, randomised, controlled, phase 2 study. *Lancet Oncol* 2016;17(12):1672–1682.
26. Palma DA, Haasbeek CJ, Rodrigues GB, et al. Stereotactic ablative radiotherapy for comprehensive treatment of oligometastatic tumors (SABR-COMET): study protocol for a randomized phase II trial. *BMC Cancer* 2012;12(1):305.
27. Salama JK, Milano MT. Radical irradiation of extracranial oligometastases. *J Clin Oncol* 2014;32(26):2902–2912.
28. Postow MA, Callahan MK, Barker CA, et al. Immunologic correlates of the abscopal effect in a patient with melanoma. *N Engl J Med* 2012;366(10):925–931.
29. Golden EB, Demaria S, Schiff PB, et al. An abscopal response to radiation and ipilimumab in a patient with metastatic non–small cell lung cancer. *Cancer Immunol Res* 2013;1(6):365–372.
30. Shaverdian N, Lisberg AE, Bornazyan K, et al. Previous radiotherapy and the clinical activity and toxicity of pembrolizumab in the treatment of non-small-cell lung cancer: a secondary analysis of the KEYNOTE-001 phase 1 trial. *Lancet Oncol* 2017;18(7):895–903.
31. Benedict SH, Yenice KM, Followill D, et al. Stereotactic body radiation therapy: the report of AAPM Task Group 101. *Med Phys* 2010;37:4078–4101.
32. Solberg TD, Balter JM, Benedict SH, et al. Quality and safety considerations in stereotactic radiosurgery and stereotactic body radiation therapy: executive summary. *Pract Radiat Oncol* 2012;2:2–9.
33. Yeung YP, Lo CM, Liu CL, et al. Natural history of untreated nonsurgical hepatocellular carcinoma. *J Gastroenterol* 2005;100:1995–2004.
34. Ruzzenente A, Capra F, Pachera S, et al. Is liver resection justified in advanced hepatocellular carcinoma? Results of an observational study in 464 patients. *J Gastrointest Surg* 2009;13:1313–1320.
35. Meng M, Cui Y, She B, et al. Transcatheter arterial chemoembolization in combination with radiotherapy for unresectable hepatocellular carcinoma: a systematic review and meta-analysis. *Radiother Oncol* 2009;92:184–194.
36. Tse RV, Hawkins M, Lockwood G, et al. Phase I study of individualized stereotactic body radiotherapy for hepatocellular carcinoma and intrahepatic cholangiocarcinoma. *J Clin Oncol* 2008;26:657–664.
37. Méndez Romero A, Wunderink W, Hussain SM, et al. Stereotactic body radiation therapy for primary and metastatic liver tumors: a single institution phase i-ii study. *Acta Oncol* 2006;45(7):831–837.
38. Choi BO, Choi BI, Jang HS, et al. Stereotactic body radiation therapy with or without transarterial chemoembolization for patients with primary hepatocellular carcinoma: preliminary analysis. *BMC Cancer* 2008;8:351.
39. Son SH, Choi BO, Ryu MR, et al. Stereotactic body radiotherapy for patients with unresectable primary hepatocellular carcinoma: dose-volumetric parameters predicting the hepatic complication. *Int J Radiat Oncol Biol Phys* 2010;78:1073–1080.

40. Seo YS, Kim M-S, Yoo S, et al. Preliminary result of stereotactic body radiotherapy as a local salvage treatment for inoperable hepatocellular carcinoma. *J Surg Oncol* 2010;102:209–214.
41. Cardenes HR, Price TR, Perkins SM, et al. Phase I feasibility trial of stereotactic body radiation therapy for primary hepatocellular carcinoma. *Clin Transl Oncol* 2010;12:218–225.
42. Andolino DL, Johnson CS, Maluccio M, et al. Stereotactic body radiotherapy for primary hepatocellular carcinoma. *Int J Radiat Oncol Biol Phys* 2011;81:e447–e453.
43. Bibault JE, Dewas S, Vautravers-Dewas C, et al. Stereotactic body radiation therapy for hepatocellular carcinoma: prognostic factors of local control, overall survival, and toxicity. *PLoS One* 2013;8(10):e77472.
44. Su TS, Liang P, Liang J, et al. Long-term survival analysis of stereotactic ablative radiotherapy versus liver resection for small hepatocellular carcinoma. *Int J Radiat Oncol Biol Phys* 2017;98(3):639–646.
45. Herfarth KK, Debus J, Wannenmacher M. Stereotactic radiation therapy of liver metastases: update of the initial phase-I/II trial. *Front Radiat Ther Oncol* 2004;38:100–105.
46. Wulf J, Guckenberger M, Haedinger U, et al. Stereotactic radiotherapy of primary liver cancer and hepatic metastases. *Acta Oncol* 2006;45:838–847.
47. Hoyer M, Roed H, Traberg-Hansen A, et al. Phase II study on stereotactic body radiotherapy of colorectal metastases. *Acta Oncol* 2006;45:823–830.
48. van der Pool AE, Mendez-Romero A, Wunderink W, et al. Stereotactic body radiation therapy for colorectal liver metastases. *Br J Surg* 2010;97:377–382.
49. Rusthoven K, Kavanagh BD, Cardenes H, et al. Mature results of a multi-institutional phase I/II trial of stereotactic body radiation therapy for liver metastases. *J Clin Oncol* 2009;27:1572–1578.
50. Lee MT, Kim JJ, Dinniwell R, et al. Phase I study of individualized stereotactic body radiotherapy of liver metastases. *J Clin Oncol* 2009;27:1585–1591.
51. Goodman KA, Wiegner EA, Maturen KE, et al. Dose-escalation study of single-fraction stereotactic body radiotherapy for liver malignancies. *Int J Radiat Oncol Biol Phys* 2010;78:486–493.
52. Rule W, Timmerman R, Tong L, et al. Phase I dose-escalation study of stereotactic body radiotherapy in patients with hepatic metastases. *Ann Surg Oncol* 2011;18:1081–1087.
53. Scorsetti M, Comito T, Tozzi A, et al. Final results of a phase II trial for stereotactic body radiation therapy for patients with inoperable liver metastases from colorectal cancer. *J Cancer Res Clin Oncol* 2015;141(3):543–553.
54. Chang DT, Swaminath A, Kozak M, et al. Stereotactic body radiotherapy for colorectal liver metastases: a pooled analysis. *Cancer* 2011;117:4060–4069.
55. Schefter TE, Kavanagh BD. Radiation therapy for liver metastases. *Semin Radiat Oncol* 2011;21:264–270.
56. Høyer M, Swaminath A, Bydder S, et al. Radiotherapy for liver metastases: a review of evidence. *Int J Radiat Oncol Biol Phys* 2012;82:1047–1057.
57. Schefter TE, Kavanagh BD, Timmerman RD, et al. A phase I trial of stereotactic body radiation therapy (SBRT) for liver metastases. *Int J Radiat Oncol Biol Phys* 2005;62:1371–1378.
58. Yeas RJ, Kalend A. Local stem cell depletion model for radiation myelitis. *Int J Radiat Oncol Biol Phys* 1988;14:1247–1259.
59. Herfarth KK, Hof H, Bahner ML, et al. Assessment of focal liver reaction by multiphasic CT after stereotactic single-dose radiotherapy of liver tumors. *Int J Radiat Oncol Biol Phys* 2003;57:444–451.
60. Olsen CC, Welsh J, Kavanagh BD, et al. Microscopic and macroscopic tumor and parenchymal effects of liver stereotactic body radiotherapy. *Int J Radiat Oncol Biol Phys* 2009;73(5):1414–1424.
61. Blomgren H, Lax, I, Goranson, H, et al. Radiosurgery for tumors in the body: clinical experience using a new method. *J Radiosurg* 1998;1:63–74.
62. Fakiris AJ, McGarry RC, Yiannoutsos CT, et al. Stereotactic body radiation therapy for early-stage non-small-cell lung carcinoma: four-year results of a prospective phase II study. *Int J Radiat Oncol Biol Phys* 2009;75:677–682.
63. Baumann P, Nyman J, Hoyer M, et al. Outcome in a prospective phase II trial of medically inoperable stage I non–small-cell lung cancer patients treated with stereotactic body radiotherapy. *J Clin Oncol* 2009;27:3290–3296.
64. Timmerman R, Paulus R, Galvin J, et al. Stereotactic body radiation therapy for inoperable early stage lung cancer. *JAMA* 2010;303:1070–1076.
65. Ricardi U, Filippi AR, Guarneri A, et al. Stereotactic body radiation therapy for early stage non-small cell lung cancer: results of a prospective trial. *Lung Cancer* 2010;68(1):72–77.
66. Nyman J, Hallqvist A, Lund JÅ, et al. SPACE–A randomized study of SBRT vs conventional fractionated radiotherapy in medically inoperable stage I NSCLC. *Radiother Oncol* 2016;121(1):1–8.
67. Bezjak A, Paulus R, Gaspar LE, et al. Primary study endpoint analysis for NRG Oncology/RTOG 0813 trial of stereotactic body radiation therapy (SBRT) for centrally located non-small cell lung cancer (NSCLC). *Int J Radiat Oncol Biol Phys* 2016;1(94):5–6.
68. Videtic GM, Donington J, Giuliani M, et al. Stereotactic body radiation therapy for early-stage non-small cell lung cancer: executive summary of an ASTRO Evidence-Based Guideline. *Pract Radiat Oncol* 2017;7(5):295–301.
69. Schefter TE, Kavanagh BD, Raben D, et al. A phase I/II trial of stereotactic body radiation therapy (SBRT) for lung metastases: initial report of dose escalation and early toxicity. *Int J Radiat Oncol Biol Phys* 2006;66(4S):S120–S127.
70. Rusthoven K, Kavanagh BD, Burri SH, et al. Multi-institutional phase I/II trial of stereotactic body radiation therapy for lung metastases. *J Clin Oncol* 2009;27:1579–1584.
71. Hamilton AJ, Lulu BA, Fosmire H, et al. LINAC-based spinal stereotactic radiosurgery. *Stereotact Funct Neurosurg* 1996;66:1–9.
72. Ryu S, Fang Yin F, Rock J, et al. Image-guided and intensity-modulated radiosurgery for patients with spinal metastasis. *Cancer* 2003;97(8):2013–2018.
73. Ryu S, Rock J, Rosenblum M, et al. Patterns of failure after single-dose radiosurgery for spinal metastasis. *J Neurosurg* 2004;101(Suppl 3):402–405.
74. Chang EL, Shiu AS, Lii MF, et al. Phase I clinical evaluation of near-simultaneous computed tomographic image-guided stereotactic body radiotherapy for spinal metastases. *Int J Radiat Oncol Biol Phys* 2004;59:1288–1294.
75. Chang EL, Shiu AS, Mendel E, et al. Phase I/II study of stereotactic body radiotherapy for spinal metastasis and its pattern of failure. *J Neurosurg Spine* 2007;7:151–160.
76. Nelson JW, Yoo DS, Sampson JH, et al. Stereotactic body radiotherapy for lesions of the spine and paraspinal regions. *Int J Radiat Oncol Biol Phys* 2009;73(5):1369–1375.
77. De Salles AA, Pedroso AG, Medin P, et al. Spinal lesions treated with Novalis shaped beam intensity-modulated radiosurgery and stereotactic radiotherapy. *J Neurosurg* 2004;101(S3):435–440.
78. Gerszten PC, Burton SA, Ozhasoglu C, et al. Radiosurgery for spinal metastases: clinical experience in 500 cases from a single institution. *Spine* 2007;32:193–199.
79. Gibbs IC, Kamnerdsupaphon P, Ryu MR, et al. Image-guided robotic radiosurgery for spinal metastases. *Radiother Oncol* 2007;82:185–190.
80. Yamada Y, Bilsky MH, Lovelock DM, et al. High-dose, single fraction image-guided intensity-modulated radiotherapy for metastatic spinal lesions. *Int J Radiat Oncol Biol Phys* 2008;71:484–490.
81. Rose PS, Laufer I, Boland PJ, et al. Risk of fracture after single fraction image-guided intensity-modulated radiation therapy to spinal metastases. *J Clin Oncol* 2009;27(30):5075–5079.
82. Boehling NS, Grosshans DR, Allen PK. Vertebral compression fracture risk after stereotactic body radiotherapy for spinal metastases. *J Neurosurg Spine* 2012;16(4):379–386.
83. Sahgal A, Ma L, Gibbs I, et al. Spinal cord tolerance for stereotactic body radiotherapy. *Int J Radiat Oncol Biol Phys* 2010;77:548–553.
84. Sahgal A, Ma L, Weinberg V, et al. Reirradiation human spinal cord tolerance for stereotactic body radiotherapy. *Int J Radiat Oncol Biol Phys* 2012;82:107–116.
85. Cox BW, Spratt DE, Lovelock M, et al. International Spine Radiosurgery Consortium consensus guidelines for target volume definition in spinal stereotactic radiosurgery. *Int J Radiat Oncol Biol Phys.* 2012;83(5):e597–e605.
86. Thibault I, Chang EL, Sheehan J, et al. Response assessment after stereotactic body radiotherapy for spinal metastasis: a report from the SPIne response assessment in Neuro-Oncology (SPINO) group. *Lancet Oncol* 2015;16(16):e595–e603.
87. Madsen BL, His RA, Pham HT, et al. Stereotactic hypofractionated accurate radiotherapy of the prostate (SHARP), 33.4 Gy in five fractions for localized disease: first clinical trial results. *Int J Radiat Oncol Biol Phys* 2007;67:1099–1105.
88. Pham HT, Song G, Badiozamani K, et al. Five-year outcome of stereotactic hypofractionated accurate radiotherapy of the prostate (SHARP) for patients with low-risk prostate cancer. *Int J Radiat Oncol Biol Phys* 2010;78:S58.
89. Katz A, Santoro M, Ashley R, et al. Stereotactic body radiotherapy for organ-confined prostate cancer. *BMC Urol* 2010;10:1.
90. Jabbari S, Weinberg VK, Kaprealian T, et al. Stereotactic body radiotherapy as monotherapy or post-external beam radiotherapy boost for prostate cancer: technique, early toxicity, and PSA response. *Int J Radiat Oncol Biol Phys* 2012;82:228–234.
91. King CR, Brooks JD, Harcharan G, et al. Long-term outcomes from a prospective trail of stereotactic body radiotherapy for low-risk prostate cancer. *Int J Radiat Oncol Biol Phys* 2012;82(2):877–882.
92. King CR, Freeman D, Kaplan I, et al. Stereotactic body radiotherapy for localized prostate cancer: pooled analysis from a multi-institutional consortium of prospective phase II trials. *Radiother Oncol* 2013;109(2):217–221.
93. King CR, Collins S, Fuller D, et al. Health-related quality of life after stereotactic body radiation therapy for localized prostate cancer: results from a multi-institutional consortium of prospective trials. *Int J Radiat Oncol Biol Phys* 2013;87(5):939–945.
94. Boike TP, Lotan Y, Chinsoo Cho L, et al. Phase I dose-escalation study of stereotactic body radiation therapy for low-and intermediate-risk prostate cancer. *J Clin Oncol* 2011;29:2020–2026.
95. Kim DN, Cho LC, Straka C, et al. Predictors of rectal tolerance observed in a dose-escalated phase 1-2 trial of stereotactic body radiation therapy for prostate cancer. *Int J Radiat Oncol Biol Phys* 2014;89(3):509–517.
96. Ruggieri R, Naccarato S, Stavrev P, et al. Dosimetric impact of a rectal spacer and an increased near maximum target dose in VMAT prostate SBRT. *Int J Radiat Oncol Biol Phys* 2015;93(3):E552–E553.
97. Loehrer Sr PJ, Feng Y, Cardenes H, et al. Gemcitabine alone versus gemcitabine plus radiotherapy in patients with locally advanced pancreatic cancer: an Eastern Cooperative Oncology Group trial. *J Clin Oncol* 2011;29(31):4105–4112.
98. Hammel P, Huguet F, van Laethem JL, et al. Effect of chemoradiotherapy vs chemotherapy on survival in patients with locally advanced pancreatic cancer controlled after 4 months of gemcitabine with or without erlotinib: the LAP07 randomized clinical trial. *JAMA* 2016;315(17):1844–1853.
99. Hoyer M, Roed H, Sengelov L, et al. Phase II study on stereotactic radiotherapy of locally advanced pancreatic carcinoma. *Radiother Oncol* 2005;76(1):48–53.
100. Schellenberg D, Quon A, Minn AY, et al. ^{18}Fluorodeoxyglucose PET is prognostic of progression-free and overall survival in locally advanced pancreas cancer treated with stereotactic radiotherapy. *Int J Radiat Oncol Biol Phys* 2010;77(5):1420–1425.
101. Polistina F, Constantin G, Cassamissima F, et al. Unresectable locally advanced pancreatic cancer: a multimodal treatment using neoadjuvant chemoradiotherapy (gemcitabine plus stereotactic radiosurgery) and subsequent surgical exploration. *Ann Surg Oncol* 2010;17:2092–2101.
102. Mahadevan A, Jain S, Goldstein M, et al. Stereotactic body radiotherapy and gemcitabine for locally advanced pancreatic cancer. *Int J Radiat Oncol Biol Phys* 2010;78(3):735–742.
103. Murphy JD, Christman-Skieller C, Kim J, et al. A dosimetric model of duodenal toxicity after stereotactic body radiotherapy for pancreatic cancer. *Int J Radiat Oncol Biol Phys* 2010;78(5):1420–1426.
104. Herman JM, Chang DT, Goodman KA, et al. Phase 2 multi-institutional trial evaluating gemcitabine and stereotactic body radiotherapy for patients with locally advanced unresectable pancreatic adenocarcinoma. *Cancer* 2015;121(7):1128–1137.

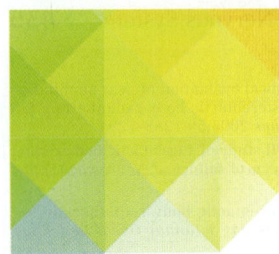

CHAPTER 19

Stereotactic Radiation Therapy Techniques

Mark J. Amsbaugh and Shiao Y. Woo

AN INTRODUCTION TO STEREOTACTIC RADIOSURGERY

The tools used by the surgeon must be adapted to the task, and where the human brain is concerned they cannot be too refined.

—Lars Leksell (Stereotaxis and Radiosurgery)

The tools of radiosurgery have been constantly refined and adapted from their humble beginnings to some of the most precise and impressive in all of modern medicine. Remarkably, at the time of their conception, many techniques we take for granted in modern stereotactic radiosurgery treatment planning and delivery had not yet been developed. Parts of the planning process as integral as 3D imaging were not available to early adopters of this new treatment modality. Therefore, both the capabilities and applications of stereotactic radiosurgery have evolved over its history and continue to change as technology and our understanding of these tools improve.

A Definition for Stereotactic Radiosurgery

Stereotactic radiosurgery and its various derivations, such as fractionated stereotactic radiotherapy (fSRT), stereotactic body radiotherapy (SBRT), and stereotactic ablative body radiotherapy (SABR), are treatment techniques, which require precise localization of the patient and the target, combined with the ability to safely deliver large biologically effective radiation doses.[1] When Lars Leksell conceptualized radiosurgery, he saw a role for this new therapy to minimize the toxicity of traditional neurosurgical techniques of the day by causing "the non-invasive destruction of intracranial tissues that may be inaccessible or unsuitable for open surgery."[2] This definition has evolved and a modern consensus was formulated in 2007:

(a) Stereotactic radiosurgery is a distinct discipline that utilizes externally generated ionizing radiation in certain cases to inactivate or eradicate a defined target(s) in the head and spine without the need to make an incision. The target is defined by high-resolution stereotactic imaging. To assure quality of patient care the procedure involves a multidisciplinary team consisting of a neurosurgeon, radiation oncologist, and medical physicist.

(b) Stereotactic radiosurgery typically is performed in a single session, using a rigidly attached guiding device, or other immobilization technology and/or a stereotactic image-guidance system but can be performed in a limited number of sessions, up to a maximum of five.

(c) Technologies that are used to perform stereotactic radiosurgery include linear accelerators, particle beam accelerators, and multi source Cobalt 60 units. In order to enhance precision, various devices may incorporate robotics and real time imaging.

—AANS Position Statement[3]

Despite this comprehensive definition put forward, the role of stereotactic radiosurgery continues to evolve as the pace of clinical and technologic innovation increases. The first stereotactic radiosurgical procedure was the treatment of trigeminal neuralgia using an orthovoltage x-ray tube by Lars Leksell.[4] Many of the first patients to receive radiosurgery were similarly treated for nonmalignant purposes including trigeminal neuralgia, pituitary adenomas, and refractory pain (Fig. 19.1). In contrast, today, the majority of patients in the United States receiving intracranial radiosurgery are undergoing treatment for metastatic cancer to the brain (Fig. 19.1).[5]

The History and Development of the Stereotactic Method for Radiotherapy Delivery

In addition to increasing computational power and dose planning algorithms, technical advances have been made in two main areas: development and improvement of stereotactic localization, and transformation and specialization of known radiotherapy sources for radiosurgical applications. These two paths of development began very separately but have, over the last 50 years, been integrated into complete systems with incredible precision, accuracy, and efficacy for treating human disease.

The first devices for stereotactic localization were developed by Victor Horsley and Robert H. Clarke for the purpose of precisely localizing electrodes in the primate brain by relying on external fixation referenced to a coordinate systems in the early 1900s.[6,7] Expanding on this work, Ernest A. Spiegel and Henry T. Wycis developed a stereotactic localization device for use in humans in the 1940s.[8] By 1947, this headframe was being used to guide surgery on the thalamus and other deep brain structures in an effort to limit the toxicity by traditional, nonstereotactic approaches. It was clear by the 1950s that Speiegel's stereotactic localization device and others like it were allowing neurosurgeons to reduce the operative morbidity and mortality of traditional open approaches.[9] However, neurosurgeons of the day soon realized that any invasive approach had significant morbidity and mortality associated with it, and some began to search for a way to accomplish the same disease control rates while improving toxicity.

Lars Leksell, the father of stereotactic radiosurgery, began experimenting with a 250-kVp x-ray tube attached to a stereotactic headframe for the treatment of function brain disorders in the early 1950s.[10] The first patient was treated by Leksell in 1951 to the gasserian ganglion for trigeminal neuralgia.[10,11] Although his work showed promise, the application of this new treatment technique was limited by the poor dosimetry of such a low-energy beam.[10] Despite this limitation, the radical concept of inactivating or obliterating a target but not removing it would prove extremely provocative to many neurosurgeons of the time.

Leksell's desire was to develop a system that could be used by general neurosurgeons in a hospital operating room, similar to other surgical tools.[2] Although cross-fired protons were tried for a short time, they were dismissed due to difficulty of use in the clinic.[12,13] It was Kurt Liden, head of the Department of Radiation Physics at Lund University, who recommended a 10- to 20-MV photon source for future radiosurgery applications after performing a preliminary analysis of the physical possibilities. Although linear accelerators were briefly

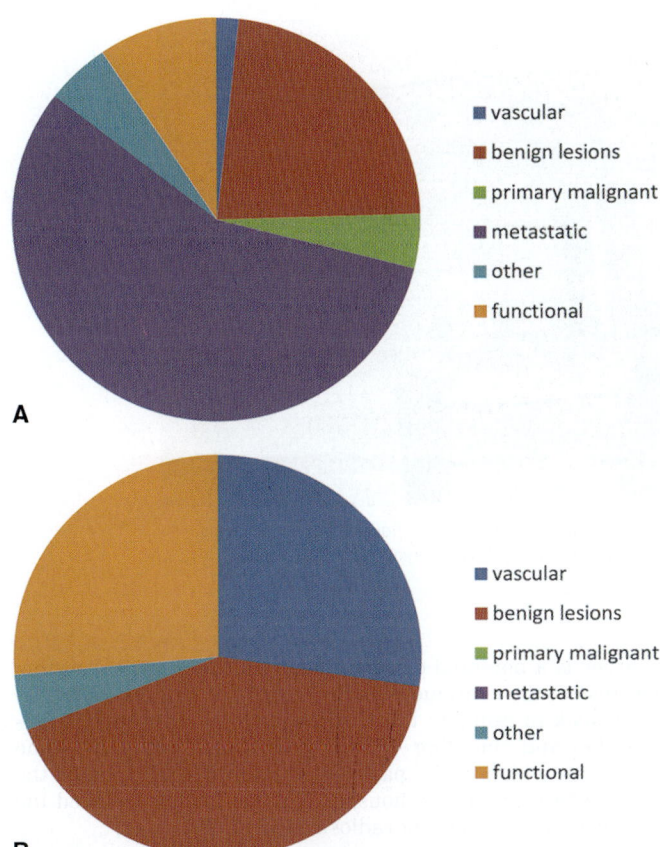

■ vascular
■ benign lesions
■ primary malignant
■ metastatic
■ other
■ functional

A

■ vascular
■ benign lesions
■ primary malignant
■ metastatic
■ other
■ functional

B

FIGURE 19.1. Indications for radiosurgery **(A)** in the RSSearch Registry from 2008 through 2013[5] and **(B)** at the Karolinska from 1968 through 1982.[2] (Reproduced from Leksell L. Stereotactic radiosurgery. *J Neurol Neurosurg Psychiatry*. 1983;46[9]:797–803, with permission from BMJ Publishing Group Ltd.)

TABLE 19.1 INDICATIONS FOR EXTRACRANIAL RADIOSURGERY FROM 2008 TO 2013 IN THE RSSEARCH REGISTRY

Indication	Number (%)
Lung/bronchus	1,973 (30.9)
Prostate	1,165 (18.3)
Pancreas	108 (1.7)
Liver	50 (0.8)
Metastatic site	1,722 (27)
Other	1,359 (21.3)

Davis JN, Medbery C 3rd, Sharma S, et al. The RSSearch Registry: patterns of care and outcomes research on patients treated with stereotactic radiosurgery and stereotactic body radiotherapy. *Radiat Oncol* 2013;8:275.

considered, because of the limited precision that was achievable at the time, ^{60}Co sources were ultimately chosen for this new surgical tool.[11]

Leksell's first "gamma unit" was built in 1967 and treated the first patient with ^{60}Co-based radiosurgery in November of 1967.[14] After improvements to the design were made, the second "gamma unit" was installed in 1974 at the Karolinska Hospital in Stockholm.[2] From 1968 to 1982, 762 patients were treated with radiosurgery using the "gamma unit." By the early 1980s, radiosurgery was offering an outstanding alternative to traditional surgery for many patients with small tumors. Dade Lunsford and others completed the installation of the first American Gamma Knife for clinical use (the fifth in the world) at the University of Pittsburgh in 1984.[15] This new gamma knife model U held 201 ^{60}Co sources, weighed 22 tons, and had many targeting improvements over earlier models.[15] There was increasing international interest in this new technique; however, many investigators began to look for alternatives to a cobalt-based system, which could be heavy and have high cost resulting in limited availability.

By the 1980s, great advances had been made in the precision of linear accelerators. Additionally, with the clinical availability of computed tomography (CT) and later magnetic resonance (MR), increasing target localization was now much easier. This combination of technical advantages increasingly made linear accelerator systems more attractive for radiosurgery.[16] Groups in Italy and Argentina independently developed and implemented linear accelerator–based systems in the early 1980s.[17,18] Many other groups quickly developed their own systems, but there was a lack of standardization across the field. This was addressed by Ken Winston and Wendell Lutz who described a radiosurgical system using a commercially available stereotactic frame in 1988,[19,20] resulting in

the increasing adoption of radiosurgery by confirming safety through a rigorous description of a proven quality assurance and testing process with commonly available technology. Shortly after publication of their techniques and others, linear accelerator–based radiosurgery began gaining acceptance as a reliable alternative to ^{60}Co-based techniques.[21]

With the gaining popularity of intracranial radiosurgery and the ability to deliver fractionated treatment with some linear accelerator–based systems, interest began moving toward delivering radiosurgery outside of the cranium. After spending a fellowship year with Lars Leksell in 1985, the neurosurgeon John Adler began to develop a method for delivering radiosurgery without a stereotactic frame at Stanford University.[16] The first patient was treated with the CyberKnife in 1994, as Adler's creation was named. This system used a 6-MV linear accelerator mounted on an industrial robot allowing a theoretically infinite number of beam angles for treatment of a target.[22] Other systems were being developed or modified to allow for extracranial radiosurgery at the same time. Hamilton and colleagues described the first spine radiosurgery system in 1995, the first truly extra cranial site treated with radiosurgery.[23]

Although the system described by Hamilton and colleagues was the first designed for extracranial treatments, it required the patient to be placed prone and a clamp to be placed on the spinous process.[16] There was increasing desire to develop a system that allowed for treatment of sites outside of the central nervous system. Ingmar Lax developed a mobilization frame that incorporated stereotactic fiducial markers, which allowed for targeting of thoracic and abdominal tumors using axial CT imaging. The device was subsequently commercially produced by Elekta.[11] This frame was quickly adopted as investigators such as Robert Timmerman began to use it for the treatment of early-stage lung tumors at Indiana University.[24] The indications for extracranial radiosurgery have continued to expand (Table 19.1).

MODERN TECHNOLOGIES FOR THE DELIVERY OF HIGHLY CONFORMAL RADIOTHERAPY

A multitude of modern systems exist, with new systems constantly under development, for the delivery of radiosurgery to both intracranial and extracranial targets. Although specifics may vary significantly, and each system has comparative advantages and disadvantages, the current systems can be grouped into similar types that have common guiding principles.

Gamma Knife
Common Principles for Gamma Knife Radiosurgery
The gamma knife's development has been closely tied with the evolution of the field of radiosurgery since its inception. In essence, any gamma knife facilitates the positioning of a target at the focal point of many ^{60}Co beams for the delivery

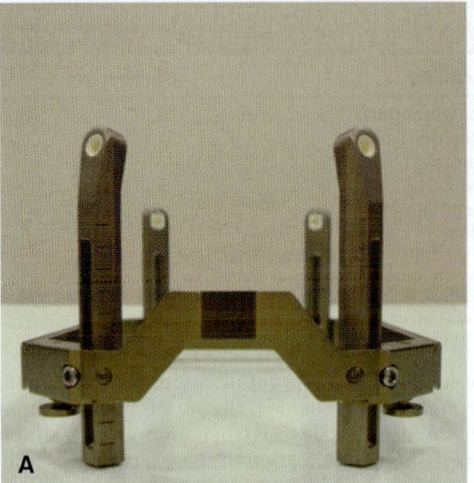
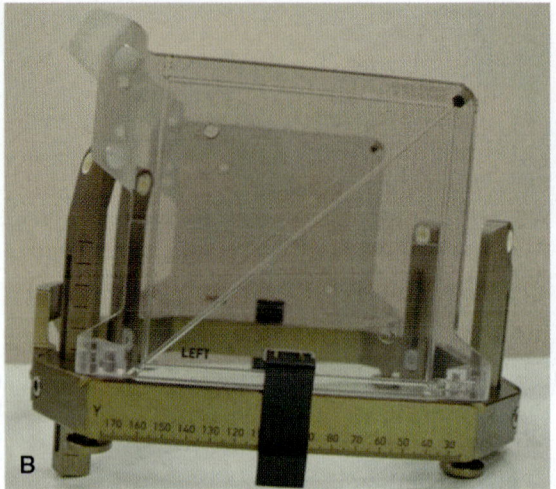

FIGURE 19.2. The Leksell headframe **(A)** and the Leksell headframe with an attached fiducial box for imaging **(B)**. (From Rojas-Villabona A, Miszkiel K, Kitchen N, et al. Evaluation of the stability of the stereotactic Leksell Frame G in Gamma Knife radiosurgery. *J Appl Clin Med Phys* 2016;17[3]:75–89.)

of high doses of radiation. This focal point is known as an isocenter.

The primary components of gamma knife treatment are precision and conformality of radiation delivery. This requires an accurate radiation field, immobilization of the region of interest, and reproducible localization. The stereotactic headframe developed by Lars Leksell[25] (Fig. 19.2) when appropriately attached to the head can immobilize patients with a high level of certainty.[26,27] This immobilization combined with high-quality axial imaging allows for reproducible localization using a three-dimensional coordinate system.

Once the target is localized and the patient is immobilized, both accurate and precise radiation delivery is essential. This is accomplished using collimated ^{60}Co sources in all gamma knife models. Depending on the model, 192 to 201 ^{60}Co sources are positioned around the head with an isocenter that is aligned with the target and then shifted to the next target after that portion of the treatment is complete. The accuracy and reproducibility of the alignment of the machine isocenter with the target is essential for successful radiosurgery. The use of small collimators combined with multiple beam angles results in a high-dose fall of at the 50% isodose line. This allows the treatment of targets to high doses while respecting the tolerance of the surrounding brain and critical structures. Much of the technical development and improvement of various gamma knife units has been related to the ability to better spare critical structures by creating more conformal isodose distributions surrounding the target, from selective blocking to now more sophisticated techniques.[28]

Gamma knife systems use ^{60}Co sources, which emit two photons, one with an energy of 1.17 MeV and one with an energy of 1.33 MeV. The resulting average energy of 1.25 MeV is relatively low when compared to modern day radiotherapy machines, and the dose rate is ultimately determined by the source activity, which degrades according to a half-life of 5.27 years.[29] The initial dose rate is around 3 Gy per minute[28] and decreases as the source continues to decay. This combined with the time required to move the patient into the correct position, change out collimators, and the use of a number of isocenters can result in long treatment times. Recent gamma knife systems have been able to minimize this by reducing the setup and patient positioning times despite using a similar source activity for radiotherapy.[28]

All gamma knife systems must conform to radiation safety principles and limit unnecessary dose both to other parts of the patient's body and to radiosurgery staff. Using radioactive sources is a potential disadvantage of a radiosurgical system because of the continuous radioactivity, but gamma knife systems seek to mitigate this disadvantage by appropriate collimation and shielding. Newer models also automate some functions, which in the past have required staff to enter the room where the unit is housed. This has further reduced the unnecessary exposure of radiosurgical staff.

Early Units

The first larger production gamma knife unit was branded as the Model U. There was also a similar model called the B model, which had a slightly different helmet shape and positioning. These units arranged 201 sources in a hemispheric array and later a circular configuration. In these early gamma knife units, a frame was affixed to the patient's head, a helmet with various collimators was placed on the frame, which was then attached to an adapter through a trunnion system or, later, an automatic positioning system, resulting in movement of the target to the focal point of the machine.

Gamma Knife Perfexion

The gamma knife Perfexion makes several key improvements over previous gamma knife units. Launched in 2006, it contains an array of 192 ^{60}Co sources arranged in a configuration differing from the previous hemispheric arrangement behind a solid tungsten collimator with multiple holes drilled directly into it (Fig. 19.3). As a result, no helmet is needed to attach the headframe and patient to the gamma knife. The patient positioning system uses the headframe attached to the motorized treatment couch, which moves the target into the planned treatment position.

This system has improvements in speed and isocenter reproducibility over previous gamma knife units.[28,30,31] A new method for collimator selection has been developed as well. The 14 mm and 18 mm collimators that existed in the previous models have been replaced with a 16 mm collimator. Beam collimation can be set to intermediate values by alternating selection of different size collimators. This is accomplished by moving the radiation sources between one of five positions by servo-motors (home position, 4 mm collimator, 8 mm collimator, 16 mm collimator, off position) (Fig. 19.3).[29] By generating a single isocenter made of different beam diameters, a composite shot is formed, and each isocenter can be planned to an optimized shape increasing dose conformality.[28] The ability to block sectors that contain beams passing through these volumes at risk has improved treatment conformity around critical structures.[31]

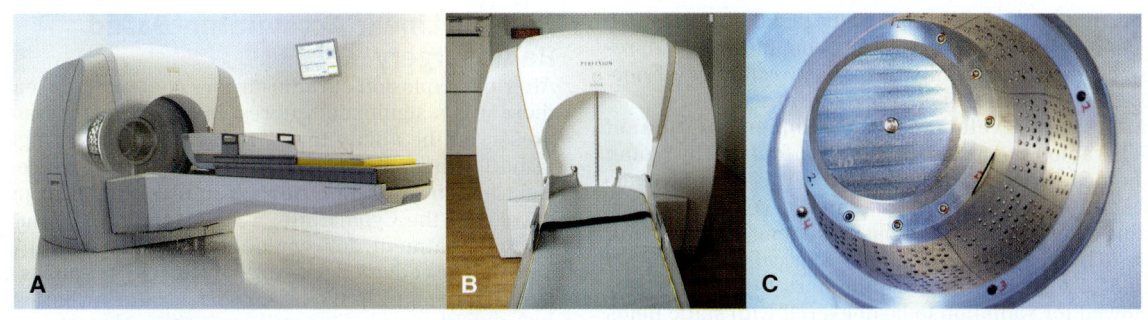

FIGURE 19.3. Leksell Gamma Knife® Perfexion™ unit with tungsten collimator shown from the side **(A)** and from the treatment couch with the shielded doors closed **(B)**. The tungsten collimator is shown removed from device **(C)**. (Reprinted with permission from Elekta AB, Stockholm, Sweden.)

Procedure of a Gamma Knife Treatment

The first step is application of the Leksell headframe to the patient's head. Before attachment, previous imaging should be reviewed to determine the optimal location for the headframe. The headframe should be attached with the target closest to the center of the frame as possible using one of several described techniques.[16] This can be difficult for the case of multiple brain metastases, especially with cerebellar metastases, but is made less critical by the improvements in newer models that allow for treatment in larger range of area. It is also essential to place the frame in a way that allows for the fiducial box to be firmly affixed.

After frame placement, stereotactic imaging must be performed in order to aid in target identification and delineation. The most common modern imaging modalities used with radiosurgery are CT, MR, and angiography. CT is often used with other methods because of the additional three-dimensional information when combined with angiography and because of the concern of image distortion with 1.5 and 3.0 T MR scanners. Although the reported variations are less than a millimeter in the center of the field, more peripheral lesions have been shown to have clinically significant distortion.[32] However, MR, especially with fine cut sequences, is the usually preferred imaging modality because of improved target delineation.

Following imaging, treatment planning occurs while the patient waits with the headframe intact. Many experienced physicians proceed with planning immediately, but target definition and identification of any at risk structures nearby are highly recommended. Often for difficult to define targets such as arteriovenous malformations, the input of a radiologist or other specialized personnel is needed. Once the target is defined, the planning process can occur.

After the final plan has been created, reviewed, and approved, the patient is brought into the treatment vault and docked to the machine. The therapists will then perform the quality assurance process to ensure collisions do not occur and that the plan will proceed with as few interruptions as possible. Following plan delivery, the stereotactic headframe is removed and the patient is discharged from the clinic.

Gantry-Mounted Linear Accelerator–Based Systems

Common Principles for Radiosurgery with Gantry-Mounted Systems

Linear accelerator systems use multiple beam entry points to sufficiently spread out the dose in a way that geometrically sums to a high dose with as rapid dose falloff as possible. With linear accelerator–based radiosurgery, 4 to 5 rotational arcs are chosen based on the target location. The gantry will rotate through an entire arc, the couch will rotate to a new plane, and another arc will be delivered by a gantry rotation. These arcs can be circular collimators, shaped conformal collimators with or without microleaf collimators, or even intensity-modulated fields.[11]

As frameless systems continue to develop, these systems now have precision approaching traditional frame-based approaches.[33,34] One of the major advantages of a gantry-based system is the availability of onboard imaging for localization and monitoring of both intrafraction and interfraction movement. Various systems exist using orthogonal kV radiographs, cone beam CT, electromagnetic transponders, infrared markers, or skin contours. Each of these imaging options are combined with immobilization techniques to ensure treatment accuracy. A very common immobilization approach is a custom thermoplastic mask with a stiffness intended for radiosurgery applications. Sometimes, a bite block to further immobilize the skull is used.

An advantage of omitting an invasive headframe is the ability to deliver fractionated radiosurgery treatments. Although there is significant controversy regarding fractionation of intracranial radiosurgery, there seems to be a clinical benefit for large lesions that may be difficult to control with doses that can be safely delivered in a single fraction such as brain metastases.[35] Fractionation combined with the open nature of linear accelerators also allows for the delivery of high biologic effective doses to extra cranial targets such as lung tumors.[24]

Development of Modern Linear Accelerator–Based Systems

One of the first linear accelerator systems developed was reported by Oswaldo Betti and colleagues in 1984.[18] A 10-MV photon linear accelerator was used with a secondary collimator system with circular inserts ranging from 6 to 25 mm. The patient was seated in a chair while attached to a rotating headframe. Working separately and at the same time Frederico Columbo and colleagues reported their technique using a modified 4-MV photon linear accelerator using multiple converging arcs.[17]

The first reports of linear accelerator–based radiosurgery were soon followed by an explosion of different solutions for delivering intracranial radiosurgery using a modified linear accelerator. Some degree of standardization was introduced when Winston and Lutz described a radiosurgical system using a 6-MV linear accelerator equipped with a special collimator. A Brown-Roberts-Wells (BRW) stereotactic headframe was affixed to the patient and photon beam arcs were used in four positions. Although this system was able to deliver very conformal treatment plans, the most significant advance was a system of extensive testing and quality assurance, which later became standard for many clinics.[19]

With the increasing accuracy in many systems, it soon became clear that circular collimators originally designed for small regular shaped targets were severely limited when larger or grossly irregular targets were treated. To address this, Dennis Leavitt first described a method of dynamic field shaping for arc-based radiosurgery. A circular collimator was chosen for a target lesion and four independent vanes were used to trim the circular field to a trapezoidal shape, which was more conformal to the target projection in that arc increment. This resulted in an ability to reduce irradiation of normal brain tissue surrounding an irregular target.[36]

Soon after the development and implementation of dynamic field radiosurgery, a new company, founded by Stefan Vilsmeier named Brainlab, partnered with Varian to produce small micromultileaf collimator system that could be added on to existing linear accelerator–based systems or used with the purpose to build 6-MV linear accelerator called Novalis.[11,37] The addition of micromultileaf collimators to radiosurgery systems allowed for radiation to be delivered with static fields or dynamic arcs. These principles would later be expanded to allow for intensity modulation during radiosurgery treatment deliver, leading to even more conformal treatment plans for linear accelerator–based radiosurgery.[38]

Procedure of Linear Accelerator–Based Radiosurgery

The procedure of radiosurgery starts with imaging to identify a target. This usually occurs with MR imaging, angiography, or CT imaging. This imaging, regardless of modality, will need to be coregistered to images taken at the time of CT simulation for most systems.

After CT simulation and target localization imaging are coregistered, segmentation of targets and at risk structures occurs. The quality of coregistration should always be checked before beginning this process as it is a common source of error in radiosurgical planning. Once target structures and organs at risk are identified, the treatment planning processes begins. This process can take several hours.

Following the creation and approval of a treatment plan, a quality assurance process ensuring the "tightness" of the isocenter is usually performed. After that the patient returns to the clinic and is placed in the treatment position on the couch with the head immobilized. Once the patient is determined to be in the appropriate position, the treatment is delivered. Following treatment delivery, the patient is discharged from the clinic.

Robotic Linear Accelerator–Based Radiosurgery

After the explosion of radiosurgery centers in the early 1990s, there was a significant interest in developing a system, which preserved the ability to deliver very conformal high doses of radiation but allowed patients to avoid the placement of a rigid headframe. John Adler a neurosurgeon from Stanford developed the CyberKnife, a radiosurgical system that integrated treatment delivery and localization in an innovative way.[22,39] The radiation delivered by the CyberKnife is generated by a lightweight 6-MV linear accelerator, which is mounted on a robotic arm with 6 degrees of freedom. The robotic arm moves the linear accelerator in three-dimensional space to any of 100 nodes for delivery of radiation beam resulting in an extremely conformal dose distribution. At those nodes, the radiation beam is collimated in several ways. A traditional cone-based secondary collimator can be used (12 cones are included with sizes from 5 to 60 mm). Additionally, an iris-based collimator is included in the linear accelerator to reduce the treatment time attributed to cone switching. Newer models offer the option of a true multileaf collimator that can increase the ability to collimate the beam and higher dose rates to help decrease treatment times.

Traditional gantry-mounted linear accelerator–based radiosurgical systems and the gamma knife deliver radiation to a fixed isocenter usually in a spherical pattern. This is extremely effective for simple spherical targets, but different approaches must be used for more complex target shapes. The CyberKnife allows for isocentric and nonisocentric treatment modes to help improve the conformity and dose delivery to these targets (Fig. 19.4).[40]

The CyberKnife has two primary onboard imaging systems. Orthogonal kV x-ray tubes are used with a real-time, flat panel amorphous silicon digital x-ray imager.[41,42] This system establishes initial patient position and ensures tracking of intrafraction movement by comparing the images captured at the time of treatment with previously generated digitally reconstructed radiographs. When small movement of the

FIGURE 19.4.   A: With standard radiosurgery-dispersed isocentric beams, all beams intersect a common region. Because multiple spherical volumes are needed to cover irregular lesions, the resulting dose distributions tend to be inhomogeneous. **B:** Nonisocentric beams from various directions. Beams do not all cross in a single point; therefore, dose distributions tend to be less inhomogeneous than in **A**.

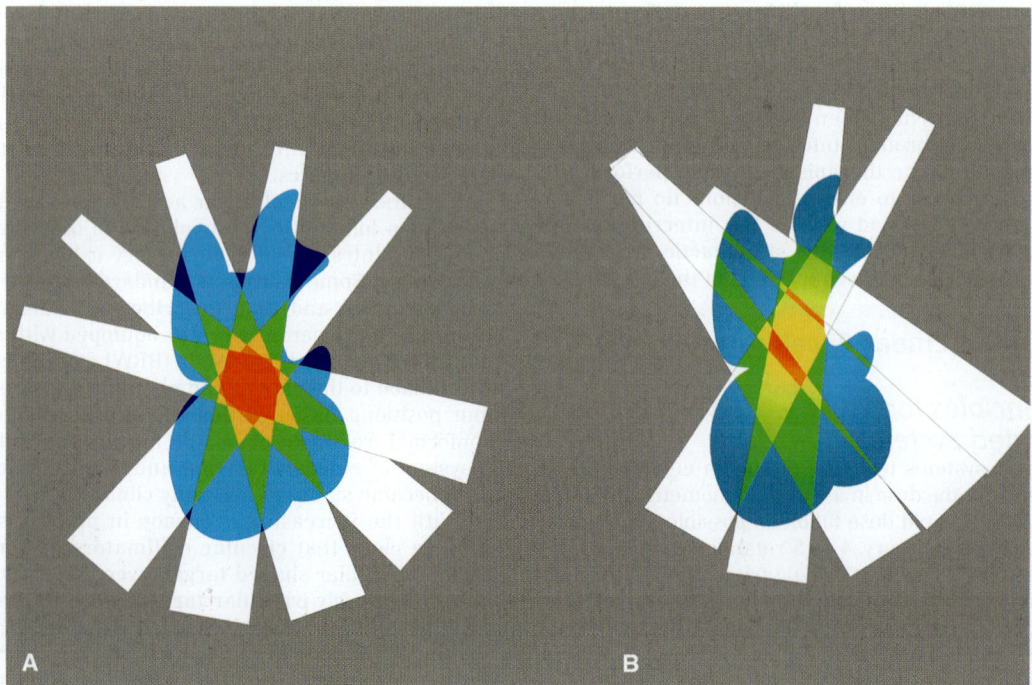

target is detected, the robotic arm can adjust the position of the linear accelerator to a new position in order to reduce inaccuracy by compensating for the movement. The second imaging system uses infrared markers to track patient chest wall movement caused by respiration and is called Synchrony. This system starts by constructing a model predicting the location of the tumor in real time based on chest wall movement with respiration correlated to x-ray verification of target at eight different points in the respiratory cycle.[43]

TREATMENT PLANNING FOR RADIOSURGERY

Target Delineation and Dose Selection for Radiosurgery

Target Delineation for Intracranial Radiosurgery

Target delineation and the segmentation of organs at risk are an essential part of modern planning for traditional fractionated external beam radiotherapy. By identifying both targets and avoidance structures, beam angles can be selected, and dose tolerances can be evaluated for conformal radiotherapy plans. For intensity-modulated radiotherapy and other techniques, which utilize an inverse planning method, segmentation of these structures is required for planning.

The original radiosurgery techniques were developed by neurosurgeons in collaboration with medical physicists,[11] and it can be helpful to conceptualize the treatment planning process including target delineation for radiosurgery as a surgeon would think of any other minimally invasive surgical technique. The concepts of gross tumor volume (GTV), clinical target volume (CTV), and planning target volume are interpreted somewhat differently in radiosurgery than in traditional fractionated external beam radiotherapy. Typically, a tumor is contoured as target, and for well-defined tumors, no expansion is made for subclinical tumor spread.[44]

Intracranial radiosurgery has always made the assumption that targets retained a fixed position in relation to skull anatomy. Systems using this principle have continued to be refined, so now, errors are typically on the order of 1 to 2 mm.[45] This is further improved to submillimeter accuracy with kV imaging and a robotic couch[33] or with a rigid headframe.[26] Therefore, intrafraction motion management has primarily been accomplished by either attaching a fixed rigid headframe to the skull or by imaging the bony structures of the head. Many physicians do not place a margin for motion on intracranial targets in an attempt to lower the risk of subsequent toxicity by making the target as small as possible and allowing dose falloff to account for slight variations in patient positioning. Still others have included a margin on some targets including brain metastases in an attempt to improve local control by ensuring all of the lesion is included in a high-dose region.[46]

Target Delineation for Extracranial Radiosurgery

The concept of delivering ablative doses to areas outside of the cranium is a relatively new one and its implementation is often more technically difficult. Unlike for intracranial radiosurgery, there is rarely an opportunity to use rigid fixation for extracranial body sites. As a result of high-dose gradients next to radiosensitive structures and large doses required to ablate target lesions, fractionation is often employed when treating patients with Stereotactic Ablative Body Radiotherapy (SABR).

Target delineation varies significantly by body site for SABR. Gross tumor is of course contoured on simulation scans. For most body sites, a CTV is not added. It is instead assumed that dose falloff from the prescription isodose line will cover the areas of microscopic disease spread.[47] Although margin is not typically added for subclinical tumor spread, motion must be accounted for in the process. This is accomplished by the addition of an internal target volume (ITV). These can be relatively small for sites such as prostate, but very large for other sites such as lower lobe of the lung. The effect of motion can be reduced or eliminated by using techniques such as gaiting; however, assuming these techniques are not used, most physicians will segment the tumor on multiple phases of a four-dimensional CT scan and combine contours to make an ITV.

Because the majority of body radiosurgery is fractionated, unlike single-fraction intracranial radiosurgery, most physicians will add an additional margin on the GTV or ITV to account for setup uncertainty. This is especially true when time passes from simulation for body sites that do not allow for rigid fixation where targets or organs at risk may have moved or changed in size. Treatments can take course over three to five fractions, which may be delivered over 10 days or longer. Expansions therefore should be as small as possible to minimize the normal tissue exposed to ablative doses of radiation therapy while covering setup uncertainties that would lead to underdosing the target.[44] Ideally, these expansions would be based on measured uncertainties specific to the individual radiosurgery system, technique, and clinic where the radiosurgery is being delivered.

Prescribing Doses for Radiosurgery

There is a clear and convincing dose–response and dose–toxicity relationship for radiosurgery.[48,49] This fact underlines the importance of dose selection when planning radiosurgery. In early cases, radiosurgery was used for functional neurosurgery, and there was often no predefined lesion to target.[50-52] Furthermore, because of the limited number and type of systems designed to deliver radiosurgery, dose was commonly described as a single maximum dose because doses were prescribed to the isocenter with the dose distributions commonly known in the community.[4] As treatment systems continued to evolve and multiply in both number and complexity, it was apparent that describing dose to the isocenter was not sufficient for reporting radiosurgery procedures. Other dose statistics were soon adopted as it became clear that some, such as peripheral lesion dose, mattered as much or more than maximum dose.[53]

Traditionally, the peripheral isodose is normalized to value that corresponds with the steepest portion of the dose curve. This is typically around the 80% isodose line for one isocenter plans[4] but can range between 90% and 40%.[54] With multiple isocenter, lower prescription isodose lines are used, resulting in higher maximum doses. Because of the heterogeneity, conformality of dose is a significantly more important metric than it is for traditional fractionated radiotherapy.

It is also important to note that body sites often have large tissue inhomogeneity adjacent to the target. Heterogeneity corrections can therefore have significant effect on the calculated dose and generally should be used when treating body sites with body radiosurgery. Furthermore, when referencing doses used in clinical trials from the literature, great care must be taken to determined whether heterogeneity calculations were employed or not, for example, the original Indiana University lung SBRT data.[24]

This is not to say that common dose prescriptions do not exist for radiosurgery; many of the doses used in the modern era are based on clinic outcome data painstakingly collected over the last several decades. These dosing guidelines however can be somewhat complicated and difficult to interpret. For example, the Radiation Therapy Oncology Group performed a phase I dose escalation trial to determine the maximum tolerated dose for single-fraction radiosurgery in patients with recurrent brain tumors.[55] This trial described peripheral dose for brain tumors by lesion size; targets 20 mm or less received 24 Gy as a maximal tolerated dose, targets between 21 and 30 mm received 18 Gy, and targets between 31 and 40 mm received 15 Gy. As discussed earlier, however, the prescription isodose line was left up to the discretion of the treating physician, so resulting maximum doses did differ even within set dose arms. Given that dose and control of brain metastases are tightly correlated with radiosurgery,[35] today, larger lesions are treated with fractionated radiosurgery at many institutions.[56]

Developing the Treatment Plan
Common Principles of Treatment Planning

The single isocenter technique was the first used for stereotactic radiosurgery. Originally used on the gamma knife platform, this technique involves the geometric summation of multiple beams in a small "focal point" at the isocenter of the machine. This can also be accomplished on gantry-mounted linear accelerator systems using multiple rotating arcs with circular collimators, producing a sphere of high dose with extremely quick dose falloff outside of the isocenter. The size of the sphere is determined by the diameter of the collimators used for the individual beams; larger collimator sizes result in larger high-dose spheres. These spherical dose distributions are often viewed in a cross-sectional axial plane and appear as circles. Therefore, the single isocenter technique is ideal for small spherical targets for which conformality and equal dose falloff are desired for planning. Treatment systems, which have multileaf collimators, are able to add additional conformality to single isocenter techniques by collimating the beam using either conformal collimation or intensity modulation.

For irregular targets, the single isocenter approach without multileaf collimators requires a much larger dose sphere than would normally be necessary to provide adequate target coverage. Therefore, these cases are usually planned out using different techniques. One such technique is known as sphere packing.[57] Sphere packing provides more conformal dose coverage of an irregular target by using multiple single isocenter techniques to pack the target with spherical dose (Fig. 19.5). Typically, the largest diameter sphere that will fit within a target is chosen first. Additional smaller isocenters are added, and the dose is summed over the entire target to produce the final dose distribution. Gamma knife uses the Leksell GammaPlan software for planning radiosurgery. A sphere-packing plan can be created either by contouring the target and using an inverse dose planning algorithm, which can be manually adjusted at the end of the process, or by a completely manual process. The gamma knife Perfexion allows for several newer treatment planning modes including an automatic dynamic shaping ability to shape the dose in a way to protect structures contoured as avoidance structures. Also, beam shape can be changed as the system now allows for single isocenters composed of different collimated beam diameters including completely blocked.

Although linear accelerators are capable of a single isocenter dose distribution as described above, using multiple rotational arcs with cone-based collimators, several other isocentric techniques can be used for irregularly shaped or large targets using linear accelerators using either fixed or rotational fields. For simple targets, fixed noncoplanar fields with multileaf collimators can be used for a deliver that is analogous to 3D conformal radiotherapy. Each field is shaped to a conformal beam's eye view of the target, and with sufficient beams, plans can be adequate for treatment delivery. Conformality can be an issue with this technique[58]; however, using intensity-modulated radiotherapy methods can significantly increase the conformality. Rotational techniques include combining the dosimetric advantages of arc-based therapy with the increased conformity of multileaf collimator techniques by using dynamic conformal arcs and volume-modulated arc therapy, which additionally uses intensity-modulated radiotherapy. These can produce plans with similar conformality as traditional ^{60}Co-based multisource techniques but at the cost of low-dose spillage.[59,60]

Irregular targets can also be conformally treated using nonisocentric techniques. Used primarily by the CyberKnife robotic radiosurgery system but also by other linear accelerator based systems, this technique uses narrow beams from multiple noncoplanar directions to cover the target (Fig. 19.4). Because the beams do not cross in a single point, the dose does not become heterogenous, which can occur with other techniques such as sphere packing. This approach allows for a virtually limitless number of beam positions and can produce very conformal homogenous dose distributions over irregular targets. This further allows for specific shaping of where the hot spot occurs.[61] Given the complexity and sheer number of iterations that exist using nonisocentric techniques, inverse planning is nearly always used. The CyberKnife uses the multiplan software for treatment planning. Although over 300 possible linear accelerator positions are possible, most CyberKnife plans choose between 110 nodes arranged in a hemisphere surrounding the target.[16] For isocentric plans, the linear accelerator is pointed toward the isocenter at each node position; however, for nonisocentric plans, there are 12 discrete pointing directions at each node called vectors. The treatment plan is formed from a combination of different nodes and vectors and by weighting each of the resulting beams accordingly. By designating the treatment site, the system selects a group of nodes, which is ideally used to treat that body site called paths.[16] Different collimator sizes can be used for each beam,[62] and in addition to traditional circular collimators, the CyberKnife has a variable collimator that can change the aperture size between 5 and 60 mm. After contouring, a sequential optimization algorithm is commonly employed, which performs a series of individual optimization steps in a defined order.[63]

Extracranial radiosurgery treatment planning is similar to that used for intracranial targets with several key differences. Although conformality is extremely important for both intracranial and extracranial radiosurgery, extracranial targets can often be positioned next to sensitive structures in one direction with considerable distance to sensitive structures in other directions. In this case, avoidance of dose-limiting structures is

FIGURE 19.5. With an irregularly shaped target, the process of adding shots to construct a multi-isocenter treatment is shown. Panels **A** through **C** demonstrate the reduced heterogeneity and increasing coverage with the addition of more shots.

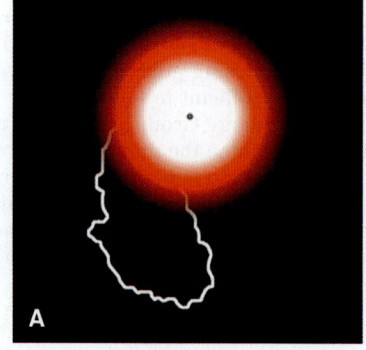
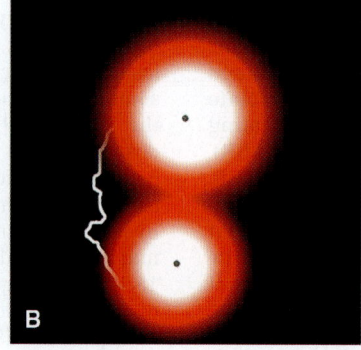
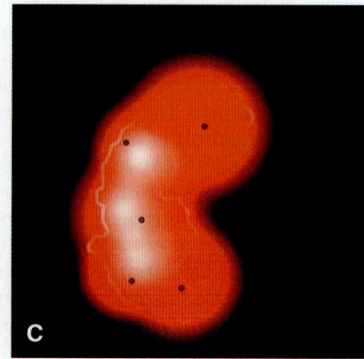

prioritized above strict uniform conformality. Geometry of the patient, couch, and treatment machine much more frequently come into play with the multiple beams or multiple dynamic arcs that are used for the majority of extracranial radiosurgery. Care must be taken to avoid choosing beam angles or positions, which are not deliverable in the actual patient without causing a collision. Finally, although intracranial targets are rarely deep enough to prompt the selection of high-energy beams, body sites sometimes lead themselves toward treatment with higher-energy beams for better dosimetry at depth. This should be avoided in radiosurgery given neutron contamination and increasing penumbra size with higher-energy photon beams.

Dose calculation was originally performed for the gamma knife system using a standard beam profile combined with the inverse square law and the linear attenuation of the beam. By summing all beams at the focal point, a dose calculation can be completed.[57,64] A similar approach can be used for arc-based linear accelerator radiosurgery. Individual arcs can be estimated as individual beams, calculated, and then summed for the total contribution of a specific arc. The density of the medium for intracranial radiosurgery is usually assumed to be that of water, and heterogeneity corrections are not typically employed where the magnitude of error from not taking in to account the skull is generally <1%.[16] Even older dose calculation algorithms appear to be sufficient.[65] For extracranial targets, differences can be more pronounced, even >10% depending on what algorithm is used for dose calculation.[66] Older algorithms can overestimate dose in low-density tissues.[67] These differences can have clinically significant effects and can vary depending on beam energy, technique, and geometric position of beams. Today, the Monte Carlo algorithm is being increasingly used for dose calculation, especially for extracranial radiosurgery as computing power becomes more available in reducing the computational time needed for this extremely accurate dose calculation method.[68,69]

Radiosurgery Plan Evaluation

Once the plan has been created, it must be reviewed by the radiosurgery team before delivery. Confirmation of the dose prescription should be followed by a visual inspection of the isodose lines of the plan on the target imaging. Coverage of the target should be confirmed. The isodose lines should be visualized in the axial, coronal, and sagittal plane through all slices in and surrounding the target. Careful attention should be paid to the relationship of these isodose lines to the target and other critical structures surrounding. Following visual inspection of the plan in the treatment planning system, a dose–volume histogram should be generated and reviewed. The dose–volume histogram is a way to convey three-dimensional information in two dimensions by plotting target and avoidance structure volume against dose received. Doses and volumes can be either relative to the total or absolute. Both these methods for plotting the dose–volume histogram can be useful in evaluating a radiosurgery plan. This can be used to determine target coverage, ensure any hot or cold spots are within plan tolerances, and determine volumetric doses to avoidance structures. It is important to note, however, that a limitation of the dose–volume histogram is that it does not provide spatial information for where these things occur in the plan, for that the actual isodose lines are needed. A sample radiosurgery plan is shown in Figure 19.6.

In addition to visually inspecting the isodose plot and the dose–volume histogram, a number of additional parameters are available to determine the quality of a given radiosurgical plan. It is important to remember, however, that in actual patient's plans, it will often not be able to meet all dose parameters and often compromises will have to be made. It is the role of an experience radiosurgical team to determine when and how these compromises are made in order to best serve the patient.

The most basic parameter is coverage. Coverage is a measure of what isodose line completely encompasses the target. Generally, it is desirable to have 90% of the prescription isodose line encompass the target whenever possible.[1] Another parameter of radiosurgical plans is the homogeneity index. This index measures how high the maximum dose is compared to the prescription for a given plan and is calculated by dividing the global maximum dose by the prescription isodose line. Ideally, the homogeneity index is <2.0 (or another way to think of this is that the prescription isodose line is normalized to 50% or higher).[1] The conformity index is used to measure the conformality of the dose distribution. This is calculated by dividing the prescription isodose volume by the target volume. Ideally, this will range from 1.0 to 2.0.[1] Other dose indices have been reported,[30,70–72] but are not commonly used outside of specific clinical scenarios.

FIGURE 19.6. A radiosurgery plan for delivery using the CyberKnife robotic linear accelerator to an acoustic neuroma. Shown in *left panel* are the isodose curves for the 12-Gy prescription normalized to 81% and delivered using a nonisocentric technique. In *right panel*, a dose–volume histogram is shown.

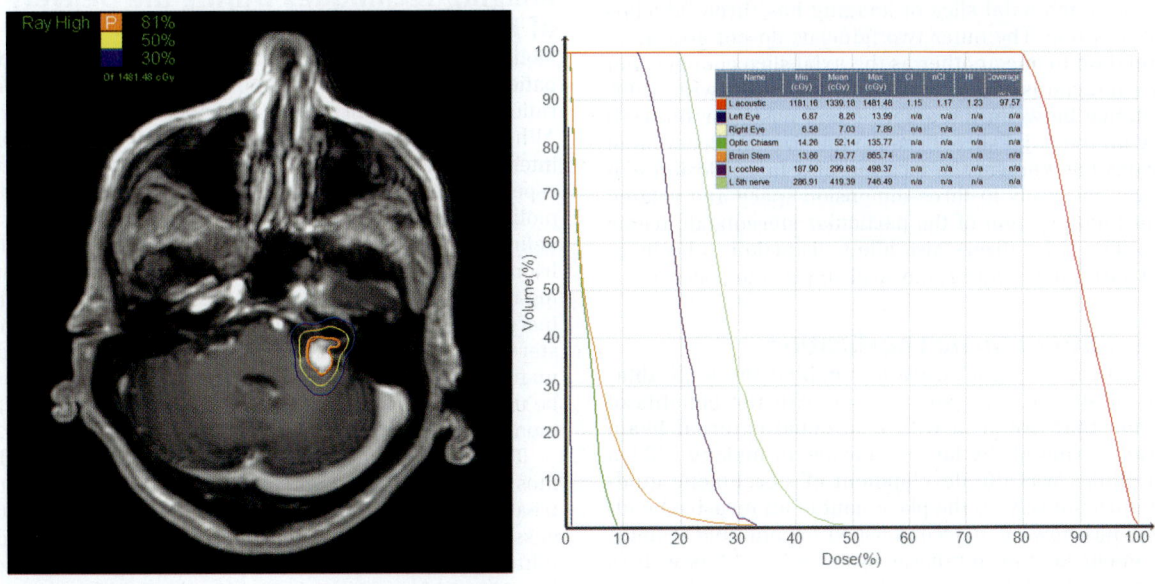

LOCALIZATION AND MOTION MANAGEMENT TECHNOLOGIES

Localization of target lesions is of the upmost importance for stereotactic radiosurgery. Regardless of how precisely and conformally the radiation can be delivered, if it is delivered to the wrong location, the patient can suffer significant harm. In fact, mechanical accuracy of modern radiosurgical systems is submillimeter making imaging the largest source of radiosurgery error.[42,64,73] Devices for stereotactic localization of targets in the brain have been in use since the early 1900s for research purposes[7] and since the 1940s for therapeutic use.[8] Today, the tools for stereotactic localization continue to evolve, but the general goal remains the same as when the first devices were designed and implemented. Any system used for stereotactic localization in radiosurgery must use a reproducible system for knowing the precise location of objects in three-dimensional space from the time of lesion localization through the delivery of treatment using one of several methods.[74]

Stereotactic Localization with a Rigid Headframe

Stereotactic localization for the gamma knife has historically been based on the use of a rigid headframe, which was developed by Lars Leksell[25] (Fig. 19.2). The Leksell stereotactic headframe is attached to the skull with four pins, which provide relatively fixed position throughout the treatment planning and delivery process, with submillimeter immobilization.[26,27] The frame has a three coordinate positioning system comprised of an x, y, and z-axis. The y-axis runs from posterior to anterior, the x-axis runs from side to side, and the z-axis runs superior to inferior. By convention, zero for each of the planes is placed right, posterior and superior. A frame cap is used for the Perfexion model to ensure no collisions will occur with the patient or the headframe once affixed. Other headframes exist for use with the linear accelerator–based radiosurgery. The BRW system was developed at the University of Utah in 1977.[75] This was later improved by Wells and Cosman as the Cosman-Roberts-Wells (CRW) frame by simplifying the design. Other frame systems exist for radiosurgery including some that allow for fractionated stereotactic radiosurgery such as the TALON system.[76]

Many systems that use rigid headframes for patient immobilization and stereotactic localization make use of an "N-localizer."[77] This is an essential piece of equipment for these systems, which allows for imaging to be performed with the headframe in place and fiducial markers to be present in that imaging. Each axial slice of imaging has three fiducials visualized in a line. The outer two fiducials do not appear to move in relation to one another as the axial slice changes, but the middle fiducial is always in a different place (with a different distance between the anterior and posterior fiducial) depending on the axial slice. Because the size and location of the N-localizer is known, the location of a target lesion can be measured precisely in three-dimension space and related to the coordinate system of the particular stereotactic frame (Fig. 19.2). The N-localizers also allow distortion to be measured and corrected before radiosurgical planning occurs.

Frameless Stereotactic Localization

There has always been a desire to combine the high ablative doses of stereotactic radiosurgery with the benefits of fractionation that are seen with traditional external beam radiotherapy.[78] One of the largest hurdles to making fSRT a reality in clinics was the development of stereotactic guidance that does not rely on the placement of an invasive headframe. This has now been accomplished for multiple systems including linear accelerator–based systems[22,34,39,79,80] as well as ^{60}Co systems.[81,82] In addition to the benefits of reduced patient discomfort, better workflow, and less procedural time, this development finally allowed for multiple radiosurgery treatment to be given to the same target lesion in a patient on different days without the need for repeat headframe placement.

Intracranial Sites

Image-guided radiosurgery without a stereotactic frame for intracranial targets relies on concept of a fixed position of intracranial lesions with the skull anatomy. Therefore, it is the bony anatomy of the skull that is of primary importance. Cone beam CT can be used to accurately position the patient, as can infrared light–emitting diods,[83,84] but the advent of dedicated radiosurgical systems such as the CyberKnife and Novalis allows for a quicker method.[85,86] Computed tomography scans with fine cuts taken at simulation time are reconstructed into a digitally reconstructed radiograph. This digitally reconstructed radiograph is then used as a reference for orthogonal kV x-rays taken before treatment. By comparing the orthogonal kV x-rays, which are taken from a fixed position in the room, a stereotactic coordinate system is formed.[58,87] The patient can therefore be shifted to the desired position, and the treatment can proceed. This method has been demonstrated to be extremely accurate, with average setup errors <1 mm.[34,42,58,87] When a frame is not used for stereotactic localization, a thermoplastic mask or other immobilization device is typically used to limit patient movement after correct positioning and during the delivery of radiotherapy. This technique has shown to be extremely effective for limiting motion during treatment.[88]

Extracranial Sites

For radiosurgery outside of the skull, there are several approaches that can provide stereotactic guidance information. The traditional technique is to implant radiopaque fiducial markers. These markers, which are present at the time of simulation, can be used to compare orthogonal kV images at the time of treatment with the original planning images much in the same way that kV imaging is compared to digitally reconstructed radiographs of the skull for the creating of stereotactic space.[41,89] For extracranial sites near the spine, some radiosurgery systems have specific techniques that can be used to improve accuracy and allow for the delivery of radiosurgery without the implantation of fiducial markers.[90] The CyberKnife Xsight system uses deformable modeling of bony spinal anatomy with a hierarchical mesh tracking system to create the stereotactic information needed to localize a target lesion in three-dimensional space.[41,91]

Imaging Techniques During the Delivery of Radiosurgery

Motion does not cease after initial stereotactic localization. Both patient motion and internal motion (from the heart beat, respiration, and bowel peristalsis) contribute to intrafraction motion. Although patient motion can be limited with immobilization, internal motion can significantly contribute to the target motion, especially respiration.[92] Targeting is further complicated as this motion is often irregular[93] and is overestimated using imaging defined at respiratory extremes.[94] With increasing adoption of frameless techniques and proportion of extracranial sites making up delivered radiosurgery cases every year, there has been increasing interest in extending the concept of image-guided stereotactic localization to intrafraction imaging and motion management. Several of the methods previously discussed can be used to establish stereotactic guidance for radiosurgery and monitor movement during the delivery of radiosurgery.

Techniques using orthogonal kV imaging are perhaps the most commonly used way to monitor patient motion during treatment. This approach used technology previously discussed for stereotactic localization but will continue intermittent assessment during the delivery of radiosurgery. The frequency of assessment can be changed by the therapists during treatment delivery, so less frequent imaging can be used if minor corrections are being made or the frequency can be increased if more motion is observed. In addition to orthogonal kV imaging, some systems make use of an infrared bite block for intracranial stereotactic radiosurgery.[79,80,83,95] These systems can track motion using an optical camera focused on several optical tracking spheres fixed to a bite block inserted into the mouth, much in a similar way to optical guidance for invasive otolaryngology and neurosurgery procedures. Benefits to these systems include more frequent position determination and no need to use ionizing radiation to determine position.

The ideal system for intrafraction motion management provides near instantaneous location information constantly without the need to use ionizing radiation. In an effort to meet these goals, the Calypso system has been used to monitor motion during radiosurgical treatment.[96,97] Calypso uses an electromagnetic transponder fiducial implanted in or near the target that is monitored by an electromagnetic detector. The detector's position is monitored by optical cameras tracking infrared fiducials placed on the detector to discern its position in the room. This allows for the benefits of near real-time continuous tracking without using ionizing radiation but requires an invasive procedure for implantation. Furthermore, although various sites are undergoing active investigation, electromagnetic transponder–guided radiosurgery is not available for many of the common body sites treated with radiosurgery.

Perhaps the greatest contribution to intrafraction motion during radiosurgery procedures when appropriate immobilization devices are used is respiration. One of the first systems clinically used for this purpose relied on kV imaging connected to the linear accelerator that would image up to 30 times a second and shut the beam off when fiducial markers placed in the tumor were outside a predefined volume.[98] Therefore, the beam is delivered in a "gated" manner, only during specific phases of the respiratory cycle. Similar systems can be combined with infrared monitoring of the chest wall as a surrogate marker for respiratory tumor movement.[42,99] These systems use infrared light–emitting diodes or passive markers. Some systems are able to take this tumor tracking data and update a dynamic model to continuously deliver a radiosurgery treatment. The CyberKnife has the ability to track respiratory movement using the Synchrony system. This system creates a model from kV imaging taken at the time of treatment combined with chest wall movement seen using infrared makers and then uses external infrared imaging to allow the linear accelerator to target different positions in the lung automatically within a specific tolerance. The model is continuously updated with information from the kV imaging, which can verify the internal position.

THE FUTURE OF RADIOSURGERY IS BRIGHT

Advances in radiosurgery over the last 60 years have been astounding. Many conditions that were unable to be treated using standard surgical techniques because of size or location are now common in radiosurgery programs across the world. Designers continue to innovate, constantly improving machine tolerances and quality of delivered treatment. These new and improved technologic systems allow for investigators to continue pushing the limits for what is able to be accomplished.

Advances will continue to be made in localization and tracking of the target. It is likely that methods not involving ionizing radiation for localization will continue to grow in popularity, especially those that can provide multiple verifications per second and help form predictive models for motion. By decreasing treatment times as a result of more "beam-on" time, and potentially limiting toxicity by reducing margin for uncertainty, the patient's experience will continue to improve.

As systemic therapies continue to improve survival for a patient with metastatic disease and radiosurgical systems become easier to use by traditional radiation oncology clinics, it is likely that the number of patients receiving radiosurgery will increase. Hopefully as the numbers of patients receiving radiosurgery increase, it will only serve to spark innovation and development. The future of radiosurgery is bright. Many of the advances that are now essential to the field could not even be conceptualized by Leksell when he first described the technique. Hopefully, similar gains will be made within the next 60 years, thereby increasing our ability as physicians to care for our patients.

REFERENCES

1. Shaw E, Kline R, Gillin M, et al. Radiation Therapy Oncology Group: radiosurgery quality assurance guidelines. *Int J Radiat Oncol Biol Phys* 1993;27(5):1231–1239.
2. Leksell L. Stereotactic radiosurgery. *J Neurol Neurosurg Psychiatry* 1983;46(9):797–803.
3. Barnett GH, Linskey ME, Adler JR, et al. Stereotactic radiosurgery—an organized neurosurgery-sanctioned definition. *J Neurosurg* 2007;106(1):1–5.
4. Pollock B. *Contemporary stereotactic radiosurgery: technique and evaluation.* Armonk, NY: Futura Publishing, 2002.
5. Davis JN, Medbery C III, Sharma S, et al. The RSSearch Registry: patterns of care and outcomes research on patients treated with stereotactic radiosurgery and stereotactic body radiotherapy. *Radiat Oncol* 2013;8:275.
6. Horsley V, Clarke R. The structure and functions of the cerebellum examined by a new method. *Brain* 1908;31(1):45–124.
7. Clarke R, Horsley V. On a method of investigating the deep ganglia and tracts of the central nervous system (cerebellum). *Clin Orthop Relat Res* 2007;463:3–6.
8. Spiegel EA, Wycis HT, Marks M, et al. Stereotaxic apparatus for operations on the human brain. *Science* 1947;106(2754):349–350.
9. Lasak JM, Gorecki JP. The history of stereotactic radiosurgery and radiotherapy. *Otolaryngol Clin North Am* 2009;42(4):593–599.
10. Leksell L. The stereotaxic method and radiosurgery of the brain. *Acta Chir Scand* 1951;102(4):316–319.
11. Benedict SH, Bova FJ, Clark B, et al. Anniversary Paper: the role of medical physicists in developing stereotactic radiosurgery. *Med Phys* 2008;35(9):4262–4277.
12. Larsson B, Leksell L, Rexed B, et al. The high-energy proton beam as a neurosurgical tool. *Nature* 1958;182(4644):1222–1223.
13. Larsson B, Leksell L, Rexed B. The use of high energy protons for cerebral surgery in man. *Acta Chirurgica Scandinavica (Sweden)* 1963;125.
14. Niranjan A, Lunsford LD. Radiosurgery: where we were, are, and may be in the third millennium. *Neurosurgery* 2000;46(3):531–543.
15. Lunsford LD, Flickinger J, Lindner G, et al. Stereotactic radiosurgery of the brain using the first United States 201 cobalt-60 source gamma knife. *Neurosurgery* 1989;24(2):151–159.
16. Chin L, Regine W. *Principles and practice of stereotactic radiosurgery.* New York: Springer, 2015.
17. Colombo F, Benedetti A, Pozza F, et al. External stereotactic irradiation by linear accelerator. *Neurosurgery* 1985;16(2):154–160.
18. Betti O, Derechinsky V. Hyperselective encephalic irradiation with linear accelerator. *Advances in stereotactic and functional neurosurgery 6.* Springer, 1984:385–390.
19. Winston KR, Lutz W. Linear accelerator as a neurosurgical tool for stereotactic radiosurgery. *Neurosurgery* 1988;22(3):454–464.
20. Lutz W, Winston KR, Maleki N. A system for stereotactic radiosurgery with a linear accelerator. *Int J Radiat Oncol Biol Phys* 1988;14(2):373–381.
21. Loeffler JS, Shrieve DC, Wen PY, et al. Radiosurgery for intracranial malignancies. *Semin Radiat Oncol* 1995;5(3):225–234.
22. Adler JR Jr, Chang S, Murphy M, et al. The Cyberknife: a frameless robotic system for radiosurgery. *Stereotact Funct Neurosurg* 1998;69(1–4):124–128.
23. Hamilton AJ, Lulu BA, Fosmire H, et al. Preliminary clinical experience with linear accelerator-based spinal stereotactic radiosurgery. *Neurosurgery* 1995;36(2):311–319.
24. Timmerman R, Papiez L, McGarry R, et al. Extracranial stereotactic radioablation: results of a phase I study in medically inoperable stage I non-small cell lung cancer. *Chest* 2003;124:1946–1955.
25. Leksell L. A stereotaxic apparatus for intracerebral surgery. *Acta Chir Scand* 1950;99(3):229–233.
26. Otto K, Fallone BG. Frame slippage verification in stereotactic radiosurgery. *Int J Radiat Oncol Biol Phys* 1998;41(1):199–205.
27. Rojas-Villabona A, Miszkiel K, Kitchen N, et al. Evaluation of the stability of the stereotactic Leksell Frame G in Gamma Knife radiosurgery. *J Appl Clin Med Phys* 2016;17(3):75–89.
28. Lindquist C, Paddick I. The Leksell Gamma Knife Perfexion and comparisons with its predecessors. *Neurosurgery* 2008;62(Suppl 2):721–732.
29. Ganz J. *Gamma knife neurosurgery.* 1st ed. New York: Springer-Wien, 2011.
30. Yomo S, Tamura M, Carron R, et al. A quantitative comparison of radiosurgical treatment parameters in vestibular schwannomas: the Leksell Gamma Knife Perfexion versus Model 4C. *Acta Neurochir (Wien)* 2010;152(1):47–55.
31. Regis J, Tamura M, Guillot C, et al. Radiosurgery with the world's first fully robotized Leksell Gamma Knife PerfeXion in clinical use: a 200-patient prospective, randomized, controlled comparison with the Gamma Knife 4C. *Neurosurgery* 2009;64(2):346–355; discussion 355–346.

Section II

32. Yu C, Apuzzo ML, Zee CS, et al. A phantom study of the geometric accuracy of computed tomographic and magnetic resonance imaging stereotactic localization with the Leksell stereotactic system. *Neurosurgery* 2001;48(5):1092–1098; discussion 1098–1099.

33. Takakura T, Mizowaki T, Nakata M, et al. The geometric accuracy of frameless stereotactic radiosurgery using a 6D robotic couch system. *Phys Med Biol* 2010;55(1):1–10.

34. Wurm RE, Erbel S, Schwenkert I, et al. Novalis frameless image-guided noninvasive radiosurgery: initial experience. *Neurosurgery* 2008;62(5 Suppl):A11–A17; discussion A17–A18.

35. Amsbaugh MJ, Boling W, Woo S. Tumor bed radiosurgery: an emerging treatment for brain metastases. *J Neurooncol* 2015;123(2):197–203.

36. Leavitt DD, Gibbs FA Jr, Heilbrun MP, et al. Dynamic field shaping to optimize stereotactic radiosurgery. *Int J Radiat Oncol Biol Phys* 1991;21(5):1247–1255.

37. Yin FF, Zhu J, Yan H, et al. Dosimetric characteristics of Novalis shaped beam surgery unit. *Med Phys* 2002;29(8):1729–1738.

38. Benedict SH, Cardinale RM, Wu Q, et al. Intensity-modulated stereotactic radiosurgery using dynamic micro-multileaf collimation. *Int J Radiat Oncol Biol Phys* 2001;50(3):751–758.

39. Murphy MJ. An automatic six-degree-of-freedom image registration algorithm for image-guided frameless stereotaxic radiosurgery. *Med Phys* 1997;24(6):857–866.

40. Webb S. Conformal intensity-modulated radiotherapy (IMRT) delivered by robotic linac—testing IMRT to the limit? *Phys Med Biol* 1999;44(7):1639–1654.

41. Gibbs IC. Frameless image-guided intracranial and extracranial radiosurgery using the Cyberknife robotic system. *Cancer Radiother* 2006;10(5):283–287.

42. Chang SD, Main W, Martin DP, et al. An analysis of the accuracy of the CyberKnife: a robotic frameless stereotactic radiosurgical system. *Neurosurgery* 2003;52(1):140–146; discussion 146–147.

43. Ozhasoglu C, Saw CB, Chen H, et al. Synchrony—cyberknife respiratory compensation technology. *Med Dosim* 2008;33(2):117–123.

44. Benedict SH, Yenice KM, Followill D, et al. Stereotactic body radiation therapy: the report of AAPM Task Group 101. *Med Phys* 2010;37(8):4078–4101.

45. Schell MC, Bova FJ, Larson D, et al. *Stereotactic radiosurgery. Report of Task Group 42.* Woodbury, NY, 1995.

46. Choi CY, Chang SD, Gibbs IC, et al. Stereotactic radiosurgery of the postoperative resection cavity for brain metastases: prospective evaluation of target margin on tumor control. *Int J Radiat Oncol Biol Phys* 2012;84(2):336–342.

47. Arvidson NB, Mehta MP, Tome WA. Dose coverage beyond the gross tumor volume for various stereotactic body radiotherapy planning techniques reporting similar control rates for stage I non-small-cell lung cancer. *Int J Radiat Oncol Biol Phys* 2008;72(5):1597–1603.

48. Flickinger JC. An integrated logistic formula for prediction of complications from radiosurgery. *Int J Radiat Oncol Biol Phys* 1989;17(4):879–885.

49. Kjellberg RN, Hanamura T, Davis KR, et al. Bragg-peak proton-beam therapy for arteriovenous malformations of the brain. *N Engl J Med* 1983;309(5):269–274.

50. Larsson B, Liden K, Sarby B. Irradiation of small structures through the intact skull. *Acta Radiol Ther Phys Biol* 1974;13:512–534.

51. Leksell L. Cerebral radiosurgery. I. Gammathalanotomy in two cases of intractable pain. *Acta Chir Scand* 1968;134(8):585–595.

52. Leksell L. Stereotaxic radiosurgery in trigeminal neuralgia. *Acta Chir Scand* 1971;137:311–314.

53. Steiner L, Leksell L, Forster DM, et al. Stereotactic radiosurgery in intracranial arterio-venous malformations. *Acta Neurochir (Wien)* 1974;(Suppl 21):195–209.

54. Friedman WA, Bova FJ. The University of Florida radiosurgery system. *Surg Neurol* 1989;32(5):334–342.

55. Shaw E, Scott C, Souhami L, et al. Single dose radiosurgical treatment of recurrent previously irradiated primary brain tumors and brain metastases: final report of RTOG protocol 90–05. *Int J Radiat Oncol Biol Phys* 2000;47:291–298.

56. Minniti G, Scaringi C, Paolini S, et al. Single-fraction versus multifraction (3 × 9 Gy) stereotactic radiosurgery for large (>2 cm) brain metastases: a comparative analysis of local control and risk of radiation-induced brain necrosis. *Int J Radiat Oncol Biol Phys* 2016;95(4):1142–1148.

57. Flickinger JC, Lunsford LD, Wu A, et al. Treatment planning for gamma knife radiosurgery with multiple isocenters. *Int J Radiat Oncol Biol Phys* 1990;18(6):1495–1501.

58. Verhey LJ, Smith V, Serago CF. Comparison of radiosurgery treatment modalities based on physical dose distributions. *Int J Radiat Oncol Biol Phys* 1998;40(2):497–505.

59. Liu H, Andrews DW, Evans JJ, et al. Plan quality and treatment efficiency for radiosurgery to multiple brain metastases: non-coplanar rapidArc vs. gamma knife. *Front Oncol* 2016;6:26.

60. McDonald D, Schuler J, Takacs I, et al. Comparison of radiation dose spillage from the Gamma Knife Perfexion with that from volumetric modulated arc radiosurgery during treatment of multiple brain metastases in a single fraction. *J Neurosurg* 2014;121(Suppl):51–59.

61. Amsbaugh MJ, Dunlap NE, Boling W, et al. Simultaneous integrated boost using stereotactic radiosurgery for resected brain metastases: rationale, dosimetric parameters, and preliminary clinical outcomes. *J Community Support Oncol* 2015;13(6):214–218.

62. Poll JJ, Hoogeman MS, Prevost JB, et al. Reducing monitor units for robotic radiosurgery by optimized use of multiple collimators. *Med Phys* 2008;35(6):2294–2299.

63. Schlaefer A, Schweikard A. Stepwise multi-criteria optimization for robotic radiosurgery. *Med Phys* 2008;35(5):2094–2103.

64. Wu A, Lindner G, Maitz AH, et al. Physics of gamma knife approach on convergent beams in stereotactic radiosurgery. *Int J Radiat Oncol Biol Phys* 1990;18(4):941–949.

65. Yuan J, Lo SS, Zheng Y, et al. Development of a Monte Carlo model for treatment planning dose verification of the Leksell Gamma Knife Perfexion radiosurgery system. *J Appl Clin Med Phys* 2016;17(4):190–201.

66. Haedinger U, Krieger T, Flentje M, et al. Influence of calculation model on dose distribution in stereotactic radiotherapy for pulmonary targets. *Int J Radiat Oncol Biol Phys* 2005;61(1):239–249.

67. Wilcox EE, Daskalov GM, Lincoln H. Stereotactic radiosurgery-radiotherapy: Should Monte Carlo treatment planning be used for all sites? *Pract Radiat Oncol* 2011;1(4):251–260.

68. Kubsad SS, Mackie TR, Gehring MA, et al. Monte Carlo and convolution dosimetry for stereotactic radiosurgery. *Int J Radiat Oncol Biol Phys* 1990;19(4):1027–1035.

69. Chaves A, Lopes MC, Alves CC, et al. A Monte Carlo multiple source model applied to radiosurgery narrow photon beams. *Med Phys* 2004;31(8):2192–2204.

70. Wagner TH, Bova FJ, Friedman WA, et al. A simple and reliable index for scoring rival stereotactic radiosurgery plans. *Int J Radiat Oncol Biol Phys* 2003;57(4):1141–1149.

71. Paddick I, Lippitz B. A simple dose gradient measurement tool to complement the conformity index. *J Neurosurg* 2006;105(Suppl):194–201.

72. Paddick I. A simple scoring ratio to index the conformity of radiosurgical treatment plans. Technical note. *J Neurosurg* 2000;93(Suppl 3):219–222.

73. Rahimian J, Chen JC, Rao AA, et al. Geometrical accuracy of the Novalis stereotactic radiosurgery system for trigeminal neuralgia. *J Neurosurg* 2004;101(Suppl 3):351–355.

74. Lightstone AW, Benedict SH, Bova FJ, et al. Intracranial stereotactic positioning systems: Report of the American Association of Physicists in Medicine Radiation Therapy Committee Task Group no. 68. *Med Phys* 2005;32(7):2380–2398.

75. Roberts T. The BRW/CRW stereotactic apparatus. In: Lozano AM, Gildenberg PL, eds. *Textbook of functional and stereotactic neurosurgery.* New York: McGraw-Hill, 1998:65–71.

76. Salter BJ, Fuss M, Vollmer DG, et al. The TALON removable head frame system for stereotactic radiosurgery/radiotherapy: measurement of the repositioning accuracy. *Int J Radiat Oncol Biol Phys* 2001;51(2):555–562.

77. Brown RA, Nelson JA. The invention and early history of the N-localizer for stereotactic neurosurgery. *Cureus* 2016;8(6):e642.

78. Adler JR Jr, Colombo F, Heilbrun MP, et al. Toward an expanded view of radiosurgery. *Neurosurgery* 2004;55(6):1374–1376.

79. Keshavarzi S, Meltzer H, Ben-Haim S, et al. Initial clinical experience with frameless optically guided stereotactic radiosurgery/radiotherapy in pediatric patients. *Childs Nerv Syst* 2009;25(7):837–844.

80. Nath SK, Lawson JD, Wang JZ, et al. Optically-guided frameless linac-based radiosurgery for brain metastases: clinical experience. *J Neurooncol* 2010;97(1):67–72.

81. Dong P, Perez-Andujar A, Pinnaduwage D, et al. Dosimetric characterization of hypofractionated Gamma Knife radiosurgery of large or complex brain tumors versus linear accelerator-based treatments. *J Neurosurg* 2016;125(Suppl 1):97–103.

82. Zeverino M, Jaccard M, Patin D, et al. Commissioning of the leksell gamma knife(R) icon. *Med Phys* 2017;44(2):355–363.

83. Meeks SL, Bova FJ, Wagner TH, et al. Image localization for frameless stereotactic radiotherapy. *Int J Radiat Oncol Biol Phys* 2000;46(5):1291–1299.

84. Ryken TC, Meeks SL, Pennington EC, et al. Initial clinical experience with frameless stereotactic radiosurgery: analysis of accuracy and feasibility. *Int J Radiat Oncol Biol Phys* 2001;51(4):1152–1158.

85. Jaffray DA, Drake DG, Moreau M, et al. A radiographic and tomographic imaging system integrated into a medical linear accelerator for localization of bone and soft-tissue targets. *Int J Radiat Oncol Biol Phys* 1999;45(3):773–789.

86. Murphy MJ, Cox RS. The accuracy of dose localization for an image-guided frameless radiosurgery system. *Med Phys* 1996;23(12):2043–2049.

87. Gall KP, Verhey LJ, Wagner M. Computer-assisted positioning of radiotherapy patients using implanted radiopaque fiducials. *Med Phys* 1993;20(4):1153–1159.

88. Menke M, Hirschfeld F, Mack T, et al. Photogrammetric accuracy measurements of head holder systems used for fractionated radiotherapy. *Int J Radiat Oncol Biol Phys* 1994;29(5):1147–1155.

89. Chang Z, Liu T, Cai J, et al. Evaluation of integrated respiratory gating systems on a Novalis Tx system. *J Appl Clin Med Phys* 2011;12(3):3495.

90. Yu C, Main W, Taylor D, et al. An anthropomorphic phantom study of the accuracy of Cyberknife spinal radiosurgery. *Neurosurgery* 2004;55(5):1138–1149.

91. Ho AK, Fu D, Cotrutz C, et al. A study of the accuracy of cyberknife spinal radiosurgery using skeletal structure tracking. *Neurosurgery* 2007;60(2 Suppl 1):ONS147–ONS156; discussion ONS156.

92. Winer-Muram HT, Jennings SG, Meyer CA, et al. Effect of varying CT section width on volumetric measurement of lung tumors and application of compensatory equations. *Radiology* 2003;229(1):184–194.

93. Seppenwoolde Y, Shirato H, Kitamura K, et al. Precise and real-time measurement of 3D tumor motion in lung due to breathing and heartbeat, measured during radiotherapy. *Int J Radiat Oncol Biol Phys* 2002;53(4):822–834.

94. Stevens CW, Munden RF, Forster KM, et al. Respiratory-driven lung tumor motion is independent of tumor size, tumor location, and pulmonary function. *Int J Radiat Oncol Biol Phys* 2001;51(1):62–68.

95. Jin JY, Yin FF, Tenn SE, et al. Use of the BrainLAB ExacTrac X-Ray 6D system in image-guided radiotherapy. *Med Dosim* 2008;33(2):124–134.

96. James J, Cetnar A, Dunlap NE, et al. Technical Note: validation and implementation of a wireless transponder tracking system for gated stereotactic ablative radiotherapy of the liver. *Med Phys* 2016;43(6):2794.

97. Wen N, Snyder KC, Scheib SG, et al. Technical Note: evaluation of the systematic accuracy of a frameless, multiple image modality guided, linear accelerator based stereotactic radiosurgery system. *Med Phys* 2016;43(5):2527.

98. Shirato H, Shimizu S, Kitamura K, et al. Four-dimensional treatment planning and fluoroscopic real-time tumor tracking radiotherapy for moving tumor. *Int J Radiat Oncol Biol Phys* 2000;48(2):435–442.

99. Baroni G, Ferrigno G, Pedotti A. Implementation and application of real-time motion analysis based on passive markers. *Med Biol Eng Comput* 1998;36(6):693–703.

CHAPTER 20

Intraoperative Radiotherapy

Timothy J. Kinsella

INTRODUCTION

Intraoperative radiotherapy (IORT) involves the delivery of radiation during surgery using various types of radiation sources/technologies, including intraoperative electron radiation therapy (IOERT), high dose rate brachytherapy (HDR-IORT), and electronic brachytherapy/low-kilovoltage x-rays (KV-IORT). The major advantage of IORT is the potential for delivery of higher effective radiation doses to a tumor or, more ideally, to the bed of a grossly resected tumor, while limiting the radiation dose to adjacent, dose-limiting, normal tissues or organs. This normal tissue sparing is accomplished by the dosimetric features of these different IORT technologies and by surgical approaches and/or customized lead shielding to exclude/limit normal tissues during IORT. Although IORT may be used alone following resection of certain primary or recurrent cancers, it is more often (and ideally) combined with external beam radiotherapy (EBRT), typically administered preoperatively with or without concurrent chemotherapy. Indeed, based on clinical IORT data generated over the last three decades, one can conclude that the acute and late normal tissue toxicities and local tumor control rates are quite acceptable in patients with a variety of solid cancers treated with curative intent combining EBRT (± chemotherapy) with gross total resection and IORT. Effective use of IORT requires a multidisciplinary approach, including close cooperation with surgical oncology, medical physics, and surgical nursing personnel. However, despite encouraging clinical data and more widespread use of IORT throughout the world over the last decade, level 1 evidence based on large phase III trials is lacking, with the possible exception of its use in the treatment of breast cancer.

This chapter begins with an overview of the radiobiology of IORT, based largely on comprehensive preclinical experiments using canine models that established normal tissue and organ-specific guidelines, principally for IOERT ± EBRT. Using American foxhounds and beagles as models, acute and late normal tissue responses to IOERT ± EBRT were categorized using experimental designs that mimicked thoracic and abdominal cavity surgeries where IOERT was anticipated to be used clinically. Next, the physics and technical applications of IORT are described with details regarding the specific uses of IOERT, HDR-IORT, and KV-IORT. Finally, a summary of the available clinical IORT data is presented for some tumor sites where IORT has shown efficacy as a component of multimodality treatment. A discussion of potential future clinical uses of IORT is also presented in this final section.

RADIOBIOLOGY PRINCIPLES AND EXPERIMENTAL STUDIES OF IORT

Radiobiologic Modeling for the Determination of Equivalent Single-Fraction IORT Doses

The principal advantage of IORT is the ability to maximally exclude adjacent normal tissues by surgical mobilization and/or the use of customized lead wafer shielding in the cases of IOERT and HDR-IORT. However, the clinical application of IORT to treat minimal gross (R_2 resection) or suspected microscopic residual disease (R_1 resection) in a resected tumor bed necessitates inclusion of partial volumes of adjacent normal tissues or organs based on tumor location, tumor size, and extent of infiltration of adjacent normal tissues, including regional lymph node basins. Based on typical *in vitro* clonogenic studies and *in vivo* small animal studies, where large single doses of 5 to 20 Gy have often been used, it is evident that IORT doses of 15 to 25 Gy could provide a theoretical disadvantage with respect to IORT-related tumor cell kill (or local control) versus normal tissue toxicities.

Typically, the radiation dose–response curve for acute-reacting normal tissues, such as gastrointestinal epithelium and bone marrow, is very steep, and a small change in the radiation dose near the tissue tolerance level can result in a significant risk of toxicity. In contrast, the radiation dose–response curve for late-reacting normal tissues, such as heart muscle, peripheral nerve, large arterial blood vessels, and bone, is less steep and correlates directly with the volume of tissue included within the irradiated field. Extrapolating from the linear-quadratic model using clonogenic survival data, one can extrapolate the shape of the radiation survival curve for tumor and normal tissues using the α/β ratio. A late-reacting normal tissue has a low α/β ratio (usually <5 Gy), whereas acute-reacting normal tissues, as well as most solid tumors, have α/β ratio of >7 Gy. Using these α/β ratios, one can estimate the single-fraction IORT dose (compared to conventional fractionated EBRT) to control tumor while limiting specific normal tissue toxicities. For example, for a squamous cell carcinoma with minimal residual disease following surgery, an EBRT dose of 60 Gy using 2-Gy fractions ($D_{2Gy} = 60$) is required, and the α/β ratio for squamous cell carcinoma cells is 10 Gy. We can use the linear-quadratic (LQ) formula to calculate the equivalent D_{IORT} to be 22.3 Gy, which is supported by multiple single-institution IORT clinical studies that included patients with recurrent or locally advanced head and neck cancers.[1] Similarly, such an equivalent IORT dose can be calculated for a late-reacting normal tissue, such as peripheral nerve, using $D_{2Gy} = 70$ and α/β ratio = 2 Gy. The calculated D_{IORT} is 16 Gy, which is again supported by experimental canine and human clinical data.[2]

Although the D_{IORT} calculation has some clinical utility, as these two examples illustrate, many other clinical variables are not factored into the calculation, such as prior or recent EBRT ± chemotherapy, the inclusion of multiple types and volumes of acute- and late-reacting normal tissues within the IORT field, and other patient-specific comorbidities, for example, cardiovascular disease, diabetes, and connective tissue disease. Indeed, in patients treated with preoperative or postoperative EBRT ± chemotherapy, the IORT boost dose calculation should include these additional treatment effects, particularly with regard to both acute- and late-reacting normal tissues. There are experimental canine data, specifically from the beagle dog model, to assist in the $D_{IORT\ boost}$ calculation, which is often in the 10- to 15-Gy range. In addition, from a radiobiologic perspective, it is recognized that tumor cell hypoxia is the major factor determining tumor radioresponse, as other biologic factors, such as repair, reoxygenation, and repopulation, are not operative with single-fraction treatment.

Another radiobiologic effect that is not included within the D_{IORT} calculation for normal tissue toxicity is the risk of a radiation-induced cancer. Radiation-induced cancers are typically a late effect, often occurring a decade or more after radiation therapy. For an IORT-induced cancer, the cancer should arise within the IORT field and should have a different histology than the original primary. In the canine studies of normal tissue tolerance to varying IORT doses, long-term follow-up (up to 5 years) demonstrated IORT-induced sarcomas of bone and soft tissue, evident at autopsy, in up to 20% to 25% of animals receiving >25 Gy.[3] No IORT-induced cancers have been reported in humans, although many IORT-treated patients have very aggressive primary or recurrent cancers and often die from progressive metastatic disease within 1 to 2 years after IORT without autopsy evaluation of the IORT volume. Because IORT is being used for some pediatric oncology cases, it will be especially important to follow these patients closely for the potential risk of an IORT-induced cancer as a late effect.

Experimental Studies of IOERT with or without EBRT to Establish Normal Tissue Tolerance Guidelines

Comprehensive studies of acute and late normal tissue responses to IOERT ± EBRT were performed using two canine models. The American foxhound model was principally used for IOERT studies at the National Cancer Institute (NCI), whereas a beagle dog model was used for IOERT ± EBRT studies at Colorado State University (CSU). Both canine species are large enough to allow surgical procedures in the thoracic and abdominal cavities that mimic surgeries for human cancers for which IORT may be applied. The goal of these studies was to establish dose guidelines of IOERT alone (NCI) and IOERT ± EBRT (CSU) to reduce acute and late normal tissue toxicities in selected intact and surgically manipulated tissues that mimicked clinical situations in which IOERT might be used. After IOERT ± EBRT, dogs were closely followed clinically and by various sequential diagnostic studies for up to 5 years. All dogs were subjected to complete autopsy with detailed histologic analyses of irradiated tissues.

A description of the NCI IOERT studies is presented in Table 20.1. A more comprehensive overview of these studies is summarized in two reviews.[4,5] A total of 13 sites or target tissues were studied using escalating IOERT doses and a fixed IOERT volume based on the target site. In total, these NCI studies involved 227 dogs, with 196 receiving IOERT and 31 receiving sham IOERT (0 Gy). At CSU, adult beagles were randomized to receive IOERT alone (5 × 8-cm field; 6 MeV; dose range 17.5 to 55 Gy), EBRT alone (5 × 10-cm field; 6-MV photons; dose range 60, 70, and 80 Gy in 30 fractions of 2, 2.33, and 2.67 Gy,

respectively), or initial EBRT (5 × 10-cm field; 6-MV photons; dose 50 Gy in 25 fractions of 2 Gy) followed by IOERT (5 × 8-cm field; 6 MeV; dose range 10 to 45.5 Gy). A summary of the clinical and pathologic data regarding normal tissue tolerance from these collective NCI and CSU canine studies is presented in Table 20.2 and briefly described below.

Vascular Tissues

Because the vasculature determines, in large measure, the viability and functionality of all normal tissue systems, an understanding of the tolerance thresholds of IORT on blood vessels is critically important. Intact large vessels (aorta, vena cava) appear to tolerate large single IOERT doses without significant clinical sequelae, based on serial follow-up radiographic studies for up to 5 years.[6] At autopsy, no pathologic changes were found following a 20-Gy dose, and only mild to moderate subintimal fibrosis was found after 30- and 40-Gy doses, respectively. However, the combination of 50-Gy EBRT and >20-Gy IOERT resulted in an IOERT dose–related luminal narrowing with thrombus formation and moderate mural fibrosis pathologically, with up to 2 years of follow-up.[7] To evaluate the IORT tolerance of intraoperatively mandated vascular repairs and anastomoses, a transection and end-to-end reanastomosis of the infrarenal abdominal aorta was performed, followed by IOERT doses of 20 to 45 Gy.[6] Pathologically, moderate medial wall fibrosis was found at doses >30 Gy. Although anastomotic integrity was maintained at all doses, follow-up arteriograms showed anastomotic occlusion at doses >30 Gy within 6 to 12 months. However, occlusion was sufficiently slow to allow formation of arterial collaterals around the occlusion, preventing any clinical or pathologic signs of ischemia distal to the anastomosis. At 45 Gy, development of a late arteriovenous fistula at the anastomotic site in one dog suggested the potential for IORT dose–limiting, clinically relevant, toxicity.

The tolerance of vascular grafts to IORT was investigated in beagles, for which a segmental resection of the infrarenal aorta was performed with reconstruction using a polyfluorotetraethylene graft.[8] IOERT up to 30 Gy was immediately delivered following the prosthetic grafting, and half of the dogs were randomized to receive postoperative EBRT to 36 Gy in 10 fractions over 4 weeks. Arterial graft occlusion occurred acutely in both treatment groups but was correctable by thrombectomy. During clinical follow-up, most dogs receiving ≥30-Gy IOERT ± EBRT developed late graft

TABLE 20.1 NATIONAL CANCER INSTITUTE INTRAOPERATIVE ELECTRON RADIATION THERAPY STUDIES OF NORMAL TISSUE TOLERANCE

Sites	Surgical Procedure	IOERT Field; Electron Energy (MeV)	Dose Range (Gy): Number Treated
Retroperitoneal soft tissues, aorta, vena cava, left ureter, lower pole left kidney	LAP; exposure to unilateral retroperitoneum	4 × 15 cm; 11	0:4; 20:4; 30:4; 40:4; 50:4
Aortic anastomosis and small bowel suture line	LAP; transection and reanastomosis of aorta; Roux-en-y with blind loop	4 × 15 cm; 11	0:1; 20:1; 30:1; 45:1
Aortic anastomosis	LAP; transection and reanastomosis	4 × 15 cm; 11	0:1; 20:4; 30:3; 45:3
Small bowel suture line; retroperitoneal soft tissues	LAP; Roux-en-y with small bowel blind loop	4 × 15 cm; 11	0:1; 20:5; 30:5; 45:5
Intact extrahepatic bile duct	LAP; mobilization of biliary tree	5-cm circle; 11	0:1; 20:3; 30:2; 45:2
Extrahepatic bile duct with jejunal anastomosis	LAP; biliary–jejunal anastomosis	5-cm circle; 11	0:2; 20:3; 30:2; 45:2
Trigone of the bladder	LAP; cystotomy	5-cm circle; 12	0:3; 20:3; 25:3; 30:3; 35:3; 40:7
Arterial vascular graft to infrarenal aorta	LAP; segmental resection and immediate grafting	4 × 15 cm; 9	0:6; 20:8; 25:8; 30:8
Peripheral nerve; lumbosacral plexus (L4-L5)	LAP; exposure of unilateral lumbosacral plexus	9-cm circle; 11	0:3; 10:4; 15:4; 20:8; 25:4; 30:3; 35:3; 40:4; 50:2
Spinal cord	LAP; exposure of retroperitoneum over lumbar spine	4 × 15 cm; 11	0:3; 20:7; 25:7; 30:8
Right upper lobe lung and mediastinum including right atrium	Right thoracotomy	5-cm circle; 9	0:3; 20:7; 30:7; 40:7
Left bronchial stump, pulmonary artery and vein, left atrium	Left pneumonectomy	5-cm circle; 13	0:3; 20:4; 30:4; 40:4
Esophagus	Right thoracotomy and mobilization of the esophagus	6-cm circle; 9	0:1; 20:7; 30:5

IOERT, intraoperative electron radiation therapy; LAP, laparotomy.

TABLE 20.2 TOLERANCE DOSES TO INTRAOPERATIVE RADIOTHERAPY IN CANINE MODELS

System	Organ	Maximum Tolerated IORT Dose (Gy)	Maximum Follow-up Period (Months)	Comments
Cardiothoracic	Aorta	30	60	Threshold for fibrosis, patency to 60 Gy
	Vena cava	30	60	Threshold for fibrosis, patency to 60 Gy
	Arterial anastomosis	30	36	Threshold for stenotic occlusion
	Arterial graft	30	24	Threshold for occlusion
	Heart	30	60	Threshold for fibrosis, no clinical effects to 40 Gy
	Tracheobronchus	30	60	Threshold for fibrosis, no clinical effects to 40 Gy
	Bronchial suture line	40	60	Intact to 40 Gy, bronchovascular fistulae at 20 Gy
	Lung	20	60	Threshold for fibrotic pneumonitis, no clinical effects to 40 Gy
	Esophagus	20	60	Ulceration and stricture with full-thickness exposure, no sequelae to 40-Gy partial thickness
Gastrointestinal	Duodenum	18	6	Threshold for ulceration, obstruction, or perforation
	Small intestine diverted loop	45	60	Defunctionalized bowel loop, no clinical effects, fibrosis at ≥20 Gy
Hepatobiliary–pancreatic	Bile duct	20	60	Threshold for fibrosis and stenosis
	Bile duct anastomosis	<20	12	Dehiscence at all doses ≥20 Gy
Urinary	Kidney	15	60	Threshold for tubular loss
	Ureter	30	60	Threshold for fibrosis and stenosis
	Bladder	30	60	Threshold for ureterovesical junction stenosis, normal contractility to 40 Gy
Nervous	Peripheral nerve	15	60	Threshold for motor neuropathy

IORT, intraoperative radiotherapy.
Adapted from Sindelar WF, Kinsella TJ. Normal tissue tolerance to intraoperative radiotherapy. *Surg Oncol Clin North Am* 2003;12(4):925–942. Copyright © 2003 Elsevier. With permission.

occlusion (within 12 months) but again showed evidence of progressive collateralization by arteriography, preventing distal ischemia–related complications.

Gastrointestinal Tissues

Because of its rapidly proliferating mucosa and rich blood supply, the small and large intestines are among the most radiosensitive normal tissues. As such, the intestine needs to be surgically mobilized and excluded from IORT portals. NCI investigators assessed the IORT tolerance of small intestinal suture lines where a jejunal blind loop was created surgically and intestinal continuity maintained by distal jejunojejunostomy.[9] The IOERT field encompassed the suture line and the full thickness of the intestinal wall, and doses of 20 to 45 Gy were delivered. No immediate histologic changes were seen, and no clinical evidence of suture line dehiscence was found with 5 years of follow-up. However, internal interloop fistulae occurred following 45 Gy. Thus, whereas acute IOERT tolerance of a defunctionalized bowel loop was acceptable to 45 Gy, chronic complications suggest a maximum of 30 Gy. However, functional small and large bowel showed clinical and pathologic manifestations of ulceration, stricture, and perforations following doses as low as 15 to 20 Gy.

Hepatobiliary Tissues

Bile duct tolerance to IOERT was studied at the NCI using a 5-cm IORT portal to the subhepatic space, which encompassed the extrahepatic bile duct.[10] When using a dose range of 20 to 45 Gy, no acute complications were noted, but progressive and IOERT dose–related chemical evidence of partial biliary obstruction was seen within 2 to 8 months of follow-up. Frank biliary cirrhosis developed in one-half of dogs receiving 30 Gy or more that were followed for a minimum of 12 months. The tolerance of biliary–enteric anastomoses was also studied using a similar IOERT dose range. After laparotomy and formation of a jejunal biliary loop, the bile duct was transected and anastomosed to the jejunal loop, followed by immediate IOERT to the anastomotic site. All animals developed acute complications within several weeks, with either anastomotic disruption or subacute anastomotic obstruction, resulting in cholangitis or bile duct necrosis. Thus, although the intact bile duct may tolerate doses of up to 20 Gy, a bile duct anastomosis cannot be included within an IORT field.

Urinary Tract Tissues

In the IOERT study involving the intact unilateral retroperitoneum,[6] a 12-cm segment of ureter, as well as the inferior pole of one kidney, was irradiated to IOERT doses as high as 50 Gy. Dogs were followed clinically with renal function testing and radiographic pyelography. The kidney showed dose-related fibrosis and hyalinization. Acute obstructive nephropathy secondary to ureteral obstruction was evident with 50 Gy, whereas subacute obstructive nephropathy was evident at 2 to 3 months of follow-up in the 40-Gy dogs and at 6 to 12 months following 30 Gy. In the 20-Gy–treated dogs, no clinical or pathologic changes in the irradiated ureter were evident. A CSU study showed that shorter (≤4 cm) segments of the ureter would tolerate doses of 30 Gy.[11] Typically, the ureter can be surgically mobilized and excluded from the IORT field, but segments at high risk of residual microscopic disease may be included, and prophylactic ureteral stenting may reduce the risk of narrowing/obstruction as a subacute complication.

Bladder tolerance to IOERT was studied using the foxhound model at the NCI.[12,13] Following laparotomy and cystotomy, a 5-cm circular IORT portal, including the trigone and both ureteral orifices, was treated with doses of 20 to 40 Gy. Dogs were then followed for up to 5 years with clinical evaluation, kidney function tests, intravenous pyelography, and cystometry. Although no acute complications were noted, some dogs who received 25 Gy or greater developed fibrotic strictures at the ureterovesical junction within 2 years, which became more frequent at 5 years in the ≥30-Gy–treated dogs. Whereas pathologic changes of fibrosis and microvascular changes in the bladder wall were evident at 30 Gy or greater, follow-up cystometric studies showed little difference in post-IOERT bladder contractility from baseline at all IOERT doses.

Cardiothoracic Tissues

In the NCI studies of IOERT to the canine mediastinum, atrial appendages of the heart received doses up to 40 Gy.[14,15] Dense fibrosis of the myocardium was found pathologically following IOERT doses of 30 Gy or greater, with early (within 1 month) medial hyaline degeneration followed by radiation vasculopathy and infarction within 12 months. However, because of the limited irradiated volume of cardiac muscle, no clinical signs of cardiac failure were evident with up to 5 years of follow-up.

Segments of the trachea and mainstem bronchi also received IOERT of 20 to 40 Gy in the NCI mediastinal IOERT studies.[14,15] Pathologic changes of fibrosis in the tracheobronchial wall were evident at doses of 30 Gy or greater, with infrequent development of chondronecrosis of the tracheal rings at doses of <40 Gy; however, most animals showed no clinical respiratory symptoms. In addition, the canine pneumonectomy study found normal healing of the bronchial stump following IOERT to 20 to 40 Gy, and no clinical sequelae were observed through 5 years of follow-up.[16] However, when limited amounts of lung tissue received IOERT, acute confluent pneumonitis progressing to interstitial fibrosis and pulmonary arteriolar sclerosis developed at all doses within 12 months.[14,16]

IOERT tolerance of the esophagus was also evaluated in the NCI mediastinal studies, with both full-thickness and partial-thickness (<50% of circumference) treatment.[14,15] Clinical examinations, barium swallows, and esophagoscopies were performed for up to 2 years following doses to 30 Gy for full-thickness irradiation and to 40 Gy for partial-thickness irradiation. With full-thickness esophageal IOERT, all animals receiving 20 Gy or more showed acute clinical toxicity with signs of dysphagia and weight loss. Acute, but transient, inflammatory changes to esophageal mucosa were found at 20 Gy, but progressive severe inflammatory changes leading to ulceration and stricture by 2 to 3 months were found following 30 Gy. With partial esophageal wall IOERT, no severe clinical or radiographic sequelae occurred at doses up to 40 Gy, with dose-related fibrosis but no mucosal ulcers or strictures.

Nervous Tissue

Whereas peripheral nerves were traditionally considered to be relatively radioresistant, clinical IORT trials at the NCI reported a significantly increased risk of lumbosacral neuropathy following IOERT + EBRT in patients with localized but technically resectable retroperitoneal sarcomas.[17] In this clinical trial, patients were randomized to receive postoperative EBRT alone (initial 40 Gy, followed by a 14- to 16-Gy boost) or IOERT (20 Gy using multiple abutting fields based on tumor bed size/location) followed by postoperative EBRT (36 Gy). Subacute (within 1 to 3 months) and late (>6 months) clinical motor and/or sensory neuropathies to the lower trunk and/or lower extremity were found in 9 of 15 patients randomized to IOERT + EBRT and in 1 of 20 patients randomized to postoperative EBRT alone ($P < .01$).[18]

To further establish the tolerance of peripheral nerve trunks to IORT, a series of studies was conducted at the NCI and CSU.[2,19] In the initial NCI study using foxhounds, the lumbosacral plexus was surgically exposed and IOERT doses of 20 to 75 Gy were delivered. Hind limb motor changes developed in 90% of treated dogs within 12 months, ranging in severity from slight motor strength weakness to complete motor paralysis, with an approximately inverse relationship between IOERT dose and the time to onset and severity of neurologic signs. However, no threshold dose for neuropathy was found, even with the use of nerve conduction times as a measure. Pathologically, loss of large nerve fibers and perineural fibrosis with radiation vasculopathy in perineural connective tissue were seen. A follow-up NCI trial attempted to establish a threshold dose for IORT-induced neuropathy in the lumbosacral plexus. No animal receiving IOERT doses of up to 15 Gy developed clinical neuropathy by exam and nerve conduction testing for more than 3 years following IOERT, whereas all animals receiving 20 Gy developed hind leg paresis with lower nerve conduction testing within 12 months. With up to 5 years of follow-up, dogs treated with IORT doses of up to 15 Gy showed continued lack of neurotoxicity.[18]

Studies assessing lumbar nerve injury following IOERT alone, EBRT alone, and combined IOERT plus EBRT were performed at CSU using a beagle dog model.[19] Similar neurologic and nerve conduction testing as used in the NCI studies was performed for up to 2 years of follow-up. Although no neurologic complications were found using EBRT alone, dose- and time-related neuropathy was seen in IOERT alone and in IOERT + EBRT–treated dogs with an IOERT dose threshold of 15 Gy. Radiation-induced changes to Schwann cells and nerve vasculature were found, similar to the NCI findings, and ultrastructural studies suggested microvascular damage causing regional hypoxia and subsequent nerve fiber loss. Thus, peripheral nerve appears to be a dose-limiting tissue for IORT, in contrast to the relative radioresistance of peripheral nerves to EBRT.

IORT-Induced Malignancies

As mentioned previously, radiation-induced malignancies are infrequent following conventionally fractionated EBRT and are most commonly seen several to many years after the successful treatment of childhood cancers. Although IORT-induced cancers have not been reported in humans, the canine data support a potential risk in humans. Again, an IORT-induced cancer should fulfill several criteria, including occurring within the IORT field, developing after an appropriate latency period (e.g., a few years in canines), and being histologically confirmed and of a histologic type that develops infrequently in the particular dog species.

In studies of IOERT-related toxicity to the bone at CSU, a 21% incidence of osteosarcoma was noted, with at least 4 years of follow-up following IOERT alone to >25 Gy with or without EBRT.[20] In dogs treated with EBRT alone for spontaneous soft tissue tumors, a 3% incidence of osteosarcoma within the EBRT volume was seen. IOERT-induced tumors were also seen in the NCI canine trials.[3,21] Among 59 animals followed for 2 or more years, 12 tumors were pathologically confirmed at complete necropsy. Three tumors did not meet the criteria for being radiation induced, including 2 benign fibrous tumors and a mammary carcinoma. The 9 IORT-related tumors included a bladder rhabdomyosarcoma, a soft tissue malignant fibrous histiocytoma, and 7 sarcomas of the bone or cartilage. In dogs receiving >25-Gy IOERT, the overall incidence of radiation-induced neoplasms was 25%, consistent with the CSU data.

In summary, the validity of the canine tissue tolerance models as described in this section and Table 20.2 as representative of the human tissue response to IORT is supported by clinical IORT data from human trials. Although the tolerance to IORT-induced acute and late toxicities can vary considerably between tissues, doses up to 20 Gy are generally tolerated. The general principle providing the rationale for IORT should always be practiced, that is, maximize the radiation dose to the tumor or, ideally, the bed of a grossly resected tumor while minimizing dose exposure to adjacent normal tissues.

PHYSICS AND TECHNICAL ASPECTS OF IORT

Definition of Techniques

IORT involves the use of a single fraction of radiation therapy delivered while the patient is under anesthesia. Three different technologies can be used to deliver IORT, including electrons (IOERT), high dose brachytherapy with iridium 192 (^{192}Ir; HDR-IORT), and low-kV x-rays (KV-IORT). IOERT is delivered by a linear accelerator electron beam in the 6- to 15-MeV dose range. Although the use of a conventional linear accelerator in the radiation oncology department was the standard for IOERT delivery in the 1970s and early 1980s, the subsequent development of mobile linear accelerators that are transported to the operating room (OR), or the installation of a dedicated accelerator in an OR, improved the efficiency and use of IOERT, no longer requiring the patient to be transported under anesthesia. At present, there are three commercial mobile linear accelerators designed for IOERT, including the Mobetron

(4- to 12-MeV electrons; IntraOp Medical, Sunnyvale, CA), the Novac 7 (4- to 10-MeV electrons; NRT SpA, Rome, Italy), and the LIAC (4- to 10-MeV electrons; Sordina SpA, Saonara, Italy). HDR-IORT uses a high dose rate afterloader with ^{192}Ir that decays via β or electron capture, and the daughter isotopes are short lived, emitting γ-rays of various energies. The β decay is absorbed by the source capsule, and the average photon energy emitted is 370 keV with a 74-day half-life. HDR-IORT is feasible only after a near gross total resection, as the maximum depth of coverage is typically 0.5 cm deep from the surface of the resected tumor bed. Several ^{192}Ir HDR remote afterloaders are commercially marketed by Nucletron (Veenendaal, Netherlands) and by Varian Medical Systems (Crowley, United Kingdom). A shielded OR is required for HDR-IORT. Over the last decade, mobile IORT devices using low-kV x-rays (KV-IORT) have been developed. Low-kV x-rays (20 to 50 kV) have the advantage of a steep dose gradient, not requiring specially shielded ORs, but have a major disadvantage in that the target (tumor bed) should ideally be spherical in shape with a maximum tissue treatment radius of 1 to 2 cm. Two commercial low–KV-IORT devices are available, including the Zeiss Intrabeam (Zeiss Surgical, Oberkochen, Germany) and the Xoft S700 Axxent System (Zoft, Medford, MA).

IOERT: Physics and Technical Applications

With the development of mobile linear accelerators as described earlier, no permanent OR shielding is required, unlike a fixed OR-based linear accelerator, because the maximum electron beam energy is 12 MeV or less and these mobile linear accelerators are designed without bending magnets. In addition, neutron contamination is not a problem for OR personnel or patients. The Mobetron has a fixed beam stopper, whereas the Novac 7 and LIAC accelerators are equipped with mobile beam stoppers. The 90% depth dose in water ranges from 1.1 cm for 4-MeV electrons to 3.5 cm for 12-MeV electrons. A variety of applicator shapes (e.g., circular, rectangular) and sizes are available from the manufacturers. However, to commission a machine for IORT, a minimum set of dosimetry measurements is required for each applicator and each electron energy including percentage depth dose, beam profiles in two orthogonal planes, isodose curves in two orthogonal planes, and applicator ratios. The applicator ratios are compared to a reference applicator for which the accelerator output is calibrated.

Quality assurance (QA) procedures for mobile IOERT linear accelerators are outlined in detail in the reports of the American Association of Physicists in Medicine (AAPM) Radiation Therapy Task Groups 48 and 72.[22,23] Because any malfunction of these mobile accelerators could result in a patient not receiving the scheduled IOERT treatment or in having a patient's surgery delayed, a high level of QA requires calibration of all electron energies early on the day of surgery, in addition to a rigorous process of periodic checks similar to the QA for a standard linear accelerator. Unique factors to the mobile IOERT linear accelerators are the lack of adjustable collimators and bending magnets. QA checks are necessary of the alignment of the soft docking system as used in the Mobetron and of a hard docking system for the two other mobile accelerators. Although *in vivo* dosimetry using TLDs or silicon diodes is not feasible for placement in a sterile surgical resection bed during IOERT, offline procedures such as the use of radiochromic films or real-time methods such as the use of metal oxide semiconductor field-effect transistors are being applied to breast cancer.[24,25] IORT may be applied to other tumor sites.

Mobile IOERT accelerators, however, have limited mobility, requiring the patient and OR table to be moved to the accelerator in the OR and sometimes requiring a change in the patient's position. The use of special OR tables with fine movement capabilities superiorly, inferiorly, laterally, and pitch and roll positioning, as well as Trendelenburg and reverse Trendelenburg movements, makes IOERT patient positioning and docking much easier and faster. The soft docking process required for the Mobetron is facilitated by a set of lasers in the accelerator head. The hard docking system used with the Novac 7 and LIAC accelerators involves a two-part applicator. Once the appropriate field size and applicator shape are determined, the superior part of the applicator is fixed to the linear accelerator head and then physically mated with the inferior part, which is in contact with the target (tumor bed). Once aligned, a rigid interlocking of the two parts is made prior to IOERT delivery. Typically, the process of soft or hard docking requires <10 to 15 minutes.

However, prior to docking, a detailed determination of the IOERT treatment volume is required, involving close collaboration between the surgical oncologist and the radiation oncologist. Typically, surgical sutures or clips are placed by the surgeon to better visualize the tumor bed, and at least a 1-cm margin is added. Next, the size, shape, and degree of bevel for the suitable applicator are determined, as well as determining whether one or more IOERT fields are necessary to cover the tumor bed. Although the IOERT applicators can function as a normal tissue retractor, additional surgical packing is often required to further exclude certain normal tissues, for example, bowel. In the clinical situation in which sensitive normal tissues cannot be physically displaced from the IOERT field, secondary shielding using sterilized lead sheets can be placed with appropriate thickness to attenuate 90% or more of the dose. Lead shielding is also essential to prevent any dose overlap, if multiple IOERT fields are required to cover the tumor bed with at least 1-cm margins. Finally, to reduce the accumulation of serous fluid in the tumor bed during IOERT (which would attenuate the dose), placement of suction adjacent to the IOERT applicator is recommended.

HDR-IORT: Physics and Technical Applications

HDR-IORT involves the use of an ^{192}Ir HDR afterloader to deliver a large single fraction of brachytherapy to a grossly resected tumor bed with necessary retraction and physical shielding of adjacent normal tissues, similar to the guidelines for IOERT as described. Because of the high activity of ^{192}Ir afforded by computer-controlled remoter afterloading, HDR-IORT treatment times of 30 to 60 minutes can be accomplished, based on the target (tumor bed) size. The desired dose distribution is generated by superimposing a large number of single-source radiation distributions at different locations and different dwell times. Two AAPM publications from Task Group 43 summarize in detail the dose calculations for ^{192}Ir in air and water.[26,27] A recent review of HDR-IORT is also recommended.[28]

Construction of an HDR-IORT–dedicated facility requires a shielded OR equipped with door interlocks, room radiation monitors, and additional adjacent space for the OR team (surgeon, radiation oncologist, nurses) to remain sterile during HDR-IORT, should any emergency reentry be needed. Anesthesia and surgical monitoring via video cameras must also be available in this adjacent OR space. Ideally, construction of a HDR-IORT facility in the hospital OR complex allows for most efficient use of OR personnel and equipment. The QA program for HDR-IORT follows guidelines outlined by AAPM task groups.[29] Typically, a series of QA checks is performed 24 hours prior to each HDR-IORT procedure and involves determination of source positioning and source strength, verification of proper functioning of room radiation monitors, and checking of equipment for use in the event of emergency source retraction.

For HDR-IORT, the applicator must be rigid enough to secure the afterloader catheters in a fixed and reproducible position while also conforming to the tumor bed contour. The applicator design must provide adequate thickness to maintain a 0.5-cm distance between the source plane and the treatment surface.[28] Prior to HDR-IORT delivery, the radiation oncologist must confirm that the applicator is in direct contact with the tissue surface throughout the entire target area, as a separation of only 0.5 cm can reduce dose delivery by up to 30%. Treatment planning for HDR-IORT is greatly facilitated by creating a plan atlas of clinically anticipated tumor volumes.[30] Plans incorporating optimized dwell times enhance efficiency and reduce risks of error. However, a plan atlas cannot anticipate the need to spare an adjacent normal tissue in certain patients, but customized lead wafers of 0.3 cm thickness can be used at the applicator–tissue interface.

KV-IORT: Physics and Technical Applications

The Zeiss Intrabeam has a miniature x-ray source at the end of a 10-cm-long, 3-mm-wide probe, where electrons are accelerated at a gold target in the probe tip, resulting in a nearly isotronic distribution of low-kV x-rays in the 30- to 50-kV range. Because these x-rays are of such low energy, no special shielding is required in a standard OR, which normally has adequate shielding for the intraoperative use of diagnostic radiology equipment. The Intrabeam is small, lightweight, and designed with a floor stand and can be easily accommodated in a standard OR. A dose rate of 2 Gy/min at 1 cm in water from the center of the target is possible with a 50-kV setting. However, the dose decreases in tissue as the inverse cube of the distance. It has an extended lifetime of over 10 years.

The Xoft S700 Axxent System is an electronic brachytherapy apparatus with a Wolfram target that operates at x-ray energies of 20 to 50 kV. As with the Intrabeam, the 50-kV energy is most commonly used. A miniature x-ray tube is located within a flexible, disposable sheath, which permits water cooling of the x-ray tube. The Xoft source is more adaptable in the OR compared to the Intrabeam source and has a higher depth–dose rate of 0.6 Gy/min at 3 cm in water. In addition, because of heavier filtration, the dose falls off less slowly in tissue than the Intrabeam source. However, the typical Xoft source lifetime is only 2.5 hours, and it has been used clinically for a much shorter time period, compared to more than a decade for Intrabeam.

A recent comprehensive review of these two KV-IORT systems is available.[31] Both units are potentially suited for IORT treatment of breast cancer, either as a boost or as definitive treatment, although most of the current clinical data involve the use of the Intrabeam. Both manufacturers are expanding the clinical use of their respective low–kV-IORT systems to superficial skin tumors and vaginal applications for endometrial cancers. The main applicators for the Intrabeam are spherical, with diameters ranging from 1.5 to 5 cm, and are composed of solid biodegradable material with a 2.8-mm central cavity where the source is placed. A homogeneous surface dose is generated with the addition of an aluminum flattening filter for applicators >3.5 cm in diameter. The Xoft system uses inflatable balloons, similar to MammoSite (Hologic, Bedford, MA) for breast irradiation, with spherical or ellipsoidal balloon shapes. The balloon sizes vary from 3 to 6 cm for spherical balloons and 5 × 7 cm and 6 × 7 cm for ellipsoidal balloons. Both systems have a number of safety features to alert the user to the emission of x-rays and allow monitoring of the output dose. QA procedures involving pretreatment checks, monthly checks, and yearly checks are reviewed.[32]

Comparison of IORT Technical Applications

A comprehensive comparison of the technical applications of the three IORT approaches is published.[32] The potential advantages of IOERT compared to HDR-IORT include better dose homogeneity, faster treatment times, requirement for less OR shielding, and the ability to treat gross residual disease based on depth-dose characteristics. Potential disadvantages include surface dose of <90% with 6- to 9-MeV electrons (compensated with the use of bolus) and difficulty in treating anatomic areas such as the low pelvis, abdominal side walls, retropubic areas, subdiaphragmatic areas, thoracic side walls, and skull base. Low–kV-IORT requires a small target (tumor) volume, where the depth in tissue at risk is 0.5 to 1.0 cm or less from the surface of the applicator.

CLINICAL RESULTS OF IORT WITH OR WITHOUT EBRT: AN OVERVIEW

A comprehensive review of the clinical experience of IORT ± EBRT (± chemotherapy) is beyond the scope of this chapter, and the reader is referred to a published textbook of IORT in which the clinical data by tumor site are presented in detail.[33] In addition, some of the IORT clinical data are discussed in this textbook in chapters devoted to specific cancers and tumor sites. The general conclusions from these mostly nonrandomized studies in selected cancers will be discussed here, in addition to a brief overview of the limited clinical data from a few prospective, randomized trials. A general conclusion is that IORT, as a component of a multidisciplinary approach for typically locally advanced primary and recurrent cancers, is feasible and appears to improve local control, as well as overall survival in some cancers, with acceptable acute and late toxicities based on the normal tissue tolerance guidelines previously presented (Table 20.2). The clinical use of IORT in a larger number of institutions across the world over the last 10 to 15 years has been aided by improvements in IORT technology as described in the last section. The more widespread use and the promising nonrandomized, generally single-institution, clinical data, as well as data from a few prospective, randomized trials, will, it is hoped, facilitate the design and implementation of prospective, randomized trials in specific tumor sites in the next decade.

Colorectal Cancer

The clinical experience with the use of IOERT and HDR-IORT as part of a multidisciplinary approach to locally advanced colorectal cancer was recently summarized.[34,35] More than 900 patients have been treated with IOERT and 59 patients with HDR-IORT, usually following preoperative combined modality treatment with EBRT (45 to 54 Gy) and concomitant infusional 5-fluorouracil (5-FU). These data are derived from multiple, nonrandomized, single-institution studies in the United States and Europe. No randomized, prospective studies are available or ongoing. Most patients had clinical T4 or tethered T3 lesions in these IORT studies, making direct comparison to large prospective, randomized trials, such as the German Rectal Cancer Study, difficult, because, certainly, the clinical T4 lesions would not be included in the phase III trial. The 3- to 5-year local control rates for IORT-treated patients were, respectively, 85% to 90% for R_0 patients and 50% to 75% for R_1/R_2 resections, with a 5% to 10% risk of grade 2 or 3 normal tissue toxicities to peripheral nerve or ureter. The 3- to 5-year disease-free survivals were in the 50% to 60% range for R_0 patients but dropped to 25% to 35% for R_2 patients. Thus, these data suggest some benefit to IORT in these clinically tethered T3 and T4 patients, but systemic relapse remains a major problem.

A similar general conclusion can be reached for the use of IORT in patients with recurrent colorectal cancer, based on a recent summary of the literature.[36] For this patient group, many will have already received EBRT ± 5-FU–based chemotherapy at the time of presentation, making the use of further EBRT (± chemotherapy) somewhat limited. The largest experience with IOERT in this patient group is from the Mayo Clinic. In a group of 140 patients with prior EBRT, the subsequent use of 30-Gy preoperative EBRT followed by IOERT (10 to 20 Gy based on extent of resection) resulted in a 3-year local control rate of 70% and overall survival rate of 30%. Again, no randomized, prospective data are available to more accurately assess the role of IORT in this patient group, but the single-institution data are encouraging.

Gastric Cancer

The clinical data regarding the integration of IORT as a component of combined modality treatment of resectable gastric cancer were recently summarized in detail.[37,38] Three randomized prospective trials of IOERT have been reported. In 1988, M. Abe from Kyoto University, Japan, reported a trial in which more than 200 patients with stage I to IV stomach cancer (using the Japanese Surgical Staging System) were randomized to surgery alone versus surgery + IOERT (28 to 35 Gy).[39] A nonstatistically significant trend toward improved 5-year overall survival was seen in stage II to IV patients. However, two smaller phase 3 studies did not show a survival benefit. At the NCI, 40 stage III and IV (American Joint Committee on Cancer) patients were randomized to surgery + IORT (20 Gy) versus surgery + EBRT (50 Gy), whereas at the University of Freiburg (Freiburg, Germany), 115 patients were randomized to surgery versus surgery + IORT (28 Gy).[40,41] Data from other single-institution, nonrandomized studies suggest a benefit to IORT or IORT + EBRT compared to surgery alone.[37] The present standard of care for locally advanced (node positive and/or margin positive) gastric cancer includes postoperative chemoradiation or perioperative chemotherapy alone, based on recent phase 3 trial experience.[42] Thus, any future trial testing the integration of IORT in locally advanced gastric cancer must include these approaches.

Pancreatic Cancer

The results of many single-institution, nonrandomized clinical trials in patients with pancreas cancer were recently summarized.[43,44] For patients found to have localized but technically unresectable disease, the use of IORT ± EBRT ± chemotherapy is associated with better long-term epigastric pain control but with no effect on median or overall survival. In patients with resectable pancreatic cancer, the combination of preoperative EBRT (± chemotherapy) followed by IORT appears to increase local control and overall survival modestly. Any future trials of IORT in pancreatic cancer will require the integration of more effective systemic therapy.

Sarcomas

IORT has played a role in the management of adult soft tissue sarcomas arising in the retroperitoneum, trunk, and extremities as a component of combined modality treatment.[45] IORT has also been used in the treatment of some primary bone sarcomas in adolescents. Both IOERT and HDR-IORT techniques have been used.

Retroperitoneal soft tissue sarcomas, although rare, are an appropriate tumor for using IORT because these tumors are typically large (>10 to 15 cm) and locally invasive, making wide excisions with negative margins very difficult to achieve. A comprehensive review of the IORT studies in retroperitoneal sarcomas is published.[46] In the only randomized, prospective trial, a small group of 35 patients with technically resectable retroperitoneal sarcomas were randomized to receive postoperative EBRT (50 to 55 Gy; control group; 20 patients) or IOERT (20 Gy to multiple abutting fields) plus reduced-dose postoperative EBRT (30 to 35 Gy; study group; 15 patients).[17] With a minimum follow-up of 5 years, in-field local recurrences occurred in 20% of the study group and in 80% of the controls (*P* < .001). However, there were no differences in overall survival or risk of distant metastases, which were correlated primarily with pathologic stage. Differences in the type of acute and late normal tissue complications were found with significantly increased gastrointestinal toxicities in the control group and significantly increased peripheral nerve toxicities in the study group. Multiple nonrandomized, single-institution studies support an improved local control rate with less peripheral nerve toxicities using IOERT doses of 15 Gy or less.[46] Two institutions have published their experience using combinations of EBRT and HDR-IORT for primary or locally recurrent retroperitoneal sarcomas. A prospective, nonrandomized trial at Memorial Sloan-Kettering Cancer Center (MSKCC) included 32 patients (12 with primary disease and 20 with recurrent disease) who each received 14 Gy at 0.5 cm deep to the resected tumor bed using HDR-IORT. The MSKCC group reported a 5-year local control rate of 74% and 54% and a 5-year overall survival rate of 55% and 30%, respectively, in the primary and recurrent tumor patient groups.[47] A second series of 46 patients with primary or recurrent retroperitoneal sarcomas from the Curie Cancer Center in France received 20-Gy HDR-IORT following a gross total resection (30 patients with R_0 resection and 16 patients with R_1 resection). These patients experienced actuarial 5-year overall survival and local recurrence survival rates of 55% and 51%, respectively.[48]

The IORT literature for extremity and truncal soft tissue sarcomas is summarized.[49] Although local recurrence risks using surgery and EBRT (either preoperative or postoperative) are low (5% to 8%) with R_0 resections, patients with positive margins or gross residual disease require higher EBRT doses, with an increased risk of acute and late normal tissue toxicities. For these patients, IOERT or HDR-IORT treatments have been used as a treatment boost while maintaining the EBRT dose at 45 to 50 Gy. In general, local control is excellent (≥85%), and normal tissue complications and functional outcomes are acceptable.[50]

The more limited experience with IORT in bone sarcomas is also reviewed.[51] Typically, IOERT has been used for marginally resected Ewing sarcomas and osteosarcomas in adolescents at centers in Germany, Spain, and Japan. Although local control is excellent in these high-risk patients, the risks of late normal tissue complications, including IORT-induced second cancers, are of concern, and long-term follow-up is needed before an endorsement of the role of IORT in these patient groups can be made.

Breast Cancer

IORT is playing a major role in the curative treatment of early-stage breast cancer throughout the world, as reviewed.[52] Based on several prior single-institution, nonrandomized studies, two large phase III studies have been designed for patients with early-stage disease to test the concept of IORT as full-dose, single-dose partial breast irradiation treatment compared to standard, conventionally fractionated whole-breast radiation therapy (WBRT). In addition, the concept of using IORT as a boost followed by WBRT for patients with adverse pathologic features is being evaluated by the European Group of the International Society of Intraoperative Radiotherapy (ISIORT Europe). A brief description of the two large phase III studies of definitive IORT and the ongoing single-arm IORT boost study is given later. A more detailed discussion of these trials is provided in the chapter of this book on breast cancer.

The Targeted Intraoperative Radiotherapy Trial enrolled and randomized more than 2,200 early-stage (T1, T2; N0) breast cancer patients with invasive ductal carcinoma without evidence of lobular carcinoma and older than 45 years of age to single-fraction, orthovoltage IORT to 20 Gy (surface dose) or conventionally fractionated WBRT to 50 Gy.[53] Only in the case of specific risk factors was the IORT complemented with WBRT. An interim analysis, published in February 2014, with a median follow-up of 5 years, reported a higher local recurrence risk at 4 years (3.3% in IORT arm vs. 1.3% in the WBRT arm, *P* = .042).[54] Longer follow-up is needed before definitive conclusions may be drawn. Although TARGIT-IORT is included in national guidelines for breast cancer treatment in Europe and Asia, it is not considered a national guideline in the United States. Two recent editorials have presented arguments that support or criticize the TARGIT-A trial design and data interpretation.[55,56]

Section II

Other Cancer Types

The clinical data regarding the use of IORT for lung cancers, head and neck cancers, CNS malignancies, and pediatric cancers were recently reviewed in detail,[33] and the reader is referred to chapters in this textbook on specific tumor sites for additional information. No prospective, randomized trials of IORT for these cancers are available or in development.

REFERENCES

1. Hu K, Yom S, Kaplan M, et al. Head and neck cancer. In: Gunderson L, Willett C, Calvo F, et al., eds. *Intraoperative irradiation. techniques and results.* 2nd ed. Totowa, NJ: Humana Press, 2011:163–168.

2. Kinsella TJ, DeLuca AM, Barnes M, et al. Threshold dose for peripheral neuropathy following intraoperative radiotherapy (IORT) in a large animal model. *Int J Radiat Oncol Biol Phys* 1991;20(4):697–701.

3. Barnes M, Duray P, DeLuca A, et al. Tumor induction following intraoperative radiotherapy: late results of the National Cancer Institute canine trials. *Int J Radiat Oncol Biol Phys* 1990;19(3):651–660.

4. Sindelar WF, Kinsella TJ. Normal tissue tolerance to intraoperative radiotherapy. *Surg Oncol Clin N Am* 2003;12(4):925–942.

5. Vujaskovic Z, Willett CG, Tepper J, et al. Normal tissue tolerance to IOERT, EBRT, or both: animal and clinical studies. In: Gunderson L, Willett CG, Calvo F, et al., eds. *Intraoperative irradiation: techniques and results.* Totowa, NJ: Humana Press, 2011:119–138.

6. Sindelar WF, Tepper JE, Kinsella TJ, et al. Late effects of intraoperative radiation therapy on retroperitoneal tissues, intestine, and bile duct in a large animal model. *Int J Radiat Oncol Biol Phys* 1994;29(4):781–788.

7. Gillette EL, Powers BE, McChesney SL, et al. Response of aorta and branch arteries to experimental intraoperative irradiation. *Int J Radiat Oncol Biol Phys* 1989;17(6):1247–1255.

8. Johnstone PA, Sprague M, DeLuca AM, et al. Effects of intraoperative radiotherapy on vascular grafts in a canine model. *Int J Radiat Oncol Biol Phys* 1994;29(5):1015–1025.

9. Tepper JE, Sindelar W, Travis EL, et al. Tolerance of canine anastomoses to intraoperative radiation therapy. *Int J Radiat Oncol Biol Phys* 1983;9(7):987–992.

10. Sindelar WF, Tepper J, Travis EL. Tolerance of bile duct to intraoperative irradiation. *Surgery* 1982;92(3):533–540.

11. Gillette EL, Gillette S, Powers BE. Studies at Colorado State University of normal tissue tolerance of beagles to IOERT, EBRT or a combination. In: Gunderson L, Willett CG, Calvo F, et al., eds. *Intraoperative irradiation: techniques and results.* 1st ed. Totowa, NJ: Humana Press, 1999:147–163.

12. DeLuca AM, Johnstone PA, Ollayos CW, et al. Tolerance of the bladder to intraoperative radiation in a canine model: a five-year follow-up. *Int J Radiat Oncol Biol Phys* 1994;30(2):339–345.

13. Kinsella TJ, Sindelar WF, DeLuca AM, et al. Tolerance of the canine bladder to intraoperative radiation therapy: an experimental study. *Int J Radiat Oncol Biol Phys* 1988;14(5):939–946.

14. Barnes M, Pass H, DeLuca A, et al. Response of the mediastinal and thoracic viscera of the dog to intraoperative radiation therapy (IORT). *Int J Radiat Oncol Biol Phys* 1987;13(3):371–378.

15. Tochner ZA, Pass HI, Sindelar WF, et al. Long term tolerance of thoracic organs to intraoperative radiotherapy. *Int J Radiat Oncol Biol Phys* 1992;22(1):65–69.

16. Pass HI, Sindelar WF, Kinsella TJ, et al. Delivery of intraoperative radiation therapy after pneumonectomy: experimental observations and early clinical results. *Ann Thorac Surg* 1987;44(1):14–20.

17. Sindelar WF, Kinsella TJ, Chen PW, et al. Intraoperative radiotherapy in retroperitoneal sarcomas. Final results of a prospective, randomized, clinical trial. *Arch Surg* 1993;128(4):402–410.

18. Johnstone PA, DeLuca AM, Bacher JD, et al. Clinical toxicity of peripheral nerve to intraoperative radiotherapy in a canine model. *Int J Radiat Oncol Biol Phys* 1995;32(4):1031–1034.

19. Vujaskovic Z, Gillette SM, Powers BE, et al. Intraoperative radiation (IORT) injury to sciatic nerve in a large animal model. *Radiother Oncol* 1994;30(2):133–139.

20. Gillette SM, Gillette EL, Powers BE, et al. Radiation-induced osteosarcoma in dogs after external beam or intraoperative radiation therapy. *Cancer Res* 1990;50(1):54–57.

21. Johnstone PA, Laskin WB, DeLuca AM, et al. Tumors in dogs exposed to experimental intraoperative radiotherapy. *Int J Radiat Oncol Biol Phys* 1996;34(4):853–857.

22. Beddar AS, Biggs PJ, Chang S, et al. Intraoperative radiation therapy using mobile electron linear accelerators: report of AAPM Radiation Therapy Committee Task Group No. 72. *Med Phys* 2006;33(5):1476–1489.

23. Palta JR, Biggs PJ, Hazle JD, et al. Intraoperative electron beam radiation therapy: technique, dosimetry, and dose specification: report of task force 48 of the Radiation Therapy Committee, American Association of Physicists in Medicine. *Int J Radiat Oncol Biol Phys* 1995;33(3):725–746.

24. Avanzo M, Rink A, Dassie A, et al. In vivo dosimetry with radiochromic films in low-voltage intraoperative radiotherapy of the breast. *Med Phys* 2012;39(5):2359–2368.

25. Consorti R, Petrucci A, Fortunato F, et al. In vivo dosimetry with MOSFETs: dosimetric characterization and first clinical results in intraoperative radiotherapy. *Int J Radiat Oncol Biol Phys* 2005;63(3):952–960.

26. Nath R, Anderson LL, Luxton G, et al. Dosimetry of interstitial brachytherapy sources: recommendations of the AAPM Radiation Therapy Committee Task Group No. 43. American Association of Physicists in Medicine. *Med Phys* 1995;22(2):209–234.

27. Rivard MJ, Butler WM, DeWerd LA, et al. Supplement to the 2004 update of the AAPM Task Group No. 43 Report. *Med Phys* 2007;34(6):2187–2205.

28. Furhang EE, Sillanpaa JK, Hu KS, et al. HDR-IORT: physics and techniques. In: Gunderson L, Willett CG, Calvo F, et al., eds. *Intraoperative irradiation: techniques and results.* 2nd ed. Totowa, NJ: Humana Press, 2011:73–84.

29. Kutcher GJ, Coia L, Gillin M, et al. Comprehensive QA for radiation oncology: report of AAPM Radiation Therapy Committee Task Group 40. *Med Phys* 1994;21(4):581–618.

30. Anderson LL, Hoffman MR, Harrington PJ, et al. Atlas generation for intraoperative high dose rate brachytherapy. *J Brachyther Int* 1997;13:333–340.

31. Kraus-Tiefenbacher U, Biggs PJ, Vaidya J, et al. Electronic brachytherapy/Low KV IORT: physics and techniques. In: Gunderson L, Willett CG, Calvo F, et al., eds. *Intraoperative irradiation: techniques and results.* 2nd ed. Totowa, NJ: Humana Press, 2011:85–98.

32. Nag S, Willett CG, Gunderson L, et al. IORT with electron-beam, high-dose-rate brachytherapy or low-KV/electronic brachytherapy: methodological comparisons. In: Gunderson L, Willett CG, Calvo F, et al., eds. *Intraoperative irradiation: techniques and results.* 2nd ed. Totowa, NJ: Humana Press, 2011:99–115.

33. Gunderson L, Willett CG, Calvo F, et al. *Intraoperative irradiation: techniques and results.* 2nd ed. Totowa, NJ: Humana Press, 2011.

34. Nils D, Arvold ND, Hong TS, et al. Primary colorectal cancer. In: Gunderson L, Willett CG, Calvo F, et al., eds. *Intraoperative irradiation: techniques and results.* 2nd ed. Totowa, NJ: Humana Press, 2011:297–322.

35. Mirnezami R, Chang GJ, Das P, et al. Intraoperative radiotherapy in colorectal cancer: systematic review and meta-analysis of techniques, long-term outcomes, and complications. *Surg Oncol* 2013;22(1):22–35.

36. Haddock MG, Nelson H, Valentini V, et al. Recurrent colorectal cancer. In: Gunderson L, Willett CG, Calvo F, et al., eds. *Intraoperative irradiation: techniques and results.* 2nd ed. Totowa, NJ: Humana Press, 2011:323–351.

37. Martinez-Monge R, Gaztanaga M, Alvarez-Cienfuegos J, et al. Gastric cancer. In: Gunderson L, Willett CG, Calvo F, et al., eds. *Intraoperative irradiation: techniques and results.* 2nd ed. Totowa, NJ: Humana Press, 2011:223–248.

38. Bacalbasa N, Balescu I, Calin M, et al. Intraoperative radiation therapy in gastric cancer. *J Med Life* 2014;7(2):128–131.

39. Abe M, Takahashi M, Ono K, et al. Japan gastric trials in intraoperative radiation therapy. *Int J Radiat Oncol Biol Phys* 1988;15(6):1431–1433.

40. Kramling HJ, Willich N, Cramer C, et al. Early results of IORT in the treatment of gastric cancer. *Front Radiat Ther Oncol* 1997;31:157–160.

41. Sindelar WF, Kinsella TJ, Tepper JE, et al. Randomized trial of intraoperative radiotherapy in carcinoma of the stomach. *Am J Surg* 1993;165(1):178–186; discussion 186–177.

42. Ajani JA, D'Amico TA, Almhanna K, et al. Gastric cancer, version 3.2016, NCCN clinical practice guidelines in oncology. *J Natl Compr Canc Netw* 2016;14(10):1286–1312.

43. Miller RC, Valentini V, Moss A, et al. Pancreas cancer. In: Gunderson L, Willett CG, Calvo F, et al., eds. *Intraoperative irradiation: techniques and results.* 2nd ed. Totowa, NJ: Humana Press, 2011:249–271.

44. Krempien R, Roeder F. Intraoperative radiation therapy (IORT) in pancreatic cancer. *Radiat Oncol* 2017;12(1):8.

45. Roeder F, Krempien R. Intraoperative radiation therapy (IORT) in soft-tissue sarcoma. *Radiat Oncol* 2017;12(1):20.

46. Czito B, Donohue J, Willett CG, et al. Retroperitoneal sarcomas. In: Gunderson LL, Willett CG, Calvo F, et al., eds. *Intraoperative irradiation: techniques and results.* 2nd ed. Totowa, NJ: Humana Press, 2011:353–386.

47. Alektiar KM, Hu K, Anderson L, et al. High-dose-rate intraoperative radiation therapy (HDR-IORT) for retroperitoneal sarcomas. *Int J Radiat Oncol Biol Phys* 2000;47(1):157–163.

48. Dziewirski W, Rutkowski P, Nowecki ZI, et al. Surgery combined with intraoperative brachytherapy in the treatment of retroperitoneal sarcomas. *Ann Surg Oncol* 2006;13(2):245–252.

49. Petersen IA, Krempien R, Beauchamp C, et al. Extremity and trunk soft-tissue sarcomas. In: Gunderson LL, Willett CG, Calvo F, et al., eds. *Intraoperative irradiation: techniques and results.* 2nd ed. Totowa, NJ: Humana Press, 2011:387–405.

50. Kunos C, Colussi V, Getty P, et al. Intraoperative electron radiotherapy for extremity sarcomas does not increase acute or late morbidity. *Clin Orthop Relat Res* 2006(May):247–252.

51. Calvo F, Sierrasesumaga L, Patino A, et al. Bone sarcomas. In: Gunderson LL, Willett CG, Calvo F, et al., eds. *Intraoperative irradiation: techniques and results.* 2nd ed. Totowa, NJ: Humana Press, 2011:407–429.

52. Sedlmayer F, DuBois J-B, Reitsamer R, et al. Breast cancer. In: Gunderson LL, Willett CG, Calvo F, et al., eds. *Intraoperative irradiation: techniques and results.* 2nd ed. Totowa, NJ: Humana Press, 2011:189–200.

53. Vaidya JS, Joseph DJ, Tobias JS, et al. Targeted intraoperative radiotherapy versus whole breast radiotherapy for breast cancer (TARGIT-A trial): an international, prospective, randomised, non-inferiority phase 3 trial. *Lancet* 2010;376(9735):91–102.

54. Vaidya JS, Wenz F, Bulsara M, et al. Risk-adapted targeted intraoperative radiotherapy versus whole-breast radiotherapy for breast cancer: 5-year results for local control and overall survival from the TARGIT-A randomised trial. *Lancet* 2014;383(9917):603–613.

55. Hepel J, Wazer DE. A flawed study should not define a new standard of care. *Int J Radiat Oncol Biol Phys* 2015;91(2):255–257.

56. Vaidya JS, Bulsara M, Wenz F, et al. Pride, prejudice, or science: attitudes towards the results of the TARGIT-A trial of targeted intraoperative radiation therapy for breast cancer. *Int J Radiat Oncol Biol Phys* 2015;92(3):491–497.

CHAPTER 21

Proton Therapy

Nancy P. Mendenhall and Zuofeng Li

INTRODUCTION

The potential to improve the therapeutic ratio in radiation therapy has fueled interest in proton therapy. This chapter will touch on the rationale, evolving technology, applications and outcomes, and current challenges associated with proton therapy.

RATIONALE

Therapeutic Ratio

With any medical intervention, there is an optimal balance between the potential to benefit and the potential to harm a patient, known as the therapeutic ratio. In radiation oncology, it is the balance between radiation effects on the tumor and radiation effects on normal, nontargeted tissues. This ratio informs every physician and patient decision. Different priorities may drive different decisions in certain clinical situations. One physician might recommend a treatment that results in a lower probability of disease control but minimizes the risk of optic nerve damage, whereas another physician might recommend a treatment that results in a higher probability of disease control but carries a greater risk of optic nerve damage. In another example, the potential risks of low-dose radiation exposure to a large volume of the brain tissue may be of great concern to the parents of a young child, but not of concern to an elderly patient with a short life expectancy. In evaluating new radiation modalities, the first question is whether there exists a potential to improve the therapeutic ratio.

The Impact of Dose Distribution on the Therapeutic Ratio

Many factors influence radiation effects and the therapeutic ratio: total dose, dose intensity (the overall time and number of fractions), relative biologic effectiveness (RBE), and modifying factors, such as chemotherapy, patient age, and comorbidities. No factor is as important as dose distribution—the dose to the target compared with the dose to nontargeted normal tissues—because radiation therapy is a nonspecific intervention that affects both normal and cancerous cells. A basic principle in radiation oncology is that the higher and/or more intense the radiation dose, the greater the probability of tumor control. Similarly, the higher and/or more intense the radiation dose to a normal tissue, the greater the probability of injury. A second less well-understood principle is that the volume of tumor or normal tissue exposed to various radiation dose levels impacts the effect. For example, a higher dose of radiation to an organ may be tolerated if the absolute or relative volume of exposure to the organ at risk (OAR) is limited. In addition, there may be critical components of either an OAR or a tumor that require a higher or lower dose for a clinical response. For example, the hypoxic section or the positron-emission tomography (PET)-avid portion of a tumor may require a higher dose than the rest of the tumor for disease control. These principles of dose and volume response relationships have been observed in both malignancies and normal tissues but may not always be apparent if effective doses are not delivered to critical volumes (of tumor or a normal tissue), if adequate tools for measuring response (toxicity or functional compromise) are not available, or if observation time is insufficient for manifestation of the effect.

The primary barrier to maximizing local tumor control through dose escalation or intensification is the risk of damaging normal tissues, either by delivering too high a dose to a critical tissue or by exposing too great a volume of the critical normal tissue to a potentially harmful dose of radiation. *The most direct means of improving the therapeutic ratio is by reducing radiation dose and exposure to nontargeted tissues, which both reduce toxicity and facilitate dose escalation for increased tumor control: herein lies the rationale for proton therapy.*

The Problem with Photons (X-Rays) and the Promise and Challenge of Protons

The pattern of dose deposition with photon-based external beam radiotherapy (Fig. 21.1) is problematic because the dose to tissues along the beam entrance path is always higher than the dose to the target and additional dose is deposited in nontargeted tissues along the exit path of the beam. *Thus, most of the radiation dose with photon-based therapy is deposited outside the target.*

Many elegant strategies have been developed for offsetting this basic problem (4-field box technique, stereotactic radiosurgery and stereotactic radiation therapy [SRT], three-dimensional conformal radiation therapy [3DCRT], intensity-modulated radiation therapy [IMRT], tomotherapy, volumetric modulated arc therapy [VMAT], etc.), but with these technologies, radiation to nontargeted tissues is primarily redistributed rather than reduced. Because the total dose to a given tissue is one of the key determinants of toxicity, certain toxicities are reduced when using these sophisticated techniques. It is likely, however, that

FIGURE 21.1. As shown here, the shapes of the depth-dose curves for electrons (*tan*), photons/x-rays (*orange*), a pristine proton Bragg peak (*purple*), and an SOBP comprised of multiple pristine Bragg peaks (*blue*) differ significantly. Compared to photons or electrons, the entrance dose with protons is constant and reduced relative to the target dose and there is no exit dose. The depth of penetration is much greater and the dose falloff at the end of the proton range much sharper for protons than for electrons. The depth of the proton Bragg peak can be varied according to acceleration energy; current cyclotrons and synchrotrons accelerate protons to energies sufficient to place the Bragg peak at 30- to 35-cm depth in tissue for coverage of deep-seated tumors. Because of the entrance and exit doses with photons, most of the radiation energy is deposited outside of the target, whereas with protons, most of the radiation energy is deposited inside of the target.

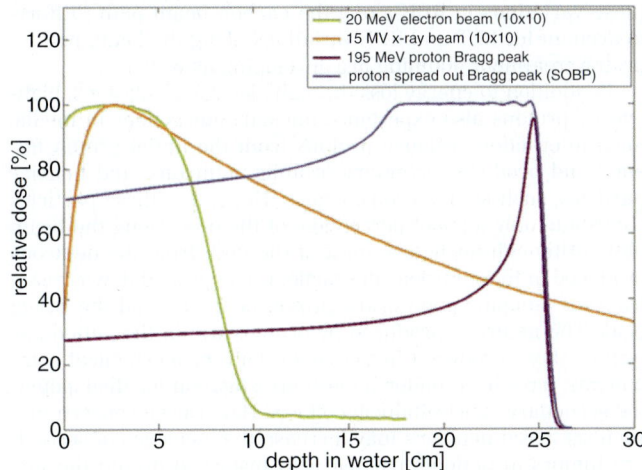

other toxicities will increase owing to methods that redistribute integral dose and expose greater volumes of normal tissue to lower doses of radiation. Some effects from low-dose exposure may require more time for clinical manifestation (second malignancies), and some may require more subtle tools for detection (neurocognitive testing), leading to an early underestimation of toxicity with these sophisticated photon delivery methods.

The pattern of dose deposition with protons differs significantly from that of photons. A proton carries a positive charge, which means it can be accelerated and directed by magnets; the proton has mass, which means it will not travel an infinite distance but rather only to the range or depth in tissue determined by its acceleration energy. In a patient, protons can be made to stop at a depth corresponding to the tumor depth. As protons traverse matter, they lose energy primarily through interactions with atomic electrons. Because of the significantly larger mass of protons (~1800×) relative to electrons, protons lose only a small portion of their energy in each interaction (in contrast to x-rays) and experience only small directional changes.

As protons traverse matter, the rate of energy loss in electronic interactions is described by the linear stopping power, $S(E)$, defined as dE/dx, where dE is the mean energy lost by a proton in electronic collisions over a distance of dx in media. A more commonly used function is the mass stopping power, $s = S(E)/\rho$, which denotes the energy loss dE when protons travel through a distance of dx in a media of mass density ρ.[1]

Linear energy transfer (LET) is closely related to stopping power. Although stopping power indicates energy lost by the protons, LET denotes the energy transferred to a medium as the protons traverse it. LET therefore represents the density of energy deposition in media and is directly related to the local RBE of the radiation. At higher energies (e.g., along the beam's entrance path), protons have a small stopping power and low LET values; their LET values increase sharply by up to two orders of magnitude as the protons' energy decreases just before coming to a complete stop. This phenomenon creates a characteristic pattern of dose deposition with protons known as the Bragg peak: a small, nearly constant rate of dose deposition along the entrance path followed by a sharp peak immediately before the protons stop in media. Because RBE values are related to LET values, the RBE values also rise sharply near the end of a proton-beam range. Much work has been done to determine *in vitro* and *in vivo* proton-beam RBE values.[1] Currently in proton therapy treatment planning, an RBE multiplicative factor of 1.10 is uniformly applied to the physical dose[2] without explicitly accounting for the increased RBE values near the end of a proton-beam range. The actual RBE-corrected dose at the very end of the range may exceed the physical dose by up to 25%, thus producing an RBE value up to 1.3 at the very end of the proton range.[3] Enhanced RBE effects are more significant in heavier ions like carbon, and nascent carbon ion treatment planning systems are attempting to account for these variations in RBE along the carbon beam path.[4] Efforts to account for LET and RBE variations along the beam path in proton treatment planning are developing as well.[5]

In addition to energy loss through electronic collisions, high-energy protons also experience nuclear interactions in media. Such interactions remove protons from the initial proton fluence and produce secondary protons, neutrons, and heavier particles, such as deuterons, tritons, He, and α; these particles contribute only a small percentage of the dose along the beam path.[6] Although negligible, most of the dose from the neutrons produced in these nuclear interactions is deposited downstream from the stopping point of the proton beam, beyond the Bragg peak. The neutrons produced by protons within the patient, as well as those produced in the beam delivery mechanical components, have been under intense investigation for their potential secondary cancer-inducing effects. Hall[7] raised concern that such scattered neutrons may increase the incidence of secondary tumors in patients treated with historical proton therapy systems, similar to the transition from conventional 3DCRT to

IMRT.[8] Much research has been performed to estimate secondary cancer risks from contemporary proton therapy systems using either scattering beam techniques or scanning-beam techniques.[9] Consistent reductions in secondary cancer induction have been predicted with protons compared to photons in studies of medulloblastoma, prostate cancer, and liver cancer.[10–12] A clinical outcome study comparing actual secondary cancers between a cohort of patients treated with protons at the Harvard Cyclotron and a cohort of photon-treated patients matched by age and tumor type from the Surveillance, Epidemiology, and End Results database has shown nearly twice as many secondary cancers in the photon cohort.[13] Modern proton therapy equipment produces fewer neutron contaminants than the early proton therapy sources in physics research laboratories, so it appears that neutron production should be of much less concern for late effects than excess integral dose from photons.

The primary rationale for an improved therapeutic ratio with protons, compared with photons, is thus the significant reduction in integral dose (dose to nontargeted tissues) related to a significantly reduced entrance path dose and the absence of any exit path dose, which should translate into a lower risk of complications for a given target dose and greater probability of tumor control. A lower risk of complications could also be leveraged to permit dose escalation or intensification (yielding higher disease control in certain settings) or to facilitate hypofractionation (reducing patient inconvenience and treatment costs in other settings).

There is emerging evidence of another difference between proton and photon radiation therapy, which may provide a second rationale for an increased therapeutic ratio from proton therapy. The predominant pattern of DNA damage with photon therapy is isolated double-stranded DNA breaks; however, after proton radiation, most DNA lesions are clustered double-stranded breaks, which may be more difficult to repair and require slower repair processes, possibly homologous rather than nonhomologous repair pathways. It is possible that these differences in DNA damage and tissue repair responses provide part of the explanation for apparent RBE differences and a rationale to expect higher disease control rates but also potentially higher complication rates with proton therapy.[14–18] Some tumors and host conditions may have genetic variations that impact responses to radiation in general and proton therapy specifically.[18]

TECHNOLOGY

Beam Production and Transport

Protons are produced either from hydrogen gas obtained from electrolysis of deionized water or from commercially available high-purity hydrogen gas. Application of a high-voltage electric current to the hydrogen gas strips the electrons from the hydrogen atoms, leaving positively charged protons. The protons are then accelerated to energies applicable for clinical proton therapy with either a cyclotron or a synchrotron (Fig. 21.2). Energies on the order of 230 MeV are required for penetrating approximately 32 cm into a tissue. Cyclotrons produce a continuous beam of nearly monoenergetic and unidirectional protons. The beam must then be degraded to meet specific requirements for each treatment field in each patient. This process takes place shortly after the beam exits the cyclotron in a device known as the "energy degrader," which is composed of a material of variable thickness with a low atomic number. The proton beam exiting the energy degrader will have a spread of energies centered around the final energy spread necessary for coverage of the target. An energy selection system (ESS), consisting of energy slits, bending magnets, and focusing magnets, is then used to eliminate protons with excessive energy or deviations in angular direction. Cyclotrons can produce a large proton-beam current of up to 800 nA and thus deliver proton therapy at a high dose rate using either a double-scattering technique or a scanning technique.

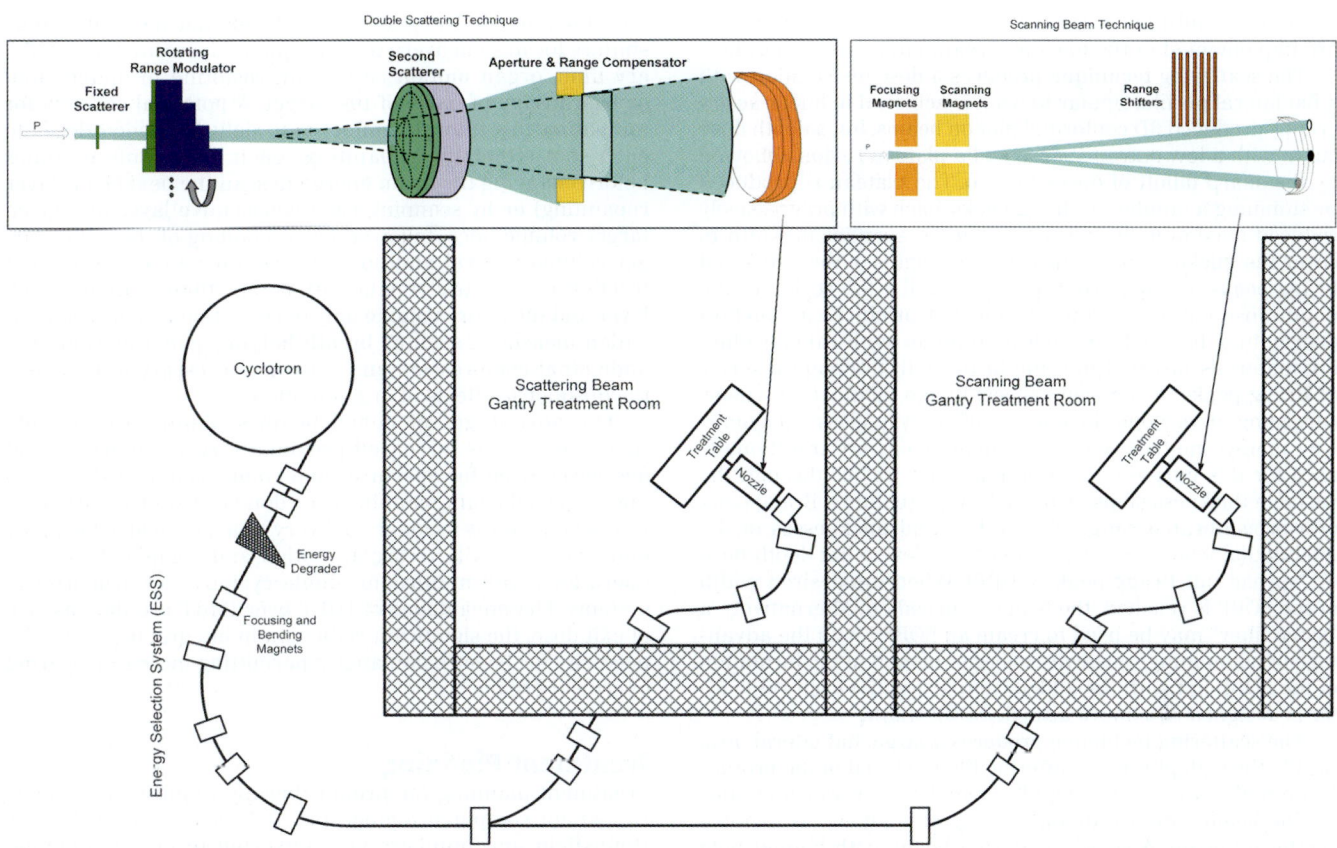

FIGURE 21.2. A proton therapy system with a cyclotron, ESS, beamline, gantry, and nozzle. Scattering is illustrated in the nozzle on the left and scanning in the nozzle on the right.

Synchrotrons, however, produce proton beams of varying energies, which can be selected, thereby eliminating the need for the energy degrader and energy selection devices. A proton pulse exiting a preaccelerator, with energy typically up to 7 MeV, is injected into the ring-shaped accelerator. Each complete circuit of the proton pulse through the accelerator ring structure incrementally increases the proton pulse energy. When the desired beam energy is reached, the proton pulse is extracted from the accelerator. The time segment between pulses depends on the final energy required of the proton beam, ranging from subseconds to several seconds for the highest beam energy. The pulsed nature of the beam introduces additional complexity in certain treatment delivery scenarios, such as gated treatment of mobile targets and intensity-modulated proton therapy (IMPT).[19] Beam currents from synchrotrons are typically much lower than with cyclotrons, thus limiting the maximum dose rates that can be used for patient treatment, especially for larger field sizes. The maximum dose rate available from a commercially available synchrotron-based proton therapy system for a 25×25-cm^2 field has been specified at 0.8 Gy/min.[20] The elimination of the energy degrader and selection system removes a major source of neutron production and thus subsequent activation of beamline components in the accelerator vault. A synchrotron vault is therefore accessible immediately after the beam is stopped for maintenance, whereas for a cyclotron vault, approximately 30 minutes is necessary to allow the neutron-activated parts of the accelerator and ESS to "cool down" before maintenance can be performed, sometimes longer if access to internal parts of the cyclotron is required. The shielding requirements for cyclotrons are also higher than for synchrotrons because of the higher neutron radiation produced by the ESS. However, the overall footprint of a cyclotron vault, including the additional shielding required, is actually similar to or smaller than that of a synchrotron vault because of the smaller physical dimensions of cyclotrons.

The proton beam, on exiting the ESS for a cyclotron-based system or exiting the accelerator for a synchrotron-based system, is transported to the treatment room(s) via the beam transport system. Maintenance of beam focusing, centering, spot size, and divergence throughout the beam transport system is critical to maintaining a high-quality proton beam for treatment delivery. Paganetti et al.[21] performed Monte Carlo calculations of the dosimetric effect of proton-beam energy spread, spot size, and angular energy spread on the shape of the Bragg peak. They found that small deviations in these parameters from their nominal values result in a widening of the Bragg peak and increased entrance doses. Beam transport systems in clinical proton facilities therefore include bending and focusing magnets and beam profile monitors so that the proton-beam quality may be monitored and adjusted ("tuned") as it is transported through the beam transport system.

Recent progress in accelerating and control technologies has led to new designs of proton therapy systems in the form of single-treatment room systems with small cyclotrons that may be mounted on a gantry, as well as dielectric wall accelerators and laser-accelerated accelerators.[22] Single-room proton therapy systems are currently available from a number of commercial vendors, each with its own strengths and weaknesses. Dielectric wall accelerators and laser-accelerated systems are currently under development. One of the primary drivers for development of these single-room proton therapy solutions is facility cost reduction (see "Challenges" below).

Beam Delivery

The proton beam exiting the transport system (Fig. 21.2) is a pencil-shaped beam with minimal energy and direction spread. The beam has a small spot size in its lateral direction and forms a narrow Bragg peak in its depth direction in water. Two basic techniques have been developed to convert this narrow pencil beam into a dose distribution suitable for treatment of a 3D target, broadly categorized into the "scattering technique" and the "scanning technique." These techniques are implemented in the machine treatment head or "nozzle."

The scattering technique produces a dose distribution with a flat lateral profile, similar to what is achieved in linear accelerator–produced 3D conformal photon beams, but a depth dose curve with a low entrance dose and a plateau region, followed by the sharp falloff of doses to zero. The plateau is produced by summing a number of Bragg peaks, each with progressively reduced maximum energy and range, to a sufficient width to cover the thickness of the target. The weights of the individual Bragg peaks are optimized to achieve a flat top region of the depth-dose curve. A proton beam that produces a constant energy may be used for such treatments, with range-reducing materials inserted into the beam path to create a series of Bragg peaks of reduced ranges. Range modulation wheels consisting of variable thicknesses of "acrylic glass" (polymerized methyl methacrylate) or graphite steps are traditionally used for this purpose.[21] The proton beam travels through the variable thickness steps, with each step creating a Bragg peak of a precalibrated range. The widths and thicknesses of the modulation wheels are calibrated to achieve a flat depth dose or "spread-out Bragg peak" (SOBP). When the desired width of the SOBP is reached, the beam is turned off. Alternatively, a "ridge filter" may be used to create an SOBP[23] with the advantage of eliminating sensitivity to organ motion in the formation of the SOBP but with the added complexity that each ridge filter is designed to achieve a single SOBP width.

The scattering technique produces a large, flat lateral dose profile through physical scattering filters placed in the proton-beam path.[21] One scattering filter may be used, which creates a wide beam with a Gaussian dose profile known as a single scattering beam. A single scattering beam, with limited field sizes, is used primarily in dedicated eye treatment rooms for proton therapy of eye tumors, such as choroidal melanoma, and proton stereotactic radiosurgery treatments of brain lesions. Alternatively, and more often, a second scattering filter can be added into the beam that flattens the lateral dose profile, known as a double-scattering beam. Apertures fabricated out of brass or other metals are used to confine the treatment field to the target. A tissue-equivalent range compensator, or bolus, is designed to adjust the beam range within the field to conform to the distal profile of the target.[24] With the scattering technique, it is not possible to achieve conformity of the dose distribution to the proximal contour of the target.

In the scanning technique, as the pencil beam exits the transport system, it is magnetically steered laterally to deliver dose to the treatment field.[25–27] The proton-beam intensity may be modulated as the beam is moved across the field, resulting in intensity-modulated proton beam therapy, or IMPT, technique delivery. Current implementation of IMPT uses the "spot-scanning" technique, in which the beam is moved from one spot, where a prescribed dose is delivered, to the next spot. In the beam axis direction, IMPT treatments are delivered using a layer-stacking technique. A pencil beam with a pristine peak is scanned through the deepest layer of the target to deliver the intensity-modulated dose distribution for the layer before a range shifter—effectively an energy degrader of predetermined thickness—is inserted into the beam path to deliver dose to a depth immediately proximal to the deepest layer. Doses to each subsequent layer are delivered by inserting additional range shifters. The size of the spot, represented by the sigma of the Gaussian function describing the pencil beam profile, is a critical parameter of the pencil beam. Smaller beam sigma values allow intricate sculpting of the intensity-modulated dose distribution but require increased control system complexity and delivery time; larger beam sigma values result in faster dose delivery but produce a greater lateral penumbra and a reduced dose gradient at interface regions of target and critical organs.

Similar to the interplay effect reported for IMRT,[28–30] scanning techniques are sensitive to organ motion because time is required for moving the pencil beam across the treatment field for dose delivery to a given layer and inserting range shifters for dose delivery to subsequent layers; over the delivery time, organ motion can occur, resulting in under- and/or overdosage of parts of the target. A potential strategy for mitigating this interplay effect is to deliver divided doses to each spot either by "repainting" each layer multiple times before changing the beam energy to scan the next layer (layer repainting) or by scanning each consecutive layer of a given target volume once, followed by rescanning of the entire target volume several additional times during each treatment fraction (volumetric repainting), rather than scanning each layer and the entire volume only once.[31] Standard motion mitigation measures, such as breath holding, gated therapy, and abdominal compression, may also be necessary to minimize the dosimetric effects of organ motion.

The advantages of pencil beam scanning over double scattering are its increased proximal target conformity and decreased need for apertures and compensators A disadvantage of pencil beam scanning over double scattering with current technology is its longer delivery time per field, which may enhance sensitivity to organ motion and complicate system operations with multiroom, single cyclotron or synchrotron systems. The advantages of IMPT over IMRT are the absence of exit dose, the significant reduction in integral dose, and the necessity for fewer beam angles permitting increased sparing of critical organs.

Treatment Planning

Treatment planning for proton therapy requires a volumetric patient computed tomography (CT) scan dataset. The CT Hounsfield unit numbers are converted to proton stopping power values for calculating the proton range required for the treatment field.[32,33] Unlike the relatively reliable conversion of CT numbers to relative electron density for photon dose calculations, errors and uncertainties in the conversion of CT numbers to proton stopping power in proton dose calculations translate linearly into proton range calculation uncertainties and errors. In clinical practice, these uncertainties are handled during the treatment planning process by bracketing the intended SOBP with a distal margin beyond the target and a proximal margin before the target in the range calculation of each treatment field.[34] Other considerations in determining the values for distal and proximal margins include target motion, daily setup errors, beam delivery uncertainties, and uncertainties in patient anatomy and physiology changes throughout treatment that could affect the water-equivalent depth of the target. It is worth noting that the concept of PTV, as defined in the various International Commission on Radiation Units and Measurements reports,[35,36] does not strictly apply to proton therapy. Generally, a planning target volume (PTV) expansion, with either uniform or nonuniform margins, is used for photon planning, which accommodates maximum target motion and setup error in each of the patient axes (longitudinal, lateral, and anterior/posterior). In contrast to photon planning, the PTV for proton therapy is specific for each treatment field. In the lateral direction of the beam's eye view of a proton field, margins are identical to traditional definitions, but the distal and proximal margins along the beam axis are calculated to account for proton-specific uncertainties. The lower entrance dose and absence of exit dose of a proton beam afford additional flexibility in selection of beam angles for which lateral target motion and setup error are minimal; thus, the PTV expansion margin may be less for a given proton-beam angle than would be required with IMRT to account for uncertainties for all beam angles. Commercial proton treatment planning systems have been designed to allow for the definition of beam-specific PTV volumes such that the range and modulation width (or SOBP width) of each beam may be calculated with adequate consideration of the varying distal and proximal target margins.

The pencil beam scanning treatment technique, with its additional ability to modulate dose intensity within and outside of the target region, requires additional considerations in treatment plan optimization. The single-field uniform dose (SFUD), or single-field optimization technique, allows the treatment planning system optimizer algorithm to optimize the treatment plan on a field-by-field basis, so that each field will deliver a nearly uniform dose that covers the target to the extent that OAR protection constraints permit. The SFUD technique provides the most plan robustness after a proper passive-scattering treatment plan, despite various physical and physiologic uncertainties that may significantly perturb dose delivery accuracy, including the interplay effect of moving organs, with potential compromises in plan quality of conformity and OAR protection. The multifield uniform dose (MFUD) optimization technique, on the other hand, allows each treatment field to deliver a heavily modulated dose distribution to a subvolume of the target and relies on the accurate delivery and combination of all fields to achieve plan goals. This MFUD optimization technique can therefore achieve the highest plan quality, but potentially increases sensitivity to the effects of delivery uncertainties, and should therefore be applied judiciously. IMPT plans may use either SFUD or MFUD or a combination of the two. Pencil beam treatment plans can additionally be optimized with consideration for various sources and magnitudes of delivery uncertainties, such as range uncertainties and setup errors, resulting in the so-called robust optimization, which allows optimization of a treatment plan over the 10 breathing phases of a four-dimensional CT scan of a moving target. The effectiveness of these newer optimization techniques must be carefully evaluated, disease site by disease site, before they are broadly accepted for treatment planning.

State-of-the-art proton therapy dose calculations use pencil beam algorithms,[37–40] which model proton interactions and scattering in various media of the beam path, including the nozzle, range compensators, and patient. Monte Carlo calculations have been used to study the accuracy of such dose calculation algorithms, with results indicating errors near tissue interfaces, particularly near interfaces of media differing in density and composition, such as the air cavity and bone in head and neck treatments.[41,42] Several fast Monte Carlo calculation algorithms have been proposed to improve proton therapy dose calculation accuracy,[43–46] which will soon be available in commercial proton treatment planning systems.

As of yet, there are no clear class solutions to treatment planning, although it is agreed that beams that stop at the interface of a critical organ should generally be avoided because of range uncertainties and our current inability to account for changes in RBE at the end of the range. Concerns regarding dose delivery time, intrafraction organ motion, potential changes in beam path length and composition, and adjacency of critical organs impact decisions regarding the number of fields to use, overall plan robustness, scanning versus scattering delivery modes, single-field versus multifield optimization of the treatment plan with scanning modes, and clinical operations.

Even with strategies to account for proton range uncertainties, comparisons of treatment plans involving proton and photon techniques generally demonstrate a striking advantage with protons for reducing the volume of nontargeted normal tissue receiving low- to medium-range radiation doses. In some cases, the volume of nontargeted tissue receiving moderate- to high-dose irradiation is also reduced. With double-scattered proton delivery modes currently in common usage, the target dose homogeneity and conformality index can sometimes, but not always, be inferior to that of IMRT. With scanned proton delivery modes, IMPT plans can, in addition to reducing low and moderate integral doses, also improve dose homogeneity and conformality indexes when compared with IMRT. However, depending on spot size and specific machine characteristics, the penumbra of scanned proton beams may be greater than that of double-scattered proton beams, making IMPT less useful, particularly in patients with adjacent critical structures. This concern can be addressed with beam collimating apertures, identical to those used in passive-scattering proton therapy, to reduce the beam penumbra. Each case within each tumor type is different, and until comparative plans are performed, it remains unclear whether protons are preferable to IMRT, VMAT, or 3DCRT and, further, whether IMPT would be more beneficial than double-scattering proton delivery. The clinical impact of improvements in physical dose distribution achievable with proton therapy may not be fully appreciated or even anticipated at this time; therefore, how to achieve the maximum benefits from proton therapy will require time, careful trial design, and detailed outcome assessments to define.

Applications and Outcomes

Many publications have reported significant differences in dose distribution between proton treatment plans and photon-based treatment plans in a wide range of malignancies and benign lesions throughout the body, including the eye,[47] brain,[48–55] skull base,[56,57] advanced head and neck sites,[58] sinonasal structures,[59,60] oropharynx[61,62] and nasopharynx,[63,64] lung,[65–68] lymphoma,[69–73] pancreas,[74–76] esophagus,[77–79] rectum[80] and anal canal,[81,82] seminoma,[83] prostate,[12,84,85] cervix,[86–91] breast,[92–95] sarcomas,[96] and standard target volumes, such as pelvic lymph nodes[97] and craniospinal irradiation,[98] and complex cases requiring reirradiation.[99]

Despite the existence of only a few facilities with technology capable of proton delivery to most cancers, the efficacy and safety of proton therapy have already been demonstrated in a variety of malignancies including retinoblastomas[100]; melanomas of the eye[101–107] and other sites[108,109]; bone and soft tissue sarcomas of the base of skull, lumbosacral, spine, extremities, and retroperitoneal space[110–124]; brain[125–129] and spinal cord tumors[130]; head and neck cancers including paranasal sinus tumors[108,109,131–139]; oropharyngeal carcinoma,[140–142] nasopharyngeal cancer,[143,144] ipsilateral head and neck tumors,[145] and adenoid cystic carcinoma[146–148]; gastrointestinal malignancies including esophageal cancer[78,149–153]; thoracic malignancies including early- and advanced-stage lung cancer,[154–164] thymoma,[165,166] and mesothelioma[167]; urologic malignancies including bladder cancer[168] and low-, intermediate-, and high-risk prostate cancer[169–182]; breast cancer[183–186]; Hodgkin and other lymphomas[69,73,187–196]; upper abdominal malignancies including hepatocellular carcinoma[197–204]; pancreatic cancer[205–209]; cholangiocarcinoma[201,210]; liver metastases[211]; cervical cancer[212]; a variety of pediatric brain tumors,[213–227] and other pediatric malignancies[123,195,196,228–237]; benign lesions like pituitary tumors[238]; acoustic neuroma,[239,240] age-related macular degeneration,[241–243] non–age-related macular degeneration choroidal neovascularization[244]; and hemangiopericytoma,[245] craniopharyngiomas,[224,226] paragangliomas,[246] and meningioma.[247,248] In addition, protons have been used in situations requiring re-irradiation.[249,250]

Figures 21.3 through 21.12 illustrate comparative treatment plans for 10 examples of clinical settings that could benefit from proton therapy. The examples are not comprehensive but representative. Currently, some proton facilities provide only double-scattering proton therapy (DS PT), some provide only pencil beam scanning proton therapy, and a few provide both. Where differences between IMPT and DS PT were anticipated, both plans were provided. The term "IMPT" used in examples below refers to PBS using SFUD and/or multifield optimization. Treatment planning techniques, particularly with IMPT and VMAT, are rapidly evolving. Current methods of dose prescription and treatment planning are not standardized across the field, so it may be possible to improve upon some of the treatment plans depicted below with other techniques, delivery modes, and better treatment planning systems.

Skull Base Sarcomas

Skull base sarcomas typically are not amenable to complete resection and require very high-radiation doses for disease control. Their adjacency to the brainstem, optic chiasm, and optic nerves often precludes delivery of optimal tumor doses for fear of fatal or severe functional radiation injuries. Proton therapy in these cases can achieve dose distributions that often provide better target coverage and permit the delivery of potentially curative doses of radiation to the tumor with minimal risk of brainstem necrosis or blindness; in some cases, proton therapy may offer the patient the only realistic chance of cure. Outcomes from several institutions suggest that up to 81% of chordomas and 94% of chondrosarcomas of the skull base can be controlled with proton therapy with a low risk of serious toxicity like brain necrosis.[111,113,118,119]

Figure 21.3A shows axial, coronal, and sagittal color wash displays of the dose distributions for IMPT, DS PT, and

FIGURE 21.3. A: Axial, sagittal, and coronal displays of the dose distributions achieved with pencil beam scanning proton therapy, also known as IMPT, with a 3-mm spot size, double-scatter delivery of proton therapy (DS PT), and photon-based IMRT using the volumetric arc treatment planning system (VMAT) for a **skull base chondrosarcoma of the clivus**. The *thick red line* indicates the target volume containing gross residual tumor (GRTV), the *thin yellow line* indicates the spinal cord, and the *thin red line* indicates the brainstem. The color wash indicates the radiation dose levels achieved with each treatment plan; the inner bright blue wash and line indicate the isodose volume receiving 104% of the prescribed radiation dose. The colored shaded areas indicate the following volumes: *red*, isodose volume receiving the prescribed dose of 73.8 Gy (RBE); *bright green*, volume receiving 98% of the prescribed dose; *magenta*, volume receiving 95% of the prescribed dose; *yellow*, volume receiving 90% of the prescribed dose; *aqua*, volume receiving 80% of the prescribed dose; *dark green*, volume receiving 50% of the prescribed dose; and *orange*, volume receiving 10% of the prescribed dose.

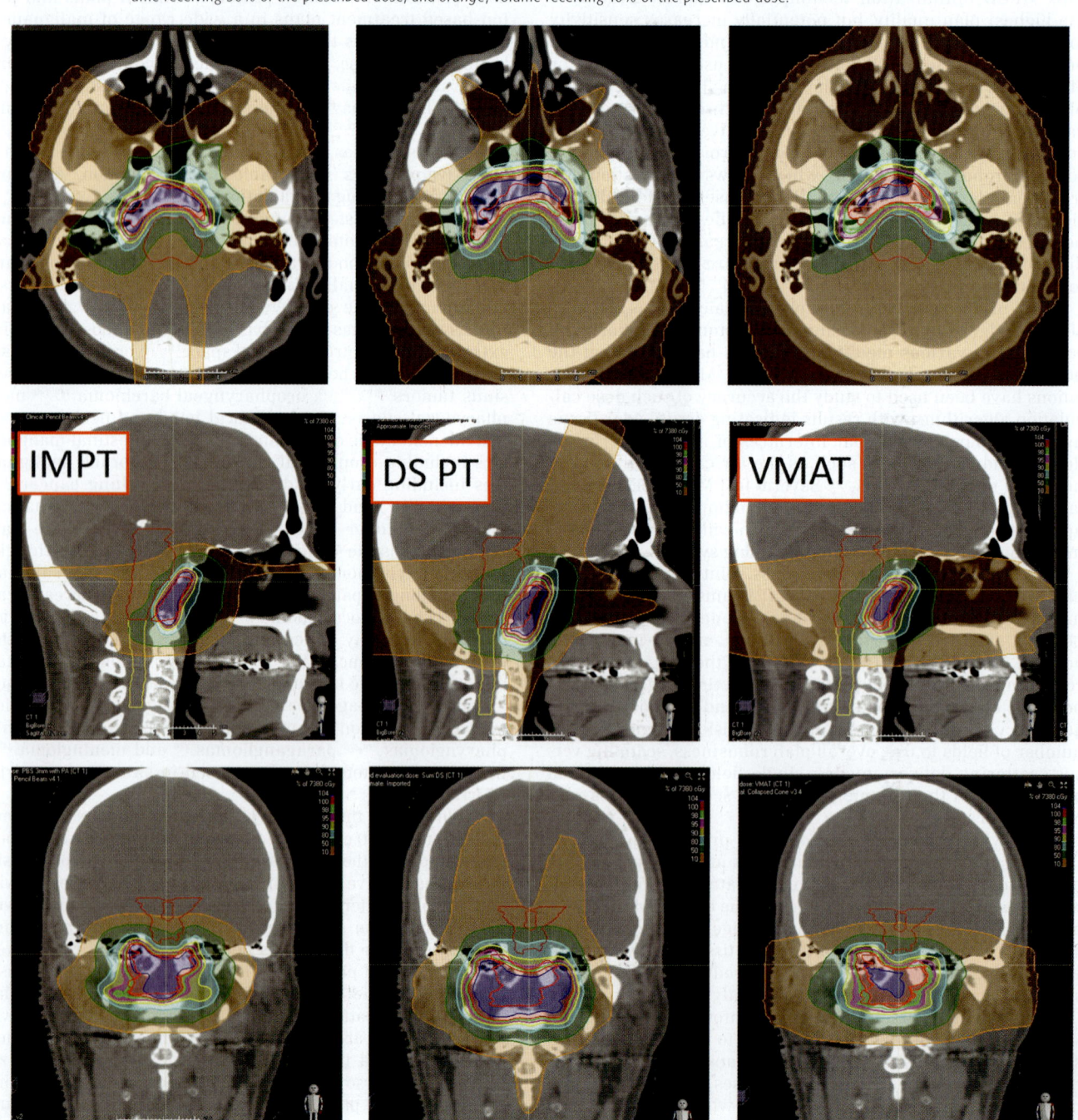

Targets	Goal Value	IMPT	DS PT	VMAT
PTV1	V50.4 Gy ≥95%	99.40%	99.97%	99.76%
PTV1	D95% ≥50.4 Gy	54.52	59.77	54.62
PTV2	V73.8 Gy ≥95%	65.4%	74.6%	46.0%
PTV2	D95% ≥73.8 Gy	66.33	66.39	62.11
GTV	V73.8 Gy ≥99%	96%	92%	79%
GTV	D99% ≥70.1 Gy	71.31	69.09	60.52

OARs	Goal Value	IMPT	DS PT	VMAT
Brainstem	D0.1 cc ≤55 Gy	59.32	64.22	62.74
Brainstem	Max dose ≤60 Gy	67.85	68.12	68.16
Brainstem core	D0.1 cc ≤50 Gy	47.98	60.01	52.63
Brainstem surface	D0.1 cc ≤55 Gy	59.30	64.23	62.72
Cochlea, left	Mean dose ≤36 Gy	18.40	30.85	41.38
Cochlea, right	Mean dose ≤36 Gy	57.30	65.92	67.10
HippoHead, left	Mean dose ≤5 GY	0.94	4.59	2.36
HippoHead, right	Mean dose ≤5 GY	8.12	28.83	9.73
HippoTail, left	Mean dose ≤20 Gy	10.88	26.44	9.37
HippoTail, right	Mean dose ≤20 Gy	0.48	7.01	2.19
Hypothalamus	Mean dose ≤5 Gy	0.78	13.39	2.81
Optic chiasm	D0.1 cc ≤55 Gy	6.54	35.38	11.46
Optic nerve, left	D0.1 cc ≤55 Gy	11.11	23.72	14.32
Optic nerve, right	D0.1 cc ≤55 Gy	8.11	33.59	15.78
Pituitary	Mean dose ≤30 Gy	54.79	61.81	57.72
Spinal cord	D0.1 cc ≤50 Gy	49.66	51.02	48.37
Temporal lobe, left	V20 Gy ≤10%	9%	12%	12%
Temporal lobe, right	V20 Gy ≤10%	10%	17%	15%
Brain	Mean dose (Gy)	3.09	8.93	5.78
Conformity index	GTV2	0.62	0.35	0.62
Homogeneity index	GTV2	0.53	0.68	0.71

B

FIGURE 21.3. (*Continued*) **B:** Dose distribution goals for skull base tumors. Different institutions use different dose distribution goals for evaluating skull base tumor plans. In this case, the target coverage goals were to deliver a dose of 50.4 Gy (RBE) to at least 95% of the planning target volume PTV1, a dose of 73.8 Gy (RBE) to at least 95% of the PTV2, and a dose of 73.8 Gy (RBE) to at least 99% of the GTV. As is apparent in the goal sheet above, target coverage goals for the PTV1 were met with all three plans, but target coverage goals for PTV2 could not be achieved with any of the plans. The goals for the GTV likewise were not achieved with any of the plans but were better met with the proton plans than the VMAT plan and best met with the pencil beam scanning proton therapy plan, with the GTV receiving 96%, 92%, and 79% of the prescribed dose with IMPT, DS PT, and VMAT plans, respectively. With respect to OARs, several parameters must be considered simultaneously, including "hot spots" reflected by the D0.1 cm³ and max dose, mean organ doses, and various relative or absolute volumes of an organ receiving certain doses. The DS PT plan involved the use of matched "patch" fields that treat partial target volumes to achieve better coverage of the target but can result in hot spots or higher mean organ doses in some cases. In this case, all three plans produced "hot spots" in the brainstem that exceeded the very conservative planning goal of D0.1 cm³ ≤ 55Gy. Using a volumetric definition of the outer 3-mm rim of the brainstem as the "brainstem surface" and the remaining volume inside the brainstem surface as the "brainstem core," it was felt that all plans would carry only a very small risk of brainstem injury, because the "hot spots" were small. None of the plans could avoid a significant risk of injury to the right cochlea, but both proton plans provided a good chance of preserving the left cochlea, with mean doses to the left cochlea of 18 Gy (RBE), 31 Gy (RBE), and 41 Gy (RBE) with IMPT, DS PT, and VMAT, respectively. Considering both target coverage and OAR protection, the best plan for this patient was the IMPT plan. Although mean and maximum doses of some structures were better with VMAT than DS PT, the improved target coverage with DS PT would generally warrant selection of the DS PT plan over VMAT, if IMPT were not available. (GTV, gross tumor volume visible on treatment planning imaging; CTV [not shown], GTV plus expansion including area at risk for subclinical disease; PTV1, planning target volume for the first phase of a sequential treatment involving more than one treatment volume, in this case a volume that included not only the GTV but also the CTV, as well as a margin or expansion to account for daily setup variations; PTV2, the planning target volume for the second phase of treatment, which, in this case, includes only the GTV plus a margin or expansion for daily setup variation; V, volume; D, dose; Gy, gray [RBE], a dose prescribed for protons intended to be radiobiologically equivalent [RBE] to the prescribed photon dose and to the physical photon dose divided by a factor of 1.1; IMPT, pencil beam scanning delivery of proton therapy using single-field uniform dose [SFUD] optimization and/or multifield uniform dose [MFUD] optimization treatment planning techniques; DS PT, double-scatter delivery of proton therapy; OARs, organs at risk; VMAT, photon-based intensity-modulated volumetric arc treatment planning; IMRT [not shown], photon-based intensity-modulated radiation therapy; V50.4 Gy and V73.8 Gy, the percentage of a target volume or OAR receiving a dose of 50.4 Gy [RBE] or 73.8 Gy [RBE]; D95% and D99%, the doses to 95% and 99%, respectively, of a target or OAR.)

photon-based VMAT treatment plans for a skull base chondrosarcoma. Figure 21.3B shows an analysis of dose–volume histogram data for the three plans. The IMRT plan delivers low-dose irradiation to a much larger volume of nontargeted tissue than either proton plan, specifically to the nose and posterior fossa, and provided inferior target coverage compared with the proton plans. With a goal of delivering ≥70 Gy (RBE) to the gross residual tumor volume, the doses achieved were 71 Gy (RBE) with IMPT, 69 Gy (RBE) with DS PT, and 60 Gy with photons (VMAT). Sparing of all OARs was best with IMPT. Conformality was similar between IMPT and VMAT, whereas homogeneity was similar between DS PT and VMAT.

Additional factors in comparing plans include the complexity of delivery, the robustness of the treatment plan, and the number of fields and time required for delivery. DS PT generally requires more fields and treatment delivery time;

"through and patch" fields, which cover only parts of the target volume, are often necessary, with some fields treating "through" the target whereas others are "patched" in to fill gaps in dose coverage. Care must be taken to avoid placing potential hot spots in critical structures.

Advantages of IMPT over DS PT proton therapy are the avoidance of patch fields, less need for apertures and compensators, increased dose homogeneity within the target, and reduced utilization of room time; however, depending on spot size, the penumbra of the scanned beams for IMPT may preclude its use in some cases. In this case, with minimal concern for organ motion, IMPT provided the best treatment plan. In other skull base sarcomas, the benefits from proton therapy may differ or differ in degree.

Paranasal Sinus Tumors

Paranasal sinus tumors frequently extend into the orbit or anterior cranial fossa adjacent to critical optic structures, such as the chiasm, optic nerves, retinae, lacrimal glands, cornea, and lens. With photon-based therapy, it is often difficult to deliver adequate doses to the entire tumor target without injury to at least one of the critical optic structures.[251] The physician often must choose between prioritizing tumor control and preserving vision. Figure 21.4 shows a comparison of IMRT and proton plans with both DS PT and IMPT delivery in a patient with a paranasal sinus tumor. All three plans were specified to deliver the prescribed dose of 50.4 Gy to the volume at standard risk for clinical and subclinical disease and 74.4 Gy to the high-risk volume containing gross disease.

As indicated in Figure 21.4A and B, target coverage with the IMRT1 plan (which was optimized for OAR protection) is inferior to both proton plans; the doses of 95% of the PTV1, 95% of PTV2, 99% of the gross tumor volume (GTV) were only 44, 53, and 62 Gy with the IMRT1 plan compared to 53, 71, and 74 Gy (RBE) with the DS PT plan and 53, 70, and 75 Gy (RBE) with the IMPT plan. The IMRT2 plan, which was optimized for target coverage, produced excellent target coverage but was considered unacceptable because of OAR exposures and hot spots in the PTV. As apparent in Figure 21.4A, compared with both proton plans, the IMRT plan exposes a much larger volume of nontargeted tissue to low-dose radiation, which includes the right temporal lobe, posterior fossa, oral cavity, and supratentorial brain. For example, the volumes of left and right temporal lobes receiving 20 Gy are 54% and 31% with the IMRT2 plan, 46% and 26% with the IMRT1 plan, 17% and 5% with the DS PT plan, and 11% and 5% with the IMPT plan.

All four plans struggle with the difficulty of target coverage and sparing of the critical structures. With each of these plans, there is only a small risk of brainstem and optic chiasm injury. However, none were able to sufficiently spare the left optic nerve to avoid a high risk of loss of vision in the left eye. Despite the addition of apertures to the IMPT plan to increase the sharpness of the dose gradient between the optic nerve and target volume, the DS PT plan still offered the best chance of preserving the right optic nerve. Although the proton plans both offer obvious advantages over the photon-based plan, neither avoids the necessity of prioritizing either tumor control or avoidance of injury to a critical organ.

Dagan et al.[134] from the University of Florida (Jacksonville, FL) have reported on 84 adult patients with a variety of sinonasal tumors treated with proton therapy, most with accelerated hyperfractionated regimens and chemotherapy. Local control, disease-free survival, and overall survival rates were 83%, 63%, and 68% at 3 years with a grade 3 or higher unilateral vision loss rate of 2%. Russo et al.[137] from the Massachusetts

General Hospital (Boston, MA), reported on 54 patients with nasal cavity and paranasal sinus tumors treated with proton therapy with a median follow-up of 82 months; 2- and 5-year local control rates were 80% and 2- and 5-year survival rates were 67% and 47%.

Oropharyngeal Cancers

Oropharyngeal carcinoma is the most common head and neck cancer. There is a rising incidence of p16-positive oropharyngeal carcinomas related to human papillomavirus exposure. In contrast to tobacco-related carcinomas, this p16+ population is generally younger and healthier, has a better chance for disease control, and is thus more likely to experience the late effects of radiation than their tobacco-related p16-negative counterpart.

Figure 21.5A depicts IMRT, DS PT, and IMPT plans in a patient with oropharyngeal carcinoma. As apparent in Figure 21.5A, there is significant sparing of the oral cavity, posterior neck, and contralateral parotid with both proton plans compared with the IMRT plan, likely impacting the risks of acute mucositis, alopecia, and xerostomia and the need for a feeding tube. The mean OAR doses (Gy [RBE]) for the IMRT, DS PT, and IMPT plans were 39, 22, and 10 for the esophagus; 26, 26, and 5 for the right cochlea; 53, 27, and 18 for the left submandibular gland; 46, 18, and 11 for the larynx; 58, 45, and 38 for the pharyngeal constrictors; 39, 19, and 16 for the oral cavity; 40, 20, and 17 for the mandible; 22, 11, and 10 for the left parotid; and 51, 48, and 40 for the right parotid. Although there are some advantages to DS PT over IMRT, the benefits with IMPT are more striking and consistent and suggest the possibility of significant improvements in xerostomia and swallowing compared with IMRT.

An early report from Slater et al.[140] from the Loma Linda University suggested better tolerance of oropharyngeal radiation therapy with the use of protons for a portion of the treatment. Gunn et al.[141] from the MD Anderson Cancer Center (Houston, TX) have reported 2-year overall and progression-free survival rates in advanced oropharyngeal cancer (98% stage III/IV) of 94.5% and 88.6% using IMPT. Blanchard et al.[142] reported a case-matched analysis of patients treated for oropharyngeal cancer at the MD Anderson Cancer Center with either IMRT or IMPT and showed equal disease control and survival rates but reduced rates of feeding tube dependency and severe weight loss among the patients treated with IMPT.

Pediatric Benign and Malignant Brain Tumors

Craniopharyngioma

Craniopharyngioma is usually diagnosed in children and adolescents. Its suprasellar location places the temporal lobes, hippocampi, hypothalamus, optic chiasm, and optic nerves at risk for radiation injury. Figure 21.6 shows IMRT, SRT, and DS PT plans in an adolescent patient. All three plans achieve target coverage goals of 54 Gy. Mean body and brain doses are 2.2 Gy and 9.2 Gy with IMRT, 2.2 Gy and 8.1 Gy with SRT, and 0.5 Gy (RBE) and 3.2 Gy (RBE) with DS PT. Some of the differences in relative mean organ doses with IMRT, SRT, and DS PT are as follows: in the right temporal lobe, 17%, 20%, and 8%; left temporal lobe, 18%, 22%, and 10%; left hippocampus, 50%, 61%, and 16%; right cochlea, 16%, 7%, and 0%; and left cochlea, 14%, 16%, and 1%, respectively. These reductions in dose to nontargeted brain tissues with proton therapy are likely to result in reduced loss in neurocognitive and auditory function.

A number of investigators have reported early outcomes in medulloblastoma, ependymoma, craniopharyngioma, and other tumors. Indelicato et al.[226] reported on a variety of

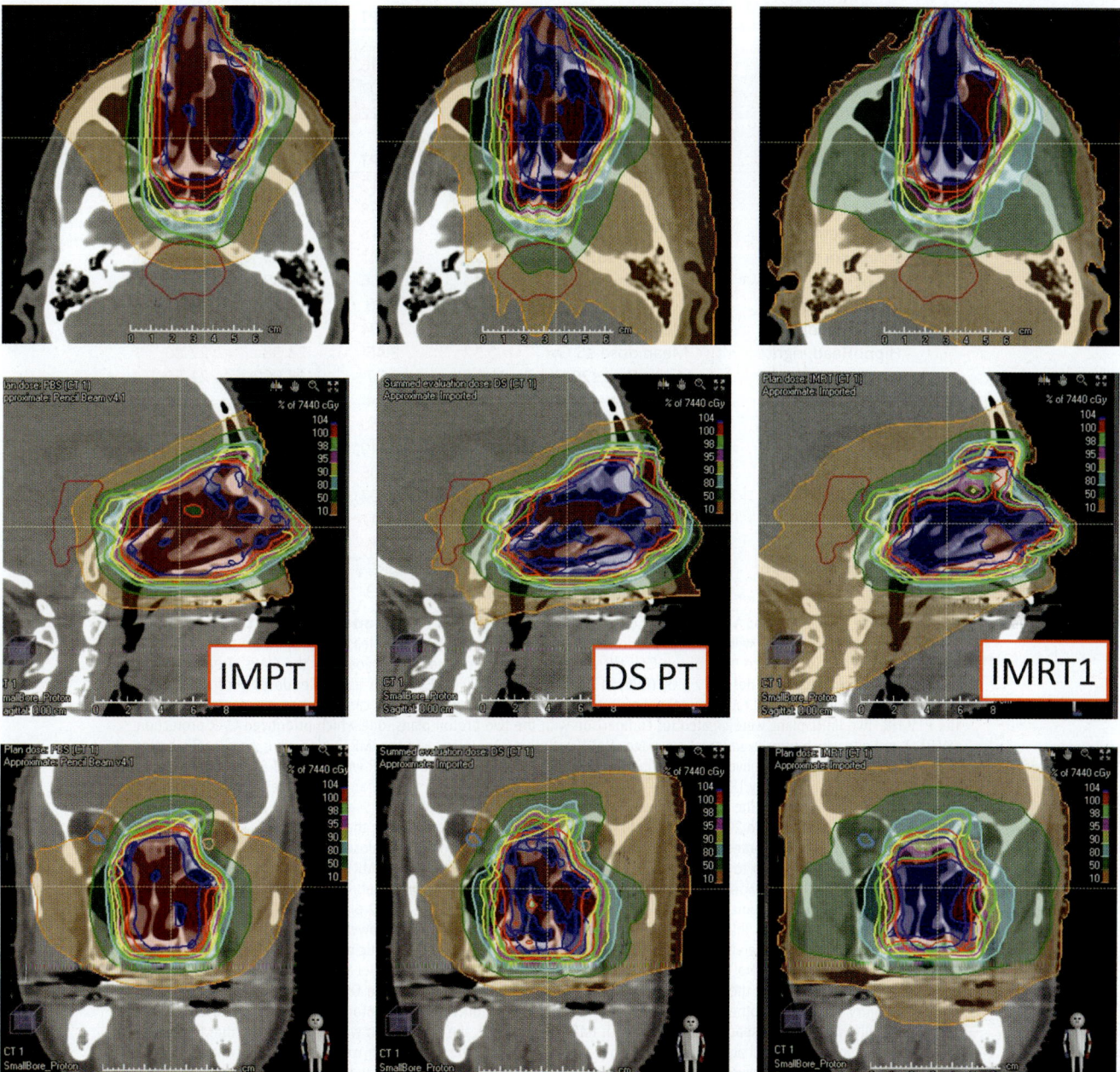

FIGURE 21.4. A: Axial, sagittal, and coronal displays of the dose distributions achieved with IMPT, DS PT, and IMRT for a **paranasal sinus tumor**. The *thick red line* indicates the GTV and the *thin red line* indicates the brainstem. The *color wash* indicates the radiation dose levels achieved with each treatment plan; the inner *bright blue wash* and *line* indicate the isodose volume receiving 104% of the prescribed radiation dose. The remaining colored regions indicate the following: *red*, isodose volume receiving the prescribed dose of 74.4 Gy (RBE); *bright green*, volume receiving 98% of the prescribed dose; *magenta*, volume receiving 95% of the prescribed dose; *yellow*, volume receiving 90% of the prescribed dose; *aqua*, volume receiving 80% of the prescribed dose; *dark green*, volume receiving 50% of the prescribed dose, and *orange*, volume receiving 10% of the prescribed dose. The goals of the plans were to deliver at least 50.4 Gy (RBE) to the PTV SR, at least 74.4 Gy (RBE) to the PTV HR, and a dose of 74.4 Gy (RBE) to 99% of the CTV HR while respecting dose constraint goals for organs at risk (OAR). The treatment plan delivered a total daily dose of 2.4 Gy (RBE) divided in 2 fractions of 1.2 Gy (RBE) delivered at least 6 hours apart. Two IMRT plans were created for comparison with the two proton plans, one prioritizing OAR protection (IMRT1) and one prioritizing target coverage (IMRT2), which is not shown. (IMPT, pencil beam scanning delivery of proton therapy using single-field uniform dose [SFUD] optimization and/or multifield uniform dose [MFUD] optimization treatment planning techniques; DS PT, double-scatter delivery of proton therapy; IMRT, photon-based intensity-modulated radiation therapy ; CTV SR, clinical target volume including both gross tumor and an area at "standard risk" for subclinical disease; CTV HR, clinical target volume at "high risk" for gross tumor and a high burden of subclinical disease; PTV, clinical target volume plus a margin or expansion for daily setup variations; OARs, organs at risk; PRV, planning risk volume, an OAR volume plus an expansion to account for daily setup variations.)

(Continued)

Targets	Goal Value	IMPT	DS PT	IMRT1	IMRT2*
PTV SR (N/A PT)	D95% ≥50.4 Gy	53.35	53.22	44.45	67.08
PTV HR (N/A PT)	D95% ≥74.4 Gy	69.91	71.46	53.34	76.68
CTV SR	D99% ≥50.4 Gy	58.11	58.07	55.58	66.10
CTV HR	D99% ≥74.4 Gy	74.70	74.22	62.41	74.22

OARs	Goal Value	IMPT	DS PT	IMRT1	IMRT2
Brainstem	D0.1 cc <55 Gy	46.83	59.12	48.55	57.74
Brainstem	D0.01 cc <60 Gy	51.64	61.58	51.04	60.69
Brainstem core	D0.1cc ≤50 Gy	35.14	56.18	43.64	51.69
Brainstem surface	D0.1 cc ≤55 Gy	46.86	59.03	48.45	57.62
Cochlea, left	Mean dose < 36 Gy	3.49	12.66	26.37	31.36
Cochlea, right	Mean dose < 36 Gy	1.28	4.38	20.82	24.75
HippoHead, left	Mean dose ≤5 Gy	20.81	32.94	41.61	49.48
HippoHead, right	Mean dose ≤5 Gy	6.32	8.45	23.38	27.80
HippoTail, left	Mean dose ≤20 Gy	1.16	8.37	18.08	21.50
HippoTail, right	Mean dose ≤20 Gy	0.20	0.14	8.50	10.11
Hypothalamus	Mean dose ≤5 Gy	13.76	15.60	22.13	22.13
Optic chiasm	D0.1 cc ≤55 Gy	43.76	49.49	43.23	51.42
Optic nerve, left	D0.1 cc ≤55 Gy	66.96	64.06	68.49	81.46
Optic nerve, right	D0.1 cc ≤55 Gy	57.22	54.07	56.37	67.03
Pituitary	Mean dose ≤30 Gy	58.09	64.47	55.06	65.48
Temporal lobe, left	V20 Gy ≤10%	11%	17%	46%	54%
Temporal lobe, right	V20 Gy ≤10%	5%	5%	26%	31%
Brain	Mean dose (Gy)	3.25	5.13	10.60	12.61

FIGURE 21.4. *(Continued)* **B:** A DVH analysis of IMPT, DS PT, and IMRT for the **paranasal sinus tumor** depicted in **(A)**. The goals of the plans were to deliver at least 50.4 Gy (RBE) to the PTV SR, at least 74.4 Gy (RBE) to the PTV HR, and a dose of 74.4 Gy (RBE) to 99% of the CTV HR while respecting dose constraint goals for the OARs. Treatment was planned to deliver a total daily dose of 2.4 Gy (RBE) in 2 fractions of 1.2 Gy (RBE) per day as smaller doses per fraction have been associated with improved radiation tolerance in the optic structures, which, in this case, are partially contained within the PTV HR. Two IMRT plans were created for comparison with the two proton plans, one which prioritized OAR protection (IMRT1) and one which prioritized target coverage (IMRT2). Both proton plans and the IMRT2 plan were significantly better able than the IMRT1 plan to deliver the prescribed dose of 50.4 Gy (RBE) to the PTV SR with doses of 53 Gy (RBE), 53 Gy (RBE), 44 Gy (RBE), and 67 Gy (RBE) to 95% of the PTV SR with IMPT, DS PT, IMRT1, and IMRT2, respectively. Although the IMRT2 plan best achieved the goal of delivering at least 74.4 Gy (RBE) to at least 95% of the PTV HR, it did so with a "hot spot" of 98.85 Gy (RBE) to 2% of the PTV HR [not shown]. Although not achieving the PTV HR goal, the proton plans both provided acceptable coverage of the PTV HR, in contrast to the IMRT1 plan, with doses of 70 Gy (RBE), 71 Gy (RBE), 53 Gy (RBE), and 77 Gy (RBE) to 95% of the PTV HR with IMPT, DS PT, IMRT1, and IMRT2, respectively. With respect to OAR protection, all four plans would likely preserve optic chiasm function but result in left optic nerve injury and unilateral blindness. Therefore, preservation of the right optic nerve was a high priority. The IMRT2 plan would almost certainly result in right optic nerve injury and thus bilateral blindness; the DS PT plan provided the lowest dose to the right optic nerve and thus the best hope of preserving unilateral vision. The better sparing of the right optic nerve with DS PT compared with IMPT is related to the penumbra at a depth of even a 3-mm pencil beam scanning spot size and the sharper penumbra achievable with apertures with the DS PT. The best preservation of unilateral vision with DS PT would carry a small risk of brainstem injury. Most of the other OARs show significant dose reduction with both proton plans compared to both IMRT plans, generally with the best sparing achievable with IMPT. In this case, the IMRT2 plan would be rejected due to the risk of bilateral blindness and an unacceptable hot spot of 98.85 Gy (RBE). The IMRT1 plan would be rejected due to inferior target coverage. The choice between IMPT and DS PT would be difficult but probably favors DS PT for the best chance of unilateral vision preservation with only a very small risk of brainstem injury. (IMPT, pencil beam scanning delivery of proton therapy using single-field uniform dose [SFUD] optimization and/or multifield uniform dose [MFUD] optimization treatment planning techniques; DS PT, double-scatter delivery of proton therapy; IMRT, photon-based intensity-modulated radiation therapy; CTV SR, clinical target volume including both gross tumor and an area at "standard risk" for subclinical disease; CTV HR, clinical target volume at "high risk" for gross tumor and a high burden of subclinical disease; PTV, clinical target volume plus a margin or expansion for daily setup variations; N/A PT, not applicable to proton therapy; D95%, the minimum dose to 95% of the volume of a target or OAR ; D99%, the minimum dose to 99% of the volume of a target or OAR. OARs, organs at risk; PRV, planning risk volume, an OAR volume with an expansion to account for daily setup variations; Gy, gray; Gy [RBE], a dose prescribed for protons intended to be radiobiologically equivalent to the prescribed photon dose and to the physical photon dose divided by a factor of 1.1.)

pediatric brain tumors referred for treatment from overseas; within this cohort, the 3-year disease control rate for craniopharyngioma was 100%. Extensive work from Merchant et al.[219] at the St. Jude Children's Research Hospital in a variety of pediatric brain tumors has correlated the risk of radiation-related neurocognitive decline to radiation dose level and distribution; there is emerging evidence that proton therapy may cause less neurocognitive decline than conventional radiation consistent with dosimetric predictions; however, long-term data will be necessary to fully understand potential benefits.[215]

Craniospinal Axis Irradiation

Craniospinal axis irradiation is required in most medulloblastomas and occasionally in other brain tumors, such as advanced or metastatic germ cell tumors, primitive neuroectodermal tumors, and ependymomas. Most patients with these tumors are young and at risk for late effects of radiation.

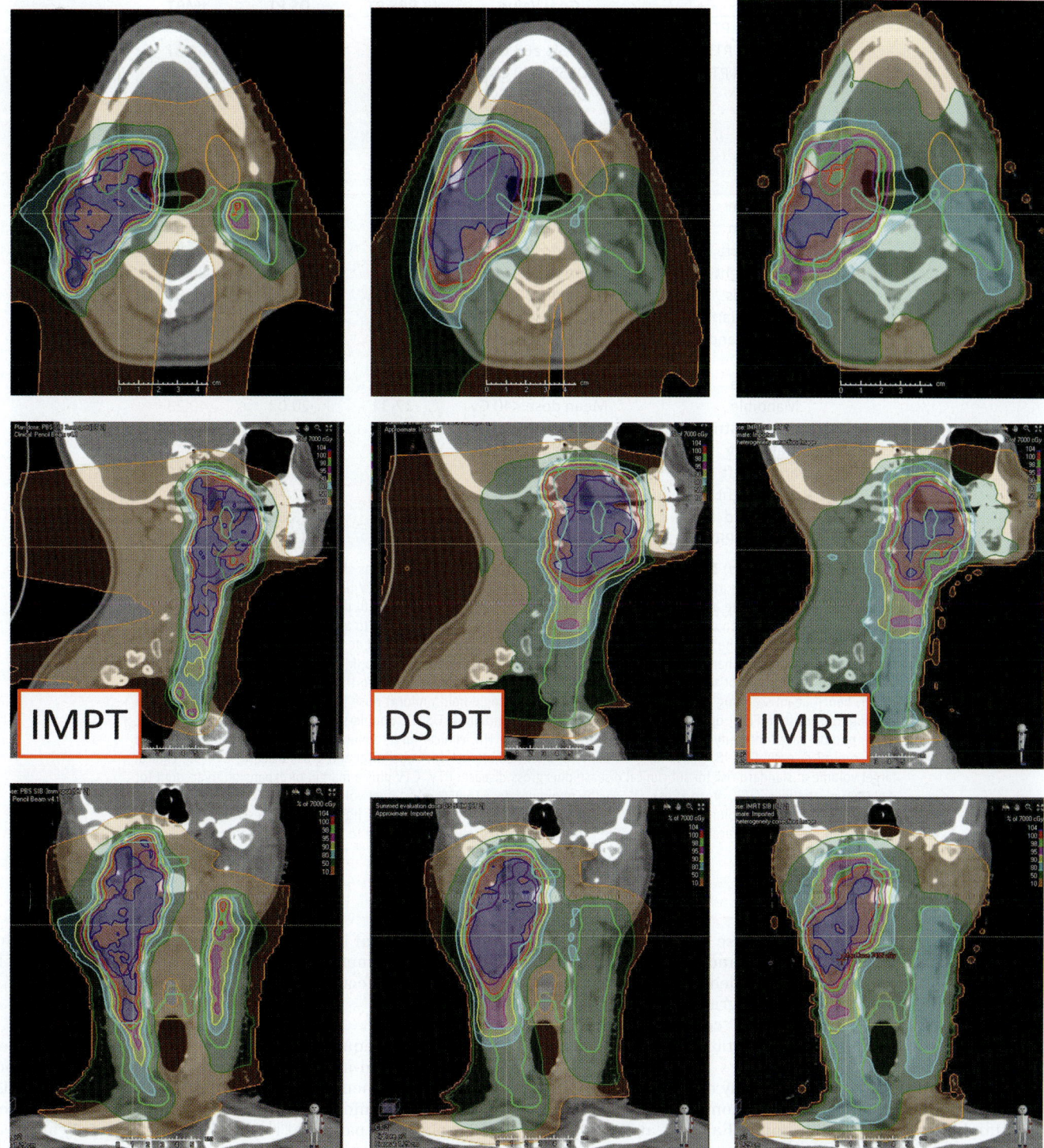

FIGURE 21.5. A: IMPT, DS PT, and IMRT plans for a patient with a node-positive right-sided **oropharyngeal cancer**. The CTV HR is indicated by the *thick red line*. The goals of the treatment plans were to deliver at least 50 Gy (RBE) to the PTV SR, 63 Gy (RBE) to the PTV IR, and 70 Gy (RBE) to the PTV HR. (IMPT, pencil beam scanning delivery of proton therapy using single-field uniform dose [SFUD] optimization and/or multifield uniform dose [MFUD] optimization treatment planning techniques; DS PT, double-scatter delivery of proton therapy; IMRT, photon-based intensity-modulated radiation therapy; CTV HR, clinical target volume at high risk for subclinical and gross clinical disease; CTV IR, clinical target volume at intermediate risk for subclinical and gross disease; CTV SR, clinical target volume at standard risk for subclinical disease plus gross disease; PTV, CTV plus a margin or expansion to account for daily setup variations; Gy [RBE], a dose prescribed for protons intended to be radiobiologically equivalent to the prescribed photon dose and to the physical photon dose divided by a factor of 1.1.)

(Continued)

Targets	Goal Value	PBS PT	DS PT	IMRT
PTV SR (N/A PT)	D95% ≥50 Gy	48.54	51.21	56.50
PTV IR (N/A PT)	D95% ≥63 Gy	61.31	66.48	64.07
PTV HR (N/A PT)	D95% ≥70 Gy	69.55	71.61	70.00
CTV SR	D99% ≥50 Gy	51.49	51.36	56.73
CTV IR	D99% ≥63 Gy	65.35	66.09	64.28
CTV HR	D99% ≥70 Gy	70.00	71.54	70.05

OARs	Goal Value	PBS PT	DS PT	IMRT
Brainstem	D0.1 cc <55 Gy	15.08	37.32	36.29
Brainstem	D0.01 cc <60 Gy	16.13	39.98	37.96
Cochlea, left	Mean dose <36 Gy	0.05	0.00	7.38
Cochlea, right	Mean dose <36 Gy	4.85	25.89	26.42
Esophagus	Mean dose <50 Gy	9.61	22.36	39.35
Submandibular gland, left	Mean dose <40 Gy	18.28	27.25	53.37
Submandibular gland, right	Mean dose <40 Gy	70.24	73.35	68.71
Larynx	Mean dose <36 Gy	11.19	18.10	46.13
Mandible	V70 Gy <10%	0.39%	6.79%	1.25%
Mandible	Mean dose <40 Gy	17.32	20.07	40.23
Pharyngeal Constrictors	Mean dose <50 Gy	37.73	45.39	57.70
Oral cavity	Mean dose <36 Gy	16.34	19.21	39.45
Parotid, left	Mean dose <26 Gy	10.07	10.94	22.26
Parotid, right	Mean dose <26 Gy	39.61	47.76	50.81
Spinal cord	V0.1 cc <50 Gy	16.88	38.68	44.79
Spinal cord, PRV	V0.1 cc <55 Gy	19.20	43.98	48.12

B

FIGURE 21.5. (*Continued*) **B:** DVH comparison for the IMPT, DS PT, and IMRT plans shown in **A**. The goals of the treatment plans were to deliver at least 50 Gy [RBE] to the PTV SR, 63 Gy [RBE] to the PTV IR, and 70 Gy [RBE] to the PTV HR. All plans provided adequate and similar doses to the PTV SR, PTV IR, and PTV HR, with the IMPT plan slightly below goals. However, with the exception of the right (ipsilateral) submandibular gland, the doses to all OARs were significantly reduced with IMPT compared with the DS PT and IMRT plans. The DS PT plan provided reduced doses to the esophagus, left submandibular gland, mandible, pharyngeal muscle constrictors, and larynx compared to the IMRT plan. In this case, both proton plans appear to be superior to the IMRT plan, but the IMPT plan was also superior to the DS PT plan for OAR protection. (IMPT, pencil beam scanning delivery of proton therapy using single-field uniform dose [SFUD] optimization and/or multifield uniform dose [MFUD] optimization treatment planning techniques; DS PT, double-scatter delivery of proton therapy; IMRT, photon-based intensity-modulated radiation therapy; CTV HR, clinical target volume at high risk for subclinical and gross clinical disease; CTV IR, clinical target volume at intermediate risk for subclinical and gross disease; CTV SR, clinical target volume at standard risk for subclinical disease plus gross disease; PTV, CTV plus a margin or expansion to account for daily setup variations. OAR, organ at risk; D95%, the minimum dose to 95% of a target volume or OAR; D99%, the minimum dose to 99% of a target volume or OAR; DVH, dose–volume histogram; Gy, gray; Gy [RBE], a dose prescribed for protons intended to be radiobiologically equivalent [RBE] to the prescribed photon dose and to the physical photon dose divided by a factor of 1.1.)

As shown in Figure 21.7, the exit dose from photon therapy exposes the thyroid, heart, lung, gut, and gonads to functional and neoplastic risks that can be avoided with proton therapy. The total-body V_{10} and total-body integral dose in this case are 37.2% and 0.223 Gy-m^3 with 3DCRT compared with 28.7% and 0.185 Gy-m with DS PT, a reduction likely to result in a lower risk of second malignancy.

In a multi-institutional cohort study of 88 children treated with chemotherapy and either photon or proton radiation for standard-risk medulloblastoma, Eaton et al.[220] found no significant difference in disease control, survival, or patterns of failure between proton and photon radiation, suggesting equivalent efficacy. Barney et al.[252] reporting on 50 patients treated with proton craniospinal irradiation at the MD Anderson Cancer Center between 2007 and 2011, documented extremely low median radiation doses to the thyroid of 0.003 Gy (RBE); the lung 1.1 Gy (RBE), heart 0.002 Gy (RBE), kidney 0.04 Gy (RBE), bowel 0.02 Gy (RBE), testicles 0.003 Gy (RBE), and ovaries 0.003 Gy (RBE). Treatment-related morbidity in this series included grade 3 leukopenia in 9%, thrombocytopenia in 2%, and median weight loss of 1.1 kg or 1.6% loss from baseline. Progression-free survival rates at 2 and 5 years were 82% and 68%, with 80% of treatment failures involving a local recurrence. These data suggest that craniospinal irradiation with proton therapy is effective but potentially much less toxic acutely and much less likely to result in late effects.

Lymphomas

Lymphomas frequently involve the mediastinum and often require a low-to-moderate dose of radiation therapy in conjunction with chemotherapy for maximum probability of disease control. Unfortunately, even low-to-moderate radiation doses place the patient at risk for late cardiac injury and second cancers, particularly breast cancers. Figure 21.8 shows a comparison of 3DCRT, IMRT, and DS PT plans in a young woman with Hodgkin lymphoma. The proton plan shows a significant reduction in the volume of the heart, lung, breast, spinal cord, and other soft tissues exposed to low-dose irradiation. Mean lung V_4 and lung V_{20} are 59% and 25% with 3DCRT, 62% and 10% with IMRT, and 31% and 16% with DS PT. Mean cardiac V_4 and cardiac V_{20} are 79% and 54% with 3DCRT, 76% and 26% with IMRT, and 40% and 26% with DS PT, respectively. These reductions are likely to result in lower risks of late cardiac injury and second malignancy.

In a variety of settings in a single institution as well in a multi-institutional registry study, Hoppe et al.[188–193,195,196,229] have reported minimal acute toxicity and excellent early disease

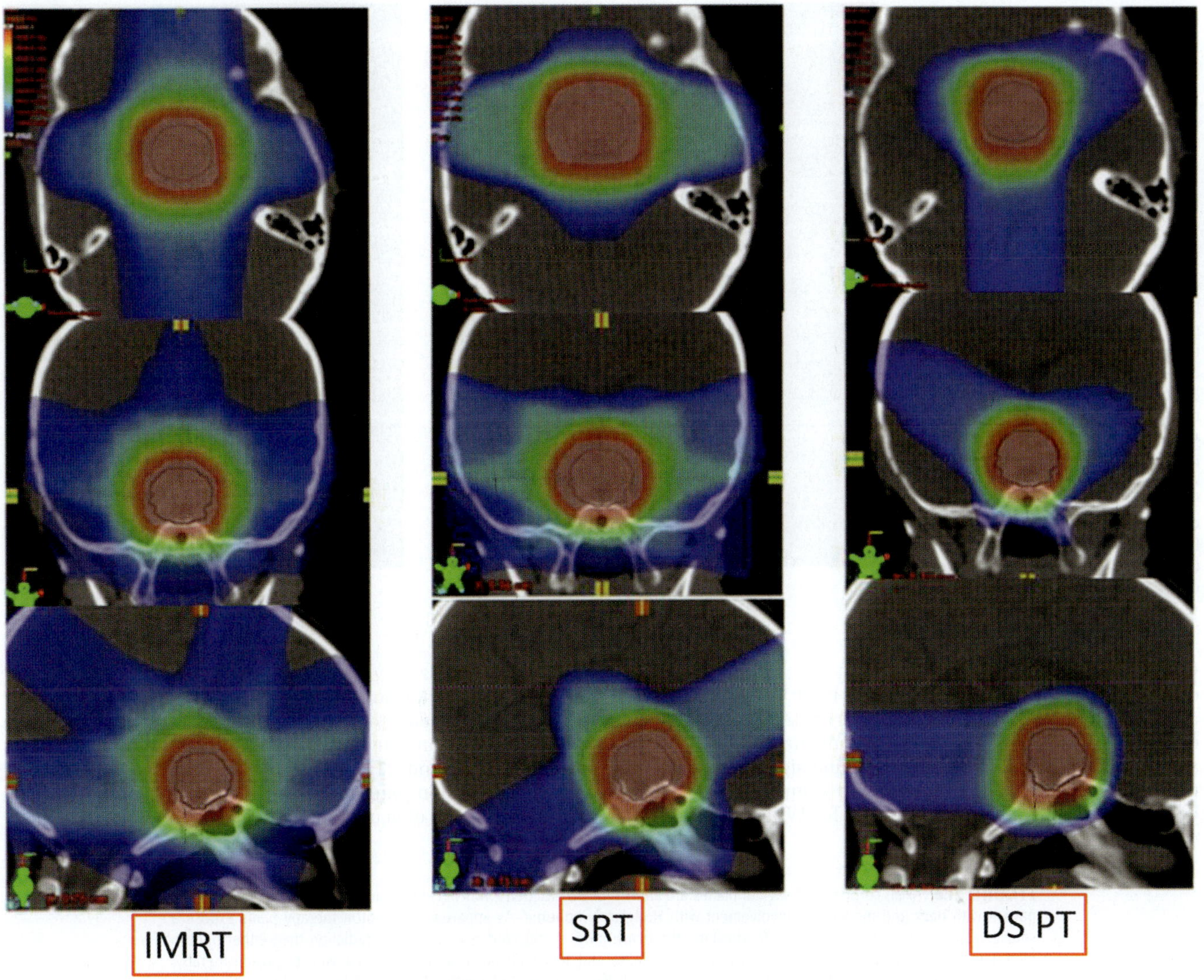

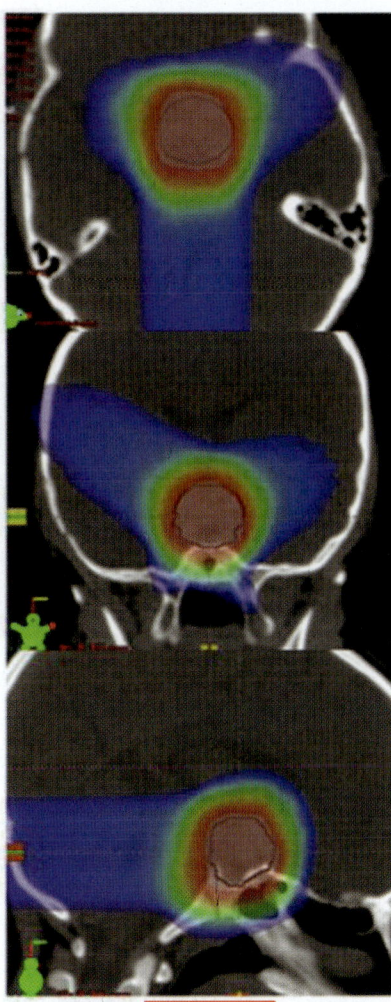

IMRT　　　SRT　　　DS PT

FIGURE 21.6. Axial, coronal, and sagittal displays of the dose distributions achieved with IMRT (*left*), SRT (*center*), and DS PT (*right*) plans for a small **craniopharyngioma**. The prescription dose was 54 Gy (RBE) to the PTV. All treatment techniques provided excellent conformal coverage of the target. As apparent, the volume of tissue exposed to low- and intermediate-dose irradiation is reduced with the DS PT plan. A DVH comparison of doses to OARs showed mean body and mean brain doses, excluding the PTV, of 233 cGy and 888 cGy with IMRT, 215 cGy and 810 cGy with SRT, and 63 cGy (RBE) and 358 cGy (RBE) with PT, respectively. The mean right temporal lobe doses are 904 cGy with IMRT, 1,090 cGy with SRT, and 297 cGy (RBE) with PT. The mean left temporal doses are 951 cGy with IMRT, 1200 cGy with SRT, and 370 cGy (RBE) with PT. The mean left hippocampal doses are 2,749 cGy with IMRT, 3,299 cGy with SRT, and 815 cGy (RBE) with PT. The mean right cochlear doses are 807 cGy with IMRT, 388 cGy with SRT, and 7 cGy (RBE) with PT. The mean left cochlear doses are 792 cGy with IMRT, 887 cGy with SRT, and 5 cGy (RBE) with PT. (IMRT, photon-based intensity-modulated radiation therapy; SRT, photon-based stereotactic radiation therapy; DS PT, double-scatter delivery of proton therapy. GTV, gross residual tumor volume; CTV, GTV plus volume at risk for subclinical disease; PTV, CTV plus a margin or expansion to account for daily setup variations. OAR, organs at risk for radiation injury. Gy, gray; cGy, 1/100th of a Gy; Gy [RBE], a dose prescribed for protons intended to be radiobiologically equivalent [RBE] to the prescribed photon dose and to the physical photon dose divided by a factor of 1.1.)

control outcomes with proton therapy in lymphoma. Pinnix et al.[253] from the MD Anderson Cancer Center have reported that small doses to large volumes of lung had the greatest influence on the risk of radiation pneumonitis in patients receiving IMRT for lymphoma, so it is likely that the reductions in volumes of lung receiving low doses with PT, compared with IMRT, will result in lower rates of pulmonary injury.

Lung Cancers

Lung cancers typically are diagnosed at an advanced stage and often occur in patients with underlying lung damage. Consequently, concern for protection of unaffected lung tissue often mandates compromise in the tumor dose. Figure 21.9 shows IMRT and proton plans in a patient with stage III lung cancer. As apparent, a smaller volume of nontargeted lung tissue, spinal cord, esophagus, and heart is exposed to radiation with proton therapy. With 3DCRT, IMRT, and DS PT, the mean lung doses were 11.7 Gy, 14.2 Gy, and 8.2 Gy (RBE); lung V5s were 36%, 50%, and 21%; lung V20s were 23%, 22%, and 13%; mean heart doses were 11.6 Gy, 7.1 Gy, and 5.5 Gy (RBE); and mean esophageal doses were 34 Gy, 26.2 Gy, and 21.7 Gy (RBE).

Chun et al.[254] reporting secondary analyses from RTOG 0617, a randomized trial of 60 Gy versus 74 Gy with concurrent chemotherapy using carboplatin and paclitaxel with

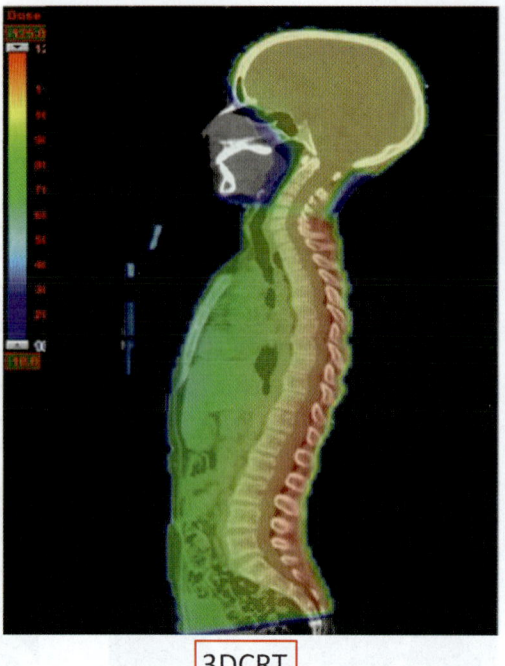

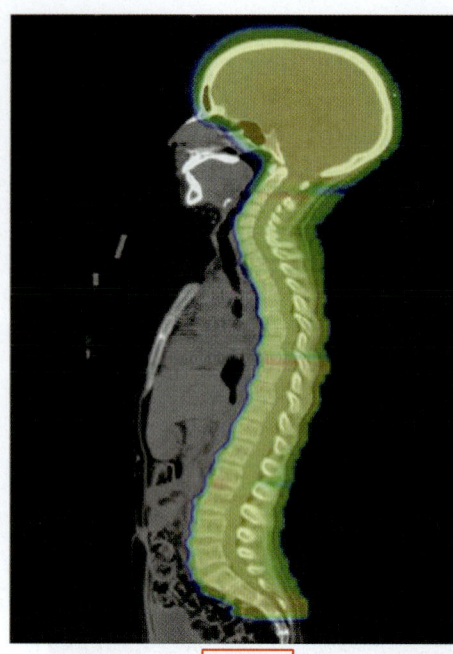

3DCRT **DS PT**

FIGURE 21.7. Sagittal planes from 3DCRT plans (*left*) and DS PT plans (*right*) for **craniospinal irradiation** necessary in a variety of brain tumors, most of which occur in young patients at risk for late effects. As apparent in the figure, the risks for functional and neoplastic effects in the thyroid, heart, lungs, breast, gut, and gonads from photon therapy can be avoided with proton therapy because of the lack of an exit dose. The total-body V10 and total-body integral doses are 37.2% and 0.223 Gy-m³ with 3DCRT compared with 28.7% and 0.185 Gy-m³ with proton therapy. (3DCRT, photon-based three-dimensional conformal radiation therapy; DS PT, double-scatter delivery of proton therapy. Total-body V10 = the relative percentage of total body receiving a dose of 10 Gy.)

or without cetuximab, showed that lung V20 was associated with increased ≥3 pneumonitis risk (*P* = .026) and the cardiac V40 was associated with overall survival (*P* < .05). In a retrospective study, Wang et al.[255] found significant associations between mean heart doses and symptomatic cardiac events in an analysis that accounted for WHO/International Society of Hypertension scores and history of coronary artery disease; the 2-year competing risk-adjusted event rates for patients with heart mean doses of <10, 10 to 20 Gy, and ≥20 Gy were 4%, 7%, and 21%, respectively. In the case illustrated above, the proton plan produces a dose distribution that carries a lower risk of acute (potentially fatal) pneumonitis, likely

FIGURE 21.8. Axial, coronal, and sagittal planes are shown for 3DCRT (*left*), IMRT (*center*), and DS PT (*right*) for a female patient with neck and mediastinal involvement with Hodgkin lymphoma. As apparent, the proton therapy plans expose a smaller volume of nontargeted tissue (particularly the heart, lung, spinal cord, and breast) to radiation than either photon plan. Lung V4 and V20 are 59% and 25% with 3DCRT, 62% and 10% with IMRT, and 32% and 16% with proton therapy, respectively. Heart V4 and V20 are 79% and 54% with 3DCRT, 76% and 26% with IMRT, and 40% and 26% with proton therapy, respectively. (3DCRT, photon-based three-dimensional conformal radiation therapy; IMRT, photon-based intensity-modulated radiation therapy; DS PT, double-scatter delivery of proton therapy; V, volume; V4, the relative volume [%] of an organ receiving 4 Gy; V20, the relative volume [%] of an organ receiving 4 Gy.)

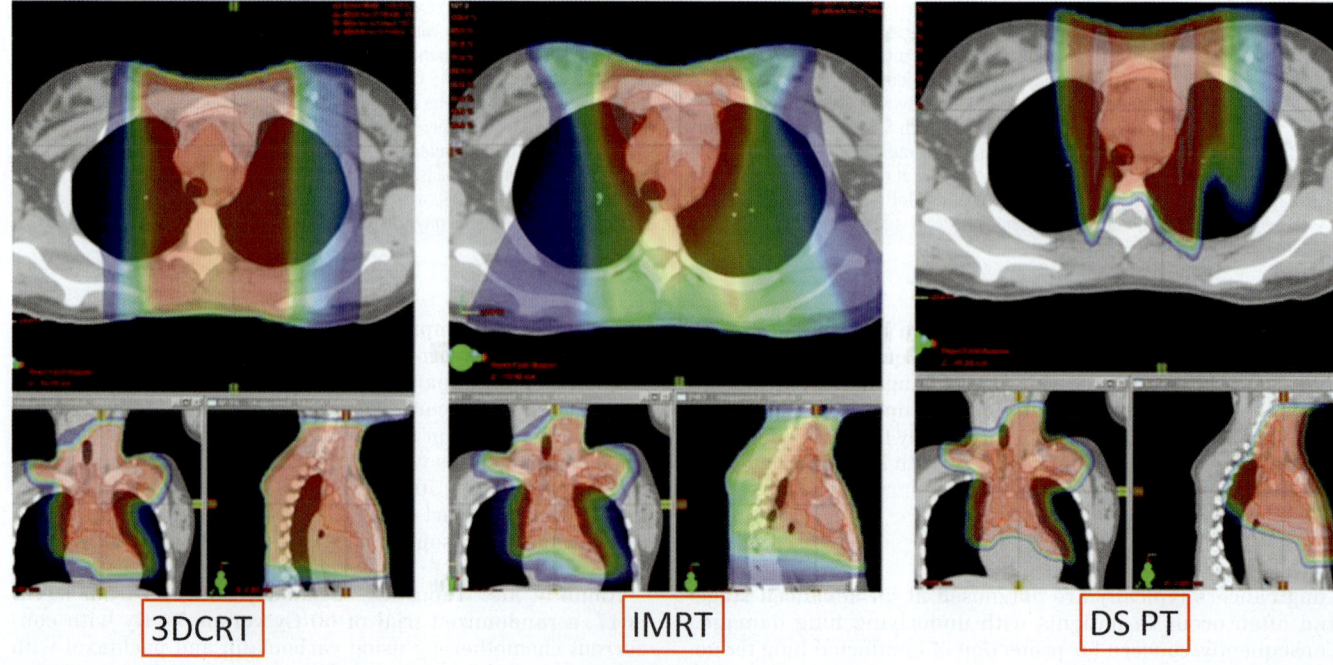

3DCRT **IMRT** **DS PT**

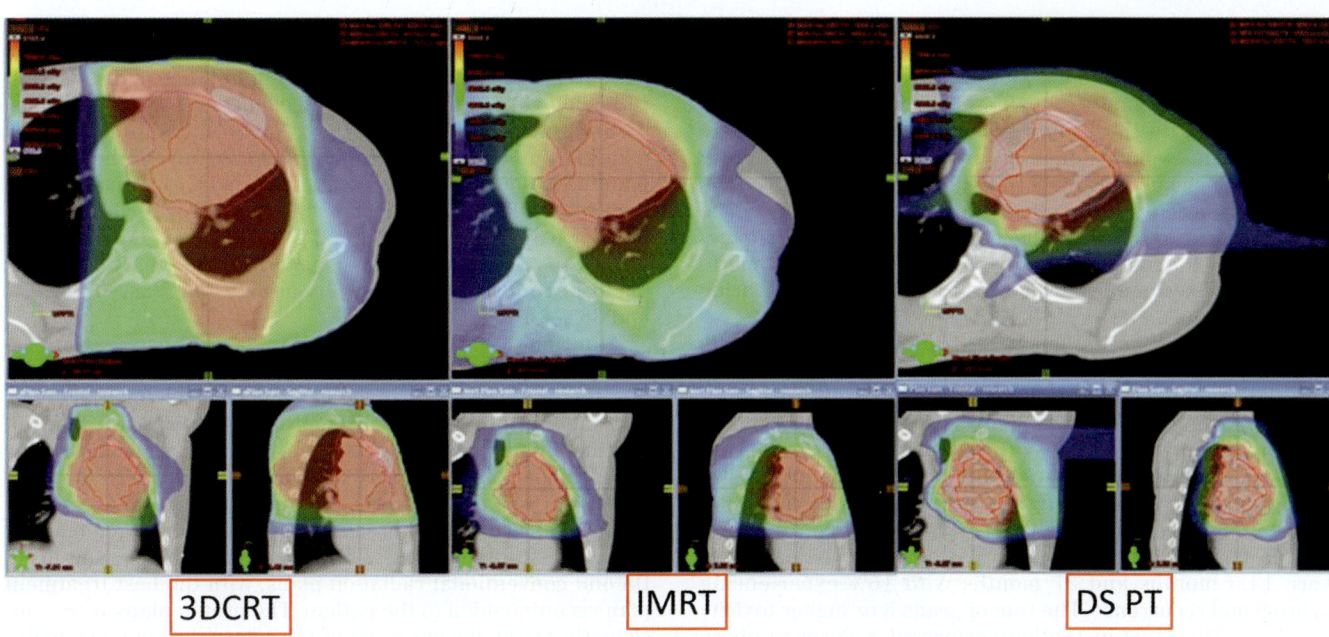

3DCRT IMRT DS PT

FIGURE 21.9. Axial, coronal, and sagittal planes are shown for 3DCRT (*left*), IMRT (*center*), and DS PT (*right*) for a patient with lung cancer. As apparent, both the IMRT and DS PT plans reduce the volume of nontargeted tissue receiving high-dose irradiation. The DS PT plan further reduces the volume of nontargeted tissue receiving low- and intermediate-dose irradiation compared to both the 3DCRT and IMRT plans. 3DCRT, IMRT, and DS PT plans, respectively, produced mean lung doses of 11.7 Gy, 14.2 Gy, and 8.2 Gy (RBE); lung V5 of 36%, 50%, and 21%; lung V10 of 27%, 37%, and 18%; lung V20 of 23%, 22%, and 13%; mean heart doses of 11.6 Gy, 7.1 Gy, and 5.5 Gy (RBE); and mean esophageal doses of 34 Gy, 26.2 Gy, and 21.7 Gy (RBE). (3DCRT, photon-based three-dimensional conformal radiation therapy; IMRT, photon-based intensity-modulated radiation therapy; DS PT, double-scatter delivery of proton therapy; V, volume; V5, the relative volume or percentage of an organ receiving 5 Gy; V10, the relative volume or percentage of an organ receiving 10 Gy; V20, the relative volume or percentage of an organ receiving 20 Gy; Gy [RBE], a dose prescribed for protons intended to be radiobiologically equivalent [RBE] to the prescribed photon dose and to the physical photon dose divided by a factor of 1.1.)

impacting the delivery of chemotherapy; the proton therapy plan also lowers the cardiac exposure, possibly correlating with a greater chance of survival.

Pancreatic Cancers
Pancreatic cancers have an extremely low therapeutic ratio with radiation alone or combined with surgery and

chemotherapy. The disease is frequently localized for a window of time before spreading, providing a potential opportunity to improve the overall outcome by intensifying local therapy. Figure 21.10 shows IMRT and proton therapy plans for a patient with cancer in the pancreatic head. As apparent, there is much less low-to-intermediate dose to the bowel, kidney, and liver with the proton plan. Mean doses with IMRT

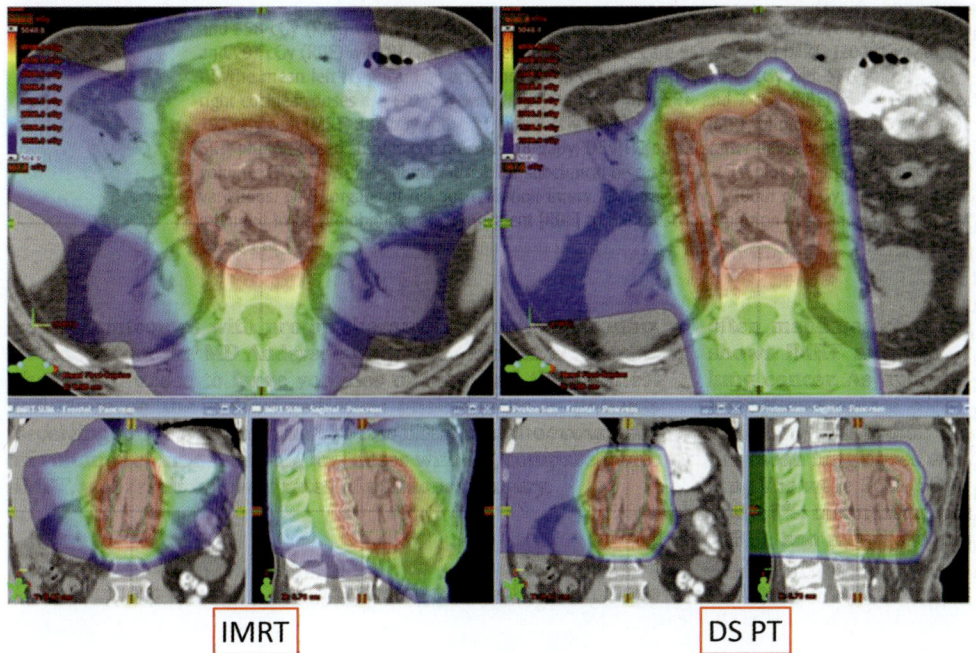

IMRT DS PT

FIGURE 21.10. Axial, coronal, and sagittal planes of IMRT (*left*) and DS PT (*right*) plans for a **pancreatic head carcinoma**. As apparent, there is much less low-to-intermediate dose to the bowel, kidney, and liver with the proton plan. Mean doses with IMRT and proton therapy are 1,174 cGy and 760 cGy (RBE) to the liver and 1,705 cGy and 443 cGy (RBE) to the small bowel, respectively. Although mean right and left kidney doses are similar for the IMRT and proton therapy plans, over 40% of the left kidney tissue is unirradiated with the proton therapy plan. (IMRT, photon-based intensity-modulated radiation therapy; DS PT, double-scatter delivery of proton therapy; Gy, gray; Gy [RBE], a dose prescribed for protons intended to be radiobiologically equivalent to the prescribed photon dose and to the physical photon dose divided by a factor of 1.1.)

and DS PT are 1,174 cGy and 760 cGy (RBE) to the liver and 1,705 cGy and 443 cGy (RBE) to the small bowel, respectively. Although mean right and left kidney doses are similar for the IMRT and DS PT plans, over 40% of the left kidney tissue is unirradiated with the proton therapy plan. This savings in normal-tissue exposure may be leveraged to permit either radiation or chemotherapy dose escalation or intensification, potentially increasing the opportunity for complete surgical resection, cure, or both. It is unclear whether motion management of upper abdominal organs is sufficient at this time to employ IMPT techniques, which may provide further sparing of critical organs.

Hong et al.[208] reported phase 1/2 trial from Massachusetts General Hospital of neoadjuvant short-course proton therapy with capecitabine followed by surgery and adjuvant gemcitabine. Proton therapy was delivered to the pancreas and draining lymphatics to 25 Gy (RBE) in 5 fractions. Surgery was performed in 37 of the 50 patients with the findings of positive nodes in 81%, positive margins in 16%, and no pathologic complete responses. The median progression-free and overall survival times in the 37 patients who had surgery were 14.5 months and 27 months with 16% experiencing locoregional recurrence. The rate of grade 3 or higher toxicity was 4.1%. The same institution performed a separate phase 1 trial of photon-based stereotactic body radiation therapy using the same treatment volumes and dose fractionation regimen; this study was terminated early because of intraoperative toxicity.[209] The investigators concluded that preoperative proton therapy was feasible and well tolerated and that it did not delay surgical resection. Nichols et al.[206] reported on the University of Florida experience with 22 patients treated with concomitant capecitabine and proton therapy for resected ($n = 5$), marginally resectable ($n = 5$), and inoperable ($n = 12$) pancreatic and ampullary carcinomas. Doses ranged from 50.4 to 59.4 Gy (RBE). No grade 3 or higher toxicity was observed. Median weight loss was 1.3 kg or 1.75% of the body weight, and 99% of the prescribed chemotherapy doses were given. Two of the twelve patients with inoperable disease achieved excellent radiographic responses, including one pathologically documented complete response. Despite the much higher radiation dose delivered in the University of Florida experience, the University of Florida experience confirmed the low rate of gastrointestinal toxicity with proton therapy observed by Hong et al.,[208] suggesting the potential for improvement in efficacy through dose escalation to accomplish complete pathologic responses. Neither proton experience delayed surgery or resulted in increased surgical complications, suggesting an additional potential value of proton therapy in facilitating both surgical resection and chemotherapy intensification.

Breast Cancer

Among breast cancer patients, there is level I evidence for treating all regional nodes, including internal mammary nodes and axillary nodes, in patients at risk for residual disease after surgery because of positive axillary nodes, tumor size, and in some cases tumor location and grade.[256-264] There is also growing interest in minimizing dose to the heart and lung as increases in late cardiac and pulmonary morbidity and mortality continue to be documented.[256,257,265-268] The excess in cardiac disease has primarily been associated with left-sided breast cancer patients[256,266,268] presumably because a greater volume of the heart is exposed to radiation with left-sided breast cancers compared with right-sided breast cancers. More recently, evidence suggests that the risk of heart disease may be related to dose–volume histogram parameters,[265] which has led groups to recommend minimizing heart exposure to radiation as much as possible.[269,270]

Figure 21.11A shows comparative treatment plans for a breast cancer patient receiving left-sided breast and regional node irradiation using IMRT, DS PT, and IMPT plans. As indicated in Figure 21.11B, there is excellent coverage of the breast with all plans. Coverage of the axillary and supraclavicular nodes is similar among the plans, but coverage of the internal mammary nodes is inferior with IMRT (44 Gy) compared with both the DS PT and IMPT plans (50 Gy [RBE]). Striking differences are apparent among the IMRT, DS PT, and IMPT plans in heart V10s, 23%, 2%, and 3%; mean heart doses, 7, <1, and 1; mean LAD doses, 14, 2, and 2; and left lung V5s, 85%, 27%, and 38%.

MacDonald et al.[186] from the Massachusetts General Hospital reported the acute toxicity and feasibility of proton therapy in a prospective trial of 12 postmastectomy patients; at a median follow-up of 6 months, there were no cases of pneumonitis and maximum skin toxicity was grade 2. Bradley et al.[185] from the University of Florida have reported a pilot study of proton therapy for right- and left-sided cancers (stage IIA to IIIB) after either breast-conserving therapy or mastectomy. The study included a treatment plan comparison of PT DS and conventional radiation plans, with the best treatment plan recommended to the patient. The proton plans were consistently better for coverage of the internal mammary nodes ($P = .0005$), minimization of cardiac V5 ($P < .0001$), and minimization of ipsilateral lung V5 and V20 ($P < .0001$). The only grade 3 toxicity was radiation dermatitis observed in 22% of patients.

Prostate Cancer

The recent ProtecT trial has underscored (1) the importance of early definitive treatment for prostate cancer in men with a ≥10-year life expectancy to maximize freedom from distant metastases[271] and (2) documented increased toxicity with surgery compared to radiation therapy without an attendant increase in disease control.[272] These findings are likely to change patterns of care by increasing the role of radiation therapy in prostate cancer. Prostate cancer results with radiation therapy are generally excellent, but dose escalation trials indicate that increasing the dose to the prostate is associated with improved disease control.[171,273-275] Dose escalation photon-based trials from the RTOG also show that increasing dose, dose per fraction, and the volume of the rectum exposed to a high-radiation dose are associated with an increased risk of rectal toxicity.[276] Analysis of outcome data with proton therapy indicates a similar correlation between increasing volume of rectal wall receiving high doses and the risk of gastrointestinal toxicity.[277] Hypofractionation of the treatment regimen is of great interest in prostate cancer, and studies have demonstrated similar outcomes[278,279] but often more toxicity[280] so that attention to radiation exposure of the OARs is critically important.[281] Most physician-reported gastrointestinal toxicity has been temporary rectal bleeding or ulceration.[277] However, rectal urgency, frequency, and incontinence have been identified as problems that may occur later, persist, and significantly impact long-term patient-reported quality of life.[282-285] This symptom complex has been found to be related to reduced rectal elasticity and sphincter tone,[282,286] and these symptoms have been associated with the volumes of anus and rectum receiving 5 to 40 Gy.[281,287,288] Comparative IMRT and proton dosimetry studies[84,289] have shown that with historical techniques for prostate stabilization, the volumes of the rectum and rectal wall receiving high-radiation doses associated with rectal bleeding and ulceration are similar; however, the volume of the rectum and rectal wall receiving low-to-moderate doses is significantly less with proton therapy compared to IMRT. It is likely that strategies to create distance between the anterior rectal wall and posterior prostate[290,291] will reduce the risk of rectal bleeding and/or ulceration in eligible patients receiving either photon- or proton-based radiation, so the main gastrointestinal issue will become rectal urgency and frequency. At this point, bladder and urethral toxicities with photon- and proton-based external beam radiation have not clearly been associated with dose–volume parameters; however, with dose escalation or hypofractionation of treatment, this may change.

The most controversial indication for proton therapy at this time is prostate cancer. More than 20,000 men with prostate cancer have been treated with proton therapy or a combination of proton therapy and photon therapy with excellent results; however, it is unclear whether outcomes with proton therapy in prostate cancer are superior to outcomes with photon-based therapy. Tables 21.1 and 21.2 show disease control and toxicity rates for early dose escalation trials and

contemporary proton and photon experiences with standard and hypofractionated radiation regimens.[170–173,182,273–275,278,279,298,299] Disease control and toxicity rates with proton experiences compare favorably with contemporaneous photon experiences. A comparison of prospectively collected patient-reported quality of life data from cohorts of men treated with IMRT and proton therapy has shown similar overall functional summary scores but significant differences in selected questions that potentially reflect radiation injuries associated with the volume of the rectum receiving low-to-moderate doses,[300] perhaps providing the first evidence of anticipated differences in functional outcomes related to proton and photon therapy reported directly by patients.

Figure 21.12 shows VMAT, DS PT, and IMPT plans for two patients with low-risk prostate cancer, the first with a large median lobe and the second with more typical prostate anatomy. As apparent, the rectal volumes receiving 25 Gy and

Section II

FIGURE 21.11. A: IMPT, DS PT, and IMRT plans for a woman with a left-sided node-positive breast cancer. Targets included the internal mammary; levels I, II, and III axillary; and supraclavicular nodal areas as well as the breast. The prescribed dose is 50 Gy to the breast PTV and nodal PTV. (IMPT, pencil beam scanning delivery of proton therapy using single-field uniform dose [SFUD] optimization and/or multifield uniform dose [MFUD] optimization treatment planning techniques; DS PT, double-scatter delivery of proton therapy; IMRT, photon-based intensity-modulated radiation therapy; PTV, the clinical target volume, which includes the volume at risk for clinical and subclinical disease, plus a margin or expansion to account for daily setup variations.)

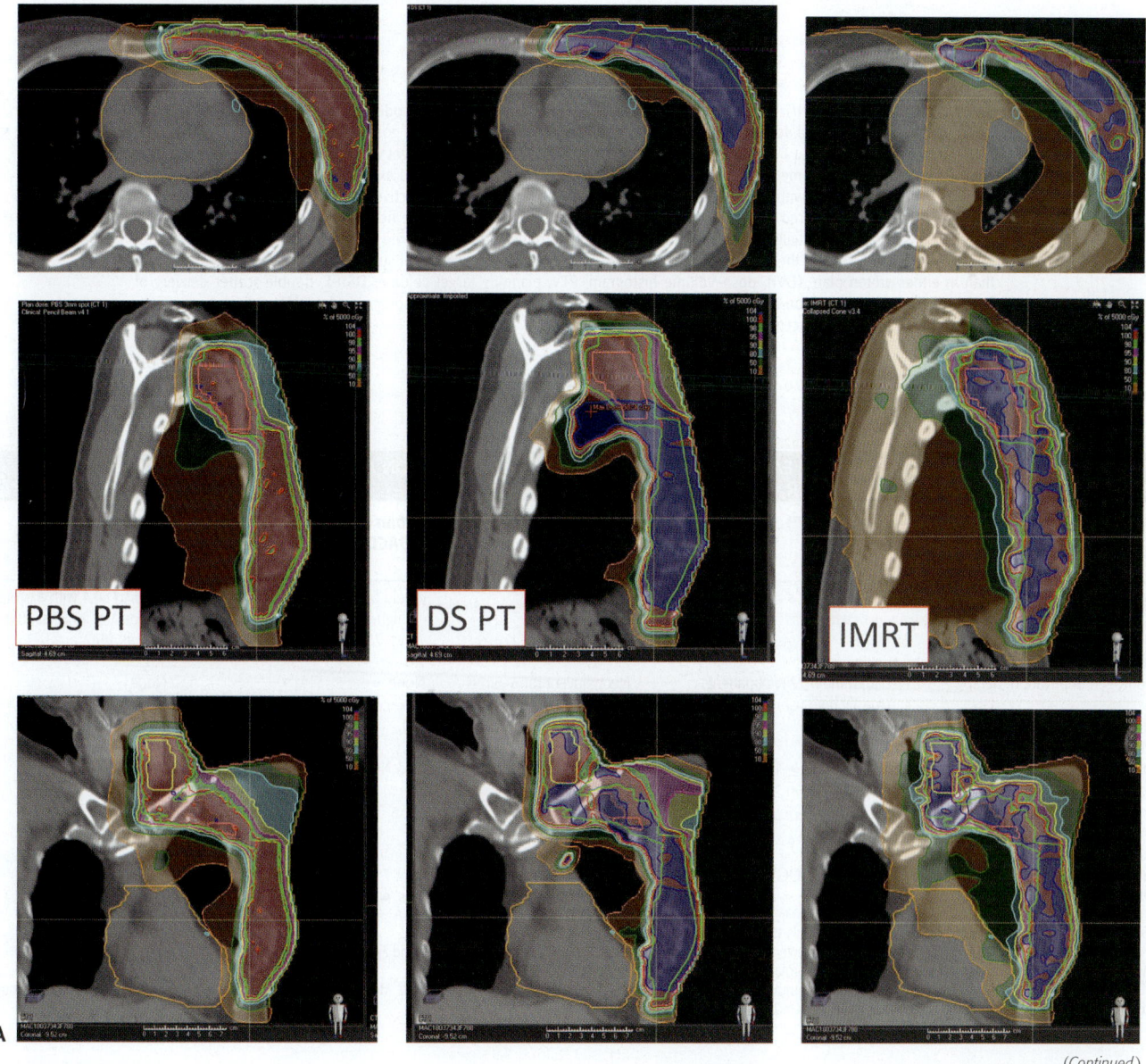

A

(Continued)

Targets	Goal Value	PBS PT	DS PT	IMRT
Breast PTV	V47.5 Gy ≥95%	99.92%	99.91%	98.13%
Breast PTV	D50% ≤54 Gy	50.83	52.66	52.06
Breast PTV	Max dose ≤54 Gy	53.36	57.05	64.39
SCV Nodes	D95% ≥45 Gy	50.06	49.82	49.54
Level I axillary	D95% ≥45 Gy	50.26	50.26	50.85
Level II axillary	D95% ≥45 Gy	50.18	50.62	50.84
Level III axillary	D95% ≥45 Gy	50.12	50.66	50.89
IMN nodes	D95% ≥45 Gy	50.03	50.54	44.91

OARs	Goal Value	PBS PT	DS	IMRT
Brachial plexus	D0.1 cc ≤55 Gy	51.93	52.48	55.20
Heart	V25 Gy ≤5%	0.92%	0.58%	3.89%
Heart	V10 Gy ≤10%	3.31%	1.53%	22.63%
Heart	D5% ≤25 Gy	5.94	0.44	22.48
Heart	Mean dose ≤4 Gy	1.03	0.47	6.93
LAD	Mean dose ≤3 Gy	2.03	1.79	13.82
Lung, left	D20 Gy ≤30%	15.74%	18.52%	35.10%
Lung, left	D10 Gy ≤50%	28.10%	23.05%	61.11%
Lung, left	D5 Gy ≤65%	38.25%	26.83%	85.15%
Ventricles	D25 Gy ≤1%	0.74%	0.33%	3.34%
Ventricles	D5 Gy ≤20%	4.43%	1.32%	18.13%
Skin	D1 cc (Gy)	50.59	54.46	55.18
Skin	Mean dose (Gy)	7.41	7.33	10.72
Skin	V50 Gy (cc)	3.50	72.00	9.70

B

FIGURE 21.11. (*Continued*) **B:** Comparison of treatment plans for left-sided node-positive breast cancer shown in Figure 21.10A. The prescribed dose is 50 Gy to the breast PTV and nodal PTV. The DVH goals were to deliver a dose of 47.5 Gy to at least 95% of the breast PTV and to deliver at least 45 Gy to 95% of the nodal target volumes. As apparent from the DVH comparison, all three plans met the target coverage goals for the breast and SCV and axillary nodal targets. The DS PT and IMRT plans had "hot spots" within the breast volume of 57 Gy (RBE) and 64 Gy, respectively. The IMRT plan provided inferior coverage of the IMN compared with either proton plan. With respect to the OARs, the heart V10, mean heart dose, and LAD mean dose were all substantially higher with the IMRT plan than either proton plan. The volume of lung receiving a dose of 20 Gy, 10 Gy, and 5 Gy and the volume of ventricles receiving a dose of 5 Gy were all substantially greater in the IMRT plan than in either proton plan. (DVH, dose–volume histogram; PTV, planning target volume; DS PT, double-scatter delivery of proton therapy; IMRT, photon-based intensity-modulated radiation therapy; SCV, supraclavicular; IMN, internal mammary nodes; LAD, left anterior descending artery.)

TABLE 21.1 CLINICAL OUTCOMES IN THE EARLY DOSE ESCALATION TRIALS WITH PHOTON AND COMBINED PHOTON AND PROTON RADIATION THERAPY IN PROSTATE CANCER

	Peeters (2006)[273] Dutch 3DCRT	Dearnaley (2005)[292] Creak, 2013[284] MRC	Kuban (2008)[274] MDACC	Zietman (2010)[171] PROG 95
Technique	3DCRT	3DCRT	4-field box with 3DCRT boost on high-dose arm	3CRT to 50.4 with a proton boost of 19.8 vs. 28.8
Dose (Gy or Gy [RBE])	68 vs. 78	64 vs. 74	70 vs. 78	70.2 vs. 79.2
Dose (Gy or Gy [RBE])/fraction	2.0	2.0	2.0	1.8
Androgen deprivation therapy	Neoadjuvant in 22% of patients (mostly high risk) for 6 mo or 3 y	Neoadjuvant for 3–6 mo in all patients	None	None
No. of patients	664	126	301	393
Median follow-up	51 mo	6.2/13.7 y	8.7 y	8.9 y
Stage I–III included[a]	PSA <60 and CS ≥ T1c or T1b with PSA >4 and Gleason ≥6	T1b-T3BN0M0	T1-3 N0M0	T1-T2B and PSA ≤15
Freedom from biochemical progression[b]	54 vs. 64 at 5 y	59 vs. 71/at 5 y 45 vs. 49 at 10 y	59 vs. 78 at 8 y	68 vs. 82.6
Grade 3 or higher toxicity[c]				
Gastrointestinal	4 vs. 5 (MOD RTOG)	0 vs. 5 at 2 y	1 vs. 7	0 vs. 1
Urologic	12 vs. 13	No difference at 3 y	5 vs. 4	2 vs. 2

[a]Staging is based on the American Joint Committee on Cancer's 1997 guidelines.[293]
[b]ASTRO definition of 3 consecutive PSA rises after nadir for Peeters, 2 consecutive rises for Creak, 2 ng/mL over nadir for Kuban and Zietman.
[c]Modified Radiation Therapy Oncology Group–Late Effects Normal Tissue (RTOG-LENT).[285,294,295]
3DCRT, three-dimensional conformal radiation therapy; m, months; MDACC, M. D. Anderson Cancer Center; MOD, modified; MRC, Medical Research Council; PROG, Proton Radiation Oncology Group; RBE, relative biologic effectiveness; RTOG, Radiation Therapy Oncology Group; y, years.

TABLE 21.2 FIVE-YEAR CLINICAL OUTCOMES WITH CONTEMPORARY PROTON THERAPY AND PHOTON-BASED INTENSITY-MODULATED RADIATION THERAPY

	Spratt (2013)[296] MSKCC IMRT	Vora (2013)[297] Mayo IMRT	Mendenhall (2014)[172] UF DS PT	Bryant (2016)[182] UF DS PT	Lee (2016)[278] RTOG IMRT	Catton (2017)[279] OCOG[6] IMRT	Henderson (2017)[173] UF DS PT
Dose (Gy or Gy [RBE])/no. of fractions	86/48	75.6/41	78/39	78/39	70/28	60/20	70–72.5/28–29
Dose (Gy or Gy[RBE])/fraction	1.8	1.8	2.0	2.0	2.5	3.0	2.5
No. of patients	1002	302	211	1327	550	1206	216
Median follow-up (y)	5.5	7.6	5.2	5.5	5.8	6.0	5.2
Freedom from biochemical progression							
Low risk	98%	77%	99%	99%	86%	–	99%
Intermediate risk	86%	70%	99%	94%	–	85%	93%
High risk	68%	53%	76%	74%	–	–	–
Grade 3 or higher toxicity per CTCAE v 4							
Gastrointestinal	0.7%	0	0.5%	0.6%	4.1%		0.5%
Urologic	2.2%	0.7%	1.0%	2.9%	3.5%	5.4%	1.7%

CTCAE, Common Terminology Criteria for Adverse Events; DS PT, double-scatter delivery of proton therapy; IMRT, intensity-modulated radiation therapy; Mayo, Mayo Clinic, Arizona; MSK, Memorial Sloan Kettering Cancer Center; OCOG, Ontario Clinical Oncology Group; RBE, relative biologic effectiveness; RTOG, Radiation Therapy Oncology Group; UF, University of Florida; y, years.

FIGURE 21.12. A: Axial, sagittal, and coronal planes of treatment plans with VMAT, DS PT, and IMPT for a **prostate cancer** patient with a very large median lobe, which protruded into the bladder, making it difficult to meet dose constraints to the bladder wall. The target volume is shown in the heavy *magenta line*, the bladder is outlined in *aqua*, and the rectum in *yellow*. A rectal balloon was used to stabilize the prostate and reduce the dose to the posterior portion of the rectum. As apparent, the VMAT plan delivered a low dose to a larger volume of nontargeted pelvic tissue, including the rectum. (VMAT, photon-based intensity-modulated volumetric arc treatment planning; DS PT, double-scatter delivery of proton therapy; IMPT, pencil beam scanning delivery of proton therapy using single-field uniform dose [SFUD] optimization and/or multifield uniform dose [MFUD] optimization treatment planning techniques.) **B:** Comparison of IMRT, DS PT, and IMPT treatment plans for a prostate cancer patient with a large median lobe. The target coverage goals were to deliver 100% of the prescribed dose to 95% of the PTV and to deliver 95% of the prescribed dose to 100% of the PTV. As apparent, all plans met both target coverage goals with a high degree of dose homogeneity. The OAR protection goals for the volume of bladder wall receiving 30 and 80 Gy could not be met with the IMRT (VMAT) plan; the DS PT plan met the goal for the volume of bladder receiving 80 Gy, but not the volume receiving 30 Gy. The IMPT plan met all bladder protection goals. All plans met the relative rectal wall dose goals, but not the rectum absolute dose goals. A gel spacer may have helped in this case to meet the rectum dose constraint. (IMRT, photon-based intensity-modulated radiation therapy; DS PT, double-scatter delivery of proton therapy; IMPT, pencil beam scanning delivery of proton therapy using single-field uniform dose [SFUD] optimization and/or multifield uniform dose [MFUD] optimization treatment planning techniques; VMAT, photon-based intensity-modulated volumetric arc treatment planning; PTV, planning target volume; OAR, organ at risk.)

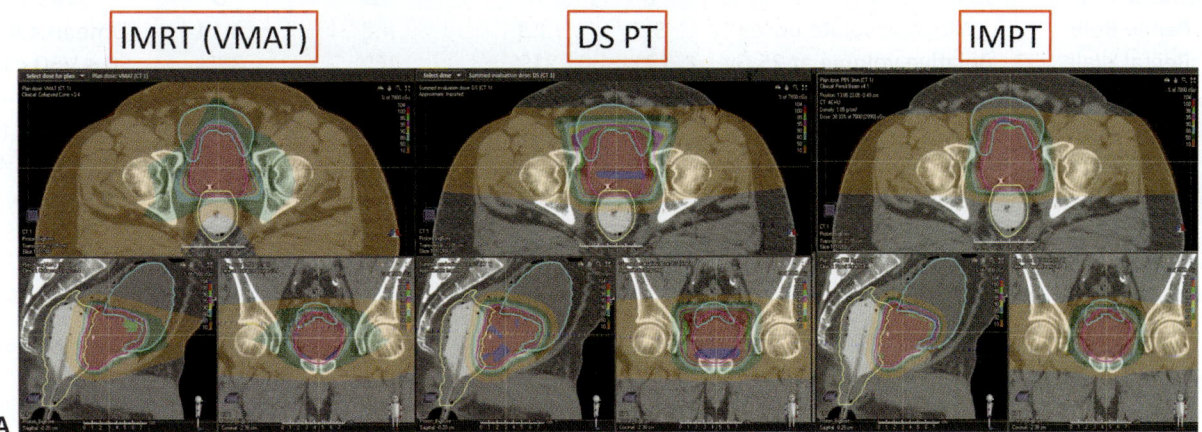

IMRT (VMAT) **DS PT** **IMPT**

A

Target	Goal Value	PBS	DS	IMRT	Goals
PTV	Relative dose at 95% volume	100%	100%	100%	
PTV	Relative dose at 2% volume	105%	105%	104%	
OARs	**Goal Value**	**PBS**	**DS**	**IMRT**	
Bladder	Relative volume at 30 Gy (cc)	26%	39%	33%	
BladderWall	Absolute volume at 30 Gy (cc)	33.3	43.1	40.7	35 ≤ V30 < 45 cc
BladderWall	Absolute volume at 80 Gy (cc)	6.1	7.7	7.3	8 ≤ V80 < 10 cc
BladderWall	Absolute volume at 82 Gy (cc)	1.3	0	0	7 ≤ V82 < 8.5 cc
BowelLarge	Absolute volume at 60 Gy (cc)	0	0.1	0	
FemoralHeads	Absolute dose at 0.1cc (Gy)	36	36	48	
FemoralHeads	Absolute volume at 55 Gy	0	0	0	1 ≤ V55 < 2 cc
PenileBulb	Mean absolute dose (Gy)	1.49	2.6	3.7	Dmean ≤ 40 Gy
RectalWall	Relative volume at 30 Gy	23%	29%	30%	
RectalWall	Relative volume at 40 Gy	22%	27%	26%	
RectalWall	Relative volume at 50 Gy	20%	24%	22%	50 ≤ V50 < 60%
RectalWall	Relative volume at 70 Gy	16%	18%	17%	30 ≤ V70 < 40%
Rectum1	Absolute volume at 70 Gy	13.6	18.6	15.1	V70 < 10 cc
UreteralOrificeLeft	Maximum absolute dose	79.1	80.8	78.4	
UreteralOrificeRight	Maximum absolute dose	80	81.1	81.1	
Integral Dose	Joule	76.4	102.8	145.2	

B

(Continued)

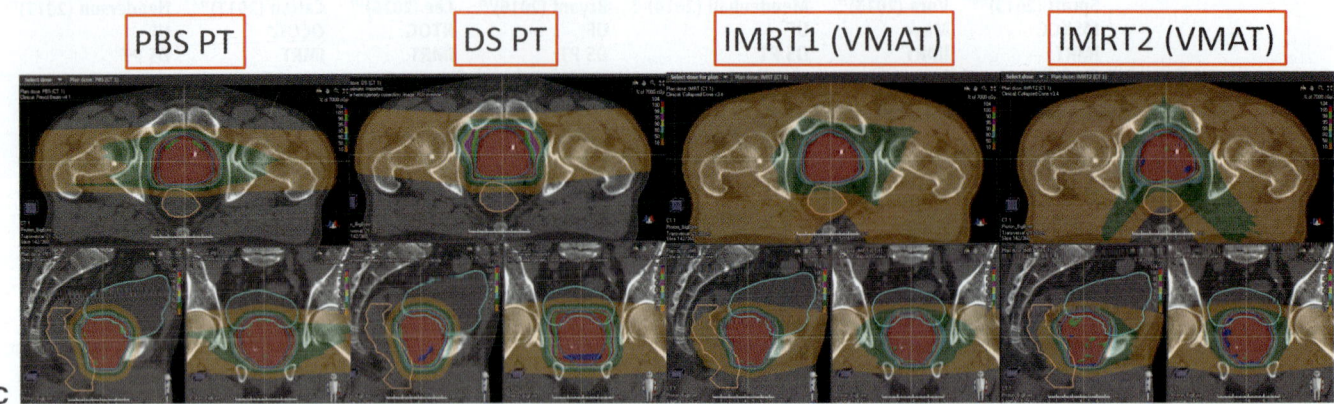

Target	Goal Value	PBS PT	DS PT	IMRT1	IMRT2	Goals
Prostate PTV	Relative dose at 95% volume	100%	100%	100%	100%	
Prostate PTV	Relative dose at 2% volume	102%	105%	102%	105%	
OARs	**Goal Value**	**PBS**	**DS**	**IMRT1**	**IMRT2**	**Goals**
Bladder	Relative volume at 27.5 Gy	18%	29%	25%	28%	
Bladder Wall	Absolute volume at 27.5 Gy	19.7	27.5	27.3	29.5	35 ≤ V27.5 < 45 cc
Bladder Wall	Absolute volume at 70 Gy	9.3	11.7	9	9.6	13 ≤ V70 < 15 cc
Bladder Wall	Absolute volume at 72.5 Gy	0	0.2	0	1.1	8 ≤ V72.5 < 10 cc
Large Bowel	Absolute volume at 60 Gy	0%	0%	0%	0%	
Femoral Heads	Absolute dose at 0.1 cc	41.9	30.6	44.8	29.8	-
Femoral Heads	Absolute volume at 45 Gy (cc)	0	0	0.1	0	1 ≤ V45 < 2 cc
Penile Bulb	Mean absolute dose	3.2	3.8	4.2	4.14	Dmean < 40 Gy
Rectal Wall	Relative volume at 25 Gy	17%	21%	26%	32%	50 ≤ V50 < 60 %
Rectal Wall	Relative volume at 35 Gy	14%	18%	18%	23%	30 ≤ V70 < 40 %
Rectal Wall	Relative volume at 45 Gy	11.57	15.46	12.83	15.2	50 ≤ V45 < 60 %
Rectal Wall	Relative volume at 65 Gy	5.76	7.73	6.28	6.06	30 ≤ V65 < 40 %
Rectum	Absolute volume at 70 Gy	1.5	1.1	1.4	1.5	
L Ureter Orifice	Maximum absolute dose	59	70.1	61.7	59.9	
R Ureter Orifice	Maximum absolute dose	59.6	70.7	60.2	62.15	
Integral Dose	Joule	63.7	72.2	111.5	112.8	

FIGURE 21.12. *(Continued)* **C:** Comparative plans using pencil beam scanning delivery of proton therapy, double-scatter delivery of proton therapy, photon-based intensity-modulated volumetric arc treatment planning (VMAT) prioritizing rectal sparing, and VMAT prioritizing hip sparing for a patient with a normal-sized prostate and a rectal spacer. The major difference is the substantial low-to-moderate dose bath in both VMAT plans compared with both proton plans. **D:** Although all plans met all dose constraints, the IMPT plan provided the best sparing for low-to-moderate doses of both the bladder wall (27.5 Gy) and the rectal wall (25 to 45 Gy) as well as the lowest overall integral dose. The DS PT plan was better than the IMRT1 plan for hip sparing and better than the IMRT2 plan for sparing of the rectal wall for low-to-moderate doses as well as providing a lower integral dose. (IMRT, photon-based intensity-modulated radiation therapy; IMPT, pencil beam scanning delivery of proton therapy using single-field uniform dose [SFUD] optimization and/or multifield uniform dose [MFUD] optimization treatment planning techniques.)

45 Gy are generally lower with both proton plans than with the VMAT plan and lowest with the IMPT plan. Treatment planning is rapidly evolving for both VMAT and IMPT, and the relative value of high-dose conformality versus minimization of integral dose in prostate cancer will require further investigation.

Comparative Effectiveness of Proton and Photon Therapy

In medical interventions, level I evidence of comparative effectiveness is desirable but frequently difficult to generate. Currently in the United States, fewer than 5% of adults participate in clinical trials. Among the reasons cited for low clinical trial participation are restrictive eligibility criteria, insurance coverage, distrust of physicians or the medical system, patient preference for either the "tried and true" or the "new"

approach, physician equipoise, and institutional disincentives. In radiation therapy, randomized trials were not conducted to compare orthovoltage and cobalt, cobalt and x-rays, or 3DCRT with either SRT or IMRT before the general adoption of each of these technologies; each technology was adopted based on improved radiation dose distribution and the expectation of consequent improved clinical outcomes. However, many entities have called for comparative effectiveness evidence before adoption of proton therapy.

With respect to the design of comparative effectiveness studies in proton therapy, the basic difference between protons and photons is the difference in beam entrance dose and exit dose that leads to significant differences in integral dose to nontargeted tissues. The essence of a randomized clinical trial of proton therapy and photon-based therapy thus would be to test whether changes in integral dose result in clinical outcomes that can be measured, that is, toxicity or functional loss from injury to nontargeted tissue. Altruism, therefore, would be the primary motivation for patient participation. It is unclear how willing patients would be to participate in such trials. Given the relatively few sites providing proton therapy at this point in time (~26 in the United States compared with ~4,000 photon facilities), there are also practical issues affecting comparative effectiveness research in protons. For example, some patients would not be able to travel to receive proton therapy, and others who might travel to receive proton therapy might withdraw from a randomized study if assigned to receive conventional radiation therapy, which could be delivered more conveniently in their hometown. Insurance coverage with proton therapy has been unpredictable, often not verified in a time frame that would permit study participation. Finally, the numbers of patients and resources required for randomized controlled trials raise concerns regarding the best use of currently available proton therapy treatment slots. Some investigators believe that more questions could be answered in the same time frame as a randomized controlled trial with a series of well-designed sequential studies aimed at optimizing proton therapy through dose escalation and hypofractionation or comparative effectiveness cohort studies.

Despite these challenges, there are a few completed or ongoing randomized trials comparing photon and proton-based therapy in lung cancer,[298,299,301] prostate cancer,[302] oropharyngeal carcinoma,[303] glioblastoma,[304] and breast cancer[305] and a trial comparing proton and carbon-based therapy in skull base sarcomas.[306]

In pediatric cancer survivors, increased risks of second malignancies and cardiovascular disease have been associated with radiation doses as low as 4 to 15 Gy.[307] In addition, elegant dose modeling studies at St. Jude Children's Research Hospital (Memphis, TN) have suggested no threshold dose for radiation injury in the childhood brain.[221] Thousands of children and many years of follow-up would be required to assess the results of a hypothetical controlled trial of proton therapy and conventional radiation to determine whether the reduction in low-dose exposure to the brain and total body with proton therapy would indeed result in a lower incidence of second malignancies or late cardiac injury. In the process, many children would intentionally be exposed to low-dose radiation in nontargeted tissues in the brain, likely resulting in permanent decreased neurocognitive function. Therefore, comparative trials will likely not be done in pediatric patients. Similar arguments may follow for Hodgkin lymphoma, which also affects relatively young patients with a high cure rate, long life expectancy, and substantial risks for second malignancy and late cardiac injury.

Comparative Cost-Effectiveness

Many factors must be accounted for in comparing the costliness and cost-effectiveness of different radiation technologies. Some of these include facility and equipment costs, operating and maintenance costs, patient throughput, clinical outcomes, and the global and individual impact of those clinical outcomes.

Current proton therapy equipment and facilities are up to 10-fold more expensive to construct than current conventional radiation therapy facilities capable of treating a similar patient volume. In addition, operating costs are higher by one- to threefold. There are substantial differences between patient throughput in conventional radiation and proton facilities, however, that may offset differences in initial costs. Typically, conventional radiation equipment is used for a single daily work shift and is replaced every 7 to 10 years. Most proton therapy facilities, however, operate two shifts a day and equipment is expected to last 20 or more years. The Harvard

Cyclotron was in use for over 40 years and closed primarily because of the availability of a new gantry-based clinical facility. The Loma Linda University (Loma Linda, CA) synchrotron and most of its gantries have been in continuous operation for over 27 years. Proton therapy equipment appears to be substantially more durable than linear accelerators. Thus, the actual patient throughput (*for a given patient mix*) in a proton facility may be substantially higher than typical for a conventional radiation therapy facility, perhaps double the patients per day (because of double shifts) for 2 to 6 times as many years of operation, leading to a 4- to 12-fold increased throughput with proton facilities compared to photon facilities. Proton therapy throughput may be further enhanced if hypofractionation is more feasible with proton therapy than with x-rays. Although initial cost of the facilities and equipment is a known factor, ultimate throughput and clinical outcomes evolve over time, so that the true cost-effectiveness of proton therapy relative to conventional radiation will not be known until there are long-term facility performance and clinical outcome data.

The impact of a particular clinical outcome may affect stakeholders differently. For example, if there is no intervention (cost) associated with a radiation injury that affects a patient's quality of life, that particular clinical outcome may be valued differently by a patient and that patient's insurer. Currently, there is no objective way to resolve such valuation differences. Meaningful cost-effectiveness analyses must account for a number of variables that are ill-defined and difficult to reduce to financial units. Regardless of the outcomes of cost and cost-effectiveness analyses, a shift to proton therapy as a predominant radiation modality will likely require a paradigm shift in philosophy about both profit and daily operations.

CHALLENGES

The multiple challenges facing proton therapy are complex and interrelated.

The first involves **technical developments** necessary to realize the full clinical outcome potential of proton therapy, including the following:

- *Improved treatment planning systems that better account for proton stopping power and biologic effects of variations in LET and RBE along the beam path.*
- *Online volumetric imaging and real-time range verification to assure accuracy.*
- *Real-time treatment plan adaptation to changes in tumor and/or normal tissue.*
- *Increased delivery speed to minimize motion mitigation and improve operational workflow.*

The second challenge is the generation of **reasonable evidence of improved clinical outcomes** that are anticipated with improved dose distributions. The development of reasonable evidence requires a critical mass of treatment facilities, a sufficient number of patients, sufficient technology maturation to reflect the modality's potential for outcome improvements, sufficient physician expertise to employ optimal techniques, and clinical trials that are scientifically credible, appealing to patients, nondisruptive to general clinical operations, and supported by funding agencies. The larger the anticipated clinical difference between treatment arms, the less likely a physician would have equipoise and a patient would consent to randomization, making accrual to a randomized study difficult. With smaller anticipated differences, accrual might be feasible, but larger numbers of subjects would be required to assess the difference. A full assessment of clinical outcome typically involves long follow-up to document differences in late effects, as well as early outcomes. Thus, comparative studies of proton and photon therapy will likely require large numbers of patients, possibly nonrandomized study designs, and long-term follow-up, making the funding of such studies challenging.

The third challenge is the development of **less expensive equipment** to lower the cost of participation in proton therapy by patients, providers, hospitals, and payors. Despite the paucity of comparative effectiveness data for proton therapy, the compelling dosimetric rationale is driving increased capacity, although not as rapidly as commonly perceived. Although proton therapy facilities have been described as increasing in number exponentially, studies by Miller et al.[308] and Waddle et al.[309] have shown minimal diffusion. The primary barrier to more rapid diffusion has been the cost of facilities. Vendors' current solutions to lowering the cost of proton therapy have converged on developing one-room facilities. Instead of installing a single large cyclotron or synchrotron that provides a proton beam for three to five treatment rooms, a smaller cyclotron could service only a single room, permitting access to the technology for 30% to 40% of the cost of a full facility but at a commensurate reduction in capacity. It is likely that true cost reduction will require significant technology development, which may only be driven by a significant increase in market demands.

Finally, the fourth challenge to progress in proton therapy is attaining a **critical mass of facilities**. In 2005, there were just three proton facilities treating nonocular tumors in the United States. In 2015, just a decade later, there were 5 times as many facilities in operation in the United States treating approximately 5,000 patients per year.[310] Today, in 2017, despite an eightfold increase in the number of facilities over the past 12 years, there are currently only 26 centers in operation, compared with >4,000 conventional radiation facilities. A critical mass of facilities, physicians, and physicists is necessary to collaborate with industry on technologic developments, conduct sound clinical research, and drive significant market-driven cost reduction developments.

CONCLUSIONS

Proton therapy offers the promise of reduced toxicity to patients compared with photon therapy—by reducing the radiation dose to nontargeted tissues—and possibly enhanced disease control through differential tumor effects and normal tissue biologic responses. Reduced toxicity may be leveraged to increase disease control through dose escalation or intensification (hypofractionation). Hypofractionation may result in lower health care costs as well as increased disease control and reduced toxicity. Additional clinical research and technical development are needed to optimize treatment planning and delivery of proton therapy, to document and maximize its potential clinical benefits, and to understand its full impact on health care economics.

REFERENCES

1. Paganetti H, Niemierko A, Ancukiewicz M, et al. Relative biological effectiveness (RBE) values for proton beam therapy. *Int J Radiat Oncol Biol Phys* 2002;53(2):407–421.
2. DeLuca P, Wambersie A, Whitmore G. Prescribing, recording, and reporting proton-beam therapy (ICRU Report 78). *J ICRU* 2007;7.
3. Paganetti H, Goitein M. Radiobiological significance of beamline dependent proton energy distributions in a spread-out Bragg peak. *Med Phys* 2000;27(5):1119–1126.
4. Combs SE, Bohl J, Elsasser T, et al. Radiobiological evaluation and correlation with the local effect model (LEM) of carbon ion radiation therapy and temozolomide in glioblastoma cell lines. *Int J Radiat Biol* 2009;85(2):126–137.
5. Giovannini G, Bohlen T, Cabal G, et al. Variable RBE in proton therapy: comparison of different model predictions and their influence on clinical-like scenarios. *Radiat Oncol* 2016;11:68.
6. Paganetti H. Nuclear interactions in proton therapy: dose and relative biological effect distributions originating from primary and secondary particles. *Phys Med Biol* 2002;47(5):747–764.
7. Hall EJ. Intensity-modulated radiation therapy, protons, and the risk of second cancers. *Int J Radiat Oncol Biol Phys* 2006;65(1):1–7.
8. Hall EJ, Wuu CS. Radiation-induced second cancers: the impact of 3D-CRT and IMRT. *Int J Radiat Oncol Biol Phys* 2003;56(1):83–88.
9. Xu XG, Bednarz B, Paganetti H. A review of dosimetry studies on external-beam radiation treatment with respect to second cancer induction. *Phys Med Biol* 2008;53(13):R193–R241.
10. Newhauser WD, Durante M. Assessing the risk of second malignancies after modern radiotherapy. *Nat Rev Cancer* 2011;11(6):438–448.
11. Yoon M, Ahn SH, Kim J, et al. Radiation-induced cancers from modern radiotherapy techniques: intensity-modulated radiotherapy versus proton therapy. *Int J Radiat Oncol Biol Phys* 2010;77(5):1477–1485.
12. Fontenot JD, Lee AK, Newhauser WD. Risk of secondary malignant neoplasms from proton therapy and intensity-modulated x-ray therapy for early-stage prostate cancer. *Int J Radiat Oncol Biol Phys* 2009;74(2):616–622.
13. Chung CS, Yock TI, Nelson K, et al. Incidence of second malignancies among patients treated with proton versus photon radiation. *Int J Radiat Oncol Biol Phys* 2013;87(1):46–52.
14. Friedland W, Schmitt E, Kundrat P, et al. Comprehensive track-structure based evaluation of DNA damage by light ions from radiotherapy-relevant energies down to stopping. *Sci Rep* 2017;7:45161.
15. Tommasino F, Friedrich T, Scholz U, et al. A DNA double-strand break kinetic rejoining model based on the local effect model. *Radiat Res* 2013;180(5):524–538.
16. Fontana AO, Augsburger MA, Grosse N, et al. Differential DNA repair pathway choice in cancer cells after proton- and photon-irradiation. *Radiother Oncol* 2015;116(3):374–380.
17. Grosse N, Fontana AO, Hug EB, et al. Deficiency in homologous recombination renders Mammalian cells more sensitive to proton versus photon irradiation. *Int J Radiat Oncol Biol Phys* 2014;88(1):175–181.
18. Liu Q, Ghosh P, Magpayo N, et al. Lung cancer cell line screen links fanconi anemia/BRCA pathway defects to increased relative biological effectiveness of proton radiation. *Int J Radiat Oncol Biol Phys* 2015;91(5):1081–1089.
19. Tsunashima Y, Vedam S, Dong L, et al. The precision of respiratory-gated delivery of synchrotron-based pulsed beam proton therapy. *Phys Med Biol* 2010;55(24):7633–7647.
20. Smith A, Gillin M, Bues M, et al. The M. D. Anderson proton therapy system. *Med Phys* 2009;36(9):4068–4083.
21. Paganetti H, Jiang H, Lee SY, et al. Accurate Monte Carlo simulations for nozzle design, commissioning and quality assurance for a proton radiation therapy facility. *Med Phys* 2004;31(7):2107–2118.
22. Schippers JM, Lomax AJ. Emerging technologies in proton therapy. *Acta Oncol* 2011;50(6):838–850.
23. Akagi T, Higashi A, Tsugami H, et al. Ridge filter design for proton therapy at Hyogo Ion Beam Medical Center. *Phys Med Biol* 2003;48(22):N301–N312.
24. Urie M, Goitein M, Wagner M. Compensating for heterogeneities in proton radiation therapy. *Phys Med Biol* 1984;29(5):553–566.
25. Pedroni E, Bacher R, Blattmann H, et al. The 200-MeV proton therapy project at the Paul Scherrer Institute: conceptual design and practical realization. *Med Phys* 1995;22(1):37–53.
26. Pedroni E, Bearpark R, Bohringer T, et al. The PSI Gantry 2: a second generation proton scanning gantry. *Z Med Phys* 2004;14(1):25–34.
27. Kooy HM, Clasie BM, Lu HM, et al. A case study in proton pencil-beam scanning delivery. *Int J Radiat Oncol Biol Phys* 2010;76(2):624–630.
28. Yu CX, Jaffray DA, Wong JW. The effects of intra-fraction organ motion on the delivery of dynamic intensity modulation. *Phys Med Biol* 1998;43(1):91–104.
29. Bortfeld T, Jokivarsi K, Goitein M, et al. Effects of intra-fraction motion on IMRT dose delivery: statistical analysis and simulation. *Phys Med Biol* 2002;47(13):2203–2220.
30. Paganetti H, Jiang H, Adams JA, et al. Monte Carlo simulations with time-dependent geometries to investigate effects of organ motion with high temporal resolution. *Int J Radiat Oncol Biol Phys* 2004;60(3):942–950.
31. Zenklusen SM, Pedroni E, Meer D. A study on repainting strategies for treating moderately moving targets with proton pencil beam scanning at the new Gantry 2 at PSI. *Phys Med Biol* 2010;55(17):5103–5121.
32. Schneider U, Pedroni E, Lomax A. The calibration of CT Hounsfield units for radiotherapy treatment planning. *Phys Med Biol* 1996;41(1):111–124.
33. Szymanowski H, Oelfke U. CT calibration for two-dimensional scaling of proton pencil beams. *Phys Med Biol* 2003;48(7):861–874.
34. Moyers MF, Miller DW, Bush DA, et al. Methodologies and tools for proton beam design for lung tumors. *Int J Radiat Oncol Biol Phys* 2001;49(5):1429–1438.
35. *Prescribing, recording, and reporting proton-beam therapy (ICRU Report 50). Contract No. 50.* Bethesda, MD: International Commission on Radiation Units & Measurements; 1993.
36. *Prescribing, recording, and reporting photon-beam therapy (ICRU Report 62). Contract No. 62.* Bethesda, MD: International Commission on Radiation Units & Measurements; 1999.
37. Schaffner B, Pedroni E, Lomax A. Dose calculation models for proton treatment planning using a dynamic beam delivery system: an attempt to include density heterogeneity effects in the analytical dose calculation. *Phys Med Biol* 1999;44(1):27–41.
38. Szymanowski H, Oelfke U. Two-dimensional pencil beam scaling: an improved proton dose algorithm for heterogeneous media. *Phys Med Biol* 2002;47(18):3313–3330.
39. Bortfeld T. An analytical approximation of the Bragg curve for therapeutic proton beams. *Med Phys* 1997;24(12):2024–2033.

40. Hong L, Goitein M, Bucciolini M, et al. A pencil beam algorithm for proton dose calculations. *Phys Med Biol* 1996;41(8):1305–1330.

41. Ciangaru G, Polf JC, Bues M, et al. Benchmarking analytical calculations of proton doses in heterogeneous matter. *Med Phys* 2005;32(12):3511–3523.

42. Paganetti H, Jiang H, Parodi K, et al. Clinical implementation of full Monte Carlo dose calculation in proton beam therapy. *Phys Med Biol* 2008;53(17):4825–4853.

43. Newhauser W, Fontenot J, Zheng Y, et al. Monte Carlo simulations for configuring and testing an analytical proton dose-calculation algorithm. *Phys Med Biol* 2007;52(15):4569–4584.

44. Fippel M, Soukup M. A Monte Carlo dose calculation algorithm for proton therapy. *Med Phys* 2004;31(8):2263–2273.

45. Yepes P, Randeniya S, Taddei PJ, et al. Monte Carlo fast dose calculator for proton radiotherapy: application to a voxelized geometry representing a patient with prostate cancer. *Phys Med Biol* 2009;54(1):N21–N28.

46. Hotta K, Kohno R, Takada Y, et al. Improved dose-calculation accuracy in proton treatment planning using a simplified Monte Carlo method verified with three-dimensional measurements in an anthropomorphic phantom. *Phys Med Biol* 2010;55(12):3545–3556.

47. Weber DC, Bogner J, Verwey J, et al. Proton beam radiotherapy versus fractionated stereotactic radiotherapy for uveal melanomas: A comparative study. *Int J Radiat Oncol Biol Phys* 2005;63(2):373–384.

48. Beltran C, Roca M, Merchant TE. On the benefits and risks of proton therapy in pediatric craniopharyngioma. *Int J Radiat Oncol Biol Phys* 2012;82(2):e281–e287.

49. Boehling NS, Grosshans DR, Bluett JB, et al. Dosimetric comparison of three-dimensional conformal proton radiotherapy, intensity-modulated proton therapy, and intensity-modulated radiotherapy for treatment of pediatric craniopharyngiomas. *Int J Radiat Oncol Biol Phys* 2012;82(2):643–652.

50. Adeberg S, Harrabi SB, Bougatf N, et al. Intensity-modulated proton therapy, volumetric-modulated arc therapy, and 3D conformal radiotherapy in anaplastic astrocytoma and glioblastoma: a dosimetric comparison. *Strahlenther Onkol* 2016;192(11):770–779.

51. Brodin NP, Munck af Rosenschold P, Blomstrand M, et al. Hippocampal sparing radiotherapy for pediatric medulloblastoma: impact of treatment margins and treatment technique. *Neuro Oncol* 2014;16(4):594–602.

52. Brower JV, Indelicato DJ, Aldana PR, et al. A treatment planning comparison of highly conformal radiation therapy for pediatric low-grade brainstem gliomas. *Acta Oncol* 2013;52(3):594–599.

53. Dennis ER, Bussiere MR, Niemierko A, et al. A comparison of critical structure dose and toxicity risks in patients with low grade gliomas treated with IMRT versus proton radiation therapy. *Technol Cancer Res Treat* 2013;12(1):1–9.

54. Takizawa D, Mizumoto M, Yamamoto T, et al. A comparative study of dose distribution of PBT, 3D-CRT and IMRT for pediatric brain tumors. *Radiat Oncol* 2017;12(1):40.

55. Harrabi SB, Bougatf N, Mohr A, et al. Dosimetric advantages of proton therapy over conventional radiotherapy with photons in young patients and adults with low-grade glioma. *Strahlenther Onkol* 2016;192(11):759–769.

56. Harding R, Trnkova P, Weston SJ, et al. Benchmarking of a treatment planning system for spot scanning proton therapy: comparison and analysis of robustness to setup errors of photon IMRT and proton SFUD treatment plans of base of skull meningioma. *Med Phys* 2014;41(11):111710.

57. Hall DC, Trofimov AV, Winey BA, et al. Predicting patient-specific dosimetric benefits of proton therapy for skull-base tumors using a geometric knowledge-based method. *Int J Radiat Oncol Biol Phys* 2017;97(5):1087–1094.

58. Cozzi L, Fogliata A, Lomax A, et al. A treatment planning comparison of 3D conformal therapy, intensity modulated photon therapy and proton therapy for treatment of advanced head and neck tumours. *Radiother Oncol* 2001;61(3):287–297.

59. Chera BS, Malyapa R, Louis D, et al. Proton therapy for maxillary sinus carcinoma. *Am J Clin Oncol* 2009;32(3):296–303.

60. Mock U, Georg D, Bogner J, et al. Treatment planning comparison of conventional, 3D conformal, and intensity-modulated photon (IMRT) and proton therapy for paranasal sinus carcinoma. *Int J Radiat Oncol Biol Phys* 2004;58(1):147–154.

61. Apinorasethkul O, Kirk M, Teo K, et al. Pencil beam scanning proton therapy vs rotational arc radiation therapy: a treatment planning comparison for postoperative oropharyngeal cancer. *Med Dosim* 2017;42(1):7–11.

62. Holliday EB, Kocak-Uzel E, Feng L, et al. Dosimetric advantages of intensity-modulated proton therapy for oropharyngeal cancer compared with intensity-modulated radiation: a case-matched control analysis. *Med Dosim* 2016;41(3):189–194.

63. Widesott L, Pierelli A, Fiorino C, et al. Intensity-modulated proton therapy versus helical tomotherapy in nasopharynx cancer: planning comparison and NTCP evaluation. *Int J Radiat Oncol Biol Phys* 2008;72(2):589–596.

64. Noel G, Boisserie G, Dessard-Diana B, et al. Comparison with dose-volume histograms of two conformal irradiation techniques used for the treatment of T2N0M0 nasopharyngeal cancer, one with association of photons and protons and another with photons alone. *Cancer Radiother* 2002;6(6):337–348.

65. Chang JY, Zhang X, Wang X, et al. Significant reduction of normal tissue dose by proton radiotherapy compared with three-dimensional conformal or intensity-modulated radiation therapy in Stage I or Stage III non-small-cell lung cancer. *Int J Radiat Oncol Biol Phys* 2006;65(4):1087–1096.

66. Zhang X, Li Y, Pan X, et al. Intensity-modulated proton therapy reduces the dose to normal tissue compared with intensity-modulated radiation therapy or passive scattering proton therapy and enables individualized radical radiotherapy for extensive stage IIIB non-small-cell lung cancer: a virtual clinical study. *Int J Radiat Oncol Biol Phys* 2010;77(2):357–366.

67. Berman AT, Teo BK, Dolney D, et al. An in-silico comparison of proton beam and IMRT for postoperative radiotherapy in completely resected stage IIIA non-small cell lung cancer. *Radiat Oncol* 2013;8:144.

68. Giaddui T, Chen W, Yu J, et al. Establishing the feasibility of the dosimetric compliance criteria of RTOG 1308: phase III randomized trial comparing overall survival after photon versus proton radiochemotherapy for inoperable stage II-IIIB NSCLC. *Radiat Oncol* 2016;11:66.

69. Hoppe BS, Flampouri S, Su Z, et al. Consolidative involved-node proton therapy for Stage IA-IIIB mediastinal Hodgkin lymphoma: preliminary dosimetric outcomes from a Phase II study. *Int J Radiat Oncol Biol Phys* 2012;83(1):260–267.

70. Chera BS, Rodriguez C, Morris CG, et al. Dosimetric comparison of three different involved nodal irradiation techniques for stage II Hodgkin's lymphoma patients: conventional radiotherapy, intensity-modulated radiotherapy, and three-dimensional proton radiotherapy. *Int J Radiat Oncol Biol Phys* 2009;75(4):1173–1180.

71. Jorgensen AY, Maraldo MV, Brodin NP, et al. The effect on esophagus after different radiotherapy techniques for early stage Hodgkin's lymphoma. *Acta Oncol* 2013;52(7):1559–1565.

72. Hoppe BS, Flampouri S, Su Z, et al. Effective dose reduction to cardiac structures using protons compared with 3DCRT and IMRT in mediastinal Hodgkin lymphoma. *Int J Radiat Oncol Biol Phys* 2012;84(2):449–455.

73. Hoppe BS, Flampouri S, Li Z, et al. Cardiac sparing with proton therapy in consolidative radiation therapy for Hodgkin lymphoma. *Leuk Lymphoma* 2010;51(8):1559–1562.

74. Bouchard M, Amos RA, Briere TM, et al. Dose escalation with proton or photon radiation treatment for pancreatic cancer. *Radiother Oncol* 2009;92(2):238–243.

75. Ding X, Dionisi F, Tang S, et al. A comprehensive dosimetric study of pancreatic cancer treatment using three-dimensional conformal radiation therapy (3DCRT), intensity-modulated radiation therapy (IMRT), volumetric-modulated radiation therapy (VMAT), and passive-scattering and modulated-scanning proton therapy (PT). *Med Dosim* 2014;39(2):139–145.

76. Nichols RC, Jr., Huh SN, Prado KL, et al. Protons offer reduced normal-tissue exposure for patients receiving postoperative radiotherapy for resected pancreatic head cancer. *Int J Radiat Oncol Biol Phys* 2012;83(1):158–163.

77. Welsh J, Gomez D, Palmer MB, et al. Intensity-modulated proton therapy further reduces normal tissue exposure during definitive therapy for locally advanced distal esophageal tumors: a dosimetric study. *Int J Radiat Oncol Biol Phys* 2011;81(5):1336–1342.

78. Chuong MD, Hallemeier CL, Jabbour SK, et al. Improving outcomes for esophageal cancer using proton beam therapy. *Int J Radiat Oncol Biol Phys* 2016;95(1):488–497.

79. Ling TC, Slater JM, Nookala P, et al. Analysis of intensity-modulated radiation therapy (IMRT), proton and 3D conformal radiotherapy (3D-CRT) for reducing perioperative cardiopulmonary complications in esophageal cancer patients. *Cancers (Basel)* 2014;6(4):2356–2368.

80. Blanco Kiely JP, White BM. Robust proton pencil beam scanning treatment planning for rectal cancer radiation Therapy. *Int J Radiat Oncol Biol Phys* 2016;95(1):208–215.

81. Ojerholm E, Kirk ML, Thompson RF, et al. Pencil-beam scanning proton therapy for anal cancer: a dosimetric comparison with intensity-modulated radiotherapy. *Acta Oncol* 2015;54(8):1209–1217.

82. Anand A, Bues M, Rule WG, et al. Scanning proton beam therapy reduces normal tissue exposure in pelvic radiotherapy for anal cancer. *Radiother Oncol* 2015;117(3):505–508.

83. Efstathiou JA, Paly JJ, Lu HM, et al. Adjuvant radiation therapy for early stage seminoma: proton versus photon planning comparison and modeling of second cancer risk. *Radiother Oncol* 2012;103(1):12–17.

84. Vargas C, Fryer A, Mahajan C, et al. Dose-volume comparison of proton therapy and intensity-modulated radiotherapy for prostate cancer. *Int J Radiat Oncol Biol Phys* 2008;70(3):744–751.

85. Scobioala S, Kittel C, Wissmann N, et al. A treatment planning study comparing tomotherapy, volumetric modulated arc therapy, sliding window and proton therapy for low-risk prostate carcinoma. *Radiat Oncol* 2016;11(1):128.

86. Slater JD, Slater JM, Wahlen S. The potential for proton beam therapy in locally advanced carcinoma of the cervix. *Int J Radiat Oncol Biol Phys* 1992;22(2):343–347.

87. Clivio A, Kluge A, Cozzi L, et al. Intensity modulated proton beam radiation for brachytherapy in patients with cervical carcinoma. *Int J Radiat Oncol Biol Phys* 2013;87(5):897–903.

88. Dinges E, Felderman N, McGuire S, et al. Bone marrow sparing in intensity modulated proton therapy for cervical cancer: efficacy and robustness under range and setup uncertainties. *Radiother Oncol* 2015;115(3):373–378.

89. Hashimoto S, Shibamoto Y, Iwata H, et al. Whole-pelvic radiotherapy with spot-scanning proton beams for uterine cervical cancer: a planning study. *J Radiat Res* 2016;57(5):524–532.

90. Marnitz S, Wlodarczyk W, Neumann O, et al. Which technique for radiation is most beneficial for patients with locally advanced cervical cancer? Intensity modulated proton therapy versus intensity modulated photon treatment, helical tomotherapy and volumetric arc therapy for primary radiation—an intraindividual comparison. *Radiat Oncol* 2015;10:91.

91. Xu M, Maity A, Kirk ML, et al. Proton therapy reduces normal tissue dose compared to intensity modulated radiation therapy in extended field pelvic radiation therapy for gynecologic malignancies. *Int J Radiat Oncol Biol Phys* 2016;96(2 Suppl):E634.

92. Moon SH, Shin KH, Kim TH, et al. Dosimetric comparison of four different external beam partial breast irradiation techniques: three-dimensional conformal radiotherapy, intensity-modulated radiotherapy, helical tomotherapy, and proton beam therapy. *Radiother Oncol* 2009;90(1):66–73.

93. Ares C, Khan S, Macartain AM, et al. Postoperative proton radiotherapy for localized and locoregional breast cancer: potential for clinically relevant improvements? *Int J Radiat Oncol Biol Phys* 2010;76(3):685–697.

94. Xu N, Ho MW, Li Z, et al. Can proton therapy improve the therapeutic ratio in breast cancer patients at risk for nodal disease? *Am J Clin Oncol* 2014;37(6):568–574.

95. Lin LL, Vennarini S, Dimofte A, et al. Proton beam versus photon beam dose to the heart and left anterior descending artery for left-sided breast cancer. *Acta Oncol* 2015;54(7):1032–1039.

96. Swanson EL, Indelicato DJ, Louis D, et al. Comparison of three-dimensional (3D) conformal proton radiotherapy (RT), 3D conformal photon RT, and intensity-modulated RT for retroperitoneal and intra-abdominal sarcomas. *Int J Radiat Oncol Biol Phys* 2012;83(5):1549–1557.

97. Chera BS, Vargas C, Morris CG, et al. Dosimetric study of pelvic proton radiotherapy for high-risk prostate cancer. *Int J Radiat Oncol Biol Phys* 2009;75(4):994–1002.

98. Krejcarek SC, Grant PE, Henson JW, et al. Physiologic and radiographic evidence of the distal edge of the proton beam in craniospinal irradiation. *Int J Radiat Oncol Biol Phys* 2007;68(3):646–649.

99. Eekers DB, Roelofs E, Jelen U, et al. Benefit of particle therapy in re-irradiation of head and neck patients. Results of a multicentric in silico ROCOCO trial. *Radiother Oncol* 2016;121(3):387–394.

100. Mouw KW, Sethi RV, Yeap BY, et al. Proton radiation therapy for the treatment of retinoblastoma. *Int J Radiat Oncol Biol Phys* 2014;90(4):863–869.

101. Caujolle JP, Mammar H, Chamorey E, et al. Proton beam radiotherapy for uveal melanomas at nice teaching hospital: 16 years' experience. *Int J Radiat Oncol Biol Phys* 2010;78(1):98–103.

102. Damato B, Kacperek A, Chopra M, et al. Proton beam radiotherapy of choroidal melanoma: the Liverpool-Clatterbridge experience. *Int J Radiat Oncol Biol Phys* 2005;62(5):1405–1411.

103. Dendale R, Lumbroso-Le Rouic L, Noel G, et al. Proton beam radiotherapy for uveal melanoma: results of Curie Institut-Orsay proton therapy center (ICPO). *Int J Radiat Oncol Biol Phys* 2006;65(3):780–787.

104. Desjardins L, Levy-Gabriel C, Lumbroso-Lerouic L, et al. Prognostic factors for malignant uveal melanoma. Retrospective study on 2,241 patients and recent contribution of monosomy-3 research. *J Fr Ophtalmol* 2006;29(7):741–749.

105. Lane AM, Kim IK, Gragoudas ES. Long-term risk of melanoma-related mortality for patients with uveal melanoma treated with proton beam therapy. *JAMA Ophthalmol* 2015;133(7):792–796.

106. Petrovic A, Bergin C, Schalenbourg A, et al. Proton therapy for uveal melanoma in 43 juvenile patients: long-term results. *Ophthalmology* 2014;121(4):898–904.

107. Choi EC, Park J, Shin D, et al. Clinical and volumetric outcomes of gated proton beam therapy for choroidal melanoma in Korea. *Int J Radiat Oncol Biol Phys* 2016;96(2 Suppl 1):E370.

108. Fuji H, Yoshikawa S, Kasami M, et al. High-dose proton beam therapy for sinonasal mucosal malignant melanoma. *Radiat Oncol* 2014;9:162.

109. Zenda S, Akimoto T, Mizumoto M, et al. Phase II study of proton beam therapy as a nonsurgical approach for mucosal melanoma of the nasal cavity or paranasal sinuses. *Radiother Oncol* 2016;118(2):267–271.

110. Demizu Y, Mizumoto M, Onoe T, et al. Proton beam therapy for bone sarcomas of the skull base and spine: a retrospective nationwide multicenter study in Japan. *Cancer Sci* 2017;108(5):972–977.

111. Deraniyagala RL, Yeung D, Mendenhall WM, et al. Proton therapy for skull base chordomas: an outcome study from the University of Florida Proton Therapy Institute. *J Neurol Surg B Skull Base* 2014;75(1):53–57.

112. Di Maio S, Temkin N, Ramanathan D, et al. Current comprehensive management of cranial base chordomas: 10-year meta-analysis of observational studies. *J Neurosurg* 2011;115(6):1094–1105.

113. Grosshans DR, Zhu XR, Melancon A, et al. Spot scanning proton therapy for malignancies of the base of skull: treatment planning, acute toxicities, and preliminary clinical outcomes. *Int J Radiat Oncol Biol Phys* 2014;90(3):540–546.

114. Mima M, Demizu Y, Jin D, et al. Particle therapy using carbon ions or protons as a definitive therapy for patients with primary sacral chordoma. *Br J Radiol* 2014;87(1033):20130512.

115. Holliday EB, Mitra HS, Somerson JS, et al. Postoperative proton therapy for chordomas and chondrosarcomas of the spine: adjuvant versus salvage radiation therapy. *Spine (Phila Pa 1976)* 2015;40(8):544–549.

116. Rotondo RL, Folkert W, Liebsch NJ, et al. High-dose proton-based radiation therapy in the management of spine chordomas: outcomes and clinicopathological prognostic factors. *J Neurosurg Spine* 2015;23(6):788–797.

117. Ciernik IF, Niemierko A, Harmon DC, et al. Proton-based radiotherapy for unresectable or incompletely resected osteosarcoma. *Cancer* 2011;117(19):4522–4530.

118. Ares C, Hug EB, Lomax AJ, et al. Effectiveness and safety of spot scanning proton radiation therapy for chordomas and chondrosarcomas of the skull base: first long-term report. *Int J Radiat Oncol Biol Phys* 2009;75(4):1111–1118.

119. Hayashi Y, Mizumoto M, Akutsu H, et al. Hyperfractionated high-dose proton beam radiotherapy for clival chordomas after surgical removal. *Br J Radiol* 2016;89(1063):20151051.

120. Indelicato DJ, Keole SR, Shahlaee AH, et al. Spinal and paraspinal Ewing tumors. *Int J Radiat Oncol Biol Phys* 2010;76(5):1463–1471.

121. DeLaney TF, Liebsch NJ, Pedlow FX, et al. Phase II study of high-dose photon/proton radiotherapy in the management of spine sarcomas. *Int J Radiat Oncol Biol Phys* 2009;74(3):732–739.

122. DeLaney TF, Chen YL, Baldini EH, et al. Phase 1 trial of preoperative image guided intensity modulated proton radiation therapy with simultaneously integrated boost to the high risk margin for retroperitoneal sarcomas. *Adv Radiat Oncol* 2017;2(1):85–93.

123. Indelicato DJ, Rotondo RL, Begosh-Mayne D, et al. A Prospective Outcomes Study of Proton Therapy for Chordomas and Chondrosarcomas of the Spine. *Int J Radiat Oncol Biol Phys* 2016;95(1):297–303.

124. Nikoghosyan AV, Rauch G, Munter MW, et al. Randomised trial of proton vs. carbon ion radiation therapy in patients with low and intermediate grade chondrosarcoma of the skull base, clinical phase III study. *BMC Cancer* 2010;10:606.

125. MacDonald SM, Safai S, Trofimov A, et al. Proton radiotherapy for childhood ependymoma: initial clinical outcomes and dose comparisons. *Int J Radiat Oncol Biol Phys* 2008;71(4):979–986.

126. Matsuda M, Yamamoto T, Ishikawa E, et al. Prognostic factors in glioblastoma multiforme patients receiving high-dose particle radiotherapy or conventional radiotherapy. *Br J Radiol* 2011;84(Spec No 1):S54–S60.

127. Shih HA, Sherman JC, Nachtigall LB, et al. Proton therapy for low-grade gliomas: Results from a prospective trial. *Cancer* 2015;121(10):1712–1719.

128. Mizumoto M, Tsuboi K, Igaki H, et al. Phase I/II trial of hyperfractionated concomitant boost proton radiotherapy for supratentorial glioblastoma multiforme. *Int J Radiat Oncol Biol Phys* 2010;77(1):98–105.

129. Mizumoto M, Yamamoto T, Ishikawa E, et al. Proton beam therapy with concurrent chemotherapy for glioblastoma multiforme: comparison of nimustine hydrochloride and temozolomide. *J Neurooncol* 2016;130(1):165–170.

130. Kahn J, Loeffler JS, Niemierko A, et al. Long-term outcomes of patients with spinal cord gliomas treated by modern conformal radiation techniques. *Int J Radiat Oncol Biol Phys* 2011;81(1):232–238.

131. Weber DC, Chan AW, Lessell S, et al. Visual outcome of accelerated fractionated radiation for advanced sinonasal malignancies employing photons/protons. *Radiother Oncol* 2006;81(3):243–249.

132. Nakamura N, Zenda S, Tahara M, et al. Proton beam therapy for olfactory neuroblastoma. *Radiother Oncol* 2017;122(3):368–372.

133. Nakamura T, Azami Y, Ono T, et al. Preliminary results of proton beam therapy combined with weekly cisplatin intra-arterial infusion via a superficial temporal artery for treatment of maxillary sinus carcinoma. *Jpn J Clin Oncol* 2016;46(1):46–50.

134. Dagan R, Bryant C, Li Z, et al. Outcomes of Sinonasal Cancer Treated With Proton Therapy. *Int J Radiat Oncol Biol Phys* 2016;95(1):377–385.

135. Fukumitsu N, Okumura T, Mizumoto M, et al. Outcome of T4 (International Union Against Cancer Staging System, 7th edition) or recurrent nasal cavity and paranasal sinus carcinoma treated with proton beam. *Int J Radiat Oncol Biol Phys* 2012;83(2):704–711.

136. Okano S, Tahara M, Zenda S, et al. Induction chemotherapy with docetaxel, cisplatin and S-1 followed by proton beam therapy concurrent with cisplatin in patients with T4b nasal and sinonasal malignancies. *Jpn J Clin Oncol* 2012;42(8):691–696.

137. Russo AL, Adams JA, Weyman EA, et al. Long-term outcomes after proton beam therapy for sinonasal squamous cell carcinoma. *Int J Radiat Oncol Biol Phys* 2016;95(1):368–376.

138. Truong MT, Kamat UR, Liebsch NJ, et al. Proton radiation therapy for primary sphenoid sinus malignancies: treatment outcome and prognostic factors. *Head Neck* 2009;31(10):1297–1308.

139. Akimoto T, Zenda S, Nakamura N, et al. A retrospective multi-institutional study of proton beam therapy for head and neck cancer with non-squamous cell histologies. *Int J Radiat Oncol Biol Phys* 2016;96(2 Suppl):E337.

140. Slater JD, Yonemoto LT, Mantik DW, et al. Proton radiation for treatment of cancer of the oropharynx: early experience at Loma Linda University Medical Center using a concomitant boost technique. *Int J Radiat Oncol Biol Phys* 2005;62(2):494–500.

141. Gunn GB, Blanchard P, Garden AS, et al. Clinical outcomes and patterns of disease recurrence after intensity modulated proton therapy for oropharyngeal squamous carcinoma. *Int J Radiat Oncol Biol Phys* 2016;95(1):360–367.

142. Blanchard P, Garden AS, Gunn GB, et al. Intensity-modulated proton beam therapy (IMPT) versus intensity-modulated photon therapy (IMRT) for patients with oropharynx cancer—a case matched analysis. *Radiother Oncol* 2016;120(1):48–55.

143. Lewis GD, Holliday EB, Kocak-Uzel E, et al. Intensity-modulated proton therapy for nasopharyngeal carcinoma: decreased radiation dose to normal structures and encouraging clinical outcomes. *Head Neck* 2016;38(Suppl 1):E1886–E1895.

144. McDonald MW, Liu Y, Moore MG, et al. Acute toxicity in comprehensive head and neck radiation for nasopharynx and paranasal sinus cancers: cohort comparison of 3D conformal proton therapy and intensity modulated radiation therapy. *Radiat Oncol* 2016;11:32.

145. Romesser PB, Cahlon O, Scher E, et al. Proton beam radiation therapy results in significantly reduced toxicity compared with intensity-modulated radiation therapy for head and neck tumors that require ipsilateral radiation. *Radiother Oncol* 2016;118(2):286–292.

146. Bhattasali O, Holliday E, Kies MS, et al. Definitive proton radiation therapy and concurrent cisplatin for unresectable head and neck adenoid cystic carcinoma: a series of 9 cases and a critical review of the literature. *Head Neck* 2016;38(Suppl 1):E1472–E1480.

147. Gentile MS, Yip D, Liebsch NJ, et al. Definitive proton beam therapy for adenoid cystic carcinoma of the nasopharynx involving the base of skull. *Oral Oncol* 2017;65:38–44.

148. Deraniyagala RL, Bryant CM, Morris CG, et al. Proton therapy for head and neck adenoid cystic carcinoma. *Int J Radiat Oncol Biol Phys* 2016;96(2):e369–e370.

149. Mizumoto M, Sugahara S, Okumura T, et al. Hyperfractionated concomitant boost proton beam therapy for esophageal carcinoma. *Int J Radiat Oncol Biol Phys* 2011;81(4):e601–e606.

150. Lin SH, Komaki R, Liao Z, et al. Proton beam therapy and concurrent chemotherapy for esophageal cancer. *Int J Radiat Oncol Biol Phys* 2012;83(3):e345–e351.

151. Takada A, Nakamura T, Takayama K, et al. Preliminary treatment results of proton beam therapy with chemoradiotherapy for stage I–III esophageal cancer. *Cancer Med* 2016;5(3):506–515.

152. Zeng YC, Vyas S, Dang Q, et al. Proton therapy posterior beam approach with pencil beam scanning for esophageal cancer: clinical outcome, dosimetry, and feasibility. *Strahlenther Onkol* 2016;192(12):913–921.

153. Ishikawa H, Saito T, Iizumi T, et al. Concurrent chemo-proton therapy for esophageal cancer. *Int J Radiat Oncol Biol Phys* 2016;96(2 Suppl):E192.

154. Chang JY, Komaki R, Lu C, et al. Phase 2 study of high-dose proton therapy with concurrent chemotherapy for unresectable stage III nonsmall cell lung cancer. *Cancer* 2011;117(20):4707–4713.

155. Bush DA, Slater JD, Shin BB, et al. Hypofractionated proton beam radiotherapy for stage I lung cancer. *Chest* 2004;126(4):1198–1203.

156. Bush DA, Cheek G, Zaheer S, et al. High-dose hypofractionated proton beam radiation therapy is safe and effective for central and peripheral early-stage non-small cell lung cancer: results of a 12-year experience at Loma Linda University Medical Center. *Int J Radiat Oncol Biol Phys* 2013;86(5):964–968.

157. Chang JY, Zhang W, Komaki R, et al. Long-term outcome of phase I/II prospective study of dose-escalated proton therapy for early-stage non-small cell lung cancer. *Radiother Oncol* 2017;122(2):274–280.

158. Colaco RJ, Huh S, Nichols RC, et al. Dosimetric rationale and early experience at UFPTI of thoracic proton therapy and chemotherapy in limited-stage small cell lung cancer. *Acta Oncol* 2013;52(3):506–513.

159. Gomez DR, Tucker SL, Martel MK, et al. Predictors of high-grade esophagitis after definitive three-dimensional conformal therapy, intensity-modulated radiation therapy, or proton beam therapy for non-small cell lung cancer. *Int J Radiat Oncol Biol Phys* 2012;84(4):1010–1016.

160. Harada H, Fuji H, Ono A, et al. Dose escalation study of proton beam therapy with concurrent chemotherapy for stage III non-small cell lung cancer. *Cancer Sci* 2016;107(7):1018–1021.

161. Hoppe BS, Flampouri S, Henderson RH, et al. Proton therapy with concurrent chemotherapy for non-small-cell lung cancer: technique and early results. *Clin Lung Cancer* 2012;13(5):352–358.

162. Westover KD, Seco J, Adams JA, et al. Proton SBRT for medically inoperable stage I NSCLC. *J Thorac Oncol* 2012;7(6):1021–1025.

163. Badiyan SN, Hartsell WF, Cahlon O, et al. Clinical outcomes of patients with stage II–III non-small cell lung cancer (NSCLC) treated with proton beam therapy (PBT) on the Proton Collaborative Group (PCG) Prospective Registry Trial. *Int J Radiat Oncol Biol Phys* 2016;96(2 Suppl):E434–E435.

164. Zhu HJ, Nichols RC Jr, Henderson RH, et al. Impact of unfavorable factors on outcomes among inoperable stage II–IV non-small cell lung cancer patients treated with proton therapy. *Int J Radiat Oncol Biol Phys* 2017;98(1):225.

165. Figura N, Hoppe BS, Flampouri S, et al. Postoperative proton therapy in the management of stage III thymoma. *J Thorac Oncol* 2013;8(5):e38–e40.

166. Vogel J, Berman AT, Lin L, et al. Prospective study of proton beam radiation therapy for adjuvant and definitive treatment of thymoma and thymic carcinoma: early response and toxicity assessment. *Radiother Oncol* 2016;118(3):504–509.

167. Pan HY, Jiang S, Sutton J, et al. Early experience with intensity modulated proton therapy for lung-intact mesothelioma: a case series. *Pract Radiat Oncol* 2015;5(4):e345–e353.

168. Takaoka EI, Miyazaki J, Ishikawa H, et al. Long-term single-institute experience with trimodal bladder-preserving therapy with proton beam therapy for muscle-invasive bladder cancer. *Jpn J Clin Oncol* 2017;47(1):67–73.

169. Mendenhall NP, Li Z, Hoppe BS, et al. Early outcomes from three prospective trials of image-guided proton therapy for prostate cancer. *Int J Radiat Oncol Biol Phys* 2012;82(1):213–221.

170. Slater JD, Rossi CJ Jr, Yonemoto LT, et al. Proton therapy for prostate cancer: the initial Loma Linda University experience. *Int J Radiat Oncol Biol Phys* 2004;59(2):348–352.

171. Zietman AL, Bae K, Slater JD, et al. Randomized trial comparing conventional-dose with high-dose conformal radiation therapy in early-stage adenocarcinoma of the prostate: long-term results from proton radiation oncology group/american college of radiology 95-09. *J Clin Oncol* 2010;28(7):1106–1111.

172. Mendenhall NP, Hoppe BS, Nichols RC, et al. Five-year outcomes from 3 prospective trials of image-guided proton therapy for prostate cancer. *Int J Radiat Oncol Biol Phys* 2014;88(3):596–602.

173. Henderson RH, Bryant C, Hoppe BS, et al. Five-year outcomes from a prospective trial of image-guided accelerated hypofractionated proton therapy for prostate cancer. *Acta Oncol* 2017;56(7):963–970.

174. Kim YJ, Cho KH, Pyo HR, et al. A phase II study of hypofractionated proton therapy for prostate cancer. *Acta Oncol* 2013;52(3):477–485.

175. McGee L, Mendenhall NP, Henderson RH, et al. Outcomes in men with large prostates (≥60 cm³) treated with definitive proton therapy for prostate cancer. *Acta Oncol* 2013;52(3):470–476.

176. Pugh TJ, Munsell MF, Choi S, et al. Quality of life and toxicity from passively scattered and spot-scanning proton beam therapy for localized prostate cancer. *Int J Radiat Oncol Biol Phys* 2013;87(5):946–953.

177. Talcott JA, Rossi C, Shipley WU, et al. Patient-reported long-term outcomes after conventional and high-dose combined proton and photon radiation for early prostate cancer. *JAMA* 2010;303(11):1046–1053.

178. Taneja SS. Re: five-year biochemical results, toxicity, and patient-reported quality of life after delivery of dose-escalated image guided proton therapy for prostate cancer. *J Urol* 2017;197(1):149–152.

179. Yonemoto LT, Slater JD, Rossi CJ Jr, et al. Combined proton and photon conformal radiation therapy for locally advanced carcinoma of the prostate: preliminary results of a phase I/II study. *Int J Radiat Oncol Biol Phys* 1997;37(1):21–29.

180. Rossi CJ Jr, Slater JD, Yonemoto LT, et al. Influence of patient age on biochemical freedom from disease in patients undergoing conformal proton radiotherapy of organ-confined prostate cancer. *Urology* 2004;64(4):729–732.

181. Cuaron JJ, Harris AA, Chon B, et al. Anterior-oriented proton beams for prostate cancer: a multi-institutional experience. *Acta Oncol* 2015;54(6):868–874.

182. Bryant C, Smith TL, Henderson RH, et al. Five-year biochemical results, toxicity, and patient-reported quality of life after delivery of dose-escalated image guided proton therapy for prostate cancer. *Int J Radiat Oncol Biol Phys* 2016;95(1):422–434.

183. Chang JH, Lee NK, Kim JY, et al. Phase II trial of proton beam accelerated partial breast irradiation in breast cancer. *Radiother Oncol* 2013;108(2):209–214.

184. Cuaron JJ, Chon B, Tsai H, et al. Early toxicity in patients treated with postoperative proton therapy for locally advanced breast cancer. *Int J Radiat Oncol Biol Phys* 2015;92(2):284–291.

185. Bradley JA, Dagan R, Ho MW, et al. Initial report of a prospective dosimetric and clinical feasibility trial demonstrates the potential of protons to increase the therapeutic ratio in breast cancer compared with photons. *Int J Radiat Oncol Biol Phys* 2016;95(1):411–421.

186. MacDonald SM, Patel SA, Hickey S, et al. Proton therapy for breast cancer after mastectomy: early outcomes of a prospective clinical trial. *Int J Radiat Oncol Biol Phys* 2013;86(3):484–490.

187. Li J, Dabaja B, Reed V, et al. Rationale for and preliminary results of proton beam therapy for mediastinal lymphoma. *Int J Radiat Oncol Biol Phys* 2011;81(1):167–174.

188. Hoppe BS, Tsai H, Larson G, et al. Proton therapy patterns-of-care and early outcomes for Hodgkin lymphoma: results from the Proton Collaborative Group Registry. *Acta Oncol* 2016;55(11):1378–1380.

189. Hoppe BS, Flampouri S, Zaiden R, et al. Involved-node proton therapy in combined modality therapy for Hodgkin lymphoma: results of a phase 2 study. *Int J Radiat Oncol Biol Phys* 2014;89(5):1053–1059.

190. Sachsman S, Hoppe BS, Mendenhall NP, et al. Proton therapy to the subdiaphragmatic region in the management of patients with Hodgkin lymphoma. *Leuk Lymphoma* 2015;56(7):2019–2024.

191. Sachsman S, Flampouri S, Li Z, et al. Proton therapy in the management of non-Hodgkin lymphoma. *Leuk Lymphoma* 2015;56(9):2608–2612.

192. Hoppe BS, Hill-Kayser CE, Tseng YD, et al. The use of consolidative proton therapy after first-line therapy among patients with Hodgkin lymphoma at academic and community proton centers. *Int J Radiat Oncol Biol Phys* 2016;96(2 Suppl):S39.

193. Plastaras JP, Vogel J, Elmongy H, et al. First clinical report of pencil beam scanned proton therapy for mediastinal lymphoma. *Int J Radiat Oncol Biol Phys* 2016;96(2 Suppl):E497.

194. Rutenberg MS, Flampouri S, Hoppe BS. Proton therapy for Hodgkin lymphoma. *Curr Hematol Malig Rep* 2014;9(3):203–211.

195. Holtzman A, Flampouri S, Li Z, et al. Proton therapy in a pediatric patient with stage III Hodgkin lymphoma. *Acta Oncol* 2013;52(3):592–594.

196. Figura NB, Flampouri S, Hopper K, et al. Consolidative proton therapy following high-dose chemotherapy and autologous stem cell transplant in an adolescent with relapsed Hodgkin lymphoma. *J Adolesc Young Adult Oncol* 2011;1(2):103–106.

197. Bush DA, Hillebrand DJ, Slater JM, et al. High-dose proton beam radiotherapy of hepatocellular carcinoma: preliminary results of a phase II trial. *Gastroenterology* 2004;127(5 Suppl 1):S189–S193.

198. Bush DA, Kayali Z, Grove R, et al. The safety and efficacy of high-dose proton beam radiotherapy for hepatocellular carcinoma: a phase 2 prospective trial. *Cancer* 2011;117(13):3053–3059.

199. Chiba T, Tokuuye K, Matsuzaki Y, et al. Proton beam therapy for hepatocellular carcinoma: a retrospective review of 162 patients. *Clin Cancer Res* 2005;11(10):3799–3805.

200. Fukuda K, Okumura T, Abei M, et al. Long-term outcomes of proton beam therapy in patients with previously untreated hepatocellular carcinoma. *Cancer Sci* 2017;108(3):497–503.

201. Hong TS, Wo JY, Yeap BY, et al. Multi-institutional phase ii study of high-dose hypofractionated proton beam therapy in patients with localized, unresectable hepatocellular carcinoma and intrahepatic cholangiocarcinoma. *J Clin Oncol* 2016;34(5):460–468.

202. Kimura K, Nakamura T, Ono T, et al. Clinical results of proton beam therapy for hepatocellular carcinoma over 5 cm. *Hepatol Res* 2017.

203. Qi WX, Fu S, Zhang Q, et al. Charged particle therapy versus photon therapy for patients with hepatocellular carcinoma: a systematic review and meta-analysis. *Radiother Oncol* 2015;114(3):289–295.

204. Mizumoto M, Okumura T, Hashimoto T, et al. Proton beam therapy for hepatocellular carcinoma: a comparison of three treatment protocols. *Int J Radiat Oncol Biol Phys* 2011;81(4):1039–1045.

205. Hong TS, Ryan DP, Blaszkowsky LS, et al. Phase I study of preoperative short-course chemoradiation with proton beam therapy and capecitabine for resectable pancreatic ductal adenocarcinoma of the head. *Int J Radiat Oncol Biol Phys* 2011;79(1):151–157.

206. Nichols RC Jr, George TJ, Zaiden RA Jr, et al. Proton therapy with concomitant capecitabine for pancreatic and ampullary cancers is associated with a low incidence of gastrointestinal toxicity. *Acta Oncol* 2013;52(2):498–505.

207. Hitchcock KE, Nichols RC, Morris CG, et al. Feasibility of pancreatectomy following high-dose proton therapy for unresectable pancreatic cancer. *World J Gastrointest Surg* 2017;9(4):103–108.

208. Hong TS, Ryan DP, Borger DR, et al. A phase 1/2 and biomarker study of preoperative short course chemoradiation with proton beam therapy and capecitabine followed by early surgery for resectable pancreatic ductal adenocarcinoma. *Int J Radiat Oncol Biol Phys* 2014;89(4):830–838.

209. Wo JY, Mamon HJ, Ferrone CR, et al. Phase I study of neoadjuvant accelerated short course radiation therapy with photons and capecitabine for resectable pancreatic cancer. *Radiother Oncol* 2014;110(1):160–164.

Section
II

210. Makita C, Nakamura T, Takada A, et al. Clinical outcomes and toxicity of proton beam therapy for advanced cholangiocarcinoma. *Radiat Oncol* 2014; 9:26.

211. Colbert LE, Cloyd JM, Koay EJ, et al. Proton beam radiation as salvage therapy for bilateral colorectal liver metastases not amenable to second-stage hepatectomy. *Surgery* 2017;161(6):1543–1548.

212. Kagei K, Tokuuye K, Okumura T, et al. Long-term results of proton beam therapy for carcinoma of the uterine cervix. *Int J Radiat Oncol Biol Phys* 2003;55(5):1265–1271.

213. MacDonald SM, Trofimov A, Safai S, et al. Proton radiotherapy for pediatric central nervous system germ cell tumors: early clinical outcomes. *Int J Radiat Oncol Biol Phys* 2011;79(1):121–129.

214. Hauswald H, Rieken S, Ecker S, et al. First experiences in treatment of low-grade glioma grade I and II with proton therapy. *Radiat Oncol* 2012; 7:189.

215. Kahalley LS, Ris MD, Grosshans DR, et al. Comparing intelligence quotient change after treatment with proton versus photon radiation therapy for pediatric brain tumors. *J Clin Oncol* 2016;34(10):1043–1049.

216. Jimenez RB, Sethi R, Depauw N, et al. Proton radiation therapy for pediatric medulloblastoma and supratentorial primitive neuroectodermal tumors: outcomes for very young children treated with upfront chemotherapy. *Int J Radiat Oncol Biol Phys* 2013;87(1):120–126.

217. MacDonald SM, Yock TI. Proton beam therapy following resection for childhood ependymoma. *Childs Nerv Syst* 2010;26(3):285–291.

218. McGovern SL, Okcu MF, Munsell MF, et al. Outcomes and acute toxicities of proton therapy for pediatric atypical teratoid/rhabdoid tumor of the central nervous system. *Int J Radiat Oncol Biol Phys* 2014;90(5):1143–1152.

219. Merchant TE, Kiehna EN, Li C, et al. Radiation dosimetry predicts IQ after conformal radiation therapy in pediatric patients with localized ependymoma. *Int J Radiat Oncol Biol Phys* 2005;63(5):1546–1554.

220. Eaton BR, Esiashvili N, Kim S, et al. Endocrine outcomes with proton and photon radiotherapy for standard risk medulloblastoma. *Neuro Oncol* 2016;18(6):881–887.

221. Sethi RV, Giantsoudi D, Raiford M, et al. Patterns of failure after proton therapy in medulloblastoma; linear energy transfer distributions and relative biological effectiveness associations for relapses. *Int J Radiat Oncol Biol Phys* 2014;88(3):655–663.

222. Eaton BR, Esiashvili N, Kim S, et al. Clinical outcomes among children with standard-risk medulloblastoma treated with proton and photon radiation therapy: a comparison of disease control and overall survival. *Int J Radiat Oncol Biol Phys* 2016;94(1):133–138.

223. Eaton BR, Goldberg S, Gaudet D, et al. Radiation dosimetry and health-related quality of life in pediatric brain tumor survivors treated with proton therapy at ≤3 years of age. *Int J Radiat Oncol Biol Phys* 2016;96(2 Suppl):S121.

224. Indelicato DJ, Bradley JA, Rotondo RL, et al. Single-institution outcomes following proton therapy for children with central nervous system tumors referred overseas. *Int J Radiat Oncol Biol Phys* 2016;96(2 Suppl):E551.

225. Indelicato DJ, Flampouri S, Rotondo RL, et al. Incidence and dosimetric parameters of pediatric brainstem toxicity following proton therapy. *Acta Oncol* 2014;53(10):1298–1304.

226. Indelicato DJ, Bradley JA, Sandler ES, et al. Clinical outcomes following proton therapy for children with central nervous system tumors referred overseas. Pediatr Blood Cancer 2017.

227. Mizumoto M, Oshiro Y, Takizawa D, et al. Proton beam therapy for pediatric patients with ependymoma. *Pediatr Int* 2015;57(4):567–571. doi: 10.1111/ped.12624. [Epub ahead of print].

228. Lucas JT Jr, Ladra MM, MacDonald SM, et al. Proton therapy for pediatric and adolescent esthesioneuroblastoma. *Pediatr Blood Cancer* 2015;62(9):1523–1528.

229. Wray J, Flampouri S, Slayton W, et al. Proton therapy for pediatric Hodgkin lymphoma. *Pediatr Blood Cancer* 2016;63(9):1522–1526.

230. Amsbaugh MJ, Grosshans DR, McAleer MF, et al. Proton therapy for spinal ependymomas: planning, acute toxicities, and preliminary outcomes. *Int J Radiat Oncol Biol Phys* 2012;83(5):1419–1424.

231. Oshiro Y, Mizumoto M, Okumura T, et al. Clinical results of proton beam therapy for advanced neuroblastoma. *Radiat Oncol* 2013;8:142.

232. Oshiro Y, Okumura T, Mizumoto M, et al. Proton beam therapy for unresectable hepatoblastoma in children: survival in one case. *Acta Oncol* 2013;52(3):600–603.

233. Rombi B, Vennarini S, Vinante L, et al. Proton radiotherapy for pediatric tumors: review of first clinical results. *Ital J Pediatr* 2014;40:74.

234. Mizumoto M, Murayama S, Akimoto T, et al. Long-term follow-up after proton beam therapy for pediatric tumors: a Japanese national survey. *Cancer Sci* 2017;108(3):444–447.

235. Harrell LM, Paulino AC, Mahajan A, et al. Clinical outcomes and toxicity following proton radiation therapy for head and neck rhabdomyosarcoma. *Int J Radiat Oncol Biol Phys* 2016;96(2):E549–E550.

236. Leiser D, Malyapa RS, Albertini F, et al. Clinical outcome of pencil beam scanning proton therapy for children with rhabdomyosarcoma. *Int J Radiat Oncol Biol Phys* 2016;96(2 Suppl):E547–E548.

237. Hill-Kayser C, Tochner Z, Both S, et al. Proton versus photon radiation therapy for patients with high-risk neuroblastoma: the need for a customized approach. *Pediatr Blood Cancer* 2013;60(10):1606–1611.

238. Wattson DA, Tanguturi SK, Spiegel DY, et al. Outcomes of proton therapy for patients with functional pituitary adenomas. *Int J Radiat Oncol Biol Phys* 2014;90(3):532–539.

239. Vernimmen FJ, Mohamed Z, Slabbert JP, et al. Long-term results of stereotactic proton beam radiotherapy for acoustic neuromas. *Radiother Oncol* 2009;90(2):208–212.

240. Bush DA, McAllister CJ, Loredo LN, et al. Fractionated proton beam radiotherapy for acoustic neuroma. *Neurosurgery* 2002;50(2):270–273; discussion 273–275.

241. Zambarakji HJ, Lane AM, Ezra E, et al. Proton beam irradiation for neovascular age-related macular degeneration. *Ophthalmology* 2006;113(11):2012–2019.

242. Ciulla TA, Danis RP, Klein SB, et al. Proton therapy for exudative age-related macular degeneration: a randomized, sham-controlled clinical trial. *Am J Ophthalmol* 2002;134(6):905–906.

243. Zur C, Caujolle JP, Chauvel P, et al. Proton therapy of occult neovessels in age-related macular degeneration. *J Fr Ophtalmol* 2001;24(9):949–954.

244. Chen L, Kim IK, Lane AM, et al. Proton beam irradiation for non-AMD CNV: 2-year results of a randomised clinical trial. *Br J Ophthalmol* 2014;98(9):1212–1217.

245. Gear HC, Kemp EG, Kacperek A, et al. Treatment of recurrent orbital haemangiopericytoma with surgery and proton beam therapy. *Br J Ophthalmol* 2005;89(1):123–124.

246. Chowdhury I, Nead KT, Lustig RA, et al. First report of paragangliomas treated with proton therapy. *Int J Radiat Oncol Biol Phys* 2016;96(2 Suppl):E126.

247. Slater JD, Loredo LN, Chung A, et al. Fractionated proton radiotherapy for benign cavernous sinus meningiomas. *Int J Radiat Oncol Biol Phys* 2012;83(5):e633–e637.

248. Noel G, Bollet MA, Calugaru V, et al. Functional outcome of patients with benign meningioma treated by 3D conformal irradiation with a combination of photons and protons. *Int J Radiat Oncol Biol Phys* 2005;62:1412–1422.

249. Chao HH, Berman AT, Simone CB II, et al. Multi-institutional prospective study of reirradiation with proton beam radiotherapy for locoregionally recurrent non-small cell lung cancer. *J Thorac Oncol* 2017;12(2):281–292.

250. McAvoy SA, Ciura KT, Rineer JM, et al. Feasibility of proton beam therapy for reirradiation of locoregionally recurrent non-small cell lung cancer. *Radiother Oncol* 2013;109(1):38–44.

251. Mendenhall WM, Amdur RJ, Morris CG, et al. Carcinoma of the nasal cavity and paranasal sinuses. *Laryngoscope* 2009;119(5):899–906.

252. Barney CL, Brown AP, Grosshans DR, et al. Technique, outcomes, and acute toxicities in adults treated with proton beam craniospinal irradiation. *Neuro Oncol* 2014;16(2):303–309.

253. Pinnix CC, Smith GL, Milgrom S, et al. Predictors of radiation pneumonitis in patients receiving intensity modulated radiation therapy for Hodgkin and non-Hodgkin lymphoma. *Int J Radiat Oncol Biol Phys* 2015;92(1):175–182.

254. Chun SG, Hu C, Choy H, et al. Impact of intensity-modulated radiation therapy technique for locally advanced non-small-cell lung cancer: a secondary analysis of the NRG Oncology RTOG 0617 Randomized Clinical Trial. *J Clin Oncol* 2017;35(1):56–62.

255. Wang K, Eblan MJ, Deal AM, et al. Cardiac toxicity after radiotherapy for stage iii non-small-cell lung cancer: pooled analysis of dose-escalation trials delivering 70 to 90 Gy. *J Clin Oncol* 2017;35(13):1387–1394.

256. Cuzick J, Stewart H, Rutqvist L, et al. Cause-specific mortality in long-term survivors of breast cancer who participated in trials of radiotherapy. *J Clin Oncol* 1994;12(3):447–453.

257. Clarke M, Collins R, Darby S, et al. Effects of radiotherapy and of differences in the extent of surgery for early breast cancer on local recurrence and 15-year survival: an overview of the randomised trials. *Lancet* 2005;366(9503):2087–2106.

258. Whelan TJ, Olivotto IA, Parulekar WR, et al. Regional nodal irradiation in early-stage breast cancer. *N Engl J Med* 2015;373(4):307–316.

259. Overgaard M, Hansen PS, Overgaard J, et al. Postoperative radiotherapy in high-risk premenopausal women with breast cancer who receive adjuvant chemotherapy. Danish Breast Cancer Cooperative Group 82b Trial. *N Engl J Med* 1997;337(14):949–955.

260. Overgaard M, Jensen MB, Overgaard J, et al. Postoperative radiotherapy in high-risk postmenopausal breast-cancer patients given adjuvant tamoxifen: Danish Breast Cancer Cooperative Group DBCG 82c randomised trial. *Lancet* 1999;353(9165):1641–1648.

261. Ragaz J, Olivotto IA, Spinelli JJ, et al. Locoregional radiation therapy in patients with high-risk breast cancer receiving adjuvant chemotherapy: 20-year results of the British Columbia randomized trial. *J Natl Cancer Inst* 2005;97(2):116–126.

262. Darby S, McGale P, Correa C, et al. Early Breast Cancer Trialists' Collaborative Group. Effect of radiotherapy after breast-conserving surgery on 10-year recurrence and 15-year breast cancer death: meta-analysis of individual patient data for 10,801 women in 17 randomised trials. *Lancet* 2011;378(9804):1707–1716.

263. McGale P, Taylor C, Correa C, et al. Early Breast Cancer Trialists' Collaborative Group. Effect of radiotherapy after mastectomy and axillary surgery on 10-year recurrence and 20-year breast cancer mortality: meta-analysis of individual patient data for 8135 women in 22 randomised trials. *Lancet* 2014;383(9935):2127–2135.

264. Poortmans PM, Collette S, Kirkove C, et al. Internal mammary and medial supraclavicular irradiation in breast cancer. *N Engl J Med* 2015;373(4):317–327.

265. Darby SC, Ewertz M, McGale P, et al. Risk of ischemic heart disease in women after radiotherapy for breast cancer. *N Engl J Med* 2013;368(11):987–998.

266. Bouillon K, Haddy N, Delaloge S, et al. Long-term cardiovascular mortality after radiotherapy for breast cancer. *J Am Coll Cardiol* 2011;57(4):445–452.

267. Harris EE, Correa C, Hwang WT, et al. Late cardiac mortality and morbidity in early-stage breast cancer patients after breast-conservation treatment. *J Clin Oncol* 2006;24(25):4100–4106.

268. Borger JH, Hooning MJ, Boersma LJ, et al. Cardiotoxic effects of tangential breast irradiation in early breast cancer patients: the role of irradiated heart volume. *Int J Radiat Oncol Biol Phys* 2007;69(4):1131–1138.

269. National Clinical Trials Network. NRG Oncology/Radiation Therapy Oncology Group 1005: a phase III trial of accelerated whole breast irradiation with hypofractionation plus concurrent boost versus standard whole breast irradiation plus sequential boost for early-stage breast cancer 2014; https://www.rtog.org/clinicaltrials/protocoltable/studydetails.aspx?study=1005. Accessed September 5, 2017.

270. National Surgical Adjuvant Breast and Bowel Project (NSABP). Protocol B-51/Radiation Therapy Oncology Group 1304: a randomized phase III clinical trial evaluating post-mastectomy chest wall and regional nodal XRT and post-lumpectomy regional nodal XRT in patients with positive axillary nodes before neoadjuvant chemotherapy who convert to pathologically negative axillary nodes after neoadjuvant chemotherapy 2013; http://meetinglibrary.asco.org/content/132077-144. Accessed September 5, 2017.

271. Hamdy FC, Donovan JL, Lane JA, et al. 10-Year outcomes after monitoring, surgery, or radiotherapy for localized prostate cancer. *N Engl J Med* 2016;375(15):1415–1424.

272. Donovan JL, Hamdy FC, Lane JA, et al. Patient-reported outcomes after monitoring, surgery, or radiotherapy for prostate cancer. *N Engl J Med* 2016;375(15):1425–1437.

273. Peeters ST, Heemsbergen WD, Koper PC, et al. Dose-response in radiotherapy for localized prostate cancer: results of the Dutch multicenter randomized phase III trial comparing 68 Gy of radiotherapy with 78 Gy. *J Clin Oncol* 2006;24(13):1990–1996.

274. Kuban DA, Tucker SL, Dong L, et al. Long-term results of the M. D. Anderson randomized dose-escalation trial for prostate cancer. *Int J Radiat Oncol Biol Phys* 2008;70(1):67–74.

275. Dearnaley DP, Sydes MR, Graham JD, et al. Escalated-dose versus standard-dose conformal radiotherapy in prostate cancer: first results from the MRC RT01 randomised controlled trial. *Lancet Oncol* 2007;8(6):475–487.

276. Michalski JM, Bae K, Roach M, et al. Long-term toxicity following 3D conformal radiation therapy for prostate cancer from the RTOG 9406 phase I/II dose escalation study. *Int J Radiat Oncol Biol Phys* 2010;76(1):14–22.

277. Colaco RJ, Hoppe BS, Flampouri S, et al. Rectal toxicity after proton therapy for prostate cancer: an analysis of outcomes of prospective studies conducted at the university of Florida Proton Therapy Institute. *Int J Radiat Oncol Biol Phys* 2015;91(1):172–181.

278. Lee WR, Dignam JJ, Amin MB, et al. Randomized phase III noninferiority study comparing two radiotherapy fractionation schedules in patients with low-risk prostate cancer. *J Clin Oncol* 2016;34(20):2325–2332.

279. Catton CN, Lukka H, Gu CS, et al. Randomized trial of a hypofractionated radiation regimen for the treatment of localized prostate cancer. *J Clin Oncol* 2017;35(17):1884–1890.

280. Sanguineti G, Arcidiacono F, Landoni V, et al. Macroscopic hematuria after conventional or hypofractionated radiation therapy: results from a prospective phase 3 study. *Int J Radiat Oncol Biol Phys* 2016;96(2):304–312.

281. Hoffman KE, Voong KR, Pugh TJ, et al. Risk of late toxicity in men receiving dose-escalated hypofractionated intensity modulated prostate radiation therapy: results from a randomized trial. *Int J Radiat Oncol Biol Phys* 2014;88(5):1074–1084.

282. Krol R, Smeenk RJ, van Lin EN, et al. Impact of late anorectal dysfunction on quality of life after pelvic radiotherapy. *Int J Colorectal Dis* 2013;28(4):519–526.

283. Resnick MJ, Koyama T, Fan KH, et al. Long-term functional outcomes after treatment for localized prostate cancer. *N Engl J Med* 2013;368(5):436–445.

284. Creak A, Hall E, Horwich A, et al. Randomised pilot study of dose escalation using conformal radiotherapy in prostate cancer: long-term follow-up. *Br J Cancer* 2013;109(3):651–657.

285. Cox JD, Stetz J, Pajak TF. Toxicity criteria of the Radiation Therapy Oncology Group (RTOG) and the European Organization for Research and Treatment of Cancer (EORTC). *Int J Radiat Oncol Biol Phys* 1995;31(5):1341–1346.

286. Yeoh EK, Holloway RH, Fraser RJ, et al. Pathophysiology and natural history of anorectal sequelae following radiation therapy for carcinoma of the prostate. *Int J Radiat Oncol Biol Phys* 2012;84(5):e593–e599.

287. Peeters ST, Lebesque JV, Heemsbergen WD, et al. Localized volume effects for late rectal and anal toxicity after radiotherapy for prostate cancer. *Int J Radiat Oncol Biol Phys* 2006;64(4):1151–1161.

288. al-Abany M, Helgason AR, Cronqvist AK, et al. Toward a definition of a threshold for harmless doses to the anal-sphincter region and the rectum. *Int J Radiat Oncol Biol Phys* 2005;61(4):1035–1044.

289. Trofimov A, Nguyen PL, Coen JJ, et al. Radiotherapy treatment of early-stage prostate cancer with IMRT and protons: a treatment planning comparison. *Int J Radiat Oncol Biol Phys* 2007;69(2):444–453.

290. Song DY, Herfarth KK, Uhl M, et al. A multi-institutional clinical trial of rectal dose reduction via injected polyethylene-glycol hydrogel during intensity modulated radiation therapy for prostate cancer: analysis of dosimetric outcomes. *Int J Radiat Oncol Biol Phys* 2013;87(1):81–87.

291. Uhl M, Herfarth K, Eble MJ, et al. Absorbable hydrogel spacer use in men undergoing prostate cancer radiotherapy: 12 month toxicity and proctoscopy results of a prospective multicenter phase II trial. *Radiat Oncol* 2014;9:96.

292. Dearnaley DP, Hall E, Lawrence D, et al. Phase III pilot study of dose escalation using conformal radiotherapy in prostate cancer: PSA control and side effects. *Br J Cancer* 2005;92(3):488–498.

293. American Joint Committee on Cancer. *AJCC Cancer Staging Manual.* 5th ed. Philadelphia, PA: Lippincott Raven, 1997.

294. Pavy JJ, Denekamp J, Letschert J, et al. EORTC Late Effects Working Group. Late effects toxicity scoring: the SOMA scale. *Int J Radiat Oncol Biol Phys* 1995;31(5):1043–1047.

295. Hanlon AL, Schultheiss TE, Hunt MA, et al. Chronic rectal bleeding after high-dose conformal treatment of prostate cancer warrants modification of existing morbidity scales. *Int J Radiat Oncol Biol Phys* 1997;38(1):59–63.

296. Spratt DE, Pei X, Yamada J, et al. Long-term survival and toxicity in patients treated with high-dose intensity modulated radiation therapy for localized prostate cancer. *Int J Radiat Oncol Biol Phys* 2013;85(3):686–692.

297. Vora SA, Wong WW, Schild SE, et al. Outcome and toxicity for patients treated with intensity modulated radiation therapy for localized prostate cancer. *J Urol* 2013;190(2):521–526.

298. M.D. Anderson Cancer Center. Trial of image-guided adaptive conformal photon vs proton therapy, with concurrent chemotherapy, for locally advanced non-small cell lung carcinoma: treatment related pneumonitis and locoregional recurrence 2009; https://clinicaltrials.gov/ct2/show/NCT00915005.

299. M. D. Anderson Cancer Center. Intensity-Modulated Scanning Beam Proton Therapy (IMPT) With Simultaneous Integrated Boost (SIB) 2012; https://clinicaltrials.gov/ct2/show/NCT01629498.

300. Hoppe BS, Bryant C, Sandler HM. Radiation for prostate cancer: intensity modulated radiation therapy versus proton beam. *J Urol* 2015;193(4):1089–1091.

301. Radiation Therapy Oncology Group. Comparing Photon Therapy to Proton Therapy to Treat Patients with Lung Cancer 2013; https://clinicaltrials.gov/ct2/show/NCT01993810.

302. Massachusetts General Hospital. Proton Therapy vs. IMRT for Low or Intermediate Risk Prostate Cancer (PARTIQoL) 2012; https://clinicaltrials.gov/ct2/show/NCT01617161.

303. M. D. Anderson Cancer Center. Randomized Trial of Intensity-Modulated Proton Beam Therapy (IMPT) Versus Intensity-Modulated Photon Therapy (IMRT) for the Treatment of Oropharyngeal Cancer of the Head and Neck 2013; https://clinicaltrials.gov/ct2/show/NCT01893307.

304. NRG Oncology. Dose-Escalated Photon IMRT or Proton Beam Radiation Therapy Versus Standard-Dose Radiation Therapy and Temozolomide in Treating Patients with Newly Diagnosed Glioblastoma 2014; https://clinicaltrials.gov/ct2/show/NCT02179086.

305. University of Pennsylvania. Pragmatic Randomized Trial of Proton vs. Photon Therapy for Patients with Non-Metastatic Breast Cancer: A Radiotherapy Comparative Effectiveness (RADCOMP) Consortium Trial. https://clinicaltrials.gov/ct2/show/NCT02603341.

306. Habl G, Uhl M, Katayama S, et al. Acute toxicity and quality of life in patients with prostate cancer treated with protons or carbon ions in a prospective randomized phase ii study—the IPI Trial. *Int J Radiat Oncol Biol Phys* 2016;95(1):435–443.

307. Mulrooney DA, Yeazel MW, Kawashima T, et al. Cardiac outcomes in a cohort of adult survivors of childhood and adolescent cancer: retrospective analysis of the Childhood Cancer Survivor Study cohort. *BMJ* 2009;339:b4606.

308. Miller RC, Van Houten H, Foote RL, et al. Photon and proton radiation therapy utilization in a population of over 100 million commercially insured patients. *Int J Radiat Oncol Biol Phys* 2015;93(3 Suppl):E358.

309. Waddle MR, Sio TT, Van Houten HK, et al. Photon and proton radiation therapy utilization in a population of more than 100 million commercially insured patients. *Int J Radiat Oncol Biol Phys* 2017.

310. Hartsell W. Proton treatment patterns in the US from 2012 to 2015. *Int J Particle Ther* 2016;3(2):341.

Section II

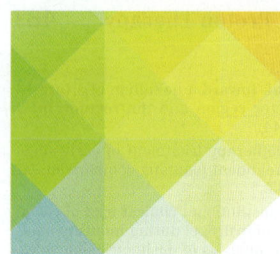

CHAPTER 22

Neutron Therapy and Boron Neutron Capture Therapy

George E. Laramore

INTRODUCTION

The neutron was discovered by Sir James Chadwick at the Cavendish Laboratory in 1932 as a neutral particle that was produced by naturally produced α-particles interacting with the nuclei of various elements. At approximately the same time, E. O. Lawrence invented the cyclotron at the Radiation Laboratory of the University of California thus paving the way for the generation of higher-energy particle beams. The first cyclotron was only 11 inches across and could accelerate protons to 80 keV. Lawrence built a series of larger cyclotrons, one of which was used by Robert Stone to treat 240 patients with "fast" neutrons at the Crocker Radiation Laboratory, the forerunner of the Lawrence Berkeley Laboratory.[1] In Stone's era, the radiobiology of fast neutrons was poorly understood and almost all of his patients suffered severe radiation sequelae. A subsequent review of the work by Brennan and Phillips[2] showed that the majority of Stone's patients had been significantly overdosed. Catterall et al.[3-5] at the Hammersmith Hospital in London resumed clinical trials with fast neutrons in the 1960s and, after treating several hundred patients, concluded that with appropriate fractionation schemes, neutron radiotherapy was well tolerated and many advanced tumors responded amazingly well. Following these initial reports, clinical trials using fast neutrons were instituted at many other facilities throughout the world, and to date, over 41 centers have been involved in fast neutron radiotherapy with over 35,000 patients treated. Although fast neutron radiotherapy has been shown to have significant clinical utility in many situations, it has not proven to be the panacea that was initially hoped for. In what follows, I will describe the important elements of the historical development and discuss the important areas of current clinical use.

An alternate way of using neutrons to treat cancer is via neutron capture therapy. Although several isotopes have a high cross-section for capturing low-energy neutrons leading to an energy-releasing reaction, the great majority of laboratory and clinical work involves boron-10 (^{10}B). The concept of using a low-energy thermal neutron to target cancer cells via a capture reaction involving ^{10}B nuclei was first proposed by Locher in 1936.[6] This is a binary process requiring a source of thermal or epithermal neutrons and a carrier compound both having adequate specificity for tumor cells and being able to deliver sufficient ^{10}B. The beam of low-energy neutrons is broad, and so, tumor selectivity comes almost entirely from the ^{10}B carrier. Because carrier agents are typically cleared from the body via the liver or the kidneys, there is an advantage to using an intrinsically nontoxic compound rather than tagging the carrier with a toxic moiety such as ricin. The first human clinical trials using boron neutron capture therapy (BNCT) took place in the 1950s at the Brookhaven National Laboratory using ^{10}B-enriched boric acid derivatives to treat patients with high-grade brain tumors.[7,8] This compound produced high levels of ^{10}B in the blood and low absolute levels of ^{10}B in the tumors resulting in substantial blood vessel damage and no therapeutic benefit. Several other trials were conducted in the 1960s, but interest in the technique waned until Hatanaka and others[9,10] in Japan began using a different compound, ^{10}B–sodium mercaptoundecahydrododecaborate (BSH), to treat brain tumors. This produced a better tumor-to-blood ratio than the boric acid derivatives and resulted in less damage to normal brain tissue. Favorable reports on patient outcomes have generated renewed worldwide interest in the technique. To date, all treatments have been carried out using beams from nuclear reactors, but there is active ongoing work to develop accelerator-based neutron sources suitable for a medical center environment. I will discuss the important elements in the historical development of this technique with emphasis on current areas of active investigation.

BASIC RADIOBIOLOGY

The rate of energy transferred by ionizing radiation along its path is referred to as *linear energy transfer* (LET). Conventional photon and electron beams used in therapy typically have LETs in the range of 0.2 to 2.0 keV/μ, whereas a high LET form of radiation such as a fast neutron typically has an LET in the range of 20 to 100 keV/μ. The biologic effect of radiation is highly dependent on its LET. This is characterized by the relative biologic effectiveness (RBE) factor, which is the ratio of the dose of ^{60}Co radiation to the dose of particle radiation producing the same biologic end point. The RBE of a given type of radiation is, of course, dependent upon many factors such as the tissue type, chosen end point, dose fractionation schema, etc. However, for practical clinical work using common fractionation schedules, one can use a set of simple numbers in comparing the effective doses of the various types of particle radiation. Fast neutrons have RBEs in the range of 3.0 to 3.5 in terms of most normal tissue late effects, in the range of 4.0 to 4.5 in terms of damage to the central nervous system (CNS), and in the range of 8.0 for salivary gland malignancies.[11-13] In the BNCT reaction shown in Figure 22.7, the emitted α-particle and ^7Li nucleus are also high LET forms of radiation. It is the different radiobiology of high LET radiation that makes it interesting in the treatment of certain cancers.

Low LET radiation primarily kills cells via an indirect, free radical–mediated mechanism.[12] For this to be effective, a long free radical lifetime is required. Oxygen acts as an electron scavenger; hence, free radical lifetimes are longer in cells that are well oxygenated. Oxygen also acts to stabilize the free radical damage. In hypoxic cells, the free radical lifetimes are shorter; hence, these cells are "protected" from much of the damage. Thus, it takes a higher radiation dose in hypoxic cells to achieve the same biologic end point compared to the required dose in well-oxygenated cells. High LET radiation causes a higher proportion of direct damage to the critical cellular targets and therefore is not as dependent on a free radical intermediary. The oxygen enhancement ratio (OER) is the ratio of the radiation dose required to produce a specific biologic effect under anoxic conditions to the dose required to produce the same effect under well-oxygenated conditions. For most mammalian cells, the OER for conventional low LET radiation is in the range of 2.5 to 3.0, whereas for clinically used high LET radiation, the OER is in the range of 1.4 to 1.7. Although the lower OER was one of the primary motivating factors in using high LET radiation, its actual importance in most clinical settings may not be that great because of reoxygenation during a course of fractionated radiotherapy.

Another potential advantage to high LET radiation relates to the reduced ability of cells to repair the radiation damage it produces. The dense chain of ionization events produced by high LET radiation causes simultaneous damage to both strands of the cellular deoxyribonucleic acid (DNA) and also nonrepairable damage to other targets within the cell. Cell survival curves for low LET radiation characteristically exhibit a shoulder at low radiation doses, indicating the ability of the cells to repair this "sublethal" damage. High LET radiation, however, exhibits a very reduced shoulder, resulting in a cell survival curve that is almost log-linear in shape over the range of radiation doses of clinical relevance.[12,14] One therefore would expect tumors having a large capacity for radiation damage repair to be among those better treated with high LET radiation. Another type of radiation damage is "potentially lethal" damage, which occurs in cells that are in a noncycling, plateau phase.[12,15] This has been demonstrated in the laboratory and may be important in tumors having a large fraction of cells in the G0 phase of the cell cycle. This type of repair is less important for high LET radiation than for low LET radiation.

A final point relates to the variation of radiosensitivity across the cell cycle. Mammalian cells are more radiosensitive in M and late G1/early S phase than in early G1 and G2. If radiation is given to an asynchronously dividing cell population, then cells in the sensitive portions of the cycle are killed preferentially. Over a course of fractionated radiotherapy, cells continue through the cycle, and when other fractions of radiation are delivered, many of the formerly resistant cells are in the more sensitive phases of the cycle. The variation in radiosensitivity across the cell cycle is about a factor of four less with high LET radiation.[12,16] Hence, tumors with long cell cycle times theoretically would be better treated with high LET radiation.

FAST NEUTRON RADIOTHERAPY

At one time or another, 41 different centers in North America, Europe, Asia, and Africa treated patients with fast neutrons. To date, over 35,000 patients have received neutron radiotherapy as all or part of their cancer therapy. Although neutron radiotherapy has demonstrated clinical utility in the treatment of certain tumors, it has not proven to be a panacea as was originally hoped, and current indications are limited. There are currently four operating neutron radiotherapy facilities, which are listed in Table 22.1 along with some of their more important characteristics. The more important conclusions from the neutron clinical trials are discussed later in this chapter. Because space does not permit us to be all inclusive, we will emphasize the areas where neutrons show therapeutic benefit compared to conventional radiotherapy.

Salivary Gland Tumors

Although fast neutron radiotherapy has been used in the treatment of many different types of tumors, its major therapeutic advantage has been demonstrated for salivary gland tumors. In retrospect, this could have been predicted from the early radiobiologic work of Battermann and associates,[11] in which the RBE for fractionated radiotherapy was found to be approximately 8, compared to values in the range of 3 to 3.5 expected for late damage in most normal tissues. With appropriate field shaping, one can deliver neutron radiation doses of approximately 20 $Gy_{n\gamma}$ (by convention the γ-rays produced by the neutron interactions are included in the physical dose measurement) to the head and neck region with blocking to reduce the dose to the spinal cord. This roughly corresponds to an equivalent photon dose of 60 to 70 Gy equivalent (Gy equivalent = physical dose × RBE) as far as normal tissues are concerned but approximately 160 Gy equivalent as far as the tumor is concerned. Thus, the therapeutic gain factor for salivary gland tumors is in the range of 2.3 to 2.6.

Early single-institution series seemed to confirm this therapeutic advantage, and the Radiation Therapy Oncology Group (RTOG) and the Medical Research Council of Great Britain conducted a prospective randomized trial for this disease site. A final report on this study showed improved locoregional control at 10 years (56% vs. 17%, P = .009) but no improvement in long-term survival because of distant metastases.[17] This study was stopped early for ethical reasons when 2-year survival data showed a strong trend in favor of the neutron patients. At the 10-year end point, there was a slight (but not statistically significant) benefit to median patient survival on the neutron arm of about 8 months, but with the patients living longer as a result of controlled locoregional disease, the subsequent development of distant metastases became the dominant cause of death. The final locoregional control curve from this study is shown in Figure 22.1.

More recent single-institution data continue to support the efficacy of fast neutron radiotherapy in the treatment of salivary gland tumors. Douglas et al.[18] have analyzed their results for tumors of the major salivary gland (all histologies) and found that if the overall tumor size was <4 cm, the local control rate at 9 years was 78%. The control rate was about 40% for the larger tumors. Figure 22.2 shows actuarial local control probabilities as a function of tumor size as taken from this analysis.

FIGURE 22.1. Actuarial locoregional control rates for patients with unresectable salivary gland tumors who were treated on the RTOG/MRC randomized trial (80–01). The neutron curve is shown as the dashed line and the photon curve is shown as the solid line. The difference between the two curves is statistically significant at the P = .009 level. (Reprinted from Laramore GE, Krall JM, Griffin TW, et al. Neutron versus photon irradiation for unresectable salivary gland tumors: final report of an RTOG-MRC randomized clinical trial. *Int J Radiat Oncol Biol Phys* 1993;27[2]:235–240. Copyright © 1993 Elsevier. With permission.)

TABLE 22.1 LOCATION OF OPERATING FAST NEUTRON RADIOTHERAPY CENTERS—2017		
Location	**Beam Reaction**	**Comments**
United States		
University of Washington Medical Center–Seattle, WA	50 MeV p→Be	Isocentric gantry and multileaf collimator
Europe		
Tomsk Polytechnical University–Tomsk, Russia	Cyclotron	Mean neutron energy 6.3 MeV
Technisch Universtät Munich–Munich, Germany	Fission neutrons	FRMII reactor, horizontal beam with multileaf collimator, mean neutron energy 1.9 MeV
Institute of Physics and Power Engineering–Obninsk, Russia	Fission neutrons	Horizontal beam

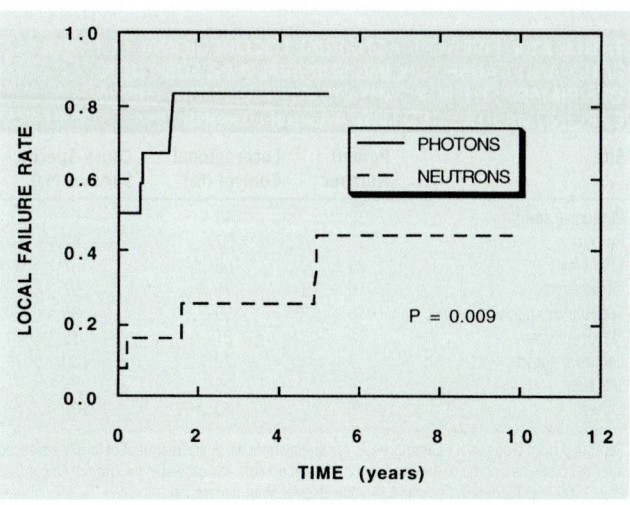

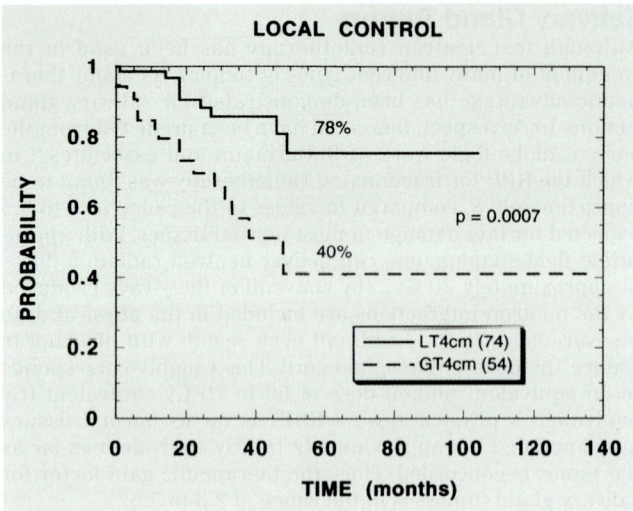

FIGURE 22.2. Actuarial locoregional control rates for patients with major salivary gland tumors who were treated at the University of Washington Fast Neutron Radiotherapy facility. On both univariate and multivariate analysis, tumor size was a predictive factor for locoregional control. The *solid line* depicts the results for patients with tumors <4 cm in extent, whereas the *dashed line* depicts the results for tumors >4 cm in extent. (From Douglas JD, Lee S, Laramore GE, et al. Neutron radiotherapy for the treatment of locally advanced major salivary gland tumors. *Head Neck* 1999;21[3]:255–263. Copyright © 1999 John Wiley & Sons, Inc. Reprinted by permission of John Wiley & Sons, Inc.)

Tumor size and location (parotid vs. submandibular and sublingual) were also factors affecting locoregional control and survival. Another analysis of Douglas et al.[19] focused specifically on patients with adenoid cystic carcinomas. Control rates and cause-specific survival as a function of tumor location are given in Table 22.2. The lower locoregional control rates for tumors arising in the paranasal sinuses or nasopharynx are attributable to tumors invading the cavernous sinus or skull base where the proximity of critical CNS structures limited the neutron dose that could be given relative to tumors in other sites. On multivariate analysis, the presence of base of skull involvement was found to be a statistically significant adverse factor for locoregional control at the $P \leq .01$ level. The risk of developing distant metastases was approximately 50% at 2 years for node-positive patients. For node-negative patients, the metastatic risk also reached approximately 50% but took 10 years to do so. Clearly, better systemic therapy is needed for this tumor.

The poorer outcomes associated with skull base invasion appears to be due to the necessity of reducing the neutron dose to the upper part of the tumor to avoid damage to the CNS, which has an RBE in the range of 4 to 4.5. In an

TABLE 22.2 FIVE-YEAR ACTUARIAL LOCOREGIONAL CONTROL RATES AND CAUSE-SPECIFIC SURVIVAL AS A FUNCTION OF PRIMARY SITE FOR PATIENTS WITH ADENOID CYSTIC CARCINOMAS TREATED WITH FAST NEUTRONS

Site	Patient Number	Locoregional Control (%)	Cause-Specific Survival (%)
Paranasal sinus	32	43	67
Parotid	27	67	82
Oral cavity	26	68	87
Oropharynx	19	75	92
Submandibular/sublingual	15	59	83
Nasopharynx	15	21	35
Lacrimal gland	7	80	100
Trachea	4	25	75
Other	6	100	100

Reprinted from Douglas JD, Laramore GE, Austin-Seymour M, et al. Treatment of locally advanced adenoid cystic carcinoma of the head and neck with neutron radiotherapy. *Int J Radiat Oncol Biol Phys* 2000;46(3):551–557. Copyright © 2000 Elsevier. With permission.

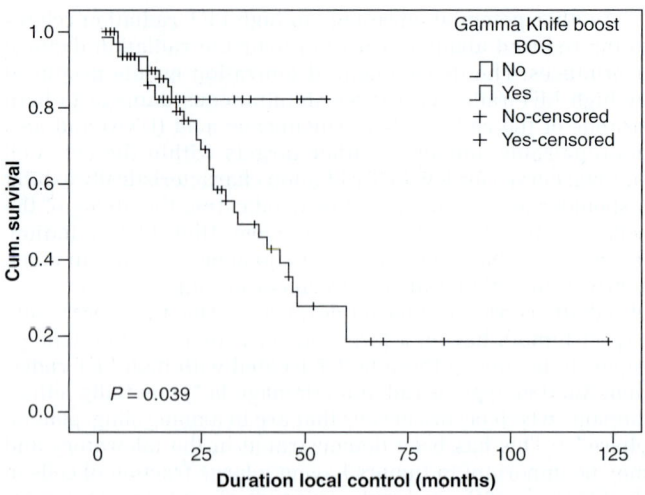

FIGURE 22.3. Kaplan-Meier plots comparing 34 patients with skull base invasion treated with neutron radiotherapy and a gamma knife boost versus 61 patients with skull base invasion treated with neutron radiotherapy alone ($P = .039$). (From Douglas JG, Goodkin R, Laramore GE. Gamma knife stereotactic radiosurgery for salivary gland neoplasms with base of skull invasion following neutron radiotherapy. *Head Neck* 2008;30[4]:492–496. Copyright © 2007 Wiley Periodicals, Inc. Reprinted by permission of John Wiley & Sons, Inc.)

attempt to compensate for this, a stereotactic boost to the superior aspect using a gamma knife has been instituted at the University of Washington. Figure 22.3 shows the dramatic improvement in local tumor control compared to an earlier cohort of patients with skull base tumors treated without the gamma knife boost.[20] The use of a proton boost in an attempt to obtain better coverage for large, irregular tumor volumes at the skull base is currently being explored.

Late effects associated with any high LET form of radiotherapy are always a concern. A study of the University of Washington patient population was conducted in collaboration with the Department of Dentistry, evaluating 140 patients with either minor salivary gland tumors of the oral cavity or tumors of the submandibular and sublingual glands where substantial amounts of the oral cavity were irradiated.[21] The study population was treated between 1997 and 2006, and so, there was a minimum of 10 years at risk at the time of analysis. Because of the wide geographic referral region and the intervening time, only 27 patients could be located for an updated quality of life assessment. Otherwise, the data in the existing medical records were utilized. In terms of acute effects, xerostomia and significant mucositis occurred, respectively, in 88% and 89% of patients, which is about the same as would be expected with patients treated with concurrent chemotherapy and photon radiotherapy using the same treatment fields. The actuarial locoregional control at 6 years was 72.2%, and the overall survival was 58%. In terms of late effects, 15 patients reported significant trismus, and 8 patients had osteoradionecrosis of the mandible.

To reduce the side effects associated with the poorly penetrating properties of the early beams, early neutron work often involved treating patients with a combination of neutrons and photons (known as a "mixed beam" regimen) rather than with neutrons alone. There is a concern that this approach also might reduce the tumor control probability in the case of adenoid cystic carcinomas where there is a high therapeutic gain factor. Huber and colleagues[22] reported on a series of patients with adenoid cystic carcinomas treated at the Heidelberg neutron facility and found a 5-year local control rate of 75% for patients treated with neutrons alone compared to 32% for groups of patients treated with a "mixed beam" regimen or with photons alone. In settings where treatment morbidity is not a major problem, it appears advantageous to use the more effective modality, for example neutrons, for the entire treatment. A high rate of distant metastases prevented improved locoregional control from being translated into improved survival.

Neutron radiotherapy has also been used to treat high-risk, multiply recurrent, pleomorphic adenomas of the major salivary glands.[23] For 16 patients with a median time of 96 months from completion of treatment until analysis, the 15-year locoregional control was 76% for patients with gross disease and 100% for patients with microscopic disease at the time of treatment. The 15-year actuarial risk for grade >3 complications (RTOG/EORTC [European Organization of Radiation Treatment Centers]) was 21%. There were no facial nerve injuries as a result of the neutron treatment.

Squamous Cell Tumors of the Head and Neck

The results for the more common squamous cell tumors of the head and neck have not paralleled those of salivary gland tumors. Early reports by Duncan and associates[24,25] did not confirm the findings of Catterall and colleagues.[4,5] In an attempt to more rigorously evaluate the results of the Hammersmith group, the RTOG conducted a randomized trial comparing conventional photon irradiation with a mixed beam (neutron/photon) fractionation schedule for patients with inoperable tumors.[26,27] Although there was no improvement in terms of local control of the primary tumor or in survival, there was an apparent benefit in terms of improved regional control in the neck for patients presenting with clinically positive adenopathy. In contrast to the results of Catterall and colleagues,[4,5] many patients who had an initial apparent complete locoregional response with fast neutrons developed failures within the radiation fields with passage of time—just as occurred for those patients on the photon control arm. The results of this trial were criticized because its neutron arm did not correspond to the particular regimen used at Hammersmith Hospital. Instead, it was "diluted" with photon irradiation and also had a substantially longer overall treatment time of 7 weeks compared to the 4-week fractionation schema used at Hammersmith. The Neutron Therapy Cooperative Working Group (NTCWG) therefore repeated this study using the second-generation, hospital-based facilities located in the United States and Great Britain with the experimental neutron treatment regimen being identical to that used by Catterall. The results of this second randomized trial also showed no benefit in either locoregional control or survival for the neutron-treated patients.[28] There was a suggestion of improved regional control of clinically positive nodes with fast neutrons, but it did not achieve clinical significance. Late complications graded "severe or greater" according to the joint RTOG/EORTC scoring schema were 40% on the neutron arm compared to 17% on the photon arm (P = .008). Hence, it currently is felt that neutron radiotherapy is of limited utility in the treatment of head and neck squamous cell tumors with the possible exception of patients with massive cervical adenopathy.

Non–Small Cell Lung Cancer

The first reported experience using fast neutron radiotherapy for non–small cell lung cancer was by Eichhorn,[29] who utilized a very low–energy neutron beam. Autopsy rates showed higher rates of tumor sterilization as the percentage of the dose given with neutrons increased: photons alone produced a 33% sterilization rate in 149 patients, mixed beam (20% neutrons and 80% photons) produced a sterilization rate of 48% in 75 patients, and mixed beam (37% neutrons and 63% photons) produced a sterilization rate of 57% in 49 patients. There have been two reported series that showed exceptionally high local control rates for Pancoast or superior sulcus tumors: Komaki and associates[30] found a 91% local control rate, which translated into improved survival relative to a

group of photon-treated patients, and Sawada and colleagues[31] found a mean survival of 11.5 months for 18 patients treated with neutrons compared to 4 months for five patients treated with conventional photon irradiation.

There have been two randomized, clinical trials for inoperable, non–small cell lung cancer. The first was a three-armed study comparing conventional photon radiation versus mixed (neutron/photon) radiation versus neutron radiation alone.[32] The complication rate was higher on the neutron-only arm (perhaps due in part to the relatively low-energy neutron beams in use at that time), and there was no difference in overall survival. A second randomized trial was conducted using the modern hospital-based facilities, which compared a neutron-only regimen with conventional photon irradiation.[33] For the entire cohort of patients, there was no difference in overall survival. However, there was a statistically significant survival advantage for the subset of patients having squamous cell histology. The survival curves for this subset of patients are shown in Figure 22.4. There was also a nonsignificant trend toward increased survival (P = .15) for patients of all histologies having favorable prognostic factors (no pleural effusion, not T4 or N3 in stage, weight loss <5% of normal body weight). Except for skin and subcutaneous changes, which were more severe on the neutron arm, acute and late toxicities were comparable.

The overall results are consistent with the conclusions of conventional photon therapy—namely, that a more aggressive form of radiation treatment delivering higher doses resulting in improved local control will only affect survival in a favorable subgroup of patients that are not prone to early distant metastases. There have been no reported studies in which chemotherapy was used along with neutron irradiation.

Prostate Cancer

There have been two important randomized clinical trials comparing neutron radiotherapy versus conventional photon radiotherapy for patients with locally advanced prostate cancer. In the late 1970s and early 1980s, the RTOG conducted a study (77–04) comparing mixed (neutron/photon) beam radiation with standard external beam radiotherapy for patients with stages C and D_1 tumors.[34] At the 10-year end

FIGURE 22.4. Actuarial survival curves in patients having squamous cell carcinomas of the lung treated on NTCWG study 85–24. The neutron-treated group is shown as the *dotted line*, and the photon-treated group is shown as the *solid line*. The difference between the two curves is statistically significant at the P = .02 level. (Reprinted from Koh WJ, Krall JM, Peters LJ, et al. Neutron vs. photon radiation therapy for inoperable regional non-small cell lung cancer: results of a multicenter randomized trial. *Int J Radiat Oncol Biol Phys* 1993;27[3]:499–505. Copyright © 1993 Elsevier. With permission.)

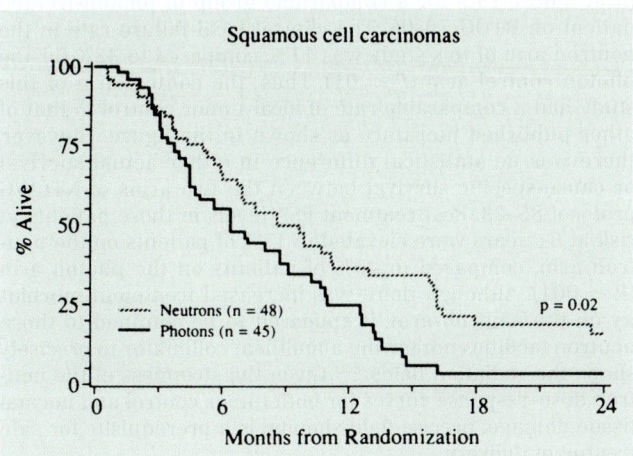

Squamous cell carcinomas

········ Neutrons (n = 48)
—— Photons (n = 45)

p = 0.02

% Alive

Months from Randomization

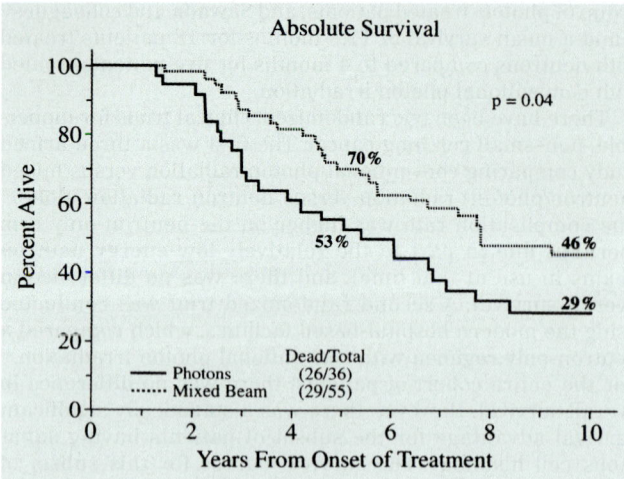

FIGURE 22.5. Actuarial survival curves for patients with locally advanced prostate cancer treated on RTOG protocol 77-04. The curve for the mixed beam (neutron/photon) group is shown as the *dashed line*, and the curve for the photon group is shown as the *solid line*. The difference between the two curves is statistically significant at the *P* = .04 level. (Reprinted from Laramore GE, Krall JM, Griffin TW, et al. Fast neutron radiotherapy for locally advanced prostate cancer. Final report of Radiation Therapy Oncology Group randomized clinical trial. *Am J Clin Oncol* 1993;16[2]:164–167. With permission.)

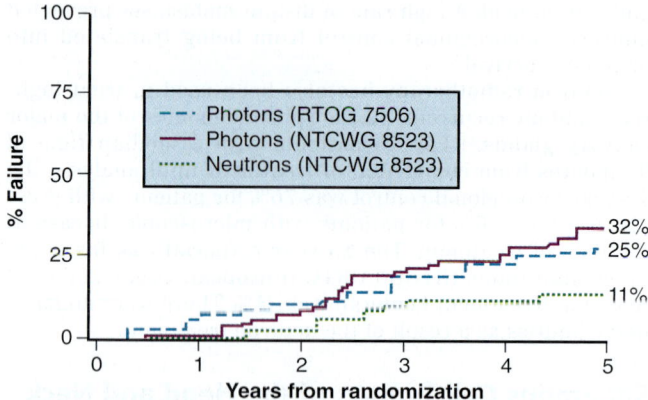

FIGURE 22.6. Actuarial local failure curves for patients with locally advanced prostate cancer treated on Neutron Therapy Collaborative Working Group (NTCWG) protocol 85-23. For comparison, the local failure curve for patients treated on an earlier RTOG protocol 75-06 is also shown. The improved local control for the neutron-treated group is significant at the *P* < .01 level. (Reprinted from Russell KJ, Caplan RJ, Laramore GE, et al. Photon versus fast neutron external beam radiotherapy in the treatment of locally advanced prostate cancer: results of a randomized prospective trial. *Int J Radiat Oncol Biol Phys* 1994;28[1]:47–54. Copyright © 1994 Elsevier. With permission.)

point, there were both improved locoregional control (70% vs. 58%, *P* = .03) and survival (46% vs. 29%, *P* = .04) in favor of the mixed beam arm. The survival curves from this study are reproduced in Figure 22.5. There was no difference in the rate of significant complications between the two arms. This is one of the few published studies showing improved survival, as opposed to local control, with an experimental form of treatment for prostate cancer. This study was criticized because of its relatively small size (91 evaluable patients), its unbalanced randomization (3:2 in favor of the experimental arm), and the fact that the photon control group appeared to do somewhat worse than would have been expected for supposedly comparable patients based on historical results. Hence, although this study was maturing, a second randomized trial comparing fast neutron radiotherapy alone versus conventional photon radiotherapy was initiated by the NTCWG for patients with high-grade T_2 or any grade T_3–T_4, N_0–N_1, M_0 tumors. One hundred seventy-two evaluable patients were entered into the study, and 5-year data have been reported.[35] A routine, posttreatment biopsy was designed into the study to assay for local control in the pre-PSA (prostate-specific antigen) era, but unfortunately, all patients at risk for failure at the 2-year end point did not undergo this biopsy. Figure 22.6 shows local failure rates for the two arms of this study as well as the local failure rate for a comparable group of photon-treated patient on RTOG 75–06. The clinical local failure rate in the neutron arm of this study was 11%, compared to 32% for the photon control arm (*P* < .01). Thus, the control arm of this study had a comparable rate of local tumor control to that of other published literature as shown in the figure. However, there was no statistical difference in either actual survival or cause-specific survival between the two arms of NTCWG protocol 85-23. Posttreatment PSA levels in those patients at risk at 5+ years were elevated in 17% of patients on the neutron arm, compared to 45% of patients on the photon arm (*P* < .001). Although there was increased treatment morbidity on the neutron arm, it appeared to be confined to those neutron facilities not having a multileaf collimator to precisely shape the radiation fields.[35,36] Given the steepness of the neutron dose–response curves for both tumor control and normal tissue damage, precise field shaping is a prerequisite for safe treatment delivery.

Considerable work has been done by the Wayne State University group using a combination of neutrons and photons (mixed beam) to treat prostate cancer. This work was done using a multirod collimator for field shaping and achieved an acceptable level of morbidity with over 1,500 patients having been treated at the present time. Forman et al. have summarized this work and discussed the sequence of studies that were undertaken.[37,38] Following dose escalation studies to determine the maximum safe radiation doses, the Wayne State group compared two different treatment schemas: (a) giving the neutron portion of the treatment before the photon portion and (b) giving the photon portion prior to the neutron portion. Interestingly, they found a higher therapeutic advantage when the neutron radiotherapy was given prior to the photon radiotherapy with disease-free survival being 93% if the neutron radiation was given initially versus 73% if the photon radiation was given initially. Furthermore, they found that the overall complication rate was about the same as that expected using conventional photon irradiation delivered via a three-dimensional conformal schema.

There also have been several reported single-institution studies from Europe[39,40] and Asia[41,42] that showed high local control rates with fast neutrons and support the results of the two randomized trials. Among these was a major review of prostate cancer patients treated at the Universite Catholique de Louvain reported by Scalliet et al.[39] Five hundred thirty-three patients were treated between 1978 and 1998 with a mixed beam combination of neutrons and photons with three neutron treatments of 0.7 $Gy_{n\gamma}$ and 2 photon treatments of 2 Gy given per week on a daily basis. The total dose was felt to be equivalent to 66 Gy photon based upon RBE estimates for their neutron beam. Prior to 1992, only simple field blocking was available; after 1992, a multileaf collimator was used for more precise field shaping. The review group consisted of 308 consecutive patients treated from 1990 to 1996 with either the mixed beam regimen or photon radiotherapy alone. Of these, 262 were presumed alive and QOL questionnaires mailed to them. There were 230 responses: 20 in the photon group and 210 in the mixed beam group. Bowel problems, nocturia, urinary incontinence, and loss of sexual potency were present in each group. There were more patient-reported side effects in the mixed beam group with the difference in bowel problems felt to be significant (*P* = .003). The authors acknowledge that this was likely due to unsophisticated rectal blocking utilized for the lateral fields.

Although there is certainly increased risk of rectal complications with the use of high LET neutron radiotherapy, the aggregate data showed improved locoregional control compared to contemporaneously treated photon patients. This is consistent with more recent radiobiologic models showing a low α/β ratio in the range of 1.5 to 3 for prostate cancer based upon fits to clinical data.[43,44] High values of β indicate tumor ability to repair sublethal damage from conventional photon irradiation, and it is exactly this situation where high LET radiotherapy would be of benefit. It should also be noted that the neutron studies were generally done in the absence of antiandrogen therapy, which has been shown to be advantageous in improving survival in photon-treated patients.

Sarcomas

Sarcomas generally are thought to be "radioresistant" and have many of the characteristics noted by Battermann and associates[11] as being favorable for neutron radiotherapy. A review of this historical data for neutron radiotherapy seems to show a probable benefit for high LET radiotherapy with comparative local control rates (neutrons vs. photons) for patients treated for inoperable gross disease being 53% versus 38% for soft tissue sarcomas, 55% versus 21% for osteogenic sarcomas, and 49% versus 33% for chondrosarcomas.[45] Schwarz and colleagues[46] have summarized the results of 1,171 patients treated between 1972 and 1990 at 11 European neutron radiotherapy centers. For patients treated following primary resection with either clear or microscopically positive margins (categories R0–R1), the local control rate was about 90%—about the same as would be expected for conventional postoperative photon irradiation. For patients with unresectable tumors (category R2), the approximate control rate was 47%. Complication rates ranged between 7% and 29% and were correlated with field size and the limited degree of technical sophistication available at some of the treatment centers. Clearly, the results are inferior to those expected using a "clean" resection followed by conventional postoperative radiotherapy, but neutron radiotherapy appears to be more effective than photon radiation alone for those tumors where a surgical resection is not an option.

Other Cancers

Adenoid cystic carcinomas can arise in glandular elements located at nontraditional head and neck sites, and we would expect the radiobiology of such tumors to be similar to those arising in salivary glands. Examples are larynx, trachea, lacrimal glands, and breast. Small patient series treating tumors in these sites with fast neutrons report control rates similar to those expected for salivary gland tumors. Bittner et al. reported on 20 patients with adenoid cystic carcinomas of the trachea treated with neutron radiotherapy and found the 5-year actuarial survival to be 89.4%, although the 5-year local control rate was only 54.1%.[47] Six of the patients were given a brachytherapy boost following the neutron radiotherapy, but this did not statistically improve the local control rate. Gensheimer et al.[48] reported on 11 patients with lacrimal gland tumors who were treated with neutrons with gross residual disease present in 8 patients. With a median follow-up of 6.2 years, the Kaplan-Meier locoregional control rate at 5 years was 80%, and the median overall survival was 11.1 years. Anecdotal data from patients with adenoid cystic carcinomas of the breast

treated at the University of Washington also show the efficacy of neutron radiotherapy.

Neutron radiotherapy may have a role to play in the treatment of other relatively radioresistant tumors in the head and neck region. Liao et al.[49] evaluated 14 patients with mucosal melanomas treated with fast neutrons. Local control was achieved in 79% of patients until death or last follow-up. Unfortunately, 50% of patients developed distant metastases. Neutron radiotherapy has also been utilized to treat advanced thyroid malignancies in certain clinical situations.[50] Sixty-two consecutive patients with advanced thyroid cancers were treated with external beam radiotherapy between 1985 and 2015 with 23 receiving neutron radiotherapy and 39 receiving conventional photon irradiation. There was no overall survival difference between the groups, but interestingly, patients with low-grade subtypes (papillary and follicular) did better with standard photon radiation while there was a trend toward improved survival with fast neutrons for the more aggressive medullary and anaplastic histologies.

BORON NEUTRON CAPTURE THERAPY (BNCT)

The key to BNCT is the development of a boron compound that selectively localizes on or within the tumor cells in sufficient concentration to have a high probability of eradicating them when irradiated by a low-energy neutron beam. The boron neutron capture reaction is shown schematically in Figure 22.7. Currently, only three boron carrier compounds have been approved for human clinical trials: sodium mercaptoundecahydro-*closo*-dodecaborate (BSH), (L)-4-di-hydroxy-borylphenylalanine (BPA), and sodium decaborane (GB10). Unfortunately, with the possible exception of BPA being concentrated in cells, which synthesizes melanin, these compounds do not exhibit tumor-specific uptake. ^{18}F can be incorporated into BPA thus allowing for positron emission tomography (PET) imaging to ascertain boron concentration. There is considerable work taking place on the development of more effective compounds, and for a synopsis, the reader is referred to the article by Barth et al.[51] The low-energy neutron beams used in BNCT are currently produced using nuclear reactors, and at one time or another, 14 centers have been involved in clinical BNCT work. There is increasing interest in developing accelerator-based sources suitable for hospital environments. Actual, as opposed to idealized, epithermal beams contain γ-ray and fast neutron components, which have markedly different radiobiologic properties. In addition, there are capture reactions via naturally occurring isotopes in biologic material—^1H, ^{16}O, ^{14}Ni, ^{12}C, ^{35}Cl, etc. The resulting radiation field is complicated, but for clinical work, the dose is expressed as a single, RBE-weighted dose, Gy_w, with the weighting factors based upon experiments in animal models. This is specific to the boron carrier used because the effectiveness of the BNCT reaction is dependent upon the cellular location of the ^{10}B.[52,53] Monte Carlo calculations are required for the dose calculations because of the complex nature of neutron transport through matter. Boron levels are measured in the patient's blood and the boron concentration in tumor and surrounding tissue inferred based upon prior experimental studies. The depth-dose properties of epithermal neutron beams limit their effective treatment depth to around 10 cm with currently available boron compound, which restricts the classes of tumors that can be treated.[54] BNCT treatment plans give combined RBE-weighted doses for the entire region of interest using boron concentrations with different weighting factors being used for tumor and normal tissue under

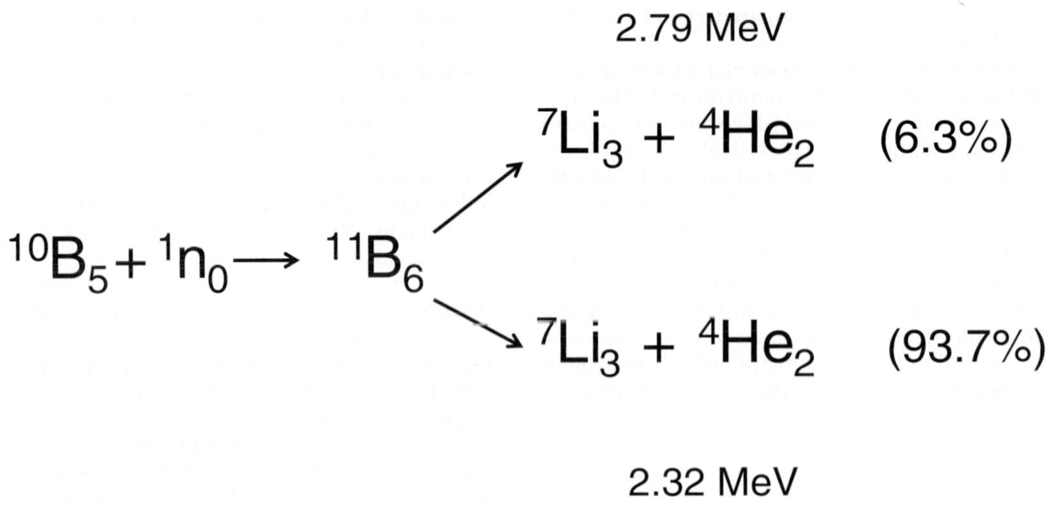

$$2.79 \text{ MeV}$$

$$^{10}B_5 + {}^1n_0 \longrightarrow {}^{11}B_6 \nearrow {}^7Li_3 + {}^4He_2 \quad (6.3\%)$$

$${}^7Li_3 + {}^4He_2 \quad (93.7\%)$$

$$2.32 \text{ MeV}$$

FIGURE 22.7. The boron neutron capture process. The atomic nucleus ^{10}B captures a thermal neutron, going into an excited state, which then decays into a ^1He nucleus and a ^7Li nucleus, which have respective ranges of approximately 10 μ and 6 μ, respectively. A 0.47 MeV γ-ray is also emitted on the higher probability branch of the decay.

the assumption that microscopic tumor extension may occur well outside the image detectable tumor volume. An example of this calculation for tumor and normal brain is shown in Figure 22.8.

High-Grade Gliomas

The second generation of BNCT trials for high-grade gliomas of the brain took place in Japan using BSH as the boron carrier.[9,10,55] These studies were not randomized and were not controlled for prognostic factors important in predicting outcomes.[56] An analysis of a subset of these patients who came from the United States was undertaken, and for this subset, there was no difference in outcomes compared to what would have been expected with the standard therapy of the time.[57] Many aspects of this early work were suboptimal, including the use of a poorly penetrating thermal neutron beam requiring an open craniotomy procedure to expose the tumor bed. The relatively low neutron flux meant that treatment times in the range of 4 to 8 hours were required to deliver a surface fluence in the range of 10^{13} neutrons/cm^2, which was necessary for treatment given the tumor boron dose being in the range of 15 to 25 µg/g. After approximately a 30-year hiatus, a BNCT clinical program resumed in the United States using the Harvard-MIT reactor and the Brookhaven National Laboratory Medical Reactor using BPA as the boron delivery agent. Using a single BNCT treatment, medial survival times were comparable to those achieved with more prolonged, conventionally fractionated radiotherapy.[58,59]

Kawabata and Miyatake et al. have utilized a higher-energy epithermal beam along with either BPA alone or in combination with BSH to treat patients with either *de novo* or recurrent glioblastoma multiforme (GBM).[60–63] The patients with recurrent tumors had received on the order of 60 Gy previously, and so, radiation necrosis and/or symptomatic pseudoprogression were major issues. *De novo* tumors are a better test for BNCT efficacy, and Figure 22.9 shows survival curves for patients treated either with BNCT alone or in combination with standard photon radiotherapy. Compared with a historical control group from their institution, median survival was better for the BNCT-treated group. While interesting, it is important to note that this was not a randomized, controlled trial.

Recurrent Head and Neck Cancer

There is a small body of work using BNCT to retreat recurrent head and neck tumors using BPA as the B-carrier. Kankaanranta et al.[64] have reported on 29 patients with recurrent head and neck tumors treated at the FiR 1 TRIGA reactor in Helsinki, Finland, with a single radiation fraction. ^{18}F-L-BPA PET imaging was used to determine the tumor background normal tissue boron levels, and it was estimated that approximately 91% of the tumor dose came from the BNCT reaction. With a median follow-up of 31 months, the 2-year local control was 27%, the 2-year overall survival was 30%, and the 2-year progression-free survival was 27%. Acute side effects included mucositis and oral pain in 54% of patients and fatigue in 32% of patients. Late effects included grade 3 osteoradionecrosis in 3 patients and grade 4 soft tissue necrosis in 1 patient. A subsequent report by the Finnish group on 9 patients treated with BNCT for recurrent or persistent laryngeal cancer showed a median time to progression after BNCT of 6.6 months with a median overall survival of only 13.3 months.[65]

Wang et al.[66] treated 17 patients with recurrent head and neck tumors at the THOR reactor facility in Taiwan using 2 radiation fractions spaced 28 days apart using BPA. With a median follow-up time of 19.7 months, there were 6 patients with partial tumor responses and 6 patients with complete tumor responses, and at 2 years, the Kaplan-Meier plots showed a local control rate of 28% and an overall survival rate of 47%. There was a 29% incidence of acute grade 3 mucositis, and 1 patient had grade 4 laryngeal edema and carotid hemorrhage. Late effects included 2 patients with grade 3 neuropathy, 1 patient with grade 3 soft tissue necrosis, and 1 patient with grade 3 local pain.

The overall results using BPA-based BNCT in the retreatment setting appear to be about the same as with other retreatment methods.

Other Cancers

BPA acts as a dopamine analogue in the melanin synthesis pathway, and Mishima et al. utilized it to treat malignant melanoma skin nodules and lymph node metastases.[67–70] Good regression was found in the 12 patients who were

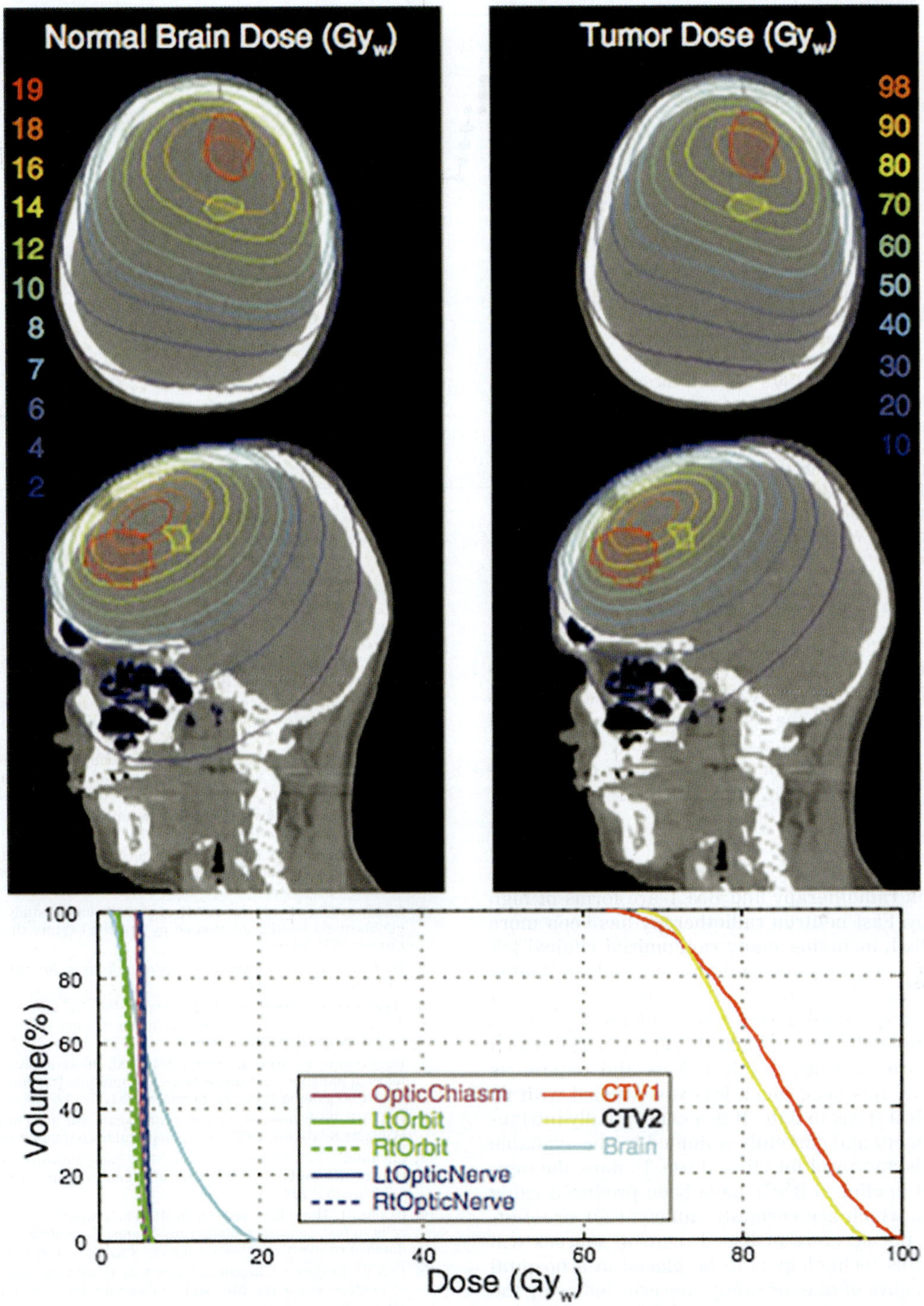

FIGURE 22.8. A treatment plan for a GBM patient using three treatment fields. The prescription is for a mean brain dose of 7.7 Gy$_w$ with isodoses calculated for tumor (*right*) and normal brain (*left*) shown on axial and sagittal slices. (Reprinted from Barth RF, Vicente MGH, Harling OK, et al. Current status of boron neutron capture therapy of high grade gliomas and recurrent head and neck cancer. *Radiat Oncol* 2012;7:146–166, with permission.)

treated. A larger series of 104 extremity skin nodules in 7 patients has been treated at the Centro Atomico Bariloche in Argentina.[71] The authors found a high control rate of >80% when the tumor volume was <0.1 cm³ when 20 Gy$_w$ was given but <40% for larger tumors even when doses >40 Gy$_w$ were given.

BNCT has also been used to treat patients with malignant meningiomas that were either nonresponsive or recurrent to conventional treatment. Miyatake et al. reported on 32 consecutively treated cases with 20 cases at risk for more than 4 years.[72,73] For these 20 patients, the medial survival time was 14.1 months, but only 3 patients had infield failures.

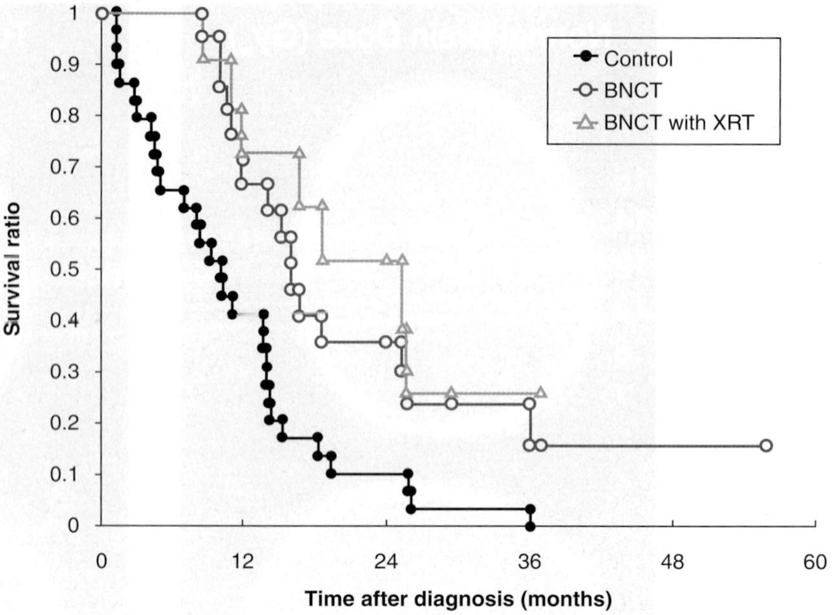

FIGURE 22.9. Kaplan-Meier survival curves for patients with *de novo* glioblastoma patients treated BNCT compared with a historical control group of 27 patients treated at the same institution with surgery, photon radiotherapy, and ACNU-based chemotherapy (medial survival 10.3 months). There are two groups of BNCT patients, those treated with BNCT alone (median survival 15.6 months) and those treated using a combination of BNCT and photon radiotherapy (median survival 23.5 months). (Reprinted from Miyatake S, Kawabata S, Hiramatsu R, et al. Boron Neutron Capture Therapy for Malignant Brain Tumors. *Neurol Med Chir* [*Tokyo*] 2016; 56[7]:361–371. Copyright © 2016 The Japan Neurosurgical Society. With permission.)

A very interesting approach to the treatment of liver metastases was begun at the University of Pavia in Italy.[74] The patient is infused with BPA, and the diseased liver is extirpated and irradiated in the reactor and then reimplanted into the patient. Two patients have been treated in this manner, with one long-term survivor who eventually died of distant metastases 4 years from the time of the procedure.

SUMMARY

Both fast neutron radiotherapy and BNCT are forms of high LET radiotherapy. Fast neutron radiotherapy has been more extensively studied, including many randomized clinical trials comparing it to conventional radiotherapy. Only in limited clinical settings has it been shown to be more effective than standard radiotherapy. Work is in progress to develop a form of intensity-modulated neutron radiotherapy (IMNT), which may reduce treatment-related side effects and extend its applicability. BNCT has been much less well studied with no randomized clinical trials to date. It is a conceptually intriguing, binary treatment and currently is limited by the available boron compounds approved for clinical use. To date, the neutron beams used in clinical BNCT have been produced using nuclear reactors, which are certainly sufficient for proof-of-concept studies, but accelerator-based neutron sources will be necessary if this technology is to be placed in a hospital environment. Because of reactor safety concerns following the Fukushima incident, the Japanese BNCT program is switching to accelerator-based neutron sources. Currently, there are only three operating reactor-based programs, the THOR reactor in Taiwan, an in-hospital neutron irradiator at the Third Xiangya Hospital of Central South University in Beijing, and the Centro Atomico Bariloche reactor in Argentina, that are actually treating patients. Programs at other centers are in the planning stage.

REFERENCES

1. Stone RS. Neutron therapy and specific ionization. *Am J Roentgenol* 1948;59:771–785.
2. Brennan JT, Phillips TL. Evaluation of past experience with fast neutron teletherapy and its implication for future applications. *Eur J Cancer Clin Oncol* 1971;7:219–225.
3. Catterall M. The treatment of advanced cancer by fast neutrons from the Medical Research Council's cyclotron at Hammersmith Hospital, London. *Eur J Cancer Clin Oncol* 1974;10:343–347.
4. Catterall M, Sutherland I, Bewley DK. First results of a randomized clinical trial of fast neutrons compared with x or gamma rays in treatment of advanced tumors of the head and neck. *Br Med J* 1975;2:653–656.
5. Catterall M, Bewley DK, Sutherland I. Second report on results of a randomized clinical trial of fast neutrons compared with x or gamma rays in treatment of advanced tumors of head and neck. *Br Med J* 1977;1:1642.
6. Locher GL. Biological effects and therapeutic possibilities of neutrons. *Am J Roentgenol Radium Ther* 1936;36:1–13.
7. Farr LE, Sweet WH, Robertson JS, et al. Neutron capture therapy with boron in the treatment of glioblastoma multiforme. *Am J Roentgenol Radium Ther Nucl Med* 1954;71:279–291.
8. Goodwin JT, Farr LE, Sweet WH, et al. Pathological study of eight patients with glioblastoma multiforme treated by neutron capture therapy using boron 10. *Cancer* 1956;8:601–615.
9. Hatanaka H. *Boron neutron capture therapy for tumors.* Niigata, Japan: Nishimura Press, 1986.
10. Hatanaka H, Nakagawa N. Clinical results of long surviving brain tumor patients who underwent boron neutron capture therapy. *Int J Radiat Oncol Biol Phys* 1994;28.1061–1066.
11. Battermann JJ, Breur K, Hare GAM, et al. Observations on pulmonary metastases in patients after single doses and multiple fractions of fast neutrons and cobalt-60 gamma rays. *Eur J Cancer* 1981;17:539–548.
12. Hall EJ. *Radiobiology for the radiologist.* 4th ed. Philadelphia: Lippincott Williams & Wilkins, 1992. (See in particular Chapters 9 and 14.)
13. Laramore GE, Austin-Seymour MM. Fast neutron radiotherapy in relation to the radiation sensitivity of human organ systems. *Adv Radiat Biol* 1992;15:153–193.
14. Gragg RL, Humphrey RM, Meyn RE. The response of Chinese hamster ovary cells to fast neutron radiotherapy beams. II. Sublethal and potentially lethal damage recovery capabilities. *Radiat Res* 1977;71:461–470.
15. Hall EJ, Kraljevic J. Repair of potentially lethal radiation damage: comparison of neutron and x-ray RBE and implications for radiation therapy. *Radiology* 1976;121:731–735.
16. Gragg RL, Humphrey RM, Meyn RE. The response of Chinese hamster ovary cells to fast neutron radiotherapy beams. III. Variations in relative biological effectiveness with position in the cell cycle. *Radiat Res* 1978;76:283–291.
17. Laramore GE, Krall JM, Griffin TW, et al. Neutron versus photon irradiation for unresectable salivary gland tumors. Final report of an RTOG-MRC randomized clinical trial. *Int J Radiat Oncol Biol Phys* 1993;27:235–240.
18. Douglas JG, Lee S, Laramore GE, et al. Neutron radiotherapy for the treatment of locally-advanced major salivary gland tumors. *Head Neck* 1999;21:255–263.
19. Douglas JG, Laramore GE, Austin-Seymour M, et al. Treatment of locally advanced adenoid cystic carcinoma of the head and neck with neutron radiotherapy. *Int J Radiat Oncol Biol Phys* 2000;46:551–557.
20. Douglas JG, Goodkin R, Laramore GE. Gamma Knife stereotactic radiosurgery for salivary gland neoplasms with base of skull invasion following neutron radiotherapy. *Head Neck* 2008;30:492–496.
21. Davis C, Sikes J, Namaranian P, et al. Neutron beam radiation therapy: an overview of treatment and oral complications when treating salivary gland malignancies. *J Oral Maxillofac Surg* 2016;74:830–835.

22. Huber PE, Debus J, Latz D, et al. Radiotherapy for advanced adenoid cystic carcinoma: neutrons, photons, or mixed beam? *Radiother Oncol* 2001;59:161–167.

23. Douglas JG, Einck J, Austin-Seymour M, et al. Neutron radiotherapy for recurrent pleomorphic adenomas of major salivary glands. *Head Neck* 2001;23:1037–1042.

24. Duncan W, Arott SJ, Batterman JJ, et al. Fast neutrons in the treatment of head and neck cancers: the results of a multi-centre randomly controlled trial. *Radiother Oncol* 1984;2:293–300.

25. MacDougall RH, Orr JA, Kerr GR, et al. Fast neutron treatment for squamous cell carcinoma of the head and neck: final report of the Edinburgh randomized trial. *BMJ* 1990;301:1241–1242.

26. Griffin TW, Davis R, Laramore GE, et al. Fast neutron radiotherapy of metastatic cervical adenopathy: the results of a randomized RTOG study. *Int J Radiat Oncol Biol Phys* 1983;9:1267–1270.

27. Griffin TW, Pajak TF, Maor MH, et al. Mixed neutron/photon irradiation of unresectable squamous cell carcinomas of the head and neck. The final report of a randomized cooperative trial. *Int J Radiat Oncol Biol Phys* 1989;17:959–965.

28. Maor MH, Errington RD, Caplan RJ, et al. Fast-neutron therapy in advanced head and neck cancer: a collaborative international randomized trial. *Int J Radiat Oncol Biol Phys* 1995;32:599–604.

29. Eichhorn HJ. Results of a pilot study on neutron radiotherapy with 600 patients. *Int J Radiat Oncol Biol Phys* 1981;8:1561–1565.

30. Komaki R, Mountain C, Holbert J, et al. Superior sulcus tumors: treatment selection and results of 85 patients without metastases (M0) at presentation. *Int J Radiat Oncol Biol Phys* 1990;19:31–36.

31. Sawada K, Fukuma S, Seki Y. Clinical experience with Pancoast tumor treated by fast neutron radiotherapy. *Gan No Rinsho* 1983;A7;111–114 (abstr).

32. Laramore GE, Bauer M, Griffin TW, et al. Fast neutron and mixed beam radiotherapy for inoperable non-small cell carcinoma of the lung. *Am J Clin Oncol* 1986;9:233–243.

33. Koh W-J, Krall JM, Peters LJ, et al. Neutron vs photon radiation therapy for inoperable regional non-small cell lung cancer: results of a multicenter randomized trial. *Int J Radiat Oncol Biol Phys* 1993;27:499–505.

34. Laramore GE, Krall JM, Griffin TW, et al. Fast neutron radiotherapy for locally advanced prostate cancer. Final report of Radiation Therapy Oncology Group randomized clinical trial. *Am J Clin Oncol* 1993;16:164–167.

35. Russell KJ, Caplan RJ, Laramore GE, et al. Photon versus fast neutron external beam radiotherapy in the treatment of locally advanced prostate cancer: results of a randomized prospective trial. *Int J Radiat Oncol Biol Phys* 1993;28:47–54.

36. Austin-Seymour M, Caplan R, Russell K, et al. Impact of a multileaf collimator on treatment morbidity in localized carcinoma of the prostate. *Int J Radiat Oncol Biol Phys* 1994;30:1065–1071.

37. Forman JD. Neutron radiotherapy for prostate cancer. *Pros J* 1999;1:8–14.

38. Forman JD, Yudelev M, Bolton S, et al. Fast neutron irradiation for prostate cancer. *Cancer Metastasis Rev* 2002;21:131–135.

39. Scalliet PG, Remouchamps V, Lhoas F, et al. A retrospective analysis of the results of p(65)+BE neutron therapy for the treatment of prostate adenocarcinoma at the cyclotron of Louvain-la-Neuve. Part I: survival and progression-free survival. *Cancer Radiother* 2001;5:262–272.

40. Schwarz R, Krull A, Heyer D, et al. Present results of neutron therapy. The German experience. *Acta Oncol* 1994;33:281–287.

41. Fuse H, Katayama T, Akimoto S, et al. Radiotherapy of prostatic carcinoma [in Japanese]. *Hinyokika Kiyo* 1991;37:801–808.

42. Tsunemoto H, Morita S, Shimazaki J. Fast neutron therapy for carcinoma of the prostate. In: Karr JP, Yamanaka H, eds. *Prostate cancer: the second Tokyo symposium*. New York: Elsevier Science Publishing, 1989:383–391.

43. Brenner DJ, Hall EJ. Fractionation and protraction for radiotherapy of prostate carcinoma. *Int J Radiat Oncol Biol Phys* 1999;43:1095–1101.

44. Wang JZ, Guerrero M, Li XA. How low is the α/β ratio for prostate cancer? *Int J Radiat Oncol Biol Phys* 2003;55:194–203.

45. Laramore GE, Griffith JT, Boespflug M, et al. Fast neutron radiotherapy for sarcomas of soft tissue, bone, and cartilage. *Am J Clin Oncol* 1989;1:320–326.

46. Schwarz R, Krull A, Heyer D, et al. Neutron therapy in soft tissue sarcomas: a review of European results. *Bull Cancer Radiother* 1996;83(Suppl):110–114.

47. Bittner N, Koh W-J, Laramore GE, et al. Treatment of locally advanced adenoid cystic carcinoma of the trachea with neutron radiotherapy. *Int J Radiat Oncol Biol Phys* 2008;72:410–414.

48. Gensheimer MF, Rainey D, Douglas JG, et al. Neutron radiotherapy for adenoid cystic carcinoma of the lacrimal gland. *Ophthal Plast Reconstr Surg* 2013;29:256–260.

49. Liao JJ, Parvathaneni U, Laramore GE, et al. Fast neutron radiotherapy for primary mucosal melanomas of the head and neck. *Head Neck* 2013;36:1162–1167.

50. Chapman TR, Laramore GE, Bowen SR, et al. Neutron radiotherapy for advanced thyroid cancers. *Adv Radiat Oncol* 2016;1:148–156.

51. Barth RF, Vicente MGH, Harling OK, et al. Current status of boron neutron capture therapy of high grade gliomas and recurrent head and neck cancer. *Radiat Oncol* 2012;7:146–146.

52. Coderre JA, Morris GM. The radiation biology of boron neutron capture therapy. *Radiat Res* 1999;151:1–18.

53. Coderre JA, Turcotte JC, Riley KJ, et al. Boron neutron capture therapy: cellular targeting of high linear energy transfer radiation. *Technol Cancer Res Treat* 2003;2:355–375.

54. Nigg D. *Private Communication*.

55. Nakagawa N. Recent study of boron neutron capture therapy for brain tumors. In: Nigg DW, Wiersema RT, eds. *Proceedings of the first international workshop on accelerator-based neutron sources for boron neutron capture therapy, vol 1,* U.S. Department of Energy Report CONF-940976, 1994:11–23.

56. Curran WJ, Scott CB, Horton J, et al. Recursive partitioning analysis of prognostic factors in three Radiation Therapy Group malignant glioma trials. *J Natl Cancer Inst* 1993;85:704–710.

57. Laramore GE, Spence AA. Boron neutron capture therapy (BNCT) for high grade gliomas of the brain: a cautionary note. *Int J Radiat Oncol Biol Phys* 1996;36:241–246.

58. Diaz AZ. Assessment of the results from the phase I/II boron neutron capture therapy trials at the Brookhaven National Laboratory from a clinician's point of view. *J Neurooncol* 2003;62:101–109.

59. Busse PM, Harling OK, Palmer MR, et al. A critical examination of the results from the Harvard-MIT NCT program phase I trial of neutron capture therapy for intracranial disease. *J Neurooncol* 2003;62:111–121.

60. Miyatake S, Kawabata, S, Kajimoto Y, et al. Modified boron neutron capture therapy for malignant gliomas performed using epithermal neutron and two boron compounds with different accumulation mechanisms: an efficacy study based upon findings on neuroimages. *J Neurosurg* 2005;103:1000–1009.

61. Kawabata S, Miyatake S, Kuroiwa T, et al. Boron neutron capture therapy for newly diagnosed glioblastoma. *J Radiat Res* 2009;50:51–60.

62. Miyatake S, Kawabata S, Yokoyama K, et al. Survival benefit for boron neutron capture therapy for recurrent malignant gliomas. *J Neurooncol* 2009;91:199–206.

63. Miyatake S, Kawabata S, Hiramatsu R, et al. Boron neutron capture therapy for malignant brain tumors. *Neurol Med Chir (Tokyo)* 2016;56:361–371.

64. Kankaanranta L, Seppälä T, Koivunoro H, et al. Boron neutron capture therapy in the treatment of locally recurred head-and-neck cancer: final analysis of a phase I/II trial. *Int J Radiat Oncol Biol Phys* 2012;82:e67–e75.

65. Haapaniemi A, Kankaanranta L, Saat R, et al. Boron neutron capture therapy in the treatment of recurrent laryngeal cancer. *Int J Radiat Oncol Biol Phys* 2016;95:404–410.

66. Wang L-W, Chen Y-W, Ho C-Y, et al. Fractionated boron neutron capture therapy in locally recurrent head and neck cancer: a prospective phase I/II trial. *Int J Radiat Oncol Biol Phys* 2016;95:396–403.

67. Mishima Y, Honda C, Ichihashi M, et al. Treatment of malignant melanoma by single neutron capture treatment with melanoma-seeking 10B-compound. *Lancet* 1989;2:388–389.

68. Mishima Y, Honda C, Ichihashi M, et al. Selective melanoma thermal neutron capture therapy for lymph node metastases. In: Soloway AH, Barth RF, Carpenter DE, eds. *Advances in neutron capture therapy*. New York: Plenum Press, 1993:705–710.

69. Ichihasi I. Boron neutron capture therapy for malignant melanoma—retrospective and perspective of clinical trials. In: *Program and abstracts, ninth international symposium on neutron capture therapy for cancer, Osaka, Japan,* 2000:3–4.

70. Mishima Y. Selective thermal neutron capture therapy of cancer cells using their specific metabolic activities—melanoma as prototype. In: Mishima Y, ed. *Cancer neutron capture therapy*. New York: Plenum Press, 1996:1–26.

71. Gonzalez SJ, Casal M, Pereira MD, et al. Tumor control and normal tissue complications in BNCT treatment of nodular melanoma: a search for predictive quantities. *Appl Radiat Isot* 2009;67:S153–S156.

72. Miyatake S, Tamura Y, Kawabata S, et al. Boron neutron capture therapy for malignant tumors related to meningiomas. *Neurosurgery* 2007;61:82–90.

73. Kawabata S, Hiramatsu R, Kuroiwa T, et al. Boron neutron capture therapy for recurrent high-grade meningiomas. *J Neurosurg* 2013;119:837–844.

74. Pinelli T, Zonta A, Alteri S, et al. TAOrMINA: from the first idea to the application to the human liver. In: Sauerwein W, Moss R, Wittig A, eds. *Research and development neutron capture therapy*. Bologna, Italy: Moduzzi Editore, 2002:1065–1072.

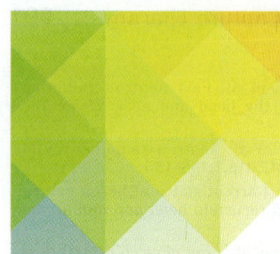

CHAPTER 23
Carbon Ions

Pascal Pommier, Stephanie E. Combs, and Tadashi Kamada

INTRODUCTION: PRESENT STATUS AND PERSPECTIVE FOR CARBON IONS

Carbon ion therapy is an innovative radiotherapy modality mostly dedicated to cancers considered as unresectable and radioresistant to photons, thanks to its radiobiologic properties combining the advantages of the high dose distribution conformity of protons for deep tumors (superior to photons and neutrons) and of the higher biologic effectiveness (compared to photons and protons) of high linear energy transfer (LET) particles such as neutrons. Moreover, the combination of the biologic and ballistic properties of carbon ions also permits to greatly reduce the treatment period compared with photon or proton radiotherapy. Long-term clinical data based on phase I and II large studies are now available, allowing to consider carbon ions as an alternative (see a referent therapy in some specific situations), and phase III trials are ongoing to measure the expected benefit of the radiotherapy modality and favor its diffusion.

Lawrence Berkeley Laboratory

The use of charged particles (protons and ions) for clinical applications has been first proposed in 1946 by R.R. Wilson.[1] A decade after, the Lawrence Berkeley Laboratory (LBL) in California started patients' irradiation, first with protons (1954) and then with light ions, helium from 1957 to 1974 (more than 2,000 patients) and higher particles, mainly neon ions (433 patients from 1975 to 1992, date of the closure of the center). Few patients were treated with carbon ions at the LBL. Miscellaneous cancer types were treated with neon ions, mainly base of skull tumors with several pathologic types including chordoma, chondrosarcoma, meningioma, adenoid cystic carcinomas (ACCs) as well as osteosarcomas, sacral chordoma, glioblastoma, cholangiocarcinoma, head and neck squamous cell carcinoma, and prostate cancer. Despite severe limitations in terms of beam application (fixed horizontal beam only), quality of imaging modalities available at that time, and limited periods for clinical applications (30% of the Bevalac running time), the LBL experience permitted first to report a high local tumor control in radioresistant tumors, especially with neon particle, and to demonstrate the feasibility and the safety of high-LET particle therapy.[2-6]

National Institute of Radiological Science

The heavy ion radiotherapy project in Japan started in 1984. A unique double-synchrotron ring heavy ion accelerator system dedicated to the project was designed and constructed. It consists of two ion sources, an RFQ (radiofrequency quadrupole) linear accelerator, an Alvarez linear accelerator, two synchrotron rings, a high-energy beam transport system, and an irradiation system. It was completed in October 1993 at the National Institute of Radiological Sciences (NIRS), Chiba, Japan, and named the Heavy Ion Medical Accelerator in Chiba (HIMAC). There are three treatment rooms with fixed vertical and horizontal beam lines. The accelerated energy of the vertical carbon ion beam is 290 or 350 MeV/u and that of the horizontal beam is 290 or 400 MeV/u. The range of the 290-MeV/u carbon ion beam is approximately 15 cm in water, that of the 350-MeV/u beam is 20 cm, and that of the 400-MeV/u carbon ion beam is 25 cm. Maximum field size is 15 cm by 15 cm.[7] To produce uniform irradiation fields, a passive beam delivery system was employed with a pair of wobbler magnets and a scatterer. The range shifter is applied for adjusting the residual range of carbon ions in the patient and the ridge filter to spread out the Bragg peak in the depth dose distribution of carbon ions. After commissioning of the system including preclinical biologic study, in June 1994, NIRS started heavy ion radiotherapy using carbon ion beams generated by HIMAC.[8]

Since then, clinical studies to develop safe and secure irradiation technologies such as respiration gating and optimized dose fractionation for various cancers have been conducted. All the carbon therapies have been performed as prospective phase I/II and II clinical trials in an attempt to identify tumor sites suitable for this treatment including radioresistant tumors and to determine optimal dose fractionation, especially for hypofractionation in common cancers. In the phase I/II studies to confirm the safety of carbon ion therapy and to obtain a clue to an antitumor effect, the number of fractions and treatment period were fixed for each disease, and the total dose was gradually increased by 5% to 10%. When the recommended dose was determined in the phase I/II studies, they were incorporated into the phase II studies. At NIRS, more than 10,000 patients have been treated with carbon ion beams for the last 23 years, and the clinical efficacy of carbon ion therapy has been demonstrated for many malignant diseases.

A new medical facility at HIMAC, using the existing synchrotron, has been opened in 2011. It comprises three rooms, two with a robotic arm–controlled patient table for fixed horizontal and vertical scanning irradiation ports, and the third one is equipped with a lightweight rotating gantry with the superconducting magnets. NIRS completed installation of scanning equipment including compact rotating gantry and commissioning of the system and started the clinical trial using compact rotating gantry in May 2017.

Present Status and Perspective for Carbon Ions in Japan

At present, 10 carbon ion therapy facilities are operating around the world, 5 of them in Japan. In 1984, Japanese government decided to embark on a program of carbon ion therapy at Chiba. Clinical studies, started in 1994, have been showing the promising outcomes in general. They have lead to other carbon ion therapy facilities in Japan.

Hyogo Ion Beam Medical Center (HIBMC) was established in 2001 and was the world's first ion beam facility that provided both proton and carbon ion beams. Since then, a total of 2,367 patients were treated with carbon ion beam by the end of September 2010 at Hyogo (PTCOG data). Its lower energy (320 Mev/u) and smaller field size (10 cm by 10 cm) for carbon ion beam compared with other Japanese facilities (more than 400 Mev/u) restricted indications of carbon ion therapy for smaller and shallower tumors. HIBM increased the energy up to 375 Mev/u recently.

The third carbon ion therapy facility was completed in March 2010 at Gunma University Heavy Ion Medical Center. It is a concise carbon ion therapy accelerator, complex realized almost one-third of size and construction cost of HIMAC with same performance.

The fourth facility, named SAGA HIMAT (heavy ion medical accelerator in Tosu), a concise Gunma-type system, located southern part of Japan, was completed in August 2013 and started treatment. The fifth is in Kanagawa Prefecture near Tokyo and begun treatment using scanning beam with fixed beam lines in December 2015. Another two facilities are under construction in Osaka and Yamagata using scanning beam, and Yamagata will be equipped with more compact rotating gantry.

Data from Germany: Gesellschaft für Schwerionenforschung and Heidelberg Ion Therapy Center

In Germany, the unique possibility to perform carbon ion research and treatment was possible at a basically preclinical research institution. At the GSI in Darmstadt, Germany, patients were treated with carbon ions from 1997 on by the Department of Radiation Oncology in Heidelberg, Germany. Within the research context of GSI, three beam time blocks per year were provided for patient treatment. As a collaborative effort consisting of clinicians, biologist, physicist, and engineers from the University Hospital of Heidelberg; the German Cancer Research Center (DKFZ) in Heidelberg, Germany; the Forschungszentrum Rossendorf in Dresden; and the Biophysics Group at GSI, patient treatment could be realized accompanied by extensive preclinical research.

For beam delivery provided by a synchrotron, the intensity-modulated raster scanning technique was developed, and biologic dose calculation was refined using the local effect model (LEM) developed by Scholz and coworkers.[9–11] Clinical efficacy of this approach was shown and validated in over 600 patients with special focus on radioresistant tumors such as chordomas and chondrosarcomas of the skull base, ACCs, and high-grade meningiomas.

In Europe, the first medical center treating patients with carbon ion radiotherapy was the Heidelberg Ion Therapy Center (HIT) in Heidelberg, Germany. The center is equipped with a synchrotron providing different particle species for three treatment rooms. Two rooms are equipped with a horizontal beam line, and in one room, the world's first carbon ion gantry has been realized. Since November of 2009, the center is in clinical operation offering particle treatment for about 1,300 patients per year. The center is directly connected to the existing department of radiation oncology to allow for streamlined work flow; patients can be treated as in- and outpatients.[12,13] The center delivers particle treatments via active raster scanning, which has been developed at the Gesellschaft für Schwerionenforschung (GSI), and treatment planning and biologic plan optimization have been adopted from the work performed also previously at GSI.[14]

Uptake of clinical routine was based on the indications treated at GSI, focusing on skull base chordomas, chondrosarcomas, as well as ACCs. Subsequently, a number of clinical studies on varying indications started recruiting with different treatment concept including randomized trial comparing carbon ions versus proton radiotherapy.[15–17]

On December 2015, more than 2,000 patients received carbon ion at the HIT (PTCOG data). Initial clinical experience included predominantly brain and skull base tumors. Especially important are long-term data on skull base chordomas and chondrosarcomas including both patients treated at GSI and in Heidelberg. Most patients are treated within clinical trials, some of the comparing protons to carbon ions, and come providing evidence for dose escalation concepts.

Marburg Ion-Beam Therapy Centre

The Marburg Ion-Beam Therapy Centre (MIT), located in Marburg, Germany, is in clinical operation since October 2015 for protons and carbon ion therapy.

The accelerator facility consists of a LINAC and synchrotron provided by Siemens Healthcare/Danfysik and is equipped with the raster scanning technique.

National Centre of Oncology Hadrontherapy, Italy

The Italian National Center of Oncologic is operational since 2011 in Pavia.[18] National Centre of Oncology Hadrontherapy (CNAO) is provided with an accelerator (synchrotron P-C 400 MeV/u) working with the same technology of one of CERN and is able to produce protons and carbon ions.

The Center has three treatment rooms (equipped with horizontal, vertical, and oblique beams) with 6-DOF robotic couches and 3-D in room imaging.

The total number of patients treated is 1,365 (up to November 2015). The treatments with carbon ions are about three times those with protons. Treatment of moving targets with gating and rescanning technology, such as treatment of pancreatic adenocarcinomas and hepatocellular carcinomas, is ongoing.

China

In China, two facilities are in operation. Institute of modern physics in Lanzhou started their treatment in 2006, and 213 patients were treated with passive beam until December 2015. Shanghai Proton and Heavy Ion Center is affiliated to Fudan University also in operation using scanning beam since 2014 and treated 149 patients.

MedAustron (Austria)

In Austria, the carbon facility at Wiener Neustadt has completed the certification process and will offer proton and carbon ion treatments in 3 medical rooms (2 rooms for carbon ions with fixed beam lines, horizontal only and vertical + horizontal, respectively).

TECHNICAL ASPECTS: PRESENT STATUS AND PERSPECTIVE

Beam Delivery

The current passive beam delivery system used in Chiba is a quite reliable and robust system and had proven stable performance at HIMAC since 1994. A respiratory-gated irradiation technique was also put into practical use for the treatment of moving targets with the passive beam delivery system.[19] The similar systems are adopted at Hyogo and Gunma University.

A scanning irradiation method, which uses "narrow" pencil beams of carbon ions to cover a target volume by superimposing the spot beams of carbon ions slice by slice, has been developed and applied at GSI and then at HIT. The new facilities at HIMAC, Pavia, Shanghai, Kanagawa, Germany, and Austria are (will be) equipped with this system. Compared to passive methods, the scanning irradiation techniques permit a more conformal irradiation of the target volume especially with a better sparing of the normal tissue located in the beam channel entrance (i.e., skin) and are therefore more appropriate for the treatment of complex-shaped lesions that cannot be adequately irradiated by the passive beams. The scanning also permits to eliminate the need for constructing compensation filters as well as patient-specific collimators. The motion management is usually more complex and difficult in scanning treatment; however, respiratory gating, high-speed rescanning, and sophisticated target volume definition like field-specific target volume (FTV) were developed to realize the clinical application of scanning for the moving target.[20,21]

Gantry

The world's first carbon ion gantry was designed and constructed at HIT (total weight of over 600 t of steel; about 420 t precisely turning around the patient; length 25 m with a diameter of 13 m). Clinical operation of the gantry started in 2012.

A lightweight rotating gantry using superconducting magnets has been designed and was installed in the new HIMAC facility in 2015. The compact gantry was put into clinical use in May 2017 at NIRS.

Gating and Tracking

To reduce the enlargement of irradiated volume with respiration, a respiratory-gated irradiation technique was developed for carbon ion therapy at HIMAC.[22] In this technique, the irradiation-gate signal is generated only when the target is located at the designed position and the synchrotron can extract a beam. Thus, one of the key technologies for the respiratory-gated irradiation is the beam-extraction method from the synchrotron according to the gate signal. For this purpose, the RF-KO slow extraction method, which utilizes a transverse beam heating by an RF-field tuned with a wave number of a horizontal betatron oscillation, was developed[23] as well as the respiratory-gated irradiation system.[18] In this system, the respiration signal is generated by observation of movement of an LED set on the surface of the patient's body through a position-sensitive detector. The respiratory-gated irradiation system has been utilized for treatments mainly for liver and lung tumors since 1996 and very effective for reduction of fraction number in these tumors moving along with respiration.

Treatment of moving organs with ions applied with the raster scanning technique confronts the physicist and clinical with novel challenges. Because of the interplay effect of the scanning beam and the moving target substantial over- and underdosage within the target volume is generated, therefore, it cannot be precisely calculated and guaranteed that the planned dose will be applied homogeneously.[24] Therefore, effective compensation mechanisms are necessary for the treatment of moving targets.

Several approaches are currently under investigation: Monitoring breathing motion and using the information for gating strategies (irradiating during set gating windows) can significantly reduce interaction.[24] Another approach is the rescanning technique: The volume is not scanned one by the beam with the whole calculated dose, that is, particle number, but the volume is scanned several times, and the particles (or dose) are divided onto the scanning runs. With this concept, a more homogeneous spread of the particles and dose over the volume can be achieved, with increasing homogeneity with the number of scanning runs.[25] A sophisticated concept is monitoring organ motion and making the beam follow the movement of the target volume; this required fast communication between the beam scanning system and the monitoring setup, to provide real-time tracking of the volume.[24]

All three concepts are currently under evaluation; potentially, the technique used may be depending on the tumor type or anatomical region treated; additionally, target volume concepts might help compensate for some minor organ movement. However, using only compensatory target volumes, such as internal target volumes (ITVs) as used in photon radiotherapy, will not suffice.[24] Variation of spot scanning size and reduction of grid size can also help compensate organ motion. It is most likely that a combination of several approaches, that is, specific target volume, modification of spot size, and perhaps gating, will provide optimal and clinically applicable dose distributions.

Beam Imaging (TEP)

As a by-product of particle radiotherapy, β⁺ activity is generated and can be monitored using conventional PET scanners to *in vivo* monitoring of dose application. Several centers offering particle therapy have established this possibility.

At GSI, an online PET imager had been built into the treatment cave allowing for online monitoring of β⁺ activity during each fraction, enabling later correlation with the planned and calculated treatment plan for passive beam delivery centers, such as Mass General in Boston or Centers in Japan.

Promising experience in PET imaging of proton and carbon ion therapy has been so far obtained for more than 50 patients monitored after passive proton treatments in the United States and Japan, as well as more than 400 patients monitored during scanned carbon ion beam irradiation at GSI Darmstadt, Germany. At the GSI pilot project, the value of PET for improving the accuracy of the semiempirical CT-range calibration curve employed by the treatment planning system as well as for detecting and quantifying deviations between planned and actual treatment delivery because of patient misalignments or anatomical changes over the course of fractionated therapy could be demonstrated.[26] At HIT, a commercial PET/CT scanner has been installed in a dedicated room adjacent to the treatment area and implemented in clinics.[27–29]

CARBON IONS' RADIOBIOLOGIC PROPERTIES: RATIONALE FOR PATIENTS' SELECTION

Carbon ions for clinical applications are characterized by two main properties: (a) a depth dose distribution with a sharp maximal energy deposition at a definite depth (the "Bragg peak") related to the beam incidence energy, with almost no dose deposited beyond this peak (Fig. 23.1), and (b) a biologic efficiency increasing at the end of the beam's range, within the Bragg peak.

Although not demonstrated by large prospective randomized clinical trials, the potential clinical gains achievable by these ballistic advantages led to the definition of several "standard" indications for protons and carbon ion therapy.[30,31]

Dose Distribution: Bragg Peak and Spread-Out Bragg Peak

Although similar, there are some notable differences between the dose-depth distribution of protons and carbon ions that may have clinical impacts, the presence of a "fragmentation tail" for carbon ions because of nuclear interactions, allowing high-quality PET imaging, and a very narrow penumbra for carbon ions compared to protons.[31]

Similarly to protons, carbon ion beams are spread out to conform to the target, resulting in the spread-out Bragg peak (SOBP) after a low dose "plateau" within the entrance channel

FIGURE 23.1. Bragg peak (protons vs. carbon ions vs. photons).

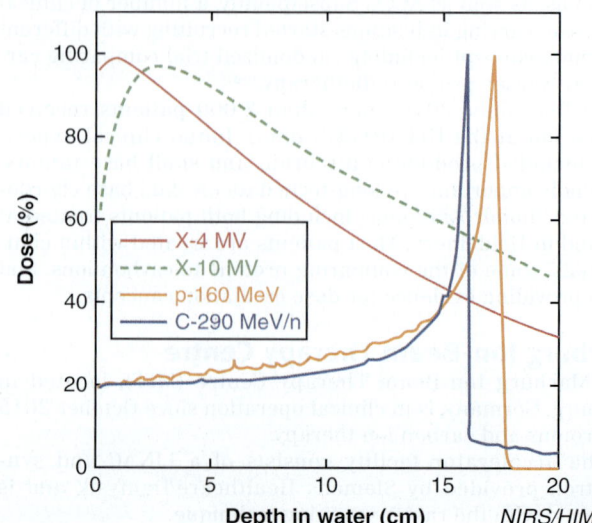

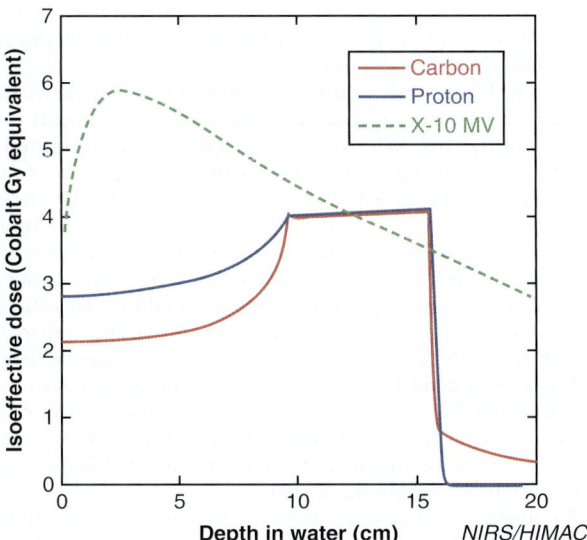

FIGURE 23.2. Spread-out Bragg peak (protons vs. carbon ions vs. photons).

beyond the target (Figs. 23.2 and 23.3). This can be achieved by several techniques, mainly with passive scattering, but also with more advanced techniques (pencil beam and wobbling or uniform scanning), achieving a lower dose deposit within the normal tissue in the entrance of the beam (proximally to the tumor volume) while optimizing the distal dose distribution and therefore a higher dose distribution conformation.

Treatment Plan Intercomparisons

Several treatment planning comparative studies between carbon ions and protons or photons have been so far published.

For similar and strict constraints to critical organs at risk, carbon ions alone or a combination of carbon ions and photon intensity–modulated radiotherapy (IMXT) was superior to IMXT alone or proton therapy for spinal chordomas or sarcomas.[32,33]

FIGURE 23.3. Design of a carbon ion spread-out Bragg peak (SOBP). The high-LET region of the carbon ion beam is located in the distal part of the Bragg peak, and the SOBP becomes a weighted function of several Bragg peaks at various energies, which results in a dilution of the dose-average LET in the target volume. Therefore, the physical dose (*gray*) has to be decreased as the relative biologic effectiveness (RBE) value rises so as to have a flat biologically effective dose across the SOBP.

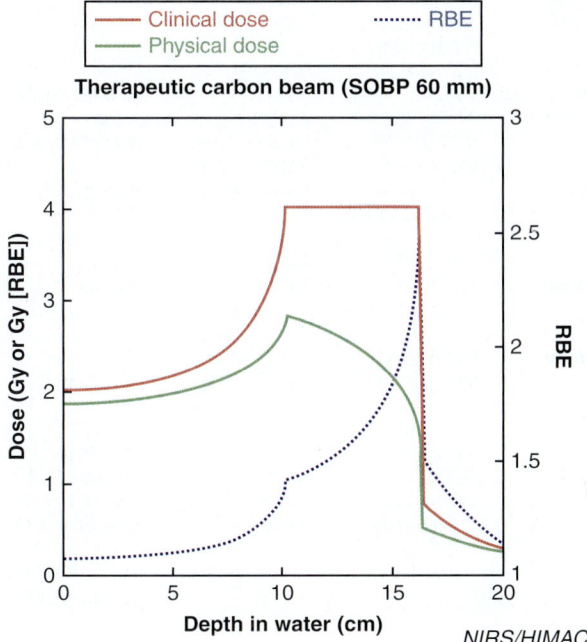

Similar results have been reported for selected head and neck tumor and ACC with infiltration of the skull base[34,35] with carbon ion versus photons both for tumor coverage and OAR preservation. More recently, the ROCOCO multicentric in silico trial also demonstrated a benefit with carbon ions over photons but also over protons in reducing at-risk organs' mean dose in reirradiation.[36] However, as expected, particle therapy (protons or carbon ions) were less effective to protect the bladder and rectal wall compared to brachytherapy for prostate cancer.[37]

Based on meta-analysis, a tumor control probability (TCP) model has been developed and validated in prostate cancer treated by photons, protons, or carbon ions and should be of interest for future prospective clinical evaluation.[38]

Integral Dose

Another advantage of particle beams is that fewer fields are required to achieve an acceptable dose distribution for difficult cases, which lead to a dramatic decrease of the integral dose (and potentially a lower incidence of radio-induced cancer, especially in pediatric indications) compared to IMXT.[39]

Biologic Effectiveness and Equivalent Biologic Rate

Similarly to neutrons, carbon ion interactions are characterized by a high LET that provides for a given physical dose a higher biologic effect compared to low-LET irradiation modalities (photons and protons). Therefore, the dose delivered with high-LET particles is prescribed in gray equivalents (GyE) or cobalt gray equivalents (CGE) equal to the measured physical dose in gray multiplied by a relative biologic effectiveness (RBE) factor.

Interestingly for clinical applications, this higher biologic efficiency may lead to a higher TCP for "radioresistant tumors" but may also increase the normal tissue complication probability (NTCP), which is limited to the Bragg peak (though to the SOBP). Within the "entrance" channel where the main proportion of the organs at risk should be, there is no additional biologic effect.

The RBE of carbon ions is difficult to calculate, and for dose-reporting purposes, a value of 3 is often utilized based on neutron experience. However, several other parameters should be taken into account such as dose per fraction, fractionation, tissue type, target volume, and pO_2 value at each point in the irradiated volume and in addition the variation in RBE along the SOBP (higher at the distal part than at the proximal part)[31] (Fig. 23.3). In NIRS, the LET dependency is taken into account in the design of clinical dose distribution by choosing the 10% survival of the HSG tumor cells as end points, and it was evaluated through the TCP analysis for non–small cell lung cancer (NSCLC).[40,41] The LEM, a generic model allowing for RBE calculation in various tissue types and for various end points, has been developed and applied in GSI and is in use for biologic treatment planning in the HIT.

Dose Fractionation

The capacity for normal and cancer tissues to repair sublethal radiation injury is sharply reduced with high-LET radiation both for normal tissues and cancer cells. This leads to question the need for dose fractionation (applying standard fractionation scheme with low dose per fraction) justified in low-LET therapy (photons and protons) by a higher kinetics of sublethal radiation injury repair for normal tissue versus "radiosensitive" tumors.

Experimental data with high-LET particles did not find any differences in RBE values between tumor and normal cell lines in standard culture condition.[42,43] However, experiments conducted with fast neutrons and carbon ions have demonstrated that increasing the dose per fraction tends to lower the RBE of both the tumor and normal tissues but with a more important decrease for the normal tissue given a higher therapeutic ratio for short-course hypofractionation schemes with carbon ion RT.[42,44] At the NIRS in Chiba, Japan, hypofractionated carbon ion RT has been investigated systematically for a variety of tumor entities, and it seems that a significant reduction of overall treatment time can be accomplished for many tumor entities without enhancing toxicity.[7]

Applications for Patients' Selection and Radiotherapy Schemes

To summarize, the best indications for carbon ions based on its biologic advantages over low-LET radiation (photons and protons) and poor dose-depth distribution (photons and neutrons) are tumors that demonstrate low radiosensitivity when treated with photons, particularly if the tumor is surrounded by radiosensitive normal tissue.

Carbon ions' biologic and physical properties also justify the use of a larger fraction dose than in conventional radiotherapy schemes with an impact on patients' quality of life (shorter overall treatment time) and also a major economical impact (reduction of the cost for the health insurance).

CLINICAL DATA

Mainly based on the clinical experience of the NIRS and the GSI, several clinical data are available to assess the efficacy and tolerance of carbon ion radiotherapy in miscellaneous tumor locations and pathologies.

To date, medical data on carbon ion therapy rely on prospective phase I (dose escalation and hypofractionation assessments) and II trials conducted in more than 20,000 patients mostly at the NIRS, GSI and HIT[45] (*PTCOG data*). The main clinical data are summarized for each tumor sites in Tables 23.1 to 23.10.

Head and Neck Cancers (Table 23.1)

Carbon ion therapy has been applied in several tumor types for head and neck primary or recurrent cancers (unresectable or R1-R2 tumors) in phase I and II prospective studies and in some selected case as a second irradiation.[46]

Data from Japan (NIRS, Hyogo, and multicenter studies)[47–55] and from Germany (HIT)[56–60] have been recently updated and are summarized in Table 23.1.

The most impressive data with carbon ion only or with an mixed treatment beam (using carbon ions as a boost) have been obtained for ACC with high local control obtained at 5 years and even later, however, with the exception of very locally advanced tumor with brain involvement (T4b). Similar results have been obtained for non-ACC malignant tumors. Regarding mucosal melanoma, despite a high local control, the prognostic is still very poor because of the frequent occurrence of distant metastases. The benefit of adding an adjuvant and concomitant chemotherapy has been suggested in the Japan Carbon Ion Radiation Oncology Study Group (J-CROS).[53]

When compared to their historical data, a dose response was observed for head and neck sarcoma in the NIRS experience in terms of 3-year local control and 3-year overall survival.[61] These results have been confirmed in a large multicentric analysis (Sulaiman, 2018).

The feasibility of dose escalation with carbon ions used as a boost has been demonstrated, thanks to the prospective phase II trial COSMIC for malignant salivary gland tumors.[56] In addition, the comparison of the clinical outcome for locally advanced ACC treated within the same period by the Heidelberg radiotherapy team either with a combination of photon IMRT with a carbon ion boost (39 pts) (total median dose 72 GyE) or with photon IMRT alone (29 pts) (median dose 66 Gy) was in favor of the dose escalation carbon ion boost versus photons only.[57]

A prospective trial has been launched at the HIT to evaluate the association with cetuximab for these tumors.[62]

Another unresolved question would be to compare the two main strategies developed for these tumors: exclusive carbon ion irradiation (applied at NIRS and CNAO) versus carbon ions as a boost, associated with photon IMRT (standard protocol at HIT).

A large literature review performed in 2011 by the Maastricht group[63] on head and neck cancer comparing photons, protons, and carbon ions was also in favor of carbon

TABLE 23.1 HEAD AND NECK CANCERS (ADENOID CYSTIC CARCINOMA, MUCOSAL MELANOMA, ADENOCARCINOMA, SARCOMA)

Author/Year	Type of Study (Pts)	Treatment (No. of Pts)	Median Follow-Up	Tumor Characteristics	OS	LC/DFS/LRFS	Toxicity (Late ≥ Gr. 2)
Mizoe 2012[48] **(NIRS)**	Phase II 236 pts (1997–2006)	CI: 57.6 GyE (215) or 64.0 GyE[21] 16 fr/4 wk Post-op: 52 Post CT: 27 Post-op + CT: 8	54 mo. (3–162)	Locally advanced tumors ACC: 69 MM: 85 Adenoca: 27 Sarcomas: 14 Papillary adeno: 13 SCC: 12 Others: 16	5-y OS: All: 47% ACC: 68% MM: 35% Adeno: 56% Sarcomas: 36% Papillary adeno: 31% SCC: 17%	5-y LC: ACC: 73% MM: 75% Adeno: 77% Sarcomas: 24% Papillary adeno: 61% SCC: 61%	Gr. 3: 0 Skin: Gr. 2: 3% Mucosa: Gr. 2: 2%
Koto 2017[52] **(NIRS)**	Retrospective 46 pts (1997–2012)	CI: 57.6 GyE[26] or 64.0 GyE (20) 16 fr/4 wk	62 mo. (4–186)	**Parotid gland** Inoperable or refusal of surgery ACC: 16 Adenoca: 8 Mucoepidermoid: 8 Acinic cell: 6 Others: 8	5-y OS: All: 70.1% MVA: poor PS Base-of-Skull invasion vs. (44% vs. 81%)	5-y LC: All: 74.5% Local rec: 10 pts Regional rec: 7 5 y. PFS: 49.2%	Facial nerve palsy: 5 pts Ipsilateral blindness: 1 pt Hearing Gr. 3: 5 pts ORN: 1
Hasegawa 2011[47] **(NIRS)**	Phase II 134 pts (04/1997–02/2010)	CI: 57.6 GyE or 64.0 GyE in 16 fr/4 wk	42.5 mo.	**ACC (all)** 108: unresec. or rec. or R2	5-y OS: 70% T1-3: 91% T4, rec or R2: 67%	5-y LC: 80% T1-3: 96% T4, rec or R2: 78%	Gr. 3: 0 Brain tox Gr. 2: 9%
Koto 2016[51] **(NIRS)**	Retrospective 18 pts (2002–2014)	CI: 57.6 GyE (10) or 64.0 GyE (8) 16 fr/4 wk	57 mo. (10–132)	**ACC tongue base** Primary treatment T4a: 17 N+: 7	5-y OS: 72% MVA: GTV vol.	5-y LC: 92% 5 y. DFS: 70% (MVA: GTV vol)	ORN: Gr. 3: 2 pts Gr. 2: 1 pt
Takagi 2014[49] **(Hyogo)**	Retrospective 80 pts (2002–2012)	CI: 40 Protons: 40 57.6 GyE–16 fr (9) or 65.0 GyE–26 fr (47) 50.2 GyE–26 fr (20)	38 mo. (6–115) Pr: 53 CI: 26	**ACC** Primary treatment N0 Nasal–paranasal: 51%	5-y OS: All: 63% (no sign diff. between Pr and CI)	5-y LC: All: 75% 5 y. PFS: All: 39%	Gr. 3: 36 pts Mucositis: Gr. 3: 2 Gr. 4: 1 Brain: Gr. 3: 2: Gr. 4: 1 Eye: Gr. 3: 2: Gr. 4: 7 Hemorrhage Gr. 5: 3

TABLE 23.1 HEAD AND NECK CANCERS (ADENOID CYSTIC CARCINOMA, MUCOSAL MELANOMA, ADENOCARCINOMA, SARCOMA) (*Continued*)

Author/Year	Type of Study (Pts)	Treatment (No. of Pts)	Median Follow-Up	Tumor Characteristics	OS	LC/DFS/LRFS	Toxicity (Late ≥ Gr. 2)
Sulaiman (submitted) (Japan)	Multicenter retrospective 289 pts (11/2003–12/2014)	CI	30 mo.	ACC Median GTV: 35.5 mL (0.5–493.1)	5-y OS: 74%	5-y LC: 68%, 5-y PFS: 44%	Gr. 3: 15%
Jensen 2015[56] (HIT)	Prospective 53 pts (07/2010–08/2011)	**COSMIC** trial CI boost: 24 GyE-8 fr X-IMRT: 50 Gy-25 fr	42 mo.	**Malignant salivary gland** **ACC**: 47 Mucoepidermoid: 3 Others: 3 T4: 57% R1: 20; R2: 17; inoperable: 16	3-y OS: 78.4%	3-y LC: 81.9%, (in field 79%) 3-y PFS: 57.9%	Gr. 3: 0 Gr. 4: 1 (hemorrhage)
Jensen 2016[58] (HIT)	Retrospective 309 pts (1998–2013)	CI boost: 23.9 GyE (median)–3 GyE/fr. X-IMRT: 50 Gy (median)–25 fr Total dose: 74 GyE	33.9 mo.	Head and neck **ACC** T4:`60%; rec.: 66 pts R1: 89; R2: 135; inoperable: 85	5-y OS: 74.6%	5-y LC: 58.5% T1: 100; T2: 80; T3: 72.5; T4a: 70.9; T4b: 38.6% 5 y. DFS: 56.1%	ORN: Gr. 3: 2 pts Gr. 2: 1 pt
Jensen 2015[57] (HIT)	**Comparative** Retrospective 95 pts (1997–2009)	**CI** boost: up to 18 GyE–(3 GyE/fr) + X-IMRT: 54 Gy (58 pts) Or **X-IMRT**: 66 Gy (37 pts)	CI boost: 74 mo. Photons: 63 mo.	Head and neck **ACC** **Inoperable–R2**	Median CI boost: 102.1 mo Photons: 73.7 mo 10-y OS: CI boost: 42.2% Photons: 27.4%	5-y LC: CI boost: 59.6% Photons: 39.9% Median LC CI boost: 73 mo. Photons: 37.6 mo. 5-y PFS: Median PFS CI boost: 59.1 mo. Photons: 32 mo.	NA
Jensen 2016[59] (HIT)	Retrospective 40 pts (2009–2013)	CI boost: 23.9 GyE (median)–3 GyE/fr X-IMRT: 50 Gy (median)–25 fr Total dose: 74 GyE.	25.5 mo.	**Non-ACC malignant salivary gland** Mucoepidermoid: 18 Adenoca: 8 Acinic cell: 3 Others: 11 T4: 45%; N+: 40% R1: 17; inoperable or R2: 23 pts	3-y OS: 72.8%	3-y LC: 81.5%, 3-y PFS: 66.8%	No Gr. ≥ 3
Mohr 2016[60] (HIT)	Retrospective 18 pts (2009–2013)	CI boost: 23.9 GyE (median)–3 GyE/fr X-IMRT: 50 Gy (median)–25 fr Total dose: 74 GyE. No chemo	18 mo.	**Paranasal MM** T4: 94% R2 or unresectable: 78%	3-y OS: 16.2%	3-y LC: 58.3%, 3-y PFS: 0%	Gr. 3: 0
Koto 2017[53] (Japan–multicenter)	Multicenter retrospective 260 pts (2003–2014)	CIRT (57.6 GyE, 16 fr to 70.4 Gy/32 fr) ± DTIC chemotherapy (60%)	22 mo. (1–132 mo)	MM Unresectable surgery refusal Nasal cavity: 68% Median GTV: 25.4 mL (0.4–325.8)	5-y OS: 44.6%	5-y LC: 72.3%, 5-y PFS: 27.2%	Gr. ≥ 3: 13% Visual: 18 pts
Saitoh 2017[54] (Japan–multicenter)	Multicenter retrospective 47 pts (11/2003–12/2014)	CIRT	51 mo.	Adenoca Median GTV: 44.6 mL (1.8–227.7)	5-y OS: 60.4%	5-y LC: 79.3%, 5-y PFS: 44.3%	Gr. 3: 26%
Shirai 2017[55] (Japan–multicenter)	Multicenter retrospective 26 pts (11/2003–12/2014)	CIRT	34 mo.	Mucoepidermoid ca Median GTV: 21 mL (3–191)	3-y OS: 89%	3-y LC: 95%, 3-y PFS: 73%	Gr. 3: 14%
Jingu 2012[61] NIRS	Phase II 27 pts (2001–2008)	CI: 70.4 GyF/16 fr	37 mo.	Unresectable bone and soft-tissue sarcoma	3-y OS: 74.1%,	3-y LC: 91.8%	Visual loss: 1 pt Bone gr. 3: 4 pts
Koto 2016[50] (NIRS)	Retrospective 13 pts (2002–2014)	CI: 57.6 GyE (8 pts) or 64.0 GyE (5 pts) 16 fr/4 wk	12 mo.	**SCC** external auditory canal and middle ear T3-T4 N+: 3	3-y OS: 40%	3y-LC: 54%	ORN: Gr. 3: 2 pts

ACC, adenoid cystic carcinoma; adenoca, adenocarcinoma; CI, carbon ions; CT, chemotherapy; DAV, dacarbazine (DTIC), nimustine hydrochloride (ACNU), and vincristine (VCR); DFS, disease-free survival; LC, local control; LRFS, locoregional relapse-free survival; MM, mucosal melanoma; mo., months; ORN, osteoradionecrosis; OS, overall survival; PFS, progression-free survival; Postop, postoperative; SCC, squamous cell carcinoma; X, photons.

ions. Based on these data, a prospective randomized study (PHRC–ETOILE) has been launched in France in 2017 to compare carbon ions and low-LET radiotherapy (either by photons or protons) in terms of progression-free survival and also in terms of medicoeconomics benefit for unresectable or R2 head and neck ACC (and sarcoma).

Sarcoma (Soft Tissue and Osteosarcoma) and Chordomas (Tables 23.2 and 23.3)

The initial phase I trial (64 pts) conducted at NIRS from June 1996 and February 2000 has established a referent dose and fractionation of 70.4 GyE delivered with 16 fractions in

TABLE 23.2 SKULL BASE (AND SPINAL) CHORDOMA AND CHONDROSARCOMA

Author/Year	Type of Study (Number of Pts)	Treatment	Follow-Up	Tumor Characteristics	OS	LC/DFS/LRFS	Toxicity (Late ≥ Gr. 3)
Mizoe 2009[65]	33 pts (34 cases[a]) Phase I/II (06/1995–07/2003)	16 fr, 4 wk 48.0: 5 pts 52.8: 3 pts 57.6: 7 pts 60.8 GyE: 5 pts	Mean 53 mo.	**Chordoma** **Skull base:** 27 pts **Paracervical spine:** 7 pts Biopsy or 1 resection: 21 pts >2 resections: 13 pts	5-y OS: 87.7% 10-y OS: 67%	5-y LC: 85.1% 10-y LC: 63.8% Dose 60.8: LC: 100%	Gr. 3: 0 1 brain Gr. 2 Tox. (steroids)
	Phase II (04/2010–06/2007)	60.8 GyE (14 pts)		CTV vol. med. 51 cc [2–328 cc]			
Uhl 2014[68] (HIT)	Retrospective (155 pts) 1998–2008	CIRT: Median 60 GyE (20 fr/3 w)	Mean 72 mo. (12–165)	**Base-of-skull chordoma** (gross tumor) Median boost vol.: 70 cc (2–294) Primary: 101 pts, Rec: 54 pts	5-y OS: 85% 10-y OS: 75%	5-y LC: 72% 10-y LC: 54%	Grading: NA
Uhl 2014[67] (HIT)	Retrospective (79 pts) 1998–2008	CIRT: Median 60 GyE (20 fr/3 w)	Med. 91 mo. (3–175)	**Skull base low-grade and intermediate-grade chondrosarcomas**	5-y OS: 96.1% 10-y OS: 78.9%	5-y LC: 88% 10-y LC: 88%	Grading: NA

[a]1 pt treated twice for a marginal recurrence.
CIRT, carbon ion radiotherapy; CTV, clinical target volume; DS, disease-free survival; LC, local control; LRFS, locoregional relapse-free survival; OS, overall survival.

TABLE 23.3 UNRESECTABLE BONE/SOFT TISSUE SARCOMAS AND SACRAL CHORDOMA (HEAD AND NECK AND SKULL BASE EXCLUDED)

Author/Year	Type of Study/ Number of Pts/ Years Inclusion	Treatment	Median Follow-Up (Months)	Tumor Characteristics	OS	LC/DFS/LRFS	Toxicity (Late ≥ Gr. 3)
Kamada 2002[64] (NIRS)	Phase I/II 57 pts (64 lesions) 1996–1999	CIRT: 52.8–73.6 GyE, 16 fr/4 wk	21 (2–60)	**Sarcoma** Median CTV: 559 cc (20–2,290)	5 y: 37%	5-y LC: 63%	Gr. 3 skin/soft tissue toxicity: 6
Demizu 2017[84] (HIBMC)	Retrospective 91 pts 2005–2014	Protons: 52 pts CI: 39 pts 70.4 GyE 32 fr (55 pts) or 16 fr (36 pts)	32 (3–112)	Pelvic sarcoma Bone and soft tissue Chordoma: 53; Chondrosarc.: 14; Osteosarcoma 10; MFH: 5	3 y: 83%	3-y LC: 92% 3-y PFS: 72% Prn factors: Chordoma; PTV < 500 cc	23 pts
Imai 2011[77] (NIRS)	Retrospective 95 pts 1996–2007	CIRT: 52.8–73.6 GyE (med. 70.4 GyE), 16 fr/4 wk	42 (13–112)	Medically **unresectable sacral chordomas** Primary T: 84 Local rec. > surgery: 11 Med. CTV vol: 370 cc	5-y OS: 86%	5-y LC: 88%	2 pts (skin necrosis) 15 pts "severe sciatic nerve toxicity" (medication)
Uhl 2015[79] (HIT)	Retrospective 56 pts 2009–2012	CIRT (15–24 GyE) + XIMRT (50 Gy): 23 Exclusive CIRT (60–66 GyE/3 Gy): 33	25	**Sacral chordoma** Primary treatment: 41: Biopsy: 20; R2: 11; R0/1: 10 Recurrent disease: 15 Med CTV vol: 244 cc	100%	2-y LC: All: 76% Primary: 85% Recurrent: 47% 3-y LC: 53%	No grade ≥ 3
Mima 2013[78] (HIBMC)	Retrospective 23 pts 2005–2011	Protons: 7 pts CI: 16 pts 70.4 GyE 32 fr (9 pts) or 16 fr (14 pts)	38 (7–78)	**Sacral chordoma** Median CTV vol: 264 cc	3 y: 83%	3 y LC: 94% 3-y PFS: 68%	Dermatitis Gr. 4: 5 pts Neuropathy Gr. 3: 4 pts
Serizawa 2009[83] (NIRS)	Phase I/II 24 pts 1997–2006	CIRT: 52.8–73.6 GyE, 16 fr/4 wk	36 (6–143)	**Unresec. retroperitoneal sarcoma** MFH: 6, lipoS: 3, MPNST: 3, Ewing/PNET: 2, misc.: 10 Median CTV: 525 cm³ (57–1,194)	2 y: 75% 5 y: 50%	2-y: 77% 5-y: 69%	No grade 3
Sugahara 2012[93] (NIRS)	Phase I–II 17 pts 2000–2010	CIRT: 70.4 GyE 16 fr/4 wk	37 (11–97)	**Sarcoma of extremities (surgery refusal)**	5-y OS: 56%	5-y LC: 76%	Gr. 3: 1 pt (fracture)
Matsumoto 2013[94] (NIRS)	Phase I–II 47 pts 1996–2011	CIRT: 52.8–73.6 GyE (med. 64 GyE), 16 fr/4 wk	25 (11–97)	**Spinal sarcoma (sacral excluded)**	5-y OS: 52%	5-y LC: 79% 5-y PFS: 48%	Gr. 3–4 skin toxicity: 2 pts Gr. 3 spinal cord reaction
Iwata 2013[95] (NIRS)	Retrospective 5 pts 1999–2009	CIRT: 70.4–73.6 GyE, 16 fr/4 wk Chemotherapy: 4 pts	(12–160)	**Unresectable Ewing sarcoma family tumors**	NA	Local rec: 1 pt Metastases: 3 pts	Paraplegia: 1 pt
Matsunobu 2012[90] (NIRS)	Phase I–II 78 pts 1996–2009	CIRT: 52.8–73.6 GyE (med. 70.4 GyE), 16 fr/4 wk	24 (14–166)	**Unresectable osteosarcoma of the trunk** **Mean T diameter: 10 cm** (<500 cc: 38 pts)	5-y OS: All: 33% <500 cc: 46% >500 cc: 19%	5-y LC: 62% <500 cc: 87% >500 cc: 31%	Gr. 3 skin toxicity: 4
Imai 2016[80] (NIRS)	Retrospective 188 pts 1996–2012	CIRT: 64.0–73.6 GyE (med. 70.4 GyE), 16 fr/4 wk	42 (13–112)	**Medically unresectable sacral chordomas** **Primary T: 188**	5-y OS: 81%	5-y LC: 77%	Gr. 4 skin toxicity: 2 Gr. 3 neurotoxicity: 6

CIRT, carbon ion radiotherapy; CTV, clinical target volume; DS, disease-free survival; LC, local control; lipoS, liposarcoma; LRFS, locoregional relapse-free survival; MFH, malignant fibrous histiocytoma; Misc, miscellaneous; MPNST, malignant peripheral nerve sheath tumor; OS, overall survival; osteoS, osteosarcoma; PNET, primitive neuroectodermal tumor.

4 weeks.[64] Since then, more than 1,000 patients have been treated at the NIRS for bone and soft tissue sarcoma, accounting for 13% of the treated patients.[45]

Many data have been recently updated, with to date large retrospective and prospective phase I to II study, with a median follow-up of more than 5 years for the NIRS and the HIT experience.

Base-of-Skull Chordoma and Chondrosarcoma (Table 23.2)

A dose–response relationship has been observed by the NIRS and HIT with a 5-year local control of 60% and 100% for dose less or above than 60 GyE, respectively.[65,66]

Results from the HIT have been updated in 2014.[67,68] Five- and 10-year overall survival was similar for both histologies, whereas chondrosarcoma was associated with a higher long-term local control compared to chordoma (respectively, 88% and 54% at 10 years).

Two phase III randomized studies have been launched by the HIT to prospectively compare protons versus carbon ion radiotherapy in these indications.[15,16]

Interestingly, the HIT teams have shown that reirradiation with carbon ions via active raster scanning may be offered in some selected patients with skull base–relapsed chordoma and chondrosarcoma.[69,70]

Combs et al. published their experience in 17 young adults and children (median age 18)[5–21] treated with carbon ions for a primary (14 pts) or a recurrent (3 pts) chordoma (10 pts) or chondrosarcoma (10 pts).[71] With a median 49-month follow-up, no severe toxicity has been observed and only 1 patient experienced a recurrence marginal to the treated volume.

Sacral Chordoma and Chondrosarcoma

CIRT appears effective and safe in the management of patients with sacral chordoma and offers a promising alternative to surgery with a high local control; similarly, see superior to surgical procedures alone[72–74] or with adjuvant proton therapy[75] and a higher functional outcome with few or no severe toxicity regarding urinary and anorectal function.[73,76–80] The occurrence of severe neuropathy was related to the dose level (more than 73.6 GyE).[77] In the series of the HIT, local control was significantly higher when carbon ions were delivered for primary tumors versus at the time of recurrence after a previous surgery.[79]

The application of particle radiotherapy for tumors adjacent to the gastrointestinal tract may be restricted because of the low tolerance of the intestine. In that situation, a surgical spacer may be placed before the particle radiotherapy.[81,82] To note, more than 10% of tumor volume increase at the end of the radiotherapy without further progression was described in 50% of cases.[83]

The HIBMC has recently published its results at 3 years for bone and soft tissue unresectable or R2 sarcomas of the pelvic (mainly chordoma and chondrosarcoma) using protons or carbon ions, with to date no significant differences between both modalities.[84] As expected, chordoma and tumor volume < 500 mL were associated with higher overall survival and progression-free survival.

A randomized phase II trial has been launched by the HIT to compare hypofractionated protons versus carbon ion radiotherapy in sacrococcygeal chordoma.[85]

Osteosarcoma

Several series with protons and photons have demonstrated that high dose irradiation may lead to a relatively high local control at 5 years (~70%) in unresected or incompletely resected osteosarcoma, with a 5-year overall survival of 40% to 67%.[76,86,87]

Similar results have been reported by the NIRS in a series of 78 patients treated with exclusive carbon ion therapy for an unresectable osteosarcoma of the trunk (median diameter of 9 cm), a location known as having the worst prognostic.[88,89] The authors reported a 5-year local control and overall survival of 62% to 33%, respectively.[90] Tumor volume was a major prognostic factor (5-year local control and overall survival of 87% and 31% for volume less or more than 500 cc, respectively).

A prospective nonrandomized study has been launched at the HIT for nonresectable osteosarcoma.[91]

Other Locations and Histology for Sarcomas

Phase I and II studies have been reported by the NIRS with exclusive carbon ion therapy for unresectable (or refusal of surgery) retroperitoneal sarcoma[92] and extremity[93] and spinal[94] sarcomas, with a high local control (respectively, 69%, 76%, and 79% at 5 years) and a 5-year overall survival of 50% to 56%, with no or limited severe late toxicities.

The role of carbon ion is still debated in unresectable Ewing family of tumors. Results in 5 patients have been reported. With a 12- to 160-month follow-up, only 1 patient experienced a local failure 22 months after the radiotherapy completion, but 3 developed distant metastases.[95]

Meningioma

The Heidelberg team demonstrated the feasibility in terms of tolerance of a protocol with carbon ions used as a boost (18 GyE) after photon therapy (50.4 Gy) even when used as a second irradiation.[96–99] However, the data are still not mature to assess a potential benefit compared to their own experience with high standard fractionation photon and proton therapy or to stereotaxic photon therapy.[100] The long-term results of a prospective protocol in patients with atypical meningiomas after incomplete resection or biopsy are still awaiting.[101]

Astrocytoma and Glioblastoma (Table 23.4)

A dose effect has been observed in a phase I/II series of 48 patients treated at the NIRS with a combination of photons, boost with carbon ion (dose escalation), and concomitant chemotherapy for malignant gliomas.[102] The NIRS also reported their experience in 14 diffuse grade 2 astrocytoma patients treated with exclusive carbon ion therapy, also reporting a high local control for high carbon ion dose and no severe toxicities.[103]

Two prospective randomized protocols are ongoing at the HIT for glioblastoma: a randomized phase II trial evaluating a carbon ion boost applied after a combined radiochemotherapy with temozolomide versus a proton boost after

TABLE 23.4 BRAIN TUMORS: ASTROCYTOMA AND GLIOBLASTOMA							
Author/Year	**Type of Study (Number of Pts)**	**Treatment**	**Median Follow-Up**	**Tumor Characteristics**	**OS**	**LC/DFS/LRFS**	**Toxicity (Late ≥ Gr. 3)**
Hasegawa 2012[103]	Phase I/II 14 pts (10/1994–02/2002)	46.2–50.4 GyE (9 pts) 55.2 GyE (5 pts) 24 fr/6 wk	Mean 62 mo (10–152)	**Astrocytomas** WHO Grade 2 Diffuse	Median OS: dose ≤ 50.4 GyE: 28 mo Dose 55.2: NA	Median PFS: dose ≤ 50.4 GyE: 18 mo Dose 55.2: 91 mo	No grade ≥ 3
Mizoe 2007[102]	Phase I/II 48 pts (10/1994–02/2002)	XRT 50 Gy/25 fr/5 wk CRT: 16.8–24.8 GyE, 8 fr/2 wk ACNU conc.	n.a.	**Malignant gliomas** (AA: 16, GBM: 32)	MST: AA: 35 mo GBM: 17 mo	GBM High dose: Median PFS: 14 mo MST: 26 mo	No grade ≥ 3 Gr. 2 brain tox: 4 pts

AA, anaplastic astrocytoma; ACNU, nimustine hydrochloride; CRT, chemoradiation; DFS, disease-free survival; GBM, glioblastoma multiforme; LC, local control; LRFS, locoregional relapse-free survival; OS, overall survival.

TABLE 23.5 STAGE I NON–SMALL CELL LUNG CANCER

Author/Year	Type of Study	Treatment	Median Follow-Up	Tumor Characteristics	OS	LC/CSS/LRFS	Toxicity (Late ≥ Gr. 3)
Miyamoto 2003[107]	Phase I/II 47 pts (48 lesions) (10/1994–08/1998)	CIRT 59.4–95.4 GyE, 18 fr/3 wk	37.5 mo	Mean T diam. 2.92 cm (0.5–6) Mean PTV 59.1 mL (4.8–290)	5 y: 42% 5-y CSS: 60%	5-y LC: 64%	0
	Phase I/II 34 pts (09/1997–02/1999)	CIRT 68.4–79.2 GyE, 9 fr/3 wk		Mean tumor size 3.57 cm (1.2–8) Mean PTV: 112.2 mL (16.9–467.4)		5-y LC: 84%	0
Miyamoto 2007[108]	Phase II 50 pts (51 lesions) (04/1999–12/2000)	CIRT: 72 GyE, 9 fr/3 wk	59.2 mo (6–83)	Mean PTV: 117.5 mL (9.8–424.4) Mean tumor diam: 2.96 cm (1–7)	5 y: 50%	5-y LC: 94.7%	Gr. 3 pulmonary Radiographic reactions: 15 Gr. 3 skin toxicity: 1
Miyamoto 2007[109]	Phase II 79 pts (80 lesions) (12/2000–11/2003)	CIRT: IA: 52.8 GyE/4 fr IB: 60 GyE/4 fr	38.6 m0 (2.5–72.2)	Mean PTV: 86.74 mL ± 50.71	5 y: 45% 5-y CSS: 68%	5-y LC: 90%	0
Yamamoto 2017[105]	Phase I/II 218 pts (04/2003–02/2012)	CIRT: Single fractionation 28–50 GyRBE	57.8 mo (1.6–160.7)	Mean PTV: 86.5 mL (24.9–357.8) Mean tumor diam: 2.8 cm (0.5–8.5) T1: 123 pts T2: 95 pts	5 y: All 49.4% 5 y: 69.2% (48–50 GyRBE)	5-y LC: All: 72.7% 5-y LC: 95.0% (48–50 GyRBE)	Grade 3 chest wall pain: 1

CIRT, carbon ion radiotherapy; CSS, cause-specific survival; DS, disease-free survival; LC, local control; LRFS, locoregional relapse-free survival; OS, overall survival; PTV, planning target volume.

radiochemotherapy with temozolomide in patients with primary glioblastoma[14] and a phase I/II trial reirradiation using carbon ions compared to fractionated stereotactic radiotherapy (FSRT) in patients with recurrent gliomas.[104]

Reirradiation (Brain, Skull Base, Head and Neck, and Sacral Region)

Thanks to its ballistic and biologic properties, carbon ion therapy has been performed for reirradiation after local recurrence following photon (or carbon ions) therapy.

The HIT reported their experience in patients with recurrent tumors of the brain, skull base, head and neck, and sacral region (mainly skull base chordoma).[46,69] Survival after reirradiation was 86% at 24 months and 43% at 60 months. For skull base tumors, local tumor control after reirradiation was 92% at 24 months and 64% at 36 months.[69]

Lung Cancer (Table 23.5)

Stage I NSCLC has been a model for the NIRS to assess the feasibility of dose escalation and hypofractionation with exclusive carbon ion therapy.[105]

From 1994 to 1999, phase I/II trials established two standard radiotherapy protocols leading to more than 95% local control with a low severe toxicity (grade 3 pneumonitis in 2.7%) established: 90 GyE in 18 fractions over 6 weeks and 72 GyE in 9 fractions over 3 weeks.[106,107] The results of the latter fractionation were confirmed in a phase II trial including 50 patients.[108] At the same time, another phase II trial permitted to validate another radiotherapy schedule using only 4 fractions with two levels of dose according to the tumor size (52.8 and 60 GyE, respectively, for stages IA and IB).[109]

These results led to initiate a phase I/II single-fraction dose escalation protocol. The total dose was raised from 28 to 50 Gy RBE. In 20 patients irradiated with 48 to 50 Gy RBE, LC at 5 years was 95.0%, OS was 69.2%, and progression-free survival (PFS) was 60.0% (median follow-up was 58.6 months). As for adverse reactions of the lung and skin, there were no patients with grade 3 or higher, and grade 2 was <2%.[105]

On multivariate analysis, overall survival outcome obtained with carbon ions was significantly better when compared with conventional radiotherapy and similar to those obtained by stereotactic radiotherapy and protons.[110]

Liver (Table 23.6)

From 1995 to 2001, phase I dose escalation and hypofractionation studies (110 pts) have been conducted at the NIRS,[111] resulting to a phase II study (47 pts) with 52.8 GyE delivered

TABLE 23.6 HEPATOCARCINOMA

Author/Year	Type of Study	Treatment (CIRT)	Median Follow-Up	Tumor Characteristics	OS	LC/DFS/LRFS	Toxicity
Imada 2010[114]	Phases I and II (64 pts) 04/2000–03/2003	52.8 GyE, 4 fr/1 wk	39.6 mo (5.7–97.8)	**Hepatocarcinoma** Stage: II: 36%, IIIA: 50%, IVA: 14% Tumor diam: med 4 cm (1.2–12) Primary: 49%, Rec: 51% <2 cm MPV: 18 Child-Pugh: A: 77%, B: 23%	5-y OS Distance from the MPV <2 cm: 22.2% >2 cm: 34.8%	5-y LC: 94% Distance from the MPV <2 cm: 87.8% >2 cm: 95.7%	Increase of Child-Pugh score ≥2: 10% (no grade 4)
Imada 2011[112]	Phases I and II (117 pts) 04/2003–04/2006	32–38.8 GyE, 2 fr	28.9 mo (6–84.4)	**Hepatocarcinoma** Tumor diam: med 4.4 cm (1.4–14)	NA	3-y LC: Dose > 42.8: 94.5% Dose < 42.8: 73.7%	Increase of Child-Pugh score ≥2: Diam <5 cm: 5% >5 cm: 7% (no grade 4)
Kasuya 2017[113]	Phases I and II Phase II (combined study) (124 pts) 04/1997–02/2003	Phases I and II 54.0–69.6 GyE 12 fr/3 wk 48.0–58.0 GyE 8 fr/2 wk 48–52.8 GyE 4 fr/1 wk Phase II 52.8 GyE 4 fr/1 wk	27.1 mo (0.9–154.8)	**Hepatocarcinoma** Tumor diam: med 4.0 cm (1–12) Child-Pugh: A: 77%, B: 23%	Overall 1 y 90.3 % 3 y 50%, 5 y 25%	Overall 3 y 91.4 % Phase II 3 y 95.5%	Late grade 3 skin 3 pt pleural effusion 1 pt (no grade 4)

DS, disease-free survival; LC, local control; LRFS, locoregional relapse-free survival; OS, overall survival.

in 4 sessions (1 week).[112,113] A high local control was obtained (96% at 3 and 5 years), without severe toxicity (≥2 increase of the Child-Pugh score in 10%), however, with a low overall survival related to the poor general status of these patients. Recently, these detailed results of stepwise dose escalation and hypofractionation in 2 combined prospective trials were published.[113]

An even more hypofractionated scheme with only 2 fractions within a phase I and then a phase II study was then developed, showing a dose effect and for the high dose group (>40.8 GyE) also a high local control rate (94.5% at 3 years), whatever the diameter of the tumor (100% for tumor > 5 cm), and a low rate of severe toxicity (≥2 increase of the Child-Pugh score in 5% to 7%),[112,114] which may be due to a compensatory enlargement in the nonirradiated liver after CIRT that contributes to the improvement of prognosis.[115]

Taking into account the alternative therapies, the optimal candidates for carbon ion therapy would be Child-Pugh A or B liver functions, tumor diameter more than 3 cm, and tumor adjacent to the porta hepatis (size and locations more difficult to treat with radiofrequency ablation or percutaneous ethanol injection).[114]

A phase I study is also planned at the HIT.[116]

Locally Recurrent Rectal Cancer (Table 23.7)

Phase I/II studies have been conducted at the NIRS since 2001 and a phase II study is still ongoing, delivering 73.6 Gy (RBE) in 16 fractions for postoperative locally recurrent rectal cancer (no previous radiotherapy). Although most of the patients had tumors considered as unresectable, results in 180 patients (186 lesions) including 151 patients treated with the highest dose were comparable than the best published surgical results.[117] A dose effect has been observed for the 5-year local control, 35%, 77%, and 88%, respectively, for 67.2, 70.4, and 73.6 Gy (RBE).

In addition, the clinical outcomes of 34 patients treated with carbon ions (48 to 52.8 Gy [RBE]) for isolated paraaortic lymph node metastasis from colorectal cancer showed a high local control rate (2 y: 70.1%) and overall survival (2 y: 83.3%) without any grade 3 to 5 toxicity.[118]

Some data are also available for carbon ion therapy reirradiation for rectal carcinoma pelvic recurrence. The preliminary results in 62 patients treated at the NIRS demonstrated a high local control (87% at 3 and 5 years) and overall survival (5 y: 43%) for carbon ions (70.4 GyE in 16 fractions) used as a second irradiation after local rectal cancer recurrence, however, with a late grade 3 toxicity in 11 patients (skin toxicity and infection) and a grade 2 peripheral neuropathy in 9 patients.[119]

The HIT is conducting a prospective phase I/II prospective study with carbon ion therapy for recurrent rectal cancer and previously treated with photons,[120] and the first results in 19 patients most of them treated with relatively low doses (median 36 Gy RBE) have been published.[121] With a limited median follow-up of 8 months, 4 experienced a local progression and 3 developed distant metastases. No grade 3 late toxicities were observed.

Pancreatic Cancer (Table 23.8)

Carbon ion therapy has been assessed as a neoadjuvant therapy in radiographically resectable pancreatic cancer[122] within a phase I dose escalation study (30 to 36.8 GyE with 8 fractions in 2 weeks). With a median follow-up time of 33.8 months, there has been no local failure in postoperative patients (21/26 pts), however, with a high rate of metastases (65%). Two patients experienced a grade 3 to 4 toxicity unrelated to carbon ion radiotherapy.

The NIRS also demonstrated the feasibility of carbon ion RT combined with gemcitabine in locally advanced pancreatic cancers, resulting in a low toxicity rate and a high local control and survival for the highest radiotherapy dose compared to historical data.[123]

The carbon ion RT facilities in Japan conducted a retrospective observational study to confirm the treatment outcome for locally advanced pancreatic cancer, which was the first multi-institutional study of carbon ion RT for pancreatic cancer. In total, 72 patients from 3 institutions in Japan were enrolled in the analysis. The data revealed that clinical outcome was comparable to historical data and toxicity was limited as well.[124]

Prostate Cancer (Table 23.9)

More than 2,700 patients have been treated with carbon ion beam for prostate cancer (mainly high and intermediate risk) at the NIRS, with three main fractionations (20, 16, and 12 fractions).[125-127] Results indicate a higher disease-free survival especially in high-risk patient and a lower incidence of radiation toxicity when compared with standard alternative

TABLE 23.7	RECTAL ADENOCARCINOMA						
Author/Year	**Type of Study**	**Treatment (CIRT)**	**Median Follow-Up**	**Tumor Characteristics**	**OS**	**LC/DFS/LRFS**	**Toxicity**
Yamada 2016[117] **(NIRS)**	Phases I and II (180 pts) 04/2001–08/2012	67.2–73.6 Gy(RBE) 16 fr/4 wk 73.6 Gy(RBE): 151 pts	42.0 mo (7–131)	**Locally recurrent rectal cancer** No prior radiotherapy Tumor diam: med 3.4 cm (1.0–14.0) Presacral: 71 pts; pelvic sidewalls 82; perineum 28; colorectal anastomosis: 5	3- and 5-y OS 67.2 Gy(RBE) 20%–20% 70.4 Gy(RBE): 53%–26% 73.6 Gy(RBE): 78%–59%	5-y LC 67.2 Gy(RBE): 35% 70.4 Gy(RBE): 77% 73.6 Gy(RBE): 88%	Late Gr. 3: 3 pts (no grade 4)
Yamada 2016[119] **(NIRS)**	Phase II (62 pts)	70.4 Gy(RBE) 16 fr/4 w	NA	**Reirradiation for locally recurrent rectal cancer** Previous X-rays: median 49.8 Gy [20–74] Median interval: 52 mo [41–157]	3 y: 69% 5 y: 43%	5-y LC: 87%	Late Gr. 3: 11 pts (infections, skin), grade 2 peripheral neuropathy: 9 pts
Habermehl 2015[121] **(HIT)**	Phases I and II (19 pts) 2010–2013	3 GyRBE/fr 36 Gy in 13 pts 39–51 Gy in 6 pts	7.8 mo	**Locally recurrent rectal cancer** Previous pelvic irradiation x rays		Local progression: 4 pts Distant metastases: 3 pts	No grade 3
ISOZAKI 2017[118] **(NIRS)**	Phases I and II (34 pts) 06/2006–08/2015	48.0–52.8 Gy(RBE) 12 fr/3 wk 73.6 Gy(RBE): 151 pts	24.4 mo (7–82.8)	**Paraaortic lymph node metastasis** Tumor diam: med 2.0 cm (1.0–4.6)	2- and 3-y OS 83.3%, 63.3%	2- and 3-y LC 70.1%, 70.1%	No grade ≥ 3

DS, disease-free survival; LC, local control; LRFS, locoregional relapse-free survival; OS, overall survival.

TABLE 23.8 PANCREATIC CANCER

Author/Year	Type of Study	Treatment (CIRT)	Median Follow-Up	Tumor Characteristics	OS	LC/DFS/LRFS	Toxicity
Shinoto 2011[122]	Phase I 10/2003–07/2010 25 pts	Preop. CIRT: 30.0 GyE–36.8 GyE	Median 13.9 mo (3.2–73.1)	**Resectable pancreatic cancer** 21: surgery	5-y OS All: 39% Post-op: 48%	No local failure (postop) Metastases: 68%	Gr. 3–4: 2 pts (unrelated to CIRT)
Shinoto 2016[123]	Phase I 04/2007–02/2012 72 pts	a. 43.2 Gy(RBE), 12 fr/3 wk + GEM 400–1,000 mg/m^2 b. 45.6–55.2 Gy(RBE), 12 fr/3 wk + GEM 1,000 mg/m^2	NA	**Locally advanced pancreatic cancer** Stage III: 65; IV: 7 pts	Median survival: 19.6 mo 2-y OS All: 35% ≥45.6 Gy(RBE): 48%	2-y LC: All: 30% ≥45.6 Gy(RBE): 40%	Late Gr. 3: 1 pt
Kawashiro 2016[124]	Retrospective 04/2012–12/2014	52.8 Gy(RBE) or 55.2 Gy(RBE), 12 fr/3 wk	13.6 mo (2.8–37.9)	**Locally advanced pancreatic cancer** Stage III: 69; IV: 3 pts	Median survival: 21.5 mo 2-y OS All: 46% 55.2 Gy(RBE): 60%	2-y LC: All: 69%	Late Gr. 3: 1 pt

CIRT, carbon ion radiotherapy; DS, disease-free survival; LC, local control; LRFS, locoregional relapse-free survival; OS, overall survival.

therapies. A multi-institutional analysis of four Japanese institutes performing carbon ion therapy for prostate cancer was conducted, and similar results to those reported at the NIRS were obtained, with a 5-year biochemical relapse-free survival of high-risk group was more than 90% without any grade 3 or worse radiation toxicity.[128]

The HIT has conducted a prospective randomized phase II study comparing protons and carbon ions using hypofractionation (66 GyRBE with 20 fractions) in both arms in 92 patients.[129] With a 22-month median follow-up, no statistical differences in acute toxicity were reported.

Gynecologic Tumor (Table 23.10)

Carbon ion therapy has been applied in locally advanced squamous cell and adenocarcinoma advanced cervix carcinomas,[130–133] within phase I to II trials. As previous studies show, carbon ion therapy produces high local control without administration of brachytherapy for locally advanced bulky cervical squamous cell carcinoma. Recent phase I/II study, with dose escalation of carbon ion radiotherapy for cervical adenocarcinoma, was accomplished without severe toxicities except 1 case, and a 5-year local control rate (55%) was observed.[133] A new clinical trial of carbon ion radiotherapy with concurrent chemotherapy for locally advanced cervical adenocarcinoma is ongoing.

Carbon ion therapy has been also applied in gynecologic melanoma. Primary melanoma of the gynecologic organs is extremely rare; it has as yet not been possible to establish an optimum treatment modality. A total of 23 patients were treated with carbon ion radiotherapy; the 3-year local control and overall survival rates were 49.9% and 53.0%, respectively.[134] Thus, carbon ion radiotherapy may become a noninvasive treatment option for gynecologic melanoma.

Choroidal Melanoma

A hundred and sixteen choroidal melanoma patients were treated with carbon ions between 2001 and 2012, and the similar local control rate (92.8% at 5 years) and survival rate (80.4% at 5 years) to the proton therapy was obtained. Although most patients had locally advanced or unfavorably located tumor, eye retention rate (92.8% at 5 years) was quite high.[135,136]

Miscellaneous

Several other tumor sites and pathology have been treated with carbon ions within phase I/II trial, the skin and[137] esophagus,[138] which need continued investigation to confirm therapeutic efficacy.

CONCLUSIONS AND PERSPECTIVES

The accumulated clinical experience has indicated that certain types of tumors such as advanced radioresistant head and neck tumors (ACC, adenocarcinoma, and mucosal

TABLE 23.9 PROSTATE CANCER

Author/Year	Type of Study	Treatment	Median Follow-Up	Tumor Characteristics	OS	LC/DFS/LRFS	Toxicity (Late ≥ Gr. 3)
Tsuji 2005[125]	Phase II 1,005 2000–2011	CIRT +/− HT 63–66 GyE/20 fr: 466 pts 57.6/16 fr: 539 pts	Min 12 mo	NA	5-y OS: 95.4%	5 years DFS: 90.6% T1-2 vs. T3: 94% vs. 84% PSA > 20 vs. >20: 92% vs. 89% GS < 6 vs. 7 vs. >8: 92 vs. 94% vs. 84%	NA
Ishikawa 2012[126]	Phases I/II and II 1,342 pts 1995–2011	CIRT +/− HT	43 mo	NA	5-y OS: 95.3%	5-y DFS: Low-risk: 90% Intermediate-risk: 97% High-risk: 88%	Rectum; 0%, GU; 0.1%
Kasuya 2016[127]	Phase II High risk 324 pts 2000–2007	CIRT +/− HT 63–66 GyE/20 fr	107 mo	NA	10 y 76.1%	Prostate cancer–specific mortality 5 y 2.2%, 10 y 4.6%	NA
Nomiya 2016[128]	Multicenter 2,157 2003–2014	CIRT +/− HT 63–66 GyE/20 fr: 291 pts 57.6/16 fr: 1,296 pts 51.6/12 fr: 570 pts	Min 12 mo	NA	NA	5-y DFS: Low-risk: 92% Intermediate-risk: 89% High-risk: 92%	Rectum; 0%, GU; 0%

CIRT, carbon ion radiotherapy; DS, disease-free survival; HT, hormonal therapy; LC, local control; LRFS, locoregional relapse-free survival; OS, overall survival.

TABLE 23.10 GYNECOLOGIC TUMOR

Author/Year	Type of Study	Treatment	Median Follow-Up	Tumor Characteristics	OS	LC/DFS/LRFS	Toxicity (Late ≥ Gr. 3)
Uterus cervical cancer (squamous cell carcinoma and adenocarcinoma)							
Nakano 1999[130]	Phase I/II 1995–1997	CIRT: 52.8–72.0 Gy(RBE)/24 fr	NA	Stage IIIB: 20 Stage IVA: 10	2-y OS: 62%	2-y LC Stage IIIB: 53% Stage IVA: 75%	GI: 2 pts
Uterus squamous cell carcinoma							
Kato 2006[131]	Phase I/II 1995–2000	CIRT: 1. 52.8–72.0 Gy(RBE)/24 fr, 30 pts 2. 68.8–72.8 Gy(RBE)/20 fr, 14 pts	27 mo	Stage IIIB: 30 Stage IVA: 14 Median tumor size: 6.5 cm (range: 4.2–11.0 cm)	5-y OS: 1. 37% 2. 43%	5-y LC: 1. 45% 2. 79%	GI: 1. 8 pts 2. 0 pt
Wakatsuki 2014[132]	Phase I/II 2000–2006	CIRT: 64.0–72.0 Gy(RBE)/20 fr, 22 pts	47 mo	Stage IIB: 1 Stage IIIB: 18 Stage IVA: 3 Median tumor size: 6.2 cm (range: 4.0–12.0 cm)	5-y OS: 50%	5-y LC: 68% *All patients who received 72.0 Gy(RBE) maintained local control.	GI: 0 pt GU: 0 pt
Uterus adenocarcinoma							
Wakatsuki 2014[133]	Phase I/II 1998–2010	CIRT: 62.4–74.4 Gy(RBE)/20 fr, 58 pts	38 mo	Stage IIB: 20 Stage IIIB: 35 Stage IVA: 3 Median tumor size: 5.5 cm (range: 3.0–11.8 cm)	5-y OS: 38%	5-year LC: 55%	GI: 2 pt GU: 0 pt
Gynecologic melanoma							
Karasawa 2014[134]	Phase I/II 2004–2012	CIRT: 57.6–64.0 Gy(RBE)/16 fr, 23 pts	17 mo	Vagina: 14 Vulva: 6 Cervix uteri: 3	5-y OS: 53%	5-year LC: 50%	GI: 0 pt GU: 1 pt

CIRT, carbon ion radiotherapy; DS, disease-free survival; LC, local control; LRFS, locoregional relapse-free survival; OS, overall survival.

malignant melanoma), large skull base tumors, rectal cancer (postoperative pelvic recurrence), and sarcomas can only be appropriately controlled and cured by carbon ion therapy with high probability. It has also been made clear that this therapy is capable of suppressing several types of tumors such as peripheral type NSCLC, liver cancer, and prostate cancer safely in a relatively short period of time through these clinical trials. Patients with these types of tumors can be remarkably healed by this therapy within a few days or weeks with minimal discomfort.

To date, no randomized clinical trial has shown the superiority of carbon ion beams to protons or photon radiotherapy. Therefore, in the future, not only evaluation of carbon ions alone in specific tumor types but also comparing to advanced photon and proton techniques are required to exploit the full advantage of high-LET particle therapy and to stratify patients for specific treatments.

REFERENCES

1. Wilson R. Radiological use of fast protons. *Radiology* 1946;47:487–491.
2. Castro JR, Linstadt DE, Bahary JP, et al. Experience in charged particle irradiation of tumors of the skull base: 1977–1992. *Int J Radiat Oncol Biol Phys* 1994;29:647–655.
3. Castro JR, Phillips TL, Prados M, et al. Neon heavy charged particle radiotherapy of glioblastoma of the brain. *Int J Radiat Oncol Biol Phys* 1997;38:257–261.
4. Linstadt DE, Castro JR, Phillips TL. Neon ion radiotherapy: results of the phase I/II clinical trial. *Int J Radiat Oncol Biol Phys* 1991;20:761–769.
5. Schoenthaler R, Castro JR, Petti PL, et al. Charged particle irradiation of sacral chordomas. *Int J Radiat Oncol Biol Phys* 1993;26:291–298.
6. Schoenthaler R, Castro JR, Halberg FE, et al. Definitive postoperative irradiation of bile duct carcinoma with charged particles and/or photons. *Int J Radiat Oncol Biol Phys* 1993;27:75–82.
7. Sato K, Yamada S, Ogawa K, et al. Performance of HIMAC. *Nucl Phys A* 1995;588:229–234.
8. Tsujii H, Mizoe JE, Kamada T, et al. Overview of clinical experiences on carbon ion radiotherapy at NIRS. *Radiother Oncol* 2004;73(Suppl 2):S41–S49.
9. Elsasser T, Kramer M, Scholz M. Accuracy of the local effect model for the prediction of biologic effects of carbon ion beams in vitro and in vivo. *Int J Radiat Oncol Biol Phys* 2008;71:866–872.
10. Elsasser T, Weyrather WK, Friedrich T, et al. Quantification of the relative biological effectiveness for ion beam radiotherapy: direct experimental comparison of proton and carbon ion beams and a novel approach for treatment planning. *Int J Radiat Oncol Biol Phys* 2010;78:1177–1183.
11. Weyrather WK, Ritter S, Scholz M, et al. RBE for carbon track-segment irradiation in cell lines of differing repair capacity. *Int J Radiat Biol* 1999;75:1357–1364.
12. Combs SE, Ellerbrock M, Haberer T, et al. Heidelberg Ion Therapy Center (HIT): initial clinical experience in the first 80 patients. *Acta Oncol* 2010;49:1132–1140.
13. Combs SE, Jakel O, Haberer T, et al. Particle therapy at the Heidelberg Ion Therapy Center (HIT)—integrated research-driven university-hospital-based radiation oncology service in Heidelberg, Germany. *Radiother Oncol* 2010;95:41–44.
14. Rieken S, Habermehl D, Nikoghosyan A, et al. Assessment of early toxicity and response in patients treated with proton and carbon ion therapy at the Heidelberg ion therapy center using the raster scanning technique. *Int J Radiat Oncol Biol Phys* 2011;81:e793–e801.
15. Combs SE, Kieser M, Rieken S, et al. Randomized phase II study evaluating a carbon ion boost applied after combined radiochemotherapy with temozolomide versus a proton boost after radiochemotherapy with temozolomide in patients with primary glioblastoma: the CLEOPATRA trial. *BMC Cancer* 2010;10:478.
16. Nikoghosyan AV, Rauch G, Munter MW, et al. Randomised trial of proton vs. carbon ion radiation therapy in patients with low and intermediate grade chondrosarcoma of the skull base, clinical phase III study. *BMC Cancer* 2010;10:606.
17. Nikoghosyan AV, Karapanagiotou-Schenkel I, Munter MW, et al. Randomised trial of proton vs. carbon ion radiation therapy in patients with chordoma of the skull base, clinical phase III study HIT-1-study. *BMC Cancer* 2010;10:607.
18. Rossi S. The National Centre for Oncological Hadrontherapy (CNAO): status and perspectives. *Phys Med* 2015;31:333–351.
19. Minohara S, Kanai T, Endo M, et al. Respiratory gated irradiation system for heavy-ion radiotherapy. *Int J Radiat Oncol Biol Phys* 2000;47:1097–1103.
20. Mori S, Zenklusen S, Inaniwa T, et al. Conformity and robustness of gated rescanned carbon ion pencil beam scanning of liver tumors at NIRS. *Radiother Oncol* 2014;111:431–436.
21. Knopf AC, Boye D, Lomax A, et al. Adequate margin definition for scanned particle therapy in the incidence of intrafractional motion. *Phys Med Biol* 2013;58:6079–6094.
22. Miki K, Mori S, Shiomi M, et al. Gated carbon-ion scanning treatment for pancreatic tumour with field specific target volume and organs at risk. *Phys Med* 2016;32:1521–1528.
23. Noda K, Kanazawa M, Itano A, et al. Slow beam extraction by a transverse RF field with AM and FM. *Nucl Instrum Methods A* 1996;374:269–277.
24. Bert C, Gemmel A, Saito N, et al. Gated irradiation with scanned particle beams. *Int J Radiat Oncol Biol Phys* 2009;73:1270–1275.
25. Furukawa T, Inaniwa T, Sato S, et al. Moving target irradiation with fast rescanning and gating in particle therapy. *Med Phys* 2010;37:4874–4879.
26. Parodi K, Saito N, Chaudhri N, et al. 4D in-beam positron emission tomography for verification of motion-compensated ion beam therapy. *Med Phys* 2009;36:4230–4243.
27. Bauer J, Unholtz D, Sommerer F, et al. Implementation and initial clinical experience of offline PET/CT-based verification of scanned carbon ion treatment. *Radiother Oncol* 2013;107:218–226.

28. Kurz C, Bauer J, Unholtz D, et al. Initial clinical evaluation of PET-based ion beam therapy monitoring under consideration of organ motion. *Med Phys* 2016;43:975–982.

29. Nischwitz SP, Bauer J, Welzel T, et al. Clinical implementation and range evaluation of in vivo PET dosimetry for particle irradiation in patients with primary glioma. *Radiother Oncol* 2015;115:179–185.

30. Schulz-Ertner D, Tsujii H. Particle radiation therapy using proton and heavier ion beams. *J Clin Oncol* 2007;25:953–964.

31. Suit H, DeLaney T, Goldberg S, et al. Proton vs carbon ion beams in the definitive radiation treatment of cancer patients. *Radiother Oncol* 2010; 95:3–22.

32. Schulz-Ertner D, Nikoghosyan A, Didinger B, et al. Treatment planning intercomparison for spinal chordomas using intensity-modulated photon radiation therapy (IMRT) and carbon ions. *Phys Med Biol* 2003;48:2617–2631.

33. Matsumoto K, Nakamura K, Shioyama Y, et al. Treatment planning comparison for carbon ion radiotherapy, proton therapy and intensity-modulated radiotherapy for spinal sarcoma. *Anticancer Res* 2015;35:4083–4089.

34. Schulz-Ertner D, Didinger B, Nikoghosyan A, et al. Optimization of radiation therapy for locally advanced adenoid cystic carcinomas with infiltration of the skull base using photon intensity-modulated radiation therapy (IMRT) and a carbon ion boost. *Strahlenther Onkol* 2003;179:345–351.

35. Amirul IM, Yanagi T, Mizoe JE, et al. Comparative study of dose distribution between carbon ion radiotherapy and photon radiotherapy for head and neck tumor. *Radiat Med* 2008;26:415–421.

36. Eekers DB, Roelofs E, Jelen U, et al. Benefit of particle therapy in re-irradiation of head and neck patients. Results of a multicentric in silico ROCOCO trial. *Radiother Oncol.* 2016;121:387–394.

37. Georg D, Hopfgartner J, Gòra J, et al. Dosimetric considerations to determine the optimal technique for localized prostate cancer among external photon, proton, or carbon-ion therapy and high-dose-rate or low-dose-rate brachytherapy. *Int J Radiat Oncol Biol Phys* 2014;88:715–722.

38. Walsh S, Roelofs E, Kuess P, et al. A validated tumor control probability model based on a meta-analysis of low, intermediate, and high-risk prostate cancer patients treated by photon, proton, or carbon-ion radiotherapy. *Med Phys* 2016;43:734–747.

39. Miralbell R, Lomax A, Cella L, et al. Potential reduction of the incidence of radiation-induced second cancers by using proton beams in the treatment of pediatric tumors. *Int J Radiat Oncol Biol Phys* 2002;54:824–829.

40. Kanai T, Endo M, Minohara S, et al. Biophysical characteristics of HIMAC clinical irradiation system for heavy-ion radiation therapy. *Int J Radiat Oncol Biol Phys* 1999;44:201–210.

41. Kanai T, Matsufuji N, Miyamoto T, et al. Examination of GyE system for HIMAC carbon therapy. *Int J Radiat Oncol Biol Phys* 2006;64:650–656.

42. Ando K, Kase Y. Biological characteristics of carbon-ion therapy. *Int J Radiat Biol* 2009;85:715–728.

43. Suzuki M, Kase Y, Yamaguchi H, et al. Relative biological effectiveness for cell-killing effect on various human cell lines irradiated with heavy-ion medical accelerator in Chiba (HIMAC) carbon-ion beams. *Int J Radiat Oncol Biol Phys* 2000;48:241–250.

44. Denekamp J, Waites T, Fowler JF. Predicting realistic RBE values for clinically relevant radiotherapy schedules. *Int J Radiat Biol* 1997;71:681–694.

45. Kamada T, Tsujii H, Blakely EA, et al. Carbon ion radiotherapy in Japan: an assessment of 20 years of clinical experience. *Lancet Oncol* 2015;16: e93–e100.

46. Jensen AD, Nikoghosyan A, Ellerbrock M, et al. Re-irradiation with scanned charged particle beams in recurrent tumours of the head and neck: acute toxicity and feasibility. *Radiother Oncol* 2011;101:383–387.

47. Hasegawa A, Koto M, Takagi R, et al. Carbon Ion Radiotherapy for Adenoid Cystic Carcinoma of the Head and Neck. *Int J Radiat Oncol Biol Phys* 2011;81:S77–S78.

48. Mizoe JE, Hasegawa A, Jingu K, et al.; Organizing Committee for the Working Group for Head Neck Cancer. Results of carbon ion radiotherapy for head and neck cancer. *Radiother Oncol* 2012;103:32–37.

49. Takagi M, Demizu Y, Hashimoto N, et al. Treatment outcomes of particle radiotherapy using protons or carbon ions as a single-modality therapy for adenoid cystic carcinoma of the head and neck. *Radiother Oncol* 2014;113: 364–370.

50. Koto M, Hasegawa A, Takagi R, et al.; Organizing Committee for the Working Group for Head and Neck Cancer. Carbon ion radiotherapy for locally advanced squamous cell carcinoma of the external auditory canal and middle ear. *Head Neck* 2016;38:512–516.

51. Koto M, Hasegawa A, Takagi R, et al.; Organizing Committee for the Working Group for Head and Neck Cancer. Evaluation of the safety and efficacy of carbon ion radiotherapy for locally advanced adenoid cystic carcinoma of the tongue base. *Head Neck* 2016;38:S2122–S2126.

52. Koto M, Hasegawa A, Takagi R, et al.; Organizing Committee for the Working Group for Head and Neck Cancer. Definitive carbon-ion radiotherapy for locally advanced parotid gland carcinomas. *Head Neck* 2017;39: 724–729.

53. Koto M, Demizu Y, Saitoh JI, et al. Multicenter study of carbon-ion radiation therapy for mucosal melanoma of the head and neck: subanalysis of the Japan Carbon-Ion Radiation Oncology Study Group (J-CROS) Study (1402 HN). *Int J Radiat Oncol Biol Phys* 2017;97:1054–1060.

54. Saitoh JI, Koto M, Demizu Y, et al. A multicenter study of carbon-ion radiotherapy for head and neck adenocarcinoma. *Int J Radiat Oncol Biol Phys* 2017;99(2):442–449.

55. Shirai K, Koto M, Demizu Y, et al. Multi-institutional retrospective study of mucoepidermoid carcinoma treated with carbon-ion radiotherapy. *Cancer Sci* 2017;108(7):1447–1451.

56. Jensen AD, Nikoghosyan AV, Lossner K, et al. COSMIC: a regimen of intensity modulated radiation therapy plus dose-escalated, raster-scanned carbon ion boost for malignant salivary gland tumors: results of the Prospective Phase 2 Trial. *Int J Radiat Oncol Biol Phys* 2015;93:37–46.

57. Jensen AD, Nikoghosyan AV, Poulakis M, et al. Combined intensity-modulated radiotherapy plus raster-scanned carbon ion boost for advanced adenoid cystic carcinoma of the head and neck results in superior locoregional control and overall survival. *Cancer* 2015;121(17):3001–3009.

58. Jensen AD, Poulakis M, Nikoghosyan AV, et al. High-LET radiotherapy for adenoid cystic carcinoma of the head and neck: 15 years' experience with raster-scanned carbon ion therapy. *Radiother Oncol* 2016;118:272–280.

59. Jensen AD, Poulakis M, Vanoni V, et al. Carbon ion therapy (C12) for high-grade malignant salivary gland tumors (MSGTs) of the head and neck: do non-ACCs profit from dose escalation? *Radiat Oncol* 2016;11:90.

60. Mohr A, Chaudhri N, Hassel JC, et al. Raster-scanned intensity-controlled carbon ion therapy for mucosal melanoma of the paranasal sinus. *Head Neck* 2016;38:S1445–S1451.

61. Jingu K, Tsujii H, Mizoe JE, et al. Carbon ion radiation therapy improves the prognosis of unresectable adult bone and soft-tissue sarcoma of the head and neck. *Int J Radiat Oncol Biol Phys* 2012;82:2125–2131.

62. Jensen AD, Nikoghosyan A, Hinke A, et al. Combined treatment of adenoid cystic carcinoma with cetuximab and IMRT plus C12 heavy ion boost: ACCEPT [ACC, Erbitux(R) and particle therapy]. *BMC Cancer* 2011;11:70.

63. Ramaekers BL, Pijls-Johannesma M, Joore MA, et al. Systematic review and meta-analysis of radiotherapy in various head and neck cancers: comparing photons, carbon-ions and protons. *Cancer Treat Rev* 2011;37:185–201.

64. Kamada T, Tsujii H, Tsuji H, et al. Efficacy and safety of carbon ion radiotherapy in bone and soft tissue sarcomas. *J Clin Oncol* 2002;20:4466–4471.

65. Mizoe JE, Hasegawa A, Takagi R, et al. Carbon ion radiotherapy for skull base chordoma. *Skull Base* 2009;19:219–224.

66. Schulz-Ertner D, Nikoghosyan A, Hof H, et al. Carbon ion radiotherapy of skull base chondrosarcomas. *Int J Radiat Oncol Biol Phys* 2007;67:171–177.

67. Uhl M, Mattke M, Welzel T, et al. High control rate in patients with chondrosarcoma of the skull base after carbon ion therapy: first report of long-term results. *Cancer* 2014;120:1579–1585.

68. Uhl M, Mattke M, Welzel T, et al. Highly effective treatment of skull base chordoma with carbon ion irradiation using a raster scan technique in 155 patients: first long-term results. *Cancer* 2014;120:3410–3417.

69. Combs SE, Kalbe A, Nikoghosyan A, et al. Carbon ion radiotherapy performed as re-irradiation using active beam delivery in patients with tumors of the brain, skull base and sacral region. *Radiother Oncol* 2011;98:63–67.

70. Uhl M, Welzel T, Oelmann J, et al. Active raster scanning with carbon ions: reirradiation in patients with recurrent skull base chordomas and chondrosarcomas. *Strahlenther Onkol* 2014;190:686–691.

71. Combs SE, Nikoghosyan A, Jaekel O, et al. Carbon ion radiotherapy for pediatric patients and young adults treated for tumors of the skull base. *Cancer* 2009;115:1348–1355.

72. Fuchs B, Dickey ID, Yaszemski MJ, et al. Operative management of sacral chordoma. *J Bone Joint Surg Am* 2005;87:2211–2216.

73. Nishida Y, Kamada T, Imai R, et al. Clinical outcome of sacral chordoma with carbon ion radiotherapy compared with surgery. *Int J Radiat Oncol Biol Phys* 2011;79:110–116.

74. Outani H, Hamada K, Imura Y, et al. Comparison of clinical and functional outcome between surgical treatment and carbon ion radiotherapy for pelvic chondrosarcoma. *Int J Clin Oncol* 2016;21:186–193.

75. Park L, Delaney TF, Liebsch NJ, et al. Sacral chordomas: impact of high-dose proton/photon-beam radiation therapy combined with or without surgery for primary versus recurrent tumor. *Int J Radiat Oncol Biol Phys* 2006;65:1514–1521.

76. Imai R, Kamada T, Tsuji H, et al. Effect of carbon ion radiotherapy for sacral chordoma: results of Phase I-II and Phase II clinical trials. *Int J Radiat Oncol Biol Phys* 2010;77:1470–1476.

77. Imai R, Kamada T, Sugahara S, et al. Carbon ion radiotherapy for sacral chordoma. *Br J Radiol* 2011;84:S48–S54.

78. Mima M, Demizu Y, Jin D, et al. Particle therapy using carbon ions or protons as a definitive therapy for patients with primary sacral chordoma. *Br J Radiol* 2014;87:20130512.

79. Uhl M, Welzel T, Jensen A, et al. Carbon ion beam treatment in patients with primary and recurrent sacrococcygeal chordoma. *Strahlenther Onkol* 2015;191:597–603.

80. Imai R, Kamada T, Araki N. Carbon ion radiation therapy for unresectable sacral chordoma: an analysis of 188 Cases. *Int J Radiat Oncol Biol Phys* 2016;95:322–327.

81. Takahashi M, Fukumoto T, Kusunoki N, et al. Particle beam radiotherapy with a surgical spacer placement for unresectable sacral chordoma. *Gan To Kagaku Ryoho* 2010;37:2804–2806.

82. Lorenzo C, Andrea P, Barbara V, et al. Surgical spacer placement prior carbon ion radiotherapy (CIRT): an effective feasible strategy to improve the treatment for sacral chordoma. *World J Surg Oncol* 2016;14:211.

83. Serizawa I, Imai R, Kamada T, et al. Changes in tumor volume of sacral chordoma after carbon ion radiotherapy. *J Comput Assist Tomogr* 2009;33:795–798.

84. Demizu Y, Jin D, Sulaiman NS, et al. Particle therapy using protons or carbon ions for unresectable or incompletely resected bone and soft tissue sarcomas of the pelvis. *Int J Radiat Oncol Biol Phys* 2017;98:367–374.

85. Uhl M, Edler L, et al. Randomized phase II trial of hypofractionated proton versus carbon ion radiation therapy in patients with sacrococcygeal chordoma-the ISAC trial protocol. *Radiat Oncol* 2014;9:100.

86. Ciernik IF, Niemierko A, Harmon DC, et al. Proton–based radiotherapy for unresectable or incompletely resected osteosarcoma. *Cancer* 2011;117:4522–4530.

87. Oertel S, Blattmann C, Rieken S, et al. Radiotherapy in the treatment of primary osteosarcoma—a single center experience. *Tumori* 2010;96:582–588.

88. Bielack SS, Wulff B, Delling G, et al. Osteosarcoma of the trunk treated by multimodal therapy: experience of the Cooperative Osteosarcoma study group (COSS). *Med Pediatr Oncol* 1995;24:6–12.

89. Bielack SS, Kempf-Bielack B, Delling G, et al. Prognostic factors in high-grade osteosarcoma of the extremities or trunk: an analysis of 1,702 patients treated on neoadjuvant cooperative osteosarcoma study group protocols. *J Clin Oncol* 2002;20:776–790.

90. Matsunobu A, Imai R, Kamada T, et al. Impact of carbon ion radiotherapy for unresectable osteosarcoma of the trunk. *Cancer* 2012;118:4555–4563.

91. Blattmann C, Oertel S, Schulz-Ertner D, et al. Non-randomized therapy trial to determine the safety and efficacy of heavy ion radiotherapy in patients with non-resectable osteosarcoma. *BMC Cancer* 2010;10:96.

92. Serizawa I, Kagei K, Kamada T, et al. Carbon ion radiotherapy for unresectable retroperitoneal sarcomas. *Int J Radiat Oncol Biol Phys* 2009;75:1105–1110.

93. Sugahara S, Kamada T, Imai R, et al.; Working Group for the Bone and Soft Tissue Sarcomas. Carbon ion radiotherapy for localized primary sarcoma of the extremities: results of a phase I/II trial. *Radiother Oncol* 2012;105:226–231.

94. Matsumoto K, Imai R, Kamada T, et al.; Working Group for Bone and Soft Tissue Sarcomas. Impact of carbon ion radiotherapy for primary spinal sarcoma. *Cancer* 2013;119:3496–3503.

95. Iwata S, Yonemoto T, Ishii T, et al. Efficacy of carbon-ion radiotherapy and high-dose chemotherapy for patients with unresectable Ewing's sarcoma family of tumors. *Int J Clin Oncol* 2013;18:1114–1118.

96. Combs SE, Hartmann C, Nikoghosyan A, et al. Carbon ion radiation therapy for high-risk meningiomas. *Radiother Oncol* 2010;95:54–59.

97. Adeberg S, Hartmann C, Welzel T, et al. Long-term outcome after radiotherapy in patients with atypical and malignant meningiomas-clinical results in 85 patients treated in a single institution leading to optimized guidelines for early radiation therapy. *Int J Radiat Oncol Biol Phys* 2012;83:859–864.

98. Combs SE, Welzel T, Habermehl D, et al. Prospective evaluation of early treatment outcome in patients with meningiomas treated with particle therapy based on target volume definition with MRI and 68Ga-DOTATOC-PET. *Acta Oncol* 2013;52:514–520.

99. Mozes P, Dittmar JO, Habermehl D, et al. Volumetric response of intracranial meningioma after photon or particle irradiation. *Acta Oncol* 2017;56:431–437.

100. Kessel KA, Fischer H, Oechsner M, et al. High-precision radiotherapy for meningiomas: long-term results and patient-reported outcome (PRO). *Strahlenther Onkol* 2017;193(11):921–930.

101. Combs SE, Edler L, Burkholder I, et al. Treatment of patients with atypical meningiomas Simpson grade 4 and 5 with a carbon ion boost in combination with postoperative photon radiotherapy: the MARCIE trial. *BMC Cancer* 2010;10:615.

102. Mizoe JE, Tsujii H, Hasegawa A, et al. Phase I/II clinical trial of carbon ion radiotherapy for malignant gliomas: combined X-ray radiotherapy, chemotherapy, and carbon ion radiotherapy. *Int J Radiat Oncol Biol Phys* 2007;69:390–396.

103. Hasegawa A, Mizoe JE, Tsujii H, et al. Experience with Carbon Ion Radiotherapy for WHO Grade 2 Diffuse Astrocytomas. *Int J Radiat Oncol Biol Phys* 2012;83:100–106.

104. Combs SE, Burkholder I, Edler L, et al. Randomised phase I/II study to evaluate carbon ion radiotherapy versus fractionated stereotactic radiotherapy in patients with recurrent or progressive gliomas: the CINDERELLA trial. *BMC Cancer* 2010;10:533.

105. Yamamoto N, Miyamoto T, Nakajima M, et al. A dose escalation clinical trial of single-fraction carbon-ion radiotherapy for peripheral stage I non-small-cell lung cancer. *J Thorac Oncol* 2017;12:673–680.

106. Koto M, Miyamoto T, Yamamoto N, et al. Local control and recurrence of stage I non-small cell lung cancer after carbon ion radiotherapy. *Radiother Oncol* 2004;71:147–156.

107. Miyamoto T, Yamamoto N, Nishimura H, et al. Carbon ion radiotherapy for stage I non-small cell lung cancer. *Radiother Oncol* 2003;66:127–140.

108. Miyamoto T, Baba M, Yamamoto N, et al. Curative treatment of Stage I non-small-cell lung cancer with carbon ion beams using a hypofractionated regimen. *Int J Radiat Oncol Biol Phys* 2007;67:750–758.

109. Miyamoto T, Baba M, Sugane T, et al. Carbon ion radiotherapy for stage I non-small cell lung cancer using a regimen of four fractions during 1 week. *J Thorac Oncol* 2007;2:916–926.

110. Grutters JP, Kessels AG, Pijls-Johannesma M, et al. Comparison of the effectiveness of radiotherapy with photons, protons and carbon-ions for non-small cell lung cancer: a meta-analysis. *Radiother Oncol* 2010;95:32–40.

111. Kato H, Tsujii H, Miyamoto T, et al. Results of the first prospective study of carbon ion radiotherapy for hepatocellular carcinoma with liver cirrhosis. *Int J Radiat Oncol Biol Phys* 2004;59:1468–1476.

112. Imada H, Yasuda S, Yamada S, et al. Carbon ion radiotherapy for liver cancer. *Proceedings of NIRS-ETOILE 2nd Joint Symposium on carbon ion radiotherapy, November 25–27, 2011*; 2011.

113. Kasuya G, Kato H, Yasuda S, et al. Progressive hypofractionated carbon-ion radiotherapy for hepatocellular carcinoma: combined analyses of 2 prospective trials. *Cancer* 2017;123(20):3955–3965.

114. Imada H, Kato H, Yasuda S, et al. Comparison of efficacy and toxicity of short-course carbon ion radiotherapy for hepatocellular carcinoma depending on their proximity to the porta hepatis. *Radiother Oncol* 2010;96:231–235.

115. Imada H, Kato H, Yasuda S, et al. Compensatory enlargement of the liver after treatment of hepatocellular carcinoma with carbon ion radiotherapy—relation to prognosis and liver function. *Radiother Oncol* 2010;96:236–242.

116. Combs SE, Habermehl D, Ganten T, et al. Phase I study evaluating the treatment of patients with hepatocellular carcinoma (HCC) with carbon ion radiotherapy: the PROMETHEUS-01 trial. *BMC Cancer* 2011;11:67.

117. Yamada S, Kamada T, Ebner DK, et al. Carbon-Ion Radiation Therapy for Pelvic Recurrence of Rectal Cancer. *Int J Radiat Oncol Biol Phys* 2016;96:93–101.

118. Isozaki Y, Yamada S, Kawashiro S. et al. Carbon-ion radiotherapy for isolated para-aortic lymph node recurrence from colorectal cancer. *J Surg Oncol* 2017;116(7):932–938.

119. Yamada S, Kamada T, Ebner DK, et al. Carbon ion radiation therapy for locally recurrent rectal cancer in patients with prior conventional pelvic irradiation. *Int J Radiat Oncol Biol Phys* 2016;96:S203.

120. Combs SE, Kieser M, Habermehl D, et al. Phase I/II trial evaluating carbon ion radiotherapy for the treatment of recurrent rectal cancer: the PANDORA-01 trial. *BMC Cancer* 2012;12:137.

121. Habermehl D, Wagner M, Ellerbrock M, et al. Reirradiation using carbon ions in patients with locally recurrent rectal cancer at HIT: first results. *Ann Surg Oncol* 2015;22:2068–2074.

122. Shinoto M, Yamada S, Yasuda S, et al. Phase 1 trial of preoperative, short-course carbon-ion radiotherapy for patients with resectable pancreatic cancer. *Cancer* 2013;119:45–51.

123. Shinoto M, Yamada S, Terashima K, et al. Carbon ion radiation therapy with concurrent gemcitabine for patients with locally advanced pancreatic cancer. *Int J Radiat Oncol Biol Phys* 2016;95:498–504.

124. Kawashiro S, Yamada S, Okamoto M, et al. Multi-institutional study of carbon ion radiation therapy for locally advanced pancreatic cancer: Japan Carbon Ion Radiation Oncology Study Group (J-CROS) Study 1403. *Int J Radiat Oncol Biol Phys* 2016; 96:S140–S141.

125. Tsuji H, Yanagi T, Ishikawa H, et al.; Working Group for Genitourinary Tumors. Hypofractionated radiotherapy with carbon ion beams for prostate cancer. *Int J Radiat Oncol Biol Phys* 2005;63:1153–1160.

126. Ishikawa H, Tsuji H, Kamada T, et al. Carbon-ion radiation therapy for prostate cancer. *Int J Urol* 2012;19:296–305.

127. Kasuya G, Ishikawa H, Tsuji H, et al. Significant impact of biochemical recurrence on overall mortality in patients with high-risk prostate cancer after carbon-ion radiotherapy combined with androgen deprivation therapy. *Cancer* 2016;122:3225–3231.

128. Nomiya T, Tsuji H, Kawamura H, et al. A multi-institutional analysis of prospective studies of carbon ion radiotherapy for prostate cancer: a report from the Japan Carbon Ion Radiation Oncology Study Group (J-CROS). *Radiother Oncol* 2016;121:288–293.

129. Habl G, Uhl M, Katayama S, et al. Acute toxicity and quality of life in patients with prostate cancer treated with protons or carbon ions in a prospective randomized phase II study—the IPI Trial. *Int J Radiat Oncol Biol Phys* 2016;95:435–443.

130. Nakano T, Suzuki M, Abe A, et al. The phase I/II clinical study of carbon ion therapy for cancer of the uterine cervix. *Cancer J Sci Am* 1999;5:362–369.

131. Kato S, Ohno T, Tsujii H, et al. Dose escalation study of carbon ion radiotherapy for locally advanced carcinoma of the uterine cervix. *Int J Radiat Oncol Biol Phys* 2006;65:388–397.

132. Wakatsuki M, Kato S, Ohno T, et al. Dose-escalation study of carbon ion radiotherapy for locally advanced squamous cell carcinoma of the uterine cervix (9902). *Gynecol Oncol* 2014;132:87–92.

133. Wakatsuki M, Kato S, Ohno T, et al. Clinical outcomes of carbon ion radiotherapy for locally advanced adenocarcinoma of the uterine cervix in phase 1/2 clinical trial (protocol 9704). *Cancer* 2014;120:1663–1669.

134. Karasawa K, Wakatsuki M, Kato S, et al. Clinical trial of carbon ion radiotherapy for gynecological melanoma. *J Radiat Res* 2014;55:343–350.

135. Tsuji H, Ishikawa H, Yanagi T, et al.; Working Group for Ophthalmologic Tumors. Carbon-ion radiotherapy for locally advanced or unfavorably located choroidal melanoma: a Phase I/II dose-escalation study. *Int J Radiat Oncol Biol Phys* 2007;67:857–862.

136. Toyama S, Tsuji H, Mizoguchi N, et al. Long-term results of carbon ion radiation therapy for locally advanced or unfavorably located choroidal melanoma: usefulness of CT-based 2-port orthogonal therapy for reducing the incidence of neovascular glaucoma. *Int J Radiat Oncol Biol Phys* 2012;86:270–276.

137. Zhang H, Li S, Wang XH, et al. Results of carbon ion radiotherapy for skin carcinomas in 45 patients. *Br J Dermatol* 2012;166:1100–1106.

138. Akutsu Y, Yasuda S, Nagata M, et al. A phase I/II clinical trial of preoperative short-course carbon-ion radiotherapy for patients with squamous cell carcinoma of the esophagus. *J Surg Oncol* 2012;105:750–755.

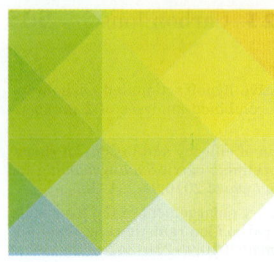

CHAPTER 24

Patient Positioning Methods: Immobilization, Stabilization, and Monitoring

Josh Evans, Bruce Libby, Laura Padilla, and Stanley H. Benedict

OVERVIEW OF EXTERNAL BEAM IMMOBILIZATION AND STABILIZATION

Rationale for Patient Immobilization and Stabilization

The success or failure of a radiotherapy treatment hinges on the accuracy with which the radiation is delivered. There are many sources of uncertainty in the radiation therapy delivery process that can result in a geometric miss of the intended target volume. A geometric miss of the intended target volume will not only decrease the probability of tumor control but also increase the volume of normal tissue that is irradiated, which can increase the probability of a treatment-related complication. Geometric uncertainties may be broadly classified as mechanical inaccuracies, localization inaccuracies, and positioning inaccuracies. Mechanical inaccuracies include the coincidence of the light and radiation fields, mechanical stability of the couch, laser alignment, and correspondence of the simulation and treatment isocenters. Localization error relates to the difficult nature of defining the location and extent of the target volume during both planning and treatment delivery. The most undesirable result of patient positioning uncertainties, the focus of this chapter, is movement of the target volume out of the treatment field.

The goal of daily patient setup is to reproduce the position at the time of simulation as best as possible; however, setup variations will inevitably occur, which is generally appreciated as a tangible problem and has earned considerable attention in the literature. In an early example, Dunscombe et al.[1] assessed components of positioning accuracy in head and neck patients and concluded that observed field placement errors were primarily attributable to patient motion. Patients may fidget from being uncomfortable or anxious during the treatment delivery. Furthermore, organs can move internally with respect to bony anatomy, skin marks, and other soft tissues because of normal and unavoidable physiologic processes such as breathing, swallowing, and peristalsis.

The focus of this chapter is to describe devices and methods for immobilization and stabilization of the radiotherapy patient, in which the goal is to reduce positioning uncertainties during each fraction (intrafraction error) and to increase the reproducibility of the patient setup for each fraction (interfraction error). In addition, immobilization devices can decrease the time needed for daily setup and target localization, thus increasing a clinic's throughput. Certain immobilization devices may also allow setup marks to be made directly on the device instead of the patient's skin, which can improve the patient's psychological well-being while under treatment, and some devices may even confer dosimetric advantages in treatment planning. The immobilization system should be lightweight for ease of setup and transport, yet strong and durable so that the device does not break during the patient's course of treatment. Furthermore, the device should be made of materials that minimally affect the megavoltage treatment beam and do not cause imaging artifacts that could impact three-dimensional (3D) visualization of the patient's anatomy for target identification or imaging used for patient alignment.

The devices and techniques for patient immobilization and stabilization described in this chapter have been shown to improve interfraction setup reproducibility as well as reduce intrafraction uncertainties. The overall accuracy of any immobilization system, however, is dependent on the skill and patience of the personnel forming the device at the time of simulation and setting the patient up on the treatment table for each fraction. Adequate training should be provided for each immobilization system employed in a given clinic, and adequate time should be scheduled for proper patient setup and immobilization. Furthermore, some patients will be more challenging to reproducibly align than others such as patients in pain and/or with mobility issues. A variety of devices and positions should be available for each treatment indication to help create a treatment position that maximizes both inter- and intrafraction reproducibility for each patient.

Surface imaging technologies for aiding in the initial setup and for real-time monitoring of the patient during treatment have begun to gain clinical adoption, and a new section has been added to this chapter to introduce these systems in the context of reducing patient positioning uncertainties. Finally, it must be noted that in some cases, even the most robust techniques for patient immobilization and monitoring do not guarantee accurate daily localization of the tumor volume and should not be a substitute for image guidance when indicated. Tumors are well known to change position relative to other soft tissue anatomy, the external surface, and bony anatomy. Thus, strategies for daily target localization, described elsewhere in this textbook, are also important and are intimately tied to patient immobilization.

Simple Immobilization Devices

Simple methods to reduce intrafraction positioning uncertainty because of patient motion have been in use for decades to ensure that the patient is comfortable. Figure 24.1 illustrates a variety of simple devices currently available that can be used to enhance the patient's comfort. For patients treated in a supine position, a wedge or roll underneath the knees (Fig. 24.1A) can help to reduce stress on the lower back. For arm-down positioning, a ring for the patient to grip (Fig. 24.1D) can increase comfort. For lung and liver treatments, it may be preferable to position the patient with the arms above the head. In these cases, the arms may be supported under the shoulder by foam wedges (Fig. 24.1B) to help the patient attain a restful position. For some head and neck patients, the patient's shoulders may block the inferior portion of lateral treatment fields. In this case, a simple strap (Fig. 24.1C) can be used to pull the shoulders down and out of the treatment fields. A headrest is almost always used with supine positioning to elevate the head and reduce strain on the neck. Standard sets of "Timo" and "Silverman" headrests (Fig. 24.1E) come in a variety of shapes, sizes, and materials. For those not adequately accommodated by the standard set of headrests, several manufacturers offer customizable head

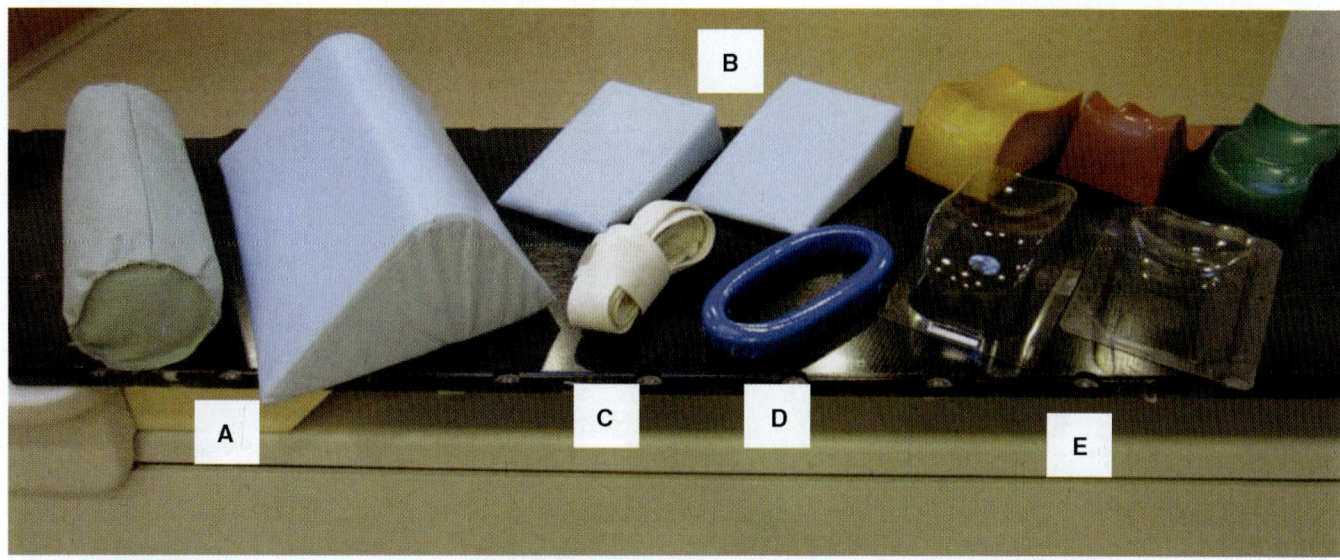

FIGURE 24.1. Simple devices to improve patient comfort. Simple devices are cost-effective and can reduce intrafraction positioning errors by increasing patient comfort. Shown here are (*A*) rolls and wedges that can be placed under the knees and (*B*) wedges to support the arms and shoulders. (*C*) A simple strap can be used to suppress the shoulders in head and neck patients and (*D*) grip rings can be used for the patient to hold on to. (*E*) Headrests are available in a wide range of shapes and sizes. (Image taken at UVA by the author—September 2011.)

cushions that can be molded to the patient's head contour. All of these devices are relatively inexpensive and are often reusable if they can be covered and/or cleaned between uses.

Immobilization Features of a Dedicated Radiation Oncology Computed Tomography Simulator

Simple devices incorporated during initial simulation can improve patient comfort and reduce intrafraction motion because of patient movement. However, they may not address day-to-day variations of overall patient setup and positioning accuracy. A major objective of a robust immobilization system is to reproduce the patient's anatomical geometry at the time of simulation for all subsequent treatment fractions. An example of a robust immobilization system to treat a patient with breast cancer is shown in Figure 24.2 to illustrate some of the desired features of a dedicated radiation oncology computed tomography (CT) simulator. With this immobilization system, the patient lies supine with an ergonomic wedge (Fig. 24.2E) under the knees. The arms are positioned above the head and out of the tangential treatment fields. A custom-formed, reusable vacuum-lock bag (Fig. 24.2C), described in more detail in the following body conformal section, helps to support the patient's arms, and a T-bar (Fig. 24.2B) may be used for the patient to grip. The angled baseboard (Fig. 24.2C) on which the vacuum-lock bag rests utilizes gravity to help the breasts fall into a more reproducible position and can be adjusted to minimize skin folds. Many of these devices provide indexing systems for the therapists to record the geometry used for each patient at the time of simulation. This example of a breast setup, where one or both arms may be positioned above the head, highlights the advantage of a wide bore (e.g., >85-cm diameter) CT scanner (Fig. 24.2B) for radiation oncology treatment simulation, as opposed to the more common 70-cm bore diameter, which may limit the options for positioning certain patients.

Flat couches are favored for radiation oncology treatments to accommodate a wide range of patient sizes, setup positions, and immobilization devices. Diagnostic CT scanners feature a curved couch for patient comfort; the geometry

of a patient simulated on a curved diagnostic couch top will be challenging to reproduce on a flat treatment couch. Flat couch top inserts are offered by numerous vendors to reproduce the couch geometry of the treatment unit. An important feature of a couch top insert is the indexing system (Fig. 24.2D), which allows an assortment of immobilization devices to be rigidly affixed in concert to both the simulator and treatment tables with high accuracy. The indexing system improves the interfraction reproducibility of the patient setup and can also decrease the amount of time to set up a patient.

External marks placed on either the patient's skin or the immobilization devices are used for initial laser alignment on the treatment machine as a surrogate for the internal target anatomy. An in-room laser system in the CT simulator suite (Fig. 24.2A) is a necessary feature to provide external reference points that correlate to the internal reference point location. After the simulation CT scan is acquired, the isocenter(s) is(are) defined and the coordinates are transferred to the in-room laser system. The laser system and CT table are then moved to the defined setup point and external setup marks can be made, thus correlating the position of an internal setup point to the external markings.

HEAD AND NECK IMMOBILIZATION DEVICES

Thermoplastic Masks

Adequate immobilization is particularly critical in the treatment of head and neck (H&N) cancers as the target is frequently located in close proximity to critical structures. Thermoplastic masks have replaced traditional plaster-casting methods in most clinics. Thermoplastic masks are heated to approximately 70°C in a water bath or a dry heat oven. At this temperature, the thermoplastic material becomes malleable and can be stretched and shaped to conform to the patient's face, head, and neck. The patient's head and neck is supported by a simple preformed cushion, like those previously described and illustrated in Figure 24.1, or a custom-formed cushion may be made. The mask is connected to a base plate, which is attached to the couch via

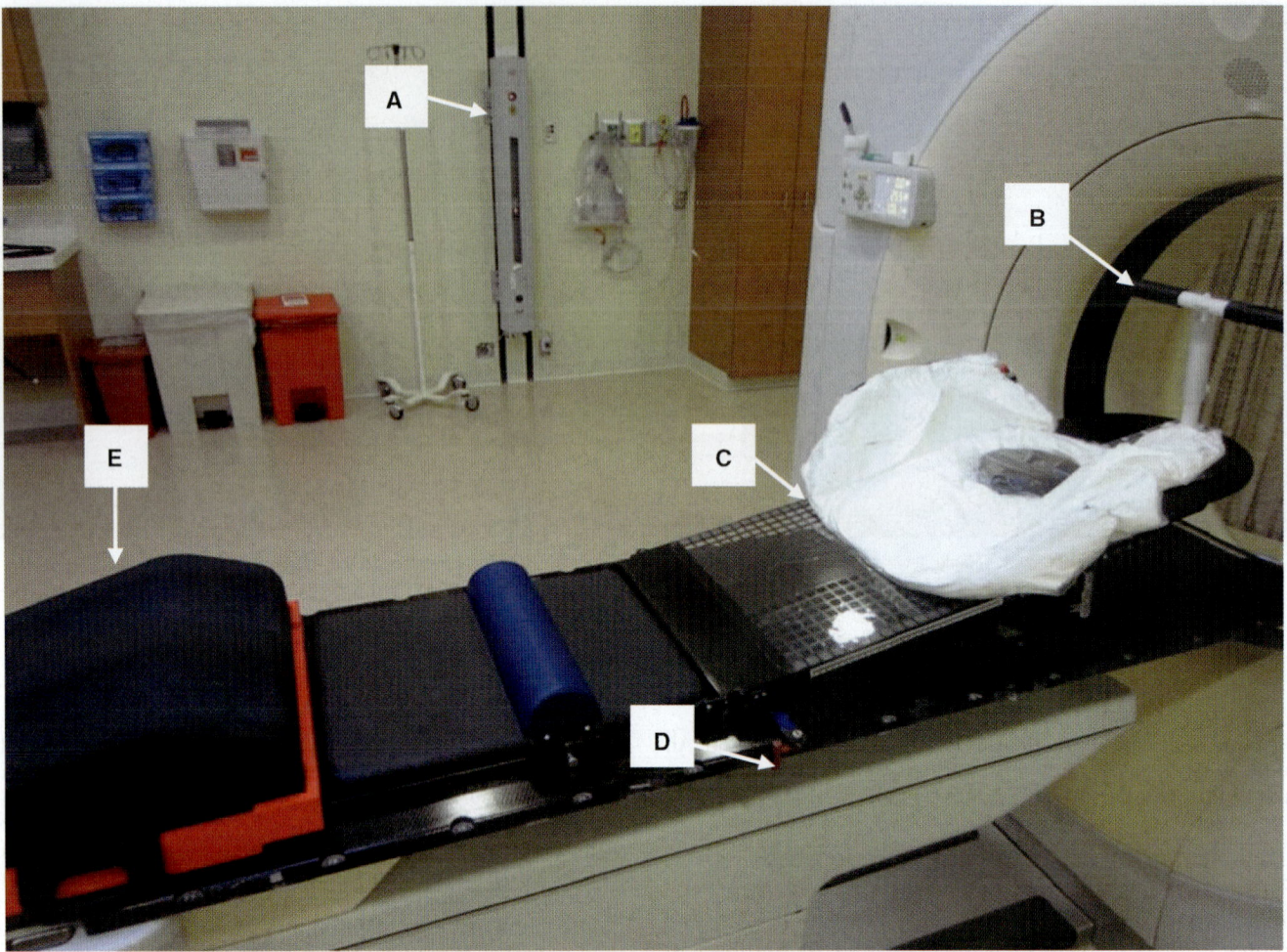

FIGURE 24.2. Dedicated radiation oncology CT simulator. Displayed here is an immobilization system for a breast cancer patient in the simulator suite at the University of Virginia. Some key features of a dedicated radiation oncology CT simulator are (A) an in-room laser system to mark the reference point position, (B) a wide patient bore (85 cm diameter) to allow more flexibility in patient positioning, and (D) an indexed flat couch-top overlay to reproduce the geometry of the treatment table. (C) An angled breast board can improve patient comfort and provide optimal positioning of the breast for radiotherapy. (D) An indexing bar is used to attach the breast board to the flat couch-top overlay. A vacuum-lock mattress and a T-bar (B) support the patient's arms above the head. An ergonomic knee support (E) can reduce stress on the lower back. (Image taken at UVA by the author—September 2011.)

the indexing system. Setup marks can be made directly onto the thermoplastic mask, eliminating the need for unsightly marks to be placed on the patient's face for the duration of the treatment.

Early work with thermoplastic mask immobilization for H&N cancer by Bentel showcased the efficacy of the thermoplastic mask in comparison to the traditional plaster three-strip immobilization technique.[2] In terms of the rate of physician-requested shifts from port films, the thermoplastic mask had a frequency of 6.2% compared to 16.1% for the plaster-casting method. However, this advantage was only observed when the mask was rigidly affixed to the couch, highlighting the importance of the couch indexing system.[2] Since then, numerous studies quantifying the accuracy of patient setup for H&N cancer have appeared in the literature. The bulk of these studies utilized two-dimensional (2D) portal imaging to quantify setup displacements, though studies utilizing 3D cone-beam CT data have become more common as this technology has recently gained widespread clinical adoption. Generally, systematic and random errors have been reported to have standard deviations ranging from 1 to 4 mm.[3-5] Based on a review of studies assessing setup errors using portal imaging, Hurkmans et al. suggest that random and systematic errors of 2 mm or less should be a practically achievable goal for H&N patients given current immobilization technology and methods.[4]

Figure 24.3 illustrates the flexibility of patient positioning options with thermoplastic masks. Masks can encompass the head only or can extend inferiorly to cover the shoulders (Fig. 24.3A). Gilbeau et al.[3] compared the setup accuracy of the short and long thermoplastic masks in the treatment of head and neck cancer. Portal images were acquired for isocenters placed at the level of the head, neck, and shoulders. Their results show similar setup accuracy with the long and short mask for the isocenters in the head and neck. For isocenter placement at the shoulder level, the use of the long mask resulted in a random setup error of around 1.0 mm, which was significantly less ($P = .01$) than the 2.3 mm error of the short mask.[3] Thus, a long mask to immobilize the shoulders is recommended for patients receiving supraclavicular treatment in which the isocenter will be placed at the level of the shoulders.

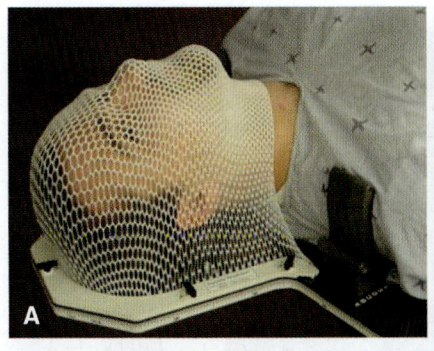
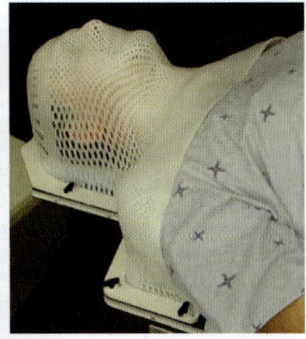
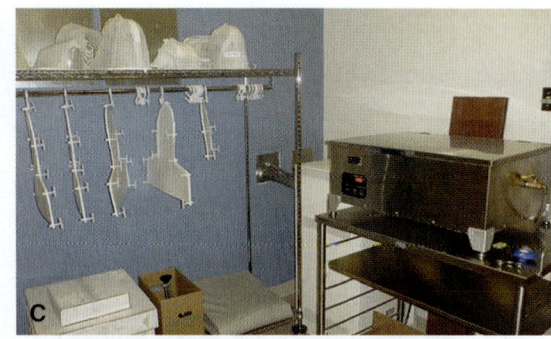

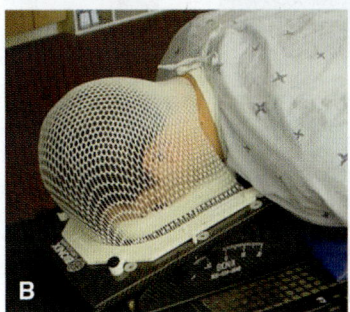
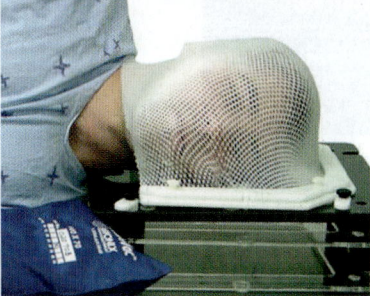

FIGURE 24.3. Thermoplastic masks for H&N patients. For treatment of targets in the head and neck, thermoplastic masks are routinely used for custom immobilization. **A:** Thermoplastic sheets are commercially available in short versions that cover only the head, as well as longer versions that extend over the patient's shoulders. **B:** They can also be used to treat patients in the prone and lateral positions. **C:** Additional space is needed to accommodate the water bath used to warm the thermoplastic sheets. (Images **A** and **B** courtesy of BionixRT. Image **C** taken at UVA by the author.)

Thermoplastic mask systems are available with a myriad of features including multilayer masks to increase rigidity and masks with cutouts for the patient's eyes to reduce anxiety and accommodate optically guided setup. They can also accommodate prone or lateral setups when these positions may be indicated (Fig. 24.3B). Some commercially available base plates can be angled to allow for the patient to be set up with the neck in an extended or flexed position, which may be used to avoid critical structures such as the eyes. Neck extension can be used with prone positioning for craniospinal irradiation. For prone setup, a donut-shaped cushion supports the patient's face in the base plate and the thermoplastic mask is formed around the posterior aspect of the head to hold the patient's face in the donut. A potential disadvantage of treatment with a flexed or extended neck position is the need for registration with different imaging modalities (e.g., PET-CT or MR-CT) in which the PET or MR were not performed in the patient treatment position.

Every clinic must consider space limitations when selecting particular immobilization and stabilization systems. Thermoplastic H&N systems necessitate more equipment and thus more space in the simulation suite. The water bath or dry heat oven used to heat the thermoplastic sheets for the long H&N masks can be large (Fig. 24.3C). For clinics with insufficient space to house a large heating device, smaller devices are commercially available that will fit the short head-only masks. Furthermore, some commercially available base plates (e.g., VersaBoard; Bionix Radiation Therapy, Toledo, OH) incorporate shoulder suppression systems, which consist of rigid plastic panels to push down on the shoulders. When a long thermoplastic mask is not indicated or not available, a base plate with shoulder suppression panels can help to keep the shoulders out of the beam path for lateral head and neck beams (Fig. 24.3A). In lieu of long thermoplastic masks or base plates with shoulder suppression panels, the patient can pull on a simple shoulder strap (Fig. 24.1C) to move the shoulders inferior and avoid unnecessary irradiation of the shoulders when opposed lateral beams are used to treat the neck.

Thermoplastic masks have been observed to shrink as they cool in the 24-hour period after formation, and this has been shown to lead to systematic setup errors if not taken into consideration.[6] Furthermore, a mask that has shrunk after the simulation process may be uncomfortable for the patient and may require a full resimulation. BionixRT has attempted to address this problem with the Klarity Green line of thermoplastic material, which is designed to have reduced shrinkage coupled with increased rigidity. As with any immobilization system, the thermoplastic manufacturer's recommendations should be carefully followed, and adequate time should be allowed during simulation for the mask to harden properly while on the patient to minimize the effect of shrinkage.

Bite Blocks as an Alternative to Masks

Thermoplastic masks are widely used for H&N treatment indications; however, they are not well tolerated by all patients, particularly patients with claustrophobia. For these patients, bite block systems that do not incorporate a mask may be an acceptable alternative. Elekta offers a bite block system, the HeadFIX, which is illustrated in Figure 24.4. A custom dental mold is formed to the patient's maxillary teeth, and a vacuum system creates suction of the mold to the hard palate. A custom cushion is placed under the patient's head, neck, and shoulders. The mouthpiece is attached to a carbon fiber frame, which is fixed to the treatment table's indexing system. The head is thus rigidly immobilized via the connection of the mouthpiece to the head frame. The carbon fiber design of the HeadFIX product allows for the use of in-room kV image guidance systems for target localization. The mold can be quickly released from the frame if the patient feels claustrophobic. Setup accuracy has been shown to be similar to thermoplastic masks, on the order of 1 to 3 mm.[7] These stand-alone bite block systems, however, require a high level of patient compliance and may not be suitable for patients with poor dentition or with edentulism. Bite blocks formed with a patient's false teeth are highly discouraged and may

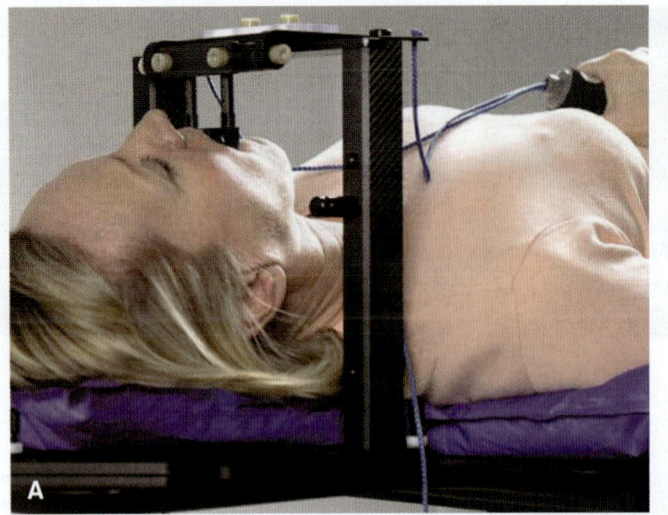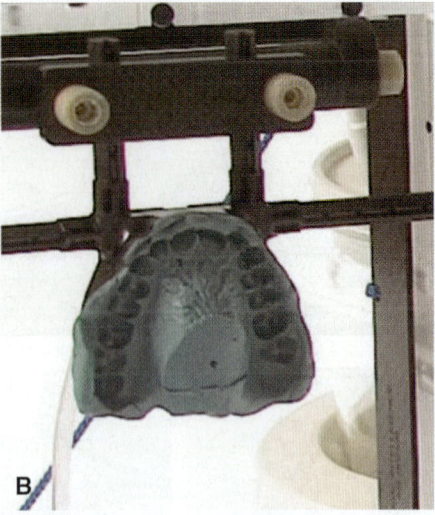

FIGURE 24.4. Bite block system. **A:** The Elekta HeadFIX® (Stockholm, Sweden) is an example of a bite block system that can provide an alternative method for immobilizing head and neck patients who are not able to tolerate a thermoplastic mask because of anxiety or claustrophobia. A custom dental mold **(B)** is formed for each patient and is suctioned to the patient's hard palate. The dental mold is attached to a carbon fiber frame featuring a quick-release handle. (Images courtesy of Elekta, Stockholm, Sweden.)

result in inaccurate setups or breakage of the patient's dentures. Custom-formed dental molds can also be incorporated in the conventional thermoplastic mask systems described above to provide an additional point of support for the patient. A custom bite block may also be formed with primary goals other than immobilization, for example, to separate the tongue from the roof of the mouth. This can be useful in treatment of sinus/nasal cavity tumors to decrease dose to the tongue and vice versa. Table 24.1 includes a top level summary of the pros and cons of available intracranial immobilization devices.

BODY CONFORMAL IMMOBILIZATION DEVICES

Numerous commercial body conformal immobilization devices are available for a variety of treatment indications. One type of body conformal system uses a two-part foaming agent to form a permanent mold of the patient's body. One such system, the Alpha Cradle, is illustrated in Figure 24.5A. Forms are available for treatment of patients with a variety of disease sites, including the head and neck, breast, thorax, abdomen, pelvis, and extremities. At the time of simulation, the appropriate body form is chosen and placed in a polyvinyl bag where the two-part chemical foaming agents are mixed together, initiating the chemical reaction that causes the foam to expand. The mixed foaming agent is distributed evenly throughout the body form and sealed inside the polyvinyl bag, and the patient is positioned inside the form as the foaming agent expands and conforms to the patient's body contour. The foam continues to expand for approximately 10 to 15 minutes during which the therapists will need to vigilantly guide the foam around the patient to prevent the foam from escaping the bag and moving into locations of least resistance that may contribute little to immobilizing the patient. As with any immobilization device, adequate training is needed to form a high-quality customized patient mold and the manufacturer's instructions should be carefully followed. Chemical foaming agent systems generally require two therapists to form at the

time of simulation, and the process can require approximately 30 minutes. Obviously, great care is needed to prevent any of the chemicals from having direct contact on the skin as this may cause irritation.

Another class of body conformal systems, commonly referred to as "vacuum-lock bags," is comprised of a bag filled with plastic mini-spheres. These bags are available in a variety of sizes to accommodate different treatment sites and patient positioning techniques. At the time of simulation, the bag is first conformed to the patient's body contour by pushing the mini-spheres to fill in around the patient. A vacuum pump is then connected to the bag and the air is evacuated from the bag, causing the plastic mini-spheres to lock together to rigidly retain the device's shape. During the evacuation, the therapists will maneuver the mini-spheres within the immobilization device to provide optimal fit and stabilization of the patient's body contour. These vacuum-lock bags are made of a durable nylon material to resist tears or punctures and can be expected to retain their shape for 6 weeks or more. They are reusable and may require less time to generate a customized mold than the expanding foam systems. Another advantage of the vacuum-lock bag is that if during the simulation process the device is found not to provide the intended level of immobilization or is found to be uncomfortable for the patient, it can be reinflated and remolded to achieve the desired shape as many times as necessary. The vacuum-lock systems, however, do require a time commitment to clean and remove any setup marks prior to use with subsequent patients. Also, if a tear or puncture occurs during the course of treatment, a new vacuum-lock bag would need to be formed and the simulation and treatment planning process may need to be repeated to deliver the remaining fractions. Each clinic should consider the benefits and drawbacks of each system and it is not uncommon to see both types of body conformal systems used within one institution.

As body conformal devices are used to treat a wide range of sites throughout the entire body, careful thought should be given to each specific case to ensure that the treatment site is properly immobilized, that the setup is reproducible

TABLE 24.1 INTRACRANIAL IMMOBILIZATION DEVICE SUMMARY

Device Name	Description	Pros	Cons	Typical Sites	Reusable?	Indexed?	Relative Cost
Timo and Silverman head rests	Foam and plastic head rests with various sizes for a range of body habitus	Inexpensive and reusable.	Not custom formed.	H&N, craniospinal, thoracic, abdominal, pretty much all supine patients	Yes	Some clip to baseplate, which is indexed to the couch, others do not clip to couch.	$
Custom-formed head rests	Vacuum-lock or water activated custom formed head rests	Custom- formed to patient. Some are re-usable	Added time to simulation process. Some are not reusable	H&N, craniospinal, thoracic, abdominal	Some Yes Some No	Can be molded around baseplate for reliable placement	$$
Thermoplastic masks	Thermoplastic mask material is warmed in a water bath until pliable and then is stretched over the patient's face to create a customized device.	Accurate, custom formed immobilization. Can cut-out treatment portals to reduce blousing.	Potential for mask shrinkage. Patient anxiety or claustrophobia. Bolusing effect.	H&N, craniospinal	No	Yes. Clip to baseplate	$$
Elekta HeadFIX	Bite block for image guided Tx. Advantageous for claustrophobic patients.	Non-invasive, relocatable. Does not require thermoplastic mask material to be tightly molded to patient's face.	Requires operator skill to create custom maxillary dentition molds. May not be best option for patients with poor dentition.	H&N	Frame = Yes; bite block = No	Yes—stereotactic	$$$
Elekta eXtend	Relocatable bite block system designed for fractionated stereotactic radiotherapy.	Non-invasive, relocatable. Does not require thermoplastic mask material to be tightly molded to patient's face. Allows for fractionated SRS. High degree of patient setup accuracy.	Requires operator skill to create custom maxillary dentition molds. May not be best option for patients with poor denitition.	Intracranial and some extracranial SRS targets in neck	Frame = Yes; bite block = No	No	$$$
Invasive, nonrelocatable stereotactic intracranial immobilization devices. E.g.: Leksell Stereotactic Coordinate Frame G, Radionics BRW Frame system	Frame is attached to the patient's skull with four screws. Used for single fraction radiosurgery.	Excellent accuracy in patient repositioning.	Typically requires sedation. Risk of infection and bleeding. Patient discomfort.	Intracranial	Frame = Yes; skull screws = No	Rigidly attached directly to treatment machine (Gamme knife), table or floor mounted stand.	$$$
Non-invasive, relocatable intracranial mask based immobilization (e.g.: Brainlab non-invasive mask system)	3 thermoplastic shells custom molded to patient's head and face, which are attached to U shaped frame via two posts on either side of the patient's head.	Does not require placement of screws into the patient's skull. Allow for fractionated SRS. High degree of patient set up accuracy.	Thermoplastic mask may be undesirable in certain patients, such as those with claustrophobia or anxiety.	Intracranial	Yes = frame and posts. No = thermoplastic mask	Attach to treatment table.	$$$
Non-invasive, relocatable intracranial mask-less immobilization (e.g., Gill-Thomas-Cosman Relocatable head ring, Stereoadapter 5000)	Variety of frame based, non-invasive techniques for reproducible immobilization of the head. May be used for single fraction and fractionated SRS.	Do not require placement of screws in to the patient's skull. Allow for fractionated SRS. No thermoplastic mask required. High degree of set up accuracy.	May require bite block in some systems. Some systems require additional time for setup verification (e.g.: Depth Helmet).	Intracranial	Yes = frame. No = custom headrests, bite blocks.	Attach to treatment table or floor mounted stand.	$$$

from day to day, and that the patient is able to maintain the position for the duration of each fraction. An immobilization device that extends well beyond the treatment site to encompass adjacent anatomy can be more effective than a more local device that focuses only on the treatment region. For example, Bentel[8] has shown that for Hodgkin lymphoma, a cradle that extends below the pelvis is more effective than a cradle that only includes the upper torso. Devices that extend around the patient also give the ability to make setup marks directly on the immobilization device for alignment. Aligning the beam to setup marks on the immobilization device can increase the daily setup reproducibility by reducing the reliance on skin marks, which can be especially troublesome for larger or older patients where the skin can be more mobile over the underlying anatomy. Marks can then be made on the patient to help align the patient within the immobilization device. Longer devices also allow for longer setup marks to be made in the superior–inferior direction, which can help detect rotational setup errors.

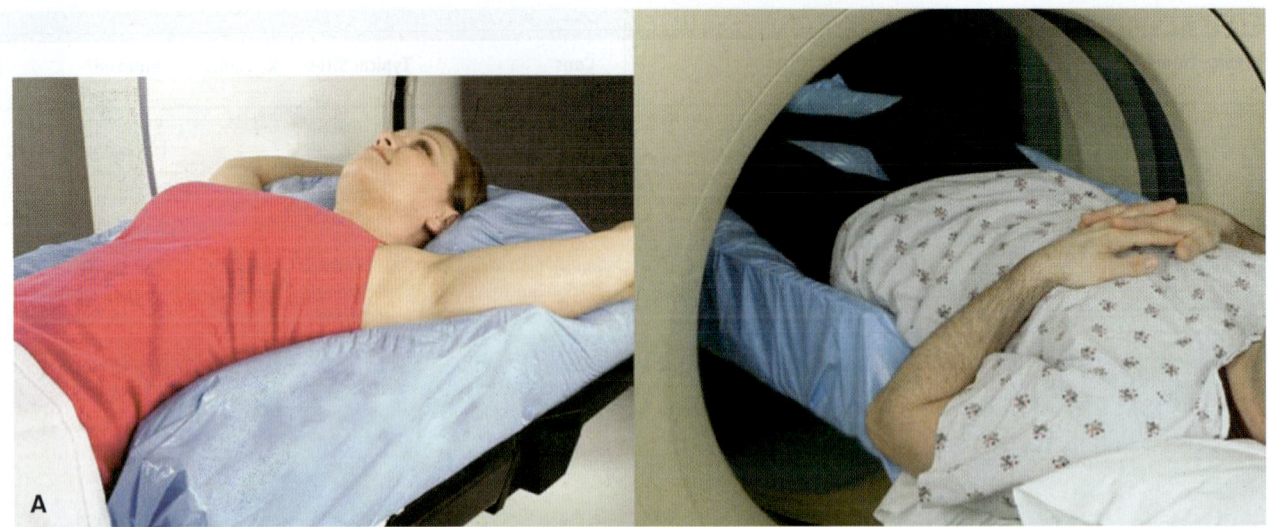

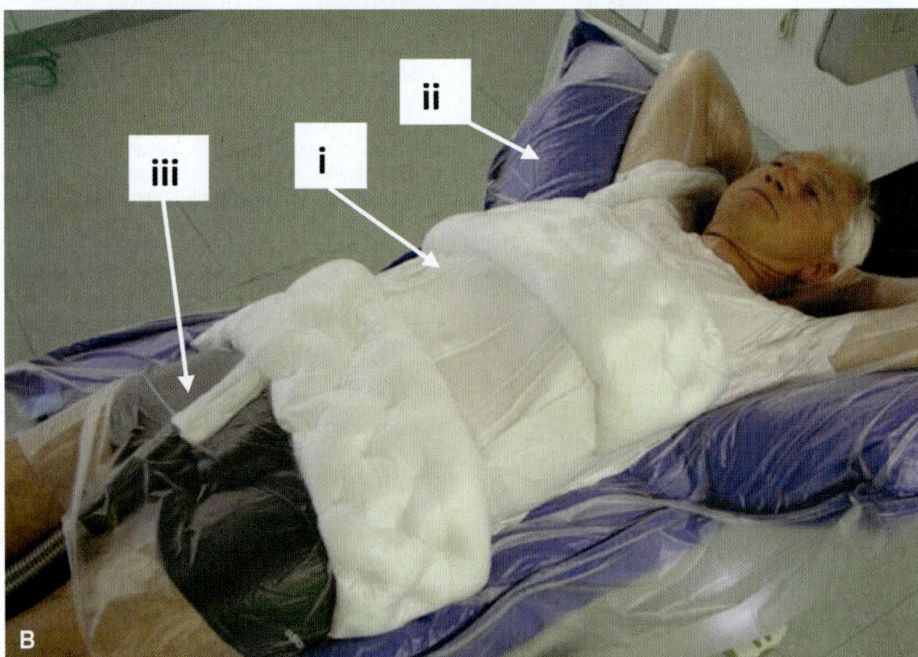

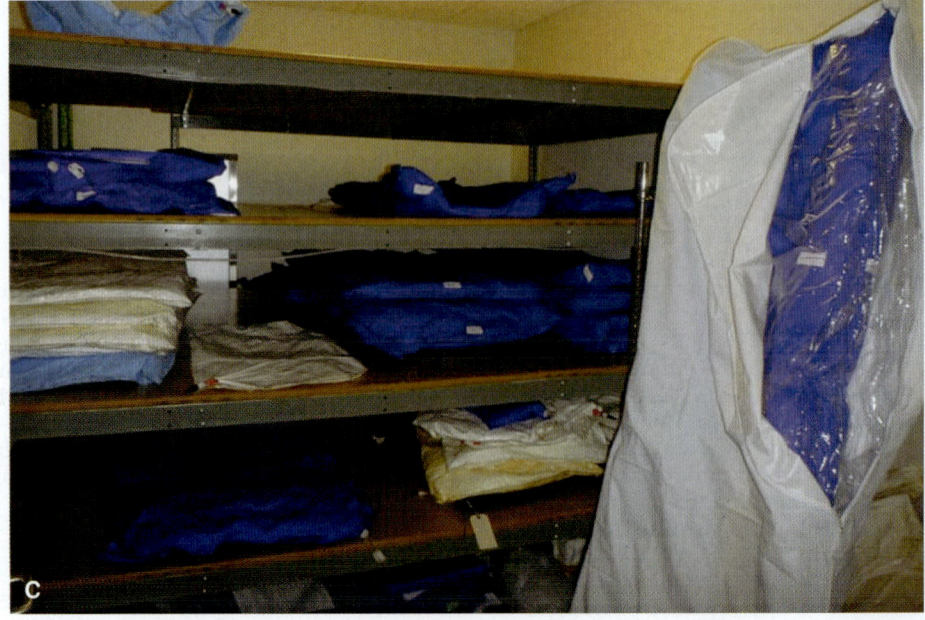

FIGURE 24.5. Body conformal systems. Body conformal systems are used for treatment indications throughout the body. **A:** Shown here are two patients in treatment position with the Alpha Cradle, which uses a two-part foaming agent to create customized conformal body immobilization. (Images courtesy of Smithers Medical Products, Inc. Alpha Cradle is a registered trademark of Smithers Medical Products, Inc., South Canton, OH.) **B:** In the Elekta BodyFIX® system, a cover sheet (*i*) is placed over the patient after being positioning inside the vacuum-lock bag (*ii*) that was formed at the time of simulation. A separate vacuum system (*iii*) evacuates the air between the cover sheet and the patient. The pressure from the cover sheet can help reduce patient motion and improve setup reproducibility. (Image courtesy of Elekta, Stockholm, Sweden.) **C:** Shown here is a room used for storing vacuum-lock bags in the simulation suite at the University of Virginia. The simulation suite services multiple treatment machines at satellite locations. After simulation, the immobilization devices are transported to the satellite treatment sites (pictured on the *right*) via a courier service. (Image taken at UVA by the author, October 2011.)

The Elekta BodyFIX is a unique immobilization system that utilizes a dual vacuum system as illustrated in Figure 24.5B. For simulation, the patient is first placed in a vacuum-lock bag system. A thin plastic cover sheet is then placed over the patient, which is attached to the vacuum-lock bag via special adhesive strips. A vacuum pump is then used to evacuate the air under the cover sheet creating a continuous pressure of up to 600 mbar. The additional pressure created by the cover-sheet vacuum system helps the patient settle into the vacuum-lock bag, which is molded to the patient and then evacuated with a second vacuum system to create the body conformal device. For all subsequent treatment fractions, the pressure from the cover-sheet vacuum system helps the patient settle reproducibly in the vacuum-lock bag. The BodyFIX's vacuum sheet can also provide a degree of abdominal compression, which may help decrease the respiratory excursion of certain tumors. Internal target motion management is discussed further in the stereotactic immobilization section. Patients tolerate the BodyFIX dual vacuum system very well, with infrequent complaints of claustrophobia or discomfort. If the patient feels that the pressure from the cover sheet is uncomfortable, the vacuum pressure for the cover sheet can be turned down or the vacuum-lock bag can be used by itself.

As an early example of body conformal immobilization's efficacy, Bentel and colleagues at Duke University showed that immobilization with the Alpha Cradle expanding foam system reduced the frequency of physician-requested setup corrections based on portal images for a variety of treatment indications, including Hodgkin lymphoma and prostate, lung, and breast cancer.[8,9] It should be noted, however, that not all studies show a clear-cut advantage in setup accuracy with body conformal immobilization devices. For example, an early study by Song et al.[10] showed no statistical advantage of using

immobilization in the treatment of prostate cancer in terms of the number of deviations > 5 mm as quantified on portal images. They did show that obese patients tend to have larger setup errors[10] highlighting the fact that certain subpopulations of patients may be more difficult to set up than others.

Hurkmans' assessment of setup accuracy based on portal imaging provides a good review of the available data up to 2001.[4] This work concludes that with current patient setup, portal imaging, and immobilization techniques, systematic and random setup errors on the order of 2.5 to 3.5 mm should be achievable for treatments of the thorax, abdomen, and pelvis. The integration of cone-beam CT units with treatment machines is an excellent tool for assessing setup accuracy and is being used in an increasing number of studies comparing and evaluating various immobilization systems. CBCT has been especially helpful to study the setup accuracy of stereotactic immobilization devices, the subject of a later section in this chapter. It should again be emphasized that the degree of interfraction setup accuracy achievable by a particular institution will depend on the skill and knowledge of the personnel involved in forming patient immobilization devices, setting up patients for daily treatments, making adjustments based on verification imaging, and the understanding of the limitations of each step of the process. Table 24.2 provides a top level summary of the pros and cons of commonly available body conformal immobilization systems.

Prone Positioning for Pelvic and Breast Treatments

The body conformal devices described above can help provide reproducible patient setup from day to day for a wide range of disease sites. The patient is most often positioned supine in these devices. For certain treatment indications, a prone setup

TABLE 24.2 EXTRACRANIAL IMMOBILIZATION DEVICE SUMMARY							
Device Name	**Description**	**Pros**	**Cons**	**Typical Sites**	**Reusable ?**	**Indexed?**	**Relative Cost**
Alpha Cradle	Expanding foam device custom-molded to patient body contour.	Rigid immobilization for wide range of body sites.	One time use. One-shot to achieve adequate and comfortable immobilization.	Thorax, abdomen, pelvis, extremities	No	No	$$
Vacuum-lock bags	Nylon bag filled with plastic minispheres. Upon evacuation mini-spheres lock together to form a custom mold of the patient body contour	Re-usable. Can quickly re-inflate and re-form during simulation if necessary.	Punctures, tears or loss of vacuum may necessitate re-simulation of the patient.	Thorax, abdomen, pelvis, extremities	Yes	Potentially. An indexing bar can be used to make indentations in the bottom of the bag for later setup with the indexing bar.	$$
Elekta BodyFix	Vacuum-lock bag with plastic cover sheet. Dual vacuum system for increased immobilization	Re-usable. Cover sheet may provide abdominal compression.	Some patients may find cover sheet uncomfortable.	Thorax, abdomen, pelvis	Vacuum-lock bag = yes; cover sheet = no	Potentially. An indexing bar can be used to make indentations in the bottom of the bag for later setup with the indexing bar.	$$$
Prone breast board	Prone breast board can improve dosimetry for patients with large, pendulous breasts.	Separates target tissue from chest wall to minimize skin folds and lung dose.	May not be tolerated by all patients. Poor visualization of treatment field alignment. Not suitable for regional nodal irradiation.	Breast	Yes	Yes	$$
Prone belly board	Prone board to help the small bowel fall out of the treatment fields.	Displacement of bowel out of treatment field can reduce toxicity.	May not be tolerated by all patients. Variability in bowel sparing.	Pelvis	Yes	Yes	$$
Modular stereotactic body immobilization systems. E.g.: Elekta Stereotactic Body Frame, Civco Body-Pro Lok, Bionix Omni V	Indexed base board with a wide range of attachments for immobilization, localization and motion management	Flexibility to treat variety of disease sites with SBRT. Attachment of devices for abdominal compression	More room for storage. More time for setup and indexing of attachments.	Spine, lung, liver, abdomen, pelvis, neck	Yes	Yes	$$$

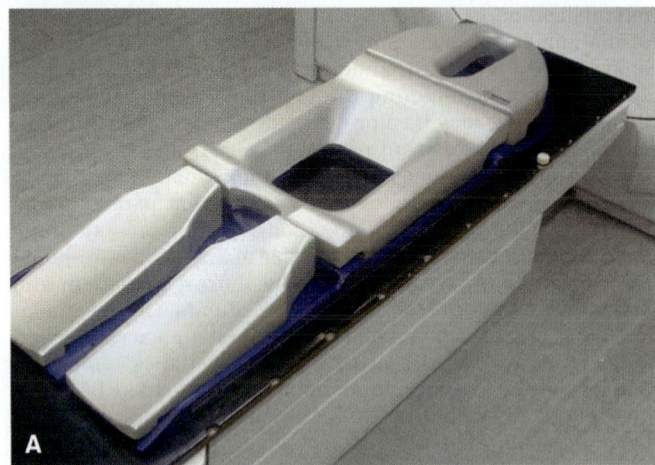

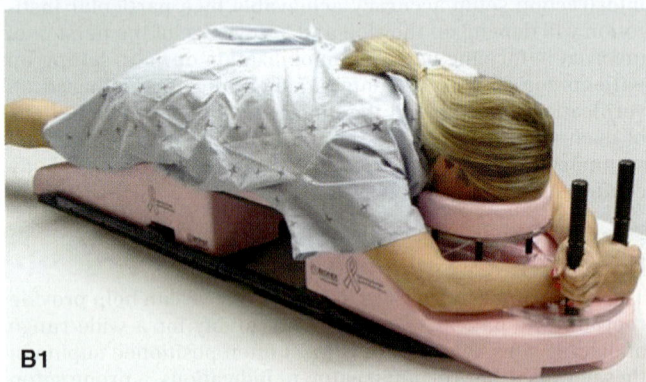

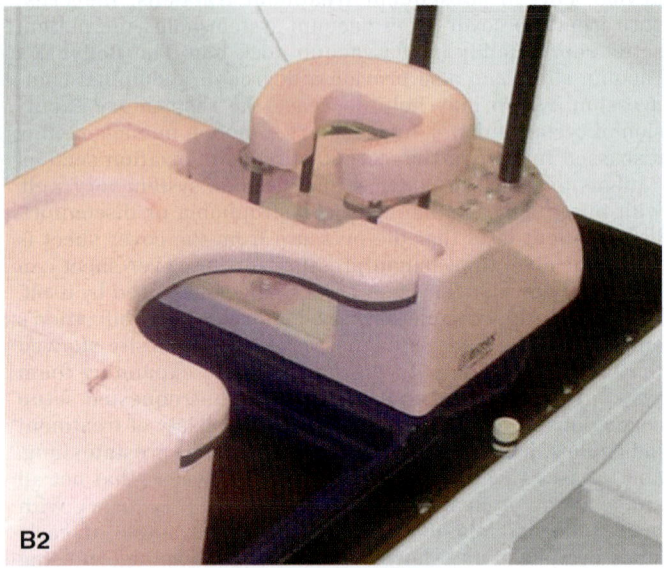

FIGURE 24.6. Specialized prone immobilization devices. Immobilization devices specifically designed for prone position-ing. **A:** A prone bellyboard can be used in treating targets in the pelvis. Gravity assists small-bowel migration out of the treat-ment fields, which can reduce treatment-related toxicity. **B:** A prone breast board offered by BionixRT can be advantageous for patients with large, pendulous breasts. The board features a cutout that is easily reversible for treatment of either breast. (Images courtesy of BionixRT, Toledo, OH.)

may provide a dosimetric advantage. In pelvic and abdominal irradiation, the small bowel is an important organ at risk, and acute toxicity is correlated with the amount of small bowel that receives a high dose. For patients receiving pelvic irra-diation, a popular method is to use a bellyboard (Fig. 24.6A) on which the patient lies prone with their stomach positioned over the cutout region. With the aid of gravity, the small bowel will fall into the board's cutout and can reduce the amount of bowel in the treatment fields. The use of a prone bellyboard has been demonstrated to reduce the volume of small bowel at all dose levels.[11–13] Even with IMRT, the use of a belly-board technique has been shown to further reduce the small-bowel dose.[11]

The magnitude of the small-bowel reduction with prone bellyboard positioning can be highly patient dependent. Kim et al.[11] correlated the amount of small bowel at the 50% isodose level with a patient's age, weight, and gender. For example, this work showed a larger amount of small bowel (total volume in cc) at the 50% isodose level for the subgroups of patients over 56 years old, female patients, and patients weighing <65 kg (143 pounds). It must also be noted that some investigators have reported that the use of a bellyboard worsened the reproducibility of patient setup. For example, Martin et al. reported having to reposition the patient based on portal imaging 68% of the time with a prone belly-board system, compared to 23% of the time with supine positioning.[12] In contrast, Acht et al.[13] reports similar setup reproducibility between prone positioning with a bellyboard and patients in the supine position. Each patient should be assessed at the time of simulation for the efficacy of the bellyboard method to

displace small bowel as intended, as well as the patient's abil-ity to tolerate lying on the bellyboard itself.

Another site where prone positioning has been used is in the treatment of breast cancer. Figure 24.6B illustrates a patient positioned on a prone breast board offered by BionixRT. The patient is positioned on the cushioned plat-form with her face resting in a donut-shaped cushion. The patient can hold the hand posts to help improve reproducibil-ity and comfort. The prone positioning is most efficacious for patients with large, pendulous breasts, though it may also be an effective option for patients with severe arthritis that may be unable to hold their arms over their head.[14] Patients with large breasts tend to have larger tissue separation, larger treatment volumes, worse surface irregularity, and an accen-tuated inframammary fold, which can cause these patients to have higher reported rates of toxicities such as high-grade dermatitis and fibrosis.[15]

The goal of prone positioning for breast treatment is to minimize the lateral tissue separation and thus improve dose homogeneity. Improved dose homogeneity may decrease the rate of late toxicities such as fibrosis, an undesirable cos-metic outcome, and decreased tissue separation can reduce the entrance dose needed to provide target coverage at depth, which may decrease the overall hot spot for the treat-ment plan, particularly at the skin surface.[14] Improved dose homogeneity and decreased skin dose from prone position-ing may also prove to be advantageous for hypofractionated breast regimens where larger doses per fraction are deliv-ered. Five-year follow-up data from Stegman et al.[14] have shown that the prone position offers comparable local control to traditional supine positioning for whole-breast irradiation, with lower levels of toxicity. With the breast hanging in the prone setup, it may also be possible to reduce the dose to other nearby normal tissues. The increased separation of the breast tissue from the chest wall has been shown to decrease the amount of irradiated lung in whole-breast irradiation.[16] Dose to the heart is more variable; for left-breast patients, most heart doses (20 to 30 Gy levels) are decreased in the prone position, though some patients did exhibit higher heart doses when prone.[16]

It can be difficult to set up patients with large or pendulous breasts in a supine position because the breast can lie in a different position each day. In the supine position, a ring or tube can be used to keep the pendulous breast from folding over. With the aid of gravity, daily setup can be more reproducible with the breast hanging in the prone position. There are, however, potential disadvantages to the prone setup for breast patients, for example, reduced visibility of the breast for alignment purposes. Furthermore, the prone positioning may not be tolerable for elderly or obese patients. And finally, the prone position may not be logistically suitable for patients requiring regional nodal irradiation as the prone position would severely limit visual alignment of an anterior supraclavicular field.

Space Considerations

Whole body expanding foam or vacuum-lock bag systems can provide excellent patient comfort and immobilization, but they are large devices making the issue of space very relevant. Adequate space is required to store each patient's custom-formed device for up to 6 weeks or more while a patient is under treatment. At the Emily Couric Clinical Cancer Center at the University of Virginia, a dedicated room next to the simulation suite and large closets in each treatment room are used for storing patient's body conformal immobilization devices (Fig. 24.5C). For clinics where one simulation suite is used to support multiple satellite clinics, the logistics of transporting the immobilization device must also be considered. At the University of Virginia and Virginia Commonwealth University, a courier service is used to transport the large body conformal devices from the simulation site to satellite treatment facilities. Each clinic must assess space availability when deciding which system to adopt in patient care.

DOSIMETRIC EFFECTS OF IMMOBILIZATION DEVICES

Any material placed between the patient and the radiation source can modify dosimetric characteristics of the treatment beam. Modern immobilization devices made of low-density materials have little impact on the depth-dose characteristics of megavoltage energy treatment beams; however, electrons liberated within the immobilization device can lead to a measurable increase in the patient's surface dose, that is, a bolusing effect. Clinical experience supports this effect and has shown that skin reactions are more frequent and tend to occur earlier in the treatment course, when beams are delivered through an immobilization device. The magnitude of the bolus effect can vary greatly depending on the composition, density, and thickness of the immobilization device as well as beam energy, field size, and geometric arrangement.

AAPM Task Group 176 has published an excellent report regarding the dosimetric effects of couch tops and immobilization devices including the basic physics rationale, a well-rounded literature review of relevant studies, and techniques that can be utilized to reduce and better model the dosimetric effects of these devices.[17] Body conformal immobilization devices have been reported to exhibit dosimetric behavior

similar to an additional 0.2 to 0.5 cm of water equivalent thickness for physical device thicknesses of 2 to 5 cm, respectively, a roughly 1:10 ratio for low-density vac-loc bags.[18] Thermoplastic masks show similar effects; for example, Hadley et al. reported increased surface dose using 6-MV photons from 16% without a mask to 61% with a mask.[19]

For thermoplastic head and neck masks, the bolus effect is reduced when the masks are stretched more as the thickness of material in the beam's path is subsequently reduced. The clinician may also cut out parts of the mask to remove material in the beam path to reduce skin reactions. Care must be taken, however, to ensure that the integrity of the mask and its ability to provide rigid immobilization is not compromised. With proper skill and attention, thermoplastic masks with cutouts to improve skin sparing have been shown to achieve similar setup accuracy as unmodified masks.[5] For custom-made foam body conformal systems, such as the Alpha Cradle, foam lying in the beam path can be shaved away to reduce the thickness along the beam path. Reusable vacuum-lock bags are commercially available with treatment beam portals for standard beam arrangements to avoid bolusing. Regardless of the immobilization device chosen for treatment and methods employed to reduce the bolusing effect, AAPM TG-176 recommended best practices are to include any patient-specific devices in the dose calculation to support more realistic clinical plan assessment. The TG-176 report also provides details for measuring skin dose and bolusing effect in order to verify the accuracy of the planning system's skin dose calculation.

STEREOTACTIC IMMOBILIZATION AND STABILIZATION

Introduction

Hypofractionated stereotactic techniques enable the radiation oncologist to deliver high-dose conformal radiation therapy with a sharp dose falloff to both intracranial and extracranial targets. Here, we describe radiation therapy delivered as a single high-dose fraction as stereotactic radiosurgery (SRS), and therapy delivered over a small number of high-dose fractions stereotactic radiotherapy (SRT). Delivering a high dose to the target volume in only a few fractions increases the requirements for precise delivery of the radiation. Advances in online image guidance have enabled the delivery of high-dose extracranial stereotactic treatments, and improvements in patient immobilization have accompanied to help decrease interfractional variation in patient setup and intrafractional patient and target motion. Intrafraction target motion occurs in lung and liver tumors because of normal physiologic processes such as respiration, and longer treatment times associated with high-dose SRT may further reduce intrafractional treatment accuracy.[20] Numerous immobilization-based strategies to minimize this motion are discussed later in this section. In general, intrafraction error from patient movement within the device during treatment can be reduced by improving the comfort and stability of the immobilization system. As with all immobilization methods and devices, patients with poorer performance status may have worse interfractional setup reproducibility and more intrafraction motion within the immobilization device,[21] so patient-specific immobilization options may need to be considered.

Intracranial Immobilization Devices

Intracranial immobilization devices can generally be classified into two categories: invasive and noninvasive, which are reviewed in the following sections. Other important characteristics include if the device is relocatable or not, and what system is used to align the patient for treatment.

Invasive Cranial Immobilization

Invasive cranial immobilization devices enabled intracranial SRS treatments prior to the widespread adoption of in-room image guidance and are exemplified by rigid metal frames attached to metal pins driven directly into the skull. Generally, two long posts are placed anterior and two shorts posts are placed posterior in the patient's skull. The patient then undergoes imaging (either CT or MRI, depending on device compatibility) with a fiducial-based system attached to the frame to provide stereotactic localization of the tumor position within the frame. A treatment plan is then developed, and at the time of treatment, the head frame is connected to either a floor-mounted stand or the treatment table to provide rigid cranial immobilization. The fiducial-based stereotactic localization system is then used to align the target to the machine isocenter and the treatment is delivered, usually in a single fraction. The primary advantage of the invasive, frame-based, nonrelocatable stereotactic head frame is the rigid immobilization it provides with accuracy generally reported on the order of <1 mm.[22,23]

The Leksell Stereotactic Coordinate Frame G (Elekta, Stockholm, Sweden) (Fig. 24.7) is an example of an invasive cranial immobilization frame that is compatible with gamma knife or linear accelerator platforms. A phantom study of the Leksell Frame G on the gamma knife system using GafChromic film found the overall accuracy (mean ± standard deviation) of an MR-defined target to be 0.21 ± 0.32 mm and 0.15 ± 0.26 mm in the x and y axes and 0.06 ± 0.09 mm and 0.04 ± 0.09 mm for a CT-based target.[22] The Brown-Roberts-Wells (BRW) frame by Integra is another invasive cranial device for linac-based SRS. The BRW localizer frame features a set of vertical and diagonal indicator rods to facilitate stereotactic localization and alignment. Ramakrishna et al.[24] used stereoscopic kV x-ray imaging to evaluate setup accuracy and intrafraction motion using the BRW system and reported a mean deviation between frame-based and image-guided positioning of 1.0 ± 0.5 mm and a mean intrafraction deviation of 0.4 ± 0.3 mm.

A disadvantage of these invasive, nonrelocatable devices is that they are for the most part limited to single-fraction SRS, requiring frame placement, imaging, planning, quality assurance, and delivery to occur in the same day before the frame can be removed. One invasive immobilization device designed to accommodate fractionated SRT is the TALON removable head frame system designed by Best Nomos. The TALON system is a relocatable invasive stereotactic head frame that utilizes two self-tapping titanium screws inserted into the patient's skull at the vertex. The detachable TALON assembly is then attached to the screws for patient positioning on imaging and treatment tables. After each fraction is delivered, the frame can be removed and the patient can leave with the two screws remaining in the skull. Salter et al. evaluated repositioning accuracy of the system with CT imaging and reported a mean isocenter deviation of 0.99 ± 0.28 mm in patients treated with SRS and a mean isocenter deviation of 1.38 ± 0.48 mm in patients treated over 6 weeks of treatment.[25]

Noninvasive Cranial Immobilization

Invasive cranial immobilization devices have been successfully used for many years to deliver intracranial SRS, but these systems require placing of screws into the patient's head, which carries the risk of bleeding and infection and requires premedication and dedicated nursing support.[24] The compressed treatment planning time required for nonrelocatable systems may also be less desirable in certain scenarios. Numerous relocatable and noninvasive systems have been developed that can provide accurate and reproducible immobilization of the head without the use of screws driven into the skull and provide the flexibility to deliver multifraction SRT. Some of these systems, as described below, utilize traditional fiducial-based localizer systems, and others have leveraged the widespread adoption of in-room image guidance systems for patient positioning.

The Stereoadapter 5000 is a noninvasive and relocatable immobilization device commercially available through Sandstrom Trade & Technology, Inc. The device is attached to the patient's head with two earplugs that are secured in place by tightening a screw on the nasal bridge support. Side arms connect to a vertex stabilizer and a band is fastened against the occiput to provide additional stabilization. Millimeter scales on the Stereoadapter components are used to reproduce the setup, and the device is compatible with both MRI and CT imaging. Kalapurakal et al.[26] evaluated setup reproducibility of this immobilization system using portal images coregistered with the CT scout image and reported mean

FIGURE 24.7. Stereotactic–invasive intracranial. The Leksell® Coordinate Frame G is **(A)** fixed to the patient's head via four self-tapping screws. At the time of treatment delivery **(B)**, the frame is attached to the treatment table. (Images courtesy of Elekta, Stockholm, Sweden.)

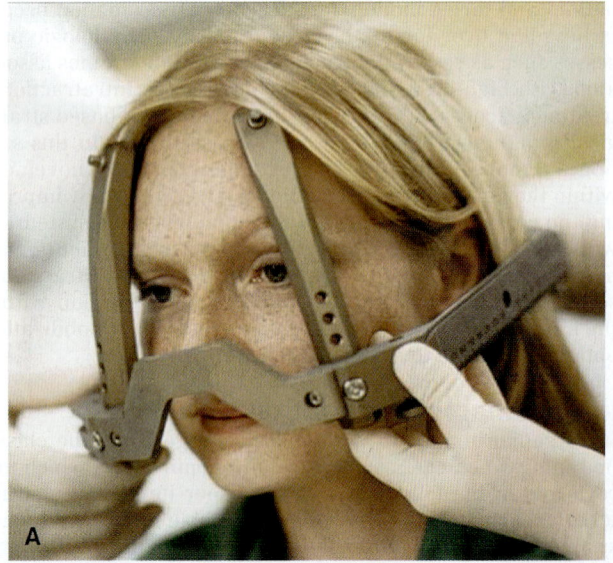
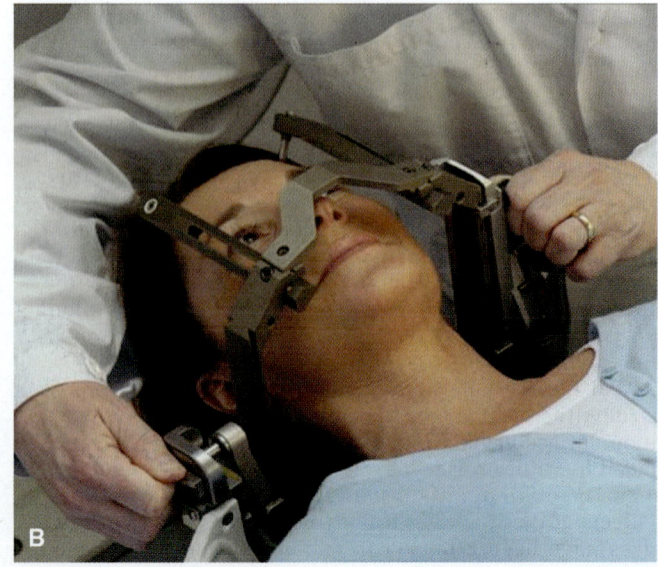

isocenter shifts of 1.0 ± 0.7 mm, 0.8 ± 0.8 mm, and 1.7 ± 1.0 mm in the x, y, and z axes.

The Gill-Thomas-Cosman (GTC) Relocatable Head Ring (Integra) is a noninvasive, relocatable cranial immobilization device that is compatible with the BRW stereotactic localizer system. A custom mold of the patient's upper dentition is formed and mounted to the head ring anteriorly, and a custom-formed headrest is mounted to the ring posteriorly. Setup accuracy is verified with the XKnife Depth Helmet, a clear plastic device that is placed over the head ring. A rod with millimeter scale is inserted into holes in the depth helmet and measurements obtained to ensure accurate placement. Das et al. measured the daily relocation error of the GTC frame using the Depth Helmet prior to each fraction and found a mean radial displacement of 1.03 ± 0.34 mm.[27] Kumar et al.[28] evaluated daily setup reproducibility with daily pretreatment portal imaging coregistered to the planning CT digitally reconstructed radiograph (DRR) and found a total 3D mean displacement of 1.8 ± 0.8 mm.

The Elekta (Stockholm, Sweden) eXtend frame system (Fig. 24.8) is a relocatable, noninvasive cranial immobilization device for fractionated SRT. Similar to the previously described HeadFIX system, a custom dental mold is formed and is attached to a carbon fiber frame that is connected to the treatment couch. Active suction to the hard palate aids in immobilizing the patient. Similar to the Depth Helmet described above, the repositioning check tool (RCT) is used to confirm that the patient is accurately relocated within the frame (Fig. 24.8B). Ruschin et al.[29] evaluated the setup accuracy of the eXtend frame using the RCT, reporting a mean 3D setup error of 0.8 mm and 1.3 mm in patients treated on a linear accelerator and a Gamma Knife Perfexion, respectively. The mean intrafraction motion was measured at 0.4 ± 0.3 mm, leading the authors to conclude that the RCT was adequate to confirm frame repositioning and that the system provided excellent intrafraction immobilization.

Systems like those above are able to provide accurate patient setup by defining the tumor's stereotactic location within the coordinate system of a rigid localizer frame. An alternative strategy is to align the patient using daily x-ray image guidance. One example is the Brainlab mask system (Fig. 24.9) that utilizes a U-shaped frame, two vertical posts, a three-piece thermoplastic mask, and an optional bite-block

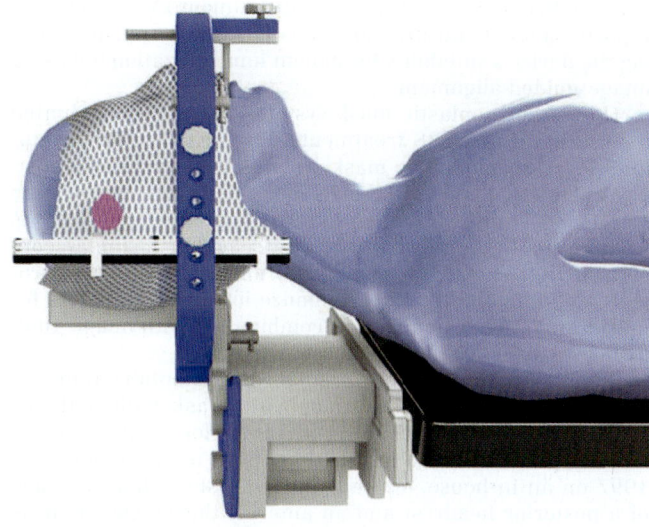

FIGURE 24.9. Intracranial stereotactic–relocatable Brainlab mask (Brainlab, Munich, Germany). The Brainlab noninvasive mask system utilizes three pieces of thermoplastic mask custom molded to the patient's head and attached to vertical posts on either side of the patient's head. These posts are then attached to a U-shaped frame, which is attached to the treatment couch, thus providing rigid immobilization of the head. A stereotactic localizer box may be used for target localization. (Image courtesy of Brainlab.)

attachment for cranial immobilization. At the time of simulation, three thermoplastic shells are formed to the anterior and posterior aspects of the patient's head. The shells are fastened to the vertical posts, which are attached to the head ring that is mounted to the CT or treatment couch. A stereotactic localizer device is available, though studies have shown it may not achieve the desired positioning accuracy. Ali et al.[30] evaluated the setup accuracy of the Brainlab mask system with the localizer device by acquiring verification onboard kV images and reported mean shifts of 0.7 ± 2.0 mm, 1.6 ± 2.6 mm, and 0.1 ± 2.2 mm in the x, y, and z dimensions. The random setup errors exhibited by standard deviations larger than 2 mm supports the argument for daily pretreatment image guidance as opposed to relying solely on the localizer device. Ramakrishna et al.[24] evaluated intrafraction motion

FIGURE 24.8. Intracranial stereotactic–relocatable Elekta Extend™ system. The Elekta Extend™ system is a relocatable immobilization device designed for fractionated stereotactic radiotherapy. A custom mold of the maxillary dentition **(A)** is fixated to the hard palate with suction and then attached to a carbon fiber frame to provide rigid immobilization to the couch. Setup accuracy is assessed with the RCT **(B)** prior to the delivery of each treatment. (Images courtesy of Elekta, Stockholm, Sweden.)

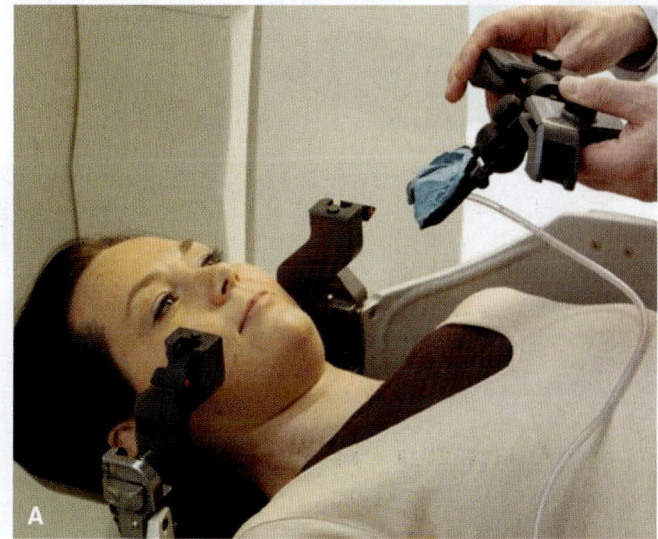

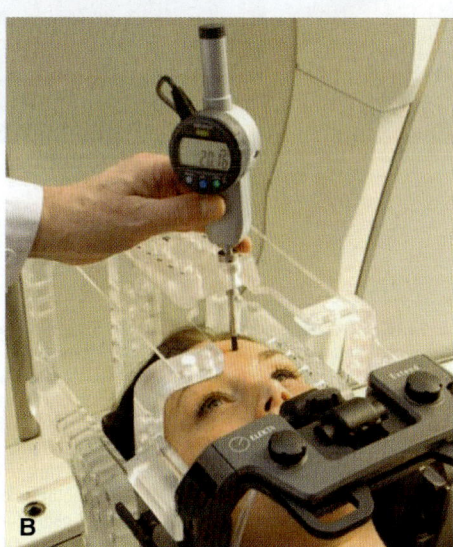

with the Brainlab system using posttreatment kV imaging and reported a mean intrafraction shift of 0.7 ± 0.5 mm, highlighting the device's suitability for patient immobilization following image-guided alignment.

Other thermoplastic mask systems have been evaluated for use in cranial SRS treatments. Tryggestad et al.[31] evaluated four thermoplastic mask systems using pre- and posttreatment CBCT. They reported a mean interfraction deviation of 2.1 to 2.7 mm, and mean intrafraction deviation of 0.7 to 1.1 mm for the four-mask systems, reaching a similar conclusion that certain thermoplastic mask systems can provide rigid immobilization to minimize intrafraction errors for intracranial SRS, when used in combination with image guidance to reduce interfractional setup errors.

Another option for intracranial SRS immobilization and positioning is to use a thermoplastic mask with optically guided fiducial markers for daily target localization and to monitor patient motion in real time. Bova et al.[32] reported in 1997 on an in-house, optically guided system that consisted of a posterior headrest and an anterior thermoplastic mask extending from the forehead to the upper lip for immobilization and a physically separate custom bite plate with a set of six infrared light-emitting diodes attached for stereotactic localization with an infrared camera system. They reported the bite plate could be positioned and repositioned to within 0.5 ± 0.3 mm and the system allowed for real-time tracking of the infrared markers, and thus patient motion. In a similar fashion, Peng et al.[33] evaluated the accuracy of using the Varian SonArray system with optically guided fiducials for setup by acquiring a verification CBCT, reporting a mean setup error of 1.2 ± 0.7 mm.

Extracranial Immobilization Devices

In 1995, Hamilton and colleagues from the University of Arizona published their preliminary clinical experience with linear accelerator–based SRS of the spine in five patients.[34] For immobilization, clamps were secured transcutaneously to the spinous processes one to two vertebral levels above and below the target volume under local or general anesthesia,

through a 2-cm incision. The spine was rigidly immobilized by attaching the clamps to a frame consisting of a rigid box with two semicircular metal arches. After CT simulation and treatment planning, the patient and frame were transferred to a modified linear accelerator and setup according to stereotactic coordinates derived from the planning CT. Although this invasive device was important in demonstrating the feasibility of extracranial stereotactic body radiation therapy (SBRT), the overwhelming majority of modern immobilization systems for extracranial SBRT utilize noninvasive customizable devices like the previously described body conformal vacuum-lock bags, with added features to allow for more precise positioning and the attachment of specialized devices such as compression plates.

Examples of modular immobilization systems for extracranial SBRT included the Body Pro-Lok from CIVCO Medical Solutions (Coralville, IA), the Bionix Omni V SBRT positioning system, and the Elekta Stereotactic Body Frame all depicted in Figure 24.10. SBRT-specific frames like these include indexing along the entire length of a lightweight carbon fiber platform allowing reproducible isocenter localization and for accessories to be attached. Attachment options typically include headrests, forehead restraints, upper arm supports, shoulder restraints, thigh and foot positioners, external fiducial arches, and abdominal compression devices.

Numerous investigators have assessed the reproducibility of these extracranial SBRT immobilization systems. Gutierrez et al. evaluated the CIVCO Body Pro-Lok system using TomoTherapy with pretreatment megavoltage CT (MVCT) to determine the mean interfractional setup error of twenty liver and lung SBRT patients[35] and reported mean localization errors of 0.9 ± 3.1 mm, 1.2 ± 5.5 mm, and 6.5 ± 2.6 mm in the x, y, and z dimensions, and a mean composite displacement vector of 8.2 ± 2.0 mm. Purdie et al.[20] evaluated the intrafraction positioning reproducibility by comparing pretreatment localization CT to a mid- or posttreatment CBCT with the Elekta Stereotactic Body Frame in 28 lung SBRT patients. The mean 3D tumor position was within 2.2 ± 1.2 mm of planned when repeat imaging was performed within 34 minutes of

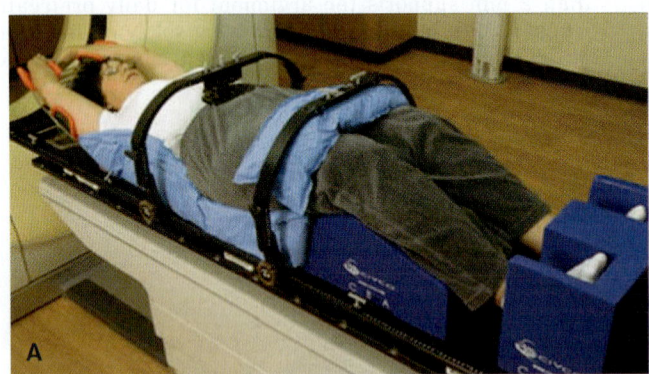

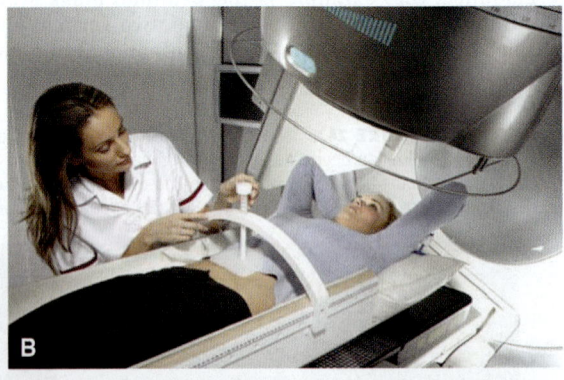

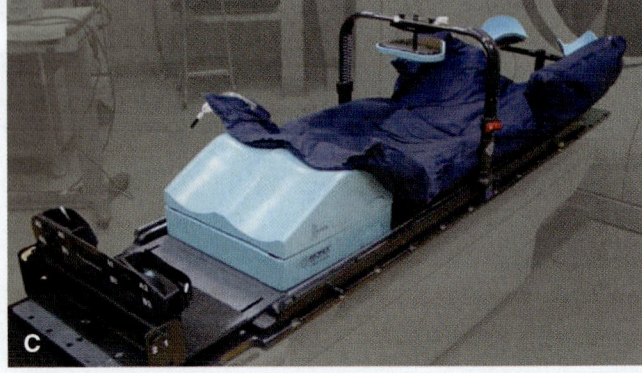

FIGURE 24.10. Stereotactic body frames. **A:** The Body Pro-Lok is a modular immobilization system that can be used of stereotactic body radiotherapy (SBRT). Multiple attachments are available to build a device customized to the needs of each patient. This particular setup utilizes an abdominal compression plate. (Image courtesy of Civco Medical Solutions, Coralville, IA.) **B:** The Stereotactic Body Frame has a reference system that runs along the length of the device. (Image courtesy of Elekta, Stockholm, Sweden.) **C:** The Omni V is another modular system with a variety of options to provide customized patient immobilization. (Image courtesy of Bionix Radiation Therapy, Toledo, OH.)

target localization, and 5.3 ± 3 mm when performed more than 34 minutes after target localization ($P < .01$). While this particular device is no longer commercially available, this study highlights the important consideration that longer treatment times can increase the intrafractional positioning error.

The Elekta BodyFIX is another example of a body conformal system with features specifically designed for SBRT. As described in the preceding section and illustrated in Figure 24.5B, the distinguishing characteristic of the BodyFIX system is the thin clear plastic cover sheet that uses an active vacuum pump to create negative pressure providing additional immobilization of the patient. A study of 126 lung SBRT patients used pre- and posttreatment cone-beam CT (CBCT) to determine intrafractional stability of the BodyFIX system and reported the intrafraction variation of mean tumor position to be 2.7 ± 2.6 mm.[36]

Immobilization and Internal Motion Management

In addition to intrafractional error because of patient movement within the immobilization device, internal target motion because of breathing must be accounted for in SBRT, particularly in treatment of lung and liver tumors. The report of AAPM Task Group 76[37] addressed the management of respiratory motion in radiation therapy and presented the results of a variety of studies evaluating the motion of lung and liver tumors under respiration. Lung and liver targets exhibit a wide variation in motion amplitude across patients and for targets in different regions of the lungs and liver. For lung tumors, mean tumor motion amplitudes from various studies ranged between 2.4 and 7.3 mm (left to right), 3.9 and 12.5 mm (sup to inf), and 2.4 and 9.4 mm (ant to post). For liver tumors, reports of superior–inferior mean motion amplitude ranged between 10 and 25 mm for shallow breathing and between 37 and 55 mm for deep breathing. Working from this wealth of available motion data, the report of AAPM Task Group 101 recommends that all thorax and abdomen SBRT patients undergo tumor motion assessment[38] and some immobilization devices have been designed to help mitigate or regularize respiratory motion.

Multiple strategies have been developed to account for or control internal target motion from respiration, including deep inspiration breath hold (DIBH), active breathing control, respiratory gating, real-time tumor tracking, and abdominal compression devices. Relevant to this chapter, some extracranial immobilization systems offer the ability to use abdominal compression devices to control respiratory excursion. This technique may also be referred to as forced shallow breathing. Abdominal compression devices typically consist of a plate attached to an arch that is indexed to a stereotactic body frame or the treatment couch. The plate is placed a few centimeters below the patient's xiphoid process and a screw is tightened until the desired amount of internal motion control is achieved. The screw is marked so that it can be reproducibly tightened for multiple fractions. Abdominal compression devices are available from a variety of companies, including CIVCO Medical Solutions for use on the Pro-Lok immobilization system, and from Bionix for use on the Omni V system.

Studies report varied results with the use of abdominal compression in reducing lung and liver tumor motion amplitude. Negoro et al.[39] studied lung tumor motion in 18 patients treated with SBRT and found the mean tumor motion in the superior–inferior dimension measured with fluoroscopy to decrease from 12.3 to 7.0 mm (range 2 to 11 mm) with the use of abdominal compression. The mean amplitude for liver motion measured with fluoroscopy was shown to decrease from 40 mm with free breathing to 11 mm with the use of abdominal compression.[40] Another study showed that while abdominal compression reduced the superior–inferior and anterior–posterior motion, an increased motion amplitude in the left–right dimension of

15% on average (maximum 1.6 mm) was observed,[41] indicating that compression may also be redistributing breathing motion. It should also be noted that the abdominal forces required to mitigate motion are often reported to be uncomfortable and may not be suitable for all patients.[42]

OPTICAL SURFACE IMAGING FOR MONITORING OF PATIENT POSITIONING

Introduction

Optical surface imaging (OSI) is a new technology used in radiation oncology for patient positioning and monitoring. As it has been established throughout this chapter, immobilization devices are a crucial tool for the appropriate delivery of radiation treatments. They promote consistent setups throughout the radiotherapy course and help patients hold their treatment position for the duration of each fraction. However, these systems have their limitations and it can sometimes be cumbersome to replicate the planned position just based on these devices and skin marks. Moreover, these tools oftentimes must balance patient comfort with motion restriction. Hence, although immobilization devices conform to the patient and limit their mobility, patients can still move during treatment increasing the delivery uncertainty. This becomes progressively worrisome as margins are reduced and fraction doses escalate. Under these conditions, patient monitoring during treatment to detect undesired motion becomes especially important. Surface imaging systems can help facilitate patient setup and allow for intrafraction monitoring without the use of additional ionizing radiation, in what is currently known as Surface-Guided Radiation Therapy (SGRT) or Surface Image-Guided Radiation Therapy (SIGRT).

OSI can be useful for initial positioning of any site, but internal imaging must be performed when the target location might not properly correlate with the surface. Intrafraction monitoring with these systems can be used to detect external motion or even track breathing,[43] but this does not necessarily reflect the true target motion as not all internal involuntary movements will be revealed by the patient's surface. It is important to understand the technology and the information these systems provide in order to ensure they are utilized correctly and to their full potential. This section aims to give the reader a general overview of these systems, their characteristics, and some typical clinical uses.

Overview of Selected Commercial Systems

Surface imaging systems acquire the patient's surface in the treatment room and compare it to the patient's planned surface position, known as the reference surface. The reference surface is typically generated using the DICOM structure and plan file information from the treatment planning system. The external CT contours from the DICOM structure file are used to create the reference surface, and the location of the reference surface within the treatment room is determined based on the treatment isocenter coordinates from the DICOM plan information. The treatment isocenter coordinates are read, and the reference surface is translated to place that point at the machine isocenter. Surface imaging systems are calibrated so that their origin coincides with the machine isocenter. The approach to obtain the real-time patient surface and its registration with the reference surface varies depending on the specific surface imaging system.

There are two main manufacturers of surface imaging equipment for radiotherapy: Vision RT (London, UK) who manufactures the AlignRT system (also available through Varian as the Optical Surface Monitoring System, OSMS) and C-RAD (Uppsala, Sweden) who manufactures the Sentinel and Catalyst systems. Each system uses a different approach in both physically acquiring the current surface and registering the acquired and reference surfaces. Details of these two systems

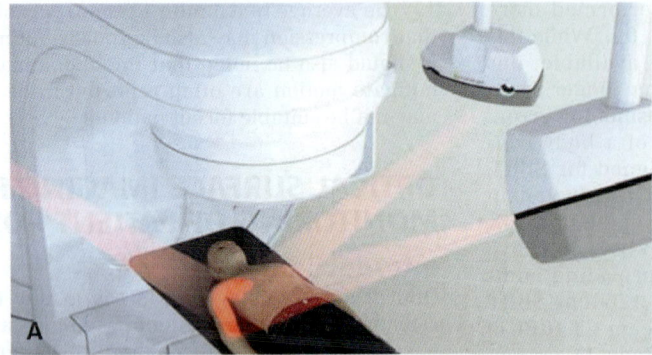
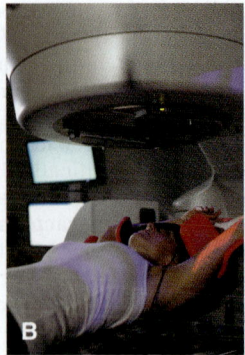

FIGURE 24.11. C-RAD surface imaging system. **A:** The C-RAD Catalyst HD OSI system consists of three ceiling-mounted camera pods to acquire patient's surface in the treatment room with a vendor-quoted accuracy of 0.5 mm. **B:** The system projects a visible pattern of light on the patient's surface to guide the therapists in aligning the patient to the reference surface. (Images courtesy of C-RAD, Uppsala, Sweden.)

are presented in the following sections. This list is not meant to be a comprehensive description of all available options but merely an introduction to a few examples that illustrate the current state of technology in OSI.

C-RAD Systems

This family of OSI systems includes Sentinel 4DCT, and a variety of Catalyst products. Sentinel is used at the CT simulator for respiratory tracking during 4DCTs and other gated scans, whereas the Catalyst family of systems is used for patient positioning and monitoring during treatment. Both the breathing trace and reference surface acquired by Sentinel at the simulator can be read by Catalyst systems for use during treatment. Sentinel is comprised of a sweeping visible red laser (635 to 690 nm wavelength) and a camera that captures the reflected light as the laser sweeps across the patient at discrete intervals to read his/her surface. It takes approximately 1 to 2 seconds to scan a length of 40 cm with a measurement reproducibility of 0.2 mm, and it detects respiratory signal with a frequency of 15 Hz. The maximal scan volume is $80 \times 130 \times 70$ cm³. Although this system is most commonly used at simulation, it can also be used for patient positioning and monitoring during treatment.[44,45]

The Catalyst system can be comprised of 1 or 3 pods, for the standard and HD versions respectively, mounted on the ceiling of the treatment room and facing the machine isocenter. In contrast with Sentinel, Catalyst uses light in the near-invisible violet range (405 nm). This allows the full patient surface to be read at once, instead of with discrete laser sweeps, which allows for a scan speed of up to 80 frames-per-second (fps) for the standard system and 200 fps for HD. Catalyst provides 6 degree-of-freedom (DOF) isocentric shift information by comparing the real-time surface of the patient to that from simulation using deformable registration. A visible pattern of red or green light is projected directly on the patient's skin to indicate to the therapists how the patient's position needs to be adjusted (see Fig. 24.11). The position and motion detection accuracy is quoted as 1 mm for the standard system and 0.5 mm for the HD system. Both maximum scan volume and measurement reproducibility match that of the Sentinel system. Details of the performance of these systems can be found in the literature.[46-48]

Vision RT Systems/Varian Optical Surface Monitoring System

Vision RT provides a family of surface imaging systems that allow for patient positioning and monitoring during treatment (AlignRT), respiratory tracking at simulation for 4DCT acquisition (GateCT), and gating during treatment delivery (GateRT). AlignRT is typically a 3-pod system mounted on the ceiling of the treatment room facing the machine isocenter as shown in Figure 24.12A below. For surface acquisition, each pod contains two cameras and a projector that casts a red

FIGURE 24.12. AlignRT surface imaging system. **A:** AlignRT's three ceiling-mounted camera pods acquire the patient's surface in the treatment room by projecting a structured light speckle pattern onto the patient. **B:** Monitors in the control and treatment rooms provide the therapists with real-time feedback about the current alignment of the patient's current and reference surfaces including rigid translations and rotations to help align the patient prior to treatment and track intrafraction surface motion during treatment. (Images taken at Virginia Commonwealth University by the author–May 2017.)

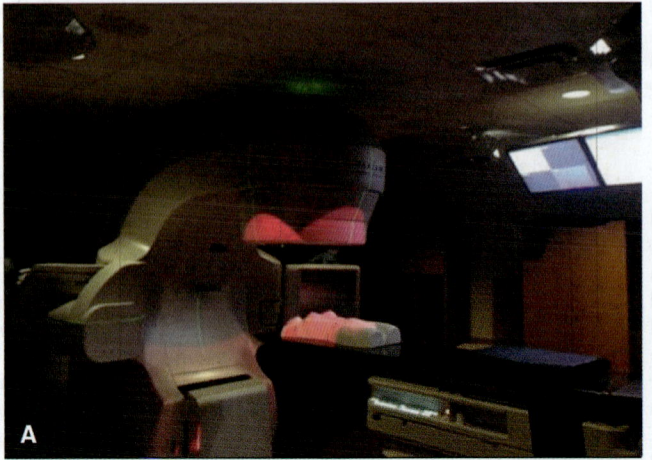
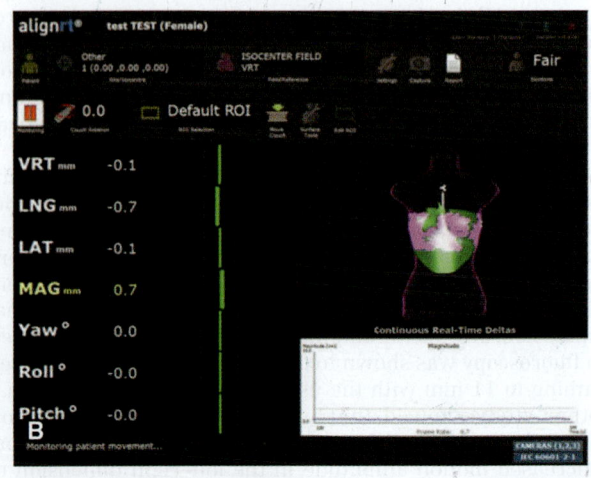

light speckle pattern on the patient. The stereoscopic cameras read the structured light projection pattern and reconstruct the patient's surface based on the deformation of the known pattern. The patient's current acquired surface is then rigidly registered to the reference surface. The reference surface is derived either from the external contours of the planning CT or from a reference capture acquired in the treatment room with the system, for example, after CBCT imaging and alignment. The reference surface for the first fraction is always based on the planning CT. The three rigid translations and three rotations needed to best align the two surfaces are then displayed on the system's screen (see Fig. 24.12B). The rigid registration is only performed in the area defined by the user as the region of interest (ROI). The frame rate for this system depends on the size of the ROI and is typically around 1 to 3 fps for thorax ROIs. There is literature on its use in radiation therapy for all treatment sites, but especially in left-sided breast DIBH treatments[49–51] and SRS.[52–54] This same equipment is commercially available through Varian Medical Systems (Palo Alto, CA) under the name of Optical Surface Monitoring System (OSMS).

The GateRT system uses the same technology, but the software display presents information optimized for respiratory tracking and beam gating. The GateCT package typically includes a single pod installed in the CT simulation room for respiration and motion tracking of the patient during 4DCT scans to provide a reference trace for treatment gating.

Current Clinical Applications

Current commercially available systems use a reference surface of the patient to guide therapists during setup. The reference surface for daily alignment is generated from the CT planning data contours, acquired from an OSI system at the time of simulation, or acquired during an earlier treatment fraction, typically following x-ray image-guided alignment. As the patient's current surface is read and compared to the reference surface in real time, visual feedback is either projected on the patient's skin or shown on a screen, informing therapists what adjustments are needed to achieve the desired surface position. Six degree-of-freedom shift information is also displayed as three translations (vertical, longitudinal, lateral) and three rotations (yaw, roll, pitch). Once the desired external position has been achieved, anatomical alignment can be confirmed with internal image guidance techniques.

Surface imaging systems give users the option to acquire a new reference surface with the optical cameras. These surfaces tend to capture a larger extent of the patient's external anatomy when compared to the DICOM reference. The purpose of updating the reference surface is twofold: (a) having a reference with extended external anatomy may facilitate setup for subsequent fractions, for example, of the elbows in arms-up positioning, and (b) rebaselining the reference position will allow for better intrafraction monitoring. Although ideally the patient's external surface should exactly match the planning position every time, this is often not the case. If the patient's current position is found to be acceptable as confirmed with internal imaging, acquiring a new reference surface will zero out any residual surface offsets between the patient's approved treatment position and the original patient surface from the time of simulation. Hence, any motion throughout the fraction will become more obvious in the displayed shift values. This is even more important if the surface imaging system interfaces with the treatment machine to gate the beam. Removing the inherent shifts between the current approved treatment surface and the original reference will allow for tighter monitoring thresholds for any given fraction and less beam interruptions from false large readings. It is important to note that for most commercial systems, the original reference surface based on the DICOM information remains available for selection throughout the course, giving the option to perform initial alignment with either reference surface at any time.

Although surface imaging may be used for the initial positioning and monitoring of patients treated to any anatomical site, it has shown special utility for DIBH breast treatments and SRS because of the close correlation between surface and target positions.

Deep Inspiration Breath Hold Treatments for Breast Radiotherapy

DIBH treatments for left-sided breast cancer patients can provide cardiac sparing because the heart moves further away from the chest wall, and hence from the treatment volume, as the lungs inflate.[49] Surface imaging has emerged as a useful tool for voluntary DIBH treatments. The use of this technology can achieve reproducible patient setups and reasonably consistent distances between the heart and the chest wall during breath holds, reliably minimizing cardiac side effects from radiotherapy.[49,50] When using OSI for this purpose, the external surfaces from both a free-breathing and a DIBH scan are sent to the system. The patient is initially setup to the free-breathing scan, and the breath hold reproducibility is checked with the DIBH surface. This is the surface used for treatment, and the radiation is only delivered when the patient's current surface is within a preset tolerance of the DIBH reference surface.

Intracranial Stereotactic Radiosurgery

Intracranial SRS patients can also benefit from OSI setup and monitoring. Conventional masks used for frameless SRS are not suitable for OSI because they cover the patient's entire face; OSI technology requires uncovered skin for proper tracking. Open masks, such as the one shown in Figure 24.13, allow for immobilization of the patient while maintaining part of the face exposed for surface monitoring. Open mask immobilization in this scenario has the advantage of both allowing continuous tracking the patient's surface directly, instead of monitoring infrared markers on an array or mask, and providing increased patient comfort. Several authors have published on the feasibility and accuracy of this technique for radiosurgery.[54–56] Whereas initial positioning is always confirmed with internal imaging to ensure the target alignment is satisfactory, the use of OSI for these treatments allow for real-time, uninterrupted monitoring of the patient without the delivery of any additional ionizing radiation dose.

Conclusions and Future Applications

OSI is an emerging technology that can improve setup efficiency of patients and provide intrafraction monitoring without the use of additional radiation dose. Patient

FIGURE 24.13. Example of an open-faced thermoplastic mask for OSI-guided intracranial SRS applications. (Image courtesy of Vision RT, London, UK.)

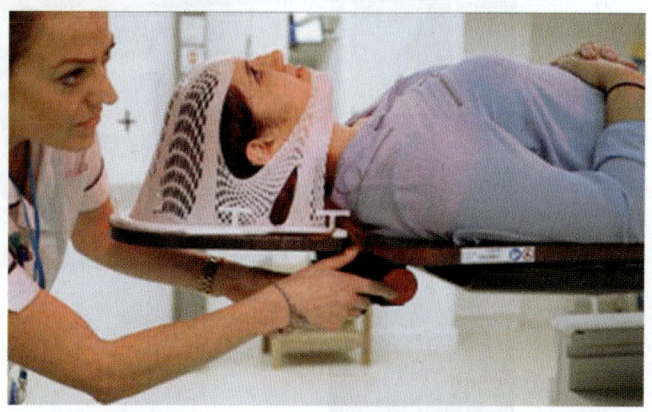

monitoring has become increasingly popular in stereotactic treatment settings where the prescribed dose per fraction is increased and treatment margins are reduced. Although surface imaging provides the means to externally ensure the patient remains in position, it is important to remember that it does not directly relay information about internal motion. Movement from involuntary processes such as digestion will not be readily detected by this technology. Despite this limitation, these systems have benefits beyond what has already been described. They intrinsically offer the possibility of increased patient safety by reading a larger range of the patient's anatomy when compared to internal imaging. This can help avoid confusion during setup and consequently reduce mistreatment of lesions because of problems identifying the correct vertebral level or accidental couch movements between imaging and treatment. Additionally, surface imaging could be utilized in the future for automatic facial recognition of patients before treatment and identification and tracking of anatomical changes such as swelling or weight loss based on the changes of the patient's surface.

IMMOBILIZATION METHODS IN BRACHYTHERAPY

Introduction

Historically, the focus in brachytherapy has been on immobilization of the applicator, leaving the patient to move freely. For example, manufacturers such as Nucletron and Varian sell brachytherapy stands that clamp onto the applicator. Whereas advancement in design has made these stands CT and MR compatible, the patient can still move and possibly change the position of the applicator with respect to the organ that is to be treated. Additionally, patient flow issues can cause difficulties in brachytherapy treatments. An applicator typically is placed in the patient in an operating room. The patient is then moved to either the radiology or radiation oncology department for imaging and then to the brachytherapy treatment room. Each time the patient is moved, the applicator can become displaced from the optimal position. While the development of integrated brachytherapy suites has lessened this workflow in academic centers, it is still common in community practices. Thus, proper patient and applicator immobilization is still important in brachytherapy.

Immobilization for Genitourinary Treatment

Brachytherapy treatment is common for prostate cancer for men and various gynecologic malignancies for women. Image-guided brachytherapy (IGBT) allows the imaging of the patient during applicator placement, analogous to image-guided radiotherapy for external beam patients. This imaging can be done by various means, including ultrasound, CT, or MR systems. The most common IGBT system is the use of ultrasound for the prostate brachytherapy. Shown in Figure 24.14 is a diagram of an ultrasound probe mounted in a stepper that is used to localize the prostate during low-dose rate (seed implant) or high-dose rate brachytherapy treatments.[57] It has been well established

FIGURE 24.14. Prostate stabilizing needles. **A:** Stabilizing needles used in prostate brachytherapy. Note the barb (inset) that is deployed in the prostate. **B:** A diagram illustrating the prostate brachytherapy implantation procedure using transrectal ultrasound for prostate visualization and a template for guiding the needle-loading process. (**A**, taken at University of Virginia, December 2011. **B**, figure reprinted from Pisansky TM, Gold DG, Furutani KM, et al. High dose-rate brachytherapy in the curative treatment of patients with localized prostate cancer. *Mayo Clin Proc* 2008;83[12]:1364–1372. Copyright © 2008 Mayo Foundation for Medical Education and Research. With permission.)

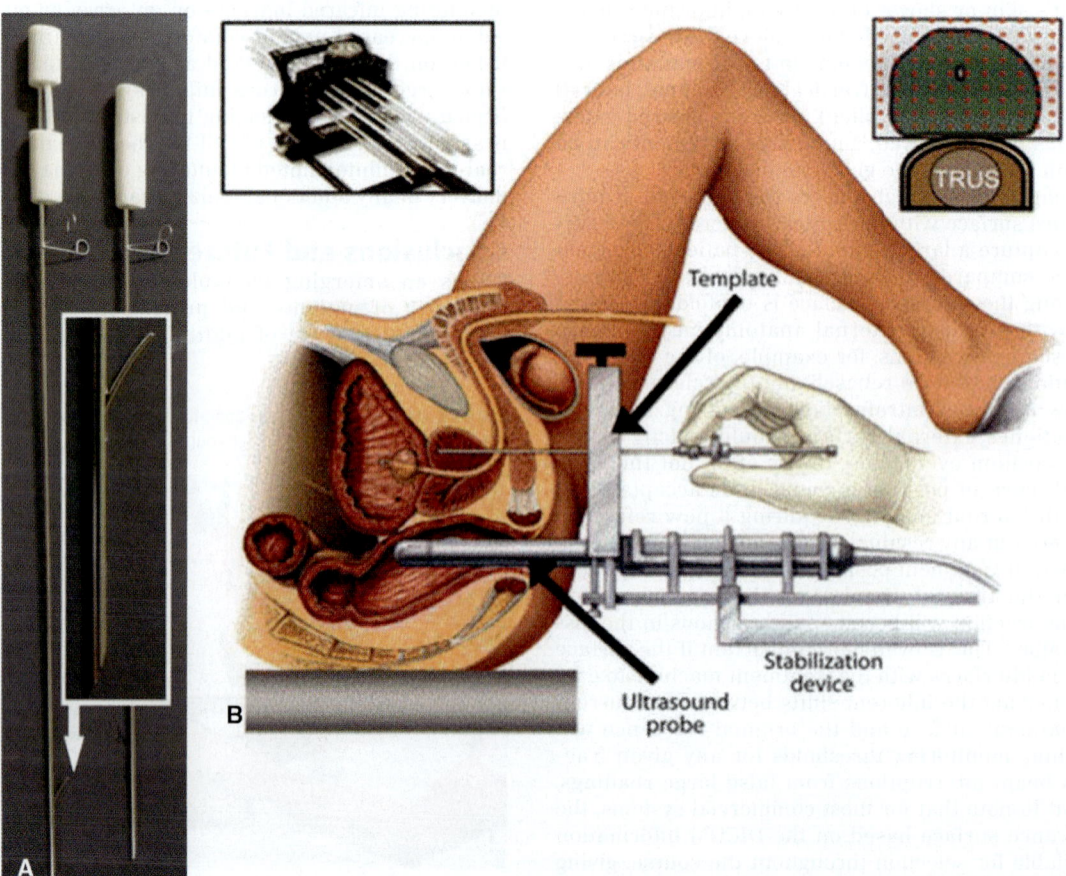

that insertion of needles into the prostate for brachytherapy treatment can cause both motion and deformation of the prostate.[58] The stabilizing needle (Fig. 24.14) is designed to reduce the amount of prostate movement from the insertion of the needles used to deposit seeds throughout the prostate. Stabilizing needles are commercially available from RPD, Inc., as well as the Mick Radio-Nuclear Morgenstern needle. Immobilization of the prostate is accomplished by deploying a side barb into the prostate tissue. The stabilizing needle is then secured with a "lock spring" to the proximal side of the implantation template. Two stabilizing needles are used in the periphery of the prostate to provide adequate stabilization.

More advanced imaging for prostate cancer is the use of MR to image the placement of needles within the prostate as well as for treatment planning purposes. Rather than the dorsal lithotomy position most common for ultrasound imaging, MR imaging usually requires the patient to be immobilized in a lateral decubitus position as shown in Figure 24.15.[59] The use of Aquaplast material can be used to prevent the patient from moving during needle placement, planning, and treatment. In addition to immobilization of the patient, a rectal coil used for imaging is connected to the template used for needle placement. In this way, patient, coil, and template are connected together, as shown in Figure 24.15. The patient can be withdrawn from the MR for needle placement and then reinserted for imaging.[59,60]

The issue of immobilization of applicators for brachytherapy of gynecologic malignancies has been known for many years. Maintenance of the relative position of the applicator to the target and normal tissue, such as bladder and rectum, can determine the quality of the outcome. Vaginal packing

and waistbands have commonly been used to immobilize the applicator but are physician-dependent and may often be unsatisfactory.[61] An early study measured the displacement of tandem and ovoid applicators of up to 5 mm because of movement of the patient from simulation to the treatment room and then back to simulation.[62] This movement caused a change in dose of up to 10% to Point A, and 9% and 17% to the rectal and bladder points, respectively. More recently, a comparison of immobilization methods for vaginal cuff brachytherapy was undertaken, showing that even when the cylinder insertion was performed by the same physician with the same immobilization method and identical patient setup position, variations occurred in the cylinder geometry between simulation and subsequent insertions.[63] The magnitude of the deviation was smaller for stand-type applicator immobilization as opposed to a skirt-type system. It has been shown that the angle of the applicator in vaginal brachytherapy can have a large effect on the normal tissue (bowel) dose and that the applicator should be held in a horizontal position.[64] Additionally, as vaginal cuff brachytherapy has migrated from a single-applicator insertion for LDR brachytherapy to multiple-applicator insertions used in high–dose rate HDR treatments, the positional variation of the applicator geometry has been documented, along with variations in the dose to the normal tissue.[65] Furthermore, because of the steeper dose gradient around HDR sources, the variation of the applicator position magnifies the variation of the dose.

The ideal situation to mitigate motion in brachytherapy would be to scan, plan, and treat in a single room without having to move the patient from the treatment position. The development of integrated brachytherapy suites, such as the

FIGURE 24.15. MR-guided prostate brachytherapy. Two MR-guided prostate HDR procedure examples from the literature. **Left:** As shown in this image from Lakosi et al.'s report, a large sheet of thermoplastic material can be formed around the pelvis to help stabilize the patient in the lateral decubitus position. The rigid connection between the rectal coil and the needle template is also well illustrated. Reprinted by permission from Springer: Lakosi F, Antal G, Vandulek C. et al.Open MR-guided high-dose-rate (HDR) prostate brachytherapy: feasibility and initial experiences open MR-guided high-dose-rate (HDR) prostate brachytherapy. *Pathol Oncol Res* 2011;17(2):315–324. Copyright © 2010 Arányi Lajos Foundation. **Right:** This image from Menard et al.'s report highlights the clinical value in MR visualization for prostate HDR implantation. (Reprinted from Menard C, Susil RC, Choyke P et al. MRI-guided HDR prostate brachytherapy in standard 1.5T scanner. *Int J Radiat Oncol Biol Phys* 2004; 59[5]:1414–1423. Copyright © 2004 Elsevier. With permission.)

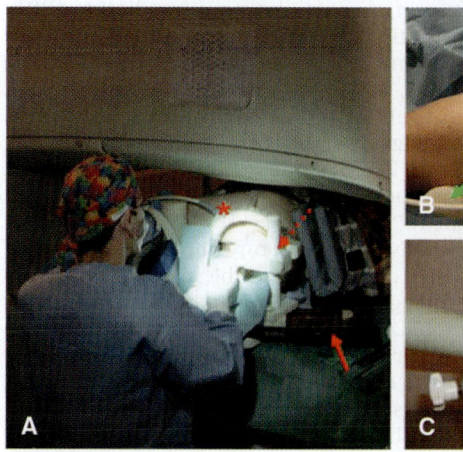
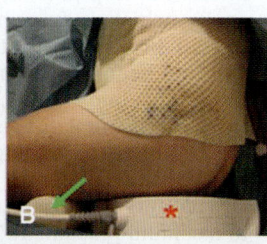
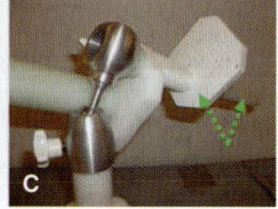
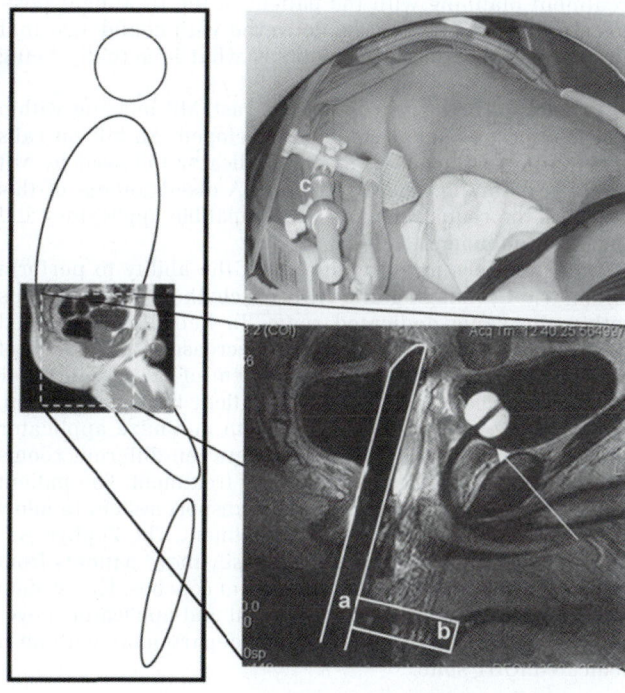

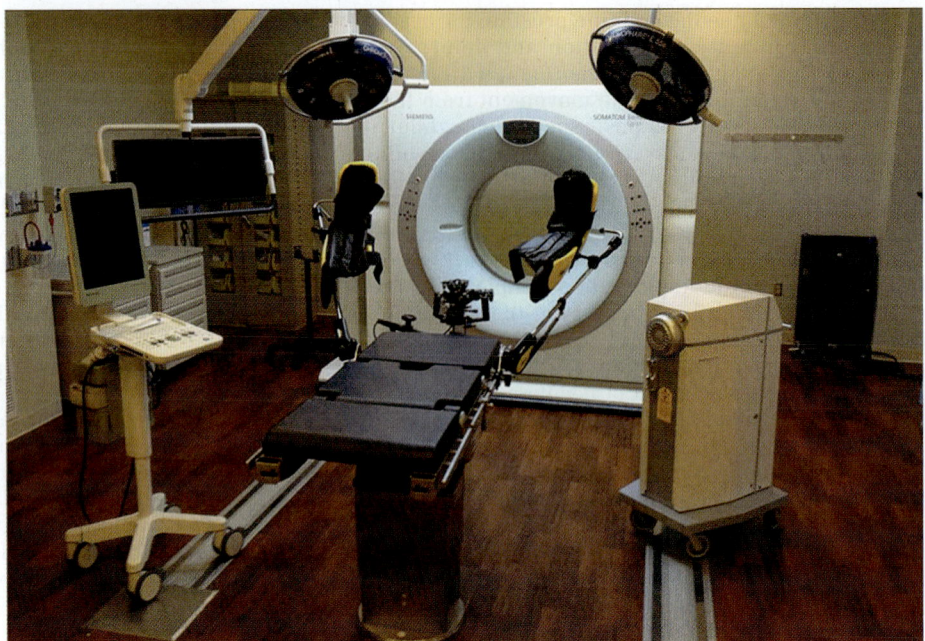

FIGURE 24.16. Image-guided brachytherapy suite at University of Virginia. The brachytherapy suite at the Emily Couric Clinical Cancer Center features a CT on rails for image guidance. The rails are on either side of the table on the floor along which the CT scanner translates over the patient. The room is equipped with high-quality operating room lights and has full anesthesia capabilities. The operating room table allows for numerous attachments to be mounted; illustrated here are leg stirrups for placement of the legs in the dorsal lithotomy position and a transrectal ultrasound stepper. Note the HDR afterloader to the right side of the table. (Image taken at University of Virginia, December 2011.)

Nucletron Integrated Brachytherapy Unit (IBU) or the Varian Acuity Suite, allows for the placement of applicators, imaging, and treatment all in the same room. These suites utilize an in-room cone-beam CT system for image guidance. At the University of Virginia (UVA), the IGBT suite (Fig. 24.16) features CT on rails for in-room patient imaging and 3D treatment planning. Contrary to conventional CT in which the patient translates through the scanner, in this setup, the scanner itself translates over the patient while he or she is immobilized on the table. The image-guided suite at UVA is also designed to accommodate a full anesthesia team. With in-room imaging capabilities, if the imaging study shows that the applicator is not optimally placed, it can be readily adjusted. Furthermore, in-room imaging allows for real-time treatment planning with the patient in the treatment position. Treatment can then be delivered with confidence that the planned treatment geometry is what is actually being delivered.

Because of better soft tissue contrast, MR imaging within a brachytherapy suite has been developed. An MR on rails system allows placement of the applicator followed by MR imaging, planning, and treatment.[66] A disadvantage of this system is the requirement of MR compatible applicators and ancillary equipment.

Unfortunately, most facilities lack the ability to perform volumetric CT imaging and HDR brachytherapy treatments within the same dedicated room. In lieu of a dedicated image-guided suite, one strategy to decrease displacement of the applicator is to minimize movement of the patient after applicator placement. The Zephyr patient transport system, shown in Figure 24.17, is designed to minimize applicator motion when the patient is moved between different rooms during the course of a brachytherapy treatment. The patient is kept in the same position on the transport system to allow for CT scanning and subsequent treatment. The Zephyr system uses air-bearing technology to easily move patients from the transport bed to the CT or treatment couches. This system has the potential to minimize logistical and applicator movement issues of patient transport for departments without a dedicated IGBT suite.[67]

Immobilization for Breast Brachytherapy

The use of brachytherapy to treat breast cancer has become more common since the introduction of balloon-based catheter systems, such as the MammoSite or the Contura, along with the related SAVVI applicator. Traditionally, breast irradiation has been delivered to the whole breast over 6 to 7 weeks after the tumor has been removed. Implanted catheters or balloons have allowed the use of accelerated regimens decreasing this time to 5 treatment days.[68,69] These implanted devices are simpler to administer, compared to the more complicated interstitial implants, in which catheters were placed through the breast tissue to treat the lumpectomy cavity.[70,71] The implanted balloon or SAVVI applicators, along with the interstitial implants, are used to only treat the lumpectomy cavity, which is known as partial breast irradiation (PBI). Partial breast irradiation can also be accomplished with external beam radiation. The arrangement of beams to treat the lumpectomy cavity, however, is much more complicated than the normal tangential arrangement for whole-breast irradiation. Breast bridges, such as the one manufactured by Varian shown in Figure 24.18, made the interstitial placement of catheters more reproducible between patients, as opposed to freehand placement.[71]

A more recent development for noninvasive breast brachytherapy (NIBB), as opposed to the insertion of catheters or balloons, which can lead to infection, is the AccuBoost system, which immobilizes the breast for imaging and subsequent high–dose rate brachytherapy treatment.[72] NIBB using the AccuBoost system consists of a three-step process. In the first step, the breast is immobilized between two mammographic paddles, achieving a stable position for imaging and treatment. This immobilization of the breast aids in the delivery of the PBI without the uncertainties that can arise from delineating the target with a CT scan. Additionally, respiratory motion and daily setup errors can also affect the treatment if external beam radiation is used for the PBI. After the mammogram has been performed, the lumpectomy cavity is delineated, typically using radio-opaque clips placed at the time of surgery. The brachytherapy treatment

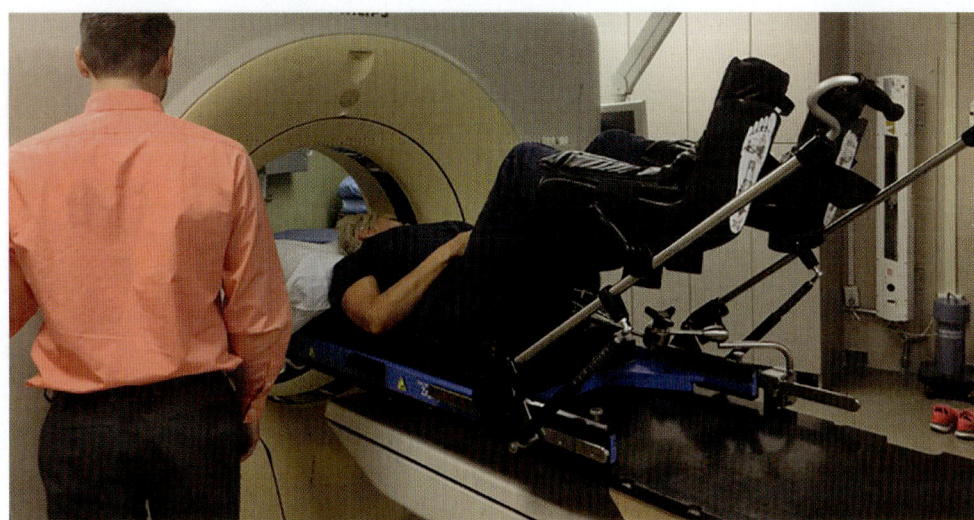

FIGURE 24.17. Zephyr patient transport system. The Zephyr patient transport system used to minimize patient movement during brachytherapy scanning, planning, and treatment. (Image provided courtesy of Diacor, Inc., Salt Lake City, UT.)

is then delivered in a parallel-opposed technique from each orthogonal direction, creating dose distributions shown in Figure 24.19.[73]

TOTAL BODY IRRADIATION IMMOBILIZATION

Several devices are available for clinical programs that include total body irradiation (TBI) with photons, generally utilized in preparation for bone marrow transplantation.

These devices can also be designed to rotate and may also support total skin irradiation (TSI) treatments for mycosis fungoides. Features of these systems generally include a beam spoiler, because a maximum dose at the skin entrance is preferred for TBI; systems for positioning partial lung blocks; and methods to keep the patient stable while standing for the treatments, which may take from 10 to 40 minutes, depending upon the treatment protocol. The major disadvantage for these systems is identifying storage in the treatment room; they are large and often take up vital space in the treatment area. It is important to note that these systems

FIGURE 24.18. Breast bridge system. The advanced breast bridge system **(left)** used for interstitial catheter placement and a CT scan showing a breast bridge along with the demarcated lumpectomy cavity **(right)** (*yellow*). (Top photo Courtesy of Varian, Palo Alto, CA. Bottom photo reprinted from Major T, Fröhlich G, Lövey K, et al. Dosimetric experience with accelerated partial breast irradiation using image-guided interstitial brachytherapy. *Radiother Oncol* 2007;90[1]:48–55. Copyright © 2007 Elsevier Ireland Ltd. With permission.)

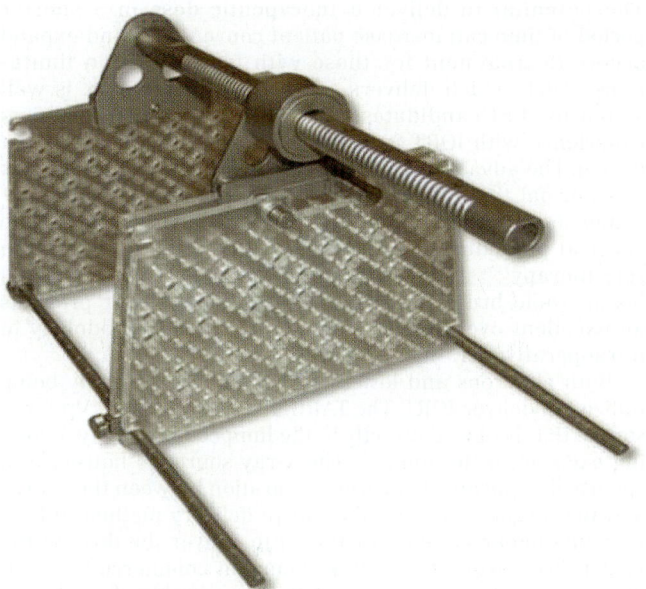

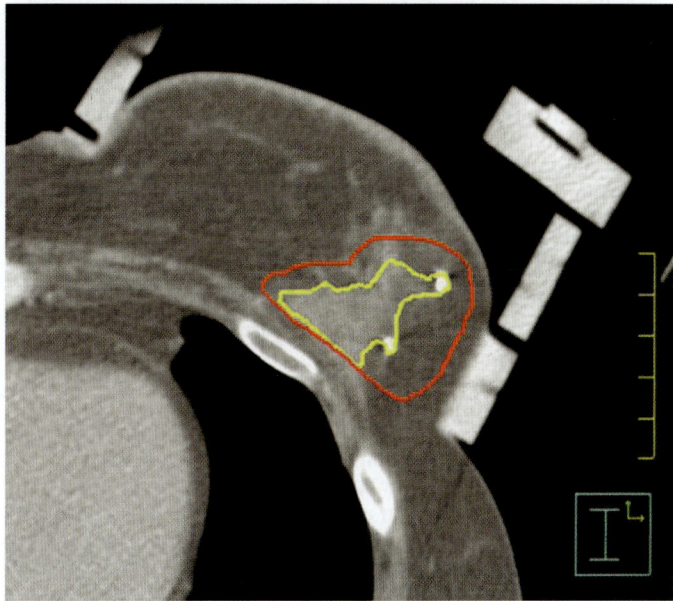

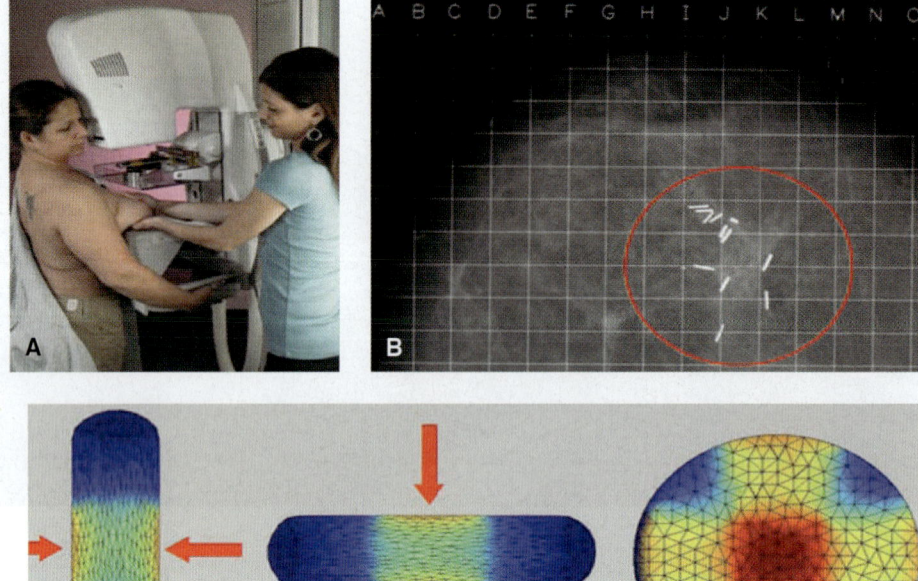

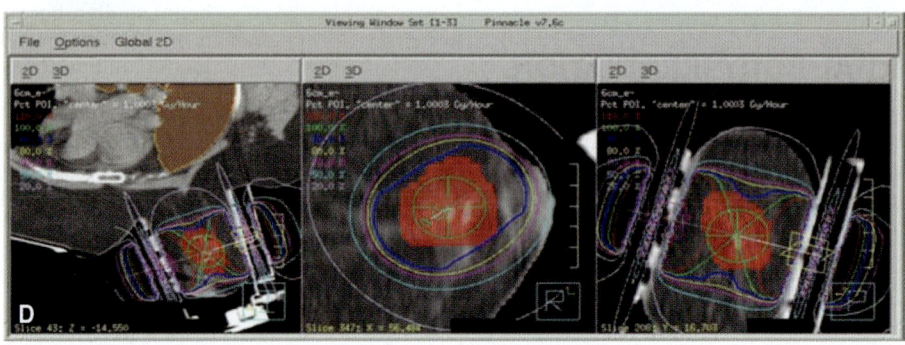

FIGURE 24.19. AccuBoost (Tyngsborough, MA) noninvasive image-guided breast brachytherapy. **A:** The breast is immobilized with mild compression and **(B)** kV image is obtained for tumor bed targeting and appropriate applicator selection. **C:** Schematic demonstrating breast compression and treatment in a parallel-opposed fashion sequentially along two orthogonal axes. **D:** Three-dimensional dose distribution covering the tumor bed using parallel-opposed applicators along a single-compression axis. (Reprinted from Hapel JT, Wazer DE. A comparison of brachytherapy techniques for partial breast irradiation. *Brachytherapy* 2012; 11[3]:163–175. Copyright © 2012 American Brachytherapy Society. With permission.)

usually operate at a distance of about 5 m from the target, with the gantry at a horizontal angle (90 or 270 degrees). Figure 24.20 shows two representative TBI devices from Radiation Products Design, Inc. and Mick Radio-Nuclear Instruments, Inc. Features such as a bicycle seat, handgrips, and shoulder stabilizers are used to help support the patient. Some photon TBI stands offer a harness that will provide an additional measure of security to prevent the patient from falling over in case the patient succumbs to fatigue and faints.

IMMOBILIZATION STRATEGIES FOR INTRAOPERATIVE RADIOTHERAPY

In intraoperative radiotherapy (IORT), a single high-dose fraction of radiation is delivered directly to the tumor bed immediately following surgical resection. The dose delivery occurs in the operating room while the patient is still under anesthesia. There is growing evidence that many low-risk breast cancer patients can achieve comparable local control with PBI as with traditional whole-breast radiotherapy.[68] Smaller volumes of irradiated tissue in PBI allows for treatment courses to be delivered on an accelerated schedule.

The potential to deliver a therapeutic dose in a shorter period of time can increase patient convenience and expand access to treatment for those with transportation limitations. IORT, which delivers a highly localized dose, is well suited for PBI candidates; and hence, most of the clinical experience with IORT is in the treatment of low-risk breast cancer. The advantages of IORT are lower rates of toxicity, as less normal tissue is irradiated, and enhanced patient convenience, as a therapeutic dose can be delivered during the surgical procedure.[74] IORT is currently being used as both sole therapy[75,76] and also as an upfront boost with external beam whole-breast therapy to follow.[77] Reitsamer presents an excellent overview of the rationale and methodology of intraoperative RT.[74]

Both electrons and low-kVp photons are currently being utilized to deliver IORT. The TARGIT trial uses a 50-kVp x-ray source that is placed directly in the lumpectomy cavity following excision of the tumor.[75] The x-ray source is housed in a spherical applicator to provide separation between the source and the target tissue. An alternative delivery method utilizes a mobile linear accelerator (linac) to deliver the dose to the target tissue with electrons. The current commercially available accelerators designed for IORT are capable of producing

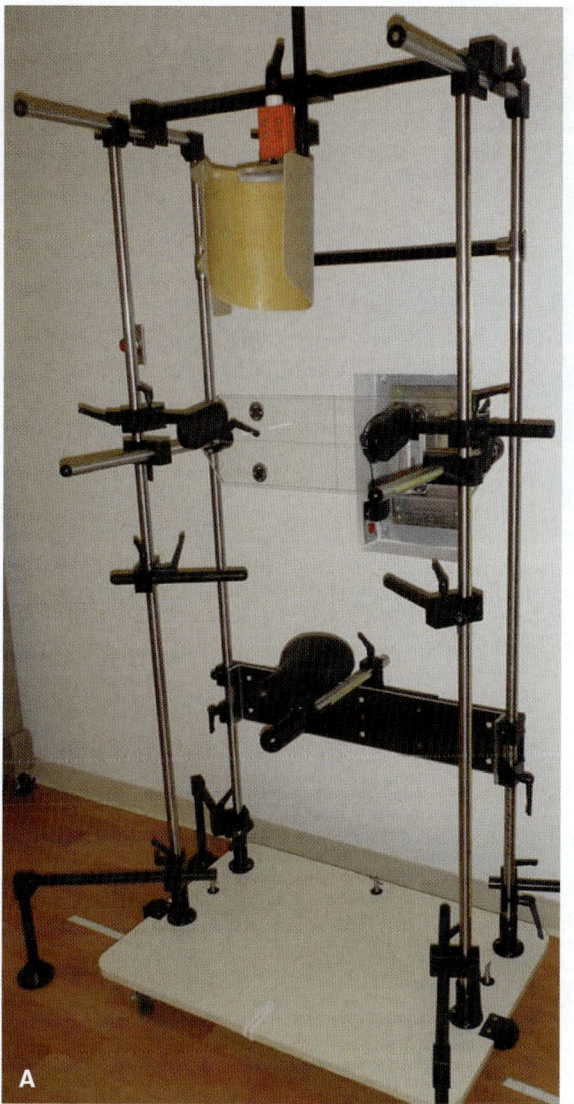
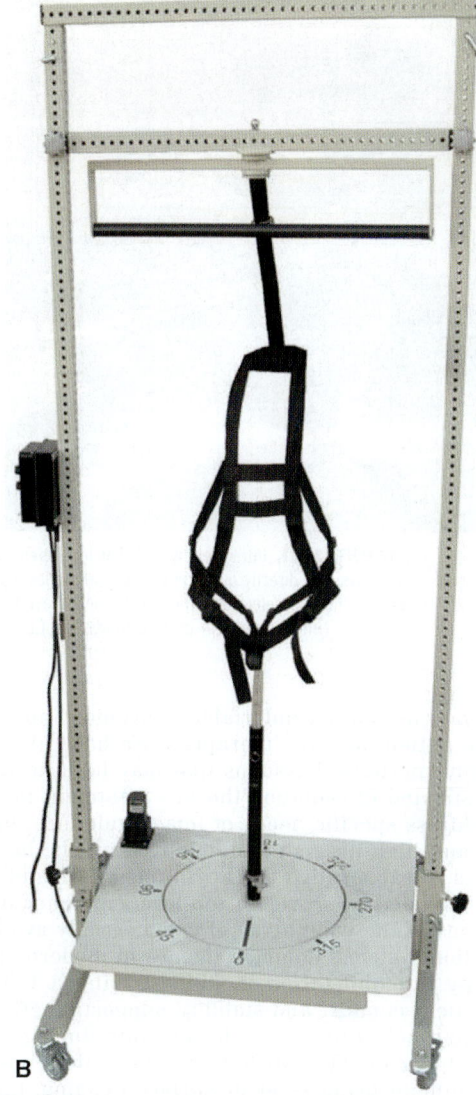

FIGURE 24.20. Total body irradiation (TBI) stand. A stand is commonly used to help position patients for TBI with photons and electrons. Common features of TBI stands include **(A)** handgrips and a seat to help support the patient. Note **(B)** the harness used to prevent the patient from falling in the case of fatigue and/or fainting. (**A** taken at University of Virginia, December 2011. **B**, courtesy of Radiation Products Design, Inc.)

electrons with energies up to 12 MeV, giving therapeutic ranges of up to roughly 3 cm in tissue. When using a linear accelerator–based delivery method for electron IORT, a collimator cone must be placed on the target tissue and then aligned with the electron beam exiting the linac.

One mobile accelerator system, the Mobetron, has an interesting method to immobilize and stabilize the irradiation geometry, illustrated in Figure 24.21. Following excision of the tumor, the tissue surrounding the lumpectomy cavity that is to be irradiated is sewn together by the surgeon. A metal shield is placed downstream of the target tissue to protect the thoracic wall and underlying lung tissue. The appropriate diameter collimator cone is chosen and placed by the physician directly over the target tissue. The linac is then rolled into place to be connected to the collimator cone. For most mobile accelerator systems, the linac must then be rigidly connected to the cone, a process termed "hard-docking," which requires great care and skill to properly align the linac while maintaining the physician's cone positioning. In

this situation, the end result is that the cone is attached to the linac itself. For the Mobetron system, the cone is immobilized following physician placement via a rigid arm clamped to the surgical table. A unique feature of the Mobetron is the "soft-docking" system in which an internal laser-guided system uses a mirror on the top of the cone to precisely align the radiation beam; the linac never actually contacts the collimating cone. The entire procedure is performed while the patient is under anesthesia.

SUMMARY: THE EVOLUTION OF PATIENT IMMOBILIZATION

Strategies to immobilize patients for radiotherapy have been developed since it was introduced as a treatment modality over 100 years ago. In this chapter, we have presented a wide array of simple devices that have continued to be used for decades, albeit with new designs and materials

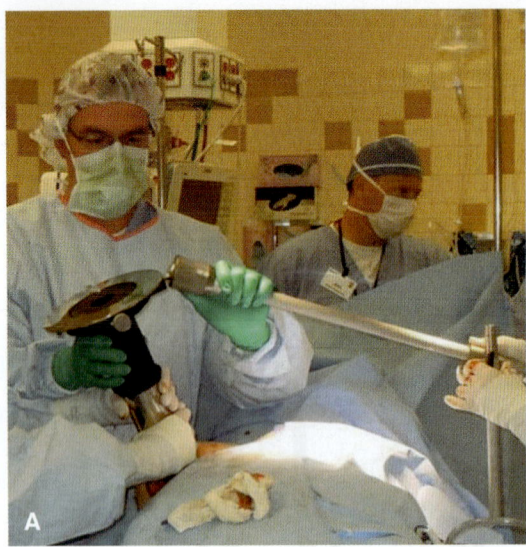
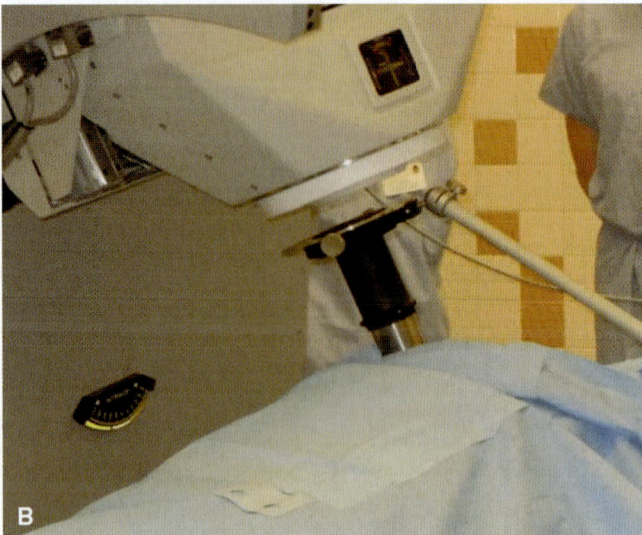

FIGURE 24.21. Intraoperative RT. For intraoperative radiotherapy with the Mobetron system **(A)**, the cone is placed by the physician directly over the target tissue following lumpectomy. The cone is fastened to the surgical table by a rigid arm. **B:** The linear accelerator is then positioned above the cone and automatically aligned using laser guidance with the mirror on the cone. (Images courtesy of IntraOp Medical Corporation, Sunnyvale, CA.)

that make their use more comfortable, convenient, and sanitary for the patient and the therapists. We have also presented highly specialized systems that may be used in the most sophisticated of radiation therapy treatment modalities that address specific needs of image guidance, highly conformal and high-dose stereotactic treatments, brachytherapy, and intraoperative therapy. Tables 24.1 and 24.2 have been included to provide a top level summary of the pros and cons of the wide array of commercially available immobilization systems. Common themes in modern radiation therapy immobilization include striking a balance between patient comfort and stability, supporting effective and safe approaches for target localization during treatment, and supporting systems to verify the patient position prior to treatment using x-ray or surface imaging. Image-guided radiation therapy (IGRT) and immobilization are interlinked, and IGRT is proving to play an increasing role with every type of treatment. It is therefore not surprising that the radiation therapy commercial industry will continue to focus on providing safe and effective immobilization that is compatible in both CT and MRI.

The importance of patient and applicator immobilization has begun to be integrated into brachytherapy treatments, especially with the development of IGBT, analogous to IGRT, in which the applicator is placed, simulation is performed, and the patient is treated with minimal motion of the patient or applicator. The advances that have been made in immobilization devices for external beam radiation, such as CT and MR compatibility, are finding increased use in brachytherapy. Integrated brachytherapy suites, which can combine imaging and treatment modalities, are becoming increasingly common.

In conclusion, effective radiation treatment is dependent on both the proper localization of the tumor as well as proper immobilization of the patient. As radiation therapy has evolved, so too have the strategies for immobilization of the patient. IGRT, including hypofractionated SBRT, as well as IGBT, require that the patient be comfortably immobilized to ensure that the radiation is properly delivered to the tumor. This is especially necessary as the dose per fraction is increased, which could lead to serious complications should the normal tissue surrounding the tumor receive excessive dose because of poor localization and immobilization.

REFERENCES

1. Dunscombe PB, et al. The investigation and rectification of field placement errors in the delivery of complex head and neck fields. *Int J Radiat Oncol Biol Phys* 1993;26(1):155–161.
2. Bentel GC, et al. Comparison of two head and neck immobilization systems. *Int J Radiat Oncol Biol Phys* 1997;38(4):867–873.
3. Gilbeau L, et al. Comparison of setup accuracy of three different thermoplastic masks for the treatment of brain and head and neck tumors. *Radiother Oncol* 2001;58(2):155–162.
4. Hurkmans CW, et al. Set-up verification using portal imaging; review of current clinical practice. *Radiother Oncol* 2001;58(2):105–120.
5. Velec M, et al. Cone-beam CT assessment of interfraction and intrafraction setup error of two head-and-neck cancer thermoplastic masks. *Int J Radiat Oncol Biol Phys* 2010;76(3):949–955.
6. Tsai JS, et al. A non-invasive immobilization system and related quality assurance for dynamic intensity modulated radiation therapy of intracranial and head and neck disease. *Int J Radiat Oncol Biol Phys* 1999;43(2):455–467.
7. Olch AJ, Lavey RS. Reproducibility and treatment planning advantages of a carbon fiber relocatable head fixation system. *Radiother Oncol* 2002;65(3):165–168.
8. Bentel GC, et al. Comparison of two repositioning devices used during radiation therapy for Hodgkin's disease. *Int J Radiat Oncol Biol Phys* 1997;38(4):791–795.
9. Carter DL, Marks LB, Bentel GC. Impact of setup variability on incidental lung irradiation during tangential breast treatment. *Int J Radiat Oncol Biol Phys* 1997;38(1):109–115.
10. Song PY, et al. A comparison of four patient immobilization devices in the treatment of prostate cancer patients with three dimensional conformal radiotherapy. *Int J Radiat Oncol Biol Phys* 1996;34(1):213–219.
11. Kim JY, et al. Intensity-modulated radiotherapy with a belly board for rectal cancer. *Int J Colorectal Dis* 2007;22(4):373–379.
12. Martin J, et al. Treatment with a belly-board device significantly reduces the volume of small bowel irradiated and results in low acute toxicity in adjuvant radiotherapy for gynecologic cancer: results of a prospective study. *Radiother Oncol* 2005;74(3):267–274.
13. Olofsen-van Acht M, et al. Reduction of irradiated small bowel volume and accurate patient positioning by use of a bellyboard device in pelvic radiotherapy of gynecological cancer patients. *Radiother Oncol* 2001;59(1):87–93.
14. Stegman LD, et al. Long-term clinical outcomes of whole-breast irradiation delivered in the prone position. *Int J Radiat Oncol Biol Phys* 2007;68(1):73–81.
15. Moody AM, et al. The influence of breast size on late radiation effects and association with radiotherapy dose inhomogeneity. *Radiother Oncol* 1994;33(2):106–112.
16. Griem KL, et al. Three-dimensional photon dosimetry: a comparison of treatment of the intact breast in the supine and prone position. *Int J Radiat Oncol Biol Phys* 2003;57(3):891–899.
17. Olch AJ, et al. Dosimetric effects caused by couch tops and immobilization devices: report of AAPM Task Group 176. *Med Phys* 2014;41(6):061501.
18. Lee KW, et al. Skin dose impact from vacuum immobilization device and carbon fiber couch in intensity modulated radiation therapy for prostate cancer. *Med Dosim* 2009;34(3):228–232.
19. Hadley SW, Kelly R, Lam K. Effects of immobilization mask material on surface dose. *J Appl Clin Med Phys* 2005;6(1):1–7.

20. Purdie TG, et al. Cone-beam computed tomography for on-line image guidance of lung stereotactic radiotherapy: localization, verification, and intrafraction tumor position. *Int J Radiat Oncol Biol Phys* 2007;68(1):243–252.

21. Li W, et al. Effect of immobilization and performance status on intrafraction motion for stereotactic lung radiotherapy: analysis of 133 patients. *Int J Radiat Oncol Biol Phys* 2011;81(5):1568–1575.

22. Heck B, et al. Accuracy and stability of positioning in radiosurgery: long-term results of the Gamma Knife system. *Med Phys* 2007;34(4):1487–1495.

23. Hong LX, et al. Clinical experiences with onboard imager KV images for linear accelerator-based stereotactic radiosurgery and radiotherapy setup. *Int J Radiat Oncol Biol Phys* 2009;73(2):556–561.

24. Ramakrishna N, et al. A clinical comparison of patient setup and intrafraction motion using frame-based radiosurgery versus a frameless image-guided radiosurgery system for intracranial lesions. *Radiother Oncol* 2010;95(1):109–115.

25. Salter BJ, et al. The TALON removable head frame system for stereotactic radiosurgery/radiotherapy: measurement of the repositioning accuracy. *Int J Radiat Oncol Biol Phys* 2001;51(2):555–562.

26. Kalapurakal JA, et al. Repositioning accuracy with the Laitinen frame for fractionated stereotactic radiation therapy in adult and pediatric brain tumors: preliminary report. *Radiology* 2001;218(1):157–161.

27. Das S, et al. Accuracy of relocation, evaluation of geometric uncertainties and clinical target volume (CTV) to planning target volume (PTV) margin in fractionated stereotactic radiotherapy for intracranial tumors using relocatable Gill-Thomas-Cosman (GTC) frame. *J Appl Clin Med Phys* 2010; 12(2):3260.

28. Kumar S, et al. Treatment accuracy of fractionated stereotactic radiotherapy. *Radiother Oncol* 2005;74(1):53–59.

29. Ruschin M, et al. Performance of a novel repositioning head frame for gamma knife perfexion and image-guided linac-based intracranial stereotactic radiotherapy. *Int J Radiat Oncol Biol Phys* 2010;78(1):306–313.

30. Ali I, et al. Evaluation of the setup accuracy of a stereotactic radiotherapy head immobilization mask system using kV on-board imaging. *J Appl Clin Med Phys* 2010;11(3):3192.

31. Tryggestad E, et al. Inter- and intrafraction patient positioning uncertainties for intracranial radiotherapy: a study of four frameless, thermoplastic mask-based immobilization strategies using daily cone-beam CT. *Int J Radiat Oncol Biol Phys* 2011;80(1):281–290.

32. Bova FJ, et al. The University of Florida frameless high-precision stereotactic radiotherapy system. *Int J Radiat Oncol Biol Phys* 1997;38(4):875–882.

33. Peng LC, et al. Quality assessment of frameless fractionated stereotactic radiotherapy using cone beam computed tomography. *Int J Radiat Oncol Biol Phys* 2010;78(5):1586–1593.

34. Hamilton AJ, et al. Preliminary clinical experience with linear accelerator-based spinal stereotactic radiosurgery. *Neurosurgery* 1995;36(2):311–319.

35. Gutierrez AN, et al. Clinical evaluation of an immobilization system for stereotactic body radiotherapy using helical tomotherapy. *Med Dosim* 2011;36(2):126–129.

36. Shah C, et al. Intrafraction variation of mean tumor position during image-guided hypofractionated stereotactic body radiotherapy for lung cancer. *Int J Radiat Oncol Biol Phys* 2012;82(5):1636–1641.

37. Keall PJ, et al. The management of respiratory motion in radiation oncology report of AAPM Task Group 76. *Med Phys* 2006;33(10):3874–3900.

38. Benedict SH, et al. Stereotactic body radiation therapy: the report of AAPM Task Group 101. *Med Phys* 2010;37(8):4078–4101.

39. Negoro Y, et al. The effectiveness of an immobilization device in conformal radiotherapy for lung tumor: reduction of respiratory tumor movement and evaluation of the daily setup accuracy. *Int J Radiat Oncol Biol Phys* 2001;50(4).889–898.

40. Eccles CL, et al. Interfraction liver shape variability and impact on GTV position during liver stereotactic radiotherapy using abdominal compression. *Int J Radiat Oncol Biol Phys* 2011;80(3):938–946.

41. Wunderink W, et al. Reduction of respiratory liver tumor motion by abdominal compression in stereotactic body frame, analyzed by tracking fiducial markers implanted in liver. *Int J Radiat Oncol Biol Phys* 2008;71(3):907–915.

42. Heinzerling JH, et al. Four-dimensional computed tomography scan analysis of tumor and organ motion at varying levels of abdominal compression during stereotactic treatment of lung and liver. *Int J Radiat Oncol Biol Phys* 2008;70(5):1571–1578.

43. Li G, et al. Characterization of optical-surface-imaging-based spirometry for respiratory surrogating in radiotherapy. *Med Phys* 2016;43(3):1348–1360.

44. Pallotta S, et al. A phantom evaluation of Sentinel™, a commercial laser/camera surface imaging system for patient setup verification in radiotherapy. *Med Phys* 2012;39(2):706–712.

45. Wikström K, et al. A comparison of patient position displacements from body surface laser scanning and cone beam CT bone registrations for radiotherapy of pelvic targets. *Acta Oncol* 2014;53(2):268–277.

46. Schonecker S, et al. Treatment planning and evaluation of gated radiotherapy in left-sided breast cancer patients using the Catalyst™/Sentinel™ system for deep inspiration breath-hold (DIBH). *Radiat Oncol* 2016;11(1):143.

47. Crop F, et al. Surface imaging, laser positioning or volumetric imaging for breast cancer with nodal involvement treated by helical TomoTherapy. *J Appl Clin Med Phys* 2016;17(5):6041.

48. Walter F, et al. Evaluation of daily patient positioning for radiotherapy with a commercial 3D surface-imaging system (Catalyst™). *Radiat Oncol* 2016;11:154.

49. Zagar TM, et al. Utility of deep inspiration breath hold for left-sided breast radiation therapy in preventing early cardiac perfusion defects: a prospective study. *Int J Radiat Oncol Biol Phys* 2017;97(5):903–909.

50. Tang X, et al. Clinical experience with 3-dimensional surface matching-based deep inspiration breath hold for left-sided breast cancer radiation therapy. *Pract Radiat Oncol* 2014;4(3):e151–e158.

51. Gierga DP, et al. A voluntary breath-hold treatment technique for the left breast with unfavorable cardiac anatomy using surface imaging. *Int J Radiat Oncol Biol Phys* 2012;84(5):e663–e668.

52. Manger RP, et al. Failure mode and effects analysis and fault tree analysis of surface image guided cranial radiosurgery. *Med Phys* 2015;42(5):2449–2461.

53. Li G, et al. Motion monitoring for cranial frameless stereotactic radiosurgery using video-based three-dimensional optical surface imaging. *Med Phys* 2011;38(7):3981–3994.

54. Cerviño LI, et al. Initial clinical experience with a frameless and maskless stereotactic radiosurgery treatment. *Pract Radiat Oncol* 2012;2(1):54–62.

55. Li G, et al. Clinical experience with two frameless stereotactic radiosurgery (fSRS) systems using optical surface imaging for motion monitoring. *J Appl Clin Med Phys* 2015;16(4):5416.

56. Pan H, et al. Frameless, real-time, surface imaging-guided radiosurgery: clinical outcomes for brain metastases. *Neurosurgery* 2012;71(4):844–852.

57. Pisansky TM, et al. High-dose-rate brachytherapy in the curative treatment of patients with localized prostate cancer. *Mayo Clin Proc* 2008;83(12):1364–1372.

58. Stone NN, et al. Prostate gland motion and deformation caused by needle placement during brachytherapy. *Brachytherapy* 2002;1(3):154–160.

59. Lakosi F, et al. Open MR-guided high-dose-rate (HDR) prostate brachytherapy: feasibility and initial experiences open MR-guided high-dose-rate (HDR) prostate brachytherapy. *Pathol Oncol Res* 2011;17(2):315–324.

60. Menard C, et al. MRI-guided HDR prostate brachytherapy in standard 1.5T scanner. *Int J Radiat Oncol Biol Phys* 2004;59(5):1414–1423.

61 Nag S, et al. Proposed guidelines for image based intracavitary brachytherapy for cervical carcinoma: report from Image-Guided Brachytherapy Working Group. *Int J Radiat Oncol Biol Phys* 2004;60(4):1160–1172.

62. Pham HT, et al. Changes in high-dose-rate tandem and ovoid applicator positions during treatment in an unfixed brachytherapy system. *Radiology* 1998;206(2):525–531.

63. Yaparpalvi R, et al. Skirt vs. stand applicator immobilization system in vaginal cylinder HDR brachytherapy. *Brachytherapy* 2008;7(2):152.

64. Hoskin PJ, Bownes P, Summers A. The influence of applicator angle on dosimetry in vaginal vault brachytherapy. *Br J Radiol* 2002;75(891):234–237.

65. Datta NR, et al. Variations of intracavitary applicator geometry during multiple HDR brachytherapy insertions in carcinoma cervix and its influence on reporting as per ICRU report 38. *Radiother Oncol* 2001;60(1):15–24.

66. Jaffray DA, et al. A facility for magnetic resonance-guided radiation therapy. *Semin Radiat Oncol* 2014;24(3):193–195.

67. Nag S. Zephyr—a novel "Airchusion" patient transportation system for transferring brachytherapy patients for imaging and treatment while minimizing risk of applicator displacement. *Brachytherapy* 2011;10:S97–S98.

68. Arthur DW, Vicini FA. Accelerated partial breast irradiation as a part of breast conservation therapy. *J Clin Oncol* 2005;23(8):1726–1735.

69. Arthur DW, et al. Accelerated partial breast irradiation: an updated report from the American Brachytherapy Society. *Brachytherapy* 2003;2(2):124–130.

70. Baglan KL, et al. The use of high-dose-rate brachytherapy alone after lumpectomy in patients with early-stage breast cancer treated with breast-conserving therapy. *Int J Radiat Oncol Biol Phys* 2001;50(4):1003–1011.

71. Major T, et al. Dosimetric experience with accelerated partial breast irradiation using image-guided interstitial brachytherapy. *Radiother Oncol* 2009;90(1):48–55.

72. Sioshansi S, et al. Dose modeling of noninvasive image-guided breast brachytherapy in comparison to electron beam boost and three-dimensional conformal accelerated partial breast irradiation. *Int J Radiat Oncol Biol Phys* 2011;80(2):410–416.

73. Hepel J, Wazer DE. A comparison of brachytherapy techniques for partial breast irradiation. *Brachytherapy* 2012;11(3):163–175.

74. Reitsamer R, et al. Concepts and techniques of intraoperative radiotherapy (IORT) for breast cancer. *Breast Cancer* 2008;15(1):40–46.

75. Vaidya JS, et al. The novel technique of delivering targeted intraoperative radiotherapy (Targit) for early breast cancer. *Eur J Surg Oncol* 2002;28(4):447–454.

76. Veronesi U, et al. Full-dose intraoperative radiotherapy with electrons during breast-conserving surgery: experience with 590 cases. *Ann Surg* 2005;242(1):101–106.

77. Reitsamer R, et al. The Salzburg concept of intraoperative radiotherapy for breast cancer: results and considerations. *Int J Cancer* 2006;118(11): 2882–2887.

Section II

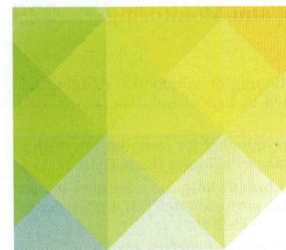

CHAPTER 25

Physics and Biology of Brachytherapy

Jeffrey F. Williamson and David J. Brenner

Brachytherapy (BT) (*brachy* is from the Greek for short distance) consists of placing sealed radioactive sources very close to or in contact with the target tissue. Because the absorbed dose falls off rapidly with increasing distance from the sources, high doses may be delivered safely to a localized target region over a short time. This chapter reviews the properties and applications of commonly used sealed radionuclides and sources, the basic biologic principles governing clinical response to BT, methods of dose calculation and source strength specification, and principles of implant design and dose specification for interstitial and intracavitary BT.

BASIC TERMINOLOGY

Implantation techniques may be classified in terms of surgical approach to the target volume (interstitial, intracavitary, transluminal, or mold techniques); the means of controlling the dose delivered (temporary or permanent implants); the source loading technology (preloaded, manually afterloaded, or remotely afterloaded); and the dose rate (low, medium, or high).

Intracavitary insertion consists of positioning applicators (bearing the radioactive sources) into a body cavity in close proximity to the target tissue. Intracavitary BT is used most widely for treatment of localized gynecologic malignancies and postoperative treatment in early-stage conservatively managed breast cancer. All intracavitary implants are *temporary implants*; they are left in the patient for a specified time to deliver the prescribed dose. With a few exceptions, during temporary implantation, the patient must be confined to a controlled, if not shielded, area in the hospital to manage the radiation safety hazard posed by the large ambient exposure rates around the implant.

Interstitial brachytherapy consists of surgically implanting small radioactive sources directly into the target tissues. A *permanent* interstitial implant remains in place indefinitely and is not removable; the initial source strength is chosen so that the prescribed dose is fully delivered only when the implanted radioactivity has decayed to a negligible level.

Surface-dose applications (sometimes called plesiocurie therapy or mold therapy) uses an applicator containing an array of radioactive sources, usually designed to deliver a uniform dose distribution, that is placed on the skin or mucosal surface immediately adjacent to the target tissue.

Transluminal brachytherapy consists of inserting a single line source into a body lumen to treat its surface and adjacent tissues.

Until the early 1960s, radioactive sources (needles for interstitial therapy or preloaded applicators for intracavitary therapy) were implanted directly into the patient. Radiation exposure to the brachytherapist and operating room staff was reduced significantly with the advent of *afterloading* technology.[1,2] *Manual afterloading* consists of implanting nonradioactive tubes or intracavitary applicators into the patient. Following transport of the patient to his or her room, sources are manipulated into the applicators by means of forceps and other handheld tools. Exposure to staff responsible for source loading and the care of BT patients can be greatly reduced or eliminated by the use of a *remote afterloading system*, which consists of a pneumatically driven or motor-driven source transport system for robotically transferring radioactive material between a shielded safe and each treatment applicator.

According to Report No. 38 of the International Commission on Radiation Units and Measurements (ICRU),[3] *low–dose rate* (*LDR*) implants deliver doses at the rate of 40 to 200 cGy/h (0.4 to 2 Gy/h), requiring treatment times of 24 to 144 hours, during which the patient is confined to an inpatient treatment room. At the other extreme, *high–dose rate* (*HDR*) BT uses dose rates in excess of 0.2 Gy/min (12 Gy/h). In fact, modern iridium-192 (^{192}Ir) HDR remote afterloaders deliver instantaneous dose rates as high as 0.12 Gy/s (430 Gy/h) at a distance of 1 cm, resulting in treatment times of a few minutes. Such treatments must be delivered in heavily shielded vaults using remote afterloading devices, but allow fractionated BT to be delivered on an outpatient basis. Medium–dose rate delivery, defined as the 2 to 12 Gy/h range, rarely is used. Although not recognized by ICRU Report No. 38, the ultralow dose rate (ULDR) range (0.01 to 0.3 Gy/h) is of great importance; it is the dose-rate domain used in permanent implants with ^{125}I and ^{103}Pd seeds.

PROPERTIES OF BRACHYTHERAPY SOURCES AND RADIONUCLIDES

The clinical utility of any radionuclide depends on physical properties such as half-life, radiation output per unit activity, specific activity (Ci/g), and photon energy. In addition, the methods of producing the radionuclide and its physical or chemical form strongly influence cost-effectiveness, safety, and toxicity. Detailed properties of BT radionuclides are listed in Table 25.1.

Photon Spectrum and Dosimetric Characteristics of Brachytherapy Sources

The dose delivered by a BT procedure depends on the individual source strengths, source arrangement, and implant duration as well as the dosimetric characteristics of the implanted sources. These dosimetric characteristics are described by specifying the distribution of dose rates per unit strength about the source, often in terms of an "away-and-along" table[4] in cartesian coordinates or in terms of the Task Group 43 protocol[5] described later in this chapter. The single-source dose distribution is of central importance to treatment planning because commercial computer planning systems estimate dose distribution from the spatial coordinates of the implanted sources using the principle of superposition. The source superposition algorithm estimates the contribution of each source, given its tip-and-end coordinates and the single-source dose-rate array, to each point of interest. These contribution estimates are summed to estimate the total dose rate at each point. Often, total dose rates are calculated over a two-dimensional (2D) grid of points and are represented as isodose rate curves.

For conventional BT, for which the therapeutically relevant distance range is 3 to 20 mm, only photons (γ-rays or characteristic x-rays) with energies in excess of 15 keV (kiloelectron volts) contribute to the therapeutic effect. In general, four factors influence the single-source dose distribution

Section
II

TABLE 25.1 PHYSICAL PROPERTIES AND USES OF BRACHYTHERAPY RADIONUCLIDES

Element	Isotope	Energy (MeV)	Half-Life	HVL-Lead (mm)	Exposure Rate Constant^a Γ_δ	Source Form	Clinical Application
Obsolete Sealed Sources of Historical Significance							
Radium	^{226}Ra	0.83 (average)	1,626 y	16	8.25^b	Tubes and needles	LDR intracavitary and interstitial
Radon	^{222}Rn	0.83 (average)	3.83 d	16	8.25^b	Gas encapsulated in gold tubing	Permanent interstitial Temporary molds
Currently Used Sealed Sources							
Cesium	^{137}Cs	0.662	30 y	3.28		Tubes and needles	LDR intracavitary and interstitial
Cesium	^{131}Cs	0.030	9.69 d	0.030	0.64	Seeds	LDR permanent implants
Iridium	^{192}Ir	0.397 (average)	73.8 d	6	4.69	Seeds in nylon ribbon; metal wires	LDR temporary interstitial Intravascular brachytherapy; cardiac
						Encapsulated source on cable	HDR interstitial and intracavitary Intravascular brachytherapy: peripheral
Cobalt	^{60}Co	1.25	5.26 y	11	13.07	Encapsulated spheres	HDR intracavitary
Iodine	^{125}I	0.028	59.6 d	0.025	1.45	Seeds	Permanent interstitial
Palladium	^{103}Pd	0.020	17 d	0.013	1.48	Seeds	Permanent interstitial
Gold	^{198}Au	0.412	2.7 d	6	2.35	Seeds	Permanent interstitial
Strontium/Yttrium	^{90}Sr–^{90}Y	2.24 β_{max}	28.9 y	–	–	Plaque Seeds	Treatment of superficial ocular lesions Intravascular brachytherapy
Electronic x-ray source	–	0.034	–	<0.03	–		Intracavitary breast brachytherapy
Developmental Sealed Sources							
Americium	^{241}Am	0.060	432 y	0.12	0.12	Tubes	LDR intracavitary
Ytterbium	^{169}Yb	0.093	32 d	0.48	1.80	Seeds	HDR interstitial
Californium	^{252}Cf	2.4 (average) neutron	2.65 y	–	–	Tubes	High-LET LDR intracavitary
Samarium	^{145}Sm	0.043	340 d	0.060	0.885	Seeds	LDR temporary interstitial

^{a}No filtration in units of R·cm²·mCi⁻¹·h⁻¹.
^{b}0.5-mm platinum filtration; units of R·cm²·mg⁻¹·h⁻¹.
HDR, high-dose rate; HVL, half-value layer; LDR, low-dose rate; LET, linear energy transfer.

for photon-emitting sources: (a) distance (inverse-square law), (b) absorption and scattering in the source core and encapsulation, (c) photon attenuation, and (d) scattering in the surrounding medium (Fig. 25.1). Encapsulation prevents radioactive material from leaking out of the source and absorbs nonpenetrating radiation (β-rays, α-rays, and low-energy photons), which would otherwise give rise to high surface doses while contributing nothing to the therapeutic effect.

Each voxel of radioactive core material shown in Figure 25.1 can be assumed to be an isotropic point source (Fig. 25.2). Because of the straight-line emission of photons with equal likelihood in all directions, photon intensity or

FIGURE 25.1. Typical cylindrical brachytherapy source, consisting of an active core (inner cylinder within which radioactivity is uniformly distributed) and the surrounding encapsulation (usually stainless steel or titanium for modern sources). The four principal factors influencing the relative dose distribution include (*1*) distance, (*2*) attenuation and scattering of photons by the source structure, and two competing effects of the surrounding medium: attenuation of primary photons (*3*) and accumulation of scattered photons (*4*) originating throughout the medium.

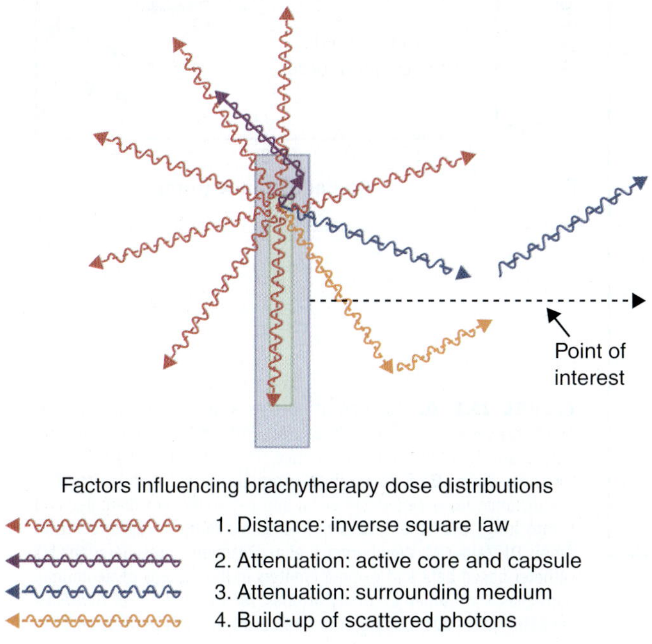

FIGURE 25.2. An *isotropic point source* of activity, A. To illustrate the derivation of inverse-square law, the source is surrounded by vacuum and placed at the center of two concentric spherical surfaces of radii r_1 and r_2. By definition, an *isotropic point source* has no extension and radiates photons with equal likelihood in all directions in straight-line paths.

Factors influencing brachytherapy dose distributions

1. Distance: inverse square law
2. Attenuation: active core and capsule
3. Attenuation: surrounding medium
4. Build-up of scattered photons

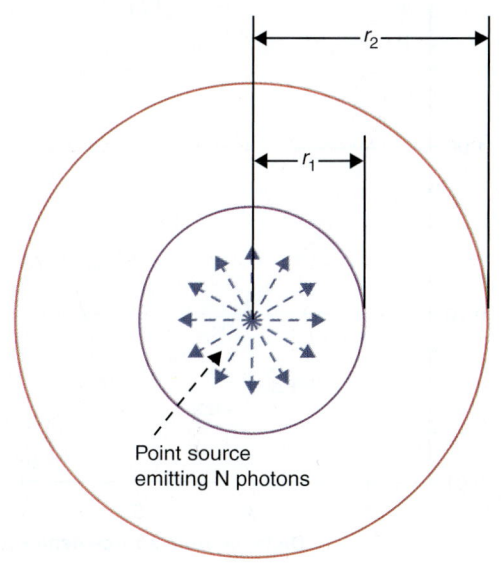
Point source
emitting N photons

fluence, $\Phi(r)$, at any point is proportional to the inverse square of its distance, r:

$$\Phi(r) = \frac{\text{no. of incident photons}}{\text{unit area irradiated}}$$
$$= \frac{\text{no. of photons emitted}}{4\pi r^2} \propto \text{dose}\,(r) \propto \text{exposure}\,(r) \qquad (1)$$

assuming that attenuation and scattering can be neglected.

As a result of this purely geometric effect, the absorbed doses $D(r_1)$ and $D(r_2)$ at the two distances r_1 and r_2 (Fig. 25.2) are related by:

$$\frac{D(r_1)}{D(r_2)} = \frac{\Phi(r_1)}{\Phi(r_2)} = \left(\frac{r_2}{r_1}\right)^2 \qquad (2)$$

This fundamental law applies exactly to each point of the radioactive core of the source shown in Figure 25.1 assuming that there is no attenuation and scattering of photons by the surrounding medium. However, Eq. (2) will not accurately describe the "collective" dose falloff arising from the combined action of the point sources distributed throughout the core, unless both r_1 and r_2 are large relative to the active source dimensions. Of the four factors influencing the dose distribution (Fig. 25.1), inverse-square law is by far the most important. For a pure isotropic point source, dose will decrease by a factor of 100 between the distances of 0.5 and 5 cm. The influence of the remaining factors over the same distance range rarely exceeds a factor of 2 or 3. Consequently, the dosimetric characteristics of implants (e.g., the heterogeneous dose distribution within the target tissue and rapid falloff of dose outside the implanted volume) can be accounted for by applying inverse-square law to each pointlike element of radioactivity within the implant. Control of intersource spacing and positioning relative to the target and dose-limiting tissues is the most challenging issue in delivering BT.

Although inverse-square law dominates BT dose distributions, the surrounding medium and the source structure do significantly affect the dose distribution (Fig. 25.1). The source

core and surrounding capsule reduce dose at the point of interest through absorption and scattering of primary photons. Primary photons contributing dose to points located near the longitudinal source axis (cylindrical axis of the source or axis of rotation) must traverse longer pathlengths of capsule and core material and therefore experience more attenuation than do photons contributing dose to equidistant points on the transverse source axis (plane perpendicular to the longitudinal source axis that bisects its active core). For any fixed distance from the source center, doses near the longitudinal axis are usually smaller than on the transverse axis. This phenomenon is known as *oblique filtration* and is the main cause of dose *anisotropy* (variation of dose as a function of polar angle at each fixed distance relative to the source center) characteristic of extended BT sources. Because BT sources are cylindrically symmetric, the dose distribution will be equatorially isotropic (constancy of dose as a function of azimuthal angle for each fixed polar angle and distance).

The tissue-equivalent medium surrounding the source affects the dose distribution in two competing ways (factors 3 and 4 of Fig. 25.1). At each point of interest, the intervening medium reduces the dose distribution by attenuating primary photons (deflecting them from their straight-line trajectories). At the same time, photons are being emitted in all directions from the source and interacting with the medium by means of Compton scattering and photoelectric absorption. Thus, each volume element of tissue is effectively radiating scattered photons in all directions, many of which contribute to dose at the point of interest. This mechanism, known as scattered-photon buildup, enhances the dose. The overall influence of the surrounding medium is the combined effect of these two competing processes: photon attenuation and scattered-photon build-up. In contrast to external beam therapy, in which the scattering volume is limited to a narrow cone, scattered photons dominate BT dose distributions at distances >2 cm. Photon scattering is the main source of complexity in BT dose measurement and algorithm development.

Figure 25.3 demonstrates that the relative dose versus distance from the source is nearly independent of its photon

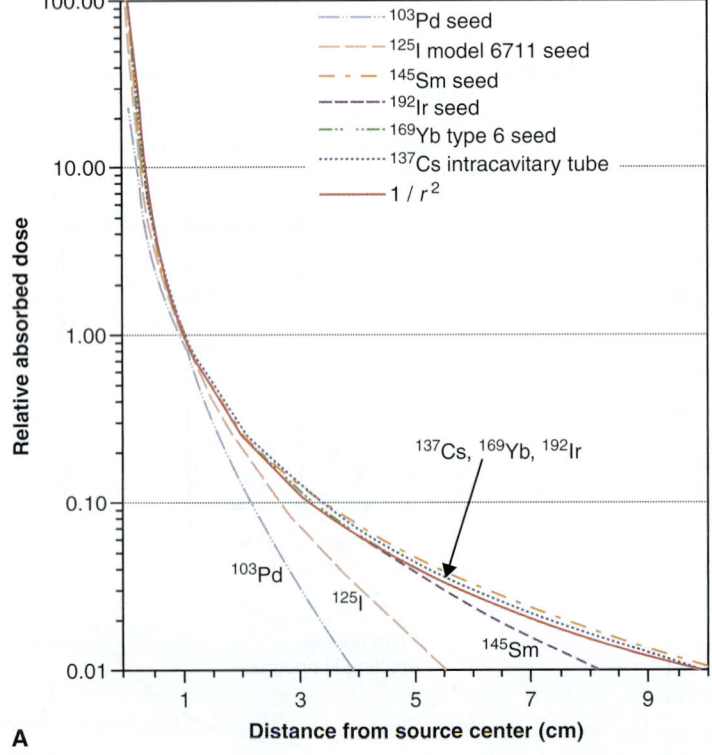

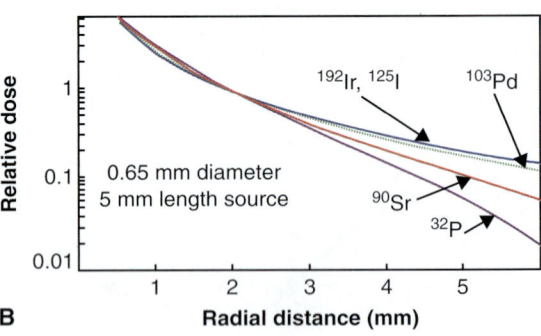

FIGURE 25.3. A: Variation of dose as a function of distance for point sources of ^{60}Co, ^{226}Ra, ^{137}Cs, ^{198}Au, ^{192}Ir, and ^{125}I. The results are normalized to 100% at 1-cm distance. The function $(1/r^2)$ is plotted for comparison. **B:** Relative dose (normalized to 1.0 at 1 mm) versus distance for various cylindrical sources (0.65 mm diameter and 5 mm long) over the 1 to 5 mm distance range. (Reprinted from Amols HI, Zaider M, Weinberger J, et al. Dosimetric considerations for catheter-based beta and gamma emitters in the therapy of neointimal hyperplasia in human coronary arteries. *Int J Radiat Oncol Biol Phys* 1996;36[4]:913–921. Copyright © 1996 Elsevier. With permission.)

energy so long as the average photon energy is >200 keV. In this energy range, dose deviates from inverse-square law by <5% over the 1- to 5-cm distance range. All of the "radium-equivalent" isotopes, including ^{137}Cs, ^{192}Ir, and [198]Au, fall into this energy range. This behavior, which greatly simplifies BT dosimetry, is the result of equilibrium between primary photon attenuation and buildup of scattered photons. Only for low-energy sources (e.g., [103]Pd and ^{125}I) does the depth–dose curve significantly deviate from inverse-square law. Because photon absorption rather than Compton scattering dominates energy deposition below 40 keV, scatter buildup is unable to compensate for loss of dose resulting from attenuation.

For radium-equivalent radionuclides, Figure 25.4A and B shows that both absolute dose rates (cGy/h to fat or water tissue per mgRaEq or unit air-kerma strength [S_K]) and relative dose distributions are nearly independent of energy and composition of the surrounding medium above 100 keV. Compton scattering, which dominates photon absorption and scattering above 100 keV, depends mainly on electron density (electrons/g) of the medium, which is nearly constant for all biologic materials. Below this energy range, absolute and relative dose distributions vary significantly with energy and composition (atomic number) of the surrounding medium. Implanting an ^{125}I seed in fat medium (effective atomic number of Z_{eff} = 6) will deliver about half the absorbed dose at 1 cm, compared to the expected dose in water (Z_{eff} = 7.5). This is because energy absorption per unit mass from photoeffect interactions is proportional to the cube of the atomic number ($Z_{eff}{}^3$) of the medium. Despite the significant impact

of tissue composition heterogeneities on low-energy seed BT dose delivery, only recently have treatment planning and dose measurement practices began to address tissue and applicator inhomogeneities.[6]

Figure 25.4B demonstrates that the inverse-square law actually underestimates relative dose at 5 cm by as much as a factor of 2 in the 60- to 100-keV energy range. In this narrow energy range, called the intermediate low-energy range, photoelectric effect is negligible, whereas Compton scattering transfers most of the colliding primary photon energy to the scattered photon rather than to the Compton electron. As a result of this imbalance between energy absorption and photon scattering, buildup of scattered photons overcompensates for loss of dose as a result of primary photon attenuation out to distances of 4 to 6 cm.

Above the 100-keV threshold, the photon energy spectrum is much less important to optimizing BT dose-rate distributions than in external beam therapy. Because artificial BT radionuclides in this energy range (^{60}Co, ^{137}Cs, ^{192}Ir, [198]Au) have dose-rate distributions nearly identical to those of [226]Ra in the 1- to 5-cm distance range, they are referred to as radium substitutes.

Figure 25.3C demonstrates that although photon energy is a relatively unimportant determinant of radium-equivalent tissue dosimetry, it significantly influences the cost, weight, and thickness of shielding required to protect critical anatomic structures in the patient and personnel involved in patient care. The half-value layer (HVL) in lead varies from 0.5 mm for a 100-keV source to 12 mm for ^{60}Co BT sources. Thus, for classical radium-equivalent BT, a radionuclide with

Section II

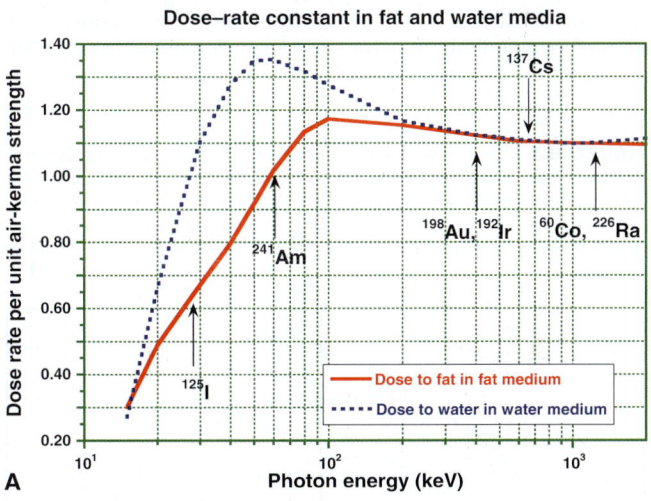

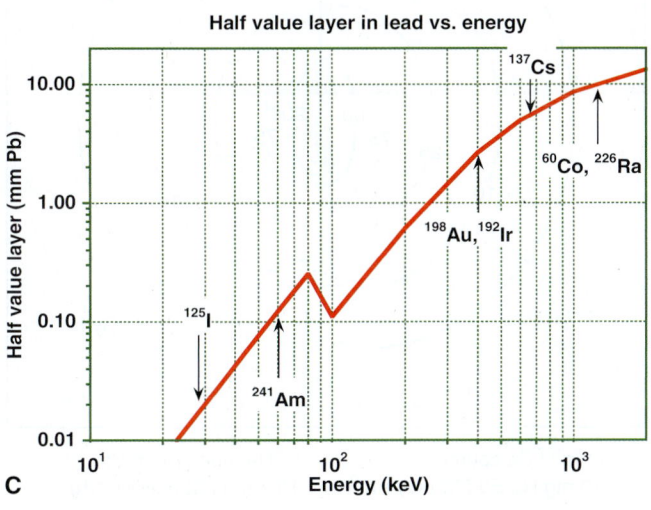

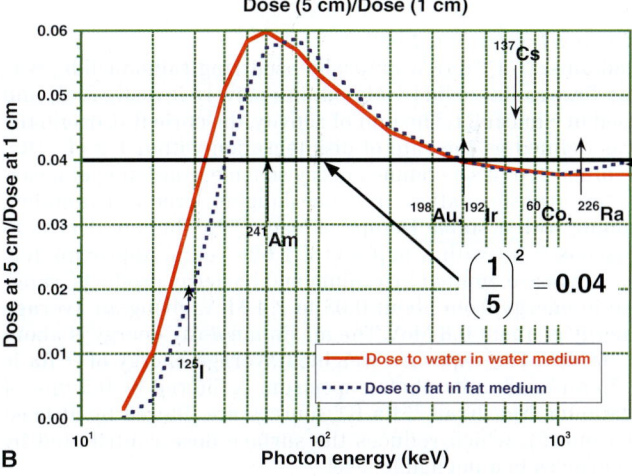

FIGURE 25.4. Variation of dosimetric properties of monoenergetic point sources as a function of photon energy. The location (in terms of average energy) of commonly used radionuclides is indicated by the labeled *vertical arrows*. **A:** Absolute dose rate per unit source strength in fat and water media at 1-cm distance. Source strength is specified in terms of output in air. **B:** Dose at 5 cm as a fraction of dose at 1 cm in fat and water media. The effect of inverse-square law, (1/5)² = 0.04, is shown for comparison as a *broken line*. **C:** Half-value layer in lead, the thickness (mm) in lead required to reduce primary dose by a factor of 2.

a mean energy of about 100 to 200 keV is optimal. The major benefit of ^{125}I and ^{103}Pd as a BT source is the ability to provide complete protection by thin lead foils (0.1 to 0.2 mm), greatly reducing exposure to physicians during the implant procedure and allowing permanent-implant patients to be released from medical confinement without posing a radiation safety hazard to the general public. Recently, interest has been expressed in using radionuclides in the intermediate low-energy range (60 to 120 keV).[7-9] Tissue dose distributions are still approximately radium equivalent in this energy range, and thin layers of lead provide significant sparing of dose-limiting normal tissues near the implanted volume.

Intracavitary Sources for Low–Dose Rate Gynecologic Brachytherapy

Since the 1930s, sources for classical LDR intracavitary BT have taken the form of "tubes" having a physical length of 2 to 2.5 cm and an external diameter of about 3 mm. For treatment systems influenced by the Manchester[10] and M.D. Anderson[11] treatment techniques, active lengths of 1.3 to 1.5 cm are typical. Radionuclides for intracavitary applications should have a half-life long enough to support a 5- to 10-year working life without large variations in prescription dose rate so that the high cost of these reusable sources can be amortized over a large number of patient treatments. The average photon energy should be at least 60 to 100 keV, as the dose falloff for lower-energy sources (e.g., ^{125}I) is too rapid to adequately treat the target-volume periphery (2 to 5 cm from the applicator center) without overtreating the mucosal tissues in contact with the applicator system.

Radium-226 Sources

Radium-226 (^{226}Ra), a naturally occurring radionuclide, was the first radionuclide isolated, intensively investigated, and used in clinical BT. The unit of activity, the curie (Ci), originally was defined as the rate of disintegration within 1 g of ^{226}Ra. Radium-226 has a complex decay scheme, consisting of a cascade of transformations from one daughter product to another, ending with a stable isotope of lead, $^{206}_{82}$Pb. Radium decays to gaseous ^{222}Rn with a half-life of 1,626 years. Approximately 75 γ-rays are emitted by radium and its decay products, ranging in energy from about 0.05 to 2.4 MeV, giving an average energy of about 0.8 MeV. The maximum β-ray energy is about 3.26 MeV. The exposure-weighted average energy of ^{226}Ra is 1.25 MeV when its photon spectrum is filtered by 0.5 mm of platinum. Nearly all ^{226}Ra BT sources are filtered by at least 0.5 mm Pt, which reduces the surface dose contributed by β particles to a negligible level.

Clinical ^{226}Ra sources consisted of discrete cells of radium salt (radium sulfate plus filler) placed in needles or tubes with platinum walls of thickness of 0.5 and 1.0 mm, respectively. Intracavitary radium tubes were usually 22 mm long, containing 5 to 30 mg of radium (S_K = 30 to 200 μGy·m^2·h^{-1}), with active lengths of 15 mm. For interstitial BT, the full-, half-, and quarter-intensity needles popularized by the Manchester LDR implant system typically contain 0.66, 0.33, or 0.165 mg of radium per centimeter of active length, respectively.

The clinical use of radium has disappeared and is now only of historic interest. The potential of damaged sources to leak radioactive salts or emit radon gas (^{222}Rn) is the major reason for its decline, and the exposure hazard to interstitial BT practitioners.[12] Further, the long half-life and disposal costs of spent ^{226}Ra sources present a significant financial liability. However, because of its many years of therapeutic use, several widely used quantities for source strength specification and prescription of intracavitary treatment are derived from the early experience with ^{226}Ra.

Cesium-137 Sources

Cesium-137, a fission by-product, was a popular radium substitute because of its 30-year half-life, dominating gynecologic intracavitary brachytherapy from 1970 to 2000. Its single γ-ray (0.66 MeV) is less penetrating (HVL$_{Pb}$ = 0.65 cm) than the γ-rays from radium (HVL$_{Pb}$ = 1.4 cm) or ^{60}Co (HVL$_{Pb}$ = 1.1 cm). Because ^{137}Cs decays to solid barium 137, ^{137}Cs sources have virtually replaced ^{226}Ra intracavitary tubes in LDR gynecologic applications.

Cesium-137 BT sources were introduced in the early 1960s.[13,14] Recently marketed sources, for example, the Amersham model CDCS-J tube and 3M model 6500 intracavitary tube, consist of radioactive cesium distributed within an insoluble glass or ceramic matrix,[4] which produces far less radiochemical hazard from ruptured sources than does the radon gas or cesium salts. These sources are encapsulated in stainless steel sheaths with wall thicknesses of 0.5 to 1.0 mm, active lengths of 13.5 to 15 mm, diameters of 2.6 to 3.1 mm, and total lengths of about 20 mm. Figure 25.5 shows that cesium and radium sources produce nearly identical transverse-axis dose–rate distributions when their active lengths and source strengths are the same. However, the ^{226}Ra tube isodose curves exhibit significant retraction along the longitudinal source axis as a result of oblique filtration of ^{226}Ra γ-rays through the dense (ρ = 21 g·cm^{-3}) 1-mm-thick platinum capsule. In contrast, lightly filtered ^{137}Cs tubes produce nearly elliptical isodose curves. Consequently, vaginal applicator systems containing modern ^{137}Cs sources with their axes positioned perpendicular to the coronal patient plane (e.g., the Fletcher colpostat) always will give rise to higher bladder and rectal doses than when loaded with ^{226}Ra tubes.[15] However, LDR brachytherapy has been largely abandoned in favor of HDR BT using high-intensity ^{192}Ir sources, with 85% of respondents in a recent survey reporting use of HDR

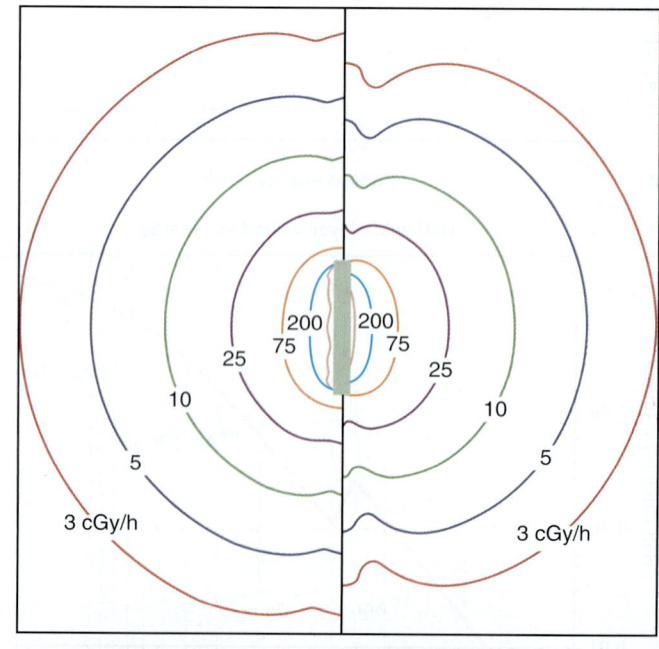

FIGURE 25.5. Comparison of isodose curves for a modern steel-clad ^{137}Cs source *(left)* containing radioactive ceramic pellets (From Williamson JF. Dose calculations about shielded gynecological colpostats. *Int J Radiat Oncol Biol Phys* 1990;19:167–178, with permission) and a ^{226}Ra tube *(right)* consisting of a RaSO$_4$ core encapsulated in 1-mm thick Pt. Both sources have an air-kerma strength of 72 μGy·m^2·h^{-1} (10 mgRaEq).

Oris^{137}Cs source
10 mg Ra Eq (72 μGy • m^2/h)

^{226}Ra tube (1 mm Pt)
10.7 mg (72 μGy • m^2/h)

or pulsed dose-rate (PDR) BT.[16] [137]Cs intracavitary tubes and other source configurations ceased to be commercially available in 2014. Recently manufactured but "orphaned" sources still in clinical use include intracavitary tubes produced by Isotope Product Laboratories[17] and Eckert & Ziegler BEBIG.[18]

Experimental Intracavitary Brachytherapy Radionuclides

Californium-252 is a unique radionuclide that decays by α-emission with a half-life of 2.65 years and emits neutrons by spontaneous fission with average energies of 2.1 to 2.3 MeV. Depending on the distance from the source, one-half to two-thirds of the total dose is the result of the neutron component. Assuming a relative biologic effectiveness (RBE) of 6 for the neutron component, approximately 90% of the biologically effective dose derives from the neutron component. The radiobiologic rationale for using [252]Cf, especially in treating bulky gynecologic malignancies, is that the high linear energy transfer (LET) neutron component more effectively depopulates the tumor's radioresistant hypoxic core, thereby improving local control, while the rapid dose falloff maintains an acceptable level of late complications.[19] Californium-252 tube sources[20] require carefully designed radiation protection and source handling procedures to reduce radiation exposure hazards to an acceptable level, because of the high neutron quality factor of 10 to 20 that is assumed by radiation protection standards.[21] Oak Ridge National Laboratory ceased fabrication of [252]Cf sources for medical use in 1997. To date, [252]Cf medical sources are not being manufactured elsewhere in the world. However, [252]Cf brachytherapy continues to be of clinical interest. Two groups who are actively practicing brachytherapy have recently reported long-term clinical experiences[22,23] based on cohorts of locally advanced cervical cancer patients treated relatively recently with orphan [252]Cf intracavitary sources and remote afterloading systems.

Ytterbium-169 ([169]Yb)[8] and americium-241 ([241]Am)[7] are examples of so-called intermediate low-energy photon emitters, giving rise to 60- and 100-keV photons, respectively. The emitted photon energy is low enough that relatively thin lead foils can be used to shield personnel and dose-limiting tissues in the patient, but high enough that the resultant dose distributions in tissue remain approximately radium equivalent.[24] Because relatively thin lead sheets can be used to shield critical structures (e.g., 0.4-mm-thick lead for 50% dose reduction from [169]Yb), customized rectal and bladder shielding can be more easily fabricated. Ytterbium-169 seeds[8] (100-keV mean energy, 32-day half-life) have been investigated as a possible substitute for ^{192}Ir in interstitial implants[25] and for intracavitary treatment. In addition, [169]Yb has an extremely high specific activity. Despite recent efforts to design and fabricate [169]Yb sources and accessories for both LDR[26] and HDR remote afterloading[9] brachytherapy, none of these systems has been commercially realized. Other promising medium-energy photon–emitting radionuclides under investigation for brachytherapy applications include [57]Co,[27] [153]Gd,[28] and [101]Rh.[29]

Sources for Low–Dose Rate Temporary Interstitial Brachytherapy

The main additional requirement for radionuclides used in temporary interstitial BT is a specific activity sufficient to support fabrication of miniaturized sources (<2 mm external diameter) so as to minimize trauma to the implanted tissues. Current interstitial implantation techniques favor disposable sources containing short-lived radionuclides that support afterloading and customization of active length.

Nonafterloading ("Preloaded") Sources: Radium and Cesium Needles

Radium-226 needles were the mainstay of interstitial BT until about 1970. These sources had external diameters of 1.5 to 2 mm, active lengths ranging from 3 mm to 4.5 cm, and Pt–Ir alloy encapsulation ranging from 0.5 to 0.65 mm in thickness. Because needle implantation can result in large exposures to the radiation oncologist's fingers, as well as whole-body exposure to operating room and implant imaging staff, neither interstitial implantation of [226]Ra nor ^{137}Cs needles is currently practiced.

Afterloading Interstitial Sources: [192]Ir Ribbons and Wires

Temporary interstitial BT experienced a renaissance in the 1960s because of the introduction of [192]Ir.[12] This useful radionuclide is produced by bombarding nonradioactive [191]Ir with thermal neutrons in a nuclear reactor, which is available in relatively pure form, has an extremely large neutron capture cross section, and produces no significant contaminant radioisotopes. Because of these properties, very high specific activities can be achieved. Miniaturized interstitial sources can be fabricated relatively cheaply. The use of ^{192}Ir in BT was pioneered by Ulrich Henschke,[30] who developed a family of widely used afterloading techniques, and to Pierquin and Dutreix,[31] who developed the ^{192}Ir-based Paris interstitial system in the early 1960s.

Iridium-192 has a 73.8-day half-life and a complex decay scheme, dominated by β decay to [192]Pt, but also including some electron capture and β+ decay. Its photon spectrum includes characteristic x-rays and γ-rays ranging from 63 keV to 1.4 MeV and has an exposure-weighted average energy of 397 keV. Compared with higher-energy ^{137}Cs, the thicknesses of lead and concrete shielding can be reduced by 33% and 20%, respectively.[32] More important advantages of ^{192}Ir sources are compatibility with afterloading techniques, technical flexibility, and patient comfort.

In the United States, ^{192}Ir is still available (but rarely used) in the form of seeds, 0.5 mm in diameter and 3 mm long, for LDR BT. The seeds are encapsulated in a 0.8-mm-diameter nylon ribbon and spaced at 1- or 0.5-cm center-to-center intervals and are available in strengths of 1 to 150 μGy·m²·h⁻¹ (0.1 to 20 mgRaEq). In Europe, ^{192}Ir was used in the form of a wire (0.3- or 0.6-mm outer diameter) consisting of an iridium–platinum radioactive core encased in a 0.1-mm sheath of platinum. In addition to eliminating radiation exposure hazards in the operating room, ^{192}Ir ribbons and wires can be trimmed to the appropriate active length for each catheter. Manual and remotely afterloading LDR interstitial brachytherapy utilization has markedly declined in the developed world over the last two decades. A recent survey[33] indicates that in high-income European countries, only 11% of brachytherapy procedures performed in 2007 used LDR techniques compared to HDR (52%), PDR (10%), and permanent seed implants (21%).

Low-Energy Sources for Temporary Interstitial Brachytherapy

High-intensity ^{125}I sources[34] have been proposed for temporary interstitial implantation at classical dose rates. High-intensity ^{125}I seeds[35,36] now are used routinely as temporary interstitial sources for episcleral plaque treatment of intraocular choroidal melanoma.[37] By placing a 0.5-mm-thick gold shield over the episcleral plaque, tissues posterior to the eye are shielded, and radiation directed toward the tumor is partially collimated.[38] A disadvantage of high-intensity ^{125}I seed therapy is their high cost relative to ^{192}Ir seeds.

Section II

Sources for Permanent Interstitial Brachytherapy

There are two basic approaches to permanent implantation. Classical LDR permanent BT originally used ^{222}Rn seeds, and more recently ^{198}Au seeds, both of which have half-lives of a few days. To manage the radiation hazard as a result of the high-energy γ-rays emitted by these sources, the patient must be confined to the hospital until the source strength decays to a safe level (two to three half-lives or about 10 days). The contemporary approach to permanent implantation, ULDR BT, uses longer-lived but low-energy photon emitters (e.g., ^{103}Pd and ^{125}I). The patient's tissues or a thin lead foil is sufficient to limit ambient exposure rates to negligible levels, eliminating the need to hospitalize patients solely for radiation protection. During the implant procedure, low-energy photon sources markedly reduce radiation exposure to operating room personnel and to the radiation oncologist's hands.

Mathematics of Radioactive Decay

The phenomenon of exponential decay results in a reciprocal relationship between dose rate achieved and radionuclide half-life. The total activity, $A(t)$, present in the implant after an interval of time t has elapsed after source insertion is given by Figure 25.6:

$$A(t) = A(0) \cdot e^{-\ln 2 \cdot t / T_{1/2}} \qquad (3)$$

where $A(0)$ is the activity at the time of insertion, ln 2 is the natural logarithm of 2 (equal to 0.693), and $T_{1/2}$ is the half-life of the radionuclide. The quantity ln $2/T_{1/2}$, represented by the symbol λ, is called the decay constant. Equation (3) is applicable to any measure of source strength (S_K, equivalent mass of radium, etc.). Because dose rate, $\dot{D}(t)$, at time t is proportional to activity, that is, $\dot{D}(t) \propto A(t)$, we can write:

$$\dot{D}(t) = \dot{D}(0) \cdot e^{-t \cdot \ln 2 / T_{1/2}} \qquad (4)$$

where $\dot{D}(0)$ is the dose rate at the time of source insertion. The total dose, $D(T)$, accumulated over time interval T after source insertion, is the shaded area under the curve of Figure 25.6 and can be obtained by integrating Eq. (4):

$$D(T) = \dot{D}(0) \cdot \int_0^T e^{-t \cdot \ln 2 / T_{1/2}} \cdot dt$$
$$= \dot{D}(0) \cdot T_{1/2} \cdot 1.443 \left[1 - e^{-T \cdot 0.693 / T_{1/2}} \right] \qquad (5)$$

FIGURE 25.6. Illustration of exponential decay of source strength and dose rate. The area of the shaded region is the total dose administered to the patient over treatment time, T.

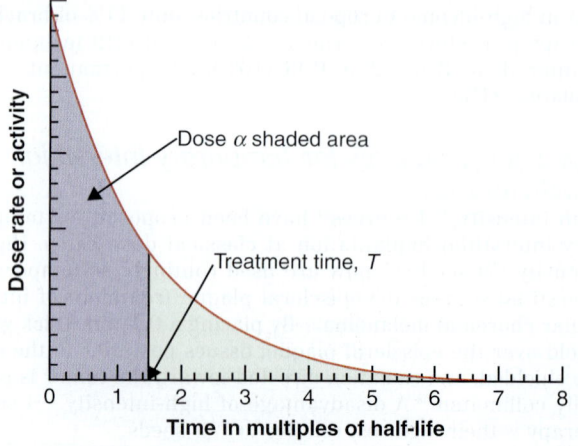

The product $T_a = 1.443 T_{1/2}$ is called the average life of the radionuclide and is the time required for all radioactive atoms to decay assuming the rate of decay remains fixed at its initial value, $A(0)$. Equation (5) should be used to calculate the total dose delivered by any implant when the treatment time, T, is more than 5% of the half-life. For shorter treatment times (<4 days for ^{192}Ir or <3 days for ^{125}I), the approximate expression:

$$D(T) = \dot{D}(0) \cdot T \qquad (6)$$

is accurate within 2%.

For permanent implants, the total dose administered to the patient, D_{tot}, resulting from complete decay of the implant can be obtained from Eq. (5):

$$D_{tot} = \lim_{T \to \infty} D(T) = 1.443 \cdot T_{1/2} \cdot \dot{D}(0) = T_a \cdot \dot{D}(0) \qquad (7)$$

This equation demonstrates that initial dose rate and radionuclide half-life are in reciprocal relationship with one another: the longer the half-life, the lower the dose rate will be. Typical total dose rates and total doses are given in Table 25.2 for commonly used permanent implant sources. These sources fall into two categories: short-lived radium-substitute sources with initial dose rates within the classical LDR range and longer-lived low-energy sources with dose rates below the classical range (ULDR).

Classical Low–Dose Rate Permanent Implant Sources: ^{198}Au

Seeds consisting of ^{222}R gas encapsulated in thin-walled gold tubes[39] were used for permanent implantation for many years. Institutions[40] that are still practicing classical LDR permanent interstitial BT use a reactor-produced radionuclide, ^{198}Au, which emits monoenergetic 412-keV γ-rays and has a half-life of 2.7 days. Its decay product is a nontoxic solid, thereby eliminating the contamination hazards associated with production and use of ^{222}Rn. ^{198}Au seed implantation is not widely practiced (although sources are commercially available) because of exposure hazards to operating room personnel (especially the brachytherapist), the need to confine the patient to the hospital for radiation protection reasons, and the logistic problems associated with maintaining an appropriate inventory of such short-lived sources.

Ultra Low–Dose Rate and Energy Permanent Implant Sources: ^{125}I and ^{103}Pd

An important development was the introduction of interstitial seeds using electron-capture decay radionuclides, which have moderately long half-lives (10 to 60 days) and emit cascades of low-energy (20 to 40 keV) characteristic x-rays and γ-rays. The first practical K-capture source, the titanium-encapsulated ^{125}I seed (half-life, 59.6 days; mean energy, 28 keV), was developed by Donald C. Lawrence[41] in the early 1960s, and its clinical applications were developed in the late 1960s by Basil Hilaris and his colleagues[42–44] at Memorial Sloan Kettering

TABLE 25.2	TOTAL DOSE AND INITIAL DOSE RATES FOR PERMANENTLY IMPLANTED RADIONUCLIDES			
Radionuclide	Mean Photon Energy	$T_{1/2}$	Typical Prescribed Dose (Gy)	Initial Dose Rate (cGy/h)
^{222}Rn	1.2 MeV	3.83 d	100	75
^{198}Au	412 keV	2.70 d	100	107
^{131}Cs	29 keV	9.7 d	115	34.2
^{125}I	28 keV	59.6 d	145	7.0
^{103}Pd	22 keV	17 d	125	21.2

Hospital. Iodine-125 is produced by neutron activation in a specially equipped reactor designed to minimize activation of the contaminant radioisotope, ^{126}I. It decays by electron capture, producing a single 35-keV γ-ray. The captured K-shell electron produces a cascade of 27- to 32-keV characteristic x-rays. In addition, 93% of the γ-rays are internally converted, producing a second characteristic x-ray cascade. Thus, ^{125}I is an "x-ray emitter" because 95% of the useful primary photons are characteristic x-rays of atomic rather than nuclear origin.

Other important radionuclides are ^{103}Pd (^{103}palladium, 19.0-day half-life and mean energy: 22 keV), commercially realized in 1987, and ^{131}Cs (^{131}Cs, 9.6-day half-life and 29-keV mean energy), which was initially proposed by Lawrence and Henschke[45] but became available as commercial product in 2006.[46,47] The low-energy photons emitted by these radionuclides dramatically reduce external exposure hazards: an 8-cm thickness of tissue reduces exposure 10-fold. Thin (0.2 mm) lead foils also produce almost complete shielding. Thus, there is usually no need to confine patients to the hospital solely for radiation safety reasons. The rapid growth trajectory of transperineal ultrasound (TRUS)-guided permanent seed brachytherapy[48,49] in the 1990s for definitive treatment of low- and intermediate-risk prostate cancer[50,51] resulted in the introduction of approximately 25 different models of ^{125}I and ^{103}Pd to the market from 1997 to 2005 (see the American Association of Physicists in Medicine [AAPM] revised TG-43

Report[5,52,53] for a review of many of the available sources). Although brachytherapy remains a widely elected treatment modality for localized prostate cancer, its utilization has fallen from 24% in 2002 to 12% in 2010.[54] As a result, there has been consolidation in the low-energy seed market. The Joint Imaging and Radiation Oncology Core (IROC)-Houston QA Center (IROC-Houston, formerly the Radiological Physics Center)/AAPM brachytherapy source registry[55,56] lists all commercially available and clinical used orphan sources that meet the AAPM dosimetric prerequisites for clinical use.[57] According to the IROC-Houston/AAPM Registry, six ^{125}I, four ^{103}Pd, and one ^{131}Cs seed models are commercially available.

Most of low-energy interstitial seeds are encapsulated in thin (0.05- to 0.10-mm-thick) titanium tubing (exception: polymer-encapsulated Civa ^{103}Pd source[58]) with external dimensions of approximately 0.8 × 4.5 mm. Most of the available ^{125}I seed products are variations on the Model 6711 seed[61] design. This source, the only ^{125}I source available from 1983 to 1998, contained a 3-mm-long silver rod on which radioactive iodine is absorbed and is available in strengths of 0.5 to 13 μGy·m²·h⁻¹ (0.5 to 9 mCi) (Fig. 25.7A, top). The radiopaque silver rod enables seeds to be visualized on orthogonal or stereo shift radiographs.

^{103}Pd decays by K-electron capture and emits characteristic x-rays of 21 keV. It has all of the radiation protection advantages of ^{125}I along with a significantly shorter half-life

FIGURE 25.7. A: Design characteristics of three commercially available low-energy interstitial seed types. *Top:* A generic ^{125}I seed with silver rod radiographic marker derived from Model 6711 source (previously marketed by GE Healthcare, Amersham, and 3M) and now offered by several seed manufacturers. (From Williamson JF, Rivard MJ. Quantitative dosimetry methods for brachytherapy. In: Thomadsen BR, Rivard MJ, Butler WM, eds. *Brachytherapy Physics.* 2nd ed. Madison, WI: Medical Physics Publishing, 2005:233–294. Reprinted by permission of Medical Physics Publishing.) *Middle:* Theragenics Model 200 ^{103}Pd seed. (From Monroe JI, Williamson JF. Monte carlo-aided dosimetry of the theragenics TheraSeed® Model 200 103Pd interstitial brachytherapy seed. *Med Phys* 2002;29[4]:609–621. Copyright © 2002 American Association of Physicists in Medicine. Reprinted by permission of John Wiley & Sons, Inc.) *Bottom:* the IsoRay Medical Inc. Model CS-1 (Rev 2) ^{131}Cs seed. (From IROC-Houston, "Joint AAPM/IROC Houston Registry of Brachytherapy Sources Meeting the AAPM Dosimetric Prerequisites," (2017), Vol. 2017. Reprinted by permission of American Association of Physicists in Medicine.) (Figures reproduced with permission from references Williamson [2005],[59] Monroe [2002],[60] and IROC-Houston.[55]) **B:** Isodose curves for a ^{198}Au seed (*left half*) and Model 6711 ^{125}I seed (*right half*) both with air-kerma strengths of 72 μGy·m²·h⁻¹ (equivalent to 35 mCi of ^{198}Au and 57 mCi of ^{125}I)

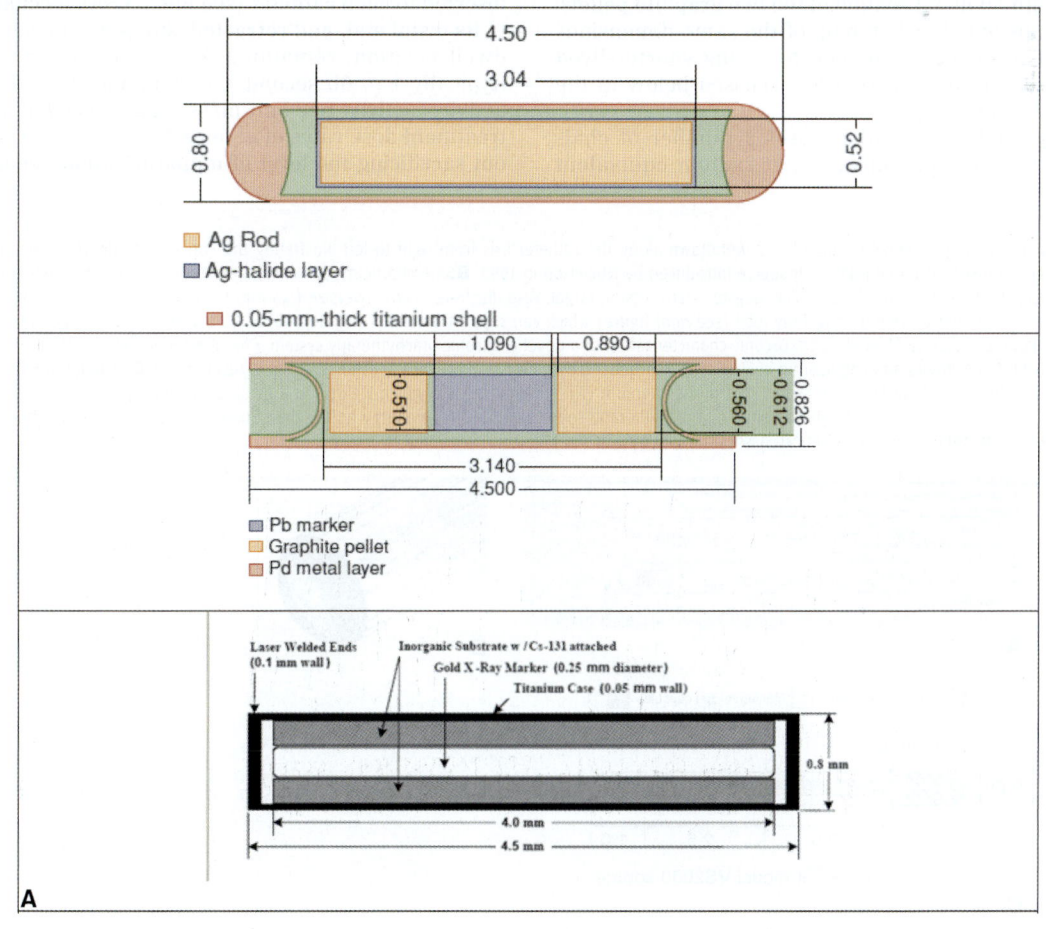

4.50
3.04
0.80
0.52

☐ Ag Rod
☐ Ag-halide layer
☐ 0.05-mm-thick titanium shell

1.090   0.890
0.510   0.560   0.826   0.612
3.140
4.500

☐ Pb marker
☐ Graphite pellet
☐ Pd metal layer

Laser Welded Ends (0.1 mm wall)
Inorganic Substrate w /Cs-131 attached
Gold X-Ray Marker (0.25 mm diameter)
Titanium Case (0.05 mm wall)
0.8 mm
4.0 mm
4.5 mm

A

(Continued)

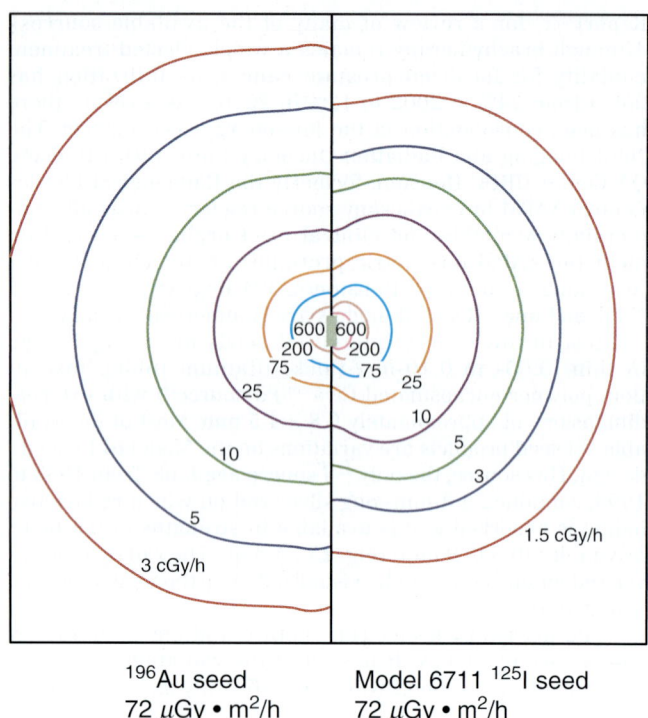

^{196}Au seed
72 μGy • m²/h
B   (10 mg Ra Eq)

Model 6711 ^{125}I seed
72 μGy • m²/h
(57 mCi)

FIGURE 25.7. *(Continued)*

of 17 days. With this source, an implant can deliver 112 Gy (90% of prescribed dose) in approximately 8 weeks at an initial peripheral dose rate of 21 cGy/h. The Model 200 seed (Fig. 25.7A, middle) was the only commercially available ^{103}Pd seed from 1988 to 1999. The radioactive palladium is distributed within a thin Pd metal coating of the two graphite pellets, which are encapsulated in Ti tubing of the same dimensions as ^{125}I seeds. The biologic rationale for using shorter-lived ^{103}Pd and ^{131}Cs interstitial sources is discussed below in the Biology section of this chapter.

Low-energy seed implantation poses a number of challenges. Their dose distributions are not radium equivalent

(Fig. 25.7B), falling off more rapidly with distance. Dose estimation is inherently more complex, depending significantly on photon energy and composition of the surrounding medium (Fig. 25.4),[62,63] and is more sensitive to the internal seed geometry.[59,60] Because of shifts in calibration standards, large uncertainties in dose measurement, and questionable applicability of classical dose calculation model, ^{125}I and ^{103}Pd dosimetry has been uncertain and variable over most of the clinical life of these products.[12] For example, between 1975 and 1999, the ^{125}I dose-rate constant was revised downward, in several steps, by nearly 50%.[12] Only with development and validation of more sophisticated experimental and computation dosimetry techniques in the past 10 to 15 years can we claim to know low-energy seed dose-rate distributions with an uncertainty of 3% to 7%.[64] Because of the low dose rates used, low-energy seed implantation is effectively a different therapeutic modality than classical LDR BT. In addition, 20- to 30-keV photons have a significantly higher LET spectrum, which results in an RBE for ^{125}I of 1.3 to 2.1 in *in vitro* systems compared with unity for radium-substitute photon spectra.[65–67] Thus, classical LDR clinical experience cannot be used to guide therapeutic decision-making for ^{125}I permanent implantation. Despite these limitations, low-energy source permanent implantation has been demonstrated to be a highly effective and convenient treatment for prostate cancer,[68,69] which produces tumor control rates comparable or superior to those of competing modalities.

Sources for High–Dose Rate Brachytherapy

Radionuclide Sources

In contrast to inpatient-based LDR BT, HDR BT uses high-intensity sources to deliver discrete fractions ranging from 3 to 10 Gy in an outpatient setting. As described in more detail in Chapter 21, a remote afterloading device must be used. Typically, a cable-mounted HDR source is sequentially inserted to each catheter (see Fig. 25.8A), mechanically driven to its distal end, and retracted, stopping at each programmed dwell position, remaining for the programmed dwell time (typically 1 to 60 seconds). A radionuclide with high specific activity (activity per unit mass; Ci/g) is needed so that overall treatment dose rates of at least 12 Gy/h can be achieved without sacrificing the level of miniaturization needed to support

FIGURE 25.8. A: *Top*: A single stepping source being withdrawn along the catheter axis from right to left illustrating the concepts of discrete dwell positions. *Bottom*: geometry of the original pulsed dose rate (PDR) ^{192}Ir source introduced by Nucletron in 1993. **B:** Geometric model (*left*) of the Xoft electronic brachytherapy source consisting of an inner catheter terminated by a 0.07-μm-thick tungsten transmission target. Also illustrated is the oversize (5.3 mm OD) outer catheter is needed to water cool the approximately 2.25-mm-diameter by 15-mm-long x-ray tube (see *right* figure) which can support an air-kerma rate of 170,000 μGy·m²·h⁻¹ when operated at 50 kVp and 300 μA.[70,71] (From Liu D, Poon E, Bazalova M, et al. Spectroscopic characterization of a novel electronic brachytherapy system. *Phys Med Biol* 2008;53[1]:61–75. doi:10.1088/0031-9155/53/1/004. © Institute of Physics and Engineering in Medicine. Reproduced by permission of IOP Publishing. All rights reserved.[71a]) **C:** A modern HDR source, consisting of a 0.34 mm diameter by 5-mm long Pt-Ir core sealed in a nickel–titanium (Ni–Ti) alloy capsule which welded to a flexible Ni–Ti alloy cable.[72] (From Perez-Calatayud J, Ballester F, Das RK, et al. Dose calculation for photon-emitting brachytherapy sources with average energy higher than 50 keV: report of the AAPM and ESTRO. *Med Phys* 2012;39[5]:2904–2929. Copyright © 2012 by American Association of Physicists in Medicine. Reprinted by permission.)

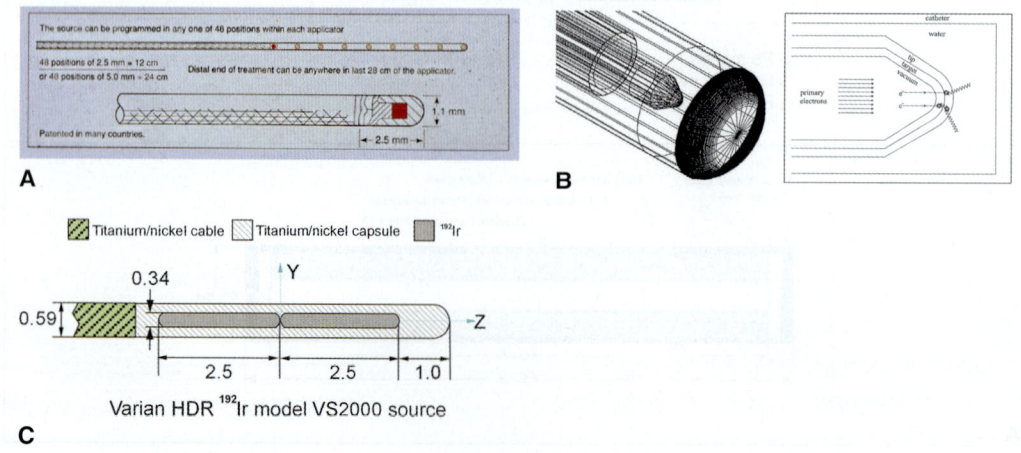

intracavitary and interstitial BT. A source no larger than 1 mm diameter by 4 mm long with an exposure rate of at least 1 R/s at 1 cm is required. Figure 25.8A and C illustrates typical PDR and HDR sources, respectively.

The upper limit on specific activity of any substance, achieved when 100% of its atoms are radioactive, is a fundamental property that depends on its number of atoms per gram:

$$\text{atoms/g} = \left(\frac{\text{Avogadro's no. } (6.023 \times 10^{23} \text{ atoms/mole})}{\text{Atomic Weight}} \right) \quad (8)$$

For radionuclides produced by neutron activation, competition with radioactive decay precludes activating 100% of the target atoms. The theoretically achievable maximum Ci/g (Table 25.3) depends on the neutron capture cross section of the target and the neutron flux in the reactor.[73] The extent to which this limit can be reached in practice depends on isotopic purity of the target, limits on reactor activation time, and the time required for shorter-lived contaminant radioisotopes to decay to an acceptable level. Finally, the exposure rate achieved by a small source (e.g., a 1 × 4-mm cylinder as shown in Table 25.3) depends on the chemical form (i.e., relative mass of nonradioactive atoms) of the source, its density, exposure-rate constant of the radionuclide, and photon self-absorption.

Table 25.3 shows that ^{226}Ra cannot support HDR BT radionuclide and that ^{137}Cs is, at best, a marginal choice. Cobalt 60 (5.26-year half-life and γ-rays of 1.17 and 1.33 MeV) has been widely used as an intracavitary HDR source in the form of small spherical pellets. Based solely on specific activity considerations, ^{192}Ir is the optimal choice for HDR BT and is the most widely used radionuclide for this application. Sources with external diameters as small as 0.6 mm (see Fig. 25.8C) are now available for use in single-stepping source remote afterloading devices. In contrast to ^{60}Co, the lower-energy ^{192}Ir photons are shielded effectively by the scatter and leakage barriers present in most existing ^{60}Co teletherapy and linear accelerator vaults. Because of their short half-lives, ^{192}Ir HDR sources usually are replaced at quarterly intervals. Because of the relative ease with which its low-energy photons can be shielded, ^{169}Yb source has been proposed for HDR intraoperative and intravascular BT.[9]

Electronic Brachytherapy Sources

Currently, there are two brachytherapy delivery systems on the market that use miniaturized low kilovoltage x-ray tubes to eliminate radionuclide sources of radiation. The Zeiss INTRABEAM system uses magnetic focusing and steering to transport externally accelerated 50-keV electrons down a long 3.2-mm diameter drift tube, which collide with a thin gold transmission target at the end of the implanted catheter.[74,75] In contrast, the Xoft Axxent electronic brachytherapy

(EBT) system[76] is based upon miniaturizing the entire x-ray tube (see Fig. 25.8B), which is placed in a somewhat larger diameter (5.4 mm) intracavitary catheter to allow for water cooling of the system. Although the intrabeam system has used several tumor sites, including skin cancer,[77] the main application for both systems has been intraoperative accelerated partial breast irradiation (APBI). Although the use of EBT as an APBI modality is supported by a randomized, phase III prospective noninferiority trial,[78] its equivalence to ^{192}Ir-based APBI remains controversial.[79] However, because of the lower penetration and more rapid falloff of 50 kVp x-rays compared to ^{192}Ir, for a fixed level of APBI PTV coverage, EBT gives rise to larger $V_{150\%}$ and $V_{200\%}$ values.[80] A recently published debate[81] highlights many of the operational and physical differences between the two classes of HDR sources.

BRACHYTHERAPY DOSIMETRY AND SOURCE-STRENGTH SPECIFICATION

Two eras of BT dosimetry can be distinguished. The *classical era* (1940 to 1980) encompassed the maturation of the classical BT systems, the transition from ^{226}Ra to artificial radionuclide sources, and the rise of modern BT. It began with the successful application of Bragg-Gray cavity theory[82] to the calibration of ^{226}Ra and other high-energy sources in terms of exposure,[83] which allowed BT treatment intensity to be quantified using the same system of units and quantities as the external orthovoltage beam therapy of the day. Classical or semiempirical dose-computation models are based on the dose distribution about an idealized point source. Dose rates around needle and tube sources were calculated by integrating the basic point-source model over their extended radio-activity distributions. Because of the technical difficulties in measuring absorbed dose in the presence of steep dose gradients, BT treatment planning relied largely on calculated rather than measured dose distributions.

The modern or *quantitative* era of BT dosimetry began in the 1980s and continues to the present. Quantitative dosimetry relies on measurement of source-specific dose distributions by means of small thermoluminescent dosimeters (TLDs) or silicon diode dosimeters.[84] Alternatively, radiation transport calculations in the form of three-dimensional (3D) Monte Carlo simulations are accepted as an accurate and reliable source of clinically useful dosimetry data.[84] These technical developments were motivated by concerns that semiempirical dose-calculation algorithms were not valid in the low-energy regimen of ^{125}I and ^{103}Pd sources. To clinically utilize dose measurements and Monte Carlo calculations, and empirical dose-calculation formalism, the TG-43 protocol[5] was developed. Both the classical and quantitative dosimetry methods are based on the principle that BT source strength should be specified in terms of radiation output in free air.

Source-Strength Specification Quantities and Units

Brachytherapy calibration is an unnecessarily confusing topic because of the multitude of quantities that have been used to specify source strength throughout its history. Many of the historically obsolete but still widely used quantities (e.g., apparent activity and equivalent mass of radium) were defined in terms of ^{226}Ra properties, the only BT radionuclide intensively studied until about 1940. Such quantities obscure the experimental origin of calibration measurements by describing output measurements in activity units. Finally, the BT literature has added to the lack of conceptual clarity by obscuring the important distinction between quantities and units. A *quantity*

TABLE 25.3 SPECIFIC ACTIVITIES AND MAXIMUM EXPOSURE RATES ACHIEVABLE FOR DIFFERENT RADIONUCLIDES

Radionuclide	Maximum Ci/g Possible	Fraction Practicably Achievable (%)	Exposure Rate[a] (R/s) at 1 cm From 1 mm × 4 mm Seed
^{226}Ra	0.98	100	0.04 R·cm^2·s^{-1}
^{137}Cs	87	23	0.22 R·cm^2·s^{-1}
^{60}Co	1,020[b]	49	50 R·cm^2·s^{-1}
^{192}Ir	7,760[b]	35	248 R·cm^2·s^{-1}
^{169}Yb	33,700[b]	14	51 R·cm^2·s^{-1}

[a]Neglecting self-absorption.
[b]Reactor produced by neutron activation: a flux $\phi = 10^{14}$ n·cm^{-2}·s^{-1} and 100% target purity are assumed.

is a property of nature that is directly or indirectly measurable (e.g., kerma, equivalent mass of radium, length, time), whereas a *unit* is a selected sample of a quantity to which the magnitude unity (1.0) is assigned (e.g., gray, mgRaEq, meter, second). A quantity such as absorbed dose can have many units (e.g., rad, cGy, Gy, J/kg).

Regardless of the units and quantity chosen to describe a calibration, all photon-emitting sealed BT sources are calibrated in terms of output (kerma rate, dose rate, or exposure rate) in air at a specific reference point on the transverse bisector of the source. Much like superficial x-ray beam calibration, a calibrated ion chamber (Fig. 25.9) is used to measure the BT source output in a free-air geometry in which the source and chamber are suspended in air in a large room.

Air-Kerma Strength

In North America, photon-emitting source strength is specified in terms of air-kerma strength, denoted by S_K, a practice that was introduced by the AAPM in 1987.[85] The AAPM[5] currently defines S_K as the air-kerma rate, $\dot{K}_{\delta,\mathrm{air}}(d)$ at distance d,

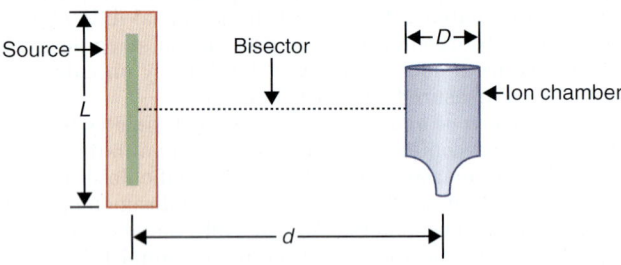

FIGURE 25.9. A: Illustration of a free-air geometry for measuring brachytherapy source strength in terms of a radiation output quantity such as air kerma. In practice, the source and cavity chamber are suspended in air in a large room and separated by 20-cm to 100-cm distance (which must be large in relation to the detector and source dimensions). The measured air-kerma must be corrected for photon scattering from walls, floor, and ceiling and for photon scattering and attenuation by the intervening air. **B:** Definition of air-kerma strength. For an actual source, the air-kerma rate must be measured at a distance, *d*, which is large in relation to the source dimensions.

Output specification

Conditions
1. Large distance d: $L \ll d$, $D \ll d$
2. Free in space
   - Measured in air
   - Corrected for air attenuation
   - Corrected for scattering from air, walls, etc.

A

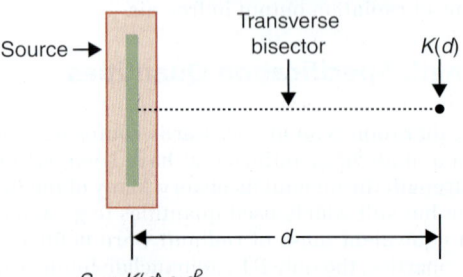

Air-kerma strength: S_k

$S_k = K(d) \cdot d^2$
where $K(d)$ is air-kerma rate in free space on transverse bisector of source at large distance
$d \gg L$

B   Units: $1\ \mu Gy \cdot m^2 \cdot h^{-1} = 1\ cGy \cdot cm^2 \cdot h^{-1} = 1\ U$

in vacuo and due to photons of energy greater than δ, multiplied by the square of this distance, d^2.

$$S_K = \dot{K}_{\delta,\mathrm{air}}(d) \cdot d^2 \qquad (9)$$

The distance d is the distance from the source center to the point of air-kerma rate specification (usually but not necessarily the point of measurement), which must be in the transverse plane of the source (the plane normal to the long axis of the source, which bisects its radioactivity distribution). S_K is independent of specification distance so long as d is large relative to the maximum linear dimension of the radioactivity distribution. $\dot{K}_{\delta,\mathrm{air}}(d)$ is usually inferred from transverse-plane air-kerma rate measurements performed in a free-air geometry (see Fig. 25.9) at distances large in relation to the maximum linear dimensions of the detector and source, typically of the order of 1 m. The "*in vacuo*" qualifier (equivalent in meaning to "in free space") means that $\dot{K}_{\delta,\mathrm{air}}(d)$ must be specified as if the source and small mass of air, producing ionization at distance d, were immersed in a vacuum. Air-kerma rate measurements must be corrected for photon attenuation and scattering by the surrounding air as well as for scattering from nearby objects. The energy cutoff, δ, is intended to exclude low-energy or contaminant photons (e.g., characteristic x-rays originating in the outer layers of steel or titanium source cladding[86]) that increase $\dot{K}_{\delta,\mathrm{air}}(d)$ without contributing significantly to dose at distances >0.1 cm in tissue. The value of δ is typically 5 keV for low-energy photon–emitting BT source. The unit of air-kerma strength is $\mu Gy \cdot m^2 \cdot h^{-1}$ and is often denoted in the literature by the symbol "U:" where $1\ U = 1\ cGy \cdot cm^2 \cdot h^{-1} = 1\ \mu Gy \cdot m^2 \cdot h^{-1}$.

Air-kerma strength is numerically (but not dimensionally) equal to the quantity reference air-kerma rate, $\dot{K}_{\mathrm{ref}}$, a very similar quantity defined by the ICRU[3] and used outside North America. $\dot{K}_{\mathrm{ref}}$ is defined as the air-kerma rate in free space at a reference distance, l (taken to be 1 m), on the transverse axis; it has units of $\mu Gy \cdot h^{-1}$ at 1 m. Thus, $\dot{K}_{\mathrm{ref}} = S_K / l^2$. The procedures for standardizing and measuring $\dot{K}_{\mathrm{ref}}$ and S_K are identical.

The U.S. National Institute of Standards and Technology (NIST) maintains primary S_K standards for commercially available ^{137}Cs sources,[87] LDR ^{192}Ir seeds,[88] and all ^{103}Pd, ^{131}Cs, and ^{125}I seeds.[89] A *primary standard* is an instrument against which all other S_K measurement devices, called secondary or tertiary standards, must be intercompared. Such instruments are designed to permit inference of air-kerma values from the measured charge and instrument design using first principles. For ^{137}Cs and ^{192}Ir sources, the S_K standard is based on transverse-axis air-kerma measurements using spherical ion chambers with carbon walls[87,88]—the same instruments used to maintain the ^{60}Co teletherapy air-kerma standard. For low-energy interstitial seeds, a special free-air chamber,[89] called the wide-angle free-air chamber (WAFAC), is used. Brachytherapy sources calibrated directly by the NIST standard or one of the AAPM-Accredited Dosimetry and Calibration Laboratories (ADCL) are said to have *directly NIST-traceable calibrations*. Sources that are calibrated against sources or ion chambers, which themselves have directly traceable NIST calibrations, are said to have *indirectly NIST-traceable calibrations*. The Xoft EBT has its own air-kerma standard based on the Lamperti free-air chamber for low-energy x-ray beams.[90] Because accurate estimation of the air attenuation correction for 50-kVp x-rays is conceptually and technically challenging, NIST chose to specify EBT source strength in terms of $\dot{K}_{\mathrm{air}}(50\ cm)$, the air-kerma rate in air (rather than free space) at 50-cm source-to-surface distance, rather than S_K. For a more detailed description of air-kerma–based standards, measurement techniques, and traceability requirements, the reader is referred to a recent review by Sander.[91] The AAPM recommends[92] that individual clinics using BT sources maintain instrumentation able to make indirectly traceable calibration measurements for verification of vendor-supplied calibrations.

Kerma (kinetic energy released in the medium), K_x, is the ratio $\Delta E_{tr}/\Delta m$, where ΔE_{tr} is the total kinetic energy transferred to charged particles by photon interactions with atoms in small mass, Δm, of medium x.[93] For photons, ΔE_{tr} includes the initial kinetic energies of any secondary charged particles (e.g., Compton electrons, photoelectrons, and positrons) liberated by Compton, photoelectric, and pair production interactions. Kerma is defined only for indirectly ionizing radiations (e.g., photons and neutrons) and quantifies the transfer of energy from these radiation fields to matter. It takes the same units (cGy and Gy) as the related quantity absorbed dose. Although kerma can be specified in any medium x, usually air medium (x = air) is assumed for radiation metrology. K_{air} replaces the obsolete quantity exposure and is closely related to absorbed dose, D: the ratio, $\Delta E_{ab}/\Delta m$, where ΔE_{ab} is the energy imparted to Δm by the radiation field. Because the secondary electrons released by photon collisions may travel a significant distance before depositing their energy and may convert some of their kinetic energy to bremsstrahlung radiation, D_{air} and K_{air} are not necessarily equal. When kerma remains relatively constant over the range of the secondary electrons, a special condition, secondary charged particle equilibrium (CPE), exists.[73,94] When the CPE is achieved, the rates of energy absorption and energy transfer are approximately equal, so that kerma closely approximates absorbed dose:

$$D_{air} = X \cdot \left(\frac{W}{e}\right) = K_{air} \cdot (1 - g) \tag{10}$$

where X represents the quantity exposure. The quantity (W/e) is the average energy imparted to air per ion pair created and is a constant, independent of photon energy: (W/e) = 33.97 eV/ion pair = 33.97 J/C = 0.876 cGy/R.[95] The factor g is the fraction of kinetic energy transferred to the medium converted back to radiant energy (photons) by the bremsstrahlung process; g is <0.001 at BT energies and usually is ignored, further simplifying Eq. (10). Most BT dose-calculation algorithms and dosimetric analyses assume that CPE obtains and that dose, D_{med}, can be well approximated by kerma, K_{med}, everywhere. Although generally valid, CPE can be expected to break down in the presence of steep dose gradients near sources,[96] near metal–tissue interfaces,[97] and within the active elements of thin, bounded detectors.[98] The combination of CPE failure and beta ray transmission give rise to (D_{med}/K_{med}) ratios that deviate from unity by 10% to 50% 0.4 to 1.5 mm from the surface of lightly encapsulated HDR ^{192}Ir sources.[99]

Activity

To define the obsolete quantities for describing source output, the quantity activity, A, must be introduced. It is defined as the rate of nuclear disintegration or transformation within a radioactive source. The contemporary unit of activity is the Becquerel (1 Bq = 1 disintegration/s). We will freely use the more traditional but obsolete unit, the curie (1 Ci = 3.7 × 10[10] disintegrations/s = 3.7 × 10[10] Bq). A more convenient multiple of the curie, the millicurie, is defined as 1 mCi = 10[−3] Ci = 3.7 × 10[7] disintegrations/s. Each disintegration represents the spontaneous transformation of an atom from one nuclear state to another. For most BT radioisotopes, such transformations of nuclear state give rise to photons in the form of unconverted γ-rays, annihilation photons, characteristic x-rays, and bremsstrahlung photons. Activity is measured by counting the number of photons, β particles, or other particles emitted by an unencapsulated point source of the radionuclide by means of scintillation or coincidence counters, from which its activity

is inferred.[100] For sealed BT sources, A refers to activity contained inside the sealed source.

Activity, as defined in this strict sense, is no longer used in BT dosimetry. However, activity continues to serve as the basis for treatment specification and dosimetry of unsealed radiopharmaceuticals used for diagnosis and therapy and may play a future role in dosimetry of sealed beta-emitting sources for intravascular BT and other clinical applications. NIST maintains contained activity standards for a wide variety of radionuclides in aqueous solution.[101]

Relationship Between Activity and Exposure Rate

The activity, A, of a radioactive nuclide emitting photons and the air-kerma rate in free space, $\dot{K}_\delta(r)$ (in Gy/s) at distance r (in meters) because of photons of energy greater than δ, are related by a fundamental quantity, the air-kerma rate constant, $(\Gamma_\delta)_K$, defined as follows[93]:

$$(\Gamma_\delta)_K = \frac{\dot{K}_\delta(r) \cdot r^2}{A} \quad \text{air-kerma rate constant} \, (m^2 \cdot Gy \cdot Bq^{-1} \cdot s^{-1})$$
$$(\Gamma_\delta)_X = \frac{\dot{X}_\delta(r) \cdot r^2}{A} \quad \text{exposure-rate constant} \, (cm^2 \cdot R \cdot mCi^{-1} \cdot h^{-1}) \tag{11}$$

Even though it is obsolete, this chapter will freely use the closely related and familiar quantity exposure rate constant, $(\Gamma_\delta)_X$, with units of R cm²·mCi⁻¹·h⁻¹. $(\Gamma_\delta)_X$ is equal to the exposure rate in R/h at 1 cm from a 1-mCi point source. It describes the rate at which air is ionized as a result of the emission of photons resulting from radioactive decay. The energy cutoff δ eliminates low-energy bremsstrahlung and characteristic x-rays from consideration that are always absorbed within any practical source. The precise value of δ depends on the application; it usually is assumed to be about 10 keV. Because $(\Gamma_\delta)_X$ is defined in terms of an isotropic point source with exposure rates corrected for air attenuation and scattering, inverse-square law applies exactly. Thus, $(\Gamma_\delta)_X$ is independent of the distance r used in Eq. (11).

$(\Gamma_\delta)_X$ depends only on the number and energy of the photons emitted per disintegration. Suppose there are N different photons emitted per disintegration with energies E_1, E_2, ..., E_N in units of MeV. We assume that each nuclear decay emits P_i photons of energy E_i where $i = 1, ..., N$. The list $\{E_i, P_i\}_{i=1}^N$ is the photon spectrum of the radionuclide. If the spectrum is known, then $(\Gamma_\delta)_X$ can be calculated by:

$$(\Gamma_\delta)_X = 193.7 \cdot \sum_{i=1}^{N} P_i \cdot E_i \cdot (\mu_{en}/\rho)_i^{air} \tag{12}$$

where $(\mu_{en}/\rho)_i^{air}$ is the mass–energy absorption coefficient (in units of cm²/g) for air at energy E_i. A detailed derivation of this fundamental relationship is given elsewhere.[24,102] $(\Gamma_\delta)_X$ is the fundamental property of the radionuclide's unencapsulated photon spectrum; applies only to an ideal point source; and neglects many significant properties of real sources such as self-absorption, filtration, and extension.

[226]Ra is an exception to this practice. First, radium source strength is specified by the quantity—mass of [226]Ra contained inside the source—denoted by M_{Ra}. M_{Ra} excludes the nonradioactive core components as well as radioactive decay products. Historically, M_{Ra} was introduced and widely used before the more general activity standards were available. Indeed, the unit curie originally was defined as the number of disintegrations produced by 1 g of [226]Ra. M_{Ra} standards were prepared by carefully weighing pure [226]Ra samples in an analytic balance. The first M_{Ra} standard was prepared by Marie Curie in 1913, and the currently used NIST standard was prepared by Hönigschmidt in 1934.[103] To calibrate a user's source in M_{Ra}, its radiation output is compared with that of the NIST radium

standard by means of an ion chamber. NIST no longer offers an M_{Ra} calibration service. In contrast to the other radionuclides, exposure-rate constant of ^{226}Ra—denoted by the special symbol $(\Gamma_\delta)_{Ra,t}$ in this chapter—is tabulated as a function of its effective capsule thickness, t, in millimeters of platinum.[104] $(\Gamma_\delta)_{Ra,t}$ is normalized to the mass of radium contained in the source and has units of R cm$^2\cdot$mg$^{-1}\cdot$h^{-1}.

Obsolete Quantities for Specifying Source Output

Because of the close association of early BT with ^{226}Ra, it is not surprising that the measured output of BT sources continues to be expressed as multiples of the output of a 1-mg radium needle. This quantity, equivalent mass of radium (M_{eq}), was introduced when artificial radioisotopes, such as ^{60}Co and ^{137}Cs, were developed as radium replacements. It allowed old implant and radium needle dosimetry tables, which gave dose per milligram-hour (mg-h) of ^{226}Ra, to be used without modification for these new sources. M_{eq} is that mass of ^{226}Ra filtered by 0.5 mm Pt that has the same S_K as that of the given source. Because M_{eq} is simply a statement of S_K relative to that of a hypothetic radium needle, the given source being quantified need not contain ^{226}Ra, be encapsulated in Pt, nor have a wall thickness of 0.5 mm. Because $K_{air} = X \cdot (W/e)$ and $(\Gamma_\delta)_{Ra,0.5} = 8.25$ R $\cdot$ cm$^2\cdot$ mg$^{-1}\cdot$ h^{-1} for ^{226}Ra filtered by 0.5 mm Pt,[105] S_K and M_{eq} are related by:

$$S_K = M_{eq} \cdot (\Gamma_\delta)_{Ra,0.5} \cdot (W/e) = M_{eq} \cdot 7.223$$

$$M_{eq} = \frac{S_K}{(\Gamma_\delta)_{Ra,0.5} \cdot (W/e)} = \frac{S_K}{7.223} \quad (13)$$

where $(W/e) = 33.97$ eV/ion pair. Until relatively recently, M_{eq} was widely used to specify strength of intracavitary and interstitial BT radium-substitute sources such as ^{137}Cs and ^{192}Ir.

Similar to the philosophy of M_{eq}, apparent activity, A_{app}, is a statement of source output relative to that of a hypothetic unfiltered point source. A_{app} is the activity of a hypothetic unfiltered point source of the same radionuclide has the same S_K as that of the given source:

$$A_{app} = \frac{S_K}{(\Gamma_\delta)_X \cdot (W/e)} \quad (14)$$

Apparent activity in units of mCi continues to be widely used for specifying strength for permanent interstitial implants (e.g., ^{125}I and ^{103}Pd sources). In contrast to M_{eq}, which is based on the universally accepted $(\Gamma_\delta)_{Ra,0.5}$ value of 8.25 R$\cdot$cm$^2\cdot$mCi$^{-1}\cdot$h^{-1}, no consensus as to $(\Gamma_\delta)_X$ values for the other radionuclides exists. Often, different vendors will assume different $(\Gamma_\delta)_X$ values for the same radionuclide. Thus, A_{app} is an inherently ambiguous means of describing source strength. In an effort to reduce low-energy dose-calculation errors associated with this ambiguity, the AAPM recommends[106] that the $(\Gamma_\delta)_X$ values of 1.476 and 1.45 R$\cdot$cm$^2\cdot$mCi$^{-1}\cdot$h^{-1} for ^{103}Pd and ^{125}I sources, respectively, be used universally for specification of A_{app}. For many years, virtually all scientific societies involved in BT[3,92,107] have recommended that M_{eq} and A_{app} be abandoned in favor of S_K for source ordering, dose calculation, and implant prescription.

Milligram/Hours and Integrated Reference Air-Kerma

In gynecologic intracavitary therapy, the quantities M_{Ra} and M_{eq} were widely used to describe source loadings and to prescribe individual treatments. For prescribing therapy, these quantities, in units of milligrams of ^{226}Ra or mgRaEq, are integrated over treatment time yielding the so-called quantities mg-h and mgRaEq-h. As the product of total source strength and treatment time, mg-h and mgRaEq-h represent the total exposure or air-kerma accumulated at a distance of 1 m from the implant, under the assumptions that the implant is a point source and that tissue attenuation is negligible. The ICRU[108] recommends that mg-h be abandoned as a prescription or reporting quantity in favor of total reference air kerma (TRAK), which is defined in terms of air-kerma strength. TRAK, symbolized by K_{ref} is given by:

$$K_{ref} = \sum_{i=1}^{N} (S_{K,i}/l^2) \cdot t_i \quad (15)$$

where $S_{K,i}$ and t_i are the air-kerma strength and treatment time in hours, respectively, of the i-th source and l is the reference distance (taken to be 1 m or 1 cm). Thus, 1 U of TRAK = 1 cGy at 1 cm = 1 μGy at 1 m. TRAK is related to mg-h and mgRaEq-h:

$$K_{ref} = \begin{cases} \text{mg-h} \cdot 6.754 & \text{for filtration } t = 1 \text{ mm Pt} \\ \text{mgRaEq-h} \cdot 7.227 & \text{for filtration } t = 0.5 \text{ mm Pt} \end{cases} \quad (16)$$

Intracavitary treatment systems[11] historically based on ^{226}Ra tubes (1 mm Pt encapsulation) typically use mg-h, whereas systems based on ^{137}Cs or other radium substitutes prescribe therapy in units of mgRaEq-h. Because of the difference in platinum filtration assumed by these two milligram-based quantities, numerically identical prescriptions can deliver quantities of TRAK that differ by 7%. The use of TRAK as an integrated output reporting quantity eliminates this 7% ambiguity that has confused comparison of different implant systems since the appearance of radium-substitute sources for BT.

Classical Dose-Calculation Formalism: Isotropic Point Source

Consider an unencapsulated point source with an air-kerma strength of S_K, illustrated in Figure 25.10. Because this source has no extension, there is no attenuation of the emitted radiation by the source itself. Isotropy (Fig. 25.2) implies that photons are emitted with equal likelihood in all directions and travel in straight lines. In reality, actual BT sources are

FIGURE 25.10. Unencapsulated point source of strength S_K immersed in an unbounded water-equivalent medium.

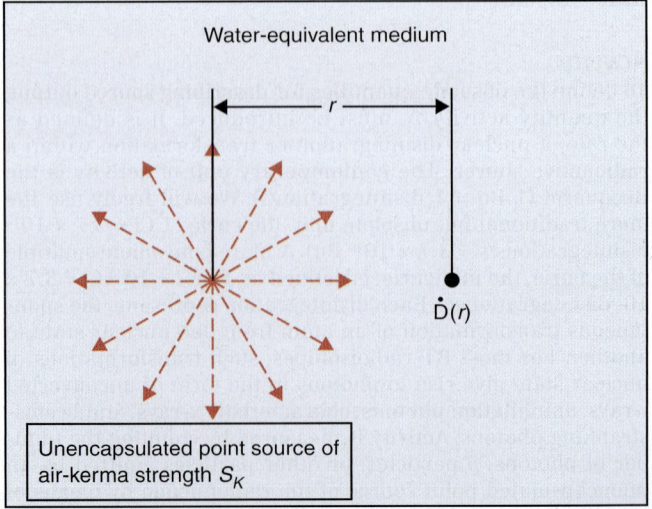

encapsulated, have finite dimensions, and usually are cylindrically rather than spherically symmetric. The dose rate, $\dot{D}(r)$ (cGy/h), at distance r (cm) in the water-equivalent medium surrounding the source is given by:

$$\dot{D}_{med}(r) = S_K \cdot \frac{\overline{(\mu_{en}/\rho)}_{air}^{med}}{r^2} \cdot T(r) \tag{17}$$

The inverse-square law term corrects for the difference in dose-specification distance, r, and the 1-cm reference point assumed by the units of air-kerma strength. The quantity $\overline{(\mu_{en}/\rho)}_{air}^{med}$ is the ratio of mass–energy absorption coefficients in medium to that in air averaged over the photon spectrum in free space. This correction, equal to $\bar{K}_{med}/\bar{K}_{air}$ in free space, is a consequence of the fundamental relationship between particle fluence and dose.[24,102] It corrects for the efficiency with which the medium extracts energy from the emitted photons compared with air. For all radionuclides emitting photons with energies >200 keV, including all radium substitutes, $\overline{(\mu_{en}/\rho)}_{air}^{med}$ has the value 1.11 in water medium.

The last term of Eq. (17)—the kerma-to-dose conversion factor, $T(r)$—describes the net influence of primary photon attenuation and buildup of scattered photons in the surrounding medium. Sometimes, this factor is termed the effective attenuation factor or the scatter buildup factor:

$$T(r) = \frac{\text{Dose in medium}}{\text{Medium} - \text{kerma in free space}}$$
$$= \frac{\text{Exposure in medium}}{\text{Exposure in air}} \Big\rbrace \begin{array}{l}\text{at distance } r \\ \text{from a point source}\end{array} \tag{18}$$

Figure 25.11 shows $T(r)$ for several radium-substitute radionuclides as well as for a few low-energy radionuclides. For ^{226}Ra-equivalent radionuclides, $T(r)$ deviates <5% from unity (1.00) out to distances, r, of 5 cm. Numerous tabulations of $T(r)$ are available in the literature; those of Meisberger and colleagues,[109] Berger,[112] and Van Kleffens and Star[113] are among the best known. Most of these data are derived

FIGURE 25.11. Photon attenuation and scatter factors, $T(r)$, for a number of brachytherapy radionuclides. The data for ^{137}Cs, ^{198}Au, and ^{60}Co are from the classic paper by Meisberger et al.[109] The HDR ^{192}Ir, Model 6702 ^{125}I, and Xoft 50 kVp x-ray $T(r)$ are from Daskalov et al.,[110] Dolan et al.,[111] and Hiatt et al.[70]

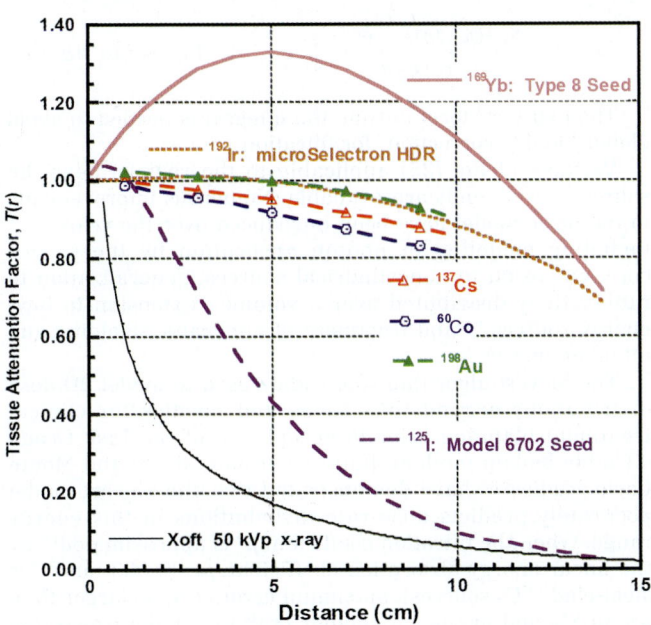

from theoretic photon transport calculations. The classical semiempirical model assumes that $T(r)$ is a function only of the radionuclide photon spectrum and that a single data set (e.g., for ^{192}Ir) can be used for all ^{192}Ir sources regardless of their construction.

By solving Eqs. (13) and (14) for S_K and substituting the results into Eq. (18), one can derive equations relating the dose rate at distance r to equivalent mass of radium and apparent activity for the same unfiltered point source:

$$\dot{D}_{med}(r) = M_{eq} \cdot \frac{(\Gamma_\delta)_{Ra,0.5} \cdot f_{med}}{r^2} \cdot T(r) \text{ Equivalent Mass of } ^{226}\text{Ra} \tag{19a}$$

$$\dot{D}_{med}(r) = A_{app} \cdot \frac{(\Gamma_\delta)_X \cdot f_{med}}{r^2} \cdot T(r) \qquad \text{Apparent Activity} \tag{19b}$$

where f_{med} is the dose-to-exposure conversion factor given by:

$$f_{med} = \frac{D_{med}}{X} = (W/e) \cdot \left[\frac{\overline{(\mu_{en}/\rho)}^{med}}{\overline{(\mu_{en}/\rho)}^{air}} \right]$$
$$= 0.876 \frac{cGy}{R} \cdot \overline{(\mu_{en}/\rho)}^{med}_{air} \Big\rbrace \text{ in free space} \tag{20}$$

For radionuclides with photon energies of more than 200 keV, f_{med} has the value 0.974 cGy·R^{-1} for water and 0.966 cGy·R^{-1} for muscle medium.[73]

Equations (17) and (19) give the dose rate, $\dot{D}_{med}(r)$, for a point source surrounded by an arbitrary medium that has been specified in terms of equivalent mass of radium, apparent activity, and S_K. Assuming that the same exposure rate constants, $(\Gamma_\delta)_{Ra,0.5}$ and $(\Gamma_\delta)_X$, were used to evaluate absorbed dose as were used to convert the measured air-kerma strength to M_{eq} and A_{app} via Eqs. (13) and (14), all three equations should give numerically identical dose rates. This demonstrates that Γ_δ is, in fact, a "dummy" constant that plays no physical role in the dosimetry of output-calibrated sealed sources because any arbitrary, but consistently used, value will yield identical dose-rate distributions. Because these unit conversions may be performed by different individuals at various stages of the calibration and clinical treatment planning processes, the potential for significant dose-calculation errors exists. The use of S_K for clinical source-strength specification eliminates these dummy constants, thereby eliminating errors resulting from inconsistent conventional choices.

Modeling of Source Anisotropy: The Anisotropy Factor

Despite its simplicity, the classical isotropic point-source model, Eq. (17), accurately predicts the transverse-axis dose-rate distributions of most actual radium-substitute sources. Simply by using an output quantity to calibrate the source, rather than contained activity, A, the influence of its internal structure (filtration and self-absorption) has been implicitly accounted for. Had true activity, A, instead of A_{app} been used in Eq. (19b), then the expression for $(\Gamma_\delta)_X$ (Eq. [12]) would require correction for attenuation and scattering in the radioactive core and surrounding encapsulation. Any uncertainties in $\{E_i, P_i\}_{i=1}^N$ (which are large for many radionuclides) and filtration corrections would directly degrade dose-calculation accuracy. In addition, fundamental activity measurements are technically difficult for the high-intensity sources used in BT. For these reasons, contained activity does not play a role in photon BT dosimetry. In contrast, Eq. (17) infers dose rate from a quantity measured outside the source, which is not influenced significantly by knowledge of the unfiltered photon spectrum. The required quantities, $\overline{(\mu_{en}/\rho)}^{med}_{air}$ and $T(r)$, are ratios and are therefore insensitive to errors in the assumed spectrum.

Section II

Practically all BT sources are cylindrical, giving rise to anisotropic dose distributions. In addition, some sources, especially those used in intracavitary BT, have active lengths that are comparable to typical calculation distances. Thus, the dose rate, $\dot{D}(r,\theta)$, around a BT source depends both on distance r and polar angle, θ (Fig. 25.8B). $\dot{D}(r,\theta)$ may deviate significantly from the transverse-axis dose rate, $\dot{D}(r,\pi/2)$, predicted by Eq. (17), especially near the long axis of the seed.

In the case of implants consisting of many randomly oriented seeds with active lengths less than the minimum distance of interest, Eq. (17) will accurately represent the multiple-seed dose distribution if an average correction for single-seed dose anisotropy is applied.[114] This correction factor, which the TG-43 protocol refers to as the "1D anisotropy function," $\phi_{an}(r)$, is defined by averaging the dose at each fixed distance r with respect to solid angle, Ω:

$$\phi_{an}(r) = \frac{\text{Average dose at } r}{\text{Transverse-axis dose at } r} = \frac{\int_{4\pi} \dot{D}(r,\theta) \cdot d\Omega}{4\pi \dot{D}(r,\pi/2)} \cdot$$
$$= \frac{\int_0^\pi \dot{D}(r,\theta) \cdot \sin\theta \cdot d\theta}{2 \cdot \dot{D}(r,\pi/2)} \quad (21)$$

Often, a distance-independent average value of $\phi_{an}(r)$, called the anisotropy constant, $\overline{\phi}_{an}$, is used. Incorporating this average correction into Eq. (17) leads to:

$$\dot{D}_{med}(r) = \frac{S_K \cdot \overline{(\mu_{en}/\rho)}_{air}^{med}}{r^2} \cdot T(r) \cdot \overline{\phi}_{an} \quad (22)$$

For early radium-substitute sources, $\overline{\phi}_{an}$ was often evaluated by measuring relative photon fluence in air at relatively large distances (30 to 100 cm) using a NaI or GeLi scintillation detector.[61,115]

Equation (22) implies that source strength should be increased by a constant fraction ranging from 2% (^{192}Ir seeds) to 10% (^{103}Pd seeds) to correct for polar anisotropy effects. Lindsay et al.[116] compared prostate implant 3D dose distributions derived from the isotropic point-source model, $\dot{D}(r)$, to those derived from the full 2D single-source dose-calculation model, $\dot{D}(r,\theta)$. Based on voxel-by-voxel comparisons, they found that the isotropic point-source model introduced errors exceeding 10% of the D_{90} (see section on dose specification) in 8% and 33% of the target volume for the Model 6711 ^{125}I and Model 200 ^{103}Pd sources. Corbett and colleagues[117] found that despite local large local dose-distribution differences, including 2D anisotropy effects did not alter the dose/volume histogram (DVH): neither the V_{100} nor the margin between D_{100} and prostate boundary was altered significantly. For volume implants consisting of parallel arrays of ^{192}Ir seeds, a similar finding has been reported.[114]

Dose Calculation for Extended Sources: The Sievert Integral Model

Dose distributions around larger sources, such as intracavitary tubes and interstitial needles, are calculated by partitioning the extended source into a set of point sources to which corrections for distance, oblique filtration, attenuation, and scattering are applied separately. By summing these point-source contributions, the dose at point P can be estimated. This class of algorithms, first described by Rolf Sievert in 1921,[118] is known as the Sievert integral algorithm or, more generally, the 1D pathlength model.[24,119]

Assume that the source illustrated in Figure 25.12 has an air-kerma strength, S_K, and contained activity, A. The classical Sievert model approximates the cylindrical active core by a line of radioactivity positioned along its axis. The axial length of the core is called the active length, L. Oblique filtration is

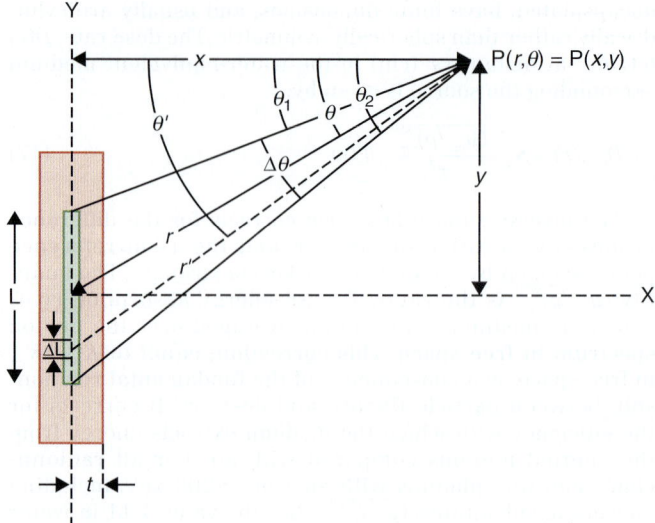

FIGURE 25.12. A typical encapsulated line source, illustrating calculation of dose rate at point P at (x,y) relative to the source center by the Sievert integral method. The active length and radial encapsulation thickness are denoted by L and t, respectively. The distances x and y are referred to as "distance away" and "distance along," respectively, in the literature.

modeled by assuming that the capsule reduces dose by exponential attenuation using an effective filtration coefficient, μ'. The dose rate $\Delta\dot{D}(x,y)$ at point (x,y) from the incremental source ΔL located at angle θ is

$$\Delta\dot{D}(x,y) = A \cdot \frac{\Delta L}{L} \cdot \frac{(\Gamma_\delta)_X \cdot f_{med}}{(x/\cos\theta)^2} \cdot T(x/\cos\theta) \cdot e^{-\mu' \cdot t/\cos\theta} \quad (23)$$

where $(\Gamma_\delta)_X$ is the exposure rate constant of the unfiltered source material. Because $S_K = A \cdot (W/e) \cdot (\Gamma_\delta)_X \cdot e^{-\mu' t}$, Eq. (23) becomes:

$$\Delta\dot{D}(x,y) = S_K \cdot \frac{\Delta L}{L} \cdot e^{\mu' t} \cdot \frac{\overline{(\mu_{en}/\rho)}_{air}^{med}}{(x/\cos\theta)^2} \cdot T(x/\cos\theta) \cdot e^{-\mu' \cdot t/\cos\theta} \quad (24)$$

By summing over all these incremental sources (i.e., integrating with respect to θ) and transforming to polar coordinates, we obtain the Sievert integral:

$$\dot{D}(r,\theta) = \frac{S_K \cdot \overline{(\mu_{en}/\rho)}_{air}^{med} \cdot e^{\mu' t}}{L \cdot r \cdot \cos\theta} \cdot \int_{\theta_1}^{\theta_2} e^{-\mu' t \cdot \sec\theta} \cdot T(x \cdot \sec\theta) \cdot d\theta \quad (25)$$

The extra $e^{\mu' t}$ term outside the integral is needed to avoid global "double correction" for filtration.

Variants of Eq. (25) applicable to the regions near the source capsule ends are available. Numerous improvements to the basic model have been introduced over the years,[104,120] including modeling of photon absorption by the source core, extension to noncylindrical sources, generalization to radioactivity distributed over a volume,[4] extension to low-energy sources,[119] and treatment of applicator shielding and attenuation.[121,122]

The Sievert algorithm was widely used to model 2D dose distributions around ^{137}Cs tubes and needles for clinical treatment planning prior to acceptance of the Task Group 43 table lookup method. Both experimental[123,124] and Monte Carlo studies[4,125] have demonstrated that the Sievert model accurately predicts dose-rate distributions in this energy range. When the filtration coefficient μ' is approximated[126] by the linear energy absorption coefficient, μ_{en} (0.023 mm^{-1} for steel-clad ^{137}Cs sources), maximum errors are no larger than 5% to 8% and are much smaller (<3%) near the transverse axis. Published dose-rate distributions derived from the Sievert model, tabulated in terms of distances away and along, are available for several types of ^{137}Cs sources[4,125] and [226]Ra sources.[127] Williamson[119] showed that the classical Sievert integral gives rise to large errors (20% to 37% maximum error, 7% to 16% average error) when applied to lower-energy sources of ^{192}Ir, [169]Yb, and [125]I. Although accuracy can be improved by modifying the basic model,[119] classical semiempirical models should be used cautiously at photon energies below [137]Cs. Tabulated dose-rate distributions derived from direct measurement or Monte Carlo simulation are preferable for these sources.

If the encapsulation thickness is set to zero ($t = 0$) in Eq. (25), the Sievert integral reduces to a simple closed-form analytic expression:

$$\dot{D}(x,y) = S_K \cdot \overline{(\mu_{en}/\rho)}_{air}^{med} \cdot \frac{\Delta\theta}{L \cdot x} \qquad (26)$$

where $\Delta\theta$ is the angle, in radians, subtended by the active length, L, with respect to the point of interest (Fig. 25.12). When the interest point lies on the transverse axis ($y = 0$), then $\Delta\theta = 2 \cdot \tan^{-1}(L/2x)$, where $\tan^{-1}$ denotes the inverse tangent or arctan function. Angles must be specified in units of radians rather than degrees (180 degrees = π radians). This approximation is extremely useful as a manual calculation aid and is highly accurate near the transverse axis of lightly encapsulated ^{137}Cs sources.

Figure 25.13 shows that as the distance $r = \sqrt{(x^2 + y^2)}$ becomes large in relation to active length, L, Eq. (26) reduces to the point-source formula. For distances less than L (1.5 cm for intracavitary tubes), use of Eq. (17) will yield errors of at least 10%. For distances >1.5 L (2 to 2.5 cm for gynecologic tubes), the point-source approximation is accurate within 5%.

Modern Quantitative Dosimetry

In contrast to classical dose-calculation models, which assume that the parameters $T(r)$ and $\overline{(\mu_{en}/\rho)}_{air}^{wat}$ depend only on the radionuclide used, quantitative dosimetry methods assume that dosimetry parameters are source-geometry specific and should be measured or calculated specifically for each type of source. Classical approaches to BT dosimetry began to break down with the introduction of ^{125}I interstitial seeds in the early 1970s, as this 30-keV x-ray emitter clearly fell outside the

scope of validated analytic models.[12] Although ^{125}I dose distributions derived from semiempirical models were published[128] and widely used, it was recognized[61] that internal seed structure could modulate the emitted photon spectrum and have significantly alter the absorbed dose distribution. The growing use of ^{125}I and the introduction of a primary exposure standard in 1985[129] motivated investigation of more quantitative dosimetry methods. For a more detailed discussion of early of ^{125}I dosimetry, the reader is referred to Appendix C of the original TG-43 report.[130] Currently, both experimental methods and sophisticated computational dosimetry approaches are routinely used to derive such source-specific parameters. Both the classical and quantitative dosimetry approaches are based on the NIST air-kerma strength standards.

Experimental Brachytherapy Dosimetry

Clinical acceptance of measured dose rates in BT is a relatively recent phenomenon, beginning in the mid-1980s. Historically, this is due not only to the difficulties and labor-intensity attending such measurements, but to a consensus that dose measurement was so difficult and intrinsically inaccurate that even simplistic theoretic models were more reliable. Brachytherapy dose measurement does indeed place severe demands on detectors because the dose distributions are characterized by large dose gradients, a large range of dose rates, and relatively low photon energies. The most severe measurement artifact is the exquisite sensitivity of detector response to positioning errors; measurement of dose near a point source with 2% accuracy requires that the source-to-detector distance be specified with accuracy of 20, 50, 100, and 200 μm, respectively, at distances of 2, 5, 10, and 20 mm.

Commonly used dose detectors include thermoluminescent detectors (TLDs), small ion chambers, diode detectors, and silver-halide radiographic film. Radiochromic film[131-133] and plastic scintillator detectors[134,135] show promise as planar dose measurement systems. Three-dimensional dose measurement technologies under investigation include liquid scintillation cocktails[136] and polymer gel dosimetry[137,138] using either magnetic resonance imaging (MRI) or reconstructed by optical transmission tomography to quantify the detector signal. One consideration in selecting a detector for BT dosimetry is minimizing energy response artifacts, which arise from compositional differences between water and the detector and can result in variation of detector reading/unit dose in medium as the photon spectrum changes with position. Silicon diodes are useful detectors for measuring relative dose distributions around ultra-low-energy sources (e.g., [103]Pd and ^{125}I) because diode sensitivity is nearly independent of measurement point location[139,140] but are not recommended for higher-energy BT sources, as variations in sensitivity with position in the phantom as large as 15% for ^{137}Cs and 75% for ^{192}Ir have been reported.[141]

Among the established dosimetric techniques, LiF TLD dosimetry is considered to offer the best compromise between sensitivity, small size, and freedom from energy-response artifacts[84,142] and is currently considered to be standard of practice.[5] The acceptance of TLD dosimetry owes much to a 3-year (1987 to 1989) multi-institutional contract to perform a definitive review of low-energy seed dosimetry that was funded by the National Cancer Institute. The three institutions, collectively called the Interstitial Collaborative Working Group (ICWG), consisted of Memorial Sloan Kettering, Yale, and UCSF.[142] Using TLD-100 thermoluminescent chips and powder capsules, embedded in machined solid-water phantoms, the ICWG developed the procedures used to this day, including TLD dose calibration and energy response correction, for making quantitative estimates of absolute dose rates in water.

FIGURE 25.13. Error in the isotropic point source model relative to the line-source model Eq. (26) as a function of transverse-axis distance expressed in multiples of active length.

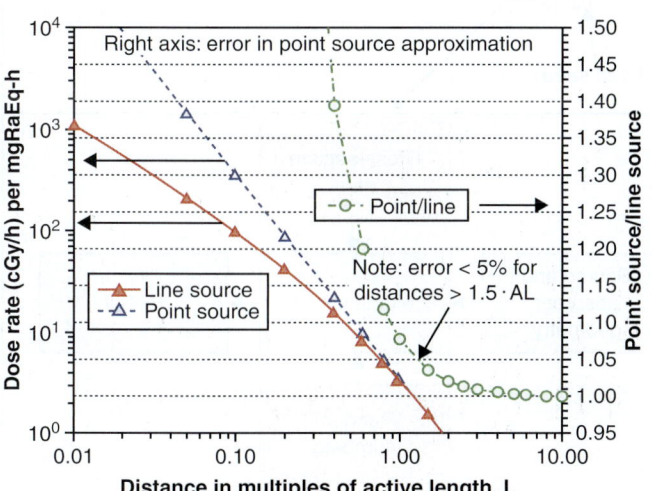

Right axis: error in point source approximation

- ○ Point/line

Note: error < 5% for distances > 1.5 · AL

- ▲ Line source
- △ Point source

Dose rate (cGy/h) per mgRaEq-h

Point source/line source

Distance in multiples of active length, L

Each investigator groups independently measured transverse-axis dose distributions for the ^{125}I and ^{192}Ir sources than available to validate their TLD measurement methodology.[142] This was followed by more complete 2D dose distributions about ^{125}I, ^{192}Ir, and [103]Pd BT sources then available.[139,143,144] The results showed good agreement among the different measurements and overall, substantial differences between measured and classically computed dose rates for ^{125}I seeds (when normalized to the air-kerma strength standard,[129] $S_{K,N85}$, then available), but good agreement between the classical and experimental approaches for [192]Ir. With careful correction for TLD linearity, perturbation of the photon field by the detectors, and relative energy response, absolute dose rate (cGy/h in tissue per unit S_K) can be measured with a total uncertainty of 6% to 9% in the 1- to 5-cm distance range.[5,84,111]

Measured dose-rate distributions using TLD detectors are available for many common BT sources, including nearly all commercially available ^{125}I and [103]Pd sources (see the revised TG-43 Report[5] and a recent review article[84] for more comprehensive discussions); many LDR ^{192}Ir sources for LDR, HDR, and PDR sources, as well as for many investigational sources. For radium-substitute sources, the measurements are in close agreement with the classical semiempirical models: isotropic point source and Sievert integral models.[4,24,119] For ^{125}I sources normalized to the 1984 Loftus[129] S_K standard, measured dose rates were found to be 10% to 20% lower than those predicted by Eq. (17).[5,145] Better agreement[84] was observed between classical models and measurements with calibrations traceable to the 1999 WAFAC standard ($S_{K,N99}$).[89] However, classical models such as the Sievert integral are not recommended for the low-energy source regimen as they poorly predict low-energy source anisotropy and do not take into account modulation of the dose distribution by internal source geometry.[119]

Computational Dosimetry Methods: Monte Carlo Photon Transport Simulation

Concurrently with the development of TLD dosimetry in the 1990s, other investigators were investigating the use of Monte Carlo photon-transport techniques as tools for quantitative evaluation of single-source dose distributions. Based on an accurate and detailed mathematical model of the internal structure of the source, photon histories can be generated and then evaluated to assess absorbed dose. Monte Carlo techniques are now accepted as a reliable and probably the most accurate source of BT dosimetry data.[5,84] As illustrated in Figure 25.14, this theoretical method uses a digital computer to randomly select a small number (10^5 to 10^7) of photon trajectories or "histories." A geometric model defining the location of all media boundaries and photon sources must be available. By using probability distributions derived from total and differential cross sections, a photon history is randomly constructed by following each photon from birth through successive scattering events and, eventually, to absorption or escape from the system. At each decision point, random sampling is used to decide the fate of the photon. The process of randomly constructing photon trajectories is equivalent to selecting photon histories from the set of all those possible by random sampling. To statistically estimate the dose rate at a specified point, the dose contributed by each simulated collision is estimated and then averaged over all collisions. Monte Carlo simulation techniques are reviewed in more detail elsewhere.[84] Because particle histories can be accurately and efficiently

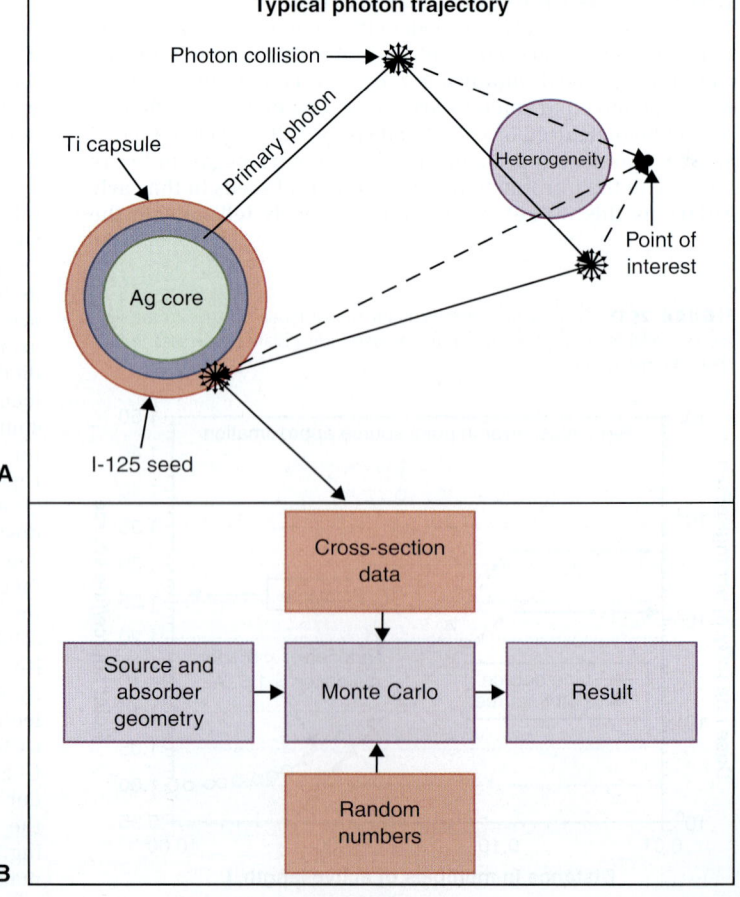

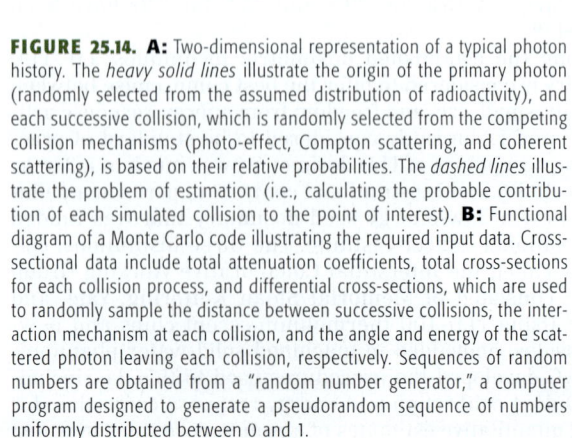

FIGURE 25.14. A: Two-dimensional representation of a typical photon history. The *heavy solid lines* illustrate the origin of the primary photon (randomly selected from the assumed distribution of radioactivity), and each successive collision, which is randomly selected from the competing collision mechanisms (photo-effect, Compton scattering, and coherent scattering), is based on their relative probabilities. The *dashed lines* illustrate the problem of estimation (i.e., calculating the probable contribution of each simulated collision to the point of interest). **B:** Functional diagram of a Monte Carlo code illustrating the required input data. Cross-sectional data include total attenuation coefficients, total cross-sections for each collision process, and differential cross-sections, which are used to randomly sample the distance between successive collisions, the interaction mechanism at each collision, and the angle and energy of the scattered photon leaving each collision, respectively. Sequences of random numbers are obtained from a "random number generator," a computer program designed to generate a pseudorandom sequence of numbers uniformly distributed between 0 and 1.

constructed even in the presence of complex 3D geometries, approximation-free but statistically inexact solutions, derived from first principles, are possible for a wide range of geometrically complex but clinically relevant BT problems.

The dosimetric accuracy of Monte Carlo simulation has been confirmed across the entire energy spectrum from ^{125}I to [137]Cs. Agreement between Monte Carlo and TLD measurement ranges from 2% to 6%, both in homogeneous medium and in the presence of tissue and applicator heterogeneities.[8,63,141,146,147] In contrast to experimental methods, Monte Carlo accuracy is not limited by dosimeter artifacts such as energy response and volume averaging. Because the geometric model can be specified exactly, detector positioning error is not an issue in Monte Carlo. Recent analyses[5,64,84] have shown that the uncertainty (including all known systematic and random error sources) of Monte Carlo absolute dose-rate estimates on the transverse axis of ^{125}I seeds is 2.5% to 5% over the 1- to 5-cm distance range. Unlike dose measurements, Monte Carlo dose calculations cannot account for unsuspected deviations from the design specifications of the problem (e.g., a contaminant radionuclide in the source or an error in measuring its source strength). A recent analysis,[148] which compared 25 sets of published TLD-100 low-energy seed measurements with parallel Monte Carlo calculations performed using a single EGSnrc-based Monte Carlo code,[149] found average differences between measurement and calculation 3.8% and 2.8% for ^{125}I and [103]Pd seeds, respectively, based upon treating TLD intrinsic energy corrections as best fit parameters.

Historically, the most important role of Monte Carlo simulation was calculation of reference-quality transverse-axis dose-rate distributions and anisotropy functions for low- and medium-energy BT sources. For low-energy interstitial seeds for routine clinical use, both experimental and Monte Carlo-based published dosimetry studies in peer-reviewed journal are required for developing AAPM-approved consensus datasets or posting the interstitial seed product on the Joint IROC-H/AAPM Source Registry.[55] Monte Carlo simulation is a useful alternative to dose measurement in many other applications such as characterizing the effects of applicator shielding materials[8] and tissue heterogeneities[63] on BT dose distributions, validating heuristic dose calculation algorithms,[150] and optimizing new source and applicator designs.[151]

AAPM Task Group 43 Report: A Table-Based Dose-Calculation Formalism

An important milestone in modern BT dosimetry is the publication of the original AAPM Task Group 43 Report in 1995[130] and a substantially revised and expanded version in 2004,[5] including two recent supplements.[52,53] The TG-43 approach consists of using measured and Monte Carlo-generated dose-rate distributions directly for clinical dose calculation aided by a standard table-lookup formalism. The revised TG-43 report and its supplements include the following:

1. A recommended table-based dose-calculation formalism for representing 2D and 1D dose distributions around interstitial sources specifically designed to use a sparse matrix of Monte Carlo or measured dose rates as its input.
2. A critically reviewed set of 2D dose-distribution data for a total of 27 ^{125}I, [103]Pd, and [131]Cs seed models that satisfy the AAPM dosimetric prerequisites.[57] For each of these source types, a consensus dose-distribution in TG-43 formalism format is recommended based upon "merging" published TG-43-compliant Monte Carlo and experimental dosimetry datasets.
3. A history of air-kerma strength primary standards,[89,129] which summarizes previous AAPM guidance,[152,153] including the impact of calibration shifts on the delivered-to-prescribed dose ratio.

4. Methodologic recommendations for obtaining TG-43 dosimetry parameters from TLD measurements or Monte Carlo simulations, including uncertainty analyses.
5. Guidance on clinical implementation of TG-43 report recommendations.

The TG-43 report recommends that all treatment-planning software systems utilize the TG-43 formalism as the basis of dose calculation or at least for data entry, allowing users to easily input the new data into their systems. With the introduction of the new WAFAC-based air-kerma strength standard by NIST and over 20 low-energy interstitial BT sources into the marketplace at various times, the radiotherapy community has embraced the TG-43 dose-calculation formalism as well as many AAPM recommendations associated with TG-43 implementation. Most important among these are the AAPM dosimetric prerequisites for routine non–IRB-approved BT procedures.[57] Only low-energy sources with NIST-traceable S_K calibrations supported by annual intercomparisons among NIST, the ADCLs, and the vendor[154] and two independent Monte Carlo and experimental dosimetry studies published in the peer-reviewed literature will be posted on the Joint IROC-Houston/AAPM Registry website[55] or included in future TG-43 supplements. In 2012, a similar dosimetry validation process was introduced for higher-energy sources.[72]

Because embracing new calibration standards and dosimetry parameters alters prescribed-to-delivered dose ratios, radiation oncologists must understand the implications for selection of prescribed dose, interpreting published outcome studies, and consistently reproducing their clinical experience through time. AAPM reports provide detailed discussions and recommendations on managing these changes. For example, in ^{125}I monotherapy for prostate cancer, the Pre-TG43 prescribed dose of 160 Gy is equivalent to 145 Gy using the TG-43 dosimetry parameters.[152,155] Managing the up to 10% variations in prescribed-to-administered dose ratios because of the complex dosimetric history of [103]Pd monotherapy is reviewed in a 2005 AAPM report.[155]

General Formalism for the Two-Dimensional Case

For a cylindrically symmetric source of strength S_K (Fig. 25.15), dose rate, $\dot{D}(r,\theta)$, at the point (r,θ), is calculated in the TG-43 formalism as follows:

$$\dot{D}(r,\theta) = S_K \cdot \Lambda \cdot \frac{G_L(r,\theta)}{G_L(r_0,\theta_0)} \cdot g_L(r) \cdot F(r,\theta) \qquad (27)$$

FIGURE 25.15. Illustration of TG-43 formalism for calculation of absorbed dose rate, $\dot{D}(r,\theta)$, at (r,θ), in a polar coordinate system centered about the source active core.

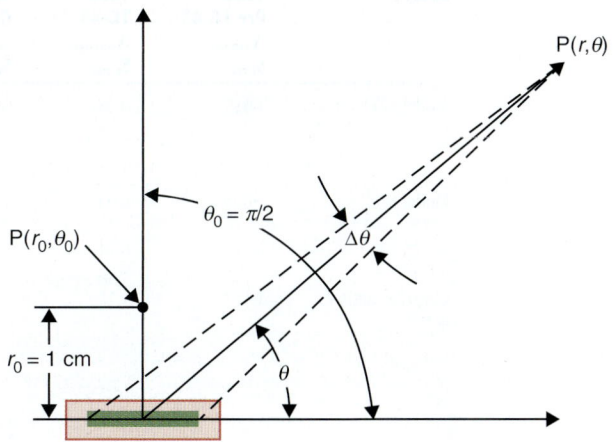

where r denotes the distance (in cm) from the center of the active source to the point of interest, θ denotes the polar angle specifying the point of interest relative to the source longitudinal axis, r_0 denotes the reference distance (specified to be 1 cm), and θ_0 is the reference angle (90° or $\pi/2$ radians) that defines the source transverse plane. For ^{125}I and ^{103}Pd sources, AAPM guidance[155] uses the symbols $S_{K,N99}$ and $S_{K,N85}$ to designate the 1999 WAFAC-based NIST standard[89] and the prior Loftus[129] free-air standard introduced in 1985. The other symbols in (27) denote the following quantities:

$G_L(r,\theta)$ is the line-source geometry function in units of cm^{-2}.

Λ is the dose-rate constant of the source type in units of cGy·h^{-1}·U^{-1}.

$F(r,\theta)$ is the dimensionless 2D anisotropy function that takes the value unity for θ_0 at all r.

$g(r)$ is the dimensionless radial dose function that takes the value unity at $r = r_0$.

The dose-rate constant in liquid-water medium is defined by:

$$\Lambda = \frac{\dot{D}(r_0,\theta_0)}{S_K} = \frac{\dot{D}(1\,\text{cm},90°)}{S_K} \qquad (28)$$

where $\dot{D}(r_0,\theta_0)$ is the measured dose rate at the reference point. Λ includes the effects of source geometry, spatial distribution of radioactivity, encapsulation, self-filtration in the source, and attenuation and scattering of photons in the surrounding medium. It also depends on the standardization measurements to which the S_K calibration of the source is traceable. For radium-substitute point sources, $\Lambda \approx (\mu_{en}/\rho)_{air}^{med} \cdot T(r) \cdot G_L(1\,\text{cm},\pi/2)$. Table 25.4 shows that during the $S_{K,N85}$ era (1984 to 1999), the classical point-source model overestimated absolute doses by as much as 15% for ^{125}I sources relative to TLD measurements and Monte Carlo calculations. In 1999, the WAFAC ($S_{K,N99}$) standard replaced $S_{K,N85}$, which required an upward adjustment of these Λ values, bringing the classical and quantitative values closer together. The old and new dose calculations are in close agreement for ^{192}Ir and other radium substitutes.

The purpose of the geometry function, $G_X(r,\theta)$ (where the subscript "X" denotes point (P) or line source (L)), is to improve the accuracy with which dose rates can be estimated by interpolation from data tabulated at discrete points. Physically, $G_X(r,\theta)$ neglects scattering and attenuation and provides an effective inverse-square law correction based upon an *approximate model* of the spatial radioactivity distribution within the source. Because the geometry function is used only to interpolate between tabulated dose-rate values at defined points, highly simplistic approximations yield

sufficient accuracy for treatment planning.[5] To improve the accuracy of linear interpolation near the source, the AAPM protocol requires use of (r,θ) for 2D calculations and prefers $G_L(r,\theta)$ over $G_P(r,\theta)$ for 1D calculations. For small cylindrical seeds, $G_X(r,\theta)$ is approximated by a line source:

$$G_P(r,\theta) = r^{-2} \qquad \text{point-source approximation}$$

$$G_L(r,\theta) = \begin{cases} \dfrac{\Delta\beta}{Lr\sin\theta} & \text{if } \theta \neq 0° \\ (r^2 - L^2/4)^{-1} & \text{if } \theta = 0° \end{cases} \quad \text{line-source approximation}$$

$$\qquad (29)$$

where $\Delta\beta = \theta_2 - \theta_1$ is the angle subtended by the active source with respect to the point (r,θ). For sources where the radioactivity is distributed over or within a right cylindrical volume or annulus, L can be taken as the length of this cylinder. For sources containing uniformly spaced multiple radioactive components, L should be taken as the effective length, L_{eff}, given by $L_{eff} = \Delta S \times (N)$, where N represents the number of discrete pellets contained in the source with a nominal pellet center-to-center spacing, ΔS.

The 2D anisotropy function $F(r,\theta)$ gives the angular variation of dose about the source at each distance as a result of self-filtration, oblique filtration of primary photons through the encapsulating material, and photon attenuation and scattering in the surrounding medium:

$$F(r,\theta) = \frac{\dot{D}(r,\theta)}{\dot{D}(r,\theta_0)} \frac{G_L(r,\theta_0)}{G_L(r,\theta)} \qquad (30)$$

where the dose rates, $\dot{D}(r,\theta)$, are obtained by measurement or Monte Carlo simulation. The line-source geometry function is used to suppress the influence of inverse-square law on the angular dose distribution at short distances. Thus, $F(r,\theta)$ need be tabulated only at a few distances, r, to facilitate accurate interpolation at all distances. Examples of anisotropy functions for various interstitial sources are illustrated in Figure 25.16 and in Table 25.6.

The radial dose function, $g_X(r)$, accounts for the fall-off of dose along the transverse axis as a result of attenuation and scattering in the medium, capsule filtration, and self-absorption:

$$g_X(r) = \frac{\dot{D}(r,\theta_0)}{\dot{D}(r_0,\theta_0)} \frac{G_X(r_0,\theta_0)}{G_X(r,\theta_0)} \qquad (31)$$

$g_X(r)$ is normalized to unity at 1 cm distance and is illustrated by Table 25.5. For 2D dose calculations, TG-43 recommends that X = L.

TABLE 25.4 DOSE–RATE CONSTANTS FOR SELECTED INTERSTITIAL SEEDS Λ (CGY·CM^2·U^{-1})

Source	1983 Pre TG-43 $\Lambda_{83D,N85S}$ $S_{K,N85}$	1995 TG-43[130] $\Lambda_{95D,N85S}$ $S_{K,N85}$	2000 AAPM Guidance[153] $\Lambda_{95D,N99S}$ $S_{K,N99}$	2004 TG-43[155] $\Lambda_{04D,N99S}$ $S_{K,N99}$	Modern values $\Lambda_{>06D,N99S}$ $S_{K,N99}$
Model 6711 I-125	1.035	0.88	0.981	0.964	0.954 (130.002: TG-43 2017[55]) 0.940 (I25.S17+: TG-43 2017[53]) 0.952 (AgX100: TG-43 2017[55]) 0.956 (6711: Dolan 2006[111])
Model 6702 I-125	1.035	0.93	1.037	1.036	–
Model 200 Pd-103	–	0.74 $S_{K,T88}$	0.665	0.686	–
LDR/HDR sources Ir-192	1.12	1.12	1.12	1.12	1.109 (Elekta mHDR-v2) 1.100 (Varian VS2000) 1.117 (Gamma Med HDR+) 1.124 (Gamma Med PDR+) 1.110 (Best LDR seed) (from AAPM HEBD Report 2012[72])

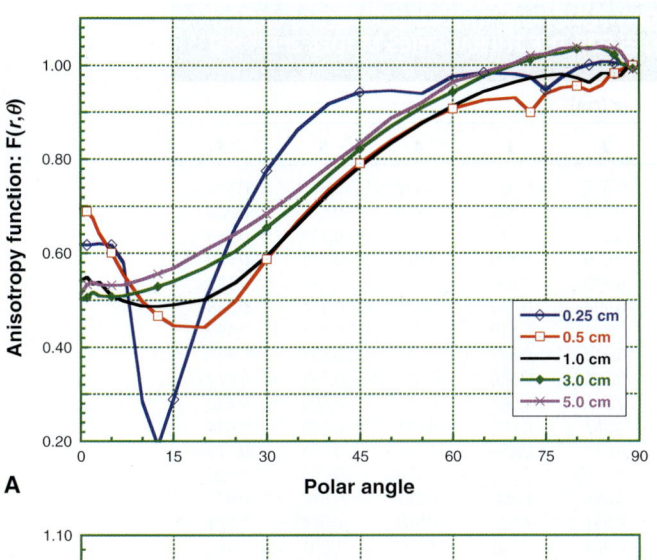

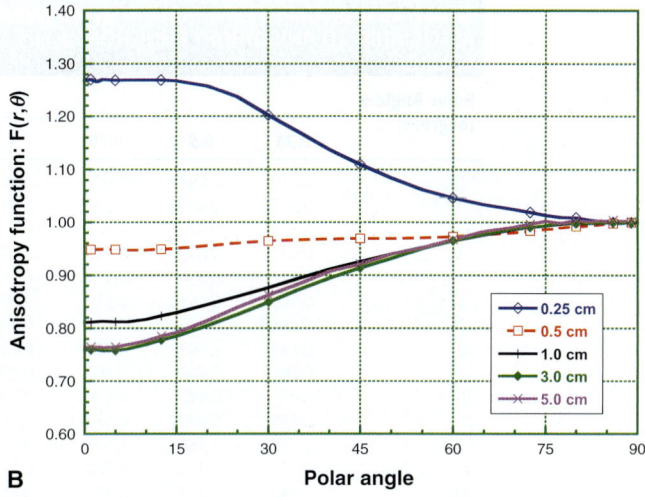

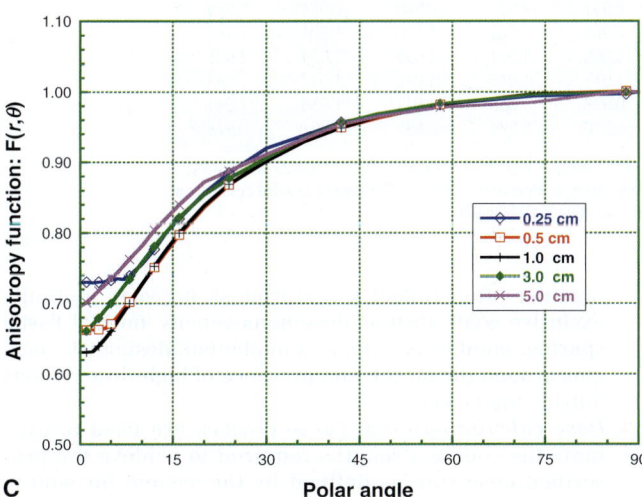

FIGURE 25.16. Examples of anisotropy functions evaluated for three different interstitial sources by the author's group. **A:** Theragenics Model 200 "light seed" [103]Pd source.[156] **B:** DRAXIMAGE Model LS-1 ^{125}I seed.[157] **C:** Nucletron MicroSelectron Model V2 high-dose-rate ^{192}Ir source.[69]

One-Dimensional Isotropic Source Approximation

Most commercial treatment planning systems used for permanent implant dose computation support only 1D isotropic point-source calculations. Thus, the TG-43 formalism includes a 1D equation analogous to the classical isotropic point-source model, Eq. (22):

$$\dot{D}(r) = S_K \cdot \Lambda \cdot \frac{G_L(r, \theta_0)}{G_L(r_0, \theta_0)} \cdot g_L(r) \cdot \phi_{an}(r) \tag{32}$$

TABLE 25.5 LINE-SOURCE RADIAL DOSE FUNCTIONS FOR VARIOUS LOW-ENERGY PHOTON–EMITTING SEED SOURCES

r (cm)	BEBIG S17plus	Elekta 130.002	Theragenics AgX100	CivaTech CS10	IsoAid 1APd-103A	IsoRay CS-1 Rev2
	[125]I	[125]I	[125]I	[103]Pd	[103]Pd	[131]Cs
0.10	1.059	1.042	1.066	1.010	0.788	0.960
0.15	1.080	**1.062**	1.086	1.164	1.080	0.971
0.25	1.092	**1.085**	1.098	1.263	1.254	0.989
0.50	1.073	1.078	1.076	1.232	1.238	1.006
0.75	1.040	**1.044**	1.042	1.124	1.122	1.009
1.00	1.000	1.000	1.000	1.000	1.000	1.000
1.50	0.909	0.907	0.908	0.770	0.758	0.962
2.00	0.814	0.808	0.813	0.580	0.569	0.908
3.00	0.635	0.627	0.633	0.320	0.313	0.777
4.00	0.482	0.477	0.482	0.1726	0.1686	0.642
5.00	0.363	0.357	0.361	0.0924	0.0911	0.518
6.00	0.270	0.265	0.269	0.0496	0.0487	0.411
7.00	0.1995	0.1963	0.1990	0.0268	0.0265	0.323
8.00	0.1467	0.1442	0.1470	0.01471	0.01472	0.251
9.00	0.1087	0.1058	0.1080	0.00816	0.00841	0.1931
10.00	0.0792	0.0776	0.0790	0.00473	0.00504	0.1481

Bolded entries indicate interpolated values.
From Rivard MJ, Ballester F, Butler WM, et al. Supplement 2: 2004 update of the AAPM Task Group No. 43 Report: Joint recommendations by the AAPM and GEC-ESTRO. *Med Phys* 2017;44(9):e297–e338. Copyright © 2017 American Association of Physicists in Medicine. Reprinted by permission of John Wiley & Sons, Inc.

TABLE 25.6 EXAMPLE OF A TABULATED 2D ANISOTROPY FUNCTION, $F(R,\Theta)$ TABLE, ALONG WITH ITS ASSOCIATED 1D ANISOTROPY FUNCTION, $\phi_{an}(r)$, VALUES FOR THE THERAGENICS MODEL 200 [103]PD SOURCE

Polar Angle θ (degrees)	r (cm)								
	0.25	0.5	0.75	1	2	3	4	5	7.5
0	0.619	0.694	0.601	0.541	0.526	0.504	0.497	0.513	0.547
1	0.617	0.689	0.597	0.549	0.492	0.505	0.513	0.533	0.580
2	0.618	0.674	0.574	0.534	0.514	0.517	0.524	0.538	0.568
3	0.620	0.642	0.577	0.538	0.506	0.509	0.519	0.532	0.570
5	0.617	0.600	0.540	0.510	0.499	0.508	0.514	0.531	0.571
7	0.579	0.553	0.519	0.498	0.498	0.509	0.521	0.532	0.568
10	0.284	0.496	0.495	0.487	0.504	0.519	0.530	0.544	0.590
12	0.191	0.466	0.486	0.487	0.512	0.529	0.544	0.555	0.614
15	0.289	0.446	0.482	0.490	0.523	0.540	0.556	0.567	0.614
20	0.496	0.442	0.486	0.501	0.547	0.568	0.585	0.605	0.642
25	0.655	0.497	0.524	0.537	0.582	0.603	0.621	0.640	0.684
30	0.775	0.586	0.585	0.593	0.633	0.654	0.667	0.683	0.719
40	0.917	0.734	0.726	0.727	0.750	0.766	0.778	0.784	0.820
50	0.945	0.837	0.831	0.834	0.853	0.869	0.881	0.886	0.912
60	0.976	0.906	0.907	0.912	0.931	0.942	0.960	0.964	0.974
70	0.981	0.929	0.954	0.964	0.989	1.001	1.008	1.004	1.011
75	0.947	0.938	0.961	0.978	1.006	1.021	1.029	1.024	1.033
80	0.992	0.955	0.959	0.972	1.017	1.035	1.046	1.037	1.043
85	1.007	0.973	0.960	0.982	0.998	1.030	1.041	1.036	1.043
$\phi_{an}(r)$	1.130	0.880	0.859	0.855	0.870	0.884	0.895	0.897	0.918

Italicized entries indicate extrapolated values. Reproduced from Rivard MJ, Butler WM, DeWerd LA, et al. Supplement to the 2004 update of the AAPM Task Group No. 43 Report. *Med Phys* 2007;34(6):2187–2205; based on Monte Carlo data from Monroe JI, Williamson JF. Monte carlo-aided dosimetry of the theragenics TheraSeed® Model 200 [103]Pd interstitial brachytherapy seed. *Med Phys* 2002;29(4):609–621.

where $\phi_{an}(r)$ is the 1D anisotropy function defined by Eq. (21) and illustrated by Table 25.6.

INTERSTITIAL IMPLANTATION

The traditional implant systems (Manchester, Quimby, and Paris) that arose early in the 20th century were developed to guide the radiation oncologist in arranging and positioning radium needles within the surgically identified target volume. In contrast, the most frequently practiced implant procedure today, transperineal permanent implants of the prostate, uses image guidance to position the sources. In place of nomograms and classical system lookup tables, 3D computerized planning is used to prescribe dose and to optimize the implant geometry. However, even the most sophisticated commercially available dwell-weight optimization software used with single-stepping source remote afterloaders (see Chapters 26, 27, and 28) requires the operator to specify the source and needle locations. To guide source positioning, we continue to rely on the classical systems of BT and their later variants.

Classical Systems for Interstitial Brachytherapy with Radium-Substitute Sources

The Manchester and Quimby systems were developed before the advent of computer-aided dosimetry in implant therapy, whereas the Paris system is based on multiplanar isodose distributions. All interstitial implant systems consist of the following components:

1. *Distribution rules:* Given a target volume, the distribution rules determine how to distribute the radioactive sources and applicators in and around the target volume.
2. *Dose-specification and implant-optimization criteria:* At the heart of each system is a dose-specification criterion (i.e., a definition of prescribed dose). In the Manchester system, for example, the prescribed dose is the modal dose in the volume bounded by the peripheral sources. The distribution rules and dose-specification criterion

together often reflect a compromise between mutually exclusive goals such as dose homogeneity, normal tissue sparing, number of catheters implanted, dosimetric margins around the target, and presence of high-dose regions outside the target.

3. *Dose calculation aids:* These devices are used to estimate the source strengths required to achieve the prescribed dose rate as defined by the system for source arrangements satisfying its distribution rules. Older systems (Manchester and Quimby) use tables that give dose delivered per mgRaEq-h as a function of treatment volume or area. The more recent Paris system makes extensive use of computerized treatment planning to relate absorbed dose to source strength and treatment time.

The Manchester System

The Manchester system was developed by Ralston Paterson (radiation oncologist) and Herbert Parker (physicist) in the 1930s[158–161] and often is called the Paterson-Parker (P-P) system. The P-P system remains relevant to today's practice patterns: Its distribution rules, anticipating the "peripheral loading technique," were designed to maximize dose homogeneity inside the implanted volume for volume implants and in the treatment plane (plane parallel to the needles at the treatment distance) for mold or planar implants (Fig. 25.17). Its volume and area lookup tables remain useful as QA tools for optimized HDR volume implants.

The P-P system rules preferentially concentrate radioactivity in the rind or periphery of the implant, compensating for the dose falloff characteristic of a uniform density implant, thereby improving dose uniformity. After deriving the optimal fraction of radioactivity to be implanted in the rind and core (4:2 ratio) using a radioactive fluid model, Parker coalesced the continuous radioactivity distribution into several concentric cylindrical surfaces and then further discretized these surfaces into individual needles. A more detailed discussion of the mathematical derivation of the Manchester system is given by Anderson and Presser.[162] Table 25.7 lists the rules of the Manchester system, and

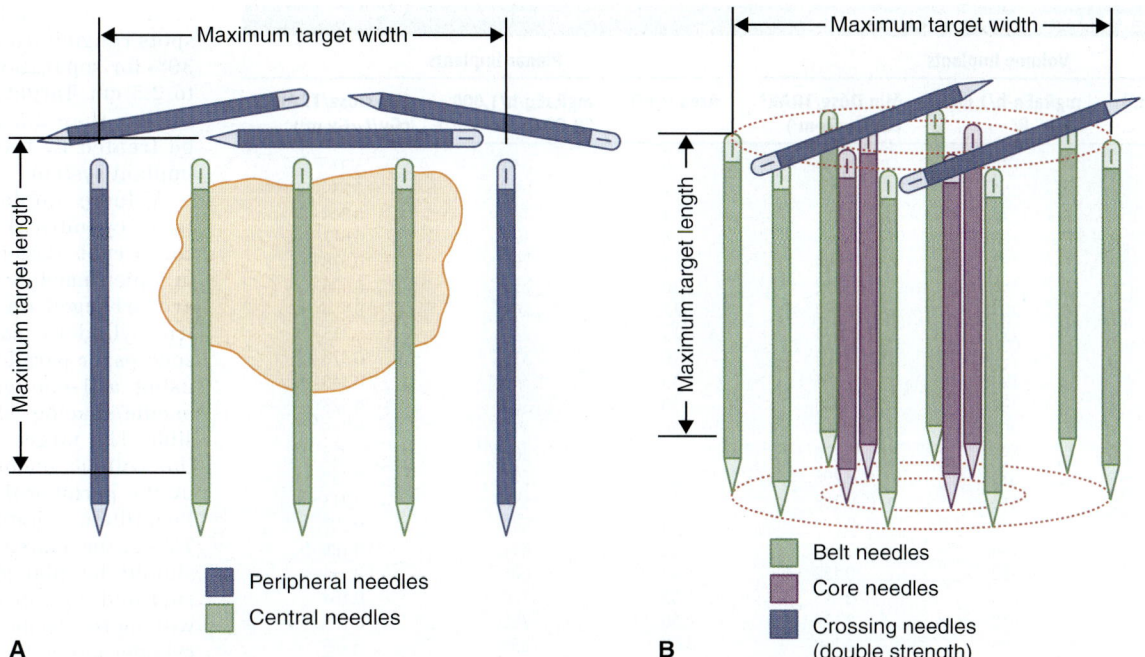

FIGURE 25.17. A: Relationship between target volume or area and peripheral needles (*solid color active regions*) and central needles (*green active regions*). Notice that peripheral needles always are placed on the boundary of the target region. **B:** For a cylindrical volume implant, the peripheral needles distributed on the cylindrical surface of the target are called *belt* needles, whereas those at right angles are called *end* or *crossing* needles. Because the inferior end of the implant is uncrossed, the target volume effectively treated is 7.5% shorter than the active length of the belt needles.

Table 25.8 lists the stated dose per mgRaEq-h and unit TRAK as a function-treated area or volume.

The P-P rules are designed to yield target area or volume dose distribution that deviates by no more than ±10% of the stated dose, excluding cold spots in the corners and local hot spots at distances <5 mm from the source centers. For planar implants, the target or treatment surface (Fig. 25.17) is that area bounded by the peripheral needles, which is parallel to and 5 mm from the needle plane. For volume implants, the target volume is that region bounded by the peripheral sources. The distribution rules assume that both planar and volume implants will be crossed at both ends

TABLE 25.7 MANCHESTER SYSTEM RULES					
Feature	**Paterson and Parker (Manchester System) Rules**				
Dose and dose rate	6,000–8,000 R in 6–8 d (1,000 R/d; 40 R/h)				
Dose specification criterion	Effective minimum dose is 10% above the absolute minimum dose in treatment plane or volume.				
Dose gradient	Dose in treatment volume or plane varies by no more than ±10% from stated dose except for localized hot spots.				
	For double-plane implants with a separation >1 cm, dose is specified on interior plane 0.5 cm from implanted plane resulting in 10%–30% midplane cold spot. Single-plane mgRaEq-h is multiplied by a separation factor to obtain total double-plane mgRaEq-h.				
Linear activity	Variable: 0.66 and 0.33 mgRaEq/cm				
Source strength distribution: planar	Area < 25 cm²:	2/3 periphery; 1/3 center			
	25 < Area < 100 cm²:	1/2 periphery; 1/2 center			
	Area >100 cm²:	1/3 periphery; 2/3 center			
Source strength distribution: volume	Cylinder:	belt : core : end : end = 4:2:1:1			
	Sphere:	belt : core = 6:2			
	Cube:	1/8 of the activity in each face			
		2/8 of the activity in the core			
Source implant pattern and spacing between sources	Constant uniform spacing: 1-cm separation between sources recommended. Smaller spacings must be used to satisfy distribution rules for small implants.				
Crossing needles	Perpendicular to and at the active ends of the parallel needles; if placed beyond the active ends of the needles, should be double strength. Crossing needles used when possible.				
	Planar implant: Target area effectively treated is reduced in length by 10% per uncrossed end.				
	Volume implant: Target volume effectively treated is reduced by 7.5% per uncrossed end.				
	1 uncrossed end : belt : core = 4:2:1				
	2 uncrossed end : belt : core = 4:2				
Elongation corrections	Long : Short Dimension: 1.5:1 2:1 2.5:1 3:1 4:1				
	Correction factors (Applied to mgRaEq-h, not area or volume)				
	Planar 1.025 1.05 1.07 1.09 1.12				
	Volume 1.03 1.06 1.10 1.15 1.23				
Relation between implanted volume/area and treated (target) volume/area	Peripheral and crossing needles placed on the target-volume boundaries. Active length determines target length.				

TABLE 25.8 MANCHESTER IMPLANT TABLES

Volume Implants			Planar Implants		
Volume (cm³)	mgRaEq-h/1,000 "P-P" R[a]	Min Dose/TRAK[b] cGy/(μGy·m²)	Area (cm²)	mgRaEq-h/1,000 "P-P" R[a]	Min Dose/TRAK[b] cGy/(μGy·m²)
1	34	3.49	0	30	3.97
2	54	2.20	2	97	1.23
3	70	1.68	4	141	0.844
4	85	1.38	6	177	0.672
5	99	1.194	8	206	0.578
10	158	0.752	10	235	0.506
15	207	0.574	12	261	0.456
20	251	0.474	14	288	0.413
25	291	0.408	16	315	0.378
30	329	0.361	18	342	0.348
40	398	0.298	20	368	0.323
50	462	0.257	24	417	0.285
60	522	0.228	28	466	0.255
70	579	0.206	32	513	0.232
80	633	0.188	36	558	0.213
90	684	0.174	40	603	0.197
100	734	0.162	44	644	0.185
110	782	0.152	48	685	0.174
120	829	0.143	52	725	0.164
140	919	0.129	56	762	0.156
160	1,005	0.118	60	800	0.149
180	1,087	0.110	64	837	0.142
200	1,166	0.102	68	873	0.136
220	1,242	0.0958	72	908	0.131
240	1,316	0.0904	76	945	0.126
260	1,389	0.0857	80	981	0.121
280	1,459	0.0815	84	1,016	0.117
300	1,528	0.0779	88	1,052	0.113
320	1,595	0.0746	92	1,087	0.109
340	1,661	0.0716	96	1,122	0.106
360	1,725	0.0690	100	1,155	0.103
380	1,788	0.0665	120	1,307	0.0910
400	1,851	0.0643	140	1,463	0.0813
—	—	—	160	1,608	0.0740
—	—	—	180	1,746	0.0682
—	—	—	200	1,880	0.0633
—	—	—	220	2,008	0.0593
—	—	—	240	2,132	0.0558
—	—	—	260	2,256	0.0527
—	—	—	280	2,372	0.0502
—	—	—	300	2,495	0.0477

[a]Original Manchester values from Paterson R, Parker HM. A dosage system for interstitial radium therapy. *Br J Radiol* 1938;11:313–339.
[b]Modified from original values for Ir-192 assuming 860 cGy minimum peripheral dose per 1,000 "P-P" R and 7.227 μGy·m²/mgRaEq-h.

by needles placed orthogonal to the predominant direction of insertion and at the level of the belt needle active tips. Fixed 1-cm needle spacing is recommended, with full-intensity sources placed on the periphery of planar implants and partial-strength needles used as central needles. For volume implants, these two groups of sources are called "belt" and "core" sources, respectively. The stated or prescribed dose is the modal dose in the target region and is approximately 10% higher than the minimum peripheral dose (minimum dose to the implanted volume or area) and 10% below the effective maximum dose.

In effect, single-plane interstitial implants with crossed ends treat a 1-cm-thick target volume with an area equal to that bounded by the peripheral sources. Target volumes thicker than 1 cm must be treated by using two parallel planes of needles placed on the target-volume boundaries (double-plane implant), with source strength arranged in each plane according to the single-plane rules. The mgRaEq-h is calculated from the 0.5-cm single-plane table, multiplied by the appropriate two-plane separation factor, and divided between the two planes. The dose actually is delivered to the inner plane 0.5 cm from each needle plane,

resulting in midplane cold spots ranging from 10% to 30% for separations of 1.5 to 2.5 cm. Target volumes thicker than 2.5 cm must be treated by the volume implant system.

Volume implants can treat cylindrical, spherical, or cubic target volumes in which needles or seeds are arranged on concentric cylinders, concentric spheres, or parallel planes, using a 1-cm needle-to-needle spacing when possible. The target region is the volume encompassed by the peripheral sources. Regardless of implant size, 75% of the source strength should be placed in the rind and 25% in the core, with more specific rules for cylinder implants.

To apply the P-P system, the relationship between target volume, implanted volume (region enclosed by peripheral sources), and treated volume (region receiving 90% of the stated dose) must be appreciated for crossed and uncrossed end cases. The treated volume may be larger than the target volume but always should contain the latter. When both ends are crossed, the active length (AL) required and target length (TL) are identical. For volume implants, AL should be at least 7.5% longer than TL for each uncrossed end. For planar implants, the AL:

$$
\begin{aligned}
\text{Two crossed ends} \quad & \text{AL} = \text{TL planar and volume} \\
\text{One crossed end} \quad & \text{AL} = \begin{cases} \text{TL}/0.90 & \text{planar} \\ \text{TL}/0.925 & \text{volume} \end{cases} \\
\text{No crossed ends} \quad & \text{AL} = \begin{cases} \text{TL}/0.81 & \text{planar} \\ \text{TL}/0.85 & \text{volume} \end{cases}
\end{aligned}
\tag{33}
$$

Conversely, given AL, the length of the treated volume always can be calculated by solving the appropriate Eq. (33) for TL. The area and volume used for looking up dose per mgRaEq-h from Table 25.8 should be calculated using the treated length. For example, for a single-plane implant with two uncrossed ends, width (W) and needles of active length (AL), the area, A, used for table lookup is given by A = W × AL × 0.81.

To apply P-P tables to modern implants using ^{192}Ir wires or ribbons, several corrections must be applied. The 1938 P-P tables assumed a Γ value of 8.4, ignored attenuation and scattering, neglected oblique filtration, and specified treatment in terms of exposure rather than absorbed dose. For [226]Ra needles, an average correction of 0.90[127] is needed to convert exposure in the original P-P tables to absorbed dose. Modifying these corrections for ^{137}Cs needles and ^{192}Ir seeds and adding an additional factor of 10% to convert from stated (modal target dose) to minimum target volume dose, we obtain the following equivalencies:

$$1'P\text{–}P'R = \begin{Bmatrix} 0.97 \cdot \dfrac{8.25}{8.4} & 0.98 & 0.98 & 0.90 \\ 0.97 \cdot \dfrac{8.25}{8.4} & 1.00 & 0.98 & 0.90 \\ 0.97 \cdot \dfrac{8.25}{8.4} & 1.00 & 1.00 & 0.90 \\ (\text{cGy/R}) \cdot \left(\dfrac{\Gamma_{\text{new}}}{\Gamma_{\text{old}}}\right) & (\text{filtration}) & (\text{attenuation/buildup}) & \left(\dfrac{\text{min}}{\text{stated}}\text{dose}\right) \end{Bmatrix}$$

$$\tag{34}$$

$$= \begin{Bmatrix} 0.82 \text{ cGy radium needles} \\ 0.84 \text{ cGy cesium needles} \\ 0.86 \text{ cGy iridium ribbons} \end{Bmatrix} \left(\dfrac{\text{Modern cGy}}{'P\text{–}P'\,R}\right)$$

Using the 0.90 cGy/P-P R conversion factor, Stovall and Shalek[127] found excellent agreement between computer calculations and the P-P tables for a variety of planar and cylindrical implants following the Manchester distribution rules. For single-plane implants, 90% of the stated dose in cGy covers 94% to 99% of the target area. For cubic arrays of seeds using fixed 1-cm spacing, agreement between the tables and computer calculations is excellent for treatment volumes of more than 100 cm^3,[163,164] but results in errors ranging from 10% to 40% for smaller arrays. These discrepancies probably result from deviations from the 4:2 activity ratio and use of a dose-specification criterion incompatible with the Manchester system.

The classical implant systems are based on ^{192}Ir wires or interstitial needles, consisting of continuous distributions of radioactivity (i.e., line sources) with well-defined active lengths. To apply the classical systems to modern interstitial sources consisting of discrete equispaced seeds or single-stepping source dwell positions, the dosimetric equivalence between linear arrays of discrete seed sources and line sources must be appreciated (Fig. 25.18). An array consisting of N seeds with center-to-center separations, S, has a dose distribution that closely approximates that of a continuous line source of length, AL, and strength $(S_K)_{\text{line}}$[114,165]:

$$\left.\begin{aligned} AL &= N \cdot S \\ (S_K)_{\text{line}} &= N \cdot (S_K)_{\text{seed}} \end{aligned}\right\} \tag{35}$$

This equivalence tends to break down at distances less than S/2: the cylindrical isodose curves break up into ellipsoidal shapes centered about each seed. In addition, the ribbon isodose curves undulate significantly at distances comparable with or less than the gap, S, between adjacent seeds, although on average the equivalence remains accurate.

FIGURE 25.18. Relationship between a linear array of equally spaced discrete seeds and its dosimetrically equivalent line source. Both sources are assumed to have the same total strength. Common errors in defining this equivalence are illustrated.

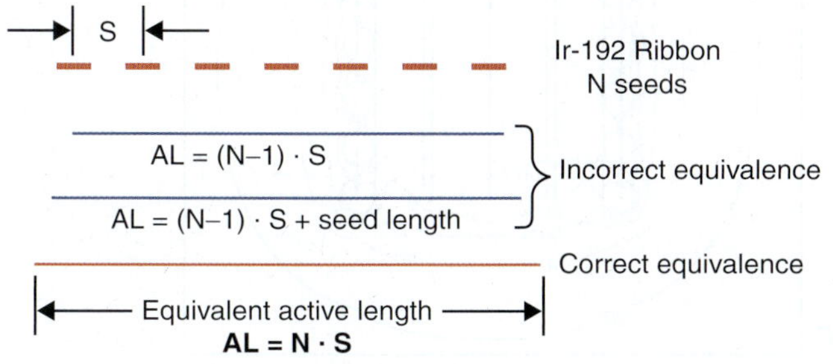

Because the P-P system uses 1-cm interneedle spacing, the fraction of sources in the core (vs. periphery) increases as volume increases. Thus, using uniform-strength ^{192}Ir ribbons and fixed spacing results in underloading the core for very small implants and overloading the core for very large implants, relative to the P-P distribution rules. In the latter case, the gap between minimum peripheral dose and central maximum dose widens. An alternative to the differential loading method is to vary the ribbon spacing with implant size, using smaller (<1 cm) spacing for very small implants and larger spacing (up to a limit of 1.5 cm) for larger implants, so that the relative number of central ribbons complies approximately with the P-P rules, allowing uniform seed strengths to be used. Two examples of this strategy are given in the next section.

To use the Manchester tables for verification of computerized dose calculations requires a method for objectively identifying the computer-generated isodose surface that corresponds to the minimum peripheral dose rate predicted by the Manchester system. For volume implants, mean central dose (MCD), a quantity proposed by the ICRU Report 58 on dose specification in interstitial BT, is useful[166] (Fig. 25.19). In the authors' experience, the maximum dose (110% of stated dose) of the Manchester system is closely approximated by MCD. Minimum peripheral dose and stated dose are given by 80% and 89%, respectively, of MCD. For planar implants, the minimum dose/MCD ratio varies from 55% to 70%, depending on catheter spacing and is of limited value.

Manchester Volume Implant Example

A 5-cm-high by 5-cm-diameter cylindrical target volume is to be treated using ^{192}Ir ribbons with seed-to-seed and intercatheter spacings of 1 and 1.3 cm, respectively (Fig. 25.20). Calculate the (a) minimum ribbon length needed, (b) the required ribbon arrangement, and (c) the strength/seed needed to deliver 45 cGy/h to the P-P minimum dose specification volume.

a. There are two approaches: treating the ribbons as needles with uncrossed ends or treating the proximal and distal seeds of each ribbon as crossing sources. In the uncrossed end approach, Eq. (33) implies that

   AL = target length/0.925^2 = 5 cm/0.85 = 5.9 cm

   Equation (35) implies that N = 6 seeds/ribbon are required.

   In the crossed-end approach, the first and last seeds must be placed at the target volume surfaces, again requiring 6 seeds/ribbon.

b. To satisfy the 1.3-cm ribbon-spacing requirement, 12 ribbons must be placed on the cylindrical target boundary, 6 ribbons must be placed on an inner cylindrical surface, and there should be 1 central ribbon. Treating the ends as uncrossed and assuming that the ribbons have uniform strengths, the belt-to-core ratio is 0.63:0.37, which is close to the P-P 4:2 ratio. Again, assuming all seeds have the same strength, Figure 25.20 shows that the required crossed-end ratios are also closely approximated. This illustrates ribbon spacing can be manipulated to adhere to the P-P distribution rules with uniform strength sources.

c. Assuming the uncrossed end point of view:

   TL = AL × 0.85 = (1 cm) × 0.85 = 5.1 cm

   Treated (lookup) Volume = $\pi \times (2.5)^2 \times 5.1 = 100.1$ cm^3

Hence:

$$\frac{734 \text{ mg} - \text{h}}{1000'P - P'R} = \frac{734 \text{ mg} - \text{h}}{860 \text{ cGy minimum dose}} = \frac{1 \, \mu\text{Gy} \cdot \text{m}^2}{0.162 \text{ cGy}}$$

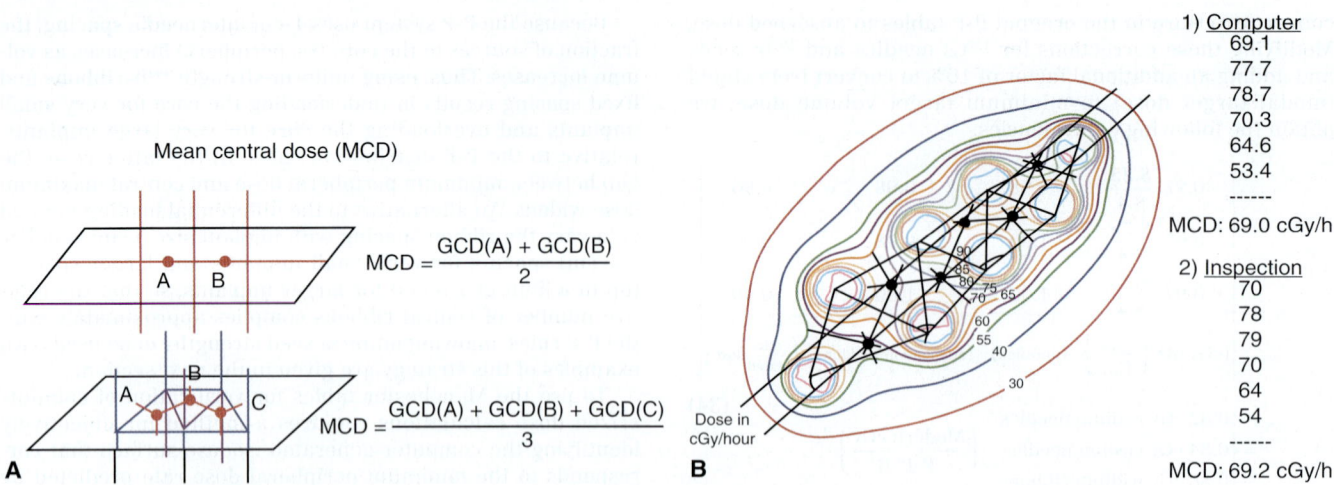

Mean central dose (MCD)

$$MCD = \frac{GCD(A) + GCD(B)}{2}$$

$$MCD = \frac{GCD(A) + GCD(B) + GCD(C)}{3}$$

Dose in cGy/hour

1) <u>Computer</u>
69.1
77.7
78.7
70.3
64.6
53.4

MCD: 69.0 cGy/h

2) <u>Inspection</u>
70
78
79
70
64
54

MCD: 69.2 cGy/h

FIGURE 25.19. A: Calculation of mean central dose (MCD) as the arithmetic mean of the doses at mid-distance between each pair of adjacent sources for single-plane implants and the mean of the local minimum doses between each group of three adjacent sources in a multiple-plane implant. All local minimum doses are specified in the "central transverse" plane, which is normal to and bisects the source axes. Practical specification of MCD for a computer plan is illustrated in **(B)**.

FIGURE 25.20. A: Cylindrical volume implant, example (C), using uniform-strength ^{192}Ir ribbons spaced at 1.3-cm intervals. Central transverse **(B)** and coronal **(C)** isodose curves are plotted normalized to the mean central dose (MCD) = 58.9 cGy/h = 100%: 115% (68 cGy/h), 100% (59 cGy/h), 90% (53 cGy/h), 80% (47 cGy/h), 60% (35 cGy/h), 40% (24 cGy/h), 20% (12 cGy/h). Note that 80% of MCD, 47 cGy/h, agrees closely with the minimum peripheral dose rate of 45 cGy/h predicted by the Paterson-Parker tables.

(C) Paterson-Parker volume implant: Ir-192 seeds

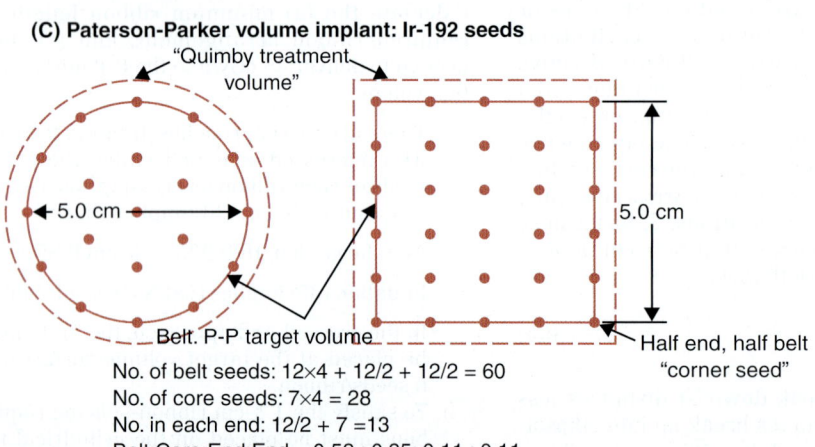

"Quimby treatment volume"

5.0 cm

5.0 cm

Belt. P-P target volume

Half end, half belt "corner seed"

No. of belt seeds: 12×4 + 12/2 + 12/2 = 60
No. of core seeds: 7×4 = 28
No. in each end: 12/2 + 7 =13
Belt:Core:End:End = 0.53 : 0.25: 0.11 : 0.11
vs 0.50: 0.25: 0.125: 0.125 for Paterson-Parker

A

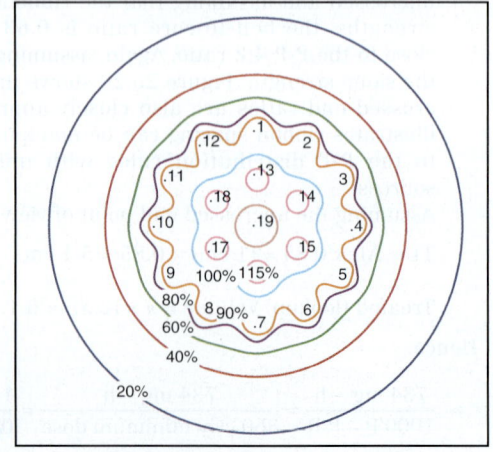

B

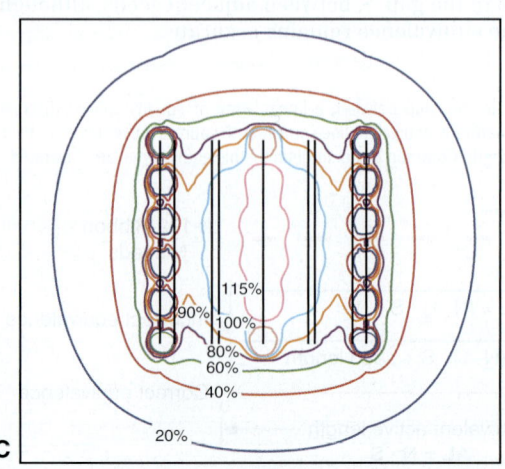

C

Differential Loading:

$$S_{K/seed} = \frac{45\,\text{cGy/h}}{0.162\,\text{cGy}} \cdot \times$$

$$\begin{cases} \dfrac{2}{3} \cdot \dfrac{1\,\mu\,\text{Gy}\cdot\text{m}^2}{12\,\text{ribbons} \times 6\,\text{seeds/ribbon}} = 2.6\,\mu\,\text{Gy}\cdot\text{m}^2\cdot\text{h}^{-1}\ \text{periphery} \\[2ex] \dfrac{1}{3} \cdot \dfrac{1\,\mu\,\text{Gy}\cdot\text{m}^2}{7\,\text{ribbons} \times 6\,\text{seeds/ribbon}} = 2.2\,\mu\,\text{Gy}\cdot\text{m}^2\cdot\text{h}^{-1}\ \text{core} \end{cases}$$

Uniform Loading:

$$S_{K/seed} = \frac{45\,\text{cGy/h}}{0.162\,\text{cGy/h}} \cdot \frac{1\,\mu\,\text{Gy}\cdot\text{m}^2}{19\,\text{ribbons} \times 6\,\text{seeds/ribbon}}$$
$$= 2.4\,\mu\,\text{Gy}\cdot\text{m}^2\cdot\text{h}^{-1}$$

The Quimby System

The Quimby system was developed by Edith Quimby and colleagues[167–169] at New York Memorial Hospital from 1920 to 1940. Unlike the Manchester system, equal linear intensity (mgRaEq/cm) needles are distributed uniformly (fixed spacing) in each implant. Like the Manchester system, the associated Quimby tables give the mgRaEq-h needed to deliver a stated exposure of 1,000 R as a function of target volume or area.

The so-called planar implant tables were intended for surface molds; none of the early Memorial publications suggest that it was used for single-plane interstitial implants. In part because Quimby's stated dose is the maximum dose in the treatment plane, Quimby planar implants deliver 30% to 40% less radiation (TRAK) per unit stated dose than an equivalent Manchester implant delivers. Rules for distributing radium needles (relationship to target-area boundaries, crossed ends, spacing, etc.) are not clearly described. Volume implant needle arrangements are similar to their Manchester counterparts; both systems recommend crossed ends and placing peripheral needles on or beyond the target-volume boundaries. However, Quimby allows the needle spacing to vary with implant size and specifies dose as the absolute minimum to the target volume. The physical and mathematical origins of the widely cited Quimby volume implant table are obscure; the tables published in the 1951 edition of *Physical Foundations of Radiology*[168] deliver 25% to 90% more mgRaEq-h per unit dose than P-P volume implants of similar size. Because they are evenly spaced, uniform-strength sources approximate the Manchester distribution rules for medium-size volumes, and these differences are likely a result of differences in the definition of "minimum dose" used by the two systems. Although vague on the subject, Quimby appears to specify minimum dose at a point located 3 to 5 mm from the peripheral needles (and therefore outside the target volume) near their active tips.[169] This corresponds to a treatment volume (volume encompassed by prescription isodose surface) that is 6 to 10 mm larger than the implanted volume (used for table lookup) in each linear dimension. The Quimby planar and volume dose specification criteria are clearly inconsistent, and a detailed derivation of the associated tables is lacking. For these reasons, we do not recommend Quimby tables for clinical use.

The Paris System

The Paris system was developed in the early 1960s by Pierquin, Chassagne, Dutreix, and Marinello[170,171] and was motivated by the ^{192}Ir afterloading techniques developed by Henschke. Outside the United States, the Paris system is widely used for definitive BT of localized lesions in the head and neck, breast, and many other sites. An up-to-date summary of the system has been published by Gillin and coworkers.[172]

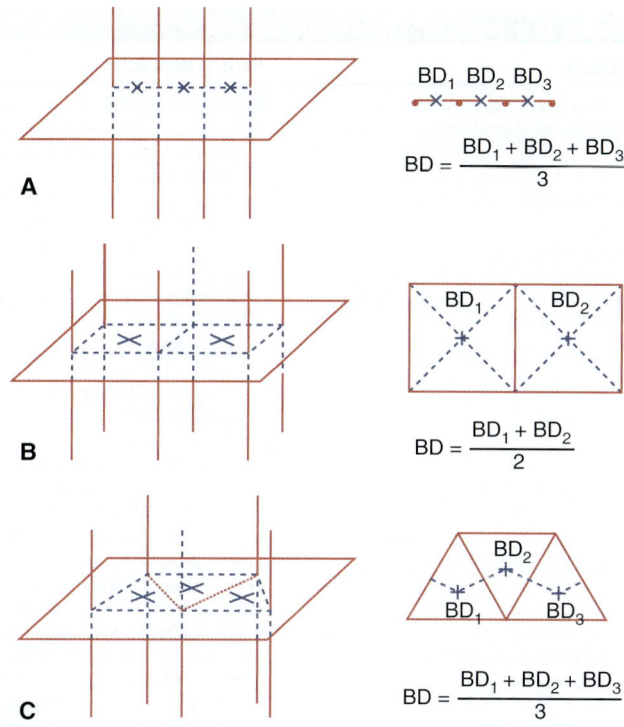

FIGURE 25.21. The three central plane configurations allowed by the Paris system: **(A)** single-plane implant, **(B)** double-plane implant using the pattern of squares; and **(C)** double-plane implant using the pattern of equilateral triangles. The calculation of basal dose rate at a point equidistant from each group of adjacent sources is illustrated for each configuration. (From Gillin MT, Albano KS, Erickson B. Classical systems II for planar and volume temporary interstitial implants: The Paris and other systems. In: Williamson JF, Thomadsen BR, Nath R, eds. *Brachytherapy physics*. Madison, WI: Medical Physics Publishing, 1995:232–343. Reprinted by permission of Medical Physics Publishing.)

The starting point of the Paris system is the definition of the target volume, which is described in terms of thickness (T), length (L), and width (W). The system provides rules for constructing implants, which, if followed, guarantee that the target volume is completely covered by the prescription isodose surface (Table 25.10). The prescription dose level, called the "reference dose," is a fixed percentage (85%) of the basal dose (see Fig. 25.21), which closely resembles the more general concept of MCD in Figure 25.19. ^{192}Ir wire sources are arranged in parallel rectilinear arrays with their centers located in the central plane, which is perpendicular to the sources. Adjacent sources must be equidistant from one another, resulting in single-plane implants with equal spacing and double-plane implants with groups of adjacent sources arranged in equilateral triangles or squares in the central plane. The linear density (μGy·m²·h⁻¹/cm) must be uniform and the same for all sources. Interneedle spacing scales with the thickness, T, of the target volume. The number of sources is determined largely by the relative shape of the target volume cross-sectional area, W × T. In contrast, the Manchester system uses fixed spacing and increases the number of sources as the cross-sectional area of the target volume increases.

Table 25.9 shows that the location of the peripheral sources relative to the treated volume (region encompassed by the reference isodose-rate surface, as shown in Fig. 25.22) differs from the Manchester system, which implants to the boundary of the treated tissue. In the transverse plane, the peripheral sources lie 2 to 4 mm (the lateral margin distance, M) inside the treatment surface, whereas longitudinally, the AL extends 15% to 20% beyond the distal and proximal margins of the target volume. In practice, the margin, M, is treated as a safety margin, and the peripheral needles are implanted along the margins of the clinical target volume (CTV). The maximum

TABLE 25.9 PARIS SYSTEM CHARACTERISTICS

Feature	Paris System Rules
Dose and dose rate	6,000–7,000 cGy in 3–11 d (25–90 cGy/h).
Dose specification criterion	Reference dose (prescribed dose) is 85% of the basal dose and encompasses the target volume when distribution rules are followed. Basal dose is the average of the minimum doses between pairs or groups of adjacent sources in the central transverse plane.
Dose gradient	Fixed 15% gradient between reference dose and basal dose. The "hyperdose sleeve" (region receiving at least twice the reference dose) diameter should be <8–10 mm.
Linear activity	Constant (4–14 μGy m²·h⁻¹/cm) linear density Ir-192 wires used.

Source arrangement geometry for target volume of thickness, width, and length of T × W × L	Only single- and double-plane implants allowed. Spacing, S, and lateral margin (called "safety margin" for double-plane case), M, are fixed fractions of T and constant within a given implant. Active length, AL, is a fixed fraction of L, which varies with S.
	Single plane:
	   $T = 12$ mm
	   $S = 2 \times T$ (2 sources)
	   $S = 1.67 \times T$ (3 sources)
	   $M = 0.37 \times T$
	   $AL = (1.3 - 1.49) \times T$
	Double plane: (square pattern)　　　　　(triangle pattern)
	   　　　$S = 0.62 \times T$　　　　　$S = 0.77 \times T$
	   　　　$M = 0.27 \times T$　　　　　$M = 0.15 \times T$
	   　　　$AL = (1.37 - 1.62) \times L$　　$AL = (1.33 - 1.49) \times L$

Source spacing, S, limits	Short sources (1–4 cm): Long sources ($\leq$10 cm): 15 mm $\leq$ S $\leq$ 22 mm
Crossing needles	Generally not used; AL ~ 1.45 × L to compensate for uncrossed ends. For oral cavity implants, hairpins are common, which approximate crossed ends.
Relation between target volume and implanted volume	W = distance between outermost sources + 2 × M $L = (1.3 - 1.62) \times L$ $T = \begin{cases} S/1.67 & \text{Single plane} \\ S + 2 \times M & \text{Double plane : squares} \\ S \times \cos 30° + 2 \times M & \text{Double plane : triangles} \end{cases}$

thickness, T, of a target volume treatable in the Paris system is about 2.5 cm. An example of a double-plane implant arranged in squares is shown in Figure 25.23.

To apply the Paris system, the target thickness T must be known, which defines the spacing and determines whether single-plane or double-plane geometry is required. The number of sources and selection of a square or triangular arrangement are defined by the relative cross-sectional shape of the target volume in the central plane perpendicular to the sources. Finally, the active length is calculated. The source tip and end coordinates are reconstructed from orthogonal

radiographs, and the dose distribution and basal dose are calculated by computer for the actual implant geometry realized in the patient, not the idealized implant of clinical intention. This approach differs from the classical Manchester method, which bases dose prescription on the P-P table and, in general, ignores deviations of the actual implant geometry from the ideal. The Paris system addresses only single- and double-plane implants; large-volume implants for treating pelvic masses and brain tumors were not part of the original system. Extensions of Paris system principles to large-volume implants are discussed by Leung[173] and Gillin and coworkers.[174]

FIGURE 25.22. Relationship of the reference isodose, source locations, and target-volume dimensions for each of the basic implant configurations allowed by the Paris system. The concept of safety margin (lateral margin, M) is illustrated. (Adapted from Pierquin B, Wilson JF, Chassange D. Modern brachytherapy. New York: Masson, 1987.)

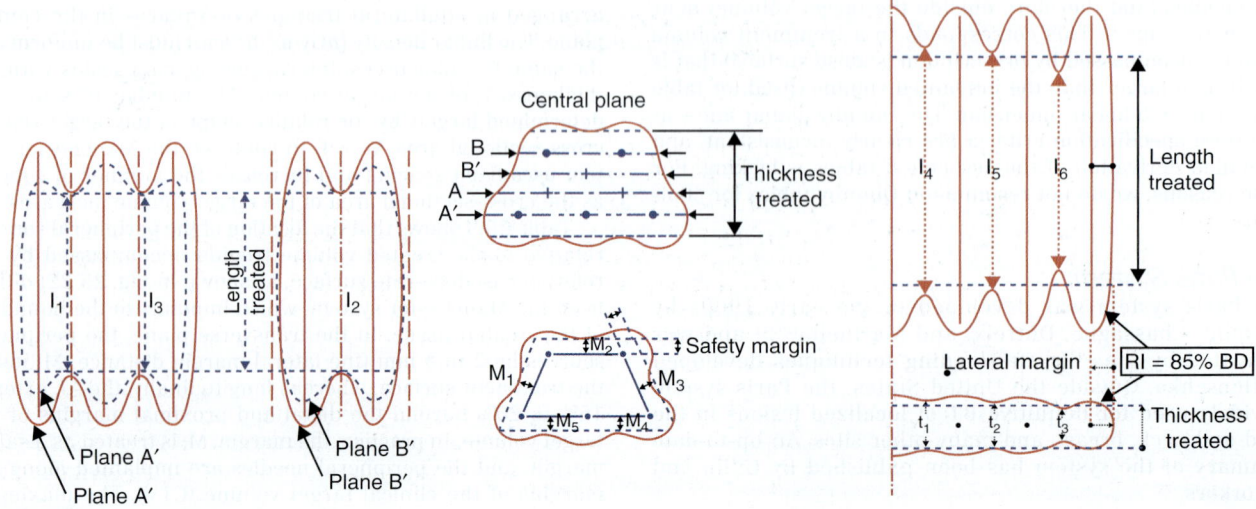

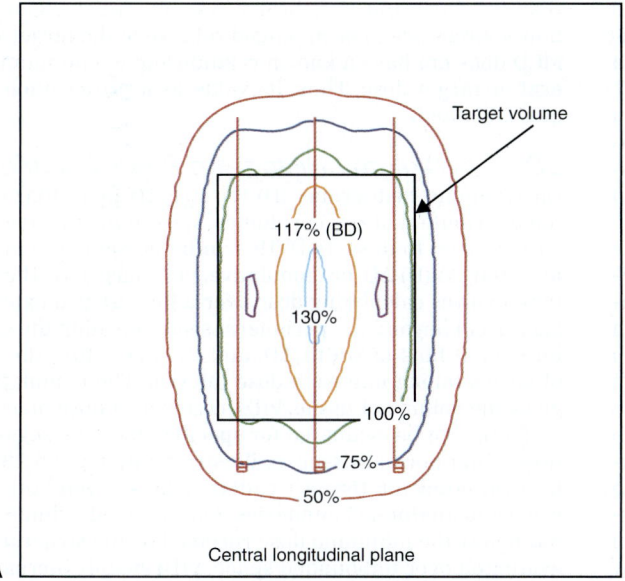

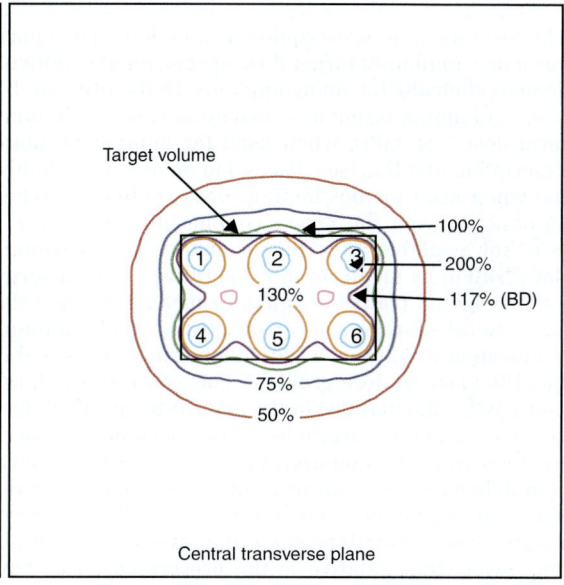

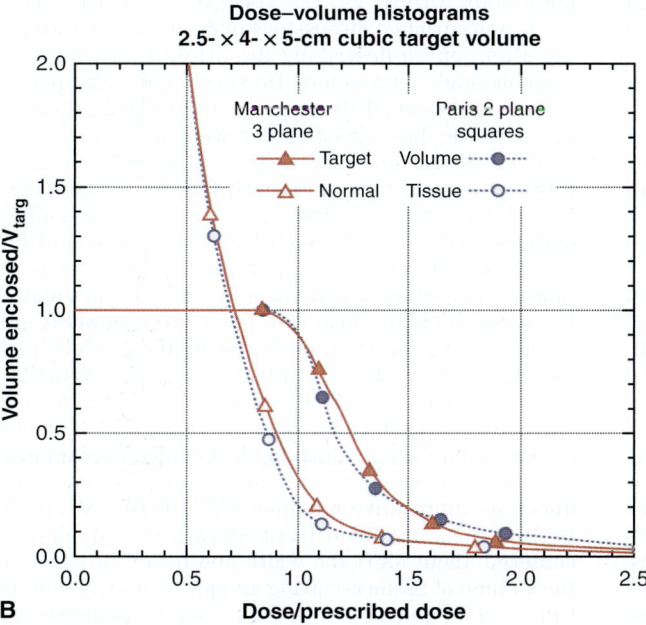

FIGURE 25.23. A: Isodose curves of a Paris system double-plane implant arranged "in squares" to treat a 2.5-cm × 4-cm × 5-cm target volume (*heavy lines*). The separation and active lengths of the ^{192}Ir wires are 1.6 and 7.3 cm, respectively. A linear strength of 6 μGy·m^2·h^{-1}/cm gives reference (100%) and basal (117%) dose rates of 60 and 70.6 cGy/h, respectively. **B:** Comparison of dose/volume histograms (DVHs) calculated separately for the 2.5-cm × 4-cm × 5-cm target volume and the tissue outside the target for the Paris implant shown and a Manchester implant consisting of 3 planes, 15 ^{192}Ir ribbons with 6 seeds each, and 1.25-cm spacing between planes and ribbons. Each graph shows volume of tissue (in multiples of volume of the target) receiving at least the specified dose (in multiples of prescribed dose). For the Paris and Manchester implants, respectively, the prescribed dose is calculated reference dose and minimum target dose predicted by the Paterson-Parker volume table. In both systems, the prescription isodose surface covers about 90% of the target. Surprisingly, both normal tissue sparing and dose homogeneity in the target are slightly better for the Paris implant.

Dose Specification in Interstitial Brachytherapy

Many of the differences between the Manchester, Paris, and Quimby systems can be attributed to fundamental differences in dose specification. Because of the high-dose gradients near the peripheral sources or the target volume boundary, reproducible specification of dose and evaluation of implant quality are difficult. Conversely, small differences in dose-specification criteria can lead to large differences in treatment time or in the geometric relationship between implanted and treated volume. The term "dose specification" means objective identification of a spatial volume or location for evaluating absorbed dose for the purposes of prescription (defining the dose that the radiation oncologist intends to deliver), for describing the quantity of radiation actually delivered to the patient, or for reporting. The "specified dose" sometimes is called "reference dose." The dose that an implant actually delivers to the patient, based on postinsertion treatment planning, may differ significantly from the dose prescribed for a variety of reasons. For example, anatomic or technical constraints may preclude accurate positioning of sources at their intended locations, resulting in a partial geometric miss or underdose of the specified volume. Dose specification for reporting purposes usually refers to efforts to develop reproducible and system-independent specification schemes to promote comparison of different implantation systems so as to minimize patient-to-patient and operator-to-operator variability in level of treatment delivered. The ability to objectively compare different interstitial implant plans as to target volume coverage, normal-tissue sparing, and dose homogeneity depends on dose specification. Several divergent and rather abstract approaches to dose specification have been developed and promoted by various national and international advisory groups; no single approach to dose specification has been widely accepted within the BT community.

Minimum Dose to an Anatomically Defined Target Volume

The minimum dose to the anatomically defined target volume harboring malignant cells is conceptually attractive because it is based on the intuitively satisfying premise that local tumor control will be determined by the minimum dose received by tumor cells. The American Brachytherapy Society (ABS)[175] recommends that minimum dose should be identified as accurately as possible by the best means available and should be used for dose prescription, evaluation, and reporting. In practice, minimum target dose specification is difficult to implement clinically for many implants. In the prostate BT literature,[176] minimum target dose usually is called "minimum peripheral dose," or mPD, when used for implant preplanning prescription and D_{100} (see discussion on dose/volume histograms) when used for postimplant dose evaluation. When imaging data showing the target volume in relation to the sources is not available, the ABS recommends approximate target localization by means of intraoperatively placed surgical clips, orthogonal planar imaging, or measurements relative to peripheral sources. A clear disadvantage of minimum dose specification is that the target-volume surface lies within the zone of the largest dose gradient. This can result in large patient-to-patient fluctuations in the central-to-specified dose ratio because of small variations in the peripheral source locations relative to the apparent target boundary or uncertainties in delineating the target volume. As discussed in the "Permanent Implantation" section, reviews of CT-based prostate implant dose evaluations show that absolute minimum delivered doses (D_{100}) relative to the prescribed dose show large patient-to-patient variabilities and average 30% to 60%.[177,178] The minimum dose covering at least 99% (or 95%) of the target volume was found to be much less sensitive to small changes in the peripheral seed locations or uncertainties in the target volume surface location.

Minimum Implant Dose Relative to Sources

Traditional treatment planning uses planar radiographs for 3D reconstruction of radioactive source positions, yielding accurate dose estimates relative to the sources but not relative to an anatomic target volume.[24,179] Thus, it is natural to prescribe treatment to a point or surface that has a fixed relationship to the peripheral sources. The minimum implant dose, or MID, is the minimum dose received by the "target" volume defined relative to the implanted volume, the smallest regular geometric shape circumscribing the peripheral sources. Often, this specification volume is taken to be that volume that is 2 to 5 mm larger in each linear dimension relative to the implanted volume, as in the Paris and Quimby systems. Prior to acceptance image-guided BT, MID was perhaps the most widely used specification approach and is the basis of the classical systems and the US practice of selecting prescription isodose surfaces from 2D isodose curve plots. However, MID yields information about tumor coverage only to the extent that the radiation oncologist has implanted peripheral sources at known distances from the anatomic target volume boundaries. In addition, MID lies in the zone of maximum dose gradient and can be difficult to evaluate objectively for an implant of irregular shape, again leading to large patient-to-patient variations and variations in the central-to-prescribed dose ratio. The Paris and Manchester systems eliminate the possibility of subjective isodose selection by rigidly specifying dose rate by means of basal dose rate and implant tables, respectively.

Mean Central Dose

The ICRU report on dose specification in interstitial BT[166] emphasizes reporting mean central dose (MCD; see Fig. 25.19), although it recommends reporting the prescribed dose, the peripheral dose (minimum target dose), and a description of dose uniformity as well. MCD specifies dose in the low-gradient regions located between adjacent source locations in the central plane of the implant. Thus, MCD is relatively free of the variability inherent in minimum peripheral or target dose specification. It is a generalization of the Paris system basal dose. As a reporting parameter, MCD can be reproducibly estimated from 2D central transverse-plane isodoses and should be very useful for comparing implants performed using different clinical systems. However, for systems other than the Paris and Manchester systems (which rigidly specify how sources are to be arranged relative to the target volume), MCD does not have a known relationship to minimum peripheral or target dose. Thus, its value as a prescription parameter is limited.

3D Dose/Volume Histogram Representations

Dose/volume histograms (DVHs) are 1D plots that describe the distribution of tissue volumes, V, irradiated by the implant with respect to dose, D. DVHs can be presented in either differential, $\Delta V(D)/\Delta D$, or cumulative, $V(D)$, forms. DVH computation involves calculating dose over a fine 3D grid extending at least 2 cm beyond the peripheral seeds, dividing the dose axis into small bins of width ΔD, and then counting the number of voxels falling into each dose interval. The cumulative DVH gives the volume of tissue, $V(D)$, receiving a dose of at least D.

DVHs can be evaluated for specific anatomic regions (e.g., target and normal tissue as illustrated by Fig. 25.23) or can be evaluated for tissue irradiated by the implant without regard to anatomic boundaries. For bounded volumes, $V(D)$ is flat below the minimum dose received by the structure. When evaluated over unbounded space, $V(D)$ steeply increases with decreasing dose and asymptotically approaches the central point-source DVH, $V_{point}(\dot{D}) = (4\pi/3) \cdot [S_K \cdot \Lambda/\dot{D}]^{3/2}$. The use of DVHs has enriched discussions of dose specification by focusing attention on describing the 3D dose distribution rather than on single parameters. However, in the absence of target volume and normal-tissue geometry, DVHs in themselves do not solve the dose-specification problem.

Because 3D anatomic models were often lacking until recently, several figures of merit (FOMs) derived from DVHs have been proposed that do not require an anatomically defined target volume. Such FOMs may be useful for ranking the quality of competing implant geometries in terms of uniformity and normal-tissue sparing or for optimally selecting a specification dose rate for a given implant geometry. An important contribution is the "natural" DVH introduced by Anderson.[180,181] The natural DVH is a plot $\Delta V(u)/\Delta u$ where $u = D^{-3/2}$. The natural DVH plots as a horizontal line for a central point source. It suppresses r^{-2} effects, which dominate the conventional $V(D)$ plot, making its detailed implant geometry–specific structure more evident. Low and Williamson[182] introduced an alternative modified DVH, $R_p(D) = V_{impl}(D)/V_{point}(D)$. Both of these modified DVHs show a sharply defined peak centered about MCD, the width and height of which quantify the volume of tissue receiving an approximately uniform dose. Other useful quality measures include the uniformity index[183] and the dose nonuniformity ratio (DNR).[184] The DNR, usually plotted as a function of reference dose, D_r, is defined as the ratio of volume receiving a specified multiple of D_r (usually 1.25 or 1.5) to that receiving at least D_r.

Target-volume–dependent DVH quality indices were introduced into brachytherapy by Saw and Suntharalingam.[185] For single- and double-plane implants designed to cover specified cubic target volumes, respectively, they defined three indices as a function of reference dose D_r. The coverage index, $CI(D_r)$, is that fraction of the target tissue receiving a dose greater than or equal to D_r. The homogeneity index, $HI(D_r)$, is the fraction of target volume receiving doses between D_r and 1.5 D_r. The external volume index, $EI(D_r)$, is the volume of tissue outside the target volume, expressed in multiples of the target volume, receiving dose rates greater than or equal to D_r. When these indices are plotted (Fig. 25.24), the trade-offs among these clinical end points are evident. If a prescription dose rate is selected to maximize dose homogeneity (i.e., maximize HI), then 85% to 95% coverage of the target must be accepted. To minimize irradiation of tissue outside the target, both target coverage and dose homogeneity must be compromised. Low and Williamson[182] suggested ranking competing implant geometries by specifying the HI achieved for the maximum reference dose level that yields a CI of unity.

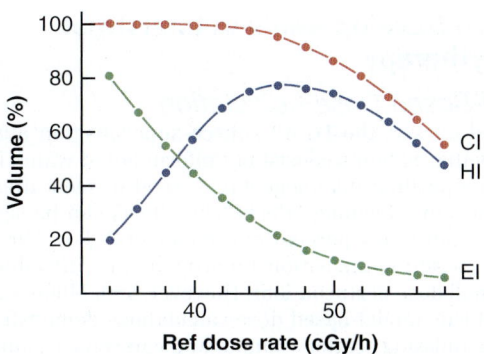

FIGURE 25.24. Plot of coverage index (CI), external index (EI), and homogeneity index (HI) as a function of reference dose rate for double-plane implant consisting of five ^{192}Ir ribbons with seven 1-mCi seeds in each plane and a 6-cm × 6-cm × 2.5-cm target volume. Ribbon and plane spacings of 1.5 cm were used. (From Saw CB, Suntharalingam N. Reference dose rates for single and double plane ^{192}Ir implants. *Med Phys* 1988;15[3]:391–396. Copyright © 1988 American Association of Physicists in Medicine. Reprinted by permission of John Wiley & Sons, Inc.)

For TRUS-guided prostate implantation, DVH metrics such as D_{100}, D_{99}, and D_{90}, denoting the minimum doses administered to the highest dose volumes covering 100%, 99%, and 90% of the contoured CTV or PTV (planned target volume), respectively, have become widely accepted as reporting parameters.[186,187] Volumetric indices, such as the V_{150}, V_{100}, and V_{90}, which denote the fraction of the CTV or PTV receiving at least 150%, 100%, and 90%, respectively, of the prescribed dose, are recommended to assess dose homogeneity and to assess adequacy with which the prescription has been fulfilled.

Permanent Implantation

In contrast to temporary implantation, in which treatment time is varied to control the total dose delivered, the dose delivered by a permanent implant is determined by the initial geometric arrangement of sources and S_K per source: once the patient is implanted, neither the total dose delivered nor the relative distribution can be modified easily. Up through the mid-1980s, manual planning and dose-calculation tools were used widely to estimate the number and density of sources needed to deliver the prescribed dose or to intraoperatively correct for deviations between the planned actual source locations. For radium-substitute sources (e.g., ^{198}Au), the Manchester, Laughlin,[163] or Shalek[164] tables and associated distribution rules have been used for this purpose. Although 3D treatment planning and dose calculation have replaced manual preplanning tools, manual aids are still widely used for verifying the correctness of patient treatment plans.

Manual planning aids for high-energy sources cannot be applied to low-energy seed (^{125}I and ^{103}Pd) implants because of the importance of tissue attenuation in this energy range. The influence of photon energy on the relationship between dose rate, $\dot{D}$, and implanted volume, V, is illustrated by Figure 25.25. Parker[158] recognized that this relationship can be described accurately by a power-law formula, of the form:

$$\dot{D} = \alpha \cdot S_K \cdot V^{-\beta} \tag{36}$$

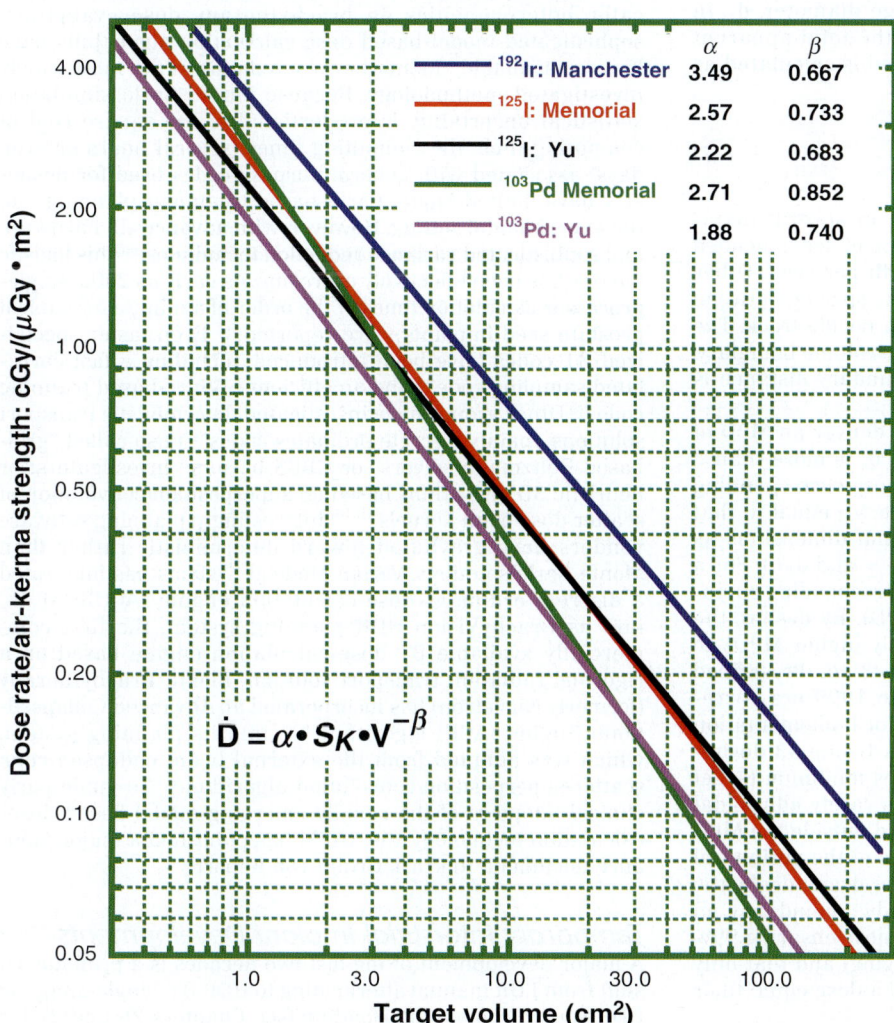

	α	β
^{192}Ir: Manchester	3.49	0.667
^{125}I: Memorial	2.57	0.733
^{125}I: Yu	2.22	0.683
^{103}Pd Memorial	2.71	0.852
^{103}Pd: Yu	1.88	0.740

$$\dot{D} = \alpha \cdot S_K \cdot V^{-\beta}$$

FIGURE 25.25. Comparison of reference dose rate per unit air-kerma strength versus volume of the target volume for Manchester volume implants and ^{103}Pd and ^{125}I permanent prostate implants. The inset gives the exponents and proportionality constants needed to describe these relationships in terms of a simple power law Eq. (36). The data in the figure are from the following references: Yu,[188] Memorial,[189] and Manchester.[158]

Section II

In fact, the original Manchester table (Table 25.8), converted to modern units and quantities, can be derived from Eq. (36) by setting $\alpha = 3.49$ and $\beta = 2/3$. Although ^{103}Pd and ^{125}I volume implants also can be described by the power law formula, they have somewhat larger exponents, β, demonstrating that dose rate falls off faster with increasing volume than for radium-substitute sources.[188,189] The proportionality constants, α, are substantially lower, indicating that low-energy seed implants require higher source strengths to achieve a stated dose rate. The author-to-author variations in α values for the same radionuclide are due, in part, to differences in dose specification and implant construction. Anderson's analysis,[189] based on the pre-TRUS era Memorial nomogram, assumes that dose is specified in terms of matched peripheral dose (MPD) and that all seeds are implanted 2 to 5 mm inside the target (prostate) boundary, whereas the Yu nomogram assumes[188] that peripheral seeds are implanted on or outside the boundary and that minimum target dose is specified. Before using a nomogram or lookup table for QA checks or preplanning, readers should assess carefully its consistency with dose calculation and planning methods used in their clinical practices.

The best-known manual planning tool for permanent ^{125}I implantation is the Memorial dimension averaging method.[189,190] The associated nomogram was used for manual intraoperative planning of implants delivered by directly implanting seeds into the surgically exposed prostate retropubic approach. After surgical exposure of the target volume (prostate), the three orthogonal dimensions of target volume are measured, and the arithmetic mean of these measurements, or average diameter, d_a, in units of centimeter, is calculated. Next, the total apparent activity, A_{app} (in mCi units), to be implanted is calculated as follows:

$$A_{app} = \begin{cases} 5 \cdot d_a & d_a < 3 \text{ cm} \\ 1.34 \cdot d_a^{2.2} & d_a \geq 3 \text{ cm} \end{cases} \qquad (37)$$

By means of a nomogram consisting of several juxtaposed logarithmic scales, the total number of seeds needed is estimated graphically given the strength per seed. Other nomogram scales were used to estimate the spacing between needles given the seed spacing along each needle track. The seeds are to be implanted inside the target-volume boundary, such that peripheral needle-to-target boundary distance is <50% of the interneedle spacing.

The calculation method is designed to deliver an MPD of 160 Gy over the life of the implant when d_a is more than 3 cm.[189] MPD is defined as the dose level whose corresponding 3D isodose surface encompasses a volume, V_E, equal to that of an ellipsoid having the same orthogonal dimensions as the originally measured target volume ($V_E = \pi d_x d_y d_z/6$). For a given implant, MPD is derived from the corresponding cumulative DVH, V(D), according to $V_E = V(MPD)$. By design, the Memorial nomogram delivers significantly higher MPDs to target volumes with average dimensions <3 cm. Prescribed doses of 160 Gy delivered in the 1985 to 1999 era correspond to doses of 144 Gy when corrected for implementation of the WAFAC primary standard and Task Group 43 dosimetry parameters.[155] The MPD overestimates minimum target dose (mPD) because the prostate gland is rarely ellipsoidal and has small protrusions that may extend outside the MPD isodose surface. Likewise, small deviations of the peripheral seeds from their planned locations can alter dramatically the shape of the MPD isodose surface. One study[191] found that, on average, MPD was twice the D_{99} level (the dose ensuring 99% target coverage on postoperative CT imaging) and that only 69% to 89% of the target volume received a dose equal to or greater than MPD.

Modern Developments in Interstitial Brachytherapy

Model-Based Dose Calculation

As noted earlier, the TG-43 source-superposition algorithm[5] assumes that patients consist of uniform liquid water, ignoring tissue-composition inhomogeneities, seed-to-seed attenuation, and applicator-shielding effects. The effects can be significant ranging from a few percent to a factor of 2. For ^{192}Ir brachytherapy, tissue composition heterogeneities introduce relatively small dose perturbations. However, both Monte Carlo and deterministic model-based dose calculations demonstrate skin contours (missing scatter volume) and can reduce skin and rib doses by 4% to 8% for breast brachytherapy,[192] whereas shielded vaginal applicators can reduce bladder and rectal doses by 8% to 25%.[193,194] In contrast, doses delivered by low-energy permanent seed BT and EBT are very sensitive to deviations of target tissues and organs at risk from water equivalence, since photoelectric dominates energy deposition in this energy range. Using standard ICRP[195] bulk tissue compositions for prostate tissue, Carrier et al.[196] found that TG-43 underestimated D_{90} from ^{125}I seed implants by 9% relative to Monte Carlo studies, with 18/28 prostate cancer patients showing a 10% effect or more. Calcifications as small as 1% to 2% of the prostate mass perturb DVH metrics by as much as 35%.[197] Even larger and highly variable (4% to 50%) deviations of Monte Carlo D_{90} estimates from corresponding TG-43 estimates[198,199] were found for low-energy seed breast implants, because the breast tissue consists of a mixture of adipose and glandular tissues which varies significantly from patient to patient.

To address the potentially large impact of tissue and applicator heterogeneities on brachytherapy dose evaluation, sophisticated model-based dose calculation algorithms have become available.[6] Monte Carlo simulation is the most widely investigated methodology. Because Monte Carlo simulation statistical uncertainty is proportional to the square root of computing time, the computing times (several hours or even days) associated with general purpose codes used for dosimetry have limited Monte Carlo–based treatment planning[200] to the experimental setting. However, with advances in hardware and sophisticated variance reduction techniques,[201] this logistic barrier has been effectively overcome. As early as 2005, single-processor calculation times of the order of a minute for clinical prostate seed implants were reported.[197] Even faster specialized BT codes have been introduced, including a fast correlated sampling code[199] and an efficient EGSnrc-based planning code.[202] Other groups have investigated deterministic transport solutions, mainly discrete ordinates codes[203] (also called "grid-based Boltzmann solvers" or GBBS by some investigators) or heuristic 3D algorithms based on superposition/convolution of scatter dose point kernels.[150,204] Interestingly, planning software vendors have gravitated toward deterministic rather than Monte Carlo solutions. Varian Medical Systems has integrated a discrete ordinates dose-calculation engine (ACUROS)[156,205] into its BrachyVision HDR planning system, the first commercially available BT dose-calculation engine based on a rigorous radiation transport solution. Elekta Brachytherapy (formerly Nucletron) has incorporated an Advanced Collapsed-Cone Engine (ACE) algorithm[150,206] into its planning system, which was adapted from the external beam collapsed-cone scatter-superposition/convolution algorithm.[207] To guide early clinical adopters of the rapidly emerging model-based dose-calculation technology, the AAPM has published a major guidance document, the Task Group 186 Report.[6]

Temporary Interstitial Implant Developments

A major development of the last two decades is a pronounced shift from LDR manual afterloading to HDR BT. Single-stepping HDR source remote afterloading (see Chapters 26 and 27 for a detailed treatment) allows the treatment time (dwell time) to be individually specified at each treatment (dwell) position in the catheter. This permits the use of dwell-weight optimization as a tool for improving dose uniformity and target coverage within implants. In contrast to the classical systems, which assume that ribbons and needs are of uniform linear density, dwell-weight optimization supports far more elaborate nonuniform source-strength distributions than those envisioned by the Manchester system rules. The published experience, confined largely to Paris-like double-plane breast implants, demonstrates that geometric optimization[208] preferentially increases the dwell times at dwell positions near the catheter ends. The most striking finding is that optimization allows the active-to-target length (AL/TL) ratio to be reduced from 1.33–1.5 to 1.1–1.25.[209-211] In the transverse plane, target coverage remains unchanged, whereas dose homogeneity is improved modestly, depending on the figure of merit used to quantify this effect. When dose-point optimization (specifying dose constraints at dose calculation points throughout the treatment volume) is used, acceptable dose homogeneity results with even smaller AL/TL ratios, even when all peripheral dwell positions are placed inside the target volume (AL/TL = 1.0)[182,212] for idealized volume implants and clinical volume implants.[210] These early efforts did not address the practical problem of how to distribute dose constraint points in clinical volume implants with irregular catheter spacings and how to select dwell positions to be activated in each catheter. While dwell-weight optimization techniques have the potential to reduce AL/TL ratios to near unity with good CI and HI, it is influenced by the direction and location of the catheters relative to the target, and thus requires distribution rules drawn from the classical systems or one's own clinical experience.

The use of 3D imaging to preplan implants or intraoperatively guide catheter or seed insertion is growing rapidly. The most widely practiced form of image-guided BT is the use of intraoperative TRUS to guide transperineal insertion of needles used to implant the prostate gland with low-energy seeds.[48,49] However, image-guided implant methodologies have been developed for HDR multicatheter interstitial[213] and balloon-applicator intracavitary[214] implants for APBI following lumpectomy and HDR interstitial implantation for prostate cancer.[215] All of these approaches require delineation of the target volume and critical structure surfaces from 3D imaging studies. Then, catheter or needle trajectories and, ultimately, seed or dwell position locations can be selected to improve target-volume coverage while minimizing unnecessary dose to critical structures. The issues involved in utilizing image-guided and image-based BT in HDR interstitial brachytherapy, including treatment planning, selection of imaging modality, and impact on clinical workflow, are covered in detail elsewhere.[179]

As practiced by most brachytherapists, image-guided, intraoperatively planned implants continue to rely on the planner's judgment for selecting source locations. These decisions are guided by a "loading approach," or set of guidelines that specify margins, seed locations relative to the target boundary, spacings, and approximate periphery-to-core loading ratios.[216,217] Dose calculations and DVH quality indices often are used to guide manual source position adjustments to improve target-volume coverage, improve dose homogeneity, and select source strengths (or dwell times) and the prescription isodose.

An important advance upon standard dose-point optimization is anatomy-based optimization in which constraints and treatment goals are defined in terms of doses to the CTV or normal tissues contoured from 3D imaging studies rather than surfaces defined relative to dwell positions. The simulated annealing HDR dwell-time optimization technique developed by Lessard and Pouliot[218] illustrates the general features of the various optimization approaches[219-222] that have been brought to bear on this problem (see Ezzell's review[223] for a highly readable introduction to BT optimization techniques).

An objective function, consisting of penalty factors summed over dose calculation points in the CTV, urethra, rectum, and other organs, is minimized. The penalty factors are functions that, by increasing in value, penalize candidate dose distributions deviate from constraints and planning goals specified by the planner. The inverse planning technique of Pouliot and colleagues[218] reduces CTV dose heterogeneity (V150 of 29% vs. 50%) and urethral doses in clinical prostate implants compared to geometric optimization[224] and solves the problem of selecting active dwell positions and locations for dose constraint points faced by the older dose-point optimization algorithms. Although anatomy-based inverse planning does not optimize catheter trajectories, its proponents argue[225] that it reduces the dependence of implant quality on the number and accurate positioning of the catheters relative to the CTV boundary. If true, inverse planning could reduce the dependence of implant quality on operator skill and reduce the need to follow system-based needle-insertion rules.

In summary, computerized dose calculation, dwell-weight optimization, and image-guided BT have made anatomy-based dose specification and meaningful implant optimization a reality in some clinical settings. However, as currently available, these innovations still require users to conceptually plan implants in terms of specified source and needle-distribution patterns, implant-target-volume margins, and loading ratios. Specific rules borrowed from the classical systems (e.g., AL/TL ratios) may require significant modification when adapted to these modern technologies

Permanent Implant Developments

The most important advance in permanent implantation in the last two decades is the rise of image-based and image-guided techniques in prostate BT, currently its only widely practiced indication. The retropubic approach has been abandoned in favor of the transperineal approach using intraoperative TRUS,[48,226] which typically consists[179] of (a) preplanning using a TRUS examination, or "volume" study, obtained 2 to 3 weeks before the scheduled implant; (b) inserting the needles using interactive real-time TRUS imaging; and (c) followed by CT-based postprocedure planning 0 to 30 days after the procedure. During preplanning, the PTV often is defined as the contoured prostate gland plus a discretionary margin. Most brachytherapists practice some form of peripheral loading to improve uniformity and reduce dose to the urethra. For example, the modified uniform loading as defined by Butler[216] distributes about 75% of the source activity in the periphery and emphasizes insertion of peripheral needles on or near the PTV boundary. Typically, needle locations and seed strengths are manipulated to achieve a prescribed minimum target dose (mPD or $D_{100\%}$) of 145 Gy for ^{125}I monotherapy. For ^{103}Pd monotherapy, the ABS[227] recommends retaining the prescribed dose of 125 Gy (compared to 115 Gy used before 2000) following implementation of the NIST $S_{K,N99}$ standard and recently revised TG-43 parameters, based on the AAPM's most recent analysis[155] of ^{103}Pd prescribed-to-administered dose ratios because of changes in calibration standards and dosimetry practice.

Dose specification, for recording and reporting doses actually administered by a permanent implant, is based on post-implant dose evaluation.[176] Following the implant procedure, a CT exam is obtained; the prostate gland, rectum, and bladder are contoured; and the seed locations are identified from the transverse images. The choice of dose-specification parameter for this purpose has been the subject of intense investigation. Based on analysis of both idealized and actual implants, Yu and colleagues[188] found that the postinsertion D_{100} was very sensitive to small random displacements of the seeds from their intended positions, which resulted in underdoses of 15% or more to small volumes in the target periphery. However, they found that the mPD of the idealized implant (no seed displacement) covered at least 90% of the target (i.e., $D_{90} \geq$ mPD and

$V_{100} \geq 90\%$), even in the face of 6-mm seed displacements. In a study of 60 consecutive implant patients, Merrick and associates[177] found mean V_{100} and D_{90} values of 94% of the CT prostate volume and 108% of the prescribed dose (mPD of preplanned implant), respectively. Of the patients, 82% had a D_{90} exceeding the preplanned mPD and no patient had a D_{90} smaller than 90% of mPD. In contrast, D_{100} was only 68% of the prescribed mPD, on average. Two groups[228,229] have found a correlation between prostate-specific antigen (PSA) relapse-free survival at 4 years and D_{90}. In particular, Potters and colleagues[228] found a D_{90} dose–response cutoff of 90% of the prescribed dose but could find no statistically significant cutoffs for D_{100} and V_{100}.

An important contemporary development is "intraoperative planning"[179,230] in which TRUS-based planning (and post-implant dose evaluation as well, in some implementations) is performed during the procedure itself rather than on a volume study acquired weeks before. Intraoperative planning eliminates uncertainties due to differences in planning and treatment anatomy due to probe positioning errors, impact of hormone ablation, or external beam therapy. An extension of intraoperative planning is dose-guided implantation[179,231] or "dynamic dose planning,[232]" in which intraoperative planning is repeated one or more times during the implantation procedure, thereby allowing optimized insertion of needles yet to be implanted to overcome errors in previously inserted sources.

INTRACAVITARY BRACHYTHERAPY

In contrast to the comparatively uniform dose distributions of interstitial BT, the unidirectional source arrangements used in gynecologic intracavitary BT give rise to dose distributions that fall off rapidly with distance from the applicator surface, producing large dose gradients across the target volume. Such large dose gradients make target volume–based dose specification difficult and give this treatment modality a highly empirical character. Numerous parameters have been used to prescribe, constrain, or report intracavitary therapy applications, including mg-h, mgRaEq-h, reference point doses (points A and B), bladder and rectal reference point doses, vaginal surface dose, treatment time, and the ICRU Report No. 38[3] 60-Gy reference volume. This section will emphasize the physical relationships among these parameters and their dependence on applicator characteristics. Systems for treating carcinoma of the cervix, the most intensively studied form of intracavitary therapy, will be reviewed. Our focus will be further restricted to applicator geometries and treatment systems (e.g., Fletcher and Washington University/Mallinckrodt systems) derived from the Manchester system. This limited focus is justified by the fact that Manchester- or Fletcher-style applicators continue to be the dominant choice across the world for both HDR and LDR treatments.

The Manchester Family of Intracavitary Therapy Systems

The Manchester system, developed in 1938 by Tod and Meredith,[10] has heavily influenced intracavitary treatment practice patterns throughout the world, especially in North America. The widely used Fletcher-Suit applicator system, the Fletcher loadings, and the point A and B reference points are all derived from the Manchester system. This system was the first to use applicators and loadings designed to satisfy specific dosimetric constraints.[10,233] It was the first system to use a radiation field quantity, exposure at point A, rather than mg-h, to specify treatment.

The Classical Manchester System

The original Manchester applicator system consisted of a rubber intrauterine tandem and two vaginal "ovoids," whose ellipsoidal shape was designed to conform to the isodose curves arising from ^{226}Ra tubes placed along their long axes. The applicators were designed for use with ^{226}Ra tubes 2.2 cm long with 1-mm platinum filtration and an active length between 1 and 1.5 cm. The small, medium, and large ovoid minimum diameters were 2, 2.5, and 3 cm, respectively, and are the same as Fletcher's small, medium, and large colpostats.[234] The preloaded ovoids contained no shielding and relied on extensive anterior and posterior packing to spare bladder and rectal tissue.

The reference point A (Fig. 25.26) originally was defined as the point "2 cm lateral to the center of the uterine canal

FIGURE 25.26. Definition of points A and B in an ideal application (*left*) and a distorted application (*right*), which is displaced to the left of the patient's midline, and a uterus, which is tilted toward the right. Note that point A is carried with the uterus, whereas points B and P are defined to be 5 and 6 cm, respectively, to the right and left of patient midline. Point P is used by the Mallinckrodt Institute of Radiology system to specify minimum dose to the pelvic lymph nodes. (Adapted from Meredith WJ. Dosage for cancer of cervix uteri. In: Meredith WJ, eds. Radium dosage: *The Manchester System*. 2nd ed. Edinburgh: E. & S, Livingston, Ltd, 1967;42–50.)

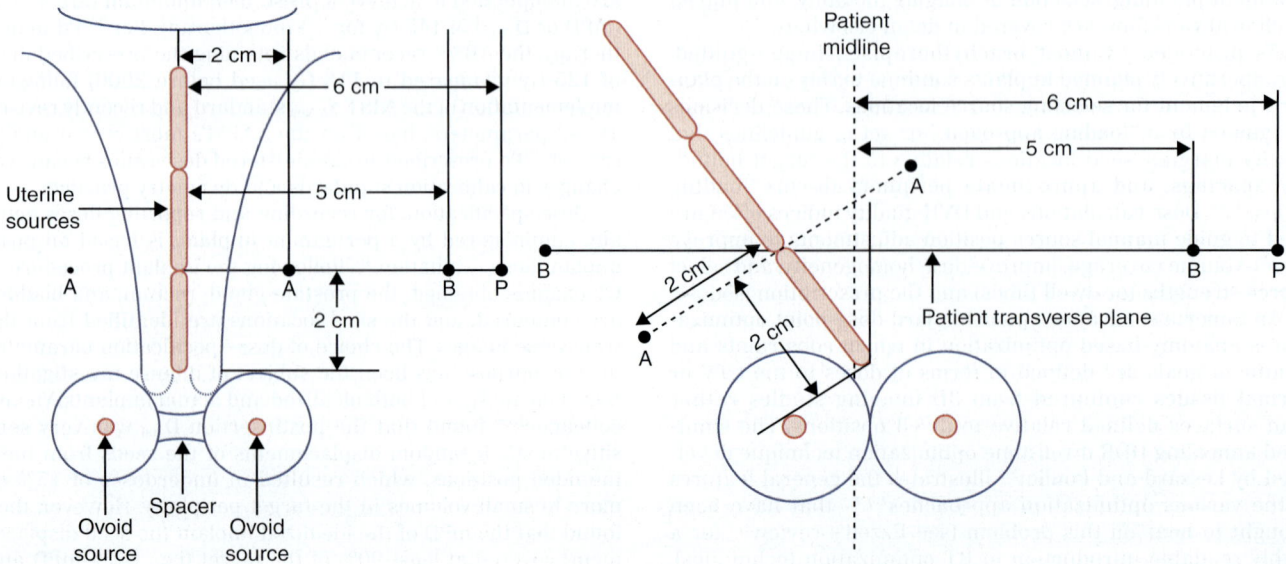

and 2 cm from the mucous membrane of the lateral fornix in the plane of the uterus."[10] This seemingly arbitrary definition reflected the system developers' view that "radiation necrosis is not the result of direct effects of radiation on the bladder and rectum, but high dose effects in the area in medial edge of the broad ligament where the uterine vessels cross the ureter."[235] They believed the radiation tolerance of this area, termed "the paracervical triangle," to be the limiting factor in the treatment of cervical cancer and used point A exposure to represent its average dose. In current practice, point A dose is used to approximate the average or minimum dose to the tumor. Point B, defined to be 5 cm from the patient's midline at the same level as point A, was intended to quantify the dose delivered to the obturator lymph nodes.

The Manchester ovoid dimensions and applicator loadings were designed to ensure that the point A dose rate, about 0.52 Gy/h in modern units, remained constant for all allowed applicator loadings and combinations. The design also ensured that the vaginal contribution to point A was limited to 40% of the total dose. Small, medium, and large ovoids were loaded with 17.5, 20, and 22.5 mg of radium, respectively, to compensate for the greater source-to-point A treatment distances with the larger ovoids. Medium (4 cm long) and long (6 cm) tandems were loaded, os to fundus, with source trains consisting of 10- and 15-mg sources and 10-, 10-, and 15-mg sources, respectively, whereas the short tandem (used for cervical stump cancer) was loaded with a single 20-mg radium tube. With the exception of the short tandem, these loadings satisfied the dosimetric constraints within 2%. The point B dose, determined largely by inverse-square law, is approximately 9 Gy for every 4,000 mg-h administered.

Without external-beam treatment to the whole pelvis, a total point A exposure of 8,000 R (72.8 Gy) in 140 hours split between two applications was prescribed.[233] Because the point A dose rate is constant whether the application contains 60 mg of ^{226}Ra (small ovoids, medium tandem) or 80 mg (large ovoids, long tandem), delivery of a fixed point A dose amounts to using time, not milligram-hours, as the factor that terminates the treatment. In contrast to the Paris and Stockholm systems, which prescribed a fixed number of milligram-hours, equivalent Manchester treatment regimens could deliver from 8,400 to 11,200 mg-h—a variation of 33%.

As the size of an intracavitary application (i.e., colpostat diameter and tandem length) increases, the penetration or "lateral throw-off" of the dose distribution increases. As colpostat diameter increases from 2 to 3 cm, the vaginal surface dose decreases by 35% relative to the dose 2 cm from the applicator surface; this is simply a consequence of increasing the source-to-surface distance. Similarly, increasing the tandem length increases the point B contribution relative to the uterine cavity surface dose; the radioactivity near the ends of the long tandem contributes little to the surface dose (because of inverse-square law), whereas each tandem segment makes roughly equal contributions to points remote from the applicator. These physical principles underlie the practice of using the largest colpostats and longest tandem that the patient's anatomy can accommodate.[11,233]

Modern Fletcher-Suit Applicator Systems

The Fletcher applicator system (Fig. 25.27A) adhered to the basic Manchester design while incorporating many improvements including internal shielding. These shields are located on the medial aspects of the anterior and posterior colpostat faces (Fig. 25.27B) and consist of 180-degree and 150-degree disk-shaped 3- to 5-mm-thick tungsten sectors to shield the rectum and bladder, respectively.[234] The cylindrical colpostat body has a diameter of 2 cm that can be increased to 2.5 and 3 cm by the use of small and large slip-on plastic caps, thereby retaining the Manchester ovoid dimensions. Afterloading

capability was added to the Fletcher applicator by Suit and coworkers.[2] The Fletcher loadings—15, 20, and 25 mg for small, medium, and large colpostats, respectively—are similar to those of the Manchester system, whereas tandem loadings are identical to their Manchester counterparts. Because of the similarity of Fletcher loadings (55 to 85 mg) to the Manchester loadings, point A dose rates are nearly independent of applicator dimensions.

The shielded Fletcher colpostat was designed to reduce dose to the bladder trigone and the anterior rectal wall without decreasing irradiation to the uterosacral and broad ligaments, thereby reducing the need for the extensive vaginal packing characteristic of Manchester insertions.[234] For a single colpostat (Fig. 25.27B–D), the maximum dose reduction varies from 40% to 50%.[15,236,237] When the effects of the intrauterine tandem and the contralateral colpostat are included, applicator shielding reduces midline rectal and bladder doses by 21% to 34% relative to conventional treatment planning calculations, which ignore shielding and include only the effects of source encapsulation.[194] CT-based dose evaluation studies reveal that colpostat shielding modestly reduces rectal doses, reducing the rectal $D_{2\%}$ by 2% to 11%[238] and D_{2cc} by 10%.[239] Modern versions of the shielded Fletcher colpostat for LDR BT include the LDR 3M Fletcher-Suit-Delclos (FSD)[15] and reproductions of the round-handled Fletcher-Suit[236] colpostats. For HDR BT, the Fletcher-Williamson[240] applicator duplicates the original Fletcher shielding configuration. Weeks and Montana[241] have designed a CT-compatible version with afterloadable shields and an aluminum body having the same dimensions as the FSD applicator.

Dose Specification in Intracavitary Brachytherapy

Point A Dose and Milligram/Hours

Two quantities are used widely to prescribe intracavitary BT: mg-h (or its modern equivalent, TRAK) is used in practices influenced by the M.D. Anderson Cancer Center system,[11,242,243] whereas some form of the Manchester point A dose specification is used by most other practitioners. Efforts to unify these two prescription practices by identifying a linear relationship between the two quantities are misguided[244] from the perspective of the Manchester system. The Manchester-like loadings specified by the Washington University (WU)/Mallinckrodt Institute of Radiology clearly show (Fig. 25.28) that despite a twofold variation in source strength loaded into the smallest versus the largest applicator system, the point A dose rate varies by only 15%. To deliver a fixed point A dose of 65 Gy with WU loadings, a constant total treatment time of approximately 100 hours is needed, resulting in delivery of mgRaEq-h ranging from 5,200 to 10,000 in any sample of patients characterized by a range of applicator sizes. Conversely, for fixed mgRaEq-h, prescription would result in a nearly twofold variation in total treatment time and point A dose.

The proportionality of point A dose and treatment time applies only to the classical (Manchester) definition of point A. Many radiation oncologists use a revised definition of point A (Fig. 25.29) that references its location to the cervical os (tandem collar, proximal aspect of the most caudal tandem source, or a gold seed implanted in the cervix) rather than to the lateral fornix. This practice obscures the relationship between point A and milligram/hour prescription philosophies. Potish and Gerbi's[244] study of 90 Fletcher applications demonstrates that the revised point A dose rates vary widely from patient to patient and are, on average, significantly higher than the classical Manchester value. Because point A is fixed to the tandem and the vertical tandem-to-colpostat displacement varies with each patient, the vaginal contribution to point A is highly variable. In contrast, classically defined point A

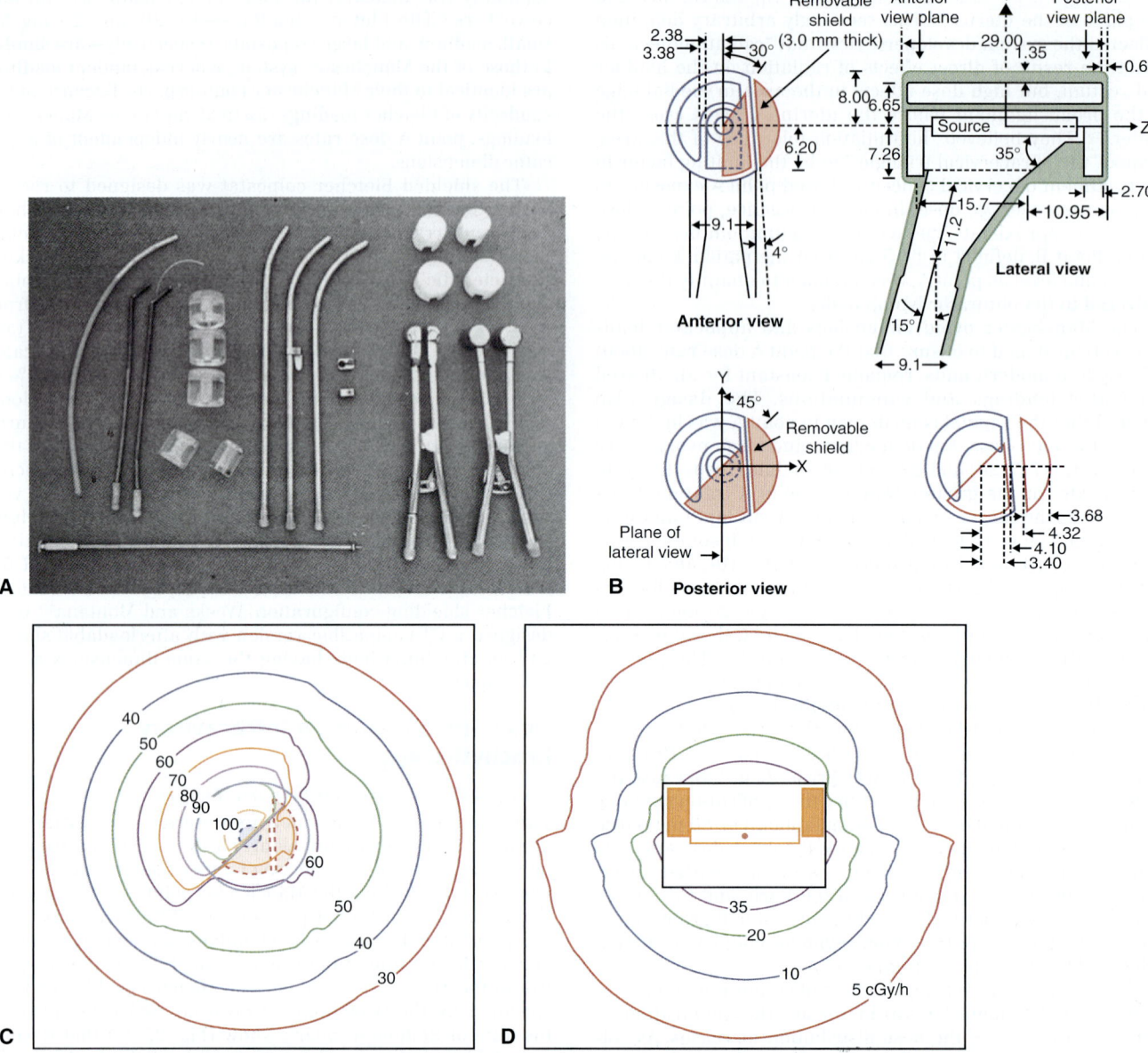

FIGURE 25.27. A: Fletcher-Suit applicator system. From *left* to *right* are tandem insert loaded with dummy sources, colpostat source holders, vaginal cylinder sleeves, three curvatures of intrauterine tandems, cervical collars, Delclos mini-colpostats, and round-handled Fletcher-Suit colpostats with small and medium caps. The tube-like instrument in the left foreground is a cervical localization seed implanter. (From Fletcher GH, Hamberger AD. Squamous cell carcinoma of the uterine cervix: Treatment techniques according to size of the cervical lesion and extension. In: Fletcher GD, ed. *Textbook of radiotherapy.* 3rd ed. Philadelphia: Lea & Febiger, 1980:732–772. With permission.) **B:** Three orthogonal views of the 3M Fletcher-Suit-Delclos colpostat, consisting of a stainless steel body. The removable parts of the tungsten alloy shield, which allow conversion of the applicator to a shielded Delclos mini-colpostat, are inserted into a nylon cap (not shown) with an outer diameter of 2 cm. Shown are isodose curves **(C)** in the coronal plane 10 mm from the posterior face of the applicator and **(D)** in the transverse plane of the colpostat for a 72 μGy·m^{2}·h^{-1} ^{137}Cs tube. (Figures **B–D** reprinted from Williamson JF. Dose calculations about shielded gynecological colpostats. *Int J Radiat Oncol Biol Phys* 1990;19[1]:167–178. Copyright © 1990 Elsevier. With permission.)

dose rates are tightly grouped, are independent of the loading, and are in close agreement with the Tod-Meredith value. The vaginal contribution to classical point A is fixed by definition, whereas the intrauterine contribution is insensitive to colpostat-to-tandem displacement because of the parallel tandem isodose curves. Thus, the revised point A definition does not have the physical significance of the classical quantity. The use of revised point A dose to prescribe therapy for "free-floating" tandem and colpostat insertions may introduce large patient-to-patient fluctuations in treatment times because of small, clinically insignificant variations in implant geometry.

Significantly, the recent ICRU Report 90[108] on prescribing and reporting brachytherapy for cervical cancer has endorsed the classical point A definition.

The previous discussion is applicable only to the Fletcher applicator system with relative loadings approximating those of the Manchester system. As the intrauterine-to-vaginal loading ratio (1:1 for the Manchester system) increases, and the maximum width of the pear-shaped reference isodoses falls and the rectal dose increases.[245] Appreciation of how loading influences isodose shape and normal-tissue doses is especially important in HDR BT as dwell-weight optimization invites

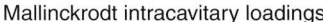

Mallinckrodt intracavitary loadings

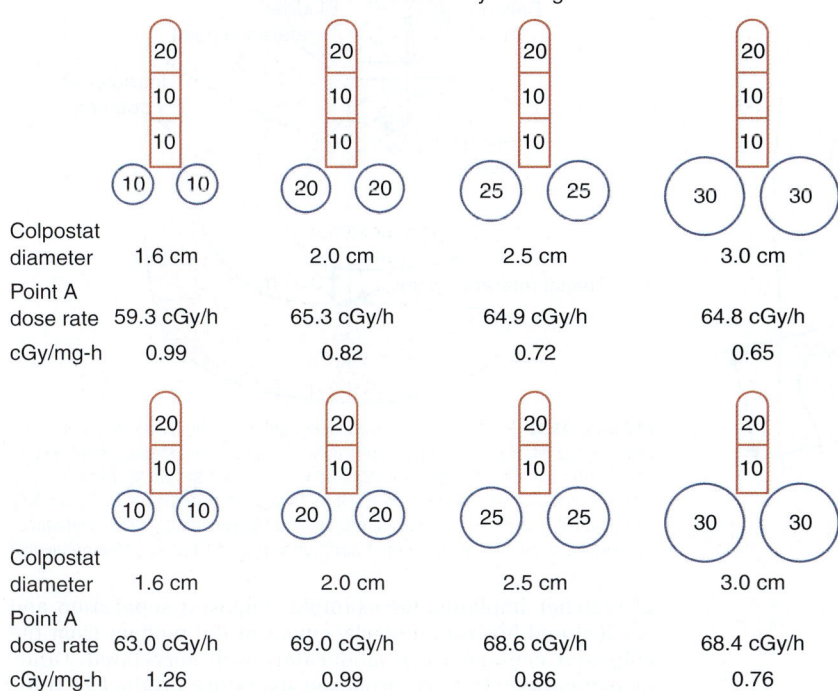

FIGURE 25.28. Mallinckrodt Institute of Radiology/Washington University (WU) applicator loadings used with Fletcher-Suit applicators for treatment of cervix carcinoma. Because the WU system uses Model 6500 3M ^{137}Cs tubes, equivalent mass of radium is used to specify loadings and mgRaEq-h, rather than mg-h, to prescribe intracavitary therapy. The point A dose rates assume the classical Manchester definition and average colpostat separations and tandem colpostat alignments.

deviation from classical loading rules. Using judiciously placed dose points to control the relative dimensions of the point A isodose surface, Mai[246] was able to increase tapering near the cephalad aspect of the tandem, to reduce the vaginal surface dose, and to modestly reduce the rectal dose with only slight loss of the maximum width of the pear-shaped isodose. These considerations suggest that dose-point driven optimization of the dwell-weight distribution should be accompanied by a geometric analysis of the point A isodose surface so that changes to target coverage can be assessed at least approximately.

Other applicators in current use include the HDR tandem and ring applicator[247] and the LDR Henschke applicator.[1] The latter consists of hemispheric colpostats rigidly attached to the tandem with the vaginal source axes parallel to the intrauterine sources rather than transverse as in the Fletcher system.

FIGURE 25.29. Radiographic definition of classical point A (2 cm above the cephalic-most aspect of the colpostat in the tilted coronal plane) and the revised point A (2 cm above the cervical collar top or center). Because the distance from caudal-most intrauterine source tip to colpostat center (tandem-to-colpostat displacement) varies from patient to patient, the vaginal contribution to revised point A is highly variable. (Reproduced with permission from Potish RA, Gerbi BJ. Role of point A in the era of computerized dosimetry. *Radiol* 1986;158:827–831.) The revised definition was suggested by Tod and Meredith in their 1953 paper.[233]

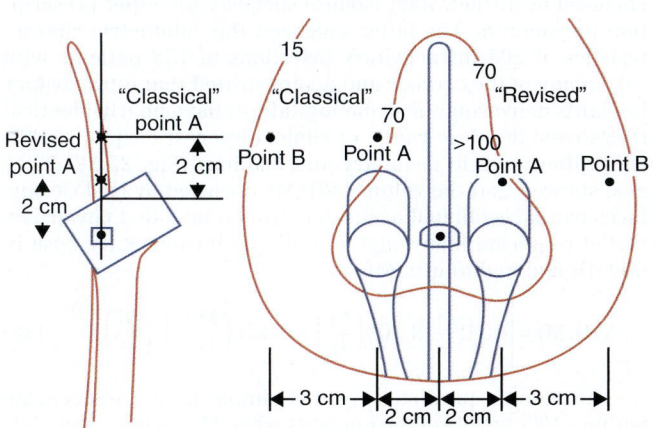

Henschke colpostats with internal shielding[248] are available. The vaginal ring applicator consists of a circular guide tube (usually 34 mm outer diameter) with its plane fixed rigidly normal to the tandem. It is placed up against the cervix and vaginal fornices with a donut-shaped cap attached, which increases the distance between the vaginal mucosa and the circular array of dwell positions (of which only the lateral dwell positions are activated) to 7 mm (compared to 10 to 15 mm for the Fletcher colpostat). Thus, the fraction of source strength loaded into the ring must be reduced to avoid overdosing the vaginal mucosa.[246,249] Although rectal and vaginal vault doses relative to the point A dose similar to that of the Fletcher system can be achieved through careful optimization, the lateral coverage (i.e., maximum coronal width of the point A isodose) is reduced.[246] Care must be taken in positioning the applicator system to avoid underdosing the gross tumor volume (GTV). Applicator geometry and loading practices should be changed only after extensive comparative evaluation of the old and new dose distributions to avoid dose distribution changes that would invalidate the evaluated clinical experience on which the brachytherapist's knowledge of dose response rests. Finally, for applicator systems that deviate from the classical Manchester geometry or relative loading rules, one cannot assume that point A dose is proportional to treatment time over all allowed variations of applicator sizes and loadings.

Volumetric Specification of Intracavitary Treatment: ICRU Report No. 38 Recommendations

The ICRU[3] introduced the concept of reference volume enclosed by the reference isodose surface for reporting and comparing intracavitary treatments performed in different centers regardless of the applicator system, insertion technique, and method of treatment prescription used. Specifically, ICRU Report No. 38 recommended that the reference volume be taken as the 60-Gy isodose surface, resulting from the addition of dose contributions from any external-beam whole-pelvis irradiation and all intracavitary insertions. The ICRU proposed that this pear-shaped reference volume (Fig. 25.30) be described in terms of its three orthogonal maximal dimensions, height (d_h), width (d_w), and thickness (d_t), measured in

Plane A

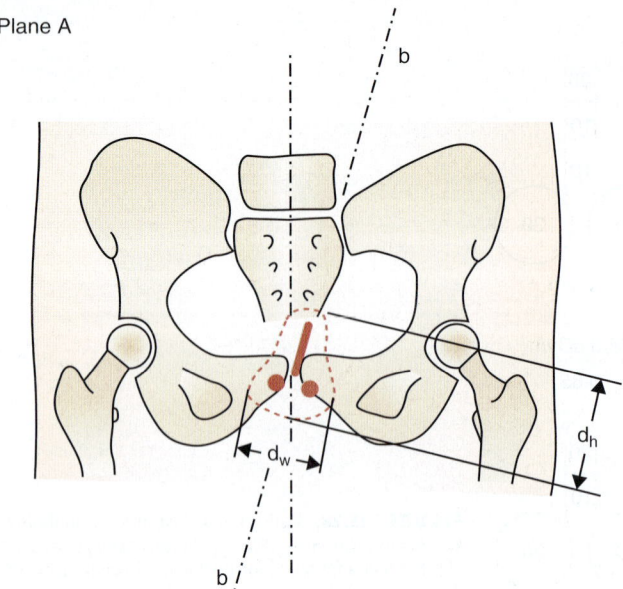

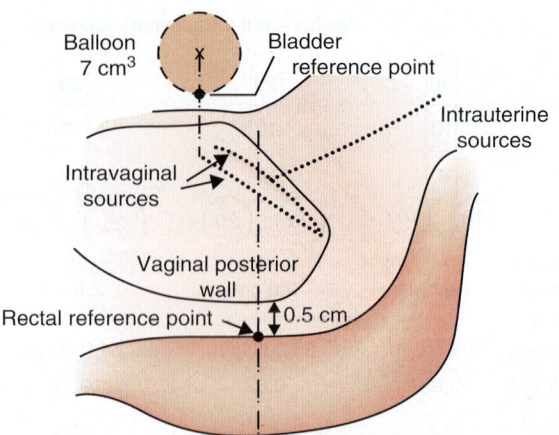

FIGURE 25.31. Reference points for bladder and rectal brachytherapy doses proposed by the International Commission on Radiation Units and Measurements Report 38.[3] (From Chassagne D, Dutreix A, Almond P, et al. ICRU Report 38. *Dose and volume specification for reporting intracavitary therapy in gynecology.* Bethesda, MD: International Commission of Radiation Units and Measurements, 1985. Reproduced by permission of International Commission on Radiation Units and Measurements.)

Plane B

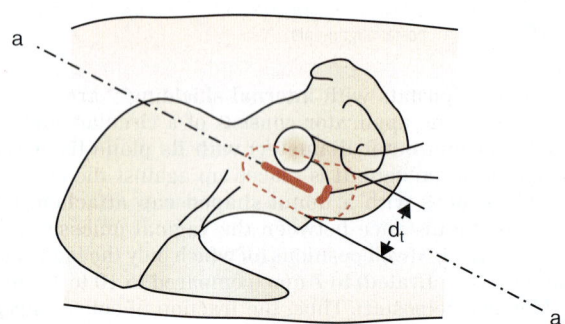

FIGURE 25.30. Geometry for measuring of the three orthogonal dimensions of the pear-shaped ICRU (International Commission on Radiation Units and Measurements) reference isodose surface (*broken line*) in a typical treatment of cervix carcinoma using one rod-shaped uterine applicator and two vaginal applicators. *Plane A* is the "oblique" frontal plane that contains the intrauterine device. The oblique frontal plane is obtained by rotation of the frontal plane around a transverse axis. *Plane B* is the "oblique" sagittal plane that contains the intrauterine device. The oblique sagittal plane is obtained by rotation of the sagittal plane around the AP axis. The height (d_h) and the width (d_w) of the reference volume are measured in *plane A* as the maximal sizes parallel and perpendicular to the uterine applicator, respectively. The thickness (d_t) of the reference volume is measured in *plane B* as the maximal size perpendicular to the uterine applicator. (From Chassagne D, Dutreix A, Almond P, et al. *ICRU Report 38. Dose and volume specification for reporting intracavitary therapy in gynecology.* Bethesda, MD: International Commission of Radiation Units and Measurements, 1985. Reproduced by permission of International Commission on Radiation Units and Measurements.)

the oblique coronal and sagittal planes containing the intrauterine sources. Figure 25.31 illustrates the bladder and rectal reference points recommended by the ICRU.

In contrast to point A dose and mgRaEq-h, the ICRU proposal is only a means of describing or reporting treatment. No guidance is given as to how to prescribe treatment, use these measurements to evaluate implant quality, or correlate reference volume dimensions with clinical outcome. The 60-Gy dose-level choice appears to have been motivated by the preoperative radiotherapy regimen popular within the French school of radiotherapy.[250] Descriptions of institution-specific treatment techniques for early-stage cervical cancer patients include rules for evaluating the 60-Gy reference volume dimensions and offsets relative to the applicator system for the allowed combinations of applicator dimensions and loadings.[250] Within North America, Potish et al.[251,252] and later Eisbruch et al.[253] found that the individual ICRU reference volume dimensions and various geometric characteristics

of Fletcher implants, for example, colpostat separation and vertical and horizontal displacement of the tandem from the colpostat centers, were moderately well correlated. Other investigators[254–256] have proposed using the product of ICRU dimensions, $V_{ICRU} = d_t \times d_w \times d_h$, as a surrogate for relative volume contained within the reference isodose surface. Esche et al.[255] found that V_{ICRU} was directly proportional to mg-h, whereas Nath[256] pointed out that V_{ICRU} increased steeply with increasing whole-pelvis dose. In a retrospective clinical study,[254] grade 3 rectal complications were correlated with high $d_t \times d_w \times d_h$ product, whereas severe bladder complications were associated with the combination of high bladder doses and large V_{ICRU} on a 2D scattergram. The rationale for studying the product of ICRU reference volume dimensions is the well-established correlation between the volume of tissue irradiated by external irradiation and clinical outcome.[257] In agreement with these authors, the current ICRU Report 89[108] discards the concept of a reference isodose surface for a single fixed-dose level, in favor of a more flexible system, for example, for 2D dosimetry specifying the volume enclosed by total dose isodose surfaces determined by prescribed doses (typically 85 and 60 Gy) to the high-risk and intermediate-risk CTVs (CTV-HR and CTV-IR, respectively). The ICRU no longer endorses measuring and reporting the three orthogonal dimensions of these reference isodose surfaces. The ICRU 38 and 89 reference volume concepts appropriately emphasize that the volume of tissue irradiated, as well as dose, is an important predictor of clinical response to intracavitary irradiation. Wilkinson and Ramachandran[258] and Eisbruch et al.[253] used DVHs to study the correlation between volume enclosed by intracavitary isodose surfaces and other prescription parameters. The latter analyzed the volumetric characteristics of 204 intracavitary insertions in 128 patients with carcinoma of the cervix s and demonstrated that intracavitary implants delivering the same mgRaEq-h have nearly identical DVHs over the dose range of clinical interest despite significant differences in geometry and loadings (Fig. 25.32). They also showed that the volume, V(D,M), enclosed by isodose surfaces can be estimated accurately from a modified power-law model requiring knowledge of only the intracavitary dose in cGy (D) and mgRaEq-h (M):

$$V(D,M) = \left[104.8 - 8.103\left(\frac{M}{D}\right) + 0.437\left(\frac{M}{D}\right)^2\right] \cdot \left(\frac{M}{D}\right)^{1.635} \quad (38)$$

The volume predicted by this simple model is accurate within ±10% in 95% of the implants when M/D is more than 0.8, which corresponds to an intracavitary dose of 100 Gy for 8,000

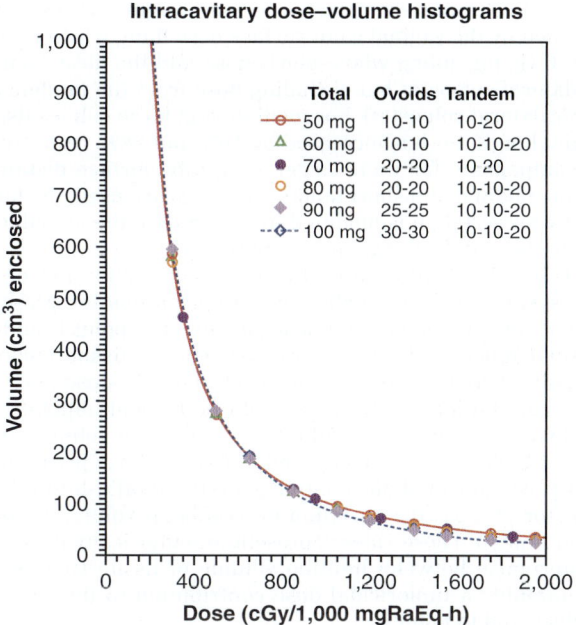

Intracavitary dose–volume histograms

Total	Ovoids	Tandem
50 mg	10-10	10-20
60 mg	10-10	10-10-20
70 mg	20-20	10 20
80 mg	20-20	10-10-20
90 mg	25-25	10-10-20
100 mg	30-30	10-10-20

FIGURE 25.32. Dose/volume histograms for seven WU intracavitary insertions using 1.4-cm active length ^{137}Cs sources. The strength of each source was determined by the loading rules for WU schema C (20 Gy, whole pelvis plus 8,000 mgRaEq-h) and then was scaled down to 1,000 mgRaEq-h. Note that as the size of the insertion increases, the volume of tissue encompassed by the high-dose isosurfaces decreases. Point A doses ranged from 8.28 to 11.35 Gy.

mgRaEq-h of intracavitary therapy. In addition, the ratio of ICRU dimension product to the true volume given by DVH analysis, $d_t \times d_w \times d_h / V(D, M)$, varied widely from patient to patient and differed systematically from one implant type to another.

The consequences of Eq. (38) can be summarized as follows:

1. Volumetrically, an intracavitary implant behaves like a central point source: $V(D, M) \propto (M/D)^{3/2}$
2. Describing an implant in terms of volume contained within its isodose curves carries no more information content than a statement of mgRaEq-h or total reference air-kerma.
3. The volume of tissue irradiated to a specified dose is closely related to total exposure given by the implant in terms of mgRaEq-h or TRAK.

Consequence (2) suggests that the correlation between clinical outcome, in terms of tumor control and complications and isodose surface volume, should be no better or worse than the correlation between clinical outcome and mgRaEq-h for a fixed external pelvis dose. Consequence (3) suggests a new and fundamental physical interpretation of mgRaEq-h or its derivative, TRAK. Prescribing intracavitary BT by mgRaEq-h is equivalent to treating until each specified isodose surface achieves a fixed volume independent of the underlying implant geometry. The use of mgRaEq-h to constrain intracavitary treatment therefore limits the volume of tissue irradiated to high doses. This observation may help explain the clinical utility of mgRaEq-h as a dose-specification parameter. Finally, the individual reference isodose dimensions, which are more strongly influenced by implant geometry than their product, clearly convey additional information about the spatial extension of the reference isodose surface in their respective planes and cannot be reduced to a statement of total exposure from the implant and may have additional prognostic significance.

Practical Systems for Intracavitary Prescription and Reporting

For Manchester-like loadings and applicators, if treatment were to be prescribed as a fixed number of mgRaEq-h or TRAK without regard to the diameter and length of the applicators, the treatment times and total point A doses would differ by the ratio of total source strengths in the applications. Small applications would have unacceptably high point A and vaginal vault surface doses and excessively long treatment times. In contrast, large applications treated to a fixed mgRaEq-h prescription would underdose these reference points. In contrast, the ICRU reference volume for fixed levels of whole-pelvis irradiation and mgRaEq-h would be independent of the loading because the mgRaEq-h is constant. Conversely, when the point A dose is held constant, the mgRaEq-h needed to deliver these doses will vary significantly, introducing corresponding variations in the volume of the ICRU reference isodose.

Clearly, no TRAK-based system would endorse such a naive approach. Actual mgRaEq-h–based systems use a combination of parameters. Physically, mgRaEq-h or TRAK controls the volume of tissue treated to high doses, and parameters such as time, colpostat surface dose, and point A are used to control doses at points near the applicator to ensure that normal tissue tolerance is not exceeded and that the tumor is not undertreated. For each applicator combination and choice of external-beam dose, a compromise between volume of tissue treated and dose delivered near the applicator must be reached. For example, the Fletcher system[11,252] specifies both a maximum treatment time and maximum milligram/hour constraint for each combination of external-beam and intracavitary therapy (Table 25.10). Whichever constraint is reached first terminates the application. Small applications tend to be terminated by the maximum time constraint, which limits

TABLE 25.10 SIMPLIFIED FLETCHER SYSTEM PRESCRIPTIONS[a]

Treatment Scheme	Indications	External Beam		Intracavitary Maximum		Range: Smallest to Largest Insertion		
		Whole Pelvis	Split Field	mg-h[b]	Time (h)	Point A	Point B[c]	mg-h[b]
A	<1-cm tumor	0 Gy	0 Gy	6,000 4,000	72 48	59–63 Gy	17–22	6,600–10,000
B	IB/IIB 1–3-cm tumor	0	<40	5,400 3,600	72 48	56–59	57–60	6,600–9,000
C		20	<20	3,600 3,900	48 52	67–69	54–56	5,500–7,500
D	Endocervical tumor; Ib/IIb moderate bulk (3–6 cm) disease; IIB/IIIB bulky (>6 cm) tumor with good regression	40	<10[c]	3,250 3,250	48 48	81–90	63–64	5,280–6,500
E	Bulky disease with poor regression	50	0	2,500 2,500 or 5,000	48 48 or 72	81–94	62	5,000

[a]Adapted from Potish RA, Gerbi BJ. Cervical cancer intracavitary dose specification and prescription. *Radiology* 1987;165:555–560.
[b]Radium tubes with 1 mm platinum filtration.
[c]With maximum split field dose.

the milligram-hours and prevents tissues near the applicator from exceeding tolerance doses, whereas larger applications are terminated by the milligram-hour constraint, ensuring adequate dose to the tumor. Although the historical Fletcher system does not use point A dose either for prescription or reporting, the total point A dose is constant within 12% for allowed tandem and colpostat loadings within each treatment scheme (A–E) of Table 25.10. The reader should note that the Fletcher system is a complex, highly individualized treatment system that resists formulation in terms of a few rules. Table 25.10 is a highly condensed and simplified summary derived from the literature, not from observation of current M.D. Anderson Cancer Center practice patterns.

The Washington University (WU)/Mallinckrodt Institute of Radiology system prescribing intracavitary therapy illustrates another empirical approach for ensuring adequate dose delivery to the tumor while limiting the volume of tissue treated to high doses. Like the Fletcher system, intracavitary BT prescriptions are stated in mgRaEq-h. Historically, the WU system used Manchester-like applicators and loadings preloaded with ^{226}Ra or ^{60}Co tubes, until the late 1950s when the Ter-Pogossian applicator was introduced. The system changed with the introduction of high-energy x-ray external-beam therapy in 1958, the adoption of the Fletcher-Suit applicator in 1965, and the acquisition of ^{137}Cs tubes in 1971.[243] Because of the long association of the WU system with artificial radionuclides, equivalent mass of radium rather than mass of radium is used to specify source strength; hence, 1 mgRaEq-h in the WU system is equivalent to 1.07 mg-h in the Fletcher system, which, in turn, is equivalent to a TRAK of 0.00723 mGy at 1 m.

Manchester-like applicator loadings (Fig. 25.28) currently are used for LDR applications, yielding an approximately constant point A dose rate of 65 cGy/h. For HDR applications, the dwell weights are selected to duplicate the relative Manchester loadings, and the TRAK per insertion is reduced to reflect the increased radiobiologic effectiveness of the HDR fractionation schedule relative to the LDR regimen. Classically defined point A doses are calculated for reporting purposes for all patients, although this quantity plays no role in prescribing therapy. Dose to the pelvic lymph nodes is calculated at point P, located 2 cm superior to the lateral fornix and 6 cm lateral to the patient's midline. The 2013 ICRU Report 89[108] continues to recommend the ICRU Report No. 38[3] Bladder and rectal reference points (Fig. 25.31) for conventional 2D orthogonal film dosimetry. The prescribed doses for the external-beam and intracavitary (delivered in two LDR insertions) components of treatment are listed in Table 25.11 as a function of extent and stage of disease. The mgRaEq-h prescription is divided equally between the vaginal and uterine components and is delivered exactly as prescribed only in the case of the standard 80-mgRaEq application (2-cm diameter colpostats and long tandem, loaded 20-10-10). For nonstandard loadings using mini-colpostats, the vaginal and intrauterine TRAK prescriptions are modified independently.

When Delclos mini-colpostats are used, vaginal TRAK is constrained by the vaginal vault surface dose limit, which for LDR is 150 Gy (including whole-pelvis dose and the dose from the ipsilateral colpostat but excluding dose from the tandem and contralateral colpostat). For medium and large colpostats, the vaginal mgRaEq-h is increased by 16% and 28%, respectively, to compensate for their larger source-to-surface distances. When medium and short tandem loadings are used, the target TRAK prescription is modified by the ratio of the actual loading to the standard loading (80 mgRaEq-h).

Table 25.12 illustrates the detailed application of the WU system to three applicator configurations for prescription schema C, listing total doses for point A, point P, and the vaginal mucosa along with the volumes of tissue enclosed by point A and 60-Gy total dose reference isodose surfaces. The mgRaEq-h actually delivered by equivalent implants varies by a factor of 1.62, leading to a reference volume variation of 2.08. However, compared to fixed point A prescription 65 Gy, which would allow administered mgRaEq-h to vary by a factor of 2.31, the variation of irradiated volume is somewhat limited. These rules represent an empirically developed compromise between limiting volume of tissue treated and maintaining a tumoricidal dose contribution to the colpostat surface and to point A.

Table 25.11 shows that as tumor size increases and therapeutic emphasis shifts from intracavitary insertions to external-beam therapy, the point A dose increases, from 58 Gy for small IB lesions (schema A) to 94 Gy for stage 4 lesions (schema E). The mgRaEq-h actually administered within a given treatment group may deviate from the target mgRaEq-h prescriptions by as much as −30% to +40% for very small and large insertions, respectively. Despite reliance on the mgRaEq-h prescription philosophy, treatment times are approximately constant, and total point A doses are nearly independent of applicator size, the defining features of the Manchester system.

Summary Principles: Intracavitary Brachytherapy Dose Specification

The most widely used intracavitary BT systems in North America are based on Manchester-type loadings and applicators, in which the point A dose rate is approximately constant and independent of loading, leading to a linear relationship between point A dose and time, not mgRaEq-h. Practical mgRaEq-h systems use various dose-specification parameters to constrain and guide treatment and are far more Manchester-like than the "strict" milligram-hour philosophy would suggest. These parameters have the following roles: (a) TRAK limits the volume of tissue treated to a high dose; (b) point A dose ensures that tumor periphery receives adequate dose; (c) vaginal surface dose ensures that dose to mucosal surfaces in contact with applicator system remains within tolerance; and (d) treatment time ensures indirect control of point A dose.

TABLE 25.11 WASHINGTON UNIVERSITY PRESCRIPTIONS FOR CARCINOMA OF THE CERVIX

Treatment Scheme	Indication	External Beam Treatment		Intracavitary Treatment		Range: Smallest to Largest Insertion		
		Whole Pelvis (Gy)	Split Field (Gy)	Target mgRaEq-h	Maximum Vaginal Vault Dose (Gy)	Point A Dose (Gy)	Point P Dose (Gy)	mgRaEq-h
A	IB < 2 cm	0	45	7,000	150	58–60	56–60	5,580–7,980
B	IB 2–4 cm	10	40	7,500	150	71–72	61–66	5,580–8,550
C	IB/IIA/IIB/IIIA bulky (>4 cm) limited parametrial extension	20	30	8,000	150	84–86	61–67	5,600–9,100
D	IIB/IIB bulky extensive parametrial extension	20	40	8,000	150	84–86	71–77	5,600–9,100
E	IIB, IIIB, IV poor anatomy, poor regression	40	20	6,500	150	92–94	69–74	4,610–7,410

TABLE 25.12 WASHINGTON UNIVERSITY SCHEMA C: 8,000 MG-H, 20 GY WHOLE PELVIS, AND 30 GY SPLIT PELVIS

Applicator	Loading	Time	mgRaEq-h	Vaginal[a] Surface Dose	Total Point A Dose (Volume)	Total Point P Dose (Gy)	ICRU[b] Volume (40 Gy)
Small tandem	20 10	×100 h =	3,000				
Miniovoids	10 10	×130 h =	2,600 / 5,600	152.3 Gy	83.5 Gy (85 cm³)	61.0	165 cm³
Standard tandem	20 10 10	×100 =	4,000				
2-cm colpostats	20 20	×100 h =	4,000 / 8,000	150.1 Gy	86.3 Gy (131 cm³)	65.2	281 cm³
Standard tandem	20 10 10	×100 =	4,000	98.6 Gy	85.6 Gy (160 cm³)	66.9 Gy	343 cm³
3-cm colpostats	30 30	×85 h =	5,100 / 9,100				

[a]On surface of single colpostat, neglecting other sources.
[b]ICRU, International Commission on Radiation Units and Measurements.

Although the traditional treatment specification quantities have clear physical meanings and interrelationships, these concepts can be applied to patient treatment only within a clinical system supported by a base of evaluated clinical experience. In current practice, implant placement is guided by direct visualization and palpation, and treatment prescription is guided by the radiation oncologist's knowledge of treatment outcome averaged over groups of uniformly treated patients with similar tumor size and location and medical condition. This implies that the implant system must be applied as a whole: Mixing dose specification methods, insertion techniques, and normal-tissue dose–response relationships from different clinical systems is a dangerous practice that can lead to suboptimal or indeterminate clinical outcomes. For example, use of the WU-recommended rectal tolerance dose (75 to 80 Gy) to guide prescription in a system using higher whole-pelvis doses will not guarantee an acceptable level of complications. Second, because classical dose-specification quantities incompletely describe the dose distribution, a radiation oncologist must be trained in all details of an intracavitary system to duplicate the results of its developers. Finally, for the clinical physicist, consistency of current dosimetric practice with past clinical experience maybe more important than absolute dose-computation accuracy or compliance with a practice standard external to the treatment system.

Image-Guided Intracavitary Brachytherapy

Classical intracavitary BT, with its empirically based rules, prescription practices, and feedback derived from patient follow-up to shape and position intracavitary dose distributions, demonstrates that even massive cervical cancers are potentially curable with concomitant chemoradiation therapy. In an effort to improve clinical outcomes in locally advanced cervical cancer and to reduce the significant incidence of local failure and late normal-tissue toxicity, anatomy-based dose specification using 3D x-ray CT or magnetic resonance (MR) imaging studies acquired with the applicator system in place has been intensively investigated. Early studies[259–261] consistently demonstrated that conventional orthogonal film-based reference points (2D planning) overestimate minimum doses to the cervix and underestimate maximum doses to critical structures by factors of 1.5 to 2.3 with large patient-to-patient variations. Because MR imaging has been shown to be far superior to CT for distinguishing tumor from normal cervical stroma[262] and for delineating surrounding critical structures, advisory

groups[263,264] recommend using T2-weighted MR imaging studies acquired prior to initiating treatment and after each intracavitary insertion for BT planning and dose reconstruction. This has culminated in the publication of a revised ICRU report[108] that provides detailed guidance for planning, prescribing, and reporting intracavitary brachytherapy in the MRI-guided era. An important innovation is a widely accepted target-volume nomenclature (high-risk, intermediate-risk, and low-risk CTVs, denoted by CTV_{HR}, CTV_{IR}, and CTV_{LR}, respectively) and specific DVH parameters[265] for assessing the correlation between clinical outcome and the delivered dose distribution. The CTV_{HR} includes the entire cervix along with all palpable or presumed residual gross tumor volume (GTV_{res}) at the time of each intracavitary insertion. ICRU Report 89 recommends a dynamic adaptive treatment philosophy: the goal of each insertion to deliver the prescribed D_{90} dose (roughly comparable to point A dose) to the "residual" CTV_{HR} for a total (external beam and brachytherapy) $D_{2Gy,90}$ dose (in 2 Gy fraction equivalents) of 85 to 90 Gy. The CTV_{IR} consists of the initial CTV_{HR} (based on the pretreatment GTV_{init} plus a margin for microscopic disease (typically 5 mm anterior–posteriorly and 10 mm elsewhere). It typically receives a total D_{90} dose (D_{2Gy}) of 65 to 70 Gy for locally advanced disease. In addition to recommending tracking the classical dose specification quantities (TRAK and point A, bladder, and rectal reference doses), ICRU Report 89[108] recommends tracking D_{90} and D_{98} for CTV_{HR} and CTV_{IR} coverage and D_{2cm^3} and $D_{0.1cm^3}$ for assessing bladder and rectal doses. The report also provides a simplified linear-quadratic model for converting LDR, HDR, and external beam doses into equivalent 2-Gy fractionated doses.

Early reports of image-based conformal therapy in locally advanced cervical cancer are promising. For example, the use of intensity-modulated radiation therapy (IMRT) to replace traditional whole- and split-pelvis fields[266,267] suggests that grade 3/4 late toxicity is significantly reduced relative to historical controls without increasing local recurrence. The most extensively reported experience with MRI-based intracavitary BT planning (156 patients at Medical University of Vienna), achieved excellent 3-year local control rates of 86% to 100% (FIGO Ib-IIIb) with 3 grade 2/4 late toxicities of 4% or less, and[268] demonstrated a robust dose–response relationship between CTV_{HR} D_{90} and D_{100} for large tumors[269] and a good correlation between bladder and rectal DVH parameters, for example, D_{2cm^3}, and major late complications.[270] Challenges to image-guided intracavitary therapy include substantial soft-tissue displacement and deformation due to applicator insertion and removal, tumor regression, and bladder and rectal filling variations (all ignored by clinical experiences cited above), making it difficult to meaningfully evaluate cumulative dose distributions. An important area of research is application of deformable image registration to account explicitly for the temporal sequence of deforming 3D anatomies needed to accurately characterize a multiple insertion course of intracavitary and external beam therapy.[271] Using dose summation over weekly MR image sets that had been contoured and

Section II

nonrigidly registered, Lim et al.[272] demonstrated that 5-mm PTV expansion of CTV_{IR} for the IMRT component of treatment was adequate for most patients, although large variations between planned and cumulative normal-tissue doses were observed for some patients. As IMRT is used to create more conformal external-beam dose distributions and to address peripheral CTV_{HR} underdoses by the intracavitary treatment components, the need to accurately account for local tissue deformation will become more acute.[273]

THE RADIOBIOLOGY OF BRACHYTHERAPY

The development of high-strength remote-afterloading stepping sources and low-energy permanently implantable sources has resulted in clinical utilization of dose rates and dose-time-fractionation patterns that can differ radically from conventional LDR BT protocols, making it logistically easier to combine BT with external beam radiation therapy (EBRT). A clear understanding of the principles governing selection of dose-time-fractionation protocols in BT or combined EBRT–BT has become an essential clinical tool.

The highly conformal dose distribution characteristic of BT sources significantly reduces the exposed volume, and, often, the maximum dose in adjacent normal tissues, compared to EBRT.[273,274] As well as diminishing late-responding normal-tissue complications, such dose sparing keeps early-responding normal-tissue sequelae to acceptable levels, dose sparing also makes the short treatment times commonly used in temporary implant BT tolerable. This is in contrast to EBRT where the risk of early-responding tissue sequelae requires treatment times to be prolonged for up to 8 weeks, potentially reducing tumor control through repopulation. The short overall treatment times used in temporary implants are likely to contribute significantly to clinical efficacy and social–economic benefits for those tumor sites (e.g., cervix, head and neck, and lung) where long overall treatment time is associated with reduced local control.

Biophysical Modeling of Brachytherapy

Along with a clear understanding of the radiobiologic basis of BT, biophysical models for predicting responses to alternative temporal dose-delivery schemes have been developed. In the 1970s, before the differential response of early- and late-responding tissues was understood, the most widespread approach for designing alternative fractionation schemes was the nominal standard dose (NSD) equation,[275] which was based on data from early-responding tissues only. By contrast, the currently used linear-quadratic (LQ) model unequivocally distinguishes between early and late responses and is based on mechanistic notions about how cells are killed by radiation. After several decades of investigation and use, the basic ideas and parameters in the LQ model have been well supported by clinical experience and outcome data.

The Linear-Quadratic Model and Its Mechanistic Basis

Central to the LQ approach is a biologic model of radiation action, which was spelled out in detail more than 50 years ago by Lea and Catcheside,[276,277] based on a mechanistic analysis of radiation-induced chromosome aberration induction. The application of the LQ formalism to radiation therapy has been reviewed by Thames and Hendry,[278] Dale,[279] Fowler,[280] and many others. The LQ model assumes that radiotherapeutic response is primarily related to cell survival (or survival of groups of cells). Although not the sole determinant of biologic response, there is now a wealth of evidence that cell killing, that is, loss of reproductive integrity, is the dominant determinant of radiotherapeutic response, both for early- and late-responding end points.[278]

In the most basic LQ approach, cellular survival, S, from dose D given in a single acute exposure or fraction, is written as

$$S(D) = \exp(-\alpha D - \beta D^2) \tag{39}$$

The mechanistic interpretation of Eq. (39) is that cell killing results from the interaction of two elementary damaged species, most often DNA double-strand breaks (DSB), to produce species that cause cell lethality, such as dicentric chromosomal aberrations. The first term in (39), which is linear in dose, describes production of two DSBs by the same ionizing radiation quantum (usually a charged particle), whereas the second term, quadratic in dose, describes production of multiple DSBs by two independent quanta. If the radiation is delivered over a protracted period rather than delivered acutely, the two DSBs may be formed at different times. Therefore, it is possible that the first may be repaired before it has a chance to interact with the second. This will not affect the first term in Eq. (39), because the two DSBs are formed simultaneously from a single particle track, but DSB repair during a prolonged exposure will result in a reduction of the second, quadratic term in Eq. (39) by a factor denoted by "G"[276,277]:

$$S(D) = \exp(-\alpha D - G \times \beta D^2), \tag{40}$$

where, for acute exposures, $G \to 1$, and for very long exposures, $G \to 0$. In this context, "acute" and "long" are defined relative to the half-time (T_r) for DSB repair of sublethal damage. In general, G will depend on the detailed temporal distribution of dose delivery, as well as on T_r. For many simple cases, G can be calculated analytically. For example, for a permanent exponentially decaying implant, G can be approximated as $\lambda/(\mu+\lambda)$ where $\lambda = \ln 2/T_{1/2} = 0.693/T_{1/2}$ is the decay constant of the radionuclide and μ (=$0.693/T_r$) is the sublethal damage repair rate. In the case of our two DSB damage models, μ describes repair of single DSBs. Formulae for G for many other standard schemes also have been derived,[277,281] as has a general formalism for any possible protraction scheme.[282]

The LQ formalism, described by Eqs. (39) and (40), is not simply a convenient formula for fitting cellular survival curves, but can be derived from a variety of underlying mechanistic models via first-order time–dependent perturbation theory when the dose or dose rate is not too high, a constraint that includes most clinically and experimentally relevant doses and dose rates.[283] For example, the theory of dual radiation action[284] is only one of several different approaches to describing radiobiology damage mechanistically. The approach devised by Lea and his coworkers[276,277] deals instead with the kinetics of damage development. Typical kinetic models track the temporal evolution of lesions as a cell gradually repairs or misrepairs initial damage.[285–287] Many different molecular mechanisms have been studied kinetically, such as pairwise misrepair of DNA DSBs, direct one-hit induction of lethal lesions, and saturable repair pathways in which the repair enzyme system can be overloaded.

Practical Applications of the LQ Model

Equation (40) can be used either to design "equivalent" dose protraction protocols (i.e., design a regimen with the same tumor response, or the same late complications, as a "tried and tested" regimen) or to predict absolute radiotherapeutic responses. We will discuss both approaches here, although we will argue that designing equivalent protraction schemes is a considerably more robust procedure.

In order to design a new dose protraction protocol (labeled "2"), which will have the same effect as a current protocol (labeled "1"), based on Eq. (40), we need to ensure the quantity $(\alpha D + G\beta D^2)$ is equal for the two protocols, that is

$$D_1(1 + G_1 D_1 /(\alpha/\beta)) = D_2(1 + G_2 D_2 /(\alpha/\beta)) \tag{41}$$

The quantity on either side of (41) is often called the biologically effective dose (BED),[280] so generating a new "equivalent" regimen amounts to matching BEDs for the old and new regimens.

By contrast, to use the LQ model to calculate absolute tumor-control probabilities (TCP) or normal-tissue complication probabilities (NTCP), we need additional models relating cellular survival (S) with TCP or with NTCP. The simplest approach, originating with Munro and Gilbert,[288] equates TCP with the probability that after radiation treatment, there are no remaining tumor stem cells capable of initiating tumor regrowth. Let us suppose that a dose, D, delivered in a given protraction pattern produces a stem-cell survival probability, S. Let K be the initial number of potential stem cells in the tumor. Then, the probability that any given stem cell will be unable to initiate tumor regrowth is (1 − S). Thus, the TCP for the irradiated tumor is simply $(1 − S)^K$, which, for small values of S, can be approximated as:

$$TCP = \exp(-S \cdot K) \tag{42}$$

Thus, if cell survival, S, is described by Eq. (40), then:

$$\begin{aligned} TCP(D) &= \exp(-K \cdot \exp[-\alpha D - G \cdot \beta D^2]) \\ &= \exp(-\exp[\ln K - \alpha D - G \cdot \beta D^2]) \end{aligned} \tag{43}$$

Equation (43) may also be used to calculate NTCP, except that now, the parameter K does not refer to the number of tumor cells that need to be sterilized, but rather to the number of groups of cells in the normal tissue ("tissue-rescuing units"),[289] whose destruction would result in the late complication.

A problem with Eq. (43), or similar approaches to estimate clinical outcomes de novo, is that absolute values of TCP or NTCP are exquisitely sensitive to the parameter values, particularly the K parameter. In contrast, using the LQ model to compare competing protraction regimens (Eq. (41) and its extensions described below) makes no assumptions about the relationship between surviving fraction and clinical outcome, and, therefore, is much less sensitive to the LQ parameter values.[290]

To improve the clinical utility of TCP or NTCP models, extensive efforts have been made to fit these models to clinical data, yielding tumor-/tissue-specific model parameters, for example, for head-and-neck tumors,[291,292] breast tumors,[293,294] prostate cancer,[295,296] brain tumors,[297] rectal cancer,[298] and liver cancer.[299]

Use of the Linear-Quadratic Model in Brachytherapy

Quantifying the Rationale for Low–Dose Rate Brachytherapy

It has long been known that lowering the dose rate generally reduces biologic damage[300] because of increased opportunity to repair sublethal damage.[276,277] It also has been clear since the pioneering work of Coutard and colleagues[301] that fractionating or protracting a radiotherapeutic exposure improves the "therapeutic ratio" (ratio of tumor control to complications). However, the exact link between these observations was not clearly made until the 1980s by Withers and colleagues.[302,303]

To understand their insight, consider the isoeffect curves in Figure 25.33 representing "equivalent" schemes for either early- or late-responding end points as a function of treatment time. For higher-dose rates, the dose reduction needed to match late effects is larger than the dose reduction needed to match tumor control. For any selected dose, increasing the dose rate will increase late effects much more than it will increase tumor control. Conversely, decreasing the dose rate will decrease late effects much more than it will decrease

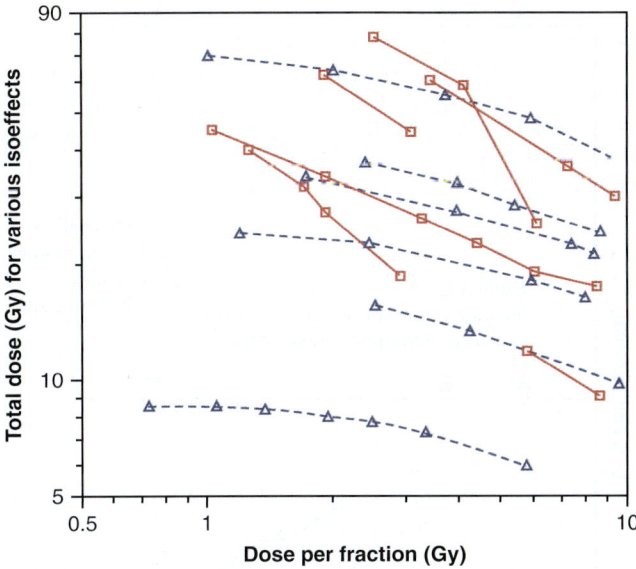

FIGURE 25.33. Isoeffect curves showing the total dose to produce a given end point, plotted against dose per fraction, a surrogate, in this context, for dose rate. The triangles, joined by *dashed lines*, refer to a variety of different early-responding end points (of which tumor control is an example), whereas the squares, joined by solid lines, refer to a variety of different late-responding sequelae. Note the generally steeper slopes of the solid lines, suggesting that late-responding tissues are more sensitive than early-responding tissues to changes in the protraction of a given radiation dose. (Adapted with permission from Withers HR, Taylor JMG, Maciejewski B. The hazard of accelerated tumor clonogen repopulation during radiotherapy. *Acta Radiol* 1988;27[2]:131–146. Copyright © 1988 SAGE Publications.)

tumor control. Thus, the therapeutic ratio increases as the dose rate decreases.

These observations can be interpreted in terms of the α/β ratio[302] in the LQ Eq. (41). In terms of survival curves (Fig. 25.34), the α/β ratio essentially describes the degree of "curviness" of the acute survival curve. A small value of α/β means that the β (dose squared) term dominates cell killing at radiotherapeutic doses, resulting in a curvy survival curve (Fig. 25.34). A large value of α/β means that the linear-in-dose α term dominates, resulting in a straighter semilog survival curve. Now, as a first approximation, the dose–response relation for a fractionated (or LDR) regimen can be thought of as simply the result of multiple repeats of the initial part of the survival curve. It is clear that repeating the early part of a curvy survival curve many times will result in far more sparing than repeating the early part of a straighter survival curve.

Thus, late effects, which are very sensitive to changes in fractionation, are characterized by small values of α/β (a typical value is 3 Gy), and early effects (tumor control or early-responding normal sequelae) are characterized by large values of α/β, a typical value for most tumors being about 10 Gy. As clinical data from which α/β ratios can be derived have accumulated, the dichotomy between α/β ratios for early and late effects has held up remarkably well. Consequently, when using the LQ model, it is essential to be clear about whether the calculation is designed to refer to early- or late-responding tissue and to then use the appropriate α/β value. From Eq. (41), it is clear that the use of different values of α/β will result in different predictions for the isoeffect dose.

Modeling the Effect of Treatment Time

For temporary implants or HDR, the effect of tumor cell repopulation is generally small, but this is not necessarily the case with longer permanent implants. Equation (40) can be simply modified to take into account repopulation, that is, the effects of overall time. Following the original formulation by

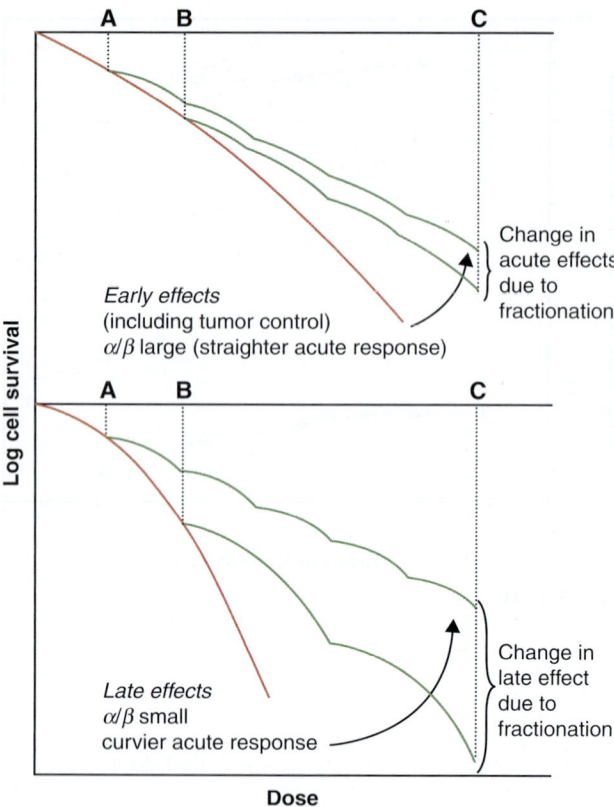

FIGURE 25.34. Illustrating the differing effects of protraction on early- and late-responding tissues, as elucidated by Thames and colleagues.[302] (Reprinted from Thames HD Jr, Withers HR, Peters LJ, et al. Changes in early and late radiation responses with altered dose fractionation: implications for dose-survival relationships. *Int J Radiat Oncol Biol Phys* 1982;8[2]:219–226. Copyright © 1982 Elsevier. With permission.)

Travis and Tucker,[305] repopulation is taken into account by increasing the surviving fraction by a factor $\exp(\gamma T)$, where T is the overall treatment time. One can also take into account delay in the onset of accelerated repopulation, by replacing T with $(T–T_D)$, where T_D is the delay after the beginning of the treatment before tumor–cell proliferation begins[280]). Then, the surviving fraction is given by:

$$S = \exp\left(-\alpha D - G \cdot \beta D^2 + \gamma\left[T - T_D\right]\right) \tag{44}$$

The parameter γ determines the speed of repopulation and is given by $\gamma = 0.693/T_P$, where T_P is the effective doubling time of cells in the tumor. If we can ignore cell loss, T_P is the same as T_{POT}, which is the measurable[306] *in vitro* doubling time of the tumor cells.

If tumor repopulation is relevant, then, in order to designed a new equivalent regimen, rather than match the quantity $(\alpha D + G \cdot \beta D^2)$, we need to match the quantity $(\alpha D + G \cdot \beta D^2 - \gamma[T - T_D])$, and Eq. (41) or (43) can be modified correspondingly.

Redistribution and Reoxygenation

Radiobiologic response is dominated by the four "Rs": repair, repopulation, redistribution, and reoxygenation.[307] Equation (40) describes repair, which is extended using Eq. (44) to include repopulation. The LQ model can be further extended to include the remaining two "Rs"[308] by treating both redistribution cell cycle progression during irradiation and reoxygenation as aspects of a single phenomenon, termed resensitization, which occurs when a radiation exposure preferentially kills the more radiosensitive cells in a diverse population, leaving a cell population with decreased average radiosensitivity. Subsequent biologically driven changes then tend to gradually restore the original population

average radiosensitivity. The resultant LQR model uses two additional adjustable parameters—an overall resensitization rate τ_S (analogous to sublethal damage repair rate) and overall resensitization amplitude $\frac{1}{2}\sigma^2$. The LQR model replaces the LQ Eq. (40) with:

$$S(D) = \exp(-\alpha D - G\beta D^2 + \frac{1}{2}\sigma^2 \hat{G}D^2) \tag{45}$$

The new term, $\frac{1}{2}\sigma^2\hat{G}D^2$, is the product of $\frac{1}{2}\sigma^2$ (representing the average of the dominant resensitization effects over the heterogeneous tumor), whereas the factor $\hat{G}$ models the influence of fractionation on resensitization. In fact, $\hat{G}$ has exactly the same form as the sublethal damage repair function, G, except that μ replaced by τ_S. In contrast to repair, resensitization tends to increase radiosensitivity as the overall time increases. For example, tumor cells in a resistant part of the cell cycle at the beginning of the treatment, and thus were spared preferentially, may move to a more sensitive part of the cell cycle as the treatment progresses. Although mechanistically driven, LQR is sufficiently simple that it can be used for isoeffect calculations in radiation therapy and supporting reasonable fits to relevant experimental data.[308]

If reoxygenation or repopulation is relevant, then, in order to designed a new equivalent regimen, rather than match the quantity $(\alpha D+G\beta D^2)$, we need to match the quantity $(\alpha D + G\beta D^2 - \frac{1}{2}\sigma^2 \hat{G}D^2)$, and Eqs. (41) or (43) can be modified correspondingly.

The Effects of Tumor Shrinkage

If the reference surface to which dose is prescribed diminishes in size as the tumor shrinks during the treatment, then the physical dose rate and total dose will increase as cells near the dose-specification surface are closer to the implanted sources. This phenomenon has been described using the LQ formalism by Dale and colleagues.[309,310] For permanent implants in tumors with long doubling times, tumor shrinkage may significantly enhance the clinical potential of longer-lived permanent implant radionuclides such as I-125, but would have much less effect for short-lived radionuclides such as Pd-103 or Cs-131, or for rapidly growing tumors. In fact, this is one argument against the use of long-lived nuclides for permanent-implant BT, in that the outcome may depend on shrinkage parameters that we are not able to predict.

Nonuniform Dose Distributions

Many implementations of the LQ and other radiobiologic models assume that an implant dose delivery can be approximated by a single uniformly administered prescribed dose, an assumption that ignores the highly nonuniform dose distributions produced by BT. A simple scalar metric for quantifying impact of such nonuniform dose is the equivalent uniform dose (EUD) concept proposed by Niemierko[311] or the corresponding equivalent uniform biologically effective dose (EUBED).[186,312–314] EUD is defined as the uniform dose, which, if delivered with the same dose protraction regimen as the nonuniform dose distribution of interest, yields the same radiobiologic effect. The related concept, EUBED,[186,312,314] addresses both spatially nonuniform dose distributions and spatially variable temporal dose distributions, by replacing physical dose with BED (biologically effective dose; see Eq. [41]). Suppose the dose distribution over an organ or tumor is described by a DVH, $\{D_i, \nu_i\}_{i=1}^{N}$ where ν_i is the fractional volume of dose bin D_i. Then, EUBED is given by:

$$EUBED = -\frac{1}{\alpha} \ln\left(\sum_i \nu_i e^{-\alpha \cdot BED_i}\right) \tag{46}$$

where ν_i is the fraction of the tumor target receiving the ith physical or biologically effective dose, D_i and BED_i.

Alternatively, dose inhomogeneity may be taken into account using other measures of cell survival, S, also weighted with the DVH[315-317]:

$$S = \sum_i v_i S(BED_i). \tag{47}$$

This equation can also be used to estimate the overall TCP or to estimate equivalences between different treatments.[315-317]

To extend the concept of EUD to normal tissues, Niemierko (1999) proposed a phenomenologic formula referred to as the generalized EUD or gEUD:

$$gEUD = \left(\sum_i v_i D_i^a \right)^{1/a} \tag{48}$$

where v_i is the fractional organ volume receiving a dose D_i and a is a tissue-specific parameter that describes the volume effect. For $a \to -\infty$, gEUD approaches the minimum dose; thus, negative values of a are used for tumors. For $a \to +\infty$, gEUD approaches the maximum dose (serial organs). For $a = 1$, gEUD is equal to the arithmetic mean dose. For $a = 0$, gEUD is equal to the geometric mean dose. The original EUD concept has a more mechanistic interpretation than the empirical gEUD (described below). However, the gEUD is often used in plan comparison and optimization metric for EBRT and may be used for comparing different protraction schemes in BT because the same functional form can be applied to both targets and OARs with a single parameter capturing (it is hoped) the dosimetric "essence" of the biologic response. By replacing the physical dose DVH $\{D_i, v_i\}_{i=1}^N$ with biologically equivalent counterpart, $\{BED_i, v_i\}_{i=1}^N$, the related metric, gEUBED,[274] is obtained.

The NTCP and TCP formalisms can also be generalized to accommodate nonuniform dose distributions. To compare different inhomogeneous dose distributions, TCP and NTCP can be computed by substituting Eq. (47) into the Poisson TCP model, Eq. (43), yielding:

$$TCP(\{D_i, v_i\}) = \exp\left(-K \cdot \sum_i v_i S(BED_i) \right)$$
$$= \prod_i [\exp(-K \cdot S(BED_i))]^{v_i} = \exp(-K \cdot e^{-\alpha \cdot EUBED}) \tag{49}$$

The second equation shows that inhomogeneous dose TCP, $TCP(\{D_i, v_i\})$, is the product of exponentially scaled (by volume fraction, v_i) TCPs, each describing uniform tumor irradiation by dose bin D_i. The third equation shows that substituting the EUBED value derived from the DVH $\{D_i, v_i\}_{i=1}^N$ into the uniform dose TCP also reproduces $TCP(\{D_i, v_i\})$. Several authors[313,316,317] have extended this approach to spatial dose inhomogeneity to also include the possibility of inhomogeneous distributions of target cells within the tumor and radiosensitivities over the population of tumors.

Similar approaches for accounting for dose heterogeneity can also be applied to NTCP models[318] based on the survival of functional subunits (FSUs). Many organs are best modeled by FSUs organized with a parallel architecture such that a complication results only if or when sufficiently large number of FSUs are inactivated,[319] although serial architectures such as the spine can also be modeled.[316]

The literature suggests that dose nonuniformity can have a large impact on biophysical surrogates of clinical outcome. For example, for permanent seed prostate implants, Ling et al.[314] demonstrated that doses between 100% and 130% of the D_{99} prescribed dose enhanced EUBED by 20% to 70%, whereas Fatyga et al.[274] found that dose inhomogeneity enhanced EUBED by 22% for HDR prostate implants. In a population of 423 prostate cancer patients with minimum follow-up of 3 years and individual 3D dose distributions, Haworth et al.[320] were able to identify a TCP cutpoint (TCP

> 0.62) that was significantly correlated with freedom from biochemical failure at 5 and 8 years. In contrast, conventional D_{90} doses were not significantly correlated with outcomes in this population. Lindsey et al.[321] found that α/β values derived by equating external beam and ^{125}I monotherapy TCPs ranged from 1.9 to 5.9 Gy when postimplant dose heterogeneity was accounted for compared to $\alpha/\beta \approx 1.5$ Gy for assumed uniform brachytherapy dose distributions. However, they cautioned that in their spatially uniform clonogen density model, α/β estimates for individual patients were highly sensitive to peripheral cold spots.

Although the above studies leave no doubt that brachytherapy dose heterogeneity can profoundly impact the results of biophysical model predictions, a major source of uncertainty is the sensitivity of TCP, NTCP, and EUBED calculations to the ubiquitous focal hot and cold spots characteristic of brachytherapy. Most applications of TCP and EUBED to 3D brachytherapy dose distributions assume a spatially uniform clonogen density and employ a cutoff (typically 110 Gy[322] or D_{99}[314]) which excludes low-dose voxels from the calculation, thereby avoiding unrealistically low estimates for clinical implant geometries. In a study of 613 postprocedure ^{125}I prostate implant dose distributions, Miksys et al.[323] found that the mean EUBED ranged from 78 to 122 Gy for BED cutoffs ranging from 30 to 130 Gy (e.g., EUBED = 108 Gy for BED > 110 Gy). The corresponding range of mean TCP was 0.20 to 1.0 (e.g., TCP = 0.92 for BED > 110 Gy). In a study of 10 HDR prostate boost dose distributions, Fatyga et al.[274] found that gEUBED for bladder and rectal tissue was highly sensitive to focal hot spots, requiring the use of a high BED cutoff taken to be the prescribed BED[98]. Including higher-dose focal hot spots for rectal complications was found to reverse the relative ranking of HDR and IMRT plans. This result is significant, because the gEUD formalism is equivalent to the DVH reduction scheme employed by the widely used Lyman-Kutcher-Burman (LKB) NTCP model.[324,325] In summary, straightforward application of EUBED and TCP to 3D dose calculations without arbitrary dose cutoffs requires patient-specific GTV and realistic spatially variant clonogen density models. Avoiding arbitrary high-dose cutoffs for normal-tissue response modeling requires a yet-to-be-advanced model for predicting local injury saturation.

The Relative Effectiveness of Different Radioisotopes Used in Brachytherapy

As discussed earlier in this chapter, the mean photon energies of currently used BT radionuclides range from 398 keV (^{192}Ir) down to 21 keV (^{103}Pd). It is well established that biologic effectiveness varies with photon energy, as a result of different patterns of energy deposition produced by the different photon spectra.[67,326] It is possible, however, to estimate the RBE of these different isotopes directly from the energy deposition patterns—the subject matter of microdosimetry.[327] In this approach, the response per unit dose at low-dose rates (or low doses), R_i, to a particular radiation, i, can be written as[328]:

$$R_i = \int w(y) \cdot d_i(y) \cdot dy \tag{50}$$

where y is the stochastic quantity, lineal energy,[327] defined as the energy imparted to a cellular target arising from all ionizing radiation events caused by a single photon track and its secondary particles, divided by the target's mean chord length. The quantity $d_i(y)$ is the dose-weighted probability that a photon will deposit lineal energy y in the target volume of interest. The quantity $d_i(y)$ often is referred to as the microdosimetric single-event spectrum. It can be measured using a low-pressure proportional counter or calculated.[327] The quantity $w(y)$ describes the response of an individual cellular target to a lineal energy deposition, y. For sparsely ionizing radiations, for example, photons and electrons, it is reasonable to assume that w(y) is proportional to y.[327] Thus, at low-dose rates:

$$RBE_i \propto \int y \cdot d_i(y) \cdot dy \qquad (51)$$

where $d_i(y)$ is the dose-averaged lineal energy. Based on this approach, RBE values have been estimated from measured or calculated microdosimetric spectra.[67,329] For example, Wuu et al.[67] report low-dose rate RBE values relative to ^{60}Co of 1.3, 2.1, 2.1, and 2.3, respectively, for ^{192}Ir, ^{241}Am, ^{125}I, and ^{103}Pd, respectively. These values are comparable to those obtained experimentally. The approach outlined above is applicable only to LDR BT, but it can be generalized to HDR regimens.[328] Incorporating the low-dose–rate RBE into the LQ equations is surprisingly easy (Dale and Jones 1988), requiring a simple modification of Eq. (41):

$$BED = D[RBE + G \cdot D/(\alpha/\beta)] \qquad (52)$$

The LQ Model for Permanent Implants

To use the LQ model to predict the total dose that a permanent implant needs to deliver to a repopulating tumor with an effective doubling time of T_p, we need to match the quantity $(\alpha D + G \cdot \beta D^2 - \gamma[T - T_D])$ (see Eq. [44] to an appropriate reference regimen.). However, as shown by Dale,[330] the effective treatment time, T_{eff}, for a permanent implant is not infinite, but achieves a finite value when the dose rate becomes sufficiently low that the rate of cell kill equals the number tumor cells created per unit time by repopulation. At this point, the treatment is effectively over, and any subsequent dose is wasted. This can be expressed mathematically by $\alpha(\partial BED(T_{eff})/\partial t) = \alpha \dot{D}_0 e^{-\lambda T_{eff}} \approx \gamma$ assuming that G ≈ 1 at low-dose rates and $T_D \ll T_{eff}$. Thus:

$$T_{eff} = -\frac{1}{\lambda} \ln\left[\frac{0.693}{\alpha \dot{D}_0 T_p}\right] = -\frac{1}{\lambda} \ln\left[\frac{\gamma}{\alpha \dot{D}_0}\right] \qquad (53)$$

where λ is the radioactive decay constant of the particular nuclide used and T_{pot} is the potential doubling time of the tumor. At time T_{eff}, the dose that has been delivered is not the total dose, D, but rather a smaller effective dose, given by:

$$D_{eff} = D(1 - e^{-\lambda T_{eff}}) \qquad (54)$$

As an example, using reasonable parameters for prostate tumors, the effective dose for a 145 Gy I-125 permanent seed implant is actually 139 Gy, which is the value that would be used in LQ-based calculations.

The LQ model can be used to optimize the choice of radionuclide for a permanent implant.[157,331,332] The most common sources in current use are I-125 and Pd-103 (with half-lives of 59 and 17 days, respectively), although Cs-131 (half-life 10 days) is being increasingly considered.[333] The optimal radionuclide for a given tumor depends on, among other factors, its growth rate, α/β value, radiosensitivity (α), and DSB repair rate. Generally speaking, short-lived radionuclides are more advantageous for treating fast-growing tumors, whereas longer-lived radionuclides are more optimal for slow-growing tumors. However, short-lived radionuclides can effectively treat both fast- and slow-growing tumors[157,331] and, in addition, are less sensitive to the tumor properties and LQ parameter values assumed than is the case for long-lived radionuclides.

HDR Intracavitary Brachytherapy for Cervical Cancer

There has been a trend in the past few years toward the increased use of HDR BT in some tumor sites, driven largely by the economic and logistical benefits of outpatient-based fractionated HDR BT. While sometimes delivered in a single fraction, more often 3 to 12 HDR fractions are used. In some situations, such as palliative or intraoperative BT, the therapeutic ratio between tumor control and late sequelae is not a primary consideration; but, in general for curative intent treatments, increasing the dose rate is likely to *decrease* the therapeutic advantage between tumor control and late sequelae. However, there are two curative applications (intracavitary implants for cancer of the uterine cervix and implant therapy for prostate cancer) where, for differing reasons, HDR BT is as effective, or potentially even more effective, compared to LDR BT.

The radiobiologic principles involved in converting LDR to HDR intracavitary insertions are illustrated schematically in Figure 25.35, which shows typical dose–response relationships for early- and late-responding tissues. As we have discussed, the dose–response relations for late effects are significantly "curvier" (smaller α/β ratio) than for early-responding tissues such as tumors, which have larger α/β ratios. Suppose that we want to replace a LDR treatment delivering dose D by an HDR treatment that gives identical tumor control. As illustrated in the left panel, we need to reduce the dose by a dose reduction factor (DRF) (see left panel). From the right panel, however,

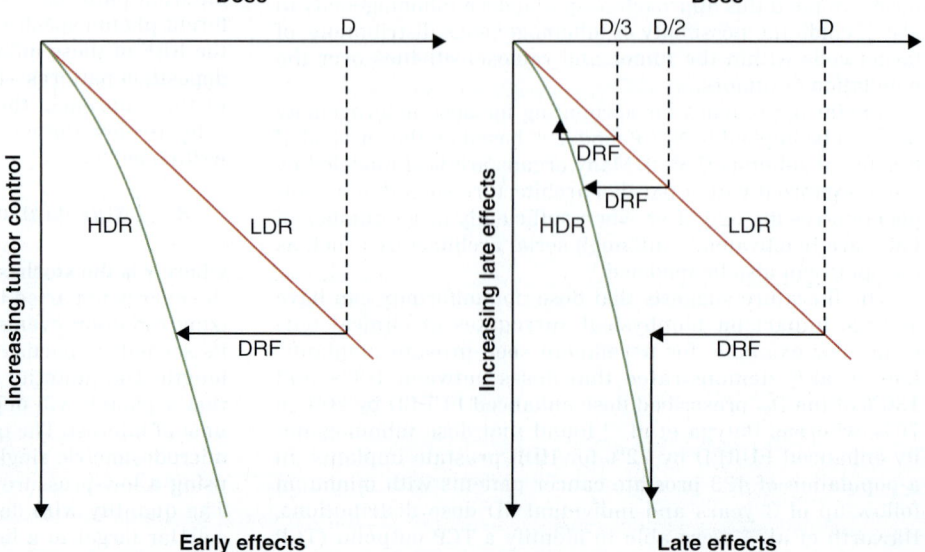

FIGURE 25.35. Illustration of the interplay between early and late effects for low–dose rate (LDR) and high–dose rate (HDR) brachytherapy for cervical cancer. DRF is the dose reduction factor that produces the same early effects (tumor control) for HDR as LDR. If D is the LDR dose giving rise to late effects, then reducing D by DRF for HDR will result in more late effects than at LDR. As the HDR dose to late-responding tissue is reduced by treatment planning, then reducing that dose by the factor DRF no longer produces worse late effects than at LDR.

it can be seen that this adjusted dose, DRF × D, will result in increased late effects, i.e., lower late responding tissue cell survival, compared to LDR. But now, let us suppose that the LDR dose to organ at risk (OAR) giving rise to the late effects is not the treatment dose D, but some lower dose. This is the case for cervical BT because the bladder and rectum are generally some significant distance from the cervical implant. To be specific, let us suppose that this OAR dose is half the treatment dose, that is, D/2. From the right-hand panel in Figure 25.35, we see that if HDR preserves the LDR level of dose sparing, that is, delivers dose DRF × D/2 to the OAR, where DRF matches tumor control, we will *not* get more late effects for HDR compared to LDR, but actually a similar late-effect probability because we are further up the survival curve. Indeed, if the rectal dose were an even smaller fraction of the treatment dose (say D/3, in Fig. 25.35), HDR would have even *less* late effects than the equivalent LDR regimen. In fact, if the cervical BT results in a dose to the bladder/rectum which is less than about three-fourths of the treatment dose, then if the HDR dose is reduced to give equal tumor control compared with LDR, the HDR late effects should not be worse than the LDR late effects.[282,334]

Of course, there is another related factor to consider, which is that the short treatment time characteristic of HDR allows packing and retraction of the sensitive organs, which typically results in a 20% further decrease in the rectal/bladder dose compared to that achievable with LDR.[335] This gives an extra physically based advantage to HDR, in addition to the biologic factors discussed here.

The following recommendations can be made based on radiobiologic consideration about the appropriate usage of HDR versus LDR for cervical cancer BT: when the dose to the dose-limiting critical normal tissues (bladder/rectum) is less than about three-fourths of the prescribed dose, HDR (with at least about five fractions to ensure adequate tumor reoxygenation) results in comparable (or less) late effects than LDR—for the same level of tumor control. These considerations are supported by a number of clinical studies.[336–342] These reports generally show that HDR and LDR for cervical BT produce similar local control and late complications.

As BT is often combined with pelvic EBRT, different time-dose patterns of EBRT and intracavitary BT should be taken into account to calculate the combined effects to tumor and OARs. For a given BED of BT, the equivalent EBRT dose expressed in conventional fractionation of 2 Gy/d (EQD2) can be calculated as EQD2 = BED/(1 + 2/(α/β)). Also, the dose from EBRT has to be recalculated if a fractionation schedule different from 2 Gy/d is used. EQD2 from EBRT and BT may be summed up assuming that the volumes and points of interest of BT receive the full EBRT dose. This estimate serves as a worst-case assumption for OARs and is reasonable for the target volume of BT which is often a boost volume of the PTV of EBRT. A more appropriate calculation should consider highly heterogeneous dose of BT, which will be demonstrated in the next section.

Brachytherapy for Prostate Cancer

Optimized Dose Protraction for Prostate Cancer Brachytherapy

As discussed above, one of the main reasons for protracting any radiotherapeutic exposure is that late sequelae are characterized by relatively low α/β ratios (3 Gy is typical) and, therefore, are spared more than tumor control, for which higher α/β ratios (10 Gy is typical), by lowering the dose rate, generally spares late-responding tissues more than the tumor. Such higher α/β ratios (10 Gy is typical) are thought to be due to the larger proportion of cycling cells in tumors compared with normal tissues. Because prostate tumors contain unusually small fractions of cycling cells,[306] it has been hypothesized that they may have α/β ratios and responses to protraction

more typical of late-responding normal tissues.[343,344] If so, much of the rationale for low dose rate, or highly fractionated regimens, would disappear.

A first estimate of α/β for prostate cancer was made in 1999,[343] by comparing results from EBRT with those from permanent seed I-125 BT. Consistent with the theoretical hypotheses (see above), the estimated value of α/β was 1.5 Gy [95% CI, 0.8–2.2 Gy], indeed comparable to α/β values for late-responding normal tissues, and much smaller than those for most tumors.

The problem with this α/β estimate, and almost all subsequent ones,[296,345–350] is that they involved comparing or equating EBRT results with permanent implantation results. There are many pertinent differences between EBRT and BT (different dose distributions, different RBEs, different overall times, different institutions, different PSA distributions, hypoxia), any or all of which could bias the α/β estimate. Much debate has been centered on the significance of these biases and how to take them into account. For example, it has been reported that the consideration of hypoxia can significantly impact the α/β estimate[351] Despite these problems, most of the analyses above support the hypothesis that the α/β value for prostate cancer is indeed quite low, probably in the 1 to 4 Gy range, which is similar to the values for most late-responding tissues.

One analysis,[352] which avoids many, though not all, of the potential biases involved in comparing EBRT and BT. Here, EBRT + two HDR boost fractions were compared with EBRT + three HDR boost fractions—all done with the same technique at the same institution. The resulting estimated α/β ratio for prostate cancer was 1.2 Gy [95% CI, 0.03–4.1 Gy], again comparable with α/β values for late-responding normal tissues. A meta-analysis of four reports summarizing 21 studies yielded an estimated α/β ratio of 1.3 Gy.[353] A recent analysis of pooled multi-institutional datasets[354] led to α/β = 1.4. A critical review of α/β ratio estimation methodologies and clinical analyses has been published by Oliveira et al.[355]

If the α/β value for prostate cancer is indeed similar to that for the surrounding late-responding normal tissue, HDR or hypofractionated external beam therapy regimens could be employed to match conventional fractionated regimens with respect to tumor control and late sequelae while reducing early urinary sequelae[356] and improving cost-effectiveness and patient convenience.

The arguments presented here really relate to the α/β value for prostate cancer in relation to the α/β value for the relevant late-responding normal tissue. Brenner reported an α/β value for RTOG grade ≥2 late rectal toxicity of 5.4 ± 1.5 Gy based on an analysis of clinical data.[357] Another recent analysis of RTOG 94-06 data suggested that the α/β value for grade ≥2 late rectal toxicity was 4.8 Gy.[358] These α/β values, which are larger than that of most late-responding tissues, are higher than recent estimates of prostate tumor α/β ratio. This suggests that HDR prostate BT, as well as being logistically convenient, might actually improve the therapeutic outcome of prostate cancer BT.

HDR (or hypofractionation) in a curative setting, even when the dose is appropriately lowered, is a prima facie unsettling idea. However, there is now a significant body of clinical evidence suggesting that these approaches do not lead to increased early or late sequelae after prostate radiotherapy, either for EBRT or for BT, providing further evidence to support the underlying radiobiologic rationale. For EBRT, in those hypofractionation studies that have reported on potential late sequelae, there is to date little indication of any unexpected late sequelae after median follow-up periods of 21 months,[359] 31 months,[360] 48 months,[361] 59 months,[362] 66 months,[363] and 97 months.[364] HDR has been used in prostate BT both as a monotherapy[365,366] and, more commonly, as a boost to external beam radiotherapy.[367–370] In both cases, the results are promising with no evidence for excessive normal-tissue complications.

Section II

Summary: Biophysical Outcome Models in Brachytherapy

This survey of biophysical models for predicting clinical outcomes from brachytherapy regimens shows that the basic LQ model is sufficiently supported by clinical experience to be used for developing equivalent fractionation regimens or to optimizing therapeutic ratios in many clinical settings. More sophisticated NTCP and TCP models, although not sufficiently robust for use in clinical planning, are able to semiquantitatively account for the LDR and HDR brachytherapy clinical outcomes in several sites in terms of underlying descriptive radiobiologic mechanisms.

CONCLUSIONS

This chapter has focused on several basic topics including physical source properties, single-source dosimetry, source-strength specification, classical interstitial and intracavitary brachytherapy systems and dose specification, and their impact on biologic effects and clinical utility. Many topics usually covered in an introductory survey have been omitted. For a review of radiographic imaging and localization of brachytherapy sources, the reader is referred to more specialized reviews.[371,372] For discussions on quality assurance of manual and remote afterloading brachytherapy and treatment planning, the reader is referred to Chapters 26, 27, and 28 of this text as well as a number of excellent reviews[92,373–377] including appropriate chapters from *Brachytherapy Physics, 2nd Edition*.[378] For useful reviews of the radiobiology of brachytherapy, the reader is referred to excellent reviews by Dale,[379] King,[380] and Carlson.[381] For a discussion of brachytherapy licensing and regulatory issues, the review by Glasgow[382] is suggested.

REFERENCES

1. Henschke UK. "Afterloading" applicator for radiation therapy of carcinoma of the uterus. *Radiology* 1960;74:834.
2. Suit HD, Moore EB, Fletcher GH, et al. Modification of the Fletcher ovoid system for afterloading, using standard sized radium tubes. *Radiology* 1963;81:126–131.
3. ICRU. *Dose and volume specification for reporting intracavitary therapy in gynecology: report 38*. Bethesda, MD: International Commission of Radiation Units and Measurements, 1985.
4. Williamson JF. Monte Carlo-based dose-rate tables for the Amersham CDCS.J and 3M model 6500 137Cs tubes. *Int J Radiat Oncol Biol Phys* 1998;41(4):959–970.
5. Rivard MJ, Coursey BM, DeWerd LA, et al. Update of AAPM Task Group No. 43 Report: A revised AAPM protocol for brachytherapy dose calculations. *Med Phys* 2004;31(3):633–674 .
6. Beaulieu L, Tedgren AC, Carrier JF, et al. Report of the Task Group 186 on model-based dose calculation methods in brachytherapy beyond the TG-43 formalism: Current status and recommendations for clinical implementation. *Med Phys* 2012;39(10):6208–6236.
7. Nath R, Gray L. Dosimetric studies on a prototype 241Am source for brachytherapy. *Int J Radiat Oncol Biol Phys* 1987;13:897.
8. Perera H, Williamson JF, Li Z, et al. Dosimetric characteristics, air-kerma strength calibration and verification of Monte Carlo simulation for a new Ytterbium-169 brachytherapy source. *Int J Radiat Oncol Biol Phys* 1994;28:953–971.
9. Medich DC, Tries MA, Munro JJ II. Monte Carlo characterization of an ytterbium-169 high dose rate brachytherapy source with analysis of statistical uncertainty. *Med Phys* 2006;33(1):163–172.
10. Tod MC, Meredith WJ. A dosage system for use in the treatment of cancer of the uterine cervix. *Br J Radiol* 1938;11:809.
11. Fletcher GH, Hamberger AD. Squamous cell carcinoma of the uterine cervix: treatment techniques according to size of the cervical lesion and extension. In: Fletcher GD, ed. *Textbook of radiotherapy*. 3rd ed. Philadelphia: Lea & Febiger, 1980:732–772.
12. Williamson JF. Brachytherapy technology and physics practice since 1950: a half-century of progress. *Phys Med Biol* 2006;51:R1–R23.
13. Horsler AFC, Jones JC, Stacey AJ. Cesium-137 sources for use in intracavitary and interstitial radiotherapy. *Br J Radiol* 1964;37:385.
14. Horwitz H, Kereiakes JG, Bahr GK, et al. An after-loading system utilizing cesium 137 for the treatment of carcinoma of the cervix. *Am J Roentgenol Radium Ther Nucl Med* 1964;91:176–191.
15. Williamson JF. Dose calculations about shielded gynecological colpostats. *Int J Radiat Oncol Biol Phys* 1990;19:167–178.
16. Viswanathan AN, Creutzberg CL, Craighead P, et al. International brachytherapy practice patterns: a survey of the Gynecologic Cancer Intergroup (GCIG). *Int J Radiat Oncol Biol Phys* 2012;82(1):250–255.
17. Meigooni AS, Wright C, Koona RA, et al. TG-43 U1 based dosimetric characterization of model 67-6520 Cs-137 brachytherapy source. *Med Phys* 2009;36(10):4711–4719.
18. Perez-Calatayud J, Granero D, Casal E, et al. Monte Carlo and experimental derivation of TG43 dosimetric parameters for CSM-type Cs-137 sources. *Med Phys* 2005;32(1):28–36.
19. Maruyama Y, Vtyurin BM, Kaneta K, et al. Californium-252 brachytherapy. In: Nag S, ed. *Principles and practice of brachytherapy*. Armonk, NY: Futura, 1997:649–687.
20. Rivard MJ. Dosimetry for Cf-252 neutron emitting brachytherapy sources: protocol, measurements, and calculations. *Med Phys* 1999;26(8):1503–1514.
21. Wierzbicki J, Maruyama Y, Feola JM, et al. Facility and clinical handling of Californium-252 sources for brachytherapy. *Endocuriether Hypertherm Oncol* 1992;8:131–135.
22. Lei X, Qian C-Y, Qing Y, et al. Californium-252 brachytherapy combined with external-beam radiotherapy for cervical cancer: long-term treatment results. *Int J Radiat Oncol Biol Phys* 2011;81(5):1264–1270.
23. Zhang M, Xu H-D, Pan S-D, et al. Low-dose-rate californium-252 neutron intracavitary afterloading radiotherapy combined with conformal radiotherapy for treatment of cervical cancer. *Int J Radiat Oncol Biol Phys* 2012;83(3):966–971.
24. Williamson JF. Semi-empirical dose-calculation models in brachytherapy. In: Thomadsen BR, Rivard MJ, Butler WM, eds. *Brachytherapy physics*. 2nd ed. Madison, WI: Medical Physics Publishing, 2005:201–232.
25. Piermattei A, Azario L, Montemaggi P. Implantation guidelines for Yb-169 seed interstitial treatments. *Phys Med Biol* 1995;40:1331–1338.
26. Leonard KL, DiPetrillo TA, Munro JJ, et al. A novel ytterbium-169 brachytherapy source and delivery system for use in conjunction with minimally invasive wedge resection of early-stage lung cancer. *Brachytherapy* 2011;10(2):163–169.
27. Enger SA, Lundqvist H, D'Amours M, et al. Exploring Co-57 as a new isotope for brachytherapy applications. *Med Phys* 2012;39(5):2342–2345.
28. Enger SA, Fisher DR, Flynn RT. Gadolinium-153 as a brachytherapy isotope. *Phys Med Biol* 2013;58(4):957–964.
29. Pakravan D, Ghorbani M, Meigooni AS. Evaluation of Rh-101 as a brachytherapy source. *J Contemp Brachytherapy* 2015;7(2):171–180.
30. Henscke UK, Hilaris BS, Mahan GD. Afterloading in interstitial and intracavitary radiation therapy. *AJR Am J Roentgenol* 1963;90:386–395.
31. Pierquin B, Dutreix A. Towards a new system in curietherapy endocurietherapy and plesiotherapy with non-radioactive preparation. *Br J Radiol* 1967;40:184.
32. NCRP. *Structural shielding design and evaluation for medical use of X-rays and gamma rays up to 10 MeV, Report No. 49*. Bethesda, MD: National Council on Radiation Protection and Measurements, 1976.
33. Guedea F, Venselaar J, Hoskin P, et al. Patterns of care for brachytherapy in Europe: Updated results. *Radiother Oncol* 2010;97(3):514–520.
34. Ling CC, Yorke ED, Schell MC, et al. Physical advantages of using Iodine-125 in temporary implants of the breast. *Endocuriether Hypertherm Oncol* 1986;2:216–217.
35. Pantelis E, Papagiannis P, Anagnostopoulos G, et al. New ^{125}I brachytherapy source IsoSeed I25.S17plus: Monte Carlo dosimetry simulation and comparison to sources of similar design. *J Contemp Brachytherapy* 2013;5(4):240–249.
36. Meigooni AS, Hayes JL, Zhang H, et al. Experimental and theoretical determination of dosimetric characteristics of IsoAid ADVANTAGE™ ^{125}I brachytherapy source. *Med Phys* 2002;29(9):2152–2158.
37. Chiu-Tsao S-T. Episcleral eye plaques for treatment of intra-ocular malignancies and benign diseases. In: Thomadsen BR, Rivard MJ, Butler WM, eds. *Brachytherapy physics*. 2nd ed. Madison, WI: Medical Physics Publishing, 2005:673–706.
38. Kline RW, Yeakel PD. Ocular melanoma I-125 plaques. *Med Phys* 1987;14:475.
39. Duane W. Methods of preparing and using radioactive substances in the treatment of malignant disease and estimating suitable doses. *Boston Med Surg J* 1917;177:787–799.
40. Teh BS, Berner BM, Carpenter LS, et al. Permanent gold-198 implant for locally recurrent adenocarcinoma of the prostate after failing initial radiotherapy. *J Brachytherapy Int* 1998;14:233–240.
41. Lawrence DC, Sondhaus CA, Feder B, et al. Soft x-ray seeds for cancer therapy. *Radiology* 1966;86:143.
42. Hilaris BS, Henschke UK, Holt JG. Clinical experience with long half-life and low-energy encapsulated radioactive sources in cancer radiation therapy. *Radiology* 1968;91:1163–1167.
43. Hilaris BS, Holt GJ, St Germain J. *The use of iodine-125 for interstitial implants*. Rockville, MD: Department of Health, Education and Welfare, Publication (FDA) 76-8022, 1975.
44. Hilaris BS, Nori D, Anderson LL. *Atlas of brachytherapy*. New York: MacMillan Publishing Co., 1988.
45. Henschke UK, Lawrence DC. Cesium-131 seeds for permanent implants. *Radiology* 1965;85:1117–1119.
46. Wang J, Zhang H. Dosimetric characterization of model Cs-1 Rev2 cesium-131 brachytherapy source in water phantoms and human tissues with MCNP5 Monte Carlo simulation. *Med Phys* 2008;35(4):1571–1579.
47. Murphy MK, Piper RK, Greenwood LR, et al. Evaluation of the new cesium-131 seed for use in low-energy x-ray brachytherapy. *Med Phys* 2004;31(6):1529–1538.
48. Holm HH, Juul N, Pederson JF. Transperineal Iodine-125 seed implantation in prostatic cancer guided by transrectal ultrasonography. *J Urol* 1983;130:283–286.
49. Blasko JC, Radge H, Schumacker D. Transperineal percutaneous Iodine-125 implantation for prostatic carcinoma using transrectal ultrasound and template guidance. *Endocuriether Hypertherm Oncol* 1987;3:131–139.
50. Grimm PD, Blasko JC, Sylvester JE, et al. 10-year biochemical (prostate-specific antigen) control of prostate cancer with (125)I brachytherapy. *Int J Radiat Oncol Biol Phys* 2001;51(1):31–40.

51. Sylvester JE, Blasko JC, Grimm PD, et al. Ten-year biochemical relapse-free survival after external beam radiation and brachytherapy for localized prostate cancer: the Seattle experience. *Int J Radiat Oncol Biol Phys* 2003;57(4):944–952.
52. Rivard MJ, Butler WM, DeWerd LA, et al. Supplement to the 2004 update of the AAPM Task Group No. 43 Report. *Med Phys* 2007;34(6):2187–2205.
53. Rivard MJ, Ballester F, Butler WM, et al. Supplement 2: 2004 update of the AAPM Task Group No. 43 Report: Joint recommendations by the AAPM and GEC-ESTRO. *Med Phys* 2017;44(9):e297–e338.
54. Martin JM, Handorf EA, Kutikov A, et al. The rise and fall of prostate brachytherapy: use of brachytherapy for the treatment of localized prostate cancer in the National Cancer Data Base. *Cancer* 2014;120(14):2114–2121.
55. IROC-Houston. *Joint AAPM/IROC houston registry of brachytherapy sources meeting the AAPM dosimetric prerequisites.* vol. 2017, 2017.
56. Li ZF, Das RK, DeWerd LA, et al. Dosimetric prerequisites for routine clinical use of photon emitting brachytherapy sources with average energy higher than 50 kev. *Med Phys* 2007;34(1):37–40.
57. Williamson JF, Coursey BM, DeWerd LA, et al. Dosimetric prerequisites for routine clinical use of new low energy photon interstitial brachytherapy sources. *Med Phys* 1998;25(12):2269–2270.
58. Rivard MJ, Reed JL, DeWerd LA. ^{103}Pd strings: Monte Carlo assessment of a new approach to brachytherapy source design. *Med Phys* 2014;41(1):011716.
59. Williamson JF, Rivard MJ. Quantitative dosimetry methods for brachytherapy. In: Thomadsen BR, Rivard MJ, Butler WM, eds. *Brachytherapy physics* 2nd ed. Madison, WI: Medical Physics Publishing, 2005:233–294.
60. Monroe JI, Williamson JF. Monte carlo-aided dosimetry of the theragenics TheraSeed® Model 200 ^{103}Pd interstitial brachytherapy seed. *Med Phys* 2002;29:609–621.
61. Ling CC, Yorke ED, Spiro IJ. Physical dosimetry of I-125 seeds of a new design for interstitial implant. *Int J Radiat Oncol Biol Phys* 1983;9:1747.
62. Dale RG. Some theoretical deviations relating to the tissue dosimetry of brachytherapy nuclides, with particular reference to Iodine-125. *Med Phys* 1983;10:176.
63. Das RK, Keleti D, Zhu Y, et al. Validation of Monte Carlo dose calculations near I-125 brachytherapy sources in the presence of bounded tissue heterogeneities. *Int J Radiat Oncol Biol Phys* 1997;38:843–853.
64. DeWerd LA, Ibbott GS, Meigooni AS, et al. A dosimetric uncertainty analysis for photon-emitting brachytherapy sources: report of AAPM Task Group No. 138 and GEC-ESTRO. *Med Phys* 2011;38(2):782–801.
65. Ling CC, Roy JN. Radiobiophysical aspects of brachytherapy. In: Williamson J, Thomadsen BR, Nath R, eds. *Brachytherapy physics: American Association of Physicists in Medicine, 1994 summer school.* Madison, WI: Medical Physics Publishing, 1995:39–71.
66. Lehnert S, Reniers B, Verhaegen F. Relative biologic effectiveness in terms of tumor response of ^{125}I implants compared with ^{60}Co gamma rays. *Int J Radiat Oncol Biol Phys* 2005;63(1):224–229.
67. Wuu CS, Kliauga P, Amols HI. Microdosimetric evaluation of relative biological effectiveness for ^{103}Pd, ^{125}I, ^{241}Am, and ^{192}Ir brachytherapy sources. *Int J Radiat Oncol Biol Phys* 1996;36(3):689–697.
68. Grimm P, Billiet I, Bostwick D, et al. Comparative analysis of prostate-specific antigen free survival outcomes for patients with low, intermediate and high risk prostate cancer treatment by radical therapy. Results from the Prostate Cancer Results Study Group. *BJU Int* 2012;109:22–29.
69. Zelefsky MJ, Kuban DA, Levy LB, et al. Multi-institutional analysis of long-term outcome for stages T1-T2 prostate cancer treated with permanent seed implantation. *Int J Radiat Oncol Biol Phys* 2007;67(2):327–333.
70. Hiatt JR, Davis SD, Rivard MJ. A revised dosimetric characterization of the model S700 electronic brachytherapy source containing an anode-centering plastic insert and other components not included in the 2006 model. *Med Phys* 2015;42(6):2764–2776.
71. Hiatt JR, Rivard MJ, Hughes HG. Simulation evaluation of NIST air-kerma rate calibration standard for electronic brachytherapy. *Med Phys* 2016;43(3):1119–1129.
71a. Liu D, Poon E, Bazalova M, et al. Spectroscopic characterization of a novel electronic brachytherapy system. *Phys Med Biol* 2008;53(1):61–75.
72. Perez-Calatayud J, Ballester F, Das RK, et al. Dose calculation for photon-emitting brachytherapy sources with average energy higher than 50 keV: report of the AAPM and ESTRO. *Med Phys* 2012;39(5):2904–2929.
73. Johns HE, Cunningham JR. *The physics of radiology*. Springfield, IL: Charles C. Thomas, 1983.
74. Armoogum KS, Parry JM, Souliman SK, et al. Functional intercomparison of intraoperative radiotherapy equipment—Photon Radiosurgery System. *Radiat Oncol* 2007;2:11.
75. Beatty J, Biggs PJ, Gall K, et al. A new miniature x-ray device for interstitial radiosurgery: Dosimetry. *Med Phys* 1996;23(1):53–62.
76. Rivard MJ, Davis SD, DeWerd LA, et al. Calculated and measured brachytherapy dosimetry parameters in water for the Xoft Axxent X-Ray Source: an electronic brachytherapy source. *Med Phys* 2006;33(11):4020–4032.
77. Goubert M, Parent L. Dosimetric characterization of INTRABEAM((R)) miniature accelerator flat and surface applicators for dermatologic applications. *Phys Med* 2015;31(3):224–232.
78. Vaidya JS, Wenz F, Bulsara M, et al. Risk-adapted targeted intraoperative radiotherapy versus whole-breast radiotherapy for breast cancer: 5-year results for local control and overall survival from the TARGIT-A randomised trial. *Lancet* 2014;383(9917):603–613.
79. Hepel J, Wazer DE. A flawed study should not define a new standard of care. *Int J Radiat Oncol Biol Phys* 2015;91(2):255–257.
80. Dickler A, Kirk MC, Seif N, et al. A dosimetric comparison of MammoSite high-dose-rate brachytherapy and Xoft Axxent electronic brachytherapy. *Brachytherapy* 2007;6(2):164–168.
81. Holt RW, Thomadsen BR, Orton CG. Miniature x-ray tubes will ultimately displace Ir-192 as the radiation sources of choice for high dose rate brachytherapy. *Med Phys* 2008;35(3):815–817.
82. Gray LH. An ionization method for the absolute measurement of gamma-ray energy. *Proc R Soc Lond* 1936;A156:578.
83. Laurence GC. Measurement of extra hard x-rays and gamma rays in roentgens. *Can J Res Sect* 1937;A15:67–78.
84. Williamson JF, Rivard MJ. Thermoluminescent detector and monte carlo techniques for reference-quality brachytherapy dosimetry. In: Rogers DWO, Cygler J, eds. *Clinical dosimetry measurements in radiotherapy (AAPM 2009 summer school)*, Madison, WI: Medical Physics Publishing, 2009:437–499.
85. Nath R, Anderson L, Jones D, et al. *Specification of brachytherapy source strength: a report by Task Group 32 of the American Association of Physicists in Medicine, Report No. 21*. New York: American Institute of Physics, 1987.
86. Williamson JF. Monte Carlo evaluation of specific dose constants in water for ^{125}I seeds. *Med Phys* 1988;15:686.
87. Loftus TP. Standardization of Cesium-137 gamma-ray sources in terms of exposure units (roentgens). *J Res Natl Bureau Stand* 1970;74:1–6.
88. Loftus TP. Standardization of Iridium-192 gamma-ray sources in terms of exposure. *J Res Natl Bureau Stand* 1980;85:19–25.
89. Seltzer SM, Lamperti PJ, Loevinger R, et al. New national air-kerma-strength standards for ^{125}I and ^{103}Pd brachytherapy seeds. *J Res Natl Inst Stand Technol* 2003;108:337–358.
90. Seltzer SM, O'Brien M, Mitch MG. New national air-kerma standard for low-energy electronic brachytherapy sources. *J Res Natl Inst Stand Technol* 2014;119:554–574.
91. Sander T. Air kerma and absorbed dose standards for reference dosimetry in brachytherapy. *Br J Radiol* 2014;87(1041).
92. Nath R, Anderson LL, Meli JA, et al. Code of practice for brachytherapy physics: report of the AAPM Radiation Therapy Committee Task Group No. 56. American Association of Physicists in Medicine. *Med Phys* 1997;24(10):1557–1598.
93. ICRU. Report 85: fundamental quantities and units for ionizing radiation. *J ICRU* 2011;11(1):1–33.
94. Attix FH. *Introduction to radiological physics and radiation physics*. New York: Wiley, 1986.
95. ICRU. Key data for ionizing-radiation dosimetry: measurement standards and applications: report 90. *J ICRU* 2014;14(1):1–110.
96. Roesch WC. Dose for nonelectronic equilibrium conditions. *Radiat Res* 1958;9:399–410.
97. Nath R, Yue N, Liu L. On the depth of penetration of photons and electrons for intravascular brachytherapy. *Cardiovasc Radiat Med* 1999;1:72–79.
98. Burlin TE. A general theory of cavity ionization. *Br J Radiol* 1966;39:361.
99. Baltas D, Karaiskos P, Papagiannis P, et al. Beta versus gamma dosimetry close to Ir-192 brachytherapy sources. *Med Phys* 2001;28(9):1875–1882.
100. Pomme S. Methods for primary standardization of activity. *Metrologia* 2007;44(4):S17–S26.
101. Coursey BM. Needs for radioactivity standards and measurements in the life sciences. *Appl Radiat Isot* 2000;52(3):609–614.
102. Williamson JF, Brenner DA. Physics and radiobiology of brachytherapy. In: Perez CA, Brady LW, Halperin E, et al., eds. *Principles and practice of radiation oncology*. 4th ed. Philadelphia: J.B. Lippincott Company, 2003:472–537.
103. Coursey BM, Colle R, Coursey JS. Standards of radium-226: from Marie Curie to the International Committee for Radionuclide Metrology. *Appl Radiat Isot* 2002;56(1–2):5–13.
104. Shalek RJ, Stovall M. The MD Anderson method for the computation of isodose curves around interstitial and intracavitary radiation sources. I. Dose from linear sources. *Am J Roentgenol Radium Ther Nucl Med* 1968;102:662–672.
105. Attix FH, Ritz VH. A determination of the gamma-ray emission of radium. *J Res Natl Bureau Stand* 1957;59:293–305.
106. Williamson JF, Coursey BM, DeWerd LA, et al. On the use of apparent activity (A_{app}) for treatment planning of ^{125}I and ^{103}Pd interstitial brachytherapy sources: recommendations of the American Association of Physicists in Medicine radiation therapy committee subcommittee on low-energy brachytherapy source dosimetry. *Med Phys* 1999;26(12):2529–2530.
107. Specification of brachytherapy sources. Memorandum from the British Committee on Radiation Units and Measurements. *Br J Radiol* 1984;57:9411984.
108. ICRU. Prescribing, recording, and reporting brachytherapy for cancer of the cervix: report 90. *J ICRU* 2013;13(1):1–258.
109. Meisberger LL, Keller RJ, Shalek RJ. The effective attenuation in water of the g-rays of gold-198, iridium-192, cesium-137, radium-226, and cobalt-60. *Radiology* 1968;90:953.
110. Daskalov GM, Loffler E, Williamson JF. Monte Carlo-aided dosimetry of a new high dose-rate brachytherapy source. *Med Phys* 1998;25(11):2200–2208.
111. Dolan J, Li Z, Williamson JF. Monte Carlo and experimental dosimetry of an 1251 brachytherapy seed. *Med Phys* 2006;33(12):4675–4684.
112. Berger MJ. Energy deposition in water by photons from point isotropic sources. *J Nucl Med* 1968;(Suppl 1):17–25.
113. Van Kleffens HJ, Star WM. Application of stereo x-ray photogrammetry (SRM) in the determination of absorbed dose values during intracavitary radiation therapy. *Int J Radiat Oncol Biol Phys* 1979;5:557.
114. Williamson JF. The accuracy of the line and point dose approximation in Ir-192 dosimetry. *Int J Radiat Oncol Biol Phys* 1986;12:409.
115. Ling CC, Anderson LL, Shipley WU. Dose inhomogeneity in interstitial implants using ^{125}I seeds. *Int J Radiat Oncol Biol Phys* 1979;5:419–425.
116. Lindsay P, Battista J, Van Dyk J. The effect of seed anisotropy on brachytherapy dose distributions using ^{125}I and ^{103}Pd. *Med Phys* 2001;28(3):336–345.
117. Corbett JF, Jezioranski JJ, Crook J, et al. The effect of seed orientation deviations on the quality of ^{125}I prostate implants. *Phys Med Biol* 2001;46(11):2785–2800.
118. Sievert RM. Die intensitatsverteilung der primaren: strahlung in der nahe medizinischer radiumpraparate. *Acta Radiol* 1921;1:89–128.

119. Williamson JF. The Sievert integral revised: evaluation and extension to low energy brachytherapy sources. *Int J Radiat Oncol Biol Phys* 1996;36:1239–1250.

120. Gooden TJ. *Physical aspects of brachytherapy (Medical physics handbook 19).* Bristol, UK: Adam Hilger, 1988.

121. Van der Laars R, Meertens H. An algorithm for ovoid shielding of a cervix applicator. In: Cunningham JR, Ragan D, Van Dyke D, eds. *Proceedings of the proceedings of 8th international conference on the use of computers in radiation therapy, Toronto, Canada.* Los Angeles, CA: IEEE Computer Society, 1984.

122. Weeks KJ, Dennett JC. Dose calculation and measurements for a CT-compatible version of the Fletcher applicator. *Int J Radiat Oncol Biol Phys* 1990;18:1191–1198.

123. Diffey BL, Levenhagen SC. An experimental and calculated dose distribution in water around CDC-K type cesium-137 sources. *Med Phys* 1975;20:446.

124. Klevenhagen SL. An experimental study of dose distribution in water around ^{137}Cs tubes used in brachytherapy. *Br J Radiol* 1973;46:1073.

125. Williamson JF. Monte Carlo and analytic calculation of absorbed dose near ^{137}Cs intracavitary sources. *Int J Radiat Oncol Biol Phys* 1988;15:227–237.

126. BIR/IPSM. *Recommendations for brachytherapy dosimetry: report of a joint BIR/IPSM working party.* London: British Institute of Radiology and Institute of Physical Sciences in Medicine, 1993.

127. Stovall M, Shalek RJ. The MD Anderson method for the computation of isodose curves around interstitial and intracavitary radiation sources. III. Roentgenograms for input data and the relation of isodose calculations to the Paterson-Parker system. *Am J Roentgenol Radium Ther Nucl Med* 1968;102:677–687.

128. Krishnaswamy V. Dose distribution around an I-125 seed source in tissue. *Radiology* 1978;126:489.

129. Loftus TP. Exposure standardization of Iodine-125 seeds used for brachytherapy. *J Res Natl Bureau Stand* 1984;89:295–303.

130. Nath R, Anderson LL, Luxton G, et al. Dosimetry of interstitial brachytherapy sources: recommendations of the AAPM Radiation Therapy Committee Task Group No. 43. *Med Phys* 1995;22(2):209–234.

131. Dempsey JF, Low DA, Mutic S, et al. Validation of a precision radiochromic film dosimetry system for quantitative two-dimensional imaging of acute exposure dose distributions. *Med Phys* 2000;27(10):2462–2475.

132. Chiu-Tsao S-T, Napoli JJ, Davis SD, et al. Dosimetry for ^{131}Cs and ^{125}I seeds in solid water phantom using radiochromic EBT film. *Appl Radiat Isot* 2014;92:102–114.

133. Sarfehnia A, Kawrakow I, Seuntjens J. Direct measurement of absorbed dose to water in HDR Ir-192 brachytherapy: Water calorimetry, ionization chamber, Gafchromic film, and TG-43. *Med Phys* 2010;37(4):1924–1932.

134. Lambert J, Nakano T, Law S, et al. In vivo dosimeters for HDR brachytherapy: a comparison of a diamond detector, MOSFET, TLD, and scintillation detector. *Med Phys* 2007;34(5):1759–1765.

135. Bambynek M, Fluhs D, Quast U. A high-precision, high-resolution and fast dosimetry system for beta sources applied in cardiovascular brachytherapy. *Med Phys* 2000;27(4):662–667.

136. Kirov AS, Shrinivas S, Hurlbut C, et al. New water equivalent liquid scintillation solutions for 3D dosimetry. *Med Phys* 2000;27(5):1156–1164.

137. Massillon-JL G, Minniti R, Mitch MG, et al. High-resolution 3D dose distribution measured for two low-energy x-ray brachytherapy seeds: ^{125}I and ^{103}Pd. *Radiat Meas* 2011;46(2):238–243.

138. De Deene Y, Reynaert N, De Wagter C. On the accuracy of monomer/polymer gel dosimetry in the proximity of a high-dose-rate ^{192}Ir source. *Phys Med Biol* 2001;46(11):2801–2825.

139. Chiu-Tsao S-T, Anderson LL, O'Brien K, et al. Dose rate determination for I-125 seeds. *Med Phys* 1990;17:815–825.

140. Li Z, Williamson JF, Perera H. Monte Carlo calculation of kerma to a point in the vicinity of media interfaces. *Phys Med Biol* 1993;38:1825–1840.

141. Williamson JF, Perera H, Li Z, et al. Comparison of calculated and measured heterogeneity correction factors for ^{125}I, ^{137}Cs and ^{192}Ir brachytherapy sources near localized heterogeneities. *Med Phys* 1993;20:209–222.

142. Anderson LL, Nath R, Weaver KA, et al. *Interstitial brachytherapy: physical, biological and clinical considerations.* New York: Raven, 1990.

143. Chiu-Tsao S-T. Thermoluminescent dosimetry for Pd-103 seeds (model 200) in solid water phantom. *Med Phys* 1991;18:449–452.

144. Nath R, Meigooni AS, Muench P, et al. Anistropy functions for ^{103}Pd, ^{125}I, and ^{193}Ir interstitial brachytherapy sources. *Med Phys* 1993;20:1465–1473.

145. Williamson JF. Comparison of measured and calculated dose rates in water near I-125 and Ir-192 seeds. *Med Phys* 1991;28:776–786.

146. Kirov AS, Williamson JF, Meigooni AS. Measurement and calculation of heterogeneity correction factors for an Ir-192 high dose-rate brachytherapy source behind tungsten alloy and steel shields. *Med Phys* 1996;23:911–916.

147. Meigooni AS, Bharucha Z, Yoe-Sein M, et al. Dosimetric characteristics of the bests double-wall ^{103}Pd brachytherapy source. *Med Phys* 2001;28(12):2568–2575.

148. Rodriguez M, Rogers DWO. Effect of improved TLD dosimetry on the determination of dose rate constants for I-125 and Pd-103 brachytherapy seeds. *Med Phys* 2014;41(11).

149. Taylor RE, Yegin G, Rogers DW. Benchmarking brachydose: voxel based EGSnrc Monte Carlo calculations of TG-43 dosimetry parameters. *Med Phys* 2007;34(2):445–457.

150. Carlsson AK, Ahnesjo A. The collapsed cone superposition algorithm applied to scatter dose calculations in brachytherapy. *Med Phys* 2000;27(10):2320–2332.

151. Candela-Juan C, Niatsetski Y, van der Laarse R. Design and characterization of a new high-dose-rate brachytherapy Valencia applicator for larger skin lesions. *Med Phys* 2016;43(4):1639–1648.

152. Williamson JF, Coursey BM, DeWerd LA, et al. Guidance to Users of Nycomed Amersham and North American Scientific, Inc. I-125 interstitial sources: dosimetry and calibration changes: recommendation of the American Association of Physicists in Medicine Radiation Therapy Committee Ad Hoc Subcommittee on Low-Energy Seed Dosimetry. *Med Phys* 1999;26:570–573.

153. Williamson JF, Coursey BM, DeWerd LA, et al. Recommendations of the American Association of Physicists in Medicine on ^{103}Pd interstitial source calibration and dosimetry: implications for dose specification and prescription. *Med Phys* 2000;27:634–642.

154. DeWerd LA, Huq MS, Das IJ, et al. Procedures for establishing and maintaining consistent air-kerma strength standards for low-energy, photon-emitting brachytherapy sources: recommendations of the Calibration Laboratory Accreditation Subcommittee of the American Association of Physicists in Medicine. *Med Phys* 2004;31(3):675–681.

155. Williamson JF, Butler W, Dewerd LA, et al. Recommendations of the American Association of Physicists in Medicine regarding the impact of implementing the 2004 task group 43 report on dose specification for ^{103}Pd and ^{125}I interstitial brachytherapy. *Med Phys* 2005;32(5):1424–1439.

156. Zourari K, Pantelis E, Moutsatsos A, et al. Dosimetric accuracy of a deterministic radiation transport based ^{192}Ir brachytherapy treatment planning system. Part I: single sources and bounded homogeneous geometries. *Med Phys* 2010;37(2):649–661.

157. Armpilia CI, Dale RG, Coles IP, et al. The determination of radiobiologically optimized half-lives for radionuclides used in permanent brachytherapy implants. *Int J Radiat Oncol Biol Phys* 2003;55(2):378–385.

158. Parker HM. A dosage system for interstitial radium therapy. II Physical aspects. *Br J Radiol* 1938;11:252–266.

159. Paterson R. *The treatment of malignant disease by radiotherapy.* 2nd ed. London: Edward Arnold, 1963.

160. Paterson R, Parker HM. A dosage system for g-ray therapy. *Br J Radiol* 1934;7:592.

161. Paterson R, Parker HM. A dosage system for interstitial radium therapy. *Br J Radiol* 1938;11:313–339.

162. Anderson LL, Presser JE. Classical systems I for temporary interstitial implants: Manchester and Quimby systems. In: Williamson JF, Thomadsen BR, Nath R, eds. *Brachytherapy physics.* Madison, WI: Medical Physics Publishing Company, 1995:301–323.

163. Laughlin JS, Siler WM, Holodny EI. A dose description system for interstitial radiation therapy: seed implants. *Am J Roentgenol Radiat Ther Nucl Med* 1963;89:470.

164. Shalek RJ, Stovall MA, Sampiere VA. The radiation distribution and dose specification in volume implants of radioactive seeds. *Am J Roentgenol Radium Ther Nucl Med* 1957;77:863–868.

165. Marinello G, Valero M, Levng S, et al. Comparative dosimetry between iridium wire and seed ribbons. *Int J Radiat Oncol Biol Phys* 1985;11:1733.

166. ICRU. *Dose and volume specification for reporting interstitial therapy.* Bethesda, MD: International Commission on Radiation Units and Measurements, 1997.

167. Quimby EH. Physical factors in interstitial radium therapy. *Am J Roentgenol Radium Ther Nucl Med* 1935;33:306–316.

168. Quimby EH. Dosage calculations in radium therapy. In: Glasser O, Quimby EH, Taylor LS, et al., eds. *Physical foundations of radiology.* New York: Paul B. Hoeker, 1952:339–372.

169. Quimby EH, Castro V. The calculation of dosage in interstitial radium therapy. *AJR Am J Roentgenol* 1953;70:739–749.

170. Dutriex A, Marinello G. The Paris system. In: Pierquin B, Wilson JF, Chassagne D, eds. *Modern brachytherapy.* New York: Masson, 1987:25–42.

171. Pierquin B, Wilson JF, Chassange D. *Modern brachytherapy.* New York: Masson, 1987.

172. Gillin MT, Mourtada F. Manchester planar and volume implants and the Paris system. In: Thomadsen BR, Rivard MJ, Butler WM, eds. *Brachytherapy physics.* 2nd ed. Madison, WI: Medical Physics Publishing, 2005:351–372.

173. Leung S. Perineal template techniques for interstitial implantation of gynecological cancers using the Paris system of dosimetry. *Int J Radiat Oncol Biol Phys* 1990;19:769–774.

174. Gillin MT, Albano KS, Erickson B. Classical systems II for planar and volume temporary interstitial implants: the Paris and other systems. In: Williamson JF, Thomadsen BR, Nath R, eds. *Brachytherapy physics.* Madison, WI: Medical Physics Publishing, 1995:232–343.

175. Anderson LL, Nath R, Olch AJ, et al. American Endocurietherapy Society recommendations for dose specification in brachytherapy. *Endocuriether Hypertherm Oncol* 1991;7:1–12.

176. Yu Y, Anderson LL, Li Z, et al. Prostate seed implant brachytherapy: report of the American Association of Physicists in Medicine Task Group No. 64. *Med Phys* 1999;26:2054–2076.

177. Merrick GS, Butler WM, Dorsey AT, et al. Potential role of various dosimetric quality indicators in prostate brachytherapy. *Int J Radiat Oncol Biol Phys* 1999;44(3):717–724.

178. Waterman FM, Dicker AP. Impact of postimplant edema on V-100 and D-90 in prostate brachytherapy: can implant quality be predicted on day 0?. *Int J Radiat Oncol Biol Phys* 2002;53(3):610–621.

179. Williamson J, Cormack R. Three-dimensional conformal brachytherapy: current trends and future promise. In: Timmerman R, Xing L, eds. *Image guided and adaptive radiation therapy.* Philadelphia: Wolters Kluwer-Lippincott Williams & Wilkins, 2010:99–188.

180. Anderson LL. A natural volume-dose histogram for brachytherapy. *Med Phys* 1986;13:898–903.

181. Anderson LL. Dose specification and quantification of implant quality. In: Williamson JF, Thomadsen BR, Nath R, eds. *Brachytherapy physics.* Madison, WI: Medical Physics Publishing Company, 1995:343–361.

182. Low DA, Williamson JF. Objective evaluation of optimized planar implants. *Med Phys* 1995;22:1477–1485.

183. Paul JM, Koch RF, Philips PC, et al. Uniformity of dose distribution in interstitial implants. *Endocuriether Hypertherm Oncol* 1986;2:107.

184. Saw CB, Suntharalingam N. Quantitative assessment of interstitial implants. *Int J Radiat Oncol Biol Phys* 1991;20:135–139.

185. Saw CB, Suntharalingam N. Reference dose rates for single and double plane ^{192}Ir implants. *Med Phys* 1988;15:391.

186. Nath R, Bice WS, Butler WM, et al. AAPM recommendations on dose prescription and reporting methods for permanent interstitial brachytherapy for prostate cancer: report of Task Group 137. *Med Phys* 2009;36(11):5310–5322.

187. Davis BJ, Horwitz EM, Lee WR, et al. American Brachytherapy Society consensus guidelines for transrectal ultrasound-guided permanent prostate brachytherapy. *Brachytherapy* 2012;11(1):6–19.

188. Yu Y, Waterman FM, Suntharalingham N, et al. Limitations of the minimum peripheral dose as a parameter for dose specification in permanent ^{125}I prostate implants. *Int J Radiat Oncol Biol Phys* 1996;34:717–725.

189. Anderson LL, Moni JV, Harrison LB. A nomograph for permanent implants of palladium-103 seeds. *Int J Radiat Oncol Biol Phys* 1993;27:129–135.

190. Anderson LL. Spacing nomograph for interstitial implants of I-125 seeds. *Med Phys* 1976;3:48.

191. Roy JN, Wallner KE, Harrington PJ, et al. A CT-based evaluation method for permanent implants: application to prostate. *Int J Radiat Oncol Biol Phys* 1993;26:163–169.

192. Hofbauer J, Kirisits C, Resch A, et al. Impact of heterogeneity-corrected dose calculation using a grid-based Boltzmann solver on breast and cervix cancer brachytherapy. *J Contemp Brachytherapy* 2016;8(2):143–149.

193. Mikell JK, Klopp AH, Price M, et al. Commissioning of a grid-based Boltzmann solver for cervical cancer brachytherapy treatment planning with shielded colpostats. *Brachytherapy* 2013;12(6):645–653.

194. Markman J, Williamson JF, Dempsey JF, et al. On the validity of the superposition principle in dose calculations for intracavitary implants with shielded vaginal colpostats. *Med Phys* 2001;28(2):147–155.

195. ICRP. *ICRP Publication 89: basic anatomical and physiological data for use in radiological protection: reference values. Report No., International Commission on Radiological Protection.* Oxford, UK: Pergamon Press, 2003.

196. Carrier JF, D'Amours M, Verhaegen F, et al. Postimplant dosimetry using a Monte Carlo dose calculation engine: a new clinical standard. *Int J Radiat Oncol Biol Phys* 2007;68(4):1190–1198.

197. Chibani O, Williamson JF. MCPI: a sub-minute Monte Carlo dose calculation engine for prostate implants. *Med Phys* 2005;32(12):3688–3698.

198. Afsharpour H, Pignol JP, Keller B, et al. Influence of breast composition and interseed attenuation in dose calculations for post-implant assessment of permanent breast Pd-103 seed implant. *Phys Med Biol* 2010;55(16):4547–4561.

199. Sampson A, Le Y, Williamson JF. Fast patient-specific Monte Carlo brachytherapy dose calculations via the correlated sampling variance reduction technique. *Med Phys* 2012;39(2):1058–1068.

200. DeMarco JJ, Smathers JB, Burnison CM, et al. CT-based dosimetry calculations for ^{125}I prostate implants. *Int J Radiat Oncol Biol Phys* 1999;45(5):1347–1353.

201. Hedtjärn H, Alm Carlsson G, Williamson JF. Accelerated Monte Carlo-based dose calculations for brachytherapy planning using correlated sampling. *Phys Med Biol* 2002;47:351–376.

202. Chamberland MJP, Taylor REP, Rogers DWO, et al. egs_brachy: a versatile and fast Monte Carlo code for brachytherapy. *Phys Med Biol* 2016;61(23):8214–8231.

203. Daskalov GM, Baker RS, Rogers DW, et al. Multigroup discrete ordinates modeling of ^{125}I 6702 seed dose distributions using a broad energy-group cross section representation. *Med Phys* 2002;29:113–124.

204. Williamson JF, Baker R, Li Z. A convolution algorithm for brachytherapy dose computations in heterogeneous geometries. *Med Phys* 1991;18:1256–1265.

205. Gifford KA, Price MJ, Horton JL, et al. Optimization of deterministic transport parameters for the calculation of the dose distribution around a high dose-rate (192)Ir brachytherapy source. *Med Phys* 2008;35(6):2279–2285.

206. Ahnesjo A, van Veelen B, Tedgren AC. Collapsed cone dose calculations for heterogeneous tissues in brachytherapy using primary and scatter separation source data. *Comput Methods Programs Biomed* 2017;139:17–29.

207. Ahnesjo A. Collapsed cone convolution of radiant energy for photon dose calculation in heterogeneous media. *Med Phys* 1989;16(4):577–592.

208. Edmundson GK. Geometry-based optimization for stepping source implants. In: Martinez AA, Orton CG, Mould RF, eds. *Brachytherapy: HDR and LDR.* Columbia, MD: Nucletron Corporation, 1992.

209. Anacak Y, Esassolak M, Aydin A, et al. Effect of geometrical optimization on the treatment volumes and the dose homogeneity of biplane interstitial brachytherapy implants. *Radiother Oncol* 1997;45:71–76.

210. Kolkman-Deurloo IKK, Visser AG, Niel CGJH, et al. Optimization of interstitial volume implants. *Radiother Oncol* 1994;31:229–239.

211. Pieters BR, Saarnak AE, Steggerda MJ, et al. A method to improve the dose distribution of interstitial breast implants using geometrically optimized stepping source techniques and dose normalization. *Radiother Oncol* 2001;58:63–70.

212. Ezzell GA. Clinical implementation of dwell-time optimization techniques. In: Williamson JF, Thomadsen BR, Nath R, eds. *Brachytherapy physics: American Association of Physicists in Medicine, 1994 summer school.* Madison, WI: Medical Physics Publishing Corporation, 1995:617–639.

213. Das RK, Patel R, Shah H, et al. 3D CT-based high-dose-rate breast brachytherapy implants: treatment planning and quality assurance. *Int J Radiat Oncol Biol Phys* 2004;59(4):1224–1228.

214. Keisch M, Vicini F, Kuske RR, et al. Initial clinical experience with the MammoSite breast brachytherapy applicator in women with early-stage breast cancer treated with breast-conserving therapy. *Int J Radiat Oncol Biol Phys* 2003;55(2):289–293.

215. Galalae RM, Martinez A, Mate T, et al. Long-term outcome by risk factors using conformal high-dose-rate brachytherapy (HDR-BT) boost with or without neoadjuvant androgen suppression for localized prostate cancer. *Int J Radiat Oncol Biol Phys* 2004;58(4):1048–1055.

216. Butler WM, Merrick GS, Lief JH. Comparison of seed loading approaches in prostate brachytherapy. *Med Phys* 2000;27:381–392.

217. Edmundson GK, Yan D, Martinez A. Intraoperative optimization of needle placement and dwell times for conformal prostate brachytherapy. *Int J Radiat Oncol Biol Phys* 1995;33:1257–1263.

218. Lessard E, Pouliot J. Inverse planning anatomy-based dose optimization for HDR-brachytherapy of the prostate using fast simulated annealing algorithm and dedicated objective function. *Med Phys* 2001;28:773–779.

219. Lahanas M, Baltas D, Giannouli S. Global convergence analysis of fast multiobjective gradient-based dose optimization algorithms for high-dose-rate brachytherapy. *Phys Med Biol* 2003;48(5):599–617.

220. Milickovic N, Lahanas M, Papagiannopoulo M, et al. Multiobjective anatomy-based dose optimization for HDR-brachytherapy with constraint free deterministic algorithms. *Phys Med Biol* 2002;47(13):2263–2280.

221. Yu Y, Zhang JBY, Brasacchio RA. Automated treatment planning engine for prostate seed implant brachytherapy. *Int J Radiat Oncol Biol Phys* 1999;43:647–652.

222. Lee EK, Gallagher RJ, Silvern D, et al. Treatment planning for brachytherapy: an integer programming model, two computational approaches and experiments with permanent prostate implant planning. *Phys Med Biol* 1999;44(1):145–165.

223. Ezzell GA. Optimization in Brachytherapy. In: Thomadsen BR, Rivard MJ, Butler WM, eds. *Brachytherapy physics.* 2nd ed. Madison, WI: Medical Physics Publishing, 2005:415–434.

224. Lachance B, Beliveau-Nadeau D, Lessard E, et al. Early clinical experience with anatomy-based inverse planning dose optimization for high-dose-rate boost of the prostate. *Int J Radiat Oncol Biol Phys* 2002;54(1):86–100.

225. Pouliot J, Lessard E, Hsu IC. Advanced 3D planning. In: Thomadsen BR, Rivard MJ, Butler WM, eds. *Brachytherapy physics.* 2nd ed. Madison, WI: Medical Physics Publishing, 2005:233–294.

226. Blasko JC, Mate T, Sylvester JE, et al. Brachytherapy for carcinoma of the prostate: techniques, patient selection, and clinical outcomes. *Semin Radiat Oncol* 2002;12(1):81–94.

227. Rivard MJ, Butler WM, Devlin PM, et al. American Brachytherapy Society recommends no change for prostate permanent implant dose prescriptions using iodine-125 or palladium-103. *Brachytherapy* 2007;6(1):34–37.

228. Potters L, Cao Y, Calugaru E, et al. A comprehensive review of CT-based dosimetry parameters and biochemical control in patients treated with permanent prostate brachytherapy. *Int J Radiat Oncol Biol Phys* 2001;50:605–614.

229. Stock RG, Stone NN, Tabert A, et al. A dose-response study for I-125 prostate implants. *Int J Radiat Oncol Biol Phys* 1998;41:101–108.

230. Zelefsky MJ, Yamada Y, Cohen GN, et al. Intraoperative real-time planned conformal prostate brachytherapy: post-implantation dosimetric outcome and clinical implications. *Radiother Oncol* 2007;84(2):185–189.

231. Cormack RA, Tempany CM, D'Amico AV. Optimizing target coverage by dosimetric feedback during prostate brachytherapy. *Int J Radiat Oncol Biol Phys* 2000;48(4):1245–1249.

232. Nag S, Ciezki JP, Cormack R, et al. Intraoperative planning and evaluation of permanent prostate brachytherapy: report of the American Brachytherapy Society. *Int J Radiat Oncol Biol Phys* 2001;51(5):1422–1430.

233. Tod M, Meredith WJ. Treatment of cancer of the cervix uteri: a revised Manchester method. *Br J Radiol* 1953;26:252–257.

234. Fletcher GH. Cervical radium applicators with screening in the direction of bladder and rectum. *Radiology* 1953;60:77.

235. Meredith WJ. Dosage for cancer of cervix uteri. In: Meredith WJ, ed. *Radium dosage: the Manchester system.* 2nd ed. Edinburgh, Scotland: E & S, Livingston, Ltd, 1967:42–50.

236. Delclos L, Fletcher GH, Sampiere V. Can the Fletcher gamma ray colpostat system be extrapolated to other systems. *Cancer* 1978;41:970.

237. Haas JS, Dean RD, Mansfield CM. Dosimetry comparison of the Fletcher family of gynecologic colpostats 1950-1980. *Int J Radiat Oncol Biol Phys* 1985;11:1317–1321.

238. Steggerda MJ, Moonen LM, Damen EM, et al. An analysis of the effect of ovoid shields in a selectron-LDR cervical applicator on dose distributions in rectum and bladder. *Int J Radiat Oncol Biol Phys* 1997;39(1):237–245.

239. Gifford KA, Horton JL Jr, Pelloski CE, et al. A three-dimensional computed tomography-assisted Monte Carlo evaluation of ovoid shielding on the dose to the bladder and rectum in intracavitary radiotherapy for cervical cancer. *Int J Radiat Oncol Biol Phys* 2005;63(2):615–621.

240. Price MJ, Horton JL, Gifford KA, et al. Dosimetric evaluation of the Fletcher-Williamson ovoid for pulsed-dose-rate brachytherapy: a Monte Carlo study. *Phys Med Biol* 2005;50(21):5075–5087.

241. Weeks KJ, Montana GS. Three-dimensional applicator system for carcinoma of the uterine cervix. *Int J Radiat Oncol Biol Phys* 1997;37(2):455–463.

242. Horiot JC, Pigneux J, Pourquier H, et al. Radiotherapy alone in carcinoma of the intact uterine cervix according to G. H. Fletcher guidelines: a French cooperative study of 1383 cases. *Int J Radiat Oncol Biol Phys* 1988;14(4):605–611.

243. Perez CA, Camel HM, Kuske RR, et al. Radiation therapy alone in treatment of the uterine cervix: a 20 year experience. *Gynecol Oncol* 1986;23:127.

244. Potish RA, Gerbi BJ. Role of point A in the era of computerized dosimetry. *Radiology* 1986;158:827–831.

245. Cetingoz R, Ataman OU, Tuncel N, et al. Optimization in high dose rate brachytherapy for utero-vaginal applications. *Radiother Oncol* 2001;58(1):31–36.

246. Mai J, Erickson B, Rownd J, et al. Comparison of four different dose specification methods for high-dose- rate intracavitary radiation for treatment of cervical cancer. *Int J Radiat Oncol Biol Phys* 2001;51(4):1131–1141.

247. Houdek PV, Schwade JG, Abitbol AA, et al. Optimization of high dose-rate cervix brachytherapy; part I: dose distribution. *Int J Radiat Oncol Biol Phys* 1991;21(6):1621–1625.

248. Mohan R, Ding IY, Martel MK. Measurement of radiation dose distribution of shielded cervical applicators. *Int J Radiat Oncol Biol Phys* 1985;11:861.

249. Noyes WR, Peters NE, Thomadsen BR, et al. Impact of optimized treatment planning for tandem and ring, and tandem and ovoids, using high dose rate brachytherapy for cervical cancer. *Int J Radiat Oncol Biol Phys* 1995;31(1):79–86.

250. Pierquin B. Cervix. In: Pierquin B, Marinello G, eds. *A practical manual of brachytherapy.* Madison, WI: Medical Physics Publishing, 1997:165–196.

251. Potish RA. The effect of applicator geometry on dose specification in cervical cancer. *Int J Radiat Oncol Biol Phys* 1990;18:1513–1520.

252. Potish RA, Gerbi BJ. Cervical cancer intracavitary dose specification and prescription. *Radiology* 1987;165:555–560.

253. Eisbruch A, Williamson JF, Dickson R, et al. Estimation of tissue volume irradiated by intracavitary implants. *Int J Radiat Oncol Biol Phys* 1993;25:733–744.

254. Crook JM, Esche BA, Chaplain G, et al. Dose-volume analysis and the prevention of radiation sequelae in cervical cancer. *Radiother Oncol* 1987;8:321–332.

255. Esche BA, Crook JM, Isturiz J, et al. Reference volume, milligram-hours and external irradiation for the Fletcher applicator. *Radiother Oncol* 1987;9:255–261.

256. Nath R, Urdaneta N, Bolanis N, et al. A dosimetric analysis of Morris, Fletcher and Henschke systems for treatment of uterine cervix carcinoma. *Int J Radiat Oncol Biol Phys* 1991;21:995–1003.

257. Letschet JGJ, Lebesque JV, de Boer RW, et al. Dose-volume correlation in radiation-related late small-bowel complications: a clinical study. *Radiother Oncol* 1990;18:307–320.

258. Wilkinson JM, Ramachandran TP. The ICRU recommendations for reporting intracavitary therapy in gynaecology and the Manchester method of treating cancer of the cervix uteri. *Br J Radiol* 1989;62:362–365.

259. Fellner C, Potter R, Knocke TH, et al. Comparison of radiography- and computed tomography-based treatment planning in cervix cancer in brachytherapy with specific attention to some quality assurance aspects. *Radiother Oncol* 2001;58(1):53–62.

260. Gebara WJ, Weeks KJ, Hahn CA, et al. Computed axial tomography tandem and ovoids (CATTO) dosimetry: three-dimensional assessment of bladder and rectal doses. *Radiat Oncol Investig* 1998;6(6):268–275.

261. Schoeppel SL, La Vigne ML, Martel MK, et al. 3-D treatment planning of intracavitary gynecologic implants: analysis of ten cases and implications for dose specification. *Int J Radiat Oncol Biol Phys* 1993;28:277–283.

262. Greco A, Mason P, Leung AWL, et al. Staging of carcinoma of the uterine cervix: MRI-surgical correlation. *Clin Radiol* 1989;40:401–405.

263. Haie-Meder C, Potter R, Van Limbergen E, et al. Recommendations from Gynaecological (GYN) GEC-ESTRO Working Group (I): concepts and terms in 3D image based 3D treatment planning in cervix cancer brachytherapy with emphasis on MRI assessment of GTV and CTV. *Radiother Oncol* 2005;74(3):235–245.

264. Nag S, Cardenes H, Chang S, et al. Proposed guidelines for image-based intracavitary brachytherapy for cervical carcinoma: report from Image-Guided Brachytherapy Working Group. *Int J Radiat Oncol Biol Phys* 2004;60(4):1160–1172.

265. Potter R, Haie-Meder C, Van Limbergen E, et al. Recommendations from gynaecological (GYN) GEC ESTRO working group (II): concepts and terms in 3D image-based treatment planning in cervix cancer brachytherapy-3D dose volume parameters and aspects of 3D image-based anatomy, radiation physics, radiobiology. *Radiother Oncol* 2006;78(1):67–77.

266. Kidd EA, Siegel BA, Dehdashti F, et al. Clinical outcomes of definitive intensity-modulated radiation therapy with fluorodeoxyglucose-positron emission tomography simulation in patients with locally advanced cervical cancer. *Int J Radiat Oncol Biol Phys* 2010;77(4):1085–1091.

267. Hasselle MD, Rose BS, Kochanski JD, et al. Clinical outcomes of intensity-modulated pelvic radiation therapy for carcinoma of the cervix. *Int J Radiat Oncol Biol Phys* 2011;80(5):1436–1445.

268. Potter R, Georg P, Dimopoulos JCA, et al. Clinical outcome of protocol based image (MRI) guided adaptive brachytherapy combined with 3D conformal radiotherapy with or without chemotherapy in patients with locally advanced cervical cancer. *Radiother Oncol* 2011;100(1):116–123.

269. Dimopoulos JCA, Potter R, Lang S, et al. Dose-effect relationship for local control of cervical cancer by magnetic resonance image-guided brachytherapy. *Radiother Oncol* 2009;93(2):311–315.

270. Georg P, Lang SF, Dimopoulos JCA, et al. Dose-volume histogram parameters and late side effects in magnetic resonance image-guided adaptive cervical cancer brachytherapy. *Int J Radiat Oncol Biol Phys* 2011;79(2):356–362.

271. Christensen GE, Carlson B, Chao KS, et al. Image-based dose planning of intracavitary brachytherapy: registration of serial-imaging studies using deformable anatomic templates. *Int J Radiat Oncol Biol Phys* 2001;51(1):227–243.

272. Lim K, Kelly V, Stewart J, et al. Pelvic radiotherapy for cancer of the cervix: is what you plan actually what you deliver?. *Int J Radiat Oncol Biol Phys* 2009;74(1):304–312.

273. Williamson JF. Integration of IMRT and brachytherapy. In: Bortfeld T, Schmidt-Ullrich R, DeNeve W, et al., eds. *Image-Guided IMRT*. Heidelberg, Germany: Springer-Verlag, 2006:423–438.

274. Fatyga M, Williamson JF, Dogan N, et al. A comparison of HDR brachytherapy and IMRT techniques for dose escalation in prostate cancer: a radiobiological modeling study. *Med Phys* 2009;36(9):3995–4006.

275. Ellis F. Dose, time and fractionation in radiotherapy. In: Ebert M, Howard A, eds. *Current topics in radiation research*. Amsterdam, The Netherlands: North Holland Publishing Company, 1968:359–397.

276. Lea DE. *Actions of radiations on living cells*. London: Cambridge University Press, 1946.

277. Lea DE, Catcheside DG. The mechanism of the induction by radiation of chromosome aberrations in Tradescantia. *J Genet* 1942;44:216–245.

278. Thames HD, Hendry JH. *Fractionation in radiotherapy*. London: Taylor and Francis, 1987.

279. Dale RG. The use of small fraction numbers in high dose-rate gynecological afterloading: some radiobiological considerations. *Br J Radiol* 1990;63:290.

280. Fowler JF. The linear-quadratic formula and progress in fractionated radiotherapy. *Br J Radiol* 1989;62:679–694.

281. Dale RG. The application of the linear-quadratic dose-effect equation to fractionated and protracted radiotherapy. *Br J Radiol* 1985;58:515–528.

282. Brenner DJ, Hall EJ. Fractionated high dose-rate versus low dose-rate brachytherapy of the cervix. I General considerations based on radiobiology. *Br J Radiol* 1991;64:133.

283. Brenner DJ, Hlatky LR, Hahnfeldt PJ, et al. The linear-quadratic and most other common radiobiological models predict similar time-dose relationships. *Radiat Res* 1998;150:83–88.

284. Kellerer AM, Rossi HH. The theory of dual radiation action. *Curr Top Radiat Res Q* 1972;8:85–158.

285. Fertil B, Reydellet I, Deschavanne PJ. A benchmark of cell survival models using survival curves for human cells after completion of repair of potentially lethal damage. *Radiat Res* 1994;138:61–69.

286. Sachs RK, Hahnfeldt PJ, Brenner DJ. Review: the link between low-LET dose-response relations and the underlying kinetics of damage production/repair/misrepair. *Int J Radiat Oncol Biol Phys* 1997;72:351–374.

287. Tobias CA. The repair-misrepair model in radiobiology: comparison to other models. *Radiat Res* 1985;8:S77–S95.

288. Munro TR, Gilbert CW. The relation between tumour lethal doses and the radiosensitivity of tumour cells. *Br J Radiol* 1961;34:246–251.

289. Hendry JH, Thames HD. The tissue rescuing unit. *Br J Radiol* 1986;59:628–630.

290. Dubray BM, Thames HD. The clinical significance of ratios of radiobiological parameters. *Int J Radiat Oncol Biol Phys* 1996;35(5):1099–1111.

291. Roberts SA, Hendry JH. The delay before onset of accelerated tumor-cell repopulation during radiotherapy—a direct maximum-likelihood analysis of a collection of worldwide tumor-control data. *Radiother Oncol* 1993;29(1):69–74.

292. Wu PM, Chua DTT, Sham JST, et al. Tumor control probability of nasopharyngeal carcinoma: a comparison of different mathematical models. *Int J Radiat Oncol Biol Phys* 1997;37(4):913–920.

293. Brenner DJ. Dose, volume, and tumor-control predictions in radiotherapy. *Int J Radiat Oncol Biol Phys* 1993;26(1):171–179.

294. Guerrero M, Li XA. Analysis of a large number of clinical studies for breast cancer radiotherapy: estimation of radiobiological parameters for treatment planning. *Phys Med Biol* 2003;48(20):3307–3326.

295. Brenner DJ, Hall EJ. Conditions for the equivalence of continuous to pulsed low-dose rate brachytherapy. *Int J Radiat Oncol Biol Phys* 1991;20(1):181–190.

296. Wang JZ, Guerrero M, Li XA. How low is the alpha/beta ratio for prostate cancer? *Int J Radiat Oncol Biol Phys* 2003;55(1):194–203.

297. Qi XS, Schultz CJ, Li XA. An estimation of radiobiologic parameters from clinical outcomes for radiation treatment planning of brain tumor. *Int J Radiat Oncol Biol Phys* 2006;64(5):1570–1580.

298. Suwinski R, Wzietek I, Tarnawski R, et al. Moderately low alpha/beta ratio for rectal cancer may best explain the outcome of three fractionation schedules of preoperative radiotherapy. *Int J Radiat Oncol Biol Phys* 2007;69(3):793–799.

299. Tai A, Erickson B, Khater KA, et al. Estimate of radiobiologic parameters from clinical data for biologically based treatment planning for liver irradiation. *Int J Radiat Oncol Biol Phys* 2008;70(3):900–907.

300. Hall EJ, Bedford JS. Dose-rate: its effect on the survival of HeLa cells irradiated with gamma-rays. *Radiat Res* 1964;22:305–315.

301. Coutard H. Roentgentherapy of epitheliomas of the tonsillar region, hypopharynx and larynx, from 1920-1926. *AJR Am J Roentgenol* 1932;28:313–331, 343–348.

302. Thames HD, Withers HR, Peters LJ, et al. Changes in early and late radiation responses with altered dose fractionation: implications for dose-survival relationships. *Int J Radiat Oncol Biol Phys* 1982;8(2):219–226.

303. Withers HR. Biologic basis for altered fractionation schemes. *Cancer* 1985;55:2086–2095.

304. Withers HR, Taylor JMG, Maciejewski B. The hazard of accelerated tumor clonogen repopulation during radiotherapy. *Acta Radiol* 1988;27:131–146.

305. Travis EL, Tucker SL. Isoeffect models and fractionated radiation therapy. *Int J Radiat Oncol Biol Phys* 1987;13(2):283–287.

306. Haustermans KM, Hofland I, Van Poppel H, et al. Cell kinetic measurements in prostate cancer. *Int J Radiat Oncol Biol Phys* 1997;37(5):1067–1070.

307. Withers HR. Biological basis of radiation therapy for cancer. *Lancet* 1992;339:156–159.

308. Brenner DJ, Hlatky LR, Hahnfeldt PJ, et al. A convenient extension of the linear-quadratic model to include redistribution and reoxygenation. *Int J Radiat Oncol Biol Phys* 1995;32:379–390.

309. Dale RG, Jones B. The effect of tumour shrinkage on biologically effective dose, and possible implications for fractionated high dose rate brachytherapy. *Radiother Oncol* 1994;33:125–132.

310. Dale RG, Jones B, Coles IP. The effect of tumour shrinkage on biologically effectiveness of permanent brachytherapy implants. *Br J Radiol* 1994;67:639–647.

311. Niemierko A. Reporting and analyzing dose distributions: a concept of equivalent uniform dose. *Med Phys* 1997;24(1):103–110.

312. Jones LC, Hoban PW. Treatment plan comparison using equivalent uniform biologically effective dose (EUBED). *Phys Med Biol* 2000;45(1):159–170.

313. Afsharpour H, Reniers B, Landry G, et al. Consequences of dose heterogeneity on the biological efficiency of (1)(0)(3)Pd permanent breast seed implants. *Phys Med Biol* 2012;57(3):809–823.

314. Ling CC, Roy J, Sahoo N, et al. Quantifying the effect of dose inhomogeneity in brachytherapy: application to permanent prostatic implant with ^{125}I seeds. *Int J Radiat Oncol Biol Phys* 1994;28(4):971–978.

315. Brahme A. Dosimetric precision requirements in radiation therapy. *Acta Radiol Oncol* 1984;23(5):379–391.

316. Niemierko A, Goitein M. Implementation of a model for estimating tumor control probability for an inhomogeneously irradiated tumor. *Radiother Oncol* 1993;29(2):140–147.

317. Webb S, Nahum AE. A model for calculating tumour control probability in radiotherapy including the effects of inhomogeneous distributions of dose and clonogenic cell density. *Phys Med Biol* 1993;38(6):653–666.

318. Yorke ED. Modeling the effects of inhomogeneous dose distributions in normal tissues. *Semin Radiat Oncol* 2001;11(3):197–209.

319. Jackson A, Kutcher GJ, Yorke ED. Probability of radiation-induced complications for normal tissues with parallel architecture subject to non-uniform irradiation. *Med Phys* 1993;20(3):613–625.
320. Haworth A, Williams S, Reynolds H, et al. Validation of a radiobiological model for low-dose-rate prostate boost focal therapy treatment planning. *Brachytherapy* 2013;12(6):628–636.
321. Lindsay PE, Moiseenko VV, Van Dyk J, et al. The influence of brachytherapy dose heterogeneity on estimates of alpha/beta for prostate cancer. *Phys Med Biol* 2003;48(4):507–522.
322. King CR, DiPetrillo TA, Wazer DE. Optimal radiotherapy for prostate cancer: predictions for conventional external beam, IMRT, and brachytherapy from radiobiologic models. *Int J Radiat Oncol Biol Phys* 2000;46(1):165–172.
323. Miksys N, Haidari M, Vigneault E, et al. Coupling I-125 permanent implant prostate brachytherapy Monte Carlo dose calculations with radiobiological models. *Med Phys* 2017;44(8):4329–4340.
324. Kutcher GJ, Burman C. Calculation of complication probability factors for non-uniform normal tissue irradiation: the effective volume method. *Int J Radiat Oncol Biol Phys* 1989;16(6):1623–1630.
325. Burman C, Kutcher GJ, Emami B, et al. Fitting of normal tissue tolerance data to an analytic function. *Int J Radiat Oncol Biol Phys* 1991;21(1):123–135.
326. Brenner DJ, Leu CS, Beatty JF, et al. Clinical relative biological effectiveness of low-energy x-rays emitted by miniature x-ray devices. *Phys Med Biol* 1999;44(2):323–333.
327. Rossi HH, Zaider M. *Microdosimetry and its applications*. Berlin, Germany: Springer-Verlag, 1996.
328. Brenner DJ, Zaider M. Estimating RBEs at clinical doses from microdosimetric spectra. *Med Phys* 1998;25(6):1055–1057.
329. Zellmer DO, Gillin MT, Wilson JF. Microdosimetric single event spectra of Ytterbium-169 compared with commonly used brachytherapy sources and teletherapy beams. *Int J Radiat Oncol Biol Phys* 1992;23(3):627–632.
330. Dale RG. Radiobiological assessment of permanent implants using tumour repopulation factors in the linear-quadratic model. *Br J Radiol* 1989;62(735):241–244.
331. Dicker AP, Lin CC, Leeper DB, et al. Isotope selection for permanent prostate implants? An evaluation of ^{103}Pd versus ^{125}I based on radiobiological effectiveness and dosimetry. *Semin Urol Oncol* 2000;18(2):152–159.
332. Yaes RJ. Late normal tissue injury from permanent interstitial implants. *Int J Radiat Oncol Biol Phys* 2001;49(4):1163–1169.
333. Bice WS, Prestidge BR, Kurtzman SM, et al. Recommendations for permanent prostate brachytherapy with ^{131}Cs: a consensus report from the Cesium Advisory Group. *Brachytherapy* 2008;7(4):290–296.
334. Brenner DJ, Huang Y-P, Hall EJ. Fractionated high dose-rate versus low dose-rate regimens for intracavitary brachytherapy of the cervix: equivalent regimens for combined brachytherapy and external irradiation. *Int J Radiat Oncol Biol Phys* 1991;21:1415–1423.
335. Orton C. High and low dose-rate brachytherapy for cervical carcinoma. *Acta Radiol* 1998;37(2):117–125.
336. Demanes DJ, Rodriguez RR, Bendre DD, et al. High dose rate transperineal interstitial brachytherapy for cervical cancer: high pelvic control and low complication rates. *Int J Radiat Oncol Biol Phys* 1999;45(1):105–112.
337. Hareyama M, Sakata K, Oouchi A, et al. High-dose rate versus low-dose-rate intracavitary therapy for carcinoma of the uterine cervix: randomized trial. *Cancer* 2002;94(1):117–124.
338. Kucera H, Potter R, Knocke TH, et al. High-dose versus low-dose rate brachytherapy in definitive radiotherapy of cervical cancer. *Wien Klin Wochenschr* 2001;113(1-2):58–62.
339. Potter R, Knocke TH, Fellner C, et al. Definitive radiotherapy based on HDR brachytherapy with iridium 192 in uterine cervix carcinoma: report on the Vienna University Hospital findings (1993-1997) compared to the preceding period in the context of ICRU 38 recommendations. *Cancer Radiother* 2000;4(2):159–172.
340. Leborgne F, Leborgne JH, Zubizarreta E, et al. High-dose-rate brachytherapy at 14 Gy per hour to point A: preliminary results of a prospectively designed schedule for cancer of the cervix based on the linear-quadratic model. *Int J Gynecol Cancer* 2001;11(6):445–453.
341. Falkenberg E, Kim RY, Meleth S, et al. Low-dose-rate vs. high-dose-rate intracavitary brachytherapy for carcinoma of the cervix: the University of Alabama at Birmingham (UAB) experience. *Brachytherapy* 2006;5(1):49–55.
342. Ferrigno R, Nishimoto IN, Novaes PE, et al. Comparison of low and high dose rate brachytherapy in the treatment of uterine cervix cancer. Retrospective analysis of two sequential series. *Int J Radiat Oncol Biol Phys* 2005;62(4):1108–1116.
343. Brenner DJ, Hall EJ. Fractionation and protraction for radiotherapy of prostate carcinoma. *Int J Radiat Oncol Biol Phys* 1999;43(5):1095–1101.
344. Duchesne GM, Peters LJ. What is the alpha/beta ratio for prostate cancer? Rationale for hypofractionated high-dose-rate brachytherapy. *Int J Radiat Oncol Biol Phys* 1999;44(4):747–748.
345. Fowler J, Chappell R, Ritter M. Is alpha/beta for prostate tumors really low?. *Int J Radiat Oncol Biol Phys* 2001;50(4):1021–1031.
346. Logue JP, Cowan RA, Hendry JH. Hypofractionation for prostate cancer. *Int J Radiat Oncol Biol Phys* 2001;49(5):1522–1523.
347. King CR, Fowler JF. A simple analytic derivation suggests that prostate cancer alpha/beta ratio is low. *Int J Radiat Oncol Biol Phys* 2001;51(1):213–214.
348. Lee WR. In regard to Brenner et al. Direct evidence that prostate tumors show high sensitivity to fractionation (low alpha/beta ratio) similar to late-responding normal tissue. *Int J Radiat Oncol Biol Phys* 2002;53(5):1392; author reply 1393.
349. Kal HB, Van Gellekom MP. How low is the alpha/beta ratio for prostate cancer?. *Int J Radiat Oncol Biol Phys* 2003;57(4):1116–1121.
350. Wang JZ, Li XA, Yu CX, et al. The low alpha/beta ratio for prostate cancer: what does the clinical outcome of HDR brachytherapy tell us? *Int J Radiat Oncol Biol Phys* 2003;57(4):1101–1108.
351. Nahum AE, Movsas B, Horwitz EM, et al. Incorporating clinical measurements of hypoxia into tumor local control modeling of prostate cancer: implications for the alpha/beta ratio. *Int J Radiat Oncol Biol Phys* 2003;57(2):391–401.
352. Brenner DJ, Martinez AA, Edmundson GK, et al. Direct evidence that prostate tumors show high sensitivity to fractionation (low alpha/beta ratio), similar to late-responding normal tissue. *Int J Radiat Oncol Biol Phys* 2002;52(1):6–13.
353. Loblaw DA, Cheung P. External beam irradiation for localized prostate cancer—the promise of hypofractionation. *Can J Urol* 2006;13(Suppl 1):62–66.
354. Miralbell R, Roberts SA, Zubizarreta E, et al. Dose-fractionation sensitivity of prostate cancer deduced from radiotherapy outcomes of 5,969 patients in seven international institutional datasets: α/β = 1.4 (0.9-2.2) Gy. *Int J Radiat Oncol Biol Phys* 2012;82(1):e17–e24.
355. Oliveira SM, Teixeira NJ, Fernandes L. What do we know about the alpha/beta for prostate cancer?. *Med Phys* 2012;39(6):3189–3201.
356. Brenner DJ. Toward optimal external-beam fractionation for prostate cancer. *Int J Radiat Oncol Biol Phys* 2000;48(2):315–316.
357. Brenner DJ. Fractionation and late rectal toxicity. *Int J Radiat Oncol Biol Phys* 2004;60(4):1013–1015.
358. Tucker SL, Thames HD, Michalski JM, et al. Estimation of α/β for late rectal toxicity based on RTOG 94-06. *Int J Radiat Oncol Biol Phys* 2011;81(2):600–605.
359. Kupelian PA, Reddy CA, Carlson TP, et al. Preliminary observations on biochemical relapse-free survival rates after short-course intensity-modulated radiotherapy (70 Gy at 2.5 Gy/fraction) for localized prostate cancer. *Int J Radiat Oncol Biol Phys* 2002;53(4):904–912.
360. Akimoto T, Muramatsu H, Takahashi M, et al. Rectal bleeding after hypofractionated radiotherapy for prostate cancer: correlation between clinical and dosimetric parameters and the incidence of grade 2 or worse rectal bleeding. *Int J Radiat Oncol Biol Phys* 2004;60(4):1033–1039.
361. Livsey JE, Cowan RA, Wylie JP, et al. Hypofractionated conformal radiotherapy in carcinoma of the prostate: five-year outcome analysis. *Int J Radiat Oncol Biol Phys* 2003;57(5):1254–1259.
362. Lukka H, Hayter C, Julian JA, et al. Randomized trial comparing two fractionation schedules for patients with localized prostate cancer. *J Clin Oncol* 2005;23(25):6132–6138.
363. Kupelian PA, Thakkar VV, Khuntia D, et al. Hypofractionated intensity-modulated radiotherapy (70 gy at 2.5 Gy per fraction) for localized prostate cancer: long-term outcomes. *Int J Radiat Oncol Biol Phys* 2005;63(5):1463–1468.
364. Lloyd-Davies RW, Collins CD, Swan AV. Carcinoma of prostate treated by radical external beam radiotherapy using hypofractionation. Twenty-two years' experience (1962-1984). *Urology* 1990;36(2):107–111.
365. Yoshioka Y, Nose T, Yoshida K, et al. High-dose-rate interstitial brachytherapy as a monotherapy for localized prostate cancer: treatment description and preliminary results of a phase I/II clinical trial. *Int J Radiat Oncol Biol Phys* 2000;48(3):675–681.
366. Martin T, Baltas D, Kurek R, et al. 3-D conformal HDR brachytherapy as monotherapy for localized prostate cancer. A pilot study. *Strahlenther Onkol* 2004;180(4):225–232.
367. Pellizzon AC, Salvajoli JV, Maia MA, et al. Late urinary morbidity with high dose prostate brachytherapy as a boost to conventional external beam radiation therapy for local and locally advanced prostate cancer. *J Urol* 2004;171(3):1105–1108.
368. Shigehara K, Mizokami A, Komatsu K, et al. Four year clinical statistics of iridium-192 high dose rate brachytherapy. *Int J Urol* 2006;13(2):116–121.
369. Galalae RM, Martinez A, Nuernberg N, et al. Hypofractionated conformal HDR brachytherapy in hormone naive men with localized prostate cancer. Is escalation to very high biologically equivalent dose beneficial in all prognostic risk groups? *Strahlenther Onkol* 2006;182(3):135–141.
370. Nickers P, Thissen B, Jansen N, et al. ^{192}Ir or ^{125}I prostate brachytherapy as a boost to external beam radiotherapy in locally advanced prostatic cancer: a dosimetric point of view. *Radiother Oncol* 2006;78(1):47–52.
371. Lief EP. Localization I: radiographic methods and accuracy. In: Thomadsen BR, Rivard MJ, Butler WM, eds. *Brachytherapy physics*. 2nd ed. Madison, WI: Medical Physics Publishing, 2005:173–186.
372. Rownd J. Localization II: volume imaging techniques. In: Thomadsen BR, Rivard MJ, Butler WM, eds. *Brachytherapy physics*. 2nd ed. Madison, WI: Medical Physics Publishing, 2005:187–200.
373. Fraass B, Doppke K, Hunt M, et al. American Association of Physicists in Medicine Radiation Therapy Committee Task Group 53: quality assurance for clinical radiotherapy treatment planning. *Med Phys* 1998;25(10):1773–1829.
374. Kubo HD, Glasgow GP, Pethel TD, et al. High dose-rate brachytherapy treatment delivery: report of the AAPM Radiation Therapy Committee Task Group No. 59. *Med Phys* 1998;25(4):375–403.
375. Kutcher GJ, Coia L, Gillin M, et al. Comprehensive QA for radiation oncology: report of AAPM Radiation Therapy Committee Task Group 40. *Med Phys* 1994;21(4):581–618.
376. Thomadsen B, NetLibrary Inc. Achieving quality in brachytherapy vital issues in the classics. In: *Medical science series*. Philadelphia: Institute of Physics Pub., Bristol, 2000:xiv, 252.
377. Williamson JF, Thomadsen BR, Ibbott GS, et al. Failure modes and effects analysis (FMEA) for accelerated partial breast irradiation delivered via high dose-rate intracavitary brachytherapy. In: Thomadsen BR, ed. *Quality and safety in radiotherapy: learning the new approaches in task group 100 and beyond*. Madison, WI: Medical Physics Publishing, 2013:273–349.
378. Thomadsen BR, Rivard MJ, Butler WM. *Brachytherapy physics*. 2nd ed. Madison, WI: Medical Physics Publishing, 2005:965.
379. Dale RG, Jones B. The clinical radiobiology of brachytherapy. *Br J Radiol* 1998;71(845):465–483.
380. King CR. LDR vs. HDR brachytherapy for localized prostate cancer: the view from radiobiological models. *Brachytherapy* 2002;1(4):219–226.
381. Carlson DJ, Chen ZJ, Hoskin P, et al. Radiobiology for brachytherapy. In: Venselaar JLM, Baltas D, Meigooni AS, et al., eds. *Comprehensive brachytherapy: physical and clinical aspects*. Boca Raton, FL: Crc Press-Taylor & Francis Group, 2013:253–270.
382. Glasgow GP. An apercu of codes, directives, guidances, notices, and regulations in brachytherapy. In: Thomadsen BR, Rivard MJ, Butler WM, eds. *Brachytherapy physics*. 2nd ed. Madison, WI: Medical Physics Publishing, 2005:173–186.

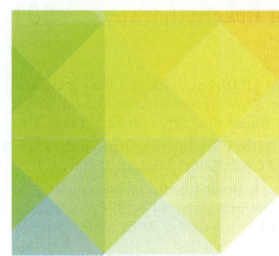

CHAPTER 26

Clinical Applications of Brachytherapy: Low Dose Rate and Pulsed Dose Rate

Sophie J. Otter, Caroline Holloway, Phillip M. Devlin, and Alexandra J. Stewart

Brachytherapy was the first form of conformal radiation therapy, utilizing placement of radioactive sources within or very close to a tumor, allowing high cancer to normal tissue dose ratios. From the time that Roentgen discovered radiography, the effects of ionizing radiation on the skin were noticed. Those exposed to the early cathode ray tubes, both patients and radiographers, developed radiation dermatitis and hair loss. After the isolation of radium, Henri Becquerel and Pierre Curie reported radium burns similar to those experienced by the early x-ray users. Radium was first used to treat skin lesions and superficial tumors using boxes and tubes as applicators. From there, radium in metal needles or radon gas in glass seeds was placed in direct contact with tumors using surface applicators and intracavitary and interstitial implants.[1] Source positioning within the tumor allowed high doses within the cancer with small volumes of normal tissue irradiated and a sufficient dose at the margin between cancer and normal tissue to eradicate microscopic tumor foci. Early results were promising and revolutionized cancer treatment.

In the 1950s, the use of brachytherapy was widespread; however, at that time brachytherapy had a number of disadvantages. Classic radium needles were rigid with a wide outer diameter (≥ 1.5 mm^2). Brachytherapists had to have a high level of surgical skill to site the needles accurately and to achieve good dosimetry quickly to minimize their own and others' radiation exposure. Therefore, the emergence of teletherapy with the advantages of decreased staff radiation exposure and radiation accessibility to more areas of the body with no dependence on surgical techniques led to a decrease in the use of brachytherapy.

However, brachytherapy has experienced a revival as a result of the emergence of newer artificial high-activity isotopes, afterloading systems, and improved radiologic imaging with more sophisticated dose planning techniques. Modern radiotherapy techniques have focused on dose escalation to the target and decreasing the dose to normal tissues. Brachytherapy can deliver both of these objectives in a highly conformal manner over a wide variety of disease sites. One advantage includes patient convenience. For example, prostate brachytherapy requires one or two hospital visits compared with 7 to 8 weeks with prostate external beam radiotherapy (EBRT). Reimbursement can have a marked impact on technique uptake with high reimbursement in non-nationalized health care systems playing a part in the resurgence of brachytherapy. However, it can also have a negative impact with a drop in uptake of prostate brachytherapy boost treatments corresponding to a fall in reimbursement rates using this approach.

Early texts describe the important principles of brachytherapy as uniformity in cross section, uniformity in depth, and uniformity in opportunity (time).[2] These principles remain the cornerstone of modern brachytherapy practice, though modern techniques allow better assessment of these. Computed tomography (CT), ultrasound, and magnetic resonance imaging (MRI) scanning have enabled enhanced imaging in brachytherapy, allowing more accurate target definition, superior determination of applicator position, and improved evaluation of the position of normal tissues. In combination with computerized dosimetry, this has allowed better determination of the dosimetric coverage of a brachytherapy implant and an estimation of the subsequent risk of normal tissue toxicity.

DOSE RATE DEFINITIONS

Three categories of brachytherapy were defined in Report 38 of the International Commission on Radiation Units and Measurements[3]:

- Low Dose Rate (LDR): a range of 0.4 to 2 Gy/hour. In clinical practice, the usual range is 0.4 to 1 Gy/hour.
- Medium Dose Rate (MDR): a range of 2 to 12 Gy/hour.
- High Dose Rate (HDR): over 12 Gy/hour.

Permanent seed implants deliver a high total dose at a very low dose rate (vLDR), usually at < 0.4 Gy/hour. Pulsed dose rate (PDR) brachytherapy was developed in an effort to simulate the radiobiologic advantages and dosimetric properties of LDR, but with the advantages of computer optimization of dose, a stepping source, and remote afterloading usually achieved by HDR. PDR is a misnomer; in fact, the dose rate is often high but the pulse intervals are short so that the radiobiologic effect is similar to LDR. A source with activity in the realm of one-tenth of HDR activity is used. Generally, the same total dose and total time as LDR are prescribed but the radiation is administered in a large number of small fractions, usually a pulse every 1 to 4 hours. Published series in a variety of tumor sites indicate that the clinical efficacy and the toxicity of PDR are similar to those of LDR/HDR.[4] It also has the advantage of a single afterloaded source compared to an inventory of LDR sources of different strengths. This will become increasingly important as manufacture of traditional LDR sources ceases and disposal costs of existing LDR sources rise. Traditional LDR sources iridium-192 and cesium-137 are no longer available in Europe and are becoming scarce in the rest of the world. Table 26.1 demonstrates the advantages and disadvantages of LDR and PDR brachytherapy.

CLINICAL USES OF BRACHYTHERAPY ISOTOPES

Brachytherapy uses radioactive isotopes to deliver therapeutic doses of radiation. The ideal radioisotope for brachytherapy should have a relatively short half-life in order to deliver the radiation in as short a time as possible and a high specific activity so that the source is small and therefore more versatile to implant. The emissions produced should have an adequate penetration to deliver the dose to the depth desired with rapid falloff to prevent damage to the surrounding normal tissue. Particular source characteristics such as half-life or specific activity can be tailored to the tumor and the surrounding organs at risk (OAR).

Temporary Implants

Cobalt-60 (^{60}Co) was one of the first artificial radionuclides used, available in interstitial needles and wires, but its usefulness for brachytherapy was limited by its low activity and short half-life, though it is still used in afterloaders in the

TABLE 26.1 THE ADVANTAGES AND DISADVANTAGES OF LDR AND PDR BRACHYTHERAPY

Advantages		Disadvantages	
LDR	**PDR**	**LDR**	**PDR**
>100 years of data	Source easily available	Often inpatient treatment with pro-	One machine per patient used for 3–5 days
Standardized doses	Standard source strength	longed bed rest	More intense maintenance
Standardized treatment plans	Minimal staff exposure	Radiation exposure to staff	Requires more physician/physicist time in certain
Less source changes needed	Dose optimization of normal tissues	Limited by available source strength	locations
(depending on isotope used)	Radiation-free periods aid nursing care	Many LDR sources no longer being	More expensive than LDR[279]
Less shielding needed during	No source inventory required	manufactured	Caution with conversion of dose from LDR to
treatment	With short pulse intervals uses long held		PDR especially as intervals increase
	doses with known safety and efficacy		May require prolonged bed rest depending on
			implant location

developing world with the advantage of decreased pressures on quality assurance and cost.[5,6] Cesium-137 (^{137}Cs) sealed into a ceramic or glass pellets was in use from the 1960s. From the 1970s, ^{137}Cs was the predominant isotope used worldwide for intracavitary gynecologic implants. However, production of this isotope ceased in 2002, and most departments wishing to continue using LDR-style dose and characteristics have switched to isotopes more suitable for remote afterloading, often using PDR techniques. Strontium-90 (^{90}Sr) is a pure beta emitter and therefore is suitable for very superficial applications; it is commonly used for coronary brachytherapy and ophthalmic problems such as pterygium. It has a half-life of 28.1 years, so many departments are still using applicators purchased in the 1980s. Ruthenium-106 (^{106}Ru) is also a beta emitter but with a much shorter half-life (1 year), making disposal concerns less and treatment delivery faster.

Iridium-192 (^{192}Ir) has been used since the 1960s in afterloading systems—both manual and remote. Its high specific activity makes it extremely suitable for remote afterloading because of the increased flexibility available with a smaller source. The small source size has enabled implants in areas where cesium sources would be too large, and the afterloading machine allows implants into much longer applicators, such as esophagus and bronchus, than was easily attainable with manually afterloaded ^{192}Ir wires.

Permanent Implants

The artificial isotopes iodine-125 (^{125}I), palladium-103 (^{103}Pd), and cesium-131 (^{131}Cs) are all used in modern permanent vLDR implants. The isotope used can be chosen according to individual characteristics that may be desirable in different implants; for example, slower dose delivery may decrease normal tissue toxicity or a tumor with a higher alpha/beta ratio may theoretically have more cell kill using an isotope with a shorter half-life. All three isotopes are almost completely shielded with 0.2 cm of lead foil, making radiation protection easier.

Clinical Suitability for Brachytherapy

Cancers with clinically and radiologically well-defined margins with a low risk of regional and metastatic spread are the most suitable for brachytherapy as a single modality. However, brachytherapy is becoming increasingly important when integrated with EBRT to give a highly localized boost. EBRT is used to sterilize a larger area of possible microscopic or nodal spread, with brachytherapy used for areas of gross macroscopic or microscopic residual disease. This ensures that high doses are achieved within tumors whereas normal tissues are not taken beyond recognized organ tolerance levels. It also has the potential for highly conformal localized dose escalation to areas at high risk of tumor recurrence.

In EBRT, the dosimetric goal is a homogeneous dose distribution with doses ranging from 95% to 107% of the prescribed amount.[7] In contrast, brachytherapy has an extremely heterogeneous dose distribution with isolated areas receiving in excess of 200% of the dose. The steep gradients are a consequence of the proximity of the clinical target volume (CTV) to the sources and decreasing dose with distance secondary to the inverse square law. The very high doses in the center of the implant contribute to additional cell kill, and the normal tissues also benefit from the inherent heterogeneity of the brachytherapy dose. As the dose falls off with distance, the normal tissue experiences not only a reduced dose but also a reduced dose rate that results in enhanced cell sparing. The sharp dose falloff with brachytherapy contrasts with the more gradual dose falloff seen with photon-based EBRT.

Brachytherapy can be given over a short duration (e.g., using PDR, a radical head and neck treatment course can be administered over 5 to 6 days compared to 5 to 7 weeks for a conventional EBRT head and neck regimen). Brachytherapy can also be used as a method of retreatment when a patient has received irradiation to normal tissue tolerance using EBRT. Using the principles described previously of sharp dose falloff and highly conformal dosing, a clinically useful radiation dose can be administered while minimizing the risk of increased late toxicity resulting from reirradiation.

Brachytherapy can be used anywhere in the body that can be accessed for direct source placement. For many years, surface applicators and intracavitary gynecologic brachytherapy were the predominant modes of brachytherapy. However, with the advent of modern surgical techniques and interventional radiology, many more areas of the body are now accessible to the brachytherapist.

Brachytherapy applicators can be placed within tubular organs in the body, either under direct vision (e.g., cervix or vagina) or with the use of radiologic or endoscopic guidance (e.g., bile ducts or esophagus). Interstitial implants can be placed with or without image guidance (e.g., prostate implants using rectal ultrasound guidance and a template or a freehand extremity sarcoma implant). Interstitial implants can take the form of free seeds, seeds within linked strands, or catheters that will be afterloaded with the radioactive source. Of course, surface applicator techniques are still used, with the added benefits of modern imaging and dosimetry techniques to ensure target coverage.

LDR sources can be placed directly into the body; however, with higher activity sources and large implants, this can result in a high radiation exposure to the brachytherapist and operating room staff. To overcome this problem, afterloading techniques were developed. Initial techniques required applicator placement in the operating room and manual afterloading of sources in a shielded room at a later time. This has mainly been supplanted by remote afterloading techniques, where the patient has the applicators placed in the operating room and is later connected to a remote afterloading machine in a shielded room. The sources will only enter the patient when all personnel are at a safe distance from the patient; this can be used for LDR and is essential for PDR.

When using afterloaded LDR or PDR, it is important that the patient can be safely left in a room without direct supervision, because during the period of source excursion, radiation dose to staff must be kept to a minimum. During an LDR implant, careful monitoring of the sources must be maintained to detect source displacement. During a PDR implant, the patient should be monitored for applicator displacement between pulses; this may be under direct vision or using radiologic confirmation. Devices aiding local protection of OAR may be used (e.g., leaded gum shield during lip brachytherapy). An analysis of 1,300 PDR treatments showed that patients received their dose as originally planned in 98% of treatments, with a deviation of 1.1% due to technical reasons and 0.9% due to coexisting medical illness. The error rate was very dependent on tumor site, with errors up to 14.9% for orbital tumors.[8] Errors due to malfunctioning catheters were often resolved during the treatment course by replanning the patient.

Target Definition

Many of the same definitions for delineation of treatment volumes in EBRT are used for brachytherapy.[7,9] There may be delineation of high-risk and low-risk areas if discrete areas of dose escalation are required within the CTV. The high-risk area has the highest risk of local recurrence, usually due to the presence of gross residual disease. An intermediate area may be defined that corresponds to areas where there was macroscopic tumor at the time of diagnosis that has regressed by the time of brachytherapy implant. The low-risk area includes potential microscopic spread, that is, the traditionally defined CTV. In EBRT, the planning target volume (PTV) traditionally consists of the CTV plus a margin that will allow for physiologic movement and setup uncertainty. Generally in brachytherapy these variations are minimized, and therefore the PTV is usually the same as the CTV.

In a brachytherapy implant there will be *high dose regions* around each source. Generally, the volume of the region receiving over 150% of dose is reported (V_{150}).[3] *Low dose regions* are those within the CTV receiving <90% of the prescribed dose. Because of the heterogeneity of dose in brachytherapy, the average dose within the prescribed volume is usually far higher than the prescribed dose at the reference isodose point on the periphery of the implant. This is tolerated because of the volume–effect relationship: very small normal tissue volumes (e.g., 1 to 2 cm³) can tolerate very high radiation doses that larger volumes would not tolerate. The dose to OAR should be reported, either as a total dose or as a ratio of volume. Parameters such as the minimum dose received by the most irradiated 2 cm³ (D2cc) of tissue or the volume receiving over 90% of the dose (V_{90}) or dose received by 90% of the CTV (D_{90}) are assessed.

RADIOBIOLOGIC CONSIDERATIONS

Radiobiologic principles are important in the daily clinical use of all forms of brachytherapy. Brachytherapy was initially developed empirically with doses being determined by clinical effect. These correspond to many of the LDR and PDR dose schedules in current use. In the modern era, radiobiologic modeling is used to predict the biologic effect of varying dose prescriptions. The importance of radiobiology and its use within brachytherapy was emphasized by the move from LDR treatment to PDR and fractionated HDR treatment. Of course,

it must be remembered that applicator and source placement remains the single most important factor in brachytherapy, such that in an implant with poor geometry, changing radiobiologic parameters, such as fractionation or dose rate, will not improve the outcome.

Factors contributing to the response of tissues to radiotherapy have been labeled the "4 Rs of radiotherapy."[10] These are repair, reassortment, repopulation, and reoxygenation. The way in which these radiobiologic characteristics relate clinically to the use of LDR and PDR either alone or in comparison to HDR is as follows:

Repair

Sublethally damaged cells are capable of repair if they are allowed sufficient time and if the cell contains all of the necessary DNA repair proteins and enzymes. If sublethally damaged cells are exposed to further irradiation before repair occurs, the damage may become lethal. Late-reacting normal tissues seem more capable of repair than tumor cells, so, at a given therapeutic dose, tumor is preferentially killed over normal tissue. This is probably a result of a loss of repair fidelity in addition to a lack of relevant repair proteins and enzymes in the tumor cell. The lower the dose rate of radiation that a cell is exposed to, the more likely it is that repair of normal tissues will occur within that cell before a second injury occurs.

The time course of LDR or PDR treatment over several days allows time for sublethal damage repair in normal tissues. In contrast, the short treatment time of HDR treatment prohibits this repair during the actual irradiation. Using PDR, generally the same total dose and total time as LDR are prescribed. If PDR is given at a pulse width of 10 minutes and a 1-hour pulse interval, the dose is equivalent to LDR 0.6 Gy/hour.[11,12] If the dose per pulse is small (≤0.5 Gy) and the normal tissue repair half-time is over 30 minutes, the differential effect to LDR is <10%. If the dose per pulse is over 2 Gy or the tissue repair half-time is under half an hour, this is not the case and the PDR effect becomes biologically closer to a highly fractionated HDR treatment, especially in close proximity to the source.[13] In this situation, a lower total PDR dose than LDR can be given in the same overall time to achieve equivalent clinical effect. Sometimes PDR is prescribed using an "extended office hours" schedule (i.e., 8 a.m. to 8 p.m.). This is commonly to overcome regulatory issues where a physicist and physician must be present for every source excursion. One general rule when transferring LDR to PDR dose is to not exceed the overall dose rate that would be delivered by LDR in a day (e.g., at a dose rate of 0.5 Gy/hour, LDR delivers a total dose of 12 Gy over 24 hours); thus, using a daytime-only PDR schedule providing a similar biologic effect and normal tissue complication probability, the overall treatment time will commonly be slightly extended.[14]

Dose rate is a key factor in determining the biologic effects of brachytherapy. In general, the effects of radiotherapy increase as the dose rate increases, predominantly because of a decrease in repair. It has been suggested that the total dose of LDR prescribed should be corrected for overall time of the implant[15] though some investigators have found no difference in local control with the same total dose administered using a dose rate ranging from 0.05 to 0.167 Gy/minute.[16] A randomized study in cervix carcinoma showed no difference in overall survival or local control for an LDR dose rate of 0.4 versus 0.8 Gy/hour.[17,18] However, there was a significant increase in late complications in the higher dose rate group. A similar trend has also been seen in LDR brachytherapy for breast cancer and head and neck carcinoma.[19,20] Therefore, it is recommended that the LDR dose rate (and PDR equivalence) should be in the range of 0.3 to 1 Gy/hour because of the effects on late complications rather than local control.

If the dose rate exceeds 1 Gy/hour, a reduction in the total dose can be calculated using the biologically equivalent dose (BED) equation.

Reassortment

In normal cells, proliferation occurs in a sequence of events termed the cell cycle.[21] There is a theoretical advantage of an improved effect on reassortment using LDR treatment because, during the overall treatment time, cells will pass out of the relatively radioresistant cell cycle phases of late S and early G_2 into the more radiosensitive phases of late G_2 and M. This has been shown *in vitro*,[22] but *in vivo*, the effect of reassortment has not been shown to give a true advantage, possibly because of a disruption of the mechanisms of the cell cycle in cancer cells.[21]

Repopulation

In squamous cell carcinoma, studies have shown improved tumor control and increased survival when a radiotherapy course is given in the shortest overall time.[23-26] This may be because shorter treatment times allow less time for tumor cell repopulation or for accelerated repopulation to occur. The continuous administration of LDR and PDR probably prevents repopulation during treatment.

Reoxygenation

The response of cells to radiation is strongly dependent on oxygen. Radiation results in free radical formation within a tumor, and oxygen reacts with these free radicals to make DNA damage irreparable. The effect of hypoxia on tumor control has been well documented, with decreased survival in certain patients with a low initial hemoglobin level.[27-29] There are two hypoxic cell populations within tumors, chronic and transient. As a tumor outgrows its blood supply, a proportion of cells will become necrotic. Viable cells near this necrotic zone will be chronically hypoxic. Transient hypoxia may occur over minutes to hours as small vessels within the tumor open and close or small tumor emboli intermittently block blood vessels. When using LDR and PDR, transient hypoxia may correct during the treatment time,[30] which is not possible during the short duration of HDR brachytherapy. If the brachytherapy is fractionated, tumor shrinkage and reoxygenation of areas of chronic hypoxia may occur between insertions.

MEASUREMENT OF BRACHYTHERAPY DOSE

Dosimetry systems aim to give the brachytherapist a set of guidelines to follow that result in a prescribed dose being delivered to a patient in a predictable fashion. Initial brachytherapy dosimetry systems were developed for LDR implants using an empirical approach toward source placement and dose calculation. More modern techniques use computer programs to generate isodose distributions that can then be analyzed in two dimensions, three dimensions, and volumetrically. To achieve the best ratio of cancer to normal tissue dose, the selection of an appropriate prescription point is essential. Again applicator positioning is of primary importance, as differential loading cannot compensate for a poorly sited implant.

The Manchester dosimetry system was one of the first published dosimetry systems, with origins dating from the 1930s.[31] Guidelines for the use of LDR wires and tubes are set out for surface molds, interstitial planar implants, and volume implants. However, it required a range of isotope activities to be available, and at that time, the available radium sources in the United States had a more limited range of activity.

Therefore, the Quimby system modified the Manchester system to allow uniform source strengths to be used throughout the implant.[32] The Paris dosimetry system developed guidelines in the 1970s for modern LDR brachytherapy sources such as flexible ^{192}Ir wires.[33] It is difficult to achieve an implant that conforms exactly to the Paris rules without the use of a template.

Whereas LDR uses fixed source positions and strengths to calculate the dose at the prescription point, afterloading machines and computerized dosimetry systems allow optimization of source dwell times to customize dose delivery to the patient's individual anatomy and tumor volume. PDR takes advantage of this dose optimization in a way that LDR cannot. Optimization results in nonuniform source loadings that give greater dose uniformity and CTV coverage that is often similar to an idealized Manchester dosimetry system implant.[34] Prior to the introduction of computerized dosimetry, the dosimetry of an implant was based on the intended source position rather than the actual source position. This could be highly dependent on the expertise of the individual brachytherapist. Improved radiologic imaging has allowed more accurate definition of the CTV and associated normal tissues, giving dose specification according to patient anatomy rather than applicator position. This is more likely to correlate with patient outcome than previous dosimetry systems. This may result in not only better tumor control but also decreased risk of late complications.

Now that computerized dosimetry is available, brachytherapists may be tempted to abandon knowledge of the previous dosimetric systems and place sources as they see fit, using the computer to calculate dose distribution. This approach risks overdosing part of the volume. There is a steep dose gradient around each wire/catheter, and widely spaced sources may form large high dose regions and increase the risk of necrosis. The maximum source separations and treatment thickness in the Paris system are useful rules to remember to decrease this risk. The principle of extending the sources beyond the target or crossing at the ends should also be remembered, to overcome the inherent dose falloff at the end of the source, though this can be achieved routinely with HDR and to some extent using optimization with PDR brachytherapy. The rules from individual systems should not be mixed, even if computerized dosimetry is used for dose calculation.

Brachytherapy dose delivery traditionally was thought not to be affected by alterations in the treatment position. Although this may be true for dose delivery to the target volume, the position of OAR in relation to the brachytherapy implant may be altered, thereby increasing the dose delivered; for example a patient undergoes simulation lying flat on a CT scanner with a breast implant that falls laterally with gravity. On sitting up, this applicator may then fall more medially potentially changing cardiac, lung, and skin doses. Therefore for temporary implants, treatment should take place in the planning position to allow accurate OAR dose determination.

CLINICAL SITES

There are areas where LDR techniques continue to predominate (e.g., vLDR prostate brachytherapy) and areas where HDR techniques predominate (e.g., esophageal brachytherapy). In some disease sites, the use of HDR and LDR was generally equal (e.g., cervix cancer), but now HDR predominates with a small but significant proportion of centers worldwide using PDR treatment. Next is presented an overview of clinical uses for LDR and PDR with an emphasis on the brachytherapy dose rate rather than the treatment technique. Individual indications will be described in the site-specific chapters.

Section II

Cervix Cancer

The use of LDR for cervix cancer treatment was first described with intracavitary implants in 1903 and with interstitial implants in 1913.[35] Brachytherapy has withstood technologic innovations to remain an essential part of curative cervix cancer treatment[36,37] for all but the very earliest stages of the disease. The use of LDR has many years of safety and efficacy data, and physicians can be confident in their choice of brachytherapy dose. These doses have been shown to be biologically equivalent using PDR so long as the rules governing pulse length and pulse interval are carefully followed.[14,38] In contrast, a wide variety of HDR dose and fractionation schemes are used,[39] with shorter follow-up data for efficacy and toxicity. Randomized clinical trials have shown the equivalence of HDR brachytherapy and LDR brachytherapy,[40] and some of these studies suggested a lower morbidity with HDR brachytherapy, which could be postulated to be due to the ability to optimize the dose away from normal tissues.[41,42]

Several trials demonstrated the superiority for chemoradiotherapy over radiotherapy alone in cervix cancer treatment.[43] All of these trials used LDR brachytherapy, and there are no prospective randomized safety data on the use of HDR brachytherapy and chemoradiotherapy. PDR brachytherapy utilizes the dose and scheduling of LDR and thus should have a similar efficacy profile while allowing the dose optimization capability of HDR, which may improve normal tissue toxicity. Studies have shown this to be the case in clinical practice.[44–46]

With the use of CT and MRI-based target volume and organ at risk definition, dose reporting in cervix cancer brachytherapy has changed from point-based to volume-based.[47–49] This means that tumor coverage is improved and the doses to normal tissues can be decreased. This method relies on the use of dose optimization and thus moves away from LDR and toward PDR as an equivalent treatment modality.[50,51] The longer time taken to deliver one overall fraction of PDR versus HDR is important when optimizing dose away from normal tissues, and it is important to recognize that the dose delivered to normal tissues over the whole treatment time may differ from that predicted, by up to 33% more.[52] Rectal volume has been shown to increase during the course of delivery of PDR, and therefore serial imaging and adaptive planning may be necessary as the cumulative rectal dose correlates with late rectal toxicity better than the planned dose.[53]

A recent randomized controlled trial has shown that there is no significant difference between late rectal, bladder, and vaginal toxicity and survival when comparing PDR with HDR brachytherapy.[54] American Brachytherapy Society (ABS) guidelines for the use of LDR and PDR in cervix cancer[55] incorporate the volume-based dosimetry and updated quality control recommendations.

The applicator is generally placed under operative conditions. Review of preoperative imaging is essential to determine which applicator is most appropriate. The patient may require a general anesthetic, but spinal anesthesia (see Fig. 26.1) has been shown to provide excellent analgesia, which can be maintained throughout the length of the implant using a spinal catheter.[56] Spinal anesthesia does not affect tumor oxygenation during an HDR implant[57] and thus is unlikely to do so during the whole duration of an LDR or PDR implant. A variety of commercial applicators are available for intracavitary brachytherapy (see Fig. 26.2) with the tandem and ring applicator becoming increasingly popular for tumors <5 cm. For tumors over this size, the addition of interstitial needles into specialized applicators is becoming more common because it has brought the ability to deliver interstitial brachytherapy to a wider group. Interstitial template applicators such as the Syed-Neblett[58] or the MUPIT[59] can be used to treat disease with lateral extension, though it is important to maintain a degree of central dose heterogeneity (in contrast

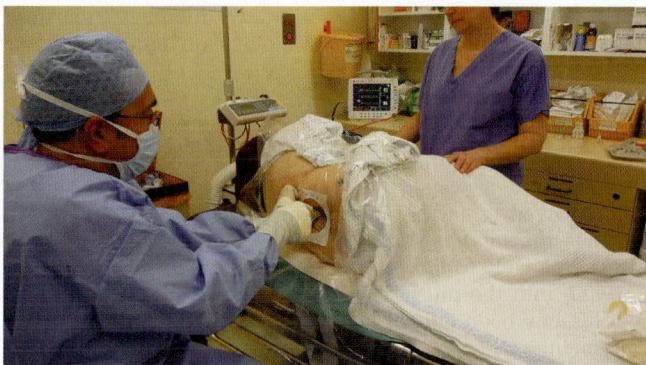

FIGURE 26.1. Administration of a spinal anesthetic prior to a pelvic brachytherapy procedure.

to the heterogeneity preferred in interstitial implants in other areas of the body) to maintain the central cervix doses needed for cure[60] (see Figs. 26.3 and 26.4). Customized vaginal molds can be used and are particularly prevalent in France,[61] offering truly customized brachytherapy dosing.

An LDR applicator is typically manually afterloaded once the patient returns to the shielded isolated patient room. The patient will undergo CT scanning and computerized planning before dose delivery. When the patient is receiving the dose she will be nursed lying flat with prophylaxis against venous thromboembolism. Typically, agents are given to slow bowel motility, and it may be preferable to follow a low-irritant fiber diet before and during implantation. A urinary catheter is maintained throughout treatment. Prophylactic antibiotics are not routinely required but can be considered for interstitial implants. Pain and discomfort may be managed by epidural or intravenous patient-controlled analgesia. During LDR, care is taken to minimize exposure to the medical staff caring for the patient with the use of mobile shielding placed around the bed and by training of the staff in the time/distance radiation safety rules. The use of pregnant staff is not allowed so as to minimize risk of dose to fetus.

FIGURE 26.2. Anteroposterior simulator radiograph demonstrating low dose rate tandem and ovoid insertion with dummy sources *in situ*.

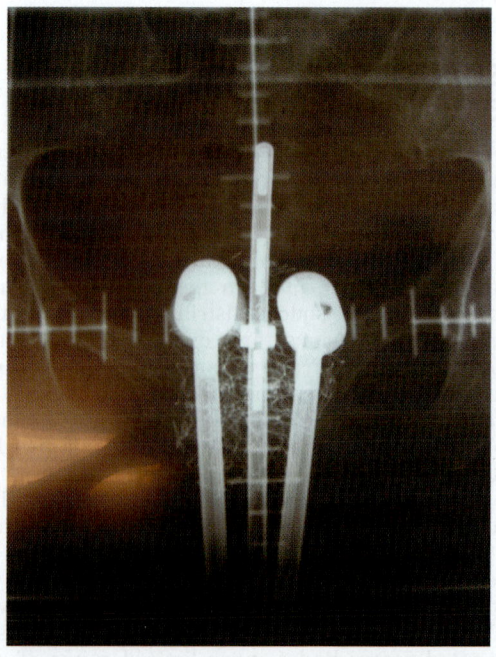

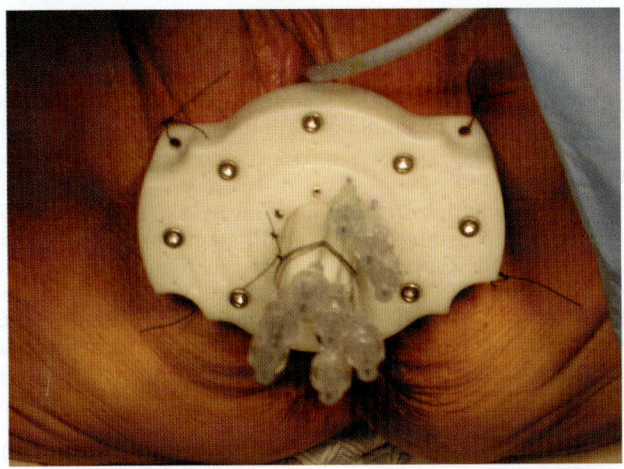

FIGURE 26.3. Low dose rate (LDR) template interstitial implant for a vaginal vault recurrence of cervical carcinoma.

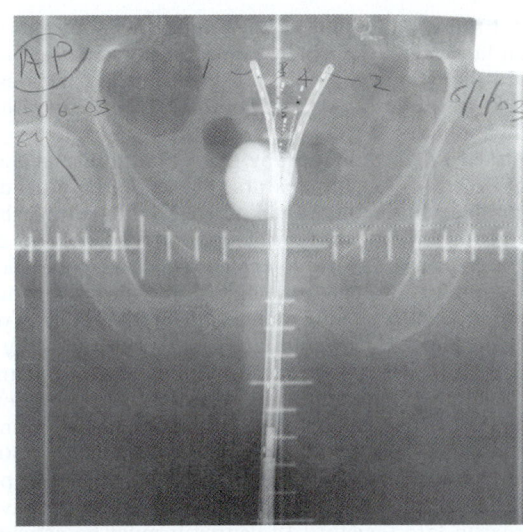

FIGURE 26.5. Double tandem Martinez applicator in place with three Heyman capsules placed within the uterus.

Endometrium

Endometrial carcinoma is the most common female pelvic malignancy in Western countries.[62,63] Brachytherapy for the management of endometrial carcinoma was first described by Heyman in 1935, prior to the routine use of hysterectomy for uterine cancer.[64] The majority of endometrial cancer patients now present at an early stage, and the use of radiation alone has evolved. The primary treatment for endometrial cancer is surgery (total abdominal hysterectomy and bilateral salpingo-oophorectomy) with or without adjuvant radiotherapy and chemotherapy, based on the histology of the tumor and stage of presentation. Pelvic lymph node sampling or lymphadenectomy is also used to give prognostic information and direct adjuvant treatment. As endometrial carcinoma is linked to obesity and hypertension, some patients have medical comorbidities that preclude surgery; for those, radiation therapy may be the definitive treatment of choice. In this group, treatment is delivered via intracavitary uterine brachytherapy, with or without EBRT.[65–67]

For definitive treatment, packing the uterus with capsules allows excellent coverage of the entire endometrial cavity that can be adapted to every patient's individual anatomy.[68,69] Standardized applicators may provide more straightforward and reproducible dosimetry. Double-channel applicators such as the Rotte applicator (Elekta AB, Stockholm, Sweden)[70] can be used with CT planning, and computerized optimization with HDR delivers a very similar dose to the serosa[71]; this could be replicated with PDR (see Figs. 26.5 and 26.6). Various whole uterus prescription points have been described[72,73]; however, CT planning allows contouring of the outer contour of the uterus for volume-based dose prescription. A typical dose is 70 to 80 Gy prescribed to the outer contour of the uterus alone or 35 to 50 Gy in combination with 30 to 45 Gy EBRT.[74] The Groupe Européen de Curiethérapie and the European Society for Radiotherapy & Oncology (GEC-ESTRO) have published guidelines on converting LDR schedules to PDR schedules for all gynecologic cancers.[75]

Vaginal vault brachytherapy can be used in the adjuvant treatment of endometrial cancer and vaginal vault recurrence of endometrial carcinoma and also in other gynecologic malignancies such postoperative early-stage cervical cancer or early stage vaginal cancer.[63,76–78] The target for adjuvant vaginal vault brachytherapy is the vaginal mucosa and the operative scar. Ninety percent of recurrences occur at the vaginal vault and 10% in the distal vagina[79]; therefore, in the majority of cases the upper third to half of the vagina is treated. This decreases the morbidity associated with treating the whole vagina, such as vaginal dryness or shortening.[74] However, for certain clinical situations such as clear cell or serous histology or lymphovascular invasion, some centers

FIGURE 26.6. Axial CT slice demonstrating the Martinez applicator *in situ*. The high-risk CTV is outlined in *red*, sigmoid in *blue*, and bowel in *orange*.

FIGURE 26.4. Axial computed tomography slice demonstrating the target volume and dosimetry of an LDR vaginal vault template interstitial implant.

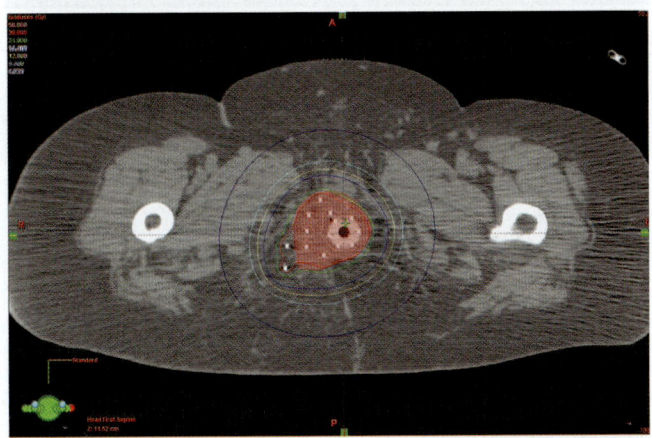

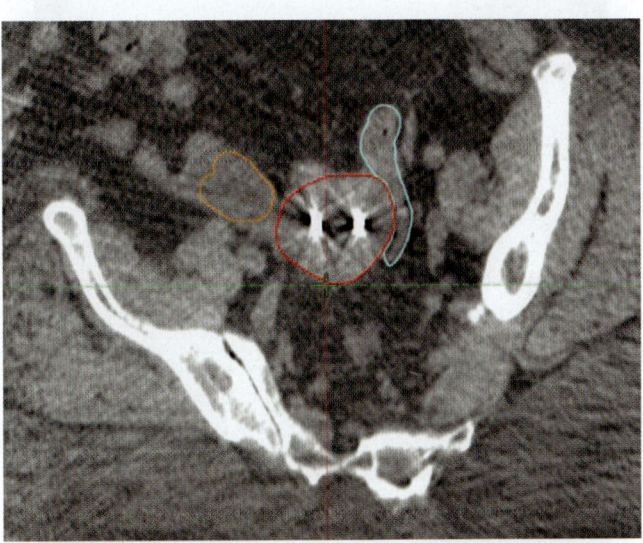

will treat the whole length of the vagina. A balance is made between late vaginal morbidity and the risk of distal vaginal relapse. Brachytherapy can be prescribed at the cylinder surface or at 5 mm into tissue, a depth that approximates the vaginal lymphatics.

Vaginal vault brachytherapy can be administered using a variety of different applicators. The commonly used single channel cylinder comes in a variety of widths chosen according to patient anatomy and comfort (see Fig. 26.7). This may be a less favorable choice when using LDR as the lack of optimization leads to effects from source anisotropy. The vaginal apex is located along the longitudinal axis of the source; therefore, the vaginal apex is exposed to the greatest effects of source anisotropy. It is important that planning systems contain modifications for source anisotropy. Li et al.[80] used Monte Carlo simulations to show that not accounting for anisotropy can result in underdosing by as much as 30% at the vaginal apex. The use of optimization with PDR to points off the cylinder apex can overcome this problem and may lead to decreased late toxicity.[81] Of course it must be considered that the doses we commonly prescribe for brachytherapy to the vaginal apex are those formulated using years of empirical dosing and the received dose at the vaginal apex may have actually been much higher than the prescribed dose. If the same prescribed dose is now used but with a lowering of the actual dose received by the vaginal mucosa using methods such as optimization to the cylinder apex or anisotropy correction, it is possible that this could be detrimental to tumor control. A vaginal colpostat is an alternative applicator that delivers a dose more localized to the vaginal vault and less dose to the mid-lower vagina.

Adjuvant primary vaginal vault irradiation has been shown to decrease the incidence of vaginal apex recurrence in early-stage endometrial cancer from 12% to 15% to as low as 0% in selected patients although it has no impact on overall survival.[76,82] The dose for LDR vaginal vault alone is 50 Gy prescribed at 5 mm over 4 to 5 days or 0.5 Gy/hour and

approximately 15 Gy when combined with 45 Gy EBRT.[74] The radiation dose received by the pelvic organs varies according to physiologic variations (e.g., the bladder dose may vary according to the extent of bladder filling, which may also affect the amount of small bowel in the field).[83,84]

Prostate

Prostate brachytherapy has become part of the treatment paradigm in prostate cancer for all stages of localized disease (see Table 26.2). It can be used as monotherapy or in combination with EBRT and/or hormone therapy for higher risk disease. A Surveillance, Epidemiology, and End Results (SEER) database analysis of men <60 years of age has shown that prostate cancer–specific mortality (PCSM) was reduced in those treated with brachytherapy (+/–EBRT) compared to those treated with EBRT alone.[85]

The most common application for monotherapy is still LDR permanent seeds, although more recently single-dose HDR monotherapy has been shown to be effective.[86] When used as a boost, LDR,[87] HDR,[88] and PDR[89,90] techniques can be used. Prostate brachytherapy is also being investigated as salvage therapy after external beam radiation[91,92] and is currently under investigation through the Radiation Therapy Oncology Group (RTOG) study RTOG-0526, which is now closed to accrual.

A transrectal ultrasound-guided transperineal technique is the most popularized technique for implanting the prostate. Other modalities incorporating MRI[93] and MRI spectroscopy imaging have also been proposed.[94] The techniques for implanting ^{125}I and ^{103}Pd have been well described.[95–97] The patient criteria for selection include ability to undergo a general, spinal, or less commonly local anesthetic[98]; prostate volume <60 cm^3 [87]; favorable anatomy (minimal or no pubic arch interference, median lobe); and minimal obstructive uropathy. Significant transurethral resection of prostate defect is also a relative contraindication to a seed implant.[99]

Tumor criteria depend on whether monotherapy or boost therapy is planned. Typically, monotherapy is reserved for patients with so-called favorable risk disease (e.g., low- to intermediate-risk disease: T1 to T2b disease, Gleason < 7, PSA < 15 ng/mL). However, there is emerging evidence that intermediate-risk disease may also be treated effectively with monotherapy[100]; therefore, boost therapy may be reserved for patients with unfavorable intermediate-risk and high-risk disease.[99,101]

The role of EBRT and hormone therapy in combination with LDR brachytherapy is unclear and under investigation. Adjuvant androgen deprivation therapy (ADT) is used for prostatic cytoreduction in patients who do not have ideal

FIGURE 26.7. Lateral image of a digitally reconstructed radiograph demonstrating a vaginal cylinder *in situ* and its relationship to surrounding normal tissues.

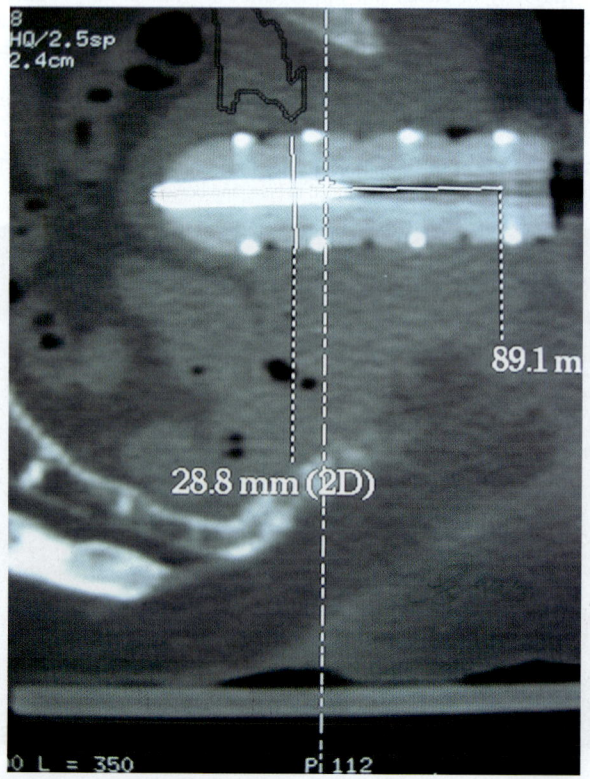

TABLE 26.2 INCLUSION CRITERIA FOR PROSTATE BRACHYTHERAPY
Selection Criteria for Prostate Brachytherapy
Patient Factors
Life expectancy > 5 years
IPSS < 15
Prostate volume < 60 cc
No defect if previous TURP
Minimal pubic arch interference
Tumor Factors
Monotherapy: T1-T2b, Gleason ≤ 7, PSA ≤ 15[a]
Boost therapy: ≥T2c, Gleason ≥ 7, PSA ≥ 10

[a]Gleason 7 and PSA > 10 may be considered for either monotherapy or boost therapy.
IPSS, International Prostate Symptom Score; TURP, Transurethral resection of prostate.
Reprinted from Ash D, Flynn A, Battermann J, et al. ESTRO/EAU/EORTC recommendations on permanent seed implantation for localized prostate cancer. *Radiother Oncol* 2000;57(3):315-321. Copyright © 2000 Elsevier Science Ireland Ltd. and Expert Panel on Radiation Oncology-Prostate, et al. American College of Radiology Appropriateness Criteria permanent source brachytherapy for prostate cancer. *Brachytherapy* 2011;10(5):357–362. Copyright © 2011 American Brachytherapy Society. With permission.

prostatic geometry.[99,102] Cytoreduction may be achieved with use of luteinizing hormone–releasing hormone agonists and antiandrogens or antiandrogen in combination with 5α reductase inhibitors.[102] ADT is also considered in patients thought to be at higher risk of prostate cancer recurrence; however, the benefit of ADT in this setting is not well defined.[103–106] A systematic review has reported no benefit of ADT in low-risk and favorable intermediate-risk patients but up to 15% improvement in biochemical progression-free survival in patients with suboptimal dosimetry or unfavorable intermediate-risk or high-risk disease.[107] None of the studies included showed an improvement in overall survival, but three did show a reduction in overall survival due to cardiovascular disease. There are several randomized controlled trials addressing this issue, and the results of RTOG 0815 are awaited.

In transperineal techniques, treatment planning can be done either as a preplan or intraoperatively. In the preplan technique, a volume study is acquired prior to the procedure, and the prostate volume and pubic arch interference are assessed. Axial images (5 mm) of the prostate from the base to the apex are taken and then used for brachytherapy planning (see Fig. 26.8A and B). Sagittal imaging can be used to help identify the base and apex. Reproducibility of the prostate position on the day of insertion must be ensured in this technique. Intraoperative techniques are defined as intraoperative preplanning, interactive planning, and dynamic dose calculation. Intraoperative preplanning avoids two separate ultrasound studies and involves the creation of a plan at the time of the implant procedure. It, like preplanned techniques, does not account for deviations of needle position or prostate geometry changes from the preplan.[108] The time required for the implant tends to be more prolonged using this technique compared to the preoperative technique. Interactive planning allows for refinement of the treatment plan based on needle-position feedback and estimation of seed placement. Modifications can then be made to needle position, or additional seeds can be added to optimize the plan. Dynamic dose calculation allows constant updating of the dose distribution based on the actual seed positions and takes into account changes in the prostate volume.[109,110]

TABLE 26.3 PRESCRIPTION DOSE FOR PERMANENT LDR BRACHYTHERAPY WHEN USED AS MONOTHERAPY OR AS A BOOST COMBINED WITH 40 TO 50 Gy EXTERNAL BEAM RADIATION THERAPY		
	Monotherapy (Gy)	**Boost (Gy)**
125I	145	110
103Pd	125	100
131Cs	115	85

Current permanent LDR techniques involve implanting 125I or 103Pd seeds. 131Cs is also approved for prostate brachytherapy and is used at some institutions. These isotopes have differing energies and half-lives and therefore differing initial dose rates (see Table 26.1). It had been postulated that 103Pd compared with 125I was more effective at treating dedifferentiated tumors as the dose rate is higher; however, studies evaluating clinical outcomes for patients with prostate cancer have shown no difference.[111–113] Studies evaluating the toxicity to OAR including rectum, bladder, and sexual function have shown no difference in acute or long-term toxicity or difference in sexual function.[114–116] There is a difference in the time for the International Prostate Symptom Score (IPSS) score to return to the preimplant baseline with 103Pd returning to baseline faster.[117] 131Cs has not been studied as extensively. Commercially 125I and 103Pd seeds are available either loose or stranded. Dosimetrically, the two are similar. The incidence of seed migration is decreased with stranded seeds as compared with that of loose seeds with the greatest difference being in migration to the lung and perineum.[118]

The prescription dose for permanent LDR brachytherapy is dependent on the isotope and the indication for the implant: either monotherapy or as a boost. Table 26.3 describes the recommended doses for 125I, 103Pd, and 131Cs when used as monotherapy or when combined with 40- to 50-Gy external beam radiation.[119–121] The prescription dose covers the entire prostate (CTV) and typically includes a margin. The dose for 131Cs is still investigational.

FIGURE 26.8. Prostate volume study with prostate and CTV defined **(A)**, preplan with peripheral loading technique **(B)**.

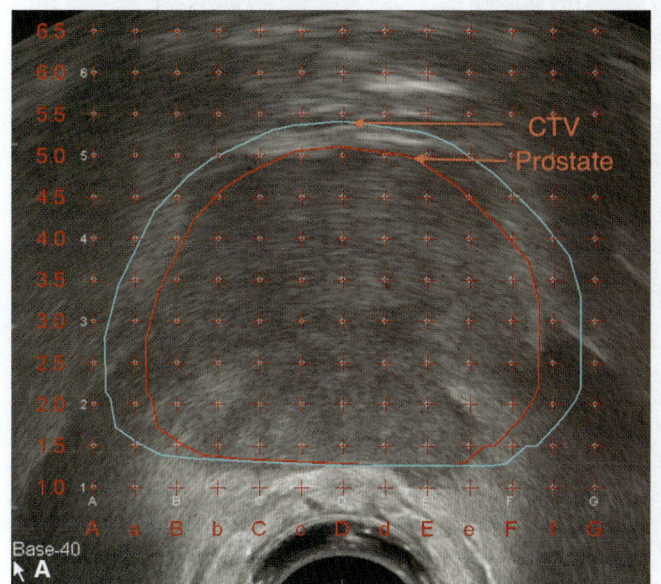

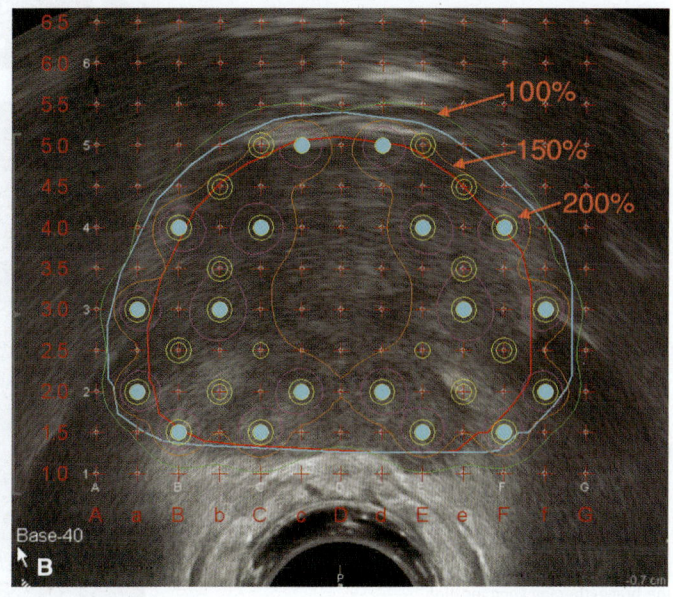

In the preoperative technique, the dose to the target volume as well as the OAR is evaluated. Different loading techniques are used to achieve these goals based on the needle placement, spacing of seeds, and seed energy.[122] A peripheral loading technique is common to avoid excess dose to the urethra with ^{125}I and a modified uniform loading with [103]Pd.[123] The source placement with [131]Cs has different guidelines to ^{125}I and [103]Pd with needles placed further from the urethra and rectum.[120] Good preimplantation dosimetry and toxicity levels correlate with a $V_{100} > 95\%$ of CTV, $D_{90} > 100\%$, $V_{150} \leq 50\%$ of CTV, rectum D2cc < reference prescription dose, $D_{max} < 150\%$ of reference prescription dose, prostatic urethra $D_{10} < 150\%$, and $D_{30} < 130\%$.[110] Dose limits to structures such as the penile bulb and neurovascular bundles are under investigation.

Postimplant dose reporting in a structured quality assurance program is highly recommended and should include dose parameters to both the target as well as the OAR.[121,124] Timing of the postimplant imaging varies at different centers but ideally should relate to the time at which edema is at a minimum. Evaluation at either day 0 or day 30 is most common. Seed localization is crucial as is the contouring of the prostate and normal structures. CT/MRI fusion if possible allows for both identification of the seeds and accurate definition of the prostate, particularly at the apex and base, which tend to be difficult to delineate on CT (see Fig. 26.9A and B). Primary parameters to report and evaluate include the intended dose, D_{90}, D_{100}, V_{100}, V_{150} to the prostate gland, and rectal volume and dose and urethral doses. For patients with unacceptably cold implants, consideration for reimplantation should be given.

There are no parameters at present for penile bulb and neurovascular bundles.

Studies have shown that prostate brachytherapy is associated with a "learning curve" effect.[125–127] As with any brachytherapy technique, outcomes and toxicities are dependent on where the radiation has been delivered. With permanent seed brachytherapy, there can be no dose optimization once the seeds are placed. A quality assurance process that enables closing the feedback loop for optimizing subsequent implants therefore is crucial. Peer review; assessments of dosimetry, toxicity, and outcomes; as well continuing education should be part of any prostate brachytherapy program.[128–132]

Under spinal or general anesthetic the patient is positioned supine in the lithotomy position. If a preplan was used, the same couch angle and ultrasound probe angle must be reproduced. Contrast agent is typically injected into the bladder for visualization under fluoroscopy. Visualization of the urethra is essential and can be accomplished by injecting foamed Mucogel into the urethra during the procedure. Alternatively, a urethral catheter can be inserted and left in place during the implant; however, some clinicians avoid the latter technique to avoid changing the shape of the prostate. The prostate, bladder, seminal vesicles, and pubic arch are identified on ultrasound. The base and apex of the prostate gland are also identified. Preloaded needles are kept within a shielded vault or sleeve until the physician is ready to insert the individual needles. Each hollow-bore needle has a beveled edge and central stylet. Ultrasound images in both the axial and sagittal views (if available) guide the

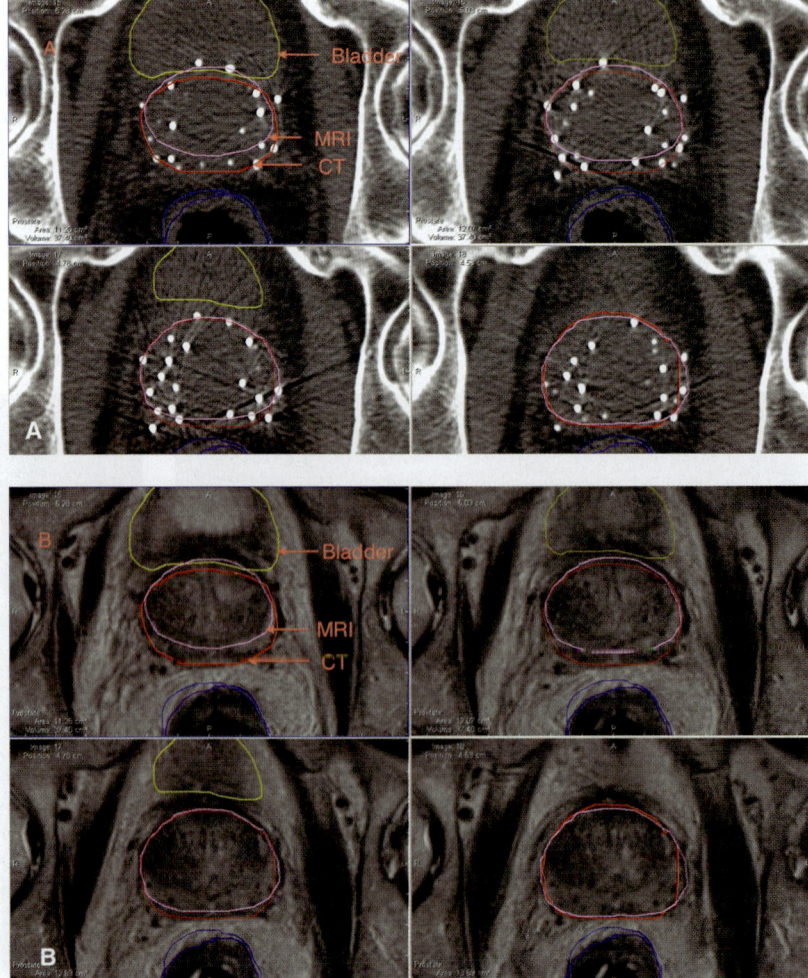

FIGURE 26.9. Prostate brachytherapy post plan with computed tomography and magnetic resonance (CT-MRI) fusion. The prostate volumes were drawn independently on the CT **(A)** and MRI **(B)** to show the difference in contours at the base of the prostate. The MRI images are better able to delineate the prostate, whereas the CT scan is better able to give information on the brachytherapy seed location.

placement of the needle. Once the first needle is in the correct position (in three-dimensional coordinates), the retraction plane is set for positioning of the remaining needles. To drop the seeds within the prostate, the central stylet is held securely in place and the outer needle is slowly pulled back along the stylet. On-demand fluoroscopy can be taken to check seed position relative to bony and organ anatomy. Additional seeds may be placed at the end of the procedure as required. Bladder irrigation and cystoscopy can be performed to evacuate migrated seeds in the bladder. Patients are conveniently discharged home the same day of the procedure; the majority of patients do not require a urinary catheter on discharge.

In intermediate- to high-risk prostate cancer, brachytherapy in combination with EBRT has been evaluated with both LDR permanent seeds and HDR brachytherapy.[133–136] The same techniques used in HDR boost brachytherapy can be applied to temporary implants with LDR ^{192}Ir strands or PDR brachytherapy with special attention to techniques that insure that the apparatus stays in place over the treatment time. PDR boost brachytherapy is not as extensively studied as HDR or permanent implants, but preliminary studies[90,137] show acceptable toxicity and tumor control with limited follow-up. In the Pieters et al. study, the patients were treated with ≤1.2 Gy/pulse at short time intervals ≤2.2 hours. The doses in their study are relatively low with an equivalent dose at 2 Gy per fraction (EQD$_2$) between 68.8 and 74.4 Gy. They note that the tumor control at 5 years is comparable to that in many HDR studies and that there are large areas of prostate receiving >20% of the prescription dose because of the heterogeneous nature of brachytherapy. They recorded low rectal and urinary toxicity and the IPSS returned to baseline by 12 weeks post brachytherapy. Further dose escalation with PDR was felt to be worth pursuing because of the low rectal and urinary toxicity. Studies evaluating ^{192}Ir LDR for boost have also been done but are not commonly used.[138–140]

Penile Cancer

Penile Cancer is rare in Western countries, representing only 1% of male malignancies. Squamous cell carcinoma is the predominant histology. Brachytherapy is used as an organ-sparing technique in T1, T2, and select T3 lesions (<4 cm) that do not involve the shaft of the penis.[141–143] Both surface mold techniques (lesions < 5 mm)[144,145] and interstitial techniques (see Fig. 26.10)[146–150] have been described. The 5-year local control with interstitial brachytherapy is 70% to 86%

with penile preservation of 72% to 88%. Typical doses range from 50 to 65 Gy delivered in 4 to 7 days. Typically, at least two planes of catheters are required as it is difficult to assess the depth of disease. Crook et al.[151] describe their implantation technique in detail for 75 cases implanted between 1989 and 2009 with both ^{192}Ir wire/seeds and PDR techniques. The implants are based on the Paris system using rigid templates with spacing between 12 and 18 mm. Computerized dosimetry mimics the Paris system and allows for visualization of dose to the target and OAR. They prescribed 60 Gy at a dose rate of 0.5 to 0.6 Gy/hour with manually afterloaded ^{192}Ir or 0.5 to 0.6 Gy in hourly fractions when using PDR. Treatment takes approximately 5 days.[143] Penile preservation was 88% at 5 years and 67% at 10 years with actuarial survival of 59% at 10 years and cause specific survival of 83.6%.[147] They reported a soft tissue necrosis rate of 12% and urethral stenosis rate of 9%. The soft tissue necrosis rate quoted in the literature ranges from 12% to 26% and increases with dose > 60 Gy, T3 disease, large volume implants (>30 cm^3), and >2 needle planes.[147–150,152] If conservative measures fail to manage soft tissue necrosis, hyperbaric oxygen therapy has shown success prior to resorting to surgical interventions such as debridement or amputation.[153] Urethral stenosis is reported in 10% to 45%[147–150,154] of cases and relates to the proximity of the needles to the urethra and the number of treatment planes. Using PDR brachytherapy allows manual optimization of dose around the urethra and may decrease the rate of stenosis. It is recommended that all men undergo circumcision prior to brachytherapy as this exposes the tumor, potentially removes disease allowing for a smaller implant, and decreases the risk of ulceration and necrosis to the foreskin.[149,151] Dose to the urethra and testes should be recorded. In men wishing to retain fertility, lead shielding around the testes can be placed.

Urethra

Brachytherapy may be used in the treatment of both male and female urethral cancers. Intraluminal, intracavitary, and interstitial techniques have been described. Intraluminal brachytherapy is limited to superficial lesions and involves a single catheter into the urethra.[155] Interstitial implants for the penile urethra are similar to penile implants. In treatment of the female urethra, an interstitial implant may be used in combination with a molded vaginal applicator[155] or alone (see Fig. 26.11). The dose with LDR as a monotherapy is 60 to 70 Gy in 3 to 5 days (0.5 to 1 Gy/hour PDR) and 20 to 25 Gy if used as a boost. Milosevic et al.[156] published their experience of 34 patients who were treated with radiation.

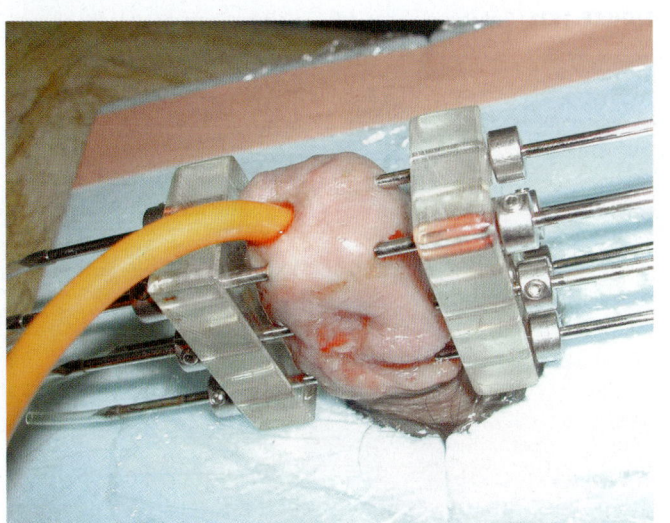

FIGURE 26.10. Low dose rate interstitial multiplane penile implant.

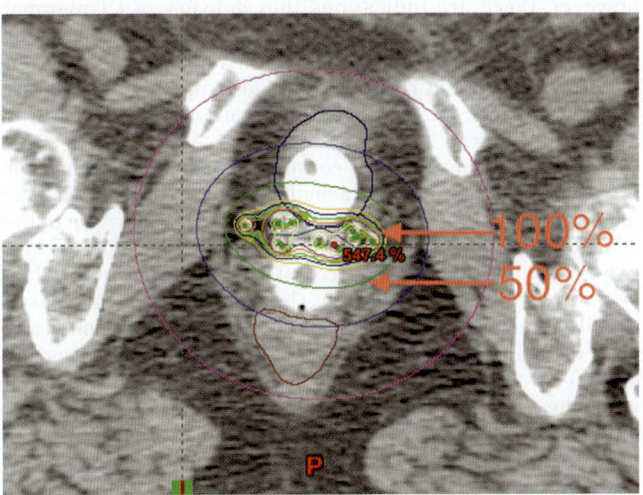

FIGURE 26.11. Low dose rate interstitial multiplanar urethral implant.

Twenty of these patients received brachytherapy (5 brachytherapy alone, 15 EBRT + brachytherapy). The tumors treated with brachytherapy tended to be ≤4 cm, involve the distal urethra, and did not invade adjacent organs. The majority of the patients underwent volume implants. Patients who had brachytherapy as part of their treatment had better local control with 7-year local relapse-free rates of 77% versus 32% with EBRT alone. There was no difference in cause-specific survival and 7-year actuarial overall survival (41%). The risk of vesicovaginal fistulas was reported as 15%.

Bladder Cancer

Bladder cancer can be treated either with radical cystectomy or with chemoradiotherapy for an organ-preserving approach.[157,158] Several studies have shown good results with the addition of brachytherapy to EBRT.[159,160] Aluwini et al.[159] reported on 192 patients with muscle-invasive bladder cancer (MIBC) who were treated with EBRT followed by surgical exploration (with or without partial cystectomy) and interstitial brachytherapy (LDR or PDR). Salvage cystectomy-free survival at 5 and 10 years was 93% and 85%. The 5- and 10-year overall survival rates were 65% and 46%, whereas cancer-specific survival at 5 and 10 years was 75% and 67%. The distant metastases-free survival rate was 76% and 69% at 5 and 10 years. Multivariate analysis revealed no independent predictors of local recurrence-free survival. RTOG grade ≥3 late bladder and rectum toxicity were recorded in 11 patients (5.7%) and 2 patients (1%), respectively.

GEC-ESTRO guidelines have recently been published and recommend that EBRT and brachytherapy are reserved for patients with a solitary tumor <5 cm, T2 to T3, no additional carcinoma in situ, and not located at the bladder neck or prostatic urethra.[161] Radiotherapy doses and schedules vary, but a typical schedule is 40 Gy in 20 fractions EBRT followed by 25- to 30-Gy brachytherapy (HDR or PDR). The implant can be sited by open surgery (retropubic approach) or endoscopically (simultaneous laparoscopy and cystoscopy). The catheters are passed through the abdominal wall into the detrusor muscle and out to the opposite side of the abdominal wall.

Head and Neck

Brachytherapy can be used to treat head and neck cancers either as definitive treatment or as a boost following EBRT. Use of brachytherapy may avoid disfiguring or mutilating surgery and allow organ conservation. Brachytherapy can also be used as a method of reirradiation for localized recurrence.[162] There are many years of safety and efficacy data for LDR brachytherapy, and PDR appears to replicate these results.[163–167] Intensity-modulated radiation therapy (IMRT) is becoming increasingly standard for head and neck cancer; however, there are indications that delivery of CT-planned optimized brachytherapy continues to deliver superior results over IMRT.[168,169] Aspects of plan quality that are important for local control and risk of toxicity are similar to interstitial implants elsewhere—quality index, volume gradient ratio, and tube distance.[170]

GEC-ESTRO have issued consensus recommendations for the use of head and neck brachytherapy[171,172] with a particular focus on dose, treatment selection, and quality assurance in the 2017 update. Data support the use of both hourly pulses and two-hourly pulses, with a dose of 0.4 Gy/pulse (24 pulses/day) or 0.8 Gy/pulse (12 pulses/day). The overall dose is decreased slightly when using 12 pulses/day—for example a monotherapy dose for a T1N0 cancer would be 70 Gy using 24 pulses/day and 60 Gy using 12 pulses/day. The ABS have recently updated guidelines for head and neck brachytherapy focusing on treatment selection in the era of advanced EBRT techniques.[173]

Patient selection is key for head and neck brachytherapy. Patients who are unfit for radical surgery may still be poor candidates for brachytherapy. PDR may allow the use of brachytherapy for patients with more complex nursing needs in whom LDR would have been contraindicated. It is important that the patient is fully assessed prior to brachytherapy. Dental assessment is essential, tooth extractions may be required, and for implants encompassing the oral cavity customized leaded mandibular shields decrease the risk of osteoradionecrosis. Feeding needs should be assessed and where necessary nasogastric or percutaneous gastrostomy feeding tubes placed before the implant. For base of tongue implants, the patient should be prepared to have a tracheostomy, which can be reversed as soon as the postimplant edema subsides. The patient should be assessed regularly during the duration of the implant for displacement of the sources or applicators. Analgesia should be administered, and mouthwashes are often helpful.

The majority of head and neck implants are placed in an operative procedure by freehand technique in a multiplane implant (see Figs. 26.12 and 26.13). These can be sited using a variety of techniques with use of afterloading catheters being preferred in the modern era for radiation safety reasons.[174] Standard applicators such as the Rotterdam applicator that can be sited under local anesthetic without image guidance are also available (see Figs. 26.14 and 26.15). Similar to other sites described below, interstitial ^{125}I seed implants can be used in cases of unresectable disease with favorable rates of control and toxicity.[175–178]

Brachytherapy is indicated in the majority of lip cancers, either as sole modality in tumors 0.5 to 5 cm or as a boost following EBRT in tumors over 5 cm. For very superficial tumors, a surface applicator may be appropriate (see Fig. 26.16), thus preventing scars from puncture wounds. However, the majority of tumors require the placement of 2 to 3 interstitial catheters across the tumor (see Fig. 26.17); these can be placed freehand under local anesthetic. Typical doses are 45 to 75 Gy at the 85% reference isodose (higher doses for larger tumors, though at the risk of decreased cosmesis). Five-year local control rates with LDR are 90% to 95%[174,179] and 94% with PDR.[180,181]

For oral tongue tumors, brachytherapy offers similar control rates to surgery with the benefit of organ and function preservation. Brachytherapy alone can be used for smaller lesions or as a boost for larger lesions. Interstitial implants are preferred, placed under general anesthetic using a metal trocar and threading the afterloading catheters through these. Looped catheters were popular when using ^{192}Ir ribbons, but with optimized PDR, it is difficult for the source to pass into the curved tube; therefore, individual button-ended catheters

FIGURE 26.12. Catheters placed to deliver a brachytherapy boost to the pharynx.

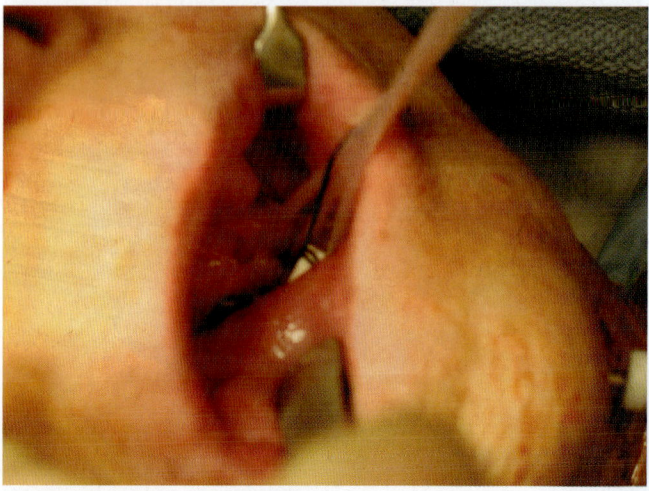

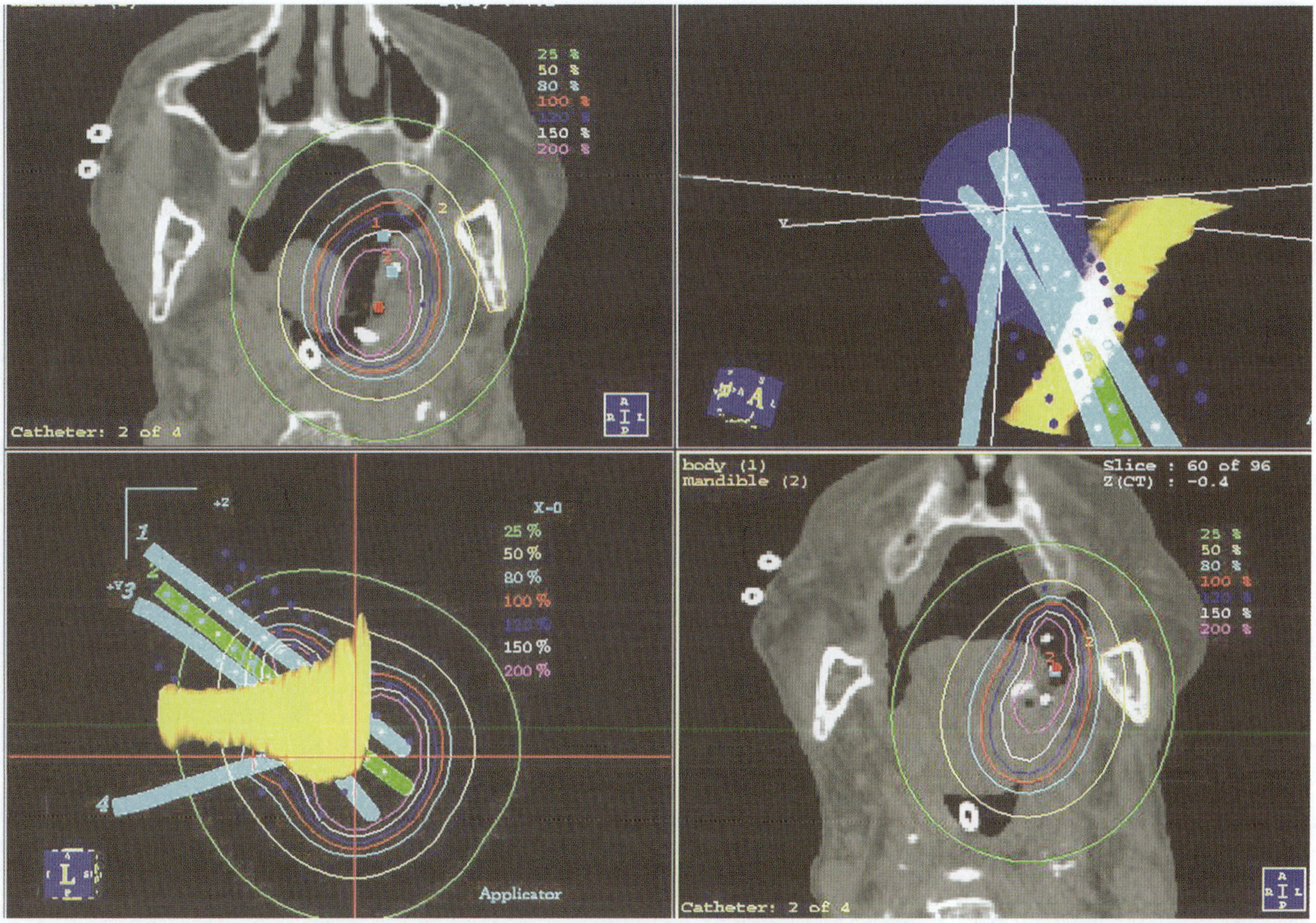

FIGURE 26.13. Three-dimensional computer-optimized dosimetry of the pharynx implant.

are preferred for source excursion (see Fig. 26.18). To prevent a cold spot on the tongue, an extra spacer can maintain the catheter above the tongue or dose optimization can be used, taking care not to cause a localized hot spot. Mandibular shielding is preferred. A dose of 65 Gy is typical as sole treatment and 20 to 25 Gy as a boost.[182] Local control compares well with surgery with small superficial tumors showing local

FIGURE 26.14. Patient with a Rotterdam applicator *in situ* within the nasopharynx.

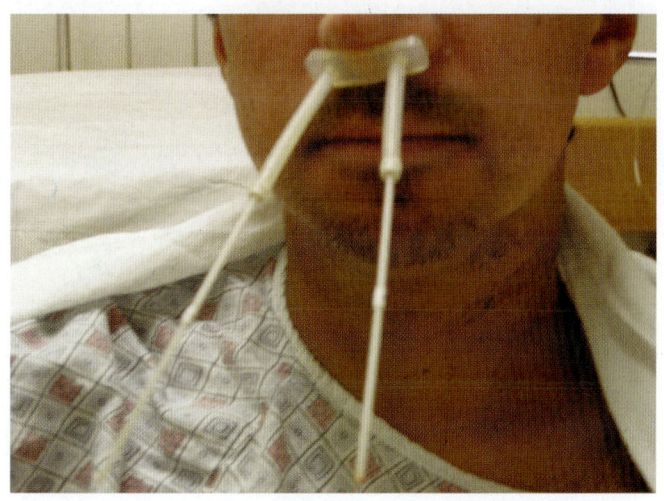

control rates over 90%.[20] When combined with EBRT, a PDR boost for base of tongue tumors gives results at least equivalent to LDR with 5-year local control of 89%.[183]

Floor of mouth tumors are also best treated with interstitial implants with similar technique to tongue implants. Distance to the mandible is critical to prevent osteoradionecrosis. It may be preferable to perform surgery with reconstruction rather than risk late sequelae. Elective nodal dissection may be preferable to EBRT in advanced cases.[184] A dose of 65 Gy for sole treatment and 20 to 30 Gy boost is recommended, keeping overall treatment time as short as possible. Control rates range from 50% to 92% depending on tumor size, but bone necrosis is more common than other sites up to 30%.[174,184]

Oropharyngeal cancers traditionally present at an advanced stage because of their location in an area that is not visible with few pain fibers. Surgery can be very debilitating; therefore, EBRT and localized boost techniques are favored. A boost of 20 to 30 Gy is delivered using an interstitial implant. The implant is performed under general anesthetic with nasal intubation, and a covering tracheostomy is usually required. Hemorrhage may occur in implant removal, so it is important to remove the catheters under controlled conditions with wide-bore venous access, suction, and surgical support.

Most nasopharyngeal tumors are inoperable because of their position at the base of the skull. However, the nasopharynx is easily accessible to brachytherapy catheters. These can be placed under topical anesthetic—for example, the Rotterdam applicator—or under direct vision using a Le Fort osteotomy. The main role of brachytherapy is as a localized

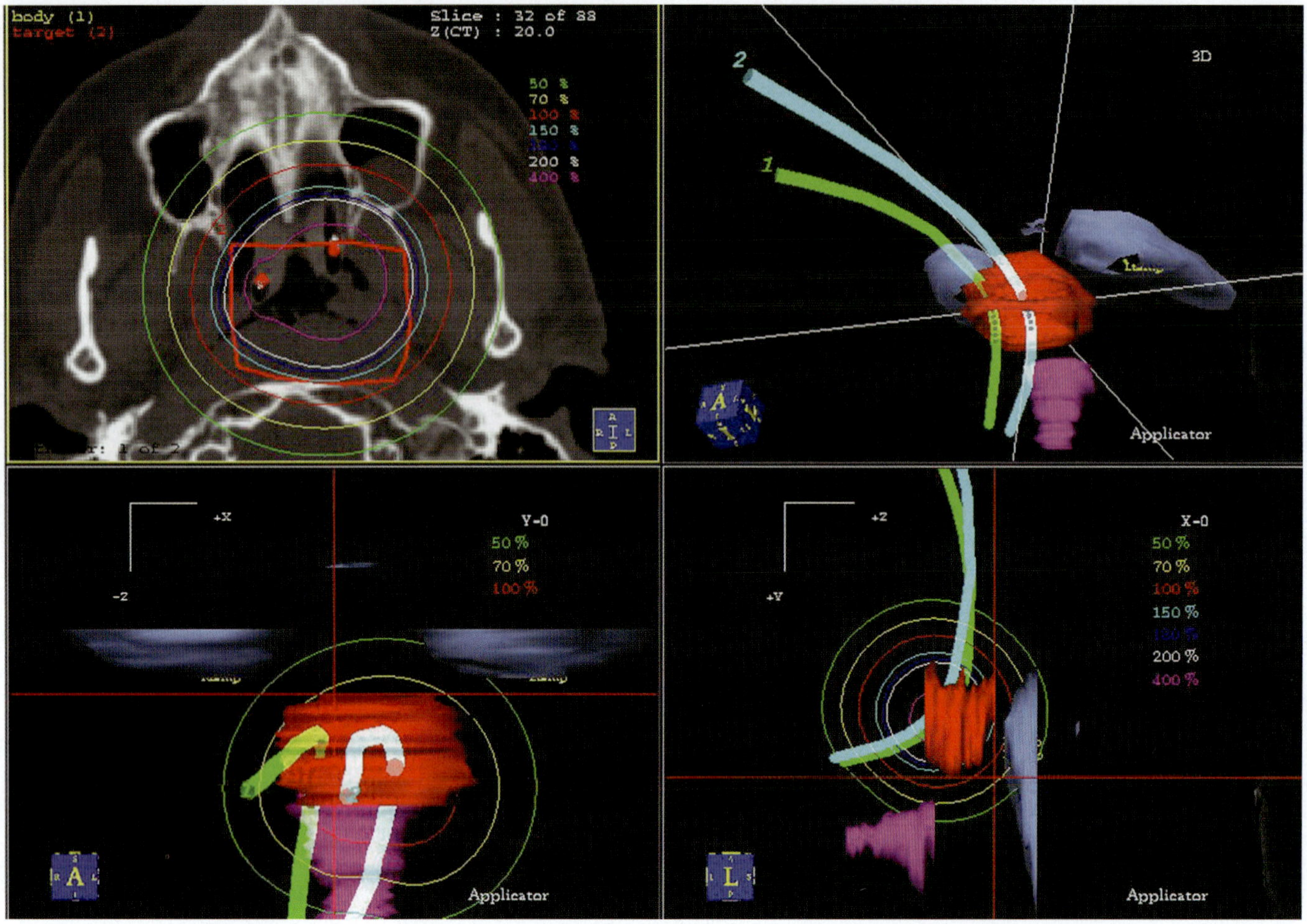

FIGURE 26.15. Three-dimensional dosimetry of the Rotterdam applicator, delivering computer-optimized brachytherapy.

boost or as a sole reirradiation technique with typical doses of 12 to 20 Gy and 60 Gy, respectively. Local control is excellent even in reirradiation where control rates of at least 50% are reported.[174]

Brachytherapy is particularly suitable for reirradiation of head and neck cancer, administered with curative intent. A series of 104 patients with recurrent head and neck cancer were treated with brachytherapy alone (81) or a brachytherapy boost (23), often with concomitant chemotherapy (56%) or hyperthermia (32%). At a median follow-up of 60 months, 5-year local control was 82% with acceptable rates of late toxicity, only requiring surgery for toxicity in 3% of cases.[185]

FIGURE 26.16. Surface applicator technique used to deliver a boost dose to a lower lip sarcoma following external beam radiation therapy. The wax mouth bite was used to displace the tongue and could be placed for every pulse of the pulsed dose rate.

FIGURE 26.17. Multicatheter single-plane cheek implant. The metal gum shield can be placed for every pulse of the pulsed dose rate.

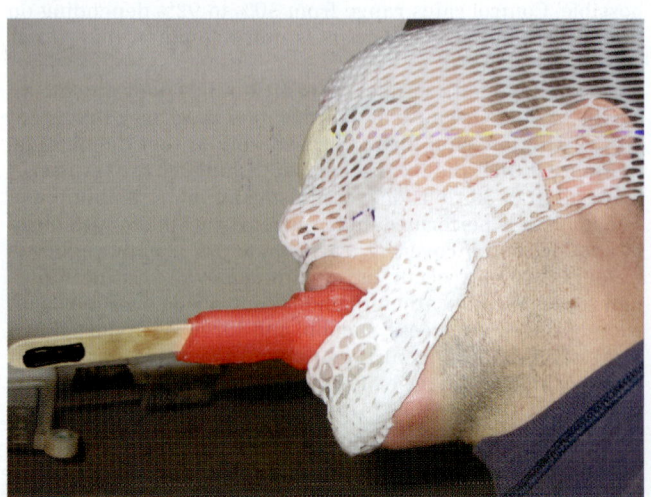

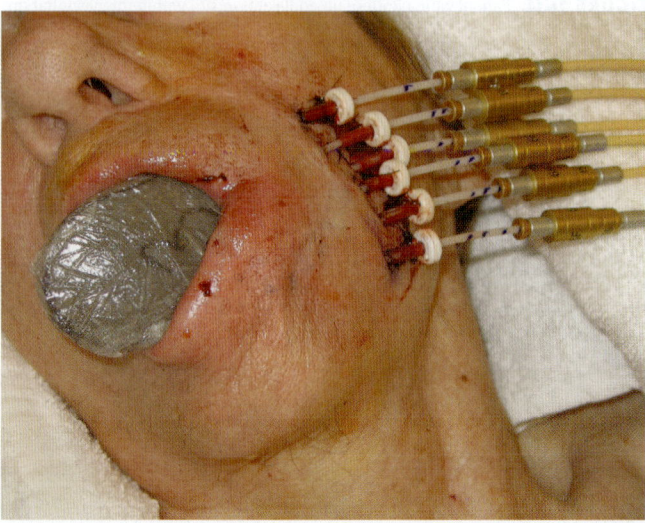

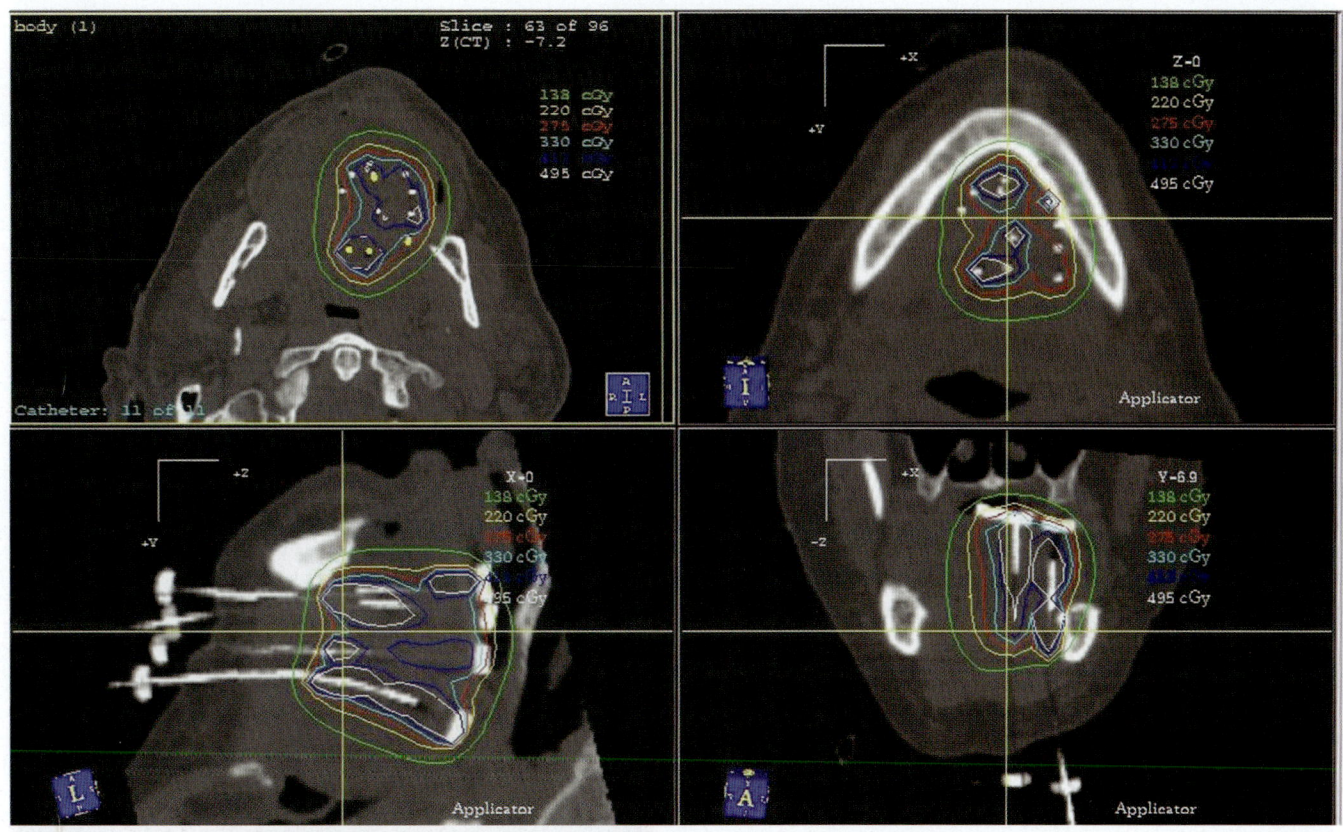

FIGURE 26.18. Three-dimensional computer-optimized dosimetry of a tongue implant using button-ended catheters.

Thoracic Seed Implants

Intraoperative permanent radioactive ^{125}I seed implantation can be used in the treatment of malignant thoracic tumors when resection margins are close or macroscopically or microscopically involved with tumor[186–201] or for palliation of inoperable disease.[202] The surgeon selects patients preoperatively when there is a concern of incomplete tumor resection or close or positive margins and refers to the brachytherapist. The patient is consented in advance for a permanent implant to be placed intraoperatively if required. Details of previous radiotherapy and chemotherapy treatment are carefully reviewed prior to surgery. The brachytherapy team is on call for the surgical procedure. Frozen section analysis of margins may be needed to assess whether an implant is needed. Seeds are placed directly into a tumor as a volume implant, or woven in a grid pattern in a planar implant. Volume implants require the use of an applicator or preloaded needles to deliver the seeds directly to the tumor. A planar implant can be ordered ready-made in advance (see Fig. 26.19) or custom-made intraoperatively[203] (see Fig. 26.20). ^{125}I seeds set into Vicryl suture with 1 cm spacing between seeds can be woven into a mesh or sutured directly to the area at risk. The Vicryl suture and accompanying mesh degrades naturally after approximately 60 days;

FIGURE 26.20. Custom-made 6-by-10-cm mesh implant using iodine-125 seeds in Vicryl carrier. The steel rings used to shield the isotope in transit can be seen at the *top left* of the picture.

FIGURE 26.19. Premade seed mesh.

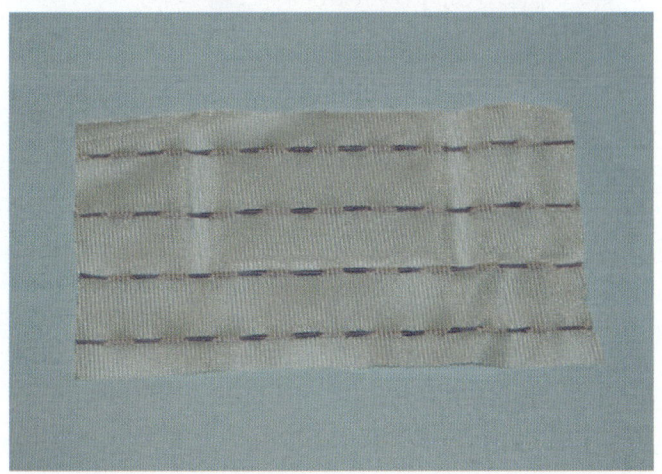

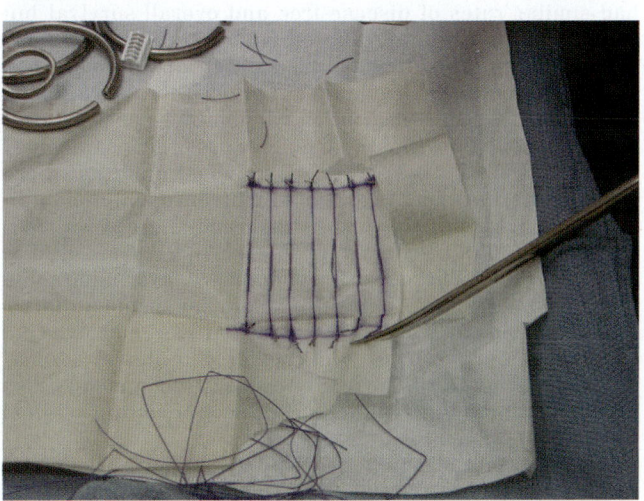

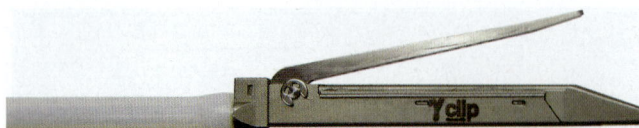

FIGURE 26.21. Seed staple gun.

at this point, much of the dose has been delivered and the seeds are often held in position by local fibrotic reactions. The mesh can be used in open surgery, thoracoscopically, or utilizing a robotic system.[204] Seeds can be placed at equally spaced intervals into a layer of foam,[193,205] but this implant may be more difficult to suture in place, as the seeds are not easily visible and are therefore at risk of being displaced or damaged by the suture needle. Alternative seed placement devices may aid seed placement such as the customized suture gun (see Fig. 26.21). Radiation exposure during the procedure to the implanting radiation oncologist and surgeon is very low[206] and well within occupational radiation exposure guidelines. When the implant has been sited, the operating room is surveyed for the presence of radiation. The patient is surveyed at the outer body surface over the implant, at 0.5 m and 1 m. In the immediate postoperative period no change in patient care is required, subject to standard post-vLDR implant precautions of preventing exposure to children or pregnant women.[207]

For sublobar resection the dose recommended is 100 Gy, at 5 mm from the mesh or 7 mm from the central axis of the implant. For incomplete resection of tumor or positive margins, the dose chosen will depend on many factors such as adjacent structures or previous radiation; the type of surgery performed must also be considered in case there is an increased risk of late normal tissue toxicity.[208] The curvature of the implant should also be assessed because over a curved surface dose penetration is asymmetric compared to a linear implant.[209] Isodoses on the concave side of a curvature are further from the implant surface, potentially decreasing the dose delivered. The asymmetry increases with decreasing radii of curvature (see Fig. 26.22). Interestingly, *in vitro* studies have shown that selected human lung cancer cell lines show a greater sensitivity to ^{125}I seed brachytherapy than HDR irradiation, an effect that was further potentiated with the use of radiosensitizers.[210]

Lobectomy is the standard of care for patients with operable Stage I non-small cell lung cancer; however, intraoperative ^{125}I seed placement has been used in conjunction with sublobar resection in patients with lung cancer who are medically unfit for lobar resection.[191,194,195,197–201] Retrospective studies showed that patients undergoing sublobar resection had similar rates of disease-free and overall survival but that patterns of relapse differed with higher rates of local recurrence in the sublobar resection group.[211] Thus intraoperative permanent seed implant brachytherapy was been evaluated in a multi-institution randomized phase III prospective trial by the American College of Surgeons Oncology Group (ACOSOG) Z4032.[212,213] This demonstrated that there was no difference in 5-year local recurrence with the addition of brachytherapy (17% with brachytherapy vs. 14% without, $P = .59$). There was no difference in disease-free or overall survival. There was a trend toward favoring brachytherapy in patients with positive staple line cytology. Better than expected rates of negative margins were achieved, so the trial may have been underpowered to detect a small difference. Therefore, the ABS consensus recommendations do not recommend this outside the confines of a clinical trial.[214]

For intrathoracic tumors with incomplete resection or microscopic close margins, retrospective and prospective

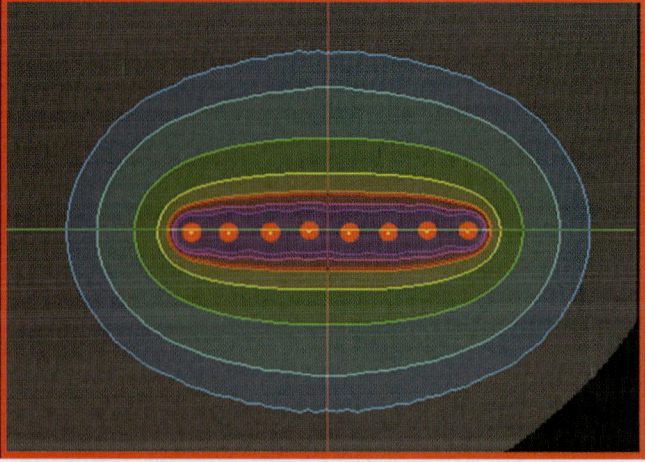

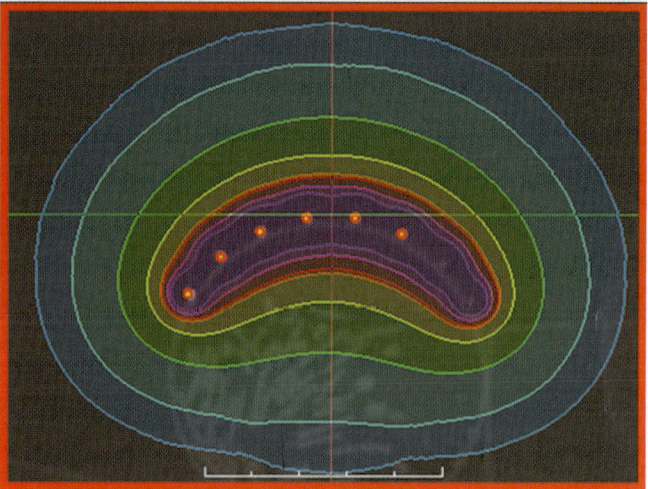

FIGURE 26.22. Effect of curvature on the dosimetry of a single planar mesh seed implant.

series have shown that disease-free and overall survival rates with the addition of an intraoperative permanent seed implant are improved over those that would be expected with incomplete resection alone[186–189,192] (see Fig. 26.23).

FIGURE 26.23. Intraoperative photograph of a custom-made mesh interstitial vLDR brachytherapy implant placed at the apex of the thoracic cavity following resection of a Pancoast tumor with close resection margins. The surgically collapsed lung can be seen at the base of the image.

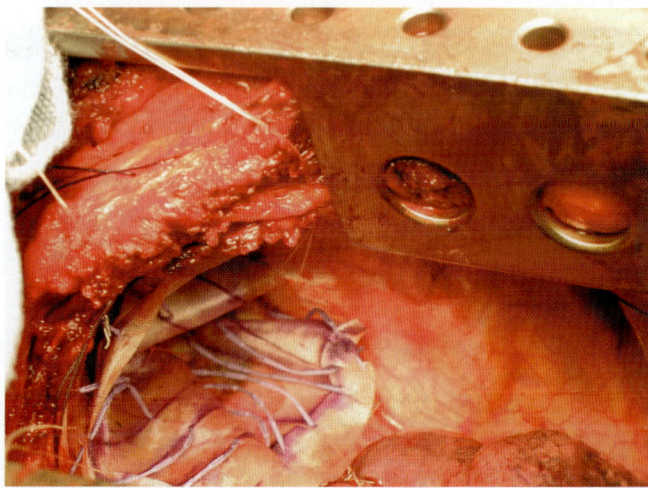

Breast

Breast-conserving surgery is a proven alternative to mastectomy in patients with early-stage breast cancer, offering equivalent disease-free and overall survival.[215–217] Adjuvant radiotherapy is required because it results in a significant reduction in the risk of death from breast cancer, Unfortunately, this is offset by an increase in deaths due to other causes.[217] In the nonirradiated breast, recurrences tend to occur in the tumor bed with an elsewhere recurrence rate of up to 3.5%.[215,216,218,219] Accelerated partial breast irradiation (APBI) has similar ipsilateral breast recurrence and survival rates to whole breast IMRT but lower acute and late toxicities and better cosmetic outcome.[220] ABPI can be delivered with brachytherapy, localized radiotherapy, or intraoperatively with electrons[221] or photons.[222]

Postoperative APBI using brachytherapy was initially developed using interstitial implants. A number of needles or tubes are placed across the tumor bed usually under general anesthetic, either using a template or freehand (see Figs. 26.24 and 26.25). The treatment volume is generally the tumor cavity plus a 1- to 2-cm margin. The dose is custom-shaped to this treatment volume. The dose can be delivered using LDR or PDR brachytherapy, typically over 4 to 5 days. The large number of catheters in an interstitial implant allows more control over skin and chest wall doses than do single catheter techniques, especially with PDR dose optimization. The dose within the tumor is more homogenous with lots of smaller hot spots, compared to one large hot spot with single catheter techniques.[223] Single-catheter technique for left-sided tumors has also been shown to have a higher mean heart dose than deep inspiration breath-hold whole breast radiotherapy,[224] whereas this is less likely to happen with multicatheter brachytherapy.

Interstitial implants have been in use for over 10 years. Phase 3 trials have shown that PDR or HDR APBI is noninferior to whole breast radiotherapy with respect to 5-year local control, disease-free survival, and overall survival in low-risk invasive or ductal carcinoma *in situ* (DCIS).[225] Early toxicity was dramatically reduced in the brachytherapy ABPI arm (86% vs. 21% for grades 1 and 2 early skin toxicity).[226] Five-year toxicity and cosmetic outcomes were similar between the groups although grade 2 and 3 late skin toxicity was significantly reduced in the brachytherapy arm.[227] APBI with LDR, PDR, or HDR brachytherapy after lumpectomy is also an option for patients with ipsilateral local recurrence with an overall survival rate equivalent to salvage mastectomy.[228]

Permanent interstitial seed implant has been described for APBI[229] (see Fig. 26.26). [103]Pd seeds were implanted using ultrasound guidance and a dose of 90 Gy prescribed to the tumor cavity plus a 1.5-cm margin. In a group of 134 patients from 3 clinical trials, the observed local recurrence rate was 1.2% at 63 months, which is similar to the estimate for whole breast irradiation. Toxicity rates were acceptable. A radiobiologic dosimetric modeling study predicts that for APBI using brachytherapy, toxicity will be lower for a seed implant than for a multicatheter interstitial technique.[230]

Sarcoma

In the modern era, sarcoma surgery has become more refined, moving away from disfiguring, disabling surgery and towards a multidisciplinary approach combining surgery and EBRT and, in certain tumors, chemotherapy.[231,232] The use of LDR brachytherapy for soft tissue sarcoma (STS) was first described in 1963[233] using a variety of isotopes including [226]Ra and [192]Ir. Brachytherapy offers several advantages over EBRT; the catheters can be placed at the time of initial resection and loaded 5 days postoperatively, enabling the whole STS treatment to be completed within 10 to 14 days. Placement under direct vision allows accurate coverage of the resection cavity. There may be less hypoxia immediately postoperatively, enabling the radiotherapy to be more effective. The heterogeneity of dose delivery allows high doses to the tumor bed whilst minimizing the dose to surrounding normal tissues, thus minimizing toxicity.

The ABS issued consensus recommendations for the use of brachytherapy in patients with STS.[234,235] Table 26.4 presents a summary of the general principles for STS brachytherapy. Catheters are placed at the time of surgery, using either a single-entry sealed-end catheter (see Fig. 26.27), or double-entry button-ended catheters. The catheter is secured with plastic buttons that do not produce artifact in CT or MRI scanning. The CTV is the tumor bed plus a margin of 2 cm craniocaudally and 1 to 2 cm laterally.[234] The catheters can then be used for afterloaded LDR ^{192}Ir strands or connected to an afterloading PDR machine. A mesh implant can also be used with similar technique to that described in the thoracic vLDR section.[186] The doses recommended in the updated ABS guidelines are LDR/PDR 45 to 50 Gy for monotherapy and 15 to 25 Gy for

FIGURE 26.24. Template interstitial breast implant. **A:** Intraoperative photograph of insertion of needles for a multiplane template interstitial breast implant. **B:** Photograph to demonstrate catheter position after template removal. (Courtesy of Dr. Bob Kuske.)

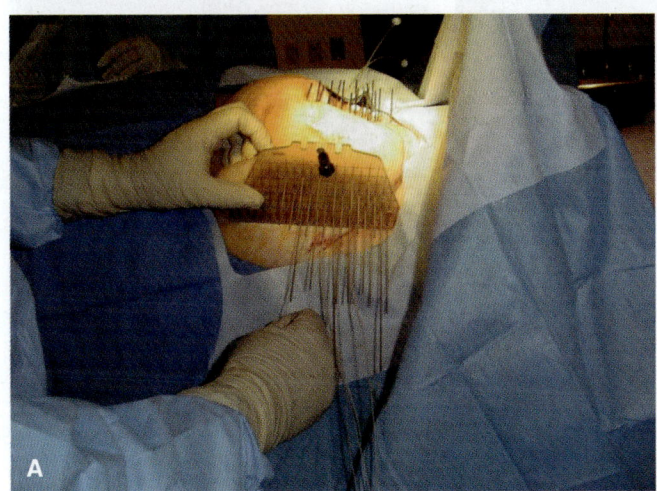

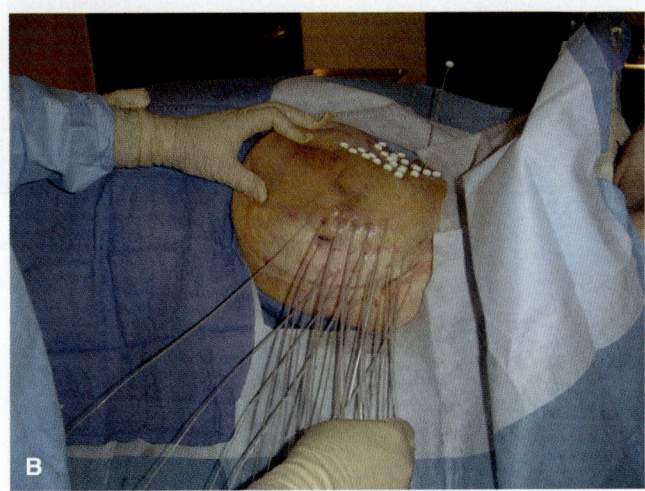

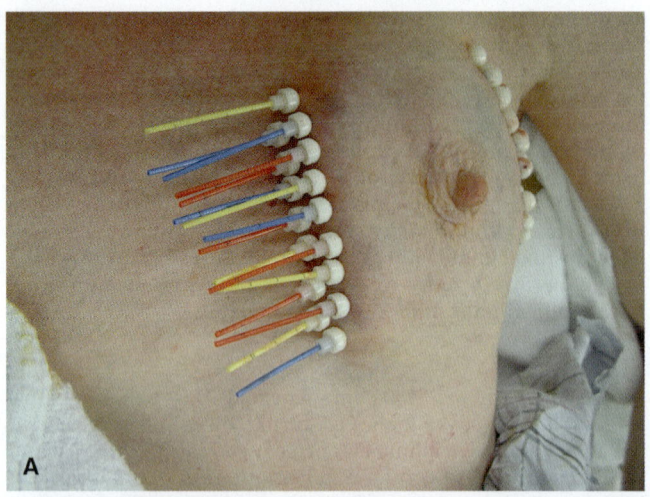

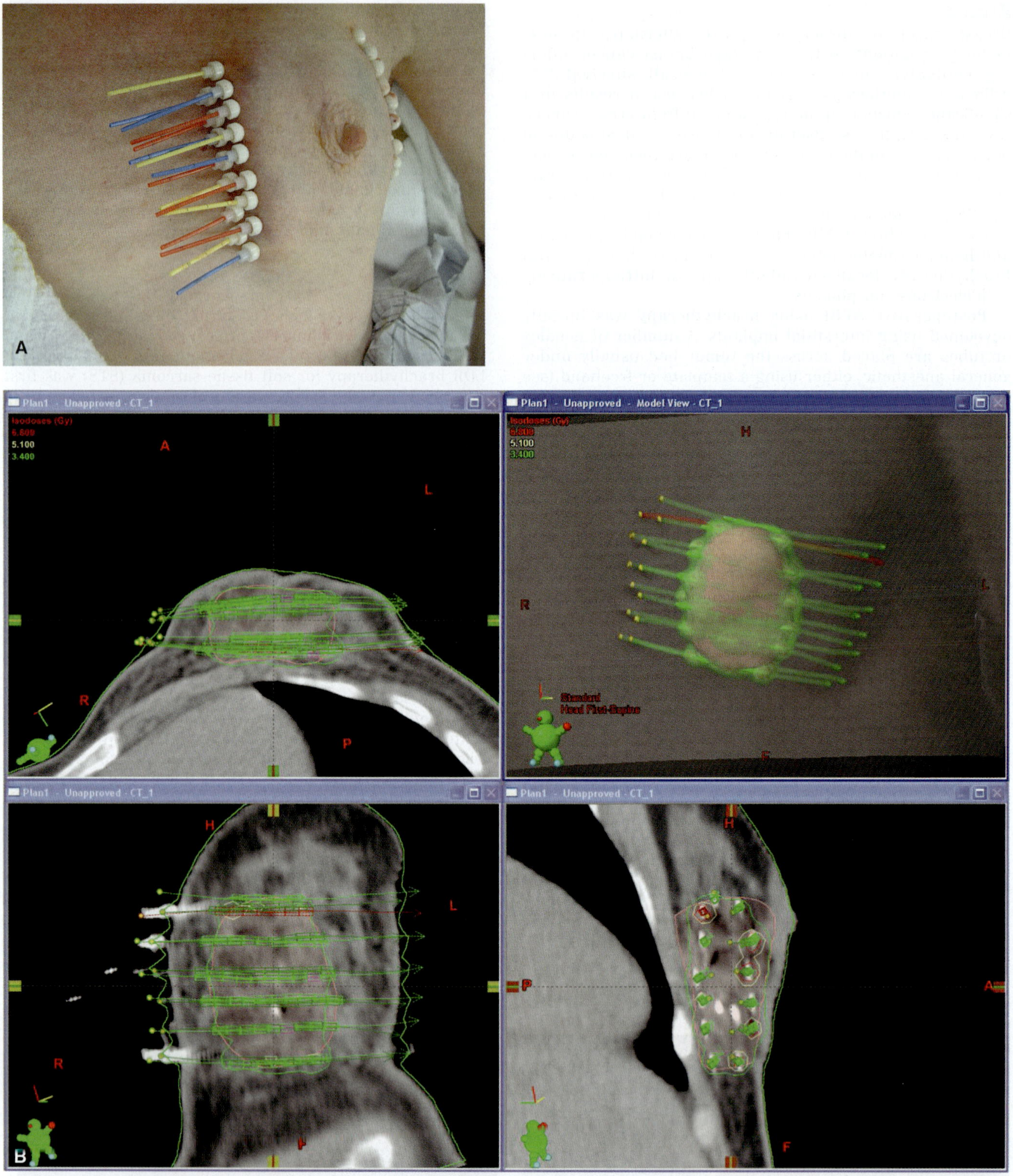

FIGURE 26.25. Freehand breast implant. **A:** Catheter position of a 2-plane breast implant. **B:** CT images demonstrating the dosimetry of the implant. The 100% isodose is marked in *green* (3.4 Gy). (Courtesy Dr. David Wazer and Dr. Dorin Todor.)

boost (PDR pulses 0.45 to 0.5 Gy/hour or equivalent).[236] The doses for a typical radical mesh implant are 100 to 150 Gy at 5 mm and 50 to 70 Gy for a boost dose, depending on previous EBRT dose administered.

Phase 2 trials showed the utility of LDR brachytherapy for postoperative STS treatment,[189,237] and therefore a randomized phase 3 trial was conducted.[238] One hundred and seventeen

patients were randomized to brachytherapy or no brachytherapy following R0 or R1 resection; patients were stratified by various factors including size and grade. Five-year actuarial local control for all patients was 82% vs. 69% (*P* = .04) but on subgroup analysis no effect seen in the patients with low-grade tumors. With longer follow-up of the high-grade tumors only, local control was 89% versus 66% (*P* = .0025) but

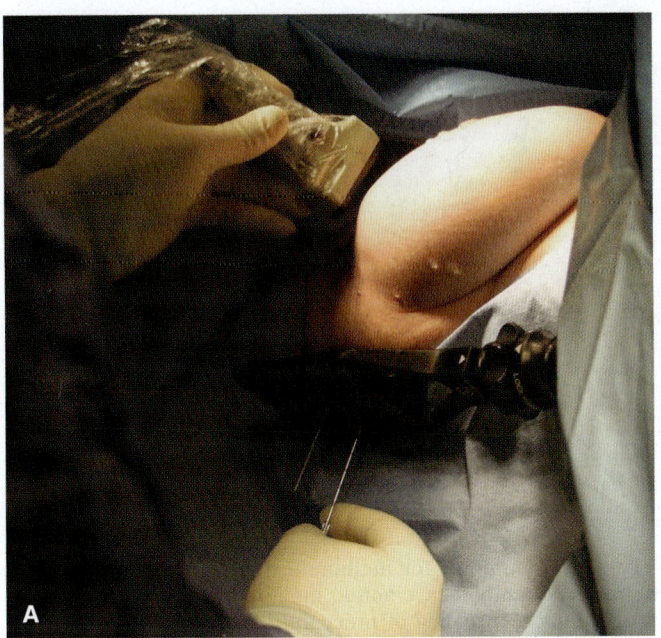
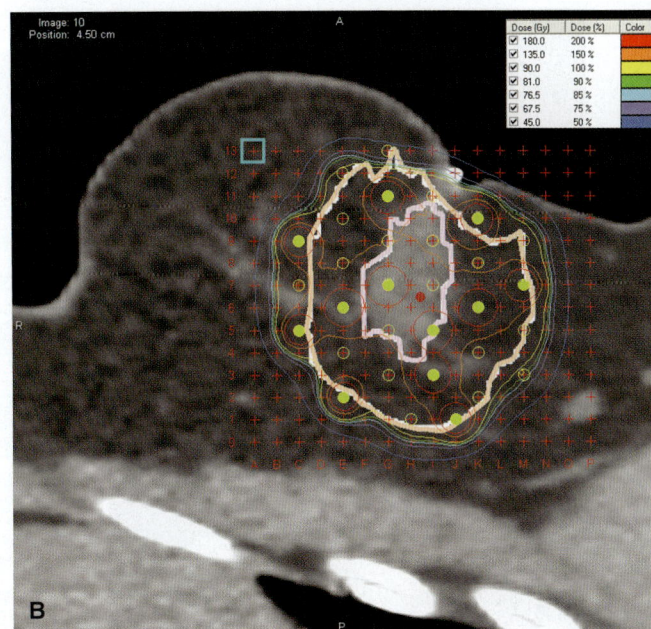

FIGURE 26.26. A: Intraoperative photograph demonstrating a template partial breast implant using iodine-125 seeds under ultrasound guidance. **B:** Sagittal computed tomography image to demonstrate the postoperative dosimetry of the implant. (Courtesy Dr. Jean-Phillipe Pignol.)

no effect was seen on distant metastases or overall survival. Functional parameters were well maintained post brachytherapy. PDR brachytherapy has been used in adults and children, either as a boost (for large tumors where compartmental surgery proved difficult) or as radical treatment.[239–241] Studies report excellent local control with good cosmetic results and acceptable toxicity, comparable to results achieved with LDR. However, a retrospective study of adjuvant LDR brachytherapy to pre- or postoperative IMRT in primary extremity sarcoma showed 5-year local control with IMRT to be better than that with brachytherapy (92% vs. 81%, $P = .04$). This is despite the fact that the IMRT group had significantly higher rates of adverse features (e.g., tumors over 10 cm in size and close or positive surgical margins).

Surface Applicators

Brachytherapy surface applicators can be used to treat a variety of superficial targets using LDR or PDR. For curved or irregular surface or thicker lesions a customized mold can be constructed, often using an acrylic or thermoplastic cast (see Fig. 26.28). The brachytherapy catheters can be laid directly onto the mold or used with a spacer to ensure uniform catheter distribution. When used with computerized optimization, this surface applicator technique has been shown to give dose distributions that are more homogeneous than those for conventional electron techniques.[242] A survey of members of ABS showed that many respondents preferred brachytherapy over EBRT because of shorter overall treatment times, conformality of treatment for irregular-shaped targets, and shallow dose deposition.[243] PDR carries the benefit of dose optimization, which allows the treatment depth to vary along different points of an individual catheter for lesions of varying thickness. Suitable superficial targets can also be treated with interstitial implants, which can give greater penetration of dose beneath the skin surface.

Surface applicator techniques have been used to treat primary tumors in both the radical and the palliative setting. A meta-analysis has shown that radiotherapy following surgery yields a lower keloid recurrence rate compared

---

TABLE 26.4 GENERAL RECOMMENDATIONS FOR STS BRACHYTHERAPY (INCORPORATING ABS GUIDELINES)
Discuss patient preoperatively in a multidisciplinary setting
Determine CTV by radiographic, surgical, and pathologic findings
Place catheters to encompass CTV, demarcate CTV with surgical clips if possible
Identify and demarcate normal structures that are at risk for complications
Cover tenuous wounds with well-vascularized flaps
Place microvascular anastomoses away from radiation target area
Use drains over catheters to act as a spacer to increase the distance of the wound from the implant
Use spacers (e.g., Gelfoam) to increase the distance between catheters and critical normal structures
Ensure catheters enter skin at least 1 cm from surgical incision
Space catheters at 1–1.5 cm intervals in parallel arrays
Secure catheters carefully, immobilizing extremity if necessary
Use CT to determine the CTV and OAR
Do not load catheters until after the 5th day postoperatively

Reprinted from Nag S, Shasha D, Janjan N, et al., The American Brachytherapy Society recommendations for brachytherapy of soft tissue sarcomas. *Int J Radiat Oncol Biol Phys* 2001;49(4):1033–1043. Copyright © 2001 Elsevier. With permission; Raut CP and Albert M. Soft Tissue Sarcoma Brachytherapy. In: Devlin PM, ed. *Brachytherapy: Applications and Techniques*. Philadelphia: Lippincott Williams and Wilkins, 2007:269–310. Reprinted by permission of Phillip M. Devlin.

FIGURE 26.27. Intraoperative photograph of a multicatheter interstitial pulsed dose rate brachytherapy implant following excision of a sarcoma of the upper back.

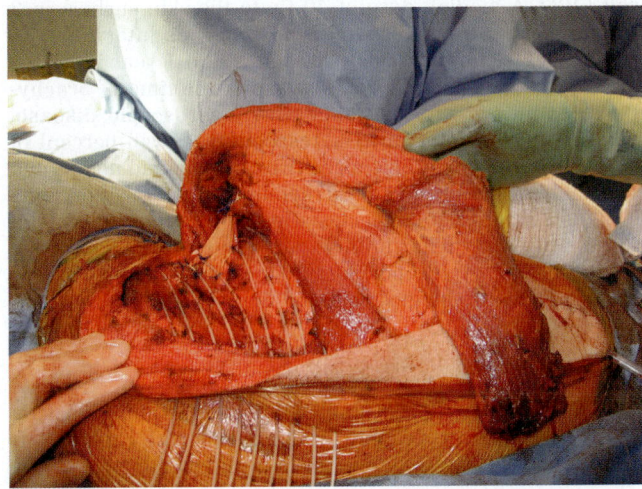

Section II

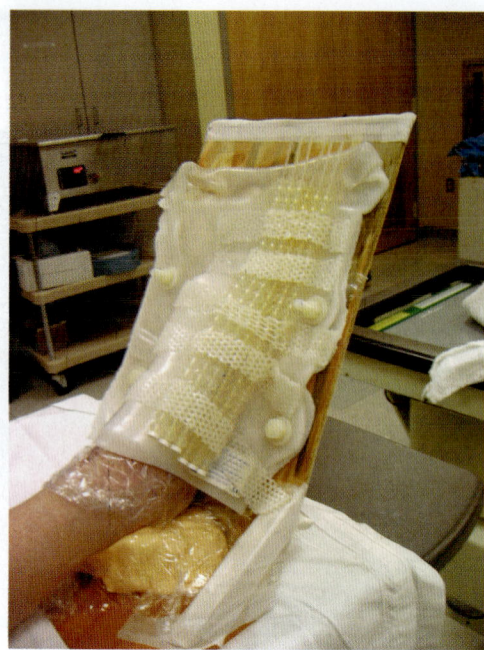

FIGURE 26.28. Surface applicator mold used to administer brachytherapy to the dorsum of the foot following incomplete excision of an STS.

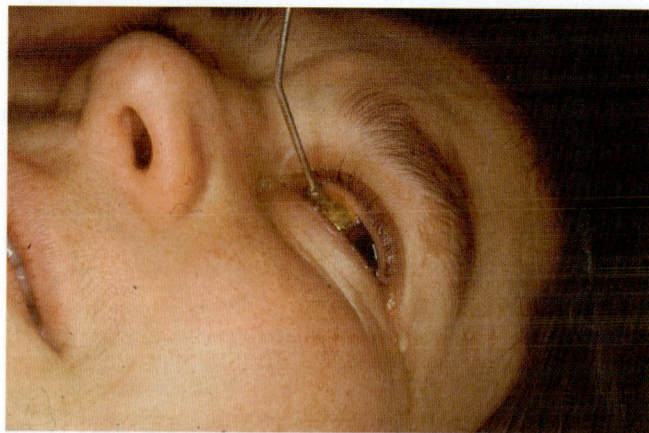

FIGURE 26.29. Patient receiving a strontium ophthalmic application. (Courtesy Dr. Steve Whitaker.)

to radiotherapy alone and that brachytherapy had the lowest recurrence rate when comparing radiotherapy modalities (15% for brachytherapy compared to 23% for photons and 23% for electrons).[244] There does not appear to be a difference in recurrence rate between LDR or HDR.[245]

Surface applicator brachytherapy techniques have been used to treat locally recurrent breast cancer following previous chest wall irradiation. Using LDR ^{192}Ir implanted into flexible silicone sheets delivered in 2 to 3 fractions at monthly intervals to administer a total dose of 65 Gy 2 to 4 mm below the skin surface, Delanian et al.[246] showed a complete regression of tumor in 9 of 11 patients. The two patients who did not respond died from pulmonary lymphangitis 4 and 5 months after brachytherapy. One patient developed a necrotic ulcer in the skin, which healed after 8 weeks of symptomatic treatment. One patient died from respiratory failure that may have been related to cumulative pulmonary toxicity, which must be considered as a treatment complication. Some patients also received interstitial implants in the chest wall, which would have increased the dose at depth to the previously irradiated tissue and to the underlying lung.

Harms et al. used PDR brachytherapy and flexible rubber surface applicator moulds in 58 patients with local recurrence of breast cancer who had received previous breast or chest wall EBRT. A median dose of 40 Gy to the skin surface in 2 fractions was administered at a median time interval of 31 days.[247] The local recurrence-free survival at 1 year was 96% for patients with microscopic disease at the time of brachytherapy and 89% for patients with macroscopic disease, and at 3 years, 75% and 71%, respectively. Seven percent of patients developed chronic ulcer, two of whom had undergone surgical treatment prior to reirradiation, and 50% of patients developed grade 3 telangiectasia in the treatment field. The skin toxicity was higher in this study, but this may have been a result of improved reporting of skin complications because the incidence of telangiectasia and fibrosis was not reported in the LDR study.

Ophthalmic Plaques

Ophthalmic brachytherapy applicators can be applied directly to the eye to deliver a highly localized dose with rapid falloff (see Fig. 26.29). These deliver dose to the conjunctiva of the eye, most commonly for malignant tumors of the conjunctiva such as squamous carcinoma, melanoma, and lymphoma or to prevent recurrence of pterygium following surgical excision. [125]I seeds are inserted into plaques formed of silicone, rubber inner seed holder with a gold exterior shield, and are then sutured to the sclera. [90]Sr and [106]Ru are manufactured as curved applicators, ^{90}Sr as a fixed diameter applicator (typically 12 mm) (see Fig. 26.30), and [106]Ru in a range of diameters. The eye is anesthetized with installation of local anesthetic eye drops. The applicator is soaked in an antiseptic solution, followed by double-rinsing in sterile saline. Sterile lubricant is then applied to the active surface of the applicator to lessen trauma to the cornea and sclera. The applicator is then gently applied over the area of bare sclera, adjacent limbus, and affected cornea and held in place by the operator for short applications or sutured to the sclera for longer applications. Undue pressure must be avoided, as this increases trauma and reduces the distance from the applicator to the lens, which is the dose-limiting normal tissue. If necessary, two treated fields can be overlapped if the area to be treated exceeds that of the active surface of the applicator though this, inevitably, carries a risk of increased acute and chronic sequelae. After treatment, the patient wears an eye patch for 2 hours until the local anesthetic wears off. Some degree of conjunctivitis is common and if mild, can be treated with antibiotic eye drops. If moderate to severe, steroid-containing eye drops should be used. Long-term sequelae are unusual but

FIGURE 26.30. Strontium ophthalmic applicator.

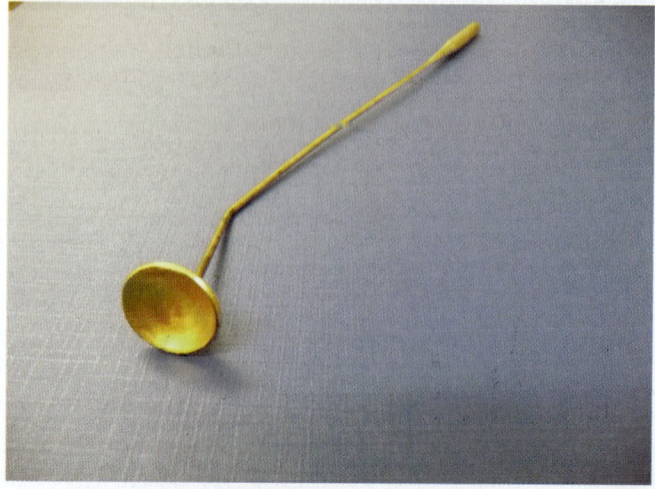

more likely with higher fraction size and higher total dose. Scleral ulceration is the most common complication in doses up to 52 Gy, with a small percentage of eyes developing symblepharon—fusion of the eyelid to the globe. Surgical trauma also plays a part in these sequelae. A small percentage of eyes will develop radiation-induced cataracts, again at higher doses (>45 Gy).

The Collaborative Ocular Melanoma Study (COMS) group conducted 2 randomized trials in North America, examining the use of ^{125}I for choroidal melanoma. The study, examining the use of ^{125}I brachytherapy versus enucleation for tumors of 3- to 8-mm depth, demonstrated no difference in survival and similar rates of toxicity[248,249] for the two techniques, thus supporting the use of [125]I. A SEER database analysis has shown similar survival outcomes for plaque brachytherapy compared to EBRT for choroidal melanoma.[250]

The use of Palladium-103 and Cesium-131 seeds has also been investigated with promising dosimetric results.[251,252] In fact, [103]Pd has similar efficacy to ^{125}I, but patients have an improved visual acuity following treatment with [103]Pd.[253] Modern dosimetry planning is being employed to investigate whether side effects may be lessened with optimal planning techniques.[252,254,255]

Strictly speaking, ^{90}Sr delivers high-dose-rate brachytherapy (a beta emitter with a typical dose rate of 100 Gy/hour compared to ^{125}I, a gamma emitter with a dose rate of 0.5 to 1 Gy/hour). Thus, ^{90}Sr delivers a single fraction treatment dose over 2 to 3 hours whereas ^{125}I delivers a treatment dose over 30 to 300 hours. The percentage depth dose in tissue falls from 100% at the surface to 4% at 4 mm, 1% at 6.5 mm, and 0.9% at 8 mm (corresponding to the anterior surface of the lens, equator, and posterior surface of the lens, respectively). Van Ginderdeuren et al. demonstrated a 90% 15-year tumor control for sclera melanoma using a ^{90}Sr applicator with a proportion of the recurrences at the edges possibly due to the small applicator size, using doses of 450 to 800 Gy at the sclera.[256] There was a 45% preservation of good vision, which was generally dependent on tumor position rather than dose delivered. Ruthenium-106 eye plaques can also be used and may become the beta emitter of choice as ^{90}Sr eye plaques gradually decay beyond useful dose delivery. They deliver similar results to ^{90}Sr and have even been used with thermotherapy to deliver improved outcomes.[257,258]

Pterygium is a benign proliferation of the conjunctiva over the cornea, occurring most commonly in areas with high sun exposure. Surgery can be performed for irritative symptoms, effects on vision, or cosmesis but carries a high recurrence rate. Locally applied ^{90}Sr has been used to decrease the rate of recurrence to as low as 0.5%,[259] using doses varying from 20 to 60 Gy in 1 to 6 fractions. The incidence of sclera complications is lower with fractionated treatment (4.5% vs. 1%). However, alternative treatments such as topical chemotherapy and conjunctival autografting are replacing ophthalmic plaque brachytherapy.[260,261] Brachytherapy should not be combined with topical chemotherapy because of the risk of scleral melting.

[90]Sr has been used in the treatment of neovascular age-related macular degeneration (AMD), visual impairment caused by neovascularization beneath the retinal pigment of the retina. However, a phase 3 trial comparing patients with active AMD who were already on a vascular endothelial growth factor (VEGF) inhibitor to either vitrectomy followed by 24-Gy brachytherapy (and continuing prn anti-VEGF treatment) to anti-VEGF treatment on an as-required basis alone showed that visual acuity and disease activity was actually better in the as-required anti-VEGF arm.[262]

Anus

Squamous cell carcinoma of the anus is a rare cancer that is usually treated with chemoradiotherapy with good rates of sphincter preservation. The most common site of relapse is

locally, and thus methods of local dose escalation have been explored. EBRT, preferably with chemotherapy, is necessary to treat the tumor and wider nodal area, and then the tumor boost can be delivered using brachytherapy.[263] Interstitial brachytherapy implants typically consist of a single-plane catheter implant using a plastic perineal template curved around the anus. Catheter placement may be optimized by the use of advanced imaging techniques such as three-dimensional endoluminal ultrasound.[264,265] Papillon described an LDR boost using ^{192}Ir to deliver 20 to 30 Gy in 221 patients 2 months after completing EBRT. Local control rates were comparable to surgical techniques, and 90% of patients with no evidence of relapse remained colostomy free.[266] It has been suggested that when using a split-course technique, if treatment time is extended over 80 days a brachytherapy boost may provide better local control than EBRT.[267] PDR techniques have been described with similar rates of disease control and toxicity to LDR.[268–270]

Esophagus

A phase 3 randomized trial of conventional stents versus stents loaded with ^{125}I seeds showed that median overall survival was increased in the irradiation stent arm compared to the conventional stent arm whereas side effects were similar.[271]

Biliary

Stent insertion with insertion of ^{125}I seeds for malignant obstructive jaundice has been shown to increase the mean stent patency time (191 days vs. 88 days) and the median survival (241 days vs. 142 days).[272]

Central Nervous System

Although initial treatment for glioblastoma has improved over the past decade, most glioblastomas recur, the majority of these within 2 cm of the original tumor cavity. Because the majority of patients will have received 60 Gy to the tumor at the time of initial diagnosis, retreatment techniques may be limited; ^{125}I seeds can be used to deliver a conformal dose of reirradiation. At the time of recurrence the surgeon will perform the maximal resection possible and implant ^{125}I seeds in the excision cavity at 0.5 to 1 cm intervals. This gives a highly localized boost, assuming the volume of disease residual is small because the dose falloff is rapid. The procedure appears to be well tolerated, and survival compares favorably to that of similar patients who did not receive brachytherapy.[253,273,274] The use of ^{125}I seeds at the time of initial radiotherapy has been investigated but no difference was seen in randomized trials.[275,276] Thus, if a boost is required, this technique has generally been supplanted by stereotactic radiosurgery, which does not require a second invasive surgical procedure. GliaSite balloon brachytherapy (GBST) is a technique in which a balloon is sited in the resection cavity and liquid ^{125}I is injected through a subcutaneous port for either primary or recurrent glioblastoma.[277] Results appear favorable.

[125]I seed placement has also been described in patients with paraspinal tumors with a low rate of toxicity and good local control rates.[190,196] The procedure was well tolerated, and no myelitis was seen despite cumulative cord doses of up to 167 Gy.

Customized yttrium-90 dural plaques have been used intraoperatively in patients with spinal or paraspinal sarcomas to deliver a high localized dose to the dura whilst minimizing the dose delivered to the underlying spinal cord (see Fig. 26.31). Local control rates are promising, and there were no acute or late complications from brachytherapy.[278]

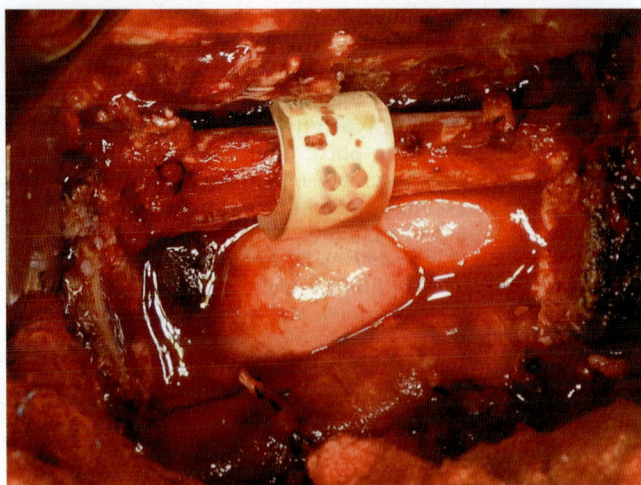

FIGURE 26.31. A dural plaque utilizes phosphorus-32 chemically bonded to a flexible polymeric film. The film is 0.5 mm thick and is backed by 4.5 mm of polycarbonate. Typical dose rates at time of treatment are in the 1.5 to 2.5 Gy/minute range.

CONCLUSIONS

The dosimetry of LDR brachytherapy treatment planning has evolved from estimation of dose delivered to accurate image-guided computer-optimized determinations of dose. Exact knowledge of the position of OAR and of the conformation of target volumes combined with dose optimization achievable with PDR computerized afterloading source delivery allows the brachytherapist to tailor dose delivery to highly specific ideals and deliver with great fidelity. This has allowed improved prediction of late toxicity and the possibility for dose escalation in areas with a high tumor burden.

Brachytherapy is particularly suited to subvolume dose escalation because of the ability to deliver a highly localized dose with rapid dose falloff in the surrounding tissue. This could allow increased dose to subvolumes within a CTV without a corresponding increase in dose to surrounding normal tissues. It is important with the advent of these new techniques that the accepted methods of practice are constantly reexamined to ensure that the patient receives the optimum treatment with the lowest risk of complications in the future.

Dosimetry remains critically important within modern brachytherapy practice. Knowledge of the established dosimetry systems is critical to prevent late complications resulting from suboptimal catheter placement with reliance on computerized optimization to overcome this. Modern imaging techniques can provide three-dimensional information about a target volume and surrounding normal structures. It is important to generate methods of incorporating this new knowledge with existing practice.

LDR and PDR brachytherapy often require indwelling applicators or catheters that necessitate hospitalization for the duration of the brachytherapy course. Surgical procedures are often required to place the brachytherapy seeds and applicators. Special skill and training are required to perform brachytherapy, much of which is not generally a part of oncology training rotations. Fellowships in brachytherapy are valuable but unfortunately rare.

LDR brachytherapy may result in a radiation exposure to medical staff, though remote afterloaders and PDR techniques minimize this exposure. HDR techniques are more prevalent than PDR due in part to the ability to treat more patients each day with a single machine. However, PDR still appeals to many centers, especially those with a high throughput of interstitial brachytherapy cases. Such a highly localized treatment can result in little or no dose to adjacent areas at risk of tumor spread, risking marginal misses and tumor recurrence if case selection is not carefully considered.

Brachytherapy also requires a high initial capital outlay. The choice of brachytherapy as a radiotherapeutic modality must be made carefully with consideration of many factors: patient centered, tumor centered and resource centered.

ACKNOWLEDGMENTS

We thank Dr. Juanita Crook, Mrs. Melanie Cunningham, Dr. George Dundas, Mr. Jorgen Hansen, Dr. Mira Keyes, Mr. Desmond O'Farrell, Dr. Howard Pai, Dr. Akila Viswanathan, Dr. Steve Whittaker, Dr. David Wazer, Dr. Dorin Todor, and Dr. Bob Kuske.

REFERENCES

1. Aronowitz J. Buried emanation; the development of seeds for permanent implantation. *Brachytherapy* 2002;1(3):167–178.
2. Souttar HS, *Radium and cancer*. London: William Heinemann, 1934.
3. International Commission on Radiation Units and Measurements. *Dose and volume specifications for reporting intracavitary therapy in gynecology (report 38)*. Bethesda, MD: International Commission on Radiation Units and Measurements, 1985:1–23.
4. Balgobind BV, et al. A review of the clinical experience in pulsed dose rate brachytherapy. *Br J Radiol* 2015;88:20150310.
5. Richter J, Baier K, Flentje M. Comparison of 60cobalt and 192iridium sources in high dose rate afterloading brachytherapy. *Strahlenther Onkol* 2008;184(4):187–192.
6. Pesee M, Krusun S, Padoongcharoen P. High dose rate cobalt-60 afterloading intracavitary therapy for cervical carcinoma in Srinagarind hospital—analysis of survival. *Asian Pac J Cancer Prev* 2010;11(6):1469–1471.
7. International Commission on Radiation Units and Measurements. *Prescribing, recording and reporting photon beam therapy (report 50)*. Bethesda, MD: International Commission on Radiation Units and Measurements, 1993.
8. Koedooder K, et al. Safety aspects of pulsed dose rate brachytherapy: analysis of errors in 1,300 treatment sessions. *Int J Radiat Oncol Biol Phys* 2008;70(3):953–960.
9. International Commission on Radiation Units and Measurements. *ICRU report 62: prescribing, recording and reporting photon beam therapy (supplement to ICRU report 50)*. Bethesda, MD: International Commission on Radiation Units and Measurements Inc., 1999.
10. Withers HR. The four Rs of radiotherapy. *Adv Radiat Biol* 1975;5:241–247.
11. Dale RG, Jones B. The clinical radiobiology of brachytherapy. *Br J Radiol* 1998;71:465–483.
12. Fu KK, et al. Radiobiology of brachytherapy. In: *Interstitial brachytherapy*. New York: Raven Press Ltd, 1990.
13. Fowler JF, van Limbergen EFM. Biological effect of pulsed dose rate brachytherapy with stepping sources if short half-times of repair are present in tissues. *Int J Radiat Oncol Biol Phys* 1997;37(4):877–883.
14. Visser AG, van den Aardweg GJ, Levendag PC. Pulsed dose rate and fractionated high dose rate brachytherapy: choice of brachytherapy schedules to replace low dose rate treatments. *Int J Radiat Oncol Biol Phys* 1996;34(2):497–505.
15. Paterson R. Studies in optimum dosages. *Br J Radiol* 1952;25:505–516.
16. Pierquin B, et al. Clinical observations on the time factor in interstitial radiotherapy using iridium-192. *Clin Radiol* 1973;24(4):506–509.
17. Haie-Meder C, et al. Analysis of complications in a prospective randomized trial comparing two brachytherapy low dose rates in cervical carcinoma. *Int J Radiat Oncol Biol Phys* 1994;29(5):953–960.
18. Lambin P, et al. Phase III trial comparing two low dose rates in brachytherapy of cervix carcinoma: report at 2 years. *Int J Radiat Oncol Biol Phys* 1993;25(3):405–412.
19. Mazeron JJ, et al. Influence of dose rate on local control of breast carcinomas treated by external beam irradiation plus iridium 192 implant. *Int J Radiat Oncol Biol Phys* 1991;21(5):1173–1177.
20. Mazeron JJ, et al. Prognostic factors of local outcome for T1, T2 carcinomas of oral tongue treated by Iridium 192 implantation. *Int J Radiat Oncol Biol Phys* 1990;19:281–286.
21. Slingerland JM, Tannock IF. Cell proliferation and cell death. In: Tannock IF, Hill RP, eds. *The basic science of oncology*. Singapore: McGraw Hill, 1998.
22. Ning S, Knox SJ. G2/M-phase arrest and death by apoptosis of HL60 cells irradiated with exponentially decreasing low-dose-rate gamma radiation. *Radiat Res* 1999;151(6):659–669.
23. Perez CA, et al. Carcinoma of the uterine cervix. Impact of prolongation of overall treatment time and timing of brachytherapy on outcome of radiation therapy. *Int J Radiat Oncol Biol Phys* 1995;32(5):1275–1288.
24. Pettereit DG, et al. The adverse effect of treatment prolongation in cervical carcinoma. *Int J Radiat Oncol Biol Phys* 1995;32(5):1301–1307.
25. Barton MB, et al. The effect of treatment time and treatment interruption on tumor control following radical radiotherapy of laryngeal cancer. *Radiother Oncol* 1992;23:137–143.
26. Cox JD, et al. Interruptions of high-dose radiation therapy decrease long-term survival of favorable patients with unresectable non small cell carcinoma of the lung: analysis of 1244 cases from 3 Radiation Therapy Oncology Group (RTOG) trials. *Int J Radiat Oncol Biol Phys* 1993;27:493–498.

27. Kapp DS, et al. Pretreatment prognostic factors in carcinoma of the uterine cervix: a multivariate analysis of the effect of age, stage, histology and blood counts on survival. *Int J Radiat Oncol Biol Phys* 1983;9:445–455.

28. Prosnitz RG, et al. Pretreatment anemia is correlated with the reduced effectiveness of radiation and concurrent chemotherapy in advanced head and neck cancer. *Int J Radiat Oncol Biol Phys* 2005;61(4):1087–1095.

29. Fyles AW, et al. Prognostic factors in patients with cervix cancer treated by radiation therapy: results of a multiple regression analysis. *Radiother Oncol* 1995;35(2):107–117.

30. Ling CC, et al. The variation of OER with dose rate. *Int J Radiat Oncol Biol Phys* 1985;11(7):1367–1373.

31. Meredith WJ. *Radium dosage: the manchester system*. Baltimore, MD: Williams and Wilkins, 1949.

32. Quimby E, Castro V. Calculation of dosage in interstitial radium therapy. *Am J Roentgenol* 1953;70(5):739–749.

33. Pierquin B, et al. The Paris system in interstitial radiation therapy. *Acta Radiol Oncol Radiat Phys Biol* 1978;17(1):33–48.

34. Hoskin PJ, Rembowska A. Dosimetry rules for brachytherapy using high dose rate remote afterloading implants. *Clin Oncol (R Coll Radiol)* 1998;10:226–230.

35. Cheron H, Rubens-Duval H. Apercu sur les resultants de la radiumtherapie des cancers d l'uterus et du vagin. *Bull Soc de'Obst et de Gynec de Par* 1913;2:418–429.

36. Lanciano RM, et al. Pretreatment and treatment factors associated with improved outcome in squamous cell carcinoma of the uterine cervix: a final report of the 1973 and 1978 patterns of care studies. *Int J Radiat Oncol Biol Phys* 1991;20:667–676.

37. Georg D, et al. Image-guided radiotherapy for cervix cancer: high-tech external beam therapy versus high-tech brachytherapy. *Int J Radiat Oncol Biol Phys* 2008;71(4):1272–1278.

38. Polo A. Pulsed dose rate brachytherapy. *Clin Transl Oncol* 2008;10:324–333.

39. Nag S, et al. The American Brachytherapy Society Survey of brachytherapy practice for carcinoma of the cervix in the United States. *Gynecol Oncol* 1999;73:111–118.

40. Viani GA, et al. Brachytherapy for cervix cancer: low-dose rate or high-dose rate brachytherapy-a meta-analysis of clinical trials. *J Exp Clin Cancer Res* 2009;28(1):47.

41. Patel FD, et al. Low dose rate vs. high dose rate brachytherapy in the treatment of carcinoma of the uterine cervix: a clinical trial. *Int J Radiat Oncol Biol Phys* 1993;28:335–341.

42. Orton CG, Seyedsadr M, Somnay A. Comparison of high and low dose rate remote afterloading for cervix cancer and the importance of fractionation. *Int J Radiat Oncol Biol Phys* 1991;21(6):1425–1434

43. Green J, et al. Concomitant chemotherapy and radiation therapy for cancer of the uterine cervix (Review). *Cochrane Database Syst Rev.* 2005;(3):CD002225.

44. Jürgenliemk-Schulz IM, et al. MRI-guided treatment-planning optimisation in intracavitary or combined intracavitary/interstitial PDR brachytherapy using tandem ovoid applicators in locally advanced cervical cancer. *Radiother Oncol* 2009;93(2):322–330.

45. Rath GK, et al. Pulsed-dose-rate intracavitary brachytherapy for cervical carcinoma: the AIIMS experience. *Am J Clin Oncol* 2010;33(3):238–241.

46. Lindegaard JC, et al. MRI-guided 3D optimization significantly improves DVH parameters of pulsed-dose-rate brachytherapy in locally advanced cervical cancer. *Int J Radiat Oncol Biol Phys* 2008;71(3):756–764.

47. Haie-Meder C, et al. Recommendations from the gynaecological (GYN) GEC ESTRO working group: concepts and terms in 3D image based 3D treatment planning in cervix cancer brachytherapy with emphasis on MRI assessment of GTV and CTV. *Radiother Oncol* 2005;74:235–245.

48. Potter R, et al. Recommendations from gynaecological (GYN) GEC ESTRO working group (II): Concepts and terms in 3D image-based treatment planning in cervix cancer brachytherapy-3D dose volume parameters and aspects of 3D image-based anatomy, radiation physics, radiobiology. *Radiother Oncol* 2006;78:67–77.

49. International Commission on Radiation Units and Measurements. ICRU report 89: prescribing, recording and reporting brachytherapy for cancer of the cervix. *J ICRU* 2013;13(1-2).

50. Mazeron, R., et al. Impact of treatment time and dose escalation on local control in locally advanced cervical cancer treated by chemoradiation and image-guided pulsed-dose rate adaptive brachytherapy. *Radiother Oncol* 2015;114(2):257–263.

51. Mazeron R, et al. Pulsed-dose rate image-guided adaptive brachytherapy in cervical cancer: dose-volume effect relationships for the rectum and bladder. *Radiother Oncol* 2015;116(2):226–232.

52. De Leeuw AA, et al. Applicator reconstruction and applicator shifts in 3D MR-based PDR brachytherapy of cervical cancer. *Radiother Oncol* 2009;93(2):341–346.

53. Morgia M, et al. Tumor and normal tissue dosimetry changes during MR-guided pulsed-dose-rate (PDR) brachytherapy for cervical cancer. *Radiother Oncol* 2013;107(1):46–51.

54. Kumar P, et al. Pulsed-dose-rate vs. high-dose-rate intracavitary radiotherapy for locally advanced carcinoma of cervix: a prospective randomized study. *Brachytherapy* 2016;15(3):327–332.

55. Lee LJ, et al. American Brachytherapy Society consensus guidelines for locally advanced carcinoma of the cervix. Part III: Low-dose-rate and pulsed-dose-rate brachytherapy. *Brachytherapy* 2012;11;53–57.

56. Benrath J, et al. Anaesthesia for brachytherapy—5½ yr of experience in 1622 procedures. *Br J Anaesth* 2006;96(2):195–200.

57. Weitmann HD, et al. Oxygenation status of cervical carcinomas before and during spinal anesthesia for application of brachytherapy. *Strahlenther Onkol* 2003;179(9):633–640.

58. Syed AMN, et al. Long term results of low dose rate interstitial intracavitary brachytherapy in the treatment of carcinoma of the cervix. *Int J Radiat Oncol Biol Phys* 2002;54(1):67–78.

59. Martinez A, Cox RS, Edmunsen GK. A multiple site perineal applicator (MUPIT) for treatment of locally advanced or recurrent prostatic, anorectal and gynaecologic malignancies. *Int J Radiat Oncol Biol Phys* 1984;10:297–305.

60. Hsu IC, et al. A comparison between tandem and ovoids and interstitial gynecologic template brachytherapy dosimetry using a hypothetical computer model. *Int J Radiat Oncol Biol Phys* 2002;52(2):538–543.

61. Albano M, Dumas I, Haie-Meder C. Brachytherapy at the Institut Gustave-Roussy: personalized vaginal mould applicator: technical modification and improvement. *Cancer Radiother* 2008;12(8):822–826.

62. American Cancer Society. *Cancer facts and figures*. Atlanta, GA: American Cancer Society, 1998.

63. Southcott BM. Carcinoma of the endometrium. *Drugs* 2001;61(10):1395–1405.

64. Heyman J. The so-called Stockholm method and the results of treatment of uterine cancer at the Radiumhemmet. *Acta Radiol* 1935;16:129.

65. Landgren RC, et al. Radiation of endometrial cancer in patients with medical contraindication to surgery or with unresectable lesions. *Am J Roentgenol* 1976;126:148–154.

66. Taghian A, et al. Radiation therapy alone for medically inoperable patients with adenocarcinoma of the endometrium. *Int J Radiat Oncol Biol Phys* 1988;15:1135–1140.

67. Fishman DA, et al. Radiation therapy as exclusive treatment for medically inoperable patients with stage I and II endometrioid carcinoma of the endometrium. *Gynecol Oncol* 1996;61:189–196.

68. Weitmann HD, et al. Pilot study in the treatment of endometrial carcinoma with 3D image-based high-dose-rate brachytherapy using modified Heyman packing: clinical experience and dose-volume histogram analysis. *Int J Radiat Oncol Biol Phys* 2005;62(2):468–478.

69. Simon N, Silverstone SM. Afterloading miniaturized 137-sources in the treatment of carcinoma of the uterus. *Int J Radiat Oncol Biol Phys* 1976;1:1017s–1021.

70. Coon D, et al. High-dose-rate Rotte "Y" applicator brachytherapy for definitive treatment of medically inoperable endometrial cancer: 10-year results. *Int J Radiat Oncol Biol Phys* 2008;71(3):779–783.

71. Beriwal S, et al. Comparison of 2D vs. 3D dosimetry for Rotte Y applicator high dose rate brachytherapy for medically inoperable endometrial cancer. *Technol Cancer Res Treat* 2005;5:1–6.

72. Stitt J. Dose specification for inoperable endometrial cancer: the Madison system. *Brachytherapy* 1991;2.32–34.

73. Rotte K. Modified Heyman technique HDR brachytherapy for endometrial cancer. In: Mould RF, ed. *Brachytherapy in the Nordic Countries*. Venendaal, Netherlands: Nucletron, 1992:16–28.

74. Potter R, Gerbaulet A, Haie-Meder C. Chapter 15: Endometrial cancer. In: Gerbaulet A, et al., eds. *The GEC ESTRO handbook of brachytherapy*. Leuven, Belgium: ESTRO, 2002.

75. Baker S, et al. The implementation of the Gynaecological Groupe Europeen de Curietherapie - European Society for Therapeutic Radiology and Oncology radiobiology considerations in the conversion of low dose rate to pulsed dose rate treatment schedules for gynaecological brachytherapy. *Clin Oncol (R Coll Radiol)* 2013;25(4):265–271.

76. Chadha M. Gynecologic brachytherapy-II: intravaginal brachytherapy for carcinoma of the endometrium. *Semin Radiat Oncol* 2002;12(1):53–61.

77. Ogino I, et al. High dose rate intracavitary brachytherapy for recurrent or residual lesions in the vaginal cuff: results in post-hysterectomy patients with carcinoma of the cervix. *Int J Gynecol Cancer* 2001;11(1):61–68.

78. Tangjitgamol S, Manusirivithaya S, Lertbutsayanukul C. Adjuvant therapy for early-stage endometrial cancer: a review. *Int J Gynecol Cancer* 2007;17(5):949–956.

79. Creutzberg CL, et al. Survival after relapse in patients with endometrial cancer: results from a randomised trial. *Gynecol Oncol* 2003;89(2):201–209.

80. Li S, et al. Effects of prescription depth, cylinder size, treatment length and curved end on dose in high-dose-rate vaginal brachytherapy. *Int J Radiat Oncol Biol Phys* 2007;67(4):1268–1277.

81. Onsrud M, Strickert T, Marthinsen ABL. Late reactions after postoperative high-dose-rate intravaginal brachytherapy for endometrial cancer: a comparison of standardized and individualized target volumes. *Int J Radiat Oncol Biol Phys* 2001;49(3):749–755.

82. Alektiar KM, et al. Intravaginal brachytherapy alone for intermediate-risk endometrial cancer. *Int J Radiat Oncol Biol Phys* 2005;62(1):111–117.

83. Hoskin PJ, Vidler K. Vaginal vault brachytherapy: the effect of varying bladder volumes on normal tissue dosimetry. *Br J Radiol* 2000;73:864–866.

84. Stewart AJ, et al. Bladder dosimetry in high dose rate vaginal cuff brachytherapy. *Int J Radiat Oncol Biol Phys* 2005;63(1):S339–S340.

85. Ashamalla H, et al. Brachytherapy improves outcomes in young men (≤60 years) with prostate cancer: a SEER analysis. *Brachytherapy* 2017;16(2):323–329.

86. Krauss DJ, et al. Favorable preliminary outcomes for men with low- and intermediate-risk prostate cancer treated with 19-Gy single-fraction high-dose-rate brachytherapy. *Int J Radiat Oncol Biol Phys* 2017;97(1):98–106.

87. Morris WJ, et al. Androgen Suppression Combined with Elective Nodal and Dose Escalated Radiation Therapy (the ASCENDE-RT trial): an analysis of survival endpoints for a randomized trial comparing a low-dose-rate brachytherapy boost to a dose-escalated external beam boost for high- and intermediate-risk prostate cancer. *Int J Radiat Oncol Biol Phys* 2016.

88. Joseph N, et al. A combined single high-dose rate brachytherapy boost with hypofractionated external beam radiotherapy results in a high rate of biochemical disease free survival in localised intermediate and high risk prostate cancer patients. *Radiother Oncol* 2016;121(2):299–303.

89. Lettmaier S, et al. Long term results of a prospective dose escalation phase-II trial: interstitial pulsed-dose-rate brachytherapy as boost for intermediate- and high-risk prostate cancer. *Radiother Oncol* 2012;104(2):181–186.

90. Pieters BR, et al. Treatment results of PDR brachytherapy combined with external beam radiotherapy in 106 patients with intermediate- to high-risk prostate cancer. *Int J Radiat Oncol Biol Phys* 2011;79(4):1037–1042.

91. Henriquez I, et al. Salvage brachytherapy in prostate local recurrence after radiation therapy: predicting factors for control and toxicity. *Radiat Oncol* 2014;9:102.

92. Burri RJ, et al. Long-term outcome and toxicity of salvage brachytherapy for local failure after initial radiotherapy for prostate cancer. *Int J Radiat Oncol Biol Phys* 2010;77(5):1338–1344.

93. D'Amico AV, et al. Real-time magnetic resonance image-guided interstitial brachytherapy in the treatment of select patients with clinically localized prostate cancer. *Int J Radiat Oncol Biol Phys* 1998;42(3):507–515.

94. Zaider M, et al. Treatment planning for prostate implants using magnetic-resonance spectroscopy imaging. *Int J Radiat Oncol Biol Phys* 2000;47(4):1085–1096.

95. Wallner K, Roy J, Harrison L. Tumor control and morbidity following transperineal iodine 125 implantation for stage T1/T2 prostatic carcinoma. *J Clin Oncol* 1996;14(2):449–453.

96. Holm H, et al. Transperineal iodine-125 seed implantation in prostate cancer guided by transrectal ultrasonography. *J Urol* 1983;130:283–286.

97. Blasko JC, et al. Prostate specific antigen based disease control following ultrasound guided 125iodine implantation for stage T1/T2 prostatic carcinoma. *J Urol* 1995;154(3):1096–1099.

98. Wallner K. Prostate brachytherapy under local anesthesia; lessons from the first 600 patients. *Brachytherapy* 2002;1(3):145–148.

99. Davis BJ, et al. American Brachytherapy Society consensus guidelines for transrectal ultrasound-guided permanent prostate brachytherapy. *Brachytherapy* 2012;11(1):6–19.

100. Prestidge BR, Winter K, Sanda MG, et al. Initial Report of NRG Oncology/RTOG 0232: a phase 3 study comparing combined external beam radiation and transperineal interstitial permanent brachytherapy with brachytherapy alone for selected patients with intermediate-risk prostatic carcinoma. *Int J Radiat Oncol Biol Phys* 2016;(2 Suppl):S4.

101. Bittner NH, et al. The American College of Radiology and the American Brachytherapy Society practice parameter for transperineal permanent brachytherapy of prostate cancer. *Brachytherapy* 2017;16(1):59–67.

102. Gaudet M, et al. Randomized non-inferiority trial of Bicalutamide and Dutasteride versus LHRH agonists for prostate volume reduction prior to I-125 permanent implant brachytherapy for prostate cancer. *Radiother Oncol* 2016; 118(1):141–147.

103. Potters L, et al. Examining the role of neoadjuvant androgen deprivation in patients undergoing prostate brachytherapy. *J Clin Oncol* 2000; 18(6):1187–1192.

104. Ho AY, et al. Radiation dose predicts for biochemical control in intermediate-risk prostate cancer patients treated with low-dose-rate brachytherapy. *Int J Radiat Oncol Biol Phys* 2009;75(1):16–22.

105. Merrick GS, et al. Impact of supplemental external beam radiotherapy and/or androgen deprivation therapy on biochemical outcome after permanent prostate brachytherapy. *Int J Radiat Oncol Biol Phys* 2005;61(1):32–43.

106. Lee WR. The role of androgen deprivation therapy combined with prostate brachytherapy. *Urology* 2002;60(3 Suppl 1):39–44.

107. Keyes M, et al. American Brachytherapy Society Task Group Report: use of androgen deprivation therapy with prostate brachytherapy—a systematic literature review. *Brachytherapy* 2017;16(2):245–265.

108. Cormack RA, Tempany CM, D'Amico AV. Optimizing target coverage by dosimetric feedback during prostate brachytherapy. *Int J Radiat Oncol Biol Phys* 2000;48(4):1245–1249.

109. Polo A, et al. PROBATE group of the GEC ESTRO. Review of intraoperative imaging and planning techniques in permanent seed prostate brachytherapy. *Radiother Oncol* 2010;94(1):12–23.

110. Nath R, et al. AAPM recommendations on dose prescription and reporting methods for permanent interstitial brachytherapy for prostate cancer: report of Task Group 137. *Med Phys* 2009;36(11):5310–5322.

111. Wallner K, et al. 125I versus 103Pd for low-risk prostate cancer: preliminary PSA outcomes from a prospective randomized multicenter trial. *Int J Radiat Oncol Biol Phys* 2003;57(5):1297–1303.

112. Potters L, et al. The effect of isotope selection on the prostate-specific antigen response in patients treated with permanent prostate brachytherapy. *Brachytherapy* 2003;2(1):26–31.

113. Peschel RE, et al. Iodine 125 versus palladium 103 implants for prostate cancer: clinical outcomes and complications. *Cancer* 2004;101(8):1701–1709.

114. Kollmeier MA, et al. A comparison of the impact of isotope ((125)I vs. (103)Pd) on toxicity and biochemical outcome after interstitial brachytherapy and external beam radiation therapy for clinically localized prostate cancer. *Brachytherapy* 2012;11(1):271–276.

115. Merrick GS, et al. Late rectal function after prostate brachytherapy. *Int J Radiat Oncol Biol Phys* 2003;57(1):42–48.

116. Merrick GS, et al. Short-term sexual function after prostate brachytherapy. *Int J Cancer* 2001;96(5):313–319.

117. Allen ZA, et al. Detailed urethral dosimetry in the evaluation of prostate brachytherapy-related urinary morbidity. *Int J Radiat Oncol Biol Phys* 2005; 62(4):981–987.

118. Fuller DB, Koziol JA, Feng AC. Prostate brachytherapy seed migration and dosimetry: analysis of stranded sources and other potential predictive factors. *Brachytherapy* 2004;3(1):10–19.

119. Nag S, et al. American Brachytherapy Society (ABS) recommendations for transperineal permanent brachytherapy of prostate cancer. *Int J Radiat Oncol Biol Phys* 1999;44(4):789–799.

120. Bice WS, et al. Recommendations for permanent prostate brachytherapy with (131)Cs: a consensus report from the Cesium Advisory Group. *Brachytherapy* 2008;7(4):290–296.

121. Nag S. Brachytherapy for prostate cancer: summary of American Brachytherapy Society recommendations. *Semin Urol Oncol* 2000;18(2):133–136.

122. Rosenthal SA, et al. American Society for Radiation Oncology (ASTRO) and American College of Radiology (ACR) practice guideline for the transperineal permanent brachytherapy of prostate cancer. *Int J Radiat Oncol Biol Phys* 2011;79(2):335–341.

123. Butler WM, et al. Isotope choice and the effect of edema on prostate brachytherapy dosimetry. *Med Phys* 2000;27(5):1067–1075.

124. Ash D, et al. ESTRO/EAU/EORTC recommendations on permanent seed implantation for localized prostate cancer. *Radiother Oncol* 2000;57(3):315–321.

125. Han BH, et al. Patient reported complications after prostate brachytherapy. *J Urol* 2001;166(3):953–957.

126. Blasko JC, et al. Brachytherapy for carcinoma of the prostate: techniques, patient selection, and clinical outcomes. *Semin Radiat Oncol* 2002; 12(1):81–94.

127. Keyes M, et al. Decline in urinary retention incidence in 805 patients after prostate brachytherapy: the effect of learning curve? *Int J Radiat Oncol Biol Phys* 2006;64(3):825–834.

128. Gillin MT, et al. Quality assurance methods for the first radiation therapy oncology group permanent prostate implant protocol. *Brachytherapy* 2006; 5(3):152–156.

129. Yu Y, et al. Permanent prostate seed implant brachytherapy: Report of the American Association of Physicists in Medicine task group no. 64. *Med Phys* 1999;26:2054–2076.

130. Hagan MP, et al. Regulatory evaluation of prostate volume implants: pitfalls of a retrospective assessment. *Brachytherapy* 2011; 10(5):385–394.

131. Keyes M, et al. Radiation Oncologists Quality Assurance Program in British Columbia Cancer Agency Provincial Prostate Brachytherapy Program. *Brachytherapy* 2011;10(Suppl 1):S78.

132. VA Office of Inspector General. Review of Brachytherapy Treatment of Prostate Cancer, Philadelphia, Pennsylvania and Other VA Medical Centres. Report No. 09-02815-143, 2010.

133. Kalkner KM, et al. Clinical outcome in patients with prostate cancer treated with external beam radiotherapy and high dose-rate iridium 192 brachytherapy boost: a 6-year follow-up. *Acta Oncol* 2007;46(7):909–917.

134. Phan TP, et al. High dose rate brachytherapy as a boost for the treatment of localized prostate cancer. *J Urol* 2007;177(1):123–127.

135. Soto DE, McLaughlin PW. Combined permanent implant and external-beam radiation therapy for prostate cancer. *Semin Radiat Oncol* 2008;18(1):23–34.

136. Sylvester JE, et al. 15-Year biochemical relapse free survival in clinical Stage T1-T3 prostate cancer following combined external beam radiotherapy and brachytherapy; Seattle experience. *Int J Radiat Oncol Biol Phys* 2007; 67(1):57–64.

137. Izard MA, et al. Six year experience of external beam radiotherapy, brachytherapy boost with a 1Ci (192)Ir source, and neoadjuvant hormonal manipulation for prostate cancer. *Int J Radiat Oncol Biol Phys* 2006;65(1):38–47.

138. Charyulu KK. Transperineal interstitial implantation of prostate cancer: a new method. *Int J Radiat Oncol Biol Phys* 1980;6(9):1261–1266.

139. Nickers P, et al. 192Ir low dose rate brachytherapy for boosting locally advanced prostate cancers after external beam radiotherapy: a phase II trial. *Radiother Oncol* 2006;79(3):329–334.

140. Syed AM, et al. Management of prostate carcinoma. Combination of pelvic lymphadenectomy, temporary Ir-192 implantation, and external irradiation. *Radiology* 1983;149(3):829–833.

141. Crook J. Radiation therapy for cancer of the penis. *Urol Clin North Am* 2010;37(3):435–443.

142. Gerbaulet A, Lambin P. Radiation therapy of cancer of the penis. Indications, advantages, and pitfalls. *Urol Clin North Am* 1992;19(2):325–332.

143. Crook JM, et al. American Brachytherapy Society-Groupe Europeen de Curietherapie-European Society of Therapeutic Radiation Oncology (ABS-GEC-ESTRO) consensus statement for penile brachytherapy. *Brachytherapy* 2013; 12(3):191–198.

144. Akimoto T, et al. Brachytherapy for penile cancer using silicon mold. *Oncology* 1997;54(1):23–27.

145. Neave F, et al. Carcinoma of the penis: a retrospective review of treatment with iridium mould and external beam irradiation. *Clin Oncol* 1993;5(4):207–210.

146. Chaudhary AJ, et al. Interstitial brachytherapy in carcinoma of the penis. *Strahlenther Onkol* 1999;175(1):17–20.

147. Crook J, Ma C, Grimard L. Radiation therapy in the management of the primary penile tumor: an update. *World J Urol* 2009;27(2):189–196.

148. Daly NJ, Douchez J, Combes PF. Treatment of carcinoma of the penis by iridium 192 wire implant. *Int J Radiat Oncol Biol Phys* 1982;8(7):1239–1243.

149. de Crevoisier R, et al. Long-term results of brachytherapy for carcinoma of the penis confined to the glans (N- or NX). *Int J Radiat Oncol Biol Phys* 2009;74(4):1150–1156.

150. Delannes M, et al. Iridium-192 interstitial therapy for squamous cell carcinoma of the penis. *Int J Radiat Oncol Biol Phys* 1992;24(3):479–483.

151. Crook J, Jezioranski J, Cygler JE. Penile brachytherapy: technical aspects and postimplant issues. *Brachytherapy* 2010;9(2):151–158.

152. Mazeron JJ, et al. Interstitial radiation therapy for carcinoma of the penis using iridium 192 wires: the Henri Mondor experience (1970-1979). *Int J Radiat Oncol Biol Phys* 1984;10(10):1891–1895.

153. Gomez-Iturriaga A, et al. The efficacy of hyperbaric oxygen therapy in the treatment of medically refractory soft tissue necrosis after penile brachytherapy. *Brachytherapy* 2011;10(6):491–497.

154. Kiltie AE, et al. Iridium-192 implantation for node-negative carcinoma of the penis: the Cookridge Hospital experience. *Clin Oncol* 2000;12(1):25–31.

155. Gerbaulet A, et al. Brachytherapy in cancer of the urethra. *Ann Urol (Paris)* 1994;28(6-7):312–317.

156. Milosevic MF, et al. Urethral carcinoma in women: results of treatment with primary radiotherapy. *Radiother Oncol* 2000;56(1):29–35.

157. James ND, et al. Radiotherapy with or without chemotherapy in muscle-invasive bladder cancer. *N Engl J Med* 2012;366(16):1477–1488.

158. Vashistha V, et al. Radical cystectomy compared to combined modality treatment for muscle-invasive bladder cancer: a systematic review and meta-analysis. *Int J Radiat Oncol Biol Phys* 2017;97(5):1002–1020.

159. Aluwini S, et al. Bladder function preservation with brachytherapy, external beam radiation therapy, and limited surgery in bladder cancer patients: long-term results [corrected]. *Int J Radiat Oncol Biol Phys* 2014;88(3):611–617.

160. Koning CC, et al. Brachytherapy after external beam radiotherapy and limited surgery preserves bladders for patients with solitary pT1-pT3 bladder tumors. *Ann Oncol* 2012;23(11):2948–2953.

161. Pieters BR, et al. GEC-ESTRO/ACROP recommendations for performing bladder-sparing treatment with brachytherapy for muscle-invasive bladder carcinoma. *Radiother Oncol* 2017;122(3):340–346.

162. Strnad V, et al. The role of pulsed-dose-rate brachytherapy in previously irradiated head-and-neck cancer. *Brachytherapy* 2003;2(3):158–163.

163. Peiffert D, et al. Pulsed dose rate brachytherapy in head and neck cancers. Feasibility study of a French cooperative group. *Radiother Oncol* 2001; 58:71–75.

164. Ziemlewski A, et al. Preliminary report of pulsed dose rate brachytherapy in head-and-neck cancer. *Strahlenther Onkol* 2007;183(9):512–516.

165. Strnad V, et al. Role of interstitial PDR brachytherapy in the treatment of oral and oropharyngeal cancer. A single-institute experience of 236 patients. *Strahlenther Onkol* 2005;181(12):762–767.

166. Mazeron JJ, et al. How to optimize therapeutic ratio in brachytherapy of head and neck squamous cell carcinoma? *Acta Oncol* 1998;37(6):583–591.

167. Haddad A, et al. A case-control study of patients with squamous cell carcinoma of the oral cavity and oropharynx treated with pulsed-dose-rate brachytherapy. *Brachytherapy* 2014;13(6):597–602.

168. Sresty NV, et al. Acquisition of equal or better planning results with interstitial brachytherapy when compared with intensity-modulated radiotherapy in tongue cancers. *Brachytherapy* 2010;9(3):235–238.

169. Eisbruch A, et al. Can IMRT or brachytherapy reduce dysphagia associated with chemoradiotherapy of head and neck cancer? The Michigan and Rotterdam experiences. *Int J Radiat Oncol Biol Phys* 2007;69(2 Suppl):S40–S42.

170. Melzner WJ, et al. Quality of interstitial PDR-brachytherapy-implants of head-and-neck-cancers: predictive factors for local control and late toxicity? *Radiother Oncol* 2007;82(2):167–173.

171. Kovács G, et al. GEC-ESTRO ACROP recommendations for head & neck brachytherapy in squamous cell carcinomas: 1st update - Improvement by cross sectional imaging based treatment planning and stepping source technology. *Radiother Oncol* 2017;122(2):248–254.

172. Mazeron JJ, et al. GEC-ESTRO recommendations for brachytherapy for head and neck squamous cell carcinomas. *Radiother Oncol* 2009;91:150–156.

173. Takácsi-Nagy Z, et al. American Brachytherapy Society Task Group Report: Combined external beam irradiation and interstitial brachytherapy for base of tongue tumors and other head and neck sites in the era of new technologies. *Brachytherapy* 2017;16(1):44–58.

174. Han P, et al. Head and neck brachytherapy. In: Devlin PM, ed. *Brachytherapy: applications and techniques.* Philadelphia: Lippincott Williams & Wilkins, 2007:49–92.

175. Paryani SB, et al. Iodine 125 suture implants in the management of advanced tumors in the neck attached to the carotid artery. *J Clin Oncol* 1985; 3(6):809–812.

176. Jiang YL, et al. CT-guided iodine-125 seed permanent implantation for recurrent head and neck cancers. *Radiat Oncol* 2010;5:68.

177. Beitler JJ, et al. Close or positive margins after surgical resection for the head and neck cancer patient: the addition of brachytherapy improves local control. *Int J Radiat Oncol Biol Phys* 1998;40(2):313–317.

178. Stannard C, et al. Iodine-125 brachytherapy in the management of squamous cell carcinoma of the oral cavity and oropharynx. *Brachytherapy* 2014; 13(4):405–412.

179. Gerbaulet A, van Limbergen E. Lip cancer. In: Gerbaulet A, et al., eds. *The GEC ESTRO handbook of brachytherapy.* Leuven, Belgium: ESTRO, 2002:227–236.

180. Serkies K, et al. Pulsed dose rate brachytherapy of lip cancer. *J Contemp Brachytherapy* 2013;5:144–147.

181. Johansson B, et al. Long term results of PDR brachytherapy for lip cancer. *J Contemp Brachytherapy* 2011;3:65–69.

182. Ash D, Gerbaulet A. Oral tongue cancer. In: Gerbaulet A, et al., eds. *The GEC ESTRO handbook of brachytherapy.* Leuven, Belgium: ESTRO, 2002.

183. Johansson B, et al. Pulsed dose rate brachytherapy as the boost in combination with external beam irradiation in base of tongue cancer. Long-term results from a uniform clinical series. *J Contemp Brachytherapy* 2011; 3(1):11–17.

184. Gerbaulet A, Mazeron JJ, Ash D. Floor of mouth cancer. In: Gerbaulet A, et al., eds. *The GEC ESTRO handbook of brachytherapy.* Leuven, Belgium: ESTRO, 2002.

185. Strnad V, et al. Reirradiation for recurrent head and neck cancer with salvage interstitial pulsed-dose-rate brachytherapy: long-term results. *Strahlenther Onkol* 2015;191(6):495–500.

186. Mutyala S, et al. Permanent iodine-125 interstitial planar seed brachytherapy for close or positive margins for thoracic malignancies. *Int J Radiat Oncol Biol Phys* 2010;76(4):1114–1120.

187. Hilaris BS, Martini N. Interstitial brachytherapy in cancer of the lung: a 20 year experience. *Int J Radiat Oncol Biol Phys* 1979;5(11):1951–1956.

188. Hilaris BS, et al. Value of perioperative brachytherapy in the management of non-oat cell carcinoma of the lung. *Int J Radiat Oncol Biol Phys* 1983; 9:1161–1166.

189. Hilaris BS, et al. Combined surgery, intraoperative brachytherapy and post-operative external radiation in stage III non-small cell lung cancer. *Cancer* 1985;55:1226–1231.

190. Armstrong JG, et al. Paraspinal tumors: techniques and results of brachytherapy. *Int J Radiat Oncol Biol Phys* 1991;20:787–790.

191. Fleischman EH, et al. Iodine 125 interstitial brachytherapy in the treatment of carcinoma of the lung. *J Surg Oncol* 1992;49(1):25–28.

192. Aye RW, et al. Extending the limits of lung cancer resection. *Am J Surg* 1993;165(5):572–576.

193. Nori D, Li X, Pugkhem T. Intraoperative brachytherapy using Gelfoam radioactive plaque implants for resected stage III non-small cell lung cancer with positive margin: a pilot study. *J Surg Oncol* 1995;60(4):257–261.

194. D'Amato TA, et al. Intraoperative brachytherapy following thoracoscopic wedge resection of stage I lung cancer. *Chest* 1998;114:1112–1115.

195. Chen A, et al. Intraoperative 125I brachytherapy for high-risk stage I non-small cell lung carcinoma. *Int J Radiat Oncol Biol Phys* 1999;44(5):1057–1063.

196. Rogers CL, et al. Surgery and permanent 125I seed paraspinal brachytherapy for malignant tumors with spinal cord compression. *Int J Radiat Oncol Biol Phys* 2002;54(2):505–513.

197. Lee W, et al. Limited resection for non-small cell lung cancer: observed local control with implantation of I-125 brachytherapy seeds. *Ann Thoracic Surg* 2003;75(1):237–242.

198. Santos R, et al. Comparison between sublobar resection and 125Iodine brachytherapy after sublobar resection in high-risk patients with stage I non small cell lung cancer. *Surgery* 2003;134:691–697.

199. Fernando HC, et al. Lobar and sublobar resection with and without brachytherapy for small stage IA non-small cell lung cancer. *J Thorac Cardiovasc Surg* 2005;129(2):261–267.

200. Voynov G, et al. Intraoperative 125I Vicryl mesh brachytherapy after sublobar resection for high-risk stage I non-small cell lung cancer. *Brachytherapy* 2005;4:278–285.

201. Birdas TJ, et al. Sublobar resection with brachytherapy versus lobectomy for stage IB nonsmall cell lung cancer. *Ann Thorac Surg* 2006;81:434–439.

202. Heelan RT, et al. Lung tumors: percutaneous implantation of I-125 sources with CT treatment planning. *Radiology* 1987;164(3):735–740.

203. Stewart AJ, et al. Intra-operative seed placement for thoracic malignancy-a review of technique, indications and published literature. *Brachytherapy* 2009;8(1):63–69.

204. Pisch J, et al. Placement of 125I implants with the da Vinci robotic system after video-assisted thoracoscopic wedge resection: a feasibility study. *Int J Radiat Oncol Biol Phys* 2004;60(3):928–932.

205. Marchese MJ, et al. A versatile permanent planar implant technique utilizing iodine-125 seeds imbedded in gelfoam. *Int J Radiat Oncol Biol Phys* 1984; 10(5):747–751.

206. Smith RP, et al. Dosimetric evaluation of radiation exposure during I-125 vicryl mesh implants: implications for ACOSOG z4032. *Ann Surg Oncol* 2007; 14(12):3610–3613.

207. Hall EJ. Radiation protection. In: Hall EJ, Giaccia AJ, eds. *Radiobiology for the radiologist.* Philadelphia: Lippincott Williams & Wilkins, 2006:224–239.

208. Stewart AJ, et al. Case reports to describe toxicity resulting from permanent radioactive seed implantation for mediastinal carcinoid tumor. *Brachytherapy* 2007;6(1):58–61.

209. Cormack RA, et al. Permanent planar iodine-125 implants: the dosimetric effect of geometric parameters for idealized source configurations. *Int J Radiat Oncol Biol Phys* 2007;69(4):1310–1315.

210. Chen H, et al. Comparison of cellular damage response to low-dose-rate 125I seed irradiation and high-dose-rate gamma irradiation in human lung cancer cells. *Brachytherapy* 2012;11(2):149–156.

211. El-Sherif A, et al. Outcomes of sublobar resection versus lobectomy for stage I non-small cell lung cancer: a 13 year analysis. *Ann Thorac Surg* 2006; 82:408–416.

212. Fernando HC, et al. Analysis of longitudinal quality-of-life data in high-risk operable patients with lung cancer: results from the ACOSOG Z4032 (Alliance) multicenter randomized trial. *J Thorac Cardiovasc Surg* 2015; 149(3):718–726.

213. Fernando HC, et al. Impact of brachytherapy on local recurrence rates after sublobar resection: results from ACOSOG Z4032 (Alliance), a phase III randomized trial for high-risk operable non-small-cell lung cancer. *J Clin Oncol* 2014; 32(23):2456–2462.

214. Stewart AJ, et al. American Brachytherapy Society Consensus Guidelines for thoracic brachytherapy for lung cancer. *Brachytherapy* 2016;15(1):1–11.

215. Veronesi U, et al. Twenty-year follow-up of a randomized study comparing breast-conserving surgery with radical mastectomy for early breast cancer. *N Eng J Med* 2002;347(16):1227–1232.

216. Clark M, et al. Effects of radiotherapy and of differences in the extent of surgery for early breast cancer on local recurrence and 15-year survival: an overview of the randomised trials. *Lancet* 2005;366(9503):2087–2106.

217. Fisher B, et al. Twenty-year follow-up of a randomized trial comparing total mastectomy, lumpectomy and lumpectomy plus irradiation for the treatment of invasive breast cancer. *N Eng J Med* 2002;347(16):1233–1241.

218. Huang E, et al. Classifying local disease recurrences after breast conservation therapy based on location and histology. New primary tumors have more favorable outcomes than true local disease recurrences. *Cancer* 2002; 95(10):2059–2067.

219. Fisher ER, et al. Pathologic findings from the National Surgical Adjuvant Breast Project (Protocol 6): II. Relation of local breast recurrence to multicentricity. *Cancer* 1986;57:1717–1724.

220. Livi L, et al. Accelerated partial breast irradiation using intensity-modulated radiotherapy versus whole breast irradiation: 5-year survival analysis of a phase 3 randomised controlled trial. *Eur J Cancer* 2015;51(4):451–463.

221. Veronesi U, et al. Intraoperative radiotherapy versus external radiotherapy for early breast cancer (ELIOT): a randomised controlled equivalence trial. *Lancet Oncol* 2013;14(13):1269–1277.
222. Vaidya JS, et al. An international randomised controlled trial to compare TARGeted Intraoperative radioTherapy (TARGIT) with conventional postoperative radiotherapy after breast-conserving surgery for women with early-stage breast cancer (the TARGIT-A trial). *Health Technol Assess* 2016;20(73):1–188.
223. Stewart AJ, et al. Does equivalent uniform dose affect toxicity for high dose rate brachytherapy using the MammoSite applicator? *Brachytherapy* 2009;8(2):138.
224. Holliday EB, et al. Lower mean heart dose with deep inspiration breath hold-whole breast irradiation compared with brachytherapy-based accelerated partial breast irradiation for women with left-sided tumors. *Pract Radiat Oncol* 2017;7(2):80–85.
225. Strnad V, et al. 5-year results of accelerated partial breast irradiation using sole interstitial multicatheter brachytherapy versus whole-breast irradiation with boost after breast-conserving surgery for low-risk invasive and in-situ carcinoma of the female breast: a randomised, phase 3, non-inferiority trial. *Lancet* 2016;387(10015):229–238.
226. Ott OJ, et al. GEC-ESTRO multicenter phase 3-trial: accelerated partial breast irradiation with interstitial multicatheter brachytherapy versus external beam whole breast irradiation: Early toxicity and patient compliance. *Radiother Oncol* 2016;120(1):119–123.
227. Polgar C, et al. Late side-effects and cosmetic results of accelerated partial breast irradiation with interstitial brachytherapy versus whole-breast irradiation after breast-conserving surgery for low-risk invasive and in-situ carcinoma of the female breast: 5-year results of a randomised, controlled, phase 3 trial. *Lancet Oncol* 2017;18(2):259–268.
228. Hannoun-Levi JM, et al. Accelerated partial breast irradiation with interstitial brachytherapy as second conservative treatment for ipsilateral breast tumour recurrence: multicentric study of the GEC-ESTRO Breast Cancer Working Group. *Radiother Oncol* 2013;108(2):226–231.
229. Pignol JP, et al. Report on the clinical outcomes of permanent breast seed implant for early-stage breast cancers. *Int J Radiat Oncol Biol Phys* 2015; 93(3):614–621.
230. Pignol JP, Keller BM, Ravi A. Doses to internal organs for various breast radiation techniques--implications on the risk of secondary cancers and cardiomyopathy. *Radiat Oncol* 2011;6:5.
231. Rosenberg AS, et al. The treatment of soft-tissue sarcomas of the extremities: prospective evaluations of (1) limb sparing surgery plus radiation therapy compared with amputation and (2) the role of adjuvant chemotherapy. *Ann Surg* 1982;196(3):305–315.
232. D'Adamo DR. Appraising the current role of chemotherapy for the treatment of sarcoma. *Semin Oncol* 2011;38(Suppl 3):S19–S29.
233. Henschke UK, Hilaris BS, Mahan GD. Afterloading in interstitial and intracavitary radiation therapy. *Am J Roentgenol Radium Ther Nucl Med* 1963; 90:386–395.
234. Naghavi AO, et al. American Brachytherapy Society consensus statement for soft tissue sarcoma brachytherapy. *Brachytherapy* 2017;16(3):466–489.
235. Holloway CL, et al. American Brachytherapy Society (ABS) consensus statement for sarcoma brachytherapy. *Brachytherapy* 2013;12(3):179–190.
236. Naghavi AO, et al. American Brachytherapy Society consensus statement for soft tissue sarcoma brachytherapy. *Brachytherapy* 2017;16(3):466–489.
237. Collins JE, Paine CH, Ellis F. Treatment of connective tissue sarcomas by local excision followed by radioactive implant. *Clin Radiol* 1976;27(1):39–41.
238. Pisters PW, et al. Long-term results of a prospective randomized trial of adjuvant brachytherapy in soft tissue sarcoma. *J Clin Oncol* 1996;14(3):859–868.
239. Muhic A, et al. Local control and survival in patients with soft tissue sarcomas treated with limb sparing surgery in combination with interstitial brachytherapy and external radiation. *Radiother Oncol* 2008;88(3):382–387.
240. Lazzaro G, et al. Pulsed dose-rate perioperative interstitial brachytherapy for soft tissue sarcomas of the extremities and skeletal muscles of the trunk. *Ann Surg Oncol* 2005;12(11):935–942.
241. Pötter R, et al. Brachytherapy in the combined modality treatment of pediatric malignancies. Principles and preliminary experience with treatment of soft tissue sarcoma (recurrence) and Ewing's sarcoma. *Klin Padiatr* 1995;207(4):164–173.
242. Stewart AJ, et al. CT computer optimized high dose rate brachytherapy with surface applicator technique for scar boost radiation following breast reconstruction surgery. *Brachytherapy* 2005;4(3):224–229.
243. Likhacheva AO, et al. Skin surface brachytherapy: A survey of contemporary practice patterns. *Brachytherapy* 2017;16(1):223–229.
244. Mankowski P, et al. Optimizing radiotherapy for keloids: a meta-analysis systematic review comparing recurrence rates between different radiation modalities. *Ann Plast Surg* 2017;78(4):403–411.
245. De Cicco L, et al. Postoperative management of keloids: low-dose-rate and high-dose-rate brachytherapy. *Brachytherapy* 2014;13(5):508–513.
246. Delanian S, et al. Iridium 192 plesiocurietherapy using silicone elastomer plates for extensive locally recurrent breast cancer following chest wall irradiation. *Int J Radiat Oncol Biol Phys* 1992;22:1099–1104.
247. Harms W, et al. Results of chest wall reirradiation using pulsed dose rate (PDR) brachytherapy molds for breast cancer local recurrences. *Int J Radiat Oncol Biol Phys* 2001;49(1):205–210.
248. Collaborative Ocular Melanoma Study Group. The COMS randomized trial of iodine 125 brachytherapy for choroidal melanoma: V. Twelve-year mortality rates and prognostic factors: COMS report No. 28. *Arch Ophthalmol* 2006;124(12):1684–1693.
249. Hawkins BS. Collaborative ocular melanoma study randomized trial of I-125 brachytherapy. *Clin Trials* 2011;8(5):661–673.
250. Abrams MJ, et al. Brachytherapy vs. external beam radiotherapy for choroidal melanoma: Survival and patterns-of-care analyses. *Brachytherapy* 2016; 15(2):216–223.
251. Zhang H, et al. A comprehensive dosimetric comparison between (131)Cs and (125)I brachytherapy sources for COMS eye plaque implant. *Brachytherapy* 2010;9(4):362–372.
252. Thomson RM, Rogers DW. Monte Carlo dosimetry for 125I and 103Pd eye plaque brachytherapy with various seed models. *Med Phys* 2010;37(1):368–376.
253. Patel S, et al. Permanent iodine-125 interstitial implants for the treatment of recurrent glioblastoma multiforme. *Neuro-surgery* 2000;46:1123–1128.
254. Asadi SO, Masoudi SE, Shahriari MA. The effects of variations in the density and composition of eye materials on ophthalmic brachytherapy dosimetry. *Med Dosim* 2012;37(1):1–4.
255. Rivard MJ, et al. Comparison of dose calculation methods for brachytherapy of intraocular tumors. *Med Phys* 2011;38(1):306–316.
256. van Ginderdeuren R, van Limbergen E, Spileers W. 18 years' experience with high dose rate strontium-90 brachytherapy of small to medium sized posterior uveal melanoma. *Br J Opthalmol* 2005;89:1306–1310.
257. Verschueren KM, et al. Long-term outcomes of eye-conserving treatment with Ruthenium(106) brachytherapy for choroidal melanoma. *Radiother Oncol* 2010;95(3):332–338.
258. Yarovoy AA, Magaramov DA, Bulgakova ES. The comparison of ruthenium brachytherapy and simultaneous transpupillary thermotherapy of choroidal melanoma with brachytherapy alone. *Brachytherapy* 2012;11(3):224–229.
259. Smitt MC, Donaldson SS. Radiation Therapy for benign disease of the orbit. *Semin Radiat Oncol* 1999;9(2):179–189.
260. Kheirkhah A, et al. Randomized trial of pterygium surgery with mitomycin c application using conjunctival autograft versus conjunctival-limbal autograft. *Ophthalmology* 2012;119(2):227–232.
261. Ang LP, Chua JL, Tan DT. Current concepts and techniques in pterygium treatment. *Curr Opin Ophthalmol* 2007;18:308–313.
262. Jackson TL, et al. Epimacular brachytherapy for previously treated neovascular age-related macular degeneration (MERLOT): a phase 3 randomized controlled trial. *Ophthalmology* 2016;123(6):1287–1296.
263. John MJ, et al. Anal cancer: American College of Radiology. ACR appropriateness criteria. *Radiology* 2000;215 (Suppl):1501–1511.
264. Christensen AF, Nielsen BM, Engelholm SA. Three-dimensional endoluminal ultrasound-guided interstitial brachytherapy in patients with anal cancer. *Acta Radiol* 2008;49(2):132–137.
265. Doniec JM, et al. Multimodal therapy of anal cancer added by new endosonographic-guided brachytherapy. *Surg Endosc* 2006;20(4):673–678.
266. Papillon J, et al. Interstitial curietherapy in the conservative treatment of anal and rectal cancers. *Int J Radiat Oncol Biol Phys* 1989;17(6):1161–1169.
267. Hannoun-Levi JM, et al. High-dose split-course radiation therapy for anal cancer: outcome analysis regarding the boost strategy (CORS-03 study). *Int J Radiat Oncol Biol Phys* 2011;80(3):712–720.
268. López Guerra JL, et al. Twenty-year experience in the management of squamous cell anal canal carcinoma with interstitial brachytherapy. *Clin Transl Oncol* 2011;13(7):472–479.
269. Widder J, et al. Radiation dose associated with local control in advanced anal cancer: retrospective analysis of 129 patients. *Radiother Oncol* 2008; 87(3):367–375.
270. Bruna A, et al. Treatment of squamous cell anal canal carcinoma (SCACC) with pulsed dose rate brachytherapy: a retrospective study. *Radiother Oncol* 2006;79(1):75–79.
271. Zhu HD, et al. Conventional stents versus stents loaded with (125)iodine seeds for the treatment of unresectable oesophageal cancer: a multicentre, randomised phase 3 trial. *Lancet Oncol* 2014;15(6):612–619.
272. Hasimu A, et al. Comparative study of percutaneous transhepatic biliary stent placement with or without iodine-125 seeds for treating patients with malignant biliary obstruction. *J Vasc Interv Radiol* 2017;28(4):583–593.
273. Larson DA, et al. Permanent iodine 125 brachytherapy in patients with progressive or recurrent glioblastoma multiforme. *Neuro Oncol* 2004;6(2):119–126.
274. Scharfen CO, et al. High activity iodine-125 interstitial implant for gliomas. *Int J Radiat Oncol Biol Phys* 1992;24:583–591.
275. Selker RG, et al. The Brain Tumor Cooperative Group NIH Trial 87-01: a randomized comparison of surgery, external radiotherapy, and carmustine versus surgery, interstitial radiotherapy boost, external radiation therapy, and carmustine. *Neurosurgery* 2002;51(2):343–355.
276. Laperriere NJ, et al. Randomized study of brachytherapy in the initial management of patients with malignant astrocytoma. *Int J Radiat Oncol Biol Phys* 1998;41(5):1005–1011.
277. Kleinberg, L.R., et al. Outcome of Adult Brain Tumor Consortium (ABTC) prospective dose-finding trials of I-125 balloon brachytherapy in high-grade gliomas: challenges in clinical trial design and technology development when MRI treatment effect and recurrence appear similar. *J Radiat Oncol* 2015;4(3):235–241.
278. DeLaney TF, et al. Intraoperative dural irradiation by customized 192iridium and 90yttrium brachytherapy plaques. *Int J Radiat Oncol Biol Phys* 2003;57(1):239–245.
279. Remonnay R, et al. Economic assessment of pulsed dose-rate (PDR) brachytherapy with optimized dose distribution for cervix carcinoma. *Cancer Radiother* 2010;14(3):161–168.
280. Expert Panel on Radiation Oncology-Prostate, et al. American College of Radiology Appropriateness Criteria permanent source brachytherapy for prostate cancer. *Brachytherapy* 2011;10(5):357–362.
281. Nag S, et al. The American Brachytherapy Society recommendations for brachytherapy of soft tissue sarcomas. *Int J Radiat Oncol Biol Phys* 2001;49(4):1033–1043.
282. Raut CP, Albert M. Soft tissue sarcoma brachytherapy. In: Devlin PM, ed. *Brachytherapy applications and techniques*. Philadelphia: Lippincott Williams & Wilkins, 2007:269–310.

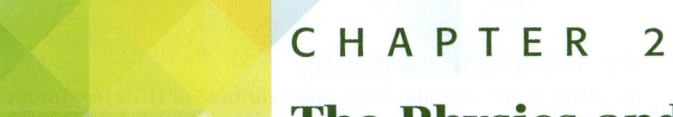

CHAPTER 27

The Physics and Dosimetry of High Dose Rate Brachytherapy

Bruce Thomadsen and Rupak K. Das

NATURE OF HIGH DOSE RATE BRACHYTHERAPY

Conventional brachytherapy was developed very soon after the discovery of radium. The limited amount of radium that could be packed into the needles and tubes dictated the use of many sources to deliver a treatment dose through a target volume, and even with many sources, the delivery of the dose required durations from 1 day to 1 week. For the most part, when new radionuclides became available, they matched the strength of the radium sources to facilitate application of the clinical experience gained through the decades of radium treatments. This conventional treatment format describes low dose rate (LDR) brachytherapy, as discussed in detail in Chapter 25.

Beginning around 1962, a new approach to brachytherapy developed. Using very intense, small sources (usually of ^{60}Co in the early machines and often three in number) on the ends of cables, a treatment unit would move the source through the volume to be treated, delivering the radiation in a relatively short time (<1 hour). The rapid treatment delivery gave these treatments the name high dose rate (HDR) brachytherapy. The original units most often oscillated the source through a catheter's treatment length, a method in common use until the modern generation of units developed in the early 1980s, described later. The treatments took so little time that the therapy proceeded on an outpatient basis. However, for reasons discussed later in this chapter, the treatment regimen usually entailed several fractions delivered over days or weeks.

The modern HDR units move a single source through the treatment volume in a stepwise fashion, moving at intervals, determined by the machine construction and the operator, to positions where the source pauses (dwell positions) for durations (dwell times) determined through optimization procedures.

Advantages and Disadvantages

Advantages of HDR brachytherapy over LDR include the following:

1. *Optimization.* The stepping-source design permits very fine control of the source position through the target volume. In most treatments, the determination of the dwell times comes from inverse planning, that is, specifying the doses desired at various locations and using some algorithm to calculate the dwell times that best fit the dose specifications. The map of how long the source dwells at each possible dwell position can be finely tailored to the geometry and needs of the particular patient because of the wide range of dwell times available. This process constitutes *optimization.* Although optimization is possible, and frequently used, with LDR applications, it forms a more natural part of the planning process with HDR brachytherapy.

2. *Immobilization and stability.* The relatively short duration of the HDR treatments allows better stability of many intracavitary treatment applicators during the treatment and, thus, higher precision in conforming the dose to the target. In addition to simply not giving much time for applicator motion, the applicator and the patient can both be immobilized with respect to the treatment table over the duration of the treatment. Such fixation is not possible with LDR brachytherapy because the patient would not tolerate the immobility for long periods. Interstitial cases may or may not exhibit better stability. The needles often tend to slide outward over the time that prostate implants remain in the patient, even with a template sutured to the patient that fixes the needles. In such a patient, the needles' positions require adjustment before each fraction but move very little during the treatment delivery. Performing the same treatment using LDR brachytherapy would include needle movement during the long, slow delivery and require larger margins around the clinical target volume (CTV). On the other hand, head and neck implants, with buttons anchoring the catheters at both ends, may allow very little movement from the time of insertion through removal. Such cases would not find improvement in stability with HDR brachytherapy.

3. *Dose reduction to normal tissue.* Again, the short duration of HDR intracavitary treatments often allows displacement of normal tissue structure to a greater extent than with LDR treatments. This holds true for gynecologic and oral intracavitary cases but not for intraluminal applications, such as endoesophageal or endobronchial treatments. Most interstitial cases cannot make use of this feature because the needles or catheters fix all the tissues in place. Exceptions are mostly in the head, where the tongue sometimes can be moved away from the treatment site.

4. *Outpatient treatment.* Most HDR patients receive treatment as an outpatient. Exceptions include patients with indwelling needles such as prostate or gynecologic implants delivered in multiple fractions. Patients containing plastic catheters that enter the patient on one end and exit the patient on the other (i.e., not with sharp needle tips poking into flesh) almost always leave the hospital between fractions. All intracavitary treatments are on an outpatient basis, unless there are medical conditions that keep the patient in the hospital between fractions. Outpatient treatments present many advantages over the inpatient treatments characteristic of LDR brachytherapy:

   - *Patient comfort.* Patients confined to a room during LDR treatments often feel closed in. Compounding the claustrophobic effects, radiation safety considerations limit the time nursing staff can spend with the patient (sometime very severely), leading the patient to feel like a pariah.

   - *Patient health.* Many LDR brachytherapy applications require the patients to stay in bed, increasing the probability of thrombosis or bedsores. Although pneumatic socks greatly reduce the likelihood of thrombosis, aching muscles from immobility still create discomfort. In many cases, patients who could not tolerate protracted LDR treatments will be able to receive their treatments using HDR techniques.

   - *Economics.* The cost of staying in the hospital greatly exceeds that of outpatient treatment. Counterbalancing the cost of hospitalization, the costs of the HDR remote afterloading equipment far exceed those for LDR applications. However, the HDR equipment costs quickly become amortized with a modest patient load, whereas the hospitalization costs remain constant, or continually increasing, for each LDR brachytherapy patient.

5. *Less discomfort due to small size.* Because the encapsulated HDR source is only 1 mm or less in diameter, the gynecologic intrauterine tandem need only be 3 mm in diameter, compared with 7 mm for the standard LDR tandem. Another way of looking at this comparison is to recognize that the diameter of the HDR tandem equals the smallest size dilator used to stretch the cervical os to accept the LDR tandem. Much of the pain and discomfort from a cervical cancer treatment come during the dilation. Eliminating that step eliminates much of that pain. Some facilities use only light sedation for the HDR tandem insertion rather than a general anesthetic, as is common with LDR procedures.

6. *Elimination of delays.* When applications fail to follow a plan or when plans have to change because of a finding in the operating room during the procedure, HDR treatments can still proceed following localization with little, if any, delay. LDR treatments likely would require ordering new sources to match the new situation and a delay in treatment to await delivery. The HDR model eliminates extra charges accruing from multiple-source orders.

7. *Intraoperative procedures.* HDR brachytherapy allows treatment intraoperatively, with suitable shielding in the operating room. With the short duration for dose delivery, a surgeon can add placement of the applicator and treatment of the patient to surgery with little additional time.

8. *Radiation safety.* HDR brachytherapy eliminates radiation exposure to personnel.

Unfortunately, HDR brachytherapy carries with it the following disadvantages:

1. *Radiobiology.* Compared with LDR brachytherapy, HDR treatments have worse therapeutic ratios, that is, the amount of damage to tumor cells compared with damage to normal tissue cells for the same dose. The damage to both types of cells per unit dose increases with dose rate, but the increase is greater for normal cells. Just as with external beam radiotherapy, which also is HDR delivery, fractionating the treatment mitigates this effect. Although LDR therapy usually entails a single session or two, most curative HDR regimens use three or more fractions. The next section discusses the radiobiology in greater detail.

2. *Error hazard.* The increased complexity of the procedures and the compressed time frame of delivery increase the probability of errors in the treatment compared with LDR therapy.

3. *Potential for very high radiation doses to patients and unit operators following failure of the source to retract.* The HDR source can deliver 7.4 Gy/min at 1 cm in the patient. If the source stops moving or separates from the drive cable, serious injury occurs in a short time.

4. *Resources.* HDR treatments demand more resources than do LDR treatments:
   - *Personnel.* Because many HDR treatments proceed quickly from placement of the treatment appliance to delivery of the treatment, all of the persons involved with the treatment must be available at the same time or in relatively quick secession. That means that the facility must have sufficient staffing to release these persons from other duties on demand of the HDR brachytherapy cases.
   - *Economics.* The HDR afterloading equipment comes with a large initial investment (at the time of writing ~$500,000 to $1,000,000), not including the significant costs of shielding the treatment room and the increased cost for all the treatment applicators and supplies.

Radiobiologic Dosimetry

Because of the radiobiologic disadvantage of HDR treatments, considerable care must be taken in planning the time course of the therapy regimen. The following discussion is intended as a supplement to that in Chapters 2, 3, 13, 14, 25, 26 and 28 of this book. One of the important tools for such planning is the linear-quadratic (LQ) model for biologic response.

The Linear-Quadratic Model

The basis for the model for biologic response to radiation stems from an approximation to the cell survival curves as shown in Figure 27.1.

Several models have been used over the years to describe the shape of the curve, each giving different insights into the interaction of the radiation and the organism irradiated. One of the more useful when investigating radiotherapy regimen is the LQ model.[1-3]

This model approximates the cell survival, S, a function of dose, D, as

$$S = e^{-\alpha D - \beta D^2} \tag{1}$$

Like any model, this equation fits the curves well over a particular range—in this case, the ranges of doses and dose rates used in radiotherapy—which makes it useful. It can also shed some light on biologic underpinnings. However, the model should not be seen as a true and complete description and explanation of a complex biologic phenomenon.

The curves shown apply to a single exposure of the cells over a short period of time at given dose rate. As can be seen, the effect of dose rate markedly changes the survival of the cells. This discussion need only consider the two components of the exponent in Eq. (1). Conceptually, the first term, αD, corresponds to damage to the cells when a single charged-particle track breaks both sides of a DNA molecule rung (e.g., both a guanine and a cytosine), referred to as a double-strand break. This form of killing the cells requires a double-strand break. The surviving fraction depends only on the dose, and the effect does not depend on the dose rate. The second term, βD^2, represents damage done when one charged-particle path breaks the bonds on one side of the DNA rung, say the guanine, and a different track breaks the other side (the cytosine). After the break on the first side, called a single-strand break, the DNA attempts repair. Because of the remaining cytosine on the opposite side, only a guanine will fit into the hole left on the damaged side. The nucleus contains many free guanine molecules, and one will be attracted to the opening and heal the wound. The repair takes place with a half-time of T_{bio}, which corresponds to a repair rate of

$$\mu = 0.693 / T_{bio}. \tag{2}$$

Because the repair takes some time, there is a window in which the second break must take place for the entire rung to be removed. If the second hit takes place after repair of the first, the damage still only forms a single-strand break, and the opposite side must be hit again to form a double-side break. Because forming a double-strand break in this way requires two independent hits, the probability follows D^2. Because the second hit must occur before the repair of the first, the incidence of double-strand breaks depends on the dose rate. Frequently, calculations use a value for T_{bio} of 1.5 hours, although most normal tissues probably have a more complicated repair pattern, with a fast component of about 20 minutes and a longer one of about 2 hours (see Chapters 3 and 14).

The surviving fraction also depends on the values of α and β. These parameters are characteristic of the tissue being irradiated and the type of tissue injury being caused. The actual values are often not well known, and large variations in most tissues have been reported. However, in general, the values of

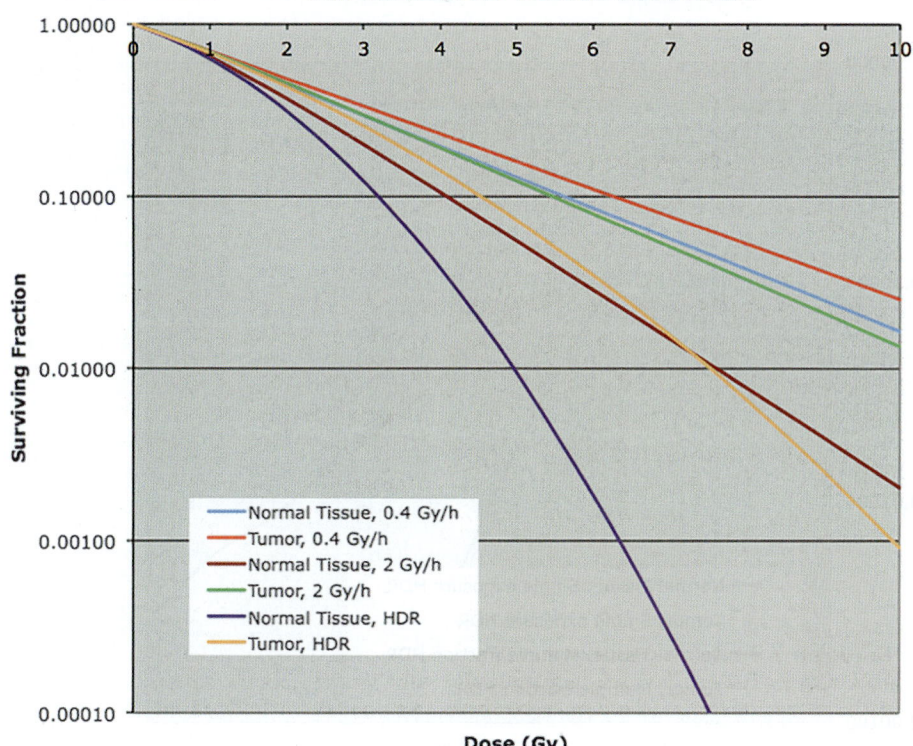

FIGURE 27.1. Typical cell survival curves with dose on the abscissa and surviving fraction on the ordinate, for three dose rates. The curves in the figure used $\alpha/\beta = 3$ Gy for normal tissue, $\alpha/\beta = 10$ Gy for the tumor, and $\alpha = 0.35$ Gy^{-1} and $\mu = 1.5$ h^{-1} for both types of tissue.

α tend to be very similar for most tissues (within the uncertainties), with most of the variations being in the β term. Although the variations in the values determined for the two parameters tend to be large, smaller variation characterizes the ratio of α/β, the quantity most often given in the literature. For the most part, this ratio tends to be on the order of 2 to 3 for late effects in normal tissues and 5 to 20 for early effects. In general, tissues exhibiting less mitotic activity show lower values. Most tumors behave similarly to normal-tissue early effects but with a much wider range of values. Prostate cancer forms a notable exception, with an α/β between 1.5 and 2.

Figure 27.1 shows that as the dose rate increases, the fraction survival decreases for a given dose, and this effect is more marked for tissues with a low value for α/β. Thus, as stated earlier, compared with LDR brachytherapy, normal tissue has a comparative disadvantage for HDR brachytherapy. The usual approach to overcome the disadvantage fractionates the dose delivery. Figure 27.2 shows a survival curve with the dose delivered in several fractions. The pauses in the delivery allow repair of those single-strand breaks not converted into double-strand breaks by a second hit. Thus, at the beginning of each fraction, the curve exhibits a new shoulder as the first single-strand breaks begin accumulating. The fractionation has no affect on the α term. Fractionation has a long history in external beam radiotherapy, which, as noted, also is HDR delivery. Understanding the repair mechanism allows for a definition of what dose rates qualify as "high": a delivery duration that remains much less than T_{bio}, or about 30 minutes.

Surviving fraction does not depend directly on dose; instead, the whole exponent forms the independent variable. Because the α tends to be constant, it is often pulled out, leaving what is called the biologically effective dose (BED) or equivalently the effective radiation dose (ERD) as

$$\text{BED} = D + \frac{D^2}{\left(\frac{\alpha}{\beta}\right)} = D\left[1 + \frac{D}{\left(\frac{\alpha}{\beta}\right)}\right]. \tag{3}$$

For the fractionated, HDR irradiations, each new fraction starts the shape of the curve over but at the surviving fraction level where it left off at the end of the previous fraction (in the absence of proliferation), and the equation becomes

$$\text{BED}_{\text{HDR}} = n\left[d\left(1 + \frac{d}{\left(\frac{\alpha}{\beta}\right)}\right)\right] = nd\left[1 + \frac{d}{\left(\frac{\alpha}{\beta}\right)}\right], \tag{4}$$

where n is the number of fractions and d is the dose per fraction.

The LDR situation becomes more complicated because repair takes place during the irradiation, reducing the effectiveness. In this case, BED becomes

$$\text{BED}_{\text{LDR}} = D\left(1 + \frac{2R}{\left(\frac{\alpha}{\beta}\right)\mu} \cdot \frac{1 - e^{-\mu T}}{\mu T}\right), \tag{5}$$

where T is the duration of the treatment and R is the dose rate. Because the BED depends on the α/β used, the convention when giving a value for BED requires that the units of gray carry a following subscript specifying the α/β. For example, the BED of 10 Gy for late-responding tissue with an α/β of 3 might be stated as BED = 10 Gy$_3$.

In fact, the equations for both modalities also contain a term, not shown in the equations,

$$\frac{0.693T}{\alpha T_{\text{pot}}} \tag{6}$$

to account for cell repopulation over the total treatment duration. T_{pot} represents the potential cell doubling time. Most applications ignore this term because of the large uncertainties in the values for α and T_{pot}. In situations comparing the

Cell Survival for Single and Multiple Fraction Exposures

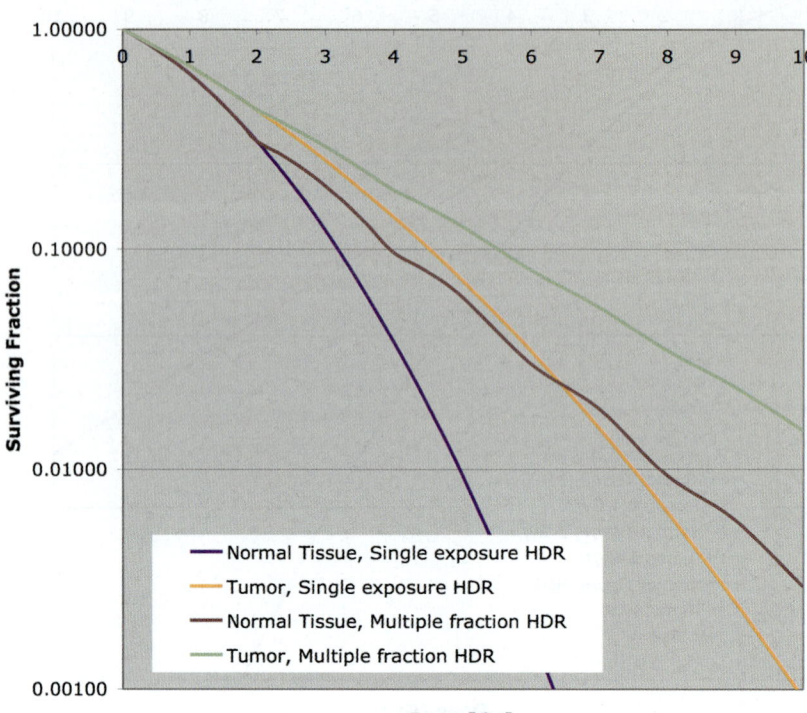

FIGURE 27.2. Survival curves illustrating the effects of fractionation. Again, the curves used $\alpha/\beta = 3$ Gy for normal tissue, $\alpha/\beta = 10$ Gy for the tumor, and $\alpha = 0.35$ Gy^{-1} and $\mu = 1.5$ h^{-1} for both types of tissue.

BED of LDR and HDR applications where the total duration of the therapy would be approximately the same, this omission probably causes no significant loss of information.

Conversion from Low to High Dose Rate Brachytherapy

Often, when beginning an HDR brachytherapy program, the biggest questions relating to treatments become how many fractions to use and what dose per fraction. The larger the number of fractions, the better is the therapeutic effect, measured as the ratio of the damage to tumor cells to the damage to normal tissue cells. This ratio improves with each additional fraction, but the amount by which the ratio increases decreases with each added fraction. For example, with the parameters used for the figures, going from 4 to 5 fractions improves the therapeutic ratio by 4%. Adding a 6th fraction improves the therapeutic ratio but only by another 3.5%. Each additional fraction carries with it costs in departmental resources (particularly the time of those persons involved) and inconvenience (and possibly discomfort) to the patient. Thus, selecting the number of fractions becomes a compromise. Most curative regimens use 5 or 6 fractions if applicator insertion procedures are involved and 8 to 12 fractions if the applicator can be left in place and the patient simply treated. Small-volume applications, such as vaginal cuff or most endobronchial treatments, may require only 3 or 4 fractions. After establishing the number of fractions, determining the dose per fraction comes next. One method that uses the LDR experience sets the BED equal for the two modalities and then solves for the dose per fraction:

$$\text{BED}_{\text{HDR}} = \text{BED}_{\text{LDR}} \tag{7a}$$

$$nd\left[1 + \frac{d}{\left(\frac{\alpha}{\beta}\right)}\right] = D_{\text{LDR}}\left\{1 + \left[\frac{2R}{\left(\frac{\alpha}{\beta}\right)\mu}\right] \bullet \left[\frac{1 - e^{-\mu T}}{\mu T}\right]\right\} \tag{7b}$$

$$d = \frac{-\left(\frac{\alpha}{\beta}\right) + \sqrt{\left(\frac{\alpha}{\beta}\right)^2 + \left(\frac{4D_{\text{LDR}}}{n}\right)\left(\frac{\alpha}{\beta}\right)\left[1 + \frac{2R}{\left(\frac{\alpha}{\beta}\right)}\left(\frac{1 - e^{-\mu T}}{\mu^2 T}\right)\right]}}{2} \tag{7c}$$

The absolute value for the dose per fraction depends on the ratio α/β, thus requiring another decision. Projecting d from the LDR experience, the normal-tissue toxicities could be held constant and an α/β of 3 used, or tumor cure could be the endpoint, suggesting an α/β of 10 (or a value of the particular type of tumor under treatment). Holding the late complications constant will lead to a BED for the tumor considerably less than was used with the LDR treatments, whereas attempting to achieve the same tumor control produces normal-tissue BED values much higher than those for the LDR regimen. For intracavitary treatments, the normal tissues sometimes can be held away from the applicator during the treatment delivery, for example, by keeping the rectal retractor in the vagina during a tandem and ovoid treatment. This would allow a dose based on equivalent tumor control. In interstitial applications, distance to the normal tissue in the implanted volume cannot be increased, but often with the improved optimization available with the HDR approach, high doses in the implant can be significantly reduced compared to conventional LDR implants, again allowing the dose based on tumor control. Seldom have HDR treatments produced more severe normal-tissue toxicities than those delivered at LDR. In general, the maximum significant dose, that is, the highest value of isodose surface that encompasses more than one catheter or needle track, should be kept to <150% of the prescription dose.[4]

High Dose Rate Devices

Remote Afterloaders

A remote afterloader (RAL) is a computer-driven system that transports the radioactive source from a shielded safe into the applicator placed in the patient. On termination or

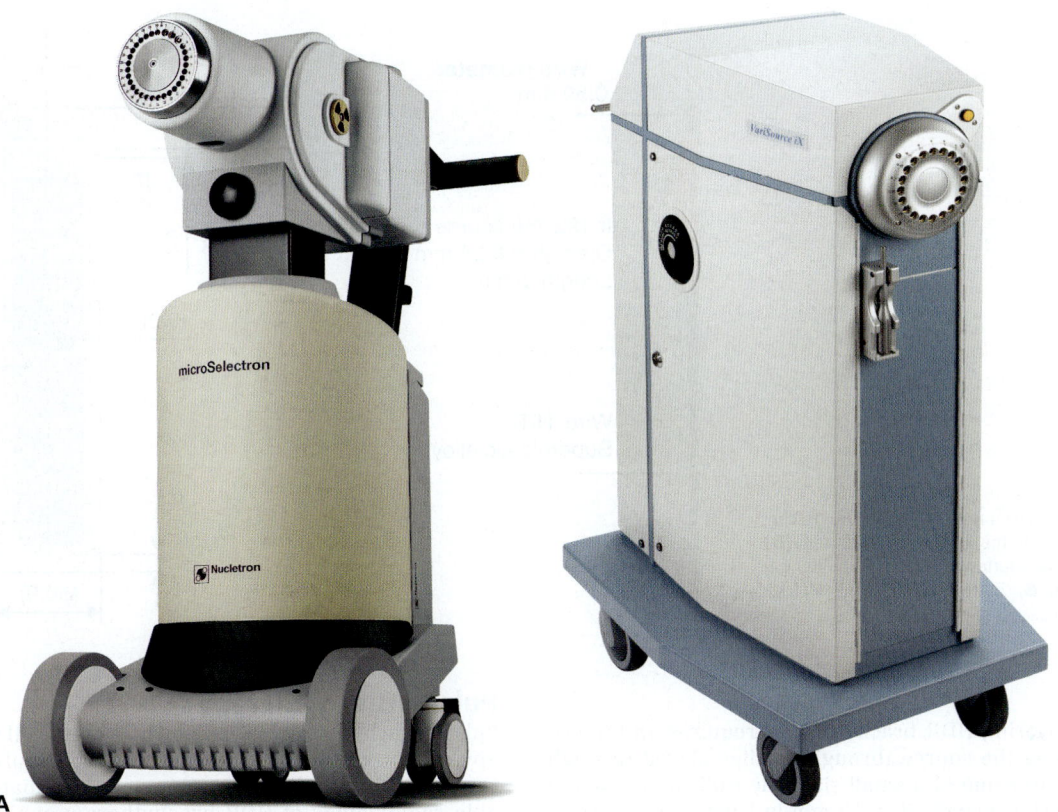

FIGURE 27.3. A: The Nucletron MicroSelectron. **B:** The Varian VariSource. (**A**, courtesy of Nucletron, an Elekta Company, Veenendaal, Netherlands; **B**, Courtesy of Varian, Palo Alto, CA.)

interruption of the treatment, the source is driven back to its safe. The device may move the source by one of several methods, most commonly pneumatic or cable drives. A stepping-source RAL is a particular design of the treatment unit that consists of a single source at the end of a cable that moves the source through applicators placed in the treated volume. The treatment unit can treat implants consisting of many needles or catheters in the patient. Multiple catheters are often required to cover the target with uniform radiation doses. Each catheter or part of an applicator is connected to the RAL through a channel. The computer drives the cable so that the source moves from the safe through a given channel to the programmed dwell position for a specific dwell time. In any applicator, there may be many dwell positions. After treating all the positions in a given catheter (channel), the source is retracted to its safe and then driven to the next channel. There can be several dwell positions per centimeter

in each channel, and the dwell time can vary from 0 to almost 1,000 seconds in 0.1-second increments, thereby giving a high level of flexibility of dose delivery. All currently available HDR RALs use the stepping-source design. Five models of HDR RALs are common. Three are marketed in the United States: Flexitron (Elekta Company, Georgia, USA) and GammaMed and VariSource (both from Varian Medical Systems, Palo Alto, CA). The MicroSelectron (Elekta Company, Georgia, USA) is no longer sold but is one of the most common units in service. In Europe, the BEBIG MultiSource (Eckert & Ziegler BEBIG, Seneffe, Belgium) is also available. Figure 27.3 shows two of the units. Even though they may vary in details, all available HDR RALs consist of the same general components: (a) shielded housing, (b) radioactive source, (c) source drive mechanism (cable, reel stepper motor), (d) indexer, (e) transfer tube, all shown in Figure 27.4, and not shown, (f) treatment control station, and (g) treatment control panel.

FIGURE 27.4. Components of a high dose rate brachytherapy remote afterloader. (Figure by Adam Uselmann after a draft by Liyong Lin.)

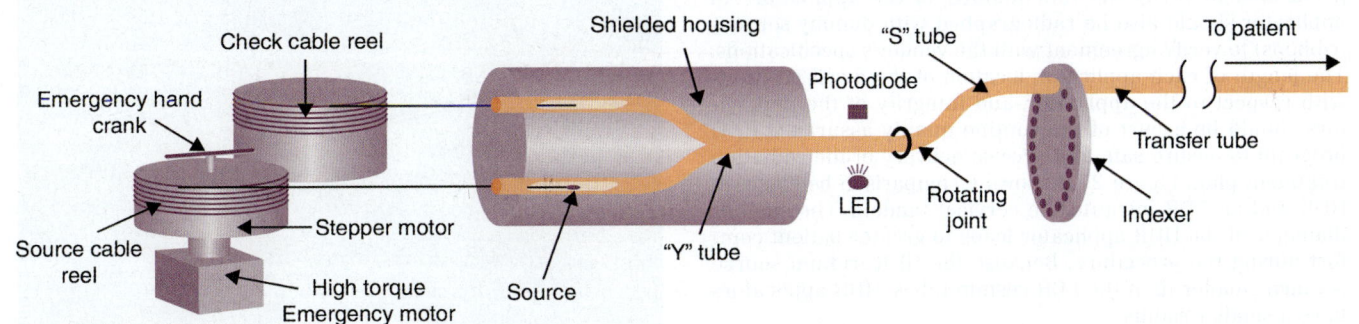

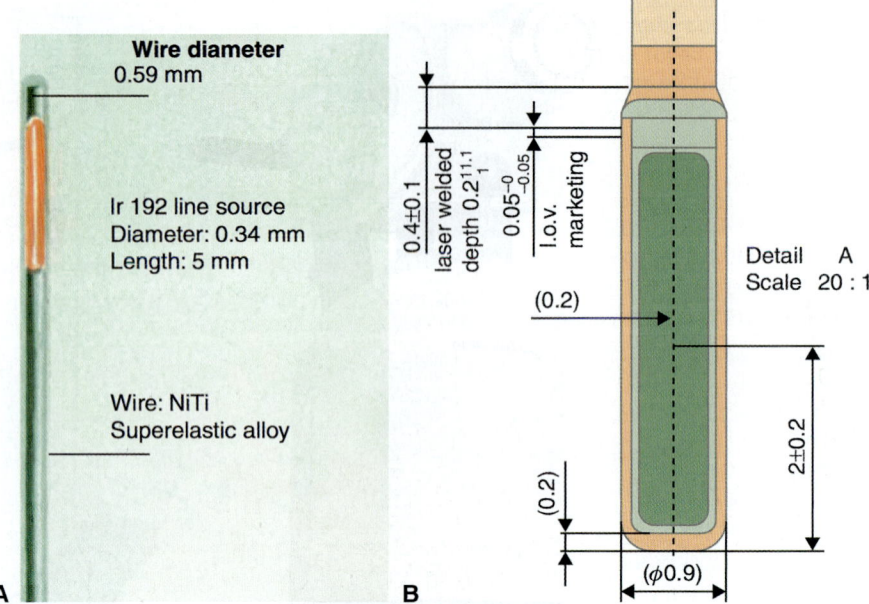

FIGURE 27.5. Diagrams of two HDR brachytherapy sources: for the **(A)** VariSource and **(B)** MicroSelectron. (**A**, courtesy of Varian, Palo Alto, CA; all rights reserved; **B**, courtesy of Nucletron, an Elekta Company, Veenendaal, Netherlands.)

Sources

Whereas delivering HDR brachytherapy requires an intense source, passing the source through needles placed through a tumor requires one of a small size. The radioactive source in an HDR RAL is usually 3 to 10 mm in length and approximately 1 mm or smaller in diameter, fixed at the end of a steel cable. The microSelectron source is placed in a stainless steel capsule and welded to the cable, whereas the Varian source is placed in a hole drilled into the cable and closed by welding. Figure 27.5 shows diagrams of the sources. Iridium-192 is now used for most HDR RALs; the BEBIG unit offers the choice of ^{192}Ir or ^{60}Co. Iridium-192 emits many photon energies, mostly between 110 and 704 keV, with an effective energy around 380 keV. A new source has an activity near 0.37 TBq (10 Ci, ~44 mGy m^2 h^{-1}). Because ^{192}Ir has a half-life of 74 days, the source should be replaced every 3 months to keep the treatment in the HDR radiobiologic regimen (see later discussion). The potential advantage of using ^{60}Co is the 5.3-year half-life, extending the time between source changes to approximately 5 years. The emissions of ^{60}Co, 1.12 and 1.33 MeV, require considerably more shielding than for devices using ^{192}Ir. A trained medical physicist calibrates the source after each installation using a reentrant, well-type ionization chamber, as discussed later. The resulting source calibration is verified against the manufacturer's source calibration.

Applicators

An array of applicators for different treatment sites is marketed by each vendor. Each vendor designs its own applicators that can only be used with its transfer tubes and HDR RALs. Before an applicator is used clinically, tests should be performed to verify the functionality of the applicator. An applicator should also be radiographed with dummy sources (ribbons) to verify agreement with the vendor's specifications. The length of each applicator, location of the dwell positions with respect to the applicator, and integrity of the applicators should be a part of the routine quality assurance (QA) program to ensure safe and precise delivery of the radiation treatment plan. Figure 27.6 shows a comparison between an HDR and an LDR intrauterine cervical tandem. The smaller diameter of the HDR applicator leads to greater patient comfort during the procedure. Because the HDR iridium source is much smaller than the LDR cesium tubes, HDR applicators have a smaller radius.

Pulsed Brachytherapy

Pulsed brachytherapy (also known as pulsed HDR brachytherapy or, not quite correctly but most commonly, pulsed dose rate [PDR] brachytherapy) attempts to eliminate the unfavorable radiobiology of HDR brachytherapy while maintaining the ability to optimize finely the dose distributions and eliminate the personnel exposure to radiation. The pulsed brachytherapy unit is the same as an HDR unit except the source can be shorter and only about one-tenth as active. The treatment also follows the same pattern as an HDR treatment, except that the patient remains in the hospital, and instead of 5 to 10 fractions, the source runs through the treatment pattern once each hour. These hourly treatment pulses last only a few minutes, but the overall treatment duration usually covers 1 or 2 days. Thus, biologically, because each fraction comes before complete repair of sublethal cellular damage, the tissues experience the radiation as almost continuous, mimicking LDR brachytherapy.

Although this approach incorporates the biologic advantages of LDR treatments and the optimization advantage of HDR brachytherapy, it also has many of the disadvantages of both modalities, including (a) inpatient treatments, (b) lack

FIGURE 27.6. HDR **(top)** and LDR **(bottom)** intrauterine tandems.

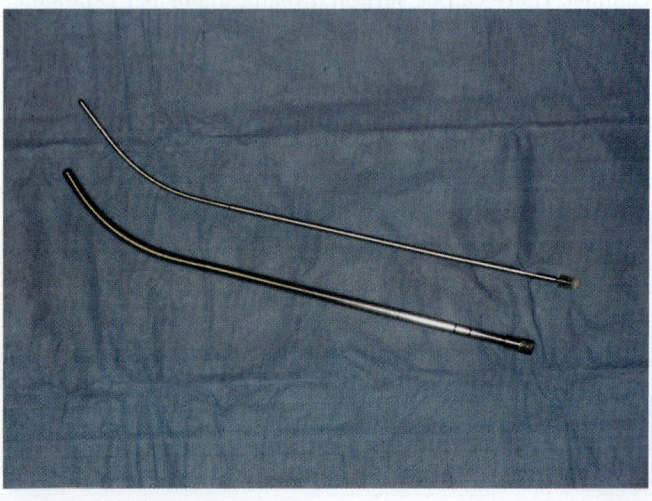

of applicator stabilization, and (c) possibility of mechanical failures. Because the source treats the patient 24 times per day, and each treatment includes three or more catheters, the number of source transits becomes quite large and many times more than for a normal HDR regimen. Such frequent source use increases the likelihood of source failure during a treatment. Should a source become caught during transit, the dose to the patient could become quite large. Unlike HDR procedures, the operator does not sit at the control panel always ready to retrieve a stuck source. Limiting the activity of the source to one-tenth of the normal HDR source allows 10 times the response time for a stuck source before significant injury to the patient. The other reason for the low activity is that, with the treatment divided into so many small fractions, the dwell times become too short for the treatment unit to control were the source very highly active. In summary, pulsed brachytherapy presents opportunities to potentially improve brachytherapy, but it also comes with detriments. PDR brachytherapy is discussed in more detail in Chapter 26.

OPERATION

Personnel Roles

The report of Task Group 59 (TG-59) of the American Association of Physicists in Medicine discusses the roles of the members of the treatment team for HDR brachytherapy.[5] For the most part, the roles follow standard procedures for any brachytherapy, with the physician inserting the treatment appliance and prescribing the treatment, the nurse monitoring the patient's condition and welfare, therapists or radiographers performing the imaging for localization, a dosimetrist or physicists performing optimization and dose calculation, a physicist checking the plan for correctness and assuring the correct calibration of the source, and the physician and physicist evaluating the plan. Who performs some of the functional roles discussed in what follows varies by institution but needs clarification so all persons involved understand the distribution of responsibilities.

Daily Quality Assurance

The tests of the treatment unit at the beginning of the treatment day often fall to the medical physicist. However, in some facilities, a therapist or dosimetrist performs the actual tests, and the medical physicist reviews the results of the tests before the first treatment.

Treatment Planning Calculation

The report of TG-59 discusses options for entering the patient data into the dose calculation computer and generating the treatment parameters (dwell positions and dwell times).[5] One model presented in that report had a dosimetrist running the program and a physicist monitoring the input to correct errors as they occur. Studies have shown that such supervision provides little protection against errors.[6] Either a physicist or a dosimetrist may perform the treatment plan generation.

Quality Assurance on the Treatment Plan

Regardless of who generates the treatment plan, a medical physicist should review the plan for appropriateness and correctness. The reviewing medical physicist should *not* be the same person who generated the plan, so in facilities with only one medical physicist, a dosimetrist should perform the planning.

Delivery of the Treatment

Several factors enter into considerations of who should staff the control panel during the treatment. In some states, regulations dictate that only therapists may deliver treatments and control treatment units. The regulations in most states and from the U.S. Nuclear Regulatory Commission are silent on the issue. At the time of writing, regulations almost uniformly require the attendance of a medical physicist at the treatment (or within unamplified voice communication of the unit operator). As a result, many facilities have the medical physicist operate in the unit during treatments. One important consideration is that at least one person in the control area during treatments must be ready and willing to enter the room and take appropriate actions in case the source becomes stuck in the patient.

Normal Procedures

When the afterloader receives a command from the treatment control panel to initiate a treatment, the source cable advances from the shielded safe through the Y tube and then the S tube to the first channel in the indexer and then along a path constrained by transfer tubes to the first treated dwell position in the applicator (see Fig. 27.4). The source dwells at that position for a predetermined duration. After completing that dwell, it goes on to the subsequent dwell positions. Some units step as the source drives out (Flexitron, MicroSelectron, and GammaMed), stopping first at the dwell position most proximal to the afterloader, whereas in the other (VariSource), the source travels first to the most distal dwell (toward the tip of the applicator) and a bit farther and then steps as the source returns toward the safe. Stepping on the outward drive obviates any concern about the effect of slack in the drive mechanism affecting the accuracy of the source position. The units that steps on the way back into the unit include correction for slack in the calibration of the source location. Regardless of the direction of stepping, on completion of the treatment for the first channel, the source is retracted into the safe and redirected to travel to the second channel. The process is repeated for all the subsequent treatment channels. The programmed movement of the source is verified by means of an optical encoder or other device that compares the angular rotation of a stepper motor or cable length ejected or retracted with the number of pulses sent to the drive motor. This system is capable of detecting catheter obstruction or constriction as increased friction in the cable movement. Under certain fault conditions, such as if the stepper motor fails to retract the source, a high-torque, direct current emergency motor will retract the source.

The confirmation of the source exit from and return to the safe is carried out by an opto-pair, consisting of a light-sensitive detector and an infrared light source, which detects the cable when its tip obstructs the light path. All the currently marketed afterloaders are also equipped with check cables, or "dummy sources." The check cable is an exact duplicate of the radioactive source along with its cable, except that it is not radioactive. Before the ejection of the radioactive source, the check cable is first ejected to check the integrity of the catheter system. After a noneventful check by this dry run with the dummy source, the radioactive source is then sent for treatment.

Emergency Procedures

Because HDR RALs are complicated devices containing very-high-activity radioactive sources, serious accidents can happen very quickly, thereby demanding many safety features and operational interlocks to prevent erroneous source movement or facilitate rapid operator response in the event of a system failure.

Door Interlock

Interlock switches prevent initiation of a treatment with the treatment-room door open. Opening the door interrupts the treatment's progress. This safety feature protects the medical personnel from radiation exposure in the event someone enters the treatment room without the knowledge of the operator. If a door is opened inadvertently during the treatment, the treatment is interrupted and the source returns to the safe. The treatment can be resumed at the same point where it was interrupted by closing the door and pressing the start or the resume button at the control panel.

Emergency Switches

Numerous emergency off switches are located at convenient places and are easily accessible in case a situation arises. One is located on the control panel for the HDR operator. Another is located on the top of the RAL treatment head. Vendors also install two or more switches in the walls of the treatment room. In the event a treatment is initiated with someone other than the patient in the treatment room, that person can stop the treatment and retract the source by pressing the emergency off button.

Emergency Crank

In the event of the failure of a source to retract normally, as well as the failure of the emergency motor, all HDR RALs have emergency cranks to retract the source cable. Using the crank requires the operator to enter the room with the source unshielded.

Emergency Service Instruments

If the radioactive source fails to retract after termination or interruption, pushing the emergency switch, or cranking the stepper motor manually, the immediate priority is to remove the source from the patient. Because the source is in contact with the patient, it can cause severe injury in a very short time. However, working at a greater distance, it is unlikely that the operator will receive a dose exceeding regulatory limits for 1 year, let alone one that would cause health problems. Once the source is removed from the patient and moved to the distance of even 1 m, the exposure rate drops drastically, and actions can then be taken to remove the patient from the room safely.

The safest approach to a source that will not retract by any of the methods is to remove the applicator from the patient as quickly as possible and place the applicator containing the source in a shielded container. If it is clear that the cable is caught in the transfer tube and not in the applicator *per se*, the applicator may be disconnected from the transfer tube and the patient removed from the treatment room. In some cases, this will be faster than removing the applicator. The reason to avoid disconnecting the applicator from the transfer tube is that a source may stay in the applicator if the source capsule shatters or come free from the cable. In that case, removing the applicator attached to the transfer tube keeps the system closed, whereas disconnecting the two opens a path for parts of a broken source to fall from the applicator into body cavities or crevices or roll onto the floor.

A situation might arise when the source needs to be detached manually from the treatment unit. Such a rare situation might occur if the unit with an unretractable source fell on a person and could not be moved by hand (perhaps by something else falling on the unit). The source could be close to the person but not inside. In this situation, the source cable should be cut from the unit and the source placed in the shielded container always present in the room. In cutting the source cable, it must be clear that the cut is *not* through the source capsule. For units with the capsule welded on the cable, the cut must be through the braided cable as opposed to the smooth steel capsule. For sources imbedded in the cable, a sufficient length of the cable must be seen to ensure that the cut occurs behind the source. Thus, emergency tools that must be present in the treatment room and always readily accessible include a wire cutter, a pair of forceps, and a shielded service container. The source should *never* be cut from the cable while the source is still in an applicator in the patient!

FACILITY DESIGN

Typically, the radioactive source in the HDR machine starts with an air kerma source strength of 44 mSv m/h, which is about at 10 Ci. According to the rules and regulations of the Nuclear Regulatory Commission (NRC), the annual limit for radiation exposure to the public is 1 mSv and the annual occupational limit is 5 mSv. (The actual limit for occupational exposure is 50 mSv/y, but following the principle of maintaining exposures as low as is reasonably achievable, the NRC usually holds licensees to exposure one-tenth of the actual limit.) In addition to the annual limit, NRC regulations requires that in an unrestricted area the dose equivalent rate should not be more than 0.02 mSv in any hour. Thus, the HDR machine needs to be housed in an adequately shielded room. To meet these requirements in an HDR suite, where the walls and the ceiling are at least 5 feet from the machine head, concrete walls of about 43 to 50 cm (or 4 to 5 cm of lead) are needed. For larger rooms, the concrete wall thickness will be lower because the exposure rate is inversely proportional to the square of the distance from the radioactive source. The tenth-value layer thicknesses for ^{192}Ir are 1.6 cm and 15 cm of lead and concrete, respectively. For details on the procedures for calculating the thickness of barriers for a particular facility, see a health physics text such as that by Cember and Johnson[7] or McGinley[8] or the report from the Nation Council on Radiation Units and Measurement.[9]

Imaging plays an important part in most brachytherapy, so consideration of required imaging modalities should enter into the room design. Having fluoroscopy and radiography in the treatment room can facilitate checking for applicator movement if moving the patient is required for CT or MRI imaging. It, of course, would be best to have the necessary imaging modalities in the procedure room. Having space and access for anesthesia in the room facilitates HDR brachytherapy for prostate cases.

All HDR brachytherapy rooms must have video and audio communication for monitoring the patient. Radiation detectors for monitoring the radiation levels in the room and indicating when the source is out of its shielding also are required.

QUALITY ASSURANCE OF THE REMOTE AFTERLOADING DEVICE

Several of the disadvantages of HDR brachytherapy concerned the probability of failure, either human or mechanical. Both aspects of the treatments require effective quality management. This section deals with quality assurance for the treatment unit. A report from the American Association of Physicists in medicine discusses this topic.[5,10–16] Williamson et al.[17] summarized much of the important material into a chapter. For a fairly comprehensive discussion, the reader is directed to Thomadsen.[18] Although most of these references are fairly old, the QA appropriate for these units has not changed.[19]

As for any piece of radiotherapy equipment, the QA begins with acceptance testing and commissioning. Periodic QA includes tests performed with each new source (approximately quarterly for most units) and those at the beginning of each treatment day. Of all of these, the daily morning checks form the basic set of essential tests.

Morning Checks

Although the list of safety checks seems long, the evaluation need not consume a great deal of time. At our facility, the entire morning routine takes about 10 to 15 minutes. Most of the items could be tested in numerous manners, but only one set of techniques will be discussed here. Individual units may differ in the exact methods. The procedure in the list often assumes the successful completion of all of the items going before. Failure of *any* item requires evaluation by the physicist of the appropriateness of continuing with patient treatments in light of the particular failure. The morning checks focus on ensuring that the unit is operating safely and correctly.

Safety Checks

The following items should be considered in a safety check:

Communication equipment. See that the television and intercom systems function.

Catheter-attachment lock. Attach a transfer tube to one of the channels of the unit, but do not lock the transfer tube in place (often accomplished by the locking ring). Program the unit to send the source to a dwell position that would be in an applicator were one attached, and initiate a source run. A program time for a single dwell of about 20 seconds would allow execution of the tests to follow. The unit should detect that the transfer tube has not been locked in place and prevent the source run. Were a treatment to take place in this condition, the source cable could push the transfer tube out of the unit and never enter the applicator.

Applicator attachment. Keeping the same program, lock the transfer tube in place but still do *not* attach an applicator to the transfer tube. Again, attempt to initiate a source run. The check cable run should detect the absence of an applicator and prevent sending out the source. Failure of the unit to detect this situation could lead to the source indicating that it treated a catheter when, in reality, the catheter was never attached. This test also checks that the unit will not send out a source if the pathway is blocked, because, for most transfer tubes, the applicators push aside a blockage of the tube when they lock in place.

Door interlock. Lock an applicator into the transfer tube. For future tests, it is convenient to use a needle in a well-type ionization chamber. Keeping the same program as in the previous tests and with the door to the room open, try to initiate a run. The unit should refuse to initiate the treatment and indicate that the door is open.

Source-out indicators. Close the door, and initiate the source run. Observe that the indication lamps operate. Most rooms have three beam-on indicator lamps: one connected to a treatment unit microswitch that triggers when the source leaves its shielded housing, one that lights when the signal on the radiation detector in the room exceeds its trip level, and one from the onboard Geiger counter. Let the exposure continue for the next test.

Room monitor audio operation. Listen through the intercom for the sound of the room radiation monitor. It should make a mild but clearly audible sound. It should not be too loud, for that would disturb the patient. There is no regulation in most states or with the NRC that the in-room monitor provides any audible signal. The presence of such a signal would alert anyone who is in the room unintentionally when the source is out. Some practitioners feel that any such signal causes concern on the part of the patient. We have tried both situations and have found that patients do not mind the signal if they have been informed that it would occur. Continue the exposure.

Room monitor visual operation. Open the door to the room and observe the visual indicators on the room monitor. The room design should provide protection to a person in the doorway until the source retracts. At the same time as this test is performed, so is the next.

Handheld monitor operation. Immediately on opening the door during the previous test, hold the handheld monitor in the doorway and see whether it indicates the presence of radiation. The handheld detector is to be carried upon entry to the treatment room any time after a source run. Alternatively, the detector could be tested with a dedicated check source at the beginning of each day. Performing the test along with the room monitor makes the treatment unit the dedicated check source.

Door interrupt. During the previous two tests, the unit should have been retracting the source, beginning from the opening of the door. The retraction should take no longer than 4 to 6 seconds to return the source to its shielded location.

Emergency stop. Close the door and reinitiate the exposure. Once the source reaches the dwell position, press the emergency off button. The unit must immediately retract the source and likely require a reset.

Treatment interrupt. Reinitiate the exposure, and once the source again reaches the dwell position, press the treatment interrupt button. Again, the unit must immediately retract the source.

Timer termination. Reinitiate the exposure and let it continue until the elapsed duration equals the time set on the timer. At that time, the unit stops the exposure and retracts the source.

Dosimetry Checks

The thrust of the dosimetry checks focuses on the delivery of the correct dose to the proper location.

Source Positioning Accuracy

Proper treatment requires that the source occupy the position along the catheter corresponding to that used in the treatment plan. The uncertainty of the determination of the dwell positions on the treatment plan is discussed elsewhere in this chapter. Here, the issue becomes duplicating the dwell locations on the treatment plan during execution. A usual criterion for coincidence with the planned treatment dwells is 2 mm, although the HDR units are able to place the source in a given location within 1 mm. Precision <0.5 mm begins to be less reproducible. To direct the source to correct locations corresponding to each dwell position, the source controller requires the distance along the catheter corresponding to the first dwell position. The distance may refer to the length from some part of the unit (such as the front face, the point of catheter insertion, or a microswitch that tells the unit when the source enters the catheter), or it may be from some fictitious point (similar in concept to the effective source for electron beams). Verifying that the unit can place the center of the source at a specified distance becomes an important part of the morning QA.

The most expeditious method uses the ruler provided with the unit. Such a ruler provides a channel for the source to follow alongside a scale marked in the distance. Using any ruler requires a high-definition television system that will be able to distinguish the source capsule clearly and resolve the markers on the ruler. The lighting of the ruler becomes an important variable. For one vendor's unit, a televised check of the source positions on a ruler forms a routine part of any treatment. For another, the ruler is just part of the unit QA equipment and requires a separate television system, such as that used to monitor the patient. To perform the check, attach the ruler as appropriate for the unit and program the source to a distance that shows on the rule. Watch on the video screen as the source moves into position. The tip of the source will be seen at some distance that should be farther than that distance programmed. From the distance of the tip, subtract the distance from the tip to the center of the source as shown in Figure 27.7. This check is performed with the source cable itself; the check

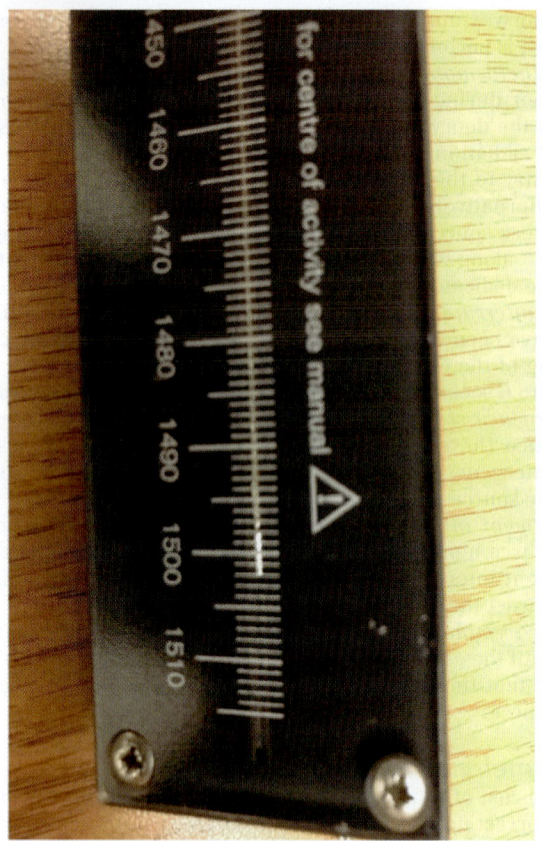

FIGURE 27.7. A typical image made to test the accuracy of the HDR unit source positioning.

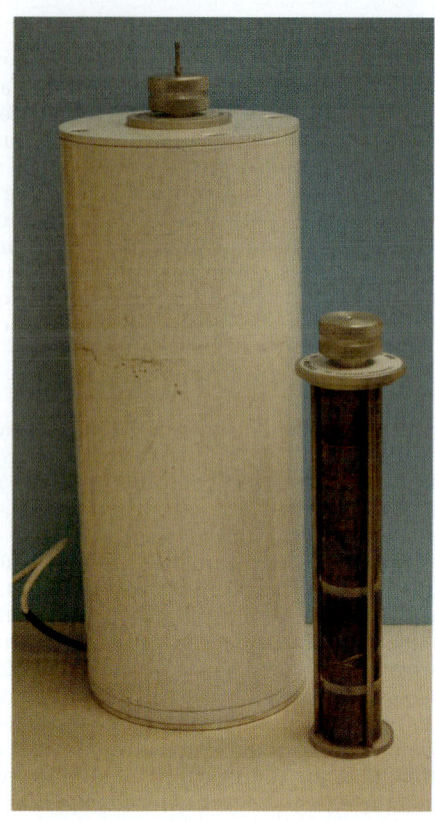

FIGURE 27.8. A special insert designed to assist in the evaluation of source positioning accuracy, with large lead cylinders separated by a plastic disc.

cable, for some units, does not go to the same distance as the source cable and would give an incorrect result.

A simpler and more precise method of verifying the positioning of the source follows the technique determined by DeWerd et al.[20] This procedure uses a well-type ionization chamber with a special insert that includes lead attenuators

and plastic transmission discs and is shown in Figure 27.8. The lead attenuators reduce the signal from the source to approximately one-third its unshielded value, whereas the plastic discs have little effect. As the source passes through the needle centered in this insert, the measured signal appears as in Figure 27.9. The peaks occur when the source is centered on the plastic discs, and the greatest gradient

FIGURE 27.9. The signal produced as the source passes through the insert shown in Figure 27.8. Notice the high signal gradient that corresponds to the source centered on the plastic–lead interface. The color of the data points correspond to the starting dwell length as indicated in the legend. Five sets of measurements are required on this unit, with different starting dwell lengths, to have measurements every quarter millimeter.

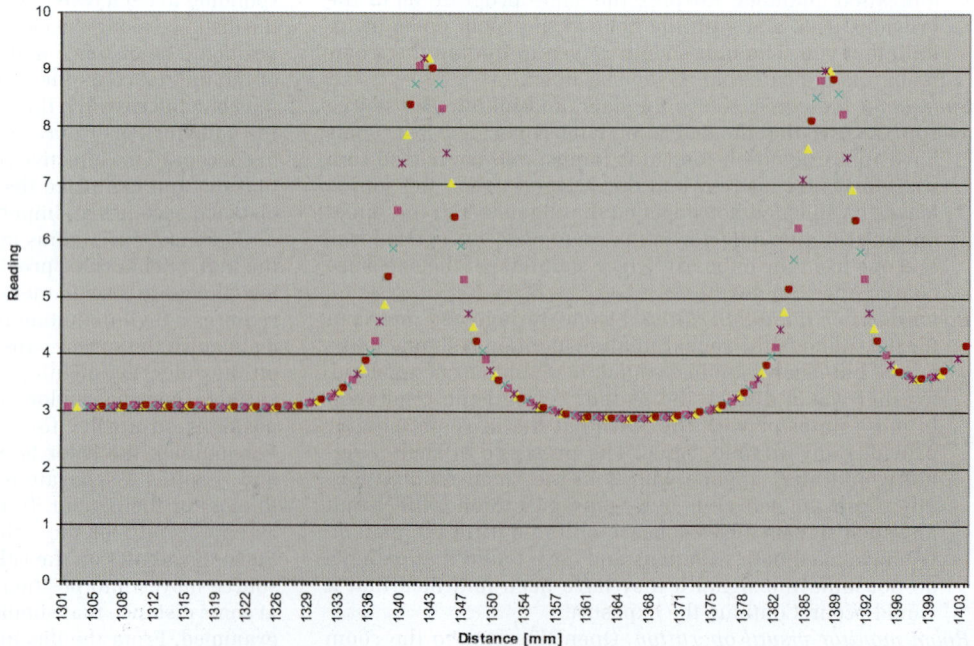

HDR Insert Profile

Reading / Distance [mm]

Legend: ■ 1399   ▲ 1400   ✳ 1401   ✶ 1402   ● 1403

occurs when half the source is shielded and half is on the plastic. At these points, the signal depends critically on the precise position of the source, with the signal changing approximately 3.5%/mm. The signal at the plateau changes little over 2 mm. Dividing the current signal at the high-gradient point by that at the plateau removes any variations in the reading due to source decay, timer miscalibration, or atmospheric density. Thus, the ratio of signals gives a sensitive indication of whether the unit accurately places the source to the correct location. Making measurements at two high-gradient points and the peak assesses not only the correct placement of the source at the one point but also the correct interval between. Use of this method requires measurement of the signal profile as a function of distance along the axis of the well chamber after initial verification of the source position using one of the other methods. Once put in place, this approach takes <1 minute. If the insert is left in the well chamber, the needle can be used for the safety checks, and this test can follow the safety checks without requiring re-entry into the room.

The source position could be checked using radiochromic film, marking the intended position of the source in a catheter using the radiographic markers and then making an autoradiograph with the source. However, this method takes more time and carries a larger uncertainty than either of the two methods discussed above.

Dose Consistency

Correct dose delivery hinges on the proper operation of the timer controlling the exposure. The proper operation does *not* depend on the timer accurately keeping true clock time. The only important features of the timer are that it operates linearly and that its operation remains consistent over time. The daily QA generally needs only check two times to evaluate timer consistency and linearity, compared with the tests performed during the source exchange. The uncertainty in the measurement should be on the order of a few tenths of a second in order to check the shorter times.

One technique for checking the timer observes the reading produced in a radiation detector as a function of the timer settings. To evaluate the timer, the measurement system must respond linearly to radiation dose and the setup provide a stable and reproducible geometry. A well chamber, such as that used for calibration, performs this function well. Such measurements in a well chamber include the effects of source decay and the source transit time. For the most part, source decay seldom deviates from the expected but should be checked because there have been sources with contaminant radionuclides that produce an anomalous decay. Because the reading varies directly with the set exposure time, these readings can form a check of the timer. The chamber reading needs a baseline, for example, a reading taken immediately after the initial calibration of the source. The expected reading can be tabulated as a function of day by correcting the initial reading by the decay factor, $e^{-0.693t/73.8 \text{ days}}$, where t is the time in days since the initial reading. The reading should remain within ±2% of the projected reading, values that also could be in the table. Deviations from the projected values indicate changes in the timer operation (linearity or consistency), changes in the unit's transit time, or anomalous decay. Further tests would be required to sort out the actual problem.

Source Strength Value

The value for the source strength at any time should be the same in the treatment planning computer as in the treatment unit computer to within 0.5%. The date and time in the treatment unit must be correct for the unit to calculate the source decay correctly. The format of the date, American or European, must be the same as that expected by the computer.

Initial Checks

Each source change requires a number of procedures in addition to the daily checks.

Safety Checks

The initial safety checks include the following:

Treatment unit backup batteries. In case of loss of power to the treatment unit, the machine has backup batteries to retract the source and save the record of the treatment up to the time of retraction. Checking the batteries entails initiating a source run, pulling the circuit breaker for power to the unit, and verifying that the source retracts; the history is then saved, and the unit resumes the program where it left off when restarted after restoring the power.

In-room radiation monitor backup batteries. The in-room radiation monitor also has backup batteries allowing it to continue functioning in case of a power loss. Continued operation at such times becomes extremely important in case the source fails to retract. Verifying operation of these batteries simply requires unplugging the unit from the wall socket and performing the usual check for the monitor.

Dosimetry Checks

The following are the initial dosimetry checks:

Calibration. The accepted method for calibration of an HDR source uses a well-type ionization chamber that has been calibrated in terms of HDR source strength per unit current. The calibration factor for the same chamber will differ for LDR and HDR ^{192}Ir sources because of differences in source construction. The uncertainty in source strength calibrations using such chambers usually runs around 1% from national standards plus an additional 5% in the national standard with respect to absolute measures of energy absorbed per unit mass. The source strength is in terms of air kerma strength, S_K, with units of μGy m^2 h^{-1}, often called U for convenience.[21] This unit gives numbers that become very large, so sometimes units of mGy m^2 h^{-1} (called U_h) are used. Most treatment planning computers accommodate units of air kerma strength; however, many practitioners still relate better to source strength converted into curies, derived simply by multiplying S_K by a constant, which must be the same as that used by the manufacture in the treatment planning program.

Timer linearity. The verification for timer linearity uses several readings, R_i, for various increasing times, t_i, taken in the well chamber. The free-running reading rate can be defined as

$$\dot{R} = \frac{R_{i+1} - R_i}{t_{i+1} - t_i} \tag{8}$$

and contains no effect from the source transit, which cancels during the subtractions. Taking approximately five readings covering the range of dwell times common in treatments gives four values for the free-running reading rate using adjacent times. These values should differ by <0.5%.

The transit time from the unit to the dwell position is hard to measure and is not important directly. What is important is that the transit time remains constant. An effective transit time can be defined as the time it would take to deliver the extra reading in the chamber because of the irradiation during the time the source moves into and then leaves the measurement dwell position, *if* the extra reading were delivered at the free-running reading rate. One expression for the effective transit time, t_e, becomes

$$t_\varepsilon = \frac{R_i}{\dot{R}} - t_i. \tag{9}$$

An alternative expression for evaluating the timer linearity calculates ζ, defined as

$$\zeta = \frac{R_i / R_{i+1}}{(t_i - t_\varepsilon) / (t_{i+1} - t_\varepsilon)}. \tag{10}$$

In general, ζ should remain between 0.99 and 1.01.

Entry of data into computers. The new source strength must be entered into the treatment planning computer and the treatment unit computer. Special attention needs to be paid to selecting the units for the source strength, particularly if the system automatically defaults to given units.

Checks Just before and during Treatment

Other than the check performed on the treatment plan just before treatment, connecting the patient also requires care and verification. For most gynecologic applicators, the three parts of a tandem and ovoid set, or the tandem and ring, have coded connectors that only allow the correct transfer tubes to attach, and the transfer tubes also can only connect to the correct holes in the indexer. However, for implants with needles or catheters, no interlocking prevents mismatches between channels and catheter or needle tracks. For large implants on older units, the treatments often require first connecting the number of catheters equal to the number of channels and delivering the part of treatment that uses those channels. Those channels are then disconnected, and the next set of catheters is then connected to the indexers starting again with channel number 1. One of the most likely errors would be connecting a channel during the second set to a catheter from the first or vice versa. Newer treatment units often have enough channels to accommodate most large implants.

Also for interstitial implants, between fractions, the catheters often move from the position they occupied during the imaging used for treatment planning. Immediately before treatment, the catheters must be returned to their original position, for example, by snugging the buttons on one side to the skin.

During the treatment, the operator needs to watch for movement by the patient that could affect the treatment and ensure that the source moves through its program.

Checks after Treatment

At the end of a treatment, the operator verifies complete source retraction by taking the following steps:

- Noting the completion of treatment as indicated by the control console
- Observing the radiation monitors in the room
- Measuring the radiation levels at the patient using the handheld radiation detector
- Measuring the radiation levels at the treatment unit with the handheld detector

The last reading should be in front of the unit in line with the source path out of the shielding container.

DOSIMETRY AND TREATMENT PLANNING

Time Course of Procedures

As with LDR brachytherapy, treatment planning for HDR cases may follow different patterns, based on the treatment approach. For example, treatments of cervical cancer using a tandem and ovoid usually have the physician place the treatment appliance, followed by localization imaging and then dosimetric calculations. Less likely than with LDR approach,

there can still be planning first based on an idealized application, such as a surface application. Some treatment planning may be interactive, such as with prostate implants, where dosimetry following needle placement can direct subsequent needle placement. Despite this range of options, in most HDR cases the treatment plan generation follows applicator placement, and that model will be assumed in this discussion.

Differences between Low and High Dose Rate Brachytherapy Treatment Planning

HDR brachytherapy treatment planning differs from LDR brachytherapy in three ways. The first difference results from the time course of the treatments. In treatments of several sites, particularly most gynecologic applications and some methods for treatment of the prostate, the patient waits in the treatment position during the treatment plan generation. Most interstitial and intraluminal treatments differ little from the LDR varieties, with treatment plan generation performed with the patient elsewhere. For those cases with the patient waiting in the treatment position, time becomes an important factor. If the plan generation takes too long, the patient will begin moving with respect to the applicator even though both may be "immobilized." Additional problems with excessively long dosimetry sessions include patient discomfort (other than leading to movement) and cost of support staff such as anesthesiologists.

A second difference entails the quantities involved with the dose calculation. LDR applications often use source strength input by the user and calculate resulting dose rates based on the source configuration. The problem in many cases, particularly in interstitial implants, becomes selecting the dose rate isodose surface on which to base the treatment duration. The case may have many sources, possibly of various strengths, but only a single duration for all sources. HDR brachytherapy has one source strength and many different dwell times. In both cases, the dose calculation algorithm uses the product of the source strength and time at a given location as the basis for the resulting dose distribution.

The third difference concerns the role of quantities as input or output. As noted earlier, LDR calculations most often input the source strengths and calculate the resultant dose rate distribution. Sometimes the treatment duration is also specified, generating a dose distribution. HDR brachytherapy planning usually reverses the process, starting with the dose pattern desired and working backward to the dwell-time distribution necessary to achieve that dose, a process termed *inverse planning*. A common part of inverse planning is *optimization*, a process to achieve a treatment plan that satisfies some criteria.

Optimization

The term *optimization* implies finding a plan that maximizes some aspects of the dose distribution. Many approaches actually only address finding a set of dwell times that deliver a specified dose to specified locations. Other approaches also try to control the dose distribution more finely and possibly limit the dose to specified organs at risk (OAR). The umbrella of optimization covers many disparate processes.

Optimization Approaches

Optimization in brachytherapy has taken many forms. The approaches fall into general categories, although considerable controversy surrounds the classifications. Ezzell[22] presents an excellent review of optimization. The discussion here can only brush the surface of the topic. One listing of the categories with examples follows.

Stochastic approaches to optimization start from a distribution of dwell times for the selected dwell positions. The starting dwell-time distribution may be arbitrary, but information on typical solutions can reduce the time to solution. Through the initial set of dwell times, the program calculates a value for an *objective function* (OF). An OF assigns a numerical value to the solution set that allows ranking the set according to quality. The OF may be as simple as the difference between the value of dose calculated at a set of points and the dose desired. OFs often become more complicated, as in the following equation:

$$OF = w_t(0.95D_{\text{pre}} - D_{\text{t,m}})_{D_{\text{t,m}} < 0.95D_{\text{pre}}}$$
$$+ \sum_i w_{\text{OAR},i}(\bar{D}_{\text{OAR},i,\text{calc}} - D_{\text{OAR},i,\text{limit}})^2_{\bar{D}_{\text{OAR},i,\text{calc}} > D_{\text{OAR},i,\text{limit}}} \quad (11)$$

In Eq. (11), D_{pre} represents the prescription dose and $D_{\text{t,m}}$ stands for the minimum dose in the planning target volume. In this example, the person running the optimization wants to evaluate whether the dwell-time set results in part of the target receiving <95% of the prescribed dose and, if so, to keep track of how much less. The second term considers the average doses ($\bar{D}$) to each of the OAR and determines for each the amount over some limiting dose assigned for that organ. The objective function, OF, in this case is a penalty paid for the dwell-time distribution. The first term would be omitted as long as the minimum target dose equaled or exceeded 95% of the prescription dose, and the term for any of the OAR would be zero as long as the dose remained below the limiting value. The power of 2 in the exponent indicates tolerance of a little excess dose but imposes serious penalties for larger values. The weighting factors, w, allow a differentiation between the importance given to achieving the desired dose distribution and limiting the dose to a given organ at risk. In addition to the OF, the dwell-time set might also be subject to *hard constraints* that would reject the set outright if the target dose fell to <90% of the prescribed dose or an organ at risk exceeded a different, maximum limit. Because the value of the OF increases as the dose distribution gets worse, the program tries to minimize this function. Keep in mind that this equation only illustrates the concepts and is not intended to serve as a model of a good OF.

The methodology for finding the best set of dwell times differs among the stochastic approaches. In *simulated annealing*,[23–26] random changes, often sizable, are made from an arbitrary initial solution for the dwell times of some or all of the dwell positions. After the changes and recalculation of the OF, the program holds on to the better of the two dwell-time sets. New random changes are made from the better set, and again, the sets are compared using the OF. As this process continues, the allowed changes become smaller, and the OF should improve as the process moves toward the solution—the set with the best OF. The process as described can fall into a local minimum for the OF, where any small change will make the OF worse, a very different solution would be better. The small changes could not get to better solution. To avoid such traps, the program periodically allows big jumps in the dwell times to investigate completely different regions of dwell times. If the new region does not seem promising because the OFs are worse, the program goes back to the better region.

Often, the value of the OF changes little with fairly large changes in individual dwell times in the neighborhood of the optimal solution. Going from a close dwell-time set to the true optimum can require a considerable amount of computer time and often more than getting close in the first place. Most programs contain a criterion for stopping the process once the OF finds an adequate solution instead of continuing to the true optimum.

Other stochastic approaches, such as the *genetic algorithm*,[27] use different search mechanisms, but the overall procedures tend to be similar.

A nonstochastic approach, *geometric optimization* solves for dwell times that would give the same doses to the vicinities around each of the dwell positions, based on several simplifying assumptions.[28] This approach recognizes that the dose near any dwell position results not only from the nearby dwell but also from the sum of the contributions from all the other sources. This method first calculates how much dose would be deposited to a dwell position from all the other dwell positions and then weights the dwell time at that dwell position under consideration by the inverse of this dose. Thus, each dwell position needs only make up for the difference between the dose it already receives from the other positions and the dose desired. The first step sets the relative dwell weight, τ_i (the relative dwell time, normalized as described later), for dwell position I, based on the dose contributions of the other dwell positions. Using the point-source formalism of AAPM Task Group 43[29,30]

$$\tau_i = \left[\sum_{j \neq i} \frac{g(r_{i \leftarrow j}) \cdot \varphi(r_{i \leftarrow j})}{r_{i \leftarrow j}^2} \right]^{-1}, \quad (12)$$

where $r_{i \leftarrow j}$ is the distance between dwell positions i and j, $g(r_{i \leftarrow j})$ is the radial dose function, and $\varphi(r_{i \leftarrow j})$ is the anisotropy factor. Commercial versions of this algorithm usually ignore the radial dose function, which remains within 2% of unity to a distance of 5 cm for ^{192}Ir, and the anisotropy factor, which falls within 3.5% of 0.98 over that same range. The errors from these omissions and the point-source approximation (inherent in the inverse-square relationship) remain smaller than errors that creep in later.

Determining the absolute dwell times then requires specifying the dose desired to a point or the average of several points. For the average dose to several points (indicated by q), the equation for the average dose to the points is

$$\bar{D}_{\text{initial pass}} = \frac{S_K \cdot \Lambda}{n} \sum_{q=n}^{1} \sum_{j=m}^{1} \frac{\tau_j \cdot g(r_{q \leftarrow j}) \cdot \varphi(r_{q \leftarrow j})}{r_{q \leftarrow i}^2}, \quad (13)$$

where S_K is the source strength in mGy m² h⁻¹, Λ is the dose rate constant in Gy cm²/unit source strength, n is the number of dose points in the average, and m is the number of dwell positions, and t_j from Eq. (12) serves as the initial estimate of the dwell time at position j.

Adjusting $\bar{D}_{\text{initial pass}}$ to become $D_{\text{prescribed}}$ requires scaling the dwell times. Letting each of the t_j be the time to deliver $D_{\text{prescribed}}$ and c be the scaling factor such that $t_j = c\tau_j$, then we have

$$c = \frac{\bar{D}_{\text{initial pass}}}{D_{\text{prescribed}}}. \quad (14)$$

This process calculated the doses to a dwell position assuming that all the dwell times were the same. That is not the case in Eq. (13), which means that the calculated dwell times are not quite correct. The uniformity could improve by iterating the process, at the sacrifice of its very high speed. The process also assumes that the implant, and particularly the dwell positions, matches the target volume.

Adjacent dwell positions along the same catheter track can produce the greatest effect on the dwell weights, resulting in isodose surfaces that tend to follow the catheters rather than conform to the shape of the implanted volume as a whole. This is especially the case if the separation between dwell positions along a catheter is much less than the separation between catheters. To reduce this effect, a version of the algorithm neglects all other dwell positions along the same catheter track when calculating the dwell weights in a given catheter. This variation is called *volume optimization* because it tends to spread the doses throughout the implanted volume. The original version, which includes the contributions of all other dwell positions for the calculation of any dwell weight, is called *distance optimization* because the isodose surfaces tend to follow a catheter at a constant distance.

The analytic approach, also known as *point optimization* or *point-dose optimization*, attempts to solve algebraically for the set of dwell times that produce the desired dose distribution, as represented by a set of points, called *optimization points*, each with its own specified desired dose. In the most basic form, the specified doses and the dwell times establish a set of simultaneous equations of the form[31,32]

$$D_i = \sum_{j=1}^{m} C_{i,j} \cdot t_j, \tag{15}$$

where D_i is the dose specified to point i, m is the number of dwell positions, t_j is the dwell time at position j, and the $C_{i,j}$ are factors that give the dose contribution at i because of the source at position j, with the sum over all sources. The source strength at each source position forms a variable (unknown), and each dose specification point yields an equation. Equal numbers of dwell times and dose points form a *determined* system with an exact solution. In more complex cases, there may be more optimization points than source positions, resulting in an *overdetermined* system (more equations than variables). This would be the situation in which optimization points were spread around the contour of a region of interest (ROI) and scattered through the volume. Faced with this situation, one can vary the source strengths to minimize the square of the differences between the desired and calculated doses at the optimization points. At the other extreme, a case may have more source positions than optimization points (more variables than equations), resulting in an *underdetermined* system. This situation most often happens with large implants and a minimum of optimization points or complicated gynecologic applicators with only a few dose control points. With this situation, the source strengths have no well-defined values; many solutions would possibly exist with the same value for the square of the difference between the doses desired and those calculated. Distinguishing between the solutions requires some other criteria. One often is a minimization of the total dwell time, under the assumption that such would also minimize the integral dose to the patient.

Determined and overdetermined systems can (and often do) generate solutions with negative dwell times. Simply truncating the negative dwell times often results in a very unsatisfactory dose distribution. Avoiding this nonphysical situation also requires an additional criterion. One possible criterion minimizes the differences between adjacent source strengths. For m dwell positions, this term becomes

$$\delta_i = \sum_{j=1}^{n-1} (t_j - t_{j+1})^2. \tag{16}$$

Including this term in the optimization limits the fluctuations between adjacent sources. To deliver a dose to the target volume requires a net positive total dwell time, and so limiting the amount of difference between the dwell times eventually results in all positive times. An additional condition for underdetermined systems selects solutions that minimize the total radiation to the patient as a whole, which depends directly on the total source strength. The final optimization becomes minimizing the chi-squared value in

$$X^2 = \sum_{i=1}^{m} w_i \left(D_i - C_{ij} \sum_{j=1}^{n} t_j \right)^2 + v \sum_{j=1}^{n-1} (t_j - t_{j+1})^2 + u \sum_{j=1}^{n} t_j, \tag{17}$$

where, in addition to those quantities defined earlier, n is the number of dose points specified, w_i is the weighting given to the dose specification at point i (how much the operator wants the correct dose there), v represents the importance in minimizing the fluctuations between adjacent sources, and u represents the importance of minimizing the integral dose to the patient.

With a large number of optimization points or source positions, or both, the running of the program solving the equations becomes long, and approximations cut the calculation time greatly without significantly compromising the accuracy of the final dose distribution. By setting the dwell time

$$t_i = \sum_{k=1}^{p} a_k \cdot F_k (j-1), \tag{18}$$

where F is a fitting function, such as a polynomial or Fourier series of order p, and a_k is the coefficient for the kth element, and substituting that into the X^2 Eq. (17), the optimization now need only solve for the fitting coefficients, presumably a much smaller set of values. An alternative approach to solving the equation follows Newton's method.[33,34]

Obviously, the selection of the optimization points becomes very important. The number of points must adequately describe the shape of the dose distribution desired. The dose distributions may satisfy the specifications established for the optimization points but leave portions of the target without dose specification points untreated. However, the points should avoid regions of large dose gradients because specification there can produce unexpected and inappropriate results.

In general, lower values for v in Eq. (17) allow better conformality of the dose distribution, and the optimum value often is that just sufficient to prevent negative dwell times. However, simply solving for the dose to specified points can produce an unwanted dose distribution, even when the points seem to follow normal guidelines. Thomadsen et al.[35] give an example similar to that in Figure 27.10. Here, the dose points mirror the basal dose points equidistant from the surrounding catheters. With a low value for v in the optimization equation, the simple solution places all of the source material in the center, bottom needle—not at all what was really desired. The situation could be avoided by limiting the dwell-time variations or using more dose points, particularly on the outside of the implant. Alternatively, performing a geometric optimization to obtain an approximate source distribution, followed by optimization on the points, also alleviates the problem.

The output of any optimization approach may leave the operator wanting to make modifications. One method commercially available works on the computer screen display of the dose distribution and allows the operator to "grab" a dose line on the display with the cursor and move the line to a desired location. These fine adjustments make changes that would be difficult to describe in the optimization routine's specifications. Most of the programs allow adjusting the impact of any change between changing all of the dwell times (scaling the distribution, making the whole larger or smaller) and changing a single dwell time (effecting very local changes). Even local changes, however, result in changes in image planes other than the one on which the change has made because the radiation carries the dose beyond the immediate locale.

Changes in the dose distribution to produce desired modifications can also produce unintended changes. Of particular concern would be expending the prescription isodose surface and inadvertently also expending the higher-dose surfaces, possibly into a significant volume. During any manipulation of the isodose surfaces, the display should also show the higher

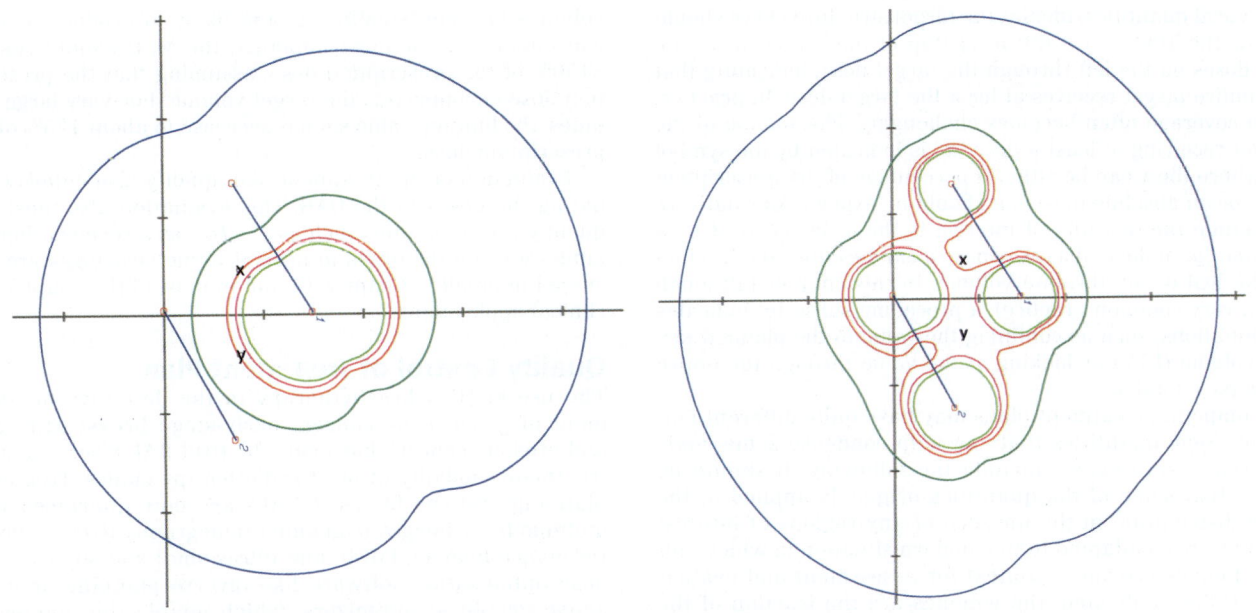

FIGURE 27.10. An example of potential optimization problem. **A:** The criterion was that the two optimization points (*X* and *Y*) receive the same dose, which was satisfied by a single active dwell position. **B:** Adding constraints on the dwell-time variation solved the problem. (Example inspired by van der Laarse R. Optimization of high dose rate brachytherapy. *Act Selectron User's Newsl* 1989;2:14–15.)

doses. Assuming that most of the manipulation occurs with the 100% surface, the 150% should also be on display.

Evaluation of Dose Distributions

Optimization calculations compute relative dose distributions and require only spatial dose information. After establishing the shape of the dose distribution, the entire distribution must be raised or lowered to give the correct absolute dose to a specified point or the average at a number of specified points. This process requires some evaluation of the dose distribution.

Other than visually examining the isodose distribution resulting from the optimization routine, there are some tools that provide quantitative assessments of various aspects. Thomadsen[18] provides a fuller discussion.

Figure 27.11 shows a typical dose–volume histogram for an implant. The histogram provides the basis for many of the

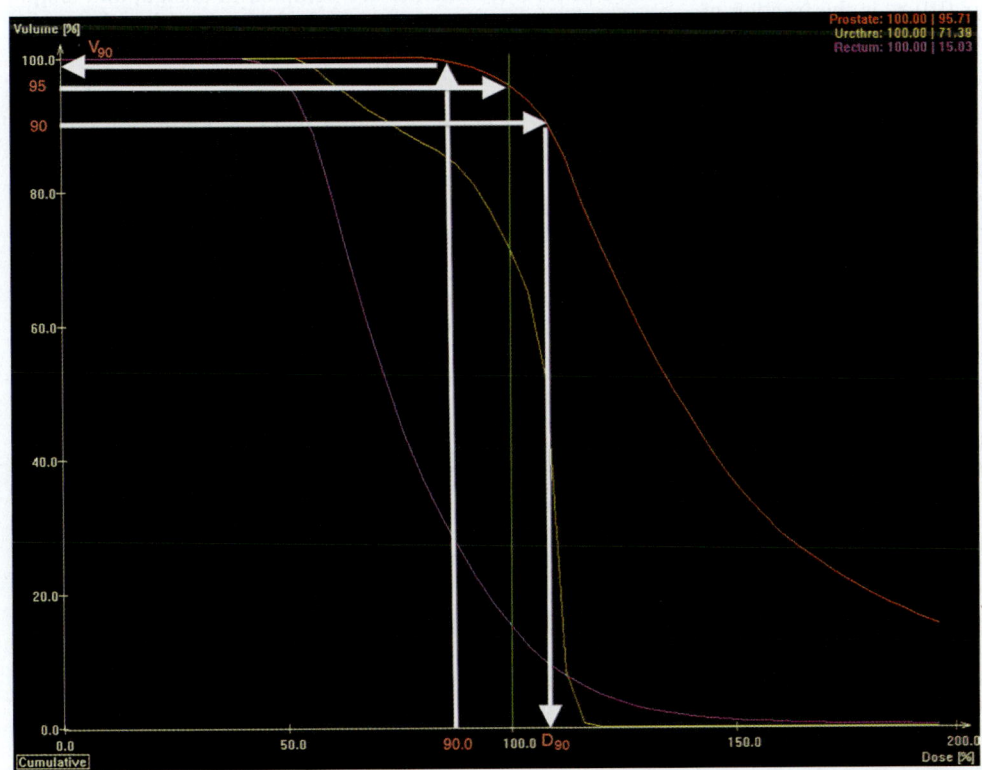

FIGURE 27.11. A dose–volume histogram (DVH) for a prostate implant. The *vertical green line* indicates that 95% of the prostate is to receive 100% of the prescribed dose. The fractional volume of the prostate receiving 90% of the prescribed dose, V_{90}, and the dose that covers 90% of the prostate, D_{90}, are also shown. This DVH also shows the volumes raised to specified fractions of the prescription dose for the rectum and bladder.

analytical quantities. Ideally, the target structure curve should follow the 100% (or 1.00) level (top of the graph) from the low doses on the left through the target dose, indicating that the entire target receives at least the target dose. In practice, such coverage often becomes challenging. The volume of the target receiving at least a dose "x" is indicated by the symbol V_x, where the x can be either a percentage of the prescription dose or an absolute dose, but should be explicit. Alternatively, sometime the quantity of interest is the dose received by a volume "y," indicated as D_y, where y can be either the fraction of the ROI or an absolute volume. In this chapter (although not a very common practice), a preceding subscript indicates delimitations, such as confining the value to the planned target volume (PTV) or looking at the value through the entire universe ("total").

Competing treatment plans may have quite different features. Some quantities that can help condense some characteristics into values include the following. It should be noted that some of the quantities originally applied to the dose distribution in the absence of any regions of interest but have been adapted to the modern situation in which volume images provide a context for assessment and evaluation. Unless indicated, the volumes are the fraction of the whole ROI.

Coverage is usually specified in terms of the faction of the CTV raised to a required dose. As an example, if it were felt that all the CTV should receive at least 95% of the prescribed dose, this would be specified as $_{\text{CTV}}V_{95\%}=100\%$. It might also be desirable that in a given fraction, 90% of the CTV receive at least 5 Gy, or $_{\text{CTV}}D_{90\%}=5$ Gy.

High-dose volume (HDV)[36–38] is the volume of an ROI raised to a dose significantly higher than the target dose, often higher by a factor of 1.5. Symbolically, we have

$$\text{HDV} = {}_{\text{ROI}}V_{150\%}. \tag{19}$$

Dose nonuniformity ratio (DNR)[38–40] is the ratio of the CTV high-dose volume to that taken to at least the target dose:

$$\text{DNR} = {}_{\text{CTV}}V_{150\%} / {}_{\text{CTV}}V_{100\%}. \tag{20}$$

Relative dose homogeneity index (HI)[38,39] is the fraction of the target volume receiving a dose between the target dose and the high-dose level:

$$\text{HI} = {}_{\text{CTV}}V_{150\%} - {}_{\text{CTV}}V_{100\%}. \tag{21}$$

Rarely are both DNR and HI used together.

Conformation number or *conformal index* (CN or COIN)[41,42] is a measure of how well the dose distribution fits the target:

$$\text{CN} = \frac{{}_{\text{CTV}}V_{100\%}}{{}_{\text{total}}V_{100\%}} \cdot \frac{{}_{\text{CTV}}V_{100\%}}{{}_{\text{CTV}}V}, \tag{22}$$

where all the volumes are absolute such as in cm³.

Each of these quantities tells a small part of the dose distribution's entire story. Each can help in the evaluation of a dose distribution, and all, taken together, give a better picture. However, none of the indices—even together—captures the complexity and nuances of the total dose distribution. Inspection of the results of the optimization remains a necessity.

The *maximum significant dose* (MSD) refers to the highest-level isodose surface that encompasses more than one needle track. The dose very close to a needle track becomes very high, but the body seems to tolerate these small local volumes. The MSD provides a convenient criterion for when the high-dose

volumes become "significant" and likely to produce biologic consequences. For most implants, the MSD should remain <150% of the prescription dose, assuming that the prescription dose encompasses the target volume. For vary large volumes, the limiting value should decrease to about 125% of the prescription dose.[4]

Evaluation of the treatment plan quality also entails evaluating the doses to the OAR. This evaluation also most frequently uses quantities such as $_{\text{rectum}}D_{2\,\text{cc}}$ as a review criterion. Limitations on the doses to normal-tissue structures are discussed in detail in Chapter 14 and in most of the chapters on clinical applications.

Quality Control of Treatment Plan

The use of HDR brachytherapy in the definitive management of gynecologic cancer,[2] early-stage breast cancer,[43,44] and prostate cancer[45] has made the HDR RAL a very common treatment modality in most radiotherapy clinics. Treatment planning systems for HDR RALs are now interfaced with multimodality images (computed tomography [CT], magnetic resonance imaging [MRI], and ultrasound) and sophisticated dose optimization software like inverse planning or interactive graphical optimizers, which enable the planner to maximize the dose uniformity while minimizing the implant volume needed to adequately cover the target volume and at the same time reduce the dose to the OAR. Such flexibility creates a challenge for the verification of the optimized calculations with practical manual calculation techniques. With the time constraint between HDR planning and the delivery of treatment while the patient is in the operating room, an efficient, precise, and easy method for checking the complex computer calculation is necessary for quality control of the treatment plan. Every institution should have an established quality control program that takes only a few minutes but at the same time gives a high probability of detecting significant errors, because the NRC considers a difference between the administered dose and calculated dose of 20% a reportable medical event.[46]

Simplistic models to verify computer calculations quickly have drawbacks because applicators or interstitial implants used in HDR treatments are complex in design, and simple point-dose or linear source calculations tend to fall apart in most circumstances.[17,47,48] Because all treatment planning systems have the capability of generating dose–volume histograms, it is logical that volume-based QA should be the choice. Das et al.[49,50] addressed this possibility and provided an easy and quick calculation check for most HDR interstitial and intracavitary implants. Because HDR treatments are delivered through a wide variety of applicators, the study was divided into three categories:

1. Single-catheter system, which includes tandem and cylinders and vaginal cylinders, as well as MammoSite balloons
2. Two- and three-catheter systems, which include tandem and ovoid pairs or ovoid pairs only
3. Multicatheter system for interstitial implants

SPECIAL CONSIDERATIONS

The following examples illustrate some of the aspects of the treatments that are unique for HDR applications. Other chapters discuss the actual therapies in more detail.

Cervical Cancer Brachytherapy

Intracavitary brachytherapy has been a major part of the treatment for cervical cancer for about 85 years, with a significant experience using HDR approaches since the mid-1980s. Of the advantages of HDR brachytherapy given earlier, several apply directly to these treatments, particularly the small size of the source and the concomitant smaller diameter of the intrauterine tandem, the greater stability of the treatment appliance and higher accuracy and relevance of the calculated dose distribution, and the ability to hold OAR away from the applicator and source track. Imaging plays a major role in these treatments, with the future likely seeing an increase in that role.[51] Ultrasound often provides guidance during the placement of the intrauterine tandem, particularly when the tumor obliterates the external cervical os and can help avoid perforation of the fundus. Fluoroscopy provides guidance during placement of the appliance, assisting in the assessment of applicator geometry (e.g., evaluating the centering of the tandem with the ovoids in both the anteroposterior and the lateral projections) and the positions of the rectum and bladder.

Imaging for gynecologic brachytherapy is evolving very rapidly, particularly for HDR approaches. Both the brachytherapy arm of the European Society for Therapeutic Radiology and Oncology (Groupe Européen de Curiethérapie [GEC-ESTRO]),[52-56] the American Brachytherapy Society (ABS) consensus guidelines for the locally advanced carcinoma to the cervix[57-59] and the International Commission on Radiation Units and Measurements (ICRU)[60] recommended moving toward image-based target prescriptions. Identifying the target, that is, tumor tissue in the uterus, requires MRI, the only form of imaging that also reliably differentiates the uterus from other pelvic tissues. GEC-ESTRO defines a high-risk clinical target volume (CTV_{HR}) as any tumor detectable by physical examination or imaging plus the entire cervix. Typically, 95% of the prescription dose should cover 95% of the CTV_{HR} volume, written as $_{CTV_{HR}}D_{95\%} = 95\% \, D_{Prescription}$. The formalism also defines an intermediate-risk clinical target volume (CTV_{IR}) based on the extent of disease at the time of diagnosis.* Generally, the CTV_{IR} should receive about two-thirds the dose of the CTV_{HR}. The recommended integrated dose to the CTV_{HR} in 2-Gy per fraction radiobiologic equivalence is 80 to 90 Gy depending on the tumor size including the external beam contribution. To maintain a connection to historic experience while prescribing the dose to a target volume, ICRU 89 recommends reporting the dose to the conventional point A, defined as per the American Brachytherapy Society.[57]

Although only MRI identifies the target and the uterus, CT images the rectum and the bladder well. Although using CT localization does not permit as detailed target information as MRI, it does allow moderate target definition and does facilitate determining the doses to the OAR when using conventional treatment prescriptions.[60] Dose calculations based on either CT or MRI often indicate that the maximum dose to the bladder falls 2 to 4 cm superior to the conventional point indicated following Report 38 of the International Commission on Radiation Units and Measurement (ICRU)[61] and may be two to four times the dose to the conventional point. The ICRU-indicated rectal point differs less than the bladder point, with the true maximum falling between 1 and 3 cm superiorly and the true maximum dose being one to three times the conventional point. The GEC-ESTRO and the ICRU 89 formalism specify the dose of interest to OAR in terms of volumes rather than points. For the rectum, bladder, and sigmoid, the point with the highest dose is found, and this point locates the volumes of interest. For each OAR, the minimum dose in the most highly irradiated 2-cm³ volume is recorded, as is the minimum dose in the most highly irradiated 0.1-cm³ volume.

The accuracy and precision of determining the dose matter much more in HDR intracavitary brachytherapy for the cervix than for LDR treatments for two reasons. The first concerns the precision of dose delivery. King et al.[62] demonstrated that the typical LDR tandem and ovoids move an average of 2 cm over the course of treatment. HDR tandems and ovoids move a maximum of 3 mm when not moving the patient.[48] Thus, the added precision of volume-imaged–based dose calculations would be lost in the general positional uncertainty of LDR intracavitary brachytherapy. In the second place, HDR applications not only can use the dosimetric accuracy, but they may require it. Because of the radiobiologic disadvantage of HDR brachytherapy, knowing the dose distribution with a high certainty is necessary to avoid complications.

Avoiding complications leads to several differences of the cervical applications with HDR compared to LDR brachytherapy. To prevent rectal complications, the dose to the rectum should remain <70% of the dose to the Manchester point A or the CTV_{HR}.[2,59]. Treating with the rectal retractor in place usually accomplishes this goal. As noted under the advantages of HDR brachytherapy, patients would not tolerate such a practice over the long durations with LDR applications. Adding distance to the bladder generally uses copious packing anterior to the ovoids, taking care not to let the packing slip between the ovoid surface and the superior or lateral fornices. An unpublished 1988 review of LDR cervical cases at the University of Wisconsin found the beginning of late complications in the superior bowel (fistulae) at about 13 years after treatment and that the prevalence increased continually with time out (unpublished). That problem with LDR treatments generated concern that the situation might be worse with HDR treatments because of the unfavorable radiobiology. With HDR, unlike LDR, the dose to the superior bowel can be reduced by not loading the tandem as high into the uterus and making the dose distribution more square than the LDR applications.[2]

Prostate Brachytherapy

Unlike most cancers, the α/β for prostate cancer is low, possibly as low as 1.2 Gy and lower than that for most normal tissues.[63,64] As discussed earlier, normally slow delivery of the radiation, such as with LDR treatments, allows normal tissues to recover better than tumors, whereas HDR causes a greater increase in the damage to the normal tissues than to tumors. When the relative size of the α/β inverts, as in prostate cancer, the advantages also invert. High doses per fraction cause a greater increase in damage to the tumor cells with an α/β of 2 than the normal-tissue cells with an α/β of 3. This situation makes HDR brachytherapy look attractive.[65,66]

Currently, the process for HDR treatments of the prostate follows the LDR model fairly closely. Ultrasound images provide guidance for the insertion of the catheters, although MRI guidance has also been reported and is likely to become more common in the future.[67-69] Generally, placement of the catheters follows a pattern such as four around the urethra and then at 1- to 1.5-cm intervals around the periphery of the gland. The square-hole pattern complicates placement at regular intervals, but the final dose distribution is relatively insensitive to the exact location of the catheters. Commercial software exists to guide the user in the placement of the catheters, but those experienced in prostate implants probably perform as well without computer assistance.

---

*The definition of the CTV_{IR} is actually more nuanced, and practitioners should study the references thoroughly before implementation.

After placement, the optimization routine calculates dwell times to achieve the criteria specified for the patient. The resultant dose distribution may still require adjustment through graphical optimization. On approval of the plan, the operator connects the needles to the treatment unit using the transfer tubes. Because the needles have no inherent numbering, great care must be taken during this process to ensure correct correlation between the needles in the patient and those in the treatment plan.

The location of the first dwell position in the needles would have been determined previously. Radiographing the needles with the x-ray markers in place forms one of the simplest methods. If the treatment unit does not seek the end of the needle to establish the first dwell position, all needles must be tested for uniformity of length.

Treating multiple fractions with the same insertion requires verification of the needle depth. Between fractions, the needles tend to work toward the surface and may need repositioning under ultrasound or fluoroscopic guidance. Marks on the needles where they enter a template also can serve as indicators of the needle for repositioning.

Breast Brachytherapy

Accelerated partial-breast irradiation (APBI) for breast cancer patients with HDR brachytherapy as monotherapy following lumpectomy has produced excellent local control rates and cosmesis.[49,70] Interstitial and intracavitary (catheter balloon) implants are used for this treatment modality. Usually within 8 weeks of lumpectomy and axillary nodal evaluation, the patient undergoes an interstitial implant with one of three methods: a prone, stereotactic, template method with digital mammographic guidance; a supine, ultrasound-guided technique; or a supine template guide CT technique, all three under local anesthesia. Because of the perceived technical challenge of multicatheter interstitial implants, alternative, intracavitary methods for APBI have been developed. One approach uses multiple catheters around the central catheter within a balloon that is placed within the lumpectomy cavity closed, often under ultrasound guidance, and inflated with saline or diluted contrast medium. Two such systems are the Contura (SenoRx, Bard Biopsy System, Tempe, AZ) and multicatheter MammoSite (Hologic, Bedford, MA). An alternative is the SAVI device (Cienna Medical, Aliso Viejo, CA) that uses six to ten struts in a configuration that looks similar to an egg whisk to hold the tylectomy cavity open instead of a balloon. The struts also serve as the paths for the source travel. A new device consisting of a double balloon (Best Industries, Springfield, VA) contains a single central treatment catheter and four peripheral treatment catheters that can be customized for radiation dosage coverage. The inner balloon can be filled with 7 to 30 cc of saline to increase the separation of the peripheral catheters and an outer balloon that can be filled with 35 to 110 cc of saline to displace the breast tissue from the peripheral catheters. The multiple catheters of each of these devices allow some shaping of the dose distribution, but not comparable to that obtainable with the multicatheter, interstitial implants. Imaging of the balloon for its integrity, as well as rotation of the multiple-catheter devices, should be performed before the initiation of each treatment.

ACKNOWLEDGMENT

We thank Adam Uselmann and Liyong Lin for the artwork they contributed to this chapter.

REFERENCES

1. Dale RG. The application of the linear-quadratic dose-effect equation to fractionated and protracted radiotherapy. *Br J Radiol* 1985;58:515–528.
2. Stitt JA, Fowler JF, Thomadsen BR, et al. High dose rate intracavitary brachytherapy for carcinoma of the cervix: the Madison system: I. Clinical and radiobiological considerations. *Int J Radiat Oncol Biol Phys* 1992;24:335–348.
3. Stitt JA, Thomadsen BR, Fowler JF. High-dose-rate brachytherapy for cervical carcinoma. *Int J Radiat Oncol Biol Phys* 1992;24:574.
4. Thomadsen BR, Shahabi S, Buchler D, et al. Differential loadings of brachytherapy templates. *Endocuriether Hyperthermia Oncol* 1990;6:197–202.
5. Kubo HD, Glasgow GP, Pethel TD, et al. High dose-rate brachytherapy treatment delivery: report of the AAPM Radiation Therapy Committee Task Group No. 59. *Med Phys* 1998;25:375–403.
6. Thomadsen B, Lin SW, Laemmrich P, et al. Analysis of treatment delivery errors in brachytherapy using formal risk analysis techniques. *Int J Radiat Oncol Biol Phys* 2003;57:1492–1508.
7. Cember H, Johnson T. *Introduction to health physics.* 4th ed. New York, NY: McGraw-Hill Medical, 2009.
8. McGinley P. *Shielding techniques for radiation oncology facilities.* 2nd ed. Madison, WI: Medical Physics Publishing, 2002.
9. National Council on Radiation Units and Measurement. *Report 151: structural shielding design and evaluation for megavoltage radiotherapy facilities.* Bethesda, MD, 2005.
10. Ezzell GA. Acceptance testing and quality assurance for high dose-rate remote afterloading systems. In: Martinez AA, Orton, CG, Mould, RF, eds. *Brachytherapy HDR and LDR.* Columbia, MD: Nucletron Corporation, 1990:138–159.
11. Ezzell G. Quality assurance in HDR brachytherapy: physical and technical aspects. *Act Selectron Brachyther J* 1991;5:59–62.
12. Chenery SG, Pla M, Podgorsak EB. Physical characteristics of the Selectron high dose rate intracavitary afterloader. *Br J Radiol* 1985;58:735–740.
13. Flynn A. Quality assurance checks on a microSelectron-HDR. *Act Selectron Brachyther J* 1990;4:112–115.
14. Grigsby PW. Quality assurance of remote afterloading equipment at the Mallinckrodt Institute of Radiology. *Act Selectron User's Newsl* 1989:1–15.
15. Jones C. Quality assurance in brachytherapy using the Selectron LDR/MDR and microSelectron-HDR. *Act Selectron Brachyther J* 1990;4:48–52.
16. Meigooni A, Williamson J, Slessinger E. Practical quality assurance tests for positional and temporal accuracy of HDR remote afterloaders. *Endocuriether Hyperthermia Oncol* 1992;9:46–48.
17. Williamson J, Ezzell G, Olch AJ, et al. Quality assurance for high dose rate brachytherapy. In: Nag S, ed. *High dose rate brachytherapy: a textbook.* Armonk, NY: Futura, 1994:147–212.
18. Thomadsen BR. *Achieving quality in brachytherapy.* London, UK: Taylor and Francis, 1999.
19. Thomadsen BR, Erickson BA, Eifel PJ, et al. A review of safety, quality management and practice guidelines for high-dose-rate brachytherapy. *Pract Radiat Oncol* 2014;4:65–70.
20. DeWerd LA, Jursinic P, Kitchen R, et al. Quality assurance tool for high dose rate brachytherapy. *Med Phys* 1995;22:435–440.
21. Nath R, Anderson LL, Jones D, et al. *Specification of brachytherapy source strength: report of AAPM Task Group No. 32.* New York, NY: American Institute of Physics, 1987.
22. Ezzell G. Optimization in brachytherapy. In: Thomadsen BR, Rivard MJ, Butler WM, eds. *Brachytherapy physics.* 2nd ed. Madison, WI: Medical Physics Publishing, 2005:415–434.
23. Pouliot J, Kim Y, Lessard E, et al. Inverse planning for HDR prostate brachytherapy used to boost dominant intraprostatic lesions defined by magnetic resonance spectroscopy imaging. *Int J Radiat Oncol Biol Phys* 2004;59:1196–1207.
24. Pouliot J, Lessard E, Hsu I-C. Number of catheters in prostate high dose rate brachytherapy: the role of inverse planning. Presented at the Joint Brachytherapy Meeting GEC/ESTRO-ABS-GLAC, Barcelona, Spain, 2004.
25. Sloboda RS. Optimization of brachytherapy dose distributions by simulated annealing. *Med Phys* 1992;19:955–964.
26. Sloboda RS, Pearcey RG, Gillan SJ. Optimized low dose rate pellet configurations for intravaginal brachytherapy. *Int J Radiat Oncol Biol Phys* 1993;26:499–511.
27. Lahanas M, Baltas D, Zamboglou N. Anatomy-based three-dimensional dose optimization in brachytherapy using multiobjective genetic algorithms. *Med Phys* 1999;26:1904–1918.
28. Edmundson GK. Geometry based optimization for stepping source implants. In: Martinez AA, Orton CG, Mould RF, eds. *Brachytherapy HDR and LDR.* Columbia, MD: Nucletron Corporation, 1990:184–192.
29. Nath R, Anderson LL, Luxton G, et al. Dosimetry of interstitial brachytherapy sources: recommendations of the AAPM Radiation Therapy Committee Task Group No. 43. American Association of Physicists in Medicine. *Med Phys* 1995;22:209–234.
30. Rivard MJ, Coursey BM, DeWerd LA, et al. Update of AAPM Task Group No. 43 Report: a revised AAPM protocol for brachytherapy dose calculations. *Med Phys* 2004;31(3):633–674. Erratum in: *Med Phys* 2004;31(12):3532–3533. PMID: 15070264.
31. van der Laarse R. Optimization of high dose rate brachytherapy. *Act Selectron User's Newsl* 1989;2:14–15.
32. van der Laarse R, Edmundson GK, Luthmann RW, et al. Optimization of HDR brachytherapy dose distributions. *Act Selectron User's Newsl* 1991;5:94–101.

33. Holmes T, Mackie TR. A comparison of three inverse treatment planning algorithms. *Phys Med Biol* 1994;39:91–106.

34. Luenberger DG. *Linear and nonlinear programming.* 2nd ed. Reading, MA: Addison and Wesley, 1989.

35. Thomadsen B, Houdek P, van der Laarse R. et al. Treatment planning and optimization. In: Nag S, ed. *High dose rate brachytherapy: a textbook.* Armonk, NY: Futura, 1994:104–108.

36. Pierquin B, Dutreix A, Paine CH, et al. The Paris system in interstitial radiation therapy. *Acta Radiol Oncol Radiat Phys Biol* 1978;17:33–48.

37. Pierquin B, Chassagne D, Chahbazian C, et al. *Brachytherapy.* St. Louis, MO: Warren H. Green, 1978.

38. Saw CB, Suntharalingam N. Reference dose rates for single- and double-plane 192Ir implants. *Med Phys* 1988;15:391–396.

39. Saw CB, Suntharalingam N. Quantitative assessment of interstitial implants. *Int J Radiat Oncol Biol Phys* 1991;20:135–139.

40. Saw CB, Waterman FM, Ayyangar K, et al. Quantitative evaluation of planar 192Ir implants [Abstract]. *Med Phys* 1986;13–580.

41. van't Riet A, Mak AC, Moerland MA, et al. A conformation number to quantify the degree of conformality in brachytherapy and external beam irradiation: application to the prostate. *Int J Radiat Oncol Biol Phys* 1997;37:731–736.

42. Baltas D, Kolotas C, Geramani K, et al. A conformal index (COIN) to evaluate implant quality and dose specification in brachytherapy. *Int J Radiat Oncol Biol Phys* 1998;40:515–524.

43. Clarke DH, Vicini FA, Jacobs H, et al. High dose rate brachytherapy for breast cancer. In: Nag S, ed. *High dose rate brachytherapy: a textbook.* Armonk, NY: Futura, 1994:321–329.

44. Kuske R, Bolton J, Wilenzick R, et al. Brachytherapy as the sole method of breast irradiation in Tis, T1, T2, N0,1 breast cancer. *Int J Radiat Oncol Biol Phys* 1994;30S1:245.

45. Martinez AA, Pataki I, Edmundson G, et al. Phase II prospective study of the use of conformal high-dose-rate brachytherapy as monotherapy for the treatment of favorable stage prostate cancer: a feasibility report. *Int J Radiat Oncol Biol Phys* 2001;49:61–69.

46. U.S. Nuclear Regulatory Commission. *Code of federal regulations—energy, Title 10, Chapter 1, Part 35, Medical use of by-product material.* Washington, DC: Government Printing Office, 2011.

47. Kubo HD, Chin RB. Simple mathematical formulas for quick-checking of single-catheter high dose rate brachytherapy treatment plans. *Endocuriether Hyperthermia Oncol* 1992;8:165–169.

48. Thomadsen BR, Shahabi S, Stitt JA, et al. High dose rate intracavitary brachytherapy for carcinoma of the cervix: the Madison system: II. Procedural and physical considerations. *Int J Radiat Oncol Biol Phys* 1992;24:349–357.

49. Das RK, Patel R, Shah H, et al. 3D CT-based high-dose-rate breast brachytherapy implants: treatment planning and quality assurance. *Int J Radiat Oncol Biol Phys* 2004;59:1224–1228.

50. Das RK, Bradley KA, Nelson IA, et al. Quality assurance of treatment plans for interstitial and intracavitary high-dose-rate brachytherapy. *Brachytherapy* 2006;5:56–60.

51. Thomadsen BR. Volume imaging in gynecological brachytherapy. In: Thomadsen BR, Rivard MJ, Butler W, eds. *Brachytherapy physics.* 2nd ed. Madison, WI: Medical Physics Publishing, 2005:785–796.

52. Haie-Meder C, Potter R, Van Limbergen E, et al. Recommendations from Gynaecological (GYN) GEC-ESTRO Working Group (I): concepts and terms in 3D image based 3D treatment planning in cervix cancer brachytherapy with emphasis on MRI assessment of GTV and CTV. *Radiother Oncol* 2005;74:235–245.

53. Potter R, Haie-Meder C, Van Limbergen E, et al. Recommendations from gynaecological (GYN) GEC ESTRO working group (II): concepts and terms in 3D image-based treatment planning in cervix cancer brachytherapy-3D dose volume parameters and aspects of 3D image-based anatomy, radiation physics, radiobiology. *Radiother Oncol* 2006;78:67–77.

54. Lang S, Nulens A, Briot E, et al. Intercomparison of treatment concepts for MR image assisted brachytherapy of cervical carcinoma based on GYN GEC-ESTRO recommendations. *Radiother Oncol* 2006;78:185–193.

55. Hellebust TP, Kirisits C, Berger D, et al. Recommendations from Gynaecological (GYN) GEC-ESTRO Working Group: Considerations and pitfalls in commissioning and applicator reconstruction in 3D image-based treatment planning of cervix cancer brachytherapy. *Radiother Oncol* 2010;96(2):153–160. doi: 10.1016/j.radonc.2010.06.004.

56. Dimopoulos JC, Petrow P, Tanderup K, Recommendations from Gynaecological (GYN) GEC-ESTRO Working Group (IV): basic principles and parameters for MR imaging within the frame of image based adaptive cervix cancer brachytherapy. *Radiother Oncol* 2012;103(1):113–122. doi: 10.1016/j.radonc.2011.12.024.

57. Viswanathan AN, Thomadsen B. American Brachytherapy Society consensus guidelines for locally advanced carcinoma of the cervix. Part I: general principles. *Brachytherapy* 2012;11(1):33–46

58. Viswanathan A, Beriwal S, Santos J, et al. American Brachytherapy Society consensus guidelines for locally advanced carcinoma of the cervix. Part II: High-dose-rate brachytherapy. *Brachytherapy* 2012;11:47-52.

59. ICRU (International Commission on Radiation Units Measurements). Report 89: Prescribing, Recording, and Reporting Brachytherapy for Cancer of the Cervix. *J ICRU* 2016;13(1–2). doi: 10.1093/jicru/ndw027.

60. Viswanathan AN, Dimopoulos J, Kirisits C, et al. Computed tomography versus magnetic resonance imaging-based contouring in cervical cancer brachytherapy: results of a prospective trial and preliminary guidelines for standardized contours. *Int J Radiat Oncol Biol Phys* 2007;68:491–498.

61. International Commission on Radiation Units and Measures. *Report 38: dose and volume specification for reporting intracavitary therapy in gynecology.* Bethesda, MD, 1985.

62. King CC, Stockstill TF, Bloomer WD, et al. Point dose variations with time in brachytherapy for cervical carcinoma. *Med Phys* 1992;19:777.

63. Brenner DJ, Hall EJ. Fractionation and protraction for radiotherapy of prostate carcinoma. *Int J Radiat Oncol Biol Phys* 1999;43(5):1095–1101.

64. Bentzen SM, Ritter MA. The alpha/beta ratio for prostate cancer: what is it, really? *Radiother Oncol* 2005;76:1–3.

65. Yamada Y, Rogers L, Demanes DJ, et al. American Brachytherapy Society consensus guidelines for high-dose-rate prostate brachytherapy. *Brachytherapy* 2012;11(1):20–32.

66. Thomadsen BR, Erickson BA, Eifel PJ, et al. A review of safety, quality management, and practice guidelines for high-dose-rate brachytherapy: executive summary. *Pract Radiat Oncol* 2014;4:65–70.

67. Cormack RA, Kooy H, Tempany CM, et al. A clinical method for real-time dosimetric guidance of transperineal 125I prostate implants using interventional magnetic resonance imaging. *Int J Radiat Oncol Biol Phys* 2000;46:207–214.

68. D'Amico A, Cormack R, Kumar S, et al. Real-time magnetic resonance imaging-guided brachytherapy in the treatment of selected patients with clinically localized prostate cancer. *J Endourol* 2000;14:367–370.

69. Menard C, Susil RC, Choyke P, et al. MRI-guided HDR prostate brachytherapy in standard 1.5T scanner. *Int J Radiat Oncol Biol Phys* 2004;59:1414–1423.

70. Patel RR, Das RK. Image-guided breast brachytherapy: an alternative to whole-breast radiotherapy. *Lancet Oncol* 2006;7:407–415.

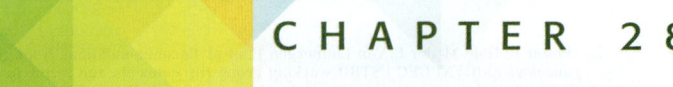

CHAPTER 28

Clinical Aspects and Applications of High Dose Rate Brachytherapy

Subir Nag, Granger R. Scruggs, and John A. Kalapurakal

Brachytherapy has the advantage of delivering a high radiation dose to the tumor while sparing the surrounding normal tissues. Brachytherapy procedures were initially performed by inserting radioactive material directly into the tumor ("hot" loading), which resulted in high radiation exposure to the physicians performing the procedure. Manually afterloaded techniques were introduced to increase accuracy and reduce the radiation hazards. In afterloaded techniques, hollow needles, catheters, or applicators are first inserted into the tumor and then loaded with radioactive materials. The introduction of remote-controlled insertion of sources eliminated radiation exposure to visitors and medical personnel. In this technique, the patient is housed in a shielded room and the radiation therapist controls the treatment from outside the room. Hollow applicators, needles, or catheters are inserted into the tumor and connected by transfer tubes to the radioactive material, which is stored in a shielded safe within the high dose rate afterloader. The radiation source is driven through the transfer tubes and into the tumor by remote control. Currently, most brachytherapy procedures are performed using remote-controlled afterloading techniques.

Remote-controlled brachytherapy can be performed using low dose rate (LDR), medium dose rate (MDR), or high dose rate (HDR) techniques. Although, the International Commission on Radiation Units and Measurements (ICRU) definition No. 38 of HDR is >12 Gy/h,[1] the usual dose rate employed in current HDR brachytherapy units is about 100 to 300 Gy/h. HDR has the added advantage that the treatments take only a few minutes, which can be given on an outpatient basis with minimal risk of applicator movement and minimal patient discomfort. Additionally, use of a single-stepping source, as used in most modern HDR afterloaders, allows finely tuned optimization of dose distribution by varying the dwell time at each dwell position. However, it should be emphasized that although optimization can improve the dose distribution, it should not be used to substitute for a poorly placed implant. Nag and Samsami[2] have provided examples of inappropriate optimization strategies that can lead to suboptimal dosimetry plans and clinical problems. HDR is normally given as a course of a number of fractionated HDR treatments, although it can be given as a single treatment, as in intraoperative HDR brachytherapy, if doses to the normal tissues can be sufficiently reduced by displacement or shielding. The advantages and disadvantages of HDR in comparison to LDR are enumerated in Table 28.1.

The advantages listed above have led to increased use of HDR worldwide; however, training and expertise are required for proper administration of these treatments. Guidelines and recommendations for the use of HDR at various sites have been published by the American Brachytherapy Society (ABS) originally between 1999 and 2001. In 2012, the ABS made updates to these guidelines and subsequently published them, much of which is summarized in this chapter[9–17] and the reader should refer to these publications for details. Controlled clinical trials are needed to critically evaluate the efficacy of these procedures.

RADIOBIOLOGIC PRINCIPLES OF HIGH DOSE RATE BRACHYTHERAPY

Most radiation oncologists are familiar with LDR brachytherapy. LDR (at 30 to 50 cGy/h) can be added to external beam radiation therapy (EBRT) doses (at 2 Gy/d) to obtain equivalent total doses. HDR brachytherapy is distinct from LDR brachytherapy, and radiation oncologists who are accustomed to LDR techniques must realize that experience in LDR cannot be automatically translated into expertise in HDR. It is important to review the current literature and survey the experiences of centers that have been performing HDR. When converting from LDR to HDR, one must keep the other parameters (chemotherapy, EBRT field/dose, dose-specification point, applicators, patient population, and so forth) the same, changing only the LDR to HDR.

Fractionation schemes for HDR are widely variable, and many radiation oncologists are not very familiar with the resultant biologic effects. Empirical methods such as the NSD (nominal standard dose), TDF (time–dose factor), or a dose reduction factor of 0.6 have been used in the past to convert HDR doses to LDR equivalent doses. The linear-quadratic (LQ) equation can be used to guide development of HDR doses and fractionation schedules.[18] However, the LQ mathematical calculations are tedious and may not be practical on a day-to-day basis. Hence, a simplified computer program was developed by Nag and Gupta[19] to obtain the isoeffective doses to be used for HDR. The clinician needs only to enter the EBRT total dose and dose/fraction, HDR dose, and the number of HDR fractions. The computer program will automatically calculate the isoeffective doses for tumor and normal tissue effects. Isoeffective doses are expressed in clinically familiar terms, as if given at 2 Gy per fraction (EQD2), rather than as biologically equivalent doses (BED), which are unfamiliar to clinicians. Furthermore, a dose-modifying factor (DMF) can be applied to the normal tissues to account for the fact that doses to normal tissues are different from the doses to the tumor, thus providing a more realistic equivalent normal tissue effect. This program can be used to determine HDR doses that are equivalent to LDR brachytherapy doses (EQD2) used to treat various cancers. Alternatively, the program may be used to express the isoeffective dose of different HDR dose-fractionation regimens as shown for cervical cancer in Table 28.2. It is remarkable that the isoeffective doses for tumor effects for the various fractionation regimens used for early-stage cervical cancers are so similar, ranging from 82 to 85 Gy, whereas those used for advanced cancers are about 90 Gy (see Table 28.2). The isoeffective dose for normal tissue late effects depends on the assumed DMF (0.6, 0.7, or 0.9). For the fractionation scheme shown in Table 28.2, row 1, the equivalent late effect on normal tissue (bladder or rectum) would be 59.5, 71, or 98 Gy, respectively, if the doses to normal tissues were 60%, 70%, or 90% of the prescribed dose to point A.

Although the LQ biomathematical model can be helpful in determining isoeffective doses, it has many limitations that must be kept in mind when using the program. The LQ model accounts for the repair of sublethal damage, but it does

TABLE 28.1 ADVANTAGES AND DISADVANTAGES OF HIGH DOSE RATE COMPARED WITH LOW DOSE RATE BRACHYTHERAPY

Advantages	Disadvantages

1. Radiation protection
  • HDR eliminates radiation exposure hazard for caregivers and visitors. Caregivers are able to provide optimal patient care without fear of radiation exposure.
  • HDR eliminates source preparation and transportation.
  • Because there is only one source, there is minimal risk of losing a radioactive source.
2. Allows shorter treatment times
  • There is less patient discomfort because prolonged bed rest is eliminated.
  • It is possible to treat patients who may not tolerate long periods of isolation and those who are at high risk for pulmonary embolism due to prolonged bed rest.
  • There is less risk of applicator movement during therapy.
  • There are reduced hospitalization costs because outpatient therapy is possible.
  • HDR may allow greater displacement of nearby normal tissues (by packing or retraction), which could potentially reduce morbidity.
  • It is possible to treat a larger number of patients in institutions that have a high volume of brachytherapy patients but insufficient inpatient facilities (e.g., in some developing countries).
  • Allow intraoperative treatments, which are completed while the patient is still in the operating room.
3. HDR sources are of smaller diameter than the cesium sources that are used for intracavitary LDR.
  • This reduces the need for dilatation of the cervix and therefore reduces the need for heavy sedation or general anesthesia.
  • High-risk patients who are unable to tolerate general anesthesia can be more safely treated.
  • HDR allows for interstitial, intraluminal, and percutaneous insertions.
4. HDR makes treatment dose distribution optimization possible
  • Variations of the dwell times of a single stepping source allow an almost infinite variation of the effective source strengths, and the source position allows for greater control of the dose distribution and potentially less morbidity.
	1. Radiobiologic
	  • The short treatment times do not allow for the repair of sublethal damage in normal tissue or the redistribution of cells within the cell cycle or reoxygenation of the tumor cells; hence, multiple treatments are required.
	2. Limited experience
	  • Few centers in the United States have long-term (>20 y) experience.
	  • Until recently, standardized treatment guidelines were not available; however, the American Brachytherapy Society (ABS) has provided guidelines for HDR at various sites.[3–8]
	3. The economic disadvantage
	  • The use of HDR brachytherapy as compared to manual afterloading techniques requires a large initial capital expenditure because the remote afterloaders cost about $400,000.
	  • There are additional costs for a shielded room, and personnel costs are higher as the procedures are more labor intensive.
	4. Greater potential risks
	  • Because a high-activity source is used, there is greater potential harm if the machine malfunctions or if there is a calculation error. The short treatment times, compared to LDR, allow much less time to detect and correct errors.

HDR, high dose rate; LDR, low dose rate.

not account for reoxygenation of hypoxic cells, reassortment within the cell cycle, or repopulation of tumor cells. These factors are generally small under normal circumstances. However, large doses per fraction do not allow reoxygenation of hypoxic tumor cells or reassortment of tumors from radioresistant S phase. Hence, a large radiation dose will preferentially kill radiosensitive cells, leaving a high number of hypoxic, radioresistant cells. Therefore, the computer program will overestimate the tumor effect of a single large dose per fraction (unless a resensitization factor is introduced).

The LQ equation does not take into account the proliferation of tumor cells. This factor is small if the treatments are performed over a short duration. However, if the treatments are highly protracted (e.g., there is a long time interval between EBRT and HDR), or in cases of tumors with high proliferation rates, the LQ model will overestimate the actual tumor effect. It also must be noted that individual α/β values are very variable. The α/β values for early reactions vary from 6 to 13 (the default in the program is set at 10); the α/β values for late reactions vary from 1 to 7 (default being set at 3), whereas α/β values for tumors vary from 0.4 to 13 (the default being set at 10). However, α/β values for a particular patient are not known and may vary even within the same tissue. The isoeffective doses obtained will therefore depend on the α/β values used for that particular calculation. The LQ model assumes complete repair between fractions. If the time interval between fractions is too short (<6 hours) or the half-time of repair is very long, the repair of normal tissues will be incomplete, and the LQ formula will underestimate the biologic effect. Hence, it is important to have sufficient time interval (at least 6 hours) between treatment fractions.

The infinite variation of the dwell times that is possible with HDR (or pulsed dose rate) allows better optimization of the doses than can be achieved with LDR. Better packing or retraction of normal tissues is possible with HDR, because of the short treatment duration. This factor is not usually taken into account in the LQ model (unless the DMF is altered). Another difference not accounted for in the LQ model is that the dose stated in brachytherapy is generally the minimum tumor dose. The doses within the tumor are much higher. Hence, the effective dose (for tumor control probability) is much higher for brachytherapy than for EBRT.

In view of the many limitations of the LQ model, it must be stressed that, as with any mathematical model, the LQ model should be used judiciously only as a guide and should always be correlated with clinical judgment and outcome results. Because of the reasons mentioned above, caution is especially warranted whenever large fraction sizes, a short time interval between fractions, or highly protracted treatments are used.

Common Uses of High Dose Rate Brachytherapy

Although HDR brachytherapy has been used in almost every site in the body, it is now most commonly used to treat cancers of the cervix, endometrium, prostate, and breast. Less

TABLE 28.2 AMERICAN BRACHYTHERAPY SOCIETY SUGGESTED DOSES OF EXTERNAL BEAM RADIATION THERAPY AND HIGH DOSE RATE BRACHYTHERAPY TO BE USED IN TREATING CERVICAL CANCER

Total EBRT Dose (Gy) at 1.8 Gy/Fraction	No. of HDR Fractions	HDR per Fraction (Gy)	Isoeffective Dose (Gy) for Tumor Effects[a]	Isoeffective Dose (Gy) for Late Effects with DMF = 0.7[b]	Isoeffective Dose (Gy) for Late Effects with DMF = 0.9[b]
45	4	7	83.9	74.2	90.1
45	5	6.0	84.3	73.4	88.6
45	6	5	81.8	70.5	83.7
45	5	5.5	79.8	69.6	82.6

[a]α/β ratio assumed for tumor = 10.
[b]α/β ratio assumed for normal tissue late effects = 3.
DMF, dose-modifying factor; EBRT, external beam radiation therapy; HDR, high dose rate.

commonly treated sites for HDR include the lung, esophagus, bile duct, rectum, head and neck, skin, soft tissues, and blood vessels (coronary and peripheral arteries). HDR is generally used as a component of multimodality treatment that includes EBRT and/or chemotherapy and surgery. A summary of the clinical uses of HDR is included in this chapter, while the details of the physics and radiobiology of HDR are provided in other chapters.

Carcinoma of the Cervix

Brachytherapy is a necessary component in the curative treatment of cervical cancers.[10,11] However, an evaluation of the SEER data by Han et al.[20] revealed an overall decline in the utilization of brachytherapy for cervical cancer between 1988 and 2009 from 83% to 58%. Furthermore, it was found that brachytherapy resulted in higher cause-specific survival and overall survival. Gill et al. reported their analysis of the National Cancer Data Base of women with cervical cancer undergoing treatment from 2004 to 2011. It demonstrated a decrease in the use of brachytherapy from 96.7% to 86.1% with a simultaneous increase with the use of intensity-modulated radiation therapy (IMRT) and stereotactic body radiation therapy (SBRT) from 3.3% to 13.9%. The use of external boost techniques resulted in inferior overall survival.[21] A practice patterns quality research study by Eifel et al.,[22] sampling 261 cases over 45 facilities between 2005 and 2007, revealed higher rates of EBRT use only without brachytherapy and protracted treatment beyond 10 weeks in nonacademic facilities compared to academic facilities. These findings across these various groups highlight our need to follow accepted treatment guidelines to provide our patients with the best possible outcome.

HDR brachytherapy has been utilized more frequently compared to LDR brachytherapy over the past few decades because of the ability to deliver therapy on an outpatient basis, avoidance of long-term bed rest, and avoidance of cervical dilation. Additionally, greater sparing of the rectum and bladder by temporary retraction, dose optimization, and integration with EBRT to the pelvis are possible.[23] These advantages must be counterbalanced with the greater number of treatments required (typically two to six treatments, lasting ~10 to 15 minutes each). An international survey published in 2012 revealed that 85% of centers now utilize HDR brachytherapy.[24] As LDR brachytherapy has been used for more than 100 years, it is imperative to analyze HDR brachytherapy, which has a much shorter history. A recent meta-analysis by Lee et al. compared treatment outcomes of LDR versus HDR for cervical cancer. Nearly 19,000 patients were analyzed, and there were no differences in 5-year overall survival, 5-year disease-free survival, pelvic recurrence, or rectal and bladder complication rates between HDR- and LDR-treated patients.[25]

The ABS recommends keeping the total duration of treatment (EBRT and HDR) to <8 weeks because prolongation adversely affects local control and survival.[10,11] To maintain this treatment duration, the HDR is interdigitated during the course of EBRT. However, it should be noted that neither EBRT nor chemotherapy is given on the day of an HDR treatment. Typically, if the tumor is small and the vaginal geometry is optimal, HDR brachytherapy begins approximately 2 to 3 weeks after starting EBRT. HDR is then continued one time per week with the EBRT given on the other 4 days of the week. If large tumor volume requires delaying the start of HDR brachytherapy, it may be necessary to perform two implants per week after the EBRT has been completed to keep the total treatment duration to <8 weeks.

The insertion of the applicator is performed under some form of sedation. The results of an international survey of gynecologic experts revealed that the most common form of sedation was general anesthesia (48%) followed by intravenous conscious sedation (28%), spinal anesthesia (27%), and oral pain medication (14%).[24] At some institutions, a Smit sleeve is placed to facilitate insertion of the central tandem. It should be emphasized that rectal and bladder retraction (by the use of packing or retractors) is essential in HDR as it is for LDR. The use of an external immobilization device (EID) to fix the position of the applicator is controversial; some centers prefer to use an EID to fix the position of the applicators, whereas others feel that the use of the EID is detrimental. Various types of applicators (tandem and ovoid or ring being the most common) have been used and depend on the preference of the radiation oncologist as well as tumor response to initial therapy to select the most appropriate device.

Treatment Planning

Traditionally, the HDR dose was prescribed to an arbitrary applicator-based definition of point A.[26,27] However, point A does not necessarily reflect the dose to the tumor. The ABS recommends the use of image-based treatment planning in brachytherapy for carcinoma of the cervix and specifically 3D imaging, where available, to optimize treatment delivery to the tumor.[10] It is well established that magnetic resonance imaging (MRI) is superior to other current imaging modalities in delineating gross tumor involving the cervix and adjacent normal tissues.[28,29] The use of MRI can lead to better delineation of the target volume, which could translate to dose escalation for better tumor control while simultaneously limiting dose to normal tissues. As MRI is not uniformly accessible, transabdominal ultrasound[30] or computed tomography (CT) scan[10] has been used as a clinically acceptable alternative to MRI.

The gynecologic working group formed by the Groupe European de Curietherapie and European Society for Therapeutic Radiology and Oncology (GEC-ESTRO) in 2000 formulated and described new terminology regarding three-dimensional (3D) image-based treatment planning in cervical cancer brachytherapy. Their recommendations are summarized in Table 28.3.[31] This working group recognized that in most patients, there is significant change of gross tumor during combined modality treatment. Because of this, a fluid description of treatment volumes during the course of treatment is required to have a better understanding of dose–volume relationships throughout treatment and to more accurately compare treatments between institutions and patients. They devised definitions of gross tumor volume (GTV) at diagnosis and at each brachytherapy procedure as well as high-risk and intermediate-risk clinical target volumes (CTV). Each of these

TABLE 28.3 GEC-ESTRO IMAGE-BASED PLANNING VOLUME DEFINITIONS FOR CERVICAL CANCER

Volume		Description
GTV_D	GTV at diagnosis	Macroscopic tumor extension at diagnosis as detected by clinical examination and visualized on MRI
$GTV_{B1,B2,B3...}$	GTV at each BT procedure	Macroscopic tumor extension at time of brachytherapy as detected by clinical examination and as visualized on MRI
HR $CTV_{B1,B2,B3...}$	High-risk CTV at each BT procedure	Includes $GTV_{B1,B2...}$, the whole cervix and presumed extracervical tumor extension at time of brachytherapy by means of clinical examination and by MRI
IR $CTV_{B1,B2,B3...}$	Intermediate-risk CTV at each BT procedure	Encompasses high-risk CTV with a safety margin of 5 to 15 mm (safety margin is chosen according to tumor size and location, potential tumor spread, tumor regression, and treatment strategy). The IR CTV is never less than GTV_D

BT, brachytherapy; CTV, clinical target volume; GEC-ESTRO, Groupe European de Curietherapie and European Society for Therapeutic Radiology and Oncology; GTV, gross tumor volume; HR, high risk; IR, intermediate risk; MRI, magnetic resonance imaging.

volumes would be determined via clinical examination and MRI (preferably T2 weighted) at their respective times during the course of treatment. The CTVs are based on tumor load and represent risk of recurrence. Thus "high risk" (HR-CTV) is that which includes macroscopic tumor, "intermediate risk" (IR-CTV) is that which includes significant microscopic disease, and "low risk" (LR-CTV) is that which includes potential microscopic tumor spread. It is assumed that the low-risk region is successfully treated with surgery and/or external beam radiotherapy. Their recommendations were expanded in 2006 to include descriptions of dose–volume parameters for organs at risk and a stepwise procedure for transition from the traditional dose prescription (i.e., point A) to the 3D image-based volume prescription.[32] The group recommended for organs at risk that the minimum dose in the most irradiated tissue volumes of 0.1, 1, and 2 cm^3 be reported. In 2010, they published recommendations pertaining to applicator reconstruction with 3D image-based treatment planning and in 2012 recommendations regarding parameters for MR imaging for adaptive cervical brachytherapy.[33,34]

As over the last several years there has been a transition from 2D to 3D planning, the Gynecology Oncology Group set out to establish a contouring atlas for both CT-based and MRI-based treatment planning. They compiled contours performed by 23 expert gynecologic radiation oncologists on both CT and MRI for three separate cases and have made available a contouring atlas at http://www.nrgoncology.org/Resources/ContouringAtlases/GYNCervicalBrachytherapy.aspx.[35]

The recommended combined EBRT and HDR dose to at least 90% (D90) of the HR-CTV is an isoeffective dose of 80 to 90 Gy.[11,31,32] The lower dose range can be utilized for early-stage disease (defined as nonbulky stage I or II < 4 cm in diameter) and the higher dose range is used for advanced stage disease (defined as stage I or IIA >4 cm in diameter or stage IIIB). The total pelvic sidewall dose recommendations are 50 to 55 Gy for smaller lesions and 55 to 60 Gy for larger ones. The ratio of EBRT to brachytherapy is dependent on the stage, with a larger EBRT dose used for the more advanced stages. Most centers use a schedule of approximately 5 to 7 Gy per fraction in four to six fractions (a smaller number of fractions is used by those using larger doses per fraction).[23,27,36,37] Some institutions use 8 to 9 Gy per fraction for two or three fractions.[38–41] These higher doses per fraction should be used with caution by experienced users. The HDR dose is also dependent on the stage of the disease and the dose of pelvic EBRT. While recognizing that many efficacious HDR fractionation schedules exist, the ABS suggestions and the isoeffective doses are given in Table 28.2 as a guide. These doses, while representing the doses to the traditional point A, correspond to the new HR-CTV D90 doses.

The University of Vienna has extensive experience with image-based dosimetry for intracavitary brachytherapy for cervical cancer. Their evaluations endorsed by the ABS have resulted in suggestions to keep the total isoeffective D2cc dose to the rectum and sigmoid <75 Gy and the bladder to <90 Gy.[42,43] As an example, in a patient who has received 45 Gy of EBRT and is planned to undergo five intracavitary brachytherapy treatments, the fractional HDR D2cc dose to the rectum and bladder should be kept to approximately <4.2 and <5.5 Gy, respectively. These doses would need to be altered based on the total EBRT dose and number of planned intracavitary brachytherapy treatments.

In certain clinical situations (e.g., a narrow fibrotic vagina, bulky tumors, the inability to enter the cervical os, extension to the lateral parametria or pelvic sidewall, lower vaginal extension, and suboptimal applicator placement), the normal tissue tolerance may be exceeded if the above doses are used. In these situations, either repacking or reoptimization may be attempted. If this fails to reduce the normal tissue doses,

the HDR fraction size can be decreased (which requires an increase in the fraction number), or the EBRT dose increased while decreasing the HDR total dose. At our centers, we prefer to use an interstitial implant in these situations. In the event of reduced vaginal capacity and if an interstitial technique is not available, Sharma et al.[44] have described an intracavitary technique that utilizes a central tandem with a single ovoid alternating with the contralateral ovoid with subsequent insertions.

Results of 3D Image-Based Treatment Planning

Over the last several years, there has been accumulating clinical evidence supporting 3D image-guided adaptive brachytherapy (IGABT) for cervical cancer. The University of Vienna has reported their results of utilization of MRI-based adaptive brachytherapy in accordance with GEC-ESTRO guidelines over the past decade. An initial report published in 2007 demonstrated improvement in complete remission and overall survival for patients with tumors > 5 cm between two separate time periods (1998–2000 and 2001–2003) reflecting the treatment planning changes employed by GEC-ESTRO guidelines.[45] Furthermore, grade 3 and 4 gastrointestinal and genitourinary (GU) complications decreased between the two time periods.[45] Dimopoulos et al.[46] performed a further analysis of this initial group of patients and found that a HRCTV D90 > 87 Gy resulted in a significantly lower local recurrence rate compared to a D90 of <87 Gy. They published updated results in 2011 evaluating 156 consecutively treated patients from 2001 to 2008. Three-year local control was 100% for IB, 96% for IIB, and 86% for IIIB. Three-year overall survival was 74% for IB, 78% for IIB, and 45% for IIIB. In addition, grade 3 + 4 late morbidity was only 3% to 4% at 5 years.[47]

The University of Pittsburgh has shown similar results. They evaluated 128 patients from 2007 to 2013 utilizing either CT or MRI after each application. Each patient was required to have at least 1 MRI for treatment planning. With a median follow-up of 24.4 months, 2-year local control was 91.6% and 2-year cancer-specific survival was 87.6%. Grade 3 or higher late toxicity at 2 years was 0.9%.[48]

Researchers at Aarhus University and Leiden University have published their comparative results of IGABT versus conventional brachytherapy (CBT). Aarhus University evaluated 140 consecutive patients treated with IGABT (2005–2011) and compared them to a prior cohort of 99 patients treated with brachytherapy based on x-ray imaging (1994–2000). Three-year actuarial local control for the IGABT group was 91%. No information regarding local control for the x-ray-based cohort was available. They also demonstrated an improvement in 3-year overall survival of 16% from 63% to 79% between the x-ray-based cohort and the IGABT cohort. There was also simultaneously a reduction in late morbidity by 50%.[49] Leiden University analyzed 126 patients of whom 43 were treated with CBT between 2000 and 2007. The remaining 83 patients were treated with image-guided brachytherapy (IGBT) between 2007 and 2012. The IGBT group demonstrated improvement in complete remission, pelvic control, overall survival, and late morbidity. Complete remission was significantly higher in the IGBT group achieving 98.8% compared to 83.7% in the CBT group. Three-year overall survival was also significantly improved from 51% in the CBT group to 86% in the IGBT group. Three-year pelvic recurrence rate was 32% in the CBT group and 7% in the IGBT group. Simultaneously, 3-year high-grade late morbidity improved from 15.4% in the CBT group down to 8.4% in the IGBT group.[50]

In 2008, GEC-ESTRO began a study on MRI-based brachytherapy for cervical cancer in a prospective multicenter setting called EMBRACE (European study on MRI-guided brachytherapy in locally advanced cervical cancer). The goal of the study was to evaluate outcomes and feasibility of GEC-ESTRO recommendations. In addition, the group started a retrospective collection of data from 12 centers treated with IGABT entitled retroEMBRACE. Results of retroEMBRACE have been recently published. With 731 patients treated, 5-year actuarial local control was 98% for stage IB, 91% for stage IIB, and 75% for stage IIIB. Five-year actuarial overall survival was 83% for stage IB, 70% for stage IIB, and 42% for stage IIIB. Late grade 3 to 5 toxicity at 5 years ranged from 5% to 7% involving the bladder, gastrointestinal tract, and vagina.[51] In their report, they suggest that overall IGBT improves pelvic control by approximately 10% compared to 2D-based imaging.[51] Analyses of 488 patients evaluating the effects of tumor dose, volume of disease, and overall treatment time on local control were also recently reported. HR-CTV D90 of ≥85 Gy administered within 7 weeks provides a 3-year local control rate of more than 94% for tumors measuring up to 20 cm^3. This drops to 93% for tumors up to 30 cm^3 and 86% for tumors measuring up to 70 cm^3. IR-CTV D98 of ≥ 60 Gy and residual GTV (Res-GTV) D98 of ≥95 Gy had a significant impact on local control. They also found that a dose of 5 Gy delivered to the HR-CTV is required to achieve similar local control when overall treatment time is increased by 1 week. Furthermore, an additional 5 Gy to the HR-CTV is required to achieve similar local control with an increase of tumor volume by 10 cm^3.[52] It should be noted that some of the patients included in the retroEMBRACE evaluation are those patients previously described above from the University of Vienna and Aarhus University.

The investigators of the EMBRACE study have recently published results regarding late rectal morbidity, late vaginal morbidity, quality of life, and early dosimetric evaluations.[53–57] In regard to late rectal morbidity, Mazeron et al. revealed that of 960 patients evaluated with a median follow-up of 25.4 months, the grade 3 rate was 1.6% and the grade 4 rate was 0.1%. There was a 12.5% risk of fistula at 3 years with a D$_{2cc}$ of ≥75 Gy. There was a two times lower risk of proctitis with a D$_{2cc}$ of <65 Gy. In regard to late vaginal morbidity, Kirchheiner et al. revealed that of 630 patients evaluated with a median follow-up of 24 months, the 2-year actuarial estimate of grade 2 or higher vaginal stenosis was 21%. The rectovaginal reference point was a risk factor with 20% risk at 65 Gy, 27% risk at 75 Gy, and 34% risk at 85 Gy. Additional risk factors included external beam radiation dose above 45 Gy and tumor extension into the vagina.

The American Brachytherapy Task Group published their review of literature of the clinical outcomes for cervical cancer patients treated with HDR brachytherapy in 16 prospective studies from 2000 to 2015. Of the patients treated with chemotherapy and radiation with HDR brachytherapy, the pelvic control, disease-free survival, and overall survival were 82%, 65%, and 70%, respectively, with at least 24-month follow-up. For these patients, the late grade 3 GU toxicity and late grade 3 gastrointestinal toxicity ranged from 2% to 20% and 1% to 11%, respectively. When comparing patients treated with chemotherapy, radiation, and image-based brachytherapy versus those utilizing the traditional point A dose prescription, there was a clinically significant improvement in both pelvic control and disease-free survival for those patients treated with image-based brachytherapy. The mean improvement was 3%.[58]

Additional studies have compared 3D IGBT to previous cohorts treated with traditional 2D planning and have shown improvements in local control[59,60] and reductions in toxicity[60,61] with 3D planning. Appropriate concerns on the feasibility of MRI-based treatment planning for brachytherapy include the increased cost of obtaining serial MRIs during a course of treatment (on average at least four to six during a normal course of treatment) and the limited availability and high cost of MRI-compatible applicator instrumentation for brachytherapy procedures. Table 28.4 summarizes the HDR fractionation and results of the published retrospective literature utilizing traditional treatment planning. Table 28.5 summarizes the results of recent literature utilizing 3D image–based treatment planning with the GEC-ESTRO recommendations. Although direct comparisons are difficult, it does give some insight to the variety of brachytherapy fractionation schedules used for cervical cancer.

In summary, the available data from recent trials suggest that 3D, image-based HDR brachytherapy of cervical cancer achieves superior tumor control with reduced morbidity.

Carcinoma of the Endometrium

HDR brachytherapy is commonly used for adjuvant treatment of the vaginal cuff after hysterectomy in patients with an intermediate or high risk for vaginal recurrence (high-grade, deep myometrial invasion or advanced stage). Additionally, brachytherapy may be used for primary treatment in inoperable endometrial carcinoma and for treatment of recurrences after hysterectomy.

TABLE 28.4 SUMMARY OF RETROSPECTIVE ANALYSIS OF HGH DOSE RATE BRACHYTHERAPY IN THE TREATMENT OF CERVICAL CANCER

Author	Stage	No. of Patients	EBRT (Gy)	HDR (Gy × Fractions)	Local Control	Survival	Late Complications
Lorvidhaya et al.[62]	I–III	1992	30–50	7–7.5 × 4 5.5–6 × 6	75.2%	68.2% (5 y)	4.8% Gr 3,4 Bowel 3.5% Gr 3,4 Bladder
Potter et al.[63]	I–IV	189	48.6–50	7 × 3–6	77.6% (3 y)	58.2% (3 y)	6% Gr 3,4 Rectal 4% Gr 3,4 Bowel 2.9% Gr 3,4 Bladder
Toita et al.[64]	I–III	88	50	6 × 3	82% (3 y)	77% (3 y)	12% Proctitis 11% Cystitis 14% Enterocolitis
Sood et al.[40]	I–III	49	45 9 Gy boost	9–9.4 × 2	77% w/o chemo 88% w/chemo (3 y)	78% (5 y)	4.1% ≥ Gr 2
Patel et al.[39]	II–III	121	Gr 1: 40 Gy (CS) Gr 2: 46 Gy	9 × 59 × 2	87.5% (5 y) 71.1% (5 y)	–	None ≥Gr 3 Rectal 1.7% ≥Gr 3 Bladder
Ferrigno et al.[65]	I–III	118	40–50	6 × 4	65% (5 y)	55% (5 y)	6% Rectal 6% Small bowel 1.7% Urinary tract
Souhami et al.[41]	I–IVA	282	45	8 × 3	75% (15 y)	57% (5 y)	6.3% Gr 3,4 Bowel 3.5% Gr 3,4 Bladder
Patel et al.[38]	II–III	52	46	9 × 2	81% (3 y)	64% (3 y)	4.5% Gr 3,4 Rectal 0% Gr 3,4 Bladder

CS, central shielding; EBRT, external beam radiation therapy; Gr, grade; HDR, high dose rate.

TABLE 28.5 SUMMARY OF 3D IMAGE BASED TREATMENT PLANNING HIGH DOSE RATE BRACHYTHERAPY IN THE TREATMENT OF CERVICAL CANCER UTILIZING GEC-ESTRO RECOMMENDATIONS

Author	No. of Patients	EBRT (Gy)	HDR (Gy × Fractions)	Stage	Local Control	Survival	Late Grade 3/4 Complications
Potter et al.[45]	145	45–50.4	7 × 4	IB–IVA	85%[a]	58%[b]	4%–5%
Potter et al.[47]	156	45–50.4	7 × 4	IB	100%[a]	74%[c]	3%–4%
				IIB	96%[a]	78%[c]	
				IIIB	86%[a]	45%[c]	
Gill et al.[48]	128	43.2–48.6	5–6 × 5	IB–IIIB	91.6%[a]	85%[d]	0.9%
Lindegaard et al.[49]	140	45–60	Pulse dosed rate	IB–IVA	91%[a]	79%[b]	7%
Rijkmans et al.[50]	83	45–50.4	7 × 3–4	IB–IVA	93%[a]	86%[b]	8.4%
Sturdza et al.[51]	123	46	Not specified	IB	98%[e]	83%[c]	5%–7%
	368			IIB	91%[e]	70%[c]	
	145			IIIB	75%[e]	42%[c]	

[a]Three-year local control.
[b]Three-year overall survival.
[c]Five-year overall survival.
[d]Two-year overall survival.
[e]Five-year local control.

Vaginal Cuff Irradiation

The standard management for operable carcinoma of the endometrium is total abdominal hysterectomy with bilateral salpingo-oophorectomy (TAH-BSO). Patients at high risk for vaginal recurrences (deep myometrial invasion, high histologic grade and stage, lymphovascular invasion, cervical or extrauterine spread, squamous cell or papillary histology) should receive radiation therapy. Two previous published randomized trials, Post Operative Radiation Therapy in Endometrial Carcinoma (PORTEC-1)[66,67] and GOG-99,[68] demonstrated general benefit of postoperative pelvic radiation therapy compared to observation in regard to local control with early-stage endometrial carcinoma and intermediate- to high-risk features for recurrence. Neither trial demonstrated improvement in survival. Following these two studies PORTEC-2[69] was undertaken to better answer how best to deliver adjuvant radiotherapy. As the majority of the recurrences in PORTEC-1 as well as GOG-99 occurred at the vaginal cuff in the observation arms, PORTEC-2 compared whole pelvic radiation therapy to vaginal cuff brachytherapy. Eligible patients for PORTEC-2 included patients 60 years or older with inner half myometrial invasion and histologic grade 3, outer half myometrial invasion, and histologic grade 1 or 2. Those with cervical glandular involvement and grade 1 or 2 histology, or cervical glandular involvement and grade 3 histology, and <50% myometrial invasion of any age were also eligible. The results of PORTEC-2 were published in 2010 and demonstrated that vaginal cuff recurrence was equal (1.8% vs. 1.6% at 5 years) in both arms. Additionally, it demonstrated that there were less acute grade one and two gastrointestinal toxicities with vaginal cuff brachytherapy (12.6% vs. 53.8%). This has led to an increase in the utilization of vaginal cuff brachytherapy alone in patients with a high intermediate risk of recurrence. A randomized study by Sorbe et al. was published in 2012 evaluating whole pelvic radiation with vaginal cuff brachytherapy versus vaginal cuff brachytherapy alone for patients with "medium-risk" endometrial cancer. "Medium-risk" was defined as FIGO stage I endometrioid histology grade 3 disease or grade 1 or 2 with ≥50% myometrial invasion or DNA aneuploidy. Five-year locoregional relapse with combined treatment was 1.5% versus 5% with brachytherapy alone, which was statistically significant. Overall survival between the two groups was equivalent. There was a significant difference in late side effects between the two groups favoring brachytherapy alone.[70] There still remains some controversy as to which patients fall into the high intermediate-risk group or medium-risk group as the four mentioned studies had subtle differences in patient eligibility. Thus, clinical judgment is needed when evaluating patients potentially eligible for vaginal cuff brachytherapy alone. The ABS released updated guidelines for vaginal brachytherapy in 2012, much of which is discussed below.[9] In addition, ASTRO with endorsement by the Society of Gynecological Oncologists published an executive summary in 2014 with regard to use of postoperative radiation for endometrial cancer with similar recommendations to the ABS as it pertains to vaginal brachytherapy.[71]

The American Brachytherapy Task Group published their review of the literature utilizing vaginal brachytherapy in various risk groups for overall early-stage endometrial cancer. Overall vaginal recurrence with the use of vaginal brachytherapy was 0% to 3.1%. In slightly higher-risk patients requiring whole pelvic radiation, the addition of vaginal brachytherapy has resulted in a vaginal recurrence rate ranging from 0% to 2.7%. Additional studies are needed though to better define when to use vaginal brachytherapy in addition to whole pelvic radiation. Although there are limited data regarding the use of vaginal brachytherapy in combination with chemotherapy and for treatment of high-risk histologies, in general, the vaginal recurrence rate is low. In regard to toxicity, their review of the literature revealed that the most common toxicity is vaginal atrophy/stenosis with a range of 0% to 5.2% for all severe toxicities.[72]

Technique

A vaginal cylinder is commonly used to deliver HDR brachytherapy. The largest diameter cylinder that comfortably fits the vagina should be used to increase the depth dose. The length of vaginal vault treated varies. Some treat the superior 3 or 5 cm, whereas others treat the superior half or two-thirds of the vagina.[9,69,73–75] For serous and clear cell histologies, treatment of the entire vaginal canal should be considered. The use of a single-line iridium 192 (^{192}Ir) source creates a dose inhomogeneity at the vaginal apex due to source anisotropy. However, the clinical significance of source anisotropy is debatable. The use of ovoids, circular rings, or an angled source may reduce the dose inhomogeneity at the apex created by the ^{192}Ir source anisotropy.[9] The applicator should be placed in the midline, as horizontal as possible and parallel to the longitudinal axis of the body for appropriate dose distribution. Placement of a radiopaque seed or clip at the vaginal apex helps to verify that the applicator is in contact with the vaginal apex on fluoroscopy or radiographs. However, these clips or seeds can sometimes fall off or migrate deep to the mucosa and, therefore, may not always indicate the position of the apex. Some centers prefer to use an EID to minimize movement; however, this is not mandatory. The use of a multichannel vaginal applicator such as the Miami applicator or the inflatable Capri balloon applicator may allow the radiation oncologist to better sculpt the desired radiation dose distribution in 3D for the individual patient compared to a single-channel device.[76]

The dose distribution should be optimized to deliver the prescribed dose either at the vaginal surface or at 0.5 cm depth, depending on the institutional policy. It is important to place dose optimization points not only along the lateral aspect of the vaginal wall but also at specified points about the dome of the vaginal cylinder to avoid higher vaginal apex doses, which can lead to vaginal vault necrosis.[2] Regardless of the prescription method, doses to both the vaginal surface and at 0.5 cm depth should be reported.[9]

The dose per fraction used has varied from 4 to 7 Gy, and the number of fractions has varied from three to six with the interval between fractions ranging from 24 to 72 hours up to 1 to 2 weeks.[73,75,77–79] The lower doses per fraction are usually given either using a larger number of fractions or in combination with EBRT to the pelvis. Sorbe et al.[80] evaluated two fractionation schemes (2.5 Gy × 6 vs. 5 Gy × 6) in a randomized trial and found no difference in locoregional recurrence rates but an increase in vaginal shortening, mucosal atrophy, and bleeding in the 5 Gy per fraction arm. The ABS dose suggestions[81] for HDR alone or in combination with 45 Gy EBRT is given in Table 28.6. Because some institutions specify the dose to the vaginal surface and others specify the dose at 0.5-cm depth, suggested HDR doses have been given for both specification methods.

From retrospective analysis, the 5-year survival rates of HDR therapy vary from 72% to 97%, depending on the stage, grade, and depth of myometrial invasion.[73,75,77,82,83] The severe (grade III or IV) late complication rate is usually <2% and depends on the dose per fraction.[74,75,77,84,85]

Petereit and Peracey[37] published a literature review analyzing 1,800 cases of postoperative HDR brachytherapy alone in patients with low- to intermediate-risk endometrial cancer. They found an overall vaginal control rate of 99.3%. Late morbidity was significantly higher with isoeffective doses for late responding tissues exceeding 100 Gy. Patient education regarding the use of frequent vaginal dilation following HDR brachytherapy is important to minimize vaginal stenosis and sexual dysfunction.[86,87] The National Forum of Gynecological Oncology Nurses (NFGON) has published best practice guidelines for the use of vaginal dilators following radiation therapy treatments.[88]

Treatment of Recurrences at the Vaginal Cuff

A combination of pelvic EBRT and brachytherapy is generally used to treat recurrences at the vaginal cuff. With distal vaginal recurrences, the entire vagina and medial inguinal nodes are included in the EBRT field. Intracavitary vaginal brachytherapy should be used only for nonbulky recurrences

(thickness < 5 mm after the completion of EBRT).[81] Interstitial brachytherapy is to be used for bulky recurrences (thickness > 5 mm after the completion of EBRT) and for previously irradiated patients.[15] Apical recurrences are often more extensive superiorly than can be judged on physical examination, thus favoring the use of interstitial brachytherapy. These patients are best treated at centers with considerable experience in interstitial brachytherapy. Radiopaque marker seeds or surgical clips should be placed at the margins of gross disease to delineate disease extent. If the relapse is limited to one wall of the vagina, consideration should be given to limiting the dose to the opposite wall. The ABS-suggested doses for HDR brachytherapy (in combination with 45 Gy EBRT) are provided in Table 28.7.[81]

Inoperable Endometrial Carcinoma

Patients with adenocarcinoma of the endometrium who are not candidates for surgery because of severe medical problems are treated with radiation therapy. A combination of pelvic EBRT and brachytherapy is preferred whenever possible. However, many of the conditions that do not allow surgery in these cases are also relative contraindications for EBRT and for LDR brachytherapy. In such cases, these patients may be treated with HDR alone.

The ABS released a consensus statement in 2015 with recommendations of treatment for medically inoperable endometrial cancer.[89] Numerous applicators can be used for treatment of primary endometrial cancer. The tandem and ovoid applicator, although often used, does not irradiate the uterine fundus homogeneously. Others have therefore used a curved tandem, turning it to the left and right in alternate insertions. A Y-shaped applicator irradiates the fundus more evenly. Other possibilities include modified Heyman capsules or multiple tandems. If CT or MRI is not available for treatment planning, then the dose is commonly specified at 2 cm from the source. However, the ABS recommends the use of CT- or MRI-based treatment planning with the latter the most preferable to ensure a more homogeneous dose to the entire myometrium. A volume-based approach is recommended with contouring the GTV as seen on T2-MRI sequences, CTV to include the entire uterus, cervix and upper 1 to 2 cm of vagina, and organs at risk. With respect to certain clinical situations, the ABS states that brachytherapy alone can be used for patients with stage I grade 1 or 2 endometrial cancer with minimal myometrial invasion as seen on MRI. In those same patients but with deep myometrial invasion, a combination of external beam radiation and brachytherapy is recommended. When MRI is not available or in patients with stage II or III disease, a combination of external beam radiation and brachytherapy is also recommended. The dose per fraction has ranged from 5 to 8.5 Gy, and three to six fractions are commonly employed.[90–93] The dose and/or the dose per fraction is reduced if EBRT is added. The ABS suggested doses for HDR brachytherapy alone or in combination with

TABLE 28.6 AMERICAN BRACHYTHERAPY SOCIETY SUGGESTED DOSES OF HIGH DOSE RATE BRACHYTHERAPY ALONE OR IN COMBINATION WITH PELVIC EXTERNAL BEAM RADIATION THERAPY TO BE USED FOR ADJUVANT TREATMENT OF POSTOPERATIVE ENDOMETRIAL CANCER

EBRT (Gy) at 1.8 Gy/Fraction	No. of HDR Fractions	HDR per Fraction (Gy)	Dose Specification Point
0	3	7.0	0.5 cm depth
0	4	5.5	0.5 cm depth
0	5	4.7	0.5 cm depth
0	3	10.5	Vaginal surface
0	4	8.8	Vaginal surface
0	5	7.5	Vaginal surface
45	2	5.5	0.5 cm depth
45	3	4.0	0.5 cm depth
45	2	8.0	Vaginal surface
45	3	6.0	Vaginal surface

EBRT, external beam radiation therapy; HDR, high dose rate.

TABLE 28.7 AMERICAN BRACHYTHERAPY SOCIETY SUGGESTED DOSES OF HIGH DOSE RATE BRACHYTHERAPY TO BE USED IN COMBINATION WITH PELVIC EXTERNAL BEAM RADIATION THERAPY FOR TREATING VAGINAL CUFF RECURRENCES FROM ENDOMETRIAL CANCER

EBRT (Gy) at 1.8 Gy/Fraction	No. of HDR Fractions	HDR per Fraction (Gy)	Dose Specification
45	3	7.0	0.5 cm depth
45	4	6.0	0.5 cm depth
45	5	6.0	Vaginal surface
45	4	7.0	Vaginal surface

EBRT, external beam radiation therapy; HDR, high dose rate.

TABLE 28.8 AMERICAN BRACHYTHERAPY SOCIETY SUGGESTED DOSES OF HIGH DOSE RATE BRACHYTHERAPY ALONE OR IN COMBINATION WITH EXTERNAL BEAM RADIATION THERAPY FOR TREATMENT OF INOPERABLE PRIMARY ENDOMETRIAL CANCER

EBRT (Gy) at 1.8 Gy/Fraction	No. of HDR Fractions	HDR per Fraction (Gy)[a]
45	2	8.5
45	3	6.3–6.5
45	4	5.2
45	5	5
50.4	2	6
50.4	6	3.75
0	4	8.5
0	5	7.3
0	6	6–6.4
0	9–10	5

[a]HDR doses are specified at 2 cm from the midpoint of the intrauterine sources.
EBRT, external beam radiation therapy; HDR, high dose rate.

45 or 50.4 Gy EBRT are given in Table 28.8.[89] The survival at 5 years for stage I disease is variable; however, some reports have revealed rates as high as 80%, which is slightly lower than that obtained by surgery.[92] Coon et al.[94] reported a 3-year overall survival of 83% for patients treated with 35 Gy HDR (treated twice a day) in five fractions without EBRT or with 20 Gy HDR in five fractions along with EBRT between 1997 and 2007. Some of these patients had higher stage disease. A later cohort treated at the same institution between 2007 and 2013 utilizing 3D image-based conformal treatment resulted in a 2-year overall survival of 94.4%.[95]

Carcinoma of the Prostate

Permanent implantation of iodine 125 (^{125}I) or palladium 103 (^{103}Pd) seeds has been the most common type of prostate brachytherapy. However, in recent years, HDR brachytherapy as a boost to EBRT has established itself as a way

for escalating dose to the prostate. Several institutions have published their results including one randomized study supporting the use of prostate HDR brachytherapy.[96–111] Table 28.9 lists these various studies. Different fractionation schemes have been used as seen in Table 28.9. In the one randomized study published to date with a median follow-up of 85 months, HDR brachytherapy boost significantly improved biochemical relapse-free survival compared to external beam radiation alone. The median time to relapse with an HDR boost was 116 months as compared to 74 months with EBRT alone.[112] One of the major advantages of HDR is that the dose distribution can be intraoperatively optimized by varying the dwell times at various dwell positions, potentially allowing reliable and reproducible delivery of the prescribed dose to the target volume while keeping the doses to normal structures (i.e., rectum, bladder, and urethra), within acceptable limits.[16,109] Another potential advantage of HDR brachytherapy in prostate cancer is the theoretical consideration that prostate cancer cells behave more like late-reacting tissue with a low α/β ratio and they should, therefore, respond more favorably to higher dose fractions rather than to the lower dose rate delivered in LDR brachytherapy.[114,115]

Patients with stages T1b to T3b prostate cancers without evidence of distant metastases are candidates for HDR brachytherapy as a boost to EBRT. Patients with distant metastases or a life expectancy of <5 years, or those who are medically unfit for anesthesia or in whom it is technically not feasible to implant the entire prostate should be excluded. Relative contraindications include large gland size (>60 cm³), significant urinary obstructive symptoms, recent transurethral resection of the prostate (TURP) within the last 6 months, large TURP defects, infiltration of the external sphincter of the bladder neck, pubic arch interference, and a rectum–prostate distance on transrectal ultrasound of <5 mm.[16,109] These patients have, however, been implanted by experienced brachytherapists by using modified techniques. Absolute contraindications to HDR brachytherapy include a preexisting rectal fistula.[16]

TABLE 28.9 RESULTS OF TREATMENT WITH INTERSTITIAL HIGH DOSE RATE BRACHYTHERAPY AS A BOOST TO EXTERNAL BEAM RADIATION THERAPY FOR PROSTATE CANCER

Author	Year	No. of Patients	EBRT Dose (Gy)	HDR (Gy × Fractions)	bNED Low	bNED Int	bNED High	FU (mo)	Grade 3 (GU/GI) Toxicity (%)
Olarte et al.[105]	2016	183	54	4.75 × 4			88.7	88.8	7.7/2.2
		56		9.5 × 2			87.8		8.9/3.6
Galalae et al.[106]	2014	122	50	15 × 2	82.6[b]	66.4[b]	72.3[b]	116.8	4.9/2.5
Boladeras et al.[107]	2014	271	60	9–15 × 1		91[a]		60	0.8/1.6
Kotecha et al.[108]	2013	229	45–50.4	5.5–7.5 × 3	95	90	57	61	4.9/0.4
Hoskin et al.[112]	2012	109	35.75	8.5 × 2		80[a]		85	9/0 (Late)
Prada et al.[110]	2012	313	46	9.5–11.5 × 2	100	88	79–91	68	0
Khor et al.[111]	2012	344	46	6.5 × 3		79.8[a]		60.5	11.8/0
Morton et al.[113]	2011	123	37.5	15 × 1		95.1		45	1.6/0 (Early)
		60	45	10 × 2		97.9		72	12/0 (Early)
Neviani et al.[103]	2011	403	45	5.5–7 × 3	94.3	86.9	86.6	48.4	2/1.3 (Early) 7.7/0.3 (Late)
Martinez et al.[102]	2011	305	46	9.5–11.5 × 2		81.1[a,b]		98.4	2.0/0.5
		167		5.5–6.5 × 3		56.9[a,b]			3/0.5
Kaprealian et al.[101]	2010	64	45	6 × 3			94	105	3.1/0
		101		9.5 × 2			84	43	1/0
Zwahlen et al.[104]	2010	196	44–50.6	5–6 × 3–4		82.5[a]		66	17.3/3 (Early) 7.1/0 (Late)
Deutsch et al.[100]	2010	160	45–50.4	5.5–7 × 3	100	98	93	47	NA
Bachand et al.[97]	2009	153	40–44	6–6.5 × 3 9–10 × 2	96.1	95.5	96	44	NA
Astrom et al.[96]	2005	214	50	10 × 2	92	87	56	48	10/0
Demanes et al.[99]	2005	209	36	5.5–6 × 4	90[b]	87[b]	69[b]	86	6.7/0
Deger et al.[98]	2005	442	40–50.4	9–10 × 2	81	65	59	60	11

[a]Authors did not report by risk group.
[b]Ten-year bNED.
bNED, biologically without evidence of recurrence; EBRT, external beam radiation therapy; GU/GI, genitourinary/gastrointestinal; HDR, high dose rate; Int, intermediate; NS, not stated; PSA, prostate-specific antigen.

TABLE 28.10 DOSE FRACTIONATION AND ISOEFFECTIVE DOSES (AS IF GIVEN AT 2 GY/FRACTION) OF COMBINED EXTERNAL BEAM RADIATION THERAPY AND HIGH DOSE RATE BRACHYTHERAPY DOSES USED FOR PROSTATE CANCER

EBRT Dose (Gy)	No. of EBRT Fractions	Total HDR (Gy)	HDR per Fraction (Gy)	No. of HDR Fractions	Isoeffective Dose (Gy) ($\alpha/\beta = 1.5$)	Isoeffective Dose (Gy) ($\alpha/\beta = 5$)	Isoeffective Dose (Gy) ($\alpha/\beta = 10$)
35.75	13	17	8.5	2	92	72	64
36	20	22–24	5.5–6	4	80–87	69–74	64–68
45	25	18	6	3	81	72	68
45	25	19	9.5	2	102	83	75
46	23	17.5–23	8.75–11.5	2	97–131	80–100	73–87
50	25	20	10	2	116	93	83
50.4	28	19.5	6.5	3	92	81	76

EBRT, external beam radiation therapy; HDR, high dose rate.

Various implant techniques and treatment planning methods have been used. As in permanent seed implantation, the procedure is performed under general or spinal anesthesia. Transrectal ultrasound is utilized for catheter placement, and cystoscopy may be performed to exclude the urethra and bladder. At some institutions, real-time transrectal ultrasound-guided treatment planning is performed. Other institutions use CT-based treatment planning. Fiducial markers are placed in the prostate so that radiographic comparison of the markers to catheter location can be confirmed prior to each delivery of each treatment.[116] Typically, 15 to 17 catheters are placed (although some institutions have used fewer) with fraction doses ranging from 3 to 15 Gy prescribed to the prostate (CTV 1—clinical target volume) depending on the clinical situation. Additionally, it is recommended to identify the peripheral zone (CTV 2) and any areas of macroscopic tumor (CTV 3) so that these areas can preferentially receive a higher fractional dose by dose painting. As in permanent seed implantation, the D90, D100, V100, V150, and V200 should be reported. Simultaneously, the organs at risk should be contoured and the D2cc of the rectum and bladder and D0.1cc of the urethra should be reported.[109] The interested reader should review the GEC-ESTRO and ABS guidelines for more specific information.[16,109]

Standard fractionation EBRT of 39.6 to 50.4 Gy or hypofractionated EBRT of 40 Gy in 16 fractions is given before, concurrently with, or after HDR brachytherapy. The minimum volume treated should include the entire prostate and seminal vesicles with a margin, with or without pelvic lymph nodes. The HDR dose is given in multiple fractions in one or two implant procedures. A variety of dose and fractionation schemes may be appropriate for same-stage disease as shown in Table 28.10.[96,98,99,101,102] The HDR fractions are generally given twice a day with a minimum of 6 hours between fractions. The most commonly encountered acute GU morbidities include urinary irritative symptoms, hematuria, hematospermia, and/or urinary retention, similar to LDR permanent implants.

HDR brachytherapy has also been used as monotherapy in a few centers, with dose fractionation ranging from 9.5 Gy × 4, 11.5 Gy × 3, 13.5 Gy × 2, and 19 Gy in a single fraction (Table 28.11).[117,118,120–122] The largest series to date is from Germany with 798 patients treated with either four fractions of 9.5 Gy each or three fractions of 11.5 Gy each. With a median follow-up of 52.8 months, the biochemical control at 60 months for low-risk patients, intermediate-risk patients, and high-risk patients was 95%, 93%, and 93%, respectively.[121] Late grade 3 GU and gastrointestinal toxicity was 3.5% and 1.6%, respectively. These results compare favorably to traditional permanent seed implant.[123]

Treatment of recurrent prostate cancer as well as treatment of de novo prostate cancer in patients who have previously received pelvic radiation is challenging. HDR brachytherapy has been used as salvage therapy post-prostatectomy, post-EBRT, as well as post permanent seed implant.[124–130] Overall patient numbers are low, so firm conclusions of its effectiveness are difficult; however, it does appear feasible in various clinical situations. Wojcieszek et al.[128] have reported their results of 83 patients utilizing HDR brachytherapy as salvage treatment for local recurrence following previous radiation therapy. Patients received three implants each delivering 10 Gy over a 4-week period. With a median follow-up of 41 months, 5-year overall survival was 86%. Late grade 3 GU toxicity was 13%, and there was no late grade 3 gastrointestinal toxicity. Yamada et al.[129] performed a phase II study evaluating salvage HDR monotherapy for patients with biopsy-proven recurrence following previous EBRT. Forty-two patients were enrolled and received a total dose of 3,200 cGy delivered over four fractions in a single implant. With a median follow-up of 36 months, the 5-year prostate-specific antigen biochemical relapse-free survival was 68.5%. One patient developed late grade 3 GU toxicity, and no patients developed late grade 3 gastrointestinal toxicity.

In a subset of men with localized focal prostate cancer, traditional definitive treatment with surgery and/or radiation

TABLE 28.11 RESULTS OF TREATMENT WITH INTERSTITIAL HIGH DOSE RATE BRACHYTHERAPY AS MONOTHERAPY FOR PROSTATE CANCER

Author (Reference)	Year	No. of Patients	HDR (Gy × Fractions)	% bNED Low	% bNED Int	% bNED High	FU (mo)	% Grade 3 Toxicity (GU/GI)
Hauswald et al.[117]	2016	448	7–7.25 × 6	98.9	95.2		78	4.9/0
Prada et al.[118]	2016	60	19 × 1		66[a]		72	0
Yoshioka et al.[119]	2016	190	6 × 8–9 6.5 × 7		93	81	92	0/0
Hoskin et al.[120]	2014	227	10.5 × 3 13 × 2		97[b]	90[b]	47	1–12.5/0[b]
Zamboglou et al.[121]	2013	718	9.5 × 4 11.5 × 3	95	93	93	52.8	3.5/1.6
Rogers et al.[122]	2012	284	6.5 × 6		94.4		35.1	0

[a]Authors did not report by risk group.
[b]Interpreted from table.
bNED, biologically without evidence of recurrence; GU/GI, genitourinary/gastrointestinal; HDR, high dose rate; NS, not stated.

may not be warranted. However, for some of these men, active surveillance is also not a desirable option. For these patients, the concept of focal therapy (destruction of the cancer with preservation of the surrounding organ) has emerged for prostate cancer just as it has been used in other disease sites. Improved imaging has allowed better localization of prostate cancer foci and thus the potential ability to better target these foci with localized treatment. Current modalities being investigated for focal therapy in prostate cancer include cryotherapy, high-intensity focused ultrasound, brachytherapy (both LDR and HDR), radiofrequency ablation, and photodynamic therapy (PDT).

HDR brachytherapy as a boost to EBRT for localized prostate cancer is being used more commonly, and its role has been well defined. Its use as monotherapy is increasing, and the early results are promising. Further studies are needed to more clearly define the role of HDR brachytherapy for recurrent disease after radical prostatectomy, previous EBRT, or permanent seed implant.

Breast

EBRT is the standard radiation modality used after lumpectomy in the conservative management of breast cancer. Over the past two decades, there has been an increase in use of brachytherapy as the sole modality of treatment[131-135] to decrease the 6-week treatment duration required for a course of EBRT to about 5 days. Table 28.12 lists the patients in whom an accelerated (4 to 5 days) brachytherapy treatment course can be an attractive alternative to 6 weeks of EBRT.[14] The ABS recommends a total dose of 34 Gy in 10 fractions to the CTV (lumpectomy site with 1 to 2 cm margin) when HDR brachytherapy is used as the sole modality.[136] The HDR treatments of 3.4 Gy are generally given at two fractions per day separated by at least 6 hours. This was also the dose used in a phase II RTOG trial[131] as well as in the phase III National Surgical Adjuvant Breast and Bowel Project (NSABP) B-39 Trial. Other prescriptive dosimetric parameters to be met recommended by the ABS include the following: (a) ≥90% of the CTV should receive ≥90% of the dose; (b) V_{150} and V_{200} should be <50 and <10 cm^3, respectively, for balloon catheters; and (c) maximum skin isodose should be <145% for balloon catheters.[126] Some investigators have evaluated ultrashort courses of accelerated partial breast irradiation. A fractionation scheme of 2,800 cGy delivered over four fractions in 2 days has been reported with acceptable toxicity rates.[137,138] Khan and colleagues[139] are planning a trial to evaluate a total dose of 2,250 cGy over three fractions in 2 to 3 days. Caution should be exercised with these ultrashort courses of accelerated partial breast irradiation until mature data are available.

The results of HDR brachytherapy as the sole modality are included in Table 28.13.[131-135,140-143,145-149] Depending on the selection criteria, final pathologic assessment is necessary to completely evaluate a patient for partial breast brachytherapy,

and, therefore, the ABS does not advocate intraoperative treatment delivery at this time.[158] There are a variety of ways to deliver HDR brachytherapy including an interstitial multicatheter implant, a single lumen incracavitary balloon, a multilumen intracavitary balloon, struts, and an electronic balloon. The use of a variety of commercially available balloon applicators has simplified the brachytherapy procedure. To date, two randomized trials have published their results of partial breast irradiation utilizing HDR brachytherapy versus whole-breast irradiation. GEC-ESTRO conducted a noninferiority trial and randomized patients to whole-breast irradiation versus partial breast irradiation utilizing multicatheter interstitial brachytherapy.[144] The 5-year risk of ipsilateral breast recurrence was equal in both arms with <2%. In a separate publication from the same trial, early side effects and patient compliance of 1,328 patients treated were reported.[159] Overall grade 3 early toxicity for all patients was limited to radiation dermatitis with a rate of 7% for whole-breast irradiation and 0.2% for partial breast irradiation. Polgar et al. reported their 10-year results of 258 patients treated on the Budapest randomized trial. A multicatheter interstitial implant was used for HDR brachytherapy. The 10-year rate of local recurrence was 5.9% for partial breast irradiation and 5.1% for whole-breast irradiation ($P = .77$). There was no difference in overall survival or cancer-specific survival or disease-free survival. An excellent or good cosmetic result was achieved in 81% of patients with partial breast irradiation versus 63% in patients treated with whole-breast irradiation ($P < .01$).[135]

In March 2005, the RTOG, in conjunction with the NSABP, opened a phase III randomized study (NSABP B-39) investigating standard whole-breast radiotherapy versus partial breast radiotherapy after lumpectomy for women with early-stage breast cancer. The partial breast treatment arm consists of three therapeutic options which are IMRT, HDR brachytherapy via MammoSite, Contura, or SAVI, and HDR brachytherapy via a multicatheter interstitial implant. The required dose for the brachytherapy treatment is 34 Gy given in 10 fractions over 5 days. The trial closed in April 2013 upon reaching its adjusted target accrual of 4,215 patients. It is hoped that over time, these large randomized studies will shed some light on the usefulness of partial breast irradiation and brachytherapy as a sole modality of treatment.

Various medical societies have published consensus statement guidelines for the selection of appropriate patients for breast brachytherapy as a sole modality treatment with slight variations.[14,160] According to the American Society of Therapeutic Radiology and Oncology (ASTRO) consensus statement, "Suitable" patients for accelerated partial breast irradiation include women 50 years of age and older, with unifocal tumors 2 cm in size or less, negative margins by at least 2 mm, and invasive ductal histology. The "Suitable" category also now includes patients with ductal carcinoma *in situ* who meet the following additional criteria: screening detected, low to intermediate nuclear grade, size ≤2.5 cm, and negative margins by at least 3 mm. The consensus statement also outlined criteria for "Cautionary" and "Unsuitable" candidates. The reader is encouraged to review the consensus statement for full details.[160] Thus far local control and cosmesis are similar to whole-breast EBRT with one group quoting 12-year follow-up.[132] However, further follow-up of clinical studies are required to define the most appropriate candidates for breast brachytherapy as a sole modality treatment and to determine the best delivery method of brachytherapy (multicatheter interstitial implant vs. balloon brachytherapy) in such patients.

A newer device, the Axxent (Xoft Inc., Sunnyvale, CA), uses a miniaturized x-ray source to deliver low-energy x-rays within a needle or catheter thereby mimicking HDR brachytherapy. The reduced radiation protection required for these devices because of limited penetration is a great advantage

---

TABLE 28.12 AMERICAN BRACHYTHERAPY SOCIETY ACCEPTABLE CRITERIA FOR ACCELERATED PARTIAL BREAST IRRADIATION

Indications for Brachytherapy as the Sole Modality	Indications for Brachytherapy as a Boost to EBRT
1. Age ≥ 50 years old	1. For patients with close, positive, or unknown margins
2. Size ≤ 3 cm	2. For patients with EIC
3. Histology: all invasive subtypes and DCIS	3. For younger patients
4. Estrogen receptor: positive or negative	4. For deep tumor location in a large breast
5. Surgical margins negative	5. For CTV of irregular thickness
6. Lymphovascular space invasion negative	
7. Nodal status negative	

CTV, clinical target volume; EBRT, external beam radiation therapy; EIC, extensive intraductal component.

TABLE 28.13 RESULTS OF BREAST-CONSERVING THERAPY WITH LUMPECTOMY PLUS HIGH DOSE RATE BRACHYTHERAPY OR AS A BOOST TO EXTERNAL BEAM RADIATION THERAPY

Author (Reference)	No. of Patients	Modality	HDR (Gy × Fractions)	Total Dose (Gy)	Median Follow-Up (mo)	Local Recurrence (%)	Good/Excellent Cosmetic Results (%)
HDR Alone							
Chen et al.[140]	79	Interstitial	4 × 8	32	76.8	1.5[a]	95–99[b]
			3.4 × 10	34			
Arthur et al.[131]	66	Interstitial	3.4 × 10	34	78.6	3	Not stated
Polgar et al.[132]	37	Interstitial	5.2 × 7	36.4	133	9.3	77.8
	8		4.33 × 7	30.3			
Strnad ct al.[133]	274	Interstitial	4 × 8	32	63	2.9	90
			PDR 0.6 Gy	49.8			
Aristei et al.[141]	100	Interstitial	4 × 8	32	60	1	98
Polgar et al.[135]	128	Interstitial	5.2 × 7	36.4	122.4	5.9[c]	81
Genebes et al.[142]	70	Interstitial	3.4 × 10	34	60.9	2.4	95.7
			4 × 8	32			
Budrukkar et al.[143]	140	Interstitial	3.4 × 10	34	60	3	77
Strnad et al.[144]	633	Interstitial	4 × 8	32	60	1.44	
			4.3 × 7	30.1			
			PDR 0.6 Gy	50			
White et al.[145]	98	Interstitial	3.4 × 10	34	145.2	5.2	
			LDR	45			
Benitez et al.[146]	43	MammoSite	3.4 × 10	34	65.2[d] (Mean)	0	83.3[d]
Harper et al.[147]	111	MammoSite	3.4 × 10	34	46	6.3	
Vicini et al.[134d]	1449	MammoSite	3.4 × 10	34	53.7	2.6	90.6
Vargo et al.[148]	157	MammoSite	3.4 × 10	34	66	2.5	93.4
Mann et al.[149]	111	Balloon	3.4 × 10	34	66	2.7	98.1
HDR Boost							
Henriquez et al.[150]	294		2–2.5 × 8–11		69.6	9	96
Polgar et al.[5]	19		4 × 3	12	63.6	7.7	88.5
	33		4.75 × 3	14.25			
Resch et al.[6]	274		7–12 × 1	7–12	104 (Mean)	1.5	38
Neumanova et al.[151]	215		8–12 × 1	8–12	69.6	1.5	73
Budrukkar et al.[152]	153		10 × 1	10	36	8	83
Guinot et al.[153]	125		4.4 × 3	13.2	84	4.2	77
Polgar et al.[154]	88		4–4.75 × 3	12–14.25	75	4.5	57
	10		8–10.35 × 1	8–10.35			
Knauerhase et al.[155]	75		8–12 × 1	8–12	93.6	5.9	Not stated
Guinot et al.[156]	167		7 × 1	7	92	4.3	97
Quero et al.[157]	621		5 × 2	10	123.6	7.4	80

[a]Reported at median follow-up of 45.6 months.
[b]Includes patients treated with LDR.
[c]Includes patients treated via partial breast irradiation with 50 Gy in 25 fractions with electrons, *n* = 128.
[d]Includes 36 patients only.
EBRT, external beam radiation therapy; HDR, high dose rate; LDR, low dose rate; PDR, pulsed dose rate.

because it allows brachytherapy to be delivered in a non-shielded procedure room or a regular (unshielded) hospital operating suite. Although longer follow-up is needed to assess the risk of recurrence, early results with the use of this device for accelerated partial breast irradiation reveal that the procedure is tolerated well and grade 3 adverse events are minimal with 93.4% excellent or good cosmetic result at 1 year in one study evaluating 69 patients.[161–163]

Brachytherapy has been used to boost the EBRT dose in select high-risk patients.[3,4] Data on the use of HDR as a boost are limited (see Table 28.13).[5,6,150–157] Polgar et al.[5] reported the results of a randomized trial involving 207 women with stage I or II breast cancer treated with breast-conserving surgery and whole-breast radiotherapy and subsequently randomized to either no further therapy or radiation boost to the tumor bed. The radiation boost consisted of either 16 Gy of electron irradiation or 12 to 14.5 Gy fractionated HDR brachytherapy. Fifty-two patients were treated with HDR brachytherapy, and the 5-year local tumor control rate was 91.4%. Excellent to good cosmesis was reported in 88.5% of patients. Similar results were noted in the group of patients receiving an electron irradiation boost. Because brachytherapy is an invasive procedure, it should be used selectively as a boosting technique. Situations in which brachytherapy may be advantageous as a boost are listed in Table 28.12. The brachytherapy boost can be given before or after EBRT, usually with a 1- to 2-week gap between EBRT and brachytherapy. The ABS recommends a dose-fractionation scheme that yields early and late effects approximately equivalent to those of 10 to 20 Gy LDR following 45 to 50 Gy EBRT.[164] Biomathematical models are often used to estimate equivalent HDR regimens.[18,19] For example, an HDR regimen of five fractions of 310 cGy per fraction should approximate the early and late effects of 20 Gy LDR delivered at 0.5 Gy/h. Although biomathematical models can be used to estimate the appropriate dose, there is no standardized HDR fractionation schedule that can be recommended for the use of HDR as a boost. Controlled clinical studies are required to further define the most appropriate doses to be used for boost treatment.

Use of interstitial HDR brachytherapy as neoadjuvant treatment in select patients not amenable to breast-conserving surgery at presentation has been reported by Roddiger et al.[165] Fifty-three patients who were unable to undergo breast-conserving surgery because of either initial tumor size or an unfavorable breast–tumor ratio were treated with systemic chemotherapy and HDR brachytherapy with 5 Gy twice per day for 3 days (total dose 30 Gy). Of these patients, 56.6% went on to receive breast-conserving surgery, and with a median follow-up of 56 months, the local recurrence rate was 2%. Further studies are needed to fully define the roll of interstitial HDR brachytherapy as neoadjuvant treatment, but these results are encouraging.

Another clinical situation in which HDR brachytherapy has been evaluated is in the setting of salvage therapy to continue maintaining the breast in previously irradiated patients.[7,166] Current standard of care of recurrent disease following breast conservation is total mastectomy. Guix et al. reported their series of 36 patients who had previously been treated with lumpectomy, external beam radiation, and HDR brachytherapy boost who subsequently developed an ipsilateral breast recurrence and underwent excision only of the recurrence. Following excision, all patients underwent a HDR brachytherapy implant delivering 30 Gy in 12 fractions over 5 days. With a median follow-up of 89 months, 10-year local control was 89.4% and 10-year disease-free survival was 64.4%. They reported a 90.4% satisfactory cosmetic result.[166] GEC-ESTRO conducted a retrospective study and reported their results of 217 patients treated with multicatheter brachytherapy (low dose rate, pulsed dose rate, or high dose rate) following second conservative management for a local recurrence. Ten-year actuarial local recurrence rate was 7.2%.[7] Again although numbers are small, the possibility of continuing to provide breast conservation in the setting of recurrent disease is encouraging.

Endobronchial Radiation

The use of HDR brachytherapy is well established for palliation of cough, dyspnea, pain, and hemoptysis in patients with advanced or metastatic lung cancer. The use of brachytherapy as a boost to EBRT in curative cases should be restricted to a select group of patients who have predominantly endobronchial disease, are medically inoperable, or have small/occult carcinomas of the lung.

An initial bronchoscopy is performed to evaluate the airway and locate the site of obstruction. The updated ABS guidelines in 2016 further recommend CT imaging to evaluate for any potential extent of tumor beyond the bronchus as brachytherapy as an adjunct to external radiation would be preferable in such cases.[13] Either a 5- or 6-French (Fr) catheter (inserted through the brush channel of the bronchoscope) can be used to deliver the brachytherapy. Use of a 6-Fr catheter allows the HDR source to negotiate tight curves, which is not possible with the 5-Fr catheter. If a 6-Fr catheter is used, a large bronchoscope (with brush channel diameter of at least 2.2 mm) is required. The bronchoscope can be connected to a teaching head or a video monitor so that the radiation oncologist can also visualize the lesion and the catheter. It is extremely important to note the distances between the proximal extent of the tumor and fixed structures such as the carina. The catheter is inserted through the brush channel of the bronchoscope, passed through the tumor, and lodged in one of the smaller bronchi. Fluoroscopic confirmation of the catheter's position is desirable. The radiation oncologist then pushes the afterloading catheter in while the pulmonologist slowly withdraws the bronchoscope. The use of fluoroscopy assists in keeping the catheter in place during this push–pull technique of bronchoscope removal. The catheter is then secured with tape at the nose, and its position is marked in ink to alert the radiation oncologist in case of displacement. As an additional precautionary measure, the external length of the catheter from the tip of the nostril is noted. If multiple catheters are to be used, the procedure is repeated, taking care to clearly label each catheter. The ABS recommends obtaining CT imaging to identify applicator location and subsequently treating the patient in the same position in which the CT was obtained. If multiple insertions are planned, then CT imaging should be obtained at each insertion. Utilization of CT for planning purposes may lead to decreased complications with better visualization of organs at risk.[167,168]

With the use of CT-based planning, the dose should be prescribed to a target volume keeping in mind dose to organs at risk. A fixed prescription point from the source is no longer recommended unless the clinical situation deems it appropriate and safe. When reporting dose, one should record the dose to the target volume, organs at risk, as well as at 1 cm from the center of the catheter.[13] Caution should be exercised when metallic stents are present as dose to the mucosa can be significantly increased from the stent surface.[169]

Palliative Endobronchial Brachytherapy

Candidates for palliative endobronchial brachytherapy include the following[13]:

1. Patients with a significant endobronchial tumor component that causes symptoms such as shortness of breath, hemoptysis, persistent cough, and other signs of postobstructive pneumonitis. Tumors with a predominantly endobronchial component are considered suitable, as opposed to extrinsic tumors that compress the bronchus or the trachea. Endobronchial brachytherapy can generally give quicker palliation of obstruction than EBRT. Furthermore, brachytherapy can be more convenient than 2 to 3 weeks of daily EBRT.
2. Patients who are unable to tolerate any EBRT because of poor lung function.
3. Patients with previous EBRT of sufficient total dose to preclude further EBRT.

A variety of doses have been successfully used by various centers. Retrospective reviews and randomized studies have found no difference in efficacy or survival with different fractionation regimens.[8,170–172] Table 28.14 lists the ABS recommended dose-fractionation schemes for endobronchial brachytherapy. These fractionation regimens have similar radiobiologic equivalence using the linear-quadratic model,[19] and there is no evidence of superiority for one regimen over the other. The benefits of fewer bronchoscopic applications should be weighed against the risks of higher dose per fraction. The interval between fractions is generally 1 to 2 weeks. If HDR is planned following palliative EBRT, then a reduced fractionation scheme is recommended. The brachytherapy dose should also be reduced when aggressive chemotherapy is given. Concomitant chemotherapy should be avoided during brachytherapy, unless it is in the context of a clinical trial.

The results from various centers (summarized in Table 28.15) show clinical improvement from 55% to 100% and bronchoscopy response from 57% to 100%.[170,171,174–183] Comparison of these results is difficult because of the differences in patient population and the variability in dose and fractionation employed. Complications of endobronchial brachytherapy include radiation bronchitis, stenosis, and fatal hemoptysis. Risk factors that increase complications include hypertension, chronic cardiac arrhythmias, chronic obstructive pulmonary disease (COPD), and cardiomyopathy.[184] Direct contact of the applicator to the tracheobronchial wall increases the risk of massive hemoptysis.[167]

TABLE 28.14 AMERICAN BRACHYTHERAPY SOCIETY SUGGESTED DOSES OF HIGH DOSE RATE ENDOBRONCHIAL BRACHYTHERAPY

HDR per Fraction (Gy)	No. of Fractions	Total Dose (Gy)
Brachytherapy alone		
10	1	10
15	1	15
7.1–10	2	14.2–20
7.5	3	22.5
6	4	24
5	6	30
Brachytherapy as a boost following EBRT[a]		
5	2	10
5	3	15

[a]EBRT of 60 Gy in 30 fractions.
HDR, high dose rate.

TABLE 28.15 SUMMARY OF HIGH DOSE RATE ENDOBRONCHIAL BRACHYTHERAPY FOR PALLIATION

Author	No. of Patients	HDR per Fraction (Gy)[a]	No. of Fractions	Percentage Improved	
				Symptoms	Bronchoscopy
Taulelle et al.[173]	189	8–10	3–4	54–74	79
Kelly et al.[174]	175	15	1–2	66	78
Celebioglu et al.[175]	95	7.5–10	2–3	100	100
Gejerman et al.[176]	41	5	3	72	54
Escobar-Sacristan et al.[177]	81	5[b]	4	85	97
Kubaszewska et al.[178]	270	8–10		76–92	80
Ozkok et al.[179]	74[c]	7.5	2	57–94	77
	41	7.5	3	55–78	72
Skowronek et al.[170]	303	7.5	3		88.4
	345	10	1		
Guarnashcelli et al.[180]	52	5–7.5	1–3	92	87
Dagnault et al.[181]	81	5	4	77–100	95
Hauswald et al.[182]	41	5	3	58	73
Niemoeller et al.[171]	60	3.8	4		57.2
	82	7.2	2		70.2
de Aquino Gorayeb et al.[183]	78	7.5	3	87.2	73.4
Totals	2008		1–4	55%–100%	57.2%–100%

[a]Dose prescribed at 1 cm.
[b]Dose prescribed at 0.5 to 1 cm.
[c]Received EBRT of 30 Gy in 10 fractions.
HDR, high dose rate; NA, not available.

A Cochrane meta-analysis published in 2012 reviewing 14 randomized studies utilizing endobronchial brachytherapy in a variety of ways found no improvement in disease-free survival or overall survival when endobronchial brachytherapy was added to EBRT.[190] Based on this, the Cochrane review does not recommend endobronchial brachytherapy for routine use of radical treatment of lung cancer. When it is used, the ABS suggests an HDR dose of 10 to 15 Gy in two to three fractions as a boost to EBRT (either 60 Gy in 30 fractions or 45 Gy in 15 fractions).[13]

Curative Endobronchial Brachytherapy

The standard, definitive therapy for unresectable lung cancer is a combination of chemotherapy and EBRT. Select patients (i.e., those with predominantly endobronchial tumor) may benefit from endobronchial brachytherapy, either alone or as a boost to EBRT.

The ideal patients for curative endobronchial radiation alone are those with occult carcinomas of the lung confined to the bronchus or trachea. Additionally, these patients tend to have early-stage disease and are medically inoperable because of decreased pulmonary function, advanced age, or refusal of surgery. Results of a few reported series are encouraging.[185–188] See Table 28.16. The largest series to date with 226 patients reported an 81% survival rate at 2 years utilizing four to six fractions of 5 to 7 Gy each.[188] Late complications did include a 5% fatal hemoptysis rate.

Endobronchial brachytherapy can be used in combination with EBRT for selected patients with inoperable non–small-cell lung carcinoma. In cases of postobstructive pneumonia or lung collapse, brachytherapy can be used to open the bronchus and aerate the lung such that the tumor volume is better defined. This allows some sparing of normal lung from the EBRT field. Muto et al.[189] performed a nonrandomized prospective study evaluating three endobronchial brachytherapy schemes concomitantly with EBRT on 320 patients with advanced inoperable non–small-cell lung cancer. Endobronchial brachytherapy consisted of either 10 Gy in one fraction, 14 Gy in two fractions, or 15 Gy in three fractions. Median survival for all patients was 11.1 months with a symptomatic response rate ranging from 82% to 94%. Complications were the least in the group of patients receiving 15 Gy in three fractions.

Brachytherapy Combined With Other Modalities

HDR brachytherapy in combination with either sublobar resection, metallic stent placement, PDT, or Yttrium-aluminum-garnet (YAG) laser has been described. McKenna et al.[191] reported their series of 48 patients who had poor pulmonary function not amenable to lobectomy who underwent wedge resection, lymph node dissection, and brachytherapy. Brachytherapy consisted of seven fractions of 350 cGy each prescribed to a depth of 1 cm delivered twice daily. Four recurrences were recorded with follow-up ranging from 1 to 27 months. Allison and colleagues[192] noted a significant improvement in Karnofsky performance status and pulmonary palliation with the use of a metallic stent placed in the endobronchial lumen followed by HDR brachytherapy of three 6 Gy fractions prescribed to a depth of 0.5 cm over a 2-week period. Finally, the use of HDR brachytherapy in combination with PDT or YAG laser has been described. Freitag et al.,[193] reported their results of 32 patients with bulky endobronchial non–small cell lung cancer treated initially with PDT followed 6 weeks later with five fractions (one per week) of 4 Gy each prescribed at a distance of 1 cm. Eighty-one percent of patients were free of endobronchial tumor at a mean follow-up of 24 months. Chella et al.[194] performed a small randomized trial comparing YAG laser alone versus YAG laser plus HDR brachytherapy in 29 patients. HDR brachytherapy consisted of three fractions (one per week) of 5 Gy each prescribed at a distance of 0.5 cm. Combination therapy resulted in a statistical improvement in period free from symptoms from 2.8 to 8.5 months. Disease progression-free period improved from 2.2 to 7.5 months as well.

TABLE 28.16 SUMMARY OF ENDOBRONCHIAL BRACHYTHERAPY WITHOUT EXTERNAL BEAM RADIATION THERAPY FOR OCCULT CARCINOMAS OF THE LUNG

Author	No. of Patients	HDR per Fraction (Gy)	Prescription Depth (cm)	No. of Fractions	Total HDR (Gy)	Cause Specific Survival (%)	Mean Follow-Up (mo)	Complications
Perol et al.[185]	19	7	1	3–5	35	78	28	NA
Marsiglia et al.[186]	34	5	0.5–1	6	30	78	24	1 PNX
Hennequin et al.[187]	106	5–7	0.5–1.5	6	30–42	67.9 (2 y) 48.5 (5 y)	NA	2 FH, 3 BN, 13 RB
Aumont-Le Guilcher et al.[188]	226	5–7	1	4–6	24–35	81 (2 y) 56 (5 y)	30.4	44 RB, 21 S, 7 BN, 10 FH

Cancer of the Esophagus

Nonoperable definitive treatment of esophageal cancer has evolved over the last two decades to now frequently include concurrent EBRT and chemotherapy. HDR brachytherapy for palliative purposes has been evaluated in a few randomized trials and is well established, but its role in conjunction with concurrent EBRT and chemotherapy is less defined. HDR brachytherapy can be used either alone or in combination with EBRT.[195-202]

Brachytherapy is relatively simple to perform, because a single catheter is used for the treatment. A nasogastric tube or a specially designed esophageal applicator is used to deliver the treatments. The largest diameter applicator that can be inserted easily (either intraorally or intranasally) should be used to minimize the mucosal dose relative to the dose at depth. The site to be irradiated, which includes the tumor and a distal and proximal margin of 2 to 5 cm, can be confirmed by fluoroscopy or endoscopy. The ABS recommends an HDR dose of 10 Gy in two fractions, prescribed at 1 cm from the source, to boost 50 Gy EBRT.[195] HDR brachytherapy can be given before, concurrently with, or after EBRT. The advantage of giving brachytherapy after EBRT is that a more uniform dose can be delivered to the residual tumor after it has been reduced by EBRT. Brachytherapy given initially provides rapid relief of dysphagia. HDR brachytherapy at doses of 16 Gy in two fractions or 18 Gy in three fractions delivered weekly or every other day has been used without additional EBRT to palliate esophageal cancers.[198,199]

A few randomized studies have evaluated esophageal HDR brachytherapy and are summarized in Table 28.17. Historically, primary treatment of esophageal cancer included definitive radiotherapy. Results with external beam radiation alone in general were poor. For medically inoperable patients with submucosal esophageal cancer, external beam radiation with the addition of intraluminal brachytherapy is an attractive approach. Ishikawa et al.,[203] demonstrated a 5-year cause-specific survival of 86% with intraluminal brachytherapy compared to 62% with EBRT alone in a cohort of 56 patients. An update published in 2012 with additional patients demonstrated again a 5-year cause-specific survival of 85% with intraluminal HDR brachytherapy.[204]

In the palliative setting to relieve dysphagia, HDR brachytherapy is more defined. As was seen in definitive therapy, the combination of EBRT and HDR brachytherapy as compared to EBRT alone has resulted in an improvement in relief of dysphagia as well as survival.

More recent studies have evaluated various HDR fractionation schemes as well as comparing HDR brachytherapy alone to combination EBRT and HDR brachytherapy. Sur et al.[199] evaluated three fractionation schemes given weekly (12 Gy in two fractions; 16 Gy in two fractions; 18 Gy in three fractions) among 172 patients with advanced esophageal

cancer. The higher dose fractionation schemes had a trend toward improved dysphagia-free survival (25% to 38% at 12 months). Subsequently, a multicenter, prospective randomized study conducted under the auspices of the International Atomic Energy Agency (IAEA) evaluated two HDR regimens in 232 patients.[198] Patients were randomized to receive 18 Gy in three fractions over 5 days or 16 Gy in two fractions over 3 days. The authors concluded that dose fractions of 6 Gy × 3 and 8 Gy × 2 within 1 week gave similar results for dysphagia-free survival (~30% at 12 months), overall survival, and incidence of strictures and fistulae.

The addition of EBRT to HDR brachytherapy has yielded mixed results. Sur et al.[197] reported on a prospective pilot-randomized trial of 60 patients comparing HDR brachytherapy alone versus HDR brachytherapy plus EBRT for palliative treatment of advanced esophageal cancer. All patients received 16 Gy in two fractions over a 3-day period and then randomized to observation (group A) versus EBRT (group B) of 30 Gy in 10 fractions. At 12 months, there was no difference in dysphagia-free survival, overall survival, or incidence of strictures and fistulas for the two groups. However, the follow-up prospective multicenter randomized study in a larger patient group as reported by Rosenblatt et al.[196] utilizing the same regimen did show a sustained improvement in dysphagia-free survival at 12 months with the combined HDR brachytherapy and EBRT. There was no difference between the complication rates or overall survival between the two treatments.

In summary, retrospective studies as well as prospective, randomized clinical trials show that there is improved local control and survival when HDR brachytherapy is added to EBRT and that HDR brachytherapy alone can be used for palliation of advanced esophageal cancers. Because a high dose is delivered to the esophageal mucosa, side effects may include ulcerations, fistulae, and esophageal strictures. Additionally, the use of HDR brachytherapy as a boost to concurrent chemotherapy and EBRT has been evaluated.[205-208] Results have varied and thus caution should be exercised with this approach.

Biliary Cancers

Cholangiocarcinomas are rare malignancies and optimal adjuvant therapy remains unclear. A Surveillance, Epidemiology and End Results (SEER) database analysis suggested that brachytherapy may improve overall survival.[209] A recent Japanese study evaluating intraluminal brachytherapy in addition to EBRT for unresectable biliary tract cancer found an improvement in local control but no difference in overall survival.[210] The Mayo Clinic has described the use of HDR biliary brachytherapy in conjunction with neoadjuvant chemoradiotherapy prior to liver transplantation for unresectable perihilar cholangiocarcinoma.[211] Tumors of the bile duct are

TABLE 28.17 SUMMARY OF ESOPHAGEAL HIGH DOSE RATE BRACHYTHERAPY							
Author	**No. of Patients**	**EBRT Dose (Gy)**	**No. of HDR Fractions**	**HDR per Fraction (Gy)**	**Relief of Dysphagia at 6 Months (%)**	**Relief of Dysphagia at 1 Year (%)**	**Survival at 1 Year**
Palliation							
Sur et al.[199]	36	—	2	6	40[a]	10[a]	9%
	68	—	2	8	52[a]	30[a]	22%
	68	—	3	6	50[a]	40[a]	35%
Sur et al.[198]	112	—	3	6	~75	~75	~25%
	120	—	2	8	~75	~60	~25%
Sur et al.[197]	30	—	2	8	>50	—	7.2 mo[b]
	30	30	2	8	>50%	—	7.5 mo[b]
Rosenblatt et al.[196]	109	—	2	8	~50%	~37%	~10%
	110	30	2	8	~70%	~45%	~18%

[a]Approximate dysphagia-free survival based on graph.
[b]Median survival.
EBRT, external beam radiation therapy; HDR, high dose rate.

Section II

often unresectable and are treated palliatively by biliary drainage and EBRT. The biliary drainage tube can be accessed to provide brachytherapy to the area of obstruction either by LDR ^{192}Ir brachytherapy or by HDR brachytherapy[212–216] alone or in combination with EBRT. Although brachytherapy is commonly delivered through a transhepatic cholangiogram catheter, it has also been delivered using an endoscopic retrograde technique. A size 12-Fr biliary drainage catheter is required to accommodate a 6-Fr HDR brachytherapy catheter. Therefore, the indwelling biliary drainage catheter is upsized to a size 12-Fr biliary drainage catheter, if required. Under fluoroscopy, the brachytherapy catheter is inserted into the biliary drainage catheter and advanced past the area of obstruction. A Tuohy-Borst (Y-shaped) adapter attached to the end of the biliary catheter allows concurrent external biliary drainage while holding the HDR catheter in place. The area of the obstruction is irradiated along with 1- to 2-cm proximal and distal margins. The dose per fraction delivered is variable, but approximately 5 Gy per fraction at a distance of 1 cm from the source is commonly used for three or four fractions (15 to 20 Gy total) to boost 45 Gy EBRT. If EBRT is not delivered, a palliative dose of 30 Gy in six fractions can be used. A phase 1 study from Italy established a recommended dose of 25 Gy in five fractions for palliative treatment.[217] Concurrent chemotherapy (5-FU) is often added. It is important to leave the biliary drainage catheter in place after therapy to minimize biliary stricture.

Head and Neck Cancers

Brachytherapy, especially using manually afterloaded ^{192}Ir, has been widely used to treat head and neck cancers. HDR brachytherapy has been used in selected cases to reduce radiation exposure and permit optimization as summarized in Table 28.18.[218–222,224–232] However, these advantages are offset by the need for multiple fractions because the head and neck area does not tolerate high doses per fraction. Both the ABS and GEC-ESTRO have separately published general recommendations of utilizing HDR brachytherapy in the various sites of head and neck cancer.[17,239]

The nasopharynx is a site within the head and neck area that is easily accessed by an intracavitary HDR applicator.[240] Levendag et al. have extensive experience in treating nasopharyngeal lesions with HDR brachytherapy. They have shown that patients most suitable for a HDR brachytherapy boost are those with T1 and T2 lesions following 60 (T1, T2a) to 70 Gy (T2b) of EBRT. HDR doses of 18 Gy in six fractions are delivered by a special nasopharynx applicator. T3 and T4 lesions are better suited to be boosted with IMRT or stereotactic external beam techniques.[240]

The use of HDR brachytherapy catheters incorporated in removable dental molds allows repeated, highly reproducible, fractionated outpatient brachytherapy of superficial (<0.5-cm thick) tumors without requiring repeated catheter insertion into the tumor.[17] Suitable sites for mold therapy include the scalp, face, pinna, lip, buccal mucosa, maxillary antrum, hard

TABLE 28.18 HIGH DOSE RATE BRACHYTHERAPY FOR HEAD AND NECK CANCERS

Author	Site	EBRT Dose (Gy)	HDR per Fraction (Gy)	No. of Fractions	Isoeffective Dose (Gy)[a]	No. of Patients	5-Year Local Control (%)
Inoue et al.[218]	Tongue	0	6	10	80	25	87
Leung et al.[219]	Tongue	0	4.5–6.3	10	54–86	19	95[b]
Guinot et al.[220]	Lip	0	4.5–5.5	8–10	54–57	39[c]	88[d]
Levendag et al.[221]	Nasal vestibule	0	3–4	14	48.3	64	92[e]
Dixit et al.[222]	Various	40–48	3	7	63–71	18	80[f]
Ozyar et al.[223]	Nasopharynx	58–74	4	3	71–86	106	86
Nag et al.[224]	Sinus	45–50	10–12.5	1	66–68	27	65
		45–63	15–20	1	94–95	7	
Lu et al.[225]	Nasopharynx	66	5	2	79	33	94[d]
Nose et al.[226]	Oropharynx	0	6	8–9	64–72	14	82
		14.4–66.6	6	3–6	62–90	68	
Ng et al.[227]	Nasopharynx	43.2–70.4	2.5–3	2–7	65–79	38	96
Nag et al.[228]	Various	45–50	7.5–20	1	61–95	65	59
Leung et al.[229]	Nasopharynx	66	10–12	2	99–110	145	95.8[g]
Yeo et al.[230]	Nasopharynx	66	10	2	99	178	91.6
Martinez-Monge et al.[231]	Oral Cavity	45	4	4	63	8	86[h]
	Oropharynx		4	6	72	31	
Guinot et al.[232]	Tongue	0	4	11	51	17	79
		55	3	6	63	33	
Takacsi-Nagy et al.[233]	Tongue	50–70	3–12	1–8	71–94	60	57
Matsumoto et al.[234]	Tongue	0	5	10[i]	62.5	33	94
		7.5–35	5	10[i]		34	
Vedasoundaram et al.[235]	Buccal	50	3.5	11	43	5	100[j]
			3.5	6	72.8	28	80–84[j]
Wan et al.[236]		50–72	2.9–5.5	2–5		213	95.9
Martinez-Monge et al.[237]	Various	0	4	8–10	37–46	46	68.6[k]
		45	4–6	4	63–76	57	83.3[k]
Teudt et al.[238]	Sinus	40–63	2.5	4–14		35	67[l]

[a]Isoeffective dose for tumor effects as if given at 2 Gy/d using the linear-quadratic model with an α/β ratio of 10.
[b]Four-year local control.
[c]One patient received 50 Gy EBRT with 3.5 Gy × 6 HDR.
[d]Three-year local control.
[e]Five-year relapse-free survival.
[f]Median follow-up of 14 months.
[g]Five-year local failure free survival.
[h]Seven-year local control.
[i]Median fractionation schedule.
[j]Median FU of 26 months.
[k]Nine-year LC.
[l]21% of patients received EBRT.
EBRT, external beam radiation therapy; HDR, high dose rate.

palate, oral cavity, external auditory canal, and the orbital cavity after exenteration. HDR can be used as the sole modality or in conjunction with EBRT. A total HDR dose equivalent to about 60 Gy LDR (prescribed at 0.5-cm depth) is recommended when used as the sole modality.[17] The HDR can also be used as a boost to 45 to 50 Gy EBRT, in which case the HDR doses are appropriately reduced to LDR equivalent doses of 15 to 30 Gy. The actual HDR dose per fraction and number of fractions can be varied to suit individual situations (including site and treatment volume). Biomathematical (LQ) modeling can be used to assist in the conversion of LDR to HDR.[19]

Local regional recurrence remains the primary pattern of failure in head and neck cancers despite advancements in surgery and concurrent chemotherapy and EBRT. Surgical salvage is generally the preferred treatment, however, is not possible in all cases. EBRT is effective as salvage treatment but comes with high toxicity. HDR brachytherapy has been used in a few limited series for recurrent disease of previously irradiated patients. Various fractionation schemes with or without EBRT or surgical resection have been utilized. Initial results appear comparable to other modalities.[241–245]

Another innovative approach is the use of intraoperative HDR brachytherapy, which permits normal tissues to be retracted or shielded during brachytherapy. Intraoperative HDR brachytherapy can reach many sites in the head and neck area that are difficult to treat or are inaccessible by either LDR brachytherapy or intraoperative electron beam radiation. The catheters are removed immediately after the single dose of radiation, hence, minimizing inconvenience and permitting the use of brachytherapy in areas such as the base of skull.[224,228] Doses of 7.5 to 15 Gy are given when EBRT of 45 to 50 Gy can be added. In recurrent tumors where no further EBRT can be given, a single intraoperative dose of 15 to 20 Gy can be given.[224,228]

An ABS Task Group recently published their review of the available literature of utilization of brachytherapy for head and neck cancers. Their review included LDR, PDR, and HDR. The most common applications of brachytherapy include the base of tongue, oral cavity, and nasopharynx. In general brachytherapy achieves good results; however, given the complexity of the anatomy, it should be performed in dedicated centers with high levels of expertise. The authors encourage the reader to review the ABS Task Group report for more details.[246]

Soft Tissue Sarcomas

Excellent results are obtained with a combination of wide excision of the tumor and adjuvant EBRT. However, irradiation of large volumes after surgery gives rise to morbidity, especially normal tissue fibrosis. To minimize morbidity, a few centers historically have used LDR brachytherapy.[247] The major problem with LDR brachytherapy of large volumes is the radiation exposure involved. Hence, a few centers have investigated the use of HDR brachytherapy for soft tissue sarcomas.[248–257] Most commonly interstitial brachytherapy catheters are placed immediately following surgical resection in the operating room, which gives the advantage of accurate tumor bed delineation as well as improved avoidance of adjacent critical normal structures. Radiopaque clips are used to indicate the margins. A 2- to 5-cm margin proximally and distally is used after gross excision of tumor along with 1 to 2 cm radially. The ABS recommends utilization of CT imaging for treatment planning purposes and using CTV D_{90} to assess the quality of the implant. In addition $D_{0.1cc}$, D_{1cc}, and D_{2cc} to critical structures should be recorded. Optimized treatment planning can be used to deliver a more homogeneous dose. Updated ABS recommendations recommend total doses of 30 to 54 Gy given twice daily in 2 to 4 Gy fractions over 4 to 7 days if the HDR is given alone.[12] If EBRT (45 to 50 Gy) is added, the brachytherapy dose is limited to 12 to 20 Gy in 2 to 4 Gy fractions over 2 to 3 days.[12] It is important to delay the start of brachytherapy for about 4 to 7 days after surgery to allow for wound healing.[12]

An alternative technique not widely available is intraoperative HDR brachytherapy (HDR-IORT).[248,258] A HDR-IORT dose of 12 to 15 Gy is given to the tumor bed in a single fraction intraoperatively to boost EBRT doses of 45 to 50 Gy. Nerve tolerance to high dose per fraction is poor, and HDR should be used with caution when catheters have to be placed in contact with neurovascular structures. The ABS suggests the following interventions to minimize morbidity in soft tissue sarcomas[12]:

1. When brachytherapy is used as adjuvant monotherapy, the source loading should start no sooner than 5 to 6 days after wound closure. However, the radioactive sources may be loaded earlier (as soon as 2 to 3 days after surgery) if doses of <20 Gy are given with brachytherapy as a supplement to EBRT.
2. Minimize dose to normal tissues (e.g., gonads, breasts, thyroid, skin) whenever possible, especially in children and patients of childbearing age.
3. Limit the allowable skin dose—the 40 Gy isodose line (LDR) to <25 cm² and the 25 Gy isodose line to <100 cm².

Outcome of nonrandomized studies using HDR doses in the range of 2 to 9 Gy per fraction given once or twice daily or single-fraction intraoperative HDR brachytherapy are outlined in Table 28.19.[248–260]

A recent nonrandomized study has demonstrated that IMRT achieved better local control over brachytherapy in patients with high-grade soft tissue sarcomas of the extremity and thus has questioned the use of brachytherapy in this patient population.[261] Despite this, HDR brachytherapy still has a role to play in the management of soft tissue sarcomas.

Pediatric Tumors

LDR brachytherapy has been used in children to reduce the deleterious effects of EBRT.[262] However, LDR brachytherapy is difficult to perform in young children and infants because they require prolonged sedation and immobilization with close monitoring, which increases the risk of radiation exposure to nursing staff and parents. HDR is therefore very appealing in infants and younger children and has undergone various trials.[263–265] The recommended dose for HDR as monotherapy is 36 Gy in 12 fractions given at 3 Gy per fraction (prescribed at 0.5 cm) twice a day.[263,265,266] The interval between fractions is at least 6 hours. Because the tissue planes are smaller in young children, catheter spacing and prescription points may have to

TABLE 28.19 OUTCOME OF NONRANDOMIZED STUDIES OF HIGH DOSE RATE BRACHYTHERAPY USED FOR PRIMARY SOFT TISSUE SARCOMAS

Author	No. of Patients	Median Follow-Up (mo)	Local Control (%)	Complications (%)
Crownover et al.[250]	10	12	100	0
Koizumi et al.[252]	16	30	50	6
Chun et al.[249]	11	31	100	9
Rachbauer et al.[258a]	39	26	100	28
Kretzler et al.[253a]	11	51[b]	91	–
Alektiar et al.[248]	12[c]	33	74	34
	20[d]		54	
Mierzwa et al.[254]	43	39	88	7
Pohar et al.[256]	17	17	94	18
Petera et al.[255]	45	38.4	74	20
Itami et al.[251]	26	49.2	78	15
San Miguel et al.[257]	60	49.2	76	30 (grade 3) 10 (grade 4)
Emory et al.[259]	49	40[b]	83–92	–
Sharma et al.[260]	52	46	100	5.7 (acute) 9.6 (late)

[a]Intraoperative single-fraction HDR.
[b]Mean follow-up.
[c]Primary disease.
[d]Recurrent disease.
HDR, high dose rate; NS, not stated.

be reduced.[263] There are no good published dose recommendations for HDR when used as a boost to EBRT. The LQ model[19] can be used to calculate a fractionation scheme equivalent to that of an LDR implant boost dose of 15 to 25 Gy (prescribed at 0.5 cm). The recommended dose for intraoperative HDR brachytherapy as a boost to EBRT is 10 to 15 Gy (prescribed at 0.5 cm), depending on the extent of residual disease.[267–269] According to the Intergroup Rhabdomyosarcoma Study (IRS), the standard EBRT dose for pediatric soft tissue sarcomas is 40 Gy for microscopic disease and 50 Gy for gross disease. Intraoperative HDR allows reduction in the dose of EBRT to 27 to 30 Gy so that concerns for impaired growth and organ function are greatly reduced.[265,268,270] The results of HDR brachytherapy in the treatment of pediatric tumors are summarized in Table 28.20.[264,268,269,271–277] Although the long-term morbidity of HDR brachytherapy in young children is not fully known, one may expect preservation of organ functions similar to that seen with LDR brachytherapy.[278] Because of the complexities involved in pediatric HDR brachytherapy, it is recommended that the use of HDR brachytherapy in pediatric tumors be limited to centers that have experience with pediatric implants.[12] The availability of proton beam does not obviate the usefulness of brachytherapy as the former produces a high entrance dose, which can be deleterious to growing tissues, whereas brachytherapy dose distribution is more localized.

Skin Cancer

The widespread availability of HDR remote afterloading brachytherapy units allows the use of surface molds as an alternative to electron beam and for cases where surface irregularity, proximity to bone, or poor intrinsic tolerance of tissues do not allow for satisfactory treatment by electron beam. In addition to melanoma and nonmelanoma skin cancers, Merkel cell lesions, benign keloids, as well as Kaposi sarcomas have been treated with HDR brachytherapy. Indications for the use of radiotherapy for skin malignancies include primary treatment of tumor after biopsy, adjuvant treatment for close or positive surgical margins, high risk of recurrence following surgery, or treatment of recurrent tumors.[279] Pretherapy imaging to determine an appropriate applicator to encompass all of the disease is important and can often be accomplished with the use of MRI or CT. Newer technologies such as optical coherence tomography and confocal microscopy can potentially play a role in determining full tumor extent.[279] For most cases, a satisfactory mold can be made from 5-mm thick sheets of wax with the HDR catheters spaced 1 cm apart. A simpler alternative is to use commercially available surface template applicators (e.g., Freiburg flab from Nucletron Corp, Columbia, MD and HAM applicator from Mick Radionuclear Instruments Inc, Bronx, NY) that are used for intraoperative HDR brachytherapy.[280,281] The use

of molds made of aquaplast allows greater conformity to curved surfaces like the scalp. Contraindications for the use of brachytherapy include invasion of the bone, extension of disease in the orbit or along facial planes, perineural invasion, and certain genetic diseases such as ataxia telangiectasia.[279]

There is a wide range of recommended doses and fractionation schemes for treating skin cancer. An ABS working group determined that common fractionation schemes for surface applicators and custom molds include 40 Gy in eight fractions and 42 Gy in six fractions. These treatments are commonly delivered two to three times a week. For interstitial brachytherapy, the recommended dose is 30 Gy in 10 fractions delivered in a twice daily fashion.[279] The linear-quadratic radiobiologic model can be used to determine the total dose for a given fractionation scheme.[19] Kuribayashi et al.[282] reported 90% control rate postkeloidectomy utilizing 20 Gy in four fractions or 15 Gy in three fractions based on the site of the keloid. Kasper et al.[283] reported 100% complete response and local control at a median follow-up of 41.4 months for patients with Kaposi sarcoma utilizing a dose of 24 to 35 Gy in four to six fractions.

The respondents of a recent survey of members of the ABS to eight clinical scenarios of cutaneous squamous cell carcinoma and basal cell carcinoma generally prefer brachytherapy to external beam radiation mainly because of shorter treatment course, conformality of treatment, and shallow dose deposition. Tumor depth >3 mm, perineural invasion, or previous radiation were typical contraindications to brachytherapy. Median treatment margin was 5 mm and hypofractionation was preferred. The fewest fractions reported was 30 Gy in 5 fractions, whereas the most was 64 Gy in 32 fractions.[284]

INTRAOPERATIVE HIGH DOSE RATE BRACHYTHERAPY

Intraoperative high dose rate brachytherapy (IOHDR) is an extreme example of reduced fractionation in that only a single HDR brachytherapy dose is applied.[285] This results in an inherent radiobiologic disadvantage because the advantages of fractionation (repair of normal tissue damage, reoxygenation of hypoxic tumor cells, and movement of tumor cells from the radioresistant S phase to the more radiosensitive mitotic phase of the cell cycle) are lost. LQ model calculations show that there has to be a dose reduction of 20% to 25% to the late-reacting normal tissues for isoeffect. However, the dose reduction achieved by 1- to 4-cm displacement of normal tissue is much more (closer to 60% to 90% reduction).[280] Hence, HDR in these situations becomes advantageous. However, if such a dose reduction cannot be achieved in normal tissues, HDR brachytherapy becomes disadvantageous. Intraoperative HDR brachytherapy also has the advantage that normal

TABLE 28.20 RESULTS OF HIGH DOSE RATE BRACHYTHERAPY USED FOR TREATMENT OF PEDIATRIC TUMORS

Author	No. of Patients	Brachytherapy	HDR (Gy)	EBRT Dose (Gy)	Median Follow-Up (mo)	Local Control (%)	Late Toxicity (%)
Nag et al.[264]	15	F-HDR	36 (3 Gy ×12)	0	120	80	20
Martinez-Monge et al.[271]	5	F-HDR	24 (4 Gy × 6)	27–45	27	100	0
Nakamura et al.[272]	16	F-HDR	10 (5 Gy × 2)	45–55	54	94	–
Viani et al.[273]	18	F-HDR	18–24	30.6–50	79.5[a]	90	16.5[a]
			21–40	0		100	
Laskar et al.[274]	21	F-HDR	36 (4 Gy × 9)	0	51	92	–
			21 (3 Gy × 7)	30.6–45		100	–
Schuck et al.[269]	20	IOHDR	10	45–55	24	65	40 (postop)
Nag et al.[268]	13	IOHDR	10–15	27–30	47	95	23
Goodman et al.[275]	66	IOHDR	4–15	0–56	12	56	12
Nag et al.[276]	13	IOERT	10–15	0–50.4	42	72	31
Folkert et al.[277]	75	IOHDR	4–17.5	0–50.4	93.6[b]	63	5.3

[a]Whole group.
[b]Surviving patients.
EBRT, external beam radiation therapy; F-HDR, fractionated high dose rate (given twice a day); IOERT, intraoperative electron beam radiation therapy; IOHDR, intraoperative high dose rate.

TABLE 28.21 ADVANTAGES OF SURGICAL DEBULKING WITH INTRAOPERATIVE HIGH DOSE RATE BRACHYTHERAPY OVER PERIOPERATIVE BRACHYTHERAPY OR ELECTRON BEAM INTRAOPERATIVE RADIATION THERAPY

Advantages over Perioperative Brachytherapy	Advantages over Electron Beam IORT
1. It is possible to use retraction or shielding to reduce the dose to normal tissues. 2. Normal structures can be temporarily moved while the radiation is given and then replaced in their normal position. For example, to access the base of skull, the maxilla can be removed and later regrafted. Ureters can be severed and then reimplanted into the bladder. During liver transplantation procedures, the liver hilum can be irradiated during the interval between the removal of the host liver and reimplantation of the donor liver. 3. The process is rapid. Using a surface applicator eliminates the needs to individually suture the catheters to the tumor bed. 4. HDR allows the treatment to be delivered at sites into which catheters cannot be sutured. 5. Because catheters are not left in the patient, there is no risk of catheter displacement, extrusion, or infection.	1. Electron beam IORT can only be delivered to areas accessible to the electron cone and, therefore, cannot treat steeply sloping surfaces, narrow cavities, or areas such as the diaphragm, pubis, and anterior abdominal wall. Intraoperative HDR brachytherapy has less anatomical constraints than electron beam IORT. 2. The HDR machine costs less than an electron beam linear accelerator. 3. Because the HDR afterloader can be transported between the radiation department and the operating room, dedicated equipment is not required.

HDR, high dose rate brachytherapy; IORT, intraoperative radiation therapy.

tissues can be temporarily displaced and/or partially shielded during irradiation.

The ABS published a consensus report in 2017 for the use of IOHDR brachytherapy.[285] In IOHDR, the surgery is performed in a shielded operating room with remote anesthesia and a video monitoring system. Maximum surgical debulking is attempted whenever possible. Appropriate patients for IOHDR include those with close, microscopic, or positive margins and/or recurrent disease in a previously resected or previously irradiated region. The tumor bed is irradiated using special intraoperative applicators containing HDR catheters that are 1 cm apart and parallel to each other. The use of a fixed geometry applicator allows the patient to be treated without delay using preplanned dosimetry for the selected applicator. Normal tissues are either retracted from the high dose area or shielded. Doses of 10 to 20 Gy depending on treatment location are usually given as a single fraction over 10 to 30 minutes.[285] Dose is typically prescribed to either the surface of the applicator or to a depth of 3, 5, or 10 mm based on treatment location. The reader is encouraged to review the consensus report for more specific treatment details based on tumor location. The advantages of IOHDR brachytherapy over perioperative brachytherapy or electron beam intraoperative radiation therapy (IORT) are listed in Table 28.21. Unfortunately, the relative scarcity of shielded operating rooms has currently limited its availability to just a few centers.[285]

Reduction of Brachytherapy Errors

The International Commission on Radiological Protection (ICRP)[286] released Publication 97 in November 2005, which outlines quality assurance (QA) procedures necessary to prevent accidents with HDR brachytherapy. The ICRP gave general

and specific recommendations for HDR brachytherapy programs which are summarized in Tables 28.22 and 28.23. The general recommendations include establishing a written comprehensive QA program, formation of a hospital radiation safety committee, external auditing of procedures, peer reviewing of each case, and reporting of every incident or accident. The specific recommendations cover a broad range of topics. Training in HDR brachytherapy should commence prior to acquisition of machines, follow a team approach, and should be sequential in the introduction of techniques with simpler techniques first followed by more complex treatments. For example, multiple plane flexible implants should not be attempted first. Transport regulations of sources should be adhered to and performed by a factory-trained and certified operator. In addition, new sources should be measured in a calibrated well chamber to verify reported activity, at which time it is advisable to do a full commissioning including physics and mechanical QA checks.

TABLE 28.23 INTERNATIONAL COMMISSION ON RADIOLOGICAL PROTECTION PUBLICATION 97—PREVENTION OF HIGH DOSE RATE BRACHYTHERAPY ACCIDENTS—SPECIFIC RECOMMENDATIONS

1. Training in an HDR center should commence prior to machine acquisition and should include the specific techniques to be used.
2. Training should be directed toward ensuring a team approach involving clinician, physicist, technician, and nurse.
3. Training and introduction of techniques should be sequential, commencing with simpler techniques before attempting more complex activities. Fixed geometry applicators and implants are less likely to result in errors.
4. Transport regulations should be adhered to and performed by a factory-trained and certified operator. This includes on-site container inspection for damage, removal of the old source and its transfer to the container, and installation of the new one in the safe.
5. New sources should be measured in a calibrated well chamber to verify the manufacturers reported activity and the results entered immediately into the software. At this time, it is advisable to do a full commissioning (physics and mechanical QA checks).
6. All systems of delivery must be closed ended (catheters, needles, and fine tubes).
7. Manual insertion of a test wire (check cable) clearly marked at the programmed treatment length before each treatment to ensure that the total length of the transfer tube plus applicator equals the programmed treatment length. A manual check cable also helps to identify any kinks or obstruction in the catheter or transfer tube.
8. The step size in a particular center should be kept constant (e.g., 5 mm) for all treatments to avoid errors of using incorrect step size.
9. Keeping all tubes outside of the body as far distant as possible from the patient's skin will help to minimize unintended doses.
10. Dedicated self-contained brachytherapy suite with adequate shielding housing all requirements is highly advisable.
11. Applicator positioning should be verified before each treatment.
12. So-called false alarms and interlock failures should be thoroughly investigated and appropriated action taken and repaired.
13. Survey of patient by portable radiation monitor after each treatment.
14. An emergency plan should be prepared and practiced with commencement of operations.
15. The person responsible for performing an emergency procedure should remain in the brachytherapy suite during the entire treatment.
16. The HDR machine and source should be kept secure at all times.

HDR, high dose rate; QA, quality assurance.

TABLE 28.22 INTERNATIONAL COMMISSION ON RADIOLOGICAL PROTECTION PUBLICATION 97—PREVENTION OF HIGH DOSE RATE BRACHYTHERAPY ACCIDENTS—GENERAL RECOMMENDATIONS

1. Written comprehensive QA program.
2. Compliance to QA procedures will contribute to minimizing the occurrence of errors, both in number and magnitude.
3. Hospital Radiation Safety committee (QA committee) needs to exist and interact with regulatory and health authorities.
4. Maintenance is an indispensable component of QA.
5. External audits of procedures reinforce good and safe practice and identify potential causes of errors.
6. Peer review of each case improves quality.
7. Every incident or accident should be reported as required to the appropriate authority.

QA, quality assurance.

It is recommended that all systems of delivery (i.e., catheters) be close ended, that the step size at a particular center be constant (i.e., 5 mm) for all treatments, and that a dedicated self-contained brachytherapy suite exist to house all equipment. Prior to initiating treatment with the HDR machine a few standard procedures should be employed. These include manual insertion of a test wire to verify programmed treatment length and identify any kinks or obstructions, verifying applicator position with an appropriate imaging modality (i.e., fluoroscopy), and ensuring that all tubes outside the patient's body are as far away as possible to minimize unintended doses. Following treatment a survey of the patient by a portable radiation monitor is essential. Finally, emergency plans and security procedures should be in place and strictly adhered to. "false alarms" and "interlock failures" should be thoroughly investigated, and persons responsible for emergency procedures should remain in the vicinity of the brachytherapy suite during the entire treatment. In some countries, it is a requirement that both the clinician and physicist remain in the vicinity of the HDR suite. The possibility of theft of an HDR source for use as a weapon for nuclear terrorism is real, and the machine and source should be kept secure at all times. Particular attention should be paid if the facility or machine is decommissioned. It is believed that if a HDR brachytherapy center follows these general and specific recommendations, errors and accidents will be minimized.

HIGH DOSE RATE BRACHYTHERAPY IN DEVELOPING COUNTRIES

HDR brachytherapy has special relevance for developing countries where resources may be scarce. In this regard, the IAEA has issued recommendations for the use of HDR brachytherapy in the developing countries.[287] A brief summary is given here; however, readers interested in the details are referred to the original article. An HDR treatment system should be purchased as a complete unit that includes the ^{192}Ir radioactive source, source loading unit, applicators, treatment planning system, and control console. Infrastructure support may require additional or improved buildings and procurement of or access to new imaging facilities. A supportive budget is needed for quarterly source replacement and the annual maintenance necessary to keep the system operational. The radiation oncologist, medical physicist, and technologist should be specially trained before HDR can be introduced. Training for the oncologist and medical physicist is an ongoing process as new techniques or sites of treatment are introduced. Procedures for QA of patient treatment and the planning system must be introduced. Emergency procedures with adequate training of all associated personnel must be in place. The decision to select HDR in preference to alternate methods of brachytherapy is influenced by the ability of the machine to treat a wide variety of clinical sites. In departments with personnel and budgetary resources to support this equipment appropriately, economic advantage

becomes evident only if large numbers of patients are treated. With HDR, it is possible to treat a large number of patients in institutions that have a high volume of brachytherapy patients but insufficient in-patient facilities for LDR brachytherapy or insufficient finances for the purchase of ^{125}I or ^{103}Pd seeds for permanent implants. Intangible benefits of source safety, personnel safety, and easy adaptation to fluctuating demand for treatments also require consideration when evaluating the need to introduce this treatment system.

Of specific interest is locally advanced cervical cancer as most of these cases occur in low-income to middle-income countries. The ABS recently published recommendations for brachytherapy treatment in cervical cancer specifically for developing countries.[288] While the basic tenants and goals of overall management of cervical cancer are the same for developed and developing countries, the ABS guidelines recognize that traditional prescription points are still very relevant in countries where 3D imaging is limited. Furthermore, an emphasis is placed on the importance of pretreatment verification and checklists particularly when overseeing experienced personnel is limited.[288]

Summary

Although brachytherapy is a very effective modality, case selection and proper patient evaluation are essential. If the tumor is very large or widely metastatic, one is doomed to fail because of the physics of dose distribution in the former case and because of the biology of the tumor in the latter case. There are some differences between various brachytherapy modalities (Table 28.24). These differences should be kept in mind when selecting the brachytherapy modality in a particular situation. When HDR brachytherapy is used, the treatments must be executed carefully because the short treatment times do not allow any time for correction of errors, and mistakes can result in harm to patients. Hence, it is very important that all personnel involved in HDR brachytherapy be well trained and constantly alert. However, with proper case selection and delivery technique, HDR brachytherapy has great promise and convenience because of avoidance of radiation exposure, short treatment times, and outpatient therapy.

One of the disadvantages of HDR brachytherapy is that it requires a shielded room. A newer device, the Axxent (Xoft Inc., Sunnyvale, CA), uses a miniaturized x-ray source to deliver low-energy x-rays within a needle or catheter thereby mimicking HDR brachytherapy. The reduced radiation protection required for these devices because of limited penetration is a great advantage because it allows brachytherapy to be delivered in a nonshielded procedure room or a regular (unshielded) hospital operating suite. Currently, the Xoft-Axxent system has only a single channel and therefore has the limitation of being able to treat only small volume tumor beds. It is being used at a few centers in the United States to treat breast cancer via a balloon device similar to the MammoSite balloon, the vaginal cuff with a single-channel cylinder applicator, and skin cancers with a surface applicator.[161,162,289,290]

There has been a recent decline in the utilization and interest and brachytherapy for various reasons including lack of facilities, training, and insufficient reimbursement. However, the inclusion of high-quality brachytherapy is imperative for good outcome in a number of malignancies. Continued education and awareness of the scope and value of brachytherapy is therefore essential.[291] It is hoped that with new

TABLE 28.24 COMPARISON OF DIFFERENT BRACHYTHERAPY TECHNIQUES						
	LDR ^{192}Ir	**LDR Remote**	**MDR**	**PDR**	**HDR**	**IOHDR**
Dose rate	Low	Low	Medium	High	High	High
Duration of each treatment	2–6 d	2–4 d	1 d	Minutes	Minutes	Minutes
Overall duration of treatment	2–6 d	2–4 d	1 d	2–4 d	3–5 wk	Minutes
Radiation hazards	High	Small	Small	Small	Small	Small
Availability (worldwide)	++	−	−	−	+	−
Ease of optimization	−	−	−	+	+	+
Dose as sole modality (Gy)	60	60	40	60	30–40	15–20
Dose as boost to EBRT (Gy)	20–40	20–40	20–30	20–40	20–30	10–15

EBRT, external beam radiation therapy; HDR, high dose rate; IOHDR, intraoperative high dose rate; LDR, low dose rate; MDR, medium dose rate; PDR, pulsed dose rate.

emphasis on value and outcome, HDR brachytherapy will continue to expand over the coming years and that refinements in the integration of imaging (computed tomography, MRI, intraoperative ultrasonography), and optimization of dose distribution will foster this expansion.[31,292] The development of well-controlled randomized trials addressing issues of efficacy, toxicity, quality of life, and costs versus benefits will ultimately define the role of HDR brachytherapy in the therapeutic armamentarium.

REFERENCES

1. International Commission on Radiation Units and Measurements. *ICRU Report 38: Dose and volume specification for reporting intracavitary therapy in gynecology.* Bethesda, MD: International Commission on Radiation Units and Measurements, 1985.

2. Nag S, Samsami N. Pitfalls of inappropriate optimization. *J Brachyther Int* 2000;16:187–198.

3. Romestaing P, Lehingue Y, Carrie C, et al. Role of a 10-Gy boost in the conservative treatment of early breast cancer: results of a randomized clinical trial in Lyon, France. *J Clin Oncol* 1997;15:963–968.

4. Poortmans P, Bartelink H, Horiot J, et al. The influence of the boost technique on local control in breast conserving treatment in the EORTC 'boost versus no boost' randomised trial. *Radiother Oncol* 2004;72:25–33.

5. Polgar C, Fodor J, Orosz Z, et al. Electron and high-dose rate brachytherapy boost in the conservative treatment of stage I-II breast cancer first results of the randomized Budapest boost trial. *Strahlenther Onkol* 2002;178:615–623.

6. Resch A, Potter R, Van Limbergen E, et al. Long-term results (10 years) of intensive breast conserving therapy including a high-dose and large-volume interstitial brachytherapy boost (LDR/HDR) for T1/T2 breast cancer. *Radiother Oncol* 2002;63:47–58.

7. Hannoun-Levi JM, Resch A, Gal J, et al. Accelerated partial breast irradiation with interstitial brachytherapy as second conservative treatment for ipsilateral breast tumour recurrence: multicentric study of the GEC-ESTRO Breast Cancer Working Group. *Radiother Oncol* 2013;108:226–231.

8. Stout R, Barber P, Burt P, et al. Clinical and quality of life outcomes in the first United Kingdom randomized trial of endobronchial brachytherapy (intraluminal radiotherapy) vs. external beam radiotherapy in the palliative treatment of inoperable non-small cell lung cancer. *Radiother Oncol* 2000;56:323–327.

9. Small W, Beriwal S, Demanes DJ, et al. American Brachytherapy Society consensus guidelines for adjuvant vaginal cuff brachytherapy after hysterectomy. *Brachytherapy* 2012;11:58–67.

10. Viswanathan A, Thomadsen B. American Brachytherapy Society consensus guidelines for locally advanced carcinoma of the cervix. Part I: General principles. *Brachytherapy* 2012;11:33–46.

11. Viswanathan A, Beriwal S, De Los Santos J, et al. American Brachytherapy Society consensus guidelines for locally advanced carcinoma of the cervix. Part II: High dose rate brachytherapy. *Brachytherapy* 2012;11:47–52.

12. Holloway CL, Delaney TF, Alektiar KM, et al. American Brachytherapy Society (ABS) consensus statement for sarcoma brachytherapy. *Brachytherapy* 2013;12:179–190.

13. Stewart A, Parashar B, Patel M, et al. American Brachytherapy Society consensus guidelines for thoracic brachytherapy for lung cancer. *Brachytherapy* 2016;15:1–11.

14. Shah C, Vicini F, Wazer D, et al. The American Brachytherapy Society consensus statement for accelerated partial breast irradiation. *Brachytherapy* 2013;12:267–277.

15. Beriwal S, Demanes DJ, Erickson B, et al. American Brachytherapy Society consensus guidelines for interstitial brachytherapy for vaginal cancer. *Brachytherapy* 2012;11:68–75.

16. Yamada Y, Rogers L, Demanes DJ, et al. American Brachytherapy Society consensus guidelines for high-dose rate prostate brachytherapy. *Brachytherapy* 2012;11:20–32.

17. Nag S, Vikram B, Demanes J, et al. The American Brachytherapy Society recommendations for HDR brachytherapy for head and neck carcinoma. *Int J Radiat Oncol Biol Phys* 2001;50:1190–1198.

18. Barendsen GW. Dose fractionation, dose rate and iso-effect relationships for normal tissue responses. *Int J Radiat Oncol Biol Phys* 1982;8:1981–1997.

19. Nag S, Gupta N. A simple method of obtaining equivalent doses for use in HDR brachytherapy. *Int J Radiat Oncol Biol Phys* 2000;46:507–513.

20. Han K, Milosevic M, Fyles A, et al. Trends in the utilization of brachytherapy in cervical cancer in the United States. *Int J Radiat Oncol Biol Phys* 2013;87:111–119.

21. Gill B, Lin J, Krivak T, et al. National cancer data base analysis of radiation therapy consolidation modality for cervical cancer: The impact of new technological advancements. *Int J Radiat Oncol Biol Phys* 2014;90:1083–1090.

22. Eifel P, Ho A, Khalid N, et al. Patterns of radiation therapy practice for patients treated for intact cervical cancer in 2005 to 2007: A quality research in radiation oncology study. *Int J Radiat Oncol Biol Phys* 2014;89:249–256.

23. Orton CG, Seyedsadr M, Somnay A. Comparison of high and low dose rate remote afterloading for cervix cancer and the importance of fractionation. *Int J Radiat Oncol Biol Phys* 1991;21:1425–1434.

24. Viswanathan A, Creutzberg C, Craighead P, et al. International Brachytherapy Practice Patterns—A Survey of the Gynecologic Cancer Intergroup (GCIG). *Int J Radiat Oncol Biol Phys* 2012;82:250–255.

25. Lee K, Lee J, Nam J, et al. High dose rate versus low dose rate intracavitary brachytherapy for carcinoma of the uterine cervix: Systematic review and meta-analysis. *Brachytherapy* 2015;14:449–457.

26. Nag S, Chao C, Erickson B, et al. The American Brachytherapy Society recommendations for low-dose rate brachytherapy for carcinoma of the cervix. *Int J Radiat Oncol Biol Phys* 2002;52:33–48.

27. Nag S, Orton C, Petereit D, et al. The American Brachytherapy Society recommendations for HDR brachytherapy of the cervix. *Int J Radiat Oncol Biol Phys* 2000;48:201–211.

28. Hricak H, Gatsonis C, Coakley F. Early invasive cervical cancer: CT and MR imaging in preoperative evaluation—ACRIN/GOG comparative study of diagnostic performance and interobserver variability. *Radiology* 2007;245:491–498.

29. Mitchell D, Snyder B, Coakley F. Early invasive cervical cancer: Tumor delineation by magnetic resonance imaging, computed tomography, and clinical examination, verified by pathologic results, in the ACRIN 6651/GOG 183 Intergroup Study. *J Clin Oncol* 2006;24(36):5687–5694.

30. van Dyk S, Kondalsamy-Chennakesavan S, Schneider M, et al. Comparison of measurements of the uterus and cervix obtained by magnetic resonance and transabdominal ultrasound imaging to identify the brachytherapy target in patients with cervix cancer. *Int J Radiat Oncol Biol Phys* 2014;88:860–865.

31. Haie-Meder C, Potter R, Van Limbergen E, et al. Recommendations from Gynaecological (GYN) GEC-ESTRO Working Group (I): concepts and terms in 3D image based 3D treatment planning in cervix cancer brachytherapy with emphasis on MRI assessment of GTV and CTV. *Radiother Oncol* 2005;74:235–245.

32. Potter R, Haie-Meder C, Van Limbergen E, et al. Recommendations from gynaecological (GYN) GEC ESTRO working group (II): concepts and terms in 3D image-based treatment planning in cervix cancer brachytherapy-3D dose volume parameters and aspects of 3D image-based anatomy, radiation physics, radiobiology. *Radiother Oncol* 2006;78:67–77.

33. Hellebust TP, Kirisits C, Berger D, et al. Recommendations from gynecological GEC-ESTRO working group: Considerations and pitfalls and conditioning and applicator reconstruction in 3D image based treatment planning of cervix cancer brachytherapy. *Radiother Oncol* 2010;96:153–160.

34. Dimopoulos J, Petrow P, Tanderup K, et al. Recommendations from gynecological GEC-ESTRO working group: Basic principles and parameters for MR imaging within the frame of image based adaptive cervix cancer brachytherapy. *Radiother Oncol* 2012;103:113–122.

35. Viswanathan A, Erickson B, Gaffney D, et al. Comparison and consensus guidelines for delineation of clinical target volume for CT and MR based brachytherapy in locally advanced cervical cancer. *Int J Radiat Oncol Biol Phys* 2014;90:320–328.

36. Nakano T, Kato S, Ohno T, et al. Long-term results of high-dose rate intracavitary brachytherapy for squamous cell carcinoma of the uterine cervix. *Cancer* 2005;103:92–101.

37. Petereit D, Peracey R. Literature analysis of high dose rate brachytherapy fractionation schedules in the treatment of cervical cancer: Is there an optimal fractionation schedule? *Int J Radiat Oncol Biol Phys* 1999;43:359–366.

38. Patel FD, Kumar P, Karunanidhi G, et al. Optimization of high-dose rate intracavitary brachytherapy schedule in the treatment of carcinoma of the cervix. *Brachytherapy* 2011;10:147–153.

39. Patel FD, Rai B, Mallick I, et al. High-dose rate brachytherapy in uterine cervical carcinoma. *Int J Radiat Oncol Biol Phys* 2005;62:125–130.

40. Sood B, Gorla G, Gupta S, et al. Two fractions of high-dose rate brachytherapy in the management of cervix cancer: clinical experience with and without chemotherapy. *Int J Radiat Oncol Biol Phys* 2002;53:702–706.

41. Souhami L, Corns R, Duclos M, et al. Long-term results of high dose rate brachytherapy in cervix cancer using a small number of fractions. *Gynecol Oncol* 2005;97:508–513.

42. Georg P, Kirisits C, Goldner G, et al. Correlation of dose-volume parameters, endoscopic and clinical rectal side effects in cervix cancer patients treated with definitive radiotherapy including MRI-based brachytherapy. *Radiother Oncol* 2009;91:173–180.

43. Georg P, Lang S, Dimopoulos JC, et al. Dose-volume histogram parameters and late side effects in magnetic resonance image-guided adaptive cervical cancer brachytherapy. *Int J Radiat Oncol Biol Phys* 2011;79:356–362.

44. Sharma V, Mahantshetty U, Menon V, et al. A modified technique for high-dose rate intracavitary brachytherapy in advanced cancer of the cervix. *Brachytherapy* 2003;2:246–248.

45. Potter R, Dimopoulos J, Georg P, et al. Clinical impact of MRI assisted dose volume adaptation and dose escalation in brachytherapy of locally advanced cervix cancer. *Radiother Oncol* 2007;83:148–155.

46. Dimopoulos JC, Lang S, Kirisits C, et al. Dose-volume histogram parameters and local tumor control in magnetic resonance image-guided cervical cancer brachytherapy. *Int J Radiat Oncol Biol Phys* 2009;75:56–63.

47. Potter R, Georg P, Dimopoulos J, et al. Clinical outcome of protocol based image MRI guided adaptive brachytherapy combined with 3D conformal radiotherapy with or without chemotherapy in patients with locally advanced cervical cancer. *Radiother Oncol* 2011;100:116–123.

48. Gill B, Kim H, Houser C, et al. MRI guided high dose rate intracavitary brachytherapy for treatment of cervical cancer: The University of Pittsburg experience. *Int J Radiat Oncol Biol Phys* 2015;91:540–547.

49. Lindegaard JC, Fokdal L, Nielsen S, et al. MRI guided adaptive radiotherapy in locally advanced cervical cancer from a Nordic perspective. *Acta Oncol* 2013;52:1510–1519.

50. Rijkmans E, Nout RA, Rutten I, et al. Improved survival of patients with cervical cancer treated with image guided brachytherapy compared with conventional brachytherapy. *Gynecol Oncol* 2014;135:231–238.

51. Sturdza AE, Potter R, Fokdal L, et al. Image guided brachytherapy in locally advanced cervical cancer: Improved pelvic control and survival in retroEMBRACE, a multicenter cohort study. *Radiother Oncol* 2016;120:428–433.

52. Tanderup K, Fokdal L, Sturdza AE, et al. Effect of tumor dose, volume and overall treatment time on local control after radiochemotherapy including MRI guided brachytherapy of locally advanced cervical cancer. *Radiother Oncol* 2016;120:441–446.

53. Jastaniyah N, Yoshida K, Tanderup K, et al. A volumetric analysis of GTVd and CTVhr as defined by the GEC ESTRO recommendations in FIGO stage IIB and IIIB cervical cancer patients treated with IGABT in a prospective multicentric trial (EMBRACE). *Radiother Oncol* 2016;120:404–411.

54. Kirchheiner K, Nout R, Tanderup K, et al. Manifestation pattern of early late vaginal morbidity after definitive radiation chemotherapy and image guided adaptive brachytherapy for locally advanced cervical cancer: an analysis from the EMBRACE study. *Int J Radiat Oncol Biol Phys* 2014;89:88–95.

55. Kirchheiner K, Nout RA, Lindegaard JC, et al. Dose effect relationship and risk factors for vaginal stenosis after definitive radio chemotherapy with image guided brachytherapy for locally advanced cervical cancer in the EMBRACE study. *Radiother Oncol* 2016;118:160–166.

56. Kirchheiner K, Potter R, Tanderup K, et al. Health-related quality of life and locally advanced cervical cancer patients after definitive chemoradiation therapy including image guided adaptive brachytherapy: an analysis from the EMBRACE study. *Int J Radiat Oncol Biol Phys* 2016;94:1088–1098.

57. Mazeron R, Fokdal L, Kirchheiner K, et al. Dose volume effect relationships for late rectal morbidity in patients treated with chemoradiation and MRI guided adaptive brachytherapy for locally advanced cervical cancer: results from the prospective multicenter EMBRACE study. *Radiother Oncol* 2016;120:412–419.

58. Mayadev J, Viswanathan A, Liu Y, et al. American Brachytherapy Task Group Report: A pooled analysis of clinical outcomes for high-dose rate brachytherapy for cervical cancer. *Brachytherapy* 2017;16:22–43.

59. Tan LT, Coles CE, Hart C, et al. Clinical impact of computed tomography-based image-guided brachytherapy for cervix cancer using the tandem-ring applicator—the Addenbrooke's experience. *Clin Oncol (R Coll Radiol)* 2009;21:175–182.

60. Kang HC, Shin KH, Park SY, et al. 3D CT-based high-dose rate brachytherapy for cervical cancer: clinical impact on late rectal bleeding and local control. *Radiother Oncol* 2010;97:507–513.

61. Narayan K, van Dyk S, Bernshaw D, et al. Comparative study of LDR (Manchester system) and HDR image-guided conformal brachytherapy of cervical cancer: patterns of failure, late complications, and survival. *Int J Radiat Oncol Biol Phys* 2009;74:1529–1535.

62. Lorvidhaya V, Tonusin A, Changwiwit W, et al. High-dose rate afterloading brachytherapy in carcinoma of the cervix: an experience of 1992 patients. *Int J Radiat Oncol Biol Phys* 2000;46:1185–1191.

63. Potter R, Knocke TH, Fellner C, et al. Definitive radiotherapy based on HDR brachytherapy with iridium 192 in uterine cervix carcinoma: report on the Vienna University Hospital findings (1993–1997) compared to the preceding period in the context of ICRU 38 recommendations. *Cancer Radiother* 2000;4:159–172.

64. Toita T, Kakinohana Y, Ogawa K, et al. Combination external beam radiotherapy and high-dose rate intracavitary brachytherapy for uterine cervical cancer: analysis of doses and fractionation schedule. *Int J Radiat Oncol Biol Phys* 2003;56:1344–1353.

65. Ferrigno R, Nishimoto IN, Novaes PE, et al. Comparison of low and high dose rate brachytherapy in the treatment of uterine cervix cancer. Retrospective analysis of two sequential series. *Int J Radiat Oncol Biol Phys* 2005;62:1108–1116.

66. Scholten AN, van Putten WL, Beerman H, et al. Postoperative radiotherapy for Stage 1 endometrial carcinoma: long-term outcome of the randomized PORTEC trial with central pathology review. *Int J Radiat Oncol Biol Phys* 2005;63:834–838.

67. Creutzberg CL, van Putten WL, Koper PC, et al. Surgery and postoperative radiotherapy versus surgery alone for patients with stage-1 endometrial carcinoma: multicentre randomised trial. PORTEC Study Group. Post Operative Radiation Therapy in Endometrial Carcinoma. *Lancet* 2000;355:1404–1411.

68. Keys H, Roberts J, Brunetto V, et al. A phase III trial of surgery with or without adjunctive external pelvic radiation therapy in intermediate risk endometrial adenocarcinoma: a Gynecologic Oncology Group study. *Gynecol Oncol* 2004;92:744-751.

69. Nout RA, Smit VT, Putter H, et al. Vaginal brachytherapy versus pelvic external beam radiotherapy for patients with endometrial cancer of high-intermediate risk (PORTEC-2): an open-label, non-inferiority, randomised trial. *Lancet* 2010;375:816–823.

70. Sorbe B, Horvath G, Andersson H, et al. External pelvic and vaginal irradiation versus vaginal irradiation alone as postoperative therapy in medium risk endometrial carcinoma—a prospective randomized study. *Int J Radiat Oncol Biol Phys* 2012;82:1249–1255.

71. Klopp A, Smith BD, Alektiar K, et al. The role of postoperative radiation therapy for endometrial cancer: Executive summary of an American Society for Radiation Oncology evidence-based guideline. *Pract Radiat Oncol* 2014;4:137–144.

72. Harkenrider MM, Block AM, Alektiar KM, et al. American Brachytherapy Task Group Report: Adjuvant vaginal brachytherapy for early-stage endometrial cancer: a comprehensive review. *Brachytherapy* 2017;16:95–108.

73. Rittenberg PV, Lotocki RJ, Heywood MS, et al. High-risk surgical stage 1 endometrial cancer: outcomes with vault brachytherapy alone. *Gynecol Oncol* 2003;89:288–294.

74. Petereit DG, Tannehill SP, Grosen EA, et al. Outpatient vaginal cuff brachytherapy for endometrial cancer. *Int J Gynecol Cancer* 1999;9:456-462.

75. Alektiar KM, Venkatraman E, Chi DS, et al. Intravaginal brachytherapy alone for intermediate-risk endometrial cancer. *Int J Radiat Oncol Biol Phys* 2005;62:111–117.

76. Kim H, Kim H, Houser C, et al. Is there any advantage to three-dimensional planning for vaginal cuff brachytherapy? *Brachytherapy* 2012;11:398–401.

77. Horowitz N, Peters W, Smith M, et al. Adjuvant high dose rate vaginal brachytherapy as treatment of stage I and II endometrial carcinoma. *Obstet Gynecol* 2002;99:235–240.

78. Townamchai K, Lee L, Viswanathan A. A novel low dose fractionation regimen for adjuvant vaginal brachytherapy in early stage endometrial cancer. *Gynecol Oncol* 2012;127:351–355.

79. Gaztanaga M, Cambeiro M, Villafranca E, et al. Long-term results of one-week intravaginal high-dose rate brachytherapy alone for endometrial cancer. *Brachytherapy* 2012;11:119–124.

80. Sorbe B, Straumits A, Karlsson L. Intravaginal high-dose rate brachytherapy for stage I endometrial cancer: a randomized study of two dose-per-fraction levels. *Int J Radiat Oncol Biol Phys* 2005;62:1385–1389.

81. Nag S, Erickson B, Parikh S, et al. The American Brachytherapy Society recommendations for HDR brachytherapy for carcinoma of the endometrium. *Int J Radiat Oncol Biol Phys* 2000;48:779–790.

82. Jolly S, Vargas C, Kumar T, et al. Vaginal brachytherapy alone: an alternative to adjuvant whole pelvis radiation for early stage endometrial cancer. *Gynecol Oncol* 2005;97:887–892.

83. Chong I, Hoskin PJ. Vaginal vault brachytherapy as sole postoperative treatment for low-risk endometrial cancer. *Brachytherapy* 2008;7:195–199.

84. Sorbe BG, Smeds AC. Postoperative vaginal irradiation with high dose rate afterloading technique in endometrial carcinoma stage I. *Int J Radiat Oncol Biol Phys* 1990;18:305–314.

85. Solhjem M, Petersen I, Haddock M. Vaginal brachytherapy alone is sufficient adjuvant treatment of surgical stage I endometrial cancer. *Int J Radiat Oncol Biol Phys* 2005;62:1379–1384.

86. Friedman LC, Abdallah R, Schluchter M, et al. Adherence to vaginal dilation following high dose rate brachytherapy for endometrial cancer. *Int J Radiat Oncol Biol Phys* 2011;80:751–757.

87. Bahng AY, Dagan A, Bruner DW, et al. Determination of Prognostic Factors for Vaginal Mucosal Toxicity Associated With Intravaginal High-Dose Rate Brachytherapy in patients With Endometrial Cancer. *Int J Radiat Oncol Biol Phys* 2012;82:667–673.

88. National Forum of Gynecological Oncology Nurses. *Best practice guidelines on the use of vaginal dilators in women receiving pelvic radiotherapy.* Brook Hill, Woodstock, Oxon, UK: Owen Mumford, 2012.

89. Schwarz J, Beriwal S, Esthappan J, et al. Consensus statement for brachytherapy for the treatment of medically inoperable endometrial cancer. *Brachytherapy* 2015;14:587–599.

90. Niazi TM, Souhami L, Portelance L, et al. Long-term results of high-dose rate brachytherapy in the primary treatment of medically inoperable stage I-II endometrial carcinoma. *Int J Radiat Oncol Biol Phys* 2005;63:1108–1113.

91. Nguyen TV, Petereit DG. High-dose rate brachytherapy for medically inoperable stage I endometrial cancer. *Gynecol Oncol* 1998;71:196–203.

92. Kucera H, Knocke TH, Kucera E, et al. Treatment of endometrial carcinoma with high-dose rate brachytherapy alone in medically inoperable stage I patients. *Acta Obstet Gynecol Scand* 1998;77:1008–1012.

93. Knocke TH, Kucera H, Weidinger B, et al. Primary treatment of endometrial carcinoma with high-dose rate brachytherapy: results of 12 years of experience with 280 patients. *Int J Radiat Oncol Biol Phys* 1997;37:359–365.

94. Coon D, Beriwal S, Heron DE, et al. High-dose rate Rotte "Y" applicator brachytherapy for definitive treatment of medically inoperable endometrial cancer: 10-year results. *Int J Radiat Oncol Biol Phys* 2008;71:779–783.

95. Gill B, Kim H, Houser C, et al. Image based 3-dimensional conformal brachytherapy for medically inoperable endometrial carcinoma. *Brachytherapy* 2014;13:542–547.

96. Astrom L, Pedersen D, Mercke C, et al. Long-term outcome of high dose rate brachytherapy in radiotherapy of localised prostate cancer. *Radiother Oncol* 2005;74:157–161.

97. Bachand F, Martin AG, Beaulieu L, et al. An eight-year experience of HDR brachytherapy boost for localized prostate cancer: biopsy and PSA outcome. *Int J Radiat Oncol Biol Phys* 2009;73:679–684.

98. Deger S, Boehmer D, Roigas J, et al. High dose rate (HDR) brachytherapy with conformal radiation therapy for localized prostate cancer. *Eur Urol* 2005;47:441–448.

99. Demanes DJ, Rodriguez RR, Schour L, et al. High-dose rate intensity-modulated brachytherapy with external beam radiotherapy for prostate cancer: California endocurietherapy's 10-year results. *Int J Radiat Oncol Biol Phys* 2005;61:1306–1316.

100. Deutsch I, Zelefsky MJ, Zhang Z, et al. Comparison of PSA relapse-free survival in patients treated with ultra-high-dose IMRT versus combination HDR brachytherapy and IMRT. *Brachytherapy* 2010;9:313–318.

101. Kaprealian T, Weinberg V, Speight JL, et al. High-Dose rate Brachytherapy Boost for Prostate Cancer: Comparison of Two Different Fractionation Schemes. *Int J Radiat Oncol Biol Phys* 2010;82:222–227.

102. Martinez AA, Gonzalez J, Ye H, et al. Dose escalation improves cancer-related events at 10 years for intermediate- and high-risk prostate cancer patients treated with hypofractionated high-dose rate boost and external beam radiotherapy. *Int J Radiat Oncol Biol Phys* 2011;79:363–370.

103. Neviani CB, Miziara MA, de Andrade Carvalho H. Results of high dose rate brachytherapy boost before 2D or 3D external beam irradiation for prostate cancer. *Radiother Oncol* 2011;98:169–174.

104. Zwahlen DR, Andrianopoulos N, Matheson B, et al. High-dose rate brachytherapy in combination with conformal external beam radiotherapy in the treatment of prostate cancer. *Brachytherapy* 2010;9:27–35.

105. Olarte A, Cambeiro M, Moreno-Jimenez M, et al. Dose escalation with external beam radiation therapy and high-dose rate brachytherapy combined with long-term androgen deprivation therapy in high and very high risk prostate cancer: Comparison of two consecutive high-dose rate schemes. *Brachytherapy* 2016;15:127–135.

106. Galalae RM, Zakikhany NH, Geiger F, et al. The 15-year outcomes of high-dose rate brachytherapy for radical dose escalation in patients with prostate cancer - a benchmark for high-tech external beam radiotherapy alone? *Brachytherapy* 2014;13:117–122.

107. Boladeras A, Santorsa L, Gutierrez C, et al. External beam radiotherapy plus single-fraction high dose rate brachytherapy in the treatment of locally advanced prostate cancer. *Radiother Oncol* 2014;112:227–232.

108. Kotecha R, Yamada Y, Pei X, et al. Clinical outcomes of high-dose rate brachytherapy and external beam radiotherapy in the management of clinically localized prostate cancer. *Brachytherapy* 2013;12:44–49.

109. Hoskin PJ, Colombo A, Henry A, et al. GEC/ESTRO recommendations on high dose rate afterloading brachytherapy for localised prostate cancer: an update. *Radiother Oncol* 2013;107:325–332.
110. Prada PJ, Gonzalez H, Fernandez J, et al. Biochemical outcome after high-dose rate intensity modulated brachytherapy with external beam radiotherapy: 12 years of experience. *BJU Int* 2012;109:1787–1793.
111. Khor R, Duchesne G, Tai KH, et al. Direct 2-arm comparison shows benefit of high-dose rate brachytherapy boost vs external beam radiation therapy alone for prostate cancer. *Int J Radiat Oncol Biol Phys* 2013;85:679–685.
112. Hoskin PJ, Rojas AM, Bownes PJ, et al. Randomised trial of external beam radiotherapy alone or combined with high-dose rate brachytherapy boost for localised prostate cancer. *Radiother Oncol* 2012;103:217–222.
113. Morton G, Loblaw A, Cheung P, et al. Is single fraction 15 Gy the preferred high dose rate brachytherapy boost dose for prostate cancer? *Radiother Oncol* 2011;100:463–467.
114. Fowler J, Chappel R, Ritter M. Is α/β for prostate tumors really low? *Int J Radiat Oncol Biol Phys* 2001;50:1021–1031.
115. Williams SG, Taylor JM, Liu N, et al. Use of individual fraction size data from 3756 patients to directly determine the alpha/beta ratio of prostate cancer. *Int J Radiat Oncol Biol Phys* 2007;68:24–33.
116. Demanes DJ, Martinez AA, Ghilezan M, et al. High-dose rate monotherapy: safe and effective brachytherapy for patients with localized prostate cancer. *Int J Radiat Oncol Biol Phys* 2011;81:1286–1292.
117. Hauswald H, Kamrava MR, Fallon JM, et al. High-dose rate monotherapy for localized prostate cancer: 10-year results. *Int J Radiat Oncol Biol Phys* 2016;94:667–674.
118. Prada PJ, Cardenal J, Blanco AG, et al. High-dose rate interstitial brachytherapy as monotherapy in one fraction for the treatment of favorable stage prostate cancer: Toxicity and long-term biochemical results. *Radiother Oncol* 2016;119:411–416.
119. Yoshioka Y, Suzuki O, Isohashi F, et al. High-Dose rate Brachytherapy as Monotherapy for Intermediate- and High-Risk Prostate Cancer: Clinical Results for a Median 8-Year Follow-Up. *Int J Radiat Oncol Biol Phys* 2016;94:675–682.
120. Hoskin P, Rojas A, Ostler P, et al. High-dose rate brachytherapy with two or three fractions as monotherapy in the treatment of locally advanced prostate cancer. *Radiother Oncol* 2014;112:63–67.
121. Zamboglou N, Tselis N, Baltas D, et al. High-dose rate interstitial brachytherapy as monotherapy for clinically localized prostate cancer: treatment evolution and mature results. *Int J Radiat Oncol Biol Phys* 2013;85:672–678.
122. Rogers CL, Alder SC, Rogers RL, et al. High dose brachytherapy as monotherapy for intermediate risk prostate cancer. *J Urol* 2012;187:109–116.
123. Demanes DJ, Ghilezan MI. High-dose rate brachytherapy as monotherapy for prostate cancer. *Brachytherapy* 2014;13:529–541.
124. Jabbari S, Hsu IC, Kawakami J, et al. High-dose rate brachytherapy for localized prostate adenocarcinoma post abdominoperineal resection of the rectum and pelvic irradiation: technique and experience. *Brachytherapy* 2009;8:339–344.
125. Lee B, Shinohara K, Weinberg V, et al. Feasibility of high-dose rate brachytherapy salvage for local prostate cancer recurrence after radiotherapy: the University of California-San Francisco experience. *Int J Radiat Oncol Biol Phys* 2007;67:1106–1112.
126. Niehoff P, Loch T, Nurnberg N, et al. Feasibility and preliminary outcome of salvage combined HDR brachytherapy and external beam radiotherapy (EBRT) for local recurrences after radical prostatectomy. *Brachytherapy* 2005;4:141–145.
127. Tharp M, Hardacre M, Bennett R, et al. Prostate high-dose rate brachytherapy as salvage treatment of local failure after previous external or permanent seed irradiation for prostate cancer. *Brachytherapy* 2008;7:231–236.
128. Wojcieszek P, Szlag M, Glowacki G, et al. Salvage high-dose rate brachytherapy for locally recurrent prostate cancer after primary radiotherapy failure. *Radiother Oncol* 2016;119:405–410.
129. Yamada Y, Kollmeier MA, Pei X, et al. A Phase II study of salvage high-dose rate brachytherapy for the treatment of locally recurrent prostate cancer after definitive external beam radiotherapy. *Brachytherapy* 2014;13:111–116.
130. Chen CP, Weinberg V, Shinohara K, et al. Salvage HDR brachytherapy for recurrent prostate cancer after previous definitive radiation therapy: 5-year outcomes. *Int J Radiat Oncol Biol Phys* 2013;86:324–329.
131. Arthur DW, Winter K, Kuske RR, et al. A Phase II trial of brachytherapy alone after lumpectomy for select breast cancer: tumor control and survival outcomes of RTOG 95-17. *Int J Radiat Oncol Biol Phys* 2008;72:467–473.
132. Polgar C, Major T, Fodor J, et al. Accelerated partial-breast irradiation using high-dose rate interstitial brachytherapy: 12-year update of a prospective clinical study. *Radiother Oncol* 2010;94:274–279.
133. Strnad V, Hildebrandt G, Potter R, et al. Accelerated partial breast irradiation: 5-year results of the German-Austrian multicenter phase II trial using interstitial multicatheter brachytherapy alone after breast-conserving surgery. *Int J Radiat Oncol Biol Phys* 2011;80:17–24.
134. Vicini F, Beitsch P, Quiet C, et al. Five-year analysis of treatment efficacy and cosmesis by the American Society of Breast Surgeons MammoSite Breast Brachytherapy Registry Trial in patients treated with accelerated partial breast irradiation. *Int J Radiat Oncol Biol Phys* 2011;79:808–817.
135. Polgar C, Fodor J, Major T, et al. Breast-conserving therapy with partial or whole breast irradiation: ten-year results of the Budapest randomized trial. *Radiother Oncol* 2013;108:197–202.
136. Keisch M, Arthur D, Patel R, et al. American Brachytherapy Society—Breast Brachytherapy Task Group—Guidelines, 2007. http://www.americanbrachytherapy.org/guidelines/abs_breast_brachytherapy_taskgroup.pdf.
137. Wallace M, Martinez A, Mitchell C, et al. Phase I/II study evaluating early tolerance in breast cancer patients undergoing accelerated partial breast irradiation treated with the mammosite balloon breast brachytherapy catheter using a 2-day dose schedule. *Int J Radiat Oncol Biol Phys* 2010;77:531–536.
138. Khan AJ, Vicini FA, Brown S, et al. Dosimetric feasibility and acute toxicity in a prospective trial of ultrashort-course accelerated partial breast irradiation (APBI) using a multi-lumen balloon brachytherapy device. *Ann Surg Oncol* 2013;20:1295–1301.
139. Khan AJ, Ahlawat S, Goyal S. Novel and Highly Compressed Schedules for the Treatment of Breast Cancer. *Semin Radiat Oncol* 2016;26:45–50.
140. Chen PY, Vicini FA, Benitez P, et al. Long-term cosmetic results and toxicity after accelerated partial-breast irradiation: a method of radiation delivery by interstitial brachytherapy for the treatment of early-stage breast carcinoma. *Cancer* 2006;106:991–999.
141. Aristei C, Palumbo I, Capezzali G, et al. Outcome of a phase II prospective study on partial breast irradiation with interstitial multi-catheter high-dose rate brachytherapy. *Radiother Oncol* 2013;108:236–241.
142. Genebes C, Chand ME, Gal J, et al. Accelerated partial breast irradiation in the elderly: 5-year results of high-dose rate multi-catheter brachytherapy. *Radiat Oncol* 2014;9:115.
143. Budrukkar A, Gurram L, Upreti RR, et al. Clinical outcomes of prospectively treated 140 women with early stage breast cancer using accelerated partial breast irradiation with 3 dimensional computerized tomography based brachytherapy. *Radiother Oncol* 2015;115:349–354.
144. Strnad V, Ott O, Hildebrandt G, et al. 5-year results of accelerated partial breast irradiation using sole interstitial multicatheter brachytherapy versus whole-breast irradiation with boost after breast-conserving surgery for low-risk invasive and in-situ carcinoma of the female breast: a randomised, phase 3, non-inferiority trial. *Lancet* 2016;387:229–238.
145. White J, Winter K, Kuske RR, et al. Long-Term Cancer Outcomes From Study NRG Oncology/RTOG 9517: A Phase 2 Study of Accelerated Partial Breast Irradiation With Multicatheter Brachytherapy After Lumpectomy for Early-Stage Breast Cancer. *Int J Radiat Oncol Biol Phys* 2016;95:1460–1465.
146. Benitez PR, Keisch ME, Vicini F, et al. Five-year results: the initial clinical trial of MammoSite balloon brachytherapy for partial breast irradiation in early-stage breast cancer. *Am J Surg* 2007;194:456–462.
147. Harper JL, Watkins JM, Zauls AJ, et al. Six-year experience: long-term disease control outcomes for partial breast irradiation using MammoSite balloon brachytherapy. *Am J Surg* 2010;199:204–209.
148. Vargo JA, Verma V, Kim H, et al. Extended (5-year) outcomes of accelerated partial breast irradiation using MammoSite balloon brachytherapy: patterns of failure, patient selection, and dosimetric correlates for late toxicity. *Int J Radiat Oncol Biol Phys* 2014;88:285–291.
149. Mann JM, Osian AD, Brandmaier A, et al. Excellent Long-term Breast Preservation Rate after Accelerated Partial Breast Irradiation Using a Balloon Device. *Clin Breast Cancer* 2016;16:217–222.
150. Henriquez I, Guix B, Tell J, et al. Long term results of high dose rate (HDR) brachytherapy boost in preserving-breast cancer patients: the experience of Radiation Oncology Medical Institute (IMOR) of Barcelona (abstract). *Radiother Oncol* 2001;60(Suppl 1):S11.
151. Neumanova R, Petera J, Frgala T, et al. Long-term outcome with interstitial brachytherapy boost in the treatment of women with early-stage breast cancer. *Neoplasma* 2007;54:413–423.
152. Budrukkar AN, Sarin R, Shrivastava SK, et al. Cosmesis, late sequelae and local control after breast-conserving therapy: influence of type of tumour bed boost and adjuvant chemotherapy. *Clin Oncol (R Coll Radiol)* 2007;19:596–603.
153. Guinot JL, Roldan S, Maronas M, et al. Breast-conservative surgery with close or positive margins: can the breast be preserved with high-dose rate brachytherapy boost? *Int J Radiat Oncol Biol Phys* 2007;68:1381–1387.
154. Polgar C, Janvary L, Major T, et al. The role of high-dose rate (HDR) brachytherapy boost in breast-conserving therapy: 10 year Hungarian experience (abstract). *Radiother Oncol* 2007;83(Suppl 1):S22.
155. Knauerhase H, Strietzel M, Gerber B, et al. Tumor location, interval between surgery and radiotherapy, and boost technique influence local control after breast-conserving surgery and radiation: retrospective analysis of monoinstitutional long-term results. *Int J Radiat Oncol Biol Phys* 2008;72:1048–1055.
156. Guinot JL, Baixauli-Perez C, Soler P, et al. High-dose rate brachytherapy boost effect on local tumor control in young women with breast cancer. *Int J Radiat Oncol Biol Phys* 2015;91:165–171.
157. Quero L, Guillerm S, Taright N, et al. 10-Year follow-up of 621 patients treated using high-dose rate brachytherapy as ambulatory boost technique in conservative breast cancer treatment. *Radiother Oncol* 2016;122(1):11–16.
158. Arthur DW, Vicini FA, Kuske RR, et al. Accelerated partial breast irradiation: an updated report from the American Brachytherapy Society. *Brachytherapy* 2003;2:124–130.
159. Ott OJ, Strnad V, Hildebrandt G, et al. GEC-ESTRO multicenter phase 3-trial: accelerated partial breast irradiation with interstitial multicatheter brachytherapy versus external beam whole breast irradiation: Early toxicity and patient compliance. *Radiother Oncol* 2016;120:119–123.
160. Correa C, Harris EE, Leonardi MC, et al. Accelerated Partial Breast Irradiation: Executive summary for the update of an ASTRO Evidence-Based Consensus Statement. *Pract Radiat Oncol* 2016;7(2):73–79.
161. Beitsch PD, Patel RR, Lorenzetti JD, et al. Post-surgical treatment of early-stage breast cancer with electronic brachytherapy: an intersociety, multicenter brachytherapy trial. *Onco Targets Ther* 2010;3:211–218.
162. Dooley WC, Algan O, Dowlatshahi K, et al. Surgical perspectives from a prospective, nonrandomized, multicenter study of breast conserving surgery and adjuvant electronic brachytherapy for the treatment of breast cancer. *World J Surg Oncol* 2011;9:30.
163. Patel RR, Beitsch PD, Nichols TD, et al. Postsurgical treatment of early-stage breast cancer with electronic brachytherapy: outcomes and health-related quality of life at 1 year. *Am J Clin Oncol* 2013;36:430–435.
164. Nag S, Kuske R, Vicini F, et al. The American Brachytherapy Society recommendations for brachytherapy for carcinoma of the breast. *Oncology* 2001;15:195–207.
165. Roddiger SJ, Kolotas C, Filipowicz I, et al. Neoadjuvant interstitial high-dose rate (HDR) brachytherapy combined with systemic chemotherapy in patients with breast cancer. *Strahlenther Onkol* 2006;182:22–29.
166. Guix B, Lejarcegui JA, Tello JI, et al. Exeresis and brachytherapy as salvage treatment for local recurrence after conservative treatment for breast cancer: results of a ten-year pilot study. *Int J Radiat Oncol Biol Phys* 2010;78:804–810.

167. Hara R, Itami J, Aruga T. Risk factors for massive hemoptysis after endobronchial brachytherapy in patients with tracheaobronchial malignancies. *Cancer* 2001;92:2623–2627.
168. Sawicki M, Kazalski D, Lyczek J. The evaluation of treatment plans in high-dose rate endobronchial brachii therapy by utilizing 2D and 3D computed tomography imaging methods. *J Contemp Brachytherapy* 2014;6:289–292.
169. Li X, Chibani O, Greenwald B. Radiotherapy dose perturbation of metallic esophageal stent. *Int J Radiat Oncol Biol Phys* 2002;54:1276–1285.
170. Skowronek J, Kubaszewska M, Kanikowski M, et al. HDR endobronchial brachytherapy (HDRBT) in the management of advanced lung cancer—comparison of two different dose schedules. *Radiother Oncol* 2009;93:436–440.
171. Niemoeller O, Pollinger B, Niyazi M, et al. Mature results of a randomized trial comparing two fractionation schedules of high-dose rate endoluminal brachytherapy for the treatment of endobronchial tumors. *Radiat Oncol* 2013;7:8.
172. Mallick I, Sharma SC, Behera D, et al. Optimization of dose and fractionation of endobronchial brachytherapy with or without external radiation in the palliative management of non-small cell lung cancer: a prospective randomized study. *J Cancer Res Ther* 2006;2:119–125.
173. Taulelle M, Chauvet B, Vincent P, et al. High dose rate endobronchial brachytherapy: results and complications in 189 patients. *Eur Respir J* 1998;11:162–168.
174. Kelly J, Delclos M, Morice C, et al. High-dose rate endobronchial brachytherapy effectively palliates symptoms due to airway tumors: the 10-year M.D. Anderson Cancer Center experience. *Int J Radiat Oncol Biol Phys* 2000;48:697–702.
175. Celebioglu B, Gurkan O, Erdogan S, et al. High dose rate endobronchial brachytherapy effectively palliates symptoms due to inoperable lung cancer. *Jpn J Clin Oncol* 2002;32:443–448.
176. Gejerman G, Mullokandov EA, Bagiella E, et al. Endobronchial brachytherapy and external-beam radiotherapy in patients with endobronchial obstruction and extrabronchial extension. *Brachytherapy* 2002;1:204–210.
177. Escobar-Sacristan J, Granda-Orive J, Gutierrez J, et al. Endobronchial brachytherapy in the treatment of malignant lung tumors. *Eur Respir J* 2004;24:348–352.
178. Kubaszewska M, Skowronek J, Chichel A, et al. The use of high dose rate endobronchial brachytherapy to palliate symptomatic recurrence of previously irriadiated lung cancer. *Neoplasma* 2008;55:239–245.
179. Ozkok S, Karakoyun-Celik O, Goksel T, et al. High dose rate endobronchial brachytherapy in the management of lung cancer: response and toxicity evaluation in 158 patients. *Lung Cancer* 2008;62:326–333.
180. Guarnaschelli JN, Jose BO. Palliative high-dose rate endobronchial brachytherapy for recurrent carcinoma: the University of Louisville experience. *J Palliat Med* 2010;13:981–989.
181. Dagnault A, Ebacher A, Vigneault E, et al. Retrospective study of 81 patients treated with brachytherapy for endobronchial primary tumor or metastasis. *Brachytherapy* 2010;9:243–247.
182. Hauswald H, Stoiber E, Rochet N, et al. Treatment of recurrent bronchial carcinoma: the role of high-dose rate endoluminal brachytherapy. *Int J Radiat Oncol Biol Phys* 2010;77:373–377.
183. de Aquino Gorayeb MM, Gregorio MG, de Oliveira EQ, et al. High-dose rate brachytherapy in symptom palliation due to malignant endobronchial obstruction: a quantitative assessment. *Brachytherapy* 2013;12:471–478.
184. Zaric B, Perin B, Jovelic A, et al. Clinical risk factors for early complications after high-dose rate endobronchial brachytherapy in the palliative treatment of lung cancer. *Clin Lung Cancer* 2010;11:182–186.
185. Perol M, Caliandro R, Pommier P, et al. Curative irradiation of limited endobronchial carcinomas with high-dose rate brachytherapy. Results of a pilot study. *Chest* 1997;111:1417–1423.
186. Marsiglia H, Baldeyrou P, Lartigau E, et al. High-dose rate brachytherapy as a sole modality for early-stage endobronchial carcinoma. *Int J Radiat Oncol Biol Phys* 2000;47:665–672.
187. Hennequin C, Bleichner O, Tredaniel J, et al. Long-term results of endobronchial brachytherapy: a curative treatment? *Int J Radiat Oncol Biol Phys* 2007;67:425–430.
188. Aumont-le Guilcher M, Prevost B, Sunyach MP, et al. High-dose rate brachytherapy for non-small-cell lung carcinoma: a retrospective study of 226 patients. *Int J Radiat Oncol Biol Phys* 2011;79:1112–1116.
189. Muto P, Ravo V, Panelli G, et al. High-dose rate brachytherapy of bronchial cancer: treatment optimization using three schemes of therapy. *Oncologist* 2000;5:209–214.
190. Reveiz L, Rueda JR, Cardona AF. Palliative endobronchial brachytherapy for non-small cell lung cancer. *Cochrane Database Syst Rev* 2012;12:Cd004284.
191. McKenna RJ, Jr, Mahtabifard A, Yap J, et al. Wedge resection and brachytherapy for lung cancer in patients with poor pulmonary function. *Ann Thorac Surg* 2008;85:S733–S736.
192. Allison R, Sibata C, Sarma K, et al. High-dose rate brachytherapy in combination with stenting offers a rapid and statistically significant improvement in quality of life for patients with endobronchial recurrence. *Cancer J* 2004;10:368–373.
193. Freitag L, Ernst A, Thomas M, et al. Sequential photodynamic therapy (PDT) and high dose brachytherapy for endobronchial tumour control in patients with limited bronchogenic carcinoma. *Thorax* 2004;59:790–793.
194. Chella A, Ambrogi MC, Ribechini A, et al. Combined Nd-YAG laser/HDR brachytherapy versus Nd-YAG laser only in malignant central airway involvement: a prospective randomized study. *Lung Cancer* 2000;27:169–175.
195. Gaspar LE, Nag S, Herskovic A, et al. American Brachytherapy Society (ABS) consensus guidelines for brachytherapy of esophageal cancer. Clinical Research Committee, American Brachytherapy Society, Philadelphia, PA. *Int J Radiat Oncol Biol Phys* 1997;38:127–132.
196. Rosenblatt E, Jones G, Sur RK, et al. Adding external beam to intra-luminal brachytherapy improves palliation in obstructive squamous cell oesophageal cancer: a prospective multi-centre randomized trial of the International Atomic Energy Agency. *Radiother Oncol* 2010;97:488–494.
197. Sur R, Donde B, Falkson C, et al. Randomized prospective study comparing high-dose rate intraluminal brachytherapy (HDRILBT) alone with HDRILBT and external beam radiotherapy in the palliation of advanced esophageal cancer. *Brachytherapy* 2004;3:191–195.
198. Sur R, Levin C, Donde B, et al. Prospective randomized trial of HDR brachytherapy as a sole modality in palliation of advanced esophageal carcinoma: an International Atomic Energy Agency study. *Int J Radiat Oncol Biol Phys* 2002;53:127–133.
199. Sur RK, Donde B, Levin VC, et al. Fractionated high dose rate intraluminal brachytherapy in palliation of advanced esophageal cancer. *Int J Radiat Oncol Biol Phys* 1998;40:447–453.
200. Nicolay NH, Rademacher J, Oelmann-Avendano J, et al. High dose rate endoluminal brachytherapy for primary and recurrent esophageal cancer: experience from a large single-center cohort. *Strahlenther Onkol* 2016;192:458–466.
201. Laskar SG, Lewis S, Agarwal JP, et al. Combined brachytherapy and external beam radiation: an effective approach for palliation in esophageal cancer. *J Contemp Brachytherapy* 2015;7:453–461.
202. Wong Hee Kam S, Rivera S, Hennequin C, et al. Salvage high-dose rate brachytherapy for esophageal cancer in previously irradiated patients: a retrospective analysis. *Brachytherapy* 2015;14:531–536.
203. Ishikawa H, Nonaka T, Sakurai H, et al. Usefulness of intraluminal brachytherapy combined with external beam radiation therapy for submucosal esophageal cancer: long-term follow-up results. *Int J Radiat Oncol Biol Phys* 2010;76:452–459.
204. Tamaki T, Ishikawa H, Takahashi T, et al. Comparison of efficacy and safety of low-dose rate vs. high-dose rate intraluminal brachytherapy boost in patients with superficial esophageal cancer. *Brachytherapy* 2012;11:130–136.
205. Brunner TB, Rupp A, Melzner W, et al. Esophageal cancer. A prospective phase II study of concomitant-boost external-beam chemoradiation with a top-up endoluminal boost. *Strahlenther Onkol* 2008;184:15–22.
206. Gaspar LE, Winter K, Kocha WI, et al. A phase I/II study of external beam radiation, brachytherapy, and concurrent chemotherapy for patients with localized carcinoma of the esophagus (Radiation Therapy Oncology Group Study 9207): final report. *Cancer* 2000;88:988–995.
207. Gaspar LE, Winter K, Kocha WI, et al. Swallowing function and weight change observed in a phase I/II study of external-beam radiation, brachytherapy and concurrent chemotherapy in localized cancer of the esophagus (RTOG 9207). *Cancer J* 2001;7:388–394.
208. Vuong T, Szego P, David M, et al. The safety and usefulness of high-dose rate endoluminal brachytherapy as a boost in the treatment of patients with esophageal cancer with external beam radiation with or without chemotherapy. *Int J Radiat Oncol Biol Phys* 2005;63:758–764.
209. Shinohara ET, Guo M, Mitra N, et al. Brachytherapy in the treatment of cholangiocarcinoma. *Int J Radiat Oncol Biol Phys* 2010;78:722–728.
210. Yoshioka Y, Ogawa K, Oikawa H, et al. Impact of intraluminal brachytherapy on survival outcome for radiation therapy for unresectable biliary tract cancer: a propensity-score matched-pair analysis. *Int J Radiat Oncol Biol Phys* 2014;89:822–829.
211. Mukewar S, Gupta A, Baron TH, et al. Endoscopically inserted nasobiliary catheters for high dose rate brachytherapy as part of neoadjuvant therapy for perihilar cholangiocarcinoma. *Endoscopy* 2015;47:878–883.
212. Lu JJ, Bains YS, Abdel-Wahab M, et al. High-dose rate remote afterloading intracavitary brachytherapy for the treatment of extrahepatic biliary duct carcinoma. *Cancer J* 2002;8:74–78.
213. Schleicher UM, Staatz G, Alzen G, et al. Combined external beam and intraluminal radiotherapy for irresectable Klatskin tumors. *Strahlenther Onkol* 2002;178:682–687.
214. Shin HS, Seong J, Kim WC, et al. Combination of external beam irradiation and high-dose rate intraluminal brachytherapy for inoperable carcinoma of the extrahepatic bile ducts. *Int J Radiat Oncol Biol Phys* 2003;57:105–112.
215. Aggarwal R, Patel FD, Kapoor R, et al. Evaluation of high-dose rate intraluminal brachytherapy by percutaneous transhepatic biliary drainage in the palliative management of malignant biliary obstruction—a pilot study. *Brachytherapy* 2013;12:162–170.
216. Jain S, Kataria T, Bisht SS, et al. Malignant obstructive jaundice—brachytherapy as a tool for palliation. *J Contemp Brachytherapy* 2013;5:83–88.
217. Mattiucci GC, Autorino R, Tringali A, et al. A Phase I study of high-dose rate intraluminal brachytherapy as palliative treatment in extrahepatic biliary tract cancer. *Brachytherapy* 2015;14:401–404.
218. Inoue T, Yoshida K, Yoshioka Y, et al. Phase III trial of high- vs. low-dose rate interstitial radiotherapy for early mobile tongue cancer. *Int J Radiat Oncol Biol Phys* 2001;51:171–175.
219. Leung TW, Wong VY, Kwan KH, et al. High dose rate brachytherapy for early stage oral tongue cancer. *Head Neck* 2002;24:274–281.
220. Guinot JL, Arribas L, Chust ML, et al. Lip cancer treatment with high dose rate brachytherapy. *Radiother Oncol* 2003;69:113–115.
221. Levendag PC, Nijdam WM, van Moolenburgh SE, et al. Interstitial radiation therapy for early-stage nasal vestibule cancer: a continuing quest for optimal tumor control and cosmesis. *Int J Radiat Oncol Biol Phys* 2006;66:160–169.
222. Dixit S, Baboo H, Rakesh V, et al. Interstitial high dose rate brachytherapy in head and neck cancers: preliminary results. *J Brachyther Int* 1997;13:363–370.
223. Ozyar E, Yildz F, Akyol FH, et al. Adjuvant high-dose rate brachytherapy after external beam radiotherapy in nasopharyngeal carcinoma. *Int J Radiat Oncol Biol Phys* 2002;52:101–108.
224. Nag S, Tippin D, Grecula J, et al. Intraoperative high-dose rate brachytherapy for paranasal sinus tumors. *Int J Radiat Oncol Biol Phys* 2004;58:155–160.
225. Lu J, Shakespeare T, Tan L, et al. Adjuvant fractionated high-dose rate intracavitary brachytherapy after external beam radiotherapy in T1 and T2 nasopharyngeal carcinoma. *Head Neck* 2004;26:389–395.
226. Nose T, Koizumi M, Nishiyama K. High-dose rate interstitial brachytherapy for oropharyngeal carcinoma: results of 83 lesions in 82 patients. *Int J Radiat Oncol Biol Phys* 2004;59:983–991.
227. Ng T, Richards GM, Emery RS, et al. Customized conformal high-dose rate brachytherapy boost for limited-volume nasopharyngeal cancer. *Int J Radiat Oncol Biol Phys* 2005;61:754–761.
228. Nag S, Koc M, Schuller DE, et al. Intraoperative single fraction high-dose rate brachytherapy for head and neck cancers. *Brachytherapy* 2005;4:217–223.

229. Leung TW, Wong VY, Sze WK, et al. High-dose rate intracavitary brachytherapy boost for early T stage nasopharyngeal carcinoma. *Int J Radiat Oncol Biol Phys* 2008;70:361–367.
230. Yeo R, Fong KW, Hee SW, et al. Brachytherapy boost for T1/T2 nasopharyngeal carcinoma. *Head Neck* 2009;31:1610–1618.
231. Martinez-Monge R, Gomez-Iturriaga A, Cambeiro M, et al. Phase I-II trial of perioperative high-dose rate brachytherapy in oral cavity and oropharyngeal cancer. *Brachytherapy* 2009;8:26–33.
232. Guinot JL, Santos M, Tortajada MI, et al. Efficacy of high-dose rate interstitial brachytherapy in patients with oral tongue carcinoma. *Brachytherapy* 2010;9:227–234.
233. Takacsi-Nagy Z, Oberna F, Koltai P, et al. Long-term outcomes with high-dose rate brachytherapy for the management of base of tongue cancer. *Brachytherapy* 2013;12:535–541.
234. Matsumoto K, Sasaki T, Shioyama Y, et al. Treatment outcome of high-dose rate interstitial radiation therapy for patients with stage I and II mobile tongue cancer. *Jpn J Clin Oncol* 2013;43:1012–1017.
235. Vedasoundaram P, Prasanna AK, Ks R, et al. Role of high dose rate interstitial brachytherapy in early and locally advanced squamous cell carcinoma of buccal mucosa. *Springerplus* 2014;3:590.
236. Wan XB, Jiang R, Xie FY, et al. Endoscope-guided interstitial intensity-modulated brachytherapy and intracavitary brachytherapy as boost radiation for primary early T stage nasopharyngeal carcinoma. *PLoS One* 2014;9:e90048.
237. Martinez-Monge R, Pagola Divasson M, Cambeiro M, et al. Determinants of complications and outcome in high-risk squamous cell head-and-neck cancer treated with perioperative high-dose rate brachytherapy (PHDRB). *Int J Radiat Oncol Biol Phys* 2011;81:e245–e254.
238. Teudt IU, Meyer JE, Ritter M, et al. Perioperative image-adapted brachytherapy for the treatment of paranasal sinus and nasal cavity malignancies. *Brachytherapy* 2014;13:178–186.
239. Mazeron JJ, Ardiet JM, Haie-Meder C, et al. GEC-ESTRO recommendations for brachytherapy for head and neck squamous cell carcinomas. *Radiother Oncol* 2009;91:150–156.
240. Levendag PC, Lagerwaard FJ, de Pan C, et al. High-dose, high-precision treatment options for boosting cancer of the nasopharynx. *Radiother Oncol* 2002;63:67–74.
241. Tselis N, Ratka M, Vogt HG, et al. Hypofractionated accelerated CT-guided interstitial (1)(2)Ir-HDR-Brachytherapy as re-irradiation in inoperable recurrent cervical lymphadenopathy from head and neck cancer. *Radiother Oncol* 2011;98:57–62.
242. Narayana A, Cohen GN, Zaider M, et al. High-dose rate interstitial brachytherapy in recurrent and previously irradiated head and neck cancers--preliminary results. *Brachytherapy* 2007;6:157–163.
243. Leung TW, Tung SY, Sze WK, et al. Salvage radiation therapy for locally recurrent nasopharyngeal carcinoma. *Int J Radiat Oncol Biol Phys* 2000;48:1331–1338.
244. Hepel JT, Syed AM, Puthawala A, et al. Salvage high-dose rate (HDR) brachytherapy for recurrent head-and-neck cancer. *Int J Radiat Oncol Biol Phys* 2005;62:1444–1450.
245. Martinez-Fernandez MI, Alcalde J, Cambeiro M, et al. Perioperative high dose rate brachytherapy (PHDRB) in previously irradiated head and neck cancer: Results of a phase I/II reirradiation study. *Radiother Oncol* 2017;122(2):255–259
246. Takacsi-Nagy Z, Martinez-Mongue R, Mazeron JJ, et al. American Brachytherapy Society Task Group Report: Combined external beam irradiation and interstitial brachytherapy for base of tongue tumors and other head and neck sites in the era of new technologies. *Brachytherapy* 2017;16:44–58.
247. Alektiar KM, Leung D, Zelefsky MJ, et al. Adjuvant brachytherapy for primary high-grade soft tissue sarcoma of the extremity. *Ann Surg Oncol* 2002;9:48–56.
248. Alektiar KM, Hu K, Anderson L, et al. High-dose rate intraoperative radiation therapy (HDR-IORT) for retroperitoneal sarcomas. *Int J Radiat Oncol Biol Phys* 2000;47:157–163.
249. Chun M, Kang S, Kim BS, et al. High dose rate interstitial brachytherapy in soft tissue sarcoma: technical aspects and results. *Jpn J Clin Oncol* 2001;31:279–283.
250. Crownover R, Marks K, Zehr R. Initial results with high dose rate brachytherapy for soft-tissue sarcomas. *Sarcoma* 1997;1:196–205.
251. Itami J, Sumi M, Beppu Y, et al. High-dose rate brachytherapy alone in postoperative soft tissue sarcomas with close or positive margins. *Brachytherapy* 2010;9:349–353.
252. Koizumi M, Inoue T, Yamazaki H, et al. Perioperative fractionated high-dose rate brachytherapy for malignant bone and soft tissue tumors. *Int J Radiat Oncol Biol Phys* 1999;43:989–993.
253. Kretzler A, Molls M, Gradinger R, et al. Intraoperative radiotherapy of soft tissue sarcoma of the extremity. *Strahlenther Onkol* 2004;180:365–370.
254. Mierzwa ML, McCluskey CM, Barrett WL, et al. Interstitial brachytherapy for soft tissue sarcoma: A single institution experience. *Brachytherapy* 2007;6:298–303.
255. Petera J, Soumarova R, Ruzickova J, et al. Perioperative hyperfractionated high-dose rate brachytherapy for the treatment of soft tissue sarcomas: multicentric experience. *Ann Surg Oncol* 2010;17:206–210.
256. Pohar S, Haq R, Liu L, et al. Adjuvant high-dose rate and low-dose rate brachytherapy with external beam radiation in soft tissue sarcoma: a comparison of outcomes. *Brachytherapy* 2007;6:53–57.
257. San Miguel I, San Julian M, Cambeiro M, et al. Determinants of Toxicity, Patterns of Failure, and Outcome Among Adult Patients With Soft Tissue Sarcomas of the Extremity and Superficial Trunk Treated With Greater than Conventional Doses of Perioperative High-Dose rate Brachytherapy and External Beam Radiotherapy. *Int J Radiat Oncol Biol Phys* 2011;81:e529–e539.
258. Rachbauer F, Sztankay A, Kreczy A, et al. High-dose rate intraoperative brachytherapy (IOHDR) using flab technique in the treatment of soft tissue sarcomas. *Strahlenther Onkol* 2003;179:480–485.
259. Emory CL, Montgomery CO, Potter BK, et al. Early complications of high-dose rate brachytherapy in soft tissue sarcoma: a comparison with traditional external-beam radiotherapy. *Clin Orthop Relat Res* 2012;470:751–758.
260. Sharma DN, Deo SV, Rath GK, et al. Perioperative high-dose rate interstitial brachytherapy combined with external beam radiation therapy for soft tissue sarcoma. *Brachytherapy* 2015;14:571–577.
261. Alektiar KM, Brennan MF, Singer S. Local control comparison of adjuvant brachytherapy to intensity-modulated radiotherapy in primary high-grade sarcoma of the extremity. *Cancer* 2011;117:3229–3234.
262. Merchant TE, Parsh N, del Valle PL, et al. Brachytherapy for pediatric soft-tissue sarcoma. *Int J Radiat Oncol Biol Phys* 2000;46:427–432.
263. Nag S, Tippin DB. Brachytherapy for pediatric tumors. *Brachytherapy* 2003;2:131–138.
264. Nag S, Tippin D, Ruymann FB. Long-term morbidity in children treated with fractionated high-dose rate brachytherapy for soft tissue sarcomas. *J Pediatr Hematol Oncol* 2003;25:448–452.
265. Nag S, Fernandes P, Martínez-Monge R, et al. Use of brachytherapy to preserve function in children with soft-tissue sarcomas. *Oncology* 1999;13:361–374.
266. Nag S, Shasha D, Janjan N, et al. The American Brachytherapy Society recommendations for brachytherapy of soft tissue sarcomas. *Int J Radiat Oncol Biol Phys* 2001;49:1033–1043.
267. Merchant TE, Zelefsky MJ, Sheldon JM, et al. High-dose rate intraoperative radiation therapy for pediatric solid tumors. *Med Pediatr Oncol* 1998;30:34–39.
268. Nag S, Tippin D, Ruymann F. Intraoperative high-dose rate brachytherapy for the treatment of pediatric soft tissue sarcomas. *Int J Radiat Oncol Biol Phys* 2001;51:729–735.
269. Schuck A, Willich N, Rube C, et al. Intraoperative high-dose rate brachytherapy after preoperative radiochemotherapy in the treatment of Ewing's sarcoma. *Front Radiat Ther Oncol* 1997;31:153–156.
270. Nag S, Martinez-Monge R, Ruymann FB, et al. Feasibility of intraoperative high-dose rate brachytherapy to boost low dose external beam radiation therapy to treat pediatric soft tissue sarcomas. *Med Pediatr Oncol* 1998;31:79–85.
271. Martinez-Monge R, Garran C, Cambeiro M, et al. Feasibility report of conservative surgery, perioperative high-dose rate brachytherapy (PHDRB), and low-to-moderate dose external beam radiation therapy (EBRT) in pediatric sarcomas. *Brachytherapy* 2004;3:196–200.
272. Nakamura R, Dos Santos Novaes P, Antoneli C, et al. High-dose rate brachytherapy as part of a multidisciplinary treatment of nasopharyngeal lymphoepithelioma in childhood. *Cancer* 2005;104:525–531.
273. Viani GA, Novaes PE, Jacinto AA, et al. High-dose rate brachytherapy for soft tissue sarcoma in children: a single institution experience. *Radiat Oncol* 2008;3:9.
274. Laskar S, Bahl G, Ann Muckaden M, et al. Interstitial brachytherapy for childhood soft tissue sarcoma. *Pediatr Blood Cancer* 2007;49:649–655.
275. Goodman KA, Wolden SL, LaQuaglia MP, et al. Intraoperative high-dose rate brachytherapy for pediatric solid tumors: a 10-year experience. *Brachytherapy* 2003;2:139–146.
276. Nag S, Tippin D, Smith S, et al. Intraoperative electron beam treatment for pediatric malignancies: The Ohio State University experience. *Med Pediatr Oncol* 2003;40:360–366.
277. Folkert MR, Tong WY, LaQuaglia MP, et al. 20-year experience with intraoperative high-dose rate brachytherapy for pediatric sarcoma: outcomes, toxicity, and practice recommendations. *Int J Radiat Oncol Biol Phys* 2014;90:362–368.
278. Blank LE, Koedooder K, van der Grient HN, et al. Brachytherapy as part of the multidisciplinary treatment of childhood rhabdomyosarcomas of the orbit. *Int J Radiat Oncol Biol Phys* 2010;77:1463–1469.
279. Ouhib Z, Kasper M, Perez Calatayud J, et al. Aspects of dosimetry and clinical practice of skin brachytherapy: The American Brachytherapy Society working group report. *Brachytherapy* 2015;14:840–858.
280. Nag S, Gunderson L, Harrison L. Techniques of intraoperative radiation therapy vs. intraoperative high dose rate brachytherapy. In: Gunderson L, et al., ed. *Intraoperative irradiation: Techniques and results*. Totowa, NJ: Humana Press, 1999:111–130.
281. Guix B, Finestres F, Tello J, et al. Treatment of skin carcinomas of the face by high-dose rate brachytherapy and custom-made surface molds. *Int J Radiat Oncol Biol Phys* 2000;47:95–102.
282. Kuribayashi S, Miyashita T, Ozawa Y, et al. Post-keloidectomy irradiation using high-dose rate superficial brachytherapy. *J Radiat Res* 2011;52:365–368.
283. Kasper ME, Richter S, Warren N, et al. Complete response of endemic Kaposi sarcoma lesions with high-dose rate brachytherapy: treatment method, results, and toxicity using skin surface applicators. *Brachytherapy* 2013;12:495–499.
284. Likhacheva AO, Devlin PM, Shirvani SM, et al. Skin surface brachytherapy: a survey of contemporary practice patterns. *Brachytherapy* 2017;16:223–229.
285. Lloyd S, Alektiar KM, Nag S, et al. Intraoperative high-dose rate brachytherapy: an American Brachytherapy Society consensus report. *Brachytherapy* 2017;16(3):446–465.
286. International Commission on Radiological Protection 2001-2005. ICRP Publication 97: prevention of high-dose rate brachytherapy accidents. *Ann ICRP* 2005;35(2):1–51.
287. Nag S, Dally M, De la Torre M, et al. Recommendations for implementation of high dose rate 192-Ir brachytherapy in developing countries by the Advisory Group of International Atomic Energy Agency. *Radiother Oncol* 2002;64:297–308.
288. Suneja G, Brown D, Chang A, et al. American Brachytherapy Society: Brachytherapy treatment recommendations for locally advanced cervix cancer for low-income and middle-income countries. *Brachytherapy* 2017;16:85–94.
289. Schneider F, Fuchs H, Lorenz F, et al. A novel device for intravaginal electronic brachytherapy. *Int J Radiat Oncol Biol Phys* 2009;74:1298–1305.
290. Dickler A, Ivanov O, Francescatti D. Intraoperative radiation therapy in the treatment of early-stage breast cancer utilizing xoft axxent electronic brachytherapy. *World J Surg Oncol* 2009;7:24.
291. Petereit DG, Frank SJ, Viswanathan AN, et al. Brachytherapy: where has it gone? *J Clin Oncol* 2015;33:980–982.
292. Li S, Frassica D, DeWeese T, et al. A real-time image-guided intraoperative high-dose rate brachytherapy system. *Brachytherapy* 2003;2:5–16.

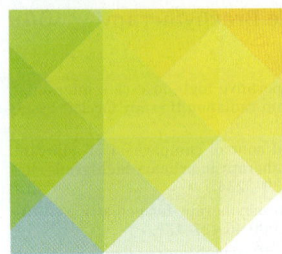

CHAPTER 29

Radioimmunotherapy and Unsealed Radionuclide Therapy

Tod W. Speer

INTRODUCTION

The concept of a "magic bullet" or targeted therapy against a tumor was first proposed by Paul Ehrlich in 1898, ultimately allowing him to garner the Nobel Prize in 1908. As testimony to the complexities and challenges of his vision, it was not until a half a century later when radiolabeled antibodies were used in the clinic to target cancer. The modern exegesis for targeting agents does not limit the use of carrier molecules to mere antibodies. Successful targeting of tumor cells, with high affinity, can also be accomplished with antibody fragments, peptides, and affinity ligands. As the research and clinical arena ever so modestly disengage from intact antibodies as the carrier molecule for the radionuclide, the impact of the immune system has been somewhat abrogated. Hence, the "immunotherapy contribution" of "radioimmunotherapy" (RIT) has become less pronounced. Perhaps, a more appropriate term for this technology would be "targeted radionuclide therapy."

To date, RIT has made significant progress secondary to advances in cell biology, immunology, radiation oncology, nuclear physics, and chemical technology. There are greater than 8 million cancer deaths worldwide and nearly 600,000 cancer deaths in the United States annually.[1,2] Millions of cancer patients each year exhaust available drug options and succumb to cancer. Current cancer drug development in the United States takes approximately 8 years and 1.3 billion dollars for FDA approval.[3] This process appears unsustainable.[4] RIT offers the potential to accelerate drug development. RIT exercises its cytotoxic action by delivering targeted molecular radiation to malignant tissue. Therefore, the success of RIT depends upon engineering a targeting construct that brings the radionuclide into close proximity of the target cell or tissue. The cytotoxic agent, the radionuclide, is always the same. Of course, there is a selected differential of energy deposition into tissue, depending upon the specific chosen radionuclide. Standard drug development relies upon identifying a different target receptor or pathway that is prevalent within a particular type of cancer. Antibodies (or blocking agents) are then designed, over months or years, to interfere with the receptor or process. A cytotoxic evaluation is then performed. Not all antibodies are initially cytotoxic. Hence, the abovementioned timeline and cost prevail.

IMMUNOLOGY AND TARGETING CONSTRUCTS

Immunity refers to protection from disease or infectious agents.[5] Our immune system is composed of the cells and molecules responsible for the immune response, which can be divided into an early (1- to 12-hour) reaction, termed *innate immunity*, and a late (1- to >7-day) reaction, termed *adaptive immunity*. The innate immune system comprises biochemical and cellular mechanisms that exist prior to the introduction of a "foreign" or infectious agent and results in a rapid response. The innate immune system consists of epithelial barriers, phagocytic cells (neutrophils, macrophages), natural killer cells, the complement system, and cytokines. The adaptive immune system develops over time, becoming more effective with subsequent exposures of antigen. It exhibits the ability to "remember" and to respond more quickly with continued exposures to the same antigen. The adaptive immune system consists of lymphocytes and secreted antibodies. The adaptive immune system can be divided into humoral immunity and cell-mediated immunity. Concerning humoral immunity, B lymphocytes secrete antibodies for protection. With cell-mediated immunity, helper T lymphocytes either activate macrophages or cytotoxic T lymphocytes, which then directly destroy pathologic (infectious or malignant) cells.

It is well known that the host's immune system is important for preventing the growth and development of cancer.[6] A large body of literature exists supporting the concept that the host immune system interacts with tumorigenesis and tumor progression. It has been shown in animal models and in the clinic that cancer immune surveillance is exceedingly important. For example, mice with an impaired innate or adaptive immune system will be more susceptible to develop chemically induced or spontaneous cancers. Additionally, the malignant transformation of cells in animals and humans, caused by the accumulation of somatic mutations and/or the deregulation of oncogenes or tumor suppressor genes, results in the expression of tumor antigens (TAs). These TAs are often recognized by the immune system as documented by TA-specific T-cell precursors and natural killer cells, found in the peripheral blood of cancer patients, capable of killing tumor cells. Further evidence of cancer immune surveillance exists in patients with genetic or drug-induced immunosuppression. Transplant patients exhibit a predisposition for certain malignancies (squamous cell carcinoma, basal cell carcinoma, Kaposi sarcoma, melanoma, and lymphoma). Patients with Chédiak-Higashi and Wiskott-Aldrich syndrome demonstrate an increased rate of lymphoproliferative malignancies. Discontinuing immunosuppressive drugs in solid organ allograph patients with occult malignant melanoma has resulted in tumor regression.

Despite the evidence of cancer genesis and progression in immune-compromised hosts, the majority of cancers develop in seemingly immune-competent individuals. The last decades of research have revealed that cancer cells have developed means to avoid immune detection and surveillance, either through the selection of nonimmunogenic tumor cells or the active suppression of the immune response. It has therefore been rightfully suggested that "tumor immune escape" be added to Hanahan and Weinberg's six hallmarks of cancer (self-sufficiency in growth signals, insensitivity to antigrowth signals, tissue invasion and metastasis, limitless replicative potential, sustained angiogenesis, and evasion of apoptosis). Interestingly, recent progress has been achieved utilizing drugs for immune checkpoint blockade therapy by targeting the programmed death protein (PD-1) with antibodies. Unfortunately, response rates have been limited.[7] Currently, the quest for the "Holy Grail" vaccine that turns the immune system against cancer remains elusive.[8]

The targets for RIT typically consist of tumor-associated antigens (TAAs) expressed on the surface of tumor cells or in the abnormal extracellular matrix. The reason for this is because the cytotoxic radionuclide must be delivered preferentially to malignant tissue and should avoid normal tissue. To date, >2,000 TAAs have been identified (http://www.re3data.org/repository/r3d100012052). One of the main methodologies used to identify TAAs is termed *SEREX* (serologic analysis of recombinant cDNA libraries). SEREX involves a bacteriophage recombinant cDNA expression library, prepared from various malignancies (isolated tumors or malignant cell lines) or testis tissue.[9] This cDNA expression library is transduced in *Escherichia coli* to produce a recombinant protein library. These various proteins (clones) are then tested against the serum from autologous cancer patients. Clones that react to IgG antibodies are identified and are then further characterized as TAAs. Many of these SEREX-identified TAAs have been elucidated by other processes and laboratories. This has led to the concept of a finite number of TAAs that are produced in cancer patients and are potentially identified by the immune system. These finite TAAs are collectively referred to as the cancer immunome. SEREX-defined antigens, representing broad categories, may be organized as follows: mutational antigens, amplified or overexpressed antigens, differentiation antigens, and cancer/testis antigens. Within these categories, only a limited number of solid tumor TAAs have been used as targets for RIT (Table 29.1).

TABLE 29.1 SELECT TUMOR ANTIGEN TARGETS AND MONOCLONAL ANTIBODIES EVALUATED FOR SOLID TUMOR RADIOIMMUNOTHERAPY

Malignancy	Antigen	Antibody
Colorectal cancer	CEA	cT84.66, hMN-14, A5B7, TFT, IMP-288, CC49
	TAG-72	B72.3, CC49, A33
	A33	huA33
	EpCAM	NR-LU-10, NR-LU-13
	DNA histone H1	chTNT-1/B
	FAP	F19
Breast cancer	MUC1	huBrE3, M170
	L6	chL6
	TAG-72	CC49
	CEA	cT84.66
	Lewis	B3
Ovarian cancer	MUC1	HMFG-1
	Folate receptor	cMov18
	TAG-72	B72.3, CC49
	Lewis	Hu3S193
Prostate cancer	PSMA	huJ591, 7E11-C5.3, PSMA-617
	TAG-72	CC49
	MUC1	M170
Lung cancer	DNA histone H1	chTNT-1/B
	TAG-72	CC49
	CEA	cT84.66
Head and neck cancer	CD44v6	U36, BIWA4
Glioblastoma	EGFR	425
	Tenascin-C	81C6, BC4
	DNA histone H1	chTNT-1/B
Melanoma	p97	96.5
	Ganglioside GD2	3F8
	Melanin	PTI-6D2
Renal cancer	CAIX/MN	cG250
Medullary thyroid cancer	CEA	cT84.66, hMN-14, NP-4, F6-734, Labetuzumab
Neuroblastoma	Ganglioside GD2	3F8
	NCAM	UJ13 A, ERIC-1
	Tenascin-C	81C6
Gastric	A33	huA33
Brain tumors	Ganglioside GD2	3F8
	4Ig-B7-H3	8H9
	DNA/histone	chTNT-1/B
Medulloblastoma	Ganglioside GD2	3F8
CEA-producing tumors	CEA	M5A
Pancreatic cancer	MUC1	hPAM4
Leptomeningeal cancer	Ganglioside GD2	3F8
Gastrointestinal	TAG-72	CC49

CAIX/MN, carbonic anhydrase IX; CEA, carcinoembryonic antigen; EGFR, epidermal growth factor receptor; EpCAM, epithelial cell adhesion molecule; FAP, fibroblast-activating protein; MUC1, mucin 1; NCAM, neural cell adhesion molecule; PSMA, prostate-specific membrane antigen; TAG-72, tumor-associated glycoprotein.
Modified from Wong YC, Williams LE, Yazaki PJ. Radioimmunotherapy of colorectal cancer. In: Speer TW, ed. *Targeted radionuclide therapy*. Philadelphia: Lippincott Williams & Wilkins, 2011:325. With permission.

The ideal target for RIT-targeting constructs would be one that is overexpressed on cancer cells, is uniformly expressed, is not found to any significant level in normal tissue, is not shed into the circulation, and exhibits an important role in tumor growth and progression.[10] TAAs, as the name implies, are antigens "associated" with tumors but are also present in normal tissue. True tumor-specific antigens have not yet been identified and utilized. Overexpression is necessary because typical targeting constructs require antigen densities $\geq 10^5$ receptors on each cell for adequate targeting. A homogenous antigen expression is desired so that a uniform activity distribution of the radionuclide will result. Nonuniform activity distributions (heterogeneity of antigen in target tissue being one potential cause) will significantly lower the effectiveness of RIT by subsequently resulting in nonuniform or heterogeneous dose distributions.[11] This is particularly important for radionuclides with short path lengths of the emitted particles (i.e., Auger and α-particle emitters). Radionuclides with longer path lengths, such as high-energy β-emitters, can partly overcome the problem of nonuniform dose distributions through the crossfire effect. If the target antigen is significantly shed into the circulation, the targeting construct may bind and "complex" with the antigen. This will result in a more rapid clearance of the RIT agent and a much less effective treatment. If the TAA has an important signaling role, then subsequent binding of the targeting construct will most likely add to the cytotoxicity of the radionuclide because of the blockade or promotion of intracellular signaling, potentially resulting in disruption of growth pathways important for tumor growth. Some TAAs (receptors) will internalize when bound by the targeting construct. In truth, most receptors internalize, although they do so at different rates. A rapid internalization process will have an impact on the type of radionuclide that is selected and potentially on the delivery strategy of the RIT agent.

A multitude of agents have been used as carriers (targeting constructs) for the targeted delivery of radiation to cancer. These consist of antibodies, antibody fragments, peptides, affibodies, aptamers, and nanostructures (i.e., liposomes, nanoparticles, microparticles, nanoshells, and minicells). By an exceedingly large margin, intact monoclonal antibodies (mAbs) have dominated the field of RIT as targeting constructs[12] (Fig. 29.1). In humans, there are five classes or isotypes of antibodies (IgA, IgD, IgE, IgG, and IgM). IgG is the most commonly used mAb for RIT because it is the most prevalent antibody in serum and has the longest serum half-life, typically measured in weeks (~23 days). IgG is further divided into four subtypes, IgG_{1-4}. IgG antibodies are large glycoprotein macromolecules, with an atomic mass of approximately 150,000 dalton (Da) or 150 kDa. The "y-shaped structure" (Fig. 29.1A) consists of two Fab fragments (antigen-binding fragment; ~50,000 Da each) and an Fc fragment (crystallizable fragment; ~50,000 Da).

The "tip" of each Fab fragment has a variable amino acid sequence, from one mAb to another. Accordingly, each tip is an antigen-binding site (ABS) and is responsible for antigen recognition. Each ABS forms a noncovalent bond (electrostatic forces, van der Waals forces, hydrophobic interactions, and hydrogen bonds) with the target or antigen. The specific region of an antigen, which binds to the ABS, is referred to as an epitope. It has been proposed that a million or more different antibodies exist in various individuals. Theoretically, $>10^9$ different antibodies can be produced. The outer core of the mAb consists of two identical light chains (outer portion of the Fab fragment) designated with an "L." The inner core, consisting of the Fc region and the inner Fab region, is designated as heavy or "H." Both the light and heavy chains contain homologous, 110 amino acid sequences that fold on one another and are connected by a disulfide bridge, resulting in "globular" motif or loop, called an Ig domain. There are three constant heavy domains ($C_H 1$-3) and only one constant

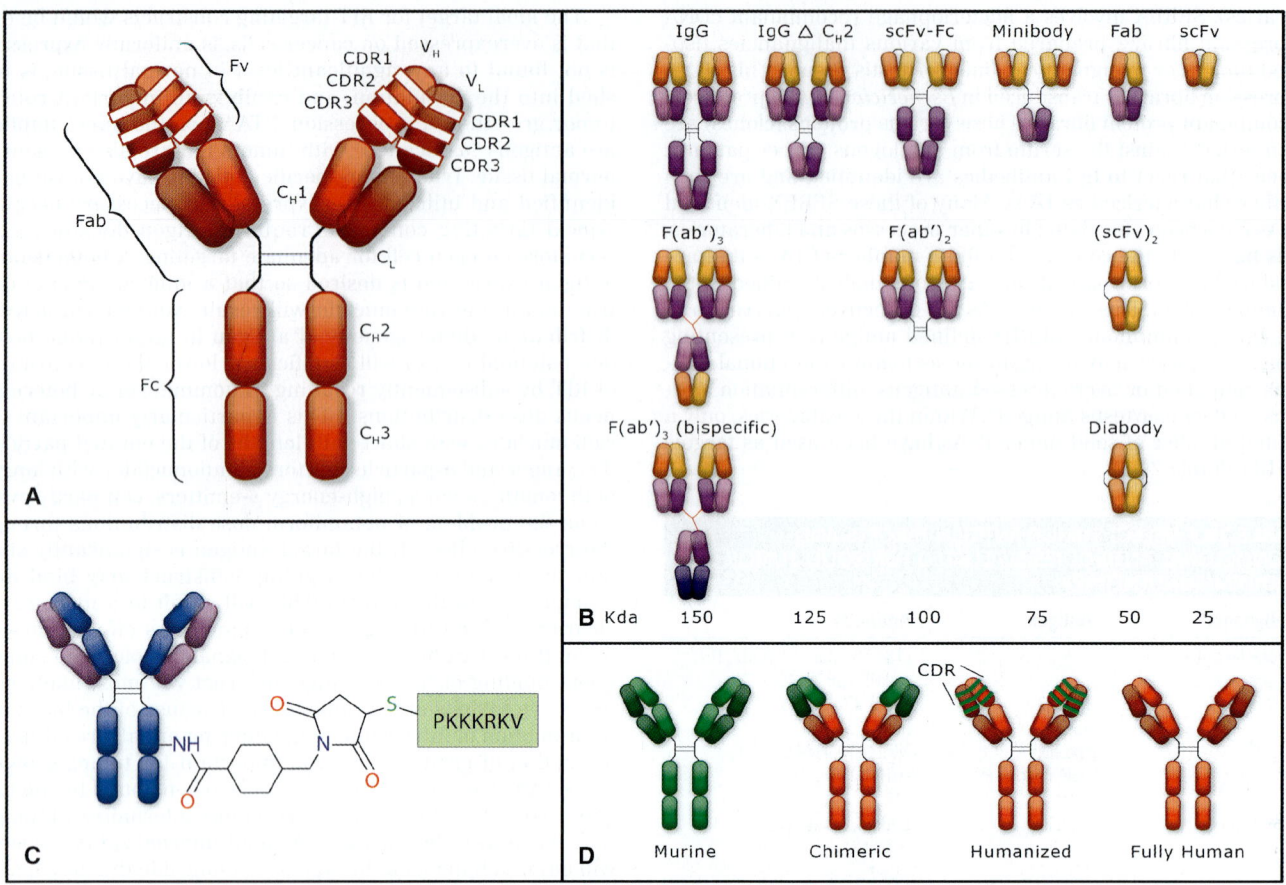

FIGURE 29.1. Antibody configurations for radioimmunotherapy. **A:** Typical structure of a humanized IgG antibody. **B:** Antibody fragments and size. **C:** Attachment of a nuclear localization signal. **D:** Humanization: *green* represents murine portion of IgG and *red* represents human portion. CDR, complementarity determining regions; CH, constant domain heavy chain; CL, constant domain light chain; Fab, antigen-binding fragment; F(ab') antigen-binding fragment (retaining a portion of the hinge region following enzymatic digestion); Fc, crystallizable fragment; Fv, variable fragment; PKKKRKV, amino acid sequence of nuclear localization signal; scFv, single-chain variable fragment.

light (C_L), one variable heavy (V_H), and one variable light (V_L) domain. The ABS consists of a V_L and a V_H region. Within each variable domain, there are three hypervariable regions (about 10 amino acid residues per hypervariable region) that form a three-dimensional surface that is "complementary" to the shape of the antigen surface; they are called complementarity determining regions (CDRs). A total of six CDRs come together to form the ABS. There are two ABS for each IgG mAb; hence, each IgG mAb is considered bivalent.

Affinity refers to the strength of the bond between the ABS and the antigen. The strength of this bond is represented by the dissociation constant (K_d). Avidity refers to the overall strength of the ABS–antigen interaction, depending on both the affinity and the valency of the interaction. It should be noted that a high-affinity interaction can improve specific delivery of the RIT agent and reduce overall dosing requirements. Increasing the affinity indefinitely, however, may decrease tumor penetration. It has been demonstrated that an affinity of 10^{-7} to 10^{-8} M is needed for tumor retention, whereas affinities in the range of $\geq 10^{-10}$ to 10^{-11} M will result in retention in normal tissue and asymmetric binding in tumor tissue, termed *binding site barrier*.[13] The binding site barrier phenomenon may be at least partially overcome by increasing the antibody mass, or the overall delivered quantity of antibody.

Unconjugated antibodies—those not attached to a radionuclide or cytotoxic agent—will also mediate biologic activities. These activities may be mediated by the Fc region of the mAb or may be Fc independent. Fc-mediated interactions are termed *effector functions* and consist of antibody-dependent cell-mediated cytotoxicity (ADCC) and complement-dependent

cytotoxicity (CDC).[5] Concerning ADCC, interaction of the Fc region of the antibody with Fc receptors (located on immune effector cells) results in the subsequent phagocytosis or lysis of the antibody-bound cancer cell. CDC is initiated by the interaction of soluble blood proteins and the Fc region. Epitope-dependent (Fc-independent) functions of the mAb may result in the inhibition of ligand binding, inhibition of ligand-induced dimerization, and inhibition of receptor shedding. These epitope-dependent functions are characteristic of modern-day biologics that target growth factor receptors, such as cetuximab and trastuzumab.

The original technology used to produce mAbs was first published by Kohler and Milstein in 1975 and is referred to as the hybridoma technique. The technique has propagated the use of murine mAbs for research and for therapy in the clinic. In fact, the two U.S. Food and Drug Administration (FDA) RIT agents used to treat non-Hodgkin lymphoma (NHL; ibritumomab tiuxetan and tositumomab) are murine mAbs. Although these agents are delivered as single instillations in patients typically with decreased immune recognition capabilities, there is a concern that human antiglobulin antibodies (HAGAs) will develop. If this phenomenon occurs in response to murine antibodies, then the resulting HAGAs will be called human antimouse antibodies (HAMAs). The formation of HAMAs will expedite blood clearance of the antibody and decrease targeting capabilities as well as potentially cause various adverse symptoms. Two main strategies, through the use of genetic engineering, have emerged[12] that reduce the immunogenicity of mAbs: (a) the production of antibody chimeras derived from both murine and human DNA and

TABLE 29.2 TARGETING AND PHARMACOKINETICS OF INTACT IgG AND ANTIBODY FRAGMENTS

	IgG	F(ab')2	CH2 deletion	Minibody	Fab	Diabody	scFv
MW	150	100	120	80	50	40–50	20–25
Serum half-life	2–3 d[a]	1 d	Hours	Hours	Hours	Hours	1 hr
Metabolism	Liver	Liver	Liver	Liver	Kidney	Kidney	Kidney
Tumor uptake[b]	*****	****	***	***	**	**	*
Time to accretion	Days	1 d	Hours	Hours	Hours	Hours	1 h

[a]Serum half-life for fully human IgG is approximately 23 days.
[b]Tumor uptake values range from large (*****) to small (*).
MW, molecular weight (kDa).

(b) the production of humanized or fully human antibodies (Fig. 29.1D). Chimeric antibodies retain murine V_H and V_L domains, whereas humanized antibodies retain murine CDRs. Fully human antibodies retain no murine components. Although the development of HAGA may not be important after a single dose of mAb in lymphoma patients, HAGA will have a greater detrimental impact for patients with solid tumors when treated with RIT.[10] It has been well proven that as the antibody changes from murine to humanized, the immunogenicity is lessened. This concept is important so that multiple doses or fractions of RIT can be delivered. Current technology allows for the production of fully human mAbs. The concept of adding a nuclear localizing signal to bring the mAb from the cell surface or cytoplasm into the cell nucleus is shown in Figure 29.1C. In this setting, Auger-emitting radionuclides will be effective.

Another factor that is critical and influences antibody targeting and pharmacokinetics is antibody molecular size (Fig. 29.1B). As stated previously, RIT has been less successful for treating solid tumors than hematologic malignancies. This is largely because of the lack of radiosensitivity of epithelial tumors (compared to hematologic malignancies) and the poor penetration of mAbs into large tumors. The decreased penetration of 150-kDa antibodies into large tumors is a direct result of increased tumor interstitial pressure, an aberrant tumor vasculature, and an abnormal tumor extracellular matrix.[14–17] Additionally, 150-kDa antibodies need longer periods of time to accrete into tumors and have long serum half-lives. When radiolabeled, a long serum half-life of the targeting construct will increase exposure of the bone marrow to radiation, which causes hematologic toxicity and limits the amount of antibody and radionuclide that can be given. To overcome some of these issues, methods have been used to generate antibody fragments of varying size and valency. These smaller fragments exhibit superior tumor penetration and clear more rapidly from the circulation. However, if clearance from the circulation is too rapid, this can further limit tumor penetration. Table 29.2 summarizes these general concepts for targeting constructs of various molecular weights.

Although mAbs and their fragments represent the most commonly used targeting constructs for the delivery of a radionuclide to malignant tissue, other agents are either in use or are being investigated, consisting of peptides,[18–20] affibody molecules,[21,22] and aptamers.[23,24] Nanostructures are also being investigated as carriers of radionuclides.[12,25,26] In their unmodified form, the targeting capabilities of nanostructures are rather nonspecific.[27]

Peptides are amino acid sequences (typically 7 to 14 amino acids) that serve as opioids, hormones, sweeteners, protein substrate inhibitors, releasing factors, antibiotics, and cytoprotectors.[28] The overexpression of receptors that are specific for various peptides has led to the development of peptide-based radiopharmaceuticals. Somatostatin is one of the most common peptides and is overexpressed in a multitude of malignancies, including breast cancer, small cell lung cancer, medullary thyroid cancer, and neuroendocrine tumors (NETs). Somatostatin is rapidly degraded; however, its derivative, octreotide, is very stable. Octreoscan (indium-111

diethylenetriamine penta-acetic acid [^{111}In-DTPA]) has been shown to be highly diagnostic for NETs. Affibody molecules[22] are classified as affinity ligands or scaffold proteins that are approximately 7 to 9 kDa. These proteins are based on a 58 amino acid residue derived from staphylococcus protein A, which binds immunoglobulin. Various applications have been applied to affibody use, including radiolabeled targeting for therapy.

Aptamers are single-stranded DND or RNA oligonucleotides (8 to 12 kDa; 10 to 100 bases) that are selected *in vitro* from a random library by a process termed *SELEX* (systemic evolution of ligands by exponential enrichment). Aptamers are an attractive alternative to larger mAbs because they are chemically synthesized (do not require a biologic system such as mAbs), have a low cost of production, exhibit high affinities, have a small size, are rapidly cleared from the circulation, have an unlimited shelf life, exhibit rapid tissue penetration, and are nonimmunogenic.[23] Aptamers fold into unique secondary and tertiary structures that not only exhibit high affinities for targets, but can also gain entry into target cells. The basic SELEX process consists of exposing a target to a random single-strand nucleic acid library, selecting candidates that bind to the target, repeating the process to further select candidates with increasing affinity for the target, and sequencing the final candidates (Fig. 29.2). Variations of SELEX include selecting aptamers that bind cells, internalize into cells, or are delivered *in vivo*, respectively, termed cell-SELEX, cell internalization SELEX, and *in vivo* SELEX. The basic configuration of an aptamer in a random library is a 5′ forward primer-binding site, a random region, and a 3′ reverse primer-binding site. The selected candidates can therefore undergo PCR amplification. The typical complexity of random library is between $1 \times 10^{13-24}$ different random sequences. For example, if the random region consists of 30 possible nucleotides, then potentially 1×10^{18} different aptamers will be available. In this particular example, 1×10^{18} represents a different aptamer or "key" for every grain of sand in the entire world. This is an amazingly large and diverse screening tool. The major detriment of using aptamers as targeting constructs for RIT is their short serum half-life (measured in minutes) secondary to nuclease degradation. Fortunately, research has shown that aptamers can be rendered nuclease resistant with the following modifications; 5′-modified uracil, 4′-thio, 2′-fluoro, 5′-α-P-borano, 2′-amino, 2′-deoxy-L-ribose, 5′-phosphorothio, 2′-methoxy, modification of bases.[29] Aptamers are amazingly versatile and can recognize nearly any type of target, from metal ions to whole cells and even entire organisms. Because of their chemical synthesis, aptamers seem to have a great chance of becoming a true tumor-specific and personalized delivery construct. Aptamers for cancer imaging or therapy are shown in Table 29.3.

THE PHYSICS AND RADIOBIOLOGY OF RADIOIMMUNOTHERAPY

RIT delivers radiation to the target tissue in a continuous, although declining, low–dose rate (LDR) fashion. Typical dose rates for RIT are in the range of 10 to 20 cGy per hour. The total dose delivered by RIT is low, in the range of 1,500 to 2,000 cGy, with an effective half-life of 24 to 72 hours. This can be compared to the high–dose rate (HDR) delivery of radiation by external beam radiation therapy (EBRT). EBRT typically will deliver radiation at a dose rate of 100 to 500

Section II

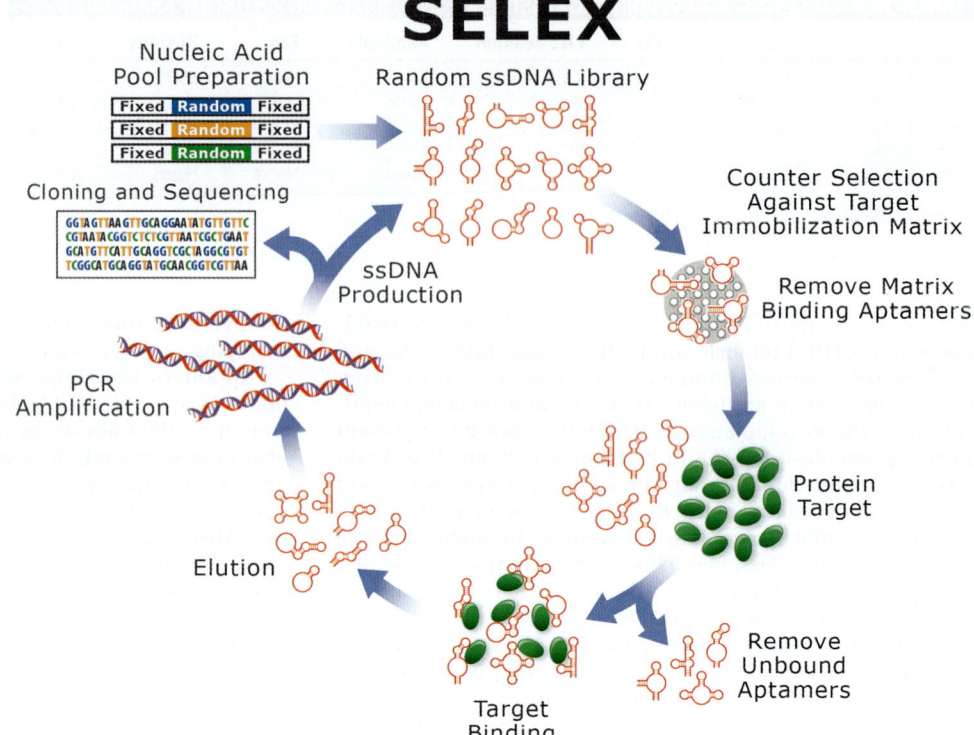

FIGURE 29.2. SELEX: A random ssDNA (or ssRNA) library is synthesized and exposed to laboratory equipment and target matrix. The aptamers that bind are considered nonspecific and are removed. The remaining aptamers are exposed to the target protein. Aptamers that don't bind are removed. Aptamers that bind the target are eluted and PCR amplified. Candidate "sense" strand aptamers are isolated and the SELEX process is repeated in order to refine the selection process. Final candidates are cloned and sequenced.

cGy per minute. This total dose range for RIT occurs despite overall very low percent injected doses (0.1% to 10.0%) that ultimately localize in target tissue.[30] Regardless, radiation-induced apoptosis still occurs.

The most radiosensitive component of a cell is the DNA. Irradiation of tissue results in DNA damage. This damage may be either repaired or result in permanent damage. Permanent damage will cause cell death. By using a target-hit model, the tissue response end point of cell death may be used to relate absorbed dose of ionizing radiation to cell death. When the log surviving fraction of irradiated cells is plotted on the ordinate and the dose (Gy) is plotted on the abscissa, a cell survival curve is generated (Fig. 29.3). The "hit" that results in most lethal event is a double-strand break (DSB) of DNA. The mathematical term, α, represents the initial slope of the cell survival curve. It is a constant for a given tumor (or tissue) and can be thought of as the probability, per unit of absorbed dose, of creating a lethal DSB.[31] The target is the resulting

TABLE 29.3 APTAMERS FOR CANCER IMAGING AND THERAPY (PRECLINICAL AND CLINICAL)

Aptamer	Target	Condition	Radionuclide	Application
AS1411	Nucleolin	Renal cell carcinoma, non–small cell lung carcinoma, leukemia	None	Therapy
AS1411	Nucleolin	Glial tumor	^{67}Ga	Imaging
Sgc8	Protein tyrosine kinase 7 (PTK-7)	Leukemia	None	Therapy
TD05	Immunoglobulin μ heavy chains (IGHM)	Lymphoma, leukemia	None	Therapy
NOX-A12	CXCL12/SDF-1	Glioblastoma, multiple myeloma, solid tumors	None	Therapy
14-16	p68	Colon cancer	None	Therapy
TTA1	Tenascin-C	Glioblastoma	^{111}In, ^{18}F	Imaging
AptA, AptB	MUC1	Breast cancer	^{99m}Tc	Imaging
A9	PSMA	Prostate cancer	^{89}Zr	Imaging
A10	PSMA	Prostate cancer	^{225}Ac	Therapy
F3	hMMP-9	Various cancers, metastases	^{99m}Tc	Imaging
U2	EGFRvIII	Glioblastoma	^{188}Re	Imaging
E07	EGFR	EGFR-expressing cells	^{111}In	Imaging
Mini 15-8	ErbB2	HER2-expressing tumors	^{99m}Tc	Imaging
Apt3, Apt3–amine	CEA	CEA-expressing tumors	^{99m}Tc	Imaging
A30	HER3	Breast cancer	None	Therapy
TTA1	Tenascin-C	Breast, colon, lung, glioblastoma	^{99m}Tc	Imaging
5TR1	O-glycan-peptide	Breast, colon, lung, ovary, pancreatic	None (photodynamic therapy agent)	Therapy
J18	EGRF	EGFR-expressing tumors	None (gold nanoparticles)	Therapy
Clone5	Sialyl Lewis X	Sialyl Lewis X–expressing tumors	None	Therapy
CTLA-4 aptamer	CTLA-4	CTLA-4 receptor	None	Therapy
A07	TGF-β	Chinese hamster ovary	None	Therapy
ST1571	PDGF β-receptor	Colon	None	Therapy
III.1	Pigpen	Glioblastoma	None	Therapy

CTLA-4, cytogenic T-cell antigen-4; CXCL2, C-X-C motif chemokine 12; EGFRvIII, epidermal growth factor receptor variant III; HER3, human epidermal growth factor-3; hMMP-9, human matrix metalloprotease-9; SDF-1, stromal cell–derived factor-1; TGF-β, transforming growth factor-β.

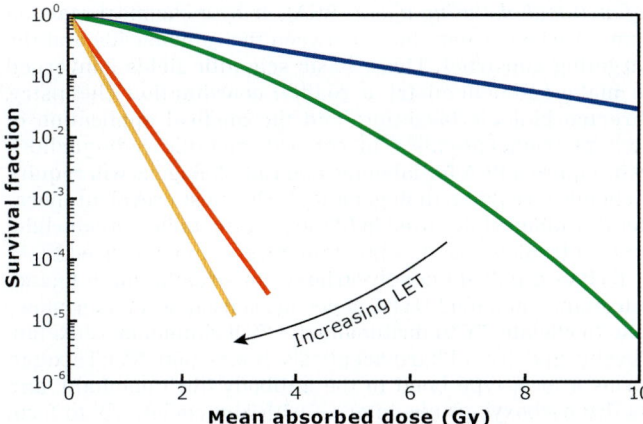

FIGURE 29.3. Cell survival curves following treatment with radiotherapy. The *blue curve* represents low–dose rate radiotherapy; the *green curve* represents high–dose rate radiotherapy. Increasing LET is represented by the *red line* (alpha particle radiation; RBE = 5) and *gold line* (Auger radiation; RBE = 7 to 9). (Adapted from Bernhardt P, Speer TW. Modeling the systemic cure with targeted radionuclide therapy. In: Speer TW, ed. *Targeted radionuclide therapy*. Philadelphia: Lippincott Williams & Wilkins, 2011:265. With permission.)

DSB, and the cell survival versus absorbed dose is a pure exponential function: $S = e^{-\alpha D}$ where S is the surviving cell fraction and D is the mean absorbed dose. Ionizing irradiation may also cause nonlethal single-strand breaks (SSBs). If these events accumulate, they may become lethal. The constant, β, is used to describe this phenomenon and represents the more distant, "linear" portion of the cell survival curve. The linear-quadratic (LQ) model combines the two processes into a continuously bending curve: $S = e^{-\alpha D - \beta D^2}$

The shoulder on the cell survival curve is typically observed when HDR radiation is employed (green line in Fig. 29.3). In RIT, the dose rate is 1,000-fold lower; therefore, the quadratic portion of the curve will have a much lower impact on survival because many SSBs, considered sublethal damage, will be repaired during the more lengthy delivery of LDR radiation. This will result in a "small" or absent observable shoulder and flattening of the cell survival curve. Thus, when estimating cell survival for RIT, α alone will define the radiosensitivity of the tumor (blue line in Fig. 29.3). Considering dose rate alone, RIT is approximately 20% less effective than HDR EBRT. Regardless, RIT does appear to be effective. This phenomenon can be attributed to many radiobiologic processes that appear to cause greater than predicted rates of apoptosis. These processes include low-dose/dose rate apoptosis, low-dose hyperradiosensitivity-increased radioresistance, inverse dose rate effect (G_2 synchronization), radiation-induced biologic bystander effect, and the crossfire effect.[30] The use of high-LET radiation, in the form of alpha particles or Auger electrons, will further increase cell kill.

Various radionuclides have been proposed for the use in RIT (Table 29.4), and their physical properties have been extensively reviewed in the nuclear medicine literature. They can be grouped into three basic categories depending on the type of emitted particulate radiation. Radionuclides that emit high-energy electrons are referred to as β-emitters. These electrons have maximum path lengths in tissue from 0.6 to 12.0 mm. This translates into a range of approximately 60 to 1,100 cell diameters. The most commonly used β-emitters for RIT are yttrium 90 [^{90}Y], iodine 131 [^{131}I], and lutetium 177 [^{177}Lu]. The maximum range of electrons in tissue for ^{90}Y and ^{131}I is 12 and 2 mm, respectively. It should be noted, however, that 90% of the electron energy is deposited over 5.2 mm for ^{90}Y and 0.7 mm for ^{131}I. This range of 90% energy deposition is referred to as the R_{90}. The most commonly used α-emitters for RIT are ^{211}At and ^{225}Ac. An α-particle is a helium nucleus that has a maximum range in tissue of 55 to 100 μm (5 to 10

TABLE 29.4 POTENTIAL RADIONUCLIDES FOR RADIOIMMUNOTHERAPY					
Radionuclide	**Physical Half-Life**	**E_{ave} (MeV)^a**	**Maximum Range in Tissue**	**LET (keV/μm)**	**Approximate Cell Diameters**
Beta-emitters		β-Particle		0.2	
Yttrium 90	2.7 d	2.19	12.0 mm		400–1,100
Iodine 131	8.0 d	0.28	2.0 mm		10–230
Lutetium 177	6.7 d	0.15	1.5 mm		4–180
Rhenium 186	3.7 d	0.36	3.6 mm		15–360
Rhenium 188	17.0 h	0.80	11.0 mm		200–1,000
Copper 67	2.6 d	0.18	2.8 mm		5–210
Phosphorus 32	14.3 d	0.70	7.6 mm		760
Phosphorus 33	25.3 d	0.08	0.6 mm		60
Holmium-166	1.1 d	1.86	8.4 mm		840
α-Emitters		α-Particle		80	
Bismuth-213	45.7 min	5.87	55–60 μm		5–6
Bismuth-212	60.6 min	6.09	60–70 μm		6–7
Astatine-211	7.2 h	5.87	55–60 μm		5–6
Actinium-225	9.92 d	5.83	60–90 μm		5–8
Terbium-149	4.12 h	3.97	30–60 μm		3–6
Low-Energy Electron Emitters		*Low-Energy Electron*		4–26	
(Auger)					
Iodine 125	60.1 d	0.030	2–500 nm		<1
Iodine 123	0.55 d	0.030	2–500 nm		<1
Gallium 67	3.26 d	0.009	2–500 nm		<1
Indium 111	2.80 d	0.026	2–500 nm		<1
Technetium 99m	6.01 h	0.018	2–500 nm		<1
Platinum-193m	4.33 d	0.053	2–500 nm		<1
Platinum-195m	4.02 d	0.063	2–500 nm		<1
Platinum-191	2.80 d	0.072	2–500 nm		<1
Antimony-119	38.9 h	0.028	2–500 nm		<1
Thallium 201	72.9 h	0.078	2–500 nm		<1
Bromine-77	57.0 h	0.012	2–500 nm		<1
Bromine-80m	4.4 h	0.013	2–500 nm		<1
Chromium 51	27.7 d	0.005	2–500 nm		<1

^{a}When appropriate.

Data were obtained from Eckerman KF, Endo A. eds. *MIRD Radionuclide Data and Decay Schemes*. 2nd ed. SNM MIRD Committee, 2008.

E_{max}, maximum energy; LET, linear energy transfer.

Section II

cell diameters). Although it has a short range, the α-particle is very destructive and has a high linear energy transfer (LET). Low-energy electron emitters also emit radiation that is high LET and have path lengths between 2 and 500 nm (width of a double-strand helix). Auger emitters, such as ^{111}In or ^{125}I, are most effective if delivered to the nucleus of a cell or incorporated into the DNA. It has been mathematically postulated that it will only take 60 decays of ^{125}I, coupled to DNA, to reduce cell survival to 50%. For a patient with 1-g circulating micrometastatic disease, 1,000 decays in the malignant cells can produce a probable cure. This amount of radiation corresponds to 0.1-MBq injected activity. This represents 5 mSv per 1 year of background radiation for the average human.[32] To further place this in perspective, Auger emitters can be safely injected into humans with an activity between 100 and 350 mCi, perhaps even at higher activities. It should be understood, 100 mCi = 3700 MBq; 1 MBq = 1,000,000 dps.

Because radionuclides have different energy spectra for their emitted particulate radiation, they will each interact with tissue and deposit their energy over varying distances. There is therefore a relation between the type of radionuclide, tumor size, absorbed dose, and ultimately tumor cure probability (TCP). If it is assumed that a tumor has a spherical volume and contains a uniform and identical activity concentration of a radionuclide, then the TCP can be calculated for different radionuclides and tumor size.[33] Figure 29.4 illustrates the relation between tumor mass and TCP for astatine-211 [[211]At], lutetium 177 [^{177}Lu], ^{131}I, and [90]Y. As can be seen, there is an optimum tumor size for the different energy spectra for each radionuclide such that the TCP is maximized. If the tumor is small relative to the emission range, then much of the energy will be lost to the surrounding tissue and the absorbed dose will be low. As the tumor size increases, more energy is absorbed until the maximum TCP is reached. As the tumor further increases in size, the absorbed energy remains high, although fewer cells are affected by the radiation and TCP begins to decrease.[33] These observations move forward the concept of using multiple radionuclides, in the RIT process, that deposit their energies over different ranges in tissue. As a result, more energy could then be deposited into tumors of various sizes, potentially improving the therapeutic ratio.

Labeling the targeting construct with the appropriate radionuclide (radiochemistry) is exceedingly important and equally complex. Radionuclides are attached to targeting constructs by either using a "linker" molecule, termed a

bifunctional chelating agent (BCA), or by a chemical reaction that forms a covalent bond between the radionuclide and the targeting construct. Three basic scientific fields converged to make radiochemistry a reality: coordination chemistry, directed biologic targeting, and the medical application of radiopharmaceuticals.[34] In general, metallic radionuclides will require a BCA for labeling, and radiohalogens will require a chemical reaction (halogenation). The most prevalent therapeutic radionuclides used in RIT are [90]Y (metallic radionuclide) and [131]I (radiohalogen). One of the most commonly used BCAs is DTPA—a polyaminopolycarboxylate straight chain ligand. Tiuxetan, a modified DTPA molecule, is used as a linker molecule to chelate ^{90}Y to ibritumomab (^{90}Y ibritumomab tiuxetan; Zevalin, Spectrum Pharmaceuticals, Henderson, NV). Tiuxetan forms a urea-type bond to the antibody (ibritumomab), and its five carboxyl groups interact with and chelate ^{90}Y to form a stable coordination sphere. The halogenation reaction that bonds ^{131}I to a protein-targeting construct (^{131}I tositumomab; Bexxar, GlaxoSmithKline, Philadelphia, PA; discontinued 2013) is called iodination. Although there are many permutations of the iodination reaction, it basically inserts ^{131}I into a tyrosine group on the mAb without the need for a chelation molecule. Regardless of the required labeling technique, it is incumbent that a reasonably high labeling yield, unaltered biodistribution, stability of the radionuclide, and immunoreactivity are preserved.

Historically, a single instillation or fraction of the RIT agent is delivered systemically (i.e., Zevalin and Bexxar). It is well known that although relatively effective for hematologic malignancies, RIT is much less effective for treating solid tumors. Therefore, a number of strategies are being developed that will potentially increase the effectiveness of RIT. These strategies include modulating the tumor microenvironment; using pretargeting techniques, extracorporeal delivery, combined modality therapy (CMT), fractionation, and multiple radionuclides (radionuclide cocktail); increasing antibody mass (the amount of antibody delivered systemically); alteration of the physical properties (size and affinity) of the targeting construct; and employing different types of LET radiation (i.e., β-emitter vs. α-emitter). These strategies are designed to deliver more radiation to the tumor, make the radiation more cytotoxic, or decrease the exposure of radiation to bone marrow. As a result, the tumor to blood ratio will increase, and ultimately, the therapeutic ratio will increase. The pretargeting strategy warrants further discussion.[35,36]

Because radiolabeled mAbs take 2 to 3 days to localize or accrete into tumors, antibody-based RIT results in a prolonged exposure of the bone marrow to radiation, causing hematologic toxicity and rendering the bone marrow as the dose-limiting normal tissue. Accordingly, the tumor/blood ratios of mAb will only slightly favor the tumor. This situation can seriously limit the successful prospects of antibody-based RIT, especially for treating solid tumors. Smaller targeting constructs (antibody fragments, peptides, aptamers) can be used for RIT, and they will exhibit pharmacokinetics that result in a more rapid blood clearance allowing for the administration of higher activities. Unfortunately, because of the lower overall tumor accretion and retention of smaller constructs, the advantage of a more rapid blood clearance is usually offset. Therefore, the ideal delivery construct would manifest the high-affinity targeting properties of an intact mAb but exhibit the blood clearance pattern of a small molecular weight construct. This conventional wisdom is based upon using beta and alpha radionuclides, both of which will be toxic with long circulation times. If targeting constructs using Auger emitters can be engineered, the circulation time becomes rather immaterial as Auger radionuclides are only cytotoxic if internalized into cells. Because no known construct manifesting all of these attributes exists today, pretargeting strategies have been developed. The basic premise of pretargeting is to separate the

FIGURE 29.4. Tumor control probability (TCP) for various radionuclides. TCP = 0.9 versus tumor mass. The optimal TCP for various tumor masses when treated with [211]At, ^{177}Lu, ^{131}I, and [90]Y. This corresponds to approximately 10^{-5}, 10^{-2}, 0.1, and 10 g, respectively. (From Bernhardt P, Speer TW. Modeling the systemic cure with targeted radionuclide therapy. In: Speer TW, ed. *Targeted radionuclide therapy.* Philadelphia: Lippincott Williams & Wilkins, 2011:266. With permission.)

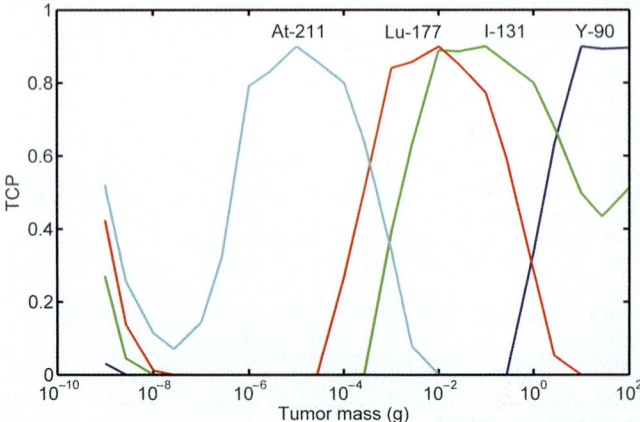

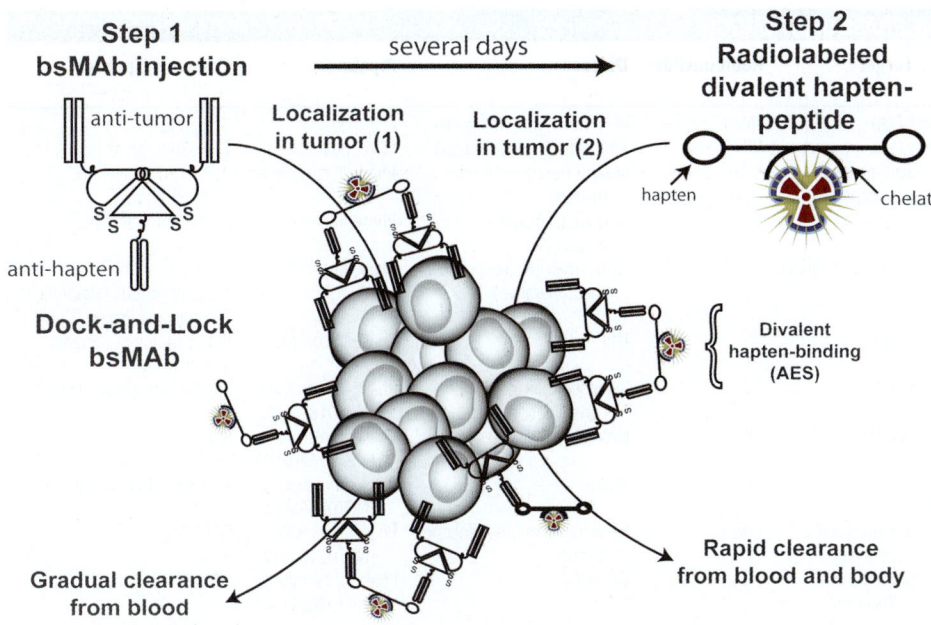

Step 1
bsMAb injection

several days

Step 2
Radiolabeled
divalent hapten-
peptide

anti-tumor

Localization
in tumor (1)

Localization
in tumor (2)

hapten

chelate

anti-hapten

Dock-and-Lock
bsMAb

Divalent
hapten-binding
(AES)

Gradual clearance
from blood

Rapid clearance
from blood and body

FIGURE 29.5. Bispecific pretargeting procedure. The bsMAb is injected, and over several days, it will localize in the tumor and clear from the blood. The bsMAb shown in this example is based on the dock-and-lock method for preparing recombinant bsMAb that has two binding arms for the tumor and one for the hapten. Once the molar concentration of the bsMAb is low enough, the radiolabeled hapten–peptide is given. The hapten–peptide has two haptens for more stable binding within the tumor, perhaps by cross-linking two adjacent bsMAb through a process known as the affinity enhancement system (AES). The peptide portion usually contains four to five D-amino acids with a single chelator bound to one of the amino acids that is used to capture the radionuclide. (From Sharkey RM, Goldenberg DM. Pretargeted radioimmunotherapy. In: Speer TW, ed. *Targeted radionuclide therapy*. Philadelphia: Lippincott Williams & Wilkins, 2011:194. With permission.)

delivery of a large, macromolecule-targeting construct (prolonged circulation time) from the delivery of a much smaller cytotoxic radioconjugate (more rapid circulation time). Two main approaches have been employed: a bispecific monoclonal antibody (bsmAb) system and a streptavidin–biotin system. In the bsmAb system (Fig. 29.5), a portion of the antibody has affinity for the tumor (antitumor), and another portion has affinity for the radionuclide carrier ligand or hapten–peptide (antihapten). Initially (step 1), a large "saturation" dose of the unlabeled bsmAb is administered, and the antibody localizes in the tumor over several days. Occasionally, a clearing step is used to facilitate the clearance of the bsmAb from the circulation. Subsequently (step 2), a radionuclide conjugated to a hapten–peptide is administered that has high affinity for the antihapten portion of the bsmAb. This step results in a rapid distribution of the radionuclide in the tumor owing to the high affinity of the hapten–peptide for the bsmAb. Because the hapten–peptide has a small molecular weight, it will clear rapidly from the body and result in a low–bone marrow exposure to radiation. In the streptavidin–biotin system, streptavidin is conjugated to the initial pretargeting macromolecule, and biotin is conjugated to the radionuclide. Streptavidin and biotin have a very high affinity for each other (10^{15} M^{-1}). When either system is used, the tumor/blood ratios of the targeting agent are significantly increased, but there may be some advantages to the bsmAB system.[37,38]

CONJUGATED THERAPY

The current state of RIT continues to improve. The basic premise has been the delivery of targeted cytotoxic radiotherapy that is low dose, LDR, sparsely ionizing and delivered in a single fraction. Initially, this reality seemed to be a natural "fit" for hematologic malignancies that were sensitive to most types of radiation. However, for RIT to ultimately impact significantly upon the world of oncology, it is clear that current approaches need to be modified so that it can be applied to carcinomas. Zevalin and Bexxar were FDA-approved in 2002 and 2003, respectively, as RIT drugs to treat relapse follicular NHL for an end point of progression-free survival. Subsequently, Zevalin received an approved frontline indication (FIT trial). Bexxar was withdrawn from production by GlaxoSmithKline (GSK) in 2013. Currently, Zevalin is greatly underutilized because it has not shown a survival benefit for

its respective indications and there are other competing drugs that are not radioactive and don't require close coordination with medical departments such as medical oncology, radiation oncology, and nuclear medicine. Table 29.5 lists FDA-approved and current phase III RIT drugs. Progress has been less sanguine for solid tumor malignancies, and phase III trials are lacking.[39,40] For the sake of clarity and brevity, this section will focus on clinically relevant phase II/III trials and U.S. FDA (or its international equivalent)-approved RIT therapeutics.

Hematologic Trials and Approved Therapeutic Agents

The National Comprehensive Cancer Network (NCCN) guidelines have recommended RIT for the following follicular lymphoma clinical situations: (1) first-line therapy for the elderly or infirm (Category 2B), (2) first-line consolidation (Category 2B), and (3) second-line (relapse/refractory) and subsequent therapy (Category 1). Initially, the NCCN guidelines rendered a Category 1 designation for first-line consolidation but downgraded this to Category 2B because of concerns about toxicity, although there is not a uniform consensus.[41] Zevalin continues to show very promising results for follicular lymphoma first-line monotherapy, diffuse large B-cell lymphoma and mantle cell lymphoma consolidation and second-line therapy, and transplantation studies. To date, however, none of these approaches have reached clinical phase III status. Zevalin has the only U.S. FDA approval for first-line consolidation and second-line therapy.

Currently, there is only one U.S. FDA-approved RIT agent in the United States: ^{90}Y ibritumomab tiuxetan (Zevalin; 2002). ^{131}I tositumomab (Bexxar; 2003) was removed from the market in 2013 by GSK. The demise of Bexxar was not because of lack of efficacy or toxicity, but because of unforeseen market pressure and financial decisions (http://www.xconomy.com/national/2013/08/26/why-good-drugs-sometimes-fail-in-the-market-the-bexxar-story/). Both will be briefly discussed as they represent common RIT paradigms. Zevalin has U.S. FDA approval for relapsed or refractory follicular NHL and as a frontline adjuvant agent for follicular NHL achieving a complete response (CR) or partial response (PR) to induction chemotherapy. Bexxar had U.S. FDA approval for the relapse or refractory setting as well as transformed NHL. Both are murine IgG mAbs that target the CD20 surface antigen on follicular NHL.[42] ^{90}Y ibritumomab tiuxetan utilizes ^{90}Y, a

Section
II

TABLE 29.5 FDA-APPROVED AND CURRENT PHASE III RIT DRUGS

Drug Name	Targeting Construct	Target	Radionuclide	Disease	Pipeline	Company/Sponsor
Zevalin (Ibritumomab Tiuxetan)	IgG1 (Murine)	CD20	^{90}Y	NHL (low-grade follicular)	FDA 2002	Biogen Idec
Bexxar[a] (Tositumomab)	IgG2a (Murine)	CD20	^{131}I	NHL (low grade follicular)	FDA 2003	GlaxoSmithKline
Lutathera (^{177}Lu–DOTATATE)	Octreotate peptide	Somatostatin receptor	^{177}Lu	Midgut neuroendocrine tumors	Phase III completed filing	Advanced Accelerator Applications
Zevalin	IgG1 (murine)	CD20	^{90}Y	Relapse DLBCL/ASC transplant	Phase III completed	Sheba Medical Center
131I–chTNT	IgG1 chimeric murine	Histone H1/DNA	^{131}I	Non–small cell lung cancer (postoperative)	Phase III complete	Guangxi Zhuang Autonomous Region Self Financing Project, China
Licartin (131I–Metuximab)	F(ab')$_2$	CD147	^{131}I	HCC with RFA	Phase III complete	Biotechnology Chengdu, China
Zevalin	IgG1 (Murine)	CD20	^{90}Y	Relapsed follicular NHL/ consolidation	Phase III recruiting (NCT01827605)	Fondazione Italiana Linfomi
Zevalin	IgG1 (Murine)	CD20	^{90}Y	Untreated follicular NHL	Phase III recruiting (NCT02320292)	Mayo Clinic
Iomab-B (BC8-I-131)	IgG1 (Murine)	CD45	^{131}I	AML	Phase III recruiting (NCT02665065)	Actinium Pharmaceuticals
^{111}In–Pentetreotide	Octreotate peptide	Somatostatin receptor	^{111}In	Resected GI neuroendocrine tumors	Phase III recruiting (NCT02465112)	GERCOR
177Lu–Edotreotide	Octreotate peptide	Somatostatin receptor	^{177}Lu	GEP-NET	Phase III recruiting (NCT03049198)	ITM Solucin GmbH

[a]Withdrawn from production by GlaxoSmithKline in 2013.

pure β-particle emitter with a physical half-life of 2.7 days. The β-particle has an energy of 2.3 MeV and a maximum tissue penetration of approximately 12.0 mm (R_{90} = 5.2 mm). Tiuxetan is a DTPA-type chelate that attaches ^{90}Y to the mAb, ibritumomab. Because there is no gamma emission in the spectrum of this isotope, it is not visualized by gamma camera scans. As a result, a biodistribution assessment cannot be performed. Therefore, a surrogate imaging radionuclide that emits gamma radiation ^{111}In is required. In contrast, ^{131}I tositumomab is a mixed β-/γ-emitter. The gamma spikes at 364 keV, and the beta emission has energy of 0.6 MeV. The maximum range in tissue of the β-particle is 2.3 mm (R_{90} = 0.7 mm). This agent can be imaged on gamma camera to calculate total body clearance.

For both agents, the treatment is delivered over 1 to 2 weeks. On day 1, both protocols deliver an infusion of nonradioactive (cold) anti-CD20 antibody (Zevalin employs rituximab; Bexxar employed tositumomab) designed to saturate the CD20 antigen sink (depletion of peripheral B cells and the binding of nonspecific sites in the liver and spleen) and provide antibody mass, which improves biodistribution and tumor targeting.[43,44] The administered activity for Zevalin is based on weight (0.4 mCi/kg for a platelet count ≥150,000; 0.3 mCi/kg for a platelet count of 100,000 to 149,000; maximum of 32 mCi). A single gamma scan (^{111}In ibritumomab tiuxetan) is used to confirm a normal biodistribution on days 3 to 4. A review of the Zevalin imaging registry reveals that only 0.6% of scans exhibited an altered biodistribution. Subsequently, the delivery of Zevalin has been simplified. Based upon the analysis of five trials, which revealed an altered biodistribution scan in only about 1% of patients, the FDA removed the requirement of the biodistribution scan. The administered activity for Bexxar was based on a calculated total body clearance (three scans over 1 week) that delivers a total-body (red bone marrow) dose of 75 cGy. This calculation is reduced to a total-body dose of 65 cGy for a platelet count <150,000. Eligible patients for Zevalin are also required to have an absolute neutrophil count (ANC) ≥1,500 and a bone marrow biopsy that reveals <25% lymphoma involvement.

Relapse Setting

Multiple prospective clinical trials have provided evidence for the use of RIT for treating relapsed or refractory follicular NHL. Together, they represent >200 patients treated with either Zevalin or Bexxar. Both agents appear to suggest an overall response rate (ORR) of 60% to 80% and a CR rate of 20% to 50%. Zevalin trials have been extensively reviewed.[45,46]

A phase III study comparing Zevalin versus rituximab for patients with relapsed or refractory low-grade follicular B-cell NHL or transformed NHL was performed.[47] Patients were randomized to either a single intravenous (IV) dose of Zevalin 0.4 mCi/kg (n = 73) or IV rituximab 375 mg/m^2 weekly for four doses (n = 70). The RIT group was pretreated with two rituximab doses (250 mg/m^2) to improve biodistribution and tumor targeting. After the first rituximab dose on day 1, ^{111}In ibritumomab tiuxetan was administered to assess biodistribution and to aide in dosimetry. No patients received the therapeutic dose of ^{90}Y ibritumomab tiuxetan (Zevalin) if >20 or 3 Gy was calculated to any nontumor organ or the red marrow, respectively. Zevalin was administered after the second rituximab dose approximately 1 week (days 7 to 9) after the first dose of rituximab and (^{111})In ibritumomab tiuxetan. The administered activity of Zevalin was capped at 32 mCi. Patients in both arms of the study received two prior chemotherapy regimens. The ORR was 80% for Zevalin and 56% for rituximab (P = .002). The CR rates were 30% and 16% (P = .04), respectively, in the Zevalin and rituximab group. Durable responses ≥6 months were 64% versus 47% (P = .030) for Zevalin versus rituximab. The conclusion of the study was that RIT with Zevalin was well tolerated and resulted in statistically significant and clinically significant higher ORRs and CRs than rituximab alone.

Frontline Therapy

Considering the concerns about RIT for treating large bulky tumors (tumor penetration, overall required dose, nonuniform dose distributions), bringing RIT into a frontline therapeutic setting after induction chemotherapy and maximum cytoreduction would be the next logical direction. A phase III first-line indolent trial (FIT) of consolidation with Zevalin compared to no additional therapy after first remission was reported for follicular B-cell NHL.[48] Patients with CD20+ stage III/IV follicular B-cell NHL who achieved a PR or CR to induction chemotherapy were randomized to Zevalin (n = 208) or to the control arm, representing no further treatment (n = 206). Prior to chemotherapy, patients had documented <25% bone marrow involvement. After induction chemotherapy, blood counts had to recover such that the ANC was ≥1.5, platelets were ≥150,000, and hemoglobin was ≥9. Patients in the

Zevalin arm were treated with an activity of 0.4 mCi/kg; a maximum activity of 32 mCi was allowed. Although two doses of rituximab (250 mg/m²) were used, an ¹¹¹In biodistribution scan was not required. The data were analyzed with a median follow-up of 3.5 years. Zevalin consolidation resulted in a median progression-free survival (PFS) advantage of 36.5 versus 13.3 months in the control arm (P < .0001). The PFS benefit was maintained in the Zevalin arm regardless if patients achieved a PR (29.3 vs. 6.2 months; P < .0001) or CR (53.9 vs. 29.5 months; P = .0154). The benefit of Zevalin consolidation was maintained across all Follicular Lymphoma International Prognostic Index (FLIPI) subgroups. In patients with a PR after induction chemotherapy, 77% were further converted to a CR when treated with Zevalin. This resulted in a final CR rate of 87% in the treatment arm, and this result compares well with established data. In the treatment arm, 90% of patients who were Bcl-2 positive converted to a negative status (90% molecular CR). Toxicity was well managed and primarily hematologic. A total of 8% of patients experienced a grade 3 to grade 4 infection. There were no treatment-related deaths. The FIT trial has been updated and with a median follow-up of 7.3 years ⁹⁰Y-ibritumomab consolidation results in a 3-year benefit in median PFS (41% vs. 22%; P < .001) and improves time to next treatment by 5.1 years (P < .001). Second malignancies were not statistically different.[49]

SOLID TUMOR TRIALS AND APPROVED THERAPEUTICS

Peptide receptor radionuclide therapy (PRRT) has been successfully used for greater than a decade to treat advanced NETs expressing somatostatin receptors. The most common PRRT agents are ¹⁷⁷Lu–DOTATATE and ⁹⁰Y–DOTATOC.[19,20] A phase III trial (NETTER-1) was performed, which randomized 229 patients with metastatic midgut NETs to either ¹⁷⁷Lu–DOTATATE (Lutathera) versus octreotide LAR (long-acting repeatable). The ¹⁷⁷Lu–DOTATATE was administered at an activity of 7.4 GBq (200 mCi) per infusion, every 8 weeks for a total of 4 doses. The ¹⁷⁷Lu–DOTATATE group exhibited a significant progression-free survival (P < .001) and overall survival (P = .004). Toxicity was acceptable.[50] Lutathera gained US FDA approval for somatostain receptor positive gastroenteropancreatic neuroendocrine tumors on 1/26/2018.

Lung cancer remains the leading cause of cancer mortality in the world. Clearly, new strategies are required to help improve local and systemic control. There are data to support the concept of targeting necrotic and hypoxic regions of tumors.[51] The selective targeting of dead or dying cells will allow a cytotoxic event of nearby malignant cells by the bystander and crossfire effect. Additionally, only one type of targeting construct needs to be manufactured to target many different types of malignancies. If the cell surface antigen does not internalize to any significant degree, then a typical targeting construct will remain on the cell surface. Because dead and dying cells (undergoing apoptosis) exhibit disruption of their cell membrane, constructs that target intracellular products of apoptosis will then be able to gain access to the cell cytoplasm and nucleus. Although several "dead cancer cell antigens" are under investigation, tumor necrosis therapy or treatment (TNT) has been investigated in human trials. TNT is an IgG₂ₐ mAb that targets nuclear histones.[52]

A pivotal trial of iodine-131–chimeric tumor necrosis treatment (¹³¹I-chTNT) in advanced lung cancer patients was performed.[53] A total of 107 patients (n = 97, non–small cell; n = 10, small cell) were enrolled from 1999 to 2002. All patients had failed at least one prior therapeutic regimen (mean = 3; range = 1 to 5), and 86.9% of the patients had stage III to stage IV disease at study entry. In all cases, the patients received two instillations of ¹³¹I-chTNT administered

over 2 to 4 weeks. Sixty-two patients received IV administrations, and 45 patients received intratumoral injections of ¹³¹I-chTNT. IV administrations were delivered at an activity 0.8 mCi/kg, and intratumoral injections were delivered at an activity of 0.8 mCi/cm³ of tumor size. In all patients (n = 107), the ORR was 34.6% (3.7% CR; 30.8% PR; 55.1% no change or stable disease; 10.3% progressive disease). Of the 62 patients receiving a systemic administration of ¹³¹I-chTNT, the ORR was 35.5% (3.2% CR; 32.2% PR). Of the 45 patients receiving intratumoral injection of ¹³¹I-chTNT, the ORR was 33.3% (5% CR; 20.9% PR). In 58 evaluable patients, the median survival was 11.7 months, and the 1-year survival rate was 41.4%. The average absorbed doses for tumor and normal lung were 8.45 and 2.35 Gy for patients receiving systemic ¹³¹I-chTNT and 30.0 and 2.65 Gy for patients receiving intratumoral ¹³¹I-chTNT. The major toxicity was hematologic and reversible. As expected, the hematologic toxicity was lower in the intratumoral injection group. In 2003, ¹³¹I-chTNT was approved by the Chinese State Food and Drug Administration to treat refractory bronchogenic carcinoma.

A phase III trial was performed randomizing patients with stage II-IIIA non–small cell carcinoma of the lung, requiring chemoradiotherapy after surgery.[54] Group A included 49 patients treated with chemotherapy (docetaxel and cisplatin) and external beam radiotherapy. Group B included 47 treated with ¹³¹I-chTNT and percutaneous microwave coagulation therapy (PMCT), with further chemotherapy. Survivals at 1 and 2 years for groups A and B were 80% and 49% versus 83% and 53% (P < .05). Adverse events and median survival were similar.

HCC, or liver carcinoma, represents a significant worldwide malignancy. Resection and orthotopic liver transplantation (OLT) represent the only potential curative options. In 1989, the Radiation Therapy Oncology Group (RTOG) reported its first and only phase III RIT trial comparing EBRT and chemotherapy to the same treatment plus ¹³¹I antiferritin antibody. None of the patients receiving EBRT and chemotherapy only were converted to a resectable state. In a separate analysis, 11 patients crossing over from the EBRT and chemotherapy arm to further therapy with ¹³¹I antiferritin antibody were converted to resection. There was, however, no significant difference in the initial "intent-to-treat" treatment arms based on response rate and survival.[55] Of course, the most promising role of RIT is in the treatment of minimal residual microscopic disease.

Licartin is an antibody fragment, F(ab')₂, that targets HAb18G/CD147, a HCC TAA. The safety and pharmacokinetics of Licartin (¹³¹I metuximab) have been investigated in phase I/II trials.[56] Realizing that TRT is most suited for treating microscopic disease, Licartin was tested in the adjuvant setting for patients with HCC undergoing OLT.[57] A total of 60 patients with HCC who were undergoing OLT were randomized to Licartin (0.42 mCi/kg) for three fractions at 28-day intervals versus placebo. Analysis at 1 year post therapy revealed that the recurrence rate was significantly decreased by 30.4% (P = .0174) and the survival rate was significantly increased by 20.6% (P = .0289) in the Licartin group. No significant toxicities were observed. The Chinese State Food and Drug Administration has approved Licartin as adjuvant therapy after OLT for HCC in 2005. To my knowledge, this trial has not been updated.

A phase III trial of radiofrequency ablation (RFA) for unresectable HCC with or without Licartin was performed.[58] Patients received RFA followed by Licartin (n = 62) or RFA alone (n = 65). Adverse events were similar and minimal in both arms. The median time to recurrence was 17 and 10 months for the RFA/Licartin group and RFA-alone group, respectively (P = .03).

Currently, the most common antigen targets for CNS malignancies consist of the epidermal growth factor receptor (EGFR), tenascin, neural cell adhesion molecule (NCAM), placental alkaline phosphatase (PLAP), and phosphatidyl inositide. The EGFR is variably amplified in malignant tissue and is also present, to some extent, in benign tissue. Tenascin is an extracellular glycoprotein that is uniformly expressed in glioma, and NCAM is present on both benign and malignant glioma cells. Clinical trials using RIT to treat CNS malignancies have been extensively reviewed.[59] A phase III trial was reported in 2002.[60] A total of 12 patients with malignant glioma were randomized to surgical resection and radiotherapy (60 Gy) ($n = 5$) versus surgical resection, radiotherapy, and RIT ($n = 7$). The RIT agent was a ^{125}I–anti–EGFR antibody 425 that was administered intravenously in three weekly doses (50 mCi) beginning during week 4 of the EBRT. All patients in the treatment arm had a recurrence at the time of publication. Considering that the EGFR was not tested in submitted tissue, the trial had a small number of patients, and the 150-kDa antibody was administered intravenously, significant conclusions could not be drawn.

Most of the CNS RIT trials to date are of "dose searching pilot" or phase I design. The evolution of the trials has seen the delivery route move from systemic (intra-arterial or IV) to local instillation of the RIT agent into a surgically created resection cavity (SCRC). Even though the blood–brain barrier (BBB) is often disrupted by a rapidly growing CNS malignancy, this phenomenon is not well defined, and 150-kDa antibodies would still not likely cross to a significant degree, although there does appear to be an element of nonspecific uptake from a systemic delivery. As a result, studies using the systemic approach often deliver EBRT in conjunction with TRT. It has been well documented that EBRT will cause an increase in the permeability of the BBB and increase vascular leakage. Regardless, it has been disappointingly estimated that only 0.001% to 0.01% of the systemically delivered antibody will penetrate each gram of solid tumor. Furthermore, biopsy data have revealed that a single systemic injection of radiolabeled anti-EGFR antibody will deliver only 0.02% of the injected activity per gram of tumor, resulting in a dose of only 100 to 200 cGy.

Direct instillation of the TRT agent into the SCRC is an attractive alternative to the systemic approach. Unlike other malignant sites where the potential for systemic spread mandates a systemic approach, this is not the case for malignant gliomas. The local approach is accomplished by injecting or instilling the RIT agent directly into the SCRC via an Ommaya or Rickham catheter. Preliminary dosimetry is performed to ensure localization within the surgical bed and that no direct communication with the ventricular system has occurred. Institutions using this technique have utilized murine, chimeric, or humanized mAbs attached to ^{131}I, ^{90}Y, [188]Re, and [211]At. Other important treatment variances include fractionation, pretargeting, and a combined modality approach using EBRT and chemotherapy. The success of this approach will depend on meaningful penetration of the RIT agent into the local brain parenchyma such that the mAbs (or targeting construct) can bind to areas of microscopic extension of malignant cells at some distance from the SCRC margin. It is still unknown as to what impact the healing process/inflammation at the surgical margin has on the success of antibody penetration. As well, it is well known that binding site barrier phenomena, interstitial tumor pressure, aberrant tumor vasculature, and a recusant extracellular tumor matrix will significantly impede antibody penetration.[61]

Hopkins et al.[62] obtained biopsy data from three patients with glioma who received two to three cycles of either ^{131}I or ^{90}Y-ERIC-1 (anti-NCAM antibody) directly instilled into a SCRC. Relevant assumptions were that the SCRCs were spherical, the radionuclide was spread evenly around the resection margin, 100% of the RIT agent was bound to its target, and diffusion into the resection margin was uniform. It was shown that "modest" diffusion occurred and the process was exponential. The peak dose occurred between 0.16 and 0.18 cm beyond the resection margin, and 4.4% to 5.8% of the peak dose was delivered to a depth of 2 cm. Of note, NCAM is expressed on benign and malignant cells and perhaps a more tumor-specific antigen would allow for greater depth of penetration. Certainly, smaller targeting constructs have been shown to penetrate to a greater depth in brain parenchyma compared to intact antibodies.[63] Using the same antibody, radiolabeled with ^{131}I and instilled into a SCRC, it was shown that diffusion occurred from 0.5 to 1.0 cm (single-photon emission computed tomography [SPECT]). The range of antibody binding to the target was 8% to 80% of total injected activity. Because the R_{95} (thickness of tissue where 95% of the β energy is deposited) for ^{131}I is only 0.992 mm, it was concluded that a more optimal radionuclide would potentially be ^{90}Y with an R_{95} of 5.94 mm.[64] Assuming a 2-cm SCRC and 100% binding, as much as 351 Gy could be delivered to the tumor with a single instillation of 18.2 mCi of ^{90}Y-ERIC-1. This calculation resulted in an impressive minimum tumor/whole-brain dose ratio of 140:1.

Using [131]I-81C6 (antitenascin mAB), dose-limiting toxicity was reached with a single injection of 80 mCi for leptomeningeal disease (intrathecal delivery), 100 mCi for heavily pretreated and recurrent glioma (into SCRC), and 120 mCi for de novo glioma (into SCRC) also receiving EBRT and chemotherapy.[65] Using a standard, fixed, mCi dose, a wide range of absorbed doses (18 to 186 Gy) will be delivered to a depth of 2 cm beyond the SCRC margin.[66] On further analysis, an optimal dose of 44 Gy to 2 cm beyond SCRC was identified. Doses <44 Gy resulted in increased recurrence rates, and doses >44 Gy resulted in a higher rate of necrosis. A trend toward significant improvement in median survival was shown for patients receiving 40 to 48 Gy versus <40 Gy.[64] Refining the technique further, it was shown that 20 of the 21 patients could be successfully dosed to 44 Gy by varying the initial injection activity and considering the volume of the SCRC.[67] Zalutsky et al.[68] showed that a high-LET, α-emitting radioconjugate ([211]At-ch81C6) could be safely delivered in a small cohort of glioma patients. Interestingly, histopathology appears to correlate with prognosis. Biopsy data from patients with a suspected recurrence, after receiving ^{131}I-labeled antitenascin 81C6 antibody, were analyzed. Three types of histologic patterns were evident: proliferative glioma, quiescent glioma, and negative for neoplasm. The median survival for each histopathologic pattern was 3.5, 15.0, and 27.5 months, respectively ($P < .0001$). Considering total dose (EBRT plus radiolabeled antibody), patients receiving <86 Gy or >86 Gy had median survivals of 7 and 19 months, respectively ($P < .002$).[69]

A review of the major RIT CNS trials[59] indicates that the range of maximum tolerated activity is between 10 and 120 mCi. There are many variables that could potentially account for the noted range. In general, by performing dosimetry for a given radionuclide delivery construct, a specific absorbed dose can be calculated to a predetermined depth from the SCRC margin. It has been shown that ^{131}I-antitenascin 81C6 can deliver 2,000, 90, and 34 Gy to the cavity interface, 1 cm depth and at 2 cm depth, respectively.[64,69] The median survival for TRT in treating glioma appears extremely favorable when compared to other treatment approaches. For de novo lesions, the median survival range is 50.9 to 57.6 months (three studies not reaching median survival at the time of the report) for anaplastic astrocytoma and 13.4 to 35.5 months for glioblastoma. For recurrent lesions, the median survival range is 13.0 to 52.0 months (one study not reaching median survival at the time of the report) for anaplastic astrocytoma and 14.0 to 25.0 months for glioblastoma.[59] Unlike sealed source brachytherapy, there appears to be a very low rate of CNS toxicity and a reduced subsequent need for surgical intervention to remove necrotic areas. Building upon Duke University research, Bradmer Pharmaceuticals developed two clinical trials using the ^{131}I-antitenascin antibody (Neuradiab) for treating glioblastoma in the de novo (phase III) and recurrent setting (phase II). Because of lack of funding, the trials were discontinued in 2010.

Cotara (Peregrine Pharmaceuticals) is a ^{131}I-chTNT-1/B mAb used to treat high-grade glioma that is continuously instilled into the SCRC with positive pressure, using a technology termed convection-enhanced delivery (CED).[70] A phase II trial was performed treating high-grade glioma (37 recurrent glioblastomas, 8 de novo glioblastomas, 6 recurrent anaplastic astrocytomas). The Cotara infusions delivered between 90% and 110% of the prescribed activity with an acceptable safety profile.[71] A phase III trial is pending collaboration with a funding partner.

Initial promising investigations evaluated the long-term survival of patients with advanced ovarian cancer treated with RIT following cytoreductive surgery and platinum-based chemotherapy.[72] Eligibility criteria included patients with histologic evidence of ovarian cancer from stage IC to IV. The conclusion of this study was that a substantial proportion of patients who achieve a CR with conventional therapy can achieve a long-term survival benefit if treated with IP ^{90}Y-HMFG1.

A phase III study was subsequently performed.[73] This multinational (74 centers, 17 countries, recruiting patients between 1998 and 2003), open-label, randomized phase III study compared ^{90}Y-HMFG1 (against the MUC 1 antigen) plus standard treatment versus standard treatment alone in patients with epithelial ovarian cancer (EOC) who had attained a complete clinical remission after cytoreductive surgery and platinum-based chemotherapy. Stage IC to stage IV patients were screened ($n = 844$), of whom 447 with a negative second-look laparoscopy (SLL) were randomly assigned to receive either a single dose of ^{90}Y-HMFG1 plus standard treatment (224 patients) or standard treatment alone (223 patients). Patients in the active treatment (RIT) arm received an IP dose of 25 mg ^{90}Y-HMFG1 to provide 666 MBq (18 mCi)/m^2. After a median follow-up of 3.5 years, 70 patients had died in the active treatment arm compared with 61 patients in the control arm. Cox proportional hazards analysis of survival demonstrated no difference between treatment arms. In the RIT arm, 104 patients experienced relapse compared with 98 patients in the standard treatment arm. No difference in time to relapse was observed between the two study arms. The conclusion was that a single IP administration of ^{90}Y-HMFG1 to patients with EOC, who had a negative SLL after primary therapy, did not extend survival or time to relapse. The reason for failure of the treatment could perhaps be explained by the choice of radionuclide. When treating microscopic disease with high-energy β-particles emitted from ^{90}Y, the electron will have too long of a range to deliver high enough energy to the tumor cell nuclei. It has been modeled that high-energy β-particle emissions will not deposit large amounts of energy (absorbed dose) into tumor spheroids below a certain size. However, there were other concerns about this study and these have been extensively reviewed.[74]

The patterns-of-failure analysis was eventually performed.[75] A total of 447 patients were included in the analysis with a median follow-up of 3.5 years. Relapse was seen in 104 of 224 patients in the RIT arm and 98 of 223 patients in the control arm. Significantly fewer IP ($P < .05$) and more extraperitoneal ($P < .05$) relapses occurred in the RIT arm. Time to IP recurrence was significantly longer ($P = .0019$), and time to extraperitoneal recurrence was significantly shorter for the RIT arm ($P < .001$). In a subset analysis, the impact of IP RIT on IP relapse-free survival was even greater and could only be seen in a subgroup of patients with residual disease after primary surgery. Although there was no survival benefit for ^{90}Y-HMFG1 IP instillation as consolidation treatment

for EOC, an improved control of IP disease was found, which appeared to be offset by increased extraperitoneal recurrences. It was proposed that the transient myelosuppression (alteration of the immune system) induced by therapy with ^{90}Y-HMFG1 indirectly caused the greater number of extraperitoneal metastases. Most likely, this observation is simply the result of an alteration in the failure pattern owing to a greater number of patients in the treatment arm benefiting from a greater IP control, as distant metastases will not be observed because of overwhelming local symptoms. In addition, for reasons mentioned previously, it is possible that the treatment arm was skewed with more advanced disease.[74] Future trials should focus on both the IP and systemic delivery of RIT, using an appropriate radionuclide to target microscopic disease.

UNSEALED RADIONUCLIDE THERAPY

Unsealed radionuclide therapy (URT) refers to the medical application of radiopharmaceuticals that are not conjugated to a targeting agent and thereby localize in diseased tissue by virtue of biologic, chemical, or physical avidity.[76] These radionuclides are considered "unsealed" because they are not confined within a container that could be inserted or implanted into a tumor, as is performed with conventional brachytherapy techniques. Because they are not conjugated to a traditional targeting construct, this class of therapeutics has also been referred to as "naked" radiopharmaceuticals. Oversight for the utilization of URT is governed by the U.S. FDA.[77] Safety issues, radioactive material shipping, and licensing are regulated by the U.S. Nuclear Regulatory Commission (NRC). A state may enter into an agreement with the NRC to perform its own regulation and to monitor of the use of radioactive material (agreement state), with the exception of fuel facilities and nuclear reactors. States that continue to allow monitoring by the NRC are referred to as nonagreement states. The NRC receives advice regarding radiopharmaceuticals from the Advisory Committee on the Medical Use of Isotopes (ACMUI). Regulations for the practice of nuclear medicine reside in U.S. NRC Title 10 of the Code of Federal Regulations, Parts 20 and 35. Part 20 largely governs the standards for radiation protection, and Part 35 governs the medical use of radioactive material.

Bone-seeking radiopharmaceuticals, used for palliation of painful bone metastases, represent one of the more common uses of URT. A few of the earlier radionuclides used for this purpose include phosphorus 32 [^{32}P], samarium 153 [^{153}Sm], and strontium 89 [(^{89})Sr];[78] however, newer agents are being investigated and are in various stages of development.[79-85] As with RIT, the radionuclides used in the application of URT can be classified as β-, α-, and Auger emitters. Many also emit gamma radiation, which can be used for imaging and dosimetry. The radionuclides used in URT target bone by either an intrinsic affinity (i.e., ^{89}Sr, radium-223 [^{223}Ra]) or by using bone-seeking phosphonate ligands attached to the radionuclide (i.e., samarium-153 ethylene diamine tetramethylene phosphonate [^{153}Sm-EDTMP] or rhenium-188 hydroxyethylidene diphosphate [^{188}Re-HEDP]).[82,86] Localization properties of individual agents and the clinical circumstances involved will determine routes of administration. These agents have been delivered by IV, intra-arterial, intracavitary, intra-articular (radiosynovectomy), and direct intralesional approaches. This variability of administration has been especially true for ^{32}P, which has been uniquely studied using IV, oral, IP, and intrathoracic routes.[87]

The initial use of a β-emitting radioisotope for the management of intractable malignant bone pain was reported in 1942. Because URT demonstrates a chemical affinity for bone, the predominant thrust of clinical investigation has been for primary and secondary malignancies of bone and bone marrow. Other target sites, however, have been considered. In some instances, these alternative uses have remained a part of the therapeutic armamentarium; however, for many indications, the use of URT has yielded to nonradioactive approaches (corticosteroids, systemic chemotherapy, hormone therapy, analgesia, and surgery) and to EBRT. The lack of access to innovative candidate radionuclides, diminished trial participation, and absence of utilization and teaching from many training programs have further exacerbated the problem.[76] Regardless, a review of 15 randomized controlled trials (1,146 analyzed patients) comparing URT to placebo or another radionuclide for the treatment of metastatic bone pain confirms the efficacy of URT for pain management. This review also provides evidence that URT resulted in significant and complete pain relief during a 1- to 6-month period.[88] Practice guidelines have been established for URT,[89] and evidence-based guidelines for palliation of bone metastases include URT as a reasonable therapeutic option.[90]

The most common malignant sites that develop bone metastases are prostate, breast, and lung cancer.[78] URT exhibits increased targeting of bone in areas of osteoblastic activity and exerts this propensity because of a chemical similarity to calcium, which is classified as an alkaline earth metal in the periodic table (as are ^{89}Sr and ^{223}Ra). These therapeutic agents may either directly substitute for stable analogues in hydroxyapatite or may be chemisorbed on the hydroxyapatite surface of the phosphate moiety of phosphonate chelates.[86] Radionuclide decay profiles that include gamma emissions may be utilized for imaging and for documentation of therapeutic uptake in regions of bone pathology. Bone scans (technetium 99m [^{99m}Tc]) are typically performed to verify disseminated osseous disease. The intensity of uptake on pretherapeutic scanning does not necessarily coincide with therapeutic efficacy, and widely disseminated disease may actually produce "dilution" of dose and potentially reduced effectiveness.[86]

Regardless of the precise method of chemical or physical affinity, the agents studied for palliation of osseous metastatic bone pain fared better than placebos in randomized trials.[90] There is, however, limited evidence that the response or morbidity profile of the different radiopharmaceuticals varies significantly among themselves. Additionally, there is little evidence that dose escalation either in individual or cumulative doses will improve effectiveness. Sequenced administration has been investigated; however, if an initial intervention has not produced a significant level or duration of response, there is little evidence that additional administrations will increase effectiveness, but they may potentially increase morbidity.[86]

Rapid and significant localization in bone by all agents will generally limit potential morbidity to myelosuppression, which in patients with adequate marrow reserve will usually be mild and be manifest initially within 1 week post administration with evidence of thrombocytopenia. Leukopenia may develop somewhat later; however, all side effects typically reverse without intervention within 8 to 10 weeks. Circulating isotope not immediately incorporated into bone is typically excreted in urine; therefore, patients with reduced renal function may not be ideal candidates for the agents and, if used, should have blood counts monitored carefully. Administration is routinely on an outpatient basis; thus, radiation protection measures for low-level radiation in urine should be practiced.

Palliative effects may be observed within 3 to 5 days but usually peak at approximately 7 to 10 days, and the beneficial effects may last for months. At this point in time, subsequent administrations may be considered. When used for manage-

ment of bone pain, all bone-seeking radiopharmaceuticals can exhibit a flare in pain within 24 to 72 hours post injection that may last for 5 to 7 days. Appropriate analgesic management must be provided during this period. In the treatment of metastatic prostate cancer, prostate-specific antigen (PSA) levels may begin to decline within several days; however, the rapidity of decline, nadir of the PSA level, and duration of PSA response are not satisfactory predictors of improved outcomes.[86]

The bone-seeking agents have been and continue to be used primarily in metastatic prostate cancer, and evidence of effectiveness in breast and lung cancer is limited with responses noted primarily in osteoblastic metastases. Plain radiographs of symptomatic metastatic sites should be obtained prior to the use of systemic agents for palliation of bone pain. If there is evidence of possible impending fracture, stabilization and/or EBRT should be initiated prior to systemic radionuclide therapy. If painful vertebral metastasis is apparent clinically, CT or magnetic resonance imaging (MRI) of the painful vertebral segments should be obtained prior to administration of isotope to ensure that no epidural disease is present. If this pathology is discovered, EBRT or surgery should be carried out prior to systemic isotope therapy. IV administration of all agents should be carried out slowly over 1 to 5 minutes, through indwelling catheters with clear and unobstructed flow clearly validated, adequate hydration, and careful radiation precautions for patients and staff.

Radiopharmaceuticals

Iodine 131

Physical Properties: $t_{1/2}$ = 8.0 days; radiation decay: β (606 keV maximum and 190 keV mean); γ (364 keV).

Clinical Utility: Radioiodine ^{131}I was first used to treat benign thyroid disease in the late 1920s and early 1930s. The first reports of using ^{131}I to treat well-differentiated thyroid cancer (WDTC) were published in the 1940s.[91] To date, ^{131}I has become the standard of care, in conjunction with surgery, for the management of WDTC; its use and indications have been extensively reviewed.[92-94] Benign thyroid tissue (follicular cells) and certain thyroid carcinomas (follicular, papillary, and Hürthle cell carcinoma) will actively transport iodine into the cell via the sodium iodide symporter to initiate the synthesis thyroid hormone. As a result, this innate targeting system has been exploited for many decades to treat locally persistent, recurrent, or metastatic thyroid carcinoma. The majority of data concerning the treatment of WDTC with ^{131}I has been generated by large retrospective series of patients, with the resulting clinical data often spanning several decades. Frequently, these institutions used unchanged protocols and fixed activities for therapy. Regardless, considerable evidence exists concerning local control, decreased metastases, and a survival benefit when ^{131}I is used as part of the treatment regimen.[95-97]

In general, ^{131}I therapy for WDTC is considered either ablation or treatment. Ablation is the use of ^{131}I to sterilize normal remnant thyroid tissue or microscopic disease that remains after thyroidectomy. Treatment refers to the therapeutic application of ^{131}I against cancer persistence, local recurrence, or distant metastatic disease. Whereas the treatment aspect of ^{131}I is well accepted, ablation is more controversial.[98] Recent decades have revealed a decrease in mortality for WDTC, owing to the early diagnosis and aggressive treatment of WDTC with near-total thyroidectomy and ^{131}I ablation in selected patients at high risk for recurrence and mortality, followed by thyroid-stimulating hormone (TSH) suppression.[99] If it is determined that ablation will be performed, patients are placed on a low-iodine diet and TSH stimulation is performed by withholding thyroid hormone.[94] Standard fixed activities of

30 to 100 mCi are used for ablation, whereas higher activities in the range of 100 to 300 mCi are used for known residual disease, recurrence, or metastatic disease. If possible, patient-specific dosimetry should be used to determine the activity in the metastatic setting.[99] Using this approach, a dose <200 cGy is calculated to the blood (bone marrow) and ≤120 mCi of ^{131}I being retained after 48 hours. This can result in administered activities between 75 and 659 mCi without the development of leukemia, permanent bone marrow suppression, or pulmonary fibrosis.[100] Diagnostic ^{131}I scanning and thyroglobulin measurement are required for follow-up.

Phosphorus 32

Physical Properties: $t_{1/2}$ = 14.3 days; radiation decay: β (1.71 MeV maximum and 1.69 MeV mean); γ (none).

Clinical Utility: Phosphorus 32 (^{32}P) represents one of the earliest agents in this class and perhaps is the most frequently studied for a wide variety of indications and routes of administration. In its aqueous form (Na_2PO_3), the agent was employed for the systemic therapy of chronic myelogenous leukemia and polycythemia vera. Orthopedic surgeons and rheumatologists have evaluated the agent for intra-articular management of persistent synovial effusions and hemarthroses secondary to hemophilia and leukemias.[101,102] The agent has been placed in indwelling catheters to treat CNS lesions.

The colloidal form of the agent (as chromic phosphate) became a standard modality for management of malignant pleural and peritoneal effusions in the 1960s and 1970s, driving numerous clinical investigations. Anecdotal reports suggesting significant activity were infrequently corroborated in randomized clinical trials. Following drainage of abdominal ascites or pleural effusions, up to 5 mCi of the agent was instilled and patients were placed in various positions to enhance distribution. The nature of the disease processes and prior therapy often predisposed patients to preinstillation adhesions with bowel or lung immobility, and distribution of the agent proved difficult. This indication has largely been replaced by instillations of various antibiotic or chemotherapeutic compounds.

Following identification of a subset of early-stage, high-risk ovarian cancer patients (FIGO stage Ia or Ib [grade 3], or stage 1c or II [any grade], or any stage I/II patient with clear cell histology), the Gynecologic Oncology Group (GOG), North Central Cancer Treatment Group (NCCTG), and Southwest Oncology Group (SWOG) undertook a randomized trial assigning patients to either a single dose of 15 mCi of IP ^{32}P or cyclophosphamide 1 g/m^2 and cisplatin 100 mg/m^2 every 21 days for three cycles. Prior to instillation of the radioactive material through multiperforated indwelling peritoneal dialysis catheters, ^{99m}Tc was instilled to ensure free flow and even distribution of the therapeutic agent. IP ^{32}P was administered within 10 days but not >6 weeks following laparotomy. Ten-year follow-up of the study population suggested a modest reduction in intra-abdominal recurrence rate for the chemotherapy population but only a small and nonsignificant improvement in survival. These findings were corroborated by other reports.[103]

(^{32})P localization in bone created interest in the use of the orthophosphate form of the isotope for painful skeletal metastases with 85% of the administered dose ultimately incorporated into bone. However, priming regimens including androgenic agents prior to isotope administration were prolonged, beneficial results modest, and myelotoxicity significant; use of the agent for this indication is not ideal[104] and has largely been abandoned.

In the 1990s, a series of patients, treated with direct intralesional infusions of ^{32}P colloidal chromic phosphate for unresectable tumors of the liver, CNS, pancreas, and head and neck, was reported. Intense activity and doses were documented; however, improvements in local control and survival were inconclusive.[105] A randomized trial was performed on 30 patients with unresectable adenocarcinoma of the pancreas. The patients were randomized to 5-FU and EBRT with or without intratumoral ^{32}P. All patients received adjuvant gemcitabine. There was more liquefaction in the ^{32}P arm (78% vs. 8%). There was no difference in survival but an increase in serious adverse events in the ^{32}P arm.[106]

Strontium-89 Chloride (Metastron, GE Healthcare, Chalfont St. Giles, UK)

Physical Properties: $t_{1/2}$ = 50.5 days; radiation decay: β (1.463 MeV maximum and 0.583 MeV mean); γ (none).

^{89}Sr, a calcium analogue, is administered as an IV injection at doses of 4 mCi.

Clinical Utility: The Trans-Canada study randomized 126 patients with painful metastatic castrate-resistant prostate cancer to EBRT to painful bone sites with either ^{89}Sr or placebo.[107] A significant improvement in the following endpoints was noted in the ^{89}Sr arm: (1) intake of analgesics, (2) progression of pain, and (3) quality of life analysis. Multiple phase II and III trials have subsequently been performed using ^{89}Sr, showing favorable results. The conclusion of the review was that ^{89}Sr should be considered for the treatment of metastatic cancer where pain control is an issue and the bone scan shows activity.[108] The TRAPEZE trial is a prospective randomized trial comparing docetaxel alone or with zoledronic acid (ZA), ^{89}Sr, or both. Results revealed that ^{89}Sr combined with docetaxel significantly improved progression-free survival.[109]

Samarium-153 Lexidronam (Quadramet, Cytogen, Princeton, NJ)

Physical Properties: $t_{1/2}$ = 46.3 hours; radiation decay: β (0.81 MeV maximum and 0.23 MeV mean); γ (maximum energy 103 keV).

Clinical Utility: Samarium-153 EDTMP (^{153}Sm) is a bone-seeking agent consisting of radioactive samarium and a telephosphonate chelator, EDTMP. The recommended therapeutic dose is 1.0 mCi/kg, administered intravenously over a period of 1 minute through a secure indwelling catheter and followed by a saline flush. Extensive preclinical and clinical investigations have demonstrated the safety and effectiveness profile of ^{153}Sm-EDTMP.[110,111] Although primarily used alone, there is increasing interest in consideration of combination therapy with the bisphosphonates and taxane-based chemotherapeutics.

The use of ^{153}Sm-EDTMP has been evaluated in osseous metastases for primary osteosarcomas. Anderson et al.[112] investigated the use of gemcitabine as a radiosensitizer to increase ^{153}Sm-EDTMP effectiveness. Using 30 mCi/kg (average of 1,640 mCi), they found acceptable toxicity and objective response in 8 of 14 patients investigated. Treatment of osteosarcoma with ^{153}Sm has been further reviewed; 153Sm used as monotherapy or in combination with chemotherapy, stem cell transplant or EBRT.[153]

Radium-223 Chloride

Physical Properties: $t_{1/2}$ = 11.4 days; radiation decay: α (6 MeV maximum); γ (270 keV maximum).

Clinical Utility: The phase III ALSYMPCA (Alpharadin in Symptomatic Prostate Cancer Patients) trial confirmed the clinical utility of ^{223}Ra (Xofigo) for the treatment of castrate-resistant adenocarcinoma of the prostate. A total of 921 patients who had received, were not eligible to receive, or declined docetaxel were randomized 2:1 to receive six instillations of Xofigo (50 kBq/kg) every 4 weeks or placebo.

Section II

Additionally, all patients received "best standard of care." The primary end point was overall survival, and the secondary end points were time to first symptomatic skeletal event and various biochemical end points (median time to increase in alkaline phosphatase [AP] and PSA; ≥30% reduction in AP; normalization of AP). Entry criterion included castrate-resistant adenocarcinoma of the prostate (serum testosterone ≤1.7 nmol/L), at least two symptomatic bone metastases, no known visceral disease, PSA ≥5 with at least two consecutive rises, ECOG performance status of 0 to 2, malignant lymphadenopathy ≤3-cm short axis, and appropriate hematologic criteria (initial criteria per Bayer; ANC ≥1.5; platelet ≥100; hemoglobin ≥10). The overall survival in the Xofigo group was 14.9 months versus 11.3 months in the placebo group ($P < .001$). All secondary end points had a benefit from Xofigo versus placebo ($P < .001$).[114] Subsequently, many questions regarding the use and sequencing of chemotherapy with Xofigo remained. In a prespecified subgroup analysis of the ALSYMPCA trial, Xofigo appeared to be equally effective before or after docetaxel, concerning overall survival.[115] A separate analysis of patients in the ALSYMPCA trial receiving chemotherapy after Xofigo was performed. The conclusion was that chemotherapy following Xofigo, regardless of prior docetaxel, is feasible and appears to be well tolerated.[116] Current areas of research include using higher activities per injection, increased overall number of doses, use in other nonprostate metastatic bone disease processes, and CMT with EBRT.

Rhenium-186 HEDP (Etidronate)

Physical Properties: $t_{1/2}$ = 3.8 days; radiation decay: β (1.07 MeV maximum and 0.336 mean); γ (0.137 MeV maximum).

Clinical Utility: Although not commercially available in the United States, [186]Rh-HEDP has been studied in phase I trials in Europe in association with autologous peripheral blood stem cell rescue in the management of hormone-refractory prostate cancer metastatic to bone. Phase I/II trials using [186]Rh-HEDP for castrate-resistant prostate cancer have indicated the potential for prolonged survival.[117]

Rhenium-188 HEDP (Etidronate)

Physical Properties: $t_{1/2}$ = 16.9 hours; radiation decay: β (2.1 MeV maximum and 0.779 mean); γ (0.155 MeV maximum and 0.061 mean).

Clinical Utility: Although not commercially available in the United States, [188]Re-HEDP has been studied in Europe for some time. The agent is produced by a generator similar to that used to produce ^{99m}Tc, enabling wide availability at relatively low cost. Liepe et al.[118] reported treatment of 46 patients with multiple bone metastases from breast and prostate cancer with pain. Thirty-one patients received [188]Re-HEDP (3,300 MBq) and 25 patients received [153]Sm-EDTMP (37 MBq/kg of body weight). All patients had a single injection of isotope. Patients with prostate cancer received hormone therapy for 6 months before isotope therapy and during the postisotope observation period. Thirty-nine patients received bisphosphonates for 6 months prior to study treatment with discontinuance of the agents 1 month prior to isotope administration. In posttherapy evaluation, only the [188]Re-HEDP group had a statistically significant improvement in the Karnofsky performance score. Pain relief within 2 weeks of treatment was noted in 77% of the [188]Re-HEDP group and in 73% of the [153]Sm-EDTMP group. These results were not statistically significant, and there was no significant difference between responses in the patients with prostate or breast cancer. A brief flare reaction was noted in 17% of patients in both groups within 14 days of therapy, and the majority of patients demonstrated a maximum of grade I anemia within 12 weeks of therapy based on the 1979 WHO criteria. Grade I thrombocytopenia was noted in 2 patients with each isotope, and 1 patient in the [188]Re-HEDP group experienced grade II thrombocytopenia. Grade I leukopenia was noted in 1 patient in each group. All cases of thrombocytopenia and leukopenia reversed within 12 weeks after therapy. Similar findings have been reported by other investigators.[119,120]

FUTURE PERSPECTIVES

In order for RIT to be successful, quite simply, an increased dose of high-LET radiotherapy must be delivered to the tumor and a lower dose delivered to normal tissue:

1. *Tumor Specificity*: To date, there are no true tumor-specific antigens or targets. This is important considering the toxicity of radionuclides. The field must move toward tumor-specific processes. This will result in greater doses to the tumor and less to normal tissue. For example, aptamers can be designed to target tumor cells and then counter selected against normal tissue to produce a "true" tumor-specific targeting construct.

2. *High-LET Radiation*: Beta radiation is sparsely ionizing and may be effective against hematologic malignancies but not against solid tumors (carcinoma). High-LET radiation will be required to combat solid tumors. Alpha radiation will be very effective but potentially toxic. Auger radiation will be very effective with limited toxicity. The caveat, the Auger radionuclide, must enter the nucleus and/or bind DNA.

3. *Fractionation*: Currently, the successful RIT agents (Zevalin, Bexxar) have been delivered in a single fraction. These agents however have treated radiosensitive hematologic malignancies. RIT must be delivered in multiple fractions for solid tumors. For example, platinum-based chemotherapy, used to treat germ cell tumors, was not curative as a single fraction. Multiple fractions were delivered with a noted "log fold" decrease in tumor markers with each fraction (cycle). Potentially survival advantageous results seem to be occurring with the multiple fraction regimens of Xofigo and Lutathera.

4. *Multiple Radionuclides*: Individual radionuclides deposit their energy over a known path length. In order to be maximally effective, radionuclides need to deposit their energy over a wide range of micrometastatic and tumor sizes. The effectiveness of multiple radionuclides seems to have come to fruition with peptide therapy (^{90}Y and [117]Lu). The use and incorporation of high-LET radionuclide are quite necessary. One can calculate that the following radionuclide combinations will encompass a subcellular level to tumor level coverage: [125]I, ^{33}P, ^{131}I, [32]P.

REFERENCES

1. Siegel RL, Miller KD, Jemal A. Cancer statistics. *CA Cancer J Clin* 2016;66:7–30.
2. Torre LA, Bray F, Siegel R, et al. Global cancer statistics, 2012. *CA Cancer J Clin* 2015;65:87–108.
3. Siddiqui M, Rajkumar SV. The high cost of cancer drugs and what we can do about it. *Mayo Clin Proc* 2012;87:935–943.
4. American Society of Clinical Oncology. Potential approaches to sustainable, long-lasting payment reform in oncology. *J Oncol Pract* 2014;10:254–258.
5. Abbas AK, Lichtman AH, Pillais S, eds. *Cellular and Molecular Immunology*. Philadelphia: Saunders Elsevier, 2007.
6. Campoli M, Ferrone S. Cancer immune surveillance and tumor escape mechanisms. In: Speer TW, ed. *Targeted Radionuclide Therapy*. Philadelphia: Lippincott Williams & Wilkins, 2011:3–21.
7. Liu X, William CC. Precision medicine in immune checkpoint blockade therapy for non-small cell lung cancer. *Clin Translat Med* 2017;6:1–4.
8. Prehn RT. On the nature of cancer and why anticancer vaccines don't work. *Cancer Cell Int* 2005;5:1–5.
9. Jeoung DI. Employing SEREX for identification of targets for anticancer targeted therapy. In: Speer TW, ed. *Targeted Radionuclide Therapy*. Philadelphia: Lippincott Williams & Wilkins, 2011:159–167.

10. Wong JYC, Williams LE, Yazaki PJ. Radioimmunotherapy of colorectal cancer. In: Speer TW, ed. *Targeted Radionuclide Therapy*. Philadelphia: Lippincott Williams & Wilkins, 2011:321–351.

11. O'Donoghue JA. Dosimetric principles of targeted radiotherapy. In: Abrams PG, Fritzberg AR, eds. *Radioimmunotherapy of Cancer*. New York: Marcel Dekker, 2000:1–20.

12. Burvenich IJG, Scott AM. The delivery construct: maximizing the therapeutic ratio of targeted radionuclide therapy. In: Speer TW, ed. *Targeted Radionuclide Therapy*. Philadelphia: Lippincott Williams & Wilkins, 2011:236–248.

13. DiCara D, Nissim A. Methods for development of monoclonal antibody therapeutics. In: Speer TW, ed. *Targeted Radionuclide Therapy*. Philadelphia: Lippincott Williams & Wilkins, 2011:22–31.

14. Jain M, Kaur S, Batra SK. Modulation of biologic impediments for radioimmunotherapy of solid tumors. In: Speer TW, ed. *Targeted Radionuclide Therapy*. Philadelphia: Lippincott Williams & Wilkins, 2011:182–190.

15. Wang Z, Dabrosin C, Yin X, et al. Broad targeting of angiogenesis for cancer prevention and therapy. *Semin Cancer Biol* 2015;35:S224–243.

16. Chauhan VP, Stylianopoulos T, Bouch Y, et al. Delivery of molecular and nanoscale medicine to tumors: transport barriers and strategies. *Annu Rev Chem Biomol Eng* 2011;2:281–298.

17. Padera TP, Kadambi A, di Tomaso E, et al. Lymphatic metastasis in the absence of functional intratumor lymphatics. *Science* 2002;296:1883–1886.

18. Zwanziger D, Beck-Sickinger AG. Malignancies treated with peptides. In: Speer TW, ed. *Targeted Radionuclide Therapy*. Philadelphia: Lippincott Williams & Wilkins, 2011:483–497.

19. Dash A, Chakraborty S, Raghavan MP, et al. Peptide receptor radionuclide therapy: an overview. *Cancer Biother Radiopharm* 2015;30:47–71.

20. Cives M, Strosberg J. Radionuclide therapy for neuroendocrine tumors. *Curr Oncol Rep* 2017;19:1–9.

21. Stahl S, Friedman M, Carlsson J, et al. Affibody molecules for targeted radionuclide therapy. In: Speer TW, ed. *Targeted Radionuclide Therapy*. Philadelphia: Lippincott Williams & Wilkins, 2011:49–58.

22. Frejd FY, Kim K. Affibody molecules as engineered protein drugs. *Exp Mol Med* 2017;49:1–8.

23. Missailidis S, Perkins A. Radiolabeled aptamers for imaging and therapy. In: Speer TW, ed. *Targeted Radionuclide Therapy*. Philadelphia: Lippincott Williams & Wilkins, 2011:59 70.

24. Gijs M, Aerts A, Impens N, et al. Aptamers as radiopharmaceuticals for nuclear imaging and therapy. *Nucl Med Biol* 2016;43:253–271.

25. Enrique MA, Mariana OR, Mirshojael SF, et al. Multifunctional radiolabeled nanoparticles: strategies and novel classification of radiopharmaceuticals for cancer treatment. *J Drug Target* 2015;23:191–201.

26. Pant K, Sedlacek O, Nadar RA, et al. Radiolabelled polymeric materials for imaging and treatment of cancer: Quo Vadis? *Adv Healthc Mater* 2017;6:1–31.

27. Maeda H, Sawa T, Konno T. Mechanism of tumor-targeted delivery of macromolecules drugs, including the EPR effect in solid tumor and clinical overview of the prototype polymeric drug SMANCS. *J Control Release* 2001;74:47–61.

28. Tesauro D, Morelli G, Pedone C, et al. Radiolabeled peptides, structure and analysis. In: Speer TW, ed. *Targeted Radionuclide Therapy*. Philadelphia: Lippincott Williams & Wilkins, 2011:32–48.

29. Zhang L. Unnatural nucleic acids for aptamer selection. In: Tan W, Fang X, eds. *Aptamers Selected by Cell-SELEX for Theranostics*. Heidelberg: Springer, 2015:35–65.

30. Murry D, McEwan AJ. Radiobiology of systemic radiation therapy. *Cancer Biother Radiopharm* 2007;22:1–23.

31. Speer TW, Khuntia D. Introduction to radiation therapy. In: Mehta MP, ed. *Principles and Practice of Neuro-oncology: A Multidisciplinary Approach*. New York: Demos Medical Publishing, 2011:719–743.

32. Lundqvist H, Stenerlow B, Gedda L. The Auger effect in molecular targeting therapy. In: Stigbrand T, Carlsson J, Adams GP, eds. *Targeted Radionuclide Tumor Therapy*. Heidelberg: Springer, 2008:195–214.

33. Bernhardt P, Speer TW. Modeling the systemic cure with targeted radionuclide therapy. In: Speer TW, ed. *Targeted Radionuclide Therapy*. Philadelphia: Lippincott Williams & Wilkins, 2011:263–280.

34. Wilson AD, Brechbiel MW. Chelation chemistry. In: Speer TW, ed. *Targeted Radionuclide Therapy*. Philadelphia: Lippincott Williams & Wilkins, 2011:88–107.

35. Patra M, Zarschler K, Pietzsch HJ, et al. New insights into the pretargeting approach to image and treat tumours. *Chem Soc Rev* 2016;45:6415–6431.

36. Sharkey RM, Goldenberg DM. Pretargeted radioimmunotherapy. In: Speer TW, ed. *Targeted Radionuclide Therapy*. Philadelphia: Lippincott Williams & Wilkins, 2011:191–208.

37. Frampas E, Rousseau C, Bodet-Milin C, et al. Improvement of radioimmunotherapy using pretargeting. *Front Oncol* 2013;3:1–8.

38. Green DJ, Frayo SL, Lin Y, et al. Comparative analysis of bispecific antibody and streptavidin-targeted radioimmunotherapy for B-cell cancers. *Cancer Res* 2016;76:6669–6679.

39. Song H, Sgouros G. Radioimmunotherapy of solid tumors: searching for the right target. *Curr Drug Deliv* 2011;8:26–44.

40. Jain M, Gupta S, Kaur S, et al. Emerging trends in radioimmunotherapy in solid tumors. *Cancer Biother Radiopharm* 2013;28:639–650.

41. Andrade-Campos MM, Lievano P, Espinosa-Lara N, et al. Long-term complication in follicular lymphoma: assessing the risk of secondary neoplasm in 242 patients treated or not with 90-yttrium-ibritumomab-tiuxetan. *Eur J Haematol* 2016;97:576–582.

42. Burdick M, Macklis RM. Radioimmunotherapy for non-Hodgkin lymphoma: a clinical update. In: Speer TW, ed. *Targeted Radionuclide Therapy*. Philadelphia: Lippincott Williams & Wilkins, 2011:426–440.

43. Sharkey RM, Karacay H, Goldenberg DM. Improving the treatment of non-Hodgkin lymphoma with antibody-targeted radionuclides. *Cancer* 2010;116:1134–1145.

44. Pandit-Taskar N, O'Donoghue JA, Morris MJ, et al. Antibody mass escalation study in patients with castration-resistant prostate cancer using 111In-J591: lesion delectability and dosimetric projections for 90Y radioimmunotherapy. *J Nucl Med* 2008;49:1066–1074.

45. Mondello P, Cuzzocrea S, Navarra M, et al. 90Y-ibritumomab tiuxetan: a nearly forgotten opportunity. *Oncotarget* 2015;7:7597–7609.

46. Rizzieri D. Zevalin (ibritumomab tiuxetan): after more than a decade of treatment experience, what have we learned? *Crit Rev Oncol Hematol* 2016;105:5–17.

47. Witzig TE, Gordon LI, Cabanillas F, et al. Randomized, controlled trial of yttrium-90-labeled ibritumomab tiuxetan radioimmunotherapy versus rituximab immunotherapy for patients with relapsed refractory low-grade, follicular, or transformed B-cell non-Hodgkin's lymphoma. *J Clin Oncol* 2002;20:2453–2463.

48. Morschhauser F, Radford J, Van Hoof A, et al. Phase III trial of consolidation therapy with yttrium-90-ibritumomab tiuxetan compared with no additional therapy after first remission in advanced follicular lymphoma. *J Clin Oncol* 2008;26:5156–5164.

49. Morschhauser F, Radford J, Van Hoof A, et al. 90Yttrium-ibritumomab tiuxetan consolidation of first remission in advanced-stage follicular non-Hodgkin lymphoma: updated results after a median follow-up of 7.3 years from the international, randomized, phase III first-line indolent trial. *J Clin Oncol* 2013;31:1977–1983.

50. Strosberg J, El-Haddad G, Wolin E, et al. Phase 3 trial of 177Lu-dototate for midgut neuroendocrine tumors. *N Engl J Med* 2017;376:125–135.

51. Al-Ejeh F, Brown MP. Combined modality therapy: relevance for targeted radionuclide therapy. In: Speer TW, ed. *Targeted Radionuclide Therapy*. Philadelphia: Lippincott Williams & Wilkins, 2011:220–235.

52. Wang H, Cao C, Li B, et al. Immunogenicity of iodine 131 chimeric tumor necrosis therapy monoclonal antibody in advanced lung cancer patients. *Cancer Immunol Immunother* 2008;57:677–684.

53. Chen S, Yu L, Jiang C, et al. Pivotal study of iodine-131-labeled chimeric tumor necrosis treatment radioimmunotherapy in patients with advanced lung cancer. *J Clin Oncol* 2005;23:1538–1547.

54. Zhao Z, Su Z, Zhang W, et al. A randomized study comparing the effectiveness of microwave ablation radioimmunotherapy and postoperative adjuvant chemoradiation in the treatment of non-small cell lung cancer. *J BUON* 2016;2:326–332.

55. Order S. Radioimmunotherapy of unresectable hepatocellular carcinoma. In: Speer TW, ed. *Targeted Radionuclide Therapy*. Philadelphia: Lippincott Williams & Wilkins, 2011:352–355.

56. Chen Z-N, Mi L, Xu J, et al. Targeting radioimmunotherapy of hepatocellular carcinoma with iodine (131I) metuximab injection: clinical phase I/II trials. *Int J Radiat Oncol Bio Phys* 2006;65:435–444.

57. Xu J, Shen Z-Y, Chen X-G, et al. A randomized controlled trial of Licartin for preventing hepatoma recurrence after liver transplantation. *Hepatology* 2007;45:269–276.

58. Bian H, Zheng JS, Nan G, et al. Randomized trial of [131I] metuximab in treatment of hepatocellular carcinoma after percutaneous radiofrequency ablation. *J Natl Cancer Inst* 2014;106:1–5.

59. Speer TW, Limmer JP, Henrich D, et al. Evolution of radiotherapy toward a more targeted approach for CNS malignancies. In: Speer TW, ed. *Targeted Radionuclide Therapy*. Philadelphia: Lippincott Williams & Wilkins, 2011:356–376.

60. Wygoda Z, Kula D, Bierzynska-Macyszyn G, et al. Use of monoclonal anti-EGFR antibody in the radioimmunotherapy of malignant gliomas in the context of EGFR expression in grade III and IV tumors. *Hybridoma* 2006;26(3):125–132.

61. Thurber GM. Kinetics of antibody penetration into tumors. In: Speer TW, ed. *Targeted Radionuclide Therapy*. Philadelphia: Lippincott Williams & Wilkins, 2011:168–181.

62. Hopkins K, Chandler C, Eatough J, et al. Direct injection of 90Y MoAbs into glioma tumor resection cavities leads to limited diffusion of the radioimmunoconjugates into normal brain parenchyma: a model to estimate absorbed radiation dose. *Int J Radiation Oncol Biol Phys* 1998;40:835–844.

63. Mamelak AN, Rosenfeld S, Bucholz R, et al. Phase I single-dose study of intracavitary-administered iodine-131-TM-601 in adults with recurrent high-grade glioma. *J Clin Oncol* 2006;24:3644–3650.

64. Akabani G, Reardon DA, Coleman RE, et al. Dosimetry and radiographic analysis of 131I-labeled anti-tenascin 81C6 murine monoclonal antibody in newly diagnosed patients with malignant gliomas: a phase II study. *J Nucl Med* 2005;46:1042–1051.

65. Reardon DA, Akabani G, Coleman RE, et al. Phase II trial of murine 131I-labeled antitenascin monoclonal antibody 81C6 administered into surgically created resection cavities of patients with newly diagnosed malignant gliomas. *J Clin Oncol* 2002;20:1389–1397.

66. Reardon DA, Akabani G, Coleman RE, et al. Salvage radioimmunotherapy with murine iodine-131-labeled antitenascin monoclonal antibody 81C6 for patients with recurrent primary and metastatic malignant brain tumors: phase II study results. *J Clin Oncol* 2006;24:115–122.

67. Reardon DA, Zalutsky MR, Akabani G, et al. A pilot study: 131I-antitenascin monoclonal antibody 81C6 to deliver a 44-Gy resection cavity boost. *Neuro Oncol* 2008;10(2):182–189.

68. Zalutsky MR, Reardon DA, Akabani G, et al. Clinical experience with α-particle-emitting 211At: treatment of recurrent brain tumor patients with 211At-labeled chimeric antitenascin monoclonal antibody 81C6. *J Nucl Med* 2008;49(1):30–38.

69. McLendon RE, Akabani G, Friedman HS, et al. Tumor resection cavity administered iodine-131-labeled antitenascin 81C6 radioimmunotherapy in patients with malignant glioma: neuropathology aspects. *Nucl Med Biol* 2007;34:405–413.

70. Bobo RH, Laske DW, Akbasak A, et al. Convection-enhanced delivery of macromolecules into the brain. *Proc Natl Acad Sci* 1994;91:2076–2080.

71. Patel SJ, Shapiro WR, Laske DW, et al. Safety and feasibility of convection-enhanced delivery of Cotara for the treatment of malignant glioma: initial experience in 51 patients. *Neurosurgery* 2005;56:1243–1252.

72. Epenetos AA, Hird V, Lambert H, et al. Long term survival of patients with advanced ovarian cancer treated with intraperitoneal radioimmunotherapy. *Int J Gynecol Cancer* 2000;10:44–46.

73. Verheijen RH, Massuger LF, Benigno BB, et al. Phase III trial of intraperitoneal therapy with yttrium-90-labeled HMFG1 murine monoclonal antibody in patients with epithelial ovarian cancer after a surgically defined complete remission. *J Clin Oncol* 2006;24:571–578.

74. Elgqvist J, Hultborn R, Lindegren S, et al. Ovarian Cancer: Background and Clinical Perspectives. In: Speer TW, ed. *Targeted Radionuclide Therapy*. Philadelphia: Lippincott Williams & Wilkins, 2011:352–355.

75. Oei AL, Verheijen RH, Seiden MV, et al. Decreased intraperitoneal disease recurrence in epithelial ovarian cancer patients receiving intraperitoneal consolidation treatment with yttrium-90-labeled murine HMFG1 without improvement in overall survival. *Int J Cancer* 2007;120:2710–2714.

76. Wallner PE. Unconjugated radiopharmaceuticals. In: Speer TW, ed. *Targeted Radionuclide Therapy*. Philadelphia: Lippincott Williams & Wilkins, 2011:294–297.

77. U.S. Food and Drug Administration. Radiation-emitting products. Available at: https://www.fda.gov/Radiation-EmittingProducts/default.htm. Accessed May 12, 2017.

78. Reisfield GM, Silberstein EB, Wilson GR. Radiopharmaceuticals for the palliation of painful bone metastases. *Am J Hosp Palliat Care* 2005;22:41–46.

79. Hindorf C, Flux GD, Ibisch C, et al. Clinical dosimetry in the treatment of bone tumors: old and new agents. *Q J Nucl Med Mol Imaging* 2011;55:198–204.

80. Jansen DR, Krijger ZI, Kolar ZI, et al. Targeted radiotherapy of bone malignancies. *Curr Drug Discov Technol* 2010;7:233–246.

81. Zafeirakis A, Zissimopoulos A, Baziotis N, et al. Introduction of a new semiquantitative index with predictive implications in patients with painful osseous metastases after (186)Re-HEDP therapy. *Q J Nucl Med Mol Imaging* 2011;55:91–102.

82. Biersack HJ, Palmedo H, Andris A, et al. Palliation and survival after repeated (188)Re-HEDP therapy of hormone-refractory bone metastases of prostate cancer: a retrospective analysis. *J Nucl Med* 2011;52:1721–1726.

83. Liu C, Brasic JR, Liu X, et al. Timing and optimized acquisition parameters for the whole-body imaging of 177Lu-EDTMP toward performing bone pain palliation treatment. *Nucl Med Commun* 2012;33:90–96.

84. Ogawa K, Kawashima H, Shiba K, et al. Development of [(90)Y]DOTA-conjugated bisphosphonate for treatment of painful bone metastases. *Nucl Med Biol* 2009;36:129–135.

85. Das T, Chakraborty S, Sarma HD, et al. (170)Tm-EDTMP: a potential cost-effective alternative to (89)SrCl(2) for bone pain palliation. *Nucl Med Biol* 2009;36:561–568.

86. Silberstein EB. Teletherapy and radiopharmaceutical therapy of painful bone metastases. *Sem Nuc Med* 2005;35:152–158.

87. Nair N. Relative efficacy of 32P and 89Sr in palliation of skeletal metastases. *J Nucl Med* 1999;40:256–261.

88. Roque I, Figuls M, Martinez-Zapata MJ, et al. Radioisotopes for metastatic bone pain. *Cochrane Database Syst Rev* 2011;(6):CD003347.

89. Spratt DE, Zaki BI, Hartford AC, et al. ACR practice parameter for the performance of therapy with unsealed radiopharmaceutical sources. *Clin Nucl Med* 2016;41:106–117.

90. Lutz S, Balboni T, Jones J, et al. Palliative radiation therapy for bone metastases: update of an ASTRO evidence-based guideline. *Pract Radiat Oncol* 2017;7:4–12.

91. Mattsson S, Johansson L, Jonsson H, et al. Radioactive iodine in thyroid medicine—how it started in Sweden and some of today's challenges. *Acta Oncol* 2006;45:1031–1036.

92. International Atomic Energy Agency. *Nuclear Medicine in Thyroid Cancer Management: A Practical Approach*. Vienna, Austria: International Atomic Energy Agency, 2009.

93. Kulkarni K, Van Nostrand D, Atkins F. 131-I ablation and treatment of well-differentiated thyroid cancer. In: Speer TW, ed. *Targeted Radionuclide Therapy*. Philadelphia: Lippincott Williams & Wilkins, 2011:281–293.

94. Reiners C, Dietlein M, Luster M. Radio-iodine therapy in differentiated thyroid cancer: indication and procedure. *Best Pract Res Clin Endocrinol Metab* 2008;22:989–1007.

95. Hay ID, McConahey WM, Goellner JR. Managing patients with papillary thyroid carcinoma: insights gained from the Mayo Clinic's experience of treating 2,512 consecutive patients during 1940 through 2000. *Trans Am Clin Climatol Assoc* 2002;113:241–260.

96. Vianello F, Mazzarotto R, Mian C, et al. Clinical outcome of low-risk differentiated thyroid cancer patients after radioiodine remnant ablation and recombinant human thyroid-stimulating hormone preparation. *Clin Oncol* 2012;24:162–168.

97. Mayson SE, Yoo DC, Gopalakrishnan G. The evolving use of radioiodine therapy in differentiated thyroid cancer. *Oncology* 2015;88:247–256.

98. Goldsmith SJ. Radioactive iodine therapy of differentiated thyroid carcinoma: redesigning the paradigm. *Mol Imaging Radionucl Ther* 2017;26:74–79.

99. Mazzaferri EL, Kloos RT. Using recombinant human TSH in the management of well-differentiated thyroid cancer: current strategies and future directions. *Thyroid* 2000;10:767–778.

100. Dorn R, Kopp J, Vogt H, et al. Dosimetry-guided radioactive iodine treatment in patients with metastatic differentiated thyroid cancer: largest safe dose using a risk-adapted approach. *J Nucl Med* 2003;44:451–456.

101. Siegel HJ, Luck JV Jr, Siegel M, et al. Advances in radionuclide therapeutics in orthopaedics. *J Am Acad Orthop Surg* 2004;12:55–64.

102. Soroa VE, del Huerto Velazquez Espeche M, Giannone C, et al. Effects of radiosynovectomy with p-32 colloid therapy in hemophilia and rheumatoid arthritis. *Cancer Biotherm Radiopharm* 2005;20:344–348.

103. Young RC, Brody MF, Nieberg RK, et al. Adjuvant treatment for early ovarian cancer: a randomized phase III trial of intraperitoneal 32P or intravenous cyclophosphamide and cisplatin—a gynecologic oncology group study. *J Clin Oncol* 2003;21:4350–4355.

104. Bouchet LG, Bolch WE, Goddu SM, et al. Considerations in the selection of radiopharmaceuticals for palliation of bone pain from metastatic osseous lesions. *J Nucl Med* 2000;41:682–687.

105. Firusian N, Dempke W. An early phase II study of intratumoral P-32 chromic phosphate injection therapy for patients with refractory solid tumors and solitary metastases. *Cancer* 1999;85:980–987.

106. Rosemurgy A, Luzardo G, Cooper J, et al. 32P as adjunct to standard therapy for locally advanced unresectable pancreatic cancer: a randomized trial. *J Gastrointest Surg* 2008;12:682–688.

107. Porter AT, McEwan AJ, Powe JE, et al. Results of a randomized phase-III trial to evaluate the efficacy of strontium-89 adjuvant to local field external beam irradiation in the management of endocrine resistant metastatic prostate cancer. *Int J Radiat Oncol Biol Phys* 1993;25:805–813.

108. Bauman G, Charette M, Reid R, et al. Radiopharmaceuticals for the palliation of painful bone metastasis-a systemic review. *Radiother Oncol* 2005;75:258–270.

109. James ND, Pirrie SJ, Pope AM, et al. Clinical outcomes and survival following treatment of metastatic castrate-refractory prostate cancer with docetaxel alone or with strontium-89, zoledronic acid, or both: the TRAPEZE randomized clinical trial. *JAMA Oncol* 2016;2:493–499.

110. Sartor O. Overview of samarium Sm 153 lexidronam in the treatment of painful metastatic disease of bone. *Rev Urol* 2004;6(Suppl 10):S3–S12.

111. Autio KA, Scer HI, Morris MJ. Therapeutic strategies for bone metastases and their clinical sequelae in prostate cancer. *Curr Treat Options Oncol* 2012;13:174–188.

112. Anderson PM, Wiseman GA, Erlandson L, et al. Gemcitabine radiosensitization after high-dose samarium for osteoblastic osteosarcoma. *Clin Cancer Res* 2005;11:6895–6900.

113. Wilky BA, Loeb DM. Beyond palliation: therapeutic applications of 153Samarium-EDTMP. *Clin Exp Pharmacol* 2013;3:1–20.

114. Parker C, Nilsson S, Heinrich D, et al. Alpha emitter radium-223 and survival in metastatic prostate cancer. *N Engl J Med* 2013;369:213–223.

115. Hoskin P, Sartor O, O'Sullivan JM, et al. Efficacy and safety of radium-223 dichloride in patients with castrate-resistant prostate cancer and symptomatic bone metastases, with or without previous docetaxel use: a prespecified subgroup analysis from the randomized, double-blind, phase 3 ALSYMPCA trial. *Lancet Oncol* 2014;15(12):1397–406.

116. Sartor O, Hoskin P, Coleman RE, et al. Chemotherapy following radium-223 dichloride treatment in ALSYMPCA. *Prostate* 2016;76:905–916.

117. Denis-Bacelar AM, Chittenden SJ, Dearnaley DP, et al. Phase I/II trials of 186Re-HEDP in metastatic castrate-resistant prostate cancer: post-hoc analysis of the impact of administered activity and dosimetry on survival. *Eur J Nucl Med Mol Imaging* 2017;44:620–629.

118. Liepe K, Runge R, Kotzerke J. The benefit of bone-seeking radiopharmaceuticals in the treatment of metastatic bone disease. *J Cancer Res Clin Oncol* 2005;131:60–66.

119. Zhang H, Tian M, Li S, et al. Rhenium-188-HEDP therapy for the palliation of pain due to osseous metastases in lung cancer patients. *Cancer Biother Radiopharm* 2003;18:719–726.

120. Erfani M, Rahmani N, Doroudi A, et al. Preparation and evaluation of rhenium-188-pamidronate as a palliative treatment in bone metastasis. *Nucl Med Biol* 2017;49:1-7.

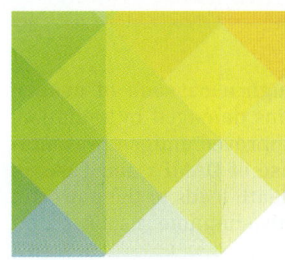

C H A P T E R   3 0

Radiation Therapy and the Immune System

Chandan Guha, James W. Hodge, and Adam P. Dicker

RADIATION AND TUMOR IMMUNITY

Radiation therapy (RT) is an essential component of cancer care that is primarily intended to eliminate tumors and destroy cancer cells through irreparable DNA damage, resulting in cell death or cell cycle arrest. RT may have a palliative or curative effect either by reducing or eliminating tumor burden or by preventing cancer recurrence and metastasis. Whether the intent is cure or palliation, the goal of RT is direct tumor cell killing and/or modulation of tumor or stromal architecture. Radiation, however, is often insufficient to kill all tumor cells in a given mass because of (a) the need to limit damage to healthy tissues, (b) resistance of the tumor cells, and (c) lack of radiation kill at distant (metastatic) sites. Preclinical studies in numerous tumor models have shown that radiation exposure of tumor cells can elicit cell death while inducing some antitumor immunity in a process described as "immunogenic cell death".[1,2] However, in clinical settings, immune responses elicited by radiation only rarely result in protective immunity.[3,4] Full and sustained clinical remissions are elusive for most patients receiving standard-of-care treatment. By contrast, immune-directed therapies can achieve clinical benefit in patients in which conventional therapy has failed. Perhaps, most strikingly, immune-based therapeutics can induce lasting or durable responses in subsets of patients with advanced diseases with no evidence of resistance development. It is expected that the demand for RT in early cancer treatment strategies will greatly increase by 2020 with the increasing age and diversity of the US population.[5] As a result, more innovative and effective RT options need to be developed that can be combined with immunotherapy (IT).

Currently, there is growing interest in combining RT with IT for treatment of a broad range of malignancies, because as monotherapies neither IT nor RT may be sufficient to fully destroy tumors. There is evidence that IT is more beneficial when employed in combination with other standard therapies.[6,7] Radiation can act synergistically with IT to enhance immune responses, inhibit immunosuppression, and/or alter the phenotype of tumor cells, increasing their susceptibility to immune-mediated cytotoxicity.[8] RT can also enhance the potency of cancer vaccine approaches by exploiting the influencing natural antigen presentation pathways that induce sustained antitumor immune responses.[7] However, RT also induces immunosuppressive pathways within the tumor microenvironment that is detrimental to the generation of antitumoral immunity.[9–11]

Cancer cells express unique tumor antigens that include mutated oncoproteins, such as p53 and Ras; unique hybrid proteins expressed from translocated oncogenes, such as bcr-c-abl; and proteins that are expressed during embryogenesis, but are not expressed by normal adult tissues.[12] Some of these "oncofetal" proteins serve as epitopes for host humoral and cellular immune response, which could potentially eradicate cancer cells. The central tenet of T-cell–mediated adaptive immunity is antigen recognition by T-cell receptors (TCR) as peptides on MHC molecules. This depends upon processing of cellular and extracellular proteins by antigen-presenting cells (APCs) and presentation on cell surface MHC molecules. In case of CD8+ cytotoxic T lymphocytes (CTL), these peptides or epitopes are displayed at the cell surface bound to class I MHC molecules that are present in almost all cells. Class I MHC molecules display a "menu" of 8 to 10 amino acids of endogenous peptides that are derived from processing and degradation of cellular proteins in proteasomes and presented directly on the peptide-binding grooves of class I MHC as it is being assembled in the endoplasmic reticulum. Direct antigen presentation of peptides represents mostly degraded "self"-proteins and occasional "foreign" proteins, such as viral antigens from an infected cell or peptides from mutated oncogenes in cancer cells. However, tumors often have central defects in antigen processing and presentation, such as down-regulation of class I MHC molecules, thereby evading recognition by T cells. In contrast to most epithelial cells, professional APCs, such as dendritic cells (DCs), have the capacity to phagocytose exogenous proteins and present them on class II MHC molecules for recognition by CD4+ T cells. In special situations, DCs can phagocytose exogenous proteins but are able to process and transport peptides to the endoplasmic reticulum for cross-presentation on class I MHC molecules. In order to induce an effective antitumoral immunity, first naïve T cells have to be primed by DCs, presenting tumor-derived peptides on class I and II MHC molecules. Upon appropriate priming and activation, CTLs would be able to recognize tumor cells if they present processed peptides on their cell surface class I MHC molecules.

Radiation-Mediated *In Situ* Vaccine

The concept that radiation-induced immune modulation may lead to the conversion of the primary tumor into an *in situ* vaccine was first described in a murine model of metastatic lung cancer where primary tumor irradiation in combination with systemic administration of Flt3 ligand (Flt3L) was able to not only control the primary tumor but result in suppression of metastatic progression and cure.[13] It was proposed that the release of putative tumor neoantigens and danger-associated molecular pattern (DAMP) signals by tumor irradiation (rather than surgical removal), synchronized with increased availability of APCs by expressing Flt3L, should prevent death of the tumor-bearing mice from distant metastasis.[13,14] Subsequently, it was shown that Flt3L can promote the abscopal effects of primary tumor irradiation in a murine breast tumor model.[15] The abscopal effect describes a condition in which the appropriate combination of host factors and tumor phenotype can lead to immune rejection of nonirradiated tumor cells or metastasis following local radiation of the primary tumor. Following irradiation of the tumor, the immune response may contribute not only to a local effect on the tumor but also to systemic rejection of metastases.[5]

Tumor antigens are released from dying tumor cells following treatment with chemotherapy or RT or from necrotic tumor cells from a growing tumor. The tumor antigens and cellular debris are normally engulfed by macrophages and neutrophils, as well as by professional APCs, such as DCs.[16] DCs are normally present as sentinels guarding the portal of entry of pathogens via skin and mucosal surfaces.[17,18] Although DCs are derived from hematopoietic stem cells, it is rarely present in circulating blood. However, systemic administration of cytokines, such as Flt3L and GM-CSF, can induce proliferation of immature DCs.[19,20] Following engulfment of the tumor antigens, the DCs process and present the peptide antigens on MHC molecules at the cell surface. Subsequently, if appropriate "danger" signals are present, the DCs are activated and antigen-loaded DCs migrate to draining lymph nodes. In lymph nodes, DCs interact with naïve CD4+ T helper cells (Th). CD40 ligand (CD40L) expressed at the surface of the helper T cells stimulates the maturation process of the DCs.[21] Costimulatory interaction between mature DCs and the Th cells results in the release of cytokines, such as, IFN-gamma and IL-2, which leads to the proliferation of neo–antigen-specific CD8+ CTL. Furthermore, mature DCs can cross-present tumor antigenic peptides via class I MHC molecules to CD8+ naïve CTLs.[22-24] The CTLs, in turn, infiltrate the tumors at primary as well as metastatic sites, inducing death of the tumor cells.

Radiation-Associated DAMP Signals

Adaptive immune responses are induced and controlled by the innate immune system. Innate immune sensors respond to infectious pathogens or endogenous tissue damage through recognition of pathogen-associated molecular patterns (PAMP) or danger-associated molecular patterns (DAMPs), respectively. Radiation-induced tumor cell death releases tumor antigens and DAMPs, which can stimulate tumor-specific adaptive immune responses.[25]

One of the primary DAMPs, calreticulin (CRT), is exposed on the cell surface at the earliest stage of cell death followed by the well-known inside-out flipping of phosphatidylserine (PS), while at the later stage of apoptosis, cytoplasmic heat shock proteins (HSP) and the nuclear nonhistone high-mobility group box 1 (HMGB1) proteins are released.[26] CRT, PS, and the complement factor C1q serve as signals for phagocytosis by macrophages via binding to the scavenger receptor SRF-1 to facilitate clearance of dying cells and also to activate a proinflammatory immune response.[27,28] HSP60, HSP72, and HMGB1 are DAMPs recognized by the pattern recognition receptor toll-like receptor-4 (TLR-4), which stimulates subtypes of DCs to increase antigen cross-presentation and initiate antitumor cytotoxic responses.[25,29] Natural killer (NK) cell–mediated destruction of tumor cells may also be stimulated through radiation-induced DNA damage pathways via ataxia telangiectasia–mutated (ATM) protein and p53, which up-regulate expression of the nonclassical MHC-I molecules, MIC-A, MIC-B, and ULBP.[30] These proteins are high-affinity ligands to the activating NK cell receptor NKG2D and promote the efficient killing of tumor cells by NK cells. In addition, restoring p53 tumor expression in p53-deficient tumors can produce complete tumor regression due to p53-mediated cellular senescence, followed by up-regulation of inflammatory cytokines and induction of tumor-specific innate immune responses rather than by inducing apoptosis.[25]

Radiation-Enhanced Antigen Presentation

A crucial result of DAMP-induced inflammation is the activation of DCs and enhanced presentation of tumor-associated antigens (TAA) to T cells. According to the current model, tumor cells undergoing immunologic cell death (ICD) release both DAMPs and a variety of TAAs that are taken up, processed, and presented by APCs, primarily mature DCs. CD11c+ myeloid DCs migrate to the tumor-draining lymph node where TAAs to CD4+ T cells are present, which can differentiate to type 1 helper (Th1) T cells and stimulate CD8+ cytotoxic T cells (CTL), NK cells, and innate phagocytic responses. Within the tumor microenvironment, CD8α+ DCs, stimulated by DAMPs, such as HSPs or HMGB1 through TLR4, up-regulate MHC-I antigen cross-presentation, which can directly activate tumor-specific CD8+ CTLs. Radiation exposure promotes alterations of multiple components of antigen presentation, including immunoproteasome subunits, peptide transporters, and protein chaperones to facilitate enhanced MHC-I–associated antigen presentation. RT also modulates the spectrum of peptides associated with MHC class I through a cascade of events, which include degradation of proteins damaged by radiation, increased peptide production, and improved antigen presentation.[31] Thus, the simultaneous release of DAMPs and TAAs in response to RT-induced tumor cell death leads to the powerful amplification of tumor-specific adaptive immune responses.

Antigen Cascade

Radiation promotes antigen cascade, or epitope spreading, described as a fundamental characteristic of the adaptive immune response in which the host responds not only to the specific peptide epitope used in the vaccine but also to other epitopes derived from the same tumor antigen. This phenomenon can also occur in ICD when DCs take up tumor-derived antigenic fragments and cross-present them with MHC class I to CTLs. Antigen cascade has been observed both in preclinical and clinical trials and, in some cases, has led to improved clinical outcome.[32]

Radiation-Induced Tumor Immune Modulation

RT in itself is not always successful at inducing tumor cell death and controlling tumor progression. Intrinsic radiosensitivity of tumor cells and limitations for dose delivery and localization often allow for survival of tumor clonogens. These constraints are sometimes dictated by the need to minimize toxicity of healthy tissue or by the inability of radiopharmaceutical agents to enter the tumor because of poor tumor vascularization.[28] Although sublethal doses of radiation by definition are unable to induce complete cell death, numerous studies have established that lower doses of radiation can initiate a wide range of phenotypic changes in the surviving tumor cell population that collectively enhance their susceptibility to CTL-mediated killing, a process termed immunogenic modulation (IM).[7]

Primary characteristics of radiation-induced IM include the up-regulation of intercellular adhesion molecules, proapoptotic TNF family member receptors, and various costimulatory molecules, the down-regulation of antiapoptotic and prosurvival genes, and an overall increase in tumor antigen presentation.[5] Increased expression of adhesion molecules, such as intercellular adhesion molecule 1 (ICAM-1/CD54) and lymphocyte function–associated antigen 3 (LFA-3/CD58), enhances the ability of CTLs to form stable immunologic synapse and kill the targets via granzyme/perforin release. Expression of the TNF receptor family member Fas/CD95 further augments killing through interaction of Fas ligand expressed on CTLs. Radiation exposure also increases expression of a broad spectrum of molecules associated with antigen presentation, such as MHC-I surface expression, the chaperone proteins CRT and calnexin, and the production of TAAs, including carcinoembryonic antigen (CEA), mucin-1 (MUC-1), HER-2/*neu*, p53, and CA125. The final effect is increased loading of TAA peptides into MHC-I complexes that are recognized by tumor-reactive CTLs. Expression of costimulatory ligands such as B7-1 and B7-2, OX-40L, and 4-1BBL is also increased in irradiated human tumor cells[33,34] and critical to overcome tumor-specific anergy and sustain productive CTL responses.[35] Some of these costimulatory molecules have also been associated with reduced levels of regulatory T cells (Tregs), which may play an additional role in curbing immunosuppression.[35] Figure 30.1 illustrates the radiation-induced phenotypic changes of tumor cells during ICD or IM and how these changes can ultimately be exploited by a variety of immunotherapy (IT)treatment strategies that enhance tumor-specific effector responses.

Radiation-Induced Activation of Inflammatory Cytokines

Inflammatory cytokines are induced in tumor and stromal cells after genotoxic stress of RT. The efficacy of RT-induced tumor ablation requires the activation of type I interferon (IFN) expression in tumor-infiltrating DCs[36] via cytosolic DNA sensor

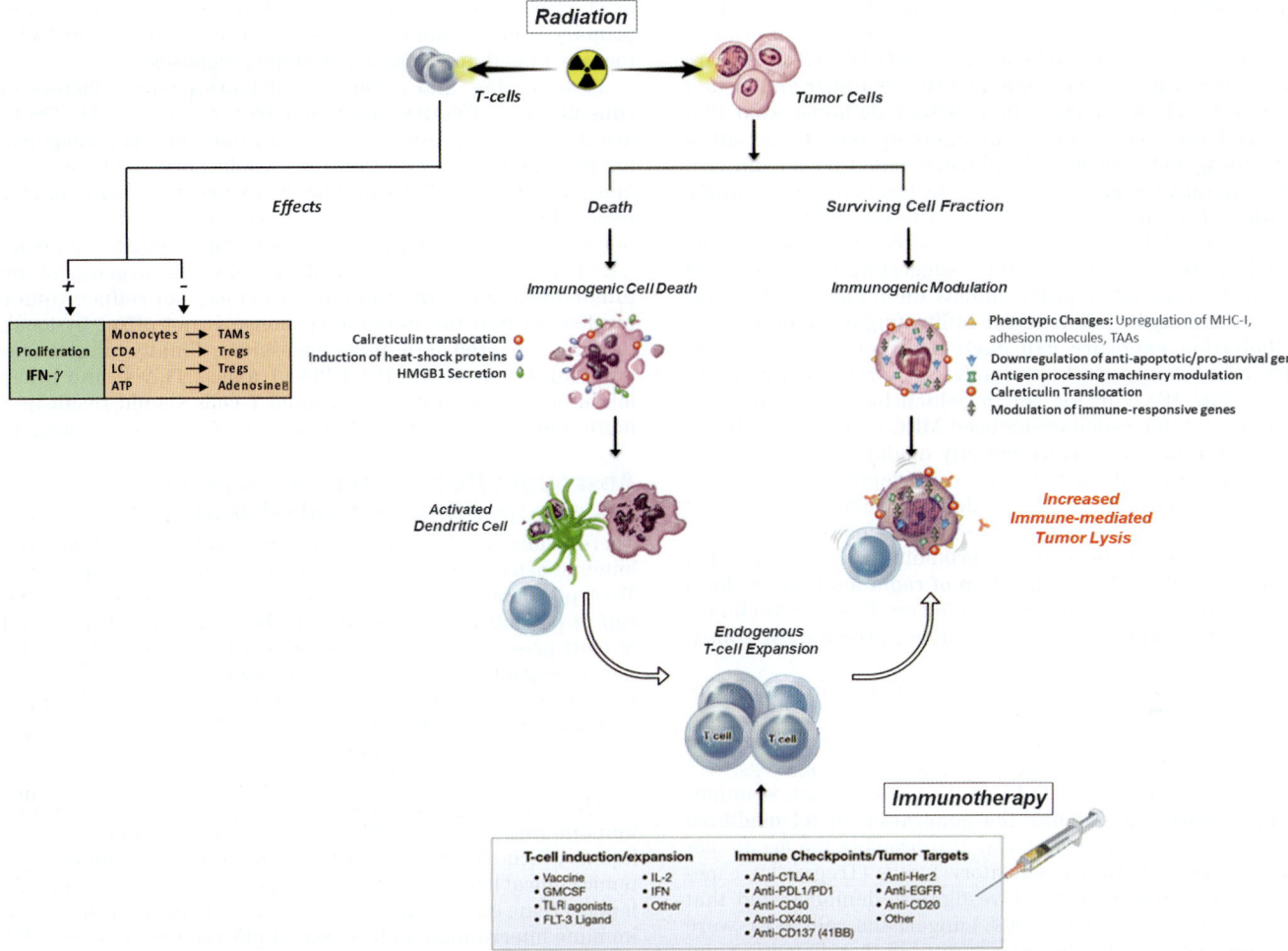

FIGURE 30.1. Radiation-induced immunogenic modulation may synergize with immunotherapy to effectively treat cancer. RT has been shown to increase T-cell proliferation as well as increase IFN-γ secretion. RT has also been shown to mediate negative effects on T-cell function: (1) RT-induced C-C chemokine receptor-2–expressing monocytes can be converted to immunosuppressive tumor-associated macrophages (TAMs) in the microenvironment; (2) RT-induced TGFβ expression could convert infiltrating CD4 T cells to suppressive regulatory T cells (Tregs); (3) RT-induced Langerhans cells (LC) could promote Tregs; and (4) ATP released from dying tumor cells could be catabolized to adenosine, which supports Treg function. On the tumor side, RT modalities can induce a myriad of phenotyping changes in tumor cells that make them more susceptible to CTL-mediated lysis. Such changes can ultimately be exploited by a variety of immunotherapy treatment strategies that enhance tumor-specific effector responses.

cyclic GMP-AMP (cGAMP) synthase (cGAS) mediated sensing of DNA from irradiated tumor cells in DCs.[37] Many tumor cells evade immunosurveillance by inhibiting cytosolic DNA sensing in DCs. For example, tumor cells express CD47 that acts as a "do-not-eat-me" signal for DCs. Inhibition of the CD47-signal regulatory protein alpha (SIRPalpha) axis by CD47 blockade activates NADPH oxidase NOX2 in DCs, thereby reducing the degradation of tumor mitochondrial DNA (mtDNA). mtDNA was recognized by cGAS in the DC cytosol, contributing to type I IFN production and antitumor adaptive immunity.[38] Recently, it was shown that a DNA exonuclease Trex1 was induced in some tumor cells after exposure to high-dose fractions (>12 to 18 Gy) of RT that attenuated their immunogenicity by degrading cytosolic DNA.[39] The cytosolic DNA sensor, cGAS, and its downstream effector, stimulator of interferon genes (STING), localize in micronuclei that are formed in irradiated cells after cell cycle progression through mitosis following double-stranded DNA breaks.[40] Inhibition of mitosis and micronuclei formation and/or cGAS–STING pathway impaired IFN signaling in tumor cells with loss of systemic tumor response after combination of RT and immune checkpoint blockade.[40] However, it is critical to note that there are redundant pathways for the activation of pattern recognition receptors (PRR) in tumor cells. For example, exosomal transfer of POL3-driven

expression of endogenous RNA, RN7SL1, from stromal fibroblasts to breast cancer cells activates the PRR RIG-I and drives an inflammatory response that enhances tumor growth, metastasis, and therapy resistance.[41,42]

THE RATIONALE OF COMBINING RT WITH IT

The rationale for combining RT and IT rests on the premise that ionizing radiation cannot only induce cell death directly but can also invoke an inflammatory response in tumor cells that will foster TAA presentation to overcome immunotolerance and stimulate a systemic immune response.[6,43,44] Evidence suggests that immune-mediated abscopal effect can be induced through a combined strategy of RT and immunotherapies, including effector cell enhancement, checkpoint inhibitors, and tumor vaccines. Radiation dose and timing are crucial elements that determine the effectiveness of tumor immunity.[6]

Local Tumor Control following RT
Traditional view of local tumor control of irradiated tumors is thought to be mediated by radiation-induced cytotoxicity. However, several investigators demonstrated that RT-induced

local tumor ablation largely depends upon T-cell immunity.[45,46] Ablative RT dramatically increases DC-induced T-cell priming in draining lymph nodes with activation of CD8+ CTLs that are essential in eradication of both the primary tumor and distant metastasis. These investigators further demonstrated that ablative RT-induced antitumoral immunity and tumor control were abrogated by conventional fractionated RT or adjuvant chemotherapy but greatly amplified by local IT.[46] Interestingly, addition of fractionated RT (3Gy × 10) to an ablative single-dose (30 Gy) RT abolished tumor control, even though the total dose was increased to 60 Gy, suggesting that protracted standard fractionation of RT inhibits the induction of antitumoral immunity by killing tumor-infiltrating lymphocytes.[45]

Radiation exposure can elicit a direct effect on MHC expression; however, TAAs stimulated by radiation can also up-regulate IFN-γ in the tumor, which has been shown to be necessary for radiation-induced MHC expression.[25] It has also been reported that RT directly modifies the phenotype of tumor cells making them more susceptible to immune-mediated cytotoxicity.[47] It has further been demonstrated that radiation promotes changes in the tumor microenvironment that reduce tumor burden and promote greater infiltration of effector cells.[48] The combination of radiation-induced local inflammation and tumor-specific effector T cells can change the tumor vasculature and phenotype, providing a robust mechanism of tumor control.

However, some reports have shown increased immunosuppressive properties of RT that include decrease in IL-12 production, leading to a negative effect on antigen presentation and an increase in the number of tumor-infiltrating Tregs.[25] RT induces the activation of TGFβ in the tumor, which is immunosuppressive and inhibits the generation of RT-mediated *in situ* tumor immunity.[49] RT can also promote the accumulation of tumor-infiltrating regulatory T cells (Treg cells), especially in melanoma.[9] These investigators demonstrated that specialized tissue-resident DCs, Langerhans cells (LC), were resistant to cell death after exposure to IR. Irradiated LCs up-regulated class II MHC molecules, migrated to draining lymph nodes, and primed the proliferation of immunosuppressive Tregs after RT. As explained above, activation of DCs is a critical effector of anti-tumoral immunity, as DCs take up antigens from dying tumor cells and present them to T cells. However, macrophages also recognize and phagocytose dying tumor cells and can rapidly remove tumor antigens from the microenvironment. Because macrophages cannot cross-present TAA with MHC class I, phagocytic clearance of tumor cells may actually enhance regrowth of tumor cells through caspase 3–dependent stimulating signals and cancel out potential beneficial local and systemic immunostimulatory effects of ICD.[25] Therefore, one has to promote the immunostimulatory properties while inhibiting the immunosuppressive features of RT[11] for effective induction of antitumoral immunity and tumor control.

Systemic Tumor Control following RT

As previously discussed, radiation-induced immune modulation can lead to the abscopal effect, which can, not only eliminate irradiated primary tumors but also reduce the growth of secondary unirradiated tumors or render them more susceptible to further treatment strategies. TAAs may be weakly immunogenic because of the inherent tolerance of the adaptive immune system to self-antigens. RT may contribute to the breakdown of tolerance to endogenous TAAs.[7] In addition, RT-associated novel TAAs can include somatically mutated proteins, which are presented as neoantigens that could induce stronger cytotoxic responses, establishing a novel strategy for personalized tumor vaccination.[6] To overcome challenges of local deficiency of APCs in the tumor microenvironment, strategies to increase functional APCs in combination with RT are being developed to enhance tumor-specific immune response. The timing of administering a second form

of IT relative to RT can be critical, as complete ablation of primary tumors could consequently remove the novel TAAs, thereby impeding sustained immune responses.[6]

Dose, timing, and schedule of RT are primary factors to consider for effective combined treatment with IT. There are many opportunities in the antitumor immune response for therapeutic intervention that would potentially enhance immune response. For example, cytokines and costimulatory molecules to enhance antigen presentation and CTL function can be introduced into the tumor environment following RT.[33] Further, physical, chemical, or molecular targeting of the tumor mass following immune response can reduce tumor burden, so that the immune response is not offset by local, tumor-associated immunosuppression.[6] Finally, pharmacologic inhibition of the PD-1/PD-L1 axis, CTLA-4, and other inhibitory checkpoints on activated T cells should result in a more intense and sustained tumor-specific immune response.

Abscopal Effects Versus Survival in RT–Immunotherapy Clinical Trials

There is substantial clinical evidence of effective radiation-induced immune activation.[7] It has also been shown that tumor-specific T-cell populations were significantly increased in most colorectal cancer patients after completion of chemoradiation therapy and in most prostate cancer patients after RT. An increased population of Treg infiltration following treatment in colorectal patients potentially suggests that there is a threshold above which immunosuppressive side effects may prevail. Still, a beneficial abscopal effect has been reported in melanoma, lymphomas, hepatocellular carcinoma, and certain adenocarcinomas.[5]

These findings indicate that RT effectively stimulates immune responses through radiation-induced immune modulation, which as a result can translate into both local and systemic clinical benefits. Still, if the tumor burden is large enough, it may create enough immunosuppression to prevent successful immune intervention. In this case, studies suggest that local RT can also sufficiently reduce tumor burden to allow for further therapeutic intervention by IT, such as tumor vaccination or checkpoint blockade of inhibitory molecules.[5] By enhancing the frequency, magnitude, and character of the immune responses induced by RT with immunomodulatory agents, cancer patients should experience further improved outcomes.

A major impediment to the abscopal effect is that lymphocytes are highly radiosensitive.[50] However, several studies have demonstrated that RT can promote productive immune-mediated responses despite lymphocyte radiosensitivity. Preclinical studies have demonstrated increase of functional T cells that secrete IFN-γ upon tumor-specific peptide stimulation within the draining lymph nodes following tumor exposure to radiation.[50]

Clinical studies have further assessed the relationships between CTL, Tregs, and RT by analyzing levels of survivin in tumor cells following RT. Survivin is associated with tumor radioresistance and proliferation.[51] The results of these studies suggest that despite the radiosensitivity of lymphocytes, productive CTL responses may be enhanced following radiation because of the focal effect of RT, which does not impair systemic immune populations. The abscopal effect is infrequent in the clinical setting, seeming largely dependent on RT dose and timing. In many cases, cancer patients treated with RT do not exhibit a sufficient enough immune response to elicit an improvement of progression-free or overall survival.[5]

RT TECHNIQUES

RT Dose and Fractionation

Traditional RT is considered locally immunosuppressive because of the rapid clearance of radiosensitive lymphocytes that reside within the field of radiation.[25,45] Fractionation lends the ability to administer a therapeutic dose of radiation to cancer cells while minimizing toxicity to surrounding healthy tissue. External beam radiation therapy (EBRT) can be delivered effectively in several ways: as a standard fractionation of 1.8 to 2.0 Gy daily for 5 to 9 weeks or as larger dose with fewer fractions (hypofractionated doses).[5] Preclinical studies have shown that conventional fractionation might diminish the immune response by eliminating infiltrating lymphocytes over time. Therefore, hypofractionated regimens have been favored to be used in combination with IT.

Normal tissue tolerance dictates the dose and fraction size of RT. With large fraction sizes, RT induces immunogenic cell death (ICD) and produces durable complete responses, which is dependent upon radiation-induced antitumoral immunity.[45,46] New RT technologies are being developed to avoid damage to healthy tissue while focusing high-dose heterogeneous radiation on the tumor. This follows the notion that a heterogeneous dose will lead to a similarly heterogeneous response by tumor cells.[8] RT-treated tumor cells can undergo several types of well-defined cell death, including necrosis, mitotic catastrophe, and ICD. However, cells that survive fractionated RT may be more susceptible to IM and therefore become better targets of tumor immunity.[9] As the dose of RT is reduced to avoid normal tissue toxicity, RT induces the cell surface expression of various immunomodulatory molecules that renders the surviving tumor cell susceptible to cytotoxic T-cell attack.[52] Therefore, subablative immunomodulatory RT doses can be combined with IT, such as tumor vaccines[52] and immune checkpoint blockade,[53] to achieve both local and systemic tumor control. It has been shown that from 1 Gy up to 25 Gy dose of radiation induces up-regulation of MHC class I expression in a dose-dependent manner. Irradiation also appears to accelerate degradation of existing proteins, leading to an increased intracellular peptide pool for MHC class I loading. Nonlethal radiation was also shown to activate the mammalian target of rapamycin (mTOR), resulting in increased protein synthesis and availability of peptides for MHC class I loading.[5] The combination of these effects results in elevated TAA presentation on the surface of the tumor, which should further enhance TAA-specific responses. In contrast to RT doses that target the tumor cells, preclinical studies have demonstrated that very low-dose irradiation (0.5 Gy × 4) can reprogram macrophages and stimulate effective T-cell immunity against tumors.[54,55] Such novel low-dose tumor microenvironment modulating RT fractionation is being investigated in clinical trials. In summary, one could consider various RT fractionations as different immunomodulatory drugs with functions ranging from immunogenic ablation and immune modulation of tumor cells to modulation of the stromal cells of the tumor microenvironment.

Ablative Versus Immunomodulatory Doses for Antitumoral Immunity

Ablative RT can be delivered as hypofractionated regimen and in some cases as a single high-dose fraction of RT.[56] Single high-dose RT provides remarkably high rates of control for tumors that are otherwise not controlled by fractionated RT. In such cases, tumor control depends upon activation of acute acid sphingomyelinase-mediated endothelial cell injury.[57,58] Significant changes in vasculature have been observed after radiosurgery where obliteration of abnormal vasculature occurs months after irradiation, but is rarely seen below a single dose of 12 Gy rising with increasing doses above this threshold.[25] In contrast to ablative fractionation of RT, subablative RT fails to control tumor growth because of the recruitment of bone marrow–derived myeloid cells and vasculogenesis, partly mediated by HIF-1–dependent stromal cell–derived factor-1 (SDF-1) and its receptor, CXCR4.[59,60] Interestingly, the myeloid cells recruited in the tumor microenvironment by hypoxia-induced up-regulation

of SDF-1 are immunosuppressive, and inhibition of CXCR4 using an inhibitor, AMD3100, inhibited tumor regrowth and lung metastasis and potentiated anti–programmed death receptor-1 immunotherapy in sorafenib-treated hepatocellular carcinoma in mice.[61] The circulating myeloid cell numbers are directly linked with tumor burden, and it correlates with primary tumor progression and recurrence. Ablative RT of tumors leads to a decline of the circulating myeloid cells and a decrease in spleen size in animals, indicating that RT may open a therapeutic window for IT at the time of minimal myeloid-induced immunosuppression.[62]

The role of dose fractionation, particularly single-fraction versus hypofractionated RT, in mediating abscopal effects of combination therapy of RT and anti–CTLA-4 immune checkpoint blockade was studied in two murine models of solid tumors, breast and colon cancer.[53] In this report, fractionated RT (8 Gy × 3, or 6 Gy × 5 fractions in consecutive days) but not single-dose RT (20 Gy × 1) induced an abscopal effect when combined with anti–CTLA-4 therapy. These investigators further discovered that high doses (>12 to 18 Gy) of RT fail to induce an abscopal effect in combination with anti–CTLA-4 checkpoint blockade because of the breakdown of intratumoral cytosolic DNA by an exonuclease, Trex, which is induced in some tumor cells with higher doses of RT.[39] Thus, the expression of Trex after radiation exposure may guide the selection of RT dose and fractionation for IT. Despite these observations, it should be noted that the dose of RT selected in these reports was not ablative, and although abscopal effects were reported, the investigators did not describe the effect of these fractionation schedules on survival from spontaneous metastatic progression in these experiments. Thus, it would be prudent to test all types of RT fractionation in combination with clinical trials of RT and IT.

Partial Tumor Irradiation: Spatially Fractionated GRID Radiotherapy

Traditional methods of RT may not fully cover tumor burden at the maximum prescribed radiation dose because of the heterogeneity of tumor burden or possible toxicity to surrounding healthy tissue. Spatially fractionated GRID radiotherapy (SFGRT) is designed to partially cover the tumor volume with the prescribed dose of radiation in order to deplete local tumor burden and stimulate systemic immune response.[5] This was first achieved using 2-dimensional grid fields with orthovoltage beams allowing spatially alternated dose distribution. By using this approach, primarily for treatment of cancers with bulky tumors, successful clinical responses have been reported. Preclinical studies using this method have reported abscopal effects, suggesting that the SFGRT tumors may have elicited inhibitory factors through immune cells preventing tumor growth.[5]

More recent preclinical studies have used SFGRT modified as 3-D GRID in a similar scheme to compare effects of high-dose RT directed at total tumor volume versus partial tumor volumes. It was shown that high-dose RT directed to partial tumor volumes may produce immune stimulation because irradiating partial tumor volume with focused high-dose beams using lattice RT (3-D SFGRT) might induce secretion of immune-related cytokines and can activate the ceramide pathway to target the nonirradiated intratumoral environment as well as distant metastases.[63]

Types of RT

Photon RT

RT is traditionally delivered by photons, or x-rays. These particles are pure energy without mass. Because photon radiation is highly penetrating and peak radiation is deposited immediately upon entry into tissue, radiation is delivered to surrounding tissues as well as the tumor, also releasing a high exit energy. Although an effective strategy of reducing or eliminating local tumors, this type of irradiation cannot easily limit damage to healthy tissues.[64]

Particle RT

In contrast to photon RT, particle therapy deposits lower energy upon tissue entry and generates Bragg peak radiation that can be targeted primarily to the tumor. As the particles travel deeper into the tissue and progressively lose speed, the radiation dose they deliver to the surrounding tissue gradually increases. When they eventually stop at the tumor, a peak energy dose is released, also known as the Bragg peak.[65] Because of its ability to selectively target tumor tissue, proton radiation is particularly favorable in situations where it is necessary to limit the damage to adjacent healthy tissue. Recent advances in carbon ion radiotherapy (CIRT) have demonstrated an ability to deliver high linear energy transfer in a focused dose with the larger mass of carbon resulting in a decreased beam scattering, yielding a sharper, more focused dose distribution. Compared with traditional photon therapy, CIRT has less cell cycle–related radiosensitivity. These characteristics show promise for future developments in potential combination treatment strategies.[66,67] Preclinical evidence for induction of systemic antitumoral immunity by carbon ion RT has been reported in mouse models.[68–70] Both photon radiation and heavy particle radiation have already demonstrated significant antitumor efficacy and have been shown to capably increase CTL lysis of prostate, breast, and lung tumor cells regardless of their p53, triple-negative, or K-Ras mutational status.[28] Both forms of RT delivery have demonstrated immune-mediated cytotoxicity of tumors in preclinical studies, and although in early stages, all three forms of RT may demonstrate effective tumor control in various combinations with IT.

Heavy particle RT may also be administered via radiopharmaceuticals. Radium-223 dichloride (^{223}Ra) has recently received approval from the U.S. Food and Drug Administration (FDA) for the treatment of bone metastases in metastatic castration-resistant prostate cancer (mCRPC), and it is now being studied in other forms of cancers that metastasize to bone. Because of its chemical similarity to calcium, ^{223}Ra forms complexes with the bone mineral hydroxyapatite at areas of increased osteoblastic activity.[64] This drug is now the preferred radionuclide for cancer therapy over the beta emitters strontium-89 (^{89}Sr) and samarium-153–EDTMP (Quadramet, ^{153}Sm), which fail to extend overall survival of patients with multifocal bone metastases.[71] Alpha particles are positively charged heavy particles, whereas beta particles are much smaller and take the form of either electrons or positrons. As a result, ^{223}Ra can deliver a greater dose of radiation in a more localized manner.[64] This is due to its shorter path length in soft tissue and bone and its higher linear energy transfer, which can be 2 to 3 orders of magnitude greater than that of beta emitters, leading to a higher frequency of complex DNA breaks that are more difficult to repair.

STRATEGIES TO COMBINE RT WITH IT

RT can be applied to several different IT strategies, including the use of costimulatory agonists and checkpoint inhibitors, cancer vaccines, and adoptive cell transfer (ACT) methods to boost effector immune responses and generate long-lasting antitumor immunologic memory. These strategies, when combined with RT, may be especially beneficial for patients who have failed RT alone or who have limited treatment options. Immunosurveillance mechanisms continuously eliminate tumor cells expressing mutated peptides on the cell surface class I MHC. During this process of immunoediting, tumors continue to evolve to evade T cells through a process of immune escape, suppression, and eventually co-option.[72]

For cancer cure, ablative treatments, such as RT, have to be combined with IT so that an effective antitumoral immunity is generated and sustained to restore the cancer immunosurveillance network. A framework for combining RT with IT can be studied as part of the cancer immunity cycle,[73] where release of TAA from irradiated tumor cells could drive the process. The various steps of the RT-mediated cancer immunity cycle include (1) RT-induced release of cancer antigens (TAA), (2) antigen presentation by CD103+ DCs, (3) T-cell priming and activation in draining lymph nodes, (4) trafficking of activated T cells from DLN to blood, (5) infiltration of T cells into tumors, and (6) recognition and killing of cancer cells. For steps 1 and 2, RT and various tumor vaccines can be combined with immune adjuvants, including TLR agonist, STING ligands, and agonist anti-CD40. For step 3, agonistic antibodies that augment T-cell activation, such as anti-OX40, anti-CD27, and anti-CD137; cytokines, such as IL2 and IL12; as well as immune checkpoint blockade, such as anti–CTLA-4 that acts in the immune priming phase, can be combined. To improve T-cell infiltration in tumors (steps 4 and 5), lowdose regimens of RT and anti-VEGF therapy can be applied. And finally, to improve cancer cell recognition and killing by tumor-infiltrating CTLs (step 6), epigenetic modulation could overcome immune ignorance and escape in tumor cells by inducing antigen presentation and class I MHC expression. At this stage, immune checkpoint blockade with anti-PD1, anti–PD-L1, anti-Tim3, and anti-LAG3 could overcome tumorevasive strategies and reinvigorate exhausted T cells, in order to sustain a robust antitumoral immune response.

Dendritic Cell Vaccines

Dendritic cells (DCs) are the regulatory cornerstones of the immune system and, therefore, are highly attractive cellular targets of immunization.[74,75] The desired TAA can be introduced into DCs by either loading with a TAA-derived peptide, protein, or TAA-reactive anti-idiotype Ab; infecting with a viral vector, which encodes the TAA or its fragments; loading with apoptotic bodies from tumor cells; or fusing directly with a tumor cell.[76–78] However, there are major time and cost constraints hindering this process. Large amounts of peripheral blood mononuclear cells (PBMCs) must be obtained from the patient via leukopheresis. DC precursors must be purified and maintained in culture several days with cytokine supplementation. The cells must be reinfused into the patient following antigen exposure/loading. This is a highly individualized and laborious procedure. However, a successful strategy approved by the FDA involves immunization with sipuleucel-T (Provenge; Dendreon), an autologous DC vaccine loaded *ex vivo* with a recombinant fusion protein consisting of the tumor antigen prostatic acid phosphatase (PAP) linked to GM-CSF for patients with mCRPC.[79,80]

Various clinical trials have shown increased tumor immunity by DC vaccines in combination with RT. One phase I study evaluated the combination of RT plus injection of autologous immature DCs in 14 patients with advanced-stage/metastatic hepatoma and demonstrated improved tumor-specific immune responses in 7 out of 10 assessable patients.[81] Another recent trial reported results from 40 patients treated with an autologous DC-based vaccine in combination with conformal RT who had recurrent, metastatic, or locally advanced tumors of the head and neck, pancreas, lung, esophagus, or uterus. Results from this study also showed that the combination of DC-based vaccine and RT induces valuable clinical responses.[82]

The systemic effect of RT through DC expansion was demonstrated in a preclinical murine model of metastatic lung cancer and hepatocellular carcinoma using direct stimulation of DC proliferation by Fms-like tyrosine kinase receptor 3 ligand (Flt3L).[13,83] Expansion of the DC compartment with Flt3L in combination with RT augmented antitumor immunity. In follow-up studies, it was shown that the addition of CD40L to the radiation and Flt3L regimen increased the long-term survival of the treated mice to 84%.[84] Similar results were reported in lymphoma and mammary carcinoma studies, indicating that radiation enhanced the systemic effect of this IT in a broad range of tumors.

Tumor Vaccines (Viral, Bacterial, and Plasmid Vectors)

Advantages of vector-based vaccines include the ability of multiple genes (including genes for costimulatory molecules and cytokines) to be inserted, their economical aspects compared with other modes of therapy, their ability to infect APCs so that the antigens they express can be efficiently processed and presented, and the characteristic of viral and bacterial vectors to act as natural adjuvants, which can stimulate the host's immune response. Known limitations of these approaches include the development of host-induced immunity to the vector itself and safety concerns related to live vectors derived from originally virulent human pathogens.[32]

Viral Vectors

One of the most studied groups of vaccine vectors is the poxvirus group. Vaccinia virus, which was derived from a benign pox disease in cows, has been administered to more than 1 billion people and is responsible for the worldwide eradication of smallpox. As a result, smallpox vaccinations in the United States and most Western countries were halted approximately 40 years ago. However, most cancer patients are older than 40 and, therefore, have some level of pre-existing immunity to vaccinia virus.[32] For this reason, recombinant vaccinia viruses cannot be given multiple times in vaccine protocols. The poxvirus family contains the replication-incompetent modified vaccinia Ankara (MVA), a derivative of vaccinia virus. MVA is thought of as a safer alternative to the smallpox vaccine because it can infect mammalian cells but cannot replicate. Other replication-defective members of the poxvirus family are the avipox vectors (fowl pox and canarypox/ALVAC). These avipox vectors infect human cells and express their transgenes for 2 to 3 weeks before cell death; they are incapable of reinfecting cells. Clinical studies have shown that avipox-based CEA vectors can be given to patients numerous times with a resulting increase in CEA-specific T-cell responses. Preclinical and clinical studies show that optimal use of recombinant vaccinia or MVA may be to prime the immune response, followed by boosting vaccinations with other vectors such as replication-defective pox vectors, peptides, or DNA.

Advantages of using vaccinia virus or the replication-incompetent MVA avipox are[7] large amounts of foreign DNA can be inserted into the vector and[5] proteins expressed in poxviruses are more immunogenic than the native protein, which is most likely a result of the inflammatory responses triggered against highly immunogenic poxvirus proteins. Several clinical trials with recombinant poxviruses containing TAAs such as CEA, MUC-1, PSA, and HPV have been completed, and others are ongoing.[32] In clinical trials, PANVAC (poxvirus-based vaccine encoding the tumor antigens CEA and MUC-1, along with three T-cell costimulatory molecules; TRICOM) demonstrated high progression-free survival relative to control groups.[85]

Adenovirus has also been proposed as a vector in recombinant vaccine design because its viral genome can be altered to accept foreign genes that are stably integrated. To produce recombinant adenovirus vectors, endogenous viral DNA sequences are typically deleted from replication-competent regions, which results in an attenuated form of the virus with potentially improved safety. A new viral vector gene delivery platform, adenovirus serotype-5 (Ad5) [E1-, E2b-], has been described. Human cells transfected with these adenovirus constructs were shown to express the encoded transgene(s)

for more prolonged time *in vivo* compared to other adenovirus vector platforms.[86] In a phase I/II clinical trial, cohorts of patients with metastatic colorectal cancer (mCRC) were vaccinated with escalating doses of the adenovirus vector carrying a gene for the GI and liver cancer–associated CEA. CEA-directed T-cell responses were induced and patients exhibited evidence of a favorable survival probability.[32]

Yeast and Bacterial Vectors

Recombinant *Saccharomyces cerevisiae* is attractive as a vaccine vector because of its nontoxic and nonpathogenic characteristic. In addition, this recombinant yeast can be engineered in large batches to express multiple antigens. *S. cerevisiae* can be propagated and purified quickly, easily, and stably. Further, it has been shown to stimulate a robust immune response from the host to non–self-antigens. Bacterial vectors, derived from intracellular pathogens, such as *Salmonella* and *Listeria*, are advantageous for their natural ability to infect APCs, such as macrophages. Once the bacterial vector is inside the cell, the exogenous tumor antigen is processed and presented with MHC class I through the natural endogenous peptide MHC class I presentation pathway without the requirement for antigen cross-presentation. Although these bacteria are potentially virulent in humans, several attenuated strains have been developed for safe clinical use.[32]

Plasmid DNA Vectors

DNA vaccination has emerged as an attractive immunotherapeutic approach against cancer because of its simplicity, stability, and safety. Results from numerous clinical trials have demonstrated that DNA vaccines are well tolerated by patients, do not trigger major adverse effects, and act as effective adjuvant CpG DNA patterns that can stimulate plasmacytoid DCs and B cells through TLR9. DNA vaccines are also very cost-effective and can be administered repeatedly for long-term protection. Despite all the practical advantages, DNA vaccines face challenges in inducing potent antigen-specific cellular immune responses as a result of immunotolerance against endogenous self-antigens in tumors. Strategies to enhance immunogenicity of DNA vaccines against self-antigens are currently being developed.[2,24]

RNA Vectors

RNA vaccines employ mRNA transcribed *in vitro* by a bacteriophage RNA polymerase and template DNA for the antigen(s) of interest. The mRNA is translated directly into the cytoplasm of host cells, and the antigens are presented to APCs in order to stimulate an immune response. DCs may also be loaded with mRNA of TAAs or tumor RNA for a more specialized response. Some RNA molecules can act as PAMP or DAMP and thereby exhibit adjuvant effects.

RNA vaccines have been employed in studies where expression of checkpoint inhibitors, such as PD-1, is silenced utilizing siRNA, showing improved vaccine efficacy. Further, RNA vaccines increased DC function in studies where tumor antigen mRNA with mRNA encoding for checkpoint molecules such as CTLA-4 and GITR were cotransfected, resulting in simultaneous TAA presentation and local checkpoint inhibition.[87]

Enhanced Effector Responses by Introduction of Cytokines or Costimulatory Molecules into the Tumor Microenvironment

Induction of antigen-specific T-cell responses requires both antigen presentation and expression of costimulatory molecules, B7-1/2, OX40L, or 41BBL, in DCs that can interact with their cognate ligands/receptors on T cells.[25] Preclinical trials have shown that exposure of human prostate cancer cells to ionizing radiation increased expression of costimulatory ligands OX40L and 41BBL and decreased expression of

PD-L1 molecules at all dose levels, thus enhancing CTL function.[33] These findings prompted the idea of localized expression of costimulatory molecules and/or cytokines within the tumor microenvironment should enhance the efficient activation of effector T cells. Introduction of B7-1/CD80, a costimulatory ligand of both the activating CD28 and inhibitory CTLA-4 receptors, into a tumor enhances antitumor immune responses. Similar positive results were achieved when cell adhesion molecules, such as ICAM-1 and (LFA)-3, were expressed in tumors. In clinical studies, recombinant vectors expressing a trio of costimulatory and cell adhesion molecules (B7-1, ICAM-1, and LFA-3; designated TRICOM) were directly injected into melanoma lesions, which enhanced tumor-specific CTL responses. Cytokines can also be introduced into the tumor mass using delivery vectors, as in the case of a recombinant vaccinia virus expressing GM-CSF directly injected into melanoma lesions.[32]

Tumor arrest and increased overall survival were shown in a murine sarcoma model when RT was administered with an agonistic antibody for OX40, which on activated T cells stimulates T-cell proliferation, effector differentiation, and expansion of the effector memory T-cell populations and also suppresses Treg function.[88] Inhibition of the inhibitory CTLA-4 engagement also enhanced effectiveness of RT in 4T1 murine mammary carcinoma resulting in diminished metastasis and increased survival. However, in this case, RT dose and timing were critical for CTLA-4 inhibition.[25]

A further study combined RT and agonist anti-CD40 antibody to treat B-cell lymphoma.[89] Although CD40 is an essential stimulatory molecule during T-/B-cell collaboration for high-affinity antibody responses, CD40 engagement is also known to play a role in macrophage activation and enhanced phagocytosis. On their own, each monotherapy was ineffective, but when RT and agonistic anti-CD40 were combined, long-term survival was reported.[89]

Recently, it has been shown that STING pathway activation is required in host APCs for spontaneous CD8+ T-cell activity targeting tumor-derived antigens. Production of IFN-β via this pathway contributes to the antitumor effect of radiation, which may be enhanced by adding a STING agonist. An *in vivo* study suggested that direct activation of the STING pathway in the tumor microenvironment by intratumoral injection of specific agonists might be an effective therapeutic strategy to promote wide range T-cell priming against an individual's tumor antigen repertoire.[90] Intratumoral injection of synthetic STING agonists induced significant regression of established tumors in mice and suggested systemic immune responses, which prevented metastases. In separate studies of a murine genetically engineered model of pancreatic cancer, combination of IGRT with a novel STING ligand synergized the control of both local and distant tumors, indicating that inflammatory pathways activated by STING ligands generate a powerful adjuvant activity for enhancing adaptive immune responses to tumor antigens released by RT.[91] Intratumoral injection of STING agonists has demonstrated significant therapeutic effects in multiple mouse tumor models, including melanoma; colon, breast, and prostate cancer; and fibrosarcoma, suggesting that development of novel pharmacologic approaches to target STING activation within the tumor microenvironment deserves attention for clinical translation.[92,93]

Another study, which employed renal carcinoma with bilateral pulmonary metastases in a mouse model, observed that combined local irradiation of one lung with systemic IL-2 therapy reduced the tumor burden in both lungs more than was achieved by either monotherapy alone.[94,95] Local tumor irradiation was also combined with intratumoral injection of a novel immunocytokine, an IL2-linked tumor-specific antibody in preclinical murine models of melanoma, neuroblastoma, and head and neck squamous cell carcinoma.[96] This treatment showed complete regression of established tumors in most

animals associated with an enhanced antibody-dependent cell-mediated cytotoxicity (ADCC) and a tumor-specific memory T-cell response. In mice bearing large primary tumors or disseminated metastases, the investigators administered a triple combination of intratumoral immunocytokine, RT, and systemic anti-CTLA-4 with eradication of large tumors and metastases and improved survival, thereby eliciting an *in situ* vaccination effect deserving potential clinical translation.[96]

Immune Checkpoint Therapy

One of the major impediments to tumor IT is the natural ability of most tumors to escape immune responses. Unlike most infectious immunity, tumor immunity must be continuously active for a long period of time, which frequently results in exhaustion of both CD4+ and CD8+ tumor-reactive T cells. Exhaustion is mediated by negative inhibitory interactions whereby either costimulatory ligands, such as B7-1/B7-2, bind to inhibitory receptor CTLA-4 or dedicated inhibitory receptors bind their cognate inhibitory ligands, as with PD-L1/PD-L2 to PD1, B7-H3 to Lag3, or Galectin to TIM3.[25] Targeted inhibition or activation of these interactions can be achieved with monoclonal antibodies (mAbs). To prevent CTL exhaustion, immune checkpoint mediators, such as CTLA-4 and PD1, on T cells and PD-L1, on tumor cells, are targeted with blocking antibodies.[97] Experimental evidence suggests that anti–CTLA-4 mAb facilitates T-cell proliferation and activation in the early phases of the response and reduces the suppressive function of Tregs. Clinical evidence has shown that fractionated RT combined with ipilimumab, an anti–CTLA-4 mAb, not only delayed tumor growth at the primary site but also significantly delayed tumor metastasis in melanoma patients. Several mAbs are also used in the clinic that block the PD-1/PD-L1/PD-L2 interactions either on T cells (anti-PD1 pembrolizumab) or on tumor cells (anti–PD-L1 avelumab). As PD1 expression is induced later in activated T cells, blockade of this pathway is particularly promising in restoring the functional competence of exhausted T cells.[97]

Fractionated RT could result in PD-L1 up-regulation on tumor cells in a variety of syngeneic mouse models of cancer via a mechanism of adaptive resistance-induced IFN-γ.[98] In a murine model of colon cancer, it was shown that the sequencing of anti–PD-L1 therapy was important for optimal therapeutic outcome, with concomitant but not sequential adjuvant administration with fractionated RT was required to improve survival. However, preclinical studies in murine models have limitations of lack of immunosurveillance in transplantation models. In a recently published phase III randomized clinical trial of consolidation therapy with anti–PD-L1 versus placebo after chemo-RT for stage II non–small cell lung cancer (NSCLC), the progression-free survival was significantly improved despite the use of anti–PD-L1 therapy after the completion of chemo-RT.[99]

Although immune checkpoint inhibitors result in impressive clinical response in a subset of patients, resistance may develop eventually. Optimal results will require combination of several immune checkpoint inhibitors. In a study of RT and anti–CTLA-4 therapy in melanoma, resistance developed due to up-regulation of PD-L1 on melanoma cells accompanied by T-cell exhaustion.[100] This highlighted the importance of combining anti–CTLA-4 and anti–PD-L1 therapy for optimal effects. Subsequent work by these investigators demonstrated that persistent type I and II IFN signaling induced PD-L1–dependent and PD-L1–independent adaptive resistance to immune checkpoint blockade. This resistance developed due to acquisition of a STAT1-related epigenomic changes in tumor cells with expression of IFN-stimulated genes and ligands for multiple T-cell inhibitory receptors, such as TIM3, LAG3, Galectin-9, and TNFRSF14 (HVEM).[101] To overcome adaptive resistance, one could either combine multiple checkpoint inhibitors or pharmacologically inhibit chronic IFN signaling in a temporal fashion.

Adoptive Cell Transfer Approaches

Adoptive cell transfer (ACT) is an innovative new IT approach that involves genetic engineering of the patients' own immune cells to treat their cancer. The two major approaches include generation of TAA-specific TCR-expressing T cells and the creation of TAA-specific chimeric antigen receptor (CAR) T cells. Patient-derived tumor-specific T cells can be isolated *in vitro* by expanding rare populations of the patient's own T cells in the presence of tumor extracts and DCs or by transducing the T cells with genetically engineered TCR reactive with the TAA associated with the patient's MHC haplotype. Although this approach is highly personalized, it is also inherently slow and complicated. Alternatively, T cells can be transduced with a genetically engineered CAR where a TAA-specific antibody is fused to the signaling subunits of the TCR. This strategy takes advantage of the high-affinity, MHC-independent nature of antigen recognition of antibodies, thus opening the way to off-the-shelf, tumor-specific, but not individual patient-restricted, reagents.[102]

CAR T cells have recently shown success in the treatment of therapy-resistant B-cell acute lymphoblastic leukemia (B-ALL) and B-cell lymphoma and have been approved by the FDA for use against B-ALL. Despite the success of CAR T cells in blood cancers, their use to treat solid tumors is challenging, because of inefficient homing of T cells to tumor sites and the shortage of unique solid TAAs.[102] A preliminary study aimed to assess the effect of local irradiation in increasing CAR T-cell infiltration in EGFR-expressing solid tumors using a murine lung cancer model. Increased infiltration of EGFR-CAR T cells was observed in tumors that were irradiated compared to tumors treated with EGFR-CAR T cells alone, suggesting that radiation improved CAR T-cell infiltration, but further research will be needed to demonstrate the broader utility of this promising new technique.

CLINICAL CONSIDERATIONS FOR RT AND THE IMMUNE SYSTEM: LEARNING TO WORK TOGETHER

Radiation therapy can have paradoxical effects on the immune system. We must learn to maximize the anti-cancer immune response when designing radiation treatments.

The excitement generated by the case reports of Postow[103] and others[104] demonstrating an abscopal effect of RT led to an unprecedented excitement of combinations with RT and immune checkpoint blockade. Other work with high-dose IL-2 suggested immune modulation combined with stereotactic body radiation could have significant clinical impact.[105] However, few reports have been able to replicate these dramatic results of Postow with RT and checkpoint inhibitors, which suggests that the clinical trial design may have significant implications when testing these combinations. However, there are retrospective data that suggest the clinical combination of RT and checkpoint inhibitor can have benefit. In this secondary analysis, patients were divided into subgroups to compare patients who previously received radiotherapy with patients who had not. Overall survival with pembrolizumab was significantly longer in patients who previously received any RT than in patients without previous radiotherapy (HR 0.58 [95% CI 0.36 to 0.94], $P = .026$; median overall survival 10.7 months [95% CI 6.5 to 18.9] vs. 5.3 months [2.7 to 7.7]) and for patients who previously received extracranial RT compared with those without previous extracranial RT (0.59 [95% CI 0.36 to 0.96], $P = .034$; median overall survival 11.6 months [95% CI 6.5 to 20.5] vs. 5.3 months [3.0 to 8.5]). Fifteen (63%) of 24 patients who had previously received thoracic RT had any recorded pulmonary toxicity versus 29 (40%) of 73 patients with no previous thoracic RT. Three (13%) patients with previous thoracic RT had treatment-related

pulmonary toxicity compared with one (1%) of those without; frequency of grade 3 or worse treatment-related pulmonary toxicities was similar (one patient in each group). This is one of the few studies that suggest that previous treatment with RT in patients with advanced NSCLC results in longer progression-free survival and overall survival with pembrolizumab treatment than that seen in patients who did not have previous RT, with an acceptable safety profile.[106]

Recently, a phase 3 study compared anti–PD-L1 antibody, durvalumab, as consolidation therapy with placebo in patients with stage II NSCLC who did not have disease progression after two or more cycles of platinum-based chemoradiotherapy.[99] After a 2:1 ratio randomization, the median progression-free survival from randomization was 16.8 months (95% confidence interval [CI], 13.0 to 18.1) with durvalumab versus 5.6 months (95% CI, 4.6 to 7.8) with placebo ($P < .001$), and the 18-month progression-free survival rate was 44.2% versus 27.0%. Without any significant increase in toxicity, the response rate was higher with durvalumab than with placebo (28.4% vs. 16.0%; $P < .001$), and the median duration of response was longer (72.8% vs. 46.8% of the patients had an ongoing response at 18 months). These impressive results will clearly set the new standard of care in NSCLC.

Clinical considerations when combining RT and IT include dose of radiation, fractions of radiation, scheduling of drug and radiation (neoadjuvant, concurrent, adjuvant), radiation field size, and concomitant use of systemic chemotherapy.[107] A review of current clinical trials from ClinicalTrials.gov combining RT and immune modulation reveals 60 trials are focused on either treatment of metastatic disease or localized disease. Within each of those categories, radiation is combined with either CTLA-4, PD-1, or both with a few trials examining the use of GM-CSF, TLR-9 agonist vaccines, or cell-based therapies.

Dose–Response Effect in Radiation Therapy

Today's radiation oncologists were bought up on the concept of "the more the better," encouraged on by Puck's seductive *in vitro* clonogenic cell survival curves that suggest an exponential relationship between radiation dose and cell kill.[108] Clinicians extrapolated these findings into the clinic, pursuing ever-higher radiation doses in the pursuit of local control and the sometimes-elusive cancer cure. In parallel to the concept of increased dose was enlarged radiation field size, seeking to destroy both the gross "macroscopic" tumor and "subclinical disease," especially small but at-risk regional lymph nodes. There is good evidence for the importance of irradiating "high-risk" lymphoid tissue in Hodgkin disease and cervical cancer, but the concept has influenced tumor planning in all cancer sites.

A number of key clinical trials from recent decades have contradicted these concepts. Although clearly a minimal dose of radiation is necessary (e.g., 60 Gy in glioblastoma and non–small cell lung cancer), attempts to escalate doses further have failed to deliver benefit in a range of cancers: esophageal, low-grade glioma, glioblastoma, and most recently non–small cell lung cancer.[109] Furthermore, large radiation fields are often poorly tolerated, especially in the context of concomitant chemotherapy. Theodore Puck succeeded in creating cell survival curves, where more radiation killed more cells, by developing techniques to grow cell monolayers *in vitro*. In doing so, he negated systemic effects and the role of the microenvironment.

What Is the Optimal Field Size? Lessons from Prostate and Pancreatic Cancer

We do not yet know the optimal dose and scheduling of radiation for combination with chemotherapy and IT. In prostate cancer, multiple randomized trials have indeed validated the concept of higher radiation dose achieving better tumor control.[110] However, the utility of larger radiation fields, that is, prophylactic irradiation of the whole pelvis, remains in doubt. A large cooperative group trial (RTOG 9413)[111] enrolled 1,323 patients in a two-by-two randomized trial seeking to assess the role of (1) whole-pelvic radiation compared to prostate radiation only and (2) neoadjuvant hormonal therapy compared to adjuvant therapy. Unfortunately, this trial did not succeed in providing clear answers, possibly because of an unexpected interaction between the size of the radiation field and hormonal therapy.[111] The trial RTOG 0924 is attempting to answer that question, which has still been elusive.

Pinkawa[112] provides important insight regarding why whole-pelvic irradiation may be less beneficial than expected in prostate cancer. Pinkawa et al. retrospectively reviewed hematologic changes during RT for prostate cancer. They noted that (1) RT significantly depressed all blood lineages in peripheral blood, especially lymphocytes, (2) these changes were prolonged—continuing at least 6 to 7 weeks following completion of therapy—(we do not know what happens at later time points), (3) whole-pelvic RT is more detrimental than prostate-only RT, and (4) neoadjuvant hormonal therapy decreased hemoglobin levels. Although endpoints in this study were confined to crude blood counts, we speculate that they reflect a detrimental impact on immune system function and tumor oxygenation, possibly explaining the disappointing results of RTOG 9413. In pancreatic cancer, the group led by Crittenden addressed this by analyzing the effect of neoadjuvant standard fractionated and hypofractionated chemoradiation on immune cells in patients with locally advanced and borderline resectable pancreatic adenocarcinoma. They found that standard fractionated chemoradiation resulted in a significant and extended loss of lymphocytes that was not explained by a lack of homeostatic cytokines or response to cytokines. By contrast, treatment with hypofractionated RT avoided the loss of lymphocytes associated with conventional fractionation.[113]

RT and the Immune System, Obstacles for Working Well Together

After many decades of basic research, the importance of the immune response in preventing and treating cancer is no longer controversial. For many years, we have known that subjects with prolonged immunosuppression are at increased risk of developing cancers.[114-116] More recently, phase III randomized trials have demonstrated the efficacy of IT in metastatic melanoma, lung cancer, head and neck cancer, Hodgkin disease, and renal cell cancer, with trials under way in almost every disease site.

The relationship between RT and the immune system is complex. On the one hand, RT may augment the immune response, for example, by (1) killing cancer cells, increasing the tumor's antigenicity, and (2) rendering surviving tumor cells more susceptible to immune-mediated killing through increased MHC class I presentation. On the other hand, the immune system may help RT, eradicating residual disease inside and outside of the radiation field. The extreme demonstration of these interactions is the occasionally observed phenomenon when radiation can also reduce tumor growth outside the treatment field, the so-called abscopal effect.

As early as 1976, the effect of radiation on lymphocyte populations was appreciated.[117] Work by Stuart Grossman has suggested another mechanism through which radiation may suppress the immune response. They noted that in a range of cancers (high-grade glioma, squamous head and neck cancer, pancreatic adenocarcinoma—in both the locally advanced and adjuvant setting—non–small cell lung cancer), radiation/chemoradiation induces severe treatment-related lymphopenia. Furthermore, they correlated severe lymphopenia with early tumor progression in each of these disease settings.[118-127]

Looking only at crude blood counts may underestimate the effect of cytotoxic therapies on the immune system. Schuler et al.[128] examined lymphocyte subtypes in patients with head and neck cancer undergoing chemoradiation.[128] They found that chemoradiation decreased the overall number of circulating CD4 helper cells, but paradoxically increased the number of CD4+ CD39+ Treg that serves to dampen the immune response. Furthermore, they found that the increase in regulatory T cells persisted years after the conclusion of therapy.

It is often assumed that the effect of RT on peripheral blood counts is the result of bone marrow irradiation, where the normal stem cells are very sensitive to DNA damage. Work by Yovino proposes an alternative mechanism: Lymphopenia is caused by apoptosis of lymphocytes passing through the radiation field.[119] The authors estimate that during 6 weeks of partial brain irradiation in glioblastoma, 99% of lymphocytes receive at least 0.5 Gy, with a mean circulating lymphocyte dose of 2 Gy, sufficient to induce apoptosis in these highly sensitive cells. A molecular mechanism has been suggested by Ellsworth et al.[123] that there is an absence of a compensatory increase in interleukin-7 levels. The failure to mount an appropriate homeostatic cytokine response may be responsible for the prolonged lymphopenia frequently observed in these patients, which may be highly dependent on field size and fractionation as the cytokine change was not observed by others.[113] RT-induced lymphopenia along with tumor-induced granulocytosis contributes to an increase in the neutrophil-to-lymphocyte (NLR) ratio, which has been validated in many studies as an independent prognosticator for overall survival in patients in clinical trials.[129]

Safety of Immune Modulation with RT

A number of reports have shown safety with the combination of immune checkpoint inhibitors and RT across different disease sites (cervix, head and neck, lung, brain[130] cancer, etc.). For single-agent PD-1/PD-L1 or CTLA-4, there appears to be no significant toxicity when added to RT. To date, there are very limited data regarding combinations of checkpoint inhibitors and RT; however, there are dozens of trials currently accruing. The diagnosis and management of immune-related adverse events in combination trials of RT and immune checkpoint blockade deserve special attention.[131]

Modulating the Immune System–Radiation Interaction

For many years, we have down-regulated the immune system by prescribing chemotherapy and steroids during RT. The expanding arsenal of immunomodulators (PD-1 inhibitors, tumor vaccines, ACT therapies) provides us with unprecedented opportunities to modulate and activate the immune system during RT. The challenges are immense, and investigators will need to choose the most appropriate patients, immunomodulators, and radiation therapies in order to succeed. Work by Pinkawa and others[112] informs us that despite the efficacy of RT in prostate cancer, its use is associated with relative lymphopenia and likely immunosuppression.

There is evidence in the metastatic disease space that a combinatorial immune approach would have the highest probability of success. One approach for designing radiation trials would be to use a neoadjuvant trial design to, first, determine optimal response by immune readout in the organ, and peripheral blood in patients with locally advanced disease, and, second, determine the clinical response in an expansion cohort of patients with oligo-/metastatic disease at presentation where appropriate. The following considerations informed the trial design.

Preoperative chemotherapy and chemoradiotherapy are components of standard treatment paradigms for several solid tumors, including muscle invasive bladder cancer (≥T2), invasive breast cancer (≥T2), esophageal cancer (T1bN+ or T2-T4a and/or N+), and rectal cancer (T3 or N+).[132-135] Pathologic responses determined at surgery provide clinical data including sensitivity to chemotherapy, potential need for adjuvant treatment, and for patients with pathologic complete response (pCR) and can correlate with survival.[132] Furthermore, intratumor and stromal molecular, hormonal, immunologic, and other changes, which evolve during preoperative therapy, can be comprehensively evaluated at the organ level following radical surgery and lymph node dissection. Fraction size should be guided by preclinical studies. One should avoid large radiation fields and prophylactic lymph node coverage or find ways to counter the radiation-induced lymphopenia. The schedule of drug and radiation should be based on data-driven preclinical experience. The primary objective for a phase I would be to determine the safety and tolerability of immune modulation combined with radiation. Secondary objectives could include evaluation of intratumoral immune responses and assessment of immune responses in peripheral blood samples. Expansion cohort would be in oligo-/metastatic patients.

Immune Profiling of Patients Undergoing Clinical Trials of RT and IT

Cancer therapy has been dictated by the histopathologic evaluation of tissue samples obtained during biopsy or surgical resection of the primary tumor. Despite traditional tumor staging using the AJCC/UICC-TNM classification, it is now recognized that clinical outcome can significantly vary among patients within the same stage. Several reports have alluded to the significance of the host immune system in controlling tumor progression. Within the same clinical stage, the type, density, and location of immune infiltrate in the tumor tissue could predict for the clinical outcome in patients with colorectal cancer.[136,137] Since this report, the immune infiltrates within tumors have been quantified by a methodology, termed an immunoscore of the tumor.[138,139] While tumor biopsies are critical to define the immunoscore, evaluation of an ongoing antitumoral immunity might require sampling of several biologic compartments, including the tumor, spleen, tumor-draining lymph nodes, bone marrow, and blood.[140] Clinical studies are beginning to define the immune profile of patients that can predict the clinical outcome of combination therapies with IT. While designing clinical trials, tumor and circulating pharmacodynamic correlates of immune modulation should be carefully considered.[141] Although blood-based immune assays are highly valued, novel immune PET imaging is being developed to monitor CD8+ T-cell infiltration in tumors[142,143] and granzyme B PET imaging to assess CTL activity.[144] Studies have also been conducted in mouse models and patients using novel immune PET imaging of PD-L1.[145-148] Finally, PD-L1 expression is being monitored in circulating tumor cells as prognostic factors for survival in patients with head and neck[149] and lung cancer.[150]

Summary

The next generation of clinical trials led by radiation oncologists should tailor their treatments and determine RT dose, fraction, and field size, based not just on tumor-ablative considerations, but also with a view to maximizing the antitumor immune response. This will be guided by a comprehensive immune profile of the patient using functional imaging of the immune effector cells and immune checkpoint molecules, immunoscore of pathology, and circulating pharmacodynamic immune markers.

REFERENCES

1. Obeid M, Panaretakis T, Tesniere A, et al. Leveraging the immune system during chemotherapy: moving calreticulin to the cell surface converts apoptotic death from "silent" to immunogenic. *Cancer Res* 2007;67(17):7941–7944.

2. Panaretakis T, Kepp O, Brockmeier U, et al. Mechanisms of pre-apoptotic calreticulin exposure in immunogenic cell death. *EMBO J* 2009;28(5):578–590.

3. Mantel F, Flentje M, Guckenberger M. Stereotactic body radiation therapy in the re-irradiation situation—a review. *Radiat Oncol* 2013;8:7.

4. Gameiro SR, Caballero JA, Hodge JW. Defining the molecular signature of chemotherapy-mediated lung tumor phenotype modulation and increased susceptibility to T-cell killing. *Cancer Biother Radiopharm* 2012;27(1):23–35.

5. Wattenberg MM, Fahim A, Ahmed MM, et al. Unlocking the combination: potentiation of radiation-induced antitumor responses with immunotherapy. *Radiat Res* 2014;182(2):126–138.

6. Ahmed MM, Hodge JW, Guha C, et al. Harnessing the potential of radiation-induced immune modulation for cancer therapy. *Cancer Immunol Res* 2013;1(5):280–284.

7. Kwilas AR, Donahue RN, Bernstein MB, et al. In the field: exploiting the untapped potential of immunogenic modulation by radiation in combination with immunotherapy for the treatment of cancer. *Front Oncol* 2012;2:104.

8. Sharp HJ, Wansley EK, Garnett CT, et al. Synergistic antitumor activity of immune strategies combined with radiation. *Front Biosci* 2007;12:4900–4910.

9. Price JG, Idoyaga J, Salmon H, et al. CDKN1A regulates Langerhans cell survival and promotes Treg cell generation upon exposure to ionizing irradiation. *Nat Immunol* 2015;16(10):1060–1068.

10. Wennerberg E, Lhuillier C, Vanpouille-Box C, et al. Barriers to radiation-induced in situ tumor vaccination. *Front Immunol* 2017;8:229.

11. Zitvogel L, Kroemer G. Subversion of anticancer immunosurveillance by radiotherapy. *Nat Immunol* 2015;16(10):1005–1007.

12. Urban JL, Schreiber H. Tumor antigens. *Annu Rev Immunol* 1992;10:617–644.

13. Chakravarty PK, Alfieri A, Thomas EK, et al. Flt3-ligand administration after radiation therapy prolongs survival in a murine model of metastatic lung cancer. *Cancer Res* 1999;59(24):6028–6032.

14. Chakravarty PK, Guha C, Alfieri A, et al. Flt3L therapy following localized tumor irradiation generates long-term protective immune response in metastatic lung cancer: its implication in designing a vaccination strategy. *Oncology* 2006;70(4):245–254.

15. Demaria S, Ng B, Devitt ML, et al. Ionizing radiation inhibition of distant untreated tumors (abscopal effect) is immune mediated. *Int J Radiat Oncol Biol Phys* 2004;58(3):862–870.

16. Fonteneau JF, Larsson M, Bhardwaj N. Dendritic cell-dead cell interactions: implications and relevance for immunotherapy. *J Immunother* 2001;24(4):294–304.

17. Steinman RM. The dendritic cell system and its role in immunogenicity. *Annu Rev Immunol* 1991;9:271–296.

18. Banchereau J, Briere F, Caux C, et al. Immunobiology of dendritic cells. *Annu Rev Immunol* 2000;18:767–811.

19. Bender A, Sapp M, Schuler G, et al. Improved methods for the generation of dendritic cells from nonproliferating progenitors in human blood. *J Immunol Methods* 1996;196(2):121–135.

20. Maraskovsky E, Brasel K, Teepe M, et al. Dramatic increase in the numbers of functionally mature dendritic cells in Flt3 ligand-treated mice: multiple dendritic cell subpopulations identified. *J Exp Med* 1996;184(5):1953–1962.

21. Schoenberger SP, Toes RE, van der Voort EI, et al. T-cell help for cytotoxic T lymphocytes is mediated by CD40-CD40L interactions [see comments]. *Nature* 1998;393(6684):480–483.

22. Albert ML, Pearce SF, Francisco LM, et al. Immature dendritic cells phagocytose apoptotic cells via alphavbeta5 and CD36, and cross-present antigens to cytotoxic T lymphocytes. *J Exp Med* 1998;188(7):1359–1368.

23. Harshyne LA, Watkins SC, Gambotto A, et al. Dendritic cells acquire antigens from live cells for cross-presentation to CTL. *J Immunol* 2001;166(6):3717–3723.

24. Heath WR, Carbone FR. Cross-presentation, dendritic cells, tolerance and immunity. *Annu Rev Immunol* 2001;19:47–64.

25. Kaur P, and Asea A. Radiation-induced effects and the immune system in cancer. *Front Oncol* 2012;2:191.

26. Tesniere A, Panaretakis T, Kepp O, et al. Molecular characteristics of immunogenic cell death. *Cell Death Differ* 2008;15(1):3–12.

27. Obeid M, Tesniere A, Ghiringhelli F, et al. Calreticulin exposure dictates the immunogenicity of cancer cell death. *Nat Med* 2007;13(1):54–61.

28. Gameiro SR, Malamas AS, Bernstein MB, et al. Tumor cells surviving exposure to proton or photon radiation share a common immunogenic modulation signature, rendering them more sensitive to T cell-mediated killing. *Int J Radiat Oncol Biol Phys* 2016;95(1):120–130.

29. Apetoh L, Ghiringhelli F, Tesniere A, et al. The interaction between HMGB1 and TLR4 dictates the outcome of anticancer chemotherapy and radiotherapy. *Immunol Rev* 2007;220:47–59.

30. Gasser S, Orsulic S, Brown EJ, et al. The DNA damage pathway regulates innate immune system ligands of the NKG2D receptor. *Nature* 2005;436(7054):1186–1190.

31. Reits EA, Hodge JW, Herberts CA, et al. Radiation modulates the peptide repertoire, enhances MHC class I expression, and induces successful antitumor immunotherapy. *J Exp Med* 2006;203(5):1259–1271.

32. Gulley JL, Arlen PM, Bastian A, et al. Combining a recombinant cancer vaccine with standard definitive radiotherapy in patients with localized prostate cancer. *Clin Cancer Res* 2005;11(9):3353–3362.

33. Bernstein MB, Garnett CT, Zhang H, et al. Radiation-induced modulation of costimulatory and coinhibitory T-cell signaling molecules on human prostate carcinoma cells promotes productive antitumor immune interactions. *Cancer Biother Radiopharm* 2014;29(4):153–161.

34. Kumari A, Cacan E, Greer S, et al. Turning T cells on: epigenetically enhanced expression of effector T-cell costimulatory molecules on irradiated human tumor cells. *J Immunother Cancer* 2013;1:1–17.

35. Garnett-Benson C, Hodge JW, Gameiro SR. Combination regimens of radiation therapy and therapeutic cancer vaccines: mechanisms and opportunities. *Semin Radiat Oncol* 2015;25(1):46–53.

36. Burnette BC, Liang H, Lee Y, et al. The efficacy of radiotherapy relies upon induction of type i interferon-dependent innate and adaptive immunity. *Cancer Res* 2011;71(7):2488–2496.

37. Deng L, Liang H, Xu M, et al. STING-Dependent Cytosolic DNA Sensing Promotes Radiation-Induced Type I Interferon-Dependent Antitumor Immunity in Immunogenic Tumors. *Immunity* 2014;41(5):843–852.

38. Xu MM, Pu Y, Han D, et al. Dendritic Cells but Not Macrophages Sense Tumor Mitochondrial DNA for Cross-priming through Signal Regulatory Protein alpha Signaling. *Immunity* 2017;47(2):363–373e5.

39. Vanpouille-Box C, Alard A, Aryankalayil MJ, et al. DNA exonuclease Trex1 regulates radiotherapy-induced tumour immunogenicity. *Nat Commun* 2017;8:15618.

40. Harding SM, Benci JL, Irianto J, et al. Mitotic progression following DNA damage enables pattern recognition within micronuclei. *Nature* 2017;548(7668):466–470.

41. Nabet BY, Qiu Y, Shabason JE, et al. Exosome RNA unshielding couples stromal activation to pattern recognition receptor signaling in cancer. *Cell* 2017;170(2):352–e66 e13.

42. Boelens MC, Wu TJ, Nabet BY, et al. Exosome transfer from stromal to breast cancer cells regulates therapy resistance pathways. *Cell* 2014;159(3):499–513.

43. Formenti SC, Demaria S. Systemic effects of local radiotherapy. *Lancet Oncol* 2009;10(7):718–726.

44. Formenti SC, Demaria S. Combining radiotherapy and cancer immunotherapy: a paradigm shift. *J Natl Cancer Inst* 2013;105(4):256–265.

45. Filatenkov A, Baker J, Mueller AM, et al. Ablative tumor radiation can change the tumor immune cell microenvironment to induce durable complete remissions. *Clin Cancer Res* 2015;21(16):3727–3739.

46. Lee Y, Auh SL, Wang Y, et al. Therapeutic effects of ablative radiation on local tumor require CD8+ T cells: changing strategies for cancer treatment. *Blood* 2009;114(3):589–595.

47. Gameiro SR, Ardiani A, Kwilas A, et al. Radiation-induced survival responses promote immunogenic modulation to enhance immunotherapy in combinatorial regimens. *Oncoimmunology* 2014;3:e28643.

48. Lugade AA, Moran JP, Gerber SA, et al. Local radiation therapy of B16 melanoma tumors increases the generation of tumor antigen-specific effector cells that traffic to the tumor. *J Immunol* 2005;174(12):7516–7523.

49. Vanpouille-Box C, Diamond JM, Pilones KA, et al. TGFbeta is a master regulator of radiation therapy-induced antitumor immunity. *Cancer Res* 2015;75(11):2232–2242.

50. Grayson JM, Harrington LE, Lanier JG, et al. Differential sensitivity of naive and memory CD8+ T cells to apoptosis in vivo. *J Immunol* 2002;169(7):3760–3770.

51. Schaue D, Comin-Anduix B, Ribas A, et al. T-cell responses to survivin in cancer patients undergoing radiation therapy. *Clin Cancer Res* 2008;14(15):4883–4890.

52. Chakraborty M, Abrams SI, Coleman CN, et al. External beam radiation of tumors alters phenotype of tumor cells to render them susceptible to vaccine-mediated T-cell killing. *Cancer Res* 2004;64(12):4328–4337.

53. Dewan MZ, Galloway AE, Kawashima N, et al. Fractionated but not single-dose radiotherapy induces an immune-mediated abscopal effect when combined with anti-CTLA-4 antibody. *Clin Cancer Res* 2009;15(17):5379–5388.

54. Klug F, Prakash H, Huber PE, et al. Low-dose irradiation programs macrophage differentiation to an iNOS(+)/M1 phenotype that orchestrates effective T cell immunotherapy. *Cancer Cell* 2013;24(5):589–602.

55. De Palma M, Coukos G, Hanahan D. A new twist on radiation oncology: low-dose irradiation elicits immunostimulatory macrophages that unlock barriers to tumor immunotherapy. *Cancer Cell* 2013;24(5):559–561.

56. Yamada Y, Bilsky MH, Lovelock DM, et al. High-dose, single-fraction image-guided intensity-modulated radiotherapy for metastatic spinal lesions. *Int J Radiat Oncol Biol Phys* 2008;71(2):484–490.

57. Garcia-Barros M, Paris F, Cordon-Cardo C, et al. Tumor response to radiotherapy regulated by endothelial cell apoptosis. *Science* 2003;300(5622):1155–1159.

58. Rao SS, Thompson C, Cheng J, et al. Axitinib sensitization of high single dose radiotherapy. *Radiother Oncol* 2014;111(1):88–93.

59. Kioi M, Vogel H, Schultz G, et al. Inhibition of vasculogenesis, but not angiogenesis, prevents the recurrence of glioblastoma after irradiation in mice. *J Clin Invest* 2010;120(3):694–705.

60. Kozin SV, Kamoun WS, Huang Y, et al. Recruitment of myeloid but not endothelial precursor cells facilitates tumor regrowth after local irradiation. *Cancer Res* 2010;70(14):5679–5685.

61. Chen Y, Ramjiawan RR, Reiberger T, et al. CXCR4 inhibition in tumor microenvironment facilitates anti-programmed death receptor-1 immunotherapy in sorafenib-treated hepatocellular carcinoma in mice. *Hepatology* 2015;61(5):1591–1602.

62. Crittenden MR, Savage T, Cottam B, et al. The peripheral myeloid expansion driven by murine cancer progression is reversed by radiation therapy of the tumor. *PLoS One* 2013;8(7):e69527.

63. Kanagavelu S, Gupta S, Wu X, et al. In vivo effects of lattice radiation therapy on local and distant lung cancer: potential role of immunomodulation. *Radiat Res* 2014;182(2):149–162.

64. Malamas AS, Gameiro SR, Knudson KM, et al. Sublethal exposure to alpha radiation (223Ra dichloride) enhances various carcinomas' sensitivity to lysis by antigen-specific cytotoxic T lymphocytes through calreticulin-mediated immunogenic modulation. *Oncotarget* 2016;7(52):86937–86947.

65. Mohan R, Grosshans D. Proton therapy—present and future. *Adv Drug Deliv Rev* 2017;109:26-44.

66. Ebner DK, Kamada T. The emerging role of carbon-ion radiotherapy. *Front Oncol* 2016;6:140.

67. Ebner DK, Tinganelli W, Helm A, et al. The immunoregulatory potential of particle radiation in cancer therapy. *Front Immunol* 2017;8:99.

68. Ando K, Fujita H, Hosoi A, et al. Intravenous dendritic cell administration enhances suppression of lung metastasis induced by carbon-ion irradiation. *J Radiat Res* 2017;58(4):446–455.

69. Matsunaga A, Ueda Y, Yamada S, et al. Carbon-ion beam treatment induces systemic antitumor immunity against murine squamous cell carcinoma. *Cancer* 2010;116(15):3740–3748.

70. Ohkubo Y, Iwakawa M, Seino K, et al. Combining carbon ion radiotherapy and local injection of alpha-galactosylceramide-pulsed dendritic cells inhibits lung metastases in an in vivo murine model. *Int J Radiat Oncol Biol Phys* 2010;78(5):1524–1531.

71. Body JJ, Casimiro S, Costa L. Targeting bone metastases in prostate cancer: improving clinical outcome. *Nat Rev Urol* 2015;12(6):340–356.

72. Dunn GP, Bruce AT, Ikeda H, et al. Cancer immunoediting: from immunosurveillance to tumor escape. *Nat Immunol* 2002;3(11):991–998.

73. Chen DS, Mellman I. Oncology meets immunology: the cancer-immunity cycle. *Immunity* 2013;39(1):1–10.

74. Banchereau J, Palucka AK, Dhodapkar M, et al. Immune and clinical responses in patients with metastatic melanoma to CD34(+) progenitor-derived dendritic cell vaccine. *Cancer Res* 2001;61(17):6451–6458.

75. Steinman RM, Dhodapkar M. Active immunization against cancer with dendritic cells: the near future. *Int J Cancer* 2001;94(4):459–473.

76. Banchereau J, Palucka AK. Dendritic cells as therapeutic vaccines against cancer. *Nat Rev Immunol* 2005;5(4):296–306.

77. Gong J, Chen D, Kashiwaba M, et al. Reversal of tolerance to human MUC1 antigen in MUC1 transgenic mice immunized with fusions of dendritic and carcinoma cells. *Proc Natl Acad Sci U S A* 1998;95(11):6279–6283.

78. Kugler A, Stuhler G, Walden P, et al. Regression of human metastatic renal cell carcinoma after vaccination with tumor cell-dendritic cell hybrids. *Nat Med* 2000;6(3):332–336.

79. Kantoff PW, Higano CS, Shore ND, et al. Sipuleucel-T immunotherapy for castration-resistant prostate cancer. *N Engl J Med* 2010;363(5):411–422.

80. Small EJ, Fratesi P, Reese DM, et al. Immunotherapy of hormone-refractory prostate cancer with antigen-loaded dendritic cells. *J Clin Oncol* 2000;18(23):3894–3903.

81. Chi KH, Liu SJ, Li CP, et al. Combination of conformal radiotherapy and intratumoral injection of adoptive dendritic cell immunotherapy in refractory hepatoma. *J Immunother* 2005;28(2):129–135.

82. Shibamoto Y, Okamoto M, Kobayashi M, et al. Immune-maximizing (IMAX) therapy for cancer: Combination of dendritic cell vaccine and intensity-modulated radiation. *Mol Clin Oncol* 2013;1(4):649–654.

83. Kawashita Y, Deb NJ, Garg M, et al. An autologous in situ tumor vaccination approach for hepatocellular carcinoma. 1. Flt3 ligand gene transfer increases antitumor effects of a radio-inducible suicide gene therapy in an ectopic tumor model. *Radiat Res* 2014;182(2):191–200.

84. Kawashita Y, Deb NJ, Garg MK, et al. An autologous in situ tumor vaccination approach for hepatocellular carcinoma. 2. Tumor-specific immunity and cure after radio-inducible suicide gene therapy and systemic CD40-ligand and Flt3-ligand gene transfer in an orthotopic tumor model. *Radiat Res* 2014;182(2):201–210.

85. Heery CR, Ibrahim NK, Mohebtash M, et al. A phase 2 randomized trial of docetaxel alone or in combination with therapeutic cancer vaccine, CEA-, MUC-1-TRICOM. *Cancer Res* 2012;72(24 Suppl):Abstract nr P5-16-06.

86. Garnett CT, Greiner JW, Tsang KY, et al. TRICOM vector based cancer vaccines. *Curr Pharm Des* 2006;12(3):351–361.

87. McNamara MA, Nair SK, Holl EK. RNA-Based Vaccines in Cancer Immunotherapy. *J Immunol Res* 2015;2015:794528.

88. Croft M, So T, Duan W, et al. The significance of OX40 and OX40L to T-cell biology and immune disease. *Immunol Rev* 2009;229(1):173–191.

89. Honeychurch J, Glennie MJ, Johnson PW, et al. Anti-CD40 monoclonal antibody therapy in combination with irradiation results in a CD8 T-cell-dependent immunity to B-cell lymphoma. *Blood* 2003;102(4):1449–1457.

90. Corrales L, Glickman LH, McWhirter SM, et al. Direct Activation of STING in the Tumor Microenvironment Leads to Potent and Systemic Tumor Regression and Immunity. *Cell Rep* 2015;11(7):1018–1030.

91. Baird JR, Friedman D, Cottam B, et al. Radiotherapy combined with novel STING-targeting oligonucleotides results in regression of established tumors. *Cancer Res* 2016;76(1):50–61.

92. Corrales L, McWhirter SM, Dubensky TW Jr, et al. The host STING pathway at the interface of cancer and immunity. *J Clin Invest* 2016;126(7):2404–2411.

93. Corrales L, Gajewski TF. Molecular pathways: targeting the stimulator of interferon genes (STING) in the immunotherapy of cancer. *Clin Cancer Res* 2015;21(21):4774–4779.

94. Dezso B, Haas GP, Hamzavi F, et al. The mechanism of local tumor irradiation combined with interleukin 2 therapy in murine renal carcinoma: histological evaluation of pulmonary metastases. *Clin Cancer Res* 1996;2(9):1543–1552.

95. Younes E, Haas GP, Dezso B, et al. Local tumor irradiation augments the response to IL-2 therapy in a murine renal adenocarcinoma. *Cell Immunol* 1995;165(2):243–251.

96. Morris ZS, Guy EI, Francis DM, et al. In situ tumor vaccination by combining local radiation and tumor-specific antibody or immunocytokine treatments. *Cancer Res* 2016;76(13):3929–3941.

97. Iwai Y, Hamanishi J, Chamoto K, et al. Cancer immunotherapies targeting the PD-1 signaling pathway. *J Biomed Sci* 2017;24(1):26-017-0329-9.

98. Dovedi SJ, Adlard AL, Lipowska-Bhalla G, et al. Acquired resistance to fractionated radiotherapy can be overcome by concurrent PD-L1 blockade. *Cancer Res* 2014;74(19):5458–5468.

99. Antonia SJ, Villegas A, Daniel D, et al. Durvalumab after chemoradiotherapy in stage III non-small-cell lung cancer. *N Engl J Med* 2017;377:1919–1929.

100. Twyman-Saint Victor C, Rech AJ, Maity A, et al. Radiation and dual checkpoint blockade activate non-redundant immune mechanisms in cancer. *Nature* 2015;520(7547):373–377.

101. Benci JL, Xu B, Qiu Y, et al. Tumor interferon signaling regulates a multigenic resistance program to immune checkpoint blockade. *Cell* 2016;167(6):1540–1554 e12.

102. Kochenderfer JN, Wilson WH, Janik JE, et al. Eradication of B-lineage cells and regression of lymphoma in a patient treated with autologous T cells genetically engineered to recognize CD19. *Blood* 2010;116(20):4099–4102.

103. Postow MA, Callahan MK, Barker CA, et al. Immunologic correlates of the abscopal effect in a patient with melanoma. *N Engl J Med* 2012;366(10):925–931.

104. Hiniker SM, Chen DS, Knox SJ. Abscopal effect in a patient with melanoma. *N Engl J Med* 2012;366(21):2035; author reply-6.

105. Seung SK, Curti BD, Crittenden M, et al. Phase 1 study of stereotactic body radiotherapy and interleukin-2—tumor and immunological responses. *Sci Transl Med* 2012;4(137):137ra74.

106. Shaverdian N, Lisberg AE, Bornazyan K, et al. Previous radiotherapy and the clinical activity and toxicity of pembrolizumab in the treatment of non-small-cell lung cancer: a secondary analysis of the KEYNOTE-001 phase 1 trial. *Lancet Oncol* 2017;18(7):895–903.

107. Crittenden M, Kohrt H, Levy R, et al. Current clinical trials testing combinations of immunotherapy and radiation. *Semin Radiat Oncol* 2015;25(1):54–64.

108. Puck TT, Marcus PI. Action of x-rays on mammalian cells. *J Exp Med* 1956;103(5):653–666.

109. Bradley JD, Paulus R, Komaki R, et al. Standard-dose versus high-dose conformal radiotherapy with concurrent and consolidation carboplatin plus paclitaxel with or without cetuximab for patients with stage IIIA or IIIB non-small-cell lung cancer (RTOG 0617): a randomised, two-by-two factorial phase 3 study. *Lancet Oncol* 2015;16(2):187–199.

110. Heemsbergen WD, Al-Mamgani A, Slot A, et al. Long-term results of the Dutch randomized prostate cancer trial: impact of dose-escalation on local, biochemical, clinical failure, and survival. *Radiother Oncol* 2014;110(1):104–109.

111. Roach M III, DeSilvio M, Lawton C, et al. Phase III trial comparing whole-pelvic versus prostate-only radiotherapy and neoadjuvant versus adjuvant combined androgen suppression: Radiation Therapy Oncology Group 9413. *J Clin Oncol* 2003;21(10):1904–1911.

112. Pinkawa M, Djukic V, Klotz J, et al. Hematologic changes during prostate cancer radiation therapy are dependent on the treatment volume. *Future Oncol* 2014;10(5):835–843.

113. Crocenzi T, Cottam B, Newell P, et al. A hypofractionated radiation regimen avoids the lymphopenia associated with neoadjuvant chemoradiation therapy of borderline resectable and locally advanced pancreatic adenocarcinoma. *J Immunother Cancer* 2016;4:45.

114. Kaplan HS. Role of immunologic disturbance in human oncogenesis: some facts and fancies. *Br J Cancer* 1971;25(4):620–634.

115. Penn I. Malignancies associated with renal transplantation. *Urology* 1977;10(1 Suppl):57–63.

116. Allison AC. Tumour development following immunosuppression. *Proc R Soc Med* 1970;63(10):1077–1080.

117. Raben M, Walach N, Galili U, et al. The effect of radiation therapy on lymphocyte subpopulations in cancer patients. *Cancer* 1976;37(3):1417–1421.

118. Balmanoukian A, Ye X, Herman J, et al. The association between treatment-related lymphopenia and survival in newly diagnosed patients with resected adenocarcinoma of the pancreas. *Cancer Invest* 2012;30(8):571–576.

119. Yovino S, Grossman SA. Severity, etiology and possible consequences of treatment-related lymphopenia in patients with newly diagnosed high-grade gliomas. *CNS Oncol* 2012;1(2):149–154.

120. Campian JL, Ye X, Brock M, et al. Treatment-related lymphopenia in patients with stage III non-small-cell lung cancer. *Cancer Invest* 2013;31(3):183–188.

121. Yovino S, Kleinberg L, Grossman SA, et al. The etiology of treatment-related lymphopenia in patients with malignant gliomas: modeling radiation dose to circulating lymphocytes explains clinical observations and suggests methods of modifying the impact of radiation on immune cells. *Cancer Invest* 2013;31(2):140–144.

122. Campian JL, Sarai G, Ye X, et al. Association between severe treatment-related lymphopenia and progression-free survival in patients with newly diagnosed squamous cell head and neck cancer. *Head Neck* 2014;36(12):1747–1753.

123. Ellsworth S, Balmanoukian A, Kos F, et al. Sustained CD4+ T cell-driven lymphopenia without a compensatory IL-7/IL-15 response among high-grade glioma patients treated with radiation and temozolomide. *Oncoimmunology* 2014;3(1):e27357.

124. Grossman SA, Ellsworth S, Campian J, et al. Survival in patients with severe lymphopenia following treatment with radiation and chemotherapy for newly diagnosed solid tumors. *J Natl Compr Canc Netw* 2015;13(10):1225–1231.

125. Wild AT, Ye X, Ellsworth SG, et al. The association between chemoradiation-related lymphopenia and clinical outcomes in patients with locally advanced pancreatic adenocarcinoma. *Am J Clin Oncol* 2015;38(3):259–265.

126. Miljkovic MD, Grossman SA, Ye X, et al. Patterns of radiation-associated lymphopenia in children with cancer. *Cancer Invest* 2016;34(1):32–38.

127. Wu ES, Oduyebo T, Cobb LP, et al. Lymphopenia and its association with survival in patients with locally advanced cervical cancer. *Gynecol Oncol* 2016;140(1):76–82.

128. Schuler PJ, Harasymczuk M, Schilling B, et al. Effects of adjuvant chemoradiotherapy on the frequency and function of regulatory T cells in patients with head and neck cancer. *Clin Cancer Res* 2013;19(23):6585–6596.

129. Kumar R, Geuna E, Michalarea V, et al. The neutrophil-lymphocyte ratio and its utilisation for the management of cancer patients in early clinical trials. *Br J Cancer* 2015;112(7):1157–1165.

130. Williams NL, Wuthrick EJ, Kim H, et al. Phase 1 study of ipilimumab combined with whole brain radiation therapy or radiosurgery for melanoma patients with brain metastases. *Int J Radiat Oncol Biol Phys* 2017;99(1):22–30.

131. Eigentler TK, Hassel JC, Berking C, et al. Diagnosis, monitoring and management of immune-related adverse drug reactions of anti-PD-1 antibody therapy. *Cancer Treat Rev* 2016;45:7–18.

132. Bonnefoi H, Litiere S, Piccart M, et al. Pathological complete response after neoadjuvant chemotherapy is an independent predictive factor irrespective of simplified breast cancer intrinsic subtypes: a landmark and two-step approach analyses from the EORTC 10994/BIG 1-00 phase III trial. *Ann Oncol* 2014;25(6):1128–1136.

133. Gerard JP, Azria D, Gourgou-Bourgade S, et al. Comparison of two neoadjuvant chemoradiotherapy regimens for locally advanced rectal cancer: results of the phase III trial ACCORD 12/0405-Prodige 2. *J Clin Oncol* 2010;28(10):1638–1644.

134. Grossman HB, Natale RB, Tangen CM, et al. Neoadjuvant chemotherapy plus cystectomy compared with cystectomy alone for locally advanced bladder cancer. *N Engl J Med* 2003;349(9):859–866.

135. van Hagen P, Hulshof MC, van Lanschot JJ, et al. Preoperative chemoradiotherapy for esophageal or junctional cancer. *N Engl J Med* 2012;366(22):2074–2084.

136. Anitei MG, Zeitoun G, Mlecnik B, et al. Prognostic and predictive values of the immunoscore in patients with rectal cancer. *Clin Cancer Res* 2014;20(7):1891–1899.

137. Galon J, Costes A, Sanchez-Cabo F, et al. Type, density, and location of immune cells within human colorectal tumors predict clinical outcome. *Science* 2006;313(5795):1960–1964.

138. Galon J, Mlecnik B, Bindea G, et al. Towards the introduction of the 'Immunoscore' in the classification of malignant tumours. *J Pathol* 2014;232(2):199–209.

139. Galon J, Pages F, Marincola FM, et al. Cancer classification using the Immunoscore: a worldwide task force. *J Transl Med* 2012;10:205.

140. Chen DS, Mellman I. Elements of cancer immunity and the cancer-immune set point. *Nature* 2017;541(7637):321–330.

141. Hegde PS, Karanikas V, Evers S. The where, the when, and the how of immune monitoring for cancer immunotherapies in the era of checkpoint inhibition. *Clin Cancer Res* 2016;22(8):1865–1874.

142. Rashidian M, Ingram JR, Dougan M, et al. Predicting the response to CTLA-4 blockade by longitudinal noninvasive monitoring of CD8 T cells. *J Exp Med* 2017;214(8):2243–2255.

143. Tavare R, Escuin-Ordinas H, Mok S, et al. An effective immuno-PET imaging method to monitor CD8-dependent responses to immunotherapy. *Cancer Res* 2016;76(1):73–82.

144. Larimer BM, Wehrenberg-Klee E, Dubois F, et al. Granzyme B PET imaging as a predictive biomarker of immunotherapy response. *Cancer Res* 2017;77(9):2318–2327.

145. Chatterjee S, Lesniak WG, Nimmagadda S. Noninvasive imaging of immune checkpoint ligand PD-L1 in tumors and metastases for guiding immunotherapy. *Mol Imaging* 2017;16:1536012117718459.

146. Gonzalez Trotter DE, Meng X, McQuade P, et al. In vivo imaging of the programmed death ligand 1 by 18F positron emission tomography. *J Nucl Med* 2017.

147. Kaira K, Higuchi T, Naruse I, et al. Metabolic activity by 18F-FDG-PET/CT is predictive of early response after nivolumab in previously treated NSCLC. *Eur J Nucl Med Mol Imaging* 2018;45(1):56–66.

148. Zhang M, Wang D, Sun Q, et al. Prognostic significance of PD-L1 expression and 18F-FDG PET/CT in surgical pulmonary squamous cell carcinoma. *Oncotarget* 2017;8(31):51630–51640.

149. Boffa DJ, Graf RP, Salazar MC, et al. Cellular expression of PD-L1 in the peripheral blood of lung cancer patients is associated with worse survival. *Cancer Epidemiol Biomarkers Prev* 2017;26(7):1139–1145.

150. Strati A, Koutsodontis G, Papaxoinis G, et al. Prognostic significance of PD-L1 expression on circulating tumor cells in patients with head and neck squamous cell carcinoma. *Ann Oncol* 2017;28(8):1923–1933.

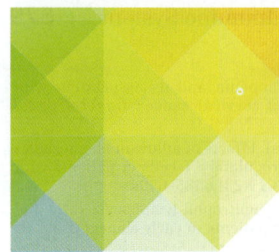

CHAPTER 31

Photodynamic Therapy

Theodore E. Yaeger

INTRODUCTION

The first report of *in vitro* cytotoxicity (in paramecium) was seen by combining visible light and an acridine drug in 1900.[1] That observation laid the foundation to begin reporting the results of combination topical eosin (a biologic stain) with visible light for treating a skin tumor.[2] Little progress in photodynamic therapy (PDT) ensued until about 1960 with the discovery—attributed to Lipson et al.[3]—of hematoporphyrin derivative (HpD). Samuel Schwartz[4] reported on a water-soluble mixture of porphyrins followed by a series of preclinical and then clinical investigations led by Dougherty et al.[5]

Despite deep historical origins and modern research investigations dating back 40 years, the clinical application of PDT still remains limited to specific clinical situations. In part, this has been due to the limited and superficial depth of cytotoxicity achieved with past photosensitizers and light delivery techniques. It is also due to the complexity of its application, requiring familiarity with safe photosensitizer administration coupled with the technical requirements for effective light delivery and, also, the optical expertise to prescribe and deliver an activating light energy for very specific indications.

Despite disadvantages, there are several compelling reasons to evaluate PDT as a major therapeutic approach in the management of cancer. PDT has the unique mechanism of action for allowing for nonoverlapping toxicities with traditional cancer therapeutics. As such, PDT does not exclude the subsequent administration of these treatment modalities. Technical advances with interstitial light delivery techniques (and advancements in modeling its dosimetry[6]) along with the clinical development of photosensitizers capable of absorbing and being activated at longer wavelengths now offer the potential for more penetrating and isolated cytotoxicity.[7] Unlike traditional chemotherapeutics and ionizing radiation therapy, there have not been any long-term genotoxic effects with the use of PDT, an observation consistent with several *in vitro* studies.[8-10] The explosion in our understanding of tumor biology and the influence of the microenvironment has also provided tremendous insights into the development of novel strategies to explore the clinical efficacy of PDT, including its combination with biologic therapeutics. This also includes the potential for PDT to enhance the effects of traditional cancer therapeutics and its promising role to more effectively induce adaptive cell-mediated immunity.

PRINCIPLES OF PHOTODYNAMIC THERAPY

Photosensitizers

PDT represents a treatment modality that combines the selective photochemical activation of photosensitizers with electromagnetic radiation in the visible energy range (i.e., visible light). Photosensitizers (PS) may be given to the cancer patient either systemically, topically, or injected locally, but its specific chemical structure can significantly influence the effectiveness of a PDT treatment. These include influencing its biodistribution and subcellular localization along with how efficiently it absorbs light (referred to as its *molar extinction coefficient*) to generate reactive oxygen species (ROS), including singlet oxygen (referred to as its *quantum yield*) (Table 31.1). A PS with a low molar extinction coefficient will require large concentrations of the PS and light energy to be effectively delivered for photoactivation.

There are now many PS that have been discovered with most under preclinical evaluation but several receiving regulatory approval for clinical application in the United States, European Union, and other countries. The first PS to receive regulatory approval was a semipurified preparation of HpD known as Photofrin (porfimer sodium). Porfimer sodium represents a complex mixture of hematoporphyrin oligomers whose chemical composition has been difficult to reproduce consistently. It has an absorption peak at 630 nm with a relatively low molar extinction coefficient, thus requiring large concentrations of drug and light energy (fluence) to be delivered. It has also been shown to have a prolonged risk of skin photosensitivity reflecting its relative lack of selectivity. Although used routinely in clinical practice, these disadvantages have spurred ongoing PS development.

Several ideal characteristics have been well articulated in the area of PS development. These include the following: PS that has a well-established structure, ideally a pure compound with a constant composition and a stable shelf life.

Without light activation, it should have little toxicity and tumor specificity when administered. With light, a PS with spectral absorption peaks demonstrates a high extinction coefficient when effectively activated. But, it is not entirely clear if the above is always desired. For example, a strong PS absorption at a specific wavelength can contribute to reduced light penetration, a phenomenon referred to as *self-shielding*. Moreover, potent PS such as temoporfin/mTHPC (Foscan) that thus require little drug and light for its efficient activation have been associated with significant complications necessitating even more vigilance to the light dosimetry (as defined below).[11] The wavelengths of a photosensitizer's absorption peaks also influence how the PS will be used clinically, with absorption at longer wavelengths (i.e., 700-nm range) offering deeper light penetration in human tissues. Lastly, some PS may undergo a process of *photobleaching*, whereby the PS in turn reacts with the singlet oxygen or other reactions created in the photoactivation process, limiting the ability to act as a PS. Typically, photobleaching decreases a photosensitizer's reactivity, which may or may not be desirable depending on the context of its clinical application.

Structurally, photosensitizers are generally classified as porphyrin-based or nonporphyrins with the former sharing a common backbone that consists of the tetrapyrrole ring. Other structural backbones that have demonstrated photosensitizing capabilities include the presence of four phenol rings and polycyclic ring compounds based on the pyrrole

TABLE 31.1 FACTORS AFFECTING THE EFFICACY OF PHOTODYNAMIC THERAPY	
Photosensitizer (PS)	Effectiveness of the tumor vasculature to deliver PS, extracellular and intracellular location of PS, PS extinction coefficient, singlet oxygen quantum yield, PS photobleaching
Light	Drug–light interval, fluence, fluence rate
Microenvironment	Oxygenation, status of immune system
Tumor response	Complex interaction between proapoptotic and prosurvival signals, angiogenic response

ring especially the tetrapyrrole PS. Extensive reviews are available regarding the specific physicochemical properties (i.e., primary structures, the presence of complexed heavy metals, and specific side chain substitutions) and the impact on its systemic biodistribution, cellular uptake, and photosensitizing properties.[7]

In general, the hydrophobic compounds with two or less negative charges have the ability to cross the plasma membrane. Otherwise, intracellular uptake is through active endocytosis. The charge of the hydrophobic PS can influence where a PS localizes with cationic charges (positive). This tends to localize to the mitochondria and anionic PS with a net charge of negative 2 or greater tending to localize in the lysosomes.[12] Cationic PS localizing to the mitochondria have been suggested to be more effective in mediating direct cytotoxicity.[13]

Tumor specificity is in part mediated by selective light administration and its natural energy attenuation. Specific extracellular and intracellular PS delivery is felt to further contribute to this process. Human tissue studies in patients receiving porfimer sodium–mediated intraperitoneal PDT have confirmed PS selectivity, even if limited.[14] Systemically administered photosensitizers (those with the tetrapyrrole backbone) will associate with serum proteins, including albumin and low-density lipoproteins (LDL). The association with LDL proteins has been suggested to be a potential mechanism that may contribute to specific tumor localization.[15] In this model, it has been proposed that tumor selectivity occurs due to a preferential up-regulation of LDL receptors in tumor cells because of the rapid plasma membrane turnover rate and the need for constituents in its biosynthesis. Alternatively, the functionally altered tumor vasculature resulting from overexpression of vascular endothelial growth factor[16] (VEGF) and its impaired lymphatic clearance of the extravasated PS have also been advanced as a functional mechanism.[17] Although it may lead to increased PS retention, the extracellular distribution of the PS can be inhomogeneous and can impact the effectiveness of a PDT treatment. The demonstrated direct tumor cell killing was a function of the distance from a tumor's vascular supply.[18] In contrast, photosensitizers that tend to be located in the intravascular space can increase the effectiveness of PDT through mediating vascular damage and tumor infarction.[19]

The subcellular localization of a PS that can similarly influence the mechanism of cellular injury has been well-studied and recently summarized.[20] In general, photosensitizers that localize to the plasma membrane and lysosomes are likely to cause injury by necrosis. Those localizing to the mitochondria and endoplasmic reticulum are likely to initiate cell death by way of direct cell apoptosis.[5,21] However, mitochondrial injury can also mediate a necrotic cell death by mitochondrial membrane damage.[20]

Most photosensitizers tend not to accumulate in the nucleus, possibly explaining the paucity of genotoxicity and observed carcinogenesis.[8,22] Although DNA damage has been reported in cell culture experiments for various photosensitizers,[8,10,23] for 5-aminolevulinic acid,[23,24] efficient DNA repair has also been observed. This suggests that the damage may not be sufficient to overwhelm a cell's repair capacity.[10,25] As PDT can mediate cell death through non-DNA targets, the potential mutagenic effects of any DNA injury are likely to be further limited by its cell death.

Photosensitizer Activation

Following photosensitizer administration, the drug–light interval (DLI) that is prescribed warrants consideration. Preclinical studies have demonstrated that varying the DLI can influence both the PS extracellular and intracellular localization.[19,26] In general, longer DLI will promote PS extravasation and intracellular uptake, provided it has a sufficient

long pharmacokinetic lifetime. However, the passive targeting of either the vascular (short DLI) or tumor compartment can be compounded by the lipophilicity of the PS and associated proteins within the vasculature. Targeting both the vascular and tumor compartment with repeat PS administration, combining both a short DLI and a long DLI, can further improve the effectiveness of PDT. However, the order of the repeat PS administration and activation may be particularly important. Prescribing an initial short DLI that targets the vasculature can create subsequent hypoxia that limits the efficacy of the repeat PS with a long DLI.[19]

PS activation involves the absorption of wavelength-specific energy, causing specific changes in the electron energy states of the PS. Energy absorption can cause a PS electron to move from its ground state to a higher energy level or excited energy state. While in the excited energy state, transition back to the ground state may occur, with energy released in the form of fluorescence or heat dissipation. Thus, some of the light absorbed by a PS may be re-emitted at a different wavelength, allowing for fluorescence detection of the PS or *photodynamic diagnosis* (PDD). Figure 31.1 demonstrates the Jablonski energy diagram. It depicts the energy transitions that may occur with PDT. Two possible excited energy states may be possible, a singlet state (S1) and the triplet state (T1), which has a longer half-life. The distinction depends on the spin direction of the excited electron relative to its paired electron in the ground state. The triplet state has both electrons parallel to each other, and its ability to return to a ground state emitting fluorescence is impeded because of this spin direction.

Transition to the triplet state through a process referred to as *intersystem crossing* is critical to the generation of cytotoxic ROS. This is largely due to the longer half-life of the triplet state that increases the probability of interacting with a nearby organic molecule (i.e., in the plasma membrane), generating reactive anions or cations that in turn may react with molecular oxygen generating ROS (referred to as a type I reaction). Alternatively, a PS in its triplet state may directly transfer its energy to molecular oxygen to form an excited state singlet oxygen ($^1O_2$) (type II reaction). Both types of reactions may occur simultaneously, though direct singlet oxygen production is felt to be the dominant mechanism of cytotoxicity.[27,28] Singlet oxygen within the cell has a limited half-life (estimated to be <0.04 µs) and thus a limited range of diffusion and activity (<0.02 µm).[22,29] As such, PS cytotoxicity is limited to its extracellular and intracellular (also, subcellular) localization and adjacent potential targets for reactivity.[22] For example, photosensitizers that tend to biodistribute or favor being localized in the vasculature will favor an antivascular necrotic mechanism of injury. The specific subcellular localization offers an added degree of specificity to its cytotoxicity.

FIGURE 31.1. Jablonski energy diagram following type II photosensitizer activation.

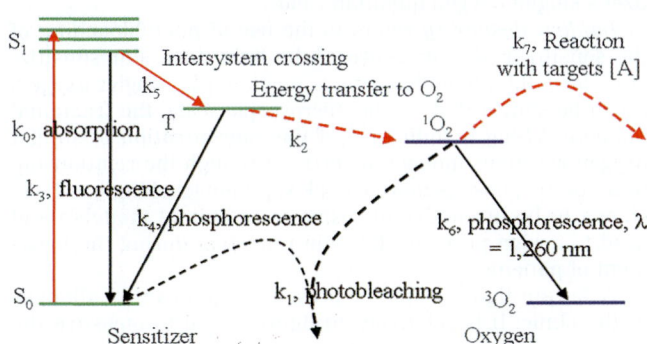

Section II

Physics of Light Dosimetry

PDT is inherently a dynamic process. All three principal components—photosensitizer, light, and oxygen—interact dynamically over the time period of a PDT prescription.[5] As light interacts with human tissue, its energy distribution is influenced by surface reflection and with absorption and scatter at depth. Light scatter in human tissues can be affected by many factors. Tissue architecture and geometry, plus heterogeneity at the histologic and cellular levels, can contribute to photon scattering, thus limiting the energy deposited at depth. Thus, it is important to recognize that light scatter is likely to be different from one tissue type to another. Although many factors remain to be fully characterized and accounted for in the prescription of PDT, it is presumed that selecting longer wavelengths for photoactivation can help to reduce photon scatter, thus increasing light penetration.

The deposition of light, or its *dosimetry*, is determined by the light source characteristics and the tissue optical properties, both on the cell surface and depth, in contrast to ionizing radiation. In turn, the tissue optical properties are influenced by the spatial distribution and concentration of both the photosensitizer and oxygen in the illuminated tissues. During illumination, the light dosimetry dynamically changes as the photodynamic process consumes oxygen and/or alters the blood flow.[30] For some photosensitizers, self-shielding can influence the light dosimetry at depth. Finally, the distribution of a photosensitizer may change as a result of photobleaching, a process whereby the photodynamic modification of the photosensitizer itself reduces the ability to further be photoactivated.

Quantifying the distribution of the light that is used in photoactivation is important biologically and for quality assurance reasons, as in the practice of ionizing radiation. The ability to relate the treatment outcome to the effective light fluence and its rate of delivery (*fluence rate*) facilitates an understanding of its relationship not only to the treatment outcome but also to any potential toxicities, as areas of high fluence and fluence rates have been associated with treatment toxicities.

Explicit dosimetry refers to the prediction of a singlet oxygen dose on the basis of measurable quantities that contribute to the photodynamic effect.[31] In clinical practice, the quantity most amenable to measurement is the PDT dose, defined as the light energy deposited to a photosensitizer. This quantity is proportional to the product of the absorption coefficient of the photosensitizer and light fluence. The absorption coefficient of the photosensitizer is, in turn, proportional to the photosensitizer concentration. PDT dose calculated in this way is a good predictor of outcome if one is operating in a drug- or light-limited situation when there is ample oxygen supply. To generally account for the oxygen effect, the concentration of reacted singlet oxygen (i.e., the concentration of reactions between singlet oxygen and molecular targets within the tumor cells) needs to be modeled as a function of PDT dose and tissue oxygenation. It has been shown that the reacted singlet oxygen concentration can be expressed as the integration of the product of the PDT dose rate and the photosensitizer's singlet oxygen quantum yield.[32]

Implicit dosimetry refers to the use of photobleaching of the sensitizer as a measure of the light dose. For sensitizers where the photobleaching is mediated by singlet oxygen, it can be shown that on the microscopic scale, the fractional photobleaching is indicative of the concentration of singlet oxygen reactions induced by PDT.[33] Although the relationship to tissue response is more complex, photobleaching has been shown to be predictive of response in animal models[34] and used to design protocols for pain reduction during the treatment of patients.[35]

Accurate light dosimetry presents significant challenges in the clinic. It is relatively straightforward to measure the irradiance of light delivered to the surface of a tissue. The light absorbed by the sensitizer also includes the light scattered by tissue not too dissimilar from ionizing radiation. Like ionizing radiation, scattered light contribution may occur on a surface and is an important concept to consider in the practice of PDT. In hollow organs or any concave surface with surface secretions that further increase the reflective index, light can be reflected from one surface to another surface, to increase the effective surface light fluence rate. This effect is often referred to as the *integrating sphere effect*. In the extreme case, multiple reflections can significantly magnify the fluence rate within a hollow organ. This integrating sphere effect has been extensively modeled in the case of bladder treatment.[36] In complex concave mucosal surfaces such as in the head and neck, scattered light photons have been demonstrated to increase the effective fluence rate by factors of three- to fourfold.[37,38]

Light scattering also occurs within tissues, leading to a significant difference between the incident fluence rate that is delivered and the fluence rate within the tissue. In practice, the integrating sphere effect and multiple scattering within the tissue occur simultaneously. Accurate dosimetry requires accounting for both of these effects, ideally through real-time measurements using an isotropic light photon detector capable of capturing both directly incident and scattered light.[39] A comparison of measurements using fiber-based isotropic detectors and photodiode detectors (that capture only incident light) indicated significant difference in the measured light dose with significant variation in the contribution from scattered light.[40] Through measurements with a series of light sources and detectors, tissue optical properties can be assessed; however, PDT treatment can significantly change the optical properties. This requires the ability to assess the optical properties in real time for an effective feedback to compensate for the influence of varying light transmission on the deposited light dose within the target tissue.[41,42] Recently, the first clinical experiences using an automated 18-channel system accommodating optical fibers for light delivery and monitoring were described in patients treated with temporfin interstitial PDT.[6]

Biology of Photodynamic Therapy

Mechanisms of Tumor Cytotoxicity

PDT can induce cytotoxicity through all three death morphologies: apoptosis, autophagy, and necrosis. The multitude of signaling pathways (apoptotic and nonapoptotic) and the molecular interplay between various cell death pathways (balanced with the induction of prosurvival signals) that are activated with cellular photodynamic oxidative stress have been the focus of intense investigations and the subject of a recent extensive review.[20] Of these modes of cell death, apoptosis is a major pathway of PDT-mediated cytotoxicity. This reflects the near ubiquitous ability of PDT to induce mitochondrial injury.[43,44]

PDT can also induce cell injury through direct damage of the vascular endothelial cells. In turn, thrombus formation and the release of various vasoactive molecules, with an increase in the vascular permeability and deterioration of vascular status, ensue. Leukocyte infiltration further compounds this response, all contributing to secondary hypoxia[45] with ischemic cell death.[46] Preclinical studies also suggest that beyond direct tumor and vascular cytotoxicity, long-term cellular (tumor) control seems to require immune-competent subjects.[47]

Influence of the Tumor Microenvironment on the Photodynamic Therapy Response

As PDT is dependent on the presence and distribution of a photosensitizer, light, and oxygen, the *normal* tissue microenvironment (within which a tumor is located) can significantly determine the treatment response of the tumor to PDT. All three key PDT components are subject to effects from the tissue microenvironment. For example, tumor vascular density, permeability, or perfusion can affect photosensitizer delivery.[48] This undoubtedly contributes to the heterogeneities detected in photosensitizer levels in different tumors among different patients.[49-52] Tumor-associated hypoxia can limit PDT-created damage.[53-56] Even the distribution of the treatment light is affected by the microenvironment because of differences in the penetration of red light as a function of the oxygenation status of hemoglobin. Compared to deoxyhemoglobin, oxygenated hemoglobin is less absorptive of red light (630 or 650 nm), thereby allowing deeper light penetration in tissues with a higher proportion of oxygenated hemoglobin.[57]

Much research has been performed on the dependence, as well as the effects, of PDT on tumor oxygenation. With conventional photosensitizers, the photochemical process can consume tissue oxygen faster than its delivery, leading to a hypoxic state that limits PDT-mediated cytotoxicity.[58-60] Moreover, intratumor heterogeneities in tumor oxygenation can have consequences to PDT-mediated cytotoxicity. This has been shown in murine studies that identify the presence of more severe PDT-created hypoxia in the base of subcutaneous tumors accompanied by a relative protection of this area from clonogenic cell death.[56]

PDT-mediated vascular effects are another cause of hypoxia during PDT. These effects can take the form of PDT-triggered vasoconstriction.[61] Additionally or alternatively, PDT can cause endothelial cell rounding, leading to intracellular gaps[62] and activation of the coagulation cascade. Ischemia then results, as leukocyte and platelet aggregation with secondary thrombosis within the vessels can further alter the blood flow.[61,63] Dynamic changes in tumor blood flow, including treatment-initiated decreases in the blood flow, have been observed for several photosensitizers including porfimer sodium, 5-aminolevulinic acid (5-ALA; Levulan), motexafin lutetium (Lutrin), verteporfin (Visudyne), palladium bacteriopherophorbide (Tookad), and 2-(1-hexyloxyethyl)-2-devinyl pyropheophorbide-a (HPPH; Photochlor).[61,64-70] In fact, PDT-triggered reductions in tumor blood flow during light delivery are not only therapy limiting but also directly correlate with outcome measures. Yu et al.[66] showed that the duration (long) and the slope (shallow) of the Photofrin-PDT-induced decrease in tumor blood flow correlated with the time-to-tumor regrowth (prolonged) in an animal. Similarly, Standish et al.[71] and Pham et al.[72] reported PDT-induced decreases in tumor blood flow and oxygen change (tissue hemoglobin oxygen saturation = %StO$_2$), respectively, correlated with developing necrosis. These findings show the value in the development and application of noninvasive approaches to measure tumor blood flow during clinical applications of PDT.[67,73,74] Although PDT-induced ischemia can limit the effectiveness of PDT, in the setting of sufficient light and drug doses, the persistent ischemia that is induced can provide incremental cytotoxicity and can improve the effectiveness.[46,75]

Experimental strategies directed at modulating the vascular response to PDT are also consistent with the importance of its contribution to the PDT effect. For example, inhibitors of nitric oxide have been effective in increasing tumor and vascular damage to porfimer sodium or ALA-PDT in a protocol-dependent manner.[76-78] Also, the vascular-disrupting agent, vadimezan (5,6-dimethylxanthenone-4-acetic acid; DMXAA), has been successful in improving PDT responses when administered in such a way as to decrease tumor perfusion after illumination.[68,79] It is even possible to deliver PDT in two fractions so that a vascular-damaging protocol follows one in which oxidative damage to tumor cells is the major cytotoxic mechanism.[19] This approach has been studied in preclinical models using verteporfin as photosensitizer by first employing a longer interval between drug administration and light delivery to allow drug accumulation in the tumor cells, leading to direct light-induced cytotoxicity, followed by a second round of drug administration and light delivery that utilizes a short DLI, which causes more extensive vascular damage because of drug localization in the blood vessels at the time of light delivery.[19] Similar observations have been reported with the photosensitizer MV6401.[26]

Tumor Stress Response to Photodynamic Therapy

The oxidative stress initiated with PDT can induce the expression of genes that can mediate various modes of cell death as well as survival signals. Using cDNA microarrays, the cellular effects of hypericin-mediated PDT were studied on the expression of a panel of genes involved in apoptosis, metabolism, and proliferation, among other cellular processes.[80] Twenty-five genes were significantly up-regulated by PDT, including dual specificity phosphatase-1 (DUSP1), which can induce apoptosis. The stress response proto-oncogene FOSB and JUN dimerize protein products to contribute transcription AP-1 (another effector - both positive and negative) to the cellular apoptosis response. Another important gene is MYC, which also codes for a proapoptotic transcription factor of c-MYC. Among the genes down-regulated by PDT were THBS1, whose protein product thrombospondin-1 is an effector of cell interaction with the extracellular matrix, angiogenesis, apoptosis, and cell migration; ADAM10, which codes for a family of cell surface proteins with roles in epithelial cell adhesion, migration, and proliferation; and several genes in the integrin family that mediate cell-to-cell and cell-to-matrix attachments, all thereby facilitating signal transduction along pathways controlling apoptosis and metastasis, among other functions.[80]

In other studies, PDT-induced apoptosis was associated with activation of p38 in the mitogen-activated protein kinase (MAPK) family,[81-83] which along with its other family members (including ERK and JNK) regulates cell proliferation, differentiation, and survival. Furthermore, expression of proapoptotic and antiapoptotic proteins of the Bcl-2 family can also be modulated by PDT in a context-dependent matter, which depends on factors such as cell type and subcellular localization of photosensitizer.[81,84,85] Similarly, PDT-induced expression and phosphorylation of "survivin" (capable of inhibiting apoptosis through inhibiting caspase-9) have also been an active area of investigation to therapeutically improve PDT cytotoxicity.[86] Signal transduction in PDT-induced apoptosis, autophagy, and necrosis is an area of expanding interest, and, for the interested reader, several comprehensive reviews[20,87,88] are available on the current state of knowledge on this topic.

Immunologic Response to Photodynamic Therapy

The altered microenvironment generated by PDT can also serve to stimulate the host immune responses. Both the activation of a nonspecific and an adaptive antigen-specific immune response may be seen following PDT. These findings have raised considerable hopes that a localized treatment with PDT may lead to broader systemic oncologic benefits. For example, PDT-induced damage is associated with the local influx of neutrophils and other cell types, such as macrophages, natural killer cells, and dendritic cells, which contribute to local damage and inflammation while initiating a general systemic immune response.[89] Both preclinical and clinical studies show this to be accompanied by the release of immune-modulating factors, such as interleukin (IL) 1-β, tumor necrosis factor (TNF)-α, IL-6, IL-10, and granulocyte colony–stimulating factor (G-CSF).[90-92]

The resulting activation of the general immune response plays a major role in tumor control after PDT. Neutrophils are key to this process. *In vitro* studies demonstrate neutrophil adhesion to an extracellular matrix exposed by PDT-mediated endothelial cell damage.[93] *In vivo* studies find neutrophils attach to PDT-treated blood vessels.[94] In contrast, various approaches toward depleting neutrophil influx into the PDT-treated tissues have caused a detriment of therapeutic outcome.[95,96] In fact, a systemic neutrophilia is known to accompany PDT of various tumor types, sites, and photosensitization protocols.[97-99] PDT can also activate the complement system with fixation of the complement C3 protein to tumor cells, which also promotes a strong neutrophilia. This serves not only to target cells for destruction by the nonspecific immune system but induces the release of proinflammatory mediators contributing to the migration of neutrophils.[100]

In addition to the induction of an innate immune response, PDT can also stimulate an adaptive cell-mediated immunity. In fact, these types of immune responses are intricately connected processes. It has been proposed that a critical aspect of PDT-induced adaptive immunity is the generation of a high antigen load causing tumor cell death. Tumor cell death is further promoted by the strong neutrophilia through the release of lysosomal enzymes, including myeloperoxidase. Strong neutrophilia also appears to be a critical factor for the development of PDT-induced adaptive immunity.[101] The AS neutrophils degranulate and release a family of mediators referred to as alarmins. *Alarmins* are a critical link between the inflammatory response and adaptive immunity as they are capable of recruiting and activating the maturation of antigen-presenting dendritic cells.[102] With a strong innate immune response, this antigen presentation can be more effectively recognized, inducing an adaptive cell-mediated immunologic response and memory.[103]

Dendritic cells (DCs) typically exist in the immature state within the tissue microenvironment. They actively survey and capture antigens and then migrate and present these to T cells in adjacent draining lymph nodes. For dendritic cells to mature and affect adaptive immunity, the expression of stimulatory molecules that are involved in antigen presentation to T cells is very important. Several aspects of the nonspecific or innate response include strong neutrophilia[101] and the release of damage-associated molecular patterns (DAMPs), which consist of various markers of normal tissue injury. Among these, the extracellular release of heat shock protein 70 (HSP-70) and its association with tumor antigens by PDT-treated cells appear to be particularly effective in being recognized by DCs through surface receptors that lead to their activation and maturation.[104]

HSPs, in particular HSP-70, have been a DAMP of particular interest in PDT for some time.[105] HSPs are molecular chaperones crucial for proper protein folding. HSPs can facilitate cell survival during intracellular functioning, but become immunostimulatory when extracellular or membrane bound.[106] In studies of PDT, HSP-70 is rapidly exposed on the surface of tumor cells treated *in vitro*,[107] and its antibody-based blockage served to inhibit maturation of dendritic cells.[108] Moreover, surface or extracellular expression of HSP-70 after PDT has been shown to correlate with curative responses in temoporfin-treated murine tumors.[109] Research in these and other aspects of PDT-generated antitumor immunity has spawned interest in the use of PDT to develop cancer vaccines, the history and progress of which have been recently reviewed.[110]

Vascular Response to Photodynamic Therapy

The therapeutic benefits to be gained from PDT-created vascular damage and inflammation come with a cost. In a post-PDT, tumor microenvironment is characterized by inflammatory infiltrates, cytokine overexpression, arachidonic acid and eicosanoid production, and hypoxia. Then, there develops a strong proangiogenic stimulus to support the growth of new tumor blood vessels.[111] Such angiogenesis can counteract the intended effects of treatment by providing a means for delivery of oxygen and nutrients to tumor cells that escaped direct (oxidative) or secondary (vascular or immune mediated) damage by PDT. VEGF is one of the most common angiogenic molecules whose expression is stimulated by PDT, and its increase has been measured following PDT with a variety of photosensitizers and tumor models.[112-114] Moreover, studies of human

tumors grown as murine xenografts find PDT to induce modest increases in host-derived (mouse) VEGF in addition to the increases in human VEGF that originate from the treated tumor.[115,116] The molecular mechanisms of PDT-initiated increases in VEGF can include increases in hypoxia-inducible factor (HIF)-1α, a transcription factor that promotes the activation of many hypoxia-responsive genes such as VEGF,[117,118] as well as activation of the p38 MAPK pathway.[119] In the case of the latter, an inhibitor of p38 MAPK significantly attenuated the PDT-induced increase in VEGF.[119]

Cyclooxygenase (COX) 2 is another proangiogenic molecule that is up-regulated by PDT under a variety of treatment conditions.[120-122] The COX-2 enzyme serves to catalyze the production of prostaglandin (PG) H_2, a substrate for multiple eicosanoid mediators (including additional prostaglandins and thromboxane) known to contribute to PDT-created ischemia.[123,124] The proangiogenic activity of COX-2 can be mediated through the enzyme's role in production of PGE_2, which in turn can promote increases in VEGF.[111] Moreover, PDT-stimulated proinflammatory cytokines such as IL-1β and TNF-α may also stimulate angiogenesis through a COX-2–dependent pathway. This is supported by findings that the decrease in PGE_2 after COX-2 inhibition is accompanied by a reduction in protein levels of IL-1β and TNF-α.[125]

Biologic Strategies to Improve Photodynamic Therapy Cytotoxicity

With improved understanding of the biologic and molecular mechanisms that underlie PDT-derived cytotoxicity has come the development of alternative, more effective approaches toward PDT delivery. These include the development of new targeted PS that exploit specific signatures or functions in diseased tissue in order to deliver, or even to activate, the PS.[126] These are commonly referred to as *PDT molecular beacons*, where the PS and a singlet oxygen–quenching or singlet oxygen–scavenging molecule are both coupled to a linker that can interact with a cancer-specific target.[127] In this way, the PS photoactivity is silenced because of the proximity of the singlet oxygen–quenching molecule. The PS is only capable of being photoactivated when the linker interacts with the cancer-specific target, which results in physical separation of the singlet oxygen–scavenging molecule from the PS. One example of a novel targeted linker includes an antisense oligonucleotide complementary to a target messenger RNA. The messenger RNA is conformationally restricted until the oligonucleotide interacts with its target.

Modulation of light delivery has also proven successful in mitigating the microenvironment limitations imposed by PDT. For example, lowering the fluence rate of light delivery can conserve tumor oxygenation during PDT, increasing direct tumor cell cytotoxicity as well as vascular and immune effects.[54,56-95,128-130] Similarly, fractionation of the light with or without repeat administration of the PS before each light fraction has improved treatment response in various preclinical protocols[45,131-135] and in early clinical studies.[136] Without repeat PS administration, preclinical studies suggest that the light fractionation is improving oxygenation[45] with more effective vascular injury[133] and necrosis.[132]

The duration of the light that is first administered[131] and the duration of time between each light fraction[132] may be particularly important in improving the oxygen delivery between light fractions. When the PS has been readministered before the second light fraction, a short DLI has demonstrated improved tumor control in preclinical models through vascular targeting with various photosensitizers such as verteporfin[19] MV6401[26] and m-tetra hydroxyphenylchlorin (mTHPC).[137]

As previously described, PDT causes cytotoxic oxidative stress and induces the expression of pleiotropic prosurvival molecules such as COX-2.[82] Understanding the mechanisms leading to prosurvival molecule induction is relevant to the design of more effective treatments. PDT in combination with various targeted agents designed to reduce the effect of the tumor stress response has demonstrated improved tumor responses in various preclinical models. Antiangiogenic agents lead to decreases in VEGF expression after PDT,[113,138–140] along with improvements in tumor response.[112,113,115,117,138,141] Inhibition of HSP increases the curative potential of PDT through decreased expression of angiogenic and prosurvival proteins in the treated tumors,[142] whereas disruption of HSP-90 function *in vitro* leads to increases in PDT-induced apoptosis.[86] The COX-2 pathway has also been targeted in combination with PDT and can improve therapeutic outcome through inhibition of post-PDT angiogenesis, as well as, under some circumstances, through increases in direct PDT cytotoxicity.[125,143–145]

PRACTICE OF PHOTODYNAMIC THERAPY

Light Delivery and Dosimetry

The ability to achieve PS activation is dependent on effective administration of light not only with a wavelength that matches the spectral absorption of the PS but also on depositing a sufficient amount of energy to the target tissue (total fluence). Wavelengths >800 nm are unable to deposit sufficient energy to activate a PS. Delivering sufficient fluence is influenced not only by the technique of its administration (i.e., surface vs. interstitial) but also by the ability of the light energy to penetrate sufficiently at depth to treat the intended target volume. As light photons interact with tissue, photons scatter and are absorbed by endogenous chromophores such as hemoglobin, myoglobin, melanin, and cytochromes. Hemoglobin is especially important to consider. Hemoglobin has spectral absorption peaks < 600 nm (i.e., hemoglobin absorbs all colors except red), and its ability to absorb light energy is affected by its oxygenation status. Oxygenated hemoglobin is less likely to absorb between 600 and 800 nm compared to deoxygenated hemoglobin. Thus, most activating light that has been used for PDT has typically been between 600 and 800 nm, depending on the spectral absorption characteristics of the PS.

The rate at which the light energy is delivered (fluence rate) is also an important treatment factor that can affect the efficacy of PDT. It primarily affects the tissue microenvironment such as the vascular flow and oxygenation. In general, it is important to recognize that high fluence rates can rapidly consume and reduce the local oxygen levels such that it limits the efficacy of the remaining light fluence.[146] The prescribed fluence rate is typically based on the power output of the light source, but surface and internal scattering of light photons may result in areas of higher fluence rates. Strategies to reduce the surface scatter effect or to modify the prescribed power output of the light source should be considered.

At present, the prescription of PDT used clinically remains limited to rudimentary power output calculations for surface illumination: That prescription dose is given in terms of the energy per unit area incident on the surface.

Various light delivery devices have been developed to perform PDT treatment. Most of them are fiberoptic based. These include linear source, endotracheal tube–modified point source, collimated light source, and flat-cut fiber (Fig. 31.2).

FIGURE 31.2. Various fiber-based light sources. These include a linear source **(A)**, an endotracheal tube–modified point source **(B)**, collimated light fiber **(C)**, and a flat-cut fiber **(D)**.

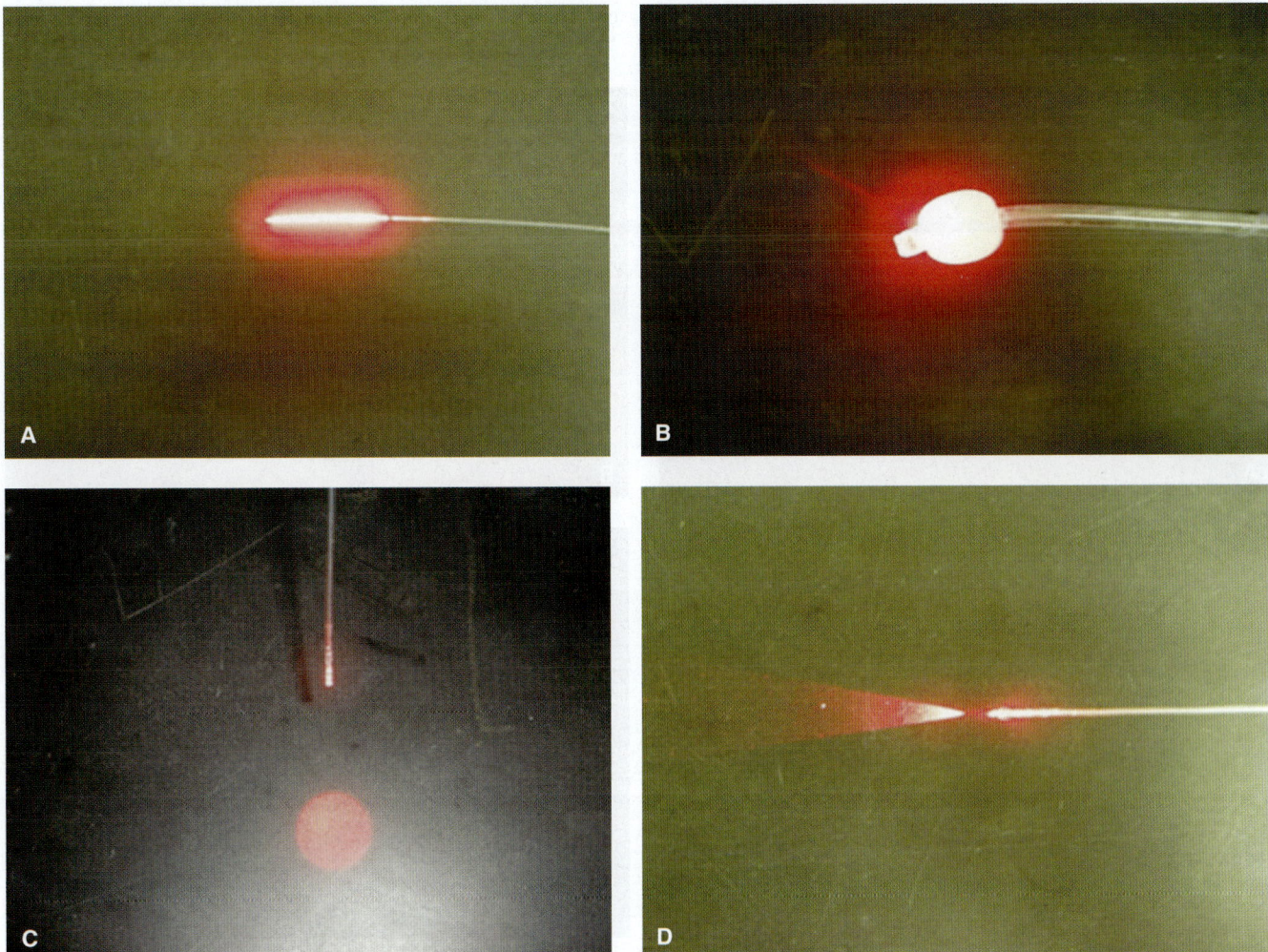

The flat-cut and linear sources are suitable for inserting into the tissue for interstitial PDT application for the treatment of bulky tumors. In contrast, the collimated light source is suitable for superficial treatment.

It is therefore helpful to recognize that various illumination techniques may be employed depending on the geometry of the target lesion that is to be treated. The most common clinical situation requires surface illumination. This is where several technical approaches may be considered. If the geometry of the target lesion is flat or may be modified to be a near flat surface, the use of a light fiber with a diffusing lens at the tip of the fiber (i.e., microlens) offers the ability to achieve homogeneous light distribution across the surface target. Inhomogeneities because of different distances between points on the surface of the target and the light source can result in different fluence rates and the total light dose (fluence) that is effectively delivered. Unlike ionizing radiation, the surface scattering of photons because of surface concavities or reflective surfaces (i.e., any adjacent metal surfaces) can further increase the risk of high surface dose inhomogeneities. In a similar manner, surface convexities may create regions of shadowing that can create regions of low fluence and fluence rate. Obviously, areas of high light fluence (and its fluence rate) could also contribute to an increased risk of normal tissue complications. But consider conversely, low fluence also decreases efficiency.

When the target lesion is cylindrical, a cylindrical diffusing fiber with the light dose prescribed along its length has commonly been used. However, it is important to note that where the target surface is not rigid (i.e., esophagus), mucosal folds that are not in apposition to the light fiber may become underdosed. To reduce this risk, the cylindrical diffusing fiber can be placed within a balloon diffuser that can be expanded to increase its surface apposition with the mucosal surface. Similar considerations can be applied to spherical surface targets such as the mucosa of the urinary bladder.

The use of a balloon diffuser may be helpful for certain complex three-dimensional surfaces, such as the lateral oral tongue and its adjacent floor of the mouth where the surface to be treated can be molded in apposition to the balloon diffuser. In such situations, it is important to verify that the mucosal surface is in direct contact with the balloon's surface before the light is delivered. Other strategies for such complex three-dimensional surfaces may include dividing the target volume into separate targets and individually treating each area with a microlens (patching technique). With this approach, it is important to bear in mind that areas of potential overlap, when illuminated, may increase the risk of normal tissue complications. Other surface illumination techniques under development include a light "blanket" that attempts to mold the light source to such complex three-dimensional surfaces.

Interstitial light fibers can also be placed when volume illumination is required. As with interstitial brachytherapy techniques, the geometry of the light fibers can significantly affect the overall distribution and amount of light that is delivered. Thus, the use of rigid templates guiding the insertion of the trocar needles (Fig. 31.3) can be very helpful in ensuring accurate interfiber spacing. These templates may be used to facilitate the advancement of rigid trocar needles whose track can then be replaced with light fibers. Alternatively, traditional low dose rate afterloading plastic catheters may be used instead to allow the use of the needle track for both light detection fibers and treatment fibers where prescription is based on light dosimetry. The placement of the catheters can also facilitate several quality assurance measures. This can include verifying the geometry of the implant, allowing

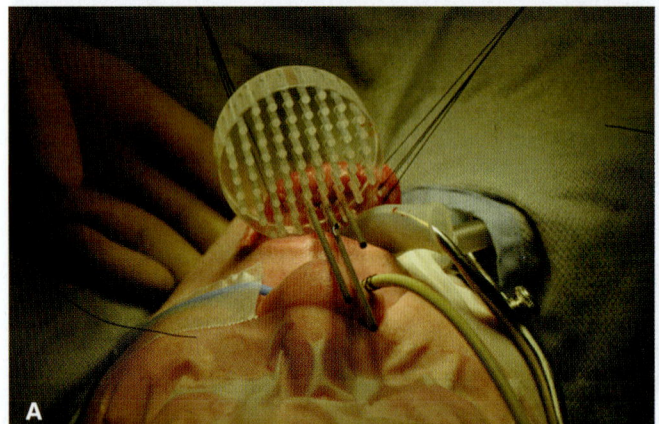

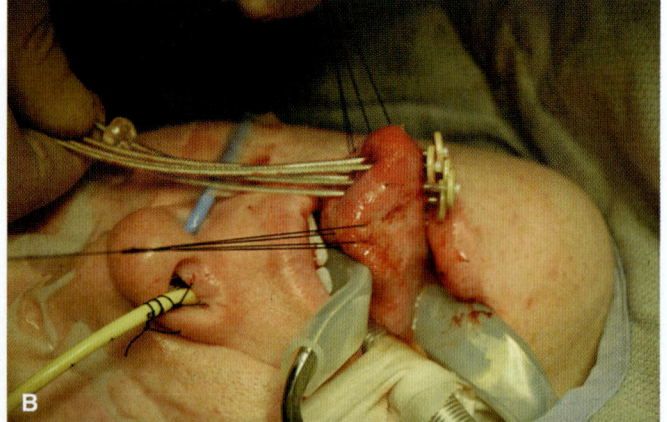

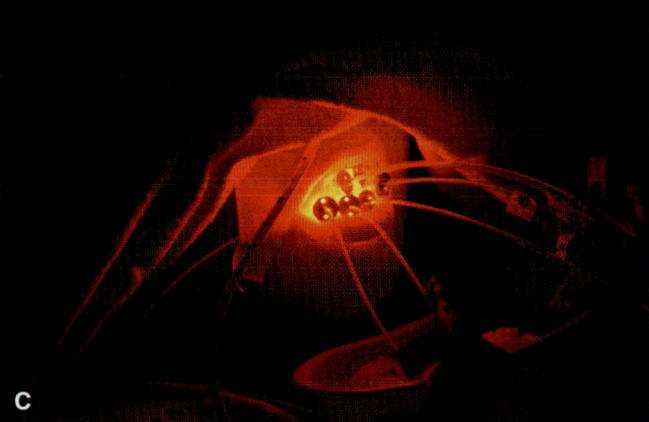

FIGURE 31.3. Example of an interstitial tongue photodynamic therapy implant. A traditional interstitial brachytherapy implant uses a template **(A)** to facilitate the placement of trocars guiding the insertion of hollow plastic catheters **(B)** that are modified for linear light sources **(C)**.

additional catheters to be placed or removed to optimize the geometry. It may also include verification or modification of the location of the light fiber in its catheter relative to the tumor volume.

Whether the optical properties of the tissue being treated are different by staging, the placement of the implant and its illumination is not clear. However, where significant tissue trauma occurs with the placement of the implant, staging the illumination may offer some potential advantages especially where significant tissue bleeding with the introduction of the trocar needles has occurred. Other theoretical advantages may also include improved oxygenation of the implanted tissue, both improving the photosensitization process and reducing hemoglobin absorption of the activating light energy.

Although the optimal interstitial PDT prescription parameters remain to be defined, it is encouraging to see successful interstitial light implants being reported. For such results to become generalizable, the development of a robust and easy-to-use dosimetry system will be needed that will facilitate characterizing the impact of different prescription factors (i.e., intercatheter distance, fluence rate) on normal tissue complications and oncologic results.

Additional Technical Considerations

A significant property of the visible light energy used for photoactivation is its ability to reflect on a surface when light is delivered with a microlens technique. This can in turn increase the fluence and fluence rate delivered especially when the surface is concave and is often referred to as the *integrating sphere effect*. Strategies to minimize variables may include manipulating the surface geometry to reduce concavities and convexities (which can reduce the fluence delivered), removing surface mucosal secretions, using anticholinergics such as glycopyrrolate, and considering alternative illumination techniques. Where the target lesion lies adjacent to reflective metal surfaces that may be used in exposing and possibly flattening the target lesion, surface reflection may be blocked by placing surgical towels over these surfaces. Alternatively, these metal surfaces may be coated with a dark pigment. Similarly, surface scatter may increase the light that is delivered to the adjacent normal skin or mucosa adjacent but outside of the target lesion.

For small surface target lesions treated with a microlens technique, movement of the light fiber because of hand tremor can have a significant impact on the light dosimetry across a small surface area. For example, this is especially a concern when the glottic laryngeal mucosa is being illuminated while working down a laryngoscope. For these reasons, adding rigidity to the flexible light fiber by fixing it to a rigid stylet and immobilizing it with various commercially available fixation devices should be considered.

CLINICAL PHOTODYNAMIC THERAPY

The clinical study of PDT has been an active area of active investigation, despite only three PS being approved for clinical use in cancer management. These include porfimer sodium for the treatment of esophageal and lung cancers and superficial papillary bladder carcinomas, temoporfin for head and neck carcinomas, and ALA for skin actinic keratosis (AK) and basal cell carcinoma (BCC). Trials have generally established clinical activity and the potential for cure in the appropriate cancer application. Despite these efforts, rigorous clinical development of PDT is generally lacking and has not evaluated important comparative questions of its activity to established treatment modalities or, where more appropriate, its value as an adjunctive modality. In general, clinical investigations have also not established the optimal PDT treatment parameters. A comprehensive evaluation of the quality of evidence supporting PDT in clinical practice is referred to in the recent systematic review by Fayter et al.[147] However, the following examples are described.

Skin

The dermatologic applications of PDT are perhaps the most established and scientifically robust of all the anatomic sites for which PDT has been evaluated, with established consensus statements regarding its use.[148] The success of PDT for skin malignancies is a testament to both its strengths and its weakness, with a multitude of randomized trials having been completed for various nonmelanomatous skin malignancies leading to its U.S. Food and Drug Administration (FDA) approval for the management of BCCs and the premalignant nonhyperkeratotic AK.

PDT has been used extensively in the treatment of both premalignant and malignant skin tumors, typically with surface illumination.[148,149] PDT of nonhyperkeratotic AK, squamous cell carcinoma *in situ* (Bowen disease), and BCC can be performed using systemically administered porfimer sodium or topically applied aminolevulinic acid (ALA) and ALA derivatives such as methyl-ALA (MAL). For example, during a placebo controlled trial of PDT for actinic keratosis (AK), ALA-PDT showed a superior complete response (CR) as compared to a sham PDT technique coupled with the same carrier vehicle. That response rate was 87% versus only 13% with the sham ($P = .001$).[150] PDT for AK shows similar efficacy with less toxicity as compared to cryotherapy, topical 5-fluorouracil cream, or curettage, for example, a study in which 119 subjects with 1,501 AK lesions of the scalp and face were randomly assigned to receive MAL-PDT to either the left- or right-sided lesions, with cryotherapy used to treat the contralateral side.[151] Twenty-four weeks after therapy, both treatment groups showed a high response rate (89% for MAL-PDT vs. 86% for cryotherapy; $P = .2$), but MAL-PDT showed superior cosmesis and patient preference. In contrast, the results for PDT of squamous cell carcinomas (SCC) of the skin using topical photosensitizers have been disappointing, with recurrence rates of >50%.[148,149] Perhaps, the most significant potential value of ALA-PDT may be its ability to prevent the development of nonmelanoma skin cancers in patients with AK, as recently demonstrated in a randomized trial of prophylactic ALA-PDT.[152]

Other indications for ALA-PDT include superficial and nodular BCC.[153–155] In a large single-institution series, high rates of local control (>90% complete response rate, <10% local failure at 3 to 5 years) can be achieved with PDT for superficial BCC. However, the response rate and local control rate for nodular BCC drop to 70% and 40%, respectively. In a multicenter randomized trial of MAL-PDT versus cryotherapy for superficial BCC, complete response rates at 3 months were 97% and 95%, with 22% and 20% 5-year recurrence rates for MAL-PDT and cryotherapy, respectively.[156] In this study, the excellent to good cosmetic outcome was 89% for MAL-PDT and 50% for cryotherapy. However, when topical PDT is compared to surgery for BCC, topical ALA or MAL-PDT consistently shows a small increase in recurrence rate as compared to surgery for both superficial and nodular BCC. However, the cosmetic outcomes for PDT are typically superior to surgery with good to excellent cosmetic outcome in >90% of PDT patients with PDT and 60% to 70% with surgery. In summary, PDT can be an appropriate and effective treatment alternative to cryosurgery or surgical excision for selected BCC. PDT is currently approved in the United States, Canada, and the European Union for the treatment of AK and approved in the European Union and Canada for treatment of BCC.

Brain

PDT has primarily been evaluated as adjunctive therapy treating the surgical bed often combined with its use for PDD as a fluorescent guide to (surgical) resection (FGR).

Yang et al.[157] demonstrated that porfimer sodium fluorescence at 640 nm could be clearly visualized in the resection bed in patients with supratentorial gliomas not seen under white light. Biopsy of these areas of fluorescence confirmed the presence of residual tumor, thus demonstrating the concept of FGR. Similar high tumor specificity was also observed with hypericin-mediated FGR for glioblastoma multiforme (GBM)[158] and protoporphyrin-IX (PpIX) fluorescence (that was produced following administration of the photosensitizer ALA) of the surgical bed in GBM patients.[159] All biopsies of fluorescent tissue contained GBM.[158,159] However, the benefits of just FGF could not be clearly demonstrated in a phase III study (n = 27) as all patients receiving ALA also had received porfimer sodium and received PDT to the surgical cavity. Eljamel et al.[159] demonstrated that the mean survival significantly increased with ALA-mediated FGR and porfimer sodium PDT (P < .01). However, in a phase III study of 322 patients with suspected malignant gliomas randomized to ALA-FGF or conventional surgery, Stummer et al.[160] reported an improved progression-free survival (41% vs. 21%, respectively; P = .0003) following a median survival of 35.5 months. No significant increased complications have been observed with photosensitizer-based PDD and FGR.[160]

Further evidence in support of PDT activity for GBM particularly comes from several institutional experiences where PDT was used to treat the resection cavity for various histologies, including newly diagnosed[161–163] and recurrent[162] GBM and anaplastic astrocytoma (AA).[161] Other histologies evaluated have also included malignant ependymomas[164] and meningiomas.[165] Muller and Wilson[163] reported the results of a retrospective institutional review of adjuvant porfimer sodium PDT (mean fluence of 58 J/cm² with only 18 patients receiving >100 J/cm²) in 96 patients with supratentorial gliomas. Of these 96 patients, 49 patients presented with either newly diagnosed (n = 12) or recurrent (n = 37) GBM; a median survival of 8.25 and 7.25 months was reported, respectively. In contrast, Stylli et al.[162] reported a median survival of 14.3 and 14.9 months, respectively, with hematoporphyrin derivative (HpD)–mediated PDT. Though Muller and Wilson indicated that such differences may have been due to selection factors, they also suggest that this may be consistent with a dose–response effect. Stylli also reported a light dose effect on overall survival for both GBM and AA. This has formed the basis for an ongoing randomized trial of low versus high light dose porfimer sodium–mediated PDT as adjuvant therapy following surgical resection for supratentorial gliomas.[166]

Head and Neck

The evaluation of PDT for head and neck malignancies has typically been for head and neck squamous cell carcinomas (HNSCC). Case reports or series have also demonstrated that PDT may have activity for other histologies such as Kaposi sarcoma and salivary gland malignancies such as adenoid cystic carcinomas.[167] Although there have been significant numbers of clinical evaluations of PDT in the management of HNSCC, the vast majority represent single-institutional experiences demonstrating activity either for definitive management or for palliation. Definitive management has typically evaluated surface illumination for premalignant dysplastic lesions or early primary invasive mucosa malignancies where the risk of nodal metastases was regarded as low. Common sites have included the oral cavity, larynx, nasopharynx,[37] and base of the tongue.[168]

Superficial premalignant mucosal lesions are attractive for PDT because of the ability to achieve wide-field mucosal ablation given the uncertainties that are commonly encountered in defining the peripheral extent of the lesion. For these reasons, treatment of the larynx is particularly attractive because of the defined nature of this anatomic site, where conservation therapies such as PDT can offer function-preserving

advantages. Contemporary clinical experience suggests that this treatment approach can be effective in obtaining a complete response for the treated lesion, but long-term follow-up is limited.[169] However, this limitation is not dissimilar from other treatment modalities that have been used for mucosal dysplasia. To date, clinical experience has also included retrospective reviews[170] and several prospective studies of porfimer sodium,[171] temoporfin, and[172,173] topical[174] and systemic[136] ALA that have demonstrated high complete response rates typically >80%. Further research efforts are needed to define both the long-term infield and out-of-field relapse risks, and the risk of malignant transformation following PDT treatments is forthcoming.

Additionally, PDT for the treatment of superficial (invasive) carcinomas has also been evaluated, typically with porfimer sodium and temoporfin, especially with the EU regulatory approval of temoporfin for the palliative management of HNSCC. Prospective studies of porfimer sodium[171,175] and temoporfin[176] have demonstrated complete response rates typically >80%, with both surface and interstitial illumination techniques used. Long-term infield control rates have also been reported in approximately 70% to 90% of treated patients.[175,176]

The head and neck site has also been the main focus for the development of interstitial illumination techniques. These include the ability to treat deeper invasive carcinomas where the risk of nodal metastases remains low, such as early tongue carcinomas (see Fig. 31.2) or the promise of less toxic salvage therapy,[177] palliation of locoregional recurrences,[178,179] and the treatment of benign tumors such as vascular malformations,[180] which would otherwise require potentially debilitating surgery or the administration of high dose radiotherapy. Lastly, a potential role for intraoperative PDT using porfimer sodium as adjuvant therapy following surgical resection for locoregionally recurrent HNSCC has been reported. With a minimum follow-up of 24 months, four of five treated patients were without locoregional recurrence or wound complications.[181]

Thorax

Since 1998, PDT has been FDA approved for the treatment of microinvasive endobronchial and advanced partially obstructing non–small cell lung cancer (NSCLC).[182] Endobronchial light delivery has typically been used limiting treatment to central lesions with techniques under development to extend PDT to treat peripheral lesions.[183] It has been used as definitive therapy in treating endobronchial occult or synchronous primary carcinomas where the bronchoscope-visible lesions are ≤1 cm in surface dimension with no clinical cartilage invasion. When PDT is attempted to treat larger tumors—without prior surgical debulking—it has largely been used for palliative indications.

Roentgenographically Occult Bronchogenic Non–Small Cell Lung Cancer

Fewer than 1% of patients with occult bronchogenic carcinoma that are endoscopically visible but lack cartilaginous invasion have metastatic lymph node involvement, indicating a potential for a less invasive focal therapy to be curative.[184] Investigators from the National Kinki Central Hospital for Chest Diseases used PDT to treat occult bronchogenic carcinoma in 25 patients with 29 lesions.[185] A complete remission was achieved in 72% of lesions, including 89% (17/19) of lesions ≤1 cm and 86% (18/21) of visible peripheral area lesions. In another series of 33 patients, with 40 clinically occult carcinomas treated with PDT, a complete response was achieved in all lesions ≤1 cm (n = 32).[186] Among the 39 occult lesions treated at Osaka Prefectural Habikino Hospital with PDT, a complete response was achieved in 64% of lesions, more in superficially infiltrating than for nodular lesions (76%

vs. 43%).[187] Tohoku University Hospital investigators treated 48 medically operable patients with occult bronchogenic SCC with tumor lengths of ≤1 cm with PDT; they observed a complete response in 94% of patients and a 10-year overall survival rate of 71%.[188]

Radiographically Visible Early-Stage and Endobronchial Non–Small Cell Lung Cancer

Similar to roentgenologically occult bronchogenic carcinomas, early-stage and endobronchial NSCLC can be effectively treated with PDT for patients unsuitable for surgical resection.

At Tokyo Medical University Hospital, 240 patients with 283 central lung cancer lesions were treated from 1980 to 1995 with PDT. The overall response rate was 99%, with a complete response in 40%. A complete response was achieved in 83% (79/95) of early-stage lesions, with a 94% (65/69) complete response rate for lesions <1 cm. Several institutional experiences also made similar observations of durable complete responses in over 75% of patients treated at a minimum of 12 months' follow-up.[189,190] However, the complete response rate fell to 54% (14/26) for lesions ≥1 cm and 38% (6/16) for lesions ≥2 cm (P = .00001).[191] A more recent report from Tokyo Medical University Hospital demonstrated that among 93 patients treated with PDT for 114 central early-stage lung cancers, as expected, the complete response rate was higher for lesions <1 cm (77/83) than ≥1 cm (18/31; 93% vs. 58%; P < .001). The recurrence rate was 12% for lesions <1 cm with an initial complete response to PDT, and many recurrences could successfully be salvaged with additional PDT.[192] In a review of 15 trials of 626 patients with 715 central early-stage bronchogenic cancers treated typically for surgery ineligibility patients, PDT-related toxicity was limited, with one PDT-related death (0.15%), photosensitivity skin reactions in 5% to 28%, respiratory complications in 0% to 18%, and nonfatal hemoptysis in 0% to 8%. A complete response was achieved in 30% to 100% of patients for a 2- to 120-month duration, and the 5-year overall survival was 61%.[193]

Synchronous multiple primary lung cancers occur in 1% to 15% of patients with lung malignancies and have been increasing in incidence because of improvements in imaging. These cases may warrant considerations for aggressive management. Incorporating PDT in the management of central lesions, especially when small in size, can significantly reduce the pulmonary morbidity. In a study of 22 patients with synchronous early lung cancers treated with PDT alone for each lesion (n = 11) or surgery for the more peripheral lesions and PDT for the more central lesions (n = 11), PDT achieved a complete response in all 39 central tumors at 2 months following therapy.[194] All patients were alive with variable follow-up of up to 5 years.

Advanced-Stage Non–Small Cell Lung Cancer

For patients with locally advanced or metastatic NSCLC, PDT has been used for palliation. In a randomized trial comparing PDT to neodymium:yttrium–aluminum–garnet (Nd:YAG) laser therapy in the NSCLC patients with an obstructed airway, both PDT and Nd:YAG laser therapy were comparable with regard to symptom relief and response rates. The time to failure (P = .03) and the median survival (P = .007) were significantly longer in the cohort receiving PDT.[195] In combination with radiotherapy, prolonged response of the luminal tumor mass may be observed and thus warrants further investigation.[196,197]

Preoperative PDT has been reported in several small institutional series of patients with NSCLC. Although small in numbers, these series have independently observed that preoperative PDT may help reduce the extent of definitive resection needed for locally advanced NSCLC by downstaging patients who would otherwise require a pneumonectomy to undergo lobectomy instead or to convert patients

originally deemed inoperable to be surgical candidates.[198–200] Okunaka et al.[198] reported on the results of 26 patients with NSCLC treated with preoperative PDT alone with the desired intent to reduce the extent of resection or convert inoperable disease to an operable status. These surgical goals were achieved in 85% of patients, with 4 of 5 originally inoperable patients converted to resectable, and 18 of 21 patients originally candidates only for pneumonectomy were able to undergo lobectomy. Ross et al.[199] reported on 41 patients with locally advanced NSCLC treated with induction PDT and chemotherapy or radiation therapy. PDT induction allowed 57% of initially unresectable patients to undergo definitive surgical resection and 27% of those initially deemed in need of pneumonectomy to undergo lobectomy. Pathologic downstaging occurred in 64%. Plus 46% of patients were alive at 3 years following therapy.

PDT has been used as part of multimodality management for patients with NSCLC with pleural spread. A phase II trial of 22 such patients at the University of Pennsylvania assessed the oncologic outcome of patients treated with surgery, achieving either a complete resection (n = 17) or partial tumor debulking (n = 3) followed by hemithoracic pleural PDT (porfimer sodium) (n = 20) or PDT alone (n = 2).[201] The 6-month local control rate for the cohort was 73.3% and the median overall survival was 21.7 months, suggesting promising activity.

Malignant Pleural Mesothelioma

The use of PDT to treat malignant pleural mesothelioma was pioneered at the National Cancer Institute in the 1980s and has since become integrated into multimodality therapy for mesothelioma.[202] In a National Cancer Institute phase I trial, 54 patients with pleural malignancies isolated to one hemithorax were evaluated, including 40 patients with mesothelioma. Among the 42 patients who underwent optimal tumor debulking to ≤5 mm of residual tumor thickness followed by PDT, the PDT was relatively well tolerated. The median survival among mesothelioma patients was 10 months.[203] In the perioperative period, however, intraoperative PDT for mesothelioma can be associated with acute bleeding, severe generalized vascular atherosclerosis, generalized edema, intrathoracic fluid accumulation, respiratory distress, and death.[204]

In a phase II study at Roswell Park Cancer Institute, 40 patients underwent extrapleural pneumonectomy or pleurectomy followed by intracavitary PDT.[205] The median survival was significantly better for stage I and II patients (n = 13) than stage III and IV patients (n = 24; 36 months vs. 10 months; P < .0001). PDT dose was found to be independent prognostic indicators for survival (P < .009).[205] Dutch investigators treated 28 predominantly advanced-stage mesothelioma patients with pleuropneumonectomy followed by intraoperative PDT. Half of the patients in the cohort had persistent local tumor control for at least 9 months following PDT, and the median overall survival of the cohort was 10 months.[204] At the University of Pennsylvania, 28 patients with malignant pleural mesothelioma, including 86% with stage III and IV diseases, were treated from 2004 to 2008 with macroscopic complete resection and intraoperative PDT. Patients who underwent radical pleurectomy (n = 14) had a significantly improved median survival compared with those who underwent modified extrapleural pneumonectomy.[206]

The only randomized phase III trial assessing the role of PDT in the management of malignant pleural mesothelioma involved 63 patients at the National Cancer Institute undergoing maximum surgery, postoperative cisplatin, interferon α-2b, and tamoxifen with or without first-generation intraoperative intrapleural PDT (630 nm, porfimer sodium, 30 J/cm² using intraoperative real-time light dosimetry). Most patients (79%) had stage III disease. The median survival for the 15 nonoptimally cytoreduced patients with >5-mm residual disease was 7.2 months, compared to 14.4 months for the remaining 48 patients. However, PDT did not influence the pattern of recurrence, median survival (14.1 vs. 14.4 months), or median progression-free time (8.5 vs. 7.7 months).[207]

Gastrointestinal Malignancies

Photodynamic Therapy for Malignancies of the Gastrointestinal Tract

Of the gastrointestinal (GI) tract tumors that can be treated with PDT, Barrett esophagus (BE) with dysplasia and early-stage esophageal cancer are the best studied.[208,209] Overholt et al.[210] demonstrated in a multicenter randomized trial that PDT for premalignant BE can eliminate dysplastic cells and is associated with a lower incidence of development of invasive carcinoma. In this trial, 208 patients were randomly assigned to receive either PDT with proton pump inhibitor (PPI) or PPI alone in a two-to-one randomization schema. PDT-treated patients received porfimer sodium (2 mg/kg) 40 to 50 hours prior to the first light delivery. Areas of BE were exposed to 130 J/cm with 630-nm light using a cylindrical fiberoptic diffuser encased in an inflated esophageal balloon so that the fiber would be centered and the esophageal folds flattened. Ninety-six to 120 hours later, a repeat endoscopy was performed to assess response, and an additional 50 J/cm could be given to areas of insufficient mucosal damage. If BE was found to persist on follow-up endoscopy, additional PDT treatments could be performed for a maximum of three total treatments given at least 3 months apart. All patients (in both arms) received omeprazole therapy at a dose of 20 mg given twice daily. The results of this trial showed that PDT plus PPI was superior to PPI alone, and the updated 5-year results confirm the long-term benefits with a 50% relative risk reduction in the incidence of invasive carcinoma.[211] At 5 years of follow-up, Overholt et al.[210] demonstrated that 77% of patients treated with PDT-PPI showed ablation of HGD versus 39% of patients treated with PPI alone (P < .0001). More significantly, 15% of the patients in the PDT-PPI arm showed progression to cancer versus 29% on the PPI arm (P < .006). The toxicity of the PDT-PPI treatment was esophageal stricture, with the majority of cases successfully managed with esophageal dilatation. Mucosal injury prior to PDT and repeat PDT treatments appears to increase this risk.[210,212]

PDT has also been studied in a variety of tumor types in the GI tract. Significant clinical efficacy has been observed in early studies of PDT for gastric,[213] early duodenal, and ampullary cancers.[214–216] Promising results have been achieved in the treatment of cholangiocarcinomas (CC). Early case reports and pilot studies of PDT for CC demonstrated significant promise.[217,218] In a randomized, controlled trial of stenting with or without PDT, the median survival of patients treated with PDT plus stenting was remarkable with 493 days compared with only 98 days in the stenting-alone group.[219] Other studies have shown similar results.[220–222] A multicenter clinical trial has been initiated to obtain regulatory approval in the United States and Canada.[223]

Other clinical applications of PDT in the GI tract have included unresectable pancreatic cancers[224] and numerous reports using PDT to eliminate colon polyps as well as to palliate bulky colon and rectal cancers.[216,225–227] In addition, PDT may have efficacy in treating hepatocellular carcinoma. Early results have been promising, and a phase III study is currently under way to evaluate the efficacy of talaporfin-mediated PDT using interstitial LEDs compared with institution-specific standard treatment.[228]

Photodynamic Therapy for Intraperitoneal Malignancies

Peritoneal carcinomatosis presents a very difficult problem for standard cancer treatment modalities. The superficial nature of PDT combined with its ability to treat large surface areas seems to lend itself to this particular problem. However, adequate and homogeneous light distribution to all peritoneal surfaces remains an ongoing technical challenge. In a phase I trial of 70 subjects with predominantly recurrent ovarian carcinomatosis, intraoperative PDT following maximal surgical debulking resulted in a 76% complete cytologic response rate with tolerable toxicity.[229] In the follow-up of a phase II study, patients were enrolled and stratified according to cancer type (ovarian, gastrointestinal, or sarcoma) and given doses of porfimer sodium and light at a phase I previously defined maximally tolerated dose.[230] Other than capillary leak syndrome and skin photosensitivity, the complication rates were similar to the complication rates typically observed after similarly extensive surgery in the absence of PDT.[231] With a median follow-up of 51 months, the median failure-free survival and overall survival rates for the patients who received PDT were 3 and 22 months in ovarian cancer patients and 3.3 and 13.2 months in gastrointestinal cancer patients, respectively. Six months after therapy, the pathologic complete response rate was 3 of 33 (9.1%) and 2 of 37 (5.4%) for the patients with ovarian cancer and gastrointestinal cancer, respectively. These results in heavily pretreated patients suggest that PDT for peritoneal carcinomatosis may have some clinical benefit.

Genitourinary Malignancies

Photodynamic Therapy for Prostate Carcinomas

The role of interstitial PDT for prostate adenocarcinoma has been investigated by several groups studying various PS including temoporfin,[6,273] motexafin lutetium,[50,230,233] and padoporfin.[234] The majority of these phase I and II trials have been in patients with locally recurrent adenocarcinoma, typically following failure of radiotherapy. Several observations are implied: Traditional brachytherapy techniques can be adopted to administer diffusing light fibers with potentially effective light delivery and oncologic efficacy. Oncologically, a dose–response relationship may exist. When higher light doses are delivered, the probability of acute tissue injury causes an increase in PSA in the first 24 hours posttreatment,[50] leading to a pathologic complete response[235] and possibly a more durable PSA response.[50]

At this time, the optimal light dose and other PDT prescription parameters remain to be determined. However, delivering a minimum and sufficient light fluence to 90% of the prostate clinical tumor volume (CTV) may be important.[235] This is further complicated by the significant patient heterogeneity[236,237] in the optical properties of the prostate that changes dynamically during the administration of the light.[6] However, analysis of the heterogeneity in the tissue injury as assessed by magnetic resonance imaging demonstrating light dosimetry may not be sufficient to completely predict for prostate and surrounding normal tissue injury or for the risk of urorectal fistulas.[238] That is, other factors such as the PS and oxygen concentrations and the effectiveness of the singlet oxygen generation along with variable patient factors may be important and remain subjects of ongoing investigation.[73] In the interim, careful attention to minimize trauma to the rectal wall[232] and the light dosimetry for interstitial PDT remains important. It may be prudent to establish a lower light fluence to the rectal wall as this tissue may have a lower intrinsic threshold for interstitial PDT injury.[238]

Photodynamic Therapy for Bladder Carcinomas

Bladder carcinomas are typically superficial and diffuse across the mucosa, lending to the application of intracavitary PDT. In fact, the first-generation photosensitizer hematoporphyrin and its derivative (HpD) were used as early as 1975. This developed the regulatory approval of the purified active component (porfimer sodium) for the treatment of recurrent superficial papillary carcinoma as seen in failed conventional intravesical therapy such as the bacille Calmette-Guérin (BCG). Several institutional experiences have demonstrated activity with HpD or porfimer sodium PDT to the whole bladder with high initial response rates of ≥70% with long-term (>2 years) control rates between 30% and 60%.[239–242] These response rates suggest comparable activity that was recently supported in a recent multicenter randomized study comparing BCG to porfimer sodium PDT in patients with superficial bladder carcinoma.[243] Bladder contracture because of fibrosis was observed to be a significant complication in the early experience of porfimer sodium PDT that was later demonstrated to be reduced by measuring the light fluence on the surface and accounting for both the incident and scattered light.[244] Other strategies that reduced the risk of late bladder injury include porfimer sodium PDT with less penetrating light (514 nm),[245] reducing the porfimer sodium dose, the light dose administered,[239] and the use of topical ALA, which is a more superficial photosensitizer.[246,247]

CONCLUSION

A significant body of preclinical and clinical evidence supports the hypothesis that PDT could have important cytotoxicity, with cure possible in limited clinical applications as applied to malignancies. There has been a tremendous body of advancement in the physics of light dosimetry, sophistication of PS development for photodiagnosis and photoactivation, and the understanding of the cellular and microenvironment effects of PDT. These achievements may offer an array of potential translational opportunities. The advances for the indications and the efficacy of PDT when used alone and in combination with traditional therapeutics continue.

ACKNOWLEDGMENTS

We would like to acknowledge Theodore E. Yaeger, MD, FACR; Professor, Radiation Oncology, Wake Forest University School of Medicine, Winston-Salem, NC.

REFERENCES

1. Raab O. Über die Wirkung fluoreszierender Stoffe auf Infusorien. *Z Biol* 1900;39:524–546.
2. von Tappeiner H, Jesionek A. Therapeutische versuche mit fluoreszierenden stoffen. *Muench Med Wochenschr* 1903;47:2042–2044.
3. Lipson RL, Baldes EJ. The photodynamic properties of a particular hematoporphyrin derivative. *Arch Dermatol* 1960;82:508–516.
4. Schwartz SK, Abolon K, Vermund H. Some relationships of porphyrins, x-rays and tumors. *Univ Minn Med Bul* 1955;27:7–8.
5. Dougherty TJ, et al. Photodynamic therapy. *J Natl Cancer Inst* 1998;90:889–905.
6. Swartling J, et al. System for interstitial photodynamic therapy with online dosimetry: first clinical experiences of prostate cancer. *J Biomed Opt* 2010;15:058003.
7. O'Connor AE, Gallagher WM, Byrne AT. Porphyrin and nonporphyrin photosensitizers in oncology: preclinical and clinical advances in photodynamic therapy. *Photochem Photobiol* 2009;85:1053–1074.
8. Halkiotis K, Yova D, Pantelias G. In vitro evaluation of the genotoxic and clastogenic potential of photodynamic therapy. *Mutagenesis* 1999;14:193–198.
9. Zenzen V, Zankl H. In vitro evaluation of the cytotoxic and mutagenic potential of the 5-aminolevulinic acid hexylester-mediated photodynamic therapy. *Mutat Res* 2004;561:91–100.
10. Rousset N, et al. Use of alkaline comet assay to assess DNA repair after m-THPC-PDT. *J Photochem Photobiol* 2000;56:118–131.
11. Grosjean P, et al. Photodynamic therapy for cancer of the upper aerodigestive tract using tetra(m-hydroxyphenyl)chlorin. *J Clin Laser Med Surg* 1996;14:281–287.
12. Woodburn KW, et al. Subcellular localization of porphyrins using confocal laser scanning microscopy. *Photochem Photobiol* 1991;54:725–732.
13. Woodburn KW, et al. Evaluation of porphyrin characteristics required for photodynamic therapy. *Photochem Photobiol* 1992;55:697–704.
14. Hahn SM, et al. Photofrin uptake in the tumor and normal tissues of patients receiving intraperitoneal photodynamic therapy. *Clin Cancer Res* 2006;12:5464–5470.
15. Jori G, Reddi E. The role of lipoproteins in the delivery of tumour-targeting photosensitizers. *Int J Biochem* 1993;25:1369–1375.

16. Roberts WG, Hasan T. Tumor-secreted vascular permeability factor/vascular endothelial growth factor influences photosensitizer uptake. *Cancer Res* 1993;53:153–157.
17. Roberts WG, Hasan T. Role of neovasculature and vascular permeability on the tumor retention of photodynamic agents. *Cancer Res* 1992;52:924–930.
18. Korbelik M, Krosl G. Cellular levels of photosensitisers in tumours: the role of proximity to the blood supply. *Br J Cancer* 1994;70:604–610.
19. Chen B, et al. Combining vascular and cellular targeting regimens enhances the efficacy of photodynamic therapy. *Int J Radiat Oncol Biol Phys* 2005;61:1216–1226.
20. Buytaert E, Dewaele M, Agostinis P. Molecular effectors of multiple cell death pathways initiated by photodynamic therapy. *Biochim Biophys Acta* 2007;1776:86–107.
21. Yang JZ, et al. Intrauterine 5-aminolevulinic acid induces selective fluorescence and photodynamic ablation of the rat endometrium. *Photochem Photobiol* 1993;57:803–807.
22. Moan J, Berg K. The photodegradation of porphyrins in cells can be used to estimate the lifetime of singlet oxygen. *Photochem Photobiol* 1991;53:549–553.
23. Fiedler DM, Eckl PM, Krammer B. Does delta-aminolaevulinic acid induce genotoxic effects? *J Photochem Photobiol* 1996;33:39–44.
24. Chu ES, et al. The cytotoxic and genotoxic potential of 5-aminolevulinic acid on lymphocytes: a comet assay study. *Cancer Chemother Pharmacol* 2006;58:408–414.
25. McNair FI, et al. A comet assay of DNA damage and repair in K562 cells after photodynamic therapy using haematoporphyrin derivative, methylene blue and meso-tetrahydroxyphenylchlorin. *Br J Cancer* 1997;75:1721–1729.
26. Dolmans DE, et al. Targeting tumor vasculature and cancer cells in orthotopic breast tumor by fractionated photosensitizer dosing photodynamic therapy. *Cancer Res* 2002;62:4289–4294.
27. Pass HI. Photodynamic therapy in oncology: mechanisms and clinical use. *J Natl Cancer Inst* 1993;85:443–456.
28. Ochsner M. Photophysical and photobiological processes in the photodynamic therapy of tumours. *J Photochem Photobiol B* 1997;39:1–18.
29. Hatz S, Lambert JD, Ogilby PR. Measuring the lifetime of singlet oxygen in a single cell: addressing the issue of cell viability. *Photochem Photobiol Sci* 2007;6:1106–1116.
30. Yu G, et al. Noninvasive monitoring of murine tumor blood flow during photodynamic therapy provides early assessment of treatment efficacy. *Clin Can Res* 2005;11:3543–3552.
31. Wilson BC, Patterson MS, Lilge L. Implicit and explicit dosimetry in photodynamic therapy: a new paradigm. *Lasers Med Sci* 1997;12:182–199.
32. Zhu TC, et al. Macroscopic modeling of the singlet oxygen production during PDT. *Proc SPIE* 2007;6427:1–12.
33. Georgakoudi I, Nichols MG, Foster TH. The mechanism of Photofrin photobleaching and its consequences for photodynamic dosimetry. *Photochem Photobiol* 1997;65:135–144.
34. Robinson DJ, et al. Fluorescence photobleaching of ALA-induced protoporphyrin IX during photodynamic therapy of normal hairless mouse skin: the effect of light dose and irradiance and the resulting biological effect. *Photochem Photobiol* 1998;67:140–149.
35. Cottrell WJ, et al. Irradiance-dependent photobleaching and pain in delta-aminolevulinic acid-photodynamic therapy of superficial basal cell carcinomas. *Clin Cancer Res* 2008;14:4475–4483.
36. van Staveren HJ, et al. Integrating sphere effect in whole-bladder-wall photodynamic therapy: III. Fluence multiplication, optical penetration and light distribution with an eccentric source for human bladder optical properties. *Phys Med Biol* 1996;41:579–590.
37. Nyst HJ, et al. Performance of a dedicated light delivery and dosimetry device for photodynamic therapy of nasopharyngeal carcinoma: phantom and volunteer experiments. *Lasers Surg Med* 2007;39:647–653.
38. Tan IB, et al. The importance of in situ light dosimetry for photodynamic therapy of oral cavity tumors. *Head Neck* 1999;21:434–441.
39. Marijnissen JP, Star WM. Performance of isotropic light dosimetry probes based on scattering bulbs in turbid media. *Phys Med Biol* 2002;47:2049–2058.
40. Vulcan TG, et al. Comparison between isotropic and nonisotropic dosimetry systems during intraperitoneal photodynamic therapy. *Lasers Surg Med* 2000;26:292–301.
41. Johansson A, et al. Realtime light dosimetry software tools for interstitial photodynamic therapy of the human prostate. *Med Phys* 2007;34:4309–4321.
42. Altschuler MD, et al. Optimized interstitial PDT prostate treatment planning with the Cimmino feasibility algorithm. *Med Phys* 2005;32:3524–3536.
43. Banihashemi B, et al. Ultrasound imaging of apoptosis in tumor response: novel preclinical monitoring of photodynamic therapy effects. *Cancer Res* 2008;68:8590–8596.
44. Zhou F, et al. Intravital imaging of tumor apoptosis with FRET probes during tumor therapy. *Mol Imaging Biol* 2010;12:63–70.
45. Curnow A, Haller JC, Bown SG. Oxygen monitoring during 5-aminolaevulinic acid induced photodynamic therapy in normal rat colon. Comparison of continuous and fractionated light regimes. *J Photochem Photobiol B* 2000;58:149–155.
46. Henderson BW, Fingar VH. Relationship of tumor hypoxia and response to photodynamic treatment in an experimental mouse tumor. *Cancer Res* 1987;47:3110–3114.
47. Korbelik M, et al. The role of host lymphoid populations in the response of mouse EMT6 tumor to photodynamic therapy. *Cancer Res* 1996;56:5647–5652.
48. Zhou X, et al. Tumor vascular area correlates with photosensitizer uptake: analysis of verteporfin microvascular delivery in the Dunning rat prostate tumor. *Photochem Photobiol* 2006;82:1348–1357.
49. Busch TM, et al. Hypoxia and Photofrin uptake in the intraperitoneal carcinomatosis and sarcomatosis of photodynamic therapy patients. *Clin Cancer Res* 2004;10:4630–4638.

50. Patel H, et al. Motexafin lutetium-photodynamic therapy of prostate cancer: short- and long-term effects on prostate-specific antigen. *Clin Cancer Res* 2008;14:4869–4876.

51. Igbaseimokumo U. Quantification of in vivo Photofrin uptake by human pituitary adenoma tissue. *J Neurosurg* 2004;101:272–277.

52. Gill KR, et al. Pilot study on light dosimetry variables for photodynamic therapy of Barrett's esophagus with high-grade dysplasia. *Clin Cancer Res* 2009;15:1830–1836.

53. Sitnik TM, Henderson BW. Effects of fluence rate on cytotoxicity during photodynamic therapy. *Proc SPIE* 1997;2972:95–102.

54. Henderson BW, Busch TM, Snyder JW. Fluence rate as a modulator of PDT mechanisms. *Lasers Surg Med* 2006;38:489–493.

55. Foster TH, et al. Fluence rate effects in photodynamic therapy of multicell tumor spheroids. *Cancer Res* 1993;53:1249–1254.

56. Busch TM, et al. Fluence rate-dependent intratumor heterogeneity in physiologic and cytotoxic responses to Photofrin photodynamic therapy. *Photochem Photobiol Sci* 2009;8:1683–1693.

57. Mitra S, Foster TH. Carbogen breathing significantly enhances the penetration of red light in murine tumours in vivo. *Phys Med Biol* 2004;49:1891–1904.

58. Busch TM. Local physiological changes during photodynamic therapy. *Lasers Surg Med* 2006;38:494–499.

59. Weston MA, Patterson MS. Calculation of singlet oxygen dose using explicit and implicit dose metrics during benzoporphyrin derivative monoacid ring A (BPD-MA)-PDT in vitro and correlation with MLL cell survival. *Photochem Photobiol* 2011;87:1129–1137.

60. Wang KK, Mitra S, Foster TH. A comprehensive mathematical model of microscopic dose deposition in photodynamic therapy. *Med Phys* 2007;34:282–293.

61. Fingar VII, et al. Vascular damage after photodynamic therapy of solid tumors: a view and comparison of effect in pre-clinical and clinical models at the University of Louisville. *In Vivo* 2000;14:93–100.

62. Chen B, et al. Vascular and cellular targeting for photodynamic therapy. *Crit Rev Eukaryot Gene Expr* 2006;16:279–305.

63. Khurana M, et al. Intravital high-resolution optical imaging of individual vessel response to photodynamic treatment. *J Biomed Opt* 2008;13:040502.

64. Standish BA, et al. Doppler optical coherence tomography monitoring of microvascular tissue response during photodynamic therapy in an animal model of Barrett's esophagus. *Gastrointest Endosc* 2007;66:326–333.

65. Busch TM, et al. Increasing damage to tumor blood vessels during motexafin lutetium-PDT through use of low fluence rate. *Radiat Res* 2010;174:331–340.

66. Yu G, et al. Noninvasive monitoring of murine tumor blood flow during and after photodynamic therapy provides early assessment of therapeutic efficacy. *Clin Cancer Res* 2005;11:3543–3552.

67. Sunar U, et al. Monitoring photobleaching and hemodynamic responses to HPPH-mediated photodynamic therapy of head and neck cancer: a case report. *Opt Express* 2010;18:14969–14978.

68. Marrero A, et al. Aminolevulinic acid-photodynamic therapy combined with topically applied vascular disrupting agent vadimezan leads to enhanced antitumor responses. *Photochem Photobiol* 2011;87:910–919.

69. Gross S, et al. Monitoring photodynamic therapy of solid tumors online by BOLD-contrast MRI. *Nat Med* 2003;9:1327–1331.

70. Madar-Balakirski N, et al. Permanent occlusion of feeding arteries and draining veins in solid mouse tumors by vascular targeted photodynamic therapy (VTP) with Tookad. *PLoS One* 2010;5:e10282.

71. Standish BA, et al. Interstitial Doppler optical coherence tomography as a local tumor necrosis predictor in photodynamic therapy of prostatic carcinoma: an in vivo study. *Cancer Res* 2008;68:9987–9995.

72. Pham TH, et al. Monitoring tumor response during photodynamic therapy using near-infrared photon-migration spectroscopy. *Photochem Photobiol* 2001;73:669–677.

73. Yu G, et al. Real-time in situ monitoring of human prostate photodynamic therapy with diffuse light. *Photochem Photobiol* 2006;82:1279–1284.

74. Becker TL, et al. Monitoring blood flow responses during topical ALA-PDT. *Biomed Opt Express* 2010;2:123–130.

75. Khurana M, et al. Drug and light dose responses to focal photodynamic therapy of single blood vessels in vivo. *J Biomed Opt* 2009;14:064006.

76. Korbelik M, et al. Nitric oxide production by tumour tissue: impact on the response to photodynamic therapy. *Br J Cancer* 2000;21:1835–1843.

77. Henderson BW, Sitnik-Busch TM, Vaughan LA. Potentiation of PDT anti-tumor activity in mice by nitric oxide synthase inhibition is fluence rate dependent. *Photochem Photobiol* 1999;70:64–71.

78. Reeves KJ, Reed MW, Brown NJ. The role of nitric oxide in the treatment of tumours with aminolaevulinic acid-induced photodynamic therapy. *J Photochem Photobiol B* 2010;101:224–232.

79. Seshadri M, Bellnier DA. The vascular disrupting agent 5,6-dimethylxanthenone-4-acetic acid improves the antitumor efficacy and shortens treatment time associated with photochlor-sensitized photodynamic therapy in vivo. *Photochem Photobiol* 2009;85:50–56.

80. Sanovic R, et al. Time-resolved gene expression profiling of human squamous cell carcinoma cells during the apoptosis process induced by photodynamic treatment with hypericin. *Int J Oncol* 2009;35:921–939.

81. Bhowmick R, Girotti AW. Signaling events in apoptotic photokilling of 5-aminolevulinic acid-treated tumor cells: inhibitory effects of nitric oxide. *Free Rad Biol Med* 2009;47:731–740.

82. Luna M, et al. Identification of MAP kinase pathways involved in COX-2 expression following photofrin photodynamic therapy. *Methods Mol Biol* 2010;635:47–63.

83. Wu RW, et al. Photodynamic therapy (PDT)—initiation of apoptosis via activation of stress-activated p38 MAPK and JNK signal pathway in H460 cell lines. *Photodiagnosis Photodyn Ther* 2011;8:254–263.

84. Kessel D, Oleinick NL. Initiation of autophagy by photodynamic therapy. *Methods Enzymol* 2009;453:1–16.

85. Liu L, Zhang Z, Xing D. Cell death via mitochondrial apoptotic pathway due to activation of Bax by lysosomal photodamage. *Free Rad Biol Med* 2011;51:53–68.

86. Ferrario A, et al. Survivin, a member of the inhibitor of apoptosis family, is induced by photodynamic therapy and is a target for improving treatment response. *Cancer Res* 2007;67:4989–4995.

87. Reiners JJ Jr, et al. Assessing autophagy in the context of photodynamic therapy. *Autophagy* 2010;6:7–18.

88. Ortel B, Shea CR, Calzavara-Pinton P. Molecular mechanisms of photodynamic therapy. *Frontiers Biosci* 2009;14:4157–4172.

89. Mroz P, et al. Stimulation of anti-tumor immunity by photodynamic therapy. *Expert Rev Clin Immunol* 2011;7:75–91.

90. Gollnick SO, et al. Role of cytokines in photodynamic therapy-induced local and systemic inflammation. *Br J Cancer* 2003;88:1772–1779.

91. Yom SS, et al. Elevated serum cytokine levels in mesothelioma patients who have undergone pleurectomy or extrapleural pneumonectomy and adjuvant intraoperative photodynamic therapy. *Photochem Photobiol* 2003;78:75–81.

92. Firczuk M, Nowis D, Golab J. PDT-induced inflammatory and host responses. *Photochem Photobiol Sci* 2011;10:653–663.

93. de Vree WJ, et al. Photodynamic treatment of human endothelial cells promotes the adherence of neutrophils in vitro. *Br J Cancer* 1996;73:1335–1340.

94. Sluiter W, et al. Prevention of late lumen loss after coronary angioplasty by photodynamic therapy: role of activated neutrophils. *Mol Cell Biochem* 1996;157:233–238.

95. Henderson BW, et al. Choice of oxygen-conserving treatment regimen determines the inflammatory response and outcome of photodynamic therapy of tumors. *Cancer Res* 2004;64:2120–2126.

96. Sun J, et al. Neutrophils as inflammatory and immune effectors in photodynamic therapy-treated mouse SCCVII tumours. *Photochem Photobiol Sci* 2002;1:690–695.

97. Grossman CE, et al. Photodynamic therapy of disseminated non-small cell lung carcinoma in a murine model. *Lasers Surg Med* 2011;43:663–675.

98. Cecic I, Stott B, Korbelik M. Acute phase response-associated systemic neutrophil mobilization in mice bearing tumors treated by photodynamic therapy. *Int Immunopharmacol* 2006;6:1259–1266.

99. Cecic I, Parkins CS, Korbelik M. Induction of systemic neutrophil response in mice by photodynamic therapy of solid tumors. *Photochem Photobiol* 2001;74:712–720.

100. Korbelik M, Cecic I. Complement activation cascade and its regulation: relevance for the response of solid tumors to photodynamic therapy. *J Photochem Photobiol* 2008;93:53–59.

101. Kousis PC, et al. Photodynamic therapy enhancement of antitumor immunity is regulated by neutrophils. *Cancer Res* 2007;67:10501–10510.

102. Yang D, et al. Alarmins link neutrophils and dendritic cells. *Trends Immunol* 2009;30:531–537.

103. Korbelik M. PDT-associated host response and its role in the therapy outcome. *Lasers Surg Med* 2006;38:500–508.

104. Todryk S, et al. Heat shock protein 70 induced during tumor cell killing induces Th1 cytokines and targets immature dendritic cell precursors to enhance antigen uptake. *J Immunol* 1999;163:1398–1408.

105. Gomer CJ, et al. Photodynamic therapy-mediated oxidative stress can induce expression of heat shock proteins. *Cancer Res* 1996;56:2355–2360.

106. Garg AD, et al. Photodynamic therapy: illuminating the road from cell death towards anti-tumour immunity. *Apoptosis* 2010;15:1050–1071.

107. Korbelik M, Sun J, Cecic I. Photodynamic therapy-induced cell surface expression and release of heat shock proteins: relevance for tumor response. *Cancer Res* 2005;65:1018–1026.

108. Etminan N, et al. Heat-shock protein 70-dependent dendritic cell activation by 5-aminolevulinic acid-mediated photodynamic treatment of human glioblastoma spheroids in vitro. *Br J Cancer* 2011;105:961–969.

109. Mitra S et al. Tumor response to mTHPC-mediated photodynamic therapy exhibits strong correlation with extracellular release of HSP70. *Lasers Surg Med* 2011;43:632–643.

110. Korbelik M. Cancer vaccines generated by photodynamic therapy. *Photochem Photobiol Sci* 2011;10:664–669.

111. Gomer CJ, et al. Photodynamic therapy: combined modality approaches targeting the tumor microenvironment. *Lasers Surg Med* 2006;38:516–521.

112. Kosharskyy B, et al. A mechanism-based combination therapy reduces local tumor growth and metastasis in an orthotopic model of prostate cancer. *Cancer Res* 2006;66:10953–10958.

113. Bhuvaneswari R, et al. Hypericin-mediated photodynamic therapy in combination with Avastin (bevacizumab) improves tumor response by downregulating angiogenic proteins. *Photochem Photobiol Sci* 2007;6:1275–1283.

114. Jiang F, et al. Angiogenesis induced by photodynamic therapy in normal rat brains. *Photochem Photobiol* 2004;79:494–498.

115. Ferrario A, Gomer CJ. Avastin enhances photodynamic therapy treatment of Kaposi's sarcoma in a mouse tumor model. *J Env Pathol Toxicol Oncol* 2006;25:251–260.

116. Bhuvaneswari R, et al. Effect of hypericin-mediated photodynamic therapy on the expression of vascular endothelial growth factor in human nasopharyngeal carcinoma. *Int J Mol Med* 2007;20:421–428.

117. Ferrario A, et al. Antiangiogenic treatment enhances photodynamic therapy responsiveness in a mouse mammary carcinoma. *Cancer Res* 2000;60:4066–4069.

118. Mitra S, et al. Photodynamic therapy mediates the oxygen-independent activation of hypoxia-inducible factor 1-alpha. *Mol Cancer Ther* 2006;5:3268–3274.

119. Solban N, et al. Mechanistic investigation and implications of photodynamic therapy induction of vascular endothelial growth factor in prostate cancer. *Cancer Res* 2006;66:5633–5640.

120. Bhuvaneswari R, et al. The effect of photodynamic therapy on tumor angiogenesis. *Cell Mol Life Sci* 2009;66:2275–2283.

121. Hendrickx N, et al. Up-regulation of cyclooxygenase-2 and apoptosis resistance by p38 MAPK in hypericin-mediated photodynamic therapy of human cancer cells. *J Biol Chem* 2003;278:52231–52239.

122. Luna M, et al. Cyclooxygenase-2 expression induced by photofrin photodynamic therapy involves the p38 MAPK pathway. *Photochem Photobiol* 2008;84:509–514.

123. Fingar VH, Wieman TJ, Doak KW. Role of thromboxane and prostacyclin release on photodynamic therapy-induced tumor destruction. *Cancer Res* 1990;50:2599–2603.

124. Fingar VH, et al. The role of microvascular damage in photodynamic therapy: the effect of treatment on vessel constriction, permeability, and leukocyte adhesion. *Cancer Res* 1992;52:4914–4921.

125. Ferrario A, et al. Celecoxib and NS-398 enhance photodynamic therapy by increasing in vitro apoptosis and decreasing in vivo inflammatory and angiogenic factors. *Cancer Res* 2005;65:9473–9478.

126. Verma S, et al. Strategies for enhanced photodynamic therapy effects. *Photochem Photobiol* 2007;83:996–1005.

127. Zheng G, et al. Photodynamic molecular beacon as an activatable photosensitizer based on protease-controlled singlet oxygen quenching and activation. *Proc Natl Acad Sci U S A* 2007;104:8989–8994.

128. Busch TM, et al. Photodynamic therapy creates fluence rate-dependent gradients in the intratumoral spatial distribution of oxygen. *Cancer Res* 2002;62:7273–7379.

129. Angell-Petersen E, et al. Influence of light fluence rate on the effects of photodynamic therapy in an orthotopic rat glioma model. *J Neurosurg* 2006;104:109–117.

130. Iinuma S, et al. In vivo fluence rate and fractionation effects on tumor response and photobleaching: photodynamic therapy with two photosensitizers in an orthotopic rat tumor model. *Cancer Res* 1999;59:6164–6170.

131. Curnow A, et al. Light dose fractionation to enhance photodynamic therapy using 5-aminolevulinic acid in the normal rat colon. *Photochem Photobiol* 1999;69:71–76.

132. Messmann H, et al. Enhancement of photodynamic therapy with 5-aminolaevulinic acid-induced porphyrin photosensitisation in normal rat colon by threshold and light fractionation studies. *Br J Cancer* 1995;72:589–594.

133. Xiao Z, et al. Fractionated versus standard continuous light delivery in interstitial photodynamic therapy of dunning prostate carcinomas. *Clin Cancer Res* 2007;13:7496–7505.

134. Estevez JP, et al. Continuous or fractionated photodynamic therapy? Comparison of three PDT schemes for ovarian peritoneal micrometastasis treatment in a rat model. *Photodiagnosis Photodyn Ther* 2010;7:251–257.

135. Middelburg TA, et al. Fractionated illumination at low fluence rate photodynamic therapy in mice. *Photochem Photobiol* 2010;86:1140–1146.

136. Quon H, et al., eds. *5-aminolevulinic acid photodynamic therapy for head and neck dysplasia.* San Francisco: SPIE Photonics West, 2012.

137. Garrier J, et al. Compartmental targeting for mTHPC-based photodynamic treatment in vivo: correlation of efficiency, pharmacokinetics, and regional distribution of apoptosis. *Int J Radiat Oncol Biol Phys* 2010;78:563–571.

138. Bhuvaneswari R, et al. Evaluation of hypericin-mediated photodynamic therapy in combination with angiogenesis inhibitor bevacizumab using in vivo fluorescence confocal endomicroscopy. *J Biomed Opt* 2010;15:011114.

139. Jiang F, et al. Combination therapy with antiangiogenic treatment and photodynamic therapy for the nude mouse bearing U87 glioblastoma. *Photochem Photobiol* 2008;84:128–137.

140. Zsebik B, et al. Photodynamic therapy combined with a cysteine proteinase inhibitor synergistically decrease VEGF production and promote tumour necrosis in a rat mammary carcinoma. *Cell Prolif* 2007;40:38–49.

141. Zhou Q, et al. Enhancing the therapeutic responsiveness of photodynamic therapy with the antiangiogenic agents SU5416 and SU6668 in murine nasopharyngeal carcinoma models. *Cancer Chemother Pharmacol* 2005;56:569–577.

142. Ferrario A, Gomer CJ. Targeting the 90 kDa heat shock protein improves photodynamic therapy. *Cancer Lett* 2010;289:188–194.

143. Ferrario A, et al. Enhancement of photodynamic therapy by 2,5-dimethyl celecoxib, a non-cyclooxygenase-2 inhibitor analog of celecoxib. *Cancer Lett* 2011;304:33–40.

144. Makowski M, et al. Inhibition of cyclooxygenase-2 indirectly potentiates antitumor effects of photodynamic therapy in mice. *Clin Cancer Res* 2003;9:5417–5422.

145. Yee KK, Soo KC, Olivo M. Anti-angiogenic effects of hypericin-photodynamic therapy in combination with Celebrex in the treatment of human nasopharyngeal carcinoma. *Int J Mol Med* 2005;16:993–1002.

146. Henderson BW, et al. Photofrin photodynamic therapy can significantly deplete or preserve oxygenation in human basal cell carcinomas during treatment, depending on fluence rate. *Cancer Res* 2000;60:525–529.

147. Fayter D, et al. A systematic review of photodynamic therapy in the treatment of pre-cancerous skin conditions, Barrett's oesophagus and cancers of the biliary tract, brain, head and neck, lung, oesophagus and skin. *Health Technol Assess* 2010;14:1–288.

148. Nestor MS, et al. The use of photodynamic therapy in dermatology: results of a consensus conference. *J Drugs Dermatol* 2006;5:140–154.

149. Braathen LR, et al. Guidelines on the use of photodynamic therapy for nonmelanoma skin cancer: an international consensus. International Society for Photodynamic Therapy in Dermatology, 2005. *J Am Acad Dermatol* 2007;56:125–143.

150. Piacquadio DJ, et al. Photodynamic therapy with aminolevulinic acid topical solution and visible blue light in the treatment of multiple actinic keratoses of the face and scalp: investigator-blinded, phase 3, multicenter trials. *Arch Dermatol* 2004;140:41–46.

151. Morton C, et al. Intraindividual, right-left comparison of topical methyl aminolaevulinate-photodynamic therapy and cryotherapy in subjects with actinic keratoses: a multicentre, randomized controlled study. *Br J Dermatol* 2006;155:1029–1036.

152. Apalla Z, et al. Skin cancer: preventive photodynamic therapy in patients with face and scalp cancerization. A randomized placebo-controlled study. *Br J Dermatol* 2010;162:171–175.

153. Taub AF. Photodynamic therapy: other uses. *Dermatol Clin* 2007;25:101–109.

154. Wolf P, Rieger E, Kerl H. Topical photodynamic therapy with endogenous porphyrins after application of 5-aminolevulinic acid. An alternative treatment modality for solar keratoses, superficial squamous cell carcinomas, and basal cell carcinomas? *J Am Acad Dermatol* 1993;28:17–21.

155. Cairnduff F, et al. Superficial photodynamic therapy with topical 5-aminolaevulinic acid for superficial primary and secondary skin cancer. *Br J Cancer* 1994;69:605–608.

156. Basset-Seguin N, et al. Topical methyl aminolaevulinate photodynamic therapy versus cryotherapy for superficial basal cell carcinoma: a 5 year randomized trial. *Eur J Dermatol* 2008;18:547–553.

157. Yang VXD, et al. A multispectral fluorescence imaging system: design and initial clinical tests in intra-operative Photofrin-photodynamic therapy of brain tumors. *Lasers Surg Med* 2003;32:224–232.

158. Ritz R, et al. Hypericin for visualization of high grade gliomas: first clinical experience. *Eur J Surg Oncol* 2012;38:352–360.

159. Eljamel MS, Goodman C, Moseley H. ALA and Photofrin fluorescence-guided resection and repetitive PDT in glioblastoma multiforme: a single centre phase III randomised controlled trial. *Lasers Med Sci* 2008;23:361–367.

160. Stummer W, et al. Fluorescence-guided surgery with 5-aminolevulinic acid for resection of malignant glioma: a randomised controlled multicentre phase III trial. *Lancet Oncol* 2006;7:392–401.

161. Kaye AH, Morstyn G, Brownbill D. Adjuvant high-dose photoradiation therapy in the treatment of cerebral glioma: a phase 1-2 study. *J Neurosurg* 1987;67:500–505.

162. Stylli SS, et al. Photodynamic therapy of high grade glioma—long term survival. *J Clin Neurosci* 2005;12:389–398.

163. Muller PJ, Wilson BC. Photodynamic therapy of brain tumors—a work in progress. *Lasers Surg Med* 2006;38:384–389.

164. Krishnamurthy S, et al. Optimal light dose for interstitial photodynamic therapy in treatment for malignant brain tumors. *Lasers Surg Med* 2000;27:224–234.

165. Kostron H, Fritsch E, Grunert V. Photodynamic therapy of malignant brain tumours: a phase I/II trial. *Br J Neurosurg* 1988;2:241–248.

166. National Cancer Institute. *Clinical trials. NCT00118222. High light and low light dose PDT in glioma.* Available from: http://www.cancer.gov/clinicaltrials/search/view?cdrid=433267&version=HealthProfessional#TrialDescription_CDR0000433267.

167. Osher J, et al. Adenoid cystic carcinoma of the tongue base treated with ultrasound-guided interstitial photodynamic therapy: a case study. *Photodiagnosis Photodyn Ther* 2011;8:68–71.

168. Quon H, et al. Transoral robotic photodynamic therapy for the oropharynx. *Photodiagnosis Photodyn Ther* 2011;8:64–67.

169. Quon H, et al. Photodynamic therapy in the management of pre-malignant head and neck mucosal dysplasia and microinvasive carcinoma. *Photodiagnosis Photodyn Ther* 2011;8:75–85.

170. Karakullukcu B, et al. Photodynamic therapy of early stage oral cavity and oropharynx neoplasms: an outcome analysis of 170 patients. *Eur Arch Otorhinolaryngol* 2011;268:281–288.

171. Rigual NR, et al. Photodynamic therapy for head and neck dysplasia and cancer. *Arch Otolaryngol Head Neck Surg* 2009;135:784–788.

172. Jerjes W, et al. Photodynamic therapy outcome for oral dysplasia. *Lasers Surg Med* 2011;43:192–199.

173. Savary JF, et al. Photodynamic therapy for early squamous cell carcinomas of the esophagus, bronchi, and mouth with m-tetra (hydroxyphenyl) chlorin. *Arch Otolaryngol Head Neck Surg* 1997;123:162–168.

174. Yu CH, et al. Comparison of clinical outcomes of oral erythroleukoplakia treated with photodynamic therapy using either light-emitting diode or laser light. *Lasers Surg Med* 2009;41:628–633.

175. Biel MA. Photodynamic therapy treatment of early oral and laryngeal cancers. *Photochem Photobiol* 2007;83:1063–1068.

176. Jerjes W, et al. Photodynamic therapy outcome for T1/T2 N0 oral squamous cell carcinoma. *Lasers Surg Med* 2011;43:463–469.

177. Lou PJ, et al. Interstitial photodynamic therapy as salvage treatment for recurrent head and neck cancer. *Br J Cancer* 2004;91:441–446.

178. Jerjes W, et al. Prospective evaluation of 110 patients following ultrasound-guided photodynamic therapy for deep seated pathologies. *Photodiagnosis Photodyn Ther* 2011;8:297–306.

179. Karakullukcu B, et al. mTHPC mediated interstitial photodynamic therapy of recurrent nonmetastatic base of tongue cancers: development of a new method. *Head Neck* 2012;34(11):1597–1606.

180. Betz CS, et al. Interstitial photodynamic therapy for a symptom-targeted treatment of complex vascular malformations in the head and neck region. *Lasers Surg Med* 2007;39:571–582.

181. Biel MA. Photodynamic therapy as an adjuvant intraoperative treatment of recurrent head and neck carcinomas. *Arch Otolaryngol Head Neck Surg* 1996;122:1261–1265.

182. Federal Drug Administration. "Medical Devices FAahwfgMdhAM, 2012.

183. Okunaka T, et al. Photodynamic therapy for peripheral lung cancer. *Lung Cancer* 2004;43:77–82.

184. Fujimura S, et al. A therapeutic approach to roentgenographically occult squamous cell carcinoma of the lung. *Cancer* 2000;89(Suppl):2445–2458.

185. Kubota K, et al. [Photodynamic therapy of roentgenographically occult lung cancer]. *Kyobu Geka* 1992;45:80–83.

186. Furuse K, et al. [Photodynamic therapy (PDT) in roentgenographically occult lung cancer by photofrin II and excimer dye laser]. *Gan To Kagaku Ryoho* 1993;20:1369–1374.

187. Imamura S, et al. Photodynamic therapy and/or external beam radiation therapy for roentgenologically occult lung cancer. *Cancer* 1994;73:1608–1614.

188. Endo C, et al. Results of long-term follow-up of photodynamic therapy for roentgenographically occult bronchogenic squamous cell carcinoma. *Chest* 2009;136:369–375.

189. Cortese DA, Edell ES, Kinsey JH. Photodynamic therapy for early stage squamous cell carcinoma of the lung. *Mayo Clin Proc* 1997;72:595–602.

190. Furuse K, et al. A prospective phase II study on photodynamic therapy with photofrin II for centrally located early-stage lung cancer. The Japan Lung Cancer Photodynamic Therapy Study Group. *J Clin Oncol* 1993;11:1852–1857.

191. Kato H, Okunaka T, Shimatani H. Photodynamic therapy for early stage bronchogenic carcinoma. *J Clin Laser Med Surg* 1996;14:235–238.

192. Furukawa K, et al. Locally recurrent central-type early stage lung cancer <1.0 cm in diameter after complete remission by photodynamic therapy. *Chest* 2005;128:3269–3275.

193. Moghissi K, Dixon K. Update on the current indications, practice and results of photodynamic therapy (PDT) in early central lung cancer (ECLC). *Photodiagnosis Photodyn Ther* 2008;5:10–18.

194. Usuda J, et al. Management of multiple primary lung cancer in patients with centrally located early cancer lesions. *J Thorac Oncol* 2010;5:62–68.

195. Diaz-Jimenez JP, et al. Efficacy and safety of photodynamic therapy versus Nd-YAG laser resection in NSCLC with airway obstruction. *Eur Respir J* 1999;14:800–805.

196. Weinberg BD, et al. Results of combined photodynamic therapy (PDT) and high dose rate brachytherapy (HDR) in treatment of obstructive endobronchial non-small cell lung cancer (NSCLC). *Photodiagnosis Photodyn Ther* 2010;7:50–58.

197. Lam S, et al. A randomized comparative study of the safety and efficacy of photodynamic therapy using Photofrin II combined with palliative radiotherapy versus palliative radiotherapy alone in patients with inoperable obstructive non-small cell bronchogenic carcinoma. *Photochem Photobiol* 1987;46:893–897.

198. Okunaka T, et al. Lung cancers treated with photodynamic therapy and surgery. *Diagn Ther Endosc* 1999;5:155–160.

199. Ross P Jr, et al. Incorporation of photodynamic therapy as an induction modality in non-small cell lung cancer. *Lasers Surg Med* 2006;38:881–889.

200. Konaka C, Usuda J, Kato H. [Preoperative photodynamic therapy for lung cancer]. *Nihon Geka Gakkai Zasshi* 2000;101:486–489.

201. Friedberg JS, et al. Phase II trial of pleural photodynamic therapy and surgery for patients with non-small-cell lung cancer with pleural spread. *J Clin Oncol* 2004;22:2192–2201.

202. Pass HI, et al. Intraoperative photodynamic therapy for malignant mesothelioma. *Ann Thorac Surg* 1990;50:687–688.

203. Pass HI, et al. Intrapleural photodynamic therapy: results of a phase I trial. *Ann Surg Oncol* 1994;1:28–37.

204. Schouwink H, et al. Intraoperative photodynamic therapy after pleuropneumonectomy in patients with malignant pleural mesothelioma: dose finding and toxicity results. *Chest* 2001;120:1167–1174.

205. Moskal TL, et al. Operation and photodynamic therapy for pleural mesothelioma: 6-year follow-up. *Ann Thorac Surg* 1998;66:1128–1133.

206. Friedberg JS, et al. Photodynamic therapy and the evolution of a lung-sparing surgical treatment for mesothelioma. *Ann Thorac Surg* 2011;91:1738–1745.

207. Pass HI, et al. Phase III randomized trial of surgery with or without intraoperative photodynamic therapy and postoperative immunochemotherapy for malignant pleural mesothelioma. *Ann Surg Oncol* 1997;4:628–633.

208. Wolfsen HC. Uses of photodynamic therapy in premalignant and malignant lesions of the gastrointestinal tract beyond the esophagus. *J Clin Gastroenterol* 2005;39:653–664.

209. Wang KK. Mucosal ablation therapy of Barrett's esophagus. *Mayo Clin Proc* 2001;76:433–437.

210. Overholt BF, et al. Photodynamic therapy with porfimer sodium for ablation of high-grade dysplasia in Barrett's esophagus: international, partially blinded, randomized phase III trial. *Gastrointest Endosc* 2005;62:488–498.

211. Overholt BF, et al. Five-year efficacy and safety of photodynamic therapy with Photofrin in Barrett's high-grade dysplasia. *Gastrointest Endosc* 2007;66:460–468.

212. Prasad GA, et al. Predictors of stricture formation after photodynamic therapy for high-grade dysplasia in Barrett's esophagus. *Gastrointest Endosc* 2007;65:60–66.

213. Nakamura H, et al. Experience with photodynamic therapy (endoscopic laser therapy) for the treatment of early gastric cancer. *Hepatogastroenterology* 2001;48:1599–1603.

214. Saurin JC, Chayvialle JA, Ponchon T. Management of duodenal adenomas in familial adenomatous polyposis. *Endoscopy* 1999;31:472–478.

215. Mlkvy P, et al. Photodynamic therapy for polyps in familial adenomatous polyposis—a pilot study. *Eur J Cancer* 1995;31A:1160–1165.

216. Abulafi AM, et al. Photodynamic therapy for malignant tumours of the ampulla of Vater. *Gut* 1995;36:853–856.

217. McCaughan JS Jr, et al. Photodynamic therapy to treat tumors of the extrahepatic biliary ducts. A case report. *Arch Surg* 1991;126:111–113.

218. Ortner MA, et al. Photodynamic therapy of nonresectable cholangiocarcinoma. *Gastroenterology* 1998;114:536–542.

219. Ortner ME, et al. Successful photodynamic therapy for nonresectable cholangiocarcinoma: a randomized prospective study. *Gastroenterology* 2003;125:1355–1363.

220. Witzigmann H, et al. Surgical and palliative management and outcome in 184 patients with hilar cholangiocarcinoma: palliative photodynamic therapy plus stenting is comparable to r1/r2 resection. *Ann Surg* 2006;244:230–239.

221. Zoepf T, et al. Palliation of nonresectable bile duct cancer: improved survival after photodynamic therapy. *Am J Gastroenterol* 2005;100:2426–2430.

222. Pereira SP, et al. Photodynamic therapy of malignant biliary strictures using meso-tetrahydroxyphenylchlorin. *Eur J Gastroenterol Hepatol* 2007;19:479–485.

223. Wolfsen HC. Carpe luz—seize the light: endoprevention of esophageal adenocarcinoma when using photodynamic therapy with porfimer sodium. *Gastrointest Endosc* 2005;62:499–503.

224. Bown SG, et al. Photodynamic therapy for cancer of the pancreas. *Gut* 2002;50:549–557.

225. Loh CS, et al. Photodynamic therapy for villous adenomas of the colon and rectum. *Endoscopy* 1994;26:243–246.

226. Nakamura T, et al. Photodynamic therapy with polypectomy for rectal cancer. *Gastrointest Endosc* 2003;57:266–269.

227. Spinelli P, Mancini A, Dal Fante M. Endoscopic treatment of gastrointestinal tumors: indications and results of laser photocoagulation and photodynamic therapy. *Semin Surg Oncol* 1995;11:307–318.

228. Wang S, et al. Talaporfin sodium. *Expert Opin Pharmacother* 2010;11:133–140.

229. Cengel KA, Glatstein E, Hahn SM. Intraperitoneal photodynamic therapy. *Cancer Treat Res* 2007;134:493–514.

230. Du KL, et al. Preliminary results of interstitial motexafin lutetium-mediated PDT for prostate cancer. *Lasers Surg Med* 2006;38:427–434.

231. Huang Z, et al. Effects of Pd-bacteriopheophorbide (TooKad)-mediated photodynamic therapy on canine prostate pretreated with ionizing radiation. *Radiat Res* 2004;161:723–731.

232. Nathan TR, et al. Photodynamic therapy for prostate cancer recurrence after radiotherapy: a phase I study. *J Urol* 2002;168:1427–1432.

233. Verigos K, et al. Updated results of a phase I trial of motexafin lutetium-mediated interstitial photodynamic therapy in patients with locally recurrent prostate cancer. *J Environ Pathol Toxicol Oncol* 2006;25:373–388.

234. Trachtenberg J, et al. Vascular targeted photodynamic therapy with palladium-bacteriopheophorbide photosensitizer for recurrent prostate cancer following definitive radiation therapy: assessment of safety and treatment response. *J Urol* 2007;178:1974–1979.

235. Trachtenberg J, et al. Vascular-targeted photodynamic therapy (padoporfin, WST09) for recurrent prostate cancer after failure of external beam radiotherapy: a study of escalating light doses. *BJU Int* 2008;102:556–562.

236. Zhu TC, et al. Optical properties of human prostate at 732 nm measured in vivo during motexafin lutetium-mediated photodynamic therapy. *Photochem Photobiol* 2005;81:96–105.

237. Svensson T, et al. In vivo optical characterization of human prostate tissue using near-infrared time-resolved spectroscopy. *J Biomed Opt* 2007;12:014022.

238. Davidson SR, et al. Treatment planning and dose analysis for interstitial photodynamic therapy of prostate cancer. *Phys Med Biol* 2009;54:2293–2313.

239. Nseyo UO, et al. Photodynamic therapy (PDT) in the treatment of patients with resistant superficial bladder cancer: a long-term experience. *J Clin Laser Med Surg* 1998;16:61–68.

240. Uchibayashi T, et al. Whole bladder wall photodynamic therapy for refractory carcinoma in situ of the bladder. *Br J Cancer* 1995;71:625–628.

241. Prout GR Jr, et al. Photodynamic therapy with hematoporphyrin derivative in the treatment of superficial transitional-cell carcinoma of the bladder. *N Engl J Med* 1987;317:1251–1255.

242. Nseyo UO, et al. Photodynamic therapy using porfimer sodium as an alternative to cystectomy in patients with refractory transitional cell carcinoma in situ of the bladder. Bladder Photofrin Study Group. *J Urol* 1998;160:39–44.

243. Jocham D, et al. [BCG versus photodynamic therapy (PDT) for nonmuscle invasive bladder cancer—a multicentre clinical phase III study]. *Aktuelle Urol* 2009;40:91–99.

244. D'Hallewin MA, Baert L. Long-term results of whole bladder wall photodynamic therapy for carcinoma in situ of the bladder. *Urology* 1995;45:763–767.

245. Nseyo UO, Merrill DC, Lundahl SL. Green light photodynamic therapy in the human bladder. *Clin Laser Mon* 1993;11:247–250.

246. Waidelich R, et al. Whole bladder photodynamic therapy with 5-aminolevulinic acid using a white light source. *Urology* 2003;61:332–337.

247. Berger AP, et al. Photodynamic therapy with intravesical instillation of 5-aminolevulinic acid for patients with recurrent superficial bladder cancer: a single-center study. *Urology* 2003;61:338–341.

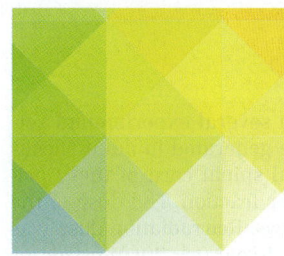

CHAPTER 32

Reirradiation

Carsten Nieder and Anthony E. Dragun

INTRODUCTION

A second course of radiotherapy to a previously treated, overlapping anatomic region poses considerable challenges if a high cumulative total dose is attempted. In palliative clinical scenarios, for example, painful bone metastases, such treatment is well established.[1,2] Occasional patients might even benefit from a third course. Reirradiation has been prescribed for locoregional relapse or second primary tumors, the latter often after very long time intervals, as well as benign diseases. Historical studies described how selected patients with cancer of the uterine cervix were reirradiated already before the Second World War.[3] The history of head and neck and brain tumor reirradiation also dates back many decades.[4,5] Despite this long-standing legacy, few prospective randomized clinical studies have provided high-level evidence clarifying the optimal approach toward previously irradiated tumors.[6] Phase II studies often included a single arm only.[7–14] Therefore, the clinical practice of reirradiation, prescribed as monotherapy or combined with other modalities,[9,13,15] is highly variable. Recent guidelines endorse repeat radiotherapy in selected patients.[16–19]

HISTORICAL PERSPECTIVE

At the Memorial Hospital New York (United States), about 11% of 1,574 patients with cervical cancer required further radiotherapy during the time period 1918 to 1931.[20] Only 2 of these patients survived more than 3 years, leading the author to conclude that "a lesion once fully and adequately irradiated cannot again be treated to advantage with radium or Roentgen therapy. Irradiation leads to tissue changes, largely in the nature of endarteritis and fibrosis, and further irradiation of such structures results in the formation of indolent chronic ulcers and sloughs, which are painful and extremely difficult to heal." In 1956, Murphy and Schmitz from Roswell Park Memorial Institute (United States) reported on treatment of failures following an apparently adequate course of radiation for cervical cancer.[3] They emphasized that "re-irradiation is particularly justified when a curative surgical approach would entail not only an appreciable mortality risk but also a high degree of permanent disability. Tissue changes resulting from previous radiotherapy do not contraindicate re-irradiation if cure or palliation is possible." This study included 46 patients with squamous cell cancer treated between 1946 and 1950. Nine patients (20%) were alive at the time of reporting with a maximum follow-up of 8 years. The absolute 5-year survival with no evidence of cancer was 16%. Subjective and objective palliation was commonly recorded. Long-term survival was achieved exclusively in patients with limited pelvic recurrence in good physical condition.

Between 1940 and 1950, selected patients with nasopharyngeal cancer were reirradiated at the University of California School of Medicine in San Francisco (United States), as later reported by Fu et al.[5] External beam radiotherapy, brachytherapy, or combination therapy was prescribed. Actuarial 5-year survival was 41%. Six of 42 patients (14%) developed soft tissue necrosis and three (7%) osteoradionecrosis,

all of whom minimally symptomatic. The authors' preferred approach in patients with local and/or nodal recurrence was surgery followed by intracavitary radium therapy. For bulky, invasive lesions, a 3-week course of external beam radiotherapy was administered first.

In 1965, Kramer (Jefferson Medical College Hospital [United States]) provided a book chapter where he summarized factors to consider during decision-making.[21] These included the natural history of the tumor, its extent, the condition of the normal tissues, the details of the previous treatment, and the objective of the proposed reirradiation. He recommended that "an attempt must be made to determine whether the initial course of therapy has failed because of inadequate doses, geographical miss or radioresistance of the tumor. Previously irradiated tissues are compromised a priori to some extent, whether this is clinically obvious or not." He advocated that radium needle implants were the first choice in certain accessible sites and concluded that "there is a definite place for re irradiation, but patients must be selected most carefully if useless therapy is to be avoided."

Stevens et al. used more modern technology in 100 patients with head and neck cancer treated with curative intent from 1964 to 1991.[22] These clinicians required presence of intact and nonulcerated mucosal surfaces and no more than minimal visible or palpable late effects from the prior irradiation. At least one-third of patients evaluated were not accepted for reirradiation. In 82 patients, external beams only were used (1.8 to 2 Gy per day, 5 days per week, planned dose at least 50 Gy). Actuarial 5-year survival was 17% in case of recurrent and 37% in case of new primary tumors.

TISSUE TOLERANCE AND RECOVERY

General Aspects

Animal studies and clinical data on reirradiation of head and neck tumors, breast cancer, lung cancer, and others showed that acute skin and mucosal reactions after reirradiation were well within the range observed after the first course of radiotherapy.[8,23–27] If the previous treatment has caused persistent severe mucosal damage, reirradiation might be poorly tolerated. Clinical data related to many cancer types revealed that late complications were more frequent than anticipated after reirradiation to high cumulative doses. The majority of data is derived from head and neck cancer retreatment. Lee et al.[28] reported the data of 654 patients with recurrent nasopharyngeal carcinoma reirradiated with now outdated technology to moderate median initial and reirradiation doses of 60 Gy and 46 Gy, respectively, with a median interval of 2 years. For all complications combined, the actuarial incidence of symptomatic late sequelae was approximately 50% at 5 years. In a later analysis, the same group found that the major determinant of postretreatment complications was the severity of damage during the initial course.[29] Severe toxicity occurred also after intensity-modulated radiotherapy (IMRT), but no prospective randomized head-to-head comparison of salvage IMRT versus 3-D conformal RT is available.[30] In the IMRT study reported by Duprez et al.,[31] 84 patients were reirradiated to a median cumulative total dose of 130 Gy (median time interval 49.5 months, median reirradiation dose 69 Gy). Late toxicity was scored in 52 patients with at least 6 months of follow-up. Eight patients developed grade 3 or 4 late dysphagia, and three developed osteoradionecrosis. Overall, 30 different grade 3 or 4 late complications were recorded. Updated results from the University of Texas MD Anderson Cancer Center ($n = 206$, IMRT) revealed actuarial rates of grade ≥ 3 toxicity of 48% at 5 years, most often dysphagia and odynophagia.[32] Increased toxicity was associated with retreatment volume >50 cm³. Stereotactic body reirradiation for recurrent head and neck cancer resulted in higher late toxicity rates if the larynx or hypopharynx was treated.[33] It is unrealistic to expect a zero risk of any severe late toxicity after IMRT or other highly conformal techniques since certain parts of the mucosal and/or connective tissues will always be part of the planning target volume and receive high cumulative doses. Overall, the available literature indicates that mesenchymal tissues recover from radiation injury less than do rapidly reacting tissues like the epidermis and mucosa, at least in the head and neck region.

Large Arteries

Recent reports of high-dose reirradiation have also identified the large arteries as critical organs at risk (OAR). Evans et al.[34] analyzed the endpoint of grade 5 aortic toxicity in 35 patients with lung cancer. The median prescribed dose was 54 Gy in 1.8-Gy fractions and 60 Gy in 2-Gy fractions, respectively. The median interval between the two courses was 32 months. The median raw composite dose to 1 cm³ of the aorta was 110 Gy. Toxicity developed in 25% of patients who received ≥ 120 Gy, but not in patients irradiated to lower cumulative doses. The issue of carotid blowout syndrome (CBOS) has been studied by Yamazaki et al..[35] They pooled data from 7 Japanese CyberKnife institutions and analyzed 381 patients. Of these, 32 (8.4%) developed CBOS after a median of 5 months from reirradiation. Twenty-two patients died (69%). Later, a predictive model (CBOS index) was developed, which includes carotid invasion of >180 degrees, presence of ulceration, and lymph node area irradiation (0 to 3 points).[36]

Lung/Thorax

In animal experiments, the lungs recover at least partially from occult injury, as reviewed in.[24] Experimental data on the trachea, bronchi, or esophagus are lacking. Most clinical series did not describe particular problems with these critical structures, except for stereotactic treatment of central lesions[37,38] and recurrent disease with infiltration or likely infiltration, where it is often difficult to determine the cause of fistula or hemoptysis (tumor progression vs. treatment toxicity). Table 32.1 shows different treatment regimens.

TABLE 32.1 PUBLISHED CONCEPTS FOR REIRRADIATION OF HEAD AND NECK (HN), LUNG, AND BRAIN TUMORS (WITH OR WITHOUT CONCOMITANT SYSTEMIC THERAPY)

Regimen	HN Tumors	Lung Tumors	Brain Tumors
External beam, conventional fractionation 1.8–2 Gy	x	x	x
External beam, hyperfractionation, twice daily	x		x
External beam, hypofractionation 2.2–2.5 Gy	x	x	x
External beam, hypofractionation 3–4 Gy		x	x
External beam, hypofractionation 5–7 Gy	x	x	x
External beam, hypofractionation 3 Gy twice daily	x		
External beam, RTOG quad shot, 3.7 Gy twice daily	x		
External beam, two fractions of 8 Gy		x	
External beam, severely hypofractionated SABR		x	
External beam, single-dose radiosurgery			x
High dose rate brachytherapy	x	x	x
Pulsed dose rate brachytherapy	x		x

RTOG, Radiation Therapy Oncology Group; SABR, stereotactic ablative body radiotherapy.

Spinal Cord

The spinal cord has been studied in several experimental settings. Clinically applicable data were generated in adult rhesus monkeys by Ang et al.[39] The cervical spinal cord of these primates was irradiated with 2.2 Gy per fraction. The dose of the initial course was 44 Gy in all monkeys. Reirradiation dose was 57.2 Gy, given after 1-year ($n = 16$) or 2-year ($n = 20$) intervals, or 66 Gy, given after 2-year ($n = 4$) or 3-year ($n = 14$) intervals. Only 4 of 45 monkeys completing the required observation period (2 to 2.5 years after reirradiation, 3 to 5.5 years total) developed myelopathy. Fitting the data with a model, assuming that all (single course and reirradiation) dose–response curves were parallel, yielded recovery estimates of 33.6 Gy (76%), 37.6 Gy (85%), and 44.6 Gy (101%) of the initial dose, after 1, 2, and 3 years, respectively, at the 5% incidence level. Another way to look at these results is to estimate the total cumulative dose that can be tolerated, expressed in EQD₂ that is equivalent dose in 2-Gy fractions calculated using the linear-quadratic approach. For a time interval of 1, 2, and 3 years between the treatment courses, cumulative doses of 150%, 156%, and 167% of the first-line setting's tolerance dose appear possible. If true in humans, an initial exposure equivalent to 46 Gy in 2-Gy fractions (arbitrarily selected to represent 100% of the tolerance dose at the 5% myelopathy risk level because many institutions limit the spinal cord dose to lower levels than true tolerance) might be followed by an additional 23 to 24 Gy in 2-Gy fractions (50% of the tolerance dose) 1 or 2 years later. Clinical data from different institutions supporting this interpretation have been published. All available data from different published series including those reporting on myelopathy[40] were analyzed by Nieder et al.[41,42] Seventy-eight patients were included and a risk prediction model was developed, based on time interval, cumulative dose, and presence or absence of any treatment course resulting in quite high spinal cord exposure. Besides cumulative dose, interval <6 months and total dose equivalent to >50 Gy in 2-Gy fractions in one of the two courses increase the risk of myelopathy. The introduction of stereotactic body radiotherapy (SBRT) has resulted in new challenges as such treatment typically is administered with few high-dose fractions or even single doses. Rather than irradiating complete spinal cord cross sections with homogeneous doses, small areas are exposed and steep dose gradients achieved. Medin et al.[43] developed a swine model where a 10-cm length of the spinal cord (C3-T1) was uniformly irradiated to 30 Gy in 10 fractions and reirradiated 1 year later with a single radiosurgery dose centered within the previously irradiated segment. Radiosurgery was delivered to a cylindrical volume approximately 5 cm in length and 2 cm in diameter, which was positioned laterally to the cervical spinal cord, resulting in a dose distribution with the 90%, 50%, and 10% isodose lines traversing the ipsilateral, central, and contralateral spinal cord, respectively. Follow-up after reirradiation was 1 year. Summarized briefly, pigs receiving radiosurgery 1 year following 30 Gy in 10 fractions were not at significantly higher risk of developing motor deficits than were pigs that received radiosurgery alone. Sahgal et al.[44] provided a recommendation of presumably safe stereotactic reirradiation doses after initial conventional radiotherapy (interval at least 5 months). A thecal sac point maximum P(max) EQD₂ of 20 to 25 Gy appeared to be safe provided the total P(max) EQD₂ does not exceed approximately 70 Gy, and the SBRT thecal sac P(max) EQD₂ constitutes no more than approximately 50% of the total normalized biologically equivalent dose. The feasibility of salvaging spinal metastases initially irradiated with SBRT, who subsequently progressed with imaging-confirmed local tumor progression, with a second SBRT course to the same level has recently been confirmed.[45]

Brain

In contrast to the spinal cord, no animal experiments on reirradiation of the brain are available. Clinical data mainly

TABLE 32.2 A COMPARISON OF SELECTED STUDIES FROM THE GLIOMA LITERATURE: RESULTS PUBLISHED BEFORE 2000 VERSUS AFTER 2010 (MEDIAN SURVIVAL)

Larson et al. (1990)[48]	13 GBM	Brachytherapy Au-198 40 Gy	9.0 mo
	20 WHO III		17.0 mo
Scharfen et al. (1992)[49]	66 GBM	Brachytherapy I-125 64.4 Gy	11.3 mo
Sneed et al. (1997)[50]	66 GBM	Brachytherapy I-125 64.4 Gy	11.7 mo
	45 WHO III		12.3 mo
Kickingereder et al. (2014)[51]	98 GBM	Brachytherapy I-125 60 Gy	10.4 mo
Schwartz et al. (2015)[52]	40 GBM	Brachytherapy I-125 50 Gy	9.3 mo
	28 WHO III		28.1 mo
Stereotactic Radiosurgery			
Shrieve et al. (1995)[53]	86 GBM	Stereotactic radiosurgery 13 Gy	10.5 mo
Cho et al. (1999)[54]	46 GBM	Stereotactic radiosurgery 17 Gy	11.0 mo
Martinez-Carrillo et al. (2014)[55]	46 GBM	Stereotactic radiosurgery	7.5 mo
	41 WHO III	Median 18 Gy (14–20 Gy)	17.0 mo
Bir et al. (2015)[56]	29 GBM	Stereotactic radiosurgery 10–20 Gy	7.9 mo
Pinzi et al. (2015)[57]	128 High grade	Stereotactic radiosurgery or hypofractionated	11.5 mo
Hypofractionated Stereotactic Radiotherapy			
Shepherd et al. (1997)[47]	33 GBM	Hypofractionated conformal radiotherapy Escalation 20–50 Gy	11.0 mo
Fogh et al. (2010)[58]	105 GBM	Stereotactic hypofractionated radiotherapy	11.0 mo
	42 WHO III	Median 35 Gy in 10 fractions	10.0 mo
Dincoglan et al. (2015)[59]	28 GBM	Stereotactic hypofractionated radiotherapy 25 Gy in 5 fractions	10.3 mo
Conventionally Fractionated (stereotactic) Radiotherapy			
Arcicasa et al. (1999)[60]	31 GBM	Fractionated conventional 2-D radiotherapy 34.5 Gy in 23 fractions (1.5Gy/F)	13.7 mo
Cho et al. (1999)[54]	25 GBM	Conventional fractionated radiotherapy 37.5 Gy in 15 fractions	12.0 mo
Lee et al. (2016)[61]	21 GBM	Conventional fractionated radiotherapy (median dose 45 Gy)	10.0 m

GBM, glioblastoma; WHO, World Health Organization.

relate to temporal lobe injury after treatment of recurrent nasopharynx cancer[46] or reirradiation of glioma and brain metastases. Shepherd et al.[47] retreated glioma with fractionated stereotactic radiotherapy (5 fractions per week, 5 Gy per fraction) after a median initial dose of 55 Gy (Table 32.2). All patients treated with more than 40 Gy developed late toxicity, whereas only 25% of those who received 30 to 40 Gy developed such adverse events. Several institutions have used reirradiation doses of 30 to 40 Gy with fraction sizes below 4 Gy with acceptable rates of toxicity,[58,62] and prospective trials with such regimens and a study comparing 5 fractions of 5 versus 7 Gy are in progress. Interstudy comparison between retrospective series is difficult because the literature is confounded by a lack of standardized recording of radiotherapy and outcome variables. In addition, some patients were treated at first and others at second or third progression. Recent prospective data from a multicenter study in 92 patients with recurrent high-grade gliomas suggest that reirradiation has no negative impact on health-related quality of life, comparable to other options such as surgery and chemotherapy.[63] Currently, there is no standard recommendation on what imaging modality has to be incorporated and what specific margins should be applied. The minimal consensus may be summarized as to confine gross tumor volume (GTV) definition to gadolinium-enhancing regions. The GLIAA (NOA 10) study (NCT01252459), an ongoing multicenter, prospective randomized, phase II clinical trial, evaluates the impact of FET-PET versus T1Gd-MRI target volume delineation on the outcome of patients with recurrent glioblastoma treated with high-precision radiation therapy (39 Gy, 3 Gy per fraction). As evident from the review of treated volumes with different modalities, such as single-dose and fractionated stereotactic irradiation, some institutions preferred hypofractionation for recurrences that others treated with a single dose. This finding reflects the lack of universally agreed dose constraints for reirradiation. In the randomized phase II NRG RTOG 1205 study of systemically administered bevacizumab with or without reirradiation, 35 Gy in 10 fractions was prescribed.[64] The maximum tumor

diameter was 6 cm and the minimum time interval from previous radiotherapy 6 months. Brainstem, optic nerves, and chiasm were expanded with 3 mm to create planning organ at risk volumes (PRV). The maximum per protocol dose to 0.03 cm^3 PRV was 24 Gy (brainstem) and 20 Gy (optic nerves and chiasm), respectively. Acceptable variations included 30 and 25 Gy, respectively. Figure 32.1 shows a clinical example of a patient treated with conventionally fractionated reirradiation.

Radiosurgery was systematically studied by the RTOG.[65,66] Adults with cerebral or cerebellar solitary non-brainstem tumors ≤40 mm in maximum diameter were eligible. Initial radiosurgical doses were 18 Gy for tumors ≤20 mm, 15 Gy for that 21 to 30 mm, and 12 Gy for that 31 to 40 mm in maximum diameter. Dose was prescribed to the 50% to 90% isodose line. Doses were escalated in 3-Gy increments providing the incidence of irreversible grade 3 or any grade 4 or 5 RTOG central nervous system toxicity was <20% within 3 months of radiosurgery. Between 1990 and 1994, 156 analyzable patients were entered, 36% of whom had recurrent primary brain tumors (median prior dose 60 Gy) and 64% recurrent brain metastases (median prior dose 30 Gy). The median interval was 11 months and minimum 3 months. The maximum tolerated doses were 24, 18, and 15 Gy for tumors ≤20 mm, 21 to 30 mm, and 31 to 40 mm in maximum diameter, respectively. However, for tumors ≤20 mm, investigators' reluctance to escalate to 27 Gy, rather than excessive toxicity, determined the maximum tolerated dose. The actuarial incidence of radionecrosis was 5%, 8%, 9%, and 11% at 6, 12, 18, and 24 months following radiosurgery, respectively. Unacceptable toxicity was more likely in patients with larger tumors. Sneed et al.[67] reported that radiosurgery followed by a second radiosurgery for recurrent brain metastases resulted in a 20% 1-year cumulative incidence of symptomatic adverse radiation effect (median reirradiation dose 18 Gy, $n = 72$, crude risk 14%). Compared to patients who had not received prior radiosurgery to the same lesion, the hazard ratio (HR) for any adverse radiation effect was 5.05 (95% confidence interval [CI] 1.9 to 13.2). Another study of 46 retreated lesions reported symptomatic radiation necrosis in 24% (actuarial 1-year rate 29%),[68] whereas local control at 1 year was 79%.

In children with diffuse intrinsic pontine glioma, reirradiation at first progression (20 to 30 Gy) provided a significant benefit in median survival compared to systemic therapy or best supportive care (13.7 vs. 10.3 months, $P = .04$) in a matched-cohort analysis ($n = 31$ and 39, respectively). Clinical improvement was observed in 77% of reirradiated patients.[69] Grade 4 to 5 toxicity was not recorded.

Heart

Wondergem et al.[70] assessed the reirradiation tolerance of the heart at intervals of up to 9 months in a rat model by measuring cardiac function ex vivo 6 months after reirradiation.

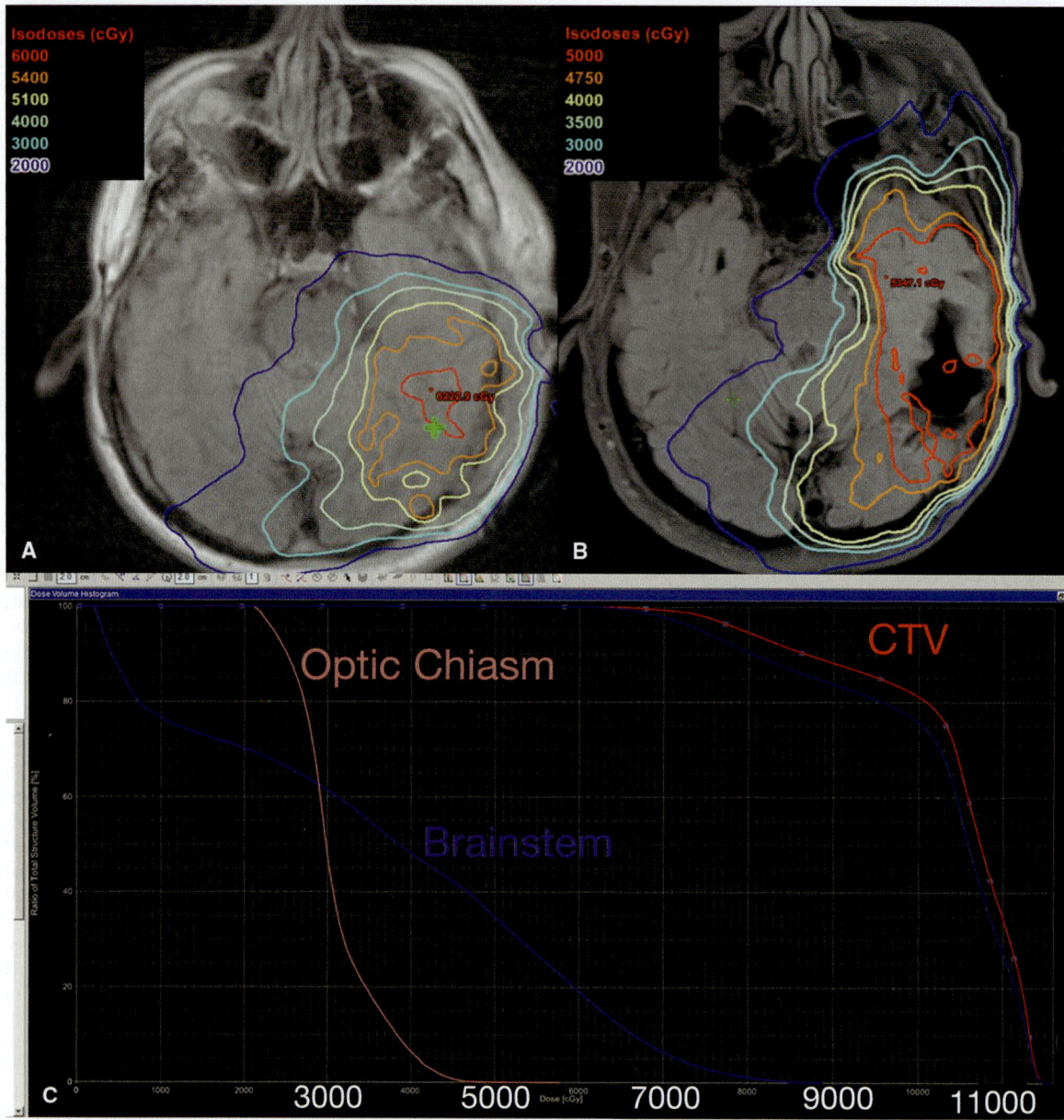

FIGURE 32.1. Representative axial slices from a T2-weighted fluid attenuation inversion recovery magnetic resonance image of a 66-year-old man with a left temporoparietal glioblastoma originally treated after surgical resection (panel **A**) to 60 Gy in 30 fractions with concurrent temozolomide. He subsequently had an in-field recurrence 4 years after the completion of his original treatment and was treated (panel **B**) to 50 Gy in 25 fractions. A dose–volume histogram is shown in panel **C**. Cumulative brainstem dose to 0.3 cm³ was limited to 80 Gy. Treatment was successfully delivered, and the patient continues to do well in follow-up. (Courtesy of Mark Amsbaugh, MD, University of Louisville School of Medicine, Louisville, KY.)

The cardiac tolerance dose was arbitrarily defined as the dose causing at least a 50% function loss in one-half of the treated animals (ED_{50}). Up to a 6-month interval, the reirradiation ED_{50} was close to the single course ED_{50} but dropped significantly when the interval was longer than 6 months. The reirradiation tolerance also decreased with an increasing priming dose. A slow progression of damage induced by the priming dose is a plausible explanation for the decrease in tolerance with increasing time from the initial course. Systematic clinical data are not available.

Kidney and Bladder

Experimental data caution also against whole-bladder reirradiation.[71] With respect to late bladder damage in mice (endpoint defined as >50% reduction in bladder volume, increased urination frequency at ≥27 weeks after reirradiation), no long-term recovery was observed in up to a 9-month interval. Unfortunately, neither

experimental data for partial organ reirradiation nor larger clinical studies on bladder reexposure are available. Studies on mouse, rat, and pig kidneys suggested that radiation-induced toxicity progresses rather than recovers with time.[72,73]

SELECTED HEAD AND NECK CANCER STUDIES

The randomized Chinese phase 2 trial by Tian et al. that included 117 patients evaluated de-escalation of the biologically effective dose (BED) for late-responding normal tissues while maintaining the same BED for nasopharynx cancer cells.[26] This was accomplished by selecting a slightly hypofractionated experimental regimen (60 Gy in 27 fractions, IMRT), which was compared to a conventional regimen with 2-Gy fractions (total dose 68 Gy, IMRT) and longer overall treatment

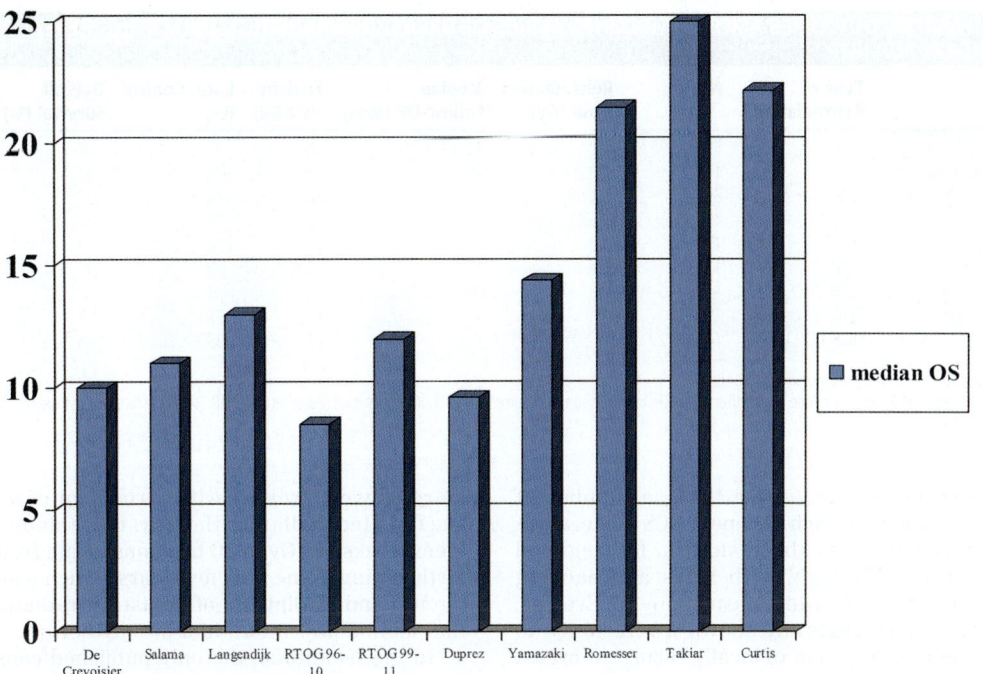

FIGURE 32.2. Median overall survival in months after reirradiation of head and neck cancers (selected studies[8,9,11,23,31,32,77–80]). The studies by Takiar et al.,[32] Romesser et al.,[78] and Curtis et al.[79] included mixed populations, that is, patients treated after salvage surgery or without resection.

time. It was assumed that normal tissue sparing would result in less life-threatening toxicity and thus better overall survival, that is, a better therapeutic ratio. In principle, the results confirmed this hypothesis, with a 5-year overall survival rate of 44% versus 30%, but the difference was not statistically significant ($P = .06$). Interestingly, the small randomized phase 2 trial by Guan et al.[74] with 69 patients compared the winner arm from the Tian et al. study,[26] that is, 60 Gy in 27 fractions, to an experimental arm, which also included weekly chemotherapy with cisplatin 30 mg/m². Only 29% of patients had received radiochemotherapy before. In the investigational arm, more patients developed mucositis and grade 3 to 4 hematologic toxicity. Late toxicity was not significantly increased. Survival was significantly better in the combined-modality arm, $P = .049$. In the absence of phase 3 studies, these results suggest that chemoreirradiation might be an effective treatment option for recurrent nasopharynx cancer. Serious toxicity was not uncommon and, therefore, continued research efforts are necessary.

The Groupe d'Oncologie Radiothérapie Tête et Cou/Groupe d'Étude des Tumeurs de la Tête et du Cou (GORTEC/GETTEC) reported on a prospective study in which 130 patients who underwent salvage surgery were randomly assigned to receive full-dose reirradiation (60 Gy) combined with concomitant chemotherapy (5-FU and hydroxyurea) versus no adjuvant treatment.[75] All patients underwent a macroscopic complete resection, and in the majority, the surgical margins were sufficient. A significant improvement with regard to the primary endpoint of locoregional tumor control (HR 2.73; 95% CI 1.66 to 4.51; $P <.001$) and disease-free survival (HR 1.68; 95% CI 1.13 to 2.50; $P = .01$) was observed in those patients that were assigned to receive postoperative chemoreirradiation compared to those that underwent surgery alone. However, this benefit in disease-free survival did not translate into a significant improvement of overall survival, which may be due to the higher incidence of distant metastases in the chemoreirradiation arm. The gain in locoregional tumor control and disease-free survival was achieved at the cost of significantly higher rates of grade 3 to 4 late side effects (39% vs. 10% at 2 years, respectively). It should be noted that participants allocated

to the wait-and-see arm could receive salvage chemoreirradiation at the time of locoregional recurrence after salvage surgery, which was the case in 25% of patients. This type of crossover reduces the likelihood of improved overall survival. Postoperative chemoreirradiation should be considered in selected cases, in particular given the very low locoregional control rate after salvage surgery alone, which was only 20% at 2 years. However, in the light of the high rate of late toxicity, the optimal postoperative regimen in the reirradiation setting has yet to be defined. Based on the results of this study, a wait-and-see policy could also be considered, in particular when patients suffer from severe late toxicities from the first course of treatment. Ho et al. in a retrospective comparison of primary closure to flap reconstruction ($n = 59$ and 37, respectively) reported that nonflap patients experienced significantly greater incidence of severe late toxicities (47.5 vs. 21.6%, $P = .02$), whereas acute toxicities and 5-year survival were comparable.[76]

As shown in Figure 32.2, median survival is limited,[8,9,11,23,31,32,77–80] but a proportion of patients experience long-term survival after reirradiation, a finding that has already been described in historical studies.[22,81] As highlighted by Stevens et al.,[22] actuarial 5-year survival was dependent on reirradiation setting, that is, 17% in case of recurrent and 37% in case of new primary tumors. Target volumes should be kept tight, and elective nodal irradiation should be avoided in order to minimize severe toxicity.[82]

BREAST CANCER

In-Breast Tumor Recurrence (IBTR) after Prior Breast-Conserving Surgery (BCS) and Whole-Breast Radiation Therapy (WBRT)

IBTR is expected to occur in approximately 5% to 10% of patients within 10 years after initial BCS + WBRT, equating to a cumulative risk of 0.5% to 1% per annum.[83] The most often recommended treatment for IBTR is salvage mastectomy, which imparts excellent locoregional control and 5-year survival rates.[84] Given the fact that there are subgroups of

TABLE 32.3 COMPARATIVE OUTCOMES AMONG PUBLISHED SERIES OF BREAST REIRRADIATION FOLLOWING REPEAT BREAST-CONSERVING SURGERY FOR IBTR

Study (Year)	Type of Reirradiation	N	Reirradiation Dose (Gy)	Median Follow-UP (Mos)	Toxicity (% ≥G3)	Local Control (%)	Overall Survival (%)	Cosmesis (% Good or Excellent)
Deutsch (2002)[88]	EBRT[a]	39	50	52	0	77	78	69
Kraus-Tiefenbacher et al. (2007)[89]	IORT	17	14–20	26	0	100	94	82
Hannoun-Levi et al. (2004)[90]	LDR	69	30–50	50	10	77	92	–
Chadha et al. (2008)[91]	LDR	15	30–45	36	0	89	100	86
Polgar et al. (2009)[92]	HDR	12	22	56	0	100	79	50
Trombetta et al. (2009)[93]	HDR	18	34	40	5	89	94	83
Giux et al. (2010)[94]	HDR	36	30	89	0	89	97	90
Kauer-Dorner et al. (2012)[95]	PDR	39	50	57	17	93	87	37
GEC-ESTRO (2013)[96]	HDR PDR LDR	102 88 27	32 50 46	47	11	93	76	85

[a]Electron beam radiotherapy directed to the postoperative tumor bed.
EBRT, external beam radiotherapy; HDR, high dose rate brachytherapy; IBTR, in-breast tumor recurrence; IORT, intraoperative radiotherapy; LDR, low dose rate brachytherapy; N, number of patients; PDR, pulsed dose rate brachytherapy.

patients who refuse mastectomy after IBTR, a number of series have described the approach of repeat BCS alone, without additional reirradiation. In these studies, locoregional recurrence is unacceptably high, with rates approaching 40%,[17,85] as opposed to 10% following mastectomy.[84,86] Even so, radiation oncologists have generally shown a reluctance to offer reirradiation in the treatment of locally recurrent breast cancer.[87] However, with increase in technologic sophistication of radiation therapy techniques over the last two decades, a number of studies have investigated the feasibility and efficacy of adding reirradiation to BCS for IBTR.

Table 32.3 shows a summary of modern series of repeat BCS and reirradiation in the setting of IBTR. The overwhelming majority of the data exists for partial breast irradiation (PBI) using interstitial, multicatheter brachytherapy with low dose rate (LDR), pulsed dose rate (PDR), or high dose rate (HDR) source techniques.[88-96] Pooled data from European experience using all three of the aforementioned methods represent the largest study of this approach published to date.[96] In a total of 217 patients, this collaborative multi-institutional analysis from high-volume centers in Europe found that interstitial brachytherapy was very well tolerated with local control rates much more comparable to salvage mastectomy (93%) as well as good to excellent cosmetic outcome in the overwhelming majority of patients (85%). Simplified interstitial techniques using single-catheter balloon brachytherapy have been described with similar outcomes.[93]

An emerging technique to address the challenge of reirradiation after second BCS for IBTR was piloted by a European cooperative group that employed intraoperative radiation therapy (IORT) at the time of salvage lumpectomy.[89] IORT was delivered using a single dose of approximately 14 to 20 Gy, 50 kV x-rays delivered to the applicator surface using the Intrabeam device (Carl Zeiss, Oberkochen, Germany). In this small study of 17 patients, the treatment was well tolerated with no grade 3 or higher toxicity, 100% local control at 2 years, and excellent or good cosmetic outcome in 82% of patients.

In terms of breast reirradiation using external beam radiation therapy (EBRT), the data are fairly scant. The largest study of its kind published to date included 39 patients treated with electron beam radiotherapy directed at the tumor bed after repeat BCS.[88] At a median follow-up of over 4 years, the therapy was generally well tolerated with local control rates at 77% and good to excellent cosmetic outcome in 69% of patients. Interest in this commonly available modality has grown, and so a multi-institutional phase II trial of the safety and efficacy of repeat PBI using three-dimensional conformal radiotherapy has recently completed accrual of its targeted sample size of approximately 60 patients (NRG Oncology/RTOG 1014).[97] In this study, patients with small invasive or preinvasive lesions completely excised with negative surgical margins were treated with a regimen of accelerated hyperfractionated radiation therapy, twice daily over three treatment weeks (45 Gy in 30 fractions). Data from this trial will be forthcoming in the next few years, which will serve to increase the use and availability of breast reirradiation among centers that do not offer interstitial brachytherapy.

In the meantime, the only published consensus guidelines that exist to inform clinicians in routine practice come from the Breast Cancer Expert Panel of the German Society of Radiation Oncology (DEGRO).[17] This panel recommends that although mastectomy is regarded as a standard of care for patients with IBRT, a subset of patients may be appropriately offered reirradiation after a second BCS. Since the largest experience to date exists for a multicatheter brachytherapy, other techniques such as EBRT or IORT should preferentially be performed on a clinical trial.

Management of Locoregional Recurrence after Prior Mastectomy and Postmastectomy Radiation Therapy (PMRT)

The Early Breast Cancer Trialists' Collaborative Group (EBCTCG) estimated that the addition of radiotherapy significantly reduced the 10-year risk of isolated local recurrence from approximately 25% to 7%.[98] The addition of modern systemic therapy has fortunately made this type of event even more rare. That does not diminish the clinical challenge that is experienced by physicians in cases of isolated chest wall or regional nodal recurrences in patients who have had prior PMRT. Published series that address this issue tend to be single institution and small experiences with heterogeneous mix of patients who are able to undergo upfront surgical resection of their disease and patients who have unresectable gross disease present at the time of therapy.[27,99-108]

A selection of the most modern published series in the reirradiation for chest wall recurrences is presented in Table 32.4. The overwhelming majority of investigators use concurrent hyperthermia (HT) combined with EBRT that is typically conventionally or hypofractionated.[27,99-104] Although HT is not available at a majority of radiotherapy centers, it does have a proven benefit in the treatment of advanced superficial local recurrences such as these. A randomized study from 2005 published by Jones et al. that examined the effect of HT found a statistically significant benefit, which was especially pronounced among the subset of patients who had been previously treated with full-dose radiation therapy.[102] In a large collaborative series published in 2002, Wahl et al. presented a cohort of 81 patients treated with reirradiation to a total median dose of 48 Gy.[103] The overwhelming majority of investigators used once-daily conventional fractionation, and just over half the patients were treated with concurrent HT and/or cytotoxic chemotherapy. The rate of grade 3 or higher

TABLE 32.4 COMPARATIVE OUTCOMES AMONG PUBLISHED SERIES OF CHEST WALL REIRRADIATION FOLLOWING LOCOREGIONAL RECURRENCE AFTER INITIAL MASTECTOMY AND PMRT

Study (Year)	Type of Reirradiation	N	Reirradiation Dose (Median, Gy)	Concurrent Treatment	Median Follow-UP (Mos)	Toxicity (% ≥G3)	Local Control (%)
Kouloulias et al. (2002)[99]	EBRT	15	30.6	HT (100%) CT (100%)	30	0	20[a]
Kouloulias et al. (2003)[100]	EBRT	30	30.6 or (4 × 1 + 8 × 3)	CT (100%)	24	0	57[a]
Li et al. (2004)[101]	EBRT	41	43	N/A	18	8	56[a]
Jones et al. (2005)[102]	EBRT	39[b]	30–66	HT (56%)	89	7	No HT: 24[a] HT: 68[a]
Wahl et al. (2008)[103]	EBRT	81	48	HT (54%) CT (54%)	12	5	66
Würschmidt et al. (2008)[27]	EBRT	29	50	CT (35%)	24	0	63
Harkenrider et al. (2011)[104]	EBRT	12	47	CT (63%)	30	8	92
Müller et al. (2011)[105]	EBRT	42	60	HT (69%)	41	0	62
Linthorst et al. (2013)[106]	EBRT	198	8 × 4	HT (100%)	42	12	78
Merino et al. (2015)[107]	EBRT	56	50	CT (12%)	17	12.5	63
Linthorst et al. (2015)[108]	EBRT	248	8 × 4	HT (100%)	32	1	40

[a]Clinical complete response rates for patients with gross disease at time of reirradiation.
[b]This trial included nonbreast superficial recurrences as well.
CT, cytotoxic chemotherapy; EBRT, external beam radiotherapy; HT, hyperthermia; N, number of patients; PMRT, postmastectomy radiotherapy.

toxicity was very low and the rate of local control at 1 year was approximately 66%.

Series that omit HT generally include fewer, more favorable patients treated for high-risk, microscopic disease post limited resection.[27,104,107] Local disease control rates are favorable, with lower rates of toxicity compared to combined hyperthermia. Although the majority of patients received concurrent cytotoxic chemotherapy, rates of distant disease failure were very high. The aforementioned DEGRO expert panel currently recommends the use of reirradiation both in cases of unresectable recurrences and after surgical resection in high-risk patients.[17] This group recommends reirradiation with doses between 45 and 50 Gy in conventional fractionation, not exceeding cumulative doses of 100 to 110 Gy, and notes that HT can further improve tumor control in this population.

Isolated Regional Nodal Recurrences after Prior Radiotherapy

Isolated supraclavicular and/or axillary recurrences are very uncommon in breast cancer, especially after appropriate adjuvant radiation therapy in the up-front setting. These clinical scenarios, however, pose the most significant clinical challenges for physicians and patients alike, because of the difficulty in early diagnosis and high-risk surgical management. In these situations, the risk of injury to clinical OAR such as the brachial plexus from repeat radiotherapy must be weighed against the certain involvement of these structures because of direct invasion of progressive disease.

In the largest series of its kind, a multi-institutional study from the Netherlands, 42 patients with isolated supraclavicular recurrence treated with a combination of systemic and locoregional radiotherapy were examined.[109] The 5-year overall survival and disease-free survival rate were significantly worse than is seen with chest wall recurrences (38% and 22%, respectively). What is more striking is that outcomes were even worse for patients who did not receive radiotherapy as a component of their salvage treatment. Given the grim prognosis, there are small emerging series that address isolated nodal recurrences with combination of either concurrent or sequential chemotherapy and reirradiation[104,110,111] using IMRT techniques to median doses of 50 Gy. Even in these most conformal techniques, point doses to the brachial plexus are well above historically cited tolerance with cumulative doses in excess of 100 Gy.[110] Since overall survival in these patients is less than half that of patients with chest wall recurrences,[104] clinicians must weigh the risks of a tumor-induced plexopathy versus iatrogenic injury in each particular case.

Patients with isolated axillary recurrences tend to fare somewhat better because of the fact that they lend themselves more often to surgical excision and reirradiation without compromising the brachial plexus. In a series of axillary recurrences from the MD Anderson Cancer Center, the authors found that durable control was able to be achieved in 31/44 patients (70%).[112] Success was most often seen in patients who were able to undergo up-front surgery and multimodality therapy. Twenty percent of these patients had prior axillary radiotherapy, and the addition of reirradiation to the axilla significantly improved local disease control (81% vs. 56%). As of now, the DEGRO expert panel acknowledges that in cases of isolated nodal recurrences, approximately 1/2 to 2/3 of patients will eventually develop distant metastatic disease. Durable locoregional control is more often achieved in patients with axillary nodal involvement only, and reirradiation improves local control and should be applied wherever feasible.[17]

DISCUSSION

Reirradiation should only be considered if the radiation tolerance of critical tissues or organs has not been exceeded during the first treatment, that is, after in-depth review of the initial plan and dose distribution, and assessment of organ status and side effects after the first treatment. Moreover, reasonable performance status, absence of other, less toxic treatment alternatives, and careful dose summation are prerequisites.[113,114] It is important to weigh the expected benefits against morbidity and compromised quality of life. Several studies, especially on lung and head and neck cancer, demonstrated that reirradiation can either cause or prevent a fatal outcome. In many scenarios including but not limited to pelvic tumors, the ability of reirradiation to palliate pain and other symptoms has repeatedly been confirmed[7,115,116] (Fig. 32.3). For many tissues, organs, and indications, an increasing body of clinical data is now emerging. These include settings with much higher single-course equivalent doses than previously prescribed, for example, stereotactic radiotherapy for early-stage lung cancer.[117] Nevertheless, little is known for a number of endpoints such as neurocognitive function, damage to endocrine organs, or reirradiation tolerance of pediatric patients.[118] Acutely responding tissues, in general, recover radiation changes practically completely within a few months and, therefore, can tolerate a repeat treatment course.

Clinical evidence suggests that fibrosis, impaired blood perfusion, and, in general, late normal tissue injury in humans continue to progress for many years and even decades. These findings have triggered a trend toward highly sophisticated, conformal image-guided reirradiation approaches aiming at better normal tissue sparing. Brachytherapy (including intraoperative administration[119–123]), stereotactic techniques, and proton and carbon ion beams are under clinical investigation.[124–127]

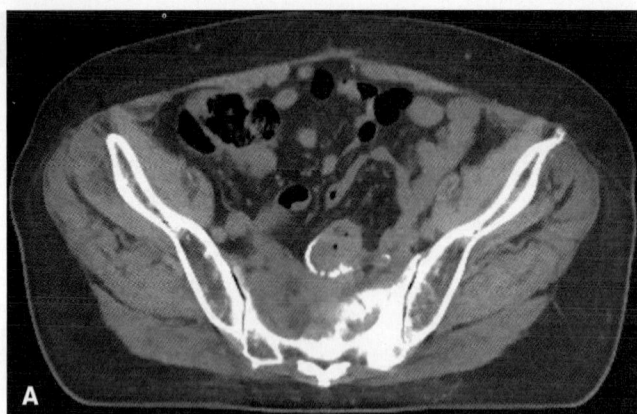
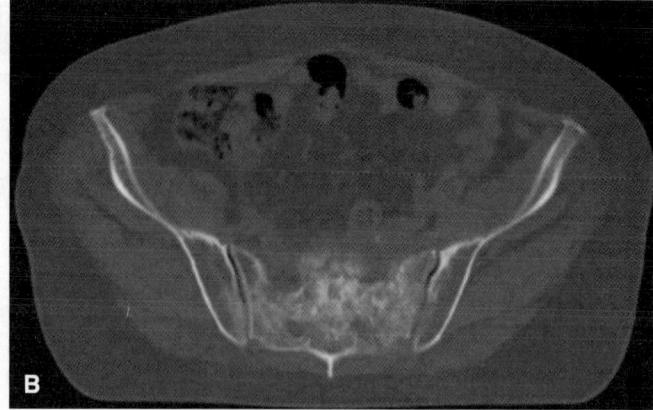

FIGURE 32.3. Representative axial slices from planning computed tomography (CT) images (soft tissue and bone window, panels **A** and **B**) of a 64-year-old female patient initially treated surgically for cancer in the sigmoid colon in 2013. She relapsed in the sacral bone in 2014 and received long-course chemoradiation (50 Gy in 25 fractions with concomitant capecitabine) without surgery. Owing to local progression, chemotherapy with an oxaliplatin/5-FU regimen was initiated in 2016. Because of increasing pain, reirradiation was offered in June 2016 (CT). A hyperfractionated regimen was chosen (1.25 Gy b.i.d., total dose 40 Gy) concomitant to capecitabine. Symptom improvement was achieved. At last follow-up in March 2017, no treatment-related toxicity was recorded.

Preliminary data suggest that these approaches are more successful than previous attempts to treat with neutrons or boron neutron capture therapy.[128–130] However, severe dysphagia and fatal bleeding might still occur after proton beam reirradiation for head and neck cancer.[78,131,132] A treatment planning study in 25 patients, which compared intensity-modulated proton therapy (IMPT) and ion therapy (IMIT) reirradiation plans to a second subsequent dose of 70 Gy to photon therapy delivered with volumetric modulated arcs, reported a dosimetric benefit favoring carbon ions above proton therapy.[133] A previous, smaller study in 7 patients suggested that IMPT was not uniformly superior to helical TomoTherapy and recommended comparative treatment planning with different techniques.[134] It is hoped that models, which predict the risk of serious complications, might contribute to optimized patient selection, for example, the model for nasopharyngeal necrosis, which should be validated in future studies.[135] Proton beam reirradiation of non–small cell lung cancer was associated with 6 grade 5 toxicities in a multi-institutional study of 57 patients.[124] Increased overlap with the central airways, mean esophagus and heart dose, and simultaneous chemotherapy were risk factors for grade ≥3 toxicity.

While small target volumes can be treated with fraction sizes above 2 Gy, radiobiologic principles and retrospective data suggest that large volume reirradiation might be less toxic if hyperfractionation is employed.[115,116,136] Despite strong rationales, this logistically difficult approach has not been studied in randomized head-to-head comparisons to conventionally fractionated reirradiation. Many institutions consider reirradiation for primary and secondary brain tumors; bone and lymph node metastases; head and neck, lung, breast, prostate, gynecologic, and rectal cancer; lymphoma; and soft tissue sarcoma. With regard to prostate cancer, several groups have started to investigate focal salvage therapies because whole-gland reirradiation has repeatedly been linked to a higher risk of late toxicity.[137] Very few reports were published regarding hepatic, pancreatic, and esophageal tumors.[138–141]

REFERENCES

1. Chow E, van der Linden YM, Roos D, et al. A randomized trial of single and multiple fractions of repeat radiation for painful bone metastases. *Lancet Oncol* 2014;15:164–171.
2. Hashmi A, Guckenberger M, Kersh R, et al. Re-irradiation stereotactic body radiotherapy for spinal metastases: a multi-institutional outcome analysis. *J Neurosurg Spine* 2016;25:646–653.
3. Murphy WT, Schmitz A. The results of re-irradiation in cancer of the cervix. *Radiology* 1956;67:378–385.
4. Brown JM, Probert JC. Early and late radiation changes following a second course of irradiation. *Radiology* 1975;115:711–716.
5. Fu KK, Newman H, Phillips TL. Treatment of locally recurrent carcinoma of the nasopharynx. *Radiology* 1975;117:425–431.
6. Nieder C, Langendijk JA, Guckenberger M, et al. Prospective randomized clinical studies involving reirradiation: lessons learned. *Strahlenther Onkol* 2016;192:679–686.
7. Cai G, Zhu J, Hu W, et al. Accelerated hyperfractionated intensity-modulated radiotherapy for recurrent/unresectable rectal cancer in patients with previous pelvic irradiation: results of a phase II study. *Radiat Oncol* 2014;9:278.
8. Langendijk JA, Kasperts N, Leemans CR, et al. A phase II study of primary reirradiation in squamous cell carcinoma of head and neck. *Radiother Oncol* 2006;78:306–312.
9. Langer CJ, Harris J, Horwitz EM, et al. Phase II study of low-dose paclitaxel and cisplatin in combination with split-course concomitant twice-daily reirradiation in recurrent squamous cell carcinoma of the head and neck: results of Radiation Therapy Oncology Group protocol 9911. *J Clin Oncol* 2007;25:4800–4805.
10. Lartigau EF, Tresch E, Thariat J, et al. Multi institutional phase II study of concomitant stereotactic reirradiation and cetuximab for recurrent head and neck cancer. *Radiother Oncol* 2013;109:281–285.
11. Spencer SA, Harris J, Wheeler RH, et al. RTOG 96-10: reirradiation with concurrent hydroxyurea and 5-fluorouracil in patients with squamous cell cancer of the head and neck. *Int J Radiat Oncol Biol Phys* 2001;94:1299–1304.
12. Valentini V, Morganti AG, Gambacorta MA, et al; Study Group for Therapies of Rectal Malignancies (STORM). Preoperative hyperfractionated chemoradiation for locally recurrent rectal cancer in patients previously irradiated to the pelvis: a multicentric phase II study. *Int J Radiat Oncol Biol Phys* 2006;64:1129–1139.
13. Vargo JA, Ferris RL, Ohr J, et al. A prospective phase 2 trial of reirradiation with stereotactic body radiation therapy plus cetuximab in patients with previously irradiated recurrent squamous cell carcinoma of the head and neck. *Int J Radiat Oncol Biol Phys* 2015;91:480–488.
14. Yamada Y, Kollmeier MA, Pei X, et al. A phase II study of salvage high-dose-rate brachytherapy for the treatment of locally recurrent prostate cancer after definitive external beam radiotherapy. *Brachytherapy* 2014;13:111–116.
15. Datta NR, Puric E, Klingbiel D, et al. Hyperthermia and radiation therapy in locoregional recurrent breast cancers: a systematic review and meta-analysis. *Int J Radiat Oncol Biol Phys* 2016;94:1073–1087.
16. Cabrera AR, Kirkpatrick JP, Fiveash JB, et al. Radiation therapy for glioblastoma: executive summary of an American Society for Radiation Oncology Evidence-Based Clinical Practice Guideline. *Pract Radiat Oncol* 2016;6:217–225.
17. Harms W, Budach W, Dunst J, et al; Breast Cancer Expert Panel of the German Society of Radiation Oncology (DEGRO). DEGRO practical guidelines for radiotherapy of breast cancer VI: therapy of locoregional breast cancer recurrences. *Strahlenther Onkol* 2016;192:199–208.
18. McDonald MW, Lawson J, Garg MK, et al; Expert Panel on Radiation Oncology-Head and Neck Cancer. ACR appropriateness criteria retreatment of recurrent head and neck cancer after prior definitive radiation expert panel on radiation oncology-head and neck cancer. *Int J Radiat Oncol Biol Phys* 2011;80:1292–1298.
19. Ryu S, Buatti JM, Morris A, et al; AANS/CNS Joint Guidelines Committee. The role of radiotherapy in the management of progressive glioblastoma: a systematic review and evidence-based clinical practice guideline. *J Neurooncol* 2014;118:489–499.
20. Healy WP. Carcinoma of cervix uteri. *JAMA* 1931;97:1680–1683.
21. Kramer S. Reirradiation: indications, technique, results. In: Buschke F, ed. *Progress in radiation therapy*. Volume 3. New York: Grune & Stratton, 1965:195–214.
22. Stevens KR, Britsch A, Moss WT. High-dose reirradiation of head and neck cancer with curative intent. *Int J Radiat Oncol Biol Phys* 1994;29:687–698.
23. De Crevoisier R, Bourhis J, Domenge C, et al. Full-dose reirradiation for unresectable head and neck carcinoma: experience at the Gustave-Roussy Institute in a series of 169 patients. *J Clin Oncol* 1998;16:3556–3562.
24. Nieder C, Milas L, Ang KK. Tissue tolerance to reirradiation. *Semin Radiat Oncol* 2000;10:200–209.

25. Tada T, Fukuda H, Matsui K, et al. Non-small-cell lung cancer: reirradiation for loco-regional relapse previously treated with radiation therapy. *Int J Clin Oncol* 2005;10:247–250.

26. Tian YM, Zhao C, Guo Y, et al. Effect of total dose and fraction size on survival of patients with locally recurrent nasopharyngeal carcinoma treated with intensity-modulated radiotherapy: a phase 2, single-center, randomized controlled trial. *Cancer* 2014;120:3502–3509.

27. Würschmidt F, Dahle J, Petersen C, et al. Reirradiation of recurrent breast cancer with and without concurrent chemotherapy. *Radiat Oncol* 2008;3:28.

28. Lee AW, Foo W, Law SC, et al. Reirradiation for recurrent nasopharyngeal carcinoma: factors affecting the therapeutic ratio and ways for improvement. *Int J Radiat Oncol Biol Phys* 1997;38:43–52.

29. Lee AW, Foo W, Law SC, et al. Total biological effect on late reactive tissues following reirradiation for recurrent nasopharyngeal carcinoma. *Int J Radiat Oncol Biol Phys* 2000;46:865–872.

30. Sulman EP, Schwartz DL, Le TT, et al. IMRT reirradiation of head and neck cancer-disease control and morbidity outcomes. *Int J Radiat Oncol Biol Phys* 2009;73:399–409.

31. Duprez F, Berwouts D, Madani I, et al. High-dose reirradiation with intensity-modulated radiotherapy for recurrent head-and-neck cancer: disease control, survival and toxicity. *Radiother Oncol* 2014;111:388–392.

32. Takiar V, Garden AS, Ma D, et al. Reirradiation of head and neck cancers with intensity modulated radiation therapy: outcomes and analyses. *Int J Radiat Oncol Biol Phys* 2016;95:1117–1131.

33. Ling DC, Vargo JA, Ferris RL, et al. Risk of severe toxicity according to site of recurrence in patients treated with stereotactic body radiation therapy for recurrent head and neck cancer. *Int J Radiat Oncol Biol Phys* 2016;95:973–980.

34. Evans JD, Gomez DR, Amini A, et al. Aortic dose constraints when reirradiating thoracic tumors. *Radiother Oncol* 2013;106:327–332.

35. Yamazaki H, Ogita M, Kodani N, et al. Frequency, outcome and prognostic factors of carotid blowout syndrome after hypofractionated re-irradiation of head and neck cancer using CyberKnife: a multi-institutional study. *Radiother Oncol* 2013;107:305–309.

36. Yamazaki H, Ogita M, Himei K, et al. Carotid blowout syndrome in pharyngeal cancer patients treated by hypofractionated stereotactic re-irradiation using CyberKnife: a multi-institutional matched-cohort analysis. *Radiother Oncol* 2015;115:67–71.

37. Binkley MS, Hiniker SM, Chaudhuri A, et al. Dosimetric factors and toxicity in highly conformal thoracic reirradiation. *Int J Radiat Oncol Biol Phys* 2016;94:808–815.

38. De Bari B, Filippi AR, Mazzola R, et al. Available evidence on re-irradiation with stereotactic ablative radiotherapy following high-dose previous thoracic radiotherapy for lung malignancies. *Cancer Treat Rev* 2015;41:511–518.

39. Ang KK, Jiang GL, Feng Y, et al. Extent and kinetics of recovery of occult spinal cord injury. *Int J Radiat Oncol Biol Phys* 2001;50:1013–1020.

40. Wong CS, van Dyk J, Milosevic M, et al. Radiation myelopathy following single courses of radiotherapy and retreatment. *Int J Radiat Oncol Biol Phys* 1994;30:575–581.

41. Nieder C, Grosu AL, Andratschke NH, et al. Proposal of human spinal cord reirradiation dose based on collection of data from 40 patients. *Int J Radiat Oncol Biol Phys* 2005;61:851–855.

42. Nieder C, Grosu AL, Andratschke NH, et al. Update of human spinal cord reirradiation tolerance based on additional data from 38 patients. *Int J Radiat Oncol Biol Phys* 2006;66:1446–1449.

43. Medin PM, Foster RD, van der Kogel AJ, et al. Spinal cord tolerance to reirradiation with single-fraction radiosurgery: a swine model. *Int J Radiat Oncol Biol Phys* 2012;83:1031–1037.

44. Sahgal A, Ma L, Weinberg V, et al. Reirradiation human spinal cord tolerance for stereotactic body radiotherapy. *Int J Radiat Oncol Biol Phys* 2012;82:107–116.

45. Thibault I, Campbell M, Tseng CL, et al. Salvage stereotactic body radiotherapy (SBRT) following in-field failure of initial SBRT for spinal metastases. *Int J Radiat Oncol Biol Phys* 2015;93:353–360.

46. Liu S, Lu T, Zhao C, et al. Temporal lobe injury after re-irradiation of locally recurrent nasopharyngeal carcinoma using intensity modulated radiotherapy: clinical characteristics and prognostic factors. *J Neurooncol* 2014;119:421–428.

47. Shepherd SF, Laing RW, Cosgrove VP, et al. Hypofractionated stereotactic radiotherapy in the management of recurrent glioma. *Int J Radiat Oncol Biol Phys* 1997;37:393–398.

48. Larson GL, Wilbanks JH, Dennis WS, et al. Interstitial radiogold implantation for the treatment of recurrent high-grade gliomas. *Cancer* 1990;66:27–29.

49. Scharfen CO, Sneed PK, Wara WM, et al. High activity iodine-125 interstitial implant for gliomas. *Int J Radiat Oncol Biol Phys* 1992;24:583–591.

50. Sneed PK, McDermott MW, Gutin PH. Interstitial brachytherapy procedures for brain tumors. *Semin Surg Oncol* 1997;13:157–166.

51. Kickingereder P, Hamisch C, Suchorska B, et al. Low-dose rate stereotactic iodine-125 brachytherapy for the treatment of inoperable primary and recurrent glioblastoma: single-center experience with 201 cases. *J Neurooncol* 2014;120:615–623.

52. Schwartz C, Romagna A, Thon N, et al. Outcome and toxicity profile of salvage low-dose-rate iodine-125 stereotactic brachytherapy in recurrent high-grade gliomas. *Acta Neurochir (Wien)* 2015;157:1757–1764.

53. Shrieve DC, Alexander E III, Wen PY, et al. Comparison of stereotactic radiosurgery and brachytherapy in the treatment of recurrent glioblastoma multiforme. *Neurosurgery* 1995;36:275–282.

54. Cho KH, Hall WA, Gerbi BJ, et al. Single dose versus fractionated stereotactic radiotherapy for recurrent gliomas. *Int J Radiat Oncol Biol Phys* 1999;45:1133–1141.

55. Martínez-Carrillo M, Tovar-Martín I, Zurita-Herrera M, et al. Salvage radiosurgery for selected patients with recurrent malignant gliomas. *Biomed Res Int* 2014;2014:657953.

56. Bir SC, Connor DE Jr, Ambekar S, et al. Factors predictive of improved overall survival following stereotactic radiosurgery for recurrent glioblastoma. *Neurosurg Rev* 2015;38:705–713.

57. Pinzi V, Orsi C, Marchetti M, et al. Radiosurgery reirradiation for high-grade glioma recurrence: a retrospective analysis. *Neurol Sci* 2015;36:1431–1440.

58. Fogh SE, Andrews DW, Glass J, et al. Hypofractionated stereotactic radiation therapy: an effective therapy for recurrent high-grade gliomas. *J Clin Oncol* 2010;28:3048–3053.

59. Dincoglan F, Beyzadeoglu M, Sager O, et al. Management of patients with recurrent glioblastoma using hypofractionated stereotactic radiotherapy. *Tumori* 2015;101:179–184.

60. Arcicasa M, Roncadin M, Bidoli E, et al. Re-irradiation and lomustine in patients with relapsed high grade gliomas. *Int J Radiat Oncol Biol Phys* 1999;43:789–793.

61. Lee J, Cho J, Chang JH, et al. Re-irradiation for recurrent gliomas: treatment outcomes and prognostic factors. *Yonsei Med J* 2016;57:824–830.

62. Combs SE, Thilmann C, Edler L, et al. Efficacy of fractionated stereotactic reirradiation in recurrent gliomas: long-term results in 172 patients treated in a single institution. *J Clin Oncol* 2005;23:8863–8869.

63. Stöckelmaier L, Renovanz M, König J, et al. Therapy for recurrent high-grade gliomas: results of a prospective multicenter study on health-related quality of life. *World Neurosurg* 2017;102:383–399. pii: S1878-8750(17)30234-6.

64. Accessed online February 27, 2017. www.rtog.org/ClinicalTrials/ProtocolTable/StudyDetails.aspx?study=1205

65. Shaw E, Scott C, Souhami L, et al. Single dose radiosurgical treatment of recurrent previously irradiated primary brain tumours and brain metastases: final report of RTOG protocol 90-05. *Int J Radiat Oncol Biol Phys* 2000;47:291–298.

66. Shaw E, Scott C, Souhami L, et al. Radiosurgery for the treatment of previously irradiated recurrent primary brain tumours and brain metastases: initial report of radiation therapy oncology group protocol (90-05). *Int J Radiat Oncol Biol Phys* 1996;34:647–654.

67. Sneed PK, Mendez J, Vemer-van den Hoek JG, et al. Adverse radiation effect after stereotactic radiosurgery for brain metastases: incidence, time course, and risk factors. *J Neurosurg* 2015;123:373–386.

68. McKay WH, McTyre ER, Okoukoni C, et al. Repeat stereotactic radiosurgery as salvage therapy for locally recurrent brain metastases previously treated with radiosurgery. *J Neurosurg* 2017;127:148–156.

69. Janssens GO, Gandola L, Bolle S, et al. Survival benefit for patients with diffuse intrinsic pontine glioma (DIPG) undergoing re-irradiation at first progression: a matched-cohort analysis on behalf of the SIOP-E-HGG/DIPG working group. *Eur J Cancer* 2017;73:38–47.

70. Wondergem J, van Ravels FJ, Reijnart IW, et al. Reirradiation tolerance of the rat heart. *Int J Radiat Oncol Biol Phys* 1996;36:811–819.

71. Stewart FA, Oussoren Y, Luts A. Long-term recovery and reirradiation tolerance of mouse bladder. *Int J Radiat Oncol Biol Phys* 1990;18:1399–1406.

72. Stewart FA, Oussoren Y, van Tinteren H, et al. Loss of reirradiation tolerance in the kidney with increasing time after single or fractionated partial tolerance doses. *Int J Radiat Biol* 1994;66:169–179.

73. Robbins ME, Bywaters T, Rezvani M, et al. Residual radiation-induced damage to the kidney of the pig as assayed by retreatment. *Int J Radiat Biol* 1991;60:917–928.

74. Guan Y, Liu S, Wang HY, et al. Long-term outcomes of a phase II randomized controlled trial comparing intensity-modulated radiotherapy with or without weekly cisplatin for the treatment of locally recurrent nasopharyngeal carcinoma. *Chin J Cancer* 2016;35:20.

75. Janot F, de Raucourt D, Benhamou E, et al. Randomized trial of postoperative reirradiation combined with chemotherapy after salvage surgery compared with salvage surgery alone in head and neck carcinoma. *J Clin Oncol* 2008;26:5518–5523.

76. Ho AS, Zumsteg ZS, Meyer A, et al. Impact of flap reconstruction on radiotoxicity after salvage surgery and reirradiation for recurrent head and neck cancer. *Ann Surg Oncol* 2016;23:850–857.

77. Salama JK, Vokes EE, Chmura SJ, et al. Long-term outcome of concurrent chemotherapy and reirradiation for recurrent and second primary head-and-neck squamous cell carcinoma. *Int J Radiat Oncol Biol Phys* 2006;64:382–391.

78. Romesser PB, Cahlon O, Scher ED, et al. Proton beam reirradiation for recurrent head and neck cancer: Multi-institutional report on feasibility and early outcome. *Int J Radiat Oncol Biol Phys* 2016;95:386–395.

79. Curtis KK, Ross HJ, Garrett AL, et al. Outcomes of patients with loco-regionally recurrent or new primary squamous cell carcinomas of the head and neck treated with curative intent reirradiation at Mayo Clinic. *Radiat Oncol* 2016;11:55.

80. Yamazaki H, Ogita M, Himei K, et al. Reirradiation using robotic image-guided stereotactic radiotherapy of recurrent head and neck cancer. *J Radiat Res* 2016;57:288–293.

81. Levendag PC, Meeuwis CA, Visser AG. Reirradiation of recurrent head and neck cancers: external and/or interstitial radiation therapy. *Radiother Oncol* 1992;23:6–15.

82. Mehanna H, Kong A, Ahmed SK. Recurrent head and neck cancer: United Kingdom national multidisciplinary guidelines. *J Laryngol Otol* 2016;130:S181–S190.

83. Fisher B, Anderson S, Bryant J, et al. Twenty-year follow-up of a randomized trial comparing total mastectomy, lumpectomy, and lumpectomy plus irradiation for the treatment of invasive breast cancer. *N Engl J Med* 2002;347:1233–1241.

84. Anderson SJ, Wapnir I, Dignam JJ, et al. Prognosis after ipsilateral breast tumor recurrence and locoregional recurrences in patients treated by breast-conserving therapy in five National Surgical Adjuvant Breast and Bowel Project protocols of node-negative breast cancer. *J Clin Oncol* 2009;27:2466–2473.

85. Harms W, Geretschläger A, Cescato C, et al. Current treatment of isolated locoregional breast cancer recurrences. *Breast Care (Basel)* 2015;10:265–271.

Section
II

86. Fowble B, Solin LJ, Schultz DJ, et al. Breast recurrence following conservative surgery and radiation: patterns of failure, prognosis, and pathologic findings from mastectomy specimens with implications for treatment. *Int J Radiat Oncol Biol Phys* 1990;19:833–842.

87. Joseph KJ, Al-Mandhari Z, Pervez N, et al. Reirradiation after radical radiation therapy: a survey of patterns of practice among Canadian radiation oncologists. *Int J Radiat Oncol Biol Phys* 2008;72:1523–1529.

88. Deutsch M. Repeat high-dose external beam irradiation for in-breast tumor recurrence after previous lumpectomy and whole breast irradiation. *Int J Radiat Oncol Biol Phys* 2002;53:687–691.

89. Kraus-Tiefenbacher U, Bauer L, Scheda A, et al. Intraoperative radiotherapy (IORT) is an option for patients with localized breast recurrences after previous external-beam radiotherapy. *BMC Cancer* 2007;7:178.

90. Hannoun-Levi JM, Houvenaeghel G, Ellis S, et al. Partial breast irradiation as second conservative treatment for local breast cancer recurrence. *Int J Radiat Oncol Biol Phys* 2004;60:1385–1392.

91. Chadha M, Feldman S, Boolbol S, et al. The feasibility of a second lumpectomy and breast brachytherapy for localized cancer in a breast previously treated with lumpectomy and radiation therapy for breast cancer. *Brachytherapy* 2008;7:22–28.

92. Polgár C, Sulyok Z, Major T, et al. Reexcision and perioperative high-dose-rate brachytherapy in the treatment of local relapse after breast conservation: an alternative to salvage mastectomy. *J Contemp Brachytherapy* 2009;1:131–136.

93. Trombetta M, Julian TB, Werts DE, et al. Long-term cosmesis after lumpectomy and brachytherapy in the management of carcinoma of the previously irradiated breast. *Am J Clin Oncol* 2009;32:314–318.

94. Guix B, Lejárcegui JA, Tello JI, et al. Exeresis and brachytherapy as salvage treatment for local recurrence after conservative treatment for breast cancer: results of a ten-year pilot study. *Int J Radiat Oncol Biol Phys* 2010;78:804–810.

95. Kauer-Dorner D, Pötter R, Resch A, et al. Partial breast irradiation for locally recurrent breast cancer within a second breast conserving treatment: alternative to mastectomy? Results from a prospective trial. *Radiother Oncol* 2012;102:96–101.

96. Hannoun-Levi JM, Resch A, Gal J, et al. Accelerated partial breast irradiation with interstitial brachytherapy as second conservative treatment for ipsilateral breast tumour recurrence: multicentric study of the GEC-ESTRO Breast Cancer Working Group. *Radiother Oncol* 2013;108:226–231.

97. Arthur DW, Winter KA, Kuerer HM, et al. NRG Oncology-Radiation Therapy Oncology Group Study 1014: 1-year toxicity report from a phase 2 study of repeat breast-preserving surgery and 3-dimensional conformal partial-breast reirradiation for in-breast recurrence. *Int J Radiat Oncol Biol Phys* 2017;98:1028–1035.

98. EBCTCG (Early Breast Cancer Trialists' Collaborative Group), McGale P, Taylor C, Correa C, et al. Effect of radiotherapy after mastectomy and axillary surgery on 10-year recurrence and 20-year breast cancer mortality: meta-analysis of individual patient data for 8135 women in 22 randomised trials. *Lancet* 2014;383:2127–2135. Erratum in: *Lancet*. 2014;384:1848.

99. Koulouulias VE, Dardoufas CE, Kouvaris JR, et al. Liposomal doxorubicin in conjunction with reirradiation and local hyperthermia treatment in recurrent breast cancer: a phase I/II trial. *Clin Cancer Res* 2002;8:374–382.

100. Koulouulias VE, Plataniotis GA, Kouvaris JR, et al. Re-irradiation in conjunction with liposomal doxorubicin for the treatment of skin metastases of recurrent breast cancer: a radiobiological approach and 2 year of follow-up. *Cancer Lett* 2003;193:33–40.

101. Li G, Mitsumori M, Ogura M, et al. Local hyperthermia combined with external irradiation for regional recurrent breast carcinoma. *Int J Clin Oncol* 2004;9:179–183.

102. Jones EL, Oleson JR, Prosnitz LR, et al. Randomized trial of hyperthermia and radiation for superficial tumors. *J Clin Oncol* 2005;23:3079–3085.

103. Wahl AO, Rademaker A, Kiel KD, et al. Multi-institutional review of repeat irradiation of chest wall and breast for recurrent breast cancer. *Int J Radiat Oncol Biol Phys* 2008;70:477–484.

104. Harkenrider MM, Wilson MR, Dragun AE. Reirradiation as a component of the multidisciplinary management of locally recurrent breast cancer. *Clin Breast Cancer* 2011;11:171–176.

105. Müller AC, Eckert F, Heinrich V, et al. Re-surgery and chest wall re-irradiation for recurrent breast cancer: a second curative approach. *BMC Cancer* 2011;11:197.

106. Linthorst M, van Geel AN, Baaijens M, et al. Re-irradiation and hyperthermia after surgery for recurrent breast cancer. *Radiother Oncol* 2013;109:188–193.

107. Merino T, Tran WT, Czarnota GJ. Re-irradiation for locally recurrent refractory breast cancer. *Oncotarget* 2015;6:35051–35062.

108. Linthorst M, Baaijens M, Wiggenraad R, et al. Local control rate after the combination of re-irradiation and hyperthermia for irresectable recurrent breast cancer: results in 248 patients. *Radiother Oncol* 2015;117:217–222.

109. van der Sangen MJ, Coebergh JW, Roumen RM, et al. Detection, treatment, and outcome of isolated supraclavicular recurrence in 42 patients with invasive breast carcinoma. *Cancer* 2003;98:11–17.

110. Chatterjee S, Lee D, Kent N, et al. Managing supraclavicular disease from breast cancer with brachial plexus-sparing techniques using helical tomotherapy. *Clin Oncol (R Coll Radiol)* 2011;23:101–107.

111. Richards GM, Tomé WA, Robins HI, et al. Pulsed reduced dose-rate radiotherapy: a novel locoregional retreatment strategy for breast cancer recurrence in the previously irradiated chest wall, axilla, or supraclavicular region. *Breast Cancer Res Treat* 2009;114:307–313.

112. Newman LA, Hunt KK, Buchholz T, et al. Presentation, management and outcome of axillary recurrence from breast cancer. *Am J Surg* 2000;180:252–256.

113. Meijneke TR, Petit SF, Wentzler D, et al. Reirradiation and stereotactic radiotherapy for tumors in the lung: dose summation and toxicity. *Radiother Oncol* 2013;107:423–427.

114. Senthi S, Griffioen GH, van Sörnsen de Koste JR, et al. Comparing rigid and deformable dose registration for high dose thoracic re-irradiation. *Radiother Oncol* 2013;106:323–326.

115. Tao R, Tsai CJ, Jensen G, et al. Hyperfractionated accelerated reirradiation for rectal cancer: an analysis of outcomes and toxicity. *Radiother Oncol* 2017;122:146–151.

116. Guren MG, Undseth C, Rekstad BL, et al. Reirradiation of locally recurrent rectal cancer: a systematic review. *Radiother Oncol* 2014;113:151–157.

117. Nieder C, De Ruysscher D, Gaspar LE, et al. Reirradiation of recurrent node positive non-small cell lung cancer after previous stereotactic radiotherapy for stage I disease: a multi-institutional treatment recommendation. *Strahlenther Onkol* 2017;193:515–524. doi:10.1007/s00066-017-1130-0.

118. Rao AD, Rashid AS, Chen Q, et al. Reirradiation for recurrent pediatric central nervous system malignancies: a multi-institutional review. *Int J Radiat Oncol Biol Phys* 2017;99(3):634–641

119. Lambers K, Hasenburg A, Stickeler E, et al. Customized treatment of recurrent gynaecological cancer—the need for intraoperative radiation therapy. *Eur J Gynaecol Oncol* 2016;37:48–52.

120. Tinkle CL, Weinberg V, Braunstein SE, et al. Intraoperative radiotherapy in the management of locally recurrent extremity soft tissue sarcoma. *Sarcoma* 2015;2015:913565.

121. Sedlmayer F, Zehentmayr F, Fastner G. Partial breast re-irradiation for local recurrence of breast carcinoma: benefit and long term side effects. *Breast* 2013;22(Suppl 2):S141–S146.

122. Backes FJ, Billingsley CC, Martin DD, et al. Does intra-operative radiation at the time of pelvic exenteration improve survival for patients with recurrent, previously irradiated cervical, vaginal, or vulvar cancer? *Gynecol Oncol* 2014;135:95–99.

123. Cambeiro M, Calvo FA, Aristu JJ, et al. Salvage surgery and radiotherapy including intraoperative electron radiotherapy in isolated locally recurrent tumors: predictors of outcome. *Radiother Oncol* 2015;116:316–322.

124. Chao HH, Berman AT, Simone CB II, et al. Multi-institutional prospective study of reirradiation with proton beam radiotherapy for locoregionally recurrent non-small cell lung cancer. *J Thorac Oncol* 2017;12:281–292.

125. Combs SE, Kalbe A, Nikoghosyan A, et al. Carbon ion radiotherapy performed as re-irradiation using active beam delivery in patients with tumors of the brain, skull base and sacral region. *Radiother Oncol* 2011;98:63–67.

126. Schulz-Ertner D, Nikoghosyan A, Thilmann C, et al. Results of carbon ion radiotherapy in 152 patients. *Int J Radiat Oncol Biol Phys* 2004;58:631–640.

127. Hayashi K, Yamamoto N, Karube M, et al. Feasibility of carbon-ion radiotherapy for re-irradiation of locoregionally recurrent, metastatic, or secondary lung tumors. *Cancer Sci* 2018. doi: 10.1111/cas.13555. [Epub ahead of print.]

128. Errington RD, Catterall M. Re-irradiation of advanced tumors of the head and neck with fast neutrons. *Int J Radiat Oncol Biol Phys* 1986;12:191–195.

129. Saroja KR, Hendrickson FR, Cohen L, et al. Re-irradiation of locally recurrent tumors with fast neutrons. *Int J Radiat Oncol Biol Phys* 1988;15:115–121.

130. Hatanaka H, Nakagawa Y. Clinical results of long-surviving brain tumor patients who underwent boron neutron capture therapy. *Int J Radiat Oncol Biol Phys* 1994;28:1061–1066.

131. Phan J, Sio TT, Nguyen TP, et al. Reirradiation of head and neck cancers with proton therapy: outcomes and analyses. *Int J Radiat Oncol Biol Phys* 2016;96:30–41.

132. Verma V, Rwigema JM, Malyapa RS, et al. Systematic assessment of clinical outcomes and toxicities of proton radiotherapy for reirradiation. *Radiother Oncol* 2017;125(1):21–30

133. Eekers DB, Roelofs E, Jelen U, et al. Benefit of particle therapy in re-irradiation of head and neck patients. Results of a multicentric in silico ROCOCO trial. *Radiother Oncol* 2016;121:387–394.

134. Stuschke M, Kaiser A, Abu-Jawad J, et al. Re-irradiation of recurrent head and neck carcinomas: comparison of robust intensity modulated proton therapy treatment plans with helical tomotherapy. *Radiat Oncol* 2013;8:93.

135. Yu YH, Xia WW, Shi JL, et al. A model to predict the risk of lethal nasopharyngeal necrosis after re-irradiation with intensity-modulated radiotherapy in nasopharyngeal carcinoma patients. *Chin J Cancer* 2016;35:59.

136. Osborne EM, Eng C, Skibber JM, et al. Hyperfractionated accelerated reirradiation for patients with recurrent anal cancer previously treated with definitive chemoradiation. *Am J Clin Oncol* 2016. doi:10.1097/COC.0000000000000338. [Epub ahead of print]

137. Duijzentkunst DA, Peters M, van der Voort van Zyp JR, et al. Focal salvage therapy for local prostate cancer recurrences after primary radiotherapy: a comprehensive review. *World J Urol* 2016;34:1521–1531. Erratum in: *World J Urol*. 2016 Dec 20.

138. Huang Y, Chen SW, Fan CC, et al. Clinical parameters for predicting radiation-induced liver disease after intrahepatic reirradiation for hepatocellular carcinoma. *Radiat Oncol* 2016;11:89.

139. Dagoglu N, Callery M, Moser J, et al. Stereotactic body radiotherapy (SBRT) reirradiation for recurrent pancreas cancer. *J Cancer* 2016;7:283–288.

140. Fernandes A, Berman AT, Mick R, et al. A prospective study of proton beam reirradiation for esophageal cancer. *Int J Radiat Oncol Biol Phys* 2016;95:483–487.

141. Nieder C, Langendijk JA, Guckenberger M, et al. Second re-irradiation: a narrative review of the available clinical data. *Acta Oncol* 2018;57(3):305–310

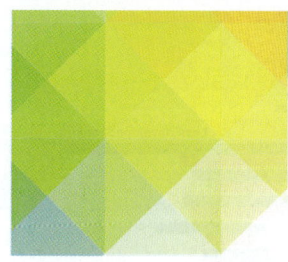

CHAPTER 33

Global Radiation Oncology

Timothy P. Hanna and C. Norman Coleman

INTRODUCTION

Global radiation oncology links the discipline of radiation oncology to global health, where the latter may be defined as "… an area for study, research, and practice that places a priority on improving health and achieving equity in health for all people worldwide."[1] This chapter will provide an overview of the unique challenges to providing radiation oncology in low-income and middle-income countries (LMIC). It will also provide reasons for hope that the global challenge of cancer can be met. Low-income countries had a 2015 per capita gross national income of US$1,025 or less, and for middle-income countries, the range was US$1,026 to $12,475.[2] Nations falling into these income groups are sometimes described as developing countries.

GLOBAL BURDEN OF DISEASE

In 2015, an estimated 16% of all deaths worldwide were due to cancer.[3] In comparison to the worldwide burden of cancer, cardiovascular disease and other chronic conditions are responsible for, respectively, 32% and 24% of deaths globally. In total, 71% of mortality worldwide is the result of noncommunicable disease. Seventy-six percent of these deaths occur in low- and middle-income countries.[3] In low-income countries, where deaths from communicable disease and other related causes are common, noncommunicable disease is already responsible for nearly 40% of all deaths.[3]

In 2012, 57% of cancers worldwide occurred in less developed countries, as did 65% of all cancer deaths.[4,5] The burden of cancer in LMIC relates to increasing life expectancy in LMIC, population growth patterns, and rising incidence of risk factors for chronic diseases in LMIC.[6,7] For example, an estimated 65% of people ≥60 years of age lived in less developed countries in 2011, and this is expected to rise to 79% by 2050.[6] The growing burden of cancer and other noncommunicable diseases in LMIC represents a significant epidemiologic transition and a dual challenge for disease control efforts.

EPIDEMIOLOGY OF CANCER WORLDWIDE

Worldwide, there were 14.1 million new cases of cancer and 8.2 million cancer deaths in 2012.[8] Lung cancer is the most common cause of cancer worldwide (1.8 million new cases in 2012), followed by breast cancer (1.7 million) and colorectal cancer (1.4 million) (Fig. 33.1).[4] Lung cancer is also the most common cause of cancer death, with 1.6 million deaths in 2012.[4] Liver cancer (0.74 million) and gastric cancer (0.72 million) are the second and third most common causes of cancer death, respectively. Age-standardized incidence rates of cancer in developed countries are nearly double the rates in LMIC, though mortality rates are far more similar. These findings reflect variation in prevalence and distribution of major risk factors and limitations in early detection and treatment resources in LMIC.[9]

Although cervix cancer is the 11th most commonly diagnosed cancer among women in developed countries, it is second only to breast cancer in developing nations.[4] This reflects a lack of sufficient prevention of cervical cancer in many LMIC. Cervix cancer is an extremely common cancer in Latin America, Sub-Saharan Africa, and parts of Asia such as India (Fig. 33.2).[4] Gastric cancer and hepatocellular carcinoma are also common in many LMIC, with 43% of all cases of gastric cancer in the world occurring in China alone (Fig. 33.2).[4] Kaposi sarcoma is a common cancer in Sub-Saharan Africa,[10] and esophageal cancer has the highest incidence rates worldwide in regions of Asia and Africa.[4] Oral cancer has a high incidence in South Asia, particularly among men.[11]

Among nine common modifiable risk factors for cancer, tobacco smoking is associated with the largest proportion of attributable risk.[12] There are one billion smokers globally, and 80% live in LMIC.[13] With large populations and high tobacco use in China and India, tobacco is an extremely important risk factor for cancer in Asia.[14] In general, many LMIC have demonstrated increased tobacco use during the past three decades. National consumption continues to rise in many countries, and in others, a peak occurred in the 1980s and 1990s.[15] History has shown a 30- to 40-year delay between the peak in smoking rates in a population and the peak in tobacco-related mortality.[16] Thus, an increasing rate of tobacco-related malignancies is expected in LMIC during the next half century.[17,18]

Over 26% of cancers in developing countries are attributed to infectious causes.[19] Hepatitis B is a major risk factor for hepatocellular carcinoma in LMIC. Other factors are hepatitis C[20] and aflatoxin produced from *Aspergillus* in certain poorly preserved foods.[21] Human papillomavirus (HPV) and *Helicobacter pylori* are important etiologic agents, and there are numerous other infectious agents relevant to cancer in the developing world. These include Epstein-Barr virus, human immunodeficiency virus (HIV), schistosomiasis, human T-cell leukemia virus type 1 (HTLV-1), and human herpesvirus 8 (HHV-8).[19,22] The prevalence of infectious causes is notable given the preventability of many of these causes through public health measures (e.g., hepatitis B, HPV vaccines).

There are a number of other factors that are relevant to patterns of global cancer incidence. Diet[23] and obesity are risk factors for some cancers.[24] This is notable given increasing trends in unhealthy diet and sedentary lifestyle among LMIC.[25] The impact of genetic polymorphisms on patterns of global cancer incidence has not been fully elucidated, but there is some suggestion of their relevance.[26,27] Similarly, the role of occupational and environmental exposures to cancer in LMIC requires continued exploration.[28]

In many LMIC, cancer often presents in advanced stages, due to factors such as lack of comprehensive screening and poor access to effective treatments.[29] As a result, case fatality rates are much higher in LMIC, with rates for breast and cervical cancer in low-income countries being more than double rates in high-income countries.[30] Overall, about half of all cancers in LMIC require radiotherapy.[31,32] With cervical cancer being so common in LMIC and the high frequency of advanced cancer presentations requiring local therapy, radiation therapy has an extremely important role in LMIC.

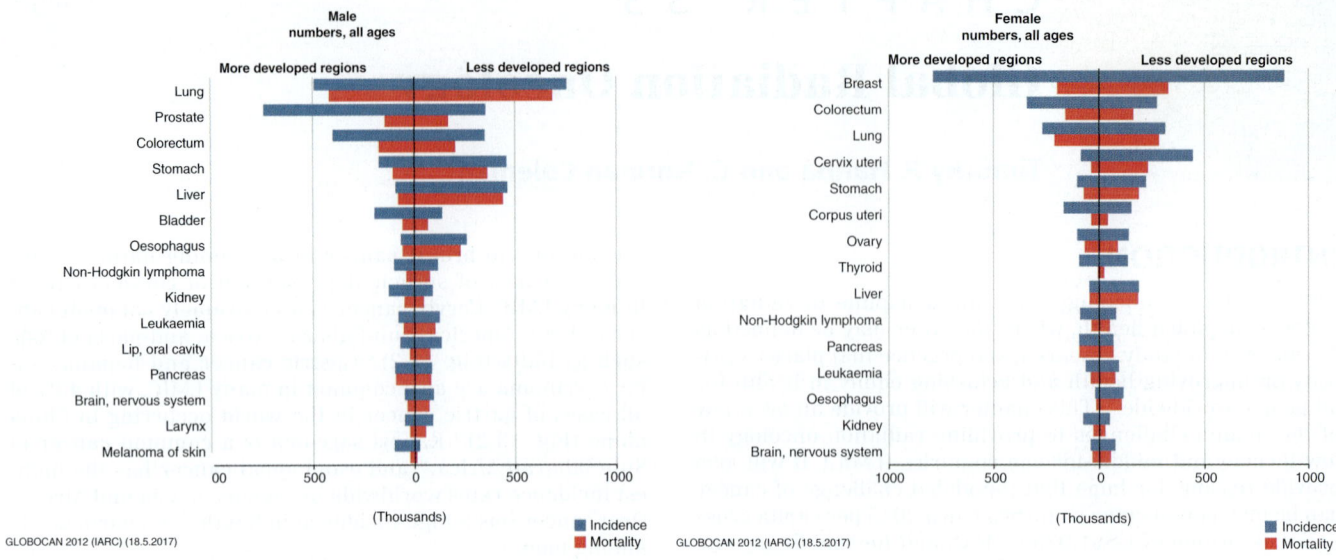

FIGURE 33.1. Estimated number of new cancer cases (incidence) and deaths (mortality) worldwide in 2012. Data are shown for more developed and less developed countries by top 15 cancer sites and sex, ranked by global cancer incidence. (Reproduced with permission from Ferlay J, Soerjomataram I, Ervik M, et al. *GLOBOCAN 2012 v1.0, Cancer Incidence and Mortality Worldwide: IARC CancerBase No. 11* [*Internet*]. Lyon, France: International Agency for Research on Cancer, 2013. Available from: http://gco.iarc.fr/today/home, accessed on 8/03/2018.)

Accordingly, the World Health Organization considers linear accelerators, remote afterloading brachytherapy systems, and their supporting technologies as priority medical devices for cancer management.[33] The following sections will describe radiation oncology in LMIC in terms of access, quality, and economics.

GLOBAL STATUS OF ACCESS TO RADIATION THERAPY

Access to radiation therapy is a multifactorial issue. Availability of machines and personnel for treatment is a key part of access to care. Other considerations include spatial

FIGURE 33.2. Global variation in estimated age-standardized cancer incidence per 10^5 in 2012 for specific cancers based on International Agency for Research on Cancer statistics. Incidence is grouped with higher incidence indicated by darker color. Rates for both sexes are shown for lung and stomach cancer. **A:** Cervix cancer rates are highest in Latin America, Sub-Saharan Africa, and parts of Asia including India. **B:** Breast cancer rates are high among high-income countries. Among low- and middle-income countries, rates are high in parts of Latin America and lower in parts of Africa and Asia. **C:** Lung cancer rates are high in both developed and developing parts of the world, including China, Southeast Asian countries, and parts of South America. **D:** Rates of stomach cancer are highest in East Asia. High rates are found in Latin America, other parts of Asia, and Eastern Europe. (Reproduced with permission from Ferlay J, Soerjomataram I, Ervik M, et al. *GLOBOCAN 2012 v1.0, Cancer Incidence and Mortality Worldwide: IARC CancerBase No. 11* [*Internet*]. Lyon, France: International Agency for Research on Cancer, 2013. Available from: http://gco.iarc.fr/today/home, accessed on 8/03/2018.)

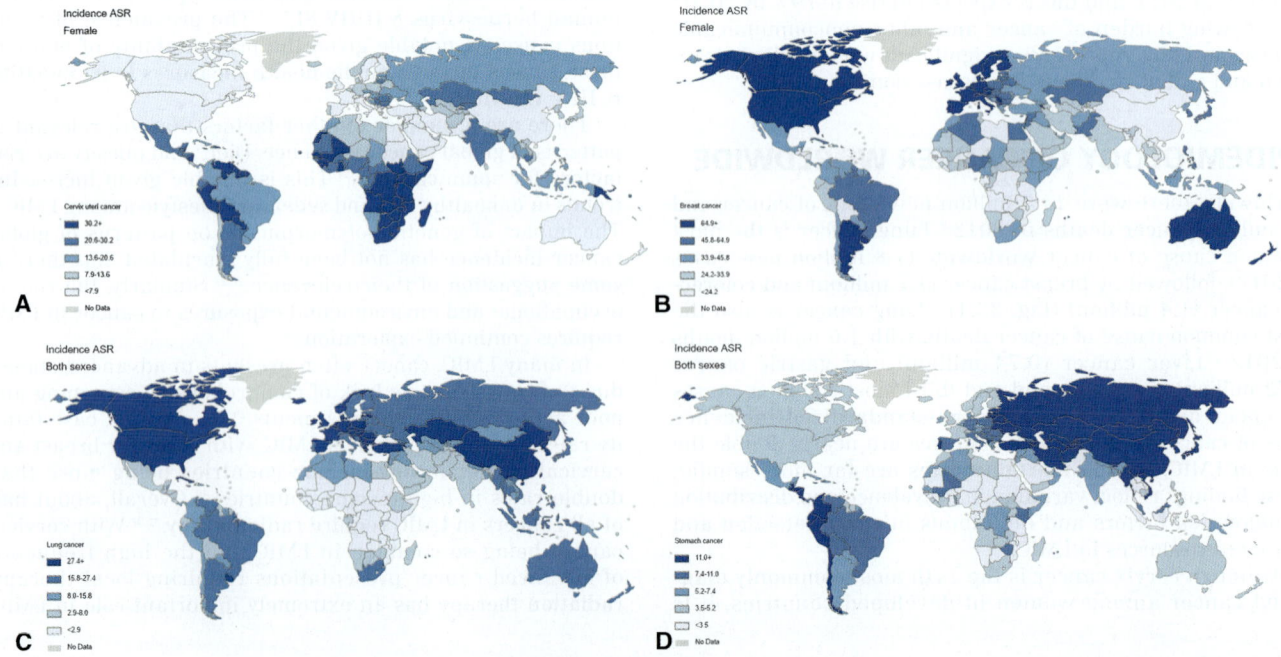

accessibility, acceptability, affordability, accommodation, and awareness.[34,35] The most pertinent elements of access to radiation therapy in LMIC are discussed here.

Availability of equipment and personnel for radiation therapy is a common limiting factor in LMIC. Less than 5% of global medical spending on cancer is in LMIC.[36] This is despite LMIC containing over 80% of the world's population[6] and almost 80% of the world's premature death, disability, and ill health from cancer.[37] Insufficient medical training programs make it difficult to address the lack of key personnel for radiation oncology.[38–42] International Atomic Energy Agency (IAEA) data suggest that LMIC only have about a third of the world's 13,136 megavoltage radiation therapy units despite an estimated need for more than double the current number.[43,44] There are currently at least 36 countries with no known machines, mostly in Africa.[44]

The greatest limitations in machine supply are strongly associated with low national economic status (Fig. 33.3).[31] Given the expected rise in cancer incidence in LMIC, these large mismatches between need and availability will only increase if current machine supply is not improved. In addition to machine availability, one must also consider the need for other physical resources. These include clinical space, bunkers, other equipment (brachytherapy, simulation, immobilization, treatment planning, beam modification, dosimetry, quality assurance), a reliable power supply for linear accelerators, and the availability of parts (and technical support) for machine maintenance and repair.[45]

The state of radiation therapy resources varies between LMIC and regions.[39,42,46,47] Some selected examples are provided for illustration. In 1999, Levin et al.[47] documented the availability and distribution of radiation therapy equipment in Africa. Only 22 of 56 countries in Africa were confidently known to have megavoltage radiation therapy facilities. In total, more than 400 million Africans had effectively no access to radiation therapy. Although machine supply has since increased, there are still dramatic shortfalls in machine supply in Sub-Saharan Africa.[43,44]

In the Asia and Pacific Region, Tatsuzaki and Levin[39] found an 82-fold variation in the number of megavoltage machines per million population for 1999. China's and India's machine supply has increased in recent years, though capacity is still well below what is needed to treat all patients (Table 33.1).[5,43,48] Workforce resources vary considerably between countries,

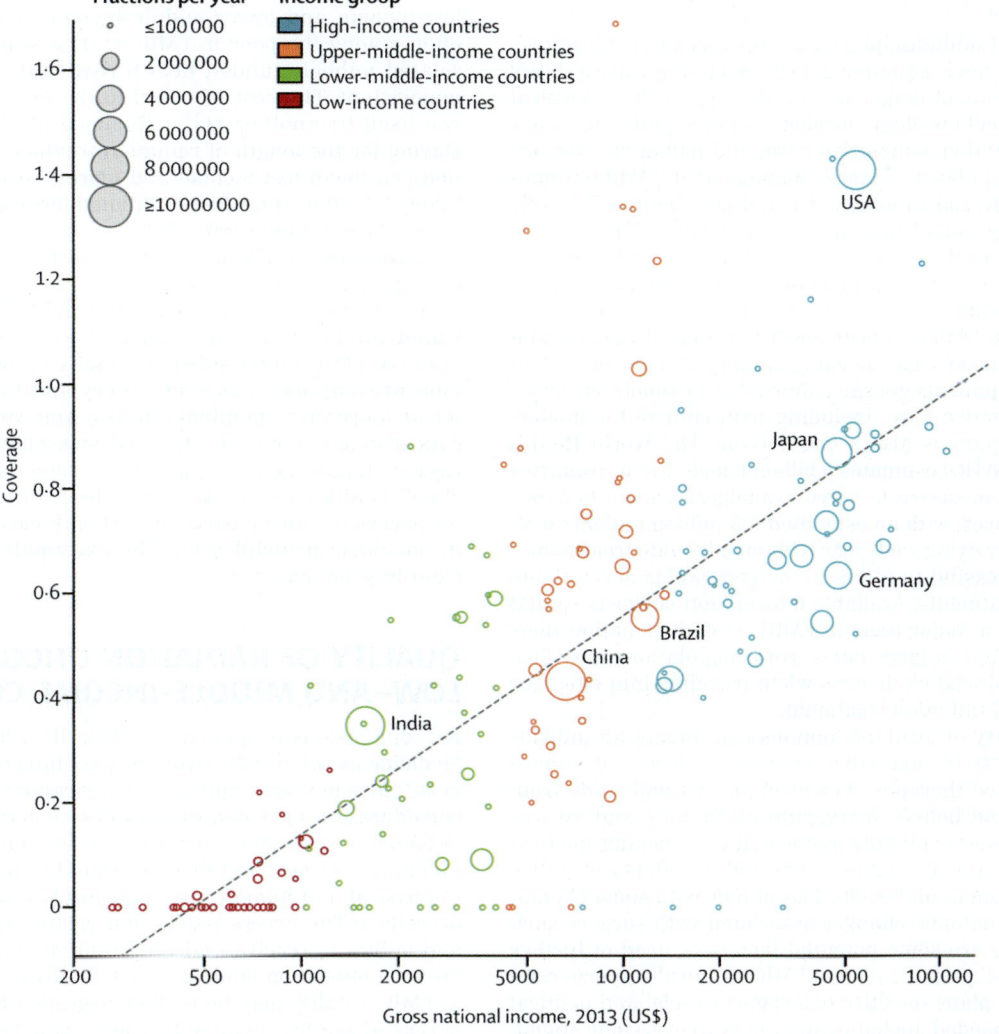

FIGURE 33.3. Radiotherapy coverage according to country gross national income per capita. Each *circle* represents a single country. The diameter corresponds to the actual annual number of fractions delivered by each country. Color corresponds to country income group. Coverage is reported assuming an 8-hour operating day. (Reprinted from Atun R, Jaffray DA, Barton MB, et al. Expanding global access to radiotherapy. *Lancet Oncol* 2015;16[10]:1153–1186. Copyright © 2015 Elsevier. With permission.)

TABLE 33.1 MEGAVOLTAGE MACHINE SUPPLY AND CANCER BURDEN IN 17 ASIA PACIFIC COUNTRIES

Country	2010 Per Capita Gross National Income (US$)	Population (Millions) 2010	Incident Cancers 2010	Megavoltage (MV) Machines 2011	Incident Cancers per MV Machine
Myanmar	n.a.	48.0	69,952	6	11,659
Bangladesh	640	148.7	150,271	15	10,018
Pakistan	1,050	173.6	147,738	44	3,358
Vietnam	1,100	87.9	119,374	32	3,730
India	1,340	1,224.6	1,001,749	477	2,100
Mongolia	1,890	2.8	4,603	2	2,302
Philippines	2,050	93.3	82,468	30	2,749
Sri Lanka	2,290	20.9	25,802	12	2,150
Indonesia	2,580	239.9	309,582	34	9,105
Thailand	4,210	69.1	118,601	66	1,797
China	4,260	1,348.9	2,978,386	1,521	1,958
Malaysia	7,900	28.4	34,386	22	1,563
Korea, Rep	19,890	48.2	179,187	108	1,659
New Zealand	29,050[a]	4.4	21,080	25	843
Singapore	40,920	5.1	14,495	12	1,208
Japan	42,150	126.5	637,963	905	705
Australia	43,740[a]	22.3	112,023	131	855
Total		3,692.6	6,007,660	3,442	

n.a., not available.

[a]2009 data. As a simple estimate, countries with more than 1,000 new cancers annually per radiation machine most likely have a shortfall of radiation machines. 2010 gross national income per capita information provided by the World Bank Group (Atlas method) (http://data.worldbank.org/about/country-classifications). 2010 population data from the World Population Prospects 2010 revision (http://esa.un.org/unpd/wpp/index.htm). Projected cancer incidence in 2010 from GLOBOCAN 2008 (http://globocan.iarc.fr/). Reported number of megavoltage radiation machines from Directory of Radiotherapy Centers (DIRAC) August 2011 (http://www-naweb.iaea.org/nahu/dirac/default.shtm).

and most countries have less than two radiation oncologists per 1,000 incident cancers annually.[5,40,43] More physicists are required if radiotherapy capacity is to expand in the Asia Pacific region.[40]

In the era of multidisciplinary cancer therapy, for instance, for head and neck squamous cell carcinoma, availability of other elements of diagnosis and therapy such as surgical oncology, medical oncology, oncology nursing, pathology, radiology, rehabilitation, supportive care, and palliative care are all important to effective cancer management.[49] Without adequate pathology and radiology, it is not possible to effectively diagnose cancer and distinguish curative from palliative cases. The need for surgical capacity is especially noted, given its central role in curative treatment of the most common cancers globally, especially in their early stages. The Lancet Oncology Commission on Global Cancer Surgery reported that despite over 80% of cancer cases needing surgery globally, less than 25% of cancer patients get safe, affordable, or timely surgery.[50] Access to palliative care, including pain control for moderate to severe pain, is also a major issue. The World Health Organization (WHO) estimates 5 billion people live in countries with limited or no access to narcotic analgesics and other controlled substances, with an estimated 5.5 million patients with terminal cancer dying each year without adequate treatment.[51]

Spatial accessibility refers to the geographic accessibility of medical treatments. Available information suggests spatial accessibility is a major issue in LMIC.[43,52] With radiation therapy centers often in large cities, rural populations may face substantial financial challenges when traveling into cities for the duration of radiation treatment.

Acceptability of available options can impact an individual's willingness to take advantage of services and adhere to recommended therapies. For example, a small study from Cameroon found beliefs, fears, cultural factors, and awareness were among explanations for delay in seeking medical attention for cancer.[53] Values surrounding effects of pelvic radiation treatment on fertility, loss of hair with some chemotherapy, and anatomic changes associated with surgery such as mastectomy are some potential factors in need of further description and quantification in LMIC. Culturally appropriate cancer control plans sensitive to a region's social and political concerns are needed, including initiatives to overcome stigma and improve awareness.[54]

Affordability of radiation therapy and other forms of cancer therapy are a major concern in LMIC.[55] Households often have limited or no health insurance coverage, especially in low-income and lower-middle-income countries and more often among the poor in LMIC.[56,57] This is notable as cancer-related publicly funded health care may be inadequate or nonexistent. The cost of travel to the nearest cancer center can itself be another major financial obstacle, and costs of staying for the length of radiation treatment in another location can mean lost income and more cost to the patient and family.[55] A family may lose additional income because of caregiver absence from work.[55,58]

Awareness of the basic cancer principles and the value of cancer screening and early detection may limit timely access to cancer services for the public in LMIC. A large Union for International Cancer Control (UICC) survey of multiple LMIC found substantial lack of awareness of common preventable causes of cancer and found that a quarter or more of respondents in Asia and Africa did not think cancer could be cured.[59] Limited awareness of principles of cancer diagnosis and appropriate referral among nonspecialist health care workers may be further limiting factors for access to cancer treatment. Health care worker training in oncologic principles may be extremely basic or insufficient in some cases.[60]

QUALITY OF RADIATION ONCOLOGY IN LOW- AND MIDDLE-INCOME COUNTRIES

Key dimensions of quality are described by the Institute of Medicine as safety, effectiveness, patient-centeredness, timeliness, efficiency, and equity.[61] Quality can be assessed through consideration of a health system's structure, process, and outcomes.[62] Elements of structure are physical resources, human resources, and organizational structure. Limitations in physical and human resources in LMIC have already been described. The access issues that relate to late presentation and failure to receive indicated treatment arguably have the greatest impact on outcomes and quality of radiation therapy in LMIC. Quality may be further degraded by the inequitable access of the few available resources between country and city and rich and poor.

The organizational structure of health care in LMIC has historically revolved around communicable disease, nutritional deficiencies, and child and maternal health. The additional burden of noncommunicable disease in LMIC, commonly cancer, cardiovascular disease, chronic lung disease, and mental illness, impose a major strain on current resources and health care models. Other issues may include political or social instability, conflict, corruption, and fragmented service provision. Challenges to the structure of cancer control in limited-resource settings may also include insufficient priority of cancer control among some governments and donor agencies with many competing priorities. Cancer infrastructure may be considered expensive. However, health investment is not a zero-sum game. There is a global need for sustainable local health care infrastructure relevant to all conditions, and focusing on cancer can help catalyze its development. Moreover, though prevention must be part of this, it is emphasized that targets set by WHO for reducing mortality from NCDs by 2025 will not be met by prevention alone.[63] Effective cancer control requires prevention, timely and accurate diagnosis, and access to treatment. The immediate need for cancer care once a diagnosis is made, and that cancer is a problem in upper-income countries altogether makes it a good focal point for investment in LMIC.

The process of health care refers to what occurs while care is provided. For radiation oncology, this includes technical elements of quality assurance, treatment prescription, treatment planning, and treatment delivery. It also includes the integration of multidisciplinary services needed alongside radiation oncology for effective cancer management. A major process issue in some countries is system-related delay in diagnosis.[64,65] This contributes to high rates of advanced disease at presentation. System-related diagnostic delay can relate to weak or nonexistent referral systems or limited resources for diagnosis. It is compounded by patient-related delay in seeking medical attention because of previously described access issues.[66] The additional impact on delay because of waiting times for radiation following radiation oncology consultation may be substantial.[67]

The technical process of radiotherapy is a vital element of quality. For this reason, the IAEA and WHO have maintained a postal dose audit program using thermoluminescent devices (TLDs). A report focusing on measurements from LMIC found acceptable results, with most machines calibrated within the ±5% dose acceptance limit. Sixteen percent of machines registered measurements outside this range in the first round of testing, with 93% measuring dose within 5% of the standard after the second round.[68] Notably, a dosimetric audit in Latin America and the Caribbean suggested an association between on-duty medical physics support and acceptable TLD results.[69] This emphasizes the importance of adequate staffing to a radiation department's quality assurance process.

Current reports are too limited to comment on the quality of general patterns of the radiation oncology clinical process in LMIC. There are most certainly specific opportunities for gains. Taking advantage of hypofractionation to increase throughput where there is supportive evidence has not always occurred, as one survey on patterns of palliative radiation for bone metastasis in Africa suggests.[70] Implementation of multidisciplinary decision-making among oncologists in LMIC is important but not always present.[71,72] Treatment refusal or nonadherence by patients can be a major issue in some cases and is an important area for quality improvement where it exists.[52,58,73] Audits of the clinical decision-making and the treatment-planning process may provide a useful means of ensuring patient safety, improving processes, and creating opportunities for continuing education.[74,75] This is particularly important with the introduction of technology at new locations. For example, initial experience with this approach in a new radiation therapy center in an Asian developing country found suboptimal management in 52% of cases.[74]

Adverse event rates in LMIC treating with radiation are largely unknown. A report examining the risk profile of radiation therapy for the WHO could not identify any detailed reports of adverse events from Africa or Asia.[76] It is important to highlight the need for adverse event recording and reporting for the purpose of patient safety and quality improvement for all countries utilizing radiation therapy.

Finally, quality of radiation oncology in LMIC relates to outcomes. Of all cancer outcomes, there is the most information on survival. Generally, overall survival for cancer patients is lower, and sometimes dramatically so, for populations in LMIC. In a large multinational series from the International Agency for Research on Cancer (IARC), 5-year age-standardized relative survival for cervix cancer was 79% in Seoul, South Korea, but 46% in Mumbai, India; 22% in The Gambia; and only 13% in Kampala, Uganda.[77] Similarly, for breast cancer, survival rates ranged from 90% in Hong Kong SAR to 13% in The Gambia. When absolute survival was stratified by extent of disease, in many cases, treatment outcomes were still inferior in regions with less developed health services compared to regions with more developed services (e.g., local and regional extent breast cancer and larynx cancer). This may reflect access and quality issues in diagnosis, treatment, and follow-up and/or limitations of the available data.

ECONOMICS OF RADIATION THERAPY IN LOW- AND MIDDLE-INCOME COUNTRIES

In 2013, The Global Task Force on Radiotherapy for Cancer Control (GTFRCC) was commissioned by the Union for International Cancer Control to determine the investment needed to achieve equitable access to radiotherapy in LMIC by 2035.[31] This was a broad collaborative effort, involving radiation oncologists, physicists, industry, economists, and global health experts. GTFRCC published their findings as a Lancet Oncology Commission, as part of the Lancet Cancer Campaign. Dramatic shortfalls in radiotherapy coverage were evident (Fig. 33.3). The cost of scaling up radiotherapy services 2015 to 2035 was estimated to be US$26.6 billion in low-income countries, $62.6 billion in lower-middle-income countries, and $94.8 billion in upper-middle-income countries. By comparison, 1 year of immunotherapy (budgeted at $295,000 per patient), for the current burden of metastatic cancer in the United States, would cost an estimated $174 billion.[78]

What could be gained by investment in radiotherapy for LMIC? The GTFRCC estimated that scaling up radiotherapy from observed levels in 2015 to 2035 could save 26.9 million life-years in LMIC over the lifetime of patients receiving treatment. Moreover, the estimated net economic benefit derived from investment in radiotherapy 2015 to 2035 was found to be substantial. These estimates utilized a full-income method, which is rooted in societal or individual willingness to pay to avoid a shortened life expectancy. Investment in radiotherapy could produce a net benefit of $265.2 million in low-income countries, $38.5 billion in lower-middle-income countries, and $239.3 billion in upper-middle-income countries.

Undoubtedly, applications of various radiation therapy techniques and modern equipment will yield opportunities to maximize the cost–benefit ratio of radiation treatment in LMIC. The GTFRCC found economic benefits from efficiency gains in radiotherapy delivery could be substantial.

These efficiency gains included automation of treatment planning and quality assurance.[31] Hypofractionation yields opportunities to treat more patients with the same supply of equipment.[79] Hypofractionation for cervical cancer and lung cancer are examples of identified areas for research.[80–82] Investigation of brachytherapy or intraoperative radiation therapy (IORT) may provide means of delivering adjuvant treatments rapidly. High–dose-rate (HDR) brachytherapy markedly increases patient throughput (e.g., for cervical cancer) compared to low–dose-rate (LDR) brachytherapy per machine.[83] An IAEA study of accelerated radiation therapy for head and neck cancer in LMIC suggests an opportunity for increasing effectiveness of treatment without increasing departmental resources, though with increased, but tolerable, acute toxicity.[84] It should be emphasized that prevention and early detection are critical to reducing the number of people diagnosed with cancer and the number of advanced cancers requiring more complex, multimodality treatments.

TRANSLATING KNOWLEDGE INTO ACTION

Recognized priorities for action fall into six categories: (a) advocacy, (b) investment, (c) planning, (d) capacity building, (e) quality, and (f) innovation.[57,85–90] The varying resources, priorities, and disease burden seen in countries at different stages of development mean that there is no single solution that will apply in all cases. In low-income countries with extreme resource limitations, a strategy focusing on cost-effective prevention, raising awareness of cancer within the population, monitoring of process and outcomes, good palliative care, and focused early detection and treatment goals would be a reasonable starting point.[87]

Advocacy

An international coalition to support cancer control and cancer care in LMIC is emerging. The UICC plays an important role as an umbrella organization for advocacy, notably commissioning the GTFRCC, whose efforts have been described above. The GTFRCC called for action on five items: (a) population-based cancer control plans, (b) expansion of access to radiotherapy, (c) human resources for radiotherapy, (d) sustainable financing to expand access to radiotherapy, and (e) align radiotherapy access with universal health coverage.[31] We will elaborate on some of these items in review of the six priority categories for action covered in this section.

Other groups involved in advocacy range from international agencies (e.g., IAEA, WHO, IARC), to national organizations (e.g., US National Cancer Institute), to professional groups (e.g., American Society for Radiation Oncology [ASTRO], European Society for Radiotherapy and Oncology [ESTRO], American Society of Clinical Oncology [ASCO], International Organization for Medical Physics [IOMP]), to nongovernmental organizations (NGOs) (e.g., International Network for Cancer Treatment and Research [INCTR], Axios International, AfrOx, American Cancer Society), to academic institutions and hospitals (e.g., the Global Task Force on Expanded Access to Cancer Care and Control in Developing Countries [GTF.CCC] convened by Harvard, St. Jude Children's Research Hospital). Through the advocacy of the UICC and many other partners (e.g., NCD Alliance), the 2011 Political Declaration[91] of the United Nations High-Level Meeting on the Prevention and Control of Noncommunicable Diseases was an important acknowledgment by governments of the global problem of cancer and other noncommunicable diseases. It was also a substantial step toward specific and concerted action by the international community.

Investment

Substantial investment is required, though the potential return on investment is substantial. The GTFRCC has called for $46 billion of investment by 2025 to establish radiotherapy infrastructure and training in LMIC.[31] Particularly in middle-income countries, incorporation of cancer care into public health insurance for those living in poverty is an important goal to meet.[57,92] The GTFRCC set a target for 80% of LMIC to include radiotherapy services as part of their universal health coverage by 2020. Given the shortage of national funding for cancer care in poorer countries, international private and public donor support and advocacy on pricing will be notably important in improving access to cancer therapy.

Planning

Development of radiation therapy capacity cannot occur in isolation. Radiation therapy resources must be integrated into a broader context of multidisciplinary cancer control and into a functional health system capable of tackling the double burden of communicable and noncommunicable diseases afflicting LMIC.[93] For this reason, the GTFRCC called for population-based cancer control plans, with a target of 80% of countries with cancer plans that include radiotherapy by 2020. A national cancer control plan and collection of cancer registry and health data are central in organizing resources in an equitable and appropriate fashion.[94] Notably, the GTF. CCC has published an important resource for planning, advocacy, and priority setting entitled *Closing the Cancer Divide: A Blueprint to Expand Access in Low and Middle Income Countries*.[95]

Prevention (e.g., tobacco control, hepatitis B and HPV vaccination) and early detection are crucial in reducing the burden of advanced cancers in LMIC. When early detection and prevention are combined with timely access to effective cancer therapy, there is great potential for dramatically reducing deaths from cancer in LMIC as well as minimizing national costs of cancer therapy.[57]

The IAEA plays a prominent role in quality assurance, safety standards, and dose calibration of radiation therapy equipment internationally. It has also been involved in numerous technical cooperation projects and radiation therapy clinical trials in LMIC. In 2004, the IAEA launched the Program of Action for Cancer Treatment (PACT) to widen the scope of its work in radiation therapy planning and capacity building. Its wide-ranging plan started with the development of sustainable demonstration radiation treatment sites in six countries throughout the developing world (Albania, Nicaragua, Sri Lanka, Tanzania, Vietnam, and Yemen).

At a global level, breast cancer guidelines stratified by availability of resources have been developed through the Breast Health Global Initiative.[96] This is a useful paradigm for developing resource-appropriate and stepwise, scalable goals and guidelines for cancer care that is being adopted for other cancers.[97] A related approach has been used by the IAEA to describe additional resource requirements, benefits, and risks for specific approaches in lung cancer treatment, including curative and palliative radiation.[98]

Developing innovative means of organizing and funding cancer services is needed. The IAEA's PACT program offers opportunities to identify successful models of service delivery and planning. A model of radiotherapy service provision utilizing geographically dispersed telemedicine-linked sites with varying levels of capacity has also been proposed by an Indian group to maximize available resources.[99] Another concept that is being explored is utilizing community health workers and primary care to expand cancer-related service provision. Proposed activities are cancer prevention, early detection, some treatment (e.g., systemic therapy), palliation, and follow-up.[57]

Capacity Building

The importance of improving human resources for radiation oncology and oncology in general cannot be overstated given the global workforce shortage of trained health care professionals. Some initial efforts have been made in developing curricula and educational approaches specific to the discipline of radiation medicine.[100-102] The IAEA has been notably involved in these efforts. The issue of loss of trained staff from developing to developed countries is especially important to consider in developing educational programs. Urban regions in LMIC may have high-level expertise that can be utilized in developing national or regional training programs. A complementary approach is online training. This is the approach of the Virtual University for Cancer Control and Regional Training Network (VUCCnet) initiative in Africa. A growing number of cancer centers, regional groups, and specific nations have been involved in twinning projects building capacity for cancer therapy in limited-resource countries. These initiatives have been particularly strong in pediatric oncology, with demonstrated success.[103,104] They provide an appealing means for broad participation in improving cancer control in LMIC.

Surge in career interest and opportunities. In the last 5 or so years, particularly following the United Nations declaration on the importance of addressing noncommunicable diseases in 2011,[91] there has been a surge in interest in radiation and clinical oncology in making global health an integral part of a career. With support from visionary senior leadership, much of the initiative has been undertaken by trainees and early career leaders in defining a career path[105,106] and for establishing resources for idea sharing and opportunities for clinical rotations.[107] The International Cancer Expert Corps (ICEC) has established an Early Career Leaders Working Group and Fund[108] to provide support for small grants for global health projects. The hurdle that must be overcome is the issue of how one supports a career in global health because it is not a revenue-generating activity. This can be surmounted with both the appreciation of the need for service as an essential component of a career in health care and also the tangible and intangible benefits to institutions and individuals that come from establishing a means of sustainable service to society. New creative paradigms have the potential to bring in interest and investment in global health from a wide range of economic sectors[109] including science, education, economics, and industry. The data from the GTFRCC[31] indicate that treating cancer provides economic as well as health benefits and is, indeed, a wise investment.

What is obvious is that visionary leaders interested in (a) innovation in career path development, (b) enhancing the capability of existing technology and creating new robust technology and connectivity, and (c) expanding the scope of what is a *bona fide* medical career are needed to address the gap in global cancer care in both capacity and capability. This will represent a paradigm shift to address an issue of health care inequality that is morally unacceptable, requiring immediate attention with effective action and a sustainable commitment to a problem that will take decades to solve.

Indigenous populations in Upper-Income Countries (UICs). Expanding the number of stakeholders in global health will benefit those in need and also may enhance the interest and investment from resource-rich countries (UICs) including a recognition that they have similar problems within their own country. Optimism for investment in global health by radiation oncology over the last few years is the result of remarkable interest by trainees and early career leaders and understanding that this is not simply a problem in the developing world. The level of interest is demonstrated by two very recent reviews, in Clinical Oncology[110] and Seminars in Radiation Oncology.[111]

Indigenous populations in UICs, particularly people living in geographically isolated or remote regions, have economic, social and societal issues that are often quite similar to the underserved in LMIC.[112] As in LMIC, there is less screening, less care and presentation with more advanced stages of disease. Although there is substantial overlap in terms of access and the need for care between indigenous and indigent populations and in the social determinants of health, a distinction is being made between indigent populations in urban centers who are near medical facilities but with limited access often because of other reasons, compared to geographically isolated indigenous people who may be many miles away and for whom physical access to facilities is limited by distance, expense and the need to be at home to care for families. Success is possible when investment is made, as demonstrated in the Walking Forward Program[113] and the Native Navigators and the Cancer Continuum (NNACC).[114] Indeed in the National Cancer Institute's Cancer Disparities Research Partnership Program, the program with the Lakota Sioux demonstrated that clinical and translational research can be accomplished.[115,116] The Union for International Cancer Control has included an indigenous populations session in its last two World Congress meetings, with participation from Australia, New Zealand, Canada and the United States.

What is critical to remember is that the health care disparities within geographically remote indigenous populations are also suffered by nonindigenous people who are neighbors of the tribes so that they, too, benefit from investment in cancer care. Addressing this common need serves to build a link among the local communities. For those seeking investment from UICs for global health, there is an advantage in including indigenous populations among the needs for LMIC. This approach serves to make the investment more immediate to those in UICs and helps address the frequently raised question as to why invest abroad when problems exist at home.

Quality

Embedded within the themes of investment, planning, and capacity building is the implicit theme of structure-related quality improvement. Process-related initiatives in quality are another very important part of ensuring optimal outcomes. These are often referred to indirectly (e.g., safety, effectiveness, patient-centeredness, timeliness, efficiency, equity).[61] Quality improvement relating to process and organizational structure is important as it holds the potential for improving some outcomes more rapidly than other drivers of health, such as economic growth.[117] One important element of quality for radiation oncology in LMIC is safety, given the potential for unsafe treatment to negate any benefit of available treatment.[118] Safety includes the clinical process and the various elements of technical quality assurance, maintenance, worker safety, public safety, and source security.[119,120] Safety requires investment in appropriate dosimetry equipment, sufficiently trained human resources, and time for quality assurance activities.[120] Internal and external audits, peer review, regulation, accreditation, certification, checklists, adverse event reporting, common protocols, quality improvement, and independent checking are examples of interventions ensuring safety and quality assurance in radiation oncology.[76,121,122]

Innovation

There are many fundamental questions that remain unanswered for cancer in LMIC. It cannot be assumed that approaches to treating cancer from developed settings will produce the same results when applied in other countries.

Considerations include potential differences in disease bulk, malnutrition, rates of chronic infections such as HIV/tuberculosis/hepatitis B, and genetic polymorphisms affecting disease biology and treatment response.[123-127] There are many unknowns in cancer epidemiology and basic science, and, as mentioned, more health services research is emphatically needed into areas such as access, quality, and economics.[94]

International research partnerships are essential in the interconnected and interdependent world we live in.[128] Many LMIC have quite advanced resources to sustain research activities; for instance, a number of clinical trials for cervical cancer radiotherapy have occurred in India (e.g., HDR vs. LDR brachytherapy, radiation vs. chemoradiation).[129,130] India is also home of the Advanced Center for Treatment, Research and Education in Cancer (ACTREC), part of the Tata Memorial Center. Regional research collaborations are developing, for example, the Forum for Nuclear Cooperation in Asia (FNCA). In addition, of note, a number of research/teaching twinning partnerships between UICs and LMIC have been formed.[103,104,131] Supporting research on cancer by investigators in the developing world is important as it can build local research capacity and provide a means of adapting scientific knowledge to local circumstances to meet national health priorities.[128] The US National Cancer Institute has also been involved with numerous international collaborations. Protocol-driven clinical research can also strengthen local treatment capacity. The INCTR has been involved in designing clinical trials relevant to developing world situations, as has the IAEA.

What should be implicit in capacity building is the capability of the workforce and also of the technology to provide state-of-the-art care. It is debated about what is the best technology for the developing world between the relative simplicity of cobalt-60 and the more sophisticated ability of linear accelerators, which are dependent on effective physical infrastructure. Logically, a range of technologies is needed[132] including brachytherapy. However, to fill the enormous gap in global cancer care, it is imperative to look forward toward longer-term solutions because although incremental steps and small projects are useful, innovative systems solutions are necessary to reach the necessary capacity and capability. This includes increasing the opportunities for a career in global health and recruiting, training, and retaining people willing to serve within challenging environments. Detailed discussions for issues raised in the sections in this chapter on capacity and capability building are in recent radiation oncology reviews mentioned above, in Clinical Oncology[110] and Seminars in Radiation Oncology.[111]

New paradigms in global health. An example of novel partnerships emerged from the White House's Interagency Working Group on Alternatives to High-Activity Radioactive Sources[133] that brought together experts interested in reducing the availability of potentially dangerous radiation sources (including medical radionuclides of cobalt-60 and cesium-137), along with radiation oncologists and medical physicists and also groups interested in nuclear nonproliferation. Pomper et al. developed a new concept "Treatment, Not Terror" that highlights the importance in providing safe alternatives to radionuclides which for cobalt-60 requires expertise for delivering linear accelerator treatment.[134] The relatively lower initial cost of cobalt-60 is offset by a very high cost of disposal of the source at the end of its useful life, a number that is often not included in the purchase price. Certainly, treatment with both cobalt and linear accelerators is important for cancer care; however, as the huge shortage of capacity is addressed, it is worthwhile to look toward the future with improvements possible in technology, telecommunications, economic models, and efficient use of expert personnel. Recognizing the need for improved infrastructure to support linear accelerators, a workshop was recently conducted by the ICEC in Geneva at CERN[135] to address this complex topic. This included people with expertise in accelerator design, technology modularization, telemedicine, industrial design, and education/training. Task groups will address unique solutions for training, education, the use of current technology, and the potential for innovative technology. Feain et al. have highlighted new approaches to radiation technology for LMIC including software, information management, and technologic solutions.[136]

CONCLUSION

Cancer in the developing world is an urgent problem, reaching critical proportions. Almost 60% of all cancer cases occur in the developing world. Vast numbers of people in LMIC have either limited access or no access to radiation therapy. At a time when new gains in oncology outcomes in the developed world are often incremental, oncologists have the chance to help make some of the largest survival gains in history in the developing world. In addition, the potential for health care gains through cancer prevention and early detection, and for the relief of suffering through palliative care is enormous. Global access to quality cancer care is a moral imperative. The challenge will now be to deliver this in a thoughtful and contextually appropriate way.

REFERENCES

1. Koplan JP, Bond TC, Merson MH, et al. Towards a common definition of global health. *Lancet* 2009;373(9679):1993–1995.
2. World Bank. World Bank Country Classifications, 2017. Available at: http://data.worldbank.org/about/country-classifications. Accessed May 20, 2017.
3. Institute for Health Metrics and Evaluation (IHME). *Global Burden of Disease Study 2015. Global Burden of Disease Study 2015 (GBD 2015) results.* Seattle, WA: Institute for Health Metrics and Evaluation (IHME), 2016. Available at: http://ghdx.healthdata.org/gbd-results-tool. Accessed May 20, 2017.
4. Ferlay J, Soerjomataram I, Ervik M, et al. *GLOBOCAN 2012 v1.0, Cancer incidence and mortality worldwide: IARC CancerBase No. 11 [Internet].* Lyon, France: International Agency for Research on Cancer, 2013. Available at: http://globocan.iarc.fr. Accessed April 26, 2017.
5. Ferlay J, Shin HR, Bray F, et al. *GLOBOCAN 2008 v1.2, Cancer incidence and mortality worldwide: IARC CancerBase No. 10 [Internet].* Lyon, France: International Agency for Research on Cancer, 2010. Available at: http://globocan.iarc.fr. Accessed July 8, 2017.
6. Population Division of the Department of Economic and Social Affairs of the United Nations Secretariat. World population prospects: the 2010 revision, 2011. Available at: http://esa.un.org/unpd/wpp/index.htm
7. Murray CJ, Lopez AD. Global mortality, disability, and the contribution of risk factors: Global Burden of Disease Study. *Lancet* 1997;349(9063):1436–1442.
8. Torre LA, Bray F, Siegel RL, et al. Global cancer statistics, 2012. *CA Cancer J Clin* 2015;65(2):87–108.
9. Jemal A, Bray F, Center MM, et al. Global cancer statistics. *CA Cancer J Clin* 2011;61(2):69–90.
10. Wabinga HR, Parkin DM, Wabwire-Mangen F, et al. Cancer in Kampala, Uganda, in 1989–91: changes in incidence in the era of AIDS. *Int J Cancer* 1993;54(1):26–36.
11. Warnakulasuriya S. Global epidemiology of oral and oropharyngeal cancer. *Oral Oncol* 2009;45(4–5):309–316.
12. Danaei G, Vander Hoorn S, Lopez AD, et al. Causes of cancer in the world: comparative risk assessment of nine behavioural and environmental risk factors. *Lancet* 2005;366(9499):1784–1793.
13. World Health Organization. Tobacco Fact Sheet. http://www.wpro.who.int/mediacentre/factsheets/fs_201203_tobacco/en/. Accessed May 20, 2017.
14. World Health Organization. WHO report on the global tobacco epidemic, 2011: warning about the dangers of tobacco. Appendix V: country profiles, 2011. Available at: http://www.who.int/tobacco/global_report/2011/en_tfi_global_report_2011_appendix_V_table_1.pdf
15. World Health Organization. *WHO report on the Global Tobacco Epidemic, 2008: the MPOWER package.* Brazil: World Health Organization, 2008.
16. Lopez AD, Collishaw NE, Piha T. A descriptive model of the cigarette epidemic in developed countries. *Tob Control* 1994;3(3):242–247.
17. Niu SR, Yang GH, Chen ZM, et al. Emerging tobacco hazards in China: 2. Early mortality results from a prospective study. *BMJ* 1998;317(7170):1423–1424.
18. World Health Organization and Center For Disease Control. *Tobacco or health: a global status report,* 1997. Available at: http://www.cdc.gov/tobacco/WHO/index.htm

19. Parkin DM. The global health burden of infection-associated cancers in the year 2002. *Int J Cancer* 2006;118(12):3030–3044.

20. Perz JF, Armstrong GL, Farrington LA, et al. The contributions of hepatitis B virus and hepatitis C virus infections to cirrhosis and primary liver cancer worldwide. *J Hepatol* 2006;45(4):529–538.

21. IARC. *IARC monographs on the evaluation of carcinogenic risks to humans: some naturally occurring substances: food items and constituents, heterocyclic aromatic amines and mycotoxins. Volume 56*. United Kingdom: World Health Organization, 1993.

22. IARC. *IARC monographs on the evaluation of carcinogenic risks to humans: schistosomes, liver flukes and helicobacter pylori*. United Kingdom: World Health Organization, 1994.

23. Key TJ, Schatzkin A, Willett WC, et al. Diet, nutrition and the prevention of cancer. *Public Health Nutr* 2004;7(1A):187–200.

24. Chow WH, Gridley G, Fraumeni JF Jr, et al. Obesity, hypertension, and the risk of kidney cancer in men. *N Engl J Med* 2000;343(18):1305–1311.

25. Popkin BM. The nutrition transition and obesity in the developing world. *J Nutr* 2001;131(3):871S–873S.

26. Liede A, Narod SA. Hereditary breast and ovarian cancer in Asia: genetic epidemiology of BRCA1 and BRCA2. *Hum Mutat* 2002;20(6):413–424.

27. Bono AV. The global state of prostate cancer: epidemiology and screening in the second millennium. *BJU Int* 2004;94(Suppl 3):1–2.

28. Vineis P, Xun W. The emerging epidemic of environmental cancers in developing countries. *Ann Oncol* 2009;20(2):205–212.

29. Kanavos P. The rising burden of cancer in the developing world. *Ann Oncol* 2006;17(Suppl 8):viii15–viii23.

30. Beaulieu N, Bloom DE, Reddy Bloom L, et al. *Breakaway: the global burden of cancer—challenges and opportunities*. Economist Intelligence Unit: The Economist, 2009.

31. Atun R, Jaffray DA, Barton MB, et al. Expanding global access to radiotherapy. *Lancet Oncol* 2015;16(10):1153–1186.

32. Yap ML, Hanna TP, Wong K, et al. The benefits of achieving equitable access to radiotherapy globally: projections to 2035. *J Med Imaging Radiat Oncol* 2015;59:30.

33. World Health Organization. *WHO list of priority medical devices for cancer management*. Geneva: World Health Organization, 2017. Available at: http://apps.who.int/iris/bitstream/10665/255262/1/9789241565462-eng.pdf?ua=1. Accessed May 18, 2017.

34. Penchansky R, Thomas JW. The concept of access: definition and relationship to consumer satisfaction. *Med Care* 1981;19(2):127–140.

35. Mackillop WJ, Hanna TP, Brundage MB. Health services research in radiation oncology: towards achieving the achievable for patients with cancer. In: Gunderson LL, Tepper JE, eds. *Clinical radiation oncology, fourth edition*. New York, NY: Churchill Livingstone, 2015.

36. Farmer P, Frenk J, Knaul FM, et al. Expansion of cancer care and control in countries of low and middle income: a call to action. *Lancet* 2010;376(9747):1186–1193.

37. World Health Organization. Projections of mortality and burden of disease, 2004–2030, 2008. Available at: http://www.who.int/healthinfo/global_burden_disease/projections/en/index.html

38. Frenk J, Chen L, Bhutta ZA, et al. Health professionals for a new century: transforming education to strengthen health systems in an interdependent world. *Lancet* 2010;376(9756):1923–1958.

39. Tatsuzaki H, Levin CV. Quantitative status of resources for radiation therapy in Asia and Pacific region. *Radiother Oncol* 2001;60(1):81–89.

40. Kron T, Cheung K, Dai J, et al. Medical physics aspects of cancer care in the Asia Pacific region. *Biomed Imaging Interv J* 2008;4(3):e33.

41. Zaidi H. Medical physics in developing countries: looking for a better world. *Biomed Imaging Interv J* 2008;4(1):e29.

42. Zubizarreta EH, Poitevin A, Levin CV. Overview of radiotherapy resources in Latin America: a survey by the International Atomic Energy Agency (IAEA). *Radiother Oncol* 2004;73(1):97–100.

43. International Atomic Energy Agency. Directory of Radiotherapy Centers (DIRAC). Available at: http://www-naweb.iaea.org/nahu/dirac/default.shtm

44. Yap ML, Zubizarreta E, Bray F, et al. Global access to radiotherapy services: have we made progress during the past decade? *J Glob Oncol* 2016;2(4):207–215.

45. Bese NS, Munshi A, Budrukkar A, et al. Breast radiation therapy guideline implementation in low- and middle-income countries. *Cancer* 2008;113(8 Suppl):2305–2314.

46. Levin V, Tatsuzaki H. Radiotherapy services in countries in transition: gross national income per capita as a significant factor. *Radiother Oncol* 2002;63(2):147–150.

47. Levin CV, El Gueddari B, Meghzifene A. Radiation therapy in Africa: distribution and equipment. *Radiother Oncol* 1999;52(1):79–84.

48. Barton MB, Frommer M, Shafiq J. Role of radiotherapy in cancer control in low-income and middle-income countries. *Lancet Oncol* 2006;7(7):584–595.

49. Sanabria A, Domenge C, D'Cruz A, et al. Organ preservation protocols in developing countries. *Curr Opin Otolaryngol Head Neck Surg* 2010;18(2):83–88.

50. Sullivan R, Alatise OI, Anderson BO, et al. Global cancer surgery: delivering safe, affordable, and timely cancer surgery. *Lancet Oncol* 2015;16(11):1193–1224.

51. Medicine Access and Rational Use, Department of Essential Medicines and Pharmaceutical Policies. Health Systems and Services. *World Health Organization briefing note—February 2009. Access to controlled medications programme. Improving access to medications controlled under international drug conventions*. World Health Organization, 2009.

52. Anyanwu SN, Egwuonwu OA, Ihekwoaba EC. Acceptance and adherence to treatment among breast cancer patients in Eastern Nigeria. *Breast* 2011;20(Suppl 2):S51–S53.

53. Ekortarl A, Ndom P, Sacks A. A study of patients who appear with far advanced cancer at Yaounde General Hospital, Cameroon, Africa. *Psychooncology* 2007;16(3):255–257.

54. Leong BD, Chuah JA, Kumar VM, et al. Trends of breast cancer treatment in Sabah, Malaysia: a problem with lack of awareness. *Singapore Med J* 2009;50(8):772–776.

55. Obi SN, Ozumba BC. Cervical cancer: socioeconomic implications of management in a developing nation. *J Obstet Gynaecol* 2008;28(5):526–528.

56. Wagner AK, Graves AJ, Reiss SK, et al. Access to care and medicines, burden of health care expenditures, and risk protection: results from the World Health Survey. *Health Policy* 2011;100(2–3):151–158.

57. Farmer P, Frenk J, Knaul FM, et al. Expansion of cancer care and control in countries of low and middle income: a call to action. *Lancet* 2010;376(9747):1186–1193.

58. Arrossi S, Matos E, Zengarini N, et al. The socio-economic impact of cervical cancer on patients and their families in Argentina, and its influence on radiotherapy compliance. Results from a cross-sectional study. *Gynecol Oncol* 2007;105(2):335–340.

59. Machlin A, Wakefield M, Spittal M, et al. *Cancer-related beliefs and behaviours in eight geographic regions*. Geneva: Union for International Cancer Control, 2009.

60. Fles R, Wildeman MA, Sulistiono B, et al. Knowledge of general practitioners about nasopharyngeal cancer at the Puskesmas in Yogyakarta, Indonesia. *BMC Med Educ* 2010;10:81.

61. Institute of Medicine Committee on Quality of Health Care in America. *Crossing the quality chasm: a new health system for the 21st century*. Washington, DC: National Academy Press, 2001.

62. Donabedian A. The quality of care. How can it be assessed? *JAMA* 1988;260(12):1743–1748.

63. World Health Organization (WHO). NCD global monitoring framework, 2013. Available at: http://www.who.int/nmh/global_monitoring_framework/en/. Accessed May 26, 2017.

64. Bright K, Barghash M, Donach M, et al. The role of health system factors in delaying final diagnosis and treatment of breast cancer in Mexico City, Mexico. *Breast* 2011;20(Suppl 2):S54–S59.

65. Khoo SP, Shanmuhasuntharam P, Mahadzir WM, et al. Factors involved in the diagnosis of oral squamous cell carcinoma in Malaysia. *Asia Pac J Public Health* 1998;10(1):49–51.

66. Dye TD, Bogale S, Hobden C, et al. Complex care systems in developing countries: breast cancer patient navigation in Ethiopia. *Cancer* 2010;116(3):577–585.

67. Kantelhardt EJ, Moelle U, Begoihn M, et al. Cervical cancer in Ethiopia: survival of 1,059 patients who received oncologic therapy. *Oncologist* 2014;19(7):727–734.

68. Izewska J, Andreo P, Vatnitsky S, et al. The IAEA/WHO TLD postal dose quality audits for radiotherapy: a perspective of dosimetry practices at hospitals in developing countries. *Radiother Oncol* 2003;69(1):91–97.

69. Izewska J, Vatnitsky S, Shortt KR. Postal dose audits for radiotherapy centers in Latin America and the Caribbean: trends in 1969–2003. *Rev Panam Salud Publica* 2006;20(2–3):161–172.

70. Sharma V, Gaye PM, Wahab SA, et al. Patterns of practice of palliative radiotherapy in Africa, Part 1: Bone and brain metastases. *Int J Radiat Oncol Biol Phys* 2008;70(4):1195–1201.

71. Cazap E, Buzaid AC, Garbino C, et al. Breast cancer in Latin America: results of the Latin American and Caribbean Society of Medical Oncology/Breast Cancer Research Foundation expert survey. *Cancer* 2008;113(8 Suppl):2359–2365.

72. El Saghir NS, El-Asmar N, Hajj C, et al. Survey of utilization of multidisciplinary management tumor boards in Arab countries. *Breast* 2011;20(Suppl 2): S70–S74.

73. Mohanti BK, Nachiappan P, Pandey RM, et al. Analysis of 2167 head and neck cancer patients' management, treatment compliance and outcomes from a regional cancer centre, Delhi, India. *J Laryngol Otol* 2007;121(1): 49–56.

74. Shakespeare TP, Back MF, Lu JJ, et al. External audit of clinical practice and medical decision making in a new Asian oncology center: results and implications for both developing and developed nations. *Int J Radiat Oncol Biol Phys* 2006;64(3):941–947.

75. Mohanti BK. Introducing radiotherapy to Oman. *Eur J Cancer* 2008;44(3):333.

76. Barton M, Shafiq J, eds. *Radiotherapy risk profile: technical manual*. Geneva: World Health Organization, Radiotherapy Safety Team within the World Alliance for Patient Safety, 2008.

77. Sankaranarayanan R, Swaminathan R, eds. *Cancer survival in Africa, Asia, the Caribbean and Central America. IARC Scientific Publications No. 162*. Lyon, France: International Agency for Research on Cancer, 2011. Available at: http://survcan.iarc.fr

78. Saltz LB. Perspectives on cost and value in cancer care. *JAMA Oncol* 2016;2(1): 19–21.

79. Vikram B. Radiation therapy for the developing countries. *J Cancer Res Ther* 2005;1(1):7–8.

80. Kitchener HC, Hoskins W, Small W Jr, et al. The development of priority cervical cancer trials: a Gynecologic Cancer InterGroup report. *Int J Gynecol Cancer* 2010;20(6):1092–1100.

81. van Lonkhuijzen L, Thomas G. Palliative radiotherapy for cervical carcinoma: a systematic review. *Radiother Oncol* 2011;98(3):287–291.

82. Kepka L, Casas F, Perin B, et al. Radiochemotherapy for lung cancer in developing countries. *Clin Oncol (R Coll Radiol)* 2009;21(7):536–542.

83. Nag S, Dally M, de la Torre M, et al. Recommendations for implementation of high dose rate ^{192}Ir brachytherapy in developing countries by the Advisory Group of International Atomic Energy Agency. *Radiother Oncol* 2002;64(3):297–308.

84. Overgaard J, Mohanti BK, Begum N, et al. Five versus six fractions of radiotherapy per week for squamous-cell carcinoma of the head and neck (IAEA-ACC study): a randomised, multicentre trial. *Lancet Oncol* 2010;11(6): 553–560.

85. Salminen EK, Kiel K, Ibbott GS, et al. International Conference on Advances in Radiation Oncology (ICARO): outcomes of an IAEA meeting. *Radiat Oncol* 2011;6:11.

86. AfrOx. *London declaration on cancer control in Africa.* London, 2007.

87. World Health Organization. National cancer control programmes: policies and managerial guidelines. Geneva: World Health Organization, 2002.

88. Anderson BO, Ballieu M, Bradley C, et al. *Access to cancer treatment in low- and middle-income countries—an essential part of global cancer control. A CanTreat Position Paper.* CanTreat, 2010. Available at: axios-group.com/index.php/download_file/view/85/151/. Accessed July 6, 2011.

89. Sloan FA, Gelband H, eds. *Cancer control opportunities in low- and middle-income countries.* Washington, DC: National Academy Press, 2007.

90. Union for International Cancer Control. The World Cancer Declaration 2008, 2011. Available at: http://www.uicc.org/declaration/download-declaration

91. United Nations General Assembly 66th Session. Political Declaration of the High-Level Meeting of the General Assembly on the Prevention and Control of Non-Communicable Diseases. A/66/L.1. New York, NY: United Nations, 2011. Available at: http://www.who.int/nmh/events/un_ncd_summit2011/political_declaration_en.pdf. Accessed April 16, 2017.

92. Harris J. Cancer: the new challenge for health care in the developing world. *HemOnc Today,* 2009.

93. Samb B, Desai N, Nishtar S, et al. Prevention and management of chronic disease: a litmus test for health-systems strengthening in low-income and middle-income countries. *Lancet* 2010;376(9754):1785–1797.

94. Hanna TP, Kangolle AC. Cancer control in developing countries: using health data and health services research to measure and improve access, quality and efficiency. *BMC Int Health Human Rights* 2010;10:24.

95. Knaul FM, Frenk J, Shulman LN; for the Global Task Force on Expanded Access to Cancer Care and Control in Developing Countries. *Closing the cancer divide: a blueprint to expand access in low and middle income countries.* Boston, MA: Harvard Global Equity Initiative, 2011.

96. Anderson BO, Shyyan R, Eniu A, et al. Breast cancer in limited-resource countries: an overview of the Breast Health Global Initiative 2005 guidelines. *Breast J* 2006;12(Suppl 1):S3–S15.

97. Collingridge D. Delivering consensus from the Asian Oncology Summit 2009. *Lancet Oncol* 2009;10(11):1029–1030.

98. Macbeth FR, Abratt RP, Cho KH, et al. Lung cancer management in limited resource settings: guidelines for appropriate good care. *Radiother Oncol* 2007;82:123–131.

99. Datta NR, Rajasekar D. Improvement of radiotherapy facilities in developing countries: a three-tier system with a teleradiotherapy network. *Lancet Oncol* 2004;5(11):695–698.

100. Coffey M, Engel-Hills P, El-Gantiry M, et al. A core curriculum for RTTs (radiation therapists/radiotherapy radiographers) designed for developing countries under the auspices of the International Atomic Energy Agency (IAEA). *Radiother Oncol* 2006;81:324–325.

101. Podgorsak EB. *Radiation oncology physics: a handbook for teachers and students.* Vienna: IAEA, 2005.

102. Turner S, Eriksen JG, Trotter T, et al. Establishing a Global Radiation Oncology Collaboration in Education (GRaCE): objectives and priorities. *Radiother Oncol* 2015;117(1):188–192.

103. Ribeiro RC, Pui CH. Saving the children—improving childhood cancer treatment in developing countries. *N Engl J Med* 2005;352(21):2158–2160.

104. Masera G, Baez F, Biondi A, et al. North-South twinning in paediatric haemato-oncology: the La Mascota programme, Nicaragua. *Lancet* 1998;352(9144):1923–1926.

105. Olson AC, Coleman CN, Hahn SM, et al. A roadmap for a new academic pathway for global radiation oncology. *Int J Radiat Oncol Biol Phys* 2015;93(3): 493–496.

106. Rodin D, Yap ML, Grover S, et al. Global health in radiation oncology: the emergence of a new career pathway. *Semin Radiat Oncol* 2017;27(2):118–123.

107. Rodin D, Longo J, Sherertz T, et al. Mobilising expertise and resources to close the radiotherapy gap in cancer care. *Clin Oncol* 2017;29(2):135–140.

108. International Cancer Expert Corps. *Ellen Lewis Stovall early career leaders,* 2017. Available at: http://www.iceccancer.org/the-international-cancer-expert-corps-establishes-the-ellen-lewis-stovall-early-career-leaders-working-group-fund/. Accessed April 16, 2017.

109. Coleman CN, Love RR. Transforming science, service, and society. *Sci Transl Med* 2014;6(259):259fs242.

110. Barton M, Zubizarreta E, eds. Special issue: radiotherapy in low and middle income countries. *Clin Oncol* 2017;29.

111. Williams T, Coleman CN, eds. Global health disparities. *Semin Radiat Oncol* 2017;27.

112. Guadagnolo BA, Petereit DG, Coleman CN. Cancer care access and outcomes for American Indian populations in the United States: challenges and models for progress. *Semin Radiat Oncol* 2017;27(2):143–149.

113. Petereit DG, Guadagnolo BA, Wong R, et al. Addressing cancer disparities among American Indians through innovative technologies and patient navigation: the walking forward experience. *Front Oncol* 2011;1:11.

114. Burhansstipanov L, Krebs LU, Dignan MB, et al. Findings from the Native Navigators and the Cancer Continuum (NNACC) study. *J Cancer Educ* 2014;29(3):420–427.

115. Wong RS, Vikram B, Govern FS, et al. National Cancer Institute's Cancer Disparities Research Partnership Program: experience and lessons learned. *Front Oncol* 2014;4:303.

116. Petereit DG, Hahn LJ, Kanekar S, et al. Prevalence of ATM sequence variants in Northern Plains American Indian cancer patients. *Front Oncol* 2013;3:318.

117. Peabody JW, Taguiwalo MM, Robalino DA, et al. Improving the quality of care in developing countries. In: Jamison DT, Breman JG, Measham AR, et al., eds. *Disease control priorities in developing countries.* Washington, DC: World Bank and Oxford University Press, 2006.

118. Borras C. Overexposure of radiation therapy patients in Panama: problem recognition and follow-up measures. *Rev Panam Salud Publica* 2006;20(2–3):173–187.

119. Barton MB. *Improving access to education and cancer care in developing countries. 14th World Conference on Lung Cancer.* Amsterdam: International Association for the Study of Lung Cancer, 2011.

120. Kutcher GJ, Coia L, Gillin M, et al. *Comprehensive QA for radiation oncology: report of AAPM Radiation Therapy Committee Task Group 40.* 1994/04/01 ed. College Park, MD: American Institute of Physics, 1994.

121. Mytton OT, Velazquez A, Banken R, et al. Introducing new technology safely. *Qual Saf Health Care* 2010;19(Suppl 2):i9–i14.

122. Newton RC, Mytton OT, Aggarwal R, et al. Making existing technology safer in healthcare. *Qual Saf Health Care* 2010;19(Suppl 2):i15–i24.

123. Negi RR, Gupta M, Kumar M, et al. Concurrent chemoradiation in locally advanced carcinoma cervix patients. *J Cancer Res Ther* 2010;6(2):159–166.

124. McArdle O, Kigula-Mugambe JB. Contraindications to cisplatin based chemoradiotherapy in the treatment of cervical cancer in Sub-Saharan Africa. *Radiother Oncol* 2007;83(1):94–96.

125. Carles J, Monzo M, Amat N, et al. Single-nucleotide polymorphisms in base excision repair, nucleotide excision repair, and double strand break genes as markers for response to radiotherapy in patients with stage I and II head-and-neck cancer. *Int J Radiat Oncol Biol Phys* 2006;66(4):1022–1030.

126. Grau C, Prakash Agarwal J, Jabeen K, et al. Radiotherapy with or without mitomycin c in the treatment of locally advanced head and neck cancer: results of the IAEA multicentre randomised trial. *Radiother Oncol* 2003;67(1):17–26.

127. Wu X, Gu J, Wu TT, et al. Genetic variations in radiation and chemotherapy drug action pathways predict clinical outcomes in esophageal cancer. *J Clin Oncol* 2006;24(23):3789–3798.

128. Frenk J, Chen L. Overcoming gaps to advance global health equity: a symposium on new directions for research. *Health Res Policy Syst* 2011;9(1):11.

129. Patel FD, Sharma SC, Negi PS, Ghoshal S, Gupta BD. Low dose rate vs. high dose rate brachytherapy in the treatment of carcinoma of the uterine cervix: a clinical trial. *Int J Radiat Oncol Biol Phys* 1994;28(2):335–341.

130. Singh TT, Singh IY, Sharma DT, et al. Role of chemoradiation in advanced cervical cancer. *Indian J Cancer* 2003;40(3):101–107.

131. Veerman AJ, Sutaryo S. Twinning: a rewarding scenario for development of oncology services in transitional countries. *Pediatr Blood Cancer* 2005;45(2):103–106.

132. Healy BJ, van der Merwe D, Christaki KE, et al. Cobalt-60 machines and medical linear accelerators: competing technologies for external beam radiotherapy. *Clin Oncol* 2017;29(2):110–115.

133. Interagency Working Group on Alternatives to High-Activity Radioactive Sources. *Transitioning from high-activity radioactive sources to non-radioisotopic (alternative) technologies,* 2017. Available at: https://obamawhitehouse.archives.gov/sites/default/files/microsites/ostp/ndrd-gars_best_practices_guide_final-.pdf. Accessed April 16, 2017.

134. Pomper MA, Dalnoki-Veress F, Moore GM. *Treatment, not terror: strategies to enhance external beam cancer therapy in developing countries while permanently reducing the risk of radiological terrorism,* 2017. Available at: http://www.stanleyfoundation.org/publications/report/TreatmentNotTerror212.pdf. Accessed April 16, 2017.

135. Pistenmaa D, Coleman CN, Dosanjh M. *Developing medical linacs for challenging region,* 2017. Available at: http://cerncourier.com/cws/article/cern/67710. Accessed April 16, 2017.

136. Feain IJ, Court L, Palta JR, et al. Innovations in radiotherapy technology. *Clin Oncol* 2017;29(2):120–128.

CHAPTER 34

Chemical Modifiers of Radiation Response

Yvonne Marie Mowery, David S. Yoo, and David M. Brizel

INTRODUCTION

Chemical agents have been administered in conjunction with radiation therapy (RT) for both the enhancement of antitumor therapeutic efficacy and the amelioration of treatment-induced toxicity. Two concepts are fundamental to understanding the rationale for chemical modification of radiation response and to interpreting the studies that have addressed this issue. The first is the therapeutic ratio (TR), which is defined as the TCP/NTCP where TCP is the tumor control probability and NTCP is the normal tissue complication probability. Both of these parameters have sigmoid dose–response curves (Fig. 34.1). The horizontal separation between these two curves for any given treatment will often determine its overall utility. As the separation between these curves increases, the likelihood becomes greater that the treatment will be effective without causing an unacceptable level of morbidity. Conversely, when the two curves are closer together, the treatment may be less effective while causing an unacceptable level of morbidity.

The second concept is the efficacy/toxicity profile of the putative chemical modifier, which can directly affect the TR. A radiosensitizing agent that exacerbates toxicity to the same extent that it improves efficacy (shifting both NTCP and TCP curves to the left) may leave the TR unchanged or worsened and not be clinically practical. Conversely, a radioprotective agent that also reduces RT efficacy against the tumor (shifting both NTCP and TCP curves to the right) also may not affect or even reduce the TR. The intrinsic toxicity of a radioprotector must also be considered when reduction of NTCP is the primary goal of a given chemical modification strategy. A compound that causes significant side effects of its own may render it unsuitable even if it can reduce the treatment-induced toxicity in question. This chapter will explore chemical radiosensitization and radioprotective strategies. The primary focus will be on treatments that have been clinically tested in head and neck cancer in order to amplify these concepts.

CHEMICAL RADIOSENSITIZATION

The Oxygen Effect

Tumor cell killing is produced by direct ionizations within critical cellular targets as well as by the indirect effect of energy deposited in other cellular molecules including water. Ionizing radiation generates free radicals, which can lead to cellular death via the creation of single-strand and double-strand breaks in DNA. This damage can be fixed or repaired by the chemical processes of oxidation and reduction, respectively.[1] The addition of molecular oxygen to target free radicals produces altered chemical structures that are potentially lethal. Tumor hypoxia reduces radiosensitivity *in vitro* and *in vivo*.[2,3] Well-oxygenated cells (partial pressure of oxygen or $Po_2 > 10$ mm Hg) are approximately 2.5 times more sensitive to a given dose of ionizing radiation than their hypoxic counterparts.

Clinical data clearly demonstrate the existence of tumor hypoxia in head and neck cancer[4,5] and extremely strong correlations between hypoxia and both infield treatment failure and overall survival (Figs. 34.2 and 34.3).[6,7] This effect is independent of presenting stage of disease.[7] Tumor hypoxia has also been correlated with local and distant recurrence in carcinoma of the cervix treated with surgery[8,9] or RT[10] and with distant failure in soft tissue sarcomas treated with surgery and adjuvant RT.[11]

Augmentation of Tumor Oxygenation

Therapeutic attempts to overcome the deleterious effect of tumor hypoxia have followed three general lines of investigation: increased delivery of oxygen to tumor, preferential sensitization of hypoxic cells with oxygen-mimetic agents, or cytotoxic agents that selectively target hypoxic tumor cells. Hemoglobin concentration is the major determinant of the oxygen delivery capability of blood to tissue. Hemoglobin oxygen saturation exceeds 90% when the arterial Po_2 is >70 mm Hg. Still, oxygen is relatively insoluble in plasma under normobaric conditions. Under hyperbaric conditions, considerable quantities of oxygen can be dissolved into plasma and thus be potentially available for delivery to hypoxic tissues.

Clinical trials of hyperbaric oxygen (HBO) and RT were conducted from the 1950s to the 1970s. Trials conducted in patients with cancers of the central nervous system,[12] lung,[13] bladder,[14] and skin[15] showed no benefit from the addition of HBO. Randomized trials conducted in carcinoma of the cervix[16] and head and neck[17,18] did, however, show improvements in locoregional control and overall survival. The cumbersome logistics associated with HBO delivery in conjunction with RT necessitated the utilization of nonconventional hypofractionated treatment regimens. This reality has prevented HBO from being incorporated into routine clinical use.

Carbogen (95% oxygen [O_2]/5% carbon dioxide [CO_2]) breathing, with or without concurrent nicotinamide administration, has also been utilized in attempts to improve tumor oxygenation and enhance RT response. The rationale for CO_2 addition in the gas breathing mixture is the generation of a mild acidosis that shifts the oxyhemoglobin association curve to the right, facilitating more unloading of oxygen into the most hypoxic tissues. The rationale for adding nicotinamide, a vitamin B derivative, is based on preclinical studies showing enhancement of tumor blood flow.[19,20] Polarographic electrode assessments in cervix and head and neck cancer have demonstrated that carbogen breathing and nicotinamide administration improve tumor oxygenation in some patients.[21–23]

A randomized trial of hyperfractionated RT with or without carbogen was conducted at the University of Florida from 1996 to 2002.[24] The study included patients with T2 to T4 squamous cell carcinoma of the oropharynx, larynx, and hypopharynx and was designed to detect a 20% improvement in a 2-year local control in the carbogen arm relative to the RT alone arm, with a 15% improvement in a 4-year cause-specific survival. Virtually all enrolled patients in both arms completed their prescribed courses of treatment. The addition of carbogen to RT did not appear to improve any of the planned end points of this trial. Most important, however, was the fact that while this trial called for the enrollment of 675 patients, only 101 were entered over a 5-year period. The trial was therefore significantly underpowered in terms of its ability to detect the desired treatment effects. The inability to accrue patients also called into question the overall viability of strategies utilizing carbogen.

The use of accelerated RT with carbogen inhalation and nicotinamide (ARCON) was tested in a phase II trial of 215

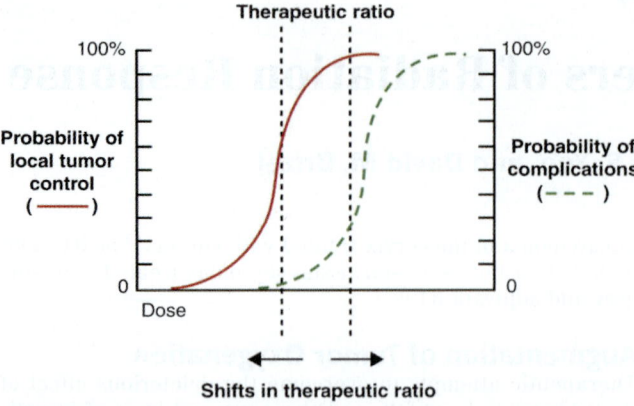

FIGURE 34.1. A graphic representation of the therapeutic index (TI). The tumor control probability (TCP) is to the left of the normal tissue complication probability (NTCP), and both are displayed as sigmoid dose–response curves. Larger separations are indicative of higher TIs. Ideally, normal tissue protection strategies would move the NTCP curve to the right without compromising TCP (moving the TCP curve to the right). Ideal therapeutic intensification strategies would move the TCP curve to the left without worsening NTCP (moving the NTCP curve to the left).

head and neck cancer patients.[25] Ninety-seven percent had stage III or IV disease, and the primary tumor site was laryngeal in 46%, hypopharyngeal in 23%, and oropharyngeal in 23%. Full compliance with carbogen breathing during RT was obtained in 88% of patients. Nicotinamide was administered 1 to 1.5 hours prior to RT at 60 to 80 mg/kg. Nicotinamide-induced nausea and vomiting necessitated discontinuation of the drug in 10% of patients receiving the lower dose and 31% of patients receiving the higher dose. Five-year locoregional control rates were 48% for hypopharynx primaries, 77% for larynx, and 72% for oropharynx primaries.[26] A subsequent phase III trial randomized 345 patients with cT2–T4 laryngeal squamous cell carcinoma to ARCON versus accelerated RT.[27] Local tumor control did not differ between treatment arms, but 5-year regional control was significantly higher with ARCON compared to accelerated RT alone (93% vs. 86%, respectively; $P = .04$). A subgroup analysis indicated that this beneficial effect of ARCON is limited to patients with tumors having a high hypoxic fraction.

FIGURE 34.2. The correlation between pretreatment head and neck tumor oxygenation and locoregional disease control after radiation therapy with or without concurrent chemotherapy. *Dashed line* represents tumor median partial pressure of oxygen (P_{O_2}) > 10 mm Hg. *Solid line* represents tumor median P_{O_2} < 10 mm Hg.

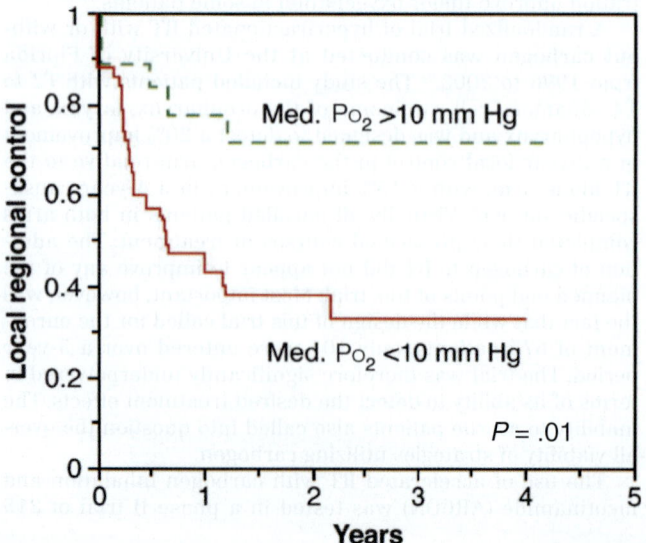

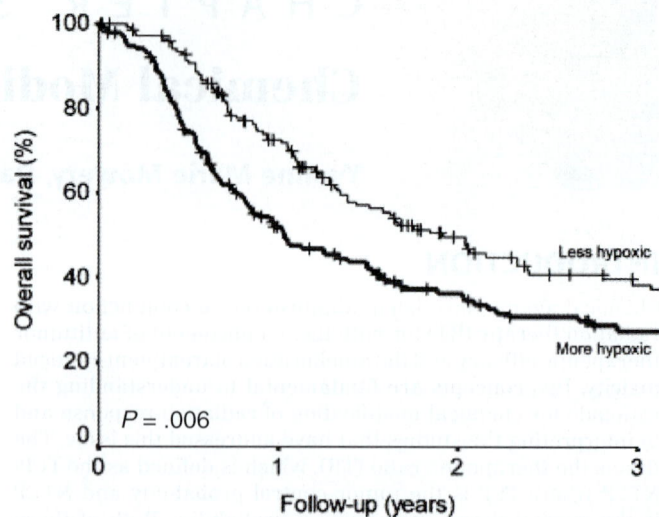

FIGURE 34.3. The correlation between actuarial overall survival for head and neck cancer patients with tumor hypoxia. Patients ($n = 397$) received definitive radiation therapy, with or without chemotherapy and/or surgical resection. *Thin line* represents patients with tumor fraction of P_{O_2} values ≤ 2.5 mm Hg ($HP_{2.5}$) below 20%. *Bold line* represents patients with $HP_{2.5}$ ≥ 20%.

Allosteric modifiers of hemoglobin structure have been identified that can shift the oxyhemoglobin dissociation curve to the right and increase O_2 delivery to hypoxic tissues.[28] One such compound, RSR13, (efaproxiral) has been tested in animal models and shown to improve tumor oxygenation[29] and enhance the effectiveness of RT.[30] A phase III open-label trial of whole-brain RT and oxygen breathing with or without daily infusion of efaproxiral was conducted in 538 patients with brain metastases.[31] Fifty-four percent of the patients had metastatic non–small cell lung cancer, and 20% had metastatic breast cancer. Overall, no improvement in survival was detected. A planned subset analysis suggested significant improvement in median survival time in breast cancer patients with sufficient levels of efaproxiral in their erythrocytes.[32] However, the phase III ENRICH trial, which examined efaproxiral and supplemental oxygen with whole-brain RT (30 Gy in 10 fractions) in 368 breast cancer patients with brain metastases, showed no significant difference in overall survival.[33]

Anemia is a very powerful adverse prognostic factor in various malignancies, including carcinomas of the lung,[34] cervix,[35] and head and neck.[36–38] Polarographic electrode oxygen measurements in head and neck cancer have demonstrated that anemic patients are significantly more likely to have poorly oxygenated tumors than nonanemic patients, but significant tumor hypoxia has also been detected in patients who are not anemic.[6,39] Whether correction or prevention of anemia with blood transfusions or erythropoiesis-stimulating agents can improve treatment outcomes has been investigated in multiple studies.

The use of blood transfusions in cervical cancer patients gained traction after an initial publication from Princess Margaret Hospital showing an improvement in pelvic control and cure rates associated with correction of anemia.[40] However, subsequent publications from the same group showed no survival benefit to transfusion when the data were critically reexamined and analyzed on an intent-to-treat basis.[41] In head and neck cancer patients, studies suggest that blood transfusions may have a negative effect on survival.[42,43]

Correction of anemia via erythropoietin (EPO) administration was evaluated in a double-blind, placebo-controlled randomized trial in 351 head and neck patients treated with RT.[44] The primary end point was locoregional progression-free survival. Eighty-two percent of patients ($n = 54$) who received

EPO maintained hemoglobin >14 g/dL (women) or 15 g/dL (men), whereas only 15% of the patients in the placebo arm attained this benchmark. The relative risk of locoregional progression, however, was 1.62 in the EPO arm compared to placebo (P = .0008), with a similar detriment seen for survival in those patients who received EPO (relative risk 1.39; P = .02). A systematic review pooling data from five randomized studies with a total of 1,397 patients showed significantly worse overall survival in head and neck cancer patients with the addition of EPO to RT (odds ratio 0.73; P = .005).[45] These poorer outcomes may have been the result of overcorrection of hemoglobin levels with increased thromboembolic events.[46] Tumor cells have also been found to express EPO receptors, with stimulation of downstream signaling pathways that may promote a more invasive phenotype.[47,48]

Sensitization of Hypoxic Cells

Electron-affinic compounds can oxidize radiation-induced free radical damage in the cell to produce increased kill.[49] The use of these agents would be particularly attractive in the hypoxic tumor microenvironment, where low oxygen concentrations impair the effectiveness of RT. The 2-nitroimidazoles are one such class of compounds that are metabolized into their active form under hypoxic conditions. Misonidazole, the prototype 2-nitroimidazole, was tested in two randomized trials. The Danish Head and Neck Cancer Study 2 (DAHANCA-2) performed a double-blind randomized trial evaluating the effect of misonidazole given in two drug schedules with split-course irradiation in the treatment of carcinoma of the larynx and pharynx.[50] Patients were stratified according to tumor site (larynx vs. pharynx), nodal status, and institution. The total misonidazole dose was 11 g/m². The study assessed 626 patients. Overall, the misonidazole group did not have significantly better local tumor control than the placebo group. Serious peripheral neuropathy, the dose-limiting toxicity of all nitroimidazole compounds, occurred in 26% of misonidazole-treated patients. The European Organisation for Research and Treatment of Cancer (EORTC) conducted a randomized study of conventional fractionation RT versus modified fractionation RT (three fractions per day) with or without misonidazole in 523 advanced head and neck cancer patients. No differences were seen in treatment outcome.[51]

Etanidazole (SR2508) is an analog of misonidazole with lower lipid solubility and less neurotoxicity in phase II studies in head and neck cancer.[52] A Radiation Therapy Oncology Group (RTOG) phase III study with etanidazole in head and neck tumors included 521 patients who received conventionally fractionated irradiation with or without etanidazole 2 mg/m² delivered three times per week.[53] Of those on the etanidazole arm, 77% received at least 14 doses of the drug. No grade 3 or 4 central nervous system or peripheral neuropathy was observed. The 2-year actuarial local tumor control was 40% in each arm, and the survival was 41% and 43%, respectively, in the irradiation alone and the irradiation plus etanidazole arms. A similar study of 374 patients performed in Europe did not show any overall benefit to treatment with etanidazole but did demonstrate increased neurotoxicity in the patients who received the drug.[54]

Nimorazole is a 5-nitroimidazole of the same structural class as metronidazole.[55] Its dose-limiting toxicity is nausea and vomiting; however, the drug can be administered with each radiation treatment. DAHANCA conducted a phase III trial of nimorazole (1.2 g/m² vs. placebo) for squamous cell cancer of the supraglottic larynx and pharynx.[56] There was a statistically significant improvement in locoregional tumor control (49% vs. 33% at 5 years; P = .002) but not for survival, which is consistent with the DAHANCA misonidazole trial. The use of nimorazole has become the standard of care (SOC) in Denmark but has not been adopted in other countries. An international multicenter phase II randomized trial

of nimorazole with accelerated radiation therapy for stage I to IV head and neck squamous cell carcinoma (excluding nasopharynx and stage I to II larynx) failed to meet accrual goals, enrolling only 104 of a planned 600 patients.[57] Although premature closure resulted in this trial being underpowered, there was a trend toward reduced 18-month locoregional failure with nimorazole (33% vs. 51% in control group, P = .1). The difference in overall death (19%; 95% CI, –3% to 42%; P = .1) also favored nimorazole but did not meet statistical significance. NIMRAD (NCT01950689) is an ongoing randomized, placebo-controlled phase III trial in the United Kingdom assessing nimorazole with a 6-week course of intensity-modulated radiation therapy for locally advanced head and neck cancer patients not suitable for concurrent cetuximab or chemotherapy.[58] Initial results are anticipated in June 2020.

Pharmacologic Targeting of Hypoxic Cells

Mitomycin C (MMC) is an alkylating agent metabolized in regions of low oxygen concentration and preferentially cytotoxic to hypoxic cells. MMC plays an integral role in conjunction with RT and 5-FU (fluorouracil) in the definitive nonsurgical management of squamous cell carcinomas of the anus.[59] Yale University investigators examined the concurrent use of MMC in 195 head and neck cancer patients treated on two randomized trials.[60] Their treatment program consisted of 68 Gy with or without MMC on days 1 and 43 of RT. Locoregional recurrence-free survival was improved with the addition of MMC from 54% to 76% (P = .003). Overall survival improved from 42% to 48%, but this was not statistically significant. The majority of patients in these trials received adjuvant postoperative or preoperative irradiation. Only 74 (38%) received definitive primary RT, and the benefit from the addition of MMC in this subset is unclear.

A three-armed randomized trial conducted by the University of Vienna compared conventionally fractionated (CF) RT (2 Gy daily to 70 Gy) against variation of continuous hyperfractionated accelerated RT with or without MMC (V-CHART + MMC and V-CHART, respectively).[61] RT was given as an initial 2.5-Gy fraction followed by 1.65 Gy twice a day to a total dose of 55.3 Gy in 17 days. MMC was given as a 20-mg/m² bolus on day 5 of RT. Of the 239 patients enrolled, 85% had T3 or T4 primaries and 79% had nodal involvement. Three-year actuarial locoregional control was 48% for V-CHART plus MMC versus 32% for V-CHART and 31% for CF (P = .05 and .03, respectively). Survival including death from all causes was also improved to 41% in the V-CHART plus MMC arm as compared with 31% for V-CHART and 24% for CF (P = .03). The incidence of confluent mucositis was 90% in both experimental arms as compared with 33% in the CF arm. The median time to complete resolution of mucositis was 6 to 7 weeks in all three arms. Grade 3 or 4 hematologic toxicity, primarily thrombocytopenia, developed in 18% of the V-CHART plus MMC patients.

Porfiromycin, a derivative of MMC, provides greater differential cytotoxicity between hypoxic and oxygenated cells *in vitro*.[62] The Yale investigators also conducted a phase III study that compared patients treated with conventionally fractionated radiation plus MMC versus radiation plus porfiromycin.[63] Hematologic and nonhematologic toxicities were equivalent in the two treatment arms. With a median follow-up >6 years, MMC was superior to porfiromycin with respect to 5-year local relapse-free survival (91.6% vs. 72.7%; P = .01), locoregional relapse-free survival (82% vs. 65.3%; P = .05), and disease-free survival (72.8% vs. 52.9%; P = .03). There were no significant differences between the two arms with respect to overall survival (49% vs. 54%) or distant metastasis-free rate (80% vs. 76%). Their data supported the continued use of MMC as an adjunct to radiation therapy in advanced head and neck cancer. However, this regimen is no longer used on a routine basis.

Tirapazamine (also known as SR-4233; WIN 59075; 3-amino-1,2,4-benzotriazine 1,4-dioxide) is a bioreductive agent preferentially cytotoxic to hypoxic cells *in vitro*. Twenty-five to 200 times more drug is required to produce the same level of cell killing in aerobic compared to anaerobic conditions.[64,65] Under hypoxic conditions, a free radical one-electron reduction product rapidly forms and is believed to be the toxic species, causing oxidative damage to pyrimidines and inducing DNA strand breaks.[66] Analysis of DNA and chromosomal breaks following hypoxic exposure to tirapazamine suggests that DNA double-strand breaks are the primary lesions involved in cell death.

This bioreductive agent differs from oxygen-mimetic sensitizers, such as the nitroimidazoles, in that it is itself cytotoxic to hypoxic tissues. Therefore, unlike the oxygen-mimetic sensitizers, tirapazamine-mediated therapeutic enhancement occurs whether the drug is given before or after irradiation.[67,68] In fractionated radiation therapy of murine tumors, tirapazamine is as effective as, if not superior to, etanidazole.[69] The efficacy of this radiation modifier depends on the number of "effective doses" that can be administered during a course of radiation therapy and the presence of hypoxic tumor cells.[70] Tirapazamine can also enhance the cytotoxicity of cisplatin.[71]

Rischin et al. investigated the use of concurrent tirapazamine, cisplatin, and RT in advanced head and neck cancer in a series of trials. A phase I trial established the dosing schedule for tirapazamine given with RT and cisplatin.[72] A randomized phase II study compared RT with cisplatin/tirapazamine versus RT with cisplatin/5-FU and suggested a benefit in the tirapazamine treatment arm (3-year locoregional failure-free survival 84% vs. 66%; $P = .07$).[73] Tumor hypoxia imaging was performed with 18-fluorodeoxyglucose-misonidazole positron emission tomography (PET) scanning in 45 of the patients on these studies.[74] Hypoxia was identified in primary or nodal sites in 71% of the patients. Eight of thirteen (62%) patients with hypoxic tumors who received cisplatin/5-FU experienced subsequent locoregional failure compared to only 1/19 (5%) patients with hypoxic tumors who received tirapazamine (hazard ratio [HR] = 15; $P = .001$). Only 1 of 10 patients with nonhypoxic tumors who received cisplatin/5-FU had a locoregional failure. These findings strongly suggested that the benefit of tirapazamine resulted from improved treatment efficacy against tumor hypoxia.

Two phase III trials were initiated to validate the use of tirapazamine in head and neck cancer. The HeadSTART study enrolled 861 patients and compared standard fractionation RT (70 Gy) with concurrent cisplatin/tirapazamine versus concurrent cisplatin alone.[75] The primary endpoint was overall survival, with 2-year rates of 65.7% in the cisplatin alone arm and 66.2% in the cisplatin/tirapazamine cohort. No differences were seen in failure-free survival, time to locoregional failure, or quality of life. Of note, the patients in this study were not selected based on the presence of tumor hypoxia. Moreover, 12% had major RT planning deficiencies, with those patients having significantly worse locoregional control and overall survival compared to those in protocol compliance.[76] A second trial with a planned enrollment of 550 patients was closed prior to completion of accrual because of an excess number of early deaths in the cisplatin/tirapazamine arm.[77]

Hyperthermia

Hyperthermia (HT) involves elevation of tissue temperature, typically to 40°C to 45°C, for a therapeutic effect.[78] Although HT monotherapy can result in some cells being killed, it has been more widely used for its radiosensitizing effect in tumors. Physiologic changes induced by HT include increased perfusion causing tissue reoxygenation and altered metabolism associated with reduced oxygen consumption. This improved oxygenation confers increased tumor radiation sensitivity and is correlated with pathologic complete response in

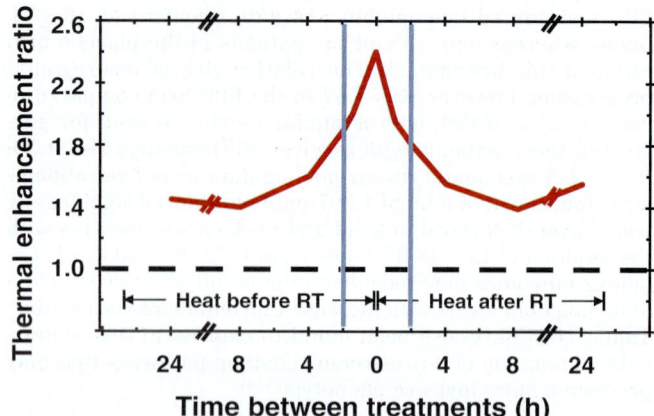

FIGURE 34.4. The effect of timing for combined hyperthermia and radiation therapy on the thermal enhancement ratio. The thermal enhancement ratio (ratio of radiation dose for radiation therapy alone and radiation therapy with hyperthermia to produce the same effect) was determined in several murine tumor models, and compiled results are shown. The greatest thermal enhancement ratio occurs when hyperthermia is performed within 2 hours before or after radiation therapy. (Adapted from Horsman MR, Overgaard J. Hyperthermia: a potent enhancer of radiotherapy. *Clin Oncol* 2007;19[6]:418–426, with permission.)

soft tissue sarcoma patients undergoing preoperative irradiation and HT.[79] In addition, cells are particularly sensitive to HT under conditions associated with radioresistance, including hypoxia, low pH, and presence in S phase of the cell cycle. Heat may also interfere with repair of radiation-induced DNA damage.[80,81] The thermal enhancement ratio (TER) quantifies the synergistic effect of HT and RT. TER is defined as the ratio of RT dose without HT to the isoeffective RT dose with HT: TER = RT dose without HT/RT dose for equivalent effect with HT. TER is >1 for most tumor types when HT is administered within 2 hours of RT (Fig. 34.4).[82]

Several randomized clinical trials have assessed RT with HT compared to RT alone. Results have been mixed, but a meta-analysis suggests overall improved tumor response with combined RT and HT for multiple tumor types (Table 34.1).[82,83] Combined RT and HT have been most widely studied for head and neck cancer and cervical cancer, largely because of the association between tumor hypoxia and poor clinical outcomes in these diseases as discussed above. The Dutch Deep Hyperthermia Group performed the largest randomized controlled trial comparing RT alone to RT with HT in patients with locally advanced bladder, cervical, or rectal cancer. HT was administered once weekly within 1 to 4 hours of RT for five total treatments. Complete response rates were significantly higher with RT and HT compared to RT alone (55% vs. 39%, respectively; $P < .001$), and local control duration was longer with combined therapy. On multivariate analysis adjusting for age, tumor site, and tumor size/stage, RT combined with HT was also associated with reduced death (relative HR, 0.74; 95% CI, 0.57 to 0.97; $P = .03$). Acute and late radiation toxicity did not differ by treatment group.[84] Although results with combined HT and RT have been promising, enthusiasm for HT has waned due in large part to technical challenges in uniformly heating tumors, particularly at deep-seated locations.[85]

Chemotherapy

Chemotherapeutic agents are often utilized in conjunction with radiation therapy for their radiosensitizing effect.[86,87] Concurrent chemoradiation with platinum agents, particularly cisplatin, improves survival in numerous malignancies including head and neck cancer,[88,89] cervical cancer,[90,91] and lung cancer.[92] Multiple potential mechanisms for platinum-induced radiosensitization have been proposed, including blocking DNA repair and inducing cell cycle arrest.[86,93] Several

TABLE 34.1 META-ANALYSIS OF RANDOMIZED CLINICAL TRIALS COMPARING RADIATION THERAPY ALONE WITH RADIATION THERAPY AND HYPERTHERMIA

Tumor Type	Number of Trials	Patient Number	LR Control, RT + HT	LR Control, RT Only	Odds Ratio (95% CI)
Advanced breast	2	143	68%	67%	1.06 (0.52–2.14)
Prostate	1	49	81%	79%	1.16 (0.28–4.77)
Mixed	3	442	39%	34%	1.24 (0.84–1.82)
Head and neck	5	274	51%	33%	2.08 (1.28–3.39)
Rectum	2	258	19%	9%	2.27 (1.08–4.76)
Chest wall	4	276	59%	38%	2.37 (1.46–3.86)
Bladder	1	101	73%	51%	2.61 (1.14–5.98)
Melanoma	1	128	56%	31%	2.81 (1.36–5.80)
Cervix	4	248	77%	52%	3.05 (1.77–5.27)
All	**23**	**1,919**	**52%**	**38%**	**1.80 (1.50–2.16)**

CI, confidence interval; HT, hyperthermia; LR, locoregional; RT, radiation therapy.
Adapted from Horsman MR, Overgaard J. Hyperthermia: a potent enhancer of radiotherapy. *Clin Oncol* 2007;19(6):418–426.

clinical trials are investigating the addition of new agents to cisplatin-based chemoradiation. For example, the ribonucleotide reductase inhibitor triapine showed promise in a phase II clinical trial for cervical cancer,[94] and a randomized phase II trial is ongoing (NCT02466971). Taxanes are also widely employed with radiation therapy for the treatment of head and neck cancer, lung cancer, and esophageal cancer. These drugs facilitate radiation-induced cell killing by synchronizing cell cycle and causing cell cycle arrest in the radiosensitive G2/M phase.[95–97] Fluoropyrimidines such as 5-fluorouracil are commonly administered concurrently with radiation therapy for gastrointestinal malignancies because of their radiosensitizing effect. Slowed repair of radiation-induced double-strand breaks and alteration of cell cycle progression by fluoropyrimidines likely result in radiosensitization.[98] Although mechanistic understanding of the interactions between radiation therapy and chemotherapy remains poorly understood, combined chemoradiation has dramatically improved outcomes for multiple malignancies.[87]

Biologic Modifiers of Radiation Response

Overexpression of the epidermal growth factor receptor 1 (EGFR-1) is associated with an adverse outcome in squamous head and neck cancer.[99] Cetuximab (C225) is a chimeric monoclonal antibody to EGFR. Preclinical studies have demonstrated that cetuximab sensitizes cells to the cytotoxic effects of ionizing irradiation.[100,101] Preliminary studies demonstrated that this drug could be safely administered in conjunction with a course of RT for head and neck cancer.[102] An open-label phase III trial tested the impact of weekly injections of cetuximab added to a course of RT alone.[103] Most patients received accelerated fractionation with concomitant boost, although hyperfractionation and standard fractionation schemes were also permitted. Oral cavity primary tumors were ineligible for enrollment. Two-year locoregional control increased from 48% with RT to 56% with RT and cetuximab (*P* = .02). The incidence of distant metastatic recurrence was the same in both treatment arms. The initial survival advantage seen with the addition of cetuximab to RT has persisted, with updated 5-year overall survival rates of 45.6% versus 36.4% (*P* = .018).[104]

This trial provided an important proof of principle that adding a biologically targeted agent to a physically targeted modality can improve therapeutic outcome, and enhanced locoregional control can lead to enhanced survival. One-third of the patients enrolled had stage III disease, however, and thus had less advanced disease with more favorable prognoses than a significant proportion of patients who typically undergo chemoradiotherapy (CRT). A more favorable prognosis and improved treatment response has also been seen in patients with oropharyngeal squamous cell cancers associated with the human papillomavirus (HPV).[105] Whether RT with cetuximab is as effective or less toxic than RT with cisplatin in this select population is being examined by the phase III RTOG 1016 study and De-ESCALaTE trial. RTOG 1016 (NCT01302834) has closed to accrual after enrollment of 987 patients, but survival results will not be available for several years. Similarly, De-ESCALaTE (NCT01874171) has enrolled 334 patients, but estimated final collection date is February 2019 for the primary outcome of acute and late toxicity. A phase II Italian trial comparing cetuximab to weekly cisplatin (40 mg/m^2) for stage III to IVB head and neck squamous cell carcinoma was closed early because of slow accrual (*n* = 70 of planned 130 patients). Serious adverse events were more common among patients receiving cetuximab compared to cisplatin (19% vs. 3%, *P* = .044). Two-year overall survival rates were similar in both arms (68% for cetuximab and 78% for cisplatin).[106]

A separate phase III study, RTOG 0522, randomized patients with locally advanced head and neck cancer to receive RT and concurrent cisplatin with or without cetuximab.[107] Treatment intensification with the addition of cetuximab to CRT did not improve 2-year progression-free or overall survival. Patients with p16-positive oropharyngeal cancer had better progression-free and overall survival than p16-negative oropharyngeal cancer patients. No significant interaction was present between p16 status and treatment, although there was a trend toward worse overall survival for p16-positive patients receiving cetuximab (HR 1.42, *P* = .13). Toxicity was more pronounced in patients who received cisplatin and cetuximab. Still, EGFR inhibition remains a very active area of investigation in head and neck cancer. Agents currently in clinical trial include fully humanized monoclonal antibodies and orally administered small molecule inhibitors of the tyrosine kinase domains of the EGFR family of receptors.

CHEMICAL RADIOPROTECTION

The protection of normal tissues from the deleterious effects of radiation is a critical component in the development of a comprehensive treatment plan. Strategies for the accomplishment of this aim include the physical manipulation of the beam, modification of the fractionation schedule, and pharmacologic manipulation of the radiation response. Physical radiation protection rests on the principle of exclusion of normal tissue from the high-dose region and may be accomplished by contouring the shape of the radiation beam, the use of multiple treatment fields, the use of different beam energies, and modulation of the dose delivery from each beam (intensity-modulated radiation therapy [IMRT]). Modified fractionation typically uses multiple fractions of treatment per day as opposed to the conventional once-daily paradigm in order to exploit the differing radiation repair capabilities of normal tissues as opposed to tumors. Physical modification of the treatment beam and altered fractionation are discussed elsewhere.

Protection

Pharmacologic radioprotection itself can be classified into three categories: protection, mitigation, and treatment. The direct cytotoxicity of ionizing irradiation results from the generation of free radicals that cause DNA strand breaks and lead to mitotic cell death. Amifostine (WR2721; Ethyol, Medimmune, Inc., Gaithersburg, MD) is the prototype pharmacologic radioprotector that functions via free radical scavenging. Amifostine is a thiol-containing prodrug that preferentially accumulates in the kidneys and salivary glands where it is metabolized to its active moiety, WR1065.[108]

An open-label phase III randomized trial was conducted from 1995 to 1997 to assess the ability of this drug to reduce the incidence of grade 2 or higher acute and late xerostomia and grade 3 or higher acute mucositis.[109] Patients enrolled in this trial received curative intent or adjuvant postoperative irradiation without concurrent chemotherapy. All treatment was delivered with conventional once-daily fractionation of 1.8 to 2.0 Gy. Curative intent delivery consisted of 66 to 70 Gy total dose, and postoperative irradiation was delivered at 50 to 60 Gy total dose depending on the patient's assessed risk for recurrence. IMRT was not utilized, and inclusion of >75% of both parotid glands was required for inclusion in the study. Those patients who were randomized to receive amifostine were given a daily dose of 200 mg/m^2 intravenously for 15 to 30 minutes every day prior to each fraction of RT.

Three hundred and three patients were enrolled in this trial, and minimum follow-up was 2 years. Amifostine did not reduce the incidence of grade 3 mucositis but did significantly reduce the incidence of acute and long-term grade >2 xerostomia. One-year post-RT, the incidence was 34% versus 56% for patients who had received amifostine versus those who had not (P = .002). Unstimulated saliva production >0.1 g was also more common in patients who had received amifostine (72% vs. 49%; P = .003). Two years post-RT, amifostine use was still associated with a significantly lower incidence of xerostomia, although the magnitude of benefit was lower (19% vs. 36%; P = .05). The lower incidences in both groups of patients also suggest some late recovery of salivary function. Reinforcing this idea of late recovery of salivary function is the fact that the percentage of patients who did not receive amifostine but who could exceed the >0.1 g of unstimulated saliva threshold had increased to 57%.[110]

Severe toxicity (CTCAE grade >3) attributable to amifostine occurred in <10% of patients in this trial and consisted of nausea and vomiting and transient hypotension. Nearly two-thirds of the patients had less severe grades of these side effects. Drug-related toxicity did cause approximately 20% of patients to discontinue amifostine prior to completing RT. Subcutaneous administration of the drug causes less nausea, vomiting, and hypotension than intravenous dosing but is associated with an increased risk of cutaneous toxicity, which again causes 15% to 20% of patients to be unable to complete a full course of amifostine in conjunction with their radiation.[111] The incidence of severe cutaneous toxicity, including erythema multiforme, Stevens-Johnson syndrome, and toxic epidermal necrolysis, is 6 to 9 in 100,000.[112]

A criticism of this trial is that it was underpowered to detect a very small compromise in survival caused by amifostine (tumor protection).[113] This argument is correct but overlooks the reality that absolute refutation of a small compromise of antitumor efficacy attributable to amifostine would have required an equivalence trial. Demonstration that amifostine reduced survival from a hypothetical 45% to 40% (P = .05; 80% power) would have necessitated >1,200 patients per study arm.[114] Such large studies have rarely been performed in head and neck cancer, because patient resources are too scarce. The largest randomized head and neck trial ever conducted, RTOG 9003, required 8 years to enroll 1,113

patients into four treatment arms.[115] A meta-analysis of amifostine that used individual patient data from 12 trials and 1,119 patients examined the impact of this drug on survival in patients treated with RT or CRT. The majority of patients (65%) had head and neck cancers, with 33% lung cancers and 2% pelvic carcinomas. The hazard ratio of death was 0.98 (95% confidence interval, 0.84 to 1.14; P = .78).[116]

The potential of amifostine as a protector against radiation-induced esophagitis during the treatment of non–small cell lung cancer was studied in a randomized trial conducted by the RTOG.[117,118] No reduction in the incidence of grade 3 esophagitis was observed, although less swallowing dysfunction occurred in the patients who received amifostine. Part of the explanation for this absence may be attributable to the study design, which utilized a hyperfractionated radiation schedule 5 days per week (69.6 Gy total dose) and concurrent carboplatin/paclitaxel. Amifostine 500 mg intravenous was delivered 4 days per week prior to the afternoon fraction only. Moreover, 28% of the patients did not complete the full course of the drug either because of toxicity or refusal. Consequently, approximately 50% of the RT was delivered in the absence of the radioprotective drug in those patients who were randomized to receive it. Preclinical study of amifostine delivered daily in conjunction with fractionated lung and esophageal irradiation has demonstrated morphologic and immunohistochemical evidence of radioprotection.[119-121]

Amifostine is approved by the U.S. Food and Drug Administration for xerostomia in the setting of RT alone. The majority of both curative intent and adjuvant postoperative RT for head and neck cancers, with large target volumes that put the parotid glands at risk, are now delivered in conjunction with concurrent chemotherapy. Small phase II and III trials suggest that amifostine has a cytoprotective benefit in the chemoradiation setting, but level 1 evidence is lacking.[122,123] Moreover, the widespread adoption of IMRT with its ability to spare one or both parotid glands and reduce the incidence of xerostomia compared to conventional, non-IMRT techniques has further reduced the role for this drug.[124] The utility of amifostine in conjunction with IMRT has been investigated in small settings with inconclusive results.[125]

Superoxide dismutase (SOD) mimetics represent a new class of radioprotectors that are currently under active investigation. These drugs convert the radiation-induced toxic reactive oxygen species superoxide anion (O_2^-) to hydrogen peroxide and molecular oxygen to mitigate radiation-induced toxicity. Similarly, these drugs interact with other potentially damaging reactive oxygen and reactive nitrogen species. A phase Ib/IIa clinical trial of the SOD mimetic GC4419 in patients with oral cavity or oropharyngeal cancer showed delayed development of oral mucositis, as well as reduced severity, incidence, and duration.[126] An ongoing randomized phase II clinical trial (NCT02508389) is assessing the effect of GC4419 administered prior to radiation therapy on oral mucositis during treatment of locally advanced head and neck cancer. Another SOD mimetic, Mn(III)meso-tetrakis (N-n-butoxyethylpyridinium-2-yl)porphyrin (MnBuOE), has been shown to mitigate oral mucositis, xerostomia, and salivary gland fibrosis in preclinical models.[127,128] Mice treated subcutaneously with MnBuOE twice daily or three times per week for 1 week prior to single-fraction radiation therapy to the oral cavity and ventral neck, followed by continued MnBuOE dosing after RT, exhibited significantly decreased incidence and severity of oral mucositis. This was demonstrated by fluorescence molecular tomography assessing cathepsin activity as a marker of mucositis (Fig. 34.5).[104] Stimulated saliva production was also significantly greater in mice treated with MnBuOE compared to saline control at 2 to 4 and 11 weeks post radiation therapy. At 6 and 12 weeks post radiation therapy, significantly decreased salivary gland fibrosis was

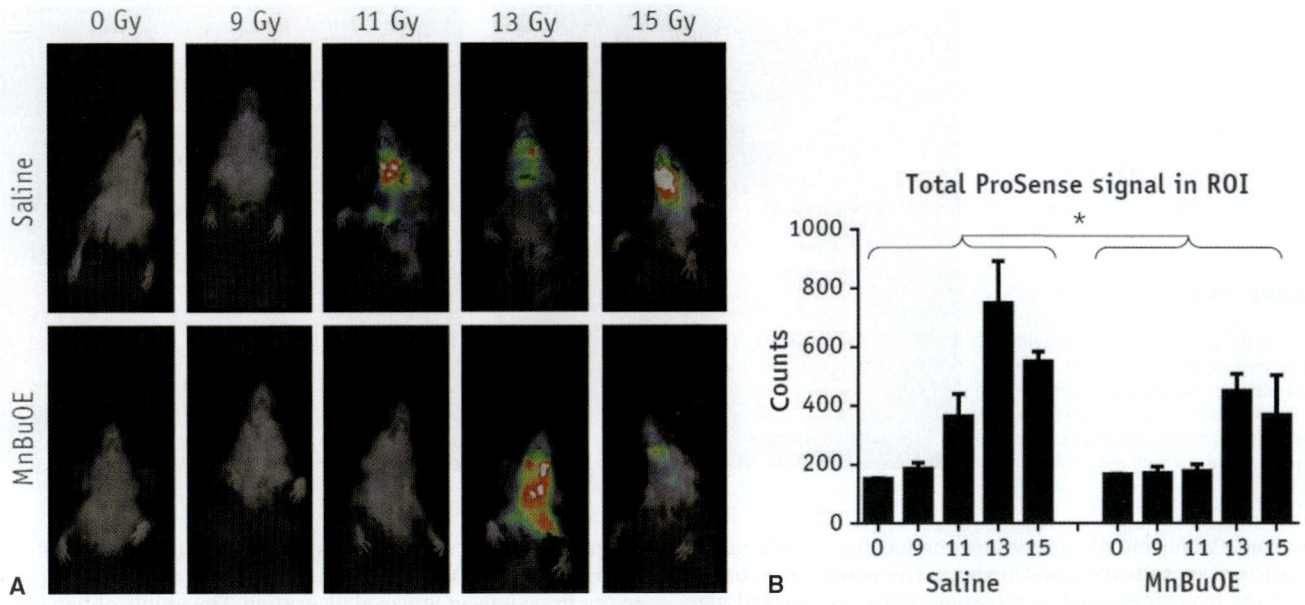

FIGURE 34.5. Reduced severity of mucositis for mice treated with MnBuOE compared to saline prior to and after single-fraction radiation therapy. **A:** Demonstrates fluorescence molecular tomography images using a probe that fluoresces after cleavage by cathepsins and plasmin as a marker for mucositis. **B:** Quantification of fluorescence in saline- and MnBuOE-treated mice. ROI, region of interest.

observed in MnBuOE-treated mice.[127,128] Importantly, MnBuOE does not appear to protect tumor cells from RT. In FaDu flank models of head and neck cancer, MnBuOE with RT resulted in further slowing of tumor growth[127] or no change in radiation-induced tumor growth delay.[128] Analogs of MnBuOE have also been shown to reduce radiation-induced erectile dysfunction[129] and pulmonary injury in mice.[130–132] A phase Ia-b clinical trial is ongoing to investigate the effect of MnBuOE (also known as BMX-001) on mucositis and xerostomia in patients with locally advanced head and neck cancer (NCT02990468). A phase I/II trial is also assessing MnBuOE in glioblastoma patients receiving concurrent RT and temozolomide to determine the maximum tolerated dose and assess median overall survival compared to historical controls (NCT02655601). Initial safety and efficacy results from the GC4419 and MnBuOE clinical trials are anticipated in early 2019.

Mitigation

Administration of compounds that mitigate damage caused by previous radiation exposure constitutes a different approach to the management of radiation-induced toxicity. This strategy contrasts to the classical free radical scavenging radioprotective mechanism of drugs such as amifostine. The leading drug under development in this category is palifermin. Palifermin is a recombinant human keratinocyte growth factor that belongs to the fibroblast growth factor (FGF-7) family of cytokines. It stimulates cellular proliferation and differentiation in a variety of epithelial tissues including mucosa throughout the alimentary tract, salivary glands, and type II pneumocytes. Palifermin also regulates intrinsic glutathione-mediated cytoprotective mechanisms. Administration of palifermin in preclinical rodent models leads to a significant thickening of oral tongue mucosa.[133] Preclinical studies of fractionated RT have revealed that the administration of palifermin leads to increases in the dose of RT necessary to induce ulcerative mucositis and to reductions in the duration of this ulceration when it does occur.[134,135] Parotid gland production of saliva is also preserved when palifermin is administered in the setting of RT in preclinical systems. Preclinical evaluation of palifermin in a rodent model has also demonstrated that

administration of a single dose of this drug after completion of a course of fractionated thoracic irradiation significantly reduces the severity and duration of pneumonitis and the severity of pulmonary fibrosis.[136]

The ability of palifermin to reduce mucositis in a clinical setting has been tested in a pivotal phase III double-blind placebo-controlled trial of patients with non-Hodgkin lymphoma undergoing bone marrow transplantation.[137] The bone marrow ablative regimen consisted of 12 Gy of total body irradiation (TBI) given at 1.5 Gy twice a day. Thereafter, etoposide (VP-16) and cyclophosphamide were administered. Palifermin was delivered prior to the initiation of TBI and again after the completion of chemotherapy, which also corresponded to 5 days after the completion of TBI. The dose schedule of palifermin was 60 mcg/kg/d three times for both administrations. This trial enrolled 212 patients who were equally divided between the placebo and palifermin arms. The World Health Organization (WHO) scoring system was used. The incidence of grade 3 or 4 mucositis approached 90% in the placebo arm as opposed to approximately 60% in the palifermin arm. For those patients who developed this level of toxicity, the duration was significantly reduced from 10.4 days in the placebo arm to 3.7 days in the palifermin arm ($P < .001$). Grade 3 mucositis developed in 62% of the placebo arm patients and only 20% of the palifermin arm patients ($P < .001$). Mean duration of grade 4 mucositis was reduced from 6.2 to 3.3 days with the use of this drug ($P < .001$).

A phase II study examined the safety and efficacy of palifermin in locally advanced head and neck cancer patients.[138] Patients were randomized 2 to 1 between palifermin and placebo. Palifermin was delivered at a dose of 60 mcg/kg. Institutions had the discretion to deliver RT via conventional once-daily 2-Gy fractions or with an accelerated hyperfractionated regimen of 1.25 Gy twice daily. One hundred patients were enrolled, of whom 34 received accelerated hyperfractionation and the remainder received standard fractionation. The first dose was delivered prior to the initiation of CRT and then every Friday afternoon after the last fraction of radiation. Two additional doses of palifermin were given 1 and 2 weeks after the completion of RT for a total of 10 doses of

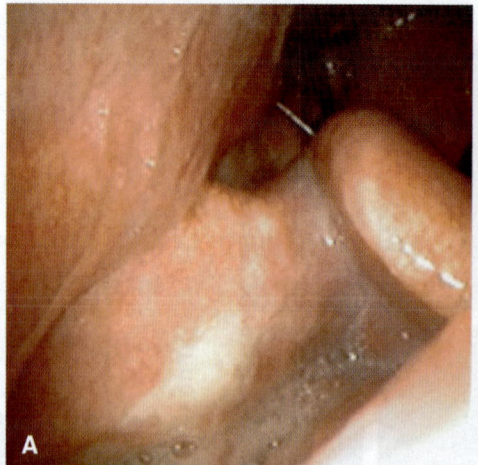
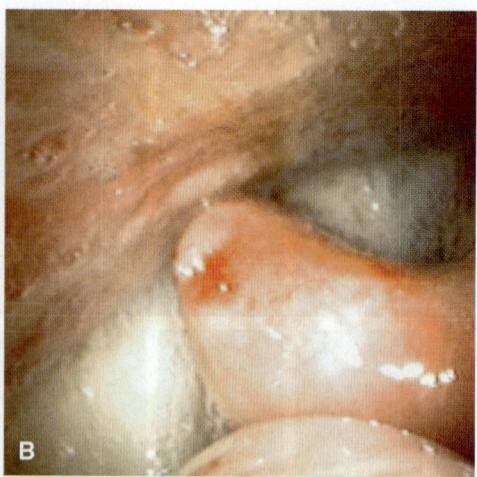

FIGURE 34.6. Confluent mucositis induced by concurrent chemoradiation in the base of tongue and supraglottic larynx regions. **A:** Demonstrates normal mucosa prior to the initiation of treatment. **B:** Demonstrates the pseudomembranous exudate, hemorrhage, and edema that are characteristic of this confluent mucositis.

the drug. Palifermin did not reduce the incidence or duration of mucosal or salivary gland toxicity. The subset of patients receiving hyperfractionated radiation, however, showed significant improvements in the duration and severity of mucositis (Fig. 34.6). They also had improved swallowing function and less salivary gland toxicity relative to patients who received placebo.

A subsequent randomized phase III study examined a higher dose of palifermin at 180 mcg/kg to reduce oral mucositis in 188 patients with locally advanced head and neck cancer treated with CRT.[139] Palifermin was administered prior to starting CRT and once weekly for 7 weeks. The incidence of severe oral mucositis, the primary endpoint, was significantly lower in the palifermin arm compared to placebo (54% vs. 69%; $P = .041$). Both overall survival and progression-free survival were similar as well. However, no statistically significant differences emerged in secondary efficacy end points such as narcotic doses and duration of treatment breaks. A similar randomized phase III study examined palifermin at 120 mcg/kg in 186 head and neck cancer patients treated with postoperative CRT.[140] Palifermin again reduced the time to development and duration of WHO grade 3 or 4 oral mucositis without differences in patient-reported pain scores, treatment breaks, or efficacy. The precise role for palifermin in the management of head and neck cancer remains to be established.

Treatment

Radioprotectors and radiation mitigators are both designed to minimize the risk of clonogenic death of normal cells and subsequent disruption of the protective mucosal barrier. Head and neck RT also initiates a local cytokine cascade, which includes interleukin-1 and interleukin-6 and tumor necrosis factor-α (TNF-α). An inflammatory response results, which contributes to the ultimate anatomic disruption of the mucosa. Secondary bacterial and fungal overgrowths are thought to exacerbate the local pathophysiology.

Sucralfate, a basic aluminum salt of sucrose, is used in the treatment of peptic ulcer disease. It provides a protective coating to ulcerated tissue by means of binding to exposed proteins in damaged cells.[141] It also stimulates mucus production, mitosis, and surface migration of cells. Sucralfate has been tested in several double-blind placebo-controlled randomized trials. Despite the attractive conceptual nature of using it to ameliorate mucositis, the clinical data do not show any benefit from sucralfate.[142–144]

Benzydamine hydrochloride is a nonsteroidal anti-inflammatory drug that also possesses antimicrobial activity.[145] It is a potent inhibitor of TNF-α.[146] Expression of this proinflammatory cytokine is upregulated in mucosal tissue

of the head and neck regions, with peak levels typically at approximately 20 Gy (conventionally fractionated) just prior to the first signs of mucosal ulceration. The ability of benzydamine to reduce mucositis during head and neck RT was tested in a randomized double-blind placebo-controlled trial.[147] The primary endpoint of this trial was the area under the curve for the mean mucositis score over a cumulative RT dose up to a total dose of 50 Gy. Secondary end points included use of concomitant pain medication, oral pain at rest and with eating, body weight, and the use of enteral nutritional support.

Benzydamine therapy resulted in a 30% reduction in mucosal erythema and ulceration. Most of this benefit was observed once doses >25 Gy had been delivered. One-third of the benzydamine patients did not develop any mucosal ulceration, compared with only 18% of the placebo-treated patients ($P = .04$). There was a nonsignificant trend toward reduction in mouth pain at rest for the patients who received benzydamine. Importantly, benzydamine was no more effective than placebo with respect to the reduction of pain during meals. Cumulative weight loss during RT was equivalent in the two treatment groups. There was no difference in the proportion of patients who required enteral nutritional support between the two treatment arms.

The data from the benzydamine trials suggest that this agent is active against mucositis but are inconclusive regarding whether it has any clinical role in treating this condition. There was no significant benefit regarding the functional sequelae of mucositis. Mucosal assessment was not performed beyond 50 Gy, and most patients received RT doses of 64 to 74 Gy. The study design may thus explain the discordance between the improvement in the anatomic assessment of mucosal integrity associated with benzydamine and the lack of any functional benefit, as the latter parameters were assessed throughout a patient's entire course of RT. The most severe mucositis during a course of head and neck RT occurs beyond the 50 Gy level. Fewer than 10% of the patients enrolled in this trial received concurrent chemotherapy, even though most of them had stage III or IV disease. Concurrent CRT has become the SOC for most patients with this extent of disease. Consequently, the clinical value of benzydamine has not been proven for patients receiving high-dose RT with or without concurrent chemotherapy.

Endogenous oral flora may exacerbate the mucosal inflammatory process once the mucosal integrity is disrupted. Secondary infections may prolong the course of mucositis and compromise overall patient well-being. Protegrins are naturally occurring peptides that have broad-spectrum antimicrobial activity.[148] Iseganan is a synthetic analog of this class of compounds. A placebo-controlled trial in patients receiving chemotherapy suggested that iseganan reduced the incidence of ulcerative stomatitis and decreased both mouth pain and swallowing difficulty.[149]

A phase III double-blind, placebo-controlled trial was subsequently conducted to test this concept in patients receiving head and neck RT.[150] This trial mandated that a minimum dose of 60 Gy be delivered but allowed different fractionation schemes. Forty percent of the patients enrolled received concurrent chemotherapy. The study contained three treatment arms: SOC oral hygiene only, placebo plus SOC, and iseganan plus SOC. Iseganan and placebo were equivalent to one another with respect to all end points in the trial. Interestingly, both iseganan and placebo arms were superior to SOC oral hygiene alone. Two-thirds of the patients in both arms had confluent mucositis compared with 79% in the SOC alone arm ($P = .02$). Only 2% of the SOC patients had no mucosal ulceration versus 9% in both the iseganan and placebo arms ($P = .04$). Peak mouth pain and difficulty swallowing were also significantly worse for the patients assigned to SOC alone. RT dose reductions were also significantly more common in the SOC patients.

The iseganan trial showed no benefit from the administration of the study drug. It did, however, reveal the importance of adherence to a strict regimen of oral hygiene during head and neck RT. Patients on both the drug and placebo arms were instructed to swish and gargle prior to each administration of study drug. They also maintained study diaries to help ensure adequate compliance with administration of the study drug. These interventions were not performed in the patients assigned to SOC alone. This trial provides an important foundation in the evaluation of new therapies for mucositis through its demonstration of the value of organized and systematic attention to the maintenance of good oral hygiene throughout a course of head and neck RT.

SUMMARY

The chemical modification of radiation response both for enhancing treatment efficacy and reducing therapy-induced toxicity remains an area of active investigation. Promising candidates identified in preclinical and early-phase trials have been less successful in randomized phase III settings. Attempts to improve treatment efficacy by augmenting tumor oxygen delivery have a mixed record of success. The use of drugs that are preferentially cytotoxic to hypoxic cells holds promise, although improved tools to identify those patients most likely to benefit from targeted therapy are needed. Proof of principle for chemical radioprotection has been established in salivary glands but not elsewhere and is associated with significant toxicity in its own right. Growth factor utilization appears to protect against treatment-induced mucositis but not to an extent to change clinical practice. As RT regimens evolve and new technologic advances continue to improve treatment delivery, investigators will continue to seek agents that optimize the TR.

REFERENCES

1. Chapman JD, Reuvers AP, Borsa J, et al. Chemical radioprotection and radiosensitization of mammalian cells growing in vitro. *Radiat Res* 1973;56(2):291–306.
2. Gray LH, Conger AD, Ebert M, et al. The concentration of oxygen dissolved in tissues at the time of irradiation as a factor in radiotherapy. *Br J Radiol* 1953;26(312):638–648.
3. Thomlinson RH, Gray LH. The histological structure of some human lung cancers and the possible implications for radiotherapy. *Br J Cancer* 1955;9(4):539–549.
4. Becker A, Hansgen G, Bloching M, et al. Oxygenation of squamous cell carcinoma of the head and neck: comparison of primary tumors, neck node metastases, and normal tissue. *Int J Radiat Oncol Biol Phys* 1998;42(1):35–41.
5. Brizel DM, Sibley GS, Prosnitz LR, et al. Tumor hypoxia adversely affects the prognosis of carcinoma of the head and neck. *Int J Radiat Oncol Biol Phys* 1997;38(2):285–289.
6. Brizel DM, Dodge RK, Clough RW, et al. Oxygenation of head and neck cancer: changes during radiotherapy and impact on treatment outcome. *Radiother Oncol* 1999;53(2):113–117.
7. Nordsmark M, Bentzen SM, Rudat V, et al. Prognostic value of tumor oxygenation in 397 head and neck tumors after primary radiation therapy. An international multi-center study. *Radiother Oncol* 2005;77(1):18–24.
8. Hockel M, Knoop C, Schlenger K, et al. Intratumoral pO$_2$ predicts survival in advanced cancer of the uterine cervix. *Radiother Oncol* 1993;26(1):45–50.
9. Hockel M, Schlenger K, Aral B, et al. Association between tumor hypoxia and malignant progression in advanced cancer of the uterine cervix. *Cancer Res* 1996;56(19):4509–4515.
10. Fyles AW, Milosevic M, Wong R, et al. Oxygenation predicts radiation response and survival in patients with cervix cancer. *Radiother Oncol* 1998;48(2):149–156.
11. Brizel DM, Scully SP, Harrelson JM, et al. Tumor oxygenation predicts for the likelihood of distant metastases in human soft tissue sarcoma. *Cancer Res* 1996;56(5):941–943.
12. Chang CH. Hyperbaric oxygen and radiation therapy in the management of glioblastoma. *Natl Cancer Inst Monogr* 1977;46:163–169.
13. Cade IS, McEwen JB. Clinical trials of radiotherapy in hyperbaric oxygen at Portsmouth, 1964–1976. *Clin Radiol* 1978;29(3):333–338.
14. Cade IS, McEwen JB, Dische S, et al. Hyperbaric oxygen and radiotherapy: a Medical Research Council trial in carcinoma of the bladder. *Br J Radiol* 1978;51(611):876–878.
15. Sealy A, Hockly J, Shepstone B. The treatment of malignant melanoma with cobalt and hyperbaric oxygen. *Clin Radiol* 1974;25(2):211–215.
16. Watson ER, Halnan KE, Dische S, et al. Hyperbaric oxygen and radiotherapy: a Medical Research Council trial in carcinoma of the cervix. *Br J Radiol* 1978;51(611):879–887.
17. Henk JM. Late results of a trial of hyperbaric oxygen and radiotherapy in head and neck cancer: a rationale for hypoxic cell sensitizers? *Int J Radiat Oncol Biol Phys* 1986;12(8):1339–1341.
18. Henk JM, Kunkler PB, Smith CW. Radiotherapy and hyperbaric oxygen in head and neck cancer. Final report of first controlled clinical trial. *Lancet* 1977;2(8029):101–103.
19. Horsman MR, Brown JM, Hirst VK, et al. Mechanism of action of the selective tumor radiosensitizer nicotinamide. *Int J Radiat Oncol Biol Phys* 1988;15(3):685–690.
20. Horsman MR, Overgaard J, Christensen KL, et al. Mechanism for the reduction of tumour hypoxia by nicotinamide and the clinical relevance for radiotherapy. *Biomed Biochim Acta* 1989;48(2–3):S251–S254.
21. Aquino-Parsons C, Lim P, Green A, et al. Carbogen inhalation in cervical cancer: assessment of oxygenation change. *Gynecol Oncol* 1999;74(2):259–264.
22. Falk SJ, Ward R, Bleehen NM. The influence of carbogen breathing on tumour tissue oxygenation in man evaluated by computerised pO$_2$ histography. *Br J Cancer* 1992;66(5):919–924.
23. Laurence VM, Ward R, Dennis IF, et al. Carbogen breathing with nicotinamide improves the oxygen status of tumours in patients. *Br J Cancer* 1995;72(1):198–205.
24. Mendenhall WM, Morris CG, Amdur RJ, et al. Radiotherapy alone or combined with carbogen breathing for squamous cell carcinoma of the head and neck: a prospective, randomized trial. *Cancer* 2005;104(2):332–337.
25. Kaanders JH, Pop LA, Marres HA, et al. ARCON: experience in 215 patients with advanced head-and-neck cancer. *Int J Radiat Oncol Biol Phys* 2002;52(3):769–778.
26. Hoogsteen IJ, Pop LA, Marres HA, et al. Oxygen-modifying treatment with ARCON reduces the prognostic significance of hemoglobin in squamous cell carcinoma of the head and neck. *Int J Radiat Oncol Biol Phys* 2006;64(1):83–89.
27. Janssens GO, Rademakers SE, Terhaard CH, et al. Accelerated radiotherapy with carbogen and nicotinamide for laryngeal cancer: results of a phase III randomized trial. *J Clin Oncol* 2012;30(15):1777–1783.
28. Teicher BA, Wong JS, Takeuchi H, et al. Allosteric effectors of hemoglobin as modulators of chemotherapy and radiation therapy in vitro and in vivo. *Cancer Chemother Pharmacol* 1998;42(1):24–30.
29. Hou H, Khan N, O'Hara JA, et al. Effect of RSR13, an allosteric hemoglobin modifier, on oxygenation in murine tumors: an in vivo electron paramagnetic resonance oximetry and bold MRI study. *Int J Radiat Oncol Biol Phys* 2004;59(3):834–843.
30. Khandelwal SR, Kavanagh BD, Lin PS, et al. RSR13, an allosteric effector of haemoglobin, and carbogen radiosensitize FSAII and SCCVII tumours in C3H mice. *Br J Cancer* 1999;79(5–6):814–820.
31. Suh JH, Stea B, Nabid A, et al. Phase III study of efaproxiral as an adjunct to whole-brain radiation therapy for brain metastases. *J Clin Oncol* 2006;24(1):106–114.
32. Stea B, Shaw E, Pinter T, et al. Efaproxiral red blood cell concentration predicts efficacy in patients with brain metastases. *Br J Cancer* 2006;94(12):1777–1784.
33. Suh JH, Stea B, Tankel K, et al. Results of the phase III ENRICH (RT-016) study of efaproxiral administered concurrent with whole brain radiation therapy (WBRT) in women with brain metastases from breast cancer. *Int J Radiat Oncol Biol Phys* 2008;72(1):S50–S51.
34. Robnett TJ, Machtay M, Hahn SM, et al. Pathological response to preoperative chemoradiation worsens with anemia in non-small cell lung cancer patients. *Cancer J* 2002;8(3):263–267.
35. Dunst J, Kuhnt T, Strauss HG, et al. Anemia in cervical cancers: impact on survival, patterns of relapse, and association with hypoxia and angiogenesis. *Int J Radiat Oncol Biol Phys* 2003;56(3):778–787.
36. Frommhold H, Guttenberger R, Henke M. The impact of blood hemoglobin content on the outcome of radiotherapy. The Freiburg experience. *Strahlenther Onkol* 1998;174(Suppl 4):31–34.

37. Lee WR, Berkey B, Marcial V, et al. Anemia is associated with decreased survival and increased locoregional failure in patients with locally advanced head and neck carcinoma: a secondary analysis of RTOG 85-27. *Int J Radiat Oncol Biol Phys* 1998;42(5):1069–1075.

38. Prosnitz RG, Yao B, Farrell CL, et al. Pretreatment anemia is correlated with the reduced effectiveness of radiation and concurrent chemotherapy in advanced head and neck cancer. *Int J Radiat Oncol Biol Phys* 2005;61(4):1087–1095.

39. Becker A, Stadler P, Lavey RS, et al. Severe anemia is associated with poor tumor oxygenation in head and neck squamous cell carcinomas. *Int J Radiat Oncol Biol Phys* 2000;46(2):459–466.

40. Bush RS, Jenkin RD, Allt WE, et al. Definitive evidence for hypoxic cells influencing cure in cancer therapy. *Br J Cancer Suppl* 1978;3:302–306.

41. Fyles AW, Milosevic M, Pintilie M, et al. Anemia, hypoxia and transfusion in patients with cervix cancer: a review. *Radiother Oncol* 2000;57(1):13–19.

42. Bhide SA, Ahmed M, Rengarajan V, et al. Anemia during sequential induction chemotherapy and chemoradiation for head and neck cancer: the impact of blood transfusion on treatment outcome. *Int J Radiat Oncol Biol Phys* 2009;73(2):391–398.

43. Hoff CM, Lassen P, Eriksen JG, et al. Does transfusion improve the outcome for HNSCC patients treated with radiotherapy? Results from the randomized DAHANCA 5 and 7 trials. *Acta Oncol* 2011;50(7):1006–1014.

44. Henke M, Laszig R, Rube C, et al. Erythropoietin to treat head and neck cancer patients with anaemia undergoing radiotherapy: randomised, double-blind, placebo-controlled trial. *Lancet* 2003;362(9392):1255–1260.

45. Lambin P, Ramaekers BL, van Mastrigt GA, et al. Erythropoietin as an adjuvant treatment with (chemo) radiation therapy for head and neck cancer. *Cochrane Database Syst Rev* 2009;(3):CD006158.

46. Bennett CL, Silver SM, Djulbegovic B, et al. Venous thromboembolism and mortality associated with recombinant erythropoietin and darbepoetin administration for the treatment of cancer-associated anemia. *JAMA* 2008;299(8):914–924.

47. Arcasoy MO, Amin K, Chou SC, et al. Erythropoietin and erythropoietin receptor expression in head and neck cancer: relationship to tumor hypoxia. *Clin Cancer Res* 2005;11(1):20–27.

48. Mohyeldin A, Lu H, Dalgard C, et al. Erythropoietin signaling promotes invasiveness of human head and neck squamous cell carcinoma. *Neoplasia* 2005;7(5):537–543.

49. Adams GE. Hypoxia-mediated drugs for radiation and chemotherapy. *Cancer* 1981;48(3):696–707.

50. Overgaard J, Hansen HS, Andersen AP, et al. Misonidazole combined with split-course radiotherapy in the treatment of invasive carcinoma of larynx and pharynx: report from the DAHANCA 2 study. *Int J Radiat Oncol Biol Phys* 1989;16(4):1065–1068.

51. Van den Bogaert W, van der Schueren E, Horiot JC, et al. The EORTC randomized trial on three fractions per day and misonidazole (trial no. 22811) in advanced head and neck cancer: long-term results and side effects. *Radiother Oncol* 1995;35(2):91–99.

52. Wasserman TH, Lee DJ, Cosmatos D, et al. Clinical trials with etanidazole (SR-2508) by the Radiation Therapy Oncology Group (RTOG). *Radiother Oncol* 1991;20(Suppl 1):129–135.

53. Lee DJ, Cosmatos D, Marcial VA, et al. Results of an RTOG phase III trial (RTOG 85-27) comparing radiotherapy plus etanidazole with radiotherapy alone for locally advanced head and neck carcinomas. *Int J Radiat Oncol Biol Phys* 1995;32(3):567–576.

54. Eschwege F, Sancho-Garnier H, Chassagne D, et al. Results of a European randomized trial of Etanidazole combined with radiotherapy in head and neck carcinomas. *Int J Radiat Oncol Biol Phys* 1997;39(2):275–281.

55. Overgaard J, Overgaard M, Nielsen OS, et al. A comparative investigation of nimorazole and misonidazole as hypoxic radiosensitizers in a C3H mammary carcinoma in vivo. *Br J Cancer* 1982;46(6):904–911.

56. Overgaard J, Hansen HS, Overgaard M, et al. A randomized double-blind phase III study of nimorazole as a hypoxic radiosensitizer of primary radiotherapy in supraglottic larynx and pharynx carcinoma. Results of the Danish Head and Neck Cancer Study (DAHANCA) Protocol 5-85. *Radiother Oncol* 1998;46(2):135–146.

57. Hassan Metwally MA, Ali R, Kuddu M, et al. IAEA-HypoX. A randomized multicenter study of the hypoxic radiosensitizer nimorazole concomitant with accelerated radiotherapy in head and neck squamous cell carcinoma. *Radiother Oncol* 2015;116(1):15–20.

58. Thomson D, Yang H, Baines H, et al. NIMRAD—a phase III trial to investigate the use of nimorazole hypoxia modification with intensity-modulated radiotherapy in head and neck cancer. *Clin Oncol* 2014;26(6):344–347.

59. Flam M, John M, Pajak TF, et al. Role of mitomycin in combination with fluorouracil and radiotherapy, and of salvage chemoradiation in the definitive nonsurgical treatment of epidermoid carcinoma of the anal canal: results of a phase III randomized intergroup study. *J Clin Oncol* 1996;14(9):2527–2539.

60. Haffty BG, Son YH, Papac R, et al. Chemotherapy as an adjunct to radiation in the treatment of squamous cell carcinoma of the head and neck: results of the Yale Mitomycin Randomized Trials. *J Clin Oncol* 1997;15(1):268–276.

61. Dobrowsky W, Naude J. Continuous hyperfractionated accelerated radiotherapy with/without mitomycin C in head and neck cancers. *Radiother Oncol* 2000;57(2):119–124.

62. Rockwell S, Hughes CS. Effects of mitomycin C and porfiromycin on exponentially growing and plateau phase cultures. *Cell Prolif* 1994;27(3):153–163.

63. Haffty BG, Wilson LD, Son YH, et al. Concurrent chemo-radiotherapy with mitomycin C compared with porfiromycin in squamous cell cancer of the head and neck: final results of a randomized clinical trial. *Int J Radiat Oncol Biol Phys* 2005;61(1):119–128.

64. Zeman EM, Brown JM, Lemmon MJ, et al. SR-4233: a new bioreductive agent with high selective toxicity for hypoxic mammalian cells. *Int J Radiat Oncol Biol Phys* 1986;12(7):1239–1242.

65. Zeman EM, Hirst VK, Lemmon MJ, et al. Enhancement of radiation-induced tumor cell killing by the hypoxic cell toxin SR 4233. *Radiother Oncol* 1988;12(3):209–218.

66. Zeman EM, Brown JM. Pre- and post-irradiation radiosensitization by SR 4233. *Int J Radiat Oncol Biol Phys* 1989;16(4):967–971.

67. Brown JM, Lemmon MJ. Potentiation by the hypoxic cytotoxin SR 4233 of cell killing produced by fractionated irradiation of mouse tumors. *Cancer Res* 1990;50(24):7745–7749.

68. Brown JM, Lemmon MJ. SR 4233: a tumor specific radiosensitizer active in fractionated radiation regimes. *Radiother Oncol* 1991;20(Suppl 1):151–156.

69. Brown JM, Lemmon MJ. Tumor hypoxia can be exploited to preferentially sensitize tumors to fractionated irradiation. *Int J Radiat Oncol Biol Phys* 1991;20(3):457–461.

70. Brown JM. Therapeutic targets in radiotherapy. *Int J Radiat Oncol Biol Phys* 2001;49(2):319–326.

71. Goldberg Z, Evans J, Birrell G, et al. An investigation of the molecular basis for the synergistic interaction of tirapazamine and cisplatin. *Int J Radiat Oncol Biol Phys* 2001;49(1):175–182.

72. Rischin D, Peters L, Hicks R, et al. Phase I trial of concurrent tirapazamine, cisplatin, and radiotherapy in patients with advanced head and neck cancer. *J Clin Oncol* 2001;19(2):535–542.

73. Rischin D, Peters L, Fisher R, et al. Tirapazamine, cisplatin, and radiation versus fluorouracil, cisplatin, and radiation in patients with locally advanced head and neck cancer: a randomized phase II trial of the Trans-Tasman Radiation Oncology Group (TROG 98.02). *J Clin Oncol* 2005;23(1):79–87.

74. Rischin D, Hicks RJ, Fisher R, et al. Prognostic significance of [18F]-misonidazole positron emission tomography-detected tumor hypoxia in patients with advanced head and neck cancer randomly assigned to chemoradiation with or without tirapazamine: a substudy of Trans-Tasman Radiation Oncology Group Study 98.02. *J Clin Oncol* 2006;24(13):2098–2104.

75. Rischin D, Peters LJ, O'Sullivan B, et al. Tirapazamine, cisplatin, and radiation versus cisplatin and radiation for advanced squamous cell carcinoma of the head and neck (TROG 02.02, HeadSTART): a phase III trial of the Trans-Tasman Radiation Oncology Group. *J Clin Oncol* 2010;28(18):2989–2995.

76. Peters LJ, O'Sullivan B, Giralt J, et al. Critical impact of radiotherapy protocol compliance and quality in the treatment of advanced head and neck cancer: results from TROG 02.02. *J Clin Oncol* 2010;28(18):2996–3001.

77. Seiwert TY, Salama JK, Vokes EE. The chemoradiation paradigm in head and neck cancer. *Nat Clin Pract Oncol* 2007;4(3):156–171.

78. Dewhirst MW, Lee CM, Ashcraft KA. The future of biology in driving the field of hyperthermia. *Int J Hyperthermia* 2016;32(1):4–13.

79. Brizel DM, Scully SP, Harrelson JM, et al. Radiation therapy and hyperthermia improve the oxygenation of human soft tissue sarcomas. *Cancer Res* 1996;56(23):5347–5350.

80. Roti Roti JL. Introduction: radiosensitization by hyperthermia. *Int J Hyperthermia* 2004;20(2):109–114.

81. Kampinga HH, Dikomey E. Hyperthermic radiosensitization: mode of action and clinical relevance. *Int J Radiat Biol* 2001;77(4):399–408.

82. Horsman MR, Overgaard J. Hyperthermia: a potent enhancer of radiotherapy. *Clin Oncol* 2007;19(6):418–426.

83. Horsman MR, Overgaard J. The impact of hypoxia and its modification of the outcome of radiotherapy. *J Radiat Res* 2016;57(Suppl 1):i90–i98.

84. van der Zee J, Gonzalez Gonzalez D, van Rhoon GC, et al. Comparison of radiotherapy alone with radiotherapy plus hyperthermia in locally advanced pelvic tumours: a prospective, randomised, multicentre trial. Dutch Deep Hyperthermia Group. *Lancet* 2000;355(9210):1119–1125.

85. Hurwitz MD. Today's thermal therapy: not your father's hyperthermia: challenges and opportunities in application of hyperthermia for the 21st century cancer patient. *Am J Clin Oncol* 2010;33(1):96–100.

86. Lawrence TS, Blackstock AW, McGinn C. The mechanism of action of radiosensitization of conventional chemotherapeutic agents. *Semin Radiat Oncol* 2003;13(1):13–21.

87. Wilson GD, Bentzen SM, Harari PM. Biologic basis for combining drugs with radiation. *Semin Radiat Oncol* 2006;16(1):2–9.

88. Pignon JP, le Maitre A, Maillard E, et al. Meta-analysis of chemotherapy in head and neck cancer (MACH-NC): an update on 93 randomised trials and 17,346 patients. *Radiother Oncol* 2009;92(1):4–14.

89. Winquist E, Agbassi C, Meyers BM, et al. Systemic therapy in the curative treatment of head and neck squamous cell cancer: a systematic review. *J Otolaryngol Head Neck Surg* 2017;46(1):29.

90. Reducing uncertainties about the effects of chemoradiotherapy for cervical cancer: individual patient data meta-analysis. *Cochrane Database Syst Rev* 2010;(1):CD008285.

91. Meng XY, Liao Y, Liu XP, et al. Concurrent cisplatin-based chemoradiotherapy versus exclusive radiotherapy in high-risk cervical cancer: a meta-analysis. *Onco Targets Ther* 2016;9:1875–1888.

92. Seiwert TY, Salama JK, Vokes EE. The concurrent chemoradiation paradigm—general principles. *Nat Clin Pract Oncol* 2007;4(2):86–100.

93. Boeckman HJ, Trego KS, Henkels KM, et al. Cisplatin sensitizes cancer cells to ionizing radiation via inhibition of non-homologous end joining. *Mol Cancer Res* 2005;3(5):277–285.

94. Kunos CA, Sherertz TM. Long-term disease control with triapine-based radiochemotherapy for patients with stage IB2–IIIB cervical cancer. *Front Oncol* 2014;4:184.

95. Golden EB, Formenti SC, Schiff PB. Taxanes as radiosensitizers. *Anticancer Drugs* 2014;25(5):502–511.

96. Milas L, Milas MM, Mason KA. Combination of taxanes with radiation: preclinical studies. *Semin Radiat Oncol* 1999;9(2 Suppl 1):12–26.

97. Hei TK, Piao CQ, Geard CR, et al. Taxol and ionizing radiation: interaction and mechanisms. *Int J Radiat Oncol Biol Phys* 1994;29(2):267–271.

98. Shewach DS, Lawrence TS. Antimetabolite radiosensitizers. *J Clin Oncol* 2007;25(26):4043–4050.

99. Ang KK, Berkey BA, Tu X, et al. Impact of epidermal growth factor receptor expression on survival and pattern of relapse in patients with advanced head and neck carcinoma. *Cancer Res* 2002;62(24):7350–7356.

100. Harari PM, Huang S. Radiation combined with EGFR signal inhibitors: head and neck cancer focus. *Semin Radiat Oncol* 2006;16(1):38–44.

101. Huang SM, Bock JM, Harari PM. Epidermal growth factor receptor blockade with C225 modulates proliferation, apoptosis, and radiosensitivity in squamous cell carcinomas of the head and neck. *Cancer Res* 1999;59(8):1935–1940.

102. Robert F, Ezekiel MP, Spencer SA. Phase I study of anti-epidermal growth factor receptor antibody cetuximab in combination with radiation therapy in patients with advanced head and neck cancer. *J Clin Oncol* 2001;19(13):3234–3243.

103. Bonner JA, Harari PM, Giralt J, et al. Radiotherapy plus cetuximab for squamous-cell carcinoma of the head and neck. *N Engl J Med* 2006;354(6):567–578.

104. Bonner JA, Harari PM, Giralt J, et al. Radiotherapy plus cetuximab for locoregionally advanced head and neck cancer: 5-year survival data from a phase 3 randomised trial, and relation between cetuximab-induced rash and survival. *Lancet Oncol* 2010;11(1):21–28.

105. Fakhry C, Westra WH, Li S, et al. Improved survival of patients with human papillomavirus-positive head and neck squamous cell carcinoma in a prospective clinical trial. *J Natl Cancer Inst* 2008;100(4):261–269.

106. Magrini SM, Buglione M, Corvo R, et al. Cetuximab and radiotherapy versus cisplatin and radiotherapy for locally advanced head and neck cancer: a randomized phase II trial. *J Clin Oncol* 2016;34(5):427–435.

107. Ang KK, Zhang Q, Rosenthal DI, et al. Randomized phase III trial of concurrent accelerated radiation plus cisplatin with or without cetuximab for stage III to IV head and neck carcinoma: RTOG 0522. *J Clin Oncol* 2014;32(27):2940–2950.

108. Yuhas JM, Spellman JM, Culo F. The role of WR-2721 in radiotherapy and/or chemotherapy. *Cancer Clin Trials* 1980;3(3):211–216.

109. Brizel DM, Wasserman TH, Henke M, et al. Phase III randomized trial of amifostine as a radioprotector in head and neck cancer. *J Clin Oncol* 2000;18(19):3339–3345.

110. Wasserman TH, Brizel DM, Henke M, et al. Influence of intravenous amifostine on xerostomia, tumor control, and survival after radiotherapy for head-and-neck cancer: 2-year follow-up of a prospective, randomized, phase III trial. *Int J Radiat Oncol Biol Phys* 2005;63(4):985–990.

111. Koukourakis MI, Kyrias G, Kakolyris S, et al. Subcutaneous administration of amifostine during fractionated radiotherapy: a randomized phase II study. *J Clin Oncol* 2000;18(11):2226–2233.

112. Boccia R, Anne PR, Bourhis J, et al. Assessment and management of cutaneous reactions with amifostine administration: findings of the ethyol (amifostine) cutaneous treatment advisory panel (ECTAP). *Int J Radiat Oncol Biol Phys* 2004;60(1):302–309.

113. Lindegaard JC, Grau C. Has the outlook improved for amifostine as a clinical radioprotector? *Radiother Oncol* 2000;57(2):113–118.

114. Simon R. Design and Analysis of Clinical Trials. In: Devita VT, Lawrence T, Rosenberg S, eds. *Cancer: principles and practice of oncology.* 8th ed. Philadelphia: Lippincott-Raven, 2008.

115. Fu KK, Pajak TF, Trotti A, et al. A Radiation Therapy Oncology Group (RTOG) phase III randomized study to compare hyperfractionation and two variants of accelerated fractionation to standard fractionation radiotherapy for head and neck squamous cell carcinomas: first report of RTOG 9003. *Int J Radiat Oncol Biol Phys* 2000;48(1):7–16.

116. Bourhis J, Blanchard P, Maillard E, et al. Effect of amifostine on survival among patients treated with radiotherapy: a meta-analysis of individual patient data. *J Clin Oncol* 2011;29(18):2590–2597.

117. Movsas B. Exploring the role of the radioprotector amifostine in locally advanced non-small cell lung cancer: Radiation Therapy Oncology Group trial 98-01. *Semin Radiat Oncol* 2002;12(1 Suppl 1):40–45.

118. Movsas B, Scott C, Langer C, et al. Randomized trial of amifostine in locally advanced non-small-cell lung cancer patients receiving chemotherapy and hyperfractionated radiation: radiation therapy oncology group trial 98-01. *J Clin Oncol* 2005;23(10):2145–2154.

119. Vujaskovic Z, Feng QF, Rabbani ZN, et al. Radioprotection of lungs by amifostine is associated with reduction in profibrogenic cytokine activity. *Radiat Res* 2002;157(6):656–660.

120. Vujaskovic Z, Feng QF, Rabbani ZN, et al. Assessment of the protective effect of amifostine on radiation-induced pulmonary toxicity. *Exp Lung Res* 2002;28(7):577–590.

121. Vujaskovic Z, Thrasher BA, Jackson IL, et al. Radioprotective effects of amifostine on acute and chronic esophageal injury in rodents. *Int J Radiat Oncol Biol Phys* 2007;69(2):534–540.

122. Antonadou D, Pepelassi M, Synodinou M, et al. Prophylactic use of amifostine to prevent radiochemotherapy-induced mucositis and xerostomia in head-and-neck cancer. *Int J Radiat Oncol Biol Phys* 2002;52(3):739–747.

123. Buntzel J, Glatzel M, Kuttner K, et al. Amifostine in simultaneous radiochemotherapy of advanced head and neck cancer. *Semin Radiat Oncol* 2002;12(1 Suppl 1):4–13.

124. Nutting CM, Morden JP, Harrington KJ, et al. Parotid-sparing intensity modulated versus conventional radiotherapy in head and neck cancer (PARSPORT): a phase 3 multicentre randomised controlled trial. *Lancet Oncol* 2011;12(2):127–136.

125. Thorstad WL, Chao KS, Haughey B. Toxicity and compliance of subcutaneous amifostine in patients undergoing postoperative intensity-modulated radiation therapy for head and neck cancer. *Semin Oncol* 2004;31(6 Suppl 18):8–12.

126. Anderson CM, Allen BG, Sun W, et al. Phase 1b/2a trial of superoxide (SO) dismutase (SOD) mimetic GC4419 to reduce chemoradiation therapy–induced oral mucositis (OM) in patients with oral cavity or oropharyngeal carcinoma (OCC). *Int J Radiat Oncol Biol Phys* 2016;94(4):869–870.

127. Ashcraft KA, Boss MK, Tovmasyan A, et al. Novel manganese-porphyrin superoxide dismutase-mimetic widens the therapeutic margin in a preclinical head and neck cancer model. *Int J Radiat Oncol Biol Phys* 2015;93(4):892–900.

128. Birer SR, Lee C, Roy Choudhury K, et al. Inhibition of the continuum of radiation-induced normal tissue injury by a redox-active Mn porphyrin. *Radiat Res* 2017;188.

129. Oberley-Deegan RE, Steffan JJ, Rove KO, et al. The antioxidant, MnTE-2-PyP, prevents side-effects incurred by prostate cancer irradiation. *PLoS One* 2012;7(9):e44178.

130. Yakovlev VA, Rabender CS, Sankala H, et al. Proteomic analysis of radiation-induced changes in rat lung: modulation by the superoxide dismutase mimetic MnTE-2-PyP(5+). *Int J Radiat Oncol Biol Phys* 2010;78(2):547–554.

131. Gauter-Fleckenstein B, Fleckenstein K, Owzar K, et al. Early and late administration of MnTE-2-PyP5+ in mitigation and treatment of radiation-induced lung damage. *Free Radic Biol Med* 2010;48(8):1034–1043.

132. Gauter-Fleckenstein B, Fleckenstein K, Owzar K, et al. Comparison of two Mn porphyrin-based mimics of superoxide dismutase in pulmonary radioprotection. *Free Radic Biol Med* 2008;44(6):982–989.

133. Potten CS, O'Shea JA, Farrell CL, et al. The effects of repeated doses of keratinocyte growth factor on cell proliferation in the cellular hierarchy of the crypts of the murine small intestine. *Cell Growth Differ* 2001;12(5):265–275.

134. Dorr W, Spekl K, Farrell CL. Amelioration of acute oral mucositis by keratinocyte growth factor: fractionated irradiation. *Int J Radiat Oncol Biol Phys* 2002;54(1):245–251.

135. Dorr W, Spekl K, Farrell CL. The effect of keratinocyte growth factor on healing of manifest radiation ulcers in mouse tongue epithelium. *Cell Prolif* 2002;35(Suppl 1):86–92.

136. Chen L, Brizel DM, Rabbani ZN, et al. The protective effect of recombinant human keratinocyte growth factor on radiation-induced pulmonary toxicity in rats. *Int J Radiat Oncol Biol Phys* 2004;60(5):1520–1529.

137. Spielberger R, Stiff P, Bensinger W, et al. Palifermin for oral mucositis after intensive therapy for hematologic cancers. *N Engl J Med* 2004;351(25):2590–2598.

138. Brizel DM, Murphy BA, Rosenthal DI, et al. Phase II study of palifermin and concurrent chemoradiation in head and neck squamous cell carcinoma. *J Clin Oncol* 2008;26(15):2489–2496.

139. Le QT, Kim HE, Schneider CJ, et al. Palifermin reduces severe mucositis in definitive chemoradiotherapy of locally advanced head and neck cancer: a randomized, placebo-controlled study. *J Clin Oncol* 2011;29(20):2808–2814.

140. Henke M, Alfonsi M, Foa P, et al. Palifermin decreases severe oral mucositis of patients undergoing postoperative radiochemotherapy for head and neck cancer: a randomized, placebo-controlled trial. *J Clin Oncol* 2011;29(20):2815–2820.

141. Martin F, Farley A, Gagnon M, et al. Comparison of the healing capacities of sucralfate and cimetidine in the short-term treatment of duodenal ulcer: a double-blind randomized trial. *Gastroenterology* 1982;82(3):401–405.

142. Makkonen TA, Bostrom P, Vilja P, et al. Sucralfate mouth washing in the prevention of radiation-induced mucositis: a placebo-controlled double-blind randomized study. *Int J Radiat Oncol Biol Phys* 1994;30(1):177–182.

143. Meredith R, Salter M, Kim R, et al. Sucralfate for radiation mucositis: results of a double-blind randomized trial. *Int J Radiat Oncol Biol Phys* 1997;37(2):275–279.

144. Pfeiffer P, Madsen EL, Hansen O, et al. Effect of prophylactic sucralfate suspension on stomatitis induced by cancer chemotherapy. A randomized, double-blind cross-over study. *Acta Oncol* 1990;29(2):171–173.

145. Segre G, Hammarstrom S. Aspects of the mechanisms of action of benzydamine. *Int J Tissue React* 1985;7(3):187–193.

146. Sironi M, Pozzi P, Polentarutti N, et al. Inhibition of inflammatory cytokine production and protection against endotoxin toxicity by benzydamine. *Cytokine* 1996;8(9):710–716.

147. Epstein JB, Silverman S Jr., Paggiarino DA, et al. Benzydamine HCl for prophylaxis of radiation-induced oral mucositis: results from a multicenter, randomized, double-blind, placebo-controlled clinical trial. *Cancer* 2001;92(4):875–885.

148. Bellm L, Lehrer RI, Ganz T. Protegrins: new antibiotics of mammalian origin. *Expert Opin Investig Drugs* 2000;9(8):1731–1742.

149. Giles FJ, Miller CB, Hurd DD, et al. A phase III, randomized, double-blind, placebo-controlled, multinational trial of iseganan for the prevention of oral mucositis in patients receiving stomatotoxic chemotherapy (PROMPT-CT trial). *Leuk Lymphoma* 2003;44(7):1165–1172.

150. Trotti A, Garden A, Warde P, et al. A multinational, randomized phase III trial of iseganan HCl oral solution for reducing the severity of oral mucositis in patients receiving radiotherapy for head-and-neck malignancy. *Int J Radiat Oncol Biol Phys* 2004;58(3):674–681.

Section II

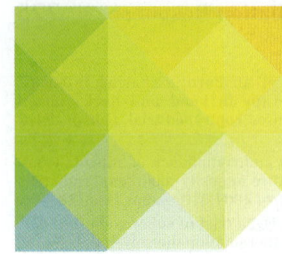

CHAPTER 35

Oncologic Imaging and Oncologic Anatomy

Junzo P. Chino, Chris R. Kelsey, Jared D. Christensen, and Lawrence B. Marks

INTRODUCTION

This chapter addresses two topics central to the management of patients with cancer: oncologic anatomy and oncologic imaging. Although these topics are relevant for all specialties involved in the treatment of cancer, they are particularly germane for radiation oncologists. A sound understanding of anatomy, especially pertaining to malignant processes, facilitates interpretation of imaging studies. Likewise, understanding the advantages and limitations of individual imaging modalities assists in defining rational clinical target volumes (CTVs) that maximize the therapeutic ratio.

Advances in diagnostic imaging have increased our ability to visualize macroscopic disease, referred to as gross tumor volume (GTV). Imaging is currently unable to identify microscopic tumor extension around a primary tumor or occult nodal involvement. A CTV is created to account for both of these uncertainties (Table 35.1). A rational definition of the CTV should reflect the clinician's knowledge regarding the patterns of spread for each particular cancer. This involves both local spread around the primary site and patterns of lymphatic drainage. Appropriate expansion of a GTV to a CTV minimizes the risk of local failure (i.e., marginal miss) while reducing the risk of complications by avoiding regions at low risk of involvement (Fig. 35.1).

Radiation treatment planning has undergone considerable evolution during the past 30 years. With conventional planning, the physician conceives of beam orientations and aperture shapes based on the interpretation of available clinical and diagnostic information, including three-dimensional (3D) imaging data such as computed tomography (CT) or magnetic resonance imaging (MRI). The beam is then applied to the patient using a fluoroscopy-based conventional simulator, relying on an understanding of tumor and normal tissue anatomy and its association with fluoroscopic bony anatomy and surface anatomy. Relatively generous margins are used to account for inherent uncertainties of the process.

With 3-D treatment planning, anatomic information from a planning CT scan is transferred to a computer where the images are segmented to define the tumor and normal tissues. Software allows this 3-D information to be displayed and viewed from any orientation. Beam orientation and shape are chosen to encompass the target, yet minimize, as much as possible, normal tissue exposure. Thus, 3-D planning tools allow the 3-D anatomy to be more accurately incorporated into the planning process than with conventional techniques.

The computer allows the planner to use beam orientations that are nonstandard (e.g., nonaxial beams). Beam apertures are typically smaller than with conventional simulation because of reduced uncertainty in the entire process. The prior specification of the beam angle and aperture by the treatment team is known as "forward planning." Current technology also allows data from other imaging modalities (MRI, positron emission tomography [PET], etc.) to be fused with the planning CT dataset and hence considered in the planning process. It is advantageous to position the patient similarly during the imaging and treatment planning scans to facilitate accurate image correlation.

Intensity-modulated radiation therapy (IMRT) and other more conformal technologies require the clinician to explicitly delineate target volumes, including elective nodal basins and avoidance structures. The introduction of IMRT has revolutionized radiation treatment planning and, in the process, has required clinicians to become more proficient in 3-D anatomy and malignant patterns of spread. The prespecification of the intended target of radiotherapy, the organs at risk of treatment, and the dosimetric goals or constraints of therapy is known as "inverse planning," as the beams' apertures and fluencies are determined afterward by an optimization algorithm.

There has been great progress in the last decade with the development of consensus guidelines for target and critical organ delineation in most disease sites (Table 35.2). While some of the volume definitions may be conceived primarily based on expert opinion, they facilitate the rational demarcation of nodal stations at risk, reporting of patterns of spread and failure, and communication with surgical colleagues. Certainly, these guidelines and atlases provide the fundament upon which future work may be built, and should be seen as living works, refined and revised on a regular basis, preferably with reference to recurrence/spread patterns (as was recently performed for bladder cancer).[1] These guidelines should complement, and not replace, the judgment of the

FIGURE 35.1. Gross disease identified with imaging is depicted, along with appropriate expansions to encompass surrounding microscopic disease (CTV) and setup/motion uncertainties (PTV). GTV, gross tumor volume.

Tumor seen on imaging: GTV

Area at risk for microscopic disease; CTV

Expansion to account for motion and setup error: PTV

TABLE 35.1 VOLUME DEFINITIONS FOR RADIATION THERAPY PLANNING

Structure	Defined	Method of Assessment
Gross tumor volume (GTV)	Palpable or visible disease	Physical examination, imaging studies
Clinical target volume (CTV)	GTV + expansion for microscopic spread	Knowledge of patterns of spread (oncologic anatomy)
Planning target volume (PTV)	CTV + expansion for setup error and organ motion	Imaging studies (fluoroscopy or 4D CT to define degree of motion) and reproducibility/stability of mobilization/localization systems

4D, four dimensional; CT, computed tomography.

TABLE 35.2 ATLASES AND GUIDELINES AVAILABLE FOR TARGET AND NORMAL TISSUE DELINEATION

Atlas	Associated Group	Availability
CNS/Brain		
Hippocampal Sparing	NRG/RTOG Legacy	www.rtog.org/CoreLab/ContouringAtlases.aspx
Head and Neck		
Cranial Nerves Atlas	NRG/RTOG Legacy	www.rtog.org/CoreLab/ContouringAtlases.aspx
Nodal Regions in the N0 Neck–2013 Update	NRG/RTOG Legacy	www.rtog.org/CoreLab/ContouringAtlases.aspx
Brachial Plexus Contouring Atlas	NRG/RTOG Legacy	www.rtog.org/CoreLab/ContouringAtlases.aspx
Breast		
Breast Cancer Atlas	NRG/RTOG Legacy	www.rtog.org/CoreLab/ContouringAtlases.aspx
Lung		
RTOG 1106 OAR (Lung)	NRG/RTOG Legacy	www.rtog.org/CoreLab/ContouringAtlases.aspx
RTOG 1106 Target Atlas (Lung)	NRG/RTOG Legacy	www.rtog.org/CoreLab/ContouringAtlases.aspx
Gastrointestinal		
Upper Abdominal Normal Organ Contouring Consensus Guidelines	NRG/RTOG Legacy	www.rtog.org/CoreLab/ContouringAtlases.aspx
Pancreas Atlas	NRG/RTOG Legacy	www.rtog.org/CoreLab/ContouringAtlases.aspx
Esophageal and Gastroesophageal Junction Cancer	ad hoc group	*Int J Radiat Oncol Biol Phys* 2015;92(4):911–920.
Anorectal	NRG/RTOG Legacy	www.rtog.org/CoreLab/ContouringAtlases.aspx
Gynecologic		
Female RTOG Normal Pelvis Atlas	NRG/RTOG Legacy	www.rtog.org/CoreLab/ContouringAtlases.aspx
GYN (postop Cervix and Uterine)	NRG/RTOG Legacy	www.rtog.org/CoreLab/ContouringAtlases.aspx
Intact Cervix	NRG/RTOG Legacy	*Int J Radiat Oncol Biol Phys* 2011;79(2):348–355.
Vulva	NRG/RTOG Legacy	*Int J Radiat Oncol Biol Phys* 2016;95(4):1191–1200
MRI contours for Image Guided Brachytherapy	GEC-ESTRO	*Radiother Oncol* 2005;74(3):235–245
Genitourinary		
Male RTOG Normal Pelvis Atlas	NRG/RTOG Legacy	www.rtog.org/CoreLab/ContouringAtlases.aspx
Post-Op Positive Apex Margins	NRG/RTOG Legacy	www.rtog.org/CoreLab/ContouringAtlases.aspx
Post-Op Positive Seminal Vesicle	NRG/RTOG Legacy	www.rtog.org/CoreLab/ContouringAtlases.aspx
Pelvic Lymph Node Volumes for Prostate Cancer Atlas	RMH & RTOG	*Int J Radiat Oncol Biol Phys* 2015;92(4):874–883
Post-cystectomy Bladder	NRG/RTOG Legacy	www.rtog.org/CoreLab/ContouringAtlases.aspx
Sarcoma		
RTOG Extremity Soft Tissue Sarcoma Atlas	NRG/RTOG Legacy	www.rtog.org/CoreLab/ContouringAtlases.aspx

treating physician, as anatomic variations, prior surgery, and unusual patterns of disease spread can invalidate the applicability of an atlas to an individual patient.

One of the risks of 3-D and IMRT is a false sense of security in the accuracy of imaging to portray the *in vivo* extent of disease. Further, imaging obtained at the time of initial treatment planning may not be representative of the *in vivo* anatomy throughout a course of therapy spanning several weeks. Indeed, there have been published examples of inferior outcomes with highly conformal treatment planning.[2,3] Modern imaging tools are clearly not perfect. The rapid embrace of newer technologies to visualize gross tumor and to address uncertainties related to organ motion and setup errors may be counterproductive if relied on too heavily in the treatment planning process. It is possible, if not likely, that microscopic tumor has been sterilized at the edge of radiotherapy fields that were expanded to account for setup errors and organ motion (i.e., not expanded with the intent of covering the microscopic disease). Further, the clinical history or examination and imaging may be discordant, and one needs to be careful not to be overly reliant on imaging when defining target volumes. For example, in a patient with cancer of the nasopharynx with cranial nerve deficits, the target volume should include the corresponding anatomic site of likely extension, even in the absence of an abnormality on imaging. Thus, a sound understanding of oncologic anatomy and imaging modalities is vital in the treatment planning process.

IMAGING MODALITIES

Radiologic imaging is an integral component in the management of cancer patients. Imaging is utilized in the diagnosis and initial staging of disease, treatment planning, and post-treatment surveillance. Radiation oncologists must be familiar with the available imaging modalities and understand the appropriate utilization and limitations of each, which often varies based on the tumor site and study indication. In particular, a general sense of the sensitivity, specificity, and positive and negative predictive values of an imaging study helps the clinician assimilate and interpret imaging information that can be misleading or even contradictory. A detailed review of each imaging modality and its associated physics is beyond the scope of this chapter; however, a general overview of the imaging modalities most frequently utilized in clinical practice is provided, with disease-specific applications addressed in the systems-based anatomy sections.

Radiography

Conventional radiography creates a two-dimensional gray-scale image produced by the differential attenuation of x-rays that pass through soft tissues of varying density. Tissues that are very dense, such as bone, will absorb (attenuate) more x-rays than tissues that are less dense, such as lung. The energy loss of source x-rays identified at the x-ray detector is directly proportional to tissue density resulting in a processed image where highly dense objects appear bright and less dense objects are dark. Radiographs are therefore best suited to detect pathology when a lesion differs greatly in density from adjacent structures, such as a soft tissue mass surrounded by aerated lung or a lytic lesion surrounded by dense bone. Radiographs have excellent spatial resolution: the ability to detect a small object within a given volume. However, they are suboptimal when there are only subtle differences in tissue density. Even large lesions can be missed if they are of similar density to surrounding structures. Further, given that radiographs are only two-dimensional, determining spatial relationships to adjacent structures is limited. Radiographs may help identify an abnormality, but additional imaging modalities are often required for further characterization. Although conventional radiography has limited utility in oncologic imaging, its basic principles underlie more advanced imaging modalities such as CT.

Cross-Sectional Imaging

CT, MRI, and ultrasound (US) generate two-dimensional cross-sectional images. The benefits of cross-sectional imaging include visualization of superimposed structures obscured on planar images, improved anatomic detail of individual organs and their precise relationship to adjacent structures, and the ability to perform multiplanar reconstructions. Some applications, such as Doppler US and cine cardiac MRI, provide functional information in addition to morphologic information and can be acquired in real time and have varying indications for image-guided procedures. For these reasons, cross-sectional modalities are the mainstay of oncologic imaging.

Computed Tomography

CT generates cross-sectional images from the transmission of radiation through tissue. A patient lies on the scanner table within a gantry that houses an x-ray generator opposite multiple rows of detectors, hence the term *multidetector CT* (MDCT). Current generation scanners (e.g., 64, 128, and 256 detector arrays) are able to acquire high-resolution image data much faster because of improvements in the number of detectors and computer processing. As the gantry rotates, the detectors measure x-ray transmission through the rotation, or slice. The patient is moved through the scanner as the gantry rotates, resulting in a helical or spiral course at a very thin slice thickness, typically 0.625 mm. The spatial and temporal data from multiple projections are then processed by a Fourier transform mechanism generating two-dimensional axial images. The thin-slice volume dataset is isotropic, meaning that images can be reconstructed in orthogonal and oblique planes without a loss in image quality. Furthermore, thin-slice acquisition improves contrast resolution and decreases partial volume artifacts, thereby improving imaging quality and accuracy.

Images are displayed within a matrix composed of voxels, each representing a volume of radiodensity that is quantified by a linear attenuation value called a Hounsfield unit (HU). Each voxel is assigned an HU in the range of −1,000 to 1,000 corresponding to a shade of gray that represents the attenuation difference between a given material and water. By convention, air is the least dense material with an HU value of −1,000, whereas water has an HU value of 0. Soft tissues have a range of attenuation with typical HU values as follows: fat (−120), blood (30), muscle (40), and bone (>300). HU analysis is more accurate than visual assessment of tissue composition and is particularly useful in characterizing enhancement postcontrast administration, a feature critical in the assessment of many solid organ lesions.

Both intravenous (IV) and oral contrast agents may be utilized to improve spatial resolution. Oral contrast agents are routinely used for abdominal and pelvic imaging to distinguish bowel from adjacent organs, lymph nodes, and tumors. The use of an intravascular contrast agent during CT depends on the study indication, target organ, and patient status. IV contrast agents contain variable concentrations of iodine compounds that attenuate, or absorb, x-rays, which allows for enhanced detection of vascular structures. Administration of IV contrast media is required for thorough assessment of vessels (e.g., aorta, pulmonary arteries), solid organs (e.g., liver, kidneys), and characterization of lesion vascularity. Contrast-enhanced CT is often necessary to detect solid organ metastases (e.g., liver, adrenal gland, brain). Contrast is usually not necessary for routine pulmonary imaging because of the inherent contrast of solid lesions within a background of aerated lung, although it does improve the characterization of hilar lymph nodes.

Given that the administration of contrast media can alter tissue attenuation, the HU value of a lesion or tissue may differ depending on whether the study was performed with or without contrast and based on the timing of image acquisition (e.g., arterial vs. portal venous phase). HUs are used during radiation treatment planning dose calculations; therefore, both IV and bowel contrast can affect these calculations. If indicated, the HU within a structure enhanced by contrast (e.g., the bladder when planning for prostate cancer treatment) can be set to an alternate value prior to dose calculations. A similar phenomenon often occurs when materials with a high atomic number are within the scanned volume. These materials (e.g., dental fillings, hip prostheses) can cause artifacts that can make it challenging to accurately segment the image or affect dose calculations. The latter can also be corrected by setting the HU within the affected area to the desired value.

IV contrast agents are excreted through the kidneys, are nephrotoxic, and are not typically administered to patients with impaired renal function (glomerular filtration rate [GFR] < 60, creatine [Cr] < 2.0, though institutional policies vary) unless on dialysis or out of emergent medical necessity. IV contrast media should also not be given to patients with a known contrast allergy resulting in anaphylaxis or laryngeal edema. More minor reactions, such as pruritus, are not an absolute contraindication, and contrast may be administered following a proper steroid pretreatment protocol. Alternative imaging modalities should be considered if a contrast-enhanced study is required in the setting of a severe contrast allergy. An allergy to shellfish is not considered a contraindication to iodinated contrast administration.[4–6]

In part because of its availability, rapid acquisition, and high-yield anatomic data, CT has become one of the most widely used medical imaging modalities in the United States, with over 85 million scans performed annually, and it serves as the core modality for oncologic imaging.[7,8] Although CT is noninvasive, it is not entirely benign. CT utilizes radiation to generate images, and although dose modulation and optimal scanning parameters can significantly reduce patient radiation exposure, the cumulative effects of CT radiation are of clinical concern. Alternative imaging modalities should always be considered and performed in lieu of CT when appropriate.

Magnetic Resonance Imaging

MRI generates cross-sectional images without ionizing radiation. MRI utilizes strong magnets to generate images, typically 1.5 or 3.0 T for clinical applications. A 3.0 T magnet is 60,000 times greater than the earth's magnetic field. The magnetic field uniformly aligns the nuclei of hydrogen protons within tissue. Applying a radiofrequency (RF) pulse sequence and gradient to the magnetic field disrupts this alignment and equilibrium. When the RF pulse is removed, the protons realign, or relax, within the field and emit a measurable resonance radio signal. The detected radio signals, referred to as *echoes* or *spin echoes*, are then used to generate an image. The most important tissue properties for image generation are the proton density, the spin-lattice relaxation time (T1), and the spin–spin relaxation time (T2). Different tissues have different proton density and relaxation times, absorbing and releasing radio wave energy at different rates, which in part accounts for the high tissue contrast obtained by MRI.

Different RF pulse sequences can accentuate different tissue characteristics by varying parameters such as the repetition time (TR)—the time between RF pulses in the sequence, which determines how much time protons have to realign within the magnetic field—and the echo time (TE)—the time between the RF pulse and the peak returning signal. TR and TE dramatically affect image contrast and determine

TABLE 35.3	MAGNETIC RESONANCE IMAGING SIGNAL INTENSITIES (SPIN-ECHO IMAGING)		
	T1WI	**T2WI**	**FLAIR**
Cerebrospinal fluid	Dark	Bright	Dark
Fat[a]	Bright	Dark	Bright
Solid mass (tumor)	Dark	Bright	Bright
Edema	Dark	Bright	Bright
Cyst	Dark	Bright	Dark

[a]Fat is bright on T2 fast spin-echo (FSE) or gradient echo sequences.
Bright, hyperintense; dark, hypointense; FLAIR, fluid-attenuation inversion recovery; T1WI, T1-weighted image; T2WI, T2-weighted image.

which tissue properties are selected. T1-weighted images, in which fluid is dark and fat is bright, are generally good at depicting anatomy; T1-weighted images are generated by selecting short TR (typically ≤800 ms) and short TE values (≤30 ms). T2-weighted images, in which fluid is bright and fat is dark, are fluid-sensitive and can depict areas of pathology; T2-weighted images are generated by selecting long TR (≥2,000 ms) and long TE values (≥60 ms) (Table 35.3). Scan sequences are composed of variations in RF pulses and TR and TE settings. Although these vary by MRI scanner manufacturer using proprietary names, the underlying principles are similar. Common sequence techniques include the following:

Spin-echo (SE) sequences produce standard T1- and T2-weighted images.

Multiple spin-echo (MSE) sequences allow for faster image acquisition and are also referred to as turbo spin echo, fast spin echo, or rapid-acquisition relaxation-enhanced imaging. The signal intensity and image quality are less than that of conventional SE sequences. Furthermore, fat is bright on MSE T2-weighted images, which can limit sensitivity for detecting pathology. Fat-suppression techniques can be used to offset this limitation. Fast low-angle acquisition with relaxation enhancement and half-Fourier acquisition single-shot turbo SE sequences are MSE variations.

Inversion recovery (IR) pulse sequences emphasize differences in T1 properties of tissues. A time of inversion (TI) is added to the sequence that can be set to target-specific tissues. Short time of IR sequences suppress tissues with short T1 relaxation times, such as fat, and enhance tissues with high T2 properties, such as fluid, resulting in added tissue contrast. The opposite effect may be achieved with fluid-attenuation IR sequences. In addition to IR, tissue suppression may be achieved with fat or fluid saturation and opposed-imaging techniques.

Gradient-recalled echo (GRE) pulse sequences are used for rapid image acquisition, which minimizes motion artifact associated with breathing, the cardiac cycle, vessel pulsation, and bowel peristalsis. GRE sequences have low tissue contrast, with the exception of flowing blood, which is bright in signal, and are therefore ideal for cardiac and vascular applications. Fast low-angle shot (FLASH) and true fast imaging with steady-state precession (FISP) are examples of this technique.

Although the inherent tissue contrast with MRI is excellent, the administration of contrast media can further improve the detection of pathology and subtle differences in tissue properties. Gadolinium chelates are the most commonly used MRI contrast agents, which, like the iodinated CT equivalents, are confined to the vasculature and do not cross an intact blood–brain barrier. Gadolinium is a heavy metal ion with paramagnetic effects that shorten T1 and T2 relaxation times. Although there are flow-related techniques for vascular imaging that do not require contrast media (e.g., time of flight imaging), the use of a contrast agent is essential for characterizing tissue perfusion. Once considered safe for patients with impaired

renal function, the use of gadolinium-based contrast agents has now been associated with nephrogenic systemic fibrosis (NSF), a debilitating and potentially fatal condition of fibrin deposition within the skin and other organs.[5,9] Although the precise mechanism is not understood, patients with severe renal dysfunction (GFR < 30) who receive gadolinium-based contrast media are at increased risk of developing NSF. Additional contributing factors may include an underlying inflammatory state, utilizing higher doses of gadolinium, or repeated dosing over short intervals.[10] Careful patient evaluation, including a risk/benefit analysis, should be performed before administering gadolinium-based contrast agents in patients with impaired renal function.

One of the advantages of MRI over CT is that it can provide functional in addition to anatomic information. This is particularly beneficial in oncologic imaging. MRI techniques allow for tissue diffusion and perfusion imaging, quantification of blood flow by velocity phase encoding, and magnetic resonance proton spectroscopy, which provides biochemical quantification of tissues. DCE (dynamic contrast-enhanced) MRI uses sequential images after contrast delivery to calculate a transfer constant k^{trans}. In situations with low vascular permeability, the constant will be driven by the rate of transfer across the vessel wall into the extracellular space; however, with high permeability, k^{trans} will be proportional to blood flow. Pretreatment k^{trans} may predict for poor outcome with head and neck cancers, though a high k^{trans} may conversely be associated with residual disease cervical cancer.[11,12] Thus, this functional imaging technique may have differing applications in clinical scenario, reflecting the complexity of the tumor and its microenvironment.

Diffusion-weighted imaging (DW or DWI) MRI measures brownian motion within the cellular microenvironment and calculates an apparent diffusion coefficient (ADC) map. A region of low intensity in an ADC map reflects restricted diffusion, a state that may correlated with increased cellularity, as seen with malignancy or fibrosis. This may improve the specificity of breast MRIs for differentiating malignancy from benign processes and even predicting the grade of the lesion.[13] DWI MRI has also improved the detection rate of hepatic lesions and differentiates between benign and malignant processes.[14] Conversely, high pretreatment ADC in cervical cancers may be associated with poorer eventual disease-free survival, again reflecting how functional imaging may be revealing a complex interaction in the tumor microenvironment.[15]

As with other imaging techniques, MRI has modality-specific artifacts that can limit image quality. Motion artifact can be problematic with MRI because of long scan times and breath-holding required with some sequences. Chemical shift artifact results in a loss of signal at the interface of tissues with highly variable contrast properties. MRI is also sensitive to magnetic field distortions that can produce artifacts. Susceptibility artifact is one of the most common problems with MRI and is frequently attributable to objects that alter the magnetic field such as metallic hardware or devices, resulting in signal voids or distortion of MRI images. The magnetization of such objects also presents a safety hazard as items can overheat or become displaced, resulting in serious harm or injury. Patients must be carefully screened to ensure that any medical devices or surgical hardware are MRI compliant.

Ultrasonography

US is an imaging modality utilizing pulse-echo techniques rather than radiation to produce an image. The US transducer coverts electrical energy into a high-frequency pulse that is transmitted through tissues. The pulse interacts at tissue interfaces, generating a reflected echo signal that is detected by the transducer. The returning sound waves are transformed into a gray-scale image in real time. Image quality is, in large part, determined by the pulse frequency. High-frequency transducers (5 to 12 MHz) produce high-resolution images but have limited ability to penetrate tissue. Therefore, they are best suited to imaging superficial structures such as the breast or thyroid. Low-frequency transducers (1 to 3.5 MHz) generate lower-quality images but have better tissue penetration and are most often used for imaging abdominal and pelvic organs. The degree to which tissues are visualized by US is called *echogenicity*. Fat is highly echogenic (bright), whereas fluid-containing structures, such as simple cysts, are anechoic (dark).

The quality of US images is highly dependent upon the user. Variability in experience can be problematic in the performance, reproducibility, and interpretation of US exams. Furthermore, US is prone to artifacts. Bone almost completely absorbs sound waves, resulting in acoustic shadowing that completely obscures tissues located beyond the bone. Air is also problematic as it almost completely reflects sound waves, leaving little pulse energy to penetrate tissues deep to the air. The application of a water-soluble gel between the transducer and the patient's skin eliminates air at the skin surface and ensures transmission of the US beam. Artifacts secondary to air markedly limit evaluation of lesions near the lung or bowel. In contrast to air, fluid readily transmits sound and makes an excellent "acoustic window" for imaging. This is the reason that patients are encouraged to drink plenty of fluids prior to a pelvic US examination—so that the bladder is fully distended.

Color Doppler US is an important adjunct to conventional gray-scale sonography. The Doppler effect is a change in frequency of returning sound waves reflected by a moving object, such as flowing blood. If blood flows away from the transducer, the echo frequency decreases, whereas if blood flows toward the transducer, the echo frequency increases. The change in frequency is directly proportional to the flow velocity and produces a color overlay in areas of flow on the standard gray-scale US image. Color Doppler US is useful in characterizing blood flow within lesions and assisting in image-guided procedures.

TABLE 35.4 ENDOSCOPIC ULTRASOUND WALL LAYERS OF THE ESOPHAGUS

Layer	EUS Characteristic	Histologic Layer	AJCC T Stage
1	Hyperechoic	Superficial mucosa	T1 *m*
2	Hypoechoic	Deep mucosa	T1 *m*
3	Hyperechoic	Submucosa	T1 *sm*
4	Hypoechoic	Muscularis propria	T2
5	Hyperechoic	Subserosa, serosa, adventitia	T3

AJCC, American Joint Committee on Cancer; EUS, endoscopic ultrasound; m, mucosa; sm, submucosa.

Endoscopic ultrasound (EUS) was introduced in the early 1980s and has become an important tool in oncologic staging. It allows for high-resolution images of internal structures not typically accessible by high-frequency transducers by passing the probe through bowel or airways. It is most widely applied in the setting of gastrointestinal (GI) malignancies, especially esophageal and rectal carcinomas. A 5 to 12 MHz transducer can readily identify five of the layers of the GI tract (Table 35.4 and Fig. 35.2).[16] Higher-frequency transducers can identify additional layers, such as the muscularis mucosa and lamina propria of the esophagus, which has important staging implications. EUS is also utilized for characterization and image-guided sampling of regional lymph nodes in GI or bronchopulmonary disease. The ability of EUS to predict the tumor (T) stage is generally superior to its ability to predict the node (N) stage, although some imaging patterns of nodal involvement are recognized. Normal lymph nodes are usually ovoid, <10 mm in short axis, and have a homogeneous but variable echogenic appearance that may be isoechoic, hyperechoic, or hypoechoic to surrounding tissues. An echogenic (bright) center is common and represents the normal fatty hilum. Suspicious lymph nodes are typically round, >10 mm in short axis, have distinct margins, and are often hypoechoic. If all four features are present, the likelihood of malignancy is 80% to 100%.[17] There is, however, considerable overlap

FIGURE 35.2. Axial endoscopic ultrasound image *(right)* and histologic specimen *(left)* from a normal esophagus. The endoscopic ultrasound layers and histologic layers of the esophagus are correlated (see Table 35.4). (Endoscopic ultrasound image courtesy of Dr. Frank Gress. Histologic image courtesy of Dr. Daniel Goodenough.)

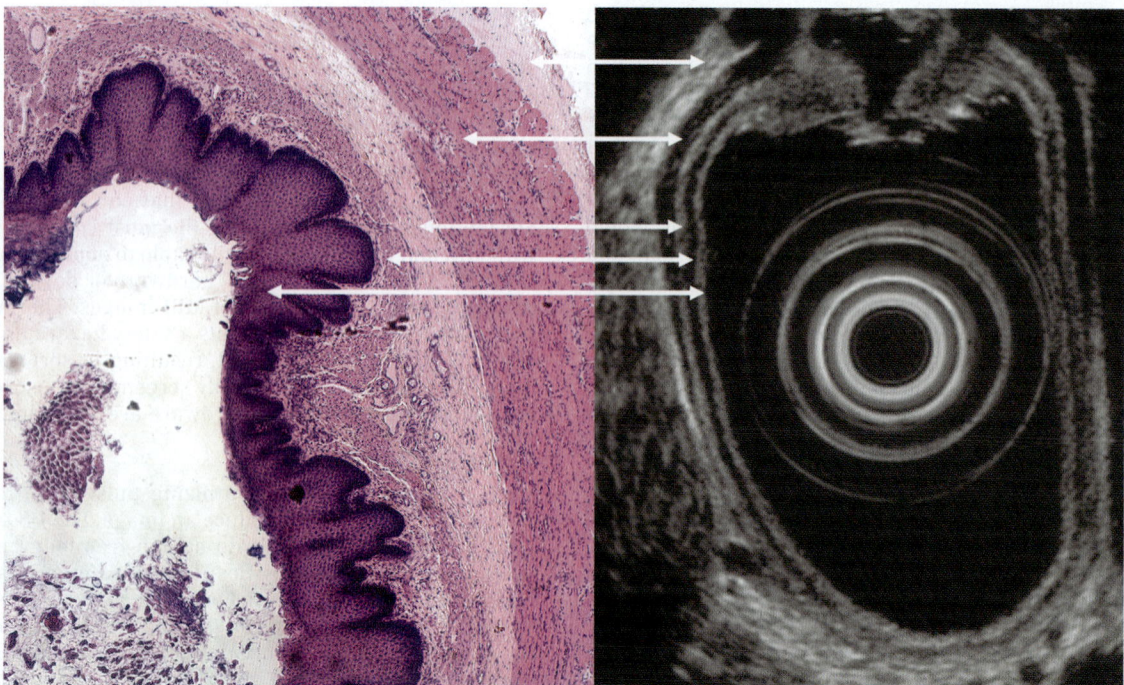

between benign and malignant features of lymph nodes on EUS in addition to wide interobserver variability. Tissue sampling is therefore recommended for accurate staging. When describing clinical T and N staging by EUS, the prefix *u* should be utilized (e.g., uT3N1).

Nuclear Imaging

Although radiographic and cross-sectional studies provide important anatomic information regarding pathologic processes, nuclear radiology provides physiologic information based on the distribution of an injected or ingested radiopharmaceutical. Radiopharmaceuticals consist of a radioactive substrate (radionuclide, radioisotope, or radiotracer) that is coupled with a physiologically active compound or analog. For example, technetium-99m is a radioisotope that is coupled to pertechnetate, water-soluble ion salt that is targeted for imaging of the thyroid, bladder, stomach, and colon, among other organs. The timing of imaging depends on the kinetics of absorption, metabolism, and half-life of the radionuclide. Gamma rays emitted by nuclear decay of the radionuclide are then detected using a γ-camera corresponding to radiotracer activity that is described in terms of uptake.

There are numerous available nuclear imaging studies that take advantage of differing radiopharmaceuticals for oncologic imaging. Many of these play a primary role in the management of oncology patients with specific malignancies. However, the primary nuclear imaging studies relevant to general oncologic imaging are PET and bone scintigraphy. These studies have broad application for many malignant processes in the diagnosis, staging, and surveillance of disease.

Positron Emission Tomography

Although several radionuclides for PET are available, the most common is 18-fluorodeoxyglucose (FDG). FDG is a glucose analog that concentrates in areas of high metabolic activity. Tumor cells are often highly metabolic, with rapid cell division and an increased number of glucose transporters. However, FDG uptake is not specific for malignancy and accumulates in any cell with increased metabolic activity, including myocardium, gastric mucosa, brain tissue, thyroid, and salivary glands, which limits PET evaluation of these organs. Furthermore, FDG tracer is excreted within the urinary system; therefore, activity within the kidneys, collecting system, and bladder can obscure malignancy of these structures. Notwithstanding these limitations, PET-CT has become the preferred imaging modality for clinical staging, facilitating the characterization of benign versus malignant pathology, detecting sites of unsuspected disease, identifying optimal sites for tissue sampling, assessing treatment response, and monitoring for recurrence for multiple malignancies.

Initially performed in isolation, PET is now routinely obtained in conjunction with CT. PET-CT combines the physiologic assessment of PET with the anatomic assessment of CT, resulting in improved diagnostic accuracy.[18] PET and CT may be obtained independently on the same day but are more commonly performed on a combined PET-CT scanner, which more precisely aligns the two imaging datasets for fusion such that the patient does not have to move between examinations. Patients must fast for 4 to 6 hours prior to scanning in order to limit metabolic activity within the GI tract. Blood glucose levels should be well controlled (<150 mg/dL) to limit glucose receptor competition with FDG, as high glucose levels can result in a false-negative scan. Speech and motion should be restricted to minimize muscle uptake, which could obscure pathology. Approximately 1 hour following FDG administration, a CT scan is performed immediately followed by PET imaging, which can take up to 60 minutes. CT and PET datasets are then reconstructed in separate axial, coronal, and sagittal series, as well as fused PET-CT images.

FDG uptake is nonspecific, localizing to any tissue with increased metabolic activity. Although most malignant tumors are hypermetabolic relative to normal tissues, nonmalignant processes also concentrate FDG, including foci of infection, inflammation, and benign neoplasms. FDG uptake is quantified by the standard uptake value (SUV). Most malignant tumors have a maximum SUV > 2.5, whereas physiologic uptake is typically <2.5. SUVs are not absolute and can be affected by the timing of imaging, improper attenuation correction, partial volume affects, patient weight, FDG dose, and factors affecting FDG uptake, as previously described. It is therefore difficult to accurately compare SUVs between scans. However, if care is taken to ensure that variables between studies are similar, such as performing the examination on the same scanner with similar patient preparation, FDG dosing, and image timing, comparing SUVs between studies may be reliable. Clinical studies to date have documented that under such uniform conditions, changes in SUV have prognostic value, indicating that most tumors responding to therapy show a 20% to 40% decrease in SUV early in course of treatment.[19–22]

The registration of CT and PET has led to novel ways of quantifying the burden of disease. Total lesion glycolysis (TLG), for example, is calculated by multiplying the mean SUV in a segmented lesion by the volume of said lesion. This metric essentially weights the volume of disease by its metabolic activity in an attempt to reflect the true burden and has been associated with worse prognosis in non–small cell lung cancer (NSCLC).[23] Metabolic tumor volume (MTV), on the other hand, is a measure of tumor volume only counting voxels above a certain SUV threshold, either relative (such as a percentage of SUVmax) or an absolute SUV value. Higher pretreatment MTV is associated with poorer eventual outcome in head and neck cancers.[24]

Other radionuclides with potential application to oncologists include ^{18}F-fluoromisonidazole (F-MISO), ^{18}F-fluoroazaomycin arabinoside (F-FAZA), and copper-64 diacetyl-bisN4-methylthiosemicarbazone (^{64}Cu-ATSM), all of which have different mechanisms of colocating to intratumoral hypoxic regions.[25] As hypoxia is a driver of both prosurvival factors such as HIF-1α, and resistance to radiotherapy, these agents are of considerable research interest, though not yet of routine clinical utility.

Bone Scintigraphy

Normal bone undergoes continuous remodeling, maintaining a balance between osteoblastic and osteoclastic activity. Most bone metastases originate as intramedullary lesions, having gained access to the bone through the vasculature. As the lesions enlarge, reactive osteoblastic and osteoclastic activity results in characteristic radiographic changes indicative of bone metastases (sclerotic, lytic, or mixed lesions). Rapidly growing metastases tend to produce lytic lesions, whereas more slowly growing metastases typically produce sclerotic (or blastic) lesions. Metastases from multiple myeloma, thyroid cancer, and renal cell carcinoma are predominantly lytic, whereas blastic lesions are associated with breast and prostate cancers. The primary utility of bone scintigraphy in oncologic imaging is the detection of osseous metastatic disease.

Bone scintigraphy or bone scan imaging utilizes radiopharmaceuticals composed of bisphosphonates, the most common of which is the radionuclide technetium-99m methylene diphosphonate (^{99m}Tc-MDP). ^{99m}Tc-MDP localizes to areas of new bone mineralization, which occurs in a wide array of bone pathology and is therefore highly sensitive to osseous disease, but is not very specific. Although a 30% to 50% reduction in bone density must occur before bone metastases are detected on radiographs, as little as 5% to 10% change is required to detect such on a bone scan.[26,27] Furthermore, bone scans are relatively inexpensive, convenient, and visualize the entire skeleton, including sites that are difficult to assess on plain films (e.g., ribs, sternum, scapula, sacrum). Reported sensitivities range from 62% to 100% with similar specificity rates (78% to 100%).[28]

Two primary patterns of radiotracer activity can be associated with malignancy: increased or decreased activity. Increased uptake occurs in areas of increased blood flow and osteoblastic activity; this is a common finding in metabolically active tumors and small sclerotic metastatic foci. Decreased radiotracer activity occurs as a "cold" area on bone scan and is associated with lytic bone disease and aggressive tumors that outgrow their blood supply. Rapidly progressing and purely lytic disease are the main causes of false-negative findings on bone scintigraphy, whereas false-positive findings can be related to trauma, healing, benign bone tumors, or arthritic changes. The false-positive rate of planar bone scintigraphy can be reduced by the use of single photon emission CT (SPECT), which can be obtained in conjunction with conventional CT or MRI for more precise localization of disease.[29,30]

Bone metastases are considered "nonmeasurable" using the Response Evaluation Criteria in Solid Tumors (RECIST).[31] Although a decrease in the intensity of radionuclide uptake is often ascribed to a response to treatment and an increase is attributed to progressive disease, several points must be considered. First, tumor treatment response may cause a "flare phenomenon," resulting in increased bone scan uptake secondary to new osteoblastic activity concomitant with new bone formation. This may be falsely attributed to progressive disease. Similarly, lytic lesions that were previously "cold" on bone scan can transform into "hot" spots (areas of uptake) after treatment. Second, rapidly progressive disease with overwhelming bone destruction without new bone formation can be misinterpreted as stable or responding disease on bone scan.

Many patients are at low risk of harboring occult osseous metastatic disease, and, in the absence of symptoms, a bone scan can be omitted from the staging workup. In prostate cancer, only approximately 1% of patients with a prostate-specific antigen (PSA) <10 will have a positive bone scan.[32,33] Patients with a Gleason score ≤7 and a PSA of 10 to 20 have a similar low risk of bone metastases.[34] In these patients, a bone scan should be omitted in the absence of symptoms. Similarly, a bone scan may be omitted in asymptomatic patients with node-negative breast cancer and lung cancer. Although studies have shown that MRI may be more sensitive than bone scans, especially for vertebral metastases, whole-body MRI is impractical and bone scintigraphy is considered sufficiently sensitive that MRI should be reserved for equivocal bone scans in the context of high clinical suspicion or for patients with positive bone scans but low clinical suspicion. Like MRI, PET has been shown to be more sensitive than scintigraphy for the diagnosis of osseous metastatic disease with sensitivity of 91% and 75% and specificity values of 96% and 95%, respectively.[35] FDG-PET also provides earlier detection of metastases than bone scans, attributable to the fact that increased glucose metabolism in neoplastic cells occurs prior to increased osteogenesis (required for bone scintigraphy uptake). PET also has the advantage of providing more comprehensive imaging in that it can detect soft tissue metastases in addition to bone disease, whereas scintigraphy only evaluates osseous structures. As a general rule, patients with isolated osteoblastic metastases may be monitored by serial bone scans, whereas other clinical scenarios are likely best suited for PET.

Radiomics

Radiomics is a burgeoning field, combining large databases of radiographic data (usually of CT, MRI, or PET orgin) with high-throughput computing capabilities to detect emergent patterns of data associated with clinically relevant outcomes.[36] It borrows its name and much of its terminology from genomics

and proteomics, utilizing similar computational techniques to detect signatures within the data, which may correlate to underlying tumor biology. An example of this is texture analysis, which derives several features of the intensity of not only a single voxel but its relationship to all neighboring voxels, which may potentially derive quantifiable measures of tumor heterogeneity, necrosis, and hypoxia.[37] However, it is worth noting that not only does it borrow its terminology with genomics, it similarly is susceptible to multiple comparisons and testing. When hundreds if not thousands of values can be derived from a finite pool of clinical data, the chances of spuriously positive correlations is quite high. It is incumbent, therefore, on all research in this promising field to externally validate all findings prior to clinical application.

BRAIN AND SPINE
Oncologic Anatomy
The Brain

The central nervous system consists of the brain and spinal cord. Both are covered with three meningeal layers—the dura mater, arachnoid mater, and pia mater. Meningiomas are the most common tumors arising from the meninges. They arise from arachnoid cells but are typically affixed to the underside of the dura mater. They are well-circumscribed tumors that do not typically invade the underlying brain parenchyma. Thus, when planning a course of radiation therapy, only minimal margins are required to account for surrounding microscopic disease extent in the direction of the brain parenchyma. Many meningiomas will have a linear area of enhancement on MRI, extending from the tumor along the dura. This so-called dural tail is generally not felt to represent direct extension of tumor but rather vascular congestion within the dura, leading to the characteristic enhancement.[38,39] Thus, enlarging the target volumes to include this linear area of enhancement is probably unnecessary unless other imaging abnormalities are apparent (e.g., nodularity).

The arachnoid mater and pia mater are considered the leptomeninges with the intervening space (subarachnoid space) filled with cerebrospinal fluid (CSF). Cancer can breach the CSF space through several routes, including hematogenous spread (via the Batson venous plexus or the arterial system) or by direct extension. Once cancer breaches the subarachnoid space, the entire craniospinal axis is at risk, and tumor deposits can lead to increased intracranial pressure, cranial nerve deficits, radiculopathies, and seizures. Leptomeningeal involvement occurs most frequently with pediatric brain tumors (e.g., medulloblastoma), acute lymphoblastic leukemia, and some solid cancers (e.g., breast cancer, melanoma, and lung cancer in particular).[40]

The major units of the brain include the cerebral hemispheres, diencephalon, cerebellum, and brainstem. The cerebral hemispheres consist of the frontal, parietal, temporal, and occipital lobes, basal ganglia, and lateral ventricles. The diencephalon includes the thalamus, hypothalamus, and third ventricle. The brainstem consists of the midbrain, the pons, and the medulla oblongata. The fourth ventricle lies between the pons and the cerebellum. Although more than half of pediatric brain tumors arise in the posterior fossa (cerebellum and brainstem), the vast majority of primary brain tumors in adults arise in the cerebral hemispheres or diencephalon.

The hippocampus is a portion of the limbic system in the deep medial temporal lobes bilaterally and plays important parts in the development and maintenance of memory. It is also a region that is seldom a site of metastatic disease and therefore a potential region that may be spared to improve the therapeutic ratio of whole-brain radiotherapy. It has been demonstrated that there is a dose-dependent atrophy of the hippocampus after radiation therapy and a dose-dependent decline in neurocognitive function.[41,42] A phase II trial from the RTOG demonstrated less cognitive decline in subjects treated with hippocampal-sparing whole-brain radiation compared to historical controls, demonstrating both feasibility and a significant signal for further study.[43]

Cranial Nerves

The cranial nerves consist of 12 paired nerves whose nuclei (with the exception of CN I) are located in the brainstem and upper spinal cord. They are termed cranial nerves because they exit the cranium through foramina in the base of skull and are encased by sheaths formed from the meninges. Nerve pathways connecting the cerebral cortex with the cranial nerves are complex. Although spinal motor neurons are innervated by the corticospinal tracts, many of the lower motor neurons in the brainstem are innervated by the corticobulbar tracts. These upper motor neurons innervate the cranial motor nuclei bilaterally (with some exceptions), in contrast to the nerves within the corticospinal tracts, which largely cross in the medulla leading to contralateral innervation.

Multiple tumors, both benign and malignant, commonly involve the cranial nerves, leading to serious neurologic deficits. Some of the more common include meningiomas involving the optic nerves (CN II), vestibular schwannomas (CN VIII), parotid gland tumors (CN VII), nasopharyngeal carcinoma (NPC) (multiple), and brainstem gliomas (multiple).

The classic presenting symptoms of diffuse pontine gliomas illustrate the intricate anatomy of the pons. A unilateral lesion in the ventral pons with involvement of the pyramidal tracts (upper motor neurons) might cause contralateral motor weakness in the arms or legs. In addition, cranial nerves within the pons might also be affected, unilaterally, without complete paralysis because of bilateral innervation of the cranial nerves by fibers in the corticobulbar tracts. Ataxia, denoting impairment of coordination without weakness, can be caused by involvement of fibers projecting from the pons to the cerebellum within the middle cerebellar peduncle. Through this pathway, the cerebellum receives a copy of the information for muscle movement that the corticospinal tracts relay to lower motor neurons, facilitating the complicated act of coordination.

The cranial nerves should also be carefully examined when evaluating a patient with NPC. One-fifth of patients with NPC present with symptoms of cranial nerve involvement (Table 35.5). The most commonly involved cranial nerves are the abducent nerve (CN VI) and the trigeminal nerve (CN V). CN VI originates in the ventral aspect of the brainstem, ascends on the clivus, and crosses the internal carotid artery near the superior aspect of foramen lacerum before entering the cavernous sinus. It then exits the skull through the superior orbital fissure. The motor and sensory nerve roots of CN V exit the pons and pass underneath the free edge of the tentorium cerebelli into the Meckel cave, forming the trigeminal (gasserian) ganglion. From the ganglion, V_1 and V_2 enter the cavernous sinus and subsequently exit the skull through the superior orbital fissure and foramen rotundum, respectively. V_3 exits the skull through foramen ovale.

The nasopharynx is in close proximity to foramen lacerum, rotundum, and ovale, explaining the frequent tumor involvement of CN V and VI. Invasion superiorly to the foramen lacerum and involvement of the trigeminal ganglion could lead to dysfunction in all three branches of CN V. In fact, most patients with NPC and CN V involvement have isolated deficits of V_2 or V_3. This occurs because of extension into foramen rotundum and ovale, respectively (Fig. 35.3). After gaining access to the middle cranial fossa, NPC may extend superiorly into the cavernous sinus. Four cranial nerves, including two branches of CN V, pass through the cavernous sinus. Within the sinus, the oculomotor nerve (CN III) is located most superiorly, whereas the maxillary nerve (CN V_2) is located most inferiorly. One

TABLE 35.5 MAJOR FORAMINA AND OTHER APERTURES IN THE CRANIAL FOSSAE AND THEIR PRIMARY CONTENTS AND CLINICAL ASSOCIATION WITH NASOPHARYNGEAL CANCER

Foramina/Opening	Contents	Frequency of Involvement by NPC (152) (%)
Anterior Cranial Fossa		
Foramina in cribriform plate	Axons of olfactory cells (CN I)	0
Middle Cranial Fossa		
Optic canal	Optic nerve (CN II)	6
	Ophthalmic artery	
Superior orbital fissure	Oculomotor nerve (CN III)	9
	Trochlear nerve (CN IV)	17
	Abducent nerve (CN VI)	44
	Ophthalmic nerve (CN V_1)	45
Foramen rotundum	Maxillary nerve (CN V_2)	67
Foramen ovale	Mandibular nerve (CN V_3)	48
Foramen spinosum	Meningeal branch of CN V_3	14
	Middle meningeal artery/vein	
Foramen lacerum	Internal carotid artery[a]	
Petrous Portion of the Temporal Bone		
Internal acoustic meatus	Facial nerve (CN VII)[b]	
	Vestibulocochlear nerve (CN VIII)	9
	Labyrinthine artery	0
Posterior Cranial Fossa		
Jugular foramen	Glossopharyngeal nerve (CN IX)	20
	Vagus nerve (CN X)	20
	Spinal accessory nerve (CN XI)	14
	Internal jugular vein (superior bulb)	
Foramen magnum	Spinal roots of spinal accessory nerve (CN XI)	14
	Medulla	
	Vertebral artery	
	Anterior/posterior spinal artery	
Hypoglossal canal	Hypoglossal nerve (CN XII)	24

[a]After entering the skull through the carotid canal.
[b]The facial nerve exits the skull through the stylomastoid foramen.
NPC, nasopharyngeal carcinoma.

FIGURE 35.3. Coronal T1 magnetic resonance image with contrast demonstrating nasopharyngeal carcinoma extending through foramen ovale into Meckel cave.

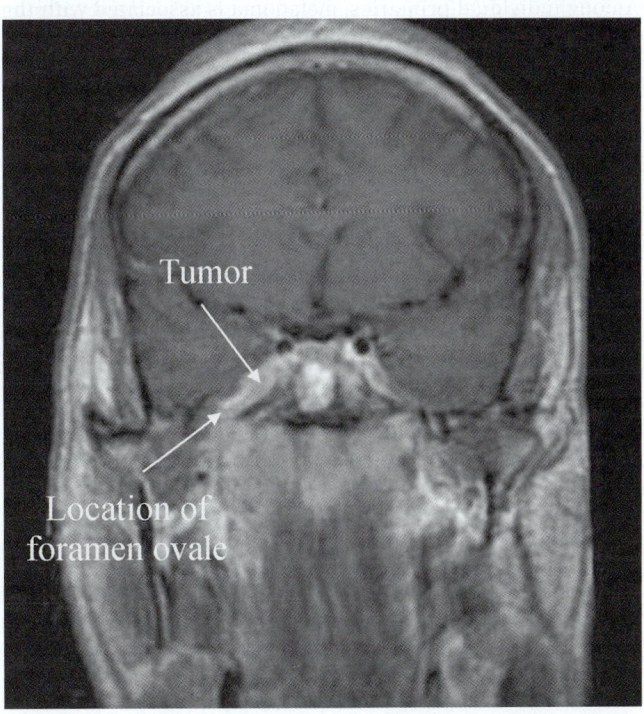

Tumor

Location of foramen ovale

would suspect that cranial nerves located more superiorly in the cavernous sinus would be involved less frequently than those located closer to the base of skull. This is consistent with what is observed clinically (see Table 35.5).

Lower cranial nerve involvement can occur without intracranial extension. The fossa of Rosenmüller is the most common site of origin of NPC. The lateral border of the fossa of Rosenmüller is the pharyngeal space. Direct tumor extension laterally into the parapharyngeal space or lymphatic metastases to high parapharyngeal lymph nodes can affect the cranial nerves exiting the jugular foramen (CN IX, X, and XI) and hypoglossal canal (CN XII). This may result in loss of the gag reflex (CN IX), hoarseness or dysphagia (CN X), atrophy or paralysis of trapezius and sternocleidomastoid (CN XI), as well as tongue deviation (CN XII).

Spine

The vertebral column typically consists of 33 bones (7 cervical, 12 thoracic, 5 lumbar, 5 sacral, and 4 coccygeal). The sacral and coccygeal vertebral bodies are fused. Although all individuals have seven cervical vertebral bodies, variations in the number of the other vertebral levels are occasionally observed. The spinal cord is housed within the spinal canal and encased by the meninges. Spinal cord levels do not correspond with levels of the vertebral column. In adults, the spinal cord typically ends at the L1-2 interspace (termed the *conus medullaris*). In an infant, the spinal cord terminates at L2 or L3. However, the spinal nerves continue to descend within the spinal canal (termed the cauda equina). The subarachnoid space, containing CSF, typically extends to the second sacral vertebral body. At this level, the meninges fuse together and extend caudally as the filum terminale, which anchors the spinal cord to the coccyx. These anatomical issues have implications when evaluating a patient with spinal cord compression, when designing craniospinal fields, and when setting up palliative spine fields.

Oncologic Imaging
Intracranial Metastases

Approximately 50% of adult intracranial neoplasms are metastatic, with lung, breast, melanoma, renal, and colon cancers being the most common, in order of decreasing frequency. Among individual primaries, melanoma is associated with the highest frequency of brain metastases.[44,45] Most metastases gain access to the brain through the vasculature and typically arise at the junction of the gray and white matter, presumably because the caliber of blood vessels decreases at this point, acting as a trap for tumor emboli.[45] Approximately 80% of brain metastases are found in the cerebral hemispheres, with less frequent involvement of the cerebellum (15%) and brainstem (5%), reflecting their smaller volume and blood flow.

The detection of brain metastases is an important part of initial staging. Furthermore, because of improved treatment strategies and overall cancer survival, the overall incidence of brain metastases is increasing. The preferred imaging modality for the diagnosis of intracranial metastasis is contrast-enhanced MRI. Brain metastases are typically well circumscribed and avidly enhance (Fig. 35.4). They are also typically associated with a disproportionate amount of surrounding edema best depicted on T2-weighted sequences. MRI is more sensitive than CT in detecting intracranial metastases, and approximately 20% of patients with solitary metastatic lesions by CT show multiple lesions on MRI.[46] Furthermore, for patients with a single brain metastasis detected with a conventional single-dose MRI-contrasted study, triple-dose studies will depict additional metastases in up to 25% of patients.[47] The detection of multiple lesions aids in directing appropriate treatment and helps to distinguish metastases from primary brain tumors, which are more commonly solitary.

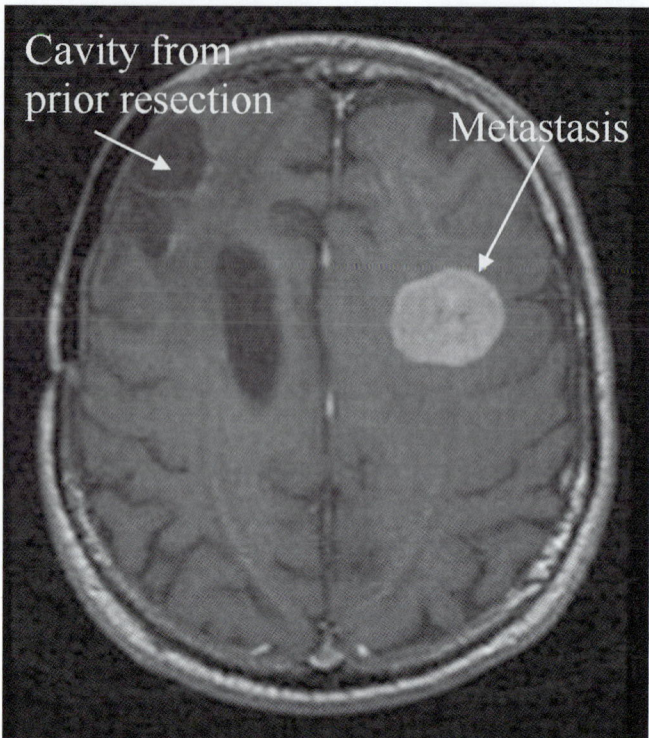

FIGURE 35.4. Axial T1 magnetic resonance image with contrast demonstrating a 2.5-cm melanoma brain metastasis in the left frontal lobe. Note the prior resection cavity in the right frontal lobe.

Primary Brain Malignancy

Primary brain tumors account for approximately 50% of adult intracranial masses, of which half are malignant. The most common malignant primary brain tumor in adults is glioblastoma multiforme (GBM), which usually arises in the cerebral hemispheres. Compared with CT, MRI is more accurate in delineating the local gross extent of disease. In a series of 52 patients with primary brain tumors, the MRI signal abnormality was larger than that identified by CT in 62% of patients. Furthermore, 10 patients with equivocal CT scans had clear abnormalities on MRI.[48] GBMs are characterized by an expansile mass that is iso- to hypointense to surrounding tissue on T1-weighted images, with central necrosis and peripheral ring enhancement postcontrast administration. T2-weighted imaging shows a heterogeneous mass with high signal of the tumor nidus and surrounding T2-signal abnormality corresponding to vasogenic edema, in which malignant cells are known to frequently reside.[49] Central areas of low signal reflect a combination of blood products, necrosis, and vascular flow voids.

GBM most commonly grows along white matter tracts and does not typically involve the dura or skull. GBM is one of two entities that may spread into the contralateral cerebral hemisphere via tracts of the corpus callosum; central nervous system lymphoma is the other. Other potential routes of spread, including subependymal extension with CSF contamination or hematogenous dissemination, are possible but unusual.

Advanced imaging techniques are also beneficial in characterizing intracranial malignancy. Magnetic resonance spectroscopy (MRS) provides metabolic and biochemical information about tumors in relation to normal brain tissue by quantifying five metabolite peaks: choline (Cho)-containing compounds, Cr, N-acetylaspartate (NAA), lactate, and lipid: the Cho peak reflects cell membrane turnover, Cr is a surrogate for energy synthesis, and NAA is a marker exclusive to neuronal cells. Lactate is detected in necrotic tumors and infarcted tissue and results from anaerobic metabolism. Lipid peaks are produced by cellular and myelin breakdown products. The hallmark spectroscopic pattern of brain tumors is an increase in Cho-containing compounds and a decrease in NAA relative to normal brain tissue. MRS can also aid in the evaluation of tumor type and grade. High-grade gliomas tend to exhibit higher Cho:Cr and Cho:NAA ratios. High-grade gliomas also typically have higher lipid and lactate peaks as the result of necrosis.[50] MRS can also distinguish metastatic disease from high-grade gliomas, particularly when combined with perfusion MRI.[51] Differentiating radiation necrosis from recurrent or progressive tumor remains a significant challenge in imaging, though delayed contrast extravasation (DCE) MRI has shown early promise in differentiating between active tumor (fast extravasation) and benign processes (slow extravasation).[52]

Conventional PET-CT has limited utility in the assessment of brain neoplasms because of the high metabolic rate of normal brain tissue. However, delayed-phase PET, performed approximately 3.5 hours following FDG injection, allows for washout of FDG from normal brain cells, whereas abnormal tissue retains FDG. Delayed phase PET has been shown to be beneficial in detecting both primary and metastatic brain lesions as well as differentiating between residual or recurrent tumor and radiation necrosis following treatment.[53,54] The development of new radioisotopes for neurologic applications, such as ^{11}C-methionine for targeting gliomas, has demonstrated clinical utility and advantages over FDG and might have similar utility in metastases. Many of these new tracers target different cellular processes such as apoptosis, angiogenesis, and hypoxia; the latter being of particular prognostic importance as hypoxic tissue is less sensitive to chemotherapies.[55] The utility of delayed phase PET may be further enhanced through fusion with MRI.[56]

Spinal Metastases

Osseous metastases are common in many malignancies, and the vertebral bodies are frequently involved because of the vascular distribution to the spine. MRI is more sensitive at detecting early vertebral body metastases than both radiographs and CT as it can image changes within the marrow space before cortical destruction occurs. Given that PET has similar sensitivity as MRI for osseous metastatic disease, is performed as part of routine staging, and can image the entire body, MRI is reserved for troubleshooting, such as determining extent of invasion into adjacent tissues. One notable exception is the use of urgent MRI for identification of cord compression in the setting of acute neurologic compromise. In this situation, it is often the T2-weighted sequences that are most useful: the high-signal CSF provides contrast to identify disease encroaching into the spinal canal. Spinal cord edema can also be identified. One should consider screening the entire spine when evaluating for cord compression.

Spinal cord compression is often considered an oncologic emergency, because the longer the duration of symptoms, the less likely the patient will regain function. Thus, therapy is often instituted emergently in these cases (e.g., with radiation, steroids, surgery, or sometimes chemotherapy in sensitive tumors). There is often discordance between the imaging and clinical examination findings. It is the *clinical* findings that determine the acuity of the situation rather than the imaging findings. A radiologic finding of cord compression certainly warrants a timley evaluation, but does not necessarily warrant emergent intervention in the absence of symptoms.

HEAD AND NECK

Oncologic Anatomy

The anatomy of the head and neck is complex, and it is important that oncologists have an intimate understanding of the location, function, and radiographic appearance of the various subsites. The potential for significant morbidity associated with local tumor progression and recurrence in the head and neck region, as well as the associated late effects of curative treatment, necessitates attention to detail. The impact of anatomy is such that the Accreditation Council for Graduate Medical Education mandates cadaver lab experience for otolaryngology residency.

Lymphatic Drainage of the Head and Neck

The lymphatics in the head and neck region largely proceed in an orderly fashion from sites in the upper aerodigestive tract into the common jugular chains, which eventually empty into systemic circulation near the junction of the internal jugular and subclavian veins. There are notable exceptions to this orderly drainage that can influence radiation treatment planning. In order to discuss this in a systematic fashion, the lymphatic basins of the neck are divided into six distinct levels, with surgical and radiographic boundaries.[57]

Level I is defined as both the submental basins (level IA) and the submandibular basins (level IB) and receive drainage from the oral cavity, although this basin may also be at risk from other sites in the setting of advanced nodal disease (N2b or greater). Level II contains the upper jugular nodes, extending from the C1 vertebral body to the hyoid bone, including the contents of the carotid sheath and the space deep to the sternocleidomastoid muscle (SCM). Level II is subdivided into anterior (level IIA) and posterior (level IIB) regions, as defined by the posterior border of the jugular vein. Level II contains the jugulodigastric node at the level of the jugular vein as it crosses the posterior belly of the digastric muscle and is a common lymphatic pathway for the majority of the upper aerodigestive tract. Level III follows the carotid sheath and space posterior to the SCM from the hyoid bone to the cricoid and receives efferent lymph drainage from level II. Level IV continues to follow the same jugular chain to the level of the clavicle. Level V contains the posterior triangle of the neck, boarded by the trapezius posteriorly, the SCM anteriorly, and the clavicle inferiorly, and is at particular risk for nasopharyngeal primaries. Level VI are the prelaryngeal lymph nodes (delphian nodes), which extend from the inferior edge of the thyroid cartilage to the sternal notch, bounded laterally by the sternal heads of the SCM. Level VI is at risk in laryngeal cancers with subglottic or transglottic extension and for hypopharyngeal cancers with esophageal extension.[58]

In addition, there are two other regions not included in this level classification that are worthy of consideration. Just superior to level II, following the carotid sheath to the skull base are the junctional or retrostyloid nodes, which may be at risk when there is ipsilateral nodal disease. Medial to these nodes and to level II lie the retropharygeal nodes (or nodes of Rouviere), which lie in the regions anterior to the prevertebral fascia, which in turn surrounds the longus capitis and the longus colli muscles. The retropharyngeal nodes extend superiorly to the skull base and inferiorly to the hyoid bone and are at risk of cancers arising from the nasopharynx, posterior pharyngeal wall, and the pyriform sinus.[59]

The Oral Cavity

The oral cavity encompasses three major subsites: the oral tongue, the floor of mouth, and the buccal mucosa. Carcinomas originating from the oral tongue have potential to spread locally through the intrinsic and extrinsic muscles of the tongue, inferiorly to the floor of mouth, and posteriorly to the anterior tonsillar pillar. For the floor of mouth, the genioglossus, geniohyoid, and root muscles of the tongue are at risk for local disease spread, as well as levels IA and IB of the neck, laterally to the alveolar ridge and mandible. Tumors of the buccal mucosa may extend superiorly to the infratemporal fossa, inferiorly to the submandibular region, anteriorly to the lip commissure, and posteriorly to the retromolar trigone.[59]

Nasopharynx, Oropharynx, and Hypopharynx

The nasopharynx is bounded superiorly and posteriorly by the sphenoid sinus, clivus, and the prevertebral fascia of C1 and C2. The parapharyngeal space lies laterally to the nasopharynx, which in turn is bounded laterally by the medial pterygoid muscle. The parapharyngeal space offers few anatomic barriers for the direct invasion of tumors superiorly and laterally to the base of skull, resulting in cranial nerve deficits as noted above. The eustachian tube empties into the nasopharynx at the torus tubarius; just posterior to the torus is the pharyngeal recess (or fossa of Rosenmüller), a fold of mucosa that is a frequent site for primary malignancies of this region.

The oropharynx anteriorly is bounded by the base of tongue, laterally by the tonsils, superiorly by the soft palate, and posteriorly by the posterior pharynx. Tumors arising from the base of tongue are often difficult to assess for extent of disease; therefore, the entire base of tongue, proximal oral tongue, and vallecula are at risk for subclinical disease. MRI may aid in delineation of the GTV for this site.[60] Tonsillar cancers may involve the base of tongue, palate, and buccal mucosa, although in locally advanced cases, they may also involve the nasopharynx, parapharyngeal space, and pterygoid muscles. Soft palate tumors may extend laterally to the tonsillar pillars and superiorly to the pterygopalatine fossa.

The pharyngeal constrictor muscles (PCM) lie along the posterior aspect of the naso- and oropharynx, bounded by the parapharyngeal space. The PCM may be further divided into (1) the superior PCM starting at the occipital condyle to the hyoid; (2) the middle PCM, starting 0.5 cm superior to the hyoid and ending at the inferior edge of the hyoid; and (3) the inferior PCM, which continues from the inferior aspect of the hyoid to the esophagus. The middle PCM was initially implicated as an organ at risk, with dose–volume metrics associated with late swallowing problems.[61] Since then, dose to other swallowing structures such as the genioglossus, mylo-geniohyoid complex, the anterior digastric, and the superior PCM have also been implicated in later dysphagia.[62]

Carcinoma arising from the posterior and lateral pharyngeal walls may spread superiorly to the nasopharynx and inferiorly to the hypopharynx. Similarly, primaries of the hypopharynx may spread superiorly through the oropharynx and nasopharynx. Malignancies of the pyriform sinus may also place the ipsilateral larynx at risk.

Larynx

The larynx is subdivided into three anatomic regions: the supraglottis (containing the epiglottis, the arytenoid and aryepiglottic folds, and the ventricular bands or false cords), the glottis (a 1-cm plane extending inferiorly from the lateral margin of the ventricle, including the true vocal cords and commissures), and the subglottis (from the inferior border of the glottis to the inferior aspect of the cricoid). The true cords have essentially no lymphatic drainage, allowing for focal treatment of a limited primary tumor without elective nodal treatment. In contrast, the supraglottic larynx has a rich and bilateral lymphatic system, requiring either dissection or elective nodal radiotherapy for even early primary tumors. The subglottis is a rare site of primary tumors and may invade locally into soft tissue as well as metastasize to laryngeal and tracheal lymphatics.

Oncologic Imaging

For cancer of the head and neck, staging relies on careful physical examination, fiberoptic and direct laryngoscopy, directed biopsies, and integration of imaging modalities.

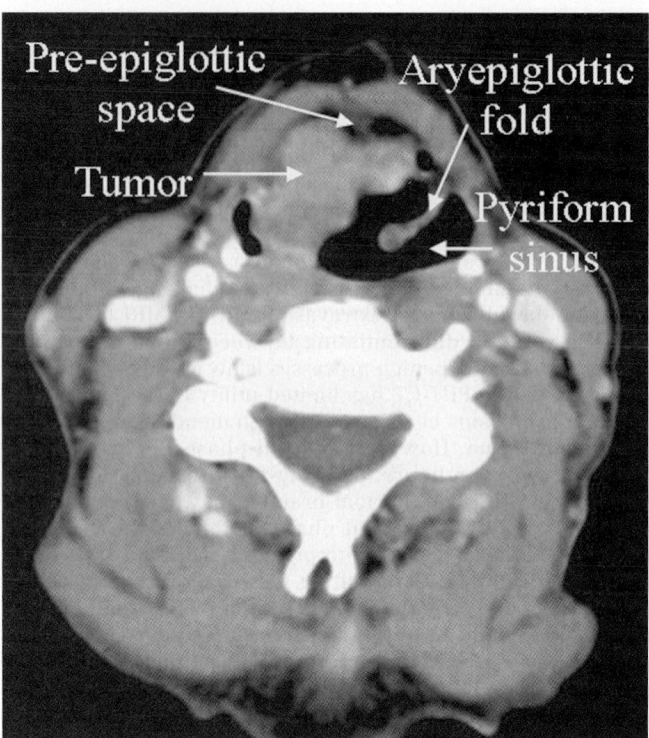

FIGURE 35.5. Axial computed tomography image demonstrating a squamous cell carcinoma involving the right aryepiglottic fold with anterior extension into the pre-epiglottic space.

Contrast-enhanced CT is the standard imaging modality for carcinomas of the head and neck region (Fig. 35.5). MRI may be a superior imaging modality for evaluating the extent of primary tumors of the oral cavity, oropharynx, and nasopharynx.[63] Novel approaches with MRI have shown promise in evaluating tumor responses to treatment by measuring physiologic changes within the tumor. Dynamic contrast-enhanced MRI may give insight into the vascular permeability (k-trans) in the tumor microenvironment; k-trans is found to be significantly higher in complete responders to concurrent chemoradiation therapy and therefore may be a predictor of treatment response.[64,65] Diffusion-weighted MRI may also provide information about the cellularity of a tumor mass or involved lymph node; an increase in the ADC (corresponding to a decrease in cellularity) during chemoradiation has been correlated with improved 2-year local control in one series.[66]

FDG-PET imaging for head and neck cancer has been useful as an adjunct to MRI and CT, particularly in clarifying the significance of intermediate lesions. In one series, the addition of FDG-PET imaging improved the accuracy of tumor delineation from 40% to 70% with MRI or CT alone to 97% to 100%, altering the management of 23% of the patient under study.[67] Another series found FDG-PET to have a sensitivity of 88% in determining the primary tumor and a sensitivity of 82% and specificity of 100% for lymph node metastases.[68] However, in initial staging, no noninvasive imaging modality has a high enough negative predictive value to forgo appropriate dissection or elective nodal irradiation when the characteristics of the primary tumor suggest a significant risk of spread. That is in contrast to the value of FDG-PET after chemoradiation for the detection of residual nodal disease. The sensitivity for detection of persistent disease was 96% with a specificity of 72% in a posttreatment series, with a negative predictive value in some series as high as 99%, allowing for the abandonment of routine posttreatment neck dissections in patients with a complete clinical and PET response.[69,70] Novel PET tracers such as Cu64-ATSM and F18-misonidasole, designed to evaluate hypoxia within the tumor, may also prove to be clinically useful.[71]

THE BRACHIAL PLEXUS

Oncologic Anatomy

The brachial plexus originates from the primary rami of the C5 through the T1 vertebral levels and joins to form three nerve trunks (upper, middle, and lower) in the neck. These trunks divide as they course beneath the clavicle, forming three cords (lateral, medial, and posterior) in close approximation to the axillary artery, posterior to the pectoralis minor. The cords then form the three primary terminal nerves for the arm (the median, ulnar, and radial nerves) as well as the musculocutaneous nerve. These peripheral nerves are of particular importance because of the significant morbidity associated with injury, either from tumor invasion or from treatment-related toxicity. As the plexus traverses the neck and axilla, it is of particular relevance when treating tumors of the head and neck, upper thorax, and breast.

Oncologic Imaging

Identifying the brachial plexus is difficult on CT imaging and may be most directly visualized on MRI.[72,73] However, one may accurately contour the position of the trunks, divisions, and cords on noncontrast CT imaging based on bony, muscular, and vascular landmarks.[74] The method put forward by Hall et al. begins contouring at the origination of the vertebral foramina of C5 through T1. The anterior and middle scalene muscles are then identified, with the trunks lying in the space between these muscles. The middle scalene will end at the superior aspect of the first rib just as the divisions of the plexus will be joining with the axillary artery as a neurovascular bundle. The artery then can be followed laterally as a surrogate for the remainder of the cords into the upper arm. Of interest to breast treatment, the course of the plexus will be brought superior and lateral with the upper arm with abduction, though still constrained by its course underneath the clavicle (Fig. 35.6).

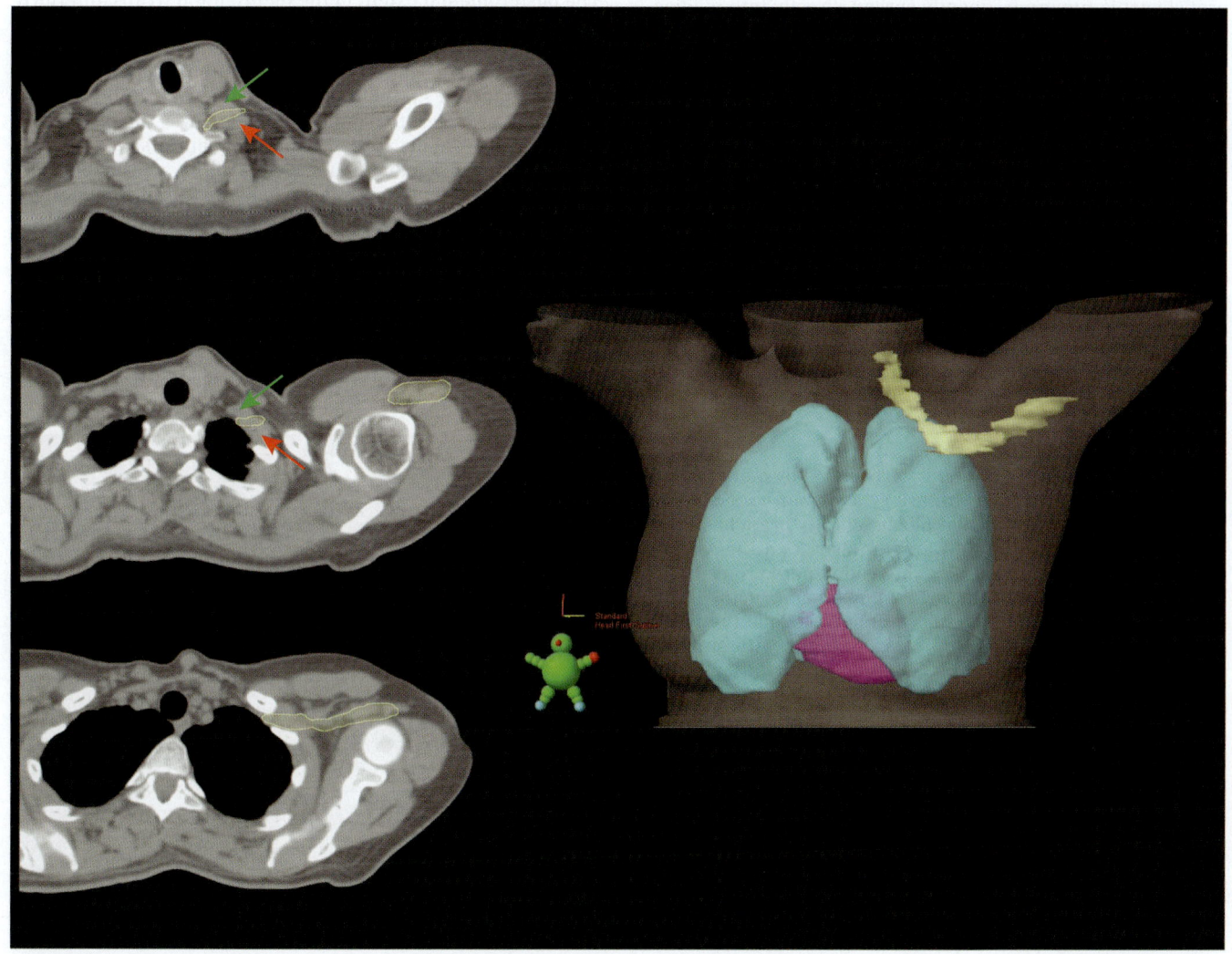

FIGURE 35.6. The brachial plexus (*yellow contour*) is delineated on axial computed tomography images on a woman undergoing treatment to the left breast. The anterior scalene (*green arrow*) and middle scalene (*red arrow*) are identified. The brachial plexus is delineated in the space between these muscles, originating at the C5-T1 roots and continuing to the axillary neurovascular bundle. The course of the plexus is contoured more distally than clinically necessary to emphasize the course and location when the arm is abducted.

THE THORAX

Oncologic Anatomy

The thorax consists of the superior part of the trunk and contains several important structures including the heart, lungs, esophagus, and pleura. Primary tumors of the heart are extremely rare. On the other hand, lung cancer is the leading cause of cancer mortality in the United States and the incidence of esophageal carcinoma is rising. Other common malignancies that arise in the thorax include malignant pleural mesothelioma, thymic malignancies, and Hodgkin lymphoma (HL) and non-Hodgkin lymphoma (NHL).

There are many clinically relevant anatomical issues when evaluating patients with cancers of the thorax, particularly lung cancer. These include (a) lobe-specific patterns of lymphatic spread, (b) the complex anatomy surrounding the lung apex, (c) the extent of the pleural space, (d) esophageal landmarks, and (e) thymic architecture.

Patterns of Lymphatic Spread

Lung cancer, both non–small cell and small cell histologies, frequently metastasize to regional lymph nodes. A basic understanding of mediastinal lymph node stations and lobe-specific lymphatic spread is helpful when evaluating and planning treatment for patients with lung cancer. The mediastinal nodes are a complex system, and it is challenging to predict where lymph node metastases will develop. However, these basic patterns provide a framework for customizing local treatment approaches (surgery and radiation therapy).

Both anatomical and clinical studies have shown that bronchogenic tumors frequently spread directly into mediastinal lymph nodes, bypassing intrapulmonary and hilar lymph nodes. This phenomenon appears to occur more frequently for upper lobe tumors.[75] For right-sided tumors, these pathways most frequently lead to ipsilateral paratracheal and subcarinal lymph node stations. For left-sided tumors, particularly those arising in the left upper lobe, direct spread to para-aortic and aortopulmonary (AP) window stations predominates. Second, right lung segments drain predominantly into the ipsilateral mediastinum. Conversely, left lung tumors commonly spread to both sides of the mediastinum,[75–77] especially left lower lobe tumors. Third, direct passageways to the supraclavicular fossa exist but are rare. Clinically, supraclavicular failures are uncommon and are usually associated with failure in upper paratracheal lymph node stations.[78] Fourth, most clinical studies have shown that subcarinal lymph nodes are frequently involved by both upper and lower lobe tumors.

The Superior Sulcus

The superior sulcus of the lung is surrounded by multiple critical structures. The subclavian artery and vein pass anterior to the lung apex, the brachial plexus and its branches cross over the apex of the lung toward the arm, and the stellate ganglia lie posteriorly alongside the exiting nerve roots of the lower cervical and upper thoracic spine. Other structures that can be involved by superior sulcus tumors include the vertebral bodies, trachea, and esophagus. Patients with superior sulcus tumors present with a variety of presentations (arm edema, hand weakness, sensory deficits, and/or Horner syndrome) related to the local extent of their disease.

The Pleura

The lungs are enclosed within a pleural sac. The visceral pleura is adherent to all of the surfaces of the lung, including the individual lobes where the pleura extends into the fissures. The parietal pleura is adherent to the thoracic wall, mediastinum, and diaphragm. The pleural recesses are potential spaces where portions of opposed parietal pleura are in contact during quiet respiration (Fig. 35.7). The inferior

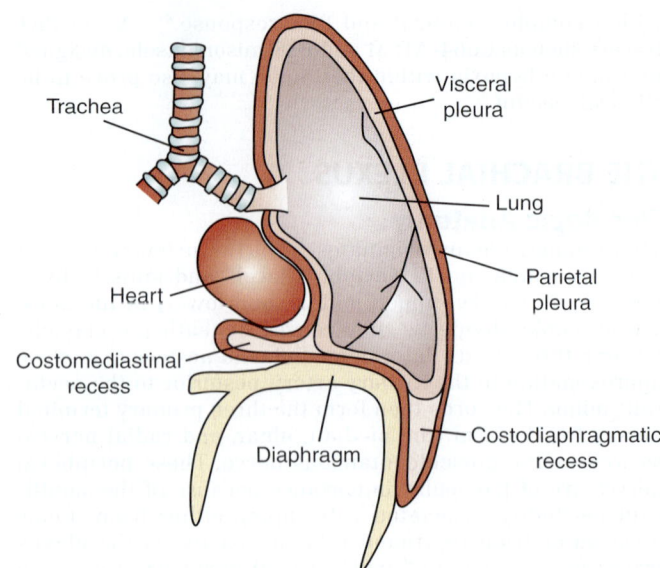

FIGURE 35.7. The extent of the pleura is illustrated. Note the inferior extension of the costodiaphragmatic recess and the medial extension of the costomediastinal recesses. (Courtesy of the University of Bristol, Centre for Applied Anatomy.)

extension of the costodiaphragmatic recess can be easily underestimated, as can the medial extent of the costomediastinal recess (see Fig. 35.7). The inferior aspect of the costodiaphragmatic recess often extends to the level of the midkidney. The posteromedial extent of the pleura often wraps anteriorly over the descending aorta.

Malignant mesothelioma is a rare pleural neoplasm associated with prior asbestos exposure. Pathologically, it can be categorized into epithelial, sarcomatoid, and mixed histologic subtypes. Mesothelioma initially involves the pleura and grows by contiguous spread from the pleural space into the lung, chest wall, mediastinum, pericardium, and diaphragm. The extent of the pleural spaces has implications for postoperative radiation target volumes (Fig. 35.8).

FIGURE 35.8. Digitally reconstructed coronal image from a treatment planning computed tomography scan illustrating the inferior extent of the costodiaphragmatic recess, which extends to the level of the midkidney. The patient had previously undergone an extrapleural pneumonectomy at which time metallic clips were placed, demarcating the inferior extent of the recess. The clinical target volume is illustrated in *red.*

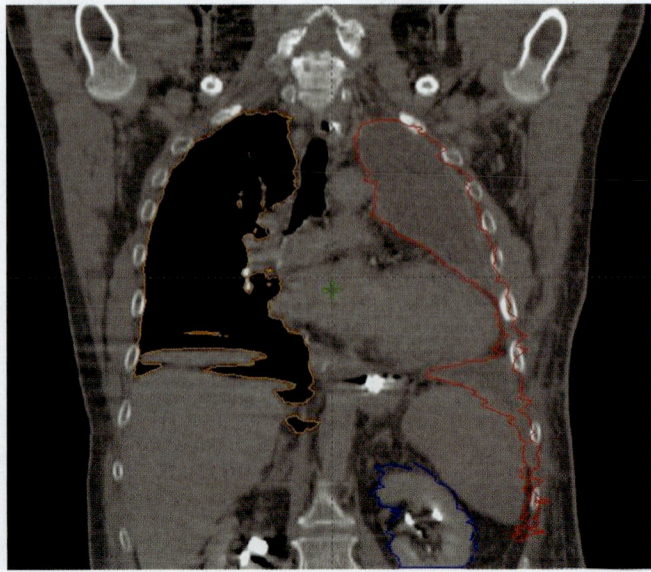

Esophageal Anatomy

The esophagus extends from the cricopharyngeus muscle at the level of the cricoid cartilage to the gastroesophageal junction in the abdomen. The cervical esophagus extends from the cricopharyngeus muscle (~15 cm from the incisors) to the level of the thoracic inlet (~18 cm from the incisors). The thoracic esophagus extends from the thoracic inlet to the diaphragm and is sometimes divided into upper, middle, and lower sections. The carina is located at approximately 25 cm from the incisors and the gastroesophageal junction is located at approximately 40 cm. These general numbers are helpful when planning radiation fields based on staging studies that include endoscopy, EUS, and PET.

Thymus Architecture

The thymus is an encapsulated, bilobed gland situated in the superior anterior mediastinum and is involved in adaptive immunity. Although prominent in size during infancy and early childhood, it begins to involute during adolescence. The thymus decreases significantly in size in most patients after administration of chemotherapy but typically regrows during the recovery phase, sometimes to a larger size than at baseline.[79]

The thymus gland is composed of both lymphocytes and epithelial cells. Thymic neoplasms are a common cause of anterior mediastinal masses. Thymomas and thymic carcinomas arise from epithelial elements within the thymus. Primary mediastinal (thymic) large B-cell lymphoma arises from B-cells within the thymus and T-cell lymphoblastic lymphomas arise from T-cells within the thymus.

Thymomas are the second most common primary mediastinal neoplasm in adults following lymphoma and are classified on a histologic spectrum from thymoma to thymic carcinoma. Once thymomas extend through the capsule, they can invade other regional structures, including the lungs and great vessels, sometimes rendering them inoperable. The thymus gland lies within the pleural envelope. The most common pattern of spread is within the pleural and pericardial spaces. Lymphatic and hematogenous metastases are rare.

Oncologic Imaging
Non–Small Cell Lung Cancer

Treatment decisions are often predicated on the status of the mediastinum in patients with operable NSCLC. Patients with operable disease, without mediastinal involvement, generally proceed directly to resection, whereas those with mediastinal lymph node involvement typically receive induction therapy or definitive chemoradiotherapy. The historical noninvasive staging tool has been CT. In general, the sensitivity and specificity of CT are less than optimal with a false-positive rate of approximately 40% and a false-negative rate of 20%[80–82] (Table 35.6). Thus, mediastinoscopy or endobronchial ultrasound (EBUS) is often utilized to pathologically stage the mediastinum. These procedures are associated with a low rate of morbidity. Nevertheless, if noninvasive studies prove to be highly accurate, invasive mediastinal staging might be avoided in some patients.

Numerous studies and meta-analyses[80–82,88,89] have assessed the ability of CT, PET, and integrated PET-CT to accurately stage the mediastinum in patients with NSCLC (see Table 35.6). Although significant heterogeneity exists among the individual studies, several conclusions can be drawn. First, the positive predictive value of CT is poor (around 50%). PET and PET-CT are somewhat better (80% to 90%). Still, 10% to 20% of patients with PET abnormalities in the mediastinum will have no evidence of disease at mediastinoscopy, although insufficient sampling may be explanatory in some cases. Therefore, many still advocate mediastinoscopy in the setting of a positive PET. The negative predictive value of PET

TABLE 35.6 "ACCURACY" OF COMPUTED TOMOGRAPHY AND POSITRON EMISSION TOMOGRAPHY FOR MEDIASTINAL STAGING OF NON–SMALL CELL LUNG CANCER					
End Point	**Toloza et al.**[83]	**Gould et al.**[84]	**Dwamena et al.**[85]	**Darling et al.**[86] **(%)**	**Bille et al.**[87] **(%)**
Computed Tomography (CT)					
Sensitivity	0.57	0.61	0.60		
Specificity	0.82	0.79	0.77		
Positive predictive value	0.56		0.50		
Negative predictive value	0.83		0.85		
Positron Emission Tomography (PET)					
Sensitivity	0.84	0.85	0.79		
Specificity	0.89	0.90	0.91		
Positive predictive value	0.79		0.90		
Negative predictive value	0.93		0.93		
Positron Emission Tomography/Computed Tomography (PET/CT)					
Sensitivity				70	54
Specificity				94	92
Positive predictive value				64	74
Negative predictive value				95	82

and PET-CT appears to be better, especially when there are no enlarged lymph nodes visible on CT.[90] Nonetheless, most guidelines recommend invasive mediastinal staging prior to resection given the inherent limitations of PET.

Localization of the esophagus is important during treatment planning of lung cancer. The esophagus is often well visualized on CT. However, its course can be tortuous and its exact location is often uncertain. Having the patient swallow dilute contrast during the planning CT can assist in localization of the esophagus. The heart and spinal canal (as a surrogate for the spinal cord) are also well seen on CT. The substructures of the heart, however, are often challenging to define on CT. If one were to try to preferentially spare or consider the dose to cardiac substructures, an MRI or nuclear medicine cardiac image might provide additional information.

Esophageal Carcinoma

The most commonly used staging tools for esophageal carcinoma are barium swallow, EUS, CT, and PET. EUS, as previously discussed, is the most accurate modality to assess depth of invasion (T stage) but is less accurate in assessing nodal involvement (N stage) (Fig. 35.9). The ability to perform fine-needle aspiration biopsies of suspicious nodes, primarily disease in the celiac axis, has increased the ability of EUS to stage regional nodes. The reported accuracy of EUS for T and N stage is approximately 85% to 90% and 75%, respectively.[91,92] CT is primarily used to assess for metastatic disease. It is fairly unreliable in predicting T or N stage. The optimal role of PET in esophageal cancer staging is undefined, but it is generally used to evaluate for local or regional nodal disease and distant metastases. However, the sensitivity of PET for local or regional nodal disease does not appear to be superior to EUS.[93] PET may be most helpful in detecting distant metastases and differentiating patients who have residual disease after neoadjuvant chemoradiotherapy, requiring surgical resection, from those who are complete responders and may be spared the morbidity of surgery.[94]

Mesothelioma

CT best evaluates suspected mesothelioma for initial diagnosis and surgical planning. The characteristic CT appearance is focal or diffuse nodular pleural thickening, which

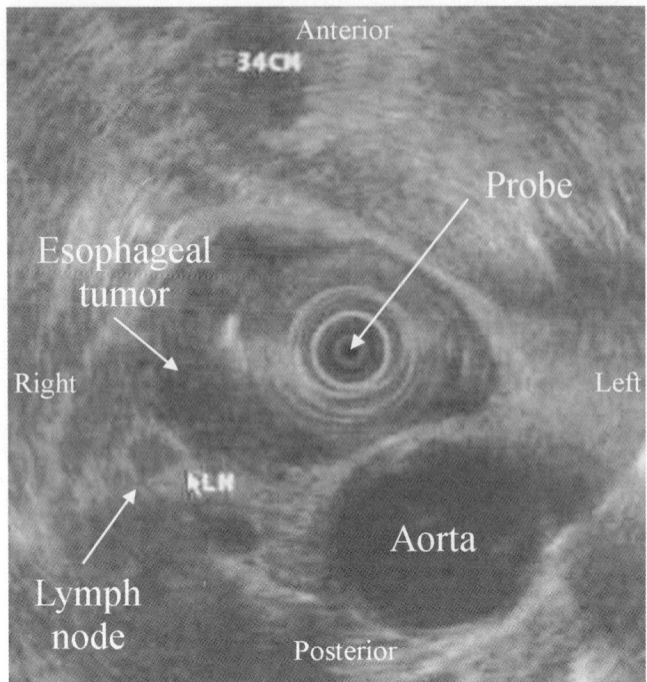

FIGURE 35.9. Endoscopic ultrasound image demonstrating a T3 esophageal tumor with an abnormal peritumoral lymph node. (Image courtesy of Dr. Frank Gress.)

demonstrates enhancement post contrast administration.[95] MRI is not routinely used in the diagnosis of mesothelioma but is a complementary modality with better sensitivity than CT for depicting chest wall, diaphragmatic, and pericardial invasion.[96] PET is often performed for staging to detect distant and nodal metastases. However, it can also be helpful in establishing the initial diagnosis when CT findings are subtle, as even small foci of disease are typically highly FDG-avid.

Superior Sulcus

Superior sulcus tumors are NSCLCs that arise in the apex of the lungs and invade surrounding structures such as the chest wall, vertebral bodies, and/or brachial plexus. Imaging plays a crucial role in the diagnosis and staging of superior sulcus tumors including CT, MRI, and/or PET-CT. CT is best to define the primary tumor and detect rib or vertebral body invasion. CT may also identify suspicious pulmonary nodules that may be below the threshold for PET detection. Contrast-enhanced MRI using T1-weighted sequences is best for determining resectability by assessing the brachial plexus.[97] The primary role of PET is to identify distant and nodal metastases.

Thymic Malignancy

Thymic neoplasms often go undetected until they are quite large and become symptomatic, at which time they may be depicted as a mediastinal mass on chest radiography. The role of imaging is to diagnose and stage patients. With respect to thymoma, this involves detecting local invasion and distant disease, thereby identifying patients who may benefit from neoadjuvant therapy prior to resection (e.g. Masaoka stage III or IV). Contrast-enhanced CT is best for characterizing thymomas and detecting local invasion. High-grade tumors tend to be larger in size, have irregular margins, enhance heterogeneously, and have regions of necrosis; mediastinal lymphadenopathy may also be present. Direct invasion into the pleura, pericardium, and vessels is often difficult to detect by CT unless extensive. A preserved fat plane between tumor and adjacent structures is a negative predictor of invasion; however, this finding has poor positive predictive value.[98]

Therefore, mere contiguity of tumor with a structure or loss of normal anatomic planes is not sufficient to preclude surgical resection. CT features that have been correlated with stage III or greater disease include primary tumor size 7 cm or larger, lobulated margins, and infiltrative changes of the mediastinal fat surrounding the mass.[99]

THE BREAST

Oncologic Anatomy

Breasts are present in both males and females, although they are only well developed in the latter with the onset of puberty. In the male, generally only a few ducts are present, which nonetheless can rarely develop into malignancy, particularly in the context of *BRCA2* mutations.[100] In the female, the breast originates from a roughly circular base or bed extending from the lateral border of the sternum to the midaxillary line from medial to lateral and from the second through sixth ribs superior to inferior. The upper outer quadrant extends along the pectoralis major toward the axilla, forming the axillary tail of Spence. This is also the most frequent quadrant for primary breast cancer (~40%), which may be simply due to the additional breast tissue associated with the tail.[101] Just posterior to the breast is the retromammary space, consisting of loose connective tissue, allowing for movement on the breast on the chest wall. Two-thirds of the breast rests on the deep pectoral fascia, which lies over the pectoralis major; the remainder rests on the fascia of the serratus anterior.

The breast tissue consists of lactiferous ducts that each drain 15 to 20 mammary gland lobules, and it is these ducts that are the origin of the majority of both noninvasive (ductal carcinoma *in situ*) and invasive disease (invasive ductal carcinoma). The breast is then anchored to the skin by suspensory ligaments (or Cooper ligaments) and interspersed with fat lobules. These ligamentous attachments to the skin become more prominent with breast edema or congestion due to tumor involving the dermal lymphatics, resulting in the characteristic appearance of peau d'orange.

The lymphatic drainage of the breast is primarily to the axilla, although the upper outer quadrant may drain to the intermediary intrapectoral nodes (or Rotter nodes) lying between the pectoralis major and pectoralis minor muscles, and the inner quadrants may drain to the internal mammary nodes (IMN). The axilla is divided into three sections with relation to the pectoralis minor muscle; the nodes found inferolateral to the muscle are termed level I, those beneath the muscle are termed level II, and those medial to the muscle are level III. Level I and II are generally removed in a standard axillary dissection, whereas the level III and the subsequent infraclavicular and supraclavicular basins are generally not considered resectable and are the target of radiotherapy if the more proximal basins have disease.

In a study of the location of sentinel nodes from various breast quadrants, the majority of drainage in all breast quadrants was to the axilla, and isolated drainage to the IMN was very rare (<6% in any quadrant).[102] However, identification of an additional IMN sentinel was found in 10% to 50% of cases dependent on quadrant (the upper outer quadrant was lowest at 10%, and the lower inner quadrant was most frequent at 52%). In surgical series in which the IMNs were routinely dissected, the incidence of isolated IMN disease was limited to 5% to 15%.[103–105] The risk of involvement increased when the axilla was also involved (20% to 55%), dependent on the axillary disease burden and location of the involved quadrant of the breast (Table 35.7). When IMNs were involved, the majority were located in the first three intercostal interspaces (first interspace 80%, second 75%, third 40%, and fourth 5%).[105] A margin of 4 mm medially and laterally to the internal mammary vessels encompasses the 90% of nodes in this region and

TABLE 35.7 RISK OF INTERNAL MAMMARY LYMPH NODE INVOLVEMENT BASED ON STATUS OF AXILLA AND LOCATION WITHIN THE BREAST

Scenario	Livingston and Arlen[106] (%)	Urban and Marjani[107] (%)	Noguchi et al.[108] (%)
Negative axilla	8	8	5
Outer quadrant primary	5	10	ns
Medial/central primary	14	16	ns
Positive axilla	33	52	35
Outer quadrant primary	23	43	ns
Medial/central primary	48	55	ns
1–3 + axillary nodes	ns	ns	20
≥4 + axillary nodes	ns	ns	52

ns, not stated.

may be a reasonable CTV for treatment.[109] That stated, irradiation of the IMN nodes remains controversial, though recent randomized data has found a modest benefit in terms of disease-free and cancer-specific survival when IMN and medial supraclavicular fields are treated.[110,111]

Oncologic Imaging

Mammography remains the preferred imaging modality for the diagnosis and follow-up of both invasive and noninvasive disease. Multiple randomized trials have shown that screening mammography reduces the risk of breast cancer mortality by 20% to 35% in women aged 50 to 69.[112–115] The efficacy of screening in younger women (aged 40 to 49) and elderly women (aged 70 or older) is less certain. Most published guidelines suggest initiating screening at age 40. Screening mammography includes two standard views of each breast: a craniocaudal (CC) view and a mediolateral oblique (MLO) view. These images are taken at approximately 45-degree angulation to each other (i.e., they are not orthogonal). Although the CC view is oriented in the long axis of the patient (i.e., superior/inferior), the MLO is oriented in the medial-superior/lateral-inferior direction. The MLO view increases visualization of the upper outer quadrant and tail of the breast, whereas the CC view ensures adequate visualization of the inferior and medial aspects of the breast. Additional views, such as spot compression, can be utilized to further evaluate suspicious lesions.

The majority of women (~95%) with abnormalities on a screening mammogram do not have breast cancer; thus, the positive predictive value is low. Overall, the sensitivity of screening mammography is approximately 75% (i.e., 25% of women diagnosed with breast cancer have a history of a normal mammogram 12 to 24 months prior to diagnosis). Sensitivity and specificity vary widely depending on breast density; for fatty versus dense fibroglandular breasts, reported sensitivities are 87% versus 63%, whereas specificities are 92% versus 68%, respectively.[116–118] Furthermore, sensitivity and specificity differ between screen-film versus digital mammography, with digital systems generally having higher diagnostic accuracy in women with dense breast tissue compared to film mammography.[119]

Systematic interpretation and unambiguous reporting is important for any screening study. Given the prevalence of breast malignancy and its clinical implications, the Breast Imaging Reporting and Data System (BI-RADS) was developed and constitutes guidelines for standardized reporting and quality assurance of screening mammography within the United States (Table 35.8). Mammographers are ahead of their radiology colleagues in this regard as the BI-RADS system affords a clear unambiguous means of quantifying the "suspiciousness" of mammographic findings. Systems similar to BI-RADS would be helpful for other imaging modalities as a means to reduce the risks of misunderstanding and miscommunication between radiologists and other care providers.

TABLE 35.8 BREAST IMAGING REPORTING AND DATA SYSTEM (BIRADS) CATEGORIES USED FOR MAMMOGRAPHY EXAMINATIONS AND RISK OF MALIGNANCY

Assessment Category	Assessment	Definition	Risk of Malignancy
0	Need additional imaging evaluation	A lesion is noted for which additional imaging is needed	n/a
1	Negative	Breasts appear normal	<0.1%
2	Benign finding	A negative mammogram result but the radiologist wishes to describe a finding	<0.1%
3	Probably benign finding; short-interval follow-up suggested	Lesion with a high probability of being benign	<2%
4	Suspicious abnormality—biopsy should be considered	A lesion is noted for which the radiologist has sufficient concern to recommend a biopsy	25%–50%
5	Highly suggestive of malignancy	A lesion is noted that has a high probability of being cancer	75%–99%

n/a, not available.

Features of concern for malignancy at mammography include a focal mass, irregular borders, and microcalcifications. Spiculation can be due to invasion into, or reactive changes within, the surrounding breast parenchyma. However, spiculated masses can also be secondary to fat necrosis, postoperative scarring, or other nonmalignant processes. Calcifications associated with ductal carcinoma *in situ* or invasive carcinoma are typically pleomorphic (heterogeneous) in appearance and clustered in a localized area (Fig. 35.10). Linear, branching calcifications are suggestive of intraductal carcinoma. Round, well-circumscribed lesions, with or without coarse calcifications, are often benign.

FIGURE 35.10. Clustered, pleomorphic calcifications visualized on mammography. The patient was found to have ductal carcinoma *in situ*.

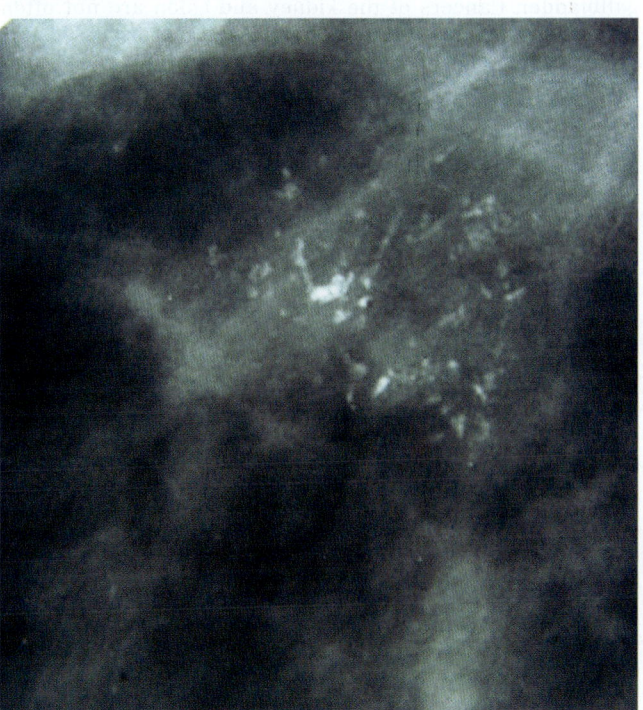

Section II

Abnormalities on screening mammogram are generally followed with a diagnostic mammogram, in which supplemental and magnified views may be obtained to detect and characterize microcalcifications. Breast US is often performed to further characterize suspicious lesions, guide core biopsy, and assess regional lymph nodes. It is most helpful in differentiating fluid-filled cysts from solid tumors. MRI is not routinely recommended for upfront screening, except in patients with dense breast tissue and those at very high risk for primary breast malignancy, including those with *BRCA* mutations or women who received chest radiation therapy at a young age (typically <30 years old).[120] In addition to T1 and T2 lesion characteristics, patterns of MRI enhancement and washout kinetics are beneficial in evaluating concerning lesions. MRI can also be used for biopsy image guidance. After biopsy confirmation of disease, MRI has been examined in an attempt to better diagnose multifocal or contralateral disease preoperatively. One trial found contralateral cancers on MRI in 3% of their cohort, at the cost of performing a biopsy in 12%.[121] Preoperative MRI, however, did not improve the requirement for reoperation in a randomized UK trial.[122] The only clinically relevant outcome that routine use of preoperative MRI appears to have changed is that more women are having mastectomies as opposed to breast conservation.[123]

Digital tomosynthesis is a method of generating three-dimensional breast imaging from several planar x-ray images taken at differing angles. It is distinct from CT in that the resolution is much higher, consistent with conventional mammography, the images are not taken in axial sections, and only a limited rotational angle is utilized. Generally, digital tomosynthesis appears to result in higher cancer detection rates, with fewer false positives, as it allows for distinguishing overlapping lesions, that may confound planar imaging.[124] As such, it is beginning to supplement screening for high-risk individuals, particularly those in follow-up after radiation treatment.[125]

THE ABDOMEN

Oncologic Anatomy

Many diverse malignancies arise from abdominal structures. The most common are epithelial cancers of the stomach, pancreas, colon, liver, kidney, and biliary tract, including the gallbladder. Cancers of the kidney and colon are not often managed with radiation therapy and are not discussed further. Several relevant anatomical issues include (a) site-specific patterns of lymphatic spread for gastric cancer, (b) local disease extension of pancreatic cancer rendering a tumor inoperable, and (c) anatomy of the biliary tree.

Gastric Cancer: Patterns of Lymphatic Spread

The stomach is a distensible organ located in the left upper abdomen. It is classically divided into four parts: the gastroesophageal junction (cardia), fundus, body, and pylorus (antrum). Although the incidence of epithelial malignancies of the distal stomach has declined in Western countries over the past century, the incidence of malignancies of the gastroesophageal junction is increasing. Lymph node involvement is common in gastric cancer, likely because of the extensive submucosal and subserosal lymphatic networks. This rich lymphatic network places all lymph node regions within the abdomen at risk of harboring regional metastases, irrespective of the part of the stomach involved. However, some general patterns have been observed, which can facilitate rational radiation treatment planning for gastric cancer.

For tumors within the stomach, the perigastric region located along the greater and lesser curvatures of the stomach are typically the initial draining lymph node basin. The other primary lymph node regions are those along the three arterial branches of the celiac axis (common hepatic, left gastric,

splenic). Secondary and tertiary drainage sites include lymph nodes in the hepatoduodenal, peripancreatic, para-aortic, mesenteric, and middle colic region.

A large surgical series from Japan demonstrated that the most common site of lymph node involvement was along the lesser and greater curvature (perigastrics), regardless of the part of the stomach involved (11% to 40%).[126] As expected, lymph node involvement around the cardia was unusual for distal stomach tumors (0% to 7%) but common for proximal tumors (13% to 31%). Similarly, infrapyloric lymph nodes were commonly involved for distant gastric cancers (49%) but rare for proximal tumors (3%). Other common sites of lymph node involvement included those along the left gastric artery (19% to 23%), common hepatic artery (7% to 25%, greatest for distal tumors), and celiac axis (8% to 13%). The risk of splenic hilar involvement has varied among surgical series but is generally highest for proximal tumors.[127,128] Based on these and other data, guidelines have been published outlining proposed radiation fields for gastric cancer based on site of involvement within the stomach.[129,130]

Pancreas

The pancreas is an elongated digestive gland posterior to the stomach. It is classically divided into four parts: the head, neck, body, and tail. The pancreatic head is nestled within the curve of the duodenum and this is where most pancreatic carcinomas arise. The pancreas has a rich lymphatic network and is in close proximity to multiple other abdominal organs and structures, making surgical resection difficult and negatively affecting long-term cure rates (resectability is the most important prognostic factor).

Biliary Tree

Hepatocytes within the liver secrete bile (an important agent for digestion) into bile canaliculi, the initial branches of the intrahepatic duct system. These canaliculi drain bile into larger and larger channels that eventually become the left and right hepatic ducts, draining bile from the left and right lobes of the liver, respectively. These exit the liver from the porta hepatis and join to form the common hepatic duct (~4 cm in length). The cystic duct joins the common hepatic duct to form the common bile duct (~10 cm in length). The common bile duct extends to, and empties into, the duodenum. It lies alongside the hepatic artery and portal vein.

Biliary tract cancers include adenocarcinomas of the gallbladder and bile ducts, the latter referred to as cholangiocarcinomas. Cholangiocarcinomas include intrahepatic, perihilar, and distant extrahepatic biliary malignancies. Klatskin tumors are perihilar tumors that involve the bifurcation of the common hepatic duct. Both resectability and prognosis increase for more distally located biliary tumors.

Oncologic Imaging
Pancreatic Cancer

The pancreas can be imaged with US, CT, and MRI. MDCT with IV contrast and thin-section reconstructions optimize pancreatic tissue characterization and allow for detection of small tumors as well as vascular and ductal invasion. CT also defines the surgical anatomy to determine resectability and can detect regional and distant metastases (Fig. 35.11).

Adenocarcinoma of the pancreas most frequently arises in the head of the gland, to the right of the superior mesenteric or portal vein. It usually appears as a hypodense mass relative to the normally enhancing pancreas. Surgical resection typically provides the only chance of cure, and CT with thin-section reconstructions and IV contrast enhancement is an important technique to assess resectability. Encasement of the superior mesenteric artery (SMA) or celiac trunk defines an unresectable T4 tumor. On the other hand, the presence

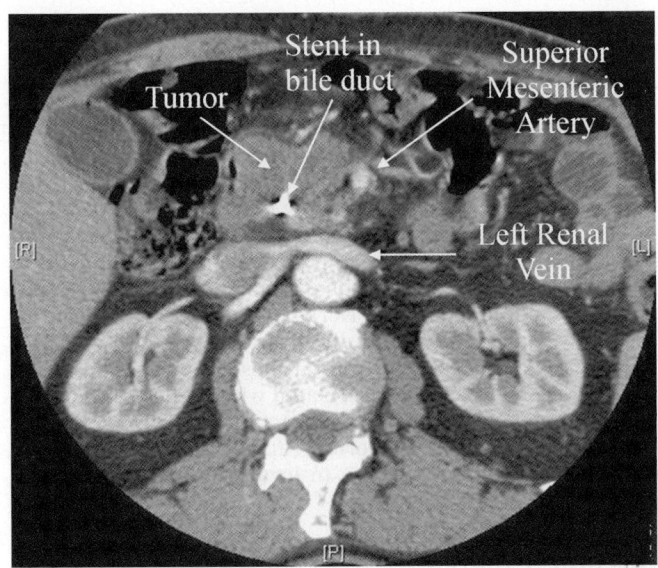

FIGURE 35.11. Axial computed tomography image demonstrating an adenocarcinoma of the pancreatic head with tumor abutting the superior mesenteric artery.

of a fat plane around the celiac trunk and SMA, along with a patent superior mesenteric or portal vein, defines potentially resectable disease. Borderline cases include those with tumor abutment on the SMA, severe unilateral superior mesenteric vein (SMV) or portal vein impingement, or adjacent organ invasion. CT does not, however, detect small volume peritoneal or surface liver metastases that can be identified with laparoscopy. Oral contrast during radiation planning scans can be helpful to define the stomach and duodenum. MRI may be performed when CT findings are equivocal or there is a contraindication to administering iodinated contrast; however, there is no diagnostic advantage of MRI over contrast-enhanced CT (sensitivity of 84% vs. 86%, respectively).[131] The role of FDG-PET for pancreatic cancer diagnosis and staging remains uncertain and is not routinely performed.

Hepatic Imaging

MDCT with IV contrast allows for morphologic characterization of the liver and biliary system. The administration of IV contrast is essential as many hepatic tumors are of similar attenuation as normal liver parenchyma and are not identifiable until central necrosis is present. MDCT with contrast is performed in both arterial and portal-venous phases of enhancement. This allows for detection of both early- and late-enhancing lesions, as well as characterization of enhancement patterns that can differentiate between benign and malignant disease. For example, hemangiomas are classically low attenuating on noncontrast images, have peripheral enhancement on the arterial phase, and demonstrate central filling on portal-venous phase imaging. Hepatocellular carcinoma is the most common primary hepatic malignancy and is characteristically hypervascular with pronounced enhancement throughout the solid tumor components on arterial phase images and diminished enhancement on the portal-venous phase. Contrast-enhanced CT can also identify invasion of tumor into the portal and hepatic veins and is frequently associated with portal vein thrombosis. As with other malignancies, PET is recommended for staging and identification of extrahepatic disease.

The liver is one of the most common sites of metastatic disease for many cancers. In patients with a known extrahepatic primary malignancy, evaluation of the liver is an important part of staging. Contrast-enhanced CT has a high sensitivity (73%) and specificity (96%) for detecting hepatic metastases.[132] MDCT of the liver for metastatic disease is typically performed with biphasic technique. Although most metastases are identified on the portal-venous phase, some hypervascular tumors (e.g., melanoma, renal cell carcinoma) may only be identified on arterial phase imaging. MRI has similar accuracy for the diagnosis of hepatic metastases as CT and may be performed in patients with an allergy to iodinated contrast media. However, CT outperforms MRI in detecting extrahepatic lesions, particularly within the lungs.

Biliary Imaging

US is typically the initial imaging study for patients with suspected biliary or pancreatic disease. The primary goals of evaluation include assessment for biliary and pancreatic ductal dilatation (abnormal is >3 mm), identify the presence of stones, characterize the gallbladder wall, and exclude a pancreatic head mass. US does not, however, image the entire pancreatic and biliary ductal system. In the presence of an US abnormality, further imaging is required.

Endoscopic retrograde cholangiopancreatography (ERCP) is a minimally invasive procedure that involves passing an endoscope into the duodenum and cannulating the main bile duct at the ampulla of Vater. Contrast is then infused to image both the biliary and pancreatic ductal system. In addition to being minimally invasive, ERCP carries risks associated with conscious sedation and can induce pancreatitis in 1.3% to 8.6% of patients.[133] Any evidence of biliary obstruction in the absence of calculi typically prompts further evaluation with cross-sectional imaging to exclude malignancy. ERCP can directly visualize ampullary carcinomas and permits tissue diagnosis achieved using needle aspiration, brush cytology, or forceps biopsy. ERCP may also provide palliation via stent placement in the setting of known obstructive biliary malignancy.

Magnetic resonance cholangiopancreatography (MRCP) is a noninvasive method of imaging the intra- and extrahepatic biliary and pancreatic ducts. MRCP does not require IV contrast; imaging relies heavily on T2-weighted sequences and high-resolution techniques resulting in the pancreatic and biliary ducts appearing very bright while surrounding tissues are dark in signal.[134] MRCP and ERCP have similar sensitivities and specificities in detecting ductal obstruction in the setting of malignancy, although MRCP is better at defining the anatomical extent and type of tumor involved (pancreatic vs. cholangiocarcinoma).[135,136]

Normal Tissue

During RT planning for cancers of the upper abdomen, consideration of the dose to the kidneys may be important. The kidneys are well visualized on CT. However, regional differences in kidney function cannot be readily assessed on CT. Nuclear medicine renal scans provide quantitative information regarding delivery of fluid into the kidneys from the bloodstream, concentration of wastes in the kidney, and excretion from the kidneys into the ureters and filling of the bladder. This information is useful when significant portions of one or both kidneys will be exposed to doses of RT expected to cause regional dysfunction. The liver, stomach, and small bowel are other organs whose location is often important to consider during RT planning. These are usually well seen on CT, although the use of oral contrast can be helpful.

THE PELVIC LYMPH NODES

Oncologic Anatomy

The lymphatic drainage of pelvic organs follows the iliac vessels throughout their branching within the pelvis. Most superiorly within the pelvis, the common iliac chains receive the majority of lymph drainage from intrapelvic organs, which then empty to the para-aortic chains superiorly in the region of the bifurcation of the abdominal aorta. The gonadal veins and arteries are notable exceptions to this orderly flow of lymph from the pelvis and are discussed separately below. Also of note, the rectum, sigmoid, and distal colon have a separate path for lymphatic metastasis via the inferior mesenteric chain to the preaortic basin.

The common iliac pathway receives lymphatic drainage from three primary routes: the external iliac chain, the internal iliac chain, and the presacral chain. The external iliac pathway begins at the point where the femoral vessels cross the inguinal ligament to become the external iliac chains, which courses more proximally to the common bifurcation. The internal iliac chain (also termed the hypogastric chain) is a more complex plexus, flowing back from the distal elaborations of the same artery. Just as these branches of the internal iliac vessels provide blood supply for the pelvic organs, the corresponding lymph node chains provide the majority of lymph drainage. The obturator nodes are part of the internal iliac system and may be found at the point in which the obturator vessels perforate the obturator internus muscle. Radiographically these nodes lay medial to the femoral head, just superior to the bony obturator foramen. The presacral chain is located just anterior to the sacrum and receives lymphatic drainage from the rectum, the cervix, and posterior vagina in the female and the prostate in the male.[137,138]

The testicles have an interesting lymphatic drainage that differs with laterality, essentially mirroring the differences in venous drainage of the two testicles. On the right, the testicle drains into the para-aortic nodes along the lower portion of the inferior vena cava at about the level of L3-L4 following the left testicular vein. On the left, the testicle drains to the renal hilar nodes following the left testicular vein.

Oncologic Imaging

CT is the current preferred means of identifying vessels within the pelvis and is an acceptable method of delineating the pelvic lymph node basins for elective radiotherapy. A 7-mm margin may be applied to the internal and external iliac vessels to arrive at a nodal CTV, with uninvolved bone, muscle (such as the psoas), and bowel excluded from the volume. The 7-mm margin was developed by investigators in London, who determined the minimum margin on CT visible vessels needed to cover 95% of all nodes identified using ultrasmall iron oxide particles (USPIO) as an MRI contrast agent.[139,140] Special care, however, should be taken to include visualized lymph nodes, even if they lie outside of this margin.

Symmetric expansion margins on vessels are not, however, adequate in the para-aortic regions or the inguinals. In the para-aortic region, the most common location for nodal involvement includes region to the left of the aorta, a basin that extends to the medial margin of the psoas muscle.[141] This region is frequently inadequately covered by a symmetric expansion. Similarly in the inguinal region, nodes lie medial to the femoral neurovascular bundle, often at a distance ≥2 cm. In this region, the space bounded by the regional musculature is the preferred CTV volume.[142]

One centimeter of soft tissue anterior to the sacrum, bridging between the common and internal nodal CTVs, should be added when presacral coverage is desired. The Radiation Therapy Oncology Group has release several atlases to aid the clinician in the contouring of pelvic CTVs that are available at its website. With 3D CT imaging, bony landmarks may not be the ideal determinant of block or multileaf collimator shapes when treating the pelvis.[143,144]

THE RECTUM
Oncologic Anatomy

The rectum is the final, straight portion of the large bowel, measuring approximately 12 cm in length, beginning at the transition from the sigmoid colon with the fusion of the tenia

into the circumferential longitudinal muscle. It terminates with the ampulla, leading to the anal canal and dentate (or pectinate) line. Posteriorly, the entire rectum is extraperitoneal, whereas anteriorly, the peritoneal reflection occurs at approximately 7 to 9 cm from the anal verge in males at the posterior aspect of the bladder (superior to the prostate) and 5 to 8 cm from the verge in females, forming the rectouterine pouch (or pouch of Douglas). Below this point, the distal third of the rectum is entirely extraperitoneal.

The mesorectum is the supportive mesentery of the rectum, lying in the extraperitoneal space between the rectum anteriorly and sacrum posteriorly. It is of critical importance as a potential area of both direct and lymphatic spread of rectal cancers. High-quality total mesorectal excision with sharp dissection has been associated with excellent local control when compared to blunt dissections. However, this has not obviated the need for perioperative radiation therapy, as demonstrated by an increase in local recurrences if this is omitted.[145-147]

Oncologic Imaging

Endorectal US is the preferred nonsurgical staging tool for determining the T stage of rectal malignancy, with an overall accuracy of approximately 85% to 90%.[148] US is probably not needed in cases where there is a large mass with clear extension into the deep portions of the wall (or surrounding tissues) based on CT or examination. There is some tendency to overstage T2 lesions as T3 (beyond the muscularis propria); however, the accuracy remains superior to other imaging modalities.[149] The nodal staging accuracy is somewhat less at approximately 80%, which is comparable to results with either MRI or CT. Accurate staging is critical when determining treatment for rectal cancer. Although surgery alone is sufficient for patients with stage I disease, surgery and chemoradiotherapy are indicated for patients with stage II or III tumors. The German Rectal Cancer Study Group showed that preoperative chemoradiotherapy is associated with improved local control with less acute and late toxicity than postoperative chemoradiotherapy.[150] In this study, 18% of patients in the immediate surgery group, believed to have stage II or III disease by EUS, were found to have stage I disease after surgical resection. Thus, further improvements in preoperative staging are needed to appropriately select patients for neoadjuvant therapy.

THE BLADDER AND URETHRA
Oncologic Anatomy

The bladder is a distensible muscular organ, which may be contained completely within the pelvis when empty or may extend far into the abdominal cavity with distention. The trigone is the posterior and inferior portion of the bladder, defined by the two ureteral orifices posteriorly and the urethral orifice inferiorly. The trigone remains fixed at the base with distension, while the superior most surface expands to accommodate urine. Because of this distensibility, this bladder is surrounded by loose connective tissue and fat. Anterior to the bladder, this loose connective tissue is termed the space of Retzius or retropubic space.

The urethra inferiorly has a short course to the introitus in the female, measuring approximately 4 to 5 cm in length. In the male, it is approximately 20 cm in length and traverses the prostate and penis to the meatus.

The lymphatic drainage of the base and posterior wall of the bladder may preferentially drain to the obturator and internal iliac basins via anterior pathways. In contrast, the external iliac chain may receive primary drainage from the lateral and superior bladder wall, and tumors arising from the bladder neck may also spread to the presacral nodal basins.

Oncologic Imaging

Bladder tumors are often inadequately evaluated with conventional imaging techniques such as radiographic IV urograms and US. CT urography is useful for the diagnosis of superficial tumors but provides limited visualization of the depth of tumor invasion within the bladder wall. PET has limited utility in the primary diagnosis because of urinary excretion of FDG that can obscure bladder disease. Notwithstanding, PET is still performed as part of staging in order to identify distant metastases. Given the imaging limitations, cystoscopy with biopsy is the preferred method of confirming diagnosis and characterizing the primary tumor stage. Regional nodal involvement is best initially characterized by contrast-enhanced CT; however, the role of MRI is evolving, particularly for evaluation of lymph nodes utilizing novel contrast agents including USPIO.[151]

CERVIX, UTERUS, AND OVARIES

Oncologic Anatomy

The uterus lies between the bladder anteriorly and the rectum posteriorly, covered by a layer of peritoneum. Laterally lie the fallopian tubes and ovaries, which are anchored medially by the ovarian ligament (or utero-ovarian ligament) and laterally by the suspensory ligament of the ovary (or infundibulopelvic [IP] ligament). The ovarian arteries originate from the abdominal aorta, just inferior to the renal vessels, following a course anterior to the psoas on the left and crossing anterior to the inferior vena cava to the psoas on the right, both sides crossing anterior to the ureter and then crossing medially with the IP ligament to the ovaries. The fold of the peritoneum over the uterus continues laterally over these structures, forming the broad ligament. Similar to the testes, the right ovarian vein drains to the inferior vena cava, whereas the left ovary drains to the left renal vein.

The uterine corpus or body is the cephalad two-thirds of the organ and is lined internally by the endometrium, which varies in thickness by the menstrual cycle and by menopausal status. The middle muscular layer, the myometrium, is primarily smooth muscle. The final outer layer is the serosa or perimetrium and is continuous with the peritoneum. The caudal one-third of the organ is the uterine cervix, which consists of firm connective tissue, approximately one-half of which extends into the vagina. The intravaginal portion is lined by nonkeratinized squamous epithelium (the ectocervix), whereas the cervical canal is lined by columnar epithelium (the endocervix).

Lateral to the uterine cervix and corpus is the parametrium that caudally consists of the paracervical tissue, including the cardinal ligament, uterine artery and vein, and the ureter as it courses anteriorly to the bladder. This caudal portion of the parametrium is of importance for evaluation of lateral spread of cervical cancer and can be staged on physical examination by the bimanual examination and, perhaps more importantly, with the rectovaginal examination, where the examining rectal finger can palpate these structures. Cephalad to this, the parametrium continues as the broad ligament, terminating at the suspensory ligament of the ovary. Posteriorly the cervix is anchored to the sacrum via the uterosacral ligament, which classically attaches at the third sacral foramen, although MRI studies would suggest a fair amount of individual variation.[152]

Oncologic Imaging

MRI of the pelvis is the most useful modality outside of the physical examination to determine the extent of disease within the uterus and cervix with an accuracy of approximately 85%.[153,154] For endometrial carcinoma, T2- and post-contrast T1-weighted sequences are beneficial in staging, such as identifying the primary tumor, extent of invasion, and

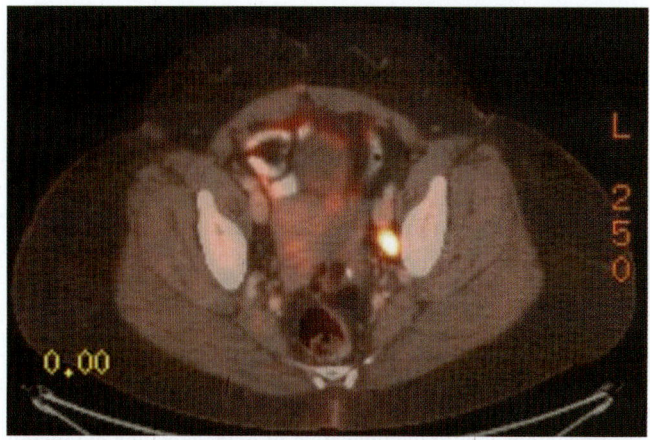

FIGURE 35.12. Positron emission tomography imaging of a patient with cervical cancer showing an 18-fluorodeoxyglucose-avid left external iliac lymph node.

involvement of regional pelvic lymph nodes. In the setting of cervical cancer, T2-weighted sequences are often the most useful in determining the extent of disease and are preferred for MRI-guided brachytherapy.[155] Either CT or MRI may be used for image-guided brachytherapy to potentially improve central disease control and reduce toxicity. However, CT systematically provides larger estimates of target size compared to MRI, particularly in the lateral extent.[156,157] US can be useful during intracavitary brachytherapy to ensure the proper placement of a uterine tandem and prevent uterine perforation.

PET-CT has been proven to be sensitive and specific in the evaluation of lymph nodes within the pelvic and para-aortic chains with squamous cell carcinoma of the cervix (sensitivity ~85%, and specificity 95% for para-aortic nodes), although it is less well studied in endometrial and other primary gynecologic sites[158] (Fig. 35.12). Investigators from Washington University have extensively studied FDG-PET in cervical cancer, showing that the initial maximum SUV of the primary tumor is predictive of response to treatment.[159] Additionally, they found that a complete metabolic response to treatment was highly predictive of progression free survival (PFS); at 3 years, with complete response, PFS was 78% versus 33% in partial responders and 0% with PET progression.[160] The prognostic significance of PET response to treatment has been confirmed by investigators in Melbourne.[83]

PROSTATE

Oncologic Anatomy

The prostate lies in the center of the male pelvis, with its widest portion, the base, in close approximation to the bladder neck superiorly, narrowing to the apex inferiorly, supported by the urogenital diaphragm (UGD). Posteriorly, the gland is closely related to the ampulla of the rectum. The seminal vesicles are located superior to the prostate and extend somewhat laterally and posteriorly and are immediately posterior to the posterior wall of the bladder. Anteriorly lies the retropubic space filled with fat.

Within the prostate five distinct zones exist: the peripheral zone, the central zone, the transitional zone, the periurethral glandular tissue, and the anterior fibromuscular stroma.[84] The peripheral zone accounts for the majority of the gland (70% of glandular tissue) as well as the majority of cancers (60% to 70%). The peripheral zone is located posteriorly and laterally within the gland. This zone is hyperintense on T2 MRI and care should be taken to include it when treatment planning with MRI. The central zone accounts for an additional 25% of glandular tissue and lies near the origin of the seminal vesicles, accounting for 10% of cancers. The transitional zone surrounds the urethra cephalad to the insertion of the ejaculatory duct, may hypertrophy with age, and is the origin of 10% to 20% of cancer within the prostate.

The Batson venous plexus is a series of valveless veins anterior to the vertebral bodies that received drainage from the deep pelvic veins and prostate gland.[85,86] It has been postulated that because of the lack of valves, this may represent a pathway of spread for metastases and provide an anatomic basis for the propensity of prostate cancer to involve the lumbosacral vertebral bodies.

The T staging of prostate cancer remains based primarily on the physical examination, where the examining rectal finger may palpate the size and extent of discrete ridges and nodules within the gland. It is important to palpate and document the presence of the lateral sulci of the gland, as evidence of effacement is highly suggestive of extracapsular extension (ECE) of disease. The examiner should also attempt to palpate the base of the seminal vesicles, although this is not always possible given body habitus and individual anatomy.

Oncologic Imaging

Transrectal US is invaluable for guiding biopsies for diagnosis of disease; however, it has limited specificity and sensitivity (~40% to 50%) for determination of seminal vesicle involvement and ECE. CT has similar limitations, as the prostate gland has similar attenuation characteristics as the anterior and lateral venous plexus, the inferior UGD, and the bladder wall superiorly. CT can detect gross extracapsular disease, identify distant metastases, and determine suspicious pelvic nodes and is currently the standard for defining pelvic radiation target volumes, if indicated. If CT alone is used for definition of the prostate for treatment planning, the penile bulb may provide a useful reference point for ascertaining the apex of the gland, which lies approximately 15 to 18 mm superior to the bulb, although there is significant interpatient variation.[87] A retrograde urethrogram can be useful to identify the inferior aspect of the UGD and aid in the delineation of the apex approximately 12 to 15 mm superiorly.

MRI may be the optimal imaging modality for evaluation of the prostate itself and is an invaluable aid in treatment planning. As noted previously, the zonal anatomy of the prostate is only visible on T2-weighted imaging, and the apex can be clearly distinguished from the UGD and other neighboring structures (Fig. 35.13). The joint maximum sensitivity and specificity of determining extraprostatic disease on MRI is approximately 70%, although this may be improved with endorectal coils.[106,107] Because of the increased tissue contrast, planning based on MRI results in a reduction of interobserver variability and a reduction in the volume of the prostate contours.[108] In general, the prostate identified on CT is larger than that identified on MRI. Therefore, with MRI-based treatment planning, the accurate delineation of the GTV is more important (compared to CT where the GTV tends be likely slightly overestimated).

Multiparametric MRI (mpMRI) consists of obtaining multiple T1, T2 weighted conventional sequences, in combination with DWI, DCE, and MR-spectroscopy. Combining the unique characteristics of each of these sequences (discussed in the MRI section above) has led to an increased specificity (>90%) of lesion location both within prostate and in detecting disease extension outside of the capsule.[161,162] As such, this collection of sequences has become useful for directing biopsies and driving treatment decisions and conceivably can be used to direct the purposeful delivery of a heterogeneous RT dose to the prostate gland.

Targeted imaging has long been of interest in prostate cancer, beginning with ProstaScint (Cytogen Corp, Princeton, NJ) imaging, which utilized a radiolabeled monoclonal antibody indium-111 capromab pendetide to identify sites of local

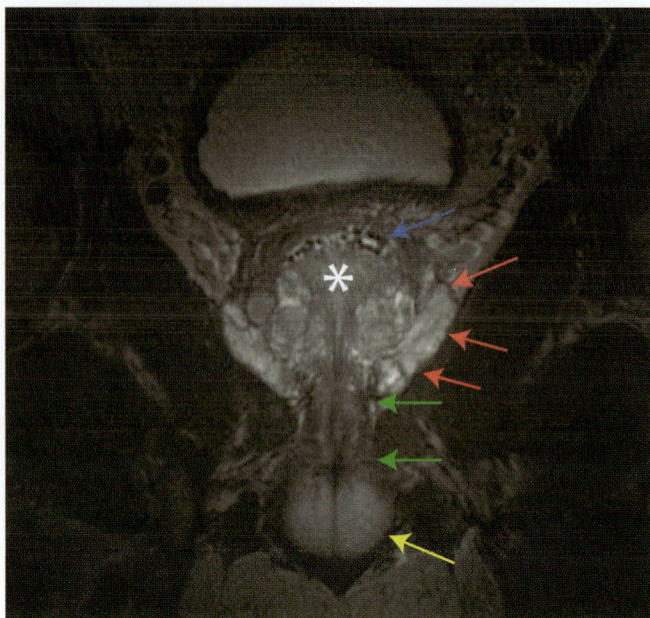

FIGURE 35.13. A coronal T2-weighted magnetic resonance image demonstrating the anatomy of the prostate. The regional anatomy is labeled as follows: the asterisk (*) is the central gland—a combination of the central zone and transitional zone; *red arrows* indicate the peripheral zone (PZ); *blue arrows* indicate the seminal vesicles (SV) and their insertion in the base; *green arrows* indicate the urogenital diaphragm (UGD); *yellow arrows* indicate the penile bulb (PB).

or metastatic disease.[163] Unfortunately, in clinical practice, it was neither sufficiently specific or sensitive to be of significant utility. However, the use of prostate-specific PET radiopharmaceuticals such as choline ^{11}C, fluciclovine ^{18}F, and ^{68}Ga prostate-specific membrane antigen (^{68}Ga-PSMA) have had more success in identifying occult metastatic prostate cancer. ^{68}Ga-PSMA PET in particular has shown promise, with both a sensitivity and specificity of 86%.[164]

Prostate imaging and pathologic analyses can be somewhat discordant. The lesions seen on imaging can often appear focal. However, prostatectomy specimens usually demonstrate the microscopic presence of cancer in multiple regions of the gland. Thus, attempts to severely restrict the therapeutic radiation dose distribution to focal areas of the prostate need to be done with care.

The normal rectum and bladder are commonly avoided structures during pelvic RT, and their location relative to surrounding tissues can be readily determined on planning CT. The interface between the bladder and prostate can be challenging and may be improved with placement of contrast agents within the bladder.

THE LYMPHATIC SYSTEM

Oncologic Anatomy

The lymphatic system is a component of the circulatory system, and wherever arteries and veins pass, lymphatic vessels are also present (with the notable exceptions of the placenta and central nervous system). In the central nervous system, lymph is carried within perivascular lymph sheaths, as opposed to actual lymphatic vessels. The lymphatic system includes lymphatic vessels, lymph nodes, lymphatic organs such as the spleen, and the lymphocytes themselves. The lymphatic system is a loosely organized system but generally follows somewhat predictable paths. Small lymphatic vessels form within the tissues of the body, drain into one or more lymph nodes, and eventually drain into larger lymph trunks. These unite to form either the thoracic duct or right lymphatic duct, which empties into the venous system at the subclavian vein–internal jugular vein junction. The lymphatics are primarily involved in returning plasma from the interstitial space to the venous system, although they are also involved in absorption and transport of fat and in defense mechanisms. Radiation oncologists must become versed in an understanding of site-specific lymphatic spread.

The primary tumors arising from the lymphatic system are leukemias and lymphomas. Leukemias are primarily managed with chemotherapy, although radiation therapy is often utilized in the setting of stem cell transplantation (total body irradiation), central nervous system involvement (cranial or craniospinal irradiation), or in palliative settings. Lymphomas consist of multiple distinct entities that are often managed with chemotherapy and/or radiation therapy.

Oncologic Imaging
Nodal Metastases

The accurate identification and characterization of lymph nodes have important diagnostic, therapeutic, and prognostic implications in patients with cancer. Prior to the advent of cross-sectional imaging, bipedal lymphangiography was the standard test for evaluating and staging nodal disease in the abdomen and pelvis. CT and PET-CT have supplanted lymphangiography.

Lymphoma

The current WHO classification of lymphoid neoplasms consists of nearly a hundred distinct entities.[165] Further, lymphomas can arise virtually anywhere in the body, including both nodal and extranodal sites. Consequently, comprehensive imaging with PET-CT plays an integral role in the staging and management of both HL and many NHL. Current guidelines recommend that PET-CT be employed for initial staging of all lymphomas that are FDG-avid.[166] CT alone is appropriate for the minority that are not, such as chronic lymphocytic leukemia/small lymphocytic lymphoma. Postchemotherapy response assessment with PET-CT is also standard and should utilize the Deauville criteria.[167] A negative (Deauville 1-3) PET-CT scan after chemotherapy does not necessarily mean

that all disease has been eradicated, simply that an excellent response was achieved (Fig. 35.14). This point has been confirmed in randomized trials of HL, where patients were randomized to observation or consolidation RT after achieving a complete response by PET-CT after chemotherapy. Even in the setting of a negative postchemo PET, consolidation RT still decreased the risk of recurrence.[168]

Summary

The term *oncoanatomy* describes the fusion of clinical oncology and anatomy, for the betterment of both. The successful practice of radiation oncology requires a thorough understanding of anatomy. Likewise, the study of malignancy and observations regarding spread of malignant tumors aids in the understanding and instruction of anatomy. Radiation oncologists have a unique opportunity to assist in the instruction of anatomy. For most medical students, gross anatomy is an early first-year course before significant clinical experience is obtained. Over the ensuing years of medical school and residency, much of this knowledge is lost as it is not routinely applied during clinical practice. It is incumbent on those who seek advanced training in fields such as surgery, radiology, and radiation oncology to again become students of anatomy, as the successful practice of such disciplines requires an in-depth understanding of anatomical principles.

A multi-institutional oncoanatomy course has been described.[169-171] It currently consists of a bimonthly conference where the anatomy of a particular disease site is reviewed along with pertinent clinical implications. Following this didactic session, the presentation continues in the gross anatomy suite where anatomy faculty demonstrate on prosections. This course is attended by medical students, residents, and faculty members from multiple disciplines. The expertise of all involved contributes to a valuable educational environment. Recently, a similar Canadian national anatomy and radiology and contouring boot camp has been developed, drawing radiation oncology residents from 10 universities, demonstrating improved understanding of anatomy and radiology, critical for successful practice.[172]

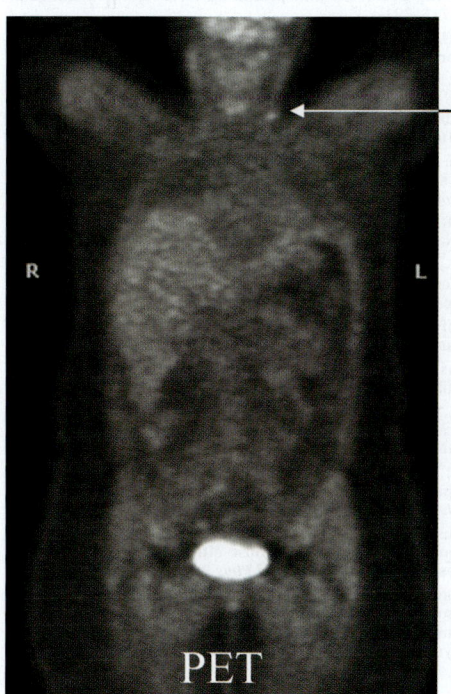
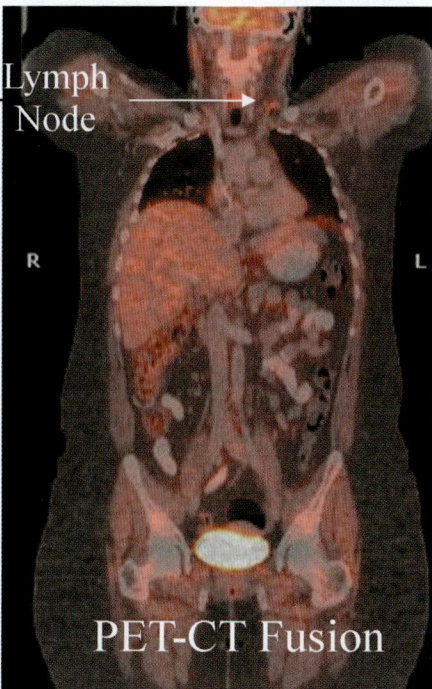

FIGURE 35.14. Postchemotherapy coronal positron emission tomography (PET) scan images of a patient with stage IVa Hodgkin disease demonstrating a hypermetabolic left supraclavicular lymph node. The lymph node was <1 cm on computed tomography (CT) and would not be considered suspicious. Biopsy confirmed persistent disease. **Left:** PET image. **Right:** PET-CT fusion image. (Image courtesy of Dr. Edward Coleman.)

REFERENCES

1. Reddy AV, Christodouleas JP, Wu T, et al. External validation and optimization of international consensus clinical target volumes for adjuvant radiation therapy in bladder cancer. *Int J Radiat Oncol Biol Phys* 2017;97:740–746.

2. Pfeffer MR, Rabin T, Tsvang L, et al. Orbital lymphoma: is it necessary to treat the entire orbit? *Int J Radiat Oncol Biol Phys* 2004;60:527–530.

3. Engels B, Soete G, Verellen D, et al. Conformal arc radiotherapy for prostate cancer: increased biochemical failure in patients with distended rectum on the planning computed tomogram despite image guidance by implanted markers. *Int J Radiat Oncol Biol Phys* 2009;74:388–391.

4. Bettmann MA. Frequently asked questions: iodinated contrast agents. *Radiographics* 2004;24(Suppl 1):S3–S10.

5. Manual on Contrast Media v10.2. American College of Radiology, 2016. Accessed April 3, 2017, at https://www.acr.org/Quality-Safety/Resources/Contrast-Manual

6. Schabelman E, Witting M. The relationship of radiocontrast, iodine, and seafood allergies: a medical myth exposed. *J Emerg Med* 2010;39:701–707.

7. Brenner DJ. Slowing the increase in the population dose resulting from CT scans. *Radiat Res* 2010;174:809–815.

8. Burke LMB, Semelka RC, Smith-Bindman R. Trends of CT utilization in North America over the last decade. *Curr Radiol Rep* 2015:78.

9. Kuo PH, Kanal E, Abu-Alfa AK, et al. Gadolinium-based MR contrast agents and nephrogenic systemic fibrosis. *Radiology* 2007;242:647–649.

10. Khawaja AZ, Cassidy DB, Al Shakarchi J, et al. Revisiting the risks of MRI with Gadolinium based contrast agents—review of literature and guidelines. *Insights Imaging* 2015;6:553–558.

11. Yoo DS, Kirkpatrick JP, Craciunescu O, et al. Prospective trial of synchronous bevacizumab, erlotinib, and concurrent chemoradiation in locally advanced head and neck cancer. *Clin Cancer Res* 2012;18:1404–1414.

12. Jalaguier-Coudray A, Villard-Mahjoub R, Delouche A, et al. Value of dynamic contrast-enhanced and diffusion-weighted MR imaging in the detection of pathologic complete response in cervical cancer after neoadjuvant therapy: a retrospective observational study. *Radiology* 2017;284:432–442.

13. Costantini M, Belli P, Rinaldi P, et al. Diffusion-weighted imaging in breast cancer: relationship between apparent diffusion coefficient and tumour aggressiveness. *Clin Radiol* 2010;65:1005–1012.

14. Parikh T, Drew SJ, Lee VS, et al. Focal liver lesion detection and characterization with diffusion-weighted MR imaging: comparison with standard breath-hold T2-weighted imaging. *Radiology* 2008;246:812–822.

15. Ho JC, Allen PK, Bhosale PR, et al. Diffusion-weighted magnetic resonance imaging as a predictor of outcome in cervical cancer after chemoradiation. *Int J Radiat Oncol Biol Phys* 2017;97:546–553.

16. Ingram M, Arregui ME. Endoscopic ultrasonography. *Surg Clin North Am* 2004;84:1035–1059, vi.

17. Catalano MF, Sivak MV Jr, Rice T, et al. Endosonographic features predictive of lymph node metastasis. *Gastrointest Endosc* 1994;40:442–446.

18. Lardinois D, Weder W, Hany TF, et al. Staging of non-small-cell lung cancer with integrated positron-emission tomography and computed tomography. *N Engl J Med* 2003;348:2500–2507.

19. Wahl RL, Jacene H, Kasamon Y, et al. From RECIST to PERCIST: evolving considerations for PET response criteria in solid tumors. *J Nucl Med* 2009;50(Suppl 1):122S–150S.

20. Francis RJ, Byrne MJ, van der Schaaf AA, et al. Early prediction of response to chemotherapy and survival in malignant pleural mesothelioma using a novel semiautomated 3-dimensional volume-based analysis of serial 18F-FDG PET scans. *J Nucl Med* 2007;48:1449–1458.

21. Adams MC, Turkington TG, Wilson JM, et al. A systematic review of the factors affecting accuracy of SUV measurements. *AJR Am J Roentgenol* 2010;195:310–320.

22. Fried DV, Mawlawi O, Zhang L, et al. Stage III non-small cell lung cancer: prognostic value of FDG PET quantitative imaging features combined with clinical prognostic factors. *Radiology* 2016;278:214–222.

23. Grootjans W, Usmanij EA, Oyen WJ, et al. Performance of automatic image segmentation algorithms for calculating total lesion glycolysis for early response monitoring in non-small cell lung cancer patients during concomitant chemoradiotherapy. *Radiother Oncol* 2016;119:473–479.

24. Schwartz DL, Harris J, Yao M, et al. Metabolic tumor volume as a prognostic imaging-based biomarker for head-and-neck cancer: pilot results from Radiation Therapy Oncology Group protocol 0522. *Int J Radiat Oncol Biol Phys* 2015;91:721–729.

25. Lopci E, Grassi I, Chiti A, et al. PET radiopharmaceuticals for imaging of tumor hypoxia: a review of the evidence. *Am J Nucl Med Mol Imaging* 2014;4:365–384.

26. Blake GM, Park-Holohan SJ, Cook GJ, et al. Quantitative studies of bone with the use of 18F-fluoride and 99mTc-methylene diphosphonate. *Semin Nucl Med* 2001;31:28–49.

27. Even-Sapir E. Imaging of malignant bone involvement by morphologic, scintigraphic, and hybrid modalities. *J Nucl Med* 2005;46:1356–1367.

28. Hamaoka T, Madewell JE, Podoloff DA, et al. Bone imaging in metastatic breast cancer. *J Clin Oncol* 2004;22:2942–2953.

29. Saha S, Burke C, Desai A, et al. SPECT-CT: applications in musculoskeletal radiology. *Br J Radiol* 2013;86:20120519.

30. Ota N, Kato K, Iwano S, et al. Comparison of (1)(8)F-fluoride PET/CT, (1)(8)F-FDG PET/CT and bone scintigraphy (planar and SPECT) in detection of bone metastases of differentiated thyroid cancer: a pilot study. *Br J Radiol* 2014;87:20130444.

31. Therasse P, Arbuck SG, Eisenhauer EA, et al. New guidelines to evaluate the response to treatment in solid tumors. European Organization for Research and Treatment of Cancer, National Cancer Institute of the United States, National Cancer Institute of Canada. *J Natl Cancer Inst* 2000;92:205–216.

32. Gleave ME, Coupland D, Drachenberg D, et al. Ability of serum prostate-specific antigen levels to predict normal bone scans in patients with newly diagnosed prostate cancer. *Urology* 1996;47:708–712.

33. Kosuda S, Yoshimura I, Aizawa T, et al. Can initial prostate specific antigen determinations eliminate the need for bone scans in patients with newly diagnosed prostate carcinoma? A multicenter retrospective study in Japan. *Cancer* 2002;94:964–972.

34. O'Sullivan JM, Norman AR, Cook GJ, et al. Broadening the criteria for avoiding staging bone scans in prostate cancer: a retrospective study of patients at the Royal Marsden Hospital. *BJU Int* 2003;92:685–689.

35. Cheran SK, Herndon JE II, Patz EF Jr. Comparison of whole-body FDG-PET to bone scan for detection of bone metastases in patients with a new diagnosis of lung cancer. *Lung Cancer* 2004;44:317–325.

36. Gillies RJ, Kinahan PE, Hricak H. Radiomics: images are more than pictures, they are data. *Radiology* 2016;278:563–577.

37. Hatt M, Majdoub M, Vallieres M, et al. 18F-FDG PET uptake characterization through texture analysis: investigating the complementary nature of heterogeneity and functional tumor volume in a multi-cancer site patient cohort. *J Nucl Med* 2015;56:38–44.

38. Kawahara Y, Niiro M, Yokoyama S, et al. Dural congestion accompanying meningioma invasion into vessels: the dural tail sign. *Neuroradiology* 2001;43:462–465.

39. Nagele T, Petersen D, Klose U, et al. The "dural tail" adjacent to meningiomas studied by dynamic contrast-enhanced MRI: a comparison with histopathology. *Neuroradiology* 1994;36:303–307.

40. Chamberlain MC. Neoplastic meningitis. *J Clin Oncol* 2005;23:3605–3613.

41. Seibert TM, Karunamuni R, Bartsch H, et al. Radiation dose-dependent hippocampal atrophy detected with longitudinal volumetric magnetic resonance imaging. *Int J Radiat Oncol Biol Phys* 2017;97:263–269.

42. Gondi V, Hermann BP, Mehta MP, et al. Hippocampal dosimetry predicts neurocognitive function impairment after fractionated stereotactic radiotherapy for benign or low-grade adult brain tumors. *Int J Radiat Oncol Biol Phys* 2013;85:348–354.

43. Gondi V, Pugh SL, Tome WA, et al. Preservation of memory with conformal avoidance of the hippocampal neural stem-cell compartment during whole-brain radiotherapy for brain metastases (RTOG 0933): a phase II multi-institutional trial. *J Clin Oncol* 2014;32:3810–3816.

44. Johnson JD, Young B. Demographics of brain metastasis. *Neurosurg Clin N Am* 1996;7:337–344.

45. Delattre JY, Krol G, Thaler HT, et al. Distribution of brain metastases. *Arch Neurol* 1988;45:741–744.

46. Sze G, Milano E, Johnson C, et al. Detection of brain metastases: comparison of contrast-enhanced MR with unenhanced MR and enhanced CT. *AJNR Am J Neuroradiol* 1990;11:785–791.

47. Sze G, Johnson C, Kawamura Y, et al. Comparison of single- and triple-dose contrast material in the MR screening of brain metastases. *AJNR Am J Neuroradiol* 1998;19:821–828.

48. Lee BC, Kneeland JB, Cahill PT, et al. MR recognition of supratentorial tumors. *AJNR Am J Neuroradiol* 1985;6:871–878.

49. Kelly PJ, Daumas-Duport C, Kispert DB, et al. Imaging-based stereotaxic serial biopsies in untreated intracranial glial neoplasms. *J Neurosurg* 1987;66:865–874.

50. Howe FA, Barton SJ, Cudlip SA, et al. Metabolic profiles of human brain tumors using quantitative in vivo 1H magnetic resonance spectroscopy. *Magn Reson Med* 2003;49:223–232.

51. Law M, Cha S, Knopp EA, et al. High-grade gliomas and solitary metastases: differentiation by using perfusion and proton spectroscopic MR imaging. *Radiology* 2002;222:715–721.

52. Zach L, Guez D, Last D, et al. Delayed contrast extravasation MRI for depicting tumor and non-tumoral tissues in primary and metastatic brain tumors. *PLoS One* 2012;7:e52008.

53. Spence AM, Muzi M, Mankoff DA, et al. 18F-FDG PET of gliomas at delayed intervals: improved distinction between tumor and normal gray matter. *J Nucl Med* 2004;45:1653–1659.

54. Horky LL, Hsiao EM, Weiss SE, et al. Dual phase FDG-PET imaging of brain metastases provides superior assessment of recurrence versus post-treatment necrosis. *J Neurooncol* 2011;103:137–146.

55. Busk M, Horsman MR. Relevance of hypoxia in radiation oncology: pathophysiology, tumor biology and implications for treatment. *Q J Nucl Med Mol Imaging* 2013;57:219–234.

56. Rosenkrantz AB, Friedman K, Chandarana H, et al. Current status of hybrid PET/MRI in oncologic imaging. *AJR Am J Roentgenol* 2016;206:162–172.

57. Som PM. Detection of metastasis in cervical lymph nodes: CT and MR criteria and differential diagnosis. *AJR Am J Roentgenol* 1992;158:961–969.

58. Harrison LB, Sessions RB, Hong W. *Head and neck cancer: a multidisciplinary approach.* 3rd ed. Philadelphia: Lippincott Williams & Wilkins, 2009.

59. Eisbruch A, Foote RL, O'Sullivan B, et al. Intensity-modulated radiation therapy for head and neck cancer: emphasis on the selection and delineation of the targets. *Semin Radiat Oncol* 2002;12:238–249.

60. Ahmed M, Schmidt M, Sohaib A, et al. The value of magnetic resonance imaging in target volume delineation of base of tongue tumours—a study using flexible surface coils. *Radiother Oncol* 2010;94:161–167.

61. Dirix P, Abbeel S, Vanstraelen B, et al. Dysphagia after chemoradiotherapy for head-and-neck squamous cell carcinoma: dose-effect relationships for the swallowing structures. *Int J Radiat Oncol Biol Phys* 2009;75:385–392.

62. MD Anderson Head and Neck Cancer Symptom Working Group. Beyond mean pharyngeal constrictor dose for beam path toxicity in non-target swallowing muscles: dose-volume correlates of chronic radiation-associated dysphagia (RAD) after oropharyngeal intensity modulated radiotherapy. *Radiother Oncol* 2016;118:304–314.

63. Dammann F, Horger M, Mueller-Berg M, et al. Rational diagnosis of squamous cell carcinoma of the head and neck region: comparative evaluation of CT, MRI, and 18FDG PET. *AJR Am J Roentgenol* 2005;184:1326–1331.

64. Kim S, Loevner LA, Quon H, et al. Prediction of response to chemoradiation therapy in squamous cell carcinomas of the head and neck using dynamic contrast-enhanced MR imaging. *AJNR Am J Neuroradiol* 2010;31:262–268.

65. Chawla S, Kim S, Dougherty L, et al. Pretreatment diffusion-weighted and dynamic contrast-enhanced MRI for prediction of local treatment response in squamous cell carcinomas of the head and neck. *AJR Am J Roentgenol* 2013;200:35–43.

66. Vandecaveye V, Dirix P, De Keyzer F, et al. Predictive value of diffusion-weighted magnetic resonance imaging during chemoradiotherapy for head and neck squamous cell carcinoma. *Eur Radiol* 2010;20:1703–1714.

67. Wong WL, Hussain K, Chevretton E, et al. Validation and clinical application of computer-combined computed tomography and positron emission tomography with 2-[18F]fluoro-2-deoxy-D-glucose head and neck images. *Am J Surg* 1996;172:628–632.

68. Hannah A, Scott AM, Tochon-Danguy H, et al. Evaluation of 18F-fluorodeoxyglucose positron emission tomography and computed tomography with histopathologic correlation in the initial staging of head and neck cancer. *Ann Surg* 2002;236:208–217.

69. Wong RJ, Lin DT, Schoder H, et al. Diagnostic and prognostic value of [(18) F]fluorodeoxyglucose positron emission tomography for recurrent head and neck squamous cell carcinoma. *J Clin Oncol* 2002;20:4199–4208.

70. Yao M, Smith RB, Hoffman HT, et al. Clinical significance of postradiotherapy [18F]-fluorodeoxyglucose positron emission tomography imaging in management of head-and-neck cancer—a long-term outcome report. *Int J Radiat Oncol Biol Phys* 2009;74:9–14.

71. Rischin D, Hicks RJ, Fisher R, et al. Prognostic significance of [18F]-misonidazole positron emission tomography-detected tumor hypoxia in patients with advanced head and neck cancer randomly assigned to chemoradiation with or without tirapazamine: a substudy of Trans-Tasman Radiation Oncology Group Study 98.02. *J Clin Oncol* 2006;24:2098–2104.

72. Todd M, Shah GV, Mukherji SK. MR imaging of brachial plexus. *Top Magn Reson Imaging* 2004;15:113–125.

73. Tharin BD, Kini JA, York GE, et al. Brachial plexopathy: a review of traumatic and nontraumatic causes. *AJR Am J Roentgenol* 2014;202:W67–W75.

74. Hall WH, Guiou M, Lee NY, et al. Development and validation of a standardized method for contouring the brachial plexus: preliminary dosimetric analysis among patients treated with IMRT for head-and-neck cancer. *Int J Radiat Oncol Biol Phys* 2008;72:1362–1367.

75. Riquet M, Hidden G, Debesse B. Direct lymphatic drainage of lung segments to the mediastinal nodes. An anatomic study on 260 adults. *J Thorac Cardiovasc Surg* 1989;97:623–632.

76. Nohl-Oser HC. An investigation of the anatomy of the lymphatic drainage of the lungs as shown by the lymphatic spread of bronchial carcinoma. *Ann R Coll Surg Engl* 1972;51:157–176.

77. Billiet C, De Ruysscher D, Peeters S, et al. Patterns of locoregional relapses in patients with contemporarily staged stage III-N2 nsclc treated with induction chemotherapy and resection: implications for postoperative radiotherapy target volumes. *J Thorac Oncol* 2016;11:1538–1549.

78. Kelsey CR, Light KL, Marks LB. Patterns of failure after resection of non-small-cell lung cancer: implications for postoperative radiation therapy volumes. *Int J Radiat Oncol Biol Phys* 2006;65:1097–1105.

79. Choyke PL, Zeman RK, Gootenberg JE, et al. Thymic atrophy and regrowth in response to chemotherapy: CT evaluation. *AJR Am J Roentgenol* 1987;149:269–272.

80. Dwamena BA, Sonnad SS, Angobaldo JO, et al. Metastases from non-small cell lung cancer: mediastinal staging in the 1990s—meta-analytic comparison of PET and CT. *Radiology* 1999;213:530–536.

81. Toloza EM, Harpole L, McCrory DC. Noninvasive staging of non-small-cell lung cancer: a review of the current evidence. *Chest* 2003;123:137S–146S.

82. Gould MK, Kuschner WG, Rydzak CE, et al. Test performance of positron emission tomography and computed tomography for mediastinal staging in patients with non-small-cell lung cancer: a meta-analysis. *Ann Intern Med* 2003;139:879–892.

83. Siva S, Herschtal A, Thomas JM, et al. Impact of post-therapy positron emission tomography on prognostic stratification and surveillance after chemoradiotherapy for cervical cancer. *Cancer* 2011;117:3981–3988.

84. Villeirs GM, L Verstraete K, De Neve WJ, et al. Magnetic resonance imaging anatomy of the prostate and periprostatic area: a guide for radiotherapists. *Radiother Oncol* 2005;76:99–106.

85. Batson OV. The function of the vertebral veins and their role in the spread of metastases. *Ann Surg* 1940;112:138–149.

86. Geldof AA. Models for cancer skeletal metastasis: a reappraisal of Batson's plexus. *Anticancer Res* 1997;17:1535–1539.

87. Plants BA, Chen DT, Fiveash JB, et al. Bulb of penis as a marker for prostatic apex in external beam radiotherapy of prostate cancer. *Int J Radiat Oncol Biol Phys* 2003;56:1079–1084.

88. Bille A, Pelosi E, Skanjeti A, et al. Preoperative intrathoracic lymph node staging in patients with non-small-cell lung cancer: accuracy of integrated positron emission tomography and computed tomography. *Eur J Cardiothorac Surg* 2009;36:440–445.

89. Darling GE, Maziak DE, Inculet RI, et al. Positron emission tomography-computed tomography compared with invasive mediastinal staging in non-small cell lung cancer: results of mediastinal staging in the early lung positron emission tomography trial. *J Thorac Oncol* 2011;6:1367–1372.

90. Pozo-Rodriguez F, Martin de Nicolas JL, Sanchez-Nistal MA, et al. Accuracy of helical computed tomography and [18F] fluorodeoxyglucose positron emission tomography for identifying lymph node mediastinal metastases in potentially resectable non-small-cell lung cancer. *J Clin Oncol* 2005;23:8348–8356.

91. Lightdale CJ, Kulkarni KG. Role of endoscopic ultrasonography in the staging and follow-up of esophageal cancer. *J Clin Oncol* 2005;23:4483–4489.

92. Rosch T. Endosonographic staging of esophageal cancer: a review of literature results. *Gastrointest Endosc Clin N Am* 1995;5:537–547.

93. van Westreenen HL, Westerterp M, Bossuyt PM, et al. Systematic review of the staging performance of 18F-fluorodeoxyglucose positron emission tomography in esophageal cancer. *J Clin Oncol* 2004;22:3805–3812.

94. Westerterp M, van Westreenen HL, Reitsma JB, et al. Esophageal cancer: CT, endoscopic US, and FDG PET for assessment of response to neoadjuvant therapy—systematic review. *Radiology* 2005;236:841–851.

95. Nickell LT Jr, Lichtenberger JP III, Khorashadi L, et al. Multimodality imaging for characterization, classification, and staging of malignant pleural mesothelioma. *Radiographics* 2014;34:1692–1706.

96. Heelan RT, Rusch VW, Begg CB, et al. Staging of malignant pleural mesothelioma: comparison of CT and MR imaging. *AJR Am J Roentgenol* 1999;172:1039–1047.

97. Bruzzi JF, Komaki R, Walsh GL, et al. Imaging of non-small cell lung cancer of the superior sulcus: part 2: initial staging and assessment of resectability and therapeutic response. *Radiographics* 2008;28:561–572.

98. Tomiyama N, Johkoh T, Mihara N, et al. Using the World Health Organization Classification of thymic epithelial neoplasms to describe CT findings. *AJR Am J Roentgenol* 2002;179:881–886.

99. Marom EM, Milito MA, Moran CA, et al. Computed tomography findings predicting invasiveness of thymoma. *J Thorac Oncol* 2011;6:1274–1281.

100. Fentiman IS, Fourquet A, Hortobagyi GN. Male breast cancer. *Lancet* 2006;367:595–604.

101. Lee AH. Why is carcinoma of the breast more frequent in the upper outer quadrant? A case series based on needle core biopsy diagnoses. *Breast* 2005;14:151–152.

102. Estourgie SH, Nieweg OE, Olmos RA, et al. Lymphatic drainage patterns from the breast. *Ann Surg* 2004;239:232–237.

103. Livingston SF, Arlen M. The extended extrapleural radical mastectomy: its role in the treatment of carcinoma of the breast. *Ann Surg* 1974;179:260–265.

104. Urban JA, Marjani MA. Significance of internal mammary lymph node metastases in breast cancer. *Am J Roentgenol Radium Ther Nucl Med* 1971;111:130 136.

105. Noguchi M, Taniya T, Koyasaki N, et al. A multivariate analysis of en bloc extended radical mastectomy versus conventional radical mastectomy in operable breast cancer. *Int Surg* 1992;77:48–54.

106. Engelbrecht MR, Jager GJ, Laheij RJ, et al. Local staging of prostate cancer using magnetic resonance imaging: a meta-analysis. *Eur Radiol* 2002;12:2294–2302.

107. Futterer JJ, Scheenen TW, Heijmink SW, et al. Standardized threshold approach using three-dimensional proton magnetic resonance spectroscopic imaging in prostate cancer localization of the entire prostate. *Invest Radiol* 2007;42:116–122.

108. Villeirs GM, De Meerleer GO, Verstraete KL, et al. Magnetic resonance assessment of prostate localization variability in intensity-modulated radiotherapy for prostate cancer. *Int J Radiat Oncol Biol Phys* 2004;60:1611–1621.

109. Jethwa KR, Kahila MM, Hunt KN, et al. Delineation of internal mammary nodal target volumes in breast cancer radiation therapy. *Int J Radiat Oncol Biol Phys* 2017;97:762–769.

110. Poortmans PM, Collette S, Kirkove C, et al. Internal mammary and medial supraclavicular irradiation in breast cancer. *N Engl J Med* 2015;373:317–327.

111. Whelan TJ, Olivotto IA, Parulekar WR, et al. Regional nodal irradiation in early-stage breast cancer. *N Engl J Med* 2015;373:307–316.

112. Alexander FE, Anderson TJ, Brown HK, et al. 14 years of follow-up from the Edinburgh randomised trial of breast-cancer screening. *Lancet* 1999;353:1903–1908.

113. Andersson I, Janzon L. Reduced breast cancer mortality in women under age 50: updated results from the Malmo Mammographic Screening Program. *J Natl Cancer Inst Monogr* 1997:63–67.

114. Miller AB, To T, Baines CJ, et al. Canadian National Breast Screening Study-2: 13-year results of a randomized trial in women aged 50–59 years. *J Natl Cancer Inst* 2000;92:1490–1499.

115. Nystrom L, Andersson I, Bjurstam N, et al. Long-term effects of mammography screening: updated overview of the Swedish randomised trials. *Lancet* 2002;359:909–919.

116. Rosenberg RD, Hunt WC, Williamson MR, et al. Effects of age, breast density, ethnicity, and estrogen replacement therapy on screening mammographic sensitivity and cancer stage at diagnosis: review of 183,134 screening mammograms in Albuquerque, New Mexico. *Radiology* 1998;209:511–518.

117. Carney PA, Miglioretti DL, Yankaskas BC, et al. Individual and combined effects of age, breast density, and hormone replacement therapy use on the accuracy of screening mammography. *Ann Intern Med* 2003;138:168–175.

118. Boyd NF, Guo H, Martin LJ, et al. Mammographic density and the risk and detection of breast cancer. *N Engl J Med* 2007;356:227–236.

119. Pisano ED, Gatsonis C, Hendrick E, et al. Diagnostic performance of digital versus film mammography for breast-cancer screening. *N Engl J Med* 2005;353:1773–1783.

120. Saslow D, Boetes C, Burke W, et al. American Cancer Society guidelines for breast screening with MRI as an adjunct to mammography. *CA Cancer J Clin* 2007;57:75–89.

121. Lehman CD, Gatsonis C, Kuhl CK, et al. MRI evaluation of the contralateral breast in women with recently diagnosed breast cancer. *N Engl J Med* 2007;356:1295–1303.

122. Turnbull L, Brown S, Harvey I, et al. Comparative effectiveness of MRI in breast cancer (COMICE) trial: a randomised controlled trial. *Lancet* 2010;375: 563–571.

123. Katipamula R, Degnim AC, Hoskin T, et al. Trends in mastectomy rates at the Mayo Clinic Rochester: effect of surgical year and preoperative magnetic resonance imaging. *J Clin Oncol* 2009;27:4082–4088.

124. Hodgson R, Heywang-Kobrunner SH, Harvey SC, et al. Systematic review of 3D mammography for breast cancer screening. *Breast* 2016;27:52–61.

125. Sia J, Moodie K, Bressel M, et al. A prospective study comparing digital breast tomosynthesis with digital mammography in surveillance after breast cancer treatment. *Eur J Cancer* 2016;61:122–127.

126. Maruyama K, Gunven P, Okabayashi K, et al. Lymph node metastases of gastric cancer. General pattern in 1931 patients. *Ann Surg* 1989;210:596–602.

127. Fly OA Jr, Waugh JM, Dockerty MB. Splenic hilar nodal involvement in carcinoma of the distal part of the stomach. *Cancer* 1956;9:459–462.

128. Gunderson LL, Sosin H. Adenocarcinoma of the stomach: areas of failure in a re-operation series (second or symptomatic look) clinicopathologic correlation and implications for adjuvant therapy. *Int J Radiat Oncol Biol Phys* 1982;8:1–11.

129. Smalley SR, Gunderson L, Tepper J, et al. Gastric surgical adjuvant radiotherapy consensus report: rationale and treatment implementation. *Int J Radiat Oncol Biol Phys* 2002;52:283–293.

130. Tepper JE, Gunderson LL. Radiation treatment parameters in the adjuvant postoperative therapy of gastric cancer. *Semin Radiat Oncol* 2002;12: 187–195.

131. Takakura K, Sumiyama K, Munakata K, et al. Clinical usefulness of diffusion-weighted MR imaging for detection of pancreatic cancer: comparison with enhanced multidetector-row CT. *Abdom Imaging* 2011;36:457–462.

132. Kinkel K, Lu Y, Both M, et al. Detection of hepatic metastases from cancers of the gastrointestinal tract by using noninvasive imaging methods (US, CT, MR imaging, PET): a meta-analysis. *Radiology* 2002;224:748–756.

133. Cheng CL, Sherman S, Watkins JL, et al. Risk factors for post-ERCP pancreatitis: a prospective multicenter study. *Am J Gastroenterol* 2006;101:139–147.

134. Mortele KJ, Ros PR. Anatomic variants of the biliary tree: MR cholangiographic findings and clinical applications. *AJR Am J Roentgenol* 2001;177: 389–394.

135. Yeh TS, Jan YY, Tseng JH, et al. Malignant perihilar biliary obstruction: magnetic resonance cholangiopancreatographic findings. *Am J Gastroenterol* 2000;95:432–440.

136. Lopera JE, Soto JA, Munera F. Malignant hilar and perihilar biliary obstruction: use of MR cholangiography to define the extent of biliary ductal involvement and plan percutaneous interventions. *Radiology* 2001;220:90–96.

137. Pano B, Sebastia C, Bunesch L, et al. Pathways of lymphatic spread in male urogenital pelvic malignancies. *Radiographics* 2011;31:135–160.

138. Myerson RJ, Garofalo MC, El Naqa I, et al. Elective clinical target volumes for conformal therapy in anorectal cancer: a radiation therapy oncology group consensus panel contouring atlas. *Int J Radiat Oncol Biol Phys* 2009;74: 824–830.

139. Taylor A, Rockall AG, Reznek RH, et al. Mapping pelvic lymph nodes: guidelines for delineation in intensity-modulated radiotherapy. *Int J Radiat Oncol Biol Phys* 2005;63:1604–1612.

140. Vilarino-Varela MJ, Taylor A, Rockall AG, et al. A verification study of proposed pelvic lymph node localisation guidelines using nanoparticle-enhanced magnetic resonance imaging. *Radiother Oncol* 2008;89:192–196.

141. Kabolizadeh P, Fulay S, Beriwal S. Are Radiation Therapy Oncology Group Para-aortic Contouring Guidelines for Pancreatic Neoplasm applicable to other malignancies—assessment of nodal distribution in gynecological malignancies. *Int J Radiat Oncol Biol Phys* 2013;87:106–110.

142. Kim CH, Olson AC, Kim H, et al. Contouring inguinal and femoral nodes; how much margin is needed around the vessels? *Pract Radiat Oncol* 2012;2:274–278.

143. Kim RY, McGinnis LS, Spencer SA, et al. Conventional four-field pelvic radiotherapy technique without computed tomography-treatment planning in cancer of the cervix: potential geographic miss and its impact on pelvic control. *Int J Radiat Oncol Biol Phys* 1995;31:109–112.

144. Chun M, Timmerman RD, Mayer R, et al. Radiation therapy of external iliac lymph nodes with lateral pelvic portals: identification of patients at risk for inadequate regional coverage. *Radiology* 1995;194:147–150.

145. Kapiteijn E, Putter H, van de Velde CJ; Cooperative investigators of the Dutch ColoRectal Cancer Group. Impact of the introduction and training of total mesorectal excision on recurrence and survival in rectal cancer in The Netherlands. *Br J Surg* 2002;89:1142–1149.

146. Kapiteijn E, Marijnen CA, Nagtegaal ID, et al. Preoperative radiotherapy combined with total mesorectal excision for resectable rectal cancer. *N Engl J Med* 2001;345:638–646.

147. Quirke P, Steele R, Monson J, et al. Effect of the plane of surgery achieved on local recurrence in patients with operable rectal cancer: a prospective study using data from the MRC CR07 and NCIC-CTG CO16 randomised clinical trial. *Lancet* 2009;373:821–828.

148. Harewood GC, Wiersema MJ, Nelson H, et al. A prospective, blinded assessment of the impact of preoperative staging on the management of rectal cancer. *Gastroenterology* 2002;123:24–32.

149. Puli SR, Bechtold ML, Reddy JB, et al. How good is endoscopic ultrasound in differentiating various T stages of rectal cancer? Meta-analysis and systematic review. *Ann Surg Oncol* 2009;16:254–265.

150. Sauer R, Becker H, Hohenberger W, et al. Preoperative versus postoperative chemoradiotherapy for rectal cancer. *N Engl J Med* 2004;351:1731–1740.

151. Deserno WM, Harisinghani MG, Taupitz M, et al. Urinary bladder cancer: preoperative nodal staging with ferumoxtran-10-enhanced MR imaging. *Radiology* 2004;233:449–456.

152. Umek WH, Morgan DM, Ashton-Miller JA, et al. Quantitative analysis of uterosacral ligament origin and insertion points by magnetic resonance imaging. *Obstet Gynecol* 2004;103:447–451.

153. Chung HH, Kang SB, Cho JY, et al. Accuracy of MR imaging for the prediction of myometrial invasion of endometrial carcinoma. *Gynecol Oncol* 2007;104:654–659.

154. Sheu MH, Chang CY, Wang JH, et al. Preoperative staging of cervical carcinoma with MR imaging: a reappraisal of diagnostic accuracy and pitfalls. *Eur Radiol* 2001;11:1828–1833.

155. Dimopoulos JC, Schard G, Berger D, et al. Systematic evaluation of MRI findings in different stages of treatment of cervical cancer: potential of MRI on delineation of target, pathoanatomic structures, and organs at risk. *Int J Radiat Oncol Biol Phys* 2006;64:1380–1388.

156. Charra-Brunaud C, Harter V, Delannes M, et al. Impact of 3D image-based PDR brachytherapy on outcome of patients treated for cervix carcinoma in France: results of the French STIC prospective study. *Radiother Oncol* 2012;103:305–313.

157. Viswanathan AN, Dimopoulos J, Kirisits C, et al. Computed tomography versus magnetic resonance imaging-based contouring in cervical cancer brachytherapy: results of a prospective trial and preliminary guidelines for standardized contours. *Int J Radiat Oncol Biol Phys* 2007;68:491–498.

158. Havrilesky LJ, Kulasingam SL, Matchar DB, et al. FDG-PET for management of cervical and ovarian cancer. *Gynecol Oncol* 2005;97:183–191.

159. Kidd EA, Siegel BA, Dehdashti F, et al. The standardized uptake value for F-18 fluorodeoxyglucose is a sensitive predictive biomarker for cervical cancer treatment response and survival. *Cancer* 2007;110:1738–1744.

160. Schwarz JK, Siegel BA, Dehdashti F, et al. Association of posttherapy positron emission tomography with tumor response and survival in cervical carcinoma. *JAMA* 2007;298:2289–2295.

161. Harvey H, deSouza NM. The role of imaging in the diagnosis of primary prostate cancer. *J Clin Urol* 2016;9:11–17.

162. Somford DM, Hamoen EH, Futterer JJ, et al. The predictive value of endorectal 3 Tesla multiparametric magnetic resonance imaging for extraprostatic extension in patients with low, intermediate and high risk prostate cancer. *J Urol* 2013;190:1728–1734.

163. Hinkle GH, Burgers JK, Neal CE, et al. Multicenter radioimmunoscintigraphic evaluation of patients with prostate carcinoma using indium-111 capromab pendetide. *Cancer* 1998;83:739–747.

164. Perera M, Papa N, Christidis D, et al. Sensitivity, specificity, and predictors of positive 68Ga-prostate-specific membrane antigen positron emission tomography in advanced prostate cancer: a systematic review and meta-analysis. *Eur Urol* 2016;70:926–937.

165. Swerdlow SH, Campo E, Pileri SA, et al. The 2016 revision of the World Health Organization classification of lymphoid neoplasms. *Blood* 2016;127:2375–2390.

166. Cheson BD, Fisher RI, Barrington SF, et al. Recommendations for initial evaluation, staging, and response assessment of Hodgkin and non-Hodgkin lymphoma: the Lugano classification. *J Clin Oncol* 2014;32:3059–3068.

167. Barrington SF, Qian W, Somer EJ, et al. Concordance between four European centres of PET reporting criteria designed for use in multicentre trials in Hodgkin lymphoma. *Eur J Nucl Med Mol Imaging* 2010;37:1824–1833.

168. Radford J, Illidge T, Counsell N, et al. Results of a trial of PET-directed therapy for early-stage Hodgkin's lymphoma. *N Engl J Med* 2015;372:1598–1607.

169. Chino JP, Lee WR, Madden R, et al. Teaching the anatomy of oncology: evaluating the impact of a dedicated oncoanatomy course. *Int J Radiat Oncol Biol Phys* 2011;79:853–859.

170. Zumwalt AC, Marks L, Halperin EC. Integrating gross anatomy into a clinical oncology curriculum: the oncoanatomy course at Duke University School of Medicine. *Acad Med* 2007;82:469–474.

171. Cabrera AR, Lee WR, Madden R, et al. Incorporating gross anatomy education into radiation oncology residency: a 2-year curriculum with evaluation of resident satisfaction. *J Am Coll Radiol* 2011;8:335–340.

172. Jaswal J, D'Souza L, Johnson M, et al. Evaluating the impact of a Canadian national anatomy and radiology contouring boot camp for radiation oncology residents. *Int J Radiat Oncol Biol Phys* 2015;91:701–707.

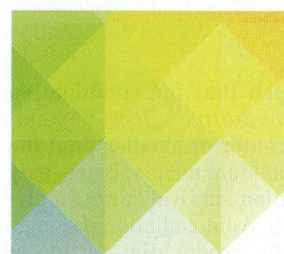

CHAPTER 36

Basic Concepts of Chemotherapy and Irradiation Interaction

D. Nathan Kim, Michael Story, and Hak Choy

For decades, radiation therapy has been a major treatment modality for locally or regionally confined cancers. The rate of treatment failure is still high, particularly for large tumors or advanced disease. Technologic improvements in radiation therapy have continuously been made that allow delivery of higher radiation doses to the tumor or lower doses to normal tissues and in the implementation of strategies that modulate the biologic response of tumors or normal tissues to radiation. These strategies include altered fractionation scheduling including extreme hypofractionation (e.g., stereotactic body radiotherapy, stereotactic radiosurgery [SRS]), combined modality treatments using chemical or biologic agents, and, more recently, targeting molecular processes and signaling pathways that have become dysregulated in cancer cells.

The combination of chemotherapeutic drugs with radiation has perhaps had one of the strongest impacts on current cancer radiation therapy practice. This is particularly true for concurrent chemoradiation therapy, which has been shown in many recent clinical trials to be superior to radiation therapy alone in controlling locoregional disease and in improving patient survival. Combining chemotherapeutic drugs with radiation therapy has a strong biologic rationale. Such agents reduce the number of cells in tumors undergoing radiation therapy by their independent cytotoxic action and by rendering tumor cells more susceptible to killing by ionizing radiation. An additional benefit of combined treatment is that chemotherapeutic drugs, by virtue of their systemic activity, may also act on metastatic disease. Most drugs have been chosen for combination with radiation therapy based on their known clinical activity in particular disease sites. Alternatively, agents that are effective in overcoming resistance mechanisms associated with radiation therapy could be chosen. There have been clinical successes with concurrent chemoradiation therapy using traditional drugs, such as cisplatin and 5-fluorouracil (5-FU), and these studies have led to extensive research on exploring newer chemotherapeutic agents for their interactions with radiation. A number of potent chemotherapeutic agents, subsequently, have entered clinical trials or practice. These agents were selected after preclinical studies demonstrated that they are potent enhancers of the radiation response and thus might further improve the therapeutic outcome of chemoradiation therapy. There are also molecular targeting strategies aimed at improving the efficacy of radiation therapy. In this era, there is significant explosion of activity revolving around the exciting and emerging data suggesting potential benefit to combining immunotherapy agents with radiation therapy. This chapter reviews the biologic rationale and principles fundamental to the use of chemotherapy, molecular targeted agents, and immunotherapy in conjunction with radiation treatments and discusses mechanistic interactions between drugs and radiation, the knowledge of which is essential in developing the optimal treatment strategies and designing appropriate clinical trials. It also provides a brief overview of current treatment applications and advances in the clinic. Owing to limited space, this review is far from comprehensive; additional information can be found in other reviews on this subject.[1–11]

THERAPEUTIC INDEX

Both radiation and chemotherapeutic drugs are cytotoxic to tumor and normal tissue cells. This lack of specificity is a major limitation in their use when applied either as individual treatments or in combination. Radiation inflicts damage to tumor and normal tissues in the radiation treatment field, whereas drugs, because of their systemic action, can affect any tissue in the body. Damage is often accentuated when the two agents are combined and when they affect the same tissue. In general, both the antitumor effectiveness and the severity of normal tissue damage produced by either radiation or drugs are increased as their dose is increased. This dose–effect relationship is sigmoidal and enables estimation of the therapeutic index (ratio), which is defined as the ratio between the doses (radiation, drug) that produce the same level (probability) of antitumor efficacy and normal tissue damage. To be therapeutically beneficial, the therapeutic ratio must be positive (>1); that is, individual agents or their combination must be more effective against tumors than normal tissues. To define therapeutic benefit in clinical settings, many factors must be taken into account, such as whether the treatment is curative or palliative, which tissues are dose limiting (critical tissues), what degree of tissue damage is acceptable, and so forth. The balance between a given level of antitumor efficacy and acceptable normal tissue complications gives a measure of the therapeutic ratio of a treatment.

EXPLOITABLE STRATEGIES IN CHEMORADIATION THERAPY

The goals of combining chemotherapeutic drugs with radiation therapy are to increase patient survival by improving locoregional tumor control, decrease or eliminate distant metastases, or both while preserving organ and tissue integrity and function. Combined modality treatment can further improve positive therapeutic outcome of individual treatments through a number of specific strategies, which Steel and Peckham[12] classified into four groups: "spatial cooperation," independent toxicity, enhancement of tumor response, and protection of normal tissues.

Spatial cooperation was the initial rationale for combining chemotherapy with radiation therapy, in which the action of radiation and chemotherapeutic drugs is directed toward different anatomic sites. Localized tumors would be the domain of radiation therapy because large doses of radiation can be given. On the other hand, chemotherapeutic drugs are likely to be more effective in eliminating disseminated micrometastases than in eradicating larger primary tumors. Thus, the cooperation between radiation and chemotherapy is achieved through the independent action of two agents. Spatial cooperation is the basis for adjuvant chemoradiation therapy, in which radiation is given first to control the primary tumor and chemotherapy is given later to cope with micrometastases. The concept of spatial cooperation is also applied in the treatment of hematologic malignancies that have spread to "sanctuary" sites, such as the brain. These sites are poorly accessible to chemotherapeutic agents, and thus, they are more appropriately treated with radiation therapy.

Independent toxicity is another important strategy for increasing the therapeutic ratio of chemoradiation therapy. Normal tissue toxicity is the main dose-limiting factor for both chemotherapy and radiation therapy. Therefore, combinations of radiation and drugs would be better tolerated if drugs were selected such that toxicities to specific cell types and tissues do not overlap with, or minimally add to, radiation-induced toxicities. This strategy requires a thorough knowledge of drug toxicity, underlying mechanisms, and drug pharmacokinetics. Another strategy in chemoradiation therapy is to exploit the ability of chemotherapeutic agents to *enhance tumor radioresponse.* The enhancement denotes the existence of some type of interaction between drugs and radiation at the molecular, cellular, or pathophysiologic (microenvironmental, metabolic) level, resulting in an antitumor effect greater than would be expected on the basis of additive actions. Many mechanisms may be involved in drug–radiation interactions leading to tumor radio enhancement, and some of them are elaborated on further in the text. The enhancement must be selective or preferential to tumors compared with critical normal tissues to achieve therapeutic gain. The ability of chemotherapeutic agents to enhance tumor radioresponse by counteracting determinants associated with tumor radioresistance is a major rationale for concurrent radiation therapy.

An additional strategy is to *protect normal tissues* so that higher doses of radiation can be delivered to the tumor. This can be achieved through technical improvements in radiation delivery or administration of chemical or biologic agents that selectively or preferentially protect normal tissues against the damage by radiation or drugs. A separate section in this chapter discusses radioprotectors in more detail.

ASSESSMENT OF DRUG–RADIATION INTERACTION

Any drug considered for use in combination with radiation therapy needs to undergo preclinical evaluation for its interaction with radiation both in *in vitro* cell culture systems and *in vivo*, with the aim of assessing antitumor activity and normal tissue toxicity. The interaction between two agents is more easily defined and quantified *in vitro* because complete cell survival curves are readily obtained. The *in vitro* cell survival assay measures the ability of cells to produce colonies of a defined minimum size. Cell survival is determined after treatment with a drug or radiation alone, given at different doses, or after treatment with both agents, in which case the cells are exposed to the drug before, during, or after irradiation. Survival curves are usually plots of the surviving fraction of cells on a logarithmic scale and the dose of radiation or drugs on a linear scale.

The cell survival curve after irradiation characteristically has a "shoulder" of varying width that denotes the capacity of cells to repair radiation damage. The curves that describe survival after chemotherapeutic agents show much more variation both in absolute sensitivity to drugs and their shape than those after radiation, all depending on the drug tested. Some curves possess shoulders, some lack them, and some show resistant "tails" at higher drug doses. The tails denote the existence of cell subpopulations resistant to chemotherapeutic agents.

To assess the effect of the drug on cell radiosensitivity, the combined drug–radiation curve is commonly plotted after the cytotoxicity produced by the drug alone is excluded ("normalized"). The radiation cell survival curve is not changed if the drug does not influence cell radiosensitivity regardless of whether the drug is cytotoxic on its own. In this case, the cytotoxicity of the drug contributes only to the overall cell killing by the combined treatment (*additive effect*) of both agents. Chemotherapeutic agents may interact with radiation

by altering cell radiosensitivity such that the combination results in a *supra-additive* or *subadditive effect*, depending on whether the cell killing is greater or smaller than the sum of cell killings produced by individual agents. Drugs may eliminate the shoulder on the radiation survival curve, implying that drugs can inhibit cell repair from radiation damage, or they may change the slope of the exponential portion of the survival curve. A steeper slope indicates increased sensitization to radiation, whereas a shallower slope indicates protection.

Because of non–linear dose-related characteristics in cell killing by both chemotherapeutic agents and radiation, the effects of the combined treatment are best assessed using the "isobologram," an isoeffect plot for the dose response to the combination of two agents[12] (Fig. 36.1). Dose–response curves are determined for each agent to generate the isobologram, an envelope of additivity, which denotes expected additive response over a range of doses of the agents used. If the interaction between drugs and radiation is supra-additive or synergistic (i.e., the effect is caused by lower doses of the two agents than the envelope of additivity would predict), the effect is shown at the left side of the envelope. In contrast, the effect of the subadditive or antagonistic interaction is shown to the right of the envelope: the effect required higher doses of the two agents than predicted. The width of the envelope of additivity depends on the degree of the nonlinearity in the dose response to individual agents. The envelope is wider as the degree of nonlinearity increases. In the case of a linear dose–response relationship for each agent, which is rare, the isobologram is also linear, represented by a single straight line.

In vitro testing is often followed by *in vivo* exploration of drug–radiation interactions, which allows assessment of the combined treatment on both tumors and normal tissues. This is essential for determination of therapeutic gain, as discussed earlier in this chapter. Syngeneic animal tumors or human tumor xenografts in nude mice are most often used for this purpose. The efficacy of the treatment is determined by the extent of tumor growth delay or the rate of tumor cure. In normal tissues, the effect of chemotherapeutic drugs on radiation response of acutely and late-responding tissues can be assessed using a variety of available assays. Some of these assays are clonogenic, such as the jejunal crypt assay, where the endpoint depends directly on the reproductive integrity

FIGURE 36.1. An isobologram for two agents when their dose–response curves are nonlinear. The isobologram shows the envelope of additivity and regions of supra-additivity and subadditivity. (Modified from Steel GG, Peckham MJ. Exploitable mechanisms in combined radiotherapy-chemotherapy: the concept of additivity. *Int J Radiat Oncol Biol Phys* 1979;5[1]:85–91. Copyright © 1979 Elsevier. With permission.)

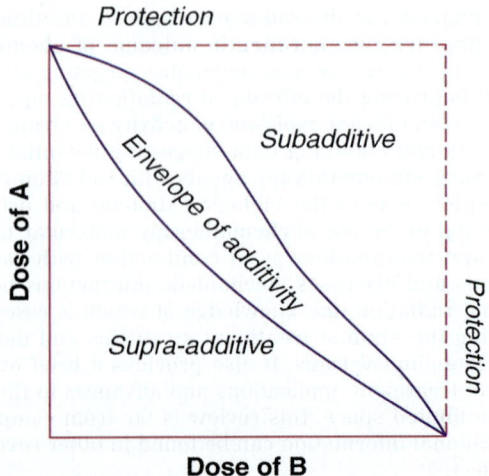

of individual cells. More frequently, however, dose–response relationships for normal tissues are based on functional endpoints (such as breathing rate in lung damage and paralysis in spinal cord damage). These endpoints tend to reflect the minimum number of functional cells remaining in tissues or organs and not the proportion of cells retaining reproductive integrity.

MECHANISTIC CONSIDERATIONS IN DRUG–RADIATION INTERACTIONS

Increasing Initial Radiation Damage
Radiation induces many different lesions in the DNA molecule, which is the critical target for radiation damage. The lesions consist of single-strand breaks (SSBs), double-strand breaks (DSBs), base damage, DNA–DNA and DNA–protein cross-links, and so forth. DSBs and chromosome aberrations that occur in association with or as a consequence of DSBs are usually considered to be the principal damage that results in cell death.[13] Any agent that makes DNA more susceptible to radiation damage may enhance cell killing. Certain drugs, such as halogenated pyrimidines, incorporate into DNA and make it more susceptible to radiation damage.[14]

Inhibition of Cellular Repair
Both sublethal[15] and potentially lethal[16,17] damage inflicted by radiation can be repaired. Although sublethal damage repair (SLDR) denotes the increase in cell survival when the radiation dose is split into two fractions of radiation separated by a time interval, potentially lethal damage repair (PLDR) designates the increase in cell survival as the result of postirradiation environmental conditions. SLDR is rapid, with a half-time of approximately 1 hour, and is complete within 4 to 6 hours after irradiation. This time between two radiation fractions allows radiation-induced DSBs in DNA to rejoin and repair. SLDR is expressed as the restitution of the shoulder on the cell survival curve for the second dose. PLDR occurs when environmental conditions prevent cells from dividing for several hours, such as keeping *in vitro* growing cells in plateau phase after irradiation. Preventing cells from division allows the completion of repair of DNA lesions that would have been lethal had DNA undergone replication within several hours after irradiation. PLDR is considered to be a major determinant responsible for radioresistance in some tumor types, such as melanomas. The repair can be achieved through restoration of damaged molecules by reducing species that donate electrons to oxidized substrates or through involvement of enzymes mediating homologous and nonhomologous recombination repair of DNA DSBs, base excision repair of base damage, and nucleotide excision repair of DNA–protein cross-links.

Many chemotherapeutic agents used in chemoradiation therapy interact with cellular repair mechanisms and inhibit repair and hence may enhance cell or tissue response to radiation. The aforementioned halogenated pyrimidines enhance cell radiosensitivity not only through increasing initial radiation damage but also by inhibiting cellular repair.[14,18] Nucleoside analogs, such as gemcitabine, are a class of chemotherapeutic agents potent in inhibiting the repair of radiation-induced DNA and chromosome damage.[19,20] They have been shown strongly to enhance tumor radioresponse in preclinical studies and have been, and are continuing to be, extensively investigated for such activity in patients with cancer.[21,22]

Cell Cycle Redistribution
Both chemotherapeutic agents and radiation are more effective against proliferating than nonproliferating cells. Their cytotoxic action further depends on the position of cells in the cell cycle. Cell cycle dependency in response to radiation was first described almost 40 years ago.[23] Terasima and Tolmach[23] reported that the sensitivity of the cell response to radiation varied widely depending on which phase of the cell cycle the cells were in at the time of irradiation and that cells in the G_2 and M cell cycle phases were approximately three times more sensitive than cells in the S-phase. The exact reason for this variability is still unknown.

The influence of the cell cycle on cell response to cytotoxic agents can be therapeutically exploited in chemoradiation therapy using cell cycle redistribution strategies. For example, some chemotherapeutic drugs, such as taxanes, can block transition of cells through mitosis, with the result that cells accumulate in the radiosensitive G_2 and M phases of the cell cycle. Radiation delivered at the time of significant accumulation of cells in both the G_2 and M phases results in enhanced radioresponse of cells *in vitro*[24,25] and of tumors *in vivo*.[26,27] However, this cell cycle mechanism of taxane-induced enhancement of tumor radioresponse is dominant only in tumors that are resistant to paclitaxel or docetaxel as a single treatment. Although tumor growth in taxane-resistant tumors is not substantially affected by the drug, tumors do exhibit significant transient accumulation of cells in mitosis 6 to 12 hours after the treatment.[27] Taxanes also enhance the radioresponse of tumors that respond by significant tumor growth delay to taxanes given as a single treatment modality, but a major mechanism for radio enhancement in such tumors is reoxygenation of radioresistant hypoxic cells, as discussed later.[26]

Elimination of the radioresistant S-phase cells by the chemotherapeutic agents may be another cell cycle redistribution strategy in chemoradiation therapy. Nucleoside analogs, such as fludarabine or gemcitabine, are good examples of the agents that become incorporated into S-phase cells and eliminate them by inducing apoptosis.[19,21] In addition to purging S-phase cells, the analogs induce the surviving cells to undergo parasynchronous movement to accumulate in the G_2 and M phases of the cell cycle between 1 and 2 days after drug administration, a time when the highest enhancement of tumor radioresponse was observed.[21] Tumors with a high cell growth fraction are likely to respond better to the cell cycle redistribution strategy in chemoradiation therapy than tumors with a low cell growth fraction.

Counteracting Hypoxia-Associated Tumor Radioresistance
Solid malignant tumors usually are characterized by defective vascularization, both in the number of blood vessels and vessel function. Because of this, blood supply to tumor cells is inadequate, cells lack oxygen and nutrients, and multiple tumor microregions become hypoxic, acidic, and eventually necrotic. Hypoxia occurs at distances from blood vessels larger than 100 to 150 μm. The hypoxic cell content in tumors varies widely and can be more than 50%. The presence of hypoxia makes tumors more aggressive (hypoxia is conducive to the emergence of more virulent tumor cell variants and stimulates metastatic spread[28,29] and more resistant to radiation as well as most chemotherapeutic agents. Hypoxic cells are 2.5 to 3 times more resistant to radiation than well-oxygenated cells. The fact that hypoxia may be a cure-limiting factor in radiation therapy, at least in some clinical situations, is suggested by the findings that reduced hemoglobin levels[30] and low tumor pO_2[31,32] are associated with higher treatment failure rates. Also, there are reports showing that local tumor control by radiation therapy can be improved by the use of hypoxic cell radiosensitizers[33] or hyperbaric oxygen.[34,35] With respect to the effects of chemotherapy, hypoxic regions are less accessible to chemotherapeutic drugs; in addition, hypoxic tumor cells are either nonproliferating or they proliferate poorly and as such do not respond well to drugs.

Section II

Combining chemotherapeutic agents with radiation therapy can reduce or eliminate hypoxia or its negative influence on tumor radioresponse. Most chemotherapeutic drugs preferentially kill proliferating cells, primarily found in well-oxygenated regions of the tumor. Because these regions are located close to blood vessels, they are easily accessible to chemotherapeutic agents. Destruction of tumor cells in these areas leads to an increased oxygen supply to hypoxic regions and hence reoxygenates hypoxic tumor cells. Massive loss of cells after chemotherapy lowers the interstitial pressure, which then allows the reopening of previously closed capillaries and the re-establishment of blood supply. It also causes tumor shrinkage so that previously hypoxic areas are closer to capillaries and thus accessible to oxygen. Finally, by eliminating oxygenated cells, more oxygen becomes available to cells that survived chemotherapy. It was recently shown that tumor reoxygenation is a major mechanism underlying the enhancement of tumor radioresponse induced by taxanes in tumors sensitive to these drugs.[26]

Another approach to counteract the negative impact of hypoxia is selective killing of hypoxic cells through bioreductive drugs, such as tirapazamine,[28] which undergo reductive activation in a hypoxic milieu, rendering them cytotoxic. A related possibility is to exploit the acidic state (low pH) of tumors, which develops as a result of hypoxia-driven anaerobic metabolism that produces lactic acid,[36] through the use of drugs that selectively accumulate in acidic environments or become activated by a low pH.[37]

The use of agents that selectively radiosensitize hypoxic cells to reduce their negative impact has been considered and tested in clinical trials. These drugs increase radiation damage by mimicking the effect of oxygen. Many clinical trials have tested these drugs, particularly misonidazole, in combination with radiation therapy, but few of them have shown an improved treatment outcome. The exception is nimorazole, which also does not elicit the neurotoxicity commonly associated with hypoxic cell sensitizers that prevented the delivery of clinically effective doses of these agents.[38]

Inhibition of Tumor Cell Repopulation

The constant balance between cell production and cell loss maintains the integrity of normal tissues. When this balance is perturbed by cytotoxic action of chemotherapeutic drugs or radiation, the integrity of tissues is re-established by an increased rate of cell production. The cell loss after each fraction of radiation during radiation therapy induces compensatory cell regeneration (repopulation), the extent of which determines tissue tolerance to radiation therapy. In contrast to normal tissues, malignant tumors are characterized by an imbalance between cell production and cell loss in favor of cell production. As with normal tissues, tumors also respond to radiation- or drug-induced cell loss with a compensatory regenerative response. Preclinical studies provided ample evidence demonstrating that the rate of cell proliferation in tumors treated by radiation or chemotherapeutic drugs is higher than that in untreated tumors.[39-41] This increased rate of treatment-induced cell proliferation is commonly termed *accelerated repopulation*. Accelerated repopulation of tumor clonogens has been shown to occur during clinical radiation therapy as well. Withers et al.[42] showed that the total dose of radiation needed to control 50% of head and neck carcinomas progressively increased with time whenever radiation therapy treatment was prolonged beyond 1 month. This increase in radiation dose required to achieve tumor control was greater than what would be anticipated based on the pretreatment tumor volume doubling time of approximately 60 days for head and neck tumors. The increase was attributed to accelerated repopulation, and it was estimated to average approximately 0.6 Gy/day[42] but may be as high as 1 Gy/day.[43]

Although accelerated cell proliferation is beneficial for normal tissues because it spares them from radiation damage, it has an adverse impact on tumor control by radiation therapy or chemotherapy. Chemotherapeutic drugs, because of their cytotoxic or cytostatic activity, can reduce the rate of proliferation when given concurrently with radiation therapy and hence increase the effectiveness of the treatment. Caution must be taken to select drugs that preferentially affect rapidly proliferating cells and preferentially localize in malignant tumors. However, the main limitation of concurrent chemoradiation therapy is the enhanced toxicity of rapidly dividing normal tissues because most available chemotherapeutic agents show poor tumor selectivity. Moreover, accelerated repopulation induced by chemotherapeutic drugs may have a negative influence on the outcome of tumor response to radiation when drugs are used in induction or neoadjuvant chemotherapy protocols. In this strategy, chemotherapy precedes radiation therapy. Treatment outcomes after induction chemotherapy followed by radiation therapy have not been overly encouraging in terms of both local tumor control and patient survival, even if a large proportion of tumors initially responded with total or partial clinical regression by the time of radiation therapy implementation. Some experimental evidence suggests that the drug-induced accelerated cell repopulation can actually make the tumor more difficult to control with radiation.[39,40]

Other Potential Interactions

Modulation of Immunogenic Mechanism of Cell Death with Radiation

In the past decade, there has been significant advance in the understanding of the molecular signals involved in immunogenic cell death. Traditionally, radiation therapy was thought to have immunosuppressive potential, particularly if significant amounts of bone/bone marrow were in the treatment field. However, even as early as 1979, preclinical studies have demonstrated the potential importance of having an immune competent host to produce effective antitumor effects by radiation.[44] In another preclinical study where higher dose of radiation (15 to 20 Gy) was used to treat implanted mouse melanoma B16 tumor, it was determined that these tumors only responded when implanted in immunocompetent hosts, whereas tumors in mice that were immunocompromised (nude mice), or in mice where CD8+ T cells were depleted, failed to respond to high-dose radiotherapy.[45] Several studies have suggested the potential importance of CD8+ T-cell infiltration as it relates to radiotherapy-mediated immune effects.[8] Additional preclinical and clinical studies have demonstrated that radiotherapy therapy (RT) may also exert tumoricidal effects both in the irradiated region and outside of the radiation field, through immune-mediated mechanisms.[9] There is now evidence to suggest that radiation and some chemotherapy agents can induce steps that can lead to immunogenic cell death. It has been demonstrated that radiotherapy can release and/or lead to expression of new antigens with immune adjuvant-like effects and has been suggested that this can convert irradiated cancer into an in situ vaccine that elicits tumor-specific T cells.[9] This "vaccination" can lead to immune memory, which becomes a powerful weapon against not only the irradiated tumor but also against nonirradiated tumor sites (e.g., abscopal effect), and potentially against cancer cells that later emerge after a period from dormancy.[9]

Preclinical and clinical data supports the notion that radiation can augment innate and adaptive immune response to increase the tumoricidal effects on the antigenic cancer cells that had previously escaped immune surveillance likely through immunosuppressive mechanisms. Mechanisms for immune enhancement by RT is suggested to involve (a) increased tumor-associated antigen (TAA) release, (b) initiation of release of danger-associated molecular patterns (DAMPs—calreticulin, ATP, HMGB1), which leads to activation of antigen-presenting cell (APC), (c) improved dendritic cell (DC) function, and (d) enhanced T-cell priming.[8] Radiotherapy is thought to lead to creation of an inflammatory microenvironment that is conducive to maturation of APCs and to T-cell activation. Chemokine expressions are induced resulting in chemotaxis of T cells to the tumor microenvironment. Signals driving migration of APCs to draining lymph nodes lead to T-cell priming and initiation of systemic response.[8] Signals driving migration of APCs to draining lymph nodes lead to T-cell priming and initiation of systemic response.[8] Radiotherapy can modulate the priming of adaptive immune response against tumors by increasing antigen release by cancer cells, increased antigen uptake by DCs, and increases DC maturation. DC maturation is required in order for DCs to migrate to the draining lymph nodes to initiate an immune response. Radiation is also shown to increase recruitment of cytotoxic CD8+ T-cell infiltration by inducing chemokine expression, and by vascular normalization, which can lead to enhancement of tumor regression.[11] Inflammatory environment and recruitment of T cells to this microenvironment also may help sensitize cancers that are typically resistant to PD-L1 therapy.

Radiation can also facilitate increased recognition and killing of tumors by T cells in part by inducing MHC expression on cancer cells, and in some tumors, by up-regulation of cell death ligand Fas. In addition, radiation could increase recognition of tumor stroma and lead to destruction of this environment by cytotoxic T cells. Radiation also has been shown to sensitize cancer cells to recognition by natural killer (NK) cells.

Alternatively, radiotherapy also induces modulators of tumor immune response, by recruitment of immune suppressive factors, including myeloid-derived suppressor cells (MDSCs), tumor-associated macrophages, and regulatory T cells (Tregs). Studies would suggest that increase in myeloid cells would be protective of irradiated tumors by fostering a pro-growth environment and by inhibiting antitumor immune effects.[11] Radiotherapy can also lead to galectin-1 expression, which can lead to systemic lymphopenia,[46] and can up-regulate PD-L1 in tumor microenvironment,[47] which can lead to tumor escape mechanism from T cells. These dual effects (stimulation and suppression) of immune response by radiotherapy

likely contributed to the overall lack of significant immune response unless radiotherapy is used in conjunction with an appropriate immune modulating agent.

It is recognized that tumors can suppress the antitumor immune response by multiple mechanisms, including production of inhibitory cytokines, recruitment of immunosuppressive immune cells, and up-regulation of immune checkpoints, which are molecules that enhance (costimulatory molecules) or inhibit the immune response.[48] Different strategies for harnessing immune response to exert its effect on tumors include development of receptors that can activate or block the inhibition of the immune response and lead to T-cell stimulation (Fig. 36.2).[49] Of these strategies, significant increase in understanding of checkpoints, molecules that shuts down the immune system as a means of immune suppression in tumors, have led to development of a novel clinically relevant paradigm for cancer therapy. Checkpoint inhibition as a method for inhibiting immunosuppressing mechanisms have been investigated for potential therapeutic gain. The two most studied immune checkpoint inhibitor class are strategies that inhibit cytotoxic T lymphocyte antigen-4 (CTLA-4) and programmed death 1 (PD1).[50]

CTLA-4 is expressed on helper CD4+ T cells and T regulatory cells. It has a high affinity for binding B7-1 and B7-2 and prevents these from binding to CD28, a costimulatory receptor. CTLA-4 can also deliver inhibitory signal to CD8+ T cells and can increase the immunosuppressive activity of Tregs. Therefore, antibodies that effectively block CTLA-4 will lead to B7 ligands binding to CD28, enhance the expansion of effector CD8+ T-cell response, and prevents Treg, all of which leads to increased immune effects on tumor.[11] PD1 is expressed on effector T cells and typically acts in the tumor microenvironment. PD1 can be up-regulated by activated T cells and binds to ligands PD-L1 and PD-L2. Cytokines such as interferon gamma can induce the expression of PD-L1 on epithelial cells and tumor cells. PD-L2 are primarily expressed on DCs and macrophages. This binding can lead to apoptotic death of effector T cells, which can lead to exhaustion of antitumor response.[11] A number of preclinical studies have demonstrated that combining radiation therapy with CTLA-4 and PD1 inhibition is a promising novel strategy for cancer therapy.[11] There are preclinical data, and early clinical data suggesting that combining RT and checkpoint inhibiting immunotherapy can lead to synergistic immune effects both locally and in nonirradiated sites (synergistic enhancement

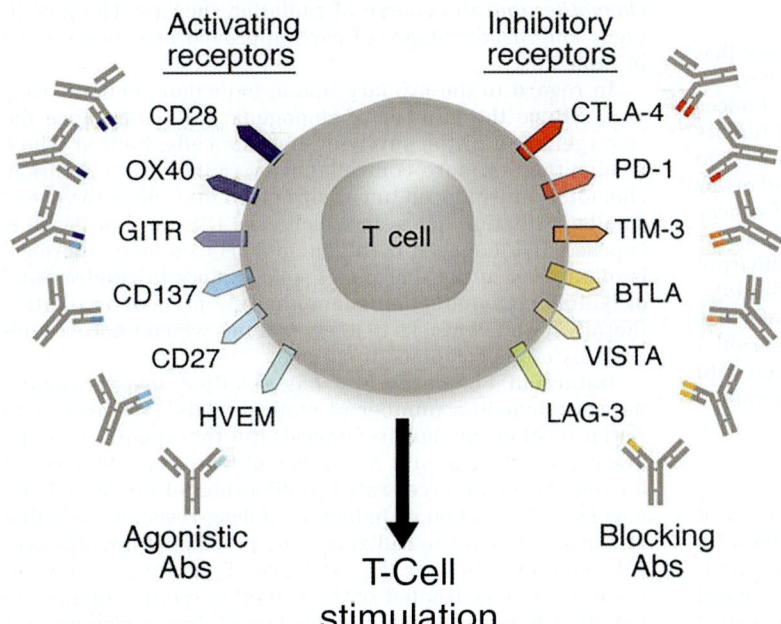

FIGURE 36.2. Potential T cell targets for development of therapeutic strategy for immunomodulation. (Reprinted by permission from Nature: Mellman I, Coukos G, Dranoff G. Cancer immunotherapy comes of age. *Nature* 2011;480(7378):480–489. Copyright © 2011 Springer Nature.)

of the abscopal effect).[10] Preclinical and early clinical studies also support continued investigation in to the use of radiation with other immune strategies including cytokine therapy (e.g., interleukin-2 [IL-2]) and vaccine therapy.[10] The furthest clinically developed CTLA-4 and PD-L1 inhibitors as these pertain to clinically applicable radiation-related immune effects are discussed in section on "Using Radiotherapy to Improve the Local and Distal Tumoricidal Effects of Immunotherapy, A Novel Paradigm in Combined Modality Therapy" below.

Molecular Signaling Pathways That May Be Responsible for Radioresistance

Significant strides have been made in elucidating molecular pathways that may be involved in resistance to cytotoxic therapy including radiation treatments. These molecular determinants are being scrutinized in preclinical and clinical settings as potential targets for cancer therapy, of which some agents are being studied for the potential for enhancing radiation effects.[51] For example, the efficacy of combining the epidermal growth factor receptor (EGFR) inhibitor cetuximab with radiation therapy has been demonstrated in randomized clinical studies in head and neck cancer patients.[52] Molecular targeting has become an immensely important topic, and effective integration of these strategies with radiation therapy to foster improved efficacy of therapy is an active area of investigation. This topic is further discussed in significant detail in the section to follow.

Targeting the Tumor Microenvironment

Tumor microenvironment has been postulated as being a potential therapeutic target for cancer therapy. Tumor microenvironment is a complex system of many cell types including endothelial cells, smooth muscle cells, fibroblasts, and cells involved with the immune system (lymphocytes, macrophages, etc.).[53] Among these different cells that make up the different components of the tumor microenvironment, the most studied preclinically and clinically are the cells that make up the tumor microvasculature. Preclinical studies have suggested the potential role for radiosensitization of the tumor microvasculature using compounds directed at targeting angiogenesis.[54] Clinical studies have been performed with efforts to combine antiangiogenic agents with radiation therapy, with mixed results.[54] Studies are ongoing, as many antiangiogenic agents are approved for cancer therapy, and are detailed in the section on antiangiogenic agents.

Cancer Stem Cells

Cancer stem cells are defined as being cells within a tumor that possess the capacity to self-renew and generate the heterogeneous lineages of cancer cells that make up the tumor.[55] Cancer stem cells as a source of radiation resistance for solid tumors is an area of active investigation. Potential for the need to eradicate cancer stem cells for effective cure by radiotherapy has been postulated, and although radioresistance of cancer stem cells has been noted in *in vitro* studies,[56] this notion has been challenged as some have demonstrated radiosensitivity of cancer stem cells.[57] But, if in fact cancer stem cells are radioresistant, one possible strategy may be to identify molecular pathways that could influence cancer stem cell radiosensitivity and investigate the use of such agents in combination with radiotherapy at different stages during the course of therapy.[58]

Combined Chemoradiation to Induce Immunogenic Cell Death Pathway

Some have proposed that achievement of immunogenic cell death may be another mechanism of improved outcomes seen with concurrent chemoradiation therapy.[9] Drug repositioning refers to the utilization of a known compound in a novel indication and new mode of activity leading to innovative

therapy.[59] It has been proposed that cancer cell immunogenicity might be recovered through "repositioning"[59,60] achieved through concurrent use of chemotherapy with radiation. In this concept, it is suggested that radiation and chemotherapy used together may complement one another and fulfill requirements for successful signaling of the immunogenic cell death pathway leading to more than additive outcomes and even noticeable improvements in nonlocoregional outcomes.

Improving Systemic Therapy Outcome by Cytoreduction of Gross Metastases with Local SBRT

Another proposed mechanism of improving outcomes with use of systemic agents with radiotherapy has been suggested involving patients with limited metastatic disease. This mechanism suggests that stereotactic body radiotherapy technique (SBRT) could be used to cytoreduce gross disease in patients with limited number of metastatic sites, at the onset of initiation of systemic therapy. This was based on studies suggesting that most failures after chemotherapy for non–small cell lung cancer (NSCLC) occur at the original gross disease and that most patients have metastases that are amenable to SBRT.[61] In a proof of principle study, a single-arm phase II trial of SBRT in patients with 6 or less metastatic site, with erlotinib systemic therapy beginning 1 week prior, and administered during, and after SBRT, was conducted.[62] This study demonstrated a remarkable progression-free survival (PFS) (14.7 months) and overall survival (OS) (20.4 months) as compared to historical patients with similar presentation. Furthermore, pattern of relapse was shifted, with failures occurring at new sites as opposed to the preexisting local sites. This suggests a potential novel mechanism for improving outcome of patients with limited metastatic disease, by combining cytoreductive SBRT with systemic treatments.

TIMING OF DRUG ADMINISTRATION IN RELATION TO RADIATION THERAPY

Most clinical chemoradiation therapy regimens evolved empirically: increasingly, information from preclinical studies is being considered in planning the optimal timing of drug administration in relation to radiation therapy. Depending on the principal aim of the therapy, drugs are administered before (*induction* or *neoadjuvant chemotherapy*), during (*concurrent* or *concomitant chemotherapy*), or after (*adjuvant chemotherapy*) the course of radiation therapy. The advantages and disadvantages of each approach are summarized in Table 36.1.

In regard to the primary tumor, induction chemotherapy may reduce the number of clonogenic cells and cause the reoxygenation of the surviving hypoxic cells, both of which render tumors more controllable by radiation. In addition, chemotherapy-induced tumor shrinkage may allow the use of smaller radiation fields, in which case less normal tissue is exposed and damaged by radiation. This treatment approach is often used in the therapy of solid tumors in children and of lymphomas. Induction chemotherapy precedes radiation therapy for a few weeks to a few months, which improves tolerability of the combined treatment.

Induction chemotherapy has resulted in therapeutic improvement in a number of clinical trials compared with radiation therapy, but in general, the therapeutic benefits are below expectations. A number of factors could account for this, including accelerated proliferation of tumor cell clonogens and selection or induction of drug-resistant cells that are cross-resistant to radiation. The preclinical findings provide solid evidence for the existence of accelerated repopulation in tumors treated with chemotherapeutic agents. On the other hand, although development of drug resistance is a

TABLE 36.1 ADVANTAGES AND DISADVANTAGES OF DIFFERENT CHEMORADIATION SEQUENCING STRATEGIES

Strategy	Advantages	Disadvantages
Sequential chemoradiation	• Least toxic • Maximizes systemic therapy • Smaller radiation fields if induction shrinks tumor	• Increased treatment time • Lack of local synergy
Concurrent chemoradiation	• Shorter treatment time • Radiation enhancement	• Compromised systemic therapy • Increased toxicity • No cytoreduction of tumor
Concurrent chemoradiation and adjuvant chemotherapy	• Maximizes systemic therapy • Radiation enhancement • Both local and distant therapy delivered up front	• Increased toxicity • Increased treatment time • Difficult to complete chemotherapy after chemoradiation
Induction chemotherapy and concurrent chemoradiation	• Maximizes systemic therapy • Radiation enhancement	• Increased toxicity • Increased treatment time • Difficult to complete chemoradiation after induction therapy

significant problem in chemotherapy, the evidence that cells that acquire drug resistance are also resistant to radiation is not convincing.

When chemotherapy is given during a course of radiation therapy, it is referred to as *concurrent chemotherapy*. This form of treatment is intended to cope with both disseminated lesions and the primary tumor, but it takes advantage of drug–radiation interactions to maximize tumor radioresponse. The drug scheduling in relation to individual radiation fractions is highly important, and the selection of optimal timing of drug administration must be based on mechanisms of tumor radio enhancement by a given drug, the drug's normal tissue toxicity, and the conditions under which the highest enhancement is achieved. The data from preclinical studies can greatly contribute to the selection of the most optimal schedules. For example, it has been demonstrated that murine tumors sensitive to taxanes show enhanced radioresponse, but the best effect is achieved if drug treatment precedes radiation by 1 to 3 days.[26] A major mechanism for tumor radio enhancement was reoxygenation of hypoxic cells. Based on this preclinical information, one would anticipate that in clinical protocols such tumors would best respond to a bolus of a taxane given once or twice weekly during radiation therapy. In contrast, tumors resistant to taxanes on their own would call for daily administration of a taxane because they show accumulation of radiosensitive G_2- and M-phase cells 6 to 12 hours after drug administration. If the objective is to counteract rapid repopulation of tumor cell clonogens induced by radiation, then administration of cell cycle–specific chemotherapeutic agents during the second half of radiation therapy, when accelerated repopulation is more expressed, might be more effective. At present, the enhancement in normal tissue complications remains the major limitation of concurrently combining chemotherapy with radiation therapy. Nevertheless, as is made evident later in the text, concurrent chemoradiation therapy has provided better clinical results both in terms of local tumor control and patient survival than have other modes of chemoradiation therapy combinations.[63,64]

Adjuvant chemotherapy designates a treatment modality in which chemotherapeutic drugs are given some time after completion of radiation therapy. The primary objective is to eradicate disseminated disease; however, the control of the primary tumor may also be improved by the ability of drugs to deal with tumor cells that survived radiation.

INTERACTION OF SPECIFIC CHEMOTHERAPIES AND RADIATION IN THE TREATMENT OF CANCER

This section provides an overview of the evidence that exists for combining particular chemotherapies with radiation. In many cases, the level of support that exists for combined therapy mirrors the age of the drug. However, as would be expected, newer drugs have generally been subject to more rigorous preclinical assessment of their efficacy before their introduction into the clinical setting (Table 36.2).

Platinum-Based Drugs

This group of compounds, distinguished from most others by its metallic element base, has come to be recognized as one of the most potent chemotherapies available to date. Cisplatin (*cis*-diamminedichloroplatinum II), which is the prototype drug, has been acknowledged to be a potent radiosensitizer for many years and has a significant role in clinical practice to date. Preclinical work done using murine models by Rosenberg et al.[80] in the late 1960s showed that cisplatin is an effective antitumor chemotherapy. Subsequent efforts have shown that its primary mechanism of inhibition of tumor growth appears to involve the inhibition of DNA synthesis by formation of DNA cross-links.[81,82] Another secondary mechanism includes the inhibition of transcription elongation by DNA interstrand cross-links.[83]

Work on nonmammalian systems first demonstrated the radiosensitizing abilities of platinum-based compounds.[84–86] This was confirmed in several mammalian systems as well.[65,87,88] This makes inherent sense because these platinum compounds have a high electron affinity and react preferentially with hydrated electrons. The exact mechanism for the increased cell death seen with combinations

TABLE 36.2 MECHANISMS OF CHEMOTHERAPY-INDUCED RADIATION SENSITIZATION

Class of Compound	Mechanism of Radiosensitization	References
Platinum-based compounds	Inhibition of DNA synthesis Inhibition of transcription elongation by DNA interstrand cross-links Inhibition of repair of radiation-induced DNA damage	65–68
Taxanes	Cellular arrest in the G_2M phase of the cell cycle Induction of apoptosis Reoxygenation of tumor cells	26,27,69,70
Topoisomerase I inhibitors	Inhibition of repair of radiation-induced DNA strand breaks Redistribution into G_2 phase of the cell cycle Conversion of radiation-induced SSBs into DSBs	71–73
Hypoxic cell cytotoxins	Complementary cytotoxicity with radiation on euoxic and hypoxic tumor cells	74,75
Antimetabolites	Nucleotide pool perturbation Lowering apoptotic threshold Cell cycle redistribution Tumor cell reoxygenation	19,20,76,77
Temozolomide	DNA repair inhibition (radiosensitization effect may be subject to MGMT status)	78,79

of ionizing radiation and platinum drugs is not known for certain; however, the evidence would seem to point to the inhibition of PLDR[66] and to the radiosensitization of hypoxic tumor cells.[89] Cisplatin-free radical–mediated sensitization may involve the ability to scavenge free electrons formed by the interaction between radiation and DNA. The reduction of the platinum moiety may serve to stabilize DNA damage that would otherwise be repairable.[90] Greater than additive effects of cisplatin and radiation are seen in tumor models most reliably when the drug is administered with fractionated radiation,[90] explained by its inhibition of SLDR. Bladder cancer, head and neck cancer, lung cancer, esophageal cancer, and cervix cancer are some of the disease sites where cisplatinum is approved for use in combination with radiation therapy.

Carboplatin, a second-generation platinum compound with a different toxicity profile, has also been studied as a radiosensitizer.[67,68] Mechanism of action also involves interfering with function of DNA by producing interstrand DNA cross-links. Carboplatin tends to have less nephrotoxic or neurotoxic effects compared to cisplatin, but hematologic toxicity is slightly increased. Its potential efficacy as a radiosensitizer has allowed for its incorporation into regimens used in several randomized trials including but not limited to landmark trials which allowed for its indication for use in esophageal cancer, head and neck cancer, and lung cancer. Oxaliplatin, although sharing a similar mode of action as other platinum compounds, has been shown to have activity in cisplatin-resistant systems *in vitro*.[4] One potential explanation for this is that oxaliplatin is not affected by loss of mismatch repair, which leads to cisplatin resistance *in vitro*,[91] and there are those who postulate that adducts formed by oxaliplatin are less well recognized by DNA repair systems.[92] Whether oxaliplatin is truly active against cisplatin-resistant cancer clinically is an area of active investigation.[93] Despite encouraging findings in phase I to II rectal cancer studies, phase III studies integrating neoadjuvant oxaliplatin with 5-FU or capecitabine with radiotherapy, with the exception of the CAO/ARO/AIO-04 study, have yielded negative findings (STAR-01, ACCORD 12, NSABP R04, PETACC-6).[94] In esophageal cancer, oxaliplatin-based chemoradiation therapy, although did not demonstrate improvement in efficacy over cisplatinum/5-FU–based regimen, was suggested to be a more convenient regimen and was not found to be more toxic.[95] Oxaliplatin-based regimens with radiation therapy are being further studied in additional randomized phase II studies in comparison to carboplatin-based regimen (NEOSCOPE and PROTECT-1402).[94,96]

Antimicrotubules

Taxanes

The radiosensitizing properties of plant-derived chemotherapeutic agents, the taxanes, have been studied extensively in both preclinical models and in clinical trials. Paclitaxel (Taxol) and docetaxel (Taxotere) act as mitotic spindle inhibitors through their promotion of microtubule assembly and inhibition of disaggregation.[97] Both taxanes bind to the *N*-terminal 31–amino-acid sequence of the β-tubulin subunit of cellular tubulin polymers, stabilizing the polymers by shifting the dynamic equilibrium that exists between tubulin dimers and microtubules in favor of the polymerized state.[98,99] Although there is preclinical evidence that docetaxel has both a higher affinity for the tubulin-binding site and greater *in vitro* cytotoxicity than paclitaxel, this has not necessarily translated into greater clinical efficacy because the toxicity profiles of the two drugs also differ.[100,101]

The administration of a taxane leads to cellular arrest in the G_2/M phase of the cell cycle, which is the precise point associated with increased sensitivity to the lethal effects of

ionizing radiation.[102] Early laboratory studies with a human lung cancer cell line[25] and human astrocytoma cells[24] bore out the prospect of significant radiosensitization, with relative enhancement ratios in the 1.48 to 1.8 range when paclitaxel was administered before irradiation.

The exact conditions used in various studies appear to determine the strength of the interaction between radiation and paclitaxel because subadditive effects have been seen in addition to the more widely reported additive and supra-additive effects.[27] In general, enhancement of radiation effects is seen when proliferating cells have been incubated with moderate concentrations of paclitaxel for 24 hours before irradiation. Conditions leading to a less-than-optimal response include paclitaxel-mediated G_1 arrest, wherein a more resistant cell subpopulation counteracts the effects of a G_2/M block; paclitaxel-induced cell cycle effects such as the G_2/M block in cells destined to die before irradiation; and incubation conditions insufficient to exert cellular effects. The fact that nonproliferating cells are also sensitized to the effects of radiation by the use of paclitaxel suggests that mechanisms other than the cell cycle arrest in the G_2/M phase underlie paclitaxel's sensitizing abilities.

Paclitaxel also acts to induce programmed cell death; work from the M.D. Anderson Cancer Center[27] has examined the relationship between mitotic arrest, apoptosis, and the antineoplastic activity of paclitaxel in 16 murine tumors. Single-dose paclitaxel (40 mg/kg) induced mitotic arrest to varying degrees in all tumors; however, apoptosis was induced in only 50% of tumors. This study also revealed that pretreatment levels of apoptosis correlated with both paclitaxel-induced apoptosis and tumor growth delay. Therefore, both the pretreatment apoptotic rate and paclitaxel-induced apoptotic rate could potentially act as predictors of the response to paclitaxel.

Milas et al.[27] summarized observations that showed that (a) there was massive loss of tumor cells though the apoptotic pathway was restricted to the perivascular region, and (b) radio enhancement occurring during this period of cell loss became even more impressive when apoptotic cells were removed from the tumor. Experiments in which tumor xenografts were treated with paclitaxel and exposed to radiation under hypoxic or air-ambient conditions were pursued.[26] It was found that the creation of hypoxic conditions greatly reduced the efficacy of paclitaxel in its enhancement of radioresponse. It appears that a combination of cell cycle effects, drug-induced reoxygenation, and drug-induced apoptosis underlies paclitaxel's radiosensitizing abilities.

Docetaxel has also been found to be a respectable radiosensitizer in both *in vitro*[69] and *in vivo* models.[70] Radiation response in the presence of docetaxel was examined in three different cell lines that have widely different responses to radiation alone.[103] Their findings suggest that the p53 status of tumor cells may have a profound effect on the radiosensitizing effects of a taxane. Other novel taxanes and analogs that continue to attract the interest of investigators for their potential to enhance radiation effects include Abraxane, paclitaxel poliglumex, larotaxel, cabazitaxel,[104,105] and orally available taxanes.[106]

Antimetabolites

5-Fluorouracil

The radiosensitizing properties of 5-FU has been known for years.[107] Several mechanisms have been proposed for the cytotoxicity of this drug:

a. Its incorporation into RNA, which leads to a disruption of RNA function
b. Inhibition of thymidylate synthase function and subsequently of DNA synthesis
c. Direct incorporation of the drug into DNA

It is believed that a combination of these effects underlies its radiosensitizing properties.[108] Optimization of its schedule of delivery is crucial to obtaining an effect with this combination, and it is accepted that cytotoxic doses of 5-FU are needed to obtain a radiosensitizing effect. In general, it is thought that a continuous infusion of the drug is needed to obtain the desired drug levels after irradiation.[109] Long-standing clinical experience with this drug bears out much of the laboratory studies of its effectiveness as a radiation sensitizer. Gastrointestinal tract cancers, bladder cancer, and head and neck cancers are some of the disease sites where 5-FU–based combined modality therapy with radiation is used as standard of care.

Capecitabine

Capecitabine is an oral prodrug of 5-FU. It is converted to its cytotoxic form in three enzymatic steps, the last of which is mediated by thymidine phosphorylase. One of the potential advantages of this mechanism for increasing tumor cytotoxicity is that thymidine phosphorylase is overexpressed in tumor tissues. Interestingly, radiation has been shown to stimulate expression of thymidine phosphorylase, which provides a further rationale for considering combined therapy with radiation treatments.[110] Capecitabine was shown to be safe to replace 5-FU in chemoradiotherapy regimen for rectal cancer.[111] It is being used in the combined modality setting as standard therapy, and in clinical trials, for many tumor types (including but not limited to rectal cancer, gastric cancer, esophageal cancer) requiring fluorouracil-based chemoradiation.

Gemcitabine

Gemcitabine is another nucleoside analog that acts as a very potent radiosensitizer. The biologic action of gemcitabine is due almost completely to its effects on DNA metabolism. Early studies of this drug in leukemic cell lines found that notable decreases in cellular deoxynucleotide triphosphates occurred with the use of the drug.[112]

Direct incorporation of the drug into DNA and drug-induced apoptosis are also thought to underlie its cytotoxicity.[112] The metabolism of gemcitabine in the cell is complex, and it is able to potentiate its cytotoxicity as a sole therapy.[112] Depending on the conditions, relative enhancement ratios in the range of 1.1 to 2.5 have been reported.

Gemcitabine is S-phase specific and as such should be selectively toxic to proliferating cells,[113] decreasing the amount of proliferation that can occur during fractionated radiation therapy. In addition, cell cycle redistribution induced by these agents may improve cell kill by allowing more cells to be treated in the more sensitive parts of the cell cycle.[114] As DNA synthesis inhibitors, these drugs may act to inhibit the repair of radiation-induced DNA damage.[19] Finally, as DNA chain terminators, they may serve to trigger the apoptotic response.[20]

There is strong preclinical evidence to suggest that the radiosensitizing abilities of gemcitabine are intimately linked to cellular deoxyadenosine triphosphate levels.[20] Interesting results from Latz et al.[76] show quite clearly that cells that are pretreated with gemcitabine no longer show a progressive increase in radioresistance as they progress toward DNA replication, and sensitization, therefore, appears to be greatest in the S-phase.

Milas et al.[21] found the largest enhancement of growth delay when gemcitabine was delivered 24 to 60 hours before irradiation in a murine sarcoma tumor model. The use of gemcitabine with radiation also decreased the risk for development of lung metastases in those mice that attained durable local control (73% in the radiation-alone group vs. 40% in the combined modality group), which was confirmed in a second study with a larger number of mice.[77] This preclinical work is supportive of the principles of combined modality therapy in that better local control translated into decreased systemic spread of tumor cells. The same authors also report a dose-dependent increase in the apoptotic rate after the administration of gemcitabine,[21] which they believe correlates with the elimination of the more radioresistant S-phase population of cells and a redistribution of the remaining cells into more radiosensitive parts of the cell cycle. They also report that reoxygenation of the resistant hypoxic fraction of tumor cells is a mechanism for the radiosensitizing action of gemcitabine.[77]

In summary, the preclinical evidence suggests that gemcitabine acts through several mechanisms (nucleotide pool perturbation, lowering of the apoptotic threshold, cell cycle redistribution, and tumor cell reoxygenation) to enhance the effect of ionizing radiation on tumors. Clinical experience has shown that this drug is indeed a potent sensitizer with the potential for significant toxicity as well as improvement in tumor control when combined with radiation.[115-121]

Pemetrexed

Pemetrexed is a novel multitargeted agent, exerting its effect via simultaneous inhibition of multiple folate-requiring enzymes, including thymidylate synthase, dihydrofolate reductase, and glycinamide ribonucleotide formyl-transferase.[122] Pemetrexed has shown synergistic activity with radiation treatments, likely because of interference with DNA synthesis.[123] There are indications that radiosensitization by pemetrexed is not cell cycle phase specific[124] *in vitro*. Others have suggested that a combination of radiation therapy and pemetrexed results in supra-additive effects, which may be in part because of apoptosis induction.[125] Phase III study in NSCLC has demonstrated nonsuperiority for pemetrexed–cisplatin with radiation, compared to cisplatin-etoposide and radiation, and although trial closed early because of futility, it is considered to be a potential alternative regimen.[126]

Topoisomerase I Inhibitors

Camptothecin is a plant alkaloid obtained from the *Camptotheca acuminata* tree. Its initial clinical evaluation in the 1960s and 1970s was abandoned because of severe and unpredictable hemorrhagic cystitis.[127,128] Camptothecin and its derivatives (e.g., irinotecan, topotecan, 9-aminocamptothecin, SN-38) target DNA topoisomerase I.[129-131] This enzyme relaxes both positively and negatively supercoiled DNA and allows for diverse essential cellular processes, including replication and transcription, to proceed. In the presence of camptothecin, a camptothecin–topoisomerase I–DNA complex becomes stabilized with the 5′-phosphoryl terminus of the enzyme-catalyzed DNA SSB bound covalently to a tyrosine residue of topoisomerase I. These stabilized cleavable complexes interact with the advancing replication fork during the S-phase or during unscheduled DNA replication after genomic stress and cause the conversion of SSBs into irreversible DNA DSBs, resulting in cell death.[130]

Several investigators have reported that camptothecin enhances the cytotoxic effect of radiation *in vitro* and *in vivo*.[71-73] Chen et al.[72] showed that cells exposed to 20(S)-10,11 methylenedioxy-camptothecin before or during radiation had sensitization ratios of 1.6, whereas those treated with the drug after radiation had substantially less enhancement of radiation-induced DNA damage. There are several hypotheses regarding the mechanism of interaction between radiation and irinotecan: (a) inhibition of topoisomerase I by irinotecan leads to inhibition of repair of radiation-induced DNA strand breaks; (b) irinotecan causes a redistribution of the cells into the more radiosensitive G_2 phase of the cell cycle; (c) topoisomerase I–DNA adducts are trapped by irinotecan at the sites of radiation-induced SSBs, leading to their conversion into DSBs.[132] Although there is currently insufficient evidence to identify the underlying mechanism with certainty, the primary mechanism involved with radiosensitization may depend on which camptothecin derivative is being used.

Data from *in vivo* experiments demonstrate that combination 9-aminocamptothecin and irradiation is more effective when fractionated, compared with single doses.[133] There is also evidence for circadian-dependent cytotoxicity and radiation sensitization when camptothecin derivatives like 9-aminocamptothecin are used as radiation sensitizers.[133] The integration of this group of drugs into clinical treatments with radiation therapy has been explored in NSCLC and brain tumors.[134–137]

Alkylating Agents

Temozolomide

Temozolomide is a second-generation alkylating agent, which is orally administered, is readily bioavailable, and demonstrates broad-spectrum activity in a variety of difficult-to-treat malignancies including glioma and melanoma.[138] It is unique in its ability to cross the blood–brain barrier (about 30% to 40% of plasma concentration found in CSF). *In vitro* studies demonstrate increased inhibition of cell growth in combination with radiotherapy.[139] Radiosensitization appears to occur via inhibition of DNA repair, leading to an increase in mitotic catastrophe.[78] It has proven efficacy as a first-line therapy for glioblastoma multiforme (GBM) patients in conjunction with radiotherapy based on a randomized phase III clinical study demonstrating survival benefit.[140] Temozolomide spontaneously converts to the reactive methylating agent 5-(3-methyl-1-triazeno)imidazole-4-carboxamide (MTIC) and transfers methyl groups to DNA, the most important one being at the O6 position of guanine, an important site for DNA alkylation.[141] The MGMT gene encodes a DNA repair protein that removes the alkyl group from the O6 position of guanine, and high MGMT activity levels abrogate the effectiveness of alkylating agents. *In vitro*, temozolomide enhances the radiation response most effectively in MGMT-negative glioblastomas, and likely because of decreased double-strand DNA repair capacity and increased DNA DSB damage, which occurs when the combination of temozolomide and radiation therapy was administered.[79] Analysis of a randomized study by the European Organization for Research and Treatment of Cancer (EORTC) and National Cancer Institute of Canada (NCIC) demonstrated that loss of MGMT expression by promoter methylation is correlated with a better outcome after treatment with radiation and temozolomide.[142] Temozolomide and radiation combination is considered the backbone standard therapy for newly diagnosed GBM, upon which combination of additional new investigational agents are being studied.

Other Agents

Mitomycin-C

Mitomycin-C is a quinone, whose mechanisms of action include inhibition of DNA and RNA synthesis.[143] When combined with radiation, the rationale for the use of mitomycin-C is based on its ability to target hypoxic cells that are known to be relatively radiation resistant.[144] There is preclinical evidence to suggest that mitomycin-C administered before irradiation leads to a supra-additive interaction.[74,145] The postulated mechanisms of action for supra-additivity include prevention of repopulation and hypoxic cell sensitization, although the definitive action is not fully elucidated. Given that normal tissues are not hypoxic, the selective targeting

of this cell population with mitomycin-C has the potential to improve cures without compromising normal tissue complication rates. The use of mitomycin-C is limited by its hematologic toxicities. Mitomycin-C combined with radiation therapy remains the standard-of-care therapy for anal carcinoma based on multiple clinical studies.[146]

Hypoxic Sensitizers

Tirapazamine

Investigators have pursued a similar strategy as outlined previously with the development of tirapazamine, a hypoxic cell cytotoxin.[28,75] Brown[75] has discovered that tirapazamine, which is a benzotriazine di-*N*-oxide, is toxic to hypoxic cells at concentrations much lower than what is needed to radiosensitize cells. It has the greatest differential toxicity known between hypoxic and well-oxygenated cells. Essentially, this drug functions through its intracellular reduction to form a highly reactive radical capable of causing both SSBs and DSBs.[147] In the presence of oxygen, a free electron is absorbed, and the compound is back-oxidized to the parent compound with the concomitant release of a superoxide radical, which is much less cytotoxic than the tirapazamine radical. Clinical trials are ongoing or have been completed in multiple tumor sites including cervix, head and neck, GBM, and lung malignancies (small cell lung cancer).[148–160] Although most studies have demonstrated a reasonable toxicity profile, several studies have suggested caution in the appropriate selection of a dose and delivery regimen when combining tirapazamine to a standard chemoradiation regimen.[152,155,161]

Fairly promising earlier phase studied led to phase III studies in head and neck and cervical cancer. A phase III study by the Trans-Tasman group (TROG 02.02) suggested no significant improvement in survival outcome in locally advanced head and neck cancer patients, unselected for hypoxia, with the addition of tirapazamine to a standard platinum-based chemoradiation regimen.[158] A subset analysis of the phase II study from the TransTasman Group suggested that tumors with a hypoxic component as assessed by 18F fluoromisonidazole positron emission tomography (FMISO-PET) imaging had a higher likelihood of locoregional failure, whereas an improvement in local control was identified for those treated with the addition of tirapazamine, suggesting that it specifically targets hypoxic tumor cells.[154] Similarly, GOG phase III trial studying the role of addition of tirapazamine to platinum-based radiation therapy in cervical cancer was closed early and demonstrated no improvement in survival outcomes with the addition of tirapazamine.[161] Study was closed early because of lack of available study drug and limits future development of this drug.[161–163]

Nimorazole

Nimorazole is another hypoxic cell radiosensitizer belonging to a class of chemical known as 5-nitroimidazoles, with less neuropathic toxicity than misonidazole; it has demonstrated improved tumor control outcome and tolerability with radiotherapy, in supraglottic laryngeal and pharyngeal tumors in the DAHANCA 5 study.[38] A randomized multicenter study, IAEA-HypoX study with nimorazole and concomitant accelerated radiotherapy in head and neck squamous cell carcinoma, was attempted but closed prematurely in 2014 because of poor recruitment (100 of the intended 600 patients were accrued).[30] Although closed early, it suggested an improvement in locoregional tumor control with the addition of nimorazole. Additional ongoing trials include NIMRAD, a phase III study of addition of nimorazole to radiotherapy in patients with locally advanced head and neck cancer not suitable for chemotherapy or cetuximab.[163] EORTC has opened a phase III multicenter study of radiation with or without nimorazole using a 15-gene signature for hypoxia in the treatment of head and neck squamous cell carcinoma. DAHANCA 30, a randomized noninferiority study of hypoxia-profile guided selection of patients who are predicted to be nonresponders to chemoradiotherapy with or without nimorazole, is recruiting patients.

EMERGING STRATEGIES FOR IMPROVEMENT OF CHEMORADIATION THERAPY

In spite of increasing therapeutic achievements of chemoradiation therapy, the use of this form of therapy is still very much restricted by its narrow therapeutic index. The available agents are either insufficiently effective on their own or in combination with radiation against tumors, or normal tissue toxicity prevents the use of effective doses of drugs or radiation. Significant research efforts, both preclinical and clinical, have been undertaken to improve chemoradiation therapy. They include developing more selective and more effective chemotherapeutic agents, incorporating additional agents into chemoradiation therapy that protect normal tissues from injury by drugs or radiation, and improving the technique of radiation therapy delivery to minimize treatment of adjacent normal tissue while maximizing tumor dose delivery.

Increasing Antitumor Efficacy of Chemotherapeutic Drugs

A number of newer chemotherapeutic agents are being developed with the goal of enhancing antitumor effects by improving on the selective targeting of tumor cells via strategies such as chemical modification of known compounds including agents currently in use with radiation therapy because of their radiosensitizing properties.

Approaches for improvement of drug safety, convenience, or efficacy could include chemical modifications or modifications of the formulation of a known drug. One example is that of Abraxane (nab-paclitaxel, ABI-007). Abraxane is a 130-nM particle form of paclitaxel that is bound to albumin and is solvent free. This avoids the need for Cremophor-based vehicles and lowers the risk of hypersensitivity reactions.[104] Such vehicles have the potential for altered pharmacokinetics by drug entrapment, leading to decreased drug clearance, decreased volume of distribution, and ultimately nonlinear pharmacokinetics. Interestingly, Abraxane has been demonstrated to have higher antitumor activity compared to Taxol in preclinical studies. This is in part mediated via utilization of albumin receptor–mediated endothelial transport, which leads to higher intracellular accumulation compared to standard paclitaxel.[164] Clinically, Abraxane has shown demonstrated efficacy in metastatic breast cancer in a phase III study.[165] Phase I/II studies in advanced NSCLC, melanoma, bladder cancer, high-risk prostate cancer, and gynecologic malignancy have been reported.[165-176] Preclinical studies have demonstrated Abraxane to have radiosensitizing properties.[177] Therefore, there is significant interest in determining the potential efficacy of Abraxane in disease sites where combined therapy with taxanes and radiation has demonstrated therapeutic advantage. Phase I and phase I/II study of nab-paclitaxel with radiation in lung cancer and head and neck cancer have been completed and reported demonstrating tolerability.[178,179]

Another approach to make current chemotherapeutic drugs more effective against tumors and at the same time less toxic to normal tissues is compound modification via conjugation with water-soluble polymeric drugs, such as polyglutamic acid. These conjugates accumulate in tumors and release the active drug into the tumor in high concentrations and for a longer time. The enhancement in uptake by and prolongation of drug release in tumors are thought to be due to the enhanced permeability and retention effect of macromolecular compounds in solid tumors.[180,181] The abnormal vasculature in tumors is porous to macromolecules, but high concentrations of drug can build up in tumors owing to inadequate lymphatic drainage, whereas polymer–drug conjugates are confined to the bloodstream in normal tissue.[180] This leads to improved spatial localization of the cytotoxic drug within tumor. A promising polyglutamic acid–paclitaxel conjugate (paclitaxel poliglumex) was developed. It is less toxic, more effective against tumors, and more enhancing of tumor radioresponse in preclinical studies than unconjugated paclitaxel.[181,182] Furthermore, there are *in vivo* laboratory data suggesting that radiation adds to the accumulation of drug within tumors by modification of tumor vasculature.[183] Therefore, multiple mechanisms for spatial localization and cooperation, including inherent drug properties, radiation modification of vasculature, and radiation-based targeting of sites within the body, could make this an attractive strategy for combining this agent with radiation treatments. Clinical trials in esophageal cancer (phase II), gastric cancer (phase I), and glioblastoma without MGMT methylation (phase II) have been reported in combination with radiation treatments.[184-186]

Normal Tissue Protection

Because normal tissue toxicity represents a major limitation of concurrent chemoradiation therapy, every effort must be taken to prevent or minimize complications. This could be achieved through the incorporation into the treatment of radioprotective or chemoprotective agents or through improvements of radiation delivery. A number of chemical and biologic compounds are available that exhibited either selective or preferential protection of normal tissues in preclinical *in vivo* testing.[187-191] In addition, there are many candidate compounds, particularly extracts from plants used in traditional medicine settings, that are undergoing *in vitro* evaluation.[192-194] The most commonly tested radioprotectors are thiol compounds, such as WR-2721 (amifostine), a prodrug that must be converted *in vivo* to its active metabolite WR-1065. Amifostine is currently the only Food and Drug Administration (FDA)-approved radioprotector. The principal mechanisms of protection by these agents include scavenging of free radicals generated by ionizing radiation and some chemotherapy agents, such as alkylating agents, and donating hydrogen atoms to facilitate direct chemical repair of DNA damage. However, amifostine modulates transcriptional regulation of genes involved in apoptosis, cell cycle regulation, and DNA repair as well.[195] The protector is taken up preferentially by normal tissues, where the entry into cells is accomplished by active transport. In contrast, the drug diffuses passively into tumors, where its availability is also reduced by deficient tumor vasculature. Amifostine has been shown to reduce normal tissue toxicity in a number of clinical settings, including protection of salivary glands in head and neck radiation therapy,[196,197] prevention of acute and late normal tissue toxicities from chemoradiation in cancers of the head and neck,[198] and the esophagus in chemoradiation therapy of lung cancer,[199,200] without adversely affecting tumor response to treatment. The drug significantly protects against cisplatin-induced nephrotoxicity, ototoxicity, and neuropathy.

Emerging Strategies to Improve Radiation Therapy

Technology-Based Strategies

Several technologic strategies to improve the efficacy and decrease the toxicity of radiation therapy have been developed. These advances include improvements in radiation therapy delivery, such as three-dimensional treatment planning, conformational radiation therapy, intensity-modulated radiation therapy (IMRT), and image-guided radiation therapy (IGRT). Use of heavy particles, such as protons or carbons, which have a more favorable beam profile, is another approach likely to minimize the toxicity, and combining such treatments with chemotherapy may lead to enhancement of the effectiveness of not only radiation therapy but also chemoradiation treatments. The principle primarily exploited with this would be that of maximizing spatial localization, with technologic advances and/or heavy particles being used to maximize radiation therapy's spatial localization. Further advances in imaging, with the advent of molecular-based imaging applications in oncology, will lead to further refinement of IGRT techniques. Because there are significant discussions of three-dimensional conformational radiation therapy (3DCRT), IMRT, IGRT, and heavy particles detailed in other chapters, we refer readers to those chapters for more in-depth discussion.

Altering Fractionation Schemes to Improve Therapeutic Ratio for Chemoradiation Treatments

Accelerated fractionation regimens are designed to counteract tumor repopulation, and accelerated fractionation with concomitant boost technique has shown superiority in terms of local control over the standard fractionation regimen in a large randomized study for head and neck cancer patients.[201] Head and neck cancer remains one of the best paradigms for effectiveness of accelerated fractionation methods in clinical use. However, when combined with chemotherapy, a benefit to accelerated fractionation over standard fractionation was not demonstrated.[202]

Hyperfractionation is another strategy aimed at increasing the tumoricidal dose by delivering smaller doses/fractions, which allows a higher total dose to be administered as smaller doses/fractions lead to improved tolerance of late-responding normal tissues.[102] The efficacy of hyperfractionation over standard fractionation has been demonstrated in several disease sites, including lung and head and neck cancer.[201,203,204] In head and neck cancer, hyperfractionated radiation therapy with chemotherapy has yielded superior outcomes compared to hyperfractionated RT alone[205]; however, there has been no trial to demonstrate superiority of hyperfractionated RT and chemotherapy compared to conventional RT and chemotherapy. Perhaps, given the limited success of concurrent therapy, methods of combining systemic agents sequentially either before or after radiation treatments with altered fractionation can be considered.

THE CLINICAL EXPERIENCE WITH CHEMORADIATION IN CANCER THERAPY

The level of clinical experience with the combination of radiation and chemotherapy has increased dramatically during the years. In many tumor types, the sequencing and method of administration of the combination have been very important in attaining improved outcomes seen in randomized trials. Improved local control and better OS rates have resulted from combination therapy in a number of diseases, including rectal cancer, limited-stage small cell lung cancer, locally advanced NSCLC, esophageal cancer, gastric cancer, cervical cancer, glioblastoma, and rhabdomyosarcomas. Equally important are the successes seen in the realm of organ preservation in sarcomas of the extremity, bladder cancers, carcinomas of the anal canal, head and neck cancers, and breast cancer.

As the role for combined modality therapy and studies leading to such for each of the tumor types are well represented in individual chapters addressing the disease site, readers will be referred to individual disease site chapters in the text for details. Briefly summarized in Table 36.3, however, are some representative disease sites in adult malignancies, where combined modality therapy with chemotherapy and/or targeted biologic agents and radiation therapy is accepted as the standard of care. The table also summarizes the commonly used systemic agent for these different disease sites. As one can see, the list, while not comprehensive, is certainly extensive and impressive, and the clinical impact that combined modality therapy has had in each of these disease sites cannot be understated.

TABLE 36.3 CHEMORADIATION THERAPY AS STANDARD OF CARE BY SELECTED DISEASE SITES

Disease Site	Commonly Used Chemotherapeutic Agents	Sequencing and Intent of Therapy	Benefit of Combined Modality Approach
Locally advanced head and neck cancer	Cisplatin, 5-FU, hydroxyurea, carboplatin, cetuximab	• Definitive concurrent • Postoperative concurrent	Definitive: organ preservation/survival benefit Postoperative: DFS/LRC benefit; OS benefit in subset of patients
Glioblastoma multiforme	Temozolomide	• Postoperative concurrent • Definitive concurrent in unresectable cases	Overall survival
Locally advanced/unresectable non–small cell lung cancer	Cisplatin, Carboplatin, Paclitaxel, Etoposide, Vinblastine	• Definitive concurrent • Sequential	Overall survival
Limited-stage small cell lung cancer	Cisplatin/etoposide	• Definitive concurrent	Overall survival
Esophageal cancer	Cisplatin/5-FU	• Preoperative concurrent • Definitive concurrent	Local control, overall survival
Gastric cancer	5-FU, Leucovorin	• Postoperative concurrent	Overall survival
Pancreatic cancer	5-FU, Gemcitabine	• Postoperative concurrent • Definitive concurrent in unresectable patients	Locoregional control, possibly survival
Locally advanced rectal cancer	5-FU, Xeloda	• Preoperative concurrent	Improved sphincter preservation, improved DFS
Anal cancer	5-FU, mitomycin C	• Definitive concurrent	Improved colostomy free survival
Cervical cancer	Cisplatin, 5-FU, hydroxyurea	• Definitive concurrent	Overall survival benefit
Bladder cancer	Cisplatin, 5-FU, mitomycin C	• Definitive concurrent	Bladder preservation

TABLE 36.4 REPRESENTATIVE LONG-TERM TOXICITY OF COMBINED CHEMORADIATION THERAPY

Agent	Toxicity	Mechanism	References
Bleomycin	Pneumonitis/pulmonary fibrosis	Undefined but related to total drug dose and effects on pulmonary macrophages, type I and II alveolar cells; effects/lethality exacerbated by the administration of radiation.	206–208
Actinomycin D	Hepatopathy	Altered liver function postradiation leads to decreased metabolism of agents, including actinomycin, which in turn worsens the hepatopathy.	209,210
Doxorubicin	Cardiomyopathy	There is an additive interaction between doxorubicin and radiation with recall of radiation effects occurring. Primary radiation effect is on the endothelial cell, whereas doxorubicin affects the connective tissue stroma of the myocardium.	211–214
Methotrexate	Leukoencephalopathy	Methotrexate may cause this syndrome on its own. Radiation effects on the blood–brain barrier and the choroid plexus can alter methotrexate clearance, leading to higher levels in the brain. Effects are increased when both modalities are used.	215–217
Cisplatin	Sensorineural hearing loss	Although cisplatinum alone can cause this, reports suggests radiation therapy concurrently with cisplatin may contribute to sensorineural hearing loss.	218–221

Section II

As outcomes in each of the solid tumors improve with concurrent therapy, we need to become cognizant of the potential for significant long-term toxicity from combination chemoradiation and do our best to minimize the risks that these side effects pose to patient survival and quality of life. Several well-documented chemoradiation-imposed late effects are summarized in Table 36.4.

MOLECULAR TARGETED THERAPIES: NEW AGENTS AND NOVEL PARADIGMS FOR OPTIMIZING COMBINED MODALITY THERAPY

Discoveries in molecular biology have identified a number of molecular pathways involving receptors, enzymes, or growth factors that may be responsible for resistance of cancer cells to radiation or other cytotoxic agents and as such may serve as targets for augmentation of radiation response or chemotherapy response. It is becoming more evident that with advances in the understanding of the molecular processes that are associated with various malignancies, a molecular profile of a tumor may prove to be as important as its pathologic profile. Further classification of a patient's tumor molecular profile should, among other things, aid in selection of the appropriate targeted agents. The challenge for radiation oncologists in this molecular era is determining what would be the best method of integrating cytotoxic radiation treatments with a molecular-based therapeutic plan.

Among this expanding list of molecular targets are epidermal growth factor (EGF) and its receptor (EGFR); vascular endothelial growth factor (VEGF) and its receptor (VEGFR); mammalian target of rapamycin (mTOR); anaplastic lymphoma kinase (ALK) fusion proteins; heat shock protein 90 (hsp90); poly(adenosine diphosphate [ADP]-ribose) polymerase (PARP); mutated *ras*; histone deacetylase (HDAC) inhibitors; cell cycle checkpoint control proteins such as checkpoint kinase 1 (CHK1); a number of the DNA repair enzymes, including DNA-dependent protein kinase (DNA-PK), ataxia telangiectasia mutated (ATM), and RAD51; the proteasome; angiogenic molecules; and various other molecules that regulate different steps in their signal transduction pathways.[222] Several agents have now gained FDA approval for cancer therapy in patients, and many are undergoing clinical trials to determine their efficacy when used in combination with radiation therapy. Some agents are potentially single-pathway targets, and others are able to target multiple molecular signaling pathways. Some molecular strategies to improve chemoradiation therapy are shown in Table 36.5. The most clinically advanced of these strategies include agents targeting EGFR, VEGF and VEGFR, and ALK1 pathways. The scope of this section will be a discussion of some relevant molecularly targeted agents that have been FDA approved for use and which hold promise for use in conjunction with radiation treatments.

TABLE 36.5 MOLECULAR TARGETING POSSIBILITIES IN COMBINATION WITH CHEMO/RADIATION OR RADIATION

Class	Agents	Status in Combination with XRT (Published)
Epidermal growth factor receptor inhibitors	Cetuximab	HN cancer–phase III NSCLC–phase III Other sites–phase I/II
	Gefitinib	NSCLC–phase III Other sites–phase I/II
	Erlotinib	Phase I/II
	Afatinib	None reported
Antiangiogenics	Bevacizumab	GBM–phase III Other sites–phase I/II
	Thalidomide	Brain metastases–phase III Other sites–phase I/II
Multitargeted tyrosine kinase inhibitors (TKIs)	Sunitinib (inhibits PDGFR, VEGFR, KIT, RET, CSF-1R, FLT3)	Phase I, II
	Sorafenib (inhibits Raf kinase, PDGF, VEGFR2/3, cKit)	Phase I, II
	Pazopanib (inhibits VEGFR1–3, PDFR-alpha, beta, c-Kit, FGFR-1, FGFR-3, Lck, c-Fms)	Phase I
mTOR inhibitors	Temsirolimus	Phase I
	Everolimus	Phase I, II
ALK inhibitor	Crizotinib	None reported
HDAC inhibitors	Vorinostat	Phase I
DNA repair	Romidepsin	None reported
	Veliparib	Phase I
	Olaparib	None reported
	Niraparib	None reported
	Rucaparib	None reported

Epidermal Growth Factor Receptor

Targeting EGFR is one of the current model paradigms for the combination of molecular-based therapy and radiation. EGFR is also known as ErbB1, a member of the ErbB family of receptor tyrosine kinases, which also includes ErbB2 (HER2/neu). EGFR is a 170-kD transmembrane glycoprotein with an intracellular domain possessing intrinsic tyrosine kinase activity. On binding to a ligand, such as EGF or transforming growth factor-α, EGFR undergoes autophosphorylation and initiates transduction signals regulating cell division, metastases, angiogenesis, proliferation, and differentiation. EGFR plays an important role in tumor growth and response to cytotoxic agents, including ionizing radiation. The receptor is frequently expressed in high levels in many types of cancer, which is often associated with more aggressive tumors, poor patient prognosis, and tumor resistance to treatment with cytotoxic agents including radiation.[223-227] In vitro experimental studies have provided solid evidence linking EGFR with resistance to cytotoxic drugs. Although transfection of EGFR into tumor cells increases their resistance to drugs[228] and radiation,[229] the blockade of the EGFR-mediated signaling pathway with antibodies to EGFR enhances the sensitivity of tumor cells to drugs[226] and ionizing radiation.[230] In vivo studies have shown that blockade of EGFR, such as with cetuximab, anti-EGFR monoclonal antibody (mAB), or interference with its downstream signaling processes, can improve tumor treatment with both chemotherapeutic agents and radiation.[231,232] Furthermore, overexpression of constitutively active EGFR vIII has been correlated with enhanced radioresistance.[233]

Broadly speaking, the two most developed strategies for inhibiting EGFR include the use of mABs against EGFR and small molecule tyrosine kinase inhibitors (TKIs). Cetuximab and panitumumab are examples of mABs, and their mechanism includes blocking the extracellular binding domain, thus inhibiting dimer formation. TKIs such as gefitinib or erlotinib target the intracellular tyrosine kinase domain. However, the activity of EGFR is complicated by the signal diversity because of the formation of homo- and heterodimers with other members of the ErbB family and by the specific autophosphorylation patterns within each ErbB family member. This is further compounded by the identification of specific mutations within EGFR that confer sensitivity to certain EGFR inhibitors. The approach of combining an anti-EGFR therapy with cytotoxic agents including radiation in the treatment of patients with cancer remains an area of active investigation,[52,234-238] and some of these key agents warrant further discussion.

Cetuximab (Erbitux)

Cetuximab is a chimeric mouse anti-EGFR mAB and is perhaps the most widely studied and developed mAB in this class. It has been studied in a large randomized phase III trial for locally advanced head and neck squamous cell carcinoma patients. This study included 424 patients treated with either radiation therapy alone or radiation therapy with concurrent cetuximab. Median survival was nearly doubled (49 months vs. 29 months, $P = .03$), and PFS and locoregional control were both improved with the addition of cetuximab.[52] This resulted in FDA approval in 2006 for use of cetuximab in combination with radiation treatments for locoregionally advanced head and neck cancer.

However, studies of combining cetuximab with established chemoradiation regimen have been relatively unsuccessful at improving outcomes. Radiation Therapy Oncology Group (RTOG) 0522 is a randomized study comparing the addition of cetuximab to standard concurrent cisplatinum and radiation treatments in head and neck cancer patients. This study demonstrated no benefit to addition of cetuximab, increased grade 3 to 4 acute toxicity events, and more frequent interruptions in radiotherapy.[239] Outcomes also did not differ by EGFR expression in this study. For esophageal cancer, potential role of cetuximab being added to chemoradiation therapy were studied in a multicenter, phase II/III randomized trial (SCOPE1), and randomized phase III trial (RTOG 0436). SCOPE1 demonstrated worse outcomes with worse toxicities and inferior survival outcomes with cetuximab.[240] RTOG 0436 demonstrated no improvement in outcomes with addition of cetuximab.[241]

Interestingly, recent phase II studies for stage III NSCLC were reported by the RTOG 0324 and Cancer and Leukemia Group B (CALGB) groups.[120,242] In the randomized phase II CALGB study, two novel chemotherapy regimens in combination with concurrent radiation therapy were investigated in stage III NSCLC patients. The first group received carboplatin (area under the curve [AUC] = 5) and pemetrexed (500 mg/m²) every 21 days for four cycles with 70 Gy of RT. The second group received the same with the addition of cetuximab. Both groups received four cycles of pemetrexed as consolidation therapy. The primary endpoint was 18-month survival with a goal of ≥55%, at which point the regimens would be deemed worthy of further study. The carboplatin/pemetrexed/ RT arm demonstrated 18-month OS of 58% and the group with cetuximab, 54%. The combination of thoracic radiation, pemetrexed, and carboplatin, with or without cetuximab, was demonstrated to be feasible and fairly well tolerated.[120]

In the RTOG study, patients were treated with a combination of Taxol, carboplatin, and cetuximab (225 mg/m²) for six weekly cycles, with 63 Gy of daily radiation therapy. All patients received a loading dose (400 mg/m²) of cetuximab 1 week prior to RT, and patients received carboplatin/Taxol/ cetuximab for two additional cycles after completion of radiation treatments. This study demonstrated median survival of 22.7 months and 2-year OS of 49.3%.[242] Because of these very promising results, cetuximab was included in the RTOG 0617 trial, which was initially designed to compare two different radiation doses (60 Gy vs. 74 Gy) with concurrent chemotherapy. Randomization includes chemotherapy + cetuximab + RT versus chemotherapy + RT, followed by adjuvant chemotherapy versus chemotherapy + cetuximab. In addition to demonstrating 74 Gy was not better than 60 Gy, addition of cetuximab to concurrent chemoradiation and consolidation treatment provided no benefit in OS in this study. However, in a planned retrospective analysis of prospectively collected pathologic specimens, high EGFR expressing patients demonstrated OS benefit (42 months vs. 21.2 months) with the addition of cetuximab ($P = .032$), whereas low EGFR expressing patients might have had a detriment (19.5 months vs. 29.6 months) with cetuximab ($P = .056$).[243]

Therefore, cetuximab has not clearly demonstrated benefit when combined with chemoradiation therapy. Efforts are under way to determine if there may be certain subgroups of patients that may benefit from cetuximab and radiation combination, in the presence or absence of chemotherapy, such as in EGFR high expression patients, HPV+ head and neck cancer population, or HIV+ anal carcinoma patients.

Panitumumab (Vectibix)

Panitumumab is a fully human mAB to EGFR, which received FDA approval in 2006 for treatment of EGFR expressing metastatic colorectal cancer with disease progression on chemotherapy and has been determined to be noninferior to cetuximab for refractory metastatic colorectal cancer patient treatments.[244] Clinical studies of panitumumab combined with radiotherapy have been reported for esophageal, rectal, head and neck, and pancreatic cancer, most of which did not show significant improvement in outcomes or increased toxicity with the use of this agent with standard radiotherapy +/– chemotherapy regimens.[245-254] For locally advanced distal esophageal cancers, neoadjuvant use of panitumumab with docetaxel/platinum chemotherapy and radiation was found to be toxic, and evaluation in an unselected population was not recommended based on a phase II study (ACOSOG Z4051).[247] In a phase II study of resectable esophageal cancer, preoperative therapy with carboplatinum/paclitaxel/radiation was tolerated, but could not improve on the preset criterion of pCR rate of 40% (PACT study).[246] In a phase II study, the use of panitumumab with RT in preop setting, in KRAS wild-type locally advanced rectal cancer, demonstrated modest pCR rates and failed to meet the primary endpoint of this study.[248] In a preop study of panitumumab with capecitabine and radiotherapy in KRAS wild-type rectal cancer patients, high near complete or complete response rates were noted, but increased toxicity (diarrhea, anastomotic leakage).[251] In a phase II study of panitumumab with oxaliplatin/5-FU and radiotherapy as preoperative therapy for rectal cancer patients (StarPan/STAR-02 Study), toxicity was high, particularly with high incidence of grade 3 to 4 diarrhea, including one toxic death because of diarrhea.[252] In a randomized phase II trial (CONCERT-2) of panitumumab with RT versus chemoradiotherapy, cisplatinum-based chemoradiotherapy yielded better tumor control compared to the panitumumab/RT therapy.[245] The use of chemoradiotherapy with or without panitumumab was studied in locally advanced head and neck cancer patients in a randomized phase II trial (CONCERT-1), and the addition of panitumumab did not confer significant benefit to chemoradiotherapy.[249] Phase III trial of cisplatin-based chemoradiotherapy versus accelerated radiotherapy with panitumumab for locoregionally advanced head and neck cancer was reported and was not able to show a noninferiority with the panitumumab-based regimen and also did not lead to improvement in quality of life or swallowing.[255,256] Phase I trial of panitumumab addition to standard gemcitabine-based chemoradiation for locally advanced pancreatic cancer demonstrated MTD of panitumumab of 1.5 mg/kg and was found to have overall manageable toxicity with potential clinical efficacy in the treated cohorts.[250]

Gefitinib (Iressa)

Gefitinib is approved for use as a single agent in the treatment of chemotherapy-refractory NSCLC.[229] It is known to inhibit primarily the EGFR tyrosine kinase but also has shown some activity for HER-2 kinase, albeit at a much lower level.[229] This agent demonstrated promise in phase II studies ("Iressa" dose evaluation in advanced lung cancer [IDEAL-1] and IDEAL-2),[257,258] but had disappointing results in phase III trials (Iressa NSCLC trial assessing combination treatment [INTACT-1] and INTACT-2), where it failed to demonstrate additional benefit to standard chemotherapy for advanced lung cancer patients.[259,260] However, a subset of patients were noted to have a significant response to gefitinib, and subsequently this led to the discovery that mutations in the EGFR tyrosine kinase domain may predict for a positive response to gefitinib.[261,262] Since then, studies involving gefitinib and combined modality therapy have also been reported.

The Southwest Oncology Group performed a large phase III trial where stage III NSCLC patients were treated with standard chemoradiation therapy, and after consolidation with docetaxel for three cycles, patients were randomized to maintenance therapy with a placebo or gefitinib 250 mg/day. This was an unselected patient population. At interim analysis, patients on the gefitinib maintenance arm had a worse OS, and therefore the study was closed.[238] CALGB 30106[263] was a phase II study designed to evaluate the addition of gefitinib to sequential or concurrent chemoradiotherapy in patients with unresectable NSCLC. Patients were categorized into poor-risk (performance status [PS] $\geq$ 2, weight loss $\geq$ 5%) and good-risk stratum (PS 0 to 1, weight loss < 5%). All patients received induction chemotherapy with two cycles of carboplatin (AUC = 6) and paclitaxel (200 mg/m^2), plus gefitinib 250 mg

from days 1 to 21. Gefitinib was removed from induction in May 2004 when a randomized phase III trial did not demonstrate benefit to adding gefitinib with chemotherapy. The poor-risk group received 66 Gy of RT delivered in 33 fractions, with gefitinib 250 mg/day. Good-risk stratum patients received the same RT and gefitinib but also received weekly carboplatin (AUC = 2) and paclitaxel (50 mg/m^2). Consolidation gefitinib was given until progression. For the poor-risk stratum, PFS was 13.4 months, and median OS was 19 months. For the good-risk stratum, PFS was 9.2 months, and median OS was 13 months. Thirteen of 45 tumors had activating EGFR mutations, and two of 13 had T790M mutations. Seven of 45 tumors had KRAS mutations. When analyzed by these molecular phenotypes, no significant difference in outcome was noted. Interestingly, the poor-risk stratum who received radiation + gefitinib after induction chemotherapy demonstrated promising survival and PFS outcomes. This will lead to further studies designed to elucidate the role of gefitinib and radiation therapy in poor performance status patients with stage III NSCLC. Meanwhile, the good-risk stratum patients did not demonstrate a very good outcome, suggesting that the addition of gefitinib to the chemoradiation therapy regimen may not be beneficial. This is consistent with studies of erlotinib and chemoradiation therapy.[264]

Erlotinib (Tarceva)

Erlotinib is also an EGFR TKI that has been approved for use by the FDA. Erlotinib is a potent inhibitor of EGFR autophosphorylation and, like gefitinib, also has some activity against HER-2. It also seems to be a fairly potent inhibitor of signaling mediated by the mutant EGFR vIII.[229] Findings from two large phase III studies, the Tarceva Lung Cancer Investigation (TALENT)[265] and Tarceva Responses in Conjunction with Paclitaxel and Carboplatin (TRIBUTE)[266] trials, demonstrated no significant benefit of the addition of erlotinib to chemotherapy to OS in patients with advanced lung cancer.[265,266] Similar to the gefitinib studies, the lack of a demonstrable global benefit to erlotinib pointed to the need for stringent patient selection criteria. In the TRIBUTE study, addition of erlotinib to carboplatin and Taxol improved PFS and OS only in a subset of never smokers. NCIC conducted a phase III study of patients with stage IIIB or IV NSCLC who had failed one to two prior chemotherapy regimens. OS was improved with erlotinib over placebo (6.7 months vs. 4.7 months), and response rate, time to symptomatic progression, and PFS were also improved.[267] Meanwhile, erlotinib has been studied in combination with gemcitabine for advanced pancreatic cancer patients demonstrating an OS benefit (median 6.24 months vs. 5.91 months) compared to gemcitabine alone[268] by NCIC.

Because EGFR TKIs appear to be most effective in never smokers and those with EGFR mutations, these issues were studied in a phase II study (CALGB 30406), which to date has only been reported in abstract form. This study evaluated patients who were never/light smokers. Patients were randomized to erlotinib alone or erlotinib with carboplatin and paclitaxel. At a median follow-up of 30 months, there was no statistically significant difference in PFS with the addition of erlotinib. However, patients with EGFR mutations had significantly improved PFS and OS in both treatment groups compared to patients who did not harbor the EGFR mutation.[269] There have been a few phase I and II studies that examine the combination of erlotinib and radiation therapy. For instance, adding erlotinib to radiation therapy and temozolomide has been studied for GBM in a phase I/II setting. The North Central Cancer Treatment Group (NCCTG) demonstrated no significant benefit for the addition of erlotinib,[270] and Cleveland Clinic's phase II study demonstrated detrimental effects.[271] Interestingly, a phase II study by Prados et al.[272] demonstrated superior median survival compared to historical controls treated without erlotinib (19.3 months), with good tolerance to therapy. Erlotinib with chemoradiation (gemcitabine, paclitaxel, and radiation) demonstrated tolerability in a phase I study for locally advanced inoperable pancreatic cancer patients,[273,274] and another study demonstrated tolerability of IMRT-based radiation therapy with erlotinib and capecitabine for pancreatic cancer patients in the postoperative setting.[275] A phase I study of the combination of chemoradiation therapy with erlotinib has been completed in cervical squamous cell carcinoma and a phase II study in locally advanced esophageal cancer, both demonstrating the feasibility of such approaches.[276,277]

In head and neck cancer patients, the addition of erlotinib has been studied with chemoradiation both in newly diagnosed patients and in early phase trials for reirradiation of patients with recurrent head and neck cancer.[278–280] The group from the Sarah Cannon consortium has recently reported on a phase II study of erlotinib, bevacizumab, and radiation therapy and the feasibility of such an approach in a community-based setting with a high level of efficacy and tolerability.[281]

Choong et al.[264] reported on a ping-pong–design phase I study of erlotinib with chemoradiotherapy in patients with NSCLC. One group received induction carboplatin and paclitaxel followed by carboplatin/paclitaxel/radiation + erlotinib, whereas a second group received cisplatin/etoposide/radiation + erlotinib followed by Taxotere. The erlotinib dose was escalated from 50 to 150 mg in three levels in each arm. Median survival in each group was 13.7 and 10.2 months, respectively, with patients who developed rash having an improvement in OS and PFS. This study demonstrated tolerability for such a regimen but with fairly disappointing survival data, once again pointing to the need for improved patient selection when using EGFR-based treatments.

In addition to lung and head and neck cancers, erlotinib and radiation therapy has been investigated in early phase studies for other disease sites including pancreatic cancer, gliomas, brain metastases, esophageal cancer, rectal cancer.[282–284]

Afatinib (Gilotrif)

Afatinib is an orally administered irreversible inhibitor of ErbB family of tyrosine kinases. It binds to EGFR, Her2 and Her4 irreversibly inhibiting tyrosine kinase autophosphorylation. It has been approved for first-line use in metastatic NSCLC patients who have EGFR exon 19 deletions or exon 21 substitution mutations. It demonstrated benefit in PFS but not OS when compared to gefitinib for patients with EGFR mutations, and OS benefit when compared to chemotherapy in patients with exon 19 deletions. It also demonstrated benefit in second-line treatment of advanced NSCLC patients regardless of EGFR mutation status when compared to erlotinib.[285] Afatinib in combination with chemotherapy and/or radiation therapy is being investigated in head and neck cancer, GBM, and EGFR mutant NSCLC.

Summary

Several studies have demonstrated the feasibility and tolerability of combining EGFR inhibitors with chemoradiation therapy in different tumor types. Of note, the importance of molecular profiling and patient selection, such as EGFR mutation status and smoking status in predicting the efficacy of an anti-EGFR–based regimen, has become apparent. Some studies have demonstrated potential for increased toxicity when these regimens are incorporated with chemoradiotherapy. Future studies involving anti-EGFR treatments in combination with radiation treatments should also incorporate such stringent patient selection criteria to maximize the chance of providing a benefit for the appropriate patients. Finally, when combining EGFR inhibitors with radiation, the efficacy and toxicity may vary by tumor type, molecular profile, use of chemotherapy, and the sequencing of the EGFR inhibitor therapy with respect to radiation treatments.

Antiangiogenesis

The formation of tumor vasculature, a prerequisite for progressive tumor growth, is initiated and sustained by angiogenic mediators secreted by tumor cells and cells from the surrounding stroma. Many different angiogenic factors have been identified, including VEGF/vascular permeability factor, members of the fibroblast growth factor (FGF) family, platelet-derived growth factor (PDGF), interleukin-8, and prostaglandins. In addition to angiogenic factors, tumors secrete substances that inhibit angiogenesis, such as angiostatin, endostatin, thrombospondin-1, and interferons, so that the final outcome of angiogenesis (and hence tumor growth) depends on the balance between proangiogenic and antiangiogenic activities.

Inhibitors of angiogenesis have undergone extensive preclinical testing, with some agents moving into clinical trials. However, as monotherapeutic agents, the early agents have not been as promising as their preclinical evaluations had suggested.[286] Even though it was assumed that an antiangiogenic agent would impair the efficacy of radiation therapy via the enhancement of hypoxia, early evidence for radiation therapy in combination with angiostatin showed both improved oxygenation and reduced oxygenation.[287–289] However, the first clinical trial with a specific inhibitor of angiogenesis, angiostatin, showed a synergistic effect.[290] Since then, the role of specific factors in vascular growth and maintenance has become clearer. VEGF receptors, in particular, play a critical role in vascular integrity, including angiogenesis and endothelial cell survival, via their tyrosine kinase activities.[291] VEGF expression induces endothelial cell proliferation by creating a vascular sprout that subsequently organizes into a capillary tube.[292,293] VEGF also promotes angiogenesis through the formation of a hyperpermeable immature vascular network.[294] VEGF expression is enhanced following radiation, which is likely a survival response for vascular endothelial cells, ultimately in support of tumor survival. Receptor tyrosine kinases, EGFR in particular, up-regulate VEGF, and cyclo-oxygenase-2 (COX-2) inhibitors limit the up-regulation of VEGF by prostaglandins. One proposed mechanism for resistance to a specific targeted antiangiogenic agent such as VEGF or VEGF receptor inhibitors is that tumor cells may be able to up-regulate alternate angiogenic factors such as PDGF and FGF.[295] Therefore, multitargeted agents that can inhibit multiple pathways have been developed and are also under investigation.

A model of normalization of tumor vasculature has been described by Jain.[296] In this model, proangiogenic factors from tumors can cause abnormal neovascularization, and inhibition of tumor angiogenesis transiently normalizes the tumor vasculature. This, therefore, has the counterintuitive effect of decreasing tumor hypoxia and improving effectiveness of radiation therapy. Preclinical studies and a phase I study of bevacizumab, 5-FU, and radiation therapy preoperatively in locally advanced rectal cancer patients also supported this notion.[297]

There are other biologic mechanisms associated with angiogenesis that suggest combining radiation treatments with antiangiogenic agents, including induction of expression of DNA repair enzymes and targeting of the tumor microenvironment with combined modality therapy. Data from a number of preclinical studies suggest that at higher doses of radiation, tumor radiosensitivity is directly linked to efficacy of endothelial cell death[298] and that the conventional fractionation dose (~2 Gy) may not be effective at targeting endothelial cells.[54] However, in preclinical studies, endothelial cell apoptosis may be induced at lower radiation doses by the addition of antiangiogenic drugs or by blocking targets such as PI3K/AKT pathways, which are activated by ionizing radiation on endothelial cells.[299] Finally, radioresistance of some tumors is thought to be mediated in part by the presence of cancer stem cells, which secrete significant amounts of VEGF,[300] and raises the question of whether these tumor cells can become a more sensitive target to radiation treatments when combined with antiangiogenic agents.[301]

Antiangiogenic compounds can also be broadly classified as mABs or TKIs. The most clinically developed agents that have been FDA approved include the mAB bevacizumab and the TKIs sorafenib, sunitinib, and pazopanib.

Bevacizumab

Bevacizumab is a recombinant humanized mAB that targets VEGF to inhibit its interaction with the VEGF receptor.[302] It has a long circulating half-life after intravenous infusion of up to 21 days. Bevacizumab was the first drug to receive approval by FDA when used as first-line therapy with 5-FU in patients with advanced colorectal cancer. It has since demonstrated efficacy and activity in NSCLC, renal cell carcinoma, GBM, and ovarian cancer.[54] A number of studies have also been performed in different disease sites with bevacizumab in conjunction with radiation therapy.

Phase I and II studies with rectal cancer have demonstrated feasibility, and recommendations for appropriate doses to be used with radiation and 5-FU or capecitabine have been established.[303–306] A phase II study of bevacizumab, capecitabine, and radiotherapy for locally advanced rectal cancer in the preoperative setting was reported. Twenty-five patients with clinically staged T3N1 or T3N0 rectal cancer received 50.4 Gy with bevacizumab every 2 weeks (5 mg/kg) and capecitabine 900 mg/m² orally bid followed by surgery. Thirty-two percent of patients had pathologic complete response, and 24% of patients had <10% viable tumor cells in the specimen. Three wound complications required surgical interventions.[307] Thirty-two patients were enrolled in a phase I/II study of neoadjuvant bevacizumab, radiation therapy, and fluorouracil in advanced rectal cancer.[304] This treatment yielded 5-year OS and local control of 100% and 5-year disease-free survival of 75%. Toxicity was acceptable, and bevacizumab was shown to decrease tumor interstitial fluid pressure. Biomarkers showed significant correlation to outcome. Phase I and II studies by Crane et al.[308] have been performed of bevacizumab with capecitabine-based chemotherapy and radiation treatments for pancreatic cancer.[308,309] In the phase II study RTOG 0411, overall median survival was not compromised, but there was a 35.4% rate of grade 3 or greater gastrointestinal-related toxicity (22% during chemoradiation therapy and 13.4% during maintenance chemotherapy). However, there was a significant correlation with grade 3 toxicity during the chemoradiation therapy phase and protocol deviation in terms of generous treatment volumes. A need for prospective quality assurance in future trials was recommended.[308] Phase I and I/II study of bevacizumab, fluorouracil-based radiation, with erlotinib have been completed with encouraging pathologic complete response rate and with demonstration of good tolerability in neoadjuvant setting for locally advanced rectal cancer patients.[282,283]

Efforts to improve the therapeutic ratio by addition of bevacizumab to chemoradiation therapy have been attempted in multiple studies for both small cell lung cancer and NSCLC patients. Unfortunately, these studies have demonstrated that this regimen was associated with an incidence of tracheoesophageal fistula in both small cell and NSCLC settings.[310]

A number of studies using bevacizumab have been reported for CNS malignancies. Findings of phase II studies showing promise for addition of bevacizumab to temozolomide/radiation therapy regiment for gliomas[311,312] led to development of two phase III studies to investigate this approach in patients with newly diagnosed GBM. In the RTOG 0825 study, Bevacizumab or placebo began during week 4 of radiotherapy and was continued for up to 12 cycles of maintenance chemotherapy.[313] No significant difference in duration of OS between bevacizumab and placebo was found. PFS was longer in the

bevacizumab group (10.7 months vs. 7.3 months). With bevacizumab, toxicity was increased, and over time, increased symptom burden, worse quality of life, and decline in neurocognitive function. The AvaGlio study randomized patients with newly diagnosed glioblastoma to receive bevacizumab versus placebo concurrently with radiotherapy and temozolomide, and was followed by maintenance bevacizumab and temozolomide.[314] Similar to the RTOG study, bevacizumab did not improve survival and increased the rate of adverse events. However, PFS and maintenance of baseline quality of life and performance status were observed.

Studies of reirradiation of recurrent high-grade gliomas with radiotherapy/fractionated stereotactic radiotherapy have been reported demonstrating feasibility/tolerability and potential efficacy of this approach.[315–319] Additional clinical trials investigating this approach are ongoing for recurrent gliomas.

The University of Chicago group has published phase I and phase II studies combining bevacizumab with 5-FU and hydroxyurea-based radiation therapy in advanced head and neck cancer patients.[320,321] In the phase I study, bevacizumab at 10 mg/m² was reported to be integratable in this chemoradiotherapy regimen, but five patients with fistula formation and four with ulceration/tissue necrosis were reported. It was felt that the fistula and tissue necrosis could have been bevacizumab related. The randomized phase II study enrolled 26 patients with newly diagnosed T4N0/1 head and neck cancers. Patients received hydroxyurea, 5-FU, and bid radiotherapy with or without bevacizumab (10 mg/kg every 14 days). Unexpectedly, there was significant locoregional progression seen in the bevacizumab arm. Two patients died during therapy, and one died shortly after therapy. This led to study termination, and it was felt that addition of bevacizumab to chemoradiotherapy should be limited to clinical trials for head and neck squamous cell carcinoma. However, addition of bevacizumab to standard chemoradiation in nasopharyngeal carcinoma was studied in a phase II multi-institutional trial (RTOG 0615).[322] In this study, addition of bevacizumab was deemed to be feasible, with possibility of delaying progression of subclinical distant disease reported. Randomized phase III study is needed to substantiate these findings.

Thalidomide

Thalidomide is an agent that was originally marketed as a sedative and was initially taken off the market because of concerns of teratogenicity. There has been a resurgence in use and interest in this agent, as it has since been found to have potent immunomodulatory effects as well as antiangiogenic properties.[323] Although its effects are not limited to angiogenesis, there are suggestions that thalidomide stimulates vessel maturation with implications for vascular normalization, which may be an important strategy for antineoplastic therapy.[324] Therefore, the use of thalidomide with or without radiation therapy has been investigated in both preclinical and clinical settings.[325]

A phase III study (RTOG 0118) was performed to study the efficacy of WBRT (37.5 Gy in 15 fractions) when combined with thalidomide, in patients with 4 or more, or large (>4 cm) tumor, or midbrain brain metastases. Median survival was 3.4 months for both arms (with or without thalidomide), and thalidomide was not well tolerated in this population (48% of patients discontinued thalidomide because of side effects).[326] The efficacy of thalidomide, temozolomide, and 30 Gy in 10 fractions of whole-brain radiation therapy was studied in patients with brain metastases from melanoma. The efficacy was found to be low, and further therapy with this approach was not recommended.[327] A phase II study of thalidomide and radiation in children with newly diagnosed brainstem gliomas and GBM also yielded negative results.[328] A phase II study of temozolomide and thalidomide in patients with newly diagnosed GBM did not demonstrate significant improvement compared to temozolomide alone.[329] Similarly, concurrent thalidomide during radiotherapy of hepatocellular carcinoma did not demonstrate additional benefits in a phase II setting.[330] Eastern Cooperative Oncology Group (ECOG) 3598 was a randomized study comparing chemoradiation therapy ± thalidomide in patients with stage III NSCLC. There was no difference in PFS or OS with the addition of thalidomide.[331]

Summary of Antiangiogenesis Agents

It is clear from these studies that the efficacy and safety of antiangiogenic agents in combination with radiation and chemoradiation therapy, while promising in many regards, need to be approached with great caution. It also appears that the location of the tumor and agents used in combination with radiation and antiangiogenic agents such as bevacizumab may factor into determining the feasibility and tolerability of such regimens. The potential for improved efficacy over chemoradiation therapy has been raised in particular for gastrointestinal, nasopharyngeal, and CNS malignancies, and further larger studies to help clarify the potential role for antiangiogenic agents in chemoradiation therapy are needed.

Multitargeted Tyrosine Kinase Inhibitors

Several TKI agents have been developed that have demonstrable antitumor and antiangiogenesis activities. These include sorafenib (Nexavar), sunitinib (Sutent), and pazopanib (Votrient). All three agents are approved for use in treatment of patients with advanced renal cell carcinoma. Preclinical studies have demonstrated promising findings when combining multitargeted receptor TKIs with radiation therapy.[299,332–338]

Sunitinib

Sunitinib is an oral, multitargeted receptor TKI, which was approved by the FDA for treatment of advanced renal cell carcinoma, imatinib-resistant gastrointestinal stromal tumor (GIST) in January of 2006, and pancreatic cancer (unresectable progressive neuroendocrine tumors). Its targets include platelet-derived growth factor receptor (PDGFR), VEGFR, KIT, RET, CSF-1R, and flt3. Several preclinical studies have suggested that sunitinib may be an appropriate agent to consider for use in combination with radiation therapy for a number of solid tumors.[299,335–338] In the clinical setting, a few studies have been reported to date, mostly phase I and phase II studies. Some representative studies are as follows.

Wuthrick et al.[339] have completed a phase I trial of 37.5 mg of sunitinib daily with radiation therapy (doses ranged from 14 to 70 Gy [1.8 to 3.5 Gy per fraction]) in 15 patients with primary (n = 3) and metastatic (n = 12) CNS malignancies.[339] Six patients developed grade 2 or less toxicities, and grade 3 toxicities occurred in seven patients. No grade 3 to 5 intracerebral hemorrhagic events or hypertensive events were reported. Two grade 5 adverse events attributed to disease progression were reported. With a median follow-up of 34.2 months, 13% achieved partial response, 60% had stable disease, and 13% had progressive disease. Six-month PFS for patients with brain metastasis was 58%. The authors recommended consideration for further phase II studies. Phase II trial of concurrent sunitinib, temozolomide, and radiation therapy for GBM patients with an unmethylated MGMT gene promoter is currently recruiting patients in Canada. A phase I trial of sunitinib and radiation therapy for preoperative treatment of soft tissue sarcoma from the German interdisciplinary sarcoma group (GISG-03) has been reported. Two-dose levels of sunitinib (25 and 37.5 mg) were studied with radiation therapy (1.8 Gy × 28 fractions), with surgery scheduled 5 to 8 weeks postneoadjuvant treatments.[340] Of 9 patients enrolled (6 and first dose level and 3 at second dose level), 1 had partial response, 7 had stable disease, and 1 had progressive

disease. Pathologic evaluation revealed ≥95% tumor necrosis in 3/9 specimens. 37.5 mg was the recommended dose for subsequent studies. However, in another phase IB/II study of sunitinib with neoadjuvant radiation therapy (50.4 Gy in 28 fractions), combination of sunitinib at 50 mg/day for 2 weeks followed by concurrent 25 mg/day during radiation and dose level −1 where patients received 37.5 mg 2 weeks before and concurrent with RT, both resulted in unacceptable toxicities (primarily liver, hematologic) and premature study closure.[341] Addition of radiation therapy may not be completely implicated in these toxicities, particularly liver when treatment was delivered to extremity where liver was not exposed to radiation. Whether this was due to the sunitinib delivered prior to concurrent/RT is not fully clear. In nonmetastatic high-risk prostate cancer, phase I study of sunitinib with androgen deprivation therapy and radiation therapy (treatment to only prostate and seminal vesicles to 75.6 Gy in 42 fractions) demonstrated that 24 mg/day dose of sunitinib should be considered for phase II study.[342]

Kao et al.[343] reported on a phase I study designed to determine the safety and maximum-tolerated dose of concurrent sunitinib and radiation therapy using image-guided technologies for patients with oligometastases (one to five sites) from renal cell carcinoma. The most common treatment sites were bone, liver, and lung. Sunitinib was given at 25 to 37.5 mg/day with either 40 or 50 Gy of radiation therapy delivered in 10 fractions in a ping-pong design of either sunitinib or radiotherapy dose escalation. Twenty-one patients with 36 metastatic lesions were enrolled. No dose-limiting toxicity (DLT) was noted for sunitinib at 37.5 mg plus 40 Gy. At 37.5 mg sunitinib with 50 Gy, and 50 mg sunitinib with 50 Gy, one out of ten patients, and two out of five patients, respectively, experienced DLTs (grade 4 myelosuppression and grade 3 nausea). The 1-year OS rate was 75%, and PFS rate was 44%. They proceeded to a phase II trial for sunitinib at 37.5 mg/day and a 50-Gy/10 fraction dose regimen, with tumor types treated including head and neck, liver, lung, kidney, and prostate cancers.[344] Local control and distant control at 18 months were 75% and 52%, respectively, with PFS and OS of 56% and 71% reported. Incidence of acute grade ≥ 3 toxicities was 28%, most commonly myelosuppression, bleeding, and abnormal liver function test findings.

Sorafenib

Sorafenib is a small-molecule TKI that has been approved for treatment of advanced renal cell carcinoma, hepatocellular carcinoma, and thyroid cancer. It is also a multikinase inhibitor of Raf kinase, PDGF, VEGFR2 and R3, and cKit.[345] Conflicting reports of efficacy and tolerability are reported in early phase studies with radiation therapy.

Phase I trial of sorafenib and SRS for patients with 1 to 4 brain metastases has been reported.[346] In a 3 + 3 dose escalation trial design, dose level 1 (400 mg/day) and dose level 2 (400 mg twice per day) starting 5 to 7 days prior to SRS, and continued for 14 days after SRS, was tolerated. In an expansion cohort of 17 patients treated with dose level 2, 6 grade 3 toxicities were reported, all of which were attributable to sorafenib, and not to the combination treatment. Recommended phase II dose for sorafenib with SRS was 400 mg twice daily. For unresectable liver metastases, a phase I trial of radiation therapy with sorafenib was reported, for SBRT or whole liver radiotherapy (WLRT).[347] Sorafenib was delivered for 4 weeks, with radiotherapy delivered during weeks 2 to 3, and 3 escalating dose levels from 200 to 400 mg twice daily was studied. Depending on effective liver volume irradiated (<80% vs. >80%), radiation dose was either 30 or 60 Gy in 6 fractions (n = 18) versus 21.6 Gy in 6 fractions (n = 15), respectively. In both strata, MTD (defined as liver toxicity grade 3+ or grade 4+ treatment related toxicity) was not reached. Grade 3+ toxicity was seen in 33% of patients at a median of 10 days. Two patients undergoing WLRT died, from nonclassic liver toxicity in the 21.6 Gy in 6 fraction group. The investigators concluded that the Sorafenib with 21.6 Gy in 6 fractions to the whole liver was with unacceptably high rates of liver toxicity. SBRT was sorafenib was deemed tolerable, efficacy was not felt to be sufficient to merit further clinical evaluation. Similarly, phase I study of sorafenib with SBRT for hepatocellular carcinoma demonstrated significant toxicity if significant volume of liver was irradiated, and not recommended outside of a clinical trial.[348] In the only reported phase II study of sorafenib and radiation therapy for unresectable hepatocellular carcinoma, 40 patients were enrolled and sorafenib was administered at 400 mg twice daily, starting with radiation therapy (40 to 60 Gy, median 50 Gy), and continued till progression.[349] Fifty-five percent patients achieved complete or partial remission, and 2-year infield PFS was 39%. However, 6 patients (15%) developed treatment-related grade 3+ hepatic toxicity during the sequential phase, and 3 of these were fatal, and investigators advised caution with this regimen. RTOG 1112 is a phase III clinical trial investigating sorafenib versus sorafenib with SBRT for liver cancer, currently recruiting patients.

In cervical cancer patients, a phase I study of 13 patients with stage IB to IIIB cervical cancer, with sorafenib administered for 7 days prior to start of cisplatin/radiation treatments, suggested that sorafenib might increase tumor hypoxia, raising concerns for potential to impair radiation efficacy when added to standard chemo/RT regimen.[350] In high-grade glioma, sorafenib dose escalation (200 mg daily, 200 mg bid, and 400 mg bid) was studied with temozolomide and radiation therapy as first-line therapy, and MTD was established at 200 mg bid.[351] Efficacy in this limited number of patients was moderate, and therefore, further study with chemoradiation in high-grade glioma was not recommended. In pancreatic cancer, a phase I study of dose escalation of sorafenib (starting at 200 mg/day up to 400 mg twice daily), with concurrent radiation therapy and gemcitabine, enrolled 27 patients.[352] Maximum tolerated dose was 400 mg twice daily. Addition of sorafenib seemed to have modest clinical activity, except in patients with angiogenesis genes polymorphisms (VEGF-A-2578AA, -1498CC, and -1154AA), with these patients having median OS of 21.6 months versus 14.7 months for others. This study suggested that select VEGF-A/VEGF-R2 genotypes may be associated with improved outcomes.

In rectal cancer, preoperative 5-FU and sorafenib with external beam radiation therapy (50.4 Gy in 28 fractions) was studied, with sorafenib dose starting at 200 mg daily with dose escalation planned up to 400 mg po bid to determine MTD.[353] Seventeen patients were enrolled. Because of acute toxicities in the initial phase of the study, protocol was amended to administer chemotherapy and sorafenib on days 1 to 5 only. With the amended protocol, primary grade 3 toxicity was hypertension in 2 patients at the 200 mg/day dose and 1 patient at the 400 mg bid dose. One patient had grade 3 liver function elevation at 400 mg, and no grade 4 toxicities were observed. No perioperative complications were reported. Pathologic complete response rate was 33%, and downstaging observed in 85.7% of patients.

A phase I trial of sorafenib with radiation therapy delivered preoperatively to extremity soft tissue sarcoma has been reported.[354] Two dose escalation cohorts for sorafenib were 200 mg/daily and 200 and 400 mg daily, with sorafenib delivered during the entire course of radiation therapy (50 Gy in 25 daily fractions) as tolerated. All tumors in this study were located in the lower extremity. Eight patients were enrolled. Two out of five patients at second dose level developed DLT, with grade 3 rash. Other grade 3 toxicities included anemia, perirectal abscess, and supraventricular tachycardia, with total of 4/8 patients having developed grade 3 toxicities. Radiation-related toxicities and postsurgical complications

(3 grade 3 wound complications) were felt to be comparable to those treated historically without sorafenib. Complete pathologic response was noted in 38% of patients. Investigators recommended further studies using dose level 1 of sorafenib. Phase II trials of sorafenib with radiation therapy for soft tissue sarcoma are in progress.

Pazopanib

Pazopanib is also a multitargeted TKI that was approved by the FDA in October 2009 and inhibits the intracellular tyrosine kinase portion of VEGFR1–3, PDGFR-α and -β, c-Kit, FGF receptor-1 (FGFR-1), FGFR-3, Lck, and c-Fms.[355] Phase I study of preoperative radiation therapy with pazopanib in patients with locally advanced soft tissue sarcoma of the extremities has been reported.[356] Twelve patients were enrolled with 11 evaluable. Dose of pazopanib was escalated from 400 to 600 to 800 mg/day, for 6 weeks given with radiation therapy (50 Gy in 25 fractions) starting day 8. No increased toxicity inside radiation field was reported, but 2/10 patients (in the 400 and 600 mg cohorts) demonstrated delayed wound healing after surgery. Pathologic complete response was noted in 4/10 cases. Grade 3 hepatotoxicity, which led to pazopanib interruption, was noted in 27% of the cases. In these cases, liver was not in the radiation field. The same group is conducting a phase II study using once daily 800 mg oral pazopanib with radiation therapy in preoperative treatment of sarcoma in extremities, trunk chest wall, and head and neck regions (PASART-2). There is also a multigroup phase II/III trial currently recruiting patients studying the potential role of preoperative pazopanib (or chemotherapy) with radiation in adult and pediatric nonrhabdomyosarcoma soft tissue sarcoma patients (COG-NRG ARST 1321).

Mammalian Target of Rapamycin

The mTOR pathway has been shown to be dysregulated in a number of solid tumors.[357] A number of rapamycin analogs exist and have been approved by the FDA, such as temsirolimus (Torisel) or everolimus (Afinitor), which inhibits mTOR. Temsirolimus is approved for treating patients with advanced renal cell carcinoma. Everolimus is approved for treatment of patients with advanced renal cell carcinoma that has progressed after other therapies, advanced breast cancer, subependymal giant cell astrocytoma (in adults and children who have tuberous sclerosis and are not amenable to surgery), and progressive well-differentiated neuroendocrine tumors of GI or lung origin. The potential for radiosensitization effects of these agents has been studied in a preclinical setting in a number of different cancer types.[358-366]

Temsirolimus

Temsirolimus was studied in combination with chemoradiation therapy in newly diagnosed GBM patients in a dose-escalation phase I study.[367] Unfortunately, concomitant and adjuvant use of temsirolimus was associated with a high rate (3 of 12 patients) of grade 4/5 infections. This was reduced with antibiotic prophylaxis and by limiting the duration of temsirolimus therapy. Therefore, based on this study, a dose of 50 mg/week of temsirolimus combined with radiation and temozolomide is the recommended phase II dose and schedule. In a phase I study, temsirolimus was studied with thoracic radiation in patients who were candidates for palliative radiotherapy.[368] Patients who were candidates for definitive chemoradiotherapy were excluded. Temsirolimus dose levels were 20 mg/week and 25 mg/week, and –1 dose level was at 15 mg/week, using 3 + 3 design. Radiation dose was 35 Gy in 14 daily fractions. Ten patients were enrolled. Maximum tolerated dose was determined to be 15 mg/weekly. At the first dose level of 20 mg/week, 1 patient experienced grade 3 pneumonitis (day 10), grade 4 fatigue, and grade 4 lymphopenia and was able to complete radiotherapy after discontinuation of temsirolimus. Another patient died after 2 doses of temsirolimus and 3 fractions of radiation. Although death was more likely to be related to cancer progression, per protocol definition, was considered DLT. At the 15 mg/week dose level, one-third patient developed pulmonary hemorrhage from a fungating right main stem bronchus mass after only 2 radiation treatments (5 Gy). With enrollment of 3 additional patients, no additional DLTs occurred. Of the 8 evaluable patients, 3 had partial response, and 2 had stable disease.

Everolimus

The North Central Cancer Treatment Group has also reported a phase I trial of everolimus and temozolomide in combination with radiation therapy in newly diagnosed GBM patients.[369] Eighteen patients were enrolled, and everolimus was well tolerated. The recommended dose for the phase II study is 70 mg/week in combination with standard temozolomide/radiation therapy. RTOG 0913 is a phase 1 study of everolimus in combination with radiation therapy and temozolomide in patients with newly diagnosed GBM. Everolimus was escalated from 2.5 to 5 to 10 mg/day in combination with 60 Gy in 30 fractions radiation therapy and temozolomide. Adjuvant temozolomide and concurrent everolimus was then given at an established dose of 10 mg/day. In this study, everolimus dose was escalated to 10 mg/day as MTD. In a multi-institutional NCCTG phase II trial (N057K), 70 mg/week everolimus was started 1 week prior to radiation/temozolomide and given concurrently and followed by adjuvant temozolomide until disease progression.[370] One hundred patients were enrolled. Fourteen percent had grade 4 hematologic toxicities, 12% had at least one grade 3 nonhematologic toxicity, and one treatment-related death was reported. One-year OS was 64%, and median time to progression was 6.4 months. On molecular imaging response assessment, responders were less likely to have alterations within the PI3K/AKT/mTOR or tuberous sclerosis complex/neurofibromatosis type 1 pathway compared to nonresponders, which did not translate into durable outcomes, and survival benefit was not seen as compared to historical controls.

In an adjuvant therapy setting, the use of bevacizumab/everolimus after concurrent radiation/temozolomide for GBM has been reported demonstrating feasibility and efficacy, with median PFS of 11.3 months, and median OS of 13.9 months reported.[371] In head and neck cancer, phase I study of everolimus with weekly cisplatin (30 mg/kg) and IMRT-based radiation therapy was reported, with maximum tolerated dose of everolimus of 5 mg/day.[372] Phase I study of everolimus with thoracic radiation for NSCLC has been reported.[373] In this study, everolimus dose was escalated either weekly (10, 20, or 50 mg) or daily (2.5, 5, or 10 mg), with everolimus starting 1 week prior to radiation, and for 3.5 weeks after end of radiotherapy. Radiation dose was 66 Gy in 2 Gy/daily fractions. Twenty-six patients were enrolled from two centers. In the weekly group (*n* = 14), dose was escalated to MTD of 50 mg/week, with 1 patient experiencing DLT with grade 2 interstitial pneumonitis at 20 mg/week dose at week 10 of therapy. Addition of 6 patients to this dose group, and further 3 patients in the 50 mg/week group, did not demonstrate any further DLTs. In the daily group (*n* = 11), 1 DLT of grade 2 pneumonitis at week 6, with subsequent fatal outcome (1 month after interruption of treatment), was noted at 2.5 mg/day dose. Expansion at this dose level to 6 patients demonstrated no further DLTs, and dose increased to 5 mg/day. At this level, grade 3 pneumonitis at week 11, grade 4 dyspnea at week 9, and grade 3 esophagitis with associated dysphagia at week 5 were reported. Because of this (2/5 patients with DLT), further recruitment was stopped, and MTD determined to be 50 mg/week. Overall, 5 patients with grade 3 to 4 pneumonitis related to treatments were reported. Of 22 patients assessable for response, 41% partial response and 32% stable

disease, with 2-year OS and PFS of 31% and 12%, respectively, were reported. Investigators recommend for further studies, weekly dose of 50 mg/week, with caution for monitoring for pulmonary toxicity.

Further studies of mTOR inhibitors with radiation therapy are ongoing, with special emphasis in trying to determine molecular markers of response to therapy to better select patients who may have improved outcome with the use of mTOR inhibitor therapy. Studies involving the use of agents inhibiting the signaling pathway downstream of mTOR are also in development.

Anaplastic Lymphoma Kinase Inhibitors

ALK fusion protein results in constitutive activation of ALK tyrosine kinase. Although studies specifically addressing ALK inhibitors with radiation therapy have not yet been reported, because of the impact this molecular has made in the NSCLC therapy paradigm, this topic will be briefly discussed. Soda et al.[374] discovered the fusion of the ALK gene with echinoderm microtubule-associated protein like 4 (ELM4-ALK). This *ELM4–ALK* fusion oncogene has become a very important potential biomarker for patients with NSCLC. The frequency of *ALK* rearrangement ranges from 3% to 7% in unselected NSCLC patients. Furthermore, similar to EGFR mutations, this rearrangement is seen more frequently in adenocarcinomas and patients with never or light smoking history. *ALK* rearrangements appear to be mutually exclusive with *EGFR* and *KRAS* mutations.[375] Several ALK inhibitors have been identified, and the furthest developed is crizotinib. Crizotinib was initially designed as an MET inhibitor but has been found to be clinically effective as an ALK inhibitor in NSCLC patients harboring *ALK* rearrangements.[375] In a phase I trial of 82 patients selected for ALK rearrangement (out of over 1,500 patients), an impressive response rate of 57% was noted.[376] Crizotinib has demonstrated efficacy in patients with ALK rearrangement in randomized trials. When compared to pemetrexed or docetaxel single-agent chemotherapy, crizotinib demonstrated improved median PFS of 7.7 months versus 3 months in patients previously treated with platinum-based chemotherapy regimen.[377] Objective response rate was improved, but OS benefit was not seen, presumably because of cross over study design, where patients progressing on chemotherapy were allowed to cross over to crizotinib. In another study of chemotherapy naïve patients, 343 patients were randomized to crizotinib versus platinum and pemetrexed chemotherapy, with cross over permitted.[378] PFS was significantly improved with crizotinib (10.9 months vs. 7 months), once again with OS not showing significant difference, likely because of cross over being permitted to the crizotinib treatment.

Although extremely effective, patients develop resistance to crizotinib within first few years of therapy. In one-third of resistant cases, tumors have acquired a secondary mutation within the ALK tyrosine kinase domain, most commonly, L1196M mutation, followed by G1269A mutations. Other mutations also exist including the G1202R mutation, which confers significant resistance to not only crizotinib but also to next-generation ALK inhibitors. Second-generation ALK inhibitor includes ceritinib, which is approved for use in patients that have progressed or are not tolerant of crizotinib.[379] Ceritinib has been shown to yield improved outcomes in patients compared to chemotherapy both in the upfront setting[380] and in those who have progressed on crizotinib (presentation at ESMO 2016, Sacagliotti et al.).[381] Alectinib is another second-generation ALK inhibitor that has activity in crizotinib-resistant disease, and also reported to have better activity for brain metastases.[382-384] It is approved for use in crizotinib-resistant or crizotinib-intolerant patients. Brigatinib, another next-generation agent, was approved by FDA for use in patients with metastatic NSCLC progressed on crizotinib on April 2017.

There are no significant data to suggest a radiosensitizing or synergistic effect when combined with radiation therapy concurrently, but sequential use of crizotinib with a chemoradiation regimen is being explored in a randomized phase II study for stage III NSCLC patients (NCT01822496). A phase I study aimed at determining safety and activity of crizotinib with temozolomide and radiation therapy for newly diagnosed GBM is also recruiting patients in Spain.

Histone Deacetylase Inhibitors

HDACs contribute to oncogenic transformation, and involvement of acetylation and HDAC activity in cancer development provides a mechanistic rationale for considering HDAC inhibitors as an anticancer therapy. Inhibitors of HDAC relax chromatin structure. This can lead to increased radiosensitivity through enhanced DNA damage.[385,386] However, some HDAC inhibitors have also been shown to down-regulate the expression of both EGFR and ErbB2 and to inhibit PI3K and AKT signaling,[387-389] all strong potentiators of tumor cell survival and modulators of DNA DSB repair.[390] This combination of DNA damage enhancement, inhibition of DNA repair, and downregulation of strong survival highlights the utility of agents that attack multiple signaling pathways.

The most clinically developed HDAC inhibitors include vorinostat and romidepsin, both of which have FDA approval for use in cutaneous T-cell lymphoma (CTCL). Although their indications are supported by data suggesting activity in hematologic malignancies, studies in solid tumors have also been reported. Preclinical studies of radiation therapy and HDAC inhibitors have been reported in squamous cells, medulloblastoma cells, breast cancer brain metastatic cells, colorectal models, GBM cells, pancreatic cells, neuroblastoma cells, osteosarcoma, and rhabdomyosarcoma cells.[387,391-402] Of note, 18 HDAC enzymes have been identified and classified into four groups (classes I through IV).

Vorinostat is a hydroxamic acid multi-HDAC inhibitor that blocks the enzymatic activity of both class I and II HDACs at low nanomolar concentrations.[398] Vorinostat is active in inducing differentiation, cell growth arrest, or apoptosis in a wide variety of transformed cells in preclinical studies.[398] Vorinostat is FDA approved for treatment of CTCL that has persisted, progressed, or recurred after treatment with other first-line agents. Therefore, primary efficacy of vorinostat has been demonstrated in hematologic malignancies. However, it is also being studied in a number of different solid tumor types with mixed success (NSCLC, colorectal cancer, breast cancer, prostate cancer, GBM) in phase I and II clinical settings in combination with other standard cytotoxic agents, including radiation therapy.[403-407] Ree et al.[397] reported on combining vorinostat with pelvic palliative radiotherapy for gastrointestinal carcinoma patients. Sixteen patients were evaluable. Patients received palliative radiotherapy (30 Gy in 10 fractions) with escalating vorinostat dose, administered orally daily 3 hours before each radiotherapy fraction. Maximum tolerated dose was determined to be 300 mg/day. Histone hyperacetylation was detected, indicating biologic activity of vorinostat.

Phase I study of vorinostat for brain metastases has been reported.[408] Vorinostat was administered by mouth during whole-brain radiation therapy (37.5 Gy in 15 fractions), escalated from 200 to 400 mg/day. Seventeen patients were enrolled. There were no specific treatment-related grade 3+ toxicities, with one death in the 400-mg cohort because of pulmonary embolus, which was unlikely to be related, but was conservatively classified as DLT. Recommended dose for further phase II study was 300 mg/day.

Romidepsin is a novel HDAC inhibitor with recent FDA approval for treatment of CTCL, approved as second-line therapy.[409] Studies in small cell lung cancer, recurrent glioma, and castrate-resistant prostate cancer have been performed with mixed success.[410-412] As yet, there are no completed and published studies demonstrating efficacy of romidepsin in combination with radiation treatments.

Miscellaneous Molecular Targets
K-Ras

Activating mutations in the ras oncogene are found in many tumors including the lungs, colon, head and neck, glioblastoma, pancreas, and others. The overall rate of ras mutations in human cancers is 25% to 30%, but for some cancers, the mutation rate can be quite high. These activating mutations drive key intracellular signaling pathways that confer proliferative and survival advantages to tumor cells, including radioresistance, through the chronic activation of the PI3K and the Ras/MAP kinase pathways.[413-415] Ras must be prenylated in order to be membrane bound, where it becomes active. Prenylation can occur by two enzymatic processes, farnesylation and geranylgeranylation. Inhibitors of farnesylation, specifically farnesyltransferase inhibitors (FTIs), have had some success in limiting the negative impact of ras activation, particularly in inhibiting tumor cell radioresistance in vitro and in vivo.[29,413,416-418] FTIs selectively affect tumors because the ras genes in normal tissues are not mutated. The activity of FTIs has had limited success, partly because of the activity against a given ras species, H-ras versus n-Ras or K-ras, and partly because of the FTI resistance of geranylgeranylated K-ras.[413,416,419-421] However, new compounds that target both farnesylation and geranylgeranylation have been shown to be effective in preclinical studies, and new molecular targets for radiosensitization by FTIs have been identified,[415,422] which may enhance their clinical utility.

Targeting DNA

Many therapy agents target the DNA of cells, preferably tumor cells. This can be through DNA damage induction, inhibition of cell cycle traversal, or inhibition of DNA replication, for example, and targeting the enzymes that manage the integrity of the DNA of cells represents a sound therapeutic strategy. Furthermore, differences between tumor and normal cells in cell cycle checkpoint controls, DNA repair capabilities, and even chromatin architecture have been identified that could be taken advantage of by combined therapies.

There are multiple strategies to targeting DNA repair pathways with drugs or small molecules. First, DNA damage must be sensed, and there are several key enzymes that are considered damage sensors. The most established sensors are telomeric repeat-binding factor 2 (TRF2), the Mre11-Rad50-Nbs1 (MRN) complex, and ATM.[423,424] These proteins set off the cascade of events that alter chromatin, recruit repair enzymes to the break site, and initiate cell cycle checkpoint control following DNA damage. ATM inhibitors, for example, have been studied in preclinical setting showing significant radiosensitizing effects, but a challenge that remains is the potential for normal tissue toxicity when used in combined modality therapy with radiation.[425] Key regulatory proteins within each of these areas are being successfully targeted in preclinical studies. Examples include a specific inhibitor of ATM, Ku55933, which has shown enhanced radiosensitivity in in vitro experiments,[426] small molecules that reconstitute the wild-type p53 protein structure in mutant p53 molecules,[427] and radiotherapy combined with adenoviral wild-type p53 delivered in vivo by liposomal carriers in clinical trials for lung cancer.[428] Preclinical evaluations of compounds that target DNA repair components directly, particularly when combined with radiation and radiosensitizing compounds such as cisplatin or gemcitabine, are ongoing. Inhibitors of DNA-PKcs, a critical enzyme in nonhomologous end joining (NHEJ), have been successful in preclinical studies on tumor cell lines; however, a treatment advantage for normal tissue may provide a challenge.[429-434]

There are novel therapeutic targets within the DNA repair pathway known as *homologous recombination* (HR). For instance, RAD51 and BRCA1/2 defective cell lines are radiosensitive, and antisense strategies against RAD51 have been used against a number of cancer cell lines. Interestingly, targeting HR may have a distinct advantage over the NHEJ pathway. NHEJ occurs throughout the cell cycle, whereas HR is considered to be a dominant repair pathway during the S and G_2 phases of the cell cycle because of the need for a template strand of DNA. This implies that for most normal tissues, where there is little to no cellular turnover and where NHEJ is the dominant DNA repair pathway, there would be a survival advantage compared to tumors where cells are traversing the cell cycle and are more likely to be found in the S or G_2 phase. Specific inhibitors such as small interfering RNA (siRNA), antisense, small molecules, and antibodies that target DNA repair are still relatively new, and although the *in vitro* data are encouraging, clinical efficacy remains to be seen. Other DNA damage response targets include CHK1, which functions in HR repair, and WEE1, a cell cycle kinase which leads to G2 cell cycle arrest in response to DNA damage.[425] Inhibitors for WEE1 and CHK1 have been identified demonstrating promising preclinical data with radiation inhibitors have been identified. AZD1775 (MK1775), a potent WEE1 inhibitor, has been studied in solid tumors in phase I trial[435] and additional studies with phase 1 trial in combination with RT/temodar in GBM, pancreatic cancer, head and neck cancer, and younger patients with diffuse intrinsic pontine gliomas ongoing. Clinical trials studying CHK1 inhibitors, including MK-8776, SRA737, prexasertib are ongoing. PARP is an enzyme whose specific function is to repair SSBs, and with recent advances in agents that block this pathway, a discussion of such agents is warranted. PARP catalyzes the transfer of ADP-ribose units from intracellular NAD$^+$ to nuclear receptor proteins, leading to the formation of ADP-ribose polymers. Nicotinamide was the first PARP inhibitor identified, and since then second-generation PARP inhibitors have been developed. Although significant current interest is in the role of PARP inhibitors in BRCA-deficient tumors, they have also been studied as chemosensitizers. Therefore, initial studies primarily were based on nonselected tumor types to determine the efficacy of PARP inhibition in combination with chemotherapy agents. However, because radiotherapy damages cells by causing DNA breaks, and PARP inhibitors impair DNA repair mechanisms, studies in combination with radiation therapy have been performed *in vitro* and *in vivo* demonstrating effectiveness in cancer cell lines, including glioma cells.[436-439] Furthermore, with exciting preclinical data suggesting that PARP inhibitors may have a significantly and selectively high impact in BRCA-deficient cells,[440,441] a new paradigm for a clinical trial was born in which patients with BRCA mutations or BRCA-ness were selected for treatment with PARP inhibitors.[442,443] BRCA-ness refers to abnormal function of BRCA1/2 genes, or other genes implicated in similar DNA repair pathways to BRCA1 and BRCA2, which is seen in triple-negative breast cancer patients, for example, without necessarily having the hereditary mutations.[443] After encouraging preclinical data in solid tumors with chemotherapy, and particularly in selected tumor cells with BRCA deficiency, multiple PARP inhibitors have been studied or are being studied in solid tumors, including breast cancer, ovarian cancer, and lung cancer. Three PARP inhibitors have now received FDA approval, olaparib (Lynparza, AstraZeneca), rucaparib (Rubraca, Clovis Oncology), and niraparib (Zejula, Tesaro). Olaparib has been approved for advanced ovarian cancer patients who have been treated with at least three types of chemotherapy. Rucaparib is approved for use in advanced ovarian cancer patients, previously treated with two or more chemotherapy regimens, and have BRCA mutation. Niraparib is approved for ovarian, fallopian tube, or primary peritoneal cancer, to be used as maintenance treatment for patients who are in complete or partial response to platinum-based chemotherapy. Two other agents furthest along in development without FDA approval include veliparib and talazoparib. Veliparib failed to improve outcome in NSCLC and triple negative breast cancer in phase III studies, and the phase III trial of gynecologic malignancies is still recruiting patients. Talazoparib is currently undergoing phase III study for patients with BRCA mutations with locally advanced or metastatic breast cancer (EMBRACA study).

Of note, Veliparib is a PARP inhibitor that appears to cross the blood–brain barrier, and its efficacy in combination with whole-brain radiation for brain metastases and with temozolomide and radiation for patients with primary brain tumors has been investigated in phase I studies. For patients with brain metastases, veliparib's dose was escalated from 10 mg bid up to 300 mg bid given concurrently during the radiation therapy course.[444] WBRT was administered as either 37.5 Gy in 2.5 Gy/daily treatments or 30 Gy in 3 Gy/day treatments. Three DLTs occurred—two at 150 mg veliparib, one of which was grade 3 hypokalemia and the other a grade 3 hyponatremia. After review, dose escalation was continued. One DLT of grade 4 posterior reversible encephalopathy syndrome occurred at 200 mg bid. At the 300 mg bid, five of eight subjects experienced AEs of nausea and or vomiting, with two events leading to discontinuation of drug. Although not meeting criteria for DLT, because 300 mg bid was not well tolerated, recommended phase II dose for veliparib was determined to be 200 mg bid with 30 Gy in 10 fractions (the most common radiation combination at higher doses).

A phase I study of veliparib in combination with low-dose fractionated whole abdominal radiation therapy in patients with advanced solid malignancies and peritoneal carcinomatosis has been reported.[445] In this study, patients were treated with veliparib (from 40 mg bid, up to 160 mg bid) for 3 cycles. Radiation consisted of 21.6 Gy in 36 fractions (0.6 Gy twice daily on days 1 and 5 for weeks 1 to 3 of each cycle). Overall, the regimen was deemed tolerable and in some patients, particularly those with ovarian and fallopian cancer, appeared to prolong disease stability. Other disease sites studied with veliparib and radiation therapy include rectal cancer (phase I/II), inflammatory or locoregionally recurrent breast cancer (phase I), unresectable pancreatic cancer (phase I), NSCLC (phase I/II), brain metastases from NSCLC (phase II), and GBM (phase I/II).

Several phase I studies combining olaparib with radiotherapy for triple negative breast cancer, soft tissue sarcoma, head and neck cancer, esophageal cancer, and NSCLC are actively recruiting patients or under development. Niraparib is being investigated for use with Radium 223 radiopharmaceutical for hormone-resistant prostate cancer bone metastases patients in the phase I setting (NCT03076203). There are no studies reported or ongoing with rucaparib with radiation therapy.

Era of Personalized Medicine Using Molecularly Tailored Therapeutics

Although high-impact molecular discoveries and effective combined modality treatment realizations have been of significant importance in the field of oncology, another area that has made significant strides and impact on cancer therapeutics is the concept of molecular selection of patients for appropriate therapy. One of the first such examples is in the field of breast cancer where hormonal therapy and Herceptin treatments are selectively given to patients whose tumors demonstrate appropriate molecular criteria (estrogen receptor positivity and HER2/neu positivity).[446] Other examples include imatinib for treatment of patients with c-kit harboring GIST tumors,[447] anti-EGFR therapy for lung cancer patients with

EGFR tyrosine kinase mutations, crizotinib for lung cancer patients with ALK fusion gene translocation, and the predictive value of KRAS mutation status for anti-EGFR therapy for patients with metastatic colorectal cancer.[448] Meanwhile, abundant studies are in progress and/or have been performed to attempt to determine biomarkers that may provide prognostic or therapeutic information. Multigene assays (Oncotype DX),[449] for example, are already in use in clinical practice for patients with breast cancer. Genomic signatures or biomarkers of response to chemotherapy of tumor, to survival, or to metastatic potential of tumor have been studied.[450] Similarly, efforts to study and identify biomarkers for radiation response, sensitivity, resistance, or toxicity are being investigated.

USING RADIOTHERAPY TO IMPROVE THE LOCAL AND DISTAL TUMORICIDAL EFFECTS OF IMMUNOTHERAPY, A NOVEL PARADIGM IN COMBINED MODALITY THERAPY

Radiation therapy's potential to improve clinical response of immunotherapy has gained tremendous momentum for clinical trial development, based on positive results from preclinical and early clinical data. There are numerous clinical trials investigating this approach, in part because of the increasing number of novel immunotherapy agents gaining FDA approval for indications for cancer therapy. In this section, we review some key radiation issues to consider when combining immune agents with radiotherapy, and some of the agents being pursued actively for such combined modality clinical trials.

RT Factors Influencing Immune Response

When considering use of RT with immunotherapy, one must consider the optimal dose of radiotherapy, the timing of radiotherapy, and the volume of area irradiated, potential role of particle therapy, as these are all important factors that could potentially affect the ability of RT/immunotherapy combination to yield successful outcomes. In addition, one size may not fit all in terms of these parameters, and some of these may prove to be dependent on tumor histology.

When considering combining immunotherapy with RT, one must consider the volume of area that will be encompassed by RT. Radiation therapy has been traditionally used for treatment of regional areas when clinically indicated and has in many disease sites, and for many disease sites, such treatment has remained a standard of care. Although this may provide benefit for impacting regional control by treatment of microscopic or gross nodal disease burden, it may counteract the immune response, as lymph nodes, and T cells would be negatively affected by the radiation and ultimately may potentially reduce the cytotoxic effects that would be mediated by immune mechanisms. Concurrent chemotherapy could further lead to this issue. Therefore, a delicate balance may be required in considering the need to irradiate potential disease burden in the lymph node regions versus impacting immune effects. Such issues will need to be considered and studied carefully when designing clinical trials aimed at implementing immunotherapy in conjunction with standard definitive radiotherapy. A potential concept could include trials where only the gross disease is treated with RT, when studied in conjunction with immunotherapeutic agents, particularly in disease sites where ENI is already safely omitted.

Another important RT factor to consider is the appropriate dose per fraction and number of fractions that should be delivered when combined with immunotherapy. Some preclinical data would support consideration of use of higher dose/fraction as a more optimal dose regimen when considering

immune effects.[451] Some studies would suggest fractionation to some degree may be beneficial, whereas others did not. For example, when combined with anti-CTLA-4, 8 Gy × 3, and to a lesser degree 6 Gy × 5 fractions demonstrated improved local and abscopal effects compared to mice treated with single fraction of 20 Gy.[452] However, other preclinical studies have demonstrated immune response or stimulatory effects with single-fraction regimen.[453] In another preclinical study of mice-bearing murine melanoma tumors, radiation dose up to 15 Gy was studied for tumor control and immune response effects and demonstrated that 7.5 Gy/fraction gave the best tumor control and tumor immunity while maintaining low Treg numbers.[454] 5 Gy in this study was not immunostimulatory, suggesting a potential threshold dose above which immune effects are manifested. Authors proposed that the optimal immunogenic effect may be a balance of increasing cross-priming while not increasing Treg cell numbers, which in their study was best accomplished with 7.5 Gy × 2 fractions. Biologic rationale for higher dose per fraction include potential for increased induction of necrosis and senescence,[455] which are thought to be associated with inflammation, and increased release of DAMP.[456,457] Relatively larger dose of RT (8 Gy) has also been shown to induce Fas-receptors, which could lead to activation of T cells.[457] One would also need to consider the mechanism of immune agent being used in conjunction with RT. Preclinical study of anti-CD137 and anti CD-40 antibodies combined with either 12 Gy in 1 fraction, or 4 Gy × 4 fractions, or 5 Gy × 4 fractions in breast cancer preclinical model demonstrated that PD-1 expression and targeting of this checkpoint with anti-PD-1 antibodies were required for combination treatment with anti-CD137 and RT to be effective.[458,459] Furthermore, the fractionated radiation regimens were less effective than that 12 Gy regimen. Another study of 30 Gy in 1 fraction versus fractionated treatments (30 Gy in 10 fractions) demonstrated higher dose/fraction RT led to intense T-cell tumor infiltration compared to fractionated regimen in weakly immunogenic colon tumors in preclinical setting.[460] In other tumor types, such as lymphoma, prostate cancer, and renal cell bone metastases in the clinical setting, there are reports that conventional dose per fraction (2 Gy × 2 fractions, 70 Gy in 1.8 to 2 Gy/fractions, and 45 to 50 Gy in 1.8 to 2 Gy/fractions) in combination with immune therapy elicited a positive clinical response.[461–463] Therefore, preclinical and clinical studies would suggest that there is a complexity in determining optimal dose and fractions for optimal radiation/immunotherapy interactions. This may depend on the tumor type, the tumor microenvironment, and the mechanism of action of immunotherapy agent being utilized.[8,451]

Another intriguing line of investigation to determine the additional potential benefit that particle therapy may have over conventional photon-based RT as it pertains to immunomodulation/activation. Preclinical studies suggest in animal studies that DC injection and carbon ion combination conferred augmentation of immunogenicity of tumor cells through maturation of DCs, which stimulates antitumor immunity and led to reduction in lung metastases.[464] Preclinical studies and development of clinical trials to determine the potential role of particle therapy with immunotherapy are areas of active investigation.

From a practical point of view, given the potential benefit for use of hypofractionated radiation favoring a higher dose/fraction regimen that has been seen in some of the preclinical studies, clinically relevant and available radiation modality may include SRS and SBRT, which typically employs larger dose/fraction in limited total fractions (typically 1 to 5 fractions) to a smaller treatment area. Regional nodal exposure would be limited with SBRT treatments. As SBRT and SRS are also frequently being used in the setting of limited extracranial and intracranial metastases/oligometastases, respectively, combining with immunotherapy may provide not only a local control advantage but can be studied to explore improvements in distant control rates. Therefore, there is significant excitement for design and implementation of clinical trials using SRS/SBRT as well as conventional fractionated RT in combination with available immunotherapy. Given the preclinical data, the appropriate dose, fractionation, treatment volume, and timing of SRS/SBRT treatments in relation to the immune agent, tumor type, and treatment site will need to be carefully considered and preferably systematically studied in the clinical setting.

Clinical Experiences

Immune agents, most of which have received recent FDA approval for cancer therapy, include cytokines (IL-2, interferon-alpha-2b), oncolytic virus therapy (T-VEC), dendritic-cell vaccine (Sipuleucel-T), and checkpoint inhibitors (ipilimumab, nivolumab, pembrolizumab, atezolizumab, durvalumab, avelumab). These agents and their current FDA-approved indications are listed in Table 36.6. Many additional agents are in the pipeline undergoing active preclinical/and clinical studies. In terms of combined therapy with radiotherapy, a large number of clinical trials are ongoing to attempt to further elucidate the potential role of RT/SBRT with these agents. However, thus far, only a handful of studies or case reports demonstrating the potential safety or efficacy of combining immune agents with RT are published. Some of the more relevant class of immune agents and published studies in conjunction with RT are reviewed below.

Vaccines

Rationale for vaccine therapy would be to boost the immune response and to overcome the baseline established immune tolerance that provided escape for the tumor. Multiple approaches for vaccine therapy have been developed including peptide-based therapy, DNA-based vaccines, and DC-based approaches.

Few studies of peptide vaccine with radiation have been reported. A randomized phase II clinical trial of use of a standard radiotherapy with or without poxviral vaccine encoding PSA was studied in 30 patients with localized prostate cancer. RT was delivered between fourth and sixth vaccinations.[465] The vaccine regimen was safely deliverable with majority of patients demonstrating PSA-specific cellular immune response to the vaccine. However, on long-term follow-up, including patients treated with adjuvant standard or low-dose IL-2 regimen, there was no specific difference in terms of PSA outcome or toxicity with addition of vaccine, and limited long-

term immune response was seen.[466] Tecemotide (L-BLP25) is a vaccine to tumor antigen MUC-1 that has been studied in a randomized phase III study for unresectable NSCLC patients undergoing chemoradiation therapy. The outcome of the study demonstrated no survival advantage to the vaccine when evaluating all patients but suggested potential benefit for patients undergoing concurrent chemoradiotherapy but not sequential chemoradiotherapy.[467] Update of the study demonstrated continued benefit in the concurrent chemoradiotherapy arm, but not the sequential chemoradiotherapy arm, and in addition, exploratory biomarker study demonstrated that high sMUC1 and ANA, but not neutrophil/lymphocyte ratio, lymphocyte count, and HLA, correlated with possible benefit for tecemotide.[468] Further studies in NSCLC have been discontinued by manufacturers, but studies in prostate and rectal cancer are being pursued.

Combining DNA vaccines with RT is an area of investigation. INO-3112 is a novel vaccine for HPV-16 and -18, combined with a proprietary immune activator expression IL-12. This compound is being studied in conjunction with concomitant chemoradiotherapy in patients with locally advanced cervical as a randomized phase II study with a safety run-in component. ADXS11-001 is another nucleic acid vaccine based on HPV protein E7, which is being evaluated in conjunction with chemoradiotherapy for HPV-related anal cancer patients.

Dendritic cell vaccine therapy aims to elicit immune response by infusion of DCs loaded with TAAs. Although several DC vaccines have been developed, the only one with FDA approval is Sipuleucel-T (PROVENGE), which is a DC enriched with prostatic acid phosphatase/GM–CSF fusion protein and approved for use in asymptomatic men with metastatic castration-resistant prostate cancer (CRPC) based on OS benefit, despite lack of disease progression benefit.[469] Several phase II trials studying the potential role of combining RT or SBRT with Sipuleucel-T are ongoing. Other DC vaccines showing promise with standard radiotherapy include EGFRvIII-targeted DC vaccine for newly diagnosed glioma patients[470] and algenpantucel-L, an allogeneic pancreatic cancer vaccine, results of which are available for phase II experience with adjuvant radiochemotherapy for pancreatic cancer patients with promising results.[471] Algenpantucel-L has been further studied in phase III trial (IMPRESS trial) with chemoradiotherapy with initial results announced on May 2016 of unfortunately negative unimpressive findings. Another method of DC therapy being explored is use of intratumoral injection of DC with neoadjuvant radiotherapy for soft tissue sarcoma, which in phase I trial demonstrated safety and induction of antitumor immune response.[472]

TABLE 36.6 REPRESENTATIVE FDA-APPROVED IMMUNE AGENTS

Category	Immune Agent	Target or Immune Mechanism	FDA-Approved Indications
Checkpoint inhibitors	Nivolumab (Opdivo)	Anti-PD1	Urothelial carcinoma, head and neck carcinoma, classical Hodgkin lymphoma, renal cell carcinoma, non–small cell lung cancer, melanoma
	Pembrolizumab (KEYTRUDA)	Anti-PD1	Hodgkin lymphoma, non–small cell lung cancer, head and neck cancer, melanoma
	Atezolizumab (TECENTRIQ)	Anti-PD-L1	Urothelial carcinoma, non–small cell lung cancer
	Durvalumab (IMFINZI)	Anti-PD-L1	Urothelial carcinoma
	Avelumab (BAVENCIO)	Anti-PD-L1	Urothelial carcinoma, Merkel cell carcinoma
	Ipilimumab	Anti-CTLA-4	Melanoma
Cytokines	Interleukin-2	T-cell growth factor and central regulator of immune function	Melanoma, renal cell carcinoma
	Interferon-alpha-2b	Activation of immune cells	Melanoma, hairy cell leukemia, non-Hodgkin lymphoma (aggressive follicular type), AIDS-related Kaposi sarcoma
Oncolytic virus	T-VEC (IMLYGIC) (talimogene laherparepvec)	Oncolytic virus therapy that initiates systemic antitumor immune response	Unresectable/recurrent cutaneous, subcutaneous, and nodal melanoma
Vaccine	Sipuleucel-T (PROVENGE)	Stimulates T-cell response against prostatic acid phosphatase	Metastatic prostate cancer (CRPC)

Cytokines

IL-2 was approved for use in adults with metastatic melanoma in 1988 and is also approved for use in metastatic renal cell carcinoma. A small percentage of patients are found to have durable response with this agent.[473] Based on preclinical evidence of efficacy of RT with IL-2, clinical studies have been explored, and some of these have been reported. Phase I study from National Cancer Institute enrolling 14 patients with metastatic melanoma and at least two sites of measurable disease is reported. All patients received local RT of 10 to 20 Gy in 5 Gy/fraction dose given twice daily, followed by high dose IL-2. Although tolerable, this particular radiation regimen did not seem to improve antitumor effects.[474] In a phase I study of SBRT and high-dose IL2, patients with metastatic melanoma (n = 7), or renal cell carcinoma (n = 5), patients received 1 to 3 doses of SBRT (20 Gy/fraction) with IL-2 to commence 3 days after completion of SBRT. Five out of seven patients with melanoma had CR or PR, and 3/5 with renal cell had PR. One of twelve patient achieved CR. All irradiated metastases had response with none recurring at the time of their publication.

Checkpoint Inhibitors

Excitement of efficacy of immune checkpoint inhibitors and successful FDA approval of several agents in the past half-decade, along with significant preclinical studies demonstrating rationale and potential for increasing efficacy of these immune agents with the addition of radiotherapy, have led to development of multiple clinical trials. Currently, there are over 90 phase I or II studies[475] exploring this concept in a number of disease sites, predominantly in the metastatic setting. Only studies with ipilimumab have been completed and reported in publication form to date.

Ipilimumab is the first in class of anti-CTLA-4 strategy, to receive FDA approval in 2011. A case report demonstrated in a melanoma patient the potential efficacy of 9.5 Gy × 3 fractions regimen in combination with ipilimumab (anti CTLA-4 antibody).[476] Retrospective series of patients undergoing SRS for melanoma brain metastases who also received ipilimumab has been reported.[477] Of 42 patients in this series, 15 received SRS during, 19 before, and 12 after ipilimumab. Patients treated with SRS during or before ipilimumab had better OS and less regional recurrence. Interestingly, a temporary increase in tumor size was also noted.[477] Overall tolerability was felt to be reasonable, with 20% of patients having grade 3+ toxicity. Although not designed to evaluate for abscopal effect, one patient demonstrated a potential abscopal effect after SRS. Ipilimumab has been studied in metastatic prostate patients with or without 8 Gy × 1 fraction radiation therapy. In an open-label multicenter phase I/II study, ipilimumab was dose escalated from 3 to 10 mg/kg +/– radiotherapy. In the phase II portion, the 10 mg/kg dose of ipilimumab was given with (n = 34) or without (n = 16) radiotherapy. This regimen was reported to be tolerable and demonstrated efficacy.[478]

Phase III trial of patients with CRPC with bone metastases was conducted, where patients received 8 Gy × 1 fraction of radiation followed by either 10 mg/kg of ipilimumab or placebo.[478] Although clear cut OS could not be made for use of ipilimumab, there was significant signs that drug may be active, particularly in certain subset of patients with more favorable prognosis, and felt that the drug requires further investigation. Most common grade 3+ adverse events were immune related, occurring in 26% in the ipilimumab group versus 3% in the placebo group. These events included diarrhea, fatigue, anemia, and colitis. Four deaths occurred due to toxic effects of ipilimumab.

Summary

Driven by strong preclinical data, a large number of clinical trials aimed at determining safety and efficacy of combining radiation with novel immune agents are actively ongoing. With this enthusiasm will be required a careful and systemic approach to careful and deliberate design of clinical trials aimed at determining the answers to many remaining questions at hand. These include determination of tumor types and tumor sites that would benefit most from radiotherapy, determination of biomarkers for response to combined RT/immune therapy, and careful dose escalation studies to determine the appropriate total dose and dose/fraction for each disease sites being considered for immune-radiotherapy. In addition, as immune therapy agents have a significantly different toxicity profile compared to other traditional systemic agents, which when combined with RT may have less predictable events in terms of severity and timing of onset, one would have to carefully study these toxicities under the auspices of prospective clinical trials. Some of the limited available experiences of potential adverse events related to combined use of immunotherapy and SBRT has been reviewed.[479] This study overall demonstrated that there were very limited data on combined SBRT with ipilimumab, nivolumab, and pembrolizumab. We await results from currently ongoing and to be developed prospective studies to properly define the potential toxicity profiles when using immunotherapy agents in combination with RT/SBRT. The next decade should provide significant clinical data that may help define a novel paradigm for combining radiotherapy with immune therapy to impact not only local but hopefully distal disease outcomes.

CONCLUDING REMARKS

The combination of chemotherapy and radiation therapy has become a common strategic practice in the therapy of locally advanced cancers, with emphasis on the concurrent delivery of both modalities. Improvements in treatment outcome in terms of both local control and patient survival have been achieved with traditional chemotherapeutic agents such as cisplatin and 5-FU. However, there is considerable room for improvement of the combined treatment strategies. Selection of the most effective drug or the optimal treatment approach remains a significant challenge.

Newer chemotherapies, novel molecularly based targeted therapeutic agents, and immunotherapeutic agents are becoming available at an increasing rate. These agents have high potential for increasing the therapeutic effectiveness when used in conjunction with radiation therapy, and therefore, their evaluation—both in the laboratory and in the clinic, in combination with radiation therapy—is essential for improvement of cancer treatment. Preclinical studies not only provide a biologic rationale for the use of a given drug with radiation but also are able to generate information that is critical to the design of effective treatment schedules in clinical settings. Studies of the mechanisms of immune agents/molecular agents/chemotherapy–radiation therapy interaction at the genetic–molecular, cellular, distal (abscopal—in case of immunotherapy), and tumor (or normal tissue) microenvironmental levels are essential for obtaining clear insight into the radiomodulating/immunomodulating potential of these agents, and their ability to increase radiotherapeutic/immunotherapeutic effects.

Biomarkers, molecular therapeutics, immunotherapy advances, advanced imaging technology, and advances in understanding of effective chemotherapy/immunotherapy and radiation treatment integration have led to an era where personalized medicine for cancer therapy is becoming a reality. Many studies have pointed toward the need for careful patient selection when designing clinical trials incorporating molecular targeted agents. Effective biomarker development and integration of such into clinical trial design are essential as it becomes more and more clear that cancer is truly a heterogeneous entity. There are certainly challenges that we can anticipate along the way toward an era of personalized medicine. For example, once numerous biomarkers have been elucidated, how will we decide which biomarkers are most important to test for further clinical trials? Furthermore, how will these studies be financed? In the era of tenuous health care finances, will we have the funds to implement the needed studies and be able to support payment for all the novel drugs coming out of the pipeline?

Finally, despite significant improvements rendered to cancer therapy in the past decades, it is sobering to realize that cancer, particularly when advanced, remains a deadly disease for many. As we embark on this era of abundant and emerging immunotherapeutics, molecular therapeutics, novel chemotherapeutic agents, better-established chemoradiation regimens, and more sophisticated imaging technology and radiation delivery methods, it will be essential to design well-thought-out and effective combined modality-therapy clinical trials to further improve the odds in the battle against cancer.

REFERENCES

1. Herscher LL, et al. Principles of chemoradiation: theoretical and practical considerations. *Oncology (Williston Park)* 1999;13(10 Suppl 5):11–22.
2. Hill B, Bellamy A. *Antitumor drug-radiation interactions*. Boca Raton, FL: CRC Press, 1990.
3. Phillips T. Radiation-chemotherapy interactions. In: Pass HI, Johnson DH, eds. *Lung cancer: principles and practice*. Philadelphia: Lippincott-Raven, 1996.
4. Seiwert TY, Salama JK, Vokes EE. The concurrent chemoradiation paradigm—general principles. *Nat Clin Pract Oncol* 2007;4(2):86–100.
5. Mierzwa ML, et al. Recent advances in combined modality therapy. *Oncologist* 2010;15(4):372–381.
6. Reichert ZR, Wahl DR, Morgan MA. Translation of targeted radiation sensitizers into clinical trials. *Semin Radiat Oncol* 2016;26(4):261–270.
7. Wahl DR, Lawrence TS. Integrating chemoradiation and molecularly targeted therapy. *Adv Drug Deliv Rev* 2017;109:74–83.
8. Weichselbaum RR, Liang H, Deng L, et al. Radiotherapy and immunotherapy: a beneficial liaison? *Nat Rev Clin Oncol* 2017;14(6):365–379.
9. Formenti SC, Demaria S. Combining radiotherapy and cancer immunotherapy: a paradigm shift. *J Natl Cancer Inst* 2013;105(4):256–265.
10. Ishihara D, Pop L, Takeshima T, et al. Rationale and evidence to combine radiation therapy and immunotherapy for cancer treatment. *Cancer Immunol Immunother* 2017;66(3):281–298.
11. Spiotto M, Fu YX, Weichselbaum RR. The intersection of radiotherapy and immunotherapy: mechanisms and clinical implications. *Sci Immunol* 2016;1(3).
12. Steel GG, Peckham MJ. Exploitable mechanisms in combined radiotherapy-chemotherapy: the concept of additivity. *Int J Radiat Oncol Biol Phys* 1979;5(1):85–91.
13. Radford IR. Evidence for a general relationship between the induced level of DNA double-strand breakage and cell-killing after X-irradiation of mammalian cells. *Int J Radiat Biol Relat Stud Phys Chem Med* 1986;49(4):611–620.
14. Kinsella TJ, et al. Enhancement of X ray induced DNA damage by pre-treatment with halogenated pyrimidine analogs. *Int J Radiat Oncol Biol Phys* 1987;13(5):733–739.
15. Elkind MM, Sutton H. X-ray damage and recovery in mammalian cells in culture. *Nature* 1959;184:1293–1295.
16. Iliakis G. Radiation-induced potentially lethal damage: DNA lesions susceptible to fixation. *Int J Radiat Biol Relat Stud Phys Chem Med* 1988;53(4):541–584.
17. Little JB, et al. Repair of potentially lethal radiation damage in vitro and in vivo. *Radiology* 1973;106(3):689–694.
18. Wang Y, Pantelias GE, Iliakis G. Mechanism of radiosensitization by halogenated pyrimidines: the contribution of excess DNA and chromosome damage in BrdU radiosensitization may be minimal in plateau-phase cells. *Int J Radiat Biol* 1994;66(2):133–142.
19. Gregoire V, et al. Radiosensitization of mouse sarcoma cells by fludarabine (F-ara-A) or gemcitabine (dFdC), two nucleoside analogues, is not mediated by an increased induction or a repair inhibition of DNA double-strand breaks as measured by pulsed-field gel electrophoresis. *Int J Radiat Biol* 1998;73(5):511–520.
20. Lawrence TS, et al. Radiosensitization of pancreatic cancer cells by 2′,2′-difluoro-2′-deoxycytidine. *Int J Radiat Oncol Biol Phys* 1996;34(4):867–872.
21. Milas L, et al. Enhancement of tumor radioresponse in vivo by gemcitabine. *Cancer Res* 1999;59(1):107–114.
22. Pauwels B, et al. Combined modality therapy of gemcitabine and radiation. *Oncologist* 2005;10(1):34–51.
23. Terasima T, Tolmach LJ. Variations in several responses of HeLa cells to x-irradiation during the division cycle. *Biophys J* 1963;3:11–33.
24. Tishler RB, et al. Taxol sensitizes human astrocytoma cells to radiation. *Cancer Res* 1992;52(12):3495–3497.
25. Choy H, et al. Investigation of taxol as a potential radiation sensitizer. *Cancer* 1993;71(11):3774–3778.
26. Milas L, et al. Role of reoxygenation in induction of enhancement of tumor radioresponse by paclitaxel. *Cancer Res* 1995;55(16):3564–3568.
27. Milas L, Milas MM, Mason KA. Combination of taxanes with radiation: preclinical studies. *Semin Radiat Oncol* 1999;9(2 Suppl 1):12–26.
28. Brown JM, Giaccia AJ. The unique physiology of solid tumors: opportunities (and problems) for cancer therapy. *Cancer Res* 1998;58(7):1408–1416.
29. Brunner TB, et al. Farnesyltransferase inhibitors as radiation sensitizers. *Int J Radiat Biol* 2003;79(7):569–576.
30. Bush RS, et al. Definitive evidence for hypoxic cells influencing cure in cancer therapy. *Br J Cancer Suppl* 1978;3:302–306.
31. Hockel M, et al. Intratumoral pO₂ predicts survival in advanced cancer of the uterine cervix. *Radiother Oncol* 1993;26(1):45–50.
32. Nordsmark M, Overgaard M, Overgaard J. Pretreatment oxygenation predicts radiation response in advanced squamous cell carcinoma of the head and neck. *Radiother Oncol* 1996;41(1):31–39.
33. Dische S. A review of hypoxic cell radiosensitization. *Int J Radiat Oncol Biol Phys* 1991;20(1):147–152.
34. Henk JM, Smith CW. Radiotherapy and hyperbaric oxygen in head and neck cancer. Interim report of second clinical trial. *Lancet* 1977;2(8029):104–105.
35. Henk JM, Kunkler PB, Smith CW. Radiotherapy and hyperbaric oxygen in head and neck cancer. Final report of first controlled clinical trial. *Lancet* 1977;2(8029):101–103.
36. Vaupel P, Kallinowski F, Okunieff P. Blood flow, oxygen and nutrient supply, and metabolic microenvironment of human tumors: a review. *Cancer Res* 1989;49(23):6449–6465.
37. Tannock IF, Rotin D. Acid pH in tumors and its potential for therapeutic exploitation. *Cancer Res* 1989;49(16):4373–4384.
38. Overgaard J, et al. A randomized double-blind phase III study of nimorazole as a hypoxic radiosensitizer of primary radiotherapy in supraglottic larynx and pharynx carcinoma. Results of the Danish Head and Neck Cancer Study (DAHANCA) Protocol 5–85. *Radiother Oncol* 1998;46(2):135–146.
39. Stephens TJ. Regeneration of tumors after cytotoxic treatment. In: Meyn RE, Withers HR, eds. *Radiation biology in cancer research*. New York: Raven Press, 1980.
40. Milas L, et al. Dynamics of tumor cell clonogen repopulation in a murine sarcoma treated with cyclophosphamide. *Radiother Oncol* 1994;30(3):247–253.
41. Hermens AF, Barendsen GW. The proliferative status and clonogenic capacity of tumour cells in a transplantable rhabdomyosarcoma of the rat before and after irradiation with 800 rad of X-rays. *Cell Tissue Kinet* 1978;11(1):83–100.
42. Withers HR, Taylor JM, Maciejewski B. The hazard of accelerated tumor clonogen repopulation during radiotherapy. *Acta Oncol* 1988;27(2):131–146.
43. Taylor JMWH, Mendenhal WM. Dose-time considerations of head and neck squamous cell carcinomas treated with irradiation. *Radiother Oncol* 1990;17:95–102.
44. Stone HB, Peters LJ, Milas L. Effect of host immune capability on radiocurability and subsequent transplantability of a murine fibrosarcoma. *J Natl Cancer Inst* 1979;63(5):1229–1235.
45. Lee Y, Auh SL, Wang Y, et al. Therapeutic effects of ablative radiation on local tumor require CD8+ T cells: changing strategies for cancer treatment. *Blood* 2009;114(3):589–595.
46. Kuo P, Bratman SV, Shultz DB, et al. Galectin-1 mediates radiation-related lymphopenia and attenuates NSCLC radiation response. *Clin Cancer Res* 2014;20(21):5558–5569.
47. Deng L, Liang H, Burnette B, et al. Irradiation and anti-PD-L1 treatment synergistically promote antitumor immunity in mice. *J Clin Invest* 2014;124(2):687–695.
48. La-Beck NM, Jean GW, Huynh C, et al. Immune checkpoint inhibitors: new insights and current place in cancer therapy. *Pharmacotherapy* 2015;35(10):963–976.
49. Mellman I, Coukos G, Dranoff G. Cancer immunotherapy comes of age. *Nature* 2011;480(7378):480–489.
50. Pardoll DM. The blockade of immune checkpoints in cancer immunotherapy. *Nat Rev Cancer* 2012;12(4):252–264.
51. Begg AC, Stewart FA, Vens C. Strategies to improve radiotherapy with targeted drugs. *Nat Rev Cancer* 2011;11(4):239–253.
52. Bonner JA, et al. Radiotherapy plus cetuximab for squamous-cell carcinoma of the head and neck. *N Engl J Med* 2006;354(6):567–578.
53. Albini A, Sporn MB. The tumour microenvironment as a target for chemoprevention. *Nat Rev Cancer* 2007;7(2):139–147.
54. Mazeron R, et al. Current state of knowledge regarding the use of anti-angiogenic agents with radiation therapy. *Cancer Treat Rev* 2011;37(6):476–486.
55. Clarke MF. Cancer stem cells, perspectives on current status and future directions: AACR Workshop on Cancer Stem Cells. *Cancer Res* 2006;66:9339–9344.
56. Koch U, Krause M, Baumann M. Cancer stem cells at the crossroads of current cancer therapy failures—radiation oncology perspective. *Semin Cancer Biol* 2010;20(2):116–124.
57. McCord AM, et al. CD133+ glioblastoma stem-like cells are radiosensitive with a defective DNA damage response compared with established cell lines. *Clin Cancer Res* 2009;15(16):5145–5153.
58. Hittelman WN, et al. Are cancer stem cells radioresistant? *Future Oncol* 2010;6(10):1563–1576.

59. Sistigu A, Viaud S, Chaput N, et al. Immunomodulatory effects of cyclophosphamide and implementations for vaccine design. *Semin Immunopathol* 2011;33(4):369–383.

60. Menger L, Vacchelli E, Adjemian S, et al. Cardiac glycosides exert anticancer effects by inducing immunogenic cell death. *Sci Transl Med* 2012;4(143):143ra199.

61. Rusthoven KE, Hammerman SF, Kavanagh BD, et al. Is there a role for consolidative stereotactic body radiation therapy following first-line systemic therapy for metastatic lung cancer? A patterns-of-failure analysis. *Acta Oncol* 2009;48(4):578–583.

62. Iyengar P, Kavanagh BD, Wardak Z, et al. Phase II trial of stereotactic body radiation therapy combined with erlotinib for patients with limited but progressive metastatic non-small-cell lung cancer. *J Clin Oncol* 2014;32(34):3824–3830.

63. Morris M, et al. Pelvic radiation with concurrent chemotherapy compared with pelvic and para-aortic radiation for high-risk cervical cancer. *N Engl J Med* 1999;340(15):1137–1143.

64. Munro AJ. An overview of randomised controlled trials of adjuvant chemotherapy in head and neck cancer. *Br J Cancer* 1995;71(1):83–91.

65. Douple EB, Lognan ME. Therapeutic potentiation in a mouse mammary tumour and an intracerebral rat brain tumour by combined treatment with cis-dichlorodiammineplatinum (II) and radiation. *J Clin Hematol Oncol* 1977;30:585–603.

66. Carde P, Laval F. Effect of cis-dichlorodiammine platinum II and X rays on mammalian cell survival. *Int J Radiat Oncol Biol Phys* 1981;7(7):929–933.

67. Begg AC, et al. Radiosensitization in vitro by cis-diammine (1,1-cyclobutanedicarboxylato) platinum(II) (carboplatin, JM8) and ethylenediamine-malonato platinum(II) (JM40). *Radiother Oncol* 1987;9(2):157–165.

68. O'Hara JA, Double EB, Richmond RC. Enhancement of radiation-induced cell kill by platinum complexes (carboplatin and iproplatin) in V79 cells. *Int J Radiat Oncol Biol Phys* 1986;12(8):1419–1422.

69. Amorino GP, Hamilton VM, Choy H. Enhancement of radiation effects by combined docetaxel and carboplatin treatment in vitro. *Radiat Oncol Investig* 1999;7(6):343–352.

70. Mason KA, et al. Effect of docetaxel on the therapeutic ratio of fractionated radiotherapy in vivo. *Clin Cancer Res* 1999;5(12):4191–4198.

71. Omura M, Torigoe S, Kubota N. SN-38, a metabolite of the camptothecin derivative CPT-11, potentiates the cytotoxic effect of radiation in human colon adenocarcinoma cells grown as spheroids. *Radiother Oncol* 1997;43(2):197–201.

72. Chen AY, et al. Mammalian DNA topoisomerase I mediates the enhancement of radiation cytotoxicity by camptothecin derivatives. *Cancer Res* 1997;57(8):1529–1536.

73. Kim JS, et al. Radiation enhancement by the combined use of topoisomerase I inhibitors, RFS-2000 or CPT-11, and topoisomerase II inhibitor etoposide in human lung cancer cells. *Radiother Oncol* 2002;62(1):61–67.

74. Grau C, Overgaard J. Radiosensitizing and cytotoxic properties of mitomycin C in a C3H mouse mammary carcinoma in vivo. *Int J Radiat Oncol Biol Phys* 1991;20(2):265–269.

75. Brown JM. The hypoxic cell: a target for selective cancer therapy—eighteenth Bruce F. Cain Memorial Award Lecture. *Cancer Res* 1998;59:5863–5870.

76. Latz D, et al. Radiosensitizing potential of gemcitabine (2′,2′-difluoro-2′-deoxycytidine) within the cell cycle in vitro. *Int J Radiat Oncol Biol Phys* 1998;41(4):875–882.

77. Mason KA, et al. Maximizing therapeutic gain with gemcitabine and fractionated radiation. *Int J Radiat Oncol Biol Phys* 1999;44(5):1125–1135.

78. Kil WJ, et al. In vitro and in vivo radiosensitization induced by the DNA methylating agent temozolomide. *Clin Cancer Res* 2008;14(3):931–938.

79. Chakravarti A, et al. Temozolomide-mediated radiation enhancement in glioblastoma: a report on underlying mechanisms. *Clin Cancer Res* 2006;12(15):4738–4746.

80. Rosenberg B, et al. Platinum compounds: a new class of potent antitumour agents. *Nature* 1969;222(5191):385–386.

81. Taylor DM, Tew KD, Jones JD. Effects of cis-dichlorodiammine platinum (II) on DNA synthesis in kidney and other tissues of normal and tumour-bearing rats. *Eur J Cancer* 1976;12(4):249–254.

82. Howle JA, Gale GR. Cis-dichlorodiammineplatinum (II). Persistent and selective inhibition of deoxyribonucleic acid synthesis in vivo. *Biochem Pharmacol* 1970;19(10):2757–2762.

83. Corda Y, et al. Transcription by eucaryotic and procaryotic RNA polymerases of DNA modified at a d(GG) or a d(AG) site by the antitumor drug cis-diamminedichloroplatinum(II). *Biochemistry* 1991;30(1):222–230.

84. Richmond RC, Powers EL. Radiation sensitization of bacterial spores by cis-dichlorodiammineplatinum(II). *Radiat Res* 1976;68(2):251–257.

85. Richmond RC, Zimbrick JD, Hykes DL. Radiation-induced DNA damage and lethality in E. coli as modified by the antitumor agent cis-dichlorodiammineplatinum (II). *Radiat Res* 1977;71(2):447–460.

86. Zimbrick JD, Sukrochana A, Richmond RC. Studies on radiosensitization of Escherichia coli cells by cis-platinum complexes. *Int J Radiat Oncol Biol Phys* 1979;5(8):1351–1354.

87. Wodinsky I, et al. Combination radiotherapy and chemotherapy for P388 lymphocytic leukemia in vivo. *Cancer Chemother Rep* 1974;4(1):73–97.

88. Szumiel I, Nias AH. The effect of combined treatment with a platinum complex and ionizing radiation on Chinese hamster ovary cells in vitro. *Br J Cancer* 1976;33(4):450–458.

89. Stratford IJ, Williamson C, Adams GE. Combination studies with misonidazole and a cis-platinum complex: cytotoxicity and radiosensitization in vitro. *Br J Cancer* 1980;41(4):517–522.

90. Dewit L. Combined treatment of radiation and cisdiamminedichloroplatinum (II): a review of experimental and clinical data. *Int J Radiat Oncol Biol Phys* 1987;13(3):403–426.

91. Chaney SG, et al. Recognition and processing of cisplatin- and oxaliplatin-DNA adducts. *Crit Rev Oncol Hematol* 2005;53(1):3–11.

92. Huerta S, Hrom J. Oxaliplatin as a radiosensitizing agent in rectal cancer. *Anticancer Drugs* 2011;22(4):317–323.

93. Stordal B, Pavlakis N, Davey R. A systematic review of platinum and taxane resistance from bench to clinic: an inverse relationship. *Cancer Treat Rev* 2007;33(8):688–703.

94. Rodel C, Hofheinz R, Fokas E. Rectal cancer: neoadjuvant chemoradiotherapy. *Best Pract Res Clin Gastroenterol* 2016;30(4):629–639.

95. Conroy T, Galais MP, Raoul JL, et al. Definitive chemoradiotherapy with FOLFOX versus fluorouracil and cisplatin in patients with oesophageal cancer (PRODIGE5/ACCORD17): final results of a randomised, phase 2/3 trial. *Lancet Oncol* 2014;15(3):305–314.

96. Messager M, Mirabel X, Tresch E, et al. Preoperative chemoradiation with paclitaxel-carboplatin or with fluorouracil-oxaliplatin-folinic acid (FOLFOX) for resectable esophageal and junctional cancer: the PROTECT-1402, randomized phase 2 trial. *BMC Cancer* 2016;16:318.

97. Rowinsky EK. The development and clinical utility of the taxane class of antimicrotubule chemotherapy agents. *Annu Rev Med* 1997;48:353–374.

98. Rao S, et al. 3′-(p-azidobenzamido)taxol photolabels the N-terminal 31 amino acids of beta-tubulin. *J Biol Chem* 1994;269(5):3132–3134.

99. Manfredi JJ, Horwitz SB. Taxol: an antimitotic agent with a new mechanism of action. *Pharmacol Ther* 1984;25(1):83–125.

100. Diaz JF, Andreu JM. Assembly of purified GDP-tubulin into microtubules induced by Taxol and Taxotere: reversibility, ligand stoichiometry, and competition. *Biochemistry* 1993;32(11):2747–2755.

101. Ringel I, Horwitz SB. Studies with RP 56976 (taxotere): a semisynthetic analogue of Taxol. *J Natl Cancer Inst* 1991;83(4):288–291.

102. Hall EJ. *Radiobiology for the radiologist.* 4th ed. Philadelphia: Lippincott, 1994.

103. Creane M, et al. Radiobiological effects of docetaxel (Taxotere): a potential radiation sensitizer. *Int J Radiat Biol* 1999;75(6):731–737.

104. Morris PG, Fornier MN. Microtubule active agents: beyond the taxane frontier. *Clin Cancer Res* 2008;14(22):7167–7172.

105. Villanueva C, et al. Cabazitaxel: a novel microtubule inhibitor. *Drugs* 2011;71(10):1251–1258.

106. Nicoletti MI, et al. IDN5109, a taxane with oral bioavailability and potent antitumor activity. *Cancer Res* 2000;60(4):842–846.

107. Bagshaw MA. Possible role of potentiators in radiation therapy. *Am J Roentgenol Radium Ther Nucl Med* 1961;85:822–833.

108. Buchholz DJ, et al. 5-Fluorouracil-radiation interactions in human colon adenocarcinoma cells. *Int J Radiat Oncol Biol Phys* 1995;32(4):1053–1058.

109. McGinn CJ, Kinsella TJ. The experimental and clinical rationale for the use of S-phase-specific radiosensitizers to overcome tumor cell repopulation. *Semin Oncol* 1992;19(4 Suppl 11):21–28.

110. Liauw SL, Minsky BD. The use of capecitabine in the combined-modality therapy for rectal cancer. *Clin Colorectal Cancer* 2008;7(2):99–104.

111. Hofheinz RD, Wenz F, Post S, et al. Chemoradiotherapy with capecitabine versus fluorouracil for locally advanced rectal cancer: a randomised, multicentre, non-inferiority, phase 3 trial. *Lancet Oncol* 2012;13(6):579–588.

112. Plunkett W, et al. Gemcitabine: metabolism, mechanisms of action, and self-potentiation. *Semin Oncol* 1995;22(4 Suppl 11):3–10.

113. Gregoire V, et al. Chemo-radiotherapy: radiosensitizing nucleoside analogues (review). *Oncol Rep* 1999;6(5):949–957.

114. Milas L, et al. Enhancement of tumor response to gamma-radiation by an inhibitor of cyclooxygenase-2 enzyme. *J Natl Cancer Inst* 1999;91(17):1501–1504.

115. Blackstock AW, et al. Phase Ia/Ib chemo-radiation trial of gemcitabine and dose-escalated thoracic radiation in patients with stage III A/B non-small cell lung cancer. *J Thorac Oncol* 2006;1(5):434–440.

116. Choy H, et al. RTOG 0017: a phase I trial of concurrent gemcitabine/carboplatin or gemcitabine/paclitaxel and radiation therapy ("ping-pong trial") followed by adjuvant chemotherapy for patients with favorable prognosis inoperable stage IIIA/B non-small cell lung cancer. *J Thorac Oncol* 2009;4(1):80–86.

117. Divers SG, et al. Phase I/IIa study of cisplatin and gemcitabine as induction chemotherapy followed by concurrent chemoradiotherapy with gemcitabine and paclitaxel for locally advanced non-small-cell lung cancer. *J Clin Oncol* 2005;23(27):6664–6673.

118. Gagel B, et al. Gemcitabine concurrent with thoracic radiotherapy after induction chemotherapy with gemcitabine/vinorelbine in locally advanced non-small cell lung cancer: a phase I study. *Strahlenther Onkol* 2006;182(5):263–269.

119. Galetta D, et al. Multimodality treatment of unresectable stage III non-small cell lung cancer: interim analysis of a phase II trial with preoperative gemcitabine and concurrent radiotherapy. *J Thorac Cardiovasc Surg* 2006;131(2):314–321.

120. van Putten JW, et al. A phase I study of gemcitabine with concurrent radiotherapy in stage III, locally advanced non-small cell lung cancer. *Clin Cancer Res* 2003;9(7):2472–2477.

121. Zinner RG, et al. Dose escalation of gemcitabine is possible with concurrent chest three-dimensional rather than two-dimensional radiotherapy: a phase I trial in patients with stage III non-small-cell lung cancer. *Int J Radiat Oncol Biol Phys* 2009;73(1):119–127.

122. Norman P. Pemetrexed disodium (Eli Lilly). *Curr Opin Investig Drugs* 2001;2(11):1611–1622.

123. Bischof M, et al. Interaction of pemetrexed disodium (ALIMTA, multitargeted antifolate) and irradiation in vitro. *Int J Radiat Oncol Biol Phys* 2002;52(5):1381–1388.

124. Bischof M, et al. Radiosensitization by pemetrexed of human colon carcinoma cells in different cell cycle phases. *Int J Radiat Oncol Biol Phys* 2003;57(1):289–292.

125. Yoshida D, et al. Interaction of radiation and pemetrexed on a human malignant mesothelioma cell line in vitro. *Anticancer Res* 2011;31(9):2847–2851.
126. Senan S, Brade A, Wang LH, et al. PROCLAIM: randomized phase III trial of pemetrexed-cisplatin or etoposide-cisplatin plus thoracic radiation therapy followed by consolidation chemotherapy in locally advanced nonsquamous non-small-cell lung cancer. *J Clin Oncol* 2016;34(9):953–962.
127. Moertel CG, et al. Phase II study of camptothecin (NSC-100880) in the treatment of advanced gastrointestinal cancer. *Cancer Chemother Rep* 1972;56(1):95–101.
128. Muggia FM, et al. Phase I clinical trial of weekly and daily treatment with camptothecin (NSC-100880): correlation with preclinical studies. *Cancer Chemother Rep* 1972;56(4):515–521.
129. Andoh T, et al. Characterization of a mammalian mutant with a camptothecin-resistant DNA topoisomerase I. *Proc Natl Acad Sci U S A* 1987;84(16):5565–5569.
130. Hsiang YH, et al. Camptothecin induces protein-linked DNA breaks via mammalian DNA topoisomerase I. *J Biol Chem* 1985;260(27):14873–14878.
131. Hsiang YH, Liu LF. Identification of mammalian DNA topoisomerase I as an intracellular target of the anticancer drug camptothecin. *Cancer Res* 1988;48(7):1722–1726.
132. Amorino GP, et al. Preclinical evaluation of the orally active camptothecin analog, RFS-2000 (9-nitro-20(S)-camptothecin) as a radiation enhancer. *Int J Radiat Oncol Biol Phys* 2000;47(2):503–509.
133. Kirichenko AV, Rich TA. Radiation enhancement by 9-aminocamptothecin: the effect of fractionation and timing of administration. *Int J Radiat Oncol Biol Phys* 1999;44(3):659–664.
134. Takeda K, et al. Phase I/II study of weekly irinotecan and concurrent radiation therapy for locally advanced non-small cell lung cancer. *Br J Cancer* 1999;79(9–10):1462–1467.
135. Grabenbauer GG, et al. Topotecan as a 21-day continuous infusion with accelerated 3D-conformal radiation therapy for patients with glioblastoma. *Front Radiat Ther Oncol* 1999;33:364–368.
136. Fisher BJ, et al. Phase I study of topotecan plus cranial radiation for glioblastoma multiforme: results of Radiation Therapy Oncology Group Trial 9507. *J Clin Oncol* 2001;19(4):1111–1117.
137. Chakravarthy A, Choy H. A phase I trial of outpatient weekly irinotecan/carboplatin and concurrent radiation for stage III unresectable non small-cell lung cancer: a Vanderbilt-Ingram Cancer Center Affiliate Network Trial. *Clin Lung Cancer* 2000;1(4):310–311.
138. Friedman HS, Kerby T, Calvert H. Temozolomide and treatment of malignant glioma. *Clin Cancer Res* 2000;6(7):2585–2597.
139. Wedge SR, et al. In vitro evaluation of temozolomide combined with X-irradiation. *Anticancer Drugs* 1997;8(1):92–97.
140. Stupp R, et al. Radiotherapy plus concomitant and adjuvant temozolomide for glioblastoma. *N Engl J Med* 2005;352(10):987–996.
141. Hegi ME, et al. MGMT gene silencing and benefit from temozolomide in glioblastoma. *N Engl J Med* 2005;352(10):997–1003.
142. Stupp R, et al. Effects of radiotherapy with concomitant and adjuvant temozolomide versus radiotherapy alone on survival in glioblastoma in a randomised phase III study: 5-year analysis of the EORTC-NCIC trial. *Lancet Oncol* 2009;10(5):459–466.
143. Sartorelli AC, et al. Mitomycin C: a prototype bioreductive agent. *Oncol Res* 1994;6(10–11):501–508.
144. Bristow RG. Molecular and cellular basis of radiotherapy. In: Tannock IF, Hill R, eds. *The basic science of oncology*. Montreal: McGraw-Hill, 1998.
145. Dobrowsky W, Dobrowsky E, Rauth AM. Mode of interaction of 5-fluorouracil, radiation, and mitomycin C: in vitro studies. *Int J Radiat Oncol Biol Phys* 1992;22(5):875–880.
146. Jiang Y, et al. Anal carcinoma therapy: can we improve on 5-fluorouracil/mitomycin/radiotherapy? *J Natl Compr Canc Netw* 2010;8(1):135–144.
147. Lloyd RV, et al. Microsomal reduction of 3-amino-1,2,4-benzotriazine 1,4-dioxide to a free radical. *Mol Pharmacol* 1991;40(3):440–445.
148. Cohen EE, et al. Phase I trial of tirapazamine, cisplatin, and concurrent accelerated boost reirradiation in patients with recurrent head and neck cancer. *Int J Radiat Oncol Biol Phys* 2007;67(3):678–684.
149. Del Rowe J, et al. Single-arm, open-label phase II study of intravenously administered tirapazamine and radiation therapy for glioblastoma multiforme. *J Clin Oncol* 2000;18(6):1254–1259.
150. Le QT, et al. Phase I study of tirapazamine plus cisplatin/etoposide and concurrent thoracic radiotherapy in limited-stage small cell lung cancer (S0004): a Southwest Oncology Group study. *Clin Cancer Res* 2004;10(16):5418–5424.
151. Le QT, et al. Phase II study of tirapazamine, cisplatin, and etoposide and concurrent thoracic radiotherapy for limited-stage small-cell lung cancer: SWOG 0222. *J Clin Oncol* 2009;27(18):3014–3019.
152. Le QT, et al. Mature results from a randomized phase II trial of cisplatin plus 5-fluorouracil and radiotherapy with or without tirapazamine in patients with resectable stage IV head and neck squamous cell carcinomas. *Cancer* 2006;106(9):1940–1949.
153. Lee DJ, et al. Concurrent tirapazamine and radiotherapy for advanced head and neck carcinomas: a Phase II study. *Int J Radiat Oncol Biol Phys* 1998;42(4):811–815.
154. Rischin D, et al. Prognostic significance of [18F]-misonidazole positron emission tomography-detected tumor hypoxia in patients with advanced head and neck cancer randomly assigned to chemoradiation with or without tirapazamine: a substudy of Trans-Tasman Radiation Oncology Group Study 98.02. *J Clin Oncol* 2006;24(13):2098–2104.
155. Rischin D, et al. Phase 1 study of tirapazamine in combination with radiation and weekly cisplatin in patients with locally advanced cervical cancer. *Int J Gynecol Cancer* 2010;20(5):827–833.
156. Rischin D, et al. Tirapazamine, cisplatin, and radiation versus fluorouracil, cisplatin, and radiation in patients with locally advanced head and neck cancer: a randomized phase II trial of the Trans-Tasman Radiation Oncology Group (TROG 98.02). *J Clin Oncol* 2005;23(1):79–87.
157. Rischin D, et al. Phase I trial of concurrent tirapazamine, cisplatin, and radiotherapy in patients with advanced head and neck cancer. *J Clin Oncol* 2001;19(2):535–542.
158. Rischin D, et al. Tirapazamine, cisplatin, and radiation versus cisplatin and radiation for advanced squamous cell carcinoma of the head and neck (TROG 02.02, HeadSTART): a phase III trial of the Trans-Tasman Radiation Oncology Group. *J Clin Oncol* 2010;28(18):2989–2995.
159. Shulman LN, et al. Phase I trial of the hypoxic cell cytotoxin tirapazamine with concurrent radiation therapy in the treatment of refractory solid tumors. *Int J Radiat Oncol Biol Phys* 1999;44(2):349–353.
160. Smith HO, et al. Tirapazamine plus cisplatin in advanced or recurrent carcinoma of the uterine cervix: a Southwest Oncology Group study. *Int J Gynecol Cancer* 2006;16(1):298–305.
161. DiSilvestro PA, Ali S, Craighead PS, et al. Phase III randomized trial of weekly cisplatin and irradiation versus cisplatin and tirapazamine and irradiation in stages IB2, IIA, IIB, IIIB, and IVA cervical carcinoma limited to the pelvis: a Gynecologic Oncology Group study. *J Clin Oncol* 2014;32(5):458–464.
162. Hassan Metwally MA, Ali R, Kuddu M, et al. IAEA-HypoX. A randomized multicenter study of the hypoxic radiosensitizer nimorazole concomitant with accelerated radiotherapy in head and neck squamous cell carcinoma. *Radiother Oncol* 2015;116(1):15–20.
163. Thomson D, Yang H, Baines H, et al. NIMRAD—a phase III trial to investigate the use of nimorazole hypoxia modification with intensity-modulated radiotherapy in head and neck cancer. *Clin Oncol (R Coll Radiol)* 2014;26(6):344–347.
164. Desai N, et al. Increased antitumor activity, intratumor paclitaxel concentrations, and endothelial cell transport of Cremophor-free, albumin-bound paclitaxel, ABI-007, compared with Cremophor-based paclitaxel. *Clin Cancer Res* 2006;12(4):1317–1324.
165. Gradishar WJ, et al. Phase III trial of nanoparticle albumin-bound paclitaxel compared with polyethylated castor oil-based paclitaxel in women with breast cancer. *J Clin Oncol* 2005;23(31):7794–7803.
166. Green MR, et al. Abraxane, a novel Cremophor-free, albumin-bound particle form of paclitaxel for the treatment of advanced non-small-cell lung cancer. *Ann Oncol* 2006;17(8):1263–1268.
167. Reynolds C, et al. Phase II trial of nanoparticle albumin-bound paclitaxel, carboplatin, and bevacizumab in first-line patients with advanced nonsquamous non-small cell lung cancer. *J Thorac Oncol* 2009;4(12):1537–1543.
168. Rizvi NA, et al. Phase I/II trial of weekly intravenous 130-nm albumin-bound paclitaxel as initial chemotherapy in patients with stage IV non-small-cell lung cancer. *J Clin Oncol* 2008;26(4):639–643.
169. Socinski MA, et al. A dose finding study of weekly and every-3-week nab-paclitaxel followed by carboplatin as first-line therapy in patients with advanced non-small cell lung cancer. *J Thorac Oncol* 2010;5(6):852–861.
170. Stinchcombe TE, et al. Phase I trial of nanoparticle albumin-bound paclitaxel in combination with gemcitabine in patients with thoracic malignancies. *J Thorac Oncol* 2008;3(5):521–526.
171. Coleman RL, et al. A phase II evaluation of nanoparticle, albumin-bound (nab) paclitaxel in the treatment of recurrent or persistent platinum-resistant ovarian, fallopian tube, or primary peritoneal cancer: a Gynecologic Oncology Group study. *Gynecol Oncol* 2011;122(1):111–115.
172. Hersh EM, et al. A phase 2 clinical trial of nab-paclitaxel in previously treated and chemotherapy-naive patients with metastatic melanoma. *Cancer* 2010;116(1):155–163.
173. Kottschade LA, et al. A phase II trial of nab-paclitaxel (ABI-007) and carboplatin in patients with unresectable stage IV melanoma: a North Central Cancer Treatment Group Study, N057E(1). *Cancer* 2011;117(8):1704–1710.
174. McKiernan JM, et al. A phase I trial of intravesical nanoparticle albumin-bound paclitaxel in the treatment of bacillus Calmette-Guerin refractory nonmuscle invasive bladder cancer. *J Urol* 2011;186(2):448–451.
175. Shepard DR, et al. Phase II trial of neoadjuvant nab-paclitaxel in high risk patients with prostate cancer undergoing radical prostatectomy. *J Urol* 2009;181(4):1672–1677; discussion 1677.
176. Teneriello MG, et al. Phase II evaluation of nanoparticle albumin-bound paclitaxel in platinum-sensitive patients with recurrent ovarian, peritoneal, or fallopian tube cancer. *J Clin Oncol* 2009;27(9):1426–1431.
177. Wiedenmann N, et al. 130-nm albumin-bound paclitaxel enhances tumor radiocurability and therapeutic gain. *Clin Cancer Res* 2007;13(6):1868–1874.
178. Chun SG, Hughes R, Sumer BD, et al. A phase I/II study of Nab-paclitaxel, cisplatin, and cetuximab with concurrent radiation therapy for locally advanced squamous cell cancer of the head and neck. *Cancer Invest* 2017;35(1):23–31.
179. Kaira K, Tomizawa Y, Imai H, et al. Phase I study of nab-paclitaxel plus carboplatin and concurrent thoracic radiotherapy in patients with locally advanced non-small cell lung cancer. *Cancer Chemother Pharmacol* 2017;79(1):165–171.
180. Maeda H, Seymour LW, Miyamoto Y. Conjugates of anticancer agents and polymers: advantages of macromolecular therapeutics in vivo. *Bioconjug Chem* 1992;3(5):351–362.
181. Li C, et al. Tumor irradiation enhances the tumor-specific distribution of poly(L-glutamic acid)-conjugated paclitaxel and its antitumor efficacy. *Clin Cancer Res* 2000;6(7):2829–2834.
182. Li C, et al. Potentiation of ovarian OCa-1 tumor radioresponse by poly(L-glutamic acid)-paclitaxel conjugate. *Int J Radiat Oncol Biol Phys* 2000;48(4):1119–1126.
183. Tishler RB. Polymer-conjugated paclitaxel as a radiosensitizing agent—a big step forward for combined modality therapy? *Int J Radiat Oncol Biol Phys* 2003;55(3):563–564.
184. Dipetrillo T, et al. Neoadjuvant paclitaxel poliglumex, cisplatin, and radiation for esophageal cancer: a phase 2 trial. *Am J Clin Oncol* 2012;35(1):64–67.

185. Dipetrillo T, et al. Paclitaxel poliglumex (PPX-Xyotax) and concurrent radiation for esophageal and gastric cancer: a phase I study. *Am J Clin Oncol* 2006;29(4):376–379.

186. Elinzano H, Glantz M, Mrugala M, et al. PPX and concurrent radiation for newly diagnosed glioblastoma without MGMT methylation: a randomized phase II study: BrUOG 244. *Am J Clin Oncol* 2015.

187. Dittmann K, et al. Selective radioprotection of normal tissues by Bowman-birk proteinase inhibitor (BBI) in mice. *Strahlenther Onkol* 2005;181(3):191–196.

188. Hahn SM, et al. Potential use of nitroxides in radiation oncology. *Cancer Res* 1994;54(7 Suppl):2006s–2010s.

189. Liu B, et al. Live attenuated Salmonella carrying platelet factor 4 cDNAs as radioprotectors. *Radiat Res* 2006;166(2):352–359.

190. Milas L, Hanson WR. Eicosanoids and radiation. *Eur J Cancer* 1995;31A(10):1580–1585.

191. Yuhas JM, Storer JB. Differential chemoprotection of normal and malignant tissues. *J Natl Cancer Inst* 1969;42(2):331–335.

192. Arora R, et al. Radioprotective and antioxidant properties of low-altitude Podophyllum hexandrum (LAPH). *J Environ Pathol Toxicol Oncol* 2005;24(4):299–314.

193. Arora R, et al. Evaluation of radioprotective activities Rhodiola imbricata Edgew—a high altitude plant. *Mol Cell Biochem* 2005;273(1–2):209–223.

194. Arora R, et al. Radioprotection by plant products: present status and future prospects. *Phytother Res* 2005;19(1):1–22.

195. Khodarev NN, et al. Interaction of amifostine and ionizing radiation on transcriptional patterns of apoptotic genes expressed in human microvascular endothelial cells (HMEC). *Int J Radiat Oncol Biol Phys* 2004;60(2):553–563.

196. Brizel D, Wasserman TH, Henke M, et al. Final report of a phase III randomized trial of amifostine as a radioprotectant in head and neck cancer. *Int J Radiat Oncol Biol Phys* 1999;45(Suppl 3):147–148.

197. Brizel DM, et al. Phase III randomized trial of amifostine as a radioprotector in head and neck cancer. *J Clin Oncol* 2000;18(19):3339–3345.

198. Antonadou D, et al. Prophylactic use of amifostine to prevent radiochemotherapy-induced mucositis and xerostomia in head-and-neck cancer. *Int J Radiat Oncol Biol Phys* 2002;52(3):739–747.

199. Komaki R, et al. Randomized phase III study of chemoradiation with or without amifostine for patients with favorable performance status inoperable stage II-III non-small cell lung cancer: preliminary results. *Semin Radiat Oncol* 2002;12(1 Suppl 1):46–49.

200. Komaki R, et al. Effects of amifostine on acute toxicity from concurrent chemotherapy and radiotherapy for inoperable non-small-cell lung cancer: report of a randomized comparative trial. *Int J Radiat Oncol Biol Phys* 2004;58(5):1369–1377.

201. Fu KK, et al. A Radiation Therapy Oncology Group (RTOG) phase III randomized study to compare hyperfractionation and two variants of accelerated fractionation to standard fractionation radiotherapy for head and neck squamous cell carcinomas: first report of RTOG 9003. *Int J Radiat Oncol Biol Phys* 2000;48(1):7–16.

202. Ang K, Zhang Q, Wheeler RH, et al. A phase III trial (RTOG 0129) of two radiation-cisplatin regimens for head and neck carcinomas (HNC): impact of radiation and cisplatin intensity on outcome. *J Clin Oncol* 2010;28(15 Suppl): [abstr 5507].

203. Belani CP, et al. Phase III study of the Eastern Cooperative Oncology Group (ECOG 2597): induction chemotherapy followed by either standard thoracic radiotherapy or hyperfractionated accelerated radiotherapy for patients with unresectable stage IIIA and B non-small-cell lung cancer. *J Clin Oncol* 2005;23(16):3760–3767.

204. Saunders M, et al. Continuous hyperfractionated accelerated radiotherapy (CHART) versus conventional radiotherapy in non-small-cell lung cancer: a randomised multicentre trial. CHART Steering Committee. *Lancet* 1997;350(9072):161–165.

205. Brizel DM, et al. Hyperfractionated irradiation with or without concurrent chemotherapy for locally advanced head and neck cancer. *N Engl J Med* 1998;338(25):1798–1804.

206. Coppin CM, Gospodarowicz MK, James K, et al. Improved local control of invasive bladder cancer by concurrent cisplatin and preoperative or definitive radiation. The National Cancer Institute of Canada Clinical Trials Group. *J Clin Oncol* 1996;14(11):2901–2907.

207. Mansfield CM, Kimler BF, Henderson SD, et al. Development of normal tissue damage in the rat subsequent to thoracic irradiation and prior treatment with cancer chemotherapeutic agents. *Am J Clin Oncol* 1984;7(5):425–430.

208. Samuels ML, Johnson DE, Holoye PY, et al. Large-dose bleomycin therapy and pulmonary toxicity. A possible role of prior radiotherapy. *JAMA* 1976;235(11):1117–1120.

209. Tefft M, Lattin PB, Jereb B, et al. Acute and late effects on normal tissues following combined chemo- and radiotherapy for childhood rhabdomyosarcoma and Ewing's sarcoma. *Cancer* 1976;37(2 Suppl):1201–1217.

210. McVeagh P, Ekert H. Hepatotoxicity of chemotherapy following nephrectomy and radiation therapy for right-sided Wilms tumor. *J Pediatr* 1975;87(4):627–628.

211. Billingham ME, Bristow MR, Glatstein E, et al. Adriamycin cardiotoxicity: endomyocardial biopsy evidence of enhancement by irradiation. *Am J Surg Pathol* 1977;1(1):17–23.

212. Fajardo LF, Eltringham JR, Steward JR. Combined cardiotoxicity of adriamycin and x-radiation. *Lab Invest* 1976;34(1):86–96.

213. LaMonte CS, Yeh SD, Straus DJ. Long-term follow-up of cardiac function in patients with Hodgkin's disease treated with mediastinal irradiation and combination chemotherapy including doxorubicin. *Cancer Treat Rep* 1986;70(4):439–444.

214. Merrill J, Greco FA, Zimbler H, et al. Adriamycin and radiation: synergistic cardiotoxicity. *Ann Intern Med* 1975;82(1):122–123.

215. Allen JC, Thaler HT, Deck MD, et al. Leukoencephalopathy following high-dose intravenous methotrexate chemotherapy: quantitative assessment of white matter attenuation using computed tomography. *Neuroradiology* 1978;16:44–47.

216. Keime-Guibert F, Napolitano M, Delattre JY. Neurological complications of radiotherapy and chemotherapy. *J Neurol* 1998;245(11):695–708.

217. Thompson CB, Sanders JE, Flournoy N, et al. The risks of central nervous system relapse and leukoencephalopathy in patients receiving marrow transplants for acute leukemia. *Blood* 1986;67(1):195–199.

218. Hitchcock YJ, Tward JD, Szabo A, et al. Relative contributions of radiation and cisplatin-based chemotherapy to sensorineural hearing loss in head-and-neck cancer patients. *Int J Radiat Oncol Biol Phys* 2009;73(3):779–788.

219. Chan SH, Ng WT, Kam KL, et al. Sensorineural hearing loss after treatment of nasopharyngeal carcinoma: a longitudinal analysis. *Int J Radiat Oncol Biol Phys* 2009;73(5):1335–1342.

220. Chen WC, Jackson A, Budnick AS, et al. Sensorineural hearing loss in combined modality treatment of nasopharyngeal carcinoma. *Cancer* 2006;106(4):820–829.

221. Kwong DL, Wei WI, Sham JS, et al. Sensorineural hearing loss in patients treated for nasopharyngeal carcinoma: a prospective study of the effect of radiation and cisplatin treatment. *Int J Radiat Oncol Biol Phys* 1996;36(2):281–289.

222. Mason KA, Komaki R, Cox JD, et al. Biology-based combined-modality radiotherapy: workshop report. *Int J Radiat Oncol Biol Phys* 2001;2001(50):1079–1089.

223. Belani CP, et al. Combined chemoradiotherapy regimens of paclitaxel and carboplatin for locally advanced non-small-cell lung cancer: a randomized phase II locally advanced multi-modality protocol. *J Clin Oncol* 2005;23(25):5883–5891.

224. Huguenin P, et al. Concomitant cisplatin significantly improves locoregional control in advanced head and neck cancers treated with hyperfractionated radiotherapy. *J Clin Oncol* 2004;22(23):4665–4673.

225. Liang K, et al. The epidermal growth factor receptor mediates radioresistance. *Int J Radiat Oncol Biol Phys* 2003;57(1):246–254.

226. Mendelsohn J, Fan Z. Epidermal growth factor receptor family and chemosensitization. *J Natl Cancer Inst* 1997;89(5):341–343.

227. Schmidt-Ullrich RK, et al. Signal transduction and cellular radiation responses. *Radiat Res* 2000;153(3):245–257.

228. Dickstein BM, Wosikowski K, Bates SE. Increased resistance to cytotoxic agents in ZR75B human breast cancer cells transfected with epidermal growth factor receptor. *Mol Cell Endocrinol* 1995;110(1–2):205–211.

229. Harari PM, Allen GW, Bonner JA. Biology of interactions: antiepidermal growth factor receptor agents. *J Clin Oncol* 2007;25(26):4057–4065.

230. Huang SM, Bock JM, Harari PM. Epidermal growth factor receptor blockade with C225 modulates proliferation, apoptosis, and radiosensitivity in squamous cell carcinomas of the head and neck. *Cancer Res* 1999;59(8):1935–1940.

231. Huang SM, Harari PM. Modulation of radiation response after epidermal growth factor receptor blockade in squamous cell carcinomas: inhibition of damage repair, cell cycle kinetics, and tumor angiogenesis. *Clin Cancer Res* 2000;6(6):2166–2174.

232. Milas L, et al. In vivo enhancement of tumor radioresponse by C225 antiepidermal growth factor receptor antibody. *Clin Cancer Res* 2000;6(2):701–708.

233. Lammering G, et al. EGFRvIII-mediated radioresistance through a strong cytoprotective response. *Oncogene* 2003;22(36):5545–5553.

234. Baselga J, et al. Phase I studies of anti-epidermal growth factor receptor chimeric antibody C225 alone and in combination with cisplatin. *J Clin Oncol* 2000;18(4):904–914.

235. Harari PM, Huang S. Radiation combined with EGFR signal inhibitors: head and neck cancer focus. *Semin Radiat Oncol* 2006;16(1):38–44.

236. Robert F, et al. Phase I study of anti–epidermal growth factor receptor antibody cetuximab in combination with radiation therapy in patients with advanced head and neck cancer. *J Clin Oncol* 2001;19(13):3234–3243.

237. Tuccillo C, et al. Antitumor activity of ZD6474, a vascular endothelial growth factor-2 and epidermal growth factor receptor small molecule tyrosine kinase inhibitor, in combination with SC-236, a cyclooxygenase-2 inhibitor. *Clin Cancer Res* 2005;11(3):1268–1276.

238. Kelly K, et al. Phase III trial of maintenance gefitinib or placebo after concurrent chemoradiotherapy and docetaxel consolidation in inoperable stage III non-small-cell lung cancer: SWOG S0023. *J Clin Oncol* 2008;26(15): 2450–2456.

239. Ang KK, Zhang Q, Rosenthal DI, et al. Randomized phase III trial of concurrent accelerated radiation plus cisplatin with or without cetuximab for stage III to IV head and neck carcinoma: RTOG 0522. *J Clin Oncol* 2014;32(27): 2940–2950.

240. Crosby T, Hurt CN, Falk S, et al. Chemoradiotherapy with or without cetuximab in patients with oesophageal cancer (SCOPE1): a multicentre, phase 2/3 randomised trial. *Lancet Oncol* 2013;14(7):627–637.

241. Ilson D, Moughan J, Sunthralingam M, et al. RTOG 0436: a phase III trial evaluating the addition of cetuximab to paclitaxel, cisplatin, and radiation for patients with esophageal cancer treated without surgery. *J Clin Oncol* 2014;32(5s Suppl): abstract 4007.

242. Blumenschein GR Jr, et al. Phase II study of cetuximab in combination with chemoradiation in patients with stage IIIA/B non-small-cell lung cancer: RTOG 0324. *J Clin Oncol* 2011;29(17):2312–2318.

243. Bradley JD, Paulus R, Komaki R, et al. Standard-dose versus high-dose conformal radiotherapy with concurrent and consolidation carboplatin plus paclitaxel with or without cetuximab for patients with stage IIIA or IIIB non-small-cell lung cancer (RTOG 0617): a randomised, two-by-two factorial phase 3 study. *Lancet Oncol* 2015;16(2):187–199.

244. Rogers JE. Patient considerations in metastatic colorectal cancer—role of panitumumab. *Onco Targets Ther* 2017;10:2033–2044.

245. Giralt J, Trigo J, Nuyts S, et al. Panitumumab plus radiotherapy versus chemoradiotherapy in patients with unresected, locally advanced squamous-cell carcinoma of the head and neck (CONCERT-2): a randomised, controlled, open-label phase 2 trial. *Lancet Oncol* 2015;16(2):221–232.

246. Kordes S, van Berge Henegouwen MI, Hulshof MC, et al. Preoperative chemoradiation therapy in combination with panitumumab for patients with resectable esophageal cancer: the PACT study. *Int J Radiat Oncol Biol Phys* 2014;90(1):190–196.

247. Lockhart AC, Reed CE, Decker PA, et al. Phase II study of neoadjuvant therapy with docetaxel, cisplatin, panitumumab, and radiation therapy followed by surgery in patients with locally advanced adenocarcinoma of the distal esophagus (ACOSOG Z4051). *Ann Oncol* 2014;25(5):1039–1044.

248. Mardjuadi FI, Carrasco J, Coche JC, et al. Panitumumab as a radiosensitizing agent in KRAS wild-type locally advanced rectal cancer. *Target Oncol* 2015;10(3):375–383.

249. Mesia R, Henke M, Fortin A, et al. Chemoradiotherapy with or without panitumumab in patients with unresected, locally advanced squamous-cell carcinoma of the head and neck (CONCERT-1): a randomised, controlled, open-label phase 2 trial. *Lancet Oncol* 2015;16(2):208–220.

250. van Zweeden AA, van der Vliet HJ, Wilmink JW, et al. Phase I clinical trial to determine the feasibility and maximum tolerated dose of panitumumab to standard gemcitabine-based chemoradiation in locally advanced pancreatic cancer. *Clin Cancer Res* 2015;21(20):4569–4575.

251. Helbling D, Bodoky G, Gautschi O, et al. Neoadjuvant chemoradiotherapy with or without panitumumab in patients with wild-type KRAS, locally advanced rectal cancer (LARC): a randomized, multicenter, phase II trial SAKK 41/07. *Ann Oncol* 2013;24(3):718–725.

252. Pinto C, Di Fabio F, Maiello E, et al. Phase II study of panitumumab, oxaliplatin, 5-fluorouracil, and concurrent radiotherapy as preoperative treatment in high-risk locally advanced rectal cancer patients (StarPan/STAR-02 Study). *Ann Oncol* 2011;22(11):2424–2430.

253. Wirth LJ, Allen AM, Posner MR, et al. Phase I dose-finding study of paclitaxel with panitumumab, carboplatin and intensity-modulated radiotherapy in patients with locally advanced squamous cell cancer of the head and neck. *Ann Oncol* 2010;21(2):342–347.

254. Foote MC, McGrath M, Guminski A, et al. Phase II study of single-agent panitumumab in patients with incurable cutaneous squamous cell carcinoma. *Ann Oncol* 2014;25(10):2047–2052.

255. Siu LL, Waldron JN, Chen BE, et al. Effect of standard radiotherapy with cisplatin vs accelerated radiotherapy with panitumumab in locoregionally advanced squamous cell head and neck carcinoma: a randomized clinical trial. *JAMA Oncol* 2016.

256. Ringash J, Waldron JN, Siu LL, et al. Quality of life and swallowing with standard chemoradiotherapy versus accelerated radiotherapy and panitumumab in locoregionally advanced carcinoma of the head and neck: a phase III randomised trial from the Canadian Cancer Trials Group (HN.6). *Eur J Cancer* 2017;72:192–199.

257. Fukuoka M, et al. Multi-institutional randomized phase II trial of gefitinib for previously treated patients with advanced non-small cell lung cancer (The IDEAL 1 Trial) [corrected]. *J Clin Oncol* 2003;21(12):2237–2246.

258. Kris MG, et al. Efficacy of gefitinib, an inhibitor of the epidermal growth factor receptor tyrosine kinase, in symptomatic patients with non-small cell lung cancer: a randomized trial. *JAMA* 2003;290(16):2149–2158.

259. Giaccone G, et al. Gefitinib in combination with gemcitabine and cisplatin in advanced non-small-cell lung cancer: a phase III trial–INTACT 1. *J Clin Oncol* 2004;22(5):777–784.

260. Herbst RS, et al. Gefitinib in combination with paclitaxel and carboplatin in advanced non-small-cell lung cancer: a phase III trial–INTACT 2. *J Clin Oncol* 2004;22(5):785–794.

261. Lynch TJ, et al. Activating mutations in the epidermal growth factor receptor underlying responsiveness of non-small-cell lung cancer to gefitinib. *N Engl J Med* 2004;350(21):2129–2139.

262. Paez JG, et al. EGFR mutations in lung cancer: correlation with clinical response to gefitinib therapy. *Science* 2004;304(5676):1497–1500.

263. Ready N, et al. Chemoradiotherapy and gefitinib in stage III non-small cell lung cancer with epidermal growth factor receptor and KRAS mutation analysis: Cancer and Leukemia Group B (CALEB) 30106, a CALGB-stratified phase II trial. *J Thorac Oncol* 2010;5(9):1382–1390.

264. Choong NW, et al. Phase I trial of erlotinib-based multimodality therapy for inoperable stage III non-small cell lung cancer. *J Thorac Oncol* 2008;3(9):1003–1011.

265. Gatzemeier U, et al. Phase III study of erlotinib in combination with cisplatin and gemcitabine in advanced non-small-cell lung cancer: the Tarceva Lung Cancer Investigation Trial. *J Clin Oncol* 2007;25(12):1545–1552.

266. Herbst RS, et al. TRIBUTE: a phase III trial of erlotinib hydrochloride (OSI-774) combined with carboplatin and paclitaxel chemotherapy in advanced non-small-cell lung cancer. *J Clin Oncol* 2005;23(25):5892–5899.

267. Shepherd FA, et al. Erlotinib in previously treated non-small-cell lung cancer. *N Engl J Med* 2005;353(2):123–132.

268. Moore MJ, et al. Erlotinib plus gemcitabine compared with gemcitabine alone in patients with advanced pancreatic cancer: a phase III trial of the National Cancer Institute of Canada Clinical Trials Group. *J Clin Oncol* 2007;25(15):1960–1966.

269. Janne P, Wang XF, Socinski MA, et al. Randomized phase II trial of erlotinib (E) alone or in combination with carboplatin/paclitaxel (CP) in never or light former smokers with advanced lung adenocarcinoma: CALGB 30406. *J Clin Oncol* 2010;28(Suppl 15): abstr 7503.

270. Brown PD, et al. Phase I/II trial of erlotinib and temozolomide with radiation therapy in the treatment of newly diagnosed glioblastoma multiforme: North Central Cancer Treatment Group Study N0177. *J Clin Oncol* 2008;26(34):5603–5609.

271. Peereboom DM, et al. Phase II trial of erlotinib with temozolomide and radiation in patients with newly diagnosed glioblastoma multiforme. *J Neurooncol* 2010;98(1):93–99.

272. Prados MD, et al. Phase II study of erlotinib plus temozolomide during and after radiation therapy in patients with newly diagnosed glioblastoma multiforme or gliosarcoma. *J Clin Oncol* 2009;27(4):579–584.

273. Iannitti D, et al. Erlotinib and chemoradiation followed by maintenance erlotinib for locally advanced pancreatic cancer: a phase I study. *Am J Clin Oncol* 2005;28(6):570–575.

274. Duffy A, et al. A phase I study of erlotinib in combination with gemcitabine and radiation in locally advanced, non-operable pancreatic adenocarcinoma. *Ann Oncol* 2008;19(1):86–91.

275. Ma WW, et al. A tolerability and pharmacokinetic study of adjuvant erlotinib and capecitabine with concurrent radiation in resected pancreatic cancer. *Transl Oncol* 2010;3(6):373–379.

276. Nogueira-Rodrigues A, et al. Phase I trial of erlotinib combined with cisplatin and radiotherapy for patients with locally advanced cervical squamous cell cancer. *Clin Cancer Res* 2008;14(19):6324–6329.

277. Li G, et al. Phase II study of concurrent chemoradiation in combination with erlotinib for locally advanced esophageal carcinoma. *Int J Radiat Oncol Biol Phys* 2010;78(5):1407–1412.

278. Arias de la Vega F, et al. Erlotinib and chemoradiation in patients with surgically resected locally advanced squamous cell carcinoma of the head and neck: a GICOR phase I trial. *Ann Oncol* 2012;23(4):1005–1009.

279. Kao J, et al. Phase 1 trial of concurrent erlotinib, celecoxib, and reirradiation for recurrent head and neck cancer. *Cancer* 2011;117(14):3173–3181.

280. Rusthoven KE, et al. Initial results of a phase I dose-escalation trial of concurrent and maintenance erlotinib and reirradiation for recurrent and new primary head-and-neck cancer. *Int J Radiat Oncol Biol Phys* 2010;78(4):1020–1025.

281. Hainsworth JD, et al. Combined modality treatment with chemotherapy, radiation therapy, bevacizumab, and erlotinib in patients with locally advanced squamous carcinoma of the head and neck: a phase II trial of the Sarah Cannon Oncology Research Consortium. *Cancer J* 2011;17(5):267–272.

282. Blaszkowsky LS, Ryan DP, Szymonifka J, et al. Phase I/II study of neoadjuvant bevacizumab, erlotinib and 5-fluorouracil with concurrent external beam radiation therapy in locally advanced rectal cancer. *Ann Oncol* 2014;25(1):121–126.

283. Das P, Eng C, Rodriguez-Bigas MA, et al. Preoperative radiation therapy with concurrent capecitabine, bevacizumab, and erlotinib for rectal cancer: a phase 1 trial. *Int J Radiat Oncol Biol Phys* 2014;88(2):301–305.

284. Mehta VK. Radiotherapy and erlotinib combined: review of the preclinical and clinical evidence. *Front Oncol* 2012;2:31.

285. Keating G. Afatinib: a review in advanced non-small cell lung cancer. *Target Oncol* 2016;11(6):825–835.

286. O'Reilly MS. Radiation combined with antiangiogenic and antivascular agents. *Semin Radiat Oncol* 2006;16(1):45–50.

287. Murata Y, Nishimura Y, Hiraoka M. An antiangiogenic agent (TNP-470) inhibited reoxygenation during fractionated radiotherapy of murine mammary carcinoma. *Int J Radiat Oncol Biol Phys* 1997;37(5):1107–1113.

288. Lund EL, Bastholm L, Kristjansen PE. Therapeutic synergy of TNP-470 and ionizing radiation: effects on tumor growth, vessel morphology, and angiogenesis in human glioblastoma multiforme xenografts. *Clin Cancer Res* 2000;6(3):971–978.

289. Teicher BA, Dupuis N, Kusomoto T, et al. Antiangiogenic agents can increase tumor oxygenation and response to radiation therapy. *Radiat Oncol Investig* 1997;2:269–276.

290. Mauceri HJ, et al. Combined effects of angiostatin and ionizing radiation in antitumour therapy. *Nature* 1998;394(6690):287–291.

291. Petrova TV, Makinen T, Alitalo K. Signaling via vascular endothelial growth factor receptors. *Exp Cell Res* 1999;253(1):117–130.

292. Pepper MS, et al. Angiogenesis: a paradigm for balanced extracellular proteolysis during cell migration and morphogenesis. *Enzyme Protein* 1996;49(1–3):138–162.

293. Lamoreaux WJ, et al. Vascular endothelial growth factor increases release of gelatinase A and decreases release of tissue inhibitor of metalloproteinases by microvascular endothelial cells in vitro. *Microvasc Res* 1998;55(1):29–42.

294. Bates DO, et al. Vascular endothelial growth factor increases Rana vascular permeability and compliance by different signalling pathways. *J Physiol* 2001;533(Pt 1):263–272.

295. Casanovas O, et al. Drug resistance by evasion of antiangiogenic targeting of VEGF signaling in late-stage pancreatic islet tumors. *Cancer Cell* 2005;8(4):299–309.

296. Jain RK. Normalization of tumor vasculature: an emerging concept in antiangiogenic therapy. *Science* 2005;307(5706):58–62.

297. Willett CG, et al. Direct evidence that the VEGF-specific antibody bevacizumab has antivascular effects in human rectal cancer. *Nat Med* 2004;10(2):145–147.

298. Garcia-Barros M, et al. Tumor response to radiotherapy regulated by endothelial cell apoptosis. *Science* 2003;300(5622):1155–1159.

299. Kim DW, et al. Molecular strategies targeting the host component of cancer to enhance tumor response to radiation therapy. *Int J Radiat Oncol Biol Phys* 2006;64(1):38–46.

300. Bao S, et al. Stem cell-like glioma cells promote tumor angiogenesis through vascular endothelial growth factor. *Cancer Res* 2006;66(16):7843–7848.

301. Zips D, et al. Triple angiokinase inhibition, tumour hypoxia and radiation response of FaDu human squamous cell carcinomas. *Radiother Oncol* 2009;92(3):405–410.

302. Bevacizumab. Anti-VEGF monoclonal antibody, Avastin, Rhumab-VEGF. *Drugs R D* 2002;3(1):28–30.

303. Willett CG, et al. A safety and survival analysis of neoadjuvant bevacizumab with standard chemoradiation in a phase I/II study compared with standard chemoradiation in locally advanced rectal cancer. *Oncologist* 2010;15(8):845–851.

304. Willett CG, et al. Efficacy, safety, and biomarkers of neoadjuvant bevacizumab, radiation therapy, and fluorouracil in rectal cancer: a multidisciplinary phase II study. *J Clin Oncol* 2009;27(18):3020–3026.

305. Czito BG, et al. Bevacizumab, oxaliplatin, and capecitabine with radiation therapy in rectal cancer: phase I trial results. *Int J Radiat Oncol Biol Phys* 2007;68(2):472–478.

306. Koukourakis MI, et al. Phase I/II trial of bevacizumab and radiotherapy for locally advanced inoperable colorectal cancer: vasculature-independent radiosensitizing effect of bevacizumab. *Clin Cancer Res* 2009;15(22):7069–7076.

307. Crane CH, et al. Phase II trial of neoadjuvant bevacizumab, capecitabine, and radiotherapy for locally advanced rectal cancer. *Int J Radiat Oncol Biol Phys* 2010;76(3):824–830.

308. Crane CH, et al. Phase II study of bevacizumab with concurrent capecitabine and radiation followed by maintenance gemcitabine and bevacizumab for locally advanced pancreatic cancer: Radiation Therapy Oncology Group RTOG 0411. *J Clin Oncol* 2009;27(25):4096–4102.

309. Crane CH, et al. Phase I trial evaluating the safety of bevacizumab with concurrent radiotherapy and capecitabine in locally advanced pancreatic cancer. *J Clin Oncol* 2006;24(7):1145–1151.

310. Spigel DR, et al. Tracheoesophageal fistula formation in patients with lung cancer treated with chemoradiation and bevacizumab. *J Clin Oncol* 2010;28(1):43–48.

311. Gruber ML, Raza S, Gruber D, et al. Bevacizumab in combination with radiotherapy plus concomitant and adjuvant temozolomide for newly diagnosed glioblastoma: update progression-free survival, overall survival, and toxicity. *J Clin Oncol* 2009;27(Suppl 15): abstr 2017.

312. Lai A, et al. Phase II study of bevacizumab plus temozolomide during and after radiation therapy for patients with newly diagnosed glioblastoma multiforme. *J Clin Oncol* 2011;29(2):142–148.

313. Gilbert MR, Dignam JJ, Armstrong TS, et al. A randomized trial of bevacizumab for newly diagnosed glioblastoma. *N Engl J Med* 2014;370(8):699–708.

314. Chinot OL, Wick W, Mason W, et al. Bevacizumab plus radiotherapy-temozolomide for newly diagnosed glioblastoma. *N Engl J Med* 2014;370(8):709–722.

315. Back M, Gzell CE, Kastelan M, et al. Large volume re-irradiation with bevacizumab is a feasible salvage option for patients with refractory high-grade glioma. *Neurooncol Pract* 2015;2(1):48–53.

316. Cuneo KC, Vredenburgh JJ, Sampson JH, et al. Safety and efficacy of stereotactic radiosurgery and adjuvant bevacizumab in patients with recurrent malignant gliomas. *Int J Radiat Oncol Biol Phys* 2012;82(5):2018–2024.

317. Flieger M, Ganswindt U, Schwarz SB, et al. Re-irradiation and bevacizumab in recurrent high-grade glioma: an effective treatment option. *J Neurooncol* 2014;117(2):337–345.

318. Niyazi M, Ganswindt U, Schwarz SB, et al. Irradiation and bevacizumab in high-grade glioma retreatment settings. *Int J Radiat Oncol Biol Phys* 2012;82(1):67–76.

319. Gutin PH, et al. Safety and efficacy of bevacizumab with hypofractionated stereotactic irradiation for recurrent malignant gliomas. *Int J Radiat Oncol Biol Phys* 2009;75(1):156–163.

320. Salama JK, et al. A randomized phase II study of 5-fluorouracil, hydroxyurea, and twice-daily radiotherapy compared with bevacizumab plus 5-fluorouracil, hydroxyurea, and twice-daily radiotherapy for intermediate-stage and T4N0–1 head and neck cancers. *Ann Oncol* 2011;22(10):2304–2309.

321. Seiwert TY, et al. Phase I study of bevacizumab added to fluorouracil- and hydroxyurea-based concomitant chemoradiotherapy for poor-prognosis head and neck cancer. *J Clin Oncol* 2008;26(10):1732–1741.

322. Lee NY, Zhang Q, Pfister DG, et al. Addition of bevacizumab to standard chemoradiation for locoregionally advanced nasopharyngeal carcinoma (RTOG 0615): a phase 2 multi-institutional trial. *Lancet Oncol* 2012;13(2):172–180.

323. Raje N, Anderson K. Thalidomide—a revival story. *N Engl J Med* 1999;341(21):1606–1609.

324. Lebrin F, et al. Thalidomide stimulates vessel maturation and reduces epistaxis in individuals with hereditary hemorrhagic telangiectasia. *Nat Med* 2010;16(4):420–428.

325. Fanelli M, et al. Thalidomide: a new anticancer drug? *Expert Opin Investig Drugs* 2003;12(7):1211–1225.

326. Knisely JP, et al. A phase III study of conventional radiation therapy plus thalidomide versus conventional radiation therapy for multiple brain metastases (RTOG 0118). *Int J Radiat Oncol Biol Phys* 2008;71(1):79–86.

327. Atkins MB, et al. Temozolomide, thalidomide, and whole-brain radiation therapy for patients with brain metastasis from metastatic melanoma: a phase II Cytokine Working Group study. *Cancer* 2008;113(8):2139–2145.

328. Turner CD, et al. Phase II study of thalidomide and radiation in children with newly diagnosed brain stem gliomas and glioblastoma multiforme. *J Neurooncol* 2007;82(1):95–101.

329. Chang SM, et al. Phase II study of temozolomide and thalidomide with radiation therapy for newly diagnosed glioblastoma multiforme. *Int J Radiat Oncol Biol Phys* 2004;60(2):353–357.

330. Ch'ang HJ, et al. Phase II study of concomitant thalidomide during radiotherapy for hepatocellular carcinoma. *Int J Radiat Oncol Biol Phys* 2012;82(2):817–825.

331. Schiller JH, Dahlberg SE, Mehta M, et al. A phase III trial of carboplatin, paclitaxel, and thoracic radiation therapy with or without thalidomide in patients with stage III non-small cell carcinoma of the lung (NSCLC): E3598. *J Clin Oncol* 2009;27:15 [suppl; abstr 7503]).

332. Zwolak P, et al. Addition of receptor tyrosine kinase inhibitor to radiation increases tumour control in an orthotopic murine model of breast cancer metastasis in bone. *Eur J Cancer* 2008;44(16):2506–2517.

333. Suen AW, et al. Sorafenib and radiation: a promising combination in colorectal cancer. *Int J Radiat Oncol Biol Phys* 2010;78(1):213–220.

334. Plastaras JP, et al. Cell cycle dependent and schedule-dependent antitumor effects of sorafenib combined with radiation. *Cancer Res* 2007;67(19):9443–9454.

335. Cuneo KC, et al. SU11248 (sunitinib) sensitizes pancreatic cancer to the cytotoxic effects of ionizing radiation. *Int J Radiat Oncol Biol Phys* 2008;71(3):873–879.

336. Lu B, et al. Broad spectrum receptor tyrosine kinase inhibitor, SU6668, sensitizes radiation via targeting survival pathway of vascular endothelium. *Int J Radiat Oncol Biol Phys* 2004;58(3):844–850.

337. Osusky KL, et al. The receptor tyrosine kinase inhibitor SU11248 impedes endothelial cell migration, tubule formation, and blood vessel formation in vivo, but has little effect on existing tumor vessels. *Angiogenesis* 2004;7(3):225–233.

338. Schueneman AJ, et al. SU11248 maintenance therapy prevents tumor regrowth after fractionated irradiation of murine tumor models. *Cancer Res* 2003;63(14):4009–4016.

339. Wuthrick EJ, et al. A phase 1b trial of the combination of the antiangiogenic agent sunitinib and radiation therapy for patients with primary and metastatic central nervous system malignancies. *Cancer* 2011;117(24):5548–5559.

340. Jakob J, Simeonova A, Kasper B, et al. Combined sunitinib and radiation therapy for preoperative treatment of soft tissue sarcoma: results of a phase I trial of the German interdisciplinary sarcoma group (GISG-03). *Radiat Oncol* 2016;11:77.

341. Lewin J, Khamly KK, Young RJ, et al. A phase Ib/II translational study of sunitinib with neoadjuvant radiotherapy in soft-tissue sarcoma. *Br J Cancer* 2014;111(12):2254–2261.

342. Corn PG, Song DY, Heath E, et al. Sunitinib plus androgen deprivation and radiation therapy for patients with localized high-risk prostate cancer: results from a multi-institutional phase 1 study. *Int J Radiat Oncol Biol Phys* 2013;86(3):540–545.

343. Kao J, et al. Phase 1 study of concurrent sunitinib and image-guided radiotherapy followed by maintenance sunitinib for patients with oligometastases: acute toxicity and preliminary response. *Cancer* 2009;115(15):3571–3580.

344. Tong CC, Ko EC, Sung MW, et al. Phase II trial of concurrent sunitinib and image-guided radiotherapy for oligometastases. *PLoS One* 2012;7(6):e36979.

345. Escudier B, et al. Sorafenib in advanced clear cell renal cell carcinoma. *N Engl J Med* 2007;356(2):125–134.

346. Arneson K, Mondschein J, Stavas M, et al. A phase I trial of concurrent sorafenib and stereotactic radiosurgery for patients with brain metastases. *J Neurooncol* 2017;133(2):435–442.

347. Goody RB, Brade AM, Wang L, et al. Phase I trial of radiation therapy and sorafenib in unresectable liver metastases. *Radiother Oncol* 2017;123(2):234–239.

348. Brade AM, Ng S, Brierley J, et al. Phase 1 trial of sorafenib and stereotactic body radiation therapy for hepatocellular carcinoma. *Int J Radiat Oncol Biol Phys* 2016;94(3):580–587.

349. Chen SW, Lin LC, Kuo YC, et al. Phase 2 study of combined sorafenib and radiation therapy in patients with advanced hepatocellular carcinoma. *Int J Radiat Oncol Biol Phys* 2014;88(5):1041–1047.

350. Milosevic MF, Townsley CA, Chaudary N, et al. Sorafenib increases tumor hypoxia in cervical cancer patients treated with radiation therapy: results of a phase 1 clinical study. *Int J Radiat Oncol Biol Phys* 2016;94(1):111–117.

351. Hottinger AF, Aissa AB, Espeli V, et al. Phase I study of sorafenib combined with radiation therapy and temozolomide as first-line treatment of high-grade glioma. *Br J Cancer* 2014;110(11):2655–2661.

352. Chiorean EG, Schneider BP, Akisik FM, et al. Phase 1 pharmacogenetic and pharmacodynamic study of sorafenib with concurrent radiation therapy and gemcitabine in locally advanced unresectable pancreatic cancer. *Int J Radiat Oncol Biol Phys* 2014;89(2):284–291.

353. Kim R, Prithviraj GK, Shridhar R, et al. Phase I study of pre-operative continuous 5-FU and sorafenib with external radiation therapy in locally advanced rectal adenocarcinoma. *Radiother Oncol* 2016;118(2):382–386.

354. Canter RJ, Borys D, Olusanya A, et al. Phase I trial of neoadjuvant conformal radiotherapy plus sorafenib for patients with locally advanced soft tissue sarcoma of the extremity. *Ann Surg Oncol* 2014;21(5):1616–1623.

355. Keisner SV, Shah SR. Pazopanib: the newest tyrosine kinase inhibitor for the treatment of advanced or metastatic renal cell carcinoma. *Drugs* 2011;71(4):443–454.

356. Haas RL, Gelderblom H, Sleijfer S, et al. A phase I study on the combination of neoadjuvant radiotherapy plus pazopanib in patients with locally advanced soft tissue sarcoma of the extremities. *Acta Oncol* 2015;54(8):1195–1201.

357. Marinov M, Fischer B, Arcaro A. Targeting mTOR signaling in lung cancer. *Crit Rev Oncol Hematol* 2007;63(2):172–182.

358. Albert JM, et al. Targeting the Akt/mammalian target of rapamycin pathway for radiosensitization of breast cancer. *Mol Cancer Ther* 2006;5(5):1183–1189.

359. Cao C, et al. Inhibition of mammalian target of rapamycin or apoptotic pathway induces autophagy and radiosensitizes PTEN null prostate cancer cells. *Cancer Res* 2006;66(20):10040–10047.

360. Ekshyyan O, et al. Comparison of radiosensitizing effects of the mammalian target of rapamycin inhibitor CCI-779 to cisplatin in experimental models of head and neck squamous cell carcinoma. *Mol Cancer Ther* 2009;8(8):2255–2265.

361. Kim KW, et al. Autophagy upregulation by inhibitors of caspase-3 and mTOR enhances radiotherapy in a mouse model of lung cancer. *Autophagy* 2008;4(5):659–668.

362. Kim KW, et al. Autophagy for cancer therapy through inhibition of pro-apoptotic proteins and mammalian target of rapamycin signaling. *J Biol Chem* 2006;281(48):36883–36890.

Section
II

363. Manegold PC, et al. Antiangiogenic therapy with mammalian target of rapamycin inhibitor RAD001 (Everolimus) increases radiosensitivity in solid cancer. *Clin Cancer Res* 2008;14(3):892–900.

364. Schiewer MJ, et al. mTOR is a selective effector of the radiation therapy response in androgen receptor positive prostate cancer. *Endocr Relat Cancer* 2012;19(1):1–12.

365. Shinohara ET, et al. Enhanced radiation damage of tumor vasculature by mTOR inhibitors. *Oncogene* 2005;24(35):5414–5422.

366. Sukumari-Ramesh S, et al. mTOR inhibition reduces cellular proliferation and sensitizes pituitary adenoma cells to ionizing radiation. *Surg Neurol Int* 2011;2:22.

367. Sarkaria JN, et al. Combination of temsirolimus (CCI-779) with chemoradiation in newly diagnosed glioblastoma multiforme (GBM) (NCCTG trial N027D) is associated with increased infectious risks. *Clin Cancer Res* 2010;16(22):5573–5580.

368. Waqar SN, Robinson C, Bradley J, et al. A phase I study of temsirolimus and thoracic radiation in non--small-cell lung cancer. *Clin Lung Cancer* 2014;15(2):119–123.

369. Sarkaria JN, et al. North Central Cancer Treatment Group Phase I trial N057K of everolimus (RAD001) and temozolomide in combination with radiation therapy in patients with newly diagnosed glioblastoma multiforme. *Int J Radiat Oncol Biol Phys* 2011;81(2):468–475.

370. Ma DJ, Galanis E, Anderson SK, et al. A phase II trial of everolimus, temozolomide, and radiotherapy in patients with newly diagnosed glioblastoma: NCCTG N057K. *Neuro Oncol* 2015;17(9):1261–1269.

371. Hainsworth JD, Shih KC, Shepard GC, et al. Phase II study of concurrent radiation therapy, temozolomide, and bevacizumab followed by bevacizumab/everolimus as first-line treatment for patients with glioblastoma. *Clin Adv Hematol Oncol* 2012;10(4):240–246.

372. Fury MG, Lee NY, Sherman E, et al. A phase 1 study of everolimus + weekly cisplatin + intensity modulated radiation therapy in head-and-neck cancer. *Int J Radiat Oncol Biol Phys* 2013;87(3):479–486.

373. Deutsch E, Le Pechoux C, Faivre L, et al. Phase I trial of everolimus in combination with thoracic radiotherapy in non-small-cell lung cancer. *Ann Oncol* 2015;26(6):1223–1229.

374. Soda M, et al. Identification of the transforming EML4-ALK fusion gene in non-small-cell lung cancer. *Nature* 2007;448(7153):561–566.

375. Sasaki T, Janne PA. New strategies for treatment of ALK rearranged non-small cell lung cancers. *Clin Cancer Res* 2011;17(23):7213–7218.

376. Kwak EL, et al. Anaplastic lymphoma kinase inhibition in non-small-cell lung cancer. *N Engl J Med* 2010;363(18):1693–1703.

377. Shaw AT, Kim DW, Nakagawa K, et al. Crizotinib versus chemotherapy in advanced ALK-positive lung cancer. *N Engl J Med* 2013;368(25):2385–2394.

378. Solomon BJ, Mok T, Kim DW, et al. First-line crizotinib versus chemotherapy in ALK-positive lung cancer. *N Engl J Med* 2014;371(23):2167–2177.

379. Khozin S, Blumenthal GM, Zhang L, et al. FDA approval: ceritinib for the treatment of metastatic anaplastic lymphoma kinase-positive non-small cell lung cancer. *Clin Cancer Res* 2015;21(11):2436–2439.

380. Soria JC, Tan DS, Chiari R, et al. First-line ceritinib versus platinum-based chemotherapy in advanced ALK-rearranged non-small-cell lung cancer (ASCEND-4): a randomised, open-label, phase 3 study. *Lancet* 2017;389(10072):917–929.

381. Sacagliotti G, Kim T, Crino L, et al. Ceritinib vs chemotherapy in patients with advanced anaplastic lymphoma kinase (ALK)-rearranged (ALK+) non-small cell lung cancer (NSCLC) previously treated with CT and crizotinib (CRZ): results from the confirmatory phase 3 ASCEND-5 study. *Ann Oncol* 2016;27(Suppl 6):LBA42_PR.

382. Ou SH, Ahn JS, De Petris L, et al. Alectinib in crizotinib-refractory ALK-rearranged non-small-cell lung cancer: a phase II global study. *J Clin Oncol* 2016;34(7):661–668.

383. Shaw AT, Gandhi L, Gadgeel S, et al. Alectinib in ALK-positive, crizotinib-resistant, non-small-cell lung cancer: a single-group, multicentre, phase 2 trial. *Lancet Oncol* 2016;17(2):234–242.

384. Avrillon V, Perol M. Alectinib for treatment of ALK-positive non-small-cell lung cancer. *Future Oncol* 2017;13(4):321–335.

385. Camphausen K, et al. Enhancement of xenograft tumor radiosensitivity by the histone deacetylase inhibitor MS-275 and correlation with histone hyperacetylation. *Clin Cancer Res* 2004;10(18 Pt 1):6066–6071.

386. Ljungman M. The influence of chromatin structure on the frequency of radiation-induced DNA strand breaks: a study using nuclear and nucleoid monolayers. *Radiat Res* 1991;126(1):58–64.

387. Chinnaiyan P, et al. Modulation of radiation response by histone deacetylase inhibition. *Int J Radiat Oncol Biol Phys* 2005;62(1):223–229.

388. Fuino L, et al. Histone deacetylase inhibitor LAQ824 down-regulates Her-2 and sensitizes human breast cancer cells to trastuzumab, Taxotere, gemcitabine, and epothilone B. *Mol Cancer Ther* 2003;2(10):971–984.

389. Yu X, et al. Modulation of p53, ErbB1, ErbB2, and Raf-1 expression in lung cancer cells by depsipeptide FR901228. *J Natl Cancer Inst* 2002;94(7):504–513.

390. Das AK, et al. Non-small-cell lung cancers with kinase domain mutations in the epidermal growth factor receptor are sensitive to ionizing radiation. *Cancer Res* 2006;66(19):9601–9608.

391. Baschnagel A, et al. Vorinostat enhances the radiosensitivity of a breast cancer brain metastatic cell line grown in vitro and as intracranial xenografts. *Mol Cancer Ther* 2009;8(6):1589–1595.

392. Bratland A, et al. Gastrointestinal toxicity of vorinostat: reanalysis of phase 1 study results with emphasis on dose-volume effects of pelvic radiotherapy. *Radiat Oncol* 2011;6:33.

393. Deorukhkar A, et al. Inhibition of radiation-induced DNA repair and prosurvival pathways contributes to vorinostat-mediated radiosensitization of pancreatic cancer cells. *Pancreas* 2010;39(8):1277–1283.

394. Mueller S, et al. Cooperation of the HDAC inhibitor vorinostat and radiation in metastatic neuroblastoma: efficacy and underlying mechanisms. *Cancer Lett* 2011;306(2):223–229.

395. Munshi A, et al. Vorinostat, a histone deacetylase inhibitor, enhances the response of human tumor cells to ionizing radiation through prolongation of gamma-H2AX foci. *Mol Cancer Ther* 2006;5(8):1967–1974.

396. Palmieri D, et al. Vorinostat inhibits brain metastatic colonization in a model of triple-negative breast cancer and induces DNA double-strand breaks. *Clin Cancer Res* 2009;15(19):6148–6157.

397. Ree AH, et al. Vorinostat, a histone deacetylase inhibitor, combined with pelvic palliative radiotherapy for gastrointestinal carcinoma: the Pelvic Radiation and Vorinostat (PRAVO) phase 1 study. *Lancet Oncol* 2010;11(5):459–464.

398. Richon VM, Garcia-Vargas J, Hardwick JS. Development of vorinostat: current applications and future perspectives for cancer therapy. *Cancer Lett* 2009;280(2):201–210.

399. Sarcar B, Kahali S, Chinnaiyan P. Vorinostat enhances the cytotoxic effects of the topoisomerase I inhibitor SN38 in glioblastoma cell lines. *J Neurooncol* 2010;99(2):201–207.

400. Shabason JE, Tofilon PJ, Camphausen K. Grand rounds at the National Institutes of Health: HDAC inhibitors as radiation modifiers, from bench to clinic. *J Cell Mol Med* 2011;15(12):2735–2744.

401. Siegel D, et al. Vorinostat in solid and hematologic malignancies. *J Hematol Oncol* 2009;2:31.

402. Zhang Y, Jung M, Dritschilo A. Enhancement of radiation sensitivity of human squamous carcinoma cells by histone deacetylase inhibitors. *Radiat Res* 2004;161(6):667–674.

403. Fakih MG, et al. A phase I, pharmacokinetic, and pharmacodynamic study of two schedules of vorinostat in combination with 5-fluorouracil and leucovorin in patients with refractory solid tumors. *Clin Cancer Res* 2010;16(14):3786–3794.

404. Traynor AM, et al. Vorinostat (NSC# 701852) in patients with relapsed non-small cell lung cancer: a Wisconsin Oncology Network phase II study. *J Thorac Oncol* 2009;4(4):522–526.

405. Ramalingam SS, et al. Carboplatin and paclitaxel in combination with either vorinostat or placebo for first-line therapy of advanced non-small-cell lung cancer. *J Clin Oncol* 2010;28(1):56–62.

406. Bradley D, et al. Vorinostat in advanced prostate cancer patients progressing on prior chemotherapy (National Cancer Institute Trial 6862): trial results and interleukin-6 analysis: a study by the Department of Defense Prostate Cancer Clinical Trial Consortium and University of Chicago Phase 2 Consortium. *Cancer* 2009;115(23):5541–5549.

407. Munster PN, et al. A phase II study of the histone deacetylase inhibitor vorinostat combined with tamoxifen for the treatment of patients with hormone therapy-resistant breast cancer. *Br J Cancer* 2011;104(12):1828–1835.

408. Shi W, Lawrence YR, Choy H, et al. Vorinostat as a radiosensitizer for brain metastasis: a phase I clinical trial. *J Neurooncol* 2014;118(2):313–319.

409. Bertino EM, Otterson GA. Romidepsin: a novel histone deacetylase inhibitor for cancer. *Expert Opin Investig Drugs* 2011;20(8):1151–1158.

410. Otterson GA, et al. Phase II study of the histone deacetylase inhibitor romidepsin in relapsed small cell lung cancer (Cancer and Leukemia Group B 30304). *J Thorac Oncol* 2010;5(10):1644–1648.

411. Iwamoto FM, et al. A phase I/II trial of the histone deacetylase inhibitor romidepsin for adults with recurrent malignant glioma: North American Brain Tumor Consortium Study 03–03. *Neuro Oncol* 2011;13(5):509–516.

412. Molife LR, et al. Phase II, two-stage, single-arm trial of the histone deacetylase inhibitor (HDACi) romidepsin in metastatic castration-resistant prostate cancer (CRPC). *Ann Oncol* 2010;21(1):109–113.

413. Bernhard EJ, et al. Direct evidence for the contribution of activated N-ras and K-ras oncogenes to increased intrinsic radiation resistance in human tumor cell lines. *Cancer Res* 2000;60(23):6597–6600.

414. Chakravarti A, Dicker A, Mehta M. The contribution of epidermal growth factor receptor (EGFR) signaling pathway to radioresistance in human gliomas: a review of preclinical and correlative clinical data. *Int J Radiat Oncol Biol Phys* 2004;58(3):927–931.

415. Wang CC, et al. HDJ-2 as a target for radiosensitization of glioblastoma multiforme cells by the farnesyltransferase inhibitor R115777 and the role of the p53/p21 pathway. *Cancer Res* 2006;66(13):6756–6762.

416. Bernhard EJ, et al. Inhibiting Ras prenylation increases the radiosensitivity of human tumor cell lines with activating mutations of ras oncogenes. *Cancer Res* 1998;58(8):1754–1761.

417. Cohen-Jonathan E, et al. Farnesyltransferase inhibitors potentiate the antitumor effect of radiation on a human tumor xenograft expressing activated HRAS. *Radiat Res* 2000;154(2):125–132.

418. Cohen-Jonathan E, et al. The farnesyltransferase inhibitor L744,832 reduces hypoxia in tumors expressing activated H-ras. *Cancer Res* 2001;61(5):2289–2293.

419. McKenna WG, et al. Regulation of radiation-induced apoptosis in oncogene-transfected fibroblasts: influence of H-ras on the G2 delay. *Oncogene* 1996;12(2):237–245.

420. McKenna WG, et al. The role of the H-ras oncogene in radiation resistance and metastasis. *Int J Radiat Oncol Biol Phys* 1990;18(4):849–859.

421. McKenna WG, et al. Synergistic effect of the v-myc oncogene with H-ras on radioresistance. *Cancer Res* 1990;50(1):97–102.

422. Brunner TB, et al. Pancreatic cancer cell radiation survival and prenyltransferase inhibition: the role of K-Ras. *Cancer Res* 2005;65(18):8433–8441.

423. Bradshaw PS, Stavropoulos DJ, Meyn MS. Human telomeric protein TRF2 associates with genomic double-strand breaks as an early response to DNA damage. *Nat Genet* 2005;37(2):193–197.

424. Lukas J, Lukas C, Bartek J. Mammalian cell cycle checkpoints: signalling pathways and their organization in space and time. *DNA Repair (Amst)* 2004;3(8–9):997–1007.

425. Le QT, Shirato H, Giaccia AJ, et al. Emerging treatment paradigms in radiation oncology. *Clin Cancer Res* 2015;21(15):3393–3401.

426. Hickson I, et al. Identification and characterization of a novel and specific inhibitor of the ataxia-telangiectasia mutated kinase ATM. *Cancer Res* 2004;64(24):9152–9159.

427. Cuddihy AR, Bristow RG. The p53 protein family and radiation sensitivity: yes or no? *Cancer Metastasis Rev* 2004;23(3–4):237–257.

428. Swisher SG, et al. Induction of p53-regulated genes and tumor regression in lung cancer patients after intratumoral delivery of adenoviral p53 (INGN 201) and radiation therapy. *Clin Cancer Res* 2003;9(1):93–101.

429. Choudhury A, Cuddihy A, Bristow RG. Radiation and new molecular agents part I: targeting ATM-ATR checkpoints, DNA repair, and the proteasome. *Semin Radiat Oncol* 2006;16(1):51–58.

430. Durant S, Karran P. Vanillins—a novel family of DNA-PK inhibitors. *Nucleic Acids Res* 2003;31(19):5501–5512.

431. Peng Y, et al. Deficiency in the catalytic subunit of DNA-dependent protein kinase causes down-regulation of ATM. *Cancer Res* 2005;65(5):1670–1677.

432. Salles B, et al. The DNA repair complex DNA-PK, a pharmacological target in cancer chemotherapy and radiotherapy. *Pathol Biol (Paris)* 2006;54(4):185–193.

433. Veuger SJ, et al. Radiosensitization and DNA repair inhibition by the combined use of novel inhibitors of DNA-dependent protein kinase and poly(ADP-ribose) polymerase-1. *Cancer Res* 2003;63(18):6008–6015.

434. Willmore E, et al. A novel DNA-dependent protein kinase inhibitor, NU7026, potentiates the cytotoxicity of topoisomerase II poisons used in the treatment of leukemia. *Blood* 2004;103(12):4659–4665.

435. Do K, Wilsker D, Ji J, et al. Phase I study of single-agent AZD1775 (MK-1775), a Wee1 kinase inhibitor, in patients with refractory solid tumors. *J Clin Oncol* 2015;33(30):3409–3415.

436. Calabrese CR, et al. Anticancer chemosensitization and radiosensitization by the novel poly(ADP-ribose) polymerase-1 inhibitor AG14361. *J Natl Cancer Inst* 2004;96(1):56–67.

437. Dungey FA, Loser DA, Chalmers AJ. Replication-dependent radiosensitization of human glioma cells by inhibition of poly(ADP-Ribose) polymerase: mechanisms and therapeutic potential. *Int J Radiat Oncol Biol Phys* 2008;72(4):1188–1197.

438. Russo AL, et al. In vitro and in vivo radiosensitization of glioblastoma cells by the poly (ADP-ribose) polymerase inhibitor E7016. *Clin Cancer Res* 2009;15(2):607–612.

439. Chalmers A, et al. PARP-1, PARP-2, and the cellular response to low doses of ionizing radiation. *Int J Radiat Oncol Biol Phys* 2004;58(2):410–419.

440. Bryant HE, et al. Specific killing of BRCA2-deficient tumours with inhibitors of poly(ADP-ribose) polymerase. *Nature* 2005;434(7035):913–917.

441. Farmer H, et al. Targeting the DNA repair defect in BRCA mutant cells as a therapeutic strategy. *Nature* 2005;434(7035):917–921.

442. Brody LC. Treating cancer by targeting a weakness. *N Engl J Med* 2005;353(9):949–950.

443. Underhill C, Toulmonde M, Bonnefoi H. A review of PARP inhibitors: from bench to bedside. *Ann Oncol* 2011;22(2):268–279.

444. Mehta MP, Wang D, Wang F, et al. Veliparib in combination with whole brain radiation therapy in patients with brain metastases: results of a phase 1 study. *J Neurooncol* 2015;122(2):409–417.

445. Reiss KA, Herman JM, Zahurak M, et al. A phase I study of veliparib (ABT-888) in combination with low-dose fractionated whole abdominal radiation therapy in patients with advanced solid malignancies and peritoneal carcinomatosis. *Clin Cancer Res* 2015;21(1):68–76.

446. Romond EH, et al. Trastuzumab plus adjuvant chemotherapy for operable HER2-positive breast cancer. *N Engl J Med* 2005;353(16):1673–1684.

447. Dematteo RP, et al. Adjuvant imatinib mesylate after resection of localised, primary gastrointestinal stromal tumour: a randomised, double-blind, placebo-controlled trial. *Lancet* 2009;373(9669):1097–1104.

448. Tol J, Punt CJ. Monoclonal antibodies in the treatment of metastatic colorectal cancer: a review. *Clin Ther* 2010;32(3):437–453.

449. Paik S, et al. A multigene assay to predict recurrence of tamoxifen-treated, node-negative breast cancer. *N Engl J Med* 2004;351(27):2817–2826.

450. Kumar R, Amado RG. Predictive genomic biomarkers. *Curr Top Microbiol Immunol* 2012;355:173–188.

451. Demaria S, Formenti SC. Radiation as an immunological adjuvant: current evidence on dose and fractionation. *Front Oncol* 2012;2:153.

452. Dewan MZ, Galloway AE, Kawashima N, et al. Fractionated but not single-dose radiotherapy induces an immune-mediated abscopal effect when combined with anti-CTLA-4 antibody. *Clin Cancer Res* 2009;15(17):5379–5388.

453. Chajon E, Castelli J, Marsiglia H, et al. The synergistic effect of radiotherapy and immunotherapy: a promising but not simple partnership. *Crit Rev Oncol Hematol* 2017;111:124–132.

454. Schaue D, Ratikan JA, Iwamoto KS, et al. Maximizing tumor immunity with fractionated radiation. *Int J Radiat Oncol Biol Phys* 2012;83(4):1306–1310.

455. Olive PL, Vikse CM, Vanderbyl S. Increase in the fraction of necrotic, not apoptotic, cells in SiHa xenograft tumours shortly after irradiation. *Radiother Oncol* 1999;50(1):113–119.

456. Sauter B, Albert ML, Francisco L, et al. Consequences of cell death: exposure to necrotic tumor cells, but not primary tissue cells or apoptotic cells, induces the maturation of immunostimulatory dendritic cells. *J Exp Med* 2000;191(3):423–434.

457. Holler N, Zaru R, Micheau O, et al. Fas triggers an alternative, caspase-8-independent cell death pathway using the kinase RIP as effector molecule. *Nat Immunol* 2000;1(6):489–495.

458. Verbrugge I, Hagekyriakou J, Sharp LL, et al. Radiotherapy increases the permissiveness of established mammary tumors to rejection by immunomodulatory antibodies. *Cancer Res* 2012;72(13):3163–3174.

459. Kroon P, Gadiot J, Peeters M, et al. Concomitant targeting of programmed death-1 (PD-1) and CD137 improves the efficacy of radiotherapy in a mouse model of human BRAFV600-mutant melanoma. *Cancer Immunol Immunother* 2016;65(6):753–763.

460. Filatenkov A, Baker J, Mueller AM, et al. Ablative tumor radiation can change the tumor immune cell microenvironment to induce durable complete remissions. *Clin Cancer Res* 2015;21(16):3727–3739.

461. Brody JD, Ai WZ, Czerwinski DK, et al. In situ vaccination with a TLR9 agonist induces systemic lymphoma regression: a phase I/II study. *J Clin Oncol* 2010;28(28):4324–4332.

462. Lechleider RJ, Arlen PM, Tsang KY, et al. Safety and immunologic response of a viral vaccine to prostate-specific antigen in combination with radiation therapy when metronomic-dose interleukin 2 is used as an adjuvant. *Clin Cancer Res* 2008;14(16):5284–5291.

463. Brinkmann OA, Bruns F, Gosheger G, et al. Treatment of bone metastases and local recurrence from renal cell carcinoma with immunochemotherapy and radiation. *World J Urol* 2005;23(3):185–190.

464. Ando K, Fujita H, Hosoi A, et al. Intravenous dendritic cell administration enhances suppression of lung metastasis induced by carbon-ion irradiation. *J Radiat Res* 2017;58(4):446–455.

465. Gulley JL, Arlen PM, Bastian A, et al. Combining a recombinant cancer vaccine with standard definitive radiotherapy in patients with localized prostate cancer. *Clin Cancer Res* 2005;11(9):3353–3362.

466. Kamrava M, Kesarwala AH, Madan RA, et al. Long-term follow-up of prostate cancer patients treated with vaccine and definitive radiation therapy. *Prostate Cancer Prostatic Dis* 2012;15(3):289–295.

467. Butts C, Socinski MA, Mitchell PL, et al. Tecemotide (L-BLP25) versus placebo after chemoradiotherapy for stage III non-small-cell lung cancer (START): a randomised, double-blind, phase 3 trial. *Lancet Oncol* 2014;15(1):59–68.

468. Mitchell P, Thatcher N, Socinski MA, et al. Tecemotide in unresectable stage III non-small-cell lung cancer in the phase III START study: updated overall survival and biomarker analyses. *Ann Oncol* 2015;26(6):1134–1142.

469. Kantoff PW, Higano CS, Shore ND, et al. Sipuleucel-T immunotherapy for castration-resistant prostate cancer. *N Engl J Med* 2010;363(5):411–422.

470. Sampson JH, Archer GE, Mitchell DA, et al. An epidermal growth factor receptor variant III-targeted vaccine is safe and immunogenic in patients with glioblastoma multiforme. *Mol Cancer Ther* 2009;8(10):2773–2779.

471. Hardacre JM, Mulcahy M, Small W, et al. Addition of algenpantucel-L immunotherapy to standard adjuvant therapy for pancreatic cancer: a phase 2 study. *J Gastrointest Surg* 2013;17(1):94–100; discussion 100–101.

472. Finkelstein SE, Iclozan C, Bui MM, et al. Combination of external beam radiotherapy (EBRT) with intratumoral injection of dendritic cells as neo-adjuvant treatment of high-risk soft tissue sarcoma patients. *Int J Radiat Oncol Biol Phys* 2012;82(2):924–932.

473. Barker CA, Postow MA. Combinations of radiation therapy and immunotherapy for melanoma: a review of clinical outcomes. *Int J Radiat Oncol Biol Phys* 2014;88(5):986–997.

474. Lange JR, Raubitschek AA, Pockaj BA, et al. A pilot study of the combination of interleukin-2-based immunotherapy and radiation therapy. *J Immunother* 1992;12(4):265–271.

475. Schaue D. A century of radiation therapy and adaptive immunity. *Front Immunol* 2017;8:431.

476. Postow MA, Callahan MK, Barker CA, et al. Immunologic correlates of the abscopal effect in a patient with melanoma. *N Engl J Med* 2012;366(10):925–931.

477. Kiess AP, Wolchok JD, Barker CA, et al. Stereotactic radiosurgery for melanoma brain metastases in patients receiving ipilimumab: safety profile and efficacy of combined treatment. *Int J Radiat Oncol Biol Phys* 2015;92(2):368–375.

478. Slovin SF, Higano CS, Hamid O, et al. Ipilimumab alone or in combination with radiotherapy in metastatic castration-resistant prostate cancer: results from an open-label, multicenter phase I/II study. *Ann Oncol* 2013;24(7):1813–1821.

479. Kroeze SG, Fritz C, Hoyer M, et al. Toxicity of concurrent stereotactic radiotherapy and targeted therapy or immunotherapy: a systematic review. *Cancer Treat Rev* 2017;53:25–37.

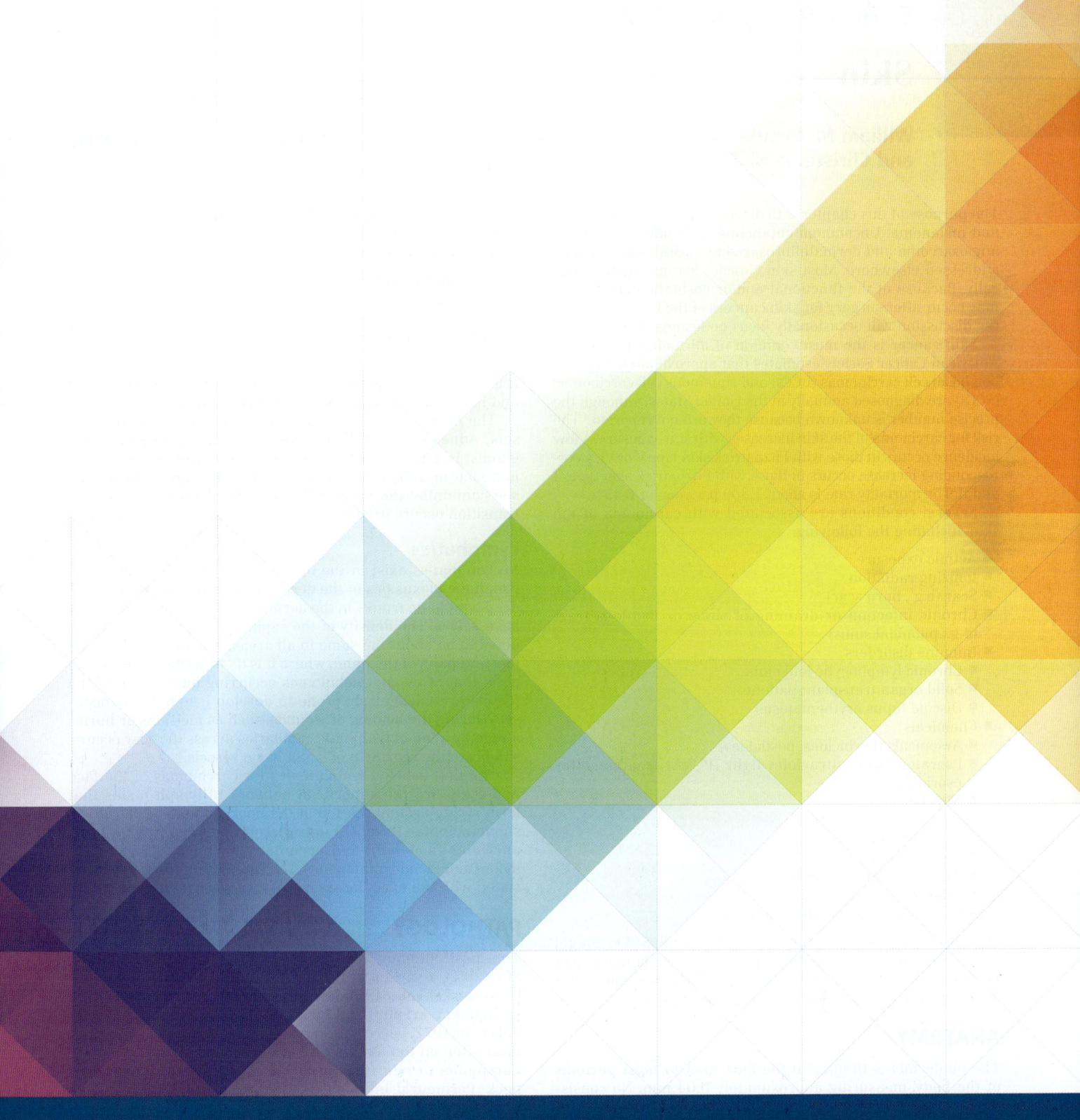

SECTION **III**

Clinical Radiation Oncology

CHAPTER 37

Skin

William M. Mendenhall, Anthony A. Mancuso, Jessica M. Kirwan, Peter T. Dziegielewski, and Christiana M. Shaw

The purpose of this chapter is to discuss cutaneous carcinoma and melanoma. Uncommon cutaneous malignancies, such as angiosarcoma and dermatofibrosarcoma protuberans, will be addressed elsewhere. Most skin cancers are managed surgically. Because of the functional and/or cosmetic deficits that may occur after surgery for skin cancers of the head and neck, the discussion will occasionally focus on lesions in this area.

Skin cancer is the most common of all malignancies. The American Cancer Society estimates that approximately two million basal cell carcinomas (BCCs) and squamous cell carcinomas (SCCs) are diagnosed annually in the United States, although the precise number is unknown because they are not reported.[1] The risk for carcinoma of the skin increases with sun exposure. A low incidence occurs in those with Fitzpatrick skin type V or VI; a corresponding increase occurs in those with Fitzpatrick skin types I and II. The mortality rate is about 1,800 per year, or 0.45%.

Several conditions are associated with carcinoma of the skin, including the following:

- Actinic exposure
- Ionizing radiation
- Scar (e.g., burn scar)
- Chronic infection or draining of sinus or fistulous tract (e.g., pilonidal sinus)
- Immune disorders
  - Chronic lymphocytic leukemia
  - Solid organ transplant patients
  - Discoid lupus erythematosus
- Chemicals
  - Arsenicals (herbicides, pesticides)
  - Psoralens and ultraviolet light (PUVA) treatment for psoriasis
  - Nitrates
  - Tars, oils, and paraffins
- Hereditary disorders
  - Xeroderma pigmentosum
  - Basal cell nevus syndrome
  - Albinism
  - Congenital epidermolysis bullosa

Melanoma is less common than BCCs and SCCs. Siegel et al.[2] estimated that approximately 76,380 melanomas will be diagnosed in the United States in 2016 and that about 10,130 deaths owing to the disease will occur.

ANATOMY

The epidermis is thinner in the face than in most portions of the body, measuring approximately 0.04 mm. No consistent change in the thickness of the epidermis occurs with increasing age, and no difference in skin thickness exists between men and women. The layers of the epidermis from superficial to deep are

- Stratum corneum
- Stratum lucidum
- Stratum granulosum
- Stratum spinosum
- Stratum basale

It is important to know these layers to understand the origin and behavior of a particular type of skin cancer.

The dermis, which contains the blood and lymphatic vessels, adnexa, hair follicles, sweat glands, and sebaceous glands, is 1 to 2 mm thick; the dermis of the eyelid is thinner, ≤0.6 mm. Beneath the dermis lies the subcutaneous tissue containing the fat and the superficial fascia. No distinct transition occurs from the dermis to the subcutaneous layer.

Lymphatics

No lymphatics exist in the epidermis. A superficial capillary lymphatic plexus lies in the dermis and is without valves.[3] The deep lymphatic trunks in the dermis and subcutaneous tissues have valves. The density of the capillary lymphatics has been noted to be about the same in all areas, except the sole of the foot and palm of the hand, where it is denser. Observation suggests that SCCs and melanomas occurring on the skin of the temple are particularly prone to develop lymphatic metastasis.[4] During the healing of wounds, such as incisions or burns, a regeneration of lymphatic capillaries across the scar occurs, similar to the regrowth of small blood vessels.[3]

The first-echelon lymph nodes for carcinomas of the face and scalp are the superficial network of lymph nodes that form a ring around the top of the neck: submental (level IA), submandibular (level IB), intraparotid or preauricular, postauricular (mastoid), and occipital lymph nodes as well as inconstant facial lymph nodes. The first echelon is highly associated with the exact location of the cancer on the face.

PATHOLOGY

The most common carcinomas of the skin are BCC (65%), SCC (30%), a variant of BCC or SCC, and the adnexal carcinomas. Merkel cell carcinoma (MCC) is a rare neuroendocrine malignancy arising in the skin that was first described by Toker[5] in 1972. Verrucous carcinoma, a variant of SCC, occurs most often on the foot and is rare in the head and neck area. Carcinoma *in situ* (CIS) occurs frequently in the head and neck. Perineural invasion (PNI) is observed in 2% to 3% of patients with BCCs and SCCs.[6]

Noncutaneous carcinomas (e.g., renal cell carcinoma) may metastasize to the skin and subcutaneous tissues.

Basal Cell Carcinoma

The common BCC, which arises from the basal layer of the epithelium, may have a variety of growth patterns merge into one another in the same tumor, and the different names applied to the gross and microscopic appearances have clinical implications. The morphea type (sclerosing BCC) shows little surface disease and a marked infiltrating pattern; it is an important subtype because of the higher risk for recurrence. Microcystic BCC is a histologic variant of BCC that exhibits the same natural history as the more common variety. Some lesions will have mixed BCC and SCC (basosquamous cell carcinoma or metatypical BCC). Melanin pigment may be seen on both gross and microscopic examination of BCC.

Squamous Cell Carcinoma

SCC and its variants (i.e., verrucous carcinoma, spindle cell SCC) are similar histologically to SCC occurring in other sites. Most are well differentiated. Evans and Smith[7] identified two categories of spindle cell tumors of skin: one was composed of SCC mixed with a spindle cell component; the other was predominantly spindle cells. The spindle cell component is similar in both groups; mitoses, giant cells, and epithelioid cells may be seen.

Keratoacanthoma

Keratoacanthoma is a benign tumor of the skin that grossly resembles a cystic BCC and microscopically resembles SCC or squamous papilloma. Part of the difficulty in histologic diagnosis is owing to an inadequate biopsy specimen. Ackerman[8] concluded that "the diagnosis of keratoacanthoma can only be made with absolute certainty by biologic behavior in the form of eventual involution."

Adnexal Carcinoma

Carcinomas may arise from the epithelium of the sweat glands, sebaceous glands, or hair follicles and microscopically resemble the tissue of origin. Carcinoma of the sweat gland can arise from either the eccrine or apocrine glands; however, no reliable histologic criteria exist to differentiate the origin. It is difficult to distinguish between benign tumors and malignant carcinomas of the sweat gland in the absence of metastases. The differential diagnosis includes adenocarcinoma metastatic to skin and BCCs and SCCs with an adenoid cystic growth pattern. They are frequently misdiagnosed at the time of the first biopsy. Malignant trichilemmoma arising from hair follicles is extremely rare.

Microcystic adnexal carcinoma (sclerosing sweat duct carcinoma) is a rare variant of adnexal carcinoma first described in 1982. The lesion usually presents on the upper lip or skin of the periorbital area as an indurated plaque without direct invasion of the overlying epidermis. It often appears as a subcutaneous nodule. It tends to be slow growing and locally invasive.[9–11] Microcystic adnexal carcinoma exhibits a propensity for local recurrence after excision and is associated with PNI; lymph node metastases are rare. The role of radiation therapy (RT) in the treatment of this rare malignancy is undefined.

Merkel Cell Carcinoma

MCC is a small cell neuroendocrine carcinoma arising in the skin. It has been found to be associated with polyomavirus infection. As in neuroendocrine carcinomas arising in other primary sites, MCC produces a neuron-specific enolase and has been found to contain membrane-bound neurosecretory granules within the tumor cell. In the past, the correct diagnosis often was not obtained until an extensive recurrence was noted. MCC was often misdiagnosed as BCC, lymphoma, adnexal carcinoma, or carcinoma metastatic to the skin from another primary site (i.e., small cell carcinoma of the lung or medullary carcinoma of the thyroid).[12]

Melanoma

Melanoma arises from melanocytes, which are present in the epidermis as well as in other parts of the body including the eye and respiratory, gastrointestinal, and genitourinary tracts.

PATTERNS OF SPREAD

The patterns of spread for individual anatomic sites are outlined in the Selection of Treatment Modality section. Some lesions remain confined to the epidermis (CIS) and may involve a large area of skin. Large *in situ* lesions occur more often on the trunk; however, small areas of CIS are common on the head and neck.

Basal Cell and Squamous Cell Carcinomas

Both BCC and SCC usually are well differentiated, and most have an indolent growth with distinct margins; a small proportion are poorly differentiated and grow rapidly. BCC occurs more frequently around the central portion of the face, whereas SCC occurs more often on the ears, preauricular and temporal area, scalp, and skin of the neck.

Most lesions remain superficial and invade the adjacent epidermis in a circumferential growth pattern. Invasion of the dermis usually is confined to the superficial (papillary) dermis. Eventually, penetration of the reticular dermis, subcutaneous tissues, and other underlying structures occurs. A few skin carcinomas tend to grow beneath the skin, and the surface lesion gives little indication of their extensive growth; this is more often seen in recurrent tumors. Most early BCCs and SCCs show an orderly invasion of the superficial dermis, which allows successful local therapy. Both BCCs and SCCs invade cartilage and bone, develop PNI, and eventually enter the lymphatics, although the latter is not common. BCC, in particular, has a low incidence of lymphatic involvement unless it is recurrent (0.05%), whereas the incidence of lymph node spread for SCC is estimated to be at least 10% to 15%. As the size and age of the lesion increase, the potential for lymphatic spread increases.

SCCs may develop distant metastases, whereas BCCs rarely produce metastases. BCC tend to be locally invasive and destructive. A variant of BCC known as basosquamous cell carcinoma acts more aggressively than does BCC and has a propensity for lymphatic spread.

Metatypical BCC is intermediate between BCC and SCC as far as recurrence rates and the risk of metastases.[13]

Spindle cell tumors of the skin have a gross appearance and growth pattern similar to SCCs.

Carcinoma of the Sweat Gland

Carcinoma of the sweat gland occurs with equal frequency in males and females. It predominantly affects elderly people, although it may occur even in early adulthood. The lesion is generally a subcutaneous nodular mass, which may be solitary or multiple, and the larger lesions may be ulcerated. Carcinoma of the sweat gland most often occurs on the eyelid, face, and scalp. The growth rate varies from indolent to rapid. The tumor may be present for several years with little change and then suddenly begin to enlarge. PNI is frequent. Regional and distant metastases may develop. Scalp lesions are the ones most likely to develop metastases to regional lymph nodes.

Recurrence after excision is frequent, and often multiple recurrences are reported.[14,15] Little information exists on the response to RT.[15] In our limited experience, carcinoma of the sweat gland is sufficiently radioresponsive to justify RT, particularly in association with excision.

Section III

The mucin-producing sweat gland adenocarcinoma is a rare tumor. The eyelid is the primary site in about one-half of cases and the face and scalp in another one-fourth of cases. The tumor presents most often in middle-aged men. Wright and Font[16] reported 21 cases that originated on the eyelid. Eight patients (38%) developed one or more local recurrences, one patient died with extensive persistent disease in the face after a 15-year interval, and only one patient had metastasis to the submandibular lymph nodes successfully treated by radical neck dissection.[16] Regional or distant metastasis is a relatively infrequent event for lesions arising in the head and neck area.

Sebaceous Gland Carcinoma

Sebaceous gland carcinoma is rare. It occurs most often on the eyelids, predominantly on the upper lid in elderly women, although the lower lid and caruncle are also sites of origin; it may occur on other parts of the head and neck skin as well. It is often indolent in its growth; however, it may be locally aggressive and develop regional and distant metastases. Local recurrence is common after excision because the lesions often have significant deep and lateral spread beyond the obvious lesion. Metastasis to regional lymph nodes is reported in about 20% of cases, and a small percentage of patients develop distant metastases.[17] Inadequate treatment often occurs because of incorrect histologic diagnosis.

Keratoacanthoma

Keratoacanthoma benign lesions start as a firm, round skin nodule and grow to 1 to 2 cm in a short time, usually a few weeks. As the lesion matures, the center becomes separate and can be removed, revealing a small crater. The lesion occurs most often in the exposed area of the head and neck. Keratoacanthoma is an unlikely diagnosis for a lesion of the lip vermilion. Typically, keratoacanthoma is twice as common in men as women. It occurs most often in patients older than 40 years of age, although it may be seen as early as the second decade of life.

Basal Cell Nevus Syndrome

The basal cell nevus syndrome (aka Gorlin syndrome) is an autosomal dominant disorder with a high level of penetrance but a variable clinical picture. The clinical syndrome may be composed of any or all of the following:

- Multiple BCCs (differing only in their tendency to develop at an early age and on unexposed skin areas)
- Jaw cysts (common)
- Palmar or plantar pits
- Skeletal abnormalities (short fingers, hypertelorism)
- Ectopic calcification
- Eye muscle palsies

- Hamartomas
- Epidermal cysts

The age at onset is frequently in the second or third decade of life, and a family history is often positive for the disorder.[18]

Merkel Cell Carcinoma

MCC occurs primarily in white men between 60 and 80 years of age.[19] The lesion often presents as a painless, raised skin nodule or mass that is red, pink, or blue and may have diffuse margins and is covered with an intact epidermis. Most lesions are ≤2 cm in size at diagnosis.[19] Human polyomavirus is thought to be etiologic in a significant proportion of patients; human polyomavirus DNA in the MCC cells may be associated with an improved prognosis.[19]

MCC displays an aggressive growth pattern. Mojica et al.[20] reported on 1,665 patients from the National Cancer Institute's Surveillance Epidemiology and End Results (SEER) database and observed the following extent of disease at diagnosis: localized, 55%; positive regional nodes, 31%; distant metastases, 6%; and no data, 8%.

Melanoma

Melanoma is more aggressive and prone to metastasize to regional lymph nodes and exhibit hematogenous dissemination compared with BCC and SCC. The likelihood of regional and/or distant metastases is related to the depth of invasion of the primary tumor. The incidence of positive sentinel lymph node biopsies (SLNBs) versus depth of penetration is depicted in Table 37.1.

Lymphatics

The overall risk of lymphatic metastases is estimated to be 10% to 15% for cutaneous SCC of the skin. The risk increases with the size of the lesion, depth of the penetration, histologic grade, and recurrence.

The risk of lymph node metastases from previously untreated BCCs is <1% and is not related to size, depth of penetration, or histologic subtype; the risk increases for recurrent BCCs, especially those with multiple recurrences over several years. Lymph node metastases, however, are seen on rare occasions without a history of recurrence, and an interval of several years may occur between the treatment of the primary lesion and the appearance of involvement in lymph nodes. When they do occur, lymph node metastases often are solitary.

CLINICAL PICTURE

Presenting Symptoms

The common history for BCC or SCC is a slowly enlarging growth on or just beneath the skin surface. Often a history exists of a sore that will not completely heal. Other symptoms such as bleeding or pain are unusual until the lesion becomes large, and even then symptoms are relatively mild and infrequent. Patients with PNI may complain of paresthesia, especially the sensation of worms crawling under skin (formication). PNI is usually observed with midface lesions and most often involves cranial nerves V2 and/or VII.[6] Advanced, neglected lesions with bone and cartilage

TABLE 37.1 PRIMARY DEPTH OF INVASION VERSUS SENTINEL LYMPH NODE BIOPSY POSITIVITY

Series	Primary Site	Depth Invasion (Number of Patients)			
		≤1 mm	1.01–2.00 mm	2.01–4.00 mm	>4.00 mm
Rousseau et al. (2003)[49] University of Texas MD Anderson Cancer Center	Various	4% (388)	12% (522)	28% (314)	44% (151)
Emery et al. (2007)[50] University of Oregon	Various	2% (41)	13% (85)	20% (35)	27% (11)
Paek et al. (2007)[51] University of Michigan	Various	–	19% (490)	32% (301)	45% (119)
Kruper et al. (2006)[52] University of Pennsylvania	Various	5% (251)	10% (228)	20% (140)	38% (63)
Leong et al. (2006)[53] Multicenter study	Head and neck	3% (134)	7% (230)	21% (160)	13% (63)
Berk et al. (2005)[54] Stanford University	Various	0% (45)	18% (115)	19% (64)	16% (32)

From Mendenhall WM, Amdur RJ, Grobmyer SR, et al. Adjuvant radiotherapy for cutaneous melanoma. *Cancer* 2008;112(6):1189–1196. Copyright © 2008 American Cancer Society. Reprinted by permission of John Wiley & Sons, Inc.

destruction, orbit invasion, and regional metastases may be seen; these advanced lesions often produce few, if any, symptoms, and patients simply delay consulting a physician.

Melanomas usually present as a pigmented skin lesion associated with a change in color, shape, and/or size. Although most probably arise de novo, some may arise in a previously benign nevus. Occasionally, patients present with regional or distant metastases without an apparent primary tumor.

Physical Examination

The site, size, and mobility of the primary lesion is always documented. Depending on location, evidence of PNI is assessed as well as any findings that might suggest involvement of underlying bone or cartilage. The regional lymph nodes must be carefully examined, even though they are not often involved. Because of the infrequent appearance of regional lymphatic metastases, and because cases of skin cancer often are not followed diligently, lymph node metastases frequently are missed. Although lymphatic metastases may appear within a few months of the management of the primary lesion, in some cases, many years intervene before the regional lymph nodes become apparent. It is not at all unusual for ≥5 years to intervene between the primary lesion and the appearance of metastases. Patients with chronic lymphocytic leukemia and concomitant skin cancer often have enlarged lymph nodes from both processes and may have elements of SCC and leukemia in the same lymph nodes.

METHODS OF DIAGNOSIS AND STAGING

Biopsy should be performed on the majority of lesions before deciding on treatment. We do not always insist on biopsy for elderly patients who have a typical skin carcinoma and are to be treated by RT.

Small lesions occurring on the free skin areas (i.e., not involving the eyelid, ear, or periorbital areas) usually can undergo biopsy and be treated simultaneously with surgical excision. Larger lesions, or those involving areas where functional or cosmetic deficit might occur from excision, first undergo biopsy with a small incisional biopsy or with a skin punch. Shave biopsies are also often used, except in pigmented lesions where a melanoma is suspected. For the diagnosis and staging of a melanoma, a full-thickness skin biopsy (such as with a punch) is needed. Biopsy with a skin punch should include the subcutaneous fat; punch biopsy is contraindicated when differentiating between keratoacanthoma and SCC because of the small sample size.

The following is a partial list of conditions to be considered in the differential diagnosis of BCC and SCC:

- Senile keratosis
- Keratoacanthoma
- Nonpigmented nevi
- Melanoma
- Cutaneous horn
- Psoriasis
- Lymphoma (mycosis fungoides)
- Soft tissue sarcomas (dermatofibrosarcoma protuberans)
- Hemangiosarcoma
- Metastatic carcinoma
- Adnexal carcinoma of skin
- MCC

Staging

The 2017 American Joint Committee on Cancer (AJCC) systems for SCC of the head and neck and melanoma are depicted in Tables 37.2 and 37.3, respectively.[21] BCC and SCC outside of the head and neck was not included in the AJCC Staging Manual for 2017. Although there is an AJCC staging

TABLE 37.2 2017 AJCC STAGING SYSTEM FOR SQUAMOUS CELL CARCINOMAS OF THE HEAD AND NECK

Primary Tumor (T)

TX	Primary tumor cannot be assessed
Tis	Carcinoma *in situ*
T1	Tumor smaller than 2 cm in greatest dimension
T2	Tumor 2 cm or larger, but smaller than 4 cm in greatest dimension
T3	Tumor 4 cm or larger in maximum dimension of minor bone erosion or perineural invasion or deep invasion[a]
T4	Tumor with gross cortical bone/marrow, skull base invasion, and/or skull base foramen invasion
T4a	Tumor with gross cortical bone/marrow invasion
T4b	Tumor with skull base invasion and/or skull base foramen involvement

Regional Nodes Lymph (N)

NX	Regional lymph cannot nodes be assessed
N0	No regional node lymph metastases
N1	Metastasis in a single ipsilateral lymph node, 3 cm or smaller in greatest dimension and extranodal extension (ENE)(−)
N2	Metastasis in a single ipsilateral node larger than 3 cm but not larger than 6 cm in greatest dimension and ENE(−); or metastases in multiple ipsilateral lymph nodes, none larger than 6 cm in greatest dimension and ENE(−); or in bilateral or contralateral lymph nodes, none larger than 6 cm in greatest dimension and ENE(−)
N2a	Metastasis in a single ipsilateral lymph node larger than 3 cm but not larger than 6 cm in greatest dimension and ENE(−)
N2b	Metastasis in multiple ipsilateral lymph nodes, none larger than 6 cm in greatest dimension and ENE(−)
N2c	Metastasis in bilateral or contralateral lymph nodes, none larger than 6 cm in greatest dimension and ENE(−)
N3	Metastasis in a lymph node larger than 6 cm in greatest dimension and ENE(−); or metastasis in any node(s) and clinically overt ENE [ENE(+)]
N3a	Metastases in a lymph node larger than 6 cm in greatest dimension and ENE(−)
N3b	Metastasis in any node(s) and ENE(+)

Distant Metastasis (M)

M0	No distant metastases		
M1	Distant metastases		

Stage	*T*	*N*	*M*
Stage 0	Tis	N0	M0
Stage I	T1	N0	M0
Stage II	T2	N0	M0
Stage III	T3	N0	M0
	T1	N1	M0
	T2	N1	M0
	T3	N1	M0
Stage IV	T1	N2	M0
	T2	N2	M0
	T3	N2	M0
	Any T	N3	M0
	T4	Any N	M0
	Any T	Any N	M1

[a]Deep invasion is defined as invasion beyond the subcutaneous fat or >6 mm (as measured from the granular layer of adjacent normal epidermis to the base of the tumor); perineural invasion for T3 classification is defined as tumor cells within the nerve sheath of a nerve lying deeper than the dermis or measuring 0.1 mm or larger in caliber, or presenting with clinical or radiographic involvement of named nerves without skull base invasion or transgression.
From Amin MB, Edge SB, Greene FL, et al., eds. *AJCC Cancer Staging Manual*. 8th ed. New York, NY: Springer; 2017. Reproduced with permission of Springer International Publishing in the format Book via Copyright Clearance Center.

system for MCC, we prefer the Yiengpruksawan system for this rare entity because of its simplicity: stage I, localized; stage II, regional lymph node metastases; and stage III, distant metastases.[22]

Diagnostic Imaging

Computed tomography (CT) and magnetic resonance imaging (MRI) are only necessary in a carefully chosen group of patients being treated for skin cancer. CT is the primary modality for showing bone invasion and nodal metastases, although MRI is often useful in determining muscular or bony

TABLE 37.3 2017 AJCC STAGING SYSTEM FOR MELANOMA

Primary Tumor (T)

T Category	Thickness	Ulceration Status
TX	Primary tumor thickness cannot be assessed (e.g., diagnosis by curettage)	
T0	No evidence of primary tumor (e.g., unknown primary or completely regressed melanoma)	
Tis	Melanoma *in situ*	
T1	<0.8 mm	Unknown or unspecified
T1a	<0.8 mm	Without ulceration
T1b	<0.8 mm	With ulceration
	0.8–1.0 mm	With or without ulceration
T2	>1.0–2.0 mm	Unknown or unspecified
T2a	>1.0–2.0 mm	Without ulceration1
T2b	>1.0–2.0 mm	With ulceration
T3	>2.0–4.0 mm	Unknown or unspecified
T3a	>2.0–4.0 mm	Without ulceration
T3b	>2.0–4.0 mm	With ulceration
T4	>4.0 mm	Unknown or unspecified
T4a	>4.0 mm	Without ulceration
T4b	>4.0 mm	With ulceration

Regional Lymph Node (N)—Extent of regional lymph node and/or lymphatic metastasis

N Category	Number of tumor-involved regional lymph node	Presence of in-transit, satellite, and/or microsatellite metastases
NX	Regional nodes not assessed (e.g., SLN biopsy not performed, regional nodes previously removed for another reason)	No
	Exception: pathologic N category is not required for T1 melanomas, use cN	
N0	No regional metastases detected	No
N1	One tumor-involved node or in-transit, satellite, and/or microsatellite metastases with no tumor-involved nodes	
N1a	One clinically occult (i.e., detected by SLN biopsy)	No
N1b	One clinically detected	No
N1c	No regional lymph node disease	Yes
N2	Two or three tumor-involved nodes or in-transit, satellite, and/or microsatellite metastases with one tumor-involved node	
N2a	Two or three clinically occult (i.e., detected by SLN biopsy)	No
N2b	Two or three, at least one of which was clinically detected	No
N2c	One clinically occult or clinically detected	Yes
N3	Four or more tumor-involved nodes or in-transit, satellite, and/or microsatellite metastases with two or more tumor-involved	
N3a	Four or more clinically occult (i.e., detected by SLN biopsy)	No
N3b	Four or more, at least one of which was clinically detected, or presence of any number of matted nodes	No
N3c	Two or more clinically occult or clinically detected and/or presence of any number of matted nodes	Yes

Distant Metastasis (M)

M Category	M Criteria	
	Anatomic site	LDH level
M0	No evidence of distant metastasis	Not applicable
M1	Evidence of distant metastasis	See below
M1a	Distant metastasis to skin, soft tissue including muscle, and/or nonregional lymph node	Not recorded or specified
M1a(0)		Not elevated
M1a(1)		Elevated
M1b	Distant metastasis to lung with or without M1a sites of disease	Not recorded or unspecified
M1b(0)		Not elevated
M1b(1)		Elevated
M1c	Distant metastasis to non-CNS visceral sites with or without M1a or m1b sites of disease	Not recorded or unspecified
M1c(0)		Not elevated
M1c(1)		Elevated
M1d	Distant metastasis to CNS with or without M1a, M1b, or M1c sites of disease	Not recorded or unspecified
M1d(0)		Normal
M1d(1)		Elevated

Prognostic Stage Groups

				Clinical					Pathologic
When T is…	And N is…	And M is…	Then the clinical stage group is…		When T is…	And N is…	And M is…	Then the clinical stage group is…	
Tis	N0	M0	0		Tis	N0	M0	0	
T1a	N0	M0	IA		T1a	N0	M0	IA	
T1b	N0	M0	IB		T1b	N0	M0	IA	
T2a	N0	M0	IB		T2a	N0	M0	IB	
T2b	N0	M0	IIA		T2b	N0	M0	IIA	
T3a	N0	M0	IIA		T3a	N0	M0	IIA	
T3b	N0	M0	IIB		T3b	N0	M0	IIB	
T4a	N0	M0	IIB		T4a	N0	M0	IIB	
T4b	N0	M0	IIC		T4b	N0	M0	IIC	
Any T, Tis	≥N1	M0	III		T0	N1b, N1c	M0	IIIB	

TABLE 37.3 2017 AJCC STAGING SYSTEM FOR MELANOMA (*Continued*)

Primary Tumor (T)

T Category	Thickness					Ulceration Status		
Any T	Any N	M1	IV		T0	N2b, N2c, N3b, or N3c	M0	IIC
					T1a/b-T2a	N1a or N2a	M0	IIIA
					T1a/b-T2a	N1b/c or N2b	M0	IIIB
					T2b/T3a	N1a-N2b	M0	IIIB
					T1a-T3a	N2c or N3a/b/c	M0	IIIC
					T3b/T4a	Any N ≥N1	M0	IIIC
					T4b	N1a-N2c	M0	IIIC
					T4b	N3a/b/c	M0	IIID
					Any T, Tis	Any	M1	IV

From Amin MB, Edge SB, Greene FL, et al., eds. *AJCC Cancer Staging Manual*. 8th ed. New York, NY: Springer; 2017. Reproduced with permission of Springer International Publishing in the format Book via Copyright Clearance Center.

Section III

invasion in large or neglected lesions, and is superior to CT for demonstrating PNI.[23] Positron emission tomography (PET) is useful to detect regional and distant metastases in patients with MCC and melanoma, but should be restricted to patients for are found to be node-positive.

SELECTION OF TREATMENT MODALITY

Basal Cell and Squamous Cell Carcinomas

The likelihood of cure is similar after surgery or RT for early-stage BCCs and SCCs.[24] Therefore, selection of one modality over another is based on other parameters such as function, cosmesis, age of the patient, convenience, cost, availability of appropriate RT equipment, and the wishes of the patient. Patients with advanced cancers are often best treated with surgery and adjuvant RT if the cancer is resectable and the functional and cosmetic outcomes are acceptable to the patient.

Radiation Therapy Alone

Small skin cancers located on "free skin," such as the cheek or forehead, may be easily excised and reconstructed with a good cosmetic result and minimal inconvenience; therefore, surgery is usually the treatment of choice for such lesions. It is also desirable to avoid RT in young patients because the late effects of irradiation progress gradually with time and, with very long-term follow-up, may be associated with a suboptimal cosmetic result compared with resection and reconstruction. In contrast, resection of an early-stage skin cancer of the eyelid, external ear, or nose may result in a significant cosmetic deformity and necessitate complex reconstruction that compares unfavorably with RT. This is particularly relevant in the case of older patients who have a limited life expectancy and who are at higher risk for a perioperative complication if the lesion is large and general anesthesia is required. In contrast, small cancers suitable for Mohs excision with local anesthesia are well treated with this technique.

Patients with locally advanced skin cancers present a difficult problem because, although the likelihood of cure may be better with combined RT and surgery in some situations, the cosmetic result is sometimes unacceptable. Patients receive postoperative RT if surgery is indicated and feasible. If surgery is not feasible, the patient is managed with RT alone. Although it might seem that the risk of bone and/or cartilage necrosis would be high after RT for a skin cancer invading these structures, the observed risk of complications is relatively low.[25,26] Exceptions are advanced cancers of the scalp and those overlying the anterior aspect of the tibia where there is little tissue between the skin surface and the bone. Following definitive RT, bone exposure is likely and

may progress to an osteoradionecrosis (ORN) requiring surgical intervention.

Patients with SCC and BCC with incidental PNI have better outcomes after Mohs surgery and postoperative RT compared with RT following a non-Mohs resection.[27] Patients with lesions associated with clinical PNI with gross tumor extending to sites that render complete resection unlikely or unfeasible, such as the cavernous sinus, are treated with RT alone. Subtotal resection does not enhance the likelihood of cure and only increases the morbidity of treatment.

Adjuvant Radiation Therapy

Postoperative RT is added after surgery if pathologic examination of the surgical specimen reveals findings indicative of a high risk for local recurrence, such as close or positive margins and/or invasion of nerve, cartilage, or bone. A significant proportion of patients with positive margins after resection of an early-stage skin cancer may never develop a local recurrence. Postoperative RT may be withheld if the lesion is a BCC, the primary site is located on the free skin, the patient is reliable and will return for close follow-up, and if salvage treatment would have a high likelihood of eradicating recurrent tumor with a good cosmetic result. BCCs of the nose, eyelid, or ear and lesions that would have immediate access to major nerve trunks are usually retreated immediately when resection margins are positive. The risk of recurrence is probably greater than for lesions of the free skin, and the consequences of recurrence may be significant. Observation is particularly attractive for the elderly patient in poor medical condition who may not live to experience a local recurrence. Metatypical BCCs behave more aggressively than BCCs, and those with positive margins after surgery should be re-excised and/or treated with postoperative RT.

Patients with BCC or SCC and focal incidental PNI involving a small nerve trunk (<0.1 mm) and widely negative margins may be safely observed.[28,29] Otherwise, patients with incidental PNI should be considered for postoperative RT, particularly if the lesion is SCC.

The usual policy for patients with positive margins from SCC is immediate retreatment by either re-excision, RT, or both, depending on the situation. There is evidence that this approach leads to a reduced risk of metastasis and reduced likelihood of death from cancer.

Management of Regional Lymph Node Metastases

Carcinoma of the skin metastatic to the parotid lymph nodes is managed as a high-grade parotid neoplasm, usually with superficial or total parotidectomy followed by postoperative RT.[24,30–32] If only one node is involved and there is no extracapsular extension, it may be safe to withhold RT. However, if the tumor recurs in the parotid area after parotidectomy, the likelihood of salvage is remote.[30] Therefore, it has been our practice to use combined treatment in all patients. If the parotid lymph node metastasis is fixed and thought to be incompletely resectable, the patient is treated with high-dose preoperative RT (6,000 to 7,000 cGy) followed by parotidectomy. RT alone is used only in patients who are inoperable because of tumor extent or poor medical condition. Patients who have positive parotid nodes and clinically negative cervical nodes may undergo a parotidectomy withholding the neck dissection followed by postoperative RT to the parotid and the neck with a high likelihood of local–regional control.[33]

Cervical lymph node metastases are managed just as they would be for other carcinomas of the head and neck. Neck dissection alone is adequate treatment if only one node is involved and there is no extracapsular extension. If two or more nodes contain tumor or if extracapsular extension is noted, neck dissection is followed by postoperative RT.

Merkel Cell Carcinoma

The preferred treatment for MCC is resection of the primary tumor with wide surgical margins (2 to 3 cm minimum) and sentinel node biopsy with completion lymph node dissection or primary dissection of any clinically positive regional nodes. Our bias is to treat both the primary site and regional lymphatics with postoperative RT. The dose fractionation schedule is the same as that employed for SCC. The role of adjuvant chemotherapy is ill defined. Patients who should be considered for adjuvant chemotherapy are those with positive nodes and/or satellite lesions. Drugs employed are often those used for small cell carcinomas and include etoposide and cisplatin.

Melanoma

The preferred treatment for melanoma is resection of the primary lesion with or without sentinel node biopsy. Patients who have lesions with a depth of invasion exceeding 1 mm and clinically negative nodes should be considered for SLNB. We also perform SLNB for lesions with depth of invasion 0.75 to 1 mm if there are high-risk features including ulceration, regression, invasion into Clark level IV or V, deep margin positive, or young age. Completion lymph node dissection for positive sentinel nodes is controversial but remains standard of care. Fine needle aspiration should be performed on any grossly positive regional nodes, followed by lymph node dissection. Patients with desmoplastic melanoma are usually suitable for surgery alone unless there is extensive PNI associated with a lesion near a named nerve, in which case postoperative RT is considered. Postoperative RT is also employed to treat the primary site when there are in-transit metastases and the margins are equivocal. Adjuvant postoperative RT is often employed for positive regional nodes. Patients who are at high risk for regional lymph node metastases and are unable to undergo SLNB and/or elective node dissection should be considered for elective nodal irradiation of the first-echelon lymphatics. The dose fractionation schedule is usually the MD Anderson Cancer Center hypofractionation technique consisting of 3,000 cGy in five fractions over 2.5 weeks with a reduction off of the spinal cord and/or central nervous system (CNS) at 2,400 cGy.[34] Alternatively, conventional fractionation (5,000 to 6,000 cGy in 200 cGy fractions) may be employed if late effects and suboptimal cosmesis are a concern.[35]

Definitive RT using orthovoltage RT or electrons may be employed for elderly patients with lentigo maligna or lentigo malignant melanoma where excision is not feasible because of cosmesis function and/or medical comorbidities.[36–38] The dose fractionation schedules are the same as those described for postoperative RT.

TREATMENT TECHNIQUES

Treatment techniques vary for primary lesions and for regional lymph node metastases.

Primary Lesion

RT of the primary lesion is usually accomplished using one of three basic external beam techniques (orthovoltage RT, electron beam, and high-energy x-rays or photons) or with an interstitial implant either alone or in combination with external beam techniques (addressed on the next page). Most early skin cancers are managed with orthovoltage RT with beam energies of 100 to 250 kVp. The advantages of this technique, compared with electron beam, are that the maximum dose is at the skin surface; bolus is not required; there is less beam constriction both at the surface and at depth so that smaller fields can be used (Fig. 37.1); shielding of the eye is easier and more effectively accomplished, particularly if electron energies ≥10 MeV are used (Table 37.4)[39]; it is less expensive; and the likelihood of tumor control may be higher, possibly as a result of increased radiobiologic effectiveness (RBE) but more likely because of technical problems that are difficult to overcome when using electrons alone. The disadvantages of orthovoltage x-rays, compared with electron beam, are that there is a higher dose to deeper tissues and to underlying bone and cartilage. The latter problem can be largely eliminated by using heavily filtered orthovoltage beams for tumors involving or overlying cartilage or bone. Another significant problem associated with orthovoltage RT is that most radiation oncology departments do not have an orthovoltage machine, and thus it is unavailable. Electron beam is usually used for lesions of the scalp to reduce the dose to the underlying brain; orthovoltage x-rays are used to treat most other skin cancers. Orthovoltage RT is particularly useful for lesions of the head and neck.

Before treatment with either electron beam or orthovoltage x-rays, a customized lead mask is constructed to collimate the beam directly on the skin surface. A 1.0- to 1.5-cm margin is adequate for a well-defined T1 lesion treated with orthovoltage RT. An additional 1 cm is added to the margin when the electron beam is used to account for beam constriction. For larger and/or ill-defined tumors, a 2-cm margin is usually necessary. If the tumor is located near the eye, a gold-plated lead eye shield is placed directly on the anesthetized cornea to minimize the irradiation dose to underlying structures (Fig. 37.2). The dose beneath the eye shield is depicted for orthovoltage x-rays and electron beams of various energies in Table 37.4. Isodose distributions for the two techniques are shown in Figure 37.1; note that the dose distribution is better for orthovoltage RT than for electron beam, particularly if a lead mask is not used with the electron beam.

Advanced skin cancers that are deeply invasive are often treated with high-energy photons to adequately cover the deep extent of the tumor. Bolus is used to ensure an adequate surface dose. Field arrangement varies with primary site. For example, a wedge-pair technique may be used for lesions involving the external ear, whereas a three-field technique (similar to that used for paranasal sinus cancer) is frequently used for skin cancers with extension proximally along the second division of the fifth cranial nerve. The target volume includes the entire course of the involved nerve, which would include the gasserian ganglion in this case, to the brain stem. Intensity-modulated radiotherapy (IMRT) may be used in some patients to produce a more conformal dose distribution to reduce the dose to surrounding normal structures. Proton beam radiotherapy may also be used to produce a very conformal dose distribution with steep dose

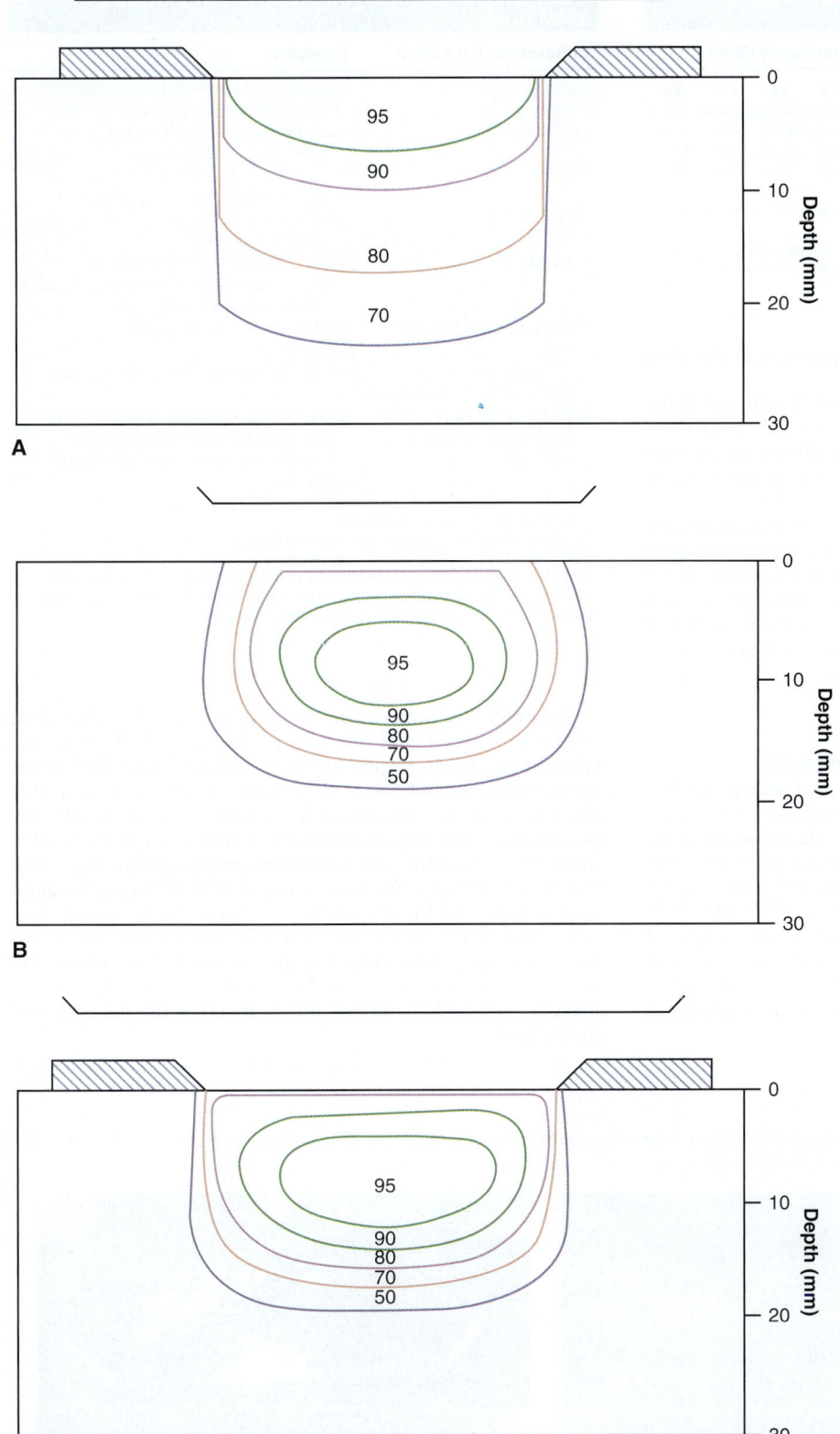

Section III

FIGURE 37.1. A: 250-kVp x-rays (HVL 1.4 mm Cu) with secondary collimation on the phantom surface. Source-to-surface distance (SSD) = 50 cm; isodose %: 95, 90, 80, and 70. **B:** 6-MeV electron beam with secondary collimation 5 cm above the phantom surface (at the level of the electron cone). Source of collimator distance (SCD) = 95 cm; SSD = 100 cm; isodose %: 95, 90, 80, 70, and 50. **C:** 6-MeV electron beam with tertiary collimation on the phantom surface. SSD = 100 cm; SCD = 100 cm; isodose %: 95, 90, 80, 70, and 50.

gradients to limit the dose to the visual apparatus and the CNS.[40,41]

The extent of RT fields for patients with PNI varies with histology and the extent of PNI. Patients with BCC or SCC and focal incidental PNI are treated with a wide local field. Those with extensive incidental PNI are treated with fields that include the at-risk nerves to the skull base, particularly if margins are positive or equivocal. The at-risk nerves receive 50 to 70 Gy depending on the extent of PNI and margin status. Patients with clinical PNI receive definitive RT to fields

TABLE 37.4 OCULAR PROTECTION: DOSE BENEATH THE EYE SHIELD

Structure (Depth)	250 kVp X-ray (HVL mm 1.4 Cu)	Electron Beam Energy (MeV)						
		6	8	10	12	14	17	20
Cornea (1 mm)	10%	18%	37%	64%	75%	93%	98%	102%
Lens (8 mm)	9%	9%	19%	36%	46%	61%	70%	87%
Retina (23 mm)	10%	19%	22%	22%	21%	23%	25%	29%

Dose is expressed as a percentage of the dose to D_{max} (depth of maximum dose deposition). HVL, half-value layer.
Reprinted from Amdur RJ, Kalbaugh KJ, Ewald LM, et al. Radiation therapy for skin cancer near the eye: kilovoltage x-rays versus electrons. *Int J Radiat Oncol Biol Phys* 1992;23(4):769–779. Copyright © 1992 Elsevier. With permission.

TABLE 37.5 GUIDELINES FOR SELECTION OF EXTERNAL BEAM DOSE

Orthovoltage Dose (cGy)[a]	Examples
6,500 over 7 wk	Large untreated lesion with bone/cartilage invasion or large recurrent tumor.[b]
6,000 over 7 wk	Large untreated lesion with minimal or suspected bone/cartilage invasion.[b]
5,500 over 6 wk	Moderate to large inner canthus, eyelid, nasal, or pinna lesions (20–30 cm² area).
5,000 over 4 wk	Small, thin lesion (<1.5 cm) around eye, nose, or ear (10 cm² area).
4,500 over 3 wk	Moderate-sized lesion on free[c] skin or postoperative treatment of moderate-sized cancer on free skin with positive margins.
4,000 over 2 wk or 3,000 over 1 wk	Small lesions (1 cm) free on skin.
The following schemes are used when the late cosmetic result is not important and travel for the patient is difficult:	
4,000 in 10 fractions or 3,000 in 5 fractions or 2,000 in 1 fraction	Rapid fractionation schemes produce a high cure rate for small lesions, although the cosmetic result may be less than optimal after 5 y.

[a]Add 10% to dose for supervoltage therapy.
[b]All or a portion of the therapy given with supervoltage photons and/or electrons.
[c]"Free" refers to not involving the ear, nose, eye, or eyelid.
From Mendenhall WM, Million RR, Mancuso AA, et al. Carcinoma of the skin. In: Million RR, Cassisi NJ, eds. *Management head of and neck cancer: a multidisciplinary approach.* 2nd ed. Philadelphia, PA: JB Lippincott, 1994:643–691. With permission.

that include the primary site and involved nerves to the skull base.

The regional lymph nodes are electively irradiated if the suspected risk of subclinical disease exceeds 10% to 15%.[42,43] Patients with SCC and PNI should be considered for elective nodal RT, particularly if the lesion is located on the head or neck.

Dose fractionation schedules used for irradiation of skin cancers are outlined in Table 37.5. We have recently used twice-daily RT with megavoltage photons or protons at 1.2 Gy per fraction to doses of 74.4 Gy in a continuous course with a minimum 6-hour interfraction interval for advanced lesions near radiosensitive structures. The suggested maximum doses for short-course orthovoltage RT are listed in Table 37.6.

Parotid Area Lymph Node Metastases

The parotid gland and upper neck are treated with an *en face* mixed beam of 6-MV x-rays and high-energy electrons (usually 20 MeV), weighted 1.0:0.67 in favor of the electron beam. The electron beam field is 1 cm larger than the x-ray field to account for the beam constriction of the electrons, except where the field abuts the low-neck field (Fig. 37.3). This field arrangement is treated to 4,600 cGy in 23 fractions, specified at a depth of 4 to 5 cm from the skin surface. An anterior field is matched to the lateral mixed beam field to treat the ipsilateral low neck and is irradiated to 5,000 cGy in 25 fractions, specified at D_{max}.

At 4,600 cGy tumor dose, the primary field is reduced off of the spinal cord, and the dose to the tumor bed is boosted with an anteriorly angled 20-MeV electron beam field or an appositional mixed beam field with an abutting posterior electron strip. The final dose for patients treated at 200 cGy per fraction with negative margins is 6,000 cGy; with positive margins, 6,600 cGy; and with gross residual disease, 7,000 cGy. If the dose per fraction is reduced to 180 cGy, the total dose is increased by 500 cGy. An alternative to the mixed electron–photon beam is a wedge-pair technique using 4- to 6-MV photon beams. IMRT may also be considered to reduce the dose to the temporal lobe and cerebellum, particularly if the margins are positive and/or tumor involves the deep lobe of the parotid.

FIGURE 37.2. A: 1-cm × 1-cm basal cell carcinoma of the midportion of the lower lid. **B:** Treatment setup that was used to irradiate the patient. *Arrows* indicate the field edge. ES, eye shield.

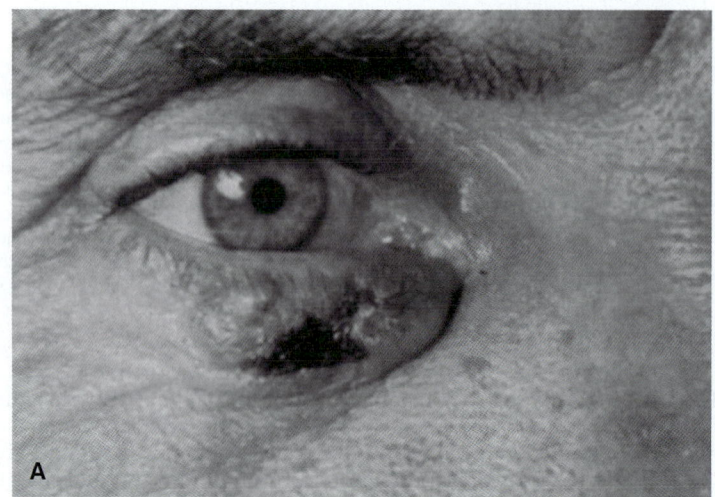
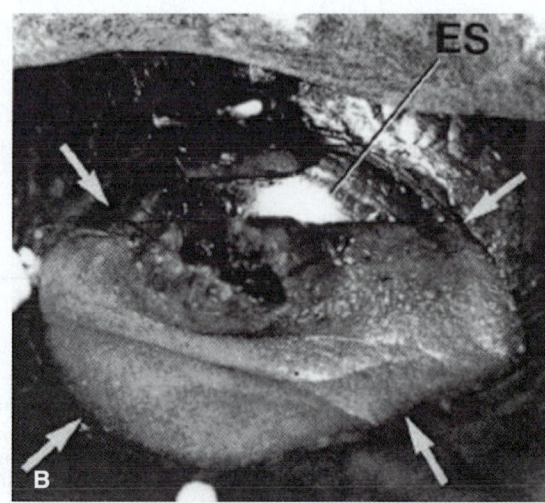

TABLE 37.6 SUGGESTED MAXIMUM SKIN DOSES*a* FOR PALLIATION WITH 250 KVP X-RAYS (BELOW MOIST DESQUAMATION LEVEL FOR THE AVERAGE PATIENT)

Field Size (Area in cm²)	Total Dose (cGy)						
	1 Day (1 Exposure)	2 Days (2 Exposures)	4 Days (4 Exposures)	5 Days (5 Exposures)	2 Weeks (10 Exposures)	3 Weeks (15 Exposures)	5 (25 Weeks Exposures)
Small fields							
10	2,000	2,750	3,500	3,750	5,000	5,500	6,000
50	1,750	2,500	3,250	3,500	4,500	5,000	5,500
Medium fields							
100	1,500	2,000	2,500	2,750	3,750	4,250	5,000
150	1,250	1,750	2,250	2,500	3,250	3,750	4,500
Large fields							
200	1,000	1,500	2,000	2,250	3,000	3,500	4,250
300	Not recommended	Not recommended	Not recommended	2,000	2,750	3,250	4,000

*a*The total doses listed are administered over a treatment course of the indicated length, divided into the indicated number of fractional treatments.
From Mendenhall WM, Million RR, Mancuso AA, et al. Carcinoma of the skin. In: Million RR, Cassisi NJ, eds. *Management head of and neck cancer: a multidisciplinary approach*. 2nd ed. Philadelphia, PA: JB Lippincott, 1994:643–691. With permission.

Axillary Metastases

Axillary lymph node metastases are irradiated with opposed anterior and posterior portals that include the supraclavicular fossa. The dose fractionation schedule is 4,500 cGy in 25 fractions with a reduction and boost depending on margin status.

Ilioinguinal Lymph Node Metastases

Ilioinguinal lymph nodes are usually irradiated with IMRT to reduce the volume of tissue irradiated, particularly small bowel. The femoral and external iliac vessels are contoured on the treatment planning CT and a 1.5- to 2-cm margin is added to obtain the clinical target volume (CTV).

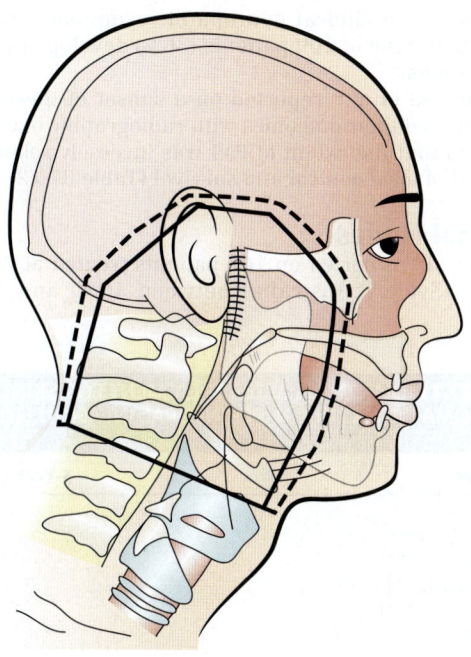

FIGURE 37.3. Typical *en face* mixed beam field used in the treatment of parotid node metastases to encompass the entire parotid bed and surgical scar. Patients are treated supine with a face mask made of low-temperature thermal plastic (polycaprolactone) for immobilization and a lead lollipop to decrease the dose to the contralateral salivary gland. A bolus of petrolatum-coated gauze is applied to all scars.

FOLLOW-UP AND MANAGEMENT OF RECURRENCE

After RT, patients are evaluated every 2 to 3 months for the first and second years, every 4 months for the 3rd year, every 6 months for the 4th and 5th years, and annually thereafter. Chest roentgenograms are obtained annually, and a follow-up CT, MRI, and/or PET-CT is obtained as needed for patients irradiated for advanced lesions.

Treatment of local–regional recurrences after RT alone or combined with surgery is usually resection. If a local recurrence is amenable to *en bloc* surgical resection with frozen section control of the margins, this may be preferable for selected cases. Local recurrences after RT may be significantly more extensive than is clinically apparent; thus, wide margins are preferred. Retreatment with RT is rarely indicated because of the high likelihood of complications. The most common scenario for recurrence in the neck nodes is failure in a solitary submandibular location; the success rate of salvage neck dissection is high in this circumstance.

RESULTS

Basal Cell and Squamous Cell Carcinomas

Most series reporting the results of treatment for skin cancer contain a preponderance of early lesions and do not employ a staging system, making it difficult to compare various series and the relative efficacy of different treatment modalities.

Primary Lesion

The likelihood of local control after irradiation for skin carcinomas of various sizes managed at the Mallinckrodt Institute of Radiology is outlined in Table 37.7.[44] The probability of local control is higher for smaller lesions, for BCC compared with SCC, and for previously untreated lesions compared with recurrent cancers. The results of RT using various beam energies are listed in Table 37.8; treatment with orthovoltage irradiation yields local control rates that are as good as, or better than, local control rates yielded by other treatment modalities.[44]

Schulte et al.[45] reported on 1,113 patients treated with orthovoltage RT for 1,267 skin cancers and followed for a median of 82 months (Table 37.9). Patients were usually treated at 5 Gy per fraction. The incidence of soft tissue necrosis was 6.3%; 83% healed with conservative treatment.[45]

Al-Othman et al.[46] reported on 85 patients with 88 clinical T4 SCCs (37), BCCs (41), and metatypical BCCs (10) treated

TABLE 37.7 LOCAL TUMOR CONTROL WITH RADIOTHERAPY ACCORDING TO SIZE, CELL TYPE, AND PRESENTATION (FROM MALLINCKRODT INSTITUTE OF RADIOLOGY—339 PATIENTS)

Size	Basal Cell, Previously Untreated	Basal Cell, Recurrent	Squamous Previously Cell, Untreated	Squamous Cell, Recurrent
≤1 cm	64/66 (97%)	22/23 (96%)	11/11 (100%)	10/12 (83%)
1.1–3 cm	71/75 (95%)	27/36 (75%)	19/21 (90%)	7/13 (54%)
3.1–5 cm	11/13 (85%)	7/9 (78%)	7/8 (88%)	6/9 (67%)
>5 cm	12/13 (92%)	1/2 (50%)	3/5 (60%)	6/11 (55%)
Size not specified	4/4 (100%)	1/1 (100%)	0/1 (0%)	4/6 (67%)
Total	**162/171 (95%)**	**58/71 (82%)**	**40/46 (87%)**	**33/51 (65%)**

Reprinted from Lovett RD, Perez CA, Shapiro DL, et al. External irradiation of epithelial skin cancer. *Int J Radiat Oncol Biol Phys* 1990;19(2):235–242. Copyright © 1990 Elsevier. With permission.

TABLE 37.8 LOCAL CONTROL RATES ACCORDING TO EXTERNAL BEAM TECHNIQUE (FROM MALLINCKRODT INSTITUTE OF RADIOLOGY—339 PATIENTS)

Modality	Size ≤1 cm (%)	1.1–5 cm (%)	>5 cm (%)	Not specified (%)
Basal Cell Carcinoma				
Superficial x-ray	69/71 (97%)	84/90 (93%)	4/4 (100%)	3/3 (100%)
Electron beam	11/12 (92%)	16/22 (73%)	4/5 (80%)	1/1 (100%)
Combination	5/5 (100%)	13/16 (81%)	5/6 (83%)	0/0
Photons (1.2–4 MV)	1/1 (100%)	3/5 (60%)	0/0	1/1 (100%)
Squamous Cell Carcinoma				
Superficial x-ray	12/12 (100%)	10/11 (91%)	1/1 (100%)	0/0
Electron beam	3/4 (75%)	7/10 (70%)	3/4 (75%)	0/1 (0%)
Combination	4/5 (80%)	19/26 (73%)	4/8 (50%)	2/4 (50%)
Photons (1.2–4 MV)	2/2 (100%)	3/4 (75%)	1/3 (33%)	2/2 (100%)

Significance levels: basal cell carcinoma 1.1–5 cm, superficial x-ray (84/90) vs. electron beam/combination (29/38), $P = .013$; squamous cell carcinoma ≤1 cm, superficial x-ray (12/12) vs. electron beam/combination (7/9), $P = .17$; squamous cell carcinoma 1.1–5 cm, superficial x-ray (10/11) vs. electron beam/combination (26/36), $P = .41$.
Reprinted from Lovett RD, Perez CA, Shapiro DL, et al. External irradiation of epithelial skin cancer. *Int J Radiat Oncol Biol Phys* 1990;19(2):235–242. Copyright © 1990 Elsevier. With permission.

TABLE 37.9 RAW AND CUMULATIVE RECURRENCE RATES OF BASAL CELL AND SQUAMOUS CELL CARCINOMAS AFTER SOFT X-RAY THERAPY

Tumor	Number	Raw	Recurrence Rates (%) Cumulative After 5 Years	10 Years	15 Years
BCCs and SCCs, total[a]	1,267	5.1	4.7	6.9	7.4
BCCs, total	1,019	4.5	4.2	6.1	6.1
T1[b]	615	2.4[c]	3.9	4.7	4.7
T2[b]	366	5.2[c]	4.2	8.6	8.6
T3[b]	22	9.1[c]	11.4	11.4	
Previously untreated (primary)	964	4.4	4.2	5.7	5.7
Previously and treated recurrent	55	7.3	4.3	13.2	13.2
SCCs, total	245	6.9	6.0	10.5	12.8
Tis[b]	13	7.7[d]	11.1		
T1[b]	79	1.3[d]	1.7	1.7	1.7
T2[b]	138	8.7[d]	7.4	14.2	19.0
T3[b]	14	21.4[d]	25.9	25.9	
Previously untreated (primary)	233	6.4	5.8	9.6	12.0
Previously and untreated recurrent	12	16.7	30.0	30.0	

[a]Including three patients with combinations of BCCs and SCCs.
[b]Multiple (>1) tumors in same irradiated field were excluded.
[c]Differences of the raw recurrence rate of BCCs Tis–T3 were statistically significant (X^2, 6.99; $P < .05$).
[d]Differences of the raw recurrence rate of SCCs Tis–T3 were statistically significant (X^2, 9.13; $P < .05$).
BCC, basal cell carcinoma; SCC, squamous cell carcinoma.
Reprinted from Schulte KW, Lippold A, Auras C, et al. Soft x-ray therapy for cutaneous basal cell and squamous cell carcinomas. *J Am Acad Dermatol* 2005;53(6):993–1001. Copyright © 2005 American Academy of Dermatology, Inc. With permission.

TABLE 37.10 OUTCOMES AFTER TREATMENT FOR SKIN CARCINOMA WITH INCIDENTAL PERINEURAL INVASION (107 PATIENTS)

Parameter	5-Year Outcome
Local control	80%
Ultimate local control	82%
Local–regional control	70%
Ultimate local–regional control	74%
Cause-specific survival	73%
Overall survival	55%

Reprinted from Balamucki CJ, Mancuso AA, Amdur RJ, et al. Skin carcinoma of the head and neck with perineural invasion. *Am J Otolaryngol* 2012;33(4):447–454. Copyright © 2012 Elsevier. With permission.

with definitive RT at the University of Florida (Gainesville, FL) between 1964 and 1997. Forty-three lesions were previously untreated, and 45 cancers were recurrent after prior surgery. The 5-year outcomes were as follows: local control, 53%; ultimate local control, 90%; regional control, 93%; ultimate regional control, 100%; distant metastasis-free survival, 95%; cause-specific survival, 76%; and overall survival, 56%. Thirteen (15%) of 85 patients developed a severe treatment-related complication.

Balamucki et al.[47] reported on 216 patients treated at the University of Florida for skin carcinomas with incidental (107 patients) or clinical (109 patients) PNI; median follow-up for living patients was 6 years (range, 0.6 to 2.3 years). One hundred eighty-five patients (86%) had SCCs, and the remainder had BCCs or metatypical BCCs. Patients with incidental PNI were treated with surgery and postoperative RT (99 patients), preoperative RT and surgery (4 patients), and RT alone (4 patients). Eight patients received adjuvant chemotherapy. Twenty-six of 107 patients (24%) presented with clinically positive nodes. The outcomes for patients treated with incidental PNI are depicted in Table 37.10. Seventeen of 107 patients (16%) developed treatment complications. Patients with clinical PNI were treated with surgery and postoperative RT (58 patients), preoperative RT and surgery (2 patients), or RT alone (49 patients). Fifteen of 109 patients (14%) presented with clinically positive nodes. The outcomes for patients treated for clinical PNI are depicted in Table 37.11. Fourteen of 62 patients (23%) who had achieved continuous local control experienced symptomatic improvement in clinical neuropathic symptoms after treatment. Thirty-nine of 109 patients (36%) developed treatment complications.

Balamucki et al.[48] reported on a subset of these patients and compared their outcomes with radiographic extent of PNI and found that the extent of PNI was inversely related to the likelihood of local control and survival (Table 37.12).

Regional Nodes

Veness et al.[30] reported on 167 patients treated at Westmead Hospital (Sydney, Australia) between 1980 and 2000 for

TABLE 37.11 OUTCOMES AFTER TREATMENT FOR SKIN CARCINOMA WITH CLINICAL PERINEURAL INVASION (109 PATIENTS)

Parameter	5-Year Outcome
Local control	54%
Ultimate local control	57%
Local–regional control	51%
Ultimate local–regional control	56%
Cause-specific survival	64%
Overall survival	54%

Reprinted from Balamucki CJ, Mancuso AA, Amdur RJ, et al. Skin carcinoma of the head and neck with perineural invasion. *Am J Otolaryngol* 2012;33(4):447–454. Copyright © 2012 Elsevier. With permission.

TABLE 37.12 CLINICAL PERINEURAL INVASION: 5-YEAR OUTCOME VERSUS PRETREATMENT RADIOGRAPHIC FINDINGS (45 PATIENTS)

| 5-Year Outcome | Radiographic Findings | | | |
	Imaging Negative (n = 11)	Minimal or Moderate Peripheral PNI (n = 18)	Central and/or Macroscopic PNI (n = 36)	P
Local control	81%	60%	47%	.2321
Cause-specific survival	100%	58%	65%	.0815
Overall survival	82%	50%	52%	.2637

PNI, perineural invasion.
Reprinted from Balamucki CJ, DeJesus R, Galloway TJ, et al. Impact of radiographic findings on for prognosis skin cancer with perineural invasion. *Am J Clin Oncol* 2015;38(3):248–251. With permission.

TABLE 37.13 MERKEL CELL CARCINOMA 5-YEAR OUTCOMES VERSUS STAGE

Outcomes	Stage 1 (n = 24)	Stage II (n = 16)	All Patients	P value
Local control	96%	87%	92%	.3240
Regional control	87%	65%	78%	.1587
Local–regional control	87%	67%	79%	.1607
Distant metastasis-free survival	71%	37%	57%	.0073
Cause-specific survival	58%	27%	45%	.0090
Overall survival	48%	18%	36%	.0037

Reprinted from Mendenhall WM, Kirwan JM, Morris CG, et al. Cutaneous Merkel cell carcinoma. *Am J Otolaryngol* 2012;33(1):88–92. Copyright © 2012 Elsevier. With permission.

cutaneous SCCs metastatic to the parotid and/or cervical nodes. Twenty-one patients (13%) were treated with surgery alone, and the remainder received surgery and adjuvant RT. The median time to recurrence after treatment was 8 months. The 5-year local–regional recurrence and disease-free survival rates were as follows: surgery and RT, 20% and 73%, and surgery alone, 43% and 54%, respectively. Multivariate analysis revealed that multiple positive nodes and treatment with surgery alone were significantly associated with decreased survival.

Hinerman et al.[31] reported on 117 patients with 121 clinically positive parotids treated at the University of Florida between 1969 and 2005. Patients were treated with preoperative RT and surgery (17 parotids), surgery and postoperative RT (87 parotids), and RT alone (17 parotids). The 5-year outcomes were as follows: local (parotid) control, 78%; local–regional control, 74%; distant metastasis-free survival, 92%; disease-free survival, 70%; and overall survival, 54%. The 5-year local–regional control rate was 83% after surgery and postoperative RT versus 47% after preoperative RT and surgery or RT alone. Three (3%) patients developed severe complications.

Merkel Cell Carcinoma

Mendenhall et al.[19] reported on 40 patients treated with RT alone (3 patients) or combined with surgery (37 patients) at the University of Florida between 1984 and 2009. Eleven patients received adjuvant chemotherapy. Twenty-four patients had stage I disease, and 16 patients had stage II MCC. Median follow-up on survivors was 4.2 years (range, 2.2 to 14.2 years). No patient was lost to follow-up. The 5-year outcomes are depicted in Table 37.13. No severe late complications were observed.

Melanoma

One of the largest experiences with adjuvant RT for melanoma has been reported by investigators from the MD Anderson Cancer Center (Houston, TX; Table 37.14). Although RT may be used to treat gross disease, this would only occur by default and in mostly palliative situations.

Mendenhall et al.[35] recently reported on 82 patients treated with surgery and postoperative RT with either conventional fractionation (40 patients) or hypofractionation (42 patients) and observed the following 5-year in-field local–regional control rates: conventional fractionation, 78% and hypofractionation, 87%. Most of those treated with hypofractionated RT received the MD Anderson schedule of 30 Gy in 5 fractions over 2.5 weeks.

Tsang et al.[36] reported on 36 patients treated between 1968 and 1988 with definitive RT for lentigo maligna at the Princess Margaret Hospital (Toronto, Canada) and followed for a median 6 years. The 5-year local control rate was 86%. Farshad et al.[38] reported on 150 patients treated at the University of Zurich with definitive RT for lentigo maligna (93 patients), lentigo maligna melanoma (54 patients), or both (3 patients). One hundred one patients were followed for at least 2 years (mean, 8 years); the local control rate was 93%.

CONCLUSIONS

RT is an effective modality for the primary treatment of skin cancer as well as in the adjuvant setting. It is used to treat the primary skin lesion when resection would result in an unacceptable functional and/or cosmetic outcome as well as in the patient who is medically unsuitable for, or who declines, surgery. Adjuvant RT is usually indicated after surgery for close or positive margins, PNI, bone and/or cartilage involvement, metastatic parotid area lymph nodes, multiple lymph node metastases, and extracapsular extension.

TABLE 37.14 OUTCOMES AFTER SURGERY AND POSTOPERATIVE RADIOTHERAPY AT THE UNIVERSITY OF TEXAS MD ANDERSON CANCER CENTER FOR LYMPH NODE–POSITIVE MELANOMA PATIENTS

Series	Number of Patients	Site	Follow-Up[a]	RC[b]	DMFS[b]	Survival[b]
Ballo, 2002[55]	89	Axilla	Median, mo 58 (range, 7–159 mo)	87% (5 y)	49% (5 y)	OS, 50% (5 y)
Ballo, 2003[56]	160	Cervical	Median, 78 mo (range, 6–224 mo)	94% (10 y)	43% (10 y)	CSS, 48% (10 y)
Ballo, 2004[57]	40	Ilioinguinal	Median, mo 23 (range, 4–107 mo)	74% (3 y)	35% (3 y)	OS, 38% (3 y)

[a]Follow-up for surviving patients.
[b]Outcome (interval).
CSS, cause-specific survival; DMFS, distant metastasis-free survival; OS, overall survival; RC, regional control.
From Mendenhall WM, Amdur RJ, Grobmyer SR, et al. Adjuvant radiotherapy for cutaneous melanoma. *Cancer* 2008;112(6):1189–1196. Copyright © 2008 American Cancer Society. Reprinted by permission of John Wiley & Sons, Inc.

REFERENCES

1. American Cancer Society. Skin Cancer: Basal and Squamous Cell. 2016. Available at: http://www.cancer.org/cancer/skincancer-basalandsquamouscell/detailedguide/index. Accessed July 12, 2016.
2. Siegel RL, Miller KD, Jemal A. Cancer statistics, 2016. *CA Cancer J Clin* 2016;66:7–30.
3. Courtice JM, Yoffrey FC. *Lymphatics, lymph and lymphoid tissue.* Cambridge, MA: Edward Arnold, 1956.
4. Taylor BW Jr, Brant TA, Mendenhall NP, et al. Carcinoma of the skin metastatic to parotid area lymph nodes. *Head Neck* 1991;13:427–433.
5. Toker C. Trabecular carcinoma of the skin. *Arch Dermatol* 1972;105:107–110.
6. Mendenhall WM, Amdur RJ, Hinerman RW, et al. Skin cancer of the head and neck with perineural invasion. *Am J Clin Oncol* 2007;30:93–96.
7. Evans HL, Smith JL. Spindle cell squamous carcinomas and sarcoma-like tumors of the skin: a comparative study of 38 cases. *Cancer* 1980;45:2687–2697.
8. Ackerman AB. Histopathology of keratoacanthoma. In: Andrade R, Gumport SL, Popkin GL, eds. *Cancer of the skin: biology, diagnosis, management.* Philadelphia, PA: WB Saunders, 1976:781–796.
9. Chow WC, Cockerell CJ, Geronemus RG. Microcystic adnexal carcinoma of the scalp. *J Dermatol Surg Oncol* 1989;15:768–771.
10. Mayer MH, Winton GB, Smith AC, et al. Microcystic adnexal carcinoma (sclerosing sweat duct carcinoma). *Plast Reconstr Surg* 1989;84:970–975.
11. Requena L, Marquina A, Alegre V, et al. Sclerosing-sweat-duct (microcystic adnexal) carcinoma—a tumor from a single eccrine origin. *Clin Exp Dermatol* 1990;15:222–224.
12. Goepfert H, Remmler D, Silva E, et al. Merkel cell carcinoma (endocrine carcinoma of the skin) of the head and neck. *Arch Otolaryngol* 1984;110:707–712.
13. Schuller DE, Berg JW, Sherman G, et al. Cutaneous basosquamous carcinoma of the head and neck: a comparative analysis. *Otolaryngol Head Neck Surg (1979)* 1979;87:420–427.
14. Fierstein JT, Thawley SE, Druck NS, et al. Metastatic sweat gland carcinoma. *Laryngoscope* 1978;88:1691–1696.
15. Harari PM, Shimm DS, Bangert JL, et al. The role of radiotherapy in the treatment of malignant sweat gland neoplasms. *Cancer* 1990;65:1737–1740.
16. Wright JD, Font RL. Mucinous sweat gland adenocarcinoma of eyelid: a clinicopathologic study of 21 cases with histochemical and electron microscopic observations. *Cancer* 1979;44:1757–1768.
17. Mellette JR, Amonette RA, Gardner JH, et al. Carcinoma of sebaceous glands on the head and neck. A report of four cases. *J Dermatol Surg Oncol* 1981;7:404–407.
18. Southwick GJ, Schwartz RA. The basal cell nevus syndrome: disasters occurring among a series of 36 patients. *Cancer* 1979;44:2294–2305.
19. Mendenhall WM, Kirwan JM, Morris CG, et al. Cutaneous Merkel cell carcinoma. *Am J Otolaryngol* 2012;33:88–92.
20. Mojica P, Smith D, Ellenhorn JD. Adjuvant radiation therapy is associated with improved survival in Merkel cell carcinoma of the skin. *J Clin Oncol* 2007;25:1043–1047.
21. Amin MB, Edge SB, Greene FL, et al. *AJCC cancer staging manual.* New York: Springer, 2017.
22. Yiengpruksawan A, Coit DG, Thaler HT, et al. Merkel cell carcinoma. Prognosis and management. *Arch Surg* 1991;126:1514–1519.
23. Mancuso AA, Hanafee WN. *Head and neck radiology.* Philadelphia, PA: Lippincott Williams & Wilkins, 2011.
24. Mendenhall WM, Million RR, Mancuso AA. Carcinoma of the skin. In: Million RR, Cassisi NJ, eds. *Management of head and neck cancer: a multidisciplinary approach.* Philadelphia, PA: JB Lippincott, 1994:643–691.
25. Million RR. The myth regarding bone or cartilage involvement by cancer and the likelihood of cure by radiotherapy. *Head Neck* 1989;11:30–40.
26. Mendenhall WM, Amdur RJ, Hinerman RW, et al. Radiotherapy for cutaneous squamous and basal cell carcinomas of the head and neck. *Laryngoscope* 2009;119:1994–1999.
27. Kropp L, Balamucki CJ, Morris CG, et al. Mohs resection and postoperative radiotherapy for head and neck cancers with incidental perineural invasion. *Am J Otolaryngol* 2013;34:373–377.
28. Ross AS, Whalen FM, Elenitsas R, et al. Diameter of involved nerves predicts outcomes in cutaneous squamous cell carcinoma with perineural invasion: an investigator-blinded retrospective cohort study. *Dermatol Surg* 2009;35:1859–1866.
29. Mendenhall WM, Ferlito A, Takes RP, et al. Cutaneous head and neck basal and squamous cell carcinomas with perineural invasion. *Oral Oncol* 2012;48:918–922.
30. Veness MJ, Morgan GJ, Palme CE, et al. Surgery and adjuvant radiotherapy in patients with cutaneous head and neck squamous cell carcinoma metastatic to lymph nodes: combined treatment should be considered best practice. *Laryngoscope* 2005;115:870–875.
31. Hinerman RW, Indelicato DJ, Amdur RJ, et al. Cutaneous squamous cell carcinoma metastatic to parotid-area lymph nodes. *Laryngoscope* 2008;118:1989–1996.
32. Andruchow JL, Veness MJ, Morgan GJ, et al. Implications for clinical staging of metastatic cutaneous squamous carcinoma of the head and neck based on a multicenter study of treatment outcomes. *Cancer* 2006;106:1078–1083.
33. Herman MP, Amdur RJ, Werning JW, et al. Elective neck management for squamous cell carcinoma metastatic to the parotid area lymph nodes. *Eur Arch Otorhinolaryngol* 2016;273:3875–3879.
34. Mendenhall WM, Amdur RJ, Grobmyer SR, et al. Adjuvant radiotherapy for cutaneous melanoma. *Cancer* 2008;112:1189–1196.
35. Mendenhall WM, Shaw C, Amdur RJ, et al. Surgery and adjuvant radiotherapy for cutaneous melanoma considered high-risk for local-regional recurrence. *Am J Otolaryngol* 2013;34:320–322.
36. Tsang RW, Liu FF, Wells W, et al. Lentigo maligna of the head and neck. Results of treatment by radiotherapy. *Arch Dermatol* 1994;130:1008–1012.
37. Khan N, Khan MK, Almasan A, et al. The evolving role of radiation therapy in the management of malignant melanoma. *Int J Radiat Oncol Biol Phys* 2011;80:645–654.
38. Farshad A, Burg G, Panizzon R, et al. A retrospective study of 150 patients with lentigo maligna and lentigo maligna melanoma and the efficacy of radiotherapy using Grenz or soft x-rays. *Br J Dermatol* 2002;146:1042–1046.
39. Amdur RJ, Kalbaugh KJ, Ewald LM, et al. Radiation therapy for skin cancer near the eye: kilovoltage x-rays versus electrons. *Int J Radiat Oncol Biol Phys* 1992;23:769–779.
40. Bhandare N, Monroe AT, Morris CG, et al. Does altered fractionation influence the risk of radiation-induced optic neuropathy? *Int J Radiat Oncol Biol Phys* 2005;62:1070–1077.
41. Monroe AT, Bhandare N, Morris CG, et al. Preventing radiation retinopathy with hyperfractionation. *Int J Radiat Oncol Biol Phys* 2005;61:856–864.
42. Garcia-Serra A, Hinerman RW, Mendenhall WM, et al. Carcinoma of the skin with perineural invasion. *Head Neck* 2003;25:1027–1033.
43. Wray J, Amdur RJ, Morris CG, et al. Efficacy of elective nodal irradiation in skin squamous cell carcinoma of the face, ears, and scalp. *Radiat Oncol* 2015;10:199.
44. Lovett RD, Perez CA, Shapiro SJ, et al. External irradiation of epithelial skin cancer. *Int J Radiat Oncol Biol Phys* 1990;19:235–242.
45. Schulte KW, Lippold A, Auras C, et al. Soft x-ray therapy for cutaneous basal cell and squamous cell carcinomas. *J Am Acad Dermatol* 2005;53:993–1001.
46. Al-Othman MO, Mendenhall WM, Amdur RJ. Radiotherapy alone for clinical T4 skin carcinoma of the head and neck with surgery reserved for salvage. *Am J Otolaryngol* 2001;22:387–390.
47. Balamucki CJ, Mancuso AA, Amdur RJ, et al. Skin carcinoma of the head and neck with perineural invasion. *Am J Otolaryngol* 2012;33:447–454.
48. Balamucki CJ, DeJesus R, Galloway TJ, et al. Impact of radiographic findings on for prognosis skin cancer with perineural invasion. *Am J Clin Oncol* 2015;38:248–251.
49. Rousseau DL Jr, Ross MI, Johnson MM, et al. Revised American Joint Committee on Cancer staging criteria accurately predict sentinel lymph node positivity in clinically node-negative melanoma patients. *Ann Surg Oncol* 2003;10:569–574.
50. Emery RE, Stevens JS, Nance RW, et al. Sentinel node staging of primary melanoma by the "10% rule": pathology and clinical outcomes. *Am J Surg* 2007;193:618–622; discussion 22.
51. Paek SC, Griffith KA, Johnson TM, et al. The impact of factors beyond Breslow depth on predicting sentinel lymph node positivity in melanoma. *Cancer* 2007;109:100–108.
52. Kruper LL, Spitz FR, Czerniecki BJ, et al. Predicting sentinel node status in AJCC stage I/II primary cutaneous melanoma. *Cancer* 2006;107:2436–2445.
53. Leong SP, Accortt NA, Essner R, et al. Impact of sentinel node status and other risk factors on the clinical outcome of head and neck melanoma patients. *Arch Otolaryngol Head Neck Surg* 2006;132:370–373.
54. Berk DR, Johnson DL, Uzieblo A, et al. Sentinel lymph node biopsy for cutaneous melanoma: the Stanford experience, 1997–2004. *Arch Dermatol* 2005;141:1016–1022.
55. Ballo MT, Strom EA, Zagars GK, et al. Adjuvant irradiation for axillary metastases from malignant melanoma. *Int J Radiat Oncol Biol Phys* 2002;52:964–972.
56. Ballo MT, Bonnen MD, Garden AS, et al. Adjuvant irradiation for cervical lymph node metastases from melanoma. *Cancer* 2003;97:1789–1796.
57. Ballo MT, Zagars GK, Gershenwald JE, et al. A critical assessment of adjuvant radiotherapy for inguinal lymph node metastases from melanoma. *Ann Surg Oncol* 2004;11:1079–1084.

Central Nervous System

CHAPTER 38

Primary Intracranial Neoplasms

Vinai Gondi, Michael A. Vogelbaum, Sean Grimm, and Minesh P. Mehta

ANATOMY

The central nervous system (CNS) is enveloped by three meningeal layers: the *dura mater* (also known as the pachymeninges), the *arachnoid mater*, and the *pia mater*. The pia and arachnoid layers are also referred to as the leptomeninges, and within them is the subarachnoid space, which is filled with cerebrospinal fluid (CSF). Dural folds separate the two hemispheres of the cerebrum (falx cerebri) and the cerebrum from the cerebellum and brainstem (tentorium or falx cerebelli). The frontal and parietal lobes are separated by a well-defined sulcus ("central sulcus"). The frontal and temporal lobes are separated by the sylvian fissure, whereas the parietal and occipital lobes are separated by the calcarine sulcus (Figs. 38.1–38.3).

The diencephalon consists of the thalamus and the pineal region and is situated between the cerebrum and the mesencephalon, adjacent to the third ventricle. Lateral to the thalamus is the internal capsule, which carries the motor fibers (upper motor neurons) from the cortex en route to the brainstem and spinal cord.

At the tentorial notch, the mesencephalon rides on the upper part of the clivus. Its interior, the tectum, is partially occupied by cranial nerve nuclei (for the oculomotor, trochlear, and proprioceptive portions of the trigeminal nerves). The dorsal plate houses the superior and inferior colliculi, which regulate eye movements and hearing impulses, respectively. The trochlear nerve is the only cranial nerve that exits from this dorsal location.

FIGURE 38.1. Coronal section through the telencephalon at the plane of the frontal horn of the lateral ventricle. (Reprinted from Paulsen F, Waschke J, Sobotta J. *Sobotta Atlas of Human Anatomy.* 15th ed. Munich: Urban & Fischer, 2011. Copyright © 2011 Elsevier GmbH. With permission.)

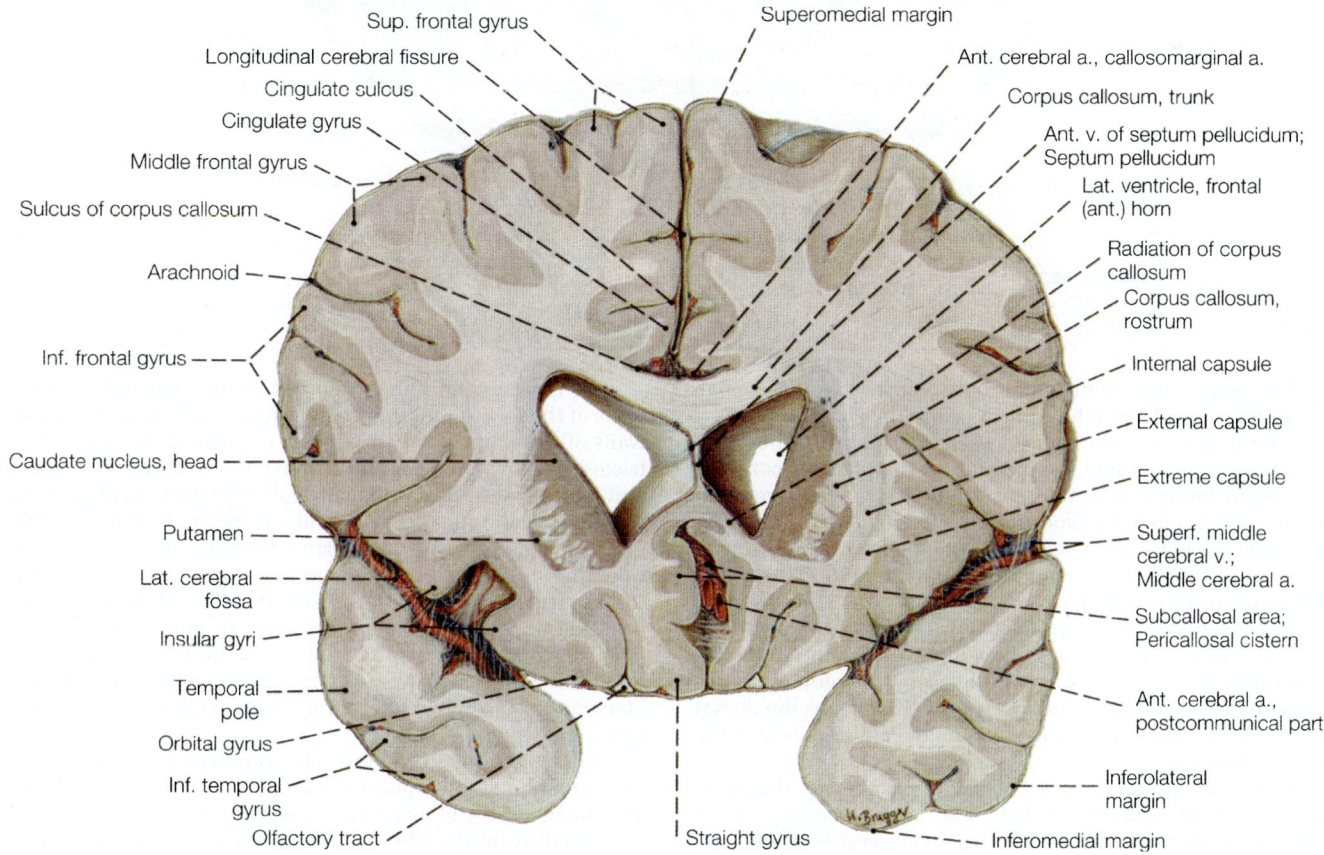

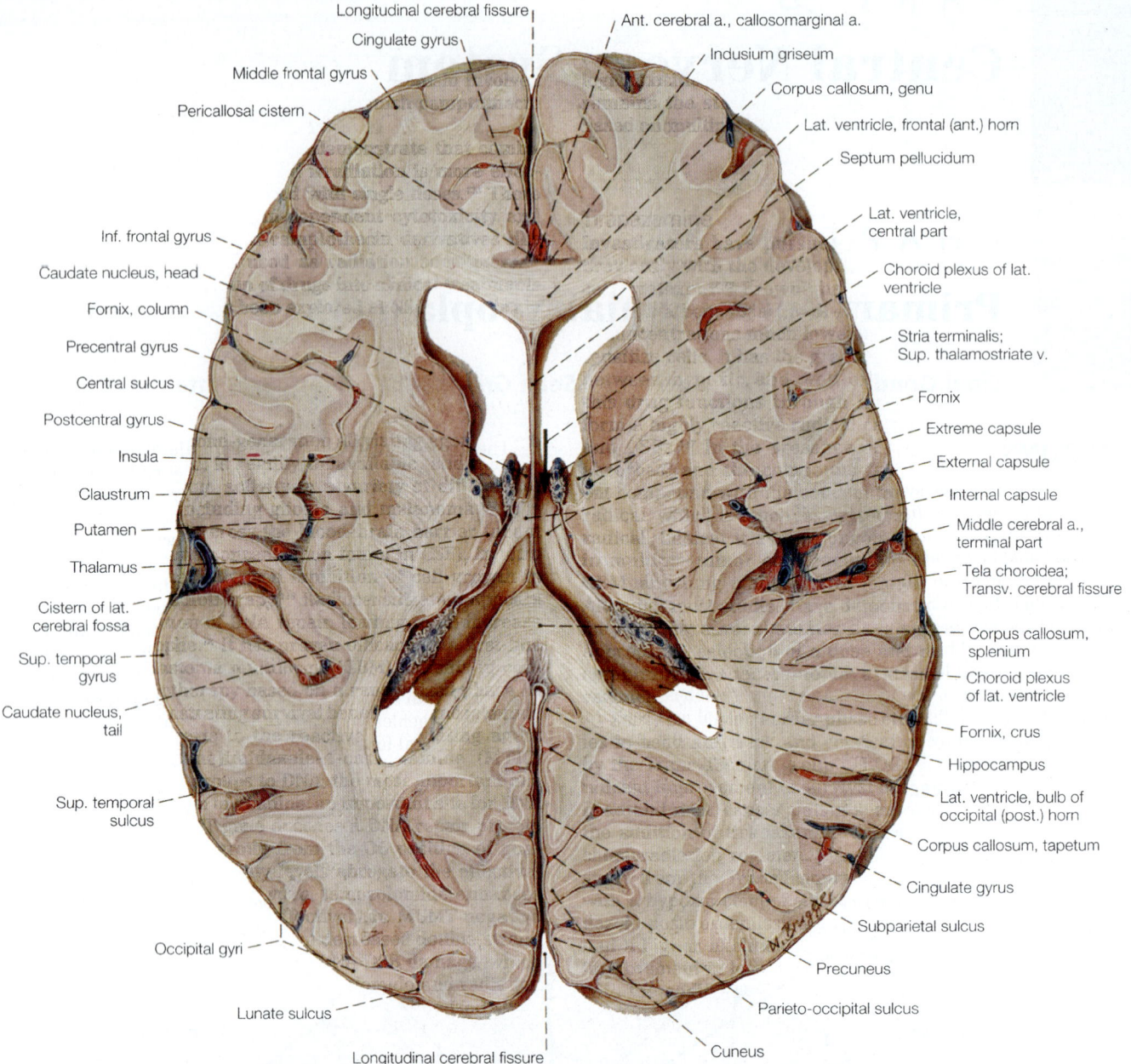

FIGURE 38.2. Transverse section at the level of the floor of the central part of the lateral ventricle. View of the superior surface of the plane of sectioning. (Reprinted from Paulsen F, Waschke J, Sobotta J. *Sobotta Atlas of Human Anatomy*. 15th ed. Munich: Urban & Fischer, 2011. Copyright © 2011 Elsevier GmbH. With permission.)

The pons relays information between the two cerebellar hemispheres and from the spinal cord to the cerebellum, carries the major ascending and descending pathways between the mesencephalon and the medulla oblongata, and contains the major motor and tactile sensory nuclei for the trigeminal nerve, which emerges from its lateral surface. The border between the pons and the medulla oblongata is noteworthy for the emergence of the abducens, facial, and vestibulocochlear (acoustic) cranial nerves.

The cerebellum develops laterally and posteriorly from the pons and differentiates into the median vermis and the bilateral hemispheres, which are flattened by the sloping tentorium on both sides. Anteriorly, the cerebellum faces the dorsal aspects of the pons and the medulla oblongata (the floor of the fourth ventricle).

The medulla oblongata forms the link between the pons, the spinal cord, and the cerebellum. It houses the majority of the cranial nerve nuclei (abducens, facial, vestibulocochlear, glossopharyngeal, vagal, accessory, and hypoglossal).

CSF is produced by the choroid plexus, which lies in the roofs of the fourth and third ventricles as well as in the medial walls of the central body and inferior horns of the lateral ventricles. The foramina of Monro transmit CSF between the third and lateral ventricles at the superolateral corners of the third ventricle. The aqueduct of Sylvius in the midbrain transmits CSF from the third to the fourth ventricles. It is the narrowest canal of the intracranial nervous system and is therefore the most common location of obstruction of flow by compression or tumor deposits, resulting in noncommunicating (obstructive) hydrocephalus. CSF in the fourth ventricle flows out of the ventricular system through the midline foramen of Magendie and the two lateral foramina of Luschka to the subarachnoid space.

CSF resorption back into the venous system occurs at arachnoid (or pacchionian) granulations, special outpouching structures from the arachnoid membrane that enhance fluid movement from the CSF space into the venous sinus system. Scarring from infection or inflammation or clogging of the

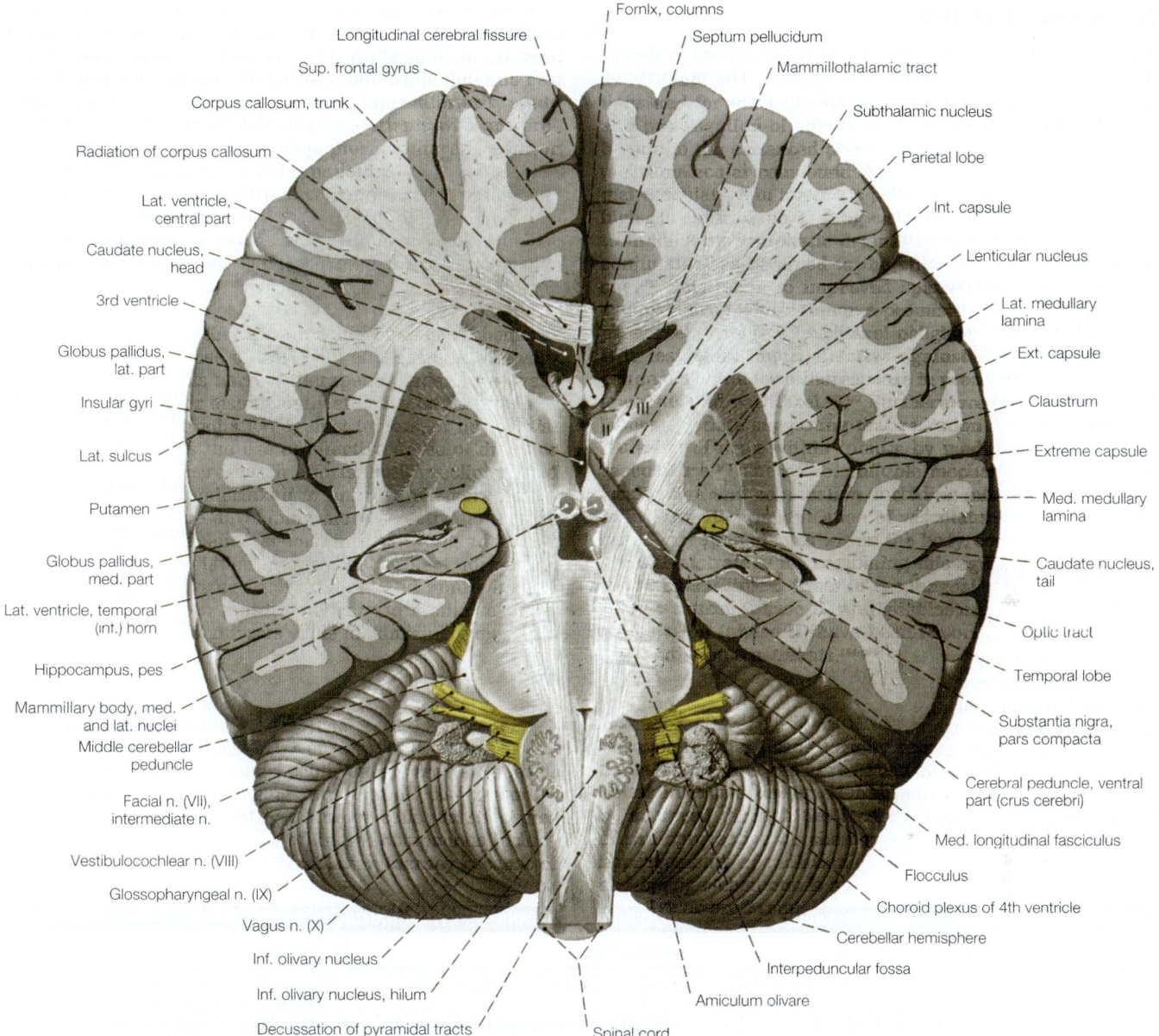

FIGURE 38.3. Section through the telencephalon and brainstem parallel with the cerebral peduncles. View of the posterior surface of the plane of sectioning. On the right side of the figure, the section reaches back to approximately the middle of the cerebral peduncle (oblique section). I to III indicate thalamic nuclei: I, medial nucleus; II, anterior nucleus; III, lateral nucleus. (Reprinted from Paulsen F, Waschke J, Sobotta J. *Sobotta Atlas of Human Anatomy.* 15th ed. Munich: Urban & Fischer, 2011. Copyright © 2011 Elsevier GmbH. With permission.)

arachnoid granulations causes increased pressure in the CSF space and communicating hydrocephalus.

EPIDEMIOLOGY

In 2016, there were an estimated 26,070 new cases of primary CNS tumors in the United States and 16,947 deaths, for an incidence of approximately 7.18 per 100,000 persons. The incidence of brain tumors increases with age.[1]

Occupational and environmental exposures have been associated with the development of CNS tumors. Farmers and petrochemical workers have been shown to have a higher incidence of primary brain tumors. A variety of chemical exposures have been linked, as reviewed by Ohgaki and Kleihues.[2] The use of cellular phones has been questioned as a contributing factor to the development of brain tumors. The World Health Organization (WHO) classified radiofrequency electromagnetic fields, such as those emitted by wireless phones, as "possibly carcinogenic to humans" (Group 2B) based on limited clinical evidence.[3] Although prior cohort, case–control, and time-trend analyses have shown no association between cell phone use and brain tumor risk,[4] more recent case–control studies have suggested a potential increased risk of glioma among individuals with the greatest cumulative lifetime cell phone use (>1,620 hours in one study).[5–9] However, significant concerns with respect to recall and selection biases in both studies prevent a causal association from being concluded.

Prior exposure to ionizing radiation is a known risk factor for development of primary CNS tumors, particularly meningiomas, but also gliomas, sarcomas, and other tumor types.[10,11] There is a 2.3% incidence of primary brain tumors in children treated with prophylactic cranial irradiation for acute leukemia, a 22-fold increase over expected.[12]

Development of intracranial malignancy is also associated with several hereditary diseases such as neurofibromatosis types 1 and 2, von Hippel-Lindau disease, and tuberous sclerosis. Other hereditary associations are with retinoblastoma and Li-Fraumeni syndrome.

NATURAL HISTORY

The natural history of a primary brain neoplasm is determined by its histology, grade, and location. The majority of adult gliomas spread invasively without forming a natural capsule. They frequently cause edema in surrounding tissue. This edema is usually vasogenic but may be cytotoxic. It is seen best on T2-weighted MRI and is responsible for at least some of the clinical symptoms and signs. The edema is a consequence of altered blood–brain barrier (BBB) permeability. Different tumors cause varying amounts of edema (in descending order, metastases, astrocytomas, meningiomas, and oligodendrogliomas).

Some high-grade neoplasms metastasize by "seeding" the subarachnoid and ventricular spaces. Because of gravity or flow, these metastatic deposits are often present in the caudal portion of the spinal canal. Tumors that have a propensity for CSF spread include medulloblastomas, germ cell tumors, and CNS lymphoma. The exact frequency of CSF spread among other histologies (e.g., germ cell tumors, ependymomas) is debated in the literature. Extracranial metastases from primary brain tumors are rare but can occur with medulloblastomas, germinomas, and high-grade astrocytomas.

CLINICAL PRESENTATION

The presenting symptoms of a primary brain tumor are classified as generalized or focal. Headache is more prevalent in patients with fast-growing, high-grade tumors. Seizures are a more common presenting feature in low-grade tumors. Focal neurologic deficits such as weakness, language dysfunction, or sensory loss are more frequent presentations of high-grade tumors. Acute events such as hemorrhage markedly alter the tempo of symptom onset regardless of tumor grade. Table 38.1 summarizes common clinical presentations of the more common CNS tumors.

Because brain parenchyma is anesthetic, headaches associated with brain tumors are due to increased intracranial pressure or to local pressure on sensitive intracranial structures (mainly dura and vessels). Headaches associated with increased intracranial pressure classically occur in the morning. Associated findings may include focal neurologic deficits, behavioral changes, and papilledema. Cushing triad is classically associated with increased intracranial pressure, but the full triad (hypertension, bradycardia, respiratory irregularity) is seen in only one-third of the cases of increased intracranial pressure. Long-standing increases in intracranial pressure may lead to optic atrophy and blindness because of transmission of the pressure to the optic nerves.

DIAGNOSTIC WORKUP

The initial workup of patients with brain tumors must include a complete history and physical examination. Information obtained from relatives and friends is helpful because many tumors cause changes in mentation not appreciated by the patient. In patients with symptoms, signs, or imaging suggestive of systemic dissemination, biopsy confirmation of the primary tumor or at least one of the extracranial metastatic sites is recommended. Solitary brain lesions in adult patients with certain types of known systemic cancer (e.g., lung, breast, or colon cancers or melanoma) are far more likely to be a cerebral metastasis than a primary CNS tumor, although this is not always the case.

Imaging Studies

MRI with a gadolinium (Gd)-containing contrast agent is the imaging modality of choice for most CNS tumors. Computed tomography (CT) is generally reserved for those situations in which MRI is contraindicated, such as implanted pacemaker, metal fragment, or paramagnetic surgical clips, or where there is a need to image the extent of calcification or hemorrhage.

TABLE 38.1 SYMPTOMS, SIGNS, AND DIAGNOSTIC CHARACTERISTICS OF VARIOUS INTRACRANIAL TUMORS

Tumor	Common Symptoms	Common Signs	Imaging Characteristics
Glioblastoma multiforme	Headache, seizure, unilateral weakness, mental changes	Focal presentation related to tumor location	Enhancing MRI or CT lesion, hypodense interior, often with associated edema
Meningioma	Localized headache	Focal presentation related to tumor location	Enhancing MRI or CT lesion associated with dura
Astrocytoma	Headache, seizure, unilateral weakness, mental changes	Focal presentation related to tumor location	May not enhance on CT or MRI
Cerebral	Headache, seizure, unilateral weakness, mental changes	Focal presentation related to tumor location	
Cerebellar	Occipital headache	Increased intracranial pressure (i.e., papilledema), abducens and oculomotor nerve deficits; coordination	
Brainstem or thalamus	Nausea, vomiting, ataxia	Increased intracranial pressure (i.e., papilledema), abducens and oculomotor nerve deficits; ataxia	May be seen only on MRI
Optic nerve	Ocular changes	Ocular changes	Uniform enhancement on MRI or CT scan
Medulloblastoma	Morning headaches, nausea, vomiting	Coordination, increased intracranial pressure (i.e., papilledema), abducens and oculomotor nerve deficits	Heterogeneously enhancing on MRI or CT, typical lateral location in adults
Ependymoma	Morning headaches, nausea, vomiting	Coordination, increased intracranial pressure (i.e., papilledema), abducens and oculomotor nerve deficits	Heterogeneous enhancement on MRI or CT with or without calcification
Neurilemoma, schwannoma, neurinomas	Unilateral deafness, vertigo	Ipsilateral acoustic and facial or trigeminal nerve deficits	Homogenous enhancing mass on MRI or CT, arising from cranial nerve
Oligodendroglioma	Insidious headache, mental changes	Focal presentation related to tumor location	Heterogeneous lesion that may or may not enhance on MRI or CT, frequently with calcification, cystic regions, or hemorrhage
Lymphoma	Focal presentation related to tumor location	Focal presentation related to tumor location	Homogeneous, intense enhancement on MRI, may have a diffuse or "cotton wool" appearance
Craniopharyngioma	Headache, mental changes, hemiplegia, seizure, vomiting, visual impairment	Cranial nerve deficits (II–VII)	Mixed cystic, calcified lesion on MRI and CT, arising from suprasellar region

CT, computed tomography; MRI, magnetic resonance imaging.

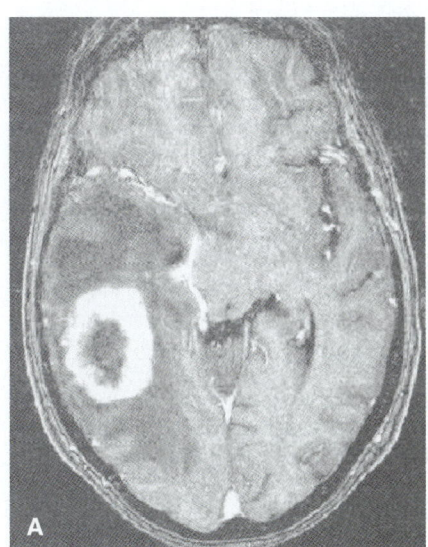
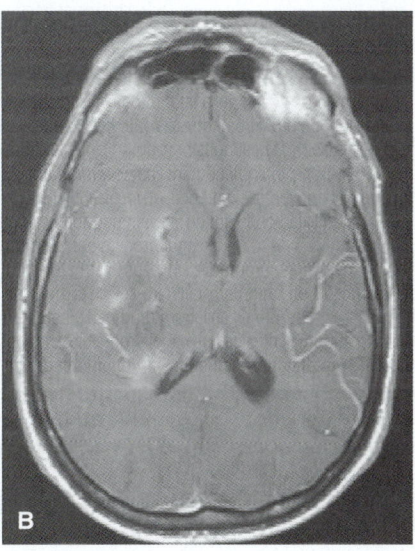

FIGURE 38.4. Magnetic resonance image of brain showing **(A)** glioblastoma, demonstrating a contrast-enhancing lesion with central necrosis and vasogenic edema; and **(B)** low-grade glioma, illustrating a nonenhancing lesion difficult to delineate from normal parenchyma.

Magnetic Resonance Imaging

The most useful imaging studies are T1-weighted sagittal images, Gd-enhanced (usually obtained in high-resolution modes such as SPGR or MP-RAGE) and non-enhanced T1 axial images, T2-weighted axial images, and FLAIR (fluid-attenuated inversion recovery) sequences.[13,14] As is the case with CT contrast agents, Gd-based contrast leaks into parenchyma in areas with BBB breakdown, and the paramagnetic properties of Gd generate hyperintense signal on T1 scans. T1 images usually are better at demonstrating anatomy and areas of contrast enhancement. T2 and FLAIR images are more sensitive for detecting edema and infiltrative tumor. Tumor appearance on T1-weighted MRI is similar to that on CT, although tumor volumes are better delineated on MRI, particularly with low-grade neoplasms that do not demonstrate contrast enhancement (Fig. 38.4). With the increasing incidence of posttreatment "pseudoprogression," additional specialized diffusion, perfusion, and spectroscopic sequences are being increasingly utilized to distinguish tumor from necrosis or pseudoprogression, and PET imaging may also have some role in this; in the United States, only FDG-PET is approved, but amino acid, FLT, and F-DOPA PET imaging is being evaluated (Fig. 38.5). Diffusion-weighted and functional MR also has utility in guiding resection.

Neuraxis Imaging

For neoplasms with high risk of CSF spread, staging of the neuraxis is essential. Gd-enhanced MRI of the spine is the

FIGURE 38.5. Oligodendroglioma imaged using an anatomic imaging technique, contrast-enhanced 3D-SPGR T1-w MRI (*top image panel*), and a functional imaging technique, FDG-PET (*bottom image panel*). The red contour delineates the extent of increased metabolic activity seen using functional imaging. Looking at the top panel, one can appreciate the fact that if the anatomic image set alone would be used for target definition it would yield a gross underestimation of the target volume as compared with the functional imaging technique.

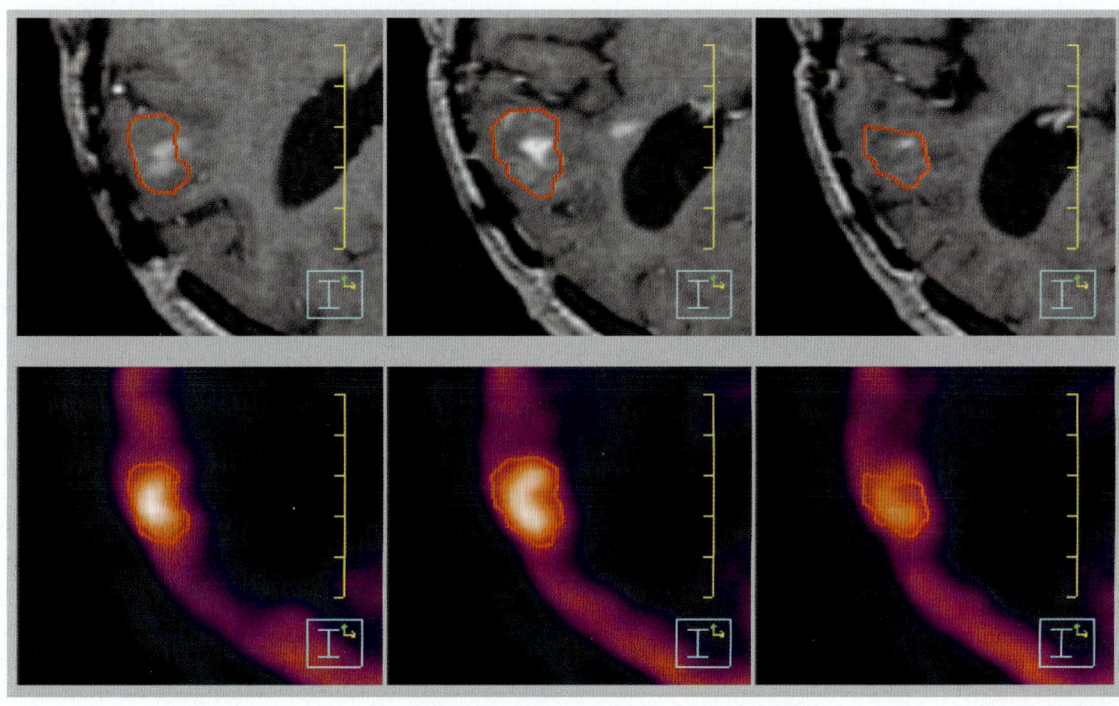

imaging modality of choice. Ideally, neuraxis imaging should be performed before surgery. In the immediate postoperative period, spinal MRI scans may be difficult to interpret because arachnoiditis and blood products in the CSF can mimic leptomeningeal metastasis. Delayed spinal MRI (>3 weeks after surgery), combined with an increased dose of intravenous Gd, is a sensitive imaging study to detect leptomeningeal disease.

Histologic Confirmation of Diagnosis

The morbidity of biopsy has decreased significantly with improvements in operative technique and anesthesia, as well as the availability of stereotactic biopsy techniques. Exception might be made in selected patients, such as those patients with known active systemic cancer and multiple lesions that are radiographically consistent with brain metastases, patients with typical clinical and MRI findings of a brainstem glioma or optic nerve meningioma, HIV-positive patients with CT or MRI findings consistent with primary CNS lymphoma (PCNSL) and positive Epstein-Barr virus PCR in the CSF, or patients with secretory germ cell tumors.

Cerebrospinal Fluid Cytology

CSF cytology is essential for staging tumors with a propensity for CSF spread (e.g., medulloblastoma, germ cell tumors, and CNS lymphoma). Sampling of the CSF in the immediate post-operative period may lead to false-positive results, however, and is best done before surgery or more than 3 weeks after surgery, as long as intracranial pressure is not elevated. CSF spread of tumor may be associated with several abnormal CSF findings. These include CSF pressure above 150 mm H_2O at the lumbar level in a laterally positioned patient, elevated protein level (>40 mg/dL in the lumbar cistern), a reduced glucose level (below 50 mg/mL), and the finding of tumor cells by cytologic examination. Tumor markers in the CSF may help in making the diagnosis.

Differential Diagnosis

Most adults with new or persistent neurologic findings (focal deficit, increased intracranial pressure, seizures, altered mentation) are investigated using CT or MRI. There are a number of classical imaging features that help refine the differential diagnosis (Table 38.2).

TABLE 38.2 DIFFERENTIAL DIAGNOSIS OF SPACE-OCCUPYING LESIONS ON COMPUTED TOMOGRAPHY OR MAGNETIC RESONANCE IMAGING

Pathology	Features on CT or MRI
Neoplasm	
Primary	Solitary, no prior cancer, thick nodular CE
Metastatic	Multiple, prior cancer, ++edema, located at gray/white junction
Infectious	
Abscess	Fever, acutely ill, ±systemic infection, cyst cavity with smooth thin walls, CE, and restricted diffusion within cavity
Cerebritis	Fever, acutely ill, ±systemic infection, diffuse T2 change, no CE mass
Meningitis	Diffuse enhancement of meninges on T1-weighted imaging (may simulate leptomeningeal metastases)
Vascular	
Infarct	Gray and white matter involvement, wedgelike vascular distribution associated with restricted diffusion and low ADC signal
Bleeding	Homogenous, clears quickly, residual hemosiderin ring
Treatment-related necrosis	Central hypodensity, ring CE, edema, >6 mo after radiation therapy or chemotherapy, metabolic scan shows low activity

ADC, apparent diffusion coefficient; CE, contrast enhancement; CT, computed tomography; MRI, magnetic resonance imaging.

PATHOLOGY

Primary intracranial tumors are of ecto- and mesodermal origin and arise from the brain, cranial nerves, meninges, pituitary, pineal, and vascular elements. In 2016, the WHO revised its classification system for pathologic subtypes of CNS tumors to combine histology with molecular parameters such as IDH1 mutation, 1p19q codeletion, and H3 K27M mutation for gliomas; RELA fusion for ependymoma; and WNT and SHH activation for medulloblastoma (Table 38.3).[15] Guidelines for assigning grade of malignancy are provided, where applicable.

GENERAL MANAGEMENT

The medical management of patients with brain tumors includes management of increased intracranial pressure, seizures, and venous thromboembolic disease.

Cerebral Edema

Glucocorticoids are used to control neurologic signs and symptoms caused by cerebral edema. Lower doses of steroids (e.g., 2 to 4 mg dexamethasone) twice daily have been shown to be as effective as higher doses, and in fact, based on pharmacokinetic properties, even once-daily dosing should be effective. Prolonged steroid use is associated with multiple medical problems, and therefore steroids should be discontinued or tapered to the lowest dose necessary, as soon as possible. Dexamethasone is the most common corticosteroid used for historical reasons and because of minimal mineral–corticoid effects. As with all corticosteroids, a taper is necessary to prevent rebound in cerebral edema and also to allow the pituitary–adrenal axis to recover.

Seizures

Patients with seizures require anticonvulsants. Because anticonvulsants such as carbamazepine, phenobarbital, and phenytoin induce hepatic cytochrome P-450 isoenzymes, which increase the metabolism and clearance of several cancer chemotherapy agents such as paclitaxel and irinotecan,[16] non–enzyme-inducing anticonvulsants, such as levetiracetam, lacosamide, lamotrigine, and pregabalin, are preferred.

Prophylactic anticonvulsant use (in patients who have never experienced a seizure) remains controversial, although practice guidelines from the American Academy of Neurology recommend against their use because of lack of data.[17,18]

SURGERY

Surgical procedures can be summarized as biopsy for diagnosis only, resection for cure, surgical debulking for management of mass effect-related symptoms, CSF diversion procedures to relieve acute symptoms caused by increased intracranial pressure or hydrocephalus, and increasingly re-resection to distinguish and manage the effects of progressive tumor from symptomatic necrosis or pseudoprogression. Other roles of surgery include the placement of chemotherapy wafers, brachytherapy devices, and catheters for interstitial drug delivery and for monitoring tumor drug concentrations and/or biologic effects. Complete resection of tumor is associated with a survival advantage for some tumor types.[19] However, for some radio- and/or chemosensitive malignancies such as PCNSL, aggressive resection is unnecessary, and the surgeon's role is limited to providing diagnostic material.

Operative Technique

Ultrasound and CT- and MRI-guidance systems provide surgeons with intraoperative navigation based upon preoperative and/or intraoperative data. In general, these consist of a workstation into which the relevant imaging studies have been

TABLE 38.3 HISTOLOGIC CLASSIFICATION OF TUMORS OF THE CENTRAL NERVOUS SYSTEM

Diffuse astrocytic and oligodendroglial tumors
  Diffuse astrocytoma, IDH mutant
    Gemistocytic astrocytoma, IDH mutant
  Diffuse astrocytoma, IDH wild type
  Diffuse astrocytoma, NOS
  Anaplastic astrocytoma, IDH mutant
  Anaplastic astrocytoma, IDH wild type
  Anaplastic astrocytoma, NOS
  Glioblastoma, IDH wild type
    Giant cell glioblastoma
    Gliosarcoma
    Epithelioid glioblastoma
  Glioblastoma, IDH mutant
  Glioblastoma, NOS
  Diffuse midline glioma, H3 K27M mutant
  Oligodendroglioma, IDH mutant and 1p/19q codeleted
  Anaplastic oligodendroglioma, NOS
  Oligoastryctoma, NOS
  Anaplastic oligoastrocytoma, NOS
Other astrocytic tumors
  Pilocytic astrocytoma
    Pilomyxoid astrocytoma
  Subependymal giant cell astrocytoma
  Pleomorphic xanthoastrocytoma
  Anaplastic pleomorphic xanthoastrocytoma
Ependymal tumors
  Subependymoma
  Myxopapillary ependymoma
  Ependymoma
    Papillary ependymoma
    Clear cell ependymoma
    Tancystic ependymoma
  Ependymoma, RELA fusion-positive
  Anaplastic ependymoma
Choroid plexus tumors
  Choroid plexus papilloma
  Angiocentric glioma
  Astroblastoma
Neuronal and mixed neuronal-glial tumors
  Dysembryoplastic neuroepithelial tumor
  Gangliocytoma
  Ganglioglioma
  Anaplastic ganglioglioma
  Dysplastic cerebellar gangliocytoma (Lhermitte-Duclos disease)
  Desmoplastic infantile astrocytoma and ganglioma
  Papillary glioneuronal tumor
  Rosette-forming glioneuronal tumor
  Diffuse leptomeningeal glioneuronal tumor
  Central neurocytoma
  Extraventricular neurocytoma
  Cerebellar liponeurocytoma
  Paraganglioma
Tumors of the pineal region
  Pineocytoma
  Pineal parenchymal tumor of intermediate differentiation
  Pineoblastoma
  Papillary tumor of the pineal region
Embryonal tumors
  Medulloblastoma, genetically defined
    Medulloblastoma, WNT-activated
    Medulloblastoma, SHH-activated and TP53 mutant
    Medulloblastoma, SHH-activated and TP53 wild type
    Medulloblastoma, non-WNT/non-SHH
      Medulloblastoma, group 3
      Medulloblastoma, group 4
  Medulloblastoma, histologically defined
    Medulloblastoma, classic
    Medulloblastoma, desmoplastic/nodular
    Medulloblastoma with extensive nodularity
  Medulloblastoma, large cell/anaplastic
  Medulloblastoma, NOS
  Embryonal tumor with multilayered rosettes, C19MC altered

Meningiomas
  Meningioma
  Meningothelial meningioma
  Fibrous meningioma
  Transitional meningioma
  Psammomatous meningioma
  Angiomatous meningioma
  Microcystic meningioma
  Secretory meningioma
  Lymphoplasmacyte-rich meningioma
  Metaplastic meningioma
  Chordoid meningioma
  Clear cell meningioma
  Atypical meningioma
  Papillary meningioma
  Rhabdoid meningioma
  Anaplastic (malignant) meningioma
Mesenchymal, nonmeningothelial tumors
  Solitary fibrous tumor/hemangiopericytoma
    Grade 1
    Grade 2
    Grade 3
  Hemangioblastoma
  Hemangioma
  Epithelioid hemangioendothelioma
  Angiosarcoma
  Kaposi sarcoma
  Ewing sarcoma/PNET
  Lipoma
  Angiolipoma
  Hibernoma
  Liposarcoma
  Desmoid-type fibromatosis
  Myofibroblastoma
  Inflammatory myofibroblastic tumor
  Benign fibrous histiocytoma
  Fibrosarcoma
  Undifferentiated pleomorphic sarcoma/malignant fibrous histiocytoma
  Leiomyoma
  Leiomyosarcoma
  Rhabdomyoma
  Rhabdomyosarcoma
  Chondroma
  Chrondrosarcoma
  Osteoma
  Osteochondroma
  Osteosarcoma
  Chondrosarcoma
  Malignant fibrous histiocytoma
  Rhabdomyosarcoma
Melanocytic tumors
  Meningeal melanocytosis
  Meningeal melanocytoma
  Meningeal melanoma
  Meningeal melanomatosis
Lymphomas
Diffuse large B-cell lymphoma of the CNS
Immunodeficiency-associated CNS lymphomas
  AIDS-related diffuse large B-cell lymphoma
  EBV-positive diffuse large B-cell lymphoma, NOS
  Lymphomatoid granulomatosis
Intravascular large B-cell lymphoma
Low-grade B-cell lymphomas of the CNS
T-cell and NK/T-cell lymphomas of the CNS
Anaplastic large-cell lymphoma, ALK-positive
Anaplastic large-cell lymphoma, ALK-negative
MALT lymphoma of the dura
Histiocytic tumors
  Langerhans cell histiocytosis
  Erdheim-Chester disease
  Rosai-Dorfman disease
  Juvenile xanthogranuloma
  Histiocytic sarcoma

(Continued)

Section III

TABLE 38.3 HISTOLOGIC CLASSIFICATION OF TUMORS OF THE CENTRAL NERVOUS SYSTEM (*Continued*)

Embryonal tumor with multilayered Rosettes, NOS	Germ- cell tumors
Medulloepithelioma	Germinoma
CNS neuroblastoma	Embryonal carcinoma
CNS ganglioneuroblastoma	Yolk-sac tumor
CNS embryonal tumor, NOS	Choriocarcinoma
Atypical teratoid/rhabdoid tumor	Teratoma
CNS embryonal tumor with rhabdoid features	Mature teratoma
Tumors of cranial and spinal nerves	Immature teratoma
Schwannoma	Teratoma with malignant transformation
Cellular schwannoma	Mixed germ cell tumor
Plexiform schwannoma	Tumors of the sellar region
Melanotic schwannoma	Craniopharyngioma
Neurofibroma	Adamantinomatous craniopharyngioma
Atypical neurofibroma	Papillary craniopharyngioma
Plexiform neurofibroma	Granulosa cell tumor of the sellar region
Perineurioma	Pituicytoma
Hybrid nerve sheath tumors	Spindle cell oncocytoma
Malignant peripheral nerve sheath tumor	Metastatic tumors
Epithelioid MPNST	
MPNST with perineurial differentiation	

The italicized entries are provisional, i.e., the WHO Working Group felt there was insufficient evidence to recognize these as distinct entities at this time.
Reprinted from Louis DN, Ohgaki H, Wieslter OD, et al. *World Health Organization histologic classificaiton of tumours of the central nervous system.* Lyon: International Agency for Research on Cancer, 2016, with permission from the WHO.

loaded, together with infrared or ultrasound detectors that recognize the 3D orientation and position in space of various tools. Once the patient is registered, the tumor's margins are "visualized" below the scalp so that the surgeon can plan the smallest and safest approach. Resection is assisted by use of the intraoperative microscope and guided by the appearance and consistency of tumor tissue compared with surrounding normal brain. Intraoperative CT, MRI, or ultrasonography can be used to evaluate the completeness of tumor resection. In the case of lesions that are in or near suspected functional cortex, cortical mapping under awake conditions can be performed to localize areas that are critical for motor or speech function. Endoscopy can be used to minimize access for resection of intraventricular lesions or pituitary tumors, as well as for reestablishing pathways of CSF flow, for example, in cases of tumors that have obstructed the cerebral aqueduct, thereby avoiding the need for a CSF shunt. In addition to intraoperative image guidance, the use of fluorescent tumor-localizing dyes such as 5-aminolevulinec acid has gained acceptance in Europe to enhance the completeness of resection and is being investigated in the United States.

Stereotactic biopsy is performed with either a stereotactic frame or scalp fiducials; a CT or MRI is performed and the data are loaded into an image-guidance system. A target and entry points are selected, and the trajectory is visualized on a workstation. The entry point is located on the patient's scalp, and a small burr hole or twist drill hole is made. The biopsy needle is oriented using the image-guidance system and passed to the appropriate depth, and tissue samples are obtained. Multiple tissue samples may be obtained along the needle tract, until the pathologist can provide an intraoperative diagnosis. The volume of tissue removed is insufficient to relieve mass effect, and patients who are symptomatic are better treated by open resection.

A more recently developed stereotactic technique for treating the mass component of brain tumors involves the use of laser interstitial thermal therapy (LITT). Briefly, this approach involves the temporary stereotactic implantation of a cooled laser probe, which can be activated and manipulated within the MRI environment. The laser is used to heat, but not coagulate, adjacent tissue, and it is progressively advanced through the target tissue as the treatment progresses. This approach takes advantage of a previously described relationship between temperature and time, which can be used to predict the likelihood of permanent injury even with relatively small

(<10°C) increases in local tissue temperature. A specialized MRI technique, called MR thermometry, is used to monitor tissue temperature, and the combination of temperature data with duration of heating is used by specialized LITT software to create a visual indication on each MRI slice of the probability of tissue death as a result of treatment. LITT for brain tumors was developed initially for the treatment of malignant tumors that would be difficult to access via conventional surgery, and its practice has expanded to include resectable and even benign pathologies. Although the LITT procedure has shown an encouraging safety profile, there have not been any randomized studies to date that have directly compared this approach to conventional surgical treatment.[20]

RADIOTHERAPY

Radiobiologic Considerations Underlying Tissue Injury

The process of radiation injury in the brain is highly complex and dependent on a variety of technical factors including dose, volume, fraction size, and the specific target cell population, as well as secondary mechanisms of expression of injury such as vascular leak causing edema, vascular endothelial loss resulting in hypoxic injury, reactive gliosis, and to-date inadequately studied host factors. Some structures (e.g., optic chiasm, hypothalamus, lacrimal gland, lenses, etc.) appear to be substantially more sensitive to radiation than others. Even focal lesions may result in widespread radiographic and/or functional perturbations. The time course for the manifestation of injury can be highly variable and the clinical picture easily confounded with tumor progression. The effect on endothelial cells often becomes manifest as an early T2 signal abnormality on MRI, possibly due to disruption of the BBB and edema formation. Metabolic perturbations observed with PET may reflect oligodendroglial demyelination. Further vascular perturbation and regeneration in response to injury results in an enhancing lesion on imaging. Delayed effects include white matter necrosis and vascular obliteration. The time course can be shortened from several months to a few weeks by increasing the volume of brain irradiated or increasing the fraction size or total dose.

Historically, late injury from radiotherapy has been reported as the "tolerance" dose at either the 5% or 50% risk level at 5 years (TD 5/5 or TD 50/5, respectively). The values for whole-brain fractionated radiotherapy at 2 Gy/fraction are 60 and 70 Gy, respectively. With partial-brain irradiation, the corresponding values are 70 and 80 Gy, respectively. In the setting of fractionated radiotherapy with a fraction size <2.5 Gy, quantitative analyses of normal tissues effect in the clinic (QUANTEC) have estimated 5% and 10% rates of symptomatic necrosis at 72 and 90 Gy maximum equivalent doses in 2-Gy fractions, respectively.[21,22]

General Concepts
Pertinent Anatomic Landmarks
With conventional simulation, radiographic and surface topographic reference points for appreciation of beam-to-head projection geometry are necessary. The external auditory meatus define anatomic reference planes such as Reid base line and the Frankfort horizontal plane, connecting points in the two external auditory meatus and one anterior infraorbital edge. Unless marked at simulation, the external auditory meatus may be difficult to see on lateral projections because of the overlying temporal bone. The two lateral parts of the anterior cranial fossa, the two anterior parts of the middle cranial fossa floors, and the two mandibular angle points, with their lateral locations, represent appropriate reference points. With CT-based planning, the need for identifying these is obviated.

In a lateral radiograph, the sella turcica is centrally located and marks the lower border of the medial telencephalon and diencephalon. The hypothalamic structures are located an additional 1 cm superior to the sellar floor, and the optic canal runs at most 1 cm superior and 1 cm anterior to that point. The pineal body (or the tentorial notch) usually sits approximately 1 cm posterior and 3 cm superior to the external auditory meatus. The cribriform plate is the most inferior part of the anterior cranial fossa; it is an important reference point for the inferior border of whole-brain irradiation fields. In most patients, little distance is found between the lateral projections of the lens and the most inferior part of the cribriform plate. The temporal lobes are situated in the middle cranial fossae, the floor of which is easily identified on lateral radiographs. Individualized blocks should always be used to delineate the field inferior border for WBRT.

On an anteroposterior radiograph with a Frankfort horizontal plane (ear markers and one inferior orbital edge in a horizontal plane), the temporal bones (pyramids) project in the orbits. This implies that the ethmoid sinuses and the sphenoid sinus will project between the orbits, the sella just above these air cavities, and the foramen magnum just below the connection line between the inferior orbital edges. The frontal and occipital lobes therefore project above the orbits, and the temporal lobes and cerebellum project in and somewhat below the orbits.

Treatment Setup
The head should be positioned so that its major axes are parallel with and perpendicular to the central axis incident beam and the treatment table. It may be preferable to fully flex or extend the neck in some patients depending on tumor location and choice of beams, although the use of noncoplanar fields and IMRT techniques makes this less necessary (Fig. 38.6).

Reproducibility of head positioning is achieved by using a fixation device. Many devices are available for this with reproducibility precision ranging from 1 to 5 mm. With the advent of image-guided radiation therapy (IGRT) and intrafraction motion detection, unprecedented accuracy can be achieved in delivering radiotherapy. This permits substantial reduction in margins for setup variability.[23]

Target Volume Definition
Two major factors drive margin selection: the inaccuracy of estimating the clinical target volume (CTV) and the specific

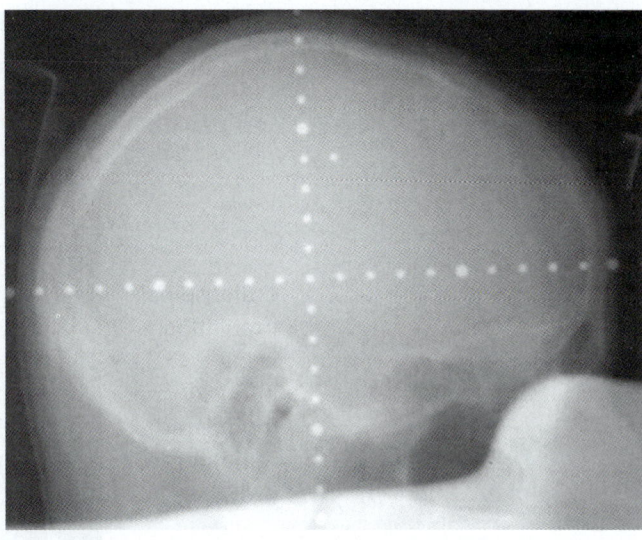

FIGURE 38.6. Lateral portal localization film of whole brain illustrating adequate inclusion of the cribriform plate and the anterior and middle cranial fossae.

dosimetric and setup variability components that are institution specific and determine the planning target volume (PTV).

Common sense and practice dictates that these CTV expansion margins should not traverse anatomically discontiguous structures or include areas unlikely to be infiltrated by tumor. Inclusion of the bony skull is unnecessary unless direct tumor extension is suspected. With some exceptions, "compartmental crossing" to the contralateral hemisphere or, for example, into the posterior fossa or the brainstem for a supratentorial cortical tumor, is not necessary, but because many infiltrating gliomas "cross" through the anterior and/or posterior corpus callosal tracts, these should be adequately included in CTV margin selection.

Radiotherapy Techniques
The most commonly employed radiotherapy techniques in the management of CNS tumors are partial-brain irradiation, whole-brain radiotherapy (WBRT), craniospinal irradiation (CSI), stereotactic radiosurgery (SRS), fractionated stereotactic radiotherapy (FSRT), less commonly brachytherapy, and, recently, emerging utilization of proton therapy. The indications for each of these techniques are discussed under the sections on the individual tumor types. CSI is more frequently used in management of pediatric CNS tumors and is discussed in detail in Chapter 82.

Whole-Brain Radiotherapy
WBRT is used most often for patients with brain metastases but also for patients with PCNSLs and as a component of CSI.

Whole-brain irradiation is administered through parallel-opposed lateral portals. The inferior field border should be inferior to the cribriform plate, the middle cranial fossa, and the foramen magnum, all of which should be distinguishable on simulation or portal localization radiographs (Fig. 38.7). The safety margin depends on penumbra width, head fixation, and anatomic factors, but should be at least 1 cm, even under optimal conditions. A special problem arises anteriorly because sparing of the ocular lenses and lacrimal glands may require blocking with <5-mm margins at the cribriform plate.

The anterior border of the field should be approximately 3 cm posterior to the ipsilateral eyelid for the diverging beam to exclude the contralateral lens. However, this results in only approximately 40% of the prescribed dose to the posterior eye. A better alternative is to angle the beam approximately 3 degrees or more (100- or 80-cm source-to-axis distance mid-

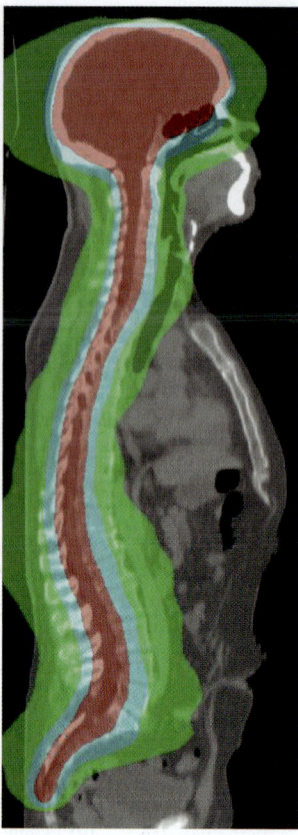

Craniospinal
irradlation
using
intensity-
modulated
radiotherapy
(IMRT)

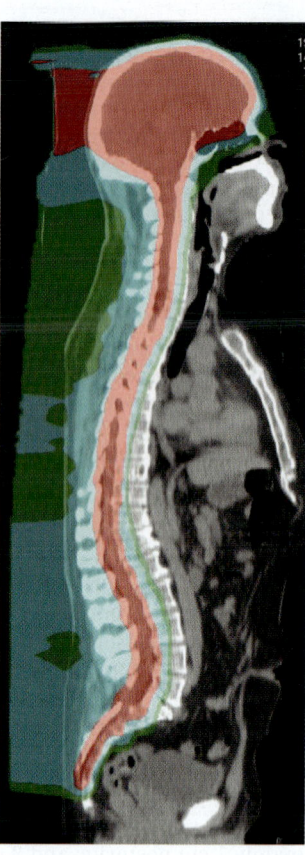

Craniospinal
irradiation
using proton
therapy

FIGURE 38.7. Comparison of proton therapy to intensity-modulated radiotherapy for craniospinal irradiation demonstrates negligent "exit" dose in visceral structures anterior to the spine and maximal sparing of vertebral body-based marrow achieved with proton therapy.

line but also field size dependent) against the frontal plane so that the anterior beam border traverses posterior to the lenses (approximately 2 cm posterior to eyelid markers). Placing a radiopaque marker on both lateral canthi and aligning the markers permits individualization in terms of the couch angle. This arrangement provides full dose to the posterior eyes. However, the eyelid-to-lens and -retina topography is individually more constant than the canthus, and lateral beam eye shielding is better individualized with the aid of CT or MRI scans.[24] When in doubt about tumor coverage or lens sparing for tumors in a subfrontal or middle cranial fossa location, CT-based contouring and planning should be considered.

Craniospinal Irradiation

Traditional CSI techniques utilize opposed lateral cranial fields and one or more posterior spinal fields depending on patient size. The junctioning of noncoplanar fields in the cervical region is potentially hazardous because of the risk of overlap resulting in radiation myelitis. Consequently, great attention needs to be paid to precise immobilization, and a variety of immobilization devices are available for this purpose. Image guidance during radiotherapy can help in ensuring day-to-day reproducibility. The prone position permits direct visualization of the light field from the linear accelerator on the patient thereby allowing daily adjustments of the junctions. However, if anesthesia or sedation is required as may be the case with young children, a supine setup may be considered safer.[25] To avoid the risk of dose overlap, at least two techniques (with numerous variations) are commonly used, and several variations of these have also been reported. In the first, a gap is employed between abutting fields such that the beam edges intersect deep to the spinal cord. This gap could result in a cold spot in a small segment of the spinal cord. If the beam intersection point were raised dorsally, a hot spot would result.

The second technique attempts to avoid this problem by using a half-beam technique in which the caudal edge of the

brain is matched precisely with the cephalad edge of the abutting spine field without cold or hot spots. This requires collimator angulation and sometimes a couch rotation as well. For both techniques, the use of moving junctions (known as "feathering") smoothens out any dose inhomogeneity.[26] Several studies have demonstrated that adequate coverage of the subfrontal region and posterior fossa and depth assessment of the cord require CT-based planning. Given the complexity of CSI, we recommend that it be delivered at centers with adequate staff, experience, and expertise.

With sophisticated techniques such as image-guided intensity-modulated helical tomotherapy and volumetric arc-modulated radiotherapy (VMAT), it is possible to treat the entire neuraxis in a single setup.[27] Increasingly, proton therapy has been used for CSI with placement of the finite distal range in the vertebral body leading to negligent "exit" dose in visceral structures anterior to the spine and maximal sparing of vertebral body-based marrow (Fig. 38.8).

Stereotactic Radiosurgery

Stereotactic radiosurgery (SRS) requires a team composed at a minimum of a radiation oncologist, neurosurgeon, and radiation oncology physicist, in addition to appropriate support staff. SRS can be delivered using a conventional or modified linear accelerator (LINAC) system, a Gamma Knife (Elekta Corp., Stockholm, Sweden) or a robotically controlled miniaturized linear accelerator (CyberKnife). In LINAC radiosurgery, circular or oval collimators ranging from 4 to 40 mm have historically been used to collimate the treatment beam into a circular pencil beam, and treatment is delivered using multiple noncoplanar arcs that intersect at a single point to treat an approximately spherical target of <4 cm in diameter. Newer miniaturized multileaf collimators allow beam shaping. Techniques incorporate multiple noncoplanar arcs with couch and jaw rotations, which permits a greater portion of the three-dimensional space subtended over the skull to be utilized for beam entry. This approach, sometimes referred

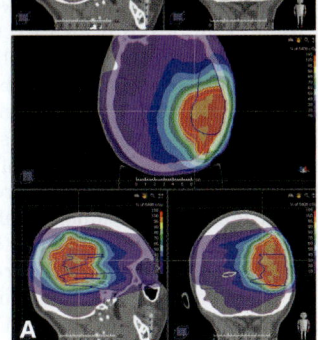

Low-Grade Glioma   **Pituitary Adenoma**

Proton Therapy

Intensity Modulated Radiotherapy

FIGURE 38.8. Comparison of proton therapy to intensity-modulated radiotherapy (IMRT) treatment plans for **(A)** left temporal oligodendroglioma and **(B)** nonfunctional pituitary adenoma, demonstrating tight target coverage and significant sparing of low-dose radiation exposure to normal tissues throughout the brain in tumor types with favorable prognosis.

to as the "hyperarc technique," allows for better dose conformality and rapid treatment of multiple intracranial lesions, without the need for selecting individual isocenters for each lesion. The legacy Gamma Knife is a fixed beam multisource radiation unit containing 201 cobalt-60 (^{60}Co) sources that are collimated using a helmet with circular apertures ranging from 4 to 18 mm that are focused onto a single target point. The newer Gamma Knife technology obviates the need for "helmet changes" and can effectively allow IMRT-like dose distributions to be created. For irregularly shaped lesions, treatments delivered using either noncoplanar arcs delivered through a single circular collimator or a single collimator helmet lead to the inclusion of a large amount of normal brain and yield inferior conformality. In these cases, it is advantageous to use multiple circular collimators or collimator helmets placed on different target points (and in the newer version of the Gamma Knife [Perfexion], different segments can be treated with different collimator diameters, and differential weighting is also possible) or to consider the use of multileaf collimated beams. The "hyperarc technique" referred above also achieves improved dose conformality because of the combination of multiple noncoplanar arcs, use of a sophisticated multileaf collimator, varying collimator rotations, and multiple couch angles. The newest version of the Gamma Knife (Icon) incorporates an on-board kV imaging tube capable of generating volumetric CT images that permit noninvasive and repetitive positioning for fractionated treatments.

Radiation Therapy Oncology Group (RTOG) study 90-05 established the maximum tolerated dose of single faction SRS to be 24, 18, and 15 Gy for tumors ≤20, 21 to 30, and 31 to 40 mm in maximum diameter, respectively, and these and other parameters are frequently used to guide prescription doses.[28] In modern practice, because the number of intracranial lesions treated in one SRS session has increased significantly, there has been a tendency toward decreasing the SRS dose; for example, in a large Japanese study of multiple brain metastases, the SRS dose was decreased to 15 Gy.[29]

Fractionated Stereotactic Radiotherapy

For lesions larger than 4 cm and/or located in critical regions, the delivery of a single large fraction treatment as in SRS is not desirable because of a high risk of CNS toxicity. FSRT is a hybrid between conventionally fractionated radiotherapy and SRS that combines fractionation with stereotactic localization and targeting techniques. Various systems for FSRT have been developed, with a reported accuracy of 1 to 3 mm.[30] As for SRS, the use of multiple arcs and circular collimators for irregularly shaped lesions leads to the inclusion of a large amount of normal tissue. The use of multiple noncoplanar fixed fields each having a unique entrance and exit pathway will be preferable because of better conformality, as multileaf collimators are almost always used.[31-33] With the Perfexion device, the use of the "Extend" frame permits FSRT as well as targeting of lower cranial lesions. With the incorporation of on-board volumetric imaging, modern LINACS and the most recent version of the Gamma Knife (Icon) also permit fractionation, using noninvasive mask-fixation systems. The CyberKnife also permits this option using repetitive 2D radiographic imaging incorporated into a sophisticated skull-anatomy based visualization software. There is increasing use of a 9 Gy x 3 fractions schedule of FSRT for larger (>3 cm) brain metastases.

Heavy Charged Particles

Heavy charged particle beams deposit their dose at a depth that depends on their energy over a distance of few millimeters when the heavy charged particles come to rest, the so-called Bragg peak. In order to cover a larger volume, the particle beam can be modulated, in effect adding up multiple Bragg peaks. The very sharp dose gradient at the distal edge permits the use of high-dose radiotherapy for tumors in critical locations, such as at the clivus and base of the skull, and provides better normal tissue sparing in other situations, especially, for example, in CSI.[24,34] Currently, a small number of European and Japanese centers are treating CNS tumors with carbon ions, which putatively have higher linear energy of transfer (LET) and presumed superior biologic effect, but no substantial clinical data are available to back these claims. There are currently no US centers utilizing these technologies, although neutron-beam irradiation, with or without coadministration of boronated agents to increase the cross-sectional area of interaction, continues to be used in some US centers.

Brachytherapy and Radiocolloid Solutions

Selection criteria for brachytherapy include tumor confined to one hemisphere, no transcallosal or subependymal spread, small size (<5 to 6 cm), well circumscribed on CT or MRI, and accessible location for the implant. A balloon-based system, GliaSite, placed into the cavity at the time of surgery has been employed in the treatment of recurrent malignant gliomas whose largest spatial dimension is <4 cm and are roughly spherical.[35] After treatment planning, the balloon is filled with a liquid that contains organically bound iodine-125 (^{125}I) and treatment is completed within 3 to 7 days. Direct infusion of radioimmunoglobulins has been used in primary and recurrent brain gliomas.[36]

CHEMOTHERAPY AND TARGETED AGENTS

Conventional Chemotherapy

Many conventional chemotherapy agents do not adequately penetrate normal or nonenhancing tumor-infiltrated brain, while some drugs, despite having a molecular weight and chemical structure that make them appear capable of crossing the BBB, are actively effluxed out of the brain parenchyma by p-glycoprotein and other active transporter substrates. Even when drug delivery is adequate, most CNS tumors are resistant to most conventional chemotherapeutic agents. Alkylating agents such as BCNU (carmustine) and CCNU (lomustine) have been the most widely studied drugs in CNS tumors. These agents cross the BBB, but prolonged use is difficult because of cumulative myelotoxicity and the dose-related risk of pulmonary fibrosis. Despite radiographic responses in 15% to 40% of patients, the impact on survival has been modest at best. Procarbazine has similar efficacy but is better tolerated. Cisplatin and carboplatin have been used as either single agents or in combination regimens. Response rates have been modest, and their impact on survival is unclear. Topoisomerase I (CPT-11, irinotecan) and topoisomerase II inhibitors (etoposide) have shown only modest activity. Taxanes, such as paclitaxel, have not demonstrated activity as single agents. Temozolomide (TMZ), an oral agent with excellent bioavailability, has a good toxicity profile and is the only agent to demonstrate a survival benefit for glioblastoma and anaplastic astrocytoma patients in randomized clinical trials.

The use of combination regimens plays a role in the management of specific CNS tumors. Radiation therapy with immediate chemotherapy utilizing the combination of procarbazine, CCNU, and vincristine (PCV) prolongs survival in patients with anaplastic oligodendroglioma and high-risk low-grade gliomas.[37] Other CNS tumors in which combination regimens are standard of care include PCNSL (high-dose methotrexate with procarbazine/vincristine, or high-dose cytarabine, or TMZ) and medulloblastoma (CCNU, cisplatin, and vincristine or cisplatin and cyclophosphamide and vincristine).

Direct Delivery of Therapeutic Agents

Methods for circumventing the BBB include implantation of slow-release chemotherapy wafers into a tumor resection cavity,[38,39] pharmacologic or osmotic BBB disruption,[40,41] and convection-enhanced drug delivery (CED). CED involves the use of intracerebrally implanted catheters to deliver a drug into the brain parenchyma or tumor, at a slow but continuous rate of flow. Unlike diffusion, in which a drug distributes along an exponentially decaying concentration gradient depending on the size of the molecule, drug distribution by CED is less size-dependent, occurs over a larger volume of brain tissue, and results in a more uniform drug concentration within the volume of distribution.[42,43] Large and/or hydrophilic agents that do not cross the BBB are ideal candidates for delivery via CED. Examples of agents used in CED studies include viruses,[44] paclitaxel,[45] topotecan,[46] and a variety of engineered, targeted protein toxins. These toxins are engineered to include a targeting ligand (e.g., interleukin-4 [IL-4], IL-13, tumor growth factor-α [TGF-α], transferrin) and a genetically altered bacterial toxin

that is effective only when internalized by a cell that expresses the target of the ligand.[47] Two phase III clinical trials have evaluated the use of CED. The PRECISE trial[48-51] studied CED of IL-13 linked to *Pseudomonas* exotoxin (cintredekin besudotox), as compared to Gliadel wafers in glioblastoma patients at first recurrence. No difference in overall survival was observed, but cintredekin besudotox was associated a higher rate of complications. The TransMID trial evaluated the efficacy of transferrin-CRM107 delivered by CED to patients with inoperable recurrent or progressive glioblastoma. The trial was terminated early in 2007 because it was deemed unlikely to meet the prespecified criteria for efficacy. Post hoc analysis of the PRECISE trial indicated that the nonspecialized delivery technology that was used in all of the prior CED studies ("off the shelf" single lumen catheters) could not be placed sufficiently close to target tissue because of concerns about backflow of infusate, or leakage into CSF spaces that would prevent effective intraparenchymal delivery. These concerns were magnified by the lack of imaging data to verify extent of delivery in real time. Recently, several specialized, backflow-resistant delivery devices have been introduced into clinical trial, and coinfusion of Gd conjugates, which are visible on MRI, has verified the ability of these devices to produce clinically relevant volumes of distribution. These devices are currently incorporated into new, early-stage therapeutic trials involving CED, and more trials are expected to open over the next few years.

BCNU impregnated in a polymer and made into a wafer has been used for local delivery, placed on the walls of the resection cavity at the time of surgery. The wafer slowly undergoes biodegradation, releasing the active drug. This local delivery system has the advantages of minimal systemic toxicity, no limitation posed by the BBB, and delivery of very high local concentrations of chemotherapy. Studies in glioblastoma (GBM) have shown only marginal benefit.[52]

Targeted Agents

Although no single defining genetic mutation has been identified for gliomas, several key proliferation and survival signaling pathways appear to be important in GBM. The vascular endothelial growth factor (VEGF), epidermal growth factor (EGF), platelet-derived growth factor (PDGF), hepatocyte growth factor (HGF), and insulin-like growth factor (IGH) pathways are thought to be particularly relevant in the growth and proliferation of GBM. These pathways are characterized by receptors associated with tyrosine kinase activities and share common mechanisms of pathway activation and intracellular signaling. Overexpression or mutations of receptors and intracellular downstream effectors have been identified in GBM, leading to constitutive activation of signaling pathways, resulting in uncontrolled cellular proliferation, survival, and invasion. The Cancer Genome Atlas Research Network demonstrated that 88% of primary GBM tumors have deregulation in the receptor tyrosine kinases and downstream RAS or PI3K pathways.[41,53] Laboratory and clinical trials have focused on targeting these pathways with a variety of agents including monoclonal antibodies, low-molecular weight tyrosine kinase inhibitors, and ligand-toxin conjugates. At the present time, the VEGF pathway inhibitor bevacizumab is the only targeted agent approved for GBM. The efficacy of others has been overwhelmingly disappointing in GBM.

The only other targeted strategy that has been successful in gliomas is the use of inhibitors of mTor for treatment of subependymal giant cell astrocytomas (SEGA), seen in association with tuberose sclerosis. Franz et al. prospectively treated 23 patients with a definite diagnosis of tuberous sclerosis and increasing SEGA lesion size with daily everolimus. Twelve (52.2%) of patients experienced SEGA volume reductions of ≥50% relative to baseline after 60 months of treatment. The proportion of patients experiencing daily seizures was reduced from 26.9% to 11.1% at 60 months.[54]

Two large randomized trials utilizing the antiangiogenic agent bevacizumab for the treatment of newly diagnosed GBM improved progression-free survival but failed to improve overall survival.[55] Because approximately a third of GBMs express an aberrant EGFR surface receptor, small molecule inhibitors, antibodies, and vaccine-mediated approaches to this have been undertaken. A phase III study of rindopepimut, an EGFRviii peptide conjugated to keyhole limpet hemocyanin failed to improve survival in newly diagnosed glioblastoma in a prospective, randomized, phase III study.[56,57] Depatuximab mafodotin is an antibody-drug conjugate that preferentially binds cells with EGFR amplification. It is internalized by targeted cells and releases a potent antimicrotubule agent, monomethylauristatin F. A non-placebo controlled Phase II clinical trial in recurrent glioblastoma with EGFR amplification demonstrated six-month progression free survival of 28.8%.[57a] A Phase III, prospective, randomized, placebo control trial of depatuximab mafodotin in newly diagnosed glioblastoma with EGFR amplification has been completed, although the results have not been reported. Investigators have studied various adoptive and active immunotherapies in the treatment of GBM. Despite limited success, there has been renewed interest recently with the development of tumor-specific vaccines and the approval of new agents for other solid tumors. The use of an active, tumor-specific immunotherapy is appealing as it could potentially maintain long-term antitumor response while limiting toxicity. In addition to Rindopepimut (EGFRvIII-targeted peptide vaccine), other vaccine strategies in clinical trials include DC Vax (autologous tumor lysate-pulsed dendritic cell vaccine), ICT-107 (dendritic cells prepared from autologous mononuclear cells that are pulsed with six synthetic peptides), and HSPPC-96 (autologous tumor-derived heat shock protein [glycoprotein 96]). The most recent investigational focus has shifted to the evaluation of immune checkpoint inhibitors, but the data are too preliminary to be considered outside the clinical trial context.

Alternating Electrical Field Therapy

Tumor-treating fields (TTFields) are a novel treatment modality approved for the treatment of either newly diagnosed or recurrent GBM. TTFields therapy involves a medical device and transducer arrays to provide targeted delivery of low-intensity, intermediate-frequency, alternating electric fields to produce antimitotic effects selective for rapidly dividing tumor cells with limited toxicity. In the phase 3 EF-14 trial, TTFields plus TMZ provided significantly longer PFS and OS compared with TMZ alone in patients with newly diagnosed GBM after initial chemoradiotherapy.[58] In the phase 3 EF-11 trial, for recurrent GBM, TTFields provided comparable efficacy as investigator's choice systemic therapy, with improved patient-reported quality of life and a lower incidence of serious adverse events.[59] Primary toxicity associated with TTFields is skin irritation generally managed with array relocation and topical treatments including antibiotics and steroids.

FOLLOW-UP

The follow-up schedule for a brain tumor patient must be frequent enough to check on side effects and to taper steroids shortly after completion of radiation therapy. Periodic MRIs are used to detect tumor recurrence at a stage when further therapy may be contemplated. Assessment of cognitive functioning and quality of life is important, and patients must be monitored for neuroendocrine and ophthalmologic side effects.

SEQUELAE OF TREATMENT

Surgery

With appropriate patient selection, diligent surgical technique and use of surgical adjuncts such as speech and/or motor mapping, the rate of complications can be minimized. Even in the best of hands, new temporary neurologic deficits can be seen

in 15% or more of patients, although the rate of permanent new deficits is typically now <5%.[60] The incidence and types of deficits seen following surgery depend upon the location of the tumor and the deficits present preoperatively. The most common complications associated with surgery are bleeding and infection, particularly in the case of reoperation in a patient who has received prior radiotherapy and/or chemotherapy or when chemotherapy wafers are placed into a resection cavity.[61] It has been suggested that the use of linear incisions (as opposed to U-shaped flaps) can help reduce the incidence of incision-related complications, such as infection.[62] Posterior fossa resections, particularly in children with medulloblastoma, may be associated with posterior fossa syndrome (mutism plus bulbar symptoms). Transient perioperative edema, within about 48 hours of surgery, may be responsible for early postoperative neurologic worsening and can often be mitigated with the use of a short course of high-dose steroid therapy.

Patients with postoperative neurologic deterioration require careful clinical assessment, and in most cases, a CT or MRI is required to determine the cause of the deterioration. MRI diffusion-weighted sequences can be used to detect the presence of a new infarct. A high index of suspicion should be maintained for postoperative infection because symptoms may be masked by perioperative steroid use, and the headache and fever associated with craniotomy may obscure the classic signs of meningitis.

Radiotherapy

The response of intracranial tissues to radiation has been classically divided into three phases based on the timing of onset of symptoms: acute, subacute, and late.

Acute Toxicity

Transient worsening of pretreatment deficits may develop during the course of treatment, and further acute toxicities may manifest up to 6 weeks following completion of irradiation. These symptoms are believed to be the consequence of a transient peritumoral edema and usually respond to a short-term increase or the institution of corticosteroids. Persistent or refractory symptoms may be caused by tumor progression, and repeat imaging while under treatment may be indicated if the clinical condition worsens despite steroids.

General symptoms such as fatigue, headache, and drowsiness may be seen, especially in individuals treated with large brain fields or with CSI. A mild dermatitis that develops in irradiated areas may be treated with topical agents if necessary. Alopecia within the irradiated areas is common and may be permanent with higher total doses. Nausea and vomiting independent of changes in intracranial pressure may occur, particularly with posterior fossa or brainstem irradiation. Otitis externa can be seen if the ear is included in the irradiation fields, and serous otitis media also may occur. Patients treated with CSI with photons are at risk for mucositis and esophagitis because of the exit dose from the spinal fields through the oropharynx and mediastinum. Hematologic toxicity may also be seen in these patients because of irradiation of the vertebral bodies, a major depot of bone marrow in adults. These GI and hematologic effects are less severe and less frequent with the use of proton therapy for CSI.[63]

Subacute Toxicity

Subacute or "early-delayed" toxicity that develops during the 6-week to 6-month period following irradiation is attributed to changes in capillary permeability as well as transient demyelination due to damage to oligodendroglial cells. Symptoms, which include headache, somnolence, fatigability, and deterioration of pre-existing deficits, usually respond to steroids. The main challenge is to distinguish the clinical and imaging findings from tumor recurrence. The phenomenon of "pseudoprogression" temporally fits within the subacute toxicity time frame.

Section III

Late Sequelae

Late sequelae of radiotherapy appear from 6 months to many years following treatment and are usually irreversible and progressive. They are thought to be due to white matter damage from vascular injury, demyelination, and necrosis. The pathophysiology of radiation-induced neurocognitive damage is complex and involves inter- and intracellular interactions between vasculature and parenchymal cells, particularly oligodendrocytes, which are important for myelination. Oligodendrocyte death occurs either because of direct p53-dependent radiation apoptosis or because of exposure to radiation-induced TNF-α.[63] Postradiation injury to the vasculature involves damage to the endothelium leading to platelet aggregation and thrombus formation, followed by abnormal endothelial proliferation and intraluminal collagen deposition.[64,65]

The most serious late reaction to radiotherapy is radiation necrosis, which has a peak incidence at 3 years. Radiation necrosis can mimic recurrent tumor clinically by the reappearance and worsening of initial symptoms and neurologic deficits and radiographically with the development of a progressive, irreversible, enhancing mass with associated edema on imaging. PET, MR spectroscopy, and nuclear and dynamic CT scanning procedures may aid in the differentiation of radiation necrosis from recurrent tumor. The best treatment for symptomatic necrosis is control of symptoms with steroids followed by surgical debulking, although even after resection necrosis may progress. Given the central role of capillary leakage to radiation necrosis, bevacizumab, an antibody against VEGF, has been tested clinically as treatment for radiation necrosis and has shown encouraging results.[66] Other measures include use of corticosteroids with anticoagulation or hyperbaric oxygen, although randomized trials have not shown these to be useful. In limited clinical series, LITT has shown utility in treating focal radiation necrosis.[67] Although focal necrosis is usually due to radiotherapy alone, diffuse leukoencephalopathy is more commonly associated with the combination of radiotherapy and chemotherapy, particularly methotrexate.

Inclusion of the middle ear may result in high-tone hearing loss and vestibular damage, especially in patients who receive cisplatin. Retinopathy or cataract formation may be seen if the eye is in the radiation field. Optic chiasm and nerve injury may manifest as a decrease in visual acuity, visual field changes, or blindness at doses >54 to 60 Gy. Onset of hormone insufficiency from irradiation of the hypothalamic–pituitary axis is variable but may be seen with doses as low as 20 Gy.

Cranial irradiation can produce neuropsychological changes and neurocognitive impairment; other factors such as tumor-related morbidity, as well as the effects of surgery and chemotherapy, may also contribute.[68] Decline in list-learning recall has been observed in prospective clinical trials of therapeutic and prophylactic cranial irradiation.[66,69] These changes are thought to be due in part to interactions between the vasculature and parenchymal cells. Hippocampal-dependent functions of new learning, memory, and spatial information processing appear to be most affected.[70–72] Doses as low as 2 Gy can induce apoptosis in the proliferating cells in the hippocampus.[73] Agents such as methylphenidate and memantine or radiotherapeutic strategies such as hippocampal avoidance may improve neurocognitive function.[74–76]

MANAGEMENT OF INDIVIDUAL TUMORS

Malignant Glioma

Malignant or high-grade gliomas account for approximately half of all primary brain tumors in adults. They are rapidly growing tumors that directly invade the brain parenchyma but almost never metastasize outside the CNS. They present in any age group, although most occur in late adulthood. Malignant gliomas correspond to anaplastic gliomas (WHO grade III) and GBM (WHO grade IV). Molecular genetics and results from clinical series have shown these to be two distinct diseases with unique behavior, response to treatment, and prognosis. Historical trials that included grade III and IV gliomas are described in the section on GBM, as patients with GBM constituted the majority of subjects, whereas anaplastic gliomas are discussed in further detail in the following section.

Glioblastoma

GBM accounts for approximately 75% of all high-grade gliomas. The histopathologic features of GBM include nuclear atypia, mitotic activity, vascular proliferation, and necrosis; any three of these suffice to make the diagnosis. GBM is diffusely infiltrative, involving large portions of the brain. MRI characteristically shows vasogenic edema and ring enhancement around central necrotic regions.

The prognosis for patients with GBM is poor with median survival time of approximately 14 months in highly selected patients receiving contemporary treatment. Pretreatment patient and tumor characteristics such as age at diagnosis, tumor histology, and Karnofsky performance status (KPS) are the best predictors of outcome. Extent of resection, duration of neurologic symptoms, and radiographic response to treatment have also been suggested as predictors of survival.

Curran et al.[79] used nonparametric recursive partitioning analysis (RPA) (a statistical tool that allows for the identification of significant prognostic factors and subsequent classification of patients into groups with similar outcomes) to analyze data from three RTOG trials that included 1,578 patients with malignant gliomas. Age was the most important predictor of survival, with patients <50 years faring best; KPS ≥ 70 was the next most significant prognostic factor. Taking into account these and other variables, patients could be divided into groups with similar outcomes with 2-year overall survival ranging from 4% to 76% and median survival ranging from 2.7 to 58.6 months (Table 38.4). Though developed in patients receiving radiotherapy alone, the RPA classification retains prognostic significance in patients treated with radiotherapy plus TMZ.[79] More recent studies have integrated molecular data from O[6]–methylguanine-DNA methyltransferase (MGMT) promoter methylation status and other novel biomarkers to develop novel risk-stratification models.[80]

Molecular Genetics

Glioblastoma may arise *de novo* (primary) or from a low-grade glioma that has transformed into a higher-grade tumor (secondary). Secondary GBM arise in younger patients and are associated with a more favorable prognosis than those with primary GBM. The more favorable prognosis may be related

TABLE 38.4 RADIATION THERAPY ONCOLOGY GROUP RECURSIVE PARTITIONING ANALYSIS OF MALIGNANT GLIOMA

Class	Patient Characteristics	Median Survival (mo)
I, II	Anaplastic astrocytoma Age ≤50 y, normal mental status or age >50 y, KPS >70, symptoms >3 mo	40–60
III, IV	Anaplastic astrocytoma Age ≤50 y, abnormal mental status Age >50 y, symptoms <3 mo Glioblastoma Age <50 Age >50 y, KPS ≥70	11–18
V, VI	Glioblastoma Age >50 y, KPS <70 or abnormal mental status	5–9

KPS, Karnofsky performance status.

to the impact of younger age and better performance status of this group. Emerging data suggest that promoter methylation of the PTEN gene in low-grade gliomas may be causally linked to secondary malignant transformation to GBM. Secondary GBM usually have a mutation in the isocitrate dehydrogenase (IDH1) gene and often have p53 mutations.

Treatment

Standard treatment consists of maximal safe surgical resection followed by radiotherapy with concurrent TMZ chemotherapy and subsequent adjuvant TMZ chemotherapy and consideration for application of TTFields. Other approaches including alterations in the delivery of radiotherapy, newer chemotherapeutic agents, immunotherapy, and other agents are the subject of ongoing research.

Radiotherapy Target Volume

Randomized trials have demonstrated a clear survival benefit to the use of radiotherapy after surgery.[81,82] Localized irradiation volumes are recommended despite the fact that GBM is usually more widely disseminated. Dandy et al.,[83] for example, identified recurrences in the contralateral hemisphere even after hemispherectomy, showing the phenomenal capability of malignant gliomas to spread along white matter tracts. Such findings as well as autopsy studies[84–86] led to recommendations that the entire intracranial contents should be irradiated. However, Hochberg and Pruitt[87] reported that in 35 patients who had a CT scan within 2 months prior to autopsy, 78% of recurrences of GBM were within 2 cm of the margin of the initial tumor bed and 56% were within 1 cm or less of the volume outlined by the CT scan. These findings were confirmed by Wallner et al.[88] who showed that 78% of unifocal tumors (25/32) recurred within 2 cm of the initial tumor volume, defined as the enhancing edge of the tumor on CT scan, and 56% of tumors (18/32) recurred within 1 cm of the initial tumor margin. No unifocal tumor recurred as a multifocal lesion, and large tumors were not more likely to recur farther from the initial tumor margin than smaller tumors.

In a correlative study, Halperin et al.[89] reviewed CT scans and pathologic sections of 15 brains of patients with GBM who received minimal or no radiotherapy. If radiation treatment portals had been designed to cover the contrast-enhancing volume and peritumoral edema with a 1-cm margin, the portals would have covered histologically identified tumor in only 6/11 cases. However, treatment of the contrast-enhancing area and all surrounding edema with a 3-cm margin around the edema would have covered histologically identified tumor in all cases.

Kelly et al.[90] reported on 40 patients with intracranial glial neoplasms who underwent CT- and MRI-guided stereotactic serial biopsies. Histologic analysis of 195 biopsy specimens showed that contrast enhancement most often corresponded to tumor tissue without intervening parenchyma and hypodensity most often corresponded to parenchyma infiltrated by isolated tumor cells, tumor in low-grade gliomas, or edema. Isolated tumor cell infiltration extended at least as far as T2 changes on MRI. T2-weighted MRI revealed much larger volumes of infiltrated parenchyma than shown by low attenuation on CT scans.

Therefore, inclusion of all radiographic evidence of tumor and associated edema with generous margins is common practice in the design of treatment portals. The extent of margin expansion remains a relatively poorly studied and controversial area, with considerable variance.[91] With advances in MRI technology, the definition of tumor margins continues to change. For example, Pirzkall et al.[92] showed metabolically active tumor extending outside the region defined on T2-weighted MRI in 88% of patients. PET imaging with methionine and/or thymidine may also prove useful.

Radiotherapy Dose

The current "standard approach" delivers a total dose of 59.4 to 60 Gy in 30 to 33 fractions of 1.8 to 2 Gy/fraction, using a "shrinking field" technique. Walker et al.[93] performed a dose–response analysis using data from 420 patients treated on Brain Tumor Cooperative Group protocols. Doses ranged from <45 to 60 Gy using daily fractions of 1.7 to 2 Gy; only one-third of the patients received <60 Gy. A significant improvement in median survival from 28 to 42 weeks in the groups treated with doses of 50 to 60 Gy was found. A Medical Research Council study of 443 patients also showed a significant survival advantage in patients who received 60 Gy compared to those who received 45 Gy (12 vs. 9 months; $P = .007$).[94]

For patients with poor pretreatment prognostic factors and a limited expected survival who are not able to tolerate conventional treatment, a shorter course of treatment may provide good palliation. Older patients (>65 years), especially those with poor performance status, have been shown to experience limited posttreatment improvement or rapid neurologic deterioration following conventional radiotherapy. Short-course radiotherapy, utilizing hypofractionated techniques, some as short as only 1 week, has been tested in older patients, and results are described below. In Europe and Canada, such hypofractionated schedules are considered "standard" for "elderly" or "poor performance" status patients, and such techniques are also being increasingly utilized in the United States.

Dose Escalation and Altered Fractionation

With the vast majority of tumor recurrences occurring within the previous irradiation field and the poor outcomes associated with standard therapy, regimens designed to deliver a larger dose have been attempted to improve local control and enhance survival.

A benefit for doses >60 Gy either without chemotherapy or with nitrosurea-based chemotherapy has not been demonstrated. The RTOG and Eastern Cooperative Oncology Group (ECOG) randomized 253 patients to either whole-brain irradiation to 60 Gy given in 6 to 7 weeks or 60 Gy plus a 10-Gy boost to a limited volume given in 7 to 8 weeks.[95] There was no benefit for the higher irradiation dose. Chan et al.[96] published the results of 34 patients with high-grade gliomas treated using 3D conformal IMRT to a dose of 90 Gy. At median follow-up of 11.7 months, median survival was found to be 11.7 months and 1- and 2-year survivals of 47.1% and 12.9%, respectively, comparable to historical controls.

Several groups have used hyperfractionated or accelerated regimens as a means to escalate dose, using twice daily, three times daily, and even four times daily fractionation.[97] Only the study of Shin et al.[98–100] showed an improvement in survival using daily fractionation. In this study, 81 patients were randomized to 61.4 Gy in 69 fractions of 0.89 Gy given three times daily over 4.5 weeks or conventional fractionation to 58 Gy in 30 fractions given once daily over 6 weeks. Median survival in the two groups was 39 and 27 weeks, respectively, and the 1-year survival rates were 41% and 20%, respectively ($P < .001$). Others have failed to confirm these results. In a prospective, randomized phase I/II trial, RTOG 83-02 examined dose escalation using twice-daily fractionation in patients with malignant gliomas. Hyperfractionated regimens studied were 64.8, 72.0, 76.8, and 81.6 Gy given in 1.2 Gy fractions twice daily, and accelerated hyperfractionated regimens were 48 and 54.4 Gy given in 1.6 Gy twice-daily fractions. Patients also received chemotherapy with BCNU. In the final report on all 747 patients, there were no significant differences between the treatment arms with regard to median survival time.[100] A phase III trial compared conventional radiotherapy to 60 Gy in 30 daily fractions to hyperfractionated radiotherapy to 72 Gy in 60 fractions of 1.2 Gy given twice daily.[101] No difference in survival was found. Several other accelerated hyperfraction-ation regimens to doses over 70 Gy have been investigated, also without significant improvement in survival.[102]

In the contemporary era of concurrent and adjuvant TMZ, escalation of both dose and dose per fraction using IMRT was tested in a prospective phase I/II study. The maximum tolerated dose with temozolomide was 75 Gy in 30 fractions (2.5 Gy/fraction). Median survival was 20.1 months, suggesting improved efficacy compared to other contemporary studies. The probability of in-field failure decreased in with increasing dose escalation. Prospective randomized trial of this dose-fractionation regimen using either IMRT or proton therapy remains ongoing.

Dose Escalation Using Radiosurgery and FSRT

A radiosurgical boost was reported as effective in patients with newly diagnosed malignant glioma in a retrospective analysis of 115 patients treated at three institutions with a combination of surgery, external beam radiotherapy, and LINAC-based radiosurgery on similar institutional protocols.[103,104] In a prospective randomized trial, Souhami et al.[105] compared conventional radiotherapy (60 Gy) plus adjuvant BCNU with and without radiosurgery in 203 patients with GBM. At a median follow-up of 61 months, no significant improvement in median survival was observed (13.5 vs. 13.6 months).

The use of a boost using FSRT was tested prospectively in RTOG 0023.[106] 76 patients with GBM with postoperative residual tumor plus tumor cavity diameter <60 mm were treated with 50 Gy standard radiotherapy in daily 2 Gy fractions, plus four FSRT treatments given once weekly during weeks 3 to 6 of radiotherapy. The FSRT dose was either 5 Gy or 7 Gy/fraction for a cumulative dose of 70 or 78 Gy in 29 treatments over 6 weeks. Overall, no survival advantage was seen when compared to the RTOG historical database.

Dose Escalation Using Brachytherapy

Laperriere et al.[107] used brachytherapy as a boost to conventional radiotherapy in patients with malignant gliomas. Patients were randomized to external beam radiotherapy (50 Gy in 25 fractions) alone (*n* = 69) or external beam radiotherapy plus a temporary stereotactic ^{125}I implant delivering a minimum peripheral tumor dose of 60 Gy (*n* = 71). Median survival was not significantly different between the two arms (13.8 vs. 13.2 months; *P* = .49).

The results of the Brain Tumor Cooperative Group National Institutes of Health Trial 8701 reported by Selker et al.[108] support these findings. In this randomized, prospective trial, 299 patients with newly diagnosed malignant glioma received surgery, external beam radiotherapy, and BCNU with or without an interstitial radiotherapy boost with ^{125}I. Treatment with an interstitial boost did not prolong survival as compared to conventional treatment.

Radiotherapy delivered by an inflatable balloon brachytherapy catheter has also been tested. Tatter et al.[109] evaluated the safety and performance of one such device (GliaSite Radiation Therapy System, Cytyc, Marlborough, MA). Twenty-one patients with recurrent malignant gliomas underwent surgical resection and implantation of a subcutaneous port. At 1 to 2 weeks following implantation, the catheter was filled with an aqueous solution of organically bound ^{125}I for delivery of a minimum of 40 to 60 Gy over 3 to 6 days, with subsequent removal of the device. Median survival was 12.7 months. Subsequent dose-finding prospective studies failed to determine a maximum tolerated dose as early imaging changes, presumed to be progression, occurred in 7 of 12 patients and interfered with the assessment of treatment-related toxicity.[36]

Dose Escalation Using Proton Therapy

Dose escalation up to 90 cobalt gray equivalent (CGE) with mixed photon and proton-beam irradiation has been tested in two prospective trials.

Fitzek et al.[110] reported on a phase II study of 23 patients with newly diagnosed GBM. Two-year overall survival was 34% and median overall survival was 20 months, which compared favorably to historical data. Recurrence was observed in regions treated to 60 to 70 CGE, but only one recurrence was observed in regions treated to 90 CGE. More recently, Mizumoto et al.[111] reported on a phase I/II study of 20 patients with supratentorial GBM treated with mixed photon and proton-beam irradiation to 96.6 Gy in 56 twice-daily fractions with concomitant nimustine chemotherapy. MRI-defined T2 enhancing region was treated to 50.4 CGE in 28 daily morning fractions. In daily evening fractions, patients were treated to 23.1 CGE for the first 14 fractions to the T1-enhancing region plus 1 cm and then 23.1 CGE for the subsequent 14 fractions to the T1-enhancing region only. Median survival was 22 months and 2-year overall survival was 45%. Late radiation necrosis was noted in one patient, and late leukoencephalopathy was observed in a second patient. As part of a prospective randomized trial, dose escalation to 75 Gy in 30 fractions using proton therapy is currently under investigation.

Radiosensitizers

Studies using radiation modifiers in conjunction with radiotherapy to overcome the hypoxia present in malignant gliomas have shown disappointing results. Chang[112] reported on 38 patients treated with hyperbaric oxygen and irradiation using fractionation schedules ranging from 36 Gy given in 3 weeks to 60 Gy given in 6 to 7 weeks and compared them with 42 patients treated with radiotherapy alone. An improvement in 18-month survival rate from 10% to 28% and an increase of median survival from 31 to 38 weeks was noted. Perfluorocarbon emulsions, such as Fluosol, which have enormous oxygen carrying capacity, have been tested as hypoxic sensitizers without significant benefit.[113] Randomized studies failed to show significant improvement with the addition of the hypoxic cell sensitizer misonidazole.[114]

Miralbell et al.[98,115] reported the results of a European Organisation for Research and Treatment of Cancer (EORTC) trial examining the addition of carbogen and nicotinamide to overcome the effects of proliferation and hypoxia presumed responsible for radioresistance in GBM. Overall survival was similar in all arms and did not differ from results of series using radiotherapy alone.

The redox-modulating radiosensitizer motexafin gadolinium (MGd) showed encouraging results in a phase I clinical trial[74]; however, results from a single-arm phase II trial, RTOG 0513, of MGd and conventional therapy in newly diagnosed GBM showed no survival improvement.

Chemotherapy

The use of cytotoxic chemotherapeutic agents for glioblastoma dates back to the 1960s when the Brain Tumor Study Group conducted a controlled study using carmustine.[116] After surgery, patients were assigned to one of four treatment groups: (1) no further therapy, (2) carmustine alone, (3) radiation therapy, and (4) radiation therapy followed by carmustine. At 18 months, 23% of patients who received radiation therapy plus carmustine were still alive as compared to 5% with carmustine or radiotherapy alone. The Food and Drug Administration (FDA) approved carmustine and lomustine for the treatment of brain tumors (including glioblastoma) in the 1970s. Subsequent prospective studies failed to demonstrate a survival advantage to carmustine or other cytotoxic chemotherapy for glioblastoma, although two meta-analyses demonstrated a small survival benefit from chemotherapy.[117]

The only chemotherapeutic agent that has demonstrated efficacy for glioblastoma and anaplastic astrocytoma in randomized trials is TMZ, an oral imidazotetrazine derivative of dacarbazine that is metabolized *in vivo* to an active agent. Like the nitrosureas, it akylates the O^6 position on guanine, producing single-strand DNA breaks. It is well tolerated by patients; fatigue, constipation, and nausea are the most common toxicities. The drug is myelosuppressive in a minority of patients. Approval for the treatment of recurrent anaplastic astrocytoma was obtained from the Food and Drug Administration (FDA) in 1999.[118,119] Its approval for use as adjuvant therapy for glioblastoma was based on a large phase III clinical trial conducted by the EORTC and National Cancer Institute of Canada (NCIC).[120] This phase III trial randomized 573 patients with newly diagnosed glioblastoma (between the ages of 18 to 70 and KPS > 70) to either radiation therapy alone (total 60 Gy in 30 fractions; control arm) or TMZ chemotherapy in combination with radiation therapy (total 60 Gy in 30 fractions; experimental arm). Patients on the experimental arm received TMZ daily during radiation therapy (because of its radiosensitization effect in preclinical studies) at a dose of 75 mg/m^2, followed by monthly TMZ at a dose of 150 to 200 mg/m^2 on a 5 out of every 28 days schedule for six cycles.

Patients randomized to the experimental arm had a median survival of 14.6 months as compared to 12.1 months for the control arm. The 2-year survival of patients treated with radiation therapy plus chemotherapy was 26%, compared to 6% for radiation alone. Toxicity with chemoradiotherapy was acceptable with 7% grade 3 or 4 hematologic toxicities, compared to none in the group treated with radiotherapy alone. Long-term survival benefit from the addition of TMZ has been demonstrated.[121,122] Five-year overall survival was 9.8% for patients who received combined TMZ and radiotherapy as compared to 1.9% for those who received radiotherapy alone.[122] The benefit of adding TMZ to radiotherapy has also been demonstrated for elderly patients (age ≥ 65) with GBM. A recently reported randomized phase III trial demonstrated that adding TMZ chemotherapy during short-course radiation therapy, followed by monthly adjuvant TMZ improved survival of elderly glioblastoma patients from 7.6 month with radiation therapy alone to 9.3 months with combination therapy.[123] Progression-free survival was 5.3 months versus 3.9 months 1-year survival rate was 37.8% versus 22.2%, and 2-year survival rate was 10.4% versus 2.8% with radiation plus TMZ versus radiation alone.

Because only a subgroup of patients benefit from TMZ, their identification is desirable to avoid exposing patients unlikely to benefit to the toxicity of a potentially ineffective therapy. Recent work has focused on identifying potential predictive laboratory markers. Epigenetic silencing of the MGMT DNA repair gene by promoter methylation has been associated with longer survival for malignant glioma patients treated with alkylating agents.[124] A retrospective analysis of assessable cases from the EORTC/NCIC TMZ study demonstrated a survival benefit for patients treated with TMZ and radiotherapy if their tumor contained a methylated MGMT promoter (median 21.7 months) as compared to patients with nonmethylated MGMT promoters (median 12.7 months).[125] In the NCIC-EORTC trial of elderly GBM patients,[123] the MGMT nonmethylated group did not achieve a statistically significant benefit in survival, and consequently, a number of new clinical trials are attempting to enroll the MGMT-unmethylated GBM patients to trials that do not mandate TMZ in the experimental, and sometimes, even in the control arm.

The RTOG completed an 1,100 patient, randomized, phase III trial comparing standard adjuvant TMZ with a dose-dense schedule in newly diagnosed glioblastoma.[126] Eight hundred and thirty-three patients were randomized to receive either standard therapy (TMZ + radiotherapy followed by 6 to 12 cycles of TMZ at a dose of 150 to 200 mg/m^2 on a 5/28 day schedule) or dose-intense TMZ (TMZ + radiotherapy followed by 6 to 12 cycles of TMZ at a dose of 150 mg/m^2 on a 21/28 day schedule). There was no statistical difference between the experimental and standard arm for overall survival (16.6 vs.14.9 months, P = .63) or progression-free survival (5.5 vs.

6.7 months, P = .06), indicating no additional benefit from dose-intense TMZ. The trial prospectively stratified for MGMT methylation status, and no survival benefit with dose-intense therapy was identified in any subgroup. Overall, MGMT methylation was associated with improved median overall survival (21.2 vs. 14 months, P < .0001), median progression-free survival (8.7 vs. 5.7 months, P < .001), and response (P = .012). As expected, the dose-intense arm resulted in increased toxicity. Thus, at the present time, there is no role for dose-intense TMZ for newly diagnosed glioblastoma patients.

In addition, though the standard for postsurgical care includes radiotherapy with concurrent TMZ followed by adjuvant TMZ for six cycles, this regimen has been adopted with variations including extending adjuvant TMZ beyond six cycles. A recent pooled analysis of patient-level data from four randomized trials of newly diagnosed glioblastoma demonstrated a slight improvement in progression-free survival (hazard ratio [HR] 0.80, P = .03), particularly in MGMT-methylated patients (HR 0.65, P < .01), with continuation of adjuvant TMZ beyond six cycles.[127] However, continuation of temozolomide beyond six cycles demonstrated no difference in overall survival in the overall population and specifically in the MGMT-methylated subgroup and, given the potential for increased toxicity, is not considered standard postsurgical care.

Other chemotherapeutic regimens, such as the combination of CPT-11 and TMZ, have shown promising results in a phase II trial with an objective response rate of 25% and 6-month progression-free rate of 38%. When tested prospectively in a single-arm RTOG trial, the regimen did not show improved survival.[128] Buckner et al.[129] reported on a phase III trial of carmustine with or without cisplatin before and concurrently with radiotherapy and observed increased toxicity but no survival benefit with the addition of cisplatin.

Tumor-Treating Fields

Tumor-treating fields (TTFields) involve the placement of noninvasive transducer arrays on the scalp and the delivery of low intensity (1 to 3 V/cm), intermediate frequency (100 to 300 kHz), alternating electric fields to the tumor. TTFields lead to tumor cell kill through their action during two phases of mitosis: (1) during metaphase, by disrupting the formation of the mitotic spindle, and (2) during cytokinesis, by dielectrophoretic dislocation of intracellular constituents resulting in apoptosis. TTFields are most effective when applied in the direction of the division axis of the dividing cell, and therefore, two sequential field directions are applied to tumors by using two perpendicular pairs of transducer arrays in order to increase the efficacy of TTFields.[130] Following preclinical studies demonstrating *in vitro* and *in vivo* activity in glioma, a prospective randomized trial of TTFields versus conventional chemotherapy for recurrent glioblastoma demonstrated no difference in overall survival, but higher patient-reported quality of life and cognitive and emotional function and less toxicity with TTFields.[130,132] This study also demonstrated improved overall with use of TTFields for 18 hours/day or longer.

Interim analysis of another prospective randomized trial demonstrated improvement in overall and progression-free survival but no difference in serious adverse events or quality of life with the addition of TTFields to conventional treatment involving maximally safe resection and adjuvant chemoradiotherapy for newly diagnosed glioblastoma.[59] Final results of this trial confirm the existence of a survival benefit with a prolongation of median overall survival from 16.0 months to 20.9 months.[132a] Additionally, tumor-treating fields was not associated with any negative influence on quality of life, except for more itchy skin.[132b] Based on these results, TTFields has been approved for the treatment of recurrent and newly diagnosed glioblastoma by the Food and Drug Administration (FDA) in the United States and have obtained a CE mark in Europe for the same indications.

Investigational Approaches

Immunotherapy

Modulation of the immune system is being explored in the setting of GBM through such therapeutic interventions as blocking naturally occurring inhibitory immune checkpoint molecules, adoptive T-cell therapeutics, or vaccine therapy against tumor-specific antigens. Nivolumab, a human IgG4 monoclonal antibody targeting PD-1, demonstrated no improvement in overall survival relative to bevacizumab for recurrent GBM in preliminary results from a phase III trial.[133] Rindopepimut, a peptide vaccine targeting EGF receptor variant III (EGFR vIII), has been tested in multicenter trials of newly diagnosed EGFvIII-expressing GBM following gross total resection and conventional radiotherapy with concurrent TMZ. Although phase II results demonstrated promising outcomes, a double-blind randomized phase III trial failed to demonstrate an improvement in overall survival with the use of rindopepimut.[134] Heat shock protein-peptide complex-96 (HSPPC-96) vaccine is an autologous treatment derived from dendritic cells extracted from the patient's tumor to induce antitumor antibodies, demonstrated no survival benefit when added to bevacizumab for recurrent GBM in preliminary results from a randomized trial.

Radioimmunotherapy

Radioimmunotherapy using monoclonal antibodies against EGFR tagged with ^{125}I has been evaluated in the treatment of high-grade gliomas. In a phase II trial by Brady et al., 25 patients with malignant gliomas (10 with anaplastic astrocytoma and 15 with GBM) were treated with surgical resection or biopsy followed by definitive external beam radiotherapy and one or multiple doses (35 to 90 mCi per intravenous or intra-arterial infusion) of ^{125}I-labeled monoclonal antibody-425. The total cumulative dose ranged from 40 to 224 mCi. At 1 year, 60% of patients were alive, and the median survival was 15.6 months. In an updated report of this study that included a total of 180 patients with a minimum follow-up of 5 years, median survival was 13.4 months for those with GBM.[135]

Another potential target is tenascin, an extracellular protein overexpressed in malignant gliomas but not found in normal tissue. Radiolabeled monoclonal antibodies to tenascin have been evaluated in phase I or II trials showing activity against newly diagnosed and recurrent malignant gliomas.[136] In a phase II trial by Reardon et al.,[137,138] ^{131}I-labeled murine antitenascin monoclonal antibody was injected directly into the surgical resection cavity in 33 patients with untreated malignant glioma. Patients were subsequently treated with external beam radiotherapy and 1 year of alkylator-based chemotherapy. Even after accounting for prognostic factors, median survival (86.7 weeks) was longer than that of historical controls. Treatment-related toxicities were mild; only one patient required reoperation for radionecrosis.

Targeted Therapies

EGFR gene amplification is seen in approximately 40% to 50% of patients with GBM. EGFR is associated with control of cell growth through autocrine and peregrine effects of growth factors. Inhibitors of EGFR tyrosine kinase such as gefitinib and erlotinib and EGFR antibodies have not been successful to date likely because of mutational resistance mechanisms, limited brain penetration of tyrosine kinase inhibitors, as well as the presence of multiple signaling bypass opportunities. Clinical trials of vaccine therapy directed against EGFRvIII are discussed above. A randomized trial of ABT-414, an antibody-drug conjugate targeting EGFR, added to conventional radiotherapy and TMZ for newly diagnosed GBM with EGFR amplification is ongoing.

Mutations and loss of the PTEN gene are encountered in approximately 70% of patients with GBM. PTEN inhibits signaling through the PI3-kinase and AKT signaling pathway.

Loss of PTEN results in loss of effectiveness of EGFR inhibitors, probably because of constitutive signaling through PI3-kinase, which bypasses any upstream EGFR inhibitor effect. Specific inhibitors such as CCI-779 and everolimus are ineffective as single agents. Although preclinical experiments suggest that these agents are potential radiosensitizers,[139-141] a prospective trial of everolimus added to conventional radiotherapy and TMZ demonstrated no survival improvement compared to historical controls in newly diagnosed GBM.[142]

Cilengitide, a selective integrin inhibitor that acts on tumor cell motility and impacts tumor interaction with brain microenvironment, demonstrated no improvement in overall survival when added to conventional radiotherapy and TMZ for newly diagnosed MGMT promoter-methylated glioblastoma in a large phase III trial.[143]

Neovascularization is a major feature of GBM, and many studies demonstrate that GBM secrete VEGF in abundance. The supporting endothelium strongly expresses receptors for VEGF. Bevacizumab, anti-VEGF antibody, has demonstrated impressive radiographic response rate and reduction in peritumoral edema in multiple phase II trials and is FDA approved for the treatment of recurrent glioblastoma (see below). However, two large phase III randomized clinical trials investigating the addition of bevacizumab to the EORTC/NCIC regimen demonstrated no improvement in overall survival.[56,57]

Treatment of Elderly Patients

Approximately one-third of patients with GBM are 65 years or older. Older age has been demonstrated to be an important adverse prognostic factor in GBM. In a population-based survey of 3,298 patients with GBM in Ontario,[144] each decade increase in age has been associated with a reduction in overall survival, with patients older than 70 years having a median survival of 4 to 5 months. In the updated results from the EORTC/NCIC trial, Stupp et al.[122] observed a survival advantage to radiotherapy with concomitant and adjuvant TMZ compared to radiotherapy alone in all age subgroups, including patients >60 years old.

However, because of concerns over the tolerance of conventional chemoradiotherapy for older patients, particularly those with poor performance status, nonconventional approaches to adjuvant therapy have been tested. A phase III ANOCEF group trial observed improved median survival (6.7 vs. 3.9 months) and progression-free survival, but equivalent toxicity, with adjuvant radiotherapy to 50 Gy compared to best supportive care in patients 70 years and older with KPS ≥ 70.[145]

Short-course radiotherapy and single-agent TMZ have also been investigated. As described previously, Roa et al. observed no difference between standard radiotherapy of 60 Gy in 30 fractions or a shorter course of 40 Gy in 15 fractions in GBM patients older than 50 years.[146] A more recent European trial compared overall survival between standard radiotherapy (60 Gy in 30 fractions), short-course radiotherapy (34 Gy in 10 fractions), and single-agent TMZ in patients ≥60 years old.[147] This trial demonstrated inferior median survival with 60 Gy radiotherapy versus TMZ in the overall population and inferior median survival with 60 Gy radiotherapy versus short-course radiotherapy in patients >70 years old. TMZ was associated with more grade 3 to 4 toxicity. The NOA-08 phase III trial demonstrated noninferior survival but higher grade 3 to 4 toxicity with 1-week-on/1-week-off TMZ compared to radiotherapy to 54 to 60 Gy in patients ≥65 years old with anaplastic astrocytoma or GBM.[148] These trials also demonstrated that when single modality therapy is being considered because of poor performance status, tolerability concerns, etc., TMZ alone is superior to radiotherapy for the MGMT-methylated patients, but the converse is true for the unmethylated patients.

A Canadian-led phase III trial demonstrated improvement in progression-free and overall survival with the addition of

TMZ during and as monthly maintenance doses following short-course radiotherapy (40 Gy in 15 fractions) in elderly (65 years or older) patients with newly diagnosed glioblastoma.[123] Median age of patients was 73 years, and two-thirds were older than 70 years. TMZ prolonged median overall survival from 7.6 months to 9.3 months and increased 1-year survival rate from 22.2% to 37.8%. This survival benefit was most marked in patients with MGMT promoter methylation where median survival was extended from 7.7 to 13.5 months, and for the MGMT-unmethylated patients, the survival difference did not reach statistical significance. Quality of life analyses demonstrated no difference in functional domains but noted more nausea, vomiting, and constipation in patients receiving TMZ. Therefore, in the elderly, and poor performance status, in the absence of statistically significant survival improvement, and the increase in toxicity, the use of TMZ for the unmethylated patient needs to be questioned.

Treatment at Recurrence

Although several therapeutic options have been considered for patients with recurrent GBM, none are curative, and therefore, the management goals should be palliative. Hospice referral for palliative care is reasonable for many patients. Palliative debulking may help selected patients by relieving mass effect and probably extends survival by about 4 to 6 months on average. Based on an impressive radiographic response rate in two nonrandomized, phase II clinical trials,[149,150] single-agent bevacizumab was approved by the FDA in 2009 for the treatment of recurrent glioblastoma. In a study of 49 glioblastoma patients, Kreisl et al.[150] reported objective response rate of 35%, 6-month progression-free survival of 29%, 3.7 month median progression-free survival, and 7.2 month median overall survival. Similarly, Friedman et al.[149] reported an objective response rate of 28%, 6-month progression-free survival of 43%, median progression-free survival of 4.2 months and median overall survival of 9.2 months in a total of 85 patients. Although approved as a single agent, controversy remains on whether bevacizumab should be combined with a cytotoxic agent as with other solid tumors.

Polymer-based local chemotherapy (carmustine wafers) has been tested in a randomized trial that included 222 patients with recurrent glioma (mostly GBM); survival increased from 44% to 64% at 6 months ($P = .02$) for patients with GBM, and median survival from 23 to 31 weeks.[53] Systemic chemotherapeutic agents have been tested mostly in the context of clinical trials and have been uniformly disappointing, as have targeted agents with the notable exception of EGFR tyrosine kinase inhibitors in patients with recurrent GBM expressing wild-type PTEN and mutant EGFR.[151] Of 37 patients with recurrent GBM treated with EGFR tyrosine kinase inhibitors at UCLA, there were seven responders, while 19 had early progression.[152] Coexpression of mutant EGFR and wild-type PTEN had 86% sensitivity, 89% specificity, and a positive predictive value of 75% for response. The BELOB trial was an open-label phase II trial that randomized patients to single-agent bevacizumab or lomustine versus combination of bevacizumab plus lomustine in recurrent bevacizumab-naïve GBM.[153] This trial demonstrated promising 9-month overall survival of 59% with combination bevacizumab plus lomustine 90 mg/m² relative to single-agent bevacizumab (38%) or lomustine (43%). During this trial, lomustine administered in combination with bevacizumab required dose reduction from 110 to 90 mg/m² because of severe thrombocytopenia. However, subsequent phase III trial of single-agent lomustine 110 mg/m² versus combination bevacizumab and lomustine 90 mg/m² for recurrent GBM at time of first progression prolonged PFS but did not confer a survival advantage.[154]

Repeat radiotherapy using one of several different methods (including radiosurgery, brachytherapy, GliaSite balloon brachytherapy, and even repeat external beam radiotherapy) may be considered for carefully selected patients. Hypofractionated re-irradiation with bevacizumab has shown promising results in small single institutional reports, with surprisingly limited toxicity, attributed to "vascular stabilization and protection" resulting from bevacizumab, and more investigations of this approach are being considered.[155] The hypofractionated approach with TMZ and bevacizumab has been extended to the newly diagnosed setting, and at the Society of Neuro-oncology 2011 meeting, investigators from MSKCC reported median survival in excess of 21 months in a small cohort of unmethylated MGMT GBM patients.[156] A prospective randomized trial of hypofractionated re-irradiation with bevacizumab has completed accrual, and results are pending.

Evidence-Based Treatment Summary

1. Maximal surgical resection, although not tested in a prospective trial, is generally recommended to establish pathologic diagnosis, provide tissue for molecular studies, and achieve cytoreduction that may improve neurologic deficits.
2. Postoperative radiotherapy has been shown to provide a survival advantage in several clinical trials. The typical radiotherapy dose is 60 Gy in 6 weeks for younger and prognostically favorable patients. Dose escalation beyond 60 Gy has not proven to be effective.
3. Temozolomide, given during and after radiotherapy for six cycles, provides a significant survival advantage that is greatest in patients with methylation of the promoter region of the MGMT gene. The benefit in the unmethylated population is questionable. Even elderly patients benefit from this approach.
4. Tumor-treating fields administered after radiotherapy and concomitant with high-dose TMZ also prolongs survival.
5. Bevacizumab confers no survival benefit for newly diagnosed glioblastoma, but can be an effective salvage therapy at time of progression, although there are no categorical data demonstrating that it prolongs survival in patients with recurrent GBM. It can also be useful in large tumors with significant cerebral edema by improving neurologic disability and sparing prolonged steroids.
6. Short-course radiotherapy is a reasonable option for elderly patients or those with poor performance status or transportation limitations.
7. If unimodality therapy is being contemplated (especially in sicker patients, less likely to tolerate combination therapy), TMZ alone for the MGMT-methylated and radiotherapy alone for the MGMT unmethylated are reasonable considerations.

Anaplastic Glioma

Anaplastic gliomas (WHO grade III gliomas: anaplastic astrocytoma and anaplastic oligoastrocytoma, Table 38.3) constitute approximately 25% of high-grade gliomas in adults, generally occurring during young to middle adulthood. Histologically, these tumors have increased cellularity, nuclear atypia and marked mitotic activity, without necrosis or neovascularization. On imaging, anaplastic gliomas may show enhancement and necrosis similar to GBM, although up to one-third of tumors may not enhance.[157]

The prognosis for patients with anaplastic glioma is heavily influenced by a number of molecular genetic factors. Patients with histologically defined anaplastic oligodendroglioma, in general, have a better prognosis. Other prognostic factors include age at diagnosis, mental status, and performance status (see Table 38.4). However, the prognosis of these patients is best defined by molecular factors, such as allelic loss of 1p and 19q and presence of IDH1 mutation (see below). The previously described mixed glioma (anaplastic oligoastrocytoma) is no longer recognized in the 2016 revised WHO criteria.

Anaplastic Oligodendroglioma

Anaplastic oligodendroglioma represents 3.5% of all malignant gliomas and 30% of oligodendroglial tumors. They occur predominantly in adults, with median age at diagnosis of 45 to 50 years, approximately 7 to 9 years older than grade II oligodendroglioma; this age difference reasonably corresponds to the average time of tumor "evolution" from grade II to grade III.

Molecular Genetics

Allelic loss of 1p and 19q is thought to be an early genetic alteration in the transformation and progression of oligodendrogliomas. Combined 1p and 19q deletions have been found in 63% of patients with anaplastic oligodendroglioma and 52% of patients with mixed anaplastic oligoastrocytoma, whereas astrocytic tumors have a lower incidence (8% to 11%) of combined 1p and 19q deletions.[158] Deletions in 1p and 19q have been associated with longer progression-free survival, overall survival, and chemo- and radiosensitivity.[158-160]

The impact of 1p19q codeletion status on outcome has been confirmed in two phase III trials. RTOG 94-02 retrospectively assessed 1p and 19q status in 263/291 enrolled patients (71%) with anaplastic oligodendroglioma/oligoastrocytoma randomized to receive chemotherapy with PCV followed by radiotherapy or radiotherapy alone.[38] Combined loss of 1p and 19q was present in 44% of patients in the PCV plus radiotherapy arm and 52% in the radiotherapy alone arm and was more frequent in anaplastic oligodendroglial tumors (76%) than in anaplastic oligoastrocytoma (24%). Combined loss of 1p and 19q resulted in a longer median survival time (14.7 vs. 2.6 years [$P < .001$] in patients receiving PCV plus radiotherapy; 7.3 vs. 2.7 years [$P < .001$] in patients radiotherapy alone). In EORTC 26951, 368 patients with anaplastic oligodendroglioma/oligoastrocytoma were randomized to receive radiotherapy followed by PCV or radiotherapy alone.[39] Presence of 1p or 19q loss was found to be the most important predictor of outcome, with a median survival of 10.3 versus 1.9 years for tumors with or without combined allelic loss of 1p and 19q, respectively.

Others molecular factors with clinical implications include somatic mutations in the isocitrate dehydrogenase 1 (IDH1) gene and MGMT promoter methylation. IDH1 mutations have been observed in 55% to 80% of grade II and III gliomas.[161] Though rarely present in primary grade IV gliomas, IDH1 mutations are frequently present in secondary grade IV gliomas that develop from lower-grade tumors, providing a biologic explanation for this clinical categorization.[162] IDH mutations generate an oncometabolite that is believed to be contributory to malignant transformation for precursor cells to gliomas and therefore is an early event. Intriguingly, in spite of the fact that the mutation generates the causative oncometabolite, prospective trials of anaplastic gliomas have demonstrated IDH1 mutations to be a strong positive prognostic factor. In EORTC 26951, IDH1 mutations were observed in 46% of patients and demonstrated prognostic significance, independent of 1p/19q codeletion, in both arms of the trial for both progression-free survival and overall survival.[163] In RTOG 9402, IDH1 mutations were observed in 74% of patients, were associated with longer overall survival (9.4 vs. 5.7 years), and identified patients without 1p19q codeletion who derived an overall survival benefit from the addition of PCV chemotherapy to radiotherapy (5.5 vs. 3.3 years).[164] This suggests that both subgroups, 1p19q codeleted (which almost always harbor IDH mutations), as well as the 1p19q noncodeleted, but with IDH mutations, should be treated with combination chemoradiotherapy, and the third subset, 1p19q noncodeleted without IDH mutations, has the worst prognosis (similar to GBM) and appears unlikely to derive benefit from the addition of chemotherapy. In both the EORTC and RTOG trials, the longest overall survival after PCV chemotherapy plus radiotherapy was observed in patients whose anaplastic oligodendroglial tumors contained both allelic loss of 1p and 19q and IDH1 mutation (overall survival 12.8 years on EORTIC trial, 14.7 years on RTOG 9402). MGMT promoter methylation has also demonstrated prognostic significance for anaplastic oligodendroglial tumors. However, unlike grade IV astrocytoma tumors, in which MGMT promoter methylation predicts survival benefit from TMZ added to radiotherapy, MGMT promoter methylation has not shown similar predictive significance for outcome to PCV chemotherapy in anaplastic oligodendroglial tumors.[165] This is to be expected because MGMT methylation provides a mechanistic opportunity for TMZ to exert its specific cytotoxicity, and the PCV regimen does not contain TMZ or a drug that creates an identical cytotoxic DNA lesion. A German multicenter phase III trial of up-front radiotherapy versus up-front chemotherapy for newly diagnosed anaplastic gliomas observed IDH1 mutations to be a stronger prognostic factor than either 1p19q codeletion or MGMT promoter hypermethylation.[162] The caveat of course is that both MGMT promoter hypermethylation and IDH1 mutations are strongly correlated with 1p19q chromosomal loss.

Treatment

The current standard of care for patients with anaplastic oligodendrogliomas is maximal surgical resection followed by postoperative radiotherapy and chemotherapy. The radiotherapy target volume includes both the postoperative cavity and any residual enhancing disease, but also the FLAIR or T2 abnormality; unlike the situation with GBM, the postoperative FLAIR abnormality from anaplastic oligodendroglioma (and for that matter low-grade, grade 2 gliomas) most likely represents predominantly residual tumor with minimal contribution from tumor-associated edema and therefore has to be included in the target volume. Indirect support for this comes from the small, but growing body of data regarding supraradical resection of lower grade gliomas, where complete resection of all MR abnormality is associated with longer survival.[166] Although the commonly used radiotherapy dose on prospective trials of anaplastic oligodendroglioma is 59.4 Gy, this never took into account molecular variability, and some have proposed that consideration could be made to lower the RT dose to 54 Gy for tumors with favorable prognostic features as outlined above, to minimize long-term toxicity (e.g., 1p19q codeleted).

Anaplastic oligodendrogliomas are generally thought of as chemosensitive primarily based on high response rates to PCV in several studies. Two large randomized trials, described above, have investigated the use of sequential chemoradiotherapy compared to radiotherapy alone with chemotherapy reserved for salvage in patients with anaplastic oligodendroglioma and oligoastrocytoma.[38,39] With 11-year follow-up on RTOG 9402, the addition of PCV chemotherapy for four cycles prior to radiotherapy did not impact overall survival for the overall cohort, but did prolong overall survival for patients with allelic loss of both 1p and 19q from 7.7 years to 14.7 years.[38] Among patients without combined allelic loss of 1p and 19q, the addition of PCV chemotherapy prior to radiotherapy prolonged survival for patients with IDH1-mutated tumors from 3.3 to 5.5 years.[164] With 11-year follow-up, the EORTC trial did observe an overall survival prolongation with the addition of PCV for six cycles after radiotherapy in the overall cohort from 2.6 to 3.5 years, with more benefit observed in tumors with combined allelic loss of 1p and 19q.[39] Therefore, currently, it would be prudent to conclude that in practice, both the 1p19q codeleted and any IDH-mutated (with or without 1p19q codeletion) patients should receive chemoradiotherapy, but the role of combinatorial therapy for the 1p19q noncodeleted and IDH wild-type tumors is questionable.

Because of the significant toxicity associated with PCV, many clinicians now use TMZ, which is much better tolerated. TMZ has produced high response rates in patients with anaplastic oligodendroglioma. Chinot et al.[167] administered TMZ to 48 patients with anaplastic oligodendroglioma/oligoastrocytoma who had previously failed PCV chemotherapy. The objective response rate was 43.8% (complete response 16.7%, partial response 27.1%). Vogelbaum et al.[168] reported the results of RTOG 01-31, a phase II trial in which TMZ was given preradiotherapy to newly diagnosed patients with anaplastic oligodendroglioma/oligoastrocytoma. In the 27 patients available for review, the objective response rate was 33.3% (complete response 3.7%, partial response 29.6%). The 6-month-progression rate was 10.3%. Toxicity was acceptable. In a retrospective series from Ducray et al.,[169] up-front temozolomide for patients older than 70 with anaplastic oligodendroglioma or anaplastic oligoastrocytoma demonstrated a median progression-free survival of 6.9 months and median survival of 12.1 months, with improved outcomes in patients with MGMT methylation. Response to temozolomide has also been shown to be significantly associated with loss of 1p in a small retrospective study.[170]

In addition, a recent international retrospective study of over 1,000 adults with anaplastic oligodendroglial tumors observed that combination chemotherapy and radiotherapy was associated with longer time to progression and overall survival than either modality alone.[171] In cases without 1p19q codeletion, Lassman et al. observed that combination chemotherapy and radiotherapy was associated with longer time to progression and overall survival than either modality alone. In cases with 1p19q codeletion, combination chemotherapy and radiotherapy was associated with longer median time to progression compared to either modality alone, but this difference was not associated with a survival advantage. In addition, longer time to progression was observed with PCV, compared to temozolomide, in codeleted cases. Therefore, although temozolomide is widely used in lieu of PCV, the data supporting this practice are weak at best, and, based on Lassman's retrospective review, possibly deleterious.

Anaplastic Astrocytoma

Molecular Genetics

Anaplastic astrocytomas can be separated into molecular subgroups based on 1p19q codeletion status and IDH mutation status. Anaplastic astrocytoma with 1p19q codeletion and IDH mutation carries the most favorable prognosis, whereas anaplastic astrocytoma without 1p19q codeletion but with IDH mutation carries an intermediate prognosis. IDH wild-type anaplastic astrocytoma carries the worst prognosis, comparable biologically to GBM.[172]

Treatment

The current standard of care for patients with anaplastic oligodendrogliomas is maximal surgical resection followed by postoperative radiotherapy and chemotherapy. The radiotherapy target volume and dose are similar to those for anaplastic oligodendroglioma.

Levin et al. randomized patients with anaplastic gliomas or GBM to receive radiotherapy with adjuvant BCNU or PCV.[173] The use of PCV was found to be associated with an improved outcome in patients with anaplastic glioma. In contrast, a retrospective review of 432 patients with newly diagnosed anaplastic astrocytoma treated with BCNU or PCV on RTOG studies showed no improvement in survival with chemotherapy.[174]

A prospective phase III trial by the United Kingdom Medical Research Council randomized 674 patients of whom 117 (17%) had anaplastic astrocytoma after surgery to radiotherapy alone or radiotherapy followed by PCV.[175] There was no advantage for adjuvant PCV in any subgroup. The median survival of patients with anaplastic astrocytoma, 13 to 15 months, was substantially lower than the median survival of

2 to 3 years reported in previous trials, which has led to debate over the applicability of these results.

Temozolomide has shown activity in patients with recurrent anaplastic astrocytoma. In a phase II trial by Yung et al.[120] 162 patients with anaplastic astrocytoma were treated with temozolomide (150 to 200 mg/m²/d on days 1 to 5 every 28 days) at first relapse. The 6-month progression-free survival was 46% and overall survival was 13.6 months. The objective response rate was 35% (complete response 8%, partial response 27%).

The effectiveness of temozolomide was further tested in a phase III trial of non–1p19q-codeleted anaplastic glioma patients (the CATNON Intergroup trial). This trial randomized patients with newly diagnosed anaplastic glioma without 1p19q codeletion to radiotherapy alone versus radiotherapy followed by adjuvant temozolomide for 12 cycles versus radiotherapy concomitant with daily temozolomide and followed by 12 cycles of adjuvant temozolomide. Preliminary results from a planned interim analysis by an independent Data Monitoring Committee demonstrated a prolongation of overall survival with the addition of adjuvant temozolomide with an increase in 5-year survival from 44.1% to 55.9%.[176] MGMT methylation was observed in 42% of patients and was prognostic for overall survival. However, MGMT methylation did not predict for prolonged survival with the addition of adjuvant temozolomide. The impact of concurrent temozolomide and IDH1 mutational status requires further follow-up.

RTOG 9813 was a phase III trial of radiotherapy plus temozolomide versus radiotherapy plus nitrosourea.[172] This study closed early because of inability to meet target accrual rate. However, with median follow-up of 10.1 years, no difference in progression-free or overall survival was observed. However, the radiotherapy plus nitrosourea arm experienced more grade 3 or higher toxicity (76% vs. 48%) primarily because of myelosuppression, which led to discontinuation of therapy in 27.6% in the nitrosurea arm versus none in the temozlomide arm. The trial demonstrated the prognostic benefit of the IDH1 mutation in AA with IDH wild type (7.9 vs. 2.8 years).

The NOA-04 trial compared radiation with two chemotherapy regimens for anaplastic gliomas, the majority of whom carried a diagnosis of anaplastic astrocytoma.[177] In a 2:1:1 randomization, 318 patients were assigned to partial-brain irradiation alone versus PCV versus temozolomide with time to treatment failure as the primary endpoint. Chemotherapy failures were salvaged with radiotherapy, and vice versa, and further, temozolomide failures were salvaged with PCV and vice versa, almost ensuring that every patient received every therapy at some point. Time to treatment failure was similar between each of the arms, as was overall survival, imputing that the sequence of radiotherapy, temozolomide or PCV might not actually matter. This study also helped to establish *IDH1* mutation as an important prognostic factor for anaplastic astrocytoma.

A North American Intergroup trial is currently enrolling patients in order to compare chemoradiotherapy with either temozolomide or PCV for both grade 3 and grade 2 gliomas.

Evidence-Based Treatment Summary

1. Maximal resection, although not tested in a prospective trial, is generally associated with more favorable outcome and is recommended whenever feasible.
2. Molecular characterization of the tumor in terms of combined allelic loss of 1p and 19q and IDH mutational analysis carries important prognostic information.
3. Postoperative radiotherapy has been shown to provide a survival advantage in several clinical trials. These trials included patients with WHO grade III and IV tumors; no trial for only grade III tumors, evaluating RT versus no RT, has been conducted. The radiotherapy dose is typically 59.4% to 60 Gy in 6 to 6.5 weeks. Although some

Section III

have proposed that tumors with prognostically favorable molecular features could be treated to a slightly lower dose of 54 Gy in 6 weeks given the potential for extended survival with the addition of chemotherapy and the desire to minimize long-term neurotoxicity.

4. In patients with anaplastic oligodendroglioma, the addition of PCV chemotherapy to radiotherapy prolongs overall survival, most notably in patients with combined allelic loss of 1p and 19q, but also in those with IDH mutation. Although temozolomide is frequently used for these patients, there has been no direct comparison between PCV and temozolomide, and limited evidence supports its use.

5. In patients with anaplastic astrocytoma, (most without combined allelic loss of 1p and 19q), the addition of adjuvant temozolomide after radiotherapy provides a survival advantage, and IDH retains prognostic significance. The exact role of concurrent temozolomide and the impact of IDH mutational status have not been fully defined. Based on the NOA-04 trial, if all three approaches, i.e., radiation, temozolomide, and PCV are to be used, sequencing may not matter.

Low-Grade Glioma

Low-grade gliomas are generally slower-growing tumors that are divided into pilocytic and nonpilocyitc subtypes. They account for 20% of gliomas and 10% of primary intracranial tumors in adults.

Pilocytic Astrocytoma

Pilocytic astrocytoma, also known as juvenile pilocytic astrocytoma, corresponds to WHO grade I. They are more common in children. On imaging, they are well circumscribed enhancing lesions, often with a cystic component. Tandem duplication of chromosome 7q34 resulting in fusion of the BRAF and KIAA1549 genes is observed in 60% to 80% of sporadic pilocytic astrocytomas.[178]

Treatment

Pilocytic astrocytomas are more amenable to total resection than other low-grade gliomas. Fenestration of the cyst and resection of the mural nodule are usually curative. In tumors in which the wall of the cyst enhances, cystic degeneration of a larger tumor is more likely, and resection of the entire cyst is necessary. Complete resection of pilocytic astrocytomas is associated with excellent survival, with the majority (>90%) of patients cured of the tumor; no adjuvant therapy is necessary. Incomplete resection is associated with long-term survival rates of 70% to 80% at 10 years.

The benefit of postoperative radiotherapy is unclear. The usual recommendation is for close follow-up following gross or subtotal resection, and utilizing radiotherapy for tumors that have recurred more than once, or for those with considerable residual disease in a critical location, where even slight progression could result in significant morbidity. NCCTG 867251 enrolled 20 patients with supratentorial pilocytic astrocytoma on a prospective trial of radiotherapy after biopsy (3 patients) or observation after gross (11 patients) or subtotal (6 patients) resection.[179] With 20-year follow-up, progression-free survival was 95% and overall survival was 90% with the cause of death in both patients being unrelated to tumor. If radiotherapy is indicated, the dose is typically 50 to 54 Gy (1.8 to 2 Gy fractions). However, there is evidence of improved progression-free survival with RT, and immediate postoperative irradiation may be appropriate in some relatively uncommon cases, depending on the location of the tumor, the extent of residual disease, the feasibility of repeated surgical excision, and availability for follow-up.

The presence of the tandem duplication of chromosome 7q34 resulting in fusion of the BRAF and KIAA1549 genes, observed in 60% to 80% of sporadic pilocytic astrocytomas,

has prompted the use of BRAF inhibitors in some of these patients, especially at recurrence, and when other options have been exhausted. Occasional tumor responses have been reported.

Evidence-Based Treatment Summary

1. Maximal surgical resection, although not tested in a prospective trial, is associated with more favorable outcome and is recommended whenever feasible. Molecular testing, especially for BRAF should be conducted, if feasible.

2. Postoperative radiotherapy may be considered in patients with incompletely resected tumors, based on risk factors for progression and consequences of progression.

3. Chemotherapy does not have an established role in pilocytic astrocytoma in adults, but BRAF inhibitors are being used in situations where other options have been exhausted.

Nonpilocytic/Diffusely Infiltrating Gliomas

Nonpilocytic or diffusely infiltrating low-grade gliomas are classified as WHO grade II tumors. They may arise from astrocytic, oligodendrocytic, or mixed lineage. Presentation usually occurs in the third or fourth decade of life and only a small percentage of patients are younger than 19 or older than 65. Approximately 80% of patients present with seizures.[180] CT typically demonstrates an ill-defined, diffuse, nonenhancing low-density region, often in the frontal or temporal lobes. Calcifications are commonly seen with oligodendrogliomas. MRI is more sensitive in detecting and defining these lesions, which are hypointense and nonenhancing on T1-weighted images and hyperintense on T2-weighted images. Because these tumors are highly infiltrative, tumor always extends beyond the abnormality observed on imaging. MR imaging analysis reveals an average growth rate of 5 mm/year.[181]

Histologically, there is increased cellularity compared to normal brain tissue with mild to moderate nuclear pleomorphism and no evidence of mitotic activity, vascular proliferative changes or necrosis. Differentiation from reactive gliosis can be difficult. Histologic subtypes are often identified in low-grade astrocytomas. Fibrillary and protoplasmic subtypes convey no specific prognostic information. Gemistocytic subtypes behave in a fashion more consistent with a malignant glioma.

Several clinical variables have been found to be of prognostic importance. Pignatti et al.[182] performed the most comprehensive of these analyses and constructed a scoring system to identify patients at low and high risk. This trial was based on data from two large European phase III trials for low-grade glioma designed to examine the dose and timing of postoperative radiotherapy, EORTC 22844 and 22845. Cox regression analysis was used to identify prognostic variables from 322 patients from EORTC 22844 and then validated on 288 patients from EORTC 22845. Multivariate analysis showed that age 40 or older, astrocytoma histology, maximum diameter 6 cm or greater, tumor crossing the midline, and presence of neurologic deficits negatively impacted survival. A prognostic scoring system was derived: patients with up to two of these factors were considered low risk (median survival 7.7 years) and patients with three or more, high risk (median survival 3.2 years). However, the data used to identify these prognostic factors predated modern clinical trials evaluating molecular genetics.

Molecular Diagnosis and Prognosis

The 2007 WHO criteria classified tumor subtype based on subjective measures that led to significant interobserver variability and suboptimal diagnostic reproducibility. Recent retrospective molecular analyses of tumors from patients enrolled on randomized clinical trials have identified important molecular alterations with prognostic implications. As described above, this has led to a fundamental shift in tumor classification using a combined histologic-genotype model, as outlined in the 2016 WHO CNS tumor grading system (Table 38.3), which gives priority to genotypic alterations over histologic appearance in order to reduce subjectivity and increase reliability.

The distinction between astrocytoma and oligodendroglioma rests on the detection of combined allelic loss of 1p and 19q, which is characteristic of oligodendroglioma, as well as additional genetic aberrations such as ATRX, TP53, and TERT mutations. 1p19q codeletion is present only with an IDH1 mutation and is the molecular signature with the most favorable overall prognosis. The prior tumor subtype of mixed oligoastrocytoma is no longer considered a distinct entity on the 2016 WHO CNS tumor grading system, as the 1p19q-codeleted and IDH-mutant grade II oligodendroglioma and the IDH-mutant grade II astrocytoma are considered mutually exclusive subtypes. 1p19q-codeleted and IDH-mutant grade II oligodendroglioma, when associated with a TERT mutation, carries a median overall survival of 11 years, whereas IDH-mutant grade II astrocytoma associated with TP53 mutation and ATRX loss carries a median survival of only 6 to 8 years. Low-grade gliomas identified as IDH wild type show clinical behavior similar to high-grade tumors with poor overall survival.[183]

Smith et al.[158] found loss of 1p and 19q in 44% of 52 patients with oligodendrogliomas, of which 34 (65%) were low grade. Combined loss of 1p and 19q was associated with an improved probability of survival, independent of other factors such as age. Fallon et al.[184] examined 139 tumor samples from 80 patients with primary and recurrent oligodendrogliomas of which 74% were grade II at initial diagnosis. Combined loss of 1p and 19q occurred in 71% of patients, more commonly in pure oligodendrogliomas (75%) than in mixed oligoastrocytomas (39%). Patients with combined loss of 1p and 19q had an overall median survival of 14.9 years compared to 4.7 years for those without 1p and 19q deletions.

Okamota et al.[185] found a similar frequency of loss of 1p and 19q of 70% in patients with low-grade oligodendrogliomas in a population-based study. In a review of 44 cases of low-grade oligodendrocytic tumors, Sasaki et al.[186] considered half of the cases classical oligodendroglioma and the remainder nonclassical oligodendroglioma with more astrocytic features on histopathology. Deletion of 1p was detected in 86% and 27% of these groups, respectively. Response to chemotherapy was assessed at time of recurrence in 13 patients. Of the 11 who responded to chemotherapy, 10 had loss of 1p. Both of the nonresponders were found not to have loss of 1p. A small prospective trial by Hoang-Xuan et al.[187] found a similar trend. Loss of 1p with or without loss of 19q, which was detected in 12/26 patients with low-grade oligodendrocytic tumors treated with temozolomide, was found to have a significant association with response to chemotherapy ($P < .004$).

IDH1 mutations may be predictive of a better prognosis in patients with low-grade gliomas, but this marker does not categorically appear to predict response to chemotherapy, with the caveat that the data testing this are dated and sparse.[188] In one prospective trial of radiotherapy with or without chemotherapy, presence of IDH1 mutation was associated with prolonged median survival from 5.1 years among patients without the mutation to 13.1 years among those with the mutation, when receiving the combined modalities.[189] Promoter methylation of the PTEN gene has been associated with poorer prognosis and a higher likelihood of malignant transformation.[190] Other smaller studies have not shown an association between other molecular findings and chemosensitivity.[191,192]

Unplanned molecular analyses of EORTC 22033-26033 demonstrated prognostic significance associated with molecular characterization.[193] Median PFS was 62 months for IDH-mutated/1p19q-codeleted tumors, 48 months for IDH-mutated/1p19q noncodeleted tumors, and 20 months for IDH

wild-type tumors. MGMT promoter was methylated in all patients with IDH-mutated/1p19-codeleted tumors, in 86% of IDH-mutated/1p19q noncodeleted tumors, and 56% of IDH wild-type tumors.

Treatment

The clinical course for patients with diffusely infiltrative low-grade tumors is variable with some patients having long survival even with treatment and others suffering from progressive deterioration despite treatment. In general, early intervention is indicated for almost all patients. Adequate tissue sampling is critical to ensure accurate diagnosis, and maximal surgical resection in this context may be advisable in appropriately selected patients. In younger patients (<40 years) who have undergone complete resection, observation with serial imaging is an option. In those who have undergone a subtotal resection or those with high-risk features, postoperative radiotherapy and chemotherapy is recommended, typically 50 to 54 Gy in 1.8 Gy fractions.

Surgery

Although surgery is considered an integral part of treatment, the goal of surgery and its timing are still debated. In practice, most patients undergo surgery at presentation in order to establish the diagnosis and to determine histology, grade, and molecular characteristics that affect treatment. However, even under the best circumstances, total resection with an adequate margin is rarely achieved because of the diffusely infiltrative nature of these tumors and involvement of eloquent regions. Although controversial, most studies have found total or subtotal (>90%) resection to be associated with improved outcome.[194] Moreover, with the advent of modern MR imaging and intraoperative electrostimulation in the awake craniotomy setting to assist in identifying critical areas of the brain, resection may be achieved with less morbidity and mortality than in the past.[194-196] Proponents of aggressive resection are also supported by studies that suggest that radical surgery results in more accurate histopathologic diagnosis.[197] In RTOG 98-02, 5-year progression-free survival in 111 good risk patients, defined as patient age <40 and gross total tumor resection, was 48%.[198] Review of postoperative MR imaging demonstrated crude recurrence rates of 26%, 68%, and 89% for <1, 1 to 2 and >2 cm residual disease, respectively.

Radiotherapy

Three recent phase III trials provide the best evidence with respect to the indications for radiotherapy as well as the dose (Table 38.5).

Patients considered favorable by the scoring system introduced by Pignatti et al.[182] are typically observed postoperatively and given radiotherapy at disease progression or recurrence. This practice is based on the results of a phase III trial by van

TABLE 38.5 PHASE III TRIALS OF PATIENTS WITH LOW-GRADE GLIOMA TREATED WITH RADIOTHERAPY

Study (Reference)	Treatment Arm	N	5-Year Survival (%)
EORTC 22845	Observation[a]	157	66
	54 Gy (30 fractions)	157	68
EORTC 22844	45 Gy (25 fractions)	171	58
	59.4 Gy (33 fractions)	172	59
NCCTG	50.4 (28 fractions)	101	72
RTOG 9802	64.8 (36 fractions)	102	64
(age ≥40 or STR)	54 Gy (30 fractions)	128	63
	54 Gy plus PCV	126	72

[a]Treatment with radiotherapy at progression.
CCNU, vincristine; EORTC, European Organization for Research and Treatment of Cancer; N, number of patients; NCCTG, North Central Cancer Treatment Group; PCV, procarbazine; RTOG, Radiation Therapy Oncology Group; TMZ, temozolomide.

den Bent et al. in EORTC 22845.[199] In this multi-institutional trial, 314 patients with low-grade gliomas were randomized to receive postoperative radiotherapy to 54 Gy in fractions of 1.8 Gy (n = 157) or radiotherapy at progression (n = 157). A significant improvement in median progression-free survival was found with early radiotherapy, 5.3 versus 3.4 years (P < .0001), but there was no difference in median survival, 7.4 versus 7.2 years (P = .872). It is of note that only 65% the patients in the delayed radiotherapy group received radiotherapy at progression. Malignant transformation occurred in 65% to 72% of patients with no difference between the two groups. Although seizure control was superior in the early radiotherapy group, adequate data on quality of life were not obtained. The authors concluded that although early radiotherapy may be appropriate in some situations, for example, patients with symptomatic lesions, withholding radiotherapy until tumor progression does not jeopardize survival.

For patients given radiotherapy postoperatively, the dose has been established by 2 phase III trials. In EORTC 22844 379, patients were randomized to receive 45 Gy in 5 weeks or 59.4 Gy in 6.6 weeks postoperatively.[200] With a median follow-up of 74 months, overall survival (58% vs. 59%) and progression-free survival (47% vs. 50%) were similar in both arms.

In a joint North Central Cancer Treatment Group (NCCTG), RTOG, and ECOG study, 203 patients were randomized to low-dose radiotherapy to 50.4 Gy in 28 fractions (n = 101) or high-dose radiotherapy to 64.8 Gy in 36 fractions.[201] There was no significant difference in progression-free survival or overall survival. Survival at 2 and 5 years was 94% and 72%, respectively, with low-dose radiotherapy and 85% and 64% with high-dose radiotherapy. Grade 3 to 5 neurotoxicity occurred in 5% of patients in the high-dose cohort and 2.5% of patients in the low-dose cohort.

Consequently low-dose radiotherapy, 50 to 54 Gy in 1.8 Gy fractions, is the standard of care for patients with low-grade gliomas. The target volume is local, with a margin of 2 cm beyond changes demonstrated on traditional MRI sequences. Using FLAIR images, which usually show abnormality beyond any enhancing or nonenhancing tumor, a smaller margin of 0.8 to 1 cm may be used.

However, this concept of dose will likely need to be revisited in light of the fact that it might be possible to decrease dose (to say 45 Gy) in the most favorable subset (1p19q codeleted, IDH mutated), but increase it (to say 59.4 Gy) in the most unfavorable subset (IDH wild type).

Chemotherapy

Multiagent chemotherapy, in particular PCV, appears promising with response rates ranging from 50 to 80% in recurrent and newly diagnosed tumors.[191,192] The publication of mature results from RTOG 9802 has significantly altered the standard of care, as the addition of PCV to radiotherapy provided a significant overall survival advantage.[189] In this phase III trial, 254 unfavorable patients (age 40 or greater with subtotal resection or biopsy) were randomized to receive radiotherapy alone to 54 Gy in 30 fractions or radiotherapy followed by six cycles of standard-dose PCV. With a median follow-up of 11.9 years, median overall survival was extended from 7.8 years following radiotherapy alone to 13.3 years following radiotherapy plus chemotherapy, and 10-year overall survival was increased from 40% with radiotherapy alone to 60% following radiotherapy plus chemotherapy. The superiority of radiotherapy plus chemotherapy over radiotherapy alone was observed with all histologic subtypes, although the difference did not reach statistical significance among patients with astrocytoma. Patients with IDH1-mutated tumors had longer survival with the addition of chemotherapy to radiotherapy. The number of events in patients with IDH1 wild-type tumors was too small to

evaluate treatment effect in this subgroup. Acute grade 3 or 4 toxicity occurred in 67% of patients who received radiotherapy plus PCV as compared with 9% of patients who received radiotherapy alone.

Temozolomide has been shown to have activity in phase II trials in newly diagnosed and recurrent low-grade gliomas.[187,202–204] RTOG 0424[205] was a phase II study of patients diagnosed with low-grade glioma with three or more risk factors for recurrence as established by the aforementioned EORTC Cog regression analysis, reported by Pignatti and colleagues[182]: (1) age ≥ 40, (2) astrocytoma histology, (3) bihemispherical tumor, (4) preoperative tumor diameter ≥6 cm, and (5) preoperative neurologic function status >1. In this study, patients were treated with radiotherapy to 54 Gy in 30 fractions with concurrent and adjuvant temozolomide for 12 cycles. With median follow-up of 4.1 years, 3-year overall survival was 73%, which was significantly improved relative to the 54% rate derived from the prespecified historical control. Median survival time had not yet been reached. Three-year PFS was 59%. Grade 3 or higher toxicities were increased from 10% to 43% with the addition of temozolomide.

Prior to the publication of the mature results of RTOG 9802, a number of efforts to exclude or delay radiotherapy in the management of low-grade glioma, based on the expectation of equivalent results from the use of temozolomide were undertaken.

EORTC 22033-26033 was a phase III intergroup trial that randomized 477 patients to either dose-dense temozolomide (75 mg/m² once daily for 21 days, repeated every 28 days (one cycle) for maximum of 12 cycles) or radiotherapy (50.4 Gy in 28 fractions) with low-grade glioma and at least one of the following high-risk features: (1) age ≥40, (2) progressive disease, (3) tumor size >5 cm, tumor crossing midline, or neurologic symptoms.[193] The primary endpoint was PFS, with the study powered to demonstrate a prolongation in PFS with the use of dose-dense temozolomide as opposed to radiotherapy. The study observed no difference in PFS with median PFS of 46 months following radiotherapy and 39 months following temozolomide. Unplanned analyses demonstrated improved PFS with radiotherapy relative to temozolomide for IDH-mutated, 1p19q noncodeleted tumors (55 vs. 36 months). Other molecular subgroups did not show treatment-related differences, although patient numbers in this unplanned analysis were small. Temozolomide was associated with higher grade 3 to 4 hematologic toxicity (9% vs. <1%) and more grade 3 to 4 infections (3% vs. 1%). With median follow-up of 3 years, no difference between health-related quality of life, assessed using the EORTC patient-reported questionnaires, and cognitive function, as assessed by the Mini-Mental Status Examination, was observed.[206] This trial, at least based on the results available to date, does not support the use of up-front temozolomide and deferral of radiotherapy for WHO grade II gliomas. Similarly, a prospective single-institution trial of 120 patients with WHO grade II gliomas proactively treated with up-front temozolomide, and deferral of radiotherapy demonstrated median survival of 9.7 years, considerably inferior to the 13.3 years noted on the chemoradiotherapy arm of RTOG 9802.[207] These data therefore should suffice to detract from the practice of radiotherapy deferral for these patients, outside the clinical trial context.[193,206]

Evidence-Based Treatment Summary

1. Maximal surgical resection, although not tested in a prospective trial, is generally associated with more favorable outcome and is recommended whenever feasible.
2. Molecular analysis of resected tumors for 1p19q codeletion, IDH1 mutation, and MGMT promoter methylation, as well as other genetic aberrations such as TP53, TERT,

and ATRX, provides important prognostic information that complements known clinical risk factors and may aid in treatment decision-making; these should be obtained whenever feasible.

3. Postoperative radiotherapy has not been shown to provide a survival advantage in the only clinical trial testing this question, although progression-free survival and seizure control were superior. The typical radiotherapy dose is 45 to 54 Gy; randomized trials do not show a survival advantage with higher doses, but dose-tailoring based on molecular features has not been tested and could be considered in future trials. In fact, based on the longevity of patients with favorable features, other attempts to reduce radiotherapy-related toxicity should also be considered, and in that vein, NRG Oncology has launched a randomized trial testing protons versus photons for grade 2 gliomas.

4. In a practice-changing phase III trial, the addition of PCV chemotherapy to radiotherapy significantly lengthened overall survival in patients with subtotally resected tumors or whose age was 40 or higher. The addition of temozolomide to radiotherapy has also improved survival in high-risk tumors relative to historical control data, but these data do not approach level 1. A randomized trial comparing temozolomide radiotherapy to PCV with radiotherapy is underway.

5. The substitution of radiotherapy with dose-dense temozolomide in high-risk tumors does not provide a PFS benefit, significantly augments hematologic toxicities, and does not impact long-term cognitive functioning or patient-reported quality of life. In IDH-mutated/1p19q noncodeleted tumors, radiotherapy is associated with improved PFS relative to dose-dense temozolomide. Retrospective comparison to a large multi-institutional experience raises concern about possible survival degradation when radiotherapy is deferred.

Gliomatosis Cerebri

Gliomatosis cerebri is a rare condition with diffuse involvement of multiple parts of the brain (greater than two lobes), frequent bilateral growth and regular infratentorial extension. This entity has been removed from the 2016 revision of the WHO classification of CNS tumors but is instead considered a special pattern of spread of diffuse glioma subtypes, and therefore, obtaining tissue and performing molecular analysis is strongly recommended.[16] On MRI, there is typically diffuse increased signal on T2-weighted and FLAIR images and low or absent signal in the affected areas on T1-weighted images.

Treatment choices remain limited. Perkins et al.[208] reviewed the treatment outcomes of 30 patients with gliomatosis cerebri treated with radiotherapy. Transient radiographic improvement or disease stabilization was achieved in 87% of patients with clinical improvement observed in 70%. Patients younger than 40 and those with nonglioblastoma histology had significantly improved overall survival.

In a French study, 63 patients with gliomatosis cerebri were treated initially with PCV or temozolomide.[209] Objective responses were observed in 33% of patients and radiologic responses in 26% with no significant difference between the two regimens. Median progression-free survival and overall survival were 16 and 29 months, respectively. Regardless of regimen, patients with an oligodendroglial component had significantly better outcomes in terms of progression-free and overall survival.

A recent German phase II trial treated 35 gliomatosis cerebri patients with procarbazine and lomustine.[210] Median progression-free survival was 14 months, and median overall survival was 30 months. Twelve patients received salvage radiotherapy at progression. IDH1 mutation was a strong independent prognostic factor.

A retrospective review of 296 patients with gliomatosis cerebri from the literature (n = 206) and the Association des Neuro-Oncologues d'Expression Francaise (ANOCEF) network (n = 90) demonstrated median survival of 14.5 months.[211] Patients younger than 42, with better KPS, low-grade histology, or oligodendroglial subtype, had better outcomes. The impact of radiotherapy on survival remained unclear.

Evidence-Based Treatment Summary

1. Maximal surgical resection is not an achievable goal.
2. Radiotherapy is considered the standard, but no trials have validated its role. Dose remains ill defined.
3. The role of chemotherapy remains ill defined.
4. In the absence of definitive data, our recommendation is therefore to treat based on histopathologic and molecular features; one such strategy includes the following:

   a. Non-GBM, IDH mutated, (grade 2 or 3): treat all visible tumor to 45 Gy with concurrent and adjuvant temozolomide.
   b. Non-GBM, IDH wild type, (grade 2 or 3): evaluate for MGMT status; if methylated, treat all visible tumor to at least 45 Gy (and consider possible focal boosting to 54 to 59.4 Gy), with concurrent and adjuvant temozolomide; if unmethylated, substitute PCV for temozolomide.
   c. GBM: if MGMT unmethylated, RT alone, and if methylated, temozolomide alone; consider adding RT for methylated patients if performance status is high, or there is significant tumor response to temozolomide.

Adult Brainstem Glioma

Brainstem gliomas account for 15% of all pediatric brain tumors but can occur in adults.[212] They can be divided into several distinct types. Diffuse midline glioma is a narrowly defined but phenotypically and molecularly distinct tumor that is characterized by K27M mutations in the histone H3 gene *HeF3A*, or less commonly in the related *HIST1H3B* gene, occurring primarily in children (but sometimes in adults), with a diffuse growth pattern and midline location (e.g., thalamus, brainstem, and spinal cord).[213,214] This entity was newly defined in the 2016 revision to the WHO classification system and includes tumors previously referred to as diffuse intrinsic pontine glioma (DIPG).[16] Although these tumors are associated with poor prognosis, their distinct molecular characteristic provides rationale for future targeted therapies.

Diffuse midline gliomas can have diverse imaging appearances, ranging from expansile masses without enhancement or necrosis to peripherally enhancing masses with central necrosis but little surrounding T2/FLAIR abnormality.[215] In contrast, focal, dorsally exophytic or cervicomedullary tumors can be low grade and have a much better prognosis, especially when found in the context of neurofibromatosis. In addition, enhancement, particularly in a focal lesion, may suggest a juvenile pilocytic astrocytoma rather than a high-grade glioma. Although rare, other aggressive tumors such as PNETs and atypical teratoid-rhabdoid tumors can occur in the brainstem.[216,217] Nonneoplastic processes that may be confused with a primary brainstem tumor include neurofibromatosis, demyelinating diseases, arteriovenous malformations, abscess, and encephalitis.

Treatment

Corticosteroids may be necessary to manage neurologic symptoms until treatment is instituted. Patients with hydrocephalus may require placement of a ventriculoperitoneal shunt. The approach to treatment should be based on the type of brainstem glioma as determined by both the clinical presentation and radiographic findings. Surgery is the treatment of choice for operable lesions (i.e., accessible focal tumors, dorsally exophytic and cervicomedullary tumors). For low-grade tumors amenable to surgical resection, as in other low-grade gliomas, the role of postoperative radiotherapy is controversial and many would advocate close observation. For unresectable low-grade tumors radiotherapy should be delivered using volumes and doses as for low-grade gliomas in other locations.

Involved field radiotherapy is the primary treatment for infiltrating pontine gliomas. The GTV is usually best defined using T2-weighted or FLAIR MRI. A margin of 1 to 1.5 cm is added to create a CTV and further expanded by 0.3 to 0.5 cm to create a PTV. Margins may not need to be uniform in all directions, particularly where bone limits tumor extension. These lesions should be treated with doses on the order of 55.8 to 60 Gy using daily fractions of 1.8 to 2.0 Gy/day. Although radiotherapy provides short-term benefits, long-term results have remained dismal. There is no benefit from radiotherapy dose-escalation. Chemotherapy has no established role. Chapter 82 provides more details as most data on intrinsic pontine gliomas come from pediatric trials.

Fewer data exist with respect to brainstem glioma in adults, but there is some evidence that these tumors may be less aggressive in adults, with overall survival that ranges from 45% to 66% at 2 to 5 years, perhaps because of a greater frequency of more favorable tumor types.[218] Kesari et al.[219] published a series of 101 adults with brainstem gliomas and observed 5- and 10-year overall survival rates of 58% and 41%, respectively. Of 24 candidate factors, they observed prognostic significance associated with ethnicity, tumor location, age of diagnosis and tumor grade. In the series from ANOCEF, 48 adult patients with brainstem gliomas were grouped on the basis of their clinical, radiologic, and histologic features.[220] Nearly half had nonenhancing diffusely infiltrative tumors and had symptoms that were present for more than 3 months. Eleven of these 22 patients underwent biopsy, and nine had low-grade histology. Nearly all underwent radiotherapy and had a median survival of 7.3 years. A second group of 15 patients who had presented with rapid progression of symptoms and had contrast enhancement on MRI were described. Fourteen of these patients underwent biopsy and anaplasia was identified in all 14 specimens. Despite radiotherapy, the median survival in this group was 11.2 months, which approximates the survival in pediatric series.

Evidence-Based Treatment Summary

1. Surgical resection is indicated for patients with favorable tumor types (based mostly on location) but is not an achievable goal in patients with intrinsic pontine gliomas; however, obtaining tissue is strongly recommended, and molecular testing should be considered.
2. The H3 K27M mutation defines a phenotypically and molecularly distinct tumor, called diffuse midline glioma, occurring in midline location and associated with an especially poor prognosis; however, this maybe a targetable driver mutation. Gliomas with diffuse growth pattern and midline location should be tested for H3 K27M mutation.
3. For diffuse midline gliomas, radiotherapy is considered the standard. The addition of chemotherapy remains undefined.

Ependymoma

Ependymoma accounts for only 1.8% of all adult brain tumors.[2] Rosette formation is a hallmark of ependymoma on pathologic specimens. WHO grade I ependymomas, including myxopapillary ependymoma, typically occur in the spine, and subependymoma.[16] In adults, the subependymomas, which are mostly intracranial, have favorable clinical outcomes. Ependymomas are otherwise divided between WHO grade II and III (anaplastic), with the latter showing increased mitotic activity, tumor necrosis, and microvascular proliferation suggests a diagnosis of anaplastic ependymoma. Unlike pediatric ependymomas, which largely arise intracranially, 75% of ependymomas in the

adult population arise in the spinal canal. Spinal ependymomas typically present with sensory deficits. Ependymomas may expand locally, extend along ependymal spaces, and occasionally disseminate through the CSF. However, the predominant pattern of relapse is local, even when anaplasia is present.[221-226]

Posterior fossa and supratentorial ependymoma are biologically different tumors but are both treated with surgery and radiotherapy. In a recent international collaborative study,[227] nine molecular subgroups of ependymoma were identified, three in each anatomic compartment: spine (SP), posterior fossa (PF), and supratentorial (ST) region. In each compartment, one molecular subgroup of WHO grade I subependymoma (ST-SE, PF-SE, and SP-SE) was observed, occurring in adults only. In the spine, the two other molecular subgroups matched the histopathologic diagnoses of myxopapillary ependymoma (SP-MPE) and WHO grade II and III ependymoma (SP-EPN). In the posterior fossa, the remaining two molecular subtypes were classified as PF-EPN-A and PF-EPN-B. PF-EPN-A occurs primarily in infants and young children (but is observed in 11% of adult patients) and because of its predominately lateral location can be difficult to completely resect and thus is associated with high relapse rates.[228] PF-EPN-B occurs primarily in older children and adults and is associated with more favorable prognosis. More than 70% of supratentorial ependymomas are characterized by fusions between *C11ORF95* and *RELA* genes.[229] Termed ST-EPN-RELA tumors, these ependymomas are can occur in both adults and children and are recognized as a distinct molecular entity by the 2016 revision of the WHO classification system. The remaining supratentorial tumors harbor fusions to the oncogene *YAP1* and have a highly favorable prognosis.

Treatment

Maximal surgical resection, including second surgery if necessary, is the initial treatment for ependymoma. Surgery alone may be sufficient in selected patients based on the results of pediatric series described in Chapter 82. However, the standard of care for most adults is postoperative irradiation. There appears to be a radiation dose response with improved tumor control with doses >50 Gy and doses of 54 to 59.4 Gy are typically prescribed. Radiation dose for spinal ependymomas can be limited by spinal cord tolerance. At 1.8 to 2 Gy/fraction, the estimated risk of radiation myelopathy is <1% at 54 Gy and <10% at 61 Gy.[230]

Historically, for posterior fossa tumors, the entire posterior fossa has been irradiated. However, Paulino[231] has shown that the pattern of failure to be "local," i.e., within the tumor bed itself. In nine patients who received radiation therapy to the tumor bed plus a 2 cm margin, the two failures in this group were within the tumor bed (i.e., there were no failures within the posterior fossa outside the tumor bed). For most patients, a more usual volume now consists of the tumor bed and any residual disease (GTV) plus an anatomically defined margin of 1 to 1.5 cm to create a CTV. Larger margins may be required in areas of infiltration, and special attention must be paid to areas of spread along the cervical spine because 10% to 30% of fourth ventricular tumors extend down through the foramen magnum to the upper cervical spine.[225,232] Radiotherapy field size for spinal ependymomas commonly includes two cranial and two caudal vertebral bodies. Lumbosacral or sacral ependymomas should include coverage of nerve roots with the caudal border extending to S4/S5 and lateral borders extending to the sacroiliac joints.

In the past, CSI was recommended for patients with high-grade and infratentorial tumors who were believed to be at an increased risk of CSF spread.[223] Modern series document that local recurrence is the primary pattern of failure and that the incidence of isolated spinal relapses is low even among the highest-risk patients, with the majority of spinal failures associated with local recurrences.[221,224] As a result, the current recommendation for patients with ependymomas is limited-field radiation if the spinal MRI scan and CSF cytology are negative. Patients with neuraxis spread (positive MRI or positive CSF cytology) should receive CSI (36 Gy) with boosts to the areas of gross disease and to the primary tumor to total doses of 50 to 59.4 Gy. One exception is spinal myxopapillary ependymomas (WHO grade I), where MR evidence of neuraxis spread can be treated with focal radiotherapy, rather than CSI.

Chemotherapy has not been proven useful in ependymoma. Randomized trials of chemotherapy in the pediatric population have failed to identify a clinically useful benefit relative to radiotherapy,[233] although a study of neoadjuvant chemotherapy to permit second-look surgery for subtotally resected tumors remains ongoing.

Results of Treatment

In modern series that utilized mostly local fields for patients with nondisseminated disease 5-year survival is on the order of 70%.[223,232,234–237]

Several authors have attempted to identify variables associated with improved outcome in adults. Ferrante et al.[235] analyzed 20 patients with fourth ventricle ependymomas. The 5-year survival rate in patients older than 16 years was 60%. The use of postoperative irradiation was associated with a markedly improved 5-year survival of 68% versus 18% without radiotherapy ($P = .011$).

Reni et al.[238] reported on a series of 70 adult intracranial ependymomas and observed 5-year overall and progression-free survival rates of 67% and 43%, respectively. Older age and supratentorial location were poor prognostic factors, and the use of postoperative radiotherapy was associated with improved progression-free survival and a trend toward improved overall survival.

Metellus et al.[239] evaluated 114 adult patients with intracranial ependymoma and observed incomplete resection and supratentorial location to be significant predictors of recurrence and poor survival. For incompletely resetected tumors, postoperative radiotherapy improved both overall and progression-free survival. In a study of spinal myxopapillary ependymomas from the Rare Cancer Network,[240] use of postoperative radiotherapy was an independent predictor of progression-free survival.

A retrospective study of 23 adult patients with supratentorial ependymomas treated at Columbia-Presbyterian Medical Center with a variety of radiotherapy field sizes and doses (including SRS) showed a 5-year survival rate of 100% for hemispheric tumors and 73% for third ventricular tumors.[237] Of interest, six patients with low-grade tumors did not receive postoperative irradiation. Five remained free of recurrence during a mean follow-up period of 69 months.

Five-year survival was 62% for a French series of 34 adult patients with ependymoma, 17 of whom had anaplastic histology.[241] Gross total resection was performed in 27 patients. Half of the 34 patients were irradiated; 13 of these received local fields to a mean dose of 56 Gy. Univariate analysis showed that anaplasia and location in the brain parenchyma predicted for poor outcome.

Evidence-Based Treatment Summary

1. Maximal surgical resection should be performed when feasible.
2. Postoperative radiotherapy is considered the standard, but no prospective trials have validated its role. CSI is used only in patients with disseminated disease.
3. The role of chemotherapy remains to be defined.

Medulloblastoma

Medulloblastoma is a relatively rare tumor in adults with an incidence of 0.5 per 100,000.[2,242] The majority arise in the 20- to 40-year age group. Adult medulloblastomas are more frequently located laterally than those in childhood (50% vs. 10%), and are more frequently desmoplastic.[243] In addition, the incidence of severe anaplasia is lower than in the pediatric population.[244] Medulloblastoma is a densely cellular tumor with small, darkly staining ovoid cells with hyperchromatic nuclei and frequent mitoses. Homer Wright rosettes (clustered cells surrounding a central eosinophilic core) are characteristic. CSF dissemination may manifest as positive cytology or macroscopic seeding of the subarachnoid space and is not uncommon. Systemic spread is seen in approximately 5% of patients, mostly to bone and bone marrow. Shunt procedures have been suggested as a cause, although modern series dispute this.[245]

In children, adverse prognostic factors include male gender and age <3 years.[246] Patients with total or near-total resections fare better than those with subtotal resection or biopsy only, and residual tumor >1.5 cm² on postoperative scans is an adverse prognostic factor. Patients with CSF spread have a worse prognosis. Patients are classified as "average risk" if there is <1.5 cm² residual tumor and no dissemination; patients with >1.5 cm² residual and/or dissemination are considered "high risk."

Molecular analyses have identified four distinct subgroups that have now been defined in the 2016 revision to the WHO classification system.[16,247] WNT tumors most frequently occur in late childhood and adolescence, are rarely metastatic, and have a favorable prognosis regardless of metastatic status. Most WNT tumors display classic medulloblastoma histology and nuclear localization of CTNNB1 (β-catenin), as detected by immunohistochemical staining.[248] Ongoing research has focused on therapeutic de-escalation for this favorable subtype, although prognosis of WNT tumors is worse in adults, relative to pediatric patients.[249] SHH tumors account for most of the infant and adult medulloblastomas and are rare in children. SHH tumors are typically found within the cerebellar hemispheres and have an intermediate prognosis. All nodular desmoplastic medulloblastomas can be characterized as SHH subgroup.[250] Non-WNT and non-SHH tumors are classified as group 3 or 4. Although there can be considerable overlap between these groups, group 3 tumors have characteristically poor prognosis. Group 3 tumors affect mostly infants and children, are rare in adults, commonly present with metastases, and are characterized by MYC amplification. Group 4 tumors can affect patients of all ages.

Treatment

All patients with nondisseminated medulloblastoma should undergo complete resection if feasible. In cases where extension into the brainstem precludes complete resection without significant morbidity, there is no benefit to complete surgical resection as compared to near-total resection.[251]

In general, the treatment guidelines for pediatric medulloblastoma detailed in Chapter 82 should probably be followed. Postoperative radiotherapy should begin within 28 to 31 days following surgical resection whenever possible. Radiotherapy is delivered to the entire craniospinal axis followed by a boost to the tumor bed for average-risk patients and to the posterior fossa and gross metastatic disease for high-risk patients. Although there may be less concern over long-term toxicity of full-dose CSI in adults as compared with children, adults treated for medulloblastoma with a mean dose to the whole brain of 35 Gy have been shown to have long-term cognitive deficits.[252] It may be reasonable to extrapolate from the pediatric experience and to treat healthy young adults with average-risk disease with reduced-dose CSI (23.4 Gy) as long as appropriate multiagent chemotherapy is administered. For average-risk patients, boost to the tumor bed plus a 1.5 cm margin as opposed to whole posterior fossa) to 54 Gy is associated with equivalent event-free survival outcomes, although reduction in CSI to 18 Gy (as opposed to 23.4 Gy) leads to inferior event-free survival.[253] Full-dose CSI (36 Gy) should be delivered in the setting of high-risk disease. This is then followed by a boost to the posterior fossa. Intracranial and spinal metastases should be boosted as well to total doses on the order of 45 to 50 Gy for spinal metastases and 50 to 54 Gy for intracranial metastases. Treatment is usually delivered at 1.8 Gy/day.

The role of adjuvant chemotherapy in children with medulloblastoma is well established but remains unclear in adults. A series of 32 adults with medulloblastoma from Germany has shown a nonsignificant trend to prolonged survival with adjuvant chemotherapy.[254] However, preliminary results from NOA-07 a prospective trial of chemoradiotherapy for adult medulloblastoma demonstrated favorable event-free survival rate of 67%.[255] Ability to complete at least four cycles of adjuvant chemotherapy was dependent on age, with leukopenia being the most common toxicity. The use of proton therapy has been associated with a meaningful reduction in hematologic and gastrointestinal toxicity and should be considered when feasible for adult medulloblastoma.[63]

Evidence-Based Treatment Summary

1. Molecular classification has identified four distinct subtypes: WNT, SHH, group 3 and group 4.
2. Maximal surgical resection should be performed, where feasible.
3. Standard treatment consists of postoperative radiotherapy to the craniospinal axis followed by a boost to the tumor bed for average-risk disease and to the posterior fossa and any intracranial/spinal metastases for high-risk disease.
4. The use of chemotherapy generally follows the pediatric indications and guidelines.

Primary Central Nervous System Lymphoma

Primary central nervous system lymphoma (PCNSL) is a non-Hodgkin lymphoma that is restricted to the central nervous system (brain, spinal cord, meninges, and eye) and accounts for <3% of primary intracranial malignancies. It occurs in two distinct patient populations: immunocompromised (HIV, post-transplant, etc.) and immunocompetent. Immunodeficiency is the only known risk factor. Immunocompetent patients present typically in the sixth and seventh decades of life, whereas immunosuppressed individuals more commonly present in the third and fourth decades of life.

The majority of PCNSLs are B-cell lymphomas of intermediate or high grade that are indistinguishable from high-grade non-Hodgkin lymphomas occurring elsewhere in the body. In immunocompetent patients, PCNSL typically presents with one or multifocal (in 30%) mass lesions primarily located in the frontal lobes, corpus callosum, and deep periventricular brain structures. Although the lesions appear focal, diffuse involvement of the parenchyma is invariably present. As a consequence of this deep localization, patients usually present with cognitive dysfunction or personality change. Other symptoms include headache or focal neurologic dysfunction such as hemiparesis or hemisensory loss; seizures are rare. Symptoms often progress over weeks to months before a diagnosis is made.

On MRI, PCNSL is hypointense on T1 and hypointense to isointense on T2/FLAIR sequences with variable surrounding edema. There is usually homogenous enhancement with IV contrast. Ring enhancement is uncommon, except in immunocompromised patients. The appearance on T2 sequences and lack of central necrosis help differentiate PCNSL from glioma.

Even with the "classic" imaging appearance, histology is essential for diagnosis. If PCNSL is suspected, stereotactic biopsy is the best approach; extensive resection does not improve survival. Corticosteroids should be held at presentation unless absolutely necessary (e.g., impending brain herniation) because their "lytic" effect on lymphoma may lead to a false-negative biopsy. Once a diagnosis of PCNSL is established, an extent of disease workup is required. At diagnosis of PCNSL, ocular disease is present in 20% (often misdiagnosed as idiopathic uveitis) and demonstrable leptomeningeal disease is present in 25% (usually asymptomatic until late). A complete staging workup consists of contrast-enhanced brain MR, lumbar puncture (for CSF cytology, flow cytometry, and Epstein-Barr virus PCR), slit-lamp ocular exam (to look for intraocular lymphoma), HIV serology, and contrast-enhanced spine MRI. Systemic staging (body CT, bone marrow biopsy) is rarely positive in patients with typical findings of CNS lymphoma but should be performed if systemic symptoms are present (weight loss, night sweats, fever).

Age and performance status are the most important prognostic factors. A RPA analysis of 338 patients at Memorial Sloan-Kettering Cancer Center led to the identification of three RPA classes: class I (age <50) was associated with median survival of 8.5 years; class II (age >50 and KPS ≥ 70) 3.2 years; and, class III (age >50 and KPS < 70) 1.1 years.[256] The International Extranodal Lymphoma Study Group evaluated 378 patients and observed age >60, ECOG >1, elevated LDH, high CSF protein and deep regions of the brain as prognostic.[257]

Molecular analyses have identified activating mutations in MYD88 and CD79B in PCNSL, which are important in the Bruton tyrosine kinase (BTK) pathway.[258] BTK integrates B-cell antigen receptor (BCR) and Toll-like receptor (TLR) signaling. Diffuse large B-cell lymphomas (DLBCL), which includes PCNSL, frequently harbor mutations in genes encoding members of the BTK pathway. These include the BCR-associated protein CD79B and myeloid differentiation primary response 88 (MYD88), a cytosolic adapter protein that links interleukin-1 and TLRs with the Nuclear factor kappa B (NF-κB).

Treatment

The role of surgery is limited to establishing the tissue diagnosis. This is best achieved by stereotactic biopsy; extensive tumor resection offers no survival benefit. Because PCNSL often responds dramatically to corticosteroid therapy, corticosteroids should be avoided unless absolutely necessary until after tissue is obtained.

PCNSL is exquisitely sensitive to radiotherapy and chemotherapy. Although never studied in a prospective fashion, WBRT is thought to be more effective than focal radiotherapy because of the extensive infiltration of lymphoma throughout the brain. The optimal dose is 45 to 50 Gy, and there is no benefit of adding a boost to the tumor site. With WBRT alone, median survival is 12 to 18 months and the five-year survival rate is only 4%.

The standard systemic lymphoma chemotherapy regimens are ineffective for PCNSL, as demonstrated in prospective clinical trials.[259-261] High-dose systemic methotrexate, administered at a high dose (1 to 8 g/m²) and at a rapid rate of infusion to overcome the blood–brain barrier, is the only agent that has demonstrated improved survival over WBRT alone. A recent randomized phase II study suggests that combination chemotherapy with methotrexate results in superior disease control and survival as compared to single-agent methotrexate.[262] High-dose methotrexate regimens produce adequate levels of drug in the CSF so that direct instillation of chemotherapy (e.g., using an Ommaya reservoir) into the CSF is not necessary, unless CSF cytology is positive.[263]

Whole-brain radiotherapy is typically used as postchemotherapy consolidation in patients younger than 60, as a salvage strategy for recurrence, or as up-front therapy alone for patients with poor performance status (KPS < 40) or renal failure. Patients ≥60 years are at high risk of developing treatment-relate neurotoxicity following treatment with methotrexate and WBRT; WBRT is often deferred in this subgroup except for recurrence.

Neurotoxicity after PCNSL treatment is characterized by dementia, ataxia, and urinary incontinence, occurring a mean of 7 months from treatment. Both methotrexate and radiotherapy can cause this syndrome, and the combination is synergistic. The risk is greatest in patients ≥60 years of age at diagnosis and when methotrexate is administered concurrently or following radiotherapy. In one phase II trial, patients ≥60 years had a 100% incidence of neurotoxicity at 24 months, whereas those <60 had a 30% incidence at 96 months.[264]

The commonly used radiotherapy schedule for PCNSL in immunocompetent patients is 40 to 45 Gy to the whole brain. The posterior orbits should be included in the whole-brain fields. In patients with ocular involvement, the whole eye can be treated to 30 to 40 Gy, with shielding of the anterior chamber and lacrimal apparatus after this dose. However, most treating physicians reserve the use of ocular radiotherapy for failure of intravitreal methotrexate and rituximab. CSI has been advocated for patients with documented CSF involvement. However, intrathecal chemotherapy is preferred because it may be equally efficacious but less toxic with less impact on bone marrow reserve.

For immunosuppressed patients with PCNSL, modification of the irradiation dose and schedule may be necessary. Patients with poor prognostic features (low KPS, CD4 counts <200, advanced AIDS) may be treated with an abbreviated course of radiotherapy (e.g., 36 to 40 Gy).

Results of Treatment

Unlike non-CNS lymphoma, there appears to be a radiotherapy dose response with a threshold between 30 and 50 Gy, with a median of 40 Gy. A study by Bessell et al.[265] showed a higher relapse rate and reduced survival rate in patients who received 30.6 Gy WBRT as compared to 45 Gy in patients who had complete response to chemotherapy. This was significant for patients younger than 60. However, radiation doses beyond 45 to 50 Gy are associated with a plateau in radiation response. The RTOG conducted a phase II study (RTOG 83-15) to evaluate WBRT as first-line treatment. Median survival was 12 months and recurrence in the brain occurred in 61% of patients, with more relapses in the 60 Gy region, suggesting no clear dose–response over 40 Gy.

The most widely used treatment regimen is based on a phase II study (RTOG 93-10) that treated 102 newly diagnosed PCNSL patients with five cycles of high-dose methotrexate (2.5 g/m^2), vincristine, and procarbazine followed by 45 Gy WBRT and high-dose cytarabine (3.0 g/m^2) postradiotherapy.[266] Approximately halfway through the study, the dose of WBRT was decreased to 36 Gy delivered by hyperfractionation to those that achieved a complete response after preradiotherapy chemotherapy. 58% of patients achieved a complete response and 36% had a partial response after preradiotherapy chemotherapy. Median progression-free and overall survival was 24 and 37 months, respectively.

Long-term results with various combination chemotherapy regimens that include intravenous and intrathecal methotrexate, cranial radiotherapy, and intravenous cytarabine have been encouraging, especially in patients younger than 50 years (5-year survival rate of 60%). In older patients (>50 years), results are poor (5-year survival of rate of <10%) and toxicity is greater with dementia and ataxia in a substantial proportion of patients.[267]

Chemotherapy has also been used without radiotherapy or as a means of delaying radiotherapy particularly in patients over age 60 because of their substantial risk to develop treatment-related neurotoxicity.[268] Complete responses occur in >50% of patients. Single-agent methotrexate using a dose of 8 g/m^2 had a high response rate, but responses were of a relatively short duration with a median progression-free survival of approximately 1 year.[269]

Eliminating WBRT from treatment regimens results in higher recurrence incidence, but this does not appear to translate into an overall survival detriment. The German PCNSL phase III trial randomized 524 patients to high-dose methotrexate-based chemotherapy with or without whole-brain radiotherapy to 45 Gy in 1.5-Gy fractions.[270] The addition of upfront WBRT significantly prolonged PFS, most prominently in patients who did not achieve a complete response following chemotherapy, but this benefit did not translate into an overall survival difference. In patients with disease less sensitive or insensitive to high-dose methotrexate, WBRT was observed to be more effective than high-dose Ara-C. The addition of upfront WBRT led to greater impact in patient-reported cognitive functioning and global health status, as well as lower values on Mini-Mental Status Examination.[271]

Current work is focusing on methods to eliminate or reduce the risk of neurotoxicity without compromising long-term disease control. Shah et al.[272] reported a phase II study that evaluated the effectiveness and toxicity of reduced-dose WBRT (23.4 Gy) in patients who achieved a complete response following methotrexate-based chemotherapy. The estimated 2-year overall survival and progression-free survival in these 19 patients was 89% and 79%, respectively. At a follow-up of 12 months, none of the patients treated with reduced-dose RT developed treatment-related dementia on neurocognitive studies. This approach was further evaluated in a multicenter phase II study of rituximab, methotrexate, procarbazine, and vincristine (R-MVP) followed by consolidative WBRT to 23.4 Gy in patients who achieve a postchemotherapy complete response.[273] Consolidative cytarabine was given after radiotherapy. Among 52 patients enrolled, 60% achieved a complete response after R-MVP with a 2-year PFS of 77% and a 3-year OS of 87%. Cognitive assessments demonstrated improvement in executive function and verbal memory after R-MVP with stability of follow-up scores.

The use of high-dose chemotherapy with autologous stem transplant (HDC/ASCT) in newly diagnosed PCNSL patients is another strategy that has been explored as an alternative to WBRT. Available data are limited to a few small, nonrandomized phase 2 studies.[274] In a single-institution study, patients who developed a complete or partial response to R-MVP proceed with HDC with thiotepa, cyclophosphamide, and busulfan, followed by ASCT.[275] In transplanted patients, two-year PFS and OS were 81%. Two ongoing clinical trials (NCT01011920; NCT00863460) randomizing patients to consolidative WBRT versus HDC/ASCT will help establish the highest tolerated and most effective consolidation strategy. Until more data are available, HDC/ASCT consolidation to primary chemotherapy can only be recommended as an experimental approach.

Ibrutinib is a first-in-class, oral inhibitor of BTK. Ibrutinib induces death of DLBCL cells with deregulated BCR signaling and has showed promising activity in a variety of B-cell malignancies, with 70% to 90% response rates in patients with Chronic Lymphocytic Leukemia, Small Lymphocytic Lymphoma, Mantle-Cell Lymphoma, and Waldenström Macroglobulinemia, but only about 25% response rates in relapsed/refractory DLBCL.[276] In a phase 1–2 study, ibrutinib was administered to 20 patients with relapsed or refractory PCNSL or secondary CNS involvement (SCNSL). Patients received ibrutinib at 560 or 840 mg once daily in the dose-escalation portion of the study and 840 mg once daily in the expansion portion. Responses were observed in 15 of 20 patients (75%); 10 of these had a complete response. For PCNSL, the response rate was 77%. Ibrutinib CSF concentrations two hours post dose were 0.77 ng/mL (1.7 nM) and 1.95 ng/mL (4.4 nM) in the 560 and 840 mg groups, respectively, demonstrating a dose-dependent increase in CSF penetration, and levels sufficient to induce cell death in CNS lymphoma cells in culture. Upon mutational analysis, many tumors harbored mutations in the BTK pathway, but tumors without such mutations also responded. Ibrutinib therefore has substantial activity in patients with relapsed or refractory B-cell lymphoma of the CNS and is being further developed for front-line testing.[277]

In patients with immunosuppression and PCNSL, results are discouraging, although selected patients (non-HIV immunosuppression, favorable-prognosis patients with AIDS) may have survival comparable with that of nonimmunosuppressed populations when treated in a standard fashion.[278]

Evidence-Based Treatment Summary

1. Surgical resection is not necessary.
2. Avoiding or deferring WBRT results in inferior PFS but without significantly impacting OS. Lower-dose WBRT is being investigated to improve the therapeutic window.
3. High-dose systemic methotrexate is the only agent that has demonstrated improved survival over WBRT alone. High-dose methotrexate-based chemotherapy followed by whole-brain radiotherapy is the standard treatment for patients <60 years of age with a good performance status. Patients who achieve complete response with high-dose methotrexate–based chemotherapy should be treated with WBRT to reduced dose of 23.4 Gy in 1.8-Gy fractions.
4. High-dose methotrexate–based chemotherapy alone with deferred radiotherapy may be preferred in elderly patients because of substantial risk of neurotoxicity associated with combined chemotherapy–radiotherapy regimens.
5. WBRT alone should be pursued for patients who are not candidates for chemotherapy.

Meningioma

Meningiomas account for approximately 30% of primary intracranial neoplasms and are the most common benign intracranial tumor in adults.[2] The peak age of incidence is in the sixth and seventh decades, although they may occur at any age. They are more common in women. Typical locations for meningiomas include the cerebral convexities, falx cerebri, tentorium cerebelli, cerebellopontine angle, and sphenoid ridge. Malignant varieties with invasive growth and aggressive behavior occasionally occur.

Grossly, meningiomas are well-circumscribed firm, tan, or grayish lesions arising from the meninges. Hyperostosis of adjacent bone may be present. Microscopically benign meningiomas usually have a bland whorled appearance with little anaplasia or mitotic activity. Psammoma bodies may be present. Histologic variants (e.g., fibrous, transitional, angiomatous) can be identified but are of little prognostic significance. Malignant varieties are identified on the basis of clinical behavior (rapid growth or recurrence, invasiveness) or pathologic features such as microscopic features of malignancy (cellular or nuclear anaplasia, mitotic figures)

or specific histologic type (rhabdoid, papillary, anaplastic). The 2007 updated WHO grading criteria incorporate mitotic activity, nuclear to cytoplasmic ratio, spontaneous necrosis, brain invasion, and certain meningioma variants to assign a grade I through III (Table 38.6).[279] Benign meningiomas (~78% to 80%) are classified as WHO grade I and associated with slower growth and lower risk of recurrence, atypical meningiomas (20%) WHO grade II with an increased likelihood of aggressive behavior, and anaplastic or malignant gliomas (3% to 5%) WHO grade III and associated with high invasiveness and the worst prognosis. The 2016 update to the WHO classification system introduced brain invasion as a criterion that, similar to mitotic count of 4 or more, can alone suffice for diagnosis of an atypical WHO grade II meningioma.[16]

Meningiomas are known to be induced by ionizing radiation, with an average interval to diagnosis of 19 to 35 years, depending on the dose of radiation. They may be multiple particularly in patients with neurofibromatosis type 2 (NF2) and in non-NF2 families with a hereditary predisposition to meningioma.

The most common cytogenetic alteration in meningiomas involves a deletion of chromosome 22. Molecular genetics findings indicate that approximately 50% of meningiomas have allelic losses that involve band q12 on chromosome 22. Allelic losses of chromosomal arms 6q, 9p, 10q, and 14q are seen in both atypical and anaplastic meningiomas. Genetic and cytogenetic alterations accumulate with progression from WHO grade I to WHO grade III lesions. Mutations in the NF2 gene have been detected in 60% of sporadic meningiomas. The cumulative effect of NF2 mutations or copy number alterations affecting chromosome 22 is the loss of activity/function of a tumor suppressor protein, Merlin (Moesin-ezrin-radixin-like protein) encoded by the gene *NF2*. More recent genomic analysis of meningiomas reveals that in the 40+% of tumors without chromosome 22 loss or NF2 mutation, other somewhat uncommon, but potentially targetable mutations can be identified. In a whole-genome or whole-exome sequencing on 17 meningiomas and focused sequencing on an additional 48 tumors, most meningiomas were found to have "simple genomes," with fewer mutations, rearrangements, and copy number alterations than reported in other CNS tumors in adults. This study confirmed focal *NF2* inactivation in 43% of tumors and found alterations in epigenetic modifiers of NF2 in an additional 8% of tumors. A subset of meningiomas lacking *NF2* alterations harbored recurrent oncogenic mutations in *AKT1* and *SMO* with immunohistochemical evidence of activation of these pathways. These mutations are linked to the potential for identifying targeted therapeutics for some meningiomas.[280] A recent analysis of 274 high-grade meningiomas compared to 456 low-grade meningiomas concluded that high-grade meningiomas actually have a higher mutation burden, but no statistically significant mutated genes other than NF2 could be identified.[281]

In a recent analysis of the histologically aggressive variant, rhabdoid meningiomas, designated in the WHO classification as high grade, sequencing of cancer-related genes from 27 meningiomas from 18 patients with rhabdoid features was performed, findings from which led to specifically evaluating the breast cancer (BRCA)1–associated protein 1 (BAP1) expression by immunohistochemistry in 336 meningiomas. The tumor suppressor gene

TABLE 38.6 WHO 2016 TUMOR GRADE

Grade I (Benign)	Grade II (Atypical)	Grade III (Anaplastic/Malignant)
Any major variant other than clear cell, chordoid, papillary, or rhabdoid	Frequent mitoses (>4 per 10 hpf)	Excessive mitotic index (>20 per 10 hpf)
OR	**OR**	**OR**
Does not fulfill criteria for grades II or III	3 or more of the following: Sheeting architecture Hypercellularity (focal or diffuse) Prominent nucleoli Small cells with high nuclear–cytoplasmic ratio Foci of spontaneous necrosis	Frank anaplasia defined as focal or diffuse loss of meningothelial differentiation resembling: Sarcoma Carcinoma or Melanoma
	OR	**OR**
	Additional subtypes/features Chordoid meningioma Clear cell meningioma Brain invasion	Additional subtypes/features Papillary meningioma Rhabdoid meningioma

b.i.d., twice daily; RT, radiotherapy.

BAP1, a ubiquitin carboxy-terminal hydrolase, was found to be inactivated in a subset of high-grade rhabdoid meningiomas. Patients with BAP1-negative rhabdoid meningiomas had reduced time to recurrence compared with patients with BAP1-retained rhabdoid meningiomas, and a subset of patients with BAP1-deficient rhabdoid meningiomas harbored germline BAP1 mutations, indicating that rhabdoid meningiomas could be a harbinger of the BAP1 cancer predisposition syndrome.[282] These findings are beginning to provide clues toward the goal of identifying actionable mutations in meningioma.

The incidental finding of a meningioma on CT or MRI is not uncommon, particularly in the elderly. Many meningioma patients are asymptomatic and may remain so for a long time.[283,284] Lesions in the cerebellopontine angle commonly present with symptoms of cranial neuropathy. Cerebral convexity meningioma may present with symptoms of headache or a seizure. Meningiomas of the sphenoid wing or optic nerve may be associated with visual loss. The differential diagnosis of meningioma in the base of the skull or spine includes bone metastasis or primary bone tumors (chondrosarcoma, chordoma, osteosarcoma). In the cerebellopontine angle, acoustic neuromas may resemble meningiomas on imaging.

Meningiomas typically grow slowly. In 47 asymptomatic patients with meningioma diagnosed incidentally by MRI, Nakamura et al.[285] reported a mean annual growth measured using serial MRI of 14.6% and a mean tumor doubling time of 21.6 years. Higher annual growth rates were seen in young patients and lower annual growth rates in patients with calcification and hypointense or isointense T2 signals on MRI. The location of the lesion, extent of surgical resection, and histopathologic features of the tumor (benign or malignant) are the most important determinants of prognosis.[286]

After surgery, the average time to recurrence is approximately 4 years. In a review of 38 patients who underwent subtotal resection, the mean diameter increase was 0.37 cm/year and mean tumor doubling time was 8 years.[287]

Treatment
Grade I Meningioma
Patients with asymptomatic lesions may be observed and followed with serial imaging. The treatment of choice for symptomatic or progressive benign meningiomas is complete surgical resection if it can be accomplished with acceptable morbidity. Resection of these typically vascular tumors may be facilitated by preoperative angiography with or without embolization. Even after complete resection, 7% to 12% of these tumors recur at 5 years and 20% to 25% recur at 10 years[288,289] so that follow-up with serial imaging is necessary.

Complete resection of skull-based, cerebellopontine angle, or cavernous sinus meningiomas may be difficult without significant morbidity. Subtotal resections are associated with higher relapse rates of 39% to 47% at 5 years and 60% to 61% at 10 years without adjuvant therapy.[288,289] For these patients, conservative subtotal resection followed by postoperative irradiation may give good local control with less morbidity than an aggressive base of skull resection. An alternative approach for patients who have undergone subtotal resection is follow-up with further surgery, if feasible, and radiotherapy delayed to time of recurrence.

In patients with subtotally excised unresectable or recurrent meningiomas, the typical radiotherapy dose is 50 to 54 Gy in 25 to 30 fractions over 5 to 6 weeks. The target volume for radiotherapy is defined by CT or MRI scan and modified according to the neurosurgeon's description of the location of residual tumor. The margin expansion for meningiomas is based on the knowledge of direction of spread, especially through neural foramina, bony invasion, dural tails, and so forth. The GTV is the enhancing abnormality on contrast-enhanced MRI. Margin expansions then incorporate setup errors and block margins; these can vary from 0.5 to 1 cm in total depending on the precision of the immobili-

zation and delivery systems. Multiple fields with wedges or rotational fields and 3-D conformal techniques are used for maximal sparing of normal brain tissue. IMRT or proton therapy may be helpful in avoiding adjacent surrounding structures.

Postoperative irradiation after less than complete resection improves local control, prolongs the interval to recurrence, and improves survival. In series by Condra et al.,[288] subtotal resection with postoperative irradiation had a local control rate of 87% at 15 years compared to 76% following total excision and 30% after subtotal excision (*P* = .0001). In modern series using MRI and CT localization, 5-year local control is reported to be >90%.[290]

Radiosurgery as the sole modality or as postoperative adjuvant therapy may be of interest for selected patients, generally those with smaller tumors. In recent series, 5-year progression-free survival rates are >80%.[291-295] In a recent single institutional study, 85 patients eligible for a potential Simpson grade 1 or 2 resection were treated with SRS (usually because of preference). These patients received SRS either because of radiographic evidence of growth (72%) or postoperative recurrence (28%). With a mean follow-up of 69 months, the estimated 2-, 5-, and 10-year local control rates were 99%, 93%, and 93%, results that compare well with surgical series.[296]

Chemotherapy has not been useful in the treatment of benign meningiomas. Given the high estrogen and progesterone receptor expression on meningiomas, progesterone receptor antagonists have been tested but have not been found beneficial.

Grade II and III Meningioma
For atypical or malignant meningiomas, the recurrence rate after surgery alone is high (41% to 100% at 5 years), even after complete surgical resection,[297] and postoperative irradiation after maximal resection is recommended for all patients. The target volume is more generous than that used for benign meningiomas. The GTV and/or resection bed is typically expanded by 0.5 to 1.0 cm along the dural margin and into brain parenchyma in cases of brain invasion. The recommended dose is on the order of 54 to 59.4 Gy in 30 to 33 fractions for atypical meningioma and 59.4 Gy in 33 fractions for malignant meningioma, although some have reported improved local control with higher doses.[298]

RTOG 0539 enrolled 52 patients into an intermediate-risk cohort comprising WHO grade II tumors with gross total resection (70%) and recurrent WHO grade I tumors (30%) and treated with fractionated radiotherapy to 54 Gy[299]. 3-year and 5-year PFS were 92% and 84%, comparable to PFS estimates following observation of resected WHO grade I meningioma observed in the same trial. In a National Cancer Database analysis, the use of adjuvant radiotherapy for subtotally resected WHO grade II meningioma improved overall survival.[300] In the setting of gross totally resected WHO grade II meningioma, two randomized trials seek to address whether adjuvant radiotherapy prolongs PFS and OS.

In a review of 38 patients with malignant meningiomas by Dziuk et al.,[297] use of postoperative radiotherapy resulted in superior local control. At 5 years, irradiation following initial resection improved 5-year disease-free survival from 15% to 80% (*P* = .002). Progression-free survival was 57% in patients treated with total resection and radiotherapy compared to 28% in patients treated with total resection alone.

Systemic therapy has no defined role. Combined chemotherapy with vincristine, adriamycin, and cyclophosphamide has shown some efficacy in patients with malignant meningiomas.[301]

Unresectable or Recurrent Meningioma
In patients in whom aggressive surgery is not an option, radiotherapy may relieve symptoms and decrease the rate of tumor progression.

Radiotherapy may be useful in the treatment of recurrent meningioma. In a review by Miralbell et al.,[302] progression-free survival at 8 years for patients treated with subtotal resection and radiotherapy at first recurrence was 78% compared to 11% in patients treated with resection alone (P = .001).

Various chemotherapy treatments that have been used in patients with recurrent meningiomas include combined doxorubicin and dacarbazine or ifosfamide and mesna.[303] Long-term low-dose daily hydroxyurea may have some activity.[304]

Hormonal manipulation, including tamoxifen and the anti-progesterone drug RU486, showed some activity in a SWOG phase II evaluation of tamoxifen in unresectable or refractory meningiomas.[305] However, a subsequent SWOG phase III study of mifepristone for unresectable meningioma was negative.[306]

The EORTC has completed accrual to a randomized open-label multicenter comparative phase II trial investigating whether trabectedin demonstrates sufficient antitumor activity against recurrent grade II or III meningioma to justify further investigation in phase III or as adjuvant therapy for newly diagnosed disease after resection and radiotherapy. Trabectedin blocks DNA binding of the oncogenic transcription factor FUS-CHOP and reverses the transcriptional program in myxoid liposarcoma. By reversing the genetic program created by this transcription factor, trabectedin promotes differentiation and reverses the oncogenic phenotype in these cells. Other than transcriptional interference, the mechanism of action of trabectedin is poorly understood. It is approved for use in sarcomas and has demonstrated anectodal responses in meningioma; results of this trial are awaited. The Alliance for Clinical Trials in Oncology is currently conducting a trial of targeted agents selected by the presence of specific mutations in recurrent/progressive meningioma. In this three-arm phase II trial, patients with NF2 would be treated with vismodegib, those with SMO mutations with the focal adhesion kinase (FAK) inhibitor GSK2256098, and those with AKT mutations with a PI3Kinase pathway inhibitor.

Evidence-Based Treatment Summary

1. Small asymptomatic meningiomas in noncritical locations, especially in the elderly or in patients with other comorbidities, can be observed.
2. The goal of surgery is to completely resect the meningioma, with negative margins as patients with WHO grade I completely resected meningiomas have low rates of relapse and can be observed postoperatively.
3. For subtotally resected or unresectable progressive meningioma, radiotherapy is frequently used but has not been tested in a prospective clinical trial. Local control appears to be improved with postoperative radiotherapy. Both radiosurgery and radiotherapy have been used in this context, but have not been directly compared.
4. For grades II and III meningioma, postoperative radiotherapy is routinely recommended.
5. Primary radiotherapy or radiosurgery could be used for unresectable, progressive meningiomas.
6. Systemic therapy does not have a defined role in meningioma.

Craniopharyngioma

Craniopharyngiomas arise from epithelial remnants of the Rathke pouch and are typically found in the suprasellar region in children or adolescents. They account for <5% of all CNS neoplasms in adults. They are slowly growing tumors that often have solid and cystic components, the latter filled with lipoid, cholesterol-laden ("crankcase oil") fluid. Although appearing well encapsulated, craniopharyngiomas typically demonstrate invaginations into adjacent brain and may provoke a vigorous glial reaction.

The cystic nature of craniopharyngiomas is usually evident on CT and MRI and helps distinguish these tumors from other base of skull lesions and pituitary adenomas. The solid portion is often calcified and enhancing, whereas the cystic portion typically demonstrates a thin rim of enhancement. The finding of multiple cysts of varying intensity on T1- and T2-weighted MRI is characteristic of craniopharyngioma.

Intrasellar lesions may compress the pituitary gland and hypothalamus, producing hormonal abnormalities, especially antidiuretic and growth hormone deficits. Prechiasmal lesions may compress the optic pathway leading to visual field cuts or decreased central visual acuity. Retrochiasmal lesions may grow into the third ventricle and cause hydrocephalus or compress the optic tracts. Craniopharyngiomas can occasionally reach enormous size and produce neurologic impairment by direct impingement on brain parenchyma. Surgical decompression is the optimal treatment for rapid symptom relief. However, the location, proximity, and adhesiveness of the tumor to adjacent structures often preclude complete resection.

Treatment

A discussion of craniopharyngioma in the pediatric context is provided in Chapter 82. Management options include complete resection, subtotal resection alone, or subtotal resection or biopsy followed by postoperative radiotherapy.

Complete surgical resection, which is applicable only to a minority of patients, is associated with local control and long-term survival in 70% to 90% of patients.[307] However, aggressive resection may be associated with significant morbidity, with up to a 10% incidence of perioperative mortality and up to 30% severe morbidity, especially diabetes insipidus or other endocrine deficits, visual impairment, obesity, and memory impairment.

Partial resection or cyst aspiration and biopsy rapidly relieve local compressive symptoms and have less operative morbidity but are associated with eventual tumor progression in most cases. Long-term survival and local control are achieved only in approximately 30% of patients. In contrast to aggressive resections, subtotal resections carry a mortality of about 1%.

With a limited surgical procedure (partial resection or cyst aspiration plus biopsy) followed by radiotherapy, local control and survival rates are nearly equivalent to those achieved with complete resection, with survival rates of 89% and 77% at 5 and 10 years, respectively, as compared with 53% to 37% for patients who have had subtotal resection alone. Typically, doses of 50.4 to 54 Gy in 28 to 30 fractions (1.8 Gy) are delivered to the postoperative residual tumor and the borders of preoperative tumor extent with a 1- to 1.5-cm margin depending on the accuracy of the imaging used for planning and the reproducibility of the treatment setup. Reduction of margins to 0.5cm can be considered when weekly MR imaging during treatment is used to monitor intra-tumoral cystic changes. In patients with compressive symptoms, surgical decompression before irradiation is essential because the tumor typically responds slowly to radiotherapy, and radiation-induced edema may worsen compressive symptoms.

With these dose recommendations (i.e., 1.8-Gy fractions to 50 to 54 Gy), the risk of visual impairment is very low (1% and 1.5%). In a retrospective analysis of patients treated with 51.3 to 70 Gy, a higher incidence of radiation-related complications was seen in those who received more than 60 Gy (with an actuarial incidence of optic neuropathy of 30% and brain necrosis of 12.5%), without any concomitant improvement in tumor control.[308]

Radiotherapy may be given as salvage rather than immediately after subtotal resection. In a series of 76 patients treated at the University of Pennsylvania, long-term survival rates were equivalent.[309] In another series, radiotherapy given at recurrence yielded a 10-year progression-free survival rate of >70%.[310] Recurrences occur from 3 to 192 months (median 12 months) after subtotal resection so that close surveillance is necessary during the first years following incomplete resection.

Other modalities used in the treatment of craniopharyngioma have included intralesional bleomycin and radioactive colloid instillations for cystic tumors. Radiosurgery may be useful in ablating small residual or recurrent tumors.[311] With radiosurgery, dose to the optic chiasm and nerves must be kept below 8 Gy, estimated to be radiobiologic tolerance for optic neuropathy with single-fraction radiosurgical doses. As a result, radiosurgery use should be restricted to tumors <3 cm in size and located >3 to 5 mm from the optic apparatus.

Evidence-Based Treatment Summary

1. Surgical resection is recommended, when feasible.
2. The use of postoperative radiotherapy has not been tested in prospective trials but reduces the risk of recurrence and improves survival in incompletely resected tumors. Cyst decompression and biopsy followed by radiotherapy may be an acceptable treatment for patients for whom resection is not considered feasible.
3. Intracavitary bleomycin or radiocolloids may be useful in cystic tumors.

Vestibular Schwannoma and Neurofibroma

Neurilemomas, also known as schwannomas and neurinomas, arise from the Schwann cells of the myelin sheath of the peripheral nerves. When occurring close to the eighth cranial nerve, they are also called vestibular schwannomas or acoustic neuromas. These tumors account for approximately 6% of CNS neoplasms in adults. They may be sporadic or associated with NF2, with bilateral vestibular schwannomas being pathognomonic of this disease. Most sporadic vestibular schwannomas are unilateral and occur in the fourth and fifth decades of life. Those arising in patients with NF2 tend to occur in the second or third decades. These tumors grow slowly in a well-circumscribed, expansile fashion, displacing adjacent nerves rather than invading them. Most arise from cranial nerve VIII in the medial internal auditory canal. Less commonly, they may arise from other cranial nerves, the trigeminal nerve being the most common alternate site.

Growth in the internal auditory canal gives rise to vestibular and hearing abnormalities in up to 95% of patients. A progressive unilateral sensorineural hearing loss is characteristic. Expansion into the cerebellopontine angle may lead to trigeminal symptoms, and a unilateral absent corneal reflex is an early sign of trigeminal involvement. Large tumors may impinge on the cerebellum and brainstem, leading to ataxia and long tract signs as well as involvement of cranial nerves IX, X, XI, and XII.

Pure tone and speech audiometry are the most useful screening tests. Selective loss of speech discrimination in excess of pure tone loss is particularly suggestive of vestibular schwannoma. Brainstem auditory evoked responses typically demonstrate a slowing of conduction, and electronystagmography may detect a decrease in caloric response on the ipsilateral side. Thin-slice Gd-enhanced MRI through the cerebellopontine angle is the imaging modality of choice for suspected vestibular schwannoma. Thin-slice, contrast-enhanced, high-resolution CT scan is an acceptable alternative when MRI is not obtainable. An intensely enhancing lesion close to the internal auditory canal is highly suggestive of this diagnosis. Patients with suspected neurofibromatosis should have complete imaging of the craniospinal axis to document other neurilemomas, neurofibromas, and meningiomas that may be present.

Neurofibromas differ from neurilemomas in their cellular composition and growth pattern. Although neurofibromas also arise from peripheral nerves, they are most commonly multiple and associated with NF1. Neurofibromas expand rather than displace the nerve of origin. Histologically, neurofibromas are composed of a hypertrophied mass of fibroblasts and Schwann cells through which run normal neurons. Symptoms are caused primarily through compression of the involved or adjacent nerves.

Treatment

Treatment should offer a high chance of local control as well as preservation of cranial nerve function. Observation alone may be appropriate in patients willing to undergo regular clinical and imaging follow-up and may allow treatment to be deferred for some time. The mainstay of treatment has been microsurgical resection. Retrosigmoid (suboccipital) middle fossa and translabyrinthine approaches offer the possibility of hearing preservation but are associated with higher incidences of seventh nerve damage and postoperative complications. The translabyrinthine approach is associated with low operative morbidity and mortality but sacrifices hearing. At centers with expertise in microsurgical resection, total or near-total resection rates of 90% are routinely obtained with a surgical mortality rate of <2%. Anatomic preservation of the facial nerve may be achieved in 90% of patients and functional preservation in more than two-thirds. Preservation of useful hearing is reported in 30% to 50%. In patients in whom a near-total or total resection is achieved, the tumor recurrence rate is <10%. In patients in whom a subtotal resection is achieved, tumor recurrence may occur in one-third to one-half. Adjuvant radiotherapy may reduce the rate of recurrence to that of complete resection.

In patients with a medical contraindication to surgery, treatment with external beam irradiation alone is an option. A dose of 50 to 55 Gy in 25 to 30 fractions over 5 to 6 weeks is recommended. Maire et al.[312] evaluated 24 patients with stage III and IV cerebellopontine angle schwannomas treated with external irradiation. With median follow-up of 60 months, there was an 88% tumor control rate with no injuries to the cranial nerve V or VIII.

Radiosurgery may be an alternative to microsurgical resection. The well-circumscribed nature of these tumors, coupled with their typical intense enhancement on MRI, facilitates their localization and treatment using stereotactic techniques. The progression-free survival rate with radiosurgery is nearly 90% at 20 years. Radiosurgical treatment with higher doses yielded high rates of tumor growth arrest (>80%) and tumor shrinkage in up to two-thirds of patients, although facial or trigeminal neuropathy develops in nearly one-third of patients as long as 2 years after therapy. The volume of the lesion is a significant risk factor for complications involving cranial nerve V, VII, or VIII. Temporary enlargement may occur up to 2 years following radiosurgery.[313]

Noren[314] reviewed the results of 669 patients with vestibular schwannoma treated with Gamma Knife radiosurgery between 1969 and 1997. Long-term growth control was achieved in 95%. Facial weakness and/or numbness occurred in approximately one-third of patients during the 1970s but <2% in the 1990s. Hearing was preserved in 65% to 70% of patients, although tinnitus was rarely changed by treatment. With dose reduction to 12 to 13 Gy, high rates of tumor control and cranial nerve preservation may be achieved. Flickinger et al.[315] reported the results of 313 patients treated with radiosurgery to median dose of 13 Gy. The actuarial 6-year tumor control rate was 98.6%. The actuarial 6-year rates for preservation of seventh nerve function, normal fifth nerve function, unchanged hearing level, and useful hearing were 100%, 95.6%, 70.3%, and 78.6%, respectively. Hayhurst et al.[316] reported on their clinical series of 200 patients treated with radiosurgery to 12 Gy and observed 5 cm³ to be the target volume threshold above which adverse treatment effects were more likely. In addition, they observed a maximum dose threshold of 9 Gy to cranial nerve V as significantly associated with trigeminal neuropathy.

Radiosurgery provides similar local control with less morbidity than surgery for small (<3 cm) unilateral tumors. In a series from the University of Pittsburgh, radiosurgery was found to have improved preservation of facial function ($P < .05$) and hearing ($P < .03$) with decreased associated morbidity ($P < .01$) when compared to surgical resection.[317]

FSRT has been shown to give local control rates of 91% to 97% with similar effects on cranial nerves V and VII.[318–321] However, in one series, FSRT resulted in 2.5-fold greater preservation of hearing compared to radiosurgery.[318] FSRT may be an option for tumors too large to receive radiosurgery.

Bevacizumab has been used in patients with progressive bilateral vestibular schwannomas associated with NF2, usually in the context of bilateral hearing loss, producing both tumor regression and restoration of hearing in some patients. This has led to this approach being actively investigated at present. Sporadic and NF2-related vestibular schwannomas express VEGF, and bevacizumab binds VEGF with high affinity. In the initial experience reported by Plotkin et al., 10 NF2 patients at risk for complete hearing loss or brainstem compression were treated with bevacizumab on a compassionate-care basis and demonstrated promising results with 6 of 10 patients experiencing ≥20% tumor volume reduction and 4 of 7 patients experiencing significantly improved hearing.[322]

Evidence-Based Treatment Summary

1. Small nonprogressive tumors can be observed.
2. Surgical resection is generally considered the standard of care for symptomatic lesions.
3. Radiosurgery produces outcomes equivalent to surgery, although these modalities have not been prospectively compared.
4. Fractionated stereotactic radiotherapy is being increasingly employed, with institutional reports suggesting a lower incidence of cranial neuropathies than radiosurgery, but this has not been prospectively validated.
5. The role of bevacizumab in NF-2-associated progressive bilateral vestibular schwannomas is being explored.

Hemangioblastoma and Hemangiopericytoma

Hemangioblastomas are benign vascular tumors that present during the third and fourth decades of life. They account for 1% to 2% of primary CNS tumors in adults. Most arise in the cerebellum, constituting the most common primary cerebellar tumors in adults. An association with von Hippel-Lindau disease is noted in 10% of patients. Histologically, the tumor consists of closely packed, thin-walled blood vessels in a stroma of large, oval foamy cells. The lesions are intensely enhancing on CT and MRI, and angiography confirms the vascular nature of the lesion. Imaging of the craniospinal axis often documents multiple lesions in patients with von Hippel-Lindau disease. Treatment is surgical and complete resection is curative. Radiosurgery has also been shown to be useful in patients with unresectable disease but is associated with higher rates of recurrence.[323-325] In von Hippel-Lindau, treatment of symptomatic hemangioblastoma is warranted, but observation of asymptomatic tumors can be considered.[326]

Hemangiopericytoma is a sarcomatous lesion developing from smooth muscle in blood vessels usually along the base of the skull, although intraparenchymal lesions may be seen. In contrast to other primary CNS tumors, hemangiopericytomas commonly develop systemic metastases. There is a 90% 9-year actuarial risk for local failure following surgical resection only. Postoperative radiotherapy to total doses of 50 to 60 Gy reduces the risk of recurrence rate and improves overall survival. Tumor control is dose dependent, with doses >50 Gy associated with superior outcomes. Radiographic response is slow. Radiosurgery has been used for recurrent hemangiopericytomas, with reported local control rates of approximately 80% following treatment.[327]

Evidence-Based Treatment Summary

1. Surgical resection is recommended, when feasible, for both of these diseases.
2. Radiotherapy is generally reserved for subtotally resected progressive hemangioblastoma, but there are no prospective data.
3. Postoperative radiotherapy is recommended for subtotally resected hemangiopericytoma, but there are no prospective data.
4. Radiotherapy or radiosurgery may be considered for unresectable tumors.

REFERENCES

1. Ostrom QT, Gittleman H, Fulop J, et al. CBTRUS Statistical Report: Primary brain and central nervous system tumors diagnosed in the United States in 2009–2013. *Neuro Oncol* 2016;18(s5):iv1–iv76.
2. *CBTRUS statistical report: Primary brain and central nervous system tumors diagnosed in 2004–2007 [Internet].* 2011. Available from: http://www.cbtrus.org/reports/reports.html
3. Ohgaki H, Kleihues P. Epidemiology and etiology of gliomas. *Acta Neuropathol* 2005;109(1):93–108. doi: 10.1007/s00401-005-0991-y.
4. Baan R, Grosse Y, Lauby-Secretan B, et al. Carcinogenicity of radiofrequency electromagnetic fields. *Lancet Oncol* 2011;12(7):624–626.
5. Inskip PD, Tarone RE, Hatch EE, et al. Cellular-telephone use and brain tumors. *N Engl J Med* 2001;344(2):79–86. doi: 10.1056/NEJM200101113440201
6. Muscat JE, Malkin MG, Thompson S, et al. Handheld cellular telephone use and risk of brain cancer. *JAMA* 2000;284(23):3001–3007.
7. Schuz J, Jacobsen R, Olsen JH, et al. Cellular telephone use and cancer risk: update of a nationwide Danish cohort. *J Natl Cancer Inst* 2006;98(23):1707–1713. doi: 10.1093/jnci/djj464.
8. Grell K, Frederiksen K, Schuz J, et al. The Intracranial Distribution of Gliomas in Relation to Exposure From Mobile Phones: Analyses From the INTERPHONE Study. *Am J Epidemiol* 2016;184(11):818–828. doi: 10.1093/aje/kww082.
9. Group IS. Brain tumour risk in relation to mobile telephone use: results of the INTERPHONE international case–control study. *Int J Epidemiol* 2010;39(3):675–694. doi: 10.1093/ije/dyq079.
10. Brain tumour risk in relation to mobile telephone use: results of the INTERPHONE international case–control study. *Int J Epidemiol* 2010;39:675–694.
11. Hardell L, Carlberg M, Hansson Mild K. Pooled analysis of case–control studies on malignant brain tumours and the use of mobile and cordless phones including living and deceased subjects. *Int J Oncol* 2011;38(5):1465–1474. doi: 10.3892/ijo.2011.947.
12. Mack EE, Wilson CB. Meningiomas induced by high-dose cranial irradiation. *J Neurosurg* 1993;79(1):28–31. doi: 10.3171/jns.1993.79.1.0028.
13. Bassal M, Mertens AC, Taylor L, et al. Risk of selected subsequent carcinomas in survivors of childhood cancer: a report from the Childhood Cancer Survivor Study. *J Clin Oncol* 2006;24(3):476–483. doi: 10.1200/JCO.2005.02.7235.
14. Neglia JP, Meadows AT, Robison LL, et al. Second neoplasms after acute lymphoblastic leukemia in childhood. *N Engl J Med* 1991;325(19):1330–1336. doi: 10.1056/NEJM199111073251902.
15. Ellingson BM, Bendszus M, Boxerman J, et al. Consensus recommendations for a standardized Brain Tumor Imaging Protocol in clinical trials. *Neuro Oncol* 2015;17(9):1188–1198. doi: 10.1093/neuonc/nov095.
16. Louis DN, Ohgaki H, Wieslter OD, et al. *World Health Organization histologic classificaiton of tumours of the central nervous system.* Lyon: International Agency for Research on Cancer, 2016.
17. Fetell MR, Grossman SA, Fisher JD, et al. Preirradiation paclitaxel in glioblastoma multiforme: efficacy, pharmacology, and drug interactions. New Approaches to Brain Tumor Therapy Central Nervous System Consortium. *J Clin Oncol* 1997;15(9):3121–3128.
18. Gilbert MR, Supko JG, Batchelor T, et al. Phase I clinical and pharmacokinetic study of irinotecan in adults with recurrent malignant glioma. *Clin Cancer Res* 2003;9(8):2940–2949.
19. Glantz MJ, Cole BF, Forsyth PA, et al. Practice parameter: anticonvulsant prophylaxis in patients with newly diagnosed brain tumors. Report of the Quality Standards Subcommittee of the American Academy of Neurology. *Neurology* 2000;54(10):1886–1893.
20. Rahmathulla G, Recinos PF, Kamian K, et al. MRI-guided laser interstitial thermal therapy in neuro-oncology: a review of its current clinical applications. *Oncology* 2014;87(2):67–82. doi: 10.1159/000362817.
21. Lacroix M, Abi-Said D, Fourney DR, et al. A multivariate analysis of 416 patients with glioblastoma multiforme: prognosis, extent of resection, and survival. *J Neurosurg* 2001;95(2):190–198. doi: 10.3171/jns.2001.95.2.0190.
22. Vunrinen V, Hinkka S, Farkkila M, et al. Debulking or biopsy of malignant glioma in elderly people—a randomized study. *Acta Neurochir (Wien)* 2003;145(1):5–10.
23. Lawrence YR, Li XA, el Naqa I, et al. Radiation dose-volume effects in the brain. *Int J Radiat Oncol Biol Phys* 2010;76(3 Suppl):S20–S27. doi: 10.1016/j.ijrobp.2009.02.091.
24. Tome WA, Meeks SL, McNutt TR, et al. Optically guided intensity modulated radiotherapy. *Radiother Oncol* 2001;61(1):33–44.
25. Karlsson U, Kirby T, Orrison W, et al. Ocular globe topography in radiotherapy. *Int J Radiat Oncol Biol Phys* 1995;33(3):705–712.
26. Thomadsen B, Mehta M, Howard S, et al. Craniospinal treatment with the patient supine. *Med Dosim* 2003;28(1):35–38. doi: 10.1016/S0958-3947(02)00239-X.
27. Kiltie AE, Povall JM, Taylor RE. The need for the moving junction in craniospinal irradiation. *Br J Radiol* 2000;73(870):650–654.
28. Bauman G, Yartsev S, Coad T, et al. Helical tomotherapy for craniospinal radiation. *Br J Radiol* 2005;78(930):548–552. doi: 10.1259/bjr/53491625.
29. Yamamoto M, Serizawa T, Shuto T, et al. Stereotactic radiosurgery for patients with multiple brain metastases (JLGK0901): a multi-institutional prospective observational study. *Lancet Oncol* 2014;15(4):387–395. doi: 10.1016/S1470-2045(14)70061-0.
30. Shaw E, Scott C, Souhami L, et al. Single dose radiosurgical treatment of recurrent previously irradiated primary brain tumors and brain metastases: final report of RTOG protocol 90–05. *Int J Radiat Oncol Biol Phys* 2000;47(2):291–298.
31. Bova FJ, Buatti JM, Friedman WA, et al. The University of Florida frameless high-precision stereotactic radiotherapy system. *Int J Radiat Oncol Biol Phys* 1997;38(4):875–882.
32. Menke M, Hirschfeld F, Mack T, et al. Photogrammetric accuracy measurements of head holder systems used for fractionated radiotherapy. *Int J Radiat Oncol Biol Phys* 1994;29(5):1147–1155.
33. Yeung D, Palta J, Fontanesi J, et al. Systematic analysis of errors in target localization and treatment delivery in stereotactic radiosurgery (SRS). *Int J Radiat Oncol Biol Phys* 1994;28(2):493–498.

34. Tome WA, Meeks SL, Buatti JM, et al. A high-precision system for conformal intracranial radiotherapy. *Int J Radiat Oncol Biol Phys* 2000;47(4):1137–1143.

35. Kirsch DG, Tarbell NJ. Conformal radiation therapy for childhood CNS tumors. *Oncologist* 2004;9(4):442–450.

36. Tatter SB, Shaw EG, Rosenblum ML, et al. An inflatable balloon catheter and liquid 125I radiation source (GliaSite Radiation Therapy System) for treatment of recurrent malignant glioma: multicenter safety and feasibility trial. *J Neurosurg* 2003;99(2):297–303. doi: 10.3171/jns.2003.99.2.0297.

37. Riva P, Arista A, Franceschi G, et al. Local treatment of malignant gliomas by direct infusion of specific monoclonal antibodies labeled with 131I: comparison of the results obtained in recurrent and newly diagnosed tumors. *Cancer Res* 1995;55(23 Suppl):5952s–5956s.

38. Cairncross G, Wang M, Shaw E, et al. Phase III trial of chemoradiotherapy for anaplastic oligodendroglioma: long-term results of RTOG 9402. *J Clin Oncol* 2013;31(3):337–343. doi: 10.1200/JCO.2012.43.2674.

39. van den Bent MJ, Brandes AA, Taphoorn MJ, et al. Adjuvant procarbazine, lomustine, and vincristine chemotherapy in newly diagnosed anaplastic oligodendroglioma: long-term follow-up of EORTC brain tumor group study 26951. *J Clin Oncol* 2013;31(3):344–350. doi: 10.1200/JCO.2012.43.2229.

40. Brem H, Ewend MG, Piantadosi S, et al. The safety of interstitial chemotherapy with BCNU-loaded polymer followed by radiation therapy in the treatment of newly diagnosed malignant gliomas: phase I trial. *J Neurooncol* 1995;26(2):111–123.

41. Westphal M, Lamszus K, Hilt D. Intracavitary chemotherapy for glioblastoma: present status and future directions. *Acta Neurochir Suppl* 2003;88:61–67.

42. Emerich DF, Dean RL, Osborn C, et al. The development of the bradykinin agonist labradimil as a means to increase the permeability of the blood–brain barrier: from concept to clinical evaluation. *Clin Pharmacokinet* 2001;40(2):105–123.

43. Kroll RA, Neuwelt EA. Outwitting the blood–brain barrier for therapeutic purposes: osmotic opening and other means. *Neurosurgery* 1998;42(5):1083–1099; discussion 99–100.

44. Groothuis DR. The blood–brain and blood-tumor barriers: a review of strategies for increasing drug delivery. *Neuro Oncol* 2000;2(1):45–59.

45. Hadaczek P, Mirek H, Berger MS, et al. Limited efficacy of gene transfer in herpes simplex virus-thymidine kinase/ganciclovir gene therapy for brain tumors. *J Neurosurg* 2005;102(2):328–335. doi: 10.3171/jns.2005.102.2.0328.

46. Lidar Z, Mardor Y, Jonas T, et al. Convection-enhanced delivery of paclitaxel for the treatment of recurrent malignant glioma: a phase I/II clinical study. *J Neurosurg* 2004;100(3):472–479. doi: 10.3171/jns.2004.100.3.0472.

47. Kaiser MG, Parsa AT, Fine RL, et al. Tissue distribution and antitumor activity of topotecan delivered by intracerebral clysis in a rat glioma model. *Neurosurgery* 2000;47(6):1391–1398; discussion 8–9.

48. Kawakami K, Kawakami M, Liu Q, et al. Combined effects of radiation and interleukin-13 receptor-targeted cytotoxin on glioblastoma cell lines. *Int J Radiat Oncol Biol Phys* 2005;63(1):230–237. doi: 10.1016/j.ijrobp.2005.05.017.

49. Sampson JH, Akabani G, Archer GE, et al. Progress report of a Phase I study of the intracerebral microinfusion of a recombinant chimeric protein composed of transforming growth factor (TGF)-alpha and a mutated form of the Pseudomonas exotoxin termed PE-38 (TP-38) for the treatment of malignant brain tumors. *J Neurooncol* 2003;65(1):27–35.

50. Weaver M, Laske DW. Transferrin receptor ligand-targeted toxin conjugate (Tf-CRM107) for therapy of malignant gliomas. *J Neurooncol* 2003;65(1):3–13.

51. Weber FW, Floeth F, Asher A, et al. Local convection enhanced delivery of IL4-Pseudomonas exotoxin (NBI-3001) for treatment of patients with recurrent malignant glioma. *Acta Neurochir Suppl* 2003;88:93–103.

52. Kunwar S, Chang S, Westphal M, et al. Phase III randomized trial of CED of IL13-PE38QQR vs Gliadel wafers for recurrent glioblastoma. *Neuro Oncol* 2010;12(8):871–881. doi: 10.1093/neuonc/nop054.

53. Brem H, Piantadosi S, Burger PC, et al. Placebo-controlled trial of safety and efficacy of intraoperative controlled delivery by biodegradable polymers of chemotherapy for recurrent gliomas. The Polymer-Brain Tumor Treatment Group. *Lancet* 1995;345(8956):1008–1012.

54. Franz DN, Agricola KD, Tudor CA, et al. Everolimus for tumor recurrence after surgical resection for subependymal giant cell astrocytoma associated with tuberous sclerosis complex. *J Child Neurol* 2013;28(5):602–607. doi: 10.1177/0883073812449904.

55. Sathornsumetee S, Rich JN. Molecularly targeted therapy in neuro-oncology. *Handb Clin Neurol* 2012;104:255–278.

56. Gilbert MR, Dignam JJ, Armstrong TS, et al. A randomized trial of bevacizumab for newly diagnosed glioblastoma. *N Engl J Med* 2014;370(8):699–708. doi: 10.1056/NEJMoa1308573.

57. Chinot OL, Wick W, Mason W, et al. Bevacizumab plus radiotherapy-temozolomide for newly diagnosed glioblastoma. *N Engl J Med* 2014;370(8):709–722. doi: 10.1056/NEJMoa1308345.

57a. van den Bent M, Gan HK, Lassman AB, et al. Efficacy of depatuxizumab mafodotin (ABT-414) monotherapy in patients with EGFR-amplified, recurrent glioblastoma: results from a multi-center, international study. *Cancer Chemother Pharmacol* 2017;80(6):1209–1217.

58. Stupp R, Taillibert S, Kanner AA, et al. Maintenance therapy with tumor-treating fields plus temozolomide vs temozolomide alone for glioblastoma: a randomized clinical trial. *JAMA* 2015;314(23):2535–2543. doi: 10.1001/jama.2015.16669.

59. Stupp R, Wong ET, Kanner AA, et al. NovoTTF-100A versus physician's choice chemotherapy in recurrent glioblastoma: a randomised phase III trial of a novel treatment modality. *Eur J Cancer* 2012;48(14):2192–2202. doi: 10.1016/j.ejca.2012.04.011.

60. Weller M, Butowski N, Tran DD, et al. Rindopepimut with temozolomide for patients with newly diagnosed EGFRvIII-expressing glioblastoma (ACT IV): a randomised, double-blind, international phase 3 trial. *Lancet Oncol* 2017;18(10):1373–1385.

61. Taylor MD, Bernstein M. Awake craniotomy with brain mapping as the routine surgical approach to treating patients with supratentorial intraaxial tumors: a prospective trial of 200 cases. *J Neurosurg* 1999;90(1):35–41. doi: 10.3171/jns.1999.90.1.0035.

62. McGovern PC, Lautenbach E, Brennan PJ, et al. Risk factors for postcraniotomy surgical site infection after 1,3-bis (2-chloroethyl)-1-nitrosourea (Gliadel) wafer placement. *Clin Infect Dis* 2003;36(6):759–765. doi: 10.1086/368082.

63. Brown AP, Barney CL, Grosshans DR, et al. Proton beam craniospinal irradiation reduces acute toxicity for adults with medulloblastoma. *Int J Radiat Oncol Biol Phys* 2013;86(2):277–284. doi: 10.1016/j.ijrobp.2013.01.014.

64. Cammer W. Effects of TNFalpha on immature and mature oligodendrocytes and their progenitors in vitro. *Brain Res* 2000;864(2):213–219.

65. Chow BM, Li YQ, Wong CS. Radiation-induced apoptosis in the adult central nervous system is p53-dependent. *Cell Death Differ* 2000;7(8):712–720.

66. Crossen JR, Garwood D, Glatstein E, et al. Neurobehavioral sequelae of cranial irradiation in adults: a review of radiation-induced encephalopathy. *J Clin Oncol* 1994;12(3):627–642.

67. Gonzalez J, Kumar AJ, Conrad CA, et al. Effect of bevacizumab on radiation necrosis of the brain. *Int J Radiat Oncol Biol Phys* 2007;67(2):323–326. doi: 10.1016/j.ijrobp.2006.10.010.

68. Missios S, Bekelis K, Barnett GH. Renaissance of laser interstitial thermal ablation. *Neurosurg Focus* 2015;38(3):E13. doi: 10.3171/2014.12.FOCUS14762.

69. Lee AW, Kwong DL, Leung SF, et al. Factors affecting risk of symptomatic temporal lobe necrosis: significance of fractional dose and treatment time. *Int J Radiat Oncol Biol Phys* 2002;53(1):75–85.

70. Chang EL, Wefel JS, Hess KR, et al. Neurocognition in patients with brain metastases treated with radiosurgery or radiosurgery plus whole-brain irradiation: a randomised controlled trial. *Lancet Oncol* 2009;10(11):1037–1044. doi: 10.1016/S1470-2045(09)70263-3.

71. Sun A, Bae K, Gore EM, et al. Phase III trial of prophylactic cranial irradiation compared with observation in patients with locally advanced non-small-cell lung cancer: neurocognitive and quality-of-life analysis. *J Clin Oncol* 2011;29(3):279–286. doi: 10.1200/JCO.2010.29.6053.

72. Brown PD, Jaeckle K, Ballman KV, et al. Effect of radiosurgery alone vs radiosurgery with whole brain radiation therapy on cognitive function in patients with 1 to 3 brain metastases: a randomized clinical trial. *JAMA* 2016;316(4):401–409. doi: 10.1001/jama.2016.9839.

73. Monje ML, Palmer T. Radiation injury and neurogenesis. *Curr Opin Neurol* 2003;16(2):129–134. doi: 10.1097/01.wco.0000063772.81810.b7.

74. Peissner W, Kocher M, Treuer H, et al. Ionizing radiation-induced apoptosis of proliferating stem cells in the dentate gyrus of the adult rat hippocampus. *Brain Res Mol Brain Res* 1999;71(1):61–68.

75. Brown PD, Pugh S, Laack NN, et al. Memantine for the prevention of cognitive dysfunction in patients receiving whole-brain radiotherapy: a randomized, double-blind, placebo-controlled trial. *Neuro Oncol* 2013;15(10):1429–1437. doi: 10.1093/neuonc/not114.

76. Gondi V, Pugh SL, Tome WA, et al. Preservation of memory with conformal avoidance of the hippocampal neural stem-cell compartment during whole-brain radiotherapy for brain metastases (RTOG 0933): a phase II multi-institutional trial. *J Clin Oncol* 2014;32(34):3810–3816. doi: 10.1200/JCO.2014.57.2909.

77. Meyers CA, Weitzner MA, Valentine AD, et al. Methylphenidate therapy improves cognition, mood, and function of brain tumor patients. *J Clin Oncol* 1998;16(7):2522–2527.

78. Gondi V, Tome WA, Mehta MP. Why avoid the hippocampus? A comprehensive review. *Radiother Oncol* 2010;97(3):370–376. doi: 10.1016/j.radonc.2010.09.013.

79. Curran WJ Jr, Scott CB, Horton J, et al. Recursive partitioning analysis of prognostic factors in three Radiation Therapy Oncology Group malignant glioma trials. *J Natl Cancer Inst* 1993;85(9):704–710.

80. Mirimanoff RO, Gorlia T, Mason W, et al. Radiotherapy and temozolomide for newly diagnosed glioblastoma: recursive partitioning analysis of the EORTC 26981/22981-NCIC CE3 phase III randomized trial. *J Clin Oncol* 2006;24(16):2563–2569. doi: 10.1200/JCO.2005.04.5963.

81. Gorlia T, van den Bent MJ, Hegi ME, et al. Nomograms for predicting survival of patients with newly diagnosed glioblastoma: prognostic factor analysis of EORTC and NCIC trial 26981-22981/CE.3. *Lancet Oncol* 2008;9(1):29–38. doi: 10.1016/S1470-2045(07)70384-4.

82. Bell EH, Pugh SL, McElroy JP, et al. Molecular-based recursive partitioning analysis model for glioblastoma in the temozolomide era: a correlative analysis based on NRG Oncology RTOG 0525. *JAMA Oncol* 2017;3(6):784–792. doi: 10.1001/jamaoncol.2016.6020.

83. Dandy WE. Removal of right cerebral hemisphere for certain tumors with hemiplegia. *JAMA* 1928;90:823–825.

84. Bull JWD, Rovit RL. The radiographic localization of intracerebral gliomata. *J Fac Radiol (Lond)* 1957;8:147–157.

85. Kramer S. Tumor extent as a determining factor in radiotherapy of glioblastomas. *Acta Radiol Ther Phys Biol* 1969;8(1):111–117.

86. Matsukado Y, Maccarty CS, Kernohan JW. The growth of glioblastoma multiforme (astrocytomas, grades 3 and 4) in neurosurgical practice. *J Neurosurg* 1961;18:636–644. doi: 10.3171/jns.1961.18.5.0636.

87. Hochberg FH, Pruitt A. Assumptions in the radiotherapy of glioblastoma. *Neurology* 1980;30(9):907–911.

88. Wallner KE, Galicich JH, Krol G, et al. Patterns of failure following treatment for glioblastoma multiforme and anaplastic astrocytoma. *Int J Radiat Oncol Biol Phys* 1989;16(6):1405–1409.

89. Halperin EC, Burger PC, Bullard DE. The fallacy of the localized supratentorial malignant glioma. *Int J Radiat Oncol Biol Phys* 1988;15(2):505–509.

90. Wernicke AG, Smith AW, Taube S, et al. Glioblastoma: Radiation treatment margins, how small is large enough? *Pract Radiat Oncol* 2016;6(5):298–305. doi: 10.1016/j.prro.2015.12.002.

91. Kelly PJ, Daumas-Duport C, Scheithauer BW, et al. Stereotactic histologic correlations of computed tomography- and magnetic resonance imaging-defined abnormalities in patients with glial neoplasms. *Mayo Clin Proc* 1987;62(6):450–459.

92. Pirzkall A, McKnight TR, Graves EE, et al. MR-spectroscopy guided target delineation for high-grade gliomas. *Int J Radiat Oncol Biol Phys* 2001;50(4):915–928.

93. Walker MD, Strike TA, Sheline GE. An analysis of dose-effect relationship in the radiotherapy of malignant gliomas. *Int J Radiat Oncol Biol Phys* 1979;5(10):1725–1731.

Section III

94. Bleehen NM, Stenning SP. A Medical Research Council trial of two radiotherapy doses in the treatment of grades 3 and 4 astrocytoma. The Medical Research Council Brain Tumour Working Party. *Br J Cancer* 1991;64(4):769–774.

95. Nelson DF, Diener-West M, Horton J, et al. Combined modality approach to treatment of malignant gliomas—re-evaluation of RTOG 7401/ECOG 1374 with long-term follow-up: a joint study of the Radiation Therapy Oncology Group and the Eastern Cooperative Oncology Group. *NCI Monogr* 1988(6):279–284.

96. Chan JL, Lee SW, Fraass BA, et al. Survival and failure patterns of high-grade gliomas after three-dimensional conformal radiotherapy. *J Clin Oncol* 2002;20(6):1635–1642.

97. Deutsch M, Green SB, Strike TA, et al. Results of a randomized trial comparing BCNU plus radiotherapy, streptozotocin plus radiotherapy, BCNU plus hyperfractionated radiotherapy, and BCNU following misonidazole plus radiotherapy in the postoperative treatment of malignant glioma. *Int J Radiat Oncol Biol Phys* 1989;16(6):1389–1396.

98. Payne DG, Simpson WJ, Keen C, et al. Malignant astrocytoma: hyperfractionated and standard radiotherapy with chemotherapy in a randomized prospective clinical trial. *Cancer* 1982;50(11):2301–2306.

99. Shin KH, Urtasun RC, Fulton D, et al. Multiple daily fractionated radiation therapy and misonidazole in the management of malignant astrocytoma. A preliminary report. *Cancer* 1985;56(4):758–760.

100. Werner-Wasik M, Scott CB, Nelson DF, et al. Final report of a phase I/II trial of hyperfractionated and accelerated hyperfractionated radiation therapy with carmustine for adults with supratentorial malignant gliomas. Radiation Therapy Oncology Group Study 83–02. *Cancer* 1996;77(8):1535–1543. doi: 10.1002/(SICI)1097-0142(19960415)77:8<1535::AID-CNCR17>3.0.CO;2–0.

101. Scott C, Curran W, Yung WK, et al. Long term results of RTOG 9006: A randomized trial of hyperfractionated radiotherapy (RT) to 72.0 Gy and carmustine vs. standard RT and carmustine for malignant glioma patients with emphasis on anaplastic astrocytoma (AA) patients. *Proc Am Soc Clin Oncol* 1998;16:384.

102. Coughlin C, Scott C, Langer C, et al. Phase II, two-arm RTOG trial (94–11) of bischloroethyl-nitrosourea plus accelerated hyperfractionated radiotherapy (64.0 or 70.4 Gy) based on tumor volume (>20 or < or = 20 cm(2), respectively) in the treatment of newly-diagnosed radiosurgery-ineligible glioblastoma multiforme patients. *Int J Radiat Oncol Biol Phys* 2000;48(5):1351–1358.

103. Prados MD, Wara WM, Sneed PK, et al. Phase III trial of accelerated hyperfractionation with or without difluromethylornithine (DFMO) versus standard fractionated radiotherapy with or without DFMO for newly diagnosed patients with glioblastoma multiforme. *Int J Radiat Oncol Biol Phys* 2001;49(1):71–77.

104. Sarkaria JN, Mehta MP, Loeffler JS, et al. Radiosurgery in the initial management of malignant gliomas: survival comparison with the RTOG recursive partitioning analysis. Radiation Therapy Oncology Group. *Int J Radiat Oncol Biol Phys* 1995;32(4):931–941.

105. Souhami L, Seiferheld W, Brachman D, et al. Randomized comparison of stereotactic radiosurgery followed by conventional radiotherapy with carmustine to conventional radiotherapy with carmustine for patients with glioblastoma multiforme: report of Radiation Therapy Oncology Group 93–05 protocol. *Int J Radiat Oncol Biol Phys* 2004;60(3):853–860. doi: 10.1016/j.ijrobp.2004.04.011.

106. Cardinale R, Won M, Choucair A, et al. A phase II trial of accelerated radiotherapy using weekly stereotactic conformal boost for supratentorial glioblastoma multiforme: RTOG 0023. *Int J Radiat Oncol Biol Phys* 2006;65(5):1422–1428. doi: 10.1016/j.ijrobp.2006.02.042.

107. Laperriere NJ, Leung PM, McKenzie S, et al. Randomized study of brachytherapy in the initial management of patients with malignant astrocytoma. *Int J Radiat Oncol Biol Phys* 1998;41(5):1005–1011.

108. Selker RG, Shapiro WR, Burger P, et al. The Brain Tumor Cooperative Group NIH Trial 87–01: a randomized comparison of surgery, external radiotherapy, and carmustine versus surgery, interstitial radiotherapy boost, external radiation therapy, and carmustine. *Neurosurgery* 2002;51(2):343–355; discussion 55–7.

109. Kleinberg LR, Stieber V, Mikkelsen T, et al. Outcome of Adult Brain Tumor Consortium (ABTC) prospective dose-finding trials of I-125 balloon brachytherapy in high-grade gliomas: challenges in clinical trial design and technology development when MRI treatment effect and recurrence appear similar. *J Radiat Oncol* 2015;4(3):235–241. doi: 10.1007/s13566-015-0210-y.

110. Fitzek MM, Thornton AF, Rabinov JD, et al. Accelerated fractionated proton/photon irradiation to 90 cobalt gray equivalent for glioblastoma multiforme: results of a phase II prospective trial. *J Neurosurg* 1999;91(2):251–260. doi: 10.3171/jns.1999.91.2.0251.

111. Mizumoto M, Tsuboi K, Igaki H, et al. Phase I/II trial of hyperfractionated concomitant boost proton radiotherapy for supratentorial glioblastoma multiforme. *Int J Radiat Oncol Biol Phys* 2010;77(1):98–105. doi: 10.1016/j.ijrobp.2009.04.054.

112. Chang CH. Hyperbaric oxygen and radiation therapy in the management of glioblastoma. *Natl Cancer Inst Monogr* 1977;46:163–169.

113. Evans RG, Kimler BF, Morantz RA, et al. Lack of complications in long-term survivors after treatment with Fluosol and oxygen as an adjuvant to radiation therapy for high-grade brain tumors. *Int J Radiat Oncol Biol Phys* 1993;26(4):649–652.

114. Bleehen NM, Wiltshire CR, Plowman PN, et al. A randomized study of misonidazole and radiotherapy for grade 3 and 4 cerebral astrocytoma. *Br J Cancer* 1981;43(4):436–442.

115. Miralbell R, Mornex F, Greiner R, et al. Accelerated radiotherapy, carbogen, and nicotinamide in glioblastoma multiforme: report of European Organization for Research and Treatment of Cancer trial 22933. *J Clin Oncol* 1999;17(10):3143–3149.

116. Posner JB, Shapiro WR. Editorial: Brain tumor. Current status of treatment and its complications. *Arch Neurol* 1975;32(12):781–784.

117. Fine HA, Dear KB, Loeffler JS, et al. Meta-analysis of radiation therapy with and without adjuvant chemotherapy for malignant gliomas in adults. *Cancer* 1993;71(8):2585–2597.

118. Stewart LA. Chemotherapy in adult high-grade glioma: a systematic review and meta-analysis of individual patient data from 12 randomised trials. *Lancet* 2002;359(9311):1011–1018.

119. Yung WK, Prados MD, Yaya-Tur R, et al. Multicenter phase II trial of temozolomide in patients with anaplastic astrocytoma or anaplastic oligoastrocytoma at first relapse. Temodal Brain Tumor Group. *J Clin Oncol* 1999;17(9):2762–2771.

120. Stupp R, Mason WP, van den Bent MJ, et al. Radiotherapy plus concomitant and adjuvant temozolomide for glioblastoma. *N Engl J Med* 2005;352(10):987–996. doi: 10.1056/NEJMoa043330.

121. Stupp R, Hegi ME, Mason WP, et al. Effects of radiotherapy with concomitant and adjuvant temozolomide versus radiotherapy alone on survival in glioblastoma in a randomised phase III study: 5-year analysis of the EORTC-NCIC trial. *Lancet Oncol* 2009;10(5):459–466. doi: 10.1016/S1470-2045(09)70025-7.

122. Perry JR, Laperriere N, O'Callaghan CJ, et al. Short-course radiation plus temozolomide in elderly patients with glioblastoma. *N Engl J Med* 2017;376(11):1027–1037. doi: 10.1056/NEJMoa1611977.

123. Esteller M, Garcia-Foncillas J, Andion E, et al. Inactivation of the DNA-repair gene MGMT and the clinical response of gliomas to alkylating agents. *N Engl J Med* 2000;343(19):1350–1354. doi: 10.1056/NEJM200011093431901.

124. Hegi ME, Diserens AC, Gorlia T, et al. MGMT gene silencing and benefit from temozolomide in glioblastoma. *N Engl J Med* 2005;352(10):997–1003. doi: 10.1056/NEJMoa043331.

125. Gilbert MR, Wang M, Aldape KD, et al. RTOG 0525: A randomized phase III trial comparing standard adjuvant temozolomide with a dose-dense schedule in newly diagnosed glioblastoma. *J Clin Oncol* 2011;29:abstr 2006.

126. Blumenthal DT, Gorlia T, Gilbert MR, et al. Is more better? The impact of extended adjuvant temozolomide in newly diagnosed glioblastoma: a secondary analysis of EORTC and NRG Oncology/RTOG. *Neuro Oncol* 2017;19(8):1119–1126. doi: 10.1093/neuonc/nox025.

127. Gilbert MR, Kuhn JG, Lamborn KR, et al. Phase I/II study of combination temozolomide (TMZ) and irinotecan (CPT-11) for recurrent malignant gliomas: a North American Brain Tumor Consortium (NABTC) study. *J Clin Oncol* 2003;22:22.

128. Buckner JC, Ballman KV, Michalak JC, et al. Phase III trial of carmustine and cisplatin compared with carmustine alone and standard radiation therapy or accelerated radiation therapy in patients with glioblastoma multiforme: North Central Cancer Treatment Group 93-72-52 and Southwest Oncology Group 9503 Trials. *J Clin Oncol* 2006;24(24):3871–3879. doi: 10.1200/JCO.2005.04.6979.

129. Kirson ED, Gurvich Z, Schneiderman R, et al. Disruption of cancer cell replication by alternating electric fields. *Cancer Res* 2004;64(9):3288–3295.

130. Lee SX, Tunkyi A, Wong ET, Swanson KD, eds. CB-17. Mitosis Interference of Cancer Cells During Anaphase By Electric Field from NovoTTF-100A. Society for Neuro Oncology Annual Meeting; 2011; Orange County, California. Neuro Oncol.

131. Kirson ED, Dbaly V, Tovarys F, et al. Alternating electric fields arrest cell proliferation in animal tumor models and human brain tumors. *Proc Natl Acad Sci U S A* 2007;104(24):10152–10157. doi: 10.1073/pnas.0702916104.

132a. Stupp R, Tailibert S, Kanner A, et al. Effect of tumor-treating fields plus maintenance temozolomide vs maintenance temozolomide alone on survival in patients with glioblastoma: a randomized clinical trial. *JAMA* 2017; 328(23): 2306–2316.

132b. Taphoorn MJB, Dirven L, Kanner AA, et al. Influence of treatment with tumor-treating fields on health-related quality of life of patients with newly diagnosed glioblastoma: a secondary analysis of a randomized clinical trial. *JAMA Oncol* 2018; 4(4): 495–504.

133. Omuro A, Vlahovic G, Lim M, et al. Nivolumab with or without ipilumumab in patients with recurrent glioblastoma: results from exploratory phase I cohorts of CheckMate 143. *Neuro Oncol* 2018;20(5):674–686.

134. Schuster J, Lai RK, Recht LD, et al. A phase II, multicenter trial of rindopepimut (CDX-110) in newly diagnosed glioblastoma: the ACT III study. *Neuro Oncol* 2015;17(6):854–861.

135. Brady LW, Markoe AM, Woo DV, et al. Iodine-125-labeled anti-epidermal growth factor receptor-425 in the treatment of glioblastoma multiforme. A pilot study. *Front Radiat Ther Oncol* 1990;24:151–160; discussion 61–65.

136. Emrich JG, Brady LW, Quang TS, et al. Radioiodinated (I-125) monoclonal antibody 425 in the treatment of high grade glioma patients: ten-year synopsis of a novel treatment. *Am J Clin Oncol* 2002;25(6):541–546. doi: 10.1097/01.COC.0000041009.06780.E5.

137. Reardon DA, Akabani G, Coleman RE, et al. Phase II trial of murine (131) I-labeled antitenascin monoclonal antibody 81C6 administered into surgically created resection cavities of patients with newly diagnosed malignant gliomas. *J Clin Oncol* 2002;20(5):1389–1397.

138. Reardon DA, Akabani G, Coleman RE, et al. Salvage radioimmunotherapy with murine iodine-131-labeled antitenascin monoclonal antibody 81C6 for patients with recurrent primary and metastatic malignant brain tumors: phase II study results. *J Clin Oncol* 2006;24(1):115–122. doi: 10.1200/JCO.2005.03.4082.

139. Raizer JJ, Giglio P, Hu J, et al. A phase II study of bevacizumab and erlotinib after radiation and temozolomide in MGMT unmethylated GBM patients. *J Neurooncol* 2016;126(1):185–192. doi: 10.1007/s11060-015-1958-z.

140. Clarke JL, Molinaro AM, Phillips JJ, et al. A single-institution phase II trial of radiation, temozolomide, erlotinib, and bevacizumab for initial treatment of glioblastoma. *Neuro Oncol* 2014;16(7):984–990. doi: 10.1093/neuonc/nou029.

141. Chakravarti A, Wang M, Robins HI, et al. RTOG 0211: a phase 1/2 study of radiation therapy with concurrent gefitinib for newly diagnosed glioblastoma patients. *Int J Radiat Oncol Biol Phys* 2013;85(5):1206–1211. doi: 10.1016/j.ijrobp.2012.10.008.

142. Rao RD, Buckner JC, Sarkaria JN. Mammalian target of rapamycin (mTOR) inhibitors as anti-cancer agents. *Curr Cancer Drug Targets* 2004;4(8):621–635.

143. Ma DJ, Galanis E, Anderson SK, et al. A phase II trial of everolimus, temozolomide, and radiotherapy in patients with newly diagnosed glioblastoma: NCCTG N057K. *Neuro Oncol* 2015;17(9):1261–1269. doi: 10.1093/neuonc/nou328.

144. Paszat L, Laperriere N, Groome P, et al. A population-based study of glioblastoma multiforme. *Int J Radiat Oncol Biol Phys* 2001;51(1):100–107.

145. Gallego Perez-Larraya J, Ducray F, Chinot O, et al. Temozolomide in elderly patients with newly diagnosed glioblastoma and poor performance status: an ANOCEF phase II trial. *J Clin Oncol* 2011;29(22):3050–3055. doi: 10.1200/JCO.2011.34.8086.

146. Roa W, Brasher PM, Bauman G, et al. Abbreviated course of radiation therapy in older patients with glioblastoma multiforme: a prospective randomized clinical trial. *J Clin Oncol* 2004;22(9):1583–1588. doi: 10.1200/JCO.2004.06.082.

147. Malmstrom A, Gronberg BH, Marosi C, et al. Temozolomide versus standard 6-week radiotherapy versus hypofractionated radiotherapy in patients older than 60 years with glioblastoma: the Nordic randomised, phase 3 trial. *Lancet Oncol* 2012;13(9):916–926. doi: 10.1016/S1470-2045(12)70265-6.

148. Wick W, Engel C, Combs SE, et al. NOA-08 randomized phase III trial of 1-week-on/1-week-off temolomide versus involved-field radiotherapy in elderly (older than age 65) patients with newly diagnosed anaplastic astrocytoma or glioblastoma. *Proc Am Soc Clin Oncol* 2010;28(18s):LBA 2001.

149. Friedman HS, Prados MD, Wen PY, et al. Bevacizumab alone and in combination with irinotecan in recurrent glioblastoma. *J Clin Oncol* 2009;27(28): 4733–4740. doi: 10.1200/JCO.2008.19.8721.

150. Kreisl TN, Kim L, Moore K, et al. Phase II trial of single-agent bevacizumab followed by bevacizumab plus irinotecan at tumor progression in recurrent glioblastoma. *J Clin Oncol* 2009;27(5):740–745. doi: 10.1200/JCO.2008.16.3055.

151. Hess KR, Wong ET, Jaeckle KA, et al. Response and progression in recurrent malignant glioma. *Neuro Oncol* 1999;1(4):282–288.

152. Mellinghoff IK, Wang MY, Vivanco I, et al. Molecular determinants of the response of glioblastomas to EGFR kinase inhibitors. *N Engl J Med* 2005;353(19):2012–2024. doi: 10.1056/NEJMoa051918.

153. Taal W, Oosterkamp HM, Walenkamp AM, et al. Single-agent bevacizumab or lomustine versus a combination of bevacizumab plus lomustine in patients with recurrent glioblastoma (BELOB trial): a randomised controlled phase 2 trial. *Lancet Oncol* 2014;15(9):943–953. doi: 10.1016/S1470-2045(14)70314-6.

154. Wick W, Gorlia T, Bendszus M, et al. Lomustine and bevacizumab in progressive glioblastoma. *N Engl J Med* 2017;377(20):1954–1963.

155. Gutin PH, Iwamoto FM, Beal K, et al. Safety and efficacy of bevacizumab with hypofractionated stereotactic irradiation for recurrent malignant gliomas. *Int J Radiat Oncol Biol Phys.* 2009;75(1):156–163. doi: 10.1016/j.ijrobp.2008.10.043.

156. Omuro A, Beal K, Gutin P et al. Phase II study of bevacizumab, temozolomide, and hypofractionated stereotactic radiotherapy for newly diagnosed glioblastoma. *Clin Cancer Res* 2014;20(19):5023–5031.

157. Henson JW, Gaviani P, Gonzalez RG. MRI in treatment of adult gliomas. *Lancet Oncol* 2005;6(3):167–175. doi: 10.1016/S1470-2045(05)01767-5.

158. Smith JS, Perry A, Borell TJ, et al. Alterations of chromosome arms 1p and 19q as predictors of survival in oligodendrogliomas, astrocytomas, and mixed oligoastrocytomas. *J Clin Oncol* 2000;18(3):636–645.

159. Bauman GS, Ino Y, Ueki K, et al. Allelic loss of chromosome 1p and radiotherapy plus chemotherapy in patients with oligodendrogliomas. *Int J Radiat Oncol Biol Phys* 2000;48(3):825–830.

160. Cairncross JG, Ueki K, Zlatescu MC, et al. Specific genetic predictors of chemotherapeutic response and survival in patients with anaplastic oligodendrogliomas. *J Natl Cancer Inst* 1998;90(19):1473–1479.

161. Parsons DW, Jones S, Zhang X, et al. An integrated genomic analysis of human glioblastoma multiforme. *Science* 2008;321(5897):1807–1812. doi: 10.1126/science.1164382.

162. Yan H, Parsons DW, Jin G, et al. IDH1 and IDH2 mutations in gliomas. *N Engl J Med* 2009;360(8):765–773. doi: 10.1056/NEJMoa0808710.

163. van den Bent MJ, Dubbink HJ, Marie Y, et al. IDH1 and IDH2 mutations are prognostic but not predictive for outcome in anaplastic oligodendroglial tumors: a report of the European Organization for Research and Treatment of Cancer Brain Tumor Group. *Clin Cancer Res* 2010;16(5):1597–1604. doi: 10.1158/1078-0432.CCR-09-2902.

164. Cairncross JG, Wang M, Jenkins RB, et al. Benefit from procarbazine, lomustine, and vincristine in oligodendroglial tumors is associated with mutation of IDH. *J Clin Oncol* 2014;32(8):783–790. doi: 10.1200/JCO.2013.49.3726.

165. van den Bent MJ, Dubbink HJ, Sanson M, et al. MGMT promoter methylation is prognostic but not predictive for outcome to adjuvant PCV chemotherapy in anaplastic oligodendroglial tumors: a report from EORTC Brain Tumor Group Study 26951. *J Clin Oncol* 2009;27(35):5881–5886. doi: 10.1200/JCO.2009.24.1034.

166. Duffau H. Long-term outcomes after supratotal resection of diffuse low-grade gliomas: a consecutive series with 11-year follow-up. *Acta Neurochir (Wien)* 2016;158(1):51–58. doi: 10.1007/s00701-015-2621-3.

167. Chinot OL, Honore S, Dufour H, et al. Safety and efficacy of temozolomide in patients with recurrent anaplastic oligodendrogliomas after standard radiotherapy and chemotherapy. *J Clin Oncol* 2001;19(9):2449–2455.

168. Vogelbaum MA, Berkey B, Peereboom D, et al. Phase II trial of preirradiation and concurrent temozolomide in patients with newly diagnosed anaplastic oligodendrogliomas and mixed anaplastic oligoastrocytomas: RTOG BR0131. *Neuro Oncol* 2009;11(2):167–175. doi: 10.1215/15228517-2008-073.

169. Ducray F, del Rio MS, Carpentier C, et al. Up-front temozolomide in elderly patients with anaplastic oligodendroglioma and oligoastrocytoma. *J Neurooncol* 2011;101(3):457–462. doi: 10.1007/s11060-010-0264-z.

170. Kouwenhoven MC, Kros JM, French PJ, et al. 1p/19q loss within oligodendroglioma is predictive for response to first line temozolomide but not to salvage treatment. *Eur J Cancer* 2006;42(15):2499–2503. doi: 10.1016/j.ejca.2006.05.021.

171. Lassman AB, Iwamoto FM, Cloughesy TF, et al. International retrospective study of over 1000 adults with anaplastic oligodendroglial tumors. *Neuro Oncol* 2011;13(6):649–659. doi: 10.1093/neuonc/nor040.

172. Chang S, Zhang P, Cairncross JG, et al. Phase III randomized study of radiation and temozolomide versus radiation and nitrosourea therapy for anaplastic astrocytoma: results of NRG Oncology RTOG 9813. *Neuro Oncol* 2017;19(2):252–258. doi: 10.1093/neuonc/now236.

173. Levin VA, Hess KR, Choucair A, et al. Phase III randomized study of postradiotherapy chemotherapy with combination alpha-difluoromethylornithine-PCV versus PCV for anaplastic gliomas. *Clin Cancer Res* 2003;9(3):981–990.

174. Prados MD, Scott C, Curran WJ Jr, et al. Procarbazine, lomustine, and vincristine (PCV) chemotherapy for anaplastic astrocytoma: A retrospective review of radiation therapy oncology group protocols comparing survival with carmustine or PCV adjuvant chemotherapy. *J Clin Oncol* 1999;17(11): 3389–3395.

175. Randomized trial of procarbazine, lomustine, and vincristine in the adjuvant treatment of high-grade astrocytoma: a Medical Research Council trial. *J Clin Oncol* 2001;19(2):509–518.

176. van den Bent MJ, Baumert, B, Erridge SC, et al. Interim results from the CATNON trial (EORTC study 26053-22054) of treatment with concurrent and adjuvant temozolomide for 1p19q non-co-deleted anaplastic glioma: a phase 3, randomised, open-label intergroup study. *Lancet* 2017;390(10103):1645–1653.

177. Wick W, Hartmann C, Engel C, et al. NOA-04 randomized phase III trial of sequential radiochemotherapy of anaplastic glioma with procarbazine, lomustine, and vincristine or temozolomide. *J Clin Oncol* 2009;27(35):5874–5880. doi: 10.1200/JCO.2009.23.6497.

178. Jones DT, Kocialkowski S, Liu L, et al. Tandem duplication producing a novel oncogenic BRAF fusion gene defines the majority of pilocytic astrocytomas. *Cancer Res* 2008;68(21):8673–8677. doi: 10.1158/0008-5472.CAN-08-2097.

179. Brown PD, Anderson SK, Carrero XW, et al. Adult patients with supratentorial pilocytic astrocytoma: long-term follow-up of prospective multicenter clinical trial NCCTG-867251 (Alliance). *Neurooncol Pract* 2015;2(4):199–204. doi: 10.1093/nop/npv031.

180. Chang EF, Potts MB, Keles GE, et al. Seizure characteristics and control following resection in 332 patients with low-grade gliomas. *J Neurosurg* 2008;108(2):227–235. doi: 10.3171/JNS/2008/108/2/0227.

181. Pallud J, Blonski M, Mandonnet E, et al. Velocity of tumor spontaneous expansion predicts long-term outcomes for diffuse low-grade gliomas. *Neuro Oncol* 2013;15(5):595–606. doi: 10.1093/neuonc/nos331.

182. Pignatti F, van den Bent M, Curran D, et al. Prognostic factors for survival in adult patients with cerebral low-grade glioma. *J Clin Oncol* 2002;20(8):2076–2084.

183. Sun H, Yin L, Li S, et al. Prognostic significance of IDH mutation in adult low-grade gliomas: a meta-analysis. *J Neurooncol* 2013;113(2):277–284. doi: 10.1007/s11060-013-1107-5.

184. Fallon KB, Palmer CA, Roth KA, et al. Prognostic value of 1p, 19q, 9p, 10q, and EGFR-FISH analyses in recurrent oligodendrogliomas. *J Neuropathol Exp Neurol* 2004;63(4):314–322.

185. Okamoto Y, Di Patre PL, Burkhard C, et al. Population-based study on incidence, survival rates, and genetic alterations of low-grade diffuse astrocytomas and oligodendrogliomas. *Acta Neuropathol* 2004;108(1):49–56. doi: 10.1007/s00401-004-0861-z.

186. Sasaki H, Zlatescu MC, Betensky RA, et al. Histopathological-molecular genetic correlations in referral pathologist-diagnosed low-grade "oligodendroglioma". *J Neuropathol Exp Neurol* 2002;61(1):58–63.

187. Hoang-Xuan K, Capelle L, Kujas M, et al. Temozolomide as initial treatment for adults with low-grade oligodendrogliomas or oligoastrocytomas and correlation with chromosome 1p deletions. *J Clin Oncol* 2004;22(15):3133–3138. doi: 10.1200/JCO.2004.10.169.

188. Taal W, Dubbink HJ, Zonnenberg CB, et al. First-line temozolomide chemotherapy in progressive low-grade astrocytomas after radiotherapy: molecular characteristics in relation to response. *Neuro Oncol* 2011;13(2):235–241. doi: 10.1093/neuonc/noq177.

189. Buckner JC, Shaw EG, Pugh SL, et al. Radiation plus procarbazine, CCNU, and vincristine in low-grade glioma. *N Engl J Med* 2016;374(14):1344–1355. doi: 10.1056/NEJMoa1500925.

190. McBride SM, Perez DA, Polley MY, et al. Activation of PI3K/mTOR pathway occurs in most adult low-grade gliomas and predicts patient survival. *J Neurooncol* 2010;97(1):33–40. doi: 10.1007/s11060-009-0004-4.

191. Stege EM, Kros JM, de Bruin HG, et al. Successful treatment of low-grade oligodendroglial tumors with a chemotherapy regimen of procarbazine, lomustine, and vincristine. *Cancer* 2005;103(4):802–809. doi: 10.1002/cncr.20828.

192. Buckner JC, Gesme D Jr, O'Fallon JR, et al. Phase II trial of procarbazine, lomustine, and vincristine as initial therapy for patients with low-grade oligodendroglioma or oligoastrocytoma: efficacy and associations with chromosomal abnormalities. *J Clin Oncol* 2003;21(2):251–255.

193. Baumert BG, Hegi ME, van den Bent MJ, et al. Temozolomide chemotherapy versus radiotherapy in high-risk low-grade glioma (EORTC 22033-26033): a randomised, open-label, phase 3 intergroup study. *Lancet Oncol* 2016;17(11):1521–1532. doi: 10.1016/S1470-2045(16)30313-8.

194. Claus EB, Horlacher A, Hsu L, et al. Survival rates in patients with low-grade glioma after intraoperative magnetic resonance image guidance. *Cancer* 2005;103(6):1227–1233. doi: 10.1002/cncr.20867.

195. Berger MS, Deliganis AV, Dobbins J, Keles GE. The effect of extent of resection on recurrence in patients with low grade cerebral hemisphere gliomas. *Cancer* 1994;74(6):1784–1791.

196. Leighton C, Fisher B, Bauman G, et al. Supratentorial low-grade glioma in adults: an analysis of prognostic factors and timing of radiation. *J Clin Oncol* 1997;15(4):1294–1301.

197. Jackson RJ, Fuller GN, Abi-Said D, et al. Limitations of stereotactic biopsy in the initial management of gliomas. *Neuro Oncol* 2001;3(3):193–200.

198. Shaw EG, Berkey BA, Coons SW, et al. Initial report of Radiation Therapy Oncology Group (RTOG) 9802: prospective studies in adult low-grade glioma. *Proc Am Soc Clin Oncol* 2006;24(18s):1500.

199. van den Bent MJ, Afra D, de Witte O, et al. Long-term efficacy of early versus delayed radiotherapy for low-grade astrocytoma and oligodendroglioma in adults: the EORTC 22845 randomised trial. *Lancet* 2005;366(9490):985–990. doi: 10.1016/S0140-6736(05)67070-5.

200. Karim AB, Maat B, Hatlevoll R, et al. A randomized trial on dose–response in radiation therapy of low-grade cerebral glioma: European Organization for Research and Treatment of Cancer (EORTC) Study 22844. *Int J Radiat Oncol Biol Phys* 1996;36(3):549–556.

201. Shaw E, Arusell R, Scheithauer B, et al. Prospective randomized trial of low-versus high-dose radiation therapy in adults with supratentorial low-grade glioma: initial report of a North Central Cancer Treatment Group/Radiation Therapy Oncology Group/Eastern Cooperative Oncology Group study. *J Clin Oncol* 2002;20(9):2267–2276.

202. Brada M, Viviers L, Abson C, et al. Phase II study of primary temozolomide chemotherapy in patients with WHO grade II gliomas. *Ann Oncol* 2003;14(12):1715–1721.

203. Quinn JA, Reardon DA, Friedman AH, et al. Phase II trial of temozolomide in patients with progressive low-grade glioma. *J Clin Oncol* 2003;21(4):646–651.

204. van den Bent MJ, Chinot O, Boogerd W, et al. Second-line chemotherapy with temozolomide in recurrent oligodendroglioma after PCV (procarbazine, lomustine and vincristine) chemotherapy: EORTC Brain Tumor Group phase II study 26972. *Ann Oncol* 2003;14(4):599–602.

205. Fisher BJ, Hu C, Macdonald DR, et al. Phase 2 study of temozolomide-based chemoradiation therapy for high-risk low-grade gliomas: preliminary results

of Radiation Therapy Oncology Group 0424. *Int J Radiat Oncol Biol Phys* 2015;91(3):497–504. doi: 10.1016/j.ijrobp.2014.11.012.

206. Reijneveld JC, Taphoorn MJ, Coens C, et al. Health-related quality of life in patients with high-risk low-grade glioma (EORTC 22033–26033): a randomised, open-label, phase 3 intergroup study. *Lancet Oncol* 2016;17(11):1533–1542. doi: 10.1016/S1470-2045(16)30305-9.

207. Wahl M, Phillips JJ, Molinaro AM, et al. Chemotherapy for adult low-grade gliomas: clinical outcomes by molecular subtype in a phase II study of adjuvant temozolomide. *Neuro Oncol* 2017;19(2):242–251. doi: 10.1093/neuonc/now176.

208. Perkins GH, Schomer DF, Fuller GN, et al. Gliomatosis cerebri: improved outcome with radiotherapy. *Int J Radiat Oncol Biol Phys* 2003;56(4):1137–1146.

209. Sanson M, Cartalat-Carel S, Taillibert S, et al. Initial chemotherapy in gliomatosis cerebri. *Neurology* 2004;63(2):270–275.

210. Glas M, Bahr O, Felsberg J, et al. NOA-05 phase 2 trial of procarbazine and lomustine therapy in gliomatosis cerebri. *Ann Neurol* 2011;70(3):445–453. doi: 10.1002/ana.22478.

211. Taillibert S, Chodkiewicz C, Laigle-Donadey F, et al. Gliomatosis cerebri: a review of 296 cases from the ANOCEF database and the literature. *J Neurooncol* 2006;76(2):201–205. doi: 10.1007/s11060-005-5263-0.

212. Smith MA, Freidlin B, Ries LA, et al. Trends in reported incidence of primary malignant brain tumors in children in the United States. *J Natl Cancer Inst* 1998;90(17):1269–1277.

213. Khuong-Quang DA, Buczkowicz P, Rakopoulos P, et al. K27M mutation in histone H3.3 defines clinically and biologically distinct subgroups of pediatric diffuse intrinsic pontine gliomas. *Acta Neuropathol* 2012;124(3):439–447. doi: 10.1007/s00401-012-0998-0.

214. Wu G, Broniscer A, McEachron TA, et al. Somatic histone H3 alterations in pediatric diffuse intrinsic pontine gliomas and non-brainstem glioblastomas. *Nat Genet* 2012;44(3):251–253. doi: 10.1038/ng.1102.

215. Aboian MS, Solomon DA, Felton E, et al. Imaging Characteristics of Pediatric Diffuse Midline Gliomas with Histone H3 K27M Mutation. *AJNR Am J Neuroradiol* 2017;38(4):795–800. doi: 10.3174/ajnr.A5076.

216. Burger PC, Yu IT, Tihan T, et al. Atypical teratoid/rhabdoid tumor of the central nervous system: a highly malignant tumor of infancy and childhood frequently mistaken for medulloblastoma: a Pediatric Oncology Group study. *Am J Surg Pathol* 1998;22(9):1083–1092.

217. Zagzag D, Miller DC, Knopp E, et al. Primitive neuroectodermal tumors of the brainstem: investigation of seven cases. *Pediatrics* 2000;106(5):1045–1053.

218. Selvapandian S, Rajshekhar V, Chandy MJ. Brainstem glioma: comparative study of clinico-radiological presentation, pathology and outcome in children and adults. *Acta Neurochir (Wien)* 1999;141(7):721–726; discussion 6–7.

219. Kesari S, Kim RS, Markos V, et al. Prognostic factors in adult brainstem gliomas: a multicenter, retrospective analysis of 101 cases. *J Neurooncol* 2008;88(2):175–83. doi: 10.1007/s11060-008-9545-1.

220. Guillamo JS, Monjour A, Taillandier L, et al. Brainstem gliomas in adults: prognostic factors and classification. *Brain* 2001;124(Pt 12):2528–39.

221. Goldwein JW, Corn BW, Finlay JL, et al. Is craniospinal irradiation required to cure children with malignant (anaplastic) intracranial ependymomas? *Cancer* 1991;67(11):2766–71.

222. Merchant TE, Jenkins JJ, Burger PC, et al. Influence of tumor grade on time to progression after irradiation for localized ependymoma in children. *Int J Radiat Oncol Biol Phys* 2002;53(1):52–7.

223. Salazar OM, Castro-Vita H, VanHoutte P, et al. Improved survival in cases of intracranial ependymoma after radiation therapy. Late report and recommendations. *J Neurosurg* 1983;59(4):652–9. doi: 10.3171/jns.1983.59.4.0652.

224. Timmermann B, Kortmann RD, Kuhl J, et al. Combined postoperative irradiation and chemotherapy for anaplastic ependymomas in childhood: results of the German prospective trials HIT 88/89 and HIT 91. *Int J Radiat Oncol Biol Phys* 2000;46(2):287–295.

225. Wallner KE, Wara WM, Sheline GE, et al. Intracranial ependymomas: results of treatment with partial or whole brain irradiation without spinal irradiation. *Int J Radiat Oncol Biol Phys* 1986;12(11):1937–1941.

226. Tensaouti F, Ducassou A, Chaltiel L, et al. Patterns of failure after radiotherapy for pediatric patients with intracranial ependymoma. *Radiother Oncol* 2017;122(3):362–367. doi: 10.1016/j.radonc.2016.12.025.

227. Pajtler KW, Witt H, Sill M, et al. Molecular classification of ependymal tumors across all CNS compartments, histopathological grades, and age groups. *Cancer Cell* 2015;27(5):728–743. doi: 10.1016/j.ccell.2015.04.002.

228. Witt H, Mack SC, Ryzhova M, et al. Delineation of two clinically and molecularly distinct subgroups of posterior fossa ependymoma. *Cancer Cell* 2011;20(2):143–157. doi: 10.1016/j.ccr.2011.07.007.

229. Parker M, Mohankumar KM, Punchihewa C, et al. C11orf95-RELA fusions drive oncogenic NF-kappaB signalling in ependymoma. *Nature* 2014;506(7489):451–455. doi: 10.1038/nature13109.

230. Kirkpatrick JP, van der Kogel AJ, Schultheiss TE. Radiation dose-volume effects in the spinal cord. *Int J Radiat Oncol Biol Phys* 2010;76(3 Suppl):S42–S49. doi: 10.1016/j.ijrobp.2009.04.095.

231. Paulino AC. The local field in infratentorial ependymoma: does the entire posterior fossa need to be treated? *Int J Radiat Oncol Biol Phys* 2001;49(3):757–761.

232. Shaw EG, Evans RG, Scheithauer BW, et al. Postoperative radiotherapy of intracranial ependymoma in pediatric and adult patients. *Int J Radiat Oncol Biol Phys* 1987;13(10):1457–1462.

233. Pajtler KW, Mack SC, Ramaswamy V, et al. The current consensus on the clinical management of intracranial ependymoma and its distinct molecular variants. *Acta Neuropathol* 2017;133(1):5–12. doi: 10.1007/s00401-016-1643-0.

234. Donahue B, Steinfeld A. Intracranial ependymoma in the adult patient: successful treatment with surgery and radiotherapy. *J Neurooncol* 1998;37(2):131–133.

235. Ferrante L, Mastronardi L, Schettini G, et al. Fourth ventricle ependymomas. A study of 20 cases with survival analysis. *Acta Neurochir (Wien)* 1994;131(1–2):67–74.

236. Garrett PG, Simpson WJ. Ependymomas: results of radiation treatment. *Int J Radiat Oncol Biol Phys* 1983;9(8):1121–1124.

237. Schwartz TH, Kim S, Glick RS, et al. Supratentorial ependymomas in adult patients. *Neurosurgery* 1999;44(4):721–731.

238. Reni M, Brandes AA, Vavassori V, et al. A multicenter study of the prognosis and treatment of adult brain ependymal tumors. *Cancer* 2004;100(6):1221–1229. doi: 10.1002/cncr.20074.

239. Metellus P, Guyotat J, Chinot O, et al. Adult intracranial WHO grade II ependymomas: long-term outcome and prognostic factor analysis in a series of 114 patients. *Neuro Oncol* 2010;12(9):976–984. doi: 10.1093/neuonc/noq047.

240. Pica A, Miller R, Villa S, et al. The results of surgery, with or without radiotherapy, for primary spinal myxopapillary ependymoma: a retrospective study from the rare cancer network. *Int J Radiat Oncol Biol Phys* 2009;74(4):1114–1120. doi: 10.1016/j.ijrobp.2008.09.034.

241. Guyotat J, Signorelli F, Desme S, et al. Intracranial ependymomas in adult patients: analyses of prognostic factors. *J Neurooncol* 2002;60(3):255–268.

242. Carrie C, Lasset C, Blay JY, et al. Medulloblastoma in adults: survival and prognostic factors. *Radiother Oncol* 1993;29(3):301–307.

243. Prados MD, Warnick RE, Wara WM, et al. Medulloblastoma in adults. *Int J Radiat Oncol Biol Phys* 1995;32(4):1145–1152.

244. Rodriguez FJ, Eberhart C, O'Neill BP, et al. Histopathologic grading of adult medulloblastomas. *Cancer* 2007;109(12):2557–2565. doi: 10.1002/cncr.22717.

245. Berger MS, Baumeister B, Geyer JR, et al. The risks of metastases from shunting in children with primary central nervous system tumors. *J Neurosurg* 1991;74(6):872–877. doi: 10.3171/jns.1991.74.6.0872.

246. Packer RJ, Rood BR, MacDonald TJ. Medulloblastoma: present concepts of stratification into risk groups. *Pediatr Neurosurg* 2003;39(2):60–67. doi: 10.1159/000071316. PubMed PMID: 12845195.

247. Northcott PA, Korshunov A, Witt H, et al. Medulloblastoma comprises four distinct molecular variants. *J Clin Oncol* 2011;29(11):1408–1414. doi: 10.1200/JCO.2009.27.4324.

248. Robinson G, Parker M, Kranenburg TA, et al. Novel mutations target distinct subgroups of medulloblastoma. *Nature* 2012;488(7409):43–48. doi: 10.1038/nature11213.

249. Remke M, Hielscher T, Northcott PA, et al. Adult medulloblastoma comprises three major molecular variants. *J Clin Oncol* 2011;29(19):2717–2723. doi: 10.1200/JCO.2011.34.9373.

250. Schwalbe EC, Lindsey JC, Straughton D, et al. Rapid diagnosis of medulloblastoma molecular subgroups. *Clin Cancer Res* 2011;17(7):1883–1894. doi: 10.1158/1078-0432.CCR-10-2210.

251. Thompson EM, Hielscher T, Bouffet E, et al. Prognostic value of medulloblastoma extent of resection after accounting for molecular subgroup: a retrospective integrated clinical and molecular analysis. *Lancet Oncol* 2016;17(4):484–495. doi: 10.1016/S1470-2045(15)00581-1.

252. Kramer JH, Crowe AB, Larson DA, et al. Neuropsychological sequelae of medulloblastoma in adults. *Int J Radiat Oncol Biol Phys* 1997;38(1):21–26.

253. Michalski JM, VEzina JG, Gajjar A, et al. Results of COG ACNS0331: a phase III trial of involved-field radiotherapy (IFRT) and low dose craniospinal irradiation (LD-CSI) with chemotherapy in average-risk medulloblastoma: a report from the Children's Oncology Group. *Int J Radiat Biol Oncol Phys* 2016;96(5):937–938.

254. Herrlinger U, Steinbrecher A, Rieger J, et al. Adult medulloblastoma: prognostic factors and response to therapy at diagnosis and at relapse. *J Neurol* 2005;252(3):291–299. doi: 10.1007/s00415-005-0560-2.

255. Beier D, Proescholdt M, Reinert C, et al. Multicenter pilot study of radiochemotherapy as first-line treatment for adults with medulloblastoma (NOA-07). *Neuro Oncol* 2018;20(3):400–410.

256. Abrey LE, Ben-Porat L, Panageas KS, et al. Primary central nervous system lymphoma: the Memorial Sloan-Kettering Cancer Center prognostic model. *J Clin Oncol* 2006;24(36):5711–5. doi: 10.1200/JCO.2006.08.2941.

257. Ferreri AJ, Blay JY, Reni M, et al. Prognostic scoring system for primary CNS lymphomas: the International Extranodal Lymphoma Study Group experience. *J Clin Oncol* 2003;21(2):266–272.

258. Vater I, Montesinos-Rongen M, Schlesner M, et al. The mutational pattern of primary lymphoma of the central nervous system determined by whole-exome sequencing. *Leukemia* 2015;29(3):677–685. doi: 10.1038/leu.2014.264.

259. Lachance DH, Brizel DM, Gockerman JP, et al. Cyclophosphamide, doxorubicin, vincristine, and prednisone for primary central nervous system lymphoma: short-duration response and multifocal intracerebral recurrence preceding radiotherapy. *Neurology* 1994;44(9):1721–1727.

260. Schultz C, Scott C, Sherman W, et al. Preirradiation chemotherapy with cyclophosphamide, doxorubicin, vincristine, and dexamethasone for primary CNS lymphomas: initial report of radiation therapy oncology group protocol 88–06. *J Clin Oncol* 1996;14(2):556–564.

261. Shibamoto Y, Tsutsui K, Dodo Y, et al. Improved survival rate in primary intracranial lymphoma treated by high-dose radiation and systemic vincristine-doxorubicin-cyclophosphamide-prednisolone chemotherapy. *Cancer* 1990;65(9):1907–1912.

262. Ferreri AJ, Reni M, Foppoli M, et al. High-dose cytarabine plus high-dose methotrexate versus high-dose methotrexate alone in patients with primary CNS lymphoma: a randomised phase 2 trial. *Lancet* 2009;374(9700):1512–1520. doi: 10.1016/S0140-6736(09)61416-1.

263. Glantz MJ, Cole BF, Recht L, et al. High-dose intravenous methotrexate for patients with nonleukemic leptomeningeal cancer: is intrathecal chemotherapy necessary? *J Clin Oncol* 1998;16(4):1561–1567.

264. Abrey LE, DeAngelis LM, Yahalom J. Long-term survival in primary CNS lymphoma. *J Clin Oncol* 1998;16(3):859–863.

265. Bessell EM, Lopez-Guillermo A, Villa S, et al. Importance of radiotherapy in the outcome of patients with primary CNS lymphoma: an analysis of the CHOD/BVAM regimen followed by two different radiotherapy treatments. *J Clin Oncol* 2002;20(1):231–236.

266. DeAngelis LM, Seiferheld W, Schold SC, et al. Combination chemotherapy and radiotherapy for primary central nervous system lymphoma: Radiation Therapy Oncology Group Study 93–10. *J Clin Oncol* 2002;20(24):4643–4648.

267. Blay JY, Conroy T, Chevreau C, et al. High-dose methotrexate for the treatment of primary cerebral lymphomas: analysis of survival and late neurologic toxicity in a retrospective series. *J Clin Oncol* 1998;16(3):864–871.
268. Ferreri AJ, Abrey LE, Blay JY, et al. Summary statement on primary central nervous system lymphomas from the Eighth International Conference on Malignant Lymphoma, Lugano, Switzerland, June 12 to 15, 2002. *J Clin Oncol* 2003;21(12):2407–2414. doi: 10.1200/JCO.2003.01.135.
269. Batchelor T, Carson K, O'Neill A, et al. Treatment of primary CNS lymphoma with methotrexate and deferred radiotherapy: a report of NABTT 96–07. *J Clin Oncol* 2003;21(6):1044–1049.
270. Korfel A, Thiel E, Martus P, et al. Randomized phase III study of whole-brain radiotherapy for primary CNS lymphoma. *Neurology* 2015;84(12):1242–1248. doi: 10.1212/WNL.0000000000001395.
271. Herrlinger U, Schafer N, Fimmers R, et al. Early whole brain radiotherapy in primary CNS lymphoma: negative impact on quality of life in the randomized G-PCNSL-SG1 trial. *J Cancer Res Clin Oncol* 2017;143(9):1815–1821. doi: 10.1007/s00432-017-2423-5.
272. Shah GD, Yahalom J, Correa DD, et al. Combined immunochemotherapy with reduced whole-brain radiotherapy for newly diagnosed primary CNS lymphoma. *J Clin Oncol* 2007;25(30):4730–4735. doi: 10.1200/JCO.2007.12.5062.
273. Morris PG, Correa DD, Yahalom J, et al. Rituximab, methotrexate, procarbazine, and vincristine followed by consolidation reduced-dose whole-brain radiotherapy and cytarabine in newly diagnosed primary CNS lymphoma: final results and long-term outcome. *J Clin Oncol* 2013;31(31):3971–3979. doi: 10.1200/JCO.2013.50.4910.
274. Ferreri AJ, Crocchiolo R, Assanelli A, et al. High-dose chemotherapy supported by autologous stem cell transplantation in patients with primary central nervous system lymphoma: facts and opinions. *Leuk Lymphoma* 2008;49(11):2042–2047. doi: 10.1080/10428190802381238.
275. Omuro A, Correa DD, DeAngelis LM, et al. R-MPV followed by high-dose chemotherapy with TBC and autologous stem-cell transplant for newly diagnosed primary CNS lymphoma. *Blood* 2015;125(9):1403–1410. doi: 10.1182/blood-2014-10-604561.
276. Wilson WH, Young RM, Schmitz R, et al. Targeting B cell receptor signaling with ibrutinib in diffuse large B cell lymphoma. *Nat Med* 2015;21(8):922–926. doi: 10.1038/nm.3884.
277. Grommes C, Pastore A, Palaskas N, et al. Ibrutinib unmasks critical role of bruton tyrosine kinase in primary CNS lymphoma. *Cancer Discov* 2017. doi: 10.1158/2159-8290.CD-17-0613.
278. de Angelis LM. Current management of primary central nervous system lymphoma. *Oncology (Williston Park)* 1995;9(1):663–671.
279. Perry A, Louis DN, Scheithauer BW, *et al.* In: Louis DN, Ohgaki H, Wieslter OD, Cavenee WK, eds. *WHO Classification of Tumours of the Central Nervous System*. Lyon, France: IARC, 2007.
280. Brastianos PK, Horowitz PM, Santagata S, et al. Genomic sequencing of meningiomas identifies oncogenic SMO and AKT1 mutations. *Nat Genet* 2013;45(3):285–289. doi: 10.1038/ng.2526.
281. Bi WL, Greenwald NF, Abedalthagafi M, et al. Genomic landscape of high-grade meningiomas. *NPJ Genom Med* 2017;2.
282. Shankar GM, Abedalthagafi M, Vaubel RA, et al. Germline and somatic BAP1 mutations in high-grade rhabdoid meningiomas. *Neuro Oncol* 2017;19(4):535–545. doi: 10.1093/neuonc/now235.
283. Go RS, Taylor BV, Kimmel DW. The natural history of asymptomatic meningiomas in Olmsted County, Minnesota. *Neurology* 1998;51(6):1718–1720.
284. Olivero WC, Lister JR, Elwood PW. The natural history and growth rate of asymptomatic meningiomas: a review of 60 patients. *J Neurosurg* 1995;83(2):222–224. doi: 10.3171/jns.1995.83.2.0222.
285. Nakamura M, Roser F, Michel J, et al. The natural history of incidental meningiomas. *Neurosurgery* 2003;53(1):62–70; discussion 70–71.
286. Forbes AR, Goldberg ID. Radiation therapy in the treatment of meningioma: the Joint Center for Radiation Therapy experience 1970 to 1982. *J Clin Oncol* 1984;2(10):1139–1143.
287. Jung HW, Yoo H, Paek SH, et al. Long-term outcome and growth rate of subtotally resected petroclival meningiomas: experience with 38 cases. *Neurosurgery* 2000;46(3):567–574; discussion 74–75.
288. Condra KS, Buatti JM, Mendenhall WM, et al. Benign meningiomas: primary treatment selection affects survival. *Int J Radiat Oncol Biol Phys* 1997;39(2):427–436.
289. Stafford SL, Perry A, Suman VJ, et al. Primarily resected meningiomas: outcome and prognostic factors in 581 Mayo Clinic patients, 1978 through 1988. *Mayo Clin Proc* 1998;73(10):936–942. doi: 10.4065/73.10.936.
290. Goldsmith BJ, Wara WM, Wilson CB, et al. Postoperative irradiation for subtotally resected meningiomas. A retrospective analysis of 140 patients treated from 1967 to 1990. *J Neurosurg* 1994;80(2):195–201. doi: 10.3171/jns.1994.80.2.0195.
291. Debus J, Wuendrich M, Pirzkall A, et al. High efficacy of fractionated stereotactic radiotherapy of large base-of-skull meningiomas: long-term results. *J Clin Oncol* 2001;19(15):3547–3553.
292. Hakim R, Alexander E III, Loeffler JS, et al. Results of linear accelerator-based radiosurgery for intracranial meningiomas. *Neurosurgery* 1998;42(3):446–453; discussion 53–54.
293. Nicolato A, Foroni R, Alessandrini F, et al. Radiosurgical treatment of cavernous sinus meningiomas: experience with 122 treated patients. *Neurosurgery* 2002;51(5):1153–1159; discussion 9–61.
294. Pollock BE, Stafford SL. Results of stereotactic radiosurgery for patients with imaging defined cavernous sinus meningiomas. *Int J Radiat Oncol Biol Phys* 2005;62(5):1427–1431. doi: 10.1016/j.ijrobp.2004.12.067.
295. Stafford SL, Pollock BE, Foote RL, et al. Meningioma radiosurgery: tumor control, outcomes, and complications among 190 consecutive patients. *Neurosurgery* 2001;49(5):1029–1037; discussion 37–38.
296. Tutunji J, Grau SJ, Rueb D, et al. Stereotactic radiosurgery for the treatment of meningiomas eligible for complete resection. *Neuro Oncol* 2017;19(Suppl 3):iii16–iii17.
297. Dziuk TW, Woo S, Butler EB, et al. Malignant meningioma: an indication for initial aggressive surgery and adjuvant radiotherapy. *J Neurooncol* 1998;37(2):177–188.
298. Hug EB, Devries A, Thornton AF, et al. Management of atypical and malignant meningiomas: role of high-dose, 3D-conformal radiation therapy. *J Neurooncol* 2000;48(2):151–160.
299. Rogers L, Zhang P, Vogelbaum MA, et al., eds. *Low-risk meningioma: Initial outcomes from NRG Oncology/RTOG 0539*. Boston, MA: American Society for Therapeutic Oncology (ASTRO), 2016.
300. Wang C, Kaprealian TB, Suh JH, et al. Overall survival benefit associated with adjuvant radiotherapy in WHO grade II meningioma. *Neuro Oncol* 2017;19(9):1263–1270. doi: 10.1093/neuonc/nox007.
301. Chamberlain MC. Adjuvant combined modality therapy for malignant meningiomas. *J Neurosurg* 1996;84(5):733–736. doi: 10.3171/jns.1996.84.5.0733.
302. Miralbell R, Linggood RM, de la Monte S, et al. The role of radiotherapy in the treatment of subtotally resected benign meningiomas. *J Neurooncol* 1992;13(2):157–164.
303. Kyritsis AP. Chemotherapy for meningiomas. *J Neurooncol* 1996;29(3):269–272.
304. Schrell UM, Rittig MG, Anders M, et al. Hydroxyurea for treatment of unresectable and recurrent meningiomas. I. Inhibition of primary human meningioma cells in culture and in meningioma transplants by induction of the apoptotic pathway. *J Neurosurg* 1997;86(5):845–852. doi: 10.3171/jns.1997.86.5.0845.
305. Goodwin JW, Crowley J, Eyre HJ, et al. A phase II evaluation of tamoxifen in unresectable or refractory meningiomas: a Southwest Oncology Group study. *J Neurooncol* 1993;15(1):75–77.
306. Grunberg SM, Rankin C, Townsend J, et al. Phase III double-blind randomized placebo-controlled study of mifepristone (RU) for the treatment of unresectable meningioma. *J Clin Oncol* 2001;20s:56.
307. Brada M, Thomas DG. Craniopharyngioma revisited. *Int J Radiat Oncol Biol Phys* 1993;27(2):471–475.
308. Flickinger JC, Lunsford LD, Singer J, et al. Megavoltage external beam irradiation of craniopharyngiomas: analysis of tumor control and morbidity. *Int J Radiat Oncol Biol Phys* 1990;19(1):117–122.
309. Stripp DC, Maity A, Janss AJ, et al. Surgery with or without radiation therapy in the management of craniopharyngiomas in children and young adults. *Int J Radiat Oncol Biol Phys* 2004;58(3):714–720. doi: 10.1016/S0360-3016(03)01570-0.
310. Jose CC, Rajan B, Ashley S, et al. Radiotherapy for the treatment of recurrent craniopharyngioma. *Clin Oncol (R Coll Radiol)* 1992;4(5):287–289.
311. Kobayashi T. Long-term results of gamma knife radiosurgery for 100 consecutive cases of craniopharyngioma and a treatment strategy. *Prog Neurol Surg* 2009;22:63–76.
312. Maire JP, Caudry M, Darrouzet V, et al. Fractionated radiation therapy in the treatment of stage III and IV cerebello-pontine angle neurinomas: long-term results in 24 cases. *Int J Radiat Oncol Biol Phys*. 1995;32(4):1137–1143.
313. Nakamura H, Jokura H, Takahashi K, et al. Serial follow-up MR imaging after gamma knife radiosurgery for vestibular schwannoma. *AJNR Am J Neuroradiol* 2000;21(8):1540–1546.
314. Noren G. Long-term complications following gamma knife radiosurgery of vestibular schwannomas. *Stereotact Funct Neurosurg* 1998;70(Suppl 1):65–73.
315. Flickinger JC, Kondziolka D, Niranjan A, et al. Acoustic neuroma radiosurgery with marginal tumor doses of 12 to 13 Gy. *Int J Radiat Oncol Biol Phys* 2004;60(1):225–230. doi: 10.1016/j.ijrobp.2004.02.019.
316. Hayhurst C, Monsalves E, Bernstein M, et al. Predicting nonauditory adverse radiation effects following radiosurgery for vestibular schwannoma: a volume and dosimetric analysis. *Int J Radiat Oncol Biol Phys* 2012;82(5):2041–2046. doi: 10.1016/j.ijrobp.2011.02.017.
317. Pollock BE, Lunsford LD, Kondziolka D, et al. Outcome analysis of acoustic neuroma management: a comparison of microsurgery and stereotactic radiosurgery. *Neurosurgery* 1995;36(1):215–224; discussion 24–29.
318. Andrews DW, Suarez O, Goldman HW, et al. Stereotactic radiosurgery and fractionated stereotactic radiotherapy for the treatment of acoustic schwannomas: comparative observations of 125 patients treated at one institution. *Int J Radiat Oncol Biol Phys* 2001;50(5):1265–1278.
319. Meijer OW, Vandertop WP, Baayen JC, et al. Single-fraction vs. fractionated linac-based stereotactic radiosurgery for vestibular schwannoma: a single-institution study. *Int J Radiat Oncol Biol Phys* 2003;56(5):1390–1396.
320. Shirato H, Sakamoto T, Takeichi N, et al. Fractionated stereotactic radiotherapy for vestibular schwannoma (VS): comparison between cystic-type and solid-type VS. *Int J Radiat Oncol Biol Phys* 2000;48(5):1395–1401.
321. Szumacher E, Schwartz ML, Tsao M, et al. Fractionated stereotactic radiotherapy for the treatment of vestibular schwannomas: combined experience of the Toronto-Sunnybrook Regional Cancer Centre and the Princess Margaret Hospital. *Int J Radiat Oncol Biol Phys* 2002;53(4):987–991.
322. Plotkin SR, Stemmer-Rachamimov AO, Barker FG II, et al. Hearing improvement after bevacizumab in patients with neurofibromatosis type 2. *N Engl J Med* 2009;361(4):358–367. doi: 10.1056/NEJMoa0902579.
323. Rajaraman C, Rowe JG, Walton L, et al. Treatment options for von Hippel-Lindau's haemangioblastomatosis: the role of gamma knife stereotactic radiosurgery. *Br J Neurosurg* 2004;18(4):338–342.
324. Tago M, Terahara A, Shin M, et al. Gamma knife surgery for hemangioblastomas. *J Neurosurg* 2005;102(Suppl):171–14.
325. Wang EM, Pan L, Wang BJ, et al. The long-term results of gamma knife radiosurgery for hemangioblastomas of the brain. *J Neurosurg* 2005;102 (Suppl):225–229.
326. Lonser RR, Butman JA, Huntoon K, et al. Prospective natural history study of central nervous system hemangioblastomas in von Hippel-Lindau disease. *J Neurosurg* 2014;120(5):1055–1062. doi: 10.3171/2014.1.JNS131431.
327. Sheehan J, Kondziolka D, Flickinger J, et al. Radiosurgery for treatment of recurrent intracranial hemangiopericytomas. *Neurosurgery* 2002;51(4):905–10; discussion 10–1.

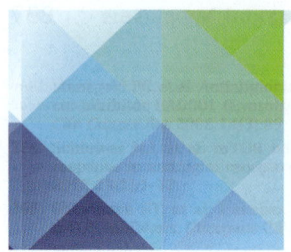

CHAPTER 39

Pituitary Gland Cancer

Theodore E. Yaeger

ANATOMIC CONSIDERATIONS

The pituitary gland, also known as the hypophysis cerebri, is an important endocrine organ. It appears as an ovoid body, the main portion of which is situated in the hypophysial fossa of the sphenoid bone (Fig. 39.1). That main portion is physically connected to the brain by the infundibulum. The diaphragma sellae forms a dural roof for the greater part of the hypophysis and is pierced by the infundibulum. In front of the infundibulum, the superior aspect of the gland is related directly to the arachnoid and pia[1] and the subarachnoid space then extends below the diaphragma.[2] The gland is completely surrounded in the fossa by a fibrous capsule that fuses with the endosteum.[3]

The hypophysis is related above to the optic chiasma and below to the intercavernous venous sinus and the sphenoid air sinus. This location conveniently allows an endonasal approach for surgical purposes[4] with laterally to the cavernous sinuses. By causing pressure on the chiasma, hypophysial tumors commonly result in visual defects such as superior temporal anopsia or bilateral temporal hemianopsia. Clinically, this is described as a profound loss of peripheral vision of varying degrees depending on achieved tumor size and chiasm affects.

The hypophysis is best divided on the embryologic basis into two main parts[5]: the adenohypophysis and the neurohypophysis. The former comprises the pars infundibularis (or pars tuberalis), the pars intermedia, and the pars distalis. The latter comprises the median eminence, the infundibular stem, and the infundibular process or neural lobe. The median eminence is frequently also classified as part of the tuber cinereum. The terms infundibulum or neural stalk is used for the median eminence and the infundibular stem. The term hypophysial stalk usually refers to the pars infundibularis and the infundibulum.

The adenohypophysis constitutes about 80% of the total volume of the pituitary gland[6] and is an embryologic diverticulum from the buccopharyngeal region. The pars distalis area secretes a number of hormones. The neurohypophysis develops as a diverticulum from the floor of the third ventricle. Specifically, it is not an actual endocrine-producing gland but more appropriately should be considered a storage gland for neurosecretions produced by the hypothalamus, which are then carried down via the axona of the supraopticohypophysial neural tracts.

Blood Supply and Innervations

The hypophysis is supplied by a series of hypophysial arteries from the internal carotids. The maintenance and regulation of the activity of the adenohypophysis are dependent on the blood supply by way of the hypophysial portal system.[7-11] Nerve fibers from the hypothalamus liberate releasing factors into the capillary beds in the infundibulum, and these substances are then carried by the portal vessels to the distal parts of the gland, causing the effects relevant to the specific secretions. The neurohypophysis receives its main nerve supply from the hypothalamus by way of fibers known collectively as the hypothalamohypophysial tract. This tract contains two main sets of fibers: the supraopticohypophysial tract and the tuberohypophysial tract.

Gross Appearance

Upon gross examination, the pituitary gland is a small, gray, rounded gland. It is developed from ingrown oral epithelium known as Rathke pouch as an extension of the developing oral cavity. As development matures, the gland is eventually cut off from its origins by the growth of the sphenoid bone and settles into what is described as a saddle-shaped, base-of-brain, bone depression formally called the sella turcica. The anterior pituitary has a portal vascular system that is the conduit for the transport of hypothalamic-releasing hormones from the hypothalamus to the anterior pituitary. Hypothalamic neurons have terminals in the median eminence where the hormones are released into the portal systems. This vascular supply traverses the pituitary stalk and then enters the anterior pituitary lobe. Most pituitary hormones are controlled predominately by releasing factors from the hypothalamus, with the exception of prolactin, which is controlled by the dopamine system via an inhibitory mechanism. It is attached to the lower surface of the hypothalamus by the infundibular stalk. The Rathke pouch portion forms the anterior lobe and the intermediate area. The posterior pituitary is embryologically derived from an outpouching from the floor of the third ventricle and grows inferiorly along the stalk of the anterior lobe. In contrast to the anterior lobe, this posterior lobe is supplied by the inferior hypophyseal artery. This will then drain into the venous sinus system for direct product release into the systemic circulation. As such, the pituitary gland has a dual circulation; one is composed of arteries and veins and the other a portal venous system that links the hypothalamus and the anterior lobe. Lastly, the neural tissue of the infundibular stalk essentially forms the posterior lobe. In general, the pituitary gland averages $1.3 \times 1.0 \times 0.5$ cm in size and weighs 0.55 to 0.6 g. It temporarily enlarges during pregnancy.[12] Overall, it is about the smallest functioning gland in the human body, but it has a critically important role in systemic physiologic regulation as demonstrated next.[6]

Physiology

There are five cell types that are revealed using specific antibody staining:

1. *Somatotrophs*. Growth hormone–producing acidophilic cells constituting about 50% of the anterior lobe
2. *Lactotrophs*. Prolactin-producing acidophilic cells (also known as mammotrophs)
3. *Corticotrophs*. Basophilic-appearing cells that produce adrenocorticotrophic hormone, pro-opiomelanocortin, melanocytic-stimulating hormone, endorphins, and lipotropin
4. *Thyrotrophs*. Very pale-appearing cells that produce thyroid-stimulating hormone
5. *Gonadotrophs*. Basophilic cells that produce follicle-stimulating hormone and luteinizing hormone

MORPHOLOGY

The most common pituitary adenoma is a small, soft, well-circumscribed lesion that may be confined to the sella turcica. Larger lesions typically extend superiorly through the diaphragm sella into the suprasellar region. This can cause

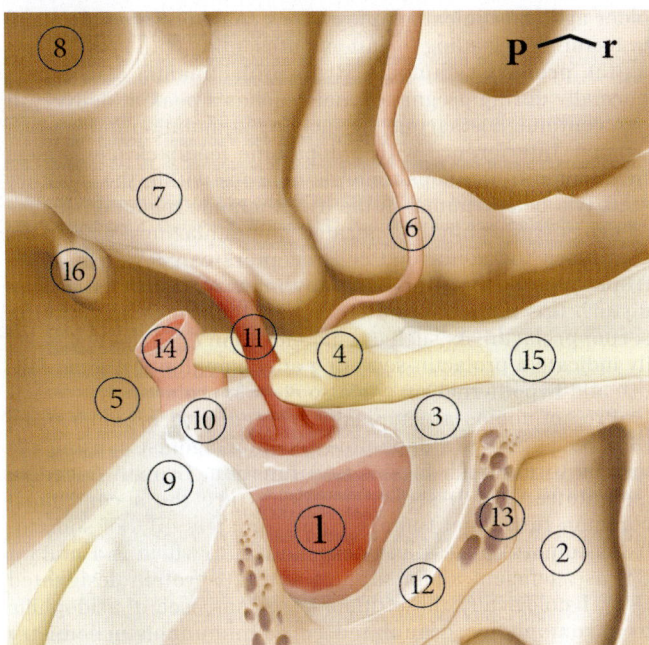

p ⌢ r

FIGURE 39.1. Posterolateral view of the pituitary gland. *P*, posterior; *r*, right. *1*, pituitary gland; *2*, sphenoid sinus; *3*, diaphragm sellae; *4*, optic chiasm; *5*, chiasmatic cistern; *6*, anterior cerebral artery; *7*, hypothalamus; *8*, third ventricle; *9*, dorsum sellae; *10*, posterior clinoid; *11*, pituitary stalk; *12*, sella turcica; *13*, cavernous sinus; *14*, internal carotid artery; *15*, right optic nerve; *16*, mamillary body.

compression of the optic chiasm and adjacent structures, including cranial nerves. Continued expansion eventually erodes the sella turcica, the anterior clinoid process, and can project into the cavernous and sphenoid sinuses. As many as 30% of cases adenomas can be nonencapsulated and infiltrate adjacent bones, dura, and rarely into the brain proper.[13] Foci of hemorrhage and necrosis are hallmarks of these invasive larger adenomas and are easily identified by imaging. Pituitary apoplexy occurs when an acute hemorrhage causes a rapidly enlarging mass. Clinically, this presents with dramatic symptomatic issues that are the result of the sudden onset of mass effects in a relatively confined space.

CLINICAL COURSE

The signs and symptoms of active pituitary adenomas can include endocrine abnormalities, mass effects, or both. Abnormalities associated with excessive secretions of anterior pituitary hormones are specific to the particular aberrant cell line, as described below. Local mass effect can be associated with any type of pituitary tumor, including a rare metastatic tumor from another site. The earliest changes in local anatomy result in radiographic changes with local deformation of the sella, the diaphragm, and bone erosions. Ultimately, compression of surrounding normal soft tissues results in visual field abnormalities with headache, nausea, and vomiting; eventually compressing the nonneoplastic pituitary and resulting in hypopituitarism. This can occur rapidly if there is hemorrhage resulting in pituitary apoplexy with excruciating headache, diplopia from pressure on the oculomotor nerves, visual defects, and eventually hypopituitarism.

The posterior pituitary or neurohypophysis consists of pituicytes—modified glial cells—and axonal processes extending from nerve cell bodies in the supraoptic and paraventricular nuclei of the hypothalamus. These cells transit through the pituitary stalk to the posterior lobe where the two posterior lobe hormones, oxytocin and vasopressin, are stored.

Hormones are secreted from the following lobes:

- *Intermediate lobe:* no effects are known in warm-blooded mammals.
- *Anterior lobe: Growth hormone*–regulating cell division and protein synthesis; *adrenocorticotrophic hormone*, which regulates the functional activity of the adrenal cortex; *thyroid-stimulating hormone*, which regulates the functional activity of the thyroid gland; *follicle-stimulating hormone*, which regulates ovarian follicles and spermatogenesis; *luteinizing hormone* (in women), which stimulates ovulation, formation of the corpus luteum, and secretion of estrogen and progesterone. In men, it can be called *interstitial cell–stimulating hormone*, which stimulates testosterone secretion. Also in women, there is *prolactin*, which induces secretion of breast milk.
- *Posterior lobe:* Hormones are secreted by the neurosecretory cells of the hypothalamus and pass through the fibers of the supraopticohypophyseal tracts in the infundibular stalk to the neurohypophysis where they are stored. These stored secretions are *oxytocin*, which acts on smooth muscles of the female uterus to increase contractility. There is also *antidiuretic hormone*, which increases water reabsorption of the renal system via the kidney tubules, and a derivative known as *vasopressin* to regulate blood pressure.

DISORDERS

Diseases of the pituitary are divided into those that affect the anterior lobe and those that affect the posterior lobe. The former are either hypersecretory or hyposecretory in nature. In most cases, hypersecretion is caused by a functioning adenoma within the anterior lobe. Hypopituitarism may be caused by a variety of destructive processes, including ischemic injury, radiation exposure (including therapeutic radiation), inflammatory responses, and nonfunctioning tumors such as a squamous "pearl" from cell rests that occurs during the embryo stage of development. Other than endocrine abnormalities, diseases of the anterior pituitary may manifest by a local mass effect. Radiographically, this can usually be seen by enlargement of the sella turcica. Clinical signs are visual field defects or vision cuts, evidence of increased intracranial pressure by optic examination or a patient's complaint of double vision, headache, and nausea. The posterior pituitary may also provide clinical evidence of antidiuretic hormone abnormalities. This can present as the symptoms of inappropriate antidiuretic hormone (SIADH) resulting in hypervolemia and hyponatremia if the gland is still in a functioning state.

Hyperpituitarism and Pituitary Anterior Adenomas

Excess production of hormones related to the anterior pituitary is often caused by a benign adenoma arising from cells in the anterior lobe. Less commonly, there can be hyperplasia or, rarely, actual carcinoma of glandular elements. Conversely, nonfunctioning adenomas may cause hypopituitarism as they grow and displace the normal functioning gland. Functional pituitary adenomas are usually composed of a single aberrant cell *type*, thus producing a single dominant hormone. Less common are adenomas that may have a single cell *line* but produce more than one hormone product; these are called plurihormal. Rarely are functional adenomas with multiple cell lines. Regardless, the vast majority of pituitary adenomas are monoclonal in origin, suggesting a single somatic cell, even when a plurihormonal diagnosis is made.[14] Some plurihormonal adenomas may arise from a primitive stem cell. This type may subsequently differentiate to develop multiple productive cell lines simultaneously. Molecular studies have identified specific mutations (such as a single base-pair missense mutations) that would stabilize one protein into an active formation while inhibiting a controlling protein, thus mimicking an active hormone. This has been identified in about 40% of growth hormone–secreting tumors. Other molecular aberrations seem more sporadic, and the pathogenesis of most pituitary tumors is still largely unknown.

PHYSIOLOGY

Hyperpituitarism of the Pituitary Lobes

Hypersecretion of the anterior lobe causes gigantism, acromegaly, and Cushing disease (pituitary basophilism). Hyposecretion of the anterior lobe causes dwarfism, Simond disease (pituitary cachexia), Sheehan syndrome (postpartum pituitary necrosis), acromicria, eunuchoidism, and hypogonadism. A posterior lobe deficiency results in a hypothalamic lesion that causes diabetes insipidus. Anterior *and* posterior lobe deficiencies *plus* a hypothalamic lesion causes Frohlich syndrome (adiposogenital dystrophy) and pituitary obesity.

Anterior Lobe

In the anterior lobe, the most common tumor, accounting for about 30% of all adenomas, is a prolactinoma (lactotroph adenoma).[15] These range from small or microadenomas (Fig. 39.2) to very large and expanded tumors associated with clinical presentations of mass effects. Microscopically, they are chromophobic or weakly acidophilic by staining.

Immunohistochemistry can identify prolactin within the cells as secretory granules. Prolactin is a very efficient hormone, and even microadenomas can produce enough excess prolactin to cause hyperprolactin syndrome. Serum concentrations of prolactin tend to be proportional with the size of the tumor. Patients between 20 and 40 years of age presenting with amenorrhea, galactorrhea, loss of libido, and infertility should be checked for serum prolactin.[16] Almost 25% of cases of female amenorrhea are related to increased prolactin. At an

older age, the clinical manifestations could be very subtle and unfortunately leading to patients presenting with mass effects as the primary symptoms. Hyperprolactinemia also occurs normally during pregnancy and reaches a peak at delivery. It can continue postpartum by suckling stimulation in lactating women. Interference with a dopamine feedback mechanism by damage to the dopaminergic neurons within the pituitary stalk (via head trauma) in the hypothalamic region or the use of drugs (reserpine, haloperidol, phenothiazines, estrogens) that block the lactotroph cell receptors can result in lactotroph hyperplasia. Moreover, any mass within the stalk can disturb this inhibition influence, causing a mild elevation in serum prolactin. As such, a mild elevation does not necessarily indicate a prolactin-secreting adenoma. Finally, renal failure and hypothyroidism can also elevate prolactin.

Prolactinomas are typically treated with bromocriptine (Box 39.1) that is a dopamine receptor agonist causing the lesions to diminish in size and function. Growth hormone (somatotroph cell)–secreting tumors are the second most common functional tumors. Approximately 40% of somatotroph tumors express an oncogene (*GSP*), which is a mutant GTPase-deficient alpha subunit of the G protein designated Gs.[17] Histologically, these tumors are composed of acidophilic to chromophobic granulated cells. Immunohistochemistry can also demonstrate growth hormone associated with small amounts of prolactin.[18] Children who develop hypersecretion adenomas before the epiphyses are closed develop clinical gigantism. If the epiphyseal plates have fused, such as in young adults, then acromegaly can occur. This is usually manifested clinically with enlarged hands and feet, increased bone density, enlarged thyroid, heart, liver, adrenals, and broadening of the lower face with jaw protrusion that can develop into prognathism. Patients often have associated prolactinemia, with gonadal dysfunction, hypertension, congestive heart failure, and a risk of gastrointestinal cancer. The goals of treatment are to control serum growth hormone and decrease mass effects of the primary adenoma while preventing deficiencies. Most commonly, the tumors are removed surgically via a transsphenoid approach in younger patients, treatment with external-beam radiotherapy (see the Radiation Techniques section), or drug therapy. Eventually, good growth hormone control over a long period allows the characteristic tissue overgrowth and related symptoms to recede, with improvement in metabolic abnormalities. It is important to remember that because clinical manifestations of growth hormone are subtle, these adenomas can usually present with mass effects from large tumor sizes. Corticotrophin cell adenomas usually

FIGURE 39.2. Photomicrograph of microadenoma. (From Damjanov I. *Histopathology: a color atlas and textbook.* Baltimore: Williams & Wilkins, 1996. With permission.)

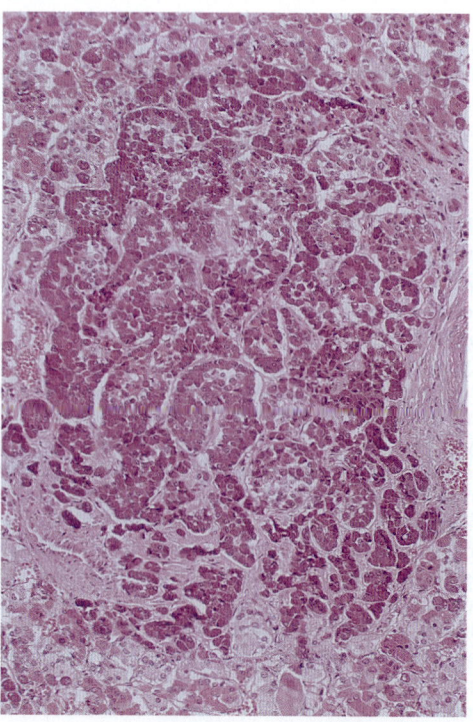

Box 39.1

Pituitary Adenoma Management Overview

Symptomatic adenomas present for medical attention as a result of hormone secretions, compression of nearby normal structures with neurologic symptoms, or compression of the pituitary stalk causing hypopituitarism. An initial therapy for most prolactinomas is with a dopamine agonist such as bromocriptine, lysuride, or pergolide. Medical intervention usually decreases adenoma function and size. Initial therapy for other pituitary adenomas is transsphenoidal surgical resection. Surgery is generally safe and reverses neurologic symptoms, with most patients normalizing hormone levels. It is mostly useful to cure microadenomas. Radiation therapy is often reserved for patients with residual disease after surgery, such as after a debulking surgery. It is also considered for recurrence after definitive surgery or for medically inoperable patients. Typically, conventional radiation delivers a dose of 45 Gy at 1.8 Gy daily fractions. At this dose, good control can usually be achieved with a very low risk of optic neuropathy. Normalization of hormone levels, however, can take months to years to achieve.

TABLE 39.1 PITUITARY ADENOMA DISTRIBUTIONS

Type	Frequency (%)
Prolactinoma	20–30
Growth hormone adenoma	5
Mixed growth/prolactin adenoma	5
Adrenocorticotrophic hormone adenoma	10–15
Gonadotroph adenoma	10–15
Null cell adenoma	20
Thyroid-stimulating hormone adenoma	1
Plurihormonal adenoma	15

Reprinted from Pituitary neoplasia. In: Berger PC, Scheithauer BW, Vogel FS, eds. *Surgical pathology of the nervous system and its coverings*. 3rd ed. New York: Churchill Livingstone, 1991. Copyright © 1991 Elsevier. With permission.

present as microadenomas. Histologically, these tumors are basophilic, but they can be chromophobic and stain for the periodic acid stain (Schiff stain) because of presence of carbohydrate in the precursor adrenocorticotrophic hormone (ACTH). Excess ACTH eventually leads to Cushing *syndrome*, with a chronic hypersecretion of cortisol from adrenal stimulation. However, when the hypercortisolism comes directly from the pituitary adenoma, the process is Cushing *disease*. Nelson syndrome (hyperpigmentation, hyporeflexia, vision loss, headache, and menstrual irregularities) occurs in most cases by a loss of inhibitory feedback of adrenal cortisol of the pituitary when hyperfunctioning adrenals are surgically excised and a subclinical pituitary corticotroph microadenoma exists. The microadenoma is stimulated, but hypercortisolism does not occur due to the absence of the adrenals. However, mass effects can still occur, and ACTH precursor molecules can also stimulate melanocytes, thus producing hyperpigmentation. It is more common in women and younger patients.

Mixed adenomas, gonadotroph, and thyrotroph adenomas can occur, but these are less frequent than nonsecreting or null-cell adenomas (Table 39.1). Mostly gonadotroph adenomas are luteinizing or follicle-stimulating producing tumors of middle-age men and women with complaints of chronic fatigue or menorrhea.[19] Like null-cell adenomas, these tumors can become substantial in size with mass effects (Table 39.2). Thyrotrophs are rare, found in about 1% of patients, and are a rare source of hyperthyroidism.[20] Primary pituitary carcinomas are quite rare, typically not functional, and have variable polymorphisms. A clinical diagnosis of an actual carcinoma requires the demonstration of metastases, usually to lymph nodes, brain, bone, or liver, and rarely elsewhere. Radiation therapy to the primary pituitary site can be palliative.

Hypopituitarism

Decreased secretions of pituitary hormones can result from diseases of the hypothalamus or the pituitary proper, which cause syndromes of hypopituitarism. Most cases of a hypofunctioning pituitary result from the destruction of more than 75% of the anterior gland. Metastatic tumors, involuted primary tumors, ischemic necrosis, or surgical or radio-ablated

Box 39.2

Craniopharyngiomas

Craniopharyngiomas are frequently calcified and can be visualized radiographically. They are usually about 3.5 cm in diameter, encapsulated, and solid but can be cystic or multilobulated. They can displace cranial nerves and the optic chiasm and protrude into the floor of the third ventricle. They are thought to be vestigial remnants of the Rathke pouch, representing about 2% of intracranial tumors, occurring about half the time in children and young adults. In children, they can cause growth retardation. Adults usually present with visual disturbances. Both can demonstrate hormonal disturbances and diabetes insipidus. Histologically, there can be two forms. The adamantinomatous form has nests or cords of squamous to columnar epithelium in a background of spongy-like reticulum. Because keratin formation occurs, these tumors are frequently calcified. A brisk glial reaction can occur if in direct contact with brain tissue. The second type is a papillary craniopharyngioma. These are usually solid sections of squamous cells typically lacking a cystic component and calcification.

pituitary can produce empty sella syndrome. A Rathke cleft cyst can accumulate proteinaceous fluids, expanding and destroying the normal pituitary. Primary necrosis can be caused by postpartum Sheehan syndrome[21] or by disseminated intravascular coagulopathy (DIC) and, more rarely, sickle cell crisis. Also causative is elevated intracranial pressure from hydrocephalus, head trauma, or severe shock. Destroying all or part of the functioning pituitary can result in a clinical diagnosis of empty sella syndrome.[22]

Histologically the empty syndrome presents as a small fibrotic nidus of tissue in a radiographically expanded sella turcica. Two distinct types are identified: primary empty syndrome, which occurs in obese women with multiple pregnancies, and a defect of the diaphragma sella, which allows arachnoid matter and cerebrospinal fluid to herniate into an expanded sella, thus compressing the pituitary gland. Hyperprolactinemia can occur due to the loss of dopamine inhibition. Only rarely does actual complete hypopituitarism occur because enough functioning residual tissue usually remains. Secondary syndromes can occur from surgical removal, radiation ablation, or spontaneous infarction. These patients express hypopituitarism syndromes. Rare congenital defects are known,[23] such as a gene that encodes Pit-1, a transcription factor related to important pituitary-specific genes such as growth hormone, prolactin, and thyroid-stimulating hormones. The genetically altered protein will bind to the appropriate cell receptors but can de-activate the expression of the gene, thus causing the patient to fail to produce the appropriate hormone(s). Less frequently, diseases of the hypothalamus or hypothalamic stalk can cause the pituitary to become dysfunctional. These can include craniopharyngiomas (Box 39.2),[24] metastases, sarcoidosis, or tuberculous meningitis and infiltrative diseases such as opportunistic infections. Radiotherapy to nearby structures such as the brain, base of brain, optic chiasm, and nasopharynx can also cause hypothalamic disorders at higher doses. Dysfunction of the adrenal cortex, thyroid, and gonads, the loss of melanocyte-stimulating hormone, atrophy of the genitalia, amenorrhea, impotency, loss of libido, and pubic and axillary hair are changes related to the cause and type(s) of deficiencies in pituitary hypofunction.

TABLE 39.2 ENDOCRINE SECRETIONS AND CLINICAL PRESENTATIONS

Type of Secretion	Frequency (%)	Symptoms	Size at Diagnosis
Prolactinoma	43	Women: amenorrhea, galactorrhea	Microadenoma
		Men: impotence, hypopituitarism	Microadenoma
Nonsecreting	30	Hypopituitarism	Microadenoma
Gonadotrophin	17	Children: gigantism	Microadenoma
Growth hormone		Adults: acromegaly	Microadenoma
Adrenocorticotrophic hormone	7	Cushing disease	Microadenoma
		Nelson disease	
Thyroid-stimulating hormone	1	Hyperthyroidism	Microadenoma or macroadenoma

From Oruckaptan HH, Senmevsim O, Ozcan OE, et al. Pituitary adenomas: results of 684 surgically treated patients and review of the literature. *Surg Neurol Int* 2000;53:211–219, with permission.

Posterior Lobe

The posterior pituitary is composed of pituicytes—modified glial cells—with associated axonal processes extending from nerve origins in the supraoptic and paraventricular nuclei within the hypothalamus. Two proteins are produced: antidiuretic hormone (ADH) and oxytocin. These hormones are stored in the posterior pituitary and released with the appropriate stimuli. Oxytocin functions to stimulate the smooth muscle contractions of the uterus during birth as well as stimulating smooth muscle of the lactiferous mammary gland ducts within the gravid breasts. No known clinical abnormalities are known for inappropriate secretions. ADH is a nonpeptide produced primarily in the supraoptic nucleus (see anatomy). ADH is released from axon terminals from the neurohypophysis directly into the general circulation secondary to appropriate stimulation(s). ADH is causative for two distinct clinical syndromes: diabetes insipidus and the syndrome of inappropriate ADH secretion (SIADH). Diabetes insipidus can result from head trauma, surgical or radiation damage, tumors, and inflammatory conditions. It causes the inappropriate oversecretion of urine and can lead to life-threatening dehydration. SIADH is causative in the absorption of excessive water, thus causing hematologic dilution (hypervolemia) and hyponatremia. The most frequent cause of SIADH is from ectopic ADH produced by malignant neoplasms such as lung carcinoma (commonly small cell) and by nonneoplastic lung disease producing a paraneoplastic syndrome. However, direct or compression injury to the hypothalamus or posterior pituitary is known in the presence of glial tumors such as primary central nervous system (CNS) neoplasms or craniopharyngiomas. These can cause direct mechanical or stimulatory effects. SIADH causes hyponatremia, cerebral edema, and neurologic dysfunction, and patients are typically initially evaluated because of sudden clinical changes in cognition.[25] Peripheral edema does not usually develop because although the blood is diluted, it retains a normal total volume except when hypervolemia occurs.

RADIATION THERAPY

Radiation therapy can be a highly effective form of intervention to control pituitary adenomas. In current practice, it is rarely the sole means of treatment and is usually reserved for patients with residual surgical disease or the medically inoperable patient. The overall 10-year control rates are consistently reported in the range of 85% or higher,[26–29] including two recent reports from the University of Florida[28,30] that report a 93% control rate at 9.2 years and the absence of "late recurrences" with long-term follow-up using doses of 45 Gy or higher. In the former report,[27] patients were analyzed as to whether they experienced surgery followed by radiation versus radiotherapy alone. Combined approaches achieved a 95% control rate, whereas radiotherapy alone achieved 90% at 10 years of follow-up. Importantly, an 80% control rate was achieved for patients treated by initial surgery who then developed a recurrence after application of delayed radiotherapy. This result is consistent with an older report from Princess Margaret Hospital analyzing 166 patients with similar treatment and results.[26]

Pediatric pituitary adenomas have similar results when comparing surgery and radiation with radiotherapy alone. In the study by Grigsby et al.,[31] 19 patients were treated who were younger than 19 years of age, and at 15 years of follow-up, only two had failed. It is a small study but that is likely due to the relative rarity of these tumors. A sentinel paper was published in 1971 that arguably solidified the use of about 45 Gy as the threshold dose for acceptable local control and tolerance.[32] This has been confirmed many times by both American and European authors.[33]

Although there can a lack of tumor progression, clinically and radiographically, many patients who have elevated hormone levels at the outset of definitive therapy do not achieve complete normalization following radiotherapy alone. The University of Heidelberg reported on 68 patients with hormone active adenomas. The complete response rate for normalization occurred in only 38%.[28] Again, Princess Margaret Hospital reported on 145 patients receiving radiation alone for hormonally active adenomas. Although the progress-free rate was 96%, the long-term biochemical remission rate (if >2 years) was only 40%.[34] Therefore, radiation alone is demonstrated to be highly effective for controlling pituitary adenoma growth and progression. However, radiotherapy alone is less effective in normalizing hormone activity when patients present with a hormone active tumors. Biochemical suppression or persistence then requires ongoing medical management as needed for symptoms and/or function. Common suppressive medications are bromocriptine or cabergoline. Insufficiencies are supplemented appropriately.

A newer technique has rapidly become available when using radiotherapy intervention for pituitary adenomas: stereotactic radiosurgery (SRS). A number of institutions have reports using SRS either as a single fraction or with a fractionated schedule, called fractionated stereotactic radiotherapy (FSRT).[35] In FSRT, conventional doses of 45 to 50 Gy are delivered using a relocatable head-frame technique over about 5 weeks. With SRS, a single fraction is delivered in doses from 10 to 27 Gy (lower for nonfunctioning, higher for functioning) and often using cranial hard-fixation techniques.[35–37] The local control rates using these advanced techniques have been reported as >90%, and the prevalent hypothesis is that the hormone response rates would be higher than with conventional doses. In an encouraging article, Yoon et al.[37] reported that 11 of 13 patients had normalization of prolactin-secreting adenomas within 1 year. Unfortunately, Mitsumori et al.[36] reported that the 3-year actuarial rate for an adverse CNS event was 38% for a single fraction versus 0% (in that study) for the FSRT technique. Presently, many radiation oncologists are using modified fraction schemes via various technologies, being acutely aware of the nearby critical anatomic structures—especially the radiosensitive optic chiasm, and the likely potential that patients will live long enough to develop late sequelae particularly for the younger population. There is an excellent and deeply referenced review in Neurosurgery Focus about early stereotactic pituitary radiotherapy.[38]

Radiation Techniques

Radiation therapy planning and delivery has evolved from a two-dimensional calculated, parallel-opposed small open or minimally blocked bitemporal fields (Fig. 39.3) to three-dimensional, computer tomographic–assisted planning (Fig. 39.4) that uses a multiple field approach with custom blocks or multileaf collimation (MLC) blocked portals designed to concentrate therapeutic doses and minimize risks to surrounding normal tissues. Intensity-modulated radiotherapy can be accomplished via several approaches using megavoltage photons with MLC or three-dimensional constructed beam modulators. Either technique essentially produces dose distributions consistent with desired treatment plans to cover the region of interest and protect surrounding normal critical structures with highly conformal energy clouds and lowered hot spots (Fig. 39.5). Radiosurgery also employs megavoltage x-rays, but typically, the beams are delivered through small tubular collimators or sources from many angles and multiple planes of approach. Two machines—Gamma Knife (Elekta

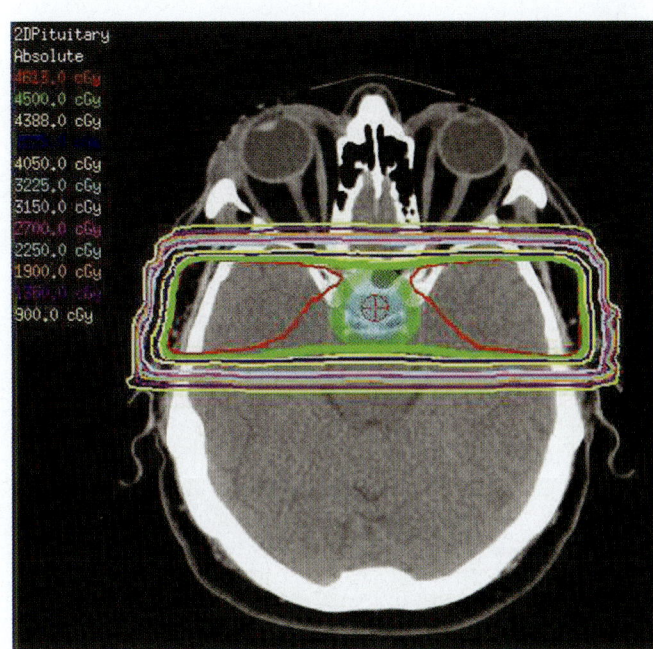

FIGURE 39.3. Two-dimensional parallel opposed pair radiotherapy planning.

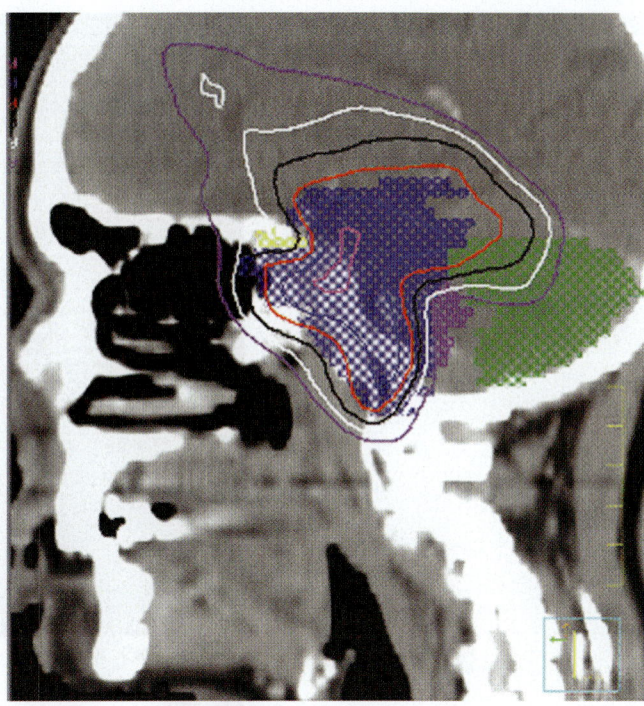

FIGURE 39.5. Intensity-modulated radiotherapy.

FIGURE 39.6. Gamma Knife.

Corp, Stockholm; Fig. 39.6) and CyberKnife (Accuray Inc., Sunnyvale, CA; Fig. 39.7)—usually deliver the desired doses through dozens to hundreds of "pencil beams." There are many newer machines available today to deliver stereotactic body radiotherapy.

At present, there are an increasing number of facilities that are investigating treatments with protons.[39] Proton therapy, while still exceedingly expensive, utilizes the unique advantage of the Bragg-Peak phenomenon to deliver doses mostly confined to the region of interest (Fig. 39.8).

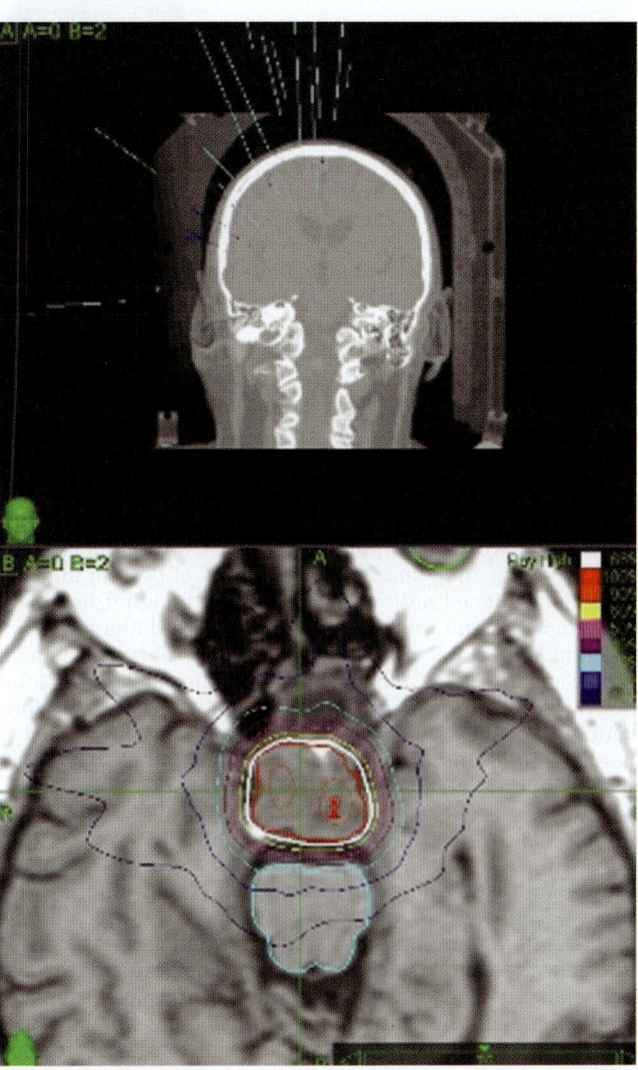

FIGURE 39.4. Three-dimensional radiotherapy planning.

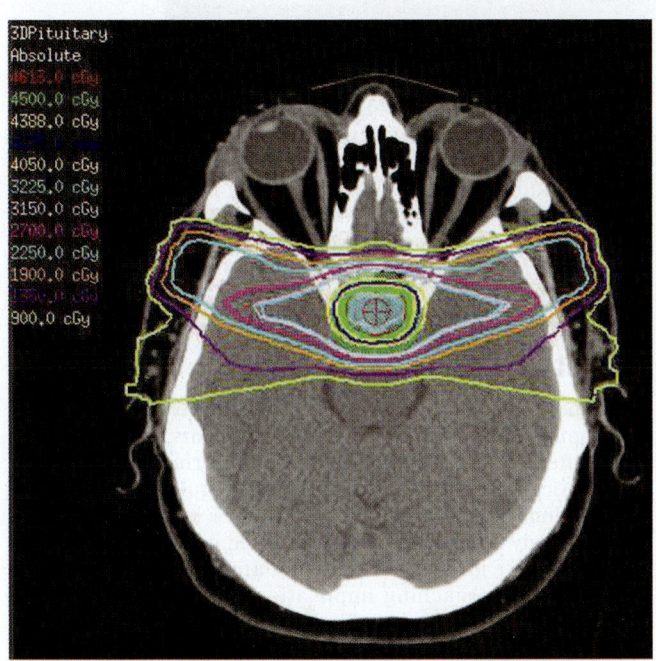

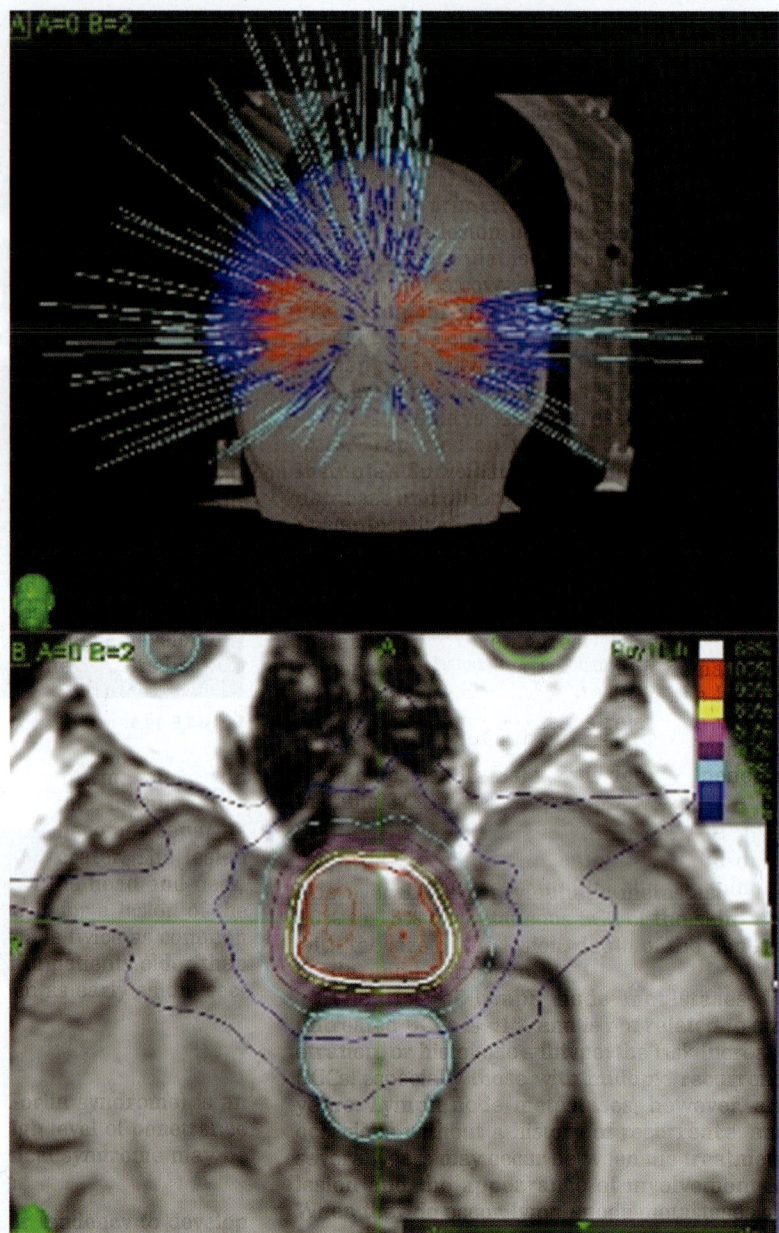

FIGURE 39.7. CyberKnife.

Late Effects

A common worrisome potential when using higher doses to a pituitary adenoma is the possibility of developing late radiation-induced optic neuropathies. Although it has been reported that the incidence of optic nerve damage is low, ranging from 0.7% to 2%, the risk of optic nerve or chiasm injury is dependent on the proximity of the chiasm, the total delivered dose and dose per fraction.[27,28,34] Even with conventional doses of 45 to 50 Gy, the risk is very low, but it is not zero. Additionally, doses ranging from 45 to 50 Gy to the whole pituitary gland carry substantial risk of causing hypopituitarism. This is reported in the range of 10% to 30% in some series,[26-29,35] and potentially half of all patients treated to 45 Gy will develop a deficiency of at least one pituitary hormone within 2 to 5+ years after definitive radiotherapy. Therefore, the patient must be followed indefinitely for this complication risk. Second malignant neoplasms are always a concern for long-term survivors who have received therapeutic doses of radiation. The Royal Marsden Hospital looked at 334 patients irradiated for pituitary adenomas to a media dose of 45 Gy. Five patients developed a secondary brain tumor, for an actuarial risk of 1.3% at 10 years and 1.9% at 20 years.[40] Thus, the relative risk of developing a second tumor compared with the normal, unexposed, population was 9.3%. Princess Margaret Hospital reported similarly with four gliomas from 306 treated patients over a latency period of 8 to 15 years. The actuarial risk was 1.7% at 10 years and 2.7% at 15 years for a relative risk of 16%.[41]

CONCLUSION

The hypophysis cerebri or pituitary gland may be the smallest functioning gland in humans, but it represents one of the most critical functioning endocrine glands for normal development, growth, organ regulation, reproductive regulation, and birthing functions as well as regulation of other hormone glands in the total body system. The physical gland may be small, but its capabilities are great. Dysfunction of any part of this hormone gland has wide-reaching implications for endocrine abnormalities and for local mass effects. The latter especially affects

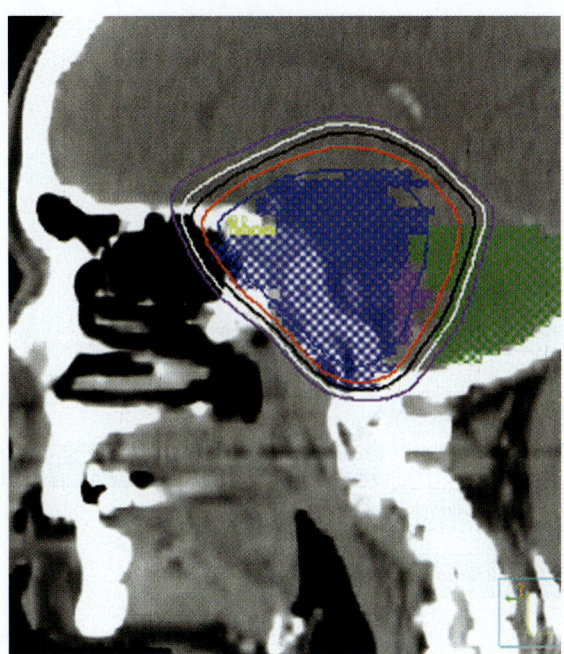

FIGURE 39.8. Proton therapy.

the optic nerves and proliferates a cascade of additional and potentially devastating hormonal dysfunctions. The former influences cellular division, protein synthesis, regulation of the adrenal cortex and the thyroid, follicle and sperm production, formation and function of the gravid uterus, testosterone secretion, and milk production. Lasting effects from chronic hypopituitarism also increased mortality from cardiac and cardiovascular events.[42,43] To summarize, adequate medical knowledge and understanding of the pituitary gland include understanding multiple feedback mechanisms required for the hormone normal-regulatory processes of the human body. Knowledge of therapy mechanisms for abnormalities plays an essential role for medical intervention, especially for the appropriate use of radiotherapy.

REFERENCES

1. Sutherland S. The meningeal relations of the human hypophysis cerebri. *J Anat* 1945;79:33.
2. Ferner H. The hypophyseal cistern of man and its relation to the pathogenesis mechanisms of secondary sella dilation. *Anat Entw Gesch* 1960;121:407.
3. Boyd WH. Pituitary. *Anat Rec* 1960;137:437.
4. Radojevic S, Jovanovic S, Lotric N. Anatomic notes on trans-sphenoidal approach to the pituitary gland. *Arch Anat Pathol* 1969;17:274.
5. McK Ricoh D, Wislocki GB, O'Leary JL. Visual effects of hypophyseal tumors. *Res Publ Assoc Nerv Ment Dis* 1940;20:3.
6. Ramzi S, Vinay K, Collins T. *Robbins pathologic basis of disease.* 6th ed. Philadelphia: WB Saunders, 1999.
7. Morin F. Pituitary blood supply. *Arch Ital Anat Embriol* 1940;45:94.
8. Xuereb GP, Pritchard ML, Daniel PM. The hypophyseal portal system of vessels in man. *Q J Exp Physiol* 1954;39:219–230.
9. Stanfield JP. The blood supply of the human pituitary gland. *J Anat* 1960;94:257.
10. Harris GW. *Neural control of the pituitary gland.* London: Arnold, 1955.
11. O'Rahilly R. Anatomy. In: *A regional study of the human structure.* 4th ed. Philadelphia: WB Saunders, 1975.
12. Craven RH Jr. *Taber's encyclopedic medical dictionary.* Philadelphia: FA Davis, 1997.
13. Yeh PJ, Chen JW. Pituitary tumors: surgical and medical management. *Surg Oncol* 1997;6:67.
14. Alexander JM. Clinically nonfunctioning pituitary tumors are monoclonal in origin. *J Clin Invest* 1990;86:336.
15. Schlechte J, Dolan K, Sherman B, et al. The natural history of untreated hyperprolactinemia. *J Clin Endocrinol Metab* 1989;68:412.
16. Mindermann T, Wilson CB. Age-related and gender-related occurrences of pituitary adenomas. *Clin Endocrinol* 1994;41:359.
17. Lyons J, Landis CA, Harsh G, et al. Two G protein oncogenes in human endocrine tumors. *Science* 1990;249:655.
18. Melmed S, Ho K, Kalbinski A, et al. Recent advances in pathogenesis, diagnosis and management of acromegaly. *J Clin Endocrinol Metab* 1995;80:3395.
19. Ho DM, Hsu CY, Ting LT, et al. The clinicopathological characteristics of gonadotroph cell adenomas: a study of 118 cases. *Hum Pathol* 1997;28:905–911.
20. Beck-Peccoz P. Thyrotropin secreting pituitary tumors. *Endocr Rev* 1997;17:610.
21. Sheehan H. Postpartum necrosis of the anterior pituitary. *J Pathol Bacteriol* 1987;45:189.
22. Barkin A. Pituitary atrophy in patients with Sheehan's syndrome. *Am J Med Sci* 1989;298:39.
23. Pfaffle RW, DeMattia GE, Parks JS, et al. Mutation of POU specific domain of Pit-1 and hypopituitarism without pituitary hypoplasia. *Science* 1992;257:1118–1121.
24. DeVile CJ, Grant DB, Hayward RD, et al. Growth and endocrine sequelae of craniopharyngioma. *Arch Dis Child* 1996;75:108–114.
25. Maesaka JK. An expanded view of SIADH. *Clin Nephrol* 1996;46:79.
26. Tsang RW, Brierley JD, Panzarella T, et al. Radiation therapy for pituitary adenoma: treatment outcome and prognosis factors. *Int J Radiat Oncol Biol Phys* 1994;30:557–565.
27. McCord MW, Buatti JM, Fennell EM, et al. Radiotherapy for pituitary adenoma: long term outcome and sequelae. *Int J Radiat Oncol Biol Phys* 1997;39: 437–444.
28. Zierhut D, Flentje M, Adolph J, et al. External radiotherapy of pituitary adenomas. *Int J Radiat Oncol Biol Phys* 1995;33:307–314.
29. Breen P, Flickinger JC, Kondziolka D, et al. Radiotherapy for non-functional pituitary adenoma: analysis of long term tumor control. *J Neurosurg* 1998;89:933–938.
30. McCollugh WM, Marcus R, Rhoton AL, et al. Long-term follow up of radiotherapy for pituitary adenomas: the absence of late recurrence after >4500 cGy. *Int J Radiat Oncol Biol Phys* 1991;21:607.
31. Grigsby PW, Thomas PR, Simpson JR, et al. Long term results of radiotherapy in the treatment of pituitary adenomas in children and adolescents. *Am J Clin Oncol* 1998;11:607.
32. Hayes TP, Davis RA, Raventos A. The treatment of pituitary chromophobe adenomas. *Radiology* 1971;98:149.
33. Zierhut D, Flentje M, Adolph J, et al. External radiotherapy of pituitary adenomas. *Int J Radiat Oncol Biol Phys* 1995;33:307.
34. Tsang RW, Brierley JD, Panzarella T, et al. Role of radiation therapy in clinical hormonally active pituitary adenomas. *Radiother Oncol* 1996;41:45.
35. Milker-Zabel S, Debus J, Thilmann C, et al. Fractionated stereotactically guided radiotherapy and radiosurgery in the treatment of functional and non-functional adenomas of the pituitary gland. *Int J Radiat Oncol Biol Phys* 2001;50:1279.
36. Mitsumori M, Shrieve DC, Alexander E III, et al. Initial clinical results of LINAC-based stereotactic radiosurgery and stereotactic radiotherapy for pituitary adenomas. *Int J Radiat Oncol Biol Phys* 1998;42:573–580.
37. Yoon SC, Suh TS, Jang HS, et al. Clinical results of 24 pituitary adenomas with LINAC-based radiosurgery. *Int J Radiat Oncol Biol Phys* 1998;42:849.
38. Witt TC. Stereotactic radiosurgery for pituitary tumors. *Neurosurgical Focus* 2003;14(5):1–12.
39. Malyapa R. *Clinical outcomes study of proton therapy for pituitary adenoma.* University of Florida Proton Therapy Institute. Protocol 0701-P101.
40. Brada M, Ford D, Ashley S, et al. Risk of second brain tumor after conservation surgery and radiotherapy for pituitary adenoma. *BMJ* 1992;304:1343.
41. Tsang RW, Laperriere NJ, Simpson WJ. Glioma arising after radiation therapy for pituitary adenoma. A report of four patients and estimation of risk. *Cancer* 1993;72:2227.
42. Bates T, Bengtsson A-G. Premature mortality due to cardiovascular disease in hypopituitarism. *Lancet* 1990;336:285.
43. Bulow B, Hagman I, Mikczy Z, et al. Increased cerebrovascular mortality in patients with hypopituitarism. *Clin Endocrinol* 1997;46:75.

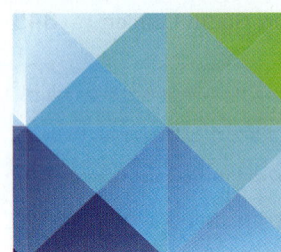

CHAPTER 40

Spinal Canal

Jiayi Huang, Clifford G. Robinson, and Jeff M. Michalski

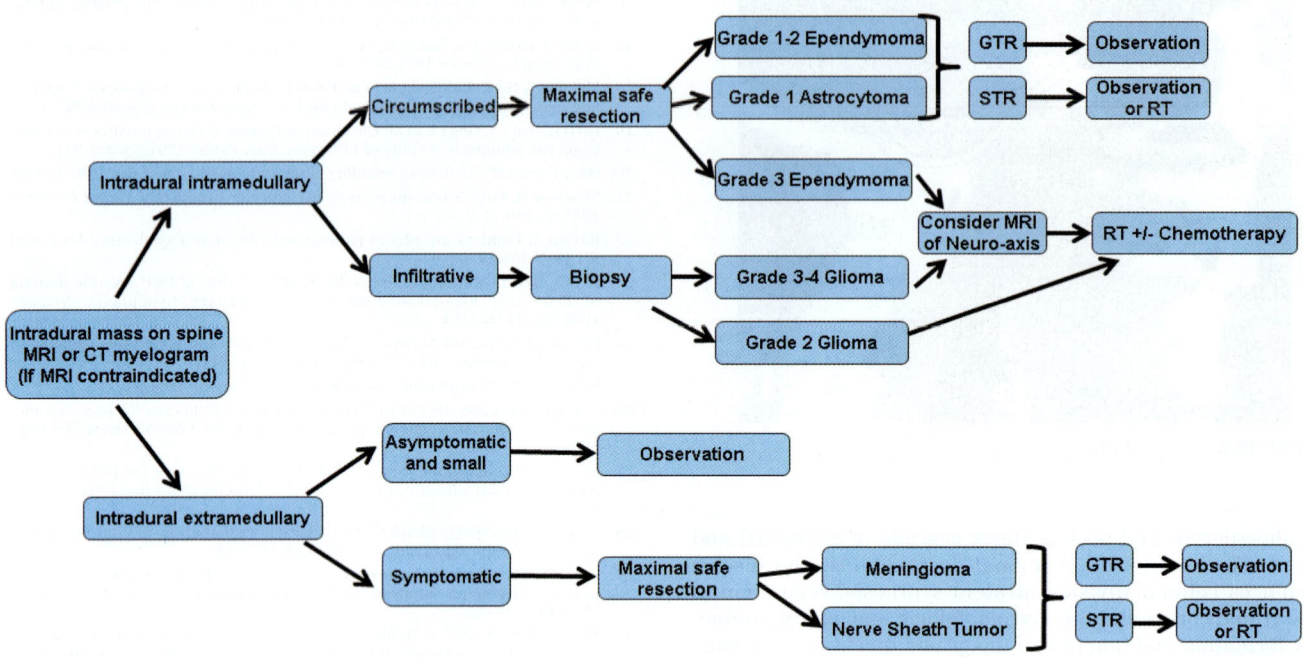

Treatment Algorithm. GTR, gross tumor resection; STR, subtotal resection.

INTRODUCTION

Tumors of the spinal cord and cauda equina account for approximately 3% of primary central nervous system (CNS) tumors overall and 4% in children.[1] Spinal canal tumors are classified by the World Health Organization (WHO) according to histologic types. Clinically, they are also characterized by their location relative to the protective layers of the spinal cord as extradural, intradural–extramedullary, or intramedullary (Fig. 40.1). Intramedullary lesions arise from the intrinsic substance of the spinal cord. Histologically, intramedullary spinal cord neoplasms include gliomas such as astrocytoma, ependymoma, and oligodendroglioma. Intradural–extramedullary tumors arise from the connective tissues, blood vessels, or coverings adjacent to the cord or cauda equina. Common histologies include nerve sheath tumor, meningioma, and ependymoma. Extradural tumors are most commonly metastatic, although primary tumors in this compartment may occur as well. Primary extradural tumors arising from the vertebral bodies may include benign tumors such as osteoid osteoma, osteoblastoma, or aneurysmal bone cysts, or as malignant tumors such as plasmacytoma or myeloma, chordoma or

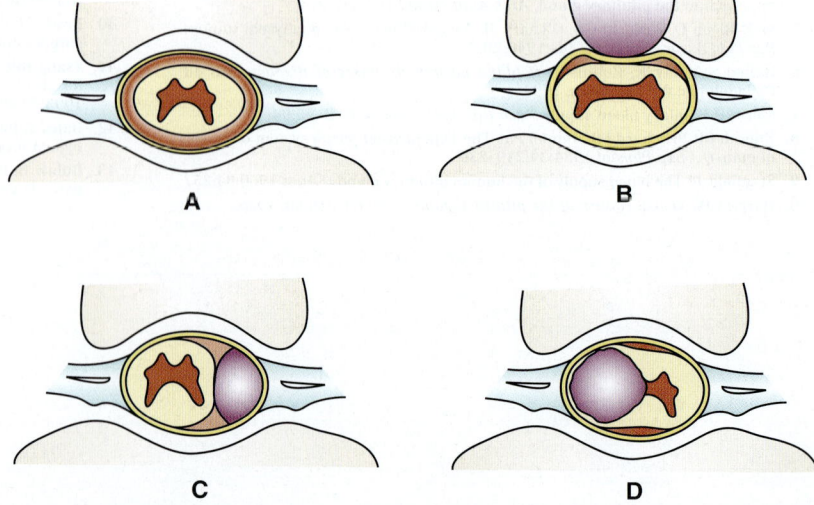

FIGURE 40.1. Neoplasms affecting the spinal cord. **A:** Normal transverse spine. The spinal cord is enveloped by the pia, arachnoid, and dura mater, which are housed in the spinal canal and surrounded by ligaments supporting the vertebral bony structures. The subarachnoid space contains cerebrospinal fluid (brown). **B:** Transverse spine with extradural mass. An extradural mass (e.g., metastasis) from the vertebral body is compressing the dural sac and the spinal cord from the anterior direction. The subarachnoid space becomes obliterated at that level, causing a myelographic block. **C:** Transverse spine with an intradural–extramedullary mass. The mass, typically a meningioma or nerve sheath tumor, is compressing the spinal cord and roots in the dural sac, causing a myelographic block with a laterally displaced cord and, at times, producing a capping contour of contrast border. **D:** Transverse spine with intramedullary mass. An intramedullary mass (astrocytoma or ependymoma) is infiltrating and expanding the spinal cord within the dural sac, causing a myelographic block.

chondrosarcoma, osteosarcoma, and Ewing sarcoma. Other primary extradural tumors arising outside of the vertebral body include epidural hemangiomas, lipomas, extradural meningiomas, nerve sheath tumors, and lymphomas.

Radiation therapy is an important modality in the management of both primary and metastatic tumors involving the spinal canal. This chapter focuses primarily on the management of primary spinal cord tumors. Primary extradural tumors are usually managed in a manner similar to histopathologically identical tumors arising at other locations and will not be discussed here in detail. The management of metastatic tumors involving the spinal canal is discussed in Chapter 96.

ANATOMY

Spinal Cord

The spinal cord is a slender cylinder composed of functional segments corresponding to 31 pairs of spinal nerves: 8 cervical, 12 thoracic, 5 lumbar, 5 sacral, and 1 coccygeal. In contrast to the brain, the white matter of the spinal cord is located in the periphery and surrounds the central gray matter. The gray matter contains the cell bodies of sensory, motor, and autonomic neurons. On cross section, the gray matter is a butterfly-shaped region with anterior horns controlling motor function, lateral horns (in the thoracic and upper lumbar region) controlling autonomic functions, and posterior horns involved in sensation. The white matter contains the axonal elements of neurons that transmit impulses to and from the brain. As in the brain, the axons of the spinal cord white matter possess a myelin sheath formed by the cytoplasmic extension of glial cells. Schwann cells sheath the spinal nerves that enter and exit the spinal cord. The spinal cord is organized into somatotopically distinct regions (Fig. 40.2). The lateral and anterior spinal cord white matter contains the nerve tracts that are involved with fine motor control and tone, including the corticospinal tracts. The spinocerebellar tracts transmit muscle stretch and tone sensation from the extremities to the cerebellum. The lateral spinal thalamic tract is located laterally near the spinal cord surface and carries ascending crossed pain fibers to the thalamus. The dorsal columns transmit fine touch and positional sensation from the extremities to the brain. Because of its serial organization, injury to the spinal cord results in characteristic neurologic findings that depend on the location of the insult.

The spinal cord is surrounded by the meninges, which is composed (from outer to inner) of the dura mater, arachnoid, and pia mater. The pia mater covers the spinal cord and its blood vessels. This layer condenses laterally into approximately 20 pair of dentate ligaments, which suspend the cord to the dura mater. The dura mater forms a dense, fibrous barrier between the bony spinal canal and the spinal cord. The dural sac ends inferiorly at S2-3, but the dura continues with the filum terminale down to the coccyx. The arachnoid mater resides between the dura mater and the pia mater. The arachnoid encloses the subarachnoid space filled with cerebrospinal fluid (CSF). The subarachnoid space follows the arachnoid down to the end of the dural sac.

The growth of the vertebral column during childhood takes place at a rate and extent greater than that of the spinal cord itself. By adulthood, the spinal cord is nearly 25 cm shorter than the vertebral column and ends near the level of the L1 vertebral body. Because of this differential growth, the exit level of each pair of spinal nerves in the spinal cord is usually higher than the corresponding vertebral body level. For example, in adults, the C8 nerve root leaves the cord at the C6 vertebral body, the T6 nerve at the T3 vertebral level, and the T12 nerve at the T9 vertebral level. All of the lumbar nerves exit the spinal cord from vertebral levels T10 through T12, and all of the sacral nerves exit the spinal cord near the L1 vertebral level. The lower lumbar, sacral, and coccygeal nerves form the cauda equina, the collection of nerves that fills the thecal sac below L1. At its most caudal extent, the cord tapers to a thin segment, the conus medullaris. It is tethered to the coccyx by the filum terminale, a dense thread of pia mater.

Spinal Canal

The posterior body surfaces and neural arches of the vertebrae form the vertebral foramina, which in continuity form the spinal canal. Vertebral foramina are triangular in the lumbar and cervical regions, where the cord is mostly mobile, and round in the thoracic region. The spinal canal is lined with ligaments, including the posterior longitudinal ligament on its anterior wall, the flaval ligaments between adjacent arches, and the interspinous ligaments between the spinous processes. At each vertebral level, a spinous process protrudes from the posterior aspect of the neural arch, and transverse processes extend from the lateral edges of each arch. The laminae are those portions of the neural arch between the spinous and transverse processes, and the pedicles lie between the transverse processes and the body. At the intersection between the laminae and pedicles are superior and inferior paired articular facets. The superior articular facets are synovial joints that articulate with the inferior articular facets of the vertebra immediately above. The paired pedicles of each vertebra are notched at their superior and inferior edges such that the notches from two contiguous vertebra form an intervertebral foramen, through which the spinal nerve courses.

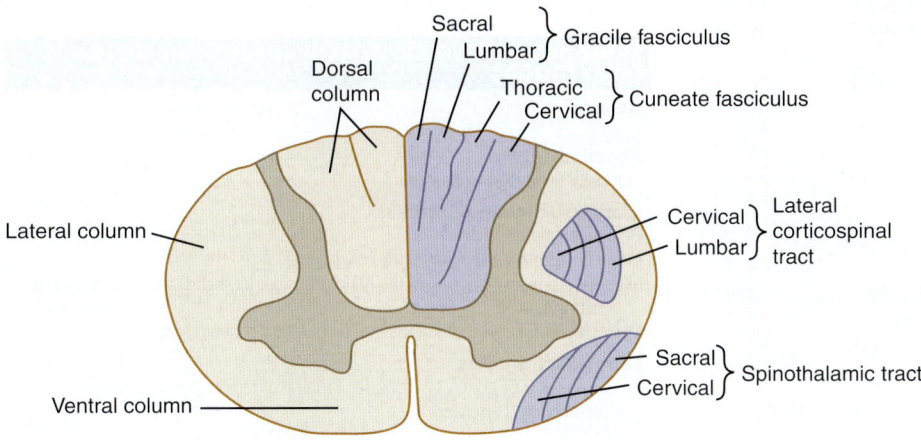

FIGURE 40.2. Somatotopic organization of the cervical spinal cord in transection. (Reprinted from Waxman S. *Clinical neuroanatomy.* 28th ed. New York: McGraw-Hill, 2017:54. Copyright © 2017 McGraw-Hill Education. All rights reserved.)

EPIDEMIOLOGY

Based on population data in the National Program of Cancer Registries (NPCR) and Surveillance, Epidemiology, and End Results (SEER) programs from 2004 to 2007, 22% of primary spinal tumors are malignant and 78% nonmalignant (62% benign and 16% with borderline behavior).[2] The most common sites are the spinal cord (60%), followed by the spinal meninges (36%), and the cauda equina (4%). Incidence appears to increase with advancing age, peaking at the seventh decade of life. Age-adjusted incidence rates are 0.76 per 100,000 persons for nonmalignant tumors and 0.22 per 100,000 persons for malignant tumors. The frequency of nonmalignant cases is higher for females (60%), whereas malignant cases are equally distributed by sex. Age-adjusted rates appear to be higher in Caucasian race and non-Hispanic ethnicity.[2] In adults, the most common histology types are meningioma (37.6%), nerve sheath tumor (23.1%), ependymoma (20.5%), and astrocytoma (4.2%). In children, the most common histology types are astrocytoma (31.4%), ependymoma (21.6%), oligodendroglioma (16.8%), nerve sheath tumor (13.3%), and meningioma (7.4%) (Table 40.1).[1]

NATURAL HISTORY

Primary spinal tumors have the capacity to cause significant neurologic morbidity. Intramedullary tumors produce neurologic damage by local invasion or cystic compression of the cord, whereas extramedullary lesions compress, stretch, or distort the cord or the spinal nerves. Primary spinal cord tumors may be focal or relatively localized in some patients but may involve nearly the entire length of the cord in others. Local tumor progression is the dominant form of treatment failure of spinal cord tumors, though leptomeningeal dissemination may occur rarely.[3,4] Spread to lymph nodes is not typically seen with spinal canal tumors. Extraneural spread is rare, occurring with an overall incidence of approximately 1%, though this risk appears to be higher than cerebral tumors.[5] The major causes of death in patients with spinal canal tumors are complications of paraplegia or quadriplegia such as infection or respiratory compromise.

CLINICAL PRESENTATION

Pain is the most common presenting symptom, affecting approximately 72% of patients.[6] Often the pain is localized to the region of involvement and may be present well before the patient manifests localizing neurologic signs. Radicular pain, a result of pressure on nerve roots, reflects the distribution of the involved root and indicates that conduction is intact. Numbness replacing pain is a more advanced sign that indicates compromise of spinal nerve or nerve tract conduction. Extramedullary tumors can cause distention of the dura with severe pain in the region of the tumor that is characteristically aggravated by recumbency because of venous congestion. Thus, pain is often worse at night. Movement or the Valsalva maneuver also may worsen pain.

Other symptoms of CNS involvement include weakness (55% of patients), sensory deficits (39%), and sphincter dysfunction (15%).[6] Low-grade tumors generally have a more prolonged duration of symptoms than high-grade tumors. Bladder and bowel dysfunction as presenting symptoms are relatively uncommon except for tumors that involve the conus medullaris and filum terminale.

Tumors involving the lumbosacral spine present with a cauda equina nerve root compression syndrome. Patients may have radicular pain in the anterior (L4), lateral (L5), or posterior (S1) thigh with corresponding paresthesias followed by muscle wasting of the glutei, hamstrings, or tibialis anterior muscles. Saddle anesthesia, absent ankle reflexes (S1), or plantar (S2) responses may be present. Impotence and loss of anal or bulbar cavernous reflexes also may occur.

DIAGNOSTIC WORKUP

History and Physical Findings

Table 40.2 shows the diagnostic workup for primary tumors of the spinal cord. A meticulous and accurate patient history and physical examination are critical aspects of the initial assessment and can often localize suspected spinal tumors. The neurologic examination should concentrate on testing motor and sensory functions and reflexes. The differential diagnosis of a patient with a spinal cord tumor may include syringomyelia, multiple sclerosis, amyotrophic lateral sclerosis, diabetic neuropathy, viral myelitis, or paraneoplastic syndromes.

A cutaneous sensory level may be definable, although the level of cord injury will be a few segments higher than the superior level of sensory loss because of pathway crossing characteristics. Loss of pain and heat and cold sensation below a specific dermatomal level indicates compromise of the spinothalamic pathway in the lateral columns. Impaired posture, gait, and coordination and loss of vibration sense indicate compromise of the posterior spinocerebellar pathways or the posterior columns.

At the level of the lesion, flaccid weakness and loss of tendon reflexes may occur. Below the lesion, the same signs are noticed in acute stages, but spastic paralysis and hyperactive tendon reflexes plus an upward Babinski toe sign ensue in subacute and chronic stages. These findings are consistent with lower and upper motor neuron involvement, respectively.

TABLE 40.1 PRIMARY SPINAL CANAL TUMORS OF ADULTS AND CHILDREN: TYPES, LOCATIONS, AND FREQUENCIES[a]

	Type	Location	Frequency (%)
Adults	Meningioma	Intradural–extramedullary	37.6
	Nerve sheath tumor	Intradural–extramedullary	23.1
	Ependymoma	Intramedullary or intradural–extramedullary	20.5
	Astrocytoma	Intramedullary	4.2
	Hemangioma	Intramedullary	3.8
	Oligodendroglioma	Intramedullary	2.5
	Others	–	8.4
Children	Astrocytoma	Intramedullary	31.4
	Ependymoma	Intramedullary or intradural–extramedullary	21.6
	Oligodendroglioma	Intramedullary	16.8
	Nerve sheath tumor	Intradural–extramedullary	13.3
	Meningioma	Intradural–extramedullary	7.4
	Hemangioma	Intramedullary	1.8
	Others	–	7.7

[a]Based on Central Brain Tumor Registry of the United States (CBTRUS) statistical Report from 2008–2012.

TABLE 40.2 DIAGNOSTIC WORKUP FOR PRIMARY SPINAL CORD TUMORS

General
History
Physical examination
Complete neurologic examination

Diagnostic Imaging Studies
Plain radiography
Magnetic resonance imaging of the entire spine
Magnetic resonance imaging of the brain (Consider for high-grade ependymomas or astrocytomas)
Myelography with computed tomography (if MRI is contraindicated)

Laboratory Studies
Cerebrospinal (CSF) cytology (consider if clinical or radiological suspicion of leptomeningeal disease)

The signs and symptoms of neurologic dysfunction may be asymmetric. In some cases, a classic Brown-Séquard syndrome may be present with ipsilateral loss of motor function and fine touch sensation and contralateral loss of pain and temperature sensation below the level of the lesion.

Autonomic reflexes (e.g., sweating) frequently are increased below the level of the lesion and may encompass the whole body if the lesion is cervical. Sweating disappears at the level of the compressed cord. Disruption of urinary and bowel function usually occurs later than sensory and motor dysfunction. Early loss of bladder function, saddle anesthesia, and later pain characterize neoplasms of the conus medullaris and filum terminale.[7]

Radiographic Studies

Although plain films are not typically used as the principal imaging modality for the evaluation of suspected spinal canal tumors, abnormalities can be detected from increased intracanal pressure including erosion of vertebral pedicles, enlargement of the anteroposterior diameter of the bony canal, or scalloping of the posterior wall of the vertebral bodies. Calcification may be seen in extramedullary tumors, especially meningiomas, and less frequently in nerve sheath tumors. Changes are more likely to be detected on plain radiographs in children than in adults, such as kyphoscoliosis or scalloping of the vertebral bodies.[8,9]

Myelography, once considered the standard examination in evaluation of the spinal cord and canal, is now used principally in patients who are unable to undergo magnetic resonance imaging (MRI) because of the presence of implanted ferromagnetic materials or for whom images at the level of concern are distorted by the presence of surgical hardware. In this situation, computed tomography (CT) scanning combined with myelography will give better spatial resolution. CT myelography may be particularly beneficial as part of radiotherapy treatment planning in the postoperative setting, where the spinal cord may be obscured by artifact on the MRI.[10]

Computed Tomography

CT is most helpful in evaluating the spine for extradural pathologic processes. Bone tumors or paraspinal soft tissue masses that secondarily involve the spinal cord (e.g., dumbbell tumors) can be imaged with contrast-enhanced CT scans. Nerve sheath tumors can enlarge the intervertebral

foramina or spinal canal and cause smooth erosion of bone. Meningiomas are occasionally calcified. Both of these neoplasms are partially outlined by CSF and produce extramedullary deformity by displacement of the spinal cord.[11]

Magnetic Resonance Imaging

MRI has replaced myelography and CT as the imaging study of choice in evaluation of tumors of the spinal canal. Sagittal and axial images give a three-dimensional appreciation of the patient's anatomy and help plan therapy. The various signal characteristics of the CSF—white and gray matter, bone and bone marrow, fat, and flowing blood—all facilitate the interpretation of the study. Some cystic tumors, vascular lesions, or lipomas can be diagnosed based on their characteristic signals on T1- and T2-weighted images without contrast injection. Intravenous gadolinium-diethylenetriamine penta-acetic acid (Gd-DTPA) administration improves the sensitivity of MRI by enhancing the solid component of intramedullary tumors and differentiating them from surrounding edema or syrinx cavities (Figs. 40.3 and 40.4). Unlike low-grade gliomas in the brain, nearly all spinal cord gliomas, regardless of grade, enhance with Gd-DTPA. Sagittal T1-weighted images usually localize intramedullary mass neoplasms along with adjacent cysts. Intradural–extramedullary lesions also show enhancement on T1-weighted images after administration of Gd-DTPA. The use of Gd-DTPA also increases the sensitivity of detecting leptomeningeal metastases.[12]

MRI of the brain should be performed in patients with high-grade ependymomas or astrocytomas to exclude the possibility of neuraxis seeding or the presence of an intracranial primary tumor.

Cerebrospinal Fluid

A patient suspected of having a spinal canal neoplasm should not be subjected to a lumbar puncture before MRI. Symptoms may be exacerbated after a spinal tap because of shifting of the spinal cord and incarceration before the tumor can be localized adequately. The CSF usually has increased protein levels and may exhibit xanthochromia, especially with extradural compression conditions, but lower values can be found in cases of intramedullary disease and with compression in the cervical region.[7] The incidence of leptomeningeal spread in patients with primary spinal cord glioma is low overall but is substantially more common with malignant tumors. Of note, two recently recognized entities have significantly higher risk of leptomeningeal dissemination: glioblastoma with primitive

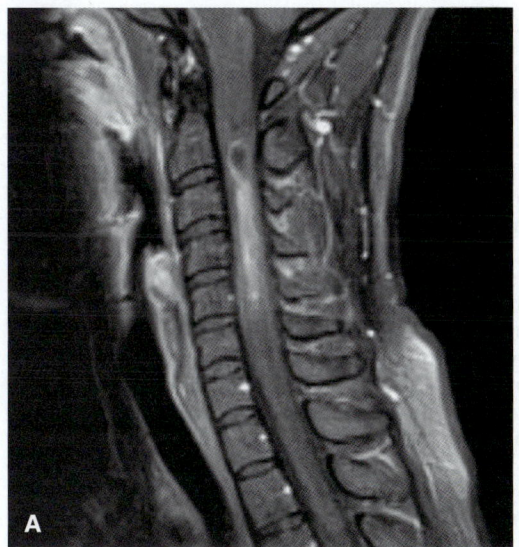
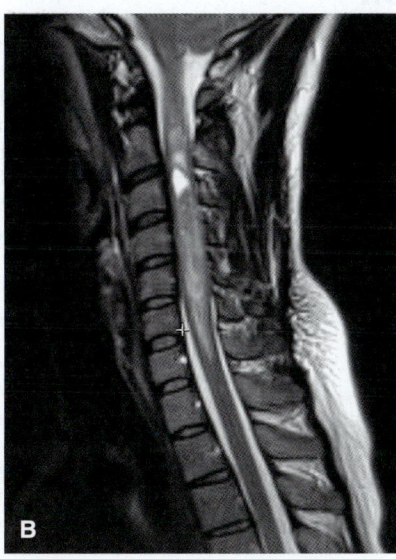

FIGURE 40.3. Sagittal magnetic resonance imaging scans of a 30-year-old female with a low-grade astrocytoma involving the cervical spine. **A:** T1-weighted image demonstrates an intramedullary lesion that expands the cord from the level of the craniocervical junction to the level of C7. The enhancing component extends from mid C2 to C5, and there is an associated cystic component at the cranial aspect of the lesion. **B:** T2-weighted image demonstrates T2 hyperintensity within the lesion suggestive of edema and hypointensity suggestive of blood products.

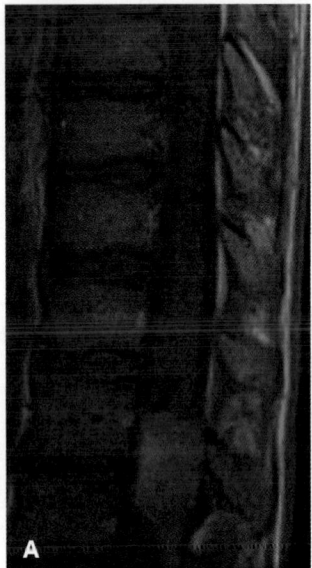
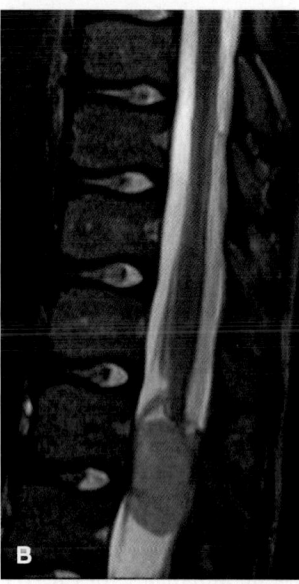

FIGURE 40.4. Sagittal magnetic resonance imaging scans of a 12-year-old male with a myxopapillary ependymoma involving the lumbar spine. **A:** T1-weighed image demonstrates a homogenously enhancing intradural extramedullary mass at the level of L1. **B:** T2-weighted image demonstrates hyperintensity of the mass. (Courtesy Aseem Sharma, MD, Mallinckrodt Institute of Radiology.)

neuronal component and diffuse leptomeningeal glioneuronal tumors (DLGT).[13,14] Cytologic examination of the CSF is not done routinely but may be considered in the presence of clinical or radiologic suspicion.

Tissue Diagnosis

Suspected primary tumors of the spinal cord and spinal canal should be pathologically confirmed whenever possible. Strong consideration should also be given to biopsy of any presumed metastatic tumors if they are the first site of disease recurrence after successful management of a previous malignant primary tumor. In rare circumstances in which emergency radiation therapy is indicated to relieve spinal cord compression in the absence of a confirmed cancer diagnosis, a patient should be made aware of the consequences of treatment in the absence of a definitive diagnosis, including the inability to tailor therapy based on histology and possible delay of appropriate treatment for nonmalignant etiologies.

PATHOLOGIC CLASSIFICATION

The current comprehensive classification system of spinal tumors was published by the WHO in 2007 and recently updated in 2016 to incorporate many molecular markers to establish histology types. The WHO classification groups CNS neoplasms by the tumor histology and provides a grading system to predict prognosis and guide therapy.[15,16] Tumor types include neuroepithelial (i.e., astrocytoma, ependymoma, ganglioglioma), nerve sheath (i.e., schwannoma, neurofibroma), meningioma, lymphoma, germ cell, and metastatic tumors. Clinically, spinal tumors are also characterized by their location as extradural, intradural–extramedullary, or intramedullary.

Intramedullary Tumors

Intramedullary spinal tumors constitute approximately 20% to 30% of all primary spinal tumors, and approximately 80% are glial in origin of which ependymoma is the most common histology (60% to 70%) followed by astrocytoma (30% to 40%).[17] Ependymomas are derived from glial cells similar to

those lining the ventricular system and can be either intramedullary or intradural extramedullary. Histologic subtypes can be classified into three grades based on histologic appearance and biologic behavior. Grade I tumors include myxopapillary ependymoma and subependymoma. Myxopapillary ependymomas typically occur around the conus medullaris and often involve the cauda equina or filum terminale. Grade II tumors include cellular (classic), papillary, clear cell, and tanycytic subtypes. Grade III tumors are defined as anaplastic ependymomas.[16,18]

In contrast to intracranial astrocytoma, the majority of spinal cord astrocytomas are low grade (WHO grade I or II), including 75% in adults and 85% to 90% in children.[6,19,20] Juvenile pilocytic astrocytomas (grade I) in particular, as in other locations in the CNS, are not infiltrative in nature. Recognition of this feature, along with advances in surgical techniques and intraoperative monitoring, has led neurosurgeons to manage these tumors with more radical resections. However, many fibrillary astrocytomas (grade II) as well as anaplastic astrocytomas (grade III) and glioblastoma multiforme (grade IV) are infiltrative, and complete resection carries a significant risk of neurologic disability. In these cases, a subtotal resection or biopsy may be the only safe surgical option.[21–23]

A discriminating feature of intramedullary spinal cord tumors is the presence or absence of a syrinx. Syringes associated with spinal cord astrocytoma occur in 20% to 40% of patients. Syringes can span the entire length of the cord, although they tend to favor more rostrally located tumors, as well as favoring the more rostral portion of the tumor itself.[24] In certain instances, a syrinx may even extend into the medulla, producing an obstructive hydrocephalus.[25] The syrinx itself can be responsible for significant neurologic deficit.

A variety of vascular neoplasms can arise from within the spinal cord, including arteriovenous malformations, hemangiomas, and hemangioblastomas. Approximately one-third of hemangioblastomas are associated with von Hippel-Lindau disease. These are benign neoplasms that are usually well circumscribed and amenable to surgery.[26] Unresectable or recurrent hemangioblastomas may be treated with stereotactic radiosurgery (SRS).[27]

Intradural–Extramedullary Tumors

Most intradural–extramedullary neoplasms are meningiomas, nerve sheath tumors, or extramedullary ependymomas such as myxopapillary ependymomas. They usually are amenable to complete surgical excision.

Meningiomas are usually benign, slow-growing, well-encapsulated neoplasms that are easily separated from the spinal cord; most can be completely excised, and they rarely recur. They may arise anywhere within the intradural space but are most commonly found in the cervicothoracic region and are uncommon in the lumbar region and rare in the sacrum. Spinal meningioma occurs more frequently in females. The peak incidence is between the sixth and eighth decades of life. The duration of symptoms before diagnosis is typically between 12 and 24 months, with longer duration as an independent predictor for a lack of improvement after surgery.[28]

Nerve sheath tumors arise from the Schwann cell, the cell responsible for insulating peripheral nerves and contributing to impulse conduction. Nerve sheath tumors have been called neurofibroma, schwannoma, neuroma, and neurilemoma in the past. More recently, a distinction between neurofibroma and schwannoma has been made. Although both tumors arise from Schwann cells, certain gross, microscopic, and clinical features help distinguish the two. Growing evidence also suggest that they arise via distinct pathogenic mechanisms.[29,30] Neurofibromas typically encase involved nerve roots, whereas schwannomas commonly displace the nerve roots because of their asymmetric growth. The plexiform neurofibroma is associated with type 1 neurofibromatosis, and the presence of multiple tumors helps establish the diagnosis of this genetic condition. In contrast, schwannoma is associated with type 2 neurofibromatosis. Patients with type 1 neurofibromatosis may be at risk for malignant tumor transformation following radiotherapy.[31,32] Nerve sheath tumors usually are solitary and may occur in any section of the spinal canal. They are evenly distributed in the cervical, thoracic, and lumbar regions; they are least common in the sacrum. They occur in men and women with equal frequency and are most commonly diagnosed in the fourth through sixth decades of life. Most of these tumors are completely intradural, although 10% to 15% may have an extradural component as well (so-called dumbbell tumors). Most nerve sheath tumors are benign, well-encapsulated lesions that are amenable to total surgical excision. The rare malignant nerve sheath tumors have a natural history similar to soft tissue sarcomas, and they should be treated as such.[33,34]

Miscellaneous Neoplasms

Unusual intradural–extramedullary tumors include lipomas, dermoids, and epidermoid tumors. They are typically benign and amenable to complete resection. Even if incompletely excised, recurrences are usually slow.

Extradural Tumors

Most extradural tumors are metastatic, and the presentation and management of these is discussed in Chapter 94. A variety of primary bone and soft tissue tumors may arise from an extradural location and involve the spinal canal. Bone tumors include osteosarcoma, chordomas, chondrosarcoma, and Ewing sarcoma. Soft tissue tumors include soft tissue sarcomas, including malignant nerve sheath tumors, lymphomas, and neuroblastomas. These tumors and their management are discussed in Chapters 82 (lymphoma), 86 (osteosarcoma/chordoma), 87 (soft tissue sarcoma), 90 (neuroblastoma), and 92 (Ewing tumor), respectively.

PROGNOSTIC FACTORS

The major prognostic factors in patients with primary spinal canal tumors are tumor type and grade, tumor extent and location, patient age, and presenting neurologic function. Treatment-related factors that influence the outcome include tumor resectability and the use of radiation therapy for certain tumor types. Many of these factors are interdependent. For example, ependymomas occur most frequently in the distal spinal canal and are more often resectable than astrocytic tumors.

Recently, Milano et al. analyzed 664 patients with spinal cord astrocytomas and 1,057 patients with spinal cord ependymomas using the SEER database. In this largest study to date on prognostic factors for long-term outcome, lower grade, younger age, and surgical resection were associated with significantly better overall survival and cause-specific survival for both astrocytomas and ependymomas. Radiotherapy was associated with worse cause-specific survival, but this is likely because of adverse selection bias. The 5-year overall survival of grades 1, 2, 3, and 4 astrocytomas was 82%, 70%, 28%, and 14% and the 5-year cause-specific survival was 89%, 77%, 36%, and 20%, respectively. The 5-year overall survival of grades 1, 2, and 3 ependymomas was 92%, 97%, and 58% and the 5-year cause-specific survival was 100%, 98%, and 64%, respectively.[35] Weber et al. analyzed the long-term outcomes of 183 patients with spinal myxopapillary ependymomas from a pooled database of the Rare Cancer Network and the MD Anderson Cancer Center and reported 10-year overall survival of 92% and 10-year progression-free survival of 61%.

Tumor recurrence occurred in 32% of patients, and 85% of the recurrences were local. On multivariate analysis, older age (≥36), adjuvant radiation therapy, and gross-total resection were associated with improved local control and progression-free survival.[36]

Several investigators have reported that patients with cervical spinal tumors have a worse survival and neurologic outcome than patients with more caudal tumors.[37–40] Guidetti et al. stated that patients with cervical lesions had a higher surgical risk and complication rate, which made thorough resection of tumors in this location difficult and sometimes inadvisable.[40] In a series of 62 patients with exclusively intramedullary ependymomas, patients with high cervical presentations (above C5) accounted for 4 of 6 postoperative deaths because of apneic respiratory complications.[38] In the Mallinckrodt Institute of Radiology experience, Garcia reported that the primary tumor location was the most important prognostic feature. It was suggested that a greater concentration of function per unit volume of the upper spinal cord compared with that of the cauda equina accounted for the worst neurologic outcome and survival in patients with rostral tumors.[39] In these studies, tumors affecting the cervical spinal cord were more likely to be astrocytomas, and tumors in the caudal spinal cord, filum terminale, or cauda equina were more likely to be ependymomas. The anatomic dependence of various tumor types may also contribute to the better prognosis seen in patients with tumors of the lower spinal canal.

Extensive involvement of the spinal cord with an ependymoma is associated with a worse outcome. Linstadt et al. reported a 93% 10-year disease-specific survival rate with localized ependymoma compared with 50% for patients with diffuse tumors.[41] Extensive tumors have a 50% local failure rate after surgery and radiation therapy, compared with only 20% for limited disease (one to three vertebral body segments).[42] However, extent of disease has not been a prognostic factor in other series.[43]

Neurologic function at diagnosis is an important clinical prognostic factor. In general, the fewer the symptoms and the better the neurologic function at presentation, the greater the likelihood the tumor will be controlled with fewer long-term adverse neurologic sequelae. Poor neurologic function in patients with spinal cord tumors is often attributable to the disease process and a prolonged delay in diagnosis rather than the effect of surgery or radiation therapy.[38,40,44]

SURGICAL MANAGEMENT

Intramedullary Tumors

Intramedullary tumors, most of which are astrocytomas and ependymomas, present a surgical challenge. Complete surgical excision is the treatment of choice if it can be achieved without compromising neurologic function. Ependymomas are more frequently amenable to gross total excision than are astrocytomas.[21,40] Myxopapillary ependymomas most commonly involve the cauda equina and are less aggressive than other ependymomas, though they have been reported to seed the CSF.[45–49] Encapsulated myxopapillary tumors of the cauda equina are frequently amenable to complete en bloc excision, and the recurrence rate is very low. Unencapsulated or adherent tumors often are removed piecemeal and are associated with a high local recurrence rate after surgery alone, and adjuvant radiation therapy should be considered.[42,49–51]

Complete resection of intramedullary tumors with preservation of neurologic function was not possible until 1940, when Greenwood introduced the bipolar coagulation forceps. Since then, other technologic advancements have emerged, including the dissecting microscope, intraoperative ultrasound, ultrasonic aspirator, contact laser scalpel, and intraoperative neurophysiologic monitoring. These modern surgical techniques have increased the complete resectability of intramedullary tumors while minimizing neurologic injury.[52–55]

Intraoperative ultrasonography is used to localize the lesion, define its extent, and assess the progress of tumor resection.[56] The ultrasonic aspirator allows removal of tissue fragments from within 1 mm of the vibrating tip, permitting dissection immediately adjacent to vital neural tissue.[57] The contact laser scalpel only delivers thermal energy to tissue upon direct contact, and the laser beam resides entirely within a coated sapphire crystal probe tip. It provides precise dissection of tumor with little mechanical or thermal injury to normal spinal cord parenchyma.[58]

Intraoperative neurophysiologic monitoring is considered standard of care for resection of intramedullary tumors. It is dependent on two key components: somatosensory-evoked potentials (SEPs) and motor-evoked potentials (MEPs). SEPs are monitored continuously during the incision of the dorsal midline of the spinal cord to avoid injuring the dorsal column, as the cord anatomy is often distorted by the tumor. MEPs are monitored once the surgeon starts to dissect the tumor to avoid irreversible damage to the corticospinal tract. MEPs should be monitored using a combination of epidural electrodes (D waves) and signals from limb muscle (mMEPs). Typically, a decrement of 50% or more of D-wave amplitude is considered a major indication to stop surgery.[59] Sala et al. reported that the use of intraoperative neurophysiologic monitoring during resection of intramedullary tumors significantly improved long-term ambulatory status as compared to historical controls.[60]

The risk of paralysis after surgery is <1% of patients with minimal or no preoperative neurologic deficits but may be much higher for those who present with more substantial deficits. Approximately one-third of patients will develop temporary motor deficits after surgery and most will have at least some postoperative deterioration in neurologic status.[61,62] If complete excision of low-grade spinal cord tumors is achieved, the local recurrence rate is low and prognosis is excellent without additional adjuvant therapy. In patients who recur, tumor regrowth is often slow and second resection may be possible.[22,63–65]

Intradural–Extramedullary Tumors

The treatment of choice for most tumors in this location is maximal surgical excision with preservation of neurologic function. Most benign nerve sheath tumors can be completely resected with low risk of recurrence. In contrast, complete resection of malignant peripheral nerve sheath tumor is difficult, and local recurrence is high and typically occurs between 7 and 15 months after surgery. For spinal meningioma, local recurrence is low after Simpson grade I resection but can be as high as 30% after Simpson grade II resection with an average time of 12 years after surgery. Thus, Simpson grade I resection is preferred for spinal meningioma if attainable.[66–68]

CHEMOTHERAPY

The reported use of chemotherapy for primary spinal canal tumors is limited. Outside of a clinical trial, chemotherapy is often reserved for patients with progression of disease following surgery and radiotherapy with no other treatment options. Combined with the low incidence of the disease, most studies are retrospective with very few patients, which limits any definitive conclusion regarding their efficacy. The use of chemotherapy for spinal canal tumors is often extrapolated based on the experience for intracranial tumors. However, such assumption requires further validation as the underlying oncogenesis and biologic pathways may be different between the two entities.[69]

Platinum and etoposide are generally considered the most active agents for ependymomas. In the setting of recurrent ependymoma, platinum-based chemotherapy has been shown to produce higher response rates than nitrosourea-based chemotherapy, but most patients in the studies had intracranial ependymomas.[70,71] In a prospective phase II study, 10 consecutive patients with recurrent cellular spinal cord ependymomas were treated with oral etoposide. Two patients had partial responses, and five patients had stable disease. The median overall survival was 17.5 months.[72]

Temozolomide is an attractive agent for primary spinal cord glioma given its success in treating intracranial astrocytoma.[73] Kim et al. reported their experience of treating two patients with primary spinal cord glioblastoma multiforme with concurrent radiotherapy and temozolomide followed by adjuvant temozolomide. The two patients survived 12 and 16 months, respectively, in contrast with a median survival time of 9 months in other reports.[74] Chamberlain reported a series of 22 patients with recurrent WHO grade II glioma treated with temozolomide. Overall, there were 18% partial response and 55% with stable disease. The median survival was 23 months, and progression-free survival at 2 years was 27%.[75]

For young children, especially those <3 years of age, there is an even greater interest in identifying effective and minimally toxic chemotherapy to delay or eliminate radiation therapy. There are two prospective cooperative group trials that have included children with primary spinal cord astrocytomas. In one clinical trial conducted by the French Society of Pediatric Oncology, eight children with unresectable or recurrent intramedullary low-grade gliomas were treated with a planned 16-month course of carboplatin, procarbazine, vincristine, cyclophosphamide, etoposide, and cisplatin. Seven of the patients had a clinical or radiographic response to the chemotherapy. Five of the patients remained progression free, with follow-up ranging from 16 to 59 months.[76] In the Children's Cancer Group 945 trial, 13 children with high-grade astrocytic spinal cord neoplasms were assigned to receive two cycles of "8-drugs-in-1-day" chemotherapy before radiation therapy, then eight additional cycles thereafter. At 5 years, 46% of the children had no progression and 54% were alive. The authors argued that more intensive therapy was necessary.[77] Mora et al. reported a small but thought-provoking study of three infants with spinal cord astrocytomas (WHO grade II or III) treated with irinotecan and cisplatin. All three infants had subtotal resection and progressed on conventional carboplatin-based chemotherapy. After switching to irinotecan and cisplatin, all three patients had remarkable radiologic and clinical response. At the time of the last follow-up, they had remained in remission at 12, 20, and 48 months after diagnosis. The authors hypothesized that irinotecan and cisplatin may provide synergistic effect without overlapping toxicities.[78] A recent phase II Children's Oncology Group clinical trial (COG-ACNS0423) treated pediatric patients with high-grade glioma with adjuvant radiation and concurrent temozolomide followed by additional temozolomide and lomustine chemotherapy, which included 5% of spinal high-grade astrocytomas. The study demonstrated improved event-free survival and overall survival as compared to historical controls of similar regimen without lomustine.[79]

RADIATION THERAPY

There are currently no randomized controlled trials to guide the role of radiation therapy for primary spinal canal tumors. Clinical use of postoperative radiation therapy is generally guided by patterns of failure and the prevailing attitude of many radiation centers.[80] Patients with completely resected low-grade astrocytomas and ependymomas typically have an excellent prognosis, with local failure rates of <10% without additional therapy.[68,81–83] Most centers do not advocate routine use of adjuvant radiation therapy in this setting, but long-term follow-up is indicated as late failures can occur.

In contrast, adjuvant radiation therapy after incomplete resection or piecemeal excision of low-grade ependymomas and astrocytomas is supported by retrospective analyses. Guidetti et al. first reported a beneficial outcome in patients receiving radiation therapy after an incomplete excision of an ependymoma.[40] Piecemeal removal of ependymoma in the region of the conus medullaris, cauda equina, and filum terminale (most commonly myxopapillary ependymoma) has high local failure rate ranging from 20% to 43%. Adjuvant radiation therapy in these patients after piecemeal excision produces similar local recurrence rate equal to that of patients undergoing gross total resection.[42,49,51,84] The long-term outcome of 183 spinal myxopapillary ependymomas from Weber et al. showed adjuvant radiation therapy improved 10-year progression-free survival from <40% to 70%. The authors advocated more liberal use of adjuvant radiation therapy for myxopapillary ependymoma patients with subtotal resection, piecemeal resection, or questionable gross-total resection.[36] In a multi-institutional series, adjuvant radiation therapy significantly improved progression-free survival in the 40 patients with low- and intermediate-grade astrocytomas.[21] After adjuvant radiotherapy, the cumulative incidence of local failure ranges from approximately 20% for low-grade ependymoma to 40% for low-grade astrocytoma.[80]

Nonetheless, there are clinical circumstances in which careful follow-up after incomplete resection is appropriate, with a second surgery or radiation therapy considered at the time of progression or recurrence. Radiation therapy of the spine in a child may produce a spinal deformity (i.e., scoliosis or kyphosis) because of retardation of bone growth from damage to epiphyseal plates of the vertebral bodies as well as soft tissue fibrosis and contracture.[85] Most spinal cord tumors in young children are either low-grade astrocytomas or well-differentiated ependymomas that have a very low growth rate. Delaying radiation therapy until recurrence or tumor progression may allow the child to grow at a normal rate for several years before receiving radiation therapy. Constantini et al. reported a series of 164 patients younger than 21 years of age treated with radical surgery alone without adjuvant radiotherapy. Gross total resection or subtotal resection was achieved in 77% and 20% of patients, respectively. The 3-month neurologic function was 60% stable, 16% improved, and 24% deteriorated compared with preoperative function. The 5-year progression-free survival rate for low-grade and high-grade tumors was 78% and 30%, respectively.[86]

The prognosis of high-grade astrocytomas and ependymomas is dismal, and multimodality treatment is recommended, ideally on a clinical trial. Adjuvant radiation therapy is routinely recommended regardless of the extent of resection. The role of concurrent and adjuvant chemotherapy for high-grade intramedullary astrocytoma remains inconclusive as discussed earlier. Despite aggressive treatments, few patients with high-grade astrocytomas survive beyond 2 years.[80,87] As with intracranial high-grade glioma, novel therapies beyond traditional radiotherapy and cytotoxic chemotherapy are desperately needed.

Relapse can occur years after treatment and is predominantly local. In a series of 37 spinal ependymomas treated with adjuvant radiotherapy, more than 50% of failures developed 5 years after diagnosis, and the extent of surgical resection correlated with time to progression.[88] These findings were confirmed in another series of patients with spinal myxopapillary ependymoma, where Chao et al. reported a median time to recurrence of 7.7 years.[89]

The prognosis is excellent for most patients with intradural–extramedullary tumors, which rarely recur after total excision. However, subtotally resected meningiomas may recur late after surgery.[90] Some investigators have advocated postoperative radiation therapy using either conventional fractionated external-beam radiotherapy or SRS.[91,92] Data supporting the routine use of radiation therapy in the management of patients with nerve sheath tumors, vascular malformations, lipomas, hemangiomas, teratomas, and dermoids are limited.

RADIATION THERAPY TECHNIQUES

Target Volume

Historically, it had been recommended that superior and inferior field borders encompass two vertebral bodies above and below a tumor defined by myelography, with the width of the field approximated between the tips of the lateral processes of the vertebral bodies. With the advancement of CT simulation and MRI fusion, the gross tumor volume (GTV) can be more accurately defined and smaller margins may be used. For low-grade astrocytomas or ependymomas, a clinical target volume (CTV) margin of 0.5 to 1 cm is appropriate. The CTV should encompass the preoperative GTV plus any associated intratumoral cysts. It is not necessary to include an intramedullary syrinx that extends above or below the primary tumor unless there is radiographic or surgical evidence of tumor extension to these regions. Planning treatment volume (PTV) margins of 0.5 cm or less may be used to account for setup error, with smaller PTV margins necessitating adequate patient immobilization and optimal daily localization techniques (orthogonal kilovoltage imaging, cone-beam CT, etc.).

High-grade astrocytomas and ependymomas can be more infiltrative, and a larger CTV margin of at least 1.5 cm craniocaudally should be used. Merchant et al. described a diffuse failure pattern in children with high-grade gliomas shortly after completing radiation therapy, suggesting that the tumor was not adequately covered in the irradiated volume and the need for larger CTV margins of 1.5 cm.[93] The intervertebral foramina should be included within the CTV if tumor extension is suspected.

For myxopapillary ependymomas involving the conus, a 1.5-cm CTV margin cephalad and caudad to the GTV is used, but not beyond the thecal sac, which is typically at the level of S2-3. If the cauda equina is involved, the CTV should extend inferiorly to encompass the entire thecal sac, with the volume widened at the sacroiliac joints to ensure adequate coverage of the meningeal sleeves in the intervertebral foramina. Failure to adequately encompass the thecal sac has been associated with an increased rate of treatment failure.[84]

Craniospinal or spinal axis irradiation usually is not indicated in the treatment of most spinal cord tumors; local failure accounts for most tumor recurrences.[21,39,41,42,82] However, neuraxis dissemination may be seen in patients with anaplastic ependymomas,[94] malignant astrocytomas,[95,96] and myxopapillary ependymomas.[46,47] Craniospinal irradiation may be considered if there is evidence of leptomeningeal dissemination.

Radiation Technique

For conventional external-beam field arrangements, cervical cord tumors are typically treated with parallel opposed lateral fields to reduce dose to the oral cavity, larynx, and pharynx. Thoracic cord tumors are commonly treated with direct posterior or posterior wedge fields to limit dose to the anterior structures such as the lungs, esophagus, and heart. Lumbar and cauda equina tumors are mostly treated with opposed anteroposterior–posteroanterior portals because of the lumbar lordosis and the deep location of the vertebral canal. Three-dimensional (3D) conformal or intensity-modulated radiation therapy (IMRT) methods may reduce normal tissue toxicity and should be considered when exit dose to the anterior midline structures of the trunk would otherwise be excessive (Fig. 40.5).[47] However, IMRT may increase the volume of normal

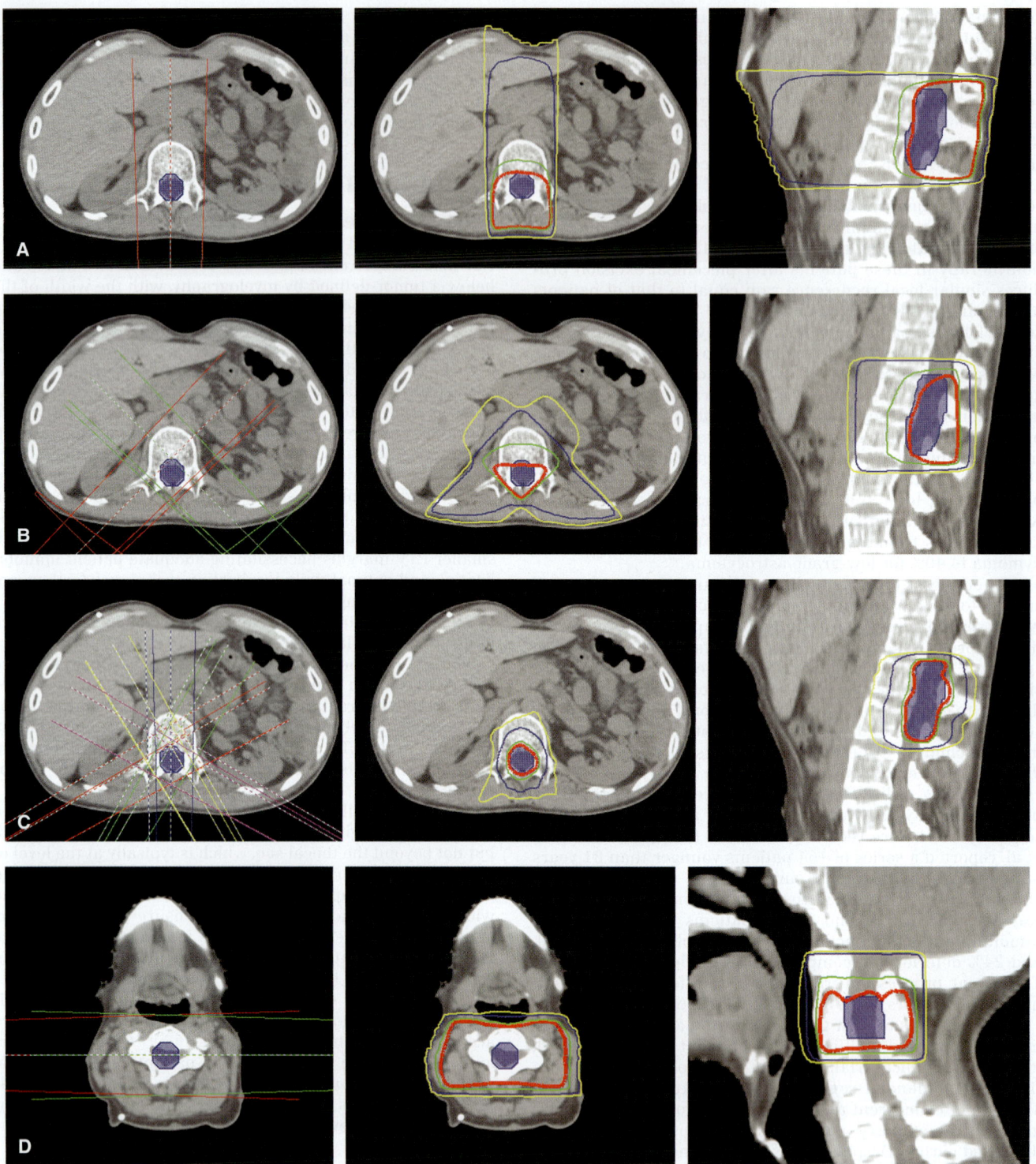

FIGURE 40.5. Treatment planning for spinal cord tumors. Planning treatment volume (PTV) in *solid blue. Red line,* prescription dose of 50.4 Gy; *green line,* 95% of prescription dose of 47.88 Gy; *blue line,* 30 Gy; *yellow line,* 20 Gy. **A:** A single posteroanterior field. The advantages of this beam arrangement include simplicity and near-universal applicability in most spinal cord radiation therapy treatments. One disadvantage of this field arrangement is the large volume of tissue that receives a significant exit dose. The axial and sagittal isodose displays reflect a 6-MV x-ray beam treated to a point just anterior to the PTV. **B:** Paired posterior oblique wedge fields. The advantage of this technique is a decrease in high exit-dose irradiation to anterior tissues with a more conformal irradiation dose distribution near the target volume. Disadvantages include more complicated treatment setup and verification. The axial and sagittal isodose displays reflect a 45-degree wedged pair of 6-MV x-ray beams treated to the same point with a 90-degree hinge angle. **C:** Intensity-modulated radiation therapy (IMRT). An advantage is a highly conformal dose distribution with excellent sparing of adjacent critical structures. Disadvantage are complexity and high integral dose. The axial and sagittal isodose displays reflect a five-field static IMRT plan with 6-MV x-rays. **D:** Opposed lateral fields. An advantage is a homogeneous dose distribution in the target volume with sparing of anterior structures from significant irradiation dose. A disadvantage is limited capplicability cervical synd lower lumbosacral sites. Exclusive use of this field arrangement in the thorax and upper abdomen is inappropriate because of limited lung and kidney tolerance. The axial isodose display reflects a pair of laterally directed 6-MV x-ray fields treated to the midplane of the cervical spine. (**C**, Courtesy Andrew Lindsey, Washington University Department of Radiation Oncology, St. Louis, MO.)

tissue receiving low doses (integral dose) and is theoretically associated with a higher risk of secondary malignancy.[97]

In female patients requiring treatment to the lumbosacral spine for cauda equina tumors, a lateral technique may be used to avoid exit irradiation to the ovaries and uterus. This technique prevents the anterior pelvic structures from receiving significant irradiation dose, which is desirable in young women and girls to minimize incidental irradiation of the ovaries. The superior aspect of this field can be matched to the divergence of a superior posteroanterior field in a fashion similar to the junction of a cranial portal to a spinal portal in craniospinal irradiation. Beam modifiers such as wedges or tissue compensators may be required with this lateral beam arrangement. Care should be taken to avoid irradiating the kidneys at the L1 through L3 levels with this technique. Arms should be positioned appropriately to avoid entrance or exit irradiation from the lateral beams.

The depth of the vertebral surface of the cord beneath the skin surface is determined from CT or MRI, and for short field lengths this depth is used for dose prescription. The treatment plan should provide a homogeneous dose distribution. For small lesions of the cervical spinal cord, where lateral fields will be used, radiation beam energies of 4 to 6 MV photons achieve a homogeneous dose distribution. Lesions involving the thoracic and lumbar spine often require combinations of low-energy (4 to 6 MV) and high-energy (18 to 25 MV) photons to achieve a homogeneous dose distribution when posterior fields are used. Attention to the exit dose delivered to anterior anatomical structures needs to be considered against dose heterogeneity in the target volume. Parallel-opposed posterior and anterior fields or paired oblique wedge fields can give homogeneous dose distributions with x-ray energies as low as 4 or 6 MV.

Radiation Dose

Low-grade astrocytomas and ependymomas should be irradiated to a total dose of 50.4 Gy, given in 1.8 Gy daily fractions. High-grade astrocytomas can be treated to a dose of 54 Gy with 1.8 Gy daily fractions. High-grade ependymomas and multifocal low-grade astrocytoma should be treated to a dose of 50.4 to 54 Gy.[80] Limited dose response data exist for spinal cord tumors. In the Mallinckrodt series of 37 patients with primary spinal cord tumors, local control and survival were significantly better for those received 40 Gy or higher.[39] Shaw et al. reported that the local failure rate of ependymomas was 35% in patients receiving 50 Gy or less compared with only 20% in patients receiving more than 50 Gy.[42] However, doses beyond 50.4 Gy have not been shown to improve local control or survival.[41,96,98] In patients with high-grade ependymomas or other spinal cord gliomas with evidence of CSF dissemination, craniospinal irradiation should be considered. Typical doses to the craniospinal axis range from 36 to 45 Gy, with a boost to sites of gross tumor to 50.4 to 54 Gy.

Stereotactic Radiosurgery

Stereotactic radiosurgery provides the ability to deliver highly conformal, high-dose radiation in such a manner as to mitigate normal tissue injury while escalating dose to the target volume. Most spine SRS reports to date have focused on its use in the management of metastatic disease to the spine. In a recent review, Hsu et al. found local control rates in excess of 80% in most series, with significant pain improvement in 43% to 97%.[99]

A few reports have also detailed spine SRS in the management of patients with intradural tumors. In the largest series reported to date, Gerszten et al. treated 73 patients with benign intradural spinal tumors (meningioma, schwannoma, neurofibroma) using CyberKnife (Accuray Inc, Sunnyvale, CA) spine SRS to doses ranging from 16 to 30 Gy in 1 to 5 fractions. At a median of 37 months follow-up, the local control rate was 98% and pain improved in 70% of meningiomas, 50% of schwannomas, and 0% of neurofibromas. Three patients

developed radiotherapy-related spinal cord toxicity 5 to 13 months after treatment.[91] Overall radiographic response rates for benign intradural tumors in the series reported to date range from 28% to 39%.[99]

Investigators from Stanford University have reported their experience treating spinal cord ependymomas and hemangioblastomas using spine SRS delivered with the CyberKnife system (Fig. 40.6). In the earliest report, 7 patients with 10 intramedullary spinal tumors (7 hemangioblastomas, 3 ependymomas) received spine SRS to a dose of 18 to 25 Gy in 1 to 3 fractions.[27] At a mean follow-up of 12 months, one ependymoma and two hemangioblastomas were smaller on follow-up imaging, with the remainder stable. No significant treatment-related complications were reported. In a follow-up study, Daly et al. reported a 3-year actuarial control rate for 27 spinal hemangioblastomas treated with spine SRS to 18 to 25 Gy in 2 to 3 sessions. One patient developed a grade 2 foot drop 4 months after SRS, and two patients developed grade 1 sensory deficits.[100]

Early results of spine SRS for intradural–extramedullary or intramedullary lesions are promising, and with the rapidly increasing availability of extracranial radiosurgery devices, SRS for these patients will no doubt increase in utilization. However, with such few reports and limited follow-up to date, caution certainly seems warranted given the potential for late toxicity in these patients with high rates of long-term survival. Issues related to spinal cord tolerance after spine SRS are discussed below.

Proton Therapy

Proton therapy is a form of particle radiation that provides very conformal radiation therapy with a lower integral dose than other forms of photon radiation therapy.[101] Due to its unique physical property, it can spare low dose exposure to the normal tissues distal to the proton beam, which theoretically should translate to reduction of late-toxicities such as secondary malignancy and cardiac disease, especially for young adults or pediatric patients.[102–104] Amsbaugh et al. reported a prospective case series of 7 pediatric patients with spinal ependymomas treated with proton therapy (ranging from 45 to 54 cobalt gray equivalents). They showed proton therapy was well tolerated and dramatically reduced dose to all normal tissues anterior to the vertebral bodies as compared to photon therapy. After relatively short median follow-up of 26 months, local control, event-free survival and overall survival were all 100%, and there were no grade 3 toxicity.[105] However, due to the relative rarity of the primary spinal tumors and the required long-term follow-up for endpoints such as secondary malignancy and cardiac disease, sufficient clinical data to support or refute the benefit of proton therapy for spinal tumors will unlikely to emerge in the near future. Individualized decision based on tumor location, patient age, and access to proton therapy will be required to consider treatment for proton therapy.

SPINAL CORD TOLERANCE

A reversible myelopathy can occur within 2 to 6 months after radiation therapy. L'Hermitte's sign, characterized by shock-like sensations radiating to the hands and feet when the neck is flexed, is the classic finding. It is believed that this phenomenon is related to transient demyelination of the treated length of the spinal cord.[106,107] This syndrome usually lasts a few weeks, and no therapy is required. It is not associated with chronic progressive myelitis.

Chronic, progressive, or delayed myelopathy can occur months to years after radiation therapy. The latency period of chronic myelopathy has been reported to be bimodal with peaks of incidence occurring at 13 and 29 months. The early peak may correspond to white matter injury with subsequent demyelination, and the latter peak may correspond to microvascular

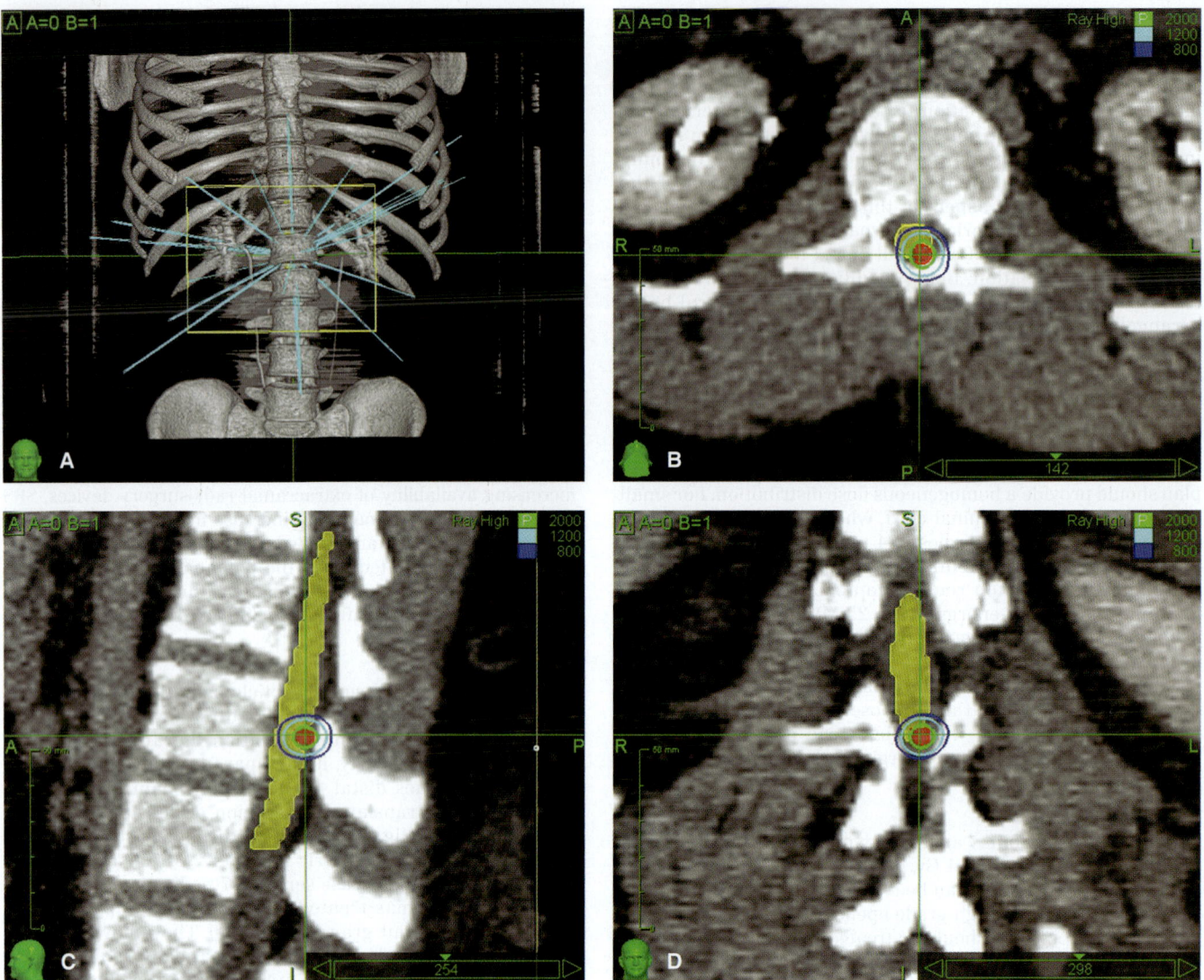

FIGURE 40.6. Stereotactic radiosurgery for an L1 hemangioblastoma. A single dose of 20 Gy was delivered with CyberKnife using 87 noncoplanar beams as shown in *blue*. As is typical of treatment delivery with this unit, the plan is nonisocentric. Gross tumor volume is shown in *solid red*, spinal cord in *solid yellow*. *Green line*, prescription dose of 20 Gy; *light blue line*, 12 Gy; *dark blue line*, 8 Gy. **A:** Three-dimensional representation of select noncoplanar beam paths. **B:** Axial isodose display reveals a sharp dose gradient between the prescription dose and the 12 and 8 Gy isodose lines. **C:** Sagittal isodose display. **D:** Coronal isodose display. (Courtesy Scott Soltys, MD, and Megan Daly, MD, Stanford University Department of Radiation Oncology, Stanford, CA.)

injury. Permanent myelopathy is characterized by progressive motor weakness, paresthesias, and loss of pain or temperature sensation. Patients ultimately lose bowel and bladder control and experience complete sensory and motor function loss.[108] Diagnosis of radiation myelopathy requires that the dominant neurologic abnormality be localized to a segment irradiated and other causes have been ruled out. MRI may assist in the diagnosis, with cord edema frequently being present in the early delayed phase. Within 8 months of the onset of symptoms, the T1-weighted images may show low intensity in the region of spinal cord injury, whereas the T2 image shows high intensity. The lesion may enhance with Gd-DTPA. Late changes in patients with permanent delayed myelopathy may include atrophy.[109] Even with modern imaging, it may be difficult to determine whether neurologic deficits after radiotherapy are related to tumor progression or treatment-induced myelopathy.

The occurrence of chronic progressive myelopathy depends on total dose, fraction size, volume, and region irradiated. Historically, the spinal cord has been limited to maximum doses of 45 to 50 Gy with fractionation schedules of 1.8 to 2 Gy per day. These estimates came from an era of inexact dose estimation with a bias toward reporting injury in highly selected populations.[110,111] More recently, data have been published from institutions that have treated large groups of patients in systematic and reliable fashion. The Quantitative Analysis of Normal Tissue Effects in the Clinic (QUANTEC) initiative comprehensively reviewed modern radiotherapy toxicity data and published guidelines on spinal cord tolerance.[112] For conventional external-beam radiation therapy at 1.8 to 2 Gy per day, a dose of 50 Gy, 60 Gy, and 69 Gy is associated with a 0.2%, 6%, and 50% rates of myelopathy, respectively. However, pediatric patients and patients receiving potentially neurotoxic chemotherapy may have decreased spinal cord tolerance, with reports of myelopathy at doses 50 Gy or less.[113–115]

Dose–volume data for myelopathy after spine SRS is evolving. In a multi-institutional review of 1,075 patients treated with spine SRS principally for metastatic disease, the rate of spinal cord toxicity was 0.6%.[116] Data from the QUANTEC initiative indicate that the rate of myelopathy will be <1% with the maximum dose to the spinal cord limited to the equivalent of 13 Gy in a single fraction or 20 Gy in 3 fractions.[112] The most commonly employed dose constraint for single fraction SRS is to keep <10% of the spinal cord (defined as 3 to 6 mm above and below the target volume) to <10 Gy.[99] Intriguing data from investigators at

Stanford University utilizing SRS for spinal hemangioblastoma suggest that spinal cord tolerance may be higher than predicted by conventional modeling.[100,117] Maximum cord dose delivered in 2 to 3 sessions in their series was an average of 22.7 Gy (range, 17.8 to 30.9 Gy) to small volumes, with only 1 of 24 treatments resulting in myelopathy. Such a phenomenon may at least in part be explained by preclinical experiments suggesting a dramatic length and partial volume effect to spinal cord tolerance after radiation. For example, in one animal study, the ED50 (dose at which 50% of animals developed limb paralysis) for single fraction full thickness radiation to the spinal cord was 20.4 Gy for a 20 mm cord length, compared with 53.7 Gy for 4 mm and 87.8 Gy for 2 mm cord lengths.[118]

Both animal and human studies have demonstrated that irradiated spinal cord may recover at least partially over time. Animal experiments of reirradiation using Rhesus monkeys estimated cord recovery of 76%, 85%, and 100% at 1, 2, and 3 years, respectively.[119,120] In human studies, where reirradiation is at least 6 months after the initial radiation course, essentially no cases of myelopathy were observed when the cumulative 2-Gy equivalent doses are 60 Gy or less.[112,121]

CONCLUSIONS

Spinal canal tumors are relatively rare and consist of diverse histological entities. Surgery remains the primary treatment modality, aided by gradual advances in neurosurgical techniques. Adjuvant radiotherapy is generally considered for incomplete resection, recurrent tumors, or high grade tumors. New radiotherapy techniques such as intensity modulated radiotherapy or SRS have shown promising potential to improve the therapeutic ratio. The role of chemotherapy is not clearly defined and is often extrapolated from intracranial counterparts. Continued long-term follow-up of clinical outcomes and innovation of novel approaches are essential for improving the management of spinal canal tumors.

REFERENCES

1. Ostrom QT, Gittleman H, Fulop J, et al. CBTRUS Statistical Report: primary brain and central nervous system tumors diagnosed in the United States in 2008–2012. *Neuro Oncol* 2015;17(Suppl 4):iv1–iv62.
2. Duong LM, McCarthy BJ, McLendon RE, et al. Descriptive epidemiology of malignant and nonmalignant primary spinal cord, spinal meninges, and cauda equina tumors, United States, 2004–2007. *Cancer* 2012;118(17):4220–4227.
3. Abel TJ, Chowdhary A, Thapa M, et al. Spinal cord pilocytic astrocytoma with leptomeningeal dissemination to the brain. Case report and review of the literature. *J Neurosurg* 2006;105(6 Suppl):508–514.
4. D'Haene N, Coen N, Neugroschl C, et al. Leptomeningeal dissemination of low-grade intramedullary gliomas: about one case and review. *Clin Neurol Neurosurg* 2009;111(4):390–394.
5. Smoll NR, Villanueva EV. The epidemiology of extraneural metastases from primary brain, spinal cord, and meningeal tumors. *Neurosurgery* 2010;67(5):E1470–E1471.
6. Raco A, Esposito V, Lenzi J, et al. Long-term follow-up of intramedullary spinal cord tumors: a series of 202 cases. *Neurosurgery* 2005;56(5):972–981; discussion 972–981.
7. Bannister R. Disorders of the spinal cord. In: Brain W, Bannister R, eds. *Clinical neurology*. London, UK: Oxford University Press, 1998.
8. DeSousa AL, Kalsbeck JE, Mealey J Jr, et al. Intraspinal tumors in children. A review of 81 cases. *J Neurosurg* 1979;51(4):437–445.
9. Reimer R, Onofrio BM. Astrocytomas of the spinal cord in children and adolescents. *J Neurosurg* 1985;63(5):669–675.
10. Uhl M, Sterzing F, Habl G, et al. CT-myelography for high-dose irradiation of spinal and paraspinal tumors with helical tomotherapy: revival of an old tool. *Strahlenther Onkol* 2011;187(7):416–420.
11. Gado M, Sartor K, Hodges F. The spine. In: Lee J, Sagel S, Stanley R, eds. *Computed body tomography*. New York: Raven Press, 1989.
12. Sze G. Neoplastic disease of the spine and spinal cord. In: Atlas SW, ed. *Magnetic resonance imaging of the brain and spine*. Philadelphia: Lippincott-Raven, 1996.
13. Perry A, Miller CR, Gujrati M, et al. Malignant gliomas with primitive neuroectodermal tumor-like components: a clinicopathologic and genetic study of 53 cases. *Brain Pathol* 2009;19(1):81–90.
14. Rodriguez FJ, Perry A, Rosenblum MK, et al. Disseminated oligodendroglial-like leptomeningeal tumor of childhood: a distinctive clinicopathologic entity. *Acta Neuropathol* 2012;124(5):627–641.
15. Louis DN, Ohgaki H, Wiestler OD, et al. The 2007 WHO classification of tumours of the central nervous system. *Acta Neuropathol* 2007;114(2):97–109.
16. Louis DN, Perry A, Reifenberger G, et al. The 2016 World Health Organization Classification of Tumors of the Central Nervous System: a summary. *Acta Neuropathol* 2016;131(6):803–820.
17. Grimm S, Chamberlain MC. Adult primary spinal cord tumors. *Expert Rev Neurother* 2009;9(10):1487–1495.
18. Celano E, Salehani A, Malcolm JG, et al. Spinal cord ependymoma: a review of the literature and case series of ten patients. *J Neurooncol* 2016;128(3):377–386.
19. Guss ZD, Moningi S, Jallo GI, et al. Management of pediatric spinal cord astrocytomas: outcomes with adjuvant radiation. *Int J Radiat Oncol Biol Phys* 2013;85(5):1307–1311.
20. Kutluk T, Varan A, Kafali C, et al. Pediatric intramedullary spinal cord tumors: a single center experience. *Eur J Paediatr Neurol* 2015;19(1):41–47.
21. Abdel-Wahab M, Etuk B, Palermo J, et al. Spinal cord gliomas: a multi-institutional retrospective analysis. *Int J Radiat Oncol Biol Phys* 2006;64(4):1060–1071.
22. Epstein FJ, Farmer JP, Freed D. Adult intramedullary astrocytomas of the spinal cord. *J Neurosurg* 1992;77(3):355–359.
23. Rossitch E Jr, Zeidman SM, Burger PC, et al. Clinical and pathological analysis of spinal cord astrocytomas in children. *Neurosurgery* 1990;27(2):193–196.
24. Samii M, Klekamp J. Surgical results of 100 intramedullary tumors in relation to accompanying syringomyelia. *Neurosurgery* 1994;35(5):865–873; discussion 873.
25. Henson JW. Spinal cord gliomas. *Curr Opin Neurol* 2001;14(6):679–682.
26. Lonser RR, Weil RJ, Wanebo JE, et al. Surgical management of spinal cord hemangioblastomas in patients with von Hippel-Lindau disease. *J Neurosurg* 2003;98(1):106–116.
27. Ryu SI, Kim DH, Chang SD. Stereotactic radiosurgery for hemangiomas and ependymomas of the spinal cord. *Neurosurg Focus* 2003;15(5):E10.
28. Setzer M, Vatter H, Marquardt G, et al. Management of spinal meningiomas: surgical results and a review of the literature. *Neurosurg Focus* 2007;23(4):E14.
29. Carroll SL. Molecular mechanisms promoting the pathogenesis of Schwann cell neoplasms. *Acta Neuropathol* 2012;123(3):321–348.
30. Rodriguez FJ, Folpe AL, Giannini C, et al. Pathology of peripheral nerve sheath tumors: diagnostic overview and update on selected diagnostic problems. *Acta Neuropathol* 2012;123(3):295–319.
31. Carroll SL. The challenge of cancer genomics in rare nervous system neoplasms: malignant peripheral nerve sheath tumors as a paradigm for cross-species comparative oncogenomics. *Am J Pathol* 2016;186(3):464–477.
32. Evans DG, Birch JM, Ramsden RT, et al. Malignant transformation and new primary tumours after therapeutic radiation for benign disease: substantial risks in certain tumour prone syndromes. *J Med Genet* 2006;43(4):289–294.
33. Grobmyer SR, Reith JD, Shahlaee A, et al. Malignant Peripheral Nerve Sheath Tumor: molecular pathogenesis and current management considerations. *J Surg Oncol* 2008;97(4):340–349.
34. James AW, Shurell E, Singh A, et al. Malignant peripheral nerve sheath tumor. *Surg Oncol Clin N Am* 2016;25(4):789–802.
35. Milano MT, Johnson MD, Sul J, et al. Primary spinal cord glioma: a Surveillance, Epidemiology, and End Results database study. *J Neurooncol* 2010;98(1):83–92.
36. Weber DC, Wang Y, Miller R, et al. Long-term outcome of patients with spinal myxopapillary ependymoma: treatment results from the MD Anderson Cancer Center and institutions from the Rare Cancer Network. *Neuro Oncol* 2015;17(4):588–595.
37. Chun HC, Schmidt-Ullrich RK, Wolfson A, et al. External beam radiotherapy for primary spinal cord tumors. *J Neurooncol* 1990;9(3):211–217.
38. Ferrante L, Mastronardi L, Celli P, et al. Intramedullary spinal cord ependymomas—a study of 45 cases with long-term follow-up. *Acta Neurochir (Wien)* 1992;119(1–4):74–79.
39. Garcia DM. Primary spinal cord tumors treated with surgery and postoperative irradiation. *Int J Radiat Oncol Biol Phys* 1985;11(11):1933–1939.
40. Guidetti B, Mercuri S, Vagnozzi R. Long-term results of the surgical treatment of 129 intramedullary spinal gliomas. *J Neurosurg* 1981;54(3):323–330.
41. Linstadt DE, Wara WM, Leibel SA, et al. Postoperative radiotherapy of primary spinal cord tumors. *Int J Radiat Oncol Biol Phys* 1989;16(6):1397–1403.
42. Shaw EG, Evans RG, Scheithauer BW, et al. Radiotherapeutic management of adult intraspinal ependymomas. *Int J Radiat Oncol Biol Phys* 1986;12(3):323–327.
43. Goh KY, Velasquez L, Epstein FJ. Pediatric intramedullary spinal cord tumors: is surgery alone enough? *Pediatr Neurosurg* 1997;27(1):34–39.
44. Nishio S, Morioka T, Fujii K, et al. Spinal cord gliomas: management and outcome with reference to adjuvant therapy. *J Clin Neurosci* 2000;7(1):20–23.
45. Chan HS, Becker LE, Hoffman HJ, et al. Myxopapillary ependymoma of the filum terminale and cauda equina in childhood: report of seven cases and review of the literature. *Neurosurgery* 1984;14(2):204–210.
46. Fassett DR, Pingree J, Kestle JR. The high incidence of tumor dissemination in myxopapillary ependymoma in pediatric patients. Report of five cases and review of the literature. *J Neurosurg* 2005;102(1 Suppl):59–64.
47. Merchant TE, Kiehna EN, Thompson SJ, et al. Pediatric low-grade and ependymal spinal cord tumors. *Pediatr Neurosurg* 2000;32(1):30–36.
48. Mork SJ, Loken AC. Ependymoma: a follow-up study of 101 cases. *Cancer* 1977;40(2):907–915.
49. Sonneland PR, Scheithauer BW, Onofrio BM. Myxopapillary ependymoma. A clinicopathologic and immunocytochemical study of 77 cases. *Cancer* 1985;56(4):883–893.
50. Miller DC. Surgical pathology of intramedullary spinal cord neoplasms. *J Neurooncol* 2000;47(3):189–194.
51. Shirato H, Kamada T, Hida K, et al. The role of radiotherapy in the management of spinal cord glioma. *Int J Radiat Oncol Biol Phys* 1995;33(2):323–328.
52. Garces-Ambrossi GL, McGirt MJ, Mehta VA, et al. Factors associated with progression-free survival and long-term neurological outcome after resection of intramedullary spinal cord tumors: analysis of 101 consecutive cases. *J Neurosurg Spine* 2009;11(5):591–599.

Section III

53. Matsuyama Y, Sakai Y, Katayama Y, et al. Surgical results of intramedullary spinal cord tumor with spinal cord monitoring to guide extent of resection. *J Neurosurg Spine* 2009;10(5):404–413.

54. McGirt MJ, Chaichana KL, Atiba A, et al. Resection of intramedullary spinal cord tumors in children: assessment of long-term motor and sensory deficits. *J Neurosurg Pediatr* 2008;1(1):63–67.

55. Sciubba DM, Liang D, Kothbauer KF, et al. The evolution of intramedullary spinal cord tumor surgery. *Neurosurgery* 2009;65(6 Suppl):84–91; discussion 91–82.

56. Epstein FJ, Farmer JP, Schneider SJ. Intraoperative ultrasonography: an important surgical adjunct for intramedullary tumors. *J Neurosurg* 1991;74(5):729–733.

57. Jallo GI. CUSA EXcel ultrasonic aspiration system. *Neurosurgery* 2001;48(3):695–697.

58. Jallo GI, Kothbauer KF, Epstein FJ. Contact laser microsurgery. *Childs Nerv Syst* 2002;18(6–7):333–336.

59. Sala F, Bricolo A, Faccioli F, et al. Surgery for intramedullary spinal cord tumors: the role of intraoperative (neurophysiological) monitoring. *Eur Spine J* 2007;16(Suppl 2):S130–S139.

60. Sala F, Palandri G, Basso E, et al. Motor evoked potential monitoring improves outcome after surgery for intramedullary spinal cord tumors: a historical control study. *Neurosurgery* 2006;58(6):1129–1143; discussion 1129–1143.

61. Jallo GI, Freed D, Epstein F. Intramedullary spinal cord tumors in children. *Childs Nerv Syst* 2003;19(9):641–649.

62. Kothbauer KF, Deletis V, Epstein FJ. Motor-evoked potential monitoring for intramedullary spinal cord tumor surgery: correlation of clinical and neurophysiological data in a series of 100 consecutive procedures. *Neurosurg Focus* 1998;4(5):e1.

63. Brotchi J, Fischer G. Spinal cord ependymomas. *Neurosurg Focus* 1998;4(5):e2.

64. Cooper PR. Outcome after operative treatment of intramedullary spinal cord tumors in adults: intermediate and long-term results in 51 patients. *Neurosurgery* 1989;25(6):855–859.

65. Epstein FJ, Farmer JP, Freed D. Adult intramedullary spinal cord ependymomas: the result of surgery in 38 patients. *J Neurosurg* 1993;79(2):204–209.

66. Conti P, Pansini G, Mouchaty H, et al. Spinal neurinomas: retrospective analysis and long-term outcome of 179 consecutively operated cases and review of the literature. *Surg Neurol* 2004;61(1):34–43; discussion 44.

67. Mattei TA, Teles AR, Mendel E. Modern surgical techniques for management of soft tissue sarcomas involving the spine: outcomes and complications. *J Surg Oncol* 2015;111(5):580–586.

68. Nakamura M, Tsuji O, Fujiyoshi K, et al. Long-term surgical outcomes of spinal meningiomas. *Spine* 2012;37(10):E617–E623.

69. Chamberlain MC, Tredway TL. Adult primary intradural spinal cord tumors: a review. *Curr Neurol Neurosci Rep* 2011;11(3):320–328.

70. Brandes AA, Cavallo G, Reni M, et al. A multicenter retrospective study of chemotherapy for recurrent intracranial ependymal tumors in adults by the Gruppo Italiano Cooperativo di Neuro-Oncologia. *Cancer* 2005;104(1):143–148.

71. Gornet MK, Buckner JC, Marks RS, et al. Chemotherapy for advanced CNS ependymoma. *J Neurooncol* 1999;45(1):61–67.

72. Chamberlain MC. Etoposide for recurrent spinal cord ependymoma. *Neurology* 2002;58(8):1310–1311.

73. Stupp R, Hegi ME, Mason WP, et al. Effects of radiotherapy with concomitant and adjuvant temozolomide versus radiotherapy alone on survival in glioblastoma in a randomised phase III study: 5-year analysis of the EORTC-NCIC trial. *Lancet Oncol* 2009;10(5):459–466.

74. Kim WH, Yoon SH, Kim CY, et al. Temozolomide for malignant primary spinal cord glioma: an experience of six cases and a literature review. *J Neurooncol* 2011;101(2):247–254.

75. Chamberlain MC. Temozolomide for recurrent low-grade spinal cord gliomas in adults. *Cancer* 2008;113(5):1019–1024.

76. Doireau V, Grill J, Zerah M, et al. Chemotherapy for unresectable and recurrent intramedullary glial tumours in children. Brain Tumours Subcommittee of the French Society of Paediatric Oncology (SFOP). *Br J Cancer* 1999;81(5):835–840.

77. Allen JC, Aviner S, Yates AJ, et al. Treatment of high-grade spinal cord astrocytoma of childhood with "8-in-1" chemotherapy and radiotherapy: a pilot study of CCG-945. Children's Cancer Group. *J Neurosurg* 1998;88(2):215–220.

78. Mora J, Cruz O, Gala S, et al. Successful treatment of childhood intramedullary spinal cord astrocytomas with irinotecan and cisplatin. *Neuro Oncol* 2007;9(1):39–46.

79. Jakacki RI, Cohen KJ, Buxton A, et al. Phase 2 study of concurrent radiotherapy and temozolomide followed by temozolomide and lomustine in the treatment of children with high-grade glioma: a report of the Children's Oncology Group ACNS0423 study. *Neuro Oncol* 2016;18(10):1442–1450.

80. Isaacson SR. Radiation therapy and the management of intramedullary spinal cord tumors. *J Neurooncol* 2000;47(3):231–238.

81. Eroes CA, Zausinger S, Kreth FW, et al. Intramedullary low grade astrocytoma and ependymoma. Surgical results and predicting factors for clinical outcome. *Acta Neurochir (Wien)* 2010;152(4):611–618.

82. Robinson CG, Prayson RA, Hahn JF, et al. Long-term survival and functional status of patients with low-grade astrocytoma of spinal cord. *Int J Radiat Oncol Biol Phys* 2005;63(1):91–100.

83. Yang S, Yang X, Hong G. Surgical treatment of one hundred seventy-four intramedullary spinal cord tumors. *Spine* 2009;34(24):2705–2710.

84. Wen BC, Hussey DH, Hitchon PW, et al. The role of radiation therapy in the management of ependymomas of the spinal cord. *Int J Radiat Oncol Biol Phys* 1991;20(4):781–786.

85. Mayfield JK. Postradiation spinal deformity. *Orthop Clin North Am* 1979;10(4):829–844.

86. Constantini S, Miller DC, Allen JC, et al. Radical excision of intramedullary spinal cord tumors: surgical morbidity and long-term follow-up evaluation in 164 children and young adults. *J Neurosurg* 2000;93(2 Suppl):183–193.

87. Kim MS, Chung CK, Choe G, et al. Intramedullary spinal cord astrocytoma in adults: postoperative outcome. *J Neurooncol* 2001;52(1):85–94.

88. Gomez DR, Missett BT, Wara WM, et al. High failure rate in spinal ependymomas with long-term follow-up. *Neuro Oncol* 2005;7(3):254–259.

89. Chao ST, Kobayashi T, Benzel E, et al. The role of adjuvant radiation therapy in the treatment of spinal myxopapillary ependymomas. *J Neurosurg Spine* 2011;14(1):59–64.

90. Mirimanoff RO, Dosoretz DE, Linggood RM, et al. Meningioma: analysis of recurrence and progression following neurosurgical resection. *J Neurosurg* 1985;62(1):18–24.

91. Gerszten PC, Burton SA, Ozhasoglu C, et al. Radiosurgery for benign intradural spinal tumors. *Neurosurgery* 2008;62(4):887–895; discussion 895–886.

92. Gezen F, Kahraman S, Canakci Z, et al. Review of 36 cases of spinal cord meningioma. *Spine* 2000;25(6):727–731.

93. Merchant TE, Nguyen D, Thompson SJ, et al. High-grade pediatric spinal cord tumors. *Pediatr Neurosurg* 1999;30(1):1–5.

94. Whitaker SJ, Bessell EM, Ashley SE, et al. Postoperative radiotherapy in the management of spinal cord ependymoma. *J Neurosurg* 1991;74(5):720–728.

95. Cohen AR, Wisoff JH, Allen JC, et al. Malignant astrocytomas of the spinal cord. *J Neurosurg* 1989;70(1):50–54.

96. Kopelson G, Linggood RM. Intramedullary spinal cord astrocytoma versus glioblastoma: the prognostic importance of histologic grade. *Cancer* 1982;50(4):732–735.

97. Hall EJ, Wuu CS. Radiation-induced second cancers: the impact of 3D-CRT and IMRT. *Int J Radiat Oncol Biol Phys* 2003;56(1):83–88.

98. Abdel-Wahab M, Corn B, Wolfson A, et al. Prognostic factors and survival in patients with spinal cord gliomas after radiation therapy. *Am J Clin Oncol* 1999;22(4):344–351.

99. Hsu W, Nguyen T, Kleinberg L, et al. Stereotactic radiosurgery for spine tumors: review of current literature. *Stereotact Funct Neurosurg* 2010;88(5):315–321.

100. Daly ME, Choi CY, Gibbs IC, et al. Tolerance of the spinal cord to stereotactic radiosurgery: insights from hemangioblastomas. *Int J Radiat Oncol Biol Phys* 2011;80(1):213–220.

101. Mohan R, Grosshans D. Proton therapy—Present and future. *Adv Drug Deliv Rev* 2017;109:26–44.

102. Merchant TE. Proton beam therapy in pediatric oncology. *Cancer J* 2009;15(4):298–305.

103. Travis LB, Fossa SD, Schonfeld SJ, et al. Second cancers among 40,576 testicular cancer patients: focus on long-term survivors. *J Natl Cancer Inst* 2005;97(18):1354–1365.

104. Tukenova M, Guibout C, Oberlin O, et al. Role of cancer treatment in long-term overall and cardiovascular mortality after childhood cancer. *J Clin Oncol* 2010;28(8):1308–1315.

105. Amsbaugh MJ, Grosshans DR, McAleer MF, et al. Proton therapy for spinal ependymomas: planning, acute toxicities, and preliminary outcomes. *Int J Radiat Oncol Biol Phys* 2012;83(5):1419–1424.

106. Fein DA, Marcus RB Jr, Parsons JT, et al. Lhermitte's sign: incidence and treatment variables influencing risk after irradiation of the cervical spinal cord. *Int J Radiat Oncol Biol Phys* 1993;27(5):1029–1033.

107. Jones A. Transient radiation myelopathy (with Reference to Lhermitte's Sign of Electrical Paraesthesia). *Br J Radiol* 1964;37:727–744.

108. Schultheiss TE, Higgins EM, El-Mahdi AM. The latent period in clinical radiation myelopathy. *Int J Radiat Oncol Biol Phys* 1984;10(7):1109–1115.

109. Rampling R, Symonds P. Radiation myelopathy. *Curr Opin Neurol* 1998;11(6):627–632.

110. Phillips TL, Buschke F. Radiation tolerance of the thoracic spinal cord. *Am J Roentgenol Radium Ther Nucl Med* 1969;105(3):659–664.

111. Wara WM, Phillips TL, Sheline GE, et al. Radiation tolerance of the spinal cord. *Cancer* 1975;35(6):1558–1562.

112. Kirkpatrick JP, van der Kogel AJ, Schultheiss TE. Radiation dose-volume effects in the spinal cord. *Int J Radiat Oncol Biol Phys* 2010;76(3 Suppl):S42–S49.

113. Chao MW, Wirth A, Ryan G, et al. Radiation myelopathy following transplantation and radiotherapy for non-Hodgkin's lymphoma. *Int J Radiat Oncol Biol Phys* 1998;41(5):1057–1061.

114. Seddon BM, Cassoni AM, Galloway MJ, et al. Fatal radiation myelopathy after high-dose busulfan and melphalan chemotherapy and radiotherapy for Ewing's sarcoma: a review of the literature and implications for practice. *Clin Oncol* 2005;17(5):385–390.

115. Townsend N, Handler M, Fleitz J, et al. Intramedullary spinal cord astrocytomas in children. *Pediatr Blood Cancer* 2004;43(6):629–632.

116. Gibbs IC, Patil C, Gerszten PC, et al. Delayed radiation-induced myelopathy after spinal radiosurgery. *Neurosurgery* 2009;64(2 Suppl):A67–A72.

117. Daly ME, Luxton G, Choi CY, et al. Normal tissue complication probability estimation by the Lyman-Kutcher-Burman method does not accurately predict spinal cord tolerance to stereotactic radiosurgery. *Int J Radiat Oncol Biol Phys* 2012;82(5):2025–2032.

118. Bijl HP, van Luijk P, Coppes RP, et al. Regional differences in radiosensitivity across the rat cervical spinal cord. *Int J Radiat Oncol Biol Phys* 2005;61(2):543–551.

119. Ang KK, Jiang GL, Feng Y, et al. Extent and kinetics of recovery of occult spinal cord injury. *Int J Radiat Oncol Biol Phys* 2001;50(4):1013–1020.

120. Ang KK, Price RE, Stephens LC, et al. The tolerance of primate spinal cord to re-irradiation. *Int J Radiat Oncol Biol Phys* 1993;25(3):459–464.

121. Milano MT, Usuki KY, Walter KA, et al. Stereotactic radiosurgery and hypofractionated stereotactic radiotherapy: normal tissue dose constraints of the central nervous system. *Cancer Treat Rev* 2011;37(7):567–578.

C H A P T E R   4 1

Tumors of the Eye and Orbit

Nicholas J. Sanfilippo and Silvia C. Formenti

Primary tumors of the eye and orbit are rare. The American Cancer Society estimates that in 2017, there will be 3,130 new cases with 330 deaths from primary eye cancers.[1] Male to female incidence is similar. In adults, melanoma is the most common primary intraocular cancer, followed by lymphoma, whereas in children, retinoblastoma is the most common tumor, followed by medulloepithelioma. Metastases, or secondary intraocular tumors, are more common than primary tumors and typically come from breast or lung cancers.[2] Numerous other tumors such as rhabdomyosarcoma, optic nerve glioma, conjunctival tumors, and eyelid carcinomas also occur in the orbit. Radiation therapy (RT) has been effective in the treatment of many of these tumors, can be delivered externally or by brachytherapy depending on the clinical situation, and can been used exclusively or in concert with other treatments such as surgery or chemotherapy. Technologic advances such as intensity-modulated radiation therapy (IMRT), proton beam therapy, and stereotactic radiotherapy (SRT) have a key role in management of these tumors given the anatomy proximity of structures in this location. This chapter will outline the most relevant malignant and benign conditions of the eye and orbit with emphasis on radiotherapeutic management. Because cancers originating in the eye require significant radiation dose for their control, exposure of normal tissue is often inevitable, with possible late toxicities that warrant therapeutic interventions. Consequently, the management of eye tumors is an exquisitely interdisciplinary field that requires successful collaboration with ophthalmologists.

ANATOMY

The eye is not an exact sphere but rather a fused two-piece unit. The smaller, more curved frontal unit is the cornea and is linked to the larger unit called the sclera. The corneal segment is typically about 8 mm in radius. The sclera constitutes the remainder of the eyeball with radius of approximately 12 mm. The cornea and sclera are connected by the limbus. The iris and the pupil are seen instead of the cornea because of the cornea's transparency. The area opposite the pupil, the fundus, shows the characteristic pale optic disc or papilla, where vessels enter the eye and optic nerve fibers depart the globe. Dimensions of the globe differ among adults by only 1 or 2 mm. The vertical measure, generally less than the horizontal distance, is about 24 mm in adults. The eye is made up of three coats or tunics, enclosing three transparent structures (Fig. 41.1). The outermost layer is composed of the cornea and sclera. The middle layer consists of the choroid, ciliary body, and iris. The innermost is the retina, which whose blood supply is from the vessels of the choroid as well as the retinal vessels. The lens is suspended to the ciliary body by the suspensory ligament, made up of fine transparent fibers.

RADIATION TOLERANCE OF OCULAR STRUCTURES

Eyelid

Acute radiosensitivity of eyelid skin is comparable to the skin at other sites, and loss of eyelashes may occur at doses as low as 20 Gy using standard fractionation.[3] Late effects can include telangiectasia and atrophy. Xerophthalmia can result from doses as low as 24 to 26 Gy and may be the result of dysfunction of the meibomian glands, lacrimal acinar cells, or both.[4] Significant xerophthalmia can cause corneal desiccation and pain. It is generally believed that smaller fraction sizes, longer treatment schedules, and smaller volumes will reduce late effects, but this must be weighed against the potential for ocular trauma when using shielding on a daily basis.[5] Optimum management of eyelid toxicity includes cleanliness, dressings for moist desquamation, healing time, and artificial tears to mitigate meibomian gland dysfunction.

Conjunctiva

Acute conjunctivitis is common with doses ≥30 Gy, and superimposed occasional bacterial or rarely viral infections may occur.[6] Conjunctivitis can be reduced by treating with an open eye with megavoltage equipment if the clinical situation permits. Treatment of acute conjunctivitis involves artificial tears to relieve symptoms and treatment of an underlying infection when indicated.

Lacrimal System

The lacrimal gland system includes the main lacrimal glands, accessory lacrimal glands, and lacrimal duct system, and symptoms of dryness can occur if any of these structures receive radiation. The most concerning late effect is "dry eye syndrome," where patients can experience tearing, redness, discharge, foreign body sensation, blurred vision, and photophobia. Moderate-dose orbital RT (30 to 45 Gy) can cause dry eye syndrome 4 to 11 years after treatment, whereas higher doses (>57 Gy) can produce it in 9 to 10 months.[7] Lacrimal shielding should be used if it does not compromise tumor control. Similarly, if clinically feasible, shielding the accessory lacrimal glands may reduce toxicity if the main gland is irradiated. IMRT can help minimize risks of RT-induced xerophthalmia, and prophylactic nasolacrimal duct intubation with silicone tubing may be considered in high-risk patients.[8,9] Treatments available for RT-induced xerophthalmia include topical lubricants, moist chamber goggles, punctual occlusion with plugs, or tarsorrhaphy.

Cornea

Although RT can directly injure the cornea, most acute corneal toxicity results from loss of the tear film with secondary

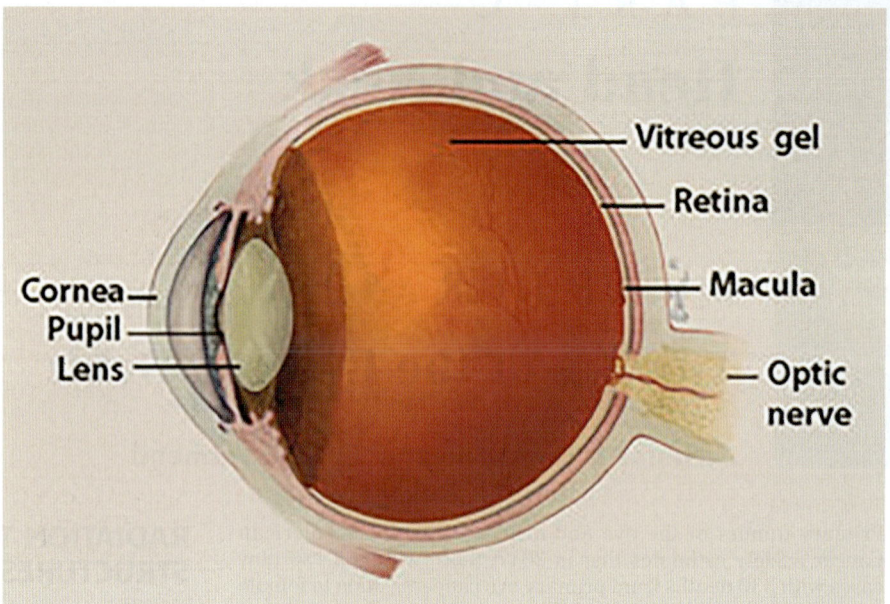

FIGURE 41.1. Normal eye anatomy. (Courtesy of National Eye Institute, National Institutes of Health.)

keratitis sicca. Punctate epithelial erosions are common after conventionally fractionated RT doses of 30 to 50 Gy.[10] They typically subside within several weeks but can persist for years. At higher doses, corneal edema (40 to 50 Gy) or perforation (60 Gy) may occur, causing pain, tearing, foreign body sensation, or reduced vision. Corneal toxicity can be reduced by using megavoltage equipment and reduce the surface dose or by using careful RT planning to minimize corneal irradiation so long as tumor dose is not compromised. Commercially available eye shields may also be used, particularly for electron beam RT.[11] There are little published data on management of corneal toxicity from RT. Close ophthalmologic follow-up is recommended, so topical treatment with steroids or antibiotics can be administered when indicated.

Iris

The iris is relatively radioresistant, and thus, acute iritis is rare. However, persistent iritis, with symptoms such as pain, red eye, and blurred vision, has been observed after hypofractionated RT doses of 30 to 40 Gy and after doses ≥70 Gy given with conventional fractionation.[12] A problematic late effect of the iris is neovascular glaucoma, where patients may present with ocular pain, headache, photophobia, decreased vision, and redness.[13] Risk factors include higher radiation dose, diabetes, vitreous hemorrhage, and retinal detachment. Whenever possible, techniques that spare the anterior chamber should be adopted. The primary treatments for iritis and neovascular glaucoma are topical steroids and cycloplegic drops, respectively. Laser panretinal photocoagulation (PRP) or peripheral cryotherapy may prevent or delay the progression of glaucoma if performed early in the course of glaucoma development. However, in many cases, more aggressive intervention such as trabeculectomy may be required. Occasionally, progression to a blind, painful eye may necessitate enucleation. Therapies such as intravitreal bevacizumab as an adjunctive treatment to retinal ablative procedure appear to be promising for the management of iris neovascularization associated with neovascular glaucoma.[14]

Lens

The lens is exquisitely radiosensitive. Age at time of treatment, total dose, and fractionation contribute to cataract formation.[15,16] Hall estimated 50% risk of cataract for 1-Gy exposure to the lens during childhood.[15] In adults, higher doses are associated with radiation-induced cataract: After 2.5 to 6.5 Gy, there is a 33%

of progressive cataract with latent period of 8 years, whereas after 6.51 to 11.5 Gy, there is a 66% risk with a latent period of 4 years.[16] Cataract risk can be reduced by using customized lens shields and lens-sparing techniques or by using more fractionated RT schedules. IMRT may be used to reduce cataract risk by reducing overall lens dose. The corrective treatment for RT-induced cataract is surgery, which yields excellent results.

Retina

Radiation retinopathy is a late effect of RT that typically presents 6 months to 3 years after treatment, although cases have been reported as far as 15 years after therapy.[17] Patients may be asymptomatic or may complain of floaters or reduced visual acuity. Clinical signs include microaneurysms, telangiectasia, hard exudates, cotton wool spots, and neovascularization. The threshold dose for retinal damage is 30 to 35 Gy: In a Cochrane database review of RT for macular degeneration, no retinopathy or optic nerve damage was reported in 1,154 patients treated with doses up to 24 Gy.[18] The risk of retinopathy increases dramatically when doses exceed 50 Gy using standard fractionation.[19] Incidence as well as severity is also increased by coexistent diabetic retinopathy, hypertension, collagen vascular disease, simultaneous chemotherapy, and pregnancy.[20] No proven therapy exists for radiation retinopathy. Local photocoagulation may improve symptoms, and there is interest in intravitreal bevacizumab, albeit with marginal results: In a recent study from the Dunedin Hospital where patients with choroidal melanoma were treated with stereotactic RT, prophylactic treatment with intravitreal bevacizumab did not lower the rate of retinopathy.[21]

Optic Nerve

Like the retina, the optic nerve manifests toxicity months or years after RT, with a peak incidence at 18 months.[22] Radiation-induced optic neuropathy (RION) has a variable presentation and is related to the nerve fibers most affected, usually causing visual field defects. In a review by investigators from the Mayo Clinic, the risk of RION was almost zero with conventionally fractionated doses ≤50 Gy and still rare with maximum dose <55 Gy. The risk of RION increases from 3% to 7% at 55 to 60 Gy and is substantial (>7% to 20%) at doses >60 Gy.[23] Parsons, in a series of 131 patients (215 optic nerves) treated with RT for extracranial head and neck tumors, found no RION in nerves that received

<59 Gy.[24] Fraction size was of primary importance: In cases where >60 Gy was received, fraction size was more important than total dose in producing RION. The 15-year actuarial risk was 11% when fraction size was <1.9 Gy compared with 47% when fraction size was >1.9 Gy. A significant exception in development of RION appears to exist for patients treated for pituitary tumors, where toxicity has been reported at doses as low as 46 Gy in 1.8-Gy fractions.[23] Because there is no known effective therapy for RION, to minimize optic nerve, dose-sophisticated treatment planning must be implemented to minimize treatment volume, total dose, and especially dose per fraction.

MANAGEMENT OF BENIGN OCULAR DISEASES

Pterygium

Pterygium is a benign growth of fibrovascular tissue on the conjunctiva that can cause irritation, erythema of the cornea, and, in advanced cases, obstruct vision. The exact cause of pterygium is unknown, but it is associated with excessive exposure to wind, sunlight, or sand. It has also been postulated that ultraviolet light exposure may increase the risk of pterygium development.[25] At present, no reliable medical treatment exists to reduce or even prevent pterygium progression. If symptoms are severe, the only definitive treatment is surgical removal, which requires removal of the head, neck, and body of the pterygium. Without adjuvant treatment, surgical resection alone carries recurrence rates of 20% to 80%.[25] Therefore, adjunctive measures are recommended, which can be broadly classified as medical methods, beta-irradiation, and surgical methods. Intraoperative and postoperative mitomycin C are the most commonly used medical adjuncts, reducing recurrence rates to 3% to 37%.[26] However, topical chemotherapy is not commonly used out of concern for late complications including scleral sclerosis, infectious scleritis, perforation, or endophthalmitis, all with consequences that can impair vision.[27] Beta-irradiation has a historical role in management of pterygium. In a prospective randomized study, 96 eyes with primary pterygium received beta-irradiation with a strontium 90 after resection or sham radiation.[25] Local control was 93.2% for the irradiated group versus 33.3% for the sham radiation group. Like topical chemotherapy, however, beta-irradiation has generally been abandoned due to the risk of sight-threatening complications such as scleral necrosis, infectious scleritis, corneal perforation, and endophthalmitis.[28] Thus, this therapy is of historic interest. Surgical adjuvant therapy is the mainstay of management for primary and recurrent pterygium. Currently, conjunctival autografting is generally regarded as the procedure of choice because of its efficacy and long-term safety, with recurrence rates of 2% to 39% without the attendant sight-threatening complications of topical chemotherapy or beta-irradiation.[29]

Choroidal Hemangiomas

Choroidal hemangiomas are benign vascular tumors of the choroid. Although probably congenital in all cases, they are frequently undetected until after the second decade of life and can have a wide range of clinical features and treatment options.[30] These tumors are characterized as either circumscribed or diffuse. Most circumscribed choroidal hemangiomas are noted first when they produce visual symptoms caused by accumulation of serous subretinal fluid, degenerative changes in the macular retina, or both. In contrast to circumscribed choroidal hemangiomas, the diffuse variety is larger and associated with Sturge-Weber syndrome, a neurologic disorder marked by a distinctive port-wine stain on the forehead, scalp, or around the eye. This stain is a birthmark caused by an overabundance of capillaries near the surface of the skin. Blood vessels on the same side of the brain as the stain may also be affected. Diffuse tumors are usually diagnosed in young patients either because of the examination of the fundus prompted by a facial hemangioma (port-wine stain) or because of the visual impairment secondary to serous retinal detachment or hyperopic amblyopia (Fig. 41.2). The clinical course of either form of choroidal hemangioma is highly variable, with visual impairment ranging from none to total blindness. Neither variety of choroidal hemangioma metastasizes or transforms to malignancy. Therefore, the primary indication for treatment is to prevent loss of visual acuity.

Treatment alternatives include laser photocoagulation, thermotherapy, photodynamic therapy, and radiotherapy. Photocoagulation is beneficial for circumscribed lesions, but diffuse lesions have high recurrence rate and retinal damage is possible.[30] Low- to moderate-dose radiation using lens-sparing external beam photon irradiation, episcleral plaque therapy, proton beam therapy, and SRT have all been used in the treatment of choroidal hemangioma.[31] Total doses of 18 to 30 Gy delivered in 10 to 18 fractions of external beam photon RT can result in partial flattening of the hemangioma, resorption of subretinal fluid, and reattachment of the retina within 6 to 12 months.[32] Heimann reported no recurrence of subretinal fluid with a mean follow-up of 3.6 years.[32] In another series with follow-up of 66 months, Kivela found that subretinal fluid had reaccumulated in only 1 of 12 patients treated, thus demonstrating response durability.[33] In very advanced cases with retinal detachment, a higher dose of 36 Gy in fractions of 1.8 Gy appear to be efficacious, but larger series with longer follow-up are needed to reliably assess response durability and delayed side effects, including retinopathy and cataract formation.[32,33] Lens-sparing techniques, including three-dimensional conformal RT with computed tomography (CT) planning, should be considered to reduce the incidence of cataract formation.[34] Brachytherapy has also been used for choroidal hemangioma treatment, particularly for circumscribed. This treatment usually achieves resolution of subretinal fluid and reattachment

FIGURE 41.2. Diffuse choroidal hemangioma with exudative retinal detachment. (From Kubicka-Trząska A, Kobylarz J. Ruthenium-106 Plaque Therapy for Diffuse Choroidal Hemangioma in Sturge-Weber Syndrome. *Case Rep Ophthalmol Med* 2011; vol. 2011, Article ID 785686, 3 pages. doi:10.1155/2011/785686. Copyright © 2011 Agnieszka Kubicka-Trząska et al.)

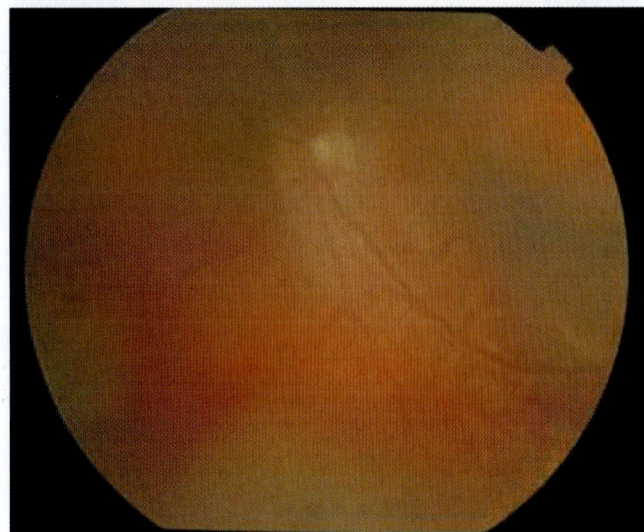

of the retina with preservation of pretreatment visual acuity.[35] Radiation dose varies with the isotope, but in a study using iodine 125 with target dose of 48 Gy to the apex of the lesion, tumor regression was noted in all 8 of 8 cases treated.[35] Long-term results of proton beam therapy have been reported from investigators at the Institut Curie: In a series of 71 cases with circumscribed choroidal hemangioma treated with 20 Cobalt Gray Equivalent, retinal reattachment occurred in all cases, and a completely flat scar was obtained in 91.5%.[36] The main complications during the surveillance period were cataract (28%) and radiation-induced maculopathy (8%). No cases of eyelid complications or neurovascular glaucoma were observed.

Capillary Hemangioma

Capillary hemangiomas are benign endothelial cell neoplasms that rarely occur on the eyelids or skin of the orbit. Retinal capillary hemangiomas may represent component of the von Hippel-Lindau syndrome (VHL), and lesions of the face that occupy the distribution of the trigeminal nerve can be a component of Sturge-Weber syndrome. The natural history of these lesions is usually spontaneous regression over 3 to 4 years, making conservative management the treatment of choice.[37] Occasionally, however, lesions may be large enough to obstruct vision and amblyopia may occur. Treatment options then include corticosteroids, interferon alfa-2a, laser therapy, embolization, immunomodulators, surgery, and systemic propranolol.[38] Because of these many alternatives, RT in the management of capillary hemangiomas is primarily of historical interest, with original studies showing that doses in the 16 to 20 Gy range provide effective local control.[39]

Orbital Pseudotumor

Orbital pseudotumor is a rare inflammatory process that affects the soft tissue components of the orbit. Clinically, it presents in the fourth and fifth decade of life with signs and symptoms including proptosis, swelling, increased orbital pressure, and restricted ocular motion.[40] The diagnosis is based on history, imaging of the orbit, and pathologic examination of tissue in accessible lesions. Characteristic imaging features include extraocular muscle enlargement, optic nerve thickening, and inflammation of retrobulbar adipose tissue. Treatment options for orbital pseudotumor include corticosteroids, external beam radiation therapy (EBRT), immunotherapy, chemotherapy, and surgery; corticosteroids are typically used as primary treatment.[41] Radiotherapy is usually reserved for cases that are refractory to corticosteroid treatment. Mathiesen recently described 20 orbits treated with a median dose of 20 Gy and at follow-up of 16.5 months found improved symptoms and/or reduction of corticosteroid dose in 87.5% with 56% able to discontinue steroid treatment completely.[42] Based on these observations, radiation appears to achieve durable control in orbital pseudotumor and is an effective strategy in patients who respond poorly to medical treatment.

Thyroid-Associated Orbitopathy

Thyroid-associated orbitopathy (TAO), frequently termed Graves ophthalmopathy, is part of an autoimmune process that can affect the orbital and periorbital tissue, the thyroid gland, and, rarely, the pretibial skin or digits (thyroid acropathy).[43] Although the use of the term thyroid ophthalmopathy is more general, the disease process is specifically an orbitopathy in which the orbital and periocular soft tissues are primarily affected with secondary effects on the eye. TAO may compromise a patient's vision by causing diplopia, decreased ocular motion, exposure keratitis, or optic neuropathy. A variety of treatments exist, starting with thyroid hormone regulation to the use of corticosteroids, external beam radiotherapy, or surgical decompression.[44] Radiation therapy with moderate doses has historically been used in cases refractory to medical therapy. Abboud reported symptom improvement in 87% of cases with doses of 20 Gy using standard fractionation.[45] However, prospective studies examining RT for TAO suggest that its role is unclear. Numerous randomized controlled trials have tested orbital RT for TAO, although studies differed with respect to severity of TAO on trial entry, radiation dose and fractionation, and inconsistent use of concurrent corticosteroids.[46-54] In controlled randomized trials, RT resulted in only a small benefit. Mourits randomized 59 patients to either 20 Gy in 10 fractions to both orbits or sham RT and found improved globe motility and elevation, but no difference in change in lid fissure, soft tissue swelling, proptosis, or clinical activity score (a measure of disease activity and propensity to progress).[50] The authors concluded that RT should be used only for motility impairment. Gorman randomized 42 subjects to orbit RT to one orbit and sham RT to the other followed by the reverse therapy 6 months later.[54] No clinically or statistically significant differences were observed at 6 months. At 12 months, muscle volume and proptosis were slightly improved in the orbit that was first irradiated. Prummel conducted a trial where 88 patients with mild TAO were randomly assigned to bilateral RT or sham RT.[53] Radiation was effective in improving motility and decreasing severe diplopia, but no differences in health-related quality of life were detected, although lack of complete quality of life data on 58% of subjects resulted in low power to detect a difference. Complications of orbital RT are rare but not insignificant. Even in the absence of known diabetes mellitus, the risk of definite retinopathy is 1% to 2% in the first 10 years after treatment.[55] Thus, based on randomized data, the role of RT for TAO remains controversial. A 2008 report on orbital RT for TAO by the American Academy of Opthhthalmology concluded that although extraocular motility may improve with RT, the evidence of treatment effect is controversial and more studies are needed to determine if improved motility translates into improved quality of life.[56] Part of difficulty in evaluating RT for TAO is that moderate to severe TAO is rare.[57] Therefore, from a practical management standpoint, a reasonable indication for RT, in combination with steroid therapy, is for patients that are refractory to steroid treatment alone.[58] Radiation technique for TAO usually involves treatment of both orbits with parallel-opposed lateral portals with low-energy (6-MV) photons. A downward 5-degree tilt or use of half-beam block should be used to avoid direct radiation of the contralateral lens.

OCULAR AND ORBITAL MALIGNANT TUMORS

Metastatic Carcinoma to the Uvea

Tumor metastases to the eye are more common than primary ocular cancers, with the uvea representing the most common site affected.[59] Shields and colleagues described a comprehensive series of usual metastases and found that within the uvea, 88% of metastases are to the choroid (Fig. 41.3), followed by metastases to the iris (9%) and ciliary body (2%).[2] This large difference is thought to reflect blood supply, which heavily favors the choroid as compared to the iris or ciliary body. The most common primary cancer sites for uveal metastasis in males were lung (40%), gastrointestinal (9%), and kidney (8%). The primary site was unknown at the time of presentation in 29% of males. In females, the most common sites included breast (68%), lung (12%), and other (4%).

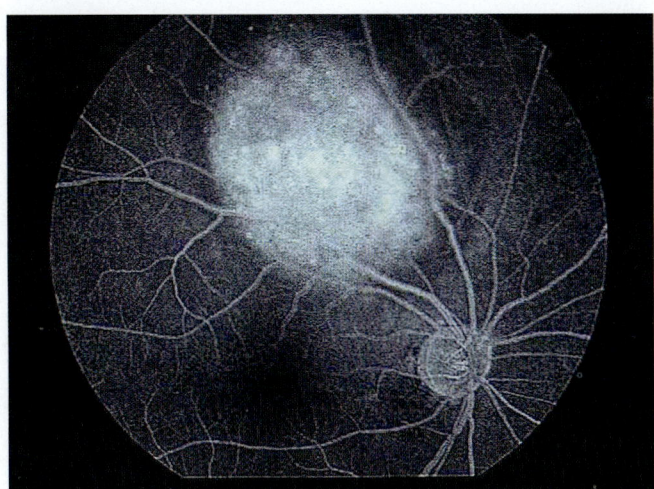

FIGURE 41.3. Fundus fluorescein angiography of choroidal metastasis from non–small cell lung cancer showing hyperfluorescence from the surface of the choroidal tumor in its late phase with the accumulation of subretinal fluid. (From Singh A, Singh P, Sahni K, et al. Non-small cell lung cancer presenting with choroidal metastasis as first sign and showing good response to chemotherapy alone: a case report. *J Med Case Rep* 2010;4:185.)

Metastases can be either unilateral or bilateral. In a study of 264 patients with uveal metastases from breast cancer reported by Demirci, 62% of patients had unilateral metastasis at presentation. Patients with breast cancer metastatic to the uvea show survival rates of 65% at 1 year, 35% at 3 years, and 24% at 5 years.[60]

Numerous treatment options exist for choroidal metastases, including systemic chemotherapy, hormonal therapy, EBRT, brachytherapy, or photodynamic therapy. Individualized treatment should be considered, taking into account disease extent and life expectancy with the primary goal of maintaining visual acuity. As systemic treatments for metastatic cancers improve, clinicians may be more frequently faced with treatment of symptomatic choroidal metastases. For cases with multifocal or diffuse presentations, external beam radiation has been effective with doses in the range of 20 to 40 Gy. Rosset described 58 patients (88 eyes) treated with external beam radiation with a median dose of 35.5 Gy (range 20 to 53 Gy) in 10 to 30 fractions.[61] Various techniques were used and lens sparing was achieved whenever possible. Visual acuity improved in 62% of patients, with significantly better results when doses >35.5 Gy were used. Complications include three cataracts, retinopathy in a single patient who underwent a biopsy, and one case of glaucoma from subretinal hemorrhage. In cases of unilateral disease undergoing bilateral radiation, the authors noted no cases of new contralateral lesions but did describe new contralateral lesions in 3 of 26 patients when unilateral technique was used. Although they recommended bilateral irradiation even for unilateral disease (Fig. 41.4), a case can be made for unilateral treatment, especially as modern techniques can more easily avoid the contralateral side and make retreatment feasible if necessary.

Plaque brachytherapy is usually reserved for solitary metastases. This modality offers precise, controlled radiation delivery to the eye and requires only 3 to 4 days of treatment, an important consideration in uveal metastases because many patients have limited survival expectancy. Clinical factors to consider for plaque therapy include the size and thickness of the lesion and the distance of the lesion from the optic nerve and foveola. Investigators from the Wills Eye Hospital studied 36 patients who received plaque radiotherapy either as primary or salvage treatment (after external radiation) for uveal metastases.[62] The mean duration of treatment was 86 hours and mean doses to the apex and base of the tumor were 68.8 and 235.6 Gy, respectively. Tumor regression was documented in 94% of cases with median follow-up of 11 months. Five of six cases where plaque therapy was used after suboptimal response to external irradiation were successfully salvaged. Complications from plaque radiotherapy are similar to those of external beam therapy, including dryness, radiation retinopathy, papillopathy, and cataract. The investigators concluded that plaque radiation is an effective, time-efficient method for treatment of selected solitary uveal metastases. Thus, both EBRT and plaque therapy are effective therapies for uveal metastases with the optimal treatment depending on the extent of intraocular disease, symptoms, and overall condition and prognosis of the patient. Close collaboration of ophthalmologists, radiation oncologists, and medical oncologists is imperative to tailor an appropriate treatment strategy for each patient.

Section III

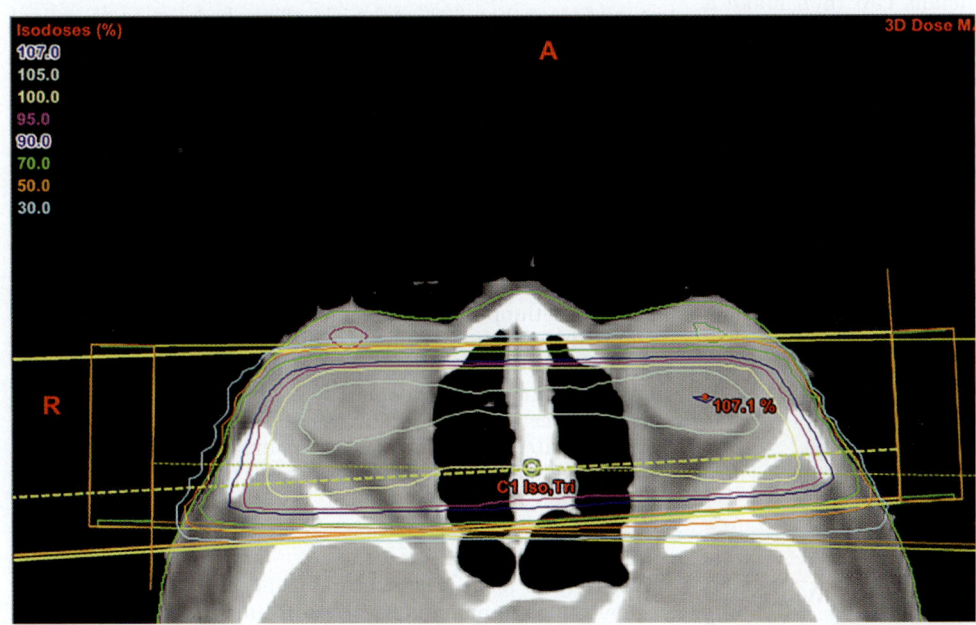

FIGURE 41.4. Bilateral radiation therapy for uveal metastases in a patient with widely metastatic lung cancer.

Malignant Melanoma of the Uvea

Uveal melanomas represent <5% of all malignant melanomas with approximately 2,580 new cases and 270 deaths per year in the United States.[63] These tumors may arise from any of the three parts of the uvea and are sometimes referred to by their location, such as iris melanoma (Fig. 41.5), ciliary body melanoma, or choroidal melanoma (Fig. 41.6). True iris melanomas, originating from within the iris as opposed to originating elsewhere and invading the iris, are distinct in their etiology and prognosis, such that the other tumors are often referred to collectively as "posterior uveal melanomas." Although uveal melanoma is rare among nonwhites, the role of sunlight and other environmental factors is unknown.[64] Detection of uveal melanoma is often by routine examination with or without symptoms; a study from the United Kingdom showed that 45% of patients were asymptomatic when their tumor was detected.[65] Advances in diagnostic techniques such as binocular indirect ophthalmoscopy, angiography, and B-scan ultrasonography have aided ocular oncologists in the evaluation and management of patients with uveal melanoma.[66]

Several treatment options exist for uveal melanoma. Most patients are treated with the goal of eradication of disease and long-term survival. There is evidence that local tumor recurrence is associated with increased mortality.[67] Factors predictive of local recurrence include epithelioid cell type, large tumor size, and posterior tumor extension.[68] When possible, curative treatment should be sought with the goal of preserving vision with acceptable cosmesis. In patients with known metastatic disease, the main objective is to preserve vision and remove any threat of the eye becoming painful within the patient's life expectancy. Many factors influence treatment selection, including tumor size, location, and extent; secondary effects, such as cataract; concurrent ocular disease, such as diabetic retinopathy; the patient's general health and life expectancy; and the cost and duration of the treatment.[69] In cases where maintaining useful vision is feasible, organ preservation therapy should be considered, and thus, RT delivered either externally or by brachytherapy has been instrumental in the primary management of uveal melanoma.

Observation

It is not uncommon for indeterminate pigmented uveal tumors to be observed without treatment until growth is documented. The probability of malignancy can be estimated according to tumor thickness, serous retinal detachment, orange pigment, and symptoms.[70] Patients and clinicians can then make a

FIGURE 41.5. Iris melanoma located at the inferonasal aspect of the eye. (From Papastefanou VP, Cohen VML. Uveal Melanoma. *J Skin Cancer* 2011; vol. 2011, Article ID 573974, 13 pages. doi:10.1155/2011/573974. Copyright © 2011 Vasilios P. Papastefanou and Victoria M. L. Cohen.)

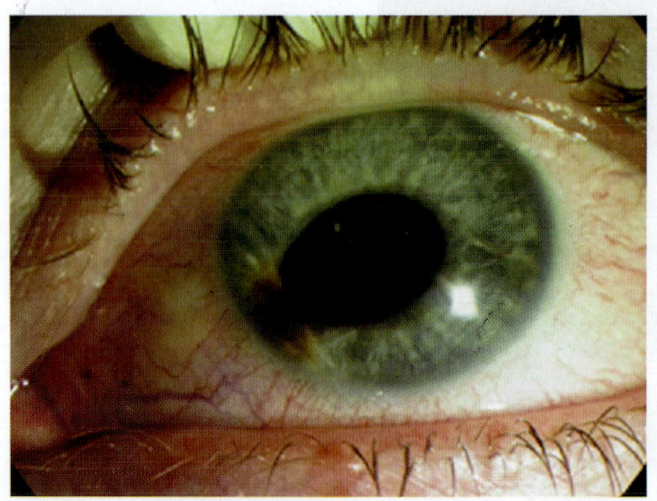

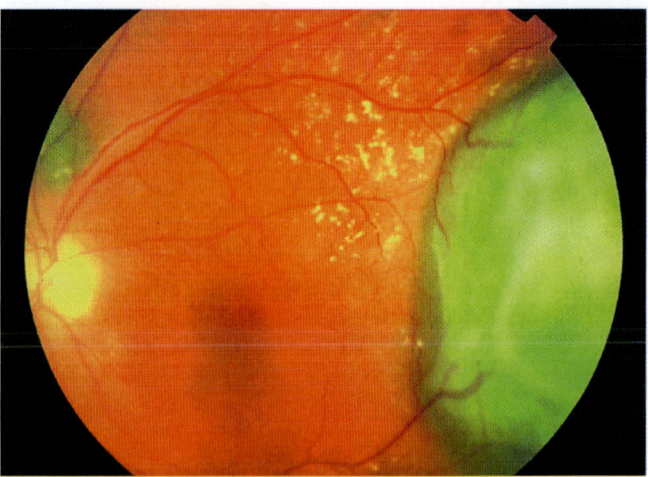

FIGURE 41.6. Typical choroidal melanoma with associated nonrhegmatogenous retinal detachment. (From Papastefanou VP, Cohen VML. Uveal Melanoma. *J Skin Cancer* 2011; vol. 2011, Article ID 573974, 13 pages. doi:10.1155/2011/573974. Copyright © 2011 Vasilios P. Papastefanou and Victoria M. L. Cohen.)

combined decision on when to commence therapy after discussion of risks and benefits.

Enucleation

Enucleation was traditionally the standard of care for choroidal melanoma since the late 19th century, but its effectiveness in improving survival has never been clearly demonstrated.[71] A study from the Helsinki University Hospital looked at the long-term prognosis of patients treated by enucleation between 1962 and 1981 and found death was attributable to melanoma in 61% of cases.[72] They also reported that cause-specific mortality (CSM) increased with longer follow-up. The 5-, 15-, 25-, and 35-year CSM was 31%, 45%, 49%, and 52%, respectively, thus illustrating that a substantial number of patients die of metastatic disease more than 5 years after enucleation. The desire to improve survival and preserve vision stimulated the development of alternative, organ-preserving therapies for uveal melanoma. Still, enucleation is required in a subset of patients, either because tumor is too extensive at presentation or if vision loss were likely to occur with conservative treatment. General guidelines for enucleation include tumor diameter >17 mm; thickness >6 to 7 mm; involvement of the optic disc; invasion of more than 30% of the iris, ciliary body, or angle; retinal perforation; or poor general health of the patient.[69]

Endoresection

Transretinal endoresection is controversial, mainly because of fears of seeding tumor cells, but has been advocated for juxtapapillary tumors up to 10 mm in diameter.[70] The operation involves vitrectomy; tumor removal with a vitrector either via a retinotomy or after lifting a retinal flap, fluid–air exchange to drain any subretinal fluid, endolaser photocoagulation to destroy any residual tumor in the sclera and to achieve retinopexy, air–silicone exchange, and, if possible, adjunctive brachytherapy.[73] Given the seemingly heightened risk of tumor seeding with endoresection, some investigators have recommended preoperative stereotactic radiation, but this practice is similarly controversial.[74] Endoresection carries approximately 10% risk of local recurrence, which can arise from microscopic disease in the scleral bed or at the margins of resection.[73]

Transscleral Resection

Transscleral local resection has been promoted for tumors >6 mm thick in patients highly motivated to retain vision and in patients with severe exudative retinal detachment after radiotherapy.[69] The procedure carries substantial operative risk. Choroidectomy and cyclochoroidectomy, for example, require hypotensive anesthesia with systolic blood pressure lowered to approximately 40 mm Hg.[75] The operation involves the preparation of a lamellar scleral flap, ocular decompression by limited pars plana vitrectomy, resection of the tumor together with the deep scleral lamella, suturing of the scleral flap, intraocular injection of balanced salt solution, and adjunctive brachytherapy either at the end of the operation or a several weeks later. This procedure has approximately 30% incidence of local relapse when performed exclusively, but this probability declines to approximately 10% when perioperative brachytherapy is delivered.[76]

Transpupillary Thermotherapy

Transpupillary thermotherapy (TTT) is a procedure in which 1-minute applications of 3-mm spots of low-energy diode laser are administered to the tumor and the surrounding choroid.[77] The objective is not immediate thermoablation but rather heating the tumor by only a few degrees so that following treatment, tumor regression occurs slowly, often resulting in a white scar. This technique may be used for indeterminate choroidal tumors. Some advocates of TTT recommend combined brachytherapy with TTT: Yaravoy and colleagues reported improved tumor regression and recurrence free survival with similar complication rates when TTT was used with brachytherapy compared with brachytherapy alone.[78]

Plaque Brachytherapy

Plaque brachytherapy is the mainstay of treatment in many centers, with iodine 125 and ruthenium-106 being the most common isotopes, although palladium 103 has also been used effectively.[79] Iodine emits gamma rays, which have a range sufficient for tumors up to 8 to 10 mm thick, whereas ruthenium delivers beta particles that have a more limited range, which is suitable for tumors <5 mm thick. Historically, the general objective with all plaques is to deliver approximately 80 Gy to the tumor apex by fixing the plaque in the exact location of the tumor (Figs. 41.7 and 41.8). However, recent data suggest lower doses may be sufficient for tumor control with less toxicity: Perez and colleagues examined 190 cases treated between 1988 and 2010 and analyzed outcome with respect to apical dose.[80] Local control and overall survival did not differ according to dose quartile (<69 Gy, 69 to 81 Gy, 81 to 89 Gy, >89 Gy). However, visual acuity and radiation complications increased

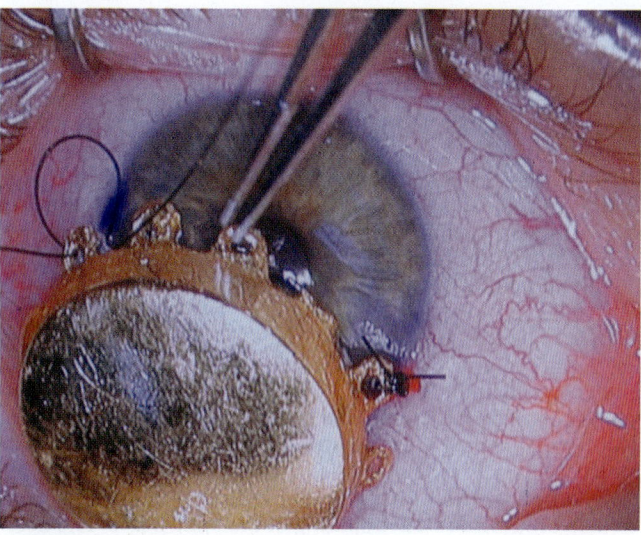

FIGURE 41.8. Plaque brachytherapy for melanoma of the iris. (From Khan MK, Khan N, Almasan A, et al. Future of radiation therapy for malignant melanoma in an era of newer, more effective biological agents. *Onco Targets Ther* 2011;4:137–148. Reproduced with permission of Dove Medical Press in the format Republish in a book via Copyright Clearance Center.)

with increasing dose and the authors concluded that doses as low as 69 Gy may be appropriate for uveal melanoma. Dedicated computer modeling has been developed for radiotherapy planning to create a three-dimensional model of the eye and determine the appropriate treatment time and estimated dose to the optic nerve, macula, and lens.[81] Tumors in approximating or overhanging the optic disc present a dosimetric challenge but may be treated with brachytherapy. Sagoo and associates reported on 141 such patients treated with plaque brachytherapy.[82] In 126 eyes, the plaque utilized a notched design, which created an elliptical dose distribution with median dose of 85 Gy. Local control was 90% and metastases developed in 13%. Visual acuity was generally poor, with 77% having final acuity of 20/200 or worse. However, given the alternative of enucleation, this technique represents a reasonable alternative.

The largest prospective experience of patients treated by plaque brachytherapy was conducted by the Collaborative Ocular Melanoma Study (COMS) group. From 1986 to 2003, COMS conducted two multicenter trials of brachytherapy with iodine 125 versus enucleation in selected patients with choroidal melanoma. Long-term results were subsequently published in COMS Report 28 in 2006, which evaluated 1,317 patients.[83] Eligible patients had unilateral choroidal melanoma with an apical height of 2.5 to 10 mm and a maximum basal tumor diameter (MBTD) of 16 mm. Patients whose tumors were contiguous with the optic disc were ineligible, as were patients with metastases from melanoma or another malignancy. Patients were followed for 5 to 15 years and within 12 years after enrollment and 471 of 1,317 (36%) died. Overall, CSM at 5 and 10 years for both treatment arms were 19% and 35%, respectively. Cumulative all-cause mortality was 43% in the iodine 125 arm and 41% in the enucleation, indicating that with long-term follow-up, no survival difference existed between plaque brachytherapy and enucleation. Age >60 years and MBTD >11 mm were the primary predictors of time to death. Local control was excellent in the COMS series with only 12.5% of patients requiring salvage enucleation.[84] Visual acuity after plaque brachytherapy depends on a number of features. Shields reported the outcome of 1,106 patients with baseline visual acuity of 20/100 or better who underwent brachytherapy for uveal melanoma and found 34% of patients had poor visual acuity at 5 years and 68% at 10 years, defined as 20/200 to no light perception.[85] Factors adversely affecting visual acuity were age >60 years, poor vision at baseline,

FIGURE 41.7. Eye anatomy and plaque placement in location of tumor. (From Chaudhari S, Deshpande S, Anand V, et al. Dosimetry and treatment planning of Occu-Prosta I-125 seeds for intraocular lesions. *J Med Phys* 2008;33:14–18. Copyright © 2008 Journal of Medical Physics. Reprinted with permission of Wolters Kluwer Medknow Publications.)

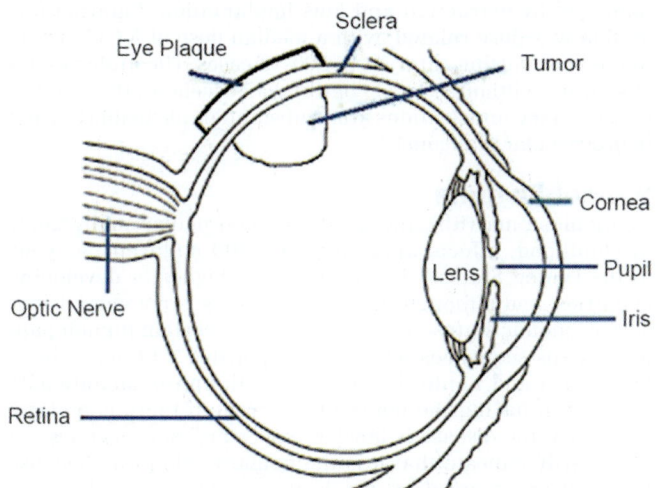

increasing tumor thickness (>8 mm), proximity to the foveola of <5 mm, recurrent tumor, subretinal fluid, and history of diabetes or hypertension. Best results were obtained in eyes with small tumors outside a radius of 5 mm from the optic disc and foveola. The American Brachytherapy Society updated their consensus guidelines on plaque therapy for uveal melanoma in 2014 and determined that brachytherapy is appropriate for the majority of uveal melanomas.[86] Exceptions include tumors with >5 mm of extraocular extension, basal diameters that exceed the limits of brachytherapy applicators, patients with blind and painful eyes, and patients with no light perception.

Proton Beam Therapy

Proton beam therapy may be used to treat uveal melanoma and is usually indicated for tumors that extend close to or are contiguous with the optic disc, referred to as parapapillary and peripapillary tumors, respectively.[87] Because of the dosimetric properties of protons, which deliver a homogeneous dose to tumor with a sharp field edge, a high tumor dose can be delivered with relative sparing of the optic nerve. The decision to use proton therapy over other forms of external beam radiation, such as helium ions or SRT, often depends on the availability of treatment facilities. One of the largest experiences in proton beam therapy for uveal melanoma is from the Harvard Medical School.[88] Treatment planning involves intraoperative examination by transillumination or indirect ophthalmoscopy, and the edges of the tumor are delineated by four tantalum rings sutured to the sclera. For tumors of the ciliary body and peripheral choroid, surgery is not performed; transillumination is instead used to define tumor margins in relation to the iris and cornea. Radiation planning is done with an interactive three-dimensional computer system to define the beam aperture and range modulation needed to adequately encompass the tumor with a 1.5 mm to allow for motion during treatment, setup error, and possible microscopic extension.[89] Patients receive a total dose of 70 Cobalt Gray Equivalents (CGE), which is delivered in five equal fractions over 7 to 10 days (63.6 proton Gy × 1.1 relative biologic effectiveness = 70 CGE).[86] The Harvard group recently reported long-term follow-up in a series of 573 patients with peripapillary and parapapillary melanomas with median surveillance of 96.3 months.[85] Local recurrence was rare, with 5- and 10-year local recurrence of 3.3% and 6%, respectively, and similarly high rates of local control have been observed in a larger series from the same institution.[90] Enucleation rates were 13.3% and 17.1% at 5 and 10 years after treatment, respectively. Of 450 patients with baseline visual acuity of 20/200 or better, two-thirds had visual acuity <20/200 years after treatment, although 56% could count fingers. The most common complications were radiation maculopathy and/or papillopathy. By 3 years, the cumulative rate of both complications was 49%, and by 10 years, it increased to 61% for papillopathy and 68% for maculopathy. The visual outcome after proton therapy depends on the height of the tumor and its location relative to the fovea and optic nerve.[88] Anterior segment severe complications, such as rubeosis iridis and neovascular glaucoma, occur less frequently, with each occurring in approximately 15% of cases at 5 years postradiation.[91] These results indicate that although visual acuity is compromised with proton beam therapy, particularly in patients with juxtapapillary lesions, some preservation is possible and eye conservation is likely with low rates of local recurrence.

Stereotactic Radiotherapy

Stereotactic radiation can be delivered by linear accelerator (LINAC) or by specialized devices for focused radiation such as the Leksell gamma knife. Because gamma knife treatment is usually done in a single fraction, the term radiosurgery is applied, whereas for LINAC-based treatment, single-fraction or multifraction treatment are possible.

Gamma knife radiosurgery (GKR) for uveal melanoma was introduced in 1998 by investigators at the Indiana University School of Medicine.[92] Nineteen patients with uveal melanoma were treated to a dose of 40 Gy prescribed to the 50% isodose line. With median follow-up of 40 months, 3- and 5-year overall survival rates were 86% and 55%, respectively. The 3- and 5-year tumor control rates were both 94%. Six of the 19 treated patients (32%) developed distant metastasis 31 to 75 months after GKR. Out of the 19 patients treated, 2 had improved, 4 had stable, and 13 had worse vision in the treated eye. Similar results were reported in a larger series of 78 patients from investigators in Milan.[93] The dose was adjusted over the treatment period: 7 patients received 50 Gy at the 50% isodose line (1994–1995), 21 patients received 40 Gy to the 50% isodose line (1995–1999), and 47 patients received 35 Gy to the 50% isodose line (2000 through 2006). Local tumor control was achieved in 91.0% of patients, and the eye retention rate was 89.7%. A significant relative reduction of visual acuity was observed during follow-up most commonly because of the exudative retinopathy (33.3%), neovascular glaucoma (18.7%), radiogenic retinopathy (13.5%), and vitreous hemorrhage (10.4%).

One theoretical disadvantage of single-dose stereotactic radiosurgery is the potential for complications. In particular, severe radiation retinopathy is dose dependent with respect to both total dose (>25 Gy) and dose per fraction (>2 Gy).[94,95] Muller and colleagues conducted a prospective study on 102 patients with uveal melanoma treated with fractionated SRT between 1999 and 2007.[96] Patients had uveal melanoma of the choroid or ciliary body with a tumor thickness smaller than 12 mm and diameter <16 mm with no metastases. The SRT technique, like GKR, utilized a fixed immobilization system, and a dose of 50 Gy was delivered in five equal fractions on 5 consecutive days using 6-MV photons with stereotactic arcs. With median follow-up of 32 months, local control was achieved in 96% of patients. Fifteen enucleations were performed 2 to 85 months after radiation, and best corrected visual acuity (defined as 20/x while using glasses if needed) decreased from a mean of 0.26 at diagnosis to 0.16 at 3 months postradiation and declined to 0.03 at 4 years after therapy. Deterioration of visual acuity was in part related to complications. Grade 3 to 4 neurovascular glaucoma occurred in 9 patients, 8 of which required enucleation. In these 9 patients, tumors were not anteriorly located, nor did they receive a high dose to the ciliary body, as one might expect, but were associated with grade 3 retinopathy. The authors hypothesized that the physical reaction of ischemic retinopathy might also affect vessels in the ciliary body. Thirteen patients (13%) developed grade 3 or 4 optic neuropathy, which was associated with posterior tumors and optic nerve dose, which was limited to 4 Gy/fraction. Grade 3 cataracts occurred in 10 patients (10%) and were managed by extraction and lens implantation. Cataract formation was dose related, with a median dose of 5 Gy/fraction to the lens causing cataract in 50% of cases. The authors concluded that although local control was excellent, the number of secondary enucleations was substantial, particularly from neurovascular glaucoma.

Retinoblastoma

Retinoblastoma (Rb), the most common ocular malignancy in childhood, affects approximately 300 children per year in the United States.[94] The incidence is higher in developing countries, and although the reason for this is not clear, lower socioeconomic status and the presence of certain human papillomavirus sequences have been implicated.[95] Rb has a heritable form and nonheritable form, with approximately 55% of children having the nonheritable form. If there is no family history, the disease is labeled "sporadic," but this does not necessarily indicate that it is the nonheritable form, because bilateral cases, most of which are heritable, also have no family history. Rb can present with unilateral disease (two-thirds of cases), with bilateral disease, or rarely with tumor in both eyes and the pineal gland, which is called trilateral disease.[97] Approximately 80% of children in Rb are diagnosed before the age of 3, with unilateral cases diagnosed at an earlier age (14 to 16 months) than those with bilateral presentations (29 to 30 months).[98] Histologically, Rb develops from immature retinal cells and replaces the retina and other intraocular tissues. Macroscopically, viable tumor cells are found near blood vessels, whereas zones of necrosis are found in relatively avascular areas. Microscopically, both undifferentiated and differentiated elements may be present. Undifferentiated elements appear as collections of small, round cells with hyperchromatic nuclei; differentiated elements include Flexner-Wintersteiner rosettes, Homer-Wright rosettes, and fleurettes from photoreceptor differentiation.[99]

The study of Rb has provided insights into the genetic basis of cancer. The Rb gene (*RB1*) is located on the long arm of chromosome 13 (13q14). In order for Rb to develop, both copies of the gene at the 13q14 locus must be lost, deleted, mutated, or inactivated. If either the maternal or paternal copy of the gene that is inherited by an individual is defective, then that individual is heterozygous for the mutant allele. Tumor formation requires both alleles of the gene to be mutant or inactive. These two mutations correlate to the two "hits" theorized by Knudson, which was based on the finding that children with bilateral Rb developed multifocal, bilateral tumors at an earlier age than those with unifocal, unilateral tumors.[100,101] The first "hit" can be inherited and would be present in all cells in the body, and the second "hit" results in loss of the remaining normal allele and occurs within a particular retinal cell or cells with dysregulation of the cell cycle.[102] In sporadic, nonheritable Rb, both hits occur within a single retinal cell after fertilization (somatic events), thus resulting in unilateral Rb. Identifying the *RB1* mutation can have management implications both in the affected child as well as siblings and future offspring. For example, if *RB1* mutation is detected, then siblings, children, and other relatives can be tested for the mutation. If they carry the mutation, they need to undergo rigorous examinations under anesthesia to rule out Rb.[103]

The most common and obvious sign of Rb is leukocoria, a discoloration of the pupil (Fig. 41.9). Less common and less specific signs and symptoms are deterioration of vision, a red or irritated eye, faltering growth, or developmental delay. Children with retinoblastoma can develop a squint, commonly referred to as "cross eyed" or "wall-eyed," indicating strabismus.[104] In developing countries, eye enlargement is a common finding of advanced disease. Funduscopy typically reveals a white-colored main tumor (Fig. 41.10), frequently with satellite lesions in the retina, subretinal space, and/or vitreous referred to as "seeds." Secondary serous retinal detachment may be associated with large lesions. To confirm these findings, a detailed examination under anesthesia through dilated pupils is performed.

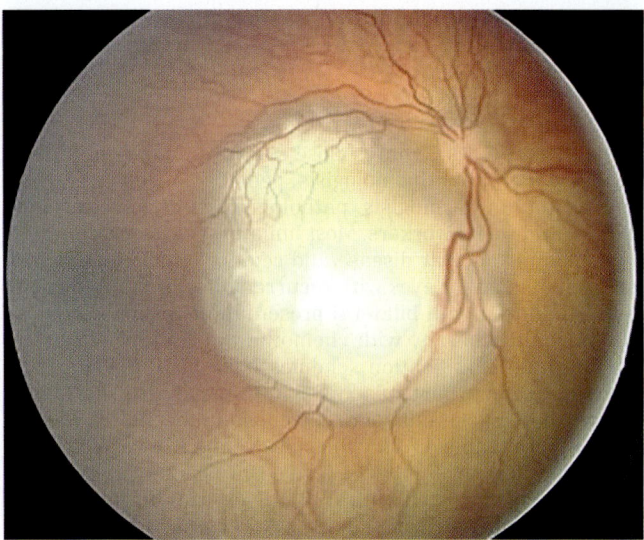

FIGURE 41.10. Retinoblastoma on funduscopic exam. (From Aerts I, Lumbroso-Le Rouic L, Gauthier-Villars M, et al. Retinoblastoma. *Orphanet J Rare Dis* 2006;1:31.)

Ultrasonography of the eyes is often performed to evaluate the intraocular mass with attention to heterogeneity and calcifications, which support a diagnosis of Rb. Ultrasonography is not as sensitive as CT, which is the ideal imaging choice to detect intraocular calcifications. Although CT raises the concern of exposure to radiation in children <1 year of age with germ line mutations,[105] it is still frequently used to confirm the diagnosis, particularly in developing countries. Magnetic resonance imaging (MRI) of the brain and orbits is the most sensitive means of evaluating for extraocular extension and also provides better delineation of the optic nerve and the pineal area.[106] MRI of the brain and spinal cord and cerebral spinal fluid examination are indicated when there is gross invasion of the optic nerve by imaging studies or evidence of microscopic involvement beyond the lamina cribrosa on histopathologic examination of the enucleated eye. A bone marrow examination and a bone scan are indicated only in cases of an abnormal blood count or clinical symptoms suggesting osseous metastases. The diagnosis of retinoblastoma is based on examination by an ophthalmologist and imaging studies. Biopsy is generally not performed due to the theoretical risk for extraocular dissemination, which could convert an intraocular, curable tumor into extraocular, metastatic disease.

Rb can spread in a variety of ways, including direct invasion of the optic nerve into the chiasm or dissemination through the subarachnoid space to the brain and spinal cord. Tumors can also invade the choroid and the vascular layer and spread via blood to the bone and bone marrow.[107,108] Anterior spread can occur and involve the aqueous

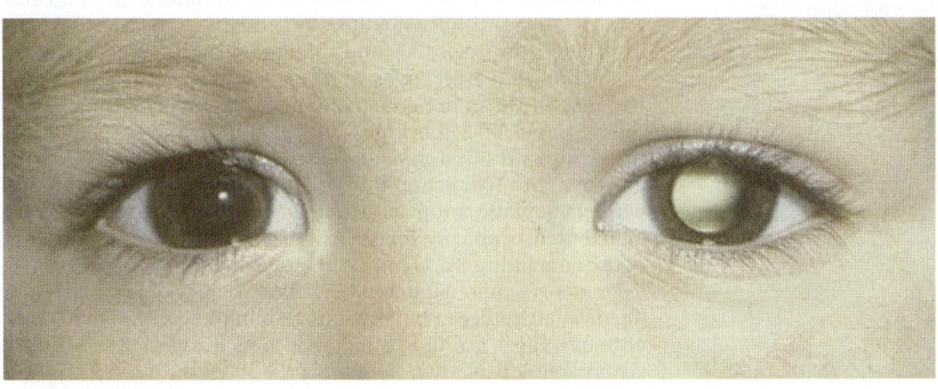

FIGURE 41.9. Leukocoria from retinoblastoma. (From Aerts I, Lumbroso-Le Rouic L, Gauthier-Villars M, et al. Retinoblastoma. *Orphanet J Rare Dis* 2006;1:31.)

venous channels, conjunctiva, and lymphatics or invade the sclera into the orbit with eventual spread to regional lymph nodes.

Treatment

Management of Rb requires close cooperation of a multidisciplinary team of ophthalmologists, pediatric oncologists, pediatric radiation oncologists, pathologists, genetic counselors, nurses, and social workers. Most unilateral cases present with advanced intraocular disease and require enucleation, which is also indicated for eyes with recurrent disease and no useful vision. Children with bilateral presentations typically require multimodality therapy with chemotherapy and local therapy. Staging and classification schemes have been developed to assess outcomes, particularly for intraocular Rb. The Reese-Ellsworth (R-E) classification, developed in the 1960s, was the first of these (Table 41.1).[109] Specifically, the R-E classification, which has five groups, was devised to predict prognosis in eyes that were treated with EBRT. Eyes with disease consistent with the lower groups have a lower risk for enucleation following EBRT, whereas group V eyes have the highest risk for enucleation. In recent years, chemotherapy has diminished the role EBRT for intraocular disease and thus the R-E classification is less useful. Alternative grouping systems have been proposed by Shields and Murphree, among others.[110,111] The International Retinoblastoma Classification, developed by a consensus panel in Paris in 2003, is used by many cooperative study groups (Table 41.2). An additional system has been proposed by Chantada designed to address extraocular disease and microscopic disease following enucleation.[112]

Enucleation

Most children with unilateral Rb present with advanced disease and require enucleation. Other indications for enucleation are cases of bilateral disease where the eye with more advanced disease does not respond to chemotherapy or other treatments, when active tumor is present in an eye with no vision, when glaucoma is present as a result of neovascularization of the iris or tumor invasion into the anterior chamber, and when direct visualization of an active tumor is obstructed by conditions including hemorrhage, corneal opacity, or cataract.[113] Enucleation is curative in >95% of patients with unilateral disease. Orbital implants are often used and connected to orbital muscles, and excellent cosmesis can be achieved.

External Beam Radiation Therapy

Rb is a highly radiosensitive tumor as first shown by Hilgartner in 1903.[114] By virtue of its radiosensitive nature, Rb was historically treated with first-line EBRT in a majority of cases, with doses of 42 to 50 Gy given in 1.5 to 2 Gy/fraction

TABLE 41.2 INTERNATIONAL CLASSIFICATION OF RETINOBLASTOMA

Group	Subgroup	Quick Reference	Features
A	A	Small tumor	Retinoblastoma ≤3 mm in size[a]
B	B	Larger tumor	Retinoblastoma >3 mm in size[a] or
		Macula	Macular retinoblastoma location (<3 mm to foveola)
		Juxtapapillary	Juxtapapillary retinoblastoma location (≤1.5 mm to disc)
		Subretinal fluid	Clear subretinal fluid ≤3 mm from margin
C		Focal seeds	Retinoblastoma with
	C1		Subretinal seeds ≤3 mm from retinoblastoma
	C2		Vitreous seeds ≤3 mm from retinoblastoma
	C3		Both subretinal and vitreous seeds ≤3 mm from retinoblastoma
D		Diffuse seeds	Retinoblastoma with
	D1		Subretinal seeds >3 mm from retinoblastoma
	D2		Vitreous seeds >3 mm from retinoblastoma
	D3		Both retinal and vitreous seeds >3 mm from retinoblastoma
E		Extensive	Extensive retinoblastoma occupying >50% globe or
			Neovascular glaucoma
			Opaque media from hemorrhage in anterior chamber, vitreous, or subretinal space
			Invasion of postlaminar optic nerve, choroid (>2 mm), sclera, orbit, anterior chamber

[a]Refers to 3 mm in basal dimension or thickness.

resulting in 87% eye preservation in R-E groups I to IV versus 29% in group V eyes.[115] In recent decades, however, the trend has been to avoid RT when possible out of concern of growth deformities of the bony orbit and mortality related to osteosarcoma development.[116,117] However, EBRT still has a viable role in the management of Rb, particularly as salvage treatment in tumors that are refractory to chemotherapy and other local therapies. Other indications include lesions that are too large, numerous or close to the optic disc or fovea for focal therapy to preserve central vision. EBRT also has a special role in treating eyes with vitreous seeds.[118] Chan reported on 36 eyes that received EBRT after incomplete response to primary chemotherapy and focal therapies in 22 patients with bilateral Rb.[119] Thirty-two received lens-sparing EBRT, and the remainder received whole eye EBRT to a dose of 40 to 44 Gy in 20 to 22 fractions. The rate of eye preservation was 83%, and 67% required no further treatment. Visual acuity was recorded for 19 eyes, of which 10 read 6/9-6/5, 3 read 6-18-6/36, and 6 read 6/60 or worse. Side effects were limited to cataracts and dry eyes although follow-up (median 40 months) was insufficient to assess second malignancies. The investigators concluded that EBRT was highly effective in preserving eyes with useful vision in bilateral Rb in cases refractory to chemotherapy and focal therapies. In a more advanced population, Kingston evaluated consolidative EBRT (40 to 44 Gy) in 14 patients with R-E group V eyes after induction chemotherapy with carboplatin, etoposide, and vincristine.[120] Four eyes were enucleated primarily for severe disease at presentation, and of the remaining 20, 6 required enucleation (4 for recurrence, 2 for neovascular glaucoma). Of the 12 surviving children, 5 have visual acuity of better than 1/60 in at least one eye. Thus, although most group V eyes could be salvaged, the resultant visual acuity was often poor.

TABLE 41.1 REESE-ELLSWORTH CLASSIFICATION OF RETINOBLASTOMA

Group 1: Very favorable for maintenance of sight
A. Solitary tumor, smaller than 4 disc diameters (DD), at or behind the equator
B. Multiple tumors, none larger than 4 DD, all at or behind the equator

Group 2: Favorable for maintenance of sight
A. Solitary tumor, 4 to 10 DD at or behind the equator
B. Multiple tumors, 4 to 10 DD behind the equator

Group 3: Possible maintenance of sight
A. Any lesion anterior to the equator
B. Solitary tumor, larger than 10 DD behind the equator

Group 4: Unfavorable for maintenance of sight
A. Multiple tumors, some larger than 10 DD
B. Any lesion extending anteriorly to the ora serrata

Group 5: Very unfavorable for maintenance of sight
A. Massive tumors involving more than one half of the retina
B. Vitreous seeding

Radiation techniques in Rb should provide uniform coverage of the entire retina approaching the ora serrata and coverage of up to 10 mm of the optic nerve while sparing the lens and bony anatomy to the extent possible.[116] In practice, the dual goals of irradiating the entire retina and protecting the lens present a difficult challenge. Historically, a single lateral field was used for the management of one eye and parallel-opposed fields for the management of both eyes. The traditional border for these "D-shaped" fields was the lateral rim of the bony orbit, which could result in underdosing of the anterior retina with associated local failure. McCormick reported local failure in two-thirds of cases when a lens-sparing lateral technique was used.[121] Based on these concerns, more sophisticated techniques were developed, such as the anterior lens-sparing technique, modified lateral field techniques using oblique angles, anterior treatment techniques using electrons, and multiple noncoplanar arcs.[122-125]

Intensity-modulated radiation therapy (IMRT) is well suited for the treatment of small tumors such as Rb. Krasin performed a planning study that favored the use of IMRT over conformal, anterior–lateral photon and anterior electron plans for the treatment of the entire globe.[126] IMRT resulted in the greatest sparing of the surrounding bony orbit and other normal tissues. As acute and late toxicity is related to volume and dose of normal tissue irradiated, proton therapy has been considered for the treatment of Rb, with the added advantage of reducing low-dose exposure of normal tissue. Lee compared protons with three-dimensional conformal RT, IMRT, and electron therapy when treating the entire retina and vitreous cavity.[127] Protons provided superior coverage with greater sparing of normal tissue, with potential for a superior therapeutic ratio. Krengli reached similar conclusions looking at target coverage and lens sparing using protons for various intraocular tumor locations and beam arrangements.[128] Mouw and colleagues from the Massachusetts General reported clinical outcomes on 49 Rb patients (66 eyes) treated with proton beam therapy between 1986 and 2012.[129] At a median follow-up of 8 years, no patients died of retinoblastoma or developed metastases. The posttreatment enucleation rate was 18% and only 11% in patients with stage A to B disease (International Classification for Intraocular Retinoblastoma). Twelve eyes (20%) required intervention for a complication (mainly cataract) and no in-field second malignancies were reported. Based on these dosimetric and clinical data, proton beam irradiation should be favored in the management of Rb. Historically, patients with hereditary disease who received EBRT have a cumulative incidence of second cancers of 35%, compared with 6% among nonirradiated patients. This risk is even higher if treatment takes place before 1 year of age.[130] Cataracts, optic nerve damage, total retinal vascular occlusion, vitreous hemorrhage, and facial and temporal bone hypoplasia are other complications associated with EBRT therapy.[131]

Brachytherapy

Brachytherapy with iodine 125, gold, and more recently ruthenium have been used in selected cases of Rb.[132] The intention is to deliver a dose of 40 to 45 Gy transsclerally to the apex of the tumor over a period of 2 to 4 days. This treatment is limited to tumors that are <16 mm in base and 8 mm in thickness and can be used as the primary treatment or, more frequently, in patients who had failed initial therapy including previous EBRT.[133] Shields described 79% local control at 5 years using this method.[134] Side effects are generally less common than with EBRT and include optic neuropathy, radiation retinopathy, and cataract formation. Second malignancies do not appear to be associated with this type of local therapy. Relative contraindications include larger tumors and those that involve the macula.

Thermotherapy

Thermotherapy involves the application of heat directly to the tumor with infrared radiation. A temperature between 45°C and 60°C is reached, which is below the coagulative threshold and therefore spares the retinal vessels from coagulation.[135] Thermotherapy alone can be used for small lesions that are ≤3 mm in diameter without vitreous or subretinal seeds. In a study of 91 tumors, 92% of the tumors that were <1.5 mm in diameter were controlled with thermotherapy alone.[133]

Chemothermotherapy and Laser Photocoagulation

Larger tumors or tumors with subretinal seeds are usually treated with a combination of thermotherapy and chemotherapy (chemothermotherapy), usually delivered within hours of each other. In one study of 188 retinoblastomas, tumor control was achieved in 86% of cases.[136] Complications included focal iris atrophy, paraxial lens opacity, sector optic disk atrophy, retinal traction, optic disk edema, retinal vascular occlusion, retinal detachment, and corneal edema. Chemothermotherapy may be especially useful for patients with small tumors adjacent to the fovea and optic nerve, where RT or laser photocoagulation may result in significant visual loss. Laser photocoagulation is recommended only for small posterior tumors with the goal of coagulating the tumor's blood supply.[137] Effective therapy usually requires 2 to 3 sessions at monthly intervals. Complications of this treatment include retinal detachment, retinal vascular occlusion, retinal traction, and preretinal fibrosis.

Cryotherapy

Cryotherapy induces tumor tissue to freeze rapidly, resulting in damage to the vascular endothelium with secondary thrombosis and infarction of the tumor tissue. It may be used as primary therapy for small peripheral tumors or for small recurrent tumors previously treated with other modalities. Tumors are typically treated three times per session, with one or two sessions at monthly intervals. Ninety percent of tumors <3 mm in diameter are cured permanently, and complications are few and rarely serious.[138] Transient conjunctival edema and transient localized serous retinal detachments can occur. Vitreous hemorrhage can be observed in large or previously irradiated tumors.

Chemotherapy

Chemotherapy has been used to treat intraocular retinoblastoma since the early 1990s. It is used to reduce the size of the tumor to allow local ophthalmologic therapies, including cryotherapy, laser photocoagulation, or thermotherapy to eradicate the remaining disease. This combination of therapies has been promoted to avoid EBRT and/or enucleation and thereby decrease the potential for long-term side effects while salvaging useful vision. The common indications for chemotherapy for intraocular Rb include tumors that cannot be effectively treated with local therapies alone, usually because of the size. Chemotherapy may be indicated in children with unilateral or bilateral disease, but many patients with unilateral disease are diagnosed with advanced disease and require enucleation. Numerous studies have been published that show that chemotherapy is effective in eliminating the need for EBRT or enucleation in R-E group I to III eyes while proving to be significantly less successful in eyes with group IV or V disease.[139-142] Carboplatin, vincristine, and etoposide are generally used, and cyclosporine has been added to the regimen in some institutions in order to reduce drug resistance.[143] Chemotherapy regimens from different investigators vary in the number and frequency of cycles, but they are generally well tolerated, with the expected side effects of myelosuppression and associated risk of infection. A risk of second malignancy also exists, especially when using etoposide.[144] Chemotherapy alone is not very effective in avoiding EBRT or enucleation in patients with R-E group V eyes, especially those with vitreous seeds. Friedman showed that only 53% of 30 group V eyes could be controlled with chemotherapy alone.[145] Based on these data, modern regimens incorporate carboplatin, vincristine, and etoposide along with sub-tenon (the virtual space between the capsule and the sclera) carboplatin for more advanced patients.[146] Eyes with diffuse vitreous seeding rarely respond to chemotherapy alone, and although EBRT is modestly successful, other approaches are needed. Therapies for patient with vitreous or subretinal seeding include intra-arterial chemotherapy (IAC) with selective catheterization of the ophthalmic artery. In a landmark study, Gobin described 78 patients (95 eyes) treated with IAC with melphalan with or without topotecan and evaluated procedure success, event-free (RT or enucleation) ocular survival, and ocular and extraocular complications.[147] The procedure succeeded in 98.5% of cases, and the ocular event-free survival rates at 2 years were 70% for all eyes, 82% for eyes that received IAC as primary treatment, and 58% for eyes that had prior treatment with chemotherapy or EBRT, and there were no permanent complications. Abramson reported similarly encouraging results in 67 patients (76 eyes) treated with IAC.[148] Among previously untreated patients, the ocular salvage rate was 83% for eyes with subretinal seeding only, 64% for eyes with vitreous seeding only, and 80% for eyes with both. Patients with persistent or recurrent vitreous seeding after primary treatment require more novel approaches. Gohssemi and colleagues tested combined intravitreal melphalan and topotecan in 9 such eyes followed by cryotherapy and control was achieved in 6 eyes (66%) using 1 to 3 injections, with 33% requiring enucleation because of the disease persistence.[149]

Management of Extraocular Disease

Patients with extraocular disease historically have had a poor prognosis, but studies using combinations of chemotherapy and EBRT have been encouraging. Chantada reported a 5-year EFS rate of 84% in 15 patients with orbital or preauricular disease treated with chemotherapy that included vincristine, doxorubicin, and cyclophosphamide or vincristine, idarubicin, cyclophosphamide, carboplatin, and etoposide.[150] These patients also received EBRT of 45 Gy administered to the optic chiasm for patients with orbital disease and to the involved nodes for those with preauricular lymphadenopathy. More recently, Chawla reported a prospective comparison of 2 neoadjuvant chemotherapy regimens followed by enucleation, EBRT, and adjuvant chemotherapy.[151] Fifty-four patients were randomized into two chemotherapy groups: Group A patients received vincristine, etoposide, and carboplatin (VEC) and group B patients received carboplatin and etoposide, alternating with cyclophosphamide, idarubicin, and vincristine. EBRT was delivered 4 to 6 weeks after enucleation and consisted of 40 Gy in 20 fractions over 4 weeks to the involved orbit. At 4 years, the survival probability for group A was higher (63% vs. 25%, $P = .05$) and the authors suggested that neoadjuvant chemotherapy with high-dose VEC be considered in these cases.

Primary Intraocular Lymphoma

Primary intraocular lymphoma (PIOL), formally known as ocular reticulum cell sarcoma, is an uncommon clinical manifestation of non-Hodgkin lymphoma, which arises in the retina or the vitreous humor.[152] It usually develops in patients in the fifth and sixth decade of life as a chronic, relapsing and steroid-resistant uveitis and vitritis. Patients often complain of blurred vision, a painless loss of vision, and floaters. Intraocular lymphoma may occur independently, prior or subsequent to a primary central nervous system lymphoma (PCNSL). PIOL progresses to intracranial involvement in 60% to 85% of cases.[153] Patients often complain of blurred vision,

a painless loss of vision, and floaters. Historically, PIOL has been difficult to diagnose, often taking several years from the onset of symptoms to establishing a diagnosis, which likely contributed to suboptimal outcome in many cases.[154] Given the tumor's rarity, the optimal treatment of PIOL is unclear. Radiation therapy has been used with durable control after 35 to 45 Gy given exclusively to both eyes in the absence of CNS disease.[151] However, concerns of CNS relapse have led investigators to use chemotherapy as initial treatment and radiation as a consolidative therapy.[155,156] Methotrexate and cytosine arabinoside are most commonly used given their ability to cross the blood–ocular barrier.

Optic Pathway Glioma

Optic pathway gliomas, with or without contiguous involvement of the hypothalamus, have an incidence of approximately 1 in 100,000, with 90% presenting in the first two decades of life.[157] Most of these neoplasms are pilocytic or low-grade astrocytomas.[158] Untreated, the clinical course is that of deterioration of visual acuity, progressive visual field deficits, endocrine or intellectual impairment, and death in up to 30% because of the local tumor progression.[159] Multiple treatment strategies exist, including surveillance, chemotherapy, RT, and surgery, of some combination of therapies. Advances in management have resulted in cause-specific survival rates of 90% to 100% except in cases associated with neurofibromatosis, which carry a worse prognosis.[160,161] Therefore, multidisciplinary management of optic pathway gliomas is critical with an emphasis on reducing treatment-related sequelae. The role of surgery is limited but may be a reasonable treatment option in patients where tumor is confined to a single optic nerve with no useful vision. Local failure rates of approximately 5% can be achieved after complete resection.[155] Radiation therapy has resulted in 10-year survival rates ranging from 40% to 93%, but with potentially severe long-term sequelae, including endocrine problems, neurodevelopmental disorders, and second malignancy.[162] Concerns of these toxicities are significant enough such that at most centers, children of any age are initially treated with chemotherapy in order to delay irradiation until progression. Investigators have found that a 2.5- to 3-year delay in RT can be achieved with this approach.[158]

The main indication of RT is for progressive disease, and radiation doses in the range from 45 to 60 Gy in 1.8- to 2.0-Gy fractions have been effective. Erkal reported on 33 cases of OPG treated between 1973 and 1994.[159] Twenty-four children had optic pathway gliomas and nine had chiasmatic–hypothalamic gliomas. Evidence of neurofibromatosis was present in six children. Subtotal resection was performed in 22 and biopsy in seven. Median total dose was 50 Gy in 25 fractions and mean follow-up was 13.6 years. Ten-year overall, progression-free, and cause-specific survival rates were 79%, 77%, and 88%, respectively. Differences in any of the survival endpoints between optic pathway and chiasmatic–hypothalamic gliomas were not statistically significant, but absence of neurofibromatosis correlated with significantly better progression-free and cause-specific survival. Grabenbauer reported a series of OPG with assessed visual outcomes.[163] Twenty-five patients received RT following surgery or biopsy. Treatment volume included a 0.5- to 1-cm margin around the tumor as depicted on CT or MRI. Age-adjusted radiation doses ranged from 45 to 60 Gy with a fraction size of 1.6 to 2 Gy. Overall survival and progression-free survival rates were 94% and 69% at 10 years, respectively. Age >10 years at time of treatment and total radiation dose >45 Gy were associated with significantly improved progression-free survival. Hypothalamic deficiency also correlated with age, with an incidence of 69% in patients <10 years old compared with 25% in patients >10 years old. As for visual acuity, 36% had an improvement, 52% remained stable, and 12% had measurable deterioration. The authors concluded that postoperative

RT with a total dose above 45 Gy should be considered for patients with progressive OPG. Lifelong yearly evaluations for levels of growth hormone, thyroid and adrenal, are warranted because there is frequent need for replacement therapy, particularly in children under 10 years of age.

As in all pediatric malignancies, radiation technique should be approached with an emphasis on normal tissue sparing. Comb reported on 15 patients treated with fractionated stereotactic RT (FSRT) to a median total dose of 50.2 Gy at 1.8 Gy/fraction.[164] The progression-free survival rate at 3 and 5 years was 92% and 72%, respectively. Functional results were encouraging with only two patients having worsening of vision after RT. Seven had preexisting endocrinopathy, but only one additional patient had endocrine dysfunction after treatment, suggesting FSRT is an effective option for OPG. Still, conformal RT, intensity-modulated radiation, and FSRT carry concerns of second malignancy due the large volume of intracranial tissue receiving a low, potentially mutagenic dose of radiation. For this reason, proton beam therapy has been advocated: Fuss and colleagues evaluated dosimetry plans for proton versus conformal plans in seven cases of OPG and found proton therapy offered substantial normal tissue sparing both at high- and low-dose areas.[165] The difference was more apparent in tumors >80 cm³, but even in tumors <20 cm³, conformal RT resulted in a larger amount of normal tissue receiving low to moderate doses of radiation.

Orbital Tumors

Primary Orbital Lymphoma

Orbital non-Hodgkin lymphomas (NHL) account for only 0.01% of NHL and are typically B-cell lymphomas.[166] Depending on the stage and grade of disease, observation, first-line chemotherapy, and chemotherapy followed by RT are treatment options. RT is generally the treatment of choice for NHL localized to the orbital cavity.[167] Local control in the rates of 90% to 100% can be achieved using doses of 30 to 36 Gy.[168] Historically, radiation was delivered with an anterior portal prescribed to the orbital apex or by wedged anterior and lateral fields. Late effects from these techniques include cataract formation, lens ulceration, glaucoma, and lacrimal impairment.[166] More recently, investigators have described the use of intensity-modulated radiation therapy (IMRT) in orbital lymphoma to reduce dose to the contralateral orbit, lacrimal gland, and lens (Fig. 41.11).[169]

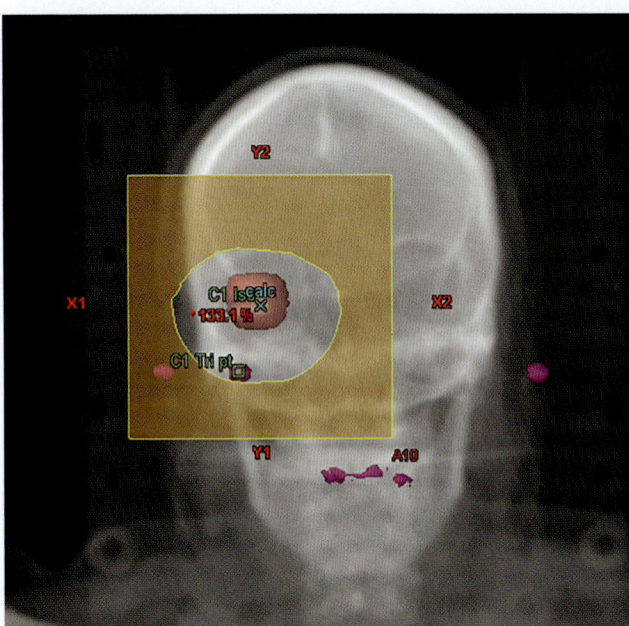

FIGURE 41.12. Electron beam therapy for mucosa-associated lymphoid tissue lymphoma of the conjunctiva. The patient received 30.6 Gy using 9-MeV electrons. Lens shielding was not used because of the extent of disease at presentation.

Conjunctival Tumors

Conjunctival tumors comprise a variety of conditions, from benign papilloma to malignant lesions such as squamous cell carcinoma (SCC). Radiotherapeutic management of these tumors is related to the histologic type, as is the case in tumors found elsewhere. MALT lymphoma, for example, has been effectively managed with exclusive RT with local control rates approaching 100%.[170] In a series of patients with MALT lymphoma of the ocular adnexa that included 37 patients with conjunctival disease, Hashimoto reported local control rates of 100% with a median dose of 30.6 Gy.[171] Electron beam therapy was frequently used with eye lens shielding when possible depending on the extent of disease (Fig. 41.12). Treatment options for SCC include excision with or without adjuvant cryotherapy or topical chemotherapy, whereas advanced cases may require orbital exenteration.[172] RT has

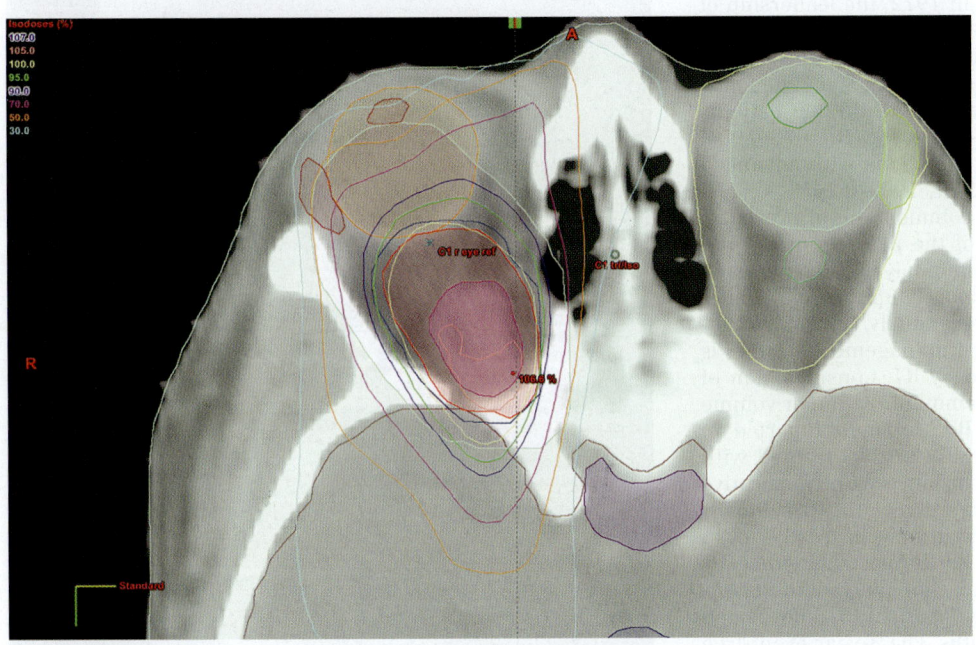

FIGURE 41.11. Primary orbital lymphoma treated with intensity-modulated radiation therapy illustrating sparing of lens, lacrimal gland, and contralateral orbit.

Section
III

been used in the primary, adjuvant, and salvage setting with a variety of methods including photon, proton, and electron beam therapy.[173,174] Most frequently, however, radiation is used in patients with relapsed disease. The treatment volume typically includes gross tumor with margins of approximately 1 cm and doses of approximately 60 Gy, as in cases of SCC from other sites.[175]

Sebaceous Carcinoma of the Eyelid

Sebaceous gland adenocarcinoma occurs in the periorbital area, usually in the eyelid.[176] It can exhibit aggressive local behavior and can metastasize to regional lymph nodes and distant organs. Older individuals tend to be affected, but it occurs with greater frequency and at an earlier age in patients with hereditary retinoblastoma treated with radiation.[177] The main systemic association is Muir-Torre syndrome, an autosomal dominant condition characterized by greater frequency of sebaceous adenoma, sebaceous carcinoma, keratoacanthoma, and gastrointestinal malignancies.[178] The most common pattern of metastasis of eyelid sebaceous carcinoma is through the lymphatic channels to regional lymph nodes. Historically, regional node metastasis occurred in about 30% of cases, but metastases have become less frequent in recent years.[179] Tumors that originate in the upper eyelid tend to metastasize to preauricular and parotid nodes. Tumors of the lower eyelid region can metastasize to submandibular and cervical nodes. Until recently, orbital exenteration was believed to be the only reasonable option in the management of sebaceous carcinoma that involved most of the conjunctiva and invaded the orbit. However, local excision with adjuvant therapies, such as topical chemotherapy or cryotherapy, is becoming more common.[180,181] EBRT, with doses of approximately 60 Gy, is rarely used for primary treatment but should be considered for patients with adverse features such as regional lymph node involvement or recurrent disease.[182]

Orbital Rhabdomyosarcoma

Rhabdomyosarcoma (RMS) affects 250 to 300 children per year in the United States.[183] In 1950, Stobbe demonstrated improvement in the outcome in head and neck sites when RT was added after incompletely resected RMS.[184] In 1961, Pinkel and Pinkren advocated adjuvant chemotherapy after complete surgical excision and postoperative RT, which was the beginning of the multimodal approach to solid tumors.[185] Recognizing the value of this multimodal approach as well as the relative rarity of these tumors, in 1972, the leadership of three US cooperative pediatric cancer research groups formed the Intergroup Rhabdomyosarcoma Study Group (IRS) to investigate the biology and treatment of RMS. Since then, five successive clinical protocols involving almost 5,000 patients have been completed: IRS-I, 1972–1978; IRS-II, 1978–1984; IRS-III, 1984–1991; IRS-IV Pilot (for patients with advanced disease only), 1987–1991; and IRS-IV, 1991–1997.[186–191] The head and neck region is the most common site of presentation and accounts for about 35% of the patients in the IRS studies.[192] These tumors are most commonly of the embryonal subtype and rarely spread to regional lymph nodes. Orbital tumors produce proptosis and, occasionally, ophthalmoplegia (Figs. 41.13 and 41.14). Modern management of RMS is multiagent chemotherapy followed by RT. Consideration of prechemotherapy as well as postchemotherapy tumor volume must be considered when planning RT. McDonald reported on 20 patients with head and neck RMS (2 orbit) treated with IMRT to total dose of 50 Gy, in accordance with cooperative group protocols.[193] The initial targeting of the prechemotherapy tumor volume with 1- to 2-cm margin to 30.6 to 36 Gy followed by a cone-down boost to the postchemotherapy tumor volume with a 0.5- to 1-cm margin allowed for significant sparing of normal tissues. Only 1 patient (5%) developed an in-field recurrence after 50 months. The 3-year event-free

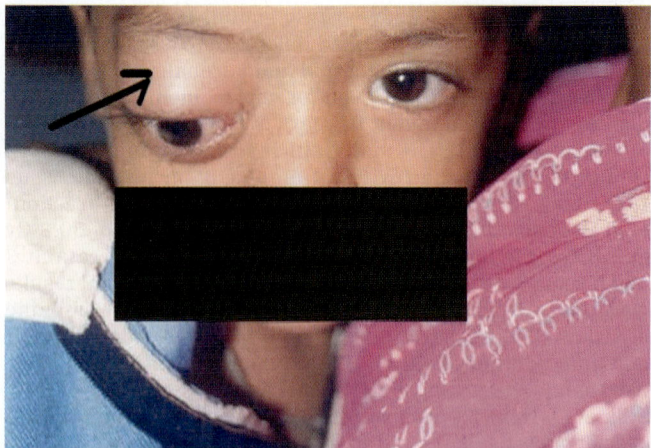

FIGURE 41.13. Orbital rhabdomyosarcoma with proptosis (*arrow* denotes tumor). (From Das JK, Tiwary BK, Paul SB, et al. Primary orbital rhabdomyosarcoma with skeletal muscle metastasis. *Oman J Ophthalmol* 2010;3:91–93. Copyright © 2010 Oman Journal of Ophthalmology. Reprinted with permission of Wolters Kluwer Medknow Publications.)

survival, overall survival, and risk of central nervous system failure were 74%, 76%, and 7%, respectively.

Periorbital Skin Cancers

Skin cancers of the eyelid and periorbital skin include most frequently basal cell carcinoma (BCC), SCC, but also rare histologies such as Merkel cell carcinoma (MCC).[194] For small BCC and SCC, single modality treatment with surgery or RT results in good local control, but RT is frequently used due to cosmetic concerns. For more advanced tumors or more aggressive histologies, such as MCC, combined surgery and RT are typically recommended. Low-energy electron beam

FIGURE 41.14. Coronal computed tomography scan of patient with orbital rhabdomyosarcoma (*arrow* denotes tumor). (From Das JK, Tiwary BK, Paul SB, et al. Primary orbital rhabdomyosarcoma with skeletal muscle metastasis. *Oman J Ophthalmol* 2010;3:91–93. Copyright © 2010 *Oman Journal of Ophthalmology.* Reprinted with permission of Wolters Kluwer Medknow Publications.)

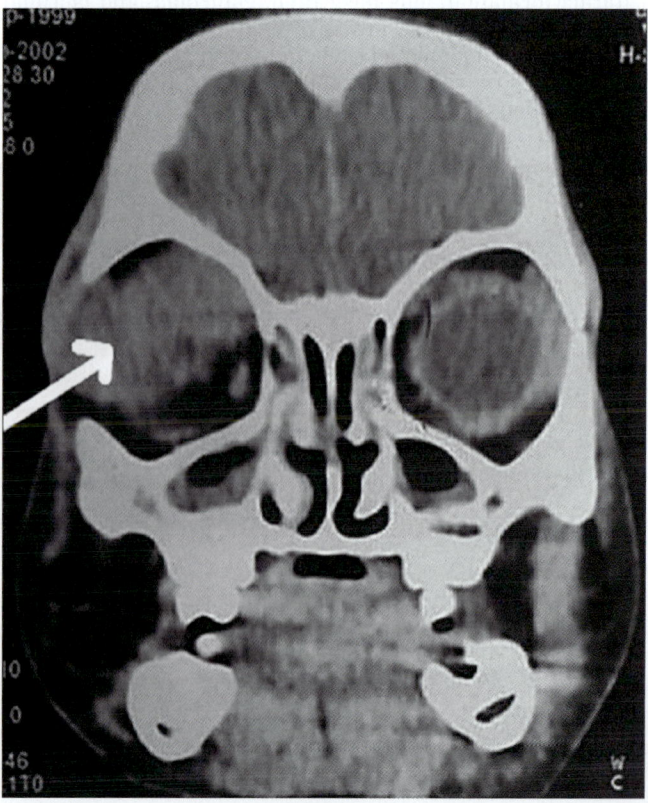

therapy or orthovoltage irradiation is useful in this setting and can be delivered with an eye shield. RT for skin tumors requires doses of 60 Gy or more for definitive treatment using standard fractionation, but altered fraction can be employed to shorten treatment duration and minimize ocular trauma of shield placement.

REFERENCES

1. http://www.cancer.org/Cancer/EyeCancer/DetailedGuide/eye-cancer-key-statistics
2. Shields CL, Shields JA, Gross N, et al. Survey of 520 eyes with uveal metastases. *Ophthalmology* 1997;104:1265–1276.
3. Karp LA, Streeten BW, Cogan DG. Radiation-induced atrophy of the Meibomian gland. *Arch Ophthalmol* 1979;97:303–305.
4. Stephens LC, Schultheiss TE, Peters LJ, et al. Acute radiation injury of ocular adnexa. *Arch Ophthalmol* 1988;106:389–391.
5. Bentzen SM, Thames HD. A 100-year Nordic perspective on the dose-time problem in radiobiology. *Acta Oncol* 1995;34:1031–1040.
6. Stafford SL, Kozelsky TF, Garrity JA, et al. Orbital lymphoma: radiotherapy outcome and complications. *Radiother Oncol* 2001;59:139–144.
7. Durkin SR, Roos D, Higgs B, et al. Ophthalmic and adnexal complications of radiotherapy. *Acta Ophthalmol Scand* 2007;85:240–250.
8. Goyal S, Cohler A, Camporeale J, et al. Intensity-modulated radiation therapy for orbital lymphoma. *Radiat Med* 2008;26:573–581.
9. de Smet MD, Buffam FV, Fairey RN, et al. Prevention of radiation-induced stenosis of the nasolacrimal duct. *Can J Ophthalmol* 1990;25:145–147.
10. Barabino S, Raghavan A, Loeffler J, et al. Radiotherapy-induced ocular surface disease. *Cornea* 2005;24:909–914.
11. Shiu AS, Tung SS, Gastorf RJ, et al. Dosimetric evaluation of lead and tungsten eye shields in electron beam treatment. *Int J Radiat Oncol Biol Phys* 1996;35:599–604.
12. Merriam GRSA, Focht EF. The effects of ionizing radiations on the eye. *Radiat Ther Oncol* 1972;6:346–385.
13. Daftari IK, Char DH, Verhey LJ, et al. Anterior segment sparing to reduce charged particle radiotherapy complications in uveal melanoma. *Int J Radiat Oncol Biol Phys* 1997;39:997–1010.
14. Douat J, Auriol S, Mahieu-Durringer L, et al. Intravitreal bevacizumab for treatment of neovascular glaucoma. Report of 20 cases. *J Fr Ophthalmol* 2009;32:652–663.
15. Hall P, Granath F, Lundell M, et al. Lenticular opacities in individuals exposed to ionizing radiation in infancy. *Radiat Res* 1999;152:190–195.
16. Bajcsay A, Kontra G, Recsan Z, et al. Lens-sparing external beam radiotherapy of intraocular metastases: our experiences with twenty four eyes. *Neoplasma* 2003;50:459–464.
17. Gupta A, Dhawahir-Scala F, Smith A, et al. Radiation retinopathy: case report and review. *BMC Ophthalmol* 2007;7:6.
18. Evans JR, Sivagnanavel V, Chong V. Radiotherapy for neovascular age-related macular degeneration. *Cochrane Database Syst Rev* 2010;5:CD004004.
19. Parsons JT, Bova FJ, Fitzgerald CR, et al. Radiation retinopathy after external-beam irradiation: analysis of time-dose factors. *Int J Radiat Oncol Biol Phys* 1994;30:765–773.
20. Kumar B, Palimar P. Accelerated radiation retinopathy in diabetes and pregnancy. *Eye (Lond)* 2000;14(Pt 1):107–108.
21. Haji Mohd Yasin NA, Gray AR, Bevin TH, et al. Choroidal melanoma treated with stereotactic fractionated radiotherapy and prophylactic intravitreal bevacizumab: the Dunedin Hospital experience. *J Med Imaging Radiat Oncol* 2016;60(6):756–763.
22. McClellan RL, el Gammal T, Kline LB. Early bilateral radiation-induced optic neuropathy with follow-up MRI. *Neuroradiology* 1995;37:131–133.
23. Mayo C, Martel MK, Marks LB, et al. Radiation dose-volume effects of optic nerves and chiasm. *Int J Radiat Oncol Biol Phys* 2010;76:S28–S35.
24. Parsons JT, Bova FJ, Fitzgerald CR, et al. Radiation optic neuropathy after megavoltage external-beam irradiation: analysis of time-dose factors. *Int J Radiat Oncol Biol Phys* 1994;30(4):755–763.
25. Jurgenliemk-Schulz IM, Hartman LJ, Roesink JM, et al. Prevention of pterygium recurrence by postoperative single-dose beta-irradiation: a prospective randomized clinical double-blind trial. *Int J Radiat Oncol Biol Phys* 2004;59(4):1138–1147.
26. Lam DS, Wong AK, Fan DS, et al. Intraoperative mitomycin C to prevent recurrence of pterygium after excision: a 30-month follow-up study. *Ophthalmology* 1998;105:901–904.
27. Rubinfeld RS, Pfister RR, Stein RM, et al. Serious complications of topical mitomycin-C after pterygium surgery. *Ophthalmology* 1992;99:1647–1654.
28. Moriarty AP, Crawford GJ, McAllister IL, et al. Severe corneoscleral infection: a complication of beta irradiation scleral necrosis following pterygium excision. *Arch Ophthalmol* 1993;111:947–951.
29. Tan DT, Chee SP, Dear KB, et al. Effect of pterygium morphology on pterygium recurrence in a controlled trial comparing conjunctival autografting with bare sclera excision. *Arch Ophthalmol* 1997;115:1235–1240.
30. Singh AD, Kaiser PK. Uveal vascular tumors. In: Singh AD, Damato BE, Pe'er J, et al., eds. *Clinical ophthalmic oncology*. Philadelphia: Saunders-Elsevier, 2007:289–299.
31. Schilling H, Sauerwein W, Lommatzsch A, et al. Long-term results after low dose ocular irradiation for choroidal haemangiomas. *Br J Ophthalmol* 1997;81:267–273.
32. Heimann H, Bornfeld N, Vij O, et al. Vasoproliferative tumours of the retina. *Br J Ophthalmol* 2000;84:1162–1169.
33. Kivela T, Tenhunen M, Joensuu T, et al. Stereotactic radiotherapy of symptomatic circumscribed choroidal hemangiomas. *Ophthalmology* 2003;110:1977–1982.
34. Zografos L, Gailloud C, Bercher L. Irradiation treatment of choroidal hemangiomas. *J Fr Ophthalmol* 1989;12:797–807.
35. López-Caballero C, Saornil MA, De Frutos J, et al. High-dose iodine-125 episcleral brachytherapy for circumscribed choroidal haemangioma. *Br J Ophthalmol* 2010;94(4):470–473.
36. Levy-Gabriel C, Rouic LL, Plancher C, et al. Long-term results of low-dose proton beam therapy for circumscribed choroidal hemangiomas. *Retina* 2009;29(2):170–175.
37. Marquileth A, Museles M. Cutaneous hemangiomas in children: diagnosis and conservative management. *JAMA* 1965;1974:523.
38. Schwartz SR, Blei F, Ceisler E, et al. Risk factors for amblyopia in children with capillary hemangiomas of the eyelids and orbit. *J AAPOS* 2006;10(3):262–268.
39. Jacobiec FA, Jones IS. Vascular tumors, malformations and degenerations. In: Duane TD, ed. *Clinical ophthalmology*. Vol. 2. Hagerstown, MD: Harper & Row, 1976:1–40.
40. Yan J, Wu Z, Li Y. A clinical analysis of idiopathic orbital inflammatory pseudotumor. *Yan Ke Xue Bao* 2000;16:208–213.
41. Leone CR Jr, Lloyd WC 3rd. Treatment protocol for orbital inflammatory disease. *Ophthalmology* 1985;92:1325–1331.
42. Matthiesen C, Bogardus C Jr, Thompson JS, et al. The efficacy of radiotherapy in the treatment of orbital pseudotumor. *Int J Radiat Oncol Biol Phys* 2011;79(5):1496–502.
43. Ing E, Abuhaleeqa K. Graves' ophthalmopathy (thyroid-associated orbitopathy). *Clin Surg Ophthalmol* 2007;25:386–392.
44. Boulos PR, Hardy I. Thyroid-associated orbitopathy: a clinicopathologic and therapeutic review. *Curr Opin Ophthalmol* 2004;15(5):389–400.
45. Abboud M, Rabi A, Ibrahim S, et al. Outcome of thyroid associated ophthalmopathy treated by radiation therapy. *Radiat Oncol* 2011;6:46.
46. Bartalena L, Marcocci C, Chiovato L, et al. Orbital cobalt irradiation combined with systemic corticosteroids for Graves' ophthalmopathy: comparison with systemic corticosteroids alone. *J Clin Endocrinol Metab* 1983;56:1139–1144.
47. Antonelli A, Saracino A, Alberti B, et al. High-dose intravenous immunoglobulin treatment in Graves' ophthalmopathy. *Acta Endocrinol (Copenh)* 1992;126:13–23.
48. Gerling J, Kommerell G, Henne K, et al. Retrobulbar irradiation for thyroid-associated orbitopathy: double-blind comparison between 2.4 and 16 Gy. *Int J Radiat Oncol Biol Phys* 2003;55:182–189.
49. Kahaly GJ, Rosler HP, Pitz S, et al. Low-versus high-dose radiotherapy for Graves' ophthalmopathy: a randomized, single blind trial. *J Clin Endocrinol Metab* 2000;85:102–108.
50. Mourits MP, van Kempen-Harteveld ML, Garcia MB, et al. Radiotherapy for Graves' orbitopathy: randomised placebo-controlled study. *Lancet* 2000;355:1505–1509.
51. Ng CM, Yuen HK, Choi KL, et al. Combined orbital irradiation and systemic steroids compared with systemic steroids alone in the management of moderate-to-severe Graves' ophthalmopathy: a preliminary study. *Hong Kong Med J* 2005;11:322–330.
52. Prummel MF, Mourits MP, Blank L, et al. Randomized double-blind trial of prednisone versus radiotherapy in Graves' ophthalmopathy. *Lancet* 1993;342:949–954.
53. Prummel MF, Terwee CB, Gerding MN, et al. A randomized controlled trial of orbital radiotherapy versus sham irradiation in patients with mild Graves' ophthalmopathy. *J Clin Endocrinol Metab* 2004;89:15–20.
54. Gorman CA, Garrity JA, Fatourechi V, et al. A prospective, randomized, double-blind, placebo-controlled study of orbital radiotherapy for Graves' ophthalmopathy. *Ophthalmology* 2001;108:1523–1534.
55. Wakelkamp IM, Tan H, Saeed P, et al. Orbital irradiation for Graves' ophthalmopathy: is it safe? A long-term follow-up study. *Ophthalmology* 2004;111:1557–1562.
56. Bradley EA, Gower EW, Bradley DJ, et al. Orbital radiation for graves ophthalmopathy: a report by the American Academy of Ophthalmology. *Ophthalmology* 2008;115(2):398–409.
57. Laurberg P, Berman DC, Bülow Pedersen I, et al. Incidence and clinical presentation of moderate to severe graves' orbitopathy in a Danish population before and after iodine fortification of salt. *J Clin Endocrinol Metab* 2012;97(7):2325–2332.
58. Tanda ML, Bartalena L. Efficacy and safety of orbital radiotherapy for graves' orbitopathy. *J Clin Endocrinol Metab* 2012;97(11):3857–3865.
59. Shields JA, Shields CL. Metastatic tumors to the intraocular structures. In: *Intraocular tumors: a text and atlas*. Philadelphia: WB Saunders Co, 1992:207–238.
60. Demirci H, Shields CL, Chao AN, et al. Uveal metastasis from breast cancer in 264 patients. *Am J Ophthalmol* 2003;136(2):264–271.
61. Rosset A, Zografos L, Coucke P, et al. Radiotherapy of choroidal metastases. *Radiother Oncol* 1998;46(3):263–268.
62. Shields CL, Shields JA, De Potter P, et al. Plaque radiotherapy for the management of uveal metastasis. *Arch Ophthalmol* 1997;115:203–209.
63. Cancer.Net, American Society of Clinical Oncology. Eye cancer: statistics. Available at: http://www.cancer.net/cancer-types/eye-cancer/statistics
64. Margo CE, Mulla Z. Incidence of surgically treated uveal melanoma by race and ethnicity. *Ophthalmology* 1998;105:1087–1090.
65. Damato B. Detection of uveal melanoma by optometrists in the United Kingdom. *Ophthalmic Physiol Opt* 2001;21:268–271.

Section III

66. Coleman DJ, Silverman RH, Rondeau MJ, et al. Noninvasive in vivo detection of prognostic indicators for high-risk uveal melanoma: ultrasound parameter imaging. *Ophthalmology* 2004;111:558–564.

67. Egan KM, Ryan LM, Gragoudas ES. Survival implications of enucleation after definitive radiotherapy for choroidal melanoma: an example of regression on time-dependent covariates. *Arch Ophthalmol* 1998;116:366–370.

68. Damato BE, Paul J, Foulds WS. Risk factors for residual and recurrent uveal melanoma after trans-scleral local resection. *Br J Ophthalmol* 1996;80:102–108.

69. Damato B. Developments in the management of uveal melanoma. *Clin Exp Ophthalmol* 2004;32(6):639–647.

70. Shields CL, Shields JA, Kiratli H, et al. Risk factors for growth and metastasis of small choroidal melanocytic lesions. *Ophthalmology* 1995;102:1351–1361.

71. Zimmerman LE, McLean IW, Foster WD. Does enucleation of the eye containing a malignant melanoma prevent or accelerate the dissemination of tumour cells? *Br J Ophthalmol* 1978;62:420–425.

72. Kujala E, Makitie T, Kivela T. Very long term prognosis of patients with malignant uveal melanoma. *Invest Ophthalmol Vis Sci* 2003;44:4651–4659.

73. Damato B, Groenewald C, McGalliard J, et al. Endoresection of choroidal melanoma. *Br J Ophthalmol* 1998;82:213–218.

74. Bornfeld N, Talies S, Anastassiou G, et al. Endoscopic resection of malignant melanomas of the uvea after preoperative stereotactic single dose convergence irradiation with the Leksell gamma knife. *Ophthalmologe* 2002;99:338–344.

75. Damato BE, Foulds WS. Surgical resection of choroidal melanomas. In: Schachat AP, Ryan SJ, eds. *Retina*. 3rd ed. St Louis, MO: Mosby, 2001:762–772.

76. Damato BE. Adjunctive plaque radiotherapy after local resection of uveal melanoma. *Front Radiat Ther Oncol* 1997;30:123–132.

77. Oosterhuis JA, Journee de Korver HG, Keunen JE. Transpupillary thermotherapy: results in 50 patients with choroidal melanoma. *Arch Otolaryngol* 1998;116:157–162.

78. Yarovoy AA, Magaramov DA, Bulgakova ES. The comparison of ruthenium brachytherapy and simultaneous transpupillary thermotherapy of choroidal melanoma with brachytherapy alone. *Brachytherapy* 2012;11(3):224–229.

79. Finger PT, Chin KJ, Duvall G; Palladium-103 for Choroidal Melanoma Study Group. Palladium-103 ophthalmic plaque radiation therapy for choroidal melanoma: 400 treated patients. *Ophthalmology* 2009;116(4):790–796, 796.e1.

80. Perez BA, Mettu P, Vajzovic L, et al. Uveal melanoma treated with iodine-125 episcleral plaque: an analysis of dose on disease control and visual outcomes. *Int J Radiat Oncol Biol Phys* 2014;89(1):127–136.

81. Astrahan MA, Luxton G, Jozsef G, et al. Optimization of 125I ophthalmic plaque brachytherapy. *Med Phys* 1990;17:1053–1057.

82. Sagoo MS, Shields CL, Mashayekhi A, et al. Plaque radiotherapy for juxtapapillary choroidal melanoma overhanging the optic disc in 141 consecutive patients. *Arch Ophthalmol* 2008;126(11):1515–1522.

83. Collaborative Ocular Melanoma Study Group. The COMS randomized trial of iodine 125 brachytherapy for choroidal melanoma: V. Twelve-year mortality rates and prognostic factors: COMS report No. 28. *Arch Ophthalmol* 2006;124(12):1684–1693.

84. Jampol LM, Moy CS, Murray TG, et al. The COMS randomized trial of iodine 125 brachytherapy for choroidal melanoma: IV. Local treatment failure and enucleation in the first 5 years after brachytherapy. COMS report no. 19. *Ophthalmology* 2002;109:2197–2206.

85. Shields CL, Shields JA, Cater J, et al. Plague radiotherapy for uveal melanoma: long term visual outcome in 1106 consecutive patients treated between 1976 and 1992. *Arch Ophthalmol* 2000;118(9):1219–1228.

86. ABS—OOTF Committee. The American Brachytherapy Society consensus guidelines for plaque brachytherapy of uveal melanoma and retinoblastoma. *Brachytherapy* 2014;13(1):1–14.

87. Lane AM, Kim IK, Gragoudas ES. Proton irradiation for peripapillary and parapapillary melanomas. *Arch Ophthalmol* 2011;129(9):1127–1130.

88. Gragoudas ES, Lane AM. Uveal melanoma: proton beam irradiation. *Ophthalmol Clin North Am* 2005;18:111–118.

89. Verhey LJ, Goitein M, McNulty P, et al. Precise positioning of patients for radiation therapy. *Int J Radiat Oncol Biol Phys* 1982;8:289–294.

90. Gragoudas E, Li W, Goitein M, et al. Evidence-based estimates of outcome in patients irradiated for intraocular melanoma. *Arch Ophthalmol* 2002;120:1665–1671.

91. Foss AJ, Whelehan I, Hungerford JL, et al. Predictive factors for the development of rubeosis following proton beam radiotherapy for uveal melanoma. *Br J Ophthalmol* 1997;81:748–754.

92. Fakiris AJ, Lo SS, Henderson MA, et al. Gamma-knife-based stereotactic radiosurgery for uveal melanoma. *Stereotact Funct Neurosurg* 2007;85:106–112.

93. Modorati G, Miserocchi E, Galli L, et al. Gamma knife radiosurgery for uveal melanoma: 12 years of experience. *Br J Ophthalmol* 2009;93:40–44.

94. Archer DB, Amoaku WM, Gardiner TA. Radiation retinopathy-clinical, histopathological, ultrastructural and experimental correlations. *Eye* 1991;5:239–251.

95. Gunduz K, Shields CL, Shields JA, et al. Radiation retinopathy following plaque radiotherapy for posterior uveal melanoma. *Arch Ophthalmol* 1999;117:609–614.

96. Muller K, Naus N, Nowak PJ, et al. Fractionated stereotactic radiotherapy for uveal melanoma, late clinical results. *Radiother Oncol* 2012;102(2):219–224.

97. American Cancer Society. Chapter 85: Neoplasms of the eye. In: *Cancer medicine*. Hamilton, ON: BC Decker Inc, 2003.

98. MacCarthy A, Birch JM, Draper GJ, et al. Retinoblastoma in Great Britain 1963-2002. *Br J Ophthalmol* 2009;93(1):33–37.

99. Kumar V, Abbas AK, Fausto N. *Robbins and cotran pathologic basis of disease*. 7th ed. Philadelphia: Elsevier Saunders, 2005:1442.

100. Knudson AG Jr. Mutation and cancer: statistical study of retinoblastoma. *Proc Natl Acad Sci U S A* 1971;68:820–823.

101. Hethcote HW, Knudson AG Jr. Model for the incidence of embryonal cancers: application to retinoblastoma. *Proc Natl Acad Sci U S A* 1978;75:2453–2457.

102. Harbour JW, Dean DC. Rb function in cell-cycle regulation and apoptosis. *Nat Cell Biol* 2000;94:E65–E67.

103. Richter S, Vandezande K, Chen N, et al. Sensitive and efficient detection of RB1 gene mutations enhances care for families with retinoblastoma. *Am J Hum Genet* 2002;72(2):253–269.

104. Shields JA, Augsburger JJ. Current approaches to the diagnosis and management of retinoblastoma. *Surv Ophthalmol* 1981;25:347–372.

105. Brenner D, Elliston C, Hall E, et al. Estimated risks of radiation-induced fatal cancer from pediatric CT. *AJR Am J Roentgenol* 2001;176:289–296.

106. Smith EV, Gragoudas ES, Kolodny NH, et al. Magnetic resonance imaging: an emerging technique for the diagnosis of ocular disorders. *Int Ophthalmol* 1990;14:119–124.

107. Karcioglu ZA, al-Mesfer SA, Abboud E, et al. Workup for metastatic retinoblastoma. A review of 261 patients. *Ophthalmology* 1997;104:307–312.

108. Kopelman JE, McLean IW, Rosenberg SH. Multivariate analysis of risk factors for metastasis in retinoblastoma treated by enucleation. *Ophthalmology* 1987;94:371–377.

109. Reese AB, Ellsworth RM. Management of retinoblastoma. *Ann N Y Acad Sci* 1964;114:958–962.

110. Shields CL, Mashayekhi A, Demirci H, et al. Practical approach to management of retinoblastoma. *Arch Ophthalmol* 2004;122:729–735.

111. Murphree AL. Intraocular retinoblastoma: the case for a new group classification. *Ophthalmol Clin North Am* 2005;18:41–53.

112. Chantada G, Doz F, Antoneli CB, et al. A proposal for an international retinoblastoma staging system. *Pediatr Blood Cancer* 2006;47:801–805.

113. Abramson DH. Treatment of retinoblastoma. In: Blodi FC, ed. *Retinoblastoma*. New York: Churchill Livingstone, 1985:3–93.

114. Hilgartner HL. Report of a case of double glioma treated with X-ray. *Tex Med* 1903;18:322–323.

115. Schipper J, Imhoff SM, Tan KE. Precision megavoltage external beam radiation therapy for retinoblastoma. *Front Radiat Ther Oncol* 1997;30:65–80.

116. Peylan-Ramu N, Bin-Nun A, Skleir-Levy M, et al. Orbital growth retardation in retinoblastoma survivors: work in progress. *Med Pediatr Oncol* 2001;37:465–470.

117. Eng C, Li FP, Abramson DH, et al. Mortality from second tumors among long-term survivors of retinoblastoma. *J Natl Cancer Inst* 1993;85:1121–1128.

118. Munier FL, Verwey J, Pica A, et al. New developments in external beam radiotherapy for retinoblastoma: from lens to normal tissue-sparing techniques. *Clin Exp Ophthalmol* 2008;36:78–89.

119. Chan MP, Hungerford JL, Kingston JE, et al. Salvage external beam radiotherapy after failed primary chemotherapy for bilateral retinoblastoma: rate of eye and vision preservation. *Br J Ophthalmol* 2009;93(7):891–894.

120. Kingston JE, Hungerford JL, Madreperla SA, et al. Results of combined chemotherapy and radiotherapy for advanced intraocular retinoblastoma. *Arch Ophthalmol* 1996;114(11):1339–1343.

121. McCormick B, Ellsworth R, Abramson D, et al. Radiation therapy for retinoblastoma: comparison of results with lens-sparing versus lateral beam techniques. *Int J Radiat Oncol Biol Phys* 1988;15:567.

122. Harnett AN, Hungerford J, Lambert G, et al. Modern lateral external beam (lens sparing) radiotherapy for retinoblastoma. *Ophthalmic Paediatr Genet* 1987;8:53–61.

123. Schipper J. An accurate and simple method for megavoltage radiation therapy of retinoblastoma. *Radiother Oncol* 1983;1:31–41.

124. Borger F, Rosenberg I, Vijayakumar S, et al. An anterior appositional electron field technique with a hanging lens block in orbital radiotherapy: a dosimetric study. *Int J Radiat Oncol Biol Phys* 1991;21:795–804.

125. Chin LM, Harter W, Svensson GK, et al. An external beam treatment technique for retinoblastoma. *Int J Radiat Oncol Biol Phys* 1988;15:455–460.

126. Krasin MJ, Crawford BT, Zhu Y, et al. Intensity-modulated radiation therapy for children with intraocular retinoblastoma: potential sparing of the bony orbit. *Clin Oncol (R Coll Radiol)* 2004;16:215–222.

127. Lee CT, Bilton SD, Famiglietti RM, et al. Treatment planning with protons for pediatric retinoblastoma, medulloblastoma, and pelvic sarcoma: how do protons compare with other conformal techniques? *Int J Radiat Oncol Biol Phys* 2005;63:362–372.

128. Krengli M, Hug EB, Adams JA, et al. Proton radiation therapy for retinoblastoma: comparison of various intraocular tumor locations and beam arrangements. *Int J Radiat Oncol Biol Phys* 2005;61:583–593.

129. Mouw KW, Sethi RV, Yeap BY, et al. Proton radiation therapy for the treatment of retinoblastoma. *Int J Radiat Oncol Biol Phys* 2014;90(4):863–869.

130. Abramson DH, Frank CM. Second nonocular tumors in survivors of bilateral retinoblastoma: a possible age effect on radiation-related risk. *Ophthalmology* 1998;105:573–579.

131. Imhof SM, Mourits MP, Hofman P, et al. Quantification of orbital and midfacial growth retardation after megavoltage external beam irradiation in children with retinoblastoma. *Ophthalmology* 1996;103:263–268.

132. Schueler AO, Fluhs D, Anastassiou G, et al. Beta-ray brachytherapy of retinoblastoma: feasibility of a new small-sized ruthenium-106 plaque. *Ophthalmic Res* 2006;38:8–12.

133. Desjardins L, Levy C, Labib A, et al. An experience of the use of radioactive plaques after failure of external beam radiation in the treatment of retinoblastoma. *Ophthalmic Paediatr Genet* 1993;14:39–42.

134. Shields CL, Shields JA, Cater J, et al. Plaque radiotherapy for retinoblastoma: long-term tumor control and treatment complications in 208 tumors. *Ophthalmology* 2001;108:2116–2121.

135. Abramson DH, Schefler AC. Transpupillary thermotherapy as initial treatment for small intraocular retinoblastoma: technique and predictors of success. *Ophthalmology* 2004;111:984–991.

136. Shields CL, Santos MC, Diniz W, et al. Thermotherapy for retinoblastoma. *Arch Ophthalmol* 1999;117:885–893.

137. Shields JA, Shields CL, Parsons H, et al. The role of photocoagulation in the management of retinoblastoma. *Arch Ophthalmol* 1990;108:205–208.

138. Abramson DH, Ellsworth RM, Rozakis GW. Cryotherapy for retinoblastoma. *Arch Ophthalmol* 1982;100:1253–1256.

139. Gallie BL, Budning A, DeBoer G, et al. Chemotherapy with focal therapy can cure intraocular retinoblastoma without radiotherapy. *Arch Ophthalmol* 1996;114:1321–1328.

140. Shields CL, De Potter P, Himelstein BP, et al. Chemoreduction in the initial management of intraocular retinoblastoma. *Arch Ophthalmol* 1996;114:1330–1338.

141. Shields CL, Honavar SG, Shields JA, et al. Factors predictive of recurrence of retinal tumors, vitreous seeds, and subretinal seeds following chemoreduction for retinoblastoma. *Arch Ophthalmol* 2002;120:460–464.

142. Gunduz K, Shields CL, Shields JA, et al. The outcome of chemoreduction treatment in patients with Reese-Ellsworth group V retinoblastoma. *Arch Ophthalmol* 1998;116:1613–1617.

143. Chan HS, DeBoer G, Thiessen JJ, et al. Combining cyclosporin with chemotherapy controls intraocular retinoblastoma without requiring radiation. *Clin Cancer Res* 1996;2:1499–1508.

144. Le Deley MC, Vassal G, Taibi A, et al. High cumulative rate of secondary leukemia after continuous etoposide treatment for solid tumors in children and young adults. *Pediatr Blood Cancer* 2005;45:25–31.

145. Friedman DL, Himelstein B, Shields CL, et al. Chemoreduction and local ophthalmic therapy for intraocular retinoblastoma. *J Clin Oncol* 2000;18:12–17.

146. Chawla B, Jain A, Seth R, et al. Clinical outcome and regression patterns of retinoblastoma treated with systemic chemoreduction and focal therapy: a prospective study. *Indian J Ophthalmol* 2016;64(7):524–529.

147. Gobin YP, Dunkel IJ, Marr BP, et al. Intra-arterial chemotherapy for the management of retinoblastoma: four-year experience. *Arch Ophthalmol* 2011;129(6):732–737.

148. Abramson DH, Marr BP, Dunkel IJ, et al. Intra-arterial chemotherapy for retinoblastoma in eyes with vitreous and/or subretinal seeding: 2-year results. *Br J Ophthalmol* 2012;96(4):499–502.

149. Ghassemi F, Shields CL, Ghadimi H, et al. Combined intravitreal melphalan and topotecan for refractory or recurrent vitreous seeding from retinoblastoma. *JAMA Ophthalmol* 2014;132(8):936–941.

150. Chantada G, Fandino A, Casak S, et al. Treatment of overt extraocular retinoblastoma. *Med Pediatr Oncol* 2003;40:158–161.

151. Chawla B, Hasan F, Seth R, et al. Multimodal therapy for stage III retinoblastoma (International Retinoblastoma Staging System): a prospective comparative study. *Ophthalmology* 2016;123(9):1933–1939.

152. Chan CC, Buggage RR, Nussenblatt RB. Intraocular lymphoma. *Curr Opin Ophthalmol* 2002;13:411–418.

153. Peterson K, Gordon KB, Heinemann M, et al. The clinical spectrum of ocular lymphoma. *Cancer* 1993;72:843–849.

154. Hoffman PM, McKelvie P, Hall AJ, et al. Intraocular lymphoma: a series of 14 patients with clinicopathological features and treatment outcomes. *Eye* 2003;17:513–521.

155. Valluri S, Moorthy RS, Khan A, et al. Combination treatment of intraocular lymphoma. *Retina* 1995;15:125–129.

156. Isobe K, Ejima Y, Tokumaru S, et al. Treatment of primary intraocular lymphoma with radiation therapy: a multi-institutional survey in Japan. *Leuk Lymphoma* 2006;47(9):1800–1805.

157. Alvord EC Jr, Lofton S. Gliomas of the optic nerve or chiasm: outcome by patients' age, tumour site, and treatment. *J Neurosurg* 1988;68:85–98.

158. Bilgic S, Erbengy A, Tinaztepe B, et al. Optic glioma of childhood: clinical, histopathological and histochemical observations. *Br J Ophthalmol* 1989;73:832–837.

159. Glaser JS, Hoyt WF, Corbett J. Visual morbidity with chiasm glioma: long-term studies of visual fields in untreated and irradiated cases. *Arch Ophthalmol* 1971;85:3–12.

160. Demaerel P, de Ruyter N, Casteels I, et al. Visual pathway glioma in children treated with chemotherapy. *Eur J Paediatr Neurol* 2002;6:207–212.

161. Erkal HS, Serin M, Cakmak A. Management of optic pathway and chiasmatic-hypothalamic gliomas in children with radiation therapy. *Radiother Oncol* 1997;45:11–5.

162. Pierce SM, Barnes PD, Loeffler JS, et al. Definitive radiation therapy in the management of symptomatic patients with optic glioma: survival and long-term effects. *Cancer* 1990;65:45–52.

163. Grabenbauer GG, Schuchardt U, Buchfelder M, et al. Radiation therapy of optico-hypothalamic gliomas (OHG)-radiographic response, vision and late toxicity. *Radiother Oncol* 2000;54:239–245.

164. Combs SE, Schulz-Ertner D, Moschos D, et al. Fractionated stereotactic radiotherapy of optic pathway gliomas: tolerance and long-term outcome. *Int J Radiat Oncol Biol Phys* 2005;62(3):814–819.

165. Fuss M, Hug EB, Schaefer RA, et al. Proton radiation therapy (PRT) for pediatric optic pathway gliomas: comparison with 3D planned conventional photons and a standard photon technique. *Int J Radiat Oncol Biol Phys* 1999;45(5):1117–1126.

166. Fitzpatrick PJ, Macko S. Lymphoreticular tumors of the orbit. *Int J Radiat Oncol Biol Phys* 1984;10:333–340.

167. Lee JL, Kim MK, Lee KH, et al. Extranodal marginal zone B-cell lymphomas of mucosa-associated lymphoid tissue-type of the orbit and ocular adnexa. *Ann Hematol* 2005;84:13–18.

168. Bolek TW, Moyses HM, Marcus RB Jr, et al. Radiotherapy in the management of orbital lymphoma. *Int J Radiat Oncol Biol Phys* 1999;44:31–6.

169. Chao CK, Lin HS, Devineni VR, et al. Radiation therapy for primary orbital lymphoma. *Int J Radiat Oncol Biol Phys* 1999;44:31–36.

170. Ejima Y, Sasaki R, Okamoto Y. Ocular adnexal mucosa associated lymphoid tissue lymphoma treated with radiotherapy. *Radiother Oncol* 2006;78:6–9.

171. Hashimoto N, Sasaki R, Nishimura H, et al. Long-term outcome and patterns of failure in primary ocular adnexal mucosa-associated lymphoid tissue lymphoma treated with radiotherapy. *Int J Radiat Oncol Biol Phys* 2012;82(4):1509–1514.

172. Soysal HG. Orbital exenteration: a 10-year experience of a general oncology hospital. *Orbit* 2010;29:135–139.

173. Hsu A, Frank SJ, Ballo MT, et al. Postoperative adjuvant external beam radiation therapy for cancers of the eyelid and conjunctiva. *Ophthal Plast Reconstr Surg* 2008;24:444–449.

174. Sinesi C, McNeese MD, Peters LJ, et al. Electron beam therapy for eyelid carcinomas. *Head Neck Surg* 1987;10:31–37.

175. Graue GF, Tena LB, Finger PT. Electron beam radiation for conjunctival squamous carcinoma. *Ophthal Plast Reconstr Surg* 2011;27(4):277–281.

176. Shields JA, Shields CL. Sebaceous adenocarcinoma of the eyelid. *Int Ophthalmol Clin* 2009;49(4):45–61.

177. Kivela T, Asko-Seljavaara S, Pihkala U, et al. Sebaceous carcinoma of the eyelid associated with retinoblastoma. *Ophthalmology* 2001;108:1124–1128.

178. Rishi K, Font RL. Sebaceous gland tumors of the eyelids and conjunctiva in the Muir-Torre syndrome: a clinicopathologic study of five cases and literature review. *Ophthal Plast Reconstr Surg* 2004;20:31–36.

179. Shields JA, Demirci H, Marr BP, et al. Sebaceous carcinoma of the ocular region. *Surv Ophthalmol* 2005;50:103–122.

180. Lisman RD, Jakobiec FA, Small P. Sebaceous carcinoma of the eyelids. The role of adjunctive cryotherapy in the management of conjunctival pagetoid spread. *Ophthalmology* 1989;96:1021–1026.

181. Shields CL, Naseripour M, Shields JA, et al. Topical mitomycin-C for pagetoid invasion of the conjunctiva by eyelid sebaceous gland carcinoma. *Ophthalmology* 2002;109:2129–2133.

182. Pardo FS, Wang CC, Albert D, et al. Sebaceous carcinoma of the ocular adnexa: radiotherapeutic management. *Int J Radiat Oncol Biol Phys* 1989;17:643.

183. Ognjanovic S, Linabery AM, Charbonneau B, et al. Trends in childhood rhabdomyosarcoma incidence and survival in the United States (1975–2005). *Cancer* 2009;115(18):4218–4226. doi:10.1002/cncr.24465.

184. Stobbe GD, Dargeon HW. Embryonal rhabdomyosarcoma of the head and neck in children and adolescents. *Cancer* 1950;3(5):826–836.

185. Pinkel D, Pickren J. Rhabdomyosarcoma in children. *JAMA* 1961;175:293–298.

186. Anderson GJ, Tom LW, Womer RB, et al. Rhabdomyosarcoma of the head and neck in children. *Arch Otolaryngol Head Neck Surg* 1990;116:428.

187. Andrassy RJ, Corpron CA, Hays D, et al. Extremity sarcomas: an analysis of prognostic factors from the intergroup rhabdomyosarcoma study (IRS) III. *J Pediatr Surg* 1996;31:191.

188. Andrassy R, Wiener ES, Raney RB, et al. Thoracic sarcomas in children. *Ann Surg* 1998;227:170.

189. Andrassy RJ, Hays DM, Raney RB, et al. Conservative surgical management of vaginal and vulvar pediatric rhabdomyosarcoma: a report from the intergroup rhabdomyosarcoma study-III. *J Pediatr Surg* 1995;30:1034.

190. Asmar L, Gehan EA, Newton WA, et al. Agreement among and within groups of pathologists in the classification of rhabdomyosarcoma and related childhood sarcomas: report of an international study of four pathology classifications. *Cancer* 1994;74:2579.

191. Burger RA, Riedmiller H, Gutjahr P, et al. Extent of surgery in rhabdomyosarcoma of urogenital structures. *Eur Urol* 1989;16:114.

192. Cofer BR, Weiner ES. Rhabdomyosarcoma. In: Andrassy RJ, ed. *Pediatric surgical oncology.* Oxford: Saunders, 1998.

193. McDonald MW, Esiashvili N, George BA, et al. Intensity-modulated radiotherapy with use of cone-down boost for pediatric head-and-neck rhabdomyosarcoma. *Int J Radiat Oncol Biol Phys* 2008;72(3):884–891.

194. Berman AT, Rengan R, Tripuraneni P. Radiotherapy for eyelid, periocular, and periorbital skin cancers. *Int Ophthalmol Clin* 2009;49(4):129–142.

Section III

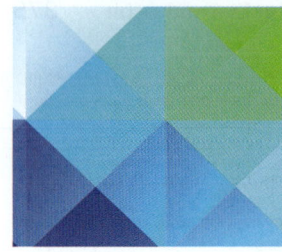

CHAPTER 42

Ear

Tony J. C. Wang and K. S. Clifford Chao

ANATOMY

The external, middle, and inner components of the ear develop from the three embryonic layers: ectoderm, mesoderm, and endoderm.

The external ear consists of the auricle or pinna, the external auditory meatus (canal), and the tympanic membrane (Fig. 42.1). The auricle is composed of elastic cartilage covered with skin. The external auditory meatus connects the tympanic membrane to the exterior and is approximately 2.4 cm long. The outer third is cartilaginous, and the inner two-thirds is bony and slightly narrower. The external auditory canal is anterior to the mastoid process and posterior to the parotid gland at the temporomandibular joint (TMJ). The inferior border of the canal lies near the jugular bulb and the facial nerve as it descends through the stylomastoid foramen. The skin lining the auditory canal is continuous with that of the auricle, and in the outer one-third of the canal, it contains hair follicles and sebaceous and ceruminous glands. The tympanic membrane, which is made of multiple layers of squamous epithelium, separates the auditory canal from the middle ear.

The middle ear houses the auditory ossicles, the tympanic cavity, and opens into the eustachian tube to communicate with the pharynx. The middle ear cavity is lined with a mucoperiosteal membrane, and the eustachian tube is lined with stratified columnar epithelium and has numerous mucous glands in the two-thirds of the tube closer to the pharynx. The overall length of the eustachian tube is 3.5 cm.[1]

The inner or internal ear lies in the petrous portion of the temporal bone and consists of the bony labyrinth and the membranous labyrinth. The membranous labyrinth, which holds the organ of hearing, is housed within the bony labyrinth. The cochlea, which is responsible for hearing, and the vestibule, which is responsible for balance, are part of the inner ear.

Blood supply to the auricle and the external auditory canal comes from branches of the posterior auricular artery and the superficial temporal artery, which arise from the external carotid artery. Blood is supplied to the middle ear region from branches of ascending pharyngeal and middle meningeal arteries and from the artery of the pterygoid canal. The inner ear is supplied by the internal auditory artery, which is a branch of the basilar artery, and from the anterior inferior cerebellar artery.

The nerves innervating the ear include cranial nerves V, VIII, IX, and X. The eighth cranial nerve or vestibulocochlear nerve is responsible for auditory and vestibular function. It exits from the brainstem between the pons and the medulla and follows the internal acoustic meatus.

For the external ear, lymphatic vessels of the tragus and anterior external portion of the auricle drain into the superficial parotid lymph nodes. The posterior and superior aspects of the auricle drain into the retroauricular lymph nodes, and the lobule drains into the superficial cervical group of lymph nodes. Lymphatics from the middle ear and the mastoid antrum pass into the parotid nodes and into the upper deep cervical lymph nodes. The lymphatics in the middle ear and eustachian tube are rather sparse, and the inner ear has no lymphatics.

EPIDEMIOLOGY

Malignant disease of the auricle is common (accounts for 6% of all skin cancer), but cancers of the middle ear and external auditory canal are rare, with an incidence of approximately 1 per million people.[2–4] Tumors of the external ear are most often cutaneous malignancies and may be related to sun

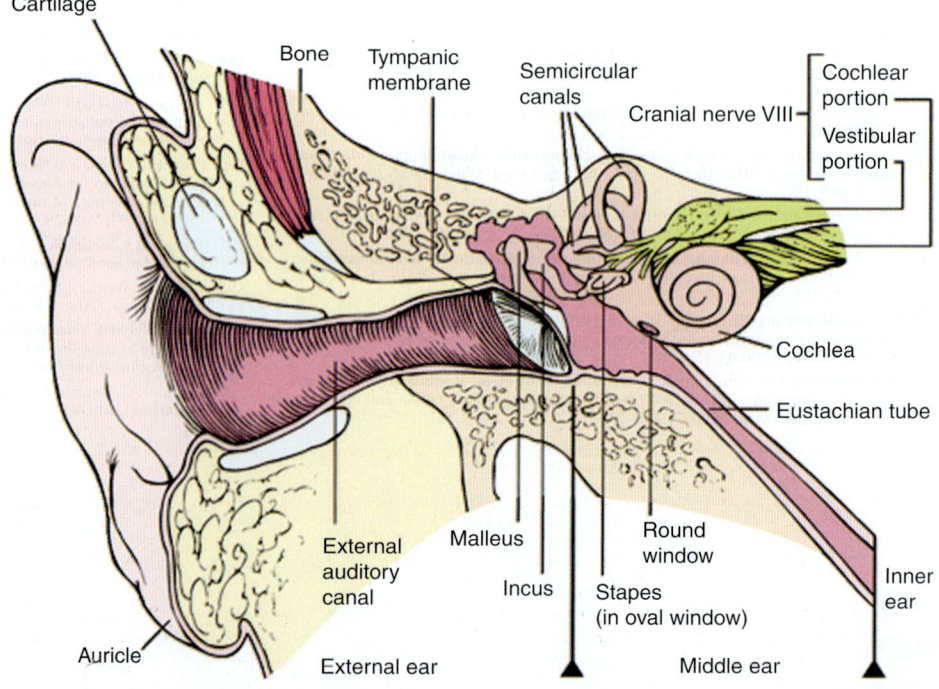

FIGURE 42.1. Ear anatomy.

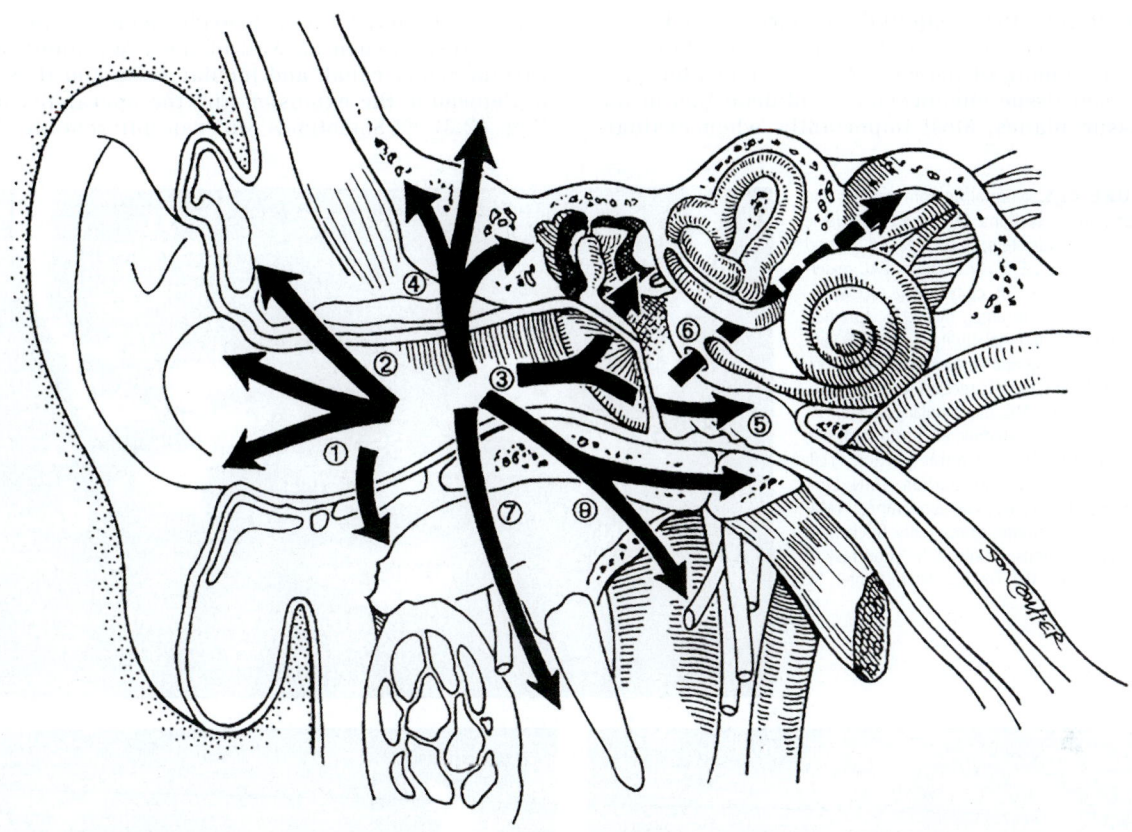

FIGURE 42.2. Coronal anatomy of pathways of spread of primary cancer of the external auditory canal. Cancer can spread (*1*) anteriorly through the cartilaginous canal into the parotid gland, (*2*) through the concha into the postauricular sulcus, (*3*) through the tympanic membrane into the middle ear, (*4*) posteriorly into the mastoid, (*5*) into the anterior mesotympanum to the carotid artery and eustachian tube, (*6*) into the inner ear through the round window or otic capsule, (*7*) along the extratemporal facial nerve into the infratemporal fossa, and (*8*) inferomedially into the jugular fossa, carotid artery, and lower cranial nerves. (Reprinted from Moody SA, Hirsch BE, Myers EN. Squamous cell carcinoma of the external auditory canal: an evaluation of a staging system. *Am J Otol* 2000;21[4]:582–588. With permission.)

exposure.[5,6] Other predisposing factors described, although their significance is in question, are otorrhea, chronic eczema, chronic dermatologic conditions, and chronic ulcerations from trauma.[7]

Tumors of the external ear most commonly occur in patients 60 to 70 years of age; tumors of the middle ear and the mastoid are more common in patients 40 to 60 years of age.[8,9] More women than men have middle ear tumors, but more men have tumors of the external ear.[10,11]

CLINICAL PRESENTATION

External Ear

Basal cell carcinomas are more common than squamous cell carcinomas in the external ear, with a ratio of 1.3 to 1.[8] They present as small ulcerations, mostly on the helix.[12,13] For squamous cell carcinomas, lymph node metastases occur in approximately 10% to 15%.[14] The common sites of lymph node metastases in order of frequency are the parotid gland, the upper deep cervical chain, and the postauricular nodes.[9,14] The rate of regional metastasis is higher in advanced disease and may involve the level 5 cervical lymph node group.[15]

External Auditory Canal

Most patients present with symptomatic lesions of the external auditory canal. Pruritus and pain are common. Swelling behind the ear, decreased hearing, and facial paralysis are seen in advanced cases. Spread of the tumor into the lymphatic areas is more common than to other areas of the ear (around 20%).[16,17] Tumors arising in the cartilaginous portion of the canal invade the cartilaginous walls and spread into the bony canal areas. However, those arising in the bony canal

have a more effective barrier (preventing spread) and therefore progress predominantly along the main axis of the canal, eventually invading the middle ear or the cartilaginous part of the canal. Local spreading route is depicted in Figure 42.2. Distant metastases are rare.

DIAGNOSTIC WORKUP

Table 42.1 summarizes workup and diagnostic procedures. A history and physical including otoscopy and careful lymph node exam should be performed. Neurologic exam finding of cranial nerve deficits may be an indication of advanced disease. A baseline audiology testing should be performed prior to any treatment.

TABLE 42.1 DIAGNOSTIC EVALUATION FOR CARCINOMA OF THE EAR

History
Physical examination
    Otoscopy
    Neurologic exam for cranial nerve function
    Careful assessment of regional lymph nodes
Laboratory tests
    Complete blood count
    Blood chemistry
Radiographic studies
    High-resolution computed tomography (standard)
    Magnetic resonance imaging (selected patients)
    Arteriography (optional)
Biopsy
Other studies
    Audiology testing

Both multidetector computed tomography (CT) and magnetic resonance imaging (MRI) play an important role in visualizing tumors of the ear.[18] CT can show abnormal soft tissue, soft tissue enhancement, and distortion of the normal tissue planes. Most importantly, when evaluat-ing EAC tumor, CT can provide accurate prediction of bone erosion, such as wall of the EAC, middle ear, TMJ, carotid artery canal, and jugular fossa and thus can help to determine the extension and the operability of tumors (Fig. 42.3).[19–21] Sometimes MRI can differentiate the tumor

FIGURE 42.3. Normal anatomy of the ear. **A–C:** Coronal sections. **D** and **E:** Transverse sections. BS, brainstem; C, cochlea; CC, carotid canal; CL, clivus; E, epitympanum; EAC, exter-nal auditory canal; ER, epitympanic recess; FC, facial canal; FO, foramen ovale; FS, foramen spinosum; IAC, internal auditory canal; JB, jug-ular bulb; LSC, lateral semicircular canal; LW, lateral wall, epitympanic recess (scutum); MAC, mastoid air cells; MC, mandibular condyle; OS, ossicles; OW, oval window; PF, posterior fossa; TLA, temporal lobe, anterior portion; TLP, temporal lobe, posterior portion; TMN, tym-panic membrane, normal appearance; TMA, tympanic membrane, abnormally thickened; SS, sphenoid sinus; V, vestibule. (Courtesy of Robert Gresick, MD, DePaul Health Center, St. Louis, MO.)

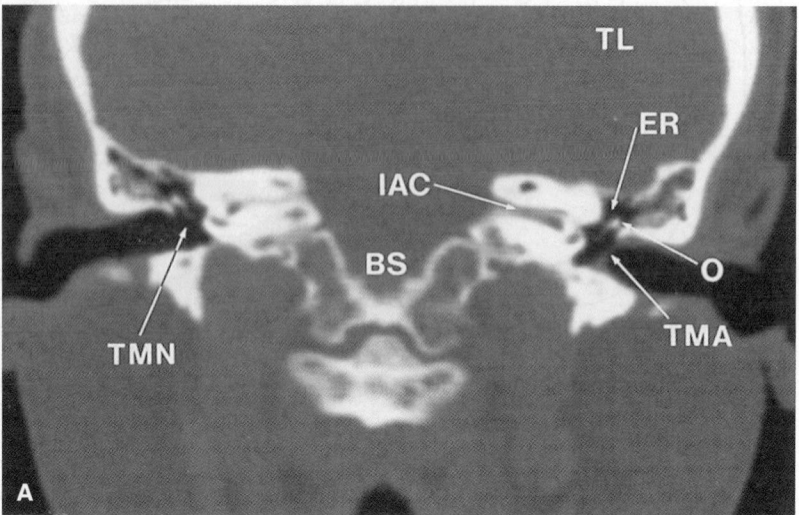

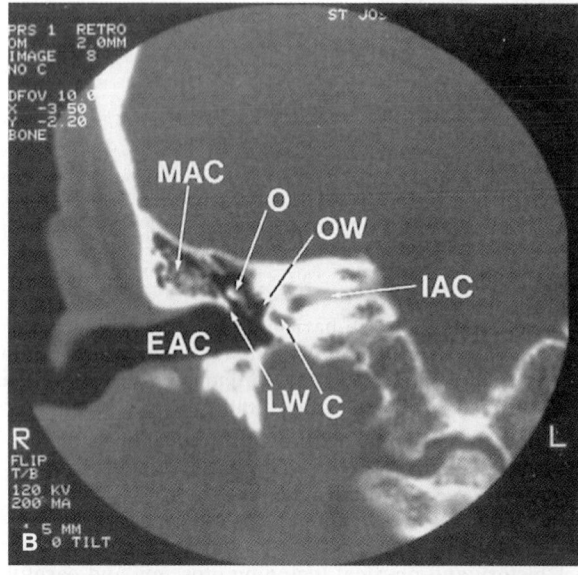

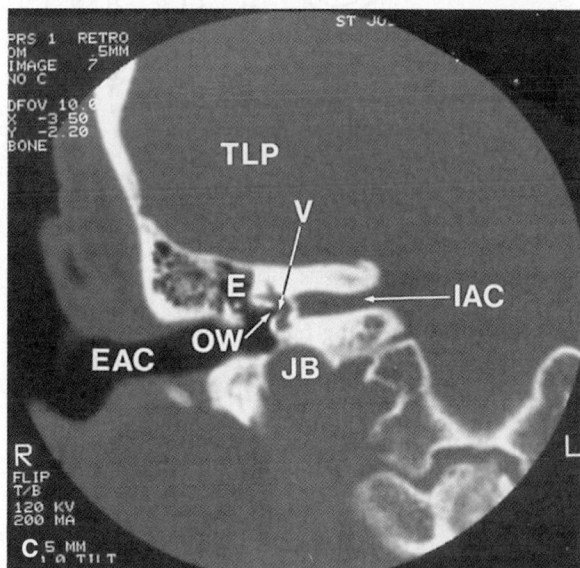

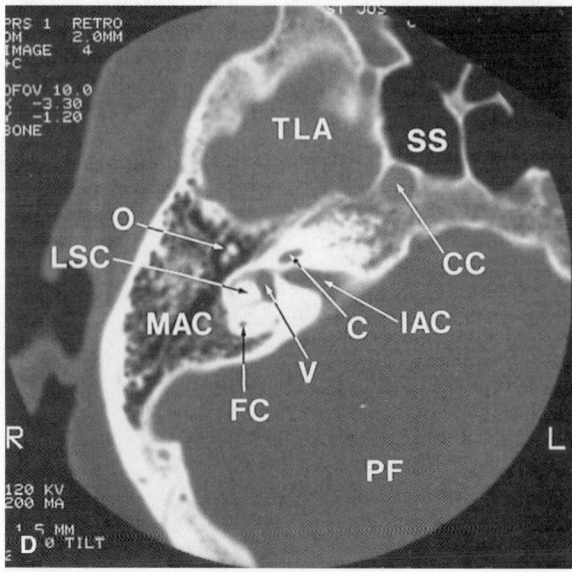

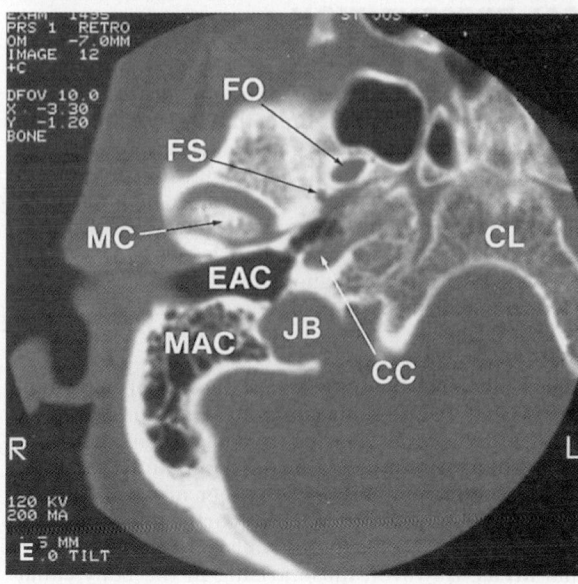

from mastoiditis and cholesteatomas and provide excellent delineation of soft tissue tumor margins, muscle infiltration, intracranial extension, dural or cerebral involvement, and vessel encasement.[21,22] Except in selected cases, angiography and jugular venography have also been abandoned in favor of CT.

Diagnosis is always established by biopsy and occasionally by aspiration of the exudative material or by surgical exploration. A bone scan may be done to determine the changes in the temporal bone around the tumor, but it provides very nonspecific information and is not a recommended method of evaluation.

PATHOLOGIC CLASSIFICATION

Approximately 85% of the tumors involving the auditory canal, middle ear, and mastoid area are squamous cell carcinomas. Infrequently, basal cell carcinomas, adenocarcinomas, adenoid cystic carcinomas, and melanomas are seen.[23] Even rarer are sarcomas, specifically embryonic rhabdomyosarcomas. Ceruminous gland tumors and papillomas rarely arise in the auditory canal.[7,23,24] Carcinoid tumor of the middle ear is rare, and only 50 cases have been reported in the literature.[25,26] Endolymphatic sac tumor or aggressive papillary middle ear tumors are distinct from middle ear adenomas and act aggressively. They are characterized by slow growth but extensive local invasion and bone destruction.[27,28]

PROGNOSTIC FACTORS

Lesions of the external ear are usually more easily controlled than are lesions of the middle ear or mastoid. External ear lesions are usually diagnosed earlier; they are mostly cutaneous, and adequate surgery or radiation therapy is usually effective.[3,9,29] Presence of large lesions involving the middle ear and those with extension into the temporal bone or soft tissue is a poor prognostic sign and more difficult to treat.[2,30,31] There does not appear to be a correlation between tumor differentiation, positive margins, or perineural disease and survival, although they may serve as a predictor for local control in tumors involving the temporal bone.[30,32,33] Seventh cranial nerve palsy associated with middle ear tumors indicates poor survival showed in pooled-data survival analysis, and have been adopted into staging system. Spread of tumors to the lymph nodes usually indicates a poor prognosis because this is often a late event in the natural history of the disease.[17,32,34] Nomogram for predicting overall survival and cause-specific survival in middle ear cancer patients has been proposed using SEER database.[35]

STAGING

The seventh edition of the American Joint Committee on Cancer (AJCC) staging manual[36] includes the external ear in its staging system under *Cutaneous Squamous Cell Carcinoma and Other Cutaneous Carcinomas* (Table 42.2). A group from the University of Pittsburgh proposed a staging system for squamous cell carcinoma of the external auditory canal and temporal bone, which was updated in 2002.[17,37–39] The primary tumor stage is determined by the level of bony erosion, size, and involvement of the middle ear. Lymph node disease is considered advanced stage with poor prognosis. This staging system has often been cited in the literature (Table 42.3).[2,17,34,38,40–46]

Section III

TABLE 42.2 THE AMERICAN JOINT COMMITTEE ON CANCER AND INTERNATIONAL UNION AGAINST CANCER STAGING SYSTEM FOR EAR CANCER

Stage	Staging Criteria
T Category	
Tx	Primary tumor cannot be assessed
T0	No evidence of primary tumor
Tis	Carcinoma *in situ*
T1	Tumor 2 cm or less in greatest dimension with fewer than two high-risk features[a]
T2	Tumor >2 cm in greatest dimension or tumor any size with two or more high-risk features[a]
T3	Tumor with invasion of maxilla, mandible, orbit, or temporal bone
T4	Tumor with invasion of skeleton (axial or appendicular) or perineural invasion of skull base
N Category	
Nx	Regional lymph nodes cannot be assessed
N0	No regional lymph node metastases
N1	Metastasis in a singly ipsilateral lymph node, 3 cm or less in greatest dimension
N2a	Metastasis in a single ipsilateral lymph node, >3 cm but not >6 cm in greatest dimension
N2b	Metastasis in multiple ipsilateral lymph nodes, none >6 cm in greatest dimension
N3c	Metastasis in bilateral or contralateral lymph nodes, none >6 cm in greatest dimension
N3	Metastasis in a lymph node, >6 cm in greatest dimension
M Category	
M0	No distant metastases
M1	Distant metastases

Stage Grouping			
0	Tis	N0	M0
I	T1	N0	M0
II	T2	N0	M0
III	T3	N0	M0
	T1	N1	M0
	T2	N1	M0
	T3	N1	M0
IV	T1	N2	M0
	T2	N2	M0
	T3	N2	M0
	T any	N3	M0
	T4	N any	M0
	T any	N any	M1

[a]High-risk features for the primary tumor (T) staging include depth of invasion >2-mm thickness, Clark level ≥ IV, and perineural invasion; anatomic location primary site on ear or hair-bearing lip; and cells that are poorly differentiated or undifferentiated.
From Edge SB, Byrd DR, Compton CC, et al., eds. *AJCC cancer staging handbook.* 7th ed. New York, NY: Springer, 2010. Copyright © 2010 American Joint Committee on Cancer. Reproduced with permission of Springer International Publishing in the format Book via Copyright Clearance Center.

TABLE 42.3 PITTSBURGH TUMOR STAGING SYSTEM (MODIFIED)[40]

Stage	CT or Pathology Findings
T1	Tumor limited to the EAC without bony erosion or evidence of soft tissue involvement
T2	Tumor with limited EAC bone erosion (not full thickness) or limited (<0.5 cm) soft tissue involvement
T3	Tumor eroding the osseous EAC (full thickness) with limited (<0.5 cm) soft tissue involvement, or tumor involving the middle ear and/or mastoid
T4	Tumor eroding the cochlea, petrous apex, medial wall of the middle ear, carotid canal, jugular foramen, or dura, or with extensive soft tissue involvement (>0.5 cm), such as involvement of TMJ or styloid process, or evidence of facial paresis

Reprinted from Cristalli G, Manciocco V, Pichi B, et al. Treatment and outcome of advanced external auditory canal and middle ear squamous cell carcinoma. *J Craniofac Surg* 2009;20(3): 816–821. With permission.

GENERAL MANAGEMENT

External Ear

Tumors of the external ear are most often treated with limited surgery or external radiation therapy. Treatment in early stages with irradiation is usually in the form of megavoltage electron beam therapy or orthovoltage.[47,48] Most radiation techniques have been fairly successful in the treatment of lesions in this area, with local control rates of 80% to 97%.[3,49-51] Caccialanza et al.[3] reported a 5-year cure rate of 78% with a mean follow-up of 2.4 years for 115 carcinomas of the pinna treated with definitive kilovoltage radiation to a total dose of 45 to 70 Gy in 2.5- to 5-Gy fractions given two to three times per week. Surgery is beneficial if the lesion has invaded the cartilage of the ear or extends medially into the auditory canal. If squamous cell carcinoma of the external ear is treated with surgery alone, there is a recurrence rate of 14% to 19%.[9,52] Mohs surgery is another option, with reported local recurrence rates of 5% to 7%.[29,53] Advanced lesions involving a significant portion of the ear canal are managed with a combination of irradiation and surgery. Palmer and Snell[54] describe the use of radical soft tissue and subtotal temporal bone excision with deltopectoral flap coverage for extensive tumors of the auricular area.

Treatment of draining lymphatics is normally not required for early stages of external ear tumors.[13] Afzelius et al.[12] indicate that lesions >4 cm and those with cartilage invasion have an increased risk of nodal spread; they recommend prophylactic neck dissection.[55] Most investigators do not agree with this approach because the overall chance of lymph node involvement in tumors of the external ear is only 16%. Osborne et al.[56] reported that parotidectomy may be unnecessary in management of advanced auricular carcinoma without clinically positive parotid disease.

Interstitial irradiation using afterloading ^{192}Ir, particularly for tumors smaller than 4 cm, is also an effective method of treatment, affording excellent local control with good cosmesis[51] (Table 42.4).

External Ear Canal and Middle Ear

Radical surgery followed by postoperative radiation therapy is an acceptable method of treatment for more advanced lesions of the external auditory canal and lesions in the middle ear and mastoid.[31,44,58] Pfreundner et al.[31] recommended a postoperative radiotherapy dose of 54 to 60 Gy for patients with negative margins. Positive margins warrant higher doses of 66 Gy because of higher recurrence rates. Except in tumors that are detected early, neither modality alone is considered optimal, and a combination of the two produces the best results.

Lesions of the outer part of the auditory canal require local excision with at least a 1-cm margin between the lesion and the tympanic membrane if there is no radiographic evidence of invasion of the mastoid. Surgery for tumors of the auditory canal is performed through a U-shaped incision with elevation of the flap from below. A split-thickness skin graft is usually required to cover the deficit along the auditory canal.

When the tumor involves the bony auditory canal and impinges on the tympanic membrane but does not involve the middle ear or the mastoid, a partial temporal bone resection may be necessary; in this procedure, the auditory canal, tympanic membrane, malleus, and incus are removed along with the TMJ, and the defect is grafted with a split-thickness skin graft. Postoperative radiation may be indicated, depending on margin status.

Middle Ear and Temporal Bone

In management of temporal bone tumors originating from the middle ear and mastoid area, surgical options include subtotal temporal bone resection, total temporal resection, lateral temporal resection, or mastoidectomy. Complete resection with clear margins may be difficult to achieve, given that important structures reside around the temporal bone.[40,55,59-61] Postoperative radiation therapy is recommended and increases local tumor control.[31,40,62] In studies that suggest limited benefit of postoperative irradiation, the results may be related to the extent of the tumor.[63] Given that total and subtotal temporal bone resection can result in significant morbidity, some investigators favor limited surgery with postoperative or perioperative radiation, or even definitive radiotherapy in early or unresectable lesions.[62,64,65] Stereotactic ablative radiotherapy (SABR) may represent a new treatment option for organ preservation. A study used 37.5 Gy/3 fractions or 40 Gy/5 fractions radiotherapy as a first-line treatment, resulting in 3-year OS rates: 69% for T1/2, 79% for T3 (95% CI, 47–93), and 0% for T4 disease with limited toxicities.[66] Masashi et al. reported their experience on treating unresectable locally advanced SCC of the external auditory canal and middle ear with carbon ion therapy. The 3-year local control was 54%.[67] Chemotherapy has been used in tumors of the ear. The common regimen includes cisplatin, docetaxel, and mitomycin via intravenous or intra-arterial.[68,69] A meta-analysis suggested that preoperative CRT followed by surgery may improve the survival of patients with external auditory canal SCC and that definitive CRT may be equivalent to surgical resection.[70] However, additional trials are necessary to determine efficacy because there was no control trial in this meta-analysis.

RADIATION THERAPY TECHNIQUES

Tumors involving the pinna can be treated with megavoltage electrons or with superficial or orthovoltage irradiation. The fields can be round or polygonal, drawn around the tumor to spare surrounding normal tissues. For small, superficial tumors, margins of 1 cm are adequate. However, more extensive lesions require large portals, which may encompass the entire pinna or external canal and require 2- to 3-cm margins around the clinically apparent tumor (Fig. 42.4). Lesions involving the pinna must be treated with slow fractionation (1.8 to 2 Gy daily) to prevent cartilage necrosis. Doses of 66 Gy over a period of 6.5 weeks are required to achieve adequate tumor control.

Large lesions of the external auditory canal are treated with radiation or combined with surgery; the portals should encompass the entire ear and temporal bone with an adequate margin (3 cm). The volume treated should include the ipsilateral preauricular, postauricular, and subdigastric lymph nodes. Treating lymphatics beyond the jugulodigastric area is usually not necessary.

TABLE 42.4 TREATMENT OF CARCINOMA OF THE EXTERNAL EAR

Result	Modality	
	Surgery	Irradiation
Cure at 3 yr[57]	330/358 (92%)[a]	141/174 (81%)
Cure at 5 yr[3]		(78%)
Local control at 2 yr[29,50]	82/87 (94%)[b]	60/62 (97%)
Local control at 2 yr[48]		(86%)[c]
Local control at 4 yr[51]		60/61 (99%)
Local control at 5 yr[49]		128/138 (93%)
Local control at 5 yr[48]		(79%)[c]

[a]Results given as number of successful outcomes/patient population.
[b]Treatment by Mohs micrographic surgery.
[c]Included advanced primary tumors.

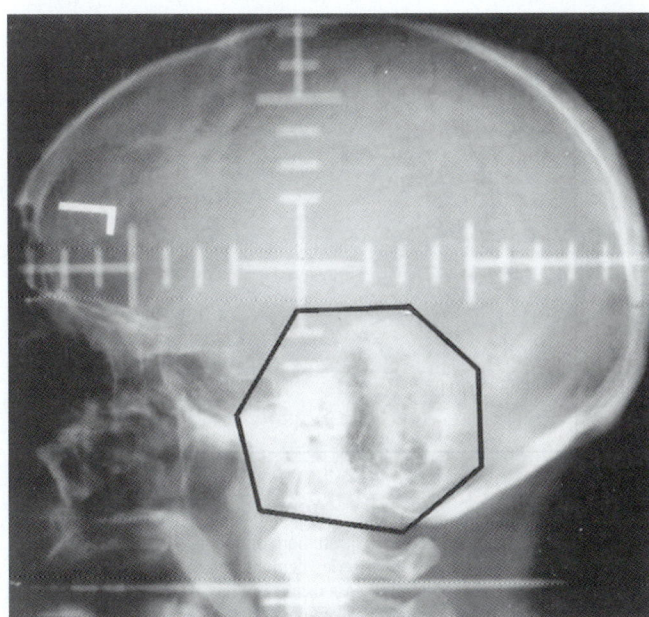

FIGURE 42.4. Example of treatment portal for tumor of the middle ear involving the petrous bone. The mastoid is included in irradiated volume.

The use of intensity-modulated radiotherapy (IMRT) can help improve target coverage and spare normal critical structures. Careful understanding of lymphatic drainage and tumor extension is crucial for target delineation and to avoid geographic miss. Pretreatment CT or MRI scans should be reviewed along with any operative or pathology reports.

In the definitive treatment of advanced external auditory canal or middle ear cancers, gross target volume (GTV) should include the clinical and radiographic gross disease (Fig. 42.5). Clinical target volume 1 (CTV1) should encompass the GTV with a 0.3- to 0.5-cm margin to a dose of 66 to 70 Gy at 2 Gy per fraction. CTV2 should include CTV1 with a 0.5- to 0.7-cm margin, as well as the preauricular nodes, postauricular nodes, ipsilateral upper cervical neck (level II), and parotid gland to a dose of 63 Gy at 1.8 Gy per fraction. A CTV3 can be considered for some patients with more advanced and aggressive tumors for treatment of the ipsilateral middle and lower neck (level III and IV) and contralateral upper neck (level II) to a dose of 56 Gy at 1.6 Gy per fraction. Planning target volumes are created with a 3- to 5-mm margin around the CTVs.

Chen et al.[62] described the target volumes for postoperative IMRT of the external auditory canal and middle ear. In the postoperative setting, CTV1 includes the original tumor region, surgical bed, soft tissue invasion, areas with positive residual disease, or positive margins to a dose of 60 to 66 Gy at 2 Gy per fraction. CTV2 includes CTV1 with a 0.5- to 0.7-cm margin, depending on the anatomy, and the ipsilateral upper neck (level II), including the parotid region, to a dose of 54 to 60 Gy at 1.8 Gy per fraction. In some patients, CTV3 is included to cover the ipsilateral middle to low neck (level III and IV) with or without the contralateral upper neck (level II) to a dose of 50 to 54 Gy at 1.6 Gy per fraction. Plans should be optimized to cover 95% of the planning target volume with 100% of the prescribed dose. In this case series, marginal failure occurred at the preauricular space and glenoid fossa of the TMJ. Caution should be taken to cover the area.

Extremely advanced tumors that are unresectable should be treated with high-energy ipsilateral electron beam therapy (16 to 20 MeV) alone or mixed with photons (4 to 6 MV), wedge pair (superior inferiorly angled beams) techniques using low-energy photons, or IMRT. IMRT is a reasonable option if nodal coverage is indicated. Doses of 60 to 70 Gy over 6 to 7 weeks are required. Doses higher than this may produce osteoradionecrosis of the temporal bone. If various types of radiation therapy beams are

FIGURE 42.5. A: Treatment plan for external auditory canal squamous cell carcinoma: gross target volume (GTV) is in red, high-risk clinical target volume (CTV1) is in green, and planning target volume (PTV) is in orange. **B:** Dose color wash of 2 full-arc volumetric modulated arc therapy (VMAT) plan.

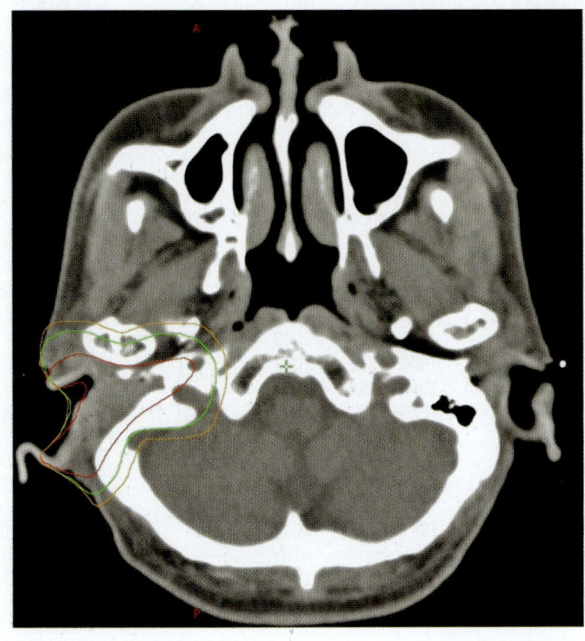

A

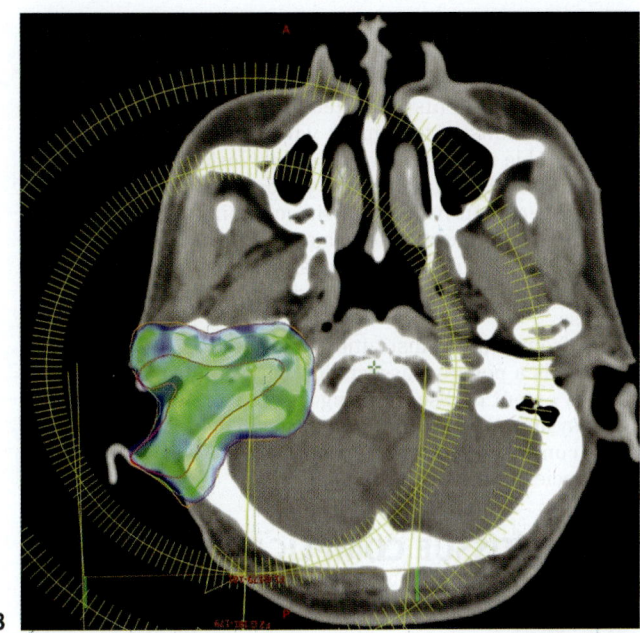

B

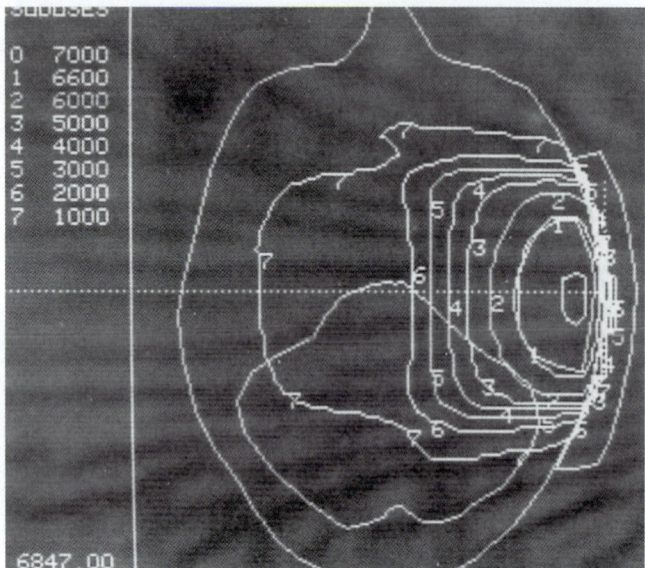

FIGURE 42.6. Computerized isodose distribution for treatment of a middle ear tumor using a combination of 4-MV photons (20%) and 16-MeV electrons (80%).

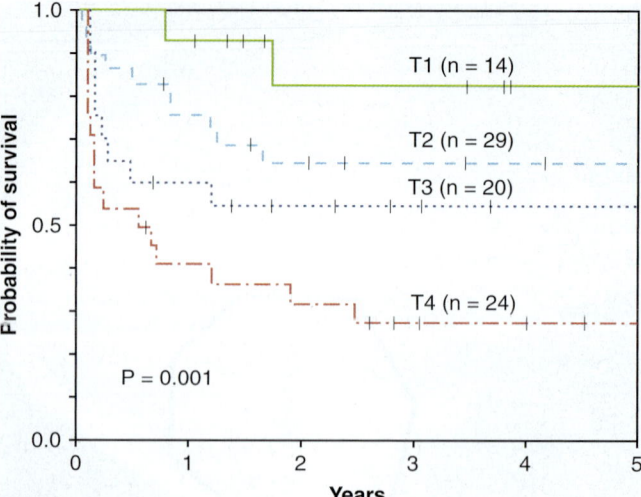

FIGURE 42.7. Data from patients with tumors of middle ear and external auditory canal from a multi-institutional series demonstrate the association between disease-free survival and extent of disease using the University of Pittsburgh staging system. (Reprinted from Ogawa K, Nakamura K, Hatano K, et al. Treatment and prognosis of squamous cell carcinoma of the external auditory canal and middle ear: a multi-institutional retrospective review of 87 patients. *Int J Radiat Oncol Biol Phys* 2007;68[5]:1326–1334. Copyright © 2007 Elsevier. With permission.)

available, individualized treatment plans should be devised (Fig. 42.6). Most patients receiving radiation therapy to the middle ear and temporal bone regions benefit from immobilization devices such as the Aquaplast system. When electron beam radiation therapy is used, use of water bolus in the external auditory canal and concha may reduce the auricular complications.

Palliative Radiation Therapy

Radiation therapy offers significant palliation in recurrent or advanced disease. Pain relief is reported in 61% of patients with tumors of the auditory canal and middle ear.[71] Recurrences developing after previous irradiation may be re-treated with low-dose radiation therapy and hope for control of tumor in approximately 20% of patients.[72] When a small-volume local recurrence occurs after previous radiation therapy, fractionated high dose rate treatment may be considered.

RESULTS OF THERAPY

The series of patients reported from several institutions are small. Results of treatment with various modalities are shown in Table 42.4. In more extensive lesions, combinations of surgery and irradiation have yielded satisfactory results. Overall 5-year survival rates with combination therapy for tumors involving the middle ear and external auditory canal range from 40% to 60%, whereas patients with early-stage tumors achieve a 70% 5-year survival rate with no evidence of disease.

Data from a multi-institutional series (Fig. 42.7) indicate that there is a negative association between disease-free survival and extent of disease using the University of Pittsburgh staging system.[44] These data also provide evidence of the success of combined surgery and postoperative irradiation for malignancies of the temporal bone.[73,74]

NORMAL-TISSUE COMPLICATIONS

Organs at risk should include the brainstem, spinal cord, cochlea, eye, optic nerve, chiasm, lens, larynx, oral cavity,

parotid glands, and temporal bone. Normal-tissue constraints are given in Table 42.5.

For conventionally fractionated radiation therapy, the mean dose to the cochlea should be limited to less or equal to 45 Gy, or more conservatively 35 Gy, to reduce sensorineural hearing loss.[85] Modeling of some of the sensorineural hearing loss data from the *Quantitative Analysis of Normal Tissue Effects in the Clinic studies* are presented in (Fig. 42.8). The phenomenological binomial equation of Zaider and Amols was used.[86] Chen et al.[89] noted that hearing loss at a

TABLE 42.5 TREATMENT OF CARCINOMA OF THE EXTERNAL AUDITORY CANAL AND MIDDLE EAR: RECENT LITERATURE

Author	Time Span	Published	Number	Result
Choi et al.[64]	1990–2013	2017	32	5-Y-OS: 57%
Gandhi et al.[75]	2001–2012	2016	43	5-Y-OS: 30%
Morita et al.[76]	1997–2015	2016	57	5-Y-OS: T1/2 OP: 100%; RT: 81.3%. T3/4 CRT: 52.1%; OP + CRT: 55.6%.
Ihler et al.[77]	1997–2013	2015	36	5-Y-OS: 59.4%
Takenaka et al.[78]	2006–2013(*)	2015	752	5-Y-OS: 57%
Xie et al.[79]	2004–2012	2015	41	2-Y-OS: 56.9%
Shen et al.[80]	1983–2011	2014	247	5-Y-OS: 47.4%
Leong et al.[81]	2001–2012	2013	35	5-Y-OS: 48.6%
Prabhu et al.[58]	1976–2003	2009	30	5-Y-OS: 74%
Madsen et al.[2]	1992–2001	2008	68	5-Y-OS: 44%
Ogawa et al.[44]	1984–2005	2007	87	5-Y-OS: 55%
Pemberton et al.[82]	1965–1988	2006	123	5-Y-LC: 56%
Nakagawa et al.[70]	1998–2004	2006	25	For T1/2, 3-Y-OS: 100%; For T3, 5-Y-OS: 80%; For T4, 5-Y-OS: 35%
Sarkar et al.[83]	1987–1996	2005	41	2-Y-OS: OP + RT: 85%; RT: 19%
Hashi et al.[84]	1980–1998	2000	20	5-Y-OS: 59%

*Meta-analysis, for published year

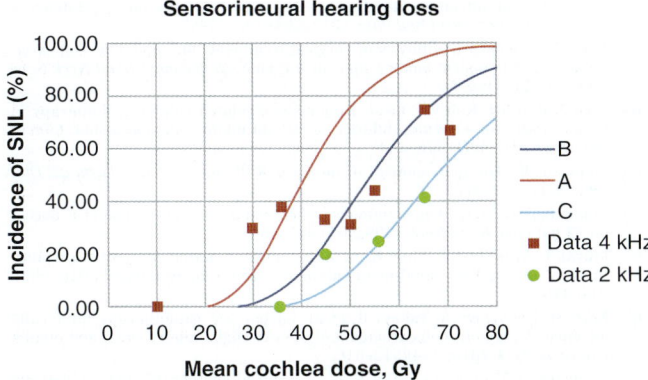

FIGURE 42.8. Modeling of quantitative analysis of normal tissue effects in the clinic sensorineural hearing loss data using the phenomenologic binomial equation of Zaider and Amols.[85-88] Data for 2 kHz are shown as circles and those for 4 kHz as squares. All points are taken from Figure 1a, b of Bhandare et al.[85,87] Theoretical curves use a simple two-parameter variant of the nested exponential equation (10) of Zaider and Amols[86,88]: $P(D) = 100 \exp[-\alpha_1 \exp(-\alpha_2 D)]$. The three curves are drawn with $\alpha_1 = 40$; the central curve has $1/\alpha_2 = 13.3$ Gy (B), and outer curves are for $1/\alpha_2 = (A)$ *green*, 10 Gy and (C) *blue*, 16 Gy. SNL, sensorineural hearing loss.[88] (From Burri RJ. Ear. In: Chao C, Perez CA, Brady LW, eds. *Radiation oncology: management decisions*. Philadelphia, PA: Lippincott Williams & Wilkins, 2011:203–209. With permission.)

given radiation dose increased as frequency of the sound increased. The data are reasonably covered by theoretical curves having a characteristic dose (parameter α_2) of about 10 Gy (Table 42.6).

SEQUELAE OF TREATMENT

Possible sequelae with surgery are hemorrhage, infection, loss of facial nerve function, and, rarely, carotid artery thrombosis. Occasionally, vertigo is reported after temporal bone resection. Vertigo may last for 2 weeks, and a period of unsteadiness may last for a few months. Permanent deafness usually occurs on the operated side.

Radiation therapy sequelae include cartilage necrosis of the external auditory canal and osteoradionecrosis of temporal bone.[13,87] Very rarely, secondary infection and meningitis are reported.[11] Because of the proximity of the brainstem and medulla oblongata, it is extremely difficult to deliver a high dose of irradiation to the temporal bone without a significant risk of injury to these structures. An overall 10% incidence of bone necrosis can be expected after administration of 60 to 65 Gy. After external ear lesions are treated with interstitial irradiation, there is a 4% incidence of late cutaneous and cartilage necrosis. Risk of necrosis increases for lesions >4 cm.[51] A majority of patients can experience acute grade 2 and 3

skin toxicities with postoperative IMRT.[62] Following definitive or postoperative radiation, there is a 30% incidence of xerostomia.[58]

REFERENCES

1. Lewis J. Cancer of the external auditory canal, middle ear, and mastoid. In: Myers E, ed. *Cancer of the head and neck.* New York: Churchill Livingstone, 1981:557–575.
2. Madsen AR, Gundgaard MG, Hoff CM, et al. Cancer of the external auditory canal and middle ear in Denmark from 1992 to 2001. *Head Neck* 2008;30(10):1332–1338.
3. Caccialanza M, Piccinno R, Kolesnikova L, et al. Radiotherapy of skin carcinomas of the pinna: a study of 115 lesions in 108 patients. *Int J Dermatol* 2005;44(6):513–517.
4. Ragi JM, Patel D, Masud A, et al. Nonmelanoma skin cancer of the ear: frequency, patients' knowledge, and photoprotection practices. *Dermatol Surg* 2010;36(8):1232–1239.
5. Gallagher RP, Hill GB, Bajdik CD, et al. Sunlight exposure, pigmentation factors, and risk of nonmelanocytic skin cancer. II. Squamous cell carcinoma. *Arch Dermatol* 1995;131(2):164–169.
6. Lewis KG, Weinstock MA. Nonmelanoma skin cancer mortality (1988–2000): the Rhode Island follow-back study. *Arch Dermatol* 2004;140(7):837–842.
7. Pulec JL. Glandular tumors of the external auditory canal. *Laryngoscope* 1977;87(10 Pt 1):1601–1612.
8. Ahmad I, Das Gupta AR. Epidemiology of basal cell carcinoma and squamous cell carcinoma of the pinna. *J Laryngol Otol* 2001;115(2):85–86.
9. Byers R, Kesler K, Redmon B, et al. Squamous cell carcinoma of the external ear. *Am J Surg* 1983;146(4):447–450.
10. Iversen T, Tretli S. Trends for invasive squamous cell neoplasia of the skin in Norway. *Br J Cancer* 1999;81(3):528–531.
11. Lewis JS. A guide to cancer of the ear. *CA Cancer J Clin* 1977;27(1):42–46.
12. Afzelius LE, Gunnarsson M, Nordgren H. Guidelines for prophylactic radical lymph node dissection in cases of carcinoma of the external ear. *Head Neck Surg* 1980;2(5):361–365.
13. Avila J, Bosch A, Aristizabal S, et al. Carcinoma of the pinna. *Cancer* 1977;40(6):2891–2895.
14. Clark RR, Soutar DS. Lymph node metastases from auricular squamous cell carcinoma. A systematic review and meta-analysis. *J Plast Reconstr Aesthet Surg* 2008;61(10):1140–1147.
15. Peiffer N, Kutz JW Jr, Myers LL, et al. Patterns of regional metastasis in advanced stage cutaneous squamous cell carcinoma of the auricle. *Otolaryngol Head Neck Surg* 2011;144(1):36–42.
16. Ouaz K, Robier A, Lescanne E, et al. Cancer of the external auditory canal. *Eur Ann Otorhinolaryngol Head Neck Dis* 2013;130(4):175–182.
17. Gaudet JE, Walvekar RR, Arriaga MA, et al. Applicability of the pittsburgh staging system for advanced cutaneous malignancy of the temporal bone. *Skull Base* 2010;20(6):409–414.
18. Nemec SF, Donat MA, Mehrain S, et al. CT-MR image data fusion for computer assisted navigated neurosurgery of temporal bone tumors. *Eur J Radiol* 2007;62(2):192–198.
19. Lane JI, Lindell EP, Witte RJ, et al. Middle and inner ear: improved depiction with multiplanar reconstruction of volumetric CT data. *Radiographics* 2006;26(1):115–124.
20. Wang Z, Zheng M, Xia S. The contribution of CT and MRI in staging, treatment planning and prognosis prediction of malignant tumors of external auditory canal. *Clin Imaging* 2016;40(6):1262–1268.
21. Horowitz SW, Leonetti JP, Azar-Kia B, et al. CT and MR of temporal bone malignancies primary and secondary to parotid carcinoma. *Am J Neuroradiol* 1994;15(4):755–762.
22. Friedman DP, Rao VM. MR and CT of squamous cell carcinoma of the middle ear and mastoid complex. *Am J Neuroradiol* 1991;12(5):872–874.
23. Lederman M. Malignant tumours of the ear. *J Laryngol Otol* 1965;79:85–119.
24. Rogers KA Jr, Snow JB Jr. Squamous cell papilloma of the external auditory canal and middle ear treated with radiation therapy. *Laryngoscope* 1968;78(12):2183–2188.
25. Ramsey MJ, Nadol JB Jr, Pilch BZ, et al. Carcinoid tumor of the middle ear: clinical features, recurrences, and metastases. *Laryngoscope* 2005;115(9):1660–1666.
26. Sahan M, Yildirim N, Arslanoglu A, et al. Carcinoid tumor of the middle ear: report of a case. *Am J Otolaryngol* 2008;29(5):352–356.
27. Bell D, Gidley P, Levine N, et al. Endolymphatic sac tumor (aggressive papillary tumor of middle ear and temporal bone): sine qua non radiology-pathology and the University of Texas MD Anderson Cancer Center experience. *Ann Diagn Pathol* 2011;15(2):117–123.
28. Gaffey MJ, Mills SE, Fechner RE, et al. Aggressive papillary middle-ear tumor. A clinicopathologic entity distinct from middle-ear adenoma. *Am J Surg Pathol* 1988;12(10):790–797.
29. Silapunt S, Peterson SR, Goldberg LH. Squamous cell carcinoma of the auricle and Mohs micrographic surgery. *Dermatol Surg* 2005;31(11 Pt 1):1423–1427.
30. Gal TJ, Futran ND, Bartels LJ, et al. Auricular carcinoma with temporal bone invasion: outcome analysis. *Otolaryngol Head Neck Surg* 1999;121(1):62–65.

TABLE 42.6 NORMAL TISSUE DOSE CONSTRAINTS

Structure	Constraints
Brainstem	Maximum <60 Gy
Spinal cord	Maximum <45 Gy
Cochlea	Mean dose <45 Gy
Optic nerve	Maximum <55 Gy
Optic chiasm	Maximum <55 Gy
Lens	Maximum <10 Gy
Larynx	Mean dose <44 Gy; maximum <66 Gy
Oral cavity	Mean dose <35 Gy
Parotid gland	Combined parotid glands mean dose <25 Gy or spare one parotid gland mean dose <20 Gy
Temporal bone	Limit to <70 Gy to reduce osteoradionecrosis chance

Section III

31. Pfreundner L, Schwager K, Willner J, et al. Carcinoma of the external auditory canal and middle ear. *Int J Radiat Oncol Biol Phys* 1999;44(4):777–788.

32. Liu FF, Keane TJ, Davidson J. Primary carcinoma involving the petrous temporal bone. *Head Neck* 1993;15(1):39–43.

33. Hammer J, Eckmayr A, Zoidl JP, et al. Case report: salvage fractionated high dose rate after-loading brachytherapy in the treatment of a recurrent tumour in the middle ear. *Br J Radiol* 1994;67(797):504–506.

34. Higgins TS, Antonio SA. The role of facial palsy in staging squamous cell carcinoma of the temporal bone and external auditory canal: a comparative survival analysis. *Otol Neurotol* 2010;31(9):1473–1479.

35. Birzgalis AR, Keith AO, Farrington WT. Radiotherapy in the treatment of middle ear and mastoid carcinoma. *Clin Otolaryngol Allied Sci* 1992;17(2):113–116.

36. American Joint Committee on Cancer. *AJCC cancer staging manual.* 7th ed. New York: Springer, 2010.

37. Arriaga M, Curtin H, Takahashi H, et al. Staging proposal for external auditory meatus carcinoma based on preoperative clinical examination and computed tomography findings. *Ann Otol Rhinol Laryngol* 1990;99(9 Pt 1):714–721.

38. Moody SA, Hirsch BE, Myers EN. Squamous cell carcinoma of the external auditory canal: an evaluation of a staging system. *Am J Otol* 2000;21(4):582–588.

39. Hirsch BE. Staging system revision. *Arch Otolaryngol Head Neck Surg* 2002;128(1):93–94.

40. Cristalli G, Manciocco V, Pichi B, et al. Treatment and outcome of advanced external auditory canal and middle ear squamous cell carcinoma. *J Craniofac Surg* 2009;20(3):816–821.

41. Gillespie MB, Francis HW, Chee N, et al. Squamous cell carcinoma of the temporal bone: a radiographic-pathologic correlation. *Arch Otolaryngol Head Neck Surg* 2001;127(7):803–807.

42. Isipradit P, Wadwongtham W, Aeumjaturapat S, et al. Carcinoma of the external auditory canal. *J Med Assoc Thai* 2005;88(1):114–117.

43. Nyrop M, Grontved A. Cancer of the external auditory canal. *Arch Otolaryngol Head Neck Surg* 2002;128(7):834–837.

44. Ogawa K, Nakamura K, Hatano K, et al. Treatment and prognosis of squamous cell carcinoma of the external auditory canal and middle ear: a multi-institutional retrospective review of 87 patients. *Int J Radiat Oncol Biol Phys* 2007;68(5):1326–1334.

45. Testa JR, Fukuda Y, Kowalski LP. Prognostic factors in carcinoma of the external auditory canal. *Arch Otolaryngol Head Neck Surg* 1997;123(7):720–724.

46. Ueda Y, Kurita T, Matsuda Y, et al. Superselective, intra-arterial, rapid infusion chemotherapy for external auditory canal carcinoma. *J Laryngol Otol Suppl* 2009(31):75–80.

47. Hunter RD, Pereira DT, Pointon RC. Megavoltage electron beam therapy in the treatment of basal and squamous cell carcinomata of the pinna. *Clin Radiol* 1982;33(3):341–345.

48. Silva JJ, Tsang RW, Panzarella T, et al. Results of radiotherapy for epithelial skin cancer of the pinna: the Princess Margaret Hospital experience, 1982-1993. *Int J Radiat Oncol Biol Phys* 2000;47(2):451–459.

49. Hayter CR, Lee KH, Groome PA, et al. Necrosis following radiotherapy for carcinoma of the pinna. *Int J Radiat Oncol Biol Phys* 1996;36(5):1033–1037.

50. Lim JT. Irradiation of the pinna with superficial kilovoltage radiotherapy. *Clin Oncol (R Coll Radiol)* 1992;4(4):236-239.

51. Mazeron JJ, Ghalie R, Zeller J, et al. Radiation therapy for carcinoma of the pinna using iridium 192 wires: a series of 70 patients. *Int J Radiat Oncol Biol Phys* 1986;12(10):1757–1763.

52. Shockley WW, Stucker FJ Jr. Squamous cell carcinoma of the external ear: a review of 75 cases. *Otolaryngol Head Neck Surg* 1987;97(3):308–312.

53. Niparko JK, Swanson NA, Baker SR, et al. Local control of auricular, peri-auricular, and external canal cutaneous malignancies with Mohs surgery. *Laryngoscope* 1990;100(10 Pt 1):1047–1051.

54. Palmer JA, Snell GE. Surgical treatment of extensive tumors of the lateral face and auricular area by radical soft tissue and subtotal temporal bone excision with deltopectoral flap coverage. *J Otolaryngol* 1979;8(6):531–536.

55. Ariyan S, Sasaki CT, Spencer D. Radical en bloc resection of the temporal bone. *Am J Surg* 1981;142(4):443–447.

56. Osborne RF, Shaw T, Zandifar H, et al. Elective parotidectomy in the management of advanced auricular malignancies. *Laryngoscope* 2008;118(12):2139–2145.

57. Schewe EJ Jr, Pappalardo C. Cancer of the external ear. *Am J Surg* 1962;104:753–755.

58. Prabhu R, Hinerman RW, Indelicato DJ, et al. Squamous cell carcinoma of the external auditory canal: long-term clinical outcomes using surgery and external-beam radiotherapy. *Am J Clin Oncol* 2009;32(4):401–404.

59. Gacek RR, Goodman M. Management of malignancy of the temporal bone. *Laryngoscope* 1977;87(10 Pt 1):1622–1634.

60. Graham MD, Sataloff RT, Kemink JL, et al. Total en bloc resection of the temporal bone and carotid artery for malignant tumors of the ear and temporal bone. *Laryngoscope* 1984;94(4):528–533.

61. Sekhar LN, Pomeranz S, Janecka IP, et al. Temporal bone neoplasms: a report on 20 surgically treated cases. *J Neurosurg* 1992;76(4):578–587.

62. Chen WY, Kuo SH, Chen YH, et al. Postoperative intensity-modulated radiotherapy for squamous cell carcinoma of the external auditory canal and middle ear: treatment outcomes, marginal misses, and perspective on target delineation. *Int J Radiat Oncol Biol Phys* 2012;82(4):1485–1493.

63. Prasad S, Janecka IP. Efficacy of surgical treatments for squamous cell carcinoma of the temporal bone: a literature review. *Otolaryngol Head Neck Surg* 1994;110(3):270–280.

64. Choi J, Kim SH, Koh YW, et al. Tumor stage-related role of radiotherapy in patients with an external auditory canal and middle ear carcinoma. *Cancer Res Treat* 2017;49(1):178–184.

65. Shaheen OH. The management of tumours of the middle ear. *J Laryngol Otol* 1983;97(4):313–317.

66. Zhang B, Tu G, Xu G, et al. Squamous cell carcinoma of temporal bone: reported on 33 patients. *Head Neck* 1999;21(5):461–466.

67. Murai T, Kamata SE, Sato K, et al. Hypofractionated stereotactic radiotherapy for auditory canal or middle ear cancer. *Cancer Control* 2016;23(3):311–316.

68. Koto M, Hasegawa A, Takagi R, et al. Carbon ion radiotherapy for locally advanced squamous cell carcinoma of the external auditory canal and middle ear. *Head Neck* 2016;38(4):512–516.

69. Fujiwara M, Yamamoto S, Doi H, et al. Arterial chemoradiotherapy for carcinomas of the external auditory canal and middle ear. *Laryngoscope* 2015;125(3):685–689.

70. Nakagawa T, Kumamoto Y, Natori Y, et al. Squamous cell carcinoma of the external auditory canal and middle ear: an operation combined with preoperative chemoradiotherapy and a free surgical margin. *Otol Neurotol* 2006;27(2):242–248; discussion 249.

71. Paaske PB, Witten J, Schwer S, et al. Results in treatment of carcinoma of the external auditory canal and middle ear. *Cancer* 1987;59(1):156–160.

72. Gabriele P, Magnano M, Albera R, et al. Carcinoma of the external auditory meatus and middle ear. Results of the treatment of 28 cases. *Tumori* 1994;80(1):40–43.

73. Lesser RW, Spector GJ, Devineni VR. Malignant tumors of the middle ear and external auditory canal: a 20-year review. *Otolaryngol Head Neck Surg* 1987;96(1):43–47.

74. Spector JG. Management of temporal bone carcinomas: a therapeutic analysis of two groups of patients and long-term followup. *Otolaryngol Head Neck Surg* 1991;104(1):58–66.

75. Gandhi AK, Roy S, Biswas A, et al. Treatment of squamous cell carcinoma of external auditory canal: a tertiary cancer centre experience. *Auris Nasus Larynx* 2016;43(1):45–49.

76. Morita S, Homma A, Nakamaru Y, et al. The outcomes of surgery and chemoradiotherapy for temporal bone cancer. *Otol Neurotol* 2016;37(8):1174–1182.

77. Ihler F, Koopmann M, Weiss BG, et al. Surgical margins and oncologic results after carcinoma of the external auditory canal. *Laryngoscope* 2015;125(9):2107–2112.

78. Takenaka Y, Cho H, Nakahara S, et al. Chemoradiation therapy for squamous cell carcinoma of the external auditory canal: a meta-analysis. *Head Neck* 2015;37(7):1073–1080.

79. Xie B, Zhang T, Dai C. Survival outcomes of patients with temporal bone squamous cell carcinoma with different invasion patterns. *Head Neck* 2015;37(2):188–196.

80. Shen W, Sakamoto N, Yang L. Prognostic models to predict overall and cause-specific survival for patients with middle ear cancer: a population-based analysis. *BMC Cancer* 2014;14:554.

81. Leong SC, Youssef A, Lesser TH. Squamous cell carcinoma of the temporal bone: outcomes of radical surgery and postoperative radiotherapy. *Laryngoscope* 2013;123(10):2442–2448.

82. Pemberton LS, Swindell R, Sykes AJ. Primary radical radiotherapy for squamous cell carcinoma of the middle ear and external auditory canal—an historical series. *Clin Oncol (R Coll Radiol)* 2006;18(5):390–394.

83. Sarkar SK, Rashid MA, Patra NB, et al. Evaluation of results of radiotherapy alone vs combined surgery and postoperative radiotherapy in carcinoma external auditory canal-10 years review. *Indian J Otolaryngol Head Neck Surg* 2005;57(4):312–314.

84. Hashi N, Shirato H, Omatsu T, et al. The role of radiotherapy in treating squamous cell carcinoma of the external auditory canal, especially in early stages of disease. *Radiother Oncol* 2000;56(2):221–225.

85. Bhandare N, Jackson A, Eisbruch A, et al. Radiation therapy and hearing loss. *Int J Radiat Oncol Biol Phys* 2010;76(3 Suppl):S50–S57.

86. Zaider M, Amols HI. Practical considerations in using calculated healthy-tissue complication probabilities for treatment-plan optimization. *Int J Radiat Oncol Biol Phys* 1999;44(2):439–447.

87. Wang CC, Doppke K. Osteoradionecrosis of the temporal bone—consideration of nominal standard dose. *Int J Radiat Oncol Biol Phys* 1976;1(9–10):881–883.

88. Burri RJ. Ear. In: Chao C, Perez CA, Brady LW, eds. *Radiation oncology: management decisions.* Philadelphia: Lippincott Williams & Wilkins, 2011:203–209.

89. Chen WC, Jackson A, Budnick AS, et al. Sensorineural hearing loss in combined modality treatment of nasopharyngeal carcinoma. *Cancer* 2006;106(4):820–829.

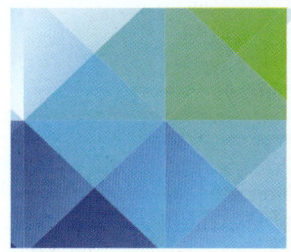

CHAPTER 43

Locally Advanced Squamous Carcinoma of the Head and Neck

David M. Brizel and Jessica L. Geiger

INTRODUCTION

Approximately 60,000 patients are diagnosed annually with squamous cell head and neck cancer (HNC) in the United States.[1] Worldwide, approximately 600,000 patients are afflicted. Nearly 60% of this population presents with locally advanced but nonmetastatic disease. Locoregional failure constitutes the predominant recurrence pattern, and most fatalities result from uncontrolled local and/or regional disease.

Historically, radiation therapy (RT) alone was the standard nonsurgical therapy for locally advanced disease. The state of the art regarding radiation dose fractionation has evolved from once-daily treatment to hyperfractionation and accelerated fractionation.[2–5] These newer strategies lead to a 7% to 10% improvement in locoregional control relative to once-daily treatment schemes. A meta-analysis of randomized trials testing modified fractionation schemes against conventional once-daily fractionation demonstrated that hyperfractionation was the most effective strategy, leading to an 8% absolute improvement in 5-year survival.[6] Nonetheless, even the most effective RT regimens result in local control rates of 50% to 70% and disease-free survivals (DFSs) of 30% to 40%.

This circumstance stimulated the investigation of treatments combining RT and chemotherapy. Review articles describe in detail the different chemotherapeutic agents and RT schemes of these treatment programs.[7,8] Randomized trials of induction cisplatin and 5-fluorouracil (5-FU) chemotherapy followed by standard fractionation versus laryngectomy and postoperative RT in advanced larynx and hypopharynx cancer performed by the Veterans Administration Cooperative Group[9] and the European Organization for the Research and Treatment of Cancer (EORTC), respectively, initially showed that larynx preservation could be achieved without compromising overall survival.

Most randomized clinical trials show the superiority of combined RT and chemotherapy to RT alone for the treatment of locally advanced, nonmetastatic HNC. A meta-analysis of individual patient data from >17,346 participants in 93 trials conducted from 1965 to 2000 (Meta-Analysis of Chemotherapy in Head and Neck Cancer [MACH-NC]) demonstrated that the use of radiotherapy and concurrent chemotherapy resulted in a 19% reduction in the risk of death and an overall 6.5% improvement in 5-year survival compared to treatment with RT alone ($P < .0001$).[10] This benefit was predominantly attributable to a 13.5% improvement in locoregional control. The 2.9% reduction in the risk of distant metastases was not statistically significant (Fig. 43.1).

The MACH-NC also demonstrated a 2% improvement in 5-year survival from the use of induction chemotherapy followed by RT, which was not significant. A subset analysis of trials that used cisplatin and 5-FU as the induction regimen did show a 4% improvement in overall survival.[11] An update of the MACH-NC meta-analysis confirmed the superiority of concurrent chemoradiotherapy (CRT) compared with RT alone across all HNC primary sites.[12]

Randomized comparisons of concurrent chemoradiation versus induction chemotherapy followed by radiotherapy alone are few but confirm that the former strategy is superior.[13,14] The Radiation Therapy Oncology Group (RTOG) conducted a three-arm trial of radiation alone versus radiation and concurrent cisplatin versus induction cisplatin followed by irradiation in larynx carcinoma. Concurrent therapy constituted the most effective means of larynx preservation and provided the best disease control, albeit without a statistically significant survival benefit.[15]

RT and concurrent chemotherapy represents the most commonly used strategy and is a biologically attractive approach because some chemotherapeutic agents may both radiosensitize cells and provide additive cytotoxicity. The superiority of concurrent CRT relative to RT alone has been demonstrated in randomized trials in squamous cell carcinoma of other anatomic sites including the esophagus and uterine cervix.[16–18]

Certain issues must be considered when evaluating randomized trials of CRT for advanced HNC. The first consideration relates to the effectiveness of the RT-alone control arm. Specifically, does it represent optimal single-modality treatment? If the CRT regimen is more effective than RT alone but the radiation is suboptimal, then it is difficult to accurately gauge whether or not the combined modality regimen represents a true improvement in therapy. The second consideration concerns the toxicity of CRT itself. Typically, both acute and late toxicities from CRT are greater than those from RT alone.[19–21]

Acute mucositis constitutes the most significant impediment to the timely delivery of concurrent therapy. Because prolongation of total treatment time adversely affects the success of RT in HNC,[22–24] a major challenge has been the development of treatment schedules that integrate RT and chemotherapy and yet do not excessively increase total treatment time. A thorough understanding of toxicity is mandatory as avoidance of the functional morbidity associated with surgery in advanced HNC is one of the main reasons for the utilization of concurrent therapy in the first place.

HISTORICAL DEVELOPMENT OF RADIATION AND CONCURRENT CHEMOTHERAPY

CRT may be administered in synchronous or alternating schemes. Synchronous administration results in the delivery of RT and chemotherapy (CT) on the same days. Typically, chemotherapy will be given for 1 or more days at the initiation of RT and then repeated in the same fashion several weeks later. Alternating regimens usually sandwich RT and CT around one another. Radiation and drugs are therefore not necessarily given on the same days. In such a scheme, CT would be given during the first week of treatment with RT following in subsequent week(s) before CT is given again.

Synchronous Radiation and Single-Agent Chemotherapy

Synchronous treatment is completed more quickly than is alternating treatment. It is therefore preferable from a theoretical standpoint in terms of addressing the issue of accelerated repopulation, albeit at the expense of increased acute side effects. Early randomized trials of conventionally fractionated RT and CT used single-agent chemotherapy. These studies are

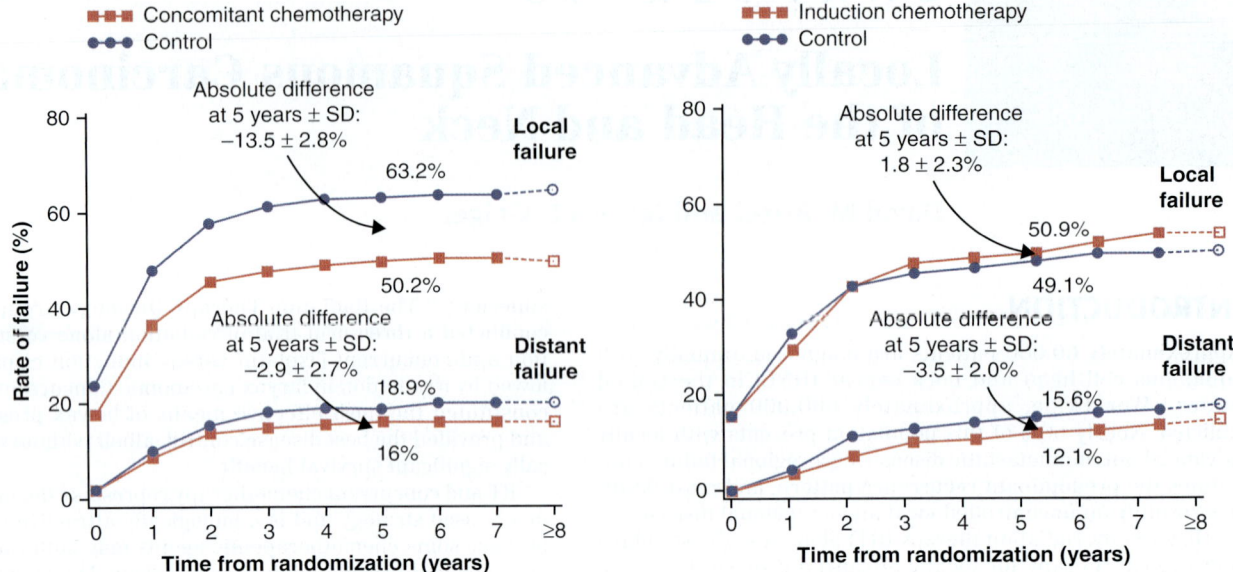

Local failure and distant failure/person-years by period

	Years 0–2	Years 3–5	Years ≥6		Years 0–2	Years 3–5	Years ≥6
Local failure							
Control	493/1,648	22/406	2/165		497/2,627	38/1,073	10/684
Chemotherapy	373/1,837	20/603	1/240		519/2,749	58/1,142	22/751
Distant failure							
Control	82/1,756	8/416	1/166		90/2,788	18/1,116	8/711
Chemotherapy	83/1,915	6/616	0/241		62/2,929	23/1,204	9/773

FIGURE 43.1. Data from the Meta-Analysis of Chemotherapy in Head and Neck Cancer (MACH-NC) illustrating that the major therapeutic benefit of platinum-based chemotherapy results from an improvement in locoregional disease control when the drugs are given concurrently with radiotherapy. No significant improvement occurs with induction chemotherapy followed by radiotherapy.

summarized in Table 43.1. The experimental arms of RTOG 90-03,[2] EORTC 22791,[4] and DAHANCA 6-7[5] are included to provide a basis for comparison with optimal regimens of RT alone.

Both the Northern California Oncology Group (NCOG) and the EORTC tested radiation and synchronous bleomycin against RT alone.[25,26] Acute toxicity was worse in the combined-modality arm in both trials, but the outcomes were quite different with respect to efficacy. The EORTC trial showed no improvement in DFS or survival, and the RT/bleomycin combination in the NCOG program led to a statistically significant doubling of locoregional control and DFS, as well as a near-significant improvement in overall survival from 24% to 43%.

Differences in study design and execution may explain the discrepancy between outcomes in the EORTC and NCOG trials. Fractionation was similar in the two studies, but patients in the EORTC trial received 15 mg of bleomycin twice weekly during the first 5 weeks of RT for a total dose of 150 mg, whereas the NCOG patients received 5 mg twice weekly for a total dose of 70 mg. Acute mucosal and skin toxicity was worse in the RT/bleomycin arm in both trials. Toxicity significantly prolonged the RT delivery time in 30% of the combined-modality patients in the EORTC trial but not in any of the RT-alone patients. This prolongation of treatment time and associated tumor repopulation in such a large proportion of patients may have negated any benefit accrued from the use of concurrent therapy. There were no differences in overall treatment time between the two treatment arms in the NCOG trial. An important lesson from these two studies is that the dose administration schedules of concurrent chemotherapy must be carefully designed so that toxicity does not adversely affect overall treatment compliance.

The Christie Hospital in Great Britain evaluated RT and 100 mg/m^2 of single-agent methotrexate (MTX) given at the commencement of and after 2 weeks of a 3-week course of treatment.[27] Most of the 313 patients in this protocol received 50 to 55 Gy in 15 or 16 fractions. Mucositis was significantly greater in the patients receiving MTX, but there was no difference in long-term toxicity. The addition of MTX increased local control from 50% to 70% (P = .02) and survival from 37% to 47% (P = .07). The greatest benefit was seen in patients with oropharyngeal primary tumors who constituted one-third of the study population. Local control with RT/MTX was 78% versus 38% with RT alone (P = .002) in this patient subset. Survival was 25% with RT alone and 50% with RT/MTX (P = .009). Unfortunately, the data from this trial are not generally applicable to current clinical practice because of the large radiation fraction sizes that were used.

5-FU has been used in conjunction with RT more frequently than any other chemotherapeutic agent. Lo et al.[28] reported the first study to show a significant improvement in local control and survival with the addition of bolus 5-FU to RT in squamous carcinoma of the oral cavity. Browman et al.[29] compared RT and continuous infusion 5-FU against RT alone in a placebo-controlled randomized trial sponsored by the National Cancer Institute of Canada. All 175 patients received 66 Gy in 2-Gy fractions. 5-FU was given at 1,200 mg/m^2/d for the first 3 days of the 1st and 3rd weeks of irradiation. Confluent mucositis was more frequent in the 5-FU arm than in the placebo arm (32% vs. 11%; P = .001), as was weight loss >15% from pretreatment baseline (41% vs. 11%; P < .0001). This increased acute toxicity did not prolong the delivery of RT in the RT/5-FU arm relative to the RT/placebo arm. Two-year DFS and survival were 30% and 50% for RT/placebo patients and 50% and 63% for RT/5-FU patients (P = .06 and .08), respectively.

TABLE 43.1 RANDOMIZED TRIALS OF ONCE-DAILY IRRADIATION AND CONCURRENT CHEMOTHERAPY IN ADVANCED HEAD AND NECK CANCER

Institution	N	Radiotherapy	Chemotherapy	Outcome RT vs. RT/CCT; *P* Value	Comments
RTOG 90-03 Accelerated fractionation	268	72 Gy/42 days	None	LC: 54% DFS: 39% S: 51%	
Hyperfractionation	263	81 Gy/49 days	None	LC: 54% DFS: 38% S: 54%	
DAHANCA 6-7	1,476	70 Gy/39 days	None	LC: 76% DFS: 73%	
EORTC 22791	356	80.5 Gy/47 days	None	LC: 59%	
NCOG	104	70 Gy (1.8 Gy/day)	Bleo 5 mg²/wk weeks 1–7; synchronous	LC: 35% vs. 70%; .001 DFS: 15% vs. 31%; .04 S: 24% vs. 43%; .11	RT/CCT → ↑ acute toxicity, but RT not delayed
EORTC	224	64 Gy (1.8–2.0 Gy/day)	Bleo 15 mg²/wk weeks 1–5; synchronous	DFS: 22% vs. 23%; NS S: 23% vs. 22%; NS	RT/CCT → ↑ acute toxicity with RT delayed in 30%
Christie Hospital	313	50–55 Gy (3.3 Gy/day)	MTX 100 mg/m² days 0, 14; synchronous	LC: 50% vs. 70%; .02 S: 37% vs. 47%; .07	Statistically significant benefit in LC and S for oropharynx
NCI Canada	175	66 Gy (2.0 Gy/day)	5-FU 1,200 mg/m² days 1–3 and 15–17; synchronous	DFS: 30% vs. 50%; .06 S: 50% vs. 63%; .08	Placebo-controlled trial
Yale University	195	68 Gy (1.8–2.0 Gy/day)	MMC 15 mg/m² days 5, 43; synchronous	LC: 54% vs. 76%; .003 S: 42% vs. 48%; NS	Predominantly postop series 1° RT in 74 patients Benefit unclear in this patient group
Cleveland Clinic	100	66–72 Gy (1.8–2.0 Gy/day)	5-FU 1,000 mg/m² CI CDDP 20 mg/m² CI Days 1–4 and 22–25; synchronous	LC: 35% vs. 55%; .02 DFS: 52% vs. 67%; .03 S: 58% vs. 58%; NS	RT/CCT ↑ toxicity but RT not delayed LC means survival with 1° site organ preservation
Princess Margaret Hospital	209	50 Gy (2.5 Gy/day)	MMC 10 mg/m² 5-FU 1,000 mg/m² CI; synchronous	LC: ~40% vs. ~40% S: ~40% vs. ~40%	RT only; continuous course RT/CCT: 4-wk break after 25 Gy
NICR Italy	157	RT/CCT: 60 Gy RT: 66 Gy	5-FU 200 mg/m² bolus CDDP 20 mg/m² bolus Days 1–5, 22–26, 43–47, and 64–68; alternating	LC: 32% vs. 64%; .04 DFS: 9% vs. 21%; .008 S: 10% vs. 24%; .01	Unresectable disease RT/CCT: RT on weeks 2, 3, 5, 6, 8, and 9 RT only: ≥2 wk delay in >30%
GORTEC 94-01	226	70 Gy (2 Gy/day)	Carboplatin (CBDCA) 70 mg/m² 5-FU 600 mg/m²/d CI	LC: 25% vs. 48%; .002 DFS: 15% vs. 27%; .01 S: 16% vs. 23%; .05	Significantly increased acute and late toxicity with RT/CCT
Intergroup Nasopharynx	193	70 Gy (2 Gy/day)	CDDP 100 mg/m² Days 1, 22, and 43 Post-RT CDDP/5-FU	DFS: 24% vs. 69%; <.001 S: 47% vs. 78%; .005	Early trial closure

5-FU, 5-fluorouracil; bid, twice daily; Bleo, bleomycin; CDDP, cisplatin; CI, continuous infusion; DFS, disease-free survival; EORTC, European Organization for the Research and Treatment of Cancer; LC, local control; MMC, mitomycin C; MTX, methotrexate; NCI, National Cancer Institute; NCOG, Northern California Oncology Group; NICR, National Institute for Cancer Research; NS, not significant; RT/CCT, radiotherapy and concurrent chemotherapy; RTOG, Radiation Therapy Oncology Group; S, survival.

The relative radioresistance of hypoxic cells *in vitro* is well understood.[28,30] Clinically, the existence of hypoxia in both head and neck primary tumors and metastatic lymph nodes has been described, and its adverse impact on the prognosis of patients treated with RT has been demonstrated.[31,32] Investigators from Yale University designed their treatment strategy around this principle. They treated 195 patients in two randomized trials with mitomycin C (MMC). This agent is predominantly metabolized in and preferentially cytotoxic to hypoxic cells. The Yale treatment program consisted of 68 Gy ± MMC on days 1 and 43 of RT. Local control was improved with the addition of MMC from 54% to 76% (*P* = .003). Survival improved from 42% to 48%, but this was not statistically significant. The majority of patients in these trials received adjuvant postoperative or preoperative irradiation, however. Only 74 (38%) received definitive, primary RT, and the benefit from the addition of MMC in this subset is unclear.[33]

Synchronous Radiation and Multiagent Chemotherapy

Cisplatin (CDDP) also has radiosensitizing properties.[34] The combination of CDDP and 5-FU is also one of the most active cytotoxic drug combinations against squamous cell HNC. Consequently, investigators have incorporated both of these drugs into a variety of concurrent treatment strategies. A randomized trial from the Cleveland Clinic assigned patients to receive 66 to 72 Gy ± two cycles of synchronous CDDP (20 mg/m²/d × 4) and infusional 5-FU (1,000 mg/m²/d × 4) during weeks 1 and 4 of RT.[35] The main objective of this study was primary site organ preservation. Surgical salvage was allowed for patients with persistent disease. Acute toxicity was significantly greater in the combined-modality treatment arm, especially with respect to weight loss. Mucosal recovery usually required 8 to 12 weeks after completion of RT and chemotherapy. There were no differences in the total time required for RT delivery, however. Three-year DFS was significantly better for the patients receiving chemoradiotherapy (67% vs. 52%; *P* = .03). Three-year survival with primary site preservation was also higher in the combined-modality group (57% vs. 35%, *P* = .02), although there was no significant difference in overall survival.

MMC and 5-FU were used together in a trial of 209 patients conducted at the Princess Margaret Hospital.[36] Patients were treated with continuous-course RT alone at 2.5 Gy/day to 50 Gy in 28 days. Patients randomized to receive RT/chemotherapy received the same dose-fractionation scheme as did those receiving RT alone but over a total time of 56 days because of a planned 4-week treatment interruption after 25 Gy. Bolus MMC (10 mg/m²) was given on days 1 and 43. Two cycles of continuous infusion 5-FU (1,000 mg/m²/d) were given on days 1 to 4 and 43 to 46. The intent of the treatment break was to maintain comparable levels of acute toxicity in the two treatment arms. Acute toxicity was, in fact, equivalent in the two groups. Unfortunately, however, there was no difference in 4-year local control (~40%) or survival (~40%).

The Princess Margaret trial raises an important question: Can one quantify the contribution provided by concurrent chemotherapy in terms of the delivery of an equivalent dose of irradiation? Approximately 0.6 Gy/day is necessary to compensate for the tumor repopulation that transpires with each day of prolongation of standard course RT.[23] Thus, the total dose in the Princess Margaret Hospital RT/chemotherapy arm would have to have been about 67 Gy [(2.5 Gy × 20) + (0.6 Gy/day × 28 days)] in order to have been isoeffective with the 50-Gy regimen in the RT-alone arm. The equivalent efficacy of the two treatments in this trial therefore suggests that the chemotherapy compensated for the tumor repopulation that occurred during the treatment break. Thus, one could argue that the chemotherapy was equivalent to approximately 17 Gy of additional irradiation. There can be no doubt as to the inferiority of the split-course fractionation scheme in this trial had it been delivered without chemotherapy and compared head to head against the continuous-course RT regimen. Conversely, if the combined-modality treatment had been given with continuous-course RT, it would quite probably have been more efficacious than the RT-only regimen.

A Spanish three-arm randomized trial ($N = 859$) provides additional information that is pertinent to the estimation of the radiotherapeutic dose equivalent provided by the delivery of concurrent chemotherapy.[37] Patients were assigned to receive one of the following regimens:

A. 2 Gy/day to 60 Gy/42 days
B. 1.1 Gy twice daily to 70.4 Gy/44 days
C. 2 Gy/day to 60 Gy/42 days with concurrent bolus 5-FU 250 mg/m² given every other day

Progression-free survival and overall survival were significantly worse in arm A as compared with arms B and C, as one would expect. Arms B and C were equally efficacious. Not accounting for the different fractionation in arms B and C and the unconventional administration of chemotherapy, it is still clear that the addition of 5-FU was comparable to dose escalation of approximately 10 Gy. A recent modeling analysis of phase III trials comparing CRT with RT only suggests that concurrent chemotherapy provides the equivalent of a 10- to 12-Gy dose escalation.[38]

Neither the Princess Margaret nor the Spanish trial delivered maximally intensive radiotherapy in their respective control arms. The rationale for treatment intensification with the addition of concurrent chemotherapy as opposed to simple RT dose escalation is weak in such a context. The situation may be dramatically different, however, when the RT-alone arm is maximally intensive such as in RTOG 90-03 or EORTC 22791. Dose escalations of 10 to 12 Gy are not possible with accelerated regimens that already deliver 72 Gy during 6 weeks or with hyperfractionated regimens delivering 79 Gy in 7 weeks (see Radiation Fractionation Scheme section). Concurrent chemotherapy, however, can be added to modified fractionation regimens ≥70 Gy.

Alternating Radiotherapy and Chemotherapy

Alternating therapy produces less acute mucosal toxicity than does synchronous therapy but may prolong the overall treatment time by several weeks. Although longer treatment times adversely affect efficacy in programs of standard RT alone because of tumor repopulation, the significance of overall treatment time (for RT) in a continuous course of alternating RT and chemotherapy is controversial. Some investigators have suggested that the usual time–dose relationships do not apply.[39]

The National Institute for Cancer Research in Italy conducted a phase III trial comparing RT with alternating RT

and chemotherapy in 157 patients with unresectable HNC.[40,41] The RT arm was designed to give 70 Gy/7 weeks via standard fractionation. The combined-therapy arm scheduled chemotherapy on weeks 1, 4, 7, and 10 and radiation (60 Gy) on weeks 2 to 3, 5 to 6, and 8 to 9. Each 2-week cycle of radiation consisted of 20 Gy/10 fractions. Each cycle of chemotherapy included 5 days of bolus CDDP (20 mg/m²/d) and bolus 5-FU (200 mg/m²/d). The incidence of grade 3/4 mucositis (18% to 19%) was the same in both treatment groups. However, RT treatment delays occurred more often in the RT-alone patients: 32% with a 1-week prolongation and 25% with a ≥2-week prolongation. Corresponding delays in the combined-modality-treatment group were 11% and 15%, respectively. The median dose of RT delivered in the combined-modality-treatment group matched the planned dose of 60 Gy, but it was only 62 Gy in the RT-alone group. Five-year actuarial survival was significantly better in the combined-modality-treatment patients (24% vs. 10%; $P = .01$), as were DFS (21% vs. 9%; $P = .008$) and local control (64% vs. 32%; $P = .04$).

Given the similar levels of acute toxicity, it is unclear why treatment times were prolonged and total doses reduced so extensively in the RT-only patients. Better protocol compliance in the control arm might well have changed the outcome of this trial. There are no other randomized trials of RT and alternating chemotherapy. Further randomized trials of alternating therapy will be necessary to determine its true value because the deficiencies of the National Institute for Cancer Research study prevent definitive conclusions.

Despite its drawbacks, the Italian study, like the Princess Margaret Hospital trial, strongly reinforces the idea that in some settings, chemotherapy counteracts tumor repopulation during treatment. The total RT treatment time was prolonged in the combined-modality arms in both studies. The fundamental difference between these two trials is that patients received no treatment during the RT break in the Princess Margaret Hospital trial and the patients in the Italian trial received chemotherapy during each interruption of RT.

CONTEMPORARY RANDOMIZED TRIALS OF RADIOTHERAPY AND CONCURRENT CHEMOTHERAPY

Curative Intent Treatment

The French cooperative group trial, GORTEC 94-01, was performed in patients who had stage III/IV oropharyngeal carcinoma.[20,42] Radiotherapy consisted of conventional 2 Gy, once-daily fractionation to 70 Gy. Patients on the CRT arm also received three cycles of concurrent carboplatin (70 mg/m²) and continuous infusion 5-FU (600 mg/m²/d × 4 days). Two hundred twenty-six patients were enrolled in the trial. CRT resulted in significant improvement in 5-year locoregional control (48% vs. 25%; $P = .002$), DFS (27% vs. 15%; $P = .01$), and survival (23% vs. 16%; $P = .05$). This improvement in efficacy was accompanied by a significant increase in acute mucositis (grade ≥ 2) from 39% to 71% ($P = .005$). Severe acute cutaneous and hematologic toxicity and worse nutritional status were also significantly more prevalent in the patients who received combined-modality therapy. Severe late toxicity, primarily cervical fibrosis, occurred in 27% of the combined-modality patients and in 12% of those treated with RT alone ($P = .04$). Severe dental complications were twice as frequent in the combined-modality patients (37% vs. 18%; $P = .01$).

Wendt et al.[43] conducted a multi-institutional trial of CRT versus RT for patients with unresectable stage III/IV HNC. CRT patients received three cycles of cisplatin, 5-FU, and leucovorin during a 7-week period. Cisplatin was given as a 60 mg/m² bolus. 5-FU was given as an initial 350 mg/m² bolus followed by a 4-day continuous infusion of 350 mg/m²/d. Leucovorin was also given for 4 days at 100 mg/m²/d. Radiotherapy was given

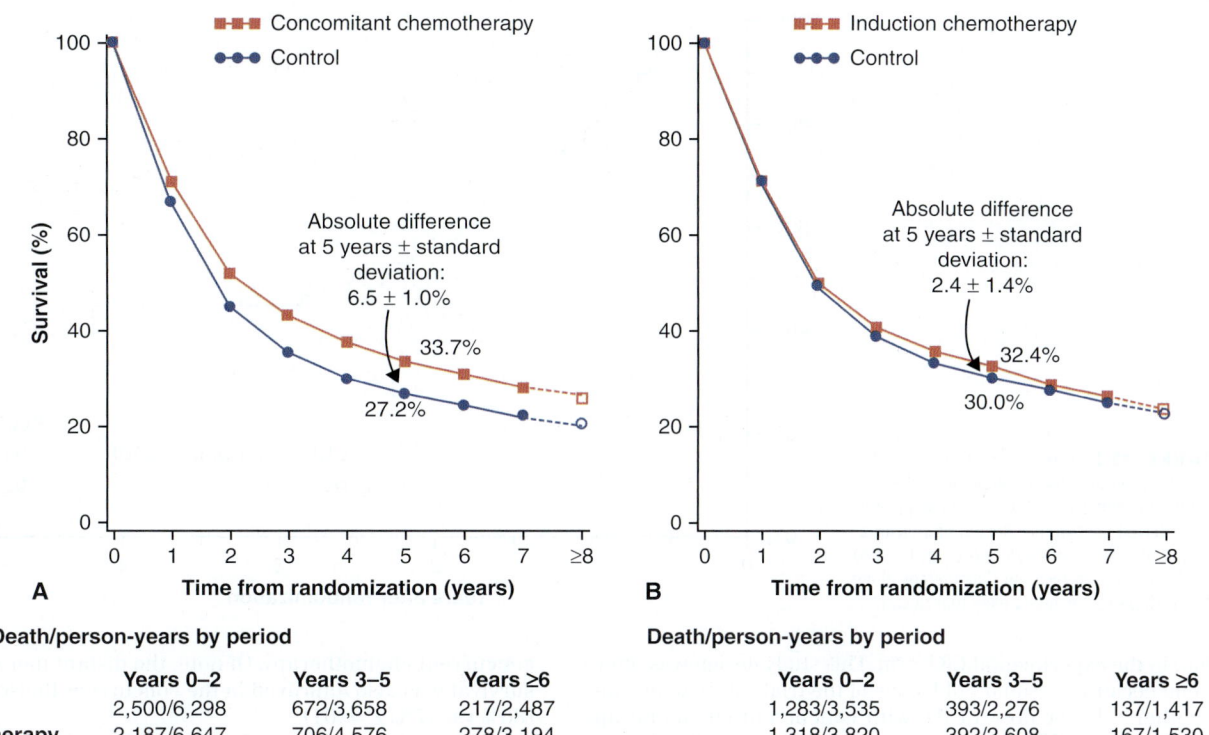

Death/person-years by period

	Years 0–2	Years 3–5	Years ≥6
Control	2,500/6,298	672/3,658	217/2,487
Chemotherapy	2,187/6,647	706/4,576	278/3,194

Death/person-years by period

	Years 0–2	Years 3–5	Years ≥6
Control	1,283/3,535	393/2,276	137/1,417
Chemotherapy	1,318/3,820	392/2,608	167/1,530

FIGURE 43.2. Data from the Meta-Analysis of Chemotherapy in Head and Neck Cancer (MACH-NC), which demonstrates that adding concurrent chemotherapy to radiotherapy provides a significant improvement in survival but that induction chemotherapy does not. **A:** Concomitant chemotherapy. **B:** Induction chemotherapy.

as three cycles of 23.4 Gy at 1.8 Gy bid in both treatment arms. It coincided with the chemotherapy on the CRT arms. Planned treatment breaks were given between the cycles of treatment to ameliorate treatment-induced mucositis. The cumulative dose of RT in both treatment arms was 70.2 Gy in 7 weeks.

One-third of the 270 patients enrolled had oropharynx primary tumors. CRT doubled both 3-year local control (35% vs. 17%; $P < .004$) and survival (49% vs. 24%; $P < .003$) (Fig. 43.2). As in the GORTEC 94-01 oropharyngeal trial, confluent mucositis was significantly higher (38% vs. 16%; $P < .001$) with the use of CRT.

Treatment of advanced nasopharynx carcinoma (NPC) with radiation and concurrent chemotherapy was the subject of an intergroup study in which patients in both arms received conventionally fractionated RT (1.8 to 2.0 Gy/day) to a total dose of 70 Gy.[44] Those patients who were randomized to concurrent chemotherapy also received three cycles of cisplatin during RT at a dose of 100 mg/m². After the completion of RT, they received an additional three cycles of adjuvant cisplatin at 80 mg/m² and 4-day continuous infusions of 5-FU at 1,000 mg/m²/d. All patients had stage III/IV, M0 disease. In spite of the initial plan of enrolling 270 patients, the trial was terminated early when an interim analysis demonstrated the superiority of the combined-modality regimen. One hundred ninety-three patients were enrolled, and the median follow-up was 2.7 years. Three-year progression-free survival favored the combined-modality patients (69% vs. 24%; $P < .001$). Similarly, 3-year survival was 78% versus 47% ($P = .005$) in favor of the patients who received concurrent chemotherapy (Fig. 43.3). Approximately, one-third of the patients in the combined modality arm did not receive some or all of their adjuvant chemotherapy.

The value of adjuvant chemotherapy in NPC has been controversial ever since the findings of this study were published. A multinational clinical trial is currently being conducted attempting to identify who might benefit from it (clinicaltrials.gov identifier NCT02135042). It is now understood that

the majority of NPC is World Health Organization (WHO) grade 2 to 3 and that serum Epstein-Barr virus deoxyribonucleic acid (EBV DNA) titers are elevated in most of these patients. Furthermore, the titers become undetectable by the completion of local therapy in most of these patients, and they have an excellent prognosis, whereas the prognosis is poor for those whose titers remain detectable. On this trial, those patients whose titers become undetectable will be randomized (phase III) to adjuvant cisplatin/5-FU versus observation with a primary endpoint of overall survival. Those patients whose titers remain detectable will be randomized (phase II) to adjuvant cisplatin/5-FU versus paclitaxel/gemcitabine with a primary endpoint of progression-free survival.

Table 43.1 summarizes the data from the trials of conventionally fractionated irradiation and concurrent chemotherapy.

One must ask not only whether CRT is more effective than conventionally fractionated RT but also whether it is superior to hyperfractionated or accelerated fractionation irradiation as these strategies represent the most efficacious single-modality treatment strategies. A prospective randomized trial from Duke University was one of the first to provide insight into this issue.[45] Patients with locally advanced HNC were randomized to hyperfractionated irradiation alone versus split-course hyperfractionation with concurrent CDDP/5-FU chemotherapy. Patients in the RT-alone arm received 1.25 Gy bid continuous course to 75 Gy in 6 weeks, whereas those patients on the CRT arm received 1.25 Gy bid split course to 70 Gy in 7 weeks. Chemotherapy was given during weeks 1 and 6 of irradiation (CDDP 12 mg/m²/d × 5 days; 5-FU continuous infusion was 600 mg/m²/d × 5 days).

The time–dose aspects of the RT in the combined-modality arm are similar to those of the previously discussed trials. The time–dose characteristics of the RT in the control arm were similar to certain aspects of both the concurrent boost arm (decreased treatment time) and the hyperfractionation arm (increased total dose) of RTOG 90-03. Most importantly, these characteristics made the RT more intensive in the control arm

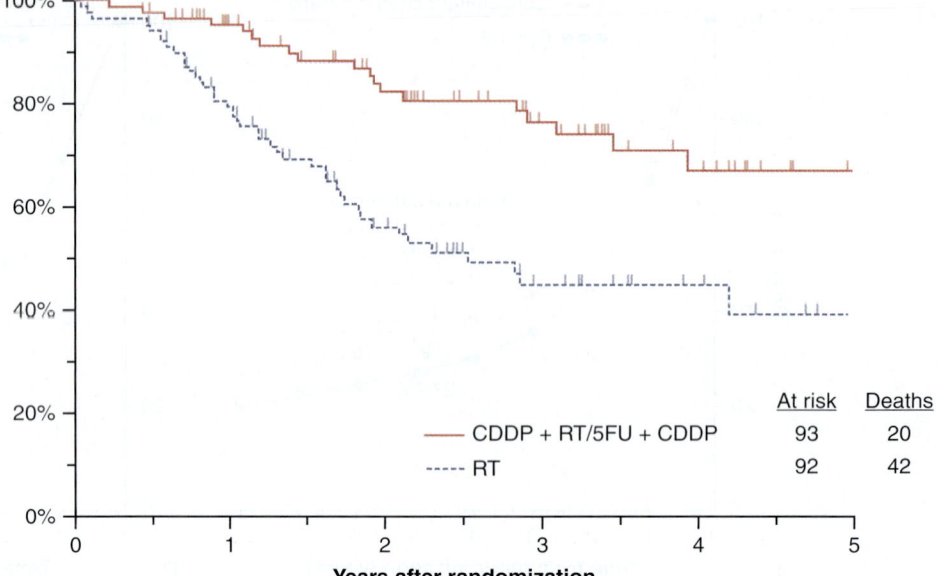

FIGURE 43.3. Three-year survival in the Intergroup Nasopharynx Carcinoma Trial was significantly better (*P* = .005) for those patients who received concurrent cisplatin and postirradiation adjuvant cisplatin/5-fluorouracil (78%) than for those who received radiotherapy alone (47%). These results led to early trial closure.

than in the experimental CRT arm. This study design was intentional because a primary objective of the trial was to determine whether a lower dose of RT with concurrent chemotherapy would be superior to maximally intensive/effective RT alone.

Fifty-four percent of the patients presented with unresectable disease, and approximately 40% of the primaries were located in the oropharynx. One hundred sixteen patients were enrolled, and the updated median follow-up now exceeds 5 years. Locoregional control was 70% versus 44% (*P* = .006), favoring the combined-modality patients. An unpublished update of the 5-year survival revealed superiority in the combined-modality patients (42% vs. 27%; *P* = .04) (Fig. 43.4). Confluent (grade 3) mucositis was seen in approximately 75% of the patients in both arms, the main difference being that the mean time to resolution of mucositis was 50% longer in the patients receiving radiation and concurrent chemotherapy (6 vs. 4 weeks).

Jeremic et al.[46] evaluated hyperfractionated irradiation (1.1 Gy bid to 77 Gy) with or without concurrent low-dose daily cisplatin (6 mg/m²) in stage III/IV patients. One hundred thirty patients were enrolled; primary tumors originated in the oropharynx in approximately one-third of the population. Fifty-nine percent presented with T3 or T4 primaries, and 80% had nodal involvement. Five-year locoregional control (50% vs. 36%; *P* = .04), progression-free survival (46% vs. 25%; *P* = .007), and overall survival (46% vs. 25%; *P* = .007) (Fig. 43.5) were all significantly improved with the addition of

concurrent chemotherapy. Of note, the distant metastasis-free survival was also improved in the concurrent therapy patients (86% vs. 57%; *P* = .01).

A German multicenter trial also confirmed that CRT is superior to maximally intensive single-modality irradiation.[19] Three hundred eighty-four patients, 93% of whom had either stage III or IV oropharyngeal or hypopharyngeal primaries, were enrolled. As in the Duke trial, the total dose of RT delivered in the CRT arm was lower than that in the RT control arm. RT patients received 77.6 Gy in 6 weeks (14 Gy at 2 Gy once daily followed by 63.6 Gy at 1.4 Gy twice daily), and CRT patients received 70.6 Gy during 6 weeks (30 Gy at 2 Gy/day followed by 40.6 Gy at 1.4 Gy twice daily). Chemotherapy consisted of mitomycin C (10 mg/m²) on days 5 and 35 and 5-FU given as a single bolus of 350 mg/m² and a 5-day continuous infusion of 600 mg/m²/d. Two-year survival was significantly better in the combined-modality arm (54% vs. 45%; *P* = .05), as was locoregional control (61% vs. 45%; *P* = .001). Acute and chronic toxicities were equivalent in the two treatment populations.

A French cooperative group (FNCLCC-GORTEC) tested a related concept in 163 patients with technically unresectable carcinomas of the oropharynx and hypopharynx.[47] RT was administered at 1.2 Gy twice daily to a total dose of

FIGURE 43.5. Five-year survival in the Yugoslavian trial of hyperfractionated irradiation alone (25%) or with daily low-dose concurrent cisplatin (46%) (*P* = .007).

FIGURE 43.4. Five-year locoregional control in the Duke University randomized trial of continuous-course accelerated hyperfractionation (44%) versus split-course accelerated hyperfractionation and concurrent cisplatin/5-fluorouracil (*P* = .01). Extended follow-up has demonstrated that the survival benefit of combined modality treatment is also statistically significant.

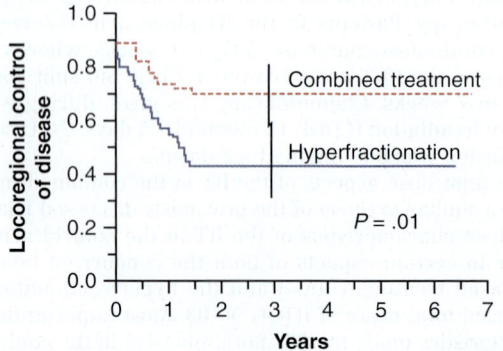

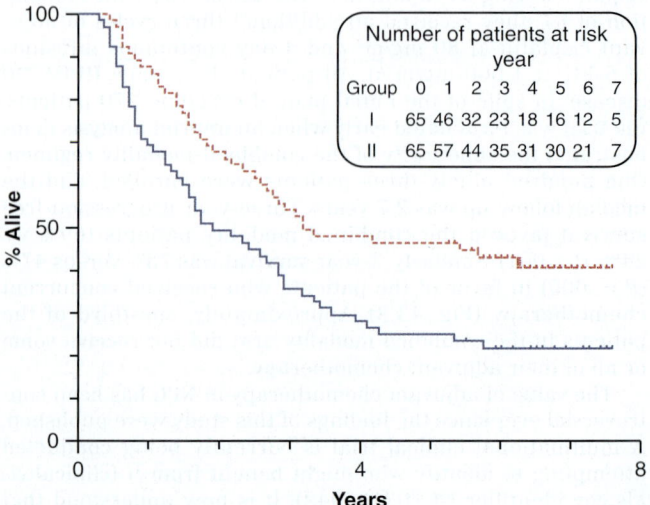

TABLE 43.2 RANDOMIZED TRIALS OF ACCELERATED OR HYPERFRACTIONATED RADIOTHERAPY AND CONCURRENT CHEMOTHERAPY IN ADVANCED HEAD AND NECK CANCER

Institution	N	Radiotherapy	Chemotherapy	Outcome RT RT/CCT *P* Value	Comments
RTOG 90-03 Accelerated fractionation and conc. boost	268	72 Gy/42 days 1.8 Gy q day and 1.5 Gy concurrent boost	None	LC: 54% DFS: 39% S: 51%	
RTOG 90-03 Hyperfractionation	263	81 Gy/49 days 1.2 Gy bid	None	LC: 54% DFS: 38% S: 54%	
University of Munich	308	70.2 Gy/51 days 1.8 Gy bid in both arms 23.4 Gy × 3 cycles 10-d split between cycles	5-FU 350 mg/m² bolus on day 2 5-FU 350 mg/m²/d × 4 CI Leucovorin 50 mg/m²/d × 4 CDDP 60 mg/m² × 1 Days 1–4, 22–25, 42–45	LC: 17% 34%; .01 S: 24% 48%; <.0003	Unresectable disease Toxicity not reported
University of Vienna	239	55 Gy/2.5 weeks for V-CHART ± MMC 70 Gy/7 weeks CF control	MMC 20 mg/m² on day 5	LC: 32% 48%; .05 S: 31% 49%; .03	V-CHART vs. V-CHART/MMC
Yugoslavian Cooperative	130	77 Gy/49 days in both arms 1.1 Gy bid	CDDP 6 mg/m²/d	LC: 36% 50%; .04 DFS: 25% 46%; .007 S: 25% 46%; .007	Daily chemotherapy
Charite' University, Berlin	384	RT/CCT: 70.6 Gy/6 weeks RT: 77.6 Gy/6 weeks	MMC 10 mg/m² days 5,36 5-FU 350 mg/m² bolus 5-FU 600 mg/m² 5 d CI	LC: 45% 61%; .001 S: 24% 29%; .009	
Duke University	116	RT/CCT: 70 Gy/48 days (1-wk break at 40 Gy) RT: 74 Gy/42 days (continuous course) 1.25 Gy bid both arms	5-FU 600 mg/m²/d CI CDDP 12 mg/m²/d bolus Days 1–5 and 36–40	LC: 44% 70%; .007 DFS: 41% 61%; .06 S: 34% 55%; .04	Acute and chronic toxicity comparable between RT and RT/CCT
FNCLCC-GORTEC	163	80 Gy/47 days (oropharynx) 76 Gy/44 days (hypopharynx)	80 Gy/47 days CDDP 100 mg/m² on days 1, 22, and 43 5-FU 750 mg/m² × 5 d cycle 1 and 430 mg/m² × 5 d cycles 2 and 3	LC: DFS: 25% 48%; .002 S: 20% 38%; .04	All patients with unresectable disease
Swiss Cooperative Group	224	74.4 Gy/44 days 1.2 Gy bid	74 Gy/40 days 1.2 Gy bid CDDP 20 mg/m²/d Two 5-d cycles	LC: 33% 51%; .04 DFS: 24% 27%; >.10 S: 32% 46%; .15	

5-FU, 5-fluorouacil; bid, twice daily; CDDP, cisplatin; CF, conventional fractionation; CI, continuous infusion; DFS, disease-free survival; LC, local controls; MMC, mitomycin C; RT/CCT, radiotherapy and concurrent chemotherapy; RTOG, Radiation Therapy Oncology Group; S, survival; V-CHART, Vienna-Continuous Hyperfractionated Accelerated Radiation Therapy.

80.4 Gy/46 days to oropharyngeal primary tumors and 75.6 Gy/44 days to hypopharyngeal primary tumors. The experimental arm received the same RT and concurrent CDDP (100 mg/m²) on days 1, 22, and 43 of RT. Three 5-day cycles of continuous infusion 5-FU were also administered. The first cycle was 750 mg/m²/d and the second and third cycles were 430 mg/m²/d. Three-year DFS favored the concurrent chemoradiation arm (48% vs. 25%; *P* = .002), as did overall survival (38% vs. 20%; *P* = .04). Post hoc subset analyses demonstrated that the larger (and statistically significant) benefit was confined to the patients with oropharyngeal carcinomas. However, the trial was not designed to compare treatment efficacy in these two different primary sites of origin.

A three-armed randomized trial from the University of Vienna compared conventionally fractionated RT (2 Gy daily to 70 Gy) against continuous hyperfractionated accelerated RT with and without mitomycin C (V-CHART + MMC and V-CHART, respectively).[48] Radiation therapy was given as an initial 2.5-Gy fraction followed by 1.65 Gy twice daily to a total dose of 55.3 Gy in 17 days. MMC was given as a 20 mg/m² bolus on day 5 of RT. Of the 239 patients enrolled, 85% had T3/4 primary tumors, and 79% had nodal involvement.

Three-year actuarial locoregional control was 48% for V-CHART + MMC versus 32% for V-CHART and 31% for conventional fractionation (CF) (*P* = .05 and .03, respectively). Survival including death from all causes was also improved to 41% in the V-CHART + MMC arm as compared with 31% for V-CHART and 24% for CF (*P* = .03).

The incidence of confluent mucositis was 90% in both experimental arms as compared with 33% in the CF arm. The median time to complete resolution of mucositis was 6 to 7 weeks in all three arms. Grade 3/4 hematologic toxicity, primarily thrombocytopenia, developed in 18% of the V-CHART +

MMC patients. Table 43.2 summarizes the data from the trials that used modified fractionation and concurrent chemotherapy and includes the RTOG 90-03 and EORTC 22791 data as a point of reference for optimally delivered RT alone.

Adjuvant Postoperative Irradiation

The role of chemotherapy for patients receiving primary resection and postoperative irradiation has been studied less extensively than in the definitive irradiation setting. The National Cancer Institute Head and Neck Contracts Program[49] conducted a three-arm trial that evaluated the addition of one cycle of preoperative cisplatin and bleomycin with or without six cycles of sequential cisplatin (80 mg/m²) maintenance chemotherapy after surgery and postoperative irradiation. The control arm consisted of surgery and postoperative irradiation alone. This trial enrolled 443 patients and demonstrated no benefit with respect to locoregional control or survival from the addition of chemotherapy. Nearly half of the patients who were randomized to receive maintenance chemotherapy never received it. Despite this flaw in study execution, the incidence of distant metastases as the site of first relapse was 9% in the patients assigned to maintenance chemotherapy as opposed to 19% in those who were not (*P* = .02).

Intergroup Study 0034 readdressed the issue of postoperative chemotherapy in a trial that randomized patients after surgery to three 21-day cycles of sequential cisplatin (100 mg/m²) and infusion 5-FU (1,000 mg/m²/d for 5 days) followed by 50 to 60 Gy versus 50 to 60 Gy alone with no chemotherapy.[50] Again, there was no significant improvement in locoregional control or overall survival associated with the use of chemotherapy, but the incidence of distant metastases was reduced from 30% to 20% (*P* = .02).

In contrast to the use of sequential postoperative RT and chemotherapy, the EORTC conducted a randomized trial in which patients were given either postoperative RT alone (2 Gy daily to 66 Gy) or the same RT with three cycles of cisplatin (100 mg/m²) on days 1, 22, and 43 of irradiation.[51] Three hundred thirty-four patients were enrolled. Two-thirds of patients in the combined-modality arm received all three cycles of chemotherapy. The median follow-up is 5 years. Three-year DFS was increased from 41% to 59% ($P = .001$), and 3-year survival was increased from 49% to 65% ($P = .006$) in favor of the group of patients receiving concurrent therapy. Acute mucosal toxicity greater than grade 3 was significantly higher in the concurrent treatment arm (41% vs. 21%; $P = .001$).

The RTOG led an intergroup trial (9501) that randomized 459 high-risk postoperative patients to receive 60 to 66 Gy with or without concurrent CDDP in the same dose and schedule as in the EORTC study.[52] Sixty-one percent of patients in the concurrent therapy arm received all three cycles of CDDP. The median follow-up for this study is 4 years; 2-year actuarial locoregional control favored the combined-modality arm by 82% versus 72% (hazard ratio [HR], 0.61; $P = .61$), with only eight local or regional recurrences occurring beyond the 2-year point. DFS also favors concurrent therapy (HR, 0.78; $P = .04$). There was no statistically significant difference in survival (HR, 0.84; $P = .19$). Acute toxicity grade 3 or higher was higher in the concurrent therapy patients (77% vs. 34%; $P < .001$), but late toxicity was similar (21% vs. 17%).

A comparative analysis of the pooled data from these two studies revealed extracapsular extension (ECE) and/or microscopically involved surgical margins were the only risk factors for which the addition of chemotherapy to postoperative radiation was significant.[53] Patients with two or more involved lymph nodes in the absence of ECE did not benefit from the addition of chemotherapy. A trend in benefit to the addition of chemotherapy was seen in patients with stage III to IV disease, perineural invasion, lymphovascular space invasion, and enlarged level IV to V lymph nodes secondary to oral cavity or oropharynx tumors. As such, concurrent chemoradiotherapy remains the standard of care for adjuvant therapy in patients with locally advanced squamous cell HNC and the presence of ECE and/or positive surgical margins. Long-term follow-up of RTOG 9501 found no significant outcome differences in analysis of all randomized patients; however, a subgroup analysis of patients with positive surgical margins and/or ECE demonstrated improved locoregional control and DFS with the addition of chemotherapy, further supporting these findings as poor risk factors in this disease.[54] Despite these recommendations, a retrospective analysis of the National Cancer Database identified a subset of patients with negative surgical margins and no ECE who still received adjuvant CRT.[55] Survival benefits of CRT versus RT alone increased in patients with multiple positive lymph nodes, despite the findings of the EORTC and RTOG studies, highlighting the need for ongoing evaluation into other poor risk factors for disease recurrence.

PRINCIPLES FOR THE CHOICE OF CONCURRENT TREATMENT REGIMENS

Three general statements can summarize the previously reviewed randomized trials:

a. RT with concurrent chemotherapy is more efficacious than conventionally fractionated RT alone in advanced HNC.
b. Concurrent therapy appears to be more effective than maximally intensive single-modality RT administered via a modified fractionation regimen.
c. Acute and late toxicities are increased with the use of concurrent chemotherapy.

No consensus exists, however, regarding either the optimal radiation dose-fractionation scheme or the optimal scheduling of chemotherapy in these concurrent regimens. These controversies pose a decision-making dilemma to the physician when it is time to devise a treatment plan. The application of certain principles may serve as a guide in this selection process, though. The radiochemotherapy regimen should be more effective than maximally effective single-modality radiation.

Radiation Fractionation Scheme

One rational approach to the choice of radiation dose fractionation within the context of concurrent chemotherapy would start with the selection of an optimal single-modality therapy and a definition of both its clinical efficacy and toxicity. Different dose-fractionation schemes in concurrent treatment programs could then be normalized to one another using the biologically equivalent dose (BED) concept.[56] The BED = $nd[1 + d/(a/b)]$, where n = the number of fractions delivered, d = the dose per fraction, and $a/b = 10$ for tumors and acute-responding normal tissues and 2 for late-responding tissues. The intent of this normalization process is to allow a comparison of these different treatment programs in order to identify those having a favorable profile in terms of maximizing the probability of tumor control while minimizing the risk of late toxicity. Kasibhatla et al.[38] evaluated prospective trials of CRT in order to estimate the radiotherapeutic dose equivalence of the concurrent chemotherapy. They concluded that, with respect to the tumor, the administration of concurrent chemotherapy was equivalent to the delivery of an additional 10 to 12 Gy. Subsequently, Lee and Eisbruch[57] estimated that concurrent chemotherapy was equivalent to the delivery of an additional 8 Gy when the development of acute mucositis was used as the endpoint.

Whether modified fractionation irradiation and concurrent chemotherapy are superior to conventionally fractionated irradiation and concurrent chemotherapy was addressed in the RTOG 0129 clinical trial.[58] Both RT and chemotherapy constituted experimental variables in this trial. Patients ($N = 743$) were randomized to receive accelerated fractionation/concomitant boost to 72 Gy/6 weeks as per RTOG 90-03 and two cycles of concurrent bolus cisplatin (100 mg/m²) or conventionally fractionated RT 70 Gy/7 weeks and three cycles of concurrent bolus cisplatin (100 mg/m²). Eight-year survival was 48% in both arms, and there were no differences observed in progression-free survival, locoregional failure, or distant metastases. The findings show that one can compensate for the elimination of the third dose of cisplatin by the more intensive radiation schedule. It should also be pointed out that on the conventionally fractionated arm, only 69% of patients could tolerate all three doses of CDDP, a common occurrence with the use of high-dose CDDP regimens. Outcome was also the same in the conventionally fractionated arm patients who only received two cycles of CDDP versus all three cycles.

Chemotherapy Scheduling Considerations

Many investigators consider 100 mg/m² bolus dosing of CDDP on days 1, 22, and 43 of RT to be standard. This schedule was originally developed for use in clinical trials of induction chemotherapy and later incorporated into CRT regimens. This traditional cyclical approach to delivery of concurrent CDDP has not been compared directly with schedules that use smaller, more frequent doses. In fact, randomized clinical trials comparing so-called nonstandard schedules of platinum-based CRT against RT alone[43–45,59,60] have treated large numbers of patients with efficacy that compares favorably with bolus CDDP CRT regimens.[14,44,61] A retrospective single-institution review of 104 patients treated in the adjuvant setting with either bolus CDDP or weekly CDDP concurrently with RT revealed no significant difference in survival outcomes by chemotherapy dosing schedule.[62]

Schedules that deliver smaller and more frequent doses of chemotherapy are also quite effective in improving outcome.[63] Given the efficacy of these nonstandard platinum schedules, they may be preferable to cyclical bolus administration on two counts. More frequent administration could provide radio-sensitizing chemotherapy during a larger proportion of the course of RT. Smaller individual doses of drug may lead to less chemotherapy-induced morbidity without compromise of efficacy.[64,65] Concurrent CRT using such schedules has proven very effective and become the standard of care in squamous carcinoma of the uterine cervix.[17,66–68]

Compliance is a significant problem with the standard three-cycle concurrent CDDP paradigm. Nearly one-third of patients do not receive all cycles, and subset analyses suggest that two cycles are as effective as three.[14,47,51,52] RTOG 0129 and other studies have suggested that there may be a mini-mum cumulative threshold dose of approximately 200 mg/m^2 of cisplatin that is required to achieve maximal benefit when used concomitantly with radiation.[69–71] Schedules that admin-ister chemotherapy more frequently throughout the course of RT deliver approximately the same cumulative dose as would result from two cycles of bolus CDDP, with treatment-related morbidity being the outcome that is most affected by drug administration schedule and cumulative dose >200 mg/m^2.[71]

Weekly cisplatin regimens have been increasingly used, in large part because of their relative ease of administration and the clinical impression of reduced toxicity. It is impor-tant to stress the limitations of this experience. No direct prospective comparison has been made between the weekly and the every-3-week regimens. The randomized data justi-fying weekly drug administration are equivocal. The North American Head and Neck Intergroup, in an older trial, com-pared radiation alone with radiation and weekly cisplatin (20 mg/m^2/wk) in patients with unresectable disease. No sur-vival difference was observed between the two treatment arms, but it is very important to recognize that the total cis-platin dose was only 140 mg/m^2.[72]

In nasopharyngeal cancer, Chan et al.[73] reported a com-parison of radiation with radiation and concurrent cisplatin (40 mg/m^2/wk). Progression-free survival was not different between the two treatment arms, and a marginal overall survival difference was only appreciated after adjustment for stage and age. This survival difference was restricted to those patients with T3 or T4 tumors, and no difference was observed in the likelihood of distant metastatic disease. Thus, despite the enthusiasm for weekly cisplatin dosing regimens, there is little objective evidence supporting their use, and the every-3-week regimen must still be considered standard.

Recently, a Chinese trial compared 70 Gy of conventionally fractionated irradiation against the same regimen given with weekly concurrent cisplatin (30 mg/m^2) in 230 patients with WHO stage II nasopharynx cancer.[74] No adjuvant chemotherapy was given. Five-year overall survival was significantly better in the combined-modality arm (95% vs. 86%; P = .007). The benefit was due to an improvement in distant metastases–free survival (95% vs. 84%; P = .007). Interestingly, concurrent chemother-apy did not improve locoregional control most likely because of the excellent results in the control arm (93% vs. 91%).

Phase III comparisons of platin- and non–platin-based concurrent treatment regimens are almost nonexistent, and the relative benefit of concurrent platin versus fluorouracil or taxane therapy is unknown. Meta-analysis data have sug-gested that fluorouracil or cisplatin regimens are more suc-cessful than carboplatin- or mitomycin-based treatments[75] and that concurrent platin monotherapy is better than non-platin monotherapy.[10] In a single small phase III trial, a weekly paclitaxel concurrent regimen appeared equivalent to a weekly cisplatin concurrent schedule.[76] Overall, however, the data must be considered limited and not definitive.

Most concurrent chemotherapy regimens use a single agent, an approach that, in general, suboptimally exploits the potential systemic adjuvant benefits of this modality. In most other diseases, multiagent chemotherapy has been consid-ered a better approach in controlling distant disease. In HNC, multiagent induction chemotherapy regimens have clearly demonstrated an impact on distant metastases, a benefit observed both from single trials and in a large meta-analy-sis.[10] This same meta-analysis demonstrated a significant but less pronounced impact on distant metastases from concur-rent treatment schedules. No clear survival difference has been identified when comparing concurrent single-agent pla-tin regimens and concurrent multiagent schedules.

Radiation has also been administered in conjunction with concurrent high-dose intra-arterial cisplatin. This approach has the hypothetical advantage of allowing selective delivery of chemotherapy to the tumor while sparing uninvolved organs and allowing for the administration of intravenous sodium thiosulfate, a systemic cisplatin neutralizing agent designed to protect the kidneys. Although the procedure proved technically challenging, a phase II multi-institutional trial proved feasi-ble.[77] However, a phase III trial comparing concurrent radia-tion and intra-arterial versus intravenous cisplatin revealed no benefit,[78] and this mode of administration is not recommended.

The most frequently utilized regimen for concurrent chemoradiotherapy remains single-agent high-dose cisplatin given every 3 weeks, despite strong feelings and consider-able rhetoric. Limited evidence suggests that cisplatin may be more effective than carboplatin.[79] Taxanes are also active agents against squamous HNC but have not been studied extensively as components of CRT regimens. The ongoing trial RTOG 1216 is a three-arm study comparing standard post-operative cisplatin–RT with single-agent docetaxel and RT as well as the combination of RT with docetaxel and cetuximab, a monoclonal antibody targeting the epidermal growth factor receptor (EGFR).

Radiotherapy and Molecularly Targeted Agents

Recent efforts to integrate radiation and systemic therapy have focused on molecularly targeted agents. The EGFR is the target most often addressed and best studied in HNC. The EGFR is up-regulated in approximately 90% of patients with squamous cell HNC and has been associated with a poor prog-nosis.[80–82] In patients with recurrent or metastatic disease, a modest response rate has been observed with the anti-EGFR monoclonal antibody cetuximab, both with and without cyto-toxic chemotherapy, as well as with the oral tyrosine kinase inhibitors gefitinib and erlotinib.[83–87] Even more impressive is the disease stability that has been identified after treatment with these agents. This experience has prompted further exploration of these agents in definitive management.

Bonner et al. reported the results of the first phase III randomized trial exploring the role anti-EGFR therapy in the definitive management of a solid tumor.[88] This trial compared the use of RT alone with radiation and concurrent cetuximab in the treatment of patients with stage III or IV nonmetastatic squamous cell carcinoma of the oropharynx, hypopharynx, or larynx. Cetuximab therapy consisted of a loading dose of 400 mg/m^2 followed by a weekly dose of 250 mg/m^2 for the duration of the RT. An updated analysis reported in 2010 con-firmed the initial results.[89] The addition of cetuximab to RT improved the median overall survival from 29 to 49 months (P = .018) and the 5-year overall survival from 36% to 46%. The incidence of grade 3 or greater toxicity including mucosi-tis did not differ between the two groups, except for a greater incidence of acneiform rash and infusion reactions in those patients treated with cetuximab. An interesting but unplanned subgroup analysis suggested that the benefit was greater in the cetuximab-treated patients with oropharynx cancers, smaller primary tumors, and more advanced nodal involve-ment. Males, patients with a better performance status, and patients who were younger also seemed to do better. This demographic distribution suggested the possibility that the drug was more effective in those patients with human papil-lomavirus (HPV)-associated disease, although HPV testing of the tumor specimens was not performed. It was also notable that survival was better in the cetuximab-treated patients who developed a cetuximab-induced rash.

It is important to recognize that the control arm of this trial, RT alone, is no longer considered a treatment standard for most patients with stage III and IV locoregionally advanced squamous cell HNC. Consequently, the relative benefit of cetuximab and radiation compared to a more standard radiation and concurrent chemotherapy combination is unknown. RTOG attempted to define this better in its 0522 trial comparing concurrent radiation, cetuximab, and cisplatin with radiation and cisplatin alone.[90] As expected, the skin reactions were worse in those patients given cetuximab, but late toxicities were not different. No differences were observed in any survival outcome including progression-free survival, overall survival, or patterns of disease failure. Given the results of this study, there is currently no justification for adding cetuximab to the standard radiation and cisplatin regimens used in definitive management outside of a clinical trial.

The findings in RTOG 0522 conflict with the observation made in the metastatic disease setting. There, a phase III randomized trial compared cisplatin and fluorouracil with cisplatin, fluorouracil, and cetuximab.[86] This study demonstrated an improvement in survival from the addition of cetuximab to standard chemotherapy, and it remains unclear why the RTOG 0522 trial did not demonstrate a similar outcome improvement. RTOG 0920 is evaluating adjuvant RT plus cetuximab with adjuvant RT alone in an intermediate-risk defined patient population without positive surgical margins or ECE. This phase III study remains ongoing.

The question also remains unanswered as to whether concurrent radiation and cetuximab is equivalent or even superior to radiation and cisplatin. This issue is currently being addressed by the RTOG 1016 study, which compares these two regimens in a more selected patient population with HPV-positive oropharynx cancer. It is anticipated that the survival outcomes on the two treatment arms will be equivalent but that a difference may emerge in terms of late toxicity, function, or quality of life. It is of note that a retrospective study reported from Memorial Sloan Kettering Cancer Center suggested the possibility that locoregional control and survival were better in patients treated with radiation and cisplatin when compared to patients given radiation and cetuximab.[91] Although these results were upheld on multivariate analysis, prospective validation is required given the very significant differences in patients selected for these treatments. The randomized phase II TREMPLIN study prospectively compared the two regimens administered after three-drug induction chemotherapy. Given the nature and size of this trial, however, it is difficult to interpret any outcome comparisons.[92] In a phase III Canadian study, locally advanced HNSCC patients were randomized to standard fractionation RT plus high-dose cisplatin versus accelerated fractionation RT plus the anti-EGFR antibody panitumumab.[93] No survival differences between the two groups were demonstrated, though intrinsic study design was flawed, including no distinction of HPV-related oropharynx tumors and low event rate. Furthermore, unlike cetuximab, panitumumab added to cytotoxic chemotherapy in the metastatic setting did not show a survival benefit compared with chemotherapy alone.[94]

DEVELOPMENTAL ASPECTS OF COMBINED-MODALITY THERAPY

Induction Chemotherapy and Sequential Chemoradiation

The use of induction chemotherapy for locoregionally advanced squamous cell HNC continues to be an attractive treatment option. The dramatic tumor shrinkage seen in previously untreated patients after cisplatin-based chemotherapy regimens would intuitively suggest that an improvement

in locoregional control and even survival should also result. Multiple phase III clinical trials, however, have failed to demonstrate any reproducible impact from induction treatment schedules on overall outcome.[95,96] A marginal survival benefit was identified by the large Meta-Analysis of Chemotherapy in Head and Neck Cancer (MACH-NC) using fluorouracil and platin induction chemotherapy, but this survival improvement was dwarfed by that obtained with the use of concurrent treatment regimens (Fig. 43.2).[10]

A frequent observation from these induction trials, however, has been a reduction in distant metastases.[9,97,98] The fact that this did not impact on overall survival likely reflects the historically limited importance of distant metastases in the natural history of this disease. Recently, however, with the increasing locoregional control achieved by concurrent treatment regimens, distant metastases have emerged as a more frequent cause of treatment failure.[99,100] This observation has led to the suggestion that there may be a role for the reintroduction of chemotherapy into current multimodality treatment schedules.[101]

Coincident with this resurgent interest in induction schedules has been the recognition that the widely used and very successful cisplatin and fluorouracil combination may not be the optimal induction regimen. Considerable phase III experience now exists demonstrating the superiority of three-drug–containing regimens (fluorouracil, cisplatin, and taxane) when compared to fluorouracil and cisplatin alone[102–105] (Table 43.3). In these studies, successful induction was followed by definitive RT with or without concurrent chemotherapy.

It is important to note that three of these studies demonstrated a survival benefit favoring the three-drug induction regimen. Long-term follow-up of TAX 324 confirmed this survival benefit of adding docetaxel to cisplatin and fluorouracil with no difference in late toxicities.[106] A meta-analysis of these studies also found the taxane-containing induction regimens to be superior to platinum-fluorouracil alone.[107] This should not be interpreted as evidence that three-drug induction chemotherapy is a new standard of care. Induction chemotherapy followed by definitive radiation or chemoradiation is not a generally established sequence of treatment modalities, and the superiority of one induction regimen over another does not define induction chemotherapy as a standard of care.

Nonetheless, there are several situations where induction chemotherapy may have a role. In the larynx preservation setting, induction fluorouracil and cisplatin followed by definitive radiation in responders has been compared directly with concurrent chemoradiation with single-agent cisplatin and with RT alone.[15] Although the laryngeal preservation and locoregional control were superior in the concurrent chemoradiotherapy arm, laryngectomy-free survival and distant metastatic control were equivalent between the two chemotherapy regimens.[15] It is of note that overall survival was unchanged by

TABLE 43.3 TAXANE, CISPLATIN, AND FLUOROURACIL (TPF) VERSUS CISPLATIN AND FLUOROURACIL (PF) INDUCTION CHEMOTHERAPY: RANDOMIZED TRIALS

	Hitt 2005[94]	Vermorken 2007[95]	Posner 2007[96]	Pointreau 2009[97]
Taxane	Paclitaxel	Docetaxel	Docetaxel	Docetaxel
Definitive treatment	Variable	Radiation	Radiation/weekly carboplatin	Variable
Response rate				
PF	68%	54%	64%	59%
TPF	80%	68%	72%	80%
P Value	<.001	.006	.07	.002
Survival	2 y	3 y	3 y	3 y
PF	54%	26%	48%	60%
TPF	67%	37%	62%	60%
P Value	.06	.02	.002	.57

the addition of chemotherapy. Thus, induction chemotherapy can be considered an acceptable larynx preservation strategy. The superiority of the three-drug docetaxel, cisplatin, and fluorouracil regimen when compared to fluorouracil and cisplatin in the larynx preservation setting has been established,[105] although the subsequent use of concurrent treatment regimens after three-drug induction has proven difficult.[92]

Of greater interest has been the use of induction chemotherapy in what has been termed *sequential treatment* regimens, that is, induction chemotherapy followed by concurrent chemoradiotherapy.[108] The rationale for this approach is that the addition of induction chemotherapy can, by improving the distant metastatic control, improve upon the overall survival achieved after concurrent chemoradiotherapy alone. These treatment schedules are intensive and require considerable commitment from both patient and physician. Toxicity, when compared to concurrent chemoradiotherapy alone, will be increased, and the administration of multiple doses of both induction and concurrent cisplatin is challenging.[92]

A preliminary report by Hitt and Lopez-Pousa from their study of three-drug induction chemotherapy followed by chemoradiotherapy compared with chemoradiotherapy alone suggested a benefit for the induction arm, though the final analysis revealed no difference in survival between the treatment groups[107,109]. A successful phase II randomized experience has been reported by Paccagnella et al.[110] comparing induction docetaxel, cisplatin, and fluorouracil before chemoradiotherapy with chemoradiotherapy alone. Another phase II study of induction chemotherapy followed by concurrent chemoradiation incorporated cetuximab in both the induction regimen and concurrent therapy.[111] The induction chemotherapy in both arms consisted of cetuximab, paclitaxel, and carboplatin, and the concurrent chemotherapy was either cetuximab, fluorouracil, and hydroxyurea or cetuximab and cisplatin. Both arms were considered successful with 2-year PFS of both arms higher than historical controls.

Two phase III studies, DeCIDE[112] and PARADIGM,[113] which compared induction chemotherapy followed by concurrent chemoradiotherapy to concurrent CRT alone failed to show a survival advantage with the sequential treatment strategy. The DeCIDE trial had a 5% incidence of treatment-induced mortality in the sequential arm compared to 0% in the CRT arm. This difference may have offset any survival benefit attributable to the lower incidence of distant metastases in the sequential arm. A meta-analysis of induction chemotherapy followed by concurrent CRT with CRT alone revealed decreased distant metastasis rate with induction chemotherapy; however, no statistically significant differences in OS, PFS, overall response rate (ORR), or locoregional recurrence rate were demonstrated.[114]

A third rationale for induction chemotherapy has been explored by the University of Michigan investigators. Their premise is that induction chemotherapy can serve as a predictive tool and allow for the appropriate selection of the subsequent definitive HNC management strategy. Patients responding to induction chemotherapy can be approached nonoperatively, whereas those in whom induction is unsuccessful should proceed to surgical resection. This strategy is based on the long-standing recognition that patients responding to induction chemotherapy are also those who respond best to RT.[115]

This approach has been used successfully in patients with advanced larynx cancer.[116,117] The treatment schedule began with a single cycle of induction cisplatin and fluorouracil, followed by concurrent chemoradiotherapy with high-dose single-agent cisplatin in responders. At least a partial response to single-cycle induction was achieved in 75% of patients, and larynx preservation ultimately proved possible in 70% of the entire patient cohort. It was of particular import that those patients requiring laryngectomy because of a failure to respond to induction chemotherapy achieved an overall survival equivalent to the chemotherapy responders.

This experience proved less successful in their patients with oropharynx and oral cavity cancer, however.[118] Furthermore, the relegation of induction chemotherapy to a purely predictive tool is disquieting to both medical and radiation oncologists. Induction adds significant cost and toxicity, and one would hope that it might provide an additional survival benefit or an improvement in distant metastatic disease control. Perhaps, other less toxic predictive "biomarkers" than responsiveness to induction chemotherapy might emerge in the future.

Thus, induction chemotherapy, particularly using the three-drug cisplatin, fluorouracil, and taxane combination, remains a very active but incompletely developed tool. Its ultimate impact on survival, distant metastases, and our treatment paradigms remains to be seen. Toxicity considerations will play an important role in the choice of therapeutic strategies. Overall, more treatment means more toxicity as treatment is escalated along the continuum from conventional once-daily RT only to the most intensive combined-modality regimens. The total toxicity burden imposed upon a patient may increase as much as fivefold.[119] These considerations are particularly relevant to sequential therapy programs. Compliance rates for an entire course of treatment with these regimens are only 65% to 70% in the most experienced hands.[102,120]

Other Targeted Agents

Other EGFR monoclonal antibodies are also being explored in the HNC patient population, both in the metastatic setting and in conjunction with radiation, including panitumumab and zalutumumab.[121,122] The oral tyrosine kinase inhibitors including gefitinib, erlotinib, and others have undergone limited phase II testing as part of definitive treatment schedules. Results from these studies have been mixed and enthusiasm is restrained.[123-126]

Treatments directed against other molecular targets, most notably the vascular endothelial growth factor receptor (VEGFR), are also now being integrated with definitive RT schedules.[127,128] Overexpression of VEGF in HNC is associated with a twofold increase in the risk of death from disease.[129] Yoo et al. performed a pilot study in 29 patients that integrated dual targeting of EGFR with erlotinib and VEGFR with the antibody bevacizumab into a regimen of platinum-based chemoradiation for newly diagnosed, locally advanced, nonmetastatic disease.[130] Three-year progression-free survival was 82%. One of the most important facets of this trial was that it utilized functional metabolic imaging with the performance of serial dynamic contrast-enhanced magnetic resonance imaging (DCE-MRI) scans to assess response to treatment. DCE-MRI quantitatively measures tumor perfusion and vascular permeability, which is expressed by the parameter K^{trans}. Patients whose disease recurred after treatment had lower baseline pretreatment median K^{trans} values, which rose during the earliest phases of therapy. Patients who did not fail, however, had higher baseline median K^{trans} values that decreased during therapy. These data suggest that K^{trans} could potentially serve as an imaging biomarker to guide initial treatment selection based on pretreatment prognosis or to guide treatment modification based on a favorable or unfavorable response to the early phases of treatment.[131]

Hypoxia is one of the most important characteristics of the aggressive malignant phenotype.[132-135] Poorly oxygenated tumors are less likely to respond to surgery,[136] radiotherapy,[31,137,138] and chemotherapy. Hypoxic primary tumors are more likely to develop distant metastases after treatment.[139] A review of 397 HNC patients who underwent tumor oxygenation measurement demonstrated that hypoxia was strongly associated with treatment failure independently of stage and therapeutic modality.[32]

Tirapazamine, a bioreductively activated compound, is one to two orders of magnitude more cytotoxic to hypoxic cells than well-oxygenated cells and also potentiates the activity of cisplatin.[140,141] Phase I/II studies in advanced squamous HNC demonstrated efficacy with acceptable toxicity when this drug was incorporated into cisplatin-containing CRT regimens and suggested that the benefit of the drug was restricted to those patients who had hypoxic tumors as assessed by ^{18}F-misonidazole positron emission tomography (PET) scanning.[142,143]

Two phase III trials were conducted to determine whether targeting of hypoxic cells with tirapazamine/cisplatin CRT was superior to cisplatin CRT. The first trial (HeadSTART) enrolled 880 patients. No benefit was observed from the addition of tirapazamine.[144] A large number of patients had significant protocol deviations with respect to the delivery of radiotherapy, however. A subset analysis of patients who correctly received all of their treatment according to the protocol guidelines did demonstrate an advantage in patients who received tirapazamine.[145] Another important consideration is that patients enrolled into this trial were not selected according to whether or not they had hypoxic tumors, which would have increased the power to detect a benefit from the drug if in fact one existed. A second trial with the same treatment schema was launched with a planned enrollment of 550 patients but was prematurely closed because of an unexplainable excess of deaths during treatment in the tirapazamine arm.

Immunotherapy

As HNC is seen as an immunosuppressive disease, immunotherapy represents an additional modality of treatment. The KEYNOTE and CHECKMATE trials were completed in patients with recurrent/metastatic disease not amenable to local therapies and refractory to platinum-based chemotherapy and studied the programmed cell death 1 (PD-1) inhibitors pembrolizumab and nivolumab, respectively. In a phase Ib expansion cohort study in patients with R/M HNSCC, half of patients demonstrated a decrease in tumor burden.[146] Nivolumab improved overall survival in a phase III randomized clinical trial enrolling patients with platinum-refractory R/M HNSCC.[147] Both therapies were granted FDA approval in 2016 for patients with R/M HNSCC with platinum-refractory disease.

There is current interest in utilizing immunotherapies in the locally advanced HNSCC setting in conjunction with radiotherapy. NRG HN003 is studying the addition of pembrolizumab to the backbone of postoperative cisplatin chemoradiotherapy in high-risk patients, in attempt to intensify therapy and improve outcomes. Using immunotherapy in place of cytotoxic chemotherapy is an attractive option for evaluation in deintensification studies for improved toxicity profiles while maintaining high cure rates in good prognosis, HPV-related oropharynx patients.

Summary

The use of modified daily fractionation as opposed to conventional once-daily fractionation improves the prognosis of patients who receive curative intent RT for advanced HNC. Radiation therapy and concurrent chemotherapy in turn are superior to both single-modality conventional and modified fractionation radiation therapies in the nonsurgical management of advanced HNC. Anti–EGFR-targeted therapy also enhances the effectiveness of RT. The role of EGFR inhibition in a chemoradiation setting is under investigation. Likewise, the benefit of adding induction chemotherapy to a platform of chemoradiation is being tested. Hypoxia-targeted therapy remains investigational.

The increased acute and late toxicity that results from combining these multiple modalities poses immediate challenges. These include the need to develop criteria for a priori selection of those patients with advanced-stage disease who can still be adequately treated with radiotherapy alone and the need to create effective strategies for toxicity prophylaxis and management. These efforts will allow for the optimal integration of radiotherapy, chemotherapy, biologically targeted therapy, and immunotherapy for those patients requiring combined modality therapy.

REFERENCES

1. Siegel RL, Miller KD, Jemal A. Cancer statistics, 2016. *CA Cancer J Clin* 2016;66(1):7–30.
2. Fu KK, et al. A Radiation Therapy Oncology Group (RTOG) phase III randomized study to compare hyperfractionation and two variants of accelerated fractionation to standard fractionation radiotherapy for head and neck squamous cell carcinomas: first report of RTOG 9003. *Int J Radiat Oncol Biol Phys* 2000;48(1):7–16.
3. Horiot JC, et al. Accelerated fractionation (AF) compared to conventional fractionation (CF) improves loco-regional control in the radiotherapy of advanced head and neck cancers: results of the EORTC 22851 randomized trial. *Radiother Oncol* 1997;44(2):111–121.
4. Horiot JC, et al. Hyperfractionation versus conventional fractionation in oropharyngeal carcinoma: final analysis of a randomized trial of the EORTC cooperative group of radiotherapy. *Radiother Oncol* 1992;25(4):231–241.
5. Overgaard J, et al. Five compared with six fractions per week of conventional radiotherapy of squamous-cell carcinoma of head and neck: DAHANCA 6 and 7 randomised controlled trial. *Lancet* 2003;362(9388):933–940.
6. Bourhis J, et al. Hyperfractionated or accelerated radiotherapy in head and neck cancer: a meta-analysis. *Lancet* 2006;368(9538):843–854.
7. Fu KK. Combined-modality therapy for head and neck cancer. *Oncology (Williston Park)* 1997;11(12):1781–1790, 1796; discussion 1796, 179.
8. Lamont EB, Vokes EE. Chemotherapy in the management of squamous-cell carcinoma of the head and neck. *Lancet Oncol* 2001;2(5):261–269.
9. Department of Veterans Affairs Laryngeal Cancer Study Group. Induction chemotherapy plus radiation compared with surgery plus radiation in patients with advanced laryngeal cancer. *N Engl J Med* 1991;324(24):1685–1690.
10. Pignon JP, et al. Meta-analysis of chemotherapy in head and neck cancer (MACH-NC): an update on 93 randomised trials and 17,346 patients. *Radiother Oncol* 2009;92(1):4–14.
11. Monnerat C, et al. End points for new agents in induction chemotherapy for locally advanced head and neck cancers. *Ann Oncol* 2002;13(7):995–1006.
12. Blanchard P, et al. Meta-analysis of chemotherapy in head and neck cancer (MACH-NC): a comprehensive analysis by tumour site. *Radiother Oncol* 2011;100(1):33–40.
13. Taylor SG, et al. Randomized comparison of neoadjuvant cisplatin and fluorouracil infusion followed by radiation versus concomitant treatment in advanced head and neck cancer. *J Clin Oncol* 1994;12(2):385–395.
14. Forastiere AA, et al. Concurrent chemotherapy and radiotherapy for organ preservation in advanced laryngeal cancer. *N Engl J Med* 2003;349(22):2091–2098.
15. Forastiere AA, et al. Long-term results of RTOG 91-11: a comparison of three nonsurgical treatment strategies to preserve the larynx in patients with locally advanced larynx cancer. *J Clin Oncol* 2013;31(7):845–852.
16. Herskovic A, et al. Combined chemotherapy and radiotherapy compared with radiotherapy alone in patients with cancer of the esophagus. *N Engl J Med* 1992;326(24):1593–1598.
17. Peters WA 3rd, et al. Concurrent chemotherapy and pelvic radiation therapy compared with pelvic radiation therapy alone as adjuvant therapy after radical surgery in high-risk early-stage cancer of the cervix. *J Clin Oncol* 2000;18(8):1606–1613.
18. Cooper JS, et al. Chemoradiotherapy of locally advanced esophageal cancer: long-term follow-up of a prospective randomized trial (RTOG 85-01). Radiation Therapy Oncology Group. *JAMA* 1999;281(17):1623–1627.
19. Budach V, et al. Hyperfractionated accelerated chemoradiation with concurrent fluorouracil-mitomycin is more effective than dose-escalated hyperfractionated accelerated radiation therapy alone in locally advanced head and neck cancer: final results of the radiotherapy cooperative clinical trials group of the German Cancer Society 95-06 Prospective Randomized Trial. *J Clin Oncol* 2005;23(6):1125–1135.
20. Denis F, et al. Final results of the 94-01 French Head and Neck Oncology and Radiotherapy Group randomized trial comparing radiotherapy alone with concomitant radiochemotherapy in advanced-stage oropharynx carcinoma. *J Clin Oncol* 2004;22(1):69–76.
21. Denis F, et al. Late toxicity results of the GORTEC 94-01 randomized trial comparing radiotherapy with concomitant radiochemotherapy for advanced-stage oropharynx carcinoma: comparison of LENT/SOMA, RTOG/EORTC, and NCI-CTC scoring systems. *Int J Radiat Oncol Biol Phys* 2003;55(1):93–98.
22. Cox JD, et al. Interruptions adversely affect local control and survival with hyperfractionated radiation therapy of carcinomas of the upper respiratory and digestive tracts. New evidence for accelerated proliferation from Radiation Therapy Oncology Group Protocol 8313. *Cancer* 1992;69(11):2744–2748.
23. Overgaard J, et al. Comparison of conventional and split-course radiotherapy as primary treatment in carcinoma of the larynx. *Acta Oncol* 1988;27(2):147–152.
24. Withers HR, Taylor JM, Maciejewski B. The hazard of accelerated tumor clonogen repopulation during radiotherapy. *Acta Oncol* 1988;27(2):131–146.
25. Eschwege F, et al. Ten-year results of randomized trial comparing radiotherapy and concomitant bleomycin to radiotherapy alone in epidermoid carcinomas of the oropharynx: experience of the European Organization for Research and Treatment of Cancer. *NCI Monogr* 1988;(6):275–278.
26. Fu KK, et al. Combined radiotherapy and chemotherapy with bleomycin and methotrexate for advanced inoperable head and neck cancer: update of a Northern California Oncology Group randomized trial. *J Clin Oncol* 1987;5(9):1410–1418.
27. Gupta NK, Pointon RC, Wilkinson PM. A randomised clinical trial to contrast radiotherapy with radiotherapy and methotrexate given synchronously in head and neck cancer. *Clin Radiol* 1987;38(6):575–581.
28. Lo TC, et al. Combined radiation therapy and 5-fluorouracil for advanced squamous cell carcinoma of the oral cavity and oropharynx: a randomized study. *AJR Am J Roentgenol* 1976;126(2):229–235.

29. Browman GP, et al. Placebo-controlled randomized trial of infusional fluorouracil during standard radiotherapy in locally advanced head and neck cancer. *J Clin Oncol* 1994;12(12):2648–2653.
30. Gray LH, et al. The concentration of oxygen dissolved in tissues at the time of irradiation as a factor in radiotherapy. *Br J Radiol* 1953;26(312):638–648.
31. Brizel DM, et al. Oxygenation of head and neck cancer: changes during radiotherapy and impact on treatment outcome. *Radiother Oncol* 1999;53(2):113–117.
32. Nordsmark M, et al. Prognostic value of tumor oxygenation in 397 head and neck tumors after primary radiation therapy. An international multi-center study. *Radiother Oncol* 2005;77(1):18–24.
33. Haffty BG, et al. Chemotherapy as an adjunct to radiation in the treatment of squamous cell carcinoma of the head and neck: results of the Yale Mitomycin Randomized Trials. *J Clin Oncol* 1997;15(1):268–276.
34. Bartelink H, et al. Therapeutic enhancement in mice by clinically relevant dose and fractionation schedules of cis-diamminedichloroplatinum (II) and irradiation. *Radiother Oncol* 1986;6(1):61–74.
35. Adelstein DJ, et al. Mature results of a phase III randomized trial comparing concurrent chemoradiotherapy with radiation therapy alone in patients with stage III and IV squamous cell carcinoma of the head and neck. *Cancer* 2000;88(4):876–883.
36. Keane TJ, et al. A randomized trial of radiation therapy compared to split course radiation therapy combined with mitomycin C and 5 fluorouracil as initial treatment for advanced laryngeal and hypopharyngeal squamous carcinoma. *Int J Radiat Oncol Biol Phys* 1993;25(4):613–618.
37. Sanchiz F, et al. Single fraction per day versus two fractions per day versus radiochemotherapy in the treatment of head and neck cancer. *Int J Radiat Oncol Biol Phys* 1990;19(6):1347–1350.
38. Kasibhatla M, Kirkpatrick JP, Brizel DM. How much radiation is the chemotherapy worth in advanced head and neck cancer? *Int J Radiat Oncol Biol Phys* 2007;68(5):1491–1495.
39. Wong WW, et al. Time-dose relationship for local tumor control following alternate week concomitant radiation and chemotherapy of advanced head and neck cancer. *Int J Radiat Oncol Biol Phys* 1994;29(1):153–162.
40. Merlano M, et al. Five-year update of a randomized trial of alternating radiotherapy and chemotherapy compared with radiotherapy alone in treatment of unresectable squamous cell carcinoma of the head and neck. *J Natl Cancer Inst* 1996;88(9):583–589.
41. Merlano M, et al. Treatment of advanced squamous-cell carcinoma of the head and neck with alternating chemotherapy and radiotherapy. *N Engl J Med* 1992;327(16):1115–1121.
42. Calais G, et al. Randomized trial of radiation therapy versus concomitant chemotherapy and radiation therapy for advanced-stage oropharynx carcinoma. *J Natl Cancer Inst* 1999;91(24):2081–2086.
43. Wendt TG, et al. Simultaneous radiochemotherapy versus radiotherapy alone in advanced head and neck cancer: a randomized multicenter study. *J Clin Oncol* 1998;16(4):1318–1324.
44. Al-Sarraf M, et al. Chemoradiotherapy versus radiotherapy in patients with advanced nasopharyngeal cancer: phase III randomized Intergroup study 0099. *J Clin Oncol* 1998;16(4):1310–1317.
45. Brizel DM, et al. Hyperfractionated irradiation with or without concurrent chemotherapy for locally advanced head and neck cancer. *N Engl J Med* 1998;338(25):1798–1804.
46. Jeremic B, et al. Radiation therapy alone or with concurrent low-dose daily either cisplatin or carboplatin in locally advanced unresectable squamous cell carcinoma of the head and neck: a prospective randomized trial. *Radiother Oncol* 1997;43(1):29–37.
47. Bensadoun RJ, et al. French multicenter phase III randomized study testing concurrent twice-a-day radiotherapy and cisplatin/5-fluorouracil chemotherapy (BiRCF) in unresectable pharyngeal carcinoma: Results at 2 years (FNCLCC-GORTEC). *Int J Radiat Oncol Biol Phys* 2006;64(4):983–994.
48. Dobrowsky W, Naude J. Continuous hyperfractionated accelerated radiotherapy with/without mitomycin C in head and neck cancers. *Radiother Oncol* 2000;57(2):119–124.
49. Adjuvant chemotherapy for advanced head and neck squamous carcinoma. Final report of the Head and Neck Contracts Program. *Cancer* 1987;60(3):301–311.
50. Laramore GE, et al. Adjuvant chemotherapy for resectable squamous cell carcinomas of the head and neck: report on Intergroup Study 0034. *Int J Radiat Oncol Biol Phys* 1992;23(4):705–713.
51. Bernier J, et al. Postoperative irradiation with or without concomitant chemotherapy for locally advanced head and neck cancer. *N Engl J Med* 2004;350(19):1945–1952.
52. Cooper JS, et al. Postoperative concurrent radiotherapy and chemotherapy for high-risk squamous-cell carcinoma of the head and neck. *N Engl J Med* 2004;350(19):1937–1944.
53. Bernier J, et al. Defining risk levels in locally advanced head and neck cancers: a comparative analysis of concurrent postoperative radiation plus chemotherapy trials of the EORTC (#22931) and RTOG (# 9501). *Head Neck* 2005;27(10): 843–850.
54. Cooper JS, et al. Long-term follow-up of the RTOG 9501/intergroup phase III trial: postoperative concurrent radiation therapy and chemotherapy in high-risk squamous cell carcinoma of the head and neck. *Int J Radiat Oncol Biol Phys* 2012;84(5):1198–1205.
55. Trifiletti DM, et al. Beyond positive margins and extracapsular extension: evaluating the utilization and clinical impact of postoperative chemoradiotherapy in resected locally advanced head and neck cancer. *J Clin Oncol* 2017;35(14):1550–1560.
56. Fowler JF. Modelling altered fractionation schedules. *BJR Suppl* 1992;24: 187–192.
57. Lee IH, Eisbruch A. Mucositis versus tumor control: the therapeutic index of adding chemotherapy to irradiation of head and neck cancer. *Int J Radiat Oncol Biol Phys* 2009;75(4):1060–1063.
58. Nguyen-Tan PF, et al. Randomized phase III trial to test accelerated versus standard fractionation in combination with concurrent cisplatin for head and neck carcinomas in the Radiation Therapy Oncology Group 0129 trial: long-term report of efficacy and toxicity. *J Clin Oncol* 2014;32(34):3858–3866.
59. Bernier J. Alteration of radiotherapy fractionation and concurrent chemotherapy: a new frontier in head and neck oncology? *Nat Clin Pract Oncol* 2005;2(6):305–314.
60. Huguenin P, et al. Concomitant cisplatin significantly improves locoregional control in advanced head and neck cancers treated with hyperfractionated radiotherapy. *J Clin Oncol* 2004;22(23):4665–4673.
61. Adelstein DJ, et al. An intergroup phase III comparison of standard radiation therapy and two schedules of concurrent chemoradiotherapy in patients with unresectable squamous cell head and neck cancer. *J Clin Oncol* 2003;21(1): 92–98.
62. Geiger JL, et al. Adjuvant chemoradiation therapy with high-dose versus weekly cisplatin for resected, locally-advanced HPV/p16-positive and negative head and neck squamous cell carcinoma. *Oral Oncol* 2014;50(4):311–318.
63. Jeremic B, et al. Hyperfractionated radiation therapy with or without concurrent low-dose daily cisplatin in locally advanced squamous cell carcinoma of the head and neck: a prospective randomized trial. *J Clin Oncol* 2000;18(7):1458–1464.
64. Kurihara N, et al. Pharmacokinetics of cis-diamminedichloroplatinum (II) given as low-dose and high-dose infusions. *J Surg Oncol* 1996;62(2):135–138.
65. Nagai N, Ogata H. Quantitative relationship between pharmacokinetics of unchanged cisplatin and nephrotoxicity in rats: importance of area under the concentration-time curve (AUC) as the major toxicodynamic determinant in vivo. *Cancer Chemother Pharmacol* 1997;40(1):11–18.
66. Morris M, et al. Pelvic radiation with concurrent chemotherapy compared with pelvic and para-aortic radiation for high-risk cervical cancer. *N Engl J Med* 1999;340(15):1137–1143.
67. Rose PG, et al. Concurrent cisplatin-based radiotherapy and chemotherapy for locally advanced cervical cancer. *N Engl J Med* 1999;340(15):1144–1153.
68. Thomas GM. Improved treatment for cervical cancer—concurrent chemotherapy and radiotherapy. *N Engl J Med* 1999;340(15):1198–1200.
69. Ang KK. Concurrent radiation chemotherapy for locally advanced head and neck carcinoma: are we addressing burning subjects? *J Clin Oncol* 2004;22(23):4657–4659.
70. Ghi MG, Paccagnella A, Floriani I, et al. Concomitant chemoradiation in locally advanced head and neck squamous cell carcinoma: A literature-based meta-analysis on the platinum concomitant chemotherapy. *J Clin Oncol* 2011;29(368s):abstr 5534.
71. Loong HH, Ma B, Mo F. The effect of cisplatin dose administered during concurrent chemoradiotherapy in patients with locoregionally advanced nasopharyngeal carcinoma. *J Clin Oncol* 2011;29(368s):abstract 5532.
72. Quon H, et al. Phase III study of radiation therapy with or without cis-platinum in patients with unresectable squamous or undifferentiated carcinoma of the head and neck: an intergroup trial of the Eastern Cooperative Oncology Group (E2382). *Int J Radiat Oncol Biol Phys* 2011;81(3):719–725.
73. Chan AT, et al. Overall survival after concurrent cisplatin-radiotherapy compared with radiotherapy alone in locoregionally advanced nasopharyngeal carcinoma. *J Natl Cancer Inst* 2005;97(7):536–539.
74. Chen QY, et al. Concurrent chemoradiotherapy vs radiotherapy alone in stage II nasopharyngeal carcinoma: phase III randomized trial. *J Natl Cancer Inst* 2011;103(23):1761–1770.
75. Budach W, et al. A meta-analysis of hyperfractionated and accelerated radiotherapy and combined chemotherapy and radiotherapy regimens in unresected locally advanced squamous cell carcinoma of the head and neck. *BMC Cancer* 2006;6:28.
76. Jain RK, et al. A comparative study of low dose weekly paclitaxel versus cisplatin with concurrent radiation in the treatment of locally advanced head and neck cancers. *Indian J Cancer* 2009;46(1):50–53.
77. Robbins KT, et al. Supradose intra-arterial cisplatin and concurrent radiation therapy for the treatment of stage IV head and neck squamous cell carcinoma is feasible and efficacious in a multi-institutional setting: results of Radiation Therapy Oncology Group Trial 9615. *J Clin Oncol* 2005;23(7):1447–1454.
78. Rasch CR, et al. Intra-arterial versus intravenous chemoradiation for advanced head and neck cancer: results of a randomized phase 3 trial. *Cancer* 2010;116(9):2159–2165.
79. Fountzilas G, et al. Concomitant radiochemotherapy vs radiotherapy alone in patients with head and neck cancer: a Hellenic Cooperative Oncology Group Phase III Study. *Med Oncol* 2004;21(2):95–107.
80. Ang KK, et al. Impact of epidermal growth factor receptor expression on survival and pattern of relapse in patients with advanced head and neck carcinoma. *Cancer Res* 2002;62(24):7350–7356.
81. Chung CH, et al. Increased epidermal growth factor receptor gene copy number is associated with poor prognosis in head and neck squamous cell carcinomas. *J Clin Oncol* 2006;24(25):4170–4176.
82. Temam S, et al. Epidermal growth factor receptor copy number alterations correlate with poor clinical outcome in patients with head and neck squamous cancer. *J Clin Oncol* 2007;25(16):2164–2170.
83. Burtness B, et al. Phase III randomized trial of cisplatin plus placebo compared with cisplatin plus cetuximab in metastatic/recurrent head and neck cancer: an Eastern Cooperative Oncology Group study. *J Clin Oncol* 2005;23(34):8646–8654.
84. Cohen EE, et al. Phase II trial of ZD1839 in recurrent or metastatic squamous cell carcinoma of the head and neck. *J Clin Oncol* 2003;21(10):1980–1987.
85. Soulieres D, et al. Multicenter phase II study of erlotinib, an oral epidermal growth factor receptor tyrosine kinase inhibitor, in patients with recurrent or metastatic squamous cell cancer of the head and neck. *J Clin Oncol* 2004;22(1):77–85.
86. Vermorken JB, et al. Platinum-based chemotherapy plus cetuximab in head and neck cancer. *N Engl J Med* 2008;359(11):1116–1127.

87. Stewart JS, et al. Phase III study of gefitinib compared with intravenous methotrexate for recurrent squamous cell carcinoma of the head and neck [corrected]. *J Clin Oncol* 2009;27(11):1864–1871.

88. Bonner JA, et al. Radiotherapy plus cetuximab for squamous-cell carcinoma of the head and neck. *N Engl J Med* 2006;354(6):567–578.

89. Bonner JA, et al. Radiotherapy plus cetuximab for locoregionally advanced head and neck cancer: 5-year survival data from a phase 3 randomised trial, and relation between cetuximab-induced rash and survival. *Lancet Oncol* 2010;11(1):21–28.

90. Ang KK, et al. Randomized phase III trial of concurrent accelerated radiation plus cisplatin with or without cetuximab for stage III to IV head and neck carcinoma: RTOG 0522. *J Clin Oncol* 2014;32(27):2940–2950.

91. Koutcher L, et al. Concurrent cisplatin and radiation versus cetuximab and radiation for locally advanced head-and-neck cancer. *Int J Radiat Oncol Biol Phys* 2011;81(4):915–922.

92. Lefebvre JL, et al. Induction chemotherapy followed by either chemoradiotherapy or bioradiotherapy for larynx preservation: the TREMPLIN randomized phase II study. *J Clin Oncol* 2013;31(7):853–859.

93. Siu LL, et al. Effect of standard radiotherapy with cisplatin vs accelerated radiotherapy with panitumumab in locoregionally advanced squamous cell head and neck carcinoma: a randomized clinical trial. *JAMA Oncol* 2017;3(2):220–226.

94. Vermorken JB, et al. Cisplatin and fluorouracil with or without panitumumab in patients with recurrent or metastatic squamous-cell carcinoma of the head and neck (SPECTRUM): an open-label phase 3 randomised trial. *Lancet Oncol* 2013;14(8):697–710.

95. Adelstein DJ. Induction chemotherapy in head and neck cancer. *Hematol Oncol Clin North Am* 1999;13(4):689–698, v–vi.

96. Cohen EE, Lingen MW, Vokes EE. The expanding role of systemic therapy in head and neck cancer. *J Clin Oncol* 2004;22(9):1743–1752.

97. Schuller DE, et al. Preoperative chemotherapy in advanced resectable head and neck cancer: final report of the Southwest Oncology Group. *Laryngoscope* 1988;98(11):1205–1211.

98. Paccagnella A, et al. Phase III trial of initial chemotherapy in stage III or IV head and neck cancers: a study by the Gruppo di Studio sui Tumori della Testa e del Collo. *J Natl Cancer Inst* 1994;86(4):265–272.

99. Adelstein DJ, et al. Maximizing local control and organ preservation in stage IV squamous cell head and neck cancer with hyperfractionated radiation and concurrent chemotherapy. *J Clin Oncol* 2002;20(5):1405–1410.

100. Vokes EE, et al. Concomitant chemoradiotherapy as primary therapy for locoregionally advanced head and neck cancer. *J Clin Oncol* 2000;18(8):1652–1661.

101. Brockstein B, et al. Patterns of failure, prognostic factors and survival in locoregionally advanced head and neck cancer treated with concomitant chemoradiotherapy: a 9-year, 337-patient, multi-institutional experience. *Ann Oncol* 2004;15(8):1179–1186.

102. Hitt R, et al. Phase III study comparing cisplatin plus fluorouracil to paclitaxel, cisplatin, and fluorouracil induction chemotherapy followed by chemoradiotherapy in locally advanced head and neck cancer. *J Clin Oncol* 2005;23(34):8636–8645.

103. Posner MR, et al. Cisplatin and fluorouracil alone or with docetaxel in head and neck cancer. *N Engl J Med* 2007;357(17):1705–1715.

104. Vermorken JB, et al. Cisplatin, fluorouracil, and docetaxel in unresectable head and neck cancer. *N Engl J Med* 2007;357(17):1695–1704.

105. Janoray G, et al. Long-term results of a multicenter randomized phase III trial of induction chemotherapy with cisplatin, 5-fluorouracil, ± Docetaxel for larynx preservation. *J Natl Cancer Inst* 2016;108(4). https://doi.org/10.1093/jnci/djv368

106. Lorch JH, et al. Induction chemotherapy with cisplatin and fluorouracil alone or in combination with docetaxel in locally advanced squamous-cell cancer of the head and neck: long-term results of the TAX 324 randomised phase 3 trial. *Lancet Oncol* 2011;12(2):153–159.

107. Blanchard P, et al. Taxane-cisplatin-fluorouracil as induction chemotherapy in locally advanced head and neck cancers: an individual patient data meta-analysis of the meta-analysis of chemotherapy in head and neck cancer group. *J Clin Oncol* 2013;31(23):2854–2860.

108. Posner MR, et al. Induction chemotherapy in locally advanced squamous cell cancer of the head and neck: evolution of the sequential treatment approach. *Semin Oncol* 2004;31(6):778–785.

109. Hitt R, et al. A randomized phase III trial comparing induction chemotherapy followed by chemoradiotherapy versus chemoradiotherapy alone as treatment of unresectable head and neck cancer. *Ann Oncol* 2014;25(1):216–225.

110. Paccagnella A, et al. Concomitant chemoradiotherapy versus induction docetaxel, cisplatin and 5 fluorouracil (TPF) followed by concomitant chemoradiotherapy in locally advanced head and neck cancer: a phase II randomized study. *Ann Oncol* 2010;21(7):1515–1522.

111. Seiwert TY, et al. Final results of a randomized phase 2 trial investigating the addition of cetuximab to induction chemotherapy and accelerated or hyperfractionated chemoradiation for locoregionally advanced head and neck cancer. *Int J Radiat Oncol Biol Phys* 2016;96(1):21–29.

112. Haddad R, et al. Induction chemotherapy followed by concurrent chemoradiotherapy (sequential chemoradiotherapy) versus concurrent chemoradiotherapy alone in locally advanced head and neck cancer (PARADIGM): a randomised phase 3 trial. *Lancet Oncol* 2013;14(3):257–264.

113. Cohen EE, et al. Phase III randomized trial of induction chemotherapy in patients with N2 or N3 locally advanced head and neck cancer. *J Clin Oncol* 2014;32(25):2735–2743.

114. Zhang L, et al. Induction chemotherapy with concurrent chemoradiotherapy versus concurrent chemoradiotherapy for locally advanced squamous cell carcinoma of head and neck: a meta-analysis. *Sci Rep* 2015;5:10798.

115. Ensley JF, et al. Correlation between response to cisplatinum-combination chemotherapy and subsequent radiotherapy in previously untreated patients with advanced squamous cell cancers of the head and neck. *Cancer* 1984;54(5):811–814.

116. Urba S, et al. Single-cycle induction chemotherapy selects patients with advanced laryngeal cancer for combined chemoradiation: a new treatment paradigm. *J Clin Oncol* 2006;24(4):593–598.

117. Worden FP, et al. Chemoselection as a strategy for organ preservation in patients with T4 laryngeal squamous cell carcinoma with cartilage invasion. *Laryngoscope* 2009;119(8):1510–1517.

118. Worden FP, et al. Chemoselection as a strategy for organ preservation in advanced oropharynx cancer: response and survival positively associated with HPV16 copy number. *J Clin Oncol* 2008;26(19):3138–3146.

119. Bentzen SM, Trotti A. Evaluation of early and late toxicities in chemoradiation trials. *J Clin Oncol* 2007;25(26):4096–4103.

120. Adelstein DJ, et al. Docetaxel, cisplatin, and fluorouracil induction chemotherapy followed by accelerated fractionation/concomitant boost radiation and concurrent cisplatin in patients with advanced squamous cell head and neck cancer: a Southwest Oncology Group phase II trial (S0216). *Head Neck* 2010;32(2):221–228.

121. Wirth LJ, et al. Phase I dose-finding study of paclitaxel with panitumumab, carboplatin and intensity-modulated radiotherapy in patients with locally advanced squamous cell cancer of the head and neck. *Ann Oncol* 2010;21(2):342–347.

122. Machiels JP, et al. Zalutumumab plus best supportive care versus best supportive care alone in patients with recurrent or metastatic squamous-cell carcinoma of the head and neck after failure of platinum-based chemotherapy: an open-label, randomised phase 3 trial. *Lancet Oncol* 2011;12(4):333–343.

123. Caponigro F, et al. A phase I/II trial of gefitinib and radiotherapy in patients with locally advanced inoperable squamous cell carcinoma of the head and neck. *Anticancer Drugs* 2008;19(7):739–44.

124. Chen C, et al. Phase I trial of gefitinib in combination with radiation or chemoradiation for patients with locally advanced squamous cell head and neck cancer. *J Clin Oncol* 2007;25(31):4880–4886.

125. Hainsworth JD, et al. Neoadjuvant chemotherapy/gefitinib followed by concurrent chemotherapy/radiation therapy/gefitinib for patients with locally advanced squamous carcinoma of the head and neck. *Cancer* 2009;115(10):2138–2146.

126. Harrington KJ, et al. Phase I study of lapatinib in combination with chemoradiation in patients with locally advanced squamous cell carcinoma of the head and neck. *J Clin Oncol* 2009;27(7):1100–1107.

127. Lee NY, et al. Addition of bevacizumab to standard chemoradiation for locoregionally advanced nasopharyngeal carcinoma (RTOG 0615): a phase 2 multi-institutional trial. *Lancet Oncol* 2012;13(2):172–180.

128. Seiwert TY, et al. Phase I study of bevacizumab added to fluorouracil- and hydroxyurea-based concomitant chemoradiotherapy for poor-prognosis head and neck cancer. *J Clin Oncol* 2008;26(10):1732–1741.

129. Kyzas PA, Cunha IW, Ioannidis JP. Prognostic significance of vascular endothelial growth factor immunohistochemical expression in head and neck squamous cell carcinoma: a meta-analysis. *Clin Cancer Res* 2005;11(4):1434–1440.

130. Yoo DS, et al. Prospective trial of synchronous bevacizumab, erlotinib, and concurrent chemoradiation in locally advanced head and neck cancer. *Clin Cancer Res* 2012;18(5):1404–1414.

131. Brizel DM. Head and neck cancer as a model for advances in imaging prognosis, early assessment, and posttherapy evaluation. *Cancer J* 2011;17(3):159–165.

132. Koukourakis MI, et al. Hypoxia-inducible factor (HIF1A and HIF2A), angiogenesis, and chemoradiotherapy outcome of squamous cell head-and-neck cancer. *Int J Radiat Oncol Biol Phys* 2002;53(5):1192–1202.

133. Graeber TG, et al. Hypoxia-mediated selection of cells with diminished apoptotic potential in solid tumours. *Nature* 1996;379(6560):88–91.

134. Koukourakis MI, et al. Hypoxia-regulated carbonic anhydrase-9 (CA9) relates to poor vascularization and resistance of squamous cell head and neck cancer to chemoradiotherapy. *Clin Cancer Res* 2001;7(11):3399–3403.

135. Moeller BJ, et al. Radiation activates HIF-1 to regulate vascular radiosensitivity in tumors: role of reoxygenation, free radicals, and stress granules. *Cancer Cell* 2004;5(5):429–441.

136. Hockel M, et al. Association between tumor hypoxia and malignant progression in advanced cancer of the uterine cervix. *Cancer Res* 1996;56(19):4509–4515.

137. Brizel DM, et al. Tumor hypoxia adversely affects the prognosis of carcinoma of the head and neck. *Int J Radiat Oncol Biol Phys* 1997;38(2):285–289.

138. Fyles A, et al. Long-term performance of interstitial fluid pressure and hypoxia as prognostic factors in cervix cancer. *Radiother Oncol* 2006;80(2):132–137.

139. Brizel DM, et al. Tumor oxygenation predicts for the likelihood of distant metastases in human soft tissue sarcoma. *Cancer Res* 1996;56(5):941–943.

140. Peters KB, Brown JM. Tirapazamine: a hypoxia-activated topoisomerase II poison. *Cancer Res* 2002;62(18):5248–5253.

141. Gatzemeier U, et al. Tirapazamine-cisplatin: the synergy. *Br J Cancer* 1998;77(Suppl 4):15–17.

142. Rischin D, et al. Phase I trial of concurrent tirapazamine, cisplatin, and radiotherapy in patients with advanced head and neck cancer. *J Clin Oncol* 2001;19(2):535–542.

143. Rischin D, et al. Tirapazamine, cisplatin, and radiation versus fluorouracil, cisplatin, and radiation in patients with locally advanced head and neck cancer: a randomized phase II trial of the Trans-Tasman Radiation Oncology Group (TROG 98.02). *J Clin Oncol* 2005;23(1):79–87.

144. Rischin D, et al. Tirapazamine, cisplatin, and radiation versus cisplatin and radiation for advanced squamous cell carcinoma of the head and neck (TROG 02.02, HeadSTART): a phase III trial of the Trans-Tasman Radiation Oncology Group. *J Clin Oncol* 2010;28(18):2989–2995.

145. Peters LJ, et al. Critical impact of radiotherapy protocol compliance and quality in the treatment of advanced head and neck cancer: results from TROG 02.02. *J Clin Oncol* 2010;28(18):2996–3001.

146. Seiwert TY, et al. Safety and clinical activity of pembrolizumab for treatment of recurrent or metastatic squamous cell carcinoma of the head and neck (KEYNOTE-012): an open-label, multicentre, phase 1b trial. *Lancet Oncol* 2016;17(7):956–965.

147. Ferris RL, et al. Nivolumab for recurrent squamous-cell carcinoma of the head and neck. *N Engl J Med* 2016;375(19):1856–1867.

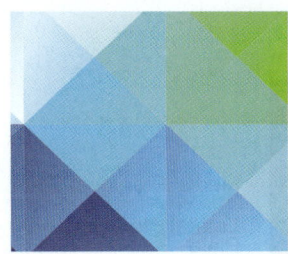

CHAPTER 44

Nasopharynx

Benjamin H. Lok, Jonathan E. Leeman, and Nancy Y. Lee

ANATOMY

The nasopharynx is a cuboidal chamber, slightly broader in the transverse dimension than the anterior–posterior dimension (Fig. 44.1). Anteriorly, it is continuous with the nasal cavity via the posterior choanae, whereas inferiorly, it communicates with the oropharynx. The roof of the nasopharynx is formed by the basilar portion of the sphenoid and occipital bones and the floor by the superior surface of the soft palate and nasopharyngeal isthmus. The lateral walls of the nasopharynx contain the pharyngotympanic tube (*Eustachian tube*) openings, which are bounded by a prominence known as the *torus tubarius*. The *torus* is formed by the cartilage of the pharyngotympanic tube elevating the mucous membrane of the lateral nasopharynx. Posterior to the *torus* is the pharyngeal recess otherwise known as the *fossa of Rosenmüller*. The lateral walls, including the pharyngeal recess (*fossa of Rosenmüller*), are the most common origin of nasopharyngeal malignancies. The posterior wall of the nasopharynx contains the superior pharyngeal constrictor muscle, pharyngobasilar fascia, and buccopharyngeal fascia.

The superior pharyngeal constrictor only extends superiorly to the skull base in the midline, and laterally the pharyngobasilar fascia serves to attach the constrictor muscle to the base of the skull at the basiocciput and petrous portion of the temporal bone. This lateral area of muscular deficiency is otherwise known as the *sinus of Morgagni*, through which the pharyngotympanic tube and levator veli palatini pass. The pharyngobasilar fascia is continuous with the foramen lacerum and is in close proximity to the foramen ovale, foramen spinosum, jugular foramen, hypoglossal canal, and carotid space. The proximity of these foramina to the *sinus of Morgagni* assumes importance in the consideration of intracranial extension (Fig. 44.2). A summary of the various foramina located in the base of skull is presented in Table 44.1.

The afferent innervation of the nasopharynx anterior to the pharyngotympanic tube orifice is provided by the maxillary division of the trigeminal nerve (V_2) and, posterior to the tubal orifice, the glossopharyngeal nerve. Motor supply is via the pharyngeal branches of the glossopharyngeal nerve, vagus nerve, and sympathetic fibers from the superior cervical ganglion. The arterial supply of the nasopharynx is provided by the ascending pharyngeal artery, sphenopalatine artery, and the artery of the pterygoid canal. Venous drainage is provided by the pharyngeal plexus that drains into the internal jugular veins directly or via communication with the pterygoid plexus.

EPIDEMIOLOGY AND ETIOLOGY

Nasopharyngeal carcinoma is an uncommon cancer in most parts of the world. The age-adjusted incidence rate (per 100,000 people per year) among men ranges from 0.6 in the United States and Japan to 5.4 in Algeria; 5.8 in the Philippines; 11.0 in Singapore; 17.2 among Eskimos, Indians, and Aleuts in Alaska to 17.8 and 26.9 in Hong Kong and Guangdong province in Southern China, respectively.[1–3]

A bimodal age distribution is observed in low-risk populations. The first peak incidence arises between 15 and 25 years of age, with the second peak at 50 and 59 years of age.[4–6] In high-risk populations, the peak incidence occurs in the fourth and fifth decade of life.[4] Both genders have a similar age distribution; however, the male to female incidence ratio is 2:1 to 3:1.[7]

This distinct racial and geographical distribution of nasopharyngeal carcinoma suggests a multifactorial cause. Current epidemiologic and experimental data identify at least three important etiologic factors: (1) genetic, (2) environmental, and (3) viral.

The high incidence of nasopharyngeal carcinoma among Southern Chinese and populations of Southern Chinese

FIGURE 44.1. A: Midsagittal magnetic resonance image (MRI) of the head, showing the nasopharynx and related structures. **B:** Axial contrast-enhanced MRI showing a small tumor in the left fossa of Rosenmüller (*arrow*) and normal structures in the rest of the nasopharynx.

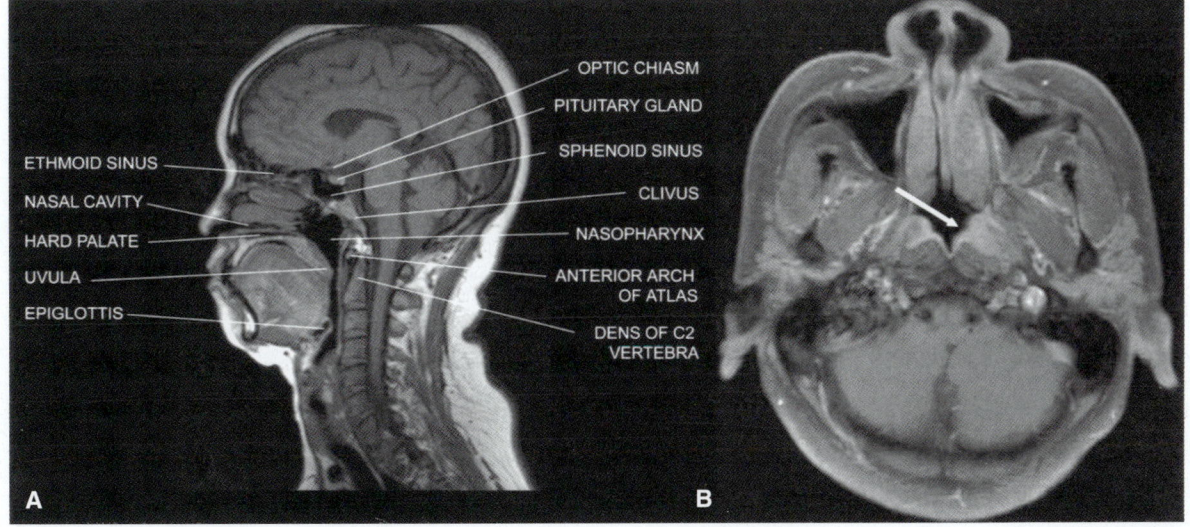

OPTIC CHIASM
PITUITARY GLAND
SPHENOID SINUS
CLIVUS
NASOPHARYNX
ANTERIOR ARCH OF ATLAS
DENS OF C2 VERTEBRA

ETHMOID SINUS
NASAL CAVITY
HARD PALATE
UVULA
EPIGLOTTIS

A   B

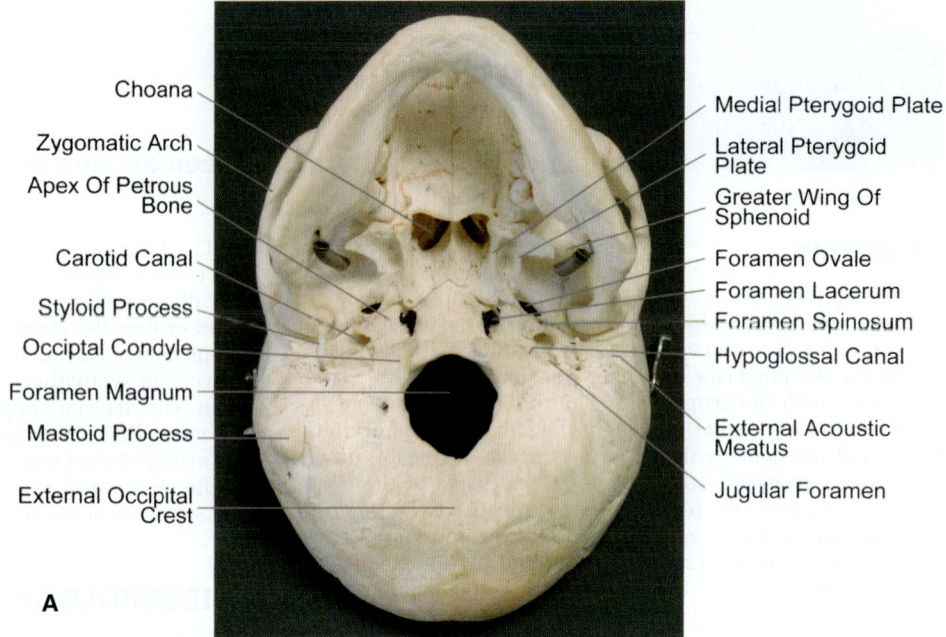

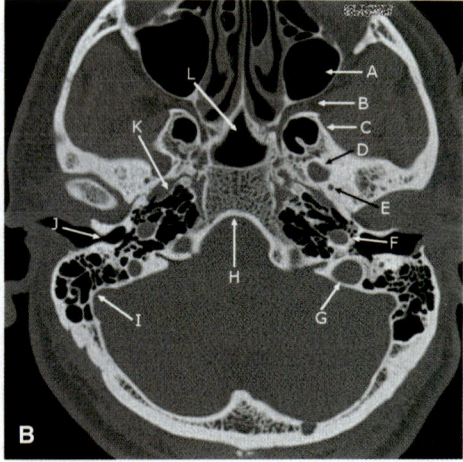

(A)- Maxillary Sinus
(B)- Pterygopalatine Fossa
(C)- Pneumatized Pterygoid Process
(D)- Foramen Ovale
(E)- Foramen Spinosum
(F)- Carotid Canal
(G)- Jugular Bulb
(H)- Clivus
(I)- Mastoid Cells
(J)- External Auditory Canal
(K)- Pneumatized Petrous Apex
(L)- Sphenoid Sinus

FIGURE 44.2. A: Basal view of skull illustrating the foramina of the base of the skull and the occupying structures. **B:** Axial computed tomography scan illustrating the bony anatomy.

TABLE 44.1 FORAMINA OF THE BASE OF THE SKULL AND ASSOCIATED ANATOMIC STRUCTURES

Foramen/Fissure	Cranial Nerve	Other Structures
Cribriform plate	Olfactory nerve (I)	Anterior ethmoidal nerve
Optic foramen	Optic nerve (II)	Ophthalmic artery
Superior orbital fissure	Oculomotor (III), trochlear (IV), ophthalmic division of trigeminal (V₁) nerve, abducent (VI) nerves	Ophthalmic vein, orbital branch of middle meningeal and recurrent branch of lacrimal arteries, sympathetic plexus, filaments from carotid plexus
Foramen rotundum	Maxillary division of trigeminal (V₂) nerve	
Foramen ovale	Mandibular division of trigeminal (V₃) nerve	Accessory meningeal artery, lesser superficial petrosal nerve
Foramen lacerum		Internal carotid, sympathetic carotid plexus, vidian nerve, meningeal branch of ascending pharyngeal artery, emissary vein
Foramen spinosum	Recurrent branch of V₃ nerve	Middle meningeal artery and vein
Stylomastoid foramen	Facial (VII) nerve	
Internal acoustic meatus	Auditory (VIII) nerve	Internal auditory artery
Jugular foramen	Glossopharyngeal (IX), vagus (X), spinal accessory (XI) nerves	Inferior petrosal sinus, transverse sinus, meningeal branches from occipital and ascending pharyngeal arteries
Hypoglossal canal	Hypoglossal (XII) nerve	Meningeal branch of ascending pharyngeal artery
Foramen magnum		Spinal cord, spinal accessory nerve, vertebral vessels, anterior and posterior spinal vessels

descent suggests a component of genetic susceptibility. A genome-wide association study of nasopharyngeal cancer found three susceptibility loci[8] and confirmed a linkage study that found a gene closely linked to the HLA locus conferred a greatly increased risk of this disease.[9] In addition, several HLA haplotypes, including A2, B46, and B17, are associated with an increased risk of developing nasopharyngeal carcinoma.[10,11]

The high consumption of salted fish in Southern China has been implicated as an important environmental factor.[12–15] Dimethylnitrosamine, a carcinogen found in salted fish, has been shown to induce carcinoma in the upper respiratory tract in rats.[13] Other potential environmental etiologic factors that have been associated with nasopharyngeal carcinoma include alcohol consumption and exposure to dust, fumes, formaldehyde, and cigarette smoke,[16,17] although definitive conclusion has been elusive. Descendents from Chinese who have migrated from endemic areas to Western countries show progressively lower risk, but their incidence remains higher than the indigenous populations.[18–20] Buell[18] observed that American-born second-generation Chinese had a lower risk than the Asian-born first generation, whereas whites born in Southeast Asia had an increased risk compared to American-born whites. Dickson and Flores[20] reported that the incidence rate in Chinese who were natively born in China was 20.5, compared with 1.3 for Chinese and 0.2 for whites born in Canada. Taken together, environmental factors appear to play a role in the etiology of nasopharyngeal cancer.

Epstein-Barr virus (EBV) has been associated with naso-pharyngeal carcinoma, especially the nonkeratinizing type, irrespective of ethnic or geographic origin.[21] Premalignant lesions of nasopharyngeal epithelium show increased levels of EBV, suggesting that EBV infection may influence the early stages of tumorigenesis in NPC.[22] Detection of a single form of EBV DNA in tumors suggests that clonal expansion from an initial EBV-infected and, ultimately, EBV-transformed cell is likely. EBV's tumorigenic potential is due to a set of latent genes, latent membrane proteins (LMP1, LMP2A, and LMP2B) and EBV-determined nuclear antigens (EBNA1 and EBNA2), which are the proteins predominantly expressed in NPC.[23] LMP1 is the principal oncogene with evidence that the C-terminal activating regions of the protein activate a variety of signaling pathways including mitogen-activated protein (MAP) kinases, phosphoinositol-3-kinase (PI3K), nuclear factor κ-B (NF-κB), and epidermal growth factor receptor (EGFR).[24,25] LMP1 is also required for cell immortalization and is present in 80% to 90% of NPC tumors.[26] This mounting evidence highlights the likely etiologic role for EBV in NPC.

NATURAL HISTORY

Local Extension

A summary of structures locally infiltrated by nasopharyngeal carcinoma at diagnosis is provided in Table 44.2.

Anterior

Anteriorly, it is common for the extension and infiltration of tumor into the nasal fossa. Invasion of the lateral wall of the nasal fossa can lead to involvement and destruction of the pterygoid plates. Beyond these structures, though less common, is invasion of the posterior ethmoid and maxillary sinuses. In advanced disease, infiltration of the orbital apex (typically through the inferior orbital fissure) can occur.

Superior and Posterior

Superiorly, tumors can directly invade the base of skull, the sphenoid sinus, and the clivus. The foramen lacerum, positioned directly above the pharyngeal recess (*Rosenmüller fossa*), is a vulnerable spot through which the tumor may enter the cavernous sinus and the middle cranial fossa to invade cranial nerves II to VI (Fig. 44.3). Figure 44.4 demonstrates

TABLE 44.2 STRUCTURES LOCALLY INFILTRATED BY NASOPHARYNGEAL CARCINOMA AT DIAGNOSIS[a]

Structures Involved	Frequency (%)
Adjacent soft tissue	
Nasal cavity	87
Parapharyngeal space, carotid space	68
Pterygoid muscle (medial, lateral)	48
Oropharyngeal wall, soft palate	21
Prevertebral muscle	19
Bony erosion/paranasal sinus	
Clivus	41
Sphenoid bone, foramina lacerum, ovale, rotundum	38
Pterygoid plate(s), pterygomaxillary fissure, pterygopalatine fossa	27
Petrous bone, petro-occipital fissure	19
Ethmoid sinus	6
Maxillary antrum	4
Jugular foramen, hypoglossal canal	4
Pituitary fossa/gland	3
Extensive/intracranial extension	
Cavernous sinus	16
Infratemporal fossa	9
Orbit, orbital fissure(s)	4
Cerebrum, meninges, cisterns	4
Hypopharynx	2

[a]Based on magnetic resonance imaging of 308 patients from Pamela Youde Nethersole Eastern Hospital, Hong Kong.
Reproduced with permission from Barnes L, Eveson JW, Reichart P, et al., World Health Organization Classification of Tumours. Pathology and Genetics of Head and Neck Tumours. Volume 9. IARC, Lyon, 2005.

involvement of the trigeminal cave (*Meckel cave*) and the maxillary branch of the trigeminal nerve (V$_2$). The foramen ovale also allows access for tumor to invade the middle cranial fossa, in addition to the petrous portion of the temporal bone, and the cavernous sinus. Posteriorly, invasion of the prevertebral (longus capitis) muscles is commonly seen.

Inferior

Extension inferiorly to the oropharynx is not unlikely, with potential involvement of the tonsillar pillars, the tonsillar fossa, and the lateral and posterior oropharyngeal walls. In advanced disease, invasion of the C1 vertebra posteriorly and inferiorly can occur. Direct invasion of the soft palate is uncommon.

Lateral

Lateral extension occurs early with involvement of the lateral parapharyngeal space along with invasion of the levator and tensor veli palatini muscles (Fig. 44.5). In advanced disease,

FIGURE 44.3. Coronal section through the sphenoid sinus and roof of the nasopharynx showing the relative positions of the cranial nerves III to VI. (Modified from Chao KSC. *Practical essentials of intensity-modulated radiation therapy.* Philadelphia, PA: Lippincott Williams & Wilkins, 2005:138.)

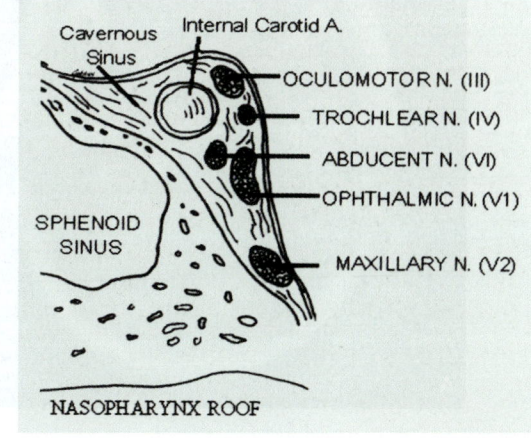

NASOPHARYNX ROOF

Section III

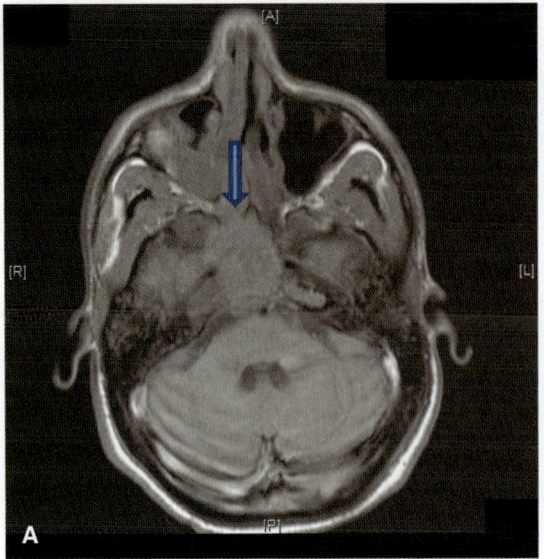

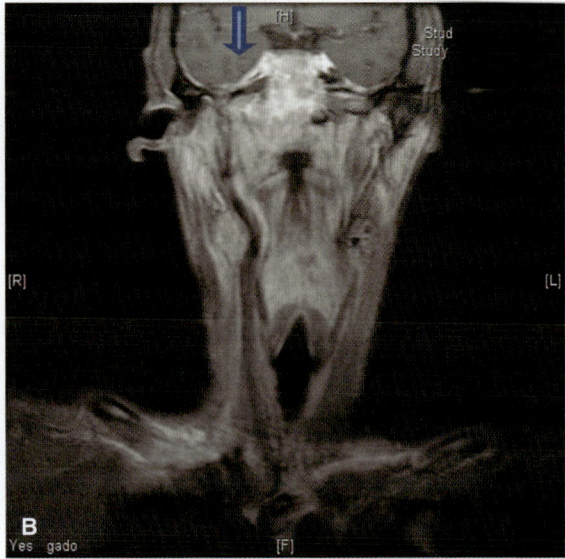

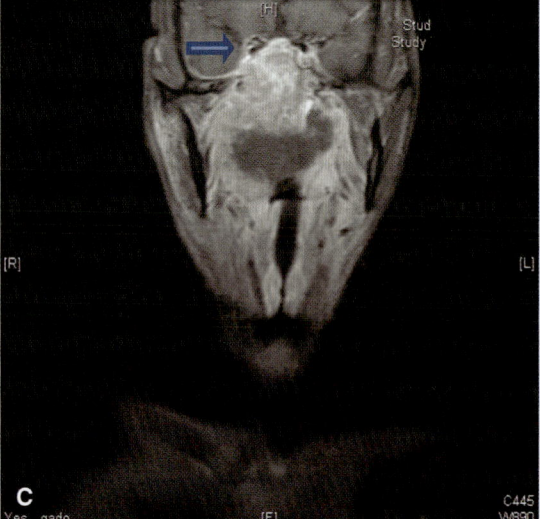

FIGURE 44.4. A: Axial T1-weighted magnetic resonance image (MRI) demonstrating involvement of the maxillary branch of the trigeminal nerve by nasopharyngeal carcinoma (V₂) (*arrow*). **B:** Coronal contrast-enhanced MRI showing involvement of the trigeminal cave (a.k.a. Meckel cave) by nasopharyngeal carcinoma (*arrow*). **C:** Coronal contrast-enhanced MRI showing involvement of the maxillary branch of the trigeminal nerve by nasopharyngeal carcinoma (V₂) (*arrow*).

FIGURE 44.5. A: Axial T1-weighted magnetic resonance image (MRI) showing tumor infiltration of the right parapharyngeal space (*left arrow*). Note the resultant serous otitis media (*right arrow*). **B:** Axial contrast-enhanced MRI showing enhanced tumor involving the parapharyngeal space and medial pterygoid muscles (*arrow*).

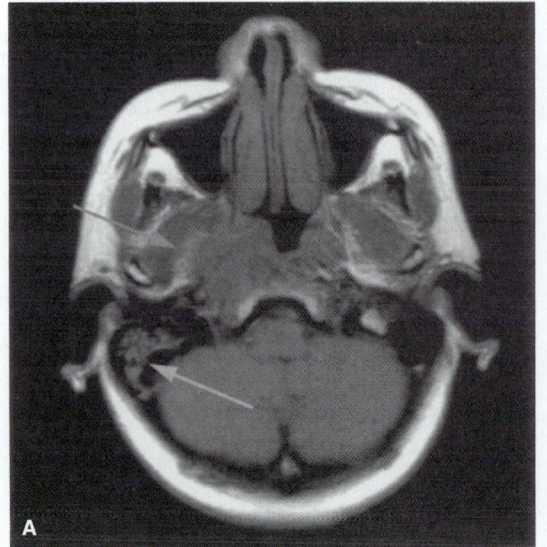

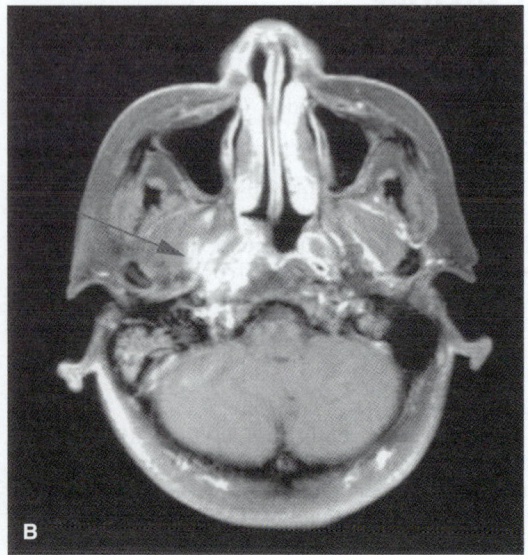

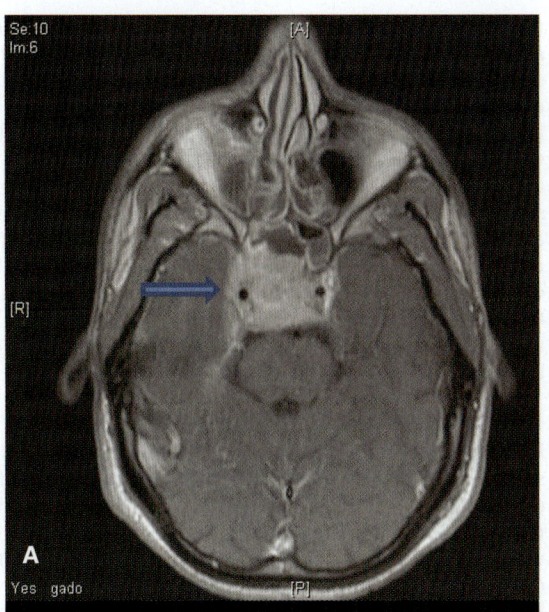
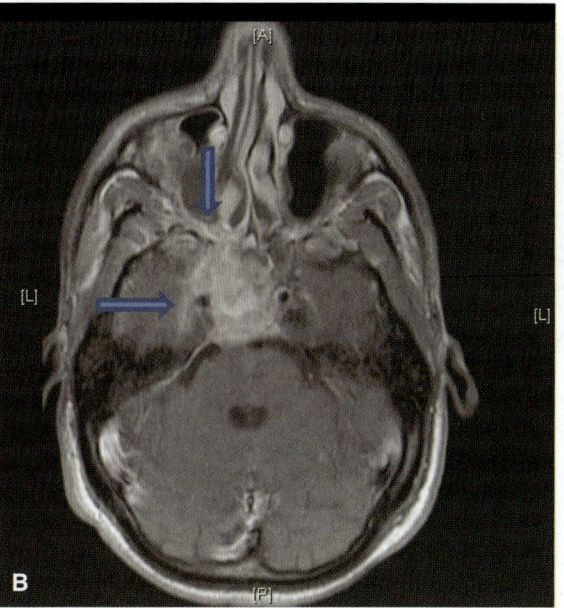

FIGURE 44.6. A: Axial contrast-enhanced magnetic resonance image (MRI) demonstrating involvement of the cavernous sinus by nasopharyngeal carcinoma. **B:** Axial contrast-enhanced MRI showing invasion of the pterygopalatine fossa (*vertical arrow*) with spread to cavernous sinus (*horizontal arrow*).

invasion of the pterygoid muscles can occur. Direct extension of the tumor or lateral retropharyngeal lymph node metastasis in the parapharyngeal space may lead to invasion or compression of cranial nerves IX to XI as they transpire the jugular foramen, cranial nerve XII as it emerges from the hypoglossal canal, and the cervical sympathetic nerves. Direct invasion or compression of the internal carotid artery can occur in advanced disease (Fig. 44.6). Tumor can directly

invade the middle ear through the pharyngotympanic tube (*Eustachian tube*).

Lymphatic Spread

The nasopharynx is comprised of a vast of avalvular lymph capillary network that exists in the mucous membrane leading to frequent involvement of regional neck nodes (Fig. 44.7). Up to 85% to 90% of cases present with lymphatic spread to

FIGURE 44.7. A: Pathways for lymphatic spread of nasopharyngeal carcinoma. (Redrawn from Rouviere H. *Anatomy of the human lymphatic system.* Ann Arbor, MI: Edward Brothers; 1938:27, with permission.) **B:** Two major lymph collectors of the nasopharynx, (i) lateral lymph collector and (ii) posterior lymph collector. *Yellow,* lymphatic vessels from the nasal cavity. *Blue,* lymphatic vessels from soft palate. *Green,* lymph nodes. Retropharyngeal nodes are numbered. *Red,* carotid artery. *Dark brown,* longus muscles. *Light brown,* remaining pharyngeal and nasal wall. (From Wei-Ren P, Suami H, Corlett RJ, et al. Lymphatic drainage of the nasal fossae and nasopharynx: Preliminary anatomical and radiological study with clinical implications. *Head Neck* 2009;31[1]:52–57. Copyright © 2008 Wiley Periodicals, Inc. Reprinted by permission of John Wiley & Sons, Inc.)

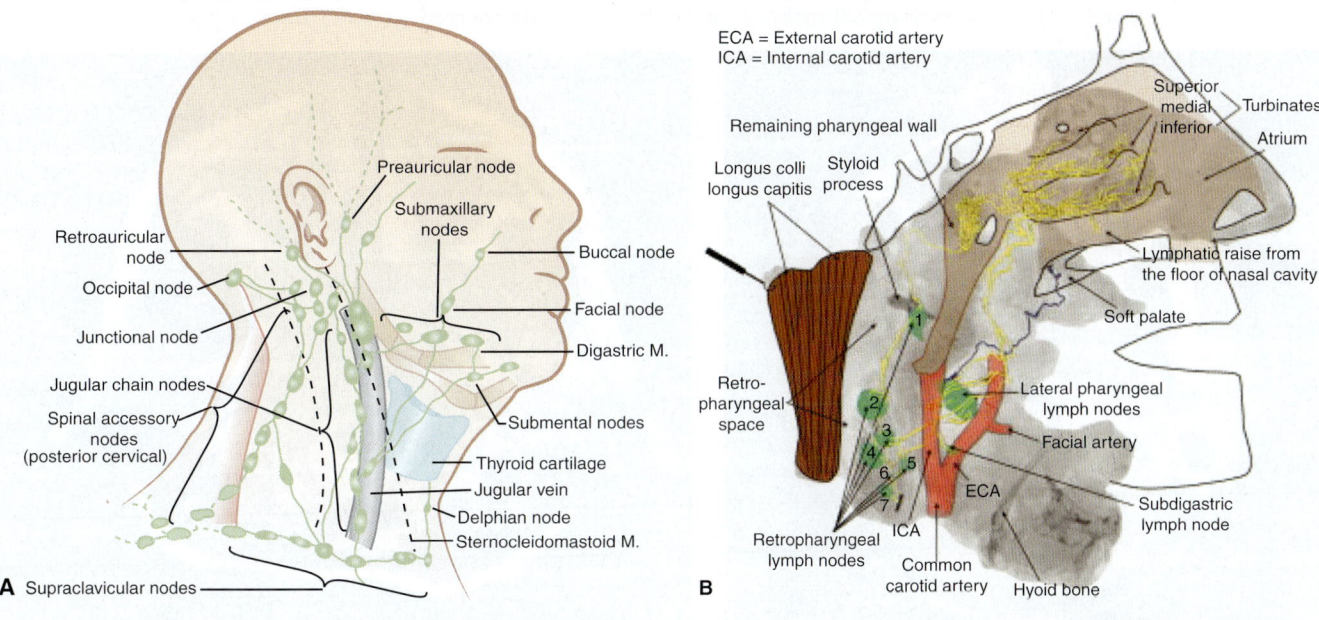

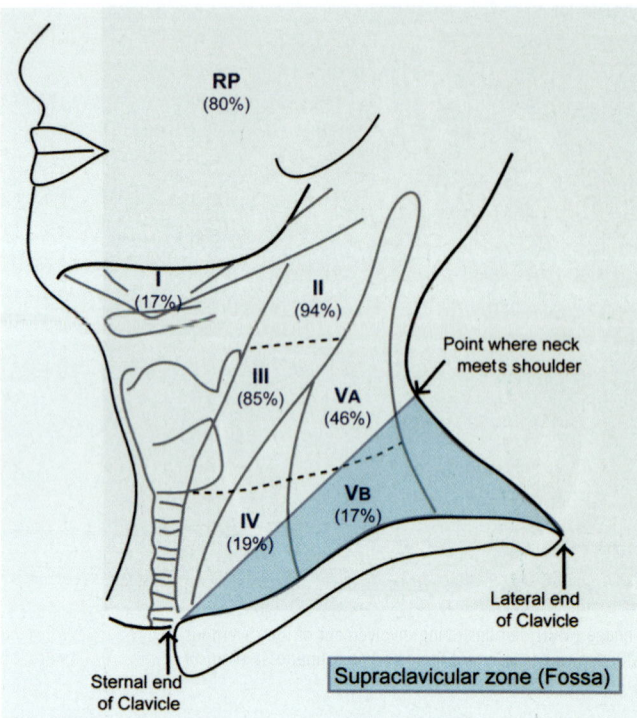

RP
(80%)

(17%)

II
(94%)

Point where neck
meets shoulder

III
(85%)

VA
(46%)

VB
(17%)

IV
(19%)

Lateral end
of Clavicle

Sternal end
of Clavicle

Supraclavicular zone (Fossa)

FIGURE 44.8. Two examples of coronal magnetic resonance images showing bilateral cervical lymphadenopathy. There is orderly downward lymphatic spread toward the supraclavicular fossa.

the ipsilateral nodes.[27–29] Bilateral spread is present in approximately 50% of cases. The distribution of NPC-involved nodes at diagnosis is shown in Figure 44.8. An anatomic and radiographic study that directly examined lymphatic vasculature concluded that there are two major lymph collectors of the nasopharynx (Fig. 44.7B).[30] One lymph collector runs along the lateral side of the pharyngeal wall, whereas the second runs more posteriorly. The lateral lymph collector empties into multiple first tier nodes, which include the lateral pharyngeal node, the jugulodigastric/subdigastric node, and the third, fourth, and fifth nodes of the retropharyngeal group.[30] The

posterior lymph collector empties into the first node (*node of Rouviere*) of the retropharyngeal group (Fig. 44.9). This direct study is corroborated clinically by frequent observation of lateral and retropharyngeal lymph node involvement by MRI of CT scans, even though they remain impalpable. Metastasis to the jugulodigastric and superior–posterior cervical nodes is also common. From these first tier nodes, further metastatic spread to the midjugular, lower jugular, and posterior cervical and supraclavicular nodes can develop. Seldom, submental and occipital nodes can be involved secondary to lymphatic obstruction caused by widespread cervical lymphadenopathy. Mediastinal lymph nodes and, occasionally, axillary nodes may be involved with the presence of supraclavicular lymphadenopathy.

Hematogenous Dissemination

Distant metastasis is present in 3% to 6% of the cases at presentation and may occur in 18% to 50% of cases during the disease course.[31–35] The rate of distant metastasis is highest in patients with advanced neck node metastasis,[27,36,37] especially with low-neck involvement.[38,39] The bone is the most common distant metastatic site followed by the lungs and liver,[40] with lung metastasis being associated with better prognosis than other sites. Brain and skin metastases rarely occur.[41,42]

CLINICAL PRESENTATION

Nasopharyngeal carcinoma presents in patients with symptoms in one or more of the following three categories: (1) neck masses, usually appearing in the upper neck, (2) presence of tumor mass in the nasopharynx (epistaxis, nasal obstruction and discharge), (3) skull base erosion and palsy of cranial nerves V and VI because of tumor extension superiorly (headache, diplopia, facial pain, and numbness).

The frequency of various presenting symptoms and signs is summarized in Table 44.3. A neck mass is the most common presenting symptom, followed by nasal and aural symptoms. The physical signs commonly present at diagnosis are enlarged neck node(s) and, less often, cranial nerve palsy. The cranial nerves V and VI are frequently involved, whereas cranial nerves I, VII, and VIII are rarely involved (Table 44.4).[29,45]

Cervical lymphadenopathy is present in up to 87% of patients.[46] Typically, a mass is observable in the upper posterior

FIGURE 44.9. A: Axial contrast-enhanced computed tomography scan showing involvement of bilateral retropharyngeal lymph nodes (*arrows*) by nasopharyngeal carcinoma. **B:** Axial T2-weighted magnetic resonance image (MRI) showing involvement of bilateral retropharyngeal lymph nodes (*arrows*) by nasopharyngeal carcinoma.

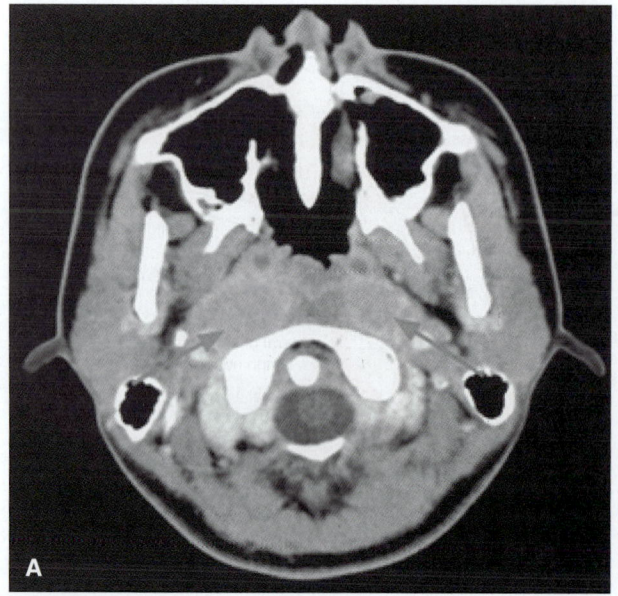

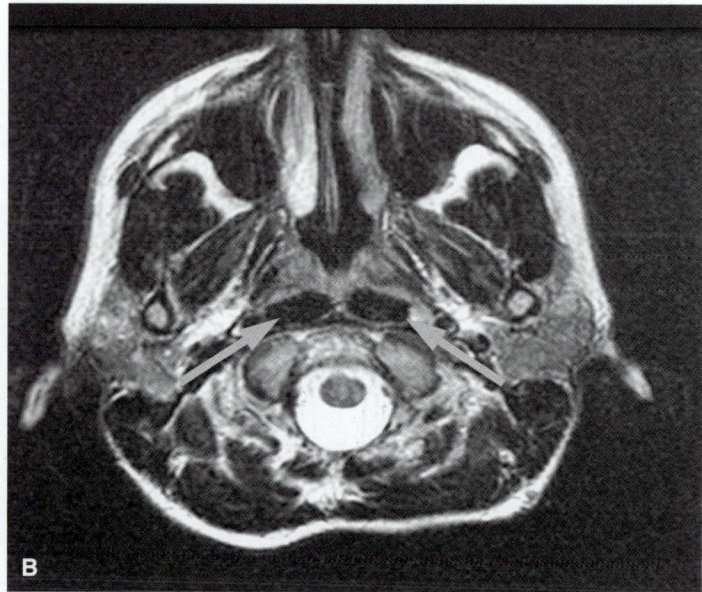

TABLE 44.3 SYMPTOMS AND PHYSICAL SIGNS OF NASOPHARYNGEAL CARCINOMA AT PRESENTATION

Symptom/Sign	Chao and Perez[43] (n = 164) (%)	Lee et al.[29] (n = 4,768) (%)
Neck mass	66	76
Enlarged neck node(s)		75
Nasal (discharge, bleeding, obstruction)	>37	73
Aural (tinnitus, hearing impairment)	41	62
Headache	40	35
Cranial nerve palsy	23	20
Neurologic symptoms		
Ophthalmic (diplopia, squint)		11
Facial numbness		8
Slurring of speech		2
Sore throat	16	
Weight loss		7
Trismus		3
Distant metastases		3
Dermatomyositis		1

neck and palpable beneath the superior portion of the sternocleidomastoid muscle close to the mastoid process. This is caused by metastasis to the parapharyngeal nodes or superior–posterior cervical nodes of the spinal accessory chain.

DIAGNOSTIC AND STAGING WORKUP

Diagnosis of nasopharyngeal carcinoma is made by biopsy of the primary tumor. This can typically be performed with local anesthesia in an outpatient setting. Biopsy by direct visualization with general anesthesia may be necessary for diagnosis when the tumor is not visible or when the patient cannot cooperate. Not uncommonly, the tumor is submucosal and not visible. For suspicious cases of a nasopharyngeal primary tumor with lack of visible tumor, random biopsies of the most commonly involved sites are warranted: pharyngeal recess (*fossa of Rosenmüller*) on each of the lateral walls and superior–posterior wall of the nasopharynx. Fine needle aspiration of a suspicious neck mass may establish the presence of metastatic nasopharyngeal carcinoma in the regional lymphatics. This may be performed prior to the biopsy of the nasopharynx when the primary tumor is not clinically detectable.

Table 44.5 lists the pretreatment diagnostic evaluations and staging evaluations that are generally recommended for NPC.

Complete physical examination should include thorough palpation of the neck, cranial nerve examination, percussion and auscultation of the chest, palpation of the abdomen for possible liver involvement, and percussion of the spine and bones for possible bone metastasis. CT and MRI of the head and neck are useful in the evaluation of tumor erosion into the bony structures of the base of skull along with retropharyngeal and cervical lymphadenopathy. However, MRI is

TABLE 44.4 INCIDENCE OF CRANIAL NERVE INVOLVEMENT BY NASOPHARYNGEAL CARCINOMA AT DIAGNOSIS

Cranial Nerve	Chao and Perez[43] (N = 164) (%)	Chan et al.[44] (N = 722) (%)
I	–	–
II	1.3	0.8
III	3.5	1.3
IV	2.4	0.6
V	7.8	V₁, 3.5; V₂, 5.8%; V₃, 3.9
VI	13.3	5.1
VII	3.6	0.1
VIII	4.8	–
IX–XII	IX, 2; X, 5.4; XI, 1.3; XII, 4.8	2.4

TABLE 44.5 RECOMMENDED PRETREATMENT DIAGNOSTIC EVALUATIONS FOR NASOPHARYNGEAL CARCINOMA

General
  Medical history
  Physical examination:
    Palpation of neck node (record size, laterality, and lowest extent of enlarged nodes)
    Testing of cranial nerve (including assessment of vision and hearing functions)
    Exclusion of gross signs of distant metastases
Fiber-optic endoscopy examination
  Nasopharyngoscopy and biopsies
  ± Panendoscopy
Otologic assessment
  Inspection of tympanic membranes (as clinically indicated)
  Baseline audiologic testing (preferable)
Laboratory studies
  Complete blood count
  Liver function tests (LFTs)
  Urinalysis
  EBV-specific serologic tests
    Immunoglobulin A (IgA)
    Antiviral capsule antigen (VCA) titers
    Serum EBV DNA levels
Radiographic studies
Assessment of locoregional extent (imaging of the nasopharynx, paranasal sinuses, base of skull, nasal cavity, and neck)
  Magnetic resonance imaging (study of choice)
  Computed tomography (acceptable alternative)
Chest radiograph (posterior–anterior and lateral)
Additional metastatic workup if clinically indicated or N3 disease
  Positron-emission tomography (study of choice)
  Computed tomography of the chest and abdomen
    In patients with abnormal LFTs or clinical suspicion of lung or liver metastasis
  Bone scan
    In patients with advanced locoregional disease, symptoms suggestive of bone metastasis, or an elevated serum alkaline phosphatase

the preferred imaging technique in the staging evaluation of nasopharyngeal carcinoma.[47–49] The current AJCC T classification requires a search for tumor invasion into the soft tissue (e.g., parapharyngeal space) and bony structures. MRI may be necessary for proper staging because CT has limitations in accurately defining tumor extension into these regions[50] and MRI was used[51] for the study that informed the updated 2017 AJCC system. MRI is superior to CT in delineating muscle and soft tissue involvement and examination of the skull base.[50,52,53] When utilizing MRI, thin slices (3 mm) should be used for accurate staging (Fig. 44.10). Thicker slices (e.g. ≥5 mm) risk misdiagnosis of what may be a higher T-stage disease.

Ng et al.[54] compared MRI and CT in assessing the extent of disease. The study found a significantly higher sensitivity of MRI for skull base involvement (60% vs. 40%), intracranial involvement (57% vs. 36%), retropharyngeal node (58% vs. 21%), and tumor infiltration of prevertebral muscles (i.e., longus colli muscles) (51% vs. 22%) compared to CT. By MRI, T-staging was modified in 27% of patients, with 22% being upstaged and 4% being downstaged.

MRI and CT scans can detect lymph node metastasis that may not be clinically evident on physical examination.[55] According to a study by Van den Brekel et al.,[56] lymph node metastasis is commonly recommended to be radiologically defined by the presence of central necrosis, extracapsular spread, shortest axial diameter ≥10 mm (11 mm for the jugulodigastric node and 5 mm for the retropharyngeal node), or a cluster of ≥3 lymph nodes that are borderline in size.

Detailed evaluation of nodal enlargement by palpation and imaging should consist of the size and location of the node, unilateral/bilateral involvement, and assessment of supraclavicular fossa involvement. Figure 44.8 defines the anatomical boundaries of the supraclavicular fossa, and Figure 44.11

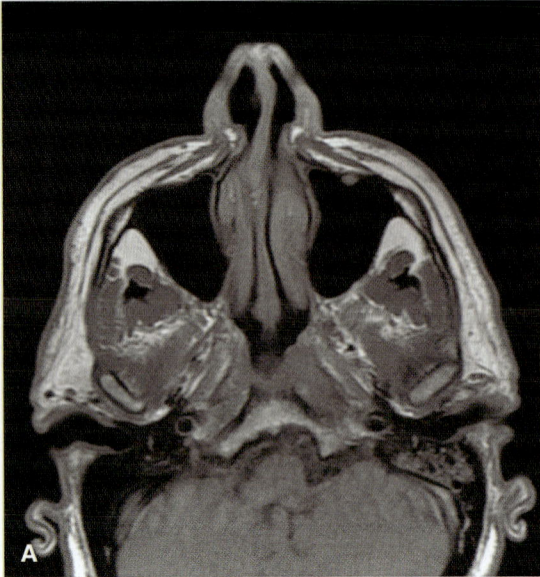
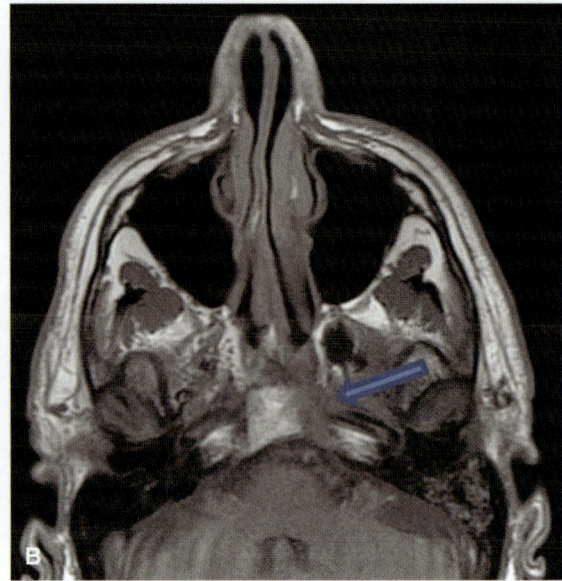

FIGURE 44.10. **A:** Axial T1-weighted magnetic resonance image (MRI) with 5-mm slices. **B:** Axial T1 MRI with 3-mm slices, skull base invasion (*arrow*) upstaged this tumor from T1 to T3.

demonstrates an example of bilateral cervical lymph node involvement seen by radiologic studies.

A complete search for distant metastasis is recommended for patients with advanced locoregional disease (e.g., N3 disease) or patients with suspicious clinical or laboratory findings. PET-CT scanning (Fig. 44.12) is now commonly utilized in place of conventional staging by CT, bone scans and ultrasound, and appears to be at least as sensitive. Chang et al.[57] demonstrated that [18F]fluorodeoxyglucose (FDG)-PET was superior to conventional workup (i.e., chest x-ray, isotope bone scan, and abdominal ultrasound) in the detection of distant metastases, where 12% of patients were upstaged to stage IVC. PET, in the study, offered a sensitivity and specificity of 100% and 90.1%, respectively. However, large comparative studies of these various staging modalities have yet to be reported.[57–59]

The intimate association of EBV with nasopharyngeal carcinoma, independent of geographic and ethnic background, has provided clinicians with a tumor marker for disease diagnosis. Immunoglobulin (Ig) A (IgA) antiviral capsid antigen (VCA) and IgG anti–early antigen (EA) antibodies are both sensitive for diagnosing nasopharyngeal carcinoma; however, IgA anti-VCA has better specificity.[60] More than 90% of untreated nasopharyngeal carcinoma patients from California, East Africa, and Hong Kong have elevated IgA antibody titers.[61–63] Elevated IgA anti-VCA and IgG anti-EA antibody titers are typically associated with nonkeratinizing carcinoma (both the differentiated and undifferentiated histologic subtype). Neel et al.[64] reported 82% and 86% of patients with nonkeratinizing carcinoma had elevated IgA anti-VCA and IgG anti-EA antibody titers, respectively, in contrast with only 16% and 35%, respectively, in patients with

FIGURE 44.11. Two examples of coronal magnetic resonance images (MRI) showing bilateral cervical lymphadenopathy. There is orderly downward lymphatic spread toward the supraclavicular fossa.

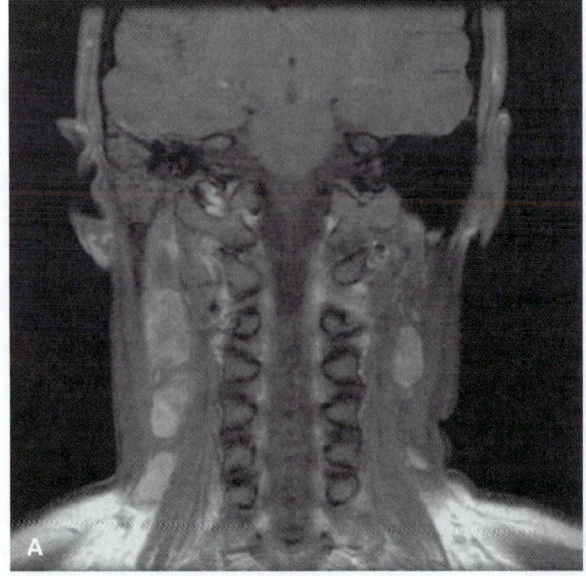
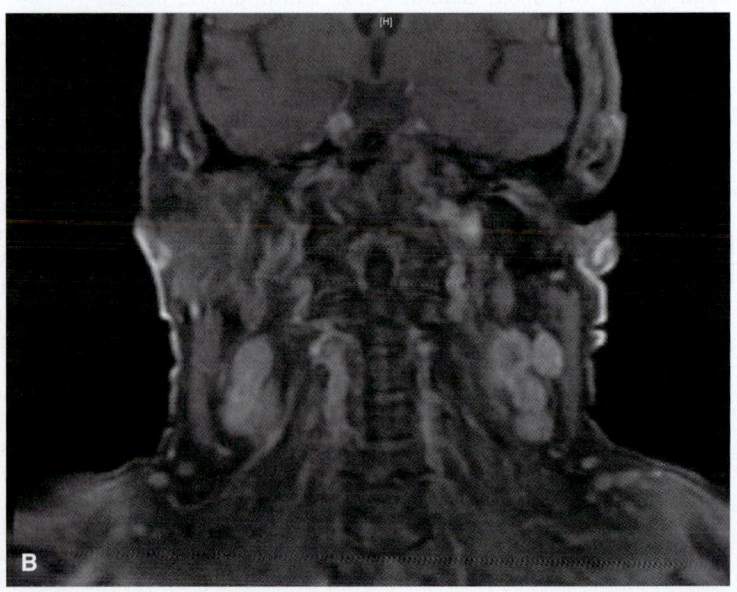

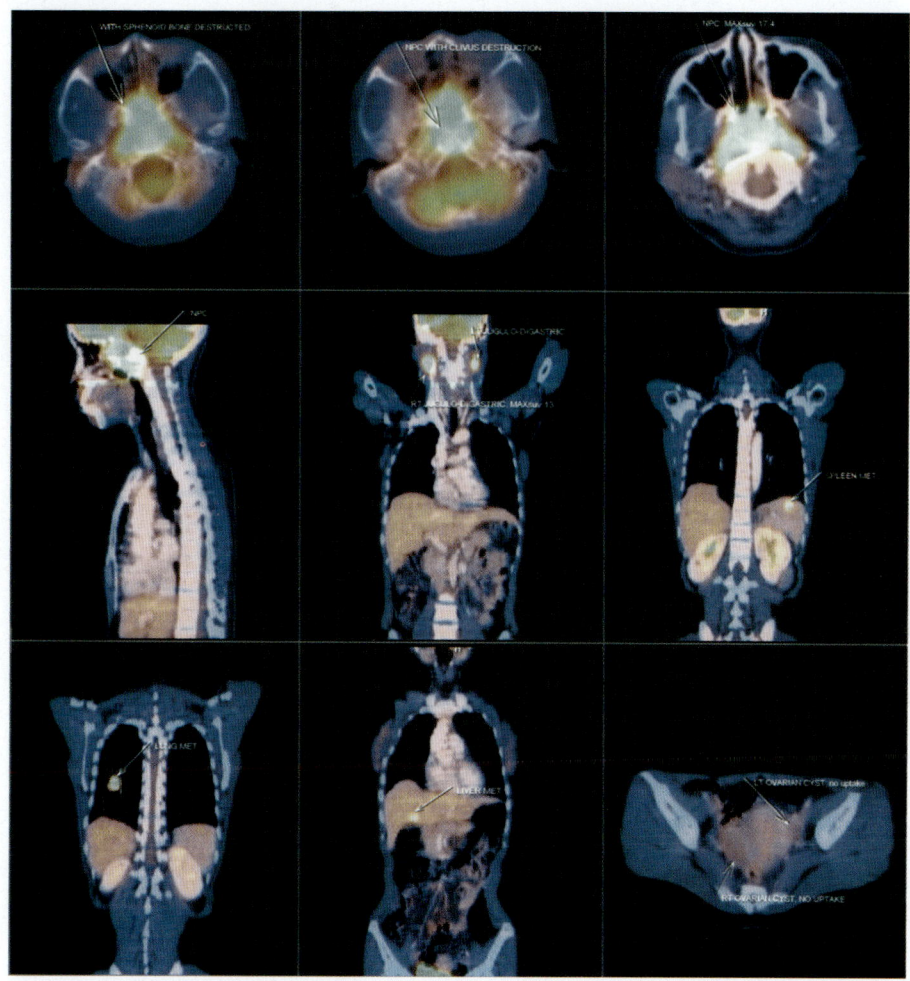

FIGURE 44.12. Positron emission tomography coupled with computed tomography (PET-CT) for a patient with nasopharyngeal carcinoma. Physical examination and biochemistry did not show any sign suggestive of distant metastases. X-ray of the chest was normal. PET-CT revealed multiple distant metastases in the lung, liver, and spleen, in addition to extensive local infiltration and bilateral cervical lymph nodes. (From Chan J, Bray F, McCarron P, et al. Nasopharyngeal carcinoma. In: Pathology and genetics of head and neck tumours. *World Health Organization Classification of Tumours*. Lyon, France: IARC Press, 2005. Copyright © Dr. A. W. M. Lee. With permission.)

the keratinizing histologic type. IgA anti-VCA antibodies may serve as a screening test in high-risk patients as it can be found elevated in patients months before the onset of symptoms.[65,66] A baseline test of plasma EBV DNA may be useful for prognosis, and levels over time can be utilized as surveillance in a posttreatment setting.[67,68]

STAGING SYSTEM

Various staging systems have been devised to predict prognosis and guide treatment strategy for patients with nasopharyngeal carcinoma.[69–72] The American Joint Committee on Cancer (AJCC), Union for International Cancer Control (UICC), and Ho staging systems are the most commonly used systems in the English literature. The AJCC and UICC systems are virtually identical in their 2002 version, and this continues in the 2010 and 2017 updates. Each system has particular limitations; however, they continually evolve and build upon each other's experience. Table 44.6 displays the 2017 AJCC staging system currently in use.[73]

It is important to understand changes to the staging system over time for interpretation of older studies, which use prior classifications. The designation "T0" has been added for an EBV-positive unknown primary with cervical lymph node involvement. Tumors confined to the nasopharynx have similar outcomes to tumors that extend to the nasal cavity and oropharynx.[20,74] From the 2002 to the 2010 system (Table 44.7 and 44.8, respectively), T2a was therefore downstaged to T1, which is defined as tumor confined to the nasopharynx or tumor that extends to the nasal cavity and/or oropharynx. Tumors with parapharyngeal involvement were classified as

T2 in the 2010 system and were no longer subdivided as T2b. Tumors with parapharyngeal space involvement are at higher risk for local and regional recurrence, as well as a high rate of distant metastasis.[76] Now, in the 2017 version, adjacent muscle involvement (including medial pterygoid, lateral pterygoid, and prevertebral muscle) is now designated as T2. Cranial nerve involvement has been shown to carry a worse prognosis than skull base involvement[27,38,77,78]; as such, T3 disease includes involvement of the bony structures of the skull base, whereas T4 includes involvement of the cranial nerves. The previous T4 criteria of extension to the "masticator space" or "infratemporal fossa" have been replaced in the 2017 by a specific description of soft tissue involvement "beyond the lateral surface of the lateral pterygoid muscle, parotid gland" to avoid ambiguity.

Nasopharyngeal carcinoma has a unique pattern of nodal spread as compared to other sites in the head and neck region, which is reflected in the nodal staging classification. Retropharyngeal nodes are the first echelon of nodal metastases,[79] and retropharyngeal lymph node involvement independent of laterality and without cervical lymph node involvement was defined as N1 beginning in the 2010 system. Spread to the low-neck correlates strongly with the development of distant metastasis.[38,39] The previous N3b criterion of supraclavicular fossa extension was changed to lower-neck involvement (as defined by nodal extension below the caudal border of the cricoid cartilage) in the 2017 update. Additionally, N3a and N3b have been merged into a single N3 category. Lastly, the previous substages IVA (T4 N0-2 M0) and IVB (any T N3 M0) are now merged to form IVA, whereas the previous IVC (any T any N M1) is now staged as IVB.

TABLE 44.6 AJCC STAGING OF NASOPHARYNGEAL CANCER, 2017

Stage	Staging Criteria		
T category			
TX	Primary tumor cannot be assessed		
T0	No evidence of primary tumor		
T1	Tumor confined to the nasopharynx or extension to oropharynx and/or nasal cavity without parapharyngeal involvement		
T2	Tumor with extension to parapharyngeal space and/or adjacent soft tissue involvement (medial pterygoid, lateral pterygoid, prevertebral muscles)		
T3	Tumor with infiltration of bony structures at skull base, cervical vertebra, pterygoid structures, and/or paranasal sinuses		
T4	Tumor with intracranial extension; involvement of cranial nerves, hypopharynx, orbit, and parotid gland; and/or extensive soft tissue infiltration beyond the lateral surface of the lateral pterygoid muscle		
N category			
NX	Regional lymph nodes cannot be assessed		
N0	No regional lymph node metastasis		
N1	Unilateral metastasis in cervical lymph node(s) and/or unilateral or bilateral metastasis in retropharyngeal lymph node(s), 6 cm or smaller in greatest dimension, above the caudal border of cricoid cartilage		
N2	Bilateral metastasis in cervical lymph node(s), 6 cm or smaller in greatest dimension, above the caudal border of cricoid cartilage		
N3	Unilateral or bilateral metastasis in cervical lymph node(s), larger than 6 cm in greatest dimension, and/or extension below the caudal border of cricoid cartilage. Metastasis in lymph node(s) >6 cm		
M category			
M0	No distant metastasis		
M1	Distant metastasis		
Stage grouping			
0	Tis	N0	M0
I	T1	N0	M0
II	T1, T0	N1	M0
	T2	N0	M0
	T2	N1	M0
III	T1, T0	N2	M0
	T2	N2	M0
	T3	N0	M0
	T3	N1	M0
	T3	N2	M0
IVA	T4	N0	M0
	T4	N1	M0
	T4	N2	M0
	Any T	N3	M0
IVB	Any T	Any N	M1

From Amin MB, Edge SB, Greene FL, et al. eds. *AJCC Cancer Staging Manual*. 8th ed. New York, NY: Springer, 2017. Reproduced with permission of Springer International Publishing in the format Book via Copyright Clearance Center.

TABLE 44.7 AJCC STAGING OF NASOPHARYNGEAL CANCER, 2002

Stage	Staging Criteria		
T category			
TX	Primary tumor cannot be assessed		
T0	No evidence of primary tumor		
Tis	Carcinoma *in situ*		
T1	Tumor confined to the nasopharynx		
T2	Tumor extends to adjacent soft tissues: Nasal cavity,[a] oropharynx[b]		
	T2a. Tumor without parapharyngeal extension[c]		
	T2b. Tumor with parapharyngeal extension		
T3	Tumor involves bony structures and/or paranasal sinuses		
T4	Tumor with intracranial extension, involvement of cranial nerves, hypopharynx, orbit, infratemporal fossa,[d] or masticator space[d]		
N category			
NX	Regional lymph nodes cannot be assessed		
N0	No regional lymph node metastasis		
N1	Unilateral metastasis in lymph node(s), ≤6 cm in greatest dimension, above the supraclavicular fossa		
N2	Bilateral metastasis in lymph node(s), ≤6 cm in greatest dimension, above the supraclavicular fossa		
N3	Metastasis in lymph node(s)		
	N3a. >6 cm in dimension		
	N3b. Extension to the supraclavicular fossa[e]		
M category			
MX	Distant metastasis cannot be assessed		
M0	No distant metastasis		
M1	Distant metastasis		
Stage grouping			
0	Tis	N0	M0
I	T1	N0	M0
IIA	T2a	N0	M0
IIB	T1	N1	M0
	T2a	N1	M0
	T2b	N0	M0
	T2b	N1	M0
III	T1	N2	M0
	T2a	N2	M0
	T2b	N2	M0
	T3	N0	M0
	T3	N1	M0
	T3	N2	M0
Stage IVA	T4	N0	M0
	T4	N1	M0
	T4	N2	M0
Stage IVB	Any T	N3	M0
Stage IVC	Any T	Any N	M1

[a]Nasal cavity: Anterior extension beyond the posterior margins of the choanal orifices.
[b]Oropharynx: Inferior extension beyond the level of the free border of the soft palate. The junction at C1/C2 level is recommended as a more consistent radiologic landmark.[75]
[c]Parapharyngeal extension: Posterior–lateral infiltration beyond the pharyngobasilar fascia.
[d]Masticator space and infratemporal fossa: Extension beyond the anterior surface of the lateral pterygoid muscle, or lateral extension beyond the posterior–lateral wall of the maxillary antrum, and the pterygomaxillary fissure.
[e]Supraclavicular fossa: Triangular region defined by the superior margin of the sternal end of the clavicle, the superior margin of the lateral end of the clavicle, and the point where the neck meets the shoulder. From Greene F, Page D, Fleming I, et al., eds. *AJCC cancer staging manual*. 6th ed. New York, NY: Springer-Verlag, 2002. Copyright © 2002 American Joint Committee on Cancer. Reproduced with permission of Springer International Publishing in the format Book via Copyright Clearance Center; and Sobin L. *International Union Against Cancer (UICC): TNM classification of malignant tumours*. 6th ed. New York: Wiley-Liss, 2002. Copyright © 2002 Wiley-Liss, New York. Reprinted by permission of John Wiley & Sons, Inc.

These modifications to the staging classifications will require continued examination to determine if they improve prognostic accuracy.

PATHOLOGIC CLASSIFICATION

The vast majority of malignant nasopharyngeal tumors are carcinoma (80% to 99%), with the remainder of these lesions (about 5%) being lymphomas.[80] Other rare malignant tumors of the nasopharynx include adenocarcinoma, plasmacytoma, melanoma, and sarcomas. Regarding nasopharyngeal carcinoma, the most current World Health Organization (WHO) pathologic classification, released in 2017,[81] includes three major types (Fig. 44.13). Keratinizing squamous cell carcinoma is distinguished by the presence of keratin pearls or intracellular keratin. Nonkeratinizing carcinoma is characterized by the complete absence of keratin formation and is further subdivided into differentiated and undifferentiated subtypes. The third type is known as basaloid squamous cell carcinoma[82] and is composed of closely packed small tumor cells that form a lobular and, at times, palisading pattern along with focal squamous carcinoma elements. Basaloid squamous cell carcinoma

is quite rare with a frequency of less than 0.2%[44] (Fig. 44.13). The nonkeratinizing type has a strong association with EBV positivity.[83] The keratinizing type may have a correlation with human papilloma virus (HPV); however, the small sample size of these studies requires continued investigation.[84]

The histologic differences between these three types are by no means distinct. Lesions can share intermediate features, and some may be histologic hybrids. Lymphoepithelioma or lymphoepithelial carcinoma is considered a morphologic variant of undifferentiated carcinoma in which many lymphocytes are found among the tumor cells. Geography, race, and national origin affect the distribution of the WHO histologic

TABLE 44.8 AJCC STAGING OF NASOPHARYNGEAL CANCER, 2010

Stage	Staging Criteria		
T category			
TX	Primary tumor cannot be assessed		
T0	No evidence of primary tumor		
Tis	Carcinoma *in situ*		
T1	Tumor confined to the nasopharynx or tumor extends to the nasal cavity[a] and/or oropharynx[b] without parapharyngeal extension[c]		
T2	Tumor with parapharyngeal extension[c]		
T3	Tumor involves bony structures of skull base and/or paranasal sinuses		
T4	Tumor with intracranial extension and/or involvement of cranial nerves, hypopharynx, and orbit or with extension to the infratemporal fossa/masticator space[d]		
N category			
NX	Regional lymph nodes cannot be assessed		
N0	No regional lymph node metastasis		
N1	Unilateral metastasis in cervical lymph node(s), ≤6 cm in greatest dimension, above the supraclavicular fossa, and/or unilateral or bilateral retropharyngeal lymph node(s), ≤6 cm in greatest dimension		
N2	Bilateral metastasis in cervical lymph node(s), ≤6 cm in greatest dimension, above the supraclavicular fossa[e,f]		
N3	Metastasis in lymph node(s)[e] >6 cm and/or to supraclavicular fossa[f]		
	N3a. >6 cm in dimension		
	N3b. Extension to the supraclavicular fossa[f]		
M category			
M0	No distant metastasis		
M1	Distant metastasis		
Stage grouping			
0	Tis	N0	M0
I	T1	N0	M0
II	T1	N1	M0
	T2	N0	M0
	T2	N1	M0
III	T1	N2	M0
	T2	N2	M0
	T3	N0	M0
	T3	N1	M0
	T3	N2	M0
IVA	T4	N0	M0
	T4	N1	M0
	T4	N2	M0
IVB	Any T	N3	M0
IVC	Any T	Any N	M1

[a]Nasal cavity: Anterior extension beyond the posterior margins of the choanal orifices.
[b]Oropharynx: Inferior extension beyond the level of the free border of the soft palate. The junction at C1/C2 level is recommended as a more consistent radiologic landmark.[75]
[c]Parapharyngeal extension: Posterior–lateral infiltration beyond the pharyngobasilar fascia.
[d]Masticator space and infratemporal fossa: Extension beyond the anterior surface of the lateral pterygoid muscle, or lateral extension beyond the posterior–lateral wall of the maxillary antrum, and the pterygomaxillary fissure.
[e]Midline nodes are considered ipsilateral nodes.
[f]Supraclavicular fossa: Triangular region defined by the superior margin of the sternal end of the clavicle, the superior margin of the lateral end of the clavicle, and the point where the neck meets the shoulder.
From Edge SB, Byrd DR, Compton CC, et al., eds. *AJCC cancer staging manual*. 7th ed. New York, NY: Springer, 2010. Copyright © 2010 American Joint Committee on Cancer. Reproduced with permission of Springer International Publishing in the format Book via Copyright Clearance Center.

types (Table 44.9). The frequency of nonkeratinizing carcinoma varies from 99% in Hong Kong to 75% in the United States.[44]

Of note, the former WHO classification remains quite commonly used and classifies the three histologic types as (I) squamous cell carcinoma, (II) nonkeratinizing carcinoma, and (III) undifferentiated carcinoma.[69] This leads to unnecessary confusion with the new WHO classification as the former classification has been used in the majority of, albeit older, studies.

PROGNOSTIC FACTORS

The extent of local invasion, regional lymphatic spread, and distant metastasis, as reflected by the TNM staging, is the

most important prognostic factor. In general, advanced T category is associated with worse local control and overall survival; advanced N category predicts increased risk of distant metastasis and worse survival. The presence of distant metastasis (M1) upon presentation usually indicates poor prognosis, and treatment has conventionally been palliative in nature. A summary of the patterns of failure and survival rate for the different stages can be found in the *Results of Treatment* section.

The association of bone erosion, cranial nerve palsy, and lower nodal level with poorer survival is largely undisputed.[85–88] However, the prognostic significance of parapharyngeal extension has been a topic of controversy. In a study of 364 patients, Chua et al.[89] showed that greater tumor extension as defined by extension to the prestyloid space or extension to the anterior part of the masticator space was associated with a worse local failure-free rate (L-FFR of 72% vs. 86%) and lower distant failure-free survival rate (D-FFR of 68% vs. 87%) compared to tumors with no extension or extension only to the retrostyloid space. Other investigators have reported similar significant findings.[76,87,90–92] Cheng et al. found parapharyngeal space extension to be the key factor in distant metastasis, even in N1 and N2 NPC.[93]

However, Teo et al. did not find parapharyngeal space involvement to be an independent significant prognosticator in a study of 903 patients.[86] Au et al.,[94] using the AJCC/UICC definition of extension beyond the pharyngobasilar fascia in a study of 1,294 patients, also found that parapharyngeal extension was not a significant factor upon multivariate analysis.

These contradictory findings may be attributed to varying definitions of parapharyngeal space and incidence in the different series,[76,86,87,90] prompting some to advocate for consideration of the degree of parapharyngeal space extension in future staging systems.[92] In addition, suboptimal imaging by CT and conflation with retropharyngeal node enlargement likely contribute to the debate.[95,96]

Nevertheless, the 2010 AJCC staging system (Table 44.8) downgraded involvement of the oropharynx and/or nasal cavity without parapharyngeal extension from T2a to T1 while designating the presence of parapharyngeal extension to be the sole determinant of T2 classification. This was in light of recent multiple large retrospective studies that found no significant difference in disease failure hazard ratios between former AJCC 2002 T2a and T1.[93,97–99]

In the current 2017 AJCC staging system,[73] further refinement to T2 stage has been defined. Soft tissue involvement of the medial and lateral pterygoid muscles was downstaged to T2 (from T4 in the 2010 AJCC system), based on a large analysis of 1,609 patients who all were staged by MRI and received IMRT.[51]

Another prognostic factor to consider is the gross volume of the primary tumor (GTV-P). Although it is highly correlated to T-stage, considerable variability in tumor volume exists within the same T-stage, and evidence increasingly suggests that tumor volume as an independent significant factor can better predict prognosis than T category as specified by both AJCC/UICC and Ho staging systems[100–104] (Fig. 44.14).

In a study of 308 patients staged with MRI, Sze et al.[102] showed that those with GTV-P <15 cm^3 had significantly higher L-FFR than those with ≥15 cm^3 (97% vs. 82% at 3 years; P < .01). Multivariate analysis confirmed GTV-P to be a strong significant factor independent of T category by 1997 AJCC/UICC fifth edition; the risk of local failure increased by 1% for every 1 cm^3 increase in volume. A similar observation between GTV and clinical outcomes has been observed in other head and neck tumors, including oropharyngeal cancers.[105] Further study is required to determine how tumor volume may be optimally incorporated into future staging systems.

Most series have found significantly better prognosis for females and younger patients.[85,94,106] In 759 patients, Sham and Choy[85] showed a higher 5-year survival rate in females compared with males (45% vs. 28%) and in patients younger than

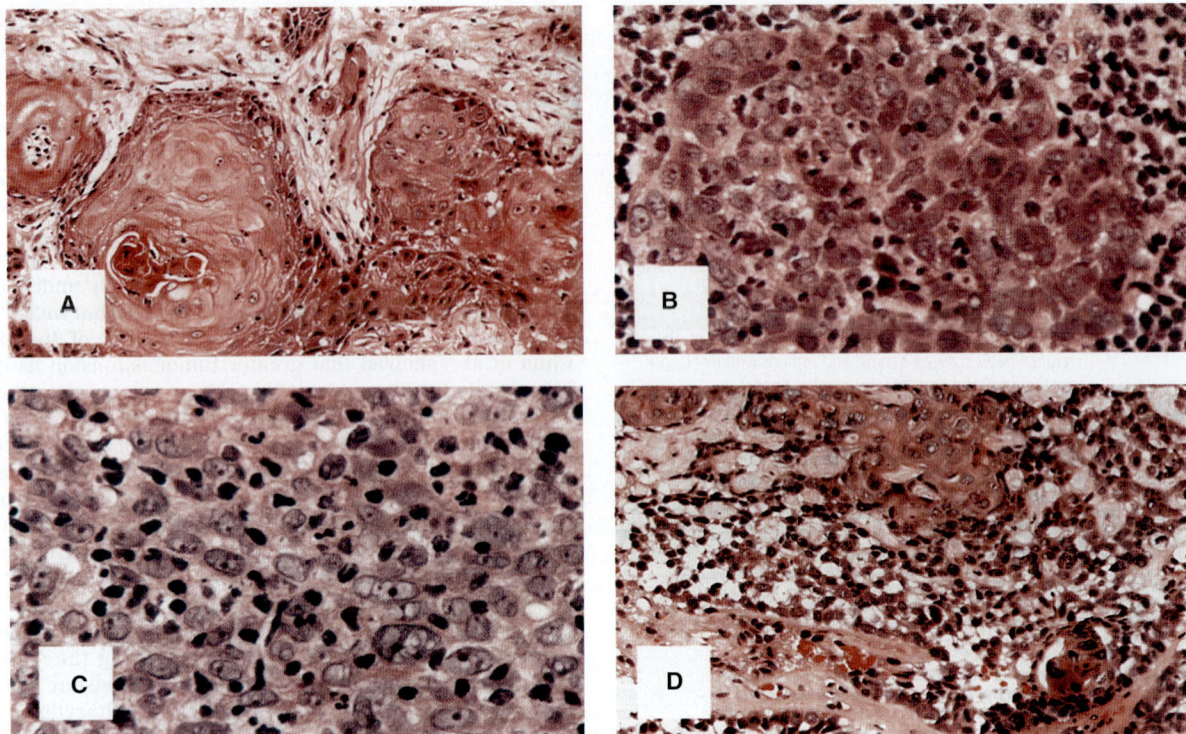

FIGURE 44.13. Photomicrographs of nasopharyngeal carcinoma. **A:** Keratinizing squamous cell carcinoma. **B:** Nonkeratinizing carcinoma, differentiated subtype. **C:** Nonkeratinizing carcinoma, undifferentiated subtype. **D:** Basaloid squamous cell carcinoma. (From Chan J, Bray F, McCarron P, et al. Nasopharyngeal carcinoma. In: Pathology and genetics of head and neck tumours. *World Health Organization Classification of Tumours.* Lyon, France: IARC Press, 2005. Copyright © Dr. J. K. C. Chan. With permission.)

40 years of age versus older than 40 (50% vs. 40%, *P* = .002). However, they did not find age to significantly affect the 10-year survival rate. Multivariate analysis of 1,294 patients by Au et al.[94] also showed worse cancer-specific death rates in males (HR = 1.28, *P* = .02) and patients older than 50 years (HR = 1.79, *P* < .001).

Although not all studies have found histology to be an independent prognostic factor,[27,107] many have found nonkeratinizing and undifferentiated carcinomas (formerly known as lymphoepitheliomas) to be more radiosensitive and offer better prognosis than keratinizing squamous cell carcinoma.[31,108,109] Of note, regarding ethnicity as a prognostic factor, a study by Corry et al.[110] showed no prognostic difference between ethnic Asian and non-Asian patients with nonkeratinizing carcinoma.

EBV, HPV, and Other Biomarkers

Because of the association of EBV with NPC, various anti-EBV antibodies have long been studied for their potential as biomarkers. Although some studies have shown that elevated level of serum anti-EBV antibodies could indicate

FIGURE 44.14. The correlation between T-category and gross volume of primary tumor (GTV-P). (UICC, International Union Against Cancer.) (Modified from Sze W, Lee A, Yau T, et al. Primary tumor volume of nasopharyngeal carcinoma: Prognostic significance for local control. *Int J Radiat Oncol Biol Phys* 2004;59:21–27.)

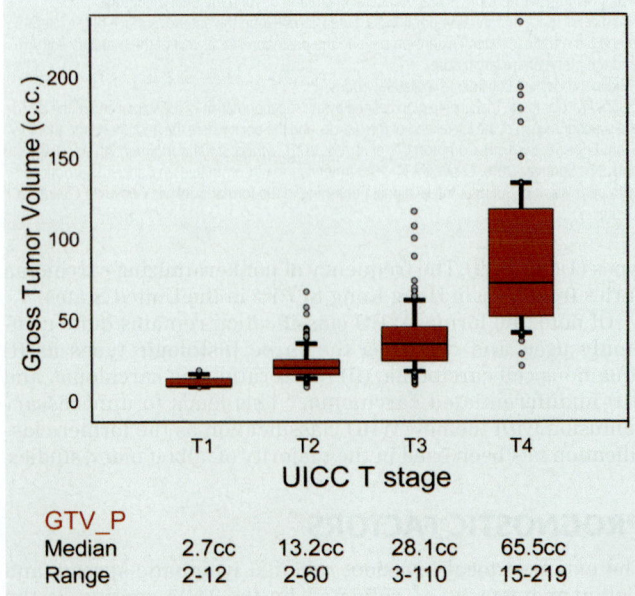

	TABLE 44.9 FREQUENCY OF DIFFERENT HISTOLOGIC SUBTYPES OF NASOPHARYNGEAL CARCINOMA		
	High-Incidence Population (%): Hong Kong	**Intermediate Population (%): Tunisia**	**Low-Incidence Population (%): United States**
Keratinizing squamous cell carcinoma	1	8	25
Nonkeratinizing carcinoma	99	92	75
Undifferentiated	92	76	NA
Differentiated	7	16	NA
Basaloid squamous carcinoma	<0.2	NA	NA

NA, not available.
Reproduced with permission from Barnes L, Eveson JW, Reichart P, et al., World Health Organization Classification of Tumours. Pathology and Genetics of Head and Neck Tumours. Volume 9. IARC, Lyon, 2005.

GTV_P

	T1	T2	T3	T4
Median	2.7cc	13.2cc	28.1cc	65.5cc
Range	2–12	2–60	3–110	15–219

the presence[63,111,112] of disease, others have shown anti-EBV antibody titers to have little value for posttreatment surveillance.[64,113,114] The prognostic value of such titers prior to treatment has also been controversial. Although Xu et al.[115] found that high EBV DNAase–specific neutralizing antibody at diagnosis predicted significantly worse event-free and overall survival, others found that a number of antibodies (VCA-IgG, VCA-IgA, EA-IgG, EA-IgA, EBNA-IgG, EBNA-IgA) could not predict prognosis.[112,116,117]

Circulating cell-free DNA of EBV in the plasma of NPC patients is a significant prognostic marker and has been found to be superior to serum anti-EBV antibodies.[117] Lo et al.[118] showed that plasma EBV DNA had high sensitivity (96%) and specificity (93%) for detecting NPC, whereas Ma et al.[119] showed that circulating EBV DNA levels correlated significantly with tumor burden. Studies by Lo et al.[120] and Lin et al.[67] found that high pretreatment levels were associated with advanced stages and poor prognosis. Meanwhile, Leung et al.[68] showed that pretreatment plasma EBV DNA load was an independent prognostic factor for OS in 376 patients and could be used to segregate early-stage patients into poor-risk and high-risk subgroups. Thus, pretreatment EBV DNA assays have the potential to complement TNM staging in guiding treatment.

The ability of posttreatment EBV DNA to prognosticate outcomes has also been studied. Le et al.[121] found no correlation between pretreatment EBV DNA levels and survival; they did find posttreatment levels to be a strong significant predictor of outcome; patients with no detectable EBV DNA had a 2-year OS rate of 94% versus 55% for patients with detectable posttreatment levels ($P < .002$).

Other studies have also consistently reported that patients with elevated posttreatment EBV DNA load have had higher risk of tumor recurrence.[67,120,122–124] Using multivariate analysis to compare various prognostic factors for NPC, Lin et al.[125] found that the combined EBV DNA load (pretreatment and 1-week posttreatment) was the single most significant factor.

The ability of posttreatment EBV DNA to influence decisions regarding adjuvant therapy is currently being investigated in the NRG Oncology cooperative group HN001 trial (NCT02135042). This phase II randomized/phase III trial offers differing treatment regimens to patients with stage IIB to IVB NPC on the basis of post-CRT EBV DNA levels. The hypothesis is that posttreatment EBV DNA can be used to risk stratify patients following a course of definitive concurrent CRT. In this way, it could serve as a biomarker potentially identifying those at the highest risk for recurrence and most likely to benefit from adjuvant chemotherapy. Therefore, in the phase III cohort, patients with undetectable post-CRT EBV DNA will be randomized to observation alone versus standard adjuvant chemotherapy consisting of cisplatin and 5-FU. The primary endpoint for this portion of the trial is OS with the hypothesis that observation will be noninferior to adjuvant chemotherapy. Patients with detectable post-CRT EBV DNA are randomized in the phase II portion of the trial to standard adjuvant chemotherapy or a non–cross-resistant, experimental doublet consisting of paclitaxel and gemcitabine with the hypothesis that experimental chemotherapy will be associated with superior PFS. The outcomes of this trial may allow for the creation of individualized treatment recommendations using post-CRT EBV DNA as a guide.

Both Wang et al.[126] and An et al.[127] demonstrated that the clearance rate of plasma EBV DNA during the first month of salvage chemotherapy could predict tumor response and overall survival in patients with metastatic/recurrent NPC; undetectable levels after the first cycle indicated significantly better survival. These data suggest that early evaluation of plasma EBV DNA can offer oncologists timely insight for potential alterations in the therapeutic regimen for patients with a slow clearance rate. In addition, Wang et al.[128] prospectively

monitored the plasma EBV DNA of 245 NPC patients in clinical remission with assays every 3 to 6 months and found the plasma EBV DNA assay to have much greater sensitivity, specificity, and accuracy than FDG-PET in predicting relapse, suggesting its utility for posttreatment surveillance.

HPV-associated oropharyngeal carcinomas are now recognized as a separate subtype in the 2017 version of AJCC.[73,129] However, the implications of HPV to NPC with respect to etiology, prognosis, and treatment are unclear. Stenmark et al.[130] reported on a 61-patient cohort from the Midwestern United States where 30% of patients were HPV-positive/EBV-negative. The patient outcomes in OS, PFS, and LRC were worse in this HPV-positive/EBV-negative subgroup, when compared to EBV-positive tumors. Lin et al.[131] evaluated NPC cases from southern China ($n = 86$) and Stanford, California, USA ($n = 108$), where no HPV-positive cases were detected in the Chinese cohort, whereas 5 of 11 EBV-negative cases in the Stanford cohort harbored HPV as confirmed by PCR. Of note, these 11 EBV-negative patients had a trend toward worse survival. Dogan et al.[132] reported on a case series of 90 patients with NPC where 6 patients with confirmed nasopharyngeal origin were HPV-positive. These HPV-positive patients had a similar OS to EBV-positive NPC, whereas EBV/HPV-negative NPC had worse OS. Because of these conflicting studies and limited patient numbers, future work will be required to determine the prognostic significance of HPV positivity in NPC.

As with other head and neck squamous cell carcinomas, epidermal growth factor receptor (EGFR) is commonly expressed in patients with NPC. Chua et al.[133] found expression of EFGR in 89% of patients, in which overexpression was associated with significantly poorer disease-specific survival. Others have reported similar findings of prognostic significance.[24,134,135] Ma et al.[134] performed multivariate analysis on several biomarkers in 78 patients, including microvessel density, Ki67 antigen, p53 oncoprotein, HER2, and EGFR, and found EGFR to be the only independent prognostic factor.

The study by Hui et al.[136] showed that 58% of NPC patients had expression of hypoxia-inducible factor 1α (HIF-1-alpha), 57% had carbonic anhydrase IX (CA IX), and 60% had VEGF. Those with positive hypoxic profile (high expression of HIF-1-alpha and CA IX) had a worse progression-free survival ($P = .04$); those with both positive hypoxic and angiogenic profile (high VEGF) were strongly associated with worse progression-free survival ($P = .0095$). Multiple other studies have also shown that overexpression of these markers, particularly VEGF, is associated with poorer survival.[137–139]

Other biologic factors that might have prognostic significance include E-cadherin and β-catenin,[140] c-erbB2,[141] p53,[142] NM23-HI,[143,144] and interleukin-10.[145] Further validation of these potential biomarkers is needed.

TREATMENT STRATEGY

Because of the anatomic location, proximity to critical structures, surgical exposure, and tumor resection with sufficient margins have been very challenging.[146] Primary surgical intervention was rare after the 1950s for these reasons, with surgical interventions employed mainly for biopsy to gain histologic confirmation and salvage therapy for persistent or recurrent cancer. Primary treatment since has typically employed radiation therapy (RT) alone and, more recently, in combination with chemotherapy.

Radiation Therapy

To achieve the best therapeutic ratio, every single step in the RT procedures (localization of gross tumor and target volumes, immobilization, optimization of dose fractionation, determination of treatment techniques, and precision in RT delivery) is important.

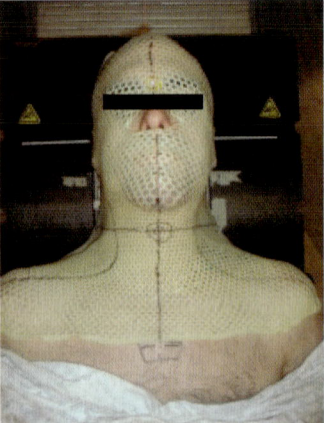
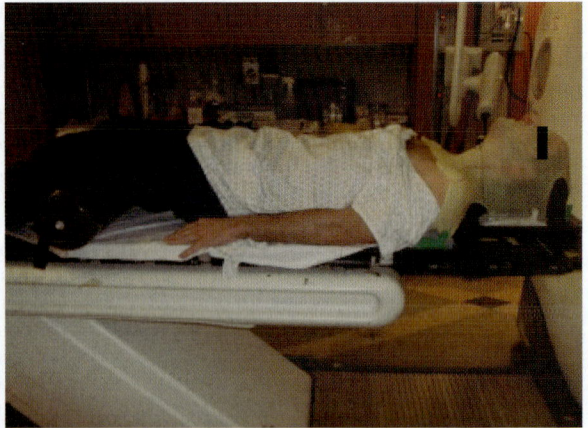
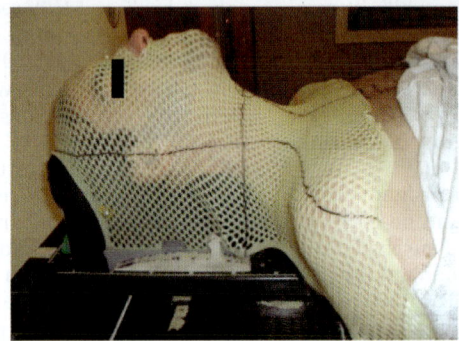
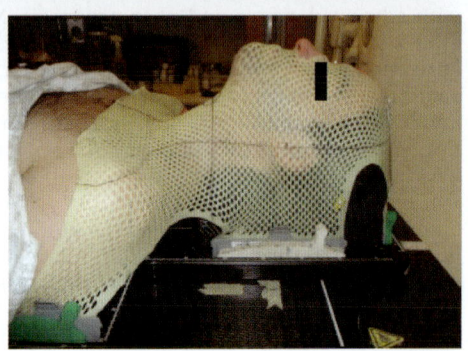

FIGURE 44.15. Immobilization of patient in a customized thermoplastic mask covering the whole head-to-shoulder region.

For planning, the patient should be set up in a supine position with head extended for adequate separation between the primary tumor/retropharyngeal nodes and the upper neck nodes. The tip of the uvula and the base of the occiput should be on a parallel plane to the beam axis. The patient is immobilized with a thermoplastic mask covering the head to shoulder region (Fig. 44.15). For patients to be treated by conventional two-dimensional (2-D) technique, a mouth bite is useful to minimize the dose to the oral cavity with enlarged neck nodes to be marked with wire before imaging.

Dose, Time, and Fractionation

A significant dose–response has been observed in the majority of retrospective studies, based on patients irradiated with 2-D techniques. Marks et al.[147] and Vikram et al.[148] showed that local control was significantly improved in patients who received >67 Gy to the tumor target. Perez et al.[27] observed that patients with T1-2 tumors had a local tumor control rate of 100% for those given >70 Gy, compared with 80% for those treated with 66 to 70 Gy. However, local control for patients with T3-4 tumors remained below 55%, even with a total dose >70 Gy. Similar findings were reported by Mesic et al.,[149] where ≥70 Gy achieved better local control for T1-2 tumors compared with 60 Gy (94% vs. 76%), but higher doses or larger fields did not significantly improve outcomes in T3-4 tumors. These observations suggest that, besides consideration of the prescribed dose, the problem of sufficient coverage has to be overcome for advanced tumors.

Lee et al.[150] reported a study of 1,008 patients with T1 tumors irradiated by four different fractionation schedules and demonstrated that total dose was the most important radiation factor (*P* = .01). Dose fraction did not affect local control; however, it was a significant risk factor for temporal lobe necrosis.[151,152] Therefore, a fractional dose of >2 Gy should be avoided[153] (see section *Sequelae of Treatment*).

The impact of the time factor is more contentious. A randomized study by Marcial et al.,[154] where 62 patients were treated with split-course irradiation (30 Gy in 10 fractions over 2 weeks, then a 3-week rest period, and followed by an additional 30 Gy in 10 fractions) compared with 59 patients with 66 Gy in 33 fractions in 6.5 to 7 weeks, demonstrated no significant difference in 5-year local control (86% vs. 80%), nodal control (86% vs. 78%), or disease-free survival (40% vs. 30%).

However, Vikram et al.[148] observed that patients with interruption of RT for ≥21 days had significantly poorer local tumor control than patients without interruptions (34% vs. 67%). Similar findings have been subsequently reported,[155,156] with the general consensus that prolongation is likely to be detrimental, even for nonkeratinizing NPC.

In general, the prescription recommended for NPC is to a total dose of about 70 Gy over 7 weeks to the gross tumor along with 50 to 60 Gy for elective treatment of potential risk sites.

Tumor Target Volumes

The GTV should encompass the primary nasopharyngeal tumor, gross retropharyngeal lymphadenopathy, and gross nodal disease as determined by clinical, endoscopic, and radiologic examinations. Lymph nodes ≥1 cm or with evidence of central necrosis are considered gross nodal disease. For patients given induction chemotherapy, it is recommended that the targets be determined by the prechemotherapy extent.

Prophylactic neck radiation is usually recommended in N0 patients because of the high incidence of occult neck node involvement. Lee et al.[35] found patients with a clinically negative neck who underwent elective neck irradiation had a significantly lower nodal recurrence rate than those untreated (11% vs. 40%). Additionally, even with successful salvage by subsequent treatment, patients with nodal recurrence had a significantly greater incidence of distant metastases than those without recurrence (21% vs. 6%).

The clinical target volume (CTV) includes the GTV, regions of microscopic disease, and potential infiltrative spread. Different centers may have different philosophies in defining the margins and dose level. For example, Table 44.10 shows the delineation criteria for the various CTVs currently

TABLE 44.10 EXAMPLE OF GUIDELINE ON ANATOMIC STRUCTURES/BOUNDARIES FOR DELINEATING CLINICAL TARGET VOLUMES (CTV) FOR INTENSITY-MODULATED RADIATION THERAPY[a]

CTV	Delineation of CTV Structures	Anatomic Boundaries
CTV_{70}	GTV + ≥5 mm margin (can be reduced to as low as 1 mm for tumors in close proximity to critical structures/neurologic structures)[b]	
$CTV_{59.4}$	CTV_{70} + ≥5 mm margin (as low as 1 mm when close to critical structures)[b]	
	Entire nasopharynx	5–10 mm from mucosal surface of nasopharynx Anterior: Junction with nasal choana Lateral: Medial border of parapharyngeal space Caudal: Caudal border of C1 vertebra
	Base of skull	Posterior: Anterior 1/2 to 2/3 of clivus (entire clivus, if involved) Lateral: Lateral border of foramen ovale
	Parapharyngeal spaces	Lateral: Lateral border of styloid processes
	Inferior sphenoid sinus	Cranial: Lower half of sphenoid sinus (in T3-T4 disease, include entire sphenoid sinus)
	Posterior nasal cavity	Anterior: Posterior fourth to third of nasal cavity
	Posterior maxillary sinuses	Anterior: Posterior fourth to third of maxillary sinuses (to ensure pterygopalatine fossae coverage)
	Cavernous sinus, include high-risk patients (T3, T4 bulky disease involving roof of nasopharynx)	
	High-risk nodal levels (include all bilaterally)	(a) Upper deep jugular (junctional, parapharyngeal) (b) Submandibular [level I]c (c) Subdigastric (jugulodigastric) [level II] (d) Midjugular [level III] (e) Low jugular and supraclavicular [level IV] (f) Posterior cervical [level V] (g) Retropharyngeal

[a]Based on guideline currently used at Memorial Sloan Kettering Cancer Center and detailed in RTOG 0615.
[b]CTV margins may also be limited to exclude the bone *not* at risk for subclinical disease or air.
[c]Bilateral IB lymph nodes can be spared if patient is node-negative. The treatment of level IB may result in the delivery of clinically significant radiation doses to normal structures such as the floor of the mouth, mandible, and upper pharyngeal mucosa above the hyoid. At the discretion of the treating radiation oncologist, level IB may also be spared or limited to the anterior border of the submandibular gland in low-risk node-positive patients. Patients presenting with isolated retropharyngeal nodes or isolated level IV nodes are considered low risk for level IB involvement. Treatment of level IB should be considered in node-negative patients with extensive involvement of the hard palate, nasal cavity, or maxillary antrum.
GTV, gross tumor volume: All gross primary tumor and involved lymph nodes.
PTV, planning target volume: CTV + 3- to 5-mm margin.
Total dose prescription at:
PTV_{70}: 70 Gy in 33 fractions (2.12 Gy per fraction). $PTV_{59.4}$: 59.4 Gy in 33 fractions (1.8 Gy per fraction).

employed at Memorial Sloan Kettering Cancer Center. A gross disease CTV (CTV_{70}) is defined as the GTV plus an additional margin of 5 mm to 1 cm surrounding all gross disease. The margin may be decreased to as small as 1 mm in critical regions near the brainstem or spinal cord. The high-risk subclinical CTV ($CTV_{59.4}$) encompasses the GTV including all potential areas of microscopic spread of disease. This volume should include at a minimum the entire nasopharynx, retropharyngeal lymph nodal regions, clivus, skull base, pterygoid fossae, parapharyngeal space, sphenoid sinus, posterior fourth to third of the nasal cavity, and posterior fourth to third of the maxillary sinuses. This $CTV_{59.4}$ should also include lymph nodal groups that are at risk of potential microscopic disease spread: bilateral upper deep jugular (junctional, parapharyngeal), submandibular, subdigastric (jugulodigastric), midjugular, posterior cervical, and retropharyngeal lymph nodes. In patients with clinically N0 neck, it is not necessary to include level I nodal regions.

The planning target volume (PTV) is defined as the CTV including a circumferential margin of typically 3 to 5 mm to all the CTVs to account for setup errors and potential patient motion. The PTV margin may be decreased to as small as 1 mm in regions near critical normal structures such as the brainstem or spinal cord.

Conventional 2-D Treatment Techniques

One of the most common RT approaches employed is comprised of two phases.[157] Phase I consists of large lateral opposing faciocervical fields that encompass the primary tumor and the upper neck nodes in one volume, with a matching lower anterior cervical field for the lower cervical lymphatics. Phase II is used after 40 Gy to limit the dose to the spinal cord. This three-field technique includes lateral opposing facial

fields coupled with anterior facial field for the primary tumor. Typical treatment fields and radiologic landmarks are shown in Figure 44.16. Shrinking treatment fields by cone down after 50 to 60 Gy should be done, when possible, to increase protection of critical structures.

The three-field technique in phase II allows the dose to be minimized to the temporomandibular joints and the bilateral temporal lobes. However, coverage may not be sufficient for tumors with extensive posterior–lateral extension to the parapharyngeal spaces or caudal extension to the oropharynx. To remedy this deficit, an additional dose is delivered by a posterior–lateral field with avoidance of neurologic structures.[158]

Three-Dimensional (3-D) Conformal Treatment Techniques

Nasopharyngeal carcinoma presents most typically as a concave tumor allowing for computerized 3-D treatment plans to be an important technical advance for improved radiation delivery. Several investigators have designed multifield conformal plans, including the seven-field technique used at Memorial Sloan Kettering Cancer Center (MSKCC) (United States)[159] and the "boomerang" technique used at Peter MacCallum Cancer Center (Australia).[160] When compared to conventional 2-D plans, 3-D planning demonstrated better tumor dose coverage while decreasing normal tissue dose in several studies.[86,161,162]

Leibel et al.[163] from MSKCC demonstrated that the target volume underdosed at the 95% isodose level was lowered with 3-D plans when compared with 2-D plans (7% vs. 22%). On average, the mean tumor dose increased 13% leading to an estimation that tumor control would increase by 15%. However, a subsequent study in which 68 patients

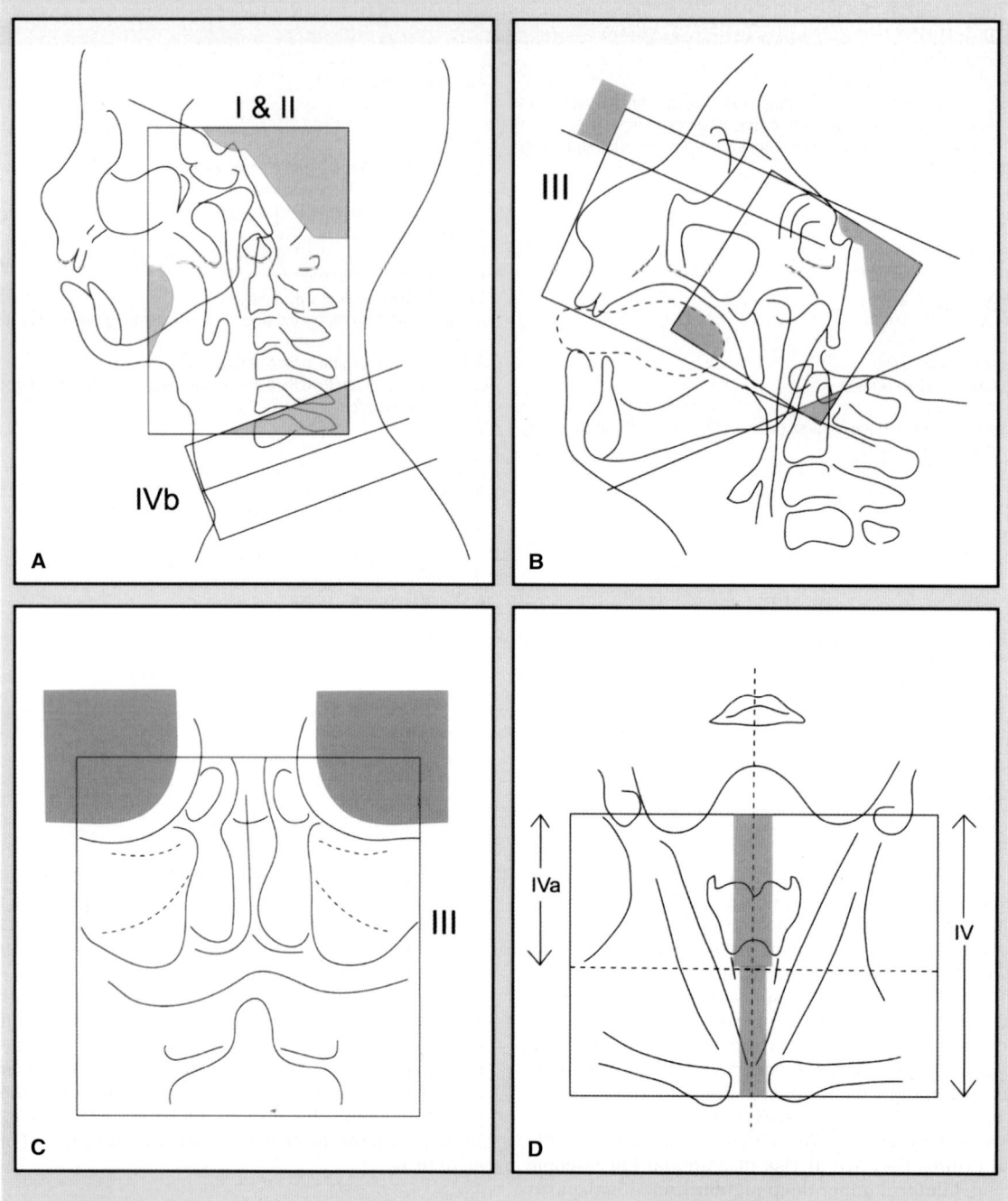

FIGURE 44.16. Conventional two-dimensional radiotherapy using Ho's technique. **A:** Phase I, lateral-opposed faciocervical fields (I–II) and lower anterior cervical field (IVb). **B:** Phase II, sagittal view showing lateral-opposed facial fields and non-coplanar anterior facial field (III). **C:** Coronal view of anterior facial field (III). **D:** Anterior cervical field for whole neck (IV).

received this technique for a boost of 19.8 to 25.2 Gy following phase I conventional 2-D treatment for 50.4 Gy to a total dose of 70.2 to 75.6 Gy did not show significant improvement; the 5-year L-FFR was 77% and late toxicity grade ≥3 was 25%.[159]

More encouraging results were obtained by Jen et al.,[164] who compared 72 patients treated with 3-D conformal technique with 108 patients treated with 2-D technique. A significant improvement in 3-year L-FFR for T4 (86% vs. 47%), and event-free survival for both stage III (80% vs. 56%) and stage IV (82% vs. 33%), was observed. Furthermore, the incidence of xerostomia at 3 years was significantly less with 3-D conformal treatment (69.2% vs. 98.0%), although for most other late toxicities, little difference was seen.

IMRT Techniques

IMRT has supplanted conventional radiotherapy in the treatment of NPC in an increasing number of institutions throughout the world. The intensity of the radiation beams can be modulated to deliver a high dose to the tumor with a superior target volume coverage while significantly limiting the dose to surrounding normal tissues.[165–170] Following the initial publication[171] and the subsequent update on IMRT for NPC from the University of California, San Francisco (UCSF),[169] several other institutions have utilized IMRT with similar excellent treatment outcomes.[172–178]

Another point of interest is the possibility of biologic enhancement by simultaneous modulated accelerated radiation therapy (SMART), also known as dose painting, as a new way of delivering an accelerated fractionation (AF) schedule, a concept that was first reported by Butler et al.[179] for the treatment of other head and neck cancers with IMRT.

These differing methods and dose fractionation regimens for IMRT are being investigated by different groups; Table 44.11 summarizes the key features along with reported results. The majority of the patients in these series received additional chemotherapy and/or enhanced RT with boosts or AF. All reported encouraging early results with local control in excess of 90% at 2 to 4 years.

At the University of California, San Francisco, patients were typically prescribed 70 Gy to the PTV$_{gross\ disease}$ and involved lymph nodes in 2.12 to 2.25 Gy fractions, whereas the PTV$_{high-risk\ subclinical}$ were prescribed 59.4 Gy in 1.8 fractions, and a clinical negative neck (PTV$_{low-risk\ subclinical}$) received 54 Gy at 1.64 Gy fractions all in conventional once-daily fractions.[169,180] Bucci et al.[180] reported the updated results of 118 patients, which confirmed excellent locoregional control of 96%. Yet, distant failure remained high (28%) despite broad use of concurrent–adjuvant CRT. OS was 74% at 4 years.

At Memorial Sloan Kettering Cancer Center, Wolden et al.[172] reported their initial experience with 74 patients, where 59 were treated with AF using the concomitant boost method and 15 by the SMART method/dose painting. For the SMART cohort, a total dose of 70.2 Gy at 2.34 Gy/fraction was given to the gross disease, and the "microscopic" PTV received 54 Gy at 1.8 Gy/fraction. There was a trend, but no statistically significant improvement in 3-year L-FFR than for patients treated by 3-D conformal boost (91% vs. 79%, $P = .11$). Updated results by Setton et al.[186] on 177 patients confirmed excellent rates of disease control (92% 3-year and 83% 5-year local control) and survival (87% 3-year and 75% 5-year OS)

with this technique. Additional dose escalation by SMART boost in 50 patients with T3 to T4 tumors was reported by Kwong et al.[182] from Queen Mary Hospital (Hong Kong). They sought to deliver a total dose of 76 Gy at 2.17 Gy/fraction to the gross tumor. The early result for locoregional control was excellent (96% at 2 years); however, serious late toxicities were observed, including 4% of patients having a life-threatening hemorrhage from carotid artery pseudoaneurysm and another 4% developing temporal lobe necrosis with a median follow-up of 2.1 years.

Two different IMRT approaches are currently being utilized by different centers: (1) an extended whole-field (EWF) IMRT technique, in which the total target volume is encompassed in the IMRT plan, or (2) a split-field (SF) IMRT technique, in which the target volumes superior to the vocal cords are treated with an IMRT plan and the lower neck nodes are treated with a conventional low anterior neck field.[187–189] Discussions among practitioners on which IMRT technique is best have been persistent. Concerns of potential failures at the SF matchline because of potential underdosing, or even complications resulting from overdosing, have caused many centers to implement EWF IMRT, even when no clinically involved neck nodes are evident in the matchline region. These concerns may be caused by the treatment delivery system that is used at centers where a perfect match between the IMRT fields and the low anterior neck field is not possible. However, with a EWF technique, an unnecessary dose of radiation is delivered to the normal glottic larynx.[190] Whereas with the SF IMRT technique, the dose to the vocal cords is minimal because of shielding by a midline Cerrobend block or the multileaf collimator (MLC). At the moment, no IMRT matchline failures or complications have been reported with the SF IMRT technique.[171]

TABLE 44.11 INTENSITY-MODULATED RADIATION THERAPY FOR NASOPHARYNGEAL CARCINOMA: METHODS AND RESULTS BY DIFFERENT CENTERS

	UCSF[169,180]	MSKCC[172]	PWH[174]	SYS[181]	QMH[173]	QMH[182]	CUHK[183]	NCCS[184]	PYNEH[185]
No. of patients	118	74	63	104	50	50	865	195	193
Patient characteristics									
Treatment period	1995–2003	1998–2004	2000–2002	2001–2004	2000–2002	2000–2004	2001–2008	2002–2005	2005–2007
T category	All	All	All	All	T1–T2	T3–T4	All	All	All
Intensity-modulated RT									
PTV-G									
Margin around GTV (mm)	–	5–10	2	–	–	–	–	3–5	5–8
Total dose (Gy)	70	70.2	66	64–70	68–70	76	68	66–70	70
Dose per fraction (Gy)	2.12	2.34	2	2.33–2.56	2–2.06	2.17	2	2–2.12	2.12
Additional treatment									
Accelerated fractionation	–	80%	–	–	–	–	–	–	62%
Boost	22% ICB		32% ICB 24% 3D	–	–	–	–	10% ICB	–
Chemotherapy (%)	90	93	30	23	0	68	65	>57	84
Median follow-up (mo)	30	35	29	19	14	25	40	36.5	30
Tumor control									
Time point (y)	4	3	3	3	2	2	5	3	2
Local-FFR (%)	96	91	92	99	100	96	90.4	89.6	95
Nodal-FFR (%)	98	93	98	99	94	–	–	–	96
Distant-FFR (%)	72	78	79	88	94	94	84	89.2	90
Overall survival (%)	74	83	90	86	NR	92	83	94.3	92
Late toxicities									
Xerostomia (grade ≥2) (%)	2[a] (2 y)	32 (1 y)	23 (2 y)	–	–	–	–	–	–
Deafness (grade >2) (%)	7[a]	>15	15	–	–	42	–	–	–
Fibrosis (grade >2) (%)	–	–	11	–	–	14	–	–	–
Dysphagia (grade >2) (%)	1[a]	–	5	–	–	–	–	–	–
Hypopituitarism (%)	–	0	23	–	–	–	–	–	–
Osteonecrosis (%)	0.8	0	2	–	–	–	–	–	–
Temporal lobe necrosis (%)	0.8	0	3	–	–	4	–	–	–
Carotid pseudoaneurysm/ epistaxis (%)	0.8[a]	–	–	–	–	4	–	–	–

[a]Based on data reported by Lee et al.[169]

3-D, three-dimensional conformal boost; FFR, failure-free rate; GTV, gross tumor volume; ICB, intracavitary brachytherapy; MSKCC, Memorial Sloan Kettering Cancer Center (United States); NR, not reported; PTV-G, planning target volume for gross tumor; PWH, Prince of Wales Hospital (Hong Kong); QMH, Queen Mary Hospital (Hong Kong); RT, radiation therapy; SYS, Sun Yat-sen Cancer Center (China); UCSF, University of California, San Francisco (United States).

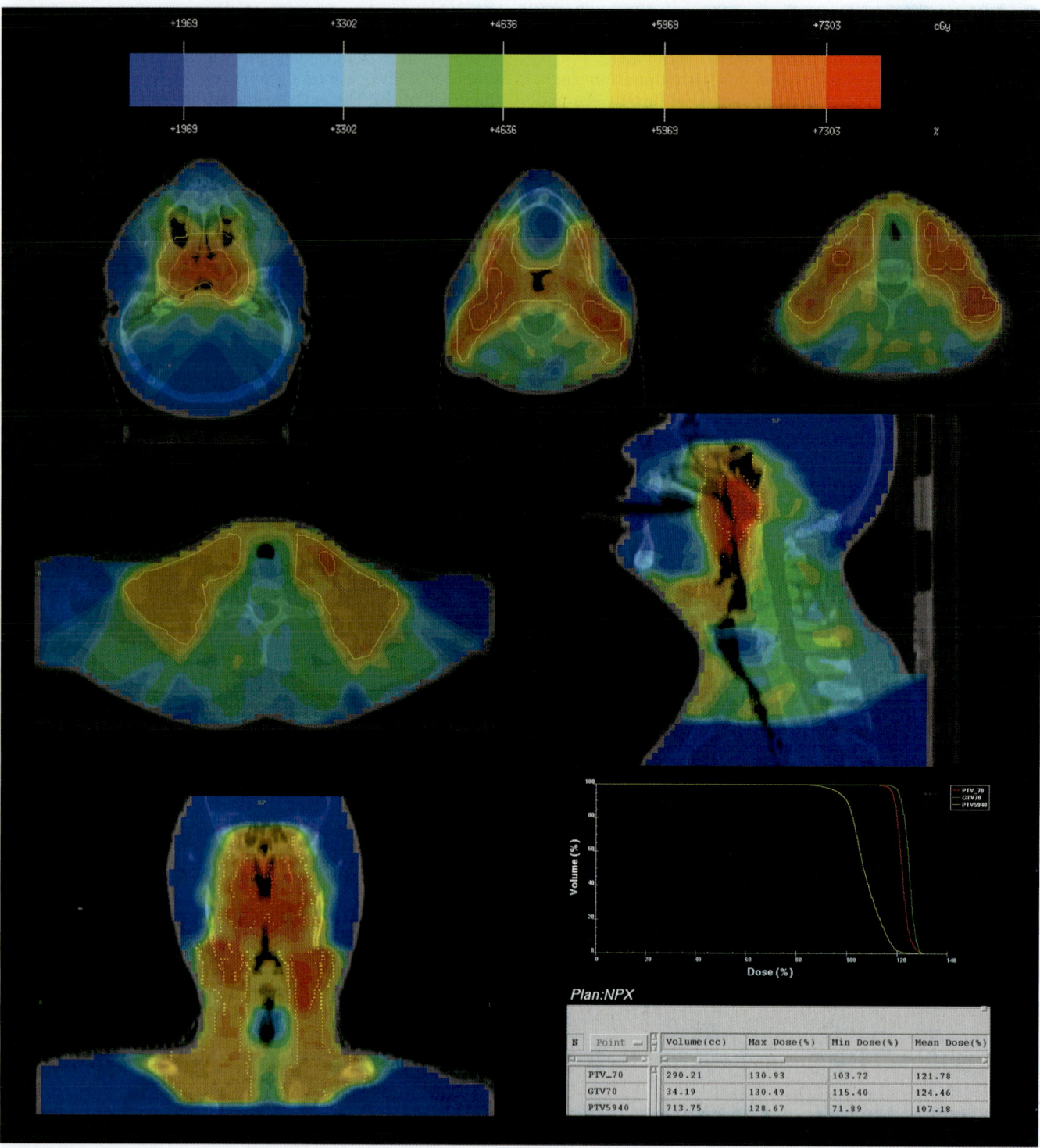

FIGURE 44.17. Intensity-modulated radiation therapy for a patient with T2N2M0 nasopharyngeal carcinoma treated at Memorial Sloan Kettering Cancer Center, showing delineation of gross tumor targets (GTV) and planning target volumes (PTV) for 70 Gy and 54 Gy, the dose distribution, and the dose volume histogram (DVH) for GTV, PTV_{70}, and $PTV_{59.4}$.

Figures 44.17 and 44.18 show examples of MSKCC IMRT plans delivered with the dynamic multileaf collimator (MLC) system using a sliding window technique to patients with early and advanced disease, respectively. A total dose of 70 Gy at 2.12 Gy/fraction to the $PTV_{gross\ disease}$ and 59.4 Gy to the $PTV_{high\text{-}risk\ subclinical}$ is given over 33 once-daily fractions (Table 44.10). For the low-neck, if split-field IMRT is used, a dose of 50.4 Gy at 1.8 Gy/fraction/day is generally prescribed. However, if the low-neck is included in the IMRT fields and is considered at low risk for nodal involvement, the $PTV_{low\text{-}risk\ subclinical}$ typically receives 54 Gy at 1.64 Gy/fraction/day.

Inverse planning involves the appropriate specification of normal tissue dose constraints. It is important to note that overstrigent use of normal tissue constraints might result in inadequate cover of tumor targets; therefore, optimal balance is essential. Different dose-constraint guidelines

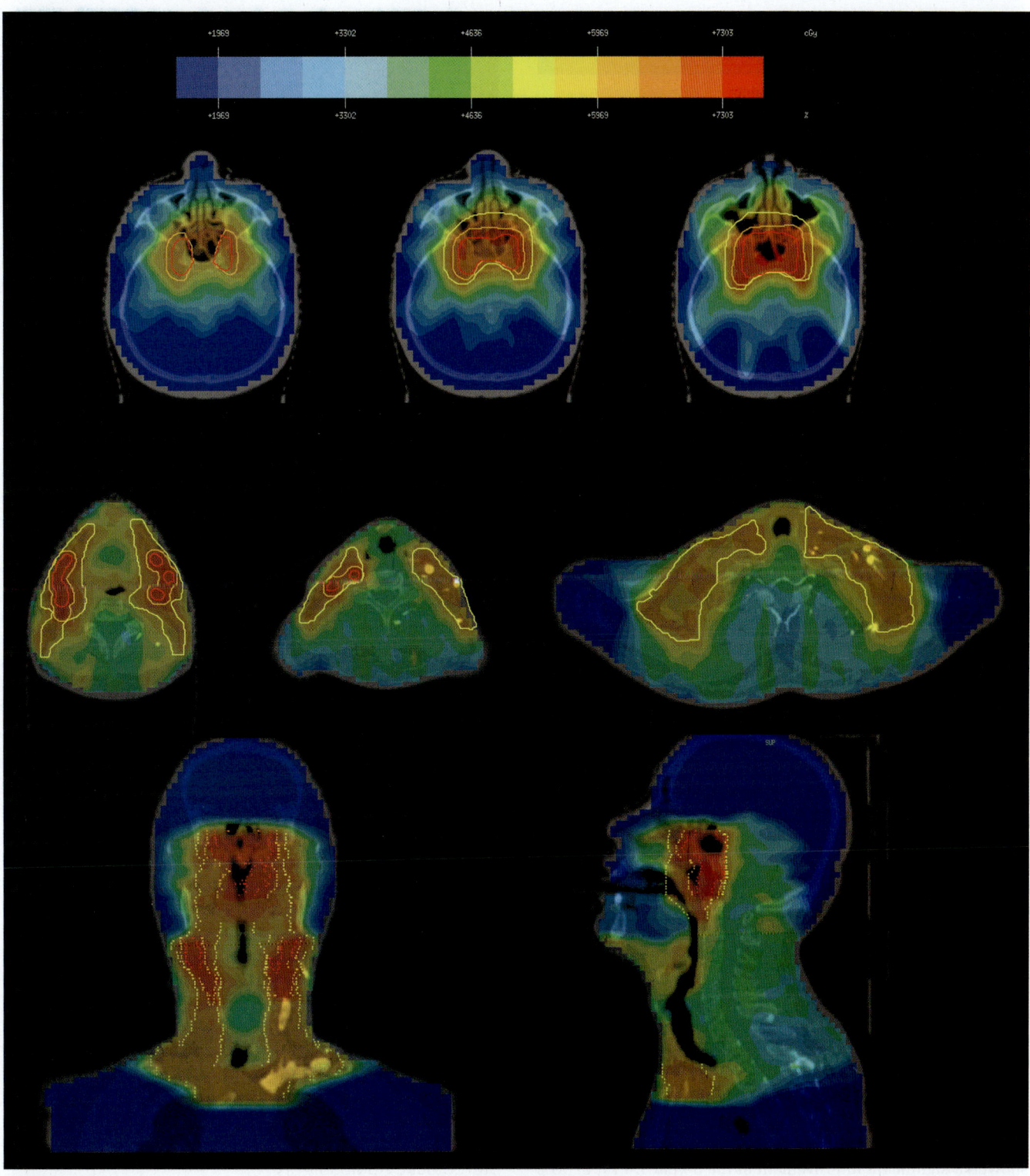

FIGURE 44.18. Intensity-modulated radiation therapy for a patient with T4N2M0 nasopharyngeal carcinoma treated at Memorial Sloan Kettering Cancer Center, showing delineation of gross tumor (GTV) and planning target volumes (PTV) for 70 Gy and 54 Gy, and the dose distribution.

have been suggested.[191,192] An example of dose-constraint guidelines is provided in Table 44.12, which displays the guidelines presently used at Memorial Sloan Kettering Cancer Center.

Dose Escalation

Excellent local tumor control has been reported by delivering an additional boost to patients with early disease treated by conventional 2-D technique.

Brachytherapy

The most commonly used method is brachytherapy. Intracavitary insertions[193–201] or interstitial implants[202–205] have been used in T1 to T3 nasopharyngeal carcinomas as a boost treatment following external beam radiation therapy (EBRT) or in the treatment of recurrent disease, either alone or in combination with EBRT. Brachytherapy is not suitable for treatment of tumors with intracranial extension because of the rapid reduction of dose as distance from the radioactive

TABLE 44.12 INTENSITY-MODULATED RADIATION THERAPY FOR NASOPHARYNGEAL CARCINOMA: AN EXAMPLE OF NORMAL TISSUE DOSE CONSTRAINTS^a

Structures	Constraints
Critical Structures	
Brainstem	Max < 5 Gy or 1% of PTV cannot exceed 60 Gy
Optic nerves	Max < 54 Gy or 1% of PTV cannot exceed 60 Gy
Optic chiasm	Max < 54 Gy or 1% of PTV cannot exceed 60 Gy
Spinal cord	Max < 45 Gy or 1 cc of the PTV cannot exceed 50 Gy
Mandible and temporomandibular joint	Max < 70 Gy or 1 cc of the PTV cannot exceed 75 Gy
Brachial plexus	Max < 66 Gy
Temporal lobes	Max < 60 Gy or 1% of PTV cannot exceed 65 Gy
Other Normal Structures	
Oral cavity	Mean < 40 Gy
Parotid gland	Mean ≤ 26 Gy (should be achieved in at least one gland) or at least 20 cc of the combined volume of both parotid glands will receive < 20 Gy or at least 50% of the gland will receive < 30 Gy (should be achieved in at least one gland)
Cochlea	V55 < 5%
Eyes	Mean < 35 Gy, max < 50 Gy
Lens	Max < 25 Gy
Glottic larynx	Mean < 45 Gy
Esophagus, postcricoid pharynx	Mean < 45 Gy

^{a}Based on guidelines presently used at Memorial Sloan Kettering Cancer Center.
PTV, planning target volume.

source increases. Since the advent of IMRT as primary radiotherapy for nasopharyngeal carcinoma and with its demonstration of excellent local control, the use of brachytherapy as a boost treatment following definitive IMRT has dramatically declined. Multiple applicators and techniques have been developed for the delivery of intracavitary brachytherapy.[195–197,199,201,206] In the past, intracavitary brachytherapy was delivered using low–dose rate (LDR) techniques. However, currently remote afterloading and fractionated high–dose rate (HDR) techniques are more commonly used (Fig. 44.19).[206]

Table 44.13 summarizes reports on the use of brachytherapy as a boost for dose escalation. Most studies demonstrated that local control up to 90% to 95% could be achieved for T1-2 tumors without excessive late damages. A retrospective comparison by Wang[196] from Massachusetts General Hospital (United States) reported that for T1 to T2 patients who received a 10- to 15 Gy, LDR brachytherapy boost after 60 to 64 Gy by EBRT had a 5-year L-FFR of 90% versus 54%, respectively, with P = .001 for patients receiving EBRT alone to 65 to 70 Gy. A similar study by Teo et al.[212] where delivery of 18 to 24 Gy in 3 fractions by HDR brachytherapy and showed a significant improvement of the 5-year L-FFR of 95% compared with a 90% 5-year L-FFR for EBRT only patients (P = .016).

However, a report by Ozyar et al.[210] of patients with T1 to T4 tumors treated with HDR brachytherapy boost of 12 Gy in 3 fractions did not show improvement over EBRT alone (3-year L-FFR: 86% vs. 94%; P = .23). More recently, a prospective trial by the International Atomic Energy Agency (IAEA) studied 275 patients with locoregionally advanced NPC disease (TNM stage III or M0 stage IV) who were all treated by induction chemotherapy followed by concurrent chemoradiotherapy to 70 Gy; then one randomized arm received a brachytherapy boost of 11 Gy LDR or 3 fractions of 3 Gy HDR. With a median follow-up of 29 months, the authors reported no additional benefit

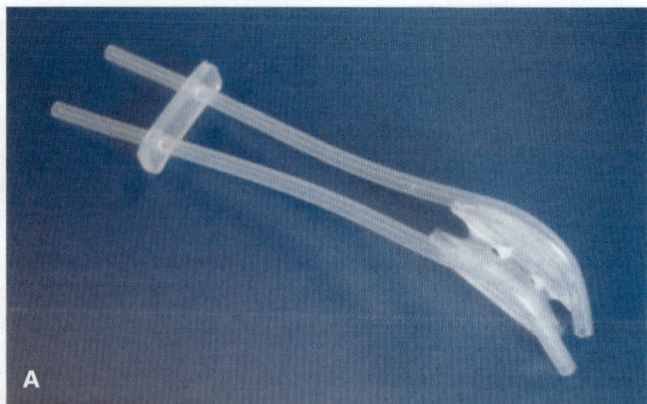

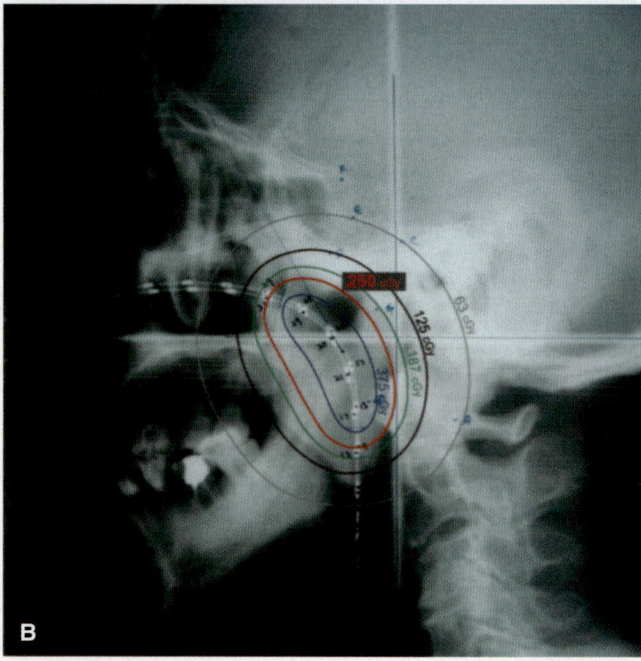

FIGURE 44.19. Endocavitary brachytherapy for nasopharyngeal carcinoma. **A:** The Rotterdam nasopharyngeal applicator. **B:** The simulator check-film showing the position of the radioactive sources and the dose distribution.

of brachytherapy boost compared with chemoradiotherapy alone toward 3-year OS (63.3% vs. 62.9%, P = .742, respectively), locoregional-FFR (54.4% vs. 60.5%, P = .647), or distant metastasis-free survival (52.6% vs. 59.8%, P = .496).[214]

One major limitation of brachytherapy is that the dose delivered is adequate only for superficial nonbulky tumors. Furthermore, optimal positioning of the applicators depends both on the individual clinician's skill and the patient's anatomic features.

Stereotactic Radiosurgery

Stereotactic radiosurgery or fractionated radiotherapy allows for precise delivery of highly conformal RT with a rapid dose falloff and provides an alternative for dose escalation. Hara et al.[215] reported a study of 82 patients with T1 to T4 tumors showing excellent 5-year L-FFR of 98% after receiving a median SRT boost of 12 Gy (range, 7 to 15 Gy) following EBRT to 66 Gy. However, despite the addition of concurrent chemotherapy in 76% of the patients, the distant failure rate was 32% and OS was 69%. With a median follow-up of 40.7 months for living patients, 12.1% of patients developed radiographic temporal lobe necrosis (only 2.4% were symptomatic with seizures) and 3.6% developed retinopathy. The risk was especially high in patients with T4 tumors.

TABLE 44.13 ADJUVANT BRACHYTHERAPY BOOST FOR PRIMARY TREATMENT OF NASOPHARYNGEAL CARCINOMA

Author	T Category[a]	External RT Dose (Gy)	Brachytherapy Modality	Dose (Gy)	Fraction	Local Control Day	Year	Rate (%)
Chang et al.[207]	T1	65–68	HDR-ICB	5–11	1–2	1–8	5	94
		65–68	HDR-ICB	15–16.5	3	15		80 vs. 74
		68–72	Control	–				(P = .01)
Lee et al.[198]	T1-3	54–72	HDR-ICB or LDR-ICB	5–7 10–54	2	1	5	89
Levendag et al.[194]	T1-2a	60	HDR-ICB	15	5	3	5	92
	T2b	70	HDR-ICB	11	2			
Lu et al.[208]	T1-2	66	HDR-ICB	10	2	8	2	94
Ng et al.[209]	T1-4	43–70	HDR-ICB	6–15	2–5	2–5	5	96
Ozyar et al.[210]	T1-4	59–71	HDR-ICB	12	3	3	5	86 vs. 94
		59–74	Control	–				(P = .23)
Ren et al.[211]	T2b	60	HDR-ICB	12–20	1	1	5	98 vs. 80
		68	Control	–				(P = .012)
Syed et al.[205]	T1-4	50–60	ICB + interstitial	33–37	1	3	5	93
Teo et al.[212]	T1-2a	60–71	HDR-ICB	18–24	3	15	5	95 vs. 90
		60–71	Control	–				(P = .17)
Vikram[213]	T1-4	60–66	Interstitial	160 in 1 yr			5	96
Wang[196]	T1-2	60–64	LDR-ICB	7–10	1	1	5	91 vs. 60
		65–70	Control	–				(P < .01)

[a]By 2002 AJCC sixth edition or 1997 AJCC fifth edition.
HDR, high–dose rate; ICB, intracavitary brachytherapy; LDR, low–dose rate; NR, not reported.

Altered Fractionation

Over the past few decades, studies have been conducted to explore the role of altered fractionation regimens in head and neck cancers, along with nasopharyngeal cancers. Hyperfractionation, accelerated fractionation, and a combination of which were explored in conjunction with concurrent chemotherapy.

Sanchiz et al.[216] conducted a large randomized trial examining twice-daily (BID) versus once-daily (QD) irradiation for head and neck cancer including tumors of the nasopharynx. 859 patients with advanced head and neck cancers (T3-T4, N0-3, M0 by UICC staging), which included 92 patients with nasopharyngeal carcinoma, were randomly assigned to QD irradiation (Group A), BID irradiation (Group B), or QD irradiation with concurrent 5-FU chemotherapy (Group C). Groups B and C showed a significant improvement in median duration of response and OS when compared to Group A. No significant differences were seen between Groups B and C.

The first randomized trial on accelerated fractionation (AF) for NPC by Teo et al.[217] used an uncommon schedule of 2.5 Gy/fraction QD for 8 fractions before randomization to an experimental arm using 1.6 Gy BID for an additional 32 fractions versus a control arm treated with 2.5 Gy QD for another 16 fractions. The trial was terminated early because of excessive neurologic toxicities in the AF arm (49% vs. 23%). For this series of 159 patients (62% with T1-2 tumors), the AF arm did not achieve a significant improvement in tumor control (5-year L-FFR, 89% vs. 85%). Jen et al.[218] reported on 222 patients where 76 patients received hyperfractionated RT at 1.2 Gy/fraction BID and 12 patients received accelerated–hyperfractionated RT at 1.6 Gy BID to a median dose of 80 Gy for these twice-daily RT groups. The remaining 134 patients are treated by conventional QD fractionation to a median dose of 70 Gy. The patients treated by BID fractionation did not demonstrate a statistically significant difference in 5-year L-FFR when compared to QD fractionation (T1-3, 93% vs. 86%; T4, 44% vs. 37%, respectively). The 1.2 Gy/fraction regimen did not cause excessive toxicity; however, patients treated with 1.6 Gy/fraction had a 27% incidence of temporal lobe necrosis.[219] See section *Sequelae of Treatment* for more details regarding the influence of dose fractionation on brain necrosis.

To minimize the risk of late damage, the more moderate AF schedule of the Danish Head and Neck Cancer Study Group 6 to 7 Trials using 2 Gy/fraction, 6 fractions per week[220] of 1,476 patients with head and neck cancer, of which 435 had pharyngeal tumors, including the nasopharynx, demonstrated accelerated fractionation resulted in significantly improved 5-year L-FFR (76% vs. 64% for 6 and 5 fractions, respectively, P = .0001) and disease-specific survival (73% vs. 66%, for 6 fractions and 5 fractions, respectively, P = .01) but not OS. This same fractionation schedule was tested retrospectively for NPC by Lee et al.[221] They reported for patients irradiated to a total dose of 66 Gy with 2-D technique when on an accelerated fractionation (AF) schedule had significantly higher L-FFR than those treated with conventional 5 fractions per week. The benefit was significant particularly for T3-4 tumors (87% vs. 62%; P < .01), and multivariate analyses confirmed that fractionation was an independent prognostic factor for overall progression (AF group, HR = 0.63, 95% CI, 0.41 to 0.98; P = .04). Additionally, no significant increase in late toxicity was observed at 3 years (20% vs. 15%).

This schedule was then used in the subsequent NPC-9902 trial initiated by the HKNPCSG,[222] which aimed to assess the therapeutic benefit of AF and/or concurrent–adjuvant chemoradiotherapy (CRT), that randomized 189 patients with locally advanced NPC (T3-T4, N0-1, M0) to four arms: (1) conventional fractionation (CF) alone, (2) AF (six fractions/week) alone, (3) CF with concurrent chemotherapy, and (4) AF with concurrent chemotherapy. Preliminary results with a median follow-up of 2.9 years showed that AF per se did not demonstrate a significant improvement in event-free survival (EFS) when compared with CF (AF vs. CF: HR 0.68, 95% CI 0.37 to 1.25, P = .22). However, AF combined with CRT (arm 4) achieved a strongly significant improvement when compared with CF alone (EFS: 94% vs. 70%, P = .008) but without an improvement in OS. A significant increase in acute and late toxicity in the AF combined with CRT arm was also noted.

From these and other experiences with altered fractionation schedules in the treatment of nasopharyngeal carcinoma, in addition to other head and neck cancers, it has been concluded that both total dose and overall treatment time are important factors in determining outcomes.[223] With the increasing use of IMRT, dose escalation—to allow ample dose delivery to the gross and subclinical disease—has become achievable without associated changes in rates of toxicity, considerably improving the therapeutic ratio

Section III

of concurrent chemoradiation and causing the above fractionation schemes to fall out of favor.

Chemotherapy

Nasopharyngeal carcinoma is generally regarded to be a highly chemosensitive disease. Although radiotherapy alone is the standard treatment for stage I NPC, concurrent chemoradiotherapy (CRT) with or without adjuvant chemotherapy is the current standard for locally advanced disease (stages III to VB) based on multiple randomized controlled trials and meta-analyses (Table 44.14). Although there is less evidence for CRT in intermediate stage (2010 AJCC stage II) disease, it is currently recommended that such patients be treated with CRT in light of pooled data from two phase III trials[236,237] and a more recent phase III trial from Chen et al.[233] In more detail, Chen and colleagues[233] demonstrated that Chinese stage II (equiv. to AJCC II-III; only 13% of the study's patients were AJCC 2010 stage III) NPC patients that received concurrent chemoradiotherapy had a superior 5-year OS compared to those treated with radiation alone (94.5% vs. 85.8%, P = .007) with improved distant control (94.8% vs. 83.9%, P = .007). Multivariate analyses found that the number of chemotherapy cycles was the only independent factor associated with improved OS, progression-free survival, and distant control. With the addition of chemotherapy, an increase in acute side effects was observed, but no significant increase in late effects was reported.

Concurrent Chemoradiotherapy

The landmark Intergroup 0099 trial was the first to document a significant survival benefit for CRT versus RT alone.[224] This trial randomized 147 patients with locally advanced NPC to either RT alone or CRT, at centers located in the United States. Chemotherapy consisted of concurrent cisplatin (CDDP; 100 mg/m² on days 1, 22, and 43), followed by three cycles of adjuvant CDDP (80 mg/m² on day 1) and 5-fluorouracil (5-FU; 1,000 mg/m²/d on days 1 to 4) every 4 weeks. Radiotherapy was delivered in 1.8 to 2 Gy fractions to a total dose of 70 Gy. The trial was closed early because of a significant overall survival benefit in favor of CRT (78% vs. 47% at 3 years). A 5-year update confirmed progression-free survival (58% vs. 29%) and overall survival (67% vs. 37%) in favor of CRT. Reactions to these findings were initially tempered by several limitations of the trial. Results achieved in the RT arm were much poorer than those generally obtained at centers treating endemic NPC. Outcomes in the CRT arm were in fact more consistent with outcomes obtained in endemic areas using RT alone. Another concern was that 24% of the enrolled patients had disease of keratinizing histology, and it was unknown whether the same benefit would be seen in endemic areas with predominantly undifferentiated disease.

Subsequent trials confirmed the benefit of concurrent CDDP-based chemotherapy in endemic populations. Wee et al.[228] reported the results of 221 stage III to IVB patients from Singapore randomized to receive either RT alone or CRT. Chemotherapy consisted of a slightly modified version of the Intergroup regimen: CDDP (25 mg/m² on days 1 to 4) for 3 cycles every 3 weeks, followed by adjuvant CDDP (20 mg/m² on days 1 to 4) and 5-FU (1,000 mg/m²/d on days 1 to 4) for 3 cycles. Radiotherapy was delivered to a dose of 70 Gy in 2-Gy fractions. Three-year overall survival for the CRT and RT arms was 85% and 65%, respectively (P = .006). CRT reduced the incidence of distant metastasis by 17% at 2 years (P = .003).

Langendijk et al.[238] performed a meta-analysis of 10 trials that randomized NPC patients to conventional RT or CRT. The 10 studies included 4 neoadjuvant trials,[239–242] 3 concurrent (+/- adjuvant) trials,[224,225,243] 2 adjuvant trials,[244,245] and 1 neoadjuvant + adjuvant trial.[246] The authors found a pooled hazard ratio for death of 0.82, with an absolute survival benefit of 4% at 5 years. Subgroup analysis revealed that the overall survival benefit was only significant for those patients receiving concurrent chemotherapy, with a hazard ratio for death of 0.48 and absolute survival benefit of 20% at 5 years. Analysis of the neoadjuvant chemotherapy trials found a significant reduction in locoregional recurrence and distant metastasis, but no overall survival benefit.

These results, in combination with results from a second meta-analysis[247] and the Singapore trial, reported by Wee et al.,[228] confirmed CRT as the standard approach in stage III, IVA, and IVB NPC. At many centers, the standard course of chemotherapy has been based on the US Intergroup regimen, which consisted of concurrent high-dose CDDP (100 mg/m² × 3 cycles) and adjuvant CDDP/5-FU for 3 cycles. This regimen is associated with significant acute and late toxicities, and patient compliance is frequently difficult to achieve. In the Intergroup 0099 trial, for example, only 63% completed all 3 cycles of concurrent chemotherapy, and only 55% were able to receive all 3 courses of adjuvant therapy.[224]

TABLE 44.14 RANDOMIZED PROSPECTIVE TRIALS WITH CONCURRENT CHEMORADIOTHERAPY

Author	Year	Patients (No.)	Control arm	Radiotherapy Dose (Gy)	Experimental Arm (Chemotherapy)			Timepoint (year)	Tumor Control (%)ᵃ		
					Induction	Concurrent	Adjuvant		LRC	DMFS	OS
Concurrent ± adjuvant chemoradiotherapy (phase III trials)											
Al-Sarraf[224]	1998	193	RT	70	–	P	PF	5	NR	NR	63 vs. 37
Lin[225]	2003	284	RT	70–74	–	PF	–	5	89 vs. 73	79 vs. 70	72 vs. 54
Kwong[226]	2004	222	RT	52.5–68	–	U	PF/VBM	3	80 vs. 72	85 vs. 71	87 vs. 77
Chan[227]	2005	350	RT	66	–	P	–	5	NR	NR	70 vs. 59
Wee[228]	2005	221	RT	70	–	P	PF	5	NR	83 vs. 63	67 vs. 49
Zhang[229]	2005	115	RT	70–74	–	O	–	2	NR	92 vs. 80	100 vs. 77
Chen[b,230]	2008	316	RT	70	–	P	PF	2	98 vs. 92	87 vs. 79	90 vs. 80
Lee[231]	2010	348	RT	70	–	P	PF	5	88 vs. 78	74 vs. 68	68 vs. 64
Lee[232]	2011	189	RT	70	–	P	PF	5	81(C)–90(A) vs. 85(C)–75(A)	75(C)–95(A) vs. 75(C)–74(A)	78(C)–85(A) vs. 66(C,A)
Chenb[233]	2011	230	RT	68–70	–	P	–	5	93 vs. 91	95 vs. 84	86 vs. 95
Induction–concurrent chemoradiotherapy (phase II trials)											
Hui[234]	2009	65	CCRT	66	DP	P	–	2	NR	NR	95 vs. 86
Fountzilas[235]	2012	141	CCRT	66–70	PET	P	–	3	NR	NR	72 vs. 67

ᵃExperimental arm versus control arm.
ᵇStage II by Chinese 1992 staging system (equivalent to stages II to III by AJCC seventh edition), 13% of patients were AJCC stage III.
A, accelerated fractionation; C, conventional fractionation; CCRT, concurrent chemoradiation; D, docetaxel; DMFS, distant metastasis-free survival; E, epirubicin; F, fluorouracil; LRC, locoregional control rate; M, methotrexate; NR, not reported; O, oxaliplatin; OS, overall survival; P, cisplatin; RT, radiotherapy alone; T, paclitaxel; U, uracil and tegafur; V, vincristine.

As a result, weekly CDDP has been adopted by many institutions, especially for patients with poor nutritional status.[248] In a phase III trial, comparing CRT versus RT alone in 350 patients with locally advanced disease, Chan et al.[227] demonstrated good efficacy and tolerability for a regimen consisting of weekly CDDP (40 mg/m²). Seventy-eight percent of patients in the CRT arm received at least 4 cycles of CDDP, and CRT was associated with a statistically significant survival benefit after adjusting for age and disease stage. A more recent randomized study by Chen et al.[249] confirmed that OS and locoregional control of weekly CRT were superior to RT alone with weekly CDDP, though it did observe greater acute (63% vs. 32%) and late (33% vs. 26%) toxicity in the CRT arm. In addition, a retrospective comparative study by Jades et al.[250] found similar clinical outcomes and toxicity profiles between concurrent weekly CDDP and the every 3 weeks schedule. Ultimately, whether weekly CDDP is equivalent to the every 3 weeks Intergroup regimen remains to be directly evaluated in a randomized fashion.

Other Chemotherapy Agents

Weekly oxaliplatin (70 mg/m²) has been demonstrated to have good tolerability and efficacy, albeit in the setting of a small phase III trial of 115 patients randomized to CRT or RT alone.[229] Carboplatin has also been employed as a substitute to high-dose CDDP, with comparable efficacy, in a noninferiority trial reported by Chitapanarux et al.[251] Two hundred and six patients were randomized to either concurrent high-dose CDDP and adjuvant CDDP/5-FU or concurrent weekly carboplatin and adjuvant carboplatin/5-FU. The trial had 80% power to detect a hazard ratio for death of 1.25 at 3 years. No significant difference in disease-free survival or overall survival was seen at a median follow-up of 26 months. Disease-free survival was 59.6% and 64.7% (P = .522) for the carboplatin and CDDP arms, respectively.

Cetuximab to target epidermal growth factor receptor (EGFR; EGFR overexpression is observed in >80% of NPC patients) has been examined in a phase II trial with optimistic findings.[252] The 2-year rates of OS, locoregional progression-free survival, distant metastasis-free survival, and progression-free survival were 89.9%, 93.0%, 82.8%, and 86.5%, respectively. Bevacizumab, to exploit the angiogenesis pathway (vascular endothelial growth factor; VEGF is overexpressed in about two-thirds of NPC patients), has been studied in a phase II trial where the agent was added to the standard chemoradiotherapy schedule and demonstrated promising results.[253] Lee et al. reported, with a median follow-up of 2.5 years, a 2-year OS, locoregional progression-free survival, distant metastasis-free survival, and progression-free survival of 90.9%, 83.7%, 90.8%, and 74.7%, respectively.

Adjuvant Chemotherapy

Although good efficacy and tolerability have been shown for select alternative regimens, the greatest body of evidence for concurrent CRT has been with the CDDP-based US Intergroup regimen of concurrent plus adjuvant chemotherapy. Nevertheless, it is unknown whether the adjuvant chemotherapy component of the US Intergroup regimen contributed to its survival benefit.

Compliance with adjuvant chemotherapy can be especially difficult, as patients are recovering from the acute effects of CRT. Randomized trials comparing RT alone to RT plus adjuvant chemotherapy have all been negative to date.[245,246] Moreover, there are data to suggest a survival benefit for concurrent CRT without adjuvant chemotherapy.[225,227]

In 2011, Chen et al.[254] reported a randomized trial that compared concurrent CRT to concurrent CRT plus adjuvant chemotherapy (CDDP/5-FU) in 508 patients. With a median follow-up of 38 months, there were fewer failures at any site in the concurrent chemoradiotherapy plus adjuvant chemotherapy group versus the chemoradiotherapy group only (14% vs. 16%); however, this difference was not statistically significant (P = .13). It is important to note that this trial was not designed as a noninferiority trial against the standard. In addition, compliance was an issue in this study, where about 18% of patients randomized to the adjuvant arm did not receive adjuvant chemotherapy.[254] Until further data emerges, adjuvant chemotherapy is considered by many to be optional in the setting of concurrent CRT. In light of these conflicting data, a biomarker such as posttreatment EBV DNA to help stratify patients for treatment with adjuvant chemotherapy versus observation would be extremely valuable. As discussed above, this is currently being investigated in the NRG Oncology HN001 trial, which randomizes patients with undetectable post-CRT EBV DNA to observation versus standard adjuvant chemotherapy consisting of cisplatin and 5-FU.

Neoadjuvant Chemotherapy

The role of adding neoadjuvant chemotherapy prior to concurrent CRT remains undefined but is an area of great interest, given predominantly distant pattern of failure experienced among patients with locally advanced NPC. Figure 44.20 demonstrates the potential value of induction chemotherapy in tumor control. Until recently, only phase II data existed regarding the use of induction chemotherapy in this setting. However, the results of three large phase III randomized trials were recently published. In a multicenter phase III study conducted by Sun Yat-sen University, 480 patients with stage III to IVB NPC were randomized to cisplatin chemoradiation with or without docetaxel, cisplatin, and fluorouracil induction therapy.[255] With median follow-up of 45 months, patients treated with induction chemotherapy had significantly improved 3-year failure-free survival (80% vs. 72%, P = .034), overall survival (92% vs. 86%, P = .029), and distant failure-free survival (90% vs. 83%, 0.031). Overall toxicity was higher in the induction arm, with 73% versus 54% of patients in the CRT alone arm experiencing a grade 3 or 4 adverse event (P < .0001). In another phase III multicenter trial reported by Cao et al.,[256] 476 patients were randomized to cisplatin chemoradiation with or without cisplatin and fluorouracil induction therapy. Patients treated with induction chemotherapy had significantly higher 3-year disease-free survival (82.0% vs. 74.1%, P = .028) with a strong trend for improved 3-year distant failure-free survival (86.0% vs. 82.0%, P = .056); however, there was no difference in overall survival, and toxicity was significantly increased during concurrent chemoradiation in patients who received induction.

The preliminary results of a phase III trial, organized by the Hong Kong Nasopharyngeal Cancer Study Group (NPC-0501), were recently reported. This study by Lee et al.[257] randomized 706 patients to one of three arms: (1) CDDP/5-FU induction chemotherapy plus concurrent CDDP-RT, (2) concurrent CDDP-RT plus adjuvant CDDP/5-FU, or (3) CDDP/capecitabine induction chemotherapy plus concurrent CDDP-RT. In addition, patients in each of these three arms were randomized to either conventional or accelerated RT. Because of the multiarmed design, patient numbers were limited in each of the six arms. Overall, the benefit of induction chemotherapy with respect to OS remains uncertain; however, the capecitabine induction arm demonstrated an improved toxicity profile that may inform future studies. Additional phase III trials are ongoing, and the OS results from the Sun Yat-sen trial must be confirmed in other studies before induction chemotherapy can be considered standard in the treatment of locally advanced NPC.

Pre-Treatment

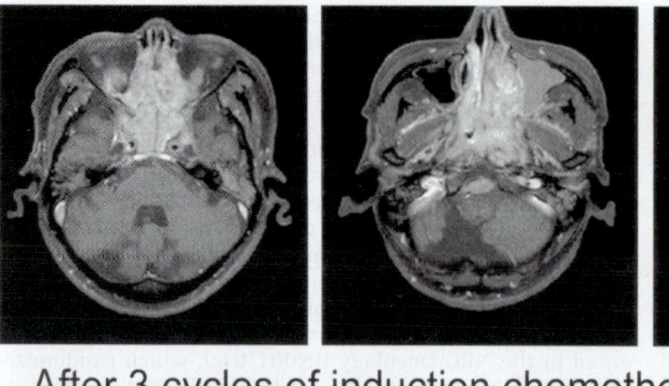
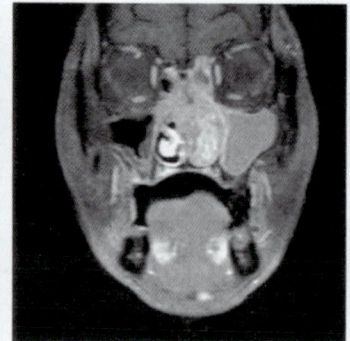
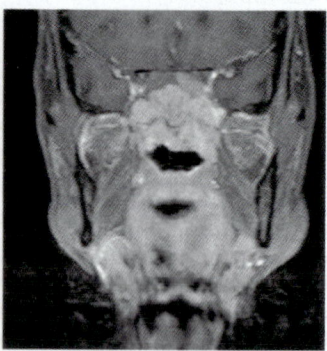

After 3 cycles of induction chemotherapy

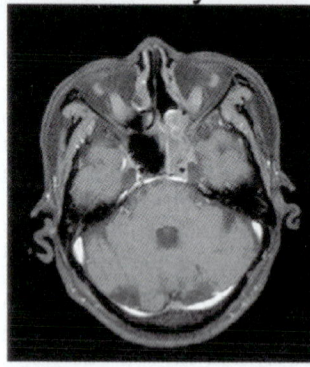
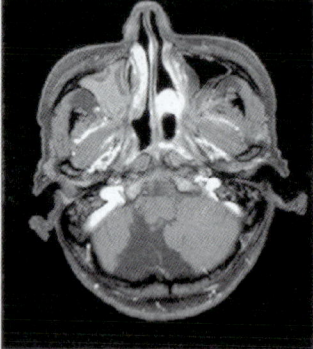
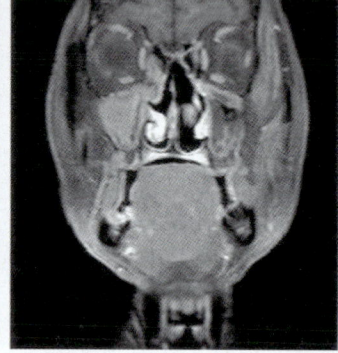
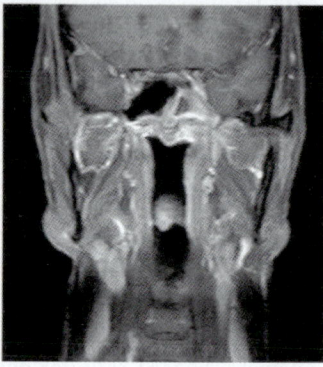

FIGURE 44.20. Magnetic resonance imaging showing shrinkage of primary tumor by induction chemotherapy using cisplatin and 5-fluorouracil before proceeding to concurrent cisplatin and radiotherapy. (Reprinted from Lee AW, Lau KY, Hung WM, et al. Potential improvement of tumor control probability by induction chemotherapy for advanced nasopharyngeal carcinoma. *Radiother Oncol* 2008;87[2]:204–210. Copyright © 2008 Elsevier Ireland Ltd. With permission.)

PERSISTENT/RECURRENT NPC

Because long-term survival can be achieved for a substantial proportion of patients with early locoregional recurrence and useful palliation for those with extensive disease, aggressive salvage treatment is usually advocated. Several approaches can be used successfully, including surgery, brachytherapy, and EBRT. Chemotherapy is generally used in conjunction with local treatment in patients with advanced disease.

Early Detection and Diagnosis

Although progress in surgical and reconstructive techniques and radiotherapy delivery methods has led to improvements in the control rate for primary treatment of NPC, local failure remains a problem for patients with advanced T category. Distinction should be made between persistent disease (tumors that do not completely regress following primary treatment) and recurrent disease (tumors that re-emerge after initial complete regression) because the prognoses and therapeutic considerations are different, with better survival and control rates for persistent disease.[258]

As tumors regress at different rates following RT, one difficult decision is when to consider residual tumors as genuine persistence and proceed with salvage treatment. In one prospective study by Kwong et al.,[259] serial biopsies of the nasopharynx were performed on 803 patients after RT treatment to observe the time course of histologic remission for NPC and determine its prognostic significance. The 5-year L-FFR was 82% for patients who achieved early histologic remission (<5 weeks) and 77% for those with delayed remission (5 to <12 weeks), but only 40% for those with persistent disease at 12 weeks, despite subsequent salvage treatment.[259] Thus, although delayed histologic remission was not a poor

prognostic factor, positive biopsies beyond 12 weeks did indicate poor prognosis. The optimal time for intervention remains uncertain, but because it is important to avoid both unnecessary overtreatment and excessive delay in treatment, the authors recommended an observation period of 10 weeks before additional treatment.[259]

Early detection of locoregional failure is crucial for a better chance of salvage, and regular follow-up after completion of primary treatment is recommended. Frequently used methods include manual palpation, rigid nasopharyngeal endoscopy and nasopharyngeal biopsies, imaging techniques (e.g., CT and MRI), and serologic tests (e.g., anti-EBV titers, plasma EBV DNA levels).

Nasopharyngoscopy is more sensitive than CT and MRI in detecting tumor persistence/recurrence and is the preferred method for initial screening.[260,261] If a patient presents with suspicious endoscopic findings or elevated anti-EBV titers, a nasopharyngeal biopsy is performed to confirm diagnosis. CT or MRI is performed upon a confirmed diagnosis to delineate the tumor extent.[262] Although MRI has limitations in separating tumor recurrence from radiation fibrosis,[263] it is superior to CT in demonstrating extent of soft tissue tumors, as well as identifying submucosal infiltration, marrow infiltration in the skull base, perineural invasion, and intracranial spread.[260,264,265]

Technetium-99m methoxyisobutylisonitrile (MIBI) single-photon emission computed tomography (SPECT) may be a useful tool for differentiating persistent or recurrent tumor from radiation fibrosis[266] and was shown by Kostakoglu et al.[267] to be superior to MRI performed at 3 to 6 months post-RT in diagnosing complete response. The advent of FDG-PET is another valuable development. FDG-PET and MRI were compared in 67 NPC patients 4 to 70 months after completion of RT and found FDG-PET superior to MRI in all aspects in detection of local recurrence, with increased sensitivity (100% vs. 62%) and specificity (93% vs. 44%).[268] It may also contribute useful information to questionable findings on MRI.[269,270]

Paraneoplastic syndrome (PNS) can signal a silent neoplasm and may precede the clinical manifestation itself of persistent or recurrent NPC. PNS can follow the course of the tumor and can sometimes be used to diagnose recurrence and monitor its evolution with the most common dermatologic manifestation being dermatomyositis and the syndrome of inappropriate antidiuretic hormone secretion (SIADH) being a common endocrinologic presentation.[271]

Circulating cell-free DNA of EBV may be another useful tool for early detection of treatment failure. A longitudinal study by Lo et al.[120] showed that elevation of EBV DNA levels was noted in patients with relapse up to 6 months before detectable clinical disease. In addition, EBV DNA copy number has been shown to predict margin status postsalvage nasopharyngectomy. Wei et al.[272] reported that in early recurrent NPC patients with elevated EBV DNA copies, surgical resection reduced the copy number of EBV DNA postoperatively and that negative surgical margins are associated with zero EBV DNA copies postoperatively.

The incorporation of plasma EBV DNA measurements as screening prior to PET in detecting posttreatment failures of NPC has been investigated. In a prospective study by Wang et al.,[128] 245 NPC patients in remission were monitored prospectively via plasma EBV DNA assay every 3 to 6 months, where 36 patients with abnormal EBV DNA tests and 5 patients with clinical suggestion signs of recurrence, but undetectable EBV DNA levels, underwent FDG-PET scans. Elevated EBV DNA levels correctly predicted all 36 recurrences, whereas the 5 patients who presented with clinical signs suggestive of recurrent disease but with undetectable EBV DNA levels did not have recurrent disease. The authors concluded that plasma EBV DNA appears to be a useful biomarker for posttreatment surveillance in NPC.

Meanwhile, the clearance rate of plasma EBV DNA during the first month of chemotherapy has also been found to predict tumor response and patient survival in 30 patients with recurrent NPC and may have potential as an early prognostic marker to help guide salvage treatment.[126]

Additional Radiation for Persistent Disease

Excellent results have been reported when using brachytherapy for locally persistent disease after a full course of EBRT (Table 44.15, part A), with 5-year L-FFR in the range of 87% to 95% for patients with initial T1 tumors (AJCC 2002 T1–2a).[212,258,273,274,276] Preliminary evidence suggests that patients with disease persisting from initial T2 tumors (AJCC 2002 T2b) could also be effectively treated by brachytherapy.[275]

Stereotactic RT is a valuable alternative for delivering additional EBRT. Yau et al.[278] studied 755 patients with T1-4 tumors and found that 7% had positive biopsies 8 weeks after completion of primary RT. Twenty-one patients were treated with fractionated stereotactic RT to a median dose of 15 Gy and achieved a 3-year L-FFR of 82%, which was similar to the corresponding L-FFR of 86% in the complete responders and was significantly better than the corresponding L-FFR of 71% in 24 patients treated with high–dose rate brachytherapy to a median dose of 20 Gy.

Reirradiation for Recurrent Disease

Various radiation therapy modalities are used to treat recurrent NPC, including intracavitary brachytherapy, external beam irradiation, interstitial implantation, particle beam radiotherapy, and stereotactic radiosurgery (Table 44.16).[195,200,201,203,204,291] IMRT has also been used with excellent preliminary results, with control rates of up to 100% for rT1-3.[287]

The most important prognostic factors are the TNM stage of the tumor at the time of recurrence and reirradiation dose. Thorough restaging, including metastatic workup, is necessary. A study of 891 patients with local recurrence from 1976 to 1985 by Lee et al.[292] showed that only 32% of reirradiated patients achieved local salvage, with 54% developing regional and/or distant failure. Most series using conventional 2-D technique showed that doses ≥60 Gy were associated with better outcome.[195,201,281,282] For IMRT, 60 to 70 Gy is recommended, taking into account factors such as previous radiation amount, overlap between previously treated area and target for reirradiation, interval between RT courses, tumor bulk, and whether concurrent chemotherapy will be given.[293]

Lee et al.[294] retrospectively compared the symptomatic late toxicity rate in 487 patients with two courses of EBRT versus 3,635 patients with one course and found that the major determinant of late complications was severity of damage during the initial course and that the sum of total biologic dose tolerated (BED-Σ) was higher than expected with a single-course treatment (BED-1). This suggested partial recovery of normal tissue (especially in patients reirradiated after 2 or more years) and higher tolerance for reirradiation when primary treatment was given with better sparing of normal tissues. Assuming an α/β ratio of 3 Gy, the BED-Σ that incurred 20% toxicity at 5 years was 129% that of BED-1.

Brachytherapy has been widely used for treatment of recurrent NPC (Table 44.15, part B) and can be used effectively on its own for early-stage recurrent NPC.[258,273] Using interstitial implants with radioactive gold grains, Kwong et al.[258] reported a 5-year L-FFR of 63%; complications included headache (28%), palatal fistula (19%), and mucosal necrosis (16%). Law et al.[273] achieved excellent local salvage up to 89% with iridium mold, but the complication rate was 53%.

The combination of brachytherapy and EBRT is useful, particularly when conventional 2-D technique is used. Lee et al.[281] showed that patients reirradiated by combined modalities had an improved 5-year L-FFR of 45% compared with 32% by EBRT alone and 29% by brachytherapy alone. The superiority of the combined method has been supported by other studies.[195,201,277,279] A study from Memorial Sloan Kettering Cancer Center

TABLE 44.15 RESULTS OF LOCALLY PERSISTENT/RECURRENT NASOPHARYNGEAL CARCINOMA TREATED WITH BRACHYTHERAPY

Author	T Category	Modality	Brachytherapy			Local Control	
			Dose (Gy)	Fraction	Day	Time (y)	Rate (%)
Part A. Local persistence							
Kwong et al.[258]	T1	Interstitial gold grain	60			5	87
Law et al.[273]	T1–2a	Iridium mold	40			5	90
Leung et al.[274]	T1–2	HDR-ICB	22.5–24	3	15	5	95
Leung et al.[275]	T2b	HDR-ICB	22.5–24	3	15	5	97
Zheng et al.[276]	T1	HDR-ICB	15–30	5–6	15–18	5	100
	T2	HDR-ICB	15–30	5–6	15–18		90
Part B. Local recurrence							
Kwong et al.[258]	rT1	Interstitial gold grain	60			5	63
Law et al.[273]	rT1–2a	Iridium mold	50–55[a]			5	89
Leung et al.[277]	rT1–2	EBRT + HDR-ICB	50 + 14.8[a]	3	15	3	72

[a]Median dose.
EBRT, external beam radiotherapy; HDR-ICB, high–dose-rate intracavitary brachytherapy.

TABLE 44.16 RESULTS ON REIRRADIATION FOR LOCAL RECURRENCE OF NASOPHARYNGEAL CARCINOMA

Author	Year	N	Reirradiation Technique	Time (y)	Treatment Outcome (Actuarial Rate)		Major Late Toxicity (Cumulative Incidence)	
					Local Control (%)	Survival (%)	Overall (%)	Brain Necrosis (%)
Fu et al.[279]	1975	39	All 2-D	5	26	41	23	NR
Yan et al.[280]	1983	219[a]	All 2-D	5	18	>29	>12	NR
Wang[195]	1987	51	All 2-D	5	NR	33	6	2
Pryzant et al.[201]	1992	53	All 2-D	5	35	18	NR	NR
Lee et al.[281]	1997	654	All 2-D	5	rT1: 35 rT2: 28 rT3-4: 11	16	26	3
Teo et al.[282]	1998	123	All 2-D	5	5	rT1: 43 rT2: 31 rT3-4: 16	rT1: 63 rT2: 48 rT3-4: 31	NR
Chua et al.[283]	1998	97	All 2-D	5	NR	rT1-2: 57 rT3: 42 rT4: 17	NR	16
Leung et al.[277]	2000	91	All 2-D	5	38	30	57	27
Chang et al.[284]	2000	186	81% 2-D, 19% 3-D	3	NR	rT1: 39 rT2: 24 rT3: 28 rT4: 4	2-D: 23 3-D: 9	2-D: 14 3-D: 0
Zheng et al.[285]	2005	86	All 3-D	5	rT1: 92 rT2: 81 rT3: 68 rT4: 41	rT1: 70 rT2: 52 rT3: 32 rT4: 10	49	16
Lu et al.[286]	2004	49	IMRT	3/4	100	NR	NR	NR
Chua et al.[287]	2005	31	IMRT	1	rT1-3: 10% rT4: 35	63	19	7
Koutcher et al.[288]	2010	29	83 % IMRT, 4% 2-D, 13% 3-D	5	52	60	31	17
Ozyigit et al.[289]	2011	51	47% SBRT, 53% 3-D	2	rT1-2: 75 rT3-4: 54	rT1-2: 85 rT3-4: 46	3-D: 48 SBRT: 21	3-D: 19 SBRT: 4
Qiu et al.[290]	2011	70	IMRT	2	66	67	36	NR

[a]Patients with regional relapse included.

2-D, conventional two-dimensional external radiotherapy and/or brachytherapy; 3-D, three-dimensional conformal radiotherapy; IMRT, intensity-modulated radiation therapy; SBRT, stereotactic body radiation therapy.

(MSKCC) associated combined modality treatment (CMT), consisting of EBRT followed by brachytherapy, achieved similar L-FFR with previous historical series. CMT also demonstrated fewer late grade 3 or higher events compared with patients receiving EBRT alone (8% vs. 73%, respectively).[288]

Stereotactic radiosurgery or fractionated stereotactic radiotherapy is another useful tool for retreatment of local recurrence, as it allows for rapid falloff of radiation dose outside tumor volume and near surrounding critical structures and can be used either alone for smaller lesions or in combination with EBRT for larger ones. Control rates ranging from 53% to 86% have been reported.[295-298] For advanced recurrence with extension beyond the nasopharynx, this method offers better dose coverage than brachytherapy. A higher salvage rate from adding stereotactic radiation as a boost after EBRT has been reported.[284,296,299] Although most series reported a low risk of complications, massive hemorrhage with potential fatal outcome has been described.[296] Radiosurgery should thus be avoided when there is direct tumor encasement of the carotid artery or when a high cumulative dose has already been delivered. Fractionated stereotactic radiotherapy has shown improved late toxicity profile compared to 3-D conformal RT[289] and single-dose radiosurgery[300] and may also give better local control rates compared with single-fraction radiosurgery.[301]

Advances in imaging technology and radiotherapy techniques have made it possible to reduce target volume without jeopardizing local control, reducing complication rates. Table 44.17 summarizes the treatment outcome and severe late complications by external beam reirradiation. Past series using 2-D technique achieved 5-year survival rates in the range of 16% to 63%, and the incidence of temporal lobe necrosis ranged from 2% to 27%. The use of 3-D conformal radiotherapy showed improving results. In one study by Chang et al.[284] none of the patients reirradiated by 3-D technique developed temporal lobe necrosis compared with 14% of those reirradiated by 2-D technique. Zheng et al.[285] reported a 5-year local salvage rate of 71% from 3-D technique, but the actuarial rate of late toxicities (grade 4) was still as high as 49%.

The use of IMRT for reirradiation has shown very encouraging short-term results. Using IMRT to deliver 68 to 70 Gy, Lu et al.[286] reported 100% salvage rate without any severe late complications in a series of 49 patients with a median follow-up of 9 months. Using IMRT to a median dose of 54 Gy in 31 patients (with or without induction chemotherapy and stereotactic boost), Chua et al.[287] reported a 1-year control rate of 100% for rT1-T3 and 35% for rT4, with late complications (> grade 3) of 25% (at 1 year). Using a median dose of 70 Gy in 70 patients, Qiu et al.[290] reported a locoregional salvage rate of 66% with similar toxicity rate at 2 years. Although rT staging did not predict control rate, original T classification remained a significant adverse prognostic factor and may serve as a strong marker for the underlying locally aggressive biology of the original disease. Longer follow-up is needed to better evaluate treatment results and sequelae resulting from IMRT.

As another alternative, proton-beam therapy (PBT) allows for delivery of radiation therapy dose distributions that are typically more conformal than can be achieved with IMRT. This is due to the physical properties of the proton beam that result in maximal dose delivery at a narrow specified

TABLE 44.17 INCIDENCE OF LATE TOXICITY FOLLOWING RADIATION WITH CONVENTIONAL TECHNIQUE (WITHOUT CONCURRENT CHEMOTHERAPY) FOR NASOPHARYNGEAL CARCINOMA

Severe Late Complication	Sanguineti et al.[28] (N = 378)	Chao and Perez[43] (N = 164)	Lee et al.[39] (N = 4,527)	Yeh et al.[302] (N = 849)	Leung et al.[303] (N = 880)[a]
Period	1954–1992	1956–1991	1976–1985	1983–1998	1990–1998
Radiotherapy					
Total dose (Gy)	61–70	56–69	65[b]	68–76	62.5–66[b]
Dose per fraction (Gy)	NR	1.8–2	2.5–4.2	1.8	2–2.5
Altered fractionation (%)	8	Nil	Nil	Nil	Nil
Sequential chemotherapy (%)	Nil	Nil	Nil	8	20
Overall incidence (%)					
Grading of toxicity	≥3	≥3	≥2	≥1	?
Crude rate	30.4	14	30.8	NR	16.5
Actuarial rate	19 (10 y)	NR	60 (10 y)	NR	14 (5 y)
Treatment mortality (%)	3.2	3	1.4	NR	0.9
Types of complications (%)					
Temporal lobe necrosis	1.1	1.2	3	6[c]	1.1
Brainstem encephalopathy/myelopathy	2.4		1		
Cranial neuropathy	4.5		5.3	3.3	6.8
Endocrine dysfunction	7.9		3.5		8.6
Severe epistaxis		1.2	0.6		0.3
Carotid rupture		0.6			
Hearing loss	2.6		8.2	54[c]	
Persistent otitis			2.5	32[c]	
Trismus	2.9	0.6	5.1	12[c]	0.7
Bone damage[d]	2.6	2.4	0.4		
Eyeball damage[e]			0.2		
Soft tissue necrosis/fistula	1.1	1.8	0.4		0.5
Pharynx stricture/dysphagia		1.2		6[c]	
Soft tissue fibrosis	4.2		15.9	25[c]	1.4
Persistent lymphedema	0.5	0.6	0.1		
Radiation-induced malignancy			<0.1		

[a]Patients with one course of radiotherapy.
[b]Median dose equivalent to 2 Gy/fraction.
[c]Five-year actuarial rate.
[d]Bone necrosis, fracture, or osteomyelitis.
[e]Cataract, retinitis, corneal ulcer.
NR, not reported.

depth in the tissue, a phenomenon known as the Bragg peak. Because of the increased precision, PBT is especially useful in the setting of reirradiation, where it is critically important to minimize overlap of radiation fields from multiple treatments, particularly for the dose to surrounding sensitive organs such as the cranial nerves and brain. An analysis of dose volume histograms from patients who underwent reirradiation with PBT for recurrent NPC found that patients with optimal dose coverage of target volumes experienced significantly improved outcomes (overall survival of 83% for optimal coverage, 17% for suboptimal coverage), highlighting the importance of high-quality radiotherapy for producing good outcomes in the recurrent setting.[304]

A multi-institutional study that included 92 patients who underwent reirradiation with PBT for multiple types of recurrent HNC found a favorable toxicity profile compared to historical controls of patients retreated with photon techniques.[305] This included a low risk of grade 3+ dermatitis (8.7%) and dysphagia (7.1%). Furthermore, locoregional failure was found to be only 25% at 1 year. However, two deaths occurred as a result of bleeding events, reflecting the increased risk of serious vascular toxicity with a second course of radiotherapy. In all cases, the risks of toxicities associated with retreatment must be weighed against the risk of uncontrolled tumor progression that is usually associated with significant morbidity and impairment in quality of life.

Chemoradiotherapy may also improve treatment outcome for recurrent NPC in certain patients, and most recent salvage radiation series have included cisplatin-based chemotherapy for advanced-stage disease.[287,288,290,306]

Using gemcitabine and cisplatin as induction chemotherapy followed by reirradiation with IMRT in 20 patients (95% rT3-4), Chua et al.[287] reported a 1-year local salvage rate of 75%. In a study of 35 patients (66% rT3-4), Poon et al.[306] reported a 1-year EFS of 42% by concurrent cisplatin followed by adjuvant chemotherapy with cisplatin and 5-fluorouracil. However, although concomitant chemoirradiation is increasingly used to treat primary NPC, it remains uncertain whether concomitant chemoirradiation is appropriate for retreatment of purely local recurrences (rT1-2), because of high rates of toxicity and potential complications.

Surgical Treatment

For patients with persistent nodal disease, radical neck dissection is the preferred treatment for persistent or recurrent lymph node involvement in the neck when there is no distant metastasis[307] and may achieve a 5-year nodal control rate of 66% and disease-free survival rate of 37%.[308] In cases with extension of disease beyond lymph nodes into nearby structures, additional afterloading brachytherapy to tumor bed may improve local control.[309]

Surgical management at the primary site is hampered by difficulties in obtaining adequate exposure and obtaining adequate surgical margins.[146,310-312] Various approaches have been employed, including an infratemporal approach from the lateral aspect[313]; transpalatal, transmaxillary, and transcervical approaches from the inferior aspect[312,314]; and an anterior–lateral approach.[315] More recently, minimally invasive techniques, such as a transnasal approach and an endoscopic approach, have also been employed successfully.[316] Although controversial, salvage surgery by nasopharyngectomy can be a viable option in certain patients in which the disease is localized in the nasopharynx, with acceptable results reported for rT1-3 tumors.[266] Wei et al.[317] reported a 5-year control rate of 62% and 5-year disease-free survival rate of 49% in 60 patients who received curative resections. Typically, all patients with recurrence have undergone prior radical RT, thereby associated complications of trismus and palatal fistula being common; however, the mortalities associated with these surgical procedures are low.

Recurrent NPC is frequently located in the pharyngeal recess on the lateral wall. Access to this region is crucial for complete tumor extirpation. Wei and Sham[318] advocated the anterior–lateral approach or maxillary swing approach for localized recurrence in the nasopharynx. After facial incisions and the necessary osteotomies, the maxilla bone is swung laterally while remaining attached to the anterior cheek flap as one

Section III

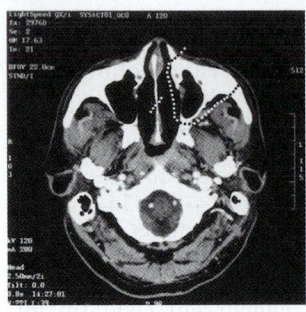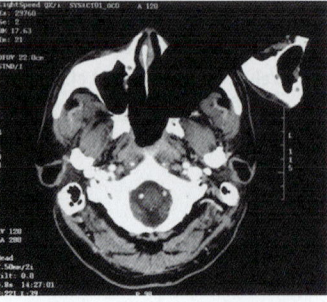

FIGURE 44.21. A: Computed tomography shows planned osteotomies of the maxilla and the posterior part of the nasal septum (*broken line*). **B:** The maxilla is swung laterally while still attached to the anterior cheek flap.

osteocutaneous entity (Figs. 44.21 and 44.22). The nasopharynx with the tumor and its surrounding area including the paranasopharyngeal region are then widely exposed for resection. Upon completion of nasopharyngectomy, the maxilla is replaced and attached to the remainder of the facial skeleton with miniplates.

Wei et al.[315] reported 161 patients with salvage nasopharyngectomy employing this approach performed at Queen Mary Hospital (Hong Kong) for recurrent NPC following primary treatment by radical RT. Twelve patients had prior brachytherapy as a salvage procedure. All patients were recurrent stage T1 with 78% of these patients achieving negative tumor resection margins, confirmed by frozen section, with the remaining patients demonstrating microscopic tumor at the internal carotid artery or the skull base during surgery, making further complete resection unattainable. All patients recovered from this anterior–lateral approach and were discharged. Regarding treatment-associated morbidities, trismus of varying grades was present in 60% and palatal fistula in 25% of patients. Recent modification of the palatal incision has eliminated the problem of palatal fistula.[319]

FIGURE 44.22. The left maxilla is swung laterally, exposing the nasopharynx (*arrow*).

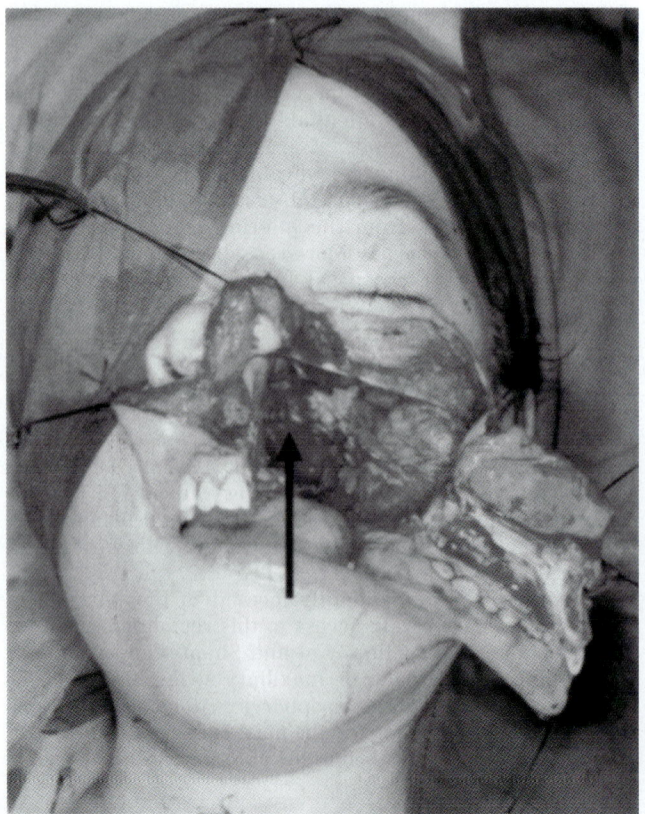

Author	Year	5-Year Local Control Rate by T-Stage[a] (%)			
		T1	T2	T3	T4
Hoppe[32]	1976	87	94	68	44
Mesic[149]	1981	97	84	73	71
Chu[51]	1984	76	79	37	55
Vikram[148]	1985		74	100[b]	63
Wang[326]	1990	76	54	34	42
		67[c]	84[c]	78[c]	52[c]
Perez[27]	1992	85[d]	75[d]	67[d]	40[d]
Bailet[327]	1992	64		61	

TABLE 44.18 LOCAL TUMOR CONTROL AFTER CONVENTIONAL RADIATION THERAPY

[a]By 1992 AJCC T-stage.
[b]With only 3 patients in this group.
[c]Treated by twice-daily accelerated fractionation.
[d]10-Year actuarial rate.
T, primary tumor stage.

Satisfactory long-term results can be achieved when persistent/recurrent tumor is completely resected. Several recent surgical series reported locoregional control and OS rates of 40% to 72% and 30% to 54%, respectively.[316,320–322] Postoperative reirradiation is recommended for patients with positive surgical margins and/or advanced disease[317,323,324] and may be beneficial even when surgical margins are negative.[266]

For recurrent tumors, margin status, adjuvant treatment type, and parapharyngeal space involvement were significant prognostic factors for local control, whereas dura or brain involvement, local recurrence, and adjuvant treatment type predicted survival.[316] Preoperative EBV DNA levels and PET-CT can assist in predicting the outcome of salvage nasopharyngectomy, and PET-CT may predict the presence of extracapsular spread of metastatic lymph nodes.[325]

RESULTS OF TREATMENT

Specific results of various treatments are mentioned in the previous respective sections. This section focuses on summarizing these results.

The local and regional control rates in select conventional radiotherapy series are listed in Tables 44.18 and 44.19. Control of the primary lesion using conventional radiotherapy varied with the T classification (Table 44.18), ranging from 64% to 97% for T1 lesions, 54% to 94% for T2 lesions, 34% to 100% for T3 lesions, and 40% to 71% for T4 lesions.[27,31,32,148,149,326,327] Dose escalation with intracavitary brachytherapy if using non-IMRT treatment techniques[196] has been shown to improve local control. Stereotactic radiosurgery boost after external beam radiotherapy (both conventional and IMRT) has also shown improved local control.[328,329] Nonkeratinizing squamous cell carcinoma (both differentiated and undifferentiated subtypes) had improved local control rates when compared to keratinizing squamous cell carcinoma in T2 to T3 lesions but not in T1 or T4 lesions.[27,224,238]

Author	Year	5-Year Nodal Control Rate by N-Stage[a] (%)			
		N0	N1	N2	N3
Hoppe[32]	1976	96	92	87	89
Mesic[149]	1981	100	90	88	82
Perez[27]	1992	82[b]	86[b]	78[b]	

TABLE 44.19 NODAL CONTROL AFTER CONVENTIONAL RADIATION THERAPY

[a]By 1992 AJCC N-stage.
[b]10-Year actuarial rate.
N, regional lymph node stage.

TABLE 44.20 OVERALL SURVIVAL AFTER CONVENTIONAL RADIATION THERAPY

Author	Year	Patients (n)	5-Year Survival Rate (%)	Analysis
Hoppe[32]	1976	82	57	Actuarial
Mesic[149]	1981	251	52	Actuarial disease-free
Chu[31]	1984	80	36	Actuarial
Vikram[148]	1985	107	56	Actuarial[a]
Wang[326]	1990	185	43	Absolute
Bailet[327]	1992	103	58	Actuarial

[a]Estimated from survival curve.
OS, overall survival.

TABLE 44.21 OVERALL SURVIVAL BY T- AND N-STAGE[a] AFTER CONVENTIONAL RADIATION THERAPY

Author	Year	5-Year Local Control Rate by T-Stage[a] (%)				5-Year Survival Rate by N-Stage[a] (%)			
		T1	T2	T3	T4	N0	N1	N2	N3
Hoppe[32]	1976	76[b]	68[b]	55[b]	0[b]	78[b]	70[b]	42[b]	39[b]
Chu[31]	1984					42[c]	27[c]	52[c]	27[c]
Wang[326]	1990	60[d]	48[d]	27[d]	29[d]	60[d]	42[d]		32[d]

[a]By 1992 AJCC T- and N-stage.
[b]Actuarial disease-free survival.
[c]Actuarial survival.
[d]Absolute survival.
N, regional lymph node stage; T, primary tumor stage.

Excellent nodal control rates in the neck have been demonstrated by conventional radiotherapy even after involvement of extensive cervical lymph node metastasis (Table 44.19). The neck nodal control rates ranged from 82% to 100% for N0, 86% to 92% for N1, and 78% to 89% for N2 to N3 disease.[27,32,149] Five-year survival rates ranged from 36% to 58% (Table 44.20).[27,31,32,149,326,327,330]

The 5-year survival rate with conventional non-IMRT radiotherapy correlated with the T-stage, as well as with the N-stage (Table 44.21), being 60% to 76% for T1, 48% to 68% for T2, 27% to 55% for T3, and 0% to 29% for T4 lesions[32,326] and 42% to 78% for N0, 27% to 70% for N1, and 32% to 52% for N2 to N3 disease. When nodes in the lower neck and/or the supraclavicular fossa are involved, prognosis is poor.

Contemporary series with IMRT, demonstrated excellent local and regional control was achieved in 97% and 98% of the patients treated at UCSF, respectively.[169] An update of the UCSF experience continued to show excellent local control of approximately 96%.[180] Subsequently, several other institutions also recently published their results, which further demonstrate excellent local control rates ranging from 82% to 100% and regional control rates ranging from 91% to 98% (Table 44.22).[153,172–174,182,184–186,252,253,331,332,334–340]

The RTOG conducted a phase II trial using IMRT+/- chemotherapy in the treatment of nasopharyngeal carcinoma where patients with ≥T2 (i.e., ≥T2b by AJCC 2002) and/or node-positive disease also received concurrent CDDP followed by adjuvant CDDP and 5-FU chemotherapies. The results showed that a multi-institutional setting can reproduce the excellent results (local control rate of 92.3%) observed from single-institution studies.[331] This reproducibility of excellent locoregional control rates in a multi-institutional trial, along with several single-institution studies, with IMRT is encouraging; however, distant metastases remain a therapeutic challenge despite extensive use of chemotherapy. The distant recurrence rate ranges from 10% to 15% at 2 years[185,331] and 4-year rates are as high as 34% (Table 44.22).[169] Novel systemic therapies or regimens are needed for improved distant control and overall survival of this disease.

SEQUELAE OF TREATMENT
Overall Incidence and Types
Because of the anatomic proximity of the nasopharynx to critical structures, and the need for high-radiation doses

TABLE 44.22 RESULTS FROM CONTEMPORARY IMRT SERIES WITH OR WITHOUT CHEMOTHERAPY

Study	Year	Stage	N	Median Follow-Up (months)	Timepoint (years)	Local Control Rate (%)	Regional Control Rate (%)	Distant Metastasis-Free Rate (%)	OS (%)
Lee et al.[169] (UCSF)	2002	All	67	31	4	97	98	66	88
Kwong et al.[173] (Hong Kong)	2004	T1 N0-1[a]	33	24	3	100	92	100	100
Kam[174] (Hong Kong)	2004	All	63	29	3	92	98	79	90
Wolden et al.[172] (MSKCC)	2006	All	74	35	3	91	93	78	83
Kwong et al.[182] (Hong Kong)	2006	III–IVB[a]	50	25	2	96	NA	94	92
Lee et al.[331] (MSKCC)	2009	All	68	31	2	93	91	85	80
Tham et al.[184] (Singapore)	2009	All	195	37	3	90	NA	89	94
Lin et al.[332] (China)	2009	II–IV[a]	323	30	3	95	98	90	90
Wong et al.[333] (China)	2010	All	175	34	3	94	93	87	87
Lin et al.[334] (China)	2010	IIB–IVB[a]	370	31	3	95	97	86	89
Kam et al.[335] (Hong Kong)	2010	All	231	59	6	82	91	75	66
Ng et al.[185] (Hong Kong)	2011	All	193	30	2	95	96	90	92
Xiao et al.[336] (China)	2011	III–IVA[a]	81	54	5	95	NA	NA	75
Bakst et al[153] (MSKCC)	2011	II–IVB[a]	25	33	3	91	91	91	89
Xiayun et al.[337] (China)	2011	IIB–IVB[b]	54	30	3	95	98	86	88
Ma et al.[252] (Hong Kong)	2011	III–IVB[b]	30	32	2	93	93	93	90
Lee et al.[253] (MSKCC)	2011	IIB–IVB[c]	42	30	2	NA	NA	91	91
Su et al.[338] (China)	2012	I–IIB[b]	198	51	5	97	98	98	NA
Sun et al.[339] (China)	2014	I–IVB[b]	868	50	5	92	96	85	NA
Setton et al.[186] (MSKCC)	2016	I–IVB[c]	177	52	5	83	91	83	74
Wu et al.[340] (China)	2017	I–IVB[c]	614	113	10	89	96	80	73

[a]By 1997 AJCC stage.
[b]By 2002 AJCC stage.
[c]By 2010 AJCC stage.
IMRT, intensity-modulated radiation therapy; M, distant metastasis stage; MSKCC, Memorial Sloan Kettering Cancer Center; N, regional lymph node stage; NA, not available; NPC, nasopharyngeal carcinoma; T, primary tumor stage; UCSF, University of California, San Francisco.

TABLE 44.23 INCIDENCE OF LATE TOXICITY FOLLOWING RADIATION WITH CONVENTIONAL TECHNIQUE (WITHOUT CONCURRENT CHEMOTHERAPY) FOR NASOPHARYNGEAL CARCINOMA

Severe Late Complication	Sanguineti et al.[28] (N = 378)	Chao and Perez[43] (N = 164)	Lee et al.[39] (N = 4527)	Yeh et al.[302] (N = 849)	Leung et al.[303] (N = 880)[a]
Period	1954–1992	1956–1991	1976–1985	1983–1998	1990–1998
Radiotherapy					
Total dose (Gy)	61–70	56–69	65[b]	68–76	62.5–66[b]
Dose per fraction (Gy)	NR	1.8–2	2.5–4.2	1.8	2–2.5
Altered fractionation (%)	8	Nil	Nil	Nil	Nil
Sequential chemotherapy (%)	Nil	Nil	8	Nil	20
Overall incidence (%)					
Grading of toxicity	≥3	≥3	≥2	≥1	?
Crude rate	30.4	14	30.8	NR	16.5
Actuarial rate	19 (10 y)	NR	60 (10 y)	NR	14 (5 y)
Treatment mortality (%)	3.2	3	1.4	NR	0.9
Types of complications (%)					
Temporal lobe necrosis	1.1	1.2	3	6[c]	1.1
Brainstem encephalopathy/ myelopathy	2.4		1		
Cranial neuropathy	4.5		5.3	3.3	6.8
Endocrine dysfunction	7.9		3.5		8.6
Severe epistaxis		1.2	0.6		0.3
Carotid rupture		0.6			
Hearing loss	2.6		8.2	54[c]	
Persistent otitis			2.5	32[c]	
Trismus	2.9	0.6	5.1	12[c]	0.7
Bone damage[d]	2.6	2.4	0.4		
Eyeball damage[e]			0.2		
Soft tissue necrosis/fistula	1.1	1.8	0.4		0.5
Pharynx stricture/dysphagia		4.2		6[c]	
Soft tissue fibrosis	4.2		15.9	25[c]	1.4
Persistent lymphedema	0.5	0.6	0.1		
Radiation-induced malignancy			<0.1		

[a]Patients with one course of radiotherapy.
[b]Median dose equivalent to 2 Gy/fraction.
[c]Five-year actuarial rate.
[d]Bone necrosis, fracture, or osteomyelitis.
[e]Cataract, retinitis, corneal ulcer.
NR, not reported.

and adequate field coverage, the risks of radiation-induced toxicities are substantial. The overall complication rate from conventional treatment ranged from 31% to 66%, with severe sequelae including temporal lobe necrosis, hearing loss, xerostomia, neck fibrosis, cranial nerve dysfunction, endocrine dysfunction, soft tissue necrosis, osteonecrosis, and transverse radiation myelitis.[28,32,39] The diagnosis of irradiation injury can be difficult, as other possible causes (tumor recurrence in particular) must be excluded.

The toxicity results of five major series using conventional irradiation for NPC are summarized in Table 44.23.

The series of 378 patients treated at MDACC during 1954 to 1992 showed an actuarial frequency rate in grade ≥4 toxicity of 16, 19, and 29% at 5, 10, and 20 years, respectively.[28] Despite the use of higher-radiation doses, Sanguineti et al. showed a reduction in the 10-year actuarial rate of severe toxicity from 14% in 1954 to 1971 to 5% in 1983 to 1992.[28] Other investigators have reported similar findings.

The decreased rates of complications over time were likely due to the use of newer oblique and opposed lateral field techniques instead of single central field, custom blocking, and image-guided (CT) treatment planning.[28]

Because of the extremely narrow therapeutic treatment margin of NPC, maximum conformity and precision in RT delivery are crucial for minimizing the risk of late damage. The emergence of IMRT is a major advance for improving physical dose distribution and has increased the potential for protecting normal tissues. Studies on patients treated with IMRT thus far have shown substantial sparing of salivary function,[169,173,174] whereas other benefits will require longer follow-up to confirm.

The improved conformity offered by IMRT has led to attempts at dose escalation in order to achieve better tumor coverage for patients with extensive locoregional infiltration. However, studies have shown that dose escalation together with concurrent chemotherapy may lead to severe toxicities.[182,341] Furthermore, extensive use of concurrent CRT independent from incorporation of dose escalation has been shown to significantly increase toxicities (grade ≥3) compared to RT alone.[222,224,228,230,231,342,343]

Temporal Lobe Necrosis

Temporal lobe necrosis (TLN) is perhaps the most troublesome complication. Studies on NPC patients treated with conventional 2D-RT found that TLN accounted for up to 65% of all irradiation-induced deaths; large fractions (>2 Gy) and overacceleration of treatment schedule greatly increased risk, with incidence as high as 33%.[39,151,152]

Diagnosis of TLN was often difficult and thus delayed. In Lee et al.'s examination of 102 patients with late TLN following conventional 2D-RT,[344] only 31% presented with classic symptoms of TLN (hallucinations, absence attacks, déjà vu), whereas 14% had headaches, confusion, convulsions, or hemiparesis. Thirty-nine percent had vague symptoms of dizziness, poor memory, or sudden changes in behavior, whereas 16% were asymptomatic.

TLN remains a serious concern in patients treated with IMRT, with incidence of 3% to 4% being reported for schedules of 70 Gy at 2.12 Gy/fraction,[180] 66 to 74 Gy at 2 Gy/fraction,[174] and 76 Gy at 2.17 Gy/fraction.[182] Series using larger fractions (70.2 at 2.34 Gy/fraction and 68 Gy at 2.27 Gy/fraction) had incidence rates as high as 12% to 14%.[153,336] According to Bakst et al.,[153] a prospective trial of hypofractionated dose-painting IMRT using 2.34-Gy fractions to deliver a total dose of 70.2 Gy had favorable disease control and survival outcomes; however, 12% of treated patients developed temporal lobe necrosis, with the conclusion that large fractional doses should be avoided to prevent infield brain radiation necrosis.

Cranial Neuropathy

Cranial nerves IX through XII, particularly XII, are the most frequently impaired by radiation.[39,303,345] This is related to marked radiation fibrosis, especially in patients who receive an additional boost dose to the parapharyngeal space. Common symptoms include slurring of speech, twitching of neck muscles, and/or dysphagia. In a study of 31 NPC patients with post-RT dysphagia, Wu et al.[346] found that 77% aspirated after the act of swallowing, raising concerns of fatal aspiration pneumonia.

Cranial nerve VI is also frequently affected, particularly in patients with TLN, whereas isolated palsy of branches of cranial nerve V is less common.[39] Optic neuropathy is rare with careful attention to the RT technique and should be considered when treating lesions with base-of-skull involvement.[347] The possibility of intracranial recurrence may confound the diagnosis of radiation injury, and exclusion of recurrence is necessary.

Oral Complications

Xerostomia is an almost universal complication from treatment with conventional RT and may lead to dental caries. Jen et al.[348] showed that the salivary flow dropped by half with a dose of 7.2 Gy, reached the nadir after 36 Gy, and then further dropped after completion of RT without recovery during the following 2 years.

However, Lee at al.[169] reported marked recovery of salivary function in patients treated with parotid-sparing IMRT (mean parotid dose, 34 Gy); the rate of grade 2 xerostomia decreased from 64% at 3 months to 2.4% at 2 years. Randomized trials comparing 2D-RT and IMRT in patients with T1-2 tumors have confirmed IMRT's advantage in this regard.[349,350] Nevertheless, it is important to rule out tumor invasion of the parotid gland prior to parotid-sparing IMRT, as recurrences have been reported. Cannon and Lee[351] concluded that PET alone may be insufficient for detection of intraparotid lymph node involvement in patients with multilevel nodal disease, including disease in level II nodes. Even with negative PET findings, these patients may require additional evaluation of any benign-appearing parotid nodules before parotid-sparing IMRT by FNA or CT-guided biopsy.

Dental sequelae frequently accompany xerostomia. In a series of 1,758 patients, 2.7% developed osteoradionecrosis at the maxilla and 1.7% at the mandible. Tong et al.[352] reported a 29% complication rate in patients who had post-RT extraction of posterior maxillary teeth, with 10.5% developing osteonecrosis. Prophylactic fluoride treatment should be employed to prevent dental decay, and decayed teeth should be extracted prior to RT to reduce this risk.[352,353]

Aural Toxicity

Hearing loss has always been a common radiation sequela, and the increasing use of cisplatin-based concurrent CRT has resulted in deafness rates as high as 42%.[354]

Sensorineural hearing loss (SNHL), particularly in the high-frequency range, was found in at least 30% of patients assessed with audiograms following RT, with higher rates in patients treated by concurrent CRT.[39,355–357] The primary determinant of high-frequency SNHL is mean cochlea dose, which should be kept below 48 Gy to minimize damage.[39,355–357] Because of the location of the primary tumor in the nasopharynx, pharyngotympanic tube (*Eustachian tube*) damage resulting in otitis media is difficult to avoid. However, lowering the dose to the external auditory canal and mastoid air cells can reduce the incidence and severity of acute external otitis and chronic serous otitis media, respectively.

Carotid Artery Injury

Carotid stenosis is a potentially fatal complication reported in patients who undergo irradiation of the head and neck region. Interval from radiotherapy was a significant independent predictor for severe carotid stenosis. Some have advocated for routine duplex ultrasound screening for high-risk patients

(older than 60 years, smoking, hypertension, hypercholesterolemia, cerebrovascular symptoms).[358,359] Severe cases may require carotid endarterectomy or endoplasty.

Massive bleeding from ruptured pseudoaneurysms at the petrous portion of the internal carotid has been reported following IMRT with dose escalation.[182,360] Urgent diagnosis and intervention with endovascular occlusion or stenting may be needed to prevent fatal consequences. Other concerns include severe telangiectasia and hypervascularization in the internal maxillary artery territory, for which emergency embolization may be considered.

Endocrine Dysfunction

The most common endocrine sequelae are amenorrhea and/or galactorrhea from hyperprolactinemia in female patients and followed by hypothyroidism and hypoadrenalism.

Lee et al.[39] observed symptomatic hypothalamic–pituitary dysfunction in 5% of patients, with a median latency of 5 years, whereas a longitudinal study by Lam et al.[361] with detailed endocrine assessment found a 5-year incidence of 62%, with dysfunction detected as early as 1 year following RT.[362] The deficiency of releasing of inhibitory factors indicated that the hypothalamus is the primary location of damage.[363,364] As many of these dysfunctions may be corrected pharmacologically, routine evaluation of hypothalamic, pituitary, and thyroid function should be considered in the follow-up examination of long-term survivors.

Shielding may help lessen endocrine dysfunction when using 2-D technique.[365] The need for maximum conformity to protect normal tissues during radiotherapy is paramount.

Second Malignancies

Radiation-induced malignancy is rare, with an incidence of 0.04% and latency period >10 years. The most common histologic types are maxillary osteosarcoma[366] and soft tissue sarcoma.[79] Surgery presents the only chance of cure, but the prognosis is often poor. Although second primary head and neck cancer is relatively uncommon for NPC patients, Teo et al.[367] reported an excessive incidence rate of tongue cancer at 0.13% per patient-year. The possibility of radiation carcinogenesis cannot be excluded.

REFERENCES

1. Lanier A, Bender T, Talbot M, et al. Nasopharyngeal carcinoma in Alaskan Eskimos Indians, and Aleuts: a review of cases and study of Epstein-Barr virus, HLA, and environmental risk factors. *Cancer* 1980;46(9):2100–2106.
2. Parkin D, Muir C, Whelan S, et al. Cancer incidence in five continents. In: Parkin D, et al., ed. *Epidemiology.* Lyon, France: IARC Scientific Publications, 1992.
3. Curado M, Edwards B, Shin H, et al. *Cancer incidence in five continents.* IARC Scientific Publications, 2007. IX(160).
4. Ferlay J, Shin H, Bray F, et al. GLOBOCAN 2008, Cancer Incidence and Mortality Worldwide: IARC Cancer Base No. 10. [Internet]. Lyon, France: International Agency for Research on Cancer, 2010.
5. Balakrishnan U. An additional younger-age peak for cancer of the nasopharynx. *Int J Cancer* 1975;15(4):651–657.
6. Singh W. Nasopharyngeal carcinoma in Caucasian children. A 25-year study. *J Laryngol Otol* 1987;101(12):1248–1253.
7. Ferlay J, Shin HR, Bray F, et al. Estimates of worldwide burden of cancer in 2008: GLOBOCAN 2008. *Int J Cancer* 2010;127(12):2893–2917.
8. Bei JX, Li Y, Jia WH, et al. A genome-wide association study of nasopharyngeal carcinoma identifies three new susceptibility loci. *Nat Genet* 2010;42(7):599–603.
9. Lu SJ, Day NE, Degos L, et al. Linkage of a nasopharyngeal carcinoma susceptibility locus to the HLA region. *Nature* 1990;346(6283):470–471.
10. Chan SH, Day NE, Kunaratnam N, et al. HLA and nasopharyngeal carcinoma in Chinese—a further study. *Int J Cancer* 1983;32(2):171–176.
11. Li X, Fasano R, Wang E, et al. HLA associations with nasopharyngeal carcinoma. *Curr Mol Med* 2009;9(6):751–765.
12. Tai TM. Descriptive epidemiology of nasopharyngeal cancer. *Curr Opin Oncol* 2001;8:114.

13. Ho JH. An epidemiologic and clinical study of nasopharyngeal carcinoma. *Int J Radiat Oncol Biol Phys* 1978;4(3–4):182–198.

14. Teo PM, Leung SF, Yu P, et al. A comparison of Ho's, International Union Against Cancer, and American Joint Committee stage classifications for nasopharyngeal carcinoma. *Cancer* 1991;67(2):434–439.

15. Yu MC, Ho JH, Lai SH, et al. Cantonese-style salted fish as a cause of nasopharyngeal carcinoma: report of a case-control study in Hong Kong. *Cancer Res* 1986;46(2):956–961.

16. Henderson BE, Louie E, SooHoo Jing J, et al. Risk factors associated with nasopharyngeal carcinoma. *N Engl J Med* 1976;295(20):1101–1106.

17. Nam JM, McLaughlin JK, Blot WJ. Cigarette smoking, alcohol, and nasopharyngeal carcinoma: a case-control study among U.S. whites. *J Natl Cancer Inst* 1992;84(8):619–622.

18. Buell P. Race and place in the etiology of nasopharyngeal cancer: a study based on California death certificates. *Int J Cancer* 1973;11(2):268–272.

19. King H, Haenszel W. Cancer mortality among foreign- and native-born Chinese in the United States. *J Chronic Dis* 1973;26(10):623–646.

20. Dickson RI, Flores AD. Nasopharyngeal carcinoma: an evaluation of 134 patients treated between 1971–1980. *Laryngoscope* 1985;95(3):276–283.

21. Vasef MA, Ferlito A, Weiss LM. Nasopharyngeal carcinoma, with emphasis on its relationship to Epstein-Barr virus. *Ann Otol Rhinol Laryngol* 1997;106(4):348–356.

22. Gulley ML. Molecular diagnosis of Epstein-Barr virus-related diseases. *J Mol Diagn* 2001;3(1):1–10.

23. Brooks L, Yao QY, Rickinson AB, et al. Epstein-Barr virus latent gene transcription in nasopharyngeal carcinoma cells: coexpression of EBNA1, LMP1, and LMP2 transcripts. *J Virol* 1992;66(5):2689–2697.

24. Kung CP, Meckes DG Jr, Raab-Traub N. Epstein-Barr Virus LMP1 Activates EGFR, STAT3, and ERK through Effects on PKCδ. *J Virol* 2011;85(9):4399–4408.

25. Mainou BA, Raab-Traub N. LMP1 strain variants: biological and molecular properties. *J Virol* 2006;80(13):6458–6468.

26. Wang D, Liebowitz D, Kieff E. An EBV membrane protein expressed in immortalized lymphocytes transforms established rodent cells. *Cell* 1985;43(3 Pt 2):831–840.

27. Perez CA, Deviveni VR, Marcial-Vega V, et al. Carcinoma of the nasopharynx: factors affecting prognosis. *Int J Radiat Oncol Biol Phys* 1992;23(2):271–280.

28. Sanguineti G, Geara FB, Garden AS, et al. Carcinoma of the nasopharynx treated by radiotherapy alone: determinants of local and regional control. *Int J Radiat Oncol Biol Phys* 1997;37(5):985–996.

29. Lee AW, Foo W, Law SC, et al. Nasopharyngeal carcinoma: presenting symptoms and duration before diagnosis. *Hong Kong Med J* 1997;3(4):355–361.

30. Pan WR, Suami H, Corlett RJ, et al. Lymphatic drainage of the nasal fossae and nasopharynx: preliminary anatomical and radiological study with clinical implications. *Head Neck* 2009;31(1):52–57.

31. Chu AM, Flynn MB, Achino E, et al. Irradiation of nasopharyngeal carcinoma: correlations with treatment factors and stage. *Int J Radiat Oncol Biol Phys* 1984;10(12):2241–2249.

32. Hoppe RT, Goffinet DR, Bagshaw MA. Carcinoma of the nasopharynx. Eighteen years' experience with megavoltage radiation therapy. *Cancer* 1976;37(6):2605–2612.

33. McNeese MD, Fletcher GH. Retreatment of recurrent nasopharyngeal carcinoma. *Radiology* 1981;138(1):191–193.

34. Moench HC, Phillips TL. Carcinoma of the nasopharynx. Review of 146 patients with emphasis on radiation dose and time factors. *Am J Surg* 1972;124(4):515–518.

35. Lee AW, Poon YF, Foo W, et al. Retrospective analysis of 5037 patients with nasopharyngeal carcinoma treated during 1976–1985: overall survival and patterns of failure. *Int J Radiat Oncol Biol Phys* 1992;23(2):261–270.

36. Frezza G, Barbieri E, Emiliani E, et al. Patterns of failure in nasopharyngeal cancer treated with megavoltage irradiation. *Radiother Oncol* 1986;5(4):287–294.

37. Johansen LV, Mestre M, Overgaard J. Carcinoma of the nasopharynx: analysis of treatment results in 167 consecutively admitted patients. *Head Neck* 1992;14(3):200–207.

38. Teo P, Shiu W, Leung SF, et al. Prognostic factors in nasopharyngeal carcinoma investigated by computer tomography—an analysis of 659 patients. *Radiother Oncol* 1992;23(2):79–93.

39. Lee AW, Law SC, Ng SH, et al. Retrospective analysis of nasopharyngeal carcinoma treated during 1976–1985: late complications following megavoltage irradiation. *Br J Radiol* 1992;65(778):918–928.

40. Hui EP, Leung SF, Au JS, et al. Lung metastasis alone in nasopharyngeal carcinoma: a relatively favorable prognostic group. A study by the Hong Kong Nasopharyngeal Carcinoma Study Group. *Cancer* 2004;101(2):300–306.

41. Luk NM, Yu KH, Choi CL, et al. Skin metastasis from nasopharyngeal carcinoma in four Chinese patients. *Clin Exp Dermatol* 2004;29(1):28–31.

42. Ngan RK, Yiu HH, Cheng HK, et al. Central nervous system metastasis from nasopharyngeal carcinoma: a report of two patients and a review of the literature. *Cancer* 2002;94(2):398–405.

43. Chao KS, Perez CA. Nasopharynx. In: *Principles and practice of radiation oncology*. Philadelphia, PA: Lippincott Williams & Wilkins, 1997:918–961.

44. Chan J, Bray F, McCarron P, et al. Nasopharyngeal carcinoma. In *Pathology and genetics of head and neck tumours. World Health Organization classification of tumours*. Lyon, France: IARC Press, 2005:85–97.

45. Li JC, Mayr NA, Yuh WT, et al. Cranial nerve involvement in nasopharyngeal carcinoma: response to radiotherapy and its clinical impact. *Ann Otol Rhinol Laryngol* 2006;115(5):340–345.

46. Lindberg R. Distribution of cervical lymph node metastases from squamous cell carcinoma of the upper respiratory and digestive tracts. *Cancer* 1972;29(6):1446–1449.

47. Poon PY, Tsang VH, Munk PL. Tumour extent and T stage of nasopharyngeal carcinoma: a comparison of magnetic resonance imaging and computed tomographic findings. *Can Assoc Radiol J* 2000;51(5):287–295, quiz 286.

48. Lanzieri CF, Bangert B. Magnetic resonance imaging of the nasopharynx. *Top Magn Reson Imaging* 1990;2(4):39–47.

49. Mancuso AA, Bohman L, Hanafee W, et al. Computed tomography of the nasopharynx: normal and variants of normal. *Radiology* 1980;137(1 Pt 1):113–121.

50. Sievers KW, Greess H, Baum U, et al. Paranasal sinuses and nasopharynx CT and MRI. *Eur J Radiol* 2000;33(3):185–202.

51. Pan JJ, Ng WT, Zong JF, et al. Proposal for the 8th edition of the AJCC/UICC staging system for nasopharyngeal cancer in the era of intensity-modulated radiotherapy. *Cancer* 2016;122(4):546–558.

52. Dillon WP, Harnsberger HR. The impact of radiologic imaging on staging of cancer of the head and neck. *Semin Oncol* 1991;18(2):64–79.

53. Glazer HS, Niemeyer JH, Balfe DM, et al. Neck neoplasms: MR imaging. Part II. Posttreatment evaluation. *Radiology* 1986;160(2):349–354.

54. Ng SH, Chang TC, Ko SF, et al. Nasopharyngeal carcinoma: MRI and CT assessment. *Neuroradiology* 1997;39(10):741–746.

55. Som PM. Detection of metastasis in cervical lymph nodes: CT and MR criteria and differential diagnosis. *AJR Am J Roentgenol* 1992;158(5):961–969.

56. van den Brekel MW, Stel HV, Castelijns JA, et al. Cervical lymph node metastasis: assessment of radiologic criteria. *Radiology* 1990;177(2):379–384.

57. Chang JT, Chan SC, Yen TC, et al. Nasopharyngeal carcinoma staging by (18) F-fluorodeoxyglucose positron emission tomography. *Int J Radiat Oncol Biol Phys* 2005;62(2):501–507.

58. Gordin A, Golz A, Daitzchman M, et al. Fluorine-18 fluorodeoxyglucose positron emission tomography/computed tomography imaging in patients with carcinoma of the nasopharynx: diagnostic accuracy and impact on clinical management. *Int J Radiat Oncol Biol Phys* 2007;68(2):370–376.

59. Liu FY, Lin CY, Chang JT, et al. 18F-FDG PET can replace conventional work-up in primary M staging of nonkeratinizing nasopharyngeal carcinoma. *J Nucl Med* 2007;48(10):1614–1619.

60. Neel HB III. Nasopharyngeal carcinoma: diagnosis, staging, and management. *Oncology (Williston Park)* 1992;6(2):87–95; discussion 99–102.

61. Wara WM, Wara DW, Phillips TL, et al. Elevated IGA in carcinoma of the nasopharynx. *Cancer* 1975;35(5):1313–1315.

62. Ho HC, Ng MH, Kwan HC, et al. Epstein-Barr-virus-specific IgA and IgG serum antibodies in nasopharyngeal carcinoma. *Br J Cancer* 1976;34(6):655–660.

63. Henle W, Ho JH, Henle G, et al. Nasopharyngeal carcinoma: significance of changes in Epstein-Barr virus-related antibody patterns following therapy. *Int J Cancer* 1977;20(5):663–672.

64. Neel HB III, Taylor WF. Epstein-Barr virus-related antibody. Changes in titers after therapy for nasopharyngeal carcinoma. *Arch Otolaryngol Head Neck Surg* 1990;116(11):1287–1290.

65. Zeng Y. Seroepidemiological studies on nasopharyngeal carcinoma in China. *Adv Cancer Res* 1985;44:121–138.

66. Zong YS, Sham JS, Ng MH, et al. Immunoglobulin A against viral capsid antigen of Epstein-Barr virus and indirect mirror examination of the nasopharynx in the detection of asymptomatic nasopharyngeal carcinoma. *Cancer* 1992;69(1):3–7.

67. Lin JC, Wang WY, Chen KY, et al. Quantification of plasma Epstein-Barr virus DNA in patients with advanced nasopharyngeal carcinoma. *N Engl J Med* 2004;350(24):2461–2470.

68. Leung SF, Zee B, Ma BB, et al. Plasma Epstein-Barr viral deoxyribonucleic acid quantitation complements tumor-node-metastasis staging prognostication in nasopharyngeal carcinoma. *J Clin Oncol* 2006;24(34):5414–5418.

69. Shanmugaratnam K, Sobin LH; World Health Organization. Histological typing of upper respiratory tract tumours / K. Shanmugaratnam, in collaboration with L. H. Sobin and pathologists in 10 countries. Geneva, Switzerland: World Health Organization, 1978.

70. Shanmugaratnam K, Sobin LH; World Health Organization. Histological typing of upper respiratory tract tumours / K. Shanmugaratnam, in collaboration with L. H. Sobin and pathologists in 8 countries. Geneva, Switzerland: World Health Organization, 1991.

71. AJCC: Pharynx. In: Beahrs OH, Hulter RVP, Kennedy BJ, et al, eds. *Manual for staging of cancer*. Vol. 31. Philadelphia, PA: JB Lippincott Company, 1992.

72. Edge SB, American Joint Committee on Cancer. *AJCC cancer staging manual*. 7th ed. New York: Springer, 2010:xiv, 648.

73. Amin MB, American Joint Committee on Cancer. *AJCC cancer staging manual*. 8th ed. New York: Springer, 2017:XVII, 1024.

74. Bedwinek JM, Perez CA, Keys DJ. Analysis of failures after definitive irradiation for epidermoid carcinoma of the nasopharynx. *Cancer* 1980;45(11):2725–2729.

75. Chong VFH, Mukherji SK, Ng S-HH, et al. Nasopharyngeal carcinoma: review of how imaging affects staging. *J Comput Assist Tomogr* 1999;23(6):984–993.

76. Xiao GL, Gao L, Xu GZ. Prognostic influence of parapharyngeal space involvement in nasopharyngeal carcinoma. *Int J Radiat Oncol Biol Phys* 2002;52(4):957–963.

77. Huang SC. Nasopharyngeal cancer: a review of 1605 patients treated radically with cobalt 60. *Int J Radiat Oncol Biol Phys* 1980;6(4):401–407.

78. Sham JS, Cheung YK, Choy D, et al. Cranial nerve involvement and base of the skull erosion in nasopharyngeal carcinoma. *Cancer* 1991;68(2):422–426.

79. King AD, Ahuja AT, Leung SF, et al. Neck node metastases from nasopharyngeal carcinoma: MR imaging of patterns of disease. *Head Neck* 2000;22(3):275–281.

80. Batsakis JG, Solomon AR, Rice DH. The pathology of head and neck tumors: carcinoma of the nasopharynx, Part 11. *Head Neck Surg* 1981;3(6):511–524.

81. El-Naggar A, Chan J, Grandis J, et al. *WHO classification of head and neck tumours*. Lyon, France: IARC Press, 2017.

82. Ferlito A, Altavilla G, Rinaldo A, et al. Basaloid squamous cell carcinoma of the larynx and hypopharynx. *Ann Otol Rhinol Laryngol* 1997;106(12):1024–1035.

83. Niedobitek G. Epstein-Barr virus infection in the pathogenesis of nasopharyngeal carcinoma. *Mol Pathol* 2000;53(5):248–254.

84. Lo EJ, Bell D, Woo JS, et al. Human papillomavirus and WHO type I nasopharyngeal carcinoma. *Laryngoscope* 2010;120(10):1990–1907.

85. Sham JS, Choy D. Prognostic factors of nasopharyngeal carcinoma: a review of 759 patients. *Br J Radiol* 1990;63(745):51–58.

86. Teo P, Yu P, Lee WY, et al. Significant prognosticators after primary radiotherapy in 903 nondisseminated nasopharyngeal carcinoma evaluated by computer tomography. *Int J Radiat Oncol Biol Phys* 1996;36(2):291–304.

87. Heng DM, Wee J, Fong KW, et al. Prognostic factors in 677 patients in Singapore with nondisseminated nasopharyngeal carcinoma. *Cancer* 1999;86(10):1912–1920.

88. Lee AW, Foo W, Law SC, et al. Staging of nasopharyngeal carcinoma: from Ho's to the new UICC system. *Int J Cancer* 1999;84(2):179–187.

89. Chua DT, Sham JS, Kwong DL, et al. Prognostic value of paranasopharyngeal extension of nasopharyngeal carcinoma. A significant factor in local control and distant metastasis. *Cancer* 1996;78(2):202–210.

90. Sham JS, Choy D. Prognostic value of paranasopharyngeal extension of nasopharyngeal carcinoma on local control and short-term survival. *Head Neck* 1991;13(4):298–310.

91. Ma J, Mai HQ, Hong MH, et al. Is the 1997 AJCC staging system for nasopharyngeal carcinoma prognostically useful for Chinese patient populations? *Int J Radiat Oncol Biol Phys* 2001;50(5):1181–1189.

92. Ho HC, Lee MS, Hsiao SH, et al. Prognostic influence of parapharyngeal extension in nasopharyngeal carcinoma. *Acta Otolaryngol* 2008;128(7):790–798.

93. Cheng SH, Tsai SY, Yen KL, et al. Prognostic significance of parapharyngeal space venous plexus and marrow involvement: potential landmarks of dissemination for stage I-III nasopharyngeal carcinoma. *Int J Radiat Oncol Biol Phys* 2005;61(2):456–465.

94. Au JS, Law CK, Foo W, et al. In-depth evaluation of the AJCC/UICC 1997 staging system of nasopharyngeal carcinoma: prognostic homogeneity and proposed refinements. *Int J Radiat Oncol Biol Phys* 2003;56(2):413–426.

95. King AD, Teo P, Lam WW, et al. Paranasopharyngeal space involvement in nasopharyngeal cancer: detection by CT and MRI. *Clin Oncol (R Coll Radiol)* 2000;12(6):397–402.

96. Ng WT, Chan SH, Lee AW, et al. Parapharyngeal extension of nasopharyngeal carcinoma: still a significant factor in era of modern radiotherapy? *Int J Radiat Oncol Biol Phys* 2008;72(4):1082–1089.

97. Liu MZ, Tang LL, Zong JF, et al. Evaluation of sixth edition of AJCC staging system for nasopharyngeal carcinoma and proposed improvement. *Int J Radiat Oncol Biol Phys* 2008;70(4):1115–1123.

98. Mao YP, Xie FY, Liu LZ, et al. Re-evaluation of 6th edition of AJCC staging system for nasopharyngeal carcinoma and proposed improvement based on magnetic resonance imaging. *Int J Radiat Oncol Biol Phys* 2009;73(5):1326–1334.

99. Lee AW, Au JS, Teo PM, et al. Staging of nasopharyngeal carcinoma: suggestions for improving the current UICC/AJCC Staging System. *Clin Oncol (R Coll Radiol)* 2004;16(4):269–276.

100. Chua DT, Sham JS, Kwong DL, et al. Retropharyngeal lymphadenopathy in patients with nasopharyngeal carcinoma: a computed tomography-based study. *Cancer* 1997;79(5):869–877.

101. Chen MK, Chen TH, Liu JP, et al. Better prediction of prognosis for patients with nasopharyngeal carcinoma using primary tumor volume. *Cancer* 2004;100(10):2160–2166.

102. Sze WM, Lee AW, Yau TK, et al. Primary tumor volume of nasopharyngeal carcinoma: prognostic significance for local control. *Int J Radiat Oncol Biol Phys* 2004;59(1):21–27.

103. Chong VF, Zhou JY, Khoo JB, et al. Correlation between MR imaging-derived nasopharyngeal carcinoma tumor volume and TNM system. *Int J Radiat Oncol Biol Phys* 2006;64(1):72–76.

104. Zhou JY, Chong VF, Khoo JB, et al. The relationship between nasopharyngeal carcinoma tumor volume and TNM T-classification: a quantitative analysis. *Eur Arch Otorhinolaryngol* 2007;264(2):169–174.

105. Lok BH, Setton J, Caria N, et al. Intensity-modulated radiation therapy in oropharyngeal carcinoma: effect of tumor volume on clinical outcomes. *Int J Radiat Oncol Biol Phys* 2012;82(5):1851–1857.

106. Perez CA, Ackerman LV, Mill WB, et al. Cancer of the nasopharynx. Factors influencing prognosis. *Cancer* 1969;24(1):1–17.

107. Bohorquez J. Factors that modify the radio-response of cancer of the nasopharynx. *AJR Am J Roentgenol* 1976;126(4):863–876.

108. Applebaum EL, Mantravadi P, Haas R. Lymphoepithelioma of the nasopharynx. *Laryngoscope* 1982;92(5):510–514.

109. Marks JE, Phillips JL, Menck HR. The National Cancer Data Base report on the relationship of race and national origin to the histology of nasopharyngeal carcinoma. *Cancer* 1998;83(3):582–588.

110. Corry J, Fisher R, Rischin D, et al. Relapse patterns in WHO 2/3 nasopharyngeal cancer: is there a difference between ethnic Asian vs. non-Asian patients? *Int J Radiat Oncol Biol Phys* 2006;64(1):63–71.

111. Lynn TC, Tu SM, Kawamura A Jr. Long-term follow-up of IgG and IgA antibodies against viral capsid antigens of Epstein-Barr virus in nasopharyngeal carcinoma. *J Laryngol Otol* 1985;99(6):567–572.

112. de-Vathaire F, Sancho-Garnier H, de-The H, et al. Prognostic value of EBV markers in the clinical management of nasopharyngeal carcinoma (NPC): a multicenter follow-up study. *Int J Cancer* 1988;42(2):176–181.

113. Fan H, Nicholls J, Chua D, et al. Laboratory markers of tumor burden in nasopharyngeal carcinoma: a comparison of viral load and serologic tests for Epstein-Barr virus. *Int J Cancer* 2004;112(6):1036–1041.

114. Shao JY, Li YH, Gao HY, et al. Comparison of plasma Epstein-Barr virus (EBV) DNA levels and serum EBV immunoglobulin A/virus capsid antigen antibody titers in patients with nasopharyngeal carcinoma. *Cancer* 2004;100(6):1162–1170.

115. Xu J, Wan XB, Huang XF, et al. Serologic antienzyme rate of Epstein-Barr virus DNase-specific neutralizing antibody segregates TNM classification in nasopharyngeal carcinoma. *J Clin Oncol* 2010;28(35):5202–5209.

116. Neel HB III, Pearson GR, Taylor WF. Antibodies to Epstein-Barr virus in patients with nasopharyngeal carcinoma and in comparison groups. *Ann Otol Rhinol Laryngol* 1984;93(5 Pt 1):477–482.

117. Twu CW, Wang WY, Liang WM, et al. Comparison of the prognostic impact of serum anti-EBV antibody and plasma EBV DNA assays in nasopharyngeal carcinoma. *Int J Radiat Oncol Biol Phys* 2007;67(1):130–137.

118. Lo YM, Chan LY, Lo KW, et al. Quantitative analysis of cell-free Epstein-Barr virus DNA in plasma of patients with nasopharyngeal carcinoma. *Cancer Res* 1999;59(6):1188–1191.

119. Ma BB, King A, Lo YM, et al. Relationship between pretreatment level of plasma Epstein-Barr virus DNA, tumor burden, and metabolic activity in advanced nasopharyngeal carcinoma. *Int J Radiat Oncol Biol Phys* 2006;66(3):714–720.

120. Lo YM, Chan LY, Chan AT, et al. Quantitative and temporal correlation between circulating cell-free Epstein-Barr virus DNA and tumor recurrence in nasopharyngeal carcinoma. *Cancer Res* 1999;59(21):5452–5455.

121. Le QT, Jones CD, Yau TK, et al. A comparison study of different PCR assays in measuring circulating plasma Epstein-Barr virus DNA levels in patients with nasopharyngeal carcinoma. *Clin Cancer Res* 2005;11(16):5700–5707.

122. Lo YM, Chan AT, Chan LY, et al. Molecular prognostication of nasopharyngeal carcinoma by quantitative analysis of circulating Epstein-Barr virus DNA. *Cancer Res* 2000;60(24):6878–6881.

123. Chan AT, Lo YM, Zee B, et al. Plasma Epstein-Barr virus DNA and residual disease after radiotherapy for undifferentiated nasopharyngeal carcinoma. *J Natl Cancer Inst* 2002;94(21):1614–1619.

124. Tan EL, Selvaratnam G, Kananathan R, et al. Quantification of Epstein-Barr virus DNA load, interleukin-6, interleukin-10, transforming growth factor-beta1 and stem cell factor in plasma of patients with nasopharyngeal carcinoma. *BMC Cancer* 2006;6:227.

125. Lin JC, Wang WY, Liang WM, et al. Long-term prognostic effects of plasma Epstein-Barr virus DNA by minor groove binder-probe real-time quantitative PCR on nasopharyngeal carcinoma patients receiving concurrent chemoradiotherapy. *Int J Radiat Oncol Biol Phys* 2007;68(5):1342–1348.

126. Wang WY, Twu CW, Chen HH, et al. Plasma EBV DNA clearance rate as a novel prognostic marker for metastatic/recurrent nasopharyngeal carcinoma. *Clin Cancer Res* 2010;16(3):1016–1024.

127. An X, Wang FH, Ding PR, et al. Plasma Epstein-Barr virus DNA level strongly predicts survival in metastatic/recurrent nasopharyngeal carcinoma treated with palliative chemotherapy. *Cancer* 2011;117(16):3750–3757.

128. Wang WY, Twu CW, Lin WY, et al. Plasma Epstein-Barr virus DNA screening followed by (1)F-fluoro-2-deoxy-D-glucose positron emission tomography in detecting posttreatment failures of nasopharyngeal carcinoma. *Cancer* 2011;117(19):4452–4459.

129. Lydiatt WM, Patel SG, O'Sullivan B, et al. Head and neck cancers-major changes in the American Joint Committee on cancer eighth edition cancer staging manual. *CA Cancer J Clin* 2017;67(2):122–137.

130. Stenmark MH, McHugh JB, Schipper M, et al. Nonendemic HPV-positive nasopharyngeal cancer: association with poor prognosis. *Int J Radiat Oncol Biol Phys* 2014;88(3):580–588.

131. Lin Z, Khong B, Kwok S, et al. Human papillomavirus 16 detected in nasopharyngeal carcinomas in white Americans but not in endemic Southern Chinese patients. *Head Neck* 2014;36(5):709–714.

132. Dogan S, Hedberg ML, Ferris RL, et al. Human papillomavirus and Epstein-Barr virus in nasopharyngeal carcinoma in a low-incidence population. *Head Neck* 2014;36(4):511–516.

133. Chua DT, Nicholls JM, Sham JS, et al. Prognostic value of epidermal growth factor receptor expression in patients with advanced stage nasopharyngeal carcinoma treated with induction chemotherapy and radiotherapy. *Int J Radiat Oncol Biol Phys* 2004;59(1):11–20.

134. Ma BB, Poon TC, To KF, et al. Prognostic significance of tumor angiogenesis, Ki 67, p53 oncoprotein, epidermal growth factor receptor and HER2 receptor protein expression in undifferentiated nasopharyngeal carcinoma—a prospective study. *Head Neck* 2003;25(10):864–872.

135. Lv X, Xiang YQ, Cao SM, et al. Prospective validation of the prognostic value of elevated serum vascular endothelial growth factor in patients with nasopharyngeal carcinoma: more distant metastases and shorter overall survival after treatment. *Head Neck* 2011;33(6):780–785.

136. Hui EP, Chan AT, Pezzella F, et al. Coexpression of hypoxia-inducible factors 1alpha and 2alpha, carbonic anhydrase IX, and vascular endothelial growth factor in nasopharyngeal carcinoma and relationship to survival. *Clin Cancer Res* 2002;8(8):2595–2604.

137. Qian CN, Zhang CQ, Guo X, et al. Elevation of serum vascular endothelial growth factor in male patients with metastatic nasopharyngeal carcinoma. *Cancer* 2000;88(2):255–261.

138. Krishna SM, James S, Balaram P. Expression of VEGF as prognosticator in primary nasopharyngeal cancer and its relation to EBV status. *Virus Res* 2006;115(1):85–90.

139. Xueguan L, Xiaoshen W, Yongsheng Z, et al. Hypoxia inducible factor-1 alpha and vascular endothelial growth factor expression are associated with a poor prognosis in patients with nasopharyngeal carcinoma receiving radiotherapy with carbogen and nicotinamide. *Clin Oncol (R Coll Radiol)* 2008;20(8):606–612.

140. Zheng Z, Pan J, Chu B, et al. Downregulation and abnormal expression of E-cadherin and beta-catenin in nasopharyngeal carcinoma: close association with advanced disease stage and lymph node metastasis. *Hum Pathol* 1999;30(4):458–466.

141. Roychowdhury DF, Tseng A Jr, Fu KK, et al. New prognostic factors in nasopharyngeal carcinoma. Tumor angiogenesis and C-erbB2 expression. *Cancer* 1996;77(8):1419–1426.

Section III

142. Masuda M, Shinokuma A, Hirakawa N, et al. Expression of bcl-2-, p53, and Ki-67 and outcome of patients with primary nasopharyngeal carcinomas following DNA-damaging treatment. *Head Neck* 1998;20(7):640–644.

143. Guo X, Min HQ, Zeng MS, et al. nm23-H1 expression in nasopharyngeal carcinoma: correlation with clinical outcome. *Int J Cancer* 1998;79(6):596–600.

144. Liu SJ, Sun YM, Tian DF, et al. Downregulated NM23-H1 expression is associated with intracranial invasion of nasopharyngeal carcinoma. *Br J Cancer* 2008;98(2):363–369.

145. Fujieda S, Lee K, Sunaga H, et al. Staining of interleukin-10 predicts clinical outcome in patients with nasopharyngeal carcinoma. *Cancer* 1999;85(7):1439–1445.

146. Wilson CP. The approach to the nasopharynx. *Proc R Soc Med* 1951;44(5):353–358.

147. Marks JE, Bedwinek JM, Lee F, et al. Dose-response analysis for nasopharyngeal carcinoma: an historical perspective. *Cancer* 1982;50(6):1042–1050.

148. Vikram B, Mishra UB, Strong EW, et al. Patterns of failure in carcinoma of the nasopharynx: I. Failure at the primary site. *Int J Radiat Oncol Biol Phys* 1985;11(8):1455–1459.

149. Mesic JB, Fletcher GH, Goepfert H. Megavoltage irradiation of epithelial tumors of the nasopharynx. *Int J Radiat Oncol Biol Phys* 1981;7(4):447–453.

150. Lee AW, Chan DK, Fowler JF, et al. Effect of time, dose and fractionation on local control of nasopharyngeal carcinoma. *Radiother Oncol* 1995;36(1):24–31.

151. Lee AW, Foo W, Chappell R, et al. Effect of time, dose, and fractionation on temporal lobe necrosis following radiotherapy for nasopharyngeal carcinoma. *Int J Radiat Oncol Biol Phys* 1998;40(1):35–42.

152. Lee AW, Kwong DL, Leung SF, et al. Factors affecting risk of symptomatic temporal lobe necrosis: significance of fractional dose and treatment time. *Int J Radiat Oncol Biol Phys* 2002;53(1):75–85.

153. Bakst RL, Lee N, Pfister DG, et al. Hypofractionated dose-painting intensity modulated radiation therapy with chemotherapy for nasopharyngeal carcinoma: a prospective trial. *Int J Radiat Oncol Biol Phys* 2011;80(1):148–153.

154. Marcial VA, Hanley JA, Chang C, et al. Split-course radiation therapy of carcinoma of the nasopharynx: results of a national collaborative clinical trial of the Radiation Therapy Oncology Group. *Int J Radiat Oncol Biol Phys* 1980;6(4):409–414.

155. Luo RX, Tang QX, Guo KP, et al. Comparison of continuous and split-course radiotherapy for nasopharyngeal carcinoma—an analysis of 1446 cases with squamous cell carcinoma grade 3. *Int J Radiat Oncol Biol Phys* 1994;30(5):1107–1109.

156. Kwong DL, Sham JS, Chua DT, et al. The effect of interruptions and prolonged treatment time in radiotherapy for nasopharyngeal carcinoma. *Int J Radiat Oncol Biol Phys* 1997;39(3):703–710.

157. Ho JHC. Nasopharynx. In: Halnan KE, ed. *Treatment of cancer.* New York: Igaku-Shoin, 1982:249–268.

158. Teo P, Tsao SY, Shiu W, et al. A clinical study of 407 cases of nasopharyngeal carcinoma in Hong Kong. *Int J Radiat Oncol Biol Phys* 1989;17(3):515–530.

159. Wolden SL, Zelefsky MJ, Hunt MA, et al. Failure of a 3D conformal boost to improve radiotherapy for nasopharyngeal carcinoma. *Int J Radiat Oncol Biol Phys* 2001;49(5):1229–1234.

160. Corry J, Hornby C, Fisher R, et al. 'Boomerang' technique: an improved method for conformal treatment of locally advanced nasopharyngeal cancer. *Australas Radiol* 2004;48(2):170–180.

161. Chau RM, Teo PM, Choi PH, et al. Three-dimensional dosimetric evaluation of a conventional radiotherapy technique for treatment of nasopharyngeal carcinoma. *Radiother Oncol* 2001;58(2):143–153.

162. Kutcher GJ, Fuks Z, Brenner H, et al. Three-dimensional photon treatment planning for carcinoma of the nasopharynx. *Int J Radiat Oncol Biol Phys* 1991;21(1):169–182.

163. Leibel SA, Kutcher GJ, Harrison LB, et al. Improved dose distributions for 3D conformal boost treatments in carcinoma of the nasopharynx. *Int J Radiat Oncol Biol Phys* 1991;20(4):823–833.

164. Jen YM, Shih R, Lin YS, et al. Parotid gland-sparing 3-dimensional conformal radiotherapy results in less severe dry mouth in nasopharyngeal cancer patients: a dosimetric and clinical comparison with conventional radiotherapy. *Radiother Oncol* 2005;75(2):204–209.

165. Nutting C, Dearnaley DP, Webb S. Intensity modulated radiation therapy: a clinical review. *Br J Radiol* 2000;73(869):459–469.

166. Xia P, Fu KK, Wong GW, et al. Comparison of treatment plans involving intensity-modulated radiotherapy for nasopharyngeal carcinoma. *Int J Radiat Oncol Biol Phys* 2000;48(2):329–337.

167. Eisbruch A, Ten Haken RK, Kim HM, et al. Dose, volume, and function relationships in parotid salivary glands following conformal and intensity-modulated irradiation of head and neck cancer. *Int J Radiat Oncol Biol Phys* 1999;45(3):577–587.

168. Eisbruch A, Ship JA, Martel MK, et al. Parotid gland sparing in patients undergoing bilateral head and neck irradiation: techniques and early results. *Int J Radiat Oncol Biol Phys* 1996;36(2):469–480.

169. Lee N, Xia P, Quivey JM, et al. Intensity-modulated radiotherapy in the treatment of nasopharyngeal carcinoma: an update of the UCSF experience. *Int J Radiat Oncol Biol Phys* 2002;53(1):12–22.

170. Kam MK, Chau RM, Suen J, et al. Intensity-modulated radiotherapy in nasopharyngeal carcinoma: dosimetric advantage over conventional plans and feasibility of dose escalation. *Int J Radiat Oncol Biol Phys* 2003;56(1):145–157.

171. Sultanem K, Shu HK, Xia P, et al. Three-dimensional intensity-modulated radiotherapy in the treatment of nasopharyngeal carcinoma: the University of California-San Francisco experience. *Int J Radiat Oncol Biol Phys* 2000;48(3):711–722.

172. Wolden SL, Chen WC, Pfister DG, et al. Intensity-modulated radiation therapy (IMRT) for nasopharynx cancer: update of the Memorial Sloan-Kettering experience. *Int J Radiat Oncol Biol Phys* 2006;64(1):57–62.

173. Kwong DL, Pow EH, Sham JS, et al. Intensity-modulated radiotherapy for early-stage nasopharyngeal carcinoma: a prospective study on disease control and preservation of salivary function. *Cancer* 2004;101(7):1584–1593.

174. Kam MK, Teo PM, Chau RM, et al. Treatment of nasopharyngeal carcinoma with intensity-modulated radiotherapy: the Hong Kong experience. *Int J Radiat Oncol Biol Phys* 2004;60(5):1440–1450.

175. Hsiung CY, Ting HM, Huang HY, et al. Parotid-sparing intensity-modulated radiotherapy (IMRT) for nasopharyngeal carcinoma: preserved parotid function after IMRT on quantitative salivary scintigraphy, and comparison with historical data after conventional radiotherapy. *Int J Radiat Oncol Biol Phys* 2006;66(2):454–461.

176. McMillan AS, Pow EH, Kwong DL, et al. Preservation of quality of life after intensity-modulated radiotherapy for early-stage nasopharyngeal carcinoma: results of a prospective longitudinal study. *Head Neck* 2006;28(8):712–722.

177. Chau RM, Teo PM, Kam MK, et al. Dosimetric comparison between 2-dimensional radiation therapy and intensity modulated radiation therapy in treatment of advanced T-stage nasopharyngeal carcinoma: to treat less or more in the planning organ-at-risk volume of the brainstem and spinal cord. *Med Dosim* 2007;32(4):263–270.

178. Taheri-Kadkhoda Z, Pettersson N, Bjork-Eriksson T, et al. Superiority of intensity-modulated radiotherapy over three-dimensional conformal radiotherapy combined with brachytherapy in nasopharyngeal carcinoma: a planning study. *Br J Radiol* 2008;81(965):397–405.

179. Butler EB, Teh BS, Grant WH III, et al. Smart (simultaneous modulated accelerated radiation therapy) boost: a new accelerated fractionation schedule for the treatment of head and neck cancer with intensity modulated radiotherapy. *Int J Radiat Oncol Biol Phys* 1999;45(1):21–32.

180. Bucci M, Xia P, Lee N. Intensity-modulated radiation therapy for carcinoma of the nasopharynx: the update of the UCSF experience [abstract]. *Int J Radiat Oncol Biol Phys* 2004;60:317–318.

181. Chong Z. Improved local control with intensity modulated radiation therapy in patients with nasopharyngeal carcinoma. *Int J Radiat Oncol Biol Phys* 2004;60(1, Suppl):S317.

182. Kwong DL, Sham JS, Leung LH, et al. Preliminary results of radiation dose escalation for locally advanced nasopharyngeal carcinoma. *Int J Radiat Oncol Biol Phys* 2006;64(2):374–381.

183. Su SF, Han F, Zhao C, et al. Treatment outcomes for different subgroups of nasopharyngeal carcinoma patients treated with intensity-modulated radiation therapy. *Chin J Cancer* 2011;30(8):565–573.

184. Tham IW, Hee SW, Yeo RM, et al. Treatment of nasopharyngeal carcinoma using intensity-modulated radiotherapy: the national cancer centre Singapore experience. *Int J Radiat Oncol Biol Phys* 2009;75(5):1481–1486.

185. Ng WT, Lee MC, Hung WM, et al. Clinical outcomes and patterns of failure after intensity-modulated radiotherapy for nasopharyngeal carcinoma. *Int J Radiat Oncol Biol Phys* 2011;79(2):420–428.

186. Setton J, Han J, Kannarunimit D, et al. Long-term patterns of relapse and survival following definitive intensity-modulated radiotherapy for non-endemic nasopharyngeal carcinoma. *Oral Oncol* 2016;53:67–73.

187. Amdur RJ, Liu C, Li J, et al. Matching intensity-modulated radiation therapy to an anterior low neck field. *Int J Radiat Oncol Biol Phys* 2007;69(2 Suppl):S46–S48.

188. Lee N, Mechalakos J, Puri DR, et al. Choosing an intensity-modulated radiation therapy technique in the treatment of head-and-neck cancer. *Int J Radiat Oncol Biol Phys* 2007;68(5):1299–1309.

189. Dabaja B, Salehpour MR, Rosen I, et al. Intensity-modulated radiation therapy (IMRT) of cancers of the head and neck: comparison of split-field and whole-field techniques. *Int J Radiat Oncol Biol Phys* 2005;63(4):1000–1005.

190. Amdur RJ, Li JG, Liu C, et al. Unnecessary laryngeal irradiation in the IMRT era. *Head Neck* 2004;26(3):257–263; discussion 263–264.

191. Hunt MA, Zelefsky MJ, Wolden S, et al. Treatment planning and delivery of intensity-modulated radiation therapy for primary nasopharynx cancer. *Int J Radiat Oncol Biol Phys* 2001;49(3):623–632.

192. Xia P, Lee N, Liu YM, et al. A study of planning dose constraints for treatment of nasopharyngeal carcinoma using a commercial inverse treatment planning system. *Int J Radiat Oncol Biol Phys* 2004;59(3):886–896.

193. Levendag PC, Schmitz PI, Jansen PP, et al. Fractionated high-dose-rate brachytherapy in primary carcinoma of the nasopharynx. *J Clin Oncol* 1998;16(6):2213–2220.

194. Levendag PC, Lagerwaard FJ, Noever I, et al. Role of endocavitary brachytherapy with or without chemotherapy in cancer of the nasopharynx. *Int J Radiat Oncol Biol Phys* 2002;52(3):755–768.

195. Wang CC. Re-irradiation of recurrent nasopharyngeal carcinoma—treatment techniques and results. *Int J Radiat Oncol Biol Phys* 1987;13(7):953–956.

196. Wang CC. Improved local control of nasopharyngeal carcinoma after intracavitary brachytherapy boost. *Am J Clin Oncol* 1991;14(1):5–8.

197. Zhang YW, Liu TF, Fi CX. Intracavitary radiation treatment of nasopharyngeal carcinoma by the high dose rate afterloading technique. *Int J Radiat Oncol Biol Phys* 1989;16(2):315–318.

198. Lee N, Hoffman R, Phillips TL, et al. Managing nasopharyngeal carcinoma with intracavitary brachytherapy: one institution's 45-year experience. *Brachytherapy* 2002;1(2):74–82.

199. Teo P, Leung SF, Choi P, et al. Afterloading radiotherapy for local persistence of nasopharyngeal carcinoma. *Br J Radiol* 1994;67(794):181–185.

200. Hwang JM, Fu KK, Phillips TL. Results and prognostic factors in the retreatment of locally recurrent nasopharyngeal carcinoma. *Int J Radiat Oncol Biol Phys* 1998;41(5):1099–1111.

201. Pryzant RM, Wendt CD, Delclos L, et al. Re-treatment of nasopharyngeal carcinoma in 53 patients. *Int J Radiat Oncol Biol Phys* 1992;22(5):941–947.

202. Harrison LB, Sessions RB, Fass DE, et al. Nasopharyngeal brachytherapy with access via a transpalatal flap. *Am J Surg* 1992;164(2):173–175.
203. Vikram B. Permanent iodine-125 (I-125) boost after teletherapy in primary cancers of the nasopharynx is safe and highly effective: long-term results. *Int J Radiat Oncol Biol Phys* 1997;38(5):1140.
204. Choy D, Sham JS, Wei WI, et al. Transpalatal insertion of radioactive gold grain for the treatment of persistent and recurrent nasopharyngeal carcinoma. *Int J Radiat Oncol Biol Phys* 1993;25(3):505–512.
205. Syed AM, Puthawala AA, Damore SJ, et al. Brachytherapy for primary and recurrent nasopharyngeal carcinoma: 20 years' experience at Long Beach Memorial. *Int J Radiat Oncol Biol Phys* 2000;47(5):1311–1321.
206. Levendag PC, Peters R, Meeuwis CA, et al. A new applicator design for endocavitary brachytherapy of cancer in the nasopharynx. *Radiother Oncol* 1997;45(1):95–98.
207. Chang JT, See LC, Tang SG, et al. The role of brachytherapy in early-stage nasopharyngeal carcinoma. *Int J Radiat Oncol Biol Phys* 1996;36(5):1019–1024.
208. Lu JJ, Shakespeare TP, Tan LK, et al. Adjuvant fractionated high-dose-rate intracavitary brachytherapy after external beam radiotherapy in Tl and T2 nasopharyngeal carcinoma. *Head Neck* 2004;26(5):389–395.
209. Ng T, Richards GM, Emery RS, et al. Customized conformal high-dose-rate brachytherapy boost for limited-volume nasopharyngeal cancer. *Int J Radiat Oncol Biol Phys* 2005;61(3):754–761.
210. Ozyar E, Yildz F, Akyol FH, et al. Adjuvant high-dose-rate brachytherapy after external beam radiotherapy in nasopharyngeal carcinoma. *Int J Radiat Oncol Biol Phys* 2002;52(1):101–108.
211. Ren YF, Gao YH, Cao XP, et al. 3D-CT implanted interstitial brachytherapy for T2b nasopharyngeal carcinoma. *Radiat Oncol* 2010;5:113.
212. Teo PM, Leung SF, Lee WY, et al. Intracavitary brachytherapy significantly enhances local control of early T-stage nasopharyngeal carcinoma: the existence of a dose-tumor-control relationship above conventional tumoricidal dose. *Int J Radiat Oncol Biol Phys* 2000;46(2):445–458.
213. Vikram B, Mishra S. Permanent iodine-125 (I-125) boost implants after external radiation therapy in nasopharyngeal cancer. *Int J Radiat Oncol Biol Phys* 1994;28(3):699–701.
214. Rosenblatt E, El-Gantiry M, Elattar I, et al. Brachytherapy boost in loco-regionally advanced nasopharyngeal carcinoma: a prospective randomized trial of the International Atomic Energy Agency. *Radiat Oncol* 2014;9:67.
215. Hara W, Loo BW Jr, Goffinet DR, et al. Excellent local control with stereotactic radiotherapy boost after external beam radiotherapy in patients with nasopharyngeal carcinoma. *Int J Radiat Oncol Biol Phys* 2008;71(2):393–400.
216. Sanchiz F, Milla A, Torner J, et al. Single fraction per day versus two fractions per day versus radiochemotherapy in the treatment of head and neck cancer. *Int J Radiat Oncol Biol Phys* 1990;19(6):1347–1350.
217. Teo PM, Leung SF, Chan AT, et al. Final report of a randomized trial on altered-fractionated radiotherapy in nasopharyngeal carcinoma prematurely terminated by significant increase in neurologic complications. *Int J Radiat Oncol Biol Phys* 2000;48(5):1311–1322.
218. Jen YM, Lin YS, Su WF, et al. Dose escalation using twice-daily radiotherapy for nasopharyngeal carcinoma: does heavier dosing result in a happier ending? *Int J Radiat Oncol Biol Phys* 2002;54(1):14–22.
219. Jen YM, Hsu WL, Chen CY, et al. Different risks of symptomatic brain necrosis in NPC patients treated with different altered fractionated radiotherapy techniques. *Int J Radiat Oncol Biol Phys* 2001;51(2):344–348.
220. Overgaard J, Hansen HS, Specht L, et al. Five compared with six fractions per week of conventional radiotherapy of squamous-cell carcinoma of head and neck: DAHANCA 6 and 7 randomised controlled trial. *Lancet* 2003;362(9388):933–940.
221. Lee AW, Sze WM, Yau TK, et al. Retrospective analysis on treating nasopharyngeal carcinoma with accelerated fractionation (6 fractions per week) in comparison with conventional fractionation (5 fractions per week): report on 3-year tumor control and normal tissue toxicity. *Radiother Oncol* 2001;58(2):121–130.
222. Lee AW, Tung SY, Chan AT, et al. Preliminary results of a randomized study (NPC-9902 Trial) on therapeutic gain by concurrent chemotherapy and/or accelerated fractionation for locally advanced nasopharyngeal carcinoma. *Int J Radiat Oncol Biol Phys* 2006;66(1):142–151.
223. Fu KK, Pajak TF, Trotti A, et al. A Radiation Therapy Oncology Group (RTOG) phase III randomized study to compare hyperfractionation and two variants of accelerated fractionation to standard fractionation radiotherapy for head and neck squamous cell carcinomas: first report of RTOG 9003. *Int J Radiat Oncol Biol Phys* 2000;48(1):7–16.
224. Al-Sarraf M, LeBlanc M, Giri PG, et al. Chemoradiotherapy versus radiotherapy in patients with advanced nasopharyngeal cancer: phase III randomized Intergroup study 0099. *J Clin Oncol* 1998;16(4):1310–1317.
225. Lin JC, Jan JS, Hsu CY, et al. Phase III study of concurrent chemoradiotherapy versus radiotherapy alone for advanced nasopharyngeal carcinoma: positive effect on overall and progression-free survival. *J Clin Oncol* 2003;21(4):631–637.
226. Kwong DL, Sham JS, Au GK, et al. Concurrent and adjuvant chemotherapy for nasopharyngeal carcinoma: a factorial study. *J Clin Oncol* 2004;22(13):2643–2653.
227. Chan AT, Leung SF, Ngan RK, et al. Overall survival after concurrent cisplatin-radiotherapy compared with radiotherapy alone in locoregionally advanced nasopharyngeal carcinoma. *J Natl Cancer Inst* 2005;97(7):536–539.
228. Wee J, Tan EH, Tai BC, et al. Randomized trial of radiotherapy versus concurrent chemoradiotherapy followed by adjuvant chemotherapy in patients with American Joint Committee on Cancer/International Union against cancer stage III and IV nasopharyngeal cancer of the endemic variety. *J Clin Oncol* 2005;23(27):6730–6738.
229. Zhang L, Zhao C, Peng PJ, et al. Phase III study comparing standard radiotherapy with or without weekly oxaliplatin in treatment of locoregionally advanced nasopharyngeal carcinoma: preliminary results. *J Clin Oncol* 2005;23(33):8461–8468.
230. Chen Y, Liu MZ, Liang SB, et al. Preliminary results of a prospective randomized trial comparing concurrent chemoradiotherapy plus adjuvant chemotherapy with radiotherapy alone in patients with locoregionally advanced nasopharyngeal carcinoma in endemic regions of china. *Int J Radiat Oncol Biol Phys* 2008;71(5):1356–1364.
231. Lee AW, Tung SY, Chua DT, et al. Randomized trial of radiotherapy plus concurrent-adjuvant chemotherapy vs radiotherapy alone for regionally advanced nasopharyngeal carcinoma. *J Natl Cancer Inst* 2010;102(15):1188–1198.
232. Lee AW, Tung SY, Chan AT, et al. A randomized trial on addition of concurrent-adjuvant chemotherapy and/or accelerated fractionation for locally-advanced nasopharyngeal carcinoma. *Radiother Oncol* 2011;98(1):15–22.
233. Chen QY, Wen YF, Guo L, et al. Concurrent chemoradiotherapy vs radiotherapy alone in stage II nasopharyngeal carcinoma: phase III randomized trial. *J Natl Cancer Inst* 2011;103(23):1761–1770.
234. Hui EP, Ma BB, Leung SF, et al. Randomized phase II trial of concurrent cisplatin-radiotherapy with or without neoadjuvant docetaxel and cisplatin in advanced nasopharyngeal carcinoma. *J Clin Oncol* 2009;27(2):242–249.
235. Fountzilas G, Ciuleanu E, Bobos M, et al. Induction chemotherapy followed by concomitant radiotherapy and weekly cisplatin versus the same concomitant chemoradiotherapy in patients with nasopharyngeal carcinoma: a randomized phase II study conducted by the Hellenic Cooperative Oncology Group (HeCOG) with biomarker evaluation. *Ann Oncol* 2012;23(2):427–435.
236. Chan AT, Felip E. Nasopharyngeal cancer: ESMO clinical recommendations for diagnosis, treatment and follow-up. *Ann Oncol* 2009;20 Suppl 4:123–125.
237. Chua DT, Ma J, Sham JS, et al. Improvement of survival after addition of induction chemotherapy to radiotherapy in patients with early-stage nasopharyngeal carcinoma: Subgroup analysis of two Phase III trials. *Int J Radiat Oncol Biol Phys* 2006;65(5):1300–1306.
238. Langendijk JA, Leemans CR, Buter J, et al. The additional value of chemotherapy to radiotherapy in locally advanced nasopharyngeal carcinoma: a meta-analysis of the published literature. *J Clin Oncol* 2004;22(22):4604–4612.
239. Chua DT, Sham JS, Choy D, et al. Preliminary report of the Asian-Oceanian Clinical Oncology Association randomized trial comparing cisplatin and epirubicin followed by radiotherapy versus radiotherapy alone in the treatment of patients with locoregionally advanced nasopharyngeal carcinoma. Asian-Oceanian Clinical Oncology Association Nasopharynx Cancer Study Group. *Cancer* 1998;83(11):2270–2283.
240. Preliminary results of a randomized trial comparing neoadjuvant chemotherapy (cisplatin, epirubicin, bleomycin) plus radiotherapy vs. radiotherapy alone in stage IV(> or = N2, M0) undifferentiated nasopharyngeal carcinoma: a positive effect on progression-free survival. International Nasopharynx Cancer Study Group. VUMCA I trial. *Int J Radiat Oncol Biol Phys* 1996;35(3):463–469.
241. Hareyama M, Sakata K, Shirato H, et al. A prospective, randomized trial comparing neoadjuvant chemotherapy with radiotherapy alone in patients with advanced nasopharyngeal carcinoma. *Cancer* 2002;94(8):2217–2223.
242. Ma J, Mai HQ, Hong MH, et al. Results of a prospective randomized trial comparing neoadjuvant chemotherapy plus radiotherapy with radiotherapy alone in patients with locoregionally advanced nasopharyngeal carcinoma. *J Clin Oncol* 2001;19(5):1350–1357.
243. Chan AT, Teo PM, Ngan RK, et al. Concurrent chemotherapy-radiotherapy compared with radiotherapy alone in locoregionally advanced nasopharyngeal carcinoma: progression-free survival analysis of a phase III randomized trial. *J Clin Oncol* 2002;20(8):2038–2044.
244. Chan AT, Teo PM, Leung TW, et al. A prospective randomized study of chemotherapy adjunctive to definitive radiotherapy in advanced nasopharyngeal carcinoma. *Int J Radiat Oncol Biol Phys* 1995;33(3):569–577.
245. Chi KH, Chang YC, Guo WY, et al. A phase III study of adjuvant chemotherapy in advanced nasopharyngeal carcinoma patients. *Int J Radiat Oncol Biol Phys* 2002;52(5):1238–1244.
246. Rossi A, Molinari R, Boracchi P, et al. Adjuvant chemotherapy with vincristine, cyclophosphamide, and doxorubicin after radiotherapy in local-regional nasopharyngeal cancer: results of a 4-year multicenter randomized study. *J Clin Oncol* 1988;6(9):1401–1410.
247. Baujat B, Audry H, Bourhis J, et al. Chemotherapy in locally advanced nasopharyngeal carcinoma: an individual patient data meta-analysis of eight randomized trials and 1753 patients. *Int J Radiat Oncol Biol Phys* 2006;64(1):47–56.
248. Chan AT. Nasopharyngeal carcinoma. *Ann Oncol* 2010;21 Suppl 7:vii, 308–312.
249. Chen Y, Sun Y, Liang SB, et al. Progress report of a randomized trial comparing long-term survival and late toxicity of concurrent chemoradiotherapy with adjuvant chemotherapy versus radiotherapy alone in patients with stage III to IVB nasopharyngeal carcinoma from endemic regions of China. *Cancer* 2013;119(12):2230–2238.
250. Jagdis A, Laskin J, Hao D, et al. Dose delivery analysis of weekly versus 3-weekly cisplatin concurrent with radiation therapy for locally advanced nasopharyngeal carcinoma (NPC). *Am J Clin Oncol* 2014;37(1):63–69.
251. Chitapanarux I, Lorvidhaya V, Kamnerdsupaphon P, et al. Chemoradiation comparing cisplatin versus carboplatin in locally advanced nasopharyngeal cancer: randomised, non-inferiority, open trial. *Eur J Cancer* 2007;43(9):1399–1406.
252. Ma BB, Kam MK, Leung SF, et al. A phase II study of concurrent cetuximab-cisplatin and intensity-modulated radiotherapy in locoregionally advanced nasopharyngeal carcinoma. *Ann Oncol* 2012;23(5):1287–1292.
253. Lee NY, Zhang Q, Pfister DG, et al. Addition of bevacizumab to standard chemoradiation for locoregionally advanced nasopharyngeal carcinoma (RTOG 0615): a phase 2 multi-institutional trial. *Lancet Oncol* 2012;13(2):172–180.

254. Chen L, Hu CS, Chen XZ, et al. Concurrent chemoradiotherapy plus adjuvant chemotherapy versus concurrent chemoradiotherapy alone in patients with locoregionally advanced nasopharyngeal carcinoma: a phase 3 multicentre randomised controlled trial. *Lancet Oncol* 2012;13(2):163–171.

255. Sun Y, Li WF, Chen NY, et al. Induction chemotherapy plus concurrent chemoradiotherapy versus concurrent chemoradiotherapy alone in locoregionally advanced nasopharyngeal carcinoma: a phase 3, multicentre, randomised controlled trial. *Lancet Oncol* 2016;17(11):1509–1520.

256. Cao SM, Yang Q, Guo L, et al. Neoadjuvant chemotherapy followed by concurrent chemoradiotherapy versus concurrent chemoradiotherapy alone in locoregionally advanced nasopharyngeal carcinoma: a phase III multicentre randomised controlled trial. *Eur J Cancer* 2017;75:14–23.

257. Lee AW, Ngan RK, Tung SY, et al. Preliminary results of trial NPC-0501 evaluating the therapeutic gain by changing from concurrent-adjuvant to induction-concurrent chemoradiotherapy, changing from fluorouracil to capecitabine, and changing from conventional to accelerated radiotherapy fractionation in patients with locoregionally advanced nasopharyngeal carcinoma. *Cancer* 2015;121(8):1328–1338.

258. Kwong DL, Wei WI, Cheng AC, et al. Long term results of radioactive gold grain implantation for the treatment of persistent and recurrent nasopharyngeal carcinoma. *Cancer* 2001;91(6):1105–1113.

259. Kwong DL, Nicholls J, Wei WI, et al. The time course of histologic remission after treatment of patients with nasopharyngeal carcinoma. *Cancer* 1999;85(7):1446–1453.

260. Chong VF, Fan YF. Detection of recurrent nasopharyngeal carcinoma: MR imaging versus CT. *Radiology* 1997;202(2):463–470.

261. Ragab SM, Erfan FA, Khalifa MA, et al. Detection of local failures after management of nasopharyngeal carcinoma: a prospective, controlled trial. *J Laryngol Otol* 2008;122(11):1230–1234.

262. Suarez C, Rodrigo JP, Rinaldo A, et al. Current treatment options for recurrent nasopharyngeal cancer. *Eur Arch Otorhinolaryngol* 2010;267(12):1811–1824.

263. Gong QY, Zheng GL, Zhu HY. MRI differentiation of recurrent nasopharyngeal carcinoma from postradiation fibrosis. *Comput Med Imaging Graph* 1991;15(6):423–429.

264. Chong VF, Fan YF. Skull base erosion in nasopharyngeal carcinoma: detection by CT and MRI. *Clin Radiol* 1996;51(9):625–631.

265. Chong VF, Fan YF, Khoo JB. Nasopharyngeal carcinoma with intracranial spread: CT and MR characteristics. *J Comput Assist Tomogr* 1996;20(4):563–569.

266. King WW, Ku PK, Mok CO, et al. Nasopharyngectomy in the treatment of recurrent nasopharyngeal carcinoma: a twelve-year experience. *Head Neck* 2000;22(3):215–222.

267. Kostakoglu L, Uysal U, Ozyar E, et al. Monitoring response to therapy with thallium-201 and technetium-99m-sestamibi SPECT in nasopharyngeal carcinoma. *J Nucl Med* 1997;38(7):1009–1014.

268. Yen RF, Hung RL, Pan MH, et al. 18-fluoro-2-deoxyglucose positron emission tomography in detecting residual/recurrent nasopharyngeal carcinomas and comparison with magnetic resonance imaging. *Cancer* 2003;98(2):283–287.

269. Ng SH, Joseph CT, Chan SC, et al. Clinical usefulness of 18F-FDG PET in nasopharyngeal carcinoma patients with questionable MRI findings for recurrence. *J Nucl Med* 2004;45(10):1669–1676.

270. Comoretto M, Balestreri L, Borsatti E, et al. Detection and restaging of residual and/or recurrent nasopharyngeal carcinoma after chemotherapy and radiation therapy: comparison of MR imaging and FDG PET/CT. *Radiology* 2008;249(1):203–211.

271. Toro C, Rinaldo A, Silver CE, et al. Paraneoplastic syndromes in patients with nasopharyngeal cancer. *Auris Nasus Larynx* 2009;36(5):513–520.

272. Wei WI, Yuen AP, Ng RW, et al. Quantitative analysis of plasma cell-free Epstein-Barr virus DNA in nasopharyngeal carcinoma after salvage nasopharyngectomy: a prospective study. *Head Neck* 2004;26(10):878–883.

273. Law SC, Lam WK, Ng MF, et al. Reirradiation of nasopharyngeal carcinoma with intracavitary mold brachytherapy: an effective means of local salvage. *Int J Radiat Oncol Biol Phys* 2002;54(4):1095–1113.

274. Leung TW, Tung SY, Sze WK, et al. Salvage brachytherapy for patients with locally persistent nasopharyngeal carcinoma. *Int J Radiat Oncol Biol Phys* 2000;47(2):405–412.

275. Leung TW, Tung SY, Wong VY, et al. Nasopharyngeal intracavitary brachytherapy: the controversy of T2b disease. *Cancer* 2005;104(8):1648–1655.

276. Zheng XK, Chen LH, Chen YQ, et al. Three-dimensional conformal radiotherapy versus intracavitary brachytherapy for salvage treatment of locally persistent nasopharyngeal carcinoma. *Int J Radiat Oncol Biol Phys* 2004;60(1):165–170.

277. Leung TW, Tung SY, Sze WK, et al. Salvage radiation therapy for locally recurrent nasopharyngeal carcinoma. *Int J Radiat Oncol Biol Phys* 2000;48(5):1331–1338.

278. Yau TK, Sze WM, Lee WM, et al. Effectiveness of brachytherapy and fractionated stereotactic radiotherapy boost for persistent nasopharyngeal carcinoma. *Head Neck* 2004;26(12):1024–1030.

279. Fu KK, Newman H, Phillips TL. Treatment of locally recurrent carcinoma of the nasopharynx. *Radiology* 1975;117(2):425–431.

280. Yan JH, Hu YH, Gu XZ. Radiation therapy of recurrent nasopharyngeal carcinoma. Report on 219 patients. *Acta Radiol Oncol* 1983;22(1):23–28.

281. Lee AW, Foo W, Law SC, et al. Reirradiation for recurrent nasopharyngeal carcinoma: factors affecting the therapeutic ratio and ways for improvement. *Int J Radiat Oncol Biol Phys* 1997;38(1):43–52.

282. Teo PM, Kwan WH, Chan AT, et al. How successful is high-dose (> or = 60 Gy) reirradiation using mainly external beams in salvaging local failures of nasopharyngeal carcinoma? *Int J Radiat Oncol Biol Phys* 1998;40(4):897–913.

283. Chua DT, Sham JS, Kwong DL, et al. Locally recurrent nasopharyngeal carcinoma: treatment results for patients with computed tomography assessment. *Int J Radiat Oncol Biol Phys* 1998;41(2):379–386.

284. Chang JT, See LC, Liao CT, et al. Locally recurrent nasopharyngeal carcinoma. *Radiother Oncol* 2000;54(2):135–142.

285. Zheng XK, Ma J, Chen LH, et al. Dosimetric and clinical results of three-dimensional conformal radiotherapy for locally recurrent nasopharyngeal carcinoma. *Radiother Oncol* 2005;75(2):197–203.

286. Lu TX, Mai WY, Teh BS, et al. Initial experience using intensity-modulated radiotherapy for recurrent nasopharyngeal carcinoma. *Int J Radiat Oncol Biol Phys* 2004;58(3):682–687.

287. Chua DT, Sham JS, Leung LH, et al. Re-irradiation of nasopharyngeal carcinoma with intensity-modulated radiotherapy. *Radiother Oncol* 2005;77(3):290–294.

288. Koutcher L, Lee N, Zelefsky M, et al. Reirradiation of locally recurrent nasopharynx cancer with external beam radiotherapy with or without brachytherapy. *Int J Radiat Oncol Biol Phys* 2010;76(1):130–137.

289. Ozyigit G, Cengiz M, Yazici G, et al. A retrospective comparison of robotic stereotactic body radiotherapy and three-dimensional conformal radiotherapy for the reirradiation of locally recurrent nasopharyngeal carcinoma. *Int J Radiat Oncol Biol Phys* 2011;81(4):e263–e268.

290. Qiu S, Lin S, Tham IW, et al. Intensity-modulated radiation therapy in the salvage of locally recurrent nasopharyngeal carcinoma. *Int J Radiat Oncol Biol Phys* 2011.

291. Lee N, Chan K, Bekelman JE, et al. Salvage re-irradiation for recurrent head and neck cancer. *Int J Radiat Oncol Biol Phys* 2007;68(3):731–740.

292. Lee AW, Law SC, Foo W, et al. Retrospective analysis of patients with nasopharyngeal carcinoma treated during 1976–1985: survival after local recurrence. *Int J Radiat Oncol Biol Phys* 1993;26(5):773–782.

293. Chen AM, Phillips TL, Lee NY. Practical considerations in the re-irradiation of recurrent and second primary head-and-neck cancer: who, why, how, and how much? *Int J Radiat Oncol Biol Phys* 2011;81(5):1211–1219.

294. Lee AW, Foo W, Law SC, et al. Total biological effect on late reactive tissues following reirradiation for recurrent nasopharyngeal carcinoma. *Int J Radiat Oncol Biol Phys* 2000;46(4):865–872.

295. Cmelak AJ, Cox RS, Adler JR, et al. Radiosurgery for skull base malignancies and nasopharyngeal carcinoma. *Int J Radiat Oncol Biol Phys* 1997;37(5):997–1003.

296. Chua DT, Sham JS, Hung KN, et al. Stereotactic radiosurgery as a salvage treatment for locally persistent and recurrent nasopharyngeal carcinoma. *Head Neck* 1999;21(7):620–626.

297. Chen HJ, Leung SW, Su CY. Linear accelerator based radiosurgery as a salvage treatment for skull base and intracranial invasion of recurrent nasopharyngeal carcinomas. *Am J Clin Oncol* 2001;24(3):255–258.

298. Pai PC, Chuang CC, Wei KC, et al. Stereotactic radiosurgery for locally recurrent nasopharyngeal carcinoma. *Head Neck* 2002;24(8):748–753.

299. Xiao J, Xu G, Miao Y. Fractionated stereotactic radiosurgery for 50 patients with recurrent or residual nasopharyngeal carcinoma. *Int J Radiat Oncol Biol Phys* 2001;51(1):164–170.

300. Wu SX, Chua DT, Deng ML, et al. Outcome of fractionated stereotactic radiotherapy for 90 patients with locally persistent and recurrent nasopharyngeal carcinoma. *Int J Radiat Oncol Biol Phys* 2007;69(3):761–769.

301. Chua DT, Wu SX, Lee V, et al. Comparison of single versus fractionated dose of stereotactic radiotherapy for salvaging local failures of nasopharyngeal carcinoma: a matched-cohort analysis. *Head Neck Oncol* 2009;1:13.

302. Yeh SA, Tang Y, Lui CC, et al. Treatment outcomes and late complications of 849 patients with nasopharyngeal carcinoma treated with radiotherapy alone. *Int J Radiat Oncol Biol Phys* 2005;62(3):672–679.

303. Leung TW, Tung SY, Sze WK, et al. Treatment results of 1070 patients with nasopharyngeal carcinoma: an analysis of survival and failure patterns. *Head Neck* 2005;27(7):555–565.

304. Lin R, Slater JD, Yonemoto LT, et al. Nasopharyngeal carcinoma: repeat treatment with conformal proton therapy—dose-volume histogram analysis. *Radiology* 1999;213(2):489–494.

305. Romesser PB, Cahlon O, Scher ED, et al. Proton beam reirradiation for recurrent head and neck cancer: multi-institutional report on feasibility and early outcomes. *Int J Radiat Oncol Biol Phys* 2016;95(1):386–395.

306. Poon D, Yap SP, Wong ZW, et al. Concurrent chemoradiotherapy in locoregionally recurrent nasopharyngeal carcinoma. *Int J Radiat Oncol Biol Phys* 2004;59(5):1312–1318.

307. Wei WI, Ho CM, Wong MP, et al. Pathological basis of surgery in the management of postradiotherapy cervical metastasis in nasopharyngeal carcinoma. *Arch Otolaryngol Head Neck Surg* 1992;118(9):923–929; discussion 930.

308. Wei WI, Lam KH, Ho CM, et al. Efficacy of radical neck dissection for the control of cervical metastasis after radiotherapy for nasopharyngeal carcinoma. *Am J Surg* 1990;160(4):439–442.

309. Wei WI, Ho WK, Cheng AC, et al. Management of extensive cervical nodal metastasis in nasopharyngeal carcinoma after radiotherapy: a clinicopathological study. *Arch Otolaryngol Head Neck Surg* 2001;127(12):1457–1462.

310. Hsu MM, Ko JY, Sheen TS, et al. Salvage surgery for recurrent nasopharyngeal carcinoma. *Arch Otolaryngol Head Neck Surg* 1997;123(3):305–309.

311. Fee WE Jr, Gilmer PA, Goffinet DR. Surgical management of recurrent nasopharyngeal carcinoma after radiation failure at the primary site. *Laryngoscope* 1988;98(11):1220–1226.

312. Fee WE Jr, Roberson JB Jr, Goffinet DR. Long-term survival after surgical resection for recurrent nasopharyngeal cancer after radiotherapy failure. *Arch Otolaryngol Head Neck Surg* 1991;117(11):1233–1236.

313. Fisch U. The infratemporal fossa approach for nasopharyngeal tumors. *Laryngoscope* 1983;93(1):36–44.

314. Morton RP, Liavaag PG, McLean M, et al. Transcervico-mandibulo-palatal approach for surgical salvage of recurrent nasopharyngeal cancer. *Head Neck* 1996;18(4):352–358.

315. Wei WI, Lam KH, Sham JS. New approach to the nasopharynx: the maxillary swing approach. *Head Neck* 1991;13(3):200–207.

316. Hao SP, Tsang NM, Chang KP, et al. Nasopharyngectomy for recurrent nasopharyngeal carcinoma: a review of 53 patients and prognostic factors. *Acta Otolaryngol* 2008;128(4):473–481.

317. Wei WI. Salvage surgery for recurrent primary nasopharyngeal carcinoma. *Crit Rev Oncol Hematol* 2000;33(2):91–98.

318. Wei WI, Sham JS. Nasopharyngeal carcinoma. *Lancet* 2005;365(9476): 2041–2054.

319. Ng RW, Wei WI. Elimination of palatal fistula after the maxillary swing procedure. *Head Neck* 2005;27(7):608–612.

320. Chang KP, Hao SP, Tsang NM, et al. Salvage surgery for locally recurrent nasopharyngeal carcinoma: a 10-year experience. *Otolaryngol Head Neck Surg* 2004;131(4):497–502.

321. Danesi G, Zanoletti E, Mazzoni A. Salvage surgery for recurrent nasopharyngeal carcinoma. *Skull Base* 2007;17(3):173–180.

322. Wei WI. Cancer of the nasopharynx: functional surgical salvage. *World J Surg* 2003;27(7):844–848.

323. Wei WI, Ho CM, Yuen PW, et al. Maxillary swing approach for resection of tumors in and around the nasopharynx. *Arch Otolaryngol Head Neck Surg* 1995;121(6):638–642.

324. Shu CH, Cheng H, Lirng JF, et al. Salvage surgery for recurrent nasopharyngeal carcinoma. *Laryngoscope* 2000;110(9):1483–1488.

325. Chan JY, Chow VL, Mok VW, et al. Prediction of surgical outcome using plasma Epstein-Barr virus dna and (18) F-FDG PET-CT scan in recurrent nasopharyngeal carcinoma. *Head Neck* 2011.

326. Wang C. Carcinoma of the nasopharynx. In: Wang CC, ed. *Radiation therapy for head and neck neoplasms: Indications, techniques, and results.* Chicago, IL: Year Book Medical Publishers, 1990:261–283.

327. Bailet JW, Mark RJ, Abemayor E, et al. Nasopharyngeal carcinoma: treatment results with primary radiation therapy. *Laryngoscope* 1992;102(9): 965–972.

328. Le QT, Tate D, Koong A, et al. Improved local control with stereotactic radiosurgical boost in patients with nasopharyngeal carcinoma. *Int J Radiat Oncol Biol Phys* 2003;56(4):1046–1054.

329. Hara W, Loo BW, Goffinet DR. Excellent local control with stereotactic radiotherapy boost after external beam radiotherapy in patients with nasopharyngeal carcinoma. *Int J Radiat Oncol Biol Phys* 2008.

330. Vikram B, Strong EW, Manolatos S, et al. Improved survival in carcinoma of the nasopharynx. *Head Neck Surg* 1984;7(2):123–128.

331. Lee N, Harris J, Garden AS, et al. Intensity-modulated radiation therapy with or without chemotherapy for nasopharyngeal carcinoma: radiation therapy oncology group phase II trial 0225. *J Clin Oncol* 2009;27(22):3684–3690.

332. Lin S, Pan J, Han L, et al. Nasopharyngeal carcinoma treated with reduced volume intensity-modulated radiation therapy: report on the 3-year outcome of a prospective series. *Int J Radiat Oncol Biol Phys* 2009;75(4):1071–1078.

333. Wong FC, Ng AW, Lee VH, et al. Whole-field simultaneous integrated-boost intensity-modulated radiotherapy for patients with nasopharyngeal carcinoma. *Int J Radiat Oncol Biol Phys* 2010;76(1):138–145.

334. Lin S, Lu JJ, Han L, et al. Sequential chemotherapy and intensity-modulated radiation therapy in the management of locoregionally advanced nasopharyngeal carcinoma: experience of 370 consecutive cases. *BMC Cancer* 2010;10:39.

335. Kam M, Leung S, Yu K, et al. Long-term treatment outcome of nasopharyngeal carcinoma (NPC) using intensity-modulated radiotherapy (IMRT). *J Clin Oncol* 2010;28(15S):Abstract 5582.

336. Xiao WW, Huang SM, Han F, et al. Local control, survival, and late toxicities of locally advanced nasopharyngeal carcinoma treated by simultaneous modulated accelerated radiotherapy combined with cisplatin concurrent chemotherapy: long-term results of a phase 2 study. *Cancer* 2010;117(9): 1874–1883.

337. Xiayun H, Ou D, Ying H, et al. Experience with combination of cisplatin plus gemcitabine chemotherapy and intensity-modulated radiotherapy for locoregionally advanced nasopharyngeal carcinoma. *Eur Arch Otorhinolaryngol* 2012;269(3):1027–1033.

338. Su SF, Han F, Zhao C, et al. Long-term outcomes of early-stage nasopharyngeal carcinoma patients treated with intensity-modulated radiotherapy alone. *Int J Radiat Oncol Biol Phys* 2012;82(1):327–333.

339. Sun X, Su S, Chen C, et al. Long-term outcomes of intensity-modulated radiotherapy for 868 patients with nasopharyngeal carcinoma: an analysis of survival and treatment toxicities. *Radiother Oncol* 2014;110(3):398–403.

340. Wu LR, Liu YT, Jiang N, et al. Ten-year survival outcomes for patients with nasopharyngeal carcinoma receiving intensity-modulated radiotherapy: an analysis of 614 patients from a single center. *Oral Oncol* 2017;69:26–32.

341. Peters LJ, Harrison ML, Dimery IW, et al. Acute and late toxicity associated with sequential bleomycin-containing chemotherapy regimens and radiation therapy in the treatment of carcinoma of the nasopharynx. *Int J Radiat Oncol Biol Phys* 1988;14(4):623–633.

342. Lee AW, Yau TK, Wong DH, et al. Treatment of stage IV(A-B) nasopharyngeal carcinoma by induction-concurrent chemoradiotherapy and accelerated fractionation. *Int J Radiat Oncol Biol Phys* 2005;63(5):1331–1338.

343. Chi KH, Chan WK, Cooper DL, et al. A phase II study of outpatient chemotherapy with cisplatin, 5-fluorouracil, and leucovorin in nasopharyngeal carcinoma. *Cancer* 1994;73(2):247–252.

344. Lee AW, Ng SH, Ho JH, et al. Clinical diagnosis of late temporal lobe necrosis following radiation therapy for nasopharyngeal carcinoma. *Cancer* 1988;61(8):1535–1542.

345. Lin YS, Jen YM, Lin JC. Radiation-related cranial nerve palsy in patients with nasopharyngeal carcinoma. *Cancer* 2002;95(2):404–409.

346. Wu CH, Hsiao TY, Ko JY, et al. Dysphagia after radiotherapy: Endoscopic examination of swallowing in patients with nasopharyngeal carcinoma. *Ann Otol Rhinol Laryngol* 2000;109(3):320–325.

347. Parsons JT, Bova FJ, Fitzgerald CR, et al. Radiation optic neuropathy after megavoltage external-beam irradiation: analysis of time-dose factors. *Int J Radiat Oncol Biol Phys* 1994;30(4):755–763.

348. Jen YM, Lin YC, Wang YB, et al. Dramatic and prolonged decrease of whole salivary secretion in nasopharyngeal carcinoma patients treated with radiotherapy. *Oral Surg Oral Med Oral Pathol Oral Radiol Endod* 2006;101(3):322–327.

349. Pow EH, Kwong DL, McMillan AS, et al. Xerostomia and quality of life after intensity-modulated radiotherapy vs. conventional radiotherapy for early-stage nasopharyngeal carcinoma: initial report on a randomized controlled clinical trial. *Int J Radiat Oncol Biol Phys* 2006;66(4):981–991.

350. Kam MK, Leung SF, Zee B, et al. Prospective randomized study of intensity-modulated radiotherapy on salivary gland function in early-stage nasopharyngeal carcinoma patients. *J Clin Oncol* 2007;25(31):4873–4879.

351. Cannon DM, Lee NY. Recurrence in region of spared parotid gland after definitive intensity-modulated radiotherapy for head and neck cancer. *Int J Radiat Biol Phys* 2008;70(3):660–665.

352. Tong AC, Leung AC, Cheng JC, et al. Incidence of complicated healing and osteoradionecrosis following tooth extraction in patients receiving radiotherapy for treatment of nasopharyngeal carcinoma. *Aust Dent J* 1999;44(3):187–194.

353. Bedwinek JM, Shukovsky LJ, Fletcher GH, et al. Osteonecrosis in patients treated with definitive radiotherapy for squamous cell carcinomas of the oral cavity and naso- and oropharynx. *Radiology* 1976;119(3):665–667.

354. Lee AW, Ng WT, Hung WM, et al. Major late toxicities after conformal radiotherapy for nasopharyngeal carcinoma-patient- and treatment-related risk factors. *Int J Radiat Oncol Biol Phys* 2009;73(4):1121–1128.

355. Grau C, Moller K, Overgaard M, et al. Sensori-neural hearing loss in patients treated with irradiation for nasopharyngeal carcinoma. *Int J Radiat Oncol Biol Phys* 1991;21(3):723–728.

356. Chen WC, Jackson A, Budnick AS, et al. Sensorineural hearing loss in combined modality treatment of nasopharyngeal carcinoma. *Cancer* 2006;106(4):820–829.

357. Chan SH, Ng WT, Kam KL, et al. Sensorineural hearing loss after treatment of nasopharyngeal carcinoma: a longitudinal analysis. *Int J Radiat Oncol Biol Phys* 2009;73(5):1335–1342.

358. Cheng SW, Ting AC, Lam LK, et al. Carotid stenosis after radiotherapy for nasopharyngeal carcinoma. *Arch Otolaryngol Head Neck Surg* 2000;126(4):517–521.

359. Lam WW, Leung SF, So NM, et al. Incidence of carotid stenosis in nasopharyngeal carcinoma patients after radiotherapy. *Cancer* 2001;92(9):2357–2363.

360. Cheng KM, Chan CM, Cheung YL, et al. Endovascular treatment of radiation-induced petrous internal carotid artery aneurysm presenting with acute haemorrhage. A report of two cases. *Acta Neurochir (Wien)* 2001;143(4):351–355; discussion 355–356.

361. Lam KS, Tse VK, Wang C, et al. Early effects of cranial irradiation on hypothalamic-pituitary function. *J Clin Endocrinol Metab* 1987;64(3):418–424.

362. Lam KS, Tse VK, Wang C, et al. Effects of cranial irradiation on hypothalamic-pituitary function—a 5-year longitudinal study in patients with nasopharyngeal carcinoma. *Q J Med* 1991;78(286):165–176.

363. Lam KS, Ho JH, Lee AW, et al. Symptomatic hypothalamic-pituitary dysfunction in nasopharyngeal carcinoma patients following radiation therapy: a retrospective study. *Int J Radiat Oncol Biol Phys* 1987;13(9):1343–1350.

364. Lam KS, Wang C, Yeung RT, et al. Hypothalamic hypopituitarism following cranial irradiation for nasopharyngeal carcinoma. *Clin Endocrinol (Oxf)* 1986;24(6):643–651.

365. Sham J, Choy D, Kwong PW, et al. Radiotherapy for nasopharyngeal carcinoma: shielding the pituitary may improve therapeutic ratio. *Int J Radiat Oncol Biol Phys* 1994;29(4):699–704.

366. Dickens P, Wei WI, Sham JS. Osteosarcoma of the maxilla in Hong Kong Chinese postirradiation for nasopharyngeal carcinoma. A report of four cases. *Cancer* 1990;66(9):1924–1926.

367. Teo PM, Chan AT, Leung SF, et al. Increased incidence of tongue cancer after primary radiotherapy for nasopharyngeal carcinoma—the possibility of radiation carcinogenesis. *Eur J Cancer* 1999;35(2):219–225.

Section
III

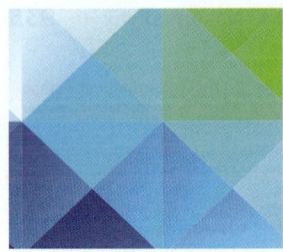

C H A P T E R   4 5

Cancer of the Nasal Cavity and Paranasal Sinuses

Steven J. Frank, Anesa Ahamad, and Carlos A. Perez

This is an update of a previous chapter published by Frank et al. in the 6th edition of Principles and Practice of Radiation Oncology.[1]

ANATOMY

Nasal Cavity

The nasal cavity extends from the hard palate inferiorly to the base of the skull superiorly. It is above and behind the vestibule and is defined anteriorly by the transition from the skin to mucous membrane and posteriorly by the choanae, which open directly into the nasopharynx.[2] The nasal cavity consists of four subsites: the nasal vestibule, the lateral walls, the floor, and the septum.

The *nasal vestibule* is the triangular space located inside the aperture of the nostril as a slight dilation that extends as a small recess toward the apex of the nose. It is defined laterally by the alae; medially by the membranous septum, the distal end of the cartilaginous septum, and columella; and inferiorly by the adjacent floor of the nasal cavity. It is lined by the skin containing hairs and sebaceous glands; therefore, tumors at this location are often those that arise from the skin, usually squamous cell cancers[3], but may occasionally be basal cell carcinoma,[4] sebaceous carcinoma,[5] melanoma,[6] or non–Hodgkin lymphoma.[7]

The *lateral walls* correspond with the medial walls of the maxillary sinuses and consist of thin bony structures that have three shell-shaped projections (superior, middle, and inferior conchae or turbinates) into the nasal cavity. The *floor* extends from the vestibule to the nasopharynx above the hard palate of the maxilla. The *septum* divides the nasal cavity into right and left halves.

Paranasal Sinuses

The paranasal sinuses are named according to the bones in which they are located: the ethmoid, maxilla, sphenoid, and frontal.

Ethmoid Sinuses

The ethmoid sinuses are composed of several small cavities, the ethmoid air cells, within the ethmoid labyrinth located below the anterior cranial fossa and between the nasal cavity and the orbit. They are separated from the orbital cavity by a thin, porous bone, the *lamina papyracea*, and from the anterior cranial fossa by a portion of the frontal bone, the *fovea ethmoidalis*. They are in close proximity to the optic nerves laterally and the optic chiasm posteriorly. The ethmoid sinuses are divided into anterior, middle, and posterior groups of air cells. The middle ethmoid cells open directly into the middle meatus. The anterior cells may drain indirectly into the middle meatus via the infundibulum. The posterior cells open directly into the superior meatus.

Maxillary Sinuses

The maxillary sinuses, the largest of the paranasal sinuses, are pyramid-shaped cavities located in the maxillae. The lateral walls of the nasal cavity form the base and the roofs correspond to the orbital floors, which contain the infraorbital canals. The floors of the maxillary sinuses are composed of the alveolar processes. The apices extend toward and frequently into the zygomatic bones. Secretions drain by mucociliary action into the middle meatus via the hiatus semilunaris through an aperture near the roof of the maxillary sinus. Ohngren line is a theoretical plane dividing each maxillary sinus into the suprastructure and infrastructure; it is defined by connecting the medial canthus with the angle of the mandible.

Sphenoid Sinus and Frontal Sinuses

The sphenoid bone forms a midline inner cavity that communicates with the nasal cavity through an aperture in its anterior wall. It is directly apposed superiorly to the pituitary gland and optic chiasm, laterally to the cavernous sinuses, anteriorly to the ethmoid sinuses and nasal cavity, and inferiorly to the nasopharynx. The paired, typically asymmetric frontal sinuses are located between the inner and outer tables of the frontal bone. They are anterior to the anterior cranial fossa, superior to the sphenoid and ethmoid sinuses, and superomedial to the orbits. They usually communicate with the middle meatus of the nasal cavity.

EPIDEMIOLOGY

Cancers of the nasal cavity and paranasal sinuses are relatively uncommon. Fewer than 7,500 cases are diagnosed each year in the United States, an incidence of 0.75 per 100,000.[8] Cancers of the maxillary sinus are twice as common as those of the nasal cavity; cancers of the ethmoid, frontal, and sphenoid sinuses are extremely rare. They generally develop after the age of 40 years, except for esthesioneuroblastoma (ENB), which has a unique bimodal age distribution[9] and occurs twice as often in men than in women.[10] These tumors are most common in Japan and South Africa.

The etiologic factors vary by tumor type and location. Adenocarcinomas of the nasal cavity and ethmoid sinus have been reported to occur more frequently in carpenters and sawmill workers who are exposed to wood dust.[11,12] Synthetic wood, binding agents, and glues may also be involved as cocarcinogens.[13] Squamous cell carcinomas (SCCs) of the nasal cavity have been seen more often in nickel workers.[14] Maxillary sinus carcinomas have been associated with radioactive thorium-containing contrast material (thorotrast) used for radiographic visualization of the maxillary sinuses in the past. Occupational exposure in the production of chromium, mustard gas, isopropyl alcohol, and radium also may increase the risk of sinonasal carcinomas.

Cigarette smoking is reported to increase the risk of nasal cancer, with a doubling of risk among heavy or long-term smokers and a reduction in risk after long-term cessation. After adjustment for smoking, a significant dose–response relationship has also been noted between alcohol consumption and risk of nasal cancer.[15]

NATURAL HISTORY

Nasal Vestibule

Nasal vestibule carcinomas can spread by direct invasion of the upper lip, gingivolabial sulcus, premaxilla (early events),

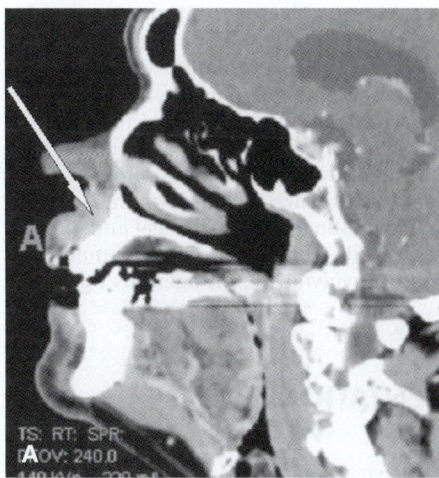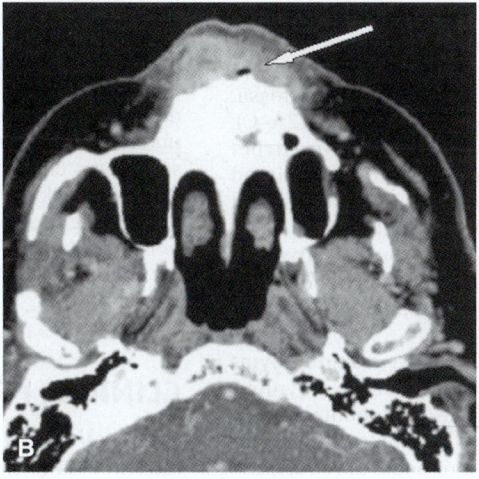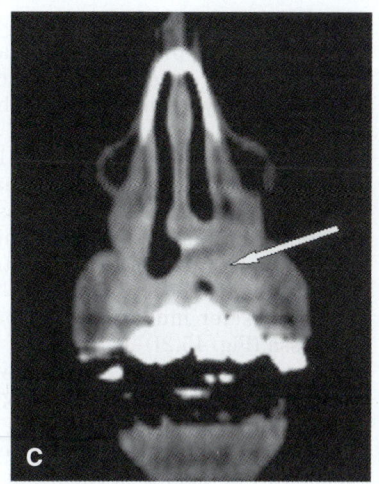

FIGURE 45.1. Computed tomography scans of a nasal vestibule SCC that has spread by direct invasion of the upper lip (*arrow* in **A**) and gingivolabial sulcus and premaxilla (*arrow* in **B** and **C**).

or nasal cavity (late events), as shown in Figure 45.1. Vertical invasion may result in septal (membranous or cartilaginous) perforation or alar cartilage destruction. Lymphatic spread from nasal vestibule carcinomas is usually to the ipsilateral facial (buccinator and mandibular) and submandibular nodes. Large lesions extending across the midline may spread to the contralateral facial or submandibular nodes. The incidence of nodal metastasis at diagnosis is approximately 5%.[16,17] Without elective nodal treatment, approximately 15% of patients develop nodal relapse. Hematogenous metastases are rare.

Nasal Cavity and Ethmoid Sinuses

The pattern of contiguous spread of carcinomas varies with the location of the primary lesion. Tumors arising in the upper nasal cavity and ethmoid cells can extend to the orbit through the thin lamina papyracea and to the anterior cranial fossa via the cribriform plate, or they may grow through the nasal bone to the subcutaneous tissue and skin. Lateral wall primaries invade the maxillary antrum, ethmoid cells, orbit, pterygopalatine fossa, and nasopharynx. Primaries of the floor and lower septum may invade the palate and maxillary antrum. Perineural extension (typically involving branches of the trigeminal nerve) is seen most often with adenoid cystic carcinomas.

Lymphatic spread of nasal cavity primaries is uncommon, although spread to retropharyngeal and cervical lymph nodes is possible. In a series of 51 patients reported by the University of Texas MD Anderson Cancer Center, only one patient had palpable subdigastric nodes at diagnosis. Of the 36 patients who did not receive elective lymphatic irradiation, two (6%) experienced subdigastric nodal relapse.[18]

The risk of nodal involvement in patients with cancer of the nasal cavity and paranasal sinuses has not been well defined and may vary depending on the histologic subtype. Current decision-making on whether to cover specific nodal regions is based on interpretation of single-institution retrospective analyses.

Ahn[19] in a review of the SEER database from 2004 to 2009 identified 1,811 patients who had local and nodal staging information, with paranasal sinus cancer as their first cancer diagnosis, defined histology (squamous, melanoma, adenocarcinoma, sinonasal undifferentiated, and ENB), and defined primary site. Of all the patients examined with information on local and nodal extent, 1,578 patients (87.1%) had no gross nodal involvement at presentation. On presentation, level 1 was involved in 5.1%, level 2 in 6.7%, level 3 in 1.8%, level 4 in 1.2%, level 5 in 1.1%, retropharyngeal nodes in 0.7%, parotid nodes in 0.6%, and facial nodes in 0.2% of all patients.

Isolated skip metastases to levels 3 or 4 occurred in 0.7% of patients. On presentation, at least 2.5% presented with bilateral or contralateral disease. In patients with SCC of the nasal cavity, there was a clear gradation in nodal risk among patients with T1 versus T4 disease (4% vs. 23%, $P < .001$); this was not evident in patients with melanoma of the nasal cavity, who had a 5% to 10% risk of nodal involvement regardless of local extension. Local extension of SCC of the maxillary sinus did not predict for nodal involvement in a significant manner, although T1 tumors showed an 11% risk of nodal involvement compared to 21% to 24% for T2+ disease. Squamous cell, small cell, and sinonasal undifferentiated carcinoma had higher rates of nodal dissemination at presentation (14.4%, 19.1%, and 25.3%, respectively), compared to adenocarcinoma, ENB, and melanoma (7.1%, 8.7%, 5.8%, respectively). Although confounded by stage and histology, maxillary sinus carries the highest risk (20.6%), followed by frontal/sphenoid (15.4%), ethmoid (11.9%), and nasal cavity (8.5%, $P < .001$).

The issue of appropriate radiation volumes in the treatment of these patients has not been entirely elucidated, although the data suggest that in some with potential higher nodal involvement, it is advisable to electively irradiate regions at risk. However, as noted by Ahn,[19] in the absence of gross neck disease, the low-neck and retropharyngeal nodes do not need to be treated.

Hematogenous dissemination is rare. In the MD Anderson Cancer Center series, for example, distant metastasis to the bone, brain, or liver occurred in only 4 of 51 patients.[20]

The olfactory region is the site of origin of ENB and, occasionally, adenocarcinomas. ENB constitutes approximately only 3% of all intranasal neoplasms. About 250 cases have been reported between 1924 and 1990.[20] The tumor typically is composed of round, oval, or fusiform cells containing neurofibrils with pseudorosette formation and diffusely increased microvascularity.[21]

Esthesioneuroblastoma may be mistaken for any other "small round cell tumor," that is, a group of aggressive malignant tumors composed of small and monotonous undifferentiated cells that include Ewing sarcoma, peripheral primitive neuroectodermal tumor (also known as extraskeletal Ewing's), rhabdomyosarcoma, lymphoma, small cell carcinoma (undifferentiated or neuroendocrine), and mesenchymal chondrosarcoma. The clinical presentations of these entities often overlap, but clinicopathologic features and immunohistochemical staining may help in distinguishing among them.

The route of contiguous spread of ENB is similar to that of ethmoid carcinomas. Lymph node involvement and distant metastasis are uncommon at diagnosis.[22,23]

Section III

Maxillary Sinuses

The pattern of spread of maxillary sinus cancers varies with the site of origin. Suprastructure tumors extend into the nasal cavity, ethmoid cells, orbit, pterygopalatine fossa, infratemporal fossa, and base of the skull (Fig. 45.2A–C). Invasion of these structures gives lesions of the suprastructure a poorer prognosis. Their treatment is also associated with greater morbidity as a consequence of craniofacial resection or radiation of intracranial and ocular structures. Infrastructure tumors often infiltrate the palate, alveolar process, gingivobuccal sulcus, soft tissue of the cheek, nasal cavity, masseter muscle, pterygopalatine space, and pterygoid fossa (Fig. 45.2D–J).

The maxillary sinuses are believed to have a limited lymphatic supply[24] and a correspondingly low incidence of lymphadenopathy at diagnosis.[25,26] Only 6 of the 73 patients (8%) in the MD Anderson Cancer Center series had palpable lymphadenopathy at diagnosis. The incidence of nodal spread, however, varies with the histologic type (17%, or 5 of 29 patients with squamous cell or poorly differentiated carcinomas, vs. 4%, or 1 of 27 for patients with adenocarcinoma, adenoid cystic carcinoma, or mucoepidermoid carcinoma). The incidence of subclinical disease, as reflected in the rate of nodal relapse in patients who did not receive elective neck treatment, also varies with histologic type (38%, or 9 of 24 patients with squamous cell or poorly differentiated carcinomas, vs. 8%, or 2 of 26 patients with adenocarcinoma, adenoid cystic carcinoma, or mucoepidermoid carcinoma). The cumulative incidence of nodal involvement (gross and microscopic) for patients with squamous cell and poorly differentiated carcinomas is about 30%. The risk of regional recurrence after treatment is 20% to 30% or higher, depending on the extent of disease and elective neck treatment.[27] Ipsilateral subdigastric and submandibular nodes are most often involved. Hematogenous spread is uncommon.

CLINICAL PRESENTATION

Nasal Vestibule

Carcinomas of the nasal vestibule usually present as asymptomatic plaques or nodules, often with crusting and scabbing. Advanced lesions may extend beyond the vestibule and may cause pain, bleeding, or ulceration. Large ulcerated lesions may become infected, leading to severe tenderness that requires anesthesia for complete clinical assessment.

FIGURE 45.2. The pattern of spread of maxillary sinus cancers. **A–C:** Suprastructure tumors are shown, with *arrows* indicating the involvement of the nasal cavity and ethmoid cells **(A)**, the orbit **(B)**, and the base of the skull **(C)**. **D–J:** Advanced tumor is shown, with *arrows* indicating alveolar process destruction with loosening of a tooth **(E)** and abutment of the orbital floor without frank intraorbital invasion **(F)**. The patient had a maxillectomy and orbital floor resection with an anterior–lateral thigh (ALT) flap (*arrow* in **G**), and titanium mesh reconstruction of the orbital floor **(H, I,** and **J)**.

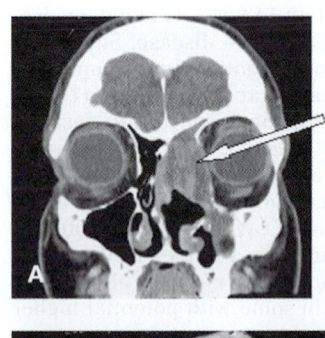
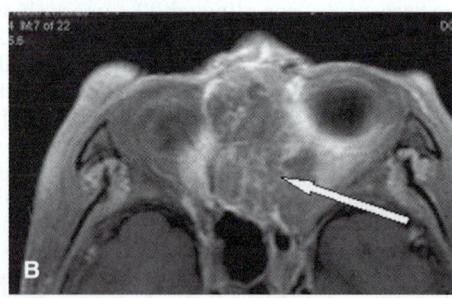
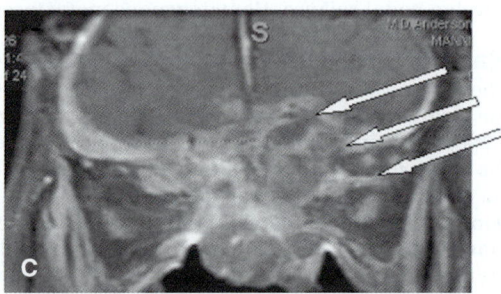
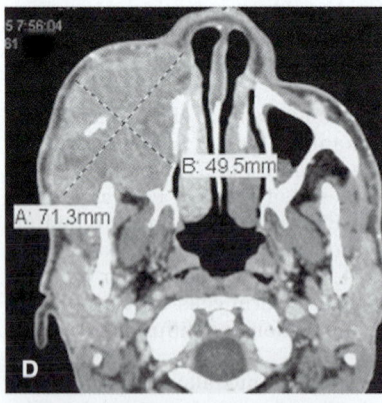
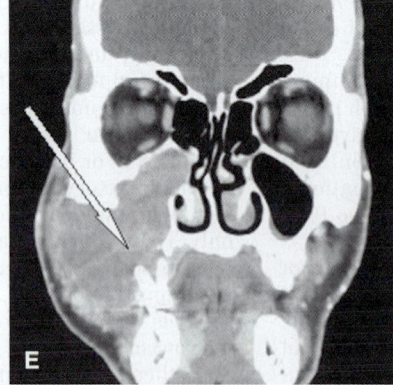
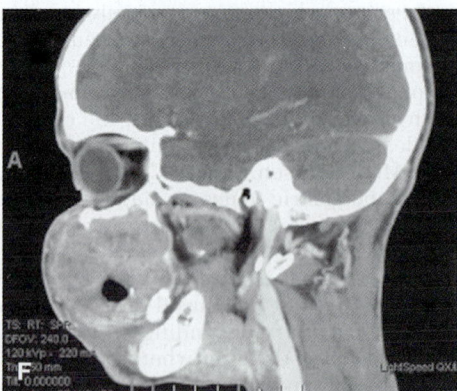
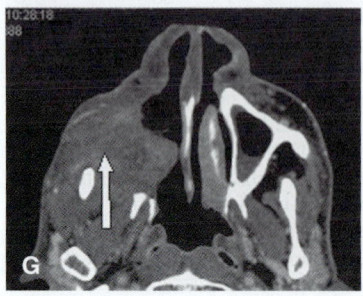
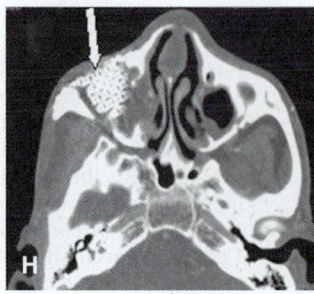
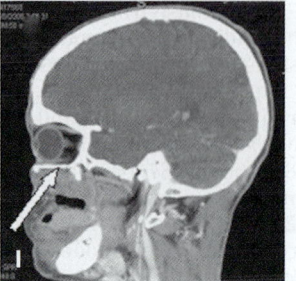
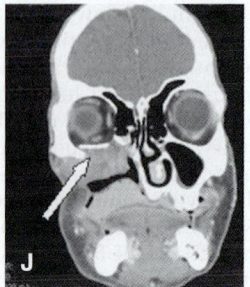

Nasal Cavity

Nasal cavity tumors present with symptoms and signs of nasal polyps (e.g., chronic unilateral discharge, ulcer, obstruction, anterior headache, and intermittent epistaxis), hence delaying the diagnosis. Additional symptoms and signs develop as the lesion enlarges: medial orbital mass, proptosis, expansion of the nasal bridge, diplopia resulting from invasion of the orbit, epiphora because of obstruction of the nasolacrimal duct, anomaly of smell or anosmia from involvement of the olfactory region, or frontal headache because of extension through the cribriform plate.

The common presenting symptoms of ENBs are nasal obstruction and epistaxis. Spaulding et al.[28] found that anosmia could precede diagnosis by many years. Other symptoms are related to contiguous disease extension into the orbit (proptosis, visual field defects, orbital pain, epiphora), paranasal sinuses (medial canthus mass, facial swelling), or anterior cranial fossa (headache) or are due to inappropriate antidiuretic hormone secretion.[28]

Ethmoid Sinuses

The presenting symptoms and signs of ethmoid sinus tumors are central or facial headaches and referred pain to the nasal or retrobulbar region, a subcutaneous mass at the inner canthus, nasal obstruction and discharge, diplopia, and proptosis. In one study of 34 patients with ethmoid sinus cancers treated at MD Anderson Cancer Center between 1969 and 1993,[29] nasal cavity symptoms (nasal obstruction, epistaxis, discharge) were reported in 25 patients (74%), orbital symptoms (diplopia, orbital pain, vision loss, proptosis, inner canthus mass, tearing) in 12 (35%), headache in 6 (18%), and hyposmia or anosmia in 5 (15%).

Maxillary Sinuses

Maxillary sinus cancers usually are diagnosed at advanced stages. Symptoms and signs are facial swelling, pain, or paresthesia of the cheek induced by disease extension to the premaxillary region, epistaxis, nasal discharge and obstruction related to tumor spread to the nasal cavity, ill-fitting dentures, alveolar or palatal mass, unhealed tooth socket after extraction from spread to the oral cavity, and proptosis, diplopia, impaired vision, or orbital pain because of orbital invasion.[30]

DIAGNOSTIC WORKUP

The recommended pretreatment physical, diagnostic, and staging evaluations are listed in Table 45.1.

Physical Examination

Inspection and palpation of the orbits, nasal and oral cavities, and nasopharynx can provide preliminary determination of tumor extent. Bimanual palpation is important in assessing contiguous extension of nasal vestibule lesions and in identifying buccinator and submandibular nodal involvement. Careful examination of cranial nerves is required. Fiber-optic nasal endoscopy after mucosal decongestion and topical analgesia allows assessment of local extent and facilitates biopsy of tumor involving the nasal cavity or nasopharynx.

Radiographic Evaluation

Imaging has a crucial role in the staging of sinonasal tumors. Magnetic resonance imaging (MRI) and computed tomography (CT) scans are complementary.[31] MRI is superior at detecting direct intracranial or perineural or leptomeningeal spread.[32] T2-weighted MRI can be helpful in distinguishing tumor (low signal) from obstructed secretions (bright).[33] CT is superior for detecting early cortical bone erosion or extension through the cribriform plate or orbital walls.

MRI, especially T1-weighted with gadolinium contrast, may be used as a supplement or alternative to CT scanning. CT provides the best information about the tumor and its local invasion into surrounding bone structures. MRI allows an estimate of tumor spread into surrounding soft tissue areas, such as the anterior cranial fossa and the retromaxillary space. Bone scintigraphy scan is useful in detecting distant metastases.

The expansile tendency of olfactory neuroblastoma is characterized by bowing of the sinus walls. The destructive aspect is manifested as tumor replacing the turbinates, septum, and sinus walls with extension into contiguous areas. The density or signal and enhancement characteristics are nonspecific of olfactory neuroblastoma.

Certain features provide clues as to the nature of the tumors in this region. Slowly progressive lesions tend to deform instead of destroy bony structures. Intermediate-grade tumors can cause sclerosis of the adjacent bone. Lymphomas tend to permeate the bone without frank destruction, and carcinomas and sarcomas infiltrate and destroy adjacent bone.

Biopsy

Transnasal biopsy is preferred for tumors arising from or extending into the nasal cavity or nasopharynx. Some paranasal sinus tumors may be more easily sampled using transoral procedures or an open Caldwell-Luc approach.

Laboratory Studies

Complete blood counts and serum chemistries can be used to screen for the presence of distant metastases. Abnormalities of these tests can be further investigated as necessary.

STAGING

The eighth edition of the American Joint Committee on Cancer's (AJCC) *AJCC Cancer Staging Manual* tumor–node–metastasis (TNM) classification includes staging for cancers of the maxillary sinus, the ethmoid sinus, and the nasal cavity.[34] Significant updates from the sixth edition affect classifications of T4 lesions and hence stage IV disease. Specifically, T4 lesions are now considered either T4a (moderately advanced local disease) or T4b (very advanced local disease), which leads to stratification of stage IV disease as either IVA (moderately advanced local or regional disease), IVB (very advanced local or regional disease), or IVC (distant metastatic disease). Definitions of anatomic stage prognostic groupings and TNM classifications are given in Table 45.2.

PATHOLOGIC CLASSIFICATION

Most nasal vestibule cancers are SCCs; the remaining tumors are basal cell or adnexal carcinomas. Most cancers of the

TABLE 45.1 PRETREATMENT EVALUATION FOR TUMORS OF THE NASAL CAVITY AND PARANASAL SINUSES

General	Complete History and Physical Examination
Radiographic	Fiberoptic endoscopic examination with biopsies
	Computed tomography/magnetic resonance imaging of the primary site and neck
	Chest x-ray; computed tomography of the thorax if adenoid cystic or neuroendocrine carcinoma
Laboratory	Complete blood count
Others	Dental evaluation with extractions/restorations as needed
	Baseline ophthalmologic examination
	Baseline speech and swallowing assessment if surgery is planned

Section III

TABLE 45.2 2017 AMERICAN JOINT COMMITTEE ON CANCER STAGING SYSTEM FOR CANCER OF THE NASAL CAVITY AND PARANASAL SINUSES

Definitions of TNM

Primary Tumor (T)

TX	Primary tumor cannot be assessed
Tis	Carcinoma *in situ*

Maxillary Sinus

T1	Tumor limited to maxillary sinus mucosa with no erosion or destruction of the bone
T2	Tumor causing bone erosion or destruction including extension into the hard palate and/or middle nasal meatus, except extension to posterior wall of maxillary sinus and pterygoid plates
T3	Tumor invades any of the following: the bone of the posterior wall of maxillary sinus, subcutaneous tissues, floor or medial wall of the orbit, pterygoid fossa, ethmoid sinuses
T4a	Moderately advanced local disease
	Tumor invades anterior orbital contents, skin of the cheek, pterygoid plates, infratemporal fossa, cribriform plate, sphenoid or frontal sinuses
T4b	Very advanced local disease
	Tumor invades any of the following: orbital apex, dura, brain, middle cranial fossa, cranial nerves other than maxillary division of trigeminal nerve (V2), nasopharynx, or clivus

Nasal Cavity and Ethmoid Sinus

T1	Tumor restricted to any one subsite, with or without bony invasion
T2	Tumor invading two subsites in a single region or extending to involve an adjacent region within the nasoethmoidal complex, with or without bony invasion
T3	Tumor extends to invade the medial wall or floor of the orbit, maxillary sinus, palate, or cribriform plate
T4a	Moderately advanced local disease
	Tumor invades any of the following: anterior orbital contents, skin of the nose or cheeks, minimal extension to anterior cranial fossa, pterygoid plates, sphenoid or frontal sinuses
T4b	Very advanced local disease
	Tumor invades any of the following: orbital apex, dura, brain, middle cranial fossa, cranial nerves other than (V2), nasopharynx, or clivus

Regional Lymph Nodes (N)

NX	Regional lymph nodes cannot be assessed
N0	No regional lymph node metastasis
N1	Metastasis in a single ipsilateral lymph node. 3 cm or less in greatest dimension, ENE neg
N2	Metastasis in a single ipsilateral lymph node, larger than 3 cm but not larger than 6 cm in greatest dimension, or in multiple ipsilateral lymph nodes or contralateral lymph nodes, none more than 6 cm in greatest dimension and ENE neg
N2a	Metastasis in a single ipsilateral lymph node, more than 3 cm but not more than 6 cm in greatest dimension and ENE neg
N2b	Metastasis in multiple ipsilateral lymph nodes, none more than 6 cm in greatest dimension and ENE neg
N2c	Metastasis in bilateral or contralateral lymph nodes, none more than 6 cm in greatest dimension and ENE neg
N3a	Metastasis in a lymph node larger than 6 cm in greatest dimension and ENE neg
N3b	Metastasis in any node(s) with clinically overt ENE (ENE positive)

Distant Metastasis (M)

M0	No distant metastasis
M1	Distant metastasis

Anatomic Stage/Prognostic Groups

Stage 0	Tis	N0	M0
Stage I	T1	N0	M0
Stage II	T2	N0	M0
Stage III	T3 T1 T2 T3	N0 N1 N1 N1	M0 M0 M0 M0
Stage IVA	T4a T4a T1 T2 T3 T4a	N0 N2 N2 N2 N2 N2	M0 M0 M0 M0 M0 M0
Stage IVB	T4b Any T	Any N N3	M0 M0
	Any T	Any N	M1

From Amin MB, Edge SB, Greene FL, et al. eds. *AJCC Cancer Staging Manual*. 8th ed. New York, NY: Springer, 2017. Reproduced with permission of Springer International Publishing in the format Book via Copyright Clearance Center.

nasal cavity and paranasal sinuses are also SCCs, although minor salivary gland neoplasms (adenocarcinoma, adenoid cystic carcinoma, and mucoepidermoid carcinoma) account for 10% to 15% of lesions in these locations. Melanoma accounts for 5% to 10% of nasal cavity malignancies but is rare in the paranasal sinuses. Neuroendocrine carcinomas of the sinonasal region (including small cell carcinoma, ENB, and sinonasal undifferentiated carcinomas), lymphomas, sarcomas, and plasmacytomas are even less common.

PROGNOSTIC FACTORS

Patient-specific factors (primarily prognostic for survival) include age and performance status. Disease-specific factors (primarily prognostic for locoregional control) include location, histology, locoregional extent (reflected in TNM stage), and perineural invasion. Extensive local disease involving the nasopharynx, base of the skull, or cavernous sinuses markedly increases surgical morbidity as well as the risk of subtotal

surgical excision. Tumor extension into the orbit may require enucleation, but minimal invasion of the floor or medial wall may be dealt with through resection and reconstruction, sparing the globe.

GENERAL MANAGEMENT

Nasal Vestibule Tumors

Nasal vestibule tumors can be treated definitively with surgery, primary radiation therapy (RT), or postoperative (adjuvant) RT when indicated because of tumor size or positive surgical findings. For small superficial tumors, standard treatment approaches are surgery or primary RT. Depending on the location and size of the primary tumor, radiation can be delivered as external beam RT, brachytherapy, or a combination of the two. Primary RT may be preferable for nasal vestibule carcinoma for better cosmetic outcome, although surgery can yield high control rates with excellent cosmetic results for selected small superficial tumors. Adjuvant radiation is indicated for cases involving positive surgical margins, positive lymph nodes, or perineural invasion. Cartilaginous invasion is not a contraindication for RT because fractionated treatment carries a low risk of necrosis.[35] For large invasive tumors with extensive tissue destruction and distortion, the combination of surgery and RT, with the radiation given either before or after surgery, is the mainstay of treatment. However, some clinicians favor primary radiation with salvage surgery for this situation.[36] Cosmesis can be enhanced by having experienced prosthodontists design aesthetically satisfactory custom-made nasal prostheses after radical surgery. Patients who are older or who have poor performance status can be treated with RT alone. No role for systemic chemotherapy has been established for tumors of this type.

Nasal Fossa Tumors

Either surgery or primary RT can produce similarly high control rates for early-stage nasal fossa lesions. The choice of treatment modality is generally guided by the size and location of the tumor as well as the anticipated cosmetic outcome. Posterior nasal septum lesions or locally advanced lesions are generally treated surgically, but small anterior–inferior septal lesions (≤ 1.5 cm) can be treated effectively with interstitial brachytherapy (iridium 192 [^{192}Ir] implant). For lateral wall lesions extending to the nasal ala, primary external beam RT may produce the best cosmetic results.

Paranasal Sinus Tumors

Surgery can produce excellent control rates for T1 and T2 tumors and is generally the mainstay of treatment. The combination of surgery and postoperative RT is the treatment of choice for patients with more advanced but resectable disease who are medically fit to undergo surgery. Maxillary sinus and ethmoid sinus tumors often present as locally advanced disease (large T3 or T4) and are commonly managed with surgery and postoperative RT. Ethmoid sinus carcinomas can be treated with radiation alone or with concurrent chemotherapy to avoid structural or functional deficits. Surgery generally involves medial maxillectomy and en bloc ethmoidectomy; a craniofacial approach is required if tumor extends superiorly to the ethmoid roof or olfactory region.[37,38] Primary RT, with or without concurrent chemotherapy, can be considered for patients who are not fit to undergo surgery owing to significant comorbid conditions or poor performance status or for patients who decline radical surgery.[39]

Early ENB lesions involving the ethmoids with little or no bony destruction or nerve invasion can be treated adequately by high-energy (photon, proton, or electron) RT with good cosmetic and functional results. Those with more extensive local disease benefit from surgery and adjuvant irradiation, although some have advocated against combined surgery and RT because of complications. Patients with locally advanced disease or high-grade tumors should receive aggressive treatment with combined modalities, such as surgery, RT, and chemotherapy. Elective nodal irradiation is not generally recommended for Kadish stage A and B because the incidence of nodal relapse is <15%. Distant metastasis is uncommon (10%) even among patients presenting with locally advanced disease.

CHEMOTHERAPY: NEOADJUVANT AND CONCOMITANT

Neoadjuvant chemotherapy (i.e., chemotherapy given before surgery) can reduce tumor volumes, which may allow a less extensive surgical resection than would be possible otherwise. Similarly, chemotherapy given before primary RT can also reduce tumor volumes and facilitate radiotherapy planning by increasing the distance between tumor borders and critical organ structures such as the brain, chiasm, optic nerve, or spinal cord. Investigations are ongoing to determine whether the response (or lack of same) to neoadjuvant chemotherapy can help in the choice of definitive treatment. For example, if neoadjuvant chemotherapy produces a complete response, then primary RT, with or without chemotherapy, can be considered; a less-than-complete response would prompt surgical excision of the lesion followed by adjuvant RT.

The optimal treatment strategy for patients with orbital encroachment of sinonasal cancer is controversial. Organ (orbital) preservation with neoadjuvant therapy may determine if patients require an orbital exenteration for locally advanced sinonasal cancer. Yusuf et al.[40] reported on 20 patients determined by a multidisciplinary team to require an orbital exenteration as part of definitive treatment of their sinonasal cancer. Neoadjuvant treatment consisted of concurrent chemoradiation (CRT) in all patients aside from two who refused chemotherapy and underwent RT alone. Six patients received primary surgery followed by adjuvant CRT. Five patients (36%) receiving neoadjuvant therapy had complete disease response at the time of surgery. Fourteen patients underwent orbital preservation (OP). With a median time of follow-up of 18.8 months, actuarial exenteration-free survival was 62% at 2 years for patients undergoing OP. No patients receiving neoadjuvant therapy required an immediate post-treatment orbital exenteration; however, one patient required salvage orbital exenteration when she experienced local failure 35 months after treatment. At 2 years, there were no significant differences in locoregional control (75% vs. 60%, $P = .997$), progression-free survival (40% vs. 36%, $P = .493$), or overall survival (40% vs. 58%, $P = .815$) between patients receiving OP or up-front surgery ($P = .815$). On multivariate analysis, tumor site predicted for locoregional control (maxillary, 86%; nasal cavity, 80%; ethmoid sinus, 40%; $P = .050$). Treatment was well tolerated in both groups. One patient treated with OP experienced grade 3 radiation-related toxicity, developing dysphagia, which improved with medical management. However, one patient developed renal failure following his first dose of cisplatin and subsequently died before completion of treatment.

Concurrent chemoradiation therapy (CRT) can also be used for patients with medical conditions that preclude surgery if those patients have good performance status. Depending on the patient's performance status and renal function, single-agent cisplatin or carboplatin can be used concurrently with external beam radiation for locally advanced, unresectable SCC. Neoadjuvant chemotherapy or concurrent chemoradiation with etoposide and cisplatin or carboplatin can be used to treat sinonasal undifferentiated carcinoma, neuroendocrine carcinoma, or small cell carcinoma. Chemotherapy is not used routinely for ENB, and its role in the management of this disease is under investigation. Chemotherapy may have a role in the management of Kadish stage C disease, and although responses to chemotherapy have been reported, they are usually of limited duration.[41] Concurrent chemotherapy during radiation may be considered for inoperable cases.

PALLIATION

Symptoms of incurable sinonasal cancer are particularly distressing. Multidisciplinary input is required even for very advanced cases, as palliation may involve limited surgery, RT, chemotherapy, investigational studies, or best supportive care. The morbidity of each modality must be balanced with the potential benefits in symptom control and improved quality of life. Particular attention is required to address the control of pain and discomfort as a first priority, and the impact of disfigurement and dysfunction, which is often present.

Chemotherapy can be given as single-agent therapy in investigational settings. If RT is given, large doses per fraction are usually given to reduce the duration of treatment. However, if concurrent chemotherapy is added, treatment with 2-Gy fractions should be considered to avoid severe acute effects. Radiation or chemotherapy is often effective in reducing tumor bulk and relieving symptoms associated with disfiguring masses, proptosis, discomfort or neuropathic pain, headache, epistaxis or other bleeding, nasal obstruction or discharge, and trismus.

RADIATION THERAPY TECHNIQUES

Tumors of the Nasal Cavity

Nasal Vestibule Tumors

Target Volumes

For small, well-differentiated lesions that are ≤1.5 cm in diameter, small fields with a 1- to 2-cm margin are appropriate. The initial target volume for all poorly differentiated tumors and well-differentiated primary tumors larger than 1.5 cm without palpable lymphadenopathy should include both nasal vestibules with at least 2- to 3-cm margins around the primary tumor (wider margins for infiltrative tumor) as well as bilateral facial, submandibular, and subdigastric nodes. When lymph node involvement is present at diagnosis, the lower neck is also irradiated. For larger nasal vestibule lesions, the lower half of the nose and the upper lip are treated as well as the regional lymphatics, including the facial lymphatics and upper neck nodes. For postoperative RT, the initial target volume includes the operative bed plus a 1- to 1.5-cm margin and the elective nodal regions.

Treatment Techniques

External Beam Radiation. Thin superficial nasal vestibule lesions can be treated with orthovoltage x-rays or electrons with skin bolus, whereas thicker lesions are generally treated with electrons, photons, or protons. In definitive therapy, the target volume is treated to a dose of 66 to 70 Gy, with a small reduction in the treatment fields after 50 Gy to boost the dose to the gross disease. For patients presenting with palpable neck adenopathy, the entire neck is treated with at least a subclinical dose of 50 Gy, and the gross disease plus a 1- to 2-cm margin is then treated with an additional 16 to 20 Gy. A technique for external beam irradiation using electrons is illustrated in Figure 45.3. The patient lies supine, immobilized with the neck slightly flexed by using a custom mask to align the anterior surface of

FIGURE 45.3. Nasal vestibule squamous cell carcinoma. **A:** *Arrows* indicate tumor expanding the columella. **B** and **C:** *Arrows* indicate invasion downward into the upper gingivobuccal sulcus on CT imaging. **D:** *Arrow* shows setup for electron-beam phase of therapy with custom lead skin collimation *in situ*. **E:** *Arrow* shows the beeswax bolus *in situ*. **F:** Dosimetry to 50 Gy resulting from an appositional electron beam with beeswax bolus (*arrow*) to compensate for surface obliquity. The primary tumor, facial, and level II nodes were treated with 50 Gy. This was followed by 25 Gy administered by an interstitial low dose rate iridium needle implant at 0.55 Gy/hour. **G:** Dummy wires are inserted into each hollow tube. Each tube has a ball anchor at the distal end of the needles, which is pushed snugly against the skin and sutured to the skin. Note the placement of transverse "moustache" needles. **H** and **I:** Orthogonal x-ray (anterior–posterior, lateral) films taken to document the placement of the needles. CT-based planning was performed. **J** and **K:** Live sources *in situ*.

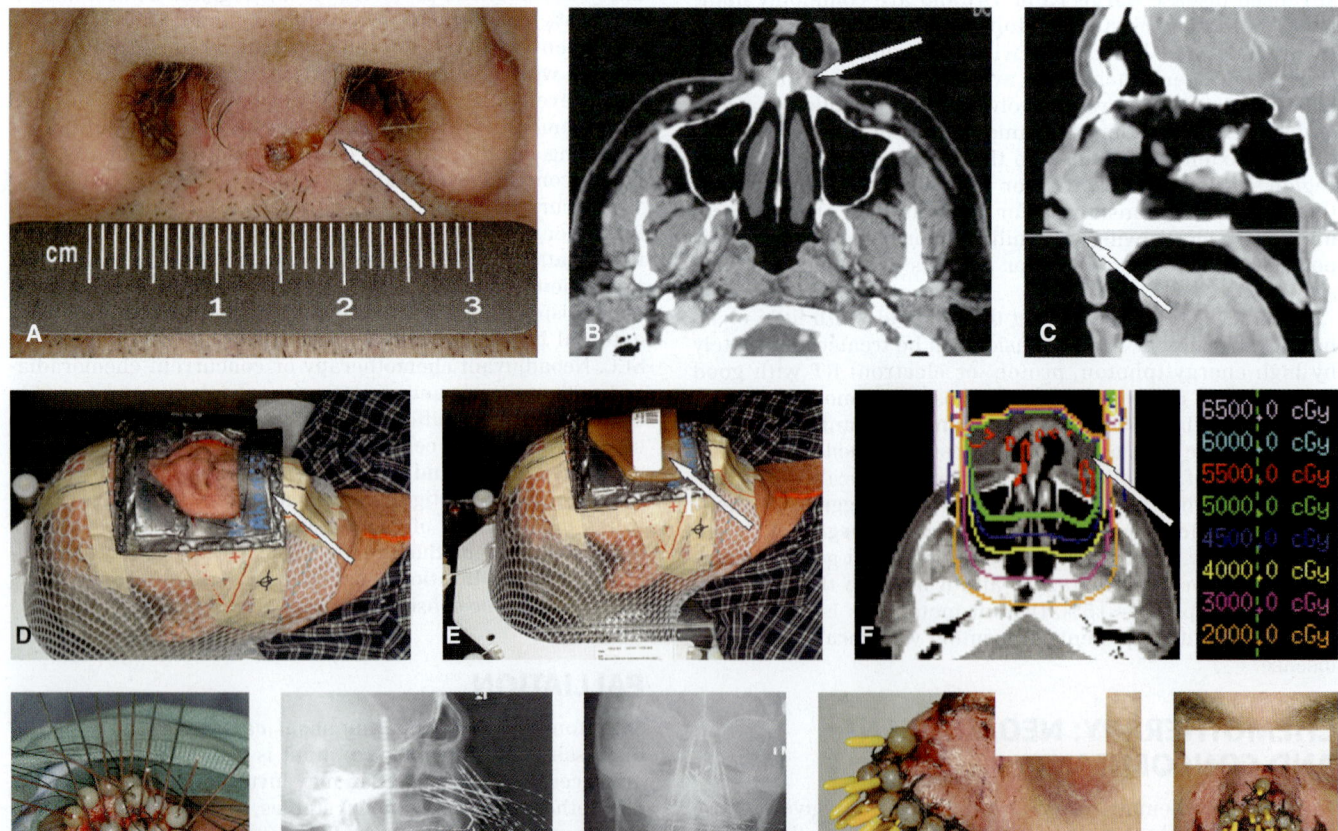

the maxilla parallel with the top of the couch. For larger nasal vestibule lesions, the lower half of the nose and the upper lip are treated with an anterior appositional field using 20-MeV electrons and 6-MV photons weighted 4 to 1. Skin collimation is used to minimize scatter irradiation to the eye and reduce the penumbra of the beam and reduce the field size required. Custom beeswax bolus material is prepared to allow a relatively flat surface contour onto which the electron beam is incident, avoiding inhomogeneity because of oblique incidence and surface irregularity. A bolus is also used to fill the nares to avoid the dose perturbation from the air cavity with electron beams. In photon treatments, the bolus is removed to spare the skin unless the overlying skin is involved. An intraoral Cerrobend-containing stent is used to displace the tongue posteriorly and partially shield the upper alveolar ridge. In proton treatments, bolus material is not required and an aperature is used instead of skin collimation to minimize scatter irradiation to the eye and reduce penumbra of the beam.

When indicated, the right and left facial lymphatics are irradiated with appositional fields; these require an approximately 15-degree gantry rotation to the respective side with 6-MeV electron fields, each abutting the appositional primary lesion portal and the upper neck fields. The medial border is matched to the lateral border of the anterior primary field. The anterior border extends down from the oral commissure to the middle of the horizontal ramus of the mandible, whereas the posterior border extends from the upper edge of the anterior field to just above the angle of the mandible. The inferior border splits the horizontal ramus of the mandible and is matched to the upper neck field. The junctions are moved twice during the course of treatment to reduce dose heterogeneity. The submandibular and subdigastric nodes are treated with lateral parallel-opposed photon fields. For patients with involved nodes, these upper neck fields are matched inferiorly to an anterior portal treating the middle and lower neck nodes.

For definitive treatment, the external beam radiation schedule for lesions up to 1.5 cm in diameter for which a combination of electrons and photons is used is typically 50 Gy in 25 fractions followed by a boost of 10 to 16 Gy in 5 to 8 fractions (prescribed at the 90% isodose line). Larger lesions to be treated by external beam radiation alone receive 50 Gy in 25 fractions plus a boost of 16 to 20 Gy in 8 to 10 fractions. The schedule for elective nodal irradiation is 50 Gy in 25 fractions. Palpable nodes are given a boost to a total dose of 66 to 70 Gy in 33 to 35 fractions, depending on the size. For postoperative treatment, the volume is reduced off the undissected nodal regions after 50 Gy (25 fractions) to deliver an additional 6 Gy to the surgical bed. At 56 Gy, a final "cone down" is done to include a 4-Gy dose to the preoperative tumor bed, for a total dose of 60 Gy. If the excision was limited or positive margins are present, the final cone down dose is 10 Gy for a total dose of 66 Gy.

Brachytherapy. Brachytherapy for small lesions is accomplished by using a ^{192}Ir wire implant or, in selected cases, by using an intracavitary ^{192}Ir mold. Hollow needles for afterloading are inserted under general anesthesia, which allows good exposure of the tumor and protects the airway in the event of bleeding from the vascular Kiesselbach plexus on the anterior nasal septum or from posterior hemorrhages originating from larger vessels near the sphenopalatine artery, behind the middle turbinate. Implantation of a T2 SCC of the columella is shown in Figure 45.3. The recommended doses for low dose rate brachytherapy have evolved empirically and range from 60 to 65 Gy delivered during 5 to 7 days.

Brachytherapy can be used instead of an external beam boost for patients with T1 or T2 nasal vestibule tumors after initial larger-field RT. After delivery of 50 Gy, the patient is assessed, and if the tumor volume has been substantially reduced, a boost of 20 to 25 Gy may be administered in about 2 days by using low dose rate brachytherapy.

High dose rate brachytherapy has also been used to deliver the boost. A custom mold of the nasal vestibule is fabricated,

and tumor is marked in the mold. Two to four plastic tubes are inserted in the mold alongside the tumor at 1-cm intervals. For tumors of the lateral part of the vestibule, two catheters are placed on the inner aspect of the nasal vestibule. For medially localized tumors, catheters are placed on both sides of the vestibule. After external beam radiation to 50 Gy in 5 weeks, high dose rate brachytherapy is delivered in week 6. The dose is typically 3 Gy per fraction, given twice a day, to a total dose of 18 Gy specifically at the center of the tumor. With a median overall treatment time (external beam radiation plus brachytherapy) of 36 days, this technique has been reported to yield 2-year local control rates of 86% and ultimate locoregional control rates of 100%.[42]

Nasal Fossa Tumors

Target Volume

The technique for primary or postoperative external beam irradiation of nasal cavity tumors depends on the depth of the neoplasm. For tumors located <3.5 or 4.0 cm from the skin of the apex of the nose, electrons can be used, as 20-MeV electrons will provide coverage up to 5 cm in depth. A margin of at least 1 cm deep to the posterior edge must be included in the full-dose volume. The technique is as previously described for nasal vestibule carcinoma. CT-based treatment planning is necessary for accurate target localization and dose calculation.

Intensity-modulated radiation therapy (IMRT) with either photons or protons are recommended for tumors of the nasal cavity in which the target volume is more than 5 cm deep or for tumors of the ethmoid sinus[43] (Fig. 45.4). This technique delivers the desired dose to the target volume while minimizing the dose to critical organs such as the cornea, lens, lacrimal glands, retina, optic nerve, optic chiasm, brain, and brainstem. For postoperative RT, the primary clinical target volume (CTV) descriptions are given in Table 45.3. The CTV_1 consists of the primary tumor bed with a 1.0- to 1.5-cm margin. A boost subvolume consisting of high-risk regions (sites of positive margins, gross macroscopic residual tumor) to be treated to higher doses may be outlined. The CTV_2 includes the entire operative bed. For ethmoid sinus tumors, this might include the frontal sinus, maxillary sinus, and sphenoid sinus. The bony orbit is part of the operative bed when orbital exenteration is performed because of tumor invasion. For lesions involving the ethmoid sinuses or olfactory region, the CTV should also include the cribriform plate. A third CTV may be delineated to encompass the tract of cranial nerve V2 to the foramen rotundum if perineural invasion is present. For primary RT given as IMRT, the CTV_1, consisting of the gross tumor volume plus a margin of 1 to 2 cm, receives the full dose of 66 to 70 Gy. For patients receiving neoadjuvant chemotherapy, target volume definition is based on the extent of disease before chemotherapy.

For three-dimensional (3-D) conformal RT, the initial target volume for postoperative radiation consists of the surgical bed with 1- or 2-cm margins, depending on the surgical pathology findings and the proximity of critical structures. The boost volume consists of areas at greatest risk of recurrence, such as close or positive resection margins or regions of perineural invasion, with 1- to 2-cm margins.

For small anterior–inferior septal lesions, brachytherapy can be accomplished by using a single-plane implant of the lesion with 2-cm margins. Elective neck irradiation is not given routinely even for patients with large tumors or early stage Kadish A or B ENB.

Setup and Field Arrangement

For target volumes <5 cm deep, an electron technique similar to that described for nasal vestibule carcinomas is used. Treatment devices include lead skin collimation to obtain a sharp penumbra as well as bolus material in the nasal cavity, in postoperative defects, and on skin scars. An intraoral stent is used to depress the tongue, provide a patent airway, and aid in immobilization. Tungsten internal eye shields may be used if the target volume approaches the orbits (see Fig. 45.3).

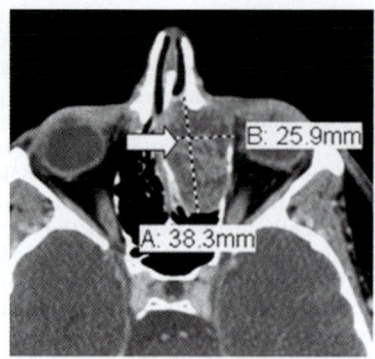
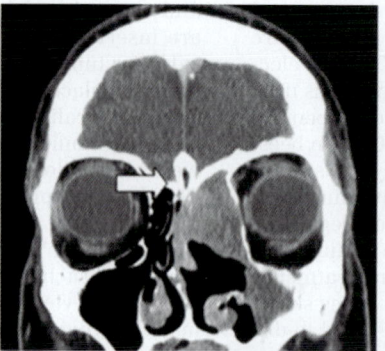
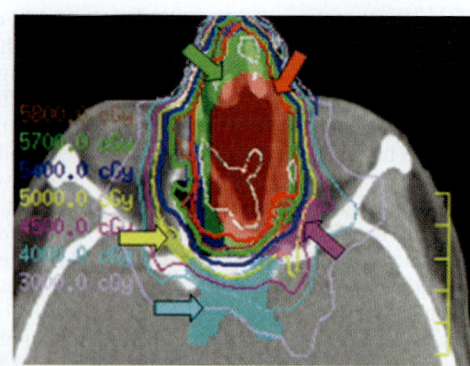

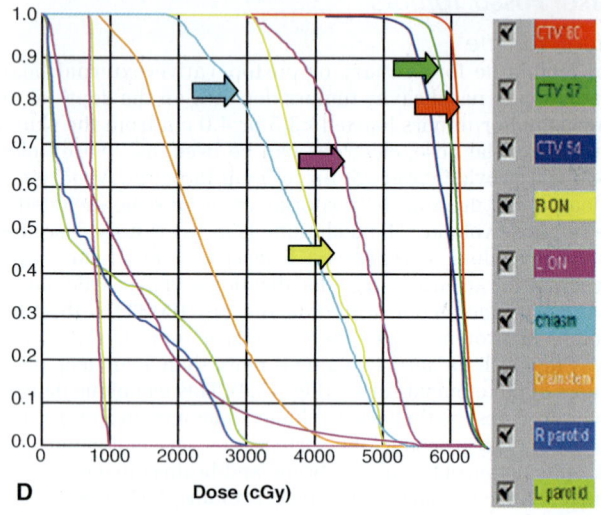
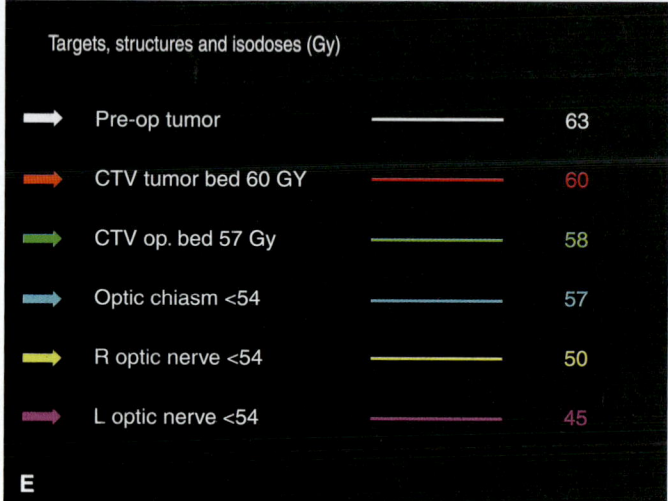

FIGURE 45.4. Intensity-modulated radiotherapy for adjuvant radiotherapy for an adenoid cystic carcinoma of the ethmoid sinus, anterior skull base, nasal cavity, and medial orbit following endoscopic anterior–posterior ethmoidectomy with resection of tumor, left maxillary antrostomy with disease removal, bilateral sphenoidotomy, and frontal sinusotomy with anterior approach to the anterior skull base including a left lateral rhinotomy and medial maxillectomy and extradural resection of anterior cranial base. **A** and **B:** Preoperative CT scans with tumor indicated by *white arrow*. **C:** Transverse section at the level of the orbit that shows sharp dose gradient at the interface of the CTV and the optic nerves and chiasm. **D** and **E:** Cumulative dose–volume (*y*-axis) histogram.

TABLE 45.3 TARGET VOLUMES FOR INTENSITY-MODULATED RADIATION THERAPY OF SINONASAL CANCERS

Target	Description	Dose (33–35 fractions) (Gy)
Primary Radiation Therapy		
GTV	GTV (= prechemotherapy volume)	66–70
CTV₁ (primary CTV)	GTV + 1.0 – 1.5 cm	66–70
CTV₂ (intermediate dose CTV)	Primary CTV + 1.0 – 1.5 cm	59–63
CTV₃ (elective CTV)	Nodal volumes, nerve tract, and base of skull margin	54–57

Target	Description	Dose (30 fractions) (Gy)
Postoperative Radiation Therapy		
CTV_HR (high-risk CTV)	Sites of suspected positive margins, gross macroscopic residual tumor, extracapsular nodal disease	66–70[a]
CTV₁ (primary CTV)	Primary tumor bed with 1.0–1.5-cm margin	60
CTV₂ (intermediate dose CTV)	Surgical bed	57
CTV₃ (low dose CTV)	Trigeminal nerve perineural invasion is present, additional skull base margin, elective nodal volume if indicated	54

[a]70 Gy may be given by adding a second boost plan or increasing the number of fractions to 35. CTV, clinical target volume; GTV, gross tumor volume.

For 3-D conformal therapy or IMRT, the patient is immobilized in a supine position with the head positioned such that the hard palate is perpendicular to the treatment couch. Scars are marked with thin radio-opaque wires, bolus and other devices are positioned, and transverse CT images are obtained from the vertex to the upper mediastinum. For IMRT, rigid immobilization is necessary, including the use of special head and shoulder thermoplastic masks that extend down to the upper thorax. The shoulders can be additionally depressed and fixed by using wrist straps tethered to a footboard. Target volumes are delineated as previously described.

For IMRT, multiple gantry angles are used based on beam optimization algorithms. An example of a 10-field noncoplanar arrangement with two vertex beams is shown in Figure 45.4. The beam angle selections are based on the same principles as for 3-D conformal therapy:

1. Preference for the shortest path to the target
2. Avoidance of direct irradiation of the critical structures (e.g., avoid beam entry through the contralateral eye after ipsilateral exenteration)
3. Use of as large a beam separation as possible

Inverse planning is usually done, and multiple iterations may be necessary to ensure that the following are accomplished:

1. Targets are covered.
2. Normal tissue constraints are respected.
3. Dose is relatively homogenous.

Dose calculations should include heterogeneity corrections because of the significant amounts of air and bone in the sinuses. Radiation oncologists must work closely with physicists and dosimetrists. It is important to realize that the criteria for accepting or rejecting the plan may not be evident from the dose–volume histogram.

For 3-D conformal RT, anterior oblique wedge-pair photon fields are appropriate for lesions located in the anterior lower half of the nasal cavity. Opposed-lateral fields can be used to treat tumors at the posterior part of the nasal fossa, provided the ethmoid cells are not involved. The optic pathway can be excluded from the radiation fields with this setup. For primaries of the upper nasal cavity and ethmoidal air cells, a three-field setup allows coverage of the ethmoid cells while sparing the optic apparatus. CT-based treatment planning is necessary to select beam and wedge angles (usually 45 to 60 degrees) and the relative loading of the fields, as well as to evaluate the dose to critical structures such as the brain, brainstem, and optic structures.

Proton beam therapy techniques for treating nasal fossa tumors are rapidly evolving and include both passive scattering and discrete spot scanning beams. Theoretically, the advantage of proton therapy (PT) derives from the unique physical properties of protons that allow deposition of most of the particle's energy at the end of its range. Descriptions of the various techniques by which PT can be delivered are beyond the scope of this chapter. Nevertheless, with optimization of dosimetry, the conformality and heterogeneity within the target volumes provided by PT should be equivalent to what can be achieved with either electron or photon therapy, with the added advantage of minimizing the unnecessary dose or "dose bath" from IMRT to the surrounding normal tissue structures.

Greenwalt et al.[44] reported on seven adult patients with primary mucosal nasal cavity,[5] ethmoid sinus,[1] and maxillary antrum[1] melanoma treated with external beam PT. Six patients underwent gross total resection before PT, and one patient underwent a biopsy of unresectable disease from intracranial extension. In the postoperative setting, PT was initiated at a median of 53 days after surgery. The primary target volume was defined as the surgical bed plus a margin for microscopic disease and set-up uncertainties. The median PT dose to the primary high-risk planning target volume was 74.4 Gy (relative biologic effectiveness [RBE]) (range, 69.6 to 74.4). Six patients were treated with elective nodal radiation to the neck to a median dose of 50 Gy (range, 48 to 50). None of the patients had neoadjuvant, concurrent, or adjuvant chemotherapy. Median follow-up was 1.4 years from the end of PT (range, 0.5 to 6.6 years). The cause-specific survival and overall survival rates were equivalent at 83% at 1 year and 67% at 1.5 years. Three patients died of metastatic disease, all died within 25 months of completing PT. One patient who was treated with 69.6 Gy (RBE) recurred locally at 2 months after completing PT and died of distant disease. The locoregional control rates at 1 and 1.5 years were both 86%, whereas the freedom from distant metastases rate was 71% at 1 and 1.5 years. One patient experienced grade 2 epiphora and grade 4 visual toxicity, leading to loss of useful vision in the treated eye. One patient with brain necrosis was found to have developed brain metastases requiring steroids following PT. Two patients reported grade 2 sinusitis, one patient had a grade 2 oral cavity fistula, and one patient reported grade 2 sensorineural hearing loss. No contralateral visual complications occurred.

Radiation Therapy Dose Fractionation Schedule

The dose schedule for low dose rate brachytherapy is 60 to 65 Gy during 5 to 7 days. The external beam regimen for primary RT is 50 Gy in 25 fractions followed by a boost of 16 to 20 Gy in 8 to 10 fractions, depending on the size of the lesion. Postoperative RT consists of 50 Gy to elective tissue, 56 Gy to the operative bed, and 60 Gy to the tumor bed, with an optional boost to close or positive surgical margins, all given at 2 Gy per fraction. Dose regimens for intensity-modulated therapy, whether with photons or protons, are summarized in Table 45.3.

Tumors of the Paranasal Sinuses

Target Volume

Because maxillary cancers are usually diagnosed at a locally advanced stage and surgery is the primary therapy, most patients receive postoperative RT. Delineation of target volumes is based on physical examination, pretreatment imaging, intraoperative findings (tumor extension relative to critical structures such as orbital wall, cribriform plate, cranial nerve foramina, and ease of resection), and pathologic findings (such as positive margin or perineural invasion).

For photon-based treatment delivery, IMRT is the preferred treatment method as it generally yields better dose distribution in terms of both tumor coverage and sparing of normal tissues than can be achieved with 3-D conformal RT.[43,45]

Jeong et al.[46] compared in 10 patients volumetric modulated arc therapy (VMAT) and noncoplanar intensity-modulated radiation therapy (IMRT) for nasal cavity and paranasal sinus cancer with regard to the coverage of planning target volume (PTV) and the sparing of organs at risk (OARs). Planning objectives were (a) to deliver 60 Gy in 30 fractions to 95% of PTV; (b) to ensure maximum dose (D_{max}) of optic nerves, optic chiasm, and brainstem to be <50 Gy, eyes to <40 Gy, and lenses to <10 Gy and the mean dose (D_{mean}) of parotid glands to <25 Gy; and (c) to reduce doses of OARs as much as possible without compromising coverage of PTV.

VMAT plan and each of noncoplanar IMRT (7-, 11-, and 15-beam) plans were evaluated by heterogeneity index (HI) and conformity index (CI) of the PTV, D_{max}, and D_{mean} of the OARs, treatment delivery time, and monitor units (MUs). The HI of PTV was defined as D5% to D95%/D_{mean}, where D5% and D95% are the minimum doses delivered 5% and 95% of the PTV. The CI of PTV was defined as VTV/VPTV, where VTV is the treatment volume enclosed by the prescribed 60-Gy isodose surface and VPTV is the volume of the PTV. The HI and CI of VMAT plan were better than each of 7-, 11-, 15-beam noncoplanar IMRT plans (mean HI, 0.07 vs. 0.10 vs. 0.09 and 0.10, respectively, $P = 0.004$, $P = 0.012$, and $P = 0.005$; mean CI, 1.05 vs. 1.13 vs. 1.10 and 1.10, respectively, $P = 0.002$, $P = 0.008$, and $P = 0.016$). In OAR-sparing effects, VMAT and each of noncoplanar IMRT (7-, 11-, and 15-beam) plans showed equivalent sparing effects for bilateral optic nerves, optic chiasm, brainstem, and bilateral parotid glands. For the eyes and lenses, VMAT achieved equivalent or better sparing effects when compared with each of noncoplanar IMRT plans. For bilateral lacrimal glands, which did not apply constraint during planning, each of the noncoplanar IMRT plans showed better D_{max} and D_{mean} than VMAT. VMAT showed lower MUs and reduced treatment delivery time when compared with noncoplanar IMRT plans. The authors concluded that in the patients with nasal cavity or paranasal sinus cancer, VMAT provided better homogeneity and conformity for PTV than each of 7-, 11-, 15-beam noncoplanar IMRT plans while achieving equal or better OAR-sparing effects and using fewer MUs and lower treatment delivery times.

Proton therapy and intensity modulated proton therapy (IMPT)[47] may offer additional advantages over IMRT in terms of further reducing the dose to normal tissues while achieving equivalent doses to the target volume. The CTV_1 consists of the primary tumor bed with 1.0- to 1.5-cm margin of normal tissue. The CTV$_2$ encompasses the operative bed, including the bony orbit after orbital exenteration and the ethmoid, frontal, or sphenoid sinuses if explored during surgery. A third CTV may be delineated to encompass the tract of cranial nerve V2 to the foramen rotundum if perineural invasion is present. A CTV for high-risk areas (CTV$_{HR}$; see Table 45.3) may also be outlined to cover, for example, gross macroscopic residual tumor or positive margins to which a higher dose may be delivered.

Radiation Therapy Dose Prescriptions

For primary RT using IMRT, VMAT, or IMPT the prescription doses are 66 to 70 Gy to the gross tumor volume (the prechemotherapy volume for those receiving systemic treatment), plus a 1- to 1.5-cm margin of normal-appearing tissue (CTV$_1$), 59 to 63 Gy to other secondary CTVs such as the rest of the involved sinus and wider region around the primary target, and 54 to 57 Gy to the tracts of nerves (if perineural invasion is present) and to elective nodal regions. An example of an IMRT plan for primary definitive RT of a T4N0 SCC is shown in Figure 45.5.

For postoperative RT using a 3-D conformal technique, the initial target volume consists of the operative bed with 1- to 2-cm margins. The boost field consists of the primary tumor bed and areas at higher risk of recurrence, such as positive resection margins or perineural invasion. Radiation is administered to the neck after node dissection if multiple nodes are involved or extracapsular extension is present. Elective radiation of ipsilateral submandibular and subdigastric nodes is given for patients with squamous cell or poorly differentiated carcinoma. An example of an intensity-modulated proton plan for postoperative RT is shown in Figure 45.6.

Setup and Field Arrangement

Patients undergoing treatment of paranasal tumors are immobilized in a supine position with the head slightly hyperextended to bring the floor of the orbit parallel to the axis of the anterior field. An intraoral stent is used to open the mouth and depress the tongue out of the radiation field. After palatectomy, the stent can be designed to hold a water-filled balloon to obliterate the large air cavity in the surgical defect to

FIGURE 45.5. Intensity-modulated radiotherapy (IMRT) for definitive radiotherapy for T4N0 SCC of the maxillary sinus. **A** and **B:** Pretreatment photographs showing the skin of cheek involvement. **C** and **D:** Magnetic resonance imaging (MRI) scans with tumor indicated by *white arrow*. **E** and **F:** MRIs following induction chemotherapy showed progressive disease involving the left maxilla, left nasoethmoid region, extending inferiorly into the premaxillary soft tissues. **G–I:** IMRT plan with sections showing coverage of the target volumes. The patient was treated using concomitant boost fractionation. The primary plan delivered 57 Gy and a concomitant boost plan administered an additional 15 Gy. **G** and **H** also show avoidance of the normal tissues, as listed in the key and illustrated further in the cumulative dose–volume histogram in **(L)**. **J** and **K:** The skin reaction during the final week of radiotherapy. **M** and **N:** MRI and patient photo at follow-up, showing healed skin with hyperpigmentation. The tumor was in complete remission at the last visit 7 months after therapy.

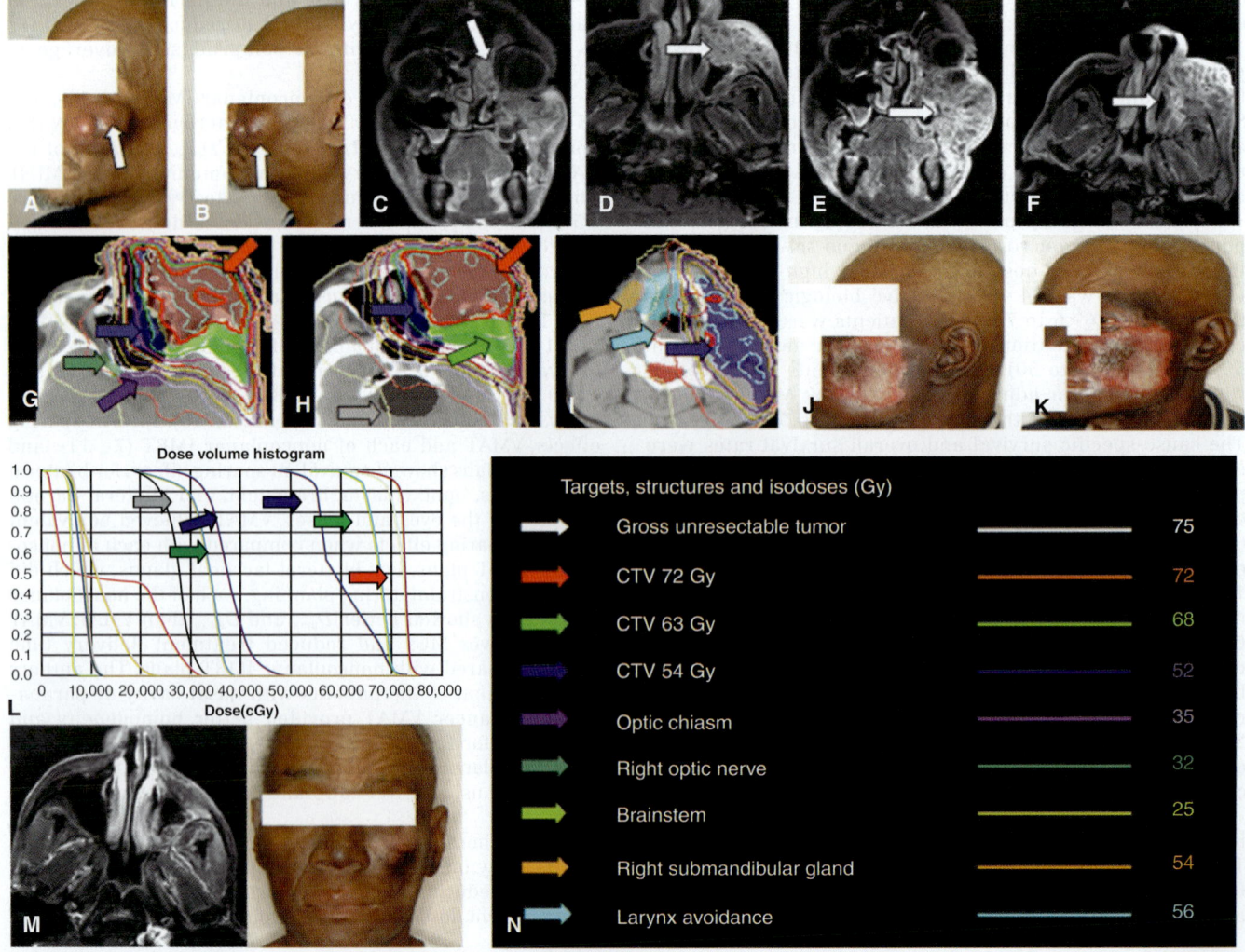

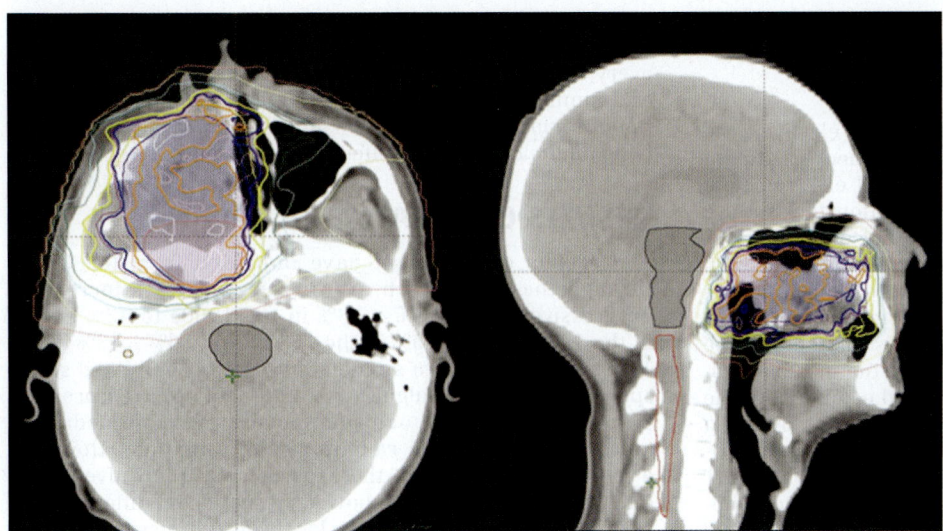

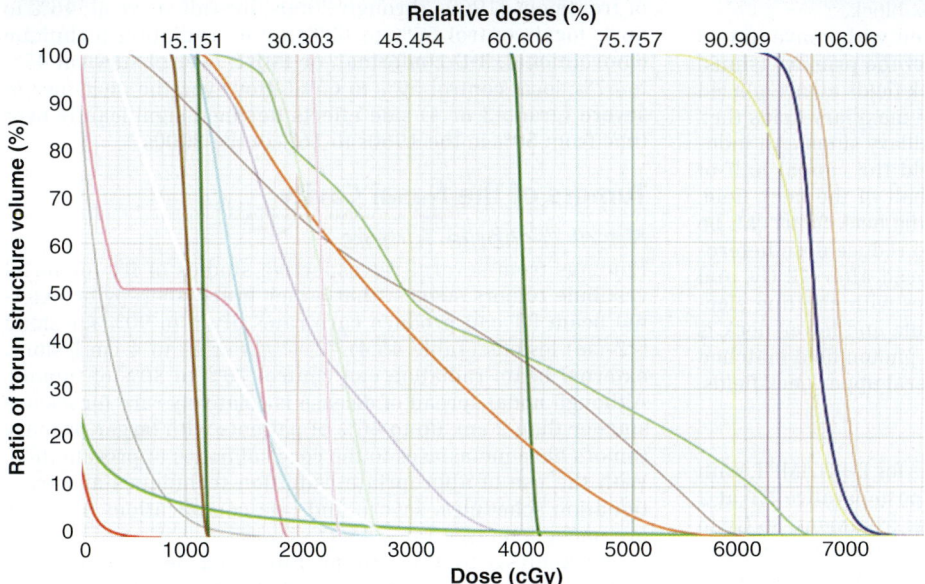

FIGURE 45.6. Proton therapy for recurrent adenoid cystic carcinoma (ACC) of the right hard palate. The patient had a palatectomy with radial forearm free flap reconstruction followed by postoperative external beam RT with IMRT to 60 Gy in 30 fractions. One year later, the ACC recurred with enhancement in right V1 and V2, involvement of the right cavernous sinus, and an enhancing mass in the infratemporal fossa and pterygopalatine fossa. Salvage surgery involved a right total maxillectomy with OP, pterygomaxillary space dissection and resection, and an extracranial dissection of Vidian nerve and cranial nerve 5, V2. With evidence of skull base and cavernous sinus involvement after surgery, he was treated with postoperative chemoradiation with IMPT and cisplatin to a dose of 66 Gy (RBE) in 33 fractions. No evidence of disease was present at 6 months after salvage therapy. The figure represents the axial, sagittal, and dose–volume histogram (DVH) of the IMPT plan. (DVH for the IMPT plan, from *left* to *right* on the graph: *red*, spinal cord; *green*, whole brain; *black*, brainstem; *pink*, left parotid; *white*, left eye; *brown*, right cochlea; *dark green*, left lens; *sky blue*, right parotid; *brown*, oral cavity; *violet*, optic chiasm; *red*, right eye; *green*, mandible; *light green*, left optic nerve; *soft pink*, right lens; *dark green*, right optic nerve; *yellow*, CTV or CTV₃; *blue*, CTV₂; *orange*, CTV₁.)

improve dose homogeneity. An orbital exenteration defect can also be filled directly with a water-filled balloon to decrease the dose delivered to the temporal lobe. Marking of the lateral canthi, oral commissures, external auditory canals, and external scars facilitates target volume delineation. The planning CT scan should include the entire head to allow the use of vertex beams. The principles of target delineation and plan evaluation for IMRT of maxillary sinus cancer are the same as those described for nasal cavity and ethmoid tumors.

For 3-D conformal radiation, a three-field technique consisting of anterior and right and left lateral fields is used for tumors involving the suprastructure or extending to the roof of the nasal cavity and ethmoid cells. The lateral fields may have a 5-degree posterior tilt and 60-degree wedges. The relative loading varies from 1:0.15:0.15 to 1:0.07:0.07 depending on the tumor location and photon energy. For the initial target volume, the superior border of the anterior portal is above the crista galli to encompass the ethmoids and, in the absence of orbital invasion, at the lower edge of the cornea to cover the orbital floor. The inferior border is 1 cm below the floor of the sinus, and the medial border is 1 to 2 cm (or more if necessary) across the midline to cover contralateral ethmoidal extension. The lateral border is 1 cm beyond the apex of the sinus or falling off the skin. The superior border of the lateral portals follows the floor of the anterior cranial fossa, the anterior border is behind the lateral bony canthus

parallel to the slope of the face, the posterior border covers the pterygoid plates, and the inferior border corresponds to that of the anterior portal. The boost volume encompasses the tumor bed while sparing the optic pathway.

Anterior and ipsilateral wedge-pair (usually 45-degree wedges) photon fields are used for tumors of the infrastructure with no extension into the orbit or ethmoids. If necessary, the lateral portal can have a 5-degree inferior tilt to avoid beam divergence into the contralateral eye. Lateral-opposed photon fields are preferred for tumors of the infrastructure spreading across the midline through the hard palate. If necessary, the fields can be slightly angled (5-degree inferior tilt from the ipsilateral side and 5-degree superior tilt from the contralateral side) to avoid irradiating the contralateral eye. The use of a half beam with the isocenter placed at the level of the orbital floor and the upper half of the fields shielded further reduces exposure of the eyes by beam divergence.

The eyes and the optic pathway are of particular concern. With 3-D conformal/IMRT/VMAT/IMPT techniques, the cornea can generally be shielded or a planned avoidance structure (to avoid keratitis) in patients with limited involvement of the medial or inferior orbital wall. If the tumor invades the orbital cavity without necessitating orbital exenteration, care should be taken to avoid irradiating the lacrimal gland to prevent xerophthalmia. It is important to keep the dose to the contralateral optic nerve as well as the optic chiasm below 54 Gy in 27 fractions to prevent bilateral blindness.

Treatment of the Neck

For squamous and undifferentiated carcinoma, elective neck irradiation is recommended. Ipsilateral upper neck treatment can be delivered using a lateral appositional electron field (usually 12 MeV). With conventional radiation techniques, careful matching is required to prevent hot or cold spots. The superior border of the field slopes up from the horizontal ramus of the mandible anteriorly to match the inferior border of the primary portal posteriorly, leaving a small triangle over the cheek untreated. The anterior border is just behind the oral commissure, the posterior border is at the mastoid process, and the inferior border is at the thyroid notch (above the arytenoids). The nodal volume can also be covered by using IMRT with sparing of the parotid gland. Alternatively, the primary tumor bed and the upper neck can be treated with IMRT with the isocenter above the arytenoids and matched to a separate unmodulated lower neck field. This allows the laryngeal structures to be spared by using a larynx block.

If the maxillary sinus is being treated with conventional non-IMRT techniques, the central axes of the primary (sinus) fields and the opposed lateral upper neck fields all are placed in the plane of the inferior border of the maxillary fields (i.e., usually 1 cm below the floor of the maxillary sinus). An independent collimator jaw is used to shield the caudal half of the maxillary fields and the cephalad half of the neck field. The junction between the primary and the neck fields can be moved during the course of treatment to reduce dose heterogeneity in this region. Portals are reduced after 42 Gy, and treatment to the posterior neck continues with abutting electron fields to the desired dose. The middle and lower neck is irradiated with an anterior appositional photon field matched to the inferior border of the opposed-lateral upper neck fields.

Dose Fractionation Schedule

Table 45.3 summarizes the dose regimens for IMRT/IMPT. With 3-D conformal techniques, the dose for postoperative RT at 2 Gy per fraction is 50 Gy for elective nodal treatment, 56 Gy to the operative bed, 60 Gy to the tumor bed if resection margins are negative, and 66 Gy if margins are positive. For primary RT, the total dose to the primary tumor at 2 Gy per fraction is 66 to 70 Gy. The contralateral optic nerve and chiasm are excluded from the field after a dose of 50 to 54 Gy. When the tumor invades structures adjacent to the optic chiasm, a dose of up to 60 Gy to the chiasm may be acceptable because of the higher probability of control and the relatively low risk of visual impairment,[36] after clear discussion with the patient.

FOLLOW-UP AND RECURRENCES

Salvage is possible for some persistent or recurrent lesions. In particular, recurrent cancers of the nasal vestibule remain curable with salvage surgery after primary radiation or occasionally with salvage radiation after primary surgery. Regional recurrences can be treated successfully with neck dissection with or without postoperative radiation depending on the pathologic features. Treatment options are limited for tumors that recur after combined modality therapy, although a few highly selected patients may qualify for reirradiation with curative intent. Cumulative doses of radiation to neural tissues (spinal cord, brainstem, brain, optic structures) are the main limitation to reirradiation.

Most oncologists recommend a second baseline physical examination together with CT, MRI, or positron emission tomography with CT for patients with nasal cavity or paranasal sinus tumors at 3 months after treatment. Common practice is to repeat clinical examination and imaging when indicated every 4 months for the first 3 years after treatment, every 6 months for the fourth and fifth years after treatment, and annually thereafter. In addition to monitoring possible tumor recurrence, these follow-up visits are critical for identifying and managing side effects of treatment.

RESULTS OF TREATMENT

The results of treatment have improved from the 1960s through the 1990s, with overall survival rates increasing progressively from 33% ± 18% in the 1960s to 42% ± 15% in the 1970s, 54% ± 15% in the 1980s, and 56% ± 13% in the 1990s ($P < .001$).[48] In a systematic review of published series spanning 40 years, Dulguerov et al.[49] demonstrated progressive improvements in outcome for all treatment modalities (surgery, surgery with radiation, and radiation). However, a more recent review of the experience at the University of California, San Francisco, showed no significant differences in 5-year overall survival rates or local control rates by a decade of treatment (1960s through 2000s; overall survival, 46% to 56%; local control 55% to 62%) or by radiation technique (conventional, 3-D conformal, or IMRT; overall survival 47% to 57%; local control 59% to 65%). However, the incidence of severe (grade 3 or 4) side effects declined significantly over time from 50% in the 1960s to 16% in the 2000s.[50]

Tumors of the Nasal Cavity

Nasal Vestibule Tumors

Findings from several retrospective studies of RT for nasal vestibule tumors suggest that either brachytherapy or external beam RT can produce cure rates of up to 90% for small (<2-cm) lesions (Table 45.4).[3,4,16,17,52-60] For 2- to 4-cm lesions, external beam radiation can control 70% to 80% of tumors. Although nodal spread of disease is relatively rare for lesions smaller than 2 cm, up to 40% of patients with larger primary tumors have metastases to the cervical nodes at presentation. With the use of appropriate radiation techniques and fractionation schedules, severe and late complications after RT are uncommon (see Table 45.4).

An analysis by the Groupe Europeen de Curietherapie of 1,676 carcinomas of the skin of the nose and nasal vestibule treated by brachytherapy or external beam irradiation revealed an overall local control rate of 93%.[4] Local control depended on tumor size (<2 cm, 96%; 2 to 3.9 cm, 88%; ≥4 cm, 81%), tumor site (external surface, 94%; vestibule, 75%), and status (new, 95%; recurrent, 88%). Local control was independent of histology for tumors <4 cm, but for those >4 cm, basal cell carcinomas were more often controlled than were SCCs. Complications were rare (necrosis, 2%). The local control rate with surgery was approximately 90%.

Nasal Fossa Tumors

Documentation of treatment outcomes for nasal fossa tumors, like nasal vestibule tumors, comes mostly from retrospective studies.[18,61,62] Results are best for lesions confined to the nasal septum, which are generally small and well controlled with primary RT. Locoregional control rates range from 60% to 85%, and the rate of isolated regional recurrence for patients who did not receive elective nodal irradiation is approximately 5%. The most common complications after RT are soft tissue necrosis, visual impairment, and nasal stenosis, seen in 5% to 11% of patients (Table 45.5).[18,59-61] Ang et al.[18] at MD Anderson Cancer Center reported better primary disease control and survival rates for patients with tumors located in the septum (86%) versus patients with tumors on the lateral wall or floor of the nasal fossa (68%). In that study, no patients with nasal septum carcinomas who underwent elective nodal irradiation

TABLE 45.4 LOCAL AND REGIONAL CONTROL RATES OF NASAL VESTIBULE CARCINOMAS TREATED BY DEFINITIVE RADIOTHERAPY

Series (Reference)	Patients	Local Control	Regional Control	Comments/Complications
MD Anderson 1967–1984[52]	32	BT: 11/11 controlled EB: 20/21 (95%) controlled	Small lesions, no ENI: 11/11 Large lesions, no ENI: 5/9 (56%) Large lesions, ENI: 12/12 (100%)	Osteonecrosis, epistaxis: 1 patient each
Princess Margaret Hospital 1958–1983[17]	54	<2 cm ($n = 34$): 97% ≥2 cm ($n = 16$) + size not reported ($n = 6$): 57%	No ENI: 51/54 (94%)	Osteonecrosis, 2 patients; nasal stenosis, 2 patients; massive epistaxis, 1 patient
Daniel den Hoed Cancer Center, Rotterdam 1968–1978[54]	32	EB, <1.5 cm, 72% (5 y); >1.5 cm, 50% (5 y) Dose <54 Gy, 37%; >54 Gy, 82%	Data not available	External beam radiotherapy was hypo-fractionated (2.5–3 Gy/fraction)
VU University, Amsterdam[41]	56	Overall at 2 y: 79% (ultimate at 5 years after salvage, 95%) <1.5 cm ($n = 32$): 83% (ultimate, 94%) ≥1.5 cm ($n = 24$): 74% (ultimate, 96%)	Routine ENI to the mustache region 2-year control rate: 87% (6 of 7 neck relapses were salvaged) 5-year ultimate control rate: 97%	Rhinorrhea: 45%; nasal dryness 39%; epistaxis 15%; adhesions 4% Skin necrosis: 3 patients (all in IDR BT group) Sarcoma in the nasal vestibule: 1 patient
University of Florida 1970–1995[57]	564	Overall at 5 years: 87% EB: 60/71 (86%) Surgery and EB: 8/8 (100%) (ultimate LC: 94%)	T1–T2: 39/43 (91%) T4: 30/36 (83%) N0 LC: 87% (ultimate, 97%) N0/no ENI: 47/54 (87%) (ultimate neck control, 97%)	Soft tissue necrosis: 15 patients-Severe complications: 3 patients
Queens Medical Centre, Nottingham, UK[53]	23	EB only: 8/13 Surgery only: 8/10	Not reported	Radionecrosis: 1 patient
DAHANCA, Denmark[50]	174	5-year locoregional control: 67% T1: 79% T2: 54% T3: 35%	No ENI: 89%	Not reported
Queensland Radium Institute, Australia[57]	28	Surgery and EB: 4/6 (66%) EB: 13/22 (59%)	Surgery and EB: 57% EB: 86%	Septal necrosis, 2 patients; nasobuc-coalveolar fistula and fistula, 1 patient each
French Groupe Europeen de Curietherapie[3]	1676	Skin of the nose and nasal vestibule carcinoma treated by BT or EB (ortho- or megavoltage) Overall LC = 93% (FU ≥2 y); <2 cm, 96%; 2–3.9 cm, 88%; ≥4 cm, 81% LC of nose skin: 94% LC of vestibule: 75% LC for previously untreated tumors: 95% vs. 88% for recurrent tumors		
Daniel den Hoed Cancer Center, Rotterdam[55]	64	Local relapse-free survival: 92% at 5 years T1: 89% T2: 100%		Not reported

BT, brachytherapy; EB, external beam; ENI, elective nodal irradiation; FU, follow-up; IDR, intermediate dose rate; LC, local control; RT, radiotherapy.

had nodal relapses, whereas two of eight patients who did not undergo nodal irradiation experienced recurrence in the ipsilateral subdigastric nodes. Distant metastasis was more common among patients with lateral wall and floor disease, and ultimately survival rates were best among patients with nasal septum tumors. However, other groups[61] found no differences in results for tumors at various sites within the nasal cavity. Results of treatment for early-stage tumors are excellent after either RT or surgery.

An analysis of 783 patients with nasal cavity cancer included in the Surveillance, Epidemiology, and End Results (SEER) database from 1988 through 1998[62] revealed SCC to be the most common tumor type (49.3%), followed by ENB (13.2%). More than half of the cases presented with a small primary tumor (T1), and only 5% had positive nodes at diagnosis. Overall mean survival time was 57 months and the 5-year

TABLE 45.5 TREATMENT OUTCOMES FOR NASAL FOSSA TUMORS

Series (Reference)	Patients	Treatments	Survival Rates at 5 Years	Late Complications
MD Anderson 1969–1985[18]	45	RT alone: 18 patients RT+ surgery: 2 patients Surgery + RT: 25 patients Median time to relapse: 9 mo	Overall: 75% Disease-specific: 83%	Radiation-induced blindness: 2 patients Surgical blindness: 2 patients Maxilla necrosis: 3 patients Nasal stenosis: 2 patients Septal perforation: 1 patient Severe dental decay: 1 patient
Roswell Memorial Park Institute 1942–1964[59]	57	RT alone: 30 patients Surgery alone: 13 patients Surgery + RT: 14 patients	Crude overall: 56% Disease-free: 56%	Not reported
University of Puerto Rico 1976[60]	40	RT alone: 34 patients Surgery alone: 6 patients	Overall: 56%	Not reported
Mallinckrodt Institute of Radiology 1969–1984[61]	56	RT alone: 28 patients RT + surgery: 18 patients Surgery + RT: 10 patients	Overall: 52%	Soft tissue necrosis: 2 patients Cataract: 1 patient Nasal synechiae: 1 patient Severe otitis media: 2 patients Hemorrhage (fatal): 2 patients Optic neuropathy: 1 patient Brain necrosis: 1 patient

RT, radiation therapy.

TABLE 45.6 TREATMENT RESULTS FOR NASAL CAVITY CANCER FROM THE SURVEILLANCE, EPIDEMIOLOGY, AND END RESULTS DATABASE FOR 1988 THROUGH 1998[g]

Tumor Type	5-Year Survival Rate (%)	T or N Classification	5-Year Survival Rate (%)
Adenocarcinoma	49.0	T1	66.4
Adenoid cystic carcinoma	59.1	T2	51.8
Melanoma	22.1	T3	45.6
Other tumors	59.5	T4	40.2
Sarcoma	78.0	Overall	56.7
Squamous cell carcinoma	61.6		
Esthesioneuroblastoma	63.6	N0	62.3
SNUC	49.5	N+	28.4

[a]Results are shown by tumor type and by T- and N-stage. Because of rounding, percentages may not total 100.
SNUC, sinonasal undifferentiated carcinoma.
Reproduced with permission from Bhattacharyya N. Cancer of the nasal cavity: survival and factors influencing prognosis. *Arch Otolaryngol Head Neck Surg* 2002;128(9):1079–1083. Copyright © 2002 American Medical Association. All rights reserved.

survival rate was 40.3%. On multivariate analysis, male sex, increasing age, T status, N status, and poorer tumor grade all adversely affected survival ($P < .05$). RT, given to 50.5% of patients, also independently predicted poorer survival ($P = .03$), probably because those patients had had poor prognostic features such as perineural invasion, positive margins, or poor performance status (medically unfit for surgery). Five-year survival rates by tumor type, T status, and N status are shown in Table 45.6.[62] Five-year survival rates also correlated with extent of tumor dedifferentiation, being 75.3%, 61.9%, 47.6%, and 36.8% for well-, moderately, poorly, and undifferentiated cancers, respectively.

Esthesioneuroblastoma

Either surgery or primary RT as single-modality therapy can produce locoregional control rates exceeding 90% for tumors that are confined to the nasal cavity (Kadish stage A).[8] Single-modality therapy has also been used for lesions involving the nasal cavity and one or more paranasal sinuses (stage B), as has surgery followed by adjuvant RT. However, the optimal therapy for stage B lesions is not clear because of the heterogeneity of these tumors. Disease that extends beyond the nasal cavity and paranasal sinuses (stage C) seems to be best treated with a combination of surgery and radiation, and the role of chemotherapy, if any, is being investigated. Elective nodal irradiation is not generally recommended because the incidence of nodal relapse is <15%. Distant metastasis is uncommon (10%) even among patients presenting with locally advanced disease. Among 783 nasal cavity cancers identified from the SEER database, 103 (13.2%) were ENBs; the median survival time for patients with these tumors was 88 months, and the overall 5-year survival rate was 63.6%.[62] Tables 45.7[63–68] and 45.8[9] summarize the results of treatment. The prognosis for patients with stage A disease is excellent. Overall, 30% of patients with stage B tumor died of the disease. About 60% of patients with stage C tumors died of the disease, primarily because of failure to control the primary tumor. As noted above, distant metastasis is uncommon (10%) even in locoregionally advanced disease.

Spaulding et al.[28] reported results for 25 patients treated at the University of Virginia Medical Center from 1959 through 1986 who were followed for 2 years after therapy. Treatment approaches had gradually evolved during that period, with progressive introduction of craniofacial resections, complex field megavoltage radiation, and, for stage C disease, the addition of chemotherapy. Therefore, patients were assigned to two groups, based on treatment era, for comparative analysis. Although this series is relatively small, it revealed two interesting findings on this rare disease: First, that extensive craniofacial resection does not seem to confer a major advantage over wide local excision for patients with stage B lesions, and second, that the addition of chemotherapy to craniofacial resection and RT for patients with stage C tumors may yield higher disease-specific survival rates.

A larger series of 72 patients with sinonasal neuroendocrine tumors treated at MD Anderson Cancer Center between 1982 and 2002[63] included a spectrum of histologies: ENB (31 patients), sinonasal undifferentiated carcinoma (SNUC, 16 patients), neuroendocrine carcinoma (18 patients), and small cell carcinoma (7 patients). The overall survival rates at 5 years were 93.1% for patients with ENB, 62.5% for those with SNUC, 64.2% for neuroendocrine carcinoma, and 28.6% for small cell carcinoma ($P = .0029$; log-rank test). The local control rates at 5 years also were superior for patients with ENB (96.2%) compared with patients who had SNUC (78.6%), neuroendocrine carcinoma (72.6%), or small cell carcinoma (66.7%) ($P = .04$). The corresponding regional failure rates at

TABLE 45.7 OVERALL TREATMENT RESULTS OF ESTHESIONEUROBLASTOMA

Series (Reference)	Patients	Local Control	Regional Control and Survival	Comments/Complications
MD Anderson 1982–2002[63]	31	5 y: 96.2%	5 y: 91.3%5-year OS: 93.1% DM: 0%	
UCLA 1970–1990[64]	26	Overall: 18/26 (69%) S alone: 1/7 (14%) RT alone: 2/5 (40%) S + RT: 10/12 (83%)	4/26 (15%) patients had nodal disease (at presentation or after initial therapy) 5-year CSS: 74% 5-year RFS: 58%	Postoperative cerebrospinal fluid leak, epiphora, radiation retinopathy (3/17 patients)
Mayo Clinic 1951–1990[65]	49	5 y: 65% (all patients) S alone: 73%S + RT: 86%	3/49 (6%) had N1 at presentation and 8/46 (17%) had regional relapse (7/8 with concurrent local failure) 5-year DFS and OS: 55% and 69% (all patients)	Osteonecrosis of trephine bone plate (4 patients)
U. of Virginia 1959–1991[66]	40	Overall: 30/40 (75%) controlled	4/40 (10%) clinically N1 at presentation and 4/36 (11%) developed regional relapse 5-year OS: 78%	–
U. of Virginia Health System, 1976–2004 treated with a standardized protocol[67a]	50	17 patients (34%) developed recurrent disease, which was locoregional in 12 patients	5-year DFS: 86.5% Possibility for surgical salvage	–
Hospital do Cancer Instituto Nacional de Cancer, Rio de Janeiro, Brazil 1983–2000[68]	36	S + RT, 18; RT only, 14; S only, 1 RT; and chemotherapy, 2	5- and 10-year DFS: 46% and 24% 5- and 10-year OS: 55% and 46% N+ and DM adversely affected prognosis ($P < .001$ and $P = .01$, respectively)	Kadish classification best predicted disease-free survival

[a]Kadish A or B received preoperative RT followed by craniofacial resection; Kadish stage C disease was treated with preoperative chemotherapy and RT followed by a craniofacial resection.
CSS, cause-specific survival; DFS, disease-free survival; DM, distant metastases; OS, overall survival; RFS, relapse-free survival; RT, radiation therapy; S, surgery.

TABLE 45.8 PATTERN OF FAILURE AND RESULTS OF SALVAGE TREATMENT OF ESTHESIONEUROBLASTOMA BY STAGE AND TREATMENT

Kadish Stage	Therapy	Local Control	Nodal Relapse	Salvage by Subsequent RT or S	Distant Metastasis	Died of Disease
A (n = 24)	RT	3/5	1/5	3/3	0/5	0/5
	S	5/9	1/9	4/4	0/9	0/9
	S + RT	9/10	2/10	2/2	1/10	1/10
	All	17/24 (71%)	4/24 (17%)	9/9	1/24 (4%)	1/24 (4%)
B (n = 33)	RT	6/7	2/7	0/1	0/7	3/7
	S	3/6	0/6	1/2	0/6	2/6
	S + RT	15/20	1/20	3/4	3/20	5/20
	All	24/33 (73%)	3/33 (9%)	4/7	3/33 (9%)	10/33 (30%)
C (n = 21)	RT	2/5	2/7	0/0	1/5	4/5
	S	1/1	0/6	0/0	0/1	0/1
	S + RT	9/15	1/20	1/1	1/15	8/15
	All	12/21 (57%)	3/33 (9%)	1/1	2/21 (10%)	12/21 (57%)

RT, radiotherapy; S, surgery.
Modified from Elkon D, Hightower SI, Lim ML, et al. Esthesioneuroblastoma. *Cancer* 1979;44:1087–1094.

5 years were 8.7% for patients with ENB, 15.6% for SNUC, 12.9% for neuroendocrine carcinoma, and 44.4% for small cell carcinoma, and distant metastasis rates were 0% for ENB, 25.4% for SNUC, 14.1% for neuroendocrine carcinoma, and 75.0% for small cell carcinoma. Moreover, local therapy alone produced excellent local and distant control rates for ENB. Among eight patients treated for ENB since 2000 with surgery and adjuvant IMRT to 60 Gy (one with stage B disease and seven with stage C [five of whom had intracranial extension]), there were no local recurrences and one nodal recurrence was salvaged surgically. All eight patients were alive with no evidence of disease at the last follow-up. Institutional experiences outcomes from several institutions are reported in Table 45.7.[63–68]

Ozsahin et al.[23] described results of treatment in 13 European and North American centers for 77 patients with olfactory neuroblastoma, 11 with Kadish stage A, 29 with stage B, and 37 with stage C; 56 patients had surgery, 44 with total tumor excision. All but 5 patients received RT (50% with 3-D CRT) and 21 had chemotherapy. With median follow-up of 72 months, locoregional tumor control was 62%, disease-free survival 57%, and overall survival 64%. Patients having total tumor resection or receiving ≥54 Gy had better overall survival than those treated with lower doses. Six of the patients treated with RT (56 to 70 Gy) developed grade 3 or 4 late complications (five osteonecrosis and one retinopathy).

Madani et al.[69] published a report on 84 patients (73 with primary and 11 with local recurrent sinonasal tumors), 9 of which were ENB, treated with IMRT (median dose of 70 Gy in 35 fractions). Mean D50 to the optic chiasm was 37.2 Gy, to ipsilateral optic nerve 49.4 Gy, to contralateral optic nerve 47.1 Gy, and to the retina 37.7 and 28.4 Gy, respectively.

Multimodality management has been correlated with improved outcomes.[70]

Modesto et al.[71] described their experience in 43 patients with ENB, 2 groups, 1 of 26 and the other of 17 patients treated at separate institutions. Five patients had stage A at diagnosis (confined to the nasal cavity), 13 stage B (tumor extending into the paranasal sinuses), 16 stage C (beyond the paranasal sinuses), and 9 stage D (cervical lymph node involvement) according to the modified Kadish classification. Neoadjuvant platinum-based chemotherapy was administered to 24 patients, leading to 70.8% response rate (6 CR and 11 PR). A total of 31 patients (72%) were treated by surgery; 39 (90.6%) underwent RT. Among them, 11 patients (28.2%) were treated using IMRT. Median dose was 64 Gy (range 30 to 70 Gy). Twelve patients (28%) received bilateral cervical lymph node irradiation (LNI) (median dose 57 Gy, range 50 to

66 Gy). Twelve patients (21%) received platinum-based CRT. After a median follow-up of 77 months, the 5-year overall survival was 65% and the 5-year progression-free survival 58%. Twelve patients (28%) developed locoregional relapse. The major prognostic factor was the modified Kadish stage with 3-year survival rates of 100% for Kadish A to B versus 48% for stage C and 22% for stage D. After adjustment for tumor stage, neither neoadjuvant chemotherapy nor LNI seemed predictive for locoregional tumor control or survival.

Protons have been used sparingly in the treatment of some of these patients. Nakamura et al.[72] reported on 42 patients with esthesioneuroblastoma treated with proton therapy and 26% receiving chemotherapy. With a median follow-up time of 69 months, the 5-year overall survival and progression-free survival was 100% and 80% for Kadish A, 86% and 65% for Kadish B, and 76% and 39% for Kadish C. Dagan et al.[73] reported on 84 adult patients without metastases receiving primary (13%) or adjuvant (87%) treatment with PT for sinonasal cancers of which 23 % (19) were olfactory neuroblastoma. Advanced stage (T3 in 25% and T4 in 69%) and high-grade histology (51%) were common. Surgical procedures included endoscopic resection alone (45%), endoscopic resection with craniotomy (12%), or open resection (30%). Gross residual disease was present in 26% of patients. Most patients received hyperfractionated PT (1.2-Gy RBE twice daily, 99%) and chemotherapy (75%). The median PT dose was 73.8 Gy (RBE), with 85% of patients receiving more than 70 Gy. The median follow-up was 2.4 years for all patients and 2.7 years among living patients. Local tumor control (LC), neck control, freedom from distant metastasis, disease-free survival, cause-specific survival, and overall survival rates were 83%, 94%, 73%, 63%, 70%, and 68%, respectively, at 3 years. The 3-year LC rate was 61% for primary RT and 59% for patients with gross disease. Late toxicity occurred in 24% of patients (with grade 3 or higher unilateral vision loss in 2%). Akimoto et al.[74] reported on 339 patients with non–squamous cell cancer in the head and neck, of which 63 were olfactory neuroblastomas, treated with protons. Median follow-up was 64 months. Overall survival, progression-free survival, and local control rate of all patients at 5 years were 61.2%, 36.8%, and 71.2%, respectively, and, for olfactory neuroblastomas, 86.2% and 79.0%. Among all patients, 254 (75%) were not suited for photon RT because doses to OARs exceeded tolerance dose in the evaluation of dose–volume histogram. However, OS at 5 years of these patients was 65.5%. Regarding treatment morbidity, 34 (10%) patients developed grade 3 or 4 late toxicities such as brain injuries and neuropathy. None experienced grade 5 toxicities.

Tumors of the Paranasal Sinuses

Five-year outcomes from studies reported since 1998 continue to illustrate that local control after treatment of paranasal sinus tumors remains problematic[75–82] (Table 45.9). For patients with carcinoma of the maxillary sinuses, the combination of surgery and radiation yields 5-year local control and survival rates ranging from 44% to 80%. These rates are better than those achieved with either surgery or RT alone. For RT alone, the 5-year local control rates range from 22% to 39% and the 5-year overall survival rates from 22% to 40%. Findings from a large multicenter retrospective

Section III

TABLE 45.9 OUTCOME OF PATIENTS WITH LOCALLY ADVANCED CANCER OF THE PARANASAL SINUSES TREATED WITH COMBINED SURGERY AND RADIATION THERAPY

Study (Reference)	Year	Patients	5-Year Survival (%)	Local Recurrence (%)	Distant Metastasis (%)
A. Results from Surgery and Conventional Radiation Therapy					
Lavertu et al.[75]	1989	54	38	52	–
Spiro et al.[76]	1989	105	38	49	15
Zaharia et al.[77]	1989	149	36	43	–
Paulino et al.[46]	1998	48	47	46	17
Le et al.[78]	1999	97	34	54	34
Myers et al.[79]	2002	141	52	56	33
Jiang et al.[30]	1991	67[a]	53[b]	24	27
Katz et al.[80]	2002	31		21	
Blanco et al.[81]	2004	106	27	42	29
Dirix et al.[42]	2007	127	54	47	20
Bristol et al.[82]	2007	90 G1(1969–1991) 56 G2(>1991–2002)			
B. Results from Surgery and Intensity-Modulated Radiation Therapy					
Duthoy et al.[84]	2005	39	2-year OS: 68 4-year OS: 59	2-year: 27 4-year: 32	–
Ahamad et al. (unpublished)[c]	2005	53	Crude: 88.6	Crude: 15.1 2-year: 20 4-year: 25	20.7
Daly et al.[62]	2007	36	45	2-year: 38	
Hoppe et al.[86]	2008	37	80	2-year: 25	
Madani et al.[69]	2009	84	58.5	41.5	18
Dirix et al.[42]	2010	40	89	2-year: 24	

C. Side Effects of Combined Surgery and Radiation Therapy in Patients with Paranasal Sinus Cancer

Vestibulocochlear	Vestibular dysfunction, persistent otitis, tinnitus, hearing impairment
Ophthalmologic (lacrimal gland, eyes, lens, optic nerves, and chiasm)	Retinopathy, xerophthalmia, keratopathy, cataracts, visual impairment
Neurologic (brain, brainstem, spinal cord, temporal lobe)	Neurocognitive impairment, cranial neuropathy, myelopathy, brain necrosis
Endocrine (pituitary gland, hypothalamus, thyroid gland if neck is irradiated)	Multiple endocrine dysfunction: hyperprolactinemia, syndromes associated with decreased GH, FSH, LH, T4, TSH, ACTH, and their downstream hormones
Oral (major salivary glands, oral mucosa, mandible, and temporomandibular joint)	Xerostomia, dental caries, dysgeusia, mandible exposure, necrosis, and trismus
Connective tissue complications (oral cavity, soft palate musculature, pharynx, larynx, skin and subcutaneous tissues, skull bones)	Soft tissue necrosis, skin changes, persistent lymphedema, subcutaneous fibrosis, cartilage necrosis, nasal dryness, choanal stenosis, swallowing and voice dysfunction, bone necrosis

[a]Patients with node-negative disease.
[b]Five-year relapse-free survival.
[c]Patients treated at MD Anderson Cancer Center with intensity-modulated radiation therapy.
ACTH, adrenocorticotropic hormone; FSH, follicle-stimulating hormone; GH, growth hormone; LH, luteinizing hormone; OS, overall survival; TSH, thyroid-stimulating hormone.

analysis of 418 patients with ethmoid sinus adenocarcinoma indicated that the size of the lesion (T4), the extent of nodal involvement (N+), and the presence of brain extension were the most significant prognostic factors for overall survival.[83] Although the authors concluded that surgery followed by postoperative RT remains the treatment of choice, they did note that 51% of the patients developed recurrences, 74% of which were local.

A 1991 review of outcomes after treatment of 73 patients with maxillary sinus carcinomas at MD Anderson Cancer Center reported 5-year local and regional control rates according to pathologic T category as follows: for T1 and T2 tumors, 91% local and 71% regional control; for T3, 77% local and 80% regional; and for T4, 65% local and 93% regional.[30] Five-year regional control rates according to N category were 84% for N0 disease and 82% for N1 or N2 disease. The most common histologic subtypes were SCC (48%) and adenoid cystic carcinoma (27%); 5-year local and regional control rates were 62% (local) and 86% (regional) for squamous cell tumors and 82% (local) and 94% (regional) for adenoid tumors. Perineural invasion and nodal disease at presentation were poor prognostic factors. An update of this report published in 2007[75] showed that increasing the radiation portals to cover the skull base for patients with perineural invasion

reduced the risk of local recurrence and that adding elective nodal irradiation for patients with squamous or undifferentiated tumors improved the rates of nodal control, distant metastasis, and recurrence-free survival.

The extent of neuroendocrine differentiation of sinonasal carcinomas also influences the patterns of failure. In one study, the 5-year actuarial rates of local, regional, and distant failure according to tumor histology were as follows: ENB 4% local failure, 9% regional failure, and 0% distant failure; neuroendocrine carcinoma 27% local, 13% regional, and 12% distant; sinonasal undifferentiated carcinoma 21% local, 16% regional, and 25% distant; and small cell carcinoma 33% local failure, 44% regional failure, and 75% distant failure.[63]

IMRT has emerged as the standard of care for tumors of the paranasal sinuses with low toxicity and high local control rates.[43,69,84-87] Madani et al.[69] reported the largest series to date, in which 105 patients (most of whom [56%] had ethmoid sinus tumors) were treated with IMRT. At a median follow-up time of 40 months, the 5-year actuarial local control and overall survival rates were 70.7% and 58.5%. In multivariate analysis, invasion of the cribriform plate was found to predict worse local control ($P < .001$) and lower overall survival ($P < .001$).

The role of proton therapy using passive scattering and IMPT in the management of sinonasal malignancies is rapidly evolving and may be preferred over IMRT when dose limiting structures may be compromised with definitive doses.[47] Resto et al.[88] reported on 102 patients with various histologies receiving surgery and post-operative proton therapy. With a median follow-up of 61 mo, the 5-year local control and overall survival were 95% and 90% for complete resection, 82% and 53% for partial resection, and 87% and 49% for biopsy-only. Toxicity was not reported. Russo et al.[89] reported on 54 patients with squamous cell carcinoma treated with proton therapy of which 69% had surgery and 39% had chemotherapy. The 5-year local regional control rate and overall survival were 73% and 47%, respectively. Wound site complications (e.g., fistulas) occurred most commonly with 9 Grade 3 and 6 Grade 4 complications. Zenda et al.[90] reported on 90 patients with various histologies of which 18% had surgery and 12% had chemotherapy. With a median follow-up of 57 months the 5-year overall survival and progression free survival rates were 64% and 44%, respectively. Linton et al.[91] reported on 26 patients with adenoid cystic carcinoma of which 77% had surgery and 23% were treated with protons alone. The 2-year local control and overall survival were 95% and 93%, respectively. There were 17 (19%) late Grade 3 and 6 (7%) late Grade 4 toxicities including 2 patients with encephalomyelitis infection and 4 patients with a optic nerve disorder. Takagi et al.[92] reported on 40 patients treated with definitive proton therapy alone for adenoid cystic carcinoma tumors, and with a median follow-up of 38 months, the 5-year local control, progression-free survival and overall survival were 76%, 30%, and 63%, respectively. There were 36 Grade 3 or higher events in 21 patients (26%). High grade toxicities included osteoradionecrosis, vision loss, and nasopharyngeal ulcers resulting in 3 Grade 5 toxicities.

Dagan et al.[93] described their experience in 84 patients treated with PT involving sinonasal sites: nasal/ethmoid (67), maxillary (15), frontal or sphenoid (2). Histologies included squamous cell carcinoma (22), adenoid cystic carcinoma (14), olfactory neuroblastoma (23), adenocarcinoma (8), sinonasal undifferentiated carcinoma (7), neuroendocrine carcinoma (4), mucoepidermoid carcinoma (3), and other histologies (3). Thirty-eight patients had intracranial tumors and 31 had orbital invasion. Eleven patients were treated after biopsy alone, 9 after subtotal resection, and 2 for recurrence after gross total resection. Twenty-two (26%) had gross tumor at the time of proton therapy. Median PT dose was 73.8 CGE (range, 56.8-74.4 CGE) at 1.2 CGE/fraction twice daily with elective nodal therapy. Sixty-six (78%) of patients were treated to the neck electively. Sixty-three patients (75%) received chemotherapy (mostly concurrent low-dose weekly cisplatin). Median follow-up was 2.4 years (range, 0.4 to 6.7 years) for all patients and 2.7 years for living patients (range, 0.6 to 6.7 years). Three-year local control and nodal controls rates were 83% and 94%, respectively. Freedom from distant mets was 73.2%, cause-specific survival was 70%, and overall survival was 68%. Grade 3-5 toxicities occurred in 24% of patients with 1 fatal central nervous system necrosis.

Truong et al.[94] described their experience with 20 patients with primary sphenoid malignancy who received proton beam to a median dose of 76 CGE with a median follow-up of 27 months. The 2-year local control, regional control, and freedom from distant metastasis rates were 86%, 86%, and 50%, respectively.

Patel et al.[95] performed a meta-analysis summarizing the retrospective data of various histologies and performed comparative effective analysis between charged particle and photon therapy. The median follow-up time was approximately 40 months for both groups, and the pooled overall survival (relative risk 1.51, 95% CI 1.14-1.99; $p = 0.0003$) and disease-free survival (1.93, 95% CI 1.36-2.75, $p = 0.0003$) was higher at 5 years for charged particle than for photon therapy.

Future Directions in Radiation Therapy

IMRT has improved the cancer care in external beam RT for sinonasal malignancies.[43,76–79] Proton beam therapy confers further benefits for nasal and paranasal sinus tumors, and investigators at MD Anderson Cancer Center and others have demonstrated the clinical feasibility of IMPT for this purpose (Fig. 45.6).[96] The additional advantages of this technique over photon-based IMRT are its ability to limit the low dose radiation received by adjacent critical OAR structures and allow escalation of dose to the target volume. Well-designed clinical trials in cooperative group setting will be necessary to provide the evidence required for widespread adoption of PT over IMRT for these rare malignancies. Finally, further improvements in the local control of sinonasal malignancies will require incorporating systemic agents as neoadjuvant or concurrent therapy. Again, the rarity of

sinonasal cancer will most likely require international cooperative group trials to facilitate timely analyses of outcomes and design of future trials.

SEQUELAE OF TREATMENT

Soft Tissue and Bone

The formation of nasal cavity synechiae (fibrous mucosal bands causing airway stenosis) can be prevented by intermittent dilation of the nasal passages with a petroleum-coated cotton swab until mucositis has resolved. Dry mucous membranes can be managed symptomatically with saline nasal spray. Soft tissue or cartilage necrosis is uncommon after therapy, at an estimated incidence of 5% to 10%.[26,66]

Eyes and Optic Pathway

Chronic keratitis and iritis (dry eye syndrome) can develop after RT if tumor extension to the orbital cavity mandates irradiation of the lacrimal gland to doses of more than 30 to 40 Gy.[97,98] Without lacrimal irradiation, fewer than 20% of patients treated with up to 55 Gy to the cornea develop chronic corneal injury. The risk of cataract formation at 5 years is approximately 5% after doses of up to 10 Gy to the lenses using conventional fractionation; this risk increases to 50% at 5 years after 18 Gy.

Radiation retinopathy generally occurs within 18 months to 5 years after treatment.[99] It is rare after doses of <45 Gy, but the incidence increases to about 50% after doses of 45 to 55 Gy.[97,98] Optic neuropathy tends to develop between 2 and 4 years after RT, but it has been reported as late as 14 years after treatment. The reported incidence of optic neuropathy is <5% after 50 to 60 Gy but increases to around 30% for doses of 61 to 78 Gy. Factors that influence the risk of radiation-induced optic neuropathy were reported in 2006 for 273 patients treated between 1964 and 2000 in whom the radiation fields included the optic nerves or chiasm.[27] The likelihood of developing optic neuropathy was primarily influenced by the total dose, but fraction size was marginally significant. The 5-year rates of freedom from optic neuropathy were 95% for doses ≤63 Gy treated once daily, 98% for doses ≤63 Gy treated twice daily, 78% for doses >63 Gy treated once daily, and 91% for doses >63 Gy treated twice daily. On multivariate analysis, the risk of optic neuropathy was found to correlate with increasing total dose ($P = .0047$) and possibly with increasing patient age ($P = .091$), once-daily versus twice-daily fractionation ($P = .068$), and overall treatment time ($P = .097$). When the target volumes include the optic pathway, special attention must be paid to hot spots and dose per fraction to avoid optic neuropathies.

Optimizing the technique for paranasal sinus tumors is crucial so that the radiation dose to the optic apparatus is limited to the greatest extent possible to minimize the risk of complications. Investigators at the University of Florida, reviewing 464 patients treated from 1964 through 2001,[100] reported a 20% incidence of ipsilateral radiation retinopathy at 5 and 10 years after conventional or 3-D RT. In that study, patients were deemed functionally blind when visual acuity dropped to 20/100 on the Snellen chart, and neovascularization (rubeosis iridis or neovascular glaucoma) was coincident with radiation retinopathy. Use of IMRT has been shown to limit the doses to the optic apparatus without compromising local control. Indeed, Chen et al.[50] reported findings for 127 patients treated between 1960 and 2005 with a variety of RT techniques that had evolved over that period, namely, conventional, 3-D conformal, and IMRT. They concluded that the incidence of severe (grade ≥ 3) complications depended on the radiation treatment technique used: 54% for conventional therapy, 22% for 3-D conformal therapy, and 13% for IMRT. Specifically, the incidence of grade 3 or 4 late ocular toxicity decreased from 20% with conventional techniques to 0% with IMRT, whereas grade 3 or 4 late auditory toxicity decreased from 15% with conventional to 4% with IMRT (*P* < .001).[50] Moreover, to date, no radiation-induced blindness has been reported among the collective experience, with 308 patients treated with IMRT as either definitive or postoperative therapy for nasal and paranasal malignancies.[43,50,61,69,84,85,87,101]

REFERENCES

1. Frank SJ, Ahamad A, Ang KK. Chapter 42: Cancer of the nasal cavity and paranasal sinuses. In: Halperin EC, Wazer DE, Perez CA, Brady LW, eds. *Principles and practice of radiation oncology.* 6th ed. Philadelphia, PA: Wolters Kluwer/Lippincott Williams & Wilkins, 2013:761–777.

2. Bridger MW, van Nostrand AW. The nose and paranasal sinuses—applied surgical anatomy. A histologic study of whole organ sections in three planes. *J Otolaryngol* 1978;7:1–33.

3. Goepfert H, Guillamondegui OM, Jesse RH, et al. Squamous cell carcinoma of nasal vestibule. *Arch Otolaryngol* 1974;100:8–10.

4. Mazeron JJ, Chassagne D, Crook J, et al. Radiation therapy of carcinomas of the skin of nose and nasal vestibule: a report of 1676 cases by the Groupe Europeen de Curietherapie. *Radiother Oncol* 1988;13:165–173.

5. Murphy J, Bleach NR, Thyveetil M. Sebaceous carcinoma of the nose: multifocal presentation? *J Laryngol Otol* 2004;118:374–376.

6. Prasad ML, Patel SG, Busam KJ. Primary mucosal desmoplastic melanoma of the head and neck. *Head Neck* 2004;26:373–377.

7. Su K, Xu J, Qiao M, et al. CT characteristics of primary nasal non-Hodgkin lymphoma. *J Clin Otorhinolaryngol* 2003;17:261–263.

8. Roush G. Epidemiology of cancer of the nose and paranasal sinuses: current concepts. *Head Neck Surg* 1979;2:3–11.

9. Elkon D, Hightower SI, Lim ML, et al. Esthesioneuroblastoma. *Cancer* 1979;44:1087–1094.

10. Lewis JS, Castro EB. Cancer of the nasal cavity and paranasal sinuses. *J Laryngol Otol* 1972;86:255–262.

11. Acheson ED, Hadfield EH, Macbeth RG. Carcinoma of the nasal cavity and accessory sinuses in woodworkers. *Lancet* 1967;1:311–312.

12. Klintenberg C, Olofsson J, Hellquist H, et al. Adenocarcinoma of the ethmoid sinuses. A review of 28 cases with special reference to wood dust exposure. *Cancer* 1984;54:482–488.

13. Schwaab G, Julieron M, Janot F. Epidemiology of cancers of the nasal cavities and paranasal sinuses. *Neurochirurgie* 1997;43:61–63.

14. Torjussen W, Solberg LA, Hogetveit AC. Histopathological changes of the nasal mucosa in active and retired nickel workers. *Br J Cancer* 1979;40:568–580.

15. Zheng W, McLaughlin JK, Chow WH, et al. Risk factors for cancers of the nasal cavity and paranasal sinuses among white men in the United States. *Am J Epidemiol* 1993;43:61–63.

16. Bars G, Visser AG, Van Andel JG. The treatment of squamous cell carcinoma of the nasal vestibule with interstitial iridium implantation. *Radiother Oncol* 1985;4:121–125.

17. Wong CS, Cummings BJ, Elhakim T, et al. External irradiation for squamous cell carcinoma of the nasal vestibule. *Int J Radiat Oncol Biol Phys* 1986;12:1943–1946.

18. Ang KK, Jiang G-L, Frankenthaler RA, et al. Carcinomas of the nasal cavity. *Radiother Oncol* 1992;24:163–168.

19. Ahn P. Risk of lymph node metastasis and nodal level involvement based on site and histology in the paranasal sinus: a SEER analysis. *Int J Radiat Oncol Biol Phys* 2013;87(2S):S59, Abstr 149.

20. Goldsweig HG, Sundaresan N. Chemotherapy of recurrent esthesioneuroblastoma. Case report and review of the literature. *Am J Clin Oncol* 1990;13:139–143.

21. Kadish S, Goodman M, Wang CC. Olfactory neuroblastoma. A clinical analysis of 17 cases. *Cancer* 1976;37:1571–1576.

22. Howell MC, Branstetter BF IV, Snyderman CH. Patterns of regional spread for esthesioneuroblastoma. *AJNR Am J Neuroradiol* 2011;32:929–933.

23. Ozsahin M, Gruber G, Olszyk O, et al. Outcome and prognostic factors in olfactory neuroblastoma: a rare cancer network study. *Int J Radiat Oncol Biol Phys* 2010;78:992–997.

24. Rouviere H, Tobias MJ. *Anatomy of the human lymphatic system.* Ann Arbor, MI: Edwards, 1938.

25. Le Q-T, Fu KK, Kaplan MJ, et al. Lymph node metastasis in maxillary sinus carcinoma. *Int J Radiat Oncol Biol Phys* 2000;46:541–549.

26. Paulino AC, Fisher SG, Marks JE. Is prophylactic neck irradiation indicated patients with squamous cell carcinoma of the maxillary sinus? *Int J Radiat Oncol Biol Phys* 1997;39:283–289.

27. Mendenhall WM, Mendenhall CM, Riggs CEJ, et al. Sinonasal undifferentiated carcinoma. *Am J Clin Oncol* 2006;29:27–31.

28. Spaulding CA, Kranyak MS, Constable WC, et al. Esthesioneuroblastoma: a comparison of two treatment eras. *Int J Radiat Oncol Biol Phys* 1988;15:581–590.

29. Jiang GL, Morrison WH, Garden AS, et al. Ethmoid sinus carcinomas: natural history and treatment results. *Radiother Oncol* 1998;49:21–27.

30. Jiang GL, Ang KK, Peters LJ, et al. Maxillary sinus carcinomas: natural history and results of postoperative radiotherapy. *Radiother Oncol* 1991;21:193–200.

31. Kondo M, Horiuchi M, Inuyama Y, et al. Value of computed tomography for radiation therapy of tumors of the nasal cavity and paranasal sinuses. *Acta Radiol Oncol Radiat Phys Biol* 1983;22:3–7.

32. Shapiro MD, Som PM. MRI of the paranasal sinuses and nasal cavity. *Radiol Clin North Am* 1989;27:447–475.

33. Som PM, Shapiro MD, Biller HF, et al. Sinonasal tumors and inflammatory tissues: differentiation with MR imaging. *Radiology* 1988;167:803–808.

34. Ahmin MB, Edge SB, Gren FL et al., eds. Nasal cavity and paranasal sinuses. In: *AJCC cancer staging manual.* 8th ed. New York: Springer, 2017:137–147.

35. Million RR. The myth regarding bone or cartilage involvement by cancer and the likelihood of cure by radiotherapy. *Head Neck* 1989;11:30–40.

36. McCollough WM, Mendenhall NP, Parsons JT, et al. Radiotherapy alone for squamous cell carcinoma of the nasal vestibule: management of the primary site and regional lymphatics. *Int J RadiatOncolBiol Phys* 1993;26:73–79.

37. Lund VJ, Howard DJ, Wei WI, et al. Craniofacial resection for tumors of the nasal cavity and paranasal sinuses. A 17 year experience. *Head Neck* 1998;20:97–105.

38. Bridger GP, Kwok B, Baldwin M. Craniofacial resection for paranasal sinus cancers. *Head Neck* 2000;22:772–780.

39. Waldron JN, O'Sullivan B, Warde P, et al. Ethmoid sinus cancer: twenty-nine cases managed with primary radiation therapy. *Int J Radiat Oncol Biol Phys* 1998;41:361–369.

40. Yusuf MB, Amsbaugh MJ, Silverman C, et al. Organ preservation in patients with orbit-invasive sinonasal cancer. *Int J Radiat Oncol Biol Phys* 2016;94:904, Abstr 183.

41. Wade PMJ, Smith RE, Johns ME. Response of esthesioneuroblastoma to chemotherapy. Report of five cases and review of the literature. *Cancer Bull* 1984;53:1036–1041.

42. Langendijk JA, Poorter R, Leemans CR, et al. Radiotherapy of squamous cell carcinoma of the nasal vestibule. *Int J Radiat Oncol Biol Phys* 2004;59:1319–1325.

43. Dirix P, Vanstraelen B, Jorissen M, et al. Intensity-modulated radiotherapy for sinonasal cancer: improved outcome compared to conventional radiotherapy. *Int J Radiat Oncol Biol Phys* 2010;78:998–1004.

44. Greenwalt JC, Dagan R, Bryant CM, Morris CG. Proton therapy for sinonasal mucosal melanoma. *Int J Radiat Oncol Biol Phys* 2015;93(3S):E 293, Abstr 2729.

45. Hoppe BS, Stegman LD, Zelefsky MJ, et al. Treatment of nasal cavity and paranasal sinus cancer with modern radiotherapy techniques in the postoperative setting—the MSKCC experienced. *Int J Radiat Oncol Biol Phys* 2007;67:691–702.

46. Jeong Y, Lee J, Kwak I. A dosimetric comparison of volumetric modulated arc therapy (VMAT) and non-coplanar intensity modulated radiation therapy (IMRT) for nasal cavity and paranasal sinus cancer. *Int J Radiat Oncol Biol Phys* 2014;90(1S):S865, Abstr 3664.

47. Frank SJ, Cox JD, Gillin M, et al. Multi-field optimization intensity modulated proton thearpy for head and neck tumors: a translation to practice. *Int J Radiat Oncol Biol Phys* 2014; 89(4):846–853.

48. Paulino AC, Marks JE, Bricker P, et al. Results of treatment of patients with maxillary sinus carcinoma. *Cancer* 1998;83:457–465.

49. Dulguerov P, Jacobsen MS, Allal AS. Nasal and paranasal sinus carcinoma: are we making progress? *Cancer* 2001;92:3012–3029.

50. Chen AM, Daly ME, Bucci MK, et al. Carcinomas of the paranasal sinuses and nasal cavity treated with radiotherapy at a single institution over five decades: are we making improvement? *Int J Radiat Oncol Biol Phys* 2007;69:141–147.

51. Agger A, von Buchwald C, Madsen AR, et al. Squamous cell carcinoma of the nasal vestibule 1993–2002: a nationwide retrospective study from DAHANCA. *Head Neck* 2009;31:1593–1599.

52. Chobe R, McNeese M, Weber R, et al. Radiation therapy for carcinoma of the nasal vestibule. *Otolaryngol Head Neck Surg* 1988;98:67–71.

53. Dowley A, Hoskison E, Allibone R, et al. Squamous cell carcinoma of the nasal vestibule: a 20-year case series and literature review. *J Laryngol Otol* 2008;122:1019–1023.

54. Levendag PC, Pomp J. Radiation therapy of squamous cell carcinoma of the nasal vestibule. *Int J RadiatOncolBiol Phys* 1990;19:1363–1367.

55. Levendag PC, Nijdam WM, van Moolenbourgh SE, et al. Interstitial radiation therapy for early stage nasal vestibule cancer: a continuing quest for optimal tumor control and cosmesis. *Int J Radiat Oncol Biol Phys* 2006;66:160–169.

56. Mak AC, Van Andel JG, van Woerkom-Eijkenboom WM. Radiation therapy of the carcinoma of the nasal vestibule. *Eur J Cancer* 1980;16:81–85.

57. Mendenhall WM, Stringer SP, Cassisi NJ, et al. Squamous cell carcinoma of the nasal vestibule. *Head Neck* 1999;21:385–393.

58. Poulsen M, Turner S. Radiation therapy for squamous cell carcinoma of the nasal vestibule. *Int J RadiatOncolBiol Phys* 1993;27:267–272.

59. Wallace A, Morris CG, Kirwan J, et al. Radiotherapy for squamous cell carcinoma of the nasal vestibule. *Am J Clin Oncol* 2007;30:612–616.

60. Lipman D, Verhoef LC, Takes RP, et al. Outcome and toxicity profile after brachytherapy for squamous cell carcinoma of the nasal vestibule. *Head and Neck* 2015; 37(9):1297–1303.

61. Hawkins RB, Wynstra JH, Pilepich MV, et al. Carcinoma of the nasal cavity results in primary and adjuvant radiotherapy. *Int J RadiatOncolBiol Phys* 1988;15:1129–1133.

62. Bhattacharyya N. Cancer of the nasal cavity: survival and factors influencing prognosis. *Arch Otolaryngol Head Neck Surg* 2002;128:1079–1083.

63. Rosenthal DI, Barker JLJ, El-Naggar AK, et al. Sinonasal malignancies with neuroendocrine differentiation. *Cancer* 2004;101:2567–2573.

64. Dulguerov P, Calcaterra T. Esthesioneuroblastoma: the UCLA experience 1970-1990. *The Laryngoscope* 1992;102(8):843–849.

65. Foote RL, Morita A, Ebersold MJ, et al. Esthesioneuroblastoma: the role of adjuvant radiation therapy. *Int J RadiatOncolBiol Phys* 1993;27:835–842.

66. Eden BV, Debo RF, Larner JM, et al. Esthesioneuroblastoma. Long-term outcome and patterns of failure—the University of Virginia experience. *Cancer* 1994;73:255–2562.

67. Loy AH, Reibel JF, Read PW, et al. Esthesioneuroblastoma: continued follow-up of a single institution's experience. *Arch Otolaryngol* 2006;132:134–138.

68. Dias FL, Sa GM, Lima RA Patterns of failure and outcomes in esthesioneuroblastoma. *Arch Otolaryngol* 2003;129:1186–1192.

69. Madani I, Bonte K, Vakaet L, Boterberg T, De Neve W. Intensity-modulated radiotherapy for sinonasal tumors: Ghent university hospital update. *Int J Radiat Oncol Biol Phys* 2009;73:424–432.

70. Sharrett JM, Jiang W, Mohamed ASR, et al. Multimodality management of patients with esthesioneuroblastoma. *Int J Radiat Oncol Bio Phys* 2015;93:E349.

71. Modesto A, Blanchard P, Tao Y, Rives M, et al Esthesioneuroblastomas: bicentric review of clinical features, multimodal treatment, and long-term outcome. *Int J Radiat Oncol Biol Phys* 2012;84:S498–S499.

72. Nakamura N, Zenda S, Tahara M, et al. Proton beam therapy for olfactory neuroblastoma. *Radiother Oncol* 2017; 122(3)368–372.

73. Dagan R, Bryant CM, Mendenhall WM. Improving local control for unresectable/incompletely resected sinonasal cancer with hyperfractionated proton therapy and concurrent chemotherapy. *Int J Radiat Oncol Biol Phys* 2016;94(4):951, Abstr 305.

74. Akimoto T, Zenda S, Nakamura N, et al. A retrospective multi-institutional study of proton beam therapy for head and neck cancer with non-squamous cell histologies. *Int J RadiatOncol Biol Phys* 2016;96:E337.

75. Lavertu P, Roberts JK, Kraus DH, et al. Squamous cell carcinoma of the paranasal sinuses: the Cleveland Clinic experience 1977–1986. *Laryngoscope* 1989;99:1130–1136.

76. Spiro JD, Soo KC, Spiro RH. Squamous carcinoma of the nasal cavity and paranasal sinuses. *Am J Surg* 1989;158:328–332.

77. Zaharia M, Salem LE, Travezan R, et al. Postoperative radiotherapy in the management of cancer of the maxillary sinus. *Int J Radiat Oncol Biol Phys* 1989;17:967–971.

78. Le QT, Fu KK, Kaplan M, et al. Treatment of maxillary sinus carcinoma: a comparison of the 1997 and 1977 American Joint Committee on cancer staging systems. *Cancer* 1999;86:1700–1711.

79. Myers LL, Nussenbaum B, Bradford CR, et al. Paranasal sinus malignancies: an 18-year single institution experience. *Laryngoscope* 2002;112:1964–1969.

80. Katz TS, Mendenhall WM, Morris GC, et al. Malignant tumors of the nasal cavity and paranasal sinuses. *Head Neck* 2002;24:821–829.

81. Blanco AI, Chao KSC, Ozyigit G, et al. Carcinoma of paranasal sinuses: long-term outcomes with radiotherapy. *Int J Radiat Oncol Biol Phys* 2004;59:51–58.

82. Bristol IJ, Ahamad A, Garden AS, et al. Postoperative radiotherapy for maxillary sinus cancer: long-term outcomes and toxicities of treatment. *Int J Radiat Oncol Biol Phys* 2007;68:719–730.

83. Choussy O, Ferron C, Vedrine P, et al. Adenocarcinoma of ethmoid: a GETTEC retrospective multicenter of 418 cases. *Laryngoscope* 2008;118:437–443.

84. Duthoy W, Boterberg T, Claus F, et al. Postoperative intensity-modulated radiotherapy in sinonasal carcinoma. *Cancer* 2005;104:71–82.

85. Daly ME, Chen AM, Bucci MK, et al. Intensity-modulated radiation therapy for malignancies of the nasal cavity and paranasal sinuses. *Int J Radiat Oncol Biol Phys* 2007;67:151–157.

86. Hoppe BS, Wolden SL, Zelefsky MJ, et al. Postoperative intensity-modulated radiation therapy for cancers of the paranasal sinuses, nasal cavity, and lacrimal glands: technique, early outcomes, and toxicity. *Head Neck* 2008;30:925–932.

87. Combs SE, Konkel S, Schultz-Ertner D, et al. Intensity-modulated radiotherapy (IMRT) in patients with carcinomas of the paranasal sinuses: clinical benefit for complex shaped target volumes. *Radiat Oncol* 2006;1:23.

88. Resto VA, Chan AW, Deschler DG, et al.. Extent of surgery in the management of locally advanced sinonasal malignancies. *Head and Neck* 2008;30(2):222–229.

89. Russo AL, Adams JA, Weyman EA, et al. Long-term outcomes after proton beam therapy for sinonasal squamous cell carcinoma. *Int J Radiat Oncol Biol Phys* 2016; 95(1):368–376.

90. Zenda S, Kawashima M, Arahira S, et al. Late toxicity of proton beam therapy for patients with the nasal cavity, para-nasal sinuses, or involving the skull base malignancy: importance of long-term follow-up. *Int J of Clinical Oncol* 2015; 20(3):447–454.

91. Linton OR, Moore MG, Brigance JS, et al. Proton therapy for head and neck adenoid cystic carcinoma: Initial clinical outcomes. *Head and Neck* 2014; 37(1):117–124.

92. Takagi M, Demizu Y, Hashimoto N. Treatment outcomes of particle radiotherapy using protons or carbon ions as a single-modality therapy for adenoid cystic carcinoma of the head and neck. *Radiotherapy and Oncology* 2014; 113:364–370.

93. Dagan R, Bryant C, Li Z, et al. Outcomes of sinonasal cancer treated with proton therapy. *Int J Radiat Oncol Biol Phys* 2016;95:377–385.

94. Truong MT, Kamat UR, Liebsch NJ, et al. Proton radiation therapy for primary sphenoid Sinus malignancies:treatment outcome and prognostic factors. *Head and Neck* 2009;31(10):1297–1308.

95. Patel SH, Wang Z, Wong WW, et al. Charged particle therapy versus photon therapy for paranasal sinus and nasal cavity malignant diseases: a systemic review and meta-analysis. *The Lancet Oncology* 2014;15(4):1027–1038.

96. Holliday E, Bhattasali O, Kies MS, et al. Post-operative Intensity-Modulated Proton Therapy for Head and Neck Adenoid Cystic Carcinoma. *Int J of Particle Therapy* 2016; 2(4):533–543.

97. Parsons JT, Bova FJ, Fitzgerald CR, et al. Radiation retinopathy after external-beam irradiation: analysis of time-dose factors. Int J *RadiatOncolBiol Phys* 1994;30:765–773.

98. Parsons JT, Bova FJ, Fitzgerald CR, et al. Severe dry-eye syndrome following external beam irradiation. *Int J RadiatOncolBiol Phys* 1994;30:775–780.

99. Takeda A, Shigematsu N, Suzuki S, et al. Late retinal complications of radiation therapy for nasal and paranasal malignancies: relationship between irradiated-dose area and severity. *Int J RadiatOncolBiol Phys* 1999;44(3):599–605.

100. Monroe AT, Bhandare N, Morris CG, et al. Preventing radiation retinopathy with hyperfractionation. *Int J RadiatOncolBiol Phys* 2005;61:856–864.

101. Bhandare N, Monroe AT, Morris CG, et al. Does altered fractionation influence the risk of radiation-induced optic neuropathy? *Int J RadiatOncolBiol Phys* 2005;62:1070–1077.

102. Monroe AT, Bhandare N, Morris CG, et al. Preventing radiation retinopathy with hyperfractionation. *Int J Radiat Oncol Biol Phys* 2005;61:856–864.

103. Bhandare N, Monroe AT, Morris CG, et al. Does altered fractionation influence the risk of radiation-induced optic neuropathy? *Int J Radiat Oncol Biol Phys* 2005;62:1070–1077.

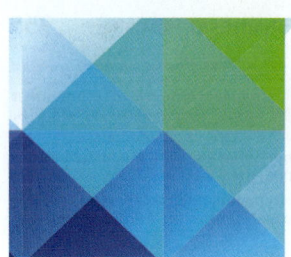

CHAPTER 46

Salivary Glands

Chris H. J. Terhaard

The salivary glands consist of the three large, paired major glands—parotid, submandibular, and sublingual (Fig. 46.1)—and many smaller, minor glands located throughout the upper aerodigestive tract. Salivary gland malignancies make up only approximately 0.4% of all cancers and account for <5% of the annual incidence of head and neck malignancies in the United States. The international variation in the incidence is between 0.4 and 2.6/100,000 per year, with a mean of approximately 1.2/100,000.[1] In the United States, the incidence of major salivary gland cancer increased from 1977 till 2009 from 1.0 to 1.6/100,000, mainly seen for the smaller tumors.[2]

ANATOMY

Major Salivary Glands

Parotid Gland

The parotid gland is located superficial to and partly behind the ramus of the mandible and covers the masseter muscle. Superficially, it overlaps the posterior part of the muscle and largely fills the space between the ramus of the mandible and the anterior border of the sternocleidomastoid muscle. One or more isthmi that wrap around the branches of the facial nerve connect the superficial and deep lobes of the gland. The nerve enters the deep surface of the gland as a single trunk, passing posterolateral to the styloid process. It usually leaves the gland as five or more branches, emerging at the anterior, upper, and lower borders of the gland. The facial nerve runs superficial to the main blood vessels that traverse the gland but is interwoven within the glandular tissue and its ducts. Thus, removal of all or part of the parotid gland demands meticulous dissection, if the nerve is to be spared.

The parotid gland contains an extensive lymphatic capillary plexus, many aggregates of lymphocytic cells, and numerous intraglandular lymph nodes in the superficial lobe. Lymphatics drain from more lateral areas on the face, including parts of the eyelids, diagonally downward and posterior toward the parotid gland, as do the lymphatics from the frontal region of the scalp. Associated with the gland, both superficially and more deeply, are parotid nodes. These drain downward along the retromandibular vein to empty in part into the superficial lymphatics and nodes along the outer surface of the sternocleidomastoid muscle and in part into upper nodes of the deep cervical chain. Lymphatics from the parietal region of the scalp drain partly to the parotid nodes in front of the ear and partly to the retroauricular nodes in back of the ear, which, in turn, drain into upper deep cervical nodes.[3]

Submandibular Gland

The submandibular gland largely fills the triangle between the two bellies of the digastric and the lower border of the mandible and extends upward deep to the mandible. It lies partly on the lower surface of the mylohyoid and partly behind the muscle against the lateral surface of the muscle of the tongue, the hypoglossus. The submandibular gland has a larger superficial part, or body, and a smaller deep process. The inferior surface is adjacent to the submandibular lymph nodes, and the deep process of the submandibular gland lies between the mylohyoid laterally and the hypoglossus medially and between the lingual nerve above and the hypoglossal nerve below.[4] Bimanual palpation with one finger in the floor of the mouth and one under the edge of the mandible facilitates clinical detection of masses in this gland.

FIGURE 46.1. Anatomy of salivary glands.

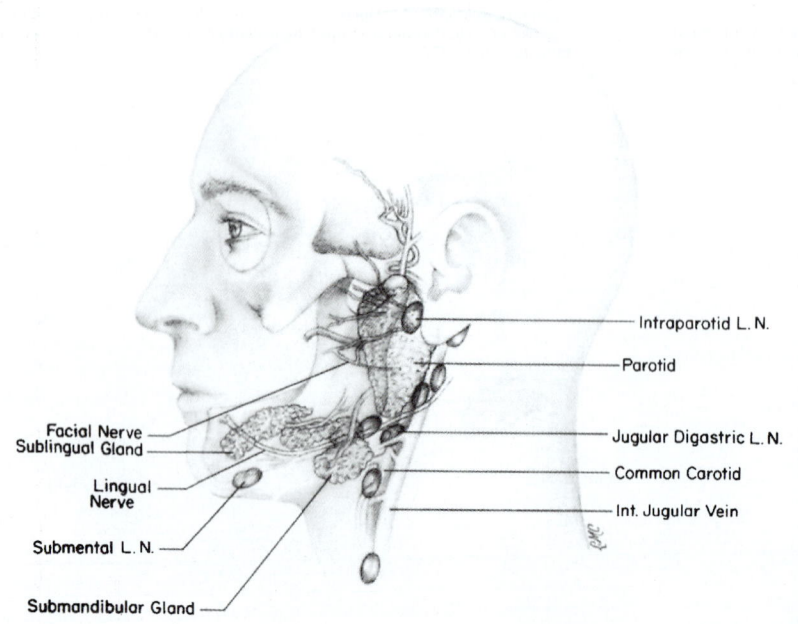

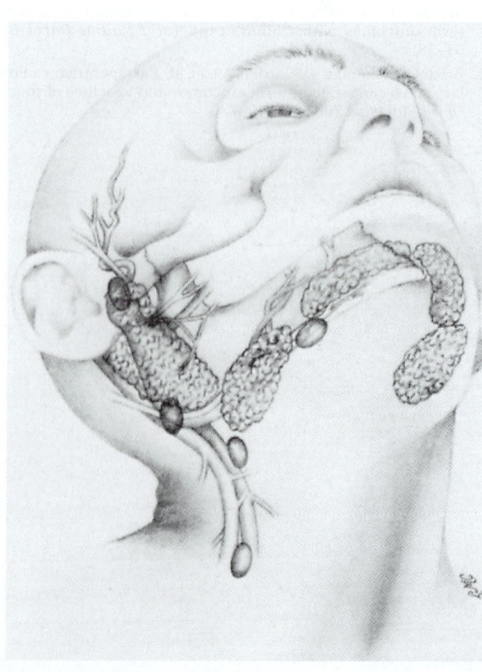

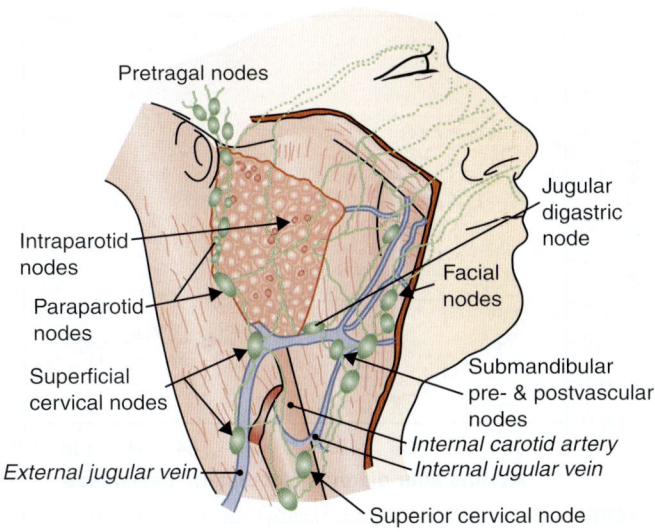

FIGURE 46.2. Lymph node distribution in and around the parotid gland.

A rich lymphatic capillary network lies in the interstitial spaces of the gland (Fig. 46.2). From the lateral and superior portions of the gland, lymph flows to the prevascular or preglandular submandibular lymph nodes. The posterior portion of the gland gives rise to one or two lymphatic trunks, which follow the facial artery and go directly to the anterior subdigastric nodes of the internal jugular chain.[5] The nodes overlying the submandibular gland, followed by the subdigastric and high midjugular lymph nodes, are those involved in nodal metastases.

Sublingual Gland

This smallest of the three major salivary glands, along with many minor salivary glands, lies between the mucous membrane of the floor of the mouth above and the mylohyoid muscle below, the mandible laterally, and the genioglossus muscles of the tongue medially. This is a rare site for malignant neoplasms; they are difficult to distinguish from cancer of the floor of the mouth accounting for fewer than 2% of all reported cases of salivary gland tumors.[1,6] The sublingual gland drains either to the submandibular lymph nodes or more posterior into the deep internal jugular chain between the digastric and omohyoid muscles. Rarely, the lymphatics of the sublingual gland drain into a submental node or supraomohyoid jugular node.

Minor Salivary Glands

Minor salivary glands are widely distributed in the upper aerodigestive tract, palate, buccal mucosa, base of tongue, pharynx, trachea, cheek, lip, gingiva, and floor of mouth, tonsil, paranasal sinuses, nasal cavity, and nasopharynx.

EPIDEMIOLOGY

Seventy percent of all salivary tumors arise in the parotid gland, 8% in the submandibular gland, and 22% in the minor salivary glands.[6] The proportion of malignant tumors increases from parotid (25%) to submandibular (43%) to minor salivary glands (65%).[6,7] There is a preponderance of benign tumors in women; malignant tumors exhibit an equal sex distribution.[1] Patients with benign tumors are younger (mean age, 46 years) compared with those with malignant tumors (mean age, 54 years), with a trend to an older age for submandibular and minor salivary gland locations.[6] Two to three percent of salivary neoplasms occur in children, in whom half of the tumors are malignant.[8] Two-thirds of the cancers are located in the

major salivary glands (parotid gland 53%, submandibular gland 12%, sublingual 1.5%), and one-third in the minor salivary glands, predominantly in the oral cavity.[1] The tumors in children are mostly less advanced, and a 95% 5-year survival is reached.[8]

Etiologic factors are not clearly defined. Nutrition may be a factor because Eskimos in the Arctic, who have low intake of vitamins A and C, have a high incidence. Cigarette smoking and alcohol consumption is in general not related with salivary gland cancer,[9] despite for Warthin tumors. In a study of de Ru et al.,[10] patients with a Warthin tumor had a smoking history in 97%; their mean age at the time of operation was 11 years higher compared to the pleomorphic adenoma group. Irradiation can also be a cause, as evidenced by the increased incidence in survivors of the atomic bombs dropped on Hiroshima and Nagasaki.[11] Saku et al.[11] studied salivary gland tumors in atomic bomb survivors of Hiroshima and Nagasaki. Two-thirds of all cases were parotid, and the remainder was equally distributed between submandibular and minor salivary glands. Mucoepidermoid cancer and Warthin tumor (benign) were particularly elevated compared with nonexposed persons and disproportionately high at high radiation doses. The incidence of subsequent salivary gland cancer after radiation in childhood is increased compared to the general population.[12] There is a dose–response relationship with an excess relative risk of 0.27 to 0.36 per Gy.[13] The majority of these tumors are mucoepidermoid cancers[12]; however, <1% of salivary gland tumors may be caused by former irradiation.[14]

Workers in various occupations experience an increased risk of salivary gland cancer.[15] For women employed as hairdressers or working in beauty shops, a significant elevated risk was observed in a study by Swanson and Burns.[16]

Women with salivary gland cancer may have a 2.5 elevated breast cancer risk.[17] After treatment for salivary gland cancer, an increased risk for subsequent cancer of the oral cavity hazard ratio (HR 3.5) thyroid (HR 2.7), lung and kidney cancer (HR 1.7), and second salivary gland cancer (HR 10), especially after acinic cell cancer (HR 31) is seen. For adenoid cystic cancer, the risk of developing nasopharyngeal is increased with a factor 17.[18]

NATURAL HISTORY

Local invasion is the initial route of spread of malignant tumors of the salivary glands, depending on location and histologic type. For parotid tumors, this may result in fixation to structures in around 20% of cases.[19] Skin invasion is more often seen in parotid tumors (8% to 10%), compared with submandibular tumors (3%).[20,21]

Approximately 18% to 25% of patients with a malignant parotid salivary gland tumor present with facial palsy from cranial nerve invasion.[6,19,21,22]

A detailed study of the Dutch Head and Neck Oncology Group (NWHHT) concerning patients with a salivary gland malignancy found an overall incidence of clinically positive nodes of 14% and clinically occult, pathologically positive nodes in an additional 11% of patients.[20] This percentage depends on the number of neck dissections performed, the tumor location, histology, and T-stage. The number of elective neck dissections performed varies between the tumor locations. Stennert et al.[23] performed a neck dissection in all malignant *parotid* tumors and found 53% unilateral positive nodes and 0% contralateral nodes. In selected patients in other studies, the percentage positive nodes varied between 20%[24] and 38%.[25] In the large National Cancer Database in 24% of 22.653 parotid cases positive nodes and in 10% occult nodes were found.[26] Three out of four involved lymph nodes in early parotid malignancies (21% occult nodes) were localized in intraparotideal nodes by Stenner et al.[27] Resection of *submandibular* tumors is combined with a (partial) neck dissection in most cases. Pathologic neck nodes may be seen in up to 42% of cases.[25] The risk of positive lymph nodes in *minor salivary gland* cancer is depending on four prognostic factors: male gender, T3-T4, pharyngeal site, and histology (high-grade mucoepidermoid and high-grade adenocarcinoma). Based on these factors, a scoring system from 0 to 4 was developed by Lloyd et al.[28] The risk of positive nodes in minor salivary gland cancer is less than 10% for score 0 to 1, 17% for score 2, 41% for score 3, and 70% for score 4. Salivary gland tumors arising in the oral cavity produce an incidence of cervical node metastases of <10%.[7,25,29,30] In nasopharyngeal salivary gland tumors, a risk around 20% has been shown.[30] In general, the risk of positive findings in the neck including *all salivary gland malignancies* may be based on a combination of T-stage, tumor localization, and histology. The highest risk is seen for squamous cell, undifferentiated cancer, and salivary duct cancer.[25,31] There is an intermediate risk for mucoepidermoid cancer and a low risk for acinic cell, adenoid cystic carcinoma, and carcinoma ex pleomorphic adenoma.[25] A 15% risk is found for T1 tumors, 26% for T2, and 33% for T3-T4.[25] An example of a rating scale to estimate the risk of positive neck nodes, based on tumor location, T-stage, and histologic type, is shown in Table 46.1.

Distant metastases overall are encountered in 3% to 4% of patients at presentation and in 33% after 10 years.[20,22] They are fairly common with adenoid cystic, salivary duct, squamous cell, and undifferentiated carcinomas; in the case of adenoid cystic carcinomas, they may occur quite late in the course of the disease, without recurrence of the primary tumor.[20,32,33] Distant metastases are primarily to lung, bone, and occasionally to the liver.[20] Reported incidence of distant metastases in patients with adenoid cystic carcinoma after 10 years of follow-up is around 40%.[20,33,34] Five years after diagnosis of distant metastases of adenoid cystic carcinoma and acinic cell cancer, more than one-third of the patients are still alive; 10% are alive after 10 years. An update of the survival data of the NWHHT study after diagnosis of distant metastases of salivary gland cancer is shown in Figure 46.3.

CLINICAL PRESENTATION

Three of four parotid masses are benign.[6] Patients most often have a painless, rapidly enlarging mass, often present for years before a sudden change in its indolent growth pattern prompts the patient to seek medical attention. Duration of clinical symptoms before diagnosis may last more than 10 years.[6,20] For malignant tumors, the median duration of clinical symptoms generally is shorter (3 to 6 months)[20,37] compared to that of benign tumors, although for some minor salivary gland tumors, median periods of 2 years have been reported.[29]

Pain is more frequently associated with malignant disease.[6] Although as many as one-third of parotid cancers may have facial nerve involvement, only 10% to 20% of patients

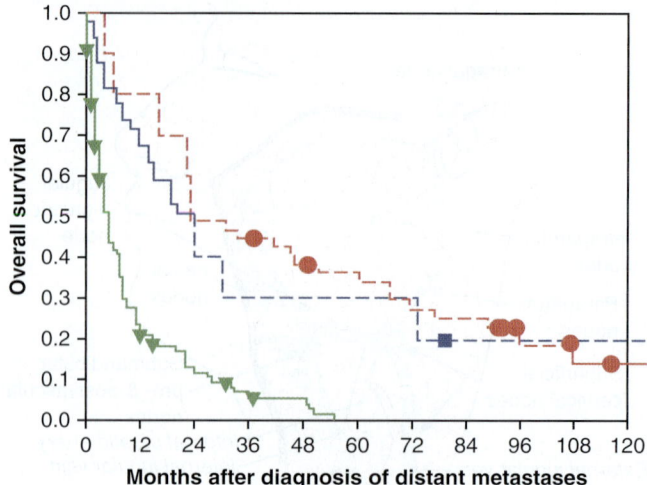

FIGURE 46.3. Survival after diagnosis of distant metastases depending on histology, update of the nationwide Dutch study. (●) adenoid cystic carcinoma[35]; (■) acinic cell carcinoma[11]; (▲) others[36]; *P* < .001. (From Terhaard CHJ, Lubsen H, Van der Tweel, et al. Salivary gland carcinoma: Independent prognostic factors for locoregional control, distant metastases, and overall survival: results of the Dutch Head and Neck Oncology Cooperative Group. *Head Neck* 2004;26[8]:681–693. Copyright © 2004 Wiley Periodicals, Inc. Reprinted by permission of John Wiley & Sons, Inc.)

complain of pain.[6,19,20] Pain may appear with involvement of deeper structures (masseter, temporal, and pterygoid muscles). Rarely, tumors of the parotid may involve the base of skull and cause intractable pain and paralysis of various cranial nerves. Asymptomatic swelling of the floor of mouth is the primary presentation in sublingual salivary gland cancer, with pain and tongue numbness as symptoms of advanced disease.[38]

The signs and symptoms associated with tumors of the minor salivary glands vary because of their diverse locations. The distribution of presenting sites and risk of malignancy for 380 cases of intraoral minor salivary gland tumors is shown in Table 46.2.[39] A painless lump is the most common presenting symptom. Almost all extraoral minor salivary gland tumors are malignant.[6] Extraoral minor salivary gland tumors are most frequently seen in the nasal cavity (52%), followed by the larynx (18%), the oropharynx (14%, mostly localized in the tonsil), nasopharynx (8%), and ethmoid (8%).[6] For tumors arising in the nasal cavity or sinuses, facial pain is the most common presenting symptom, followed by nasal obstruction. Laryngeal primary tumors most frequently cause hoarseness or voice change.

Clinical features suggesting a malignant salivary gland tumor are rapid growth rate, pain, facial nerve palsy, childhood occurrence, skin involvement, and cervical adenopathy.

TABLE 46.1 RISK ESTIMATION (%) FOR POSITIVE NECK NODES

Summation: T Score + Histologic Type Score	Parotid Gland	Submandibular Gland	Oral Cavity	Other Locations
2	4	0	4	0
3	12	33	13	29
4	25	57	19	56
5	33	60	–	–
6	38	50	–	–

T1 = 1; T2 = 2; T3-T4 = 3; acinic/adenoid cystic/carcinoma ex pleomorphic adenoma = 1; mucoepidermoid = 2; squamous/undifferentiated = 3.
Reprinted from Terhaard C, Lubsen H, Rasch C, et al. The role of radiotherapy in the treatment of malignant salivary gland tumors. *Int J Radiat Oncol Biol Phys* 2005;61(1):103–111. Copyright © 2005 Elsevier. With permission.

TABLE 46.2 DISTRIBUTION OF PRESENTING SITES OF INTRAORAL MINOR SALVARY GLAND TUMORS

Site	No. of Patients (%)	Percentage Malignant
Palate	206 (54)	43
Upper lip	64 (17)	9
Buccal mucosa	54 (14)	37
Retromolar region	20 (5)	95
Lower lip	18 (5)	56
Floor of mouth	13 (3)	69
Tongue	5 (1)	60
Total	380	41

Adapted from Buchner A, Merrell P, Carpenter W. Relative frequency of intra-oral minor salivary gland tumors: a study of 380 cases from northern California and comparison to reports from other parts of the world. *J Oral Pathol Med* 2007;36:207–214. Copyright © 2007 Blackwell Munksgaard. Reprinted by permission of John Wiley & Sons, Inc.

DIAGNOSTIC WORKUP AND STAGING

Major Salivary Glands

The diagnostic workup of major salivary gland tumors includes a careful history and physical examination, with particular attention to signs of local fixation or regional adenopathy.

For superficial lesions of the parotid gland, the submandibular gland, and sublingual gland and evaluation of the cervical lymph nodes, ultrasound (US) is the first diagnostic step, combined with fine needle aspiration cytology (FNAC). In US, signs of malignancy are ill-defined borders with heterogonous architecture, internal necrosis, and cystic changes.[40] Benign salivary tumors are well defined and hypoechoic. FNAC is very useful to differentiate between yes or no neoplastic lesions with a specificity of more than 95%. In a systematic review, Colella et al. found, for patients with a histologic diagnosis of a malignant tumor, benign tumor, or nonneoplastic lesion, concordant cytology in 80%, in 96%, and in 94%, respectively.[41] False-negative findings may be seen as a result of lack of representative material or a cyst. The next imaging tool in salivary gland tumors suspected for malignancy is magnetic resonance imaging (MRI). MRI is superior to CT, especially when malignancy is suspected, based on the excellent soft tissue contrast (Fig. 46.4). T1-weighted (W) images are excellent to assess the margins, extension into the deep tissues, and patterns of infiltration because the (fatty) background of the gland is hyperintensive. With T1-W gadolinium series, tumor infiltration and heterogeneous enhancement may be visualized, as seen in high-grade tumors.[40] With fat-suppressed T2-W images, the fluid content of a tumor is visualized. In general, benign tumors are hyperintensive, and malignant tumors show intermediate or low intensity at T2-W MR images. A low apparent diffusion coefficient (ADC), derived from diffusion-weighted MRI, using high *b*-values, is associated with malignancy.[42] However, Warthin tumors (benign) may also show low ADC values.[43] Perineural invasion of adenoid cystic carcinoma may be evaluated with both CT (foraminal enlargement) and MRI (thickened nerve with enhancement at the fat-suppressed T1-weighted images).[40] The tumor extension along the facial nerve (VII) (foramen styloideum), the cranial nerve V-3 (foramen ovale) or nerve V-2 (foramen rotundum) as seen in tumors of the deep parotid lobe, may be visualized by T1-weighted images.[42] This is of special importance for the delineation of these nerves in case of postoperative radiotherapy for extensive perineural invasion; see Figure 46.5 for the trigeminal and facial nerves. Cortical involvement will be best evaluated by CT.

Fluorodeoxyglucose (FDG) uptake in salivary glands is quite unpredictable, resulting in a low sensitivity of FDG-PET for the diagnosis of malignancy in salivary glands.[44]

The 8th edition of the manual of the American Joint Committee on Cancer and the 8th edition of the classification system of the International Union Against Cancer are identical for major salivary glands[45] (Table 46.3). They are based on size, tumor extension, nodal size, and location, and, different from the 7th edition, extranodal extension. Relative survival rates for major salivary gland cancer according to stage are shown in Figure 46.6.

Minor Salivary Glands

Various radiographic studies may be used, including plain films, to ascertain bone erosion in advanced lesions. CT and MRI scans may be used to evaluate depth, contiguous involvement, and the retropharyngeal nodes. US and FNAC may be used to examine the neck nodes. The definitive diagnostic procedure is an excisional biopsy, particularly if malignancy is clinically expected. Unplanned incisional biopsies should be avoided, and fine needle biopsies are impractical because of the polymorphism of most malignant salivary gland tumors.

A formal staging system has not been developed for minor gland tumors. The same staging system for minor salivary glands as for squamous cell carcinoma in sites other than the parotid or submandibular glands may be used.[45]

PATHOLOGIC CLASSIFICATION

Salivary glands are composed of acinar–ductal units with acinar cells on the inside of the acinic and ductal epithelial cells on the inside of the striated and excretory ducts. Myoepithelial cells are located in the outside of acini and intercalated and striated ducts. Basal (reserve) cells are found on the outside of the excretory ducts.[46] Carcinomas may arise from all these cell types, separately or combined. The histologic classification of these salivary gland tumors is very demanding for the head

FIGURE 46.4. A patient with acinic cell cancer of the left parotid gland. **A:** Axial contrast-enhanced computed tomography image. **B:** T1-weighted magnetic resonance image. Both images show an infiltrating soft tissue mass involving the deep and superficial lobe. The tumor has widened the left stylomandibular tunnel, with infiltration in the pterygoid musculature. The left internal carotid artery is displaced medially. (Courtesy of Dr. F.A. Pameyer, radiologist, University Medical Center Utrecht.)

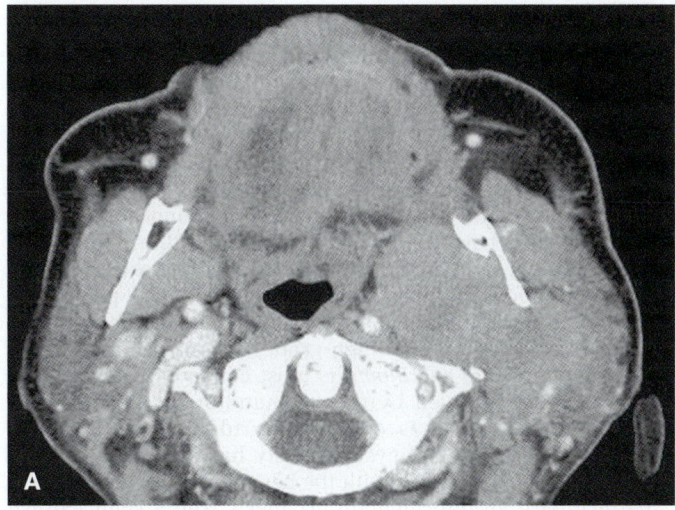
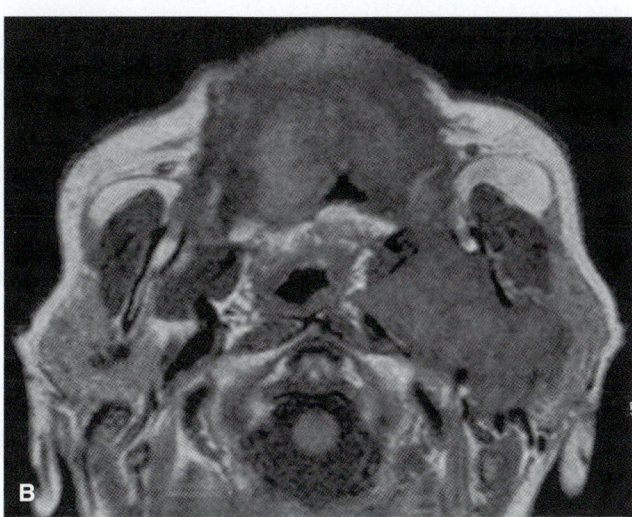

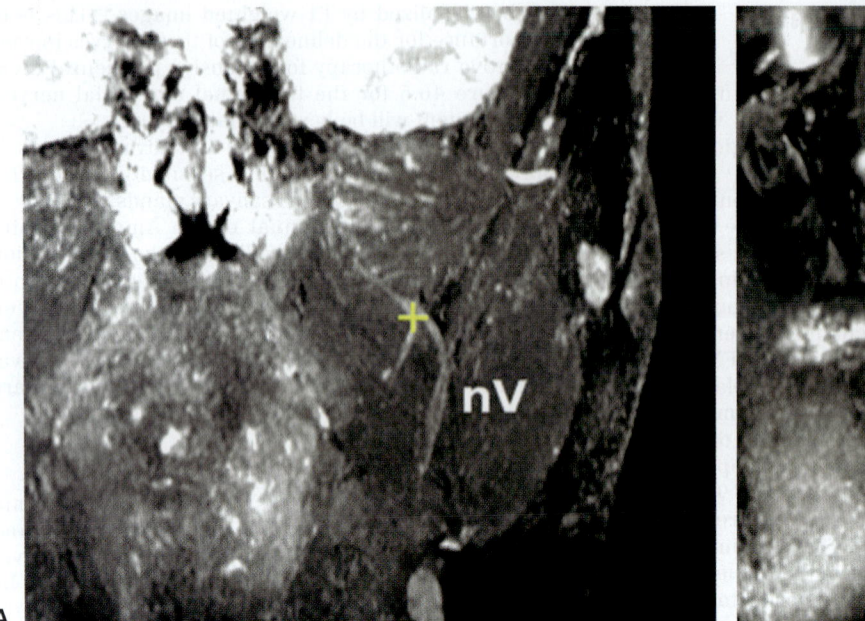
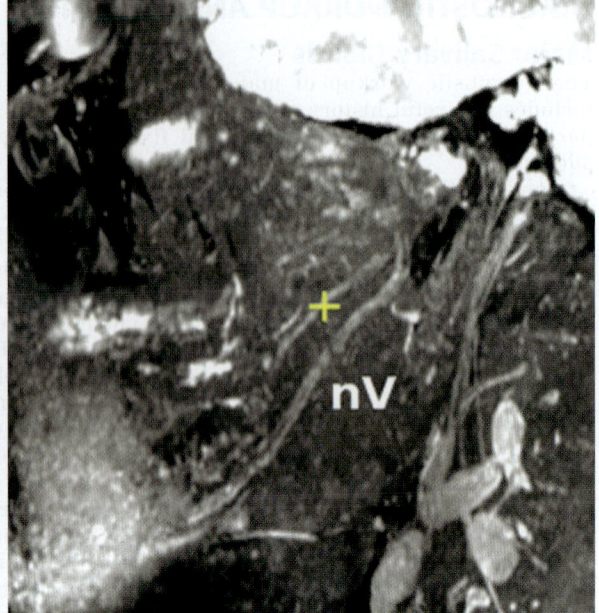
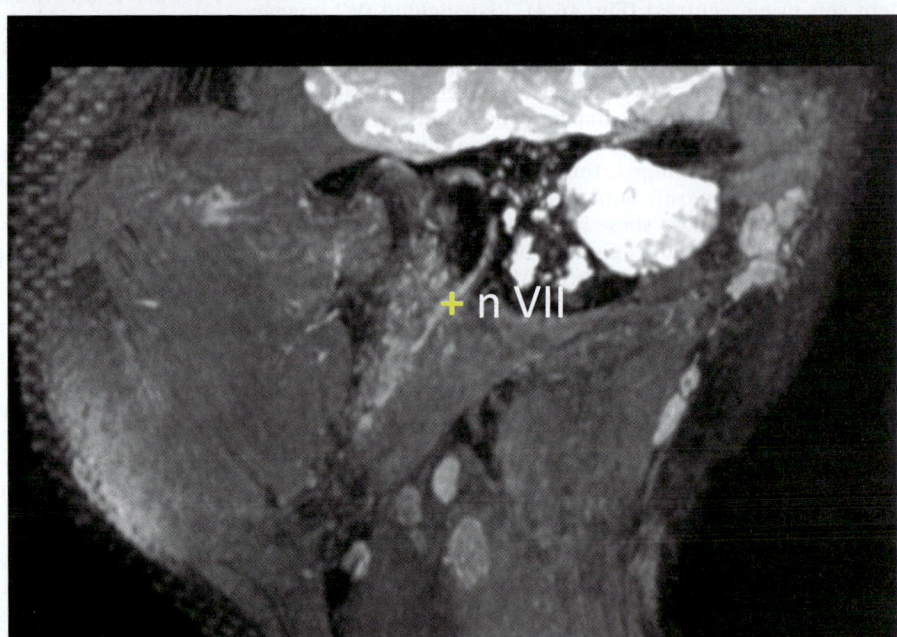

FIGURE 46.5. Three-dimensional magnetic resonance imaging, T2-FFE with binomial RF pulses for water-selective excitation: **(A)** nerve V (nV), **(B)** nerve VII (nVII).

and neck pathologist. In 1991, the World Health Organization classification for salivary gland tumors of 1972 was expanded from 7 to 20 subtypes. Various types of carcinomas were distinguished based on precise histologic definitions, prognosis, and treatment, discussed more in detail by Seifert and Sobin.[47] In 2005, the WHO classification of malignant salivary gland tumors was extended. Again, 24 subtypes were specified[46] (Table 46.4). Classification may be difficult, as shown in a reevaluation of 101 intraoral salivary gland tumors by experienced pathologists; major disagreement was seen in 8 and there was minor disagreement in 33.[48]

Most salivary gland subtypes are very rare. The percentage of the histologic subtypes varies from series to series and from the localization of the tumor (Fig. 46.7). In 666 patients with a salivary gland carcinoma in a study performed in the Netherlands, for which the pathology was revised, adenoid cystic carcinoma was most frequently diagnosed (27%), followed by mucoepidermoid carcinoma (16%), acinic cell carcinoma (14%), carcinoma ex pleomorphic adenoma (8%), undifferentiated carcinoma (7%), salivary duct carcinoma

(SDC) and adenocarcinoma NOS (both 6%), polymorph low-grade adenocarcinoma (PLGA) and squamous cell carcinoma (both 5%), and epithelial–myoepithelial carcinoma in 2%. In this large study, all other subtypes were rarely or not at all diagnosed.[20]

Salivary gland carcinomas may be graded as low and high malignant, particularly for mucoepidermoid tumors. However, there is a disparity for grading, even among experienced pathologists.[49] Low-grade mucoepidermoid, PLGA, epithelial–myoepithelial, and acinic cell carcinomas comprise a group of low-to-moderate malignancy; high-grade mucoepidermoid, malignant mixed, adenoid cystic, squamous, undifferentiated, and SDCs represent more high-grade malignancies.[49]

Adenoid cystic carcinoma is most common in minor salivary glands, followed by the submandibular gland.[7,20,35,50,51] Perineural invasion is common in adenoid cystic carcinoma.[51–53] The adenoid cystic variety has a tubular pattern that has been associated with the best prognosis, a cribriform pattern with an intermediate prognosis, and a solid pattern with the worst prognosis.[54]

TABLE 46.3 UICC CANCER STAGING SYSTEM FOR MAJOR SALIVARY GLAND CANCER (PAROTID, SUBMANDIBULAR, SUBLINGUAL), 8TH EDITION

Primary Tumor (T)

T1	≤2 cm without extraparenchymal extension[a]
T2	>2–4 cm without extraparenchymal extension
T3	>4 cm and/or extraparenchymal extension[a]
T4a	Invasion skin and/or mandible and/or ear canal and/or facial nerve
T4b	Invasion skull base and/or pterygoid plates and/or carotid artery

Regional Lymph Nodes (N)

N0	No regional lymph node metastasis
N1	Ipsilateral single lymph node, ≤3 cm, without ENE
N2a	Single ipsilateral lymph node >3 cm but <6 cm, without ENE
N2b	Multiple ipsilateral lymph nodes, none >6 cm, without ENE
N2c	Bilateral or contralateral lymph nodes, none >6 cm, without ENE
N3a	Lymph node >6 cm, without ENE
N3b	Single or multiple nodes with ENE

Distant Metastases (M)

MX	Presence of distant metastasis cannot be assessed
M0	No distant metastasis
M1	Distant metastasis

Stage Grouping

I	T1	N0	M0
II	T2	N0	M0
III	T3	N0	M0
	T1, T2, T3	N1	M0
IVA	T1, T2, T3	N2	M0
	T4a	N0, N1, N2	M0
IVB	T4b	Any N	M0
	Any T	N3	M0
IVC	Any T	Any N	M1

ENE, extranodal extension.
From Brierley J, Gospodarowicz M, and Wittekind C. TNM Classification of Malignant Tumors. 8th ed. Hoboken, NJ: Wiley-Blackwell, 2017:47–50. Copyright © 2017 UICC. Reprinted by permission of John Wiley & Sons, Inc.

TABLE 46.4 WHO 2005 CLASSIFICATION OF TUMORS OF THE SALIVARY GLANDS

Malignant Epithelial Tumors	Benign Epithelial Tumors
Acinic cell carcinoma	Pleomorphic adenoma
Mucoepidermoid carcinoma	Myoepithelioma
Adenoid cystic carcinoma	Basal cell adenoma
Polymorphous low-grade adenocarcinoma	Warthin tumor
Epithelial–myoepithelial carcinoma	Oncocytoma
Clear cell carcinoma NOS	Canalicular adenoma
Basal cell adenocarcinoma	Sebaceous adenoma
Sebaceous carcinoma	Lymphadenoma
Sebaceous lymphadenocarcinoma	Sebaceous
Cystadenocarcinoma	Nonsebaceous
Low-grade cribriform cystadenocarcinoma	Ductal papilloma
Mucinous adenocarcinoma	Inverted ductal papilloma
Oncocytic carcinoma	Intraductal papilloma
Salivary duct carcinoma	Sialadenoma papilliferum
Adenocarcinoma NOS	Cystadenoma
Myoepithelial carcinoma	
Carcinoma ex pleomorphic adenoma	**Soft tissue tumors**
Carcinosarcoma	Hemangioma
Metastasizing pleomorphic adenoma	
Squamous cell carcinoma	**Hematolymphoid tumors**
Small cell carcinoma	Hodgkin lymphoma
Large cell carcinoma	Diffuse large B-cell lymphoma
Lymphoepithelial carcinoma	Extranodal marginal zone B-cell
Sialoblastoma	lymphoma

NOS, not otherwise specified.
From Leivo I. Insights into a complex group of neoplastic disease: advances in histopathologic classification and molecular pathology of salivary gland cancer. *Acta Oncol* 2006;45:662–668. Copyright © Acta Oncologica Foundation, reprinted by permission of Taylor & Francis Ltd, www.tandfonline.com on behalf of Acta Oncologica Foundation.

Section III

In parotid tumors in children and adults, the most common malignant subtype is the *mucoepidermoid* (MEC).[8,55–57] MEC contains squamous cells, mucus-producing cells, and cells of intermediate type. Several grading criteria and cell cycle–based Ki 67 proliferation index of MEC have been published.[46] *Acinic cell* cancer derives from cells of the terminal ducts and intercalated ducts. An extensive update of the literature is published by Vander Poorten et al.[58] Most tumors (86%) are located in the parotid gland.[58] Like in MEC, Ki 67 proliferation index is a prognostic factor for disease-free survival.[46] *Carcinoma ex pleomorphic adenoma* may be localized in all salivary glands, although the majority is found in the parotid gland. In the development of carcinoma ex pleomorphic

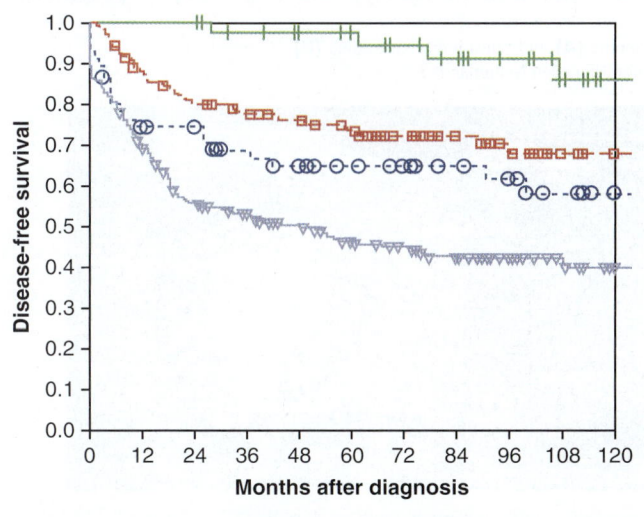

FIGURE 46.6. Disease-free survival for major salivary glands according to the 2002 classification of the American Joint Committee on Cancer. Results of the nationwide Dutch study: +, stage I; □, stage II; ○, stage III; ∇, stage IV.

adenoma, a progressive loss of heterozygosity of chromosome 8q, 12 G, and 17P is seen.[59] The prognosis is poor with a high risk of distant metastases.[20] *Undifferentiated and squamous cell carcinoma* are mainly localized in the parotid gland. The prevalence of comorbidity for patients with squamous cell carcinoma of the salivary gland is comparable to other head and neck cancers, whereas the prevalence of comorbidity in all other malignant salivary gland cancer subtypes is significantly less.[60] Also, patients with squamous cell carcinoma of the salivary glands are mostly older.[1] So squamous cell carcinoma of the salivary gland may be a different entity among salivary gland cancers. The PLGA, salivary duct, and epithelial myoepithelial carcinoma are the most common new subtypes of the World Health Organization 1991 classification. *PLGA* is a solid, ovoid, noncapsulated mass with a highly variable growth pattern (Fig. 46.8A). Most are located in the palate and are slowly growing tumors and 80% are stage I/II. The prognosis generally is good, with a tendency to local and seldom regional recurrences or distant metastases.[61] *Salivary duct carcinoma* resembles ductal breast cancer morphologically (Fig. 46.8B). They derive from excretory duct cells. They are usually located in the parotid gland and are highly aggressive.[62,63] They are frequently positive for androgen receptors and positive for HER2/neu protein.[63] However, the gene amplification is seen in <50% of the cases.[46] There is also a low-grade subtype, resembling breast atypical ductal hyperplasia and low-grade ductal carcinoma *in situ*. The prognosis is excellent.[64] *Epithelial–myoepithelial carcinoma* is mainly localized in the parotid gland. The tumors are composed of myoepithelial cells, surrounded by epithelial-lined ducts, resembling intercalated ducts. It is a low-grade tumor, and all 14 patients of the Dutch study remained disease free. However, local recurrences may be encountered.[65] *Myoepithelial carcinomas* have exclusive myoepithelial differentiation. They are commonly seen in the parotid gland and the palate. Differentiation with other salivary gland cancers may be difficult. The prognosis is poor with a 40% 5-year disease-free survival.[66] *Basal cell adenocarcinoma* is a low-grade tumor, predominantly seen in the parotid gland, with a high risk on local recurrence but a low risk on regional recurrences or distant metastases.[67] *Malignant*

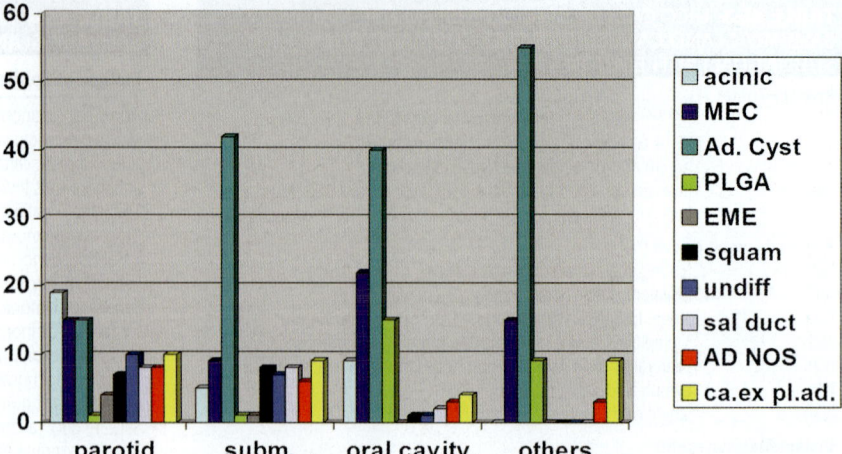

FIGURE 46.7. Distribution of various cell types (%) in series from the Dutch study, depending on site. Ad. Cyst, adenoid cystic; AD NOS, adenocarcinoma not otherwise specified; ca. ex pl. ad., carcinoma ex pleomorphic adenoma; EME, epithelial myoepithelial carcinoma; MEC, mucoepidermoid cancer; PLGA, polymorph low-grade adenocarcinoma; sal duct, salivary duct carcinoma; squam, squamous cell carcinoma; subm, submandibular. undiff, undifferentiated.

oncocytoma is a high-grade malignant tumor, characterized by oncocytes, with necrosis, perineural spread, vascular invasion, and a high risk on cervical lymph nodes.[68] Most tumors are found in the parotid or submandibular gland. Positive resection margins are a major source of poor overall survival.[68] *Salivary gland cystadenocarcinoma* is a low-grade tumor, predominantly localized in the parotid gland. It has an excellent prognosis.[69] *Mucinous adenocarcinoma* is a high-grade malignancy from the palate and floor of mouth, with a high risk for neck node and distant metastases.[70] Sebaceous carcinoma is mainly localized in the parotid gland and a slow-growing, low-grade tumor.[71] In 2017, four new entities were described by Skalova et al.[72] *Mammary analog secretory carcinoma*, mostly a low-grade tumor, in the past was mainly classified as acinic cell carcinoma. They have specific chromosomal translocations and molecular and immunohistochemical findings. Most cases are seen in the parotid gland and oral cavity. *Cribriform adenocarcinoma* mimics PLGA and is primarily seen in the tongue. It is a very rare tumor, with a high risk on positive cervical lymph nodes. *Sclerosing polycystic adenosis adenoma* involves the parotid gland and is, although benignant, associated with a high risk of local recurrence after surgery. Finally, a new myoepithelioma variant is the *mucinous (secretory) myoepithelioma*, with a benignant to low-grade malignant behavior. It is a very rare subtype mainly seen in the minor salivary glands.

So based on the high morphologic diversity of salivary gland carcinomas, the differential diagnosis is a challenging task for the pathologist. Molecular testing may serve as a powerful diagnostic tool.[73]

PROGNOSTIC FACTORS

A number of prognostic variables have been studied in the management of salivary gland cancer. In these studies, multivariate analyses have been performed considering locoregional control, distant metastases, and survival. Results of studies with sufficient number of patients and follow-up have been summarized in Table 46.5. Local control and overall survival is influenced by site, favoring tumors of the oral cavity.[20] T- and N-stages are independent variables for locoregional control, distant metastases, and survival, regardless of site.[7,20,33,55,56,74,75,78–81] As may concluded from Table 46.5 in almost all studies, histologic subtype is not an independent prognostic factor for locoregional control but plays a role in risk on distant metastases and overall survival.[20] The added prognostic value of cytology and/or histologic subtype in salivary carcinoma is limited, largely because of the combined prognostic value of other prognostic factors such as tumor size, N- and M-classification, and comorbidity.[82] Histologic subtypes may be divided into low- and high-grade tumors, although a bit subjective. Grading is associated with risk of recurrence and overall survival.[75,78] Comorbidity is associated with overall survival; however, it is not with disease-free survival.[60]

Oncogene expression has been evaluated in the search for additional prognostic factors. In a review, Stenman et al. discussed the diagnostics and therapeutic importance of new biologic markers for salivary gland cancer.[83] Overexpression of HER2/neu is related with aggressiveness, distant metastases, and poor survival in salivary gland cancer[84] especially in SDC.[85] It also has been similarly associated with poor prognosis in carcinomas of the breast, ovary, and endometrium. High Ki 67 nuclear antigen and p53 tumor suppressor expression may be related with poor prognosis. In a study of Finland, comparing both markers, only Ki 67 expression was an independent prognostic factor for overall survival.[86] Another molecular feature studied in relationship to prognosis was the DNA content in adenoid cystic carcinomas. DNA aneuploidy is correlated with the solid type and thus with poor prognosis.[54]

FIGURE 46.8. Examples of polymorphous low-grade adenocarcinoma **(A)** and salivary duct carcinoma **(B)**. (Courtesy of Prof. Dr. P. Slootweg, pathologist, Radboud University Medical Center, Nijmegen Netherlands.)

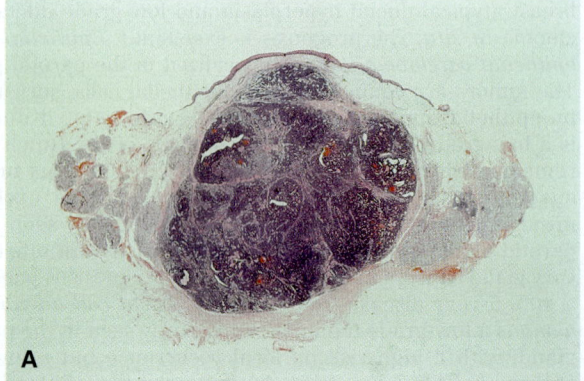
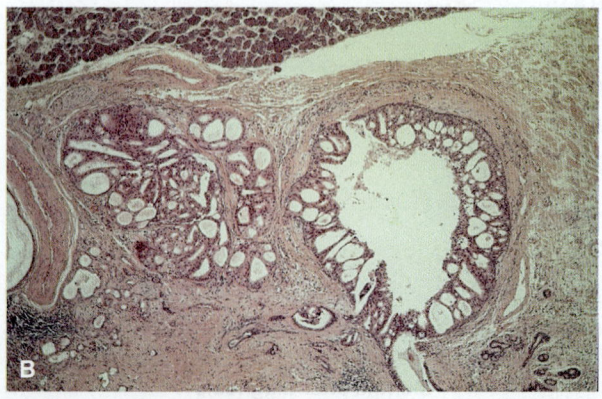

TABLE 46.5 PROGNOSTIC FACTORS FOR SALIVARY GLAND CANCER—SELECTION OF MULTIVARIATE ANALYZED STUDIES

Study (by Name of First Author)	No.	Locoregional Control	Distant Meta-Analyses	Survival
General				
Terhaard[20,60]	565	L: T, site, bone inv. R: N VII dysfunction, N L + R: Margin, therapy[a]	Gender, T, N, skin, histology, perineural inv.	OS: Gender, age, T, skin inv., bone inv., comorbidity
Holtzman[74]	291	L: T, therapy[b]	Stage	DFS + OS: Stage, clinical nerve invasion, therapy[a]
Bjorndal[75]	871	L + R: Stage, therapy[b]		
Chen, adenoid cystic[76]	140	L + R: Stage, margin, vasc. invasion, grade		OS: Age, latency, stage, margin, vasc. invasion
Chen, S alone[93]	207	L + R: T4, perineural inv., major nerve involvement, therapy[a] L + R: pN+, grade, margin, T3-T4		
Major				
Yun Li[78] (SEER)	4218			OS + DFS: Age, gender, grade, site (par > subm), T,N, therapy[a]
Parotid				
Spiro[57]	470			OS: Stage, age, histology, site
Bhattacharryya[55]	903			OS: Age, T, N, extraglandular extension
Van der Poorten[21]	237			DFS: Age, pain, T, N, perineural + skin inv., N VII dysfunction
Poulsen[77]	209	L: Age, N, margin, grade		
Submandibular				
Bhattachatyya[35]	370			OS: Age, grade
Storey[50]	83	Grade, histology, margin, early years		DS: Early years
Minor				
Jones[7]	103	L: T, N		OS: T, general condition
Lopes[29]	128	R: Stage N, histology, bone invasion		DFS: Stage, therapy[b]
Beckhardt[37]	116	Histology		DFS: Grade, T, margin
Parsons[99a]	95	L. Stage, therapy[a]		DFS: Stage, therapy[a]
Zeidan[36] (SEER)	2222			OS: Gender, T, N, therapy[a]

[a]S + RT > S.
[b]S + RT > RT
DFS, disease-free survival; inv., invasion; L, local; OS, overall survival; R, regional; SG, salivary glands.

Major Salivary Glands

The survival of patients with submandibular cancers is inferior to that of parotid cancers according to a study by Spiro et al.[57] Extraglandular extension[55,56] and skin invasion[21,79,87] in parotid cancers result in decreased disease-free survival. More advanced age was found to be a negative prognostic factor for locoregional control in some studies[19,31,80] and for disease-free and overall survival in most studies.[21,55,57,79,81] Impairment of function of the facial nerve is a known prognostic factor, not only influencing locoregional control[6,20,87] but also disease-free survival.[79,81,87,88] Pain at presentation may be associated with reduced disease-free survival.[79] Perineural invasion and pain are closely related: not pain, but perineural growth, in some studies, is an independent prognostic factor for distant metastases[20] or disease-free survival.[56,76,89]

The importance of histologic subtype for major salivary gland cancer varies in published studies. In most studies, histologic types are subdivided into low and high grade. The main prognostic significance of grading relates to disease-free survival,[55,75] although grade was not a prognostic factor in most studies. In the large SEER database of major salivary gland carcinomas, higher grade was associated with higher stage and an independent prognostic factor for overall survival in stage II to IV.[90] The best prognosis is seen for acinic cell and (low-grade) mucoepidermoid cancer,[20,57] the worst for undifferentiated[20,87] and squamous cell cancer.[20,57] At the Netherlands Cancer Institute, a prognostic score for patients with parotid carcinoma was developed and validated.[21,79] The preoperative prognostic score was based on a weighted combination of prognostic factors (age, pain, clinical T- and N-stages, skin invasion, and facial nerve dysfunction); histology and grading were not incorporated. Four subgroups were formed with markedly different prognoses. In the postoperative score, perineural invasion and positive surgical margins were also included. In adenoid cystic carcinoma, named major nerve involvement is a prognostic factor; however, this may not be true for microscopic invasion only.[91] Intraneural invasion is a more predominant prognostic factor than perineural invasion.[92] Positive or close surgical

margins result in an increase in local recurrence rate.[20,50,75,77,93] Radiation therapy in addition to surgery improves locoregional control in patients with adverse prognostic factors.[19,25,76,78,87,94,95] Improvement of overall survival by adjuvant radiotherapy has been shown in data from the national cancer database[96] and even in early-stage adenoid cystic carcinoma.[97] In a matched-pair analysis of adjuvant radiotherapy, improved overall survival was found in stage III and IV major salivary glands.[98]

Minor Salivary Glands

Tumors located in the larynx or nasal cavity/paranasal sinus have significant lower cause-specific survival compared to location in the oral cavity.[99] The poorest prognosis is associated with adenoid cystic carcinoma.[29,36] Stage, base of skull involvement, and bone invasion are risk factors for locoregional recurrence and survival in minor salivary gland cancers.[7,29,36] Locoregional control may be improved by adding postoperative radiotherapy.[36]

GENERAL MANAGEMENT

The general management of salivary gland malignancies in most patients includes surgical excision followed by radiation therapy for unfavorable prognostic factors (Table 46.5). Postoperative radiotherapy to enhance local control is recommended for T3-T4 tumors, close or incomplete resection, bone involvement, perineural invasion, high-grade cancer, and recurrent cancer.[20,37,50,56,80,87] Postoperative radiotherapy is indicated for patients with neck node lymph metastases.[20,93] Elective neck radiotherapy prevents nodal relapses in a selected group of patients; however, it is in general not indicated for acinic cell or adenoid cystic carcinoma.[100] According to Chen et al., for carcinoma ex pleomorphic adenoma of the parotid gland and adenoid cystic carcinoma, surgery and postoperative local radiotherapy are the standards.[76,95] Concurrent postoperative platinum- and/or paclitaxel-based chemoradiotherapy for high-risk patients (nodal involvement, microscopic positive margins, T3-T4, perineural involvement) may result in high locoregional control rates, although in the published data, the number of

TABLE 46.6 INDICATIONS FOR RADIOTHERAPY: SALIVARY GLAND CANCER

Local Port	Regional Port	Primary RT (≥70 Gy)	High LET RT Consider if Available
AJC Stage T3-T4	pN₁ (60 Gy)	Med. inoperable	R2 resection
High grade	ENE (66 Gy)	Funct. inoperable	Primary RT: T4
Perineural invasion	Elective (Table 46.1) 50 Gy	Irresectable	Reirradiation
Close Res. (1–5 mm) (60 Gy)		Recurrent	
Incomplete Res. (66 Gy)			

ENE, extranodal extension; Funct, functional; Med, medical; PORT, postoperative radiotherapy; Res, resection; RT, radiotherapy.

patients is small, the follow-up is short, and the acute toxicity is more severe. However, in general, there is little proof that for salivary gland cancer, concurrent postoperative chemoradiotherapy is superior to postoperative radiation alone.[101,102] For advanced, inoperable, and recurrent salivary gland cancers, high linear energy transfer (LET) radiotherapy like primary neutron therapy[103] may lead to superior local control rates, compared with primary photon therapy, without evidence of improved survival rates[104] Another treatment option in these cases is carbon ions, with the obvious advantage of a higher relative biologic effect on tumor.[105] High local control rates may be achieved with primary treatment with carbon ions or protons in adenoid cystic carcinoma.[106] In Table 46.6, indications for radiotherapy of salivary gland cancer are summarized.

Major Salivary Glands

Surgical technique depends on location and extent of primary disease and regional adenopathy. Preservation of the facial nerve, at least partially, followed by postoperative radiotherapy is the preferable treatment unless the facial nerve is involved by tumor.[107] Aggressive surgery does not improve disease-free survival. A decrease in extended surgery, resulting in a decrease of sacrifice of the facial nerve, has been shown in the course of years.[57] Cable facial nerve grafting with the greater auricular or sural nerve graft decreases the incidence of facial palsy postoperatively, especially if branches and not the main trunk are involved.[108] Adjuvant postoperative radiotherapy has no negative effect on facial nerve function.[108]

Surgical treatment includes neck dissection in cases of clinically positive nodes, followed by postoperative radiotherapy.[25] The risk of occult nodal disease depends on T-stage and histologic type.[25,100] As shown in the scoring system in Table 46.1, the decision to treat the neck for parotid tumors will be indicated by a score of at least 4.[25] When local prognostic factors indicate postoperative radiotherapy, no elective neck dissection has to be performed; the neck nodes will also be irradiated.[23,109] Parotid tumors with facial nerve weakness are associated with frequent occult neck nodes; elective treatment is also indicated.[109] The first echelon neck nodes in parotid salivary gland cancer are the intraparotideal,[27,110] followed by level II, III, and IV nodes.[100,111] Involvement of level I nodes is an independent risk factor for disease-free survival.[110] Level I and V nodes are only involved if other levels are positive.[111] Contralateral nodes are not at risk. So in case of prophylactic treatment of the clinical N₀ neck, at least level II and III should be incorporated, followed by postoperative radiotherapy in case of pathologic positive nodes of level I to V. In most cases, elective neck dissection of level I to III combined with a local resection is performed for submandibular tumors. There is no indication for neck dissection for T1 acinic or T1 adenoid cystic tumors (Table 46.1).[25,50,100]

Minor Salivary Glands

The treatment of minor salivary gland tumors varies with location but usually involves an attempt at adequate surgical excision first. Irradiation has been used in surgically inaccessible sites or combined with surgery because of locally aggressive tumor behavior and the occurrence of incomplete resection.[20,37,112] For tumors arising in the palate, tongue, floor of the mouth, oral cavity, or oropharynx, surgical exposure is readily available, and resection usually can be accomplished with acceptable morbidity. Tumors arising in the posterior nasal cavity, nasopharynx, or sphenoid region, however, are relatively inaccessible and are mostly treated with radiation therapy.[112] The indication of elective neck treatment may depend on a prognostic index (score 0 to 4) using four clinicopathologic factors associated with increased risk on positive nodes: 1/male gender, 2/stage T3/T4, 3/pharyngeal location, and 4/high grade (28). For a score of ≥2, elective treatment of the neck nodes is indicated. Adenoid cystic carcinoma is the predominant histologic subtype in minor salivary gland cancer. The risk of occult neck disease is largest for oral cavity or oropharyngeal localizations. When postoperative radiotherapy is indicated, it is advised to treat the ipsilateral neck node levels I to III.[113] Patients with adenoid cystic carcinoma can have a long natural history with late recurrences,[112] and consideration should be given to careful surgical reconstruction and rehabilitation because even patients who are not cured can live many years before dying of disease (Fig. 46.3).[20] Occasionally, a patient may present after simple excision of a lesion, and the pathologic examination shows adenoid cystic carcinoma. If reexcision would cause significant functional or cosmetic sequelae, irradiation alone may be used. However, simple excision is not recommended as the initial management of these tumors because of the potential for a significant volume of residual disease. Surgery alone may be used to treat early-stage hard palate lesions without evidence of positive margins, perineural spread, or bone invasion; simple excision must be avoided.[37]

RADIATION THERAPY TECHNIQUES

Pleomorphic Adenoma

The pleomorphic adenoma (benign mixed tumor) is histologically benign, occurs frequently in a relatively young population, and comprises 65% to 75% of all parotid epithelial tumors.[57] Standard therapy has been conservative (superficial) parotidectomy, with recurrence rates of about up to 6.5% after 2 years.[114–116] Simple excision results in a high recurrence rate of around 25% as focal capsular exposure occurs in virtually all cases.[117] Besides, local recurrence is more frequently encountered in younger patients and positive resection margins.[114,116] Indications for postoperative irradiation may include microscopically positive margins after surgical resection and large, deep-seated lesions that may not allow complete surgical excision with adequate margins or would require sacrificing the facial nerve. The risk of malignant transformation in a large Dutch study was only 0.15%; however, in recurrent cases, it is 3.2%.[116] The mean delay between surgery and the first recurrence was 7 years and only 2 years for the second recurrence. The risk of facial nerve paresis increases after repeated surgery.[117] Most recurrent pleomorphic adenomas are multinodular.[118] In a review of Witt et al., local control after surgery for recurrence was 63% after surgery alone, and 91% after surgery with postoperative radiotherapy.[118] Radiotherapy may decrease the risk of a second recurrence in case of multinodular recurrence only, not for uninodular disease.[119] The entire parotid area should be irradiated with a dose of 50 to 60 Gy in 5 to 6 weeks. In Figure 46.9, an example of a large, multicystic pleomorphic adenoma is shown, with a close safety margin and spillage during parotidectomy; postoperative radiotherapy was indicated.

Parotid Gland

The volume of irradiation is determined by pathologic findings, such as perineural invasion of a major nerve. Typically, the entire ipsilateral parotid gland is delineated on the postoperative CT scan performed in a custom-made head and neck mold.[56,120] The delineation of the clinical target volume

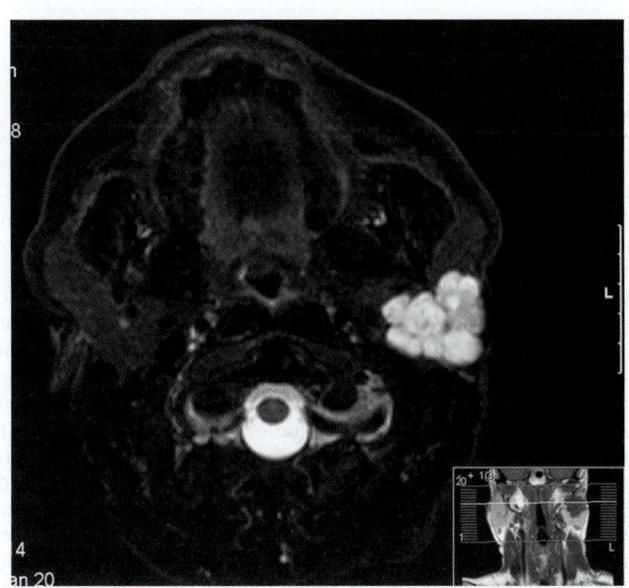

FIGURE 46.9. Multicystic pleomorphic adenoma, T2 STIR, transversal slice.

will be individualized based on the extent of the disease and surgery.[56] In case of a tumor of the deep lobe, the parapharyngeal space and the infratemporal fossa have to be covered adequately. In general, it is not necessary to treat the scar to full skin dose because only 1% of the patients have a scar failure.[80] For very superficial localized tumors and in case of skin invasion, a bolus over the scar is required. In tumors with named perineural invasion (e.g., adenoid cystic carcinoma), especially in case of intraneural invasion,[92] the nerve provides a route to the base of skull. So it is important to cover the

cranial nerve pathways from the parotid up to the base of the skull.[91] In perineural invasion, postoperative radiotherapy with a dose of 50 Gy, including the base of skull, decreased local recurrence rate from 15% with surgery alone to 5% with combined surgery and radiotherapy in a study of Chen et al.[121] Focal perineural invasion only is not an indication for routine inclusion of the nerve pathways. A clear relationship between dose and local control has only been found by Chen et al.; a dose of ≥60 Gy resulted in significant higher local control rates.[76] In general, a dose of at least 60 Gy postexcision is recommended[24,90,120] and at least 66 Gy (33 fractions) for high-risk patients with positive margins (<1 mm).[56]

The ipsilateral neck is treated after a neck dissection has been performed for positive nodes; level I to V should be included.[25] There is no indication for bilateral elective neck treatment.[23,27,100] The recommended postoperative dose for positive nodes is at least 60 Gy (30 fractions) and 66 Gy for extranodal disease.[25] Elective irradiation of the neck should be considered for advanced T-stage, certain histologic subtypes (Table 46.1), facial nerve dysfunction at presentation, and recurrent disease. The intraparotideal nodes should be included.[27,110] At least in early case, high-risk parotid cancer level II and III should be included.[27] Level I and V are seldom positive if only one positive node is diagnosed. However, because in elective treatment the number of possible positive nodes is unknown, most authors advise to treat level Ib to IV prophylactically.[25,109,122] A dose of around 46 to 50 Gy is recommended.[25,56]

Three basic radiation therapy approaches are used, depending on available equipment: conventional, three-dimensional conformal radiation therapy (3DCRT) planning procedure, and intensity-modulated radiation therapy (IMRT) planning. The first involves unilateral anterior and posterior wedged pair fields using ^{60}Co or 4- to 6-MV photons (Fig. 46.10A). Typical field boundaries are the zygomatic arch superiorly, the

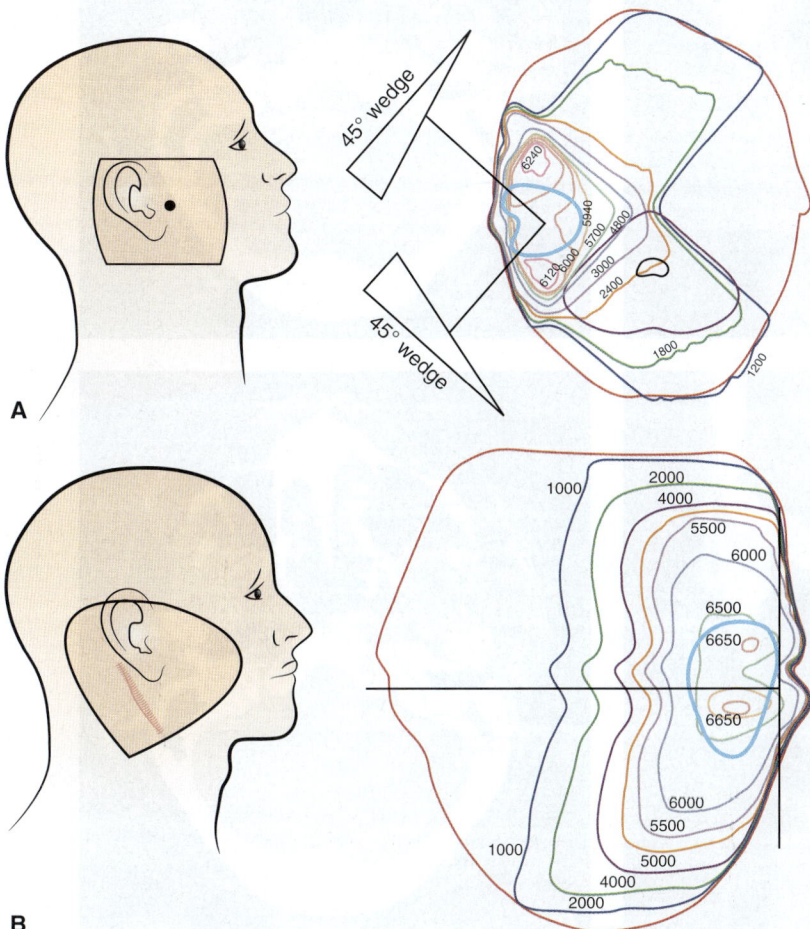

FIGURE 46.10. Conventional radiotherapy for parotid cancer. **A:** Unilateral wedge arrangement and isodose distribution using wedged pair. **B:** Ipsilateral 16-MeV electrons plus [60]Co (4:1) electron beam field.

masseter muscle anteriorly, the pterygoid muscle and ramus mandibulae laterally, the mastoid process posteriorly, and the posterior belly of the digastric muscle inferiorly.[95] A slight inferior angulation of the beams avoids an exit dose through the contralateral eye. A simpler technique uses homolateral fields with 12- to 16-MeV electrons in combination with photons.[66,123] Usually, 80% of the dose is delivered with electrons and 20% with ^{60}Co or 4- to 6-MV photons to spare the opposite salivary gland, reduce mucositis, and decrease the skin reaction produced by electrons (Fig. 46.10B). Yaparpalvi et al.[123] compared nine conventional treatment techniques. Ipsilateral wedge pair technique with 6-MV photons, wedged anterior–posterior and posterior–anterior and lateral technique with 6-MV photons, and mixed beam using 6-MV photons and 16-MeV electrons (1:4 weighted) were most optimal, considering dose homogeneity within the target and dose to normal tissues. Electron beam (9 to 12 MeV) and tangential photon fields are effective conventional techniques for sparing the underlying spinal cord (from doses more than 45 Gy) and the opposite parotid gland in elective neck irradiation. Conventional techniques do not allow for tissue heterogeneity (air cavity, dense bones, and tissues); underdose and overdose may be seen. So in modern radiotherapy, conformal techniques should be the treatment of choice.

After outlining of the target volumes and critical normal tissues on the planning CT scan, a more conformal 3DCRT plan by the use of geometrically shaped beams of uniform intensity may be reached.[119] More normal tissue may be spared with this technique.[120,124] In case of named perineural invasion, a 3-D FFE T2 MRI technique, performed in treatment position, may be used to delineate the cranial nerves (Fig. 46.5). Probably, the most conformal radiation technique is IMRT. It can produce convex dose distributions and steep dose gradients. Five- to seven-field inverse IMRT allows excellent coverage of the tumor with sparing of mandible, cochlea, spinal cord, brain, and oropharynx,[125] compared with conformal 3DCRT. Especially the dose to the cochlea and Eustachian tube should stay under 45 to 50 Gy.[126,127] Compared to 3-D conformal radiotherapy, IMRT may spare the inner ear better.[128] In the national cancer database, 5-year overall survival for major salivary gland treated postoperatively with IMRT or 3DCRT was respectively 84.7% and 80.7% (P was 0.06).[97] Figure 46.11 shows a comparison of 3DCRT and IMRT planning for a postoperative radiotherapy plan for a parotid cancer, without named nerve involvement,

FIGURE 46.11. Postoperative radiation therapy of a parotid cancer, microscopically incomplete resected. Coronal (**A** and **C**) and transversal (**B** and **D**) dose distribution for three-dimensional conformal radiation therapy (25 × 2 Gy primary field, 8 × 2 Gy boost) (**A** and **B**) and intensity-modulated radiation therapy (inverse, 7 fields and 39 segments; simultaneously moderated accelerated radiotherapy (SMART): 33 × 1.6 Gy primary field, 33 × 2 Gy boost) (**C** and **D**).

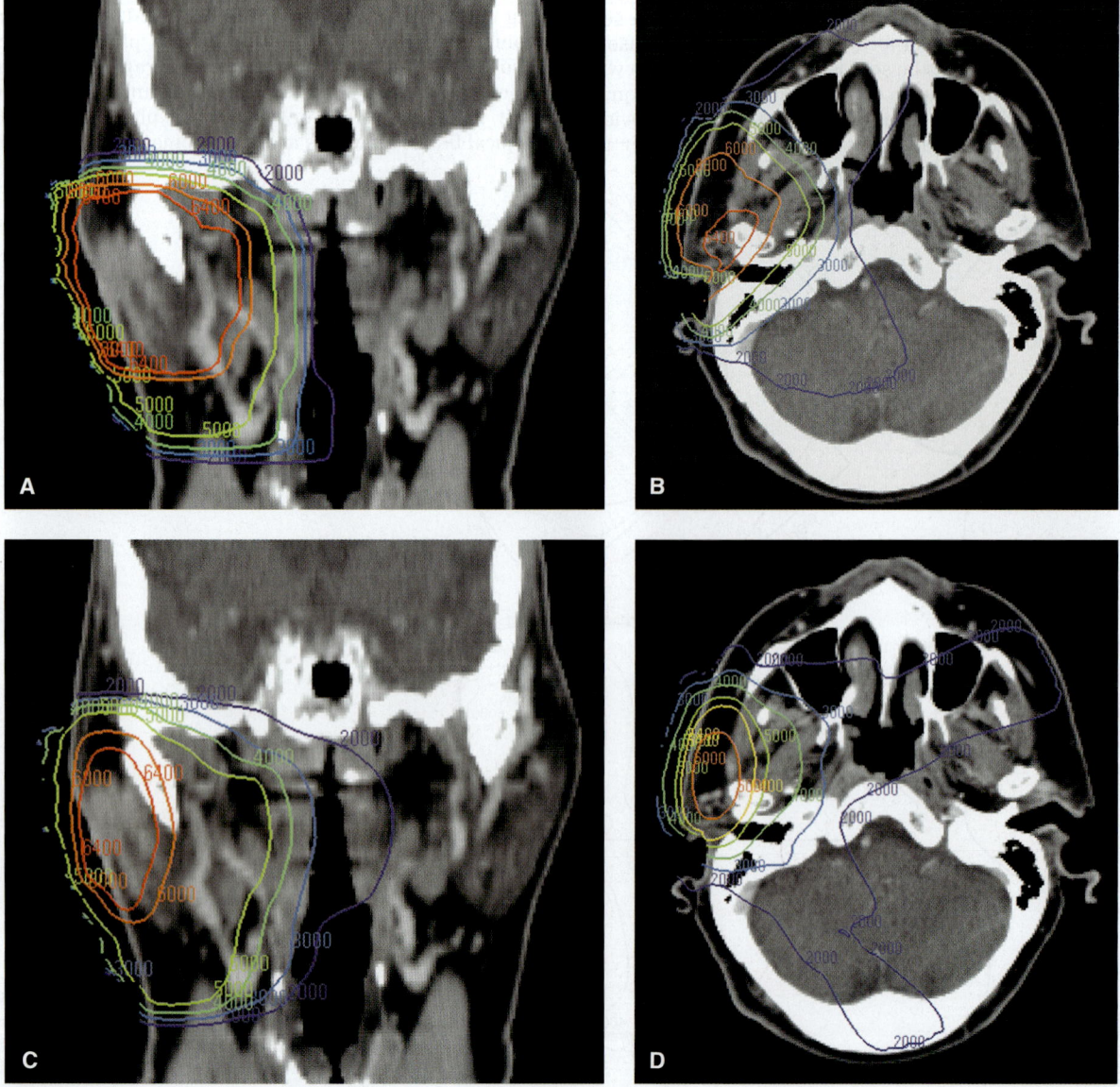

treated with a dose of 66 Gy. The mean dose to the mastoid, meatus acusticus externus, and contralateral parotid gland was 53 and 43 Gy, 57 and 51 Gy, and 1 and 9 Gy, for 3DCRT and IMRT, respectively. The maximum dose to the cochlea was 39 and 32 Gy, respectively. In Figure 46.12, a patient with a recurrent adenocarcinoma of the parotid gland with named perineural involvement, for which a total parotidectomy was performed, is shown. The resection was incomplete. The facial nerve was delineated based on MRI (Figure 46.5B). A unilateral IMRT technique was used.

Submandibular Gland

Except for small acinic cell and adenoid cystic cancer (Table 46.1), the neck node level I to IV[122] should be irradiated electively, following the indications outlined for parotid tumors; technical considerations are similar. Bilateral fields may be required for tumor extension toward the midline. Five years locoregional control was significantly higher for a dose of more than 56 Gy in a study of Mallik et al.[129] If there is named perineural invasion of a major nerve, a tumor dose of 60 to 66 Gy in 6 to 6.5 weeks is recommended, and the nerve path to the base of skull should be treated, preferably by IMRT. For an adenoid cystic carcinoma of the submandibular gland with only focal perineural invasion, an attempt to encompass the base of the skull would require a significant change in the treatment volume and may not be warranted because of potential morbidity and the low rate of relapse at that site.[112] An example of 3DCRT for a T2 adenoid cystic carcinoma of the submandibular gland is shown in Figure 46.13.

Sublingual Gland

These tumors are mostly malignant, mostly adenoid cystic carcinoma, mostly advanced disease, and high-grade, however with a low risk of positive neck nodes. Aggressive surgery is required, with postoperative local radiotherapy in almost all cases,[38,130] with elective treatment of level I to III.[130] In case of named nerve involvement, the lingual and/or hypoglossic nerve should be included in the radiation portals.

Minor Salivary Glands

The radiation therapy technique for treating minor salivary gland tumors depends on the area involved and is similar to the treatment for squamous cell carcinomas in these areas, with two significant exceptions. First, when a named branch of a cranial nerve is involved by adenoid cystic carcinoma, the nerve pathways to the base of the skull should be electively treated. Second, for tumors of the paranasal sinuses, the base of the skull is included because of its proximity to the tumor bed. In case of an adenoid cystic carcinoma with perineural invasion, IMRT may reduce the high dose volume, compared to conventional bilateral opposed fields; Figure 46.14 shows an example for a patient with a minor salivary gland cancer of the palate. IMRT is a useful strategy for irradiating minor salivary gland sites such as the ethmoid sinuses while sparing the optic pathways.[131]

Also, because the incidence of lymph node metastases is usually lower than that for squamous cell carcinomas of similar size, the radiation therapy fields are rarely extended to cover such areas if there are no palpable lymph node metastases. Indications for elective treatment of the neck nodes may depend on a scoring system.[25,28] Typically, for male patients with a $T_3/T_4 N_0$, pharyngeal site tumor neck nodes should be treated prophylactically.[112] In minor salivary gland cancers of the oral cavity, elective radiation of the neck nodes is seldom indicated. Postoperative radiotherapy is indicated after resection of metastatic neck lymphadenopathy.

For patients receiving postoperative irradiation after surgical resection, a dose of 60 Gy is given for close margins and 66

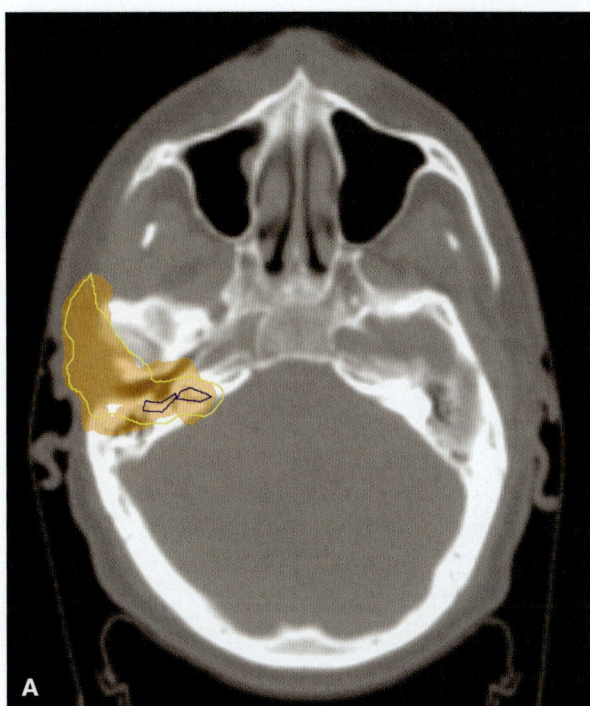
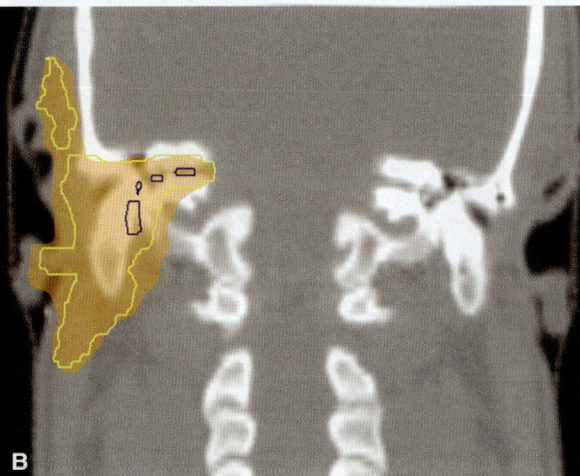
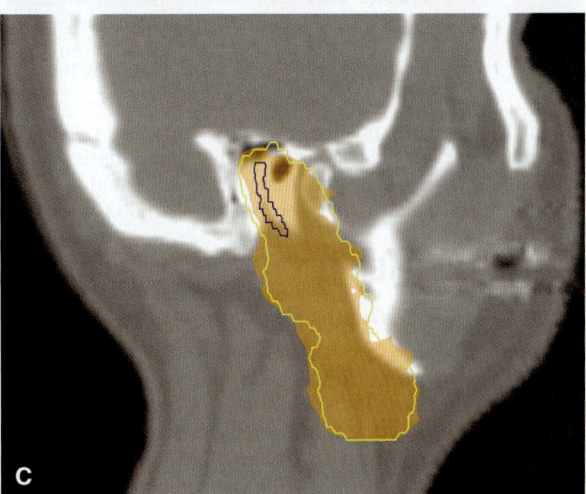

FIGURE 46.12. Recurrent adenocarcinoma of the parotid gland with named nerve involvement (nVII, in *blue*), delineated on base of MRI (Fig. 46.5B). A unilateral IMRT technique was used, in *yellow* 50 Gy isodose (boost not shown); transversal **(A)**, coronal **(B)**, and sagittal **(C)** planes.

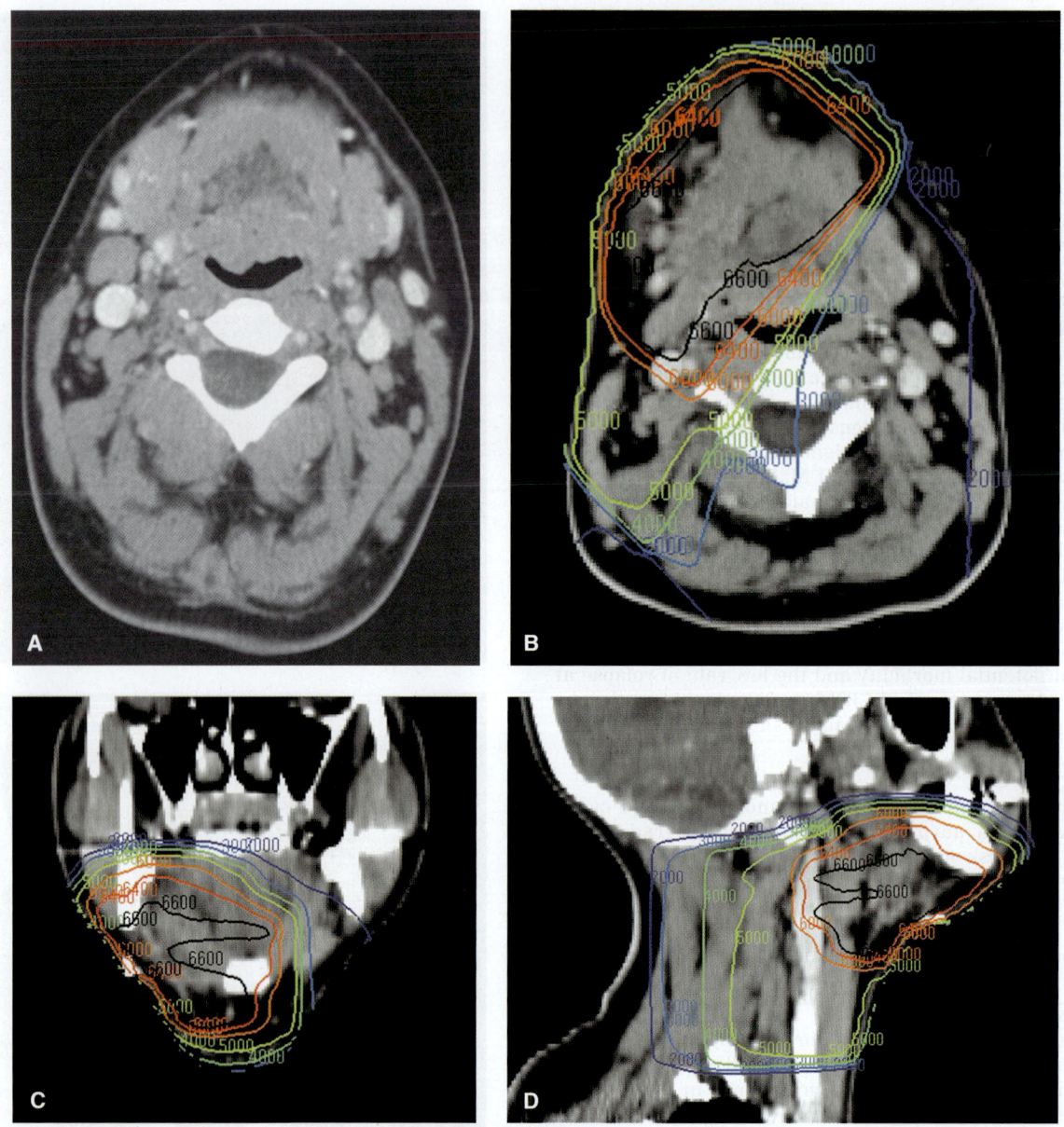

FIGURE 46.13. Dose distribution for a T2N0 adenoid cystic cancer of the right submandibular gland. Computed tomography performed before microscopically incomplete local excision **(A)**. Three-dimensional conformal radiation therapy, three fields (one right and two left oblique): 25 × 2 Gy, 5 × weekly primary tumor and level I to III nodes, 8 × 2 Gy boost; transversal **(B)**, coronal **(C)**, and sagittal **(D)** planes. Mean dose to contralateral submandibular gland is 27 Gy.

Gy for microscopically positive margins. For gross residual disease after surgery or for lesions treated with irradiation alone, a total dose of 70 Gy is recommended at 2 Gy per fraction. Elective dose to the nodal levels is in the range of 46 to 50 Gy.[25,132]

RESULTS OF THERAPY

Surgery Plus or Minus Postoperative Radiotherapy

Tables 46.7 through 46.9 list local control rates and 5- and 10-year survival rates for several series reporting the surgical, irradiation, and combination treatment of carcinomas of the major and minor salivary glands. Little adverse effect of delay between surgery and radiotherapy may be predicted for what are, in general, slow-growing salivary gland cancers. In three studies, one concerning submandibular cancer,[50] one for minor salivary gland,[112] and another for adenoid cystic cancer,[76] impaired locoregional control rates were seen for a delay of more than 6 weeks, which was not confirmed in

the Dutch study.[25] The prognosis for children with a malignant salivary gland cancer (mostly mucoepidermoid cancer of the parotid gland) is excellent, with a 5-year overall survival of more than 90%.[8] Most are treated with surgery alone because of the possible risk on radiation-induced malignancies.

Long-term follow-up is recommended because failures may appear after 5 years, especially for minor salivary gland tumors and adenoid cystic cancer.[7,20,22,76] Recurrent tumors in general are more difficult to control than are primary ones, so high initial locoregional control rates should be the goal. Because of high rates of local failure of approximately 40% for parotid, 60% for submandibular, and 65% for minor salivary glands with surgery alone in the past,[6] many institutions have advocated postoperative irradiation especially to reduce the incidence of local failure. Local tumor control appears to be improved by the combination of surgery and irradiation, although randomized, controlled trials have not been performed. Evidence of a positive role of postoperative radiotherapy is based on retrospective studies and a matched-pair analysis. In the study by Armstrong

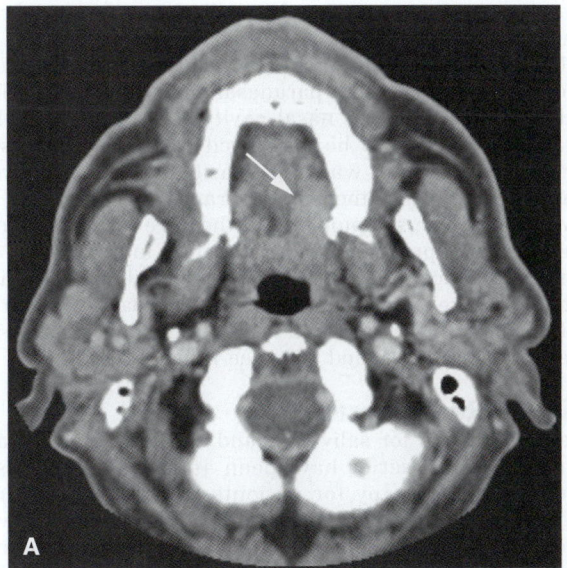

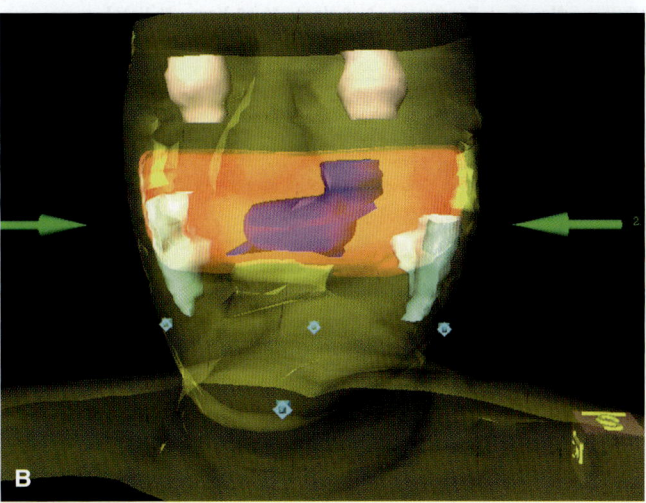

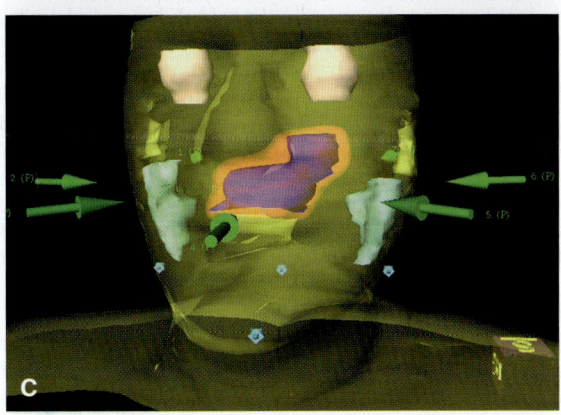

FIGURE 46.14. T2N0 adenoid cystic cancer of the palate with major perineural invasion. Computed tomography performed before local excision (**A**, *arrow:* tumor); target includes right palatinus major nerve until base of skull. Dose distribution (25 × 2 Gy primary field) in transversal planes; conventional bilateral opposed fields (**B**); intensity-modulated radiation therapy (7 fields, 40 segments) (**C**); 95% isodose of 50 Gy in *red.*

et al.,[76] postoperative radiotherapy significantly improved locoregional control (from 17% to 51% for stage III to IV), not for stage I and II major salivary gland cancer. Locoregional control for patients with positive nodes increased from 40% to 69%. In most studies, an imbalance in prognostic factors is seen comparing surgery alone with combined therapy, favoring surgery alone. Despite this imbalance, locoregional control with combined surgery and postoperative radiotherapy is superior to surgery alone for patients with negative prognostic factors, irrespective of site.[20,25,50,52,74,76,78,95,129] This was also

shown for low-grade salivary gland cancer.[133] In the nationwide Dutch study, the relative risk for surgery alone, compared with combined treatment, was 9.7 for local recurrence and 2.3 for regional recurrence.[25] Postoperative radiotherapy is particularly effective if there are close (<5 mm) or microscopic positive resection margins, enhancing local control from around 50% to 80% to 95%.[25,76,77,107] Comparable results are noted for T3-T4 tumors and pathologically confirmed bone and perineural invasion.[25,52,74,129] For adenoid cystic carcinoma with perineural invasion, postoperative radiotherapy increased 10-year local control rates from 30% to 80% in a study of Chen et al.[76] However, for a T1 or T2 tumor that was completely resected with no bone or perineural invasion, surgery alone will result in more than 90% 10-year local control rate and radiotherapy is not indicated.[25]

Treatment results also may depend on histopathologic status. However, after review, histologic type may change, even among experienced pathologists. In general, the best prognosis is shown

TABLE 46.7 RESULTS OF STANDARD THERAPY FOR CANCER OF THE PAROTID

Study (by Name of First Author)	No. of Patients	Treatment	% 5-Year Survival	% 10-Year Survival	% Local Control
Bhattacharyya[55]	903	S ± R	67	50	NA
Spiro[6]	623	S	55	47	61
Terhaard[20]	37	S	67	61	51 (10 y)
	254	S + R	65	51	88 (10 y)
Garden[56]	166	S + R	78	60	90 (10 y)
North[87]	19	S	59	NA	74
	50	S + R	75	NA	98
Poulsen[77]	209	S + R	71	65	76
Renehan[94]	37	S	77	63	57 (locoreg.)
	66	S + R	78	67	85 (locoreg.)
Pohar[19]	56	S	65	50	63 (locoreg.)
	91	S + R	55	40	89 (locoreg.)
Chen (carc,	23	S	44	NA	49 (5-y)
ex pl. ad.)[95]	40	S + R	59	NA	75 (5-y)

ad, adenoma; carc, carcinoma; locoreg., locoregional; NA, not available; pl., pleomorphic; R, irradiation; S, surgery, .

TABLE 46.8 RESULTS OF STANDARD THERAPY FOR CANCER OF THE SUBMANDIBULAR GLANDS

Study (by Name of First Author)	No. of Patients	Treatment	% 5-Year Survival	% 10-Year Survival	% Local Control
Spiro[6]	129	S	31	22	40 (loreg.)
Terhaard[20]	68	S + R	57	45	91 (10 y)
Storey[50]	83	S + R	60 (DFS)	53 (DFS)	88 (loreg.)
Bhattacharyya[49]	370	S ± R	60	NA	NA
Mallik[129]	39	S + RT			
	25	RT≤56Gy	59 (DFS)	NA	59 (loreg.)
	14	RT>56 Gy	77 (FDS)	NA	100 (loreg.)

DFS, disease-free survival; loreg., locoregional; NA, not available; R, irradiation; S, surgery.

TABLE 46.9 RESULTS OF STANDARD THERAPY FOR MINOR SALIVARY GLANDS

Study (by Name of First Author)/Site	No. of Patients	Treatment	% 5-Year Survival	% 10-Year Survival	% Local Control
Spiro[6]	526	S	48	37	35 (locoreg.)
Garden[112]	160	S + R	81	65	88 (15 y)
Terhaard[20] (oral cavity)	67	S	87	76	91
	54	S + R	85	72	98
Lopes[29] (oral cavity)	59	S	86	83	90 (locoreg.)
	32	S + R	88	56	78 (locoreg.)
	15	R	46	–	13 (locoreg.)
Beckhardt[37] (palate)	79	S	90 (DSS)	80 (DSS)	NA
	35	S + R	87 (DSS)	83 (DSS)	NA
Ali[52] (adenoid cystic, 59 minor)	28	S			42 (10 y)
	58	S+R			90 (10 y)
Salgado[132]	98	S + R	82	58	81 (10 y)
Zeidan[36]	90	S + R	76	63	88 (10 y)

DSS, disease-specific survival; locoreg., locoregional; NA, not available; R, irradiation; S, surgery.

for *acinic cell* and *mucoepidermoid* cancer, with a 15% risk of distant metastases after 10 years and a 10-year locoregional control rate of around 85%. Ten-year overall survival is around 80% and 65%, respectively.[6,20,35,58] Postoperative radiotherapy is indicated for the high-risk group.[20,58] *Squamous cell* and *undifferentiated* tumors have been associated with a 10-year overall survival of 35% or less, caused by a high risk of distant metastases (35% and 50%, respectively) and locoregional recurrence.[6,20,77] Postoperative radiotherapy is indicated in all cases to improve locoregional control. The intermediate-risk group consists of *cancer ex pleomorphic adenoma and adenoid cystic cancer*. Distant failure after 10 years is around 35%.[20,33,95] Although the risk of nodal recurrence is low (5% to 10%), local recurrence is diagnosed more often (20% to 50%). Postoperative radiotherapy is indicated in almost all cases. In cancer ex pleomorphic adenoma, 5-year local control rates were 75% and 49% for yes or no postoperative radiotherapy in a study of Chen et al.[95] A precipitous decrease in relapse-free survival is noted among 5 (around 70%), 10 (around 50%), and 15 years (around 45%) for patients with adenoid cystic carcinomas, which are well known for late recurrences.[20,52,76] Significant improvement was reported in local control for adenoid cystic cancer with combined surgery and irradiation in several studies,[53,76,93,94] regardless of site. Local tumor control rates with combined modality therapy for these tumors approach 85% to 90% at 10 years.

In the World Health Organization classification of 1991, among others, three new subtypes were described that are diagnosed relatively frequently. *PLGA* is situated predominantly in the palate. The vast majority is cured with a wide local excision, without a need for elective treatment of the neck. In the large SEER database, the 10 years disease-specific survival was >95%, only 20% of the patients were treated with postoperative radiotherapy.[61] *Salivary duct carcinoma* is a very aggressive disease, predominantly localized in the parotid gland. Postoperative locoregional radiotherapy is indicated in all cases. Most patients die of disease, despite often successful locoregional combined therapy. Postoperative radiotherapy improves locoregional control.[62,63] Because of a high percentage of distant metastases, 5-year survival is only around 30%.[62] The prognosis correlates with HER2/neu receptor status. HER2/neu overexpression correlates with decreased disease-specific survival.[63] *Epithelial–myoepithelial* cancers have a very favorite outcome with a risk on distant metastases below 5%, and a disease-free survival of more than 80% after 10 years. However, local recurrences may be seen in one out of three; postoperative local radiotherapy is indicated in case of incomplete margin, tumor necrosis, lymphatic invasion, and myoepithelial anaplasia.[65] In *basal cell*

adenocarcinoma, postoperative radiotherapy may increase overall survival for T3-T4 cases.[67]

Minor salivary gland tumors of the oral cavity have a more favorable prognosis than paranasal sinus tumors (maxillary and ethmoid sinus and nasal cavity).[112] Patients with hard palate lesions tend to be diagnosed when they have small asymptomatic lumps, which are easily detected on physical examination. On the other hand, paranasal sinus tumors usually do not cause symptoms until they are locally advanced. The surgical approach for these tumors is more difficult, with a greater chance for leaving behind residual disease, leading to high recurrence rates. A combined approach with surgery and postoperative irradiation is recommended, with 10-year local control rates around 85% (see Table 46.9).[36,112,132]

Primary Radiotherapy

The poor results for salivary gland cancer with irradiation alone in several series have been attributed to the use of primary radiotherapy for patients with locally advanced lesions or distant metastases at presentation, who were essentially treated for palliation. Locoregional control rates after conventional photon or electron therapy are around 25%.[101,104] Ten-year locoregional control depended on T-stage in a series of the University of Florida, 72% and 20% for T1-T3 and T4, respectively.[74] For treatment with photons with curative intent, a clear dose–response relationship has been described.[25,134] A dose of at least 66 to 70 Gy should be adapted, resulting in a 5-year local control of 50% to 70%, although late recurrence was observed. The generally slow rate of regression of advanced salivary gland tumors have made them a logical target for alternative radiation therapy approaches, such as high LET particles and proton therapy.

Particle Therapy

Patients with inoperable primary or recurrent major or minor salivary glands were included in the RTOG-MRC randomized phase III clinical trial. Patients were randomized between 70 Gy for 7.5 weeks or 55 Gy for 4 weeks photon therapy and neutron therapy. The study had to be stopped because of a statistically significant difference in 2-year locoregional control, after inclusion of only 32 patients. The 10-year locoregional control probability was 17% after photon therapy and 56% after neutron therapy.[104] However, survival was identical. Late morbidity was somewhat higher for neutron therapy. Primary neutron therapy in salivary gland disease is reserved for macroscopically residual disease after surgery (R2) and unresected and irresectable tumors. Stannard et al. have published results of 335 patients with neutrons.[103] The 5-year locoregional control was 80% after R2 resection, 55% for unresected cases, and 40% for irresectable cases. The risk of late grade 3 to 4 morbidity was 20%.

In an effort to improve poor results for tumors invading the base of skull, several new techniques have been developed. A combination of neutron therapy with, after a 4-week split, a gamma knife stereotactic radiosurgical boost has been used for tumors invading the base of skull.[135] Compared to a historical control group, treated with neutrons only, in 34 patients treated with combined neutrons and gamma knife, the actuarial local control rate at 40 months was 82% versus 39% for the control group. Complication grades were equal.[135]

Carbon ions have the theoretical advantage of comparable LET as neutrons, however with a higher biologic effectiveness. In Heidelberg, 309 advanced adenoid cystic carcinoma, 60% T4, and 37% paranasal location were treated with a combination of photons (median 50 Gy) and carbon ions (median 24 GyE).[136] Five-year local control for R1 (29%), R2 resection (44%), and inoperable tumors (28%) were ±80%, 56%, and 51%, respectively. Toxicity was moderate. In a subset of R2 resection and inoperable cases (>90% T4, paranasal, parotid gland with base of skull invasion, nasopharynx), combined IMRT with carbon ion boost (*n* = 58) was compared with IMRT only (*n* = 37). Although not randomized, 5-year local control with carbon ion boost was significantly better (60% vs. 40%).[137] In a series from Japan, primary carbon ion therapy (*n* = 40) was compared with primary proton therapy (*n* = 40) for advanced adenoid cystic carcinoma. Local control after 5 years for T4 and inoperable cases was equal (68%) for both treatment options.[106] However, the incidence of late grade 3 or more late complications in their study was high (61% for protons and 39% for carbon ions) and dose dependent (>72 GyE).[106] Actually, because of the favorable Brack peak, protons may be used to decrease toxicity. Because of a lower dose to organs at risk, acute toxicity was lower in a retrospective study comparing protons with photons in pediatric salivary gland tumors.[138] However, data concerning proton therapy for salivary gland cancer are scarce, and future studies are needed.

In conclusion, carbon ions or neutron beam therapy should be taken into account, if available, for unresectable, residual, or recurrent salivary gland tumors.[105] Despite high locoregional control, overall survival seems not to be improved and late toxicity is of concern. The value of proton therapy for these indications should be studied.

SYSTEMIC THERAPY

The rarity of these neoplasms and their localized nature provide limited opportunities for trials with chemotherapy. Most published studies concern small series with different histologic subtypes, using a large variety in chemotherapy regimens. Encouraging results are shown for *concurrent* postoperative chemoradiotherapy (paclitaxel, 5FU, hydroxyurea; twice a day 1.5 Gy, mean dose 65 Gy) in high-risk salivary gland cancer by Pederson et al.[139] In 24 patients, a 5-year locoregional progression-free survival of 96% and a 5-year overall survival of 59% was reached. In another small case control study of 24 patients, comparing postoperative platinum-based chemoradiotherapy (63 Gy) with postoperative radiotherapy alone, 3-year overall survival was significantly higher for the combined group (83% vs. 44%, respectively).[140] However, 3-year local progression-free survival was moderate in both groups (61% vs. 44% respectively). In the analysis of the large SEER database, postoperative chemoradiation for resected major salivary gland cancer resulted into worse overall survival compared to postoperative radiation alone, even after propensity score-matched analysis.[101] So in general, there is no proof of superiority for concurrent chemoradiotherapy in the curative setting.[102] Although there might be a case for postoperative chemoradiation in high-risk salivary gland cancer (T3-T4, positive margins, high grade, perineural extension, positive nodes),[141] this has to be proven in prospective randomized studies, like the ongoing RTOG 1008 trial.

In the *palliative* setting, chemotherapy may be beneficial in patients who have progressive, symptomatic disease with no other treatment options. Cisplatin as monotherapy shows a 20% response rate for locoregional disease and only 7% for distant failures, with duration of 6 to 9 months. In a phase 2 study, chemotherapy alone (platinum and gemcitabine) for advanced, metastatic, or locoregionally recurrent salivary gland cancer showed an objective, modest, response of 25% (*n* = 30) with a mean duration of 6 months.[142] Comparable response rates were shown for a combination of cisplatin and vinorelbine.[143] In ACC single-agent, vinorelbine, epirubicin, and mitoxantrone are first-line options; for combined regimens, cisplatin and anthracyclines are recommended, however with a response rate of 30% or less.[144]

Molecular targeting therapy is a promising cancer treatment option. A variety of drugs, targeting on specific pathways, are used in the palliative treatment of salivary gland cancer.[73,83] In a large series of 139 patients with primary, recurrent, and metastatic salivary gland cancer, treatment relevant target immunophenotyping has been performed by Locati et al.[145]

Tyrosine kinase receptors (TKRs) and EGFR were positive in 70% for all histologic subtypes. C-kit was positive in 78% of the ACC. HER2/neu was positive in 44% in SDC and in 21% adenocarcinoma NOS. Hormonal receptor status was also determined. In SDC and adenocarcinoma NOS, androgen receptor was positive in 43% and 21% respectively.[145] Her2/NEU and EGFR were positive in 26% and 70%, respectively, in a study with 66 SDC.[85] These findings could be exploited for selection of patients for molecular targeting treatment. However, the response rate of the investigated targeted therapy is, until now, limited. A promising role for antiandrogen deprivation has been shown in 17 patients with a recurrent/metastatic androgen receptor expressing salivary gland cancer. The response rate was 67% with even three complete responders and a median progression-free survival of 11 months.[146] In the future, the role of molecular-targeted therapy for these salivary gland cancers has to be further established.[147]

SEQUELAE OF TREATMENT

The most notable complication of treatment of parotid malignancies is facial nerve paralysis, which is often caused by the initial or a repeated surgical procedure. However, various series have shown that facial nerve sacrifice is rarely necessary, unless the nerve is directly involved by tumor, particularly when postoperative irradiation is given.[57,77] When facial nerve sacrifice is required, facial nerve grafting and postoperative radiation therapy achieve comparable facial nerve function compared with unirradiated graft despite more negative prognostic factors.[107] Other postoperative sequelae, such as salivary fistulae and neuromas of the greater auricular nerve, are sometimes seen. Frey syndrome (i.e., gustatory sweating) may occur in a few patients after parotid surgery, but it is rarely bothersome.[80]

Partial xerostomia after irradiation of the parotid gland is frequently observed and may be permanent. Trismus may result from radiation-induced fibrosis of the temporomandibular joint or the masseter muscles. It usually occurs when there is extensive tumor infiltration of the masseter muscle and high doses are given.

Radiotherapy to the parotid gland may result in complications along the auditory system. As late toxicity, external canal stenosis, dryness, skin atrophy, and chronic otitis externa, resulting in conductive hearing loss, although rare, may be seen. Chronic otitis media has been documented in 35% to 40%, because of damage to the muscles of the tuba of Eustachius. This may lead to conductive hearing loss, and repeated myringotomies may be indicated.[148] Radiation-induced hearing loss mostly is caused by progressive endothelial damage to the vascularization of the inner ear. This will cause sensorineural hearing loss, cognitive impairment, and, at the end, decrease quality of life. However, most hearing loss is seen above 4,000 Hz; for daily use, normal frequency ranges from 1,000 to 3,000 Hz. In a prospective study of patients treated for head and neck cancer, a ≥10 dB hearing loss 2 years after radiotherapy was seen in 40% for 8,000 Hz, and in 50% for 3,000 Hz.[127] A threshold of 45 Gy was seen at ≥2,000 Hz, also depending on age and baseline hearing loss.[127] In published results, the mean threshold dose for the cochlea and tuba of Eustachius for sensorineural hearing loss varies between 40 Gy and 50 Gy.[126,127,148] The latency is around 1.5 to 2 years. After this time, hearing loss stabilizes. The risk of sensorineural hearing loss is depending on radiation technique. From 2-D conventional to 3-D conformal radiotherapy, the mean dose to the cochlea may decrease from above 50 Gy to around 40 Gy,[120,124] and further improvement is noted with the use of IMRT.[120,128] No dose–response relationship has been published for vestibular damage.[148]

Garden et al.[112] reported complications of irradiation in 51 of 160 patients receiving postoperative *conventional 2-D* irradiation for minor salivary gland tumors. The most common complication was decreased hearing in 26 patients, 20 of whom had myringotomies or myringotomy tubes placed for serous otitis media. Bone necrosis or exposure was observed in several patients; however, this complication has been seen infrequently during the past decade with improved radiation therapy techniques and treatment of multiple, as opposed to single fields per day. Complications to the eyes or optic pathways were diagnosed in patients with paranasal sinus primary tumors. At least six cases of contralateral optic atrophy occurred.[112] Other eye complications included dry eye syndrome, nasolacrimal duct obstruction, cataract, retinopathy, and perforated globe.[112] To reduce the incidence of bilateral blindness, the dose to the optic chiasm and contralateral optic nerve is limited to 54 Gy. In patients with extensive tumor involvement of the orbit, it may be preferable to remove the eye surgically rather than to subject the entire orbit to high doses. Radiation-induced injury to the visual pathway is dose dependent. None of the patients receiving a dose of <50 Gy develop optic neuropathy or chiasm injury, whereas the 10-year actuarial incidences of optic nerve chiasm injury is 5% and 30% for patients receiving 50 to 60 Gy and 61 to 78 Gy, respectively.[149]

Radiotherapy of tumors of the pharynx, and less frequently the oral cavity, may result in permanent complaints of xerostomia. In the largest published series, the mean dose to the parotid glands that relates to 50% risk of 1-year xerostomia was 39 Gy, and no threshold was seen.[150] A dose beneath 20 Gy is preferable to reach a low risk on xerostomia.[150] This serious late complication may be significantly reduced by the use of IMRT.[151] Data on quality of life are scarce. In a prospectively scored small series of 36 patients treated for parotid carcinoma with postoperative radiotherapy, quality of life deteriorated during treatment and returned to almost baseline levels from 6 weeks to 1 year after radiotherapy.[152] In general, the risk of late toxicity is much lower using modern radiation techniques like IMRT and Vmat compared to 2 or 3DRT. Based on dose–response models for organs at risk, particle treatment may be preferred in some cases, depending on the estimated lower risk at late toxicity.[153]

TREATMENT OF RECURRENCE

Retreatment usually involves additional surgery, if feasible, and postoperative irradiation in previously irradiated patients (Fig. 46.15). In the retreatment of parotid neoplasms, preserving

facial nerve function and obtaining local control are more difficult than for the initial tumor. Therapy consisting of surgery with postoperative irradiation has demonstrated enhanced local control, and facial nerve sacrifice may be necessary less often if this combination is used. In certain histologic subtypes (e.g., adenoid cystic carcinoma), retreatment of locally recurrent disease yields prolonged survival. Aggressive local therapy for recurrent disease is indicated if the probability of long-term survival is high, as in the case of adenoid cystic carcinoma. Fractionated stereotactic reirradiation, with a dose of 5 times 6 Gy, resulted in a 50% locoregional control in a study by Karam et al.[154] Reirradiation is not advised within 1 year after the first radiotherapy and not for large tumor volumes.[154] Multimodality treatment may be beneficial for recurrence disease of minor salivary gland, if initial tumor classification is $T_{1/2}$.[155]

Chemotherapy also has been used for recurrent disease.[143,144] However, in view of its significant toxicity and modest response rates in a population that may have recurrent yet indolent progressive disease, trials of aggressive cytotoxic therapy are recommended only on carefully drafted protocols. In the future, molecular target agents may be tested in selected recurrent salivary gland cancers.

REFERENCES

 1. Bjørndal K, Krogdahl A, Therkildsen MH, et al. Salivary gland carcinoma in Denmark 1990–2005: a national study of incidence, site and histology. Results of the Danish Head and Neck Cancer Group (DAHANCA). *Oral Oncol* 2011;47:677–682.
 2. Del Signore A, Megwalu U. The rising incidence of major salivary gland cancer in the United States. *Ear Nose Throat J* 2017;96(3):E13–E16.
 3. Rosse C, Gaddum-Rosse P. *Hollingshead's textbook of anatomy*. 5th ed. Lippincott-Raven, 1997.
 4. Batsakis J. Tumors of the major salivary glands and neoplasms of the minor and "lesser" major salivary glands. In: Batsakis JC, ed. *Tumors of the head and neck: clinical and pathological considerations*. 2nd ed. Baltimore, MD: Lippincott Williams & Wilkins, 1979.
 5. Haagensen C, Feind C, Herter F. *The lymphatics in cancer*. Philadelphia: WB Saunders, 1972.
 6. Spiro R. Salivary neoplasms: overview of a 35-year experience with 2,807 patients. *Head Neck Surg* 1986;8:177–184.
 7. Jones A, Beasley N, Houghton D, et al. Tumours of the minor salivary glands. *Clin Otolaryngol* 1998;23:27–33.
 8. Sultan L, Rodriguez-Galindo C, Al-Sharabati S, et al. Salivary gland carcinomas in children and adolescents: a population-based study, with comparison to adult cases. *Head Neck* 2011;33:1476–1481.
 9. Muscatt J, Wynder E. A case/control study of risk factors for major salivary gland cancer. *Otolaryngol Head Neck Surg* 1998;118:195–198.
10. de Ru J, Plantinga R, Majoor M, et al. Warthin's tumour and smoking. *B-ENT* 2005;1(2):63–66.
11. Saku T, Hayashi Y, Takahara O, et al. Salivary gland tumors among atomic bomb survivors, 1950–1987. *Cancer* 1997;79:1465–1475.
12. Boukheris H, Stovall M, Gilbert E, et al. Risk of salivary gland cancer after childhood cancer: a report from the childhood cancer survivor study. *Int J Radiat Oncol Biol Phys* 2013;85(3):776–783.
13. Inskip P, Sigurdson A, Veiga L, et al. Radiation-related new primary solid cancers in the childhood cancer survivor study: comparative radiation dose response and modification of treatment effects. *Int J Radiat Oncol Biol Phys* 2016;94(4):800–807.
14. Beal K, Singh B, Kraus D, et al. Radiation-induced salivary gland tumors: a report of 18 cases and a review of the literature. *Cancer J* 2003;9:467–471.
15. Horn-Ross P, Ljung B, Morrow M. Environmental factors and the risk of salivary gland cancer. *Epidemiology* 1997;10:414–419.
16. Swanson G, Burns P. Cancer of the salivary gland: workplace risk among women and men. *Ann Epidemiol* 1997;7:369–374.
17. In der Maur C, Klokman W, Van Leeuwen F, et al. Increased risk of breast cancer development after diagnosis of salivary gland tumour. *Eur J Cancer* 2005;41:1311–1315.
18. Megwalu U, Shin E. Second primaries after major salivary gland cancer. *Otolaryngol Head Neck Surg* 2011;145(2):254–258.
19. Pohar S, Gay H, Rosenbaum P, et al. Malignant parotid tumors: Presentation, clinical/pathologic prognostic factors, and treatment outcomes. *Int J Radiat Oncol Biol Phys* 2005;61:112–118.
20. Terhaard C, Lubsen H, Van Der Tweel I, et al. Salivary gland carcinoma: Independent prognostic factors for locoregional control, distant metastases, and overall survival: Results of the Dutch Head and Neck Oncology Cooperative Group. *Head Neck* 2004;26:681–693.
21. Van de Poorten V, Hart A, Vauterin T, et al. Prognostic index for patients with parotid carcinoma. *Cancer* 2009;115:540–550.
22. Bjorndal K, Krogdahl A, Therkildsen M, et al. Salivary gland carcinoma in Denmark 1990–2005: outcome and prognostic factors. Results of the Danish Head and Neck Cancer Group (DAHANCA). *Oral Oncol* 2012;48:179–185.
23. Stennert E, Kisner D, Jungehuelsing M, et al. High incidence of lymph node metastasis in major salivary gland cancer. *Arch Otolaryngol Head Neck Surg* 2003;129:720–723.

FIGURE 46.15. Coronal fat-suppressed contrast-enhanced magnetic resonance image shows a recurrence of squamous cell cancer of the parotid gland after total parotidectomy. The tumor is centered in the left masticator space with perineural spread along the nV3. Retrograde perineural spread of tumor through foramen ovale on the left side. (Courtesy of Dr. F.A. Pameyer, radiologist, University Medical Center Utrecht, Netherlands.)

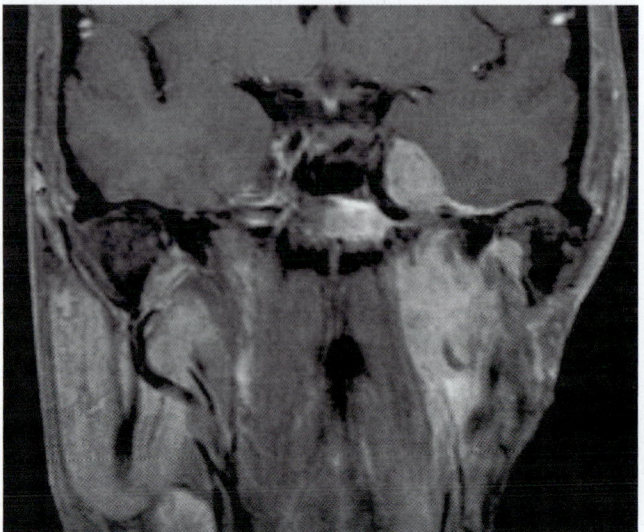

24. Zbären P, Schüpbach J, Nuyens M, et al. Elective neck dissection versus observation in primary parotid carcinoma. *Otolaryngol Head Neck Surg* 2005;132:387–391.
25. Terhaard C, Lubsen H, Rasch C, et al. The role of radiotherapy in the treatment of malignant salivary gland tumors. *Int J Radiat Oncol Biol Phys* 2005;61:103–111.
26. Xiao C, Zhan K, White-Gilbertson SJ, et al. Predictors of nodal metastasis in parotid malignancies: a national cancer data base study of 22,653 patients. *Otolaryngol Head Neck Surg* 2016;154:121–130.
27. Stenner M, Molls C, Luers J. Occurrence of lymph node metastasis in early-stage parotid gland cancer. *Eur Arch Otorhinolaryngol* 2012;269(2):643–648.
28. Lloyd S, Yu J, Ross D, et al. A prognostic index for predicting lymph node metastasis in minor salivary gland cancer. *Int J Radiat Oncol Biol Phys* 2010;76(1):169–175.
29. Lopes M, Santos G, Kowalski L. Multivariate survival analysis of 128 cases of oral cavity minor salivary gland carcinomas. *Head Neck* 1998;20:699–706.
30. Cao C, Zhang X, Luo J, et al. Primary salivary gland-type carcinoma of the nasopharynx: prognostic factors and outcome. *Int J Oral Maxillofac Surg* 2012;41:958–964.
31. Régis de Brito Santos I, Kowalski L, Cavalcante de Araujo V, et al. Multivariate analysis of risk factors for neck metastases in surgically treated parotid carcinoma. *Arch Otolaryngol Head Neck Surg* 2001;127:46–60.
32. Otsaka K, Imanishi Y, Tada Y, et al. Clinical outcomes and prognostic factors for salivary duct carcinoma: a multi-institutional analysis of 141 patients. *Ann Surg Oncol* 2016;23:2038–2045.
33. Spiro RH. Distant metastasis in adenoid cystic carcinoma of salivary origin. *Am J Surg* 1997;174:495–498.
34. Locati L, Guzzo M, Bossi P, et al. Lung metastasectomy in adenoid cystic carcinoma (ACC) of salivary gland. *Oral Oncol* 2005;41:890–894.
35. Bhattacharyya N. Survival and prognosis for cancer of the submandibular gland. *J Oral Maxillofac Surg* 2004;62:427–430.
36. Zeidan Y, Shultz D, Murphy J, et al. Long-term outcomes of surgery followed by radiation therapy for minor salivary gland carcinomas. *Laryngoscope* 2013;123:2675–2680.
37. Beckhardt R, Weber R, Zane R, et al. Minor salivary gland tumors of the palate: Clinical and pathologic correlates of outcome. *Laryngoscope* 1995;105:1155–1160.
38. Sun G, Yang X, Tang E, et al. The treatment of sublingual gland tumours. *Int J Oral Maxillofac Surg* 2010;39:863–868.
39. Buchner A, Merrell P, Carpenter W. Relative frequency of intra-oral minor salivary gland tumors: a study of 380 cases from northern California and comparison to reports from other parts of the world. *J Oral Pathol Med* 2007;36:207–214.
40. Lee Y, Wong K, King A, et al. Imaging of salivary gland tumours. *Eur J Radiol* 2008;66:419–436.
41. Colella G, Cannavale R, Flamminio F, et al. Fine-needle aspiration cytology of salivary gland lesions: a systematic review. *J Oral Maxillofac Surg* 2010;68:2146–2153.
42. Thoeny H. Imaging of salivary gland tumours. *Cancer Imaging* 2007;7:52–62.
43. Habermann C, Arndt C, Graessner J, et al. Diffusion weighted echo-planar MR Imaging of primary parotid gland tumors: is a prediction of different histologic subtypes possible? *Am J Neuroradiol* 2009;30:591–596.
44. Kendi A, Magliocca K, Corey A, et al. Is there a role for PET/CT parameters to characterize benign, malignant, and metastatic parotid tumors? *AJR Am J Roentgenol* 2016;207(3):635–640.
45. Brierley J, Gospodarowicz M, Wittekind C. *TNM classification of malignant tumors*. 8th ed. Wiley-Blackwell, 2017:47–50.
46. Leivo I. Insights into a complex group of neoplastic disease: advances in histopathologic classification and molecular pathology of salivary gland cancer. *Acta Oncol* 2006;45:662–668.
47. Seifert G, Sobin LH. The World Health Organization's histological classification of salivary gland tumors. *Cancer* 1992;70:379–385.
48. Van Der Wal J, Carter L, Klijanienko J, et al. Histological re-evaluation of 101 intraoral salivary gland tumors by an EORTC-study group. *J Oral Pathol Med* 1993;22:21–22.
49. Brandwein M, Ivanov K, Wallace D, et al. Mucoepidermoid carcinoma: a clinicopathologic study of 80 patients with special reference to histological grading. *Am J Surg Pathol* 2001;25:835–845.
50. Storey M, Garden A, Morrison W, et al. Postoperative radiotherapy for malignant tumors of the submandibular gland. *Int J Radiat Oncol Biol Phys* 2001;51:952–958.
51. Coca-Pelaz A, Rudrigo J, Bradley P, et al. Adenoid cystic carcinoma of the head and neck—an update. *Oral Oncol* 2015;51:652–661.
52. Ali S, Palmer F, Katabi N, et al. Long-term local control rates of patients with adenoid cystic carcinoma of the head and neck managed by surgery and postoperative radiation. *Laryngoscope* 2017;127(10):2265–2269.
53. Bjorndal K, Krogdahl A, Therkildsen M, et al. Salivary adenoid cystic carcinoma in Denmark 1990–2005: outcome and independent prognostic factors including the benefit of radiotherapy. Results of the Danish Head and Neck Cancer Group (DAHANCA). *Oral Oncol* 2015;51:1138–1142.
54. Enamorado I, Lakhani R, Korkmaz H, et al. Correlation of histopathological variants, cellular DNA content, and clinical outcome in adenoid cystic carcinoma of the salivary glands. *Otolaryngol Head Neck Surg* 2004;131:646–650.
55. Bhattacharyya N, Fried MP. Determinants of survival in parotid gland carcinoma: a population-based study. *Am J Otolaryngol* 2005;26:39–44.
56. Garden AS, el-Naggar AK, Morrison WH, et al. Postoperative radiotherapy for malignant tumors of the parotid gland. *Int J Radiat Oncol Biol Phys* 1997;37:79–85.
57. Spiro R, Armstrong J, Harrison L, et al. Carcinoma of major salivary glands. *Arch Otolaryngol Head Neck Surg* 1989;115:316–321.
58. Vander Poorten V, Triantafyllou A, Thompson L, et al. Salivary acinic cell carcinoma: reappraisal and update. *Eur Arch Otorhinolaryngol* 2016;273(11):3511–3531.
59. Antony J, Gopalan V, Smith R, et al. Carcinoma ex pleomorphic adenoma: a comprehensive review of clinical, pathological and molecular data. *Head Neck Pathol* 2012;6(1):1–9.
60. Terhaard C, Schroeff M, Schie K. The prognostic role of comorbidity in salivary gland carcinoma. *Cancer* 2008;113(7):1572–1579.
61. Patel T, Vazquez A, Marchiano E, et al. Polymorphous low-grade adenocarcinoma of the head and neck: a population-based study of 460 cases. *Laryngoscope* 2015;125(7):1644–1649.
62. Breinholt H, Aelhakim M, Godballe C, et al. Salivary duct carcinoma: a Danish national study. *J Oral Pathol Med* 2016;45:664–671.
63. Haderlein M, Scherl C, Semrau S, et al. Impact of postoperative radiotherapy and HER2/neu overexpression in salivary duct carcinoma: a monocentric clinicopathologic analysis. *Strahlenther Onkol* 2017;193:961–970.
64. Kuo Y, Weinreb I, Perez-Ordonez B. Low-grade salivary duct carcinoma or low-grade intraductal carcinoma? review of the literature. *Head Neck Pathol* 2013;7(Suppl 1):S59–S67.
65. Seethala R, Barnes E, Hunt L, et al. Epithelial-myoepithelial carcinoma: a review of the clinicopathologic spectrum and immunophenotypic characteristics in 61 tumors of the salivary glands and upper aerodigestive tract. *Am J Surg Pathol* 2007;31:44–57.
66. Kane S, Bagwan I. Myoepithelial carcinoma of the salivary glands. *Arch Otolaryngol Head Neck Surg* 2010;136(7):702–712.
67. Zhan K, Lentsch E. Basal cell adenocarcinoma of the major salivary glands: a population-level study of 509 cases. *Laryngoscope* 2016;126(5):1086–1090.
68. Zhan K, Lentsch E. Oncocytic carcinoma of the major salivary glands: a population-based study of 278 cases. *Head Neck* 2016;38(Suppl 1):E1981–E1986.
69. Cheng-Fu C, Jia-Yuan S, Zhen-Yu H, et al. Clinicopathological characteristics, treatment, and survival outcomes of cystadenocarcinoma of the salivary gland: a population-based study. *Onco Targets Ther* 2016;9:6569–6572.
70. Ide F, Mishima K, Tanaka A, et al. Mucinous adenocarcinoma of minor salivary glands: a high-grade malignancy prone to lymph node metastasis. *Virchows Arch* 2009;454:55–60.
71. Gnepp D. My journey into the world of salivary gland sebaceous neoplasms. *Head Neck Pathol* 2012;6(1):101–110.
72. Skalova A, Gnepp D, Lewis J, et al. Newly described entities in salivary gland pathology. *Am J Surg Pathol* 2017;41:33–47.
73. Skálová A, Stenman G, Simpson R, et al. The role of molecular testing in the differential diagnosis of salivary gland carcinomas. *Am J Surg Pathol* 2018;42:e11–e27.
74. Holtzman A, Morris C, Amdur R, et al. Outcomes after primary or adjuvant radiotherapy for salivary gland carcinoma. *Acta Oncol* 2017;56(3):484–489.
75. Bjørndal K, Krogdahl A, Therskilden H, et al. Salivary gland carcinoma in Denmark 1990–2005: outcome and prognostic factors. Results of the Danish Head and Neck Cancer Group (DAHANCA). *Oral Oncol* 2012;48:179–185.
76. Chen A, Bucci M, Weinberg V, et al. Adenoid cystic carcinoma of the head and neck treated by surgery with or without postoperative radiation therapy: prognostic features of recurrence. *Int J Radiat Oncol Biol Phys* 2006;66(1):152–159.
77. Poulsen M, Pratt G, Kynaston B, et al. Prognostic variables in malignant epithelial tumors of the parotid. *Int J Radiat Oncol Biol Phys* 1992;23:327–330.
78. Li Y, Ju J, Liu X, et al. Nomograms for predicting long-term overall survival and cancer-specific survival in patients with major salivary gland cancer: a population-based study. *Oncotarget* 2017;8:24469–24482.
79. Vander Poorten V, Balm A, Hilgers F, et al. The development of a prognostic score for patients with parotid carcinoma. *Cancer* 1999;85:2057–2067.
80. Kirkbride P, Liu FF, O'Sullivan B, et al. Outcome of curative management of malignant tumors of the parotid gland. *J Otolaryngol* 2001;30:271–279.
81. Lima R, Tavares M, Dias F, et al. Clinical prognostic factors in malignant parotid gland tumors. *Otolaryngol Head Neck Surg* 2005;133:702–708.
82. Schroef M, Terhaard C, Wieringa M, et al. Cytology and histology have limited added value in prognostic models for salivary gland carcinomas. *Oral Oncol* 2010;46(9):662–666.
83. Stenman S, Persson F, Andersson M. Diagnostic and therapeutic implications of new molecular biomarkers in salivary gland cancers. *Oral Oncol* 2014;50:683–690.
84. Hashimoto K, Hayashi R, Mukaigawa T, et al. Concomitant expression of ezrin and HER2 predicts distant metastasis and poor prognosis of patients with salivary gland carcinoma. *Hum Pathol* 2017;63:110–119.
85. Williams M, Roberts D, Kies M, et al. Genetic and expression analysis of HER-2 and EGFR genes in salivary duct carcinoma: empirical and therapeutic significance. *Clin Cancer Res* 2010;16(8):2266–2274.
86. Luukkaa H, Klemi P, Leivo I, et al. Prognostic significance of Ki-67 and p53 as tumor markers in salivary gland malignancies in Finland: an evaluation of 212 cases. *Acta Oncol* 2006;45:669–675.
87. North C, Lee D, Piantadosi S, et al. Carcinoma of the major salivary glands treated by surgery or surgery plus postoperative radiotherapy. *Int J Radiat Oncol Biol Phys* 1990;18:1319–1326.
88. Gallo O, Franchi A, Vittorio Bottai G, et al. Risk factors for distant metastases from carcinoma of the parotid gland. *Cancer* 1997;80:844–851.
89. Hocwald E, Korkmaz H, Yoo G, et al. Prognostic factors in major salivary gland cancer. *Laryngoscope* 2001;111:1434–1439.
90. Rayes H, Dezube A, Bawab I, et al. Tumor differentiation as a prognostic factor for major salivary gland malignancies. *Otolaryngol Head Neck Surg* 2017;157(3):454–461.
91. Barrett A, Speight P. Perineural invasion in adenoid cystic carcinoma of the salivary glands: a valid prognostic indicator? *Oral Oncol* 2009;45:936–940.
92. Amit M, Binenbaum Y, Trejo-Leider L, et al. International collaborative validation of intraneural invasion as a prognostic marker in adenoid cystic carcinoma of the head and neck. *Head Neck* 2015;37(7):1038–1045.
93. Chen A, Granchi P, Garcia J, et al. Local-Regional recurrence after surgery without postoperative irradiation for carcinomas of the major salivary glands: implications for adjuvant therapy. *Int J Radiat Oncol Biol Phys* 2007;67(4):982–987.

94. Renehan A, Gleave E, Slevin N, et al. Clinico-pathological and treatment-related factors influencing survival in parotid cancer. *Br J Cancer* 1999;80:1296–1300.

95. Chen A, Garcia J, Bucci K, The role of postoperative radiation therapy in carcinoma ex pleomorphic adenoma of the parotid gland. *Int J Radiat Oncol Biol Phys* 2007;67(1):138–143.

96. Bakst R, Su W, Ozbek U, et al. Adjuvant radiation for salivary gland malignancies is associated with improved survival: a National Cancer Database analysis. *Adv Radiat Oncol* 2017;2:159–166.

97. Lee A, Babak G, Osborn V, et al. Patterns of care and survival of adjuvant radiation for major salivary adenoid cystic carcinoma. *Laryngoscope* 2017;127(9):2057–2062.

98. Armstrong J, Harrison L, Spiro R, et al. Malignant tumors of major salivary gland origin. A matched pair analysis of the role of combined surgery and postoperative radiotherapy. *Arch Otolaryngol Head Neck Surg* 1990;116:290–293.

99. Baddour H, Fedewa S, Chen A. Five and 10-year cause specific survival rates in carcinoma of the minor salivary gland. *JAMA Otolaryngol Head Neck Surg* 2016;142(1):67–73.

99a. Parsons JT, Mendenhall WM, Stringer SP, et al. Management of minor salivary gland carcinomas. *Int J Radiat Oncol Biol Phys* 1996;35:443–454.

100. Chen A, Garcia J, Lee N, et al. Patterns of nodal relapse after surgery and postoperative radiation therapy for carcinomas of the major and minor salivary glands: what is the role of elective neck irradiation? *Int J Radiat Oncol Biol Phys* 2007;67(4):988–994.

101. Amini A, Waxweiler V, Brower J, et al. Association of adjuvant chemoradiotherapy vs. radiotherapy alone with survival in patients with resected major salivary gland carcinoma. Data from the national cancer data base. *JAMA Otolaryngol Head Neck Surg* 2016;142:1100–1110.

102. Gebbhardt B, Ohr J, Ferris R, et al. Concurrent chemoradiotherapy in the adjuvant treatment of high-risk primary salivary gland malignancies. *Am J Clin Oncol* 2017; in press.

103. Stannard C, Vernimmen F, Carrar H, et al. Malignant salivary gland tumors: can fast neutron therapy results point the way to carbon ion therapy? *Radiother Oncol* 2013;109:262–268.

104. Laramore G, Krall J, Griffin T, et al. Neutron versus photon irradiation for unresectable salivary gland tumors: final report of an RTOG-MRC randomized clinical trial. *Int J Radiat Oncol Biol Phys* 1993;27:235–240.

105. Orlandi E, Iacovelli N, Bonora M, et al. Salivary gland. Photon therapy and particle therapy: present and future. *Oral Oncol* 2016;60:146–156.

106. Tagaki M, Demizu Y, Hashimoto N, et al. Treatment outcomes of particle therapy using protons or carbon ions as a single-modality therapy for adenoid cystic carcinoma of the head and neck. *Radiother Oncol* 2014;113:364–370.

107. Sood S, Ncgurk M, Vaz F. Management of salivary gland tumours: United Kingdom national multidisciplinary guidelines. *J Laryngol Otol* 2016;130(Suppl S2):142–149.

108. Brown P, Eshleman J, Foote R, et al. An analysis of facial nerve function in irradiated and unirradiated facial nerve grafts. *Int J Radiat Oncol Biol Phys* 2000;48:737–743.

109. Ferlito A, Pellitteri P, Robbins T, et al. Management of the neck in cancer of the major salivary glands, thyroid and parathyroid glands. *Acta Otolaryngol* 2002;122:673–678.

110. Klussmann J, Ponert T, Mueller R, et al. Patterns of lymph node spread and its influence on outcome in respectable parotid cancer. *Eur J Surg Oncol* 2008;34:932–937.

111. Chisholm E, Elmiyeh B, Dwivedi R, et al. Anatomic distribution of cervical lymph node spread in parotid carcinoma. *Head Neck* 2011;33:513–515.

112. Garden A, Weber R, Ang K, et al. Postoperative radiation therapy for malignant tumors of minor salivary glands. Outcome and patterns of failure. *Cancer* 1994;73:2563–2569.

113. Suarez C, Barnes L, Silver C, et al. Cervical lymph node metastasis in adenoid cystic carcinoma of oral cavity and oropharynx: a collective international review. *Auris Nasus Larynx* 2016;43:477–484.

114. Dulguerov P, Todic J, Pusztaszeri M, et al. Why do parotid pleomorphic adenomas recur? A systematic review of pathological and surgical variables. *Front Surg* 2017;(4):1–7.

115. Andreasen S, Therskilden M, Bjorndal K, et al. Pleomorphic adenoma of the parotid gland 1985–2010: a Danish nationwide study of incidence, recurrence rate, and malignant transformation. *Head Neck* 2016;38:1364–1369.

116. Valstar M, de Ridder M, van den Broek E, et al. Salivary gland pleomorphic adenoma in the Netherlands: a nationwide observational study of primary tumor incidence, malignant transformation, recurrence, and risk factors for recurrence. *Oral Oncol* 2017;66:93–99.

117. Nohr A, Andreasen S, Therskilden M, et al. Stationary facial nerve paresis after surgery for recurrent parotid pleomorphic adenoma: a follow-up study of 219 cases in Denmark in the period 1985–2012. *Head Neck* 2016;273:3313–3319.

118. Witt R, Eisele D, Morton R, et al. Etiology and management of recurrent parotid pleomorphic adenoma. Contemporary review. *Laryngoscope* 2014;125:888–893.

119. Renehan A, Gleave E, Mc Gurk M. An analysis of the treatment of 114 patients with recurrent pleomorphic adenomas of the parotid gland. *Am J Surg* 1996;172:710–714.

120. Nutting C, Rowbottom C, Cosgrove V, et al. Optimisation of radiotherapy for carcinoma of the parotid gland: a comparison of conventional, three-dimensional conformal, and intensity-modulated techniques. *Radiother Oncol* 2001;60:163–172.

121. Chen A, Garcia J, Granchi P, et al. Base of skull recurrences after treatment of salivary gland cancer with perineural invasion reduced by postoperative radiotherapy. *Clin Otolaryngol* 2009;34:539–545.

122. Lombardi D, Mc Gurk M, Vander Poorten V, et al. Surgical treatment of salivary malignant tumors. *Oral Oncol* 2017;65:102–113.

123. Yaparpalvi R, Fontenla D, Tyerech S, et al. Parotid gland tumors: A comparison of postoperative radiotherapy techniques using three dimensional (3D) dose distributions and dose-volume histograms (DVHS). *Int J Radiat Oncol Biol Phys* 1998;40:43–49.

124. Jereczek-Fossa B, Rondi E, Zarowski A, et al. Prospective study on the dose distribution to the acoustic structures during postoperative 3D conformal radiotherapy for parotid tumors. *Strahlenther Onkol* 2011;187:350–356.

125. Bragg C, Conway J, Robinson M. The role of intensity-modulated radiotherapy in the treatment of parotid tumors. *Int J Radiat Oncol Biol Phys* 2002;52:729–738.

126. Van der Putten L, De Bree R, Plukker J, et al. Permanent unilateral hearing loss after radiotherapy for parotid gland tumors. *Head Neck* 2006;28:902–908.

127. Pan C, Eisbruch A, Lee J, et al. Prospective study of inner ear radiation dose and hearing loss in head-and-neck cancer patients. *Int J Radiat Oncol Biol Phys* 2005;61(5):1393–1402.

128. Lamers-Kuijper E, Schwarz M, Rasch C, et al. Intensity-modulated vs Conformal radiotherapy of parotid gland tumors: potential impact on hearing loss. *Med Dosim* 2007;32(4):237–245.

129. Mallik S, Agarwal J, Gupta T, et al. Prognostic factors and outcome analysis of submandibular gland cancer: a clinical audit. *J Oral Maxillofac Surg* 2010;68:2104–2110.

130. Andreasen S, Bjorndal K, Agander T, et al. Tumors of the sublingual gland: a national clinicopathologic study. *Eur Arch Otorhinolaryngol* 2016;273:3847–3856.

131. Claus F, De Gersem W, De Wagter C, et al. An implementation of strategy for IMRT of ethmoid sinus cancer with bilateral sparing of the optic pathways. *Int J Radiat Oncol Biol Phys* 2001;51:18–31.

132. Salgado L, Spratt D, Riaz N, et al. Radiation therapy in the treatment of minor salivary gland tumors. *Am J Clin Oncol* 2014;37(5):492–497.

133. Cho J, Lim B, Kim E, et al. Low grade salivary gland cancers: treatment outcomes, extent of surgery and indications for postoperative adjuvant radiation therapy. *Ann Surg Oncol* 2016;25:4368–4375.

134. Chen A, Bucci M, Quivey J, et al. Long-term outcome of patients treated by radiation therapy alone for salivary gland carcinomas. *Int J Radiat Oncol Biol Phys* 2006;66(4):1044–1050.

135. Douglas J, Goodkind R, Laramore G. Gamma knife stereotactic radiosurgery for salivary gland neoplasms with base of skull invasion following neutron radiotherapy. *Head Neck* 2008;30:492–496.

136. Jensen A, Poulakis M, Nikoghosyan A. et al. High-LET radiotherapy for adenoid cystic carcinoma of the head and neck: 15 years' experience with raster-scanned carbon-ion therapy. *Radiother Oncol* 2016;118:272–280.

137. Jensen A, Nikoghosyan A, Poulakis M, et al. Combined intensity modulated radiotherapy pus raster-scanned carbon ion boost for advanced adenoid cystic carcinoma of the head and neck results in superior locoregional control and overall survival. *Cancer* 2015;121:3001–3009.

138. Grant S, Grosshans D, Bilton S, et al. Proton versus conventional radiotherapy for pediatric salivary gland tumors: acute toxicity and dosimetric characteristics. *Radiother Oncol* 2015;116:309–315.

139. Pederson A, Salama J, Haraf D, et al. Adjuvant chemoradiotherapy for locoregionally advanced and high-risk salivary gland malignancies. *Head Neck Oncol* 2011;3:31.

140. Tanvetyanon T, Zin D, Padhya T. Outcomes of postoperative concurrent chemoradiotherapy for locally advanced major salivary gland carcinoma. *Head Neck Surg* 2009;135(7):687–692.

141. Cerda T, Sun X, Vignot S, et al. A rationale for chemoradiation (vs. radiotherapy) in salivary gland cancers? on behalf of the REFCOR (French rare head and neck cancer network). *Crit Rev Oncol Hematol* 2014;91:142–158.

142. Laurie S, Siu L, Winquist E, et al. A phase 2 study of platinum and gemcitabine in patients with advanced salivary gland cancer. A trial of the NCIC clinical trial group. *Cancer* 2010;116:362–368.

143. Airoldi M, Garzaro M, Pedani F, et al. Cisplatin and Vinorelbine treatment of recurrent or metastatic salivary gland malignancies (RMSGM). A final report on 60 cases. *Am J Clin Oncol* 2017;40:86–90.

144. Laurie S, Ho A, Fury M, et al. Systemic therapy in the management of metastatic or locally recurrent adenoid cystic carcinoma of the salivary glands: a systematic review. *Lancet Oncol* 2011;12:815–824.

145. Locati L, Perrone F, Loca M, et al. Treatment relevant target immunophenotyping of 139 salivary gland carcinomas (SGCs). *Oral Oncol* 2009;45:986–990.

146. Locati L, Perrone F, Cortelazzi B, et al. Clinical activity of androgen deprivation therapy in patients with metastatic/relapsed androgen receptor-positive salivary gland cancers. *Head Neck* 2016;38:724–731.

147. Keller G, Steinmann D, Quaas A, et al. New concepts of personalized therapy in salivary gland carcinomas. *Oral Oncol* 2017;69:103–113.

148. Bhide S, Harrington K, Nutting C. Otological toxicity after postoperative radiotherapy for parotid tumors. *Clin Oncol* 2006;19:77–82.

149. Jiang G, Tucker S, Guttenberger R, et al. Radiation-induced injury to the visual pathway. *Radiother Oncol* 1994;30:17–25.

150. Dijkema T, Raaijmakers C, Ten Haken R, et al. Parotid gland function after radiotherapy: the combined Michigan and Utrecht experience. *Int J Radiat Oncol Biol Phys* 2010;78(2):449–453.

151. Nutting C, Morden J, Harrington K, et al. Parotid-sparing intensity modulated versus conventional radiotherapy in head and neck cancer (PARSPORT): a phase 3 multicentre randomised controlled trial. *Lancet Oncol* 2011;12(2):127–136.

152. Al-Mamgani A, van Rooij P, Verduijn G, et al. Long-term outcomes and quality of life of 186 patients with primary parotid carcinoma treated with surgery and radiotherapy at the Daniel den Hoed cancer center. *Int J Radiat Oncol Biol Phys* 2012;84:189–195.

153. Langendijk J, Lambin P, De Ruysscher D, et al. Selection of patients for radiotherapy with protons aiming at reduction of side effects: the model-based approach. *Radiother Oncol* 2013;107(3):267–273.

154. Karam S, Snider J, Wang H, et al. Reirradiation of recurrent salivary gland malignancies with fractionated stereotactic body radiation therapy. *J Radiat Oncol* 2012;1:147–153.

155. Erovic B, Schopper C, Pammer J, et al. Multimodal treatment of patients with minor salivary gland cancer in the case of recurrent disease. *Head Neck* 2010;32:1167–1172.

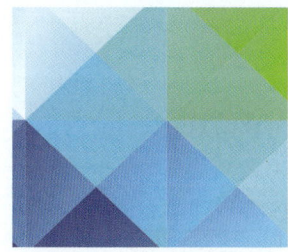

CHAPTER 47

Oral Cavity

Rafael R. Mañon, Jeffrey N. Myers, and Paul M. Harari

GENERAL PRINCIPLES

Squamous cell carcinoma of the lip and oral cavity is primarily a surgical disease. This is reflected by evidence-based practice guidelines in oncology published by the National Comprehensive Cancer Network (NCCN) that provide two clinical pathways for the management of oral cavity and lip squamous cell carcinoma: one pathway for early-stage disease and another for locally advanced disease. The NCCN guidelines recommend surgery as the preferred treatment approach for early-stage T1 or T2N0 lesions of the oral cavity or lip (Fig. 47.1).[1] For more advanced disease (T3/T4a, N0 or T1/T4a, N1/N3), NCCN guidelines recommend a combined modality approach involving surgery followed by adjuvant radiation or chemoradiation (Fig. 47.2). The functional outcomes after primary surgical management are acceptable due to advances in microvascular reconstruction techniques. Thus, particularly for oral cavity carcinoma, organ preservation approaches using primary radiotherapy have largely grown out of favor in North America. Nevertheless, definitive radiotherapy may be a treatment option for patients who are not candidates for surgery because of medical reasons or who refuse surgery.[1] A multidisciplinary approach is paramount in the evaluation and management of patients with oral cavity cancer. A team of health care providers including head and neck surgical oncology, radiation and medical oncology, plastic surgery, nursing, dentistry, dietary, speech pathology, and social work should evaluate the patient before treatment is delivered. Multidisciplinary evaluation prior to treatment disposition helps to ensure that broad consensus treatment recommendations are made and interdisciplinary coordination of care is facilitated. Once treatment has been completed, the multidisciplinary team should provide follow-up to the patient to ensure early detection of recurrent disease and adequate management of treatment sequelae.[1]

INCIDENCE, EPIDEMIOLOGY, AND ETIOLOGY

Oral cancer represents the most common noncutaneous malignancy of the head and neck.[2] Surveillance, Epidemiology, and End Results (SEER) program data estimate 49,670 new cases of cancer of the oral cavity and pharynx and 9,700 deaths for 2017.[3] The incidence rate of oral cancer continues to be more than twice as high in men than in women.[4] The estimated 5-year survival for all stages is 64.5%, whereas survival for cancer localized to the primary site is 83.7%.[3] According to American Cancer Society statistics, mortality rates from carcinoma of the oral cavity and pharynx have been stable in the United States from 2005 to 2014.[4]

Global estimates suggest 300,373 new cases of oral cancer and 145,000 deaths in 2012.[2,5] Worldwide age-standardized mortality estimates for lip and oral cavity cancer were 2.7 per 100,000 during the same year.[2,5] International Agency for Research on Cancer data indicate that the highest rates of oral cancer are found in Melanesia, South-Central Asia,

and Eastern Europe, whereas the lowest rates are in Western Africa and Eastern Asia.[5] The incidence of oral cavity cancer seems to be decreasing in many parts of the world, which parallels regional declines in the tobacco epidemic.[6]

The epidemiology of oral cancer strongly reflects exposure to certain environmental agents, particularly tobacco and alcohol. Smoking is identified as an independent risk factor in 80% to 90% of patients who present with cancer of the oral cavity.[7-9] Tobacco users have a 5-fold to 25-fold higher risk of oral cavity and oropharyngeal cancer.[10] Cessation of smoking is associated with a decline in the risk of cancer of the oral cavity.[9] In India, the habit of chewing betel nut leaves rolled with lime and tobacco (mixture known as "pan"), which results in prolonged carcinogen exposure to the oral mucosa, is thought to be the leading cause of oral cancer.[11,12] The combined use of alcohol and tobacco may have a synergistic effect on carcinogenesis.[10] International Head and Neck Epidemiology Consortium (INHANCE) pooled analysis data demonstrate a greater than multiplicative joint effect between tobacco and alcohol on head and neck cancer risk, which is most pronounced in carcinoma of the pharynx and oral cavity.[13]

Ultraviolet radiation has been associated with carcinoma of the lip. In geographic regions where there are long daily periods of sun exposure, cancer of the lip may represent up to 60% of all cancers of the oral cavity. The relationship between HPV and oropharyngeal cancer has been well established.[14,15] However, oral cavity carcinoma, unlike oropharyngeal carcinoma, does not appear to be typically associated with HPV.[16] Certain syndromes such as xeroderma pigmentosum, Li-Fraumeni, ataxia telangiectasia, Bloom syndrome, and Fanconi anemia, because of inherent genetic instability, have been associated with a predisposition to oral cancer.[17,18]

Overall, there has been a declining trend in the overall incidence of oral cavity squamous cell carcinoma over the past 30 years. However, SEER data suggest an increasing incidence of oral tongue carcinoma in young white individuals ages 18 to 44, which is most pronounced among young white women.[16,19] Past reports suggest that oral tongue carcinoma in this population is associated with a worse prognosis. Recent matched-control studies and national database reviews suggest that outcomes are similar to that in other demographics of oral cancer patients.[16,19] This young population of patients does not seem to have the traditional risk factors of tobacco and alcohol abuse. The increasing incidence of oral tongue carcinoma in young individuals is unlikely due to an HPV-related etiology and may represent a unique and emerging oral cancer patient population.[16]

In patients with cancer of the oral cavity, the risk of developing a second primary cancer is well recognized. Second primary cancers have an adverse effect on prognosis and are the major cause of treatment failure in patients with early-stage disease.[20,21] In an analysis of 851 patients with squamous cell carcinoma of the head and neck, 19% of the study population developed a secondary head and neck carcinoma 5 years after undergoing initial therapy.[21] The probability of developing a second metachronous malignancy at 5 years was 22% (18% for the subset of patients with oral cavity cancer).[21]

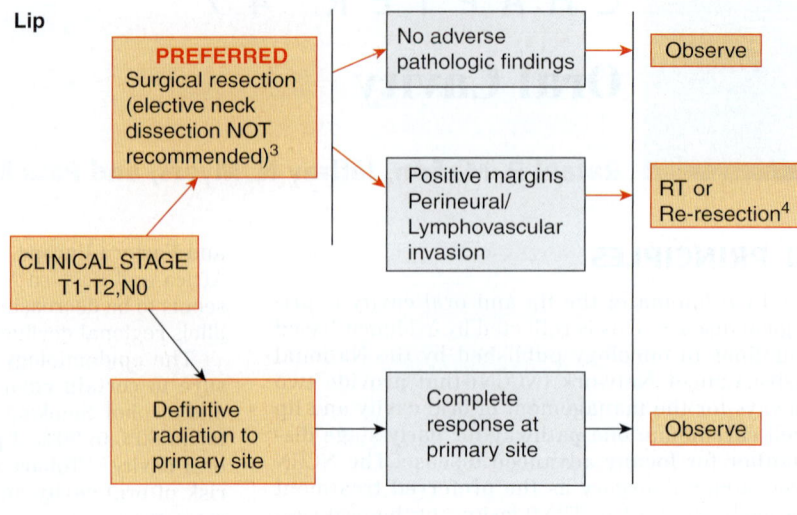

A

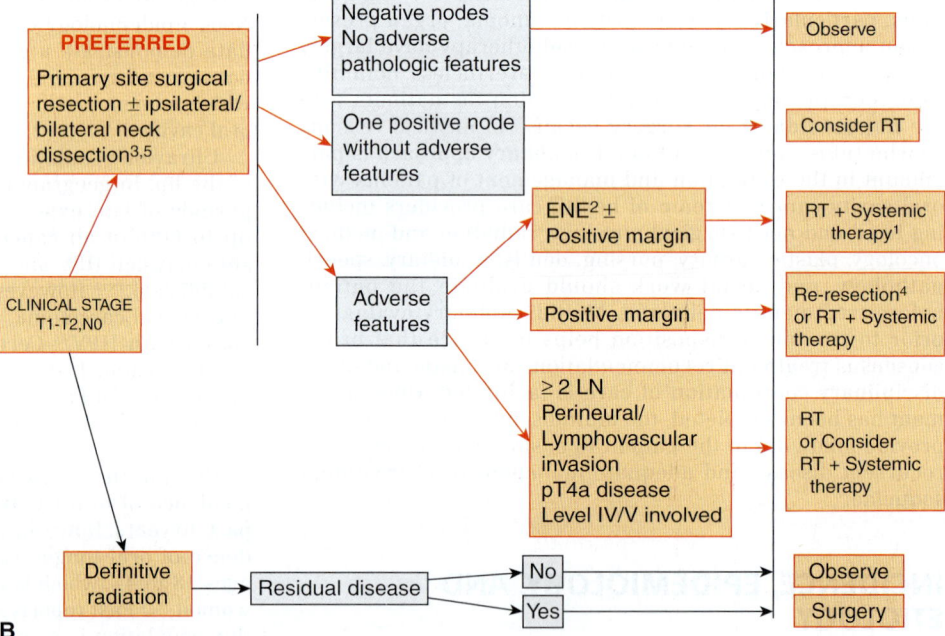

Oral tongue, floor of mouth, buccal mucosa, hard palate, alveolar ridge, retromolar trigone

B

FIGURE 47.1. This treatment algorithm is based on NCCN Guidelines Version 1.2017. **A:** Guidelines for the management of early-stage carcinoma of the lip. **B:** Guidelines for the management of early-stage carcinoma of theoral tongue, floor of mouth, buccal mucosa, hard palate, alveolar ridge, and retromolar trigone.[1] This recommendation is based upon high-level evidence and uniform NCCN consensus.[2] The acronym "ENE" stands for extranodal extension.[3] Resection of the primary site with sentinel lymph node biopsy is a treatment option.[4] In the event of a positive margin, consider reresection to achieve negative margins.[5] Tumor thickness and location of the primary drive the decision to perform a neck dissection, please refer to the section "Surgical Management of the Neck" in this chapter for details.

Quitting tobacco and alcohol use greatly reduces the risk of developing subsequent head and neck squamous cell carcinoma. Individuals that have stopped smoking for 1 to 4 years have a 30% decrease in risk of developing carcinoma of the head and neck compared to those that continue to smoke. For those that quit smoking beyond 20 years, the risk parallels that of never smokers; a similar effect is seen with stopping the use of alcohol.[22] Several chemoprevention strategies have been explored in patients who are at high risk of developing second primary cancer. These strategies include retinoids, COX2 inhibitors, EGFR inhibitors, thiazolidinediones, and green tea polyphenols.[2,22] There is no intervention that can be considered standard of care to date. Therefore, continued efforts toward tobacco and alcohol cessation are a central strategy in the management of patients with oral squamous cell carcinoma.[1,22]

ANATOMY

The oral cavity consists of the lips, oral tongue, floor of the mouth, retromolar trigone, alveolar ridge, buccal mucosa, and hard palate (Figs. 47.3–47.5). The anterior boundary of the oral cavity is the skin–vermilion junction. The superior portion of the oral cavity extends posteriorly to the junction between the hard and soft palate, whereas the inferior

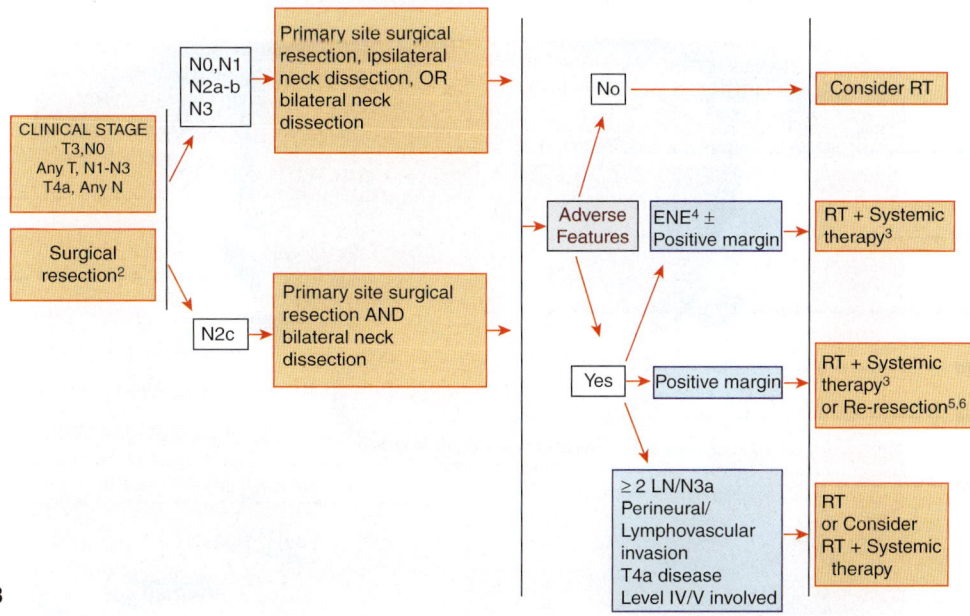

Section III

FIGURE 47.2. This treatment algorithm is based on NCCN Guidelines Version 1.2017. **A:** Guidelines for the management of locally/regionally advanced carcinoma of the lip. **B:** NCCN Guidelines for the management of locally/regionally advanced carcinoma of the oral tongue, floor of mouth, buccal mucosa, hard palate, alveolar ridge, and retromolar trigone.[1] Although surgery is the preferred initial treatment, radiation therapy is an option for local control. In the event of primary radiation, the patient will need to undergo response assessment and be evaluated for salvage surgery in the event of incomplete response to therapy.[2] For this population of patients, enrollment clinical trials involving multimodality treatment is an option.[3] This recommendation is based upon high-level evidence and uniform NCCN consensus.[4] The acronym "ENE" stands for extranodal extension.[5] In the event of a positive margin, consider reresection to achieve negative margins.[6] If negative margins are achieved after reresection, consider adjuvant radiation.

portion extends to the circumvallate papillae. The specific anatomic subsites of this region are noted below.

Lip

The lips begin at the junction of the vermilion border with the skin and form the anterior aspect of the oral vestibule. The lips are comprised of the vermilion surface, which is the portion of the lip that comes in contact with the opposing lip. The lips are well defined into an upper and lower. The primary motor control of the lips is provided by the buccal and mandibular branches of the facial nerve.

Oral Tongue

The anterior two-thirds of the tongue is mobile and considered part of the oral cavity. The oral tongue extends anteriorly from the circumvallate papillae to the undersurface of the tongue at the junction of the floor of the mouth. The fibrous septum divides the tongue into right and left halves. The oral tongue can be demarcated into four anatomic areas: the tip, lateral borders, dorsal surface, and undersurface (ventral surface). There are six pairs of muscles that form the oral tongue. Three of these muscles are extrinsic, whereas the other three are intrinsic. The extrinsic muscles include the genioglossus,

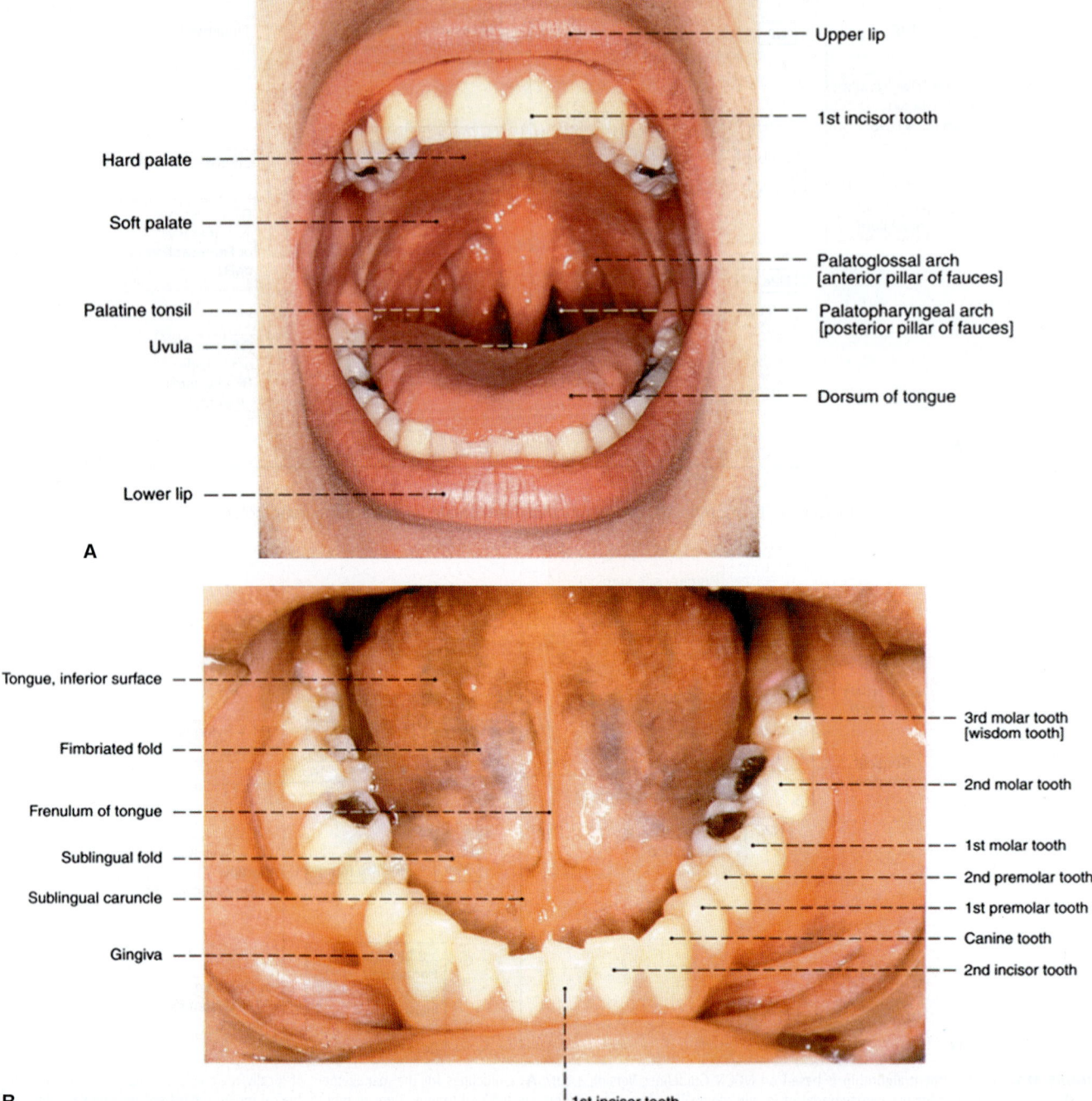

FIGURE 47.3. A: Oral cavity surface anatomy. **B:** Floor of the mouth surface anatomy. (Reprinted from Paulsen F, Waschke J, Sobotta J. *Sobotta Atlas of Human Anatomy.* 15th ed. Munich: Urban & Fischer, 2011. Copyright © 2011 Elsevier GmbH. With permission.)

hyoglossus, and styloglossus. The intrinsic muscles include the lingual, vertical, and transverse muscles. The former primarily move the body of the tongue, whereas the latter alter the shape and conformation of the tongue during speech and swallowing. The blood supply to the tongue is primarily via the lingual artery, tonsillar branch of the facial artery, and the ascending pharyngeal artery with primary drainage by the internal jugular vein. General sensation of the anterior two-thirds of the tongue is supplied by the lingual nerve. Excluding the circumvallate papillae, taste fibers from the anterior two-thirds of the tongue run in the chorda tympani branch of the facial nerve; the glossopharyngeal nerve provides sensation and taste to the posterior third of the tongue and circumvallate papillae.

Floor of the Mouth

The floor of the mouth is a semilunar space extending from the lower alveolar ridge to the undersurface of the tongue. The floor of the mouth overlies the mylohyoid and hyoglossus muscles. The posterior boundary of the floor of the mouth is the base of the anterior tonsillar pillar. This region is divided into right and left by the frenulum of the tongue and contains the ostia of the submandibular and sublingual salivary glands. A sling formed by the mylohyoid muscles medially supports the anterior floor of the mouth, and the hyoglossus supports the posterior floor of the mouth. The lingual and hypoglossal nerves are lateral to the hyoglossus, whereas the lingual artery is medial to the hyoglossus. Innervation of the floor of the mouth is provided by the lingual nerve.

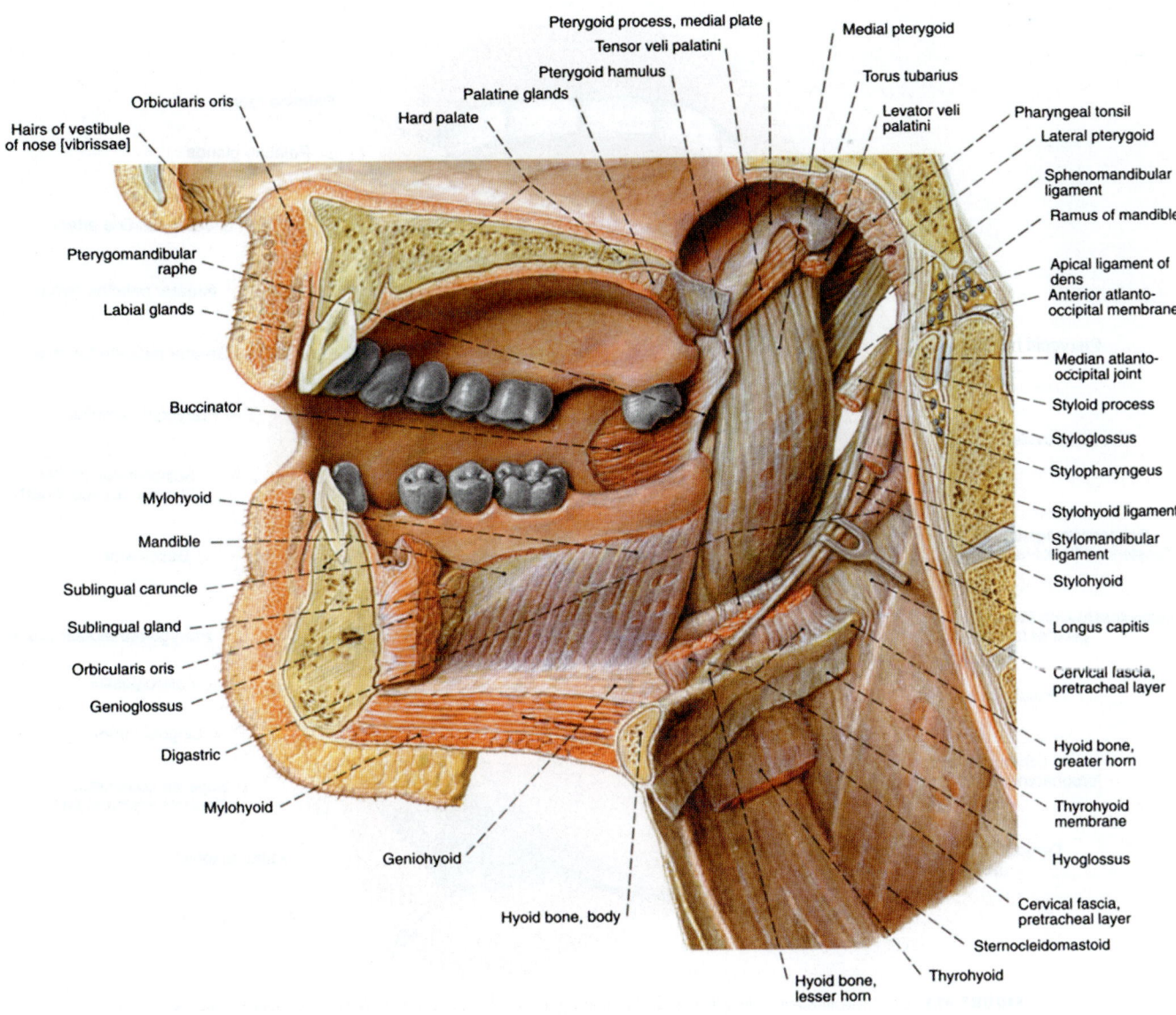

FIGURE 47.4. Oral cavity; paramedian section depicting regional anatomy. (Reprinted from Paulsen F, Waschke J, Sobotta J. *Sobotta Atlas of Human Anatomy*. 15th ed. Munich: Urban & Fischer, 2011. Copyright © 2011 Elsevier GmbH. With permission.)

Hard Palate

The hard palate extends from the inner surface of the superior alveolar ridge to the posterior edge of the palatine bone. This is a semilunar area between the superior alveolar ridge and the mucous membrane covering the palatine process of the maxillary palatine bones.

Alveolar Ridge

The alveolar ridges include the alveolar processes of the maxilla and mandible and the overlying mucosa. The mucosal covering of the lower alveolar ridge extends from the line of attachment of mucosa in the buccal gutter to the line of free mucosa of the floor of the mouth. The lower alveolar ridge extends to the ascending ramus of the mandible posteriorly. The superior alveolar ridge mucosa extends from the line of attachment of mucosa in the upper gingival buccal gutter to the junction of the hard palate. The posterior margin is the upper end of the pterygopalatine arch.

Retromolar Trigone

The retromolar trigone is the triangular area overlying the ascending ramus of the mandible. The base of the triangle is formed by the posterior most molar, and the apex lies at the maxillary tuberosity.

Buccal Mucosa

The buccal mucosa includes the mucosal surfaces of the cheek and lips from the line of contact of the opposing lips to the pterygomandibular raphe posteriorly. This extends to the line of attachment of the mucosa of the upper and lower alveolar ridge superiorly and inferiorly. Innervation is supplied by the buccal nerve, a branch of the mandibular nerve.

Nodal Levels

The neck is traditionally divided into five primary nodal levels (i.e., levels I–V) plus the retropharyngeal nodes that are relevant to the staging and management of oral cavity carcinoma. The level VI nodal station will not be discussed in this section because it is rarely pertinent for oral cavity cancer. The classification of neck nodal regions, initially popularized by Robbins et al.,[23] has served as a surgical reference system based on visible landmarks. Over the years, there have been several revisions regarding proposed boundaries of nodal stations in the neck, with refinements to include radiologic landmarks.[24,25] Gregoire et al.[26,27] published consensus guidelines

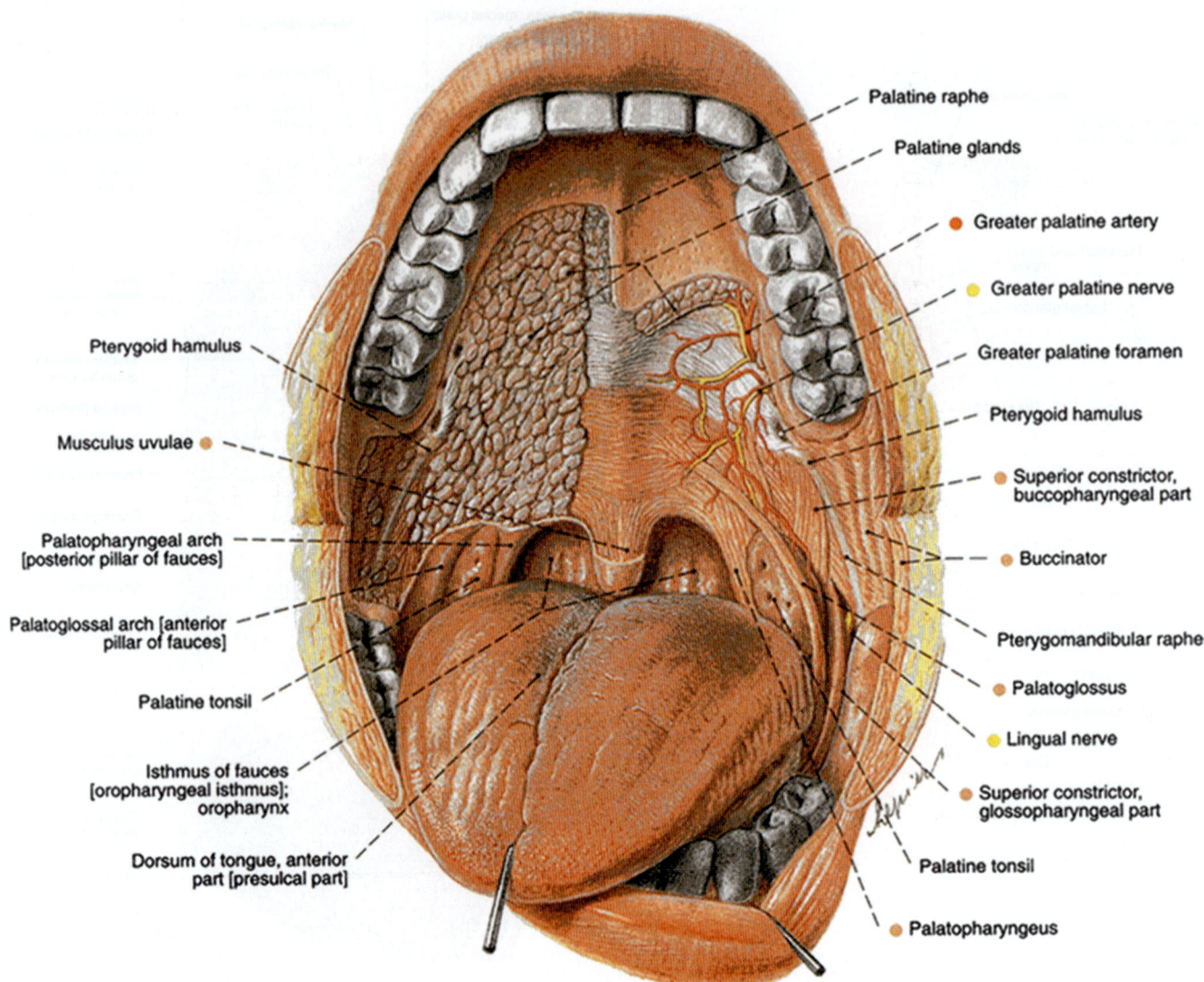

FIGURE 47.5. Oral cavity illustration depicting regional anatomy. (Reprinted from Paulsen F, Waschke J, Sobotta J. *Sobotta Atlas of Human Anatomy*. 15th ed. Munich: Urban & Fischer, 2011. Copyright © 2011 Elsevier GmbH. With permission.)

for the CT-based delineation of nodal levels in the node-negative neck that were revised in 2014 to serve as a guide in the practice of radiation oncology. In the following discussion, we incorporate radiographic landmarks and anatomic considerations from these guidelines (where relevant) along-side traditional surgical anatomic landmarks.

Level I

Level I includes the submental (Ia) and submandibular (Ib) triangles. Level Ia is limited anteriorly by the mandibular symphysis, posteriorly by the body of the hyoid bone, and cranially by the geniohyoid muscle. The medial border is virtual because this region continues to the contralateral Ia station. Level Ib is located within the space bounded by the inner table of the mandible laterally, the digastric muscle medially, the mandibular symphysis anteriorly, and the submandibular gland posteriorly.

Level II

Level II includes the upper jugular chain lymph nodes from the base of the skull to the carotid bifurcation (surgical landmark) or the caudal body of the hyoid bone (clinical landmark); this nodal station extends from the posterior edge of the submandibular gland anteriorly to the posterior border of the sternocleidomastoid posteriorly. The level II nodal region is further subdivided into IIa and IIb. The vertical plane defined by the spinal accessory nerve (surgical landmark) or the posterior edge of the internal jugular vein (radiographic landmark) defines each the subdivision within this level; level IIa lies anterior, whereas IIb lies posterior to this plane.

Robbins et al.[23] initially defined the cranial limit of level II as the base of the skull.[23] However, from a practical standpoint, during surgical management of the neck, the cranial border of level II is taken as the insertion of the posterior belly of the digastric into the mastoid.[27] It was later proposed that the bottom edge of C1 serve as the radiographic landmark for defining the cranial border of level II in the node-negative neck.[27] Consequently, the retrostyloid space is considered the cranial continuation of level II from C1 to the skull base.[26,27]

Level III

Level III is the caudal extension of level II. It includes the midjugular nodes, of which the surgical landmarks extend from the carotid bifurcation to the omohyoid muscle inferiorly, the sternohyoid medially, and the posterior aspect of the sternocleidomastoid posteriorly. The corresponding radiographic landmarks are the caudal edge of the hyoid bone superiorly and the caudal edge of the cricoid cartilage inferiorly.

Level IV

Level IV includes the inferior jugular nodes located around the inferior third of the internal jugular vein. Level IV is bounded by the omohyoid muscle superiorly, the clavicle inferiorly, and the posterior aspect of the sternocleidomastoid posteriorly.

Level V

Level V includes nodes in the posterior triangle, which are located posterior to the sternocleidomastoid muscle. This space is bordered by the base of the skull superiorly, clavicle inferiorly, and posterior aspect of the sternocleidomastoid anteriorly. The uppermost part of level V is generally thought to belong to the occipital nodal region.[26] Therefore, from a practical standpoint, the radiographic cranial border of level V has been accepted as a horizontal plane crossing the cranial edge of the hyoid bone.[27] From a surgical perspective, level V is further subdivided into Va and Vb, and the caudal edge of the cricoid arch is the anatomic landmark denoting this subdivision (Vb lies below this boundary).

Retropharyngeal Nodes

The retropharyngeal space, which contains the retropharyngeal nodes, extends from the skull base (cranially) to the hyoid bone (caudally). The anterior boundary of the retropharyngeal space is the pharyngeal constrictor muscles and the posterior boundary is the prevertebral fascia. The retropharyngeal nodes are further divided into medial and lateral groups. The lateral retropharyngeal nodes lie medial to the carotid artery and lateral to the longus capitis and longus coli muscles, whereas the medial group consists of one or two nodes intercalated along the midline lymphatics.

MOLECULAR BIOLOGY

In parallel to the Fearon and Vogelstein model describing the genetic basis of colon cancer,[28] there are a series of specific genetic events that precede the development of oral squamous cell carcinoma.[29,30] Cancer progression models describe several steps that occur during tumor development: oncogenes become activated and tumor suppressor genes become deactivated, and a series of these alterations are required for carcinogenesis. In the oral mucosa, this genetic progression is reflected histologically by the transformation from normal mucosa to dysplastic epithelium and ultimately to frankly invasive squamous cell carcinoma. Data to support this model come from studies that reveal genetic alterations in histologically normal tissues and in premalignant lesions, including loss of heterozygosity at chromosomes 3p14 and 9p21. Furthermore, mutations in the region of chromosome 17p13, which encompasses the tumor suppressor gene *TP53*, are among early events that contribute to malignant transformation. Indeed, biopsies of normal mucosa from patients with upper aerodigestive tract carcinomas frequently harbor *TP53* mutations.

Comprehensive studies of whole-genome sequencing, gene copy number analysis, and mRNA and protein expression of head and neck squamous cell carcinoma have been performed and have helped to provide an unbiased characterization of the genomic alterations seen in this disease.[31–34] Known tumor suppressor genes and oncogenes were found to be mutated, including *TP53, PIK3CA, PTEN, HRAS,* and *CDKN2A.* It was observed that HPV-positive tumors had a reduction in mutation rate of at least 50% relative to smoking-associated tumors. Moreover, they were inversely correlated with *TP53* mutations, suggesting that HPV-positive tumors are genomically distinct. However, very few oral cavity tumors (~4%) appear to be driven by high-risk HPV.[35]

The first genomic analyses have identified loss-of-function mutations in *NOTCH1* that suggest that *NOTCH* may act as a tumor suppressor gene in head and neck cancers rather than as an oncogene, as it had been identified in other malignancies.[36] The Cancer Genome Atlas (TCGA) published results validating the initially identified genomic findings[31] in head and neck cancers. Subset analysis of patients with oral cancer has found that reduced copy number alterations and activating mutations in *HRAS* or *PIK3CA* are associated with improved clinical outcomes.

The use of whole-exome sequencing has also been applied to evaluate genomic alterations in younger, nonsmoking patients, and this analysis surprisingly found no significant difference in mutation frequencies, types of mutations, or copy number between younger and older patients with oral tongue cancers.[33] Smoking was seen to have a minimal effect on genomic changes. *FAT1* and *TP53* mutations were not significantly increased in the younger cohort and may represent a novel area of study. Although the genomic characterization has allowed clinicians to better understand the molecular alterations underlying the development of oral cancers, the majority of known mutations represent nontargetable tumor suppressor genes. Therefore, further studies of these alterations as potential prognostic and predictive biomarkers and synthetic lethality approaches are needed to fully realize the immense potential of assessment of the genomic alterations in an individual oral cancer patient's tumor.

More recent analyses have focused on recurrent and metastatic head and neck cancers that suggest the potential for precision approaches to treating these advanced tumors with more than 20% showing "actionable" mutations.[37] Liquid biopsy approaches analyzing tissue fluids including saliva and blood also hold tremendous promise in the early detection of recurrence of oral cancers.[38] Furthermore, immunoprofiling of squamous cancers of the head and neck inclusive of oral cavity tumors indicates that immune-oncologic approaches to treating these tumors should be considered in future clinical investigations.[39]

NATURAL HISTORY AND PATTERNS OF SPREAD

Premalignant Lesions

Leukoplakia

Leukoplakia and erythroplakia are gross clinical descriptors that do not always correspond directly to specific pathologic entities.[18,40] The World Health Organization defines leukoplakia as a white patch or plaque that cannot be rubbed off or characterized clinically or pathologically as any other disease[40] (Fig. 47.6). Leukoplakia is not related to the presence or absence of dysplasia; however, it is the most common precursor of cancer of the oral cavity. Leukoplakia is primarily a clinical entity, with certain key pathologic features. These features include hyperkeratosis and acanthosis. Leukoplakia may begin as a thin gray or gray/white plaque that may appear translucent, is sometimes fissured or wrinkled, and typically soft and flat. They frequently have sharply demarcated borders but occasionally blend gradually into normal surrounding mucosa.

Homogenous leukoplakia is a uniform white lesion that is prevalent in the buccal mucosa; it is the most common variety of leukoplakia and has a low malignant potential. Conversely, high-risk oral leukoplakia demonstrates abnormal orientation of cells, nuclear hyperchromatism, increased mitosis, and nuclear cytoplasmic ratio.[18] Clinically, these lesions are nonhomogenous, nodular, speckled, or verrucous, with central ulceration or erosion.[40,41] Follow-up studies demonstrate that between <1% and 18% of oral leukoplakias develop into oral cancer, with the latter clinical subtype conferring a higher risk of malignant transformation.[42,43]

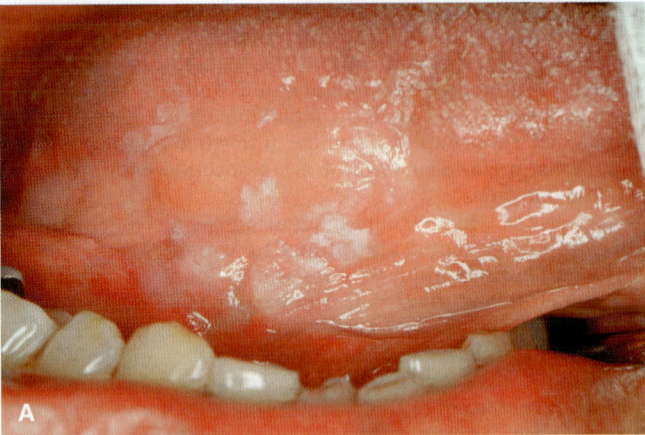
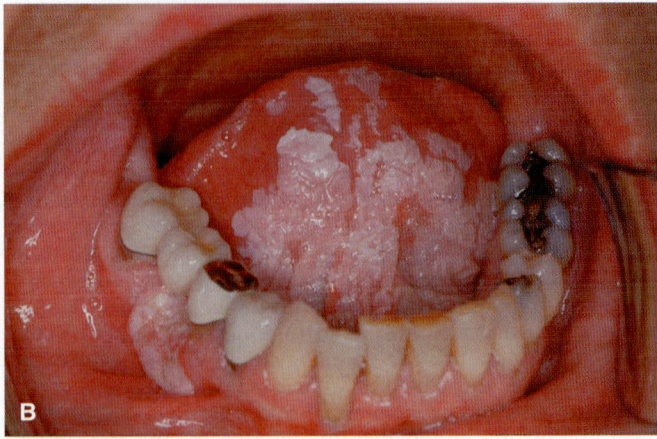

FIGURE 47.6. A: Superficial patches of leukoplakia involving the lateral and ventral surface of the oral tongue. **B:** Extensive leukoplakia involving the ventral oral tongue, floor of the mouth, and mandibular alveolus.

Leukoplakia may regress spontaneously without therapy. A baseline biopsy may be performed to establish diagnosis and rule out malignant transformation. Leukoplakia with clinically or histologically aggressive features, demonstrating dysplasia, should be excised.

Erythroplakia

Erythroplakia describes a chronic, red, generally asymptomatic lesion or patch on the mucosal surface that cannot be attributed to a traumatic, vascular, or inflammatory cause. Erythroplakia, like leukoplakia, is a clinical diagnosis of exclusion that requires the clinician to rule out all other erythematous oral lesions.[44] However, erythroplakia is associated with a higher risk of malignant transformation than leukoplakia. Transformation rates are considered to be the highest among all precancerous oral lesions and conditions.[45] Histopathologically, it has been documented that in homogenous oral erythroplakia, 51% showed invasive carcinoma, 40% carcinoma *in situ*, and 9% mild or moderate dysplasia.[45] The treatment of choice for erythroplakia is surgical excision.

Oral Submucous Fibrosis

The term describes a generalized fibrosis of the oral cavity tissues resulting in marked rigidity and trismus. At early stages, these premalignant lesions are characterized by blanching of the mucosa with a marble-like appearance. At more advanced stages, palpable fibrous bands become evident around the buccal mucosa and the mouth opening. Once oral submucous fibrosis reaches advanced stages, approximately 25% of cases biopsied demonstrate epithelial dysplasia in addition to subepithelial alterations.[10] Oral submucous fibrosis is associated with the use of betel quid (with or without tobacco) or pan masala.[10] In India, it is estimated that as many as 5 million individuals are afflicted with oral submucous fibrosis.[10]

Oral Cavity Cancer

Relative Distribution

The most common subsite for squamous cell carcinoma of the oral cavity (excluding the lip) is the oral tongue.[47] In a review of 3,308 cases of oral cavity cancer treated at the University of Texas MD Anderson Cancer Center between 1970 and 1999, 32% involved the oral tongue.[18] The floor of the mouth is the second most common subsite where oral cavity carcinomas may arise. Carcinoma of the alveolar ridge accounts for approximately 10% of oral cavity carcinomas. Squamous cell carcinoma of the retromolar trigone and hard palate is rare. Similarly, carcinoma of the buccal mucosa is rare in the United States but is the most common carcinoma of the oral cavity in Southeast Asia because of the widespread use of betel nut.[18]

Patterns of Spread

Local Spread

Carcinoma from distinct anatomic subsites may exhibit different tendencies for spread based on natural anatomic barriers and location. For instance, the majority of lip cancers are local growths that do not invade deeply into the tissues of the oral cavity or mandible.[46] However, a select few lip carcinomas may be deeply invasive with perineural involvement, posterior spread to involve cortical bone, extension to the inferior alveolar nerve, or spread to the skin of the face.[47] Squamous cell carcinoma of the floor of the mouth can secondarily involve the ventral tongue, extend along the lingual nerve and submandibular duct, or invade the cortex of the mandible. Tumors in this location can invade deeply, involving the muscles of the floor of the mouth. There is an anatomical gap between the mylohyoid and hyoglossus muscles through which a carcinoma can gain access to submandibular and sublingual areas. Carcinomas of the alveolar ridge and retromolar trigone tend to invade bone early. Tumors of the inferior alveolar ridge may access the mandibular canal and the inferior alveolar nerve, whereas tumors of the superior alveolar ridge may pass into the maxillary antrum or floor of the nose. Infiltrating lesions of the buccal mucosa can invade the buccinator muscle, extend to the buccal fat pad, and invade the subcutaneous tissue. The hard palate has a relatively dense mucoperiosteum that is relatively resistant to tumor invasion. However, the primary and secondary palates are fused at the incisive fossa, where tumors can gain access into the nasal cavity. The greater palatine foramina can allow tumors to spread posteriorly and enter the pterygopalatine fossa and skull base.

Lymphatic Metastases

The oral cavity has an extensive group of lymphatics that manifest a fairly predictable lymph node drainage pattern based on location (subsite) within the oral cavity[47] (Table 47.1).

TABLE 47.1 RELATIVE INVOLVEMENT OF LYMPH NODE REGIONS BY ORAL CAVITY SUBSITE

	Percentage Involved			
	Submaxillary	**Submental**	**Upper Jugular**	**Midjugular**
Oral tongue	18	9	73	18
FOM	64	7	43	0
RMT	25	0	63	12.5

FOM, floor of mouth; RMT, retromolar trigone.
From Byers RM, Wolf PF, Ballantyne AJ. Rationale for elective modified neck dissection. *Head Neck Surg* 1988;10(3):160–167. Copyright © 1988 Wiley-Liss, Inc., A Wiley Company. Reprinted by permission of John Wiley & Sons, Inc.

The lymphatic nodal stations most commonly involved include levels I to IV.[48,49] The retrostyloid space is potentially at risk for involvement by metastatic disease when upper level II nodes are grossly positive.[26] The medial retropharyngeal nodes are rarely a site of metastases in head and neck squamous cell carcinoma.[50] The lateral retropharyngeal nodes generally at risk in primary carcinoma of the nasopharynx and oropharynx are rarely involved in oral cavity cancer unless there is oropharyngeal involvement or a significant nodal burden.[51–53] The lymphatic drainage pattern to the upper and lower lip is distinct. The principal lymphatic drainage of the upper lip is to preauricular, periparotid, submental, and submandibular lymph nodes, which secondarily drain to deep jugular lymph nodes. The medial portion of the lower lip drains primarily to the submental lymph nodes, whereas the lateral portion drains to the submandibular triangle.

A classical study by Lindberg[54] demonstrated that the superior deep jugular nodes are most frequently involved by cancers of the oral cavity. The anterior portion of the tongue drains to the submental nodes (level Ia), and the lateral portion drains to the submandibular (level Ib) and deep jugular nodes (level II). The posterior oral tongue drains into the upper jugulodigastric group of lymph nodes (level II). The lymphatics of the oral tongue also have extensive communication across the midline; thus, carcinomas of the oral tongue can metastasize bilaterally. Studies suggest that some carcinomas of the lateral oral tongue may metastasize to level IV lymph nodes without involving levels I, II, or III.[55] This implies that there may be separate lymphatic channels draining from the oral tongue directly to level IV nodes, allowing for apparent "skip metastases."

Dye injection studies have shown that the floor of the mouth has superficial and deep lymphatic drainage systems.[55] The superficial system crosses randomly in the midline and drains into both the ipsilateral and contralateral submandibular lymph nodes. The deep lymphatic system is thought to penetrate the periosteum and drains into the submandibular and upper jugular lymph nodes. Lymphatics from the buccal mucosa drain into the periparotid, submental, and submandibular nodes. Tumors of the alveolar ridge may drain into the submental and submandibular triangles, upper deep jugular, and retropharyngeal lymph nodes. Tumors of the inferior alveolus are more likely to metastasize to the neck than tumors of the superior alveolus. The main lymphatic drainage from the retromolar trigone is into the superior deep jugular lymph nodes; however, there may be some drainage into periparotid and retropharyngeal lymph nodes. Lymphatics in the hard palate are few, but drainage is into submandibular, superior deep jugular, and retropharyngeal nodes.

The risk of neck metastases depends on several factors including site and size of the primary tumor. Overall, for patients with squamous cell carcinoma of the oral cavity, cervical metastases occur in approximately 30% of cases.[41] The rate of neck metastases for carcinoma of the lip is approximately 10%.[41] Squamous cell cancer of the oral tongue carries a higher risk of nodal metastases, the frequency ranging from 15% to 75%, depending on the size and depth of the primary lesion.[54,56] Approximately 25% of patients with carcinoma of the oral cavity will have occult nodal metastases, and 3% of patients will have contralateral metastases.[54,56] Contralateral metastases are more common in tumors that approach or cross the midline. Early tumors of the floor of the mouth have approximately a 12% to 30% incidence of occult nodal metastases depending on the thickness of the lesion, whereas larger lesions can have an incidence of nearly 50%.[57] Approximately 15% to 20% of upper alveolar ridge tumors will involve the neck at presentation; the risk of occult metastases in a clinically negative neck is approximately 15% to 20%.[54] The incidence of neck metastases in lower alveolar ridge tumors is higher than for tumors of the upper alveolar ridge.[54]

For cancers of the buccal mucosa, the incidence of positive cervical lymph nodes at diagnosis is 10% to 30%; the incidence of pathologically positive nodes in a clinically negative neck is about 15%. Similar rates of occult metastases occur for squamous cell carcinoma of the retromolar trigone; however, patients tend to present with more advanced disease, resulting in a somewhat higher rate of regional metastases.[41] The incidence of lymph node involvement from carcinoma of the hard palate is low, approximately 15%.[46,58]

Distant Metastases

Distant metastasis occurs in approximately 15% to 20% of patients who eventually die of their disease.[41] The risk of distant metastases increases with the degree of lymph node involvement. Patients with recurrent disease are also at higher risk for distant metastases.[59] Patients without clinically appreciable neck disease rarely fail distantly after treatment. In general terms, with respect to head and neck cancer, 66% of distant metastases are to the lungs, 22% to the bones, and 9.5% to the liver.[60] On rare occasion, the oral cavity will serve as a site for distant metastasis from another anatomic primary tumor site.[47]

PATHOLOGIC CLASSIFICATION

The predominant histopathologic type of cancer in the oral cavity is squamous cell carcinoma. There are several variants of squamous cell carcinoma, including basaloid and verrucous carcinoma. Basaloid squamous cell carcinoma is believed to have a worse prognosis than traditional squamous cell carcinoma. In a retrospective comparison between basaloid squamous cell carcinoma and traditional poorly differentiated squamous cell carcinoma, the former had a higher incidence of advanced disease at presentation, distant metastases, and poorer overall survival rate.[61] Verrucous carcinoma is a less common variant of squamous cell carcinoma. It is generally considered a low-grade malignancy with low metastatic potential and good overall prognosis, although often with challenges for local control in elderly patients.[18] For most cases, adjuvant radiation and elective neck dissection (END) are not indicated. Sarcomatoid carcinomas can be found in the oral cavity and larynx. This variant of squamous cell carcinoma carries a poor prognosis with a mean survival of approximately 2 years.[62]

Less than 10% of neoplasms of the oral cavity have nonsquamous histology. Most of these are minor salivary gland tumors, which tend to arise in the hard palate. Adenoid cystic carcinoma accounts for approximately 30% to 40% of minor salivary gland cancers of the oral cavity.[63] Other histologies that can occur in the oral cavity include adenocarcinomas, melanoma, ameloblastoma, lymphoma, and Kaposi sarcoma.[47] Approximately 50% of acquired immunodeficiency syndrome–related cases of Kaposi sarcoma have oral cavity involvement.[41] Most lymphomas in the head and neck arise in Waldeyer ring (tonsil, base of the tongue, and nasopharynx). Only 2% of all lymphomas are found in the oral cavity.[64] Fortunately, melanoma of the oral cavity is very rare and represents only 0.2% to 8% of all melanomas.[65] Mucosal melanomas generally have a worse prognosis than cutaneous melanomas.

CLINICAL PRESENTATION

The oral cavity is an anatomic region that is readily accessible to visual inspection and palpation. Despite this fact, many patients with oral cavity tumors present with advanced-stage disease as initial symptoms may be vague and painless. Tumors of the oral tongue often present as small ulcers and gradually invade the musculature of the tongue. Advanced lesions may be either ulcerative or exophytic and are usually quite evident. Some cancers of the oral tongue are painful

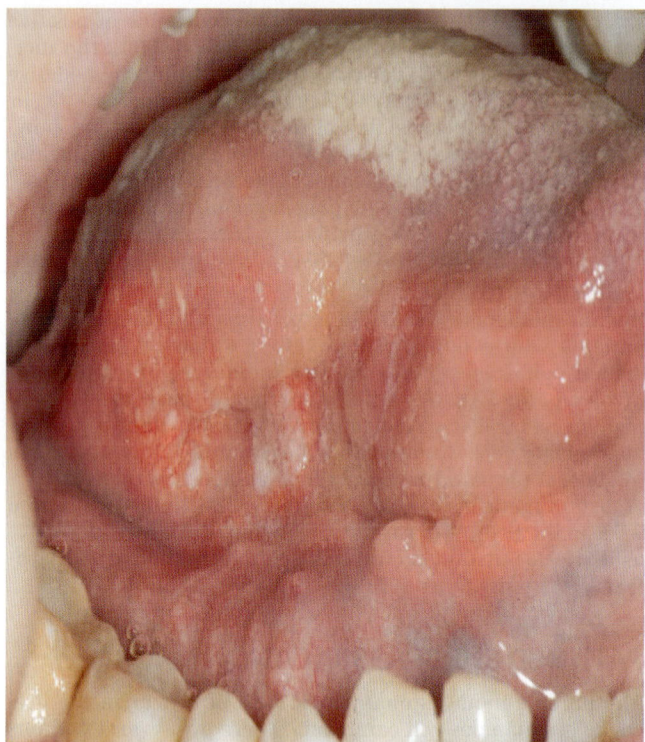

FIGURE 47.7. T2N0M0 squamous cell carcinoma involving the right lateral oral tongue.

even in their early stages. Cervical metastases occur early in the natural history of the disease, with 30% to 40% of patients harboring cervical lymph node metastases at diagnosis. Squamous cell carcinomas of the oral tongue most often arise along the lateral borders of the tongue[18] (Fig. 47.7).

Lesions of the floor of the mouth are often infiltrative and may invade bone, the muscles of the floor of the mouth, and the tongue. The frenulum is frequently a site of involvement. Clinical fixation of the tumor to the mandible suggests periosteal involvement, which may occur early.

Tumors of the alveolar ridge may present with pain while chewing, loose teeth, or ill-fitting dentures in edentulous patients. These cancers often arise in edentulous areas or along the free margin of the mandibular alveolus (Figs. 47.8 and 47.9). Anesthesia of the lower lip and teeth may indicate involvement of the mandibular canal and inferior alveolar nerve.

FIGURE 47.8. T1N0M0 squamous cell carcinoma of the mandibular alveolus. No evidence of bone invasion identified on panorex or CT imaging.

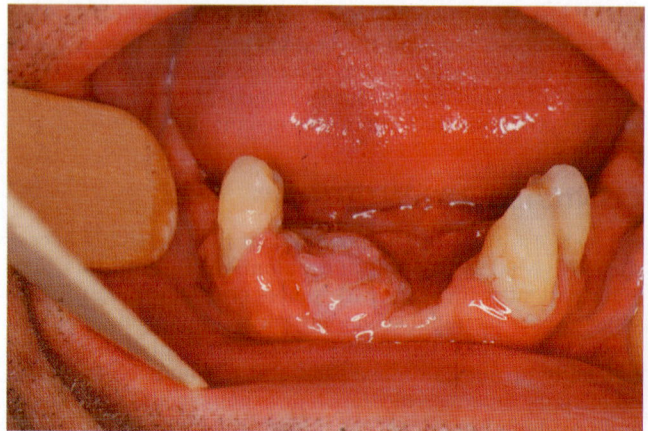

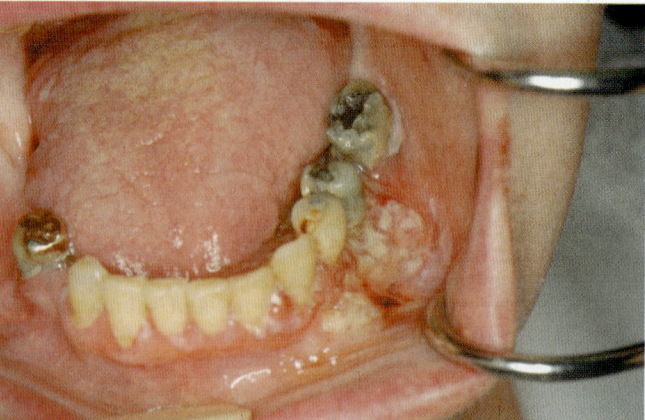

FIGURE 47.9. Squamous cell carcinoma involving the mandibular alveolus and buccogingival space.

Tumors involving the retromolar trigone region may present with an exophytic growth pattern and limited involvement of underlying bone (Fig. 47.10), or they may infiltrate cortical bone and spread along regional tissue planes to involve the pterygoid complex and parapharyngeal space. These latter lesions often induce trismus early in the clinical course.

Carcinoma of the buccal mucosa is rarely symptomatic early in its course. Lesions may be papillary or erosive and located near the dental occlusal line. These tumors are often relatively asymptotic and therefore seldom come to medical attention as T1 lesions. Often, these tumors manifest associated leukoplakia. Multiple primary sites and local recurrence are also common. These tumors most frequently arise adjacent to the lower molars along the occlusal line of the teeth.

Carcinoma of the hard palate is often painless, and the sole presenting symptom may be an irregularity in the mucosa or ill-fitting dentures. Other presenting symptoms include nonhealing ulcers of the hard palate, intermittent bleeding, and pain.

DIAGNOSTIC EVALUATION

Patients with oral cavity cancer should undergo a comprehensive history and physical examination. Detailed visual and digital examinations are particularly important for oral cavity tumors. A biopsy of lesions in question should be obtained as well as a thorough dental assessment. Computed tomography (CT) scans, panoramic radiographs, magnetic resonance imaging (MRI), and other imaging studies may also be important for accurate staging of the tumor and in treatment planning.

FIGURE 47.10. Exophytic T3 carcinoma involving the right retromolar trigone, anterior tonsillar pillar, and proximal soft palate with minimal infiltration into the right base of the tongue.

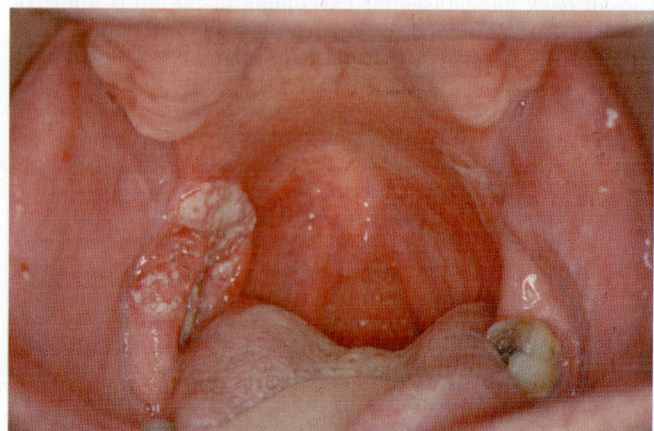

The history of present illness should address the following issues: tobacco and alcohol use; dysphagia; odynophagia; pain; trismus; difficulties with speech; hoarseness; loose teeth; ill-fitting dentures; hypoesthesia of the face, lips, or mandible; weight loss; and malnutrition. Otalgia suggests involvement of the ninth or tenth cranial nerve; facial numbness may suggest involvement of the fifth cranial nerve. Hypoesthesia usually results from perineural invasion, often from penetration of the mandible and perineural spread along the inferior alveolar nerve. The presence of trismus may indicate extension into the pterygoid musculature, signifying locally advanced disease. Other symptoms include a persistent ulcer, bleeding, drooling, or respiratory distress. A patient's comorbid illnesses must also be considered in designing the overall treatment strategy.

A detailed examination of the head and neck should be performed, with particular focus on the oral cavity and oropharynx. This usually begins with a full inspection of the oral cavity, including thorough inspection of the teeth. Palpation of the oral cavity can help assess bony involvement, tongue fixation, and depth of involvement. Deviation or fixation of the tongue suggests involvement of extrinsic muscles of the tongue. Bimanual palpation can help assess the depth of tumor invasion into musculature of the tongue and floor of the mouth. A thorough palpation of the neck is important to assess regional nodal disease.

Imaging can complement the physical examination in determining the extent of disease. A chest x-ray should be performed to exclude lung metastases or a second primary cancer. CT is the modality most commonly used to determine the extent of soft tissue and bony involvement and occult disease in the neck (Fig. 47.11). CT may be used to determine the extent of invasion into the deep musculature of the tongue and adjacent structures. Moreover, CT is a valuable modality for visualizing invasion of the mandible, palate, and pterygopalatine fossa. If CT scanning is not available, then panoramic radiographs can be used to demonstrate mandibular invasion. MRI may be used in case of contrast allergy or a lesion that is not well visualized on CT. For instance, MRI may be used if a patient has significant dental artifact that obscures visualization of the primary tumor on CT. MRI provides excellent definition of tumor involving the tongue and is a good modality for evaluating the possibility of perineural spread. Ultrasound may be used to screen for enlarged lymph nodes that are not clinically detectable. In experienced hands, the accuracy of ultrasound when combined with fine-needle aspiration may be superior to CT or MRI for staging the neck.[66]

Positron emission tomography (PET) and PET/CT have been used increasingly in head and neck cancer evaluation for staging disease in the neck, evaluation of perineural and skull base involvement, identification of distant metastases, and detection of recurrence. Several studies suggest that PET is more sensitive and specific in evaluating lymphatic metastases compared to CT and MRI.[67,68] PET/CT may improve the anatomic localization of abnormalities identified on PET and decrease the number of equivocal PET findings.[69] Liao et al.[70] prospectively evaluated 473 patients with oral cavity squamous cell carcinoma and report a sensitivity of 77.7% and a specificity of 58% for PET/CT after histopathologic correlation of nodal metastases to the neck. Maddipatla et al.,[71] in a prospective study evaluating 552 lymph nodes dissected after oral cancer surgery, report a 97% negative predictive value (NPV) for PET/CT. Pentenero et al.[72] report an accuracy of 66.7%, a specificity of 76.9%, and a NPV of 83.3% for staging of the neck with PET/CT. Despite the improved overall accuracy, clinical application of PET/CT is limited by the suboptimal detection of small metastases. Therefore, the decision to pursue a neck dissection should not be based solely on PET/CT findings.

Reports have indicated that the overall sensitivity and specificity of PET may be superior to CT and MRI for evaluating persistent or recurrent disease, particularly in patients who have received previous radiotherapy.[73,74] The accuracy of PET in detecting disease recurrence or persistence may be influenced by the time post treatment when images are acquired. It is recommended that a PET scan not be performed until 8 to 12 weeks post treatment to minimize the risk of both false-negative and false-positive interpretations.[75–78]

STAGING

The American Joint Committee on Cancer (AJCC) has established a staging system for cancer of the oral cavity. The staging guidelines apply to all forms of carcinoma and are based on the eighth edition of the AJCC Staging Manual (Table 47.2).[79] Nonepithelial malignancies and melanoma of the lip and oral cavity are not included in the staging system. There are several pertinent changes from prior editions of the AJCC Staging Manual: (a) clinical and pathologic depth of

FIGURE 47.11. A: Transverse CT image with contrast depicting infiltrative squamous cell carcinoma of the left lateral oral tongue and floor of the mouth with associated bone destruction (*arrows*). There is posterior tumor extension to involve the retromolar trigone and tonsillar complex. **B:** Corresponding CT bone window views demonstrating destruction of the mandibular body.

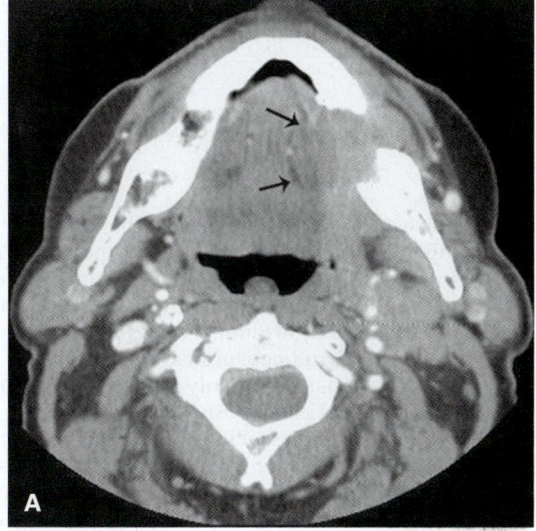
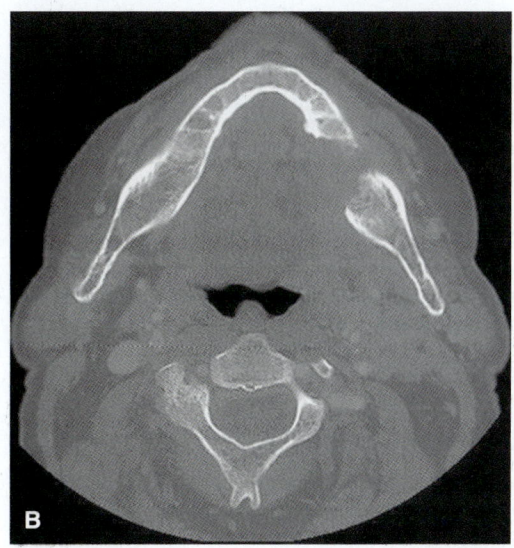

TABLE 47.2 STAGING OF ORAL CAVITY CARCINOMA

Definition of Primary Tumor

T Category	T Criteria
TX	Primary tumor cannot be assessed
Tis	Carcinoma in situ
T1	Tumor ≤2 cm in greatest dimension, ≤5 mm depth of invasion (DOI)
T2	Tumor ≤2 cm in greatest dimension, DOI > 5 mm and ≤10 mm, *or* tumor >2 cm, but ≤4 cm, and ≤10 mm of DOI
T3	Tumor >4 cm in greatest dimension
	Any tumor >10 mm DOI
T4	Moderately advanced or very advanced local disease
T4a (lip)	Tumor invades through cortical bone, inferior alveolar nerve, floor of the mouth, or skin of the face (i.e., chin or nose).
T4a (oral cavity)	Tumor invades adjacent structures (e.g., through cortical bone of the mandible or maxilla, maxillary sinus, or skin of the face).
	Note: superficial erosion of bone/tooth socket by a gingival primary is not sufficient to classify a tumor as T4.
T4b	Tumor invades masticator space, pterygoid plates, or skull base and/or encases carotid artery.

Definition of Regional Lymph Node (N)
Clinical N (cN)

N Category	N Criteria
Nx	Regional lymph nodes cannot be assessed
N0	No regional lymph node metastases
N1	Metastases in a single ipsilateral lymph node, ≤3 cm in greatest dimension, ENE (−)
N2	Metastases in a single ipsilateral lymph node >3 cm, but ≤6 cm in greatest dimension and ENE (−); in multiple ipsilateral lymph nodes, none >6 cm in greatest dimension and ENE (−); *or* in bilateral or contralateral lymph nodes, ≤6 cm in greatest dimension and ENE (−)
N2a	Metastases in a single ipsilateral lymph node >3 cm, but ≤6 cm in greatest dimension and ENE (−)
N2b	Metastases in multiple ipsilateral lymph nodes, ≤6 cm in greatest dimension, and ENE (−)
N2c	Metastases in bilateral or contralateral lymph nodes ≤6 cm in greatest dimension and ENE (−)
N3	Metastases in a lymph node >6 cm in greatest dimension and ENE (−) *or* in any node with clinically overt ENE (+)
N3a	Metastases in a lymph node >6 cm in greatest dimension and ENE (−)
N3b	Metastases in any lymph node(s) and clinically over ECE (+)

Definition of Regional Lymph Node (N)
Pathologic N (pN)

N Category	N Criteria
Nx	Regional lymph nodes cannot be assessed
N0	No regional lymph node metastases
N1	Metastases in a single ipsilateral lymph node ≤3 cm in greatest dimension and ENE (−)
N2	Metastases in a single ipsilateral lymph node ≤3 cm in greatest dimension and ENE (+); >3 but ≤6 cm in greatest dimension and ENE (−); in multiple ipsilateral lymph nodes, ≤6 cm in greatest dimension and ENE (−); *or* in bilateral or contralateral lymph nodes, ≤6 cm in greatest dimension and ENE (−)
N2a	Metastases in a single ipsilateral or contralateral lymph node ≤3 cm in greatest dimension and ENE (+), *or* in a single ipsilateral lymph node, >3 but ≤6 cm in greatest dimension and ENE (−)
N2b	Metastases in multiple ipsilateral lymph nodes ≤6 cm in greatest dimension and ENE (−)
N2c	Metastases in bilateral or contralateral lymph nodes ≤6 cm in greatest dimension and ENE (−)
N3	Metastases in a lymph node >6 cm in greatest dimension and ENE (−); in a single ipsilateral lymph node, >3 cm in greatest dimension and ECE (+); *or* multiple ipsilateral, contralateral, or bilateral lymph nodes, any with ENE (+)
N3a	Metastases in a lymph node >6 cm in greatest dimension and ENE (−)
N3b	Metastases in a single ipsilateral lymph node >3 cm in greatest dimension and ECE (+), *or* in multiple ipsilateral, contralateral, bilateral lymph nodes, any with ENE (+)

Note. A designation of "U" or "L" may be used for any N category to indicate metastases above or below the lower border of the cricoid, respectively. Similarly, clinical or pathologic extranodal extension (ENE) should be recorded as ENE (−) or ENE (+).

AJCC Prognostic Stage Groups

Stage I	T1	N0	M0
Stage II	T2	N0	M0
Stage III	T3	N0	M0
	T1-3	N1	M0
Stage IVA	T4a	N0	M0
	T4a	N1	M0
	T1-4a	N2	M0
Stage IVB	Any T	N3	M0
	T4b	Any N	M0
Stage IVC	Any T	Any N	M1

invasion are now used in indicating the T category, (b) extrinsic tongue muscle involvement is no longer denoted as T4, (c) separate N staging categories are now present for patients treated with and without neck dissection, and (d) the presence of extranodal extension (ENE) is introduced as a descriptor of HPV-negative squamous cell carcinoma.

GENERAL MANAGEMENT

Surgical resection, radiation, chemotherapy, or combined modality approaches are classical treatment options that have been employed for patients with cancer of the oral cavity. The choice of treatment modality, either singly or in combination, depends on the stage and size of the tumor and relevant patient factors such as toxicity, performance status, comorbid disease, and convenience. The overall health and functional status of the patient are important determinants in choosing between surgical and nonsurgical approaches.

Surgery is most commonly the treatment of choice for lesions of the oral cavity.[1] Surgical resection is expeditious, effective, and often associated with modest morbidity and good functional outcome particularly for patients with small-to moderate-sized lesions. Radiation therapy can be considered for patients with early-stage disease who either are not surgical candidates or refuse surgical management. For patients with advanced lesions of the oral cavity, a combined modality approach is generally recommended. In patients with high-risk pathologic features, the addition of concurrent chemotherapy during the postoperative radiation treatment course may further augment tumor control rates provided the chemotherapy can be tolerated.[80-82] High-risk features commonly include ENE and positive resection margins.[81,83-85]

PRINCIPLES OF SURGERY

All patients with oral cavity carcinoma should be evaluated by a head and neck surgical oncologist.[1] One major reason why surgery is often the primary modality in sequential therapy is that definitive high-dose radiation has been associated with higher rates of osteoradionecrosis and inferior control rates, particularly in the setting of more advanced disease.[86-89] The primary objectives of surgery are complete resection of the primary tumor with negative margins and staging and treatment of the regional lymphatics. Margin status is one of the most important variables associated with survival, as locoregional control is significantly improved with margins of 0.5 cm or greater, relative to margins of <0.5 cm (36% vs. 18%, respectively).[81,84,90]

Surgical Management of the Primary Tumor

In treating cancer of the oral tongue, it is best to obtain adequate margins during initial resection. The outcome of intraoperative positive margins followed by immediate repeat resection revised to negative margins is associated with worse survival compared to negative margins achieved with initial resection (31% vs. 49%, respectively).[91] Several strategies are being developed to enhance the ability of surgeons to detect margins intraoperatively. However, these remain largely experimental and are yet not being used in routine clinical practice.[92-94] Although surgeons and pathologists agree on the quantified distances for free margins, pathologic findings of margin status can be misclassified because of tissue shrinkage, inaccurate sampling, and improper orientation.[95] Although shrinkage is unavoidable, accurate assessment of all margins can be performed from the main specimen, as opposed to sampling from the tumor bed. How the surgeon takes the margins is also extremely important, and it is recommended that the margins be taken from the tumor specimen rather from the tumor bed, as the latter is associated with higher risks of local recurrence.[96] Furthermore, proper orientation of the specimen and communication with the pathologist are vital to assessing accurate margin status.

The ability to obtain clear, three-dimensional margins is the most important factor in selecting the surgical approach, and this is typically guided by the size and location of the tumor as well as factors related to the patient's dentition as well as the presence or absence of trismus. Most often, lesions of the anterior or lateral oral tongue and floor of the mouth can be resected transorally; however, in cases with significant posterior extent and/or in patients with trismus and/or obstructive dentition, a visor flap with lingual release—sometimes referred to as a pull-through or lip-splitting incision with mandibulotomy—may be required for optimal resection. The visor flap is an approach that avoids a facial incision and is associated with lower rates of oral incompetence and fistula.[97] Buccal resections can often be performed with a transoral approach or with a lip-split incision to allow adequate exposure for mandibular or maxillary resection. Retromolar trigone resections often require mandibulectomy because of the posterior extent and increased rate of bone invasion. The introduction of transoral robotic surgery offers a novel approach for resecting more posterior tumors without mandibulotomy.

Transoral resection is often used for excision of floor of the mouth tumors, and these excisions often involve marginal or segmental mandibulectomy because the presence of mandibular invasion is associated with worsened local control. The decision on whether to perform a marginal versus a segmental resection is based on the preoperative assessment of invasion of the periosteum and cortex.[98] However, this type of assessment remains a challenge because results of preoperative physical examination are predictive of bone invasion only two-thirds of the time. This can be enhanced through the use of imaging that has excellent specificity despite limitations in assessment of microscopic invasion.[99] For the management of small tumors with periosteal involvement, marginal mandibulectomy is associated with outcomes equivalent to those of segmental mandibulectomy. The major indications for segmental mandibulectomy include pre- or intraoperative findings of bone invasion, tooth loss with low mandibular bone height, and bone that has previously been irradiated. In cases in which both a mandibulotomy and marginal mandibulectomy are contemplated, the risk of postradiation ORN is high and should be considered with caution.[100] Transoral resection can often be employed to resect lesions of the hard palate and maxillary alveolar ridge, though larger tumors that extend into the paranasal sinuses, masticator space, or infratemporal fossa and may require a facial incision to improve access.

Surgical Management of the Neck

The relatively high rate of cervical nodal metastasis associated with oral cavity cancers warrants management of the neck in the vast majority of patients with oral tongue, floor of the mouth, buccal, and retromolar trigone tumors. The selection of type and extent of neck dissection is dependent on whether the patient is clinically node negative based on physical examination and imaging; in clinically node-negative patients, a neck dissection is considered elective. In contrast, patients with nodes that are palpable or detected on imaging require a therapeutic neck dissection. Although neck dissection is a safe procedure, it is not without morbidity; shoulder dysfunction, iatrogenic cranial nerve injuries, and vascular insult remain significant complications of neck dissection.

Therapeutic neck dissection in clinically positive disease is a well-established treatment strategy, and the extent of dissection recommended in this setting has decreased considerably over the past several decades. In the early 1900s, radical en bloc resections according to the surgical oncologic principles advanced by Dr. William Halsted were recommended. Over the intervening years, these relatively morbid operations have largely been replaced by more selective approaches to involve only the nodal basins with expected metastasis with preservation of uninvolved nonlymphatic structures including the internal jugular vein, sternocleidomastoid muscle, and spinal accessory nerve. The contemporary practice of these more limited procedures has been supported with data demonstrating that regional control and survival rates do not decrease with more selective approaches, particularly when adjuvant therapies are used to manage microscopic residual disease in high-risk patients.[101]

For patients whose preoperative examination reveals a cN-positive neck, a selective neck dissection at levels I to IV or I to V is recommended. In these cases, positive pathologic nodes are found in more than 75% with 15.8% having skip metastasis to level III or IV, without involvement of levels I or II.[47,55,101,102] The use of radical and modified neck dissections is typically reserved for patients with advanced nodal disease (N3), disease extending into level V, or invading critical structures in the neck.

The decision to proceed to END is based on a >20% probability of occult nodal disease being present for patients with early-stage tumors that are clinically node negative (cN0).[103] END can be therapeutic if no positive nodes are found at pathologic review and it can provide important staging information to guide decision about the need for adjuvant therapy in patients found to have pN-positive disease with or without ENE.

The depth of tumor invasion has been reported to be the best predictor for regional metastasis in the cN0 neck. Nevertheless, cutoffs for the extent of depth of invasion for which neck dissection is recommended remains ill defined. A meta-analysis identified a depth of 4 mm from the mucosal surface in oral tongue cancers as the cutoff most frequently cited as an indication for END, based on a NPV of 95.5%.[104] Other analyses have shown that depth of invasion >4 mm is associated with increased risk of occult metastasis and late cervical recurrences.[105-107] In floor of the mouth tumors, a depth of invasion >1.5 mm is associated with 33% occult regional metastasis, whereas in buccal carcinomas, tumors of the maxillary alveolar ridge, and tumors of the hard palate, depth has not been extensively studied, and occult metastases are rare, occurring in 9% of patients and most often associated with T4 tumors.[108,109] Therefore, END is not indicated for early-stage buccal, maxillary alveolar ridge, or hard palate cancers in cN0 cases. In addition to depth of invasion, growth type, number of mitoses, PNI, lymphovascular invasion, and poorly differentiated and infiltrative growth patterns are associated with metastasis.[107,109] There is no clear consensus regarding which of these risk factors necessitate END. Once the decision to proceed with END is made, the literature supports dissection of at least the supraomohyoid neck, including levels I to III. The notable exception is cancer of the oral tongue, for which extension to remove level IV can be considered because of the occasional identification of skip metastases, which are difficult to salvage.[55] The need to extend a neck dissection to include level IIB has been questioned because dissection of this nodal level requires dissection of spinal accessory nerve, which in turn is associated with greater morbidity. The results of several prospective studies support the exclusion of level IIB in ENDs for patients with oral cavity cancer as the incidence of nodes with occult regional disease is 11.1% in cN0 patients.[110]

Given that as many as 70% of END are found to have no pathologic lymph nodes at pathologic review and neck dissection can be both morbid and costly, alternatives to END have been explored, and these include observation, elective radiation, or sentinel lymph node biopsy (SLNB). There have been several prospective studies performed to evaluate observation versus END, with one study demonstrating a survival benefit with END.[111] The rate of nodal recurrence in the observation arms in that study performed in Brazil was 41.7% compared with 15% in the END arm. Although successful salvage was higher with observation than with END (57% vs. 16%, respectively), 66% fewer salvage attempts occurred in the END groups. Because the node-related mortality is higher with observation than with END (22% vs. 10%, respectively), END has been the standard of care for most patients with oral cavity cancers.[112]

In a recent landmark study, D'Cruz and colleagues at Tata Memorial Hospital in Mumbai evaluated 500 patients with early-stage oral cavity squamous cell carcinoma who were randomly assigned to undergo END versus observation with therapeutic neck dissection to evaluate survival differences between treatment options.[113] The unadjusted improvement in OS for END was 12.5% (END vs. observation with TND, 80% vs. 67.5%, respectively) and this result was confirmed after the investigators adjusted for other covariates (hazard ratio [HR], 0.63; P<.001). Although no difference was observed in the cohorts when patients had pN0 disease (HR, 1.2; P=.54), among pN-positive cases, significant improvement in survival was noted in the END cohort (HR, 0.52; P=.008). In addition, data from this study confirmed that depth >3 mm was a significant independent predictor of regional metastasis (HR, 2.17; P<.001). There was no difference observed for OS when patients with tumor depth <3 mm were compared across the two cohorts (P=.12); however, the study was not powered to definitively address this issue. Overall, this study's results support the practice of END for early-stage N0 OCSCC and confirm that depth is an important variable in the decision between END or observation and therapeutic neck dissection.

Another option for managing the clinically node-negative neck is SLNB, which is a less invasive approach used to accurately identify occult metastasis in early-stage oral cancer. SLNB is based on the principle that cancer spreads first to a primary echelon lymph node known as the "sentinel node" that can be readily identified and meticulously evaluated for microscopic disease. This minimally invasive technique to stage regional lymph nodes is well established in melanoma and breast cancer and allows for a more systematic and accurate pathologic assessment of regional lymph nodes for metastasis without the morbidity of END. There have been several multi-institutional prospective studies that have been performed to assess the efficacy of SLNB in oral squamous cell carcinoma. In a trial completed in Europe, sentinel lymph nodes were identified in 93% of patients with a low false-negative rate.[114] In a study performed in North America (ClinicalTrials.gov identifier: NCT00042926), SLNB was found to have a 96% NPV overall in cancers of the oral tongue.[115] A meta-analysis showed a pooled NPV of 96% in early-stage oral cavity tumors, with no difference in regional recurrence between SLNB and END (6.7% and 6%, respectively). The accuracy and consistent NPV found in most studies indicate that SLNB offers an excellent alternative to END in cN0 patients with early oral squamous cancers. Although this approach has become a standard of care for management of the cN0 neck in oral cavity cancer patient in Europe, its use in the United States has been much more limited. Factors that might explain the slow adaptation of SLNB in this country include the steep learning curve, the additional preoperative workup required, and the need for an experienced multidisciplinary team. There is no level I evidence yet available regarding survival equivalency with END.

Reconstruction

The oral cavity is a complex site made up of several structures critical for speech, swallowing, and appearance, and successful rehabilitation of these functions in patients that have undergone oral cancer extirpative surgery involves meticulous anatomic restoration post resection. A successful, reconstruction should attempt to address all three of these functions, and it must be tailored to the site of the defect. Patients with advanced-stage disease are often best reconstructed with microvascular free tissue transfer, which has become standard in head and neck reconstruction and has improved both oncologic and functional outcomes.[116] In the case of oral tongue reconstruction, which is critical to restoring function, the major goals of reconstruction are to allow obliteration of the oral cavity to minimize dead space, to maintain premaxillary contact for articulation and the oral phase of swallowing, and to optimize the mobility of the tip of the tongue to maximize tongue sweep. Postoperative measures of tongue protrusion and elevation have helped to identify objective targets for favorable speech and swallowing outcomes.[117] Also, for total glossectomy, the volume and convexity of the flap are critical to the achievement of optimal functional outcomes.[118]

For patients with oral cancers requiring mandibulectomy, mandibular reconstruction with bone ensures the best outcomes for speech, swallowing, and cosmesis and also helps to maintain symmetric temporomandibular joint articulation enabling mouth opening and maintenance of an occlusal plane for chewing. The major cosmetic goals of mandibular reconstruction include providing facial height and projection to prevent the "Andy Gump" deformity.[119] Reconstruction of maxillary and hard palate reconstruction can provide oronasal separation as well as a surface necessary for premaxillary contact and obliteration during the oral phase of swallowing. Although prosthetic palatal obturation can also help achieve these objections, the choice between prosthetic obturation and free tissue is based on the size of the defect, the location, and the number of remaining teeth.[120] The major goals for reconstruction of the floor of the mouth include separation of the oral cavity from the neck and provision of soft tissue bulk between the ventral tongue and the mandible that prevents tethering of the tongue as well as provision of a platform for tongue elevation and protrusion. Major objectives of buccal reconstruction include resurfacing the cheek with prevention of cicatricial scaring and trismus. As swallowing function is well established as one of the most important factors associated with improved quality of life, oral cavity reconstruction and swallowing therapy under the guidance of an experienced speech pathologist are the critical elements in the successful functional rehabilitation after oral cavity cancer resection.

PRINCIPLES OF RADIATION THERAPY

Primary Radiation Therapy

In considering primary radiation as a treatment option, it must be borne in mind that the keratinizing, well-differentiated histology of many oral cancers may portend radioresistance. It is also important to consider that the bony structures of the mandible and maxilla may impact the transmission of ionizing radiation. For early-stage disease, a combined approach including both external beam radiation and interstitial brachytherapy is often recommended for optimal outcome. Thus, a course of radiation can require several weeks of daily therapy followed by an interstitial implant. The normal tissue toxicity risks of xerostomia, dental and gum injury, and occasional osteoradionecrosis may render radiation therapy a less attractive option for single modality treatment of patients who are candidates for surgery. For locally advanced disease, definitive radiation or chemoradiation is not advised in patients who are candidates for surgery.[1]

Historically, sites commonly treated with single modality radiation include the lip, floor of the mouth, and oral tongue.[121,122] Early work indicates that the success rate of radiotherapy is higher if some or all of the treatment is administered with brachytherapy.[123,124] Decroix and Ghossein[125] reported outcomes in 602 patients with cancer of the oral tongue treated with radium implantation or implantation plus external beam radiation. In this series, recurrence at the primary site or at the primary site and neck was 14% and 22% for T1 and T2 lesions, respectively. The Royal Marsden Hospital reported local control rates of 90% at 5 years for T1 and T2 tumors treated with interstitial radiation with or without external beam radiation.[126] Pernot et al.[127] reported local control rates of 96% for T1, 85% for T2, and 64% for T3 lesions of the oral cavity treated with brachytherapy and neck dissection. In this series, locoregional control rates were 83%, 70%, and 44%, respectively. Retrospective studies suggest that control rates at the primary site of early oral cavity lesions treated with brachytherapy alone or a combination of brachytherapy plus external beam radiation range from approximately 70% to >95%.[125–128] For tumors that either involve the mandible or are immediately adjacent to it, definitive radiotherapy is contraindicated because it compromises control and increases the risk of osteoradionecrosis.

Intraoral cone, like interstitial brachytherapy, is a localized radiation therapy technique that has been used to boost the dose to the primary tumor in the oral cavity. Institutions with significant experience with this technique have reported results that rival those obtained by interstitial brachytherapy.[129,130] Either technique for boosting the primary tumor has resulted in improved outcomes compared to high-dose radiation therapy alone.[131,132] In general, external beam radiation therapy followed by either technique is preferable over radiation therapy alone. As with all specialized procedures, the skill and experience of the radiation oncologist are of critical importance to the successful delivery and outcome of interstitial radiation or intraoral cone therapy.

The outcomes for advanced lesions of the oral cavity (T3 and T4) are less than satisfactory with either surgery or radiation alone. In most advanced-stage cancers, single modality therapy is inferior to combined modality therapy.[124,133,134] Adjuvant radiation therapy can be delivered preoperatively or postoperatively.[129,133] Although each strategy has potential advantages and disadvantages, postoperative radiation therapy is generally preferred. Postoperative radiation treatment carries the advantage of no delay in the implementation of surgical resection and complete pathologic staging of the tumor. However, it must be borne in mind that postoperative wound complications may delay the implementation of radiation therapy.

Adjuvant Radiation

Although surgery has emerged as the preferred initial treatment approach for the majority of patients with tumors of the oral cavity, adjuvant radiation is commonly recommended to enhance the likelihood of locoregional tumor control. Robertson et al.[135] conducted a phase III study in the United Kingdom of 350 patients with T2–T4/N0–N2 oral cavity or oropharyngeal cancers comparing surgery and postoperative radiation versus radiation alone. Because a difference in survival was identified, the study was closed early. The authors found that after 23 months, overall survival, cause-specific survival, and local control were all improved in the surgery plus radiation arm. Traditionally, indications for postoperative radiation therapy include multiple cervical metastases, positive or close margins, extracapsular extension, perineural invasion, advanced T stage, and mandibular bone involvement. A phase III study conducted at the University of Texas MD Anderson Cancer Center established the relative prognostic significance of clusters of two or more clinicopathologic features.[136] The adverse clinicopathologic features in this study included (a) close or positive margins, (b) nerve involvement, (c) ≥2 positive lymph nodes, (d) largest node >3 cm, (e) treatment delay >6 weeks, and (f) Zubrod performance status ≥2. The presence of ENE was the only factor independently predictive of locoregional recurrence. Moreover, the authors concluded that escalation of dose beyond 63 Gy (in 1.8 Gy per fraction) to sites of increased risk did not yield improved locoregional control.

It is well appreciated that head and neck tumors are rapidly proliferating. Several retrospective series have demonstrated an association between diminished outcomes and a delay beyond 6 weeks in initiating postoperative radiation.[137–139] A multi-institutional prospective study by Ang et al. demonstrated that the total treatment time from the completion of surgery to the completion of radiation may affect the likelihood of ultimate disease control.[140] This study illustrated the impact of overall treatment time on 5-year locoregional control: patients with overall times <11 weeks demonstrated a locoregional control rate of 76%, compared to 62% for 11 to 13 weeks, and 38% for times beyond 13 weeks. Hence, it is recommended that adjuvant radiation proceed as soon as surgical wounds are well healed, optimally 4 to 6 weeks after completion of surgery.

There has been significant interest in the use of intensified radiation fractionation schedules to counter rapid tumor cell repopulation as a means of improving outcomes in head and neck cancer patients treated with radiation. Altered fractionation regimens such as hyperfractionation or accelerated fractionation have been considered for patients being treated with radiation alone, as this approach has been demonstrated to improve the likelihood of locoregional tumor control in the definitive setting.[141] However, the use of altered fractionation in the postoperative setting has not been resolved. Ang et al. reported a trend toward higher locoregional control and survival with a concomitant boost schedule compared to a standard fractionation schedule.[140] However, in a subsequent study, Sanguineti et al.[142] demonstrated no benefit for accelerated fractionation, except in patients for whom postoperative radiation was delayed.

There has been recent interest in postoperative chemoradiation for patients with high-risk pathologic features. The results of two randomized trials suggest that postoperative chemoradiation may be beneficial for improving locoregional control and disease-free survival among selected patients with specific high-risk features.[81,84] The impact of chemoradio-therapy appears to be most pronounced in patients with ENE and/or microscopically involved surgical margins.[83,84]

Radiation Techniques

General Considerations

Historically, carcinoma of the oral cavity has been treated with opposed lateral fields, using either two-dimensional or three-dimensional (CT-based) techniques. However, since the emergence of intensity-modulated radiation therapy (IMRT) at the turn of the millennium, there has been a dramatic shift in the radiotherapeutic management of head and neck cancer. Since that time, IMRT has gained widespread adoption and has become the de facto standard in the management of carcinoma of the head and neck.[1,88,143] The major driver for this dramatic shift away from conventional techniques has been the potential for normal tissue sparing and consequent improvement in functional outcomes, particularly in the realms of salivary function and dysphagia.

With respect to oral cavity cancer, the improvements in conformality afforded by IMRT have opened the opportunity to mitigate damage to major salivary glands (xerostomia), the mandible (osteoradionecrosis), and the pharyngeal structures (dysphagia).[50,144–148] However, it is important to bear in mind that there are instances in which IMRT may not provide significant additional benefit in the treatment of oral cavity cancer and conventional techniques may be fully adequate. It is also valuable to consider that practitioner and treating center experience may be important indicators of potential outcomes when IMRT is utilized in the treatment of head and neck cancer patients.[149,150]

Each institution should select appropriate oral cavity cases for treatment with IMRT. For instance, patients with T1/T2N0 carcinoma of the floor of the mouth or alveolar ridge that have undergone surgical staging of the neck may not benefit from IMRT because the bulk of both parotid glands can be excluded from opposed lateral portals (Fig. 47.12). Ideal candidates for IMRT include patients with T1/T4 primary lesions with ipsilateral neck disease. In patients that have ipsilateral

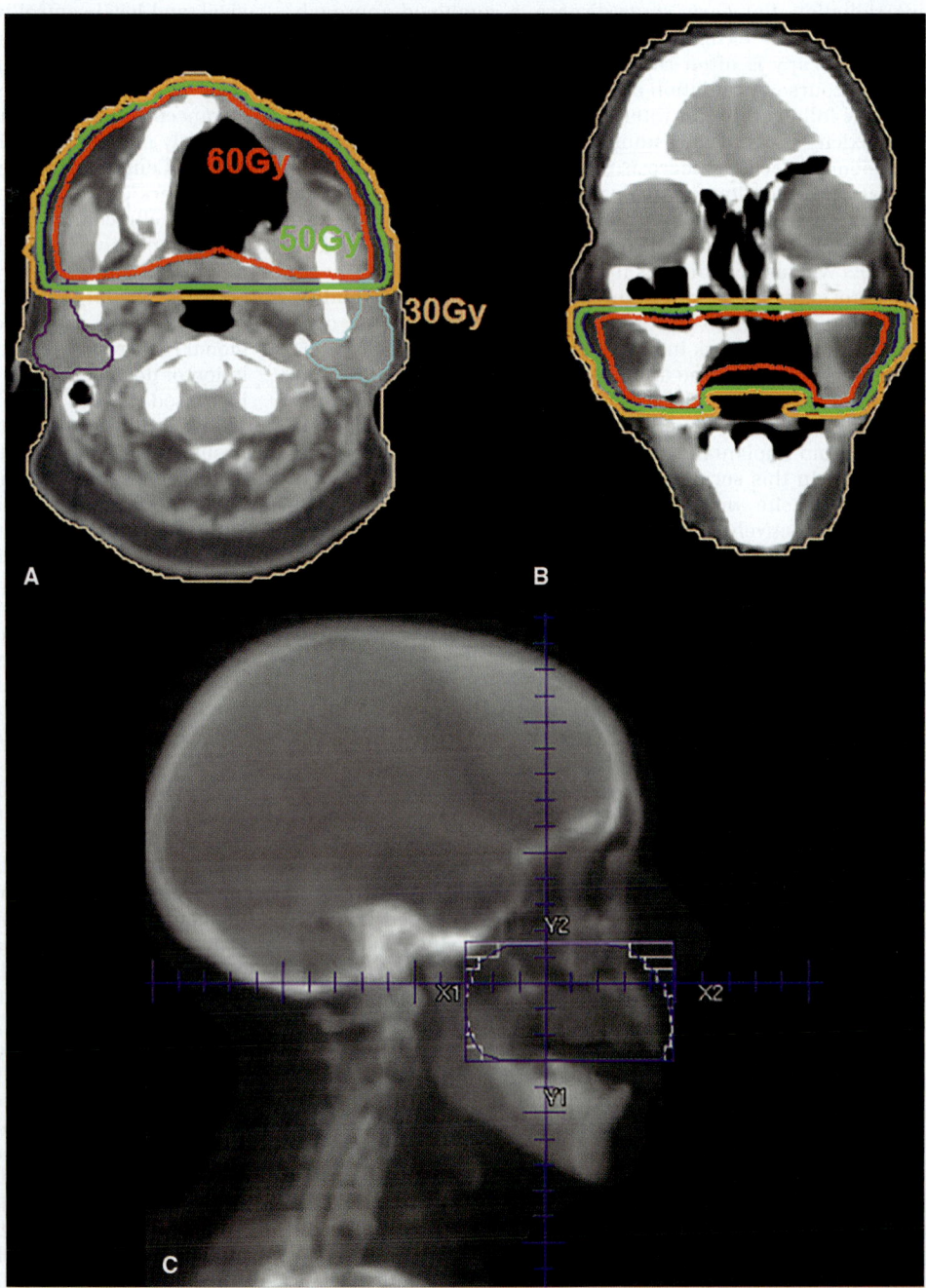

FIGURE 47.12. T4N0M0 squamous cell carcinoma of the maxillary alveolar ridge in a patient who underwent left infrastructure maxillectomy and left selective neck dissection. The figure illustrates postoperative conventional radiation field design with opposed laterals to cover the maxilla and operative bed at risk. Treatment of the neck was omitted in lieu of a negative neck dissection. **A** and **B:** Relevant isodose lines. **C:** Right lateral field DRR. The parotid tissue is nearly completely spared by this field arrangement.

positive neck nodes, IMRT may allow dose limitation to the contralateral parotid gland without compromising treatment results.[151] In patients with bilateral neck disease, it may be difficult to effectively spare the parotid glands, particularly when superior level II cervical lymph nodes are involved, because of the coverage of the retrostyloid space in this setting.[152]

Intensity-Modulated Radiation Therapy

The use of more conformal techniques may be associated with a unique set of potential pitfalls. Whereas treatment planning with two-dimensional or three-dimensional techniques does not universally mandate careful interpretation of cross-sectional imaging and attention to anatomic detail, IMRT requires precise target volume delineation. If a target volume is not included within the clinical target volume (CTV), it may receive a subtherapeutic dose of radiation and thus portend marginal recurrence. The quality of conformal radiation therapy is significantly associated with outcomes in the treatment of head and neck cancer.[149,150,153]

Most cases of oral cavity cancer will be treated postoperatively. It is important to consider that neck dissection tends to disrupt the anatomic landmarks defining borders between nodal levels. The task of distinguishing the primary tumor

resection bed and adjacent neck dissection poses a significant challenge in target volume design. Gregoire et al.[26,152] proposed guidelines for target volume delineation in the postoperative patient that are available as a reference. The authors encourage the reader to review these guidelines as they consider more selective coverage of nodal regions during target volume delineation. These guidelines serve in part as the basis for the recommendations presented in this section. Treatment considerations for each oral cavity subsite are presented in the section "Subsite Specific Treatment and Results."

The discussion to follow is relevant to target volume design in the postoperative setting. Figure 47.13 illustrates relevant target volumes for a typical postoperative oral cavity case. Figures 47.14 and 47.15 provide examples of special considerations for patients with positive margins/ENE and ipsilateral treatment, respectively. There are three classes of CTVs that can be defined based on the practice of a range of North American institutions and cooperative group guidelines.[26,27,51,152,154,155]

- The high-risk CTV (CTV$_{66}$) is defined as the volume harboring ENE or a positive margin. It is recommended that CTV$_{66}$ receives 66Gy either as a simultaneous integrated boost (SIB) (2.2 Gy per fraction over 30 fractions) or as a sequential boost.

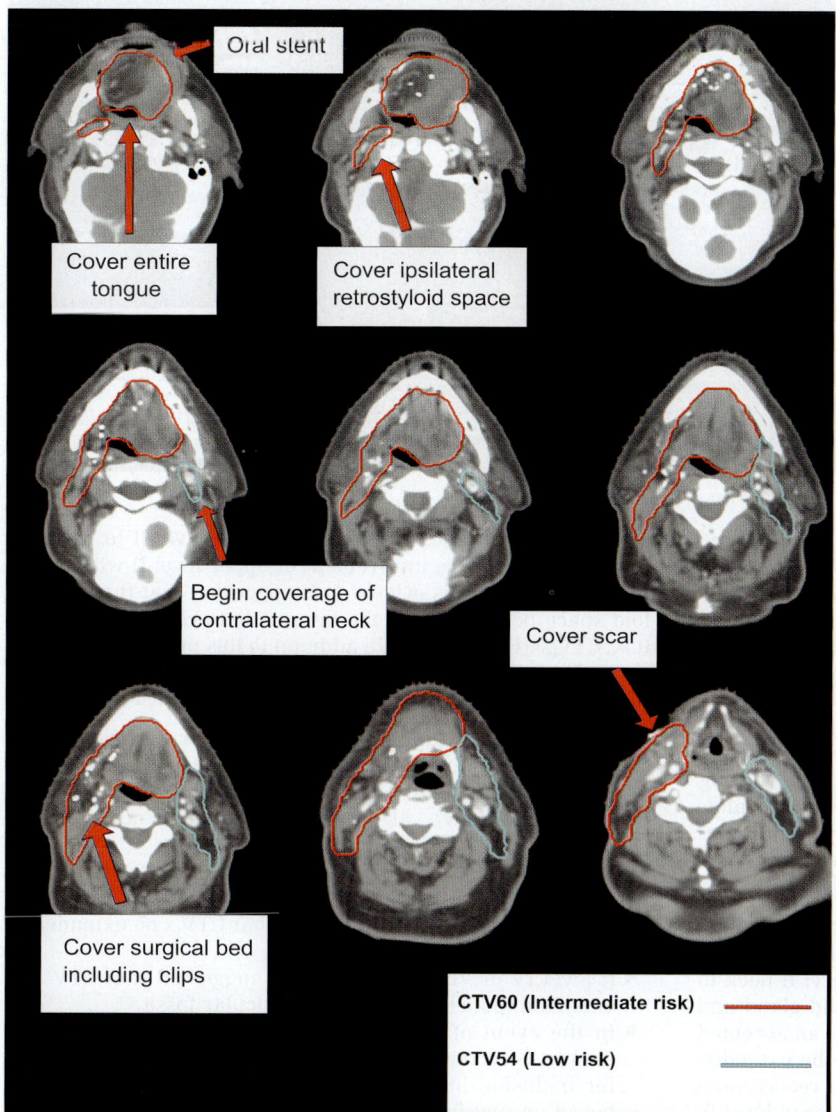

Oral stent

Cover entire tongue

Cover ipsilateral retrostyloid space

Begin coverage of contralateral neck

Cover scar

Cover surgical bed including clips

CTV60 (Intermediate risk) ———

CTV54 (Low risk) ———

FIGURE 47.13. T3N1M0 squamous cell carcinoma of the right oral tongue. The patient underwent right hemiglossectomy, including resection of the floor of the mouth; and right selective neck dissection. The tumor was 3 cm in size, with a depth of invasion of 1.3 cm, and 1/46 lymph nodes with evidence of carcinoma (no evidence of ENE). Adjuvant treatment was delivered with radiation therapy alone using IMRT with the intent of maximizing coverage to regions at risk while sparing salivary glands and pharyngeal tissues. Note that the ipsilateral retrostyloid space and entire tongue, intraoral free flap, and dissected neck are included in CTV$_{60}$. The cranial extent of CTV$_{54}$ in the contralateral neck is the bottom edge of the body of C1. The retropharyngeal nodes are not covered in this setting to allow sparing of the pharyngeal structures.

Section III

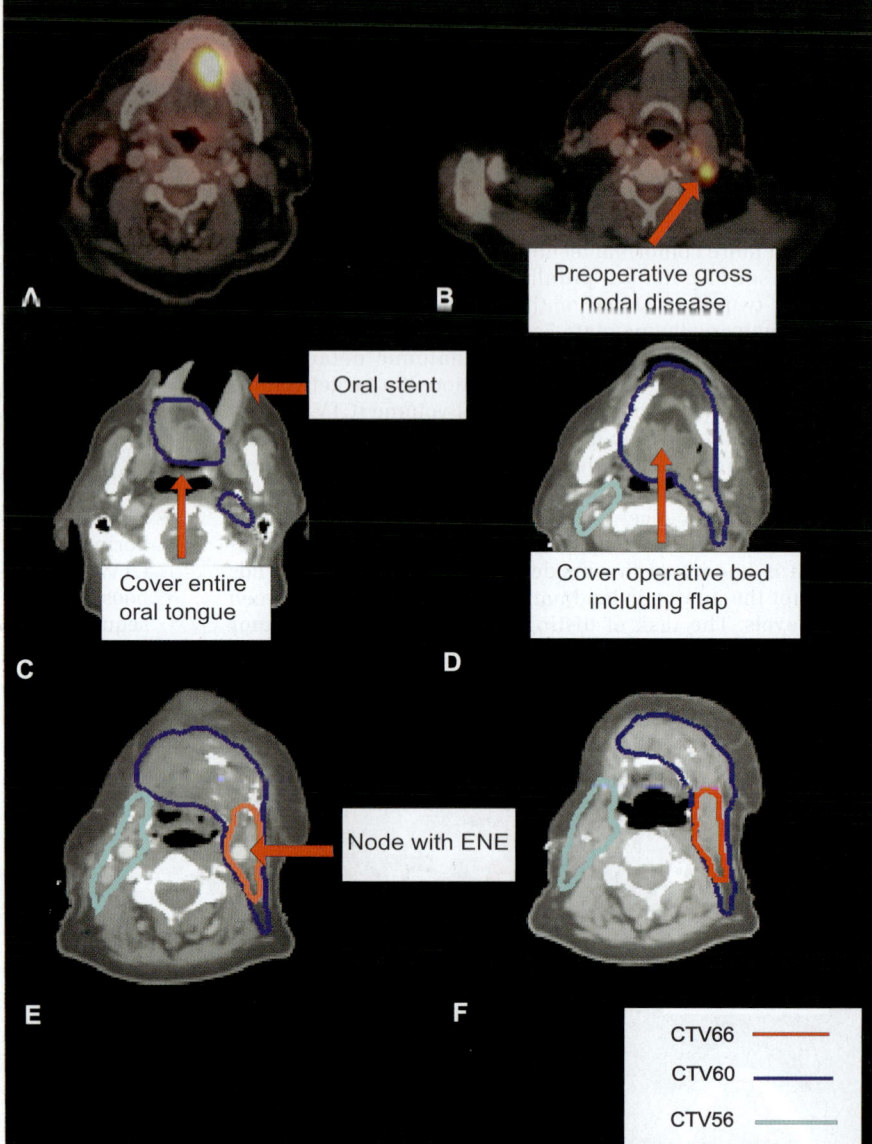

FIGURE 47.14. T4N3bM0 squamous cell carcinoma of the floor of the mouth with evidence of ENE treated on RTOG protocol 1216 (ClinicalTrials.gov identifier: NCT01810913). The patient underwent left mandibulectomy, composite resection of the floor of the mouth, left hemiglossectomy, and neck dissection. The final pathology demonstrated 3 cm primary lesion, with 6/55 lymph nodes positive for carcinoma, and ENE in a lymph node at left level II. The treatment was delivered with IMRT using an SIB concurrently with chemotherapy. The neck region with evidence of ENE received 66 Gy in 2.2 Gy per fraction, whereas the primary site, free flap, and ipsilateral neck received 60 Gy in 2.0 Gy per fraction. The contralateral neck received 56 Gy in 1.87 Gy per fraction. **A** and **B:** Preoperative PET showing primary and nodal disease. **C–F:** Postoperative target volume delineation.

- The intermediate-risk CTV (CTV_{60}) is defined as the volume that includes the primary tumor bed (based on preoperative imaging, physical exam, and operative findings) plus regions of grossly involved adenopathy. The target volume should include the entire primary surgical bed and the pathologically positive hemineck; this frequently requires coverage of nodal levels I, IIa-b, III, and IV for most cases. It is recommended that CTV_{60} receives 60 Gy in 2.0 Gy per fraction.
- The low-risk CTV (CTV_{54-56}) usually includes the prophylactically treated neck felt to have a low risk of harboring microscopic disease (e.g., the uninvolved low or contralateral neck) and should receive 54 to 56 Gy as a simultaneous integrated boost in 1.8 to 1.87 Gy per fraction.

It is common practice for the radiation oncologist to consider selective coverage of the neck and retropharyngeal nodes' order to limit dose to critical organs at risk. This generally involves limiting cranial coverage of the level II neck to the level of C1 in the N0 neck to spare the parotid gland and the upper pharyngeal structures.[51,146,147,152,156] This is an accepted standard in the N0 neck, which may potentially be extended to patients with small N1 disease.[51,152,157] Marginal recurrences near the base of the skull, above this cranial border of level II, have been reported in the node-positive neck.[151] The retrostyloid

space represents the cranial extension of level II to the skull base. In cases where involvement of upper level II with one or more lymph nodes is evident, it is suggested that the retrostyloid space be included in the intermediate-risk target volume (i.e., CTV_{60}) (Fig. 47.13).[152] In addition to this principle, there are several target volume design details specific to the postsurgical head and neck cancer patient that should be considered.

- When a metastatic lymph node abuts or infiltrates muscle (most commonly the sternocleidomastoid or paraspinal musculature), it is recommended that the muscle be included in CTV_{60}, at least for the invaded nodal station (Fig. 47.14).[152]
- When a metastatic node lies at the boundary with a nodal level that was not intended to be part of the intermediate-risk CTV, it is recommended that CTV_{60} be extended to encompass this adjacent level.[152]
- If level IV or Vb is involved, it is suggested that CTV_{60} be extended to include the supraclavicular fossa.[152]
- In the event of flap reconstruction of the oral cavity or neck, it is recommended that the entire flap be considered for inclusion in the IMRT field (either CTV_{60} or CTV_{54-56} based on physician discretion), particularly if there is evidence of ENE.[158]

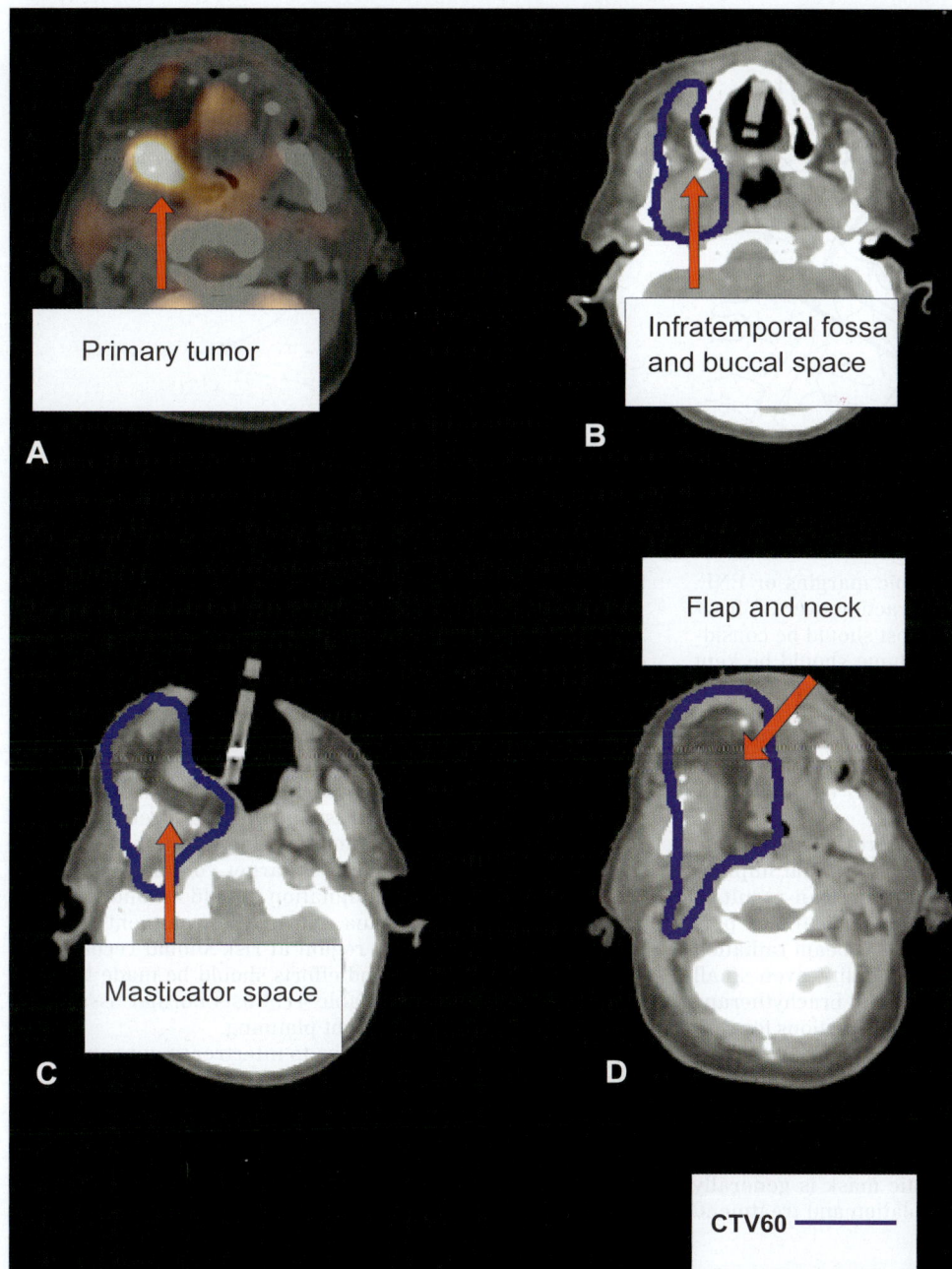

A: Primary tumor

B: Infratemporal fossa and buccal space

Flap and neck

C: Masticator space

D:

CTV60 ——————

FIGURE 47.15. T2N1M0 squamous cell carcinoma of the right retromolar trigone. The patient underwent composite resection of the right retromolar trigone, buccal mucosa, maxilla, and right neck dissection, followed by anterolateral thigh free flap reconstruction of the defect. **A:** Preoperative PET showing disease at the primary site. **B–D:** Postoperative target volume delineation of the surgical bed, masticator space, infratemporal fossa, free flap, and ipsilateral neck.

■ In the case of extensive perineural spread, it is recommended that the proximal course of the involved nerves be included in the treatment field to the level of the infratemporal fossa or skull base.[159]

Conventional Radiotherapy

For the treatment of oral cavity cancer with either two-dimensional or three-dimensional techniques, the oral cavity tumor bed and upper echelon lymph nodes are included within the initial lateral fields (Fig. 47.16). The upper border of the field is positioned to provide a 1.5- to 2.0-cm border on the tumor bed in attempt to partially spare parotid glands and hard palate without compromising coverage of the tumor bed and regional lymphatics. The inferior border of the field resides at approximately the thyroid notch, just above the true vocal cords. The posterior border is set at the midvertebral body level if level V nodal coverage is not required. The nodal volume should include levels Ia–Ib, II, and III. For patients with more advanced neck disease or positive level V lymph

nodes, where the posterior chain requires radiation, the initial fields should be set behind the C1 vertebral body spinous process. The portals are then reduced at approximately 45 Gy to spare high dose to the spinal cord. If patients harbor cervical lymph node metastases, or high-risk disease, then the lower neck will also be treated. In this case, half-beam–blocked anteroposterior (AP) or opposed anteroposterior/posteroanterior (AP/PA) fields can be matched to the inferior border of the opposed lateral fields at the level of the thyroid notch. An anterior larynx block is used, which not only protects the central larynx from unnecessary radiation dose but also protects against spinal cord overdose because of three-field overlap.

Dose and Fractionation

When postoperative radiation is used for oral cavity cancer, the most common dose fractionation in the United States is 1.8 to 2.0 Gy/day. The authors generally recommend 2.0 Gy daily fractions. Dissected tissues that harbored the original tumor should generally receive dose on the order of 60 Gy.

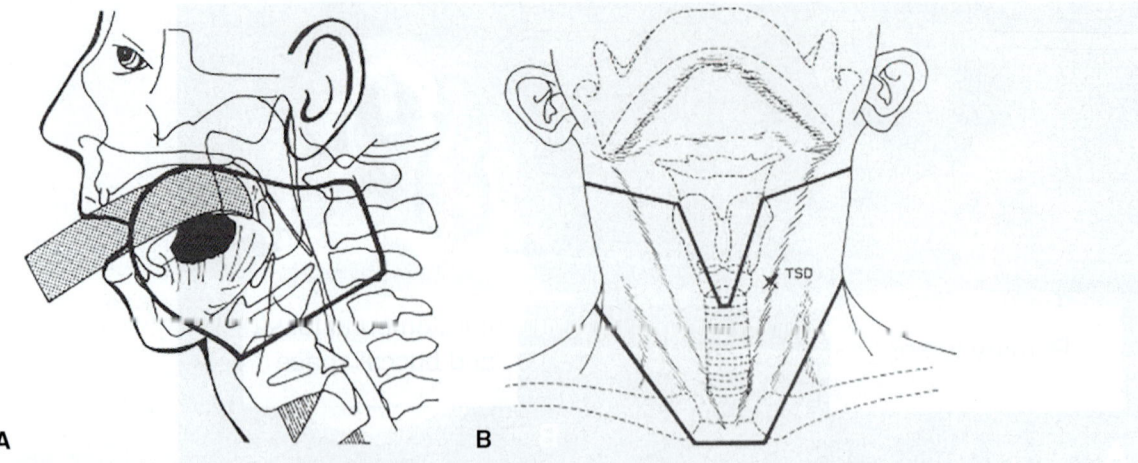

FIGURE 47.16. A: Illustration of field design for treatment of carcinoma of the oral tongue with an N0 neck. **B:** Illustration of field design for treatment of the neck for elective bilateral neck irradiation. (From Million RR, Cassisi NJ, eds. Management of head and neck cancer: *a multidisciplinary approach.* 2nd ed. Philadelphia: Lippincott, 1994. With permission.)

However, for close or positive microscopic margins or ENE, either an SIB to 66 Gy (e.g., 2.2 Gy per fraction over 30 fractions) or a sequential 6.0 Gy localized boost should be considered. In the former scenario, the SIB volume should be kept small to minimize normal tissue complications (Fig. 47.14). If there is gross residual disease, either further surgical resection or focal boosting up to 70 Gy may be necessary. Regions of somewhat lesser risk (i.e., clinically or pathologically uninvolved necks) should receive dose on the order of 54 to 56 Gy if treatment is delivered with an SIB.

When definitive radiation is used for oral cavity cancer, boosting the primary tumor with either interstitial implantation, submental, or intraoral cone therapy can result in increased tumor control and decreased complications, particularly osteoradionecrosis.[131] When external beam radiation therapy is used as the sole treatment modality, even small lesions that cannot be excised or treated with brachytherapy require doses in the range of 66 Gy in 2.0 Gy fractions for reliable control. For larger tumors, local control rates are generally unacceptable, even with the utilization of IMRT.[88,89]

Simulation and Treatment Considerations
The patient should undergo simulation in the supine position with the neck extended. A thermoplastic mask is generally used to immobilize patients during simulation and treatment.

Shoulder immobilization is important during this process, which is accomplished by using either a three-/four-point Aquaplast mask along with a shoulder immobilization device or a five-point mask that also encompasses the shoulders. For most oral cavity simulations, a bite block should be used to depress the tongue away from the hard palate; some institutions use a cork and tongue blade or a custom intraoral stent[160] for this purpose (Fig. 47.17).

CT simulation should be performed using a slice thickness of ≤3 mm, and i.v. contrast should be utilized in patients that have adequate renal function. The addition of contrast dye during simulation facilitates target volume delineation. The CT acquired during simulation should extend from the top of the head to the carina. During the treatment planning process, the PTV for each region at risk should receive 95% of the prescription dose, and efforts should be made to spare critical structures at risk. Table 47.3 lists normal tissue dose constraints for IMRT treatment planning.

IMRT may be more sensitive to intertreatment setup variations than conventional radiation therapy.[161] Daily imaging and strict immobilization protocols may decrease setup error and improve the fidelity of treatment delivery.[161–163] It is recommended that institutions use daily image-guided radiation therapy (IGRT) to enhance setup reproducibility of IMRT treatment delivery. This may be accomplished with

FIGURE 47.17. A: Lucite oral cavity mouthpiece fabricated at the University of Wisconsin for patients with oral cavity carcinomas. Upper dentition or maxillary alveolus links to U-shaped notch and tongue rests beneath smooth undersurface of mouthpiece. Note embedded solder wire in mouthpiece floor to facilitate visualization of tongue positioning at the time of simulation and beam design. **B:** Custom acrylic mouth-opening and tongue-depressing stent utilized at several centers for the treatment of oral cavity carcinoma. The posterior edge (*red arrow*) helps to immobilize the tongue, whereas the superior ridges allow the maxillary teeth to rest and secure the stent in place.

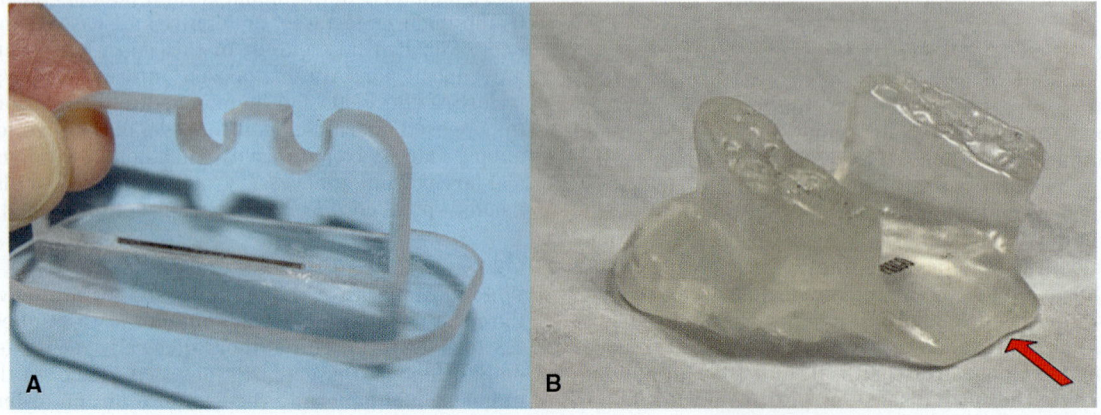

TABLE 47.3 NORMAL TISSUE DOSE–VOLUME CONSTRAINTS[a]

Organ at Risk (OAR)	Dose–Volume Constraint
Spinal cord (+5 mm)	Dose to 0.03 cc ≤ 48 Gy
Brain stem (+3 mm)	Dose to 0.03 cc ≤ 52 Gy
Parotid glands	(a) Mean dose to single gland ≤ 26 Gy
	(b) 20 cc of combined volume of both parotids < 20Gy
	(c) 50% single gland < 30 Gy
OAR pharynx	(a) Dose to 33% ≤ 50 Gy
	(b) Mean dose ≤ 45 Gy
	(c) Dose to 15% ≤ 60 Gy
Glottic/supraglottic larynx	Mean dose ≤ 44 Gy
Cochlea	Max dose < 35 Gy
Optic apparatus	Max dose < 54 Gy
Brachial plexus	Max dose < 66 Gy

[a]Dose–volume constraints for IMRT planning adapted based on Qualitative Analysis of Normal Tissue Effects in the Clinic (QUANTEC) recommendations,[217-220] practice standards, and Radiation Therapy Oncology Group protocol guidelines (RTOG 0920, ClinicalTrials.gov identifier, NCT00956007, and RTOG 1216, ClinicalTrials.gov identifier, NCT01810913).

several IGRT techniques including orthogonal kilovoltage films, kilovoltage cone beam CT, or megavoltage CT imaging. With the use of IGRT techniques, planning treatment volume (PTV) expansions on the CTV may be limited to 2 to 5 mm. However, larger margins may be necessary for target volumes subject to significant interfraction variability; examples include the tongue in the absence of an intraoral stent, a large flap in the oral cavity or neck, and some cases where there is significant shoulder motion and the low neck must be included in an extended IMRT field.[164] For these circumstances, a CTV–PTV expansion margin of 10 mm or greater may be necessary.

The delivery of a single IMRT plan throughout the course of treatment provides better dose conformality compared to the delivery of several consecutive (sequential) plans.[165] In the absence of low-lying cervical adenopathy, the low anterior neck can be treated with a single AP field or AP/PA fields matched to an upper IMRT field. The advantage of this split-field technique, compared to treating the low neck with an extended IMRT field, lies in the ability to decrease mean dose to the larynx and inferior pharyngeal constrictors.[166]

Brachytherapy

Historically, brachytherapy has played an important role in the treatment of oral cavity carcinoma. Brachytherapy has been used to boost the primary site in the oral cavity before or following external beam radiation (Fig. 47.18). This technique has also been used as a sole modality in the treatment of selected (early-stage) tumors of the oral cavity with good results.[127,128,167] When brachytherapy is used as a sole treatment modality, doses of 65 to 75 Gy are commonly prescribed over 6 to 7 days. Traditionally, radiation has been delivered using low dose rates of 0.4 to 0.6 Gy/hour to the target volume.[168,169] However, there has been recent interest in high dose rate (HDR) (Fig. 47.19) and pulsed dose rate techniques (PLDR),[170,171] although there is no compelling evidence that these techniques are superior to traditional low dose rate radiation in the treatment of head and neck cancer. There have been several dose and fractionation schedules published for HDR brachytherapy in the treatment of oral cavity cancer.[172-175] Although the American Brachytherapy Society has not provided a consensus as to optimal dose and fractionation,[176] there is concern regarding the potential morbidity with fraction sizes ≥ 6.0 Gy in this setting.[176,177]

FIGURE 47.18. **A:** T2N0M0 squamous cell carcinoma involving the left lateral oral tongue. **B:** Submental view of interstitial implantation catheters housing ^{192}Ir seeds for delivery of 25-Gy tumor boost following external beam radiation of 50 Gy. **C:** Implantation bed mucositis conforming to the tumor distribution 7 days following 25-Gy implant boost.

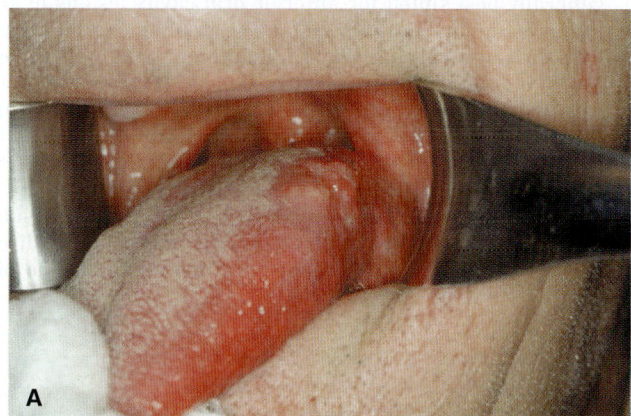

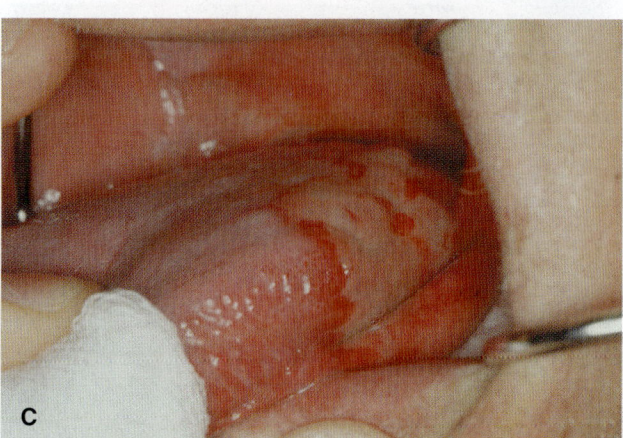

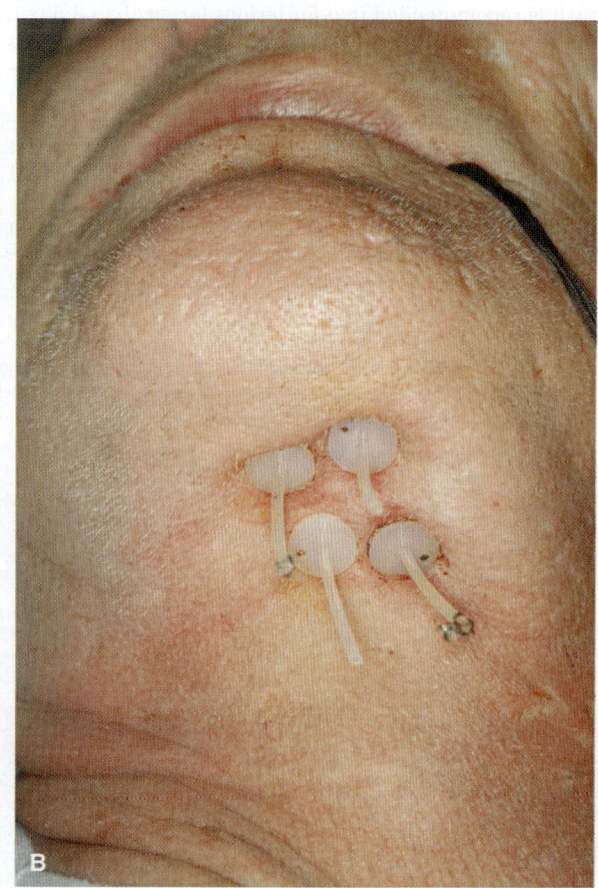

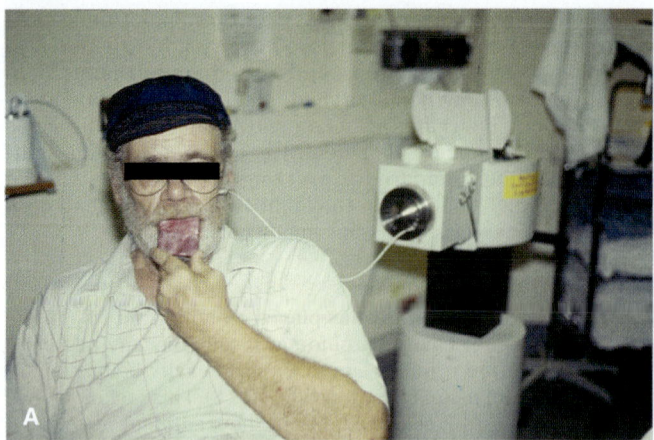
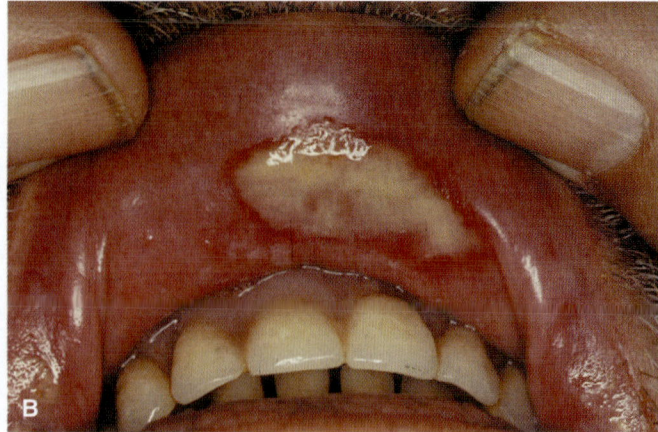

FIGURE 47.19. A: Patient undergoing high dose rate (HDR) brachytherapy for superficial T1 upper lip squamous cell carcinoma (buccal surface) using a single interstitial catheter for source delivery. **B:** Focal mucositis 1 week following completion of HDR brachytherapy treatment course.

Many techniques for brachytherapy in the oral cavity have been described.[178,179] Brachytherapy can be accomplished either with rigid cesium needles or with iridium 192 (^{192}Ir) sources afterloaded into angiocaths. The most common technique is afterloading with ^{192}Ir.[180] Guide needles can be inserted either freehand or with the aid of a custom template to help maintain optimal source spacing.

Depending on the size of the lesion, a single plane, double plane, or volume implant can be used to cover the tumor with a 1-cm margin. For tumors <1 cm in thickness, single-plane implants are adequate. Surface mold radiation can also be considered for small tumors <1 cm depth or superficial lesions of the lip, hard palate, lower gingiva, and floor of the mouth. However, when lesions exceed 2.5 cm, it is difficult to avoid significant cold spots in the implant volume. For this reason, it is recommended that for lesions larger than 2.5 cm, part of the treatment is given with external beam radiation to supplement the dose to the cold spots. In this setting, a combined treatment plan typically gives 50 Gy over 5 weeks with external beam radiation followed by 30 Gy with a brachytherapy implant. What must be borne in mind is that as tumors get too close to the mandible or are large in volume, the risk of osteoradionecrosis increases.[181]

Over the past decade or more, stepwise improvements in reconstructive surgery techniques have diminished the practice frequency of brachytherapy in the treatment of oral cavity carcinoma. In addition, a diminishing percentage of radiation oncologists remain highly skilled and experienced with the requisite implant techniques. Nevertheless, in experienced hands, the expert use of brachytherapy can provide excellent tumor control and high-quality cosmetic and functional results. An example of the use of HDR interstitial brachytherapy for a patient with an advanced T2N0 lower lip cancer is illustrated in Figure 47.20. Similar comments parallel the use of intraoral cone radiation treatment described further in the section below.

Intraoral Cone

The intraoral cone is another delivery tool to enable boosting of radiation dose to sites within the oral cavity while avoiding direct dose to the mandible (Fig. 47.21). This technique is generally best suited for anterior oral cavity lesions in edentulous patients. However, palatal arch sites can be targeted with the intraoral cone as well. Treatment with intraoral cone involves either 100 to 250 kilovolt (peak) (kvp) x-rays or electron beams in the 6 to 12 MeV range.[129,130,178] Lesions up to 3 cm are amenable to treatment with intraoral cone as long as they are accessible. Intraoral cone therapy requires careful daily positioning and verification by the physician. For this purpose, the device is equipped with a periscope to visualize the lesion. The cone abuts the mucosa and is centered directly over the lesion. Intraoral cone treatment should take place

FIGURE 47.20. A: Infiltrative T2N0 squamous cell carcinoma of the lower lip measuring 3.5 × 1.2 × 1.2 cm. **B:** Interstitial iridium 192 implant performed (2 catheters) for HDR brachytherapy delivery over 11 elapsed days as sole treatment. The patient remains with no evidence of disease at 6 years with excellent cosmetic and functional status.

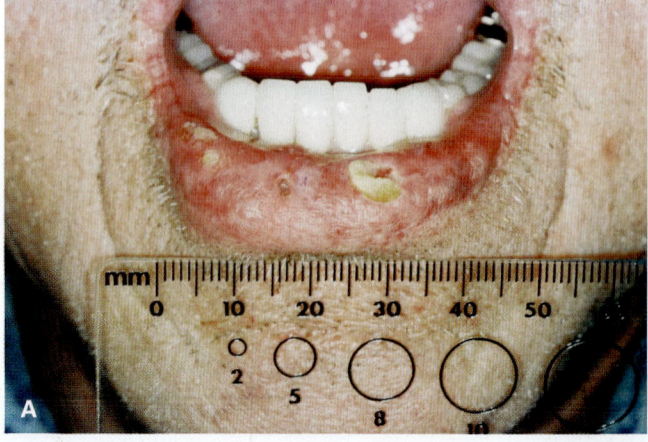
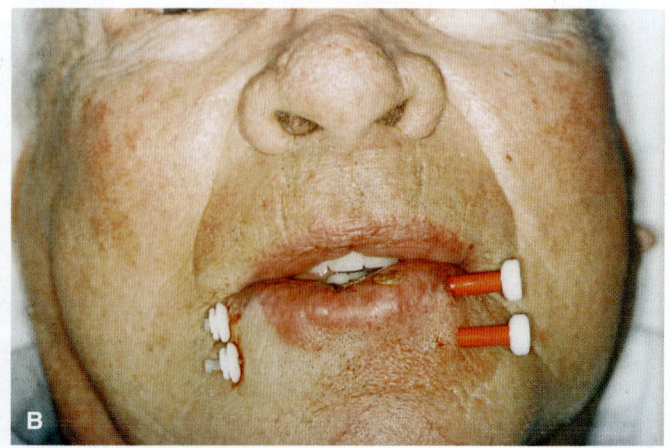

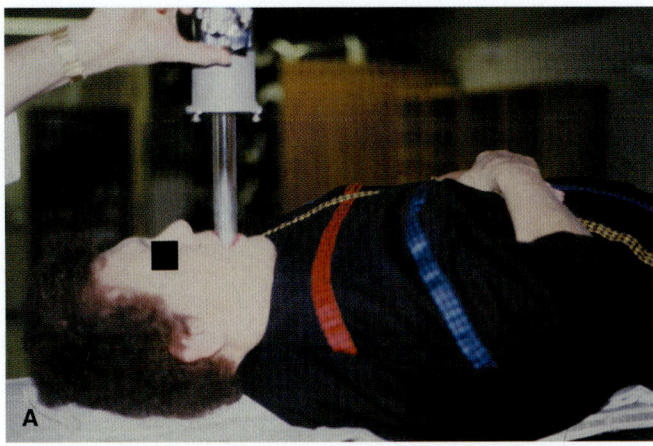
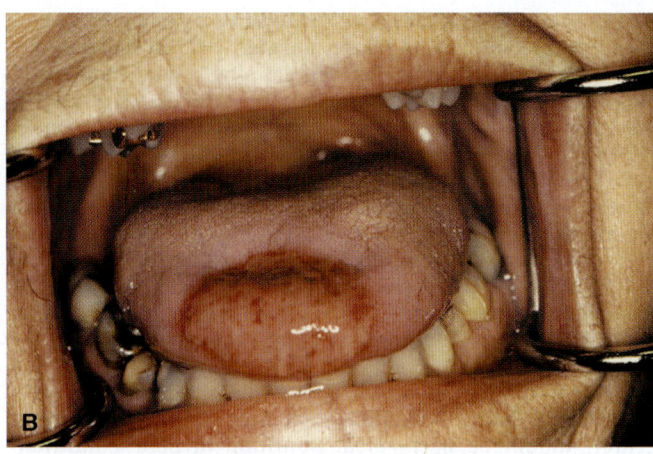

Section III

FIGURE 47.21. A: Intraoral cone boost technique at the University of Wisconsin for focal delivery of electron beam radiation. The electron cone is mounted directly to the accelerator gantry with a side view periscope enabling direct vision and positioning for daily treatment. **B:** Focal mucositis involving the distal oral tongue following treatment of a 1-cm tumor in this location with intraoral cone technique.

prior to external beam radiation so that the lesion can be adequately visualized. A major advantage of cone therapy is that it is highly focal to the tumor bed but noninvasive. Hence, when available, for suitable lesions, it may be preferred over brachytherapy. However, as noted for brachytherapy delivery, operator experience and dedication are essential to optimize outcome.

PRINCIPLES OF SYSTEMIC THERAPY

Over the decades, the role of chemotherapy has advanced from use only in the recurrent or metastatic setting to use in the definitive treatment setting. The advantage of systemic therapy was explored by the meta-analysis of chemotherapy in head and neck cancer (MACH-NC).[182,183] The study included pooled data from randomized trials of patients with a diagnosis of oral cavity, oropharynx, hypopharynx, and larynx cancer who received chemotherapy in the induction, concurrent, or adjuvant setting.[183] Although the trials included in this analysis vary with respect to radiation dose, fractionation schedule, and chemotherapy regimen, they have in common a randomized comparison between radiotherapy and radiotherapy plus chemotherapy. The updated MACH-NC report of 93 randomized trials identifies an absolute survival benefit of 4.5% at 5 years with the addition of chemotherapy, which is mainly driven by the effect of concurrent chemoradiation (6.5% at 5 years).[183] However, oral cavity patients comprised only 21% of the patient population in the pooled analysis.[86]

Several studies have focused on the use of chemoradiation in patients with high-risk pathologic features following initial surgery. Cooper et al.[81] reported the results of RTOG 9501 comparing radiation alone (60 to 66 Gy) to chemoradiation (same radiation dose plus three cycles of 100 mg/m² cisplatin) in patients with head and neck carcinoma demonstrating high-risk features after gross total resection. High-risk disease was defined as any or all of the following: two or more involved lymph nodes, extracapsular extension of nodal disease (ENE), and microscopically involved resection margins. This study demonstrated a benefit in locoregional control and disease-free survival for the chemoradiation arm, but no overall survival benefit was appreciated. A parallel study, EORTC 2931, reported by Bernier et al.[84] randomized patients to essentially equivalent treatment arms following head and neck cancer surgery. Eligibility criteria included patients with pathologic T3 or T4 disease (except T3/N0), or patients with any T-stage disease with two or more involved lymph nodes, or patients with T1/T2 and N0/N1 disease with unfavorable

pathologic findings (ENE, positive margins, perineural involvement, or vascular embolism). Local control, progression-free survival, and overall survival were superior for patients in the chemoradiation arm. In a subsequent comparative analysis using pooled data from these two studies, ENE and/or microscopically involved surgical margins were the risk factors for which the impact concurrent chemoradiation was significant.[83] There was a trend favoring concurrent chemoradiation in the subset of patients with stage III to IV disease, vascular embolism, perineural infiltration, and/or positive lymph nodes at levels IV and V with oral cavity or oropharyngeal primaries.[83] The subset of patients with two or more involved lymph nodes, without evidence of ENE, did not appear to benefit from chemotherapy in this analysis. These studies suggest that the addition of chemoradiation following surgery should be considered in patients with high-risk head and neck cancer features who are able to tolerate treatment.[1]

Neoadjuvant systemic therapy is generally not recommended in the standard management of resectable oral cavity squamous cell carcinoma.[1] In the case of technically unresectable oral cavity squamous cell carcinoma, the concept of neoadjuvant chemotherapy as a means of downstaging disease in order to enable surgical resection has been explored.[184] The engagement of an experienced head and neck surgical oncologist to explore the technical feasibility of resection is paramount due to the potential of disease progression and the consequent risk of compromising the potential for resection in borderline patients. Generally, in this context, a combination of docetaxel, cisplatin, and 5-FU is the preferred induction regimen for clinically fit patients[185] with reported response rates of 17% to 50%.[184] However, it is important to consider that the inherent toxicity of these regimens may compromise the ability to deliver local therapy.[186–188]

The use of molecular targeted therapies has steadily advanced in the field of head and neck oncology. Cetuximab is a monoclonal antibody against the epidermal growth factor receptor (EGFR) that has been approved for the management of locally advanced, recurrent, or metastatic head and neck squamous cell carcinoma.[186,189] In the context of locally advanced head and neck squamous cell carcinoma, Bonner et al. reported the results of a multinational study demonstrating the superiority of cetuximab plus radiation over radiation alone.[190] However, this study did not include patients with oral cavity squamous cell carcinoma. The RTOG launched a study (RTOG 0920, ClinicalTrials.gov identifier: NCT00956007) to evaluate the impact of cetuximab in the postoperative treatment for intermediate-risk disease. The study defines intermediate-risk disease as perineural invasion, lympho-vascular space invasion, close margins, T3/T4a disease, T2 disease with > 5 mm thickness, and single lymph node >3 cm or ≥2 or lymph nodes <6 cm without ENE. After an R0 resection, patients are randomized to radiation or cetuximab plus radiation. A parallel study (RTOG 1216, ClinicalTrials.gov identifier: NCT01810913) was launched to explore the benefit of cetuximab and docetaxel compared to standard platinum-based chemotherapy in the setting of patients with high-risk disease (ENE or positive margins). Both RTOG 0920 and RTOG 1216 are closed to accrual, but results are not yet available. The role of cetuximab in the management of locally advanced oral cavity squamous cell carcinoma remains to be defined.

Prior to the initiation of head and neck radiation, a careful oral and dental evaluation, including a panoramic radiograph, should be performed. Dentition in poor condition should be identified and considered for extraction to minimize the subsequent risk of osteoradionecrosis. Specifically, those teeth that will reside within the high-dose radiation volume that demonstrate significant periodontal disease, advanced caries, or abscess formation or are otherwise in a state of disrepair should be extracted. In addition, impacted teeth, unopposed teeth, and teeth that could potentially oppose a segment of a resected jawbone should be considered for extraction if they are anticipated to reside within the high-dose radiation treatment volume. Extraction of marginal teeth should also be considered in patients who are deemed unable to maintain adequate oral hygiene.

Radiation can induce several chronic effects in the oral cavity that warrant routine surveillance. Radiation can impair bone healing and diminish the capacity for successful recovery following trauma or oral surgery. For this reason, elective oral surgical procedures including extractions must be very carefully considered after radiation. Escalation of dental caries deriving from xerostomia following radiation is well recognized (Fig. 47.22). Radiation of the major salivary glands changes the nature of salivary secretions,[46] which can increase the accumulation of plaque and debris, reduce salivary pH, and reduce the buffering ability of saliva.[191] This creates an environment in the oral cavity, which predisposes patients to caries. During a course of radiation to the oral cavity, simple techniques such as the use of custom molds or wax to absorb electron backscatter can diminish hot spot mucositis from dental fillings and improve treatment tolerance.[47] Attention to oral hygiene with frequent dental follow-up examinations and cleanings, daily fluoride therapy (Fig. 47.23), flossing, and brushing should be an integral component of the education and postradiation care of patients who undergo radiation to the oral cavity.

FIGURE 47.22. Advanced dental caries in a patient with profound radiation xerostomia and lack of attention to dental hygiene over many years following treatment.

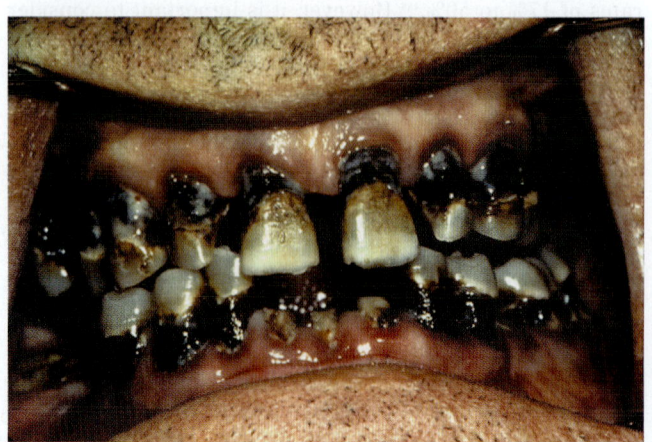

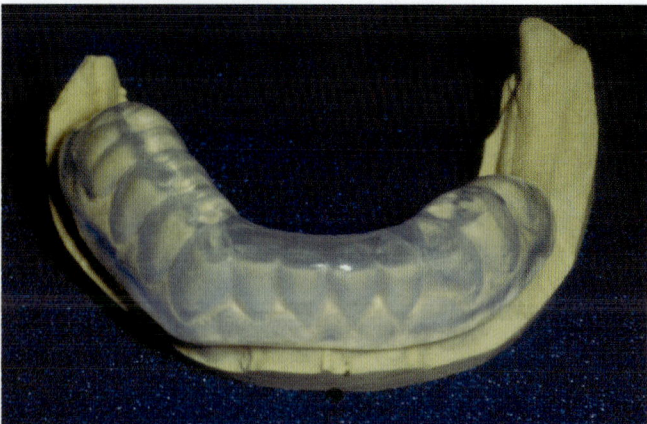

FIGURE 47.23. Custom designed fluoride carrier trays to facilitate daily fluoride application to existing dentition.

PROGNOSTIC AND PREDICTIVE FACTORS

The most significant prognostic factor for outcome in oral cavity carcinoma is the presence of cervical metastases.[192] In patients with positive cervical metastases, the 5-year survival is reduced by approximately 50% compared to those without cervical metastases.[193] The prognosis diminishes further when patients harbor multiple levels of nodal involvement or ENE. In a retrospective review, Myers et al.[192] found that 5-year disease-specific and overall survival rates for pathologically N0 patients were 88% and 75%, respectively; these decreased to 65% and 50%, respectively, if patients were node positive but without evidence of ENE. Patients who were node positive with evidence of ENE had 5-year disease-specific and overall survival rates of 48% and 30%, respectively.

Several histopathologic factors in the primary lesion are associated with adverse prognosis. Tumor thickness and depth of invasion have been shown to confer a higher risk of regional metastases.[18] Perineural invasion has been correlated with cervical lymph node metastases, extracapsular extension, and diminished survival.[194–196] Microvascular invasion has also been correlated significantly with cervical lymph node metastases.[197,198] However, lymphatic invasion has not been correlated significantly with cervical lymph node invasion.[18] The prognostic significance of grade has also been evaluated.[199] Because of the wide variation in pathologic interpretation, it is difficult to discern the independent value of histologic grading as a prognostic or predictive value.[18]

SURVEILLANCE

The NCCN recommendations for the follow-up of head and neck cancer patients are listed in Table 47.4.[1,200,201] The major goals of surveillance include early diagnosis of recurrence and second primary tumors and management of the ongoing sequelae of head and neck cancer treatment. It is advisable that follow-up be conducted by the multidisciplinary team that provided oncologic management to the patient.[202,203] All patients whom have completed radiation treatment for oral cavity cancer should undergo routine head and neck examination, imaging, and dental evaluation. In addition, it is recommended that the follow-up protocol include an assessment of thyroid function (TSH level) every 6 to 12 months. Radiation-induced hypothyroidism is detected over the subsequent years in 20% to 25% of patients who undergo neck irradiation.[1,204,205] Smoking and alcohol cessation, as well as screening for lung cancer in clinically indicated patients, are also important components of an ongoing follow-up program for all head and neck cancer patients.[1,206]

TABLE 47.4 FOLLOW-UP RECOMMENDATIONS[a]

- History and physical exam (including complete H&N examination, including mirror and fiberoptic exam as indicated)
  - Year 1, every 1–3 mo
  - Year 2, every 2–6 mo
  - Years 3–5, every 4–8 mo; >5 y every 12 mo
- Baseline imaging of primary and neck within 6 mo of therapy[a]
- Serial reimaging as clinically indicated based on signs/symptoms, continued tobacco use, and areas inaccessible to exam; routine imaging may be indicated in areas difficult to visualize on exam
- Chest imaging as clinically indicated for patient with smoking history for lung cancer screening
- TSH every 6–12 mo if neck irradiated
- Ongoing dental evaluation focused on patient education, prevention/management of caries, xerostomia, osteoradionecrosis, and oral candidiasis
- Supportive care and rehabilitation
  - Speech/hearing and swallowing evaluation as clinically indicated
  - Nutritional evaluation and rehabilitation as clinically indicated until nutritional status is stabilized
  - Ongoing surveillance for depression[b]
  - Smoking cessation and alcohol counseling
- Integration of survivorship care and care plan within 1 y, complementary to ongoing involvement by a head and neck oncologist[c]

[a]Data adapted from NCCN Guidelines for Head and Neck Cancers.[1]
[b]Refer to NCCN Guidelines for Distress Management.[200]
[c]Refer to NCCN Guidelines for Survivorship.[201]

SUBSITE-SPECIFIC TREATMENT AND RESULTS

Lip

The treatment approach for lip cancer is driven by the stage of disease and the expected functional outcome. Surgery is generally the preferred treatment modality for early-stage carcinoma of the lip although radiation therapy is an option for local tumor control (Fig. 47.1). Although the local control of T1 and T2 squamous cancers of the lip is excellent with surgical resection, disruption of the oral sphincter provided by the orbicularis muscle can lead to oral incompetence if not properly reconstructed. Therefore, several reconstructive methods have been developed to help preserve oral sphincteric function even following large excisions for T3 and T4 lesions. For these larger lesions, surgery followed by radiotherapy remains a standard therapy (Fig. 47.2). One possible exception is a superficial cancer that occupies most of the lip, which is best managed with primary radiation therapy because of the potential functional and cosmetic implications of primary surgery.[1]

The successful surgical management of lip cancers includes the eradication of the primary tumor with free margins with preservation of the oral sphincteric function of the lip. For small lesions, excision with primary closure can be highly effective in achieving both of these objectives, whereas resection of larger legions can often require complex local flap repairs to attain satisfactory oncologic, cosmetic, and functional outcomes. SLNB can also prove to be useful in the management of patients of node-negative lip cancers, but further clinical investigation in this area is needed.

When primary radiotherapy is used to treat lip cancer, the target volume should include the primary tumor plus a 1.5- to 2.0-cm margin. For early-stage lesions, photons in the orthovoltage range (100 to 200 keV) or electrons may be used. The electron energy should be chosen based on the thickness of the lesion (commonly 6 to 9 MeV). Effort should be made to shield the underlying gum, dentition, and mandible as appropriate. This can be accomplished with the use of oral shields or Cerrobend stents. The recommended dose is 50 Gy in 4.5 to 5 weeks for smaller lesions and 60 Gy in 5 to 6 weeks for larger lesions. Some institutions have used an approach where external beam radiation is given to approximately 40 to 50 Gy followed by a brachytherapy boost; however,

small to intermediate stage lesions can be treated by primary brachytherapy alone (Fig. 47.20).

An important consideration in managing lip cancer is the risk of regional metastatic disease. Generally, the risk of regional lymph node metastatic disease for T1 and T2 cancers of the lip is lower than for stage-matched tumors of other oral cavity sites. Thus, END is recommended for patients with T3 and T4 carcinomas of the lip; however, it may not be warranted for all T1 and T2 lesions. Some institutions have used a "moustache field" for elective irradiation of the perifacial lymphatics (~50 Gy) for more advanced upper lip lesions.[207]

Oral Tongue

Although primary radiation therapy and surgery are potential treatment options for early-stage carcinoma of the oral tongue, the preferred treatment for most oral tongue cancers in the United States is primary surgery (Figs. 47.1 and 47.2).[18] Surgical resection and reconstruction as appropriate is generally preferred for medically operable patients. Postoperative radiation therapy is recommended for patients with large primary tumors (T3, T4), close or positive surgical margins, evidence of perineural spread, multiple positive nodes, or ENE.[207] Postoperative chemoradiation should be considered for patients with adverse risk factors who are able to tolerate combined modality treatment[81,83–85] (Fig. 47.2). Primary radiotherapy techniques can be used for patients who refuse or are unable to tolerate surgery.

Surgical approaches to oral tongue cancers can either be transoral, transcervical, or alternatively via mandibulectomy to obtain the exposure necessary to achieve adequate margins. Partial glossectomy is the most common procedure performed for oral tongue cancers, and the extent of resection depends on the size and growth pattern of the tumor, as some lesions are relatively infiltrative, while others may be more exophytic. Because the tongue is essentially comprised of skeletal muscle covered by mucosa, the tissue is extremely elastic, and wide margins are encouraged at the onset of resection to avoid retraction of muscle fibers with microscopic tumor cells that could serve as a source of local recurrence.

Total glossectomy may be indicated for extensive tumors or those that involve the intrinsic tongue musculature. Total glossectomy, even with reconstruction, can result in difficulty with deglutition and maintenance of an adequate airway. Aspiration may be a chronic problem, and, thus, laryngectomy may be necessary in some cases. However, properly selected patients with adequate postoperative rehabilitation can be treated with total glossectomy without laryngectomy. If the larynx is preserved, laryngeal suspension and palatal augmentation may help with the rehabilitative efforts.

Tumor size and depth of invasion are currently the most reliable indicators for predicting cervical metastases in patients with oral tongue squamous cell carcinoma. Because of the high risk of nodal metastases, the neck should be addressed either with surgery or radiation in all but the earliest tumors of the oral tongue. Patients with small oral tongue cancers should be considered for neck therapy, particularly if the primary tumor exhibits extension onto the floor of the mouth or there is increased tumor thickness. Treatment of the clinically negative neck is most often accomplished by supraomohyoid neck dissection. END appears to result in better overall cancer outcome than observation. Potential pitfalls of observation include a salvage rate of only one-third for patients who do not undergo END along with resection of the oral cavity primary.

Superficial T1 lesions can be treated with brachytherapy alone. Commonly, ^{192}Ir temporary implants are used to deliver 50 to 60 Gy with dose rates of 40 to 60 cGy/hour. However, HDR techniques can also be considered. For infiltrating T1 or T2 lesions, a combined approach using external beam and a brachytherapy or intraoral cone boost should be considered. More advanced lesions should be treated with an approach

Section III

combining surgery and radiation therapy. In patients treated with IMRT, the intermediate-risk CTV (see IMRT section) should include the intrinsic and extrinsic muscles of the tongue, the floor of the mouth, base of the tongue, glosso-tonsillar sulcus, and the anterior tonsillar pillar (Fig. 47.13). The adjacent dissected neck should also be included in this volume. Patients with advanced lesions and high-risk disease (particularly with multiple positive nodes) should receive radiation treatment to the bilateral necks. In patients with early-stage disease close to midline or patients with well-lateralized disease that is deeply invasive (>4 mm), both sides of the neck should be considered for treatment. For patients with a clinically and radiographically N0 neck, with well-lateralized and superficial disease (<4 mm invasion), 50 to 54 Gy should be considered to the ipsilateral neck as elective nodal irradiation. The appropriate draining lymphatics (usually levels I to IV unilaterally or bilaterally) should be included in the low- to intermediate-risk CTV (Fig. 47.13 and Table 47.1).

Floor of the Mouth

Surgery is usually preferred in patients who are medically operable because proximity of the tumor to the mandible confers a significant risk of radiation-induced ulceration and osteoradionecrosis. Small lesions of the floor of the mouth are most commonly resected transorally. The surgical defect can be left to heal by granulation or reconstructed with a split-thickness skin graft or local flap. Advanced stage of floor of the mouth cancers is usually managed by a combination of surgery and radiation or chemoradiation.

In the surgical management of floor of the mouth cancer, special attention should be paid to mandibular invasion. A cancer that appears to involve only the periosteum or that only superficially invades the mandible can be removed via a transoral or transcervical approach in which a marginal mandibulectomy is performed. However, segmental mandibulectomy may be necessary for patients with a limited mandibular height when there is no direct bone invasion, because marginal mandibulectomy may leave these patients with insufficient bone, placing them at high risk for radionecrosis or pathologic fracture. A full-thickness segmental resection may be necessary if there is frank bone invasion. For advanced cancers, resection of the anterior arch of the mandible may be necessary. Defects of the anterior segment of the mandible require reconstruction with bone, usually with a free fibular or iliac crest graft.

Management of the neck is similar to that for other tumors of the oral cavity. Patients with lesions <2 mm thick with no adverse pathologic factors and a clinically and radiographically negative neck may be observed after primary resection and observation. Otherwise, most N0 patients should receive either selective neck dissection or radiation therapy. Patients with advanced lesions and high-risk disease (particularly with multiple positive nodes) should receive radiation treatment to bilateral necks.

Small (T1 and T2) lesions may be treated with a combination of external beam radiation and boost with interstitial implant or intraoral cone. For lesions that are very close to the mandible, brachytherapy is contraindicated because of the risk of osteoradionecrosis. Infiltrative lesions that are tethered to the mandible and advanced lesions following surgical resection should receive postoperative radiation. Target volume design considerations for postoperative treatment are similar to that for oral tongue carcinoma. In cases where IMRT is used, the intermediate-risk CTV (see IMRT section) should include genioglossus and geniohyoid muscles bilaterally, the sublingual and submandibular glands ipsilaterally (bilaterally if the tumor is midline), adjoining alveolar ridge and mandible, the muscles at the root of tongue, and the dissected necks.[157] Because of the close proximity of floor of the mouth lesions to the midline, treatment of both sides of the neck should be considered. The low- to intermediate-risk CTV (see IMRT section) should include the appropriate electively treated necks (Fig. 47.14 and Table 47.1). Another important

consideration is the presence of gross perineural invasion of the branches of the inferior alveolar nerve. In the event of extensive perineural involvement, coverage of the mandibular canal to the infratemporal fossa should be considered.[159]

Cases of floor of the mouth carcinoma in which there is no indication for neck irradiation (e.g., a T4N0M0 primary with early mandibular involvement and a negative bilateral neck dissection) may be good candidates for treatment with conventional techniques. In this setting, opposing lateral fields may be used to encompass the oral cavity tumor bed (including the mandible, floor of the mouth, and oral tongue); this volume is commonly treated to 50 to 54 Gy. High-risk areas (primary surgical bed, close margins, perineural spread) may receive additional boost treatment up to 60 to 66 Gy.

Hard Palate and Upper Alveolar Ridge

Tumors of the hard palate are quite rare, accounting for only 0.5% of all oral cancers in the United States. Most carcinomas manifest as a granular superficial ulceration of the hard palate. Initial growth tends to be superficial, although these tumors can extend through the periosteum of bone into regions adjacent to the oral cavity, such as the paranasal sinuses and floor of the nose. Surgery is the preferred modality for treatment of this subsite.

Wide local excision may be adequate to obtain surgical margins. However, infrastructure maxillectomy may in some cases be necessary. For tumors that extensively involve the adjacent bony and soft tissue structures, a total maxillectomy, with or without orbital exenteration, may be required. A defect in the maxilla results in lack of oral/nasal separation that can impair the ability to speak and swallow effectively. An obturator with or without a skin graft is the most common method used to restore oral/nasal separation. The obturator is commonly fabricated from a synthetic polymer and provides oronasal separation that can yield improved speech and swallowing function. Regional pedicled flaps and free tissue transfers may provide alternatives to obturation. One consideration in the reconstruction of palatal defects with nonremovable flaps is that they can mask local recurrences that can be more readily identified in patients whose defects are obturated.

Postoperative radiation therapy should be delivered when there are adverse features, that is, close/positive margins, perineural extension, vascular invasion, high-grade histology, multiple positive nodes, or ENE. The radiation field should encompass the entire surgical bed. In many cases, it may be feasible to treat with opposed lateral fields to cover the volume at risk (Fig. 47.12). However, for well-lateralized lesions of the upper alveolar ridge, ipsilateral radiation with a wedge pair may be adequate. Conformal treatment techniques, including IMRT, can also be used to tailor the radiation coverage to the high-risk tissue bed, draining lymphatics, surgical flap, and routes of perineural spread along V2 as deemed appropriate.

Elective treatment of the neck is controversial for hard palate region tumors. Although some series have shown lower rates of occult metastases for palatal tumors when compared to other oral cavity sites, preoperative imaging should be performed to evaluate for the presence of metastases to the retropharyngeal nodes because these are difficult to evaluate on clinical examination and are at some risk for spread from primary palatal tumors. Elective treatment of the clinically negative neck should be considered in high-grade tumors or lesions that present with advanced T stage.

Retromolar Trigone

Squamous cell carcinoma of the retromolar trigone is uncommon, and the true incidence is difficult to determine because these cancers often involve both the retromolar trigone and adjacent sites, thereby making it difficult in some cases to identify the original tumor epicenter. Cancers of the retromolar trigone may be advanced at presentation because only a thin layer of soft tissue overlies the bone in this region and invasion of the underlying bone may occur early. In addition, there are multiple pathways for spread from this site including the buccal mucosa, tonsillar fossa, glossopharyngeal sulcus, floor of the mouth, base of the tongue, hard and soft palate, masticator space, and maxillary tuberosity. As patients tend to present with advanced disease of the retromolar trigone, many have regional metastases at the time of presentation.

The treatment of carcinoma of the retromolar trigone has been controversial.[208] Traditionally, surgery and radiation have been felt to be comparable modalities of treatment. However, recent reports suggest that surgery with adjuvant or neoadjuvant radiotherapy may be associated with better outcomes compared to radiation alone.[209,210] Although early-stage T1 and T2 cancers may be treated equally effectively with surgery or radiation, the probability of osteoradionecrosis is likely higher with definitive radiation.[208] Stage III and IV lesions commonly require combined surgery and radiation. The resection of advanced cancer of the retromolar trigone usually requires a composite resection of soft tissue and bone. Transoral robotic surgery can be helpful in the management of smaller tumors in the retromolar trigone.[211] A limiting factor for the achievement of adequate surgical resection margins for tumors in this area includes extension of tumor posterosuperiorly into the pterygopalatine fossa and/or the base of the skull.

Well-lateralized lesions of the retromolar trigone can be treated by ipsilateral treatment using mixed beam techniques or angled wedge techniques. In the case of more extensive lesions that require free flap reconstruction, IMRT may be beneficial to aid in covering the postoperative tumor bed and neck (Fig. 47.15). For extensive tumors of the retromolar trigone (or those with evidence of perineural spread), the infratemporal fossa should be included in the CTV. Treatment of the contralateral neck is at the discretion of the treating physician. In considering treatment options for carcinoma of the retromolar trigone, it is important to consider that some HPV+ tonsil tumors can largely involve the retromolar trigone and are ideally managed with nonsurgical treatment, highlighting the importance of testing tumors in this area for the presence of high-risk HPV subtypes.

Buccal Mucosa

Verrucous carcinoma accounts for <5% of all oral cavity carcinomas, occurs most often in the buccal mucosa, has a more favorable prognosis, and is considered a low-grade malignancy. Surgical resection remains the preferred mode of treatment for primary lesions of the buccal mucosa. Adjuvant radiation treatment is usually not indicated in the setting of completely excised verrucous carcinoma of the buccal mucosa. Because verrucous carcinomas rarely metastasize, END is often not indicated for patients with this disease. Careful pathology review with clinical correlation is important in the categorization of verrucous carcinomas, as this diagnosis can influence subsequent treatment recommendations.

Squamous cell carcinoma of the buccal mucosa can be an especially aggressive cancer of the oral cavity, as buccal cancers have multiple potential routes of spread to adjacent areas in the head and neck. Posteriorly, they can extend to involve the pterygoid muscles, and superiorly, they can grow to involve the alveolar ridge, palate, or maxillary sinus. The majority of patients have cancer that extends beyond the buccal mucosa. Metastasis to the cervical lymph nodes most commonly affects the submandibular nodes.

Transoral resection is preferred and is most convenient for small lesions of the buccal mucosa. Tumors approximating the gingiva should be resected with the gingiva and periosteum as an additional deep margin, whereas those that involve the periosteum should be resected with an additional deep margin of bone provided by a marginal mandibulectomy. Cancers that directly invade bone should be resected with a segment of bone. Larger tumors (T3 or T4) may require surgery combined with radiation therapy or chemoradiotherapy.

When considering target volume delineation for carcinoma of the buccal mucosa, it is important to be comprehensive in covering the inner cheek and entire buccal mucosa. The CTV should extend from the orbital rim (superiorly) to the retromolar trigone (posteriorly). Moreover, in the event of extensive disease (i.e., T3/T4 or N2/N3) that is treated postoperatively, the masticator space and infratemporal fossa should be covered within the CTV. As is the case with retromolar trigone carcinoma, treatment of the contralateral neck is at the discretion of the treating physician.

MANAGEMENT OF RECURRENT DISEASE

The recurrence rates after treatment of cancer of the oral cavity are approximately 30% with local recurrence being the most common.[212] Unfortunately, the survival after salvage treatment remains quite poor at 20% to 30%.[212] The appropriate management of recurrent oral cavity cancer depends largely on the extent of disease, the prior therapy administered, and whether the recurrences are local, regional, or both. The disease-free interval between initial treatment and recurrence is among the most important factors associated with survival after salvage surgery, and a disease-free interval of more than 10 months is significantly associated with improved survival.[212] Although surgery and chemoradiotherapy have similar outcomes in the case of early recurrences, surgical salvage has been found to be superior to chemoradiotherapy for late recurrence (84.4% vs. 52% 5-year disease-specific survival, respectively).[212] In the case of small recurrences at the primary site in patients whose index therapy was surgical excision only, further excision with postoperative radiotherapy is often recommended. For larger recurrences in patients who received radiation as part of their initial management, the rate of surgical salvage is quite low. In some cases, further resection may be considered for palliation or curative treatment attempt, particularly in the setting of a clinical trial. Systemic therapy, reirradiation, and palliative care are other options for this group of patients, and the risks and benefits of each should be discussed with the individual patient.

If there is distant disease recurrence, systemic therapy approaches will likely assume primary importance. A combination of docetaxel, cisplatin, and 5-FU or a platinum doublet (plus a taxane or 5FU) combined with cetuximab are commonly used regimens for first-line treatment.[186,213] Immunomodulating agents targeting the programmed death (PD)-1 receptor and its ligand (PD-L1) represent novel and promising strategies in the treatment of metastatic and recurrent squamous cell carcinoma of the head and neck.[214,215] These agents have demonstrated a survival advantage compared to standard single agent chemotherapy in the setting of platinum refractory head and neck squamous cell carcinoma.[214] Ongoing concepts being investigated include combining these agents with standard cetuximab-containing regimens.[216]

REFERENCES

1. NCCN. Clinical Practice Guidelines in Oncology (NCCN Guidelines ™). Head and Neck Cancers. Version 1.2017, in https://www.nccn.org/professionals/physician_gls/pdf/head-and-neck.pdf, National Comprehensive Cancer Network, http://www.nccn.org
2. Chi AC, Day TA, Neville BW. Oral cavity and oropharyngeal squamous cell carcinoma—an update. *CA Cancer J Clin* 2015;65(5):401–421.
3. SEER Cancer Stat Facts. *Oral cavity and pharynx cancer*. Bethesda, MD: National Cancer Institute, 2017, http://www.seer.cancer.gov/statfacts/html/oral-cav.html
4. American Cancer Society. *Cancer Facts and Figures 2017*. Atlanta, 2017. Available from: http://www.cancer.org/Research/CancerFactsFigures/CancerFactsFigures
5. Ferlay J, et al. Cancer incidence and mortality worldwide: sources, methods and major patterns in GLOBOCAN 2012. *Int J Cancer* 2015;136(5):E359–E386.
6. Chaturvedi AK, et al. Worldwide trends in incidence rates for oral cavity and oropharyngeal cancers. *J Clin Oncol* 2013;31(36):4550–4559.
7. Boyle P, Macfarlane GJ, Scully C. Oral cancer: necessity for prevention strategies. *Lancet* 1993;342(8880):1129.

8. Kurumatani N, et al. Time trends in the mortality rates for tobacco- and alcohol-related cancers within the oral cavity and pharynx in Japan, 1950–94. *J Epidemiol* 1999;9(1):46–52.

9. Macfarlane GJ, et al. Alcohol, tobacco, diet and the risk of oral cancer: a pooled analysis of three case–control studies. *Eur J Cancer B Oral Oncol* 1995;31B(3):181–187.

10. Lambert R, et al. Epidemiology of cancer from the oral cavity and oropharynx. *Eur J Gastroenterol Hepatol* 2011;23(8):633–641.

11. Pande P, et al. Prognostic impact of Ets-1 overexpression in betel and tobacco related oral cancer. *Cancer Detect Prev* 2001;25(5):496–501.

12. Sharma DC. Betel quid and areca nut are carcinogenic without tobacco. *Lancet Oncol* 2003;4(10):587.

13. Hashibe M, et al. Interaction between tobacco and alcohol use and the risk of head and neck cancer: pooled analysis in the International Head and Neck Cancer Epidemiology Consortium. *Cancer Epidemiol Biomarkers Prev* 2009;18(2):541–550.

14. D'Souza G, et al. Case–control study of human papillomavirus and oropharyngeal cancer. *N Engl J Med* 2007;356(19):1944–1956.

15. Fakhry C, Gillison ML. Clinical implications of human papillomavirus in head and neck cancers. *J Clin Oncol* 2006;24(17):2606–2611.

16. Patel SC, et al. Increasing incidence of oral tongue squamous cell carcinoma in young white women, age 18 to 44 years. *J Clin Oncol* 2011;29(11):1488–1494.

17. Prime SS, et al. A review of inherited cancer syndromes and their relevance to oral squamous cell carcinoma. *Oral Oncol* 2001;37(1):1–16.

18. Chen AY, Myers JN. Cancer of the oral cavity. *Dis Mon* 2001;47(7):275–361.

19. Goldstein DP, Irish JC. Head and neck squamous cell carcinoma in the young patient. *Curr Opin Otolaryngol Head Neck Surg* 2005;13(4):207–211.

20. Lippman SM, Hong WK. Second malignant tumors in head and neck squamous cell carcinoma: the overshadowing threat for patients with early-stage disease. *Int J Radiat Oncol Biol Phys* 1989;17(3):691–694.

21. Schwartz LH, et al. Synchronous and metachronous head and neck carcinomas. *Cancer* 1994;74(7):1933–1938.

22. Foy JP, et al. Oral premalignancy: the roles of early detection and chemoprevention. *Otolaryngol Clin North Am* 2013;46(4):579–597.

23. Robbins KT, et al. Standardizing neck dissection terminology. Official report of the Academy's Committee for Head and Neck Surgery and Oncology. *Arch Otolaryngol Head Neck Surg* 1991;117(6):601–605.

24. Robbins KT. Integrating radiological criteria into the classification of cervical lymph node disease. *Arch Otolaryngol Head Neck Surg* 1999;125(4):385–387.

25. Robbins KT, et al. Neck dissection classification update: revisions proposed by the American Head and Neck Society and the American Academy of Otolaryngology-Head and Neck Surgery. *Arch Otolaryngol Head Neck Surg* 2002;128(7):751–758.

26. Gregoire V, et al. Delineation of the neck node levels for head and neck tumors: a 2013 update. DAHANCA, EORTC, HKNPCSG, NCIC CTG, NCRI, RTOG, TROG consensus guidelines. *Radiother Oncol* 2014;110(1):172–181.

27. Gregoire V, et al. CT-based delineation of lymph node levels and related CTVs in the node-negative neck: DAHANCA, EORTC, GORTEC, NCIC,RTOG consensus guidelines. *Radiother Oncol* 2003;69(3):227–236.

28. Fearon ER, Vogelstein B. A genetic model for colorectal tumorigenesis. *Cell* 1990;61(5):759–767.

29. Califano J, et al. Genetic progression model for head and neck cancer: implications for field cancerization. *Cancer Res* 1996;56(11):2488–2492.

30. Shavers VL, et al. Racial/ethnic patterns of care for cancers of the oral cavity, pharynx, larynx, sinuses, and salivary glands. *Cancer Metastasis Rev* 2003;22(1):25–38.

31. Cancer Genome Atlas Network. Comprehensive genomic characterization of head and neck squamous cell carcinomas. *Nature* 2015;517(7536):576–582.

32. Agrawal N, Frederick MJ, Pickering CR, et al. Exome sequencing of head and neck squamous cell carcinomas reveals mutations. *Science*. 2011;333: 1154–1157.

33. Pickering CR, et al. Squamous cell carcinoma of the oral tongue in young non-smokers is genomically similar to tumors in older smokers. *Clin Cancer Res* 2014;20(14):3842–3848.

34. Stransky N, et al. The mutational landscape of head and neck squamous cell carcinoma. *Science* 2011;333(6046):1157–1160.

35. Zafereo ME, et al. Squamous cell carcinoma of the oral cavity often overexpresses p16 but is rarely driven by human papillomavirus. *Oral Oncol* 2016;56:47–53.

36. Pickering CR, et al. Integrative genomic characterization of oral squamous cell carcinoma identifies frequent somatic drivers. *Cancer Discov* 2013;3(7): 770–781.

37. Morris LG, et al. The molecular landscape of recurrent and metastatic head and neck cancers: insights from a precision oncology sequencing platform. *JAMA Oncol* 2017;3(2):244–255.

38. Wang Y, et al. Detection of somatic mutations and HPV in the saliva and plasma of patients with head and neck squamous cell carcinomas. *Sci Transl Med* 2015;7(293):293ra104.

39. Mandal R, et al. The head and neck cancer immune landscape and its immunotherapeutic implications. *JCI Insight* 2016;1(17):e89829.

40. Monteil RA. Oral leukoplakia: clinical or histologic entity? *Ann Pathol* 1983;3(3):257–261.

41. Myers EN, Suen JY, Myers JN, et al. *Cancer of the head and neck.* 4th ed. Philadelphia, PA: Saunders, 2003.

42. Kannan S, et al. Ultrastructural variations and assessment of malignant transformation risk in oral leukoplakia. *Pathol Res Pract* 1993;189(10):1169–1180.

43. Reibel J. Prognosis of oral pre-malignant lesions: significance of clinical, histopathological, and molecular biological characteristics. *Crit Rev Oral Biol Med* 2003;14(1):47–62.

44. Shafer WG, Waldron CA. Erythroplakia of the oral cavity. *Cancer* 1975;36(3): 1021–1028.

45. Reichart PA, Philipsen HP. Oral erythroplakia—a review. *Oral Oncol* 2005;41(6):551–561.

46. Wang C. *Radiation therapy for head and neck neoplasms.* 3rd ed. New York: Wiley-Liss, 1997.

47. Byers RM, Wolf PF, Ballantyne AJ. Rationale for elective modified neck dissection. *Head Neck Surg* 1988;10(3):160–167.

48. Mukherji SK, Armao D, Joshi VM. Cervical nodal metastases in squamous cell carcinoma of the head and neck: what to expect. *Head Neck* 2001;23(11):995–1005.

49. Shah JP, Candela FC, Poddar AK. The patterns of cervical lymph node metastases from squamous carcinoma of the oral cavity. *Cancer* 1990;66(1):109–113.

50. Feng FY, et al. Intensity-modulated radiotherapy of head and neck cancer aiming to reduce dysphagia: early dose-effect relationships for the swallowing structures. *Int J Radiat Oncol Biol Phys* 2007;68(5):1289–1298.

51. Eisbruch A, et al. Intensity-modulated radiation therapy for head and neck cancer: emphasis on the selection and delineation of the targets. *Semin Radiat Oncol* 2002;12(3):238–249.

52. Kimura Y, et al. Lateral retropharyngeal node metastasis from carcinoma of the upper gingiva and maxillary sinus. *AJNR Am J Neuroradiol* 1998;19(7):1221–1224.

53. Umeda M, et al. Metastasis to the lateral retropharyngeal lymph node from squamous cell carcinoma of the oral cavity: report of three cases. *Int J Oral Maxillofac Surg* 2009;38(9):1004–1008.

54. Lindberg R. Distribution of cervical lymph node metastases from squamous cell carcinoma of the upper respiratory and digestive tracts. *Cancer* 1972;29(6):1446–1449.

55. Byers RM, et al. Frequency and therapeutic implications of "skip metastases" in the neck from squamous cell carcinoma of the oral tongue. *Head Neck* 1997;19(1):14–19.

56. Strong EW. Carcinoma of the tongue. *Otolaryngol Clin North Am* 1979;12(1): 107–114.

57. Spiro RH, et al. Predictive value of tumor thickness in squamous carcinoma confined to the tongue and floor of the mouth. *Am J Surg* 1986;152(4):345–350.

58. Shear M, Hawkins DM, Farr HW. The prediction of lymph node metastases from oral squamous carcinoma. *Cancer* 1976;37(4):1901–1907.

59. Merino OR, Lindberg RD, Fletcher GH. An analysis of distant metastases from squamous cell carcinoma of the upper respiratory and digestive tracts. *Cancer* 1977;40(1):145–151.

60. Ferlito A, et al. Incidence and sites of distant metastases from head and neck cancer. *ORL J Otorhinolaryngol Relat Spec* 2001;63(4):202–207.

61. Winzenburg SM, et al. Basaloid squamous carcinoma: a clinical comparison of two histologic types with poorly differentiated squamous cell carcinoma. *Otolaryngol Head Neck Surg* 1998;119(5):471–475.

62. Ellis GL, Corio RL. Spindle cell carcinoma of the oral cavity. A clinicopathologic assessment of fifty-nine cases. *Oral Surg Oral Med Oral Pathol* 1980;50(6):523–533.

63. Weber RS, et al. Minor salivary gland tumors of the lip and buccal mucosa. *Laryngoscope* 1989;99(1):6–9.

64. Freeman C, Berg JW, Cutler SJ. Occurrence and prognosis of extranodal lymphomas. *Cancer* 1972;29(1):252–260.

65. Smyth AG, et al. Malignant melanoma of the oral cavity—an increasing clinical diagnosis? *Br J Oral Maxillofac Surg* 1993;31(4):230–235.

66. van den Brekel MW, et al. Modern imaging techniques and ultrasound-guided aspiration cytology for the assessment of neck node metastases: a prospective comparative study. *Eur Arch Otorhinolaryngol* 1993;250(1):11–17.

67. Adams S, et al. Prospective comparison of 18F-FDG PET with conventional imaging modalities (CT, MRI, US) in lymph node staging of head and neck cancer. *Eur J Nucl Med* 1998;25(9):1255–1260.

68. Kim SY, et al. Utility of FDG PET in patients with squamous cell carcinomas of the oral cavity. *Eur J Surg Oncol* 2008;34(2):208–215.

69. Schoder H, et al. Head and neck cancer: clinical usefulness and accuracy of PET/CT image fusion. *Radiology* 2004;231(1):65–72.

70. Liao CT, et al. PET and PET/CT of the neck lymph nodes improves risk prediction in patients with squamous cell carcinoma of the oral cavity. *J Nucl Med* 2011;52(2):180–187.

71. Maddipatla S, Madero-Visbal RA, Graves T, et al. Preoperative staging of oral cavity carcinoma with FDG-PET/CT. *J Clin Oncol* 2008;26(suppl):abstr 6044.

72. Pentenero M, et al. Accuracy of 18F-FDG-PET/CT for staging of oral squamous cell carcinoma. *Head Neck* 2008;30(11):1488–1496.

73. Anzai Y, et al. Recurrence of head and neck cancer after surgery or irradiation: prospective comparison of 2-deoxy-2-[F-18]fluoro-D-glucose PET and MR imaging diagnoses. *Radiology* 1996;200(1):135–141.

74. Farber LA, et al. Detection of recurrent head and neck squamous cell carcinomas after radiation therapy with 2-18F-fluoro-2-deoxy-D-glucose positron emission tomography. *Laryngoscope* 1999;109(6):970–975.

75. Andrade RS, et al. Posttreatment assessment of response using FDG-PET/CT for patients treated with definitive radiation therapy for head and neck cancers. *Int J Radiat Oncol Biol Phys* 2006;65(5):1315–1322.

76. Greven KM, et al. Serial positron emission tomography scans following radiation therapy of patients with head and neck cancer. *Head Neck* 2001;23(11):942–946.

77. Isles MG, McConkey C, Mehanna HM. A systematic review and meta-analysis of the role of positron emission tomography in the follow up of head and neck squamous cell carcinoma following radiotherapy or chemoradiotherapy. *Clin Otolaryngol* 2008;33(3):210–222.

78. Lowe VJ, et al. Surveillance for recurrent head and neck cancer using positron emission tomography. *J Clin Oncol* 2000;18(3):651–658.

79. Ridge JA, Lydiatt WM, Patel SG, et al. *AJCC cancer staging manual.* 8th ed. New York: Springer, 2016.

80. Aviv JE, et al. Surface sensibility of the floor of the mouth and tongue in healthy controls and in radiated patients. *Otolaryngol Head Neck Surg* 1992;107(3):418–423.

81. Cooper JS, et al. Postoperative concurrent radiotherapy and chemotherapy for high-risk squamous-cell carcinoma of the head and neck. *N Engl J Med* 2004;350(19):1937–1944.
82. Day TA, et al. Oral cancer treatment. *Curr Treat Options Oncol* 2003;4(1):27–41.
83. Bernier J, et al. Defining risk levels in locally advanced head and neck cancers: a comparative analysis of concurrent postoperative radiation plus chemotherapy trials of the EORTC (#22931) and RTOG (# 9501). *Head Neck* 2005;27(10):843–850.
84. Bernier J, et al. Postoperative irradiation with or without concomitant chemotherapy for locally advanced head and neck cancer. *N Engl J Med* 2004;350(19):1945–1952.
85. Bernier J, Vermorken JB, Koch WM. Adjuvant therapy in patients with resected poor-risk head and neck cancer. *J Clin Oncol* 2006;24(17):2629–2635.
86. Huang SH, O'Sullivan B. Oral cancer: current role of radiotherapy and chemotherapy. *Med Oral Patol Oral Cir Bucal* 2013;18(2):e233–e240.
87. Scher ED, et al. Definitive chemoradiation for primary oral cavity carcinoma: a single institution experience. *Oral Oncol* 2015;51(7):709–715.
88. Sher DJ, et al. Treatment of oral cavity squamous cell carcinoma with adjuvant or definitive intensity-modulated radiation therapy. *Int J Radiat Oncol Biol Phys* 2011;81(4):e215–e222.
89. Studer G, et al. IMRT in oral cavity cancer. *Radiat Oncol* 2007;2:16.
90. Loree TR, Strong EW. Significance of positive margins in oral cavity squamous carcinoma. *Am J Surg* 1990;160(4):410–414.
91. Scholl P, et al. Microscopic cut-through of cancer in the surgical treatment of squamous carcinoma of the tongue. Prognostic and therapeutic implications. *Am J Surg* 1986;152(4):354–360.
92. Christensen A, et al. uPAR-targeted optical near-infrared (NIR) fluorescence imaging and PET for image-guided surgery in head and neck cancer: proof-of-concept in orthotopic xenograft model. *Oncotarget* 2017;8(9):15407–15419.
93. Hauff SJ, et al. Matrix-metalloproteinases in head and neck carcinoma-cancer genome atlas analysis and fluorescence imaging in mice. *Otolaryngol Head Neck Surg* 2014;151(4):612–618.
94. Warram JM, et al. Fluorescence imaging to localize head and neck squamous cell carcinoma for enhanced pathological assessment. *J Pathol Clin Res* 2016;2(2):104–112.
95. Black C, et al. Critical evaluation of frozen section margins in head and neck cancer resections. *Cancer* 2006;107(12):2792–2800.
96. Maxwell JH, et al. Early oral tongue squamous cell carcinoma: sampling of margins from tumor bed and worse local control. *JAMA Otolaryngol Head Neck Surg* 2015;141(12):1104–1110.
97. Cilento BW, et al. Comparison of approaches for oral cavity cancer resection: lip-split versus visor flap. *Otolaryngol Head Neck Surg* 2007;137(3):428–432.
98. Wax MK, Bascom DA, Myers LL. Marginal mandibulectomy vs segmental mandibulectomy: indications and controversies. *Arch Otolaryngol Head Neck Surg* 2002;128(5):600–603.
99. Arya S, Rane P, Deshmukh A. Oral cavity squamous cell carcinoma: role of pretreatment imaging and its influence on management. *Clin Radiol* 2014;69(9):916–930.
100. Wang CC, et al. Osteoradionecrosis with combined mandibulotomy and marginal mandibulectomy. *Laryngoscope* 2005;115(11):1963–1967.
101. Byers RM, et al. Selective neck dissections for squamous carcinoma of the upper aerodigestive tract: patterns of regional failure. *Head Neck* 1999;21(6):499–505.
102. Shah JP. Patterns of cervical lymph node metastasis from squamous carcinomas of the upper aerodigestive tract. *Am J Surg* 1990;160(4):405–409.
103. Weiss MH, Harrison LB, Isaacs RS. Use of decision analysis in planning a management strategy for the stage N0 neck. *Arch Otolaryngol Head Neck Surg* 1994;120(7):699–702.
104. Huang SH, et al. Predictive value of tumor thickness for cervical lymph-node involvement in squamous cell carcinoma of the oral cavity: a meta-analysis of reported studies. *Cancer* 2009;115(7):1489–1497.
105. Lim SC, et al. Predictive markers for late cervical metastasis in stage I and II invasive squamous cell carcinoma of the oral tongue. *Clin Cancer Res* 2004;10(1 Pt 1):166–172.
106. Mohit-Tabatabai MA, et al. Relation of thickness of floor of mouth stage I and II cancers to regional metastasis. *Am J Surg* 1986;152(4):351–353.
107. Sparano A, et al. Multivariate predictors of occult neck metastasis in early oral tongue cancer. *Otolaryngol Head Neck Surg* 2004;131(4):472–476.
108. Huang SF, et al. The role of elective neck dissection in early stage buccal cancer. *Laryngoscope* 2015;125(1):128–133.
109. Yang Z, et al. Cervical metastases from squamous cell carcinoma of hard palate and maxillary alveolus: a retrospective study of 10 years. *Head Neck* 2014;36(7):969–975.
110. Paleri V, et al. Dissection of the submuscular recess (sublevel IIb) in squamous cell cancer of the upper aerodigestive tract: prospective study and systematic review of the literature. *Head Neck* 2008;30(2):194–200.
111. Kligerman J, et al. Supraomohyoid neck dissection in the treatment of T1/T2 squamous cell carcinoma of oral cavity. *Am J Surg* 1994;168(5):391–394.
112. Yuen AP, et al. Prospective randomized study of selective neck dissection versus observation for N0 neck of early tongue carcinoma. *Head Neck* 2009;31(6):765–772.
113. D'Cruz AK, et al. Elective versus therapeutic neck dissection in node-negative oral cancer. *N Engl J Med* 2015;373(6):521–529.
114. Alkureishi LW, et al. Sentinel node biopsy in head and neck squamous cell cancer: 5-year follow-up of a European multicenter trial. *Ann Surg Oncol* 2010;17(9):2459–2464.
115. Civantos FJ, et al. Sentinel lymph node biopsy accurately stages the regional lymph nodes for T1-T2 oral squamous cell carcinomas: results of a prospective multi-institutional trial. *J Clin Oncol* 2010;28(8):1395–1400.
116. Hanasono MM, et al. Impact of reconstructive microsurgery in patients with advanced oral cavity cancers. *Head Neck* 2009;31(10):1289–1296.
117. Chepeha DB, et al. Rectangle tongue template for reconstruction of the hemiglossectomy defect. *Arch Otolaryngol Head Neck Surg* 2008;134(9):993–998.
118. Kimata Y, et al. Analysis of the relations between the shape of the reconstructed tongue and postoperative functions after subtotal or total glossectomy. *Laryngoscope* 2003;113(5):905–909.
119. Schrag C, et al. Complete rehabilitation of the mandible following segmental resection. *J Surg Oncol* 2006;94(6):538–545.
120. Okay DJ, et al. Prosthodontic guidelines for surgical reconstruction of the maxilla: a classification system of defects. *J Prosthet Dent* 2001;86(4):352–363.
121. Harrison LB, Fass DE. Radiation therapy for oral cavity cancer. *Dent Clin North Am* 1990;34(2):205–222.
122. Nag S, et al. The American Brachytherapy Society recommendations for brachytherapy of soft tissue sarcomas. *Int J Radiat Oncol Biol Phys* 2001;49(4):1033–1043.
123. Fu KK, et al. Time, dose and volume factors in interstitial Radium implants of carcinoma of the oral tongue. *Radiology* 1976;119(1):209–213.
124. Fu KK, et al. External and interstitial radiation therapy of carcinoma of the oral tongue. A review of 32 years' experience. *AJR Am J Roentgenol* 1976;126(1):107–115.
125. Decroix Y, Ghossein NA. Experience of the Curie Institute in treatment of cancer of the mobile tongue: I. Treatment policies and result. *Cancer* 1981;47(3):496–502.
126. Dearnaley DP, et al. Interstitial irradiation for carcinoma of the tongue and floor of mouth: Royal Marsden Hospital Experience 1970–1986. *Radiother Oncol* 1991;21(3):183–192.
127. Pernot M, et al. Evaluation of the importance of systematic neck dissection in carcinoma of the oral cavity treated by brachytherapy alone for the primary lesion (apropos of a series of 346 patients). *Bull Cancer Radiother* 1995;82(3):311–317.
128. Pernot M, et al. Epidermoid carcinomas of the floor of mouth treated by exclusive irradiation: statistical study of a series of 207 cases. *Radiother Oncol* 1995;35(3):177–185.
129. Wang CC. Radiotherapeutic management and results of T1N0, T2N0 carcinoma of the oral tongue: evaluation of boost techniques. *Int J Radiat Oncol Biol Phys* 1989;17(2):287–291.
130. Wang CC. Intraoral cone for carcinoma of the oral cavity. *Front Radiat Ther Oncol* 1991;25:128–131.
131. Emami B. Oral cavity. In: Perez HE, Brady C, Schimdt-Ullrich L, eds. *Principles and practice of radiation oncology*. Philadelphia, PA: Lippincott Williams & Wilkins, 2004.
132. Wang CC, Doppke KP, Biggs PJ. Intra-oral cone radiation therapy for selected carcinomas of the oral cavity. *Int J Radiat Oncol Biol Phys* 1983;9(8):1185–1189.
133. Shah JP, Lydiatt W. Treatment of cancer of the head and neck. *CA Cancer J Clin* 1995;45(6):352–368.
134. Vikram B, et al. Elective postoperative radiation therapy in stages III and IV epidermoid carcinoma of the head and neck. *Am J Surg* 1980;140(4):580–584.
135. Robertson AG, et al. Early closure of a randomized trial: surgery and postoperative radiotherapy versus radiotherapy in the management of intra-oral tumours. *Clin Oncol* 1998;10(3):155–160.
136. Peters LJ, et al. Evaluation of the dose for postoperative radiation therapy of head and neck cancer: first report of a prospective randomized trial. *Int J Radiat Oncol Biol Phys* 1993;26(1):3–11.
137. Byers RM, et al. Resection of advanced cervical metastasis prior to definitive radiotherapy for primary squamous carcinomas of the upper aerodigestive tract. *Head Neck* 1992;14(2):133–138.
138. Garden AS, et al. Postoperative radiation therapy for malignant tumors of minor salivary glands. Outcome and patterns of failure. *Cancer* 1994;73(10):2563–2569.
139. Vikram B, et al. Failure in the neck following multimodality treatment for advanced head and neck cancer. *Head Neck Surg* 1984;6(3):724–729.
140. Ang KK, et al. Randomized trial addressing risk features and time factors of surgery plus radiotherapy in advanced head-and-neck cancer. *Int J Radiat Oncol Biol Phys* 2001;51(3):571–578.
141. Fu KK, et al. A Radiation Therapy Oncology Group (RTOG) phase III randomized study to compare hyperfractionation and two variants of accelerated fractionation to standard fractionation radiotherapy for head and neck squamous cell carcinomas: first report of RTOG 9003. *Int J Radiat Oncol Biol Phys* 2000;48(1):7–16.
142. Sanguineti G, et al. Timing of chemoradiotherapy and patient selection for locally advanced nasopharyngeal carcinoma. *Clin Oncol* 2003;15(8):451–460.
143. Sher DJ, et al. Predictors of IMRT and conformal radiotherapy use in head and neck squamous cell carcinoma: a SEER-Medicare analysis. *Int J Radiat Oncol Biol Phys* 2011;81(4):e197–e206.
144. Caglar HB, et al. Dose to larynx predicts for swallowing complications after intensity-modulated radiotherapy. *Int J Radiat Oncol Biol Phys* 2008;72(4):1110–1118.
145. Eisbruch A, et al. Can IMRT or brachytherapy reduce dysphagia associated with chemoradiotherapy of head and neck cancer? The Michigan and Rotterdam experiences. *Int J Radiat Oncol Biol Phys* 2007;69(2 Suppl):S40–S42.
146. Eisbruch A, et al. Dysphagia and aspiration after chemoradiotherapy for head-and-neck cancer: which anatomic structures are affected and can they be spared by IMRT? *Int J Radiat Oncol Biol Phys* 2004;60(5):1425–1439.
147. Eisbruch A, et al. Salivary gland sparing and improved target irradiation by conformal and intensity modulated irradiation of head and neck cancer. *World J Surg* 2003;27(7):832–837.
148. Levendag PC, et al. Dysphagia disorders in patients with cancer of the oropharynx are significantly affected by the radiation therapy dose to the superior and middle constrictor muscle: a dose-effect relationship. *Radiother Oncol* 2007;85(1):64–73.
149. Boero IJ, et al. Importance of radiation oncologist experience among patients with head-and-neck cancer treated with intensity-modulated radiation therapy. *J Clin Oncol* 2016;34(7):684–690.
150. Wuthrick EJ, et al. Institutional clinical trial accrual volume and survival of patients with head and neck cancer. *J Clin Oncol* 2015;33(2):156–164.

151. Eisbruch A, et al. Recurrences near base of skull after IMRT for head-and-neck cancer: implications for target delineation in high neck and for parotid gland sparing. *Int J Radiat Oncol Biol Phys* 2004;59(1):28–42.

152. Gregoire V, et al. Proposal for the delineation of the nodal CTV in the node-positive and the post-operative neck. *Radiother Oncol* 2006;79(1):15–20.

153. Hong TS, Tome WA, Harari PM. Heterogeneity in head and neck IMRT target design and clinical practice. *Radiother Oncol* 2012;103(1):92–98.

154. Lee N, et al. Intensity-modulated radiation therapy for head-and-neck cancer: the UCSF experience focusing on target volume delineation. *Int J Radiat Oncol Biol Phys* 2003;57(1):49–60.

155. Yao M, et al. Intensity-modulated radiation treatment for head-and-neck squamous cell carcinoma—the University of Iowa experience. *Int J Radiat Oncol Biol Phys* 2005;63(2):410–421.

156. Eisbruch A, et al. Xerostomia and its predictors following parotid-sparing irradiation of head-and-neck cancer. *Int J Radiat Oncol Biol Phys* 2001;50(3):695–704.

157. Eisbruch A. Clinical aspects of IMRT for head-and-neck cancer. *Med Dosim* 2002;27(2):99–104.

158. Geretschlager A, et al. Outcome and patterns of failure after postoperative intensity modulated radiotherapy for locally advanced or high-risk oral cavity squamous cell carcinoma. *Radiat Oncol* 2012;7:175.

159. Yao M, et al. The failure patterns of oral cavity squamous cell carcinoma after intensity-modulated radiotherapy-the university of iowa experience. *Int J Radiat Oncol Biol Phys* 2007;67(5):1332–1341.

160. Kaanders JH, et al. Devices valuable in head and neck radiotherapy. *Int J Radiat Oncol Biol Phys* 1992;23(3):639–645.

161. Hong TS, et al. The impact of daily setup variations on head-and-neck intensity-modulated radiation therapy. *Int J Radiat Oncol Biol Phys* 2005;61(3):779–788.

162. Gregoire V, Maingon P. Intensity-modulated radiation therapy in head and neck squamous cell carcinoma: an adaptation of 2-dimensional concepts or a reconsideration of current clinical practice. *Semin Radiat Oncol* 2004;14(2):110–120.

163. Zeidan OA, et al. Evaluation of image-guidance protocols in the treatment of head and neck cancers. *Int J Radiat Oncol Biol Phys* 2007;67(3):670–677.

164. Rotondo RL, et al. Comparison of repositioning accuracy of two commercially available immobilization systems for treatment of head-and-neck tumors using simulation computed tomography imaging. *Int J Radiat Oncol Biol Phys* 2008;70(5):1389–1396.

165. Mohan R, et al. Radiobiological considerations in the design of fractionation strategies for intensity-modulated radiation therapy of head and neck cancers. *Int J Radiat Oncol Biol Phys* 2000;46(3):619–630.

166. Caudell JJ, et al. Dosimetric factors associated with long-term dysphagia after definitive radiotherapy for squamous cell carcinoma of the head and neck. *Int J Radiat Oncol Biol Phys* 2010;76(2):403–409.

167. Lefebvre JL, et al. Management of early oral cavity cancer. Experience of Centre Oscar Lambret. *Eur J Cancer B Oral Oncol* 1994;30B(3):216–220.

168. Mohanti BK, et al. Interstitial brachytherapy with or without external beam irradiation in head and neck cancer: Institute Rotary Cancer Hospital experience. *Clin Oncol (R Coll Radiol)* 2001;13(5):345–352.

169. Strnad V. Treatment of oral cavity and oropharyngeal cancer. Indications, technical aspects, and results of interstitial brachytherapy. *Strahlenther Onkol* 2004;180(11):710–717.

170. Mazeron JJ, et al. Brachytherapy in head and neck cancers. *Cancer Radiother* 2003;7(1):62–72.

171. Rudoltz MS, et al. High-dose-rate brachytherapy for primary carcinomas of the oral cavity and oropharynx. *Laryngoscope* 1999;109(12):1967–1973.

172. Donath D, et al. The potential uses of high-dose-rate brachytherapy in patients with head and neck cancer. *Eur Arch Otorhinolaryngol* 1995;252(6):321–324.

173. Inoue T, et al. Phase III trial of high and low dose rate interstitial radiotherapy for early oral tongue cancer. *Int J Radiat Oncol Biol Phys* 1996;36(5):1201–1204.

174. Lau HY, et al. Seven fractions of twice daily high dose-rate brachytherapy for node-negative carcinoma of the mobile tongue results in loss of therapeutic ratio. *Radiother Oncol* 1996;39(1):15–18.

175. Leung TW, et al. Technical hints for high dose rate interstitial tongue brachytherapy. *Clin Oncol* 1998;10(4):231–236.

176. Nag S, et al. The American Brachytherapy Society recommendations for high-dose-rate brachytherapy for head-and-neck carcinoma. *Int J Radiat Oncol Biol Phys* 2001;50(5):1190–1198.

177. Erickson BA, et al. American Society for Radiation Oncology (ASTRO) and American College of Radiology (ACR) practice guideline for the performance of high-dose-rate brachytherapy. *Int J Radiat Oncol Biol Phys* 2011;79(3):641–649.

178. Million RCN, Mancuso A. Oral cavity. In: Million RR, Cassisi NJ, eds. *Management of head and neck cancer: a multidisciplinary approach.* 2nd ed. Philadelphia, PA: JB Lippincott, 1994.

179. Pierquin B, Pierquin JW, Chassagne D. Basic techniques for endocrine therapy. In: Pierquin JW, Chassagne D, eds. *Modern brachytherapy.* New York: Masson, 1987.

180. Wang CC, Boyer A, Mendiondo O. Afterloading interstitial radiation therapy. *Int J Radiat Oncol Biol Phys* 1976;1(3–4):365–368.

181. Lozza L, et al. Analysis of risk factors for mandibular bone radionecrosis after exclusive low dose-rate brachytherapy for oral cancer. *Radiother Oncol* 1997;44(2):143–147.

182. Pignon JP, et al. Chemotherapy added to locoregional treatment for head and neck squamous-cell carcinoma: three meta-analyses of updated individual data. MACH-NC Collaborative Group. Meta-Analysis of Chemotherapy on Head and Neck Cancer. *Lancet* 2000;355(9208):949–955.

183. Pignon JP, et al. Meta-analysis of chemotherapy in head and neck cancer (MACH-NC): an update on 93 randomised trials and 17,346 patients. *Radiother Oncol* 2009;92(1):4–14.

184. Patil VM, et al. Neoadjuvant chemotherapy followed by surgery in very locally advanced technically unresectable oral cavity cancers. *Oral Oncol* 2014;50(10):1000–1004.

185. Pancari P, Mehra R. Systemic therapy for squamous cell carcinoma of the head and neck. *Surg Oncol Clin N Am* 2015;24(3):437–454.

186. Gold KA, Neskey M, William WN Jr. The role of systemic treatment before, during, and after definitive treatment. *Otolaryngol Clin North Am* 2013;46(4):645–656.

187. Lorch JH, et al. Induction chemotherapy with cisplatin and fluorouracil alone or in combination with docetaxel in locally advanced squamous-cell cancer of the head and neck: long-term results of the TAX 324 randomised phase 3 trial. *Lancet Oncol* 2011;12(2):153–159.

188. Vermorken JB, et al. Cisplatin, fluorouracil, and docetaxel in unresectable head and neck cancer. *N Engl J Med* 2007;357(17):1695–1704.

189. Wheeler S, et al. Tumor epidermal growth factor receptor and EGFR PY1068 are independent prognostic indicators for head and neck squamous cell carcinoma. *Clin Cancer Res* 2012;18(8):2278–2289.

190. Bonner JA, et al. Radiotherapy plus cetuximab for squamous-cell carcinoma of the head and neck. *N Engl J Med* 2006;354(6):567–578.

191. Keene HJ, Fleming TJ. Prevalence of caries-associated microflora after radiotherapy in patients with cancer of the head and neck. *Oral Surg Oral Med Oral Pathol* 1987;64(4):421–426.

192. Myers JN, et al. Squamous cell carcinoma of the tongue in young adults: increasing incidence and factors that predict treatment outcomes. *Otolaryngol Head Neck Surg* 2000;122(1):44–51.

193. Johnson JT, et al. The extracapsular spread of tumors in cervical node metastasis. *Arch Otolaryngol* 1981;107(12):725–729.

194. Borges AM, Shrikhande SS, Ganesh B. Surgical pathology of squamous carcinoma of the oral cavity: its impact on management. *Semin Surg Oncol* 1989;5(5):310–317.

195. Fagan JJ, et al. Perineural invasion in squamous cell carcinoma of the head and neck. *Arch Otolaryngol Head Neck Surg* 1998;124(6):637–640.

196. Soo KC, et al. Prognostic implications of perineural spread in squamous carcinomas of the head and neck. *Laryngoscope* 1986;96(10):1145–1148.

197. Close LG, et al. Microvascular invasion in cancer of the oral cavity and oropharynx. *Arch Otolaryngol Head Neck Surg* 1987;113(11):1191–1195.

198. Martinez-Gimeno C, et al. Squamous cell carcinoma of the oral cavity: a clinico-pathologic scoring system for evaluating risk of cervical lymph node metastasis. *Laryngoscope* 1995;105(7 Pt 1):728–733.

199. Anneroth G, Batsakis J, Luna M. Review of the literature and a recommended system of malignancy grading in oral squamous cell carcinomas. *Scand J Dent Res* 1987;95(3):229–249.

200. NCCN. Clinical practice guidelines in oncology (NCCN guidelines™). In: *Distress management.* https://www.nccn.org/professionals/physician_gls/pdf/distress.pdf2017, National Comprehensive Cancer Network, http://www.nccn.org

201. NCCN. Clinical Practice Guidelines in Oncology (NCCN Guidelines™). In: *Survivorship.* https://www.nccn.org/professionals/physician_gls/pdf/survivorship.pdf2017, National Comprehensive Cancer Network, http://www.nccn.org

202. Denaro N, Merlano MC, Russi EG. Follow-up in head and neck cancer: do more does it mean do better? A systematic review and our proposal based on our experience. *Clin Exp Otorhinolaryngol* 2016;9(4):287–297.

203. Kawecki A, Krajewski R. Follow-up in patients treated for head and neck cancer. *Memo* 2014;7(2):87–91.

204. Colevas AD, et al. Hypothyroidism incidence after multimodality treatment for stage III and IV squamous cell carcinomas of the head and neck. *Int J Radiat Oncol Biol Phys* 2001;51(3):599–604.

205. Tell R, et al. Long-term incidence of hypothyroidism after radiotherapy in patients with head-and-neck cancer. *Int J Radiat Oncol Biol Phys* 2004;60(2):395–400.

206. Aberle DR, et al. Reduced lung-cancer mortality with low-dose computed tomographic screening. *N Engl J Med* 2011;365(5):395–409.

207. Ang KK, Garden AS. *Radiotherapy for head and neck cancers: indications and techniques.* 2nd ed. Philadelphia, PA: Lippincott Williams & Wilkins, 2002.

208. Mendenhall WM, et al. Retromolar trigone squamous cell carcinoma treated with radiotherapy alone or combined with surgery. *Cancer* 2005;103(11):2320–2325.

209. Byers RM, et al. Treatment of squam carcinoma of the retromolar trigone. *Am J Clin Oncol* 1984;7(6):647–652.

210. Lo K, et al. Results of irradiation in the squamous cell carcinomas of the anterior faucial pillar-retromolar trigone. *Int J Radiat Oncol Biol Phys* 1987;13(7):969–974.

211. Durmus K, Apuhan T, Ozer E. Transoral robotic surgery for retromolar trigone tumours. *Acta Otorhinolaryngol Ital* 2013;33(6):425–427.

212. Liao CT, et al. Salvage therapy in relapsed squamous cell carcinoma of the oral cavity: how and when? *Cancer* 2008;112(1):94–103.

213. Gibson MK, et al. Randomized phase III evaluation of cisplatin plus fluorouracil versus cisplatin plus paclitaxel in advanced head and neck cancer (E1395): an intergroup trial of the Eastern Cooperative Oncology Group. *J Clin Oncol* 2005;23(15):3562–3567.

214. Ferris RL, et al. Nivolumab for recurrent squamous-cell carcinoma of the head and neck. *N Engl J Med* 2016;375(19):1856–1867.

215. Seiwert TY, et al. Safety and clinical activity of pembrolizumab for treatment of recurrent or metastatic squamous cell carcinoma of the head and neck (KEYNOTE-012): an open-label, multicentre, phase 1b trial. *Lancet Oncol* 2016;17(7):956–965.

216. Ferris RL. Immunology and immunotherapy of head and neck cancer. *J Clin Oncol* 2015;33(29):3293–3304.

217. Bhandare N, et al. Radiation therapy and hearing loss. *Int J Radiat Oncol Biol Phys* 2010;76(3 Suppl):S50–S57.

218. Deasy JO, et al. Radiotherapy dose-volume effects on salivary gland function. *Int J Radiat Oncol Biol Phys* 2010;76(3 Suppl):S58–S63.

219. Mayo C, et al. Radiation dose-volume effects of optic nerves and chiasm. *Int J Radiat Oncol Biol Phys* 2010;76(3 Suppl):S28–S35.

220. Mayo C, Yorke E, Merchant TE. Radiation associated brainstem injury. *Int J Radiat Oncol Biol Phys* 2010;76(3 Suppl):S36–S41.

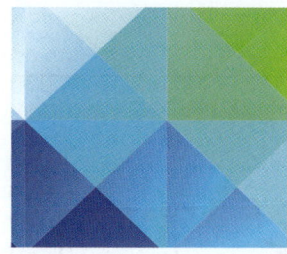

CHAPTER 48

Oropharynx

Joseph K. Salama and David M. Brizel

The incidence of oropharyngeal carcinoma is increasing, which is in contrast to the decreasing incidence of head and neck cancer arising in other anatomic sites. The classic etiologic factors of tobacco abuse and alcohol use continue to play a significant role. However, a significant increase in rates of oropharyngeal cancers in nonsmokers and nondrinkers caused by oncogenic human papillomaviruses (HPVs) is occurring, predominantly among men. Although both HPV-associated and HPV-unassociated malignancies are classified as squamous cell carcinomas, the behavior of these cancers markedly differs as HPV-associated cancers have a significantly more favorable prognosis that is treatment platform independent. The recognition that HPV-associated oropharyngeal cancer is a distinct clinical entity, and the adverse effects of standard therapies on speech, swallowing, degustation, and psychological well-being, has lead to significant multidisciplinary interest in defining different treatment paradigms for HPV-associated and HPV-unassociated oropharyngeal cancers. Treatment recommendations for these two clinical entities currently remain the same, pending the outcomes from ongoing clinical investigations.

Based on the critical role of the oropharynx in speech and swallowing, treatment of oropharyngeal carcinomas can significantly impact patients' quality of life. Appropriate treatment strategies should focus on maintaining high cure rates while minimizing long-term, treatment-induced functional morbidity. Early-stage oropharyngeal cancers are best managed with single modality therapy (radiation or surgery), with the choice based upon anticipated posttherapy consequences. Treatment of locoregionally advanced tumors involves multiple modalities, the most common strategies being either concomitant chemotherapy and radiotherapy or surgery followed by adjuvant radiotherapy with or without chemotherapy based on pathologic risk factors.

Novel approaches to surgical and radiation delivery and the incorporation of molecularly targeted chemotherapeutics are currently the focus of clinical investigation with an intent to maximize the therapeutic index for HPV-associated oropharyngeal cancers. Transoral surgical techniques including laser and robotic resection have the potential to reduce morbidity. Advances in radiotherapy allow for improved dosing to the primary tumor and involved nodes with reduced radiation exposure of normal tissues, particularly the parotid and submandibular glands and pharyngeal constrictor muscles. Further studies are needed to more completely integrate molecularly targeted agents into the treatment of oropharyngeal cancers. The use of immune-modulating agents has demonstrated improved outcomes in metastatic and recurrent head and neck cancer patients, including oropharyngeal cancer patients, establishing these agents as an integral cancer therapy.

EPIDEMIOLOGY

Oropharyngeal cancers account for approximately 10% of the annual, worldwide incidence of head and neck squamous cell carcinomas. The incidence of oropharyngeal cancer differs significantly by geography.[1] In the United States, the annual incidence of oropharyngeal squamous cell carcinoma is 4.8/100,000,[2] which is similar to other developed countries. This rate has increased by 28% from 1988 to 2004, largely because of the 225% increase in HPV-associated oropharyngeal cancer, whereas HPV-unassociated oropharyngeal cancer

has declined by 50% over the same time period.[3] The incidence of oropharyngeal cancer in developing countries is lower at approximately 3/100,000.[1] This rise in developed countries is unique as other mucosal head and neck cancer incidences have decreased over this same time period. The putative cause of this is the increasing incidence of HPV-associated cancers discussed in detail later. Worldwide, the majority of oropharyngeal cancers remain attributable to tobacco smoking and/or the excessive ingestion of alcohol. For these cases, incidence rates are generally higher for men than women (4:1), who are diagnosed more commonly in the sixth and seventh decades of life.

HUMAN PAPILLOMAVIRUS–ASSOCIATED OROPHARYNGEAL CANCER

Human Papillomavirus

The HPV is a circular, double-stranded DNA virus, first determined to be oncogenic when it was found to be the associated with cervical cancer in 1983[4] and subsequently established as a significant human carcinogen in 1996.[5] To date, approximately 150 HPV types have been identified. HPV subtypes are classified as high or low risk based upon epidemiologic associations with cervical cancer in case–control studies.[6] HPV 16 is the most common HPV type identified in human tumors and is associated with >90% of all HPV-associated related oropharyngeal cancers.[7] Infection with HPV16 confers an approximate 14-fold increase in risk for oropharyngeal cancer.[8]

The HPV genome encodes three oncoproteins (E5, E6, and E7), in addition to regulatory genes (E1 and E2) as well as capsid protein genes (L1 and L2). Oncogenesis is primarily mediated via the E6 and E7 proteins. HPV E6 complexes with E3 ubiquitin ligase and E6-associated protein, promoting ubiquitin-mediated destruction of p53. Loss of cellular p53 function results in dysregulation of the G1/S and G2/M checkpoints. An E7/cullin 2 complex ubiquitinates the Rb protein, resulting in loss of G1/S checkpoint control.[9] E7 is believed to be the major transforming oncogene during early carcinogenesis, with E6 functioning later.[10] A diagram of the pathways affecting the malignant transformation of keratinocytes by HPV is shown in Figure 48.1. Although E6 and E7 oncoprotein function is necessary for development of an HPV-associated malignancy, it is not sufficient. It is believed that as yet undefined genetic events are required for HPV malignant transformation.[11]

A number of different techniques are used to detect HPV in oropharyngeal cancer biopsy specimens. The gold standard is demonstration of HPV E6/E7 in clinical specimens. However, this approach is clinically impractical because it is very difficult to detect viral RNA from cytologic fluid and paraffin-embedded tissues. Polymerase chain reaction (PCR) of HPV DNA is a technique with high sensitivity, but low specificity, as cross-contamination or transcriptionally inactive DNA can be detected. In situ hybridization uses oligonucleotide probes designed to anneal to complementary HPV DNA in the tumor specimen. Advantages of this technique include localization of DNA within the tumor specimen and allow for identification of a single viral copy.[12] A consequence of HPV E7-mediated Rb inhibition is induction of demethylases resulting in expression of p16^{INK4A}, an upstream tumor suppressor cyclin-dependent kinase inhibitor.[13] Immunohistochemistry staining for p16^{INK4A} is frequently used as a surrogate for HPV status. There is a small (7%) discordance between HPV ISH and p16^{INK4A} IHC,

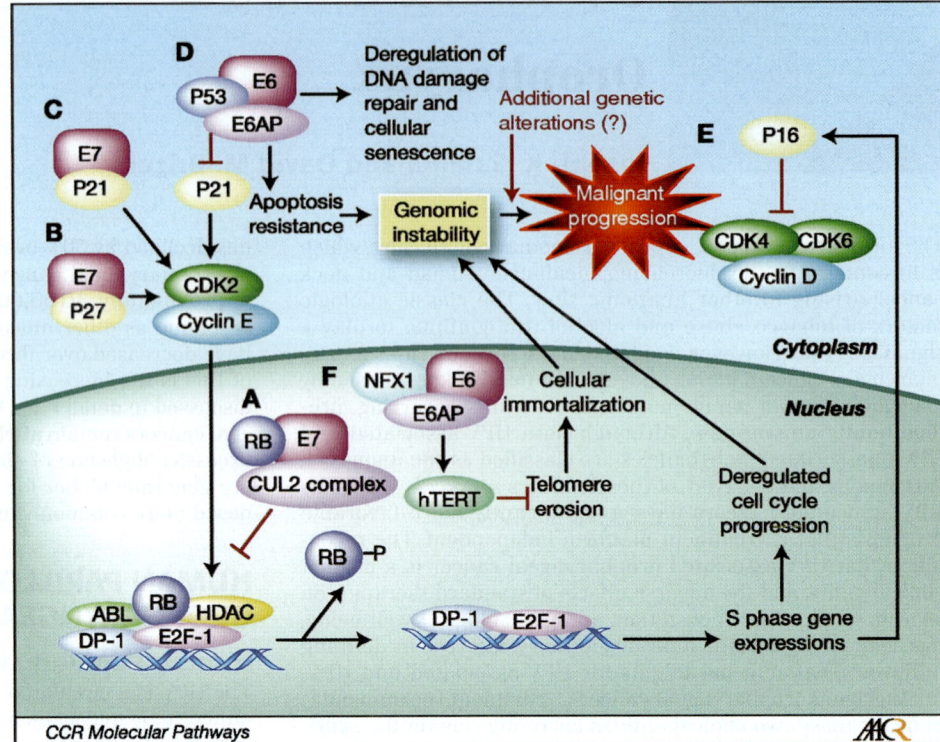

FIGURE 48.1. Diagram of malignant transformation in keratinocytes caused by the HPV oncoproteins, E6 and E7. Clockwise from *A*, ubiquitination by E7 and the cullin 2 ubiquitin ligase complex leading to pRb degradation (23, 25, 56, 57); *B*, interaction between E7 and p27[Kip1] resulting in inhibition of cell cycle arrest contributing to carcinogenesis (58); *C*, interaction between E7 and p21[Cip1] resulting in inhibition of cell cycle arrest contributing to carcinogenesis (31, 59); *D*, ubiquitination by E6 and ubiquitin ligase E6AP leading to p53 degradation (19–21); *E*, increased expression of p16[INK4A] by a consequent of feedback loops from the absence of pRb function (42); and *F*, degradation of NFX1, a transcriptional repressor of hTERT, by association with E6/E6AP resulting in hTERT activation and cellular immortalization.[60] (Reprinted from Chung CH, Gillison ML. Human papillomavirus in head and neck cancer: its role in pathogenesis and clinical implications. *Clin Cancer Res* 2009;15[22]:6758–6762. Copyright © 2009 American Association for Cancer Research. With permission from AACR.)

which is likely related to a combination of infection with non-HPV-16 subtypes or low viral copy numbers not detectable by IHC and true p16-positive/HPV-negative cases.

Clinical Characteristics of Human Papillomavirus–Associated Oropharyngeal Cancer

HPV-associated oropharyngeal cancers are more likely to occur among men than women (3:1), most of whom (80%) will not have a smoking history. These cancers are more common among white individuals than other races, are diagnosed in individuals who are 5 to 10 years younger than HPV-unassociated related oropharyngeal cancers, and are associated with higher socioeconomic status. Furthermore, when compared to patients with HPV-unassociated cancers, these patients are more likely to be married and college educated and have a median income >$55,000. The use of marijuana also elevates odds of HPV-associated oropharyngeal cancer.[14] Analogous to cervical cancers, patients with HPV-associated oropharyngeal cancer have been associated with certain sexual behaviors. These include high number of vaginal or oral sex partners, infrequent condom use, engagement in casual sex, and early age of first intercourse.[15] Whether or not HPV acts in a synergistic manner with tobacco or alcohol exposure in patients to increase risk of HPV-associated oropharyngeal cancer is a matter of ongoing controversy.

HPV-associated oropharyngeal cancers are characterized frequently as poorly differentiated, nonkeratinizing or basaloid in histopathology.[16] HPV-associated and HPV-unassociated carcinomas are also different with regard to molecular alterations.

HPV-associated oropharyngeal cancers are associated with wild-type p53, p16 expression, and infrequent amplification of cyclin D, whereas the converse is true for HPV-unassociated cancers. A subset of HPV-associated oropharyngeal cancer patients with more extensive smoking histories will have tumors exhibiting *TP53* mutations and higher epidermal growth factor receptor (EGFR) and Bcl-xL expression and have outcomes similar to those of HPV-unassociated patients.[9]

Response of Human Papillomavirus–Associated Oropharyngeal Cancer to Standard Therapy

Patients with HPV-associated oropharyngeal cancers have significantly better outcomes compared to HPV-unassociated oropharyngeal tumors.[17,18] A reanalysis of Radiation Therapy Oncology Group (RTOG) 0129, a randomized study comparing cisplatin administered with either accelerated concomitant boost radiotherapy or conventionally fractionated radiotherapy, HPV status was independently associated with improved outcomes. Three-year overall survival was 82% in HPV-positive patients compared to 54% in HPV negative. Even after adjustment for age, tumor stage, nodal stage, treatment assignment, and tobacco use, HPV status independently predicted for improved survival (Hazard ratio [HR] = 0.42, 95% confidence interval [CI] = 0.27 to 0.66). Additionally, locoregional progression (13.6% vs. 24.8%) and progression-free survival (71.8% vs. 50.4%) were significantly improved in HPV-positive cases. Other large cooperative group studies have demonstrated similar findings.[18,19] It is important to realize that the prognostic significance of HPV was independent of chemoradiotherapy platform and applies to treatment with radiotherapy alone[20] as shown in Table 48.1. In fact, HPV-related tumors have a better

TABLE 48.1	HPV STATUS AND SURVIVAL OUTCOMES IN PROSPECTIVE TRIALS							
Cooperative Group	N	Radiotherapy	Induction	Concurrent	% HPV+	Survival HPV+	Survival HPV–	P-Value
ECOG	96	70 Gy	Paclitaxel 175 mg/m² Carboplatin AUC = 6 2 cycles	Weekly paclitaxel 30 mg/m²	40%	95%	62%	0.005
TROG	195	70 Gy	None	CDDP +/– Tirapazamine	28%	94%	77%	0.007
RTOG	323	70 Gy	None	CDDP 100 mg/m²	64%	79%	46%	0.002
DAHANCA	156	62–68 Gy	None	Nimorazole 1,200 mg/m²/d	22%	62%	26%	0.003

prognosis regardless of the treatment modality (surgery,[21] radiation therapy, or chemoradiotherapy) used.

ANATOMY

The oropharynx is contiguous with the oral cavity anteriorly, the larynx and hypopharynx posterior/inferiorly, and nasopharynx superiorly. Three main subregions compose the oropharynx including the tonsil, base of tongue, and soft palate. Normal function of the oropharynx is critical for speech and swallowing.

The tonsillar region contains the anterior and posterior tonsillar pillars and the palatine tonsil. The palatine tonsils are lymphoid aggregates incompletely encapsulated with a keratinized stratified squamous epithelial mucosal lining positioned in the tonsillar bed, a part of the tonsillar cleft between the anterior (palatoglossal) and posterior (palatopharyngeal) tonsillar pillars.

The base of tongue comprises the posterior third of the tongue and is bounded anteriorly by the circumvallate papillae, sitting in front of the sulcus terminalis. It is bounded posterior–inferiorly by the hyoid and epiglottis and laterally by the glossopharyngeal sulci. Underlying the mucosa of the base of tongue are lymphatic nodules collectively known as the lingual tonsil. The vallecula is a 1-cm mucosal strip that serves as a transition between the base of tongue and epiglottis and is considered a part of the base of tongue. The sensory innervation of the base of tongue is via the glossopharyngeal nerve (CN IX) with a small aspect of the base of tongue supplied by the internal laryngeal nerve (CN X).

The soft palate is a fibromuscular structure bounded anteriorly by the hard palate, laterally coursing into the anterior tonsillar pillars and posterior/inferiorly forming a free edge, and the midline uvula. The soft palate is composed of five muscles (levator veli palatini, tensor veli palatini, palatoglossus, palatopharyngeus, and musculus uvulae) posteriorly and the palatine aponeurosis an expanded tendon of the tensor veli palatini anteriorly. The muscles of the soft palate are supplied through the pharyngeal plexus (which is composed of the pharyngeal branches of cranial nerves IX and X and sympathetic branches from the superior cervical ganglion, except for the tensor veli palatini, which is supplied by cranial nerve V2). The sensory supply is from CN IX.

The oropharynx serves many functions including that of degustation, respiration, and speech. Advanced tumors arising in the oropharynx can infiltrate muscles and nerves, significantly impeding these functions. A major goal of successful therapy is to limit the impact of treatment on long-term function.

TABLE 48.2	ANATOMIC BOUNDARIES OF NECK NODE LEVELS
I	Bounded by posterior belly of digastric, hyoid bone inferiorly, and body of mandible superiorly
II	Bounded by skull base superiorly to level of hyoid bone inferiorly
III	Bounded by hyoid bone superiorly to cricothyroid membrane inferiorly
IV	Bounded by cricothyroid membrane superiorly to clavicle inferiorly
V	Bounded by anterior border of trapezius posteriorly, posterior border of SCM anteriorly, and clavicle inferiorly
VI	Bounded by level of hyoid bone superiorly to suprasternal notch inferiorly, lateral border formed by medial border of carotid sheath

ROUTES OF SPREAD

Primary routes of oropharyngeal cancer spread include direct extension and lymphatic spread, with hematogenous metastases being less common. Oropharyngeal cancers have a predilection for submucosal extension, often visualized as raised erythematous regions without distinct borders or ulceration. This can best be appreciated by direct visualization rather than on radiographic imaging.

Lymphatic Spread of Oropharyngeal Cancer

The lymphatic drainage of the oropharynx and the neck was first described by Rouviere in 1938[22] and has since been refined since by others.[23] Originally described as lymph node chains located in particular anatomic regions, nodal groups are now classified by the level system[24] with the location of lymph nodes in the neck being defined by surgical–anatomic landmarks (Table 48.2). Recently, this system (levels I to VI) was refined with the addition of sublevels (Ia/Ib, IIa/IIb, and Va/Vb) (as shown in Table 48.2), also incorporating radiologically defined landmarks (as shown in Table 48.3 and Fig. 48.2).[25]

The most common location for lymph node metastases from oropharyngeal cancers is ipsilaterally in level II. The probability of lymphatic (regional) metastasis is related to the size and location of the primary tumor within the oropharynx. The typical order of metastatic progression is systematic, from the upper jugular chain nodes superiorly (level I/II; first echelon) to midcervical (level III) and to lower cervical nodes (level IV) inferiorly. In large series of oropharyngeal cancer patients, isolated skip metastases are rare (0.3%); level I or V involvement is usually associated with the involvement of other levels. Additionally, tumors encroaching or crossing midline or involving the posterior pharyngeal wall exhibited a higher propensity for bilateral lymphadenopathy.[26]

TABLE 48.3	RADIOGRAPHIC BOUNDARIES OF NECK NODE LEVELS					
Level	Cranial	Caudal	Anterior	Posterior	Lateral	Medial
Ia	Geniohyoid m., plane tangent to basilar edge of mandible	Plane tangent to body of hyoid bone	Symphysis menti, platysma m.	Body of hyoid bone	Medial edge of ant. belly of digastric m.	NA
Ib	Mylohyoid m., cranial edge of submandibular gland	Plane through central part of hyoid bone	Symphysis menti, platysma m.	Post. edge of submandibular gland	Inner side of mandible, platysma m., skin	Lateral edge of ant. belly of digastric m.
II	Caudal edge of lateral process of C1	Caudal edge of body of hyoid bone	Post. edge of submandibular gland; ICA; post. edge of post. belly of digastric m.	Post. edge of SCM m.	Medial edge of SCM m.	Int. edge of ICA, paraspinal m.
III	Caudal edge of body of hyoid bone	Caudal edge of cricoid cartilage	Posterolateral edge of sternohyoid m.; ant. edge of SCM m.	Post. edge of SCM m.	Medial edge of SCM m.	Int. edge of ICA, paraspinal m.
IV	Caudal edge of cricoid cartilage	2 cm cranial to sternoclavicular joint	Anteromedial edge of SCM m.	Post. edge of SCM m.	Medial edge of SCM m.	Medial edge of ICA, paraspinal m.
V	Cranial edge of body of hyoid bone	CT slice including transverse cervical vessels	Post. edge of SCM m.	Ant. border of trapezius m.	Platysma m., skin	Paraspinal m.
VI	Caudal edge of body of thyroid cartilage	Sternal manubrium	Skin, platysma m.	Separation b/w trachea and esoph	Medial edge of SCM, thyroid gland, skin	NA
RP	Base of skull	Cranial edge of body of hyoid bone	Fascia under pharyngeal mucosa	Prevertebral m.	Medial edge of ICA	Midline

Section
III

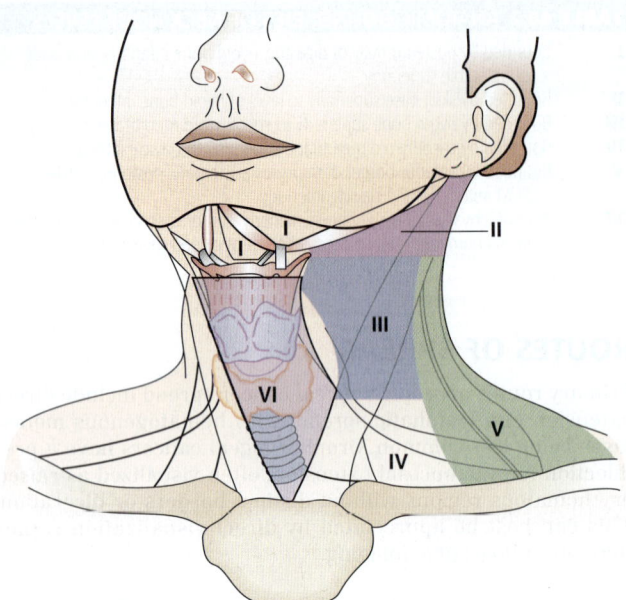

FIGURE 48.2. Schematic diagram indicating the location of the lymph node levels in the neck based on anatomic boundaries. (From Edge SB, Byrd DR, Compton CC, et al., eds. *AJCC cancer staging manual.* 7th ed. New York: Springer, 2010:25. Copyright © 2010 American Joint Committee on Cancer. Reproduced with permission of Springer in the format Book via Copyright Clearance Center.)

Knowledge of the probability of occult pathologic lymphadenopathy for each involved oropharynx anatomic subsite and extent of disease is critical to modern radiotherapy and surgery planning, as selective neck dissections and limited radiotherapy volumes, designed to preserve function, are the norm. Standardized contouring atlases have been published to aid clinicians in the development of appropriate radiotherapy volumes to cover potential occult microscopic lymphatic spread in the N0 neck.[27–29] Additionally, information regarding probabilities of occult pathologic lymphatic involvement has been compounded from series of patients undergoing elective neck dissection.[30] Use of this knowledge to develop appropriate radiotherapy volumes will be discussed in more detail in the radiotherapy planning section. The rates of pathologic lymphadenopathy for the pathologically uninvolved and involved neck are outlined in Table 48.4.

Distant Metastatic Spread of Oropharyngeal Cancer

Distant metastatic spread of oropharyngeal cancer is relatively uncommon affecting approximately 15% of all patients during the course of their disease.[31] The most common locations for distant metastatic spread of oropharyngeal cancers are the lung parenchyma[31] followed by the bone and liver. Metastases are more common in patients presenting with locoregionally advanced or recurrent tumors, with the

risk increasing with primary tumor stage and the extent of cervical lymphadenopathy (N2-N3 disease).[32] Extranodal extension, lower cervical pathologic lymphadenopathy (level IV), and lymphovascular invasion have also been associated with increased rates of distant metastases.[33]

Lung metastases typically appear radiographically as well-circumscribed, peripherally located nodules. Given different treatment and prognoses, care should be taken to differentiate between pulmonary metastases and primary pulmonary malignancies, characterized as spiculated irregularly shaped masses commonly associated with hilar and mediastinal lymphadenopathy. Often, this distinction is impossible, even after biopsy, as both can be squamous cell histology. In such instances, physically fit patients should be given the benefit of the doubt and treated as if they have two separate primary tumors. In patients with limited pulmonary metastases, who are technically resectable and fit for surgery, resection of pulmonary oropharyngeal cancer metastases may improve survival.[34] For nonsurgical candidates, hypofractionated image-guided radiotherapy to all known metastases can result in long-term disease control and should be considered for patients with limited metastatic disease.[35]

CLINICAL PRESENTATION

Oropharyngeal cancers present with a constellation of symptoms, dependent upon the location of the primary tumor, invasion of nearby organs, and extent of nodal disease. Often, patients will present with a painless neck mass, which is usually mobile, firm, and nontender, but can be fixed, indicating extranodal extension and invasion into surrounding structures. Such masses are frequently treated with an initial course of antibiotics, but persistence or growth in this context mandates further evaluation. Some patients complain of a deep-seated otalgia located within the auditory canal. This is mediated via irritation of the glossopharyngeal nerve (CN IX) with referral via the Petrosal ganglion to the tympanic nerve of Jacobson. Regurgitation of foods can occur with invasion of the soft palate, inhibiting its ability to elevate during swallowing. Trismus is seen with more advanced tumors and reflects invasion of the pterygoid fossa and/or musculature. Odynophagia and dysphagia are other common presenting symptoms that occur with invasion into the pharyngeal musculature or obstruction by pathologic lymphadenopathy.

DIAGNOSTIC EVALUATION

Physical Examination
A complete examination of all mucosal head and neck sites should be performed in any patient with a known or suspected diagnosis of oropharyngeal cancer. This process not only characterizes the primary tumor but also evaluates for synchronous malignancies given the high propensity for second primary upper aerodigestive tract tumors especially in smokers. A thorough physical examination is essential for diagnosis as understanding of the complete disease extent

Tumor Site	Patients With N+ (%)	Distribution of Metastatic Lymph Nodes per Level (Percentage of the Node-Positive Patients Ipsilateral/Contralateral)					
		I	II	III	IV	V	Other
Oral cavity (*n* = 787)	36	42/3.5	79/8	18/3	5/1	1/0	1.4/0.3
Oropharynx (*n* = 1,479)	64	13/2	81/24	23/5	9/2.5	13/3	2/1
Hypopharynx (*n* = 847)	70	2/0	80/13	51/4	20/3	24/2	3/1
Supraglottic larynx (*n* = 428)	55	2/0	71/21	48/10	18/7	15/4	2/0
Nasopharynx (*n* = 440)	80	9/5	71/56	36/32	22/15	32/26	15/10

TABLE 48.4 DISTRIBUTION OF CLINICAL METASTATIC NECK NODES FROM HEAD AND NECK SQUAMOUS CELL CARCINOMAS

Reprinted from Grégoire V, Coche E, Cosnard G, et al. Selection and delineation of lymph node target volumes in head and neck conformal radiotherapy: proposal for standardizing terminology and procedure based on the surgical experience. *Radiother Oncol* 2000;56(2):135–150. Copyright © 2000 Elsevier Science Ireland Ltd. With permission.

helps guide the surgeon on the choice of optimal biopsy site. Inspection of the oropharynx should be performed under adequate illumination, be well practiced, systematic, and reproducible. Following examination of the oral cavity, where attention should be directed to the number and health of the teeth and the mucosa, one should closely examine the anterior tonsillar pillars, the tonsillar fossae, and posterior tonsillar pillars followed by the soft palate. Proper exposure can be achieved either with gloved index fingers or two disposable tongue depressors used in unison. Palpation of the tonsillar fossa and the base of tongue should be performed since these locations can harbor occult primary tumors. The base of tongue should be palpated at the completion of the examination because of its propensity to trigger the gag reflex. Direct visualization should be followed by fiberoptic examination because this allows optimal inspection of the base of tongue, posterior-inferior tonsil, and vallecula and can detect spread to laryngeal and hypopharyngeal sites. Fiberoptic examinations should be recorded and compared to assess response during the course of therapy. Indirect mirror examination is much less informative than fiberoptic evaluation but should be performed if fiberoptic capabilities are not available and if the practitioner is skilled in this art.

Oropharyngeal tumors often appear as ulcerated masses, with surrounding erythema, neovascularization, and mucositis. Tenderness, evidence of recent bleeding, obstruction of the airway, skin invasion, alteration of gag reflex, and extent of trismus (measured from upper to lower incisors) should be documented. Bulging of the parapharyngeal space should also be noted as this could represent retropharyngeal lymphadenopathy.

Careful examination of the neck is also important for staging and management. Palpation of the neck should focus on neck levels defined by standard anatomic relationships. The neck should gently be turned to the side being examined to relax the sternocleidomastoid muscle, which facilitates the detection of smaller involved lymph nodes. Care should be taken not to palpate too firmly in older patients or those with known vascular disease, as aggressive carotid massage can be associated with syncope. Lymph nodes should be recorded in terms of the level in which they arise, their size, the character of their firmness, as well if they are fixed, and whether or not they penetrate and involve the skin.

Confirmatory biopsy of the primary site should be performed. Adequate exposure is usually possible for in-office biopsies of the proximal oropharynx. Posterior oropharyngeal tumors are often biopsied under general anesthesia in the operating room, often as part of a comprehensive examination under anesthesia as well as comprehensive endoscopic evaluation (laryngoscopy, bronchoscopy, and esophagoscopy).

Computed Tomography

Computed tomography (CT) imaging of the head and neck with intravenous contrast should be performed for all newly diagnosed oropharyngeal cancer patients to assess the extent of primary tumors and to determine the presence or absence of cervical lymph node metastases. Scan slice thickness <5 mm is necessary to optimize the detection of smaller pathologically involved lymph nodes and to provide the best anatomic delineation of both primary and nodal disease. Pathologically involved lymph nodes are characterized on CT imaging as those that are enlarged, have lost a fatty hilum, enhance with contrast, and/or have a necrotic center. Primary tumors appear as contrast-enhancing masses, distorting normal anatomic relationships. Although ulceration and invasion into surrounding organs are readily assessed, submucosal spread is often difficult to characterize with CT. As multiplanar image reconstruction is routinely available, lymph node and primary tumor size should be measured in cephalad–caudad and axial dimensions to more accurately stage patients. Unfortunately,

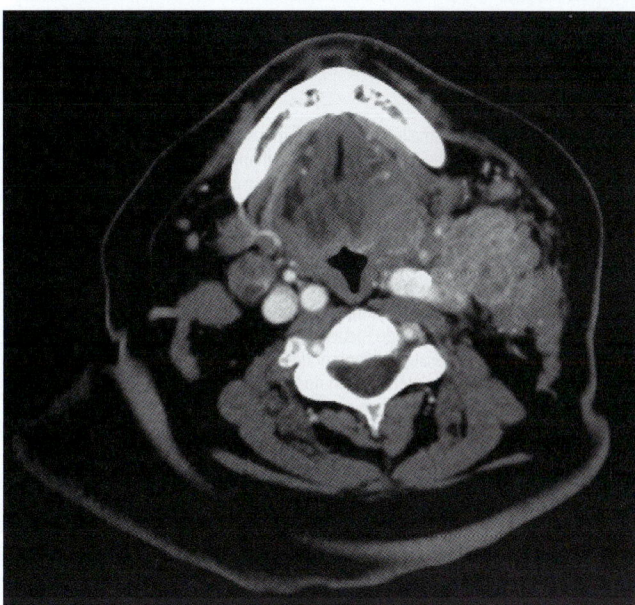

FIGURE 48.3. Diagnostic CT image demonstrating locoregionally advanced oropharyngeal cancer with extensive ipsilateral cervical lymphadenopathy.

dental artifact can affect CT imaging and may obscure complete visualization with neutral head position, requiring further scanning with an adjusted head position or use of metal artifact reducing reconstruction algorithms. Thoracic CT should be performed routinely (alone or in combination with a positron emission tomography [PET] scan) to assess for pulmonary spread of oropharyngeal cancer patients with N2 or greater nodal disease and for those with advanced primary tumors, given the risks of pulmonary metastases described above. A diagnostic CT image of a patient with locoregionally advanced head and neck cancer is shown in Figure 48.3.

Positron Emission Tomography

PET and/or PET/CT imaging incorporating tumor physiology in conjunction with anatomic information is now routinely recommended for the initial staging of oropharyngeal cancer patients. From a practical standpoint, PET-based imaging can assess not only the locoregional burden of disease but also detect and quantify the presence of distant metastases. For oropharyngeal cancer patients, the ability to detect clinically and radiographically occult pathologic cervical lymphadenopathy renders PET a powerful clinical tool, as ipsilateral radiotherapy volumes are commonly used in specific settings.[36] Although usually reported as the maximum standard uptake value (SUVmax), alternative measurements such as SUVmean may have greater prognostic value.[37] The utility of PET/CT for oropharyngeal cancer patients demonstrates high sensitivity approaching 100% but only about 60% specificity for pathologically proven tumor. Clinical status and knowledge of prior procedures is critical to PET interpretation, as recent biopsies and infections can cause artificially elevated metabolic activity.

Magnetic Resonance Imaging

Magnetic resonance imaging (MRI) can be a useful imaging tool for oropharyngeal tumors. Squamous cell carcinoma appears as low signal in T1-MRI images and corresponding high signal in T2-sequences. The ability of MRI to differentiate tumor from soft tissues is particularly useful when determination of the extent of base of tongue or oral tongue invasion is needed. Additionally, MRI is useful in patients with compromised renal function who are not able to receive iodinated-based CT contrast agents.

TABLE 48.5 AJCC/IUCC 8TH EDITION TNM STAGING SYSTEM FOR HPV-MEDIATED (P16+) OROPHARYNGEAL CANCER

Primary Tumor (T)

T0	No primary identified
T1	Tumor 2 cm or smaller in greatest dimension
T2	Tumor larger than 2 cm but not larger than 4 cm in greatest dimension
T3	Tumor larger than 4 cm in greatest dimension or extension to lingual surface of epiglottis
T4	Moderately advanced local disease; tumor invades the larynx, extrinsic muscle of tongue, medial pterygoid, hard palate, or mandible or beyond

Clinical Regional Lymph Nodes (cN)

NX	Regional lymph nodes cannot be assessed
N0	No regional lymph node metastasis
N1	One or more ipsilateral lymph nodes, none larger than 6 cm
N2	Contralateral or bilateral lymph nodes, none larger than 6 cm
N3	Lymph node(s) larger than 6 cm

Pathologic Regional Lymph Nodes (pN)

NX	Regional lymph nodes cannot be assessed
pN0	No regional lymph node metastasis
pN1	Metastasis in 4 or fewer lymph nodes
pN2	Metastasis in more than 4 lymph nodes

Distant Metastasis (M)

M0	No distant metastasis present
M1	Distant metastasis present

From Amin MB, Edge SB, Greene FL, et al., eds. *AJCC Cancer Staging Manual*. 8th ed. New York, NY: Springer, 2017. Reproduced with permission of Springer International Publishing in the format Book via Copyright Clearance Center.

PATHOLOGIC CLASSIFICATION

Squamous cell carcinomas are the most common histological subtype comprising >95% of all oropharyngeal cancers. Uncommonly, minor salivary gland tumors and mesenchymal tumors can affect this region. Given the proportionally high content of lymphoid tissue in the region within Waldeyer ring, malignant Hodgkin, and non-Hodgkin lymphomas also arise in this region. This chapter will discuss only squamous cell and related (poorly differentiated and lymphoepithelioma) histologic subtypes.

STAGING

The staging for oropharyngeal cancer has been significantly revised in AJCC/IUCC 8th edition, shown in Tables 48.5 to 48.9, given the significant differences in prognosis between HPV-associated and HPV nonassociated oropharyngeal squamous cell cancers. Clinical staging is based upon all available history, physical examination, and endoscopic, radiographic, metabolic, and scintigraphic data. For both HPV-associated and HPV nonassociated oropharyngeal cancer, the size of the primary tumor continues to define the T stage, with T1 being <2 cm, T2 >2 cm but <4 cm, and T3 > 4 cm. T4a describes tumors invading the larynx, extrinsic muscles of the tongue, medial pterygoid, hard palate, or mandible. T4b disease describes oropharyngeal tumors invading the lateral pterygoid, pterygoid plates, lateral nasopharynx, skull base, or surrounding the carotid artery.

Thus, for HPV-associated oropharyngeal cancers, T1-3 is unchanged, and T4 disease is classified as tumor invasion of the larynx, extrinsic muscles of the tongue, medial pterygoid,

TABLE 48.6 AJCC/IUCC 8TH EDITION CLINICAL STAGE GROUPING FOR HPV-ASSOCIATED (P16+) OROPHARYNGEAL CANCER

	T0	T1	T2	T3	T4
N0	N/A	I	I	II	III
N1	I	I	I	II	III
N2	II	II	II	II	III
N3	III	III	III	III	III
M1	IV	IV	IV	IV	IV

TABLE 48.7 AJCC/IUCC 8TH EDITION PATHOLOGIC STAGE GROUPING FOR HPV-ASSOCIATED (P16+) OROPHARYNGEAL CANCER

	T0	T1	T2	T3	T4
N0	N/A	I	I	II	II
N1	I	I	I	II	II
N2	II	II	II	III	III
M1	IV	IV	IV	IV	IV

hard palate, mandible, or beyond. Clinical nodal staging is simplified. N0 remains the absence of lymph nodes, N1 is one or more ipsilateral lymph node all <6 cm, N2 is contralateral or bilateral lymph nodes none <6 cm, and N3 is defined as lymph nodes >6 cm. Pathologic lymph node staging is also simplified to include pN1 with four or fewer lymph nodes and pN2 being more than 4 pathologically involved nodes.

The stage grouping of HPV-associated oropharyngeal cancers is also different from before. Clinical stage 1 now comprises T0-2, N0-1; stage 2 is now T0-2, N2 or T3, N0-2; and stage 3 is comprised of T0-4, N3 or T4, N0-2. Finally, clinical stage 4 is limited to M1 disease. The pathologic staging is similar as shown in Table 48.7.

For p16 negative tumors, the staging is similar to prior AJCC/IUCC 7th edition. The nodal staging in the 8th edition has changed to incorporate the important prognostic significance of extranodal extension. For clinically staged oropharyngeal tumors without extranodal extension, N0 indicates no clinical or radiographic evidence of pathologic lymphadenopathy, N1 indicates a single lymph node <3 cm in the ipsilateral cervical chains, N2a indicates a single lymph node >3 cm and <6 cm in the ipsilateral cervical chain, N2b indicates multiple ipsilateral cervical lymph nodes all <6 cm in size, and N2c indicates bilateral pathologically involved cervical lymph nodes with the largest node <6 cm. N3 status is now divided into two subcategories, N3a and N3b. N3a indicates the presence of at least one lymph node >6 cm and no extranodal extension, while N3b status is attained by the presence of overt clinical evidence of extranodal extension irrespective of number, size, or laterality of pathologic lymphadenopathy.

For pathologically staged nodal disease, the 8th edition now classifies a single LN (ipsilateral or contralateral) <3 cm with ENE as N2a, whereas either a single pathologic LN >3 cm with ENE or multiple lymph nodes with ENE is N3b. The presence of distant metastatic disease is classified as M1. The stage grouping for HPV nonassociated cancers is unchanged from prior editions and is shown in Table 48.9. Stage I comprises T1N0 tumors and stage II is made up of T2N0 tumors. Stage III includes patients with T3 N0-1 or T1-T2N1. Stage IV is divided into three subgroups. Stage IVa is made up of patients with T4aN0-2a-c, T1-3 N2a-c tumors. Stage IVb disease basically describes patients who are technically unresectable including patients with an extensive primary tumor (T4b) or those with any primary stage who have extensive lymphadenopathy (T any N3). Stage IVc disease is reserved for patients with distant metastases.

MANAGEMENT STRATEGIES

Functional organ preservation with minimal toxicity is the management goal for all oropharyngeal cancer patients. Based on AJCC stage, patients are usually grouped divided into two different treatment groups to help guide therapy decisions. Those with locally confined disease (T1-2, N0 tumors) are considered as early stage, whereas those with stage T3-4 or N1-3 (nonmetastatic) disease are considered as having locoregionally advanced disease. For all subsites, early-stage tumors are usually well controlled with a single local modality

TABLE 48.8 AJCC/IUCC 8TH EDITION TNM STAGING SYSTEM FOR (P16−) OROPHARYNGEAL CANCER

Primary Tumor (T)

TX	Primary tumor cannot be assessed
Tis	Carcinoma *in situ*
T1	Tumor 2 cm or smaller in greatest dimension
T2	Tumor larger than 2 cm but not larger than 4 cm in greatest dimension
T3	Tumor larger than 4 cm in greatest dimension or extension to lingual surface of epiglottis
T4	Moderately advanced or very advanced local disease
T4a	Moderately advanced local disease
	Tumor invades the larynx, extrinsic muscle of tongue, medial pterygoid, hard palate, or mandible*
T4b	Very advanced local disease
	Tumor invades lateral pterygoid muscle, pterygoid plates, lateral nasopharynx, or skull base or encases carotid artery

Clinical Regional Lymph Nodes (cN)

NX	Regional lymph nodes cannot be assessed
N0	No regional lymph node metastasis
N1	Metastasis in a single ipsilateral lymph node, 3 cm or smaller in greatest dimension and ENE(−)
N2	Metastasis in a single ipsilateral node larger than 3 cm but not larger than 6 cm in greatest dimension and ENE(−); *or* metastases in multiple ipsilateral lymph nodes, none larger than 6 cm in greatest dimension and ENE(−); *or* in bilateral or contralateral lymph nodes, none larger than 6 cm in greatest dimension and ENE(−)
N2a	Metastasis in a single ipsilateral node larger than 3 cm but not larger than 6 cm in greatest dimension and ENE(−)
N2b	Metastasis in multiple ipsilateral nodes, none larger than 6 cm in greatest dimension and ENE(−)
N2c	Metastasis in bilateral or contralateral lymph nodes, none larger than 6 cm in greatest dimension and ENE(−)
N3	Metastasis in a lymph node larger than 6 cm in greatest dimension and ENE(−); *or* metastasis in any node(s) and clinically overt ENE(+)
N3a	Metastasis in a lymph node larger than 6 cm in greatest dimension and ENE(−)
N3b	Metastasis in any node(s) and clinically overt ENE(+)

Pathologic Regional Lymph Nodes (pN)

NX	Regional lymph nodes cannot be assessed
N0	No regional lymph node metastasis
N1	Metastasis in a single ipsilateral lymph node, 3 cm or smaller in greatest dimension and ENE(−)
N2	Metastasis in a single ipsilateral lymph node, 3 cm or smaller in greatest dimension and ENE(+); *or* larger than 3 cm but not larger than 6 cm in greatest dimension and ENE(−); *or* metastases in multiple ipsilateral lymph nodes, none larger than 6 cm in greatest dimension and ENE(−); or in bilateral or contralateral lymph nodes, none larger than 6 cm in greatest dimension and ENE(−)
N2a	Metastasis in single ipsilateral or contralateral node 3 cm or smaller in greatest dimension and ENE(+); *or* a single ipsilateral node larger than 3 cm but not larger than 6 cm in greatest dimension and ENE(−)
N2b	Metastasis in multiple ipsilateral nodes, none larger than 6 cm in greatest dimension and ENE(−)
N2c	Metastasis in bilateral or contralateral lymph nodes, none larger than 6 cm in greatest dimension and ENE(−)
N3	Metastasis in a lymph node larger than 6 cm in greatest dimension and ENE(−); *or* in a single ipsilateral node larger than 3 cm in greatest dimension and ENE(+); *or* multiple ipsilateral, contralateral or bilateral nodes, any with ENE(+)
N3a	Metastasis in a lymph node larger than 6 cm in greatest dimension and ENE(−)
N3b	Metastasis in a single ipsilateral node larger than 3 cm in greatest dimension and ENE(+); *or* multiple ipsilateral, contralateral, or bilateral nodes, any with ENE(+)

Distant Metastasis (M)

M0	No distant metastasis present
M1	Distant metastasis present

*Mucosal extension to lingual surface of epiglottis from primary tumors of the base of the tongue and vallecula does not constitute invasion of the larynx

TABLE 48.9 AJCC/IUCC 8TH EDITION STAGE GROUPING FOR (P16−) OROPHARYNGEAL CANCER

	T1	T2	T3	T4a	T4b
N0	I	II	III	IVA	IVB
N1	III	III	III	IVA	IVB
N2	IVA	IVA	IVA	IVA	IVB
N3	IVB	IVB	IVB	IVB	IVB
M1	IVC	IVC	IVC	IVC	IVC

either radiotherapy or surgery. This paradigm is in flux for HPV-associated disease as some presentations that would have been considered as advanced stage in AJCC 7th edition, for example, T1N1 and T2N1, are classified as early stage in AJCC 8th edition. Selection of local modality should be based on the primary tumor size, extent of local spread, and subsite involved. Small tumors of the tonsil and small exophytic tumors of the base of tongue can be well managed surgically, whereas the morbidity of surgery on the soft palate typically favors radiotherapy. For locoregionally advanced disease, two appropriate treatment strategies are used: either surgery followed by radiation therapy with or without chemotherapy based on pathologic risk factors or radiotherapy usually given with chemotherapy.

SURGICAL TECHNIQUES, APPROACHES, AND RESULTS

Base of Tongue

Surgery plays a limited role in the management of base of tongue tumors given the inherent morbidity of a near total or total glossectomy, which is required for large and/or midline tumors. For select, well-lateralized or polypoid base of tongue tumors with minimal cervical lymphadenopathy, a partial glossectomy can be performed. Given the high propensity for occult microscopic nodal involvement, bilateral cervical lymph node dissection is often performed. Base of tongue tumors in close proximity to the laryngeal apparatus, such as those arising in the vallecula, often require a supraglottic or total laryngectomy to achieve adequate margins of resection.

Traditional surgical approaches for base of tongue tumors include the midline mandibulotomy (splitting the lip, mandible, and oral tongue midline), the lateral mandibulotomy (dividing the mandible near the angle and approaching the base of tongue from the side), and the floor drop procedure (elevating the inner periosteum from the mandible from angle to angle, which releases the entire floor of mouth and oral tongue into the neck exposing the base of tongue).

Tonsil Cancers

For small (<1 cm) early-stage tonsil cancers, confined to the anterior pillar, a wide local excision can achieve adequate tumor-free margins, whereas tumors involving the palatine tonsil often require a radical tonsillectomy. For both of these situations, the tonsil is approached transorally, with primary closure. Larger tumors with extension onto the tongue and mandible or into surrounding tissue often require a composite resection, usually including resection of the tonsil, tonsillar fossa, pillars, a portion of the soft palate, tongue, and mandible. For tumors not adjacent or adherent to the mandible, a midline mandibulotomy approach is used. For tumors adherent to the mandible, a partial mandibulectomy is used. Defects are often closed with a myocutaneous flap. Complications from surgery depend on the extent of resection, with impairment in swallowing possible with removal of part of the tongue or soft palate.

Soft Palate Cancers

Surgical resection is rarely recommended as initial therapy for soft palate tumors. Resection of the soft palate is often associated with significant reflux into the nasopharynx during swallowing, even with the use of custom prostheses. Additionally, because of the midline location, primary disease spreads bilaterally to the neck and retropharyngeal lymph nodes with frequency high enough to require elective treatment. However, when surgery is performed, the tumors are approached transorally, and a full-thickness wide local resection is performed for tumors limited to the soft palate. A more extensive composite resection is required if disease extends to surrounding structures. Flaps or prostheses are used to preserve velopharyngeal competence. Nasal speech is also often a consequence.

Transoral Surgical Approaches

Transoral surgical approaches, routinely used for limited tonsillar resections, are increasingly being increasing used for other oropharyngeal cancer operations, as an alternative to open surgical procedures. By limiting the need for open surgical exposure, these operations can have a quicker recovery time and less morbidity. More recently, endoscopic approaches have been adopted to enhance the utility of transoral surgery. However, limited prospective data support the benefit of transoral operations over traditional approaches. Prospective data are needed to further elucidate the benefits of these surgical advances and better integrate them with the other standard oncologic therapies.

Transoral Laser Surgery

Small series report favorable outcomes for selected patients with stage 1 to 2 oropharyngeal tumors treated with transoral laser microsurgery with or without neck dissection, followed by adjuvant radiotherapy or chemoradiotherapy.[38-40] Positive margin rates are variable (3% to 24%) and appear to vary based on primary site, being more common in base of tongue tumors. Complications include postoperative hemorrhage (5% to 10%). Temporary tracheostomy placement is relatively common (17% to 30%) and needed for exposure, airway control, or aspiration following extensive resection. High rates of locoregional control following this procedure have been reported, primarily for stage 1 to 2 patients (87% to 100%) although for stage 2 to 4 patients local recurrence is more common (20% to 30%). Swallowing outcomes are favorable with series reporting most patients tolerating a normal diet.[40]

Transoral Robotic Surgery

The use of a computer-aided interaction between the surgeon and the patient is commonly referred to as "robotic" surgery. The most common robotic surgical system, the da Vinci Surgical System, is comprised of three surgical instruments and a binocular endoscope controlled by robotic arms and inserted under direct or endoscopic guidance by the surgeon from a patient-side apparatus. The surgeon controls the instruments from a console separated from the patient. The operative environment is visualized virtually in a 3D environment created via a computer, which links the environment provided by the binocular endoscope to the position of the instruments. The surgeon's movements are translated into the micromovements of the instruments. The advantages of this system include motion scaling, which can increase precision, as well as reducing hand tremor and fatigue. When the system is used for transoral surgeries, an assistant is often positioned by the patient's head.

There are no prospective randomized studies supporting the use of transoral robotic surgery (TORS) for oropharyngeal tumor resection over conventional surgery. All studies to date are small single institution series. Proponents of TORS

highlight an enhanced visualization of the surgical field over traditional transoral techniques. Some have hypothesized that perhaps local control could be enhanced via TORS debulking with minimal acute sequelae. However, this claim has yet to be tested prospectively. Prospective studies have shown that TORS can be used safely with a low risk of laceration or fracture to a patient.[41] In a series of 27 patients with tonsillar cancer who underwent TORS tonsillectomy, morbidity was "acceptable," including one case of mucosal bleeding and two cases of moderate trismus, while 1 patient required a tracheostomy, and negative margins were obtained in 25/27 patients.[42]

Until mature prospective multi-institutional series and randomized data are available, the true utility of transoral laser microsurgery and TORS remains unknown. Although early results are favorable and associated with shorter hospital stays, long-term data are needed. Additionally, standard oncologic principles limiting the number of modalities used to minimize treatment-related side effects should be carefully considered prior to widespread adoption of the surgical techniques.

ADJUVANT THERAPY FOLLOWING DEFINITIVE SURGICAL RESECTION

Following surgical resection of oropharyngeal cancers, pathologic features including advanced primary T stage (T3 or T4), lymphovascular space invasion, perineural invasion, positive margins, multiple pathologically involved cervical lymph nodes, and extranodal extension place patients at high risk for locoregional recurrence.[41] In these cases, postoperative radiotherapy (PORT) often in conjunction with chemotherapy has been shown to reduce the risk of locoregional relapse.[42,43] Although the study did not specifically include oropharyngeal cancer patients, PORT was shown in RTOG 73-03 to results in superior locoregional control (70% vs. 58%) when compared to preoperative radiotherapy, but did not affect survival.[44]

Adjuvant Chemoradiotherapy for Oropharyngeal Cancer

The addition of cisplatin-based chemotherapy to postoperative radiotherapy has been compared to PORT alone for medically fit head and neck cancer patients of any site in a number of randomized studies.[45-48] All of these studies have demonstrated statistically significant[45-47] or strong statistical trends[48] for improved locoregional control and disease disease-free survival with the addition of chemotherapy to PORT. Additionally, two of these studies have demonstrated statistically significant improvements in overall survival,[48,49] whereas the other two have shown numerically improved but not statistically significant survival improvements.[50,51] A significant portion of patients in these studies had oropharyngeal cancer (EORTC 30% and RTOG 43%) generalizing these results to oropharyngeal patients with high-risk pathologic risk features.

Concurrent Chemotherapy Regimens for Adjuvant Chemoradiotherapy

The optimal chemotherapy regimen delivered with PORT is currently unknown. Schedules of bolus cisplatin 100 mg/m^2 were tested in two[45,48] randomized studies mentioned above, one tested 50 mg weekly cisplatin,[46] and the other tested cisplatin 20 mg/m^2 and 5 fluorouracil (5-FU) 600 mg/m^2 d1-5 and d29-33.[47] There have been no randomized comparisons of these cisplatin-based schedules. A recently reported study in postoperative head and neck cancer patients compared 30 mg/m^2 weekly cisplatin to 100 mg/m^2 cisplatin every 3 weeks. This study demonstrated improved locoregional control with 100 mg/m^2 cisplatin, which was the primary endpoint. However, given that the weekly regimen was only 30 mg/m^2, which many consider suboptimal and that >90% of patients were postoperative oral cavity cancer patients, the applicability of these results to the postoperative care of oropharyngeal cancer patients is questionable.[49]

Randomized studies have been attempted trying to identify the role of carboplatin-based chemotherapy concurrently with PORT compared to PORT alone.[52] Unfortunately, these studies closed before accrual goals were met, and no significant benefit was found with the addition of carboplatin to PORT. RTOG 0234 randomized high-risk postoperative patients (positive margin, extranodal extension, and/or >2 pathologically involved cervical nodes) to PORT in combination with cetuximab (400 mg/m^2 loading dose followed by 250 mg/m^2 weekly) and weekly docetaxel 15 mg/m^2 or to PORT with cetuximab (400 mg/m^2 loading dose followed by 250 mg/m^2 weekly) and weekly cisplatin 30 mg/m^2. Results of this randomized phase II study are maturing. Currently, no randomized data support the use of taxanes or cetuximab in the postoperative setting although RTOG-1216 is an ongoing randomized phase 3 trial that is designed to determine the effectiveness of both cetuximab and docetaxel relative to cisplatin in the setting of adjuvant PORT.[53] Based on the available data, many consider cisplatin 100 mg/m^2 every 3 weeks as the standard.

Adjuvant Radiation Therapy Dose

The optimal radiation therapy dose for PORT is also not well defined. Most of the randomized studies demonstrating the benefit of concurrent chemotherapy with PORT used radiotherapy doses of 60 to 66 Gy in 2 Gy daily fractions to high-risk areas (primary tumor bed with positive margin or nodal regions with extracapsular spread). Doses of 50 to 54 Gy in 2 Gy fractions were usually given to areas at risk for microscopic involvement. There is little evidence supporting the higher PORT doses used in these randomized trials over those recommended from the PORT-alone dose-finding studies of 63 Gy for extranodal extension and 57.6 Gy for all others. In three of four randomized studies testing the utility of chemotherapy concurrently with PORT, doses >65 Gy were delivered to high-risk areas.[45–47] The fourth study, RTOG 95-01 allowed a dose of 60 Gy with or without an optional 6 Gy boost.[48] As these studies were associated with significant benefits for patients with ECE and positive margins, we recommend similar dosing schedules.

Postoperative Radiotherapy Treatment Volume

The typical treatment volume used in PORT for head and neck cancer includes the bilateral neck and the primary tumor site. However, it is unclear whether both the neck and primary always need to be within the PORT volume. In those with completely resected primary tumors with negative margins whose sole indication for PORT is pathologic cervical adenopathy, some would direct therapy only to the neck. Additionally for patients with a positive margin as the sole indication for treatment in the setting of a comprehensive neck surgery without pathologically involved cervical lymph nodes, some would direct treatment to the primary resection bed only. Additionally for well-lateralized primary tumors, patterns of progression would suggest that PORT to the ipsilateral neck only may be appropriate.[50]

DEFINITIVE RADIATION THERAPY

For early-stage oropharyngeal cancers, the use of radiation therapy as a single modality is associated with good outcomes and functional preservation.[51] Although there is no consensus on the optimal dose fractionation schedule for oropharyngeal cancer patients receiving radiotherapy alone, randomized data[52–54] and meta-analyses[55,56] support an overall survival benefit with the use of accelerated fractionation or hyperfractionated radiotherapy. Therefore, for oropharyngeal cancer treated with radiotherapy alone, strong consideration should be given to altered fractionation of some sort.

Hyperfractionated Radiation Therapy

The benefit of hyperfractionated radiotherapy for oropharyngeal cancer was clearly demonstrated in EORTC 22791, in which patients with T2-3 N0-1 nonbase of tongue oropharyngeal cancers were randomized to conventionally fractionated radiotherapy at 70 Gy (2 Gy/day) or to 80.5 Gy hyperfractionated at 1.15 Gy twice daily. Hyperfractionated radiotherapy was associated with statistically significant improvements in locoregional control (5-year, 59% vs. 40%) without an increase in long-term toxicity. Additionally, there was a trend toward improved overall survival ($P = .08$) particularly in stage 3 patients.[54]

Accelerated Radiation Therapy

Accelerated radiotherapy has also been shown to benefit oropharyngeal cancer patients but may depend upon the exact regimen used. For example, a randomized study comparing an accelerated regimen of 66 to 70 Gy delivered in 2 Gy daily fractions 6 days a week to the same dose delivered 5 days a week with oropharyngeal cancer affecting the majority of patients demonstrated improved locoregional control (42% vs. 30%, $P = .004$), disease-free survival (50% vs. 40%, $P = .03$), and a trend toward improved overall survival (35% vs. 28%, $P = .07$). When analyzed as a separate subgroup, pharyngeal primary sites had improved locoregional control (HR = 0.6, 95% CI = 0.41 to 0.86).[53] Of note, accelerated fractionation improved local control for both p16-positive (HR = 0.56 [0.33 to 0.96]) and p16-negative tumors (HR = 0.77 [0.60 to 0.99]).[57] However, when a more intensive accelerated regimen of 1.8 Gy twice daily to 59.4 Gy was compared to 70 Gy in 2 Gy fractions in stage 3/4 head and neck cancer patients, no statistical benefits were seen in terms of locoregional control or overall survival.[58] It is unknown if the lack of benefit seen was due to the regimen used or due to inclusion criteria as the benefit for acceleration in some randomized studies was less significant for those with stage 4 disease as well as those with a larger nodal disease burden.[59]

Accelerated Versus Hyperfractionated Radiation Therapy

For oropharyngeal cancer patients in particular and head and neck cancer patients in general, it is not known if hyperfractionated or accelerated radiotherapy is superior. The meta-analysis of radiotherapy in carcinoma of the head and neck collaborative group pooled 15 randomized studies (including 6,515 patients) comparing conventionally fractionated radiotherapy to either accelerated radiotherapy or hyperfractionated radiotherapy. Oropharyngeal cancer patients were the largest subsite, representing 44% of all patients (1,585 patients). Altered fractionation radiotherapy regimens were associated with a 3.4% absolute improvement in 5-year overall survival. Heterogeneity in patients included on accelerated and hyperfractionated trials obscure direct comparison, although hyperfractionated patients had an absolute 8.2% improvement in overall survival at 5 years compared to a 2% absolute benefit with accelerated radiotherapy.[56]

One of the studies included in the meta-analysis, RTOG 90-03, compared conventional fractionation (70 Gy in 2 Gy/daily fractions) to hyperfractionation (81.6 Gy [1.2 Gy BID]) and to accelerated fractionation with a split course (67.2 Gy [1.6 BID with a 2-week rest after 38.4 Gy]) to accelerated fractionation with concomitant boost regimen (72 Gy in 1.8 Gy fractions for 14 fractions followed by 1.8 Gy morning and a 1.5 Gy afternoon boost to gross disease). Although all primary sites other than nasopharynx were included, 60% of patients included had oropharyngeal primary tumors. In the initial report, improved locoregional control was seen in both the hyperfractionated and accelerated concomitant boost arms.[60] These improvements resulted in trend toward improved disease-free survival for patients treated with hyperfractionation (37.6% vs. 31.7%, P = .067) and accelerated concomitant boost (39.3% vs. 31.7%, P = .054), which almost reached statistical significance at the P = .05 level. However, with longer follow-up, improved survival was seen with hyperfractionated therapy (HR 0.81, P = .05) when patients were censored at 5 years. Furthermore, less late toxicity was seen with hyperfractionation compared to accelerated fractionation. Specifically in disease-free patients, at 5 years, only 4.8% of HFX patients had feeding tubes versus 13.0% of AFX-C patients.[52] These toxicity data are difficult to interpret in a modern setting because all of the patients were treated with parallel-opposed fields. Blocking techniques were rudimentary and provided minimal sparing of parotid glands and pharyngeal constrictor muscles. Contemporary intensity-modulated radiotherapy (IMRT)/image-guided radiotherapy techniques spare these structures and probably reduce late morbidity significantly.

Simultaneous Integrated Boost Radiation Therapy

With the increasing use of IMRT, simultaneous integrated boost radiotherapy has been investigated for oropharyngeal cancer patients. The RTOG completed a study (00-22) in early-stage (T1-2, N0-2) oropharyngeal cancer patients, treated with bilateral neck radiotherapy[51] using doses of 2.2, 2, and 1.8 Gy to gross tumor and intermediate-risk and low-risk planning target volumes (PTVs), respectively. The 2-year risk of local progression was 9% and was higher in patients who had significant underdosing of known tumor. Additionally, no local recurrences, distant metastases, or second cancers were seen in never smokers, possibly representing a surrogate for HPV-related disease, compared to 7 locoregional recurrences, 5 second cancers, and 1 case of distant metastases in smokers. The 2-year overall survival was 95% and disease-free survival was 82%. Therefore, it appears for patients with early-stage oropharyngeal cancer treated with radiotherapy alone; simultaneous integrated boost radiotherapy is a viable treatment option.

CONCURRENT CHEMORADIOTHERAPY FOR LOCOREGIONALLY ADVANCED OROPHARYNGEAL CANCER

For patients with locoregionally advanced oropharyngeal cancer, concurrent chemoradiotherapy is the standard treatment. Resection when possible is generally not recommended given the associated surgical morbidity. Additionally, adjuvant chemoradiotherapy is frequently necessary and has similar morbidity to definitive intent chemoradiotherapy. Comparisons of outcomes with radiotherapy with or without neck dissection or surgery with or without adjuvant radiotherapy resulted in similar outcomes with higher complication rates with surgery.[61] With the advent of transoral and robotic surgical techniques, these findings will need to be readdressed.

Evidence for Concurrent Chemoradiotherapy

The use of concurrent chemoradiotherapy for most stages 3 and 4 (nonmetastatic) oropharyngeal cancer patients is based on the results of the meta-analysis of head and neck cancer (MACH-NC), which demonstrated a 6.2% absolute improvement in overall survival at 5 years from the use of concurrent chemoradiotherapy compared to radiotherapy alone.[62] This benefit was also observed in the oropharyngeal cancer subgroup, which showed that concurrent chemotherapy improves 5-year overall survival HR 0.78 (95% CI = 0.72 to 0.85), $P < .0001$.[63]

Additionally, level 1 evidence from multiple randomized studies restricted to oropharyngeal cancer patients supports the use of concurrent chemoradiotherapy for stage 3/4 oropharyngeal cancer.[64,65] The Groupe d'Oncologie Radiothérapie Tête et Cou (GORTEC) compared 2 Gy daily conventional radiotherapy to 70 Gy concomitantly administered with daily bolus carboplatin and continuous infusion 5-fluorouracil 600 mg/m²/d 5-day 1 to 4 every 3 weeks for three cycles. A total of 222 patients (113 assigned to radiotherapy alone and 109 assigned to combined treatment) were eligible for analysis. With a median follow-up of 5.5 years, absolute 5-year overall survival was significantly higher in the combined modality arm (15.8% with radiotherapy alone to 22.4% with chemoradiotherapy) as shown in Figure 48.4. A five-year locoregional control was also significantly improved with concomitant therapy (from 24.7% vs. 47.6%) for the combined-treatment group (P = .002).[66] Combined modality therapy was associated

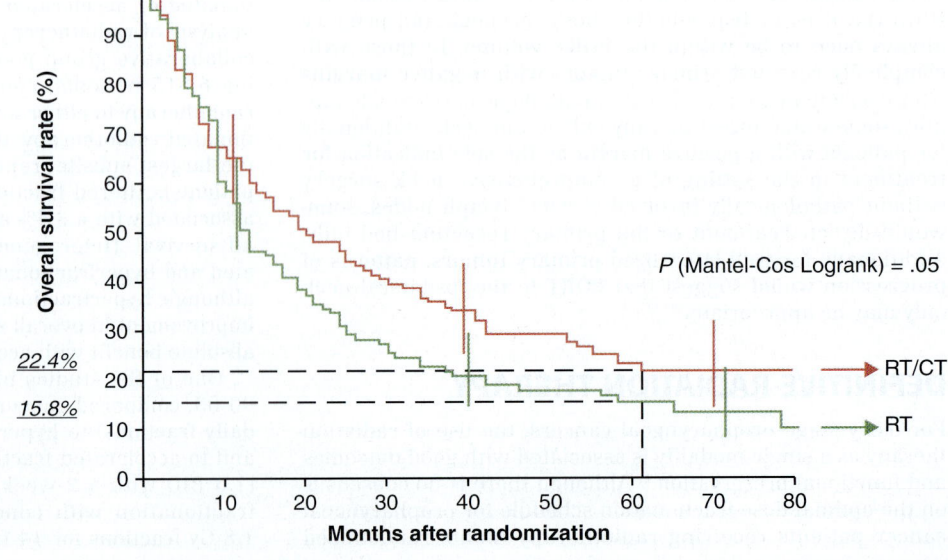

FIGURE 48.4. Overall survival among patients with oropharyngeal cancer treated with radiotherapy alone (RT) or with radiotherapy with concomitant chemotherapy (RT/CT) as analyzed by the Kaplan-Meier method on GORTEC 94-01. (From Denis F, Garaud P, Bardet E, et al. Final results of the 94-01 French Head and Neck Oncology and Radiotherapy Group randomized trial comparing radiotherapy alone with concomitant radiochemotherapy in advanced-stage oropharynx carcinoma. *J Clin Oncol* 2004;22(1):69–76. Reprinted with permission. Copyright © 2004 American Society of Clinical Oncology. All rights reserved.)

with increased hematological toxicity, increased mucositis, and weight loss. Severe late toxicity was also increased with combined modality therapy (14% vs. 9% radiotherapy alone) including increased mandibular toxicity and cervical fibrosis. These patients were treated with 2D treatment planning, typically including parallel-opposed fields with dosimetric hot spots located in the mandible and neck soft tissues. The extent to which concurrent chemotherapy contributes to these specific late toxicities in the setting of IMRT is not clearly understood.

Outcomes of locoregionally advanced oropharyngeal cancer have improved in the era of concurrent chemoradiotherapy and modern radiotherapy planning and delivery techniques. This improvement is likely influenced by newer imaging techniques leading to more informed patient selection and radiotherapy planning and the influence of a rise in HPV-related oropharyngeal cancer cases. A recent analysis of over 300 locoregionally advanced oropharyngeal cancer patients treated with primary chemoradiotherapy with a median follow-up of 34 months reported low 2-year rates of local progression (6.1%), regional progression (5.2%), and distant progression (12.2%).[67] Base of tongue cancers have historically been associated with poor outcomes when treated with surgery or radiotherapy alone or in combination (5-year disease specific and overall survival of 27.8% and 40.3%, respectively).[68] However, recent single institution series using chemoradiotherapy highlight high rates of locoregional control with the use of either 3D conformal radiotherapy (5-year 82%) or IMRT (5-year 97.4%),[69] which could represent the influence of HPV-related oropharyngeal cancer. This improvement may reflect the efficacy of chemoradiation, but it may also due to the increased incidence of HPV-associated disease compared to older series.

Acute Toxicity of Chemoradiotherapy

For oropharyngeal cancer patients, a course of concurrent chemoradiotherapy is a life-changing event given the associated toxicities, including fatigue, nausea, emesis, thickened secretions, xerostomia, mucositis, dysphagia, odynophagia, alopecia, dermatitis, anemia, neutropenia, hoarseness, Lhermitte syndrome, and infection. Dysphagia is perhaps the most difficult acute and late complication of chemoradiotherapy for oropharyngeal cancer. Oropharyngeal patients are less likely to be affected than those with laryngeal or hypopharyngeal tumors.[70] Older patients and those with worse performance status are more likely to have worsening of their swallowing following chemoradiotherapy. Those with more advanced tumors are more likely to have swallowing improvement likely due to reduction of tumor bulk.[71] Given the adverse effect of dysphagia on nutritional status, management recommendations include early therapeutic intervention with swallowing exercises designed to strengthen the pharyngeal musculature. Patients should be instructed to swallow as large a volume as possible during and after treatment and perform exercises shown to improve swallowing ability.[72] Dysphagia has been associated prospectively, with the exceeding of specific dosimetric thresholds to the pharyngeal constrictors or laryngeal apparatus, which should be incorporated into radiotherapy planning as discussed below.[73]

Late Toxicity of Chemoradiotherapy

Late toxicities of chemoradiotherapy for oropharyngeal cancer patients can also be quite significant and can include dysphagia, fibrosis, osteoradionecrosis, trismus, xerostomia, dental caries, feeding tube dependence, and neuritis. Late toxicities of chemoradiotherapy have been catalogued by the RTOG in a pooled analysis of 230 patients treated on three prospective chemoradiotherapy trials with a median follow-up of 3 years. Oropharyngeal primaries affected 34% of all

patients. Older patients and those with larger (T3, T4) tumors were more likely to experience late toxicity, as were those who underwent a posttreatment neck dissection.[74] When late toxicity was analyzed by primary tumor site, patients with oropharyngeal and oral cavity primary tumors were statistically less likely to experience late toxicity. Long-term analysis of the aforementioned GORTEC randomized trial demonstrated that 56% of patients treated with chemoradiotherapy had at least one grade 3 to 4 late toxicity compared to 30% treated with radiotherapy alone ($P = .12$). The small number of long-term survivors probably reduced the power to detect statistically significantly differences between these groups.[66] Recently, a long-term report of HPV-associated oropharyngeal cancer patients treated with chemoradiotherapy demonstrated that development of additional late toxicities beyond those present at 2 years was rare. Furthermore, long-term QOL in all domains was similar to that seen before treatment.[75]

Alternative Concurrent Chemoradiotherapy Regimens

The toxicities of concurrent chemoradiotherapy have stimulated the search for improvements in this platform. Some questions still remain unanswered, including what constitutes the optimal chemotherapy regimen. Cisplatin at 100 mg/m² is often cited as a standard regimen. The aforementioned GORTEC randomized study demonstrated an overall survival advantage using a carboplatin/5-FU regimen specifically chosen to avoid cisplatin-related tinnitus, renal dysfunction, and emesis. Randomized studies comparing alternative cisplatin dosing schedules (such as 30 to 40 mg/m² weekly, 20 mg/m²/d, d1-5, 22 to 26) to bolus cisplatin or to other chemoradiotherapy platforms have been conducted in nasopharyngeal cancer patients or in the postoperative oral cavity setting. However, multiple randomized studies that compared radiotherapy alone to concurrent chemoradiotherapy using nonbolus cisplatin schedules including daily cisplatin (6 mg/m²/d),[76] weekly cisplatin 40 mg/m²,[77] or cisplatin 20 mg/m²/d, day 1 to 5 repeated every 3 weeks[78] had comparable outcomes to bolus cisplatin. The relative merits of various chemoradiotherapy platforms will be discussed in more detail in Chapter 40.

Induction Chemotherapy Prior to Definitive Local Therapy

The use of neoadjuvant chemotherapy prior to surgical resection or radiotherapy for oropharyngeal cancer patients has been tested in randomized studies. In particular, a phase III study restricted to oropharyngeal cancer patients compared three cycles of cisplatin 100 mg/m² on day 1 and 5-fluorouracil 1,000 mg/m²/d, days 1 to 5, repeated every 3 weeks for three cycles followed by definitive local therapy to definitive local therapy alone. At the time of the study, standard local therapies included either radiotherapy alone (70 Gy to the primary, 50 Gy to the neck) or composite surgery with postoperative radiotherapy (50 to 65 Gy based on pathologic findings). Although only 318 of a planned 760 patients were enrolled, a statistically significant improvement in overall survival was seen in the induction chemotherapy arm at 5 years (5.1 years vs. 3.3 years) with a median follow-up of 5 years.[79] This study suggests a benefit to neoadjuvant chemotherapy. The applicability of this trial in the chemoradiotherapy era is questionable, however, because the patients in the control arm of the study received surgery or 70 Gy daily radiotherapy, known to be inferior to accelerated or hyperfractionated radiotherapy. The value of this treatment compared to concurrent chemoradiotherapy is also unknown.

Whether or not induction chemotherapy prior to concurrent chemoradiotherapy improves survival when compared to chemoradiotherapy was an area of active study advocated by some given distant metastases were frequently a site of first failure for patients with locoregionally advanced head and neck cancer in general,[80] This is particularly true for patients with oropharyngeal cancer patients because local regional therapy (chemoradiotherapy) has become so much more effective.[67] However, mature results from multiple randomized studies did not demonstrate improved survival with induction chemotherapy followed by concurrent chemoradiotherapy.[81,82] It is unknown if the lack of demonstrated survival benefit was due to the therapy itself or the fact that these studies were initiated prior to robust knowledge of the behavior of HPV-associated oropharyngeal cancers. Therefore, inclusion of these patients with their more favorable outcomes was not accounted for in the study design and may complicate interpretation of these studies.

Targeted Agents and Radiation therapy

A randomized study compared radiotherapy 70 to 76.8 Gy with or without weekly cetuximab (loading dose of 400 mg/m² followed by 250 mg/m²), to radiotherapy alone for locoregionally advanced head and neck cancer patients. The combination therapy was found to improve locoregional control, disease-free survival, and overall survival.[83] The majority of patients had oropharyngeal primary tumors (60%). When analyzed alone, patients with oropharyngeal cancer treated with cetuximab had demonstrated improved 2-year locoregional control (50% vs. 41%) and median locoregional disease-free duration and 23 months versus 49 months (HR 0.61) with the use of cetuximab. Furthermore, the median overall survival for oropharyngeal cancer patients treated with cetuximab and radiotherapy was >66 months compared to 30.3 months in those treated with radiotherapy alone HR 0.62, a larger difference than those with laryngeal (32.8 months vs. 31.6 months) or hypopharyngeal (13.7 vs. 13.5) primary sites. Updated analyses show that the addition of cetuximab remains beneficial regardless of p16 status[84] and presence of a prominent rash was a prognostic factor.[85] Therefore, for oropharyngeal cancer patients meeting the inclusion criteria for this study, stage 3/4, nonmetastatic, KPS > 60, and normal hematopoietic, hepatic, and renal function, cetuximab and radiotherapy is an alternative treatment platform. Consideration should be given to the use of altered radiation fractionation with cetuximab because improved overall survival was seen in patients who were treated with accelerated concomitant boost and hyperfractionated radiotherapy.

Cetuximab should be avoided in specific regions (particularly the southeastern United States) where severe anaphylactic reactions mediated by an immunoglobulin E response to the galactose-alpha-1,3-galactose oligosaccharide found on the Fab portion of the cetuximab heavy chain are seen.[86] A fully humanized monoclonal antibody to the EGFR, panitumumab, has a much lower rate of severe allergic reactions, but there is no level 1 evidence to support its equivalent efficacy in this clinical setting. Aside from these geographic limitations, it is unclear which patient populations should receive concurrent chemotherapy and which should receive cetuximab plus radiotherapy. Some physicians use cetuximab plus radiotherapy preferentially over cisplatin plus radiotherapy in patients with renal dysfunction or overall poor functional status, but there is no level 1 evidence to support this indication. In fact, these same medical conditions constituted exclusion criteria for the randomized trial proving its benefit.

Given the improved outcomes of HPV-associated oropharyngeal cancer with standard treatments, deintensification of therapy is being considered in this patient population. Randomized studies comparing standard chemoradiotherapy to combined EGFR inhibition and radiotherapy are ongoing in the cooperative group setting. RTOG 1016 is comparing bolus cisplatin 100 mg/m² d1, 23 with accelerated radiotherapy (70 Gy, 2 Gy/day 6 days per week) to the same radiotherapy and cetuximab 400 mg/m² loading dose and 250 mg/m² weekly with radiotherapy. This noninferiority study has a

primary endpoint of comparable 5-year survival. The NCIC is conducting a similar study but using panitumumab with radiotherapy given the lower rates of dermatologic and anaphylactic reactions. Other investigations are attempting radiation dose reduction aiming to keep locoregional control high while reducing acute toxicity, some using induction chemotherapy before chemoradiotherapy. Mature reports from these studies will help determine how to optimally treat this unique patient population. Need to add in HN002, as well as data from O'Sullivan, and Rad Vac.

Targeted Agents in Combination with Cytotoxins and Radiation Therapy

To date, there are no comparisons of cytotoxic agents and radiation with and without cetuximab for oropharyngeal cancer patients. Oropharyngeal cancer patients comprised 70% of RTOG 0522, which compared two concurrent cycles of 100 mg/m² cisplatin and accelerated concomitant boost to 72 Gy radiotherapy with or without the addition of a loading dose of 400 mg/m² followed by weekly 250 mg/m² cetuximab. The combination of cisplatin, cetuximab, and radiotherapy did not improve locoregional control, disease-free survival, or overall survival. However, this triplet therapy was associated with increased grade 3 to 4 mucositis (43.2% vs. 33.3%, P = .002) and skin reactions (25% vs. 15%, P < .0001) without increasing grade 3 to 4 dysphagia rates (53% vs. 57%, P = .27).[87] Fifty-one percent of oropharyngeal tumor specimens were evaluated for p16 expression, and 73% of these specimens were positive. No differences in outcome were seen as a function of HPV status.

Oropharyngeal cancer patients have also been included in studies evaluating the addition of bevacizumab to chemoradiotherapy. The addition of bevacizumab to 5-fluorouracil, hydroxyurea, and twice-daily radiotherapy (FHX) did not confer any benefit in a study of locoregionally advanced head and neck cancer patients. The study was terminated early due to toxicity and only 5 of 26 participants had oropharyngeal primary tumors.[88] Bevacizumab has also been integrated with erlotinib (synchronous dual inhibition of vascular endothelial growth factor [VEGF] and EGFR) and cisplatin (33 mg/m² cisplatin d1-3 weeks 1 and 5) together with 1.25 Gy twice-daily radiotherapy to 70 Gy. Seventy-one percent of patients had oropharyngeal primary tumors. At a median follow-up of 46 months, 3-year locoregional control and overall survival were promising at 86% and 85%, respectively, compared to historical series.[89] Soft tissue and osteoradionecrosis occurred in both series, and careful attention should be paid to the results of ongoing studies integrating bevacizumab to multiple chemoradiotherapy platforms for locoregionally advanced head and neck cancer patients including those with oropharyngeal tumors.

EXTERNAL BEAM RADIATION THERAPY SIMULATION AND TREATMENT PLANNING

Radiation Therapy Simulation

Prior to a course of radiotherapy or chemoradiotherapy, patients should undergo simulation, preferably CT based to allow for optimal radiotherapy planning. An IV should be placed prior to simulation for the delivery of low osmolar iodinated contrast to optimize the distinction between vascular structures and lymph nodes. Patients are positioned supine, with a rigid head holder cradling the posterior calvarium. Generally, an extended head position is preferable. The shoulders should be positioned as caudally as possible to allow adequate exposure of the neck. This can be achieved either with shoulder pulls or with commercially available devices. Tongue immobilization can be useful for oropharyngeal cancer patients with oral tongue involvement.

TABLE 48.10 INCIDENCE (%) OF PATHOLOGIC LYMPH NODE METASTASIS IN SQUAMOUS CELL CARCINOMAS OF THE OROPHARYNX

Tumor Site	Distribution of Metastatic Lymph Nodes per Level (Percentage of the Neck Dissection Procedures)											
	Prophylactic RND						**Therapeutic RND**					
	No. of RNDs	I	II	III	IV	V	No. of RNDs	I	II	III	IV	V
Base of tongue + vallecula	21	0	19	14	9	5	58	10	72	41	21	9
Tonsillar fossa	27	4	30	22	7	0	107	17	70	42	31	9
Total	48	2	25	19	8	2	165	15	71	42	27	9

Reprinted from Grégoire V, Coche E, Cosnard G, et al. Selection and delineation of lymph node target volumes in head and neck conformal radiotherapy: proposal for standardizing terminology and procedure based on the surgical experience. *Radiother Oncol* 2000;56(2):135–150. Copyright © 2000 Elsevier Science Ireland Ltd. With permission.

Bite blocks are also useful as they often elevate the hard palate with its minor salivary glands. This can be achieved either with shoulder-pulls or with commercially available devices. The head should be immobilized with a thermoplastic mask. Care should be taken to ensure that the mask is tight and not allow movement of the nose, chin, or forehead. Images should be taken from above the calvarium to the carina to ensure appropriate volumes can be drawn. The addition of metabolic and magnetic resonance imaging has been found to be complementary for GTV delineation.[90]

Radiation Therapy Volumes

Radiotherapy volumes for oropharyngeal cancer patients are based on ICRU 50. The gross tumor volume (GTV) includes all known primary and cervical lymph node tumor extension based on clinical, endoscopic, and imaging findings. Care should be taken to look for fat stranding, which could be indicative of extranodal extension. This is usually expanded to include a margin for microscopic extension forming the high-dose clinical target volume. The true clinical target volume (CTV) indicating the margin needed to cover microscopic extension not visible on clinical and imaging modalities is not known. Current RTOG guidelines specify an extension of 0.5 to 1 cm from the GTV to form the high-dose CTV. Nodal regions at risk for occult microscopic spread are usually included in a low-risk CTV. Many studies using clinical presentation data as well as elective surgical series have attempted to define the risk based on primary tumor site and extent of involvement as shown in Table 48.10. In general, this includes at least bilateral level II to IV. Typically, one nodal region beyond those pathologically involved is included. That is for a patient with level II pathologic lymphadenopathy, level IB should be included. The inclusion of the retropharyngeal nodes routinely in the low-risk PTV is controversial as it often increases radiation dose to the pharyngeal constrictors, which has been associated with dysphagia[91] and should depend on the extent of the primary tumor and cervical lymphadenopathy. The incidence of retropharyngeal lymphadenopathy is demonstrated in Tables 48.11 and 48.12. Coverage of the retropharyngeal nodes up to the base of skull is associated with a low risk of progression,[92] but absence of coverage is not necessarily

associated with an increased risk of recurrence. Certainly retropharyngeal coverage (i.e., extending the superior border of level II to include the retrostyloid space) should be considered for oropharyngeal tumors extending into the nasopharynx or pterygoid region, those with gross retropharyngeal nodal involvement, and those with high level II lymphadenopathy.[28]

Consensus guidelines for contouring the clinically node-negative neck have been published and endorsed by international head and neck cancer cooperative groups, including the RTOG, EORTC, DAHANCA, GORTEC, and NCIC.[29] These guidelines are clinically useful aids for delineating specific nodal treatment volumes. Similar guidelines have been proposed for the node-positive neck and postoperative patients.[28] Specific recommendations for node-positive patients include coverage of the supraclavicular fossa for patients with level IV or Vb lymphadenopathy and inclusion of the entire thickness of muscles invaded by pathological lymphadenopathy in the CTV. Additionally, pathologic lymphadenopathy spanning adjacent levels should trigger inclusion of the full extent of both levels in the CTV. For postoperative patients, coverage of the entire operative bed in the neck is recommended to account for potential tumor spillage. Coverage of the retrostyloid space was recommended for all patients with pathologic level II lymphadenopathy. Inclusion of the supraclavicular fossa in the treatment volume was recommended for those with involvement of level IV or Vb. Similar to the nondissected node-positive neck, inclusion of muscles invaded by tumor is recommended, as is coverage of all levels spanned by pathologic lymphadenopathy.

CTVs are expanded to account for organ motion and set up uncertainty ideally based on institutional specific data to form the PTV. For oropharyngeal cancer patients, consideration of movement of the base of tongue should be considered (particularly with swallowing) when designing an appropriate PTV margin. The expansion from CTV to PTV should

TABLE 48.11 INCIDENCE OF RETROPHARYNGEAL LYMPH NODES IN HEAD AND NECK PRIMARY TUMORS

Primary Site	Incidence of Retropharyngeal Lymph Nodes (Percentage of the Total Number of Patients)		
	Overall	**N0 neck**	**N+ neck**
Oropharynx			
Pharyngeal wall	18/93 (19)	6/37 (16)	12/56 (21)
Soft palate	7/53 (13)	1/21 (5)	6/32 (19)
Tonsillar fossa	16/176 (9)	2/56 (4)	14/120 (12)
Base of tongue	5/121 (4)	0/31 (0)	5/90 (6)

Reprinted from Grégoire V, Coche E, Cosnard G, et al. Selection and delineation of lymph node target volumes in head and neck conformal radiotherapy: proposal for standardizing terminology and procedure based on the surgical experience. *Radiother Oncol* 2000;56(2):135–150. Copyright © 2000 Elsevier Science Ireland Ltd. With permission.

TABLE 48.12 INCIDENCE OF PATHOLOGIC RETROPHARYNGEAL LYMPH NODE METASTASES IN HEAD AND NECK PRIMARY TUMORS

Authors	Primary Site	Incidence of Retropharyngeal Lymph Nodes (Percentage of the Total Number of Patients)		
		Overall	**pN0 neck[a]**	**pN+ neck[b]**
Ballantyne	Oropharynx (pharyngeal wall)	15/34 (44%)	n.a.	n.a.
Hasegawa and Matsuura	Oropharynx	4/11 (36%)	1/2 (50%)	3/9 (33%)
	Hypopharynx	8/13 (62%)	0/3 (0%)	9/10 (90%)
Okumura et al.	Oropharynx + hypopharynx	6/42 (14%)	Not stated	Not stated
Byers et al.	Oropharynx (pharyngeal wall)	2/45 (4%)	Not stated	Not stated

[a]Pathologically negative nodes in levels I to V.
[b]Pathologically positive nodes in levels I to V.
Reprinted from Grégoire V, Coche E, Cosnard G, et al. Selection and delineation of lymph node target volumes in head and neck conformal radiotherapy: proposal for standardizing terminology and procedure based on the surgical experience. *Radiother Oncol* 2000;56(2):135–150. Copyright © 2000 Elsevier Science Ireland Ltd. With permission.

Section III

account for imaging methods used to assess daily setup. In general, if more frequent image guidance is performed, the margin needed for setup uncertainty should be less. The RTOG currently recommends 5 to 10 mm for patients treated with standard weekly megavoltage port films and 0.25 to 5 mm if more frequent kV image or cone-beam CT guidance is used. Representative contours for a patient with locoregionally advanced oropharyngeal cancer are shown in Figures 48.5 to 48.7.

Indications for Ipsilateral Radiation Therapy

For well-lateralized tonsillar cancers, not involving the base of tongue and minimal involvement of the soft palate (>1 cm margin between medial extent of tumor and midline), the CTV can be limited to the ipsilateral neck, which will significantly limit the exposure of the contralateral parotid, submandibular gland, and pharyngeal musculature.[26] The ability to forgo treatment to the contralateral neck is based on the extremely low risk of occult contralateral neck lymph node involvement. Surgical series demonstrate that the risk of contralateral cervical lymph node involvement is due to primary tumor size (more common in T3/T4 tumors).[93,94] Additionally, an analysis of tonsillar cancer patients, mostly T1-2 (79%) and N0-1 (88%) who underwent resection of the primary tumor often with ipsilateral lymph node dissection showed that only 5% of patients progressed in the contralateral neck.[95] The low incidence of progression seen in early-stage tonsil cancers is likely due to a lack of invasion of the soft palate and base of tongue, which have richer lymphatic network and access to the contralateral nodes. Patients with contralateral cervical lymph node involvement usually have extensive involvement of ipsilateral cervical lymph nodes[96] or tumors approaching or crossing the midline.

In properly selected tonsil cancer patients, ipsilateral only radiotherapy results in low rates of contralateral neck progression. Large series of patients undergoing ipsilateral RT only demonstrated no contralateral neck progression in patients with T1 tumors and only 1% to 2% in those with T2 tumors. In the few patients with T3 tumors, contralateral nodal progression was 3% to 10%.[97,98] Further analysis of these series shows that contralateral nodal progression was associated with both base of tongue and soft palate involvement

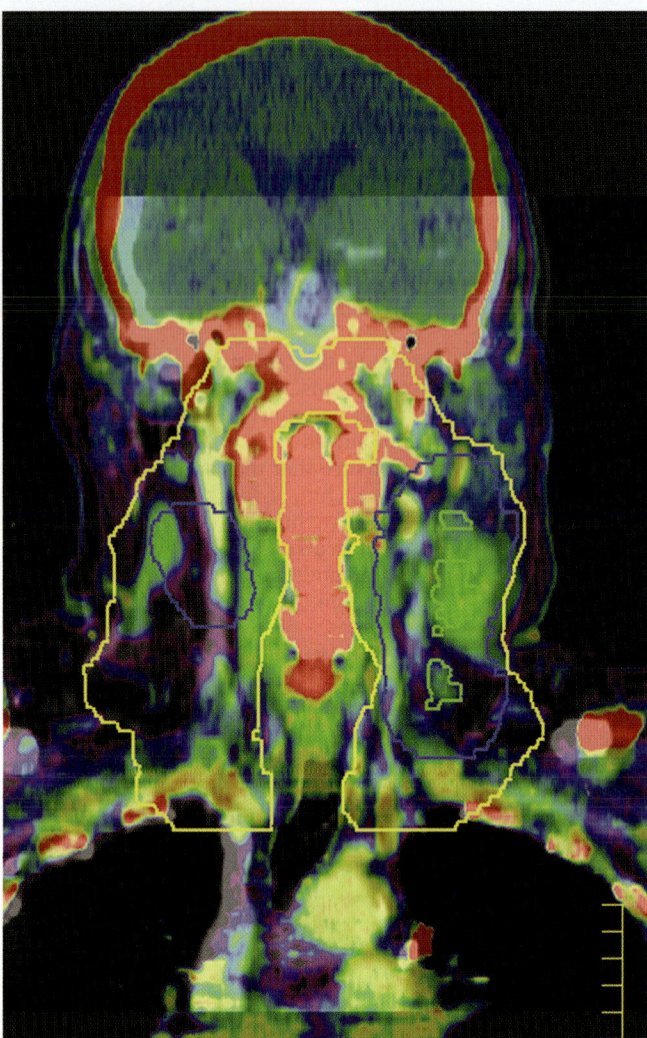

FIGURE 48.6. Coronal image of a patient with locoregionally advanced oropharyngeal cancer with gross tumor volume and planning treatment volumes.

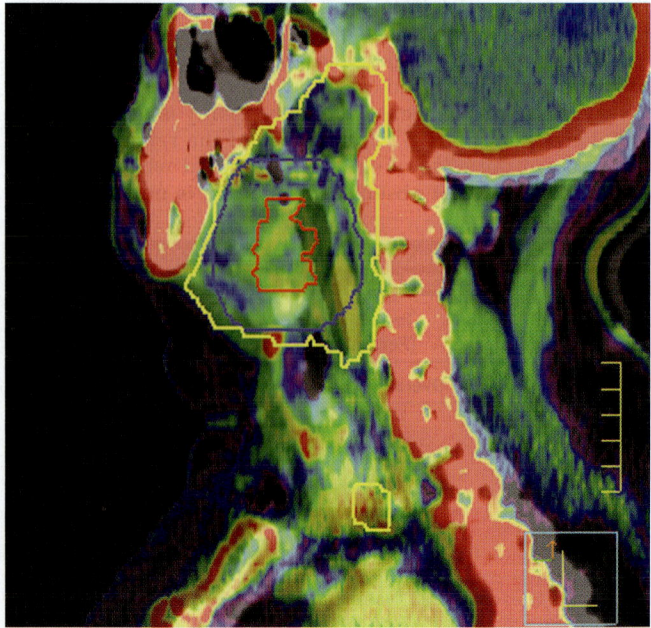

FIGURE 48.7. Sagittal image of a patient with locoregionally advanced oropharyngeal cancer with gross tumor volume and planning treatment volumes.

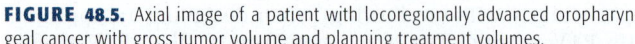

FIGURE 48.5. Axial image of a patient with locoregionally advanced oropharyngeal cancer with gross tumor volume and planning treatment volumes.

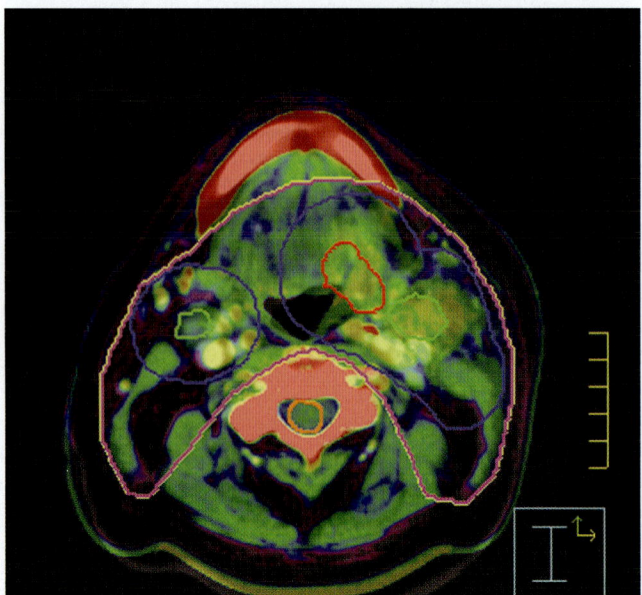

(13%), T3 stage (10%), and involvement of the midline of the soft palate (16.5%). No contralateral nodal progression was seen in patients with ≥N2b neck disease, but there were not many patients with this presentation.

Studies evaluating the role of ipsilateral treatment in the context of concurrent chemoradiation are sparse. An analysis of tonsil cancer patients treated at MD Anderson Cancer Center from 1970 to 2007 included only three patients who received concurrent systemic therapy for N2b disease. In these patients, there was no contralateral neck progression.[99] An analysis of 20 locoregionally advanced tonsillar cancer patients, with N2b nodal disease, 18 of whom received concurrent chemoradiotherapy, demonstrated high rates of primary and nodal disease control along with a low risk of contralateral nodal progression. A caveat to this study is that all of these patients were staged with a PET scan, and most of these patients underwent surgery at the primary (80%) and/or at the neck (70%).[100] There appears to be little progression in properly selected patients treated with ipsilateral only radiotherapy, but care should be taken to ensure that patients with more advanced tumors are not treated in this fashion.

Ipsilateral External Beam Radiation Therapy Planning Techniques

Techniques for ipsilateral radiotherapy traditionally include a wedge pair or mixed photon electron field arrangement. The wedge pair technique includes ipsilateral anterior and posterior oblique fields with the head hyperextended to move the orbits out of the treatment field. Adequate sparing of normal tissue with this technique is achieved as the anterior beam spares the oral cavity and the contralateral parotid gland, although usually contributes dose to the spinal cord. The posterior field aperture also spares the contralateral parotid, although it contributes dose to the spinal cord and oral cavity. With the wedge pair technique, hot spots are typically located peripherally near the surface and are between 110% and 115%. These hot spots can be reduced or eliminated if necessary with the addition of a lightly weighted (10%) third, lateral field. The contralateral parotid dose is usually negligible at 0% to 10%.

Alternatively, a combination of photons and electrons can be delivered through two ipsilateral fields. Traditional energies used 14 to 16 MeV electrons and 4 to 6 MV photons but should now be based on optimal 3D planning dosimetry. Bolus is often used to reduce dose to the temporal lobe. Often, an off-cord reduction is used to limit the spinal cord to 45 Gy with low-energy electrons supplementing the region over the spinal cord. Recently, the use of IMRT for ipsilateral only treatment has been increasing.

Bilateral External Beam Radiation Therapy Planning Techniques

Radiotherapy planning should be performed with 3D conformal radiotherapy or IMRT as available. Standard beam arrangements for 3D conformal radiotherapy are opposed lateral upper fields exactly matched to a low neck/supraclavicular field treated with either a single anterior or AP–PA fields. Once spinal cord tolerance is reached, electron fields can be used to increase dose to gross disease as needed. Caution must be exercised to ensure that AP(PA) and lateral fields do not overlap to cause an overdose to the spinal cord. Multiple techniques can be employed to prevent this complication.

Intensity-Modulated Radiation Therapy

IMRT has been widely adopted for the treatment of head and neck cancers.[101] Although theoretical consideration of second cancers exists with IMRT,[102] this technology has the ability to minimize normal organ exposure to radiation. This is particularly important for oropharyngeal cancer patients as pharyngeal constrictor dose and parotid dose are associated with dysphagia[91] and xerostomia,[103] respectively. In addition, IMRT has the potential to decrease acute dermatitis.

Care should be taken during IMRT to minimize dose to the uninvolved larynx to limit radiation-related speech disorders. Different techniques are available to achieve this objective. The two most commonly used techniques are using IMRT to cover the entire head and neck volume or to use an upper IMRT field matched to a low anterior neck field. Although comparisons of these two techniques have demonstrated reduced mean dose to the larynx and inferior pharyngeal constrictor with the use of a low anterior neck field matched to the IMRT field,[104] controversy persists. Reducing or eliminating fluence from the inferior aspect of posterior and posterior oblique fields should allow median doses to the larynx to be in the 20 to 25 Gy range. Whole-field IMRT is preferable when gross disease is present close to or below the level of the larynx as coverage is better with this technique[105] and in most other cases is simpler to deliver without the inherent difficulties of matching radiation fields.

Impact of Intensity-Modulated Radiotherapy on Xerostomia

The impact of IMRT on reduction of xerostomia in pharyngeal cancer patients (oropharynx or hypopharynx) was prospectively tested in a randomized trial. Patients with pharyngeal squamous cell carcinoma (either oro or hypo) not involving the parotid glands, with good performance status and without distant metastatic spread (T1-4 N0-3), recommended to receive either definitive or adjuvant radiotherapy without concurrent chemotherapy were randomized 1:1 to either conventional radiotherapy or intensity-modulated radiation therapy. The primary endpoint was the proportion of patients with grade 2 or worse xerostomia at 12 months, assessed via the late effects of normal tissues (LENT SOMA) scale.[103] Additionally, salivary flow was assessed preradiotherapy, during week 4 of radiotherapy and then at 2, 3, 6, 12, 18, and 24 weeks after radiotherapy. Unstimulated and sodium citrate–stimulated parotid saliva from each parotid orifice and floor of mouth was also collected. Patient reported QL was collected via the EORTC QLQC30 instrument and with the head and neck–specific instrument HN35. Patients could not receive prophylactic pilocarpine or amifostine. Radiotherapy dose was 65 Gy in 30 fractions for definitively treated patients or postoperative patients with macroscopic residual disease (2.17/fraction) or 60 Gy in 30 fractions (2 Gy/fraction) for postoperatively treated patients without macroscopic residual disease. Uninvolved nodal regions at risk for microscopic spread were treated to 50 Gy (2 Gy/fraction) in the conventional arm and 54 Gy (1.8 Gy/fraction) in the IMRT arm.

Six centers in the United Kingdom participated and recruited 94 patients (47 to each arm). Eighty-five percent of participants had oropharyngeal primary tumors. Eighty-one percent of the patients in the IMRT arm were N0-1 compared to 53% in the conventional arm. This correlated with the statistical difference in stage with 83% of the conventional arm being stage 3 to 4 compared to 68% of the IMRT group. In addition, there were numerically more patients who received PORT in the conventional group (32% vs. 17%).

IMRT significantly reduced mean radiotherapy dose to the ipsilateral (47.6 Gy vs. 61 Gy) and contralateral (25.4 Gy vs. 61 Gy) parotid glands (*P* < .0001). Median follow-up was 44 months. At each planned observation time point, a smaller proportion of IMRT patients reported grade 2 or worse LENT SOMA subjective xerostomia compared to conventional radiotherapy. At 12 months, only 38% of patients treated with IMRT had ≥grade 2 xerostomia compared to 74% in the conventional arm. These were independent of tumor site, radiotherapy indication, stage, and use of neoadjuvant chemotherapy. Additionally, both unstimulated (47% vs. 0%) and stimulated contralateral parotid saliva flow were increased in the IMRT group. Interestingly, ≥grade 2 fatigue was increased in the IMRT group 74% versus 41%. Locoregional progression (IMRT 78% conventional 80%, P = .34) and overall survival (IMRT 78% conventional 76%) were similar between the two arms.

These findings in primarily oropharyngeal patients are consistent with those found in studies of nasopharyngeal patients. It is unclear if the benefit of salivary reduction seen with IMRT continues when pharmacologic studies to reduce xerostomia such as pilocarpine and amifostine are employed. Ongoing cooperative group trials recommend limiting the mean dose to the parotids as low as possible and at least < 26 Gy. Furthermore, the mean dose to the submandibular gland is recommended to be limited to 36 Gy (RTOG 1016).

Impact of Intensity-Modulated Radiotherapy on Dysphagia

IMRT planning should also take into consideration the risk of dysphagia. Many studies have attempted to correlate dosimetric parameters with functional swallowing consequences following radiotherapy or chemoradiotherapy. As highlighted in the studies mentioned below, radiation dose to the larynx and pharyngeal constrictors should be limited as reasonable as possible to limit the risks of aspiration, feeding tube dependence, and stricture. Consensus on dosimetric parameters does not exist as the studies to date have all been retrospective, and their findings are not completely concordant.

Careful correlation of videofluoroscopic findings to radiotherapy dose to normal tissues has been performed in oropharyngeal cancer patients treated with chemoradiotherapy. Based on this analysis, the dose with a 25% or 50% risk (TD 25 or TD 50) of dysphagia to the pharyngeal constrictors was 56 and 63 Gy, respectively. Similarly, TD 25 and TD 50 were 39 and 56 Gy for the glottis and supraglottic larynx.[73] Mean dose to the esophagus was associated with the development of strictures. There were no threshold doses found in this analysis, so it is reasonable to use the TD25 as a planning goal and if not achieved trying to keep the dose to these structures as low as possible.

Others have analyzed radiotherapy doses to normal tissues and correlated to clinical outcomes, persistence use of PEG tube, aspiration rates, and stricture rates.[106] In this analysis, mean dose to the larynx and mean dose to the inferior pharyngeal constrictor predicted for persistent use of PEG tubes and aspiration. Additionally, the volume of larynx receiving 35 to 70 Gy ($V_{35} - V_{70}$) and inferior pharyngeal constrictor V_{40} through V_{65} was associated with PEG tube dependence and larynx V_{55} through V_{70} and inferior pharyngeal constrictor V_{60} and V_{65} were significantly associated with aspiration. Patients with a mean dose of approximately 50 Gy to the larynx and inferior constrictor all had PEG tubes removed by 12 months.

Concurrent Chemotherapy and Accelerated Radiation Therapy

Two recently reported randomized studies showed that there was no benefit to accelerated radiotherapy over conventionally fractionated radiotherapy when delivered with concurrent platinum-based chemotherapy. GORTEC 99-02 randomized locoregionally advanced head and neck cancer patients to either very accelerated radiotherapy 64.8 Gy (1.8 Gy twice daily), 70 Gy (2 Gy daily over 7 weeks) with concurrent carboplatin 70 mg/m² and 5-FU 600 mg/m²/d d1-4, d22-25, and d43-46 or 70 Gy (2 Gy daily to 40 Gy and then 1.5

Gy twice daily) with carboplatin 70 mg/m² and 5-FU 600 mg/m²/d d1-4, d29-33. Outcome in both chemoradiotherapy arms was similar, and both were superior to very accelerated radiotherapy with lower rates of acute toxicity and percutaneous gastrostomy tube placement during therapy and at 5 years.[107] Similarly, RTOG 0129 randomized patients to 72 Gy accelerated concomitant boost radiotherapy with two cycles of cisplatin 100 mg/m² or to 70 Gy daily radiotherapy with three cycles of cisplatin 100 mg/m². Again, there was no benefit to accelerated chemoradiotherapy seen in 8-year overall survival (accelerated 47.6% vs. conventional 47.7%), locoregional progression (36.7% vs. 38.5%), or worst grade 3 to 5 toxicity (37.9% vs. 36.5%).[108] Interestingly on an unplanned post hoc analysis, it appeared that standard fractionation patients who received fewer than three cycles of chemotherapy had worse outcomes than those who received the full-planned dose of chemotherapy. The value of acceleration via the use of a simultaneous integrated boost, a commonly used approach for IMRT delivery, must therefore be questioned when concurrent chemotherapy is being used as part of the treatment program.

Brachytherapy

Brachytherapy, the application of radioactive materials in close proximity to tumors, was developed in the pre-IMRT, preconcurrent chemoradiotherapy era as a means to deliver a tumoricidal dose to gross tumors while minimizing dose to the mandible. The advent of improved radiotherapy planning and delivery techniques in addition to a recognition that osteoradionecrosis secondary to brachytherapy is significantly underreported has corresponded to a major decrease in the utilization brachytherapy for oropharyngeal tumors.

For oropharyngeal tumors, brachytherapy has historically played a role in boosting gross disease following external beam therapy as oropharyngeal tumors have a high propensity for occult nodal spread. Typically, catheters are implanted under general anesthesia in the operating room, with two capable physicians present to handle unexpected events highlighting the fact that brachytherapy is an operator-dependent procedure. Although low–dose rate brachytherapy has previously been the most common type of brachytherapy used, high–dose rate (HDR) and pulsed–dose rate (PDR) techniques are becoming much more common and sometimes preferred given the ability to control dwell times and develop more customized dose distributions. Given the historically poor locoregional control rates for tumors of the base of tongue, intensifying the treatment with brachytherapy makes logical sense. High rates of locoregional control have been achieved using an integrated treatment approach of external beam radiotherapy directed at the primary and bilateral neck, followed by a brachytherapy boost.[109] Complications of brachytherapy for base of tongue tumors include osteoradionecrosis of the mandible. The risk of complication appears to be related to the technique of implantation but may approach 30%. There is limited information regarding the use of brachytherapy and chemotherapy concurrently; this approach should be avoided outside of a formal trial setting.

When brachytherapy is planned following external beam radiotherapy, care should be taken to delineate the pretreatment tumor extent, as regression is not always uniform. Tattoo and/or gold seed placement along the tumor border have been used to accomplish this. The CTV used is recommended by ESTRO to be 5 mm at minimum and more commonly 1 to 1.5 cm for base of tongue tumors. The PTV is usually equal to the CTV as the implanted catheters move with the tumor. Catheters are typically positioned parallel and equidistant 1 to 1.5 cm apart. Although traditional methods of calculating dose have been used in the past based on the Paris, Manchester, or New York systems, computer-derived brachytherapy plans are now routine.

Brachytherapy Guidelines

The American Brachytherapy Society (ABS) has published guidelines for the use of HDR brachytherapy for head and neck tumors and oropharyngeal tumors in particular. Prophylactic tracheostomy is recommended as posterior and large tumors are at risk to cause airway obstruction. Expert panel evidence, as well as single institution series, recommends external beam radiotherapy doses of 45 to 60 Gy followed by HDR brachytherapy boost of 3 to 4 Gy per fraction for 6 to 10 doses with locoregional control of implanted tumors reaching 82% to 94%.[110]

The European Brachytherapy Group (GEC) and the European Society for Therapeutic Radiology and Oncology (ESTRO) have also published joint guidelines for the use of brachytherapy for head and neck malignancies. Similar to the ABS, these were based on consensus recommendations reflecting limited data.[111] For oropharyngeal tumors, these guidelines recommend 45 to 50 Gy external beam radiotherapy followed by 25 to 30 Gy boost for tonsillar tumors and 30 to 35 Gy boost to base of tongue tumors. The total brachytherapy boost dose is fraction size dependent; 21 to 30 Gy in 3 Gy fractions, and 16 to 24 Gy in 4 Gy fractions. These guidelines were recently updated to reflect standardized use of CT-/MRI-based treatment planning with inhomogeneity corrections.[112] Quality of life analyses comparing a combined regimen of brachytherapy and external beam radiotherapy to surgery and postoperative radiotherapy favored a primary radiotherapy only approach,[113] suggesting that in experienced hands, this is a reasonable treatment method.

Hypofractionated Image-Guided Radiation Therapy for Oropharyngeal Cancer

Hypofractionated image-guided radiotherapy techniques, commonly referred to have stereotactic body radiotherapy (SBRT), have resulted in promising outcomes for the treatment of early-stage lung cancers[114] and limited metastases.[35] Consequently, investigators are attempting to incorporate these techniques into the treatment of oropharyngeal cancer. To date, data are limited,[115,116] and further investigations are needed to determine what role, if any, exists for this approach.

DEINTENSIFICATION OF THERAPY FOR HUMAN PAPILLOMAVIRUS–POSITIVE OROPHARYNGEAL CANCER PATIENTS

Given better outcomes of HPV-related oropharyngeal cancer patients, in combination with the known acute and late effects of surgery, chemotherapy, and radiotherapy, many are investigating strategies to maintain high rates of tumor control and survival while deintensifying curative intent treatment in locoregionally advanced patients. Many different approaches have been investigated in the prospective and pilot study arena with selected studies in Table 48.13. One such approach is altered fractionation radiation alone without chemotherapy. A retrospective analysis of HPV-related oropharyngeal cancer patients treated at a single institution with either altered fractionation radiation alone of chemoradiotherapy demonstrated that RT and CRT outcomes were similar in those patients with < 10 pack-year smoking history (3-year OS RT: 86% vs. CRT: 88%, P = .45).[117] Furthermore, locoregional control and distant metastasis rate were not different between these two approaches.

TABLE 48.13 SELECTED SERIES OF HPV-RELATED OROPHARYNGEAL CANCER TREATED WITH REDUCED RADIATION DOSE, LIMITED TREATMENT VOLUMES, OR LIMITED CHEMOTHERAPY

	PMH[a]	Multi-Inst[b]	ECOG 1308[c]	RAVD[d]
	RT Alone	CDDP Weekly/RT (60 Gy) → Bx 1° + LND	CDDP/Pacli/ Cetux × 3 CR → Cetux RT (54 Gy)	CDDP/Pacli/ Cetux × 2 GR → RT to gross disease only
2-year LRP	3 y: 95%	pCR = 86%	94%	94%
2-year PFS	3 y: DM: 8%		80%	93%
2-year OS	3 y: 86%		93%	92%

[a]O'Sullivan B, Huang SH, Perez-Ordonez B, et al. Outcomes of HPV-related oropharyngeal cancer patients treated by radiotherapy alone using altered fractionation. *Radiother Oncol* 2012;103:49–56.
[b]Chera BS, Amdur RJ, Tepper J, et al. Phase 2 trial of de-intensified chemoradiation therapy for favorable-risk human papillomavirus-associated oropharyngeal squamous cell carcinoma. *Int J Radiat Oncol Biol Phys* 2015;93:976–985.
[c]Marur S, Li S, Cmelak AJ, et al. E1308: phase II trial of induction chemotherapy followed by reduced-dose radiation and weekly cetuximab in patients with HPV-associated resectable squamous cell carcinoma of the oropharynx–ECOG-ACRIN Cancer Research Group. *J Clin Oncol* 2016; JCO2016683300.
[d]Villaflor VM, Melotek JM, Karrison TG, et al. Response-adapted volume de-escalation (RAVD) in locally advanced head and neck cancer. *Ann Oncol* 2016;27:908–913.

Other approaches are being investigated. One alternative approach being investigated is tailoring treatment based on response to induction chemotherapy. ECOG 1308 was a single-arm study basing postinduction chemotherapy radiotherapy dose on response to induction chemotherapy. Those with a complete response to cisplatin, docetaxel, and cetuximab induction chemotherapy received 54 Gy with cetuximab, and those with a partial response received 69.3 Gy with cetuximab. In those patients treated with reduced dose RT, 2-year locoregional control was 94%, and 2-year overall survival was 93%.[118] Others have deintensified therapy in patients with a good response to induction chemotherapy by keeping chemotherapy and radiation doses unchanged and instead significantly shrinking or eliminating elective nodal radiation volumes. Following induction cisplatin, paclitaxel, and cetuximab +/− everolimus, patients with >50% reduction in the sum of the tumor diameters were classified as having a good response. Those with a good response went on to receive standard dose chemoradiotherapy to gross disease only, whereas those with less than a good response received standard dose chemoradiotherapy to gross disease as well as the next elective nodal station. Interestingly, in HPV-associated cancer patients, 2-year PFS and OS in good response patients were 93.1% and 92.1%, respectively, compared to those with no response 74.0% and 95.2%, respectively,[119] indicating that this is a potential treatment strategy pending further investigation.

Another alternative is reduced dose RT concurrently with cisplatin chemotherapy. In a single-arm phase II study, HPV-associated oropharyngeal cancer patients with T0-T3, N0-N2c were treated with concurrent weekly cisplatin 30 mg/m² and 60 Gy radiation. The primary endpoint of this study was pathologic CR rate of mandatory biopsy of the primary site and dissection of involved lymph node levels irrespective of imaging response. Remarkably, 86% of patients (37 of 43) had a pathologic complete response and toxicities were reduced compared to standard course chemoradiotherapy.[120]

Although the data above are promising, deintensification of therapy in HPV-associated oropharyngeal cancer remains experimental and should not be considered standard of care. Of note, NRG is conducting HN002 randomizing these patients to 60 Gy radiotherapy with concurrent weekly cisplatin or 60 Gy accelerated radiotherapy alone (NCT02254278).

POSTTREATMENT MANAGEMENT AND SURVEILLANCE

Following definitive therapy for oropharyngeal cancer, patients should be seen regularly for clinical evaluation. Current guidelines suggest examination every 1 to 3 months for the first-year post therapy, every 2 to 4 months in the second-year post therapy and every 4 to 6 months years 3 to 5. The intensity of the examinations within the first 2 years coincides with the likelihood of recurrence in the interval. Given that radiation to the neck commonly causes hypothyroidism, TSH should be evaluated every 6 months.

Following definitive radiotherapy or chemoradiotherapy, follow-up imaging should be performed within the first 3 months of treatment completion for patients with N+ presentations. A radiographic complete response on CT imaging of the neck, defined as nonenhancing, nonnecrotic nodal tissue <1.5 cm, is associated with 100% long-term disease control in the neck, and no further therapy is needed.[121] Surveillance CT imaging of the primary site does not add additional information to physical/fiberoptic examination and should not be routinely performed.[122]

PET/CT is more widely available and is often used as the sole imaging modality following the completion of radiotherapy. An analysis of 121 node-positive predominately oropharyngeal (74%) head and neck cancer patients, prospectively followed with PET/CT at around 12 weeks post therapy (and again 4 weeks later if equivocal residual activity was present on the 12-week scan) with possible neck dissection for metabolic persistence helped to clarify the role of PET/CT scan following chemoradiotherapy. With or without residual CT abnormalities in the neck, a negative PET scan at 12 weeks, defined as the absence of metabolic activity, was associated with no isolated nodal progression.[123] Additionally, the negative predictive value of PET was 98.1% (95% CI = 93.2% to 99.8%) compared to 96.8% in CT (95% CI = 88.8% to 99.6%) However, more importantly, false-positive readings were seen in only 1.8% of PET scans compared to 38% of CT scans, resulting in a positive predictive value of 77.8% for PET/CT scan and 14% for CT. When the analysis was restricted to p16-positive patients, the results were similar with a negative predictive value of 98.2% (95% CI = 90.4% to 100%) and 66.7% (95% CI = 9.4% to 99.2%) for PET. Long-term follow-up of these patients demonstrated that PET–CT-directed posttherapy management resulted in >90% of patients were adequately spared a neck dissection, with only one patient experiencing a neck recurrence following initial metabolic resolution.[124] Of note, these patients also had a contrast-enhanced CT scan performed 6 weeks after completion of treatment. All patients who had a negative CT scan also had a negative PET. Thus, a 12-week PET may not be necessary for patients who have had a negative CT.

Since these initial evaluations, a randomized study has been reported comparing the utility of postchemoradiotherapy PET-/CT-based neck surveillance versus planned neck dissection in patients with N2 or N3 nodal disease. The trial accrued 564 patients (282 in each arm), 84% having oropharyngeal cancer, and p16 staining was positive in 75%. Patients assigned to the PET-/CT-based neck surveillance arm had 2-year overall survival rate of 84.9% (95% CI = 80.7 to 89.1) compared to 81.5% (95% CI = 76.9 to 86.3) in the planned-surgery group. Furthermore, there were no differences in locoregional control 2-year rate of 91.9% (95% CI = 88.5 to 95.3) in the surveillance group and 91.4% (95% CI = 87.8 to 95.0%) in the planned-surgery group. Finally, PET-/CT-based surveillance was more cost-effective saving an average of $2,190 per patient. Therefore, PET-/CT-based surveillance should be considered standard postchemoradiotherapy.[125]

TREATMENT OF RECURRENT AND METASTATIC OROPHARYNGEAL CANCER

Systemic Therapy for Recurrent and Metastatic Oropharyngeal Cancer

The standard therapy for patients with recurrent or metastatic oropharyngeal cancer is systemic therapy with platinum-based chemotherapy. In phase II studies, many drugs in addition to platinum agents and methotrexate have shown single-agent activity including paclitaxel,[126] docetaxel,[127] gemcitabine,[128] ifosfamide,[129] vinorelbine,[130] pemetrexed,[131] capecitabine,[132] and irinotecan.[133] Single-agent cisplatin (100 mg/m^2) has been shown to improve overall survival compared to best-supportive care.[134] Cisplatin was also shown to be superior to single-agent methotrexate.[135] Multiple randomized studies have attempted to improve survival with combination cisplatin-based regimens. The combination of cisplatin (100 mg/m^2) with 5-FU (1,000 mg/m^2/d), demonstrated improved response rates (32% vs. 17%), but not improved median survival (5.7 months) over cisplatin alone.[136] Similar results were seen when the combination of cisplatin/5-FU, carboplatin/5-FU, and methotrexate alone was randomly compared. The combination of cisplatin and 5-FU was shown to have increased response rates compared to methotrexate (32% vs. 10%) as was carboplatin and 5-FU compared to methotrexate (21% vs. 10%), but neither had improved median survival (6.6 and 5.6 months, respectively, compared to 5.0 months) to methotrexate.[137] Response rates and survival are similar with cisplatin and paclitaxel versus cisplatin/5-FU, which provides a regimen that is easier to administer.[138] For oropharyngeal cancer specifically, a planned subset analysis of a phase III trial comparing cisplatin and pemetrexed to cisplatin and placebo demonstrated that oropharyngeal cancer patients receiving the combination regimen had improved survival (9.9 months vs. 6.1 months, P = .002) and improved progression-free survival (4 months vs. 3.4 months, P = .047).[139]

The addition of agents targeted to the epidermal growth factor receptor to platinum-based systemic therapy has been shown to improve overall survival compared to platinum agents alone in a phase III study with a large proportion of oropharyngeal cancer patients. The EXTREME study randomized recurrent and metastatic head and neck cancer patients to cisplatin 100 mg/m^2 d1 or carboplatin AUC = 5 d1 along with 5-FU 1,000 mg/m^2/d 5-FU d1-4 every 3 weeks with or without cetuximab 250 mg/m^2 following a loading dose of 400 mg/m^2. Cetuximab was continued until disease progression or patient intolerance.[140] Median overall survival was improved from 7.4 months with chemotherapy alone to 10.1 months with the combination of systemic therapy and cetuximab as was median progression-free survival (3.3 to 5.6 months). No phase III data have suggested a benefit for the addition of tyrosine kinase inhibitors including gefitinib or erlotinib to platinum-based therapy. Ongoing investigations are determining the role of bevacizumab and other targeted agents.

In the platinum refractory setting, immune checkpoint inhibitors have significantly changed second-line therapy for recurrent and metastatic head and neck cancers in general and oropharyngeal cancers specifically. The checkmate 141 study randomized 361 patients (35.5% pharyngeal cancers) to nivolumab 3 mg/kg every 2 weeks or investigator choice of 40 to 60 mg/m^2 methotrexate, 30 to 40 mg/m^2 docetaxel, or 250 mg/m^2 cetuximab after a loading dose of 400 mg/m². Nivolumab treated patients had a longer median (7.5 months vs. 5.1 months) and 1-year overall survival (36% vs. 16.6%) HR = 0.98 (95% CI = 0.51 to 0.96) *P* = .01. In an exploratory analysis looking at the effect of nivolumab based on p16 status, p16-positive patients had longer median survival (9.1 months vs. 4.4 months) HR = 0.56 (95% CI = 0.32 to 0.99).[141]

Reirradiation for Locoregionally Confined Recurrent or Second Primary Disease

For the subgroup of recurrent oropharyngeal cancer patients with locoregionally confined disease, surgical resection is recommended, although this is possible only in a small proportion of patients.[142] Following surgery[143] in those with high-risk pathologic features or in those who are not surgical candidates,[144] a second course of full-dose radiotherapy with chemotherapy has been shown to result in long-term survival in approximately 20% of patients. Patients who are able to undergo surgery prior to reirradiation, as well as those who have not been exposed to prior chemotherapy and are treated to higher doses, have improved outcomes. Because of the high risk of normal tissue toxicity including up to a 20% carotid rupture rate and 15% fatal toxicity, patients undergoing a second course of chemotherapy and radiation therapy should be managed at experienced centers. It is unknown if systemic therapy alone or chemotherapy and reirradiation is a better therapy for these patients, as a phase III comparison of these modalities failed to accrue.

Recently, data has emerged demonstrating that SBRT is associated with high rates of treated tumor control in previously irradiated head and neck cancer patients with locoregionally confined recurrences.[145] This treatment is attractive as it is a much shorter course (1 to 2 weeks) compared to chemoreirradiation and has been combined with cetuximab safely.[146] However, similar to chemo-reirradiation, high-grade late toxicities including carotid blowout are possible. Patients with recurrent/second primary tumors arising in the larynx/hypopharynx were more likely to have late high-grade toxicity following SBRT reirradiation. However, the ability to offer SBRT is limited in size and location of the recurrent tumor and should be delivered by those with experience with this technique. Therefore, treatment decisions will have to be individualized based on extent of disease, performance status, and preference.

REFERENCES

1. Torre LA, Bray F, Siegel RL, et al. Global cancer statistics, 2012. *CA Cancer J Clin* 2015;65:87–108.
2. Ernster JA, Sciotto CG, O'Brien MM, et al. Rising incidence of oropharyngeal cancer and the role of oncogenic human papilloma virus. *Laryngoscope* 2007;117:2115–2128.
3. Chaturvedi AK, Engels EA, Pfeiffer RM, et al. Human papillomavirus and rising oropharyngeal cancer incidence in the United States. *J Clin Oncol* 2011;29:4294–4301.
4. Durst M, Gissmann L, Ikenberg H, et al. A papillomavirus DNA from a cervical carcinoma and its prevalence in cancer biopsy samples from different geographic regions. *Proc Natl Acad Sci U S A* 1983;80:3812–3815.
5. IARC monographs on the evaluation of carcinogenic risks to humans. 64, 1995. http://monographs.iarc.fr/ENG/Monographs/vol64/index.php
6. Munoz N, Bosch FX, de Sanjose S, et al. Epidemiologic classification of human papillomavirus types associated with cervical cancer. *N Engl J Med* 2003;348:518–527.
7. Kreimer AR, Clifford GM, Boyle P, et al. Human papillomavirus types in head and neck squamous cell carcinomas worldwide: a systematic review. *Cancer Epidemiol Biomarkers Prev* 2005;14:467–475.
8. Mork J, Lie AK, Glattre E, et al. Human papillomavirus infection as a risk factor for squamous-cell carcinoma of the head and neck. *N Engl J Med* 2001;344:1125–1131.
9. Chung CH, Gillison ML. Human papillomavirus in head and neck cancer: its role in pathogenesis and clinical implications. *Clin Cancer Res* 2009;15:6758–6762.
10. Strati K, Lambert PF. Role of Rb-dependent and Rb-independent functions of papillomavirus E7 oncogene in head and neck cancer. *Cancer Res* 2007;67:11585–11593.
11. McLaughlin-Drubin ME, Munger K. Oncogenic activities of human papillomaviruses. *Virus Res* 2009;143:195–208.
12. Singhi AD, Westra WH. Comparison of human papillomavirus in situ hybridization and p16 immunohistochemistry in the detection of human papillomavirus-associated head and neck cancer based on a prospective clinical experience. *Cancer* 2010;116:2166–2173.
13. McLaughlin-Drubin ME, Crum CP, Munger K. Human papillomavirus E7 oncoprotein induces KDM6A and KDM6B histone demethylase expression and causes epigenetic reprogramming. *Proc Natl Acad Sci U S A* 2011;108:2130–2135.
14. Gillison ML, D'Souza G, Westra W, et al. Distinct risk factor profiles for human papillomavirus type 16-positive and human papillomavirus type 16-negative head and neck cancers. *J Natl Cancer Inst* 2008;100:407–420.
15. D'Souza G, Kreimer AR, Viscidi R, et al. Case-control study of human papillomavirus and oropharyngeal cancer. *N Engl J Med* 2007;356:1944–1956.
16. Gillison ML. Human papillomavirus-associated head and neck cancer is a distinct epidemiologic, clinical, and molecular entity. *Semin Oncol* 2004;31:744–754.
17. Ang KK, Harris J, Wheeler R, et al. Human papillomavirus and survival of patients with oropharyngeal cancer. *N Engl J Med* 2010;363:24–35.
18. Fakhry C, Westra WH, Li S, et al. Improved survival of patients with human papillomavirus-positive head and neck squamous cell carcinoma in a prospective clinical trial. *J Natl Cancer Inst* 2008;100:261–269.
19. Rischin D, Young RJ, Fisher R, et al. Prognostic significance of p16INK4A and human papillomavirus in patients with oropharyngeal cancer treated on TROG 02.02 phase III trial. *J Clin Oncol* 2010;28:4142–4148.
20. Lassen P, Eriksen JG, Hamilton-Dutoit S, et al. Effect of HPV-associated p16INK4A expression on response to radiotherapy and survival in squamous cell carcinoma of the head and neck. *J Clin Oncol* 2009;27:1992–1998.
21. Broglie MA, Stoeckli SJ, Sauter R, et al. Impact of human papillomavirus on outcome in patients with oropharyngeal cancer treated with primary surgery. *Head Neck* 2017;39:2004–2015.
22. Rouvière H. *Anatomy of the human lymphatic system.* Ann Arbor, MI: Edwards Brothers, 1938.
23. Haagensen C. *The lymphatics in cancer.* Philadelphia, PA: Saunders, 1972.
24. Robbins KT, Clayman G, Levine PA, et al. Neck dissection classification update: revisions proposed by the American Head and Neck Society and the American Academy of Otolaryngology-Head and Neck Surgery. *Arch Otolaryngol Head Neck Surg* 2002;128:751–758.
25. Som PM, Curtin HD, Mancuso AA. An imaging-based classification for the cervical nodes designed as an adjunct to recent clinically based nodal classifications. *Arch Otolaryngol Head Neck Surg* 1999;125:388–396.
26. Expert Panel on Radiation Oncology–Head and Neck Cancer; Yeung AR, Garg MK, et al. ACR Appropriateness Criteria(R) ipsilateral radiation for squamous cell carcinoma of the tonsil. *Head Neck* 2012;34:613–616.
27. Gregoire V, Coche E, Cosnard G, et al. Selection and delineation of lymph node target volumes in head and neck conformal radiotherapy. Proposal for standardizing terminology and procedure based on the surgical experience. *Radiother Oncol* 2000;56:135–150.
28. Gregoire V, Eisbruch A, Hamoir M, et al. Proposal for the delineation of the nodal CTV in the node-positive and the post-operative neck. *Radiother Oncol* 2006;79:15–20.
29. Gregoire V, Levendag P, Ang KK, et al. CT-based delineation of lymph node levels and related CTVs in the node-negative neck: DAHANCA, EORTC, GORTEC, NCIC, RTOG consensus guidelines. *Radiother Oncol* 2003;69:227–236.
30. Chao KS, Wippold FJ, Ozyigit G, et al. Determination and delineation of nodal target volumes for head-and-neck cancer based on patterns of failure in patients receiving definitive and postoperative IMRT. *Int J Radiat Oncol Biol Phys* 2004;53:1174–1184.
31. Merino OR, Lindberg RD, Fletcher GH. An analysis of distant metastases from squamous cell carcinoma of the upper respiratory and digestive tracts. *Cancer* 1977;40:145–151.
32. McLeod NM, Jess A, Anand R, et al. Role of chest CT in staging of oropharyngeal cancer: a systematic review. *Head Neck* 2009;31:548–555.
33. Goodwin WJ. Distant metastases from oropharyngeal cancer. *ORL J Otorhinolaryngol Relat Spec* 2001;63:222–223.
34. Younes RN, Gross JL, Silva JF, et al. Surgical treatment of lung metastases of head and neck tumors. *Am J Surg* 1997;174:499–502.
35. Salama JK, Milano MT. Radical irradiation of extracranial oligometastases. *J Clin Oncol* 2014;32:2902–2912.
36. Schwartz DL, Ford E, Rajendran J, et al. FDG-PET/CT imaging for preradiotherapy staging of head-and-neck squamous cell carcinoma. *Int J Radiat Oncol Biol Phys* 2005;61:129–136.
37. Higgins KA, Hoang JK, Roach MC, et al. Analysis of pretreatment FDG-PET SUV parameters in head-and-neck cancer: tumor SUVmean has superior prognostic value. *Int J Radiat Oncol Biol Phys* 2012;82:548–553.
38. Grant DG, Salassa JR, Hinni ML, et al. Carcinoma of the tongue base treated by transoral laser microsurgery, part one: untreated tumors, a prospective analysis of oncologic and functional outcomes. *Laryngoscope* 2006;116:2150–2155.
39. Steiner W, Fierek O, Ambrosch P, et al. Transoral laser microsurgery for squamous cell carcinoma of the base of the tongue. *Arch Otolaryngol Head Neck Surg* 2003;129:36–43.
40. Grant DG, Hinni ML, Salassa JR, et al. Oropharyngeal cancer: a case for single modality treatment with transoral laser microsurgery. *Arch Otolaryngol Head Neck Surg* 2009;135:1225–1230.
41. Cooper JS, Pajak TF, Forastiere A, et al. Precisely defining high-risk operable head and neck tumors based on RTOG #85-03 and #88-24: targets for postoperative radiochemotherapy? *Head Neck* 1998;20:588–594.
42. Lavaf A, Genden EM, Cesaretti JA, et al. Adjuvant radiotherapy improves overall survival for patients with lymph node-positive head and neck squamous cell carcinoma. *Cancer* 2008;112:535–543.

43. Maccomb W, Fletcher G. Planned combination of surgery and radiation in treatment of advanced primary head and neck cancers. *Am J Roentgenol Radium Ther Nucl Med* 1957;77:397–414.

44. Tupchong L, Scott CB, Blitzer PH, et al. Randomized study of preoperative versus postoperative radiation therapy in advanced head and neck carcinoma: long-term follow-up of RTOG study 73-03. *Int J Radiat Oncol Biol Phys* 1991;20:21–28.

45. Bernier J, Domenge C, Ozsahin M, et al. Postoperative irradiation with or without concomitant chemotherapy for locally advanced head and neck cancer. *N Engl J Med* 2004;350:1945–1952.

46. Bachaud JM, Cohen-Jonathan E, Alzieu C, et al. Combined postoperative radiotherapy and weekly cisplatin infusion for locally advanced head and neck carcinoma: final report of a randomized trial. *Int J Radiat Oncol Biol Phys* 1996;36:999–1004.

47. Fietkau R, Lautenschläger C, Sauer R, et al. Postoperative concurrent radiochemotherapy versus radiotherapy in high-risk SCCA of the head and neck: results of the German phase III trial ARO 96-3. *J Clin Oncol* 2006;24:5507.

48. Cooper JS, Pajak TF, Forastiere AA, et al. Postoperative concurrent radiotherapy and chemotherapy for high-risk squamous-cell carcinoma of the head and neck. *N Engl J Med* 2004;350:1937–1944.

49. Noronha V, Joshi A, Patil V, et al. W3W phase III randomized trial comparing weekly versus three-weekly (W3W) cisplatin in patients receiving chemoradiation for locally advanced head and neck cancer. *J Clin Oncol* 2015;35:6007.

50. Expert Panel on Radiation Oncology--Head and Neck;, Salama JK, Saba N, et al. ACR appropriateness criteria(R) adjuvant therapy for resected squamous cell carcinoma of the head and neck. *Oral Oncol* 2011;47.554–559.

51. Eisbruch A, Harris J, Garden AS, et al. Multi-institutional trial of accelerated hypofractionated intensity-modulated radiation therapy for early-stage oropharyngeal cancer (RTOG 00-22). *Int J Radiat Oncol Biol Phys* 2010;76:1333–1338.

52. Beitler JJ, Zhang Q, Fu KK, et al. Final results of local-regional control and late toxicity of RTOG 9003: a randomized trial of altered fractionation radiation for locally advanced head and neck cancer. *Int J Radiat Oncol Biol Phys* 2014;89:13–20.

53. Overgaard J, Hansen HS, Specht L, et al. Five compared with six fractions per week of conventional radiotherapy of squamous-cell carcinoma of head and neck: DAHANCA 6 and 7 randomised controlled trial. *Lancet* 2003;362:933–940.

54. Horiot JC, Le Fur R, N'Guyen T, et al. Hyperfractionation versus conventional fractionation in oropharyngeal carcinoma: final analysis of a randomized trial of the EORTC cooperative group of radiotherapy. *Radiother Oncol* 1992;25:231–241.

55. Budach W, Hehr T, Budach V, et al. A meta-analysis of hyperfractionated and accelerated radiotherapy and combined chemotherapy and radiotherapy regimens in unresected locally advanced squamous cell carcinoma of the head and neck. *BMC Cancer* 2006;6:28.

56. Bourhis J, Overgaard J, Audry H, et al. Hyperfractionated or accelerated radiotherapy in head and neck cancer: a meta-analysis. *Lancet* 2006;368:843–854.

57. Lassen P, Eriksen JG, Krogdahl A, et al. The influence of HPV-associated p16-expression on accelerated fractionated radiotherapy in head and neck cancer: evaluation of the randomised DAHANCA 6&7 trial. *Radiother Oncol* 2011;100:49–55.

58. Poulsen MG, Denham JW, Peters LJ, et al. A randomised trial of accelerated and conventional radiotherapy for stage III and IV squamous carcinoma of the head and neck: a Trans-Tasman Radiation Oncology Group Study. *Radiother Oncol* 2001;60:113–122.

59. Overgaard J, Mohanti BK, Begum N, et al. Five versus six fractions of radiotherapy per week for squamous-cell carcinoma of the head and neck (IAEA-ACC study): a randomised, multicentre trial. *Lancet Oncol* 2010;11:553–560.

60. Fu KK, Pajak TF, Trotti A, et al. A Radiation Therapy Oncology Group (RTOG) phase III randomized study to compare hyperfractionation and two variants of accelerated fractionation to standard fractionation radiotherapy for head and neck squamous cell carcinomas: first report of RTOG 9003. *Int J Radiat Oncol Biol Phys* 2000;48:7–16.

61. Parsons JT, Mendenhall WM, Stringer SP, et al. Squamous cell carcinoma of the oropharynx: surgery, radiation therapy, or both. *Cancer* 2002;94:2967–2980.

62. Pignon JP, le Maitre A, Maillard E, et al. Meta-analysis of chemotherapy in head and neck cancer (MACH-NC): an update on 93 randomised trials and 17,346 patients. *Radiother Oncol* 2009;92:4–14.

63. Blanchard P, Baujat B, Holostenco V, et al. Meta-analysis of chemotherapy in head and neck cancer (MACH-NC): a comprehensive analysis by tumour site. *Radiother Oncol* 2011;100:33–40.

64. Fallai C, Bolner A, Signor M, et al. Long-term results of conventional radiotherapy versus accelerated hyperfractionated radiotherapy versus concomitant radiotherapy and chemotherapy in locoregionally advanced carcinoma of the oropharynx. *Tumori* 2006;92:41–54.

65. Calais G, Alfonsi M, Bardet E, et al. Randomized trial of radiation therapy versus concomitant chemotherapy and radiation therapy for advanced-stage oropharynx carcinoma. *J Natl Cancer Inst* 1999;91:2081–2086.

66. Denis F, Garaud P, Bardet E, et al. Final results of the 94-01 French Head and Neck Oncology and Radiotherapy Group randomized trial comparing radiotherapy alone with concomitant radiochemotherapy in advanced-stage oropharynx carcinoma. *J Clin Oncol* 2004;22:69–76.

67. Lok BH, Setton J, Caria N, et al. Intensity-modulated radiation therapy in oropharyngeal carcinoma: effect of tumor volume on clinical outcomes. *Int J Radiat Oncol Biol Phys* 2012;82:1851–1857.

68. Zhen W, Karnell LH, Hoffman HT, et al. The National Cancer Data Base report on squamous cell carcinoma of the base of tongue. *Head Neck* 2004;26:660–674.

69. Pederson AW, Haraf DJ, Witt ME, et al. Chemoradiotherapy for locoregionally advanced squamous cell carcinoma of the base of tongue. *Head Neck* 2010;32:1519–1527.

70. Stenson KM, MacCracken E, List M, et al. Swallowing function in patients with head and neck cancer prior to treatment. *Arch Otolaryngol Head Neck Surg* 2000;126:371–377.

71. Salama JK, Stenson KM, List MA, et al. Characteristics associated with swallowing changes after concurrent chemotherapy and radiotherapy in patients with head and neck cancer. *Arch Otolaryngol Head Neck Surg* 2008;134:1060–1065.

72. Rosenthal DI, Lewin JS, Eisbruch A. Prevention and treatment of dysphagia and aspiration after chemoradiation for head and neck cancer. *J Clin Oncol* 2006;24:2636–2643.

73. Eisbruch A, Kim HM, Feng FY, et al. Chemo-IMRT of oropharyngeal cancer aiming to reduce dysphagia: swallowing organs late complication probabilities and dosimetric correlates. *Int J Radiat Oncol Biol Phys* 2011;81:e93–e99.

74. Machtay M, Moughan J, Trotti A, et al. Factors associated with severe late toxicity after concurrent chemoradiation for locally advanced head and neck cancer: an RTOG analysis. *J Clin Oncol* 2008;26:3582–3589.

75. Vainshtein JM, Moon DH, Feng FY, et al. Long-term quality of life after swallowing and salivary-sparing chemo-intensity modulated radiation therapy in survivors of human papillomavirus-related oropharyngeal cancer. *Int J Radiat Oncol Biol Phys* 2015;91:925–933.

76. Jeremic B, Shibamoto Y, Milicic B, et al. Hyperfractionated radiation therapy with or without concurrent low-dose daily cisplatin in locally advanced squamous cell carcinoma of the head and neck: a prospective randomized trial. *J Clin Oncol* 2000;18:1458–1464.

77. Sharma A, Mohanti BK, Thakar A, et al. Concomitant chemoradiation versus radical radiotherapy in advanced squamous cell carcinoma of oropharynx and nasopharynx using weekly cisplatin: a phase II randomized trial. *Ann Oncol* 2010;21:2272–2277.

78. Huguenin P, Beer KT, Allal A, et al. Concomitant cisplatin significantly improves locoregional control in advanced head and neck cancers treated with hyperfractionated radiotherapy. *J Clin Oncol* 2004;22:4665–4673.

79. Domenge C, Hill C, Lefebvre JL, et al. Randomized trial of neoadjuvant chemotherapy in oropharyngeal carcinoma. French Groupe d'Etude des Tumeurs de la Tete et du Cou (GETTEC). *Br J Cancer* 2000;83:1594–1598.

80. Brockstein B, Haraf DJ, Rademaker AW, et al. Patterns of failure, prognostic factors and survival in locoregionally advanced head and neck cancer treated with concomitant chemoradiotherapy: a 9-year, 337-patient, multi-institutional experience. *Ann Oncol* 2004;15:1179–1186.

81. Cohen EE, Karrison TG, Kocherginsky M, et al. Phase III randomized trial of induction chemotherapy in patients with N2 or N3 locally advanced head and neck cancer. *J Clin Oncol* 2014;32:2735–2743.

82. Haddad R, O'Neill A, Rabinowits G, et al. Induction chemotherapy followed by concurrent chemoradiotherapy (sequential chemoradiotherapy) versus concurrent chemoradiotherapy alone in locally advanced head and neck cancer (PARADIGM): a randomised phase 3 trial. *Lancet Oncol* 2013;14:257–264.

83. Bonner JA, Harari PM, Giralt J, et al. Radiotherapy plus cetuximab for squamous-cell carcinoma of the head and neck. *N Engl J Med* 2006;354:567–578.

84. Rosenthal DI, Harari PM, Giralt J, et al. Association of human papillomavirus and p16 status with outcomes in the IMCL-9815 Phase III Registration Trial for patients with locoregionally advanced oropharyngeal squamous cell carcinoma of the head and neck treated with radiotherapy with or without cetuximab. *J Clin Oncol* 2016;34:1300–1308.

85. Bonner JA, Harari PM, Giralt J, et al. Radiotherapy plus cetuximab for locoregionally advanced head and neck cancer: 5-year survival data from a phase 3 randomised trial, and relation between cetuximab-induced rash and survival. *Lancet Oncol* 2010;11:21–28.

86. Chung CH, Mirakhur B, Chan E, et al. Cetuximab-induced anaphylaxis and IgE specific for galactose-alpha-1,3-galactose. *N Engl J Med* 2008;358:1109–1117.

87. Ang KK, Zhang Q, Rosenthal DI, et al. Randomized phase III trial of concurrent accelerated radiation plus cisplatin with or without cetuximab for stage III to IV head and neck carcinoma: RTOG 0522. *J Clin Oncol* 2014;32:2940–2950.

88. Salama JK, Haraf DJ, Stenson KM, et al. A randomized phase II study of 5-fluorouracil, hydroxyurea, and twice-daily radiotherapy compared with bevacizumab plus 5-fluorouracil, hydroxyurea, and twice-daily radiotherapy for intermediate-stage and T4N0-1 head and neck cancers. *Ann Oncol* 2011;22:2304–2309.

89. Yoo DS, Kirkpatrick JP, Craciunescu O, et al. Prospective trial of synchronous bevacizumab, erlotinib, and concurrent chemoradiation in locally advanced head and neck cancer. *Clin Cancer Res* 2012;18:1404–1414.

90. Thiagarajan A, Caria N, Schoder H, et al. Target volume delineation in oropharyngeal cancer: impact of PET, MRI, and physical examination. *Int J Radiat Oncol Biol Phys* 2012;83:220–227.

91. Eisbruch A, Schwartz M, Rasch C, et al. Dysphagia and aspiration after chemoradiotherapy for head-and-neck cancer: which anatomic structures are affected and can they be spared by IMRT? *Int J Radiat Oncol Biol Phys* 2004;60:1425–1439.

92. Eisbruch A, Marsh LH, Dawson LA, et al. Recurrences near base of skull after IMRT for head-and-neck cancer: implications for target delineation in high neck and for parotid gland sparing. *Int J Radiat Oncol Biol Phys* 2004;59:28–42.

93. Lim YC, Lee SY, Lim JY, et al. Management of contralateral N0 neck in tonsillar squamous cell carcinoma. *Laryngoscope* 2005;115:1672–1675.

94. Olzowy B, Tsalemchuk Y, Schotten KJ, et al. Frequency of bilateral cervical metastases in oropharyngeal squamous cell carcinoma: a retrospective analysis of 352 cases after bilateral neck dissection. *Head Neck* 2011;33:239–243.

95. Foote RL, Schild SE, Thompson WM, et al. Tonsil cancer. Patterns of failure after surgery alone and surgery combined with postoperative radiation therapy. *Cancer* 1994;73:2638–2647.

96. Cho KJ, Joo YH, Sun DI, et al. Management of cervical lymph node metastasis in tonsillar squamous cell carcinoma: is it necessary to treat node-negative contralateral neck? *Auris Nasus Larynx* 2011;38:501–507.

97. Jackson SM, Hay JH, Flores AD, et al. Cancer of the tonsil: the results of ipsilateral radiation treatment. *Radiother Oncol* 1999;51:123–128.

98. O'Sullivan B, Warde P, Grice B, et al. The benefits and pitfalls of ipsilateral radiotherapy in carcinoma of the tonsillar region. *Int J Radiat Oncol Biol Phys* 2001;51:332–343.

99. Chronowski GM, Garden AS, Morrison WH, et al. Unilateral radiotherapy for the treatment of tonsil cancer. *Int J Radiat Oncol Biol Phys* 2012;83:204–209.

100. Rusthoven KE, Raben D, Schneider C, et al. Freedom from local and regional failure of contralateral neck with ipsilateral neck radiotherapy for node-positive tonsil cancer: results of a prospective management approach. *Int J Radiat Oncol Biol Phys* 2009;74:1365–1370.

101. Mell LK, Mehrotra AK, Mundt AJ. Intensity-modulated radiation therapy use in the U.S., 2004. *Cancer* 2005;104:1296–1303.

102. Hall EJ. Intensity-modulated radiation therapy, protons, and the risk of second cancers. *Int J Radiat Oncol Biol Phys* 2006;65:1–7.

103. Nutting CM, Morden JP, Harrington KJ, et al. Parotid-sparing intensity modulated versus conventional radiotherapy in head and neck cancer (PARSPORT): a phase 3 multicentre randomised controlled trial. *Lancet Oncol* 2011;12:127–136.

104. Caudell JJ, Burnett OL III, Schaner PE, et al. Comparison of methods to reduce dose to swallowing-related structures in head and neck cancer. *Int J Radiat Oncol Biol Phys* 2010;77:462–467.

105. Lee N, Mechalakos J, Puri DR, et al. Choosing an intensity-modulated radiation therapy technique in the treatment of head-and-neck cancer. *Int J Radiat Oncol Biol Phys* 2007;68:1299–1309.

106. Caudell JJ, Schaner PE, Desmond RA, et al. Dosimetric factors associated with long-term dysphagia after definitive radiotherapy for squamous cell carcinoma of the head and neck. *Int J Radiat Oncol Biol Phys* 2010;76:403–409.

107. Bourhis J, Sire C, Graff P, et al. Concomitant chemoradiotherapy versus acceleration of radiotherapy with or without concomitant chemotherapy in locally advanced head and neck carcinoma (GORTEC 99-02): an open-label phase 3 randomised trial. *Lancet Oncol* 2012;13:145–153.

108. Nguyen-Tan PF, Zhang Q, Ang KK, et al. Randomized phase III trial to test accelerated versus standard fractionation in combination with concurrent cisplatin for head and neck carcinomas in the Radiation Therapy Oncology Group 0129 trial: long-term report of efficacy and toxicity. *J Clin Oncol* 2014;32:3858–3866.

109. Harrison LB. Applications of brachytherapy in head and neck cancer. *Semin Surg Oncol* 1997;13:177–184.

110. Nag S, Cano ER, Demanes DJ, et al. The American Brachytherapy Society recommendations for high-dose-rate brachytherapy for head-and-neck carcinoma. *Int J Radiat Oncol Biol Phys* 2001;50:1190–1198.

111. Mazeron JJ, Ardiet JM, Haie-Meder C, et al. GEC-ESTRO recommendations for brachytherapy for head and neck squamous cell carcinomas. *Radiother Oncol* 2009;91:150–156.

112. Kovacs G, Martinez-Monge R, Budrukkar A, et al. GEC-ESTRO ACROP recommendations for head & neck brachytherapy in squamous cell carcinomas: 1st update—improvement by cross sectional imaging based treatment planning and stepping source technology. *Radiother Oncol* 2017;122:248–254.

113. Levendag P, Nijdam W, Noever I, et al. Brachytherapy versus surgery in carcinoma of tonsillar fossa and/or soft palate: late adverse sequelae and performance status: can we be more selective and obtain better tissue sparing? *Int J Radiat Oncol Biol Phys* 2004;59:713–724.

114. Timmerman R, Paulus R, Galvin J, et al. Stereotactic body radiation therapy for inoperable early stage lung cancer. *JAMA* 2010;303:1070–1076.

115. Siddiqui F, Patel M, Khan M, et al. Stereotactic body radiation therapy for primary, recurrent, and metastatic tumors in the head-and-neck region. *Int J Radiat Oncol Biol Phys* 2009;74:1047–1053.

116. Kodani N, Yamazaki H, Tsubokura T, et al. Stereotactic body radiation therapy for head and neck tumor: disease control and morbidity outcomes. *J Radiat Res* 2001;52:24–31.

117. O'Sullivan B, Huang SH, Perez-Ordonez B, et al. Outcomes of HPV-related oropharyngeal cancer patients treated by radiotherapy alone using altered fractionation. *Radiother Oncol* 2012;103:49–56.

118. Marur S, Li S, Cmelak AJ, et al. E1308: phase II trial of induction chemotherapy followed by reduced-dose radiation and weekly cetuximab in patients with HPV-associated resectable squamous cell carcinoma of the oropharynx—ECOG-ACRIN Cancer Research Group. *J Clin Oncol* 2016; JCO2016683300.

119. Villaflor VM, Melotek JM, Karrison TG, et al. Response-adapted volume de-escalation (RAVD) in locally advanced head and neck cancer. *Ann Oncol* 2016;27:908–913.

120. Chera BS, Amdur RJ, Tepper J, et al. Phase 2 trial of de-intensified chemoradiation therapy for favorable-risk human papillomavirus-associated oropharyngeal squamous cell carcinoma. *Int J Radiat Oncol Biol Phys* 2015;93:976–985.

121. Liauw SL, Mancuso AA, Amdur RJ, et al. Postradiotherapy neck dissection for lymph node-positive head and neck cancer: the use of computed tomography to manage the neck. *J Clin Oncol* 2006;24:1421–1427.

122. Sullivan BP, Parks KA, Dean NR, et al. Utility of CT surveillance for primary site recurrence of squamous cell carcinoma of the head and neck. *Head Neck* 2011;33:1547–1550.

123. Porceddu SV, Pryor DI, Burmeister E, et al. Results of a prospective study of positron emission tomography-directed management of residual nodal abnormalities in node-positive head and neck cancer after definitive radiotherapy with or without systemic therapy. *Head Neck* 2011;33:1675–1682.

124. Sjovall J, Chua B, Pryor D, et al. Long-term results of positron emission tomography-directed management of the neck in node-positive head and neck cancer after organ preservation therapy. *Oral Oncol* 2015;51:260–266.

125. Mehanna H, Wong WL, McConkey CC, et al. PET-CT surveillance versus neck dissection in advanced head and neck cancer. *N Engl J Med* 2016;374:1444–1454.

126. Forastiere AA, Shank D, Neuberg D, et al. Final report of a phase II evaluation of paclitaxel in patients with advanced squamous cell carcinoma of the head and neck: an Eastern Cooperative Oncology Group trial (PA390). *Cancer* 1998;82:2270–2274.

127. Dreyfuss AI, Clark JR, Norris CM, et al. Docetaxel: an active drug for squamous cell carcinoma of the head and neck. *J Clin Oncol* 1996;14:1672–1678.

128. Catimel G, Vermorken JB, Clavel M, et al. A phase II study of Gemcitabine (LY 188011) in patients with advanced squamous cell carcinoma of the head and neck. EORTC Early Clinical Trials Group. *Ann Oncol* 1994;5:543–547.

129. Sandler A, Saxman S, Bandealy M, et al. Ifosfamide in the treatment of advanced or recurrent squamous cell carcinoma of the head and neck: a phase II Hoosier Oncology Group trial. *Am J Clin Oncol* 1998;21:195–197.

130. Saxman S, Mann B, Canfield V, et al. A phase II trial of vinorelbine in patients with recurrent or metastatic squamous cell carcinoma of the head and neck. *Am J Clin Oncol* 1998;21:398–400.

131. Pivot X, Raymond E, Laguerre B, et al. Pemetrexed disodium in recurrent locally advanced or metastatic squamous cell carcinoma of the head and neck. *Br J Cancer* 2001;85:649–655.

132. Martinez-Trufero J, Isla D, Adansa JC, et al. Phase II study of capecitabine as palliative treatment for patients with recurrent and metastatic squamous head and neck cancer after previous platinum-based treatment. *Br J Cancer* 2010;102:1687–1691.

133. Murphy BA. Topoisomerases in the treatment of metastatic or recurrent squamous carcinoma of the head and neck. *Expert Opin Pharmacother* 2005;6:85–92.

134. Morton RP, Rugman F, Dorman EB, et al. Cisplatinum and bleomycin for advanced or recurrent squamous carcinoma of the head and neck: a randomised factorial phase III controlled trial. *Cancer Chemother Pharmacol* 1985;15:283–289.

135. A phase III randomised trial of cisplatinum, methotrexate, cisplatinum + methotrexate and cisplatinum + 315-FU in end stage squamous carcinoma of the head and neck. Liverpool Head and Neck Oncology Group. *Br J Cancer* 1990;61:311–315.

136. Jacobs C, Lyman G, Velez-Garcia E, et al. A phase III randomized study comparing cisplatin and fluorouracil as single agents and in combination for advanced squamous cell carcinoma of the head and neck. *J Clin Oncol* 1992;10:257–263.

137. Forastiere AA, Metch B, Schuller DE, et al. Randomized comparison of cisplatin plus fluorouracil and carboplatin plus fluorouracil versus methotrexate in advanced squamous-cell carcinoma of the head and neck: a Southwest Oncology Group study. *J Clin Oncol* 1992;10:1245–1251.

138. Gibson MK, Li Y, Murphy B, et al. Randomized phase III evaluation of cisplatin plus fluorouracil versus cisplatin plus paclitaxel in advanced head and neck cancer (E1395): an intergroup trial of the Eastern Cooperative Oncology Group. *J Clin Oncol* 2005;23:3562–3567.

139. Urba S, van Herpen CM, Sahoo TP, et al. Pemetrexed in combination with cisplatin versus cisplatin monotherapy in patients with recurrent or metastatic head and neck cancer: final results of a randomized, double-blind, placebo-controlled, phase 3 study. *Cancer* 2012;118:4694–4705.

140. Vermorken JB, Mesia R, Rivera F, et al. Platinum-based chemotherapy plus cetuximab in head and neck cancer. *N Engl J Med* 2008;359:1116–1127.

141. Ferris RL, Blumenschein G Jr, Fayette J, et al. Nivolumab for recurrent squamous-cell carcinoma of the head and neck. *N Engl J Med* 2016;375:1856–1867.

142. Taussky D, Dulguerov P, Allal AS. Salvage surgery after radical accelerated radiotherapy with concomitant boost technique for head and neck carcinomas. *Head Neck* 2005;27:182–186.

143. Janot F, de Raucourt D, Benhamou E, et al. Randomized trial of postoperative reirradiation combined with chemotherapy after salvage surgery compared with salvage surgery alone in head and neck carcinoma. *J Clin Oncol* 2008;26:5518–5523.

144. Choe KS, Haraf DJ, Solanki A, et al. Prior chemoradiotherapy adversely impacts outcomes of recurrent and second primary head and neck cancer treated with concurrent chemotherapy and reirradiation. *Cancer* 2011;117:4671–4678.

145. Baliga S, Kabarriti R, Ohri N, et al. Stereotactic body radiotherapy for recurrent head and neck cancer: a critical review. *Head Neck* 2017;39:595–601.

146. Vargo JA, Ferris RL, Ohr J, et al. A prospective phase 2 trial of reirradiation with stereotactic body radiation therapy plus cetuximab in patients with previously irradiated recurrent squamous cell carcinoma of the head and neck. *Int J Radiat Oncol Biol Phys* 2015;91:480–488.

CHAPTER 49

Hypopharynx

Matthew E. Witek, Timothy J. Kruser, Henry T. Hoffman, Christopher J. Kandl, and Paul M. Harari

INTRODUCTION

There is a strong association between tobacco use and the development of hypopharynx cancer.[1-3] Because of the rich lymphatic network in this anatomic region, patients commonly present with regional nodal metastases. Many patients with hypopharynx cancer also carry significant medical comorbidities and social issues that present additional challenges to the successful delivery of aggressive cancer therapy. As for all complex tumors of the head and neck (H&N) region, multidisciplinary evaluation and management are critical and should involve the H&N surgeon, radiation oncologist, medical oncologist, nurse, nutritionist, speech or swallow therapist, and social worker. Although a selected cohort of early-stage tumors may be amenable to organ preservation surgery, more radical surgery such as laryngopharyngectomy is often required for patients who undergo a primary operative approach for hypopharynx cancer. This ablative procedure can induce significant cosmetic and functional changes, and postsurgical rehabilitation efforts guided by knowledgeable professionals are very important to assist in patient adaptation. Increasingly, patients with hypopharynx cancer are being considered for nonoperative treatment approaches using definitive radiation or chemoradiation as a means of obtaining tumor control with preservation of organ function. Regardless of the specific treatment approach, all patients require active rehabilitation therapy in an effort to maximize their ultimate speech and swallow function. Despite stepwise advances in the diagnosis and treatment of hypopharynx cancer, the overall outcome for these patients is relatively poor compared with other H&N cancer sites.[4] As with most tumors of the H&N region, there is significant interest in combining molecular targeted therapies with traditional cytotoxic therapy in an effort to further improve outcomes.

ANATOMY

The hypopharynx, sometimes referred to as the laryngopharynx, is contiguous superiorly with the oropharynx and

FIGURE 49.1. Posterior view of the hypopharynx shows the relationship of the pyriform sinus, pharyngeal wall, and postcricoid region within the head and neck. (From Putz R, Pabst R. *Sobotta Atlas of Human Anatomy.* 13th ed. Munich: Urban & Fischer, 2001. Copyright ©Elsevier GmbH. With permission.)

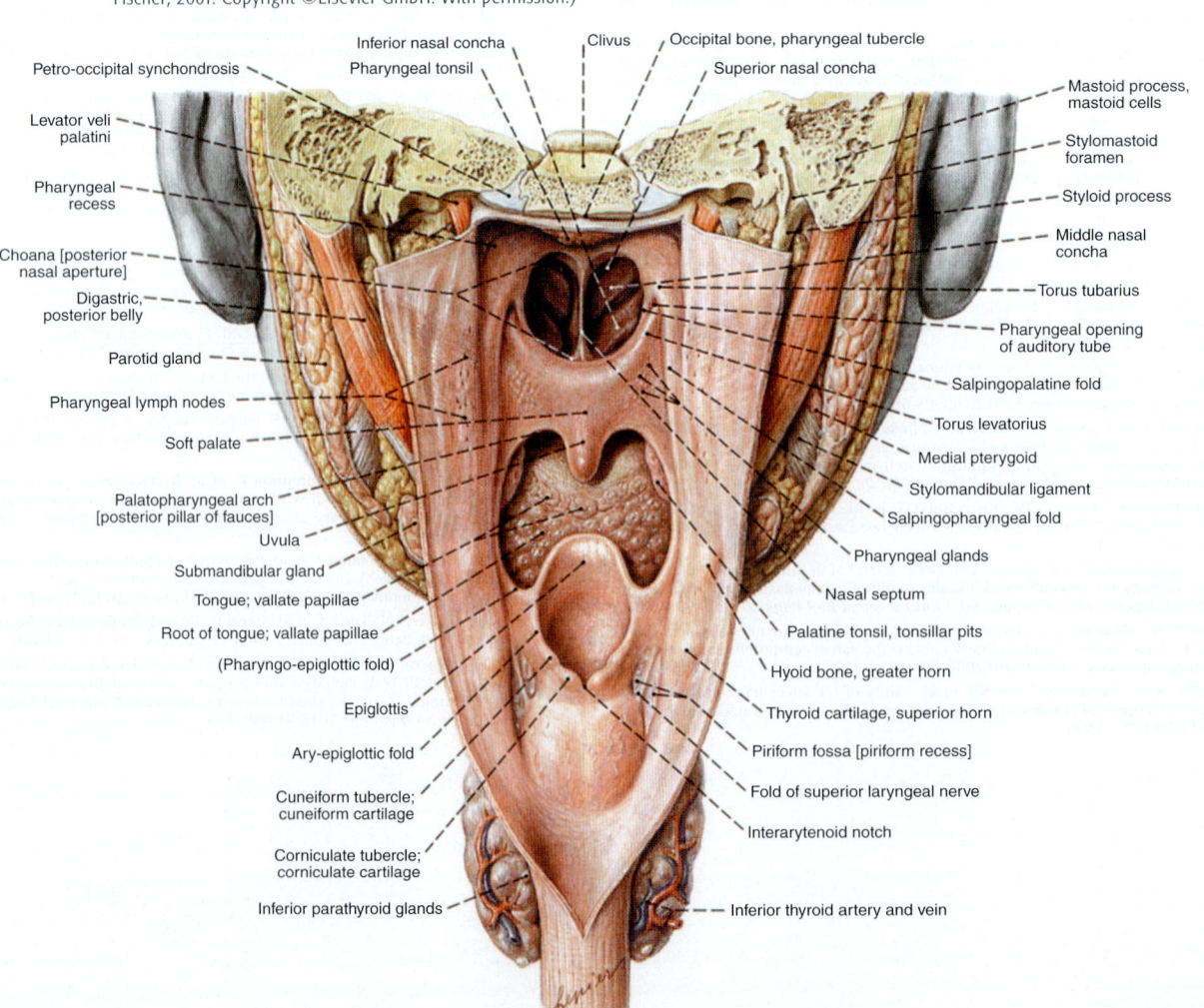

Inferior nasal concha
Pharyngeal tonsil
Clivus
Occipital bone, pharyngeal tubercle
Petro-occipital synchondrosis
Superior nasal concha
Mastoid process, mastoid cells
Levator veli palatini
Stylomastoid foramen
Pharyngeal recess
Styloid process
Choana [posterior nasal aperture]
Middle nasal concha
Digastric, posterior belly
Torus tubarius
Parotid gland
Pharyngeal opening of auditory tube
Pharyngeal lymph nodes
Salpingopalatine fold
Soft palate
Torus levatorius
Palatopharyngeal arch [posterior pillar of fauces]
Medial pterygoid
Uvula
Stylomandibular ligament
Submandibular gland
Salpingopharyngeal fold
Tongue; vallate papillae
Pharyngeal glands
Root of tongue; vallate papillae
Nasal septum
(Pharyngo-epiglottic fold)
Palatine tonsil, tonsillar pits
Epiglottis
Hyoid bone, greater horn
Ary-epiglottic fold
Thyroid cartilage, superior horn
Cuneiform tubercle; cuneiform cartilage
Piriform fossa [piriform recess]
Corniculate tubercle; corniculate cartilage
Fold of superior laryngeal nerve
Interarytenoid notch
Inferior parathyroid glands
Inferior thyroid artery and vein

inferiorly with the cervical esophagus (Fig. 49.1). As general landmarks, the superior border of the hypopharynx is demarcated by the hyoid bone and the inferior border by the cricoid cartilage. With regard to cancer diagnosis and staging, there are three primary anatomic subsites within the hypopharynx: the bilateral pyriform sinuses, the postcricoid region, and the posterior pharyngeal wall.

The pyriform sinuses are essentially inverted pyramids with the medial, lateral, and anterior walls narrowing inferiorly to form the apices. Posteriorly, the pyriform sinuses are open and contiguous with the pharyngeal walls. Superiorly, the sinuses are surrounded by the thyrohyoid membrane through which passes the internal branch of the superior laryngeal nerve. Tumor involvement of the sensory branches of this nerve can result in referred otalgia. The postcricoid region is composed of the mucosa overlying the cricoid cartilage, with the arytenoid and esophageal mucosa forming the superior and inferior borders, respectively. The posterior pharyngeal wall predominantly comprises the squamous mucosa covering the middle and inferior pharyngeal constrictor muscles and is separated from the prevertebral fascia by the retropharyngeal space. Typically, the mucosa lining the pharyngeal wall is <1 cm in thickness and provides a minimal barrier to direct tumor infiltration. The posterior pharyngeal wall is contiguous with the lateral wall of the pyriform sinus (Fig. 49.2).

Sensory innervation of the hypopharynx is provided by the internal branch of the superior laryngeal nerve as well as fibers deriving from the glossopharyngeal nerve. The recurrent laryngeal nerve and the pharyngeal plexus provide the primary motor supply. The arterial supply of the hypopharynx is derived primarily from branches of the external carotid artery: superior thyroid arteries, ascending pharyngeal arteries, and lingual arteries.

There is a rich network of lymphatics within the hypopharynx that drain directly through the thyrohyoid membrane and into the jugulodigastric lymph nodes, most commonly involving the subdigastric node. Additionally, there may be direct drainage into the spinal accessory nodes. Tumors involving the posterior pharyngeal wall can also drain to the retropharyngeal nodes, including the most cephalad retropharyngeal nodes of Rouviere.

EPIDEMIOLOGY AND ETIOLOGY

Hypopharynx cancers are relatively uncommon. Approximately 1,800 cases per year were diagnosed annually in the United States from 1990 to 2004,[4] and the population-adjusted annual incidence rate in the United States was 0.7 per 100,000 from 2000 to 2008, according to the National Cancer Institute's Surveillance, Epidemiology, and End-Results (SEER) database.[5] Hypopharyngeal cancers accounted for 5.2% of upper aerodigestive tract cancers during that time. Approximately three-fourths of hypopharyngeal cancers occur in men, with a mean age of 65 years. Over 90% of patients with hypopharynx cancer report past cigarette use.[6] Alcohol appears to potentiate the carcinogenic effects of tobacco. Additionally, alcohol consumption at medium to high levels for a long period of time can increase the likelihood of hypopharynx cancer in nonsmoking patients.[7] The index hypopharynx cancer often occurs within a field of diseased mucosa characterized by high-grade dysplasia. This "field cancerization" reflects widespread mucosal exposure to carcinogens and is responsible for the high rate of synchronous and metachronous primary tumors identified in patients with hypopharynx cancer. Successful counseling with particular emphasis on smoking cessation can enhance treatment tolerance and diminish the risk of developing subsequent cancers of the upper aerodigestive tract. Patients with occupational exposure to coal dust, steel dust, iron compounds, and fumes have also shown an increased risk for developing hypopharynx cancer.[8,9] Overall, the incidence of hypopharynx cancer has shown some gradual decline in the United States. From 1975 to 2001, the incidence decreased by approximately 35%, perhaps as a result of smoking cessation efforts.[10] Human papillomavirus (HPV) infection is well established as a risk factor for the development of squamous cell carcinoma (SCC) of the gynecologic tract, particularly the uterine cervix. The relation between HPV and H&N cancer is now becoming much better appreciated, particularly for cancers of the oropharynx, where it may approach 60% to 70% in some series. Studies have demonstrated that approximately 20% to 25% of patients with hypopharynx cancer test positive for HPV DNA,[11,12] and seropositivity for antibodies against the HPV-16

FIGURE 49.2. A: Posterior view of resected larynx and hypopharynx specimen afforded by incision through the posterior pharyngeal wall, cricopharyngeus, and cervical esophagus in the posterior midline. The aryepiglottic folds (*marked*) and arytenoids separate the pyriform sinuses (hypopharynx) from the larynx. **B:** The three primary anatomic subsites (posterior pharyngeal wall, postcricoid region, and pyriform sinuses) are revealed in this posterior view of the hypopharynx with the posterior pharyngeal wall incised.

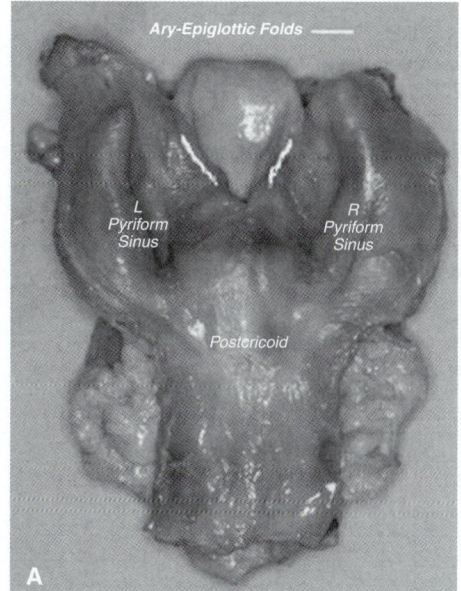

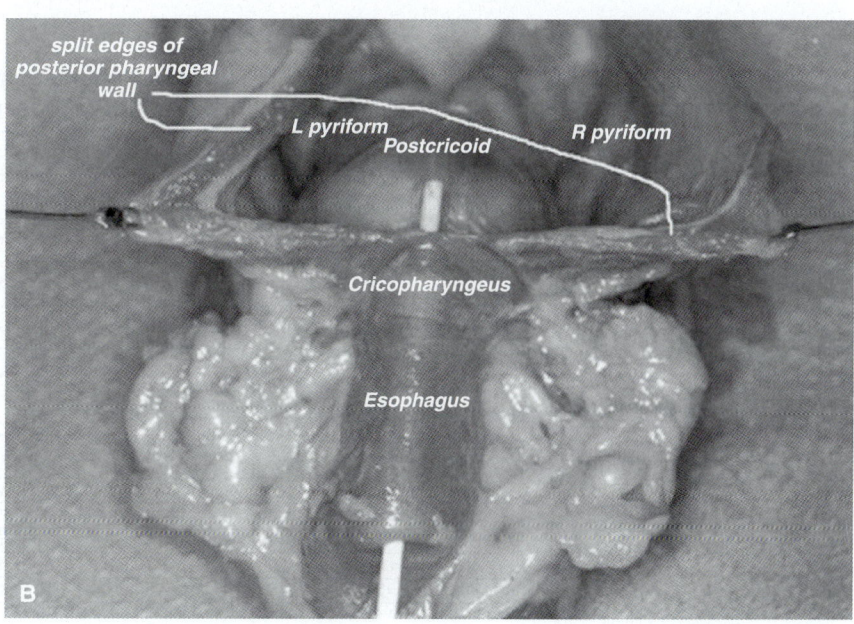

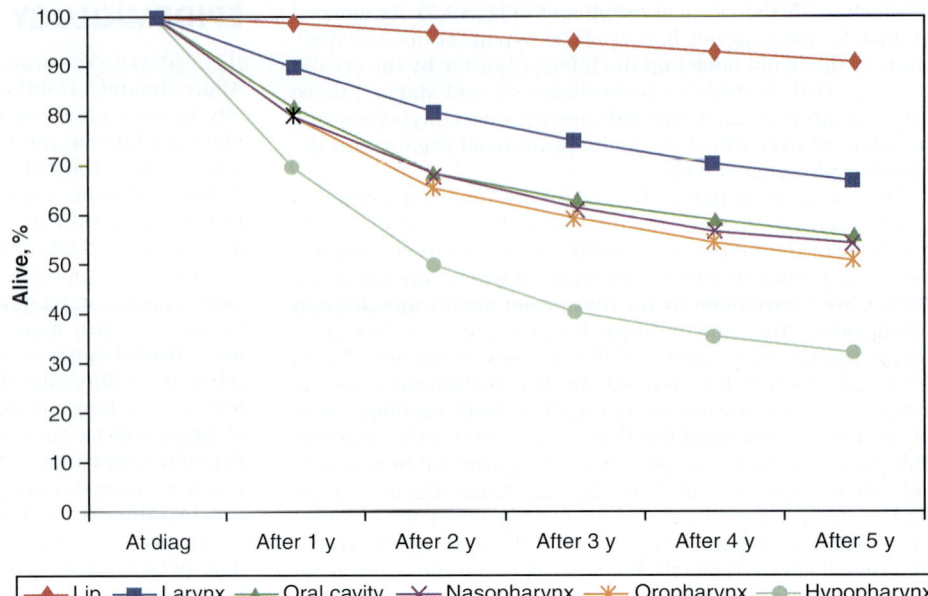

FIGURE 49.3. Five-year survival by mucosal site for head and neck cancers from 1990 to 1999 cases. (From Cooper JS, Porter K, Mallin K, et al. National Cancer Database report on cancer of the head and neck: 10-year update. *Head Neck* 2009;31[6]:748–758. Copyright © 2009 Wiley Periodicals, Inc. Reprinted by permission of John Wiley & Sons, Inc.)

E6 and E7 antibodies has been associated with a significantly elevated risk of hypopharyngeal cancer.[13] The clinical implications of the presence of HPV in hypopharynx cancer are yet to be defined.

There is a recognized increased risk of developing cancers of the postcricoid region for patients with Plummer-Vinson syndrome, characterized by iron deficiency anemia, hypopharyngeal webs, weight loss, and dysphagia.[7] Favorable changes in the epidemiology of hypopharynx cancer have resulted from changes in nutrition. The addition of iron to flour has made Plummer-Vinson syndrome quite rare in the upper Midwestern United States and Scandinavian countries where it was formerly more common. An associated decrease in hypopharynx cancer involving the postcricoid region has followed.

PROGNOSTIC FACTORS

Several prognostic factors have been identified for patients with hypopharynx cancer. Age, particularly older than 70 years, has been identified as an unfavorable predictor of outcome.[7] This may simply reflect the diminished likelihood of elderly patients to successfully tolerate the aggressive therapy approaches required for locoregionally advanced cancers of the H&N. Women have been found to achieve somewhat improved outcomes compared to men, although this may in part be a manifestation of earlier-stage disease at diagnosis.[14,15] In addition, tumor location has an impact on outcome, with cancers of the pyriform sinus generally faring better than those arising in the postcricoid or posterior pharyngeal wall regions.[14,15] As a whole, hypopharynx cancer patients fare poorly in comparison with patients harboring tumors from other H&N sites (Figs. 49.3 and 49.4).[4,16] To a lesser extent, tobacco, alcohol, medical comorbidities, and dietary factors may also have an impact on outcome.[17,18]

Biologic factors have been investigated for their potential role in hypopharyngeal cancer. The presence of p53 gene mutations has been associated with bulkier tumors and younger patients along with higher expression of the epidermal growth factor receptor (EGFR). However, p53 has not shown correlation with multiple primary tumors, tumor

FIGURE 49.4. Observed survival for hypopharyngeal cancer in the United States is calculated for new cases identified in the NCDB as an Aggregate Report from all CoC Hospitals (1233 programs) 2003 to 2009 and includes all pathologic types and the selected anatomic sites: C129, C130, C131, C132, C138, and C139. Staging according to sixth edition of the *AJCC Cancer Staging Handbook.* (From National Cancer Data Base. Commission on Cancer. American College of Surgeons for copyright from the National Cancer Database [NCDB] Survival Reports. Available at: https://m.facs.org/NCDB.SurvivalDS/app/index.html?guid=8989f6dc-9809-4603-8571-7b63548ee64e. Accessed April 17, 2017, with permission from the NCDB.)

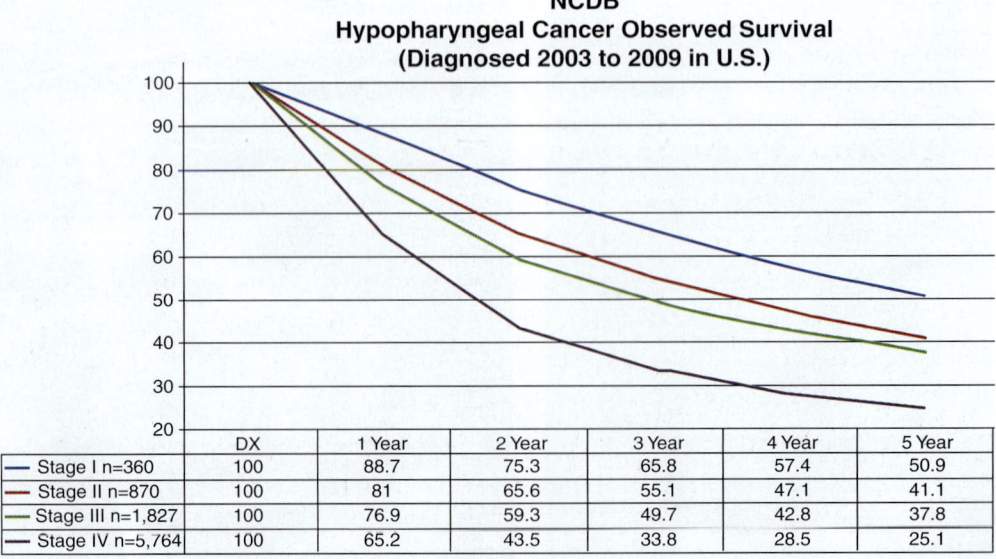

NCDB Hypopharyngeal Cancer Observed Survival (Diagnosed 2003 to 2009 in U.S.)

	DX	1 Year	2 Year	3 Year	4 Year	5 Year
Stage I n=360	100	88.7	75.3	65.8	57.4	50.9
Stage II n=870	100	81	65.6	55.1	47.1	41.1
Stage III n=1,827	100	76.9	59.3	49.7	42.8	37.8
Stage IV n=5,764	100	65.2	43.5	33.8	28.5	25.1

grade, or DNA ploidy.[19,20] Further, there are conflicting data regarding the prognostic significance of EGFR expression for patients with hypopharyngeal cancer.[21] Some studies suggest EGFR overexpression portends a worse prognosis for patients undergoing (chemo)radiotherapy but not for patients treated with primary surgical resection.[22,23]

STAGING

The primary staging system for hypopharynx cancer is the American Joint Committee on Cancer's (AJCC) 2016 eighth edition of the *AJCC Cancer Staging Handbook* and is based on a combination of clinical and radiographic data (Table 49.1).[24] There were no significant changes made between the seventh and eighth editions regarding primary tumor criteria (T-stage) and clinical stage groupings. However, in the eighth edition, the nodal group staging now incorporates extranodal extension (ENE), which constitutes N3b disease regardless of nodal size or laterality. Although AJCC staging is a very useful tool to broadly group similar cancer types, it should not be used as a blueprint for management. Patient factors, including age, comorbid medical conditions, and motivation for organ preservation, are beyond the scope of the staging system but nevertheless represent important factors for consideration with each individual patient.

PATTERNS OF SPREAD

Local Extension

It is sometimes difficult to definitively assign tumor origin to a specific subsite in the hypopharynx when the tumor overlaps more than one subsite. Of the hypopharynx cancer cases recorded in the National Cancer Institute's SEER database between 2000 and 2008, 83% of tumors with a known subsite arose in the pyriform sinus. An additional 9% arose from the posterior pharyngeal wall, and 4% originated in the postcricoid region.[5] Because of the high propensity for advanced primary disease as well as regional nodal involvement, the majority of hypopharynx cancer patients present with stages III and IV disease. In a retrospective study from Washington University, 87% of patients with cancers of the pyriform sinus and 82% of patients with posterior pharyngeal wall tumors presented with stage III or IV disease.[25]

Cancers arising from the pyriform sinus may spread superiorly to involve the aryepiglottic folds and arytenoids and invade the paraglottic and preepiglottic space. Lateral tumor extension can involve portions of the thyroid cartilage, allowing entry into the lateral compartment of the neck. High-resolution computed tomography (CT) or magnetic resonance imaging (MRI) is often useful for optimal assessment regarding the extent of tumor invasion. For tumors arising from the medial wall, the most common site of involvement for pyriform sinus tumors, there is a likelihood of tumor involvement of intrinsic muscles of the larynx resulting in vocal cord fixation. Inferior tumor extension beyond the apex can involve the thyroid gland.

Cancers arising within the postcricoid region can extend circumferentially to involve the cricoid cartilage or anteriorly to involve the larynx with resultant vocal cord fixation. Tumor involvement of the recurrent laryngeal nerve can also precipitate vocal cord fixation. Primary postcricoid tumors are often quite extensive and can involve the pyriform sinus, trachea, or esophagus. As a result, these tumors generally carry a worse prognosis in comparison to tumors from other subsites of the hypopharynx.[14] Nodal spread to the paratracheal nodes and inferior deep cervical nodes is not uncommon. Tumors arising from the posterior pharyngeal wall can extend to involve the oropharynx superiorly, the cervical esophagus inferiorly, and the prevertebral fascia and retropharyngeal space posteriorly.

Many cancers of the hypopharynx have a propensity for submucosal spread. It can therefore be difficult to accurately quantify the full microscopic extent of disease. This is particularly true for cancers of the posterior pharyngeal wall and postcricoid regions. Careful study through serial sectioning of surgical specimens has identified that 60% of hypopharynx cancers demonstrate subclinical spread with a range of 10 mm superiorly, 25 mm medially, 20 mm laterally, and 20 mm inferiorly.[26] This extensive pattern of tumor infiltration can present considerable challenge in the effort to achieve clear surgical margins or full dosimetric coverage with radiotherapy.

Regional Disease

Because of the rich lymphatic drainage of the hypopharynx, more than 50% of patients will manifest clinically positive cervical lymph nodes at the time of diagnosis, and ultimately, 65% to 80% of patients will have nodal involvement, as 30% to 40% of N0 necks harbor micrometastatic disease when electively dissected.[27] Jugular chain nodes, levels II to IV, as well as retropharyngeal nodes are all at high risk of harboring regional metastases in patients with hypopharynx cancer. Postcricoid tumors may also spread directly to pre- and paratracheal nodal basins. In light of cross-draining lymphatics, there is a significant risk of bilateral cervical node metastasis (Fig. 49.5).[28,29]

Distant Metastases

The most common site for distant metastasis to develop in patients with cancer of the hypopharynx is the lung. Previously, approximately one-quarter of patients diagnosed with hypopharynx cancer presented with distant metastases, although this incidence in more recent reports is estimated at approximately 16%.[30] For those patients not rendered free of locoregional disease following initial therapy, the incidence of distant metastases increases notably with the length of time following initial treatment.[31]

Field Cancerization

Carcinogens can induce dysplastic changes throughout the mucosa of the upper aerodigestive tract, leading to an increased risk for field cancerization that enhances the likelihood of synchronous or metachronous secondary primary tumors. Approximately 7% of patients with hypopharynx cancer will manifest a second primary tumor at initial diagnosis and between 10% and 20% will develop a secondary primary tumor over time. In fact, this second tumor risk is a significant cause of mortality in patients who survive more than 2 years following initial treatment.[6]

TABLE 49.1 AMERICAN JOINT COMMITTEE ON CANCER 2010 T STAGING FOR HYPOPHARYNX CANCER

T-Stage	Description
T1	Limited to 1 subsite of the hypopharynx and ≤2 cm in greatest dimension
T2	Tumor invades more than 1 subsite of the hypopharynx or an adjacent site, or measures >2 cm but ≤4 cm in greatest diameter without fixation of hemilarynx
T3	Tumor measures >4 cm in greatest dimension or with fixation of hemilarynx or with extension to the esophagus
T4a	Invades thyroid/cricoid cartilage, hyoid bone, thyroid gland, or central compartment soft tissue, which includes prelaryngeal strap muscles and subcutaneous fat
T4b	Tumor invades prevertebral fascia, encases carotid artery, or involves mediastinal structures

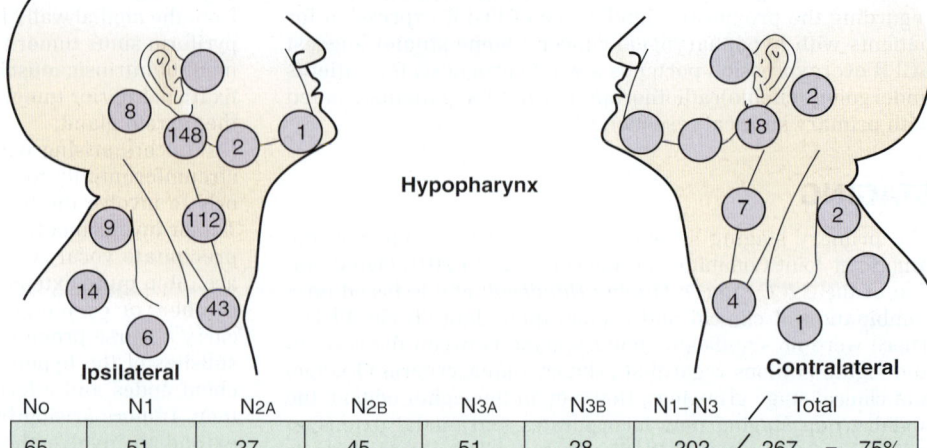

FIGURE 49.5. Nodal distribution patterns for a series of 267 patients with hypopharynx cancer as summarized by admission records at the M.D. Anderson Cancer Center. (From Lindberg R. Distribution of cervical lymph node metastases from squamous cell carcinoma of the upper respiratory and digestive tracts. *Cancer* 1972;29[6]:1446–1449. Copyright © 1972 American Cancer Society. Reprinted by permission of John Wiley & Sons, Inc.)

No	N1	N2A	N2B	N3A	N3B	N1–N3	/	Total	
65	51	27	45	51	28	202	/	267	= 75%

CLINICAL PRESENTATION

In light of the nonspecific nature of early symptoms, the majority of patients with cancers of the hypopharynx present with advanced local or regional disease. Frequently, there is a delay between presentation and diagnosis as patients are often managed for presumed infectious or gastrointestinal etiology. The majority of symptoms are related to local tumor spread, including dysphagia and odynophagia. There may be frank pharyngeal obstruction, invasion of constrictor muscles, prevertebral space invasion, or strap muscle invasion. Common presenting signs and symptoms include dysphagia, sore throat, hoarseness, weight loss >10 pounds, and neck mass. The majority of patients present with more than one of these signs and symptoms.[32] Roughly 25% of patients will present with clinical stage III disease and 50% with clinical stage IV disease; however, reflux symptoms can be a common presentation leading to diagnosis of stage I or II hypopharyngeal tumors.[6] Selected patients may first come to medical attention with complaints of unilateral ear pain (referred otalgia) due to tumor involvement of the visceral sensory nerves of the pharynx.

Pretreatment Evaluation and Staging Workup

A comprehensive workup for patients with cancers of the hypopharynx should include a detailed history focusing on the duration of symptoms, amount of weight loss, the presence of otalgia, changes in voice quality, and degree of dysphagia. A previous history of another upper aerodigestive tract malignancy and a history of tobacco smoking are commonly associated. The physical examination should include direct and indirect visualization of the full laryngopharyngeal axis with particular attention to the size, location, and anatomic positioning of the primary tumor as well as the mobility status of the true vocal cords. Dentition and oral health should be assessed. If the patient presents with cervical adenopathy, the size, number, location, texture, and mobility of these nodes should be documented.

Although cervical adenopathy associated with hypopharynx cancer may be analyzed with fine needle aspiration (FNA) biopsy, there is little value in this approach, because most patients will receive advanced radiographic imaging to further define the nodal involvement. On rare occasions, FNA may be useful to help distinguish other coexisting causes of lymphadenopathy such as lymphoma. Most patients will undergo a direct laryngoscopy under general anesthesia in conjunction with esophagoscopy. This panendoscopy allows not only biopsy confirmation of the primary tumor site but also mapping of the extent of the tumor as well as the ability to survey for synchronous primary tumors (Fig. 49.6A). Use of transnasal fiber-optic techniques makes it possible for a

FIGURE 49.6. A: Outpatient clinic photograph taken through a rigid endoscope mounted with a 35-mm camera of a newly diagnosed exophytic T2 tumor arising from the right pyriform sinus with involvement of the adjacent aryepiglottic fold. There was no compromise of vocal cord mobility, and clinical staging of the primary lesion was T2. **B:** Photographic examination 1 year following 70-Gy radiation and concurrent cisplatin chemotherapy with complete tumor regression and excellent functional status of the laryngopharynx. Note mild to moderate mucosal edema of supraglottic structures following high-dose radiation.

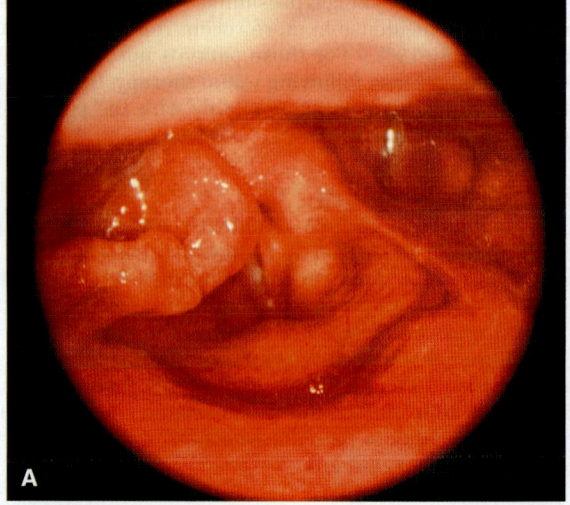

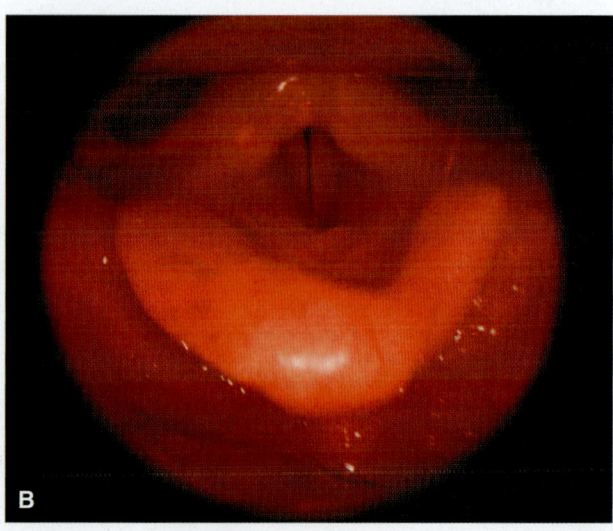

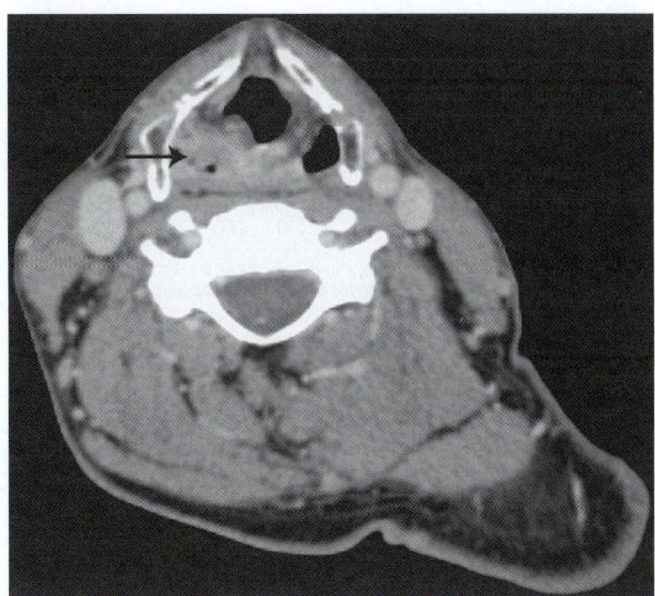

FIGURE 49.7. Axial computed tomography image from the same case as in Figure 49.6, depicting the T2 hypopharynx tumor involving the right pyriform sinus.

TABLE 49.2 COMPARISON OF VARIOUS MODALITIES FOR STAGING

	Sensitivity (%)		Specificity (%)	
	T	**N**	**T**	**N**
Panendoscopy	95	–	85	–
PET	95	84	92	90
CDDS	74	84	75	96
CT	68	84	69	88
Palpation	–	63	–	96

CDDS, color-coded duplex sonography; CT, computed tomography; PET, positron emission tomography.
Adapted with permission from Di Martino E, Nowak B, Hassan HA, et al. Diagnosis and staging of head and neck cancer: a comparison of modern imaging modalities (positron emission tomography, computed tomography, color-coded duplex sonography) with panendoscopic and histopathologic findings. *Arch Otolaryngol Head Neck Surg* 2000;126(12):1457–1461. Copyright © 2000 American Medical Association. All rights reserved.

panendoscopy to be done for selected patients without anesthesia in the clinic setting.

In addition to panendoscopy, patients should undergo either high-resolution CT with contrast or MRI extending from the skull base to below the clavicle to help assess the extent of the primary tumor and to quantitatively and qualitatively assess cervical adenopathy (Figs. 49.7 and 49.8).[29] Although a chest x-ray has traditionally been used to assess for the presence of pulmonary metastasis, 18-fluorodeoxyglucose positron emission tomography ([18]FDG-PET) imaging (with accompanying CT for coregistration) is increasingly used to assess the extent of regional adenopathy and to survey for the presence of distant metastasis. FDG-PET is becoming an increasingly valuable adjunct to CT or MRI in the radiation treatment planning process, particularly for patients treated with conformal intensity-modulated radiation therapy (IMRT) or tomotherapy

techniques. Di Martino et al.[32] compared CT, PET, color-coded duplex sonography, palpation, and panendoscopy in assessment of tumor and nodal status. The results of this study are summarized in Table 49.2 and support the promising sensitivity and specificity of PET scanning in H&N cancers. Schwartz et al.[33] examined standardized uptake value (SUV) of primary and nodal metastasis in H&N cancer patients and their relationship to clinical outcome. A primary tumor SUV >9.0 was associated with a significantly lower local recurrence-free survival and disease-free survival. However, there was no correlation between nodal SUV and clinical outcome.

A recent prospective multicenter study of 233 H&N SCC patients (including 46 hypopharyngeal cancer) highlighted the potential impact of PET imaging on H&N SCC management.[34] TNM staging and therapeutic decisions were first determined based on conventional workup, and then physicians were unblinded to FDG-PET data and asked to restage the patients and reanalyze their therapeutic decisions. PET and conventional workup revealed discordant TNM staging in 100 patients (43%). PET was deemed significantly more accurate than conventional staging and improved the staging in 20% of patients. Incorporation of PET data ultimately impacted management in 32 patients (13.7%) (Table 49.3), supporting the use of FDG-PET in H&N SCC staging.

Many patients with hypopharynx cancer present with concurrent medical and social comorbidities that require consideration before initiating cancer-directed therapy. Commonly, there is a progressive history of dysphagia and odynophagia with associated weight loss. Whether these patients are treated with surgical or nonsurgical approaches, a gastrostomy tube

FIGURE 49.8. Axial gadolinium-enhanced T1-weighted magnetic resonance image scan with fat saturation depicting metastatic lateral retropharyngeal node with evidence of central necrosis and peripheral enhancement.

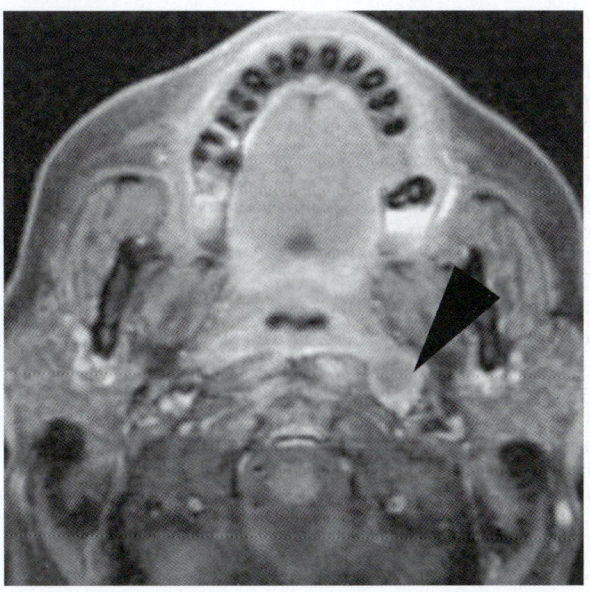

TABLE 49.3 IMPACT OF FDG-PET ON STAGING, MANAGEMENT FOLLOWING CONVENTIONAL WORKUP

End Point	Impact of FDG-PET on 233 Patients
Discordant TNM stage	100 (43%)
PET accurately upstaged	30 (13%)
PET accurately downstaged	17 (7.3%)
PET inaccurately changed stage	13 (5.6%)
No confirmed gold standard TNM	40 (17%)
***Impact on Patient Management*[a]**	
Low	188 patients (80.7%)
Medium	12 patients (5.2%)
High	20 patients (8.6%)

[a]Impact ratings: low, treatment modality and delivery unchanged; medium, change within the same treatment modality (planned procedure, dose, or mode of administration changed); high, change in treatment intent or treatment modality (e.g., curative to palliation, surgery to chemoradiation, and so on). FDG, fluorodeoxyglucose; PET, positron emission tomography; TNM, tumor–node–metastasis classification.
Adapted with permission from Lonneux M, Hamoir M, Reychler H, et al. Positron emission tomography with [18F]fluorodeoxyglucose improves staging and patient management in patients with head and neck squamous cell carcinoma: a multicenter prospective study. *J Clin Oncol* 2010;28(7):1190–1195. Copyright © 2010 American Society of Clinical Oncology. All rights reserved.

Section III

may need to be considered as a temporary measure. It is important to optimize or at least stabilize the patient's nutritional status prior to initiating definitive therapy.

It is valuable for hypopharynx cancer patients to undergo evaluation by a speech and swallow therapist to determine the degree of dysfunction prior to therapy. This may be done as a bedside study of swallowing capacity, a fiber-optic endoscopic evaluation of swallowing, or (usually preferably) through the more definitive fluoroscopic barium swallow study. This modified barium swallow study is called a cookie swallow, video pharyngogram, or oropharyngeal motility study and is most commonly done with a speech pathologist in attendance. If objective swallowing dysfunction is present, patients may be taught adaptive techniques to improve the effectiveness and safety of their oral intake. Additionally, close follow-up with the same speech and swallow therapist is highly desirable during and after therapy to maximize the patient's long-term functional capabilities.

Because many hypopharynx patients have an active history of alcohol and tobacco use, it is important to counsel accordingly and encourage all patients to take advantage of methods and programs to facilitate smoking and alcohol cessation. All patients should undergo comprehensive dental evaluation and cleaning as well as basic education regarding oral hygiene. For patients treated with conventional radiation therapy techniques, there is a significant likelihood of long-term xerostomia that can promote dental decay. If existing dentition is in poor condition, dental extractions should be considered prior to therapy, particularly for teeth that will reside within the high-dose radiation region. Typically, 10 to 14 days are required following dental extractions to allow for healing prior to the initiation of radiation therapy. Custom fluoride carrier trays should be fabricated and discussed for long-term use in an effort to diminish the rate of dental decay for patients with chronic xerostomia.

Finally, many patients with hypopharynx cancer will have social issues, including lack of family support, financial limitations, transportation issues, poor nutrition, and hygiene habits that may hamper their ability to successfully receive adequate care. Often, the involvement of a case manager or social worker is of central importance to assist patients who require support both during as well as following cancer therapy.

PATHOLOGIC CLASSIFICATION

In SEER data from 2000 to 2008, 93.9% of hypopharynx cancers were SCC, with lymphoma, sarcoma, adenocarcinoma, and adenoid cystic carcinoma each accounting for approximately 0.5% of cases.[5] Similarly, the National Cancer Data Base (NCDB) Benchmark Reports evaluated 17,654 cases of hypopharyngeal cancer in the United States between the years of 2000 and 2008. Over 90% of cases were SCC.[16]

Management

For patients presenting with early-stage, resectable disease, voice-preserving surgery and definitive radiotherapy alone are viable and acceptable treatment options. The vast majority of patients, however, present with stage III or IV disease and warrant multimodality treatment. Recent analysis of the SEER database reveals a gradual trend away from primary surgery and toward definitive radiation without a decrement in overall survival.[35] A key consideration in determining the favored approach for these patients is the likelihood and motivation to preserve laryngopharyngeal function (Table 49.4).

Primary Surgery

T1 and T2 Tumors

Contemporary indications for primary surgical management of patients with early cancers of the hypopharynx include

TABLE 49.4 GENERAL TREATMENT RECOMMENDATIONS BASED ON HYPOPHARYNX TUMOR STAGE

Stage I	Radiation alone or voice preservation surgery if feasible
Stage II	Radiation alone
Stage III and IV with functional laryngopharynx	Concurrent chemoradiation followed by selective neck dissection
Stage III and IV with dysfunctional laryngopharynx[a]	Laryngopharyngectomy with adjuvant RT or CRT

[a]Patients with bulky, destructive tumors that severely compromise the airway or destroy cartilage, bone, and deep soft tissue are often best served with immediate laryngopharyngectomy and postoperative radiation or chemoradiation.
CRT, chemoradiation therapy; RT, radiation therapy.

those with a history of previous H&N radiation, those in whom organ conservation approaches are deemed possible, and those who refuse radiation. Even for hypopharynx cancer patients who will receive nonoperative treatment approaches, it remains critical for the H&N surgeon to remain actively involved. The role of the surgeon in these cases may include endoscopic biopsy with detailed assessment of tumor extent, methods to secure the airway (tracheotomy or laser debulking), and methods to ensure adequate nutrition (gastrostomy). The surgeon will also play a vital role in multidisciplinary oncologic follow-up after nonoperative treatment.

Selected T1 and T2 hypopharynx cancers may lend themselves to surgical excision. These favorable subsites include the upper pyriform sinus and the posterior pharyngeal wall. The standard supraglottic laryngectomy encompasses the aryepiglottic fold and may be extended to include part of the arytenoids, the base of the tongue, and the upper pyriform sinus. Small cancers isolated to the posterior pharyngeal wall may be removed by endoscopic laser resection or removal using an open approach. Dysphagia requiring nothing by mouth status is common from an open approach, especially if reconstruction of the posterior wall is effected with an adynamic and insensate free flap. Relative contraindications to organ conservation surgery for hypopharynx cancers include cartilage invasion, vocal fold fixation, postcricoid invasion, deep pyriform sinus invasion, and extension beyond the larynx.

Innovations with free flap reconstruction have allowed retention of speech, swallowing, and breathing functions of the larynx despite extensive resection by way of a hemilaryngopharyngectomy. The temporoparietal flap and radial forearm free flap coupled with rigid cartilaginous support have been employed to retain function in patients with hypopharynx cancers without extension to the postcricoid region or apex of the pyriform sinus.[36]

In recent years, advancements in organ preservation surgery have included the use of transoral laser microsurgery and transoral robotic surgery (TORS). For selected cases, these approaches can achieve oncologic tumor removal while limiting normal tissue disruption, thereby potentially avoiding tracheostomy and the use of feeding tubes.[37–40] This approach may involve concurrent or delayed neck dissection following transoral resection of the primary lesion (to allow for final margin assessment). The necks in some T1N0 patients may be observed with close interval follow-up CT scans. Adjuvant (chemo)radiotherapy is utilized in the majority of patients using this approach (see "Postoperative Radiotherapy" below for indications) and should generally encompass the primary tumor site as well as bilateral necks and supraclavicular fossae. Recent results have demonstrated that appropriately selected T1 or T2 lesions can achieve negative margins by transoral laser microsurgery or TORS.[38] Oncologic outcomes appear similar to open surgical approaches using this technique and are likely accompanied by lower rates of permanent gastrostomy tube or tracheostomy placement (Table 49.5).

TABLE 49.5 FIVE-YEAR ONCOLOGIC OUTCOMES FOR TRANSORAL MICROLASER SURGERY FOR T1 OR T2 HYPOPHARYNGEAL TUMORS

Study (Reference)	T-Stage	N	Node (+)	LC	DSS	OS	Permanent Gastrostomies	Permanent Tracheostomies
Martin et al.[39]	pT1	20	62%	84%	NR	68% (stage I–II)	3.5%[a]	3.5%[a]
	pT2	48		70%	NR			
Karatzanis et al.[38]	pT1	45	56%	90%	78%	NR	0	0
	pT2	74	64%	83%	70%	NR	4%	2.5%

[a]Entire cohort, including T3 and T4 patients.

DSS, disease-specific survival; LC, local control; NR, not reported; OS, 5-year overall survival.

Transoral robotic surgery is currently approved by the Food and Drug Administration (FDA) for treatment of benign and malignant tumors classified as T1 and T2, as well as benign base of tongue resection procedures. Compared to TLM, it has the advantage of better visualization with a three-dimensional magnified camera, the option to utilized angled endoscopes, and manipulation using "wristed" instruments, which provide the means to resect tumor en bloc. Traditionally, dissection is performed with a grasping instrument and monopolar cautery; however, flexible fiber-optic CO_2 laser delivery may also be utilized via the robotic instrument cart.[41] These instruments provide the means to achieve oncologic tumor removal while limiting tissue disruption, thereby avoiding tracheostomy and feeding tubes. Neck dissection can be done concurrently or staged. Early studies demonstrated oncologic outcomes similar to open approaches.[42]

More recent literature has further supported the efficacy and safety of TORS in treating early-stage hypopharyngeal cancer and continued to demonstrate ability to achieve negative margins in the hypopharynx for T1 and T2 lesions while avoiding tracheostomy and preserving the larynx. The majority of patients in these recent series have functional swallow and voice outcomes as well.[43,44]

The main limitations in TORS are determining whether the tumor is safely resectable, and the ability to gain adequate exposure to visualize the extent of the tumor. As the technology evolves and surgeons build experience with these procedures, additional data will emerge to describe long-term outcome results for patients with early-stage hypopharyngeal cancers.[45]

T3 or T4 Resectable Tumors

Favorable T3 hypopharynx cancers that present in the upper aspect of the pyriform sinus and allow full extirpation by either an extended supraglottic laryngectomy or extended vertical partial laryngopharyngectomy with free flap reconstruction are infrequent. Most T3 and T4 hypopharynx cancers that are treated surgically will require total laryngectomy with efforts to preserve a posterior strip of the hypopharynx spanning the oropharynx to the esophagus. This preserved posterior wall of the hypopharynx may be tubed and closed on itself in selected cases. In the past, it was common practice to accept primary reconstruction of this segment as adequate for swallowing if closure over a nasogastric tube was possible. More recently, primary closure has been discouraged for cases with less than a 3- to 3.5-cm width of posterior pharyngeal wall mucosa to tube on itself. Most commonly superior swallowing results when the anterior and lateral walls of the remaining hypopharynx are reconstructed with a pedicled or free flap.

For more bulky tumors of the hypopharynx, total laryngopharyngectomy, removal of the larynx and the entire hypopharynx, is required. This procedure creates a gap between the oropharynx and esophagus that must be reconstructed with a tubed fasciocutaneous flap such as the radial forearm free flap or anterolateral thigh flap, a free jejunum, or a tubed pedicled myocutaneous flap. The myocutaneous flaps are technically difficult to tube because of the bulk of the fat and muscle underlying the skin paddle.

Laryngopharyngectomy with esophagectomy may be performed if the hypopharynx cancer extends inferior to the cricopharyngeus to ensure the inferior margin. In this case, gastric pull-up and colon interposition are reconstructive options used to restore the conduit for food and saliva extending from the oropharynx to the stomach.

Palliative Surgery

For patients with incurable, metastatic disease at presentation, or with symptomatic local recurrence not amenable to curative salvage therapy attempts, surgery can play an important role in palliation. If aspiration of secretions (despite nothing by mouth status and enteral feedings) persists, laryngopharyngectomy may afford a reasonable option to discuss with the patient and family members. Similarly, complete stenosis of the pharynx or upper esophagus due to tumor (or following treatment) may leave a patient with the constant need for suctioning his or her own secretions. In selected patients, laryngopharyngectomy with gastric pull-up may be a reasonable palliative option. Finally, gastric feeding tube placement can be considered for patients who do not wish to pursue palliative radiation therapy or surgery.

Postoperative Radiation Therapy

Most advanced hypopharynx cancers that are treated with initial surgical resection have unfavorable features that warrant the addition of postoperative radiation therapy in an effort to enhance locoregional control rates. Classical indications for postoperative radiation include T4 primary tumors, close or positive microscopic margins, cartilage or bony invasion, more than one metastatic lymph node, or the presence of extracapsular extension (ECE). Conventional therapy involves the use of a shrinking field technique to deliver 54 to 63 Gy to all areas at risk and a boost to 60 to 66 Gy to regions of ECE or positive margins. The entire cervical nodal chain from the skull base to the clavicle bilaterally should be included. IMRT techniques may be considered in an attempt to reduce radiation dose to normal tissue structures such as the contralateral parotid gland and thereby preserve better salivary function.

The Radiation Therapy Oncology Group (RTOG) and European Organization for Research and Treatment of Cancer (EORTC) have evaluated the role of concurrent chemotherapy along with postoperative radiation in prospective randomized trials. Eligibility criteria in the RTOG trial included patients with two or more positive nodes, ECE, or microscopically positive margins. All patients received 60 Gy alone or with concurrent cisplatin 100 mg/m^2 every 3 weeks. This trial demonstrated an improvement in locoregional control and disease-free survival for patients who received concurrent chemoradiotherapy. However, no significant benefit in absolute survival was confirmed (Table 49.6).[46] The EORTC conducted a similar trial that included patients with stage III (except T3N0 larynx), stage IV, and patients with stage I or II with positive margins, lymphovascular invasion, and perineural invasion. All patients received 66 Gy alone or with cisplatin at 100 mg/m^2 every 3 weeks. This trial demonstrated a significant improvement in progression-free survival and overall survival with the addition of chemotherapy (Table 49.7).[47] A subsequently published *post hoc* analysis of the combined data from these trials suggested that patients with ECE and positive margins were most likely to benefit

TABLE 49.6 RESULTS OF RTOG POSTOP CHEMORADIATION TRIAL

	Arm 1[a] (%)	Arm 2[b] (%)	P
2-yr LRC	72	82	.003
2-yr DM	23	20	NS

[a]Arm 1: 60 Gy in 6 weeks.
[b]Arm 2: 60 Gy in 6 weeks with concurrent cisplatin (100 mg/m²) days 1, 22, and 43.
DM, distant metastasis; LRC, locoregional control; NS, not significant; RTOG, Radiation Therapy Oncology Group.
From Cooper JS, Pajak TF, Forastiere AA, et al. Postoperative concurrent radiotherapy and chemotherapy for high-risk squamous-cell carcinoma of the head and neck. *N Engl J Med* 2004;350(19): 1937–1944. Copyright © 2004 Massachusetts Medical Society. Adapted with permission from Massachusetts Medical Society.

from the addition of chemotherapy, whereas those with two or more involved lymph nodes without ECE as their only risk factor did not appear to benefit from the addition of chemotherapy.[48]

Although the studies above identify that the addition of cisplatin chemotherapy to postoperative radiation can improve tumor control outcome for specific categories of high-risk patients, it is clear that this modest benefit comes at the expense of additional toxicity. Careful clinical judgment regarding the selection of patients most likely to tolerate and thereby benefit from this approach is warranted. A recently updated meta-analysis demonstrated similar modest benefit from the addition of concurrent chemotherapy in the postoperative setting as compared to the definitive setting. However, this analysis showed that patients older than 70 years of age derive little to no benefit from the addition of systemic chemotherapy to radiation in H&N cancer.[49] The inadvertent introduction of treatment breaks during the adjuvant radiation course can easily compromise the potential benefits of the combined modality therapy in this setting.

Definitive Radiation Therapy

T1 and T2 Tumors

Curative radiation therapy (RT) is generally the preferred treatment option for patients with T1 or T2 hypopharynx tumors (see Table 46.4). This approach affords good potential for organ preservation without compromise in clinical outcome. A classical course of radiation therapy for hypopharynx cancer lasts 6 to 7 weeks, with treatment delivered 5 days per week. *A review of published clinical results of definitive radiation therapy for H&N cancer suggests a significant loss of local control with prolongation of overall radiation treatment time; therefore, interruptions in treatment once underway should be avoided whenever possible.*[50,51]

Conventional treatment involves a shrinking field technique that initiates with opposed lateral fields encompassing the primary tumor and upper neck lymphatics with a matched anterior field to complete treatment of the lower neck (Table 49.8). One of the most common worldwide fractionation regimens involves the delivery of 2 Gy daily fractions to

TABLE 49.8 GENERAL ANATOMIC LANDMARKS FOR FIELD DESIGN USING CONVENTIONAL HEAD AND NECK RADIOTHERAPY FOR HYPOPHARYNX CANCER

Border	Description
Superior	Include base of skull
Posterior	Behind vertebral spinous processes (or further if required to cover metastatic cervical lymph nodes)
Inferior	Lower aspect of cricoid cartilage unless extensive caudal tumor extension
Anterior	Flash skin at level of thyroid cartilage

For T1 lesions, classical dose is 66 to 70 Gy in 2 Gy daily fractions. For T2 to T4 lesions, consider altered fractionation regimens or concurrent cisplatin-based chemotherapy, particularly for patients over 70 years of age. Gross disease should generally receive 70 Gy with concurrent chemotherapy.

70 Gy over 7 weeks. Because of the high likelihood of subclinical nodal metastases even in the clinically N0 neck, patients traditionally receive comprehensive radiation to encompass nodal regions from the skull base to the clavicle. Because of the varying thicknesses of the head and neck, custom compensators or wedges should be used for the lateral fields to improve dose homogeneity. Shrinking field techniques to spare direct spinal cord dose after approximately 45 Gy, as well as final mucosal reductions after 54 to 60 Gy, are often appropriate with posterior neck boosting, with electrons to supplement posterior chain nodal dosing without excessive dose to the spinal cord.

SCCs of the H&N are rapidly proliferating tumors. There has been significant interest over the past several decades in the use of intensified radiation fractionation schedules to counter rapid tumor cell repopulation as a means of improving outcomes in H&N cancer patients treated with radiation alone. Altered fractionation techniques, including hyperfractionation (e.g., 1.1 to 1.4 Gy twice daily) and accelerated fractionation (e.g., 6 fraction per week or concomitant boost regimens), have demonstrated improved locoregional control rates for H&N cancer patients.[52–54] A meta-analysis examined 15 trials that compared conventional fractionation to altered fractionation, either hyperfractionation or accelerated fractionation. This meta-analysis demonstrated a small but statistically significant survival benefit of 3.4% at 5 years with altered fractionation. The benefit was higher with hyperfractionation compared to accelerated fractionation and was more pronounced for patients younger than age 50.[55]

Early T-stage hypopharynx patients with N0 or N1 neck disease can be considered for treatment with radiation alone or concurrent radiation plus chemotherapy. In this setting, gross disease should receive 70 Gy and the contralateral neck (N0) should receive 50 to 54 Gy. With T1N0 lesions, patients may achieve 5-year disease-specific survival (DSS) on the order of 90%, whereas T2N0 lesions may achieve DSS above 70% (Tables 49.9 and 49.10).[56–60]

TABLE 49.7 RESULTS OF EORTC POSTOPERATIVE CHEMORADIATION TRIAL

	Arm 1[a]		Arm 2[b]		P
	Median	5 Year	Median	5 Year	
PFS	23 mo	36%	55 mo	47%	0.04
OS	32 mo	40%	72 mo	53%	0.02

[a]Arm 1: RT alone 66 Gy in 6 ½ weeks.
[b]Arm 2: 66Gy in 6½ weeks with concurrent cisplatin (100 mg/m²) days 1, 22, and 43.
EORTC, European Organization for Research and Treatment of Cancer; OS, overall survival; PFS, progression-free survival.
From Bernier J, Domenge C, Ozsahin M, et al. Postoperative irradiation with or without concomitant chemotherapy for locally advanced head and neck cancer. *N Engl J Med* 2004;350(19):1945–1952. Copyright © 2004 Massachusetts Medical Society. Adapted with permission from Massachusetts Medical Society.

TABLE 49.9 LOCAL CONTROL FOR CARCINOMA OF THE POSTERIOR PHARYNGEAL WALL TREATED WITH RADIATION ALONE

Stage	Local Control after RT		Ultimate Local Control after Salvage	
	2 Year (%)	5 Year (%)	2 Year (%)	5 Year (%)
T1	100	100	100	100
T2	79	74	86	81
T3	59	49	66	66
T4	36	36	36	36

RT, radiation therapy.
Adapted from Amdur RJ, Mendenhall WM, Stringer SP, et al. Organ preservation with radiotherapy for T1-T2 carcinoma of the pyriform sinus. *Head Neck* 2001;23(5):353–362. Copyright © 2001 John Wiley & Sons, Inc. Reprinted by permission of John Wiley & Sons, Inc.

TABLE 49.10 CAUSE-SPECIFIC AND OVERALL SURVIVAL FOR CARCINOMA OF THE PYRIFORM SINUS TREATED WITH RADIATION ALONE

Stage	5-Year Cause-Specific Survival (%)	5-Year Overall Survival (%)
I	96	57
II		61
III	62	41
IVa	49	29
IVb	33	25

Adapted from Amdur RJ, Mendenhall WM, Stringer SP, et al. Organ preservation with radiotherapy for T1-T2 carcinoma of the pyriform sinus. *Head Neck* 2001;23(5):353–362. Copyright © 2001 John Wiley & Sons, Inc. Reprinted by permission of John Wiley & Sons, Inc.

The use of three-dimensional CT-based planning has become routine in the management of H&N cancer patients (Fig. 49.9). CT-based planning allows precise delineation of target volume and visualization of dose distributions (Fig. 49.10). In recent years, there has been significant increase in the use of IMRT in H&N cancer as a means of diminishing normal tissue toxicities, particularly xerostomia resulting from irradiation of major salivary glands. Excellent candidates for IMRT include patients with unilateral T1 to T3 primary lesions with N2b or less neck disease. In light of the high-dose gradients that can accompany highly conformal plans, a critical component of successful IMRT delivery is the use of an accurate and reproducible localization system. At several centers, the optically guided localization system is used to enhance treatment precision for patients undergoing IMRT for H&N cancer.[61] The cephalad margin of the N0 contralateral neck may often be limited to the C1-C2 interspace in an effort to further improve parotid gland sparing.[62,63] A recent randomized trial of conventional radiotherapy versus IMRT in patients with T1-4N0-3 oropharyngeal and hypopharyngeal tumors at high risk for xerostomia highlighted the benefits of IMRT for parotid sparing. Patients were treated either postoperatively or definitively, and the contralateral parotid was constrained to <24 Gy to the whole gland. Grade 2 or worse

FIGURE 49.9. Digitally reconstructed radiograph depicting a classical lateral field designed to encompass the T2 pyriform sinus cancer from Figures 49.6 and 49.7 plus bilateral cervical lymphatics from skull base to cricoid, with a matching anterior low-neck field to extend the lymphatic coverage to the level of the clavicle.

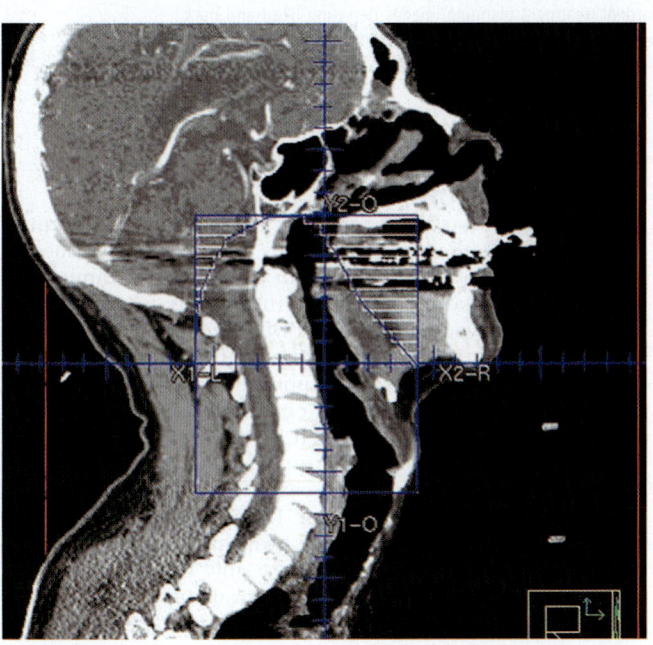

xerostomia was significantly reduced at both 12 months (74% conventional vs. 38% IMRT) and at 24 months (83% conventional vs. 29% IMRT).[64]

These benefits translated to significantly better quality-of-life scores in the IMRT group and strongly support a role for IMRT in H&N SCC radiotherapy.

T3 and T4 Tumors

There are several reasons why hypopharynx cancer patients who are technically resectable may not undergo primary surgery. These include age (e.g., patients over 70 to 80 years old), the presence of significant medical comorbidities, or patient unwillingness to accept total laryngectomy. Curative-intent radiation or chemoradiation is often pursued in these settings. Conventional radiation therapy commonly involves a shrinking three-field technique to deliver approximately 70 Gy in 2-Gy daily fractions to areas of gross disease and 50 to 60 Gy to areas of microscopic disease. If patients are scheduled to undergo postradiotherapy neck dissection, then gross nodal disease can be limited to 60 to 63 Gy. If patients are not candidates for postradiotherapy neck dissection, then gross nodal disease should be carried to 70 Gy. Altered fractionation regimens such as hyperfractionation or accelerated fractionation should be considered for patients being treated with radiation alone given the overall survival benefit observed with these approaches over standard fractionation in meta-analysis.[55]

In patients with adequate performance status, concurrent chemoradiation strategies using platinum-based chemotherapy should be considered. The updated meta-analysis to examine the benefit of chemotherapy in advanced H&N cancer confirms a significant survival advantage for the use of concomitant chemotherapy (6.5%), with the effect of single-agent platin significantly higher than other monochemotherapies.[49] However, this meta-analysis also confirms a steadily decreasing benefit for the use of chemotherapy with advancing patient age, such that no advantage is observed for patients over 70 years of age. This same loss of statistical benefit for patients over 70 years of age is also observed for the outcome gains derived from altered fractionation over conventional fractionation.[55] Therefore, once-daily radiation regimens without concurrent chemotherapy may be quite reasonable for hypopharynx patients over 70 years of age or for those patients with modest performance status.

Another alternative to concomitant chemotherapy or accelerated fractionation is the more recent introduction of molecular targeted therapies in the treatment of H&N cancer patients. The most mature clinical dataset in H&N cancer involves the use of EGFR inhibitors such as cetuximab (monoclonal antibody against the EGFR). An international phase III trial comparing high-dose radiation alone versus radiation plus cetuximab in advanced H&N cancer patients confirmed a locoregional control improvement (10% at 5 years) and overall survival advantage (10% at 5 years) with the addition of cetuximab.[65,66] A relatively small subset of patients with hypopharynx cancer was enrolled in this study of 424 patients, and this subset did not demonstrate a clear advantage with use of the EGFR inhibitor treatment. Ongoing trials to examine the potential value of adding cetuximab to concurrent chemoradiation approaches in advanced H&N cancer are in progress in both the definitive and high-risk postoperative settings.

Management of hypopharynx cancer has gradually evolved over the past decades to reflect the steady advancement of nonsurgical therapy. Data from the NCDB Benchmark Reports addressing 16,136 cases diagnosed in 2000 to 2008 reveal the combination of radiation and chemotherapy to be the most common initial treatment overall for stage II (32.6%),

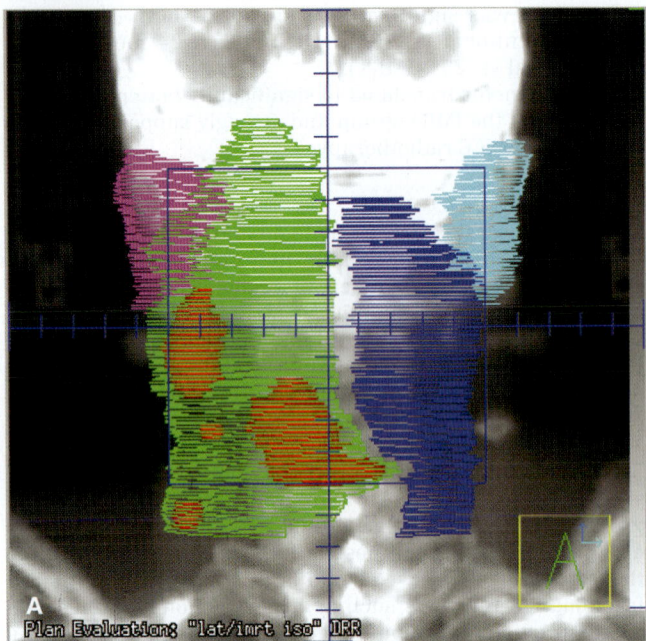
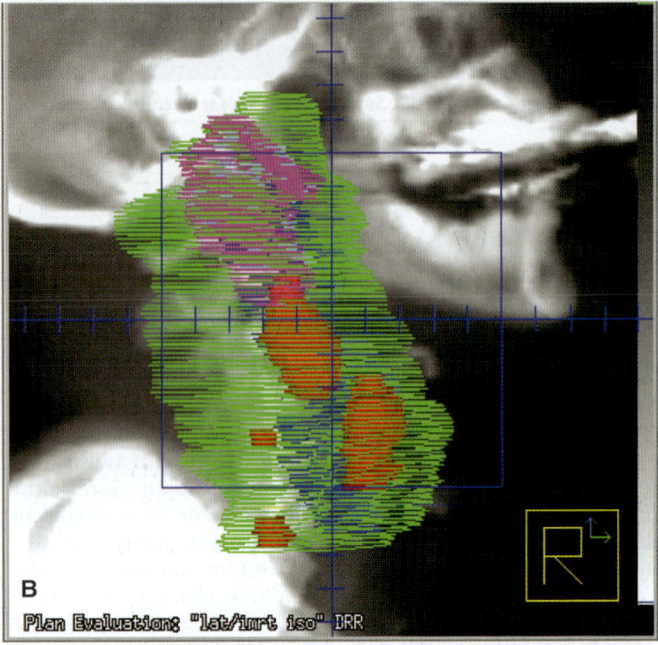

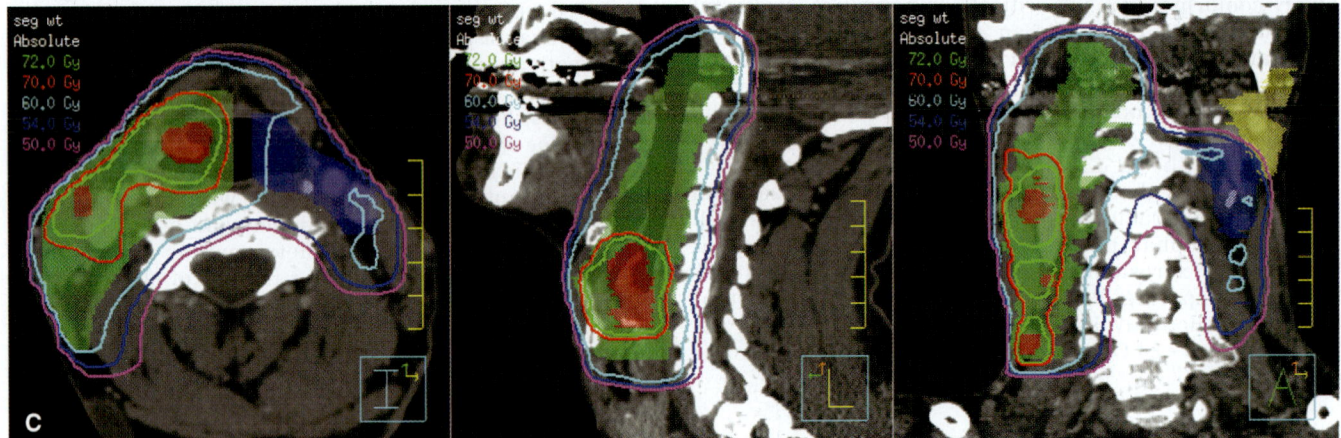

FIGURE 49.10. Beam's eye projections of intensity-modulated radiation therapy target contours for patient with T2N2bM0 tumor of the right pyriform sinus (same case as depicted in Figs. 49.6, 49.7 and 49.9). **A** and **B:** Depict anterior and lateral projections highlighting the GTV (*red,* 70 Gy), high-risk CTV1 (*green,* 60 Gy), low-risk CTV2 (*blue,* 54 Gy), and bilateral parotid glands. **C:** Demonstrates transverse, sagittal, and coronal treatment planning images depicting head and neck intensity-modulated radiation therapy isodose distributions for the same patient. The left parotid gland received a mean dose of 22 Gy.

stage III (47.8%), and stage IV (43.8%) disease (Fig. 49.11).[16] Over 50% of stage III and stage IV cases received initial treatment with chemotherapy in some form—either alone or in combination with radiation or surgery. Radiation as a single-modality therapy was the most common initial treatment for stage I hypopharynx cancer (24.4%), followed by surgery alone (21.0%) as the next most common. It has been reported that approximately 35% to 45% of patients with advanced hypopharyngeal tumors treated with concurrent chemoradiotherapy utilizing IMRT can be expected to live 5 years, with laryngeal preservation in approximately two-thirds of survivors (Table 49.11).[67–69] These survival rates from single institutions utilizing IMRT should be interpreted cautiously in light of less favorable outcomes identified through a cross-sectional analysis of patients diagnosed with hypopharyngeal cancer in the United States in 2003. Review of the NCDB data identified 5-year observed survival for the majority of hypopharyngeal cancers (stage IV) to be only 19.8% (see Fig. 49.4).[16]

Induction Chemotherapy and Sequential (Chemo)radiation

Recently, there has been renewed interest in the concept of induction chemotherapy approaches for patients with locoregionally advanced H&N cancer. In an effort to examine the potential for organ preservation in patients with advanced cancers of the hypopharynx, the EORTC conducted a randomized trial for patients with tumors that would require total laryngectomy as the surgical approach. This trial randomly allocated patients to induction chemotherapy with cisplatin and 5-florouracil (5-FU) followed by definitive radiation versus primary surgical resection and postoperative radiation. With a median follow-up of 10 years, this trial demonstrated no significant difference in 5- or 10-year overall survival or progression-free survival. Of note, two-thirds of living patients in the chemoradiotherapy arm were able to retain their larynx.[68] More recently, the introduction of taxane-containing regimens have been demonstrated to improve outcomes in

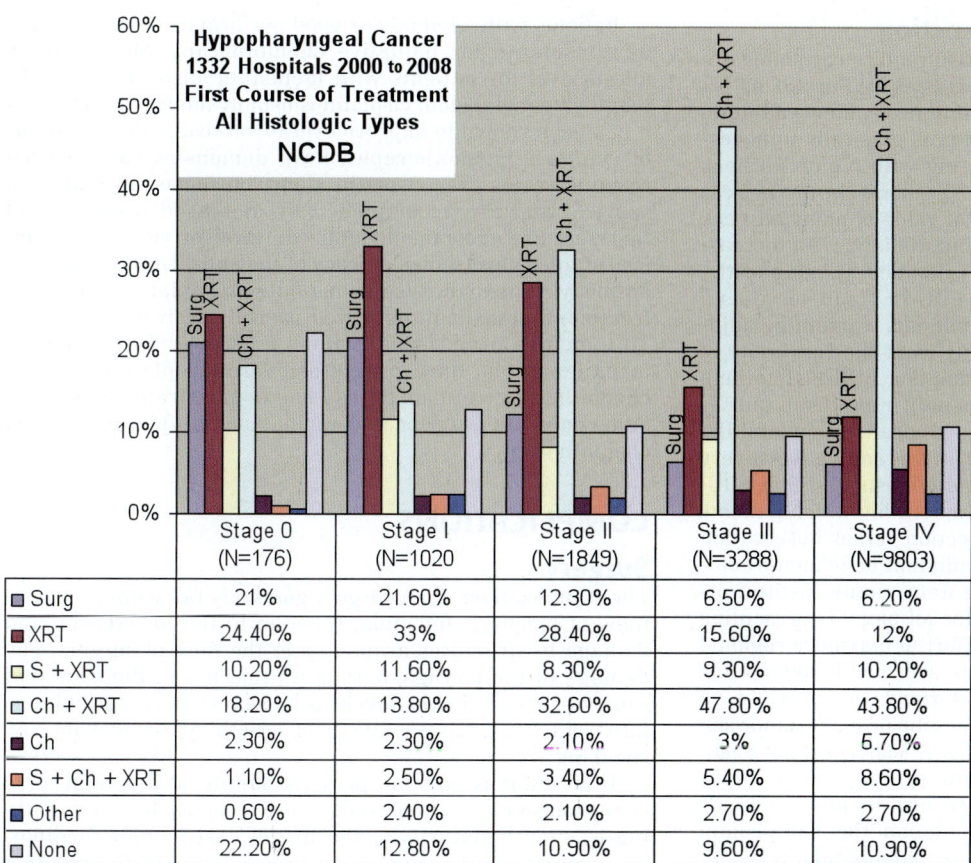

	Stage 0 (N=176)	Stage I (N=1020	Stage II (N=1849)	Stage III (N=3288)	Stage IV (N=9803)
☐ Surg	21%	21.60%	12.30%	6.50%	6.20%
■ XRT	24.40%	33%	28.40%	15.60%	12%
☐ S + XRT	10.20%	11.60%	8.30%	9.30%	10.20%
☐ Ch + XRT	18.20%	13.80%	32.60%	47.80%	43.80%
■ Ch	2.30%	2.30%	2.10%	3%	5.70%
☐ S + Ch + XRT	1.10%	2.50%	3.40%	5.40%	8.60%
■ Other	0.60%	2.40%	2.10%	2.70%	2.70%
☐ None	22.20%	12.80%	10.90%	9.60%	10.90%

FIGURE 49.11. The stage-specific first course of treatment for hypopharyngeal cancer in the United States from Commission on Cancer accredited cancer programs from 2000 to 2008 is presented with unknown stage excluded. Ch, chemotherapy; S, surgery; XRT, radiotherapy. (From National Cancer Data Base. Commission on Cancer. American College of Surgeons. Benchmark Reports. Available at: http://cromwell. facs.org/BMarks/BMPub/Ver10/bm_reports.cfm, with permission.)

patients receiving induction chemotherapy. Three randomized trials have been reported that compare induction 5-FU and cisplatin versus 5-FU, cisplatin, plus a taxane. The EORTC study (TAX-323) randomized patients with locoregionally advanced, unresectable disease to induction cisplatin and fluorouracil (PF) versus induction docetaxel, cisplatin, and fluorouracil (TPF) followed by definitive radiation alone.[70] Treatment with TPF improved the median overall survival from 14.5 to 18.8 months, with a 27% reduction in the risk of death. Similar results were noted in TAX-324, which utilized similar induction chemotherapy arms (TPF vs. PF) followed by concurrent chemoradiotherapy with carboplatin.[71] Five-year survival in the TPF arm was 52% versus 42% receiving PF, while no increased rates of gastric feeding tubes or tracheostomies were noted between groups. A subgroup analysis of larynx and hypopharynx patients demonstrated improved survival in these patients, as well as higher rates of laryngectomy-free survival.[72]

In addition to enhanced survival outcomes, a recent randomized French study demonstrated that TPF induction chemotherapy (compared to PF induction) results in superior tumor response rates (80% vs. 59%) as assessed by laryngoscopy and CT or MRI.[73] Those with response to induction chemotherapy were treated with organ-preserving (chemo) radiotherapy, whereas nonresponders underwent laryngectomy and postoperative (chemo)radiation. The higher response rates in the TPF arm translated into higher rates of laryngeal preservation (70% vs. 57% at 3 years), without a decrease in overall survival (60% at 3 years in both arms). Despite the superiority of TPF chemotherapy over PF, concerns about tolerance of postinduction chemoradiotherapy led to the TREMPLIN trial, which compared induction TPF followed by comprehensive H&N radiotherapy with either concurrent cisplatin or cetuximab.[74] Indeed, treatment compliance was challenging following completion of TPF with only 43% of patients receiving full-dose systemic therapy on the cisplatin arm and 71% on the cetuximab arm. Patients receiving concurrent cisplatin or cetuximab had similar clinical outcomes with regard to larynx preservation at 3 months (95% and 93%, respectively), larynx function preservation (87% and 82%, respectively), and overall survival at 18 months (92% and 89%, respectively). These aggressive treatment approaches certainly warrant consideration for H&N subsites such as hypopharynx where organ preservation is desirable and overall outcomes are generally poor. Patients with good performance status, no contraindications to taxanes or platins, a high tumor burden and/or advanced nodal disease may be optimal candidates for this approach.[75] Nevertheless, these strategies are toxic and costly, and prospective data support equivalent survival outcomes for patients treated with a 7-week course of concurrent chemoradiotherapy alone.[76] Therefore, careful assessment of tumor control, survival, and long-term functional outcome dovetailed with quality-of-life evaluation are important to place these regimens in best perspective for advanced H&N cancer patients.

TABLE 49.11 ONCOLOGIC OUTCOMES FOR PATIENTS UNDERGOING CONCURRENT CHEMORADIOTHERAPY AND INTENSITY-MODULATED RADIATION THERAPY FOR ADVANCED HYPOPHARYNGEAL CANCERS

Study (Reference)	Total Patients in Study (n)	Stage	# of Patients per Stage (%)	Larynx Preservation Rate (%)	5-Year OS (%)
Huang et al.[67]	33	II	2 (6%)	67	44
		III	5 (15%)		
		IV	26 (79%)		
Liu et al.[60]	27	II	5 (19%)	63	35
		III	4 (15%)		
		IV	18 (66%)		

OS, overall survival.

Section III

Postradiotherapy Neck Dissection

Patients with hypopharynx cancer also require careful evaluation regarding regional nodal metastases. For N0 or N1 patients treated with primary radiation or chemoradiation approaches, adjuvant neck dissection is generally unnecessary. However, for patients presenting with N2 or N3 neck disease, careful evaluation of tumor response in the neck is important to help gauge the potential value of adjuvant neck dissection following radiation or chemoradiation. An increasing number of reports suggest that detailed imaging of the neck 12 weeks postradiation with FDG-PET can serve as a valuable guide to help select those patients warranting adjuvant neck dissection. One such study from the University of Iowa assessed the value of a postradiation FDG-PET to help select those patients who might benefit most from subsequent neck dissection. For complete clinical responders, the Iowa study concluded that FDG-PET in this setting has a very high negative predictive value. The authors suggest that FDG-PET may be a valuable tool to help determine which patients should undergo adjuvant neck dissection versus observation following the completion of H&N radiation or (chemo)radiotherapy.[77] Despite these emerging data, many institutions mandate adjuvant neck dissection for all patients presenting with N2 or N3 neck disease in an effort to maximize regional disease control.[78-80] Both approaches are readily defendable at present. If neck dissection is performed, this provides an opportunity for the surgeon to reassess the primary tumor site under anesthesia with directed biopsy if suspicious for residual disease. If residual disease at the primary site is highly suspected or confirmed by biopsy several months following completion of radiation or chemoradiation, this will prompt consideration regarding the feasibility and advisability of salvage surgery options.

Palliative Radiotherapy

The management of patients with unresectable locoregional disease without distant metastases is dependent on patient performance status. A patient with a good performance status may be offered definitive radiotherapy, concurrent chemoradiotherapy, or induction chemotherapy with sequential (chemo)radiotherapy, as discussed above. However, patients with poor performance status who are not considered candidates for aggressive radiation or chemoradiation approaches should be managed with palliative intent. This may include short-course radiation regimens such as 4 to 5 Gy x 5 fractions over 1 to 2 weeks with consideration of the same scheme 3 weeks later if the regimen is tolerated and a favorable response is achieved. A recent study suggests using a 3.7-Gy fraction twice daily × 2 consecutive days for 3 cycles every 2 to 3 weeks, as described in RTOG-85-02, may have similar palliative efficacy with less toxicity as compared to other palliative regimens.[81] Other approaches described include 50 Gy in 16 fractions[82] and 30 Gy in 5 fractions, 2 fractions per week.[83] Systemic chemotherapy alone can be considered, although, for poor performance status patients, best supportive care with medical therapy and airway control may also be appropriate.

Palliative Chemotherapy

As many as one-quarter of hypopharynx cancer patients will develop metastatic disease at some point in their clinical course. In this setting, treatment is palliative and should be delivered to maximize or help maintain quality of life (QOL). If patients are having difficulty with local pain, bleeding, or swallowing, palliative short-course radiation therapy can be delivered, as described above. Surgery may also provide a reasonable palliative option for selected patients who have incurable disease but significant symptoms related to their localized disease, as described above. Many patients in this setting will benefit from narcotic analgesics for pain management.

Patients with adequate or good performance status should be considered for palliative chemotherapy. Median overall survival for patients with metastatic disease is 6 to 10 months.[84] Single-agent cisplatin is usually the first regimen, as it has been shown to improve overall survival.[85] Combinations of cytotoxic chemotherapies have demonstrated improved response rates over cisplatin alone, but have not improved survival and are accompanied by increased toxicity[86] and therefore are uncommonly utilized. However, recent randomized studies have shown efficacy of the anti-EGFR monoclonal antibody cetuximab. In combination with cisplatin as first-line treatment, cetuximab improved overall survival from 7.4 to 10.1 months over cisplatin alone.[87] As second-line therapy in patients who have progressed through platinum-based chemotherapy, cetuximab also has demonstrable activity as either monotherapy[88] or in combination with platinum-based chemotherapy.[89]

COMPLICATIONS

Surgery

The complications from surgery generally fall within the confines of bleeding, infection, reaction to the anesthesia, and damage to structures around or in the field of surgery. The damage to the laryngopharynx that occurs in the course of removing those tissues involved by cancer necessarily interferes with key laryngeal functions: breathing, swallowing, and speaking.

If an effort is made to preserve laryngeal function, some compromise may be required. A long-term tracheotomy, nothing by mouth status with the use of gastrostomy feedings, and significant dysphonia are not uncommon for patients with hypopharynx cancer treated with conservation laryngeal surgery. These same complications may attend the more comprehensive laryngopharyngectomy as well. Stenosis of the neopharynx, difficulty with alaryngeal speech, and stomal stenosis may compromise the same functions ordinarily ascribed to the larynx. For all open surgical approaches, the risk of a salivary fistula is greatest for those patients previously treated with radiation. Although salivary fistulas are rare with endoscopic approaches, they have occurred in cases requiring aggressive laser resection.

Radiation Therapy

During a course of H&N radiation therapy, there are predictable side effects that are experienced by the majority of patients: mucositis, fatigue, loss of taste acuity, radiation dermatitis, and xerostomia. Typically, patients will begin to experience mucositis during the 3rd week of radiotherapy. This initially manifests as mucosal blanching within the treatment field but can progress to patchy or confluent mucositis. Initially, patients can be treated with an over-the-counter pain reliever, but once patients develop grade II or III mucositis, they will commonly require narcotic analgesics for adequate pain control. The combination of dysphagia and mucositis can result in significant nutritional compromise necessitating intravenous hydration and parenteral nutritional supplementation. Nausea associated with treatment can also further complicate the nutritional status. These acute toxicities can become particularly pronounced in the setting of intensified radiation fractionation schedules or combined chemoradiotherapy. Patients may require prophylactic antiemetics. In patients receiving concurrent radiotherapy and platinum-based chemotherapy, there is clear potential for myelosuppression; therefore, blood counts should be monitored regularly. Signs or symptoms of infection should be addressed promptly. Finally, xerostomia can become problematic during the course of radiation. Ultimately, patients can be reassured that the majority of these side effects, with the exception of xerostomia, are temporary and will resolve several weeks to months following completion of therapy.

As noted, one of the acute side effects of radiotherapy that can become permanent is xerostomia. Chemical and physical modifiers of the radiation response have been utilized to reduce long-term xerostomia. The free radical scavenger amifostine has the potential to reduce radiation effects on normal tissues if administered just prior to each radiation fraction. A randomized phase III trial demonstrated a reduction in the severity of the acute and chronic grade 2 or higher xerostomia in patients who received amifostine during RT.[90] Dose-limiting toxicities commonly include hypotension and nausea. There has been concern over possible tumor-protective effects of amifostine, but a recent meta-analysis does not suggest this.[91] However, data supporting the use of amifostine to reduce xerostomia have been generated in the setting of conventional radiation, and the magnitude of benefit on xerostomia of parotid-sparing IMRT appears greater than that of amifostine.[62,64] Therefore, the ultimate value of amifostine in patients with advanced H&N cancer, especially in the setting of IMRT, has been called into question.[92] Currently, there is no universal standard recommendation across treatment centers for the use of this radioprotector.

In some cases, hypopharynx cancer patients who complete a course of radiation therapy will be noted to have persistent laryngeal edema on subsequent follow-up visits. Although in the early posttreatment phase (in fact up to 24 months), significant or newfound edema should raise suspicion regarding the possibility of persistent or recurrent disease. The majority of patients who receive high-dose radiation across major segments of the larynx and hypopharynx will manifest some degree of edema, mucosal congestion, and eventual fibrosis (see Fig. 49.6B). Generally, this collateral damage is a tolerable chronic toxicity with modest impact on patient QOL. However, in approximately 10% to 15% of patients, this edema is severe enough to cause significant airway and swallow function compromise requiring tracheostomy. Rarely, more significant complications such as osteoradionecrosis of the cervical spine may occur. In this setting, patients can present with persistent neck pain prompting imaging and biopsy. Most cases can be managed conservatively; however, progression to serious complications including epidural abscess, radiculopathy, and myelopathy has been described. Once neurologic symptoms emerge, they can progress rapidly, indicating the need to maintain vigilance in patients with cervical spine ORN.[93-95]

LONG-TERM FOLLOW-UP

Regardless of whether patients undergo primary surgery or radiation therapy, there is value in close posttreatment surveillance by H&N surgeon and radiation oncologist in a multidisciplinary fashion. Follow-up care is designed initially to survey for recurrence. As duration from time of intervention to clinic visits lengthen, the focus shifts to surveillance for second primaries (i.e., lung), to address morbidity from treatment, and to provide generalized support.

During the first 6 months after treatment, patients should be followed every 4 to 6 weeks with clinical examination, including fiber-optic nasopharyngoscopy. Recommended guidelines include a follow-up visit every 1 to 3 months during the first year, every 2 to 4 months for the second year, every 4 to 6 months for years 3 through 5, and every 6 to 12 months thereafter. Additionally, if the patient received comprehensive H&N radiation, the serum thyroid-stimulating hormone level should be measured every 6 to 12 months. Imaging evaluation of the neck, most commonly with CT or MRI scan, is obtained at 3- to 6-month intervals during the first 2 years

or as indicated based on clinical findings. Functional imaging with [18]FDG-PET can sometimes prove valuable to help differentiate posttreatment fibrosis from persistent or recurrent disease.

A study by Hermans et al.[96] examined findings on CT scan of the neck 3 to 4 months following completion of radiation therapy for patients with larynx or hypopharynx cancer to examine correlation with long-term outcome. The authors suggest that in patients achieving complete radiographic resolution of all pretreatment disease, the likelihood of subsequent local failure is very small. These patients might therefore undergo routine clinical examination, with repeat imaging reserved for instances where the clinical examination becomes suspicious for recurrence. For patients who achieved <50% reduction in tumor volume or retained a mass 1 cm or larger on the posttreatment imaging study, the likelihood of local failure was 100% and 30%, respectively. In these patients, repeat CT at 3 to 4 months, FDG-PET, or biopsy is therefore recommended. Preliminary reports indicate that the results of the first post-RT FDG-PET scan may be a strong predictor of developing locoregional disease recurrence.[77]

In the posttreatment setting of hypopharynx cancer patients, the involvement of an experienced H&N radiologist is highly desirable for optimal interpretation of imaging results. Soft tissue changes following ablative surgery and reconstruction, or following high-dose radiation or chemoradiation with resultant edema and fibrosis, can be very difficult to differentiate from tumor, particularly for the inexperienced reader.

MANAGEMENT OF RECURRENCE

After completion of treatment, patients should be followed closely for signs of recurrent or persistent disease. If recurrence is suspected, this should be confirmed by biopsy. If biopsy is confirmatory, then the patient should undergo complete restaging to assess the extent of disease. In the setting of local or regional disease alone, patients treated with initial radiation or chemoradiation can be considered for surgical salvage therapy. Although salvage surgery following comprehensive H&N radiation and chemotherapy presents several resection and reconstructive healing challenges for the surgeon, selected patients may still derive long-term benefit from this approach. Select patients with low-volume localized disease may be candidates for transoral laser microsurgery for recurrent disease following radiation.[97] Recurrent patients who initially received comprehensive H&N radiation have traditionally not been considered good candidates for repeat high-dose radiation in light of normal tissue tolerances. However, two recent prospective RTOG studies have demonstrated that reirradiation to the H&N is feasible.[98,99] With the advent of highly conformal radiation delivery techniques, selected patients may benefit from reirradiation approaches in conjunction with systemic chemotherapy.[100] A retrospective study from Memorial Sloan-Kettering Cancer Center has suggested that IMRT is beneficial for local control in this setting,[101] and a recent prospective trial of reirradiation utilizing IMRT suggests long-term disease control can be achieved in select patients with tolerable toxicity.[102] The use of stereotactic body radiosurgery (SBRT) is becoming more common in the management of head and neck cancer patients who manifest locoregional recurrence. Recent data suggest that patients with laryngeal and hypopharyngeal primaries exhibit significantly more late toxicities compared to those with oral cavity and oropharyngeal primaries, likely related to cartilage in the retreatment region. Therefore, careful consideration should be given to patient performance status, preexisting organ dysfunction, and goals of care prior to delivering ablative doses of radiotherapy in the laryngopharynx.[103]

Many patients with recurrent disease, however, are not good candidates for aggressive surgery or salvage radiation therapy and are best served with systemic chemotherapy or best supportive care approaches.

QUALITY OF LIFE

Assessment of parameters, including functional status, organ preservation, treatment cost, and patient assessment of QOL, plays an increasingly important role in the evaluation of overall treatment efficacy. For larynx and hypopharynx cancer patients, a focus of contemporary clinical investigation has been the study of treatments designed to preserve laryngeal function for patients traditionally treated with total laryngectomy. A frequently cited but somewhat controversial study by McNeil et al.[104] employed a questionnaire administered to healthy individuals and concluded that some might forgo total laryngectomy in favor of alternative therapy, even if this choice diminished their ultimate chance for cure. A more recent report by El-Deiry et al.[105] evaluated long-term QOL in a matched pair analysis comparing the surgical and nonsurgical treatment of patients with advanced H&N cancer involving the oropharynx, hypopharynx, and larynx. Although patients in the surgery arm demonstrated worse speech outcomes than those treated with chemoradiation, this difference did not carry over to the overall QOL score. These investigators concluded that, although it seems reasonable that organ preservation (nonsurgical) treatment will uniformly result in a higher QOL, the complexities of human adjustment and multitude of potential treatment effects render this assumption invalid for many patients. Alternatively, a study from the Medical University of South Carolina compared swallow-related QOL after surgery or radiotherapy for H&N cancer using a dysphagia symptom survey, the M.D. Anderson Dysphagia Inventory (MDADI). They found significantly better scores on the emotional and functional components of the MDADI for patients undergoing chemoradiation compared to those undergoing surgery followed by radiation.[106]

There have been relatively few prospective assessments of QOL following treatment for H&N cancer. In a subset of locally advanced patients requiring radical surgery, such as total laryngectomy and partial pharyngectomy, the functional deficits are predictable. However, for patients undergoing organ preservation with radiation alone or in combination with chemotherapy, it can be difficult to assess the true extent and quality of organ preservation. Regardless of the primary treatment approach, these patients often require long-term speech, swallow, and dental rehabilitation. A study from Meyer et al.[107] retrospectively assessed speech intelligibility and QOL in survivors of H&N cancer. A total of 64 patients were enrolled; 31 underwent RT alone, 5 underwent surgery alone, and 28 received both. All patients underwent comprehensive subjective and objective testing of speech function and QOL. They found significant subjective and objective deficits in speech and QOL even 5 years after completion of therapy. Terrell et al.[108] reported the results of a self-administered health survey of 570 patients at a Veterans' Administration hospital that demonstrated that the single most notable event having a negative impact on QOL was placement of a feeding tube. This was followed by medical comorbid conditions, presence of a tracheotomy tube, chemotherapy, and neck dissection.

A prospective study on QOL utilizing the EORTC QLQ-C30 and QLQ-H&N35 questionnaires was conducted in Sweden on 357 patients. This study found that QOL issues were significantly associated with the site of origin, with stage at diagnosis being the most important predictor. Additionally, patients with hypopharynx cancer exhibited the poorest QOL.[109] Similarly, another study prospectively examining swallow function in H&N cancer patients demonstrated that worse swallowing was associated with hypopharyngeal tumor sites.[110] Although the use of IMRT can have a significant impact on xerostomia and QOL measures in H&N cancer patients,[111,112] the intimate approximation of hypopharyngeal tumors to pharyngeal constrictor musculature does not allow for sparing of these structures vital to long-term swallow function, likely contributing to the poorer QOL of hypopharynx patients in comparison to other H&N cancer patients.[113]

CONCLUSION

Patients with cancers of the hypopharynx commonly present with advanced disease associated with varying degrees of compromise in speech or swallow function. Many hypopharynx cancer patients also carry significant medical and social comorbidities. Typically, small T1 or T2 lesions can be managed with either primary radiation or surgery, with similar clinical outcome. For intermediate-stage disease that would require laryngopharyngectomy for the surgical approach, an increasingly preferred treatment option is combined chemoradiation that has demonstrated equivalence to immediate surgery in cancer survival; however, with improved organ preservation and functional outcome. For bulky hypopharynx tumors with significant airway compromise, laryngeal distortion, and cartilage destruction, it is generally best to proceed with definitive surgery with postoperative radiation or chemoradiation.

Despite an aggressive approach in the overall management of hypopharynx cancer patients, ultimate cure rates remain quite poor. There are relatively few early-stage patients; and for many advanced-stage patients, it is difficult to achieve long-term control. Even for those patients with excellent response to therapy, there exists a continuous risk for the development of second malignancies, particularly of the upper aerodigestive track with long-term follow-up. Posttreatment patients often require aggressive speech and swallow therapy to maximize their functional outcome. There is significant interest in the incorporation of molecular targeted therapies in combination with traditional cytotoxic therapy and radiation in an effort to improve outcomes.

REFERENCES

1. Brugere J, Guenel P, Leclerc A, et al. Differential effects of tobacco and alcohol in cancer of the larynx, pharynx, and mouth. *Cancer* 1986;57(2):391–395.
2. Schechter GL, Kalafsky JT. Cancer of the hypopharynx and cervical esophagus: management concepts. *Oncology (Williston Park)* 1988;2(5):17–24, 34–15.
3. Spitz MR. Epidemiology and risk factors for head and neck cancer. *Semin Oncol* 1994;21(3):281–288.
4. Cooper JS, Porter K, Mallin K, et al. National Cancer Database report on cancer of the head and neck: 10-year update. *Head Neck* 2009;31(6):748–758.
5. Surveillance E and End-Results (SEER) Program. *SEER*Stat Database: Incidence-SEER 17 Regs Research Data, Nov. 2010 sub (2000-2008)*. National Cancer Institute, DCCPS, Surveillance Research Program, Cancer Statistics Branch. Released April 2011, National Institutes of Health, National Cancer Institute.
6. Hoffman HT, Karnell LH, Shah JP, et al. Hypopharyngeal cancer patient care evaluation. *Laryngoscope* 1997;107(8):1005–1017.
7. Popescu CR, Bertesteanu SV, Mirea D, et al. The epidemiology of hypopharynx and cervical esophagus cancer. *J Med Life* 2010;3(4):396–401.
8. Boffetta P, Richiardi L, Berrino F, et al. Occupation and larynx and hypopharynx cancer: an international case-control study in France, Italy, Spain, and Switzerland. *Cancer Causes Control* 2003;14(3):203–212.
9. Shangina O, Brennan P, Szszenia-Dabrowska N, et al. Occupational exposure and laryngeal and hypopharyngeal cancer risk in central and eastern Europe. *Am J Epidemiol* 2006;164(4):367–375.
10. Davies L, Welch HG. Epidemiology of head and neck cancer in the United States. *Otolaryngol Head Neck Surg* 2006;135(3):451–457.
11. Klussmann JP, Weissenborn SJ, Wieland U, et al. Prevalence, distribution, and viral load of human papillomavirus 16 DNA in tonsillar carcinomas. *Cancer* 2001;92(11):2875–2884.
12. Mineta H, Ogino T, Amano HM, et al. Human papilloma virus (HPV) type 16 and 18 detected in head and neck squamous cell carcinoma. *Anticancer Res* 1998;18(6B):4765–4768.

13. Ribeiro KB, Levi JE, Pawlita M, et al. Low human papillomavirus prevalence in head and neck cancer: results from two large case-control studies in high-incidence regions. *Int J Epidemiol* 2011;40(2):489–502.

14. Spector JG, Sessions DG, Emami B, et al. Squamous cell carcinomas of the aryepiglottic fold: therapeutic results and long-term follow-up. *Laryngoscope* 1995;105(7 Pt 1):734–746.

15. Spector JG, Sessions DG, Emami B, et al. Squamous cell carcinoma of the pyriform sinus: a nonrandomized comparison of therapeutic modalities and long-term results. *Laryngoscope* 1995;105(4 Pt 1):397–406.

16. National Cancer Data Base. Commission on Cancer. American College of Surgeons Benchmark Reports. Accessed August 24, 2011.

17. Dikshit RP, Boffetta P, Bouchardy C, et al. Lifestyle habits as prognostic factors in survival of laryngeal and hypopharyngeal cancer: a multicentric European study. *Int J Cancer* 2005;117(6):992–995.

18. Tanaka H, Takenaka Y, Nakahara S, et al. Age-adjusted Charlson comorbidity index as a prognostic factor of hypopharyngeal cancer treated with chemoradiation therapy. *Acta Otolaryngol* 2017;137(6):668–673.

19. Chang F, Syrjanen S, Syrjanen K. Implications of the p53 tumor-suppressor gene in clinical oncology. *J Clin Oncol* 1995;13(4):1009–1022.

20. Frank JL, Bur ME, Garb JL, et al. p53 tumor suppressor oncogene expression in squamous cell carcinoma of the hypopharynx. *Cancer* 1994;73(1):181–186.

21. Frank JL, Garb JL, Banson BB, et al. Epidermal growth factor receptor expression in squamous cell carcinoma of the hypopharynx. *Surg Oncol* 1993;2(3):161–167.

22. Magne N, Pivot X, Bensadoun RJ, et al. The relationship of epidermal growth factor receptor levels to the prognosis of unresectable pharyngeal cancer patients treated by chemo-radiotherapy. *Eur J Cancer* 2001;37(17):2169–2177.

23. Pivot X, Magne N, Guardiola E, et al. Prognostic impact of the epidermal growth factor receptor levels for patients with larynx and hypopharynx cancer. *Oral Oncol* 2005;41(3):320–327.

24. Amin MB, Greene FL, Edge SB, et al. The Eighth Edition AJCC Cancer Staging Manual: Continuing to build a bridge from a population-based to a more "personalized" approach to cancer staging. *CA Cancer J Clin* 2017;67(2):93–99.

25. Spector JG, Sessions DG, Haughey BH, et al. Delayed regional metastases, distant metastases, and second primary malignancies in squamous cell carcinomas of the larynx and hypopharynx. *Laryngoscope* 2001;111(6):1079–1087.

26. Ho CM, Lam KH, Wei WI, et al. Squamous cell carcinoma of the hypopharynx—analysis of treatment results. *Head Neck* 1993;15(5):405–412.

27. Koo BS, Lim YC, Lee JS, et al. Management of contralateral N0 neck in pyriform sinus carcinoma. *Laryngoscope* 2006;116(7):1268–1272.

28. Muir C, Weiland L. Upper aerodigestive tract cancers. *Cancer* 1995;75(1 Suppl):147–153.

29. Mukherji SK, Armao D, Joshi VM. Cervical nodal metastases in squamous cell carcinoma of the head and neck: what to expect. *Head Neck* 2001;23(11):995–1005.

30. Marks JE, Kurnik B, Powers WE, et al. Carcinoma of the pyriform sinus. An analysis of treatment results and patterns of failure. *Cancer* 1978;41(3):1008–1015.

31. Thawley SE. *Comprehensive management of head and neck tumors.* Philadelphia, PA: WB Saunders, 1999.

32. Di Martino E, Nowak B, Hassan HA, et al. Diagnosis and staging of head and neck cancer: a comparison of modern imaging modalities (positron emission tomography, computed tomography, color-coded duplex sonography) with panendoscopic and histopathologic findings. *Arch Otolaryngol Head Neck Surg* 2000;126(12):1457–1461.

33. Schwartz DL, Rajendran J, Yueh B, et al. FDG-PET prediction of head and neck squamous cell cancer outcomes. *Arch Otolaryngol Head Neck Surg* 2004;130(12):1361–1367.

34. Lonneux M, Hamoir M, Reychler H, et al. Positron emission tomography with [18F]fluorodeoxyglucose improves staging and patient management in patients with head and neck squamous cell carcinoma: a multicenter prospective study. *J Clin Oncol* 2010;28(7):1190–1195.

35. Newman JR, Connolly TM, Illing EA, et al. Survival trends in hypopharyngeal cancer: a population-based review. *Laryngoscope* 2015;125(3):624–629.

36. Gilbert RW, Neligan PC. Microsurgical laryngotracheal reconstruction. *Clin Plast Surg* 2005;32(3):293–301, v.

37. Boudreaux BA, Rosenthal EL, Magnuson JS, et al. Robot-assisted surgery for upper aerodigestive tract neoplasms. *Arch Otolaryngol Head Neck Surg* 2009;135(4):397–401.

38. Karatzanis AD, Psychogios G, Waldfahrer F, et al. T1 and T2 hypopharyngeal cancer treatment with laser microsurgery. *J Surg Oncol* 2010;102(1):27–33.

39. Martin A, Jackel MC, Christiansen H, et al. Organ preserving transoral laser microsurgery for cancer of the hypopharynx. *Laryngoscope* 2008;118(3):398–402.

40. Steiner W, Ambrosch P, Hess CF, et al. Organ preservation by transoral laser microsurgery in piriform sinus carcinoma. *Otolaryngol Head Neck Surg* 2001;124(1):58–67.

41. Durmus K, Kucur C, Uysal IO, et al. Feasibility and clinical outcomes of transoral robotic surgery and transoral robot-assisted carbon dioxide laser for hypopharyngeal carcinoma. *J Craniofac Surg* 2015;26(1):235–237.

42. Park YM, Kim WS, De Virgilio A, et al. Transoral robotic surgery for hypopharyngeal squamous cell carcinoma: 3-year oncologic and functional analysis. *Oral Oncol* 2012;48(6):560–566.

43. Dziegielewski PT, Kang SY, Ozer E. Transoral robotic surgery (TORS) for laryngeal and hypopharyngeal cancers. *J Surg Oncol* 2015;112(7):702–706.

44. Wang CC, Liu SA, Wu SH, et al. Transoral robotic surgery for early T classification hypopharyngeal cancer. *Head Neck* 2016;38(6):857–862.

45. Lorincz BB, Busch CJ, Mockelmann N, et al. Feasibility and safety of transoral robotic surgery (TORS) for early hypopharyngeal cancer: a subset analysis of the Hamburg University TORS-trial. *Eur Arch Otorhinolaryngol* 2015;272(10):2993–2998.

46. Cooper JS, Pajak TF, Forastiere AA, et al. Postoperative concurrent radiotherapy and chemotherapy for high-risk squamous-cell carcinoma of the head and neck. *N Engl J Med* 2004;350(19):1937–1944.

47. Bernier J, Domenge C, Ozsahin M, et al. Postoperative irradiation with or without concomitant chemotherapy for locally advanced head and neck cancer. *N Engl J Med* 2004;350(19):1945–1952.

48. Bernier J, Cooper JS, Pajak TF, et al. Defining risk levels in locally advanced head and neck cancers: a comparative analysis of concurrent postoperative radiation plus chemotherapy trials of the EORTC (#22931) and RTOG (# 9501). *Head Neck* 2005;27(10):843–850.

49. Pignon JP, le Maitre A, Maillard E, et al; Group MACH-NC. Meta-analysis of chemotherapy in head and neck cancer (MACH-NC): an update on 93 randomised trials and 17,346 patients. *Radiother Oncol* 2009;92(1):4–14.

50. Fowler JF, Lindstrom MJ. Loss of local control with prolongation in radiotherapy. *Int J Radiat Oncol Biol Phys* 1992;23(2):457–467.

51. Hansen O, Overgaard J, Hansen HS, et al. Importance of overall treatment time for the outcome of radiotherapy of advanced head and neck carcinoma: dependency on tumor differentiation. *Radiother Oncol* 1997;43(1):47–51.

52. Fu KK, Pajak TF, Trotti A, et al. A Radiation Therapy Oncology Group (RTOG) phase III randomized study to compare hyperfractionation and two variants of accelerated fractionation to standard fractionation radiotherapy for head and neck squamous cell carcinomas: first report of RTOG 9003. *Int J Radiat Oncol Biol Phys* 2000;48(1):7–16.

53. Overgaard J, Hansen HS, Specht L, et al. Five compared with six fractions per week of conventional radiotherapy of squamous-cell carcinoma of head and neck: DAHANCA 6 and 7 randomised controlled trial. *Lancet* 2003;362(9388):933–940.

54. Skladowski K, Maciejewski B, Golen M, et al. Continuous accelerated 7-days-a-week radiotherapy for head-and-neck cancer: long-term results of phase III clinical trial. *Int J Radiat Oncol Biol Phys* 2006;66(3):706–713.

55. Bourhis J, Overgaard J, Audry H, et al. Hyperfractionated or accelerated radiotherapy in head and neck cancer: a meta-analysis. *Lancet* 2006;368(9538):843–854.

56. Amdur RJ, Mendenhall WM, Stringer SP, et al. Organ preservation with radiotherapy for T1-T2 carcinoma of the pyriform sinus. *Head Neck* 2001;23(5):353–362.

57. Garden AS, Morrison WH, Clayman GL, et al. Early squamous cell carcinoma of the hypopharynx: outcomes of treatment with radiation alone to the primary disease. *Head Neck* 1996;18(4):317–322.

58. Nakamura K, Shioyama Y, Kawashima M, et al. Multi-institutional analysis of early squamous cell carcinoma of the hypopharynx treated with radical radiotherapy. *Int J Radiat Oncol Biol Phys* 2006;65(4):1045–1050.

59. Yoshimura R, Kagami Y, Ito Y, et al. Outcomes in patients with early-stage hypopharyngeal cancer treated with radiotherapy. *Int J Radiat Oncol Biol Phys* 2010;77(4):1017–1023.

60. Fein DA, Mendenhall WM, Parsons JT, et al. Pharyngeal wall carcinoma treated with radiotherapy: impact of treatment technique and fractionation. *Int J Radiat Oncol Biol Phys* 1993;26(5):751–757.

61. Hong TS, Tome WA, Chappell RJ, et al. The impact of daily setup variations on head-and-neck intensity-modulated radiation therapy. *Int J Radiat Oncol Biol Phys* 2005;61(3):779–788.

62. Eisbruch A, Ship JA, Dawson LA, et al. Salivary gland sparing and improved target irradiation by conformal and intensity modulated irradiation of head and neck cancer. *World J Surg* 2003;27(7):832–837.

63. Eisbruch A, Ten Haken RK, Kim HM, et al. Dose, volume, and function relationships in parotid salivary glands following conformal and intensity-modulated irradiation of head and neck cancer. *Int J Radiat Oncol Biol Phys* 1999;45(3):577–587.

64. Nutting CM, Morden JP, Harrington KJ, et al. Parotid-sparing intensity modulated versus conventional radiotherapy in head and neck cancer (PARSPORT): a phase 3 multicentre randomised controlled trial. *Lancet Oncol* 2011;12(2):127–136.

65. Bonner JA, Harari PM, Giralt J, et al. Radiotherapy plus cetuximab for squamous-cell carcinoma of the head and neck. *N Engl J Med* 2006;354(6):567–578.

66. Bonner JA, Harari PM, Giralt J, et al. Radiotherapy plus cetuximab for locoregionally advanced head and neck cancer: 5-year survival data from a phase 3 randomised trial, and relation between cetuximab-induced rash and survival. *Lancet Oncol* 2010;11(1):21–28.

67. Huang WY, Jen YM, Chen CM, et al. Intensity modulated radiotherapy with concurrent chemotherapy for larynx preservation of advanced resectable hypopharyngeal cancer. *Radiat Oncol* 2010;5:37.

68. Lefebvre JL, Chevalier D, Luboinski B, et al. Larynx preservation in pyriform sinus cancer: preliminary results of a European Organization for Research and Treatment of Cancer phase III trial. EORTC Head and Neck Cancer Cooperative Group. *J Natl Cancer Inst* 1996;88(13):890–899.

69. Liu WS, Hsin CH, Chou YH, et al. Long-term results of intensity-modulated radiotherapy concomitant with chemotherapy for hypopharyngeal carcinoma aimed at laryngeal preservation. *BMC Cancer* 2010;10:102.

70. Vermorken JB, Remenar E, van Herpen C, et al. Cisplatin, fluorouracil, and docetaxel in unresectable head and neck cancer. *N Engl J Med* 2007;357(17):1695–1704.

71. Lorch JH, Goloubeva O, Haddad RI, et al. Induction chemotherapy with cisplatin and fluorouracil alone or in combination with docetaxel in locally advanced squamous-cell cancer of the head and neck: long-term results of the TAX 324 randomised phase 3 trial. *Lancet Oncol* 2011;12(2):153–159.

72. Posner MR, Norris CM, Wirth LJ, et al. Sequential therapy for the locally advanced larynx and hypopharynx cancer subgroup in TAX 324: survival, surgery, and organ preservation. *Ann Oncol* 2009;20(5):921–927.

73. Pointreau Y, Garaud P, Chapet S, et al. Randomized trial of induction chemotherapy with cisplatin and 5-fluorouracil with or without docetaxel for larynx preservation. *J Natl Cancer Inst* 2009;101(7):498–506.

74. Lefebvre JL, Pointreau Y, Rolland F, et al. Induction chemotherapy followed by either chemoradiotherapy or bioradiotherapy for larynx preservation: the TREMPLIN randomized phase II study. *J Clin Oncol* 2013;31(7):853–859.

75. Budah V. TPF sequential therapy: when and for whom? *Oncologist* 2010;15(Suppl 3):13–18.

76. Haddad R, O'Neill A, Rabinowits G, et al. Induction chemotherapy followed by concurrent chemoradiotherapy (sequential chemoradiotherapy) versus concurrent chemoradiotherapy alone in locally advanced head and neck cancer (PARADIGM): a randomised phase 3 trial. *Lancet Oncol* 2013;14(3):257–264.

77. Yao M, Smith RB, Graham MM, et al. The role of FDG PET in management of neck metastasis from head-and-neck cancer after definitive radiation treatment. *Int J Radiat Oncol Biol Phys* 2005;63(4):991–999.

78. Boyd TS, Harari PM, Tannehill SP, et al. Planned postradiotherapy neck dissection in patients with advanced head and neck cancer. *Head Neck* 1998;20(2):132–137.

79. Stenson KM, Haraf DJ, Pelzer H, et al. The role of cervical lymphadenectomy after aggressive concomitant chemoradiotherapy: the feasibility of selective neck dissection. *Arch Otolaryngol Head Neck Surg* 2000;126(8):950–956.

80. Wang SJ, Wang MB, Yip H, et al. Combined radiotherapy with planned neck dissection for small head and neck cancers with advanced cervical metastases. *Laryngoscope* 2000;110(11):1794–1797.

81. Chen AM, Vaughan A, Narayan S, et al. Palliative radiation therapy for head and neck cancer: toward an optimal fractionation scheme. *Head Neck* 2008;30(12):1586–1591.

82. Al-mamgani A, Tans L, Van rooij PH, et al. Hypofractionated radiotherapy denoted as the "Christie scheme": an effective means of palliating patients with head and neck cancers not suitable for curative treatment. *Acta Oncol* 2009;48(4):562–570.

83. Porceddu SV, Rosser B, Burmeister BH, et al. Hypofractionated radiotherapy for the palliation of advanced head and neck cancer in patients unsuitable for curative treatment—"Hypo Trial". *Radiother Oncol* 2007;85(3):456–462.

84. Argiris A, Karamouzis MV, Raben D, et al. Head and neck cancer. *Lancet* 2008;371(9625):1695–1709.

85. Morton RP, Rugman F, Dorman EB, et al. Cisplatinum and bleomycin for advanced or recurrent squamous cell carcinoma of the head and neck: a randomised factorial phase III controlled trial. *Cancer Chemother Pharmacol* 1985;15(3):283–289.

86. Clavel M, Vermorken JB, Cognetti F, et al. Randomized comparison of cisplatin, methotrexate, bleomycin and vincristine (CABO) versus cisplatin and 5-fluorouracil (CF) versus cisplatin (C) in recurrent or metastatic squamous cell carcinoma of the head and neck. A phase III study of the EORTC Head and Neck Cancer Cooperative Group. *Ann Oncol* 1994;5(6):521–526.

87. Vermorken JB, Mesia R, Rivera F, et al. Platinum-based chemotherapy plus cetuximab in head and neck cancer. *N Engl J Med* 2008;359(11):1116–1127.

88. Vermorken JB, Trigo J, Hitt R, et al. Open-label, uncontrolled, multicenter phase II study to evaluate the efficacy and toxicity of cetuximab as a single agent in patients with recurrent and/or metastatic squamous cell carcinoma of the head and neck who failed to respond to platinum-based therapy. *J Clin Oncol* 2007;25(16):2171–2177.

89. Baselga J, Trigo JM, Bourhis J, et al. Phase II multicenter study of the antiepidermal growth factor receptor monoclonal antibody cetuximab in combination with platinum-based chemotherapy in patients with platinum-refractory metastatic and/or recurrent squamous cell carcinoma of the head and neck. *J Clin Oncol* 2005;23(24):5568–5577.

90. Brizel DM, Wasserman TH, Henke M, et al. Phase III randomized trial of amifostine as a radioprotector in head and neck cancer. *J Clin Oncol* 2000;18(19):3339–3345.

91. Bourhis J, Blanchard P, Maillard E, et al. Effect of amifostine on survival among patients treated with radiotherapy: a meta-analysis of individual patient data. *J Clin Oncol* 2011;29(18):2590–2597.

92. Eisbruch A. Amifostine in the treatment of head and neck cancer: intravenous administration, subcutaneous administration, or none of the above. *J Clin Oncol* 2011;29(2):119–121.

93. Cheung JP, Wei WI, Luk KD. Cervical spine complications after treatment of nasopharyngeal carcinoma. *Eur Spine J* 2013;22(3):584–592.

94. King AD, Griffith JF, Abrigo JM, et al. Osteoradionecrosis of the upper cervical spine: MR imaging following radiotherapy for nasopharyngeal carcinoma. *Eur J Radiol* 2010;73(3):629–635.

95. Lim AA, Karakla DW, Watkins DV. Osteoradionecrosis of the cervical vertebrae and occipital bone: a case report and brief review of the literature. *Am J Otolaryngol* 1999;20(6):408–411.

96. Hermans R, Pameijer FA, Mancuso AA, et al. Laryngeal or hypopharyngeal squamous cell carcinoma: can follow-up CT after definitive radiation therapy be used to detect local failure earlier than clinical examination alone? *Radiology* 2000;214(3):683–687.

97. Grant DG, Salassa JR, Hinni ML, et al. Transoral laser microsurgery for recurrent laryngeal and pharyngeal cancer. *Otolaryngol Head Neck Surg* 2008;138(5):606–613.

98. Langer CJ, Harris J, Horwitz EM, et al. Phase II study of low-dose paclitaxel and cisplatin in combination with split-course concomitant twice-daily reirradiation in recurrent squamous cell carcinoma of the head and neck: results of Radiation Therapy Oncology Group Protocol 9911. *J Clin Oncol* 2007;25(30):4800–4805.

99. Spencer SA, Harris J, Wheeler RH, et al. Final report of RTOG 9610, a multi-institutional trial of reirradiation and chemotherapy for unresectable recurrent squamous cell carcinoma of the head and neck. *Head Neck* 2008;30(3):281–288.

100. Wong SJ, Machtay M, Li Y. Locally recurrent, previously irradiated head and neck cancer: concurrent re-irradiation and chemotherapy, or chemotherapy alone? *J Clin Oncol* 2006;24(17):2653–2658.

101. Lee N, Chan K, Bekelman JE, et al. Salvage re-irradiation for recurrent head and neck cancer. *Int J Radiat Oncol Biol Phys* 2007;68(3):731–740.

102. Chen AM, Farwell DG, Luu Q, et al. Prospective trial of high-dose reirradiation using daily image guidance with intensity-modulated radiotherapy for recurrent and second primary head-and-neck cancer. *Int J Radiat Oncol Biol Phys* 2011;80(3):669–676.

103. Ling DC, Vargo JA, Ferris RL, et al. Risk of severe toxicity according to site of recurrence in patients treated with stereotactic body radiation therapy for recurrent head and neck cancer. *Int J Radiat Oncol Biol Phys* 2016;95(3):973–980.

104. McNeil BJ, Weichselbaum R, Pauker SG. Speech and survival: tradeoffs between quality and quantity of life in laryngeal cancer. *N Engl J Med* 1981;305(17):982–987.

105. El-Deiry M, Funk GF, Nalwa S, et al. Long-term quality of life for surgical and nonsurgical treatment of head and neck cancer. *Arch Otolaryngol Head Neck Surg* 2005;131(10):879–885.

106. Gillespie MB, Brodsky MB, Day TA, et al. Swallowing-related quality of life after head and neck cancer treatment. *Laryngoscope* 2004;114(8):1362–1367.

107. Meyer TK, Kuhn JC, Campbell BH, et al. Speech intelligibility and quality of life in head and neck cancer survivors. *Laryngoscope* 2004;114(11):1977–1981.

108. Terrell JE, Ronis DL, Fowler KE, et al. Clinical predictors of quality of life in patients with head and neck cancer. *Arch Otolaryngol Head Neck Surg* 2004;130(4):401–408.

109. Hammerlid E, Bjordal K, Ahlner-Elmqvist M, et al. A prospective study of quality of life in head and neck cancer patients. Part I: at diagnosis. *Laryngoscope* 2001;111(4 Pt 1):669–680.

110. Frowen J, Cotton S, Corry J, et al. Impact of demographics, tumor characteristics, and treatment factors on swallowing after (chemo)radiotherapy for head and neck cancer. *Head Neck* 2010;32(4):513–528.

111. Jabbari S, Kim HM, Feng M, et al. Matched case-control study of quality of life and xerostomia after intensity-modulated radiotherapy or standard radiotherapy for head-and-neck cancer: initial report. *Int J Radiat Oncol Biol Phys* 2005;63(3):725–731.

112. Vergeer MR, Doornaert PA, Rietveld DH, et al. Intensity-modulated radiotherapy reduces radiation-induced morbidity and improves health-related quality of life: results of a nonrandomized prospective study using a standardized follow-up program. *Int J Radiat Oncol Biol Phys* 2009;74(1):1–8.

113. Caudell JJ, Schaner PE, Desmond RA, et al. Dosimetric factors associated with long-term dysphagia after definitive radiotherapy for squamous cell carcinoma of the head and neck. *Int J Radiat Oncol Biol Phys* 2010;76(2):403–409.

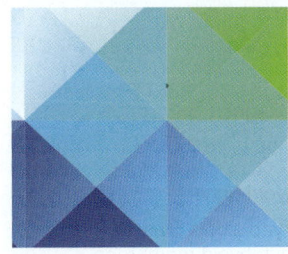

CHAPTER 50

Laryngeal Cancer

William M. Mendenhall, Anthony A. Mancuso, Robert J. Amdur,
Brian J. Boyce, and Peter T. Dziegielewski

ANATOMY

The larynx is divided into the supraglottis, glottis, and subglottis. The supraglottis consists of the epiglottis, false vocal cords, ventricles, aryepiglottic folds, and the arytenoids. The glottis includes the floor of the ventricle, interarytenoid area, true vocal cords, and the anterior commissure. The subglottis is located below the vocal cords (Figs. 50.1 and 50.2).[1]

The axial line of demarcation between the glottic and supraglottic larynx is the apex of the ventricle. The demarcation between the glottis and subglottis is ill defined, but the subglottis is considered to extend from a point 5 mm below the free margin of the vocal cord to the inferior border of the cricoid cartilage or 10 mm below the apex of the ventricle.

The vocal cords vary from 3 to 5 mm in thickness and terminate posteriorly with their attachment to the vocal process or the arytenoid cartilage. The posterior commissure is the mucosa between the arytenoids (interarytenoid area).

The shell of the larynx is formed by the hyoid bone, thyroid cartilage, and cricoid cartilage; the cricoid cartilage is the only complete ring of the upper airway. The more mobile interior framework is composed of the heart-shaped epiglottis and the arytenoid, corniculate, and cuneiform cartilages. The corniculate and cuneiform cartilages produce small, rounded bulges at the posterior end of each aryepiglottic fold.

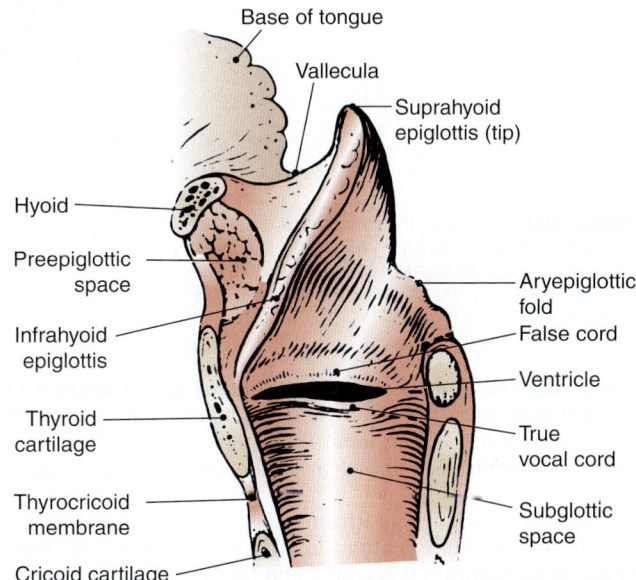

FIGURE 50.1. Diagrammatic sagittal section of the larynx. (Reprinted from Paulsen F, Waschke J, Sobotta J. *Sobotta Atlas of Human Anatomy.* 15th ed. Munich: Urban & Fischer, 2011. Copyright © 2011 Elsevier GmbH. With permission.)

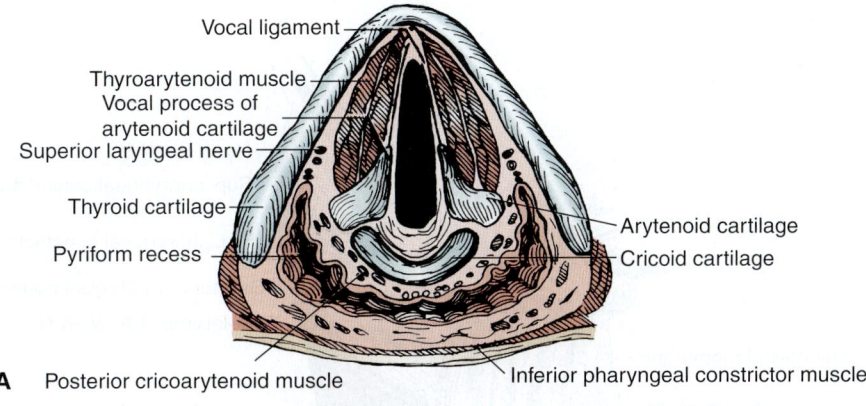

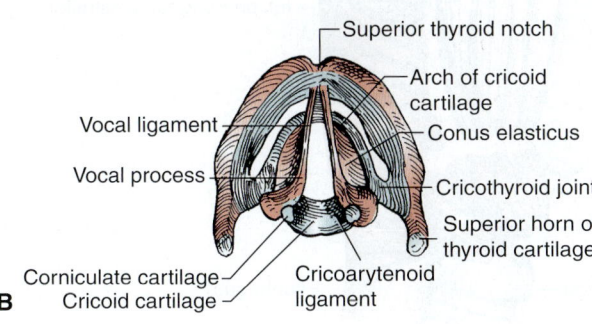

FIGURE 50.2. **A:** Cross section of the larynx at the level of the vocal cords. **B:** Framework of the larynx. (Reprinted from Paulsen F, Waschke J, Sobotta J. *Sobotta Atlas of Human Anatomy.* 15th ed. Munich: Urban & Fischer, 2011. Copyright © 2011 Elsevier GmbH. With permission.)

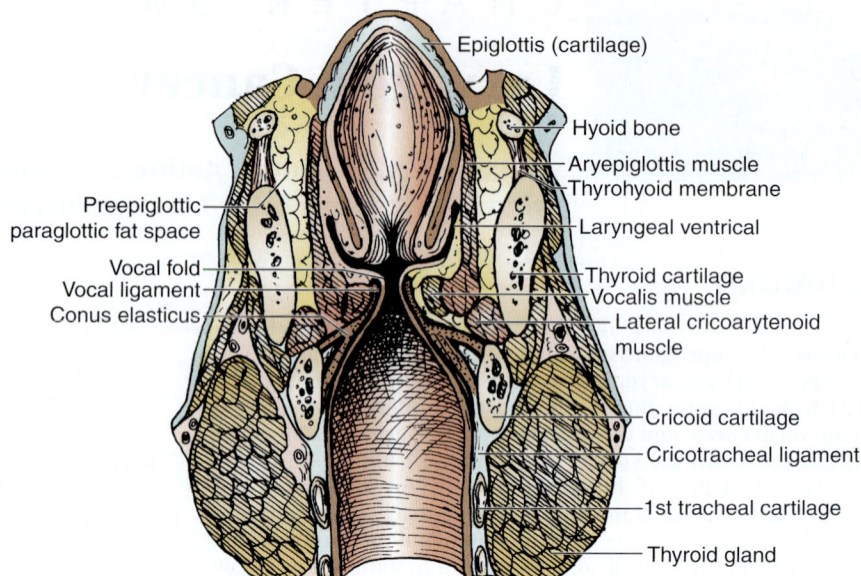

FIGURE 50.3. Diagram of the coronal view of the larynx. (Reprinted from Paulsen F, Waschke J, Sobotta J. *Sobotta Atlas of Human Anatomy.* 15th ed. Munich: Urban & Fischer, 2011. Copyright © 2011 Elsevier GmbH. With permission.)

The thyroid and the cricoid cartilages and a portion of the arytenoid cartilage are hyaline cartilage and may ossify with age, particularly in men. The epiglottis is elastic cartilage; ossification does not occur, and even focal calcification is rare.[2]

The external laryngeal framework is linked together by the thyrohyoid, the cricothyroid, and the cricotracheal ligaments or membranes (Figs. 50.3 and 50.4).[1]

The epiglottis is joined superiorly to the hyoid bone by the hyoepiglottic ligament. The epiglottis is joined to the thyroid cartilage by the thyroepiglottic ligament at a point just below the thyroid notch and above the anterior commissure. This area of attachment is the *petiole* of the epiglottis. The arrangement of the ligaments that connect the cricoid and arytenoid cartilages and form the vocal ligaments is shown in Figure 50.2B.[1] The conus elasticus (cricovocal ligament) is the lower portion of the elastic membrane that connects the inferior framework. It connects the upper surface of the cricoid, the vocal process of the arytenoid, and the lower thyroid cartilage; its free border is thickened into the vocal ligament. The quadrangular membrane is the upper portion of the elastic membrane that connects the superior framework. It connects the false vocal cords, aryepiglottic folds, and the epiglottis.

The vocal ligaments and thyroarytenoid/vocalis muscle complex attach to the vocal process of the arytenoid posteriorly and the thyroid cartilage anteriorly. The intrinsic muscles of the larynx, which primarily control the movement of the cords, are presented in Figures 50.2 and 50.3.[1] The extrinsic muscles are concerned primarily with swallowing. The

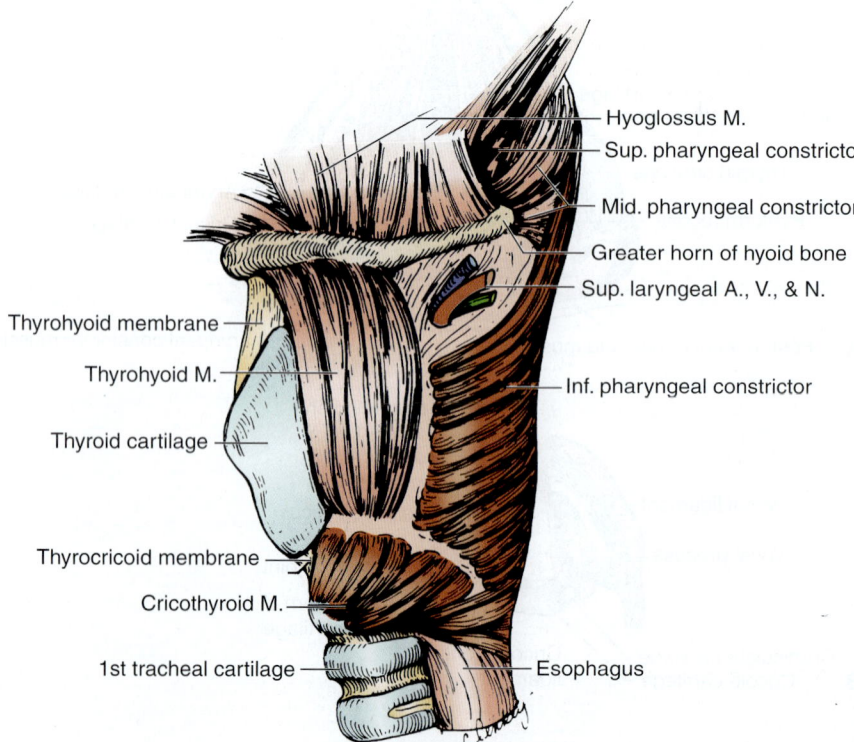

FIGURE 50.4. External view of the larynx. (Reprinted from Paulsen F, Waschke J, Sobotta J. *Sobotta Atlas of Human Anatomy.* 15th ed. Munich: Urban & Fischer, 2011. Copyright © 2011 Elsevier GmbH. With permission.)

cricothyroid muscle draws the larynx anteriorly and inferior when contracting. The consequence is increased vocal cord tension leading to increased pitch of the voice. It is innervated by the external branch of the superior laryngeal nerve (Fig. 50.4).[1] The intrinsic muscles of the larynx are innervated by the recurrent laryngeal nerve.

The preepiglottic and paraglottic fat spaces are essentially one contiguous space lying between the external framework of the thyroid cartilage and hyoid bone and the inner framework of the epiglottis and intrinsic muscles. Lam and Wong[3] showed that there are thin membranous septa between the paraglottic and preepiglottic spaces, which produce a barrier to tumor spread to a limited degree. The space is traversed by blood and lymphatic vessels as well as nerves. Because few capillary lymphatics arise in this area, invasion of the fat space seldom leads to lymph node metastases. The fat space is limited by the conus elasticus inferiorly; the thyroid ala, thyrohyoid membrane, quadrangular membrane, and hyoid bone anterolaterally; the hyoepiglottic ligament superiorly; and the fascia of the intrinsic muscles medially. Posteriorly, it is adjacent to the anterior wall of the pyriform sinus.

The laryngeal surface of the epiglottis and the free margin of the vocal cords are squamous epithelium, and the remaining mucosa is usually pseudostratified ciliated columnar epithelium. Beneath the epithelium of the free edge of the vocal cord is the lamina propria, which can be divided into three layers. There is no true submucosal layer along the free margin of the vocal fold.[4] The laryngeal arteries are branches of the superior and inferior thyroid arteries.

The supraglottic structures have a rich capillary lymphatic plexus; the trunks pass through the preepiglottic space and the thyrohyoid membrane and terminate mainly in the jugulodigastric (level II) lymph nodes; a few drain to the middle internal jugular chain (level III) lymph nodes.

There are essentially no capillary lymphatics of the true vocal cords; as a result, lymphatic spread from glottic cancer occurs only if tumor extends to supraglottic or subglottic areas.

The subglottic area has relatively few capillary lymphatics. The lymphatic trunks pass through the cricothyroid membrane to the pretracheal (delphian) lymph nodes in the region of the thyroid isthmus. The subglottic area also drains posteriorly through the cricotracheal membrane, with some trunks going to the paratracheal (level VI) lymph nodes and others continuing to the inferior jugular (level IV) chain.

EPIDEMIOLOGY AND RISK FACTORS

Cancer of the larynx represents about 2% of the total cancer burden and accounts for 0.3% of all cancer deaths. It is the second most common head and neck mucosal cancer. In 2016 in the United States, there were approximately 13,430 new cases of cancer of the larynx (10,550 men and 2,880 women) and about 3,620 deaths from laryngeal cancer.[5] Based on 1973 to 1998 US data, at diagnosis, about 51% of the cases remain localized, 29% have regional spread, and 15% have distant metastases.[6] The ratio of glottic to supraglottic carcinoma is approximately 2:1.

Cancer of the larynx is strongly related to cigarette smoking. The risk of tobacco-related cancers of the upper alimentary and respiratory tracts declines among former smokers after 5 years and is said to approach the risk of nonsmokers after 10 years of abstention.[7] The role of alcohol in provoking laryngeal cancer remains unclear.[8] Some evidence exists that heavy marijuana smoking may be associated with laryngeal cancer in young patients.

PATTERNS OF SPREAD

Local Spread

Although supraglottic and glottic lesions tend to remain confined to their original compartments, there is no anatomic barrier to growth from one area to the next. Glottic lesions tend to be slow growing, but as they increase in size, they extend to the supraglottic and subglottic areas. Supraglottic lesions do not often start near the vocal cords. Involvement of the cords on their external epithelial surface is a late phenomenon, but submucosal extension by way of the paraglottic space occurs earlier.

The fat space is an important avenue of submucosal tumor spread for infrahyoid epiglottis, false cord, and true vocal cord lesions. As the false cord and the true vocal cord lesions penetrate anteriorly and laterally, they quickly encounter the tough perichondrium of the thyroid cartilage and may eventually be shunted by the conus elasticus (lateral cricothyroid membrane) out of the larynx via the cricothyroid space. Thyroid cartilage invasion usually occurs in the ossified section of the cartilage, commonly in the region of the anterior commissure tendon or the junction of the anterior one-fourth and the posterior three-fourths of the thyroid lamina.[9]

Fixation of the vocal cord from laryngeal cancer is usually caused by invasion or destruction of the vocal cord muscle, invasion of the cricoarytenoid muscle or joint, or, rarely, invasion of the recurrent laryngeal nerve. Perineural spread is uncommon.

Supraglottic Larynx

Suprahyoid Epiglottis

A lesion of the suprahyoid epiglottis may produce a large exophytic mass with little tendency to destroy cartilage or spread to adjacent structures. Other lesions may infiltrate the tip and destroy cartilage. The destructive lesions tend to invade the vallecula and preepiglottic space, the lateral pharyngeal walls, and the remainder of the supraglottic larynx.

Infrahyoid Epiglottis

Lesions of the infrahyoid epiglottis tend to produce irregular tumor nodules and simultaneously invade the porous epiglottic cartilage and thyroepiglottic ligament into the preepiglottic fat space and extend toward the vallecula and base of the tongue. The thick hyoepiglottic ligament is an effective tumor barrier. However, the tumor may present in the vallecula and base of tongue without involving the suprahyoid epiglottis.

Lesions of the infrahyoid epiglottis grow circumferentially to involve the false cords, aryepiglottic folds, medial wall of the pyriform sinus, and the pharyngoepiglottic folds. Invasion of the anterior commissure and cords and anterior subglottic extension usually occur only in advanced lesions. Infrahyoid epiglottic lesions that extend onto or below the vocal cords are at a high risk for thyroid cartilage invasion, even if the cords are mobile.[10]

False Cord

Early false cord carcinomas, which are usually submucosal with little exophytic component, are difficult to delineate accurately. They involve the paraglottic fat space early in their development and may spread a considerable distance beneath the mucosa without producing physical signs. These carcinomas extend to the perichondrium of the thyroid cartilage quite early, but cartilage invasion is a late phenomenon. Extension to the lower portion of the infrahyoid epiglottis and invasion of the preepiglottic space are common. Submucosal extension involves the true vocal cord, which may appear normal.

Vocal cord invasion is often associated with thyroid cartilage invasion. Submucosal extension to the medial wall of the pyriform sinus occurs early.

Aryepiglottic Fold/Arytenoid

Early lesions of the aryepiglottic fold/arytenoid are usually exophytic. It may be difficult to decide whether the lesion started on the medial wall of the pyriform sinus or on the aryepiglottic fold. As the lesions enlarge, they extend to adjacent sites and eventually cause fixation of the larynx, which is usually a result of involvement of the cricoarytenoid muscle or joint or, rarely, invasion of the recurrent laryngeal nerve. Computed tomography (CT) may distinguish the cause of fixation. Advanced lesions invade the thyroid, epiglottic, and cricoid cartilages and eventually invade the pyriform sinus and postcricoid area.

Glottic Larynx

Most lesions of the true vocal cord begin on the free margin and upper surface of the cord. When diagnosed, about two-thirds are confined to the cords, usually one cord. The anterior portion of the cord is the most common site. Anterior commissure involvement, which is common, is said to occur when no tumor-free cord can be seen anteriorly; if the lesion crosses to the opposite cord, anterior commissure invasion is certain. Small lesions isolated to the anterior commissure account for only 1% to 2% of cases. Extension to the posterior commissure is uncommon, occurring only in advanced lesions.

Tumors at the anterior commissure may extend anteriorly via the anterior commissure tendon (Broyles ligament)[11] into the thyroid cartilage. Kirchner,[12] using whole-organ sections, showed that such extension is unusual unless the tumor extends off the vocal cord onto the base of the infrahyoid epiglottis and suggested that the tendon serves as more of a barrier than an avenue of tumor spread. Early subglottic extension is also associated with involvement of the anterior commissure, and tumor may grow through the cricothyroid membrane.

Lesions that arise on the posterior half of the vocal cord tend to extend along the submucosa toward the medial side of the vocal process and invade the cricoarytenoid joint and posterior commissure; this spread is difficult to appreciate by clinical examination.

Subglottic extension may occur by simple mucosal surface growth, but it more commonly occurs by submucosal penetration beneath the conus elasticus. One centimeter of subglottic extension anteriorly or 4 to 5 mm of subglottic extension posteriorly brings the border of the tumor to the upper margin of the cricoid, exceeding the anatomic limits for conventional hemilaryngectomy. Lesions may spread beneath the epithelium along the length of the vocal cord within Reinke space.[13]

As vocal cord lesions enlarge, they extend to the false cord, vocal process of the arytenoid, and subglottis. Infiltrative lesions invade the vocal ligament and muscle and eventually reach the paraglottic space and the perichondrium of the thyroid cartilage. Advanced glottic lesions eventually penetrate through the thyroid cartilage or via the cricothyroid space to enter the neck, where they may invade the thyroid gland. Lesions involving the anterior commissure often exit the larynx via the cricothyroid membrane after they extend subglottically.[13]

A fixed cord that is associated with a lesion having <1 cm of subglottic extension and no false cord involvement does not ordinarily indicate invasion of the thyroid cartilage.[12] If the false cord is also involved, cartilage invasion is likely.

Subglottic Larynx

Subglottic cancers are rare.[14] Most involve the inferior surface of the vocal cords by the time they are diagnosed, so it is difficult to know whether the tumor started on the undersurface of the vocal cord or in the true subglottic larynx. Because early diagnosis is uncommon, most lesions are bilateral or circumferential at discovery. They involve the cricoid cartilages in the early stage because there is no intervening muscle layer. Partial or complete fixation of one or both cords is common; misdiagnosis or diagnostic delay is frequent.

Lymphatic Spread

The location and stage of neck nodes detected on admission for previously untreated patients with squamous cell carcinoma of the supraglottic larynx are given in Figure 50.5.[15] The disease spreads mainly to the level II nodes. The level Ib nodes are rarely involved, and there is only a small risk of level V lymph node involvement. The incidence of clinically positive nodes is 55% at the time of diagnosis; 16% are bilateral.[15] Elective neck dissection shows pathologically positive nodes in at least 16% of cases; observation of initially node-negative necks eventually identifies the appearance of positive nodes in 33% of cases.[16,17] Spread to the pyriform sinus, vallecula, and base of the tongue increases the risk of lymph node metastases. The risk of late-appearing contralateral lymph node metastasis is 37% if the ipsilateral neck is pathologically positive, but the risk is unrelated to whether the nodes in the ipsilateral neck were palpable before neck dissection.

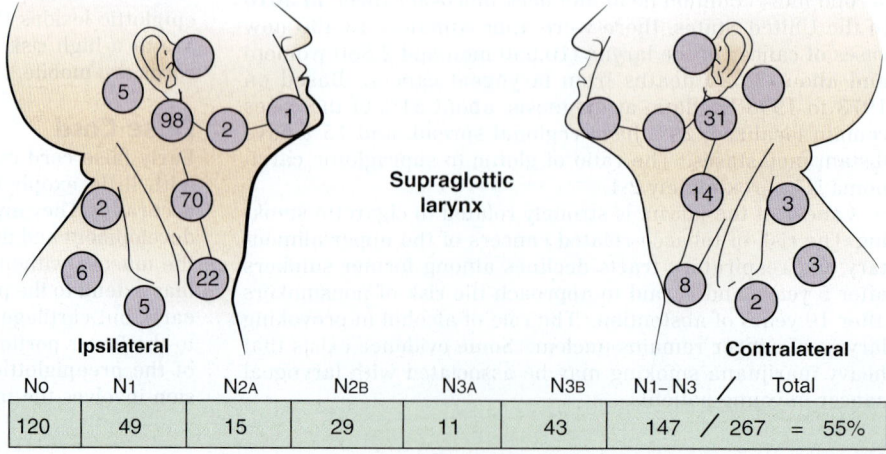

FIGURE 50.5. Nodal distribution on admission, MD Anderson Cancer Center, 1948–1965. (From Lindberg RD. Distribution of cervical lymph node metastases from squamous cell carcinoma of the upper respiratory and digestive tracts. *Cancer* 1972;29[6]:1446–1449. Copyright © 1972 American Cancer Society. Reprinted by permission of John Wiley & Sons, Inc.)

Supraglottic larynx

Ipsilateral

Contralateral

No	N1	N2A	N2B	N3A	N3B	N1–N3	/	Total
120	49	15	29	11	43	147	/ 267	= 55%

The incidence of clinically positive lymph nodes at diagnosis for vocal cord carcinoma approaches zero for T1 lesions and is <2% for T2 lesions,[18] *but it* increases to 20% to 30% for T3 and T4 lesions. Glottic spread is typically associated with metastasis to the level II nodes. Anterior commissure and anterior subglottic invasion are also associated with involvement of the midline pretracheal lymph node (level VI).

Lederman[19] reported a 10% incidence of positive lymph nodes in 73 patients with subglottic carcinoma.

CLINICAL PRESENTATION

Carcinoma arising on the true vocal cords produces hoarseness at a very early stage. Odynophagia, otalgia, pain localized to the thyroid cartilage, and airway obstruction are features of advanced lesions.

Hoarseness is not a prominent symptom of cancer of the supraglottis until the lesion becomes extensive. Odynophagia, usually mild, is the most frequent initial symptom, often described as a sore throat. Some patients report a sensation of a "lump in the throat." Pain is referred to the ear by way of the Arnold branch of the vagus nerve. A neck mass may be the first sign of a supraglottic cancer. Late symptoms include weight loss, halitosis, dysphagia, and aspiration.

DIAGNOSTIC WORKUP

Physical Examination

Flexible fiberoptic endoscopes provide the best view of the larynx, hypopharynx, and posterior oropharynx. The scope is inserted through the nasal passage and passed over the nasopharyngeal side of the soft palate to provide a "bird's-eye" view of the larynx. The mucosal surfaces of the base of the tongue, posterior pharyngeal wall, vallecula, hypopharynx, supraglottis, glottis, and subglottis are examined. Vocal cord mobility is determined by asking the patient to say "ee" (adduction) and sniff in (abduction). Subtle distinctions between paresis and paralysis may require multiple examinations or stroboscopy.

Ulceration of the infrahyoid epiglottis or fullness of the vallecula is an indirect sign of preepiglottic space invasion. Palpation of diffuse, firm fullness above the thyroid notch with widening of the space between the hyoid and the thyroid cartilages signifies invasion of the preepiglottic space. The preepiglottic fat space is a low-density area on the CT scan, and changes resulting from tumor invasion are easily seen.

Postcricoid extension may be suspected when the laryngeal click disappears on physical examination. Postcricoid tumor may cause the thyroid cartilage to protrude anteriorly, producing a fullness of the neck. Invasion of the thyroid cartilage remains a difficult clinical diagnosis. Localized pain or tenderness to palpation or a small bulge over one ala of the thyroid cartilage is suggestive.

Radiographic Studies

CT scan with contrast enhancement is often the method of choice for studying the larynx (Fig. 50.6).[20] The CT scan should be performed before biopsy so that abnormalities that may be caused by the biopsy are not confused with tumor. CT is preferred to magnetic resonance (MR) imaging because the longer scanning time for MR results in motion artifact.[21] CT slices 1 to 2 mm thick are obtained at 1- to 2-mm intervals through the larynx and at 3-mm intervals for the remainder of the study. Thinner sections (1 to 2 mm through the larynx) facilitate high-quality multiplanar reformations. The gantry is angled so that the scan slices are parallel to the plane of the true vocal cords. It is also necessary to obtain a CT scan of the entire neck to detect positive, nonpalpable lymph nodes.

Section III

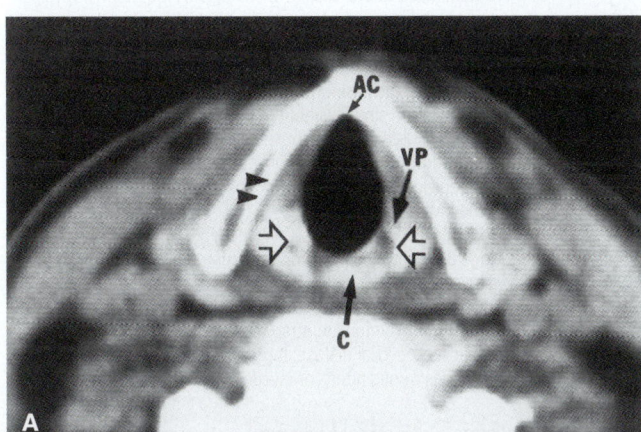

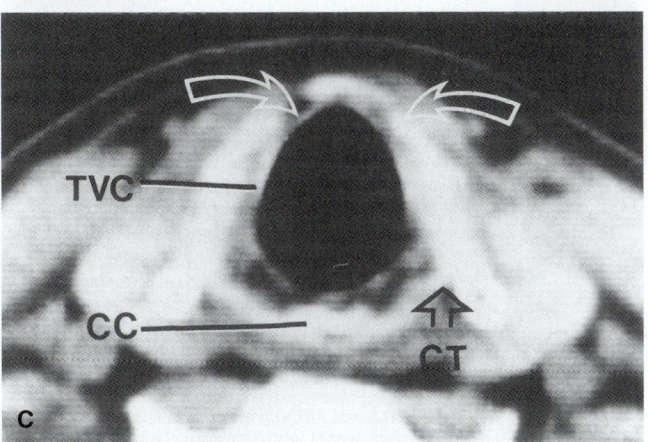

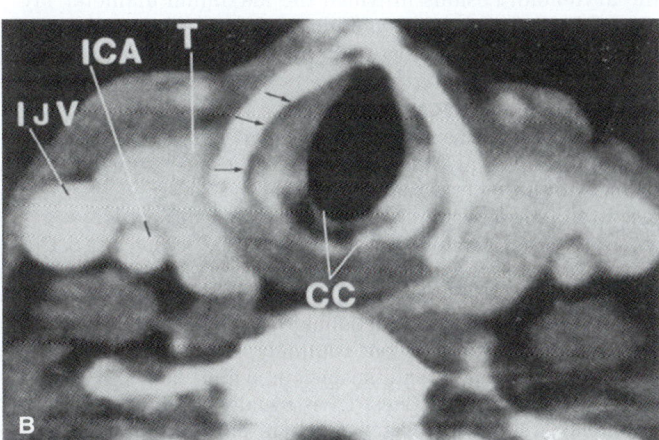

FIGURE 50.6. A: Normal CT anatomy of the midplane of the true vocal cords. *Open arrows* indicate arytenoid cartilages. The top of the cricoid cartilage (*C*) is partially visualized at this level. The vocal process (*VP*) of the left arytenoid cartilage is demonstrated. A narrow, low-density plane is seen between the right true vocal cord and the thyroid lamina (*arrowheads*); this is the inferior part of the paraglottic fat space. Notice the complete lack of tissue at the anterior commissure (*AC*). *Any tissue density here should be considered abnormal.* **B:** Normal CT anatomy just below the midplane of the vocal cords. *Arrows* indicate low-density lower paraglottic fat space. The fibrofatty tissue in this space facilitates separation of the vocal cord and the adjacent thyroid lamina. If this clear space is maintained in the face of the thyroid lamina irregularity adjacent to the tumor, the lamina abnormality can be attributed to uneven calcification rather than tumor destruction. The posterior portion (lamina) of the cricoid cartilage (*CC*) is seen. The outer and inner cortex of the cartilage is calcified; an intervening marrow space has lower density. The vertical height of the lamina is 2 to 3 cm. There is incomplete calcification of the thyroid cartilage anteriorly. ICA, internal carotid artery; IJV, internal jugular vein; T, thyroid gland. **C:** Normal CT anatomy 5 mm below the free margin of the true vocal cord (*TVC*). The vocal cord appears thin because of abduction during scanning. There is incomplete bilateral paramedian calcification and thinning of the thyroid lamina (*arrows*). Notice the normal lack of tissue density between the airway and the anterior arch of the thyroid cartilage. CC, cricoid cartilage; CT, cricothyroid joint. (From Million RR, Cassisi NJ. Larynx. In Million RR, Cassisi NJ, eds. *Management of head and neck cancer: a multidisciplinary approach.* Philadelphia: JB Lippincott, 1984:315–364. With permission.)

Positive retropharyngeal nodes may be present at diagnosis in patients with laryngeal cancer who have advanced neck disease.[22] Retropharyngeal adenopathy will not be apparent on physical examination but is usually appreciated on CT scan. Contrast enhancement helps to outline the blood vessels and the thyroid gland. Tumor is often enhanced, probably because of reactive inflammatory changes.

The value of MR imaging includes defining subtle exolaryngeal spread or early cartilage destruction as well as the extent of tracheal invasion and esophageal invasion. Sagittal MR may also be useful in detecting early invasion of the base of the tongue.

Vocal Cord Carcinoma

Although the CT scan does not show minimal mucosal lesions and is generally not helpful for well-defined and easily visualized T1 or early T2 vocal cord carcinomas, it is almost always obtained. CT is excellent for determining subglottic extension and is often used in selected T1 and most T2 lesions for this reason alone. CT scanning is useful in the diagnosis of moderately advanced and advanced lesions; it is excellent for demonstrating extension outside the larynx into the soft tissues of the neck and has potential for determining thyroid or cricoid cartilage invasion, which tends to occur at the edges of the cartilage rather than on the faces. Early cartilage involvement is difficult to detect with axial scans, but it may be demonstrated by coronal or sagittal scanning techniques. If the low-density plane of the paraglottic space is intact, cartilage is probably not invaded by tumor.

Archer et al.[23] correlated CT findings with the incidence of cartilage or bone invasion on whole-organ sections. For 12 of 14 patients with pathologic evidence of cartilage invasion, the average diameter of the tumor in two dimensions was >16 mm, and the lesion was located below the top of the arytenoid. Lesions in which the maximum diameter lay above the top of the arytenoid had a low incidence of cartilage invasion.[23]

Supraglottic Carcinoma

The CT scan provides an excellent means for viewing the preepiglottic and paraglottic fat spaces. Soft tissue extension into the neck or base of the tongue can also be seen. The CT scan is also useful for determining extension to the subglottis.[2]

Diagnostic procedures for laryngeal cancer at the University of Florida are summarized in Table 50.1.[24] A CT scan is usually performed for all patients; MR is obtained in a small subset of patients with questionable findings on CT. Positron emission tomography is not routinely obtained; although it may be useful to evaluate suspicious lymph nodes, it would change the treatment. Chest CT is usually obtained to detect pulmonary metastases, particularly in patients with positive cervical nodes. It may also be useful to identify the occasional synchronous lung cancer. Direct laryngoscopy and biopsy with frozen section are usually performed with the patient under

general anesthesia. The ventricles, subglottis, apex of the pyriform sinus, and postcricoid area must be carefully examined because these areas are not consistently seen by indirect examinations. Fiberoptic telescopes (0 and 30 degrees) are introduced through the laryngoscope for inspection of these areas. A generous biopsy specimen is taken from the obvious lesion; additional biopsy specimens may be obtained from suspicious areas and from areas grossly involved. The mucosa of the margin of the cord may be stripped to provide adequate tissue if the lesion is distributed superficially along the cord and is not obviously a carcinoma.

STAGING

The 2017 American Joint Committee on Cancer (AJCC)[25] staging system for laryngeal primary cancer is listed in Table 50.2. T2 glottic cancers are stratified into those with normal (T2A) and impaired (T2B) vocal cord mobility. For lesions arising in the supraglottis, the sites of origin include false cords, aryepiglottic folds, suprahyoid epiglottis, infrahyoid epiglottis, pharyngoepiglottic folds, and arytenoids. Only in the early T stages can one identify the specific site of origin with certainty. As the lesion enlarges, the site of origin is often an educated guess based on the location of the greatest tumor bulk/density. The major difference between the 1998 and 2010 staging systems is that a glottic cancer that invades the paraglottic space is upstaged to T3 in the latter system, even with mobile vocal

TABLE 50.1 DIAGNOSTIC WORKUP FOR CARCINOMA OF THE LARYNX

General
 History
 Physical examination
 Indirect laryngoscopy
 Direct laryngoscopy
 Biopsies
Radiographic studies
 Chest x-ray films
 Computed tomography with contrast enhancement (before biopsy)
 Magnetic resonance imaging (selected cases)

From Mendenhall WM, Parsons JT, Mancuso AA, et al. Larynx. In Perez CA, Brady LW. *Principles and practice radiation of oncology.* 4th ed. Philadelphia: Lippincott-Raven, 1998:1094–1116.

TABLE 50.2 STAGING OF LARYNGEAL CANCER

Supraglottis

TX	Primary tumor cannot be assessed
Tis	Carcinoma *in situ*
T1	Tumor limited to one subsite of supraglottis with normal vocal cord mobility
T2	Tumor invades mucosa of more than one adjacent subsite of supraglottis or glottis or region outside the supraglottis (e.g., mucosa of the base of the tongue, vallecula, medial wall of the pyriform sinus) without fixation of the larynx.
T3	Tumor is limited to the larynx with vocal cord fixation and/or invades any of the following area: postcricoid space, preepiglottic space, paraglottic space, and/or inner cortex of the thyroid cartilage
T4	Moderately advanced or very advanced
T4a	Moderately advanced local disease; tumor invades through the thyroid cartilage and/or invades tissues beyond the larynx (e.g., trachea, soft tissues of the neck including deep extrinsic muscles of the tongue, strap muscles, thyroid, or esophagus)
T4b	Very advanced local disease; tumor invades prevertebral space, encases carotid artery, or invades mediastinal structures

Glottis

TX	Primary tumor cannot be assessed
Tis	Carcinoma *in situ*
T1	Tumor limited to the vocal cord(s) (may involve the anterior or posterior commissure) with normal mobility
T1a	Tumor limited to one vocal cord
T1b	Tumor involves both vocal cords.
T2	Tumor extends to the supraglottis and/or subglottis with impaired vocal cord mobility.
T3	Tumor limited to the larynx with vocal cord fixation and/or invasion of paraglottic space and/or inner cortex of the thyroid cartilage
T4	Moderately advanced or very advanced
T4a	Moderately advanced local disease; tumor invades through the outer cortex of the thyroid cartilage and/or invades tissues beyond the larynx (e.g., trachea, cricoid cartilage, soft tissues of the neck including deep extrinsic muscle of the tongue, strap muscles, thyroid, or esophagus)
T4b	Very advanced local disease; tumor invades the prevertebral space, encases the carotid artery, or invades mediastinal structures

From Amin MB, Edge SB, Greene FL, et al., eds. *AJCC Cancer Staging Manual.* 8th ed. New York, NY: Springer, 2017. Reproduced with permission of Springer International Publishing in the format Book via Copyright Clearance Center.

cords, resulting in significant stage migration.[26] In addition, T4 has been stratified into T4A and T4B, based on resectability.

PATHOLOGIC CLASSIFICATION

Nearly all malignant tumors of the larynx arise from the surface epithelium and therefore are squamous cell carcinoma or one of its variants.

Carcinoma *in situ* occurs frequently on the vocal cords. Differentiating among dysplasia, carcinoma *in situ*, squamous cell carcinoma with microinvasion, and true invasive carcinoma is a problem that the pathologist and the clinician frequently confront.

Most vocal cord carcinomas are well or moderately well differentiated. In a few cases, an apparent carcinoma and sarcoma occur together, but most of these are actually a spindle cell carcinoma (i.e., squamous cell carcinoma with a spindle cell stromal reaction).

Verrucous carcinoma occurs in 1% to 2% of patients with carcinoma of the vocal cord. The histologic diagnosis is difficult and must correlate with the gross appearance of the lesion.

Small cell neuroendocrine carcinoma is rarely diagnosed in the supraglottic larynx, but it should be recognized because of its biologic potential for rapid growth, early dissemination, and responsiveness to chemotherapy.[27]

Minor salivary gland tumors arise from the mucous glands in the supraglottic and subglottic larynx, but they are rare.[28] Even rarer are paragangliomas, carcinoids, soft tissue sarcomas, malignant lymphomas, and plasmacytomas. Benign chondromas and osteochondromas are reported, but their malignant counterparts are rare.

PROGNOSTIC FACTORS

The extent of the primary lesion and neck disease are the major determinants of prognosis. The likelihood of local control is determined primarily by T stage; there are conflicting data pertaining to a possible inverse relationship between N stage and local control. The likelihood of local–regional control is affected primarily by the overall AJCC stage, which accounts for both T stage and N stage. AJCC stage and N stage are the major determinants of cause-specific survival. In addition, within each N stage, patients with positive nodes in the low neck below the level of the thyroid notch tend to have a lower cause-specific survival rate than do those with disease confined to the upper neck. In general, women tend to have a better prognosis than do men.

TREATMENT SELECTION AND TECHNIQUE: VOCAL CORD CARCINOMA

Selection of Treatment Modality

In treating vocal cord carcinoma, the goal is cure with the best functional result and the least risk of a serious complication. Patients may be considered to be in an early group if the chance of cure with larynx preservation is high, a moderately advanced group if the likelihood of local control is 60% to 70% but the chance of cure is still good, and an advanced group if the chance of cure is moderate and the likelihood of laryngeal preservation is relatively low.[29] The early group may be treated initially by radiotherapy (RT) or, in selected cases, by transoral laser microsurgery (TLM) or transoral robotic surgery (TORS).[30] The moderately advanced group may be treated either with RT with laryngectomy reserved for relapse or by total laryngectomy with or without adjuvant postoperative RT. The obvious advantage of the former strategy, which is used at the University of Florida, is that

there is a fairly good chance that the larynx will be preserved.[31] Although some patients may be rehabilitated with a tracheoesophageal puncture after laryngectomy, only about 20% of patients use this device long term, and the majority use an electrolarynx.[32] The advanced group is treated with total laryngectomy and neck dissection with or without adjuvant RT or by RT and adjuvant chemotherapy.[33] Data suggest that if patients whose tumors show a partial or complete response to two to three cycles of neoadjuvant chemotherapy are then given high-dose RT, the cure rates are comparable with those obtained with initial total laryngectomy.[34] Another less expensive and less toxic method to select patients likely to be cured by RT alone is to calculate the primary tumor volume on pretreatment CT or MR. Data indicate that primary tumor volume is inversely related to the probability of local control after irradiation.[35,36] Recent data indicate that whereas induction chemotherapy probably does not improve the likelihood of local–regional control and survival, concomitant chemotherapy and RT result in an improved likelihood of cure compared with RT alone.[37–39] There is a subset of patients with high-volume (>3.5 cc), unfavorable, advanced cancers who may be cured by chemoradiation but have a useless larynx and permanent tracheostomy and/or gastrostomy.[35] These patients are best treated with a total laryngectomy, neck dissection, and postoperative RT.[40]

Carcinoma *In Situ*

Lesions diagnosed as carcinoma *in situ* can be treated with TLM. However, it is difficult to exclude the possibility of microinvasion on these specimens. Recurrence is frequent if the patient continues to smoke, and the cord may become thickened and the voice hoarse with repeated treatments.

Early RT for carcinoma *in situ* often means a better chance of preserving a good voice, especially because many patients with this diagnosis eventually receive this treatment.[37]

Many patients with a diagnosis of carcinoma *in situ* have obvious lesions that probably contain invasive carcinoma. We have often proceeded with RT rather than put the patient through a repeated biopsy procedure.

Early Vocal Cord Carcinoma

In many centers, RT is the initial treatment prescribed for T1 and T2 lesions, with surgery reserved for salvage after RT failure.[18,41,42] However, TLM and TORS have shown comparable cure rates with the possibility of using RT for recurrences.[41,43,44] Supracricoid laryngectomy, as reported by Laccourreye et al.,[45] is a procedure designed to remove moderate-sized cancers involving the supraglottic and glottic larynx. The larynx may be removed with preservation of the cricoid and the arytenoid with its neurovascular innervation; the defect is closed by approximating the base of the tongue to the remaining larynx. The oncologic and functional results of this procedure in selected patients are reported to be excellent. TLM also may provide high cure rates for select patients with small, well-defined lesions limited to the mid one-third of one true cord.[46–50] A small subset of TLM surgeons successfully use this technique for moderately advanced cancers.[41] The major advantage of RT compared with partial laryngectomy is better quality of the voice. The advantages of surgical treatments include avoidance of RT, single treatment, and cost-effectiveness. However, if voice quality is important for the patient, surgery should be avoided. Open partial laryngectomy finds its major use as salvage surgery in suitable cases after RT failure. Even if the patient has a local recurrence after salvage partial laryngectomy, there is a third chance with total laryngectomy, which may still be successful.

Verrucous lesions have the reputation of being unresponsive to RT and, in some instances, converting into invasive, often anaplastic, metastasizing lesions. Partial laryngectomy is recommended for early verrucous carcinoma of the glottis, but RT is recommended if the alternative is total laryngectomy. We have observed typical verrucous lesions that have disappeared with RT and not recurred. O'Sullivan et al.[51] also made this observation. In addition, a variety of tumors that recur after unsuccessful treatment (with surgery, RT, and/or chemotherapy) are more likely to exhibit more aggressive behavior.

Moderately Advanced Vocal Cord Cancer

Fixed-cord lesions (T3) may be subdivided into relatively favorable or unfavorable lesions. Patients with unfavorable lesions usually have extensive bilateral disease with a compromised airway and are considered to be in the advanced group. Patients with favorable T3 lesions have disease confined mostly to one side of the larynx, have a good airway, and are reliable for follow-up. Some degree of supraglottic and subglottic extension usually exists. The extent of disease and tumor volume are related to the likelihood of control after RT.[35]

The patient with a favorable lesion is advised of the alternatives of RT with surgical salvage or immediate total laryngectomy. Recent data suggest that the likelihood of local–regional control is better after some altered fractionation schedules compared with conventional once-daily RT.[39,52] Follow-up examinations are recommended every 4 to 6 weeks for the 1st year, every 6 to 8 weeks for the 2nd year, every 3 months for the 3rd year, every 6 months for the 4 and 5th years, and annually thereafter. The patient must understand that total laryngectomy may be recommended purely on clinical grounds without biopsy-proven recurrence and that the risk of laryngeal osteochondronecrosis is about 5%.

Evaluation of cord mobility after 50.4 Gy or at the end of RT has not been helpful in predicting local control.[36] Some patients in whom the vocal cord remained fixed have had local tumor control of the disease for 2 years or longer after RT.

The major difficulty in using RT for the more advanced lesions is distinguishing radiation edema from local recurrence during follow-up examinations.[53] Progressive laryngeal edema, persistent throat pain, or fixation of a previously mobile vocal cord frequently signifies recurrent disease in the larynx, although a few patients with these findings remain disease free with long-term follow-up.

Extended hemilaryngectomy has been used by a few surgeons in the treatment of well-lateralized fixed-cord lesions. A permanent tracheostomy is usually required because a portion of the cricoid is resected, but a useful voice may be retained.[54]

Advanced Vocal Cord Carcinoma

Advanced lesions usually show extensive subglottic and supraglottic extension, bilateral glottic involvement, and invasion of the thyroid, cricoid, and/or arytenoid cartilages.[9,23] The airway is compromised, necessitating a tracheostomy at the time of direct laryngoscopy in approximately 30% of patients. Clinically positive lymph nodes are found in about 25% to 30% of patients.

The mainstay of treatment is total laryngectomy, with or without adjuvant RT. The most frequent sites of local failure after total laryngectomy are the tracheal stoma, the base of the tongue, the neck lymph nodes, and/or or soft tissues of the neck. If the neck is clinically negative before surgery and if postoperative RT is planned, neck dissection may be withheld, and RT may be used to treat both sides of the neck. However, in practice, most surgeons prefer to perform elective bilateral selective (levels II to IV) neck dissections in conjunction with a total laryngectomy for T3 N0 or T4 N0 laryngeal cancer, even

if postoperative RT is planned. If the lymph nodes are clinically positive, a therapeutic neck dissection is performed at the time of laryngectomy.

The indications for postoperative RT include close or positive margins, significant subglottic extension (1 cm or more), cartilage invasion, perineural invasion, lymphovascular space invasion, extension of the primary tumor into the soft tissues of the neck, multiple positive neck nodes, and extracapsular extension.[55,56] Preoperative RT is indicated for patients who have fixed neck nodes, have had an emergency tracheotomy through tumor, or have direct extension of tumor involving the skin.

Definitive RT is prescribed for the patient who refuses total laryngectomy or is medically unsuitable for major surgery.

As previously stated, there is evidence that two to three cycles of induction chemotherapy followed by RT in patients obtaining at least a partial response may provide a moderate likelihood of larynx preservation without compromising cure.[34] Data suggest that concomitant chemotherapy and RT is more efficacious than RT alone or induction chemotherapy followed by RT.[37,38] The optimal combination of concomitant chemotherapy and irradiation is unclear.[39]

A randomized intergroup trial (RTOG 91-11) compared three treatment arms: arm A, three cycles of induction cisplatin and fluorouracil followed by RT in complete and partial responders; arm B, RT and concomitant cisplatin (100 mg/m² on days 1, 22, and 43 of RT); and arm C, once-daily RT (70 Gy in 35 fractions over 7 weeks) alone.[37] Five hundred forty-seven patients were randomized and followed for a median of 3.8 years; 518 patients were evaluable. The rates of larynx preservation were as follows: arm A, 72%; arm B, 84%; and arm C, 67%. The rates of larynx presentation were significantly improved for arm B; there was no significant difference between arms A and C. The 5-year survival rates were similar for the three treatment groups: arm A, 55%; arm B, 54%; and arm C, 56%. The likelihood of developing distant metastases was lower for the two groups of patients that received adjuvant chemotherapy.

Surgical Treatment

Cordectomy is an excision of the vocal cord and may be performed by a TLM or TORS approach or externally by a thyrotomy. Its use is usually confined to small lesions of the middle one-third of the cord. After cordectomy, a pseudocord is formed, and the patient has a useful, if somewhat harsh, voice.

Vertical partial laryngectomy (i.e., hemilaryngectomy) allows removal of limited cord lesions with preservation of voice. One entire cord with as much as one-third of the opposite cord with the adjacent thyroid cartilage is the maximum cordal involvement suitable for surgery in men; women have a smaller larynx, and usually only one vocal cord may be removed without compromising the airway. Partial fixation of one cord is not a contraindication to hemilaryngectomy; a few surgeons perform a hemilaryngectomy for selected fixed-cord lesions. The maximum subglottic extension suitable for hemilaryngectomy is 8 to 9 mm anteriorly and 5 mm posteriorly; this limit is necessary to preserve the integrity of the cricoid. Tumor extension to the epiglottis, false cord, or both arytenoids is a contraindication to hemilaryngectomy.

Supracricoid partial laryngectomy is used for selected T2 and T3 glottic carcinomas and entails removal of both true and false cords as well as the entire thyroid cartilage. The cricoid is sutured to the epiglottis and hyoid (cricohyoidoepiglottopexy).

Total laryngectomy with or without neck dissection is the operation of choice for advanced lesions and as a salvage procedure for RT failures in lesions that are not suitable for conservation surgery. The entire larynx is removed, and the pharynx is reconstructed. A permanent tracheostomy is required. Speech may be reconstituted with a prosthesis or with an electrolarynx. One hundred four (63%) of 166 patients entered into the surgery and postoperative irradiation arm of the Veterans Affairs Laryngeal Cancer Study Group randomized trial were evaluable for voice rehabilitation at 2 years after treatment.[57] Ninety-six patients had undergone a total laryngectomy and communicated as follows: tracheoesophageal, 27 (28%); esophageal, 5 (5%); artificial larynx, 47 (50%); nonvocal, 7 (7%); and no data, 10 (10%).[57] One hundred seventy-three patients underwent total laryngectomy and postoperative RT at the University of Florida, and 69 patients were evaluable for 5 years or longer.[32] Voice rehabilitation was accomplished as follows: tracheoesophageal, 19%; electrolarynx, 57%; esophageal, 3%; nonvocal, 14%; and no data, 7%.

Radiation Therapy Technique

RT for T1 or T2 vocal cord cancer is delivered by small portals covering only the primary lesion.[42] The cervical lymph node chain is not electively treated. For T1 lesions, RT portals extend from the thyroid notch superiorly to the inferior border of the cricoid and fall off anteriorly. The posterior border depends on the posterior extension of the tumor.[21] For T2 tumors, the field is extended depending on the anatomic distribution of the tumor. The field size ranges from 4 × 4 cm to 5 × 5 cm (plus an additional 1.0 cm of "flash" anteriorly) and is occasionally 6 × 6 cm for a large T2 lesion. Portals larger than this increase the risk of edema without improving the cure rate. IMRT may be considered for T1 T2 glottic cancers to reduce the dose to carotid arteries.[42] The potential advantages of this technique must be weighed against the potential increased likelihood of a marginal miss.

A commonly used dose fractionation schedule at many institutions is 66 Gy for T1 lesions and 70 Gy for T2 cancers given in 2-Gy fractions. Evidence suggests that increasing the dose per fraction may improve the likelihood of local control.[58–62] Ample data suggest that 1.8 Gy once daily results in significantly lower local control rates compared with 2.0 Gy once daily.[59] Yamakazi et al.[63] reported a prospective trial in which patients with T1 N0 squamous cell carcinoma of the glottic larynx were randomized to definitive RT at 2.0 Gy per fraction or 2.25 Gy per fraction. The 5-year local control rates were 77% after 2.0 Gy per fraction and 92% after Gy per fraction (*P* = .004); there was no difference in either acute or late toxicity. Patients with T1 or T2 vocal cord cancer treated with once-a-day fractionation at the University of Florida are irradiated with 2.25-Gy fractions; the dose fractionation schemes used are as follows: Tis–T2 A, 63.0 Gy in 28 fractions, and T2B, 65.25 Gy in 29 fractions. Concomitant weekly cisplatin 30 ng/M² is considered for patients with T2B cancers.

At the University of Florida, patients are treated in the supine position; the field borders for a patient with a T1 N0 cancer are depicted in Figure 50.7.[21] The field is checked by the physician at the treatment machine according to palpable anatomic landmarks. This allows the treatment volume to be kept at a minimum and reduces the risk of geographic miss. A three-field technique, using 4- or 6-MV x-rays, is used to deliver approximately 95% of the dose through opposed lateral wedged fields weighted to the side of the lesion; the remaining dose is delivered by an anterior field shifted 0.5 cm toward the side of the lesion (Fig. 50.8).[21] The tumor dose is usually specified at the 95% normalized isodose line.

RT of T3 and T4 lesions requires larger portals, which include the levels II and III lymph nodes (Fig. 50.9).[20,64] The level IV lymph nodes are included in a separate low-neck portal. Patients treated at the University of Florida are irradiated in a continuous course twice daily at 1.2 Gy per fraction to a total dose of 74.4 Gy. The portals are reduced after 50.4 Gy in 42 fractions; the reduced portals cover only the primary lesion.

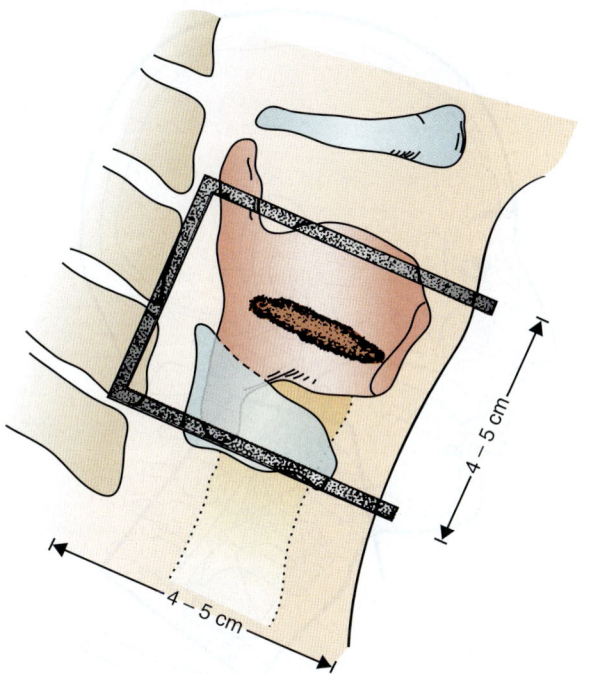

FIGURE 50.7. Conventional treatment portal for early glottic carcinoma. The top border is adjusted according to the lesion. The middle of the thyroid notch is the landmark for very early lesions, and the top of the notch is the marker for larger lesions or those with minimal supraglottic extension. The posterior border is 1 cm posterior to the back edge of the thyroid cartilage if the lesion is confined to the anterior two-thirds of the vocal cord; if the posterior one-third of the vocal cord is involved, the posterior border is placed 1.0 to 1.5 cm behind the cartilage. The inferior border is placed at the bottom of the cricoid cartilage if there is no subglottic extension. (From Million RR, Cassisi NJ, Mancuso AA. Larynx. In: Million RR, Cassisi NJ, eds. *Management head of neck and cancer: a multidisciplinary approach.* 2nd ed. Philadelphia: JB Lippincott, 1994:431–497. With permission.)

Intensity-modulated RT (IMRT) is used if there is a clear advantage associated with this technique. Disadvantages associated with IMRT include increased dose inhomogeneity, increased total body dose, and increased labor and expense.[65] The most common indications for IMRT for laryngeal cancers would be the occasional patients with a node-positive T3–T4 cancer, where the retropharyngeal nodes would be electively irradiated and the dose to the contralateral parotid

FIGURE 50.8. Normalized isodose distribution for three-field technique for treatment of a tumor involving the anterior two-thirds of one true vocal cord. The dose is specified at the 95% isodose line. (From Million RR, Cassisi NJ, Mancuso AA. Larynx. In: Million RR, Cassisi NJ, eds. *Management head of neck and cancer: a multidisciplinary approach.* 2nd ed. Philadelphia: JB Lippincott, 1994:431–497. With permission.)

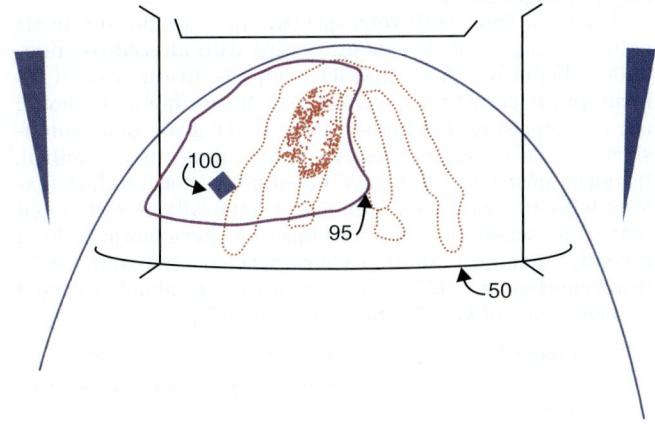

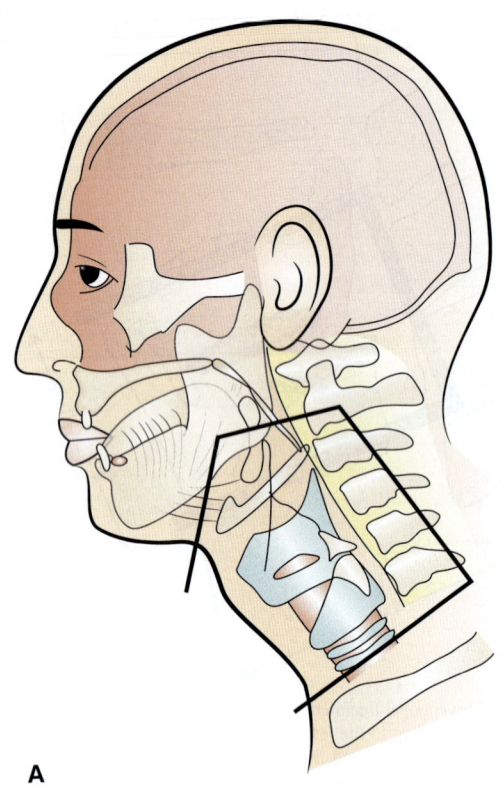

A

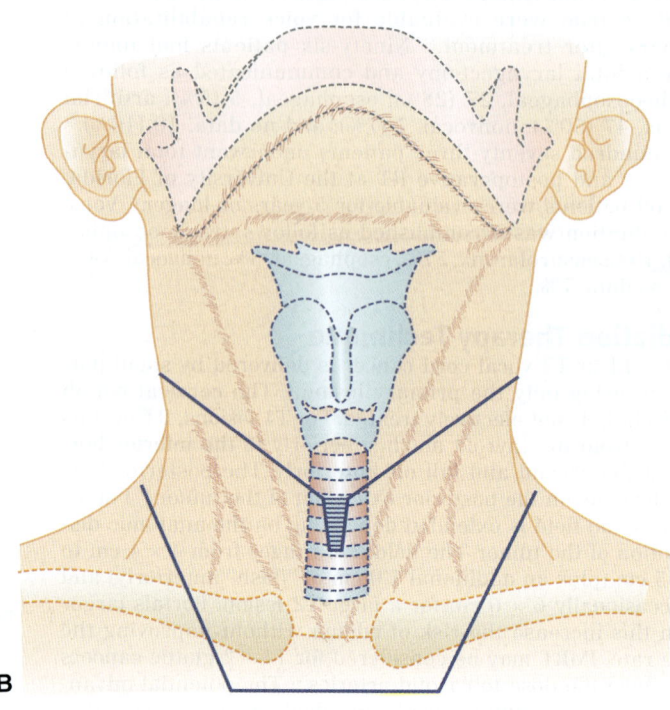

B

FIGURE 50.9. A: Radiation treatment technique for carcinoma of glottic larynx, stage T3–T4 N0. The patient is treated supine, and the field is shaped with Lipowitz metal. Anteriorly, the field is allowed to fall off. The entire preepiglottic space is included by encompassing the hyoid bone and epiglottis. The superior border (just above the angle of the mandible) includes the jugulodigastric lymph nodes. Posteriorly, a portion of the spinal cord must be included within the field to ensure adequate coverage of the midjugular lymph nodes; spinal accessory lymph nodes themselves are at little risk of involvement. The lower border is slanted to facilitate matching with the low-neck field and to reduce the length of spinal cord in the high-dose field. The inferior border is placed at the bottom of the cricoid cartilage if the patient has no subglottic spread; in the presence of subglottic extension, the inferior border must be lowered according to the disease extent. **B:** Example of a low-neck portal for T3 N0 glottic carcinoma. The main nodes at risk are the low jugular and lateral paratracheal nodes. The delphian node would be in the primary portal. A very narrow and short midline shield is used. (**A**, From Parsons JT, Mendenhall WM, Mancuso AA, et al. Twice-a-day radiotherapy for T3 squamous cell carcinoma of the glottic larynx. *Head Neck* 1989;11[2]:123–128. Copyright © 1989 Wiley Periodicals, Inc., A Wiley Company. Reprinted by permission of John Wiley & Sons, Inc.; **B**, From Million RR, Cassisi NJ, Mancuso AA, et al. Management of the neck for squamous cell carcinoma. In: Million RR, Cassisi NJ, eds. Management of head and neck a cancer: *a multidisciplinary approach*. 2nd ed. Philadelphia: JB Lippincott; 1994:75–143. With permission.)

gland reduced, and/or a difficult low match between the lateral fields used to treat the primary site and upper neck and the anterior low-neck field in a patient with a short neck and large shoulders. In the latter instance, IMRT could be used to encompass the entire target volume and avoid the problem of field junctioning entirely. IMRT is especially useful for patients with extensive subglottic invasion, where achieving an adequate inferior margin with conventional lateral portals may not be possible.

Evidence from both retrospective and randomized trials points to improved therapeutic ratios with altered fractionation schedules.[39] Given that RT is an effective treatment for head and neck primary squamous cell carcinoma, it should not be surprising that higher doses of RT given more intensively would be more effective at providing tumor control. Because most observers have noted no increase in late toxicity with the various regimens, it generally is concluded that these schedules yield an improved therapeutic ratio. A recently updated Radiation Therapy Oncology Group 90-03 trial reported on 1,073 patients who were randomly selected to receive one of four fractionation schedules[52,66,67]:

1. Standard fractionation: 2 Gy per fraction, once a day, 5 days a week, to a total dose of 70 Gy in 35 fractions over 7 weeks

2. Hyperfractionation: 1.2 Gy per fraction, twice daily (≥6 hours apart), 5 days a week, to a total dose of 81.6 Gy in 68 fractions over 7 weeks

3. Accelerated fractionation with split: 1.6 Gy per fraction, twice daily (≥6 hours apart), 5 days a week, to a total dose of 67.2 Gy in 42 fractions over 6 weeks, including a 2-week rest after 38.4 Gy

4. Accelerated fractionation with concomitant boost: 1.8 Gy per fraction, once a day, 5 days a week to a large field, plus 1.5 Gy per fraction once a day to a boost field given 6 or more hours after treatment of the large field for the last 12 treatments days, to a total dose of 72 Gy in 42 fractions over 6 weeks

The 5-year local–regional failure rates were as follows: standard fractionation, 59%; hyperfractionation, 51%; accelerated split course, 58%; and concomitant boost, 52%. Both the hyperfractionation and concomitant schedules boost yielded local–regional control rates that were significantly better than those with standard fractionation. There was a trend toward improved overall survival with hyperfractionation but no difference in cause-specific survival. Acute toxicity was increased with all three altered fractionation schedules; there was a modest increase in late effects with the concomitant boost schedule.

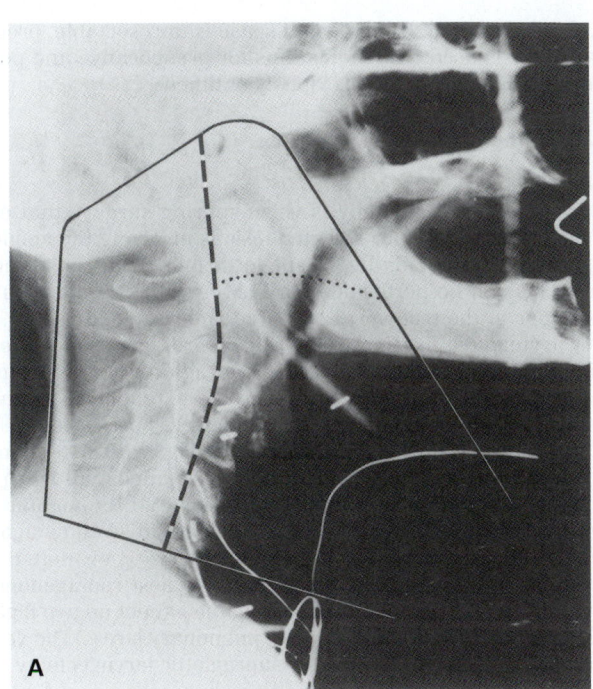

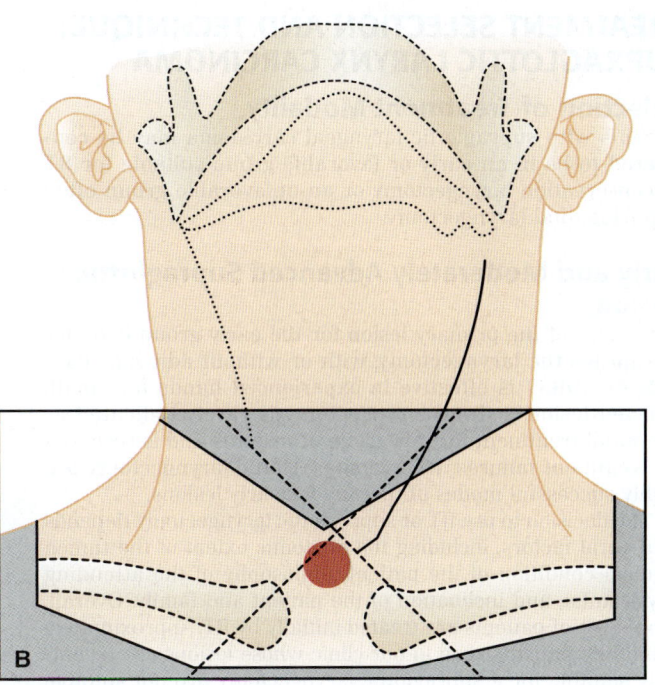

FIGURE 50.10. **A:** Typical lateral simulation film for postoperative treatment of advanced cancer of the laryngopharynx. If the neck is pathologically negative, the superior field border is lowered to 2 cm above the angle of the mandible. The initial "off-cord" reduction (50 Gy) (*broken line*) and the final reduction (*dotted line*) are indicated. Wires mark the surgical scars and stoma. The slanting line used on the lower border reduces the length of spinal cord treated by the primary field, allows better caudal coverage of the mucosal surfaces while simultaneously bypassing the shoulders, and facilitates matching of the low-neck field. **B:** Schematic diagram of the low-neck field. The rectangle (*solid line*) represents the light field. The shaded areas represent the blocked portions of the field (stacked lead blocks). The superior border of the neck field is the inferior border of the primary field. The actual line is treated only in the primary field. The upper border of the low-neck field assumes a V shape. In the midline of the patient, the apex of the V generally is at or close to the central axis (*broken lines*), so that the portal that treats the spinal cord is not divergent in its upper portion and diverges away from the primary fields in its lower portion. At the junction of the three fields, a short (2 to 3 cm) segment of the spinal cord remains untreated by any of the three fields. (Reprinted from Amdur RJ, Parsons JT, Mendenhall WM, et al. Postoperative irradiation for squamous cell carcinoma of the head and neck: an analysis of treatment results and complications. *Int J Radiat Oncol Biol Phys* 1989;16[1]:25–36. Copyright © 1989 Elsevier. With permission.)

The treatment technique used for postoperative RT after total laryngectomy is depicted in Figure 50.10.[55] The treatment technique for preoperative RT is essentially the same as that used for RT alone. Alternatively, IMRT may be employed for the indications discussed previously.

Treatment of Recurrence

Most recurrences appear within 18 months, but late recurrences may appear after 5 years. The latter are likely second primary malignancies. The risk of metastatic disease in lymph nodes increases with local recurrence.[18]

Recurrence after Radiation Therapy

With careful follow-up, recurrence is sometimes detected before the patient notices a return of hoarseness. There is often minimal lymphedema for 1 to 2 months after RT, which usually subsides or stabilizes. An increase in edema, particularly if associated with hoarseness or pain, suggests recurrence, even if there is no obvious tumor. Fixation of a previously mobile vocal cord usually implies local recurrence, but we have occasionally observed a patient who has experienced a fixed cord with an otherwise normal-appearing larynx and who has not shown evidence of recurrence.

It may be difficult to diagnose recurrence if the tumor is submucosal. Generous, deep biopsies are required. If recurrence is strongly suspected, laryngectomy may rarely be advised without biopsy-confirmed evidence of recurrence. Positron emission tomography may be useful to distinguish recurrent tumor from necrosis.

RT failures may be salvaged by cordectomy, hemilaryngectomy, supracricoid partial laryngectomy, or total laryngectomy. Biller et al.[68] reported a 78% salvage rate by hemilaryngectomy for 18 selected patients in whom RT failed; total laryngectomy was eventually required in 2 patients. Only 2 patients died of cancer. These investigators offered guidelines for using hemilaryngectomy: contralateral vocal cord is normal, arytenoid is not involved, subglottic extension does not exceed 5 mm, and vocal cord is not fixed. In our experience, 14 patients irradiated for T1 or T2 vocal cord cancers underwent a hemilaryngectomy after local recurrence, and 8 were successfully salvaged.[18]

Recurrence after Surgery

The rate of salvage by RT for recurrences or new tumors that appear after initial treatment by hemilaryngectomy is about 50%. Lee et al.[69] reported 7 successes among 12 patients; one lesion was later controlled by total laryngectomy. Total laryngectomy can be used successfully to treat hemilaryngectomy failures not suitable for RT. RT rarely cures patients with recurrence in the neck or stoma after total laryngectomy.

TREATMENT SELECTION AND TECHNIQUE: SUPRAGLOTTIC LARYNX CARCINOMA

Selection of Treatment Modality

Patients with supraglottic laryngeal carcinoma may be considered to be in an early or favorable group suitable for RT or conservation laryngectomy or an unfavorable group often requiring total laryngectomy.

Early and Moderately Advanced Supraglottic Lesions

Treatment of the primary lesion for the early group is by RT or supraglottic laryngectomy, with or without adjuvant RT.[70] TLM or TORS[71] is effective in experienced hands for small, selected lesions.[47] Total laryngectomy is rarely indicated as the initial treatment for this group of patients and is reserved for treatment failures. RT and supraglottic laryngectomy are highly successful modes of therapy for early lesions.[70]

The decision to use RT or supraglottic laryngectomy depends on several factors, including the anatomic extent of the tumor, medical condition of the patient, philosophy of the attending physician(s), and inclination of the patient and family. Overall, about 80% of patients are treated initially by RT. Approximately half of the patients seen in our clinic whose lesions are technically suitable for a supraglottic laryngectomy are not suitable for medical reasons (e.g., inadequate pulmonary status or other major medical problems); these patients are treated with RT.

Analysis of local control by anatomic site within the supraglottic larynx shows no obvious differences in local control by RT for similarly staged lesions. Invasion of the preepiglottic space is not a contraindication to supraglottic laryngectomy or RT. Primary tumor volume based on pretreatment CT is inversely related to local tumor control after RT.[35] A large, bulky (>6 cc) infiltrative lesion, especially one with extensive preepiglottic space invasion, is a common reason to select supraglottic laryngectomy.

The status of the neck often determines the selection of treatment of the primary lesion. Patients with clinically negative neck nodes have a high risk for occult neck disease and may be treated by RT or supraglottic laryngectomy and bilateral selective neck dissections (levels II to IV).

If a patient has an early-stage primary lesion but advanced neck disease (N2b or N3), combined treatment is frequently necessary to control the neck disease.[33] In these cases, the primary lesion is usually treated by definitive RT, with surgery added to the treatment of the involved neck site(s). If the same patient were treated with supraglottic laryngectomy, neck dissection, and postoperative RT, the portals would unnecessarily cover the primary site and the neck. If the patient has early, resectable neck disease (N1 or N2a) and surgery is elected for the primary site, postoperative RT is added only because of unexpected findings (e.g., positive margins, multiple positive nodes, or extracapsular extension). We prefer to avoid routine high-dose preoperative or postoperative RT in conjunction with a supraglottic laryngectomy because the lymphedema of the remaining larynx may be considerable, although it eventually subsides. However, Lee et al.[72] from the MD Anderson Cancer Center reported excellent results with combined supraglottic laryngectomy and postoperative RT for moderately advanced lesions.

Advanced Supraglottic Lesions

Although a subset of these patients may be suitable for a supraglottic or supracricoid laryngectomy, total laryngectomy is the main surgical option. Selected advanced lesions, especially those that are mainly exophytic, may be treated by RT and concomitant chemotherapy,[38] with total laryngectomy reserved for RT failures.

For patients whose primary lesion is to be treated by a total or partial laryngectomy and who have resectable neck disease, surgery is the initial treatment, and postoperative RT is added if needed. If the neck disease is unresectable, preoperative RT is used. The indications for preoperative and postoperative RT have been previously outlined.

Surgical Treatment

Supraglottic Laryngectomy

Supraglottic laryngectomy is voice-sparing surgery that can be used successfully for selected lesions involving the epiglottis, a single arytenoid, the aryepiglottic fold, or the false vocal cord. This can be performed via TLM or TORS.[30] Extension of the tumor to the true vocal cord, the anterior commissure, or both arytenoids, fixation of the vocal cord, or thyroid or cricoid cartilage invasion precludes supraglottic laryngectomy. The supraglottic laryngectomy may be extended to include the base of the tongue if one lingual artery is preserved.

All patients have difficulty swallowing, with a tendency to aspirate immediately after surgery, but almost all learn to swallow again in a short time; motivation and the amount of tissue removed are key factors in learning to swallow again. Preoperatively, adequate pulmonary reserve is evaluated by blood gas determinations, function tests, chest roentgenography, and a work test involving walking the patient up two flights of stairs to determine tolerance to pulmonary stress. The voice quality is generally normal after supraglottic laryngectomy.

Supracricoid Laryngectomy

This procedure is an option for lesions extending from the supraglottis into one or both vocal cords. However, vocal cord fixation is a relative contraindication. At least one arytenoid must be preserved for successful decannulation and phonation. Extension to the cricoid and thyroid cartilage destruction also preclude its use. Phonation and respiratory function are reconstituted by approximating the cricoid to the hyoid (cricohyoidopexy).

Wide-Field Total Laryngectomy

Total laryngectomy is performed as previously described.

Radiation Therapy Technique

The primary lesion and both sides of the neck are treated with opposed lateral portals; wedges are used to compensate for the contour of the neck (Fig. 50.11).[21] The lower neck nodes are irradiated through a separate anterior portal. IMRT may be employed to spare one or both parotids and to avoid a low match line in the occasional patient with a short neck and large shoulders. We currently use either hyperfractionation or simultaneous integrated boost (SIB). The latter schedule delivers 70 Gy in 35 fractions over 30 treatment days in 6 weeks with 1 twice-daily fraction during the last 5 weeks (with a minimum 6-hour interfraction interval). The high-risk clinical target volume (CTV) encompasses the gross disease, the intermediate-risk CTV receives 63 Gy at 1.8 Gy per fraction, and the standard-risk CTV receives 56 Gy at 1.65 Gy per fraction.

In the case of clinically positive nodes, an electron beam portal may be used to increase the dose to the posterior cervical nodes after the fields are reduced to avoid the spinal cord at 45 Gy if parallel opposed fields are employed. CT is obtained 4 weeks after completing RT, and a neck dissection is added if the residual cancer in the nodes is believed to exceed 5%; otherwise, the patient is observed and a CT is repeated in 3 months.[33] Alternatively, a PET-CT is obtained at 3 months, and a neck dissection is added if persistent positive nodes are observed.

Patients experience a sore throat, loss of taste, and moderate dryness during RT. Edema of the arytenoids may occur and give a sensation of a lump in the throat. Tracheostomy is rarely necessary, even for bulky lesions.

Edema of the larynx may persist for several months to a year. Patients who continue to smoke heighten the side effects of dryness, dysphagia, and hoarseness.

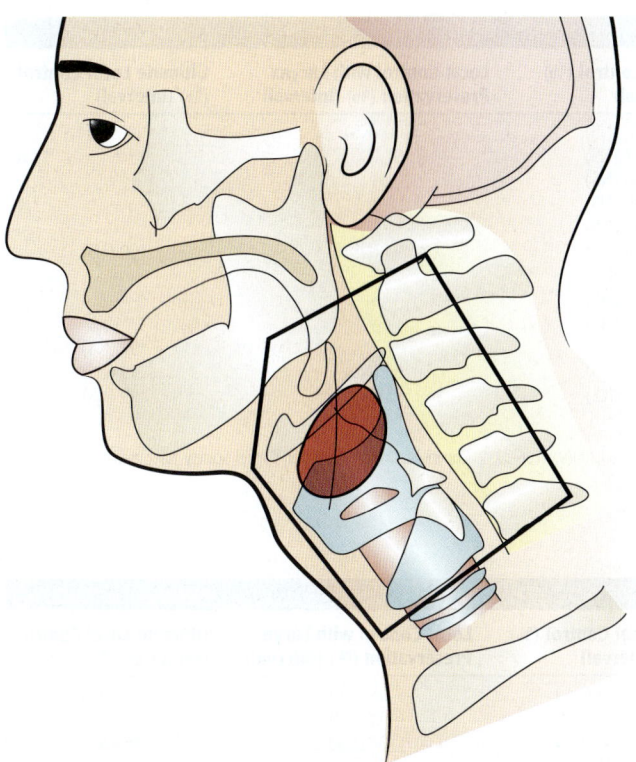

FIGURE 50.11. Example of conventional portal for a lesion of the lower epiglottis or false vocal cord and a clinically negative neck. The subdigastric nodes are included but not the junctional nodes. Depending on the anatomy and tumor extent, the anterior border may fall off (i.e., "flash") or a small strip of skin may be shielded. (From Million RR, Cassisi NJ, Mancuso AA, et al. Management of the neck for squamous cell carcinoma. In: Million RR, Cassisi NJ, eds. *Management of head and neck a cancer: a multidisciplinary approach.* 2nd ed. Philadelphia: JB Lippincott, 1994:75–143. With permission.)

Preoperative and Postoperative Treatment Technique

If total laryngectomy is required and the lesion is resectable, postoperative RT is preferred because there is no evidence that preoperative RT produces any better local–regional control or survival rates than surgery and postoperative RT. Irradiation is added for close or positive margins, invasion of soft tissues of the neck, significant subglottic extension (1 cm or more), thyroid cartilage invasion, multiple positive nodes, and extracapsular extension. The high-risk areas are usually the base of the tongue and the neck.

The dose for postoperative RT as a function of known residual disease is as follows: negative margins, 60 Gy in 30 fractions; microscopically positive margins, 66 Gy in 33 fractions; and gross residual disease, 70 Gy in 35 fractions. All patients are treated with a continuous course, one fraction per day, 5 days per week. The lower neck is treated with doses to 50 Gy in 25 fractions at D_{max}. If there is subglottic extension, the dose to the stoma is boosted with electrons (usually 10 to 14 MeV) for an additional 10 Gy in five fractions. The treatment technique is shown in Figure 50.10.[55] If postoperative RT is added after supraglottic a the laryngectomy, is dose lowered to 55.8 Gy given in 1.8-Gy fractions. This dose produces acceptable rates of local control and laryngeal edema.[72]

The treatment technique used for preoperative RT is essentially the same as that used for patients treated with RT alone, using doses of 50 to 60 Gy at 1.8 to 2.0 Gy per fraction. Thereafter, the dose is boosted to areas of unresectable disease (usually the neck) to total doses ranging from 66 to 70 Gy.

Treatment of Recurrence

Failures after supraglottic laryngectomy or RT can frequently be controlled by further treatment; therefore, recognition of recurrence should be vigorously pursued.[70] Salvage of patients with recurrence after combined total laryngectomy and RT is uncommon. Stomal recurrences are occasionally controlled by RT or surgery; however, the average life span after stomal recurrence is 6.3 months.[73]

RESULTS OF TREATMENT

Vocal Cord Cancer

The local tumor control and survival rates after treatment of early-stage glottic carcinoma are depicted in Tables 50.3 to 50.6.[41]

TABLE 50.3 LOCAL CONTROL AFTER TRANSORAL LASER EXCISION

Institution	Follow-Up[a]	Number of Patients	Stage	Local Control (%) (Interval)	Local Control with Larynx Preservation (%) (Interval)	Ultimate Local Control (%) (Interval)
University of Göttingen[47]	Median, 78 mo	159	pTis-pT2	94 (NS)	99 (NS)	—
University of Kiel[74]	Mean, 40 mo	8	pTis	100 (NS)	—	—
		88	pT1a	92 (NS)	—	—
		10	pT1b	80 (NS)	—	—
		8	pT2	88 (NS)	—	—
		114	pTis-pT2	—	96 (NS)	—
University of Brescia[75]	Mean, 76 mo	21	pTis	81 (NS)	—	95[b] (5 y)
		96	pT1	82 (NS)	—	87[b] (5 y)
		23	pT2	74 (NS)	—	91[b] (5 y)
		140	pTis-pT2	80 (NS)	97 (NS)	—
Washington University[76]	Minimum, 3 y	61	T1	77 (NS)	90 (NS)	98 (NS)
University of Naples[77]	Minimum, 5 y	321	T1	82[b] (NS)	89[c] (NS)	—
		158	T2	60[b] (NS)	67[c] (NS)	—
La Sapienza University[78]	Minimum, 3 y	12	Tis	100 (NS)	100 (NS)	—
		120	T1a	94 (NS)	100 (NS)	—
		24	T1b	91 (NS)	100 (NS)	—
Tata Memorial Hospital[79]	Minimum, 18 mo	52	T1a	90 (NS)	94 (NS)	—
		17	T1b	65 (NS)	88 (NS)	—
		13	T2	77 (NS)	92 (NS)	—

[a]Follow-up period for total number of patients.
[b]Ultimate local control with laser treatment alone.
[c]Local–regional control rate.
NS, not stated.
From Mendenhall WM, Werning JW, Hinerman RW, et al. Management of T1–T2 glottic carcinomas. *Cancer* 2004;100(9):1786–1792. Copyright © 2004 American Cancer Society. Reprinted by permission of John Wiley & Sons, Inc.

TABLE 50.4 LOCAL CONTROL AFTER OPEN PARTIAL LARYNGECTOMY

Institution	Follow-Up	Number of Patients	Stage	Local Control (%) (Interval)	Local Control with Larynx Preservation (%) (Interval)	Ultimate Local Control (%) (Interval)
Universitaire Timone[80]	NS	62	T1	100 (NS)	100 (NS)	
		65	T2	92 (NS)	92 (NS)	–
Hôpital Saint Charles[81]	Minimum, 3 y	18	T1a	100 (NS)	–	–
		40	T1b	95 (NS)	–	–
		23	T2a	83 (NS)	–	–
Mayo Clinic[82]	Median, 6.6 y	159	Tis–T1	93 (5 y)	94 (NS)	100 (NS)
Hôpital Laënnec[83]	Minimum, 3 y	295	T1	89 (NS)	–	–
		90	T2a	74 (NS)	–	–
		31	T2b	68 (NS)	–	–
		416	T1–T2b	84 (NS)	–	97 (NS)
Washington University[76]	Minimum, 3 y	404	T1	92 (NS)	93 (NS)	99 (NS)
Washington University[84]	Minimum, 5 y	71	T2	93 (NS)	93 (NS)	99 (NS)

NS, not stated.
From Mendenhall WM, Werning JW, Hinerman RW, et al. Management of T1–T2 glottic carcinomas. *Cancer* 2004;100(9):1786–1792. Copyright © 2004 American Cancer Society. Reprinted by permission of John Wiley & Sons, Inc.

TABLE 50.5 LOCAL CONTROL AFTER RADIOTHERAPY

Institution	Follow-Up[a]	Number of Patients	Stage	Local Control (%) (Interval)	Local Control with Larynx Preservation (%) (Interval)	Ultimate Local Control (%) (Interval)
University of Florida[18]	Minimum, 2 y	230	T1a	94 (5 y)	95 (5 y)	98 (5 y)
	Median, 9.9 y	61	T1b	93 (5 y)	95 (5 y)	98 (5 y)
		146	T2a	80 (5 y)	82 (5 y)	96 (5 y)
		82	T2b	72 (5 y)	76 (5 y)	96 (5 y)
Massachusetts General Hospital[85]	NS	665	T1	93 (5 y)	–	–
		145	T2a	77 (5 y)	–	–
		92	T2b	71 (5 y)	–	–
University of California, San Francisco[86]	Median, 9.7 y	315	T1	85 (5 y)	–	96[b] (5 y)
		83	T2	70 (5 y)	–	91[b] (5 y)
Princess Margaret Hospital[87]	Median, 6.8 y	403	T1a	91 (5 y)	–	–
		46	T1b	82 (5 y)	–	–
		286	T2	69 (5 y)	–	–
MD Anderson Hospital[88]	Median, 6.8 y	114	T2a	74 (5 y)	–	–
		116	T2b	70 (5 y)	–	–
		230	T2	72 (5 y)	–	91 (5 y)

[a]Follow-up period for total number of patients.
[b]Local–regional control rate.
NS, not stated.
From Mendenhall WM, Werning JW, Hinerman RW, et al. Management of T1–T2 glottic carcinomas. *Cancer* 2004;100(9):1786–1792. Copyright © 2004 American Cancer Society. Reprinted by permission of John Wiley & Sons, Inc.

TABLE 50.6 SURVIVAL DATA

Institution	Treatment	Follow-Up	Number of Patients	Stage	Cause-Specific Survival (%) (Interval)	Absolute Survival (%) (Interval)
Washington University[76]	Laser	Minimum, 3 y	61	T1	95 (5 y)	84 (5 y)
University of Göttingen[47]	Laser	Median, 6.5 y	159	pTis–T2	100 (5 y)	87 (5 y)
University of Brescia[75]	Laser	Mean, 6.3 y	140	pTis–T2	98 (5 y)	93 (5 y)
Washington University[76]	OPL	Minimum, 3 y	404	T1	97 (5 y)	84 (5 y)
Mayo Clinic[82]	OPL	Median, 6.6 y	159	Tis–T1	–	84 (5 y)
Washington University[84]	OPL	Minimum, 5 y	71	T2	–	92 (5 y)
University of Florida[18]	RT	Minimum, 2 y	230	T1a	98 (5 y)	82 (5 y)
		Median, 9.9 y	61	T1b	98 (5 y)	79 (5 y)
			146	T2a	95 (5 y)	77 (5 y)
			82	T2b	90 (5 y)	77 (5 y)
University of California, San Francisco[86]	RT	Median, 9.7 y	315	T1	96 (10 y)	65 (10 y)
			83	T2	91 (10 y)	63 (10 y)
Massachusetts General Hospital[85]	RT	NS	665	T1	98 (5 y)	–
			145	T2a	92 (5 y)	–
			92	T2b	84 (5 y)	–
MD Anderson Hospital[88]	RT	Median, 6.8 y	230	T2	92 (5 y)	73 (5 y)

NS, not stated; OPL, open partial laryngectomy; RT, radiotherapy.
From Mendenhall WM, Werning JW, Hinerman RW, et al. Management of T1–T2 glottic carcinomas. *Cancer* 2004;100(9):1786–1792. Copyright © 2004 American Cancer Society. Reprinted by permission of John Wiley & Sons, Inc.

TABLE 50.7 STAGE T3 GLOTTIC CARCINOMA TREATED WITH IRRADIATION ALONE (NO CHEMOTHERAPY)

Investigator	Institution	Number of Patients	Minimum Follow-Up (y)	Local Control (%)	Ultimate Control After Salvage Surgery (%)
Harwood et al.[91]	Princess Margaret (Toronto)	112	3	51	77
Wang[92]	Massachusetts General (Boston)	70	4	36	57
Fletcher et al.[93]	MD Anderson (Houston)	17	2	77	No data
Skolyszewski and Reinfuss[94]	15 European Centers	91	3	50	No data
Stewart et al.[95]	Manchester (England)	67	10	57	67
Mills[96]	Capetown, South Africa	18	2	44	78
Mendenhall et al.[36]	University Florida of (Gainesville)	75	2	63	86

Modified from Parsons JT, Mendenhall WM, Mancuso AA, et al. Twice-a-day radiotherapy for T3 squamous cell carcinoma of the glottic larynx. *Head Neck* 1989;11(2):123–128. Copyright © 1989 Wiley Periodicals, Inc., A Wiley Company. Reprinted by permission of John Wiley & Sons, Inc.

Sengupta et al.[89] recently reported on 37 patients treated at the University of Florida with definitive RT for carcinoma *in situ* and observed the following 5-year outcomes: local control, 91%; local control with larynx preservation, 91%; and ultimate local control, 91%. Chera et al.[42] reported on 585 patients at the University of Florida for T1–T2 N0 glottic carcinoma and observed the following 5-year local control rates: T1A1, 95%; T1B, 94%; T2 A, 81%; and T2B, 74%. The local tumor control and survival rates are similar for transoral laser excision, open partial laryngectomy, and RT. Larynx preservation rates are also comparable. Voice quality depends on the amount of tissue removed with partial laryngectomy and is probably similar for patients with limited lesions treated with laser to those undergoing RT and poorer for patients undergoing open partial laryngectomy.[41]

Foote et al.[90] reported on 81 patients who underwent laryngectomy for T3 cancers at the Mayo Clinic between 1970 and 1981. Seventy-five patients underwent a total laryngectomy and 6 underwent a near-total laryngectomy; 53 patients received a neck dissection. No patient underwent adjuvant irradiation or chemotherapy. The 5-year rates of local–regional control, cause-specific survival, and absolute survival were 74%, 74%, and 54%, respectively. The results of definitive RT patients with T3 glottic carcinoma are depicted in Table 50.7[64] and are similar to the surgical outcomes reported by Foote et al.[90]

The survival and tumor control rates of patients with T3 fixed-cord lesions treated at the University of Florida are presented in Table 50.8.[97] There was no relationship between subsequent local control and whether the vocal cord remained fixed or became mobile during irradiation. The incidence of severe complications, including those after the initial treatment and any later salvage procedures, was 15% after RT alone and 15% after surgery alone or combined with adjuvant irradiation. The vocal quality varied from fair to nearly normal. Hinerman et al.[31] recently reported an update of the University of Florida experience treating fixed-cord T3 glottic cancers with definitive RT and reported a 5-year local control rate after RT of 63%.

The results of treatment of T4 vocal cord carcinoma in four surgical series and two RT series are summarized in Table 50.9.[58] Hinerman et al.[31] observed an 81% 5-year local control rate in 22 selected patients with favorable T4 cancers treated with definitive RT at the University of Florida.

Parsons et al.[103] reviewed the literature and reported a local control rate of 62% in a series of 87 patients treated with RT alone for T4 glottic carcinoma.

Supraglottic Cancer

The proportion of patients suitable for a supraglottic laryngectomy is depicted in Table 50.10.[70] Depending on the referral patterns, a modest subset of patients is suitable for this operation. The extent of neck disease for patients treated with either surgery or RT is shown in Table 50.11.[70] In general, patients treated with supraglottic laryngectomy appropriately have earlier stage neck disease and would be anticipated to have a lower risk of distant failure and improved survival. The local control rates after transoral laser, RT, and supraglottic laryngectomy are summarized in Tables 50.12 to 50.14.[70] In general, the local control rates after transoral laser excision are fairly good for patients with T1–T2 tumors and tend to deteriorate for those with more advanced disease. The local control rate for patients selected for supraglottic laryngectomy is excellent. However, the incidence of severe complications tends to be higher after supraglottic laryngectomy compared with RT and transoral laser excision (Table 50.15).[70,126]

LARYNGECTOMY VERSUS ORGAN PRESERVATION

Treatment of advanced laryngeal cancer carries significant morbidity with deteriorations in quality of life. Thus, many centers and patients have elected to pursue organ preservation strategies. The first major breakthrough in organ preservation came with the Department of Veterans Affairs Laryngeal Cancer Study Group Trial ("The VA Trial").[34] Stage III and IV patients were randomized to total laryngectomy followed by RT versus RT or induction chemotherapy + RT. The conclusion was that induction chemotherapy + RT produced equivalent survival to total laryngectomy + RT. In 2003, the RTOG 91-11 study randomized patients to organ preservation modalities and found that concurrent chemotherapy and RT (CCRT) produced superior survival outcomes. Following these studies, the employment of CCRT for advanced laryngeal cancer has risen significantly.

TABLE 50.8 T3 GLOTTIC CARCINOMA TREATED AT THE UNIVERSITY OF FLORIDA, 1965 TO 1988: FIVE-YEAR RESULTS

Parameter	Radiotherapy Alone (53 Patients)	Surgery with or without Adjuvant Radiotherapy (65 Patients)
Local–regional control (%)	62	75
Ultimate local–regional control (%)	84	82
Absolute survival (%)	55	45
Cause-specific survival (%)	75	71

Data from Mendenhall WM, Parsons JT, Stringer SP, et al. Stage T3 squamous cell carcinoma of the glottic larynx: a comparison of laryngectomy and irradiation. *Int J Radiat Biol Oncol Phys* 1992;23:725–732.

TABLE 50.9 TREATMENT OF STAGE T4 GLOTTIC CARCINOMAS

Investigator	Tumor Stage	Number of Patients	Method of Treatment	Results: Evidence No of Disease
Jesse[98]	T4 N0–N+	48	Laryngectomy	54% at 4 y
Ogura et al.[99]	T4 N0	11	Laryngectomy	45% at 3 y
Skolnik et al.[100]	T4 N0	7	Laryngectomy	30% at 5 y
Vermund[101]	T4 N0	31	Laryngectomy	35% at 5 y
Stewart and Jackson[102]	T4 N0	13	Radiotherapy with salvage surgery	38% at 5 y
Harwood et al.[58]	T4 N0	56	Radiotherapy with salvage surgery	49% at 5 y[a]

[a]Life table method; uncorrected for deaths from intercurrent disease.
Modified from Harwood AR, Beal FA, Cummings BJ, et al. T4NOMO glottic cancer: an analysis of dose-time volume factors. *Int J Radiat Oncol Biol Phys* 1981;7(11):1507–1512. Copyright © 1981 Elsevier. With permission.

TABLE 50.10 PROPORTION OF PATIENTS SUITABLE FOR SUPRAGLOTTIC LARYNGECTOMY

Series	Number of Patients	Number of Supraglottic Laryngectomies (%)
Ogura et al., 1975[104]	263	177 (67%)
Lutz et al., 1990[105]	202	72 (36%)
Lee et al., 1990[72]	404	60 (15%)
Weems et al., 1987[106]	195	30 (15%)
Gregor et al., 1996[107]	89	26 (29%)
Spriano et al., 1997[108]	257	38 (14%)

Some values were estimated as closely as possible to fit the table format if the information was not specifically stated in the cited reference.
From Hinerman RW, Mendenhall WM, Amdur RJ, et al. Carcinoma of the supraglottic larynx: treatment results with radiotherapy alone or with planned neck dissection. *Head Neck* 2002;24(5):456–467. Copyright © 2002 Wiley Periodicals, Inc. Reprinted by permission of John Wiley & Sons, Inc.

TABLE 50.11 SUPRAGLOTTIC CARCINOMA: EXTENT OF NECK DISEASE VERSUS TREATMENT

Series	Treatment	Number of Patients	Extent of Neck Disease
Bocca, 1991[109]	SGL	537	94% N0–N1
Isaacs et al., 1998[110]	SGL	39	74% N0–N1
Ogura et al., 1975[104]	SGL	177	77% N0
Davis et al., 1991[111]	Laser	14	93% N0
Zeitels et al., 1994[112]	Laser	45	100% N0
Rudert et al., 1999[113]	Laser	34	82% N0–N1
Ghossein et al. 1974[114]	Radiation	203	53% N0
Hinerman et al., 2002[70]	Radiation	274	54% N0

Some values were estimated as closely as possible to fit the table format if the information was not specifically stated in the cited reference.
SGL, supraglottic laryngectomy.
From Hinerman RW, Mendenhall WM, Amdur RJ, et al. Carcinoma of the supraglottic larynx: treatment results with radiotherapy alone or with planned neck dissection. *Head Neck* 2002;24(5): 456–467. Copyright © 2002 Wiley Periodicals, Inc. Reprinted by permission of John Wiley & Sons, Inc.

TABLE 50.12 SUPRAGLOTTIC CANCER: LOCAL CONTROL AFTER TRANSORAL LASER EXCISION

Series	Staging	Number of Patients	Percentage of Patients with T1 or T2 Tumors	Local Control (%)			
				T1	T2	T3	T4
Davis et al., 1991[111]	P	14 R	57	100	100	50	—
Steiner,[a] 1993[47]	P	81 R	72	—	76	77	100
Zeitels et al., 1994[112]	ND	22	100	100	100	—	—
Zeitels et al., 1994[112]	ND	23 R	65	100	92	63	—
Csanády et al., 1999[115]	ND	23	100	70[b]	—	—	
Rudert et al., 1999[113]	P	34 R	50	100	75	78	38

[a]Fifty-one glottic and 30 supraglottic.
[b]Overall local control rate for T1 and T2.
ND, type of staging not provided; P, pathologic staging; R, plus or minus radiotherapy.
Some values were estimated as closely as possible to fit the table format if the information was not specifically stated in the cited reference.
From Hinerman RW, Mendenhall WM, Amdur RJ, et al. Carcinoma of the supraglottic larynx: treatment results with radiotherapy alone or with planned neck dissection. *Head Neck* 2002;24(5):456–467. Copyright © 2002 Wiley Periodicals, Inc. Reprinted by permission of John Wiley & Sons, Inc.

TABLE 50.13 SUPRAGLOTTIC CANCER: LOCAL CONTROL AFTER RADIOTHERAPY

Series	Institution	Number of Patients	Local Control (%)			
			T1	T2	T3	T4
Fletcher and Hamberger, 1974[116]	MD Anderson Hospital	173	88	79	62	47
Ghossein et al., 1974[114]	Fondation Curie	203	94	73	46[a]	52
Wang and Montgomery, 1991[117]	Massachusetts General Hospital	229 q.d.	73	60	54	26
		209 b.i.d.	89	89	71	91
Nakfoor et al., 1998[118]	Massachusetts General Hospital	164	96	86	76	43
Sykes et al., 2000[119]	Christie Hospital	331[b]	92[c]	81[c]	67[c]	73[c]
Hinerman et al., 2002[70]	University of Florida[d]	274	100	86	62	62

[a]All had cord fixation.
[b]All N0.
[c]After 17 were salvaged by total laryngectomies.
[d]1998 American Joint Committee on Cancer staging.
b.i.d., twice a day; q.d., once a day.
Some values were estimated as closely as possible to fit the table format if the information was not specifically stated in the cited reference.
From Hinerman RW, Mendenhall WM, Amdur RJ, et al. Carcinoma of the supraglottic larynx: treatment results with radiotherapy alone or with planned neck dissection. *Head Neck* 2002;24(5):456–467. Copyright © 2002 Wiley Periodicals, Inc. Reprinted by permission of John Wiley & Sons, Inc.

TABLE 50.14 LOCAL CONTROL AFTER SUPRAGLOTTIC LARYNGECTOMY

Series	Institution	Number of Patients	Patients with T1 and T2 Tumors (%)	Local Control (%) T1	T2	T3	T4
Ogura et al., 1975[104]	Washington University	177	78		94[a]		
Bocca, 1991[109]	Milan University						
Stage I		47	100	94			
Stage II		252	100		82		
Stage III		205	53		80[b]		
Stage IV		33	70		67[c]		
Lee et al., 1990[72]	MD Anderson Cancer Center	60	58	100	100	100	100
DeSanto, 1990[120]	Mayo Clinic	70	100	100	100		
Steiniger et al., 1997[121]	Albany Medical College	29	83		97[a]		
Spriano et al., 1997[108]	Varese, Italy	54	100	96[d]			
Burstein and Calcattera, 1985[122]	University of California, Los Angeles	40	58	100[d]		85	94
Isaacs et al., 1998[110]	University of Florida	33	76	100[d]		78	71
Lutz et al., 1990[105]	University of Pittsburgh	72	No data		99[d]		

[a]Overall local control rate for T1–T4.
[b]Overall local control rate for T1–T3.
[c]Overall local control rate for T2–T3.
[d]Overall local control rate for T1–T2.
Some values were estimated as closely as possible to fit the table format if the information was not specifically stated in the cited reference. T stages were not specified.
From Hinerman RW, Mendenhall WM, Amdur RJ, et al. Carcinoma of the supraglottic larynx: treatment results with radiotherapy alone or with planned neck dissection. *Head Neck* 2002;24(5):456–467. Copyright © 2002 Wiley Periodicals, Inc. Reprinted by permission of John Wiley & Sons, Inc.

In 2006, Hoffman et al.[127] used the National Cancer Data Base and found that of all cancer in the United States, laryngeal cancer is the only one with a declining survival rate. Whereas early-stage cancer maintains high survival outcomes, patients with advanced disease have a declining life span. This pattern coincides with the trend of increased use of organ preservation and decreased use of total laryngectomy for advanced laryngeal cancers.

Over the last 15 years, there has been great interest in re-examining the optimal treatment for advanced laryngeal cancers. In 2007, Chen and Halpern[128] analyzed 10,590 patients from the late 1990s and found that total laryngectomy had superior survival outcomes compared to RT or CCRT. In 2009, Gourin et al.[129] analyzed a population of patients treated between 1985 and 2002 and found that patients with stage IV disease had improved 5-year survival compared to organ preservation. In 2012, Dziegielewski et al[130] performed a population-based analysis of survival from 1998 to 2008 and found that T3 and T4a laryngeal cancers treated with total laryngectomy + RT had improved overall and disease-free survival. The 5-year survival rates for T3 cancers treated with total laryngectomy + RT, RT, and CRT were 70%, 18%, and 52%, respectively. For T4a disease, these figures were 49%, 5%, and 16%. In 2014, Megwalu and Sikora[131] found similar survival outcomes using the SEER database to analyze 5,394 patients with stage III and stage IV laryngeal carcinoma treated between 1992 and 2009. Disease-specific survival rates for surgically treated patients at 2 and 5 years were 70% and 64% versus organ preservation strategies, which yielded rates of 55% and 51%. Multivariate analysis, accounting for year of diagnosis, stage, age, sex, subsite, race, and marital status, continued to show improved disease-specific and overall survival for patients receiving primary surgery.

TABLE 50.15 SUPRAGLOTTIC CANCER: SEVERE COMPLICATIONS ACCORDING TO TREATMENT MODALITY

Series	Institution	Number of Severe Complications (%)
Radiotherapy		
Fletcher and Hamberger, 1974[116]	MD Anderson Cancer Center	10/173 (6%)
Ghossein et al., 1974[114]	Fondation Curie	8/117 (7%)
Nakfoor et al., 1998[118]	Massachusetts General Hospital	12/169 (7%)
Sykes et al., 2000[119]	Christie Hospital	7/331 (2%)
Hinerman et al., 2002[70]	University of Florida	12/274 (4%)
Supraglottic Laryngectomy		
Lee et al., 1990[72]	MD Cancer Anderson Center	9/63 (14%)
Isaacs et al., 1998[110]	University of Florida	14/34 (41%)
Burstein and Calcaterra, 1985[122]	University of California, Los Angeles	14/41 (34%)
Steiniger et al., 1997[121]	Albany Medical College	12/29 (41%)
Spriano et al., 1997[108]	Varese, Italy	13/54 (24%)
Gall et al., 1977[123]	Washington University	20/133 (15%)
Weber et al., 1993[124]	University of Pittsburgh	12/69 (17%)
Beckhardt et al., 1994[125]	University of Wisconsin	15/50 (30%)
Transoral Laser Excision		
Rudert et al., 1999[113]	University of Kiel, Germany	3/34 (9%)
Zeitels et al., 1994[112]	Massachusetts and Eye Ear Infirmary	2/45 (4%)
Steiner,[a] 1993[47]	University of Göttingen, Germany	7/240 (3%)
Davis et al., 1991[111]	University of Utah, Salt Lake City	0/14 (0%)
Csanády et al., 1999[115]	Albert Szent-Gyorgyi Medical University, Szeged, Hungary	0/23 (0%)

[a]Includes patients with glottic cancer.
Some values were estimated as closely as possible to fit the table format if the information was not specifically stated in the cited reference.
From Hinerman RW, Mendenhall WM, Amdur RJ, et al. Carcinoma of the supraglottic larynx: treatment results with radiotherapy alone or with planned neck dissection. *Head Neck* 2002;24(5):456–467. Copyright © 2002 Wiley Periodicals, Inc. Reprinted by permission of John Wiley & Sons, Inc.

Since the initial VA trial, advanced laryngeal cancer survival outcomes have deteriorated, prompting debate of whether the results of the trial can be widely applied to all advanced laryngeal cancer.[132] Population-based studies have shown that treatment strategies need to be tailored to the patient and that T stage is a better determinant of survival than overall stage.[129,130] It has become widely accepted that the majority of patients with T4a cancer will experience better survival and functional outcomes when treated with laryngectomy versus organ preservation.[129-131] However, the debate over which T3 tumors can be optimally treated with CRT continues.[133]

FOLLOW-UP POLICY

Follow-up of patients with early lesions is planned for every 4 to 8 weeks for 2 years, every 3 months for the 3rd year, and every 6 months for years 4 and 5, and then annually for life.

Follow-up of patients with vocal cord or supraglottic larynx lesions treated by RT or conservative surgery is almost more important than the treatment itself because early detection of recurrence usually results in salvage that may include cure with voice preservation.

If recurrence is suspected but the biopsy is negative, patients are re-examined at 2- to 4-week intervals until the matter is settled. The value of follow-up CT scans for detecting early local recurrence is investigational.

Wagenfeld et al.[134] studied 740 cases of glottic larynx cancer treated from 1965 to 1974 to determine the incidence of second respiratory tract malignancies. There was a minimum follow-up of 5 years. There were 48 second respiratory tract malignancies, although only 14 were expected. Twenty-five were in the lung, and 23 were scattered among other head and neck sites. Only 7 of the 23 second head and neck primary lesions resulted in death; these second lesions were frequently diagnosed in an early stage during routine follow-up for the glottic lesion.

Because the risk of a lethal lung primary lesion is nearly as great as that of dying of an early glottic carcinoma, it makes sense to obtain annual chest roentgenograms. Approximately 50% of patients who receive moderate- to high-dose RT to the entire thyroid gland will develop hypothyroidism within 5 years, and so thyroid functions are checked every 6 to 12 months and thyroid replacement is initiated if the thyroid-stimulating hormone level begins to rise.[135]

SEQUELAE OF TREATMENT

Surgical Sequelae

Neel et al.[136] reported a 26% incidence of nonfatal complications for cordectomy. Immediate postoperative complications included atelectasis and pneumonia, severe subcutaneous emphysema in the neck, bleeding from the tracheotomy site or larynx, wound complications, and airway obstruction requiring tracheotomy. Late complications included granulation tissue that had to be removed by direct laryngoscopy to exclude recurrences, extrusion of cartilage, laryngeal stenosis, and obstructing laryngeal web.

The postoperative complications and sequelae of hemilaryngectomy include chondritis, wound slough, inadequate glottic closure, and anterior commissure webs.[123] The complications associated with supraglottic laryngectomy and total laryngectomy for supraglottic carcinomas include fistula (8%), carotid artery exposure or blowout (3% to 5%), infection or wound sloughing (3% to 7%), and fatal complications (3%).[123] The risk of complication increased if tumor margins were involved by tumor; there was no change in risk associated with age, sex, race, laryngeal site, stage of primary tumor, size of primary tumor, use of low-dose preoperative RT, or status of the positive nodes.

The incidence of complications after treatment of supraglottic carcinoma is given in Table 50.15.[70]

Radiation Therapy Sequelae

The acute reactions from the treatment of early vocal cord cancer using a tumor dose of 2.25 Gy per day to administer a total dose 63 Gy (4- or 6-MV photons, five fractions per week) are relatively mild. During the first 2 to 3 weeks, the voice may improve as the tumor regresses. The voice generally becomes hoarse again because of RT-induced changes, even though the tumor continues to regress. A mild sore throat develops beginning at the end of the 2nd week, but medication is usually not required. The voice begins to improve approximately 3 weeks after completion of treatment, usually reaching a plateau in 2 to 3 months. Patients with extensive lesions often recover a normal voice, although not as frequently as those with small tumors.

Edema of the larynx is the most common sequela after RT for glottic or supraglottic lesions. The rate of clearance of the edema is related to the RT dose, volume of tissue irradiated, addition of a neck dissection, continued use of alcohol and tobacco, and size and extent of the original lesion. Edema may be accentuated by a neck dissection and may require 6 to 12 months to subside.

Soft tissue necrosis leading to chondritis occurs in <1% of patients, usually in those who continue to smoke. Soft tissue and cartilage necroses mimic recurrence, with hoarseness, pain, and edema; a laryngectomy may be recommended as a last resort for fear of recurrent cancer, even though biopsy specimens show only necrosis.

Corticosteroids such as dexamethasone (Decadron) have been used to reduce RT-induced edema after recurrence has been ruled out by biopsy. If ulceration and pain occur, administration of an antibiotic such as tetracycline may help. Of 519 patients with T1 N0 or T2 N0 vocal cord cancer treated at the University of Florida, 5 (1%) experienced severe complications,[18] including total laryngectomy for a suspected local recurrence (1 patient), permanent tracheostomy for edema (3 patients), and a pharyngocutaneous fistula after a salvage total laryngectomy (1 patient).

In patients irradiated for supraglottic carcinoma, sore throat persists 1 to 2 months after completion of treatment. There is an associated dry mouth from RT of the salivary and parotid glands, a loss of taste, and a sensation of a lump in the throat. It is unusual for patients to require a tracheotomy before RT unless severe lymphedema develops at the time of direct laryngoscopy and biopsy. However, in patients who have recovered from the direct laryngoscopy and biopsy without obstruction, a tracheotomy has rarely been required during a fractionated course of RT.

Patients treated twice a day with 1.2-Gy fractions (continuous-course technique) to a total dose of 74.4 Gy usually have more brisk acute reactions than those treated once a day with 2-Gy fractions. Approximately 30% treated with twice-a-day RT require temporary gastrostomy feeding tubes because they have difficulty in swallowing.[137]

Examples of acute chondritis requiring discontinuation of treatment have not been seen, although most epiglottic lesions exhibit cartilage invasion.

The epiglottis, both suprahyoid and infrahyoid portions, remains thicker than normal for long periods of time, but this is not often associated with difficulty in swallowing, respiratory obstruction, or aspiration. The patient is cautioned to eat and drink slowly until the edema resolves. The false cord and arytenoids may develop some edema.

Lesions of the suprahyoid epiglottis frequently destroy the tip of the epiglottis, and it may require some time for the exposed cartilage to heal. Successful RT of infrahyoid epiglottis tumors is not associated with a high rate of necrosis, even though most of these lesions penetrate the porous epiglottic cartilage.

The incidence of severe late complications in 274 patients treated with RT alone or combined with neck dissection at the University of Florida was 4%.[70]

ACKNOWLEDGMENTS

We thank the research support staff of the Department of Radiation Oncology for their help with statistics, editing, and manuscript preparation.

REFERENCES

1. Clemente CD. *Anatomy: a regional atlas of the human body.* Philadelphia: Lea & Febiger, 1975.

2. Mancuso AA, Hanafee WN. *Head and neck radiology.* Philadelphia: Lippincott Williams & Wilkins, 2010.

3. Lam KH, Wong J. The preepiglottic and paraglottic spaces in relation to spread of carcinoma of the larynx. *Am J Otolaryngol* 1983;4:81–91.

4. Hirano M. Structure and vibratory behavior of the vocal folds. In: Sawashima M, Cooper FS, eds. *Dynamic of aspects speech production: current results, emerging problems, new and instrumentation.* Tokyo, Japan: University of Tokyo Press, 1977:13–27

5. Siegel RL, Miller KD, Jemal A. Cancer statistics, 2016. *CA Cancer J Clin* 2016;66:7–30.

6. Ries LAG, Eisner MP, Kosary CL.SEER cancer statistics review, 1973–1998. 2001. Available at: http://seer.cancer.gov/archive/csr/1973_1998/.

7. Wynder EL. The epidemiology of cancers of the upper alimentary and upper respiratory tracts. *Laryngoscope* 1978;88:50–51.

8. Vincent RG, Marchetta F. The relationship of the use of tobacco and alcohol to cancer of the oral cavity, pharynx or larynx. *Am J Surg* 1963;106:501–505.

9. Archer CR, Yeager VL, Herbold DR. Computed tomography vs. histology of laryngeal cancer: their value in predicting laryngeal cartilage invasion. *Laryngoscope* 1983;93:140–147.

10. Pillsbury HR, Kirchner JA. Clinical vs. histopathologic staging in laryngeal cancer. *Arch Otolaryngol* 1979;105:157–159.

11. Broyles EN. The anterior commissure tendon. *Ann Rhinol Otol Laryngol* 1943;52:342–345.

12. Kirchner JA. Staging as seen in serial sections. *Laryngoscope* 1975;85:1816–1821.

13. Olofsson J, van Nostrand AW. Growth and spread of laryngeal and hypopharyngeal carcinoma with reflections on the effect of preoperative irradiation. 139 cases studied by whole organ serial sectioning. *Acta Otolaryngol Suppl* 1973;308:1–84.

14. Cassidy R, Morris CG, Kirwan JM, et al. Radiation therapy for squamous cell carcinoma of the subglottic larynx. *J Radiat Oncol* 2012;1:333–336.

15. Lindberg R. Distribution of cervical lymph node metastases from squamous cell carcinoma of the upper respiratory and digestive tracts. *Cancer* 1972;29:1446–1449.

16. Fletcher GH. Elective irradiation of subclinical disease in cancers of the head and neck. *Cancer* 1972;29:1450–1454.

17. Ogura JH, Biller HF, Wette R. Elective neck dissection for pharyngeal and laryngeal cancers. An evaluation. *Ann Otol Rhinol Laryngol* 1971;80:646–650.

18. Mendenhall WM, Amdur RJ, Morris CG, et al. T1-T2N0 squamous cell carcinoma of the glottic larynx treated with radiation therapy. *J Clin Oncol* 2001;19:4029–4036.

19. Lederman M. The place of radiotherapy in the treatment of cancer of the larynx. *Ann Radiol (Paris)* 1961;4:433–54.

20. Million RR, Cassisi NJ, Mancuso AA. Management of the neck for squamous cell carcinoma. In: Million RR, Cassisi NJ, eds. *Management of head and neck cancer: a multidisciplinary approach.* 2nd ed. Philadelphia: JB Lippincott, 1994:75–142.

21. Million RR, Cassisi NJ, Mancuso AA. Larynx. In: Million RR, Cassisi NJ, eds. *Management of head and neck cancer: a multidisciplinary approach.* Philadelphia: JB Lippincott, 1994:431–497.

22. McLaughlin MP, Mendenhall WM, Mancuso AA, et al. Retropharyngeal adenopathy as a predictor of outcome in squamous cell carcinoma of the head and neck. *Head Neck* 1995;17:190–198.

23. Archer CR, Yeager VL, Herbold DR. Improved diagnostic accuracy in laryngeal cancer using a new classification based on computed tomography. *Cancer* 1984;53:44–57.

24. Mendenhall WM, Parsons JT, Mancuso AA. Larynx, Chapter 42. In: Carlos A, Perez LWB, eds. *Principles and practice radiation oncology.* Philadelphia: Lippincott-Raven, 1998:1069–1093

25. American Joint Committee on Cancer. *AJCC cancer staging manual.* New York, NY: Springer, 2017.

26. Dagan R, Morris CG, Bennett JA, et al. Prognostic significance of paraglottic space invasion in T2N0 glottic carcinoma. *Am J Clin Oncol* 2007;30:186–190.

27. Coca-Pelaz A, Devaney KO, Rodrigo JP, et al. Should patients with laryngeal small cell neuroendocrine carcinoma receive prophylactic cranial irradiation? *Eur Arch Otorhinolaryngol* 2016;27310:2925–2930.

28. Gindhart TD, Johnston WH, Chism SE, et al. Carcinoma of the larynx in childhood. *Cancer* 1980;46:1683–1687.

29. Mendenhall WM, Dagan R, Bryant CM, et al. Definitive radiotherapy for squamous cell carcinoma of the glottic larynx. *Cancer Control* 2016;23:208–212.

30. Dziegielewski PT, Kang SY, Ozer E. Transoral robotic surgery (TORS) for laryngeal and hypopharyngeal cancers. *J Surg Oncol* 2015;112:702–706.

31. Hinerman RW, Mendenhall WM, Morris CG, et al. T3 and T4 true vocal cord squamous carcinomas treated with external beam irradiation: a single institution's 35-year experience. *Am J Clin Oncol* 2007;30:181–185.

32. Mendenhall WM, Morris CG, Stringer SP, et al. Voice rehabilitation after total laryngectomy and postoperative radiation therapy. *J Clin Oncol* 2002;20:2500–2505.

33. Mendenhall WM, Villaret DB, Amdur RJ, et al. Planned neck dissection after definitive radiotherapy for squamous cell carcinoma of the head and neck. *Head Neck* 2002;24:1012–1018.

34. Wolf GT, Fisher SG, Hong WK, et al. Induction chemotherapy plus radiation compared with surgery plus radiation in patients with advanced laryngeal cancer. The Department of Veterans Affairs Laryngeal Cancer Study Group. *N Engl J Med* 1991;324:1685–1690.

35. Mendenhall WM, Morris CG, Amdur RJ, et al. Parameters that predict local control after definitive radiotherapy for squamous cell carcinoma of the head and neck. *Head Neck* 2003;25:535–542.

36. Mendenhall WM, Parsons JT, Mancuso AA, et al. Definitive radiotherapy for T3 squamous cell carcinoma of the glottic larynx. *J Clin Oncol* 1997;15:2394–2402.

37. Forastiere AA, Goepfert H, Maor M, et al. Concurrent chemotherapy and radiotherapy for organ preservation in advanced laryngeal cancer. *N Engl J Med* 2003;349:2091–2098.

38. Pignon JP, Bourhis J, Domenge C, et al. Chemotherapy added to locoregional treatment for head and neck squamous-cell carcinoma: three meta-analyses of updated individual data. MACH-NC Collaborative Group. Meta-analysis of chemotherapy on head and neck cancer. *Lancet* 2000;355:949–955.

39. Mendenhall WM, Riggs CE, Vaysberg M, et al. Altered fractionation and adjuvant chemotherapy for head and neck squamous cell carcinoma. *Head Neck* 2010;32:939–945.

40. Strojan P, Haigentz M Jr, Bradford CR, et al. Chemoradiotherapy vs. total laryngectomy for primary treatment of advanced laryngeal squamous cell carcinoma. *Oral Oncol* 2013;49:283–286.

41. Mendenhall WM, Werning JW, Hinerman RW, et al. Management of T1-T2 glottic carcinomas. *Cancer* 2004;100:1786–1792.

42. Chera BS, Amdur RJ, Morris CG, et al. T1N0 to T2N0 squamous cell carcinoma of the glottic larynx treated with definitive radiotherapy. *Int J Radiat Oncol Biol Phys* 2010;78:461–466.

43. Day AT, Sinha P, Nussenbaum B, et al. Management of primary T1-T4 glottic squamous cell carcinoma by transoral laser microsurgery. *Laryngoscope* 2017;127(3):597–604.

44. O'Sullivan B, Mackillop W, Gilbert R, et al. Controversies in the management of laryngeal cancer: results of an international survey of patterns of care. *Radiother Oncol* 1994;31:23–32.

45. Laccourreye H, Laccourreye O, Weinstein G, et al. Supracricoid laryngectomy with cricohyoidoepiglottopexy: a partial laryngeal procedure for glottic carcinoma. *Ann Otol Rhinol Laryngol* 1990;99: 421–426.

46. McGuirt WF, Blalock D, Koufman JA, et al. Comparative voice results after laser resection or irradiation of T1 vocal cord carcinoma. *Arch Otolaryngol Head Neck Surg* 1994;120:951–955.

47. Steiner W. Results of curative laser microsurgery of laryngeal carcinomas. *Am J Otolaryngol* 1993;14:116–121.

48. Rodrigo JP, Suarez C, Silver CE, et al. Transoral laser surgery for supraglottic cancer. *Head Neck* 2008;30:658–666.

49. Peretti G, Piazza C, Cocco D, et al. Transoral CO(2) laser treatment for T(is)-T(3) glottic cancer: the University of Brescia experience on 595 patients. *Head Neck* 2010;32:977–983.

50. Rodel RM, Steiner W, Muller RM, et al. Endoscopic laser surgery of early glottic cancer: involvement of the anterior commissure. *Head Neck* 2009;31:583–592.

51. O'Sullivan B, Warde P, Keane T, et al. Outcome following radiotherapy in verrucous carcinoma of the larynx. *Int J Radiat Oncol Biol Phys* 1995;32:611–617.

52. Fu KK, Pajak TF, Trotti A, et al. A radiation therapy oncology group (RTOG) phase III randomized study to compare hyperfractionation and two variants of accelerated fractionation to standard fractionation radiotherapy for head and neck squamous cell carcinomas: first report of RTOG 9003. *Int J Radiat Oncol Biol Phys* 2000;48:7–16.

53. Parsons JT, Mendenhall WM, Stringer SP, et al. Salvage surgery following radiation failure in squamous cell carcinoma of the supraglottic larynx. *Int J Radiat Oncol Biol Phys* 1995;32:605–609.

54. Pearson BW, Woods RD II, Hartman DE. Extended hemilaryngectomy for T3 glottic carcinoma with preservation of speech and swallowing. *Laryngoscope* 1980;90:1950–1961.

55. Amdur RJ, Parsons JT, Mendenhall WM, et al. Postoperative irradiation for squamous cell carcinoma of the head and neck: an analysis of treatment results and complications. *Int J Radiat Oncol Biol Phys* 1989;16: 25–36.

56. Huang DT, Johnson CR, Schmidt-Ullrich R, et al. Postoperative radiotherapy in head and neck carcinoma with extracapsular lymph node extension and/or positive resection margins: a comparative study. *Int J Radiat Oncol Biol Phys* 1992;23:737–742.

57. Hillman RE, Walsh MJ, Wolf GT, et al. Functional outcomes following treatment for advanced laryngeal cancer. Part I—Voice preservation in advanced laryngeal cancer. Part II—Laryngectomy rehabilitation: the state of the art in the VA system. Research Speech-Language Pathologists. Department of Veterans Affairs Laryngeal Cancer Study Group. *Ann Otol Rhinol Laryngol Suppl* 1998;172:1–27.

58. Harwood AR, Beale FA, Cummings BJ, et al. T4N0M0 glottic cancer: an analysis of dose-time volume factors. *Int J Radiat Oncol Biol Phys* 1981;7:1507–1512.

59. Kim RY, Marks ME, Salter MM. Early-stage glottic cancer: importance of dose fractionation in radiation therapy. *Radiology* 1992;182:273–275.

60. Schwaibold F, Scariato A, Nunno M, et al. The effect of fraction size on control of early glottic cancer. *Int J Radiat Oncol Biol Phys* 1988;14:451–454.

61. Woodhouse RJ, Quivey JM, Fu KK, et al. Treatment of carcinoma of the vocal cord. A review of 20 years experience. *Laryngoscope* 1981;91:1155–1162.

62. Mendenhall WM, Riggs CE, Cassisi NJ. Treatment of head and neck cancers. In: DeVita VT, Hellman S, Rosenberg SA, eds. *DeVita, Hellman, and Rosenberg's Cancer: principles and practice of oncology.* Philadelphia: Lippincott Williams & Wilkins, 2008:809–814

63. Yamazaki H, Nishiyama K, Tanaka E, et al. Radiotherapy for early glottic carcinoma (T1N0M0): results of prospective randomized study of radiation fraction size and overall treatment time. *Int J Radiat Oncol Biol Phys* 2006;64:77–82.

64. Parsons JT, Mendenhall WM, Mancuso AA, et al. Twice-a-day radiotherapy for T3 squamous cell carcinoma of the glottic larynx. *Head Neck* 1989;11:123–128.

Section III

65. Mendenhall WM, Mancuso AA. Radiotherapy for head and neck cancer—is the "next level" down? *Int J Radiat Oncol Biol Phys* 2009;73:645–646.
66. Trotti AF, Fu FF, Pajak TF, et al. Long term outcomes of RTOG 90–03: a comparison of hyperfractionation and two variants of accelerated fractionation to standard fractionation radiotherapy for head and neck squamous cell carcinoma. *Int J Radiat Oncol Biol Phys* 2005;63:S70–S71.
67. Beitler JJ, Zhang Q, Fu KK, et al. Final results of local-regional control and late toxicity of RTOG 9003: a randomized trial of altered fractionation radiation for locally advanced head and neck cancer. *Int J Radiat Oncol Biol Phys* 2014;89:13–20.
68. Biller HF, Barnhill FR Jr, Ogura JH, et al. Hemilaryngectomy following radiation failure for carcinoma of the vocal cords. *Laryngoscope* 1970;80:249–253.
69. Lee F, Perlmutter S, Ogura JH. Laryngeal radiation after hemilaryngectomy. *Laryngoscope* 1980; 90:1534–1539.
70. Hinerman RW, Mendenhall WM, Amdur RJ, et al. Carcinoma of the supraglottic larynx: treatment results with radiotherapy alone or with planned neck dissection. *Head Neck* 2002;24:456–467.
71. Dziegielewski PT, Ozer E. Transoral robotic surgery: supraglottic laryngectomy. *Oper Tech Otolaryngol* 2013;24:86–91.
72. Lee NK, Goepfert H, Wendt CD. Supraglottic laryngectomy for intermediate-stage cancer: U.T. M.D. Anderson Cancer Center experience with combined therapy. *Laryngoscope* 1990;100:831–836.
73. Ampil F, Ghali G, Caldito G, et al. Post-laryngectomy stomal cancer recurrences, re-treatment decisions and outcomes: case series. *J Craniomaxillofac Surg* 2009;37:349–351.
74. Rudert HH, Werner JA. Endoscopic resections of glottic and supraglottic carcinomas with the CO2 laser. *Eur Arch Otorhinolaryngol* 1995;252:146–148.
75. Peretti G, Nicolai P, Redaelli De Zinis LO, et al. Endoscopic CO2 laser excision for tis, T1, and T2 glottic carcinomas: cure rate and prognostic factors. *Otolaryngol Head Neck Surg* 2000;123:124–131.
76. Spector JG, Sessions DG, Chao KS, et al. Stage I (T1 N0 M0) squamous cell carcinoma of the laryngeal glottis: therapeutic results and voice preservation. *Head Neck* 1999;21:707–717.
77. Motta G, Esposito E, Cassiano B, et al. T1-T2-T3 glottic tumors: fifteen years experience with CO2 laser. *Acta Otolaryngol Suppl* 1997;527:155–159.
78. Gallo A, de Vincentiis M, Manciocco V, et al. CO2 laser cordectomy for early-stage glottic carcinoma: a long-term follow-up of 156 cases. *Laryngoscope* 2002;112:370–374.
79. Pradhan SA, Pai PS, Neeli SI, et al. Transoral laser surgery for early glottic cancers. *Arch Otolaryngol Head Neck Surg* 2003;129:623–625.
80. Giovanni A, Guelfucci B, Gras R, et al. Partial frontolateral laryngectomy with epiglottic reconstruction for management of early-stage glottic carcinoma. *Laryngoscope* 2001;111:663–668.
81. Crampette L, Garrel R, Gardiner Q, et al. Modified subtotal laryngectomy with cricohyoidoepiglottopexy—long term results in 81 patients. *Head Neck* 1999;21:95–103.
82. Thomas JV, Olsen KD, Neel HB III, et al. Early glottic carcinoma treated with open laryngeal procedures. *Arch Otolaryngol Head Neck Surg* 1994;120:264–268.
83. Laccourreye O, Weinstein G, Brasnu D, et al. A clinical trial of continuous cisplatin-fluorouracil induction chemotherapy and supracricoid partial laryngectomy for glottic carcinoma classified as T2. *Cancer* 1994;74:2781–2790.
84. Spector JG, Sessions DG, Chao KS, et al. Management of stage II (T2N0M0) glottic carcinoma by radiotherapy and conservation surgery. *Head Neck* 1999;21:116–123.
85. Wang CC. Carcinoma of the larynx. In: Wang CC, ed. *Radiation therapy for head and neck neoplasms*. New York, NY: Wiley-Liss, 1997:221–255
86. Le QT, Fu KK, Kroll S, et al. Influence of fraction size, total dose, and overall time on local control of T1-T2 glottic carcinoma. *Int J Radiat Oncol Biol Phys* 1997;39:115–126.
87. Warde P, O'Sullivan B, Bristow RG, et al. T1/T2 glottic cancer managed by external beam radiotherapy: the influence of pretreatment hemoglobin on local control. *Int J Radiat Oncol Biol Phys* 1998;41:347–353.
88. Garden AS, Forster K, Wong PF, et al. Results of radiotherapy for T2N0 glottic carcinoma: does the "2" stand for twice-daily treatment? *Int J Radiat Oncol Biol Phys* 2003;55:322–328.
89. Sengupta N, Morris CG, Kirwan J, et al. Definitive radiotherapy for carcinoma in situ of the true vocal cords. *Am J Clin Oncol* 2010;33:94–95.
90. Foote RL, Olsen KD, Buskirk SJ, et al. Laryngectomy alone for T3 glottic cancer. *Head Neck* 1994;16:406–412.
91. Harwood AR, Beale FA, Cummings BJ, et al. T3 glottic cancer: an analysis of dose time-volume factors. *Int J Radiat Oncol Biol Phys* 1980;6:675–680.
92. Wang CC. Radiation therapy of laryngeal tumors: curative radiation therapy. In: Thawley SE, Panje WR, eds. *Comprehensive management of head and neck tumors*. Philadelphia: WB Saunders, 1987:906–919
93. Fletcher GH. Radiation therapy for cancer of the larynx and pyriform sinus. *Eye Nose Ear Throat Digest* 1969; 31:58–67.
94. Skolyszewski J, Reinfuss M. The results of radiotherapy of cancer of the larynx in six European countries. *Radiobiol Radiother (Berl)* 1981;22:32–43.
95. Stewart JG, Brown JR, Palmer MK, et al. The management of glottic carcinoma by primary irradiation with surgery in reserve. *Laryngoscope* 1975;85:1477–1484.
96. Mills EE. Early glottic carcinoma: factors affecting radiation failure, results of treatment and sequelae. *Int J Radiat Oncol Biol Phys* 1979;5:811–817.
97. Mendenhall WM, Parsons JT, Stringer SP, et al. Stage T3 squamous cell carcinoma of the glottic larynx: a comparison of laryngectomy and irradiation. *Int J Radiat Oncol Biol Phys* 1992;23:725–732.
98. Jesse RH. The evaluation of treatment of patients with extensive squamous cancer of the vocal cords. *Laryngoscope* 1975;85:1424–1429.
99. Ogura JH, Sessions DG, Ciralsky RH. Supraglottic carcinoma with extension to the arytenoid. *Laryngoscope* 1975;85:1327–1331.
100. Skolnik EM, Yee KF, Wheatley MA, et al. Carcinoma of the laryngeal glottis therapy and end results. *Laryngoscope* 1975;85:1453–1466.
101. Vermund H. Role of radiotherapy in cancer of the larynx as related to the TNM system of staging. A review. *Cancer* 1970;25:485–504.
102. Stewart JG, Jackson AW. The steepness of the dose response curve both for tumor cure and normal tissue injury. *Laryngoscope* 1975;85:1107–1111.
103. Parsons JT, Mendenhall WM, Stringer SP, et al. T4 laryngeal carcinoma: radiotherapy alone with surgery reserved for salvage. *Int J Radiat Oncol Biol Phys* 1998;40:549–552.
104. Ogura JH, Sessions DG, Spector GJ. Conservation surgery for epidermoid carcinoma of the supraglottic larynx. *Laryngoscope* 1975;85:1808–1815.
105. Lutz CK, Johnson JT, Wagner RL, et al. Supraglottic carcinoma: patterns of recurrence. *Ann Otol Rhinol Laryngol* 1990;99:12–17.
106. Weems DH, Mendenhall WM, Parsons JT, et al. Squamous cell carcinoma of the supraglottic larynx treated with surgery and/or radiation therapy. *Int J Radiat Oncol Biol Phys* 1987;13:1483–1487.
107. Gregor RT, Oei SS, Baris G, et al. Supraglottic laryngectomy with postoperative radiation versus primary radiation in the management of supraglottic laryngeal cancer. *Am J Otolaryngol* 1996;17:316–321.
108. Spriano G, Antognoni P, Piantanida R, et al. Conservative management of T1-T2N0 supraglottic cancer: a retrospective study. *Am J Otolaryngol* 1997;18:299–305.
109. Bocca E. Sixteenth Daniel C. Baker, Jr, memorial lecture. Surgical management of supraglottic cancer and its lymph node metastases in a conservative perspective. *Ann Otol Rhinol Laryngol* 1991;100:261–267.
110. Isaacs JH Jr, Slattery WH III, Mendenhall WM, et al. Supraglottic laryngectomy. *Am J Otolaryngol* 1998;19:118–123.
111. Davis RK, Kelly SM, Hayes J. Endoscopic CO2 laser excisional biopsy of early supraglottic cancer. *Laryngoscope* 1991;101:680–683.
112. Zeitels SM, Koufman JA, Davis RK, et al. Endoscopic treatment of supraglottic and hypopharynx cancer. *Laryngoscope* 1994;104:71–78.
113. Rudert HH, Werner JA, Hoft S. Transoral carbon dioxide laser resection of supraglottic carcinoma. *Ann Otol Rhinol Laryngol* 1999;108:819–827.
114. Ghossein NA, Bataini JP, Ennuyer A, et al. Local control and site of failure in radically irradiated supraglottic laryngeal cancer. *Radiology* 1974;112:187–192.
115. Csanady M, Ivan L, Czigner J. Endoscopic CO(2) laser therapy of selected cases of supraglottic marginal tumors. *Eur Arch Otorhinolaryngol* 1999;256: 392–394.
116. Fletcher GH, Hamberger AD. Causes of failure in irradiation of squamous-cell carcinoma of the supraglottic larynx. *Radiology* 1974;111:697–700.
117. Wang CC, Montgomery WW. Deciding on optimal management of supraglottic carcinoma. *Oncology (Williston Park)* 1991;5:41–46; discussion 6, 9, 53.
118. Nakfoor BM, Spiro IJ, Wang CC, et al. Results of accelerated radiotherapy for supraglottic carcinoma: a Massachusetts General Hospital and Massachusetts Eye and Ear Infirmary experience. *Head Neck* 1998;20:379–384.
119. Sykes AJ, Slevin NJ, Gupta NK, et al. 331 cases of clinically node-negative supraglottic carcinoma of the larynx: a study of a modest size fixed field radiotherapy approach. *Int J Radiat Oncol Biol Phys* 2000;46:1109–1115.
120. DeSanto LW. Early supraglottic cancer. *Ann Otol Rhinol Laryngol* 1990;99:593–597.
121. Steiniger JR, Parnes SM, Gardner GM. Morbidity of combined therapy for the treatment of supraglottic carcinoma: supraglottic laryngectomy and radiotherapy. *Ann Otol Rhinol Laryngol* 1997;106:151–158.
122. Burstein FD, Calcaterra TC. Supraglottic laryngectomy: series report and analysis of results. *Laryngoscope* 1985;95:833–836.
123. Gall AM, Sessions DG, Ogura JH. Complications following surgery for cancer of the larynx and hypopharynx. *Cancer* 1977;39:624–631.
124. Weber PC, Johnson JT, Myers EN. Impact of bilateral neck dissection on recovery following supraglottic laryngectomy. *Arch Otolaryngol Head Neck Surg* 1993;119:61–64.
125. Beckhardt RN, Murray JG, Ford CN, et al. Factors influencing functional outcome in supraglottic laryngectomy. *Head Neck* 1994;16:232–239.
126. Ganly I, Patel SG, Matsuo J, et al. Analysis of postoperative complications of open partial laryngectomy. *Head Neck* 2009;31:338–345.
127. Hoffman HT, Porter K, Karnell LH, et al. Laryngeal cancer in the United States: changes in demographics, patterns of care, and survival. *Laryngoscope* 2006;116:1–13.
128. Chen AY, Halpern M. Factors predictive of survival in advanced laryngeal cancer. *Arch Otolaryngol Head Neck Surg* 2007;133:1270–1276.
129. Gourin CG, Conger BT, Sheils WC, et al. The effect of treatment on survival in patients with advanced laryngeal carcinoma. *Laryngoscope* 2009;119:1312–1317.
130. Dziegielewski PT, O'Connell DA, Klein M, et al. Primary total laryngectomy versus organ preservation for T3/T4a laryngeal cancer: a population-based analysis of survival. *J Otolaryngol Head Neck Surg* 2012;41 Suppl 1:S56–S64.
131. Megwalu UC, Sikora AG. Survival outcomes in advanced laryngeal cancer. *JAMA Otolaryngol Head Neck Surg* 2014;140:855–860.
132. Sanabria A, Chaves AL, Kowalski LP, et al. Organ preservation with chemoradiation in advanced laryngeal cancer: The problem of generalizing results from randomized controlled trials. *Auris Nasus Larynx* 2017;44(1):18–25.
133. Riga M, Chelis L, Danielides V, et al. Systematic review on T3 laryngeal squamous cell carcinoma; still far from a consensus on the optimal organ preserving treatment. *Eur J Surg Oncol* 2017;43(1):20–31.
134. Wagenfeld DJ, Harwood AR, Bryce DP, et al. Second primary respiratory tract malignancies in glottic carcinoma. *Cancer* 1980;46:1883–1886.
135. Garcia-Serra A, Amdur RJ, Morris CG, et al. Thyroid function should be monitored following radiotherapy to the low neck. *Am J Clin Oncol* 2005;28: 255–258.
136. Neel HB, III, Devine KD, Desanto LW. Laryngofissure and cordectomy for early cordal carcinoma: outcome in 182 patients. *Otolaryngol Head Neck Surg (1979)* 1980;88:79–84.
137. Al-Othman MO, Amdur RJ, Morris CG, et al. Does feeding tube placement predict for long-term swallowing disability after radiotherapy for head and neck cancer? *Head Neck* 2003;25:741–747.

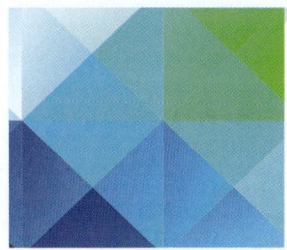

CHAPTER 51

Unusual Nonepithelial Tumors of the Head and Neck

Carlos A. Perez and Wade L. Thorstad

GLOMUS TUMORS

Anatomy

Glomus bodies are found in the jugular bulb and along the tympanic (Jacobson) and auricular (Arnold) branches of the tenth nerve in the middle ear or in other anatomic sites (Fig. 51.1). Depending on the location, glomus tumors (GTs) (chemodectoma or paraganglioma) are classified as tympanic (middle ear), jugulare, or carotid vagal or designated as originating from other locations, such as the larynx, adventitia of thoracic aorta, abdominal aorta, or the surface of the lungs (Fig. 51.2).[1]

GT or chemodectomas consist of large epithelioid (smooth muscle) cells with fine granular cytoplasm embedded in a rich capillary network and fibrous stroma with reticulin fibers, which derive from embryonic neural crest cells. Although histologically benign, they may extend along the lumen of the vein to regional lymph nodes, but rarely to distant sites. These tissues are responsive to changes in oxygen and carbon dioxide tensions and pH.

Epidemiology

The mean age at diagnosis has been reported to be 45 years for carotid body tumors and 52 years for glomus tympanicum.[2] These tumors occur three or four times more frequently in women than in men, suggesting a possible estrogen influence.[2-4] Glomus tumors may be familial; they occur in multiple sites in 10% to 20% of patients.[5] Incidence may be influenced by hereditary syndromes including PGL1-5, MEN2, and NF1.

Recent advances in genetics identified three loci associated with hereditary paragangliomas, and genetic screening may detect affected patients.[6] Multiple paragangliomas of the head and neck are rare, with an incidence of 10% of all patients, but in familial cases, it increases up to 35% to 50%.[5] In the head and neck region, the most common association is

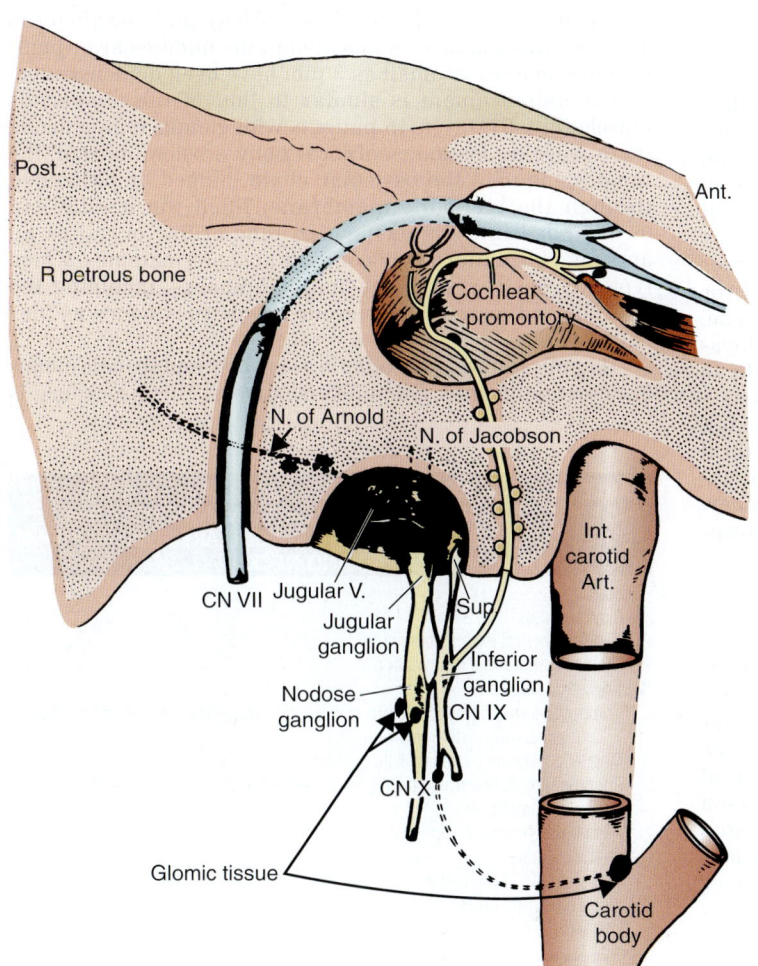

FIGURE 51.1. Anatomy of the region of the glomus jugulare. (From Hatfield PM, James AE, Schulz MN. Chemodectomas of the glomus jugulare. *Cancer* 1972;30[5]:1165–1168. Copyright © 1972 American Cancer Society. Reprinted by permission of John Wiley & Sons, Inc.)

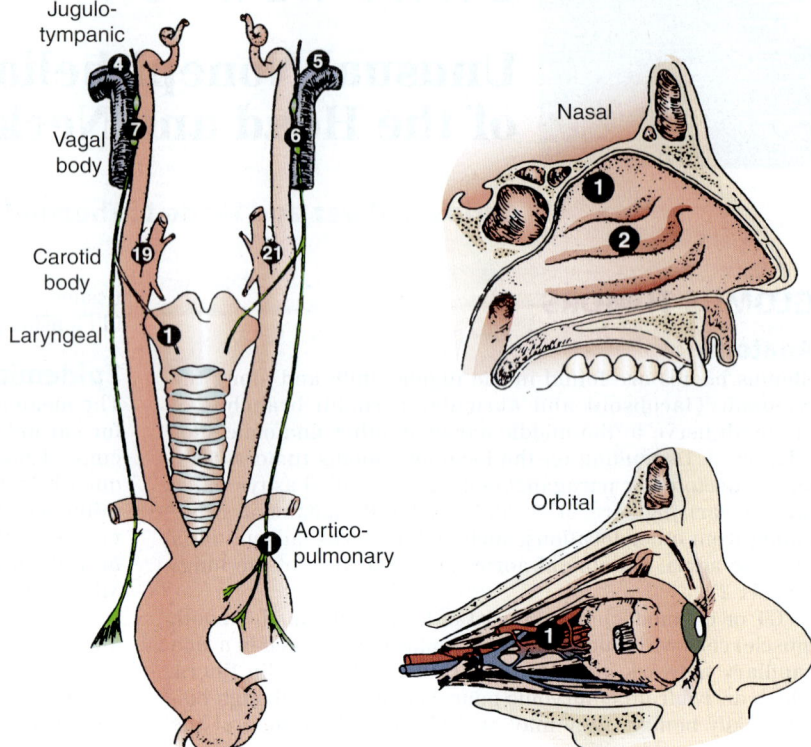

FIGURE 51.2. Distribution of paragangliomas of the head and neck region. Laterality was not specified in three patients with carotid body paragangliomas. The diagram does not include one left carotid body paraglioma that was found incidentally at autopsy and a left vagal body paraganglioma that presented in a patient who had two other paragangliomas. (From Lack EE, Cubilla AL, Woodruff JM, et al. Paragangliomas of the head and neck region. *Cancer* 1977;39[2]:397–409. Copyright © 1977 American Cancer Society. Reprinted by permission of John Wiley & Sons, Inc.)

bilateral carotid body tumors or carotid body tumor associated with tympanic–jugular glomus.[7]

Clinical Presentation

Glomus tumors may arise along the nerve roots. In the middle ear, they may initially cause earache or discomfort.[8] As they expand, eventually they produce pulsatile tinnitus, hearing loss, and, in later stages, cranial nerve paralysis resulting from invasion of the base of the skull in 10% to 15% of patients. If the tumor invades the middle cranial fossa, symptoms may include temporoparietal headache, retro-orbital pain, proptosis, and paresis of cranial nerves V and VI. If the posterior fossa is involved, symptoms may include occipital headache, ataxia, and paresis of cranial nerves V to VII, IX, and XII; invasion of the jugular foramen causes paralysis of nerves IX to XI. Chemodectoma of the carotid body usually presents as a painless, slowly growing mass in the upper neck. Occasionally, the mass may be pulsatile and may have an associated thrill or bruit. As it enlarges, the mass may extend into the parapharyngeal space and be visible on examination of the oropharynx. Very rarely, these tumors may be malignant.[9] Metastases occur in 2% to 5% of cases.[3]

Diagnostic Workup

Diagnostic evaluation for glomus tumors of the ear and base of skull is outlined in Table 51.1. In the majority of glomus tympanicum, physical examination demonstrates a red, vascular middle ear mass, although occasionally it may be bluish or white (the latter resembling a cholesteatoma).[2] Audiography may demonstrate conductive hearing loss in the ear involved by tumor as noted in 33 of 49 patients evaluated by Larson et al.[2]; 4 of 33 patients with conductive deficits also exhibited tympanic pulsations. Examination of the neck may occasionally demonstrate a mass in the neck that may be pulsatile or have a bruit or regional lymph node metastases.

Radiographic studies are invaluable in the diagnosis of these tumors. Plain mastoid radiographs never show the soft tissue mass in the middle ear, although they frequently demonstrate clouding of the mastoid air cells, suggesting

mastoiditis.[10] High-resolution computed tomography (CT) with contrast has a degree of sensitivity and specificity to diagnose this tumor when located in the middle ear or jugular bulb; masses as small as 3 mm have been demonstrated. Tumor enhancement is similar to that of the temporalis muscle (Fig. 51.3).[2] In 46 patients with glomus tympanicum, there were no instances of local bony erosion; instead, the tumors engulfed the ossicular chain, bulged or protruded through the tympanic membrane, filled the middle ear, or extended into the eustachian tube orifice or aditus ad antrum. This pattern is in contrast to cholesteatomas, which typically destroy adjacent bony landmarks, including the ossicles, and progressively erode the petrous bones as they enlarge.[2]

Magnification angiography is a sensitive and specific means of detecting glomus tympanicum tumors. This procedure is

---

TABLE 51.1 DIAGNOSTIC WORKUP FOR GLOMUS TUMORS OF THE EAR AND BASE OF THE SKULL, HEMANGIOPERICYTOMA, ESTHESIONEUROBLASTOMA, EXTRAMEDULLARY PLASMACYTOMA, AND SARCOMA OF THE HEAD AND NECK

General
  Clinical history
  General physical examination
  Ear, nose, and throat examination
Radiographic Studies
  Computed tomography scan (with contrast) to define tumor extent and possible central nervous system involvement)
  Magnetic resonance imaging with gadolinium
  Arteriography to determine bilateral involvement and collateral cerebral blood flow (optional)
  Jugular phlebography (optional)
Laboratory Studies
  Complete blood cell count
  Blood chemistry profile
  Urinalysis
Special Tests
  Audiograms to establish baseline hearing loss
  Histologic staining to determine presence of catecholamines

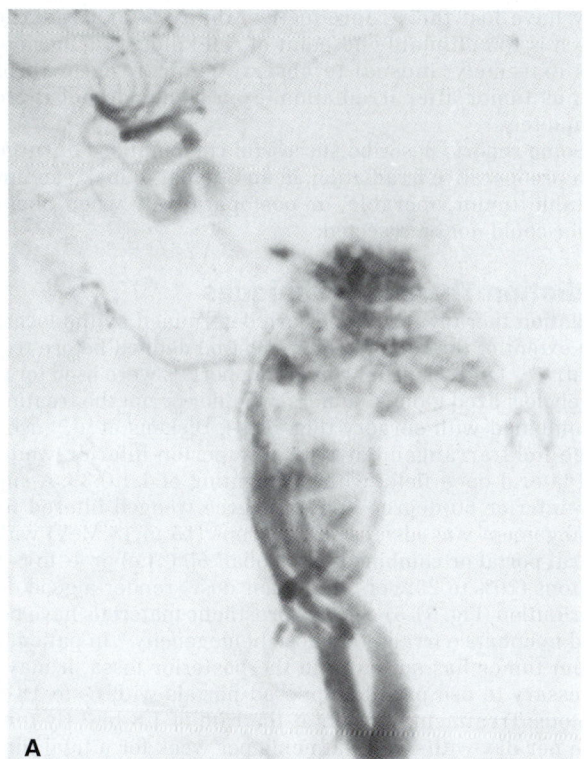

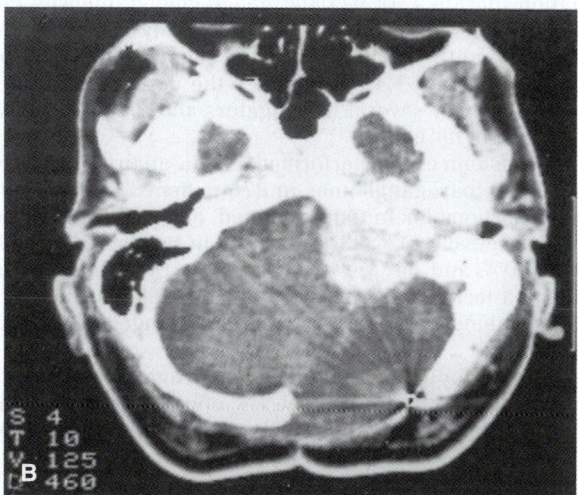

FIGURE 51.3. A: Late-phase arteriogram illustrating large glomus jugulare tumor with extension into the neck. **B:** Computed tomography scan with contrast enhancement showing intracranial component of lesion.

allowed differentiation between tumor and sinusal blood flow in all cases.

Drape et al.[12] described magnetic resonance imaging (MRI) findings in 31 patients with a clinical suspicion of glomus tumor; gadoterate meglumine was injected into 19 patients. Twenty-seven of twenty-eight pathologically confirmed glomus tumors were detected with MRI; a peripheral capsule was present in most tumors. The investigators were able to differentiate three subtypes of glomus tumors (vascular, solid, and myxoid) on the basis of relaxation times and enhancement characteristics. Multidetector CT angiography was found to be more accurate in the diagnosis of six glomus tumors, with enhancement in the arterial phase, when compared with MRI.[13]

As GTs show high levels of somatostatin receptor (SSTR) subtypes 2 and 5, fluorine-(^{18}F)-octreotate positron emission tomography (PET) may be useful for diagnostic purposes in a semiquantitative manner and for improving target volume delineation in radiation therapy planning. Astner et al.[14] noted that preliminary findings with two different PET tracers for SSTR imaging have been reported: Gallium-68 (^{68}Ga)-DOTATOC (DOTA-d-Phe(1)-Tyr(3)-octreotide [somatostatin analog]) PET was shown to detect SSTR-expressing tumors with high sensitivity and specificity. A second PET tracer, Gluc-Lys(^{18})F-TOCA, allows fast, high-contrast imaging of SSTR-positive tumors with superior biokinetics and diagnostic performance as compared with indium-111 (^{111}In)-DTPA (diethylenetriamine pentaacetic acid)-octreotide and—as far as can be determined from the literature—comparable to[15] Ga-DOTATOC.[16–18]

Cytochemical techniques demonstrate increased levels of serotonin, epinephrine, and norepinephrine in normal glomus tissue of the carotid body. Histologic staining techniques, including chromaffin and argentaffin reactions, identify patients with hormonally active tumors. This is important because the glomus tumor may coexist with a pheochromocytoma, which requires special preoperative preparation of the patient. Biopsy of glomus tumors may result in severe hemorrhage.

Staging

The prognosis of these tumors is closely related to the anatomic location and the volume of the lesion, which is reflected in the Glasscock-Jackson classification[19] shown in Table 51.2. An alternative classification proposed by McCabe and Fletcher[20] is presented in Table 51.3.

General Management

Li et al.[21] published a historical perspective of various treatment modalities used to treat glomus tumors over the past 60 years.

performed after high-resolution thin-section CT scan (with contrast material), only when there is a question regarding the nature of the lesion or the location of the carotid canal. Findings include a hypervascular middle ear mass that first appears in the middle to late arterial phase, persists through the capillary phase, and quickly disappears in the venous phase without demonstrably early draining veins. Biopsy of an aberrant internal carotid artery can result in major neurologic sequelae or death.

Vogl et al.[11] reported on 40 patients with glomus tumors of the skull; diagnostic interpretations were correlated with histologic examination, digital subtraction angiography, CT, and clinical follow-up. Sixteen of eighteen proven tumors were detected with spin-echo images alone. Although four high-flying jugular bulbs were misinterpreted as tumors because of similar signal intensity, combined evaluation

TABLE 51.2 GLASSCOCK-JACKSON CLASSIFICATION OF GLOMUS TUMORS

Glomus Tympanicum
  I. Small mass limited to promontory
 II. Tumor completely filling middle ear space
III. Tumor filling middle ear and extending into the mastoid
 IV. Tumor filling middle ear, extending into the mastoid or through tympanic membrane to fill the external auditory canal; may extend anterior to carotid

Glomus Jugulare
  I. Small tumor involving the jugular bulb, middle ear, and mastoid
 II. Tumor extending under internal auditory canal; may have intracranial canal extension
III. Tumor extending into the petrous apex; may have intracranial canal extension
 IV. Tumor extending beyond the petrous apex into the clivus or infratemporal fossa; may have intracranial canal extension

TABLE 51.3 MODIFICATION OF MCCABE AND FLETCHER CLASSIFICATION OF CHEMODECTOMAS

Group I: Tympanic Tumors
  Absence of bone destruction on x-rays of the mastoid bone and jugular fossa
  Absence of facial nerve weakness
  Intact eighth nerve with conductive deafness only
  Intact jugular foramen nerves (cranial nerves IX, X, and XI)
Group II: Tympanomastoid Tumors
  X-ray evidence of bone destruction confined to the mastoid bone and not involving the petrous bone
  Normal or paretic seventh nerve
  Intact jugular foramen nerves
  No evidence of involvement of the superior bulb of the jugular vein on retrograde venogram
Group III: Petrosal and Extrapetrosal Tumors
  Destruction of the petrous bone, jugular fossa, and/or occipital bone on x-rays
  Positive findings on retrograde jugulography
  Evidence of destruction of the petrous or occipital bones on carotid arteriogram
  Jugular foramen syndrome (paresis of cranial nerves IX, X, or XI)
  Presence of metastasis

Reprinted from Wang M-L, Hussey DH, Doornbos JF, et al. Chemodectoma of the temporal bone: a comparison of surgical and radiotherapeutic results. *Int J Radiat Oncol Biol Phys* 1988;14(4):643–648. Copyright © 1988 Elsevier. With permission.

Surgery

Surgery is generally selected for small tumors that can be completely excised. Glomus tympanicum tumors are particularly well managed with excision via tympanotomy or mastoidectomy. Percutaneous embolization of a low-viscosity silicone polymer has been used, frequently as preoperative preparation of the tumor embolization of feeding vessels allows meticulous microsurgery with virtually complete hemostasis.

Surgical treatment of a glomus tumor arising in the jugular bulb, however, often consists of piece-by-piece removal accompanied by significant intraoperative bleeding with damage to adjacent neurovascular structures and requires more complex surgical approaches involving the base of the skull. Preoperative embolization via a transarterial approach has proved beneficial but is often limited by vascular anatomy and unfavorable locations. Abud et al.[22] reported experience with preoperative devascularization using direct puncture and an intralesional injection of cyanoacrylate (acrylic glue) under fluoroscopic guidance in nine patients with head and neck paragangliomas. Ozyer et al.[23] performed devascularization with intralesional injection of N-butyl cyanoacrylate (seven carotid and three jugular paragangliomas). The tumors were subsequently surgically removed.

The local tumor control rate with surgery alone is only about 60%, and there is significant morbidity, particularly cranial nerve injury and bleeding.

In a retrospective review of all skull base surgery cases treated at Baylor University, 175 jugulotympanic glomus tumors and 9 malignant cases (5.1%) were identified.[9] The 5-year survival rate was 72%.

Radiation Therapy

Irradiation is frequently used in the treatment of glomus tumors, particularly for those in the tympanicum and jugulare bulb locations. Tumors with destruction of the petrous bone, jugular fossa, or occipital bone or patients with jugular foramen syndrome are more reliably managed with irradiation.[2,4,24,25] Some surgeons, such as Glasscock et al.,[19] have questioned the effectiveness of radiation therapy in the treatment of chemodectomas because on histologic sections, obtained even many years after irradiation, it is possible to find chromophilic cells remaining in the tumor. However, there is also evidence of fibrosis and decreased vascularity.[26] Suit and Gallager[27] demonstrated in a murine mammary carcinoma model that morphologically intact cells

may have lost their reproductive ability after irradiation, which is the ultimate end point of cell killing. Furthermore, it is extremely unusual to observe clinical regrowth of a glomus tumor after irradiation, even if they do not regress completely.

Some reports describe successful combinations of surgery with preoperative irradiation, in an attempt to make an unresectable tumor operable, or postoperatively when obvious tumor could not be resected.

Radiation Therapy Techniques

Radiation therapy techniques are determined by the location and extent of the tumor, which must be defined before treatment.[24,28,29] Limited, usually bilateral, portals were used for relatively localized glomus tumors, whether or not the treatment is combined with surgery (Fig. 51.4). Dickens et al.[30] used a three-field arrangement with a superior–inferior wedged and lateral open field, with a weighting of 1:1:0.33. A superior–inferior 60-degree and 45-degree wedged filtered field arrangement was also used. Electrons (15 to 18 MeV) with a lateral portal or combined with cobalt 60 (^{60}Co) or 4- to 6-MV photons (20% to 25% of total tumor dose) render a good dose distribution (Fig. 51.5). Several prosthetic materials have been used to enhance irradiation dose homogeneity.[31] In patients in whom tumor has spread into the posterior fossa, it may be necessary to use parallel-opposed portals with 6- to 18-MV photons. Treatment is given at the rate of 1.8 to 2 Gy tumor dose per day with five treatments per week for a total tumor dose of 45 to 55 Gy in 5 weeks. Three-dimensional conformal radiation therapy (3DCRT) and image-guided intensity-modulated radiation therapy (IMRT) are highly desirable techniques to treat these tumors, with excellent dose distributions (Fig. 51.5). Table 51.4 summarizes the doses of irradiation recommended by several investigators and the probability of tumor control for each.[24,29,37]

van Hulsteijn et al.[38] performed a meta-analysis of 283 jugulotympanic paragangliomas in 276 patients. Pooled regression proportions for initial, combined, and salvage treatment were respectively 21%, 33%, and 52% in radiosurgery studies and 4%, 0%, and 64% in external beam radiotherapy studies. Pooled local control proportions for radiation therapy as initial, combined, and salvage treatment ranged from 79% to 100%.

Radiotherapy for jugulotympanic paragangliomas results in excellent local tumor control. The effects of radiation therapy on regression of tumor volume remained ambiguous, although the data suggest that complete regression can be achieved in some patients.

Structure	Dose Range (Gy)	Mean Dose (Gy)
Planning target volume (including left neck)	38–77	70
Brain	0–59	2
Brainstem	6–35	12
Spinal cord	0–32	13

Leber et al.[39] reported on 13 patients with glomus tumors treated with radiosurgery in 6, because of recurrences after surgical removal. Histology was not available in 7 patients; diagnosis was made from neuroradiologic features only. With a mean follow-up of 42 months (range 14 to 72 months), there was no tumor progression and no clinical deterioration in any patient; 64% of the patients had improvement of symptoms, and in 36%, the volume of the lesion decreased in size. There was no radiation-related morbidity. In recent years, there have been an increasing number of reports in small series of patients with glomus tumors <2 or 3 cm treated with stereotactic radiation therapy (SRT), with tumor control over 80% and relatively minimal morbidity. The mean

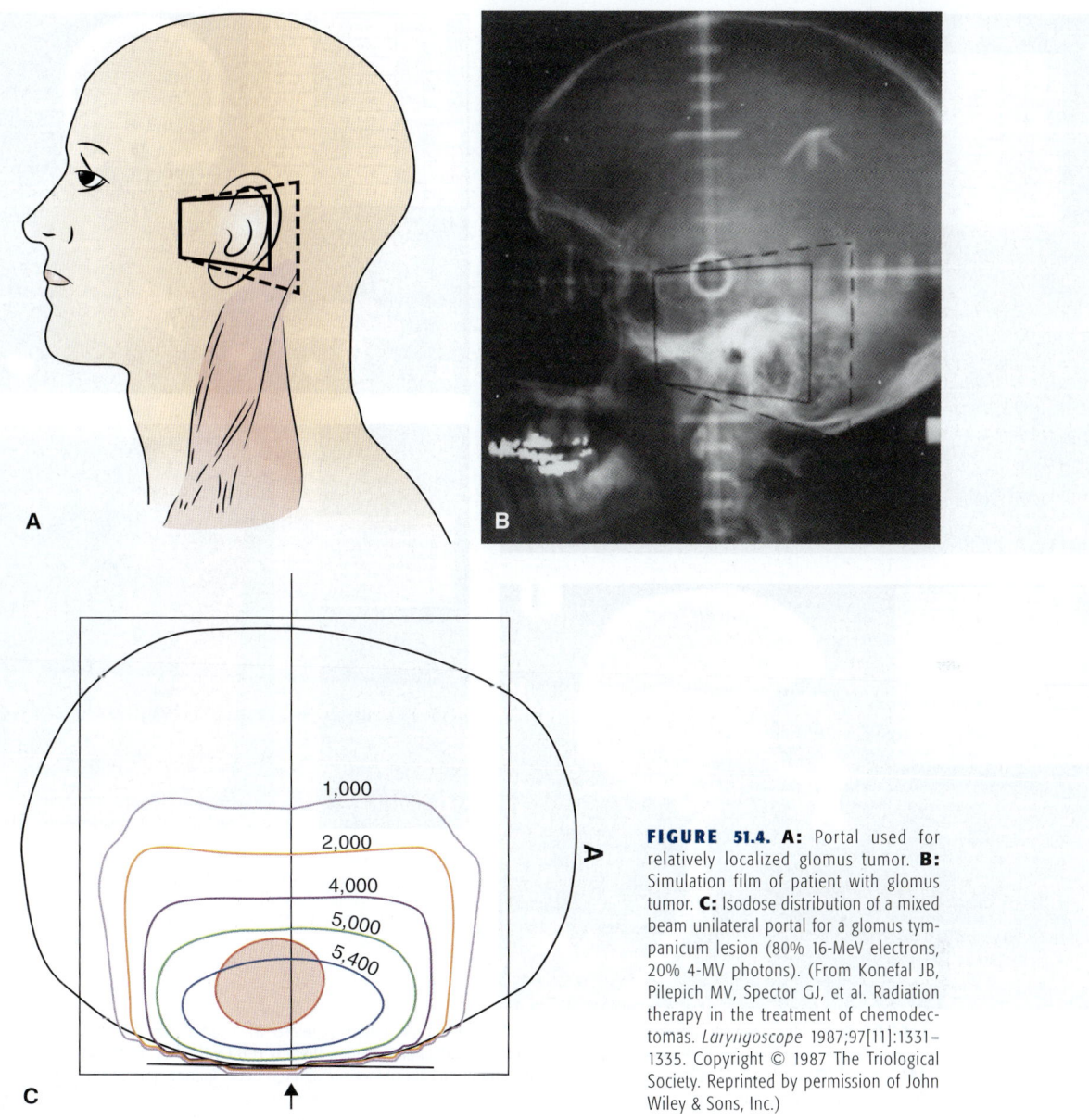

FIGURE 51.4. A: Portal used for relatively localized glomus tumor. **B:** Simulation film of patient with glomus tumor. **C:** Isodose distribution of a mixed beam unilateral portal for a glomus tympanicum lesion (80% 16-MeV electrons, 20% 4-MV photons). (From Konefal JB, Pilepich MV, Spector GJ, et al. Radiation therapy in the treatment of chemodectomas. *Laryngoscope* 1987;97[11]:1331–1335. Copyright © 1987 The Triological Society. Reprinted by permission of John Wiley & Sons, Inc.)

single dose is about 16 Gy (range 13 to 20 Gy).[40–45] A report on fractionated stereotactic irradiation (6-MV x-rays) of 17 patients has been published, with a dose of 57 Gy.[46] Pollock[47] reported on 42 glomus tumors (19 primary treatment and 23 recurrences after initial surgery) treated with Gamma Knife (Elekta Corp, Stockholm) stereotactic radiation (12 to 24 Gy single dose at 50% isodose, depending on tumor size). Twelve lesions (31%) decreased in size and 26 were unchanged. The most common complication was hearing loss (19%). Wegner et al.[48] treated 18 patients with carotid or jugular lesions with fractionated stereotactic CyberKnife (Accuray, Sunnyvale, CA) (Fig. 51.6). Fifteen patients (83%) had single glomus jugulare tumors and three patients had bilateral glomus jugulare tumors. Ten tumors were previously untreated, and eight were persistent after previous surgical resection. The median prescribed dose was 20 Gy in 3 fractions (range: 16 to 25 Gy in 1 to 5 fx) The median prescription coverage of the tumor was 93.6% (range: 83% to 98.72%).Median follow-up was 22 months. All the patients were alive at the time of the last follow-up with imaging available for review. The tumor was stable in 17 patients and decreased in size in one patient—yielding a local control rate of 100%. No patients

experienced any new or worsening treatment-related neurologic deficits.

Results of Therapy

The postirradiation change in tumor size is slow, with an increase in proliferative and perivascular fibrosis and minimal alterations in the chief epithelial cells. Histologic evaluation of tumor cell viability is not reliable.[27] Despite the persistence of tumor both clinically and angiographically, amelioration of symptoms, absence of disease progression, and occasional return of cranial nerve function have been reported. Seventeen patients were treated for glomus tympanicum tumors at Washington University.[3] In five patients, initial treatment consisted of irradiation alone, and all were tumor free at the last follow-up (4.5 years in one patient) or at death. Seven of eight patients irradiated for surgical recurrence were free of disease 4.5 to 19 years after irradiation. The remaining four patients were treated preoperatively or postoperatively; only one had recurrence and was salvaged surgically and tumor free 10 years later. Of six patients with glomus jugulare lesions treated with irradiation, two with extensive lesions died of their disease, whereas the glomus

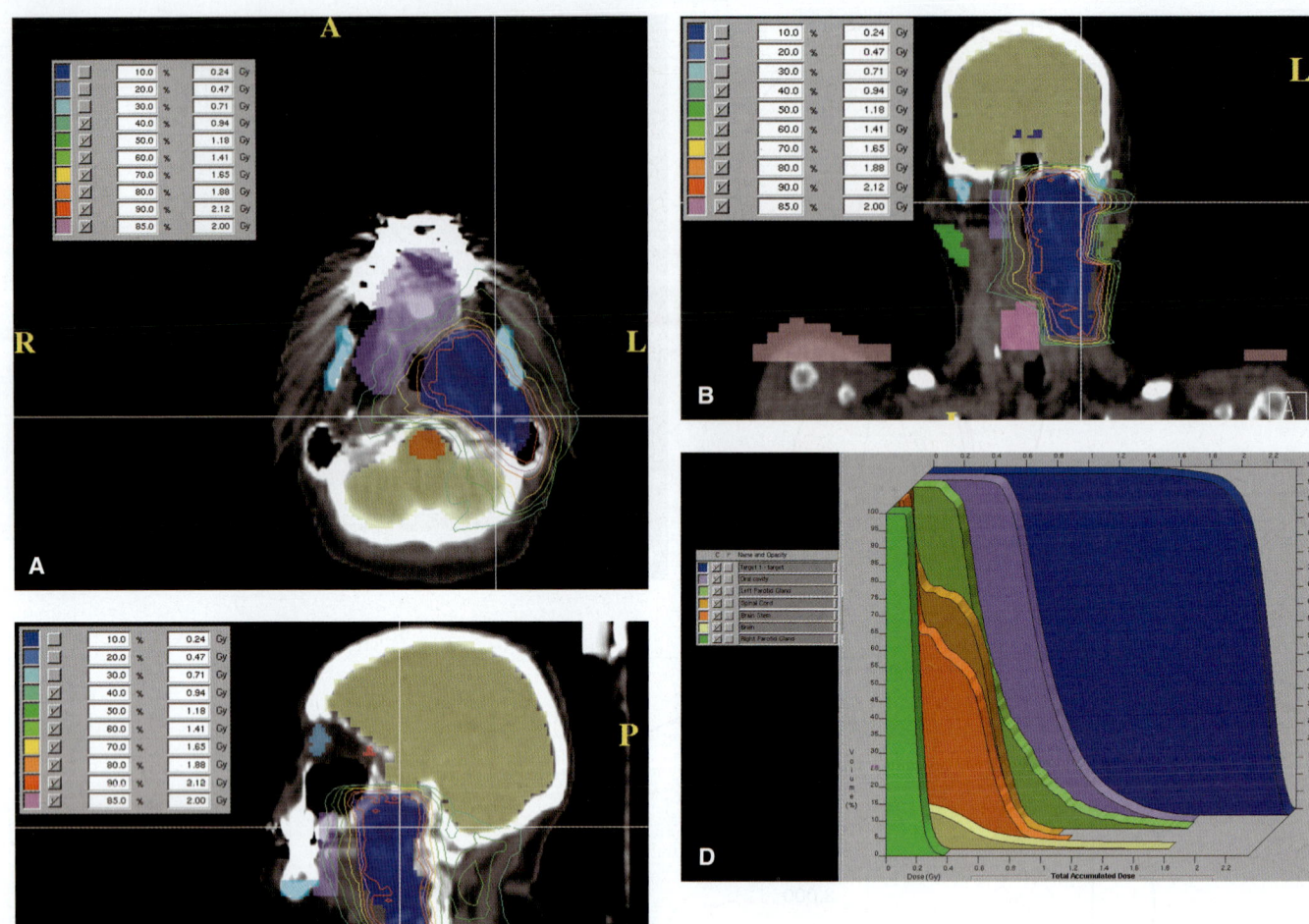

FIGURE 51.5. Fifty-nine-year-old woman with an unusual malignant left glomus jugulare, who had a metastatic left upper cervical lymph node. She was treated definitively with intensity-modulated radiation therapy (66 Gy in 2-Gy fractions). Cross **(A)**, coronal **(B)**, and sagittal **(C)** sections showing dose distributions at primary site and left neck, sparing normal structures. **D:** Dose–volume histogram.

tumor was controlled in four, including two patients with intracranial extension. Irradiation doses ranged from 46 to 52 Gy, with 86% to 100% tumor control with doses over 46 Gy and 50% (two of four) with doses below 46 Gy.

TABLE 51.4 LOCAL CONTROL WITH RADIATION THERAPY FOR CHEMODECTOMA OF THE TEMPORAL BONE (GLOMUS TYMPANICUM AND JUGULARE)

Institution (Reference)	Local Control	Nominal Dosage Schedule
Princess Margaret Hospital[32]	42/45[a]	35 Gy/3 wk
Queen Elizabeth Hospital, Birmingham[33]	19/20[b]	45–50 Gy/4–5 wk
University of Washington[34]	10/13	8–65 Gy/4–7 wk
Rotterdamsch Radio-Therapeutisch Instituut, Netherlands[35]	19/19	40–60 Gy/4–6 wk
University of Minnesota[9]	13/14	30–60 Gy/3.5–7.5 wk
University of Virginia[36]	14/17	40–50 Gy/4–5 wk
Total	117/128 (91%)	

[a]Two patients listed as failures were salvaged with further treatments.
[b]One patient listed as a failure was salvaged with further radiation therapy.
Modified from Wang M-L, Hussey DH, Doornbos JF, et al. Chemodectoma of the temporal bone: a comparison of surgical and radiotherapeutic results. *Int J Radiat Oncol Biol Phys* 1987;14:643–648; and Springate SC, Weichselbaum RR. Radiation or surgery for chemodectoma of the temporal bone: a review of local control and complications. *Head Neck* 1990;12:303–307.

Wang et al.[49] reported on 32 patients with tympanic chemodectomas; 13 are treated with surgery alone, 15 with irradiation alone, and 4 with a combination of both modalities. The initial tumor control rate was 46% with surgery alone; ultimately 84% of patients were tumor free after salvage with additional surgery. Although 78% survived 10 years, 31% developed complications. Of the patients treated with irradiation, 84% had initial local tumor control; 77% survived 10 years, and only 11% developed complications. The doses of irradiation used were slightly higher than those reported by others (mean 58.32 Gy). However, no improvement in tumor control was noted with higher doses. Complications occurred in two patients receiving 66 Gy.

Zabel et al.[50] described results in 22 patients with large chemodectomas of the skull base (8 after primary surgery and 4 after embolization), treated with fractionated stereotactic irradiation (median total dose 57 Gy with median fraction dose 1.8 Gy). With a median follow-up of 5.7 years, 5- and 10-year actuarial tumor control was 90%, with 7 patients (32%) having a partial response and 13 patients with (59%) stable tumors. No patient developed new neurologic deficit.

In a compilation of several studies, Kim et al.[51] noted a 25% local failure rate in 83 patients treated with <40 Gy and 1.4% local failure in 142 patients receiving >40 Gy.

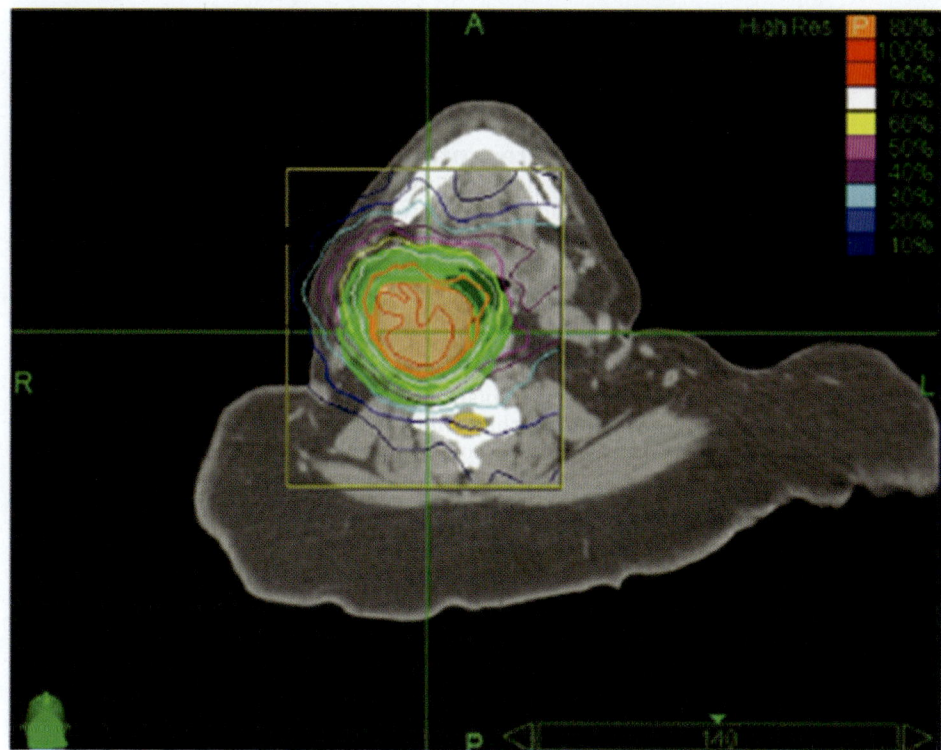

FIGURE 51.6. Dose distribution with stereotactic radiation therapy (radiosurgery) for glomus tumor. Patient was treated with 25 Gy in 5 fractions prescribed to the 80% isodose line; 98% of tumor received the prescribed dose. Thick *orange line* represents the 80% isodose. (Reprinted from Wegner RE, Rodriguez KD, Heron DE, et al. Linac-based stereotactic body radiotherapy for treatment of glomus. *Radiother Oncol* 2010;97[3]:395–398. Copyright © 2010 Elsevier Ireland Ltd. With permission.)

Powell et al.[25] reported on 84 patients with chemodectoma of the head and neck, 46 of which were in the glomus jugulare and tympanicum, treated with irradiation alone (45 to 50 Gy in 25 fractions). Local control of the lesion was 73% at 5 years. Thirty patients were treated with surgery after irradiation with no recurrences (median follow-up of 9 years). Four patients, treated with surgery alone, developed recurrences by 7 years. Four carotid body and glomus vagal tumors treated with irradiation were locally controlled at 1, 2, 8, and 11 years, respectively. In 13 patients treated with surgery alone, the 15-year local control rate was 54%.

Hinerman et al.[52,53] updated a previous report with 104 patients who had 121 chemodectomas of the temporal bone, carotid bone, or glomus vagal treated with radiation therapy alone in 104 patients or subtotal resection with or without radiation therapy (17 tumors). Seventeen patients had undergone a previous treatment (surgery 14, irradiation 1, or both 2). Eighty-nine patients were treated with megavoltage radiation therapy, 15 with stereotactic fractionated, 6 with stereotactic single dose, and 11 with IMRT. Median dose with fractionated irradiation was 45 Gy with daily fractions of 1.5 to 2 Gy delivered with[54] Co, 6-MV or 8-MV x-rays, or a combination of different beam energies.[53] There were six tumor recurrences, with a local tumor control of 95%. No severe treatment complications were noted. In the initial report,[52] 18 patients had 25 chemodectomas of carotid body and/or glomus vagal; 15 tumors originated in the carotid body and 10 in the glomus vagal. Pathologic confirmation of chemodectoma was obtained in 10 patients, and diagnosis was based on physical and radiographic findings in the remaining 8 patients. Twenty-two lesions were treated with radiation therapy alone, and two received postoperative radiation therapy after surgical resection for gross residual tumor with malignant changes and lymph node involvement. Patients with benign glomus tumors received 45 Gy in 25 fractions, in most instances, whereas patients with malignant carotid body tumors received 64.8 to 70 Gy in 1.8-Gy fractions. Local tumor control was obtained in 14 of 15 carotid body and 10 of 10 glomus vagal (overall 96% tumor control).[55]

Ivan et al.[56] published a meta-analysis based on 869 patients in 46 studies reported with glomus tumors, with follow-up ranging from 6 to 256 months. The tumor control rates were, for subtotal resection 69%, gross tumor resection (GTR) 86%, subtotal resection and radiosurgery 71%, and stereotactic radiosurgery (SRS) alone 95%. Posttreatment cranial nerve deficit was observed in 26% to 40% of patients treated with GTR and in about 10% of the SRS group. Guss et al.[57] reported on a meta-analysis of 19 studies (335 patients) with glomus tumors treated with SRT (radiosurgery), eight publications with a median follow-up of 36 months; tumor control (unchanged or reduced tumor volume) was 95% to 96%, with various SRT techniques.

In 29 patients with postsurgical recurrent glomus tumors (16 jugular, 7 carotid, 5 tympanic, and 1 thyroid) Elshaikh et al.[58] reported a 5-year tumor control of 100% in 12 treated with radiation therapy and 62% in 17 treated surgically.

Cheesman and Kelly[59] emphasized the importance of evaluating preoperatively the swallowing function of patients with glomus jugulare undergoing surgery, as it is common for these patients to develop postsurgical dysphagia.

The results of primary treatment for temporal bone chemodectoma are summarized in Table 51.5.

TABLE 51.5 TEMPORAL BONE CHEMODECTOMAS: LOCAL CONTROL AFTER RADIATION THERAPY ALONE OR RADIATION THERAPY AND SURGERY

Author (Reference)	Number of Patients	Local Control (%)	Follow-Up (Year)
Larner et al.[60]	15	93 (RT alone)	Median, 16.2
Powell et al.[25]	46	90 (RT alone)	Median, 9
Wang et al.[49]	19	84 (RT ± surgery)	5–35
Konefal et al.[3]	23	83 (RT ± surgery)	Mean, 10.5
Pryzant et al.[61]	19	95 (RT ± surgery)	Mean, 11
Cole and Beiler[62]	30	97 (RT alone)	3–27
Boyle et al.[63]	9	100 (RT alone)	1–12
Schild et al.[54]	8	100 (RT ± surgery)	Median, 7.5
de Jong et al.[64]	38	89 (RT ± surgery)	Median, 11.5
Hinerman et al.[53]	53	93 (RT ± surgery)	Mean, 15

RT, radiation therapy.
From Hinerman RW, Mendenhall WM, Amdur RJ, et al. Definitive radiotherapy in the management of chemodectomas arising in the temporal bone, carotid body, and glomus vagale. *Head Neck* 2001;23(5):363–371. Copyright © 2001 John Wiley & Sons, Inc. Reprinted by permission of John Wiley & Sons, Inc.

TABLE 51.6 CHEMODECTOMAS OF CAROTID BODY/GLOMUS VAGALE: RADIATION THERAPY ALONE OR RADIATION THERAPY AFTER SURGERY

Author (Reference)	Number of Patients	Local Control (%)	Follow-Up (Year)
Valdagni and Amichetti[65]	7	100 (RT ± subtotal resection)	1–19
Verniers et al.[55]	22	100 (RT ± subtotal resection	Mean, 10
Powell et al.[25]	4	100 (RT alone)	Median, 9
Schild et al.[54]	2	100 (Subtotal resection + RT)	Median, 7.5
Cole and Beiler[52]	30[a]	97 (RT alone)	3–27
Hinerman et al.[53]	18	96 (RT ± resection)	Mean, 9

[a]Glomus jugulare and glomus vagale.
RT, radiation therapy.
From Hinerman RW, Mendenhall WM, Amdur RJ, et al. Definitive radiotherapy in the management of chemodectomas arising in the temporal bone, carotid body, and glomus vagale. *Head Neck* 2001;23(5):363–371. Copyright © 2001 John Wiley & Sons, Inc. Reprinted by permission of John Wiley & Sons, Inc.

The initial results of treatment for carotid body or glomus vagal are summarized in Table 51.6. Complications were rare in patients treated with chemodectoma of the head and neck.

HEMANGIOPERICYTOMA

Hemangiopericytomas (HPCs) are rare soft tissue neoplasms that account for 3% to 5% of all soft tissue sarcomas and 1% of all vascular tumors. Some 15% to 30% of all HPCs occur in the head and neck, and of these, approximately 5% occur in the sinonasal area. They may resemble meningiomas in the central nervous system (CNS), clinically, and on imaging studies.[66] Vagal paragangliomas originate within the first 2 cm of the extracranial stretch of the vagus nerve and are associated with the inferior ganglion.[67] These tumors are believed to originate from the pericytes of Zimmerman extravascular cells, morphologically resembling smooth muscle, found around the capillaries or from primitive mesenchymal cells. The function of the pericyte is uncertain but is believed to provide mechanical support for the capillaries having contractile function.[68]

Epidemiology

HPC is an unusual tumor; representing approximately 1% of all vascular neoplasms; it occurs in both genders with equal frequency and is found primarily in adults. In the head and neck, the most common sites are the nasal cavity and the paranasal sinuses and, less frequently, the orbital region, the parotid gland, and the neck.[15,69–71] HPCs represent 3% to 4% of all meningeal and <1% of CNS tumors.

Pathology

HPCs are composed of a proliferation of tightly packed pericytes around thin-walled endothelial-lined vascular channels, ranging from capillary-sized vessels to large, gaping sinusoidal spaces.[69] The tumor has a tendency to grow slowly and invade locally into adjacent structures.[15,72] Although they are always well circumscribed and partially or completely surrounded by a pseudocapsule, benign tumors may be difficult to differentiate from malignant tumors. However, prominent mitoses (>4 per high-power field), foci of necrosis, and increased cellularity are suggestive of malignancy; the definitive sign is local recurrence or development of metastases. In general, tumors of the CNS, lower extremity, and mediastinum tend to be more malignant, with local recurrence occurring in up to 50% of cases.[69]

Kowalski and Paulino[73] reviewed 12 cases of HPCs. The mitotic index per 10 high-power fields varied from 0 or 1 to 15. Proliferation indices using MIB-1 (Ki-67) ranged from 2.6% to 52.5%. Clinical follow-up showed three cases with recurrence all possessing proliferation indices of approximately 10%, indicating a more aggressive subset of HPCs. Vuorinen et al.[74] found proliferation index to be a poor predictor of prognosis.

Meningeal HPCs almost always recur, despite seemingly complete removal, because of infiltrative properties of HPC cells and not just higher proliferation potential. They often metastasize.

Clinical Presentation

Soft tissue HPC is a firm, painless, slowly expanding mass that is often nodular and well localized. The skin overlying the mass does not have any discoloration or redness to indicate its vascular origin because the capillaries are emptied of the blood by compression of massive numbers of pericytes surrounding them.[67,69,75])

In the head and neck, the tumor may constitute a polypoid, soft gray or red mass that grows slowly and may cause nasal obstruction. Epistaxis and nasal obstruction are common symptoms. Orbital HPCs account for 3% of orbital malignancies and most frequently occur with painless proptosis.[76] HPC rarely originates in the lacrimal sac; it occurs in a younger age group than that of HPC of other locations. Charles et al.[77] reported on seven cases previously described and added one case.

HPC may occur intracranially. When it arises in the brain, it is a solid mass attached to the meninges that grossly resembles a meningioma. These intracranial HPCs carry a high risk of local failure (80%), as well as higher potential for dissemination. The mean time for local recurrence is 75 months.[75]

The incidence of metastasis, which depends on the site of origin, can be 50% to 80%. Late metastases occurring 10 years after diagnosis are not uncommon.

On plain radiographs, HPC appears as a soft tissue mass in the nasal cavity or other portions of the head and neck. A defect caused by pressure erosion of the surrounding bones may occur, and calcifications are rare. In the neck, the tumor appears as a well-circumscribed, homogeneously and intensely enhancing mass on CT. On MRI, the mass is iso- to slightly hyperintense to muscle on T1- and T2-weighted imaging. Multiple, branching flow voids are typically seen within the tumor on both T1- and T2-weighted images. On T2-weighted imaging, the punctate black flow voids in cross-section within the relatively bright tumor, creating a characteristic "salt-and-pepper" appearance in tumors >2 cm in diameter. Additionally, flow voids of large feeding arteries are seen at the periphery of the mass. Angiography demonstrates the characteristic appearance of a vascular tumor, with large feeding arteries, intense tumor stain, and early draining veins.[67] On arteriography, according to Yaghmai,[78] HPC is the only vascular tumor that has radially arranged or spiderlike branching vessels around and inside the tumor and a long-standing, well-demarcated tumor stain. Intracranial tumors typically have arterial blood supply from both meningeal and cerebral connections, with one to three main feeders supplying many small corkscrew-like vessels.[75] The most distinctive and constant feature of this tumor is its hypervascularity, which may be demonstrated with contrast-enhanced CT.[70] Intracranially, the diffusely enhancing tumor may closely resemble a meningioma on CT. However, some CT signs may suggest HPC rather than meningioma, such as a lack of calcification, scarce surrounding edema, and ringlike enhancement. Both CT and MRI scans are of special value in the delineation of the full extent of the tumor.

General Management

Complete surgical resection, if possible, combined with preoperative embolization of the tumor, is the treatment of choice. More extensive surgery is required in tumors that show features of malignancy. Many patients undergo surgical treatment after embolization of the feeding artery(ies).

For incompletely resected tumors, postoperative radiation therapy is used.[79,80] The role of chemotherapy in this tumor is not well determined; a few reports have described partial tumor regression in some lesions treated with cytotoxic agents. Doxorubicin, alone or in combination drug regimens, is the most effective agent for metastatic HPC, producing complete and partial remissions in 50% of cases. Other drugs prescribed when metastasis occurs are cyclophosphamide, dacarbazine, vincristine, and actinomycin D.[81] Park et al.[82] reported on 14 patients with soft tissue HPC treated with temozolomide 150 mg/m[2] orally on days 1 to 7 and days 15 to 21 and bevacizumab 5 mg/kg intravenously on days 8 and 22, repeated at 28-day intervals. Median follow-up period was 34 months. Eleven patients (79%) achieved a partial response, with a median time to response of 2.5 months. Estimated median progression-free survival (PFS) was 9.7 months, with a 6-month progression-free rate of 78.6%. The most frequently observed toxic effect was myelosuppression.

Radiation Therapy Techniques

The role of radiation therapy alone in the management of HPC is controversial. The main role of irradiation is as an adjuvant after complete excision of the lesion or postoperatively for minimal residual disease.[71,83,84] The tumor has been considered relatively radioresistant. Tumor doses of 60 to 65 Gy in 6 to 7 weeks are required to produce local tumor control in postoperative cases.[85] Orbital HPC has been cured by surgery and postoperative irradiation to 65 Gy.[76]

There appears to be a definite role for postoperative irradiation to the brain for primary HPC when radical surgery is performed because these tumors tend to recur after seemingly complete removal. Jha et al.[84] reported local tumor control in all patients treated with adjuvant external beam irradiation postoperatively. Radiation therapy also has been used as a salvage procedure after local recurrence following initial surgery or chemotherapy.

The fields of irradiation should be wide to encompass the tumor bed with a margin of at least 5 cm to safely avoid marginal recurrence. Portal arrangement and beam selection are similar to those used in treatment of malignant brain tumors or soft tissue sarcomas.

Results of Therapy

Billings et al.[86] reported on 10 patients with HPC of the head and neck; seven tumors arose from soft tissue sites and three from the mucosa. All patients underwent wide excision of the primary lesion with a local recurrence rate of 40%. Three patients developed metastatic lung disease 0 to 8 years after initial diagnosis. Each patient who developed metastatic disease had abundant mitoses on pathologic review compared with rare or absent mitoses in the lesions that took a more benign course.

Patrice et al.[87] reported on 18 primary hemangioblastoma tumors (16 had no prior surgical resection and 2 were subtotally resected lesions) and 20 lesions treated after surgical failure with stereotactic irradiation (radiosurgery). Minimum tumor doses ranged from 12 to 20 Gy (median 15.5 Gy). With a median follow-up of 24.5 months (range 6 to 77 months), the 2-year actuarial survival was 88%, and the 3-year freedom from progression was 86%. Four of twenty-two patients died. Thirty-one of thirty-six evaluable tumors (86%) were controlled locally. None of the 18 primary tumors treated with definitive stereotactic irradiation failed. Of the 18 recurrent tumors, 13 (72%) were controlled. There were no significant permanent complications attributable to the stereotactic irradiation.

Spitz et al. published a report on 36 patients with HPC. The median follow-up was 57 months. Twenty-eight patients (78%) underwent complete and potentially curative resection. Of the nine patients (32%) who had local recurrences, four (44%) had epidural tumors and three (33%) had retroperitoneal tumors,

but none had extremity tumors. Ten patients had recurrences at distant sites. Of the 13 patients who experienced any form of disease recurrence, four had recurrences after a disease-free interval of more than 5 years. The 5-year actuarial survival rate for the entire group of 36 patients was 71%.

Carew et al.[88] reviewed the records of 12 patients with HPCs of the head and neck: 5 had high- or intermediate-grade lesions and 7 had low-grade lesions. Nine patients were treated with curative intent; they underwent a variety of surgical resections dictated by tumor location and size. Four patients received postoperative radiation therapy, to a median dose of 60 Gy, for positive surgical margins (two patients), high-grade histology (one patient), or a recurrent lesion (one patient). The 5-year overall survival (OS) rate for patients treated surgically was 87.5%. A single mortality occurred in a patient with a recurrent high-grade lesion who failed at local, regional, and distant sites.

Staples et al.[89] reported on 12 patients with localized HPC, 7 treated with surgery alone (only 1 had long-term tumor control and 2 were salvaged with radiation therapy), 4 with resection and postoperative irradiation (all with long-term tumor control), and 1 with surgery and chemotherapy. Local tumor control was achieved at all sites treated with doses >55 Gy. Mitotic activity was not a reliable predictor of biologic behavior.

Kim et al.[51] evaluated 17 HPCs in nine patients treated with Gamma Knife SRT. Mean and median marginal doses were 18.1 and 20 Gy (range 11 to 22 Gy), respectively, at the 50% isodose line. Mean clinical and radiologic follow-up periods were 49 and 34 months, respectively. Successful tumor control was achieved in 14 of 17 lesions (82.4%). Actuarial local tumor control rate at 5 years was 67%. No adverse effects, such as radiation necrosis or marked peritumoral edema, were observed. Marginal dose (≥17 Gy) was the only statistically significant factor for local tumor control on univariate analysis.

Kano et al.[90] published a retrospective review of 20 patients who had undergone SRT for 29 HPCs after previous surgical resection. In addition, 12 patients underwent fractionated radiation therapy before SRT. Of the 20 patients, 16 patients had low-grade HPCs (20 tumors) and 4 had high-grade anaplastic HPCs (9 tumors). The median target volume was 4.5 cm[3] and the median marginal dose was 15 Gy (range 10 to 20 Gy). At an average of 48.2 months, the overall survival after radiosurgery was 85.9% and 13.8% at 5 and 10 years, respectively. Follow-up imaging studies demonstrated tumor control in 21 (72.4%) of 29 tumors. The PFS rate after SRT at 3 and 5 years was 89.1% for low-grade HPCs and 66.7% and 0%, respectively, for high-grade HPCs. The factors associated with improved PFS included lower grade and >14 Gy marginal radiation dose.

Olson et al.[91] published a review of 21 patients with 28 recurrent or residual HPCs on whom radiosurgery was performed. Prior treatments included embolization (6 cases), transcranial resection (39 cases), transsphenoidal resection (2 cases), and fractionated radiotherapy (8 cases). The mean prescription and maximum radiosurgical doses to the tumors were 17.0 and 40.3 Gy, respectively. Repeat radiosurgery was used to treat 13 tumors. With a median follow-up of 68 months (range 2 to 138 months), local tumor control was 47.6% (10 of 21 patients). Of the 28 tumors treated, 8 decreased in size on follow-up imaging (28.6%), 5 remained unchanged (17.9%), and 15 ultimately progressed. PFS at 5 years was 28.7%, and it improved to 71.5% after multiple radiosurgery treatments. In 4 of 21 (19%) patients, extracranial metastases developed.

Redmond et al.[92] reported on 118 patients with HPC of the CNS, 9% of whom had distant metastases at the time of initial presentation; 112 patients underwent surgical resection (23% had gross total resection, GTR, 31% had subtotal resection, and 46% had surgery not otherwise specified). Adjuvant RT was received by 31% of patients following GTR, 44% after sub-total tumor resection, and 50% of patients following surgery not otherwise specified. The 5- and 10-year overall survival for all patients was 76.7% and 50.1%, respectively. Patients receiving adjuvant RT ($n = 42$) had a significantly better over-all survival than patients who did not ($n = 67$; 10-year overall survival was 66.2% vs. 40.7%; $P = .05$). There was no differ-ence in 5- or 10-year overall survival for patients treated with subtotal resection plus RT ($n = 16$) compared with those treated with GTR alone ($n = 14$; 10-year overall survival 75% vs. 57.1%; $P = .53$)

Shaigany et al.[93] reported on a study of the Surveillance, Epidemiology, and End Results (SEER) database (1973 to 2012) encompassing 121 cases of HPC and compared results with 510 of other body sites with HPC. Head and neck HPC (HN-HPC) was most commonly located in the connective and soft tissue (18.4%), followed by the nasal cavity and paranasal sinuses (8.5%). Head and neck HPCs were smaller than other HPC and more likely to be of lower histologic grade. Primary treatment modality for HN-HPC was surgery alone 95.8% of cases. The 5-, 10-, and 20-year DSS for HN-HPC were 84.0%, 79.4%, and 69.4%, respectively. Higher histologic grade and the presence of distant metastases were poor prognostic fac-tors. Adjuvant radiotherapy did not appear to confer a sur-vival benefit for any body site.

CHORDOMAS

Anatomy
Chordomas are rare neoplasms of the axial skeleton that arise from the remnant of the primitive notochord (chorda dorsa-lis). About 50% arise in the sacrococcygeal area; 35% arise intracranially, where they typically involve the clivus, and the remaining 15% occur in the midline along the path of the notochord, primarily involving the cervical vertebrae.[93]

Epidemiology
Chordomas are more common in patients in their 50s and 60s but can occur in all age groups. In children and young adults, the prognosis and long-term survival appear to be better than in older patients. No risk factors have been identified. Male predominance is reported at a 2:1 to 3:1 ratio.

Natural History
Although slowly growing, chordomas are locally invasive, destroying bone and infiltrating soft tissues. Basisphenoidal chordomas tend to cause symptoms earlier and may be dif-ficult to differentiate histologically from chondromas and chondrosarcomas and radiographically from craniopharyn-giomas, pineal tumors, and hypophyseal and pontine gliomas. The lethality of these tumors rests on their critical location, aggressive local behavior, and extremely high local recurrence rate. The incidence of metastasis, which has been reported to be as high as 25%, is higher than previously believed and may be related to the long clinical history. The most common site of distant metastasis is the lungs, followed by the liver and bone. Lymphatic spread is uncommon.

Pathology
Chordoma is a soft, lobulated tumor that may have areas of hemorrhage, cystic changes, or calcification. It is frequently encapsulated but may be nonencapsulated or pseudoencap-sulated. Histologically, it is composed of cords or masses of large cells (physaliferous cells) with typical vacuoles and granules of glycogen in the cytoplasm and abundant intercel-lular mucoid material. Usually, there are few mitotic cells.[94] A chondroid variant of chordoma may exist, being prevalent in the spheno-occipital area. Patients with this type of histologic variant have improved survival.

Aside from the previously mentioned histologic features, the prognostic factors that most influence the choice of treat-ment are location and local extent of tumor.

Clinical Presentation
Chordomas tend to originate from the clivus and chondrosar-comas from the temporal bone.[95] Clinical symptoms vary with the location and extent of the tumor. In the head, extension may be intracranial or extracranial, into the sphenoid sinus, nasopharynx, clivus, and sellar and parasellar areas, with a resultant mass effect. In chordomas of the spheno-occipital region, the most common presenting symptom is headache. Other presentations include symptoms of pituitary insuffi-ciency, nasal stuffiness, bitemporal hemianopsia, diplopia, and other cranial nerve deficits. Volpe et al.[96] reviewed the clini-cal features of 48 patients with chordoma and 49 patients with low-grade chondrosarcoma of the skull base. Twenty-five patients (52%) with chordoma and 24 patients (49%) with chondrosarcoma had ocular symptoms (diplopia or visual impairment) as the initial manifestation of the disease. Of the 59 patients (both groups) with diplopia, it was initially inter-mittent in 25 (42%). Headache and diplopia from abducens nerve palsy occurred in 22 patients (46%) with chordoma and 23 (47%) with chondrosarcoma.

Diagnostic Workup
The diagnostic workup varies with the primary location of disease. Most patients have significant bony destruc-tion, and some may have calcifications in the tumor; hence, plain films and, specifically, CT scans or MRI are very use-ful (Table 51.7).[97] In most cases, the soft tissue component is much more extensive than initially appreciated, and a CT scan with contrast enhancement is required (Fig. 51.7A). CT and MRI are equivalent for demonstration of the presence and site of these tumors. MRI is inferior to CT in its ability to demonstrate bony destruction and intratumoral calcification (Fig. 51.7B).[98] MRI is superior to CT regarding the delinea-tion of the exact extent of the tumor, which allows for better treatment planning. Because of availability and lower cost, CT appears to be the technique of choice for routine follow-up of previously treated patients.[98]

Reliable signs of chordoma of the skull base are posterior extension to the pontine cistern; a lobulated, "honeycomb" appearance after gadolinium; the swollen appearance of the bone in the early stages; bone erosion on CT; and frequent extension to critical structures such as the circle of Willis, cav-ernous sinuses, and brainstem.[98]

General Management
Because of their surgical inaccessibility and relative resis-tance to radiation therapy, clivus chordomas represent a for-midable therapeutic challenge. The general management of the patient is dictated by the anatomic location of the tumor and the direction and extent of spread. A surgical approach is

TABLE 51.7 DIAGNOSTIC WORKUP FOR CHORDOMA

General
  History
  Physical examination
Radiologic studies
  Plain radiographs
  Computed tomography scan/magnetic resonance imaging
Laboratory studies
  Complete blood cell count
  Chemistry
  Urinalysis
Special studies
  Endocrinologic profile (clivus)
  Visual evaluations (clivus)

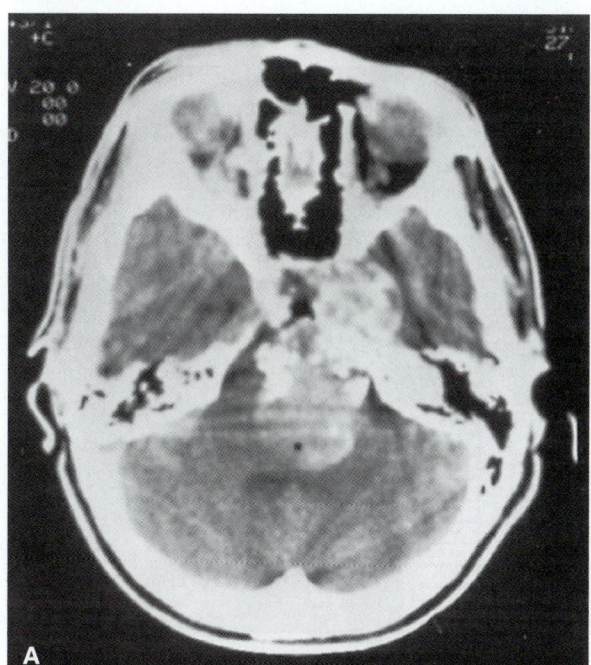

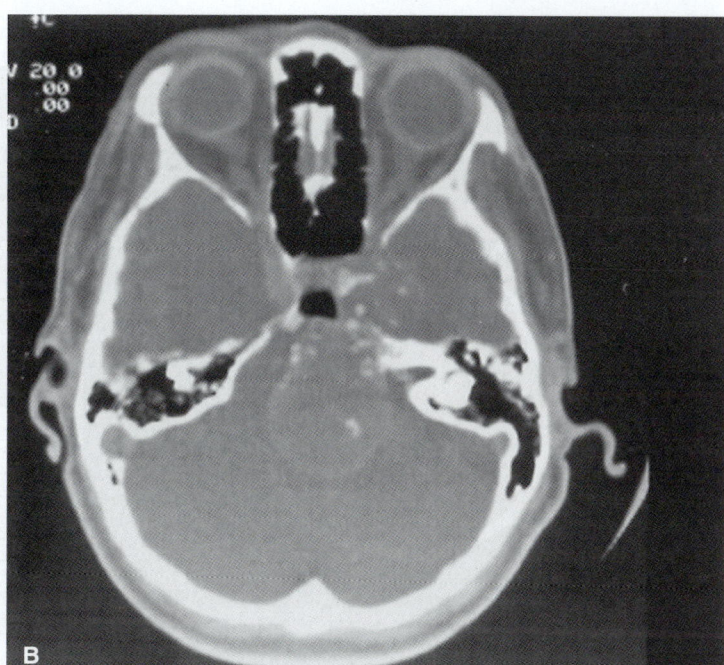

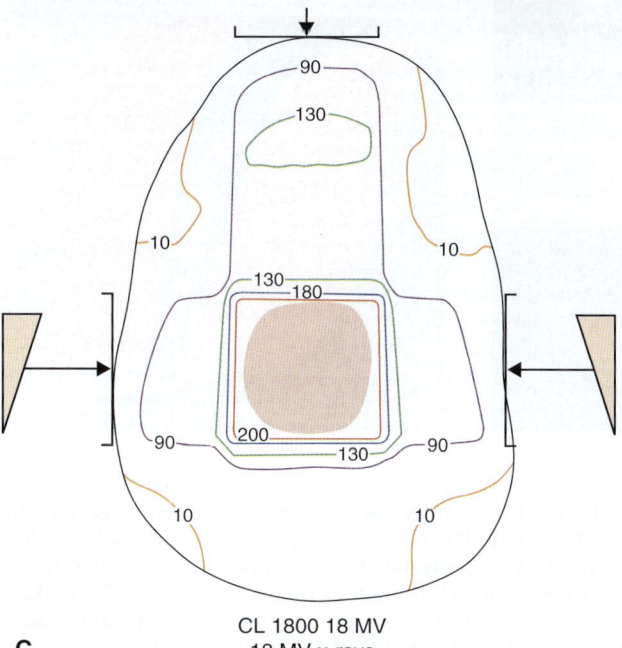

CL 1800 18 MV
18 MV x-rays

C

FIGURE 51.7. A: Contrast material–enhanced axial computed tomography scan demonstrates a large chordoma with extension into the posterior fossa and left parasellar region. **B:** Computed tomography scan photographed at bone windows shows the bony destruction and intratumoral calcifications. **C:** Treatment planning field arrangement for illustrated clivus chordoma using standard irradiation techniques with wedges on lateral ports.

recommended (when feasible), but complete surgical extirpation alone is unusual.[8] Regression of preoperative symptoms without additional postoperative morbidity could be achieved by radical transoral tumor extirpation documented by MRI. Intracranial spread usually requires steroid coverage and therapy directed to correction of neurologic deficits that may be present. Because of the high incidence of local recurrence, combined surgical excision and irradiation is frequently used. No effective chemotherapeutic agent or combination of drugs has been identified.

Radiation Therapy Techniques

Irradiation techniques vary considerably, depending on the location of the tumor along the craniospinal axis. Basisphenoidal tumors usually have been treated by a combination of parallel-opposed lateral fields, anterior wedges, photon and electron-beam combinations, and 3DCRT

or IMRT photons or protons, depending on the extent of the neoplasm. Precision radiation therapy planning, using CT and MRI, is required because high doses of external beam radiation therapy are needed. Three-dimensional CRT or IMRT with photons or protons provides optimal dose distributions.

The tumor usually surrounds the spinal cord and infiltrates vertebral bones. A combined technique using protons or electrons to boost the initial photon fields is generally applied. In the treatment of chordomas surrounding the spinal cord, IMRT can provide high-dose homogeneity and planning target volume (PTV) coverage (Fig. 51.8). Frequent 3-D (cone-beam CT, megavoltage CT) or digital portal image-based setup control reduces random positioning errors for head and neck cancer patients immobilized with conventional thermoplastic masks. Gabriele et al.[99] treated a patient with incomplete resection of a vertebral chordoma surrounding C2-C3 with a total dose of 58 Gy in 2-Gy daily fractions. Beam arrangement

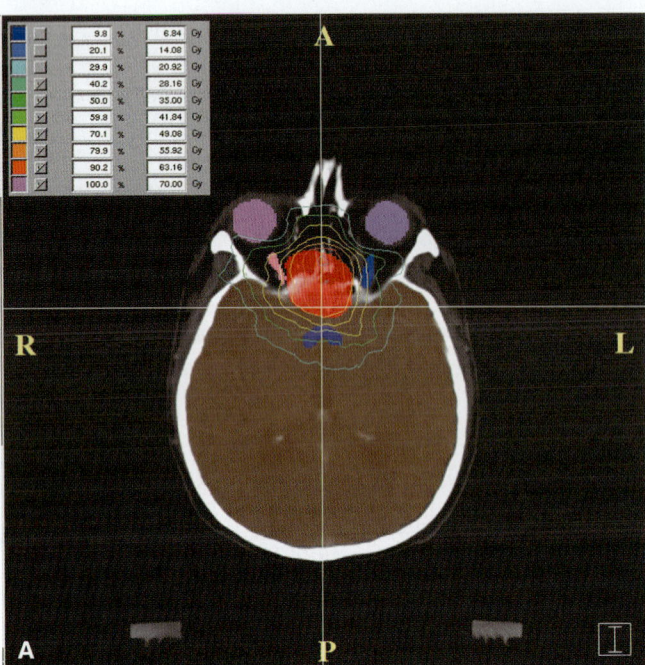

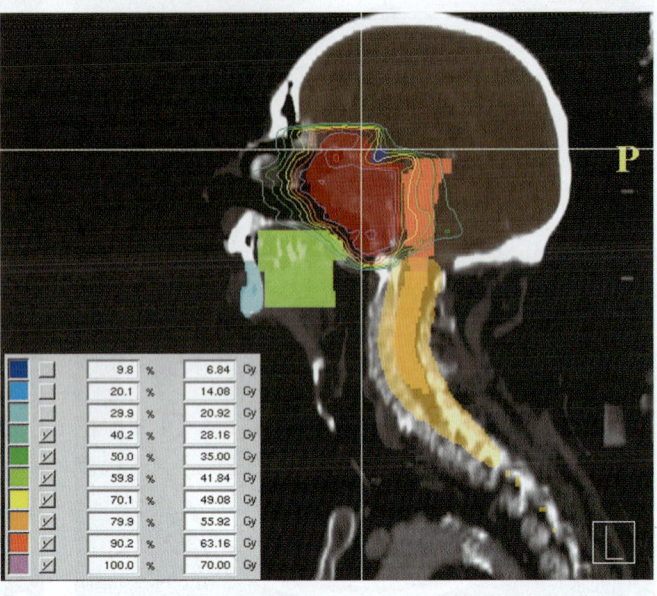

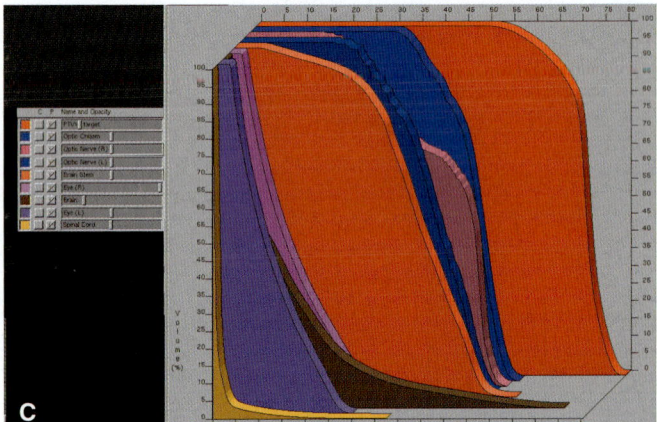

FIGURE 51.8. Chordoma of the clivus in an 81-year-old man treated with 70 Gy in 2-Gy fractions. Example of intensity-modulated radiation therapy plan: **A:** Cross-section in the upper portion of planning target volume (PTV), demonstrating coverage of target volume with sparing of ocular structures. **B:** Sagittal plane dose distribution with excellent coverage of PTV. **C:** Dose–volume histogram.

consisted of IMRT technique. The mean dose to the PTV was 57.6 Gy covering 95% of the PTV with the 95% isodose. The minimum dose to the PTV (D99) was 53.6 Gy. The maximum dose to the spinal cord was 42.2 Gy and to the spinal cord planning risk volume (8-mm margin) 53.7 Gy. The mean dose to the parotids was 37.4 Gy (homolateral gland) and 19.5 Gy (contralateral gland).

Because of the slow proliferative nature of chordomas, high linear energy transfer may prove useful in their management, as will be discussed later. Brachytherapy can be used for recurrent tumors of the base of the skull or adjacent to the spine when a more aggressive surgical exposure is offered.

Structure	Dose Range (cGy)	Mean Dose (Gy)
PTV (including left neck)	60–75	70
Optic nerves/chasm	25–50	41
Ocular globe	3–30	12

Results of Therapy

Photons

Although survival in some patients with chordoma may be long term, the salient feature of this unusual neoplasm is local recurrence with eventual death. The course may be indolent, with multiple treatments for recurrences, but the overall 5-year disease-free survival rate is <10% to 20%. Catton et al.[100] analyzed the long-term results of treatment for patients with chordoma of the sacrum, base of the skull, and mobile spine treated predominantly with postoperative photon irradiation. In 20 base-of-skull chordomas, most of them irradiated with conventionally fractionated radiation to a median dose of 50 Gy in 25 fractions for 5 weeks (range 25 to 50 Gy), median survival was 62 months (range 4 to 240 months) from diagnosis with no difference between clival and nonclival presentations. There was no survival advantage to patients receiving radiation doses >50 Gy (median 60 Gy) compared with lower doses <50 Gy (median 40 Gy). Hyperfractionation regimens did not influence the degree or duration of symptomatic response or PFS. Median survival after retreatment was 18 months.

Forsyth et al.[101] reported on 51 patients with intracranial chordomas (19 classified as chondroid) treated surgically (biopsy in 11 patients and subtotal removal or greater in 40); 39 patients received postoperative irradiation. At the time of the analysis, 17 patients were alive. The 5- and 10-year survival rates were 51% and 35%, respectively; 5-year survival was 36% for biopsy patients and 55% for those who had resection. Patients who underwent postoperative irradiation tended to have longer disease-free survival times.

Gay et al.[102] analyzed the outcome of 46 patients with cranial base chordomas and 14 with chondrosarcomas after extensive surgical resection, 50% of them treated previously and 20% received postoperative irradiation. Nine patients with chordomas and two with chondrosarcomas died during the postoperative follow-up period. The 5-year recurrence-free survival (RFS) for all patients was 76%. Chondrosarcomas had a better prognosis than chordomas (5-year RFS of 90% and 65%, respectively; $P = .09$). Patients who had undergone previous surgery had a greater risk of recurrence than did those who had not undergone previous surgery (5-year RFS rates of 64% and 93%, respectively; $P < .05$). Those with total or near-total resection had a better 5-year RFS rate (84%) than did patients with partial or subtotal resection (64%; $P < .05$). Postoperative leakage of cerebrospinal fluid was the most frequent complication (30% of patients) and was found to increase the risk of permanent disability. Patients who had undergone previous irradiation had a greater risk of death in the postoperative period (within 3 months of operation) and during follow-up.

Tai et al.[103] reviewed the results of irradiation combined with surgery, irradiation alone, and surgery alone in 159 patients reported in the literature. An analysis of the optimal biologically equivalent dose was performed using the linear-quadratic formula on 47 patients. With conventional photon irradiation, no dose–response relationship was shown. Survival improved in patients undergoing surgery followed by irradiation.

Keisch et al.[104] reported on 21 patients with chordoma treated at the authors' medical center: 5 had clival tumors, 2 had nasopharyngeal tumors, and 1 had a lumbar spine tumor. Nine patients were treated with surgery alone, eight had subtotal resection and postoperative irradiation, and four received irradiation alone after biopsy. The 5- and 10-year actuarial survivals were significantly better in patients treated with surgery alone or surgery and irradiation than in those treated with radiation therapy alone (52%, 32%, and 0%, respectively; $P = .02$). Disease-free survival of patients with base-of-skull tumors was not significantly different among the treatment groups.

Kim et al.[105] reported 14 clivus chordomas undergoing postoperative IMRT simultaneous integrated boost (SIB). Total and near-total resections were achieved in 11 patients (78.6 %) and partial in 2 patients (14.3 %), and 1 patient (7.1 %) received RT for recurrent tumor after total resection. A moderate hypofractionation schedule was used: Doses to PTV1, PTV2, and PTV3 were 3.9 Gy, 3.15 Gy, and 2.8 Gy through 15 fractions for the first two patients, and the rest received 2.5, 2.2, and 1.8 Gy through 25 fractions. The biologically equivalent dose in 2-Gy fractions (EQD2) was 65 to 68 Gy for PTV1, 52 to 56 Gy for PTV2, and 44.3 to 44.8 Gy for PTV3. Median follow-up was 41 months. Eight patients were free of disease for a median of 42.5 months (range 23 to 91 months), four patients had stable disease for a median of 60.5 months, and 1 patient showed partial response for 38 months after RT. Estimated 5-year progression-free and overall survival rates were 92.9 %. IMRT-SIB was well tolerated without lasting toxicity. Debus et al.[106] reported on 45 patients treated for chordoma or chondrosarcoma with postoperative fractionated 3-D SRT. Median dose at isocenter was 66.6 Gy for chordomas and 64.9 Gy for chondrosarcomas. All chondrosarcomas achieved and maintained local tumor and recurrence-free status at 5-years of follow-up. Local control rate of chordomas at 5 years was 50% and survival was 82%. Clinically significant late toxicity developed in only one patient.

Den et al.[107] described a multi-institutional study of 31 patients, 28 with clivus chordoma or chondrosarcoma, treated with various photon techniques (single-dose stereotactic, fractionated 3DCRT, IMRT). Median fractionated total dose was 65 Gy. Actuarial 3-year local tumor control was 68% and

overall survival 63%. Patients receiving 65 Gy or a higher dose had a 5-year tumor control of 78% and overall survival of 90%. No grade 2 or greater toxicity was observed.

Muthukumar et al.[108] published a report on 15 patients with skull base chordoma and chondrosarcoma treated with SRT (13 had previous surgical resection). Median minimum marginal tumor single dose was 18 Gy (12 to 20 Gy) and the number of isocenters ranged from 1 to 10 (average, 4). Dose to optic nerve or chiasm was ≤9 Gy. With a median follow-up of 40 months, eight patients had clinical improvement, three were stable, and four had died. No significant morbidity was noted.

Protons

The best results in the treatment of chordomas have been obtained with radical surgery followed by high-dose proton irradiation.[109] Berson et al.[110] described 45 patients with chordomas or chondrosarcomas at the base of the skull or cervical spine treated by subtotal resection and postoperative irradiation. Twenty-three patients were treated definitively by charged particles, 13 patients with photons and particles, and 9 were treated for recurrent disease. Doses ranged from 36 to 80 Gy equivalent (GyE). There appeared to be significant benefit for patients with smaller tumor volumes (80% vs. 33% actuarial survival rate at 5 years). Patients treated for primary disease had a 78% actuarial local tumor control at 2 years versus 33% for recurrent disease.

Austin et al.[111] evaluated 141 patients with chordoma and chondrosarcoma of the base of skull and cervical spine treated with proton and photon irradiation. The local disease was controlled in 111 patients. They reviewed 26 patients who had recurrent disease (21 nonchondroid chordomas, 2 chondroid chordomas, and 3 chondrosarcomas). The prescribed doses ranged from 67 to 72 Cobalt Gray Equivalent (CGE). Approximately 25% (6 of 26) of the cases failed in the prescribed dose region. More than half (15 of 26) failed in regions where tumor dose was limited by normal tissue constraints. Approximately 10% of the patients recurred in the surgical pathway and 10% were judged to be marginal misses. Overall, 75% of the patients failed in regions receiving less than the prescribed dose. All tumors that failed in the high-dose region had recurrences (10 of 26) and larger tumors (average volume of 102 cc) than those with base-of-skull disease (16 of 115) with an average volume of 63 cc.

O'Connell et al.[112] reported on 62 patients with base-of-skull chordomas treated with proton-beam irradiation (65 to 73.5 GyE); 29 patients (19 women and 10 men) experienced local failure, and 14 women (48%) and 7 men (21%) died of disease. On histologic analysis, the presence of >10% necrosis, prominent nucleoli, and tumor >70 mm were significant predictors of short-term disease-specific survival (DSS). Chondroid chordoma and conventional chordomas had equivalent outcomes.

Fagundes et al.[113] updated the Massachusetts General Hospital experience with 204 patients treated for chordoma of the base of the skull or cervical spine. Sixty-three patients (31%) had treatment failures, which were local in 60 patients (29%) and the only site of failure in 49 patients. Two patients had regional lymph node relapse, and three developed surgical pathway recurrence. Thirteen patients relapsed in distant sites (especially lungs and bones). The 5-year actuarial survival rate after any relapse was 7%. Terahara et al.[114,115] reported on 132 patients with skull base chordoma treated with combined photon and proton irradiation; in 115 patients, dose–volume data and follow-up were available. The prescribed doses ranged from 66.6 to 79.2 CGE (median 68.9 CGE). Dose to the optic structures (optic nerves and chiasm), the brainstem surface, and the brainstem center was limited to 60, 64, and 53 CGE, respectively. Local failure developed in 42 of 115 patients, with the actuarial local tumor control rates at 5 and 10 years being 59% and 44%, respectively.

In a Cox multivariate analysis, the model's equivalent uniform dose suggested that the probability of recurrence of skull base chordomas depends on gender, target volume, and target dose inhomogeneity; equivalent uniform dose was shown to be a useful parameter to evaluate dose distribution for the target volume.

Hug et al.[116] analyzed efficacy of fractionated proton radiation therapy for 33 skull base chordomas and 25 chondrosarcomas. Following various surgical procedures, residual tumor was present in 91% of patients; 59% demonstrated brainstem involvement. Target doses ranged from 64.8 to 79.2 CGE (mean 70.7 CGE). The range of follow-up was 7 to 75 months (mean 33 months). In 10 patients (17%), the treatment failed locally, resulting in local control rates of 92% (23 of 25 patients) for chondrosarcomas and 76% (25 of 33 patients) for chordomas. All tumors with volumes of ≤25 mL remained locally controlled compared with 56% of tumors >25 mL ($P = .02$). Of patients without brainstem involvement, 94% did not experience recurrence, whereas with brainstem involvement (and dose reduction because of brainstem tolerance constraints), the tumor control rate was 53% ($P = .04$). Actuarial 5-year survival rates were 100% for patients with chondrosarcoma and 79% for patients with chordoma. Grade 3 and 4 late toxicities were observed in four patients (7%) and were symptomatic in three (5%).

Ares et al.[33] treated 42 patients with chordomas and 22 with chondrosarcomas of the skull base using spot-scanning protons (median doses 73.5 and 68.4 Gy, respectively, at 1.8 to 2.0 Gy relative biologic effect). With a median follow-up of 38 months, 5-year tumor control was 81% and 94% and overall survival 100% and 91%, respectively. Late toxicity consisted of one grade 3 and one grade 4 unilateral optic neuropathy and two patients with grade 3 CNS necrosis. No patient experienced brainstem toxicity.

Noel et al.[117] reported on 49 chordomas and 18 chondrosarcomas treated with high-energy photons (two-thirds of dose) and 201-MeV protons (one-third of dose). Median total dose was 67 CGE (60 to 70 CGE). With a median follow-up of 32 months, 3-year local tumor control was 71% for chordomas and 85% for chondrosarcomas and 4-year overall survival 88% and 75%, respectively. Fourteen tumors (21%) failed locally.

Recently, heavy particles have been used to treat some of these patients.[118,119] Hasegawa et al.[81,90] reported on 54 patients with skull base or paracervical tumors (31 with chordomas) treated with carbon ions (escalating doses from 48 to 60.8 GyE in 16 fractions over 4 weeks). In the 31 chordoma patients, 5-year local tumor control and overall survival were 78% and 85%, respectively. Patients were divided into two groups; a low-dose group ($n = 10$) irradiated with doses ranging from 48 to 57.8 GyE and a high-dose group ($n = 21$) irradiated with 60.8 GyE. The 5-year local tumor control was 60% for the low-dose group and 93% for the high-dose group, and the overall survival was 90% and 84%, respectively. One late grade 2 brain sequela was noted in a patient treated with 60.8 GyE.

Likewise, Schulz-Ertner et al.[34] treated 24 chordomas and 13 chondrosarcomas with 3-D planning carbon ions (median dose 60 GyE). With a mean follow-up of 13 months, local tumor control at 2 years was 90%. PFS was 83% for chordomas and 100% for chondrosarcomas. No significant toxicity was observed.

Benk et al.[120] described results in 18 children with base-of-skull or cervical spine chordomas who received fractionated high-dose postoperative irradiation using mixed photon and 160-MeV proton beams. Median tumor dose was 69 CGE with a 1.8-CGE daily fraction. With a median follow-up of 72 months, the 5-year survival was 68%, and the 5-year disease-free survival rate was 63%. Patients with cervical spine chordomas had a worse survival rate than did those with base-of-skull lesions ($P = .008$). Treatment-related morbidity was acceptable: two cases of growth hormone deficit corrected by hormone replacement, one temporal lobe necrosis, and one fibrosis of the temporalis muscle, improved after surgery.

A report on proton therapy for base-of-skull chordoma published by the Royal College of Radiologists[121] concluded that outcome after proton irradiation is superior to that reported for conventional photon irradiation. Radiation therapy schedules involving a mixed schedule of protons and photons have achieved an approximately 60% local tumor control rate at 5 years.

Sequelae of Treatment

In patients treated with high irradiation doses, as well as with charged particles, there is an increasing probability of sequelae, including brain damage, spinal cord injury, bone or soft tissue necrosis, and xerostomia. In a report by Berson et al.,[110] three patients experienced unilateral visual loss, and four patients had radiation injury to the brainstem.

Santoni et al.[122] reported on the temporal lobe damage rate in 96 patients (75 primary and 21 recurrent tumors) treated with postoperative high-dose proton and photon irradiation for chordomas and chondrosarcomas of the base of the skull. All the patients were randomized to receive 66.6 or 72 CGE with conventional fractionation (1.8 CGE per day, 5 fractions per week) using opposed lateral fields for the photon component and a noncoplanar isocentric technique for the proton component. Of the 96 patients, 10 developed temporal lobe damage (bilateral in 2 and unilateral in 8). The cumulative temporal lobe damage incidence at 2 and 5 years was 7.6% and 13.2%, respectively. CT and MRI scans were evaluated for white matter changes; the MRI areas suggestive of temporal lobe damage in 10 patients were always separate from the tumor bed.

In patients receiving high-dose proton therapy for clivus tumors, Slater et al.[115] observed a 26% incidence of endocrine abnormalities at 3 years and 37% at 5 years, with hypothyroidism being the most frequent sequela. The dose to the pituitary in patients with abnormalities ranged from 63.1 to 67.7 GyE.

LETHAL MIDLINE GRANULOMA

Natural History and Pathology

Lethal midline granuloma (LMG) or midline malignant polymorphic reticulosis (PMR) is a clinical entity characterized by progressive, unrelenting ulceration and necrosis of the midline facial tissues.[123,124] LMG is associated with Epstein-Barr virus, which has at least two subtypes with different biologic properties that can be identified by their genomic configuration. The occurrence of the rare subtype 2 in LMG may relate to a covert immune defect.[125] Considerable controversy exists regarding various disorders characterized by a necrotizing and granulomatous inflammation of the tissues of the upper respiratory tract and oral cavity. It is now clear that if infections and other known agents such as cocaine use, sarcoidosis, environmental toxins, and various neoplasms can be excluded, three clinical–pathologic entities remain: Wegener granulomatosis, LMG, and PMR.[18] A review of the literature suggests that cases described as idiopathic midline destructive disease and PMR are a large evolutionary spectrum from almost benign to fatal malignant natural killer/T-cell lymphoma.[126,127]

Wegener granulomatosis is an epithelioid necrotizing granulomatosis with vasculitis of small vessels. Systemic involvement of the kidneys and lungs is common.

PMR is an unusual disorder with distinctive clinical and pathologic features. Histologically, PMR is characterized by an atypical mixed lymphoid infiltration of the submucosa with extensive areas of necrosis, sometimes extending to the bone or cartilage. The lesion consists of variable zones of small lymphocytes with scattered immunoblastic forms and abundant plasma cells with occasional eosinophilia and histiocytosis.[127] PMR has been considered a lymphoproliferative disorder; most, if not all, cases are peripheral T-cell lymphomas. Several authorities believe that PMR and systemic lymphomatoid granulomatosis are the same disease, with the latter predominantly involving the lungs.[128]

Idiopathic LMG describes a localized disorder not characterized by visceral lesions but by destruction of the midfacial area, which, if left untreated, is uniformly fatal. The histopathologic findings are nonspecific, with a relatively nondescript inflammatory reaction with acute and chronic inflammation and necrosis. Despite specific clinical–pathologic features, the distinction between LMG and PMR is often difficult; although controversial, they may represent two phases of the same disease, with LMG remaining histologically benign or evolving into PMR. LMG occurs more frequently in men.[99]

Ages range from 21 to 64 years; almost half of the patients are in their 50s at presentation. Most patients have involvement of the nasal cavity (including destruction of the septum) and the paranasal sinuses (particularly maxillary antrum). The primary lesion may extend into the orbits, the oral cavity (palate, gingiva), and even the pharynx.

Characteristics of the three different diseases are outlined in Table 51.8.

Clinical Features and Diagnostic Workup

Clinical manifestations include progressive nasal discharge, obstruction, foul odor emanating from the nose, and, in later stages, pain in the nasal cavity, in the paranasal areas, and even in the orbits.

Examination discloses ulceration and necrosis in the nasal cavity, perforation or destruction of nasal septum and turbinates, and even ulceration of the nose. Edema of the face and eyelids may be noted, and the bridge of the nose may be sunken. Radiographic studies initially show soft tissue swelling, mucosal thickening, and findings consistent with chronic sinusitis.

CT is invaluable in demonstrating the full extent of the tumor, including bone or cartilage destruction. In 13 patients presenting with LMG, CT proved essential for determining the extent of the disease, guiding biopsy, and planning radiation therapy.[129] MRI was also helpful for the latter because it could distinguish fluid retained within the paranasal sinuses from solid masses and tumor from granulation tissue; it was of little value for detecting bone lysis. Eight patients proved to have T-cell lymphoma, two had Crohn disease, in one the lesion was factitious, and two had granulomas without diagnostic histologic features.

General Management and Radiation Therapy Techniques

When treatment of these patients is planned, it is extremely important to exclude the diagnosis of Wegener granulomatosis, a benign process that is commonly treated with antimicrobial agents, steroids, and systemic chemotherapy.[128] *Bona fide* LMG does not respond to steroids; the treatment of choice is radiation therapy.[130–132]

Target volume should encompass all areas of involvement, including adjacent areas at risk (i.e., for a lesion of the maxillary antrum, it will include the antrum as well as all of the paranasal sinuses) with a 2- to 3-cm margin.[133] Because marginal failures are a significant problem, wide margins are necessary for treatment of these patients.[127]

Irradiation techniques are similar to those described for tumors of the paranasal sinuses, nasal cavity, or nasopharynx. Several investigators have described complete responses with doses of 30 to 50 Gy; most patients are treated with 35 to 45 Gy in 3 to 4.5 weeks.[130,134] The authors recommend 45 to 50 Gy in 4.5 to 5.5 weeks in 1.8- to 2-Gy daily fractions.

Results of Therapy

Because of the rarity of this tumor, experience is limited. Fauci et al.[134] reported on 10 patients with extensive midline granuloma treated with irradiation. Three received 10 Gy, and all failed within 2 years (retreated with 40 to 46 Gy). The remaining seven patients received 40 to 50 Gy. Local control of disease was 77%; two patients had local recurrences, one outside the initially irradiated volume.

In a study of 34 patients with PMR treated with primary radiation therapy except for one patient, Smalley et al.[127] found that a minimum dose of 42 Gy or a time–dose factor of 70 was necessary to achieve long-term local control. The most frequent failure site was within the original irradiation field. Systemic failure occurred in 25% of their patients initially presenting with limited disease. The salvage of this subset of patients requires effective systemic chemotherapy. Multimodality treatment using intensive chemotherapy and radiation therapy might improve the prognosis of these patients.

Fauci et al.[134] published a prospective study of 15 patients with systemic lymphomatoid granulomatosis. Of 13 patients treated with cyclophosphamide and prednisone, seven sustained complete remission (mean duration of remission, 5.2 ± 0.6 years). Six deaths were associated with biopsy-proven lymphoma; one was caused by a lymphoma-like illness unproven by biopsy. The eighth death was caused by adenocarcinoma in a patient with lymphoma in remission. None of these patients received radiation therapy.

Chen et al.[135] reported their experience in 92 cases of LMG or centrofacial malignant lymphoma treated with radiation therapy. Twenty-five patients received combination chemotherapy, usually containing doxorubicin, cyclophosphamide,

Section III

TABLE 51.8 DIFFERENTIAL FEATURES OF THREE CLINICAL–PATHOLOGIC ENTITIES			
	Wegener Granulomatosis	**Idiopathic Midline Granuloma**	**Polymorphic Reticulosis**
Disease features	Diffuse, inflammatory disease of the upper airway, predominately sinuses and nose	Destructive extension to the palate and facial soft tissues	Destructive lesion with destruction of the bone and extension through soft tissues
Systemic involvement	Lungs, kidneys, small-vessel vasculitis may not have airway involvement	No	No
Associated with lymphoma	No	May remain benign or progress to lymphoma	Usually evolves to lymphoma
Histologic features	Necrotizing vasculitis with epithelioid granulomas, giant cells, and fibrinoid necrosis	Inflammatory reaction, nonspecific; granulomas and giant cells are infrequent	Characteristic atypical and polymorphic lymphoreticular cellular infiltrate; angiocentric growth patterns may simulate vasculitis, but fibrinoid necrosis is absent in vessel walls
Treatment	Chemotherapy	Radiation therapy	Chemotherapy; radiation therapy and chemotherapy

vincristine, and prednisone (CHOP) or other combinations, including CHOP or nitrogen mustard, vincristine, procarbazine, and prednisone (MOPP) in some patients. The nose was the most frequently involved site at initial presentation (85% of patients). Immunophenotyping in 36 patients showed T-cell lineage in 25 (69%) and B-cell lineage in 6 (17%). The irradiation technique consisted of treating all involved and adjacent areas with doses of 30 to 75 Gy. Sixteen patients received neck irradiation (30 to 60 Gy). Daily fractions were 2 to 3 Gy in 5 weekly fractions. Actuarial survival rates were 59.5% at 5 years, 56.2% at 10 years, and 40.5% at 20 years. There was no significant difference in survival in patients receiving <50 Gy. A relapse in the midfacial region was noted in seven patients. Other relapse sites were the lung and skin in three patients, para-aortic or inguinal lymph nodes in two patients, and brain in one. Survival of patients with recurrences was poor; 73% died within 8 months.

Hatta et al.[136] reviewed 18 patients (15 males and 3 females) with LMG (PMR), about 5.6% of patients with malignant head and neck tumors. Most of the 18 patients underwent both radiation therapy and chemotherapy (cyclophosphamide, vincristine, prednisone [COP], CHOP, methotrexate, leucovorin, doxorubicin, cyclophosphamide, vincristine, bleomycin, and prednisone [MACOP-B]), but, because their disease had reached an advanced stage, three underwent radiation therapy only, three chemotherapy only, and one received no radical therapy. Of the 18 patients, 13 died of the disease; in 6 patients, progress was confined to the local lesion. The 5-year cumulative survival rate was 15.7%. Fourteen autopsy studies showed that tumor involved the liver (92.8%), lung (92.8%), and spleen (71.4%), and in all cases, it was in leukemic patterns. Five cases were positive for ubiquitin carboxyl-terminal esterase L1 (ubiquitin thiolesterase) (CD45RO), and 10 cases were positive for lysozyme. All cases were positive for Ki-1 (CD30).

Sakata et al.[137] reported on 107 patients with stage I and II non-Hodgkin lymphoma of the head and neck treated with involved field radiation therapy for orbital, nasal, or paranasal lymphoma and extended-field radiation for Waldeyer ring or neck lymphoma (39 to 48 Gy). In the latter half of the study, adjuvant chemotherapy was administered. Of 107 patients, 95 achieved complete response. Of the 12 patients who did not achieve complete response, 9 had nasal T-cell lymphoma of the lethal midline granuloma (LMG-NTL) type. Only one patient who obtained chemoradiation relapsed in a previously irradiated area. LMG-NTL was the most significant prognostic factor on multivariate analysis ($P < .001$). Older patients also experienced a higher relative risk than patients aged ≤60 years ($P = .0063$). Dose of doxorubicin reached borderline significance ($P = .0600$). Radiation therapy is excellent for obtaining local control of head and neck of non-Hodgkin lymphoma and LMG-NTL.

CHLOROMA

Natural History

Chloroma (granulocytic sarcoma, myeloblastoma) is a solid extramedullary tumor composed of early myeloid precursors usually associated with acute myelocytic or nonlymphocytic leukemia. These tumors have predilection for the skin, lymph nodes, and the spine; most common head and neck sites of presentation are in the orbit and other craniofacial bones. The name chloroma (from the Greek *chloros*, meaning green) derives from the green color of affected tissues resulting from the presence of myeloperoxidase. Because not all deposits exhibit the characteristic green tint, the term *granulocytic sarcoma* (GS) seems more appropriate.

GS, an extramedullary proliferation of malignant myeloid precursor cells, was identified in 3% of 478 patients with

acute chronic granulocytic leukemia; they can be seen with other myeloproliferative disorders, including polycythemia vera, hypereosinophilia, and myeloid metaplasia. In the absence of acute leukemia, GS is usually an ominous sign, suggesting imminent conversion to acute myelocytic leukemia or blast crisis. As survival rates for myelogenous leukemias improve, the number of patients who relapse with chloromas is increasing.

Children are affected more often than adults. Of 33 patients with orbital chloromas reported by Zimmerman and Font,[138] 75% were in their first decade of life. Chloromas are found more frequently in children with the M4 and M5 acute myeloid leukemia (AML) subtypes of the French-American-British Cooperative Group Classification and are also associated with the 8:21 translocation. Chloromas may appear during bone marrow remission before an increase in blasts is detected in the bone marrow, so they may herald relapse.

Clinical Presentation and Diagnostic Workup

Intraorbital (retrobulbar) chloroma causes progressive exophthalmos or temporal swelling. CNS involvement causes both local pressure phenomena and generalized elevation of intracranial pressure with headaches, nausea, and vomiting. Intracerebral chloromas may manifest as the rare CNS (parenchymal) involvement of acute nonlymphocytic leukemia.[139,140]

Intracranial chloromas may exhibit intermediate or high attenuation in unenhanced CT scans, with intense, uniform enhancement with contrast material.[141,142] Confusion with meningioma, hematoma, solitary metastasis, and lymphoma may occur on CT scans.[127] MRI of GS is commonly used for a spinal or cranial location that demonstrates isointensity relative to gray matter on TI-weighted images and isointensity to white matter on T2-weighted images. GS demonstrates almost uniform enhancement with gadolinium, which further aids in delineating it.

General Management

Many of these patients are treated with anthracycline-based chemotherapy, although surgical excision or radiation therapy for masses is indicated.

Radiation Therapy Techniques

Chloromas are extremely radiosensitive; however, the optimal dose of irradiation has not been established. Response rates of leukemic infiltrates have been reported with doses as low as 4 Gy, yet the need for higher doses up to 30 Gy in certain locations of extramedullary leukemic infiltrates is well recognized. Although the literature is limited regarding the maximum dose needed for treatment of chloromas, Chak et al.,[143] in a study of 23 patients with GS, reported that 20 to 30 Gy yielded 85% to 89% local tumor control. In the authors' limited experience, there appears to be a relationship between the size of the chloroma and the total dose of irradiation required for control. The target volume is the tumor mass and an adequate margin (2 to 3 cm). Irradiation techniques depend on the location of the infiltrate. For superficial lesions, electron beam is recommended. Orbital chloroma may constitute a radiation therapy emergency because visual loss is possible if the patient is not treated promptly.

Bakst et al.[142] reported on 38 patients who underwent treatment for chloromas at their institution The majority of the patients that presented with chloroma at the time of initial leukemia diagnosis (78%) did not receive radiation therapy (RT) because the tumor regressed after initial chemotherapy (CT). Yet, most patients that relapsed or remained with chloroma after CT are in the RT cohort (90%). Thirty-three courses of RT were administered to 22 patients, 39% in the head and neck. Median RT dose was 20 (6 to 36) Gy. PFS and overall survival in the RT cohort were 39% and 43%, respectively, at

5 years. The authors recommend irradiating chloromas to at least 20 Gy and propose 24 Gy in 12 fractions as an appropriate regimen.

Kuo et al.[144] described results in 43 lesions treated in 20 patients, the underlying hematologic diseases of the evaluated patients being AML in 14 (70%), chronic myeloid leukemia in 4, myelodysplastic syndrome with myeloid leukemia transformation in 1, and *de novo* GS in 1. Most patients (55%) received RT for GS at the time of relapse following bone marrow transplantation (BMT). The most common cytogenetic abnormality was t(8;21)(q22;q22). The median RT dose of 20 Gy (range, 6 to 35 Gy), administered in 1.5 to 3.5 Gy fractions, provided a 63% CR rate. One case with GS who received a hypofractionation RT regimen of 15 Gy in 5 fractions showed CR.

Hall et al.[145] reported on 90 RT courses administered for chloromas in 41 patients, 6 in the head and neck. Twelve patients were previously treated with systemic chemotherapy only, 13 with at least one prior hematopoietic stem cell transplant without TBI, and 16 with prior transplant with TBI. All patients received RT for chloroma; 27 patients also received systemic chemotherapy, 2 intrathecal chemotherapy, and 7 stem cell transplant, and 5 were treated with RT alone. Median dose was 24 (range 5 to 37) Gy. Median survival (MS) after RT was 3.6 months in patients treated with prior systemic chemotherapy alone, 10.7 months with prior chemotherapy-only transplant, and 3.4 months with prior TBI-based transplant (*P* – .66). A single course of palliative RT provided local control (LC) in 89% of patients (95% CI 0.11 to 0.54). MS for patients referred for RT for consolidation was 26.2 months compared to 3.2 months in patients referred for palliation.

ESTHESIONEUROBLASTOMA

Esthesioneuroblastomas (ENBs), first described by Berger and Luc,[146] are rare tumors thought to arise in the olfactory receptors in the nasal mucosa or the cribriform plate of the ethmoid bone. The olfactory nerves perforate grooves in the ethmoid bone in the cribriform plate and continue into the subarachnoid spaces, accounting for the high incidence of intracranial extension.[146]

Epidemiology

ENB constitutes 3% of all endonasal neoplasms. In the United States,[147] according to the data from the SEER program, 84 cases of ENB were registered from 1978 to 1990[145] and about 945 cases have been reported in the world literature.[148] The review authors' cases accounted for 198 and collaborative efforts accounted for 747 cases. Sex distribution was 53.6% male and 46.64% female. Kadish classification was applied to 563 cases: 103 (18.3%) class A, 182 (32.2%) class B, and 278 (49.4%) class C cases.

There appears to be a slight male predominance. The age incidence has a bimodal distribution, with peaks at 11 to 20 years and 40 to 60 years, the highest incidence at 51 to 60 years.

Natural History

Although others thought that ENB were of ectodermal origin, most observers believe the tumor to be of neuroectodermal origin in the olfactory epithelium.[17,146] Most of these tumors occur high in the nasal cavity or in the lateral wall adjacent to the ethmoid. The tumor may spread to the opposite ethmoid bone, superiorly to the frontal sinus and anterior cranial fossa; posteriorly to the sphenoid sinus, nasopharynx, and base of the skull; laterally to the orbits, forward to the frontonasal angle; or inferiorly to the nasal cavity and antrum (Fig. 51.9). Lymphatic spread may be to the subdigastric, posterior cervical, submaxillary, or preauricular nodes, as well as to the nodes of Rouviere. The exact incidence of distant

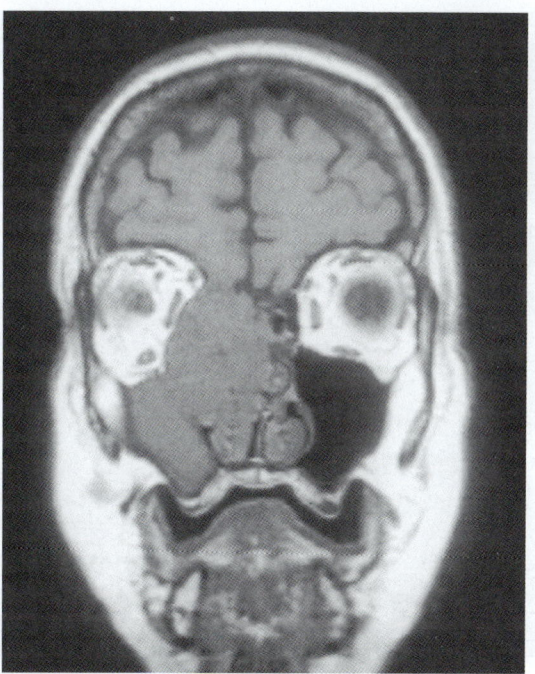

FIGURE 51.9. Coronal magnetic resonance imaging scan showing a large soft tissue mass and bone destruction in the right ethmoidal maxillary sinuses and nasal cavity secondary to extensive (Kadish stage C) esthesioneuroblastoma.

metastases is uncertain; it has been stated to be as high as 50%, but this rate is influenced by the use of chemotherapy in high-risk patients.

Clinical Presentation

These tumors tend to be friable and bleed easily. The most common clinical symptoms are epistaxis and nasal blockage. Patients also may have local pain or headache, visual disturbances, rhinorrhea, tearing, proptosis, or swelling in the cheek.[149] The symptoms may be associated with a mass in the neck.

Diagnostic Workup and Staging

Physical examination may show the inferior aspect of a polypoid friable mass in the nasal cavity. Ocular findings or a mass in the nasopharynx may be present. With early lesions, radiographs or CT or MRI may show only nonspecific opacification, soft tissue swelling, and occasionally bone destruction.[150] Octreotide is a somatostatin analog that, when coupled to a radioisotope, produces a scintigraphic image of neuroendocrine tumors (NETs) expressing somatostatin type 2 receptors. Octreotide scintigraphy may be useful in confirming the preoperative diagnosis of certain head and neck NETs, such as paragangliomas, Merkel cell carcinomas, medullary thyroid carcinomas, and ENBs. Bustillo et al.[151] carried out a retrospective study that compared the results of octreotide scintigraphy with the histopathologic diagnosis in 74 patients with head and neck NETs. Of the 60 patients undergoing evaluation for suspected paraganglioma, octreotide scintigraphy was correctly positive in 36 of 37 patients with paraganglioma and correctly negative in 19 of 23 patients who did not exhibit paraganglioma (sensitivity of 97% and a specificity of 82%). There were 14 patients in the nonparaganglioma group. Octreotide scintigraphy detected or diagnosed locoregional recurrences in two with ENB.

Table 51.1 outlines the suggested diagnostic workup. MRI, especially with gadolinium contrast, may be used as a supplement or alternative to CT scanning.[47] CT provides the best information about the tumor and its local invasion into surrounding bone structures. MRI allows an estimate of tumor

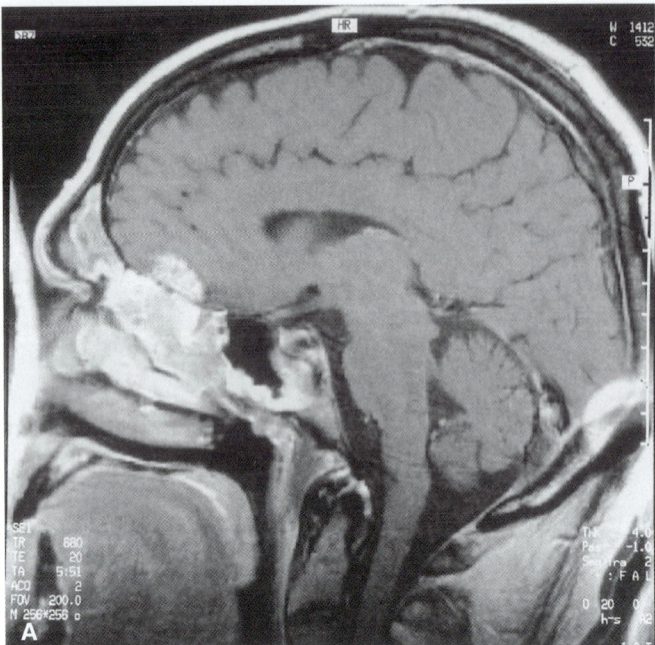
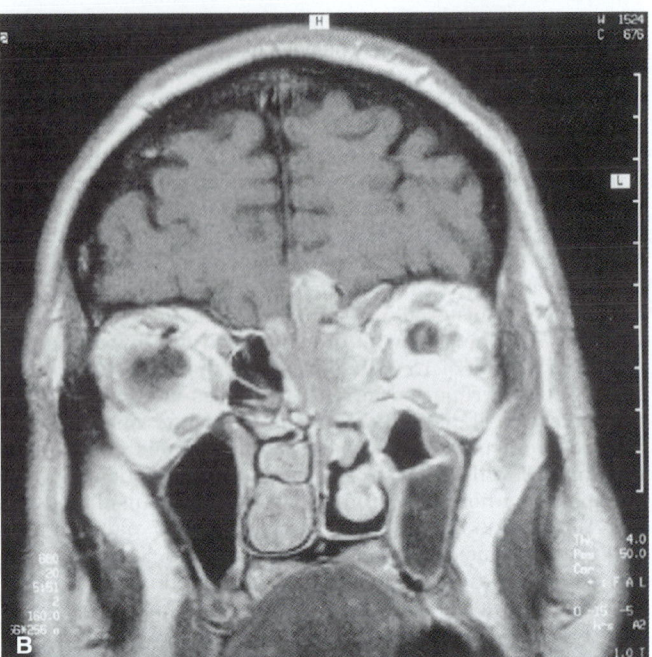

FIGURE 51.10. Sagittal **(A)** and coronal **(B)** views of preoperative magnetic resonance imaging of a 56-year-old patient who was initially seen with a Kadish stage C tumor involving left nasal cavity and extending intracranially. (From Chao KSC, Kaplan C, Simpson JR, et al. Esthesioneuroblastoma: the impact of treatment modality. *Head Neck* 2001;23[9]:749–757. Copyright © 2001 John Wiley & Sons, Inc. Reprinted by permission of John Wiley & Sons, Inc.)

spread into surrounding soft tissue areas, such as the anterior cranial fossa and the retromaxillary space. Bone scintigraphy scan is useful in detecting distant metastases.

The expansile tendency of olfactory neuroblastoma is characterized by bowing of the sinus walls. The destructive aspect is manifested as tumor replacing the turbinates, septum, and sinus walls with extension into contiguous areas (Figs. 51.9 and 51.10). The density or signal and enhancement characteristics are nonspecific of olfactory neuroblastoma.

Although dopamine β-hydroxylase and catecholamines are produced by these tumors, their measurements or vanillylmandelic acid excretion levels have not proven clinically useful.

A staging system has been proposed by Kadish et al.[149] (Table 51.9).

Pathologic Features and Prognostic Factors

ENBs are polypoid, frequently reddish, soft, and vascular tumors with neuroblasts and neurocytes. ENBs contain epithelial components serving as a supporting stroma and have a nerve component that corresponds to the olfactory cells. Rosettes are the main feature, consisting of several rows of cells arranged around the central area.[17] ENBs may be confused with lymphoma or anaplastic carcinoma and have diffuse, regular distribution. ENBs contain many fibrils, which fill the central space of the rosette (called a pseudorosette). It has been suggested that the presence of chromaffin granules indicates a derivative from primitive neural crest cells. ENB must be distinguished from other poorly differentiated neoplasms, including sinonasal undifferentiated carcinoma (SNUC), which is derived from the Schneiderian epithelium. SNUC lacks rosettes and intercellular fibrils.[17]

Extension of the primary tumor based on the Kadish staging system[149] has been identified as the most important determinant of treatment outcome, although this was not confirmed by Chao et al.[152] High-grade tumors had worse outcome in the reports from the Mayo Clinic and the University of California, Los Angeles (UCLA).[153]

Argiris et al.[154] found that in 16 patients with ENB, 11 of whom had Kadish stage C and 8 (50%) had brain involvement at presentation. Craniofacial resection was performed in 13 patients (81%); 14 received either preoperative or postoperative therapy (radiation therapy in 11 and chemotherapy in 4). The actuarial 5-year survival was 60% and disease-free survival 33%, with a median follow-up of 4.3 years. The first site of failure was locoregional alone in 10 of 12 patients who progressed, and in 6 patients involved the brain or the meninges. Two patients were successfully salvaged.

Hyams[85] proposed a histologic grading system for ENB in which grade I tumors have an excellent prognosis and grade IV tumors are uniformly fatal. The Hyams grading system predated advanced craniofacial techniques, extensive use of immunohistochemistry, and the recognition of SNUC as a distinct entity. Miyamoto et al.,[155] in a retrospective review of 12 patients with ENB and 14 with SNUC, used the Kadish clinical stage and Hyams histopathologic system. Kadish staging was available for 26 patients (2 patients with stage A tumors; 7 with stage B, and 17 with stage C). Of the eight evaluable patients with Kadish stage A or B tumors, six remained disease free for more than 2 years compared with only five of seven Kadish stage C tumors. Slides were available for Hyams grading in 21 patients (2 patients with grade I tumors, 4 with grade II, 4 with grade III, and 11 with grade IV). They concluded that both the Hyams grading and the Kadish staging system can be used as independent predictors of outcome. Papadaki et al.[156] analyzed 18 formalin-fixed paraffin-embedded olfactory neuroblastoma specimens (12 primary tumors and 6 recurrences

TABLE 51.9 KADISH SYSTEM FOR STAGING OF ESTHESIONEUROBLASTOMA	
Stage	**Characteristic**
A	Disease confined to the nasal cavity
B	Disease confined to the nasal cavity and one or more paranasal sinuses
C	Disease extending beyond the nasal cavity or paranasal sinuses; includes involvement of the orbit, base of the skull or intracranial cavity, cervical lymph nodes, or distant metastatic sites

From Kadish S, Goodman M, Wang CC. Olfactory neuroblastoma: a clinical analysis of 17 cases. *Cancer* 1976;37(3):1571–1576.

or metastases) from 14 patients and concluded that p53 point mutation does not play an important role in the initial development of olfactory neuroblastoma; however, p53 wild-type hyperexpression may occur in subsets, show local aggressive behavior, and have a tendency for recurrence.

General Management

Surgery alone (including endoscopic technique) appears to be adequate treatment for small, low-grade tumors confined to the ethmoids in which negative surgical margins can be obtained. An ethmoidomaxillary resection with or without orbital sparing is usually necessary. This procedure is combined with preoperative or postoperative irradiation.[153,157] A complete resection with preservation of vital structures is achievable by using a craniofacial approach.

Treatment, which could be classified in 898 reported cases in 1997, consisted of surgery alone in 24% (226 cases), radiation therapy alone in 18.4% (165 cases), combined surgery and radiation therapy in 43.2% (388 cases), chemotherapy in 13.2% (119 cases), and in 11 cases (1.2%) bone marrow transplant. In the reported cases, follow-up could be evaluated in 477 cases, whereas in only 234 cases, a 5-year follow-up was done; on these, 20.5% had surgery only, 11.1% radiation therapy, and 68.4% combined surgery and radiation therapy. The best survival rates were obtained by combined therapy, 72.5% versus 62.5% with surgery alone and 53.8% with radiation therapy.[40]

Dias et al.[158] reported on 35 patients with ENB treated with GTR through a transfacial approach with postoperative RT in 11 patients, craniofacial resection and postoperative RT in 7, exclusive RT in 14, craniofacial resection alone in 1, and a combination of chemotherapy and RT in 2 patients. Radiation therapy median dose was 48 Gy. Craniofacial resection plus postoperative RT provided a better 5-year disease-free survival rate (86%) compared with the other therapies (P = .05). The 5-year DSS rate was 64% and 43% for the low- and high-grade tumors, respectively (P = .20). At 5 and 10 years, disease-free survival was 46% and 24%, respectively and overall survival was 55% and 46%, respectively.

Early lesions involving the ethmoids with little or no bony destruction or nerve invasion can be treated adequately by high-energy (photon or electron) radiation therapy with good cosmetic and functional results.[10,83,104] Those with more extensive local disease benefit from surgery and adjuvant irradiation,[158,159] although some have advocated against combined surgery and radiation therapy because of complications. Patients with locally advanced disease or high-grade tumors should receive aggressive treatment with combined modalities, such as surgery, radiation therapy, and chemotherapy.

Monroe et al.[79] described treatment results in 22 patients who received RT for ENB. The modified Kadish stage was stage A in 1 patient, stage B in 4 patients, stage C in 15 patients, and stage D in 2 patients. Treatment modalities included primary RT in 6 patients, preoperative RT in 1 patient, postoperative RT after craniofacial resection in 12 patients, and salvage RT in 3 patients treated for recurrence after surgery. Elective neck RT was performed in 11 of 20 patients (2 patients had cervical metastases at presentation for RT). Rates of local tumor control, cause-specific survival, and absolute survival at 5 years were 59%, 54%, and 48%, respectively. The cause-specific survival rate at 5 years was lower after primary RT (17%) than after craniofacial resection and postoperative RT (56%). Cervical metastases occurred in 6 of 22 patients (27%). No neck recurrences occurred in 11 patients treated with elective neck RT compared with four neck recurrences in 9 patients (44%) not receiving elective neck RT (P = .02). Their data and review of the current literature suggest a higher cervical failure rate than previously recognized; elective neck RT seems to correlate with improved nodal tumor control and should be considered in the treatment of ENB.

Rosenthal et al.[157] treated 72 adults with nonmetastatic, primary sinonasal NETs (31 with ENB, 16 with SNUC, 18 with neuroendocrine carcinoma [NEC], and 7 with small cell carcinoma [SmCC]). Patients with ENB usually were treated with surgery and/or radiotherapy; only 3 of 31 patients (9.7%) received radiation to regional lymphatics, and only 5 of 31 received chemotherapy. In contrast, patients with non-ENB histologies usually received chemotherapy (10 of 16 patients with SNUC, 12 of 18 patients with NEC, and 5 of 7 patients with SmCC). With a median follow-up for surviving patients of 81.5 months, overall survival at 5 years was 93.1% for patients with ENB, 62.5% for SNUC, 64.2% for NEC, and 28.6% for SmCC (P = .0029). The local control tumor rate at 5 years also was superior for patients who had ENB (96.2%) compared with patients who had SNUC (78.6%), NEC (72.6%), or SmCC (66.7%) (P = .04). The regional failure rate at 5 years was 8.7% for patients with ENB, 15.6% for patients with SNUC, 12.9% for patients with NEC, and 44.4% for patients with SmCC. Additional late events increased the regional failure rate for patients with ENB to 31.9% at 10 years. The distant metastasis rate at 5 years was 0.0% for patients with ENB, 25.4% for patients with SNUC, 14.1% for patients with NEC, and 75.0% for patients with SmCC.

Gruber et al.[160] described 28 patients with ENB treated with RT (median dose 60 Gy). In 13 patients, total tumor resection (recommended by the authors) was performed. Chemotherapy (cisplatin, etoposide, cyclophosphamide, and vincristine) combined with RT was used in five patients. With a median follow up of 68 months, 54% of the patients were free of local tumor progression (51% at 10 years). Disease-free survival at 10 years was 25%.

Ozsahin et al.[161] described results of treatment in 13 European and North American centers for 77 patients with olfactory neuroblastoma, 11 with Kadish stage A, 29 with stage B, and 37 with stage C; 56 patients had surgery, 44 with total tumor excision. All but 5 patients received radiation therapy (50% with 3DCRT) and 21 had chemotherapy. With a median follow-up of 72 months, locoregional tumor control (LRC) was 62%, disease-free survival 57%, and overall survival 64%. Patients having total tumor resection or receiving ≥54 Gy had better overall survival than those treated with lower doses (Fig. 51.11). Six of the patients treated with RT (56 to 70 Gy) developed grade 3 or4 late complications (five osteonecrosis and one retinopathy).

Sperry et al.[162] treated 30 patients with ENB (70% with Kadish stage C) with surgery in 27 (52% craniofacial

FIGURE 51.11. Overall survival correlated with radiation therapy dose in 72 patients with olfactory neuroblastoma. (Reprinted from Ozsahin M, Gruber G, Olszik O, et al. Outcome and prognostic factors in olfactory neuroblastoma: a rare cancer network study. *Int J Radiat Oncol Biol Phys* 2010;78[4]:992–997. Copyright © 2010 Elsevier. With permission.)

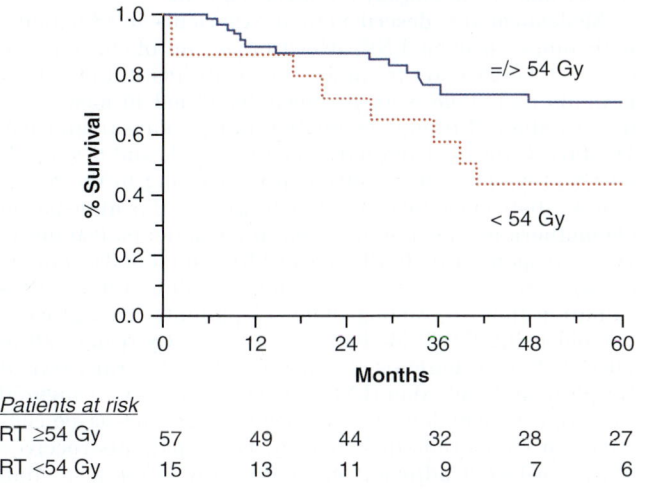

Patients at risk					
RT ≥54 Gy	57	49	44	32	28	27
RT <54 Gy	15	13	11	9	7	6

resection), combined with postoperative RT in 75.9% and chemoradiation in 23%. Local tumor failure at 5 years was 43.6% and regional failure 15.7%. The 5-year disease-free survival was 40.7% and overall survival 80%.

Madani et al.[163] published a report on 84 patients (73 with primary and 11 with local recurrent) sinonasal tumors, 9 of which were ENB, treated with IMRT (median dose 70 Gy in 35 fractions). Mean D50 to the optic chiasm was 37.2 Gy, to ipsilateral optic nerve 49.4 Gy, to contralateral optic nerve 47.1 Gy, and to the retina 37.7 and 28.4 Gy, respectively.

Kased et al.[164] reported on 17 ENB patients treated with IMRT. One patient had Kadish stage A, three B, and 11 C. Of the 15 surgical procedures, 7 had microscopically positive margins and 4 had gross residual disease. One patient received neoadjuvant chemotherapy, 7 received concurrent chemotherapy, and 4 received adjuvant chemotherapy. The median prescribed radiation dose to the gross tumor volume or clinical target volume (if tumor was grossly resected) was 66 Gy (56.7 to 70 Gy) with 2- to 2.2-Gy daily fractionation. Median follow-up was 44.5 months (7.4 to 117.3). The 5-year estimates of freedom from LRDP, PFS, and OS were 91%, 83%, and 81%. One patient developed local recurrence within the irradiation field at 25 months and died 15 months later. Another patient developed local recurrence at 72 months and was successfully salvaged with surgical resection and SRS. No regional or distant recurrences were observed. Four patients had acute grade 3 infections including meningitis (1), neutropenic sepsis (1), sinusitis requiring surgery (1), and brain abscess (1). Late complications developed in 2 patients (grade 3 brain abscesses requiring surgery).

Sharrett et al.[165] described treatment results in 75 patients with H&N ENB. Median follow-up was 105 months (range 6 to 539). Majority of the patients were men (64%) with a median age of 50.7 years at the time of diagnosis. A total of 77% had advanced-stage disease (Kadish stage C). All patients received radiation therapy (RT); 88% was postoperative and 12% definitive. Median RT dose was 60 Gy (range 42 to 70). Twenty patients (26.6%) received chemotherapy. The 5- and 10-year LC rates were 96% and 93%, whereas the 5- and 10-year locoregional tumor control were 87% and 68%, respectively. Ninety-three percent of patients were free from distant metastasis at 5-year follow-up and 81% at 10 years. Half of the total recurrences were after a 5-year follow-up. The 5- and 10-year OS rates were 87% and 74%; the 5- and 10-year DSS were 93% and 84%, respectively. On univariate analysis, younger age was associated with better RFS, DSS, and OS. On multivariate analysis, younger age was the only independent prognostic factor for improved RFS ($P = .03$), DSS ($P < .0001$), and OS ($P < .0001$).

The authors recommend surgery followed by postoperative RT and chemotherapy for advanced ENB.

Modesto et al.[166] described their experience in 43 patients with biopsy-proven ENB, two groups one of 26 and the other of 17 patients treated at separate institutions. Five patients had stage A at diagnosis (confined to nasal cavity), 13 stage B (tumor extending into paranasal sinuses), 16 stage C (beyond the paranasal sinuses), and 9 stage D (cervical lymph node involvement) according to the modified Kadish classification. Neoadjuvant platinum-based chemotherapy was administered to 24 patients, leading to 70.8% response rate (6 CR and 11 PR). A total of 31 patients (72%) were treated by surgery and 39 (90.6%) underwent radiation therapy. Among them, 11 patients (28.2%) were treated using IMRT. Median dose was 64 Gy (range 30 to 70 Gy). Twelve patients (28%) received bilateral cervical lymph node irradiation (LNI) (median dose 57 Gy range 50 to 66 Gy). Nine patients (21%) received platinum-based concomitant chemoradiation therapy. Three patients received platinum-based adjuvant chemotherapy. After a median

follow-up of 77 months, the 5-year overall survival was 65% and the 5-year progression-free survival 58%. Twelve patients (28%) developed locoregional relapse, mostly within the first two years (five locally, two regionally, and five both locally and regionally). The major prognostic factor was the modified Kadish stage with 3-year survival rates of 100% for Kadish A-B versus 48% for stage C and 22% for stage D. After adjustment for tumor stage, neither neoadjuvant chemotherapy nor LNI seemed predictive for LRC or survival. Interestingly among initial staged B and C patients ($N = 29$), 2 of them (7%) presented an isolated cervical lymph node relapse, and none occurred among patients previously treated by elective or adjuvant LNI.

Protons have been used sparingly in the treatment of some of these patients. Nishimura et al.[167] reported on 14 patients with olfactory neuroblastoma treated with proton beam (65 CGE in 2.5-GyE fractions) in 6 patients combined with surgery, sometimes combined with chemotherapy. With a median follow-up of 40 months, 5-year local PFS was 84%, disease-free survival 71%, and overall survival 93%.

Dagan et al.[168] reported on 84 adult patients without metastases receiving primary (13%) or adjuvant (87%) treatment with proton therapy for sinonasal cancers of which 23% (19) were olfactory neuroblastoma. Advanced stage (T3 in 25% and T4 in 69%) and high-grade histology (51%) were common. Surgical procedures included endoscopic resection alone (45%), endoscopic resection with craniotomy (12%), or open resection (30%). Gross residual disease was present in 26% of patients. Most patients received hyperfractionated PT (1.2 Gy [relative biologic effectiveness (RBE)] twice daily, 99%) and chemotherapy (75%). The median PT dose was 73.8 Gy (RBE), with 85% of patients receiving more than 70 Gy. The median follow-up was 2.4 years for all patients and 2.7 years among living patients. Local tumor control (LC), neck control, freedom from distant metastasis, disease-free survival, cause-specific survival, and overall survival rates were 83%, 94%, 73%, 63%, 70%, and 68%, respectively, at 3 years. The 3-year LC rate was 61% for primary radiation therapy and 59% for patients with gross disease. Late toxicity occurred in 24% of patients (with grade 3 or higher unilateral vision loss in 2%). Akimoto et al.[169] reported on 339 patients with nonsquamous cell cancer in the head and neck, of which 63 were olfactory neuroblastomas, treated with protons. Median follow-up was 64 months. Overall survival, progression-free, and local control rate of all patients at 5 years was 61.2%, 36.8%, and 71.2%, respectively, and for olfactory neuroblastomas, 86.2% and 79.0%. Among all patients, 254 (75%) were not suited for photon radiation therapy because doses to OARs exceeded tolerance dose in the evaluation of dose–volume histogram. However, OS at 5 years of these patients was 65.5%. Regarding treatment morbidity 34 (10%), patients developed grade 3 or 4 late toxicities such as brain injuries and neuropathy. None experienced grade 5 toxicities.

For advanced lesions, in which disseminated disease is likely, chemotherapy may improve tumor control and decrease the incidence of distant metastases. A combination of thiotepa, cyclophosphamide, doxorubicin, vincristine, nitrogen mustard, and actinomycin D has been used.[170,171] A retrospective review of 10 patients with recurrent ENB treated with chemotherapy at the Mayo Clinic suggested that cisplatin-based chemotherapy is active in advanced, high-grade tumors.[157] Survival from initial chemotherapy treatment was 44.5 months (range 3 to 130 months) in patients with low-grade tumors and 26.5 months (range 2 to 67 months) in patients with high-grade tumors (Table 51.10).

The optimal treatment of ENB demonstrates the benefit of adjuvant therapy, particularly radiation therapy. The largest reported series evaluated neoadjuvant chemotherapy and radiation therapy (50 Gy), resulting in improved resectability and patient survival (156 Polin).

TABLE 51.10 RESULTS OF TREATMENT CORRELATED WITH MODALITY AND STAGE FOR ESTHESIONEUROBLASTOMA

Modality[a]	Stage A			Stage B			Stage C		
	Initial Treatment	For Recurrence	Total Control Rate (%)	Initial Treatment	For Recurrence	Total Control Rate (%)	Initial Treatment	For Recurrence	Total Control Rate (%)
Radiation therapy alone	2/5	5/5	70	4/7	3/4	64	1/5	1/1	33
Surgery alone	5/9	4/4	69	3/6	1/2	50	1/1	–	–
Radiation therapy and surgery	7/10	–	70	12/30	0/1	57	7/15	–	47

[a]All results reflect treatment of 78 patients, who were observed for 6 months to 32 years.
From Elkon D, Hightower SI, Lim ML, et al. Esthesioneuroblastoma. *Cancer* 1979;44(3):1087–1094. Copyright © 1979 American Cancer Society. Reprinted by permission of John Wiley & Sons, Inc.

Elective Neck Treatment

ENB has been shown to metastasize to the neck and remote sites. Although the sites of metastases are widely variable and often atypical, Beitler et al.[172] found cervical node metastasis to be as frequent as local recurrence. Davis and Weissler[173] compiled a retrospective review of patients and found that the cumulative cervical metastasis rate reached 27% (55 of 207 patients). Noh et al.,[174] in a report of 19 patients with ENB treated with combinations of surgery, RT, and/or chemotherapy, noted that 4 patients with high-risk factors received elective neck RT (45 to 70 Gy). There were no cervical node failures in 5 patients with Kadish stages A and B, 3 of 10 in patients with Kadish stage C treated surgically, and 0 in 9 receiving chemotherapy.

Peacocky et al.[175] reported on 53 patients with ENB in the H&N; 42 (79%) underwent craniofacial resection as the definitive surgical treatment, 28 patients (53%) surgery and adjuvant radiation therapy (ART group) to the primary site only, and 25 (47%) surgery alone as treatment for the primary site (SA group). Median follow-up for the ART group was 84.5 months and for the SA group 93 months. Following initial treatment, the 5-year actuarial survival was 89% for the ART patients and 75% for the SA patients; the 5-year local RFS was 89% for the ART patients and 63% for the SA group. The 5-year cervical lymph node metastasis-free survival was 80% for the ART patients and 75% for the SA patients. Among the 18 patients with delayed cervical lymph node metastases, 10 underwent salvage neck surgery and radiation therapy, 5 had surgery alone, and 3 did not have surgery or radiation therapy, because of distant metastases or other comorbidities. Four patients recurred in the neck at following salvage treatment. With a median follow-up time of 31 months, the 2-year RFS estimate was 85% versus 74% following salvage treatment. Thus, the 5-year delayed cervical lymph node metastasis rate in patients with ENB and a clinically N0 neck undergoing local treatment is 23%. The delayed lymph node metastases were effectively salvaged in the majority of patients. The authors proposed that patients with ENB and a clinically N0 neck should not undergo elective neck radiation therapy as part of their initial treatment in order to avoid acute and late toxicity.

Yin et al.[176] published a retrospective analysis of 116 patients with naïve ENB treated in China. According to Kadish stage classification, 20% (23 patients) presented with stage B and 79% (92 patients) with stage C. Thirty-two patients showed cervical lymph node metastasis in initial staging. Among 84 patients with N0 disease, the managements of neck in 80 patients with Kadish B/C were available, treatment modalities consisting of primary radiation therapy (RT) in 27 patients, preoperative RT in 10, postoperative RT in 40, and surgery alone in 3. Fifty patients were treated with elective neck irradiation (ENI) and 30 without any prophylactic neck treatment. Thirty-two of 116 (28%) patients were N-positive at the time of initial diagnosis, most frequently involved the level II lymph nodes (81%), followed by level IB (53%), level III (28%), and the retropharyngeal nodes (RPN) (25%). Rates of overall survival, disease-free survival, and regional relapse-free survival at 5 years were 77%, 71%, and 98%, respectively,

for patients treated with ENI, compared with 62%, 50%, and 75% for those without neck treatment. The regional failure rate was 2% for patients with ENI compared with 23% without neck treatment, and distant failure rates were 20% in the ENI group versus 27% in the untreated neck group.

Neck recurrence occurred in 7 of 30 patients who were without neck treatment, all relapsed in level IB or level II. The authors concluded that the treatment target of ENI should at least cover the bilateral upper and middle neck, namely, level IB–III and RPNs.

As noted, because of the low incidence of cervical lymph node metastasis (≤10%) in early-stage ENB, elective irradiation of the neck or a dissection is not indicated. However, in patients with Kadish stage C disease, the cervical metastatic rate climbed to 44% (25 of 57 patients). As stated previously, Monroe et al.,[79] observed cervical node metastasis in 6 of 22 patients (27%). In 11 patients they treated with elective neck RT, no recurrences were noted, in contrast to 4 of 9 (44%) for patients not receiving elective neck RT. Thus, with advanced-stage disease, cervical nodes may be initially managed by irradiation, radical neck dissection, or a combination of both. Zanation et al.[177] recommend salvage of neck metastases occurring 6 months or more after treatment of the primary site to be treated with combined surgery and radiation therapy. They showed a clear disease-free survival advantage (59 vs. 14%) in patients with combined modality therapy versus single modality in the salvage setting.

Radiation Therapy Techniques

A combination of photons and electrons with conventional anterior fields provides good coverage for limited ethmoidal disease when the tumor is confined anteriorly. Beam arrangement can be modified for disease extending into the orbit or maxillary sinus. Obturator or bolus may be needed postoperatively to compensate for tissue deficit. When intracranial or posterior extension is present or tumor has spread into the maxillary sinus, a pair of perpendicular (anterior–posterior and lateral) portals with wedges or two lateral wedge fields in conjunction with an open anterior photon field will give good coverage of the treatment volume, with the dose inhomogeneity around 10% to 20%. Incorporation of a vertex field eliminates the high inhomogeneous dose along the junction line of the conventional three-field technique. Treatment techniques are similar to those described for treatment of paranasal sinuses (see Chapter 42). The orbits can be spared or treated as the degree of extension dictates. Occasionally, an anterior electron-beam field may be needed to supplement low-dose areas. When the electron beam is used over air cavities, some dosimetry problems result. Eye blocks must be positioned precisely to avoid undesirable side effects.

When combined therapy is used, preoperative doses of 45 Gy and postoperative doses of 50 to 60 Gy are indicated, depending on the status of the surgical margins. Doses of 65 to 70 Gy are delivered with irradiation alone in patients with inoperable tumors.[164] The usual fraction dose is 1.8 to 2.0 Gy. Contrast-enhanced CT or MRI scans before initiation of treatment are crucial to demarcate extension of the tumor.

Treatment planning with CT for determination of tumor extension is extremely important.[178] Because of the proximity of ENB to the optic nerves, the optic chasm, and the brainstem, the precision of treatment setup, target volume definition, and dose homogeneity dictate tumor control and the sequelae of treatment. Treatment techniques similar to those for paranasal sinuses may create "hot spots" along the optic tracks. High doses per fraction (exceeding 2 Gy) increase the possibility of late sequelae, such as blindness and bone and brain necrosis.

Three-dimensional CRT or IMRT provides alternatives to the conventional three-field technique used to treat these tumors (Fig. 51.12). Special attention should be directed to reduce unnecessary irradiation to ocular structures, including optic nerve(s) and chiasma. When occasionally a patient presents with cervical node metastasis, IMRT is very helpful to optimally treat the primary tumor and the cervical lymphatics (Fig. 51.13).

Structure	Dose Range (cGy)	Mean Dose (Gy)
Planning target volume 1	30–70	65
Planning target volume 2	40–70	58
Optic chasm and nerves	13–42	24

Results of Therapy

Surgery and Irradiation

Platek et al.,[179] in an analysis of SEER data (1973 to 2005) of 135 cases of olfactory neuroblastoma, noted that 59% of the patients were treated with surgery and RT, 23% with surgery only, 12% with RT only, and 6% with neither. No data on chemotherapy administration were available. The 5-year survival with surgery plus RT was 66%, with surgery only 51%, with RT only 26%, and with other therapy 34% (*P* = .003).

Kased et al.[164] reported on 17 patients with ENB (15 undergoing a surgical procedure, 7 receiving concurrent chemotherapy, and 4 adjuvant chemotherapy) treated with IMRT (median dose 66 Gy in 2-Gy fractions). With a median follow-up of 44.5 months, the 5-year freedom of locoregional tumor progression was 91%, PFS 83%, and overall survival 81%. Four patients had acute complications (meningitis, sepsis, sinusitis requiring surgery, and brain abscess), and two patients developed late brain abscess, requiring surgical treatment.

Radiation therapy is an important component in the management of ENB, but the optimal sequence when integrated with surgery is unknown. Eden et al.[180] observed no significant difference in survival whether preoperative or postoperative irradiation was given, but suggested improved local tumor

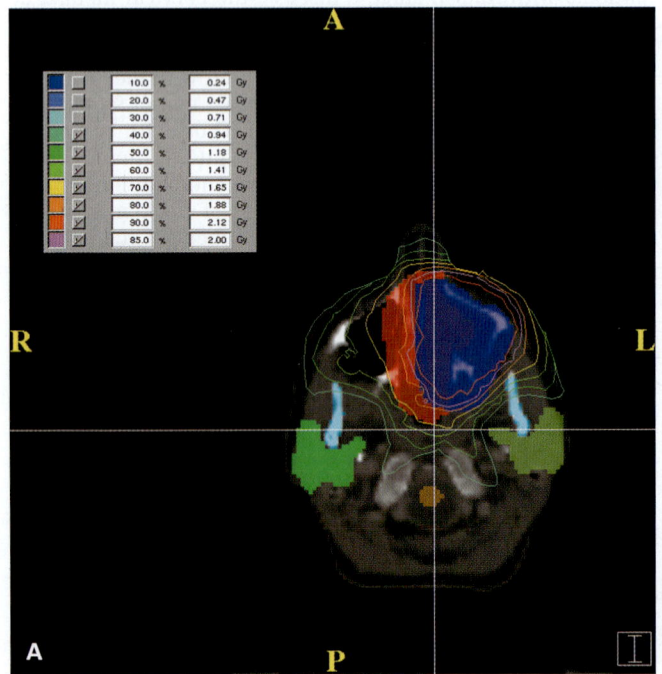

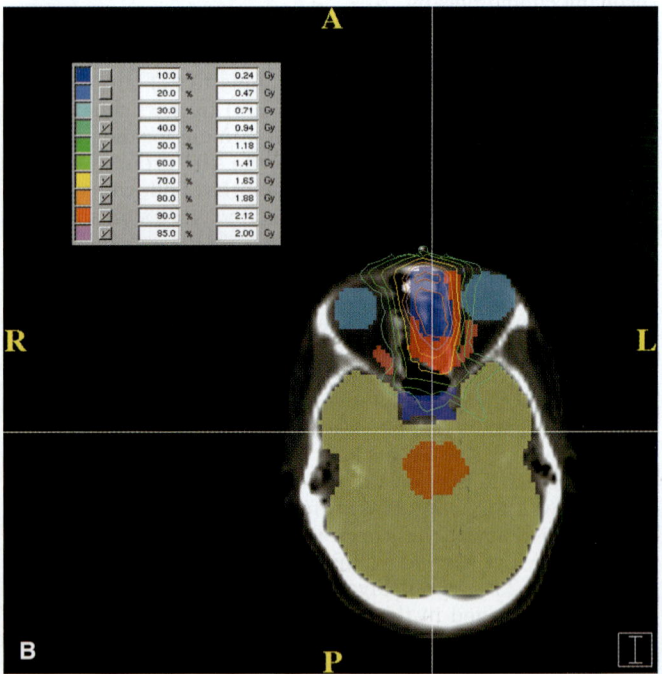

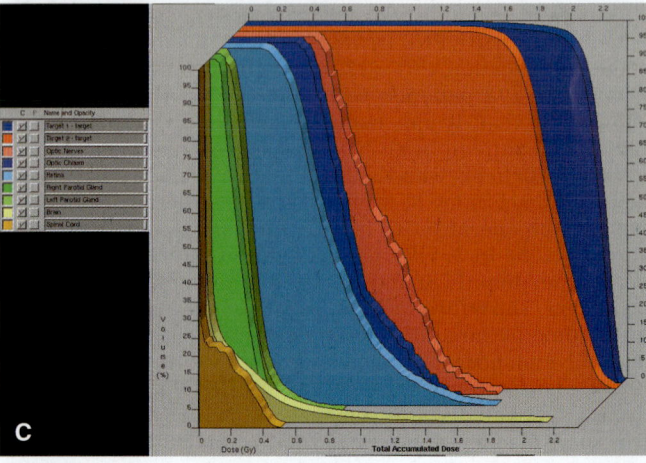

FIGURE 51.12. Esthesioneuroblastoma in a 35-year-old woman, initially treated with a craniofacial surgical resection. Patient received postoperative intensity-modulated radiation therapy (2-Gy fractions). **A:** Cross-section illustrating coverage of ethmoid nasal and left maxillary antrum volume. **B:** Cross-section showing dose distribution in target volume with excellent sparing of ocular structures. **C:** Dose-volume histogram.

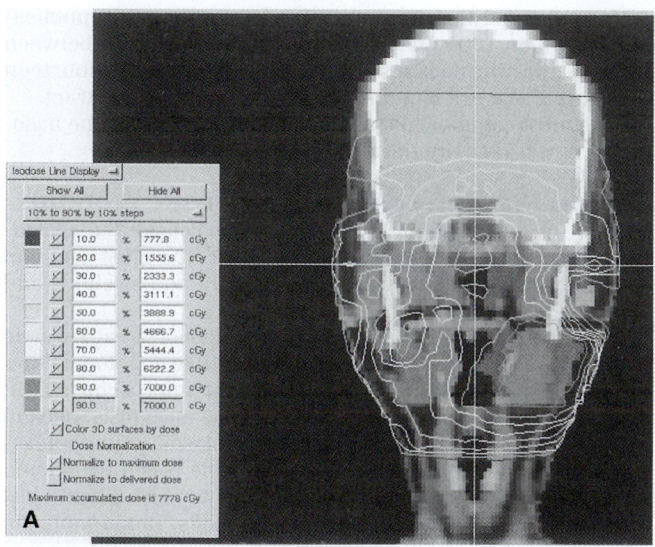

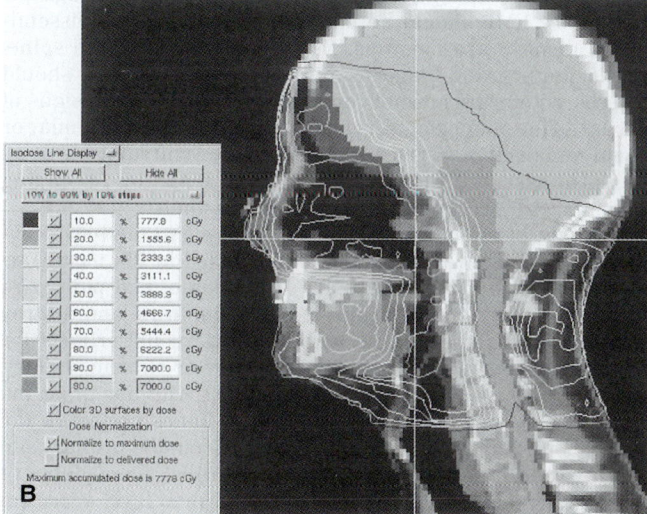

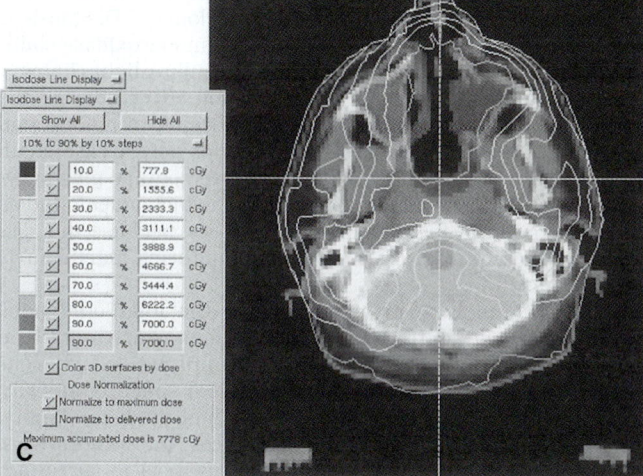

FIGURE 51.13. Patient with Kadish stage C esthesioneuroblastoma of ethmoid cells and nasal cavity who presented with a large left upper cervical lymph node metastasis. Intensity-modulated radiation therapy plans to deliver 70 Gy to primary tumor and cervical lymphadenopathy. Coronal **(A)**, sagittal **(B)**, and cross-section dose distributions illustrate excellent coverage of all target volumes **(C)**.

control with preoperative irradiation. Technical factors may have contributed to a higher incidence of postoperative radiation therapy failures because three of five postoperative cases received <50 Gy; all three patients were treated with a single anterior field, which gives less homogeneous dose distribution throughout the treatment volume.

Foote et al.[153] updated the experience of the Mayo Clinic. Seventeen patients had disease confined to the nasal cavity or paranasal sinuses (Kadish stages A and B), and 32 patients had more advanced disease. Treatment included gross total resection alone or combined with radiation therapy. The 5-year actuarial survival, disease-free survival, and local tumor control rates were 69.1%, 54.8%, and 65.3%, respectively. Local tumor control was improved in patients who received postoperative irradiation (55.5 Gy) even after complete tumor resection.

Levine et al.[181] conducted a retrospective review of 35 patients; 6% of them presented with cervical metastasis, and ultimately 25.7% developed cervical metastases. Fourteen percent of the patients had a local recurrence at an average of 6 years after diagnosis, and in 37%, at least one episode of metastatic disease occurred. The disease-free survival was 80.4% at 8 years. CNS complications occurred in 25.7% of patients, orbital complications in 22.9%, systemic posttreatment problems in 20%, and chemotoxic sequelae in 18%.

Eriksen et al.[182] carried out a retrospective review of 13 patients with ENB (Kadish stage A 1 patient, stage B 5 patients, and stage C 7 patients). The 5-year disease-free survival was 51%. Forty-six percent of the patients experienced relapse, and despite intensive salvage therapy, median survival after recurrence was only 12 months.

Chao et al.[152] reported on 25 patients with ENB (Kadish stage A in 3 patients, stage B in 13 patients, C in 8 patients, and modified D in 1 cervical nodal metastasis patient); 17 patients were treated with surgery and radiation therapy, 6 with irradiation alone, and 2 with surgery only. Eight patients received neoadjuvant chemotherapy. Median follow-up was 8 years. The 5-year actuarial overall survival, disease-free survival, and local tumor control rates were 66.3%, 56.3%, and 73%, respectively. Kadish stage was not a significant prognosticator for local tumor control or disease-free survival. Five-year local tumor control was 87.4% for combined surgery with RT and 51.2% for irradiation alone. Two patients with Kadish stages A and B disease underwent surgical resection alone; both failed locally. In contrast, only three of nine patients with Kadish stage A or B disease who received ART had a local recurrence. With ART, the surgical margin status did not influence local tumor control.

Chemotherapy and Irradiation

Eden et al.[180] described results in 16 patients with stage A or B disease and 24 patients with stage C disease treated with irradiation (median dose 50 Gy) and surgery for stage A and B diseases, with the addition of chemotherapy (cyclophosphamide and vincristine) for stage C disease. Actuarial survival rates at 5 and 10 years were 78% and 71%, respectively. Locoregional failure developed in 15 of 40 patients; 68% of the failures were locoregional (including the brain, neck, facial bone, and sinus). They had no recurrences at the primary tumor bed; all recurrences were either outside the irradiation field or at distant sites.

Preoperative neoadjuvant therapy may provide a valuable complement to radical craniofacial resection.[170]

Forty patients were treated for ENB at Institut Gustave Roussy, France.[146] Three patients had stage T1, 7 patients had T2, 15 patients had T3, and 15 patients had T4 lesions. At presentation, the cervical metastatic rate was 18% and distant metastases were detected by bone marrow biopsy and bone scan in three patients. Treatment modalities included surgery alone in 8 patients, radiation therapy alone in 3 patients, surgery plus radiation therapy in 11 patients, chemotherapy alone in 2 patients, chemotherapy plus radiation therapy in 10 patients, and chemotherapy plus surgery and radiation therapy in 6 patients. The 5-year survival rate was 51%. Multimodality treatment offered better survival (63% at 5 years). Overall local, regional, and distant failure rates were 58%, 15%, and 40%, respectively. Distant metastases commonly occurred in the bone (82%).

Noh et al.[174] summarized reports on patterns of failure of ENB treated with or without chemotherapy. Although the indications for high-dose chemotherapy and BMT must be better defined, it may be a promising alternative for patients with large tumors or those with recurrent tumor to whom no further local therapy (e.g., surgery or irradiation) can be safely given.

Konuthula et al.[183] analyzed 90 patients with Kadish stages C and D ENB in the National Cancer Database (NCDB), 55 % treated with definitive radiation (RT) (median dose 59.4 Gy) and 45 % receiving chemotherapy. Mean follow-up was 57.1 months. There was no difference in 5-year survival between the patients who received RT and those treated with RT and chemotherapy (74.8% vs. 64.4%). There was also no difference in survival between whether or not a clinically node-negative neck was treated with RT (72.9% vs. 67.0%).

Sequelae of Treatment

In a few patients, depending on the dose of irradiation, long-term sequelae include bone necrosis, brain necrosis or abscess, blindness, or painful eye reactions requiring enucleation.[183,184]

Simon et al.,[178] in 13 patients with olfactory ENB treated with surgery and radiation therapy, noted that one patient lost vision as a result of glaucoma and radiation retinopathy after 67.3 Gy in 34 fractions. One patient treated with 61.76 Gy in 34 fractions developed a visual field defect and optic atrophy; she also had a nasal cutaneous fistula. One patient sustained intraoperative rupture of the ocular globe and subconjunctival hemorrhage.

EXTRAMEDULLARY PLASMACYTOMAS

Solitary plasmacytomas are rare tumors of plasma cell origin, making up 4% of all plasma cell tumors. Multiple myeloma occurs about 40 times more frequently than solitary plasmacytoma. Monoclonal extramedullary plasmacytoma (EMP) is a rare, low-grade lymphoma found predominantly in the head and neck region. Only since the introduction of immunophenotyping techniques two decades ago has it been possible to differentiate EMP from benign polyclonal plasma cell proliferation. Hotz et al.[185] reviewed the records of 24 patients with morphologically diagnosed EMP treated at their institution; only 14 patients had true monoclonal plasmacytoma. No EMP-related deaths occurred. Two patients had local recurrence, and two patients developed multiple myeloma. Diagnostic procedures exclude a benign polyclonal plasmacytoma, multiple myeloma, and solitary bone plasmacytoma. The slow natural progression of the disease and the rarity of secondary multiple myeloma favor nonmutilating local surgery whenever possible to avoid the long-term sequelae of radiation.

Epidemiology

The annual incidence of EMP is 0.04 cases per 100,000 population.[186] They constitute only 0.5% of all upper respiratory tract malignancies. Male patients exceed female patients by a ratio of 3:1 to 4:1, and 75% of patients are 40 to 60 years of age.[187]

In a detailed literature search of more than 400 publications between 1905 and 1997, EMP mainly occurred between the 4th and 7th decades of life.[188] Seven hundred fourteen cases (82.2%) were found in the upper aerodigestive tract.

The most common sites in the head and neck are the nasopharynx, nasal cavity, paranasal sinuses, and tonsils.

Clinical Presentation and Diagnostic Workup

EMP of the head and neck area should be considered a separate entity because of its clinical behavior. The most common symptoms are nasal obstruction, local pain and swelling, and epistaxis.

Diagnosis of EMP is based on the exclusion of a systemic plasma cell proliferative disorder (multiple myeloma) and immunohistochemistry results. On light microscopy, EMP must be differentiated from a reactive plasmacytosis, plasma cell granuloma, poorly differentiated neoplasms, immunoblastic lymphoma, or extranodal marginal zone B-cell lymphoma with plasmacytic differentiation. Plasmacytoid lymphoma has a mixture of lymphocytes and plasma cells. Immunoblastic lymphomas show a cytoplasmic IgM heavy chain and express pan B-cell surface antigen, such as CD19 and CD20. Diagnosis of solitary EMP should be made only if studies for disseminated disease are negative. X-ray and/or MRI of the spine, pelvis, femurs, and humerus and bone marrow biopsy should also be within the normal range. There should be no signs of serum urine monoclonal protein, anemia, hypercalcemia, or renal impairment. A prospective study by Schirrmeister et al. has also assessed the accuracy of PET scanning in staging patients with presumed solitary plasmacytoma.

Grossly, plasmacytomas tend to be sessile in the nasal cavity and paranasal sinuses and pedunculated in the nasopharynx and larynx. The masses are soft, pliable, and pale gray. The lesion may remain localized or may infiltrate and destroy the surrounding soft tissue and bone. The usual criteria for solitary plasmacytomas, either medullary or extramedullary, include a biopsy-proven plasma cell tumor with one or, at the most, two solitary foci, absence of Bence Jones protein in the urine, bone marrow taken some distance from the primary site not involved by tumor (<10% of plasma cells), hemoglobin of 13 g/mL or more, and a normal serum protein level or serum electrophoresis at the time of the diagnosis. Basically, the diagnosis of solitary plasmacytoma is made by exclusion, that is, by eliminating the possibility of multiple myeloma.[187] Diagnosis is based on histology along with special immunoperoxidase staining for immunoglobulin-λ and immunoglobulin-κ light chains.[37]

Strict staging criteria, including normal MRI studies of the axial skeleton and the long bones and absence of monoclonal plasma cells detected by flow cytometry or polymerase chain reaction, are required for the diagnosis of solitary plasmacytoma. Careful microscopic and immunohistochemical studies are also required for the correct diagnosis, because this disease can be confused with other malignancies, particularly lymphomas.

Six patients with primary EMP in the head and neck were examined with MRI[188]; five lesions were oval and sharply demarcated without signs of infiltration, whereas the other lesion filled the parapharyngeal space bilaterally. On T2-weighted sequence, the lesions had moderate signal intensity. On plain T1-weighted sequences, the tumors were isointense or slightly hyperintense with respect to surrounding muscles; after administration of contrast medium, four lesions showed notable enhancement, with distinct central inhomogeneity.

Bone destruction is not a particularly bad prognostic sign, although some investigators report that it adversely affects prognosis.[188] Bony invasion is common in the more malignant types.[17]

Cervical lymph node metastasis from EMP varies with the site of the primary lesion and follows the same pattern of

TABLE 51.11 FAILURE PATTERNS OF ESTHESIONEUROBLASTOMA: LITERATURE REVIEW

Author (Reference)	Early Stages (Kadish A–B)						Late Stages (Kadish C–D)					
	Chemotherapy No			Chemotherapy Yes			Chemotherapy No			Chemotherapy Yes		
	Local	Regional	Distant	Local	Regional	Distant	Local	Regional	Distant	Local	Regional	Distant
Kadish et al.[149]	2/5	0/5	0/5	—	—	—	3/4	1/4	0/4	—	—	—
Elkon et al.[192]	9/42	6/42	4/42	—	—	—	9/18	2/18	2/18	—	—	—
Dulquerov[193]	1/11	1/11	1/11	—	—	—	1/4	1/4	1/4	0/1	0/1	0/1
Zappia et al.[194]	1/6	1/6	0/6	—	—	—	1/6	1/6	0/6	1/2	0/2	0/2
Eich et al.[147]	0/4	0/4	0/4	—	—	—	0/12	2/12	3/12	0/1	0/1	0/1
Eich et al.[195]	NA	1/8	0/8	NA	0/3	0/3	NA	1/13	1/13	NA	1/16	1/16
Kim et al.[196]	—	—	—	—	—	—	1/6	2/6	0/6	0/8	1/8	2/8
Noh et al.[174]	—	—	—	0/2	0/2	0/2	0/3	3/3	0/3	1/7	0/7	2/7
Total	13/68	9/76	5/76	15/53	13/66	7/66	2/19	2/35	5/35			
Percent	19	12	6.6	28	19.7	10.6	10.5	6	14.3			

NA, not available.

Modified from Noh OK, Lee S-W, Yoon SM, et al. Radiotherapy for esthesioneuroblastoma: is elective nodal irradiation warranted in the multimodality treatment approach? *Int J Radiat Oncol Biol Phys* 2011;79(2):443–449. Copyright © 2011 Elsevier. With permission.

spread as squamous cell carcinoma arising in a similar site. The reported incidence of lymph node metastasis ranges from 12% to 26%. The diagnostic workup for EMP arising in the head and neck region is shown in Table 51.1. The exact relationship between EMP and multiple myeloma is unclear; however, approximately 20% to 30% of EMP cases will convert to multiple myeloma.[185,187]

General Management

The majority of these patients are treated with multimodality therapy. Alexiou et al.[188] reviewed 714 cases in the literature published between 1905 and 1997: Radiation therapy alone was used in 44.3% of cases and surgery alone in 21.9%, with combined therapy (radiation after surgery) in 26.9% of the cases.

Pedunculated EMP lesions may be treated by surgical excision because the chance of local recurrence is low. The treatment of choice for all other lesions is radiation therapy alone or combined with other modalities.[189,190] In a review of 714 cases in the literature, the following therapeutic strategies were used to treat patients with EMP of the upper aerodigestive tract: radiation therapy alone in 44.3%, combined therapy (surgery and irradiation) in 26.9%, and surgery alone in 21.9%. The median overall survival or RFS was longer than 300 months for patients who underwent combined intervention (surgery and irradiation), for surgical intervention alone (median survival time, 156 months), and for radiation therapy alone (median survival time, 114 months). Overall, after treatment for EMP in the upper aerodigestive tract, 61.1% of all patients had no recurrence or conversion to systemic involvement (i.e., multiple myeloma); however, 22% had recurrence of EMP, and 16.1% had conversion to multiple myeloma.

Radiation Therapy Techniques

Irradiation techniques vary with the location of the primary tumor. The techniques are similar to those used for primary tumors in comparable locations (i.e., nasopharynx, tonsil, paranasal sinuses). Solitary plasmacytomas respond well to doses of 50 to 60 Gy in 2-Gy fractions. Hughes et al.[191] suggested that the optimal radiation dose is dictated by the size of the tumor, with doses in the range of 40 Gy in 20 fractions recommended for tumors <5 cm, whereas 50 Gy in 25 fractions was recommended for tumors >5 cm. The local tumor control rate with radiation therapy alone is about 85%. Harwood et al.[190] summarized the literature but could not draw a dose–response curve from the data because of a lack of cases receiving low-dose radiation therapy. Nevertheless, there is a high risk of local recurrence with tumor doses below 30 Gy and a negligible risk for those treated at or above 40 Gy (Table 51.11).

Wax et al.[37] reported on seven patients, three treated with radiation therapy (31.75 to 60 Gy). All patients have maintained local tumor control and had been followed for a minimum of 1.5 years, with an average of 3 years. One patient, treated with surgical excision, experienced a relapse at a distant site 6 years later.

The response to therapy of 32 patients with localized plasmacytoma was described by Shih et al.[197]; 22 patients had solitary plasmacytoma of the bone and 10 had EMP. Median age for EMP was 63 years. Most EMPs occurred in the oronasopharynx (six cases) and paranasal sinuses (two cases). Seven patients with EMP received radiation therapy (47 to 65 Gy), and all achieved initial local tumor control. There was one local recurrence and multiple myeloma conversion in the EMP group. Local recurrence or dissemination was associated with the appearance of or an increase in myeloma protein.

Holland et al.[198] reported on 14 cases of EMP, 8 of which were in the head and neck. With doses of 46 to 62 Gy, the complete tumor response was 72%. No dose–response effect was observed.

Liebross et al.[199] described results in 22 patients with solitary EMP, in the head or neck in 19 patients, usually in the nasal cavity or maxillary sinuses, and bone destruction was found in 10 of 11 patients. Radiation therapy was the sole treatment in 18 of 22 patients (median dose 50 Gy; range 40 to 60 Gy); 5 of 7 patients with an EMP of the oral cavity, oropharynx, nasopharynx, parotid, or larynx also received ENI. Local tumor control was achieved in 21 of 22 patients (95%), and disease never recurred in regional nodes. Disappearance of myeloma protein occurred in three of five patients with an evaluable abnormality. Multiple myeloma developed in seven patients (32%), all within 5 years. The 5-year rate of freedom from progression to multiple myeloma was 56% and the median survival was 9.5 years. Chao et al.[152] reported on 16 patients with EMP and a median follow-up of 66 months. The head and neck region accounted for the majority of presentations (88%). A serum monoclonal paraprotein was found in three patients, and bone erosion was identified in seven patients. All patients received local RT, although two patients also received elective nodal irradiation. The median RT dose was 45 Gy (range 40 to 50.4 Gy). Local tumor control was achieved in all patients (100%); however, regional recurrence outside the RT fields occurred in 2 of 16. Multiple myeloma developed in five patients (31%) all within 5 years. The 10-year myeloma-free survival was 75% and 10-year overall survival was 54%.

Galieni et al.[200] reviewed 46 cases of EMP most frequently localized in the upper airways (37 of 46 patients, 80%), with the mass being limited to a single site in all but seven patients in whom two contiguous sites were involved.

The most frequent form of treatment was local radiation therapy. Thirty-nine patients (85%) achieved complete remission, five (11%) a partial remission, and two (4%) no response to therapy. Local recurrence and recurrence at other sites occurred in 7.5% and 10%, respectively. Seven patients (15%) developed multiple myeloma. The 15-year survival rate was 78%.

Michalaki et al.[186] described 10 patients with EMP treated with radiation therapy. The disease was most frequently localized in the paranasal sinuses (50%). All nine patients who received definitive RT (40 to 50 Gy) achieved a complete response. Median follow-up period was 29 months. Four patients (40%) relapsed; three died of their disease. Two patients with paranasal sinus disease subsequently relapsed with multiple myeloma at 10 and 24 months, respectively. The relapse rate in neck nodes of 10% does not justify elective irradiation of the uninvolved neck.

Miller et al.[201] reported that tumor arose in the sinonasal or nasopharyngeal region in 11 of 20 patients (55%). The primary modality of treatment was radiation therapy (45 to 60 Gy). The mean follow-up was 60.2 months. In 15 to 20 cases, immunohistochemistry staining for immunoglobulin light-chain production was conducted. One of the two cases (50%) classified as medullary plasmacytoma demonstrated conversion to multiple myeloma, whereas only 2 of 18 cases of EMP (11%) converted to multiple myeloma.

Ozsahin et al.[184] published a compilation of solitary plasmacytoma (42 cases) in the head and neck. There were 258 patients with bone (n = 206) or extramedullary (n = 52) plasmacytomas without evidence of multiple myeloma. Most (n = 214) of the patients received RT alone; 34 received chemotherapy and RT; and 8 had surgery alone. The median radiation dose was 40 Gy. Median follow-up was 56 months (range 7 to 245 months). The median time for multiple myeloma development was 21 months (range 2 to 135 months), with a 5-year survival probability of 45% (Fig. 51.14A). The 5-year overall survival, disease-free survival, and local control rates were 74%, 50%, and 86% respectively (Fig. 51.14B). On multivariate analyses, favorable factors were younger age and tumor size <4 cm for survival; age, extramedullary localization, and RT for disease-free survival; and small tumor and RT for local control. Bone localization was the only predictor of multiple myeloma development. No dose–response relationship was found for doses >30 Gy, even for larger tumors.

Tournier-Rangeard et al.,[119] in a review of 17 patients with solitary EMP in the head and neck, noted a local tumor control of 100% for patients who received ≥45 Gy dose to the CTV versus 50% with doses <45 Gy (P = .034). Prognostic factor for 5-year DSS (81.6%) was local tumor control (P = .058). Prognostic factors for disease-free survival (64.1%) were monoclonal immunoglobulin secretion (P = .008) and CTV dose >45 Gy (P = .056).

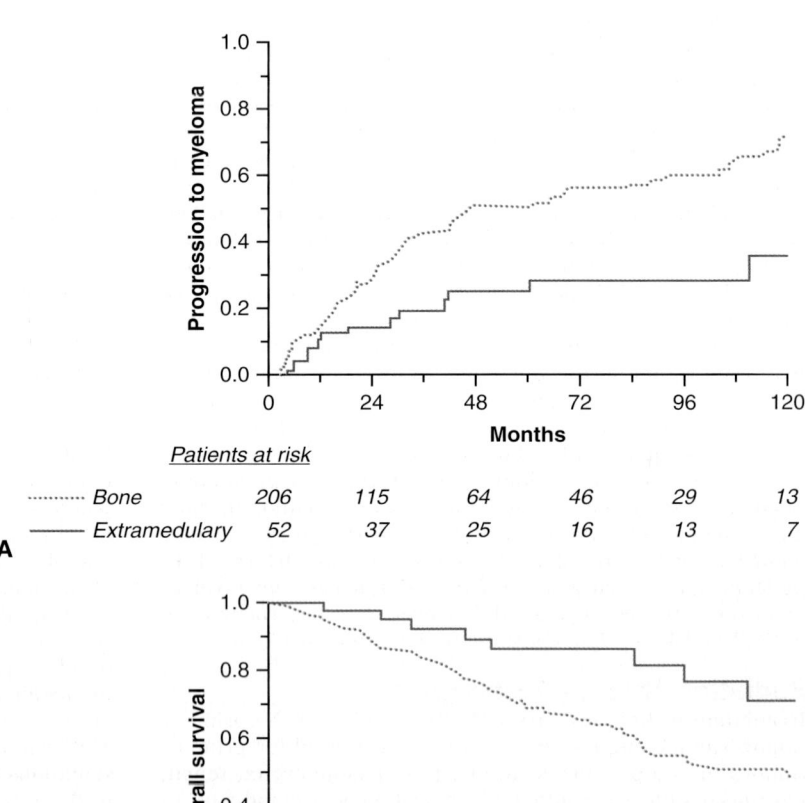

FIGURE 51.14. A: Probability of progression to multiple myeloma according to bone (*dotted line*) or extramedullary (*solid line*) solitary plasmacytoma (P = .0009). B: Overall survival correlated with bone (*dotted line*) or extramedullary (*solid line*) solitary plasmacytoma (P = .04). (Reprinted from Ozsakin M, Tsang RW, Poortmans P, et al. Outcomes and patterns of failure in solitary plasmacytoma: a multicenter rare cancer: study of 258 patients. *Int J Radiat Oncol Biol Phys* 2006;64[1]:210–217. Copyright © 2006 Elsevier. With permission.)

TABLE 51.12 EXTRAMEDULLARY PLASMACYTOMA OF HEAD AND NECK TREATED BY RADIATION THERAPY

Author (Reference)	Number of Patients	Number of Males/ Number of Females	Number <50 Years of Age	Local Control	Number with Multiple Myeloma	Recommended Tumor Dose (Gy)[a]
Kotner and Wang[204]	16	10/6	12	12/16	4	40–50
Wiltshaw[205]	14	10/4	10	11/14	N/A	–
Woodruff et al.[187]	15	8/7	11	14/15	1	40–50
Bush et al.[206]	10	5/5	5	8/10	2	50–55
Harwood et al.[190]	22	18/4	16	18/22	4	35 for 3 wk
Kapadia et al.[207]	12	9/3	10	11/12	3	–
MD Anderson Cancer Center[b]	15	12/3	12	13/15	4	50
Total	**104**	**72/32**	**76**	**87/104 (83.6)**	**18 (17.3)**	**40–50**

[a]10 Gy/wk unless otherwise stated.
[b]Updated, unpublished data of Corwin.

Bachar et al.[189] published outcomes of 68 patients with EMP of the head and neck, 39 treated with radiation (median dose 35 to 37 Gy in 15 fractions), 14 with surgery plus RT, 8 with surgery, and 3 with chemoradiation. With a median follow-up of 8 years, 5-year local RFS was 81% and survival 76%. Local recurrence was equivalent in patients treated with surgery or RT (12.5%). Multiple myeloma developed in 23% of the patients. Sasaki et al.[202,203] described results of radiation therapy in 67 patients with solitary plasmacytoma of the head and neck (in 44 combined with surgery) treated at 23 centers in Japan. Median RT dose was 50 Gy. With a median follow-up of 63 months, the 10-year local tumor control was 87% and overall survival 56%. The 10-year survival was 70% for patients treated with combined RT and surgery and 50% in those treated with RT alone (P = .004). Twelve patients (18%) developed distant metastasis and 8 (12%) converted to multiple myeloma.

Table 51.12 summarizes the doses of irradiation and probability of tumor control reported by various investigators. The authors' limited experience confirms the efficacy of tumor doses of 45 to 50 Gy for local tumor control. In patients who had extensive disease, a higher dose (50 to 60 Gy) was used, as recommended by several investigators.[208]

NASOPHARYNGEAL ANGIOFIBROMA

Epidemiology

Juvenile nasopharyngeal angiofibroma (JNPAF) is found more frequently in young pubertal boys; it has been shown to contain androgen receptors[209] and occasionally to regress with estrogen therapy. Hwang et al.,[210] in 24 nasopharyngeal angiofibromas, detected androgen receptors in 18 of 24 (75%) cases, whereas only two (8.3%) were positive to progesterone. None of the 24 cases was positive for antibodies to estrogen.

The tumor is believed to originate from the posterior–lateral wall of the nasal cavity where the sphenoidal process of the palatine bone meets the horizontal ala of the vomer and the roof of the pterygoid process because it is always involved.[211,212] Other investigators agree, because involution of tumor after irradiation usually occurs in this direction.[213]

JNPAF comprises <0.05% of head and neck tumors.[163] Patient's age at presentation ranges from 9 to 30 years,[214,215] with a median of 15 years. Females comprise <4% of the total cases.[216] Some investigators have suggested chromosomal studies in affected women because this is mainly a male disease.[212]

Clinical Presentation and Pathology

Symptoms usually occur 2 to 48 months before diagnosis.[214] The most common complaints are nasal obstruction or epistaxis, followed by nasal voice or discharge, cheek swelling, proptosis, diplopia, hearing loss, and headaches.[214] Nasopharyngeal angiofibroma may initially extend into the nasal fossae and maxillary antrum and push the soft palate downward and then through the pterygopalatine fossa and

superoanteriorly through the inferior orbital fissure or laterally through the pterygomaxillary fissure to the cheek and temporal regions.[30]

Beham et al.,[203] in a study of 32 cases of JNPAF, noted that most of the tumor vessels, which lacked elastic laminae, were characterized by vascular walls of irregular thickness and variable muscle content. In places, endothelial cells were separated from the stroma by only a single attenuated layer of contractile cells; in some more fibrotic hyaline areas, the stromal cells displayed reactivity for smooth muscle actin. The irregularity of the vascular walls, together with the lack of elastic laminae and stromal fibers, explains the pronounced tendency for hemorrhage in these lesions.

Differential diagnosis includes fibrosarcoma, rhabdomyosarcoma (RMS), chronic sinusitis, arteriovenous malformation, lymphangioma, neurofibroma, pleomorphic adenoma, lymphoma, pyogenic granuloma, polyps, and hemangioma.

Diagnostic Workup

After the history and physical examination, CT scans with and without contrast should be obtained. Characteristic findings are a mass in the posterior nasal or pterygopalatine fossa and bone erosion in the sphenopalatine foramen and extension to the pterygoid plate.[35] The pattern of enhancement in this highly vascular tumor is diagnostic,[217,218] and many investigators believe carotid angiograms are unnecessary[219] after CT diagnosis of the lesion, unless embolization, which is also controversial, is contemplated.

CT scans are especially helpful in regions involving thin bony structures (paranasal sinuses, orbits), where CT performs better than MRI. In the nasopharynx and parapharyngeal space, MRI is superior to CT. Obtaining tumor volumetric data with spiral CT or MRI facilitates 3-D treatment planning.[220]

Seventy-two patients with JNPAF were evaluated with CT or MRI.[217] Origin of the tumor was in the pterygopalatine fossa at the aperture of the pterygoid (vidian) canal. The tumor extended posteriorly along the pterygoid canal with invasion of the cancellous bone of the pterygoid base and greater wing of the sphenoid in 60% of the patients. The inability to remove the tumor in toto was principally due to deep invasion of the sphenoid; 93% of recurrences occurred with this type of tumor extension.

If intracranial extension is noted and radiation therapy is contemplated, no further studies are indicated. If the lesion is extracranial and surgery is indicated, bilateral carotid angiograms will identify the feeding vessels and delineate the boundaries of the tumor.

Biopsies are not indicated in all patients because of the potential for severe hemorrhage. It is important to perform a biopsy of the lesion when the clinical picture (sex, age, location, and behavior of the lesion) is not consistent with JNPAF because some lesions have proven to be sarcomas or chronic sinusitis.[212] Two cases of fibrosarcoma have been reported in patients in their 40s.[221]

TABLE 51.13 STUDIES REPORTING TREATMENT OUTCOME AND LATE GRADE 3 VISUAL IMPAIRMENT AFTER INTENSITY-MODULATED RADIATION THERAPY FOR SINONASAL TUMORS

Author (Reference)	Number of Patients	Treatment	Median Dose (Gy)	Follow-Up (Months)	Local Control (year)	Overall Survival	Grade 3 Visual Morbidity
Claus et al.[223]	32	IMRT+/−S	70	15	NR	80% (1 y)	0
Duthoy et al.[224]	39	IMRT+S	70	31	68% (4)	59% (4 y)	2
Combs et al.[32]	46	IMRT+/−S	64	16	81% (2)	90% (2 y)	0
Hoppe et al.[225]	30	IMRT+S	60	23	NR	NR	0
Daly et al.[226]	36	IMRT+/−S	70	39	58% (5)	45% (5 y)	0
Dirix et al.[227]	25	IMRT+S	60	27	81% (2)	88% (2 y)	0
Madani et al.[163]	84	IMRT+/−S	70	40	70% (5)	58.5% (5 y)	1

IMRT, intensity-modulated radiation therapy; S, surgery; NR, no report.
Modified from Madani I, Bonte K, Vakaet L, et al. Intensity modulated radiotherapy for sinonasal tumors: Ghent University Hospital: update. *Int J Radiat Oncol Biol Phys* 2009;73(2):424–432. Copyright © 2009 Elsevier. With permission.

Staging and Prognostic Factors

Staging schemes have been proposed by Chandler et al.,[212] a radiographic staging system by Sessions et al.,[213] and a more detailed anatomical system by Radkowski et al.[222] (Tables 51.13 and 51.14). In a retrospective review of 44 cases of JNPAF, invasion of the skull affected two-thirds of the patients, and the rate of recurrence was 27.5%.[228] Extensions to the infratemporal fossa, sphenoid sinus, base of pterygoids and clivus, the cavernous sinus (medial), foramen lacerum, and anterior fossa were correlated with more frequent recurrence. In a review of 97 cases, age at diagnosis, tumor size, and Radkowski classification were significant prognostic factors for recurrence.[229]

General Management

Optimum management of these patients remains controversial,[230] and the decision of whether surgery or radiation therapy should be used depends in part on the initial extent of the disease. In patients with extracranial tumors,[228] surgery is the treatment of choice and yields near-zero mortality or any long-term morbidity.[231] Tumor extension to the posterior infratemporal fossa or intracranially is associated with a higher risk of recurrence.[232]

Tumor remnants in symptom-free patients should be kept under surveillance by repeated CT scanning, because involution may occur. Recurrent symptoms may be treated by radiation therapy rather than by extended surgery or combined procedures.[212,228,233] When there is intracranial tumor extension (seen in about 20% of patients), the risk of surgically related death increases. Some investigators recommend preoperative intra-arterial tumor vessel embolization at the time of diagnostic bilateral carotid angiography, claiming a decrease in operative bleeding.[234] Salvage with embolization of polyvinyl alcohol has been described.[235] Others have reported anecdotal evidence of partial regression with the use of estrogens, believed to be the result of feedback inhibition of the pituitary's production of gonadotropin-releasing hormone.

Although radiation therapy is equally effective in extracranial tumors, the low but existing risk of secondary malignancies should limit its use to the more advanced tumors only, such as those involving the orbital apex or the base of the skull.[232,236] In the experience of Cummings et al.[233] covering 20 years, only two radiation-related malignancies were noted (one skin, one thyroid).

Radiation Therapy Techniques

Photon irradiation should be used for these patients, and fields must be individualized to cover the tumor completely with a margin (1 to 2 cm). Treatment portals are similar to those used in carcinoma of the nasopharynx (without irradiating the cervical lymph nodes) or carcinoma of the paranasal sinuses when these structures or the nasal cavity is involved. Opposing lateral portals are suitable in most patients, with larger fields and compensators used for tumors extending into the nose (Fig. 51.15). More extensive disease requires three-field or wedge-pair arrangements of 3DCRT or IMRT that can yield excellent dose distributions, particularly when there is nasopharyngeal or intracranial tumor extension. In all cases, the eyes are protected as much as possible.

The recommended tumor dose ranges from 30 Gy in 15 fractions in 3 weeks to 50 Gy in 24 to 28 fractions in 5 weeks.[237] A conventional setup uses 6- to 18-MV photons to treat the lesion with parallel-opposed fields to 50 Gy (2-Gy fractions).

The advantages of IMRT for the treatment of extensive or recurrent JNPAF were described in three patients on whom the tumor affected the base of the skull, pterygopalatine, infratemporal fossae, posterior orbit, and nasopharynx.[234] Tumor dose varied from 34 to 45 Gy. Chakraborty et al.[238]

FIGURE 51.15. Example of conventional lateral portal used at the Mallinckrodt Institute of Radiology for nasopharyngeal angiofibroma.

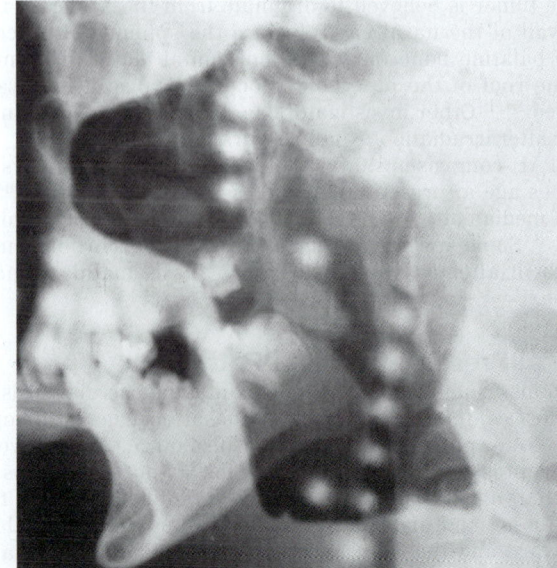

TABLE 51.14 STAGING OF NASOPHARYNGEAL ANGIOBROMA

IA	Limited to the nose or nasopharynx
IB	Extension into one or more paranasal sinuses
IIA	Minimal extension through sphenopalatine foramen medial pterygomaxillary fossa
IIB	Involvement of pterygomaxillary fossa displacing anteriorly posterior wall of maxillary antrum. Lateral or anterior displacement of maxillary artery branches or superior extension eroding orbital bones
IIC	Extension through pterygomaxillary fossa into the cheek and temporal fossa or posterior to pterygoid plates
IIIA	Erosion of skull base with minimal intracranial extension
IIIB	Erosion of skull base with extensive intracranial involvement with or without cavernous sinus involvement

Modified with permission from Radkowski D, McGill T, Healy GB, et al. Angiofibroma. Changes in staging and treatment. *Arch Otolaryngol Head Neck Surg* 1996;122(2):122–129. Copyright © 1996 American Medical Association. All rights reserved.

treated eight patients with IMRT for stage III tumors (median dose 39.6 Gy). Local control at 2 years was 87.5% and toxicity was minimal (persistent rhinitis in one patient). Significant sparing of the surrounding organs at risk was obtained. No grade 3/4 toxicities were experienced

Results of Therapy

In a surgical report, 18 patients were treated with gross tumor excision; 2 cases with intracranial involvement required a combined neurosurgical–otolaryngologic approach.[239] Recurrent intracranial disease was detected by MRI in three patients, who were treated with 35-, 36-, and 45-Gy external beam irradiation. Extracranial tumor recurrences were re-excised in seven patients. All patients (followed up with serial MRI) are living without evidence of active disease.

Cummings et al.[233] treated 42 patients primarily with irradiation and 13 for postsurgical failures; all except 6 had biopsies. Nine had stage IV disease according to Chandler's staging system. Dose was 30 to 35 Gy in 14 to 16 fractions over a 3-week period. Follow-up ranged from 3 to 26 years. The control rate was 80% and was equivalent for all dose ranges. Local control was 89% and 74%, respectively, when three fields versus two fields were used. When the field size was more than 6 × 6 cm, the control rate was 83% versus 55% for smaller portals, indicating the importance of accurately determining the target volume, including any potential tumor extension. Of 11 recurrences, 8 were controlled by a second course of irradiation and 3 by surgery. These tumors regress slowly, with 50% still present at 12 months. At 24 months, 23% of tumors were still present, and half of those recurred. Of the complete responders, only 1 of 33 had a recurrence. Robinson et al.[240] also found that objective responses after irradiation were noted within 6 months in 60% of patients and within 6 to 20 months in the other 40%. Symptoms, however, resolved in all patients within 6 months of treatment.

At the Mallinckrodt Institute of Radiology, Fields et al.[241] reviewed the authors' experience with 13 patients: 11 surgical failures and 2 primarily treated with irradiation. Intracranial extension was noted in 38% of patients. Follow-up ranged from 40 to 173 months. Doses ranged from 36 to 52 Gy, with a median of 48 Gy (1.8 to 2 Gy per fraction, 5 days a week). The control rate was 85%; patients failing irradiation were salvaged with embolization. Late morbidity was mostly xerostomia and dental decay.

Ungkanont et al.[215] described results in 20 patients treated before 1974 and 23 treated between 1975 and 1993: 31 had surgery (18 with preoperative embolization), 3 had irradiation, 7 received chemotherapy (4 combined with surgery), and 2 were observed. Disease-free survival was 67%; 28% of patients survived with residual tumor, and 4.6% died of surgical complications. Roche et al.[242] treated 15 patients with JNPAF with various maxillofacial surgical resections, combined with Gamma Knife radiosurgery in 2 patients and external RT in 4 patients. With a median follow-up of 108 months, 12 patients were tumor-free and 2 had no progression. All patients had normal or nearly normal quality of life.

Tumor regression usually occurs slowly after either irradiation[233] or chemotherapy[243]; therefore, the presence of tumor up to 2 years after treatment is not an invariable sign of failure unless it is symptomatic or progressing. McAfee et al.[244] treated 22 patients with JNPAF with definitive RT (30 to 36 Gy); with a median follow-up of 12.7 years, 20 patients (91%) had tumor control. The two patients failing were salvaged with surgery. No major treatment morbidity was noted. Kasper et al.,[245,246] in 9 patients treated with RT (30 to 35 Gy), observed 25% to 50% initial tumor regression within 1 year. Eventually, seven of the patients had complete clinical tumor regression, but on CT or MRI, only two of seven had no residual disease.

The management of large JNPAF with intracranial extension is complex. In 18 patients with JNPAF, preoperative MRI, embolization of feeding branches from the external carotid artery, and attempted complete resection were used in seven patients with intracranial disease[239]; serial MRI scans were used for follow-up. Intracranial disease that was persistent or recurrent and demonstrated subsequent growth was irradiated (35 to 45 Gy) or re-excised.

Wiatrak et al.[236] reported on three patients with extensive intracranial extension treated primarily with radiation therapy doses of 36.6, 40.0, and 50.4 Gy, respectively, without surgical tumor resection. Although there was no complete resolution of the tumors, significant improvement of symptoms was obtained without serious sequelae.

Ochoa-Carrillo et al.[218] reported on 31 patients treated with surgery or radiation therapy. Surgery was the treatment chosen in patients with stage II and III diseases, whereas radiation therapy was the treatment in stage IV, but it had low effectiveness, indicating the need to carefully investigate the value of craniofacial approaches in these tumors. Radiation therapy (30 to 55 Gy) was administered to 16 patients; seven with stage III persistent or recurrent tumor, and eight patients as initial treatment for stage IV disease. The disease-free interval of patients with stage III and IV diseases was 80.3% and 19%, respectively, after 36 months of follow-up.

Tranbahuy et al.[247] reported on seven patients with juvenile angiofibroma who underwent direct tumoral embolization. This technique induced marked devascularization and necrosis of the tumor. No neurologic sequelae were encountered.

Goepfert et al.[243] reported on five patients with aggressive nasopharyngeal angiofibromas recurrent after extracranial resection and irradiation who were treated with chemotherapy. Doxorubicin (60 mg/m[2] intravenous push for 1 day) and dacarbazine (250 mg/m[2] intravenous drip for 5 days) were given, with courses being repeated every 3 to 4 weeks. In a second regimen, vincristine, dactinomycin, and cyclophosphamide were administered at usual doses. Excellent tumor regression was noted in all patients. Patients were disease free at 2, 3, 6, and 10 years.

Sequelae of Therapy

Most investigators agree that surgical mortality increases with intracranial extension of the tumor. The most common radiation therapy sequelae include delayed growth secondary to hypopituitarism and decreased bone maturation.[159]

Malignant degeneration in JNPAF undergoing radiation therapy has been occasionally reported,[248,249] and there are several well-documented cases of radiation-induced sarcomas in these patients,[26,233] with doses ranging from 66 Gy to more than 90 Gy. Spagnolo et al.[26] reported on four patients treated with irradiation who later developed sarcoma. Cummings et al.[233] reported two neoplasms developing 13 and 14 years after irradiation, one was a basal cell carcinoma and the other metastatic thyroid carcinoma. Both patients are alive without disease. Two patients developed cataracts.

NONLENTIGINOUS MELANOMA

Malignant melanoma accounts for 11% of primary head and neck malignancies.[250] Of all malignant melanomas, 20% to 35% are located in the head and neck area.[133]

Cutaneous Melanomas

In a review of the literature, Batsakis et al.[251] found that, of all head and neck malignant melanomas, 64% to 78% were cutaneous, 6% to 8% were mucosal, and 14% to 30% were ocular. The superficial spreading and nodular types of malignant melanoma have a metastatic potential of 10% to 30% and 50%, respectively.[252] Prognosis is correlated with location and stage of the tumor.[253] Neurotropic melanoma is an uncommon variant of cutaneous melanoma, with a higher propensity to invade peripheral nerves. A thorough evaluation with CT or MRI scans should determine if there is intracranial or base of the skull involvement.

Whole-body imaging with a CT or PET-CT scan is appropriate only for patients with regional nodal metastases. CT imaging detects occult disease in 0.5% to 3.7% of patients with microscopic nodal metastases on sentinel lymph node biopsy and in 4% to 16% of patients with clinically palpable nodal disease.[254] Only one metastatic lesion was identified in over 500 patients with invasive, node-negative melanoma evaluated in two large studies.[211]

Treatment of cutaneous melanomas has typically been wide excision of the lesion with a minimum 3-cm margin.[250] More recently, margins of at least 2 cm have been used in the head and neck for stage I melanomas, with equivalent success, with local failure rate of 3% to 6%.[211] In the absence of palpable regional lymphadenopathy, the decision to proceed with lymph node sampling after excision of a primary melanoma is frequently based on the probability of detecting nodal micrometastatic disease, which increases monotonically with the depth of the primary lesion. In several large clinical trials and meta-analyses, nodal metastases were uncommon in patients with melanoma primary lesions under 1 mm thick, with positive nodes seen in only 1% to 5.6% of patients. In contrast, thick lesions with Breslow depths >4 mm were associated with nodal metastases, with estimates ranging from 35% to 45%.[211]

Radiation therapy, combined with surgery, is increasingly used in the treatment of patients with malignant melanoma (cutaneous or mucosal).[255] The Princess Margaret Hospital treated 16 patients with nodular melanomas with local excision and postoperative radiation therapy (50 Gy in 10 fractions over 2 weeks); 14 exhibited local tumor control, and 6 were alive and well 2 to 14 years after treatment. These results were comparable with those with wide local excision alone but with less morbidity and fewer cosmetic alterations. Later, at the same institution, Harwood and Cummings[252] treated five patients with definitive radiation therapy for superficial spreading melanoma of the head and neck area. All five lesions were locally controlled; one patient had a lymph node metastasis that was later controlled, and one died of distant metastases. They recommend treating these patients with 45 Gy in 10 fractions over 2 weeks to 50 Gy in 15 fractions in 3 weeks.[250,256]

Harwood and Cummings[252] also reported results in 74 patients treated with 3 fractions at 8 Gy given on days 0, 7, and 21 with shielding of the spinal cord, brain, and eye. Thirty patients were treated postoperatively after neck dissections if they had extracapsular tumor extension, multiple nodal involvement, a node >3 cm, or residual disease. Tumor control in the neck was achieved in 26 of 30 patients (86.6%) with follow-up of 1 to 4 years. In four patients with microscopic residual disease at the primary site, this postoperative regimen controlled three of four lesions with follow-up of 1 to 3.5 years. The other 40 patients were treated either for gross (13 patients) or recurrent (27 patients) cutaneous melanoma. Complete response was observed in 15 of 40 lesions (37.5%) and partial response in 12 lesions. An update of Harwood's data (personal communication, 1989) showed a neck tumor control rate of 94% in 41 adjuvantly treated patients versus 57% in 48 patients with gross residual or recurrent tumors. He concluded that irradiation alone should be considered for treatment of superficial spreading melanomas when surgery is contraindicated or after a simple excision in all cases of nodular melanoma in which a wide excision may be contraindicated because of age, location, or medical condition. For nodal disease, patients with poor prognostic pathologic factors should receive postoperative irradiation. Recurrent or unresectable tumors also should be irradiated. Harwood et al.[190] recommended high-dose fractions because the local

control rate was 71% when the dose per fraction was >4 Gy and 25% with lower fractions.

Ang et al.[257] reported on 174 patients with head and neck cutaneous melanoma high-risk features (three or more positive nodes, extracapsular tumor extension) who after surgery were treated with elective postoperative RT (30 Gy in 5 fractions of 6 Gy in 2.5 weeks). With a median follow-up of 35 months, LRC was 88%. Lesion thickness strongly affected 5-year survival (100% for <1.5 mm, 72% for >1.5 to 4.0 mm, and 30% for >4 mm). Bibault et al.[258] treated 60 patients with cutaneous melanoma with node dissection (17 in the head and neck) and postoperative RT and 26 (4 in head and neck) with surgery alone. At 5 years, the regional tumor control was better in patients receiving >50 Gy (80% vs. 35% with lower doses), which was reflected on higher overall survival. Grade 2 toxicity was noted in 9% of the patients. In 49 patients with high-risk cutaneous melanoma in the head and neck, Chang et al.[159] used postoperative RT (30 Gy in 5 fractions or 60 Gy in 30 fractions). With a median follow-up of 1.7 and 4.4 years for living patients, the 5-year LRC was 87% (no difference with either RT schedule), cause-specific survival 57%, and overall survival 46%. Two patients in the hypofractionated group developed major complications (osteonecrosis of the temporal bone and brachial plexopathy). Strojan et al.[259] reported on 83 patients with cutaneous melanoma in the head and neck, 40 treated with neck dissection only and 43 with dissection and postoperative RT (30 Gy in 5 fractions or 60 Gy in 30 fractions). In 20 patients, the primary site was included in the irradiated volume. With a median follow-up of 2.1 years, the regional tumor control at 2 years was 56% with surgery alone and 78% with surgery plus RT, with survival 58% and 51%, respectively. Late toxicity was observed in 6 of 34 (17%) of surgery-alone patients and in 10 of 36 (28%) of the surgery plus RT group. Chang et al.[159] summarized reports published on results of postoperative RT in head and neck cutaneous melanoma.

The ANZMTG 01.02/TROG 02.01 randomized controlled trial enrolled 123 patients to receive ART (48 Gy in 20 fractions, given over a maximum of 30 days) and 127 to observation after lymphadenectomy for a palpable lymph node field relapse and who were at high risk of recurrence. This study is registered with ClinicalTrials.gov, number NCT00287196. Median follow-up was 73; 23 (21%) relapses occurred in the adjuvant radiotherapy group compared with 39 (36%) in the observation group. Overall survival and relapse-free survival did not differ between the two groups. Minor, long-term toxic effects from radiotherapy (predominantly pain, and fibrosis of the skin or subcutaneous tissue) were common, and 20 (22%) of 90 patients receiving adjuvant radiotherapy developed grade 3 to 4 toxic effects. Eighteen (20%) of ninety patients had grade 3 toxic effects, mainly affecting the skin (nine [10%] patients) and subcutaneous tissue (six [7%] patients). Over 5 years, a significant increase in lower limb volumes was noted after adjuvant radiotherapy (mean volume ratio 15.0%) compared with observation (7.7%; difference 7.3%). No significant differences in upper limb volume were noted between groups. Interpretation Long-term follow-up supports our previous findings. Adjuvant radiotherapy could be useful for patients for whom lymph node field control is a major issue, but entry to an adjuvant systemic therapy trial might be a preferable first option. Alternatively, observation, reserving surgery and radiotherapy for a further recurrence, might be an acceptable strategy.

Another approach to the treatment of recurrent or unresectable cutaneous melanomas is combined hyperthermia and high-fraction radiation therapy, as reported by Emami et al.[260] and Engin et al.[261] These data support the use of high fractions for melanoma because Overgaard's complete response rate was 59% when fractions of more than 4 Gy were used and 33% for lower dose per fraction sizes.

However, a randomized study by the Radiation Therapy Oncology Group comparing 4 fractions of 8 Gy given on days 0, 7, 14, and 21 and 20 fractions of 2.5 Gy in 5 weekly fractions showed no significant difference in tumor response (24.2% and 23.4% complete response and 35% partial response).[262]

Treatment with high doses of adjuvant interferon or interleukin-2 in high-risk stage II and III melanoma reduced the risk or disease recurrence and increased the median disease-free survival in several large trials; however, the benefits were marginal and toxicity was significant. Recent developments with immune checkpoint inhibition (PD-1 receptor and CTLA-4 inhibition) and targeted therapy (MAPK inhibition) represent a new strategy for patients with metastatic and high-risk melanoma. Clinical trials integrating these treatments into treatment for patients with high-risk, advanced, or metastatic melanoma are in progress.

Mucosal Melanomas

Primary mucosal melanomas of the head and neck area comprise 2% to 8% of the cases seen each year in the United States.[251] They occur more commonly in countries such as Japan, where mucosal melanoma is found in 22% to 32% of patients with malignant melanoma.[215] Most occur in the fifth to seventh decades of life; they are extremely rare in the first two decades (0.6% of mucosal melanomas).[263] The male-to-female ratio approaches 1 to 1.[263] A review by Batsakis[17] of 204 mucosal melanomas showed 56.4% to be from the upper respiratory tract and 44% from the oral cavity and pharynx. Nasal cavity or paranasal tumors comprise <1% of malignant melanomas and 2% to 9% of head and neck melanomas.[264] Pigmentation may precede the lesion in up to 28% of patients for more than 1 year.[265] In the oral cavity, the most common location is the hard palate (up to 80%), followed in order of decreasing frequency by the upper gingiva and lower gingiva.

Diagnostic Workup

An excisional biopsy should be performed when feasible because some reports have suggested possible local or metastatic spread secondary to a punch or incisional biopsy,[246] although this has not been noted in cutaneous melanomas.[36] Batsakis[17] found that one-third of these lesions were amelanotic, and Hoki et al.[264] noted that 25% were amelanotic.

Metastatic melanoma to the mucosa of the head and neck area is less common. It can be differentiated from primary tumors by the presence of normal tissue between subepidermal tumor and the basal layer of melanocytes.[17] The larynx, tongue, and tonsils are the most common locations for metastases.

Prognostic Factors

Batsakis et al.[251] found >0.5-mm invasion to be a poor prognostic factor. Trapp et al.[266] noted this to be true only in patients with >0.7-mm invasion. Lymph node involvement is not a prognostic factor. Mucosal melanomas fare worse than their cutaneous counterparts,[149] suggesting a lack of immunologic competence.[267]

Management and Results of Therapy

Surgical excision is usually recommended for these lesions. Because of the poor results obtained and because 37% of patients had associated adjacent pigmentation, some investigators recommend prophylactic excision of all melanocytic nevi. Because the results with irradiation are comparable with those of surgical series and because of the poor survival of these patients because of distant metastases and not locoregional failure, irradiation alone, with surgery for salvage, should be seriously considered as the primary treatment for mucosal melanomas of the head and neck.[256] ENI is not indicated in all patients, as only few develop nodal metastasis.[8]

Patients with nasal cavity or paranasal mucosal melanoma have a median survival of 24 months. Five-year disease-free survival rates of 25% have been reported.[263] Patients with laryngeal melanoma had a 13% 5-year disease-free survival rate.[149] In a review of the Japanese literature, Umeda et al.[268] found a local tumor control rate for stage I and II diseases of 58% (7 of 12) in surgically treated patients with oral melanomas and a minimum follow-up of 3 years. Similar rates of failure have been reported, even with radical en bloc excisions (20% to 42%). Because the main cause of treatment failure is distant metastases and because almost no patient has clinically evident nodal metastases at presentation, an elective neck node dissection is not consistently recommended. This subject is still controversial, as 30% to 60% of patients may later develop nodal disease.[269]

Harwood and Cummings[252] treated 12 cases and added 12 cases from the literature for a total of 24 patients and 25 lesions. Local tumor control was achieved in 11 of 24 (9 to 54 months' follow-up). Six of seven tumors treated with 4-Gy fractions or larger were controlled, versus 5 of 18 treated with smaller fractions. Saigal et al.[8] treated 17 patients with mucosal melanomas (sinonasal tract in 11, oral cavity in 6) with surgery (16 combined with RT) and 1 with RT. Seven patients received adjuvant immunotherapy. With a median follow-up of 35.2 months, local tumor control at 5 years was 81%, disease-free survival 44.5%, and overall survival 51.5%. Krengli et al.[270] reported on 74 patients with upper aerodigestive tract mucosal melanomas (31 nasal and 12 oral), 17 treated with surgery alone, 42 with surgery and RT (median dose 60 Gy, 2-Gy fractions), 11 with RT alone, and 4 with chemoimmunotherapy. At 3 years, the local recurrence was 43% with surgery alone and 29% with surgery plus RT. Grade 3 mucositis was noted in nine patients.

Kingdom and Kaplan[271] described results in 13 patients with mucosal melanoma of the nasal cavity and paranasal sinuses treated with surgical resection. Eight had microscopically negative margins. Seven patients received postoperative irradiation (30 to 62 Gy). The neck was treated in three patients with doses of 30 to 50 Gy. The local tumor recurrence rate was 85% (11 of 13), with a mean interval from primary tumor treatment to recurrence of 16 months. Metastatic neck disease developed in two patients and distant metastases in four. Patients receiving postoperative irradiation had increased disease-free interval and prolonged survival. Negative surgical margins were not predictive of a more favorable outcome. The investigators recommend resection of tumor with negative margins and postoperative irradiation for the treatment of all patients with mucosal malignant melanoma.

Zenda et al.[254] treated 14 patients with head and neck mucosal melanomas using protons (60 Gy in 15 fractions, 3 fractions per week). With a median follow-up of 36.7 months, the 3-year local tumor control was 85.7% and overall survival 58%. The most frequent failure site was the cervical nodes (six patients). Two patients developed late decreased visual acuity. Carbon ion therapy was used by Yanagi et al.[272] in the primary treatment of 72 patients with mucosal melanomas of the head and neck (dose ranging from 52.8 to 64 GyE in 16 fractions). With a median follow-up of 49 months, local tumor control at 5 years was 84%, cause-specific survival 39.6%, and overall survival 27%. No grade 3 morbidity was observed. Jingu et al.[273] treated 37 patients with head and neck melanomas with carbon ions (57.6 GyE in 16 fractions) and chemotherapy. With a median follow-up of 19 months, the local tumor control at 3 years was 65.3% and overall survival 81%. MRI minimum apparent diffusion coefficient was a prognostic factor for survival.

Section III

LENTIGO MALIGNA MELANOMA

Natural History

Lentigo maligna (Hutchinson melanotic freckle[274] or circumscribed precancerous melanosis of Dubreuilh) and its invasive counterpart, lentigo maligna melanoma (LMM), are well-recognized clinical–pathologic entities. LMM comprises about 10% of all melanomas in the head and neck, occurs predominantly on the face and ears of elderly persons, and generally has a very long natural history, frequently reaching a large size before diagnosis. Approximately one-third of lentigo maligna lesions, if left untreated, will eventually transform into invasive LMM.

Tannous et al.[275] hypothesized that lentigo maligna can be divided into two categories: one represents a pigmented lesion that is a precursor to melanoma and the other melanoma *in situ*. Also, they hypothesized that in some patients, there is a progression to malignant melanoma.

Clinical Presentation and Diagnostic Workup

These lesions appear as circumscribed and later as more diffuse areas of hyperpigmentation of the skin. They may develop some superficial nodularity and eventual ulceration as they become more invasive. In 10% of the latter patients, regional and distant metastases eventually develop. The 10% metastatic spread in LMM contrasts with the 25% metastatic tendency in nodular melanomas arising in superficial spreading melanomas and a 50% metastatic spread in nodular melanomas arising *de novo*.

The diagnostic workup of these patients is similar to that of patients suspected of having malignant melanoma. Biopsies of the lesion are required to obtain histopathologic confirmation of the diagnosis. Careful physical examination must rule out any areas of extension or regional or distant spread.

General Management

The usual treatment of lentigo maligna and LMM has been surgery, with approximately 5- to 10-mm margin of normal skin or Mohs surgery, although larger margins may be required for ill-defined lesions.[276] Radiation therapy is used for more extensive lesions or for postsurgical recurrences.[276] Hill and Gramp[277] reported on 66 cases of LMM, 38% of which required two excisions or more to clear the tumor and 32% of cases showed evidence of invasive melanoma. Only one case has recurred thus far, and none have developed metastatic disease. For larger lesions, wider surgical excision with skin grafting has been reported to give poor cosmetic results.

Cohen et al.[278] reported their experience with Mohs microsurgery, which was performed in 26 patients with lentigo maligna and 19 patients with LMM. After a median follow-up of 58 months (214.3 patient-years), there was one recurrence, in a patient with five prior recurrences before Mohs micrographic surgery. Kuflik and Gage[279] treated 30 patients with cryosurgery. Lesions ranged from 1.3 to 4.5 cm in diameter. Lesions recurred in two patients (recurrence rate of 6.6%) who were successfully retreated with cryosurgery. Eleven patients observed for more than 5 years showed no recurrences.

Because of the low incidence of regional lymph node metastases, elective lymph node dissection is not indicated.

Radiation therapy with various techniques has been frequently used in the treatment of these patients, particularly those with larger lesions, because of minimal morbidity and generally excellent cosmetic results (Fig. 51.16).

Radiation Therapy Techniques

As in other skin lesions, the portals should be carefully designed to include the entire tumor with adequate margin (1 cm for lesions <2 cm and 2 cm for larger tumors). Because Miescher irradiation technique used very superficial x-rays, with 50% depth dose being at approximately 1 mm, there is the possibility of local recurrence if dermal extension is unrecognized. Therefore, Harwood and Lawson[256] recommend using minimum x-ray energies of 100 keVp and preferably 140 to 175 keVp to treat these patients. Superficial x-rays (100 to 200 keVp) with adequate filtration or electrons (6 to 9 MeV)

FIGURE 51.16. Lentigo maligna melanoma of the face before **(A)** and 6 years after **(B)** 50 Gy in 25 fractions delivered with 9-MeV electrons and bolus.

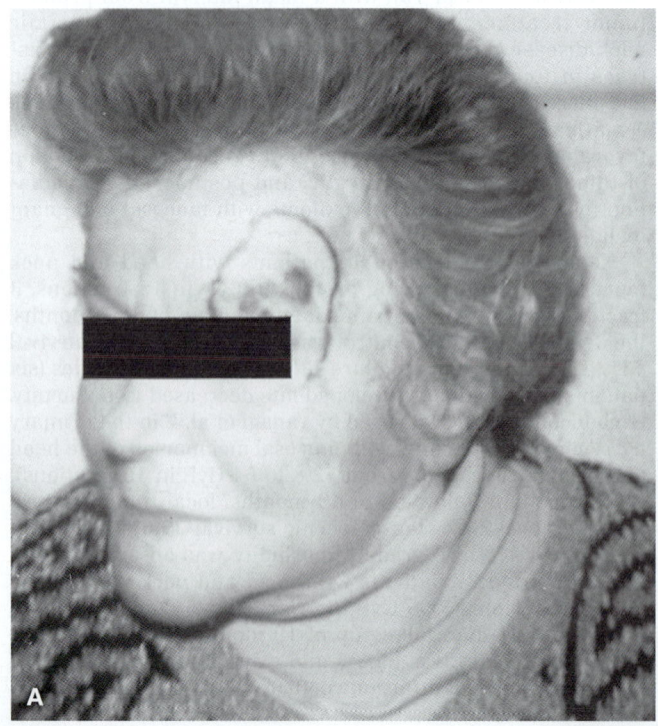
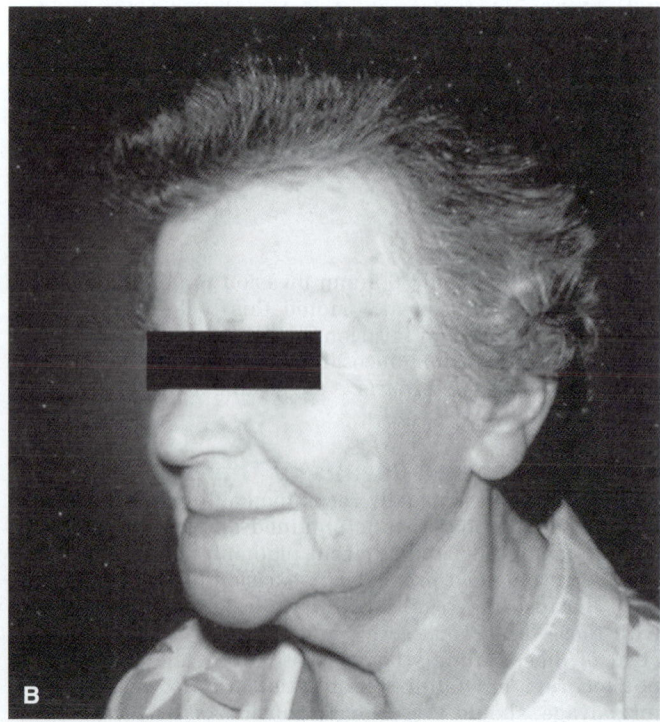

with appropriate thickness of bolus (1 to 1.5 cm) are adequate for most patients. Doses of 45 to 50 Gy in 15 to 25 fractions delivered over 3 to 5 weeks will control the disease in most patients. The authors recommend delivering 3 to 3.5 Gy, 3 times weekly, every other day, to a total of 50 Gy, depending on the size and thickness of the lesion. Elective irradiation of the regional lymphatics is not necessary. Traditionally, high dose rate (HDR) brachytherapy (BT) scalp molds have been considered the ultimate conformal therapy. Santos et al.[279a] described a new technique, tangential volumetric modulated arc therapy (TVMAT), that gives superior dosimetry to brachytherapy and conventional VMAT (cVMAT). TVMAT treats with the beam tangential to the surface of the scalp. The collimating jaws protect dose-sensitive tissue in close proximity to the PTV. Not all the PTV is within the beam aperture as defined by the jaws during all the beam-on time. TVMAT gave the best homogeneity and conformality; the PTV 98% volume was covered by 99.85% prescription dose. The conformity number for the BT, cVMAT, and TVMAT was 0.30, 0.69, and 0.83 respectively.

Careful follow-up with clinical examinations and photographs of the lesion is essential to ascertain the continuing regression of the tumor.

In patients on whom surgical excision is performed, postoperative irradiation is recommended if positive margins are found.[113] Doses are similar to those stated earlier.

Results of Therapy

Harwood and Lawson[266] described 13 patients with lentigo maligna treated with radiation therapy: 11 had local tumor control, 1 had an edge recurrence salvaged by irradiation, and 1 had residual tumor (alive and well 11 years after treatment for the recurrence). One patient alive at 2 years refused further treatment. Of 19 patients irradiated for LMM, 17 had tumor control with radiation therapy alone for periods ranging from 6 months to 6 years. One patient had a central recurrence that was salvaged by surgery (alive and well 5 years after treatment of recurrence). No patient has developed lymph node or distant metastases in either group.

Tsang et al.[263] described results in 54 patients treated with radiation therapy or surgery. Younger patients with smaller lesions were treated with surgical excision (18 patients) and achieved actuarial tumor control of 94% at 3 years. Older patients with larger lesions located in the head and neck area were treated by radiation therapy (36 patients), with an actuarial tumor control rate of 86% at 5 years. No patient developed metastatic melanoma. The late cosmetic appearance was acceptable in the majority of irradiated patients, with 11% showing poor cosmesis because of progressive skin pallor, atrophy, and telangiectasia in the treated area.

SARCOMAS OF THE HEAD AND NECK

Natural History

Sarcomas account for <1% of malignant neoplasms in the head and neck. The most frequent histologic type is malignant fibrohistiocytoma (29%), whereas the least common is liposarcoma (1%). The histology is complex and requires immunochemical analysis including angiosarcoma, chondrosarcoma, hemangiosarcoma, leiomyosarcoma, liposarcoma, malignant fibrous sarcoma, neurofibrosarcoma, osteosarcoma, RMS, malignant schwannoma, and synovial sarcoma. Fibrosarcoma, angiosarcoma, leiomyosarcoma, and RMS are the most common types, but this varies in published reports. Distribution of these sarcomas was 33% in the scalp or face, 26% in the orbit or paranasal sinuses, 14% arising from upper aerodigestive tract including the larynx, and 27% in the neck. Synovial sarcomas are rare soft tissue malignancies in the head and neck region; they account for 3% to 5% of head and neck tumors.

Histologic, immunohistochemical, and characteristic chromosomal translocation findings are necessary for diagnosis. The poor prognosis of this sarcoma justifies radical surgery with postoperative radiation.[280]

Radiation-induced sarcoma of the head and neck is a rare long-term complication of treatment. The rarity of this tumor is reflected in the very few series reported in the English language medical literature.[281,282] When they do occur, most appear at least 10 years following radiation therapy. There is a possibility of a postirradiation sarcoma whenever a suspicious lesion is seen, regardless of the amount of time that has passed since radiation therapy was administered. The original pathology should be re-examined to ensure that the original tumor was diagnosed correctly. Electron microscopy can be useful in differentiating sarcomatous-appearing epithelial lesions from true soft tissue sarcomas.

The incidence of radiation-induced sarcomas of the head and neck is, however, likely to increase due to progressive aging of the population combined with improved survival in head and neck cancer patients. This problem can be extremely challenging, and the overall outlook has been reported to be very bleak. Patel et al.[282] reviewed 69 cases reported in the English medical literature since 1966 and pooled this information with their experience in treatment of 10 patients. This group was compared for survival with 124 patients with a diagnosis of head and neck sarcoma registered on the Head and Neck Sarcoma database at the Royal Marsden Hospital. There was no site prediction for radiation-induced sarcoma of the head and neck, but malignant fibrous histiocytoma was the most common pathologic diagnosis. The period of latency between initial radiation therapy and diagnosis ranged from 9 to 45 years, with a median of 17 years. Surgery was the mainstay of treatment, and follow-up ranged from 6 months to 15 years with a median of 48 months. The actuarial 5-year disease-free survival rate in these patients was 60%.

Clinical Presentation and Diagnostic Workup

Clinical presentation varies with the primary site of disease. Tumors arising from the aerodigestive tract usually present with nasal bleeding, a palpable mass in the neck, or difficulty in swallowing or breathing. In tumors arising from the base of the skull or the nerve sheath, cranial nerve deficit is the most common presentation. Diagnostic workup follows that of soft tissue sarcomas of other sites in the body. With early lesions, radiographs or CT may show only nonspecific opacification, soft tissue swelling, and occasionally bone destruction. Table 51.1 outlines the suggested diagnostic workup. MRI, especially with gadolinium contrast, may be used as a supplement or alternative to CT scanning.[283,284] A CT scan of the chest is also mandatory for staging workup.

The American Joint Committee on Cancer staging system for soft tissue sarcomas is based on histologic grade, the tumor size and depth, and the presence of distant or nodal metastases. The staging system is the same as for sarcomas of the extremities, although specific staging for head and neck sarcomas is not standardized.[216]

Prognostic Factors

Prognostic factors for predicting local recurrence or disease-free survival include anatomic site, treatment modality, tumor histology and grade, tumor size, extension of disease, lymph node metastasis, and surgical margins.[280,285-287]

A report from Royal Marsden Hospital showed anatomic location and treatment modality to be independent prognostic factors for local recurrence; tumors of the head had a better local RFS than did those of the neck.[80] Patients treated with a combination of surgery and radiation therapy had a better RFS than did those treated with surgery or irradiation alone. The only significant independent prognostic factor for overall survival was the implementation of definitive surgery versus biopsy. In the above report, the prognostic impact of tumor stage and grade did not reach statistical significance. In contrast, Tran et al.[288] reported that 90% of patients with low-grade tumors were free of disease versus only 16% with high-grade lesions.

Bentz et al.[10] reviewed 111 head and neck sarcoma patients; median duration of follow-up was 51 months; the actuarial 5-year relapse-free, disease-specific, and overall survivals were 55%, 52%, and 44%, respectively. By multivariate analysis, size and grade significantly influenced all survivals, whereas margin status additionally influenced relapse-free survival.

In 109 soft tissue sarcomas of all sites, a French study demonstrated that quality of the surgery was one of the most important variables for predicting local recurrences. Tumor size, surgical margins, presence of tumor necrosis, and adequacy of the excision correlated with metastasis-free survival.[289]

General Management
Surgery is the preferred initial treatment modality for sarcomas.[237,289a] Unfortunately, it is often difficult to achieve complete resection of the tumor, and a high recurrence rate has been observed with surgery alone.[290] Extracapsular enucleation of the tumor results in 90% local recurrence because of the presence of microscopic pseudopodia, which tend to grow through the pseudocapsule into the surrounding tissue, and the presence of skipped lesions some distance from the main tumor mass. Pathologic analysis of the surgical bed often discloses microscopic extension of tumor. Farhood et al.,[290] in a review of 176 cases of adult head and neck sarcomas, reported that the pathologic margins of surgical specimens obtained by wide local excision were positive in >50% of cases. This resulted in inferior overall survival for sarcomas of the head and neck when compared with extremity sarcomas.[240] Wide local excision, with a 5-cm margin around the pseudocapsule in extremity sarcomas, is associated with better outcome, although approximately 20% will have local recurrence. The criteria for surgical resection are impractical for head and neck sarcomas because of anatomic limitations[216]; wide local excision is rarely possible because the tumors extend beyond the confines of origin and in the proximity of vital neurovascular structures. Some retrospective studies have suggested improved local tumor control when combined surgery and external irradiation are used. In 130 patients with soft tissue sarcomas of the head and neck treated with surgery alone at Royal Marsden Hospital, the overall 5-year survival was 50%; local tumor control was only 47%, and local recurrence was the cause of death in 63% of cases. Patients treated with combined modality treatment (surgery and irradiation) had less extensive surgery, yet local RFS was longer.[286]

Synovial sarcoma in the head and neck is rare. In a report of 36 patients, Al-Daraji et al.[291] noted there was a predilection for the parotid and the temporal regions, and nine involved skeletal muscle. Of 29 patients followed for a median of 14 years after surgical treatment, 11 were alive and tumor free.

A multidisciplinary discussion before the initiation of treatment is required to formulate the best approach for radiation delivery, surgical technique, and mode of reconstruction.

Radiation Therapy
Radiation therapy, by external beam or brachytherapy, plays an important adjunctive role in disease management, especially for tumors where en bloc resection with negative margin is not possible.[287,292] Chemotherapy regimens are available for soft tissue neoplasms, primarily designed to improve local tumor control.[129] A systematic review of radiation therapy trials was performed by the Swedish Council of Technology Assessment in Health Care.[292] This synthesis of the literature

on radiation therapy for soft tissue sarcomas is based on data from five randomized trials. Moreover, data from 6 prospective studies, 25 retrospective studies, and 3 other articles were used. In total, 39 scientific articles were included, involving 4,579 patients. The results were compared with those of a similar overview from 1996, which included 3,344 patients. There was evidence that adjuvant radiotherapy improves local tumor control in combination with conservation surgery with negative, marginal, or minimal microscopic positive surgical margins. There are still insufficient data to establish that preoperative radiotherapy is favorable compared to postoperative radiotherapy in patients presenting primarily with large tumors. The preoperative setting results in more wound complications. There is no randomized study comparing external beam radiotherapy and brachytherapy. These data suggest that external beam radiotherapy and low–dose rate brachytherapy result in comparable local control for high-grade tumors. Some patients with low-grade soft tissue sarcomas benefit from external beam radiotherapy in terms of local control. Brachytherapy with a low dose rate for low-grade tumors seems to be of no benefit, but data are sparse. In two small studies investigating hyperfractionation schedules, there was no indication of improvements compared to daily fractions of 2 Gy.

Mesenchymal chondrosarcoma of the sinonasal tract is a rare, malignant tumor of extraskeletal origin.[95] Thirteen patients with sinonasal mesenchymal chondrosarcoma presented with nasal obstruction ($n = 8$), epistaxis ($n = 7$), mass effect ($n = 4$), or a combination of these. The maxillary sinus was the most common site of involvement ($n = 9$), followed by the ethmoid sinuses ($n = 7$) and the nasal cavity ($n = 5$). All cases were managed by surgery with ART ($n = 4$) and/or chemotherapy ($n = 3$). The overall mean survival was 12.1 years, although five of six patients who developed local recurrences died of disease (mean survival, 6.5 years). Six patients were alive and disease free (mean survival, 17.3 years), and two patients were lost to follow-up.

Radiation Therapy Techniques
General principles for radiation therapy of head and neck sarcomas are similar to those of soft tissue sarcomas. Complete coverage of the surgical bed and scar with adequate margins (3 to 5 cm) is required.[293] However, because of the proximity of critical and radiosensitive organs (eyes, spinal cord, brainstem), selecting optimal portal margins without seriously compromising the functioning of these organs is an art. Techniques similar to those used in epithelial tumors of the head and neck can be applied to sarcomas. In general, 55 to 60 Gy is needed for postoperative adjuvant irradiation, and an additional 10- to 15-Gy boost is recommended if the surgical margins are close (≤3 mm) or involved by tumor. Some institutions prefer preoperative irradiation of 45 to 50 Gy. Special attention should be directed to limiting the dose to critical structures. Use of a 3-D or IMRT treatment technique can be considered as demonstrated in Fig. 51.8.

Results of Therapy
Because of the propensity for sarcomas to invade the surrounding tissues, complete surgical clearance may be difficult. In a series from UCLA, attempted en bloc resection left residual tumor at the surgical margins in 52 of 127 patients.[288] The incidence of local recurrence was high (60%) with surgery alone.

In a retrospective report of 73 patients with sarcomas of the head and neck treated at Princess Margaret Hospital, the 5-year cause-specific survival was 62%, with a local recurrence rate of 41% and a distant metastasis rate of 31%.[283] Extension to adjacent structures, high-grade tumor, and tumor >10 cm were associated with poor survival. Gross residual tumor after surgery was also associated with a high local recurrence rate (75%) despite the addition of radiation therapy. Patients with clear surgical margins or only microscopic involvement fared much more favorably and had a similar local tumor control rate (74% and 70%, respectively), provided adjuvant irradiation was given. Because of the difficulty in obtaining wide surgical margins, 68% of the patients died as a result of uncontrolled local disease. These data substantiate the importance of surgical margins as well as the contribution of adjuvant irradiation.[283]

Colville et al.[216] reported on 41 male and 19 female patients treated with head and neck soft tissue sarcomas, with an overall 5-year survival of 60%. Twenty-five patients had surgery alone, 20 had surgery and pre- or postoperative radiation therapy, and 15 received nonsurgical treatment. With a mean follow-up of almost 4 years, the 5-year local tumor control was 56% in the surgical group and 40% in the nonsurgical group (more advanced and aggressive tumors). The 5-year survival was 70% and 40%, respectively.

Penel et al.[294] recorded their experience with 28 adult head and neck soft tissue sarcomas. The most common subtype was RMS (seven cases). Twenty-two patients presented with previous inadequate resection performed elsewhere before admission. Nineteen patients had surgery (complete resection in 13 cases). Associated treatments were neoadjuvant chemotherapy, adjuvant chemotherapy, and postoperative radiotherapy in 4, 3, and 10 cases, respectively. The 2-year overall survival rate was 56%. Wolden et al.[295] treated 28 patients with head and neck RMS using IMRT (50 to 55 Gy in 1.8 Gy fractions) combined with chemotherapy. With a median follow-up of 24 months, local tumor control was 95% to 100% and 3-year survival. McDonald et al.[296] treated 20 children with RMS in the head and neck with IMRT (median dose 50.4 Gy, 1.8 per fraction). With a median follow-up of 29 months, the 3-year local tumor control was 100% and survival 76%.

Pandey et al.[297] reported on 22 cases of head and neck sarcomas (the neck, lower jaw, tongue, cheek, scalp, and maxilla were the most common sites affected). None of the patients had palpable neck nodes or distant metastasis at presentation. All the patients were treated with primary surgical resection, followed by adjuvant treatment in 14 cases (63.6%). After a median follow-up of 14.5 months, two patients died, six developed local recurrence, four developed metastatic disease, and another patient developed a second primary sarcoma. The overall 5-year survival was 80%, whereas the 5-year disease-free survival rate was 24.1%.

Barker et al.[16] published a review of 44 patients with nonmetastatic soft tissue sarcoma in the head and neck. The most common tumor histologies included malignant fibrous histiocytoma (15 patients), angiosarcoma (9 patients), fibrosarcoma (6 patients), and leiomyosarcoma (6 patients). The median overall survival for all patients was 79 months. The actuarial 5-year local tumor control was 55% and was highly correlated with the extent of surgical excision: 25% for subtotal resection or debulking, 65% for wide local excision, and 100% for radical excision. Local tumor control at 5 years was 60% for patients treated with both surgery and radiotherapy, 54% for surgery alone, and 43% for radiation alone. ART significantly improved the local control rates (from 25% to 54%) for patients with close (<2 mm) or positive surgical margins. Of 14 patients with locoregional failure in whom salvage was attempted, 9 (64%) were rendered disease free.

Moalikyar et al.[298] reported on 40 patients with head and neck sarcomas, histologies including undifferentiated pleomorphic sarcoma (9), fibrosarcoma (6), chondrosarcoma (6), angiosarcoma (5), spindle cell sarcoma (3), osteosarcoma (3), and others (7). Tumor sites were the scalp or skin (11), mandible or temporomandibular joint (9), skull base or paranasal sinuses (9), neck (6), or upper airways (6). Histologic grade was low for 13, intermediate for 5, high for 17, and unavailable for 5. All patients underwent gross total tumor resection; 22 treated with surgery alone (57%), whereas 18 patients received surgery and postoperative RT (43%). At a median follow-up of 14.9 months, the 2-year OS, LRC, and distant metastasis control (DC) were 68%, 73%, and 74%, respectively. Positive margins significantly reduced both 2-year LRC (52% vs. 84%; P = .01) and OS (42% vs. 81%; P = .004). The addition of adjuvant RT did not improve 2-year LC (70% vs. 77%; P > .05) or OS (58% vs. 79%; P > .05). However, among the subgroup of patients with positive margins, use of RT improved 2-year OS (73% vs. 0%; P = .03) without an associated LC benefit. Similarly, improved 2-year OS was identified for high-grade tumors treated with RT (73% vs. 0%; P = .03) with no associated LC benefit. Sarcomas of the skull base or paranasal sinuses demonstrated significantly worse 2-year LC (28% vs. 86%; P = .0002) and OS (0% vs. 83%; P = .001) than other evaluated subsites.

Huang et al.[299] extracted data from 1,525 patients from the Surveillance, Epidemiology, and End Results (SEER) database with diagnosis of head and neck sarcoma treated between 1973 and 2010. Selected patients had no prior malignancies and no distant metastatic disease. The most common histology was fibrohistiocytic tumors (18.6%), followed by unspecified sarcomas (15.5%), blood vessel tumors (14.0%), liposarcomas (12.1%), and leiomyosarcomas (11.6%). Most tumors were nonspecifically coded as connective tissue of the head, face, and neck (60.3%). After that, the most common site was the skin/scalp (19.6%), followed by nasal cavity/paranasal sinus (4.6%) and oral cavity (3.9%). Of the cohort, 576 patients (37.8%) received RT in addition to surgery.

With a median follow-up of 48 months, the 5-, 10-, and 15-year OS rates were 64%, 49%, and 42%, respectively. The median OS in patients treated with surgery and RT was 82 months, which was inferior to that of 139 months in patients with surgery only (P < .001). Multivariate analyses showed that age > 60, regional stage, high grade, and tumor size >5 cm were factors associated with worse survival. RT seemed to improve OS, but that result was not statistically significant (hazard ratio 0.90, P = .247).

Further analyses showed that patients with high-grade tumors had an improved OS by RT (hazard ratio 0.78, P = .017). The median survival was 59 months in patients with RT versus 45 months in those patients without RT. There was no significant difference in OS among patients with low-grade tumors by RT.

Brandmaier et al.[300] also analyzed the SEER database for local H&N cancers diagnosed between 1990 and 2011 that included an array of 12 sarcoma subtypes totaling 1,046 patients. Tumor size and staging data were limited. For all H&N sarcoma patients, the surgery-alone cohort had a 5-year OS of 65.4% compared to 53.3% for patients receiving surgery and adjuvant RT (P = .0009). The 5-year cancer-specific survival (CSS) in the surgery cohort was 82.4% compared to 64% in patients receiving surgery and adjuvant RT (P < .0001). Age >75 years was a negative prognostic factor for CSS, relative to age 20 to 39, with a hazard ratio of 1.61 (P = .033). High-grade histology was also a negative prognostic factor for CSS; grade 3 tumors had a hazard ratio of 8.0 relative to grade 1 (P < .0001). Among patients with grade 3 sarcomas, those receiving surgery alone had a 5-year OS of 48.2% versus 43.7% for those receiving surgery and RT (P = .81).

Among a smaller subset of stage T1N0 grade 3 sarcomas, the 5-year OS for surgery alone was 61.1% versus 51.6% for surgery and RT (P = .89). The CSS for the two groups was 77.5% and 71.6%, respectively (P = .99).

The authors hypothesized that adjuvant RT could be beneficial for grade 3 H&N sarcomas, regardless of tumor stage or margin status.

Mahmoud et al.[301] using the National Cancer Database (NCDB) evaluated radiation therapy (RT) utilization pattern and outcome of adjuvant therapies in 2,096 patients with nonmetastatic H&N sarcomas diagnosed between 2004 and 2012, who underwent tumor resection. Chi-square test assessed the cohort that included 1,366 males and 730 females with a

Section III

TABLE 51.15 TREATMENT RESULTS OF ADULT SOFT TISSUE SARCOMAS OF THE HEAD AND NECK

Author (Reference)	Number of Patients	Modalities	5-Year Actuarial Rates	
			Local Control (%)	Survival (%)
Weber et al.[302]	188	S, R, C	—	Overall: 49.4 (<5 cm) Overall: 30.4 (≥5 cm)
Greager et al.[303]	48	S, R, C	—	Disease free: 54
Farhood et al.[290]	176	S, R, C	—	Overall: 55
McKenna et al.[304]	16	S, R, C	75	Disease free: 63
Eeles et al.[286]	103[a]	S, R, C	47	Overall: 50
LeVay et al.[283]	52	S, R, C	59	Cause specific: 63
Tran et al.[288]	164	S, R, C	41	Overall: 66
Willers et al.[287]	57	S, R, C	60	Overall: 66
Chao et al.[152]	33	S, R, C	49	Disease free: 40
Colville et al.[216]	60	S, R, C	50	60

[a]Series based on adults and children, excluding angiosarcomas.
C, chemotherapy; R, radiation therapy; S, surgery.

median age of 62 years (range: 18 to 90). Fibromatous sarcoma (20%) and high grades (36%) were the most common histology and grade, respectively. RT delivery was significantly more frequent in high-grade, large tumors with positive surgical margins. At a median follow-up of 36 months, RT use did not impact survival nor did CT, which was delivered in 260 patients. Restricting the survival analysis to 752 high-grade patients, the 5-year OS improved from 43% to 54%, with RT delivery reducing mortality hazards ratio (HR) by 36% ($P < .001$).

Their analysis hinted that ART improves survival in high-grade H&N sarcomas and that chemotherapy may not be beneficial.

Reported results of treatment of soft tissue sarcomas are summarized in Table 51.15.

Protons

Protons or heavy ions have been used in selected patients.[305] Hug et al.[306] reported on 27 patients treated at Massachusetts General Hospital in Boston (18 primary and 9 recurrent sarcomas of the head and neck close or abutting critical structures with 160-MeV protons; mean dose 68.5 GyE in 2.1-GyE fractions). Local recurrence was seen in eight patients (29%) and regional recurrence in six patients (22%). Tumor grade had a significant impact on outcome. One patient developed Lhermitte sign and another hypothyroidism.

Jingu et al.[273] described results in 27 patients with head and neck unresectable bone and soft tissue sarcomas, treated with carbon ions (57.6, 64.0, or 70.4 GyE in 16 fractions). The 3-year local tumor control was 91.6% and survival 72%. Therapy was well tolerated. A comparison with historical results showed that local tumor control rate with 70.4 GyE was significantly higher than that with 57.6 or 64.0 GyE (3-year, 91.8% vs. 23.6%, $P < .0001$). Furthermore, the overall survival with 70.4 GyE tended to be higher than that with 57.6 or 64.0 GyE (3-year, 74.1% vs. 42.9%, $P = .09$).

Tumor Characteristics and Prognosis

Several series have shown that tumor grade and size dictate the outcome of patients with head and neck sarcomas such as leiomyosarcoma, RMS, and malignant fibrous sarcoma.[278] Farhood et al.,[290] in a review of 176 adult head and neck sarcomas, found that only 20% of the patients with high-grade tumors were alive 10 years after treatment, compared with 88% of patients with low-grade tumors. Weber et al.[302] described a 45% 10-year survival rate for patients with tumors <5 cm versus 10% for those with tumors ≥5 cm.

Many series have reported that chondrosarcoma is not a radiosensitive tumor, and radiation therapy has no role in its treatment. However, some reports have demonstrated the

contribution of radiation therapy in this histology. McNaney et al.[307] described a 65% survival rate at 2 years in 20 chondrosarcoma patients who received primary radiation therapy. Tumor grade was the most important prognostic factor.

Osteogenic sarcoma of the head and neck has a pattern of recurrence different from similar tumors elsewhere in the body. Head and neck osteosarcomas are usually high grade; they have a very high incidence of local recurrence but a lower risk of distant metastases. Several studies have used adjuvant irradiation and chemotherapy, which commonly results in improved locoregional tumor control and survival. Tran et al.[288] reported a 73% 5-year survival rate in patients with osteogenic sarcoma of the head and neck treated with high-dose preoperative irradiation followed by wide surgical excision.

Chemotherapy

Head and neck soft tissue sarcomas frequently metastasize; 25% of patients in a UCLA study had distant metastases.[268] The role of adjuvant chemotherapy to improve disease-free survival in sarcoma of the head and neck is controversial. Unlike with soft tissue sarcomas of the extremities, in which distant metastasis is the most common cause of death, the majority of deaths in sarcomas of the head and neck are associated with local failure. Approximately half of the distant metastases were detected after local recurrence occurred.[283] Chemotherapy did not appear to affect local tumor control.

In a series of 94 patients treated at UCLA,[247] local control was achieved in 52% of patients treated with surgery alone and 90% of those receiving adjuvant irradiation with or without chemotherapy.

For preoperative neoadjuvant chemotherapy, which supplements radiation therapy to downstage disease before surgery, satisfactory results are available only for sarcomas of extremities.[226] With the exception of RMS, postoperative adjuvant chemotherapy for head and neck sarcomas should be given only in a clinical trial setting.

REFERENCES

1. Davidson J, Gullane P. Glomus vagale tumors. *Otolaryngol Head Neck Surg* 1988;99:66–70.
2. Larson TC III, Reese DF, Baker HL Jr, et al. Glomus tympanicum chemodectomas: Radiographic and clinical characteristics. *Radiology* 1987;163:801–806.
3. Konefal JB, Pilepich MV, Spector GJ, et al. Radiation therapy in the treatment of chemodectomas. *Laryngoscope* 1987;97:1331–1335.
4. Mendenhall WM, Million RR, Parsons JT, et al. Chemodectoma of the carotid body and ganglion nodosum treated with radiation therapy. *Int J Radiat Oncol Biol Phys* 1986;12:2175–2178.
5. Magliulo G, Zardo F, Varacalli S, et al. Multiple paragangliomas of the head and neck. *An Otorrinolaringol Ibero Am* 2003;30:31–38.
6. Semaan MT, Megerian CA. Current assessment and management of glomus tumors. *Curr Opin Otolaryngol Head Neck Surg* 2008;16:420–426.
7. Gaut AW, Jay AP, Robinson RA, et al. Invasive glomus tumor of the nasal cavity. *Am J Otolaryngol* 2005;26:207–209.
8. Saigal K, Palmer J, Reis I, et al. Mucosal melanomas of the head and neck: A modern experience at the University of Miami. *Int J Radiat Oncol Biol Phys* 2010;78:S479.
9. Manolidis S, Shohet JA, Jackson CG, et al. Malignant glomus tumors. *Laryngoscope* 1999;109:30–34.
10. Bentz BG, Singh B, Woodruff J, et al. Head and neck soft tissue sarcomas: a multivariate analysis of outcomes. *Ann Surg Oncol* 2004;11:619–628.
11. Vogl TJ, Juergens M, Balzer JO, et al. Glomus tumors of the skull base: Combined use of mr angiography and spin-echo imaging. *Radiology* 1994;192:103–110.
12. Drape JL, Idy-Peretti I, Goettmann S, et al. Subungual glomus tumors: evaluation with mr imaging. *Radiology* 1995;195:507–515.
13. Christie A, Teasdale E. A comparative review of multidetector CT angiography and MRI in the diagnosis of jugular foramen lesions. *Clin Radiol* 2010;65:213–217.
14. Astner S, Essler M, Bundschuh R, et al. 18f-octreotate positron emission tomography (PET) for target volume delineation in stereotactic radiation therapy planning of glomus tumors. *Int J Radiat Oncol Biol Phys* 2007;69:S545–S546.
15. Rutkowski MJ, Sughrue ME, Kane AJ, et al. Predictors of mortality following treatment of intracranial hemangiopericytoma. *J Neurosurg* 2010;113:333–339.
16. Barker JL Jr, Paulino AC, Feeney S, et al. Locoregional treatment for adult soft tissue sarcomas of the head and neck: an institutional review. *Cancer J* 2003;9:49–57.

17. Batsakis JG. *Tumors of the head and neck: clinical and pathological considerations.* 2nd ed. Baltimore, MD: Williams & Wilkins, 1979.

18. Batsakis JG. Wegener's granulomatosis and midline (nonhealing) "granuloma". *Head Neck Surg* 1979;1:213–222.

19. Glasscock ME III, Jackson CG, Johnson GD, et al. Radiation therapy in chemodectoma treatment. *Laryngoscope* 1988;98:465–466.

20. McCabe BF, Fletcher M. Selection of therapy of glomus jugulare tumors. *Arch Otolaryngol* 1969;89:156–159.

21. Li G, Chang S, Adler JR Jr, et al. Irradiation of glomus jugulare tumors: a historical perspective. *Neurosurg Focus* 2007;23:E13.

22. Abud DG, Mounayer C, Benndorf G, et al. Intratumoral injection of cyanoacrylate glue in head and neck paragangliomas. *AJNR Am J Neuroradiol* 2004;25:1457–1462.

23. Ozyer U, Harman A, Yildirim E, et al. Devascularization of head and neck paragangliomas by direct percutaneous embolization. *Cardiovasc Intervent Radiol* 2010;33:967–975.

24. Cummings BJ, Beale FA, Garrett PG, et al. The treatment of glomus tumors in the temporal bone by megavoltage radiation. *Cancer* 1984;53:2635–2640.

25. Powell S, Peters N, Harmer C. Chemodectoma of the head and neck: results of treatment in 84 patients. *Int J Radiat Oncol Biol Phys* 1992;22:919–924.

26. Spagnolo DV, Papadimitriou JM, Archer M. Postirradiation malignant fibrous histiocytoma arising in juvenile nasopharyngeal angiofibroma and producing alpha-1-antitrypsin. *Histopathology* 1984;8:339–352.

27. Suit HD, Gallager HS. Intact tumor cells in irradiated tissue. *Arch Pathol* 1964;78:648–651.

28. Krych AJ, Foote RL, Brown PD, et al. Long-term results of irradiation for paraganglioma. *Int J Radiat Oncol Biol Phys* 2006;65:1063–1066.

29. Springate SC, Weichselbaum RR. Radiation or surgery for chemodectoma of the temporal bone: a review of local control and complications. *Head Neck* 1990;12:303–307.

30. Dickens WJ, Million RR, Cassisi NJ, et al. Chemodectomas arising in temporal bone structures. *Laryngoscope* 1982;92:188–191.

31. Onal C, Ozcelik TB, Sonmez S, et al. Radiation dose distribution in the external auditory canal with different prosthetic materials: a clinical report. *J Prosthet Dent* 2010;104:288–292.

32. Combs SE, Konkel S, Schulz-Ertner D, et al. Intensity modulated radiotherapy (IMRT) in patients with carcinomas of the paranasal sinuses: clinical benefit for complex shaped target volumes. *Radiat Oncol* 2006;1:23.

33. Ares C, Hug EB, Lomax AJ, et al. Effectiveness and safety of spot scanning proton radiation therapy for chordomas and chondrosarcomas of the skull base: first long-term report. *Int J Radiat Oncol Biol Phys* 2009;75:1111–1118.

34. Schulz-Ertner D, Haberer T, Jakel O, et al. Radiotherapy for chordomas and low-grade chondrosarcomas of the skull base with carbon ions. *Int J Radiat Oncol Biol Phys* 2002;53:36–42.

35. Lloyd G, Howard D, Lund VJ, et al. Imaging for juvenile angiofibroma. *J Laryngol Otol* 2000;114:727–730.

36. Griffiths RW, Briggs JC. Biopsy procedures, primary wide excisional surgery and long term prognosis in primary clinical stage I invasive cutaneous malignant melanoma. *Ann R Coll Surg Engl* 1985;67:75–78.

37. Wax MK, Yun KJ, Omar RA. Extramedullary plasmacytomas of the head and neck. *Otolaryngol Head Neck Surg* 1993;109:877–885.

38. van Hulsteijn LT, Corssmit EP, Coremans IE, et al. Regression and local control rates after radiotherapy for jugulotympanic paragangliomas: Systematic review and meta-analysis. *Radiother Oncol* 2013;106:161–168.

39. Leber KA, Eustacchio S, Pendl G. Radiosurgery of glomus tumors: midterm results. *Stereotact Funct Neurosurg* 1999;72(Suppl 1):53–59.

40. Bianchi LC, Marchetti M, Brait L, et al. Paragangliomas of head and neck: a treatment option with cyberknife radiosurgery. *Neurol Sci* 2009;30:479–485.

41. Chen PG, Nguyen JH, Payne SC, et al. Treatment of glomus jugulare tumors with gamma knife radiosurgery. *Laryngoscope* 2010;120:1856–1862.

42. Genc A, Bicer A, Abacioglu U, et al. Gamma knife radiosurgery for the treatment of glomus jugulare tumors. *J Neurooncol* 2010;97:101–108.

43. Hafez RF, Morgan MS, Fahmy OM. The safety and efficacy of gamma knife surgery in management of glomus jugulare tumor. *World J Surg Oncol* 2010;8:76.

44. Lim M, Bower R, Nangiana JS, et al. Radiosurgery for glomus jugulare tumors. *Technol Cancer Res Treat* 2007;6:419–423.

45. Maitz A, Grills I, Chen P, et al. Gamma knife radiosurgery: a viable therapy for glomus jugulare tumors. *Int J Radiat Oncol Biol Phys* 2007;72:S477.

46. Navarro Martin A, Maitz A, Grills IS, et al. Successful treatment of glomus jugulare tumours with gamma knife radiosurgery: clinical and physical aspects of management and review of the literature. *Clin Transl Oncol* 2010;12:55–62.

47. Pollock BE. Stereotactic radiosurgery in patients with glomus jugulare tumors. *Neurosurg Focus* 2004;17:E10.

48. Wegner RE, Rodriguez KD, Heron DE, et al. Linac-based stereotactic body radiation therapy for treatment of glomus jugulare tumors. *Radiother Oncol* 2010;97:395–398.

49. Wang ML, Hussey DH, Doornbos JF, et al. Chemodectoma of the temporal bone: a comparison of surgical and radiotherapeutic results. *Int J Radiat Oncol Biol Phys* 1988;14:643–648.

50. Zabel A, Milker-Zabel S, Huber P, et al. Fractionated stereotactic conformal radiotherapy in the management of large chemodectomas of the skull base. *Int J Radiat Oncol Biol Phys* 2004;58:1445–1450.

51. Kim JW, Kim DG, Chung HT, et al. Gamma knife stereotactic radiosurgery for intracranial hemangiopericytomas. *J Neurooncol* 2010;99:115–122.

52. Hinerman RW, Mendenhall WM, Amdur RJ, et al. Definitive radiotherapy in the management of chemodectomas arising in the temporal bone, carotid body, and glomus vagale. *Head Neck* 2001;23:363–371.

53. Hineman R, Morris C, Mendenhall W, et al. Paragangliomas of the head and neck treated with external-beam radiotherapy. *Int J Radiat Oncol Biol Phys* 2007;69:S434.

54. Schild SE, Foote RL, Buskirk SJ, et al. Results of radiotherapy for chemodectomas. *Mayo Clin Proc* 1992;67:537–540.

55. Verniers DA, Keus RB, Schouwenburg PF, et al. Radiation therapy, an important mode of treatment for head and neck chemodectomas. *Eur J Cancer* 1992;28A:1028–1033.

56. Ivan ME, Sughrue ME, Clark AJ, et al. A meta-analysis of tumor control rates and treatment-related morbidity for patients with glomus jugulare tumors. *J Neurosurg* 2011;114:1299–1305.

57. Guss ZD, Batra S, Limb CJ, et al. Radiosurgery of glomus jugulare tumors: A meta-analysis. *Int J Radiat Oncol Biol Phys* 2011;81:e497-502.

58. Elshaikh MA, Mahmoud-Ahmed AS, Kinney SE, et al. Recurrent head-and-neck chemodectomas: a comparison of surgical and radiotherapeutic results. *Int J Radiat Oncol Biol Phys* 2002;52:953–956.

59. Cheesman AD, Kelly AM. Rehabilitation after treatment for jugular foramen lesions. *Skull Base* 2009;19:99–108.

60. Larner JM, Hahn SS, Spaulding CA, et al. Glomus jugulare tumors. Long-term control by radiation therapy. *Cancer* 1992;69:1813–1817.

61. Pryzant RM, Chou JL, Easley JD. Twenty year experience with radiation therapy for temporal bone chemodectomas. *Int J Radiat Oncol Biol Phys* 1989;17:1303–1307.

62. Cole JM, Beiler D. Long-term results of treatment for glomus jugulare and glomus vagale tumors with radiotherapy. *Laryngoscope* 1994;104:1461–1465.

63. Boyle JO, Shimm DS, Coulthard SW. Radiation therapy for paragangliomas of the temporal bone. *Laryngoscope* 1990;100:896–901.

64. de Jong AL, Coker NJ, Jenkins HA, et al. Radiation therapy in the management of paragangliomas of the temporal bone. *Am J Otol* 1995;16:283–289.

65. Valdagni R, Amichetti M. Radiation therapy of carotid body tumors. *Am J Clin Oncol* 1990;13:45–48.

66. Sundaram C, Uppin SG, Uppin MS, et al. A clinicopathological and immunohistochemical study of central nervous system hemangiopericytomas. *J Clin Neurosci* 2010;17:469–472.

67. Paal E, Chung EM. Head and neck pathology-radiology classics: Vagal paraganglioma. *Head Neck Pathol* 2007;1:35–37.

68. Stout AP. Hemangiopericytoma; a study of 25 cases. *Cancer* 1949;2:1027–1054, illust.

69. Enzinger FM, Weiss SW. Hemangiopericytoma. In: Enzinger FM, Weiss WS, eds. *Soft tissue tumors.* 2nd ed. St. Louis, MO: Mosby, 1988:xi, 989.

70. Palacios E, Restrepo S, Mastrogiovanni L, et al. Sinonasal hemangiopericytomas: clinicopathologic and imaging findings. *Ear Nose Throat J* 2005;84:99–102.

71. Spitz FR, Bouvet M, Pisters PW, et al. Hemangiopericytoma: a 20-year single-institution experience. *Ann Surg Oncol* 1998;5:350–355.

72. Kanazawa T, Nishino H, Miyata M, et al. Haemangiopericytoma of infratemporal fossa. *J Laryngol Otol* 2001;115:77–79.

73. Kowalski PJ, Paulino AF. Proliferation index as a prognostic marker in hemangiopericytoma of the head and neck. *Head Neck* 2001;23:492–496.

74. Vuorinen V, Sallinen P, Haapasalo H, et al. Outcome of 31 intracranial haemangiopericytomas: poor predictive value of cell proliferation indices. *Acta Neurochir (Wien)* 1996;138:1399–1408.

75. Jaaskelainen J, Servo A, Haltia M, et al. Intracranial hemangiopericytoma: radiology, surgery, radiotherapy, and outcome in 21 patients. *Surg Neurol* 1985;23:227–236.

76. Setzkorn RK, Lee DJ, Iliff NT, et al. Hemangiopericytoma of the orbit treated with conservative surgery and radiotherapy. *Arch Ophthalmol* 1987;105:1103–1105.

77. Charles NC, Palu RN, Jagirdar JS. Hemangiopericytoma of the lacrimal sac. *Arch Ophthalmol* 1998;116:1677–1680.

78. Yaghmai I. Angiographic manifestations of soft-tissue and osseous hemangiopericytomas. *Radiology* 1978;126:653–659.

79. Monroe AT, Hinerman RW, Amdur RJ, et al. Radiation therapy for esthesioneuroblastoma: rationale for elective neck irradiation. *Head Neck* 2003;25:529–534.

80. Lee J, Kim I. Role of radiotherapy in intracranial hemangiopericytoma. *Int J Radiat Oncol Biol Phys* 2008;72:S230.

81. Hasegawa A, Mizoe J, Jingu K, et al. Carbon ion radiotherapy for skull base and paracervical chordomas. *Int J Radiat Oncol Biol Phys* 2009;75:S241.

82. Park MS, Patel SR, Ludwig JA, et al. Activity of temozolomide and bevacizumab in the treatment of locally advanced, recurrent, and metastatic hemangiopericytoma and malignant solitary fibrous tumor. *Cancer* 2011;117:4939–4947.

83. Espat NJ, Lewis JJ, Leung D, et al. Conventional hemangiopericytoma: modern analysis of outcome. *Cancer* 2002;95:1746–1751.

84. Jha N, McNeese M, Barkley HT Jr, et al. Does radiotherapy have a role in hemangiopericytoma management? Report of 14 new cases and a review of the literature. *Int J Radiat Oncol Biol Phys* 1987;13:1399–1402.

85. Hyams VJ. In: Hyams VJ, Batsakis JG, et al, eds. *Tumors of the upper respiratory tract and ear.* Washington, DC: Armed Forces Institute of Pathology: [Supt of Docs, U S G P O, distributor]: For sale by the Armed Forces Institute of Pathology, 1988:240–248.

86. Billings KR, Fu YS, Calcaterra TC, et al. Hemangiopericytoma of the head and neck. *Am J Otolaryngol* 2000;21:238–243.

87. Patrice SJ, Sneed PK, Flickinger JC, et al. Radiosurgery for hemangioblastoma: results of a multi-institutional experience. *Int J Radiat Oncol Biol Phys* 1995;32:147.

88. Carew JF, Singh B, Kraus DH. Hemangiopericytoma of the head and neck. *Laryngoscope* 1999;109:1409–1411.

89. Staples JJ, Robinson RA, Wen BC, et al. Hemangiopericytoma—the role of radiotherapy. *Int J Radiat Oncol Biol Phys* 1990;19:445–451.

90. Kano H, Niranjan A, Kondziolka D, et al. Adjuvant stereotactic radiosurgery after resection of intracranial hemangiopericytomas. *Int J Radiat Oncol Biol Phys* 2008;72:1333–1339.

91. Olson C, Yen CP, Schlesinger D, et al. Radiosurgery for intracranial hemangiopericytomas: outcomes after initial and repeat gamma knife surgery. *J Neurosurg* 2010;112:133–139.

Section III

92. Redmond K, Gullett N, Kleinberg L, et al. Hemangiopericytoma of the central nervous system: analysis of current national patterns of care. *Int J Radiat Oncol Biol Phys* 2010;78:S615.
93. Shaigany K, Fang CH, Patel TD, et al. A population-based analysis of head and neck hemangiopericytoma. *Laryngoscope* 2016;126:643–650.
94. Rich TA, Schiller A, Suit HD, et al. Clinical and pathologic review of 48 cases of chordoma. *Cancer* 1985;56:182–187.
95. Knott PD, Gannon FH, Thompson LD. Mesenchymal chondrosarcoma of the sinonasal tract: a clinicopathological study of 13 cases with a review of the literature. *Laryngoscope* 2003;113:783–790.
96. Volpe NJ, Liebsch NJ, Munzenrider JE, et al. Neuro-ophthalmologic findings in chordoma and chondrosarcoma of the skull base. *Am J Ophthalmol* 1993;115:97–104.
97. Doucet V, Peretti-Viton P, Figarella-Branger D, et al. MRI of intracranial chordomas. Extent of tumour and contrast enhancement: criteria for differential diagnosis. *Neuroradiology* 1997;39:571–576.
98. Oot RF, Melville GE, New PF, et al. The role of MR and CT in evaluating clival chordomas and chondrosarcomas. *AJR Am J Roentgenol* 1988;151:567–575.
99. Gabriele P, Macias V, Stasi M, et al. Feasibility of intensity-modulated radiation therapy in the treatment of advanced cervical chordoma. *Tumori* 2003;89:298–304.
100. Catton C, O'Sullivan B, Bell R, et al. Chordoma: Long-term follow-up after radical photon irradiation. *Radiother Oncol* 1996;41:67–72.
101. Forsyth PA, Cascino TL, Shaw EG, et al. Intracranial chordomas: a clinicopathological and prognostic study of 51 cases. *J Neurosurg* 1993;78:741–747.
102. Gay E, Sekhar LN, Rubinstein E, et al. Chordomas and chondrosarcomas of the cranial base: results and follow-up of 60 patients. *Neurosurgery* 1995;36:887–896; discussion 896–887.
103. Tai PT, Craighead P, Bagdon F. Optimization of radiotherapy for patients with cranial chordoma. A review of dose-response ratios for photon techniques. *Cancer* 1995;75:749–756.
104. Keisch ME, Garcia DM, Shibuya RB. Retrospective long-term follow-up analysis in 21 patients with chordomas of various sites treated at a single institution. *J Neurosurg* 1991;75:374–377.
105. Kim JW, Suh C-O, Hong C-K, et al. Maximum surgical resection and adjuvant intensity-modulated radiotherapy with simultaneous integrated boost for skull base chordoma. *Acta Neurochir* 2016:1–10.
106. Debus J, Schulz-Ertner D, Schad L, et al. Stereotactic fractionated radiotherapy for chordomas and chondrosarcomas of the skull base. *Int J Radiat Oncol Biol Phys* 2000;47:591–596.
107. Den R, Goldberg Y, Werner-Wasik M, et al. Photon based fractionated radiotherapy and radiosurgery for the treatment of chordomas and chondrosarcomas: A multi-institutional review. *Int J Radiat Oncol Biol Phys* 2008;72:S204.
108. Muthukumar N, Kondziolka D, Lunsford LD, et al. Stereotactic radiosurgery for chordoma and chondrosarcoma: Further experiences. *Int J Radiat Oncol Biol Phys* 1998;41:387–392.
109. Suit H, DeLaney T, Goldberg S, et al. Proton vs carbon ion beams in the definitive radiation treatment of cancer patients. *Radiother Oncol* 2010;95:3–22.
110. Berson AM, Castro JR, Petti P, et al. Charged particle irradiation of chordoma and chondrosarcoma of the base of skull and cervical spine: The Lawrence Berkeley Laboratory experience. *Int J Radiat Oncol Biol Phys* 1988;15:559–565.
111. Austin JP, Urie MM, Cardenosa G, et al. Probable causes of recurrence in patients with chordoma and chondrosarcoma of the base of skull and cervical spine. *Int J Radiat Oncol Biol Phys* 1993;25:439–444.
112. O'Connell JX, Renard LG, Liebsch NJ, et al. Base of skull chordoma. A correlative study of histologic and clinical features of 62 cases. *Cancer* 1994;74:2261–2267.
113. Fagundes MA, Hug EB, Liebsch NJ, et al. Radiation therapy for chordomas of the base of skull and cervical spine: Patterns of failure and outcome after relapse. *Int J Radiat Oncol Biol Phys* 1995;33:579–584.
114. Terahara A, Niemierko A, Goitein M, et al. Analysis of the relationship between tumor dose inhomogeneity and local control in patients with skull base chordoma. *Int J Radiat Oncol Biol Phys* 1999;45:351–358.
115. Slater JD, Austin-Seymour M, Munzenrider J, et al. Endocrine function following high dose proton therapy for tumors of the upper clivus. *Int J Radiat Oncol Biol Phys* 1988;15:607–611.
116. Hug EB, Loredo LN, Slater JD, et al. Proton radiation therapy for chordomas and chondrosarcomas of the skull base. *J Neurosurg* 1999;91:432–439.
117. Noel G, Jauffret E, de Crevoisier R, et al. Photon and proton therapy for chordoma and chondrosarcoma of the base of the skull and cervical spine: prognostic factors and patterns of failure. *Radiother Oncol* 2002;64:S81.
118. Jakel O, Land B, Combs SE, et al. On the cost-effectiveness of carbon ion radiation therapy for skull base chordoma. *Radiother Oncol* 2007;83:133–138.
119. Tournier-Rangeard L, Lapeyre M, Graff-Caillaud P, et al. Radiotherapy for solitary extramedullary plasmacytoma in the head-and-neck region: a dose greater than 45 gy to the target volume improves the local control. *Int J Radiat Oncol Biol Phys* 2006;64:1013–1017.
120. Benk V, Liebsch NJ, Munzenrider JE, et al. Base of skull and cervical spine chordomas in children treated by high-dose irradiation. *Int J Radiat Oncol Biol Phys* 1995;31:577–581.
121. Party TPTW. Proton therapy for base of skull chordoma: a report for the royal college of radiologists. *Clin Oncol* 2000;12:75–79.
122. Santoni R, Liebsch N, Finkelstein DM, et al. Temporal lobe (tl) damage following surgery and high-dose photon and proton irradiation in 96 patients affected by chordomas and chondrosarcomas of the base of the skull. *Int J Radiat Oncol Biol Phys* 1998;41:59–68.
123. Mendenhall WM, Olivier KR, Lynch JW Jr, et al. Lethal midline granuloma-nasal natural killer/t-cell lymphoma. *Am J Clin Oncol* 2006;29:202–206.
124. Rosignoli M, Pezzuto RW, Galli J, et al. [Midline granuloma and Wegener's granulomatosis]. *Acta Otorhinolaryngol Ital* 1992;12(Suppl 38):1–46.
125. Borisch B, Hennig I, Laeng RH, et al. Association of the subtype 2 of the Epstein-Barr virus with t-cell non-Hodgkin's lymphoma of the midline granuloma type. *Blood* 1993;82:858–864.
126. Berrettini S, Segnini G, Bruschini P, et al. Lethal midline granuloma: A case of ki-1 lymphoma. *Rev Laryngol Otol Rhinol (Bord)* 1993;114:37–42.
127. Smalley SR, Cupps RE, Anderson JA, et al. Polymorphic reticulosis limited to the upper aerodigestive tract—natural history and radiotherapeutic considerations. *Int J Radiat Oncol Biol Phys* 1988;15:599–605.
128. Gaulard P, Henni T, Marolleau JP, et al. Lethal midline granuloma (polymorphic reticulosis) and lymphomatoid granulomatosis. Evidence for a monoclonal t-cell lymphoproliferative disorder. *Cancer* 1988;62:705–710.
129. Mason M, Robinson M, Harmer C, et al. Intra-arterial adriamycin, conventionally fractionated radiotherapy and conservative surgery for soft tissue sarcomas. *Clin Oncol (R Coll Radiol)* 1992;4:32–35.
130. Fuller PS, Hafermann DR, Byrd RB, et al. Use of irradiation in lymphomatoid granulomatosis. *Chest* 1978;74:105–106.
131. Shank BB, Kelley CD, Nisce LZ, et al. Radiation therapy in lymphomatoid granulomatosis. *Cancer* 1978;42:2572–2580.
132. Dickson RJ. Radiotherapy of lethal mid-line granuloma. *J Chronic Dis* 1960;12:417–427.
133. Halperin EC, Dosoretz DE, Goodman M, et al. Radiotherapy of polymorphic reticulosis. *Br J Radiol* 1982;55:645–649.
134. Fauci A, Johnson R, Wolff S. Radiation therapy of midline granuloma. *Ann Intern Med* 1976;84:140–147.
135. Chen HH, Fong L, Su IJ, et al. Experience of radiotherapy in lethal midline granuloma with special emphasis on centrofacial t-cell lymphoma: a retrospective analysis covering a 34-year period. *Radiother Oncol* 1996;38:1–6.
136. Hatta C, Ishida M, Matsumoto T, et al. [Cases of lethal midline granuloma (polymorphic reticulosis) at our department in a recent 10-year period]. *Nihon Jibiinkoka Gakkai Kaiho* 1993;96:879–885.
137. Sakata K, Hareyama M, Oouchi A, et al. Treatment of localized non-Hodgkin's lymphomas of the head and neck: focusing on cases of non-lethal midline granuloma. *Radiat Oncol Investig* 1998;6:161–169.
138. Zimmerman LE, Font RL. Ophthalmologic manifestations of granulocytic sarcoma (myeloid sarcoma or chloroma). The third Pan American Association of Ophthalmology and American Journal of Ophthalmology Lecture. *Am J Ophthalmol* 1975;80:975–990.
139. Woo E, Yue CP, Mann KS, et al. Intracerebral chloromas. Report of a case and review of the literature. *Clin Neurol Neurosurg* 1986;88:135–139.
140. Byrd JC, Edenfield WJ, Shields DJ, et al. Extramedullary myeloid cell tumors in acute nonlymphocytic leukemia: a clinical review. *J Clin Oncol* 1995;13:1800–1816.
141. Pomeranz SJ, Hawkins HH, Towbin R, et al. Granulocytic sarcoma (chloroma): CT manifestations. *Radiology* 1985;155:167–170.
142. Bakst R, Wolden S, Yahalom J. Radiation therapy for chloroma (granulocytic sarcoma). *Int J Radiat Oncol Biol Phys* 2012;82:1816–1822.
143. Chak LY, Sapozink MD, Cox RS. Extramedullary lesions in non-lymphocytic leukemia: results of radiation therapy. *Int J Radiat Oncol Biol Phys* 1983;9:1173–1176.
144. Kuo S, Wan-Yu C, Chun-Wei W, et al. Clinicopathologic features and responses to radiation therapy of granulocytic sarcoma. *Int J Radiat Oncol Biol Phys* 2013;87(2):S558–S559.
145. Hall M, Chen Y, Schultheiss T, et al. Radiation therapy for chloroma: treatment outcomes and prognostic factors. *Int J Radiat Oncol Biol Phys* 2012;84:S622.
146. Berger L, Luc R. L'esthesioneuropitheliome olfacif. *Bull Cancer (Paris)* 1924;13:410–421.
147. Eich HT, Staar S, Micke O, et al. Radiotherapy of esthesioneuroblastoma. *Int J Radiat Oncol Biol Phys* 2001;49:155–160.
148. Sowers JJ, Moody DM, Naidich TP, et al. Radiographic features of granulocytic sarcoma (chloroma). *J Comput Assist Tomogr* 1979;3:226–233.
149. Kadish S, Goodman M, Wang CC. Olfactory neuroblastoma. A clinical analysis of 17 cases. *Cancer* 1976;37:1571–1576.
150. Pickuth D, Heywang-Kobrunner SH, Spielmann RP. Computed tomography and magnetic resonance imaging features of olfactory neuroblastoma: an analysis of 22 cases. *Clin Otolaryngol Allied Sci* 1999;24:457–461.
151. Bustillo A, Telischi F, Weed D, et al. Octreotide scintigraphy in the head and neck. *Laryngoscope* 2004;114:434–440.
152. Chao KS, Kaplan C, Simpson JR, et al. Esthesioneuroblastoma: the impact of treatment modality. *Head Neck* 2001;23:749–757.
153. Foote RL, Morita A, Ebersold MJ, et al. Esthesioneuroblastoma: the role of adjuvant radiation therapy. *Int J Radiat Oncol Biol Phys* 1993;27:835–842.
154. Argiris A, Dutra J, Tseke P, et al. Esthesioneuroblastoma: the northwestern university experience. *Laryngoscope* 2003;113:155–160.
155. Miyamoto RC, Gleich LL, Biddinger PW, et al. Esthesioneuroblastoma and sinonasal undifferentiated carcinoma: impact of histological grading and clinical staging on survival and prognosis. *Laryngoscope* 2000;110:1262–1265.
156. Papadaki H, Kounelis S, Kapadia SB, et al. Relationship of p53 gene alterations with tumor progression and recurrence in olfactory neuroblastoma. *Am J Surg Pathol* 1996;20:715–721.
157. Rosenthal DI, Barker JL Jr, El-Naggar AK, et al. Sinonasal malignancies with neuroendocrine differentiation: patterns of failure according to histologic phenotype. *Cancer* 2004;101:2567–2573.
158. Dias FL, Sa GM, Lima RA, et al. Patterns of failure and outcome in esthesioneuroblastoma. *Arch Otolaryngol Head Neck Surg* 2003;129:1186–1192.
159. Chang DT, Amdur RJ, Morris CG, et al. Adjuvant radiotherapy for cutaneous melanoma: comparing hypofractionation to conventional fractionation. *Int J Radiat Oncol Biol Phys* 2006;66:1051–1055.
160. Gruber G, Laedrach K, Baumert B, et al. Esthesioneuroblastoma: irradiation alone and surgery alone are not enough. *Int J Radiat Oncol Biol Phys* 2002;54:486–491.
161. Ozsahin M, Gruber G, Olszyk O, et al. Outcome and prognostic factors in olfactory neuroblastoma: a rare cancer network study. *Int J Radiat Oncol Biol Phys* 2010;78:992–997.

162. Sperry JL, Reis I, Casiano RR, et al. Esthesioneuroblastoma: a modern experience at the University of Miami. *Int J Radiat Oncol Biol Phys* 2010;78:S472–S473.

163. Madani I, Bonte K, Vakaet L, et al. Intensity-modulated radiotherapy for sinonasal tumors: Ghent University Hospital update. *Int J Radiat Oncol Biol Phys* 2009;73:424–432.

164. Kased N, El-Sayed I, Weinberg V, et al. Intensity modulated radiation therapy for esthesioneuroblastoma: clinical outcomes and toxicities. *Int J Radiat Oncol Biol Phys* 2010;78:S447.

165. Sharrett JM, Jiang W, Mohamed ASR, et al. Multimodality management of patients with esthesioneuroblastoma. *Int J Radiat Oncol Biol Phys* 2015;93:E349.

166. Modesto A, Blanchard P, Tao Y, et al. Esthesioneuroblastomas: bicentric review of clinical features, multimodal treatment, and long-term outcome. *Int J Radiat Oncol Biol Phys* 2012;84:S498–S499.

167. Nishimura H, Ogino T, Kawashima M, et al. Proton-beam therapy for olfactory neuroblastoma. *Int J Radiat Oncol Biol Phys* 2007;68:758–762.

168. Dagan R, Bryant C, Li Z, et al. Outcomes of sinonasal cancer treated with proton therapy. *Int J Radiat Oncol Biol Phys* 2016;95:377–385.

169. Akimoto T, Zenda S, Nakamura N, et al. A retrospective multi-institutional study of proton beam therapy for head and neck cancer with non-squamous cell histologies. *Int J Radiat Oncol Biol Phys* 2016;96:E337.

170. Bhattacharyya N, Thornton AF, Joseph MP, et al. Successful treatment of esthesioneuroblastoma and neuroendocrine carcinoma with combined chemotherapy and proton radiation. Results in 9 cases. *Arch Otolaryngol Head Neck Surg* 1997;123:34–40.

171. McElroy EA Jr, Buckner JC, Lewis JE. Chemotherapy for advanced esthesioneuroblastoma: the mayo clinic experience. *Neurosurgery* 1998;42:1023–1027; discussion 1027–1028.

172. Beitler JJ, Fass DE, Brenner HA, et al. Esthesioneuroblastoma: is there a role for elective neck treatment? *Head Neck* 1991;13:321–326.

173. Davis RE, Weissler MC. Esthesioneuroblastoma and neck metastasis. *Head Neck* 1992;14:477–482.

174. Noh OK, Lee SW, Yoon SM, et al. Radiotherapy for esthesioneuroblastoma: is elective nodal irradiation warranted in the multimodality treatment approach? *Int J Radiat Oncol Biol Phys* 2011;79:443–449.

175. Peacock JG, Link MJ, Olsen KD, et al. Risk of delayed lymph node metastasis in cases of esthesioneuroblastoma with a clinically no neck. *Int J Radiat Oncol Biol Phys* 2014;88:518–519.

176. Yin ZZ, Luo JW, Gao L. Patterns of regional spread and the role of elective neck irradiation for esthesioneuroblastoma. *Int J Radiat Oncol Biol Phys* 2015;93:E296–E297.

177. Zanation AM, Ferlito A, Rinaldo A, et al. When, how and why to treat the neck in patients with esthesioneuroblastoma: a review. *Eur Arch Otorhinolaryngol* 2010;267:1667–1671.

178. Simon JH, Zhen W, McCulloch TM, et al. Esthesioneuroblastoma: the University of Iowa experience 1978–1998. *Laryngoscope* 2001;111:488–493.

179. Platek M, Mashtare T, Popat S, et al. Improved survival following surgery and radiation for olfactory neuroblastoma: analysis of the seer database. *Int J Radiat Oncol Biol Phys* 2009;75:S396.

180. Eden BV, Debo RF, Larner JM, et al. Esthesioneuroblastoma. Long-term outcome and patterns of failure—the University of Virginia experience. *Cancer* 1994;73:2556–2562.

181. Levine PA, Gallagher R, Cantrell RW. Esthesioneuroblastoma: reflections of a 21-year experience. *Laryngoscope* 1999;109:1539–1543.

182. Eriksen JG, Bastholt L, Krogdahl AS, et al. Esthesioneuroblastoma—what is the optimal treatment? *Acta Oncol* 2000;39:231–235.

183. Konuthula N, Iloreta AM, Rhome RM, et al. Definitive radiation in the treatment of locally advanced esthesioneuroblastoma: an analysis of the national cancer data base. *Int J Radiat Oncol Biol Phys* 2016;96:E371.

184. Ozsahin M, Tsang RW, Poortmans P, et al. Outcomes and patterns of failure in solitary plasmacytoma: a multicenter rare cancer network study of 258 patients. *Int J Radiat Oncol Biol Phys* 2006;64:210–217.

185. Hotz MA, Schwaab G, Bosq J, et al. Extramedullary solitary plasmacytoma of the head and neck. A clinicopathological study. *Ann Otol Rhinol Laryngol* 1999;108:495–500.

186. Michalaki VJ, Hall J, Henk JM, et al. Definitive radiotherapy for extramedullary plasmacytomas of the head and neck. *Br J Radiol* 2003;76:738–741.

187. Woodruff RK, Whittle JM, Malpas JS. Solitary plasmacytoma. I: extramedullary soft tissue plasmacytoma. *Cancer* 1979;43:2340–2343.

188. Alexiou C, Kau RJ, Dietzfelbinger H, et al. Extramedullary plasmacytoma: tumor occurrence and therapeutic concepts. *Cancer* 1999;85:2305–2314.

189. Bachar G, Goldstein D, Brown D, et al. Solitary extramedullary plasmacytoma of the head and neck—long-term outcome analysis of 68 cases. *Head Neck* 2008;30:1012–1019.

190. Harwood AR, Knowling MA, Bergsagel DE. Radiotherapy of extramedullary plasmacytoma of the head and neck. *Clin Radiol* 1981;32:31–36.

191. Hughes M, Soutar R, Lucraft H, et al. *Guidelines on the diagnosis and management of solitary plasmacytoma of bone, extramedullary plasmacytoma and multiple solitary plasmacytomas: 2009 update.* London, UK: British Committee for Standards in Haematology, 2009.

192. Elkon D, Hightower SI, Lim ML, et al. Esthesioneuroblastoma. *Cancer* 1979;44:1087–1094.

193. Dulguerov P, Calcaterra T. Esthesioneuroblastoma: the UCLA experience 1970–1990. *Laryngoscope* 1992;102:843–849.

194. Zappia JJ, Carroll WR, Wolf GT, et al. Olfactory neuroblastoma: the results of modern treatment approaches at the University of Michigan. *Head Neck* 1993;15:190–196.

195. Eich HT, Hero B, Staar S, et al. Multimodality therapy including radiotherapy and chemotherapy improves event-free survival in stage c esthesioneuroblastoma. *Strahlenther Onkol* 2003;179:233–240.

196. Kim HJ, Kim CH, Lee BJ, et al. Surgical treatment versus concurrent chemoradiotherapy as an initial treatment modality in advanced olfactory neuroblastoma. *Auris Nasus Larynx* 2007;34:493–498.

197. Shih LY, Dunn P, Leung WM, et al. Localised plasmacytomas in Taiwan: comparison between extramedullary plasmacytoma and solitary plasmacytoma of bone. *Br J Cancer* 1995;71:128–133.

198. Holland J, Trenkner DA, Wasserman TH, et al. Plasmacytoma. Treatment results and conversion to myeloma. *Cancer* 1992;69:1513–1517.

199. Liebross RH, Ha CS, Cox JD, et al. Clinical course of solitary extramedullary plasmacytoma. *Radiother Oncol* 1999;52:245–249.

200. Galieni P, Cavo M, Pulsoni A, et al. Clinical outcome of extramedullary plasmacytoma. *Haematologica* 2000;85:47–51.

201. Miller FR, Lavertu P, Wanamaker JR, et al. Plasmacytomas of the head and neck. *Otolaryngol Head Neck Surg* 1998;119:614–618.

202. Sasaki R, Yasuda K, Abe E, et al. Multi-institutional analysis of solitary extramedullary plasmacytoma of the head and neck treated with curative radiotherapy. *Int J Radiat Oncol Biol Phys* 2012;82:626–634.

203. Beham A, Fletcher CD, Kainz J, et al. Nasopharyngeal angiofibroma: an immunohistochemical study of 32 cases. *Virchows Arch A Pathol Anat Histopathol* 1993;423:281–285.

204. Kotner LM, Wang CC. Plasmacytoma of the upper air and food passages. *Cancer* 1972;30:414–418.

205. Wiltshaw E. The natural history of extramedullary plasmacytoma and its relation to solitary myeloma of bone and myelomatosis. *Medicine (Baltimore)* 1976;55:217–238.

206. Bush SE, Goffinet DR, Bagshaw MA. Extramedullary plasmacytoma of the head and neck. *Radiology* 1981;140:801–805.

207. Kapadia SB, Desai U, Cheng VS. Extramedullary plasmacytoma of the head and neck. A clinicopathologic study of 20 cases. *Medicine (Baltimore)* 1982;61:317–329.

208. Creach KM, Foote RL, Neben-Wittich MA, et al. Radiotherapy for extramedullary plasmacytoma of the head and neck. *Int J Radiat Oncol Biol Phys* 2009;73:789–794.

209. Farag MM, Ghanimah SE, Ragaie A, et al. Hormonal receptors in juvenile nasopharyngeal angiofibroma. *Laryngoscope* 1987;97:208–211.

210. Hwang HC, Mills SE, Patterson K, et al. Expression of androgen receptors in nasopharyngeal angiofibroma: an immunohistochemical study of 24 cases. *Mod Pathol* 1998;11:1122–1126.

211. Algazi AP, Soon CW, Daud AI. Treatment of cutaneous melanoma: current approaches and future prospects. *Cancer Manag Res* 2010;2:197–211.

212. Chandler JR, Goulding R, Moskowitz L, et al. Nasopharyngeal angiofibromas: staging and management. *Ann Otol Rhinol Laryngol* 1984;93:322–329.

213. Sessions RB, Bryan RN, Naclerio RM, et al. Radiographic staging of juvenile angiofibroma. *Head Neck Surg* 1981;3:279–283.

214. Cummings BJ. The treatment of juvenile nasopharyngeal angiofibroma. The case for radiation therapy. *J Laryngol Otol Suppl* 1983;8:101–102.

215. Ungkanont K, Byers RM, Weber RS, et al. Juvenile nasopharyngeal angiofibroma: an update of therapeutic management. *Head Neck* 1996;18:60–66.

216. Colville RJ, Charlton F, Kelly CG, et al. Multidisciplinary management of head and neck sarcomas. *Head Neck* 2005;27:814–824.

217. Lloyd G, Howard D, Phelps P, et al. Juvenile angiofibroma: the lessons of 20 years of modern imaging. *J Laryngol Otol* 1999;113:127–134.

218. Ochoa-Carrillo FJ, Carrillo JF, Frias M. Staging and treatment of nasopharyngeal angiofibroma. *Eur Arch Otorhinolaryngol* 1997;254:200–204.

219. Bremer JW, Neel HB III, DeSanto LW, et al. Angiofibroma: treatment trends in 150 patients during 40 years. *Laryngoscope* 1986;96:1321–1329.

220. Greess H, Nömayr A, Tomandl B, et al. 2D and 3D visualisation of head and neck tumours from spiral-CT data. *Eur J Radiol* 2000;33:170–177.

221. Donald PJ. Sarcomatous degeneration in a nasopharyngeal angiofibroma. *Otolaryngol Head Neck Surg* 1979;87:42–46.

222. Radkowski D, McGill T, Healy GB, et al. Angiofibroma. Changes in staging and treatment. *Arch Otolaryngol Head Neck Surg* 1996;122:122–129.

223. Claus F, Boterberg T, Ost P, et al. Short term toxicity profile for 32 sinonasal cancer patients treated with IMRT. Can we avoid dry eye syndrome? *Radiother Oncol* 2002;64:205–208.

224. Duthoy W, Boterberg T, Claus F, et al. Postoperative intensity-modulated radiotherapy in sinonasal carcinoma: clinical results in 39 patients. *Cancer* 2005;104:71–82.

225. Hoppe BS, Stegman LD, Zelefsky MJ, et al. Treatment of nasal cavity and paranasal sinus cancer with modern radiotherapy techniques in the postoperative setting—the MSKCC experience. *Int J Radiat Oncol Biol Phys* 2007;67:691–702.

226. Daly ME, Chen AM, Bucci MK, et al. Intensity-modulated radiation therapy for malignancies of the nasal cavity and paranasal sinuses. *Int J Radiat Oncol Biol Phys* 2007;67:151–157.

227. Dirix P, Nuyts S, Vanstraelen B, et al. Post-operative intensity-modulated radiotherapy for malignancies of the nasal cavity and paranasal sinuses. *Radiother Oncol* 2007;85:385–391.

228. Herman P, Lot G, Chapot R, et al. Long-term follow-up of juvenile nasopharyngeal angiofibromas: analysis of recurrences. *Laryngoscope* 1999;109:140–147.

229. Sun XC, Wang DH, Yu HP, et al. Analysis of risk factors associated with recurrence of nasopharyngeal angiofibroma. *J Otolaryngol Head Neck Surg* 2010;39:56–61.

230. Marsot-Dupuch K, Cabane J, Raveau V, et al. Lethal midline granuloma: impact of imaging studies on the investigation and management of destructive mid facial disease in 13 patients. *Neuroradiology* 1992;34:155–161.

231. Lee JT, Chen P, Safa A, et al. The role of radiation in the treatment of advanced juvenile angiofibroma. *Laryngoscope* 2002;112:1213–1220.

232. Carrillo JF, Maldonado F, Albores O, et al. Juvenile nasopharyngeal angiofibroma: clinical factors associated with recurrence, and proposal of a staging system. *J Surg Oncol* 2008;98:75–80.

233. Cummings BJ, Blend R, Keane T, et al. Primary radiation therapy for juvenile nasopharyngeal angiofibroma. *Laryngoscope* 1984;94:1599–1605.

Section
III

234. Kuppersmith RB, Teh BS, Donovan DT, et al. The use of intensity modulated radiotherapy for the treatment of extensive and recurrent juvenile angiofibroma. *Int J Pediatr Otorhinolaryngol* 2000;52:261–268.

235. Jacobsson M, Petruson B, Svendsen P, et al. Juvenile nasopharyngeal angiofibroma. A report of eighteen cases. *Acta Otolaryngol* 1988;105:132–139.

236. Wiatrak BJ, Koopmann CF, Turrisi AT. Radiation therapy as an alternative to surgery in the management of intracranial juvenile nasopharyngeal angiofibroma. *Int J Pediatr Otorhinolaryngol* 1993;28:51–61.

237. Cormier JN, Pollock RE. Soft tissue sarcomas. *CA Cancer J Clin* 2004;54:94–109.

238. Chakraborty S, Ghoshal S, Patil VM, et al. Conformal radiotherapy in the treatment of advanced juvenile nasopharyngeal angiofibroma with intracranial extension: an institutional experience. *Int J Radiat Oncol Biol Phys* 2011;80:1398–1404.

239. Deschler DG, Kaplan MJ, Boles R. Treatment of large juvenile nasopharyngeal angiofibroma. *Otolaryngol Head Neck Surg* 1992;106:278–284.

240. Robinson M, Barr L, Fisher C, et al. Treatment of extremity soft tissue sarcomas with surgery and radiotherapy. *Radiother Oncol* 1990;18:221–233.

241. Fields JN, Halverson KJ, Devineni VR, et al. Juvenile nasopharyngeal angiofibroma: efficacy of radiation therapy. *Radiology* 1990;176:263–265.

242. Roche PH, Paris J, Regis J, et al. Management of invasive juvenile nasopharyngeal angiofibromas: the role of a multimodality approach. *Neurosurgery* 2007;61:768–777; discussion 777.

243. Goepfert H, Cangir A, Lee YY. Chemotherapy for aggressive juvenile nasopharyngeal angiofibroma. *Arch Otolaryngol* 1985;111:285–289.

244. McAfee WJ, Morris CG, Amdur RJ, et al. Definitive radiotherapy for juvenile nasopharyngeal angiofibroma. *Am J Clin Oncol* 2006;29:168–170.

245. Kasper ME, Parsons JT, Mancuso AA, et al. Radiation therapy for juvenile angiofibroma: evaluation by CT and MRI, analysis of tumor regression, and selection of patients. *Int J Radiat Oncol Biol Phys* 1993;25:689–694.

246. Rapini RP, Golitz LE, Greer RO Jr, et al. Primary malignant melanoma of the oral cavity. A review of 177 cases. *Cancer* 1985;55:1543–1551.

247. Tranbahuy P, Borsik M, Herman P, et al. Direct intratumoral embolization of juvenile angiofibroma. *Am J Otolaryngol* 1994;15:429–435.

248. Benghiat A. Juvenile nasopharyngeal angiofibroma treated by radiotherapy. *J Laryngol Otol* 1986;100:351–356.

249. Robinson AC, Khoury GG, Ash DV, et al. Evaluation of response following irradiation of juvenile angiofibromas. *Br J Radiol* 1989;62:245–247.

250. Harwood AR. Role of radiation therapy in the treatment of melanoma. In: Larson DL, Jones BA, Guillamondegui OM, eds. *Cancer in the neck: evaluation and treatment*. New York: Macmillan, 1986:243.

251. Batsakis JG, Regezi JA, Solomon AR, et al. The pathology of head and neck tumors: mucosal melanomas, part 13. *Head Neck Surg* 1982;4:404–418.

252. Harwood AR, Cummings BJ. Radiotherapy for mucosal melanomas. *Int J Radiat Oncol Biol Phys* 1982;8:1121–1126.

253. Tseng WH, Martinez SR. Tumor location predicts survival in cutaneous head and neck melanoma. *J Surg Res* 2011;167:192–198.

254. Zenda S, Kawashima M, Nishio T, et al. Proton beam therapy as a nonsurgical approach to mucosal melanoma of the head and neck: a pilot study. *Int J Radiat Oncol Biol Phys* 2011;81:135–139.

255. Khan N, Khan MK, Almasan A, et al. The evolving role of radiation therapy in the management of malignant melanoma. *Int J Radiat Oncol Biol Phys* 2011;80:645–654.

256. Harwood AR, Lawson VG. Radiation therapy for melanomas of the head and neck. *Head Neck Surg* 1982;4:468–474.

257. Ang KK, Peters LJ, Weber RS, et al. Postoperative radiotherapy for cutaneous melanoma of the head and neck region. *Int J Radiat Oncol Biol Phys* 1994;30:795–798.

258. Bibault JE, Dewas S, Mirabel X, et al. Adjuvant radiation therapy in metastatic lymph nodes from melanoma. *Radiat Oncol* 2011;6:12.

259. Strojan P, Jancar B, Cemazar M, et al. Melanoma metastases to the neck nodes: role of adjuvant irradiation. *Int J Radiat Oncol Biol Phys* 2010;77:1039–1045.

260. Emami B, Perez CA, Konefal J, et al. Thermoradiotherapy of malignant melanoma. *Int J Hyperthermia* 1988;4:373–381.

261. Engin K, Tupchong L, Waterman FM, et al. Hyperthermia and radiation in advanced malignant melanoma. *Int J Radiat Oncol Biol Phys* 1993;25:87–94.

262. Radiation therapy oncology group protocol no. 8305. William T Sause and Henry P Plenk, Co-chairmen 1988.

263. Tsang RW, Liu FF, Wells W, et al. Lentigo maligna of the head and neck. Results of treatment by radiotherapy. *Arch Dermatol* 1994;130:1008–1012.

264. Hoki K, Sambe S, Asakura K, et al. Malignant melanoma in the maxillary sinus—a case successfully treated with radiotherapy. *Auris Nasus Larynx* 1985;12:81–87.

265. Buchner A, Hansen LS. Pigmented nevi of the oral mucosa: a clinicopathologic study of 36 new cases and review of 155 cases from the literature. Part ii: Analysis of 191 cases. *Oral Surg Oral Med Oral Pathol* 1987;63:676–682.

266. Trapp TK, Fu Y, Calcaterra TC. Melanoma of the nasal and paranasal sinus mucosa. *Arch Otolaryngol Head Neck Surg* 1987;113:1086–1089.

267. Kato T, Takematsu H, Tomita Y, et al. Malignant melanoma of mucous membranes. A clinicopathologic study of 13 cases in Japanese patients. *Arch Dermatol* 1987;123:216–220.

268. Umeda M, Mishima Y, Teranobu O, et al. Heterogeneity of primary malignant melanomas in oral mucosa: an analysis of 43 cases in Japan. *Pathology* 1988;20:234–241.

269. Berthelsen A, Andersen AP, Jensen TS, et al. Melanomas of the mucosa in the oral cavity and the upper respiratory passages. *Cancer* 1984;54:907–912.

270. Krengli M, Masini L, Kaanders JH, et al. Radiotherapy in the treatment of mucosal melanoma of the upper aerodigestive tract: analysis of 74 cases. A rare cancer network study. *Int J Radiat Oncol Biol Phys* 2006;65:751–759.

271. Kingdom TT, Kaplan MJ. Mucosal melanoma of the nasal cavity and paranasal sinuses. *Head Neck* 1995;17:184–189.

272. Yanagi T, Mizoe JE, Hasegawa A, et al. Mucosal malignant melanoma of the head and neck treated by carbon ion radiotherapy. *Int J Radiat Oncol Biol Phys* 2009;74:15–20.

273. Jingu K, Mizoe J, Hasegawa A, et al. Improvement in the prognosis of unresectable bone and soft tissue sarcoma in the adult head and neck by carbon ion radiation therapy: results of a phase i/ii study. *Int J Radiat Oncol Biol Phys* 2009;75:S524.

274. Hutchinson J. Notes on cancer and cancerous processes. *Arch Surg* 1890;2:218–224.

275. Tannous ZS, Lerner LH, Duncan LM, et al. Progression to invasive melanoma from malignant melanoma in situ, lentigo maligna type. *Hum Pathol* 2000;31:705–708.

276. Erickson C, Miller SJ. Treatment options in melanoma in situ: topical and radiation therapy, excision and Mohs surgery. *Int J Dermatol* 2010;49:482–491.

277. Hill DC, Gramp AA. Surgical treatment of lentigo maligna and lentigo maligna melanoma. *Australas J Dermatol* 1999;40:25–30.

278. Cohen LM, McCall MW, Zax RH. Mohs micrographic surgery for lentigo maligna and lentigo maligna melanoma. A follow-up study. *Dermatol Surg* 1998;24:673–677.

279. Kuflik EG, Gage AA. Cryosurgery for lentigo maligna. *J Am Acad Dermatol* 1994;31:75–78.

279a. Santos D, Green JA, Bhandari N, et al. Tangential volumetric modulated radiation therapy is superior to brachytherapy for large scalp lesions: a case study in lentigo maligna. *Int J Radiat Oncol Bio Phys* 2014;90(1S):S935, Abstract 3838.

280. Van Damme JP, Schmitz S, Machiels JP, et al. Prognostic factors and assessment of staging systems for head and neck soft tissue sarcomas in adults. *Eur J Surg Oncol* 2010;36:684–690.

281. Johns MM, Concus AP, Beals TF, et al. Early-onset postirradiation sarcoma of the head and neck: report of three cases. *Ear Nose Throat J* 2002;81:402–406.

282. Patel SG, See AC, Williamson PA, et al. Radiation induced sarcoma of the head and neck. *Head Neck* 1999;21:346–354.

283. Le Vay J, O'Sullivan B, Catton C, et al. An assessment of prognostic factors in soft-tissue sarcoma of the head and neck. *Arch Otolaryngol Head Neck Surg* 1994;120:981–986.

284. Yancovitz M, Finelt N, Warycha MA, et al. Role of radiologic imaging at the time of initial diagnosis of stage t1b-t3b melanoma. *Cancer* 2007;110:1107–1114.

285. Dudhat SB, Mistry RC, Varughese T, et al. Prognostic factors in head and neck soft tissue sarcomas. *Cancer* 2000;89:868–872.

286. Eeles RA, Fisher C, A'Hern RP, et al. Head and neck sarcomas: prognostic factors and implications for treatment. *Br J Cancer* 1993;68:201–207.

287. Willers H, Hug EB, Spiro IJ, et al. Adult soft tissue sarcomas of the head and neck treated by radiation and surgery or radiation alone: patterns of failure and prognostic factors. *Int J Radiat Oncol Biol Phys* 1995;33:585–593.

288. Tran LM, Mark R, Meier R, et al. Sarcomas of the head and neck. Prognostic factors and treatment strategies. *Cancer* 1992;70:169–177.

289. Mandard AM, Petiot JF, Marnay J, et al. Prognostic factors in soft tissue sarcomas. A multivariate analysis of 109 cases. *Cancer* 1989;63:1437–1451.

289a. Ketabchi A, Kalavrezos N, Newman L. Sarcomas of the head and neck: a 10-year retrospective of 25 patients to evaluate treatment modalities, function and survival. *Br J Oral Maxillofac Surg* 2011;49:116–120.

290. Farhood AI, Hajdu SI, Shiu MH, et al. Soft tissue sarcomas of the head and neck in adults. *Am J Surg* 1990;160:365–369.

291. Al-Daraji W, Lasota J, Foss R, et al. Synovial sarcoma involving the head: analysis of 36 cases with predilection to the parotid and temporal regions. *Am J Surg Pathol* 2009;33:1494–1503.

292. Strander H, Turesson I, Cavallin-Stahl E. A systematic overview of radiation therapy effects in soft tissue sarcomas. *Acta Oncol* 2003;42:516–531.

293. Pellitteri PK, Ferlito A, Bradley PJ, et al. Management of sarcomas of the head and neck in adults. *Oral Oncol* 2003;39:2–12.

294. Penel N, Van Haverbeke C, Lartigau E, et al. Head and neck soft tissue sarcomas of adult: prognostic value of surgery in multimodal therapeutic approach. *Oral Oncol* 2004;40:890–897.

295. Wolden SL, Wexler LH, Kraus DH, et al. Intensity-modulated radiotherapy for head-and-neck rhabdomyosarcoma. *Int J Radiat Oncol Biol Phys* 2005;61:1432–1438.

296. McDonald MW, Esiashvili N, George BA, et al Intensity-modulated radiotherapy with use of cone-down boost for pediatric head-and-neck rhabdomyosarcoma. *Int J Radiat Oncol Biol Phys* 2008;72:884–891.

297. Pandey M, Chandramohan K, Thomas G, et al. Soft tissue sarcoma of the head and neck region in adults. *Int J Oral Maxillofac Surg* 2003;32:43–48.

298. Moalikyar O, Chen AM, Young J, et al. Adjuvant radiation therapy for sarcomas of the head and neck: a single-institution experience. *Int J Radiat Oncol Biol Phys* 2014;90:S762.

299. Huang P, Jacobson A, Choy E, et al. Radiation therapy improved survival in high-grade head and neck soft-tissue sarcoma: analysis from a population-based cancer registry. *Int J Radiat Oncol Biol Phys* 2014;88:520.

300. Brandmaier A, Wu X, Christos P, et al. A population-based comparative outcome of adjuvant radiation therapy in patients with soft tissue sarcoma of the head and neck. *Int J Radiat Oncol Biol Phys* 2015;93:E635-E636.

301. Mahmoud OMEE, Beck R, Kalyoussef E, et al. Survival outcome and radiation therapy utilization pattern in head and neck soft tissue sarcoma: a national cancer data base analysis. *Int J Radiat Oncol Biol Phys* 2016;96:E326-E327.

302. Weber DC, Rutz HP, Pedroni ES, et al. Results of spot-scanning proton radiation therapy for chordoma and chondrosarcoma of the skull base: the Paul Scherrer Institut experience. *Int J Radiat Oncol Biol Phys* 2005;63:401–409.

303. Greager JA, Patel MK, Briele HA, et al. Soft tissue sarcomas of the adult head and neck. *Cancer* 1985;56:820–824.

304. McKenna WG, Barnes MM, Kinsella TJ, et al. Combined modality treatment of adult soft tissue sarcomas of the head and neck. *Int J Radiat Oncol Biol Phys* 1987;13:1127–1133.

305. Laramore GE. Role of particle radiotherapy in the management of head and neck cancer. *Curr Opin Oncol* 2009;21:224–231.

306. Hug EB, Hanssens PE, Liebsch NJ, et al. Soft tissue sarcomas of the head and neck: results of combined proton and photon radiation therapy using 3-d treatment planning. *Int J Radiat Oncol Biol Phys* 1994;30:222.

307. McNaney D, Lindberg RD, Ayala AG, et al. Fifteen year radiotherapy experience with chondrosarcoma of bone. *Int J Radiat Oncol Biol Phys* 1982;8:187–190.

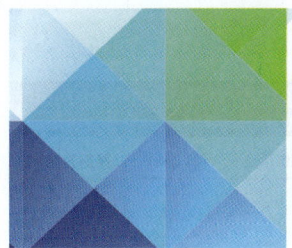

CHAPTER 52

Neck Cancer Including Carcinoma of Unknown Primary

William M. Mendenhall, Anthony A. Mancuso, Robert J. Amdur, Brian J. Boyce, and Peter T. Dziegielewski

ANATOMY

The locations of the various lymph node groups in the head and neck are shown in Figure 52.1.[1] Under normal conditions, the right and left lymphatic networks do not shunt from one side to the other.[2] The following discussion will focus on mucosal squamous cell carcinomas (SCC) unless otherwise specified.

The internal jugular chain (IJC) lymph nodes lie adjacent to the internal jugular vein and extend from the skull base to the clavicle. The most superior group of lymph nodes in this chain lies near the base of the skull in the posterior aspect of the lateral pharyngeal space and is often referred to as the parapharyngeal or junctional lymph nodes. These lymph nodes lie deep to the sternocleidomastoid muscle, the posterior belly of the digastric muscle, and the tail of the parotid gland. The remaining IJC lymph nodes are artificially divided into the subdigastric, middle jugular, and lower jugular groups.

The spinal accessory chain (SAC) lymph nodes are distributed along the course of cranial nerve XI. The superior nodes of the SAC blend with the upper IJC nodes. The supraclavicular lymph nodes merge laterally with the SAC lymph nodes and medially with the lower IJC lymph nodes.

There are typically three to six submandibular lymph nodes. They may be either preglandular or postglandular; there are no lymph nodes in the substance of the submandibular gland. Adjacent to these nodes are also the perifacial lymph nodes, which lie next to the facial artery and vein around the marginal mandibular nerve. The submental lymph nodes lie in the midline between the anterior bellies of the digastric muscles, anterior and superior to the hyoid bone and superficial to the mylohyoid muscle. There are typically 1 to 3 nodes in this area. The lateral retropharyngeal lymph nodes lie within the retropharyngeal space, which is bounded anteriorly by the pharyngeal constrictor muscles, superiorly by the skull base, and posteriorly by the prevertebral fascia. They are usually found at the level of the C1 and C2 vertebral bodies but may be found as inferiorly as C3. The medial retropharyngeal nodes are small, inconstant intercalated nodes that are located near midline and empty into the lateral retropharyngeal lymph nodes.

The neck nodes are divided into levels as follows: level I, submental (IA) and submandibular (IB) nodes; level II, upper internal jugular nodes, from the skull base to the level of the hyoid bone divided by the spinal accessory nerve into levels IIa (anterior to the nerve) and IIb (posterior to the nerve); level III, middle internal jugular nodes, from the level of the hyoid bone to the omohyoid muscle; level IV, inferior internal jugular nodes, from the level of the omohyoid muscle to the clavicle; level V, divided by the spinal accessory nerve into levels Va (superior to the nerve) and Vb (inferior to the nerve); and level VI, central neck nodes, bounded by the hyoid bone, the sternum, and the common carotid arteries. Included in level VI are the paratracheal, pretracheal, precricoid (delphian), and tracheoesophageal groove nodes.[3]

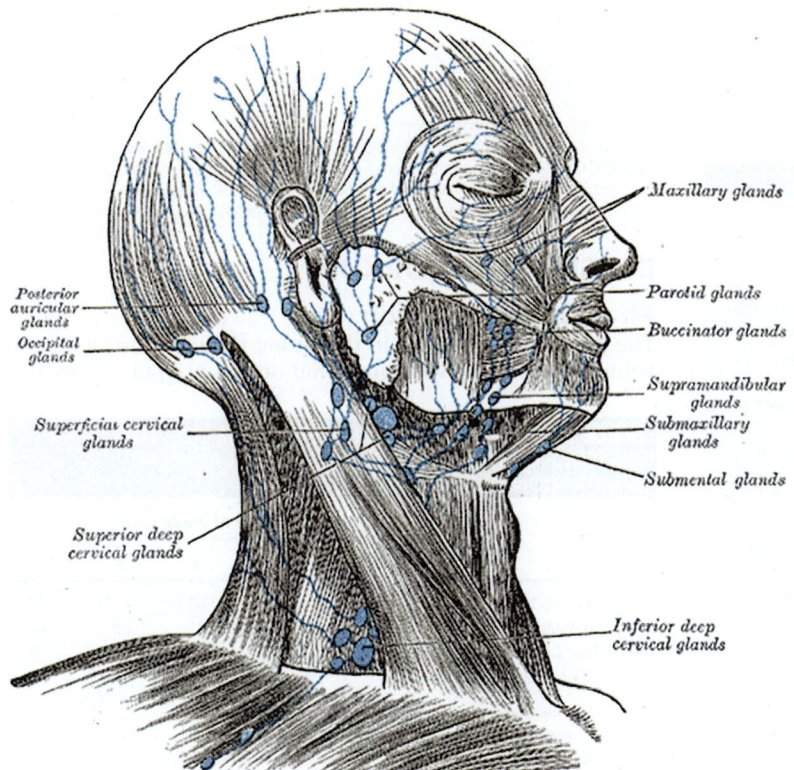

FIGURE 52.1. Arrangement of lymph nodes in the head and neck.

NATURAL HISTORY

The risk of lymph node metastases is influenced by the location of the primary tumor, histologic differentiation, size of the lesion, and the availability of capillary lymphatics.[4-7] The estimated risk of subclinical disease in the clinically negative neck as a function of primary site and tumor (T) stage is shown in Table 52.1.[4] Recurrent lesions have a higher risk of lymphatic involvement than untreated lesions. Moreover, their spread is less predictable.

The relative incidence of clinically positive lymph nodes in the neck by anatomic site and T stage is shown in Table 52.2.[5] The most commonly involved lymph nodes in the head and neck are the level II lymph nodes, followed by the level III lymph nodes. Lesions that are well lateralized almost always spread first to the ipsilateral neck nodes. Lesions on or near the midline as well as lateralized base of tongue and nasopharyngeal lesions may spread to both sides of the neck.

Patients who have clinically positive lymph nodes on the ipsilateral side of the neck may be at risk for contralateral lymph node spread if the metastatic masses produce significant obstruction of the lymphatic trunks. In addition, patients who have undergone previous surgery on one side of the neck develop shunting of lymph across the submental region to the opposite side of the neck. When contralateral lymph node metastases occur, the level II lymph nodes are most frequently involved, followed by the level III and level IV lymph node groups.

As tumor grows within a lymph node, the node becomes indurated and more rounded, and enlarges. Tumor eventually extends through the capsule of the lymph node and invades surrounding structures. Extension to neurovascular bundles is common and may produce a mass that is fixed to palpation. The incidence of tumor involvement and the likelihood of capsular penetration as a function of lymph node size are shown in Table 52.3.[6]

The risk of lateral retropharyngeal lymph node involvement is related to primary site and neck stage[7]; the medial retropharyngeal nodes are almost never the site of metastatic disease. The incidence of positive retropharyngeal nodes based on pretreatment computed tomography (CT) and, in selected cases, magnetic resonance imaging (MRI) is shown in Table 52.4.[7]

TABLE 52.2 CLINICALLY DETECTED NODAL METASTASES ON ADMISSION CORRELATED WITH T-STAGE

Primary Site	T Stage	N0 (%)	N1 (%)	N2-3 (%)
Oral tongue[a]	T1	86	10	4
	T2	70	19	11
	T3	52	16	31
	T4	24	10	66
Floor of the mouth[a]	T1	89	9	2
	T2	71	18	10
	T3	56	20	24
	T4	46	10	43
Retromolar trigone/anterior tonsillar pillar[b]	T1	88	2	9
	T2	62	18	20
	T3	46	21	33
	T4	32	18	50
Soft palate[b]	T1	92	0	8
	T2	64	12	24
	T3	35	26	39
	T4	33	11	56
Tonsillar fossa[b]	T1	30	41	30
	T2	32	14	54
	T3	30	18	52
	T4	10	13	76
Base of tongue[b]	T1	30	15	55
	T2	29	14	56
	T3	26	23	52
	T4	16	8	76
Oropharyngeal walls[b]	T1	75	0	25
	T2	70	10	20
	T3	33	22	44
	T4	24	24	52
Supraglottic larynx[c]	T1	61	10	29
	T2	58	16	26
	T3	16	25	40
	T4	26	18	41
Hypopharynx[d]	T1	37	21	42
	T2	30	20	49
	T3	21	26	54
	T4	26	15	58
Nasopharynx[e]	T1	8	11	82
	T2	16	12	72
	T3	12	9	80
	T4	17	6	78

[a]T stage defined by Lindberg.[5]
[b]T stage defined by Fletcher et al.[8]
[c]T stage defined by Fletcher et al.[9]
[d]T stage defined by MacComb et al.[10]
[e]T stage defined by Chen and Fletcher.[11]
Data are those of 2,044 patients, MD Anderson Hospital, Houston, TX, 1948–1965.
Modified from Lindberg RD. Distribution of cervical lymph node metastases from squamous cell carcinoma of the upper respiratory and digestive tracts. *Cancer* 1972;29(6):1446–1449. Copyright © 1972 American Cancer Society. Reprinted by permission of John Wiley & Sons, Inc.

DIAGNOSTIC WORKUP

Physical Examination

The patient is examined in the sitting position, the examiner behind the patient with one hand on the occiput to flex the

TABLE 52.1 DEFINITION OF RISK GROUPS

Group	Estimated Risk of Subclinical Neck Disease	Stage	Site
I: Low risk	<20%	T1	Floor of the mouth, retromolar gingiva, trigone, palate, buccal hard mucosa
II: Intermediate risk	20%–30%	T1	Oral tongue, soft palate, pharyngeal wall, supraglottic larynx, tonsil
		T2	Floor of the mouth, oral of retromolar tongue, gingiva, trigone, hard palate, buccal mucosa
III: High risk	>30%	T1–4	Nasopharynx, pyriform sinus, base of tongue
		T2–4	Soft palate, pharyngeal wall, supraglottic larynx, tonsil
		T3–4	Floor of the mouth, oral retromolar tongue, trigone, gingiva, hard palate, buccal mucosa

Reprinted from Mendenhall WM, Million RR. Elective neck irradiation for squamous cell carcinoma of the head and neck: analysis of time–dose factors and causes of failure. *Int J Radiat Oncol Biol Phys* 1986;12(5):741–746. Copyright © 1986 Elsevier. With permission.

TABLE 52.3 RELATIONSHIP BETWEEN NODE SIZE, THE PRESENCE OF TUMOR IN THE NODE, AND CAPSULAR PENETRATION IN 519 NODES[a]

	Size of Node (cm)				
	1	2	3	4	≥5
Number of nodes	177	183	84	17	58
Percentage positive	33	62	81	88	100
Percentage positive capsular with penetration	14	26	49	71	76

[a]Institut Gustave Roussy, Villejuif, France.
Modified from Richard JM, Sancho-Garnier H, Micheau C. Prognostic factors in cervical lymph node metastasis in upper respiratory and digestive tract carcinoma: study of 1713 cases during a 15-year period. *Laryngoscope* 1987;97(1):97–101. Copyright © 1987 The Triological Society. Reprinted by permission of John Wiley & Sons, Inc.

TABLE 52.4 INCIDENCE OF POSITIVE RETROPHARYNGEAL NODES FOR VARIOUS PRIMARY SITES AND CLINICAL NECK STAGES (794 TUMORS)

Primary Site	Clinical Neck Stage		
	N0 Neck (%)	N+ Neck[a] (%)	Overall (%)
Nasopharynx	2/5 (40)	12/14 (86)	74
Pharyngeal wall	6/37 (16)	12/56 (21)	19
Soft palate	1/21 (5)	6/32 (19)	13
Tonsillar region	2/56 (4)	14/120 (12)	9
Pyriform or sinus postcricoid area	0/55 (0)	7/81 (9)	5
Base of tongue	0/31 (0)	5/90 (6)	4
Supraglottic larynx	0/87 (0)	4/109 (4)	2

[a]N+ are neck nodes clinically involved (stages N1-3B).
From McLaughlin MP, Mendenhall WM, Mancuso AA, et al. Retropharyngeal adenopathy as a predictor of outcome in squamous cell carcinoma of the head and neck. *Head Neck* 1995;17(3):190–198. Copyright © 1995 Wiley Periodicals, Inc., A Wiley Company. Reprinted by permission of John Wiley & Sons, Inc.

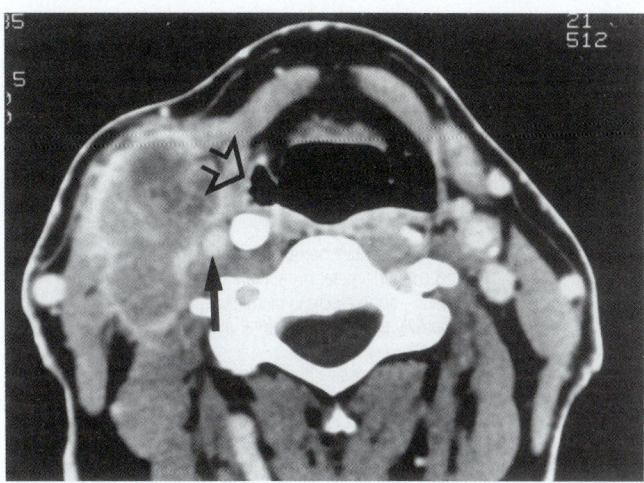

FIGURE 52.2. T1 squamous cell carcinoma of the lateral wall of the right pyriform sinus (*open arrow*) and a fixed N3B neck node that abuts but does not surround the carotid artery (*solid arrow*). (From Mendenhall WM, Parsons JT, Mancuso AA, et al. Head and neck: management of the neck. In: Perez CA, Brady LW, Halperin EC, et al., eds. *Principles practice and of radiation oncology.* Philadelphia: Lippincott Williams & Wilkins, 2004:1158–1178.)

patient's head forward and the other hand on the side of the neck to be examined. To examine the IJC lymph nodes, which lie deep to the sternocleidomastoid muscle along the internal jugular vein, place the thumb and index finger around the sternocleidomastoid muscle in the form of a "C," and then, gently proceed from the sternal notch to the angle of the mandible. Both sides of the neck should not be examined simultaneously. The level Ib and level Ia nodes may be evaluated by direct palpation of these areas as well as by a bimanual examination with the index finger placed in the floor of the mouth.[12]

The following features of metastatic lymph nodes should be recorded: anatomic location, size, consistency, mobility, and clinical impression as to whether the node is involved with cancer.

Radiographic Evaluation

CT, MRI, fluorodeoxyglucose–positron emission tomography (FDG-PET), and ultrasound may be used to evaluate cervical metastatic disease.[13] At the University of Florida, CT remains the primary method of examination of most carcinomas arising in the upper aerodigestive tract and the regional lymphatic system. MRI is the primary study only in patients with nasopharyngeal malignancies. MRI also may be used in patients who are allergic to intravenous contrast medium. Ultrasound has been used mainly in Europe to evaluate the cervical nodes. FDG-PET may be used to evaluate equivocal suspicious lymph nodes if the results of the scan would alter the treatment plan. Positive nodes <1 cm will not be reliably detected on a PET scan. FDG-PET remains unproven with regard to improving accuracy rates over those available with properly performed and interpreted CT.

Small metastases may be seen as lucent foci in normal-sized nodes. Such metastases have been identified and surgically confirmed in nodes as small as 6 to 8 mm; however, most subclinical disease in normal-sized nodes remains undetected on CT. FDG-PET has a marginal capability to improve on CT in detecting the subclinical disease in small (<1 cm) nodes.

Lucent foci in normal-sized nodes must be differentiated from hilar fat or volume-averaging artifacts. As the metastasis grows, the node becomes more spherical than elliptical. Areas of necrosis are almost always present in nodal metastases larger than 2 cm. As the metastasis enlarges, the capsule of the node becomes hyperemic and is seen radiographically as contrast-enhanced rim. When the capsule becomes indistinct and irregular along its outer margin, it is highly suggestive of early capsular penetration. Continued growth causes obliteration of the fat planes surrounding the nodes. Finally, no clear plane of normal tissue lies between the mass and the adjacent structures, at which point the clinician usually notes

fixation (Fig. 52.2). Penetration of the prevertebral fascia and fixation to the scalene muscles are uncommon in untreated patients. Largely necrotic nodes may be negative on FDG-PET examinations.

If a lymph node shows evidence of capsular penetration and envelops more than 50% of the circumference of the carotid artery, clinical evidence of fixation to the artery is likely. Ultrasound and MRI may prove useful in evaluating tumor extension to the carotid, as suggested by CT. MRI tends to be better at excluding extension to the neurovascular bundle when it is suspected on CT, whereas ultrasound can help show invasion of the vessel wall, thus confirming focal extension to the artery.

STAGING

The staging systems shown in Table 52.5 are those of the American Joint Committee on Cancer (AJCC).[14] Because all University of Florida data presented in this chapter were analyzed using the 1983 AJCC staging system,[15] both the 1983 and 2010 systems are outlined in Table 52.5. Stage N3C in the 1983 system is rare and should alert the clinician to search for another primary lesion. The 2017 AJCC staging system classifies bilateral or contralateral nodes not more than 6 cm in diameter as N2C; N3 is defined as a metastasis in a lymph node more than 6 cm in diameter.[14] The AJCC nodal staging system for head and neck cancer has not changed appreciably since the 1997 edition. The AJCC nodal staging for nasopharyngeal carcinoma differs from other head and neck primary sites and will be discussed in the chapter devoted to that topic.

SURGERY

Historically, surgical treatment of neck lymphatics involved radical neck dissection. This involves the removal of lymph nodes in levels I to V along with the spinal accessory nerve, sternocleidomastoid muscle, and internal jugular vein. This is seldom performed today, as many studies have demonstrated that structures not involved by cancer in the neck can be preserved without sacrificing survival. The only indication to remove nonlymphatic structures in the neck (nerves, muscles, internal jugular vein, etc.) is direct involvement of the structure by a cancerous node.

TABLE 52.5 1983 AND 2017 AMERICAN JOINT COMMITTEE ON CANCER STAGING FOR NECK LYMPH NODES

Stage	Definition
1983 Stage	
NX	Nodes cannot be assessed
N0	No clinically positive nodes
N1	Single clinically positive homolateral node cm 3 or less in diameter
N2	Single clinically positive homolateral node more than 3 cm but not >6 cm in diameter or multiple clinically positive homolateral nodes, none >6 cm in diameter
N2A	Single clinically positive homolateral node >3 cm but not >6 cm in diameter
N2B	Multiple clinically positive homolateral nodes, none >6 cm in diameter
N3A	Clinically positive homolateral node(s), one >6 cm in diameter
N3B	Bilateral clinically positive nodes (in this situation, each side of the neck should be staged separately) N3B (i.e., left, N23; right, N1)
N3C	Contralateral node(s) clinically positive only
2017 Stage	
NX	Regional lymph nodes cannot be assessed
N0	No lymph regional node metastasis
N1	Metastasis in a single ipsilateral lymph node, 3 cm or smaller in greatest dimension and extranodal extension (ENE)(−)
N2	Metastasis in a single ipsilateral node larger than 3 cm but not larger than 6 cm in greatest dimension and ENE (−); or metastases in multiple ipsilateral nodes, none larger than 6 cm in greatest dimension and ENE (−); or in bilateral or contralateral lymph nodes, none larger than 6 cm in greatest dimension, ENE(−)
N2a	Metastasis in single ipsilateral or contralateral node larger than 3 cm but not larger than 6 cm in greatest dimension and ENE(−)
N2b	Metastasis in multiple ipsilateral nodes, none larger than 6 cm in greatest dimension and ENE(−)
N2c	Metastasis bilateral or contralateral lymph nodes, none larger than 6 cm in greatest dimension and ENE(−)
N3	Metastasis in a lymph node larger than 6 cm in greatest dimension and ENE(−); or metastases in a single ipsilateral node ENE(+) or multiple ipsilateral, contralateral, or bilateral nodes, any with ENE(+)
N3a	Metastasis in a lymph node larger than 6 cm in greatest dimension and ENE(−)
N3b	Metastasis in a single ipsilateral node ENE(+) or multiple ipsilateral, contralateral, or bilateral nodes, any with ENE(+)

From Amin MB, Edge SB, Greene FL, et al. eds. *AJCC cancer staging manual.* 8th ed. New York: Springer, 2017. Reproduced with permission of Springer International Publishing in the format Book via Copyright Clearance Center.

Modified radical neck dissection, or functional neck dissection, involves the removal of lymph nodes in levels I to V with preservation of at least one of the following structures: spinal accessory nerve, sternocleidomastoid muscle, or internal jugular vein. This approach is used when the nodal burden is advanced with high-risk spread to level V or invasion of nonlymphatic structures.

The most commonly performed surgical neck treatment of neck lymphatics is now the selective neck dissection. This approach involves preserving all nonlymphatic structures and only removing the high-risk lymphatic levels. The advantage of this approach is that it maintains function, minimizes morbidity, and does not compromise oncologic treatment. The levels to be removed are determined by site of cancer. Levels I to III are addressed for oral cavity cancers. Levels II to IV are included for treatment of oropharyngeal, laryngeal, and hypopharyngeal cancers. If nodes suspicious for metastases are encountered in areas outside of the planned neck dissection, the selective neck dissection should be converted to a modified radical neck dissection.

Bilateral neck dissections may be performed simultaneously or separately (staged) in patients with bilateral neck disease as long as one internal jugular vein can be preserved.

TABLE 52.6 POSTOPERATIVE COMPLICATIONS OF UNILATERAL NECK DISSECTION AFTER IRRADIATION TO THE PRIMARY LESION AND NECK (143 PATIENTS)

Complications	Number of Complications	Number of Second Operations to Repair Complication	Death
Salivary fistula	1	0	0
Wound breakdown	23	15	0
Bleeding	2	1	1
Pneumonia	2	0	1
Orocutaneous fistula	1	1	0
Lymphatic fistula	2	0	0
Pulmonary embolus	1	0	0
Cardiovascular problem	2	0	1
Sepsis	1	0	1
Total complications	35[a]	17	4[b]
Incidence (%)	33/143 (23)	17/143 (12)	4/143 (3)

[a]Thirty-five complications in 33 patients.
[b]Deaths occurred 6, 7, 8, and 35 days after surgery.
Reprinted from Mendenhall WM, Million RR, Cassisi NJ. Squamous cell carcinoma of the head and neck treated with radiation therapy: the role of neck dissection for clinically positive neck nodes. *Int J Radiat Oncol Biol Phys* 1986;12(5):733–740. Copyright © 1986 Elsevier. With permission.

If both internal jugular veins need to be sacrificed, at least one should be reconstructed with a vein graft (e.g., saphenous vain or femoral vein). If both internal jugular veins are left sacrificed, the patient is at high risk of cerebral edema, extreme facial edema, and potentially blindness.

Complications of Neck Dissection

Complications of neck dissection include hematoma; seroma; lymphedema; wound infection; wound dehiscence; skin flap necrosis; chyle leak; damage to cranial nerves V, VII, X, XI, and XII; internal jugular vein rupture; and carotid rupture. The incidence of complications is higher when neck dissection is combined with resection of the primary lesion or when it follows a course of radiation therapy (RT). The postoperative mortality rate for unilateral neck dissection after RT was 3% for patients treated between 1964 and 1982.[16] This figure is now <1%.

The incidence of postoperative complications in a series of patients treated with RT to the primary lesion and neck followed by unilateral or bilateral neck dissection(s) is shown in Tables 52.6 and 52.7.[17,18] Two of 10 patients undergoing a staged bilateral neck dissection experienced a moderately severe complication compared with 4 of 40 patients undergoing a simultaneous bilateral neck dissection. None of the 10 patients who underwent a staged bilateral neck dissection experienced a severe complication, compared with 6 of 40 patients (15%) who underwent a simultaneous bilateral neck dissection (P = .24).[18]

Taylor et al.[17] analyzed the incidence of moderate (2+) and severe (3+) wound complications in a series of 205 patients

TABLE 52.7 COMPLICATIONS AFTER RADIATION THERAPY FOLLOWED BY A BILATERAL NECK DISSECTION (N = 50 PATIENTS)

Severity	Complication	Number of Patients
Moderate	Wound breakdown	2
	Bleeding	1
	Laryngeal edema	2
	Chyle fistula	1
Severe	Wound breakdown	4
	Fatal cardiac arrest	1
	Fatal acute laryngeal edema	1

Reprinted from Somerset JD, Mendenhall WM, Amdur RJ, et al. Planned postradiotherapy bilateral neck dissection for head and neck cancer. *Am J Otolaryngol* 2001;22(6):383–386. Copyright © 2001 Elsevier. With permission.

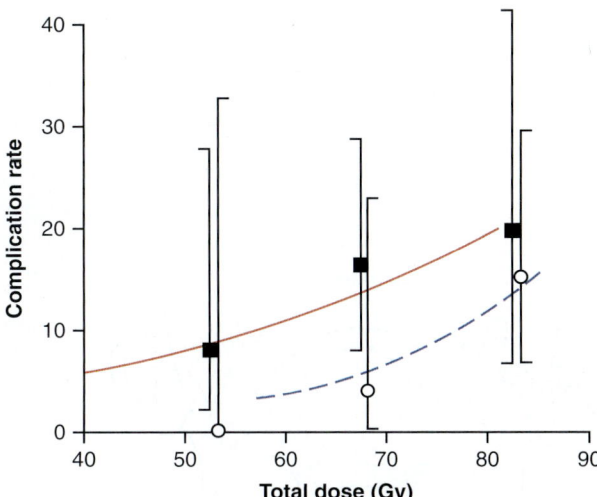

FIGURE 52.3. Complication rate (2+ or 3+) versus total dose. Separate analysis for once a day (*filled square, solid curve*) and twice a day (*circle, dashed curve*). Data are plotted at the midpoints of the range 45 to 60 Gy, 60 to 70 Gy, and 75 to 90 Gy. Error bars denote 95% confidence intervals. The curves are the results of separate logistic regression analysis. (Reprinted from Taylor JMG, Mendenhall WM, Parsons JT, et al. The influence of dose and time on wound complications following post-radiation neck dissection. *Int Radiat J Oncol Biol Phys* 1992;23[1]:41–46. Copyright © 1992 Elsevier. With permission.)

who underwent a planned unilateral neck dissection after RT at the University of Florida. RT was given once daily in 123 patients, twice daily in 80 patients, and with both techniques in the remaining two patients. The incidence of wound complications increased with total dose and dose per fraction (Fig. 52.3).

RADIATION THERAPY

RT may be used in the treatment of cervical lymph node metastases as elective treatment when there are no palpable lymph nodes, as the only treatment for clinically positive lymph nodes,[19] or as preoperative or postoperative treatment in combination with neck dissection for clinically positive lymph nodes.[20]

The regional lymph nodes are considered in the treatment planning of the primary lesion. With clinically negative neck nodes, treatment planning depends on the estimated risk of subclinical disease in the nodes. With clinically positive lymph nodes, the plan is influenced by the number of lymph nodes, size, and location.

Elective Radiation Therapy of Cervical Lymph Nodes When the Primary Tumor Is Treated by Radiation Therapy

Factors that influence the decision to irradiate the neck electively are site and size of the primary lesion, histologic grade, difficulty in neck examination, relative morbidity for adding lymph node coverage, likelihood of the patient's returning for follow-up examinations, and suitability of the patient for a radical neck dissection if the tumor appears in the neck at a later date. Patients in whom the primary lesion is to be treated by RT, who have clinically negative nodes, and in whom the risk of subclinical disease is 15% to 20% or greater receive elective neck irradiation to a minimum dose equivalent to 45 to 50 Gy over 4.5 to 5 weeks (see Table 52.1). Patients with lesions arising in the lip, nasal vestibule, nasal cavity, or paranasal sinuses have a low risk of subclinical neck disease, and the neck is not treated electively unless the lesion is recurrent, advanced, or poorly differentiated. Similarly, the risk of occult neck disease is essentially 0% for T1 and 1.7% for T2 glottic carcinomas, and elective neck radiation therapy is not indicated.[21,22]

The lateral treatment portals used to encompass cancers in the oropharynx, supraglottic larynx, and hypopharynx include the upper jugular and often the midjugular chain lymph nodes. RT portals used for primary lesions of the oral cavity, nasopharynx, glottis, nasal cavity, and paranasal sinuses must be enlarged to include the lymph nodes. The treatment portals for irradiation of the cervical lymph nodes must be designed in such a way as to minimize additional mucosal irradiation. A common error in irradiating oropharyngeal and nasopharyngeal cancers is to enlarge the lateral (primary) portals inferiorly to unnecessarily include all of the larynx in the lateral portals (Fig. 52.4).[23] Because the midneck is smaller in circumference than the upper neck, the total dose and dose per fraction are higher in the larynx than along the central axis of the beam, leading to double trouble. Although a field junction through a positive node(s) may be avoided with intensity-modulated radiation therapy (IMRT), the larynx still receives a substantially higher dose compared with a separate anterior low-neck portal with a midline laryngeal block junctioned at the thyroid notch (Figs. 52.5–52.7).[24] Treating an unnecessarily large field increases the acute and late effects of RT and, by increasing the risk of an unplanned split, reduces the probability of disease control.[23,24]

IMRT may be used to treat patients if there is a goal that can be achieved to reduce the toxicity of irradiation. These goals are usually parotid sparing to reduce the risk of long-term xerostomia, avoiding a low-neck match in patients with a low-lying larynx, and improved coverage of the poststyloid parapharyngeal space in patients with nasopharyngeal cancer.[25] If one or more of these goals cannot be achieved, the patients may be better off being treated with conventional RT because of the disadvantages of IMRT, which include increased risk of a marginal miss, less homogeneous dose distribution, and increased cost and complexity.[25]

Elective neck irradiation for early oral cavity lesions includes the level Ib and level II lymph nodes. The level III and level IV lymph nodes are treated as well by using a narrow anterior field. For primary lesions located in the oropharynx, nasopharynx, supraglottic larynx, and hypopharynx, the lower-neck nodes are also routinely included. The low neck is treated with a single anterior field (Fig. 52.8). A tapered midline larynx or trachea shield is added to protect the spinal cord, the larynx, and the pharynx. For primary lesions lying below the thyroid notch, a small midline tracheal block 1 cm wide is placed in the low-neck field, to shield the trachea, esophagus, and spinal cord.

Treatment of Clinically Positive Cervical Lymph Nodes When the Primary Tumor Is Treated by Radiation Therapy

The dose required to control a clinically positive lymph depends on the size of the lymph node[19,26] and whether concomitant chemotherapy is administered. Relatively recent data suggest that advanced disease has a better chance of cure after altered fractionation or concomitant chemotherapy.[27] Patients treated at the authors' institution routinely receive hyperfractionation on simultaneous integrated boost (SIB) combined with weekly cisplatin 30 mg/m². SIB consists of 70 Gy in 35 fractions over 30 treatment days in 6 weeks with 1 twice-daily fraction during the last 6 weeks with a minimum 6-hour interfraction interval. The high-risk planning treatment volume (PTV) receives 70 Gy at 2 Gy per fraction, intermediate-risk PTV receives 63 Gy at 1.8 Gy per fraction, and the standard-risk PTV receives 56 Gy at 1.6 Gy per fraction. Positive nodes receive approximately 70 to 74 Gy, regardless of size or rate of regression.

The decision to add a neck dissection after RT for multiple unilateral positive nodes or bilateral lymph node disease

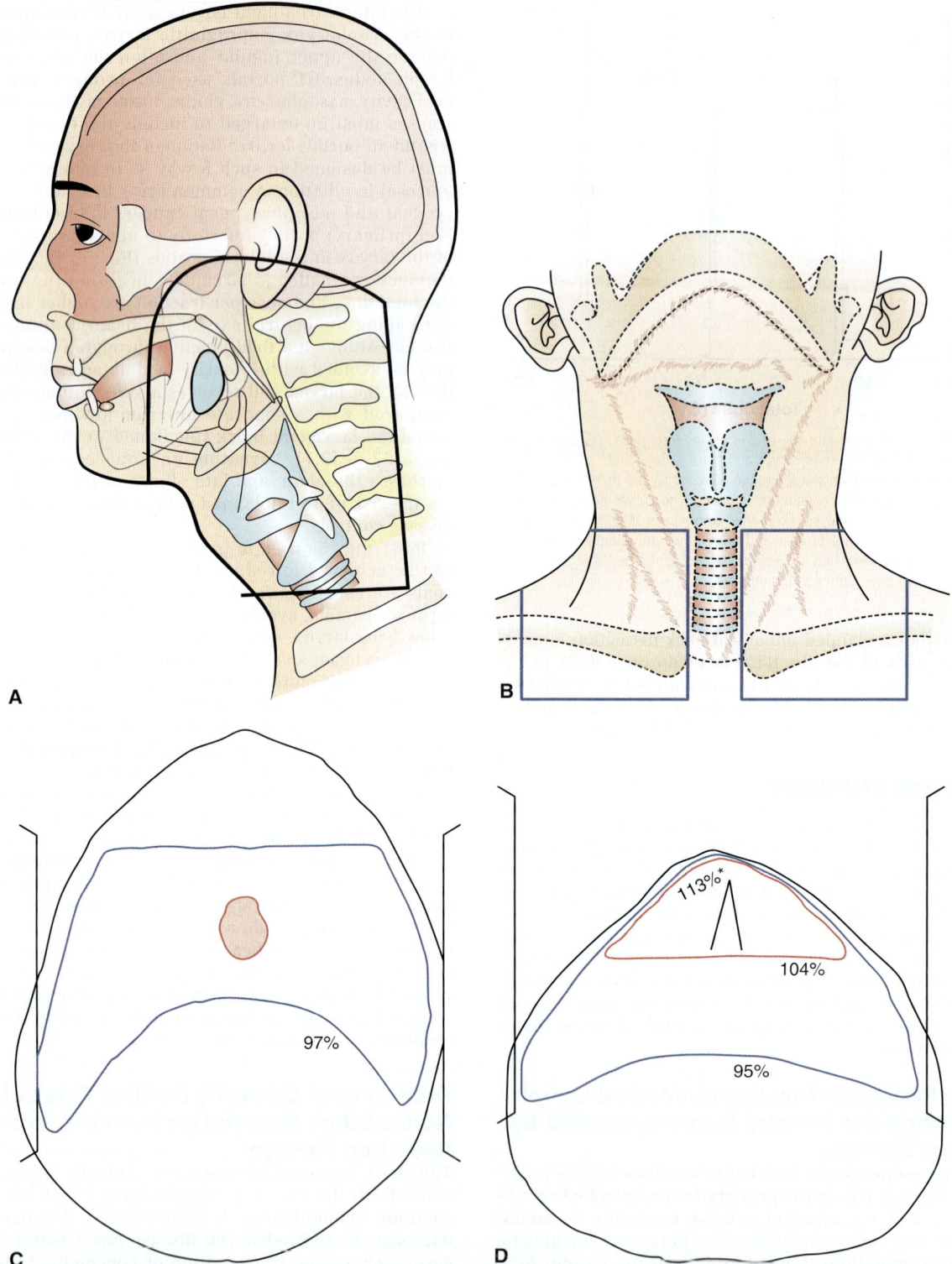

FIGURE 52.4. Carcinoma of the base of the tongue: large conventional radiation portals. **A:** Parallel-opposed lateral portals include the primary lesion, larynx, hypopharynx, most of the cervical spinal cord, and the upper portion of the trachea and cervical esophagus. Treatment through this portal tangentially irradiates the skin of the anterior neck unnecessarily. If an anterior field is not used to irradiate the low neck, the inferior border of the lateral field may be placed near the clavicle (*dashed line*). **B:** Anterior low-neck portal. The wide midline tracheal block partially shields the low internal jugular lymph nodes, which are located adjacent to the trachea. The supraclavicular lymph nodes, which are less likely to be involved with tumor than the low jugular nodes, are adequately covered. **C:** Central-axis dosimetry at the level of the base-of-tongue primary lesion. The contours were obtained from a RANDO phantom using parallel cobalt-60 fields weighted equally. The base-of-tongue tumor is outlined, and the tumor dose is specified at 97% of maximum dose. **D:** Off-axis contour through the larynx. The minimum dose to the entire larynx is 104% of the maximum dose specified at the central axis, and the maximum dose on this off-axis contour is 113%. If the base-of-tongue tumor dose is specified as 50 Gy at 2 Gy per fraction, the minimum larynx dose is 53.61 Gy at 2.14 Gy per fraction, and the maximum larynx dose is 58.25 Gy at 2.33 Gy per fraction. If the tumor dose is specified as 60 Gy at 2 Gy per fraction, the minimum larynx dose is 64.33 Gy at 2.14 Gy per fraction, and the maximum larynx dose is 69.9 Gy at 2.33 Gy per fraction. (Reprinted from Mendenhall WM, Parsons JT, Million RR. Unnecessary irradiation of the normal larynx [editorial]. *Int J Radiat Oncol Biol Phys* 1990;18[6]:1531–1533. Copyright © 1990 Elsevier. With permission.)

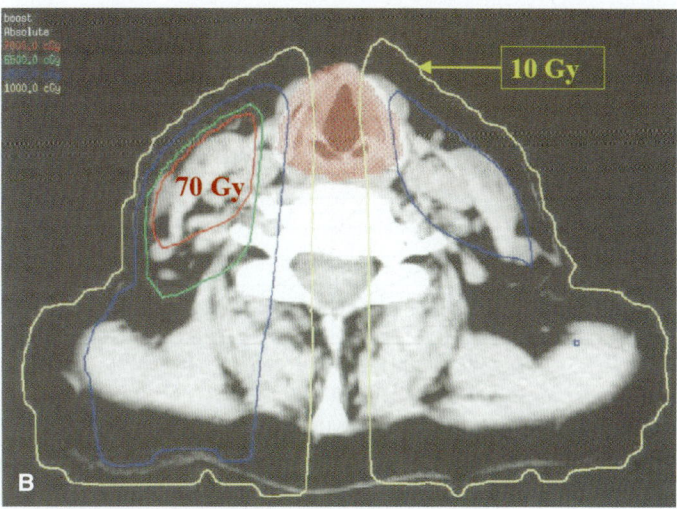

FIGURE 52.5. Laryngeal dose in a model patient with a stage T2N2b carcinoma of the tonsil with positive nodes on the right side at the level of the larynx. The primary site is irradiated with either intensity-modulated radiation therapy or conventional lateral-opposed fields. The cervical lymphatics inferior to the primary site fields are treated with an anterior low-neck field. **A:** Digitally reconstructed radiograph of the low-neck fields. The larynx was contoured and appears as a red color-wash structure. The larynx is shielded with a narrow midline block that does not cover the entire width of the larynx. In this model patient, the entire low-neck field received 50 Gy, and then the field size was reduced to boost the positive nodes on the right of the larynx to 70 Gy. Irradiation was given with a 6-MV photon beam with source to axis distance of 100 cm. **B:** Axial dose distribution at the level of the true vocal cords showing that the dose to the central portion of the larynx is extremely low when the larynx is shielded in the anterior low-neck field. (From Amdur RJ, Li JG, Liu C, et al. Unnecessary laryngeal irradiation in the IMRT era. *Head Neck* 2004;26[3]:257–264. Copyright © 2004 Wiley Periodicals, Inc. Reprinted by permission of John Wiley & Sons, Inc.)

is individualized and is based on the diameter of the largest node, node fixation, and number of clinically positive nodes in the neck. If clinically positive lymph nodes disappear completely during RT, the likelihood of control by RT alone is improved and a neck dissection may be withheld.[28–31] Peters et al.[32] reported on 100 node-positive patients with squamous cell carcinoma of the oropharynx treated with concomitant boost RT between 1984 and 1993 at the MD Anderson Cancer Center (Houston, TX). Sixty-two patients had a complete response in the neck and received no further therapy. Three patients (5%) subsequently developed an isolated recurrence in the neck, and four patients (6%) developed a recurrence in the neck in

FIGURE 52.6. Dose distribution using intensity-modulated radiation therapy as described in the text to treat the model patient with a stage T2N2b carcinoma of the tonsil with positive nodes on the right side at the level of the larynx. The plan was optimized to minimize the dose to the larynx while delivering 70 Gy to gross disease and 59.4 Gy to areas at risk for subclinical disease. **A:** Coronal projection near the middle of the larynx. **B:** Axial projection at the level of the true vocal cords. A comparison of Figures 52.5B and 52.6B shows that sparing of the central portion of the larynx is shielded in an anterior low-neck field. (From Amdur RJ, Li JG, Liu C, et al. Unnecessary laryngeal irradiation in the IMRT era. *Head Neck* 2004;26[3]:257–264. Copyright © 2004 Wiley Periodicals, Inc. Reprinted by permission of John Wiley & Sons, Inc.)

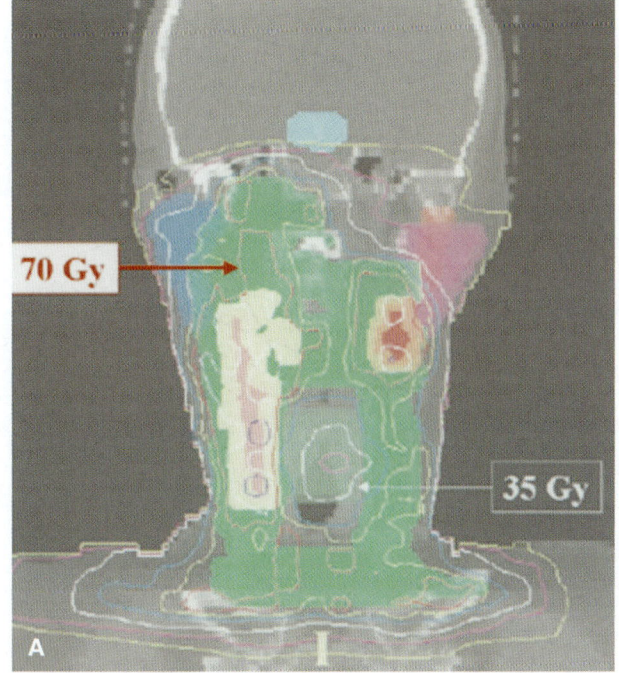

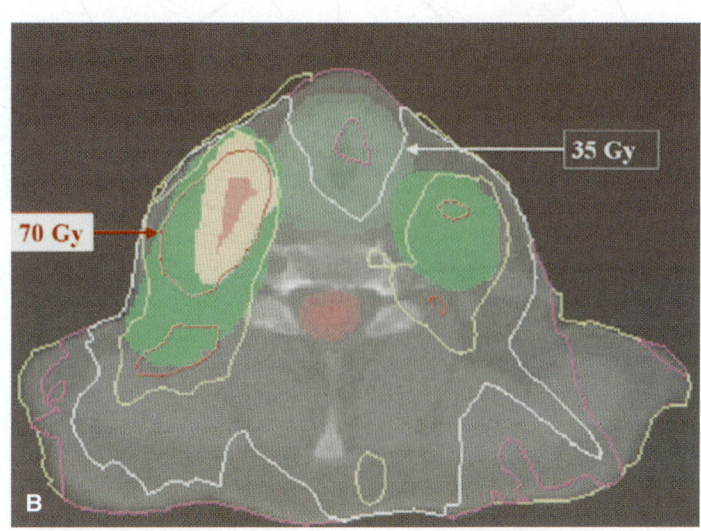

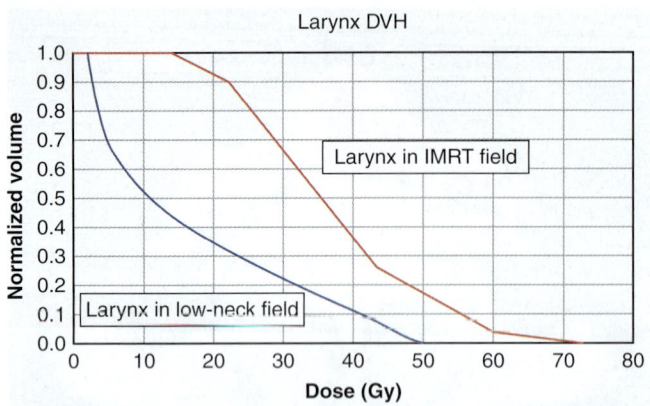

Larynx DVH

FIGURE 52.7. Dose–volume histogram (DVH) of the larynx for the model patient described in Figures 52.5 and 52.6. The thicker line is the dose–volume histogram when the larynx is included in the intensity-modulated ration therapy (IMRT) fields shown in Figure 52.6. The thinner line is the dose–volume histogram when the larynx is shielded in the anterior low-neck field shown in Figure 52.5. There is a major difference in the portion of the larynx that receives an extremely low dose. For example, when the larynx is included in the IMRT fields, the entire larynx receives more than 10 Gy, whereas when the larynx is shielded in the low-neck field, approximately 45% of the larynx receives <10 Gy. (From Amdur RJ, Li JG, Liu C, et al. Unnecessary laryngeal irradiation in the IMRT era. *Head Neck* 2004;26[3]:257–264. Copyright © 2004 Wiley Periodicals, Inc. Reprinted by permission of John Wiley & Sons, Inc.)

conjunction with other sites of relapse. The 2-year neck disease control rates did not vary significantly with pretreatment nodal size: ≤3 cm, 87%, and >3 cm, 85%. The incidence of subcutaneous fibrosis was similar following RT alone compared with another group of patients who underwent a neck dissection in addition to RT. Johnson et al.[33] reported on 81 patients with node-positive stages III and IV squamous cell carcinoma of the head and neck treated with concomitant boost accelerated hyperfractionated RT at the Medical College of Virginia (Richmond). Fifty-eight patients (72%) had a complete response in the neck and were followed; three patients (5%) subsequently developed an isolated recurrence in the neck, and one additional patient developed recurrent cancer in the neck and in the primary site. The 3-year neck disease control rates were 94% for nodes ≤3 cm compared with 86% for those >3 cm.

Both of these series of patients received aggressive altered fractionated RT, and it is unclear whether these data can be broadly extrapolated to patients with head and neck cancer from a variety of head and neck primary sites that are treated less aggressively. It is also unclear whether the addition of concomitant chemotherapy results in a lower likelihood of needing a neck dissection. However, multiple subsequent studies evaluating neck control rates after RT alone or combined with chemotherapy suggest that the likelihood of an isolated

FIGURE 52.8. Lateral and anterior conventional fields are used to irradiate a patient with a carcinoma limited to the base of tongue. **A:** Parallel-opposed fields include the primary lesion with a 2- to 3-cm inferior margin. The lower border of the field is placed at the thyroid notch and slants superiorly as the junction line proceeds posteriorly. This substantially reduces the amount of mucosa larynx and spinal cord included in the primary treatment portals. **B:** *En face* low-neck portal with tapered midline larynx and tapered midline larynx block. It is not necessary to treat the supraclavicular fossa unless clinically positive nodes are found in that particular hemineck. A 5-mm midline tracheal block may be placed in the low-neck portal (*dashed line*). (Reprinted from Mendenhall WM, Parsons JT, Million RR. Unnecessary irradiation of the normal larynx [editorial]. *Int J Radiat Oncol Biol Phys* 1990;18[6]:1531–1533. Copyright © 1990 Elsevier. With permission.)

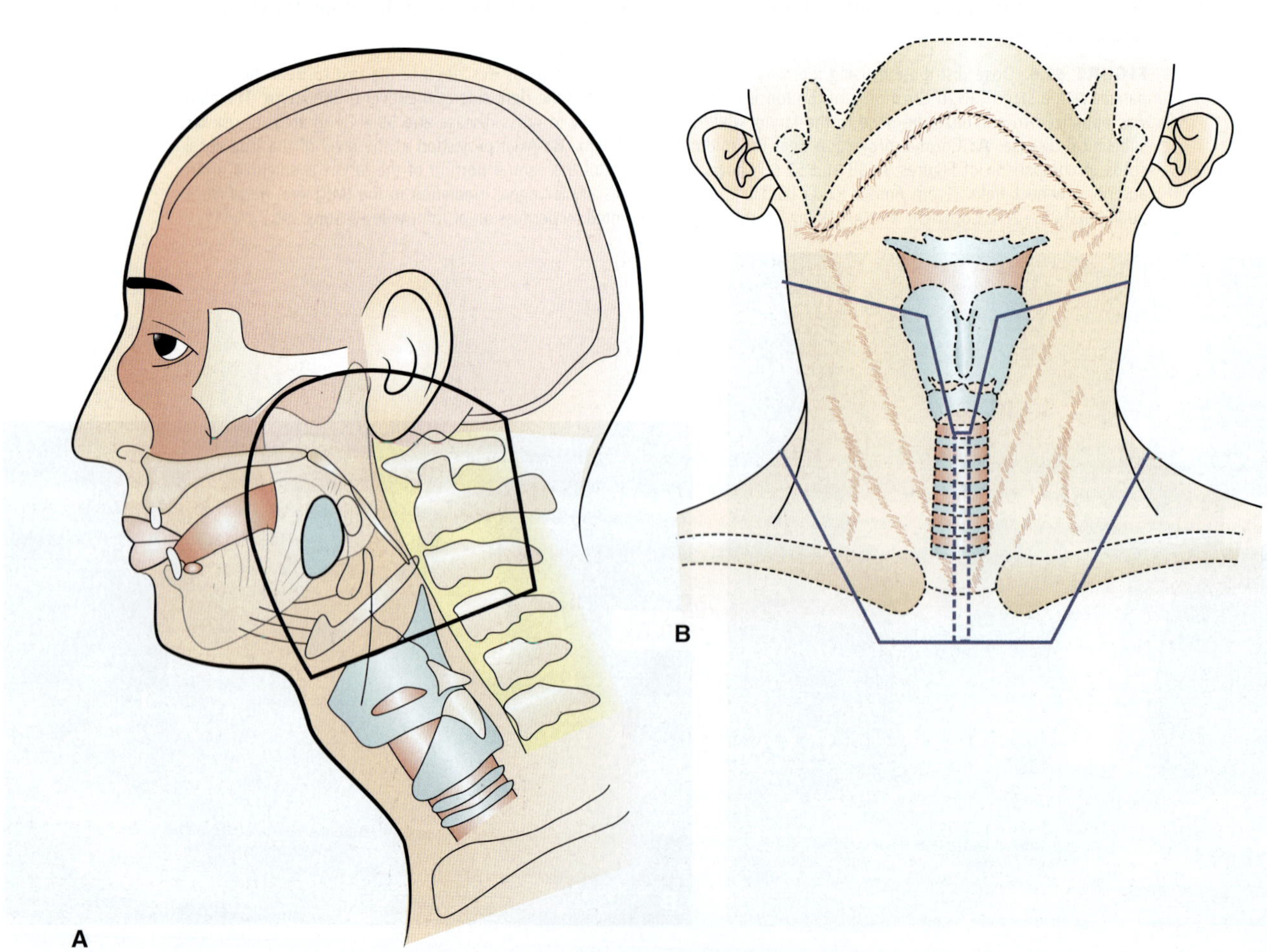

A

B

failure in the neck is low if there is a complete response after treatment.[20,34-38]

The authors' policy at the University of Florida has changed to the extent that we now evaluate patients with clinically positive nodes with CT 4 weeks after RT or a PET-CT at 3 months and withhold neck dissection in the subset of patients with a complete response thought to have ≤5% risk of residual disease.[39-46] Liauw et al.[42] evaluated a series of 550 patients treated with definitive RT at the University of Florida between 1990 and 2002; 341 patients (62%) underwent a post-RT planned neck dissection. CT images obtained at approximately 4 weeks post RT were reviewed for 211 patients; radiographic complete response (rCR) was defined as no nodes >1.5 cm and no focal abnormalities such as focal lucency, enhancement, or calcification.[36] The outcomes are depicted in Table 52.8. Thirty-two patients had an rCR and were followed and did not undergo a neck dissection; the neck control rate was 97%. Recent data published by Yeung et al.[39] suggest that for those who have a partial response to RT, neck dissection may be safely limited to only those levels that remain suspicious after RT. Post-RT selective neck dissection likely results in improved quality of life.[47] PET-CT is obtained 3 months after completion of RT to minimize the risk of a false-positive scan; those with a negative PET-CT are followed; the remainder undergo a neck dissection. Goenka et al.[45] reported on 302 patients with node-positive oropharyngeal SCCs treated with IMRT and concomitant chemotherapy at the Memorial Sloan Kettering Cancer Center between 2002 and 2009. Patients underwent a PET-CT following treatment to assess response. A clinical and radiographic complete response (CR) was observed in 260 (86.1%) patients. The neck control rate was 97.7%. Three of 4 patients who recurred in the neck were successfully salvaged. Patients who underwent a neck dissection had the following rates of pathologically visible tumor: PET-CT positive, 52%, and PET-CT negative, 25%. Mehanna et al.[46] reported on a prospective trial where 564 node-positive patients were randomized to chemoradiation followed by PET-CT and planned either neck dissection (282 patients) or observation in the event of a CR (282 patients).

Patients in the latter group underwent fewer neck dissections: the 2-year survival rates were comparable.

If a neck dissection is planned to follow RT in patients with clinically positive lymph nodes, the preoperative dose varies with the size and location of the lymph node, fixation, and response to RT. Preoperative doses of 50 Gy are sufficient for mobile lymph nodes 3 to 4 cm in size, but 60 Gy or more is recommended for 5- to 6-cm nodes and for fixed nodes. Lymph nodes measuring 7 to 8 cm are almost always fixed to adjacent structures and often require doses of 70 to 75 Gy for the surgeon to achieve a complete resection. If the lymph node lies behind the plane of the spinal cord, electrons may be used to boost the dose after the primary fields have been reduced off the spinal cord after 45 to 50 Gy.[16] Patients in whom the decision is made to add a neck dissection after completion of RT receive full-dose irradiation to the clinically positive neck nodes because the decision depends on the response to RT.

Another technique commonly used for boosting the dose to the neck mass after spinal cord tolerance has been reached, and the treatment to the primary lesion has been completed as opposed anterior and posterior fields with wedges. The final dose to the neck node (not to the entire neck) may be 70 to 80 Gy without exceeding the spinal cord tolerance (Fig. 52.9). The anterior and posterior wedge-pair technique is preferable to an appositional electron boost field because high-energy electron beams increase the skin and mucosal dose.

When the cervical lymph nodes are located superficially, sometimes within 1 cm from the skin or fixed to it, treatment with high-energy photon beams (≥ 6 MV) may underdose these nodes. Treatment should be initiated with cobalt-60 or 4-MV x-rays for the initial 45 to 50 Gy, after which a higher-energy photon beam can be used to continue RT of the primary tumor if the neck nodes are clinically negative or if a neck dissection is planned to follow RT (Fig. 52.10). Parallel-opposed 6-MV x-ray beams may adequately treat the upper neck nodes included in the primary treatment fields; however, the supraclavicular nodes in the en face low-neck field may be underdosed with a 6-MV beam in very thin patients. Although electrons alone may be used to treat cervical nodes, it is preferable to combine them with photons because of the high surface dose with high electron energies. Use of both 20-MeV electrons and 17-MV x-rays is compared with treatment by

TABLE 52.8 PREDICTIVE VALUE OF POSTRADIOTHERAPY COMPUTED TOMOGRAPHY FINDINGS AT 4 WEEKS IN THE HEMINECK CORRELATED TO NECK DISSECTION PATHOLOGY (N = 193 HEMINECKS)				
Findings	**NPV**		**PPV**	
	Number/ Total Number	**Percent**	**Number/ Total Number**	**Percent**
Any lymph node >1.5 cm	85/118	72	24/75	32
Any lymph node with focal lucency	49/57	86	49/136	36
Any focally abnormal lymph node[a]	75/98	77	34/95	36
Any lymph with node enhancement	111/147	76	21/46	46
Any lymph with node calcification	102/144	71	15/49	31
Two or more focally abnormal lymph nodes[a]	90/113	80	34/80	43
Any lymph node >1.5 cm and any focally abnormal lymph node	32/34	94	55/159	35

[a]Focally abnormal lymph nodes equal grade 3 or 4 focal lucency, focal enhancement, or focal calcification.
NPV, negative predictive value; PPV, positive predictive value.
From Liauw SL, Mancuso AA, Amdur RJ, et al. Postradiotherapy neck dissection for lymph node-positive head and neck cancer: the use of computed tomography to manage the neck. *J Clin Oncol* 2006;24(9):1421–1427. Reprinted with permission. Copyright © 2006 American Society of Clinical Oncology. All rights reserved.

FIGURE 52.9. Dose distribution for anterior and posterior wedge cobalt-60 portals, both fields weighted 1.0.

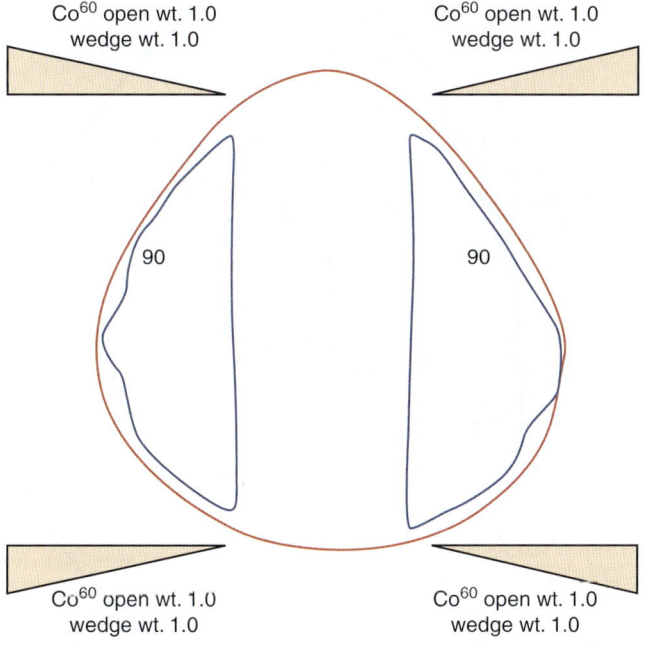

Co[60] open wt. 1.0 wedge wt. 1.0

Co[60] open wt. 1.0 wedge wt. 1.0

90   90

Co[60] open wt. 1.0 wedge wt. 1.0

Co[60] open wt. 1.0 wedge wt. 1.0

Section III

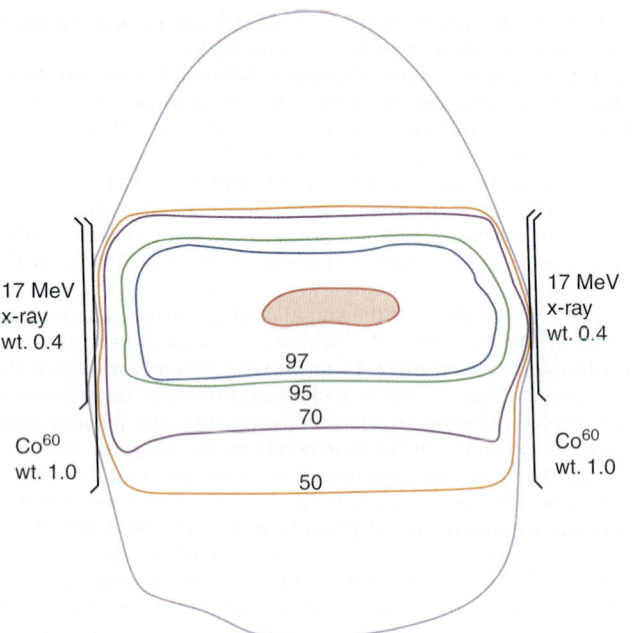

FIGURE 52.10. Dose distribution for parallel-opposed cobalt-60 portals, each weighted 1.0, with reduced 17-MV x-ray portals, each weighted 0.4.

20-MeV electrons alone in a patient with a lateralized lesion of the oropharynx (Fig. 52.11).[48] The addition of the 17-MV x-rays to the 20-MeV electrons decreases the surface dose while still adequately irradiating the cervical nodes that are within the primary field. The addition of the x-ray beam also produces a dose distribution that is less affected by bone than that from the electron beam alone.

Large lymph nodes may not show much regression during the course of RT but often show significant regression from completion of treatment to the time the patient returns

for neck dissection, usually after 4 to 6 weeks. The mass frequently has a thick capsule that facilitates its removal at the time of neck dissection.

Patients with bilateral neck disease require individualized treatment planning jointly by the radiation oncologist and the surgeon. If disease is minimal on one side, RT alone may be used to control the disease on that side of the neck, and a neck dissection may be used on the side with more disease. If major bilateral disease is present, bilateral neck dissection should follow RT.

Complications of Neck Irradiation

The complications of neck irradiation include subcutaneous fibrosis and lymphedema of the larynx and submentum. The latter complications may be minimized by sparing an anterior strip of skin when designing the parallel-opposed lateral portals used to encompass the primary lesion. The probability of complications is directly related to the radiation dose with little, if any, morbidity observed with the doses used for elective radiation therapy of the neck.

Complications of neck treatment in patients who receive RT in conjunction with resection of the primary lesion and a neck dissection are essentially the same as those occurring after neck dissection. However, they occur with an increased incidence depending on the RT dose and extent of surgery.

Treatment of the Neck after Incisional or Excisional Biopsy

Open biopsy of a clinically positive neck node before definitive treatment potentially spills tumor cells along tissue planes that may not be removed with a radical neck dissection. McGuirt and McCabe[49] reported that incisional or excisional biopsy of positive neck nodes before definitive surgery increased the risk of neck failure and worsened the prognosis for patients with squamous cell carcinoma of the head and neck. Parsons et al.[50] reported their experience with incisional or excisional biopsy of positive neck nodes followed by RT as

FIGURE 52.11. A: Dose distribution for 20-MeV electrons, field size 8.5 cm by 8.5 cm, SSD 100 cm. **B:** Dose distribution for 20-MeV electrons, field size 8.5 cm by 8.5 cm, and 17-MV x-rays, field size 7 cm by 7 cm, SSD 100 cm for both. The given doses are weighted 1 to 1. The addition of the 17-MV x-ray beam reduces the surface dose and gives a dose distribution that is affected less by bone. (From Bova FJ. Treatment planning for irradiation of head and neck cancer. In: Million RR, Cassisi NJ, eds. Management head of and neck cancer: *a multidisciplinary approach.* 2nd ed. Philadelphia: JB Lippincott, 1994:306. With permission.)

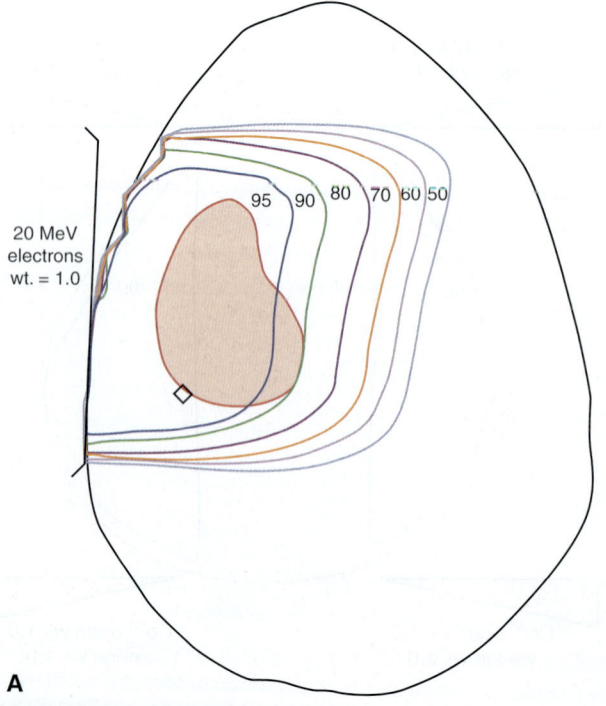

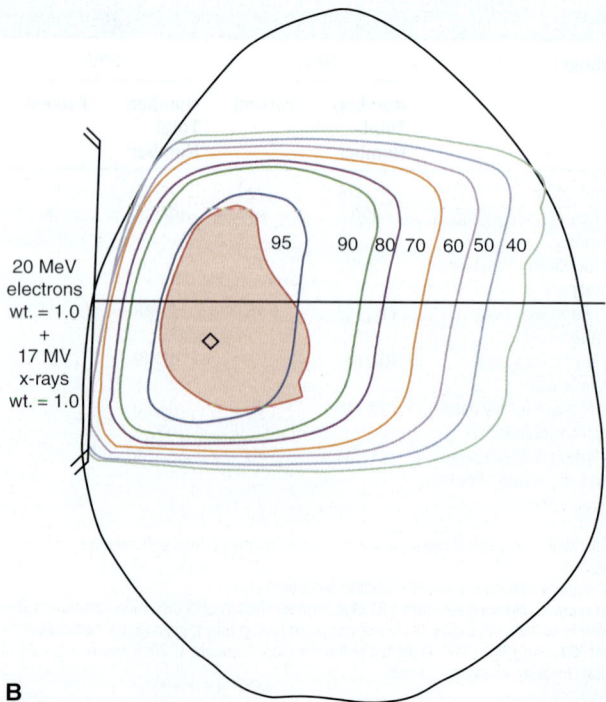

A

B

the initial step in the treatment of the patient; these data were updated by Mack et al.[51] After excisional biopsy of a single lymph node, RT alone to the primary lesion and to the neck resulted in a 95% rate of neck control.[51] If residual disease remained in the neck after biopsy, RT followed by neck dissection was more successful than RT alone for controlling neck disease (see Table 52.17).

If the primary lesion is to be treated surgically, the patient's neck is typically treated with a completion neck dissection followed by RT. If the primary lesion is to be treated with RT, the patient is treated with RT. If there is no palpable disease remaining in the neck after excisional biopsy of a positive node, the neck may be treated with RT alone. If an incisional biopsy of the node has been performed (leaving gross disease) or if other positive nodes remain after an excisional neck node biopsy, a completion neck dissection is performed with removal of skin over the biopsy site as well as any other structures involved by cancer. RT follows the surgical procedure. The dose of RT preceding a neck dissection depends on the amount of gross disease in the neck and the degree of fixation.[1]

TREATMENT OF THE NECK AFTER SURGERY

Patients treated surgically generally undergo resection of the primary cancer and a unilateral or bilateral neck dissection depending on the location and extent of the primary and presence and extent of positive neck nodes. Indications for postoperative RT include positive or close (<5 mm) margins, initially positive margins with negative separately submitted margins, extracapsular extension, multiple positive nodes, lymphovascular space invasion, perineural invasion, bone or cartilage invasion, extension into the soft tissues of the neck, invasion of the apex of the pyriform sinus, and subglottic extension of 1 cm or more.[52] The highest risk indications are positive margins and extracapsular extension and require the addition of concomitant cisplatin during the course of postoperative RT. Because of the risk of increased radioresistance due to tumor cells being in potentially hypoxic tissues, the minimum dose is 60 Gy at 2 Gy per once-daily fraction. Areas at higher risk may be boosted to doses in the range of 66 to 70 Gy. Alternatively, patients at particularly high risk may be treated with hyperfractionation at 1.2 Gy per twice-daily fraction to doses up to 74.4 Gy or 70 Gy in 35 fractions over 6 weeks treating twice daily once weekly for the last 5 weeks of RT. Consideration may be given to treating the primary site alone if the neck nodes are pathologically negative. Postoperative RT is not employed for the indication to electively treat the clinically negative neck in lieu of a neck dissection. Patients with a clinically negative neck who will require postoperative RT may forego a neck dissection and the neck irradiated in conjunction with the primary site.

RESULTS OF TREATMENT

Clinically Negative Nodes

Elective neck dissection and elective neck irradiation are equally effective in controlling subclinical disease. The decision whether to use surgery or RT for the purpose of electively treating the neck nodes depends on the method used to treat the primary lesion. Patients with a relatively early primary lesion and clinically negative nodes should be treated with one modality. Patients whose primary lesion is treated surgically may undergo an elective neck dissection, and those whose primary lesion is to be treated with RT should be considered for elective neck irradiation. Patients who develop a local recurrence or a metachronous second primary after RT for an SCC with a cN0 neck in whom the neck has been irradiated may be treated with surgery to the primary site alone and the neck observed because the likelihood of subclinical disease in the cervical lymphatics is <10%.[53,54]

TABLE 52.9 CONTROL OF DISEASE IN THE CLINICALLY NEGATIVE NECK WITH ELECTIVE NECK IRRADIATION (NUMBER CONTROLLED/NUMBER TREATED)

Risk Group	No ENI (%)	Partial ENI (%)	Total ENI (%)
I (<20%)	13/15 (87)	16/17 (94)	1/1 (100)
II (20%–30%)	6/9 (67)	34/38 (89)	10/11 (91)
III (>30%)	3/4 (75)	32/33 (97)	61/62 (98)

ENI, elective neck irradiation.
Reprinted from Mendenhall WM, Million RR. Elective neck irradiation for squamous cell carcinoma of the head and neck: analysis of time–dose factors and causes of failure. *Int J Radiat Oncol Biol Phys* 1986;12(5):741–746. Copyright © 1986 Elsevier. With permission.

The results of elective neck irradiation at the University of Florida for patients with squamous cell carcinoma of the head and neck in whom the primary lesion was controlled are shown in Table 52.9.[4,55] Patients were divided into three risk categories based on the estimated risk of subclinical disease in the neck as follows: group I, low risk (<20% likelihood of occult disease); group II, moderate risk (20% to 30% risk of occult disease); and group III, high risk (more than 30% likelihood of occult disease). There were 6 neck failures (21%) in 28 patients who did not receive elective neck irradiation and 8 neck failures (5%) in 162 patients who received elective neck irradiation. Of the eight failures in patients receiving elective neck irradiation, two occurred within the irradiation fields, one at the field margin, and five in out-of-field areas. No correlation was found between the rate of tumor control in the first-echelon lymph nodes and the irradiation dose for doses ranging from 40 to 55 Gy or greater.[4] Only one failure occurred in the first-echelon lymph nodes, and this was after 48 Gy in 25 fractions using continuous-course irradiation.[4] The low neck, defined as that part of the neck located below the treatment portals used to treat the primary lesion, received either 50 Gy in 25 fractions or 40.5 Gy in 15 fractions, specified at D_{max} (0.5 cm depth). Both dose fractionation protocols were equally effective in sterilizing subclinical disease in the low neck.[56] Elective neck irradiation is equally efficacious for squamous cell carcinoma arising from various head and neck primary sites.

In patients in whom primary failure occurs in addition to failure in the clinically negative nodes, the chances of surgical salvage are poor. In patients in whom the primary lesion is controlled and in whom failure develops in the initially negative neck, the chances of salvage with neck dissection are approximately 60%.

Although elective neck irradiation significantly reduces the risk of neck recurrence, there is no definite evidence that it improves survival. It would be necessary to conduct a large randomized trial to detect a survival difference, if one exists. Another problem is that the first-echelon lymph nodes are often included in the treatment portals used to treat the primary lesion so that it is often impossible to avoid at least partial elective neck irradiation. Therefore, such a trial would have to be restricted to primary sites where the portals would have to be enlarged to electively irradiate the neck or to patients treated with elective neck dissection rather than elective neck irradiation. Vandenbrouck et al.[57] and Fakih et al.[58] have conducted randomized trials comparing elective neck dissection with no elective neck treatment for patients with oral cavity carcinoma and oral tongue cancer, respectively. No survival advantage was noted for patients undergoing elective neck dissection in either study. However, because of the small number of patients in both trials, it is likely that even if a survival difference existed, it would have been missed. Subsequently, a randomized trial was conducted at the Tata Memorial Hospital (Mumbai) where 596 patients with T1-T2 N0 SCCs of the oral cavity were randomized to resection of the primary and observation of the neck or to resection of the primary and elective neck dissection. Those in the latter group had significantly improved overall survival at 3 years (80% vs. 68%; P = .01).[59]

Section III

Dearnaley et al.[60] reported on a series of 148 patients treated with an interstitial implant, alone or combined with external beam RT, for cancer of the tongue or floor of the mouth. Of 131 patients with negative neck nodes at diagnosis, 59 (45%) received elective neck irradiation to a dose of 40 Gy or greater. A multivariate analysis showed that elective neck irradiation significantly improved survival and reduced the risk of dying of cancer. Piedbois et al.[61] reported a series of 233 patients with T1-2N0 carcinoma of the oral cavity treated with interstitial iridium brachytherapy: 123 patients received no elective neck treatment, and 110 patients underwent elective an neck dissection. Patients who received an elective neck dissection tended to have more advanced primary lesions. Although the ultimate rates of neck control were similar, a multivariate analysis showed that elective neck dissection was significantly associated with improved survival.

Clinically Positive Nodes

The incidence of treatment failure in the neck by N stage and treatment category has been reported by the MD Anderson Cancer Center (Table 52.10) and the University of Florida (Table 52.11 and Fig. 52.12).[63,64] In patients in whom the neck is treated with combined modalities, RT precedes surgery when the primary site is to be treated with irradiation or when the node is incompletely resectable. Surgery precedes RT when the primary site is to be treated operatively and the nodes are resectable.

When the initial treatment is surgery, a neck dissection is sufficient treatment for patients with a single positive lymph node <3 cm unless there is extracapsular spread of disease. RT may be added for control of subclinical disease in the contralateral side of the neck (Table 52.12).[63] The presence of multiple positive nodes in the surgical specimen is an indication for postoperative RT of the neck, especially when positive nodes are found at more than one level.[6,65,66]

Olsen et al.[67] reported a series of 284 patients who underwent neck dissection at the Mayo Clinic for pathologic stages N1 and N2 squamous cell carcinomas of the head and neck; no patient received adjuvant therapy. Neck recurrence–free survival rates at 5 years were as follows: N1, 76%; N2, 60%; and overall, 69%. A multivariate analysis showed that four or more positive nodes (P = .005), invasion of lymphatic or vascular spaces (P = .003), invasion of soft tissue (P = .0008), and a desmoplastic stromal pattern (P = .0001) were significantly associated with an increased risk of recurrence in the neck.[67]

The postoperative dose prescribed is usually 60 Gy in 30 fractions to 65 Gy in 35 fractions over 6 to 7 weeks for patients with negative margins; higher doses may be prescribed when residual disease is present in the neck.[65,68,69] If RT is to be added after surgery, it is usually initiated within 4 to 6 weeks after the operation, although it has been reported that a delay to 10 weeks is not associated with an increased risk of neck failure.[65]

The rate of control for neck nodes treated with RT alone as a function of node size, treatment scheme, and dose is shown in Table 52.13. RT alone is sufficient for patients with N1 (up to 2 cm) disease as long as the fraction size (2 Gy) and the total dose are sufficient.[40] RT followed by neck dissection has

TABLE 52.11 FIVE-YEAR RATE OF NECK CONTROL BY 1983 AJCC STAGE AND TREATMENT (459 PATIENTS; 593 HEMINECKS)[a]

Stage	Irradiation Alone		Irradiation + Neck Dissection		Significance
	Number Heminecks	Control (%)	Number Heminecks	Control (%)	
N1	215	86	38	93	P = .28
N2A	29	79	24	68	P = .6
N2B	138	70	80	91	P < .01
N3A	29	33	40	69	P < .01

[a]Excludes 67 heminecks on which incisional or excisional biopsy was done before treatment.
AJCC, American Joint Committee on Cancer.
University of Florida data; patients treated October 1964 to October 1985; analysis December 1988 by Eric R. Ellis, MD.

provided better rates of disease control than RT alone for patients with more advanced neck disease. The rate of neck disease control for patients treated with twice-daily RT, alone or followed by neck dissection, is shown in Figure 52.12 and shows a significant improvement in the control rates when neck dissection was added in selected cases.[70,71] As shown in a multivariate analysis by Ellis et al.,[72] the addition of neck dissection after RT is independently related to a significantly decreased risk of disease-specific death. At least 50 Gy should be given preoperatively to the lymph nodes, although doses vary according to the size and degree of fixation of the lymph node. For example, large, fixed lymph nodes require 70 to 75 Gy of preoperative RT (Table 52.14). The likelihood of disease control in each side of the neck treated with irradiation and neck dissection is decreased when the node is fixed before treatment or when residual tumor is found in the pathologic specimen (Tables 52.15 and 52.16).[16] No difference is seen in the rate of control as a function of the interval between RT and neck dissection when comparing patients who have surgery within 6 weeks with those who have neck dissection more than 6 weeks after RT.[16] If a local recurrence occurs, prior combined treatment of the neck does not diminish the chance of successful surgical salvage of the patient.[73] The likelihood of disease control at the primary site was not found to be related to neck stage at diagnosis in patients treated with RT alone or followed by neck dissection at the University of Florida[74]; this finding is different from what others have reported.[75]

Results after Incisional or Excisional Biopsy

Patients who have undergone an incisional or excisional biopsy of a metastatic lymph node before referral do not have an increased risk of neck failure or a decreased cure rate if RT is the next step in treatment.[50] The likelihood of control and the cure rate are probably diminished if an operation without prior RT follows incisional or excisional biopsy of a metastatic neck node because of the risk that the biopsy procedure disseminated tumor cells into tissues not removed by neck dissection.[49]

Ellis et al.[72] reported on 508 patients with 660 positive heminecks treated at the University of Florida with RT alone or followed by a planned neck dissection. Pretreatment node

TABLE 52.10 FAILURE OF INITIAL IPSILATERAL NECK TREATMENT: 596 PATIENTS WITH CARCINOMA OF THE TONSILLAR FOSSA, BASE OF TONGUE, SUPRAGLOTTIC LARYNX, OR HYPOPHARYNX

Treatment[a]	N0			N1 (%)	N2A (%)	N2B (%)	N3A (%)	N3B (%)
	No Treatment	Partial Treatment	Complete Treatment					
Irradiation		15%	2%	15	27	27	38	34
Surgery	55% (16/29)	35%	7%	11	8	23	42	41
Combined		1/5	0/6	0	0	0	23	25

[a]MD Anderson Cancer Center data; patients treated 1948–1967.
Modified from Barkley HT Jr, Fletcher GH, Jesse RH, et al. Management of cervical lymph node metastases in squamous cell carcinoma of the tonsillar fossa, base of tongue, supraglottic larynx, and hypopharynx. Am J Surg 1972;124(4):462–467. Copyright © 1972 Elsevier. With permission.

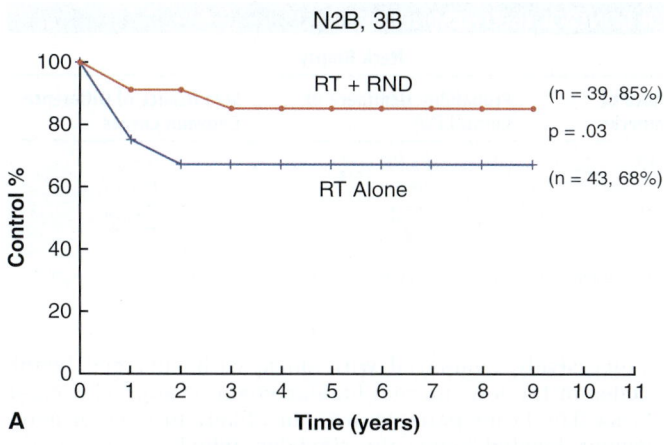
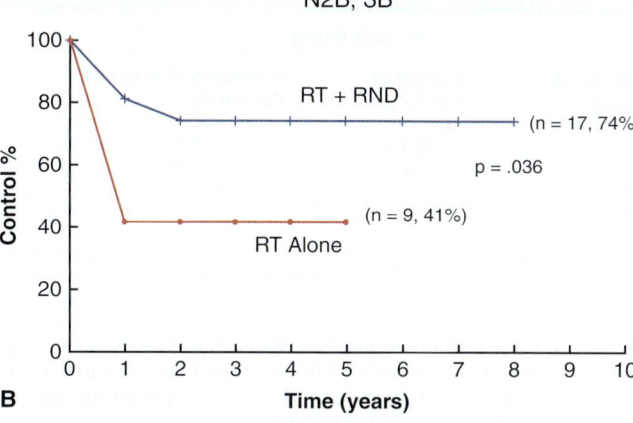

FIGURE 52.12. Rate of neck disease control (life table method[84]) for patients treated with twice-daily irradiation (RT) alone or combined with neck dissection (radiotherapy plus RND) for clinically positive neck nodes. **A:** N2B, N3B. **B:** N2A, N3A. (From Parsons JT, Mendenhall WM, Cassisi NJ, et al. Neck dissection after twice-a-day radiotherapy: morbidity and recurrence rates. *Head Neck* 1989;11[5]:400–404. Copyright © 1989 Wiley Periodicals, Inc., A Wiley Company. Reprinted by permission of John Wiley & Sons, Inc.)

TABLE 52.12 CERVICAL METASTASIS APPEARING IN THE CONTRALATERAL N0 NECK: 596 PATIENTS WITH CARCINOMA OF TONSILLAR FOSSA, BASE OF TONGUE, SUPRAGLOTTIC LARYNX, OR HYPOPHARYNX

Treatment[a]	Stage				
	N0 (%)	N1 (%)	N2A (%)	N2B(%)	N3A (%)
Irradiation	4	2	9	7	0
Surgery	25	17	23	43	33
Combined	0	0	0	11	0

[a]MD Anderson Hospital data; patients treated 1948 to 1967.
Adapted from Barkley HT Jr, Fletcher GH, Jesse RH, et al. Management of cervical lymph node metastases in squamous cell carcinoma of the tonsillar fossa, base of tongue, supraglottic larynx, and hypopharynx. *Am J Surg* 1972;124(4):462–467. Copyright © 1972 Elsevier. With permission.

TABLE 52.14 CERVICAL LYMPH NODE DISEASE CONTROL WITH RADIATION THERAPY FOLLOWED BY NECK DISSECTION, WITH PRIMARY LESION TREATED INITIALLY BY RADIATION THERAPY (NUMBER CONTROLLED/NUMBER TREATED)

Minimum Node Diameter (cm)	Minimum Node Dose (Gy)			
	<50	50–50.99	60–69.99	≥70
<3	5/5	1/2	5/5	3/3
3–4	6/8	10/14	9/9	5/7
5–6	4/7	5/5	7/8	4/4
7–8	2/3	2/4	4/6	3/4
≥9	No data	1/1	2/4	0/1

University of Florida data; patients treated 1964–1982; analysis 1984 by WM Mendenhall, MD. Ninety-one patients were treated with once-a-day fractionation, continuous- or split-course technique (100 heminecks).
Reprinted from Mendenhall WM, Million RR, Cassisi NJ. Squamous cell carcinoma of the head and neck treated with radiation therapy: the role of neck dissection for clinically positive neck nodes. *Int J Radiat Oncol Biol Phys* 1986;12(5):733–740. Copyright © 1986 Elsevier. With permission.

TABLE 52.13 LYMPH NODE DISEASE CONTROL BY RADIATION TREATMENT TECHNIQUE (NUMBER CONTROLLED/NUMBER TREATED)

Node Size (cm)	Continuous Course (%)	Split Course (%)	Excluded[a]	Total (%)
<1.0	5/5	2/2	1/1	8/8
1.0	29/35 (83)	19/23 (85)	3/4	51/62 (82)
1.5–2.0	43/49 (88)	20/24 (83)	5/9	68/82 (83)
2.5–3.0	14/19 (74)	10/18 (56)	0/3	24/40 (60)
3.5–6.0	14/20 (70)	10/17 (59)	0/1	24/38 (63)
≥7.0	0/2	0/5	0/1	0/8

[a]Less than 50 Gy for nodes equal to 1.0 cm and <55 Gy for nodes equal to 1.5 cm.
Modified from Mendenhall WM, Million RR, Bova FJ. Analysis of time-dose factors in clinically positive neck nodes treated with irradiation alone in squamous cell carcinoma of the head and neck. *Int J Radiat Oncol Biol Phys* 1984;10(5):639–643. Copyright © 1984 Elsevier. With permission.

TABLE 52.15 CONTROL OF DISEASE IN THE NECK AS A FUNCTION OF NODE MOBILITY (109 PATIENTS; 121 HEMINECKS)

Size (cm)	Proportion of Nodes Fixed (%)	Number Heminecks Controlled/ Number Treated	
		Mobile or Tethered (%)	Fixed (%)
<3	1/23 (4)	19/22 (86)	1/1 (100)
3–4	4/44 (9)	33/40 (83)	2/4 (50)
5–6	9/27 (33)	17/18 (94)	6/9 (67)
7–8	10/21 (48)	8/11 (73)	5/10 (50)
≥9	3/6 (50)	2/3 (67)	1/3 (33)

Reprinted from Mendenhall WM, Million RR, Cassisi NJ. Squamous cell carcinoma of the head and neck treated with radiation therapy: the role of neck dissection for clinically positive neck nodes. *Int J Radiat Oncol Biol Phys* 1986;12(5):733–740. Copyright © 1986 Elsevier. With permission.

TABLE 52.16 NECK DISEASE CONTROL AS A FUNCTION OF PATHOLOGIC FINDINGS IN THE NECK DISSECTION SPECIMEN (108 PATIENTS; 120 EVALUABLE HEMINECKS)[a]

Size (cm)	Number Heminecks Controlled/Number Treated		
	Proportion with Specimens Positive (%)	Negative Specimen (%)	Positive Specimen (%)
<3	10/23 (43)	13/13 (100)	7/10 (70)
3–4	22/43 (51)	20/21 (95)	14/22 (64)
5–6	10/27 (37)	17/17 (100)	6/10 (60)
7–8	12/21 (57)	8/9 (89)	5/12 (42)
≥9	4/6 (67)	2/2 (100)	1/4 (25)

[a]One patient was excluded because data were unavailable.
Reprinted from Mendenhall WM, Million RR, Cassisi NJ. Squamous cell carcinoma of the head and neck treated with radiation therapy: the role of neck dissection for clinically positive neck nodes. *Int J Radiat Oncol Biol Phys* 1986;12(5):733–740. Copyright © 1986 Elsevier. With permission.

TABLE 52.17 EFFECT OF NECK NODE BIOPSY ON 5-YEAR RATE OF NECK CONTROL (660 HEMINECKS)

	No Neck Biopsy		Neck Biopsy		
Hemineck Stage	Number of Heminecks	Probability of Hemineck Control (%)	Number of Heminecks	Probability Hemineck of Control (%)	Significance of Difference Between Curves
N1	253	87 ± 3	12	100	P = .22
N2A	53	73 ± 8	15	93 ± 6	P = .18
N2B	218	78 ± 3	23	72 ± 11	P = .86
N3A	69	54 ± 7	17	81 ± 10	P = .30

From Ellis ER, Mendenhall WM, Rao PV, et al. Incisional or excisional neck-node biopsy before definitive radiotherapy, alone or followed by neck dissection. *Head Neck* 1991;13(3):177–183. Copyright © 1991 Wiley Periodicals, Inc., A Wiley Company. Reprinted by permission of John Wiley & Sons, Inc.

biopsy did not influence outcome when RT was the next step in treatment (Table 52.17).[72] The results of the forward stepwise log-rank tests of prognostic factors for predicting time to recurrence are shown in Table 52.18.[72]

Zenga et al.[76] reported on 45 patients from 1998 to 2012 who underwent open biopsy for HPV-positive oropharyngeal cancer. All patients underwent definitive surgical treatment. Disease-specific survival was 98% versus 99% in a control group who did not undergo an open biopsy. Only 7% of the open biopsy group were found to have dermal metastases in the excised skin. It is known that hypoxic tissues, such as a scar, are increasingly resistant to RT. Thus, excision of the biopsied area along with a neck dissection will improve the efficacy of adjuvant RT. This study questions the idea that previous open biopsy adversely affects patient outcomes in this subset of patients. Neck dissection is an effective primary treatment for previously violated neck nodes. However, an adjuvant dose of RT with 60 to 70 Gy is needed to minimize recurrence rates.

CERVICAL LYMPH NODE METASTASIS WITH UNKNOWN PRIMARY TUMOR

In a small percentage of patients with enlarged cervical lymph nodes, the primary lesion cannot be found, even after extensive evaluation.[77–79] Patients with enlarged lymph nodes in the upper neck have a good prognosis when treated

TABLE 52.18 PROGNOSTIC FACTORS, IN ORDER OF THEIR IMPORTANCE, FOR PREDICTING THE TIME TO OCCURRENCE OF VARIOUS EVENTS

Event	Rank Order	Factor	Level of Significance
Recurrence in the neck (n = 660 heminecks)	1	Increasing N stage	P = .0001
	2	Treatment of the neck of with RT alone	P = .0001
	3	Fixed nodes	P = .0001
	4	T-stage[a]	P = .0350
Death with disease present (n = 508 patients)	1	Recurrence above clavicles	P = .0001
	2	Increasing N stage	P = .0003
	3	Fixed nodes	P = .0053
	4	Treatment of with neck RT alone	P = .0121
For occurrence of distant metastasis (n = 508 patients)	1	Recurrence above clavicles	P = .0001
	2	Increasing N stage	P = .0003
	3	Fixed nodes	P = .0704
	4	Nodes below the thyroid notch	P = .1023

[a]This factor is thought to be correlated with the censoring pattern.
RT, radiation therapy.
From Ellis ER, Mendenhall WM, Rao PV, et al. Incisional or excisional neck-node biopsy before definitive radiotherapy, alone or followed by neck dissection. *Head Neck* 1991;13(3):177–183. Copyright © 1991 Wiley Periodicals, Inc., A Wiley Company. Reprinted by permission of John Wiley & Sons, Inc.

aggressively, compared with those with enlarged lymph nodes in the low internal jugular chain or supraclavicular fossa. The latter patients are more likely to have primary lesions located below the clavicles, which carry a much worse prognosis. The majority of patients have either squamous cell or poorly differentiated carcinoma. Those with adenocarcinoma almost always have a primary lesion below the clavicles, although if the nodes are located in the upper neck, one must exclude a salivary gland, thyroid, or parathyroid primary tumor. This section deals with patients presenting with squamous cell or poorly differentiated carcinoma in the upper or middle neck.

Patients should be evaluated with a thorough physical examination including careful evaluation of the head and neck. A needle biopsy of the lymph node should be performed. After chest roentgenography, a CT or MRI of the head and neck is obtained to detect an unknown primary lesion arising from the mucosa of the head and neck. It is unclear whether FDG-PET scans may identify primary lesions that would not otherwise be identifiable.[80] The available data suggest that some patients will benefit from these studies. Direct laryngoscopy and examination under anesthesia are performed with directed biopsies of the nasopharynx, tonsils, base of the tongue, and pyriform sinuses and of any abnormalities noted on CT or MRI or suspicious mucosal lesions noted at laryngoscopy. Patients with adequate lymphoid tissue in their tonsillar fossae should undergo at least an ipsilateral tonsillectomy. The likelihood of bilateral tonsillar carcinomas is probably <5% and may prompt some surgeons to perform bilateral tonsillectomy. If a contralateral tonsillar malignancy is missed and the patient is treated with an ipsilateral field arrangement for an ipsilateral tonsillar cancer, salvage treatment would probably be compromised. The diagnostic evaluation for the patient with cervical metastasis from an unknown head and neck primary lesion is summarized in Table 52.19. The results of a diagnostic evaluation for an unknown primary site in 236 patients at the University of Florida are depicted in Table 52.20.[81] Overall, 132 primary sites were discovered in 126 patients (53%) and were most often located in the oropharynx: tonsillar fossa, 59 (45%); base of tongue, 58 (44%); pyriform sinus, 10 (8%); pharyngeal wall, 3 (2%); and supraglottic larynx, 1 (1%).[81]

Some patients may be cured with treatment directed only to the involved area of the neck[82]; however, the authors usually irradiate the nasopharynx and oropharynx as well as both sides of the neck. The hypopharynx and larynx were irradiated as well until 1997 when it was decided to eliminate them because they are rarely the site of the primary cancer and because irradiation of these sites significantly increases the morbidity of treatment. It is not necessary to irradiate the oral cavity unless the patient has submandibular adenopathy, in which case the authors either do a neck dissection and observe the patient or irradiate the oral cavity and oropharynx and not the nasopharynx. Patients are treated with parallel-opposed fields at 1.8 Gy per fraction to a midline dose of 64.8 Gy with reduction off the spinal cord at 45-Gy tumor dose (Fig. 52.13). An alternative is to use IMRT to spare the contralateral parotid gland in patients with ipsilateral neck

TABLE 52.19 DIAGNOSTIC WORKUP FOR CERVICAL LYMPH NODE METASTASES: UNKNOWN PRIMARY TUMOR

General
History
Physical examination
Careful examination of the neck and supraclavicular regions
Examination of the oral cavity, pharynx, and larynx (indirect laryngectomy)

Radiographic Studies
Chest roentgenogram
Computed tomography or magnetic imaging resonance scans of the head and neck (special attention to the nasopharynx, pharynx, and larynx)

Laboratory Studies
Complete cell blood count
Blood chemistry profile

Direct and Laryngoscopy-Directed Biopsies
Nasopharynx, tonsils, base of tongue, both pyriform and sinuses, any suspicious abnormal or mucosal areas
Fine needle aspirate core needle or biopsy of the cervical node
Tonsillectomy

TABLE 52.20 DETECTION OF PRIMARY SITE VERSUS PATIENT GROUP

Patient Group	Biopsy-Proven Primary of Patients Site/Number (%)
PEØ/RADØ	21/72 (29.2)
PEØ/RAD+	51/82 (62.2)
PE+/RADØ	15/25 (60.0)
PE+/RAD+	39/57 (68.4)
Total	126/236 (53.4)

PEØ, physical examination negative; PE+, physical examination suspicious, but not definitely positive; RADØ, radiologic examination negative; RAD+, radiologic examination (computed tomography and/or magnetic resonance imaging) suspicious, not definitively positive.
From Cianchetti M, Mancuso AA, Amdur RJ, et al. Diagnostic evaluation of squamous cell carcinoma metastatic to cervical lymph nodes from an unknown head and neck primary site. *Laryngoscope* 2009;119(12):2348–2354. Copyright © 2009 The American Laryngological, Rhinological, and Otological Society, Inc. Reprinted by permission of John Wiley & Sons, Inc.

nodes. The lower neck is treated through a separate en face anterior field. IMRT may be used if patients have unilateral neck disease to reduce the dose to the contralateral parotid.

Erkal et al.[78] reported on 126 patients treated with curative intent at the University of Florida between 1964 and 1997 with follow-up for at least 2 years. RT was delivered to head and neck mucosal sites and both sides of the neck in 119 patients and to the neck alone in 7 patients. Twelve patients (10%) developed squamous cell carcinoma in a head and neck mucosal site at 0.5 to 10.9 years (median, 1.8 years) after treatment. The 5-year results were as follows: head and neck mucosal failure, 13%; neck node control, 78%; distant metastases, 14%; absolute survival, 47%; and cause-specific survival, 67%. Wallace

et al.[8] reported a combined series of 179 patients treated at the University of Florida (139 patients) and the University of Wisconsin (40 patients). The 5-year mucosal control rate was 92%; the head and neck mucosa was irradiated in 174 patients (97%). For the subset of 28 patients where the mucosal RT was limited to the nasopharynx and oropharynx, the 5-year mucosal control rate was 100%. Barker et al.[77] subsequently reported on 17 patients treated with the larynx-sparing technique described above between 1997 and 2002 at the authors' institution; none of these patients developed a head and neck mucosal squamous cell carcinoma after receiving RT.

Colletier et al.[9] reported on 136 patients treated with neck dissection followed by RT to head and neck mucosal sites and bilateral lymph nodes. Six percent of patients developed carcinomas in head and neck mucosal sites within RT portals, and 4% of patients developed carcinomas in head and neck mucosal sites outside the RT portals. The absolute survival rate at

FIGURE 52.13. Conventional radiation therapy portals used starting from 1997 to treat head and neck mucosal sites and upper cervical lymph nodes **(A)** and lower cervical and supraclavicular lymph nodes **(B)**. The inferior border for lateral portals is placed at the superior anterior border of the thyroid cartilage, shielding the hypopharynx and larynx. (Reprinted from Erkal HS, Mendenhall WM, Amdur RJ, et al. Squamous cell carcinomas metastatic to cervical lymph nodes from an unknown head-and-neck mucosal site treated with radiation therapy alone or in combination with neck dissection. *Int J Radiat Oncol Biol Phys* 2001;50[1]:55–63. Copyright © 2001 Elsevier. With permission.)

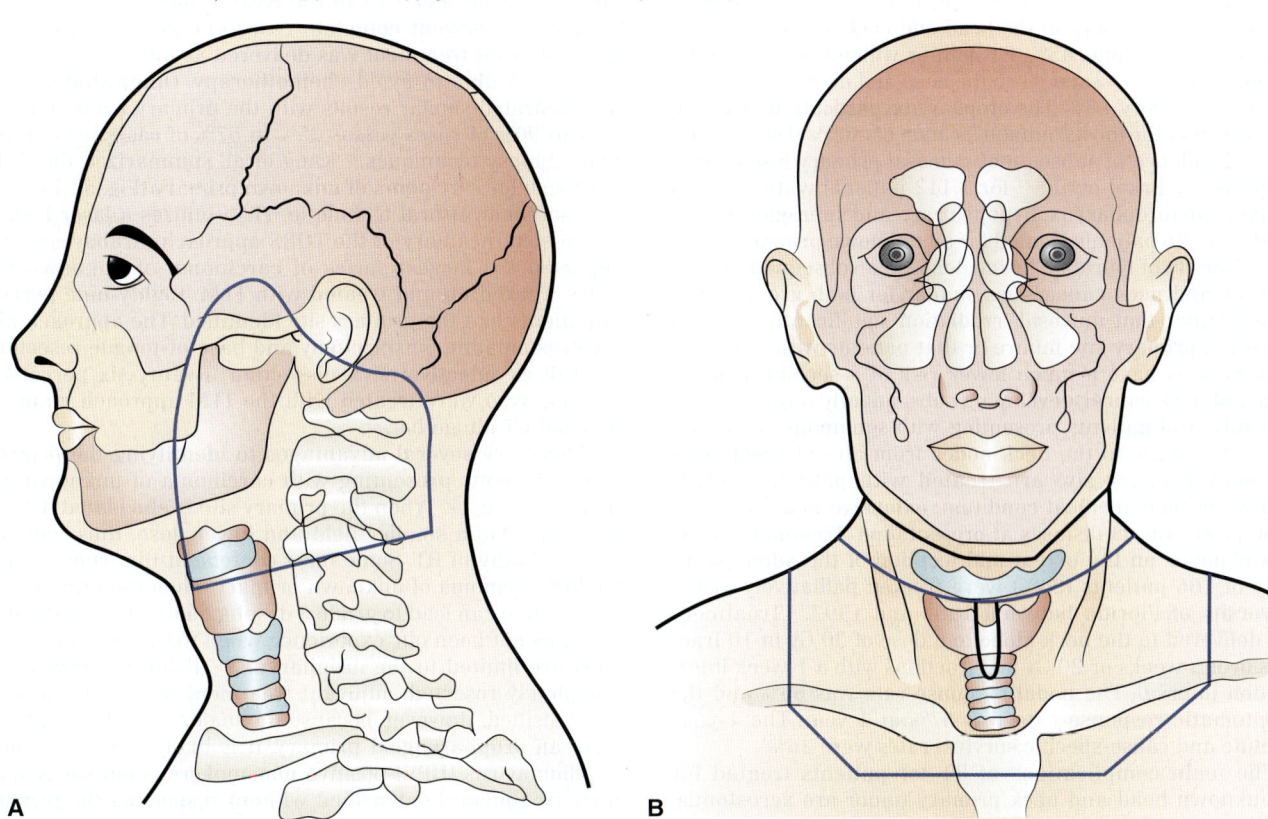

A   B

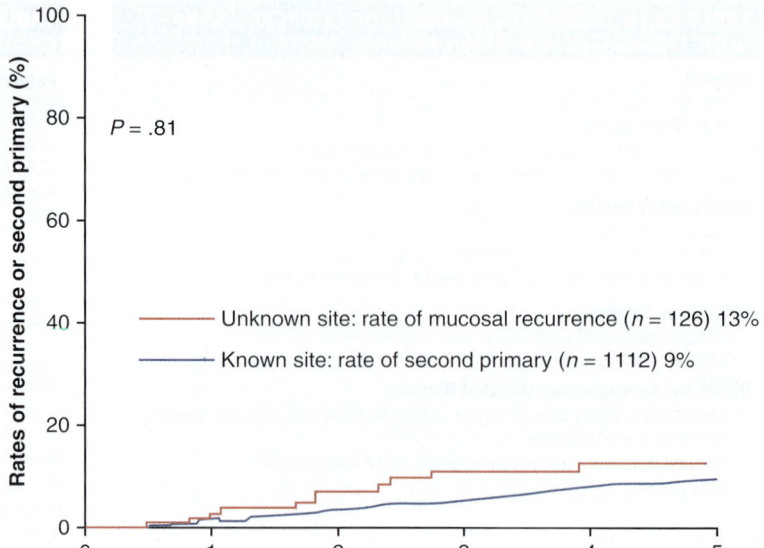

FIGURE 52.14. The rate of developing carcinomas in head and neck mucosal sites for patients treated for carcinomas with an unknown head and neck mucosal site compared to the rate of developing metachronous carcinomas in head and neck mucosal sites for patients treated for carcinomas with a known head and neck mucosal site. (Reprinted from Erkal HS, Mendenhall WM, Amdur RJ, et al. Squamous cell carcinomas metastatic to cervical lymph nodes from an unknown head-and-neck mucosal site treated with radiation therapy alone or in combination with neck dissection. *Int J Radiat Oncol Biol Phys* 2001;50[1]:55–63. Copyright © 2001 Elsevier. With permission.)

5 years was 60%. The authors recommended RT to head and neck mucosal sites. Reddy and Marks[10] reported on 16 patients with RT to ipsilateral lymph nodes and 36 patients with RT to head and neck mucosal sites and bilateral lymph nodes. The authors concluded that RT reduced the rate of developing carcinomas in head and neck mucosal sites. For patients with no RT to head and neck mucosal sites, the rate of developing carcinomas in head and neck mucosal sites was 46%, and the absolute survival rate at 5 years was 47%. For patients treated with RT to head and neck mucosal sites, the rates were 8% and 53%, respectively. Grau et al.[11] reported on 273 patients treated with curative intent at five cancer centers in Denmark between 1975 and 1995 with surgery alone (23 patients), RT to the ipsilateral neck alone or combined with surgery (26 patients), and RT to the neck and head and neck mucosa alone or combined with surgery (224 patients). The ipsilateral oropharynx unintentionally received some RT in patients treated to the ipsilateral neck alone, depending on the treatment technique. The 5-year rates of freedom from failure in the head and neck mucosa were as follows: surgery alone, 45%; RT with or without surgery to the ipsilateral neck, 77%; and RT to the head and neck mucosa with or without surgery, 87%. The oropharynx, particularly the base of tongue, was the most common location of mucosal site failure.

The incidence of subsequent mucosal primary lesions was compared by Erkal et al.[11,83] for 1,112 patients with a known primary site (oropharynx, hypopharynx, and supraglottis) and a series of 126 patients treated for an unknown primary site at the University of Florida. The incidence of a subsequent mucosal head and neck cancer was similar for both groups, suggesting either that mucosal irradiation significantly reduced the risk of primary site failure or that patients with unknown primary sites have a much lower risk of a second primary head and neck cancer developing subsequently (Fig. 52.14).[78]

A subset of patients presenting with squamous cell carcinoma metastatic to the neck nodes from an unknown head and neck primary site are treated with palliative intent because of poor medical condition, extensive nodal involvement, or distant metastases at presentation. Treatment of the neck depends on the extent and location of the adenopathy. Forty of 166 patients (24%) were treated palliatively at the University of Florida between 1964 and 1997.[62] Treatment was delivered to the neck alone to a dose of 30 Gy in 10 fractions over 2 weeks or 20 Gy in 2 fractions with a 1-week interfraction interval. The nodal response rate was 65% and the symptomatic response rate was 57% at 1 year. The 1-year absolute and cause-specific survival rates were 25%.

The main complications of RT for patients treated for an unknown head and neck primary tumor are xerostomia,

dysphagia, and neck fibrosis. The complications of treatment of the neck, which have been discussed previously, depend on whether chemotherapy and/or neck dissection is added.[62]

An alternative approach to carcinoma of unknown primary of the neck involves transoral surgery: transoral robotic surgery (TORS) or transoral laser microsurgery (TLM). The TORS approach involves using the surgical robot to access difficult-to-reach areas of the oropharynx to take more thorough directed biopsies. With the robot, the surgeon performs bilateral tonsillectomy/extended tonsillectomy as well as lingual tonsillectomy/base-of-tongue shaves. Moreover, if a primary is found on inspection or frozen section, the surgeon may perform a resection at the same time. Typically, a selective neck dissection (levels II to IV) is performed in conjunctions with the TORS procedure. Durmus et al.[84] reported on the initial experience of this method at the Ohio State University. In 77% of patients, the primary site was identified; 76% tumors were found in the palatine tonsils and 24% in the base of tongue. 77% of these patients underwent complete resection with negative margins. Adjuvant treatment was delivered as indicated with 59% of patients able to avoid chemotherapy. Other studies have demonstrated similar results with the primary being found in 72% to 90% of cases versus 25% to 57% of cases using traditional biopsy techniques.[85] Kang et al. summarized the TORS approach for carcinoma of unknown primary (Fig. 52.15).

Another transoral technique, TLM, utilizes a laser instead of the electrocautery of the TORS approach. Graboyes et al.[86] reported the largest series of carcinoma of unknown primary worked up and treated with TLM. Eighty-nine percent of patients had the primary site identified. The approach also involves palatine tonsillectomy and base-of-tongue resections as well as selective neck dissection. Twenty-six percent of patients who were treated with the TLM approach managed to avoid RT altogether.

There are several advantages to identifying the primary site in patients presenting with carcinoma of unknown primary of the neck. When the primary site is elucidated, RT can be tailored to a smaller field and lower dose, thus reducing the morbidity of RT. Some have contended that conventional RT for carcinoma of unknown primary when the primary site is not found can lead to grade 3 dysphagia in 50% of patients.[87] This has not been our experience when the targeted mucosal sites are limited to the oropharynx.[8,77] If the primary site is completely resected, adjuvant treatment may be avoided or deintensified. However, because the majority of these patients have an oropharyngeal primary, it is likely that the human papillomavirus (HPV)-positive nonsmokers could safely have their treatment deintensified without respecting the primary

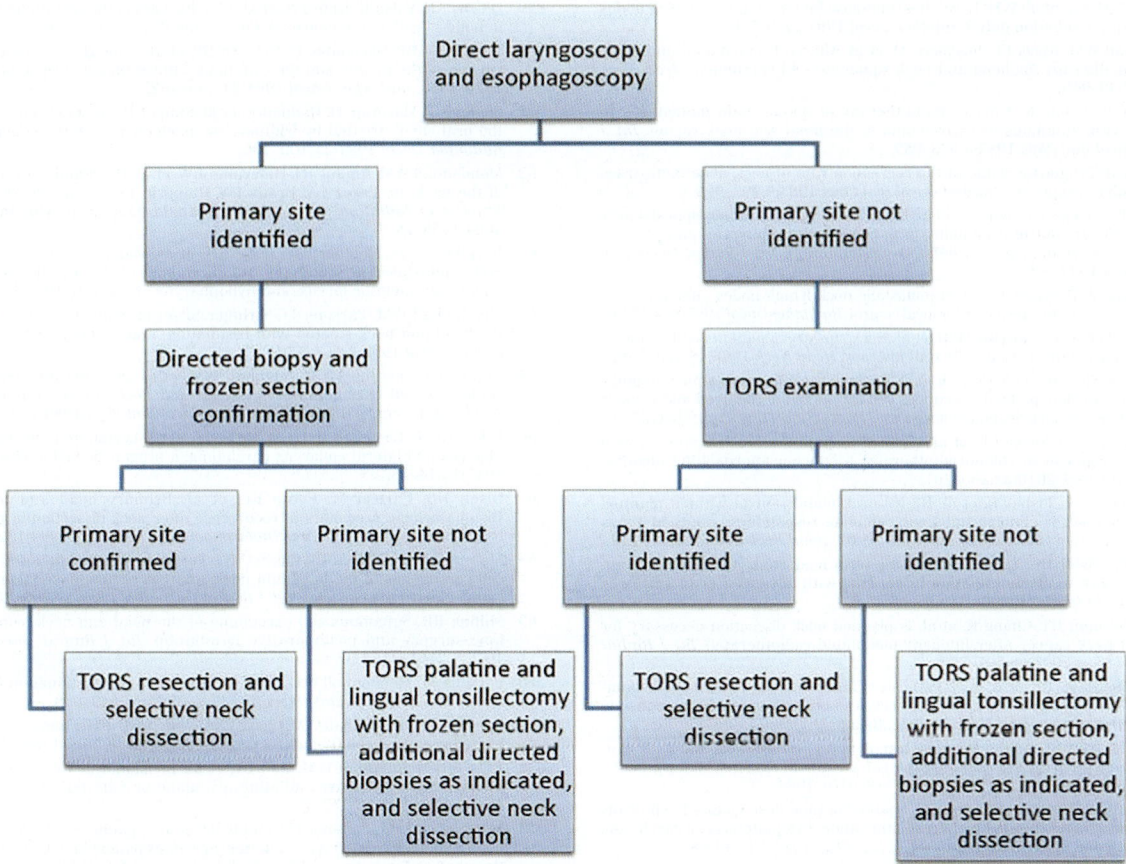

FIGURE 52.15. Treatment paradigm for cancer of unknown primary (CUP) metastatic to cervical lymph nodes. TORS, transoral robotic surgery. (From Kang SY, Dziegielewski PT, Old MO, et al. Transoral robotic surgery for carcinoma of unknown primary in the head and neck. *J Surg Oncol* 2015;112[7]: 697–701. Copyright © 2015 Wiley Periodicals, Inc. Reprinted by permission of John Wiley & Sons, Inc.)

site. Functional outcomes for this approach are excellent with a 4.5% gastrostomy rate at 1 year and return of quality of life to pretreatment baseline or better.[85] Perhaps even more significant is the potential survival advantage provided when the primary site is identified and treated appropriately.[86,88–90]

ACKNOWLEDGMENTS

We thank the research support staff of the Department of Radiation Oncology for their help with statistics, editing, and manuscript preparation.

REFERENCES

 1. Rouviére H, Tobias MJ. *Anatomy of the human lymphatic system*. Ann Arbor, MI: Edwards Brothers, 1938:1–28, 44, 56, 77, 78
 2. Fisch U. Lymphographic studies on the cervical lymphatic system. *Fortschr Hals Nasen Ohrenheilkd* 1966;14:1–196.
 3. Stringer SP. Current concepts in surgical management of neck metastases from head and neck cancer. *Oncology (Williston Park)* 1995;9:547–554; discussion 54, 57–58.
 4. Mendenhall WM, Million RR. Elective neck irradiation for squamous cell carcinoma of the head and neck: analysis of time-dose factors and causes of failure. *Int J Radiat Oncol Biol Phys* 1986;12:741–746.
 5. Lindberg R. Distribution of cervical lymph node metastases from squamous cell carcinoma of the upper respiratory and digestive tracts. *Cancer* 1972;29:1446–1449.
 6. Richard JM, Sancho-Garnier H, Micheau C, et al. Prognostic factors in cervical lymph node metastasis in upper respiratory and digestive tract carcinomas: study of 1,713 cases during a 15-year period. *Laryngoscope* 1987;97:97–101.
 7. McLaughlin MP, Mendenhall WM, Mancuso AA, et al. Retropharyngeal adenopathy as a predictor of outcome in squamous cell carcinoma of the head and neck. *Head Neck* 1995;17:190–198.
 8. Wallace A, Richards GM, Harari PM, et al. Head and neck squamous cell carcinoma from an unknown primary site. *Am J Otolaryngol* 2011;32:286–290.
 9. Colletier PJ, Garden AS, Morrison WH, et al. Postoperative radiation for squamous cell carcinoma metastatic to cervical lymph nodes from an unknown primary site: outcomes and patterns of failure. *Head Neck* 1998;20:674–681.
10. Reddy SP, Marks JE. Metastatic carcinoma in the cervical lymph nodes from an unknown primary site: results of bilateral neck plus mucosal irradiation vs. ipsilateral neck irradiation. *Int J Radiat Oncol Biol Phys* 1997;37:797–802.
11. Grau C, Johansen LV, Jakobsen J, et al. Cervical lymph node metastases from unknown primary tumours. Results from a national survey by the Danish Society for Head and Neck Oncology. *Radiother Oncol* 2000;55:121–129.
12. Million RR, Cassisi NJ, Mancuso AA, et al. Management of the neck for squamous cell carcinoma. In: Million RR, Cassisi NJ, eds. *Management of head and neck cancer: a multidisciplinary approach*. Philadelphia: JB Lippincott Company, 1994:75–142
13. Mancuso AA, Hanafee WN. *Head and neck radiology*. Philadelphia: Lippincott Williams & Wilkins, 2011.
14. Head and Neck. In: Edge SB, Byrd DR, Compton CC, Fritz AG, Greene FL, Trotti A, eds. *American Joint Committee on Cancer (AJCC) AJCC Cancer Staging Manual*. 8th ed. New York, NY: Springer, 2017:55–66.
15. Larynx. In: Beahrs OH, Myers MH, eds. *American Joint Committee on Cancer Manual for Staging of Cancer*. Philadelphia: J.B. Lippincott Company, 1983: 37–42
16. Mendenhall WM, Million RR, Cassisi NJ. Squamous cell carcinoma of the head and neck treated with radiation therapy: the role of neck dissection for clinically positive neck nodes. *Int J Radiat Oncol Biol Phys* 1986;12:733–740.
17. Taylor JM, Mendenhall WM, Parsons JT, et al. The influence of dose and time on wound complications following post-radiation neck dissection. *Int J Radiat Oncol Biol Phys* 1992;23:41–46.
18. Somerset JD, Mendenhall WM, Amdur RJ, et al. Planned postradiotherapy bilateral neck dissection for head and neck cancer. *Am J Otolaryngol* 2001;22:383–386.
19. Dubray BM, Bataini JP, Bernier J, et al. Is reseeding from the primary a plausible cause of node failure? *Int J Radiat Oncol Biol Phys* 1993;25:9–15.
20. Mendenhall WM, Villaret DB, Amdur RJ, et al. Planned neck dissection after definitive radiotherapy for squamous cell carcinoma of the head and neck. *Head Neck* 2002;24:1012–1018.
21. Mendenhall WM, Parsons JT, Stringer SP, et al. T1-T2 vocal cord carcinoma: a basis for comparing the results of radiotherapy and surgery. *Head Neck Surg* 1988;10:373–377.
22. Mendenhall WM, Parsons JT, Brant TA, et al. Is elective neck treatment indicated for T2N0 squamous cell carcinoma of the glottic larynx? *Radiother Oncol* 1989;14:199–202.
23. Mendenhall WM, Parsons JT, Million RR. Unnecessary irradiation of the normal larynx. *Int J Radiat Oncol Biol Phys* 1990;18:1531–1533.
24. Amdur RJ, Li JG, Liu C, et al. Unnecessary laryngeal irradiation in the IMRT era. *Head Neck* 2004;26:257–263; discussion 63–64.
25. Mendenhall WM, Mancuso AA. Radiotherapy for head and neck cancer—is the "next level" down? *Int J Radiat Oncol Biol Phys* 2009;73:645–646.

26. Taylor JM, Mendenhall WM, Lavey RS. Time-dose factors in positive neck nodes treated with irradiation only. *Radiother Oncol* 1991;22:167–173.
27. Mendenhall WM, Riggs CE, Vaysberg M, et al. Altered fractionation and adjuvant chemotherapy for head and neck squamous cell carcinoma. *Head Neck* 2010;32:939–945.
28. Bartelink H, Breur K, Hart G. Radiotherapy of lymph node metastases in patients with squamous cell carcinoma of the head and neck region. *Int J Radiat Oncol Biol Phys* 1982;8:983–989.
29. Bartelink H. Prognostic value of the regression rate of neck node metastases during radiotherapy. *Int J Radiat Oncol Biol Phys* 1983;9:993–996.
30. Bataini JP, Bernier J, Jaulerry C, et al. Impact of neck node radioresponsiveness on the regional control probability in patients with oropharynx and pharyngolarynx cancers managed by definitive radiotherapy. *Int J Radiat Oncol Biol Phys* 1987;13:817–824.
31. Maciejewski B. Regression rate of metastatic neck lymph nodes after radiation treatment as a prognostic factor for local control. *Radiother Oncol* 1987;8:301–308.
32. Peters LJ, Weber RS, Morrison WH, et al. Neck surgery in patients with primary oropharyngeal cancer treated by radiotherapy. *Head Neck* 1996;18:552–559.
33. Johnson CR, Silverman LN, Clay LB, et al. Radiotherapeutic management of bulky cervical lymphadenopathy in squamous cell carcinoma of the head and neck: is postradiotherapy neck dissection necessary? *Radiat Oncol Investig* 1998;6:52–57.
34. Ferlito A, Corry J, Silver CE, et al. Planned neck dissection for patients with complete response to chemoradiotherapy: a concept approaching obsolescence. *Head Neck* 2010;32:253–261.
35. Corry J, Peters L, Fisher R, et al. N2-N3 neck nodal control without planned neck dissection for clinical/radiologic complete responders-results of Trans Tasman Radiation Oncology Group Study 98.02. *Head Neck* 2008;30:737–742.
36. Rengan R, Pfister DG, Lee NY, et al. Long-term neck control rates after complete response to chemoradiation in patients with advanced head and neck cancer. *Am J Clin Oncol* 2008;31:465–469.
37. Yao M, Hoffman HT, Chang K, et al. Is planned neck dissection necessary for head and neck cancer after intensity-modulated radiotherapy? *Int J Radiat Oncol Biol Phys* 2007;68:707–713.
38. Yovino S, Settle K, Taylor R, et al. Patterns of failure among patients with squamous cell carcinoma of the head and neck who obtain a complete response to chemoradiotherapy. *Head Neck* 2010;32:46–52.
39. Yeung AR, Liauw SL, Amdur RJ, et al. Lymph node-positive head and neck cancer treated with definitive radiotherapy: can treatment response determine the extent of neck dissection? *Cancer* 2008;112:1076–1082.
40. Mendenhall WM, Million RR, Bova FJ. Analysis of time-dose factors in clinically positive neck nodes treated with irradiation alone in squamous cell carcinoma of the head and neck. *Int J Radiat Oncol Biol Phys* 1984;10:639–643.
41. Bernier J, Bataini JP. Regional outcome in oropharyngeal and pharyngolaryngeal cancer treated with high dose per fraction radiotherapy. Analysis of neck disease response in 1646 cases. *Radiother Oncol* 1986;6:87–103.
42. Liauw SL, Mancuso AA, Amdur RJ, et al. Postradiotherapy neck dissection for lymph node-positive head and neck cancer: the use of computed tomography to manage the neck. *J Clin Oncol* 2006;24:1421–1427.
43. Mabanta SR, Mendenhall WM, Stringer SP, et al. Salvage treatment for neck recurrence after irradiation alone for head and neck squamous cell carcinoma with clinically positive neck nodes. *Head Neck* 1999;21:591–594.
44. Hitchcock KE, Amdur RJ, Mendenhall WM, et al. Lessons from a standardized program using PET-CT to avoid neck dissection after primary radiotherapy for N2 squamous cell carcinoma of the oropharynx. *Oral Oncol* 2015;51:870–874.
45. Goenka A, Morris LG, Rao SS, et al. Long-term regional control in the observed neck following definitive chemoradiation for node-positive oropharyngeal squamous cell cancer. *Int J Cancer* 2013;133:1214–1221.
46. Mehanna H, Wong WL, McConkey CC, et al. PET-CT surveillance versus neck dissection in advanced head and neck cancer. *N Engl J Med* 2016;374:1444–1454.
47. Wang K, Amdur RJ, Mendenhall WM, et al. Impact of post-chemoradiotherapy superselective/selective neck dissection on patient reported quality of life. *Oral Oncol* 2016;58:21–26.
48. Bova FJ. Treatment planning for irradiation of head and neck cancer. In: Million RR, Cassisi NJ, eds. *Management of head and neck cancer: a multidisciplinary approach*. 1st ed. Philadelphia: J.B. Lippincott Company, 1984:209–230
49. McGuirt WF, McCabe BF. Significance of node biopsy before definitive treatment of cervical metastatic carcinoma. *Laryngoscope* 1978;88:594–597.
50. Parsons JT, Million RR, Cassisi NJ. The influence of excisional or incisional biopsy of metastatic neck nodes on the management of head and neck cancer. *Int J Radiat Oncol Biol Phys* 1985;11:1447–1454.
51. Mack Y, Parsons JT, Mendenhall WM, et al. Squamous cell carcinoma of the head and neck: management after excisional biopsy of a solitary metastatic neck node. *Int J Radiat Oncol Biol Phys* 1993;25:619–622.
52. Trifiletti DM, Smith A, Mitra N, et al. Beyond positive margins and extracapsular extension: evaluating the utilization and clinical impact of postoperative chemoradiotherapy in resected locally advanced head and neck cancer. *J Clin Oncol* 2017;35:1550–1560.
53. Dagan R, Morris CG, Kirwan JM, et al. Elective neck dissection during salvage surgery for locally recurrent head and neck squamous cell carcinoma after radiotherapy with elective nodal irradiation. *Laryngoscope* 2010;120:945–952.
54. Falchook AD, Dagan R, Morris CG, et al. Elective neck dissection for second primary after previous definitive radiotherapy. *Am J Otolaryngol* 2012;33:199–204.
55. Mendenhall WM, Million RR, Cassisi NJ. Elective neck irradiation in squamous-cell carcinoma of the head and neck. *Head Neck Surg* 1980;3:15–20.
56. Mendenhall WM, Parsons JT, Million RR. Elective lower neck irradiation: 5000 cGy/25 fractions versus 4050 cGy/15 fractions. *Int J Radiat Oncol Biol Phys* 1988;15:439–440.
57. Vandenbrouck C, Sancho-Garnier H, Chassagne D, et al. Elective versus therapeutic radical neck dissection in epidermoid carcinoma of the oral cavity: results of a randomized clinical trial. *Cancer* 1980;46:386–390.
58. Fakih AR, Rao RS, Borges AM, et al. Elective versus therapeutic neck dissection in early carcinoma of the oral tongue. *Am J Surg* 1989;158:309–313.
59. D'Cruz AK, Vaish R, Kapre N, et al. Elective versus therapeutic neck dissection in node-negative oral cancer. *N Engl J Med* 2015;373:521–529.
60. Dearnaley DP, Dardoufas C, A'Hearn RP, et al. Interstitial irradiation for carcinoma of the tongue and floor of mouth: Royal Marsden Hospital Experience 1970-1986. *Radiother Oncol* 1991;21:183–192.
61. Piedbois P, Mazeron JJ, Haddad E, et al. Stage I-II squamous cell carcinoma of the oral cavity treated by iridium-192: is elective neck dissection indicated? *Radiother Oncol* 1991;21:100–106.
62. Mendenhall WM, Amdur RJ, Hinerman RW, et al. Head and neck: management of the neck. In: Perez CA, Brady LW, Halperin EC, et al., eds. *Principles and practice of radiation oncology*. Philadelphia: Lippincott Williams & Wilkins, 2004:1158–78
63. Barkley HT Jr, Fletcher GH, Jesse RH, et al. Management of cervical lymph node metastases in squamous cell carcinoma of the tonsillar fossa, base of tongue, supraglottic larynx, and hypopharynx. *Am J Surg* 1972;124:462–467.
64. Mendenhall WM, Parsons JT, Stringer SP, et al. Squamous cell carcinoma of the head and neck treated with irradiation: management of the neck. *Semin Radiat Oncol* 1992;2:163–170.
65. Amdur RJ, Parsons JT, Mendenhall WM, et al. Postoperative irradiation for squamous cell carcinoma of the head and neck: an analysis of treatment results and complications. *Int J Radiat Oncol Biol Phys* 1989;16:25–36.
66. Lefebvre JL, Castelain B, De la Torre JC, et al. Lymph node invasion in hypopharynx and lateral epilarynx carcinoma: a prognostic factor. *Head Neck Surg* 1987;10:14–18.
67. Olsen KD, Caruso M, Foote RL, et al. Primary head and neck cancer. Histopathologic predictors of recurrence after neck dissection in patients with lymph node involvement. *Arch Otolaryngol Head Neck Surg* 1994;120:1370–1374.
68. Marcus RB Jr, Million RR, Cassissi NJ. Postoperative irradiation for squamous cell carcinomas of the head and neck: analysis of time-dose factors related to control above the clavicles. *Int J Radiat Oncol Biol Phys* 1979;5:1943–1949.
69. Million RR. Squamous cell carcinoma of the head and neck: combined therapy: surgery and postoperative irradiation. *Int J Radiat Oncol Biol Phys* 1979;5:2161–2162.
70. Parsons JT, Mendenhall WM, Cassisi NJ, et al. Hyperfractionation for head and neck cancer. *Int J Radiat Oncol Biol Phys* 1988;14:649–658.
71. Parsons JT, Mendenhall WM, Cassisi NJ, et al. Neck dissection after twice-a-day radiotherapy: morbidity and recurrence rates. *Head Neck* 1989;11:400–404.
72. Ellis ER, Mendenhall WM, Rao PV, et al. Incisional or excisional neck-node biopsy before definitive radiotherapy, alone or followed by neck dissection. *Head Neck* 1991;13:177–183.
73. Mendenhall WM, Parsons JT, Amdur RJ, et al. Squamous cell carcinoma of the head and neck treated with radiotherapy: does planned neck dissection reduce the change for successful surgical management of subsequent local recurrence? *Head Neck Surg* 1988;10:302–304.
74. Mendenhall WM, Parsons JT, Amdur RJ, et al. Squamous cell carcinoma of the head and neck treated with radiation therapy: the impact of neck stage on local control. *Int J Radiat Oncol Biol Phys* 1988;14:249–252.
75. Wall TJ, Peters LJ, Brown BW, et al. Relationship between lymph nodal status and primary tumor control probability in tumors of the supraglottic larynx. *Int J Radiat Oncol Biol Phys* 1985;11:1895–1902.
76. Zenga J, Graboyes EM, Haughey BH., et al. Definitive surgical therapy after open neck biopsy for HPV-related oropharyngeal cancer. *Otolaryngol Head Neck Surg* 2016;154:657–666.
77. Barker CA, Morris CG, Mendenhall WM. Larynx-sparing radiotherapy for squamous cell carcinoma from an unknown head and neck primary site. *Am J Clin Oncol* 2005;28:445–448.
78. Erkal HS, Mendenhall WM, Amdur RJ, et al. Squamous cell carcinomas metastatic to cervical lymph nodes from an unknown head-and-neck mucosal site treated with radiation therapy alone or in combination with neck dissection. *Int J Radiat Oncol Biol Phys* 2001;50:55–63.
79. Mendenhall WM. Unknown primary squamous cell carcinoma of the head and neck. *Curr Cancer Ther Rev* 2005;1:167–174.
80. Mukherji SK, Drane WE, Mancuso AA, et al. Occult primary tumors of the head and neck: detection with 2-[F-18] fluoro-2-deoxy-D-glucose SPECT. *Radiology* 1996;199:761–766.
81. Cianchetti M, Mancuso AA, Amdur RJ, et al. Diagnostic evaluation of squamous cell carcinoma metastatic to cervical lymph nodes from an unknown head and neck primary site. *Laryngoscope* 2009;119:2348–2354.
82. Coster JR, Foote RL, Olsen KD, et al. Cervical nodal metastasis of squamous cell carcinoma of unknown origin: indications for withholding radiation therapy. *Int J Radiat Oncol Biol Phys* 1992;23:743–749.
83. Erkal HS, Mendenhall WM, Amdur RJ, et al. Squamous cell carcinomas metastatic to cervical lymph nodes from an unknown head and neck mucosal site treated with radiation therapy with palliative intent. *Radiother Oncol* 2001;59:319–321.
84. Durmus K, Rangarajan SV, Old MO, et al. Transoral robotic approach to carcinoma of unknown primary. *Head Neck* 2014;36:848–852.
85. Kang SY, Dziegielewski PT, Old MO, et al. Transoral robotic surgery for carcinoma of unknown primary in the head and neck. *J Surg Oncol* 2015;112:697–701.
86. Graboyes EM, Sinha P, Thorstad WL, et al. Management of human papillomavirus-related unknown primaries of the head and neck with a transoral surgical approach. *Head Neck* 2015;37:1603–1611.
87. Madani I, Vakaet L, Bonte K, et al. Intensity-modulated radiotherapy for cervical lymph node metastases from unknown primary cancer. *Int J Radiat Oncol Biol Phys* 2008;71:1158–1166.
88. Haas I, Hoffmann TK, Engers R, et al. Diagnostic strategies in cervical carcinoma of an unknown primary (CUP). *Eur Arch Otorhinolaryngol* 2002;259:325–333.
89. Koivunen P, Laranne J, Virtaniemi J, et al. Cervical metastasis of unknown origin: a series of 72 patients. *Acta Otolaryngol* 2002;122:569–574.
90. Oen AL, de Boer MF, Hop WC, et al. Cervical metastasis from the unknown primary tumor. *Eur Arch Otorhinolaryngol* 1995;252:222–228.

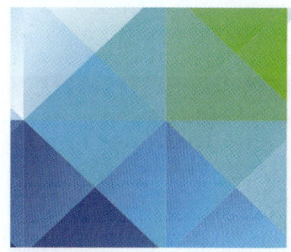

CHAPTER 53

Thyroid Cancer

Robert J. Amdur and Roi Dagan

BASIC THYROID ANATOMY AND PHYSIOLOGY

Gross Anatomy

The thyroid gland is located in the central anterior neck at the cervical–thoracic junction (Fig. 53.1). The bulk of the gland is located immediately anterior and inferior to the thyroid cartilage. It has two lateral lobes connected by a central isthmus. Approximately 50% of individuals have a pyramidal lobe that extends superiorly from the central aspect of the gland, which is a remnant of the gland's embryologic origin, the thyroglossal duct. The average adult thyroid gland measures approximately 5 × 5 cm and weighs 10 to 20 g.

The location of the gland in the central neck and its relation to critical structures explain the presenting symptoms of advanced neoplastic processes arising from the thyroid as well as potential complications of thyroid surgery and radiotherapy (Fig. 53.2). The lateral lobes extend superiorly to the level of the midthyroid cartilage overlying the larynx and inferiorly to the sixth tracheal ring. The gland wraps around 75% of the tracheal circumference, posteriorly encroaching on the esophagus. The lateral extent is just medial to the common carotid arteries. The recurrent laryngeal nerves, sympathetic trunks, vagus, and phrenic nerves are all found immediately posterior to the gland, and the gland is anteriorly bound by the strap muscles. Parathyroid glands are located posterior to the thyroid gland and vary in location and number.

Vasculature and Lymphatics

The arterial blood supply to the thyroid gland is provided by the paired superior thyroid arteries (branches of the external carotid arteries) and inferior thyroid arteries (branches of the thyrocervical trunk from the subclavian arteries). Venous blood drains via the paired superior and middle thyroid veins to the internal jugular veins and from the inferior thyroid veins to the subclavian and innominate veins. There is a dense lymphatic network draining the gland in multiple directions, and bilateral involvement of lymph node metastases is common. According to the American Joint Committee on Cancer's (AJCC) eighth edition of the *AJCC Cancer Staging Manual*, the first-echelon nodes for thyroid cancer metastases are located in level 6 (the central or "visceral" compartment) between the hyoid bone and the thoracic inlet.[1] Specifically, these are the paralaryngeal, paratracheal, and prelaryngeal (delphian) nodes. Second-echelon nodal spread is to the mid- and lower cervical nodes (levels 3 and 4), supraclavicular nodes, upper mediastinal nodes (level 7) and, to a lesser extent, the upper cervical nodes (level 2). Level 1 (submental and submandibular) lymph nodes are rarely involved.

Spread of thyroid cancer to the retropharyngeal nodes is unusual, but we see positive retropharyngeal nodes in patients with many positive nodes in the lateral cervical stations and with advanced-stage disease at the primary site. With thyroid cancer, the positive retropharyngeal nodes are often in the more inferior portion of the station (Fig. 53.3).

Microscopic Anatomy

Microscopically, the normal thyroid gland consists of numerous lobules comprising individual follicles forming the structural and functional unit of the gland (Fig. 53.4). The supporting stoma and vasculature are intertwined around the follicles. Each follicle consists of a single layer of cuboidal surface epithelium comprising thyroid follicular cells surrounding a central lumen-containing colloid, a substance rich in thyroglobulin (Tg). Separate from the follicular epithelium are the parafollicular cells, or C cells, which are neural crest–derived cells containing granules of calcitonin. The thyroid gland is incompletely surrounded by a connective tissue capsule.

Physiology

The primary physiologic role of the thyroid gland is the production of thyroid hormone, which plays an important role in metabolic homeostasis. A secondary role is the production of calcitonin, a hormone involved in calcium homeostasis. The follicular cells of the thyroid gland synthesize and secrete Tg and thyroid hormone in two biologically active forms, thyroxine ($3,5,3',5'$ iodothyronine or T_4) and tri-iodothyronine ($3,5,3'$ iodothyronine or T_3). It is useful to consider T_4 as the storage and transport form of thyroid hormone and T_3 as the metabolically active form. Most circulating thyroid hormone is bound to thyroxine-binding globulin. In peripheral tissues, where thyroid hormone executes its endocrine function, T_4 is rapidly converted to the more active form T_3 by the action of T_4 monodeiodinase. T_3 is transported to the nucleus where it binds to specific nuclear receptors and interacts with regulatory genes, influencing their expression. The gene products ultimately increase the cell's basal metabolic rate, protein synthesis, catecholamine effects, and growth of long bones and play an essential role in metabolism of proteins, fats, and carbohydrates. Thyroid hormone exerts its endocrine function on virtually all cells in the body.

Iodine is a critical component of thyroid hormone and is essential for thyroid function. The recommended daily intake is 150 μg, and at least 50 μg of daily intake is necessary to prevent deficiency, resulting in a goiter. The follicular cells of the thyroid gland possess a unique ability to actively uptake and concentrate iodine. The sodium iodine symporter (NaIS) actively transports sodium and iodine against an electrochemical gradient across the cell membrane in an energy-dependent fashion. This transmembrane protein is stimulated by thyroid-stimulating hormone (TSH or thyrotropin), which is synthesized in the anterior pituitary. Functional NaIS is present on malignant follicular cells seen in multiple variants of differentiated thyroid cancer (DTC). The unique ability to concentrate iodine within these malignant cells makes radioactive iodine, such as iodine-131 (I-131), a potent targeted therapy. The central role of TSH in driving the internalization of iodine within follicular thyroid cells is exploited in preparation for I-131. To increase the efficacy of I-131 therapy, T_4 deprivation, a low-iodine diet, and administration of recombinant human TSH (rhTSH) can be used to increase the effects of TSH on follicular thyroid cells (see the section on preparing patients for I-131). NaIS is also present in the parotid glands, breast tissues, gastric mucosa, and nasolacrimal ducts, placing them at risk for injury from I-131 therapy.

Upon entering the follicular cells, iodine is transported across the apical membrane and oxidized to a form that binds to tyrosyl residues of Tg, a large (660 kDa) glycoprotein synthesized by the follicular cells. Iodinated Tg becomes the main component of the intraluminal colloid stores of the

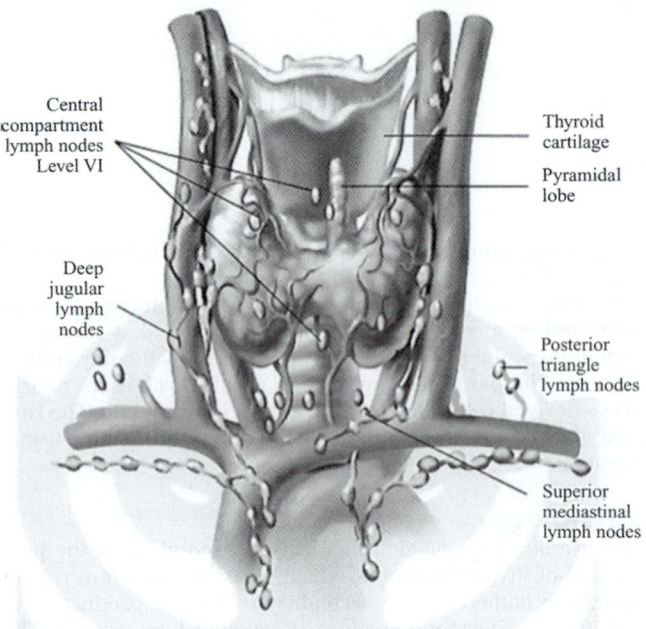

FIGURE 53.1. Anatomic location of the thyroid gland relative to the larynx, major vessels, and draining lymphatics. (Reprinted by permission from Springer: Amdur RJ, Mazzaferri EL. Basic thyroid anatomy. In: Amdur RJ, Mazzaferri EL, eds. *Essentials of thyroid cancer management*. New York: Springer, 2005:3–6. Copyright © 2005 Springer Science+Business Media, Inc.)

thyroid follicles. T_3 and T_4 are synthesized by the coupling of iodinated tyrosine. They remain attached to the Tg until leaving the gland. TSH stimulation results in endocytosis of colloid droplets from the lumen into the follicular cells where it is hydrolyzed and releases Tg, T_4, and, to lesser degree, T_3 into the circulation. Malignant differentiated follicular cells retain this function. Thus, serum Tg becomes a unique tumor marker after thyroidectomy and thyroid remnant ablation.

A feedback loop between the thyroid, pituitary, and hypothalamus regulates thyroid hormone synthesis and secretion. Thyrotropin-releasing hormone (TRH) is synthesized in the hypothalamus, and its primary function is to increase the secretion of TSH in the pituitary. Both T_3 and T_4 in turn inhibit TRH release and TSH secretion.

FIGURE 53.2. Anatomy of the thyroid gland. Contrast-enhanced axial CT slice at the level of the bottom of the cricoid cartilage (*purple*) showing the position of the thyroid gland (*blue*) relative to the esophagus (*orange*), carotid arteries (*red*), jugular vein (*lavender*), and the approximate position of the recurrent laryngeal nerves (*yellow-green*).

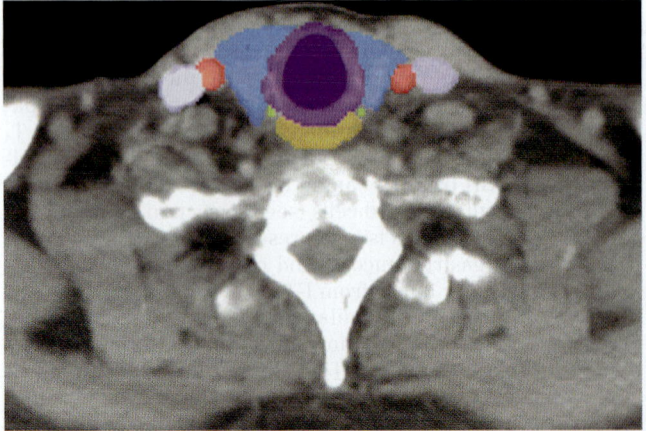

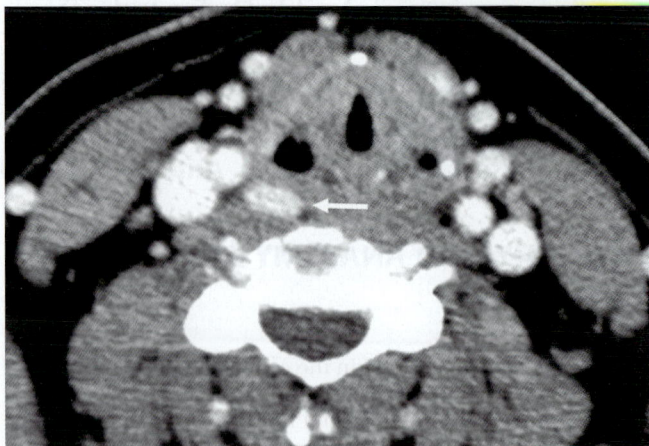

FIGURE 53.3. Axial CT image with intravenous contrast at the level of the false vocal cords in a patient with papillary thyroid cancer. The *arrow* points to a retropharyngeal node. Metastatic cancer in this node explains the avid enhancement from iodinated contrast.

CLASSIFICATIONS OF THYROID CANCER

Correct pathologic classification of thyroid carcinoma is fundamental to the appropriate clinical management of the malignancy. A system of classification is shown in Table 53.1 and discussed below. The cell of origin, cytologic features, and growth morphology determine the pathologic classification. All carcinomas of the thyroid gland are derived from the follicular epithelium, except medullary thyroid carcinoma (MTC), which is derived from the parafollicular C cells. Capsular invasion is important in the pathologic diagnosis of certain thyroid carcinomas. The diagnosis of papillary thyroid carcinoma (PTC) is entirely predicated on the presence of diagnostic nuclear features and does not require invasive growth, whereas follicular carcinoma (FC) requires the presence of capsular or vascular invasion.[2] Other rarely encountered malignant neoplasms of the thyroid gland include thyroid lymphoma and sarcomas. These two entities will not be discussed in this chapter and are better evaluated and managed under paradigms detailed in the chapters on lymphoma and sarcoma.

FIGURE 53.4. Thyroid follicle. Thyroid follicular cells produce thyroglobulin and thyroid hormone. Thyroid cells, which are normally located in the thyroid follicles and in perifollicular regions, synthesize and secrete calcitonin. (Reprinted by permission from Springer: Mazzaferri EL, Amdur RJ. Thyroid and parathyroid physiology. In: Amdur RJ, Mazzaferri EL, eds. *Essentials of thyroid cancer management*. New York: Springer, 2005:7–17. Copyright © 2005 Springer Science+Business Media, Inc.)

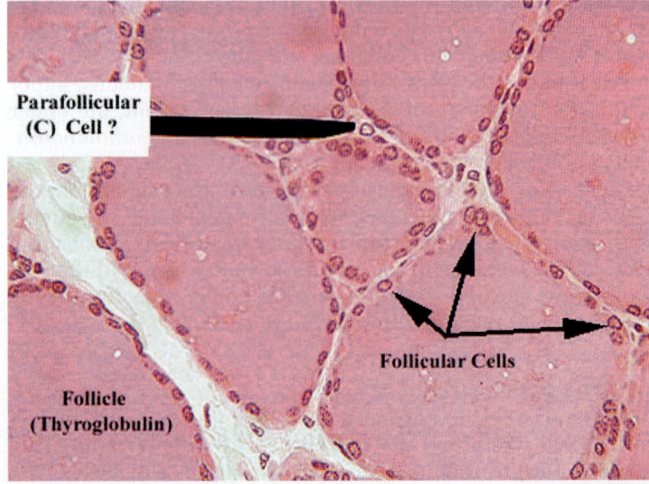

TABLE 53.1 CLASSIFICATION OF THYROID CANCER BY CELL OF ORIGIN

Follicular Epithelial Cell
Well-differentiated thyroid cancer (DTC)
    Papillary thyroid carcinoma (PTC)
        Classic
        Follicular variant
        Oncocytic variant
        Unfavorable variants
            Diffuse sclerosing
            Tall cell
            Columnar cell
            Hobnail
    Follicular thyroid carcinoma (FTC)
        Classic
        Hurthle cell carcinoma
Poorly differentiated thyroid cancer (PDTC): Insular carcinoma
Undifferentiated thyroid cancer: Anaplastic carcinoma

Parafollicular C-cell
Medullary carcinoma

Differentiated (Follicular-Derived) Thyroid Carcinoma

The two major subgroups constituting DTC are PTC and FC. They are distinguished mainly by cytologic features: in PTC, cytology is diagnostic of malignancy whereas in FC, the diagnosis of malignancy requires evidence of tumor invasion through the tumor (not the thyroid) capsule. It is for this reason that PTC is usually diagnosed by fine needle aspiration but diagnosis of FC usually requires at least a lobectomy.

Papillary Thyroid Carcinoma

The distinguishing features of PTC include nuclear enlargement, hypochromasia, intranuclear cytoplasmic inclusions (nuclear pseudoinclusions), nuclear grooves, and distinct nucleoli. After formalin fixation, nuclei may appear pale and optically clear and resemble "Orphan Annie eyes." PTC is strongly lymphotropic, and multicentric disease within the parenchyma of the gland is often present secondary to early lymphatic spread. All PTC stain strongly for Tg.[3–5]

In its classic variant, PTC has a tumor architecture comprising branching papillae with fibrovascular cores. The follicular variant of PTC differs from the classic variant by its follicular growth pattern; however, it retains the nuclear features diagnostic of PTC. The oncocytic variant of PTC has the morphology of oncocytomas elsewhere in the body with abundant pink cytoplasm. From the clinical standpoint, the distinction between classic, follicular, and oncocytic subtypes of PTC is not important because they are treated the same way and have similar prognoses. The unfavorable variants of PTC have a worse prognosis than do the above three subtypes.

Diffuse sclerosing is a rare form of PTC, with histologic features of extensive sclerosis, lymphocytic infiltrate, and psammoma bodies. A greater percentage of patients with diffuse sclerosing PTC present with extrathyroidal extension or distant metastases. Likewise, tall cell, columnar, and hobnail variants are commonly associated with poor prognostic features such as advanced age, large tumor size, aggressive histologic features with early invasion, and distant metastases. The distinguishing feature of tall cell PTC is that at least 70% of the carcinoma is composed of cells that are at least twice as tall as they are wide because of abundant cellular cytoplasm. Columnar and hobnail cell variants are rare. These carcinomas histologically show striking nuclear stratification, usually with papillary architecture. However, the usual nuclear features of PTCs may be absent; therefore, some pathologists prefer to classify columnar and hobnail cell variants as poorly differentiated carcinomas.

Follicular Carcinoma

FC, like PTC, is a DTC of follicular cell origin. This malignant thyroid neoplasm lacks the cytologic features of PTC. These carcinomas show evidence of thyroid follicle formation and are usually well circumscribed with a defined tumor capsule. They are grossly indistinguishable from follicular adenomas. The diagnosis of FC is dependent on the presence of one of two histologic features: (a) tumor invasion through the entire tumor capsule or (b) tumor invasion into a blood vessel located in the tumor capsule or immediately outside the tumor capsule. Minimally invasive forms of FC may present a pathologic challenge and often require serial sectioning to find evidence of capsular or vascular invasion, whereas widely invasive forms of FC are obviously invasive tumors on both gross and microscopic evaluation.

Hurthle Cell Carcinoma

Many references classify Hurthle cell carcinoma as a subtype of follicular thyroid cancer, but more recent molecular studies suggest it should be a separate entity.[6] An older name for Hurthle cell carcinoma is oncocytic carcinoma (not to be confused with the oncocytic variant of PTC). Hurthle cells are large and contain abundant granular eosinophilic cytoplasm. Hurthle cells may be seen in both benign and other non–Hurthle cell malignant neoplastic lesions; however, at least 75% of the tumor must be composed of Hurthle cells to designate it Hurthle cell carcinoma. Similar to FC, Hurthle cell carcinoma requires the presence of capsular or vascular invasion to classify it as a malignant neoplasm.

Poorly Differentiated Thyroid Carcinoma (Insular Carcinoma)

These follicular epithelial cell–derived tumors are intermediate between DTC and undifferentiated, or anaplastic, thyroid cancers (ATCs). Both their histologic appearance and biologic behavior are more aggressive than those of DTC. They tend to be widely invasive, and many will extend beyond the gland. Insular carcinoma is characterized by tumor cells that are arranged in discrete nests separated by a fibrous stroma. Microscopically, they are usually solid with some evidence of follicle formation. Mitoses and necrosis are often present. The presence of more differentiated areas of tumor admixed with insular carcinoma suggests that the latter represents "dedifferentiated" tumors.

Undifferentiated Thyroid Carcinoma: Anaplastic Carcinoma

ATC is the most aggressive form of thyroid carcinoma. Most patients are diagnosed at the age of 65 years or older.[7] ATC originates from the thyroid follicular epithelium but shows little to no evidence of histologic differentiation. This tumor is defined as much by its clinical behavior as its histologic appearance. When diagnosed, most ATCs are widely invasive, replacing most if not all of the normal-appearing gland, and freely infiltrate the perithyroidal tissues. They are usually accompanied by bulky metastatic lymphadenopathy and distant metastatic spread. Gross pathologic evaluation is characterized by widely infiltrative disease with areas of necrosis and hemorrhage. Various microscopic patterns have been described, including small cell, spindle cell, giant cell, squamoid cell, and pleomorphic cell. They are hypothesized to be lesions that have dedifferentiated from more benign differentiated follicular neoplasms.

Medullary Thyroid Carcinoma

MTC does not originate from the follicular epithelial cells, but from the parafollicular C cells, which are neural crest–derived cells whose function is to produce calcitonin. Cases are seen sporadically (80%) or in association with familial multiple endocrine neoplasia (MEN IIa, MEN IIb, and pure familial

TABLE 53.2 CLASSIFICATION OF THYROID CANCER BASED ON THE ABILITY TO CONCENTRATE IODINE

Usually Concentrate Iodine to a Degree That May Be Curative
Papillary thyroid carcinoma
    Classic
    Follicular variant
    Oncocytic variant
Follicular thyroid carcinoma
    Classic

Often Do NOT Concentrate Iodine to a Degree That Is Curative
Unfavorable variants of papillary thyroid carcinoma
    Diffuse sclerosing
    Tall cell
    Columnar cell
    Hobnail
Hurthle cell carcinoma

Rarely Concentrate Iodine to a Degree That Is Curative
Poorly differentiated thyroid carcinoma: insular carcinoma

Never Concentrate Iodine to a Degree That Is Curative
Anaplastic carcinoma
Medullary carcinoma

MTC) syndromes. Multifocal and bilateral MTCs are usually seen in patients with MEN, but, otherwise, familial and sporadic MTCs are indistinguishable. Grossly, these tumors are well circumscribed and nonencapsulated. Microscopically, tumors can have different appearances, including patterns that mimic other types of thyroid tumors. The most common pattern is of solid growth or nests similar to insular carcinoma. Amyloid, which is present in approximately 80% of cases, is a characteristic feature of MTC. Calcitonin stains are usually positive and specific for MTC, but up to 20% of cases may not stain for calcitonin; therefore, other neuroendocrine markers such as chromogranin may be useful.

Classification Based on the Capacity to Concentrate Iodine

Different pathologic classes of thyroid carcinoma concentrate iodine to various degrees. This characteristic is central to management decisions because the ability to concentrate iodine presents a useful therapeutic target. Table 53.2 presents a classification system that categorizes cancers based on whether they always concentrate iodine, infrequently concentrate iodine, or never concentrate iodine. Papillary and follicular carcinomas (with the exception of the more aggressive variants) usually concentrate iodine. The follicular variant of papillary cancer has the same avidity for iodine as does papillary cancer with classic morphology. Therefore, from the treatment standpoint, the distinction between these types of DTCs is not important. The aggressive variants of papillary carcinoma and Hurthle cell carcinoma can concentrate iodine, but to a lesser degree than the classic morphologies. In fact, there is often no measurable iodine uptake in metastases of these tumors. Anaplastic and medullary cancers never concentrate iodine to a clinically useful degree.

EPIDEMIOLOGY OF THYROID CANCER

The data in this section come from a recent analysis of the SEER database for the period 1974 to 2013.[8]

DTC accounted for about 90% of total thyroid cancer cases with 90% of these being papillary carcinoma. The approximate distribution of thyroid cancer cases by sex, race, histology, and age was as follows: female, 75%; white, 80%; papillary, 84%; follicular, 11%; medullary, 2%; anaplastic, 1%; and age in years <20, 2%; 20 to 39, 31%; 40 to 59, 42%; 60 to 79, 22%; and ≥80, 3%.

Between 1974 and 2013, the incidence of thyroid cancer tripled, from approximately 4.5 to 14.4 per 100,000

individuals with almost the entire increase attributable to PTC. These findings are explained by the fact that the large increase in thyroid cancer diagnosis is from the detection of early-stage tumor on neck ultrasound and other imaging studies. The extent of cancer at diagnosis was distributed as follows: localized, 59; regional, 33%; and distant, 5%.

Radiation-Induced Thyroid Cancer

Exposure to ionizing radiation is an established risk factor for thyroid nodules and cancer. Well-recognized data come from survivors of atomic bombs in Hiroshima and Nagasaki and the nuclear reactor accident in Chernobyl.[9–15] A recent analysis of the 59,687 atomic bomb survivors in the Life Span Study demonstrated that a total of 24.5% of cases of thyroid cancer in this cohort were attributed to radiation exposure with a strong dose response.[13] Women and young children appeared to be most susceptible. An estimated additional 1,000 cases of thyroid cancer throughout Europe have been attributed to the Chernobyl accident.[15] An increased risk of thyroid cancer has also been attributed to exposure to therapeutic radiation in children treated for Hodgkin lymphoma, tinea capitis, enlarged tonsils, and enlarged thymus.[16–18] Radiation-induced thyroid cancer is pathologically indistinguishable from spontaneous forms of the disease and is not associated with more aggressive biology or poorer prognosis.[19–22]

Familial Medullary Thyroid Carcinoma

Twenty-five percent of cases of MTCs are hereditary. All patients with MTC should be screened for familial disease, and genetic testing is considered the standard of care for all first-degree relatives of patients with newly diagnosed MTC. Heritable forms of MTC are associated with the familial MEN syndromes (MEN IIa, MEN IIb, and pure familial MTC) and have their own unique epidemiology. These disorders are inherited in an autosomal-dominant fashion because of a germline point mutation in the *RET* gene on chromosome 10q11.2. Men and women are affected equally given the pattern of inheritance. These patients typically present with bilateral and multifocal tumors compared to sporadic forms of MTC. The aggressiveness and age of onset of familial MTC differ depending on the specific genetic mutation. Prophylactic thyroidectomies are increasingly being performed on patients at risk for developing MTC.[23]

CLINICAL MANIFESTATIONS OF THYROID CANCER

The most common presentation of thyroid cancer is an asymptomatic thyroid nodule found incidentally by the patient or clinicians or on an imaging study performed for other reasons.[24,25]

Alternatively, locally advanced thyroid cancer presents with symptoms from involvement of the critical structures intimately associated with the thyroid gland, massive cervical lymphadenopathy, or metastatic disease. These patients present with symptoms such as hoarseness from tumor compression of the recurrent laryngeal nerve, airway compromise, dysphagia or respiratory symptoms, and pain and weight loss resulting from metastatic dissemination.

DIAGNOSTIC EVALUATION OF THYROID CANCER

Laboratory Studies

All patients with thyroid nodules should undergo a serum TSH in addition to basic metabolic, renal, and liver function tests and a complete blood count. Other lab tests, such as Tg, T_3, and T_4, are commonly obtained but are rarely useful in the initial management of thyroid cancer. Serum calcitonin can be measured during the initial evaluation of patients with MTC and is essential during follow-up for these patients.

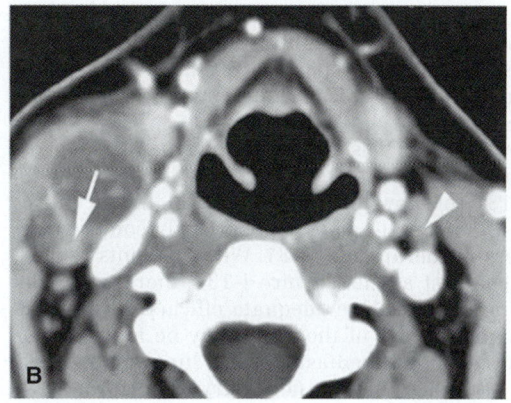

FIGURE 53.5. A patient presenting with a neck mass. **A:** CT image showing the mass to be due to a primary papillary thyroid carcinoma coming into contact with a related level 4 metastatic lymph node (*arrows*). The lymph node at level 4 and in the tracheoesophageal groove is shown by the *arrowheads*. **B:** A section more superiorly shows level 3 adenopathy that is multicystic in a pattern typical but not necessarily diagnostic of papillary thyroid carcinoma. There is upper level 4 cystic adenopathy with an enhancing mural nodule (*arrow*)—a morphology suggesting of thyroid carcinoma. A contralateral enhancing positive node with a focal low-density defect (*arrowhead*) is also present. (From Mancuso AA, Mendenhall WM, Vaysberg M. Thyroid: nodules and malignant tumors. In: Mancuso AA, ed. *Head and neck radiology*. Philadelphia, PA: Lippincott Williams & Wilkins, 2010:1457–1481. With permission.)

Ultrasound and Ultrasound-Guided Fine Needle Aspirate

Neck US with Doppler and US-FNA are the standard diagnostic approaches for evaluating thyroid nodules, both palpable and incidentally detected on imaging. US-FNA has several benefits in the evaluation of thyroid nodules over other means of obtaining a tissue diagnosis: (a) the technique is minimally invasive and is usually performed as an outpatient procedure; (b) the operator can visually verify that the biopsy needle is in the nodule(s) of suspicion; and (c) it allows for evaluation of nonpalpable nodules and, in the setting of cystic lesions, lowers the rate of inadequate specimens.

Cervical US is also an important staging tool because it is effective in identifying lymph node metastases. Cervical lymph node size, presence of calcification, and irregular diffuse intranodular blood flow are the most important US features suggestive of lymph node metastases.[26,27] Using criteria based on the ratio of largest to smallest lymph node diameter, nodule echogenicity, intranodal structure, and margin irregularity, the sensitivity and specificity of cervical US for identifying malignant cervical lesions were 90% and 82%, respectively, in a study of 112 patients followed for thyroid cancer by high-resolution US with Doppler.[28] Preoperative cervical US identified lymph node metastases that were occult on physical examination in 33% to 39% of patients in a large retrospective series.[29,30] Cervical US findings will alter the surgical approach in 14% to 24% of patients with PTC by identifying nonpalpable cervical lymph node metastases.[26,30]

Computed Tomography and Magnetic Resonance Imaging

Computed tomography (CT) and magnetic resonance imaging (MRI) commonly detect otherwise clinically occult thyroid nodules. Malignancy is likely with either imaging technique when there are findings of a mass with extrathyroidal extension, lymph node metastases, or both. In this setting, the studies are useful in presurgical planning by establishing the extent of extraglandular tumor and helping the surgeon determine the need for extended neck dissections (Figs. 53.5 and 53.6). MRI is superior to CT for establishing the local extent of a

FIGURE 53.6. The value of magnetic resonance in the detection of invasion of the trachea and cervical esophagus, especially as it pertains to treatment planning. This patient has anaplastic carcinoma of the thyroid gland. In **(A)**, T1-weighted images show distortion of the trachea (*arrow*) and esophagus (*arrowhead*), but it is difficult to determine whether invasion is present. In **(B)**, the T2-weighted image shows obvious growth of tumor replacing the normal signal of cartilage of the trachea with growth on both sides of the cartilage (*arrow*) as well as replacement of the normal muscular wall signal of the cervical esophagus (*arrowhead*), indicating esophageal wall invasion. (From Mancuso AA, Mendenhall WM, Vaysberg M. Thyroid: nodules and malignant tumors. In: Mancuso AA, ed. *Head and neck radiology*. Philadelphia, PA: Lippincott Williams & Wilkins, 2010:1457–1481. With permission.)

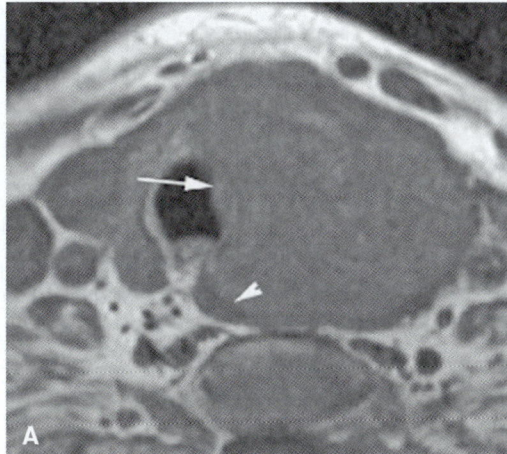
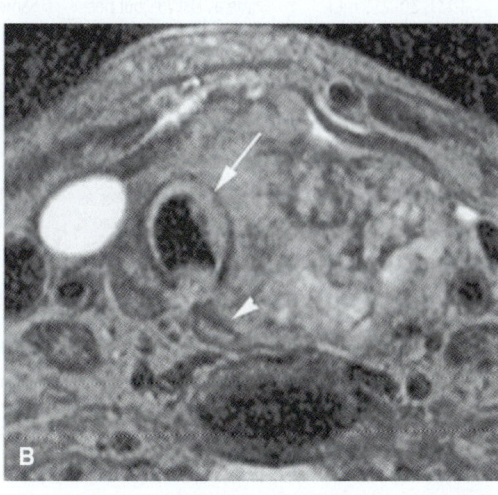

known cancer, because it will more clearly show esophageal or tracheal invasion (Fig. 53.6).[31] MRI is indicated in the presence of hoarseness, stridor, dysphagia, or other clinical signs of locally extensive thyroid cancer that cannot be adequately assessed by US.

A major downside to CT is that useful imaging of the neck requires contrast enhancement, which can interfere with subsequent I-131 therapy. Because of their high concentration of iodine, CT contrast agents can seriously compromise the effectiveness of therapeutic I-131. When patients receiving iodinated contrast agents require I-131, therapy should be delayed in order to achieve adequate efficacy. In selected cases, a noncontrasted CT of the chest may be indicated to evaluate the presence of mediastinal and lung metastases, but, generally speaking, it is not necessary to perform a CT before primary therapy of most DTCs.

Nuclear Medicine Studies

The four major nuclear medicine studies related to thyroid cancer evaluation with iodine isotopes are radioactive iodine uptake (RAIU), thyroid scan, diagnostic whole-body scan (DxWBS), and posttreatment whole-body scan (RxWBS). Table 53.3 summarizes each of these studies.

RAIU tests are used to quantify the RAI iodine-concentrating ability of remnant thyroid tissue after thyroidectomy. This value is required by federal regulation for outpatient I-131 therapy.

Thyroid scans produce images of the thyroid's ability to concentrate iodine and have a historical use in the evaluation of thyroid nodules, characterizing them as functional ("hot") or nonfunctional ("cold"). The authors do not use thyroid scans in the workup or management of patients with thyroid cancer.

The typical DxWBS involves a total-body image several days after administering approximately 3 mCi of I-131 or I-123. The current value of a DxWBS in thyroid cancer management is controversial. Some experts use a DxWBS to determine the therapeutic dose of I-131 in a patient being treated for thyroid cancer. Some experts use a DxWBS as part of the surveillance program following initial treatment. A comprehensive discussion of the issues related to DxWBS is beyond the scope of this chapter. The main arguments against doing DxWBS are low sensitivity, stunning of residual cancer cells, and unnecessary radiation exposure. The bottom line is that reasonable people will disagree about the role of DxWBS in thyroid cancer management. The authors do not use DxWBS to stage or monitor thyroid cancer patients and have not ordered a DxWBS in over 5 years.

An RxWBS should be done in every patient who receives a therapeutic dose of I-131. The optimal interval between administration and scan in most patients is approximately 7 days. The primary purposes of an RxWBS are to detect gross residual disease in the regional lymphatics or in distant sites and to determine if known disease concentrates iodine.

FDG-PET is another nuclear medicine study that is commonly used to detect metastatic disease, but the predictive value of PET in thyroid cancer is controversial.[32,33]

TSH stimulation increases the accuracy of FDG-PET in most types of DTC. A prospective trial comparing FDG-PET studies during thyroid hormone suppression to studies after administration of rhTSH showed increased detection of occult metastases in the stimulated studies.[34] Some insurers will not reimburse for FDG-PET for thyroid cancer without prior documentation of follicular-derived thyroid cancer with a suppressed or stimulated Tg over 10 ng/mL and a negative DxWBS.[35]

TABLE 53.3	NUCLEAR IMAGING STUDIES USED IN THE MANAGEMENT OF DIFFERENTIATED THYROID CARCINOMAS				
Study	**Isotope**	**Diagnostics**	**Results**	**Purpose**	**Comment**
Radioactive uptake study (RAIU)	Usually I-123 (200–400 μCi)	Counts are measured over the low neck 2–24 h after administration.	Not an image but a number. Normal findings after near-total thyroidectomy are 0.5%–3%.	Quantifies the ability of thyroid tissue and cancer to concentrate iodine and estimate the amount of remaining normal and malignant tissue. RAIU is required by federal regulation before outpatient therapy with I-131.	Performed the week before I-131 administration when prepared with T_4 deprivation and on the day of the second injection when prepared with rhTSH
Diagnostic whole-body scan (DxWBS)	I-131 (1–3 mCi) or I-123 (1.5–3 mCi)	The entire body is imaged with a gamma camera ~3 d after I-131 administration.	Records images of the distribution of radioactive iodine throughout the entire body	To detect residual cancer or normal thyroid tissue	Patients should be prepared with a low-iodine diet and TSH elevation. The value of this study is controversial. We do not use this study to plan treatment or monitor cancer status.
Posttreatment whole-body scan (RxWBS)	I-131, 30–250 mCi (therapeutic dose range)	Same as DxWBS but performed ~7 d after I-131 administration	Same as DxWBS	After remnant ablation, it documents the quality of treatment and identifies unsuspected nodal and distant metastases. When normal thyroid tissue has been previously ablated, it identifies cancer that is I-131-avid.	False positives are the only downside, and their impact is mitigated when interpreted in the appropriate clinical context.
Thyroid scan	I-123, I-131, or Tc-99	Same basic procedures as RAIU, but the thyroid is imaged with a gamma camera	Results are an image of the thyroid.	Used in the evaluation of thyroid nodules to determine if the nodule is functional (i.e., "hot" or "cold").	Thyroid scan is included in this table so that it is not confused with RAIU or whole-body scans. Thyroid scans are not used to plan cancer treatment or posttreatment surveillance.

RAIU, radioactive iodine uptake test; rhTSH, recombinant human TSH; TSH, thyroid-stimulating hormone.

TABLE 53.4 AMERICAN JOINT COMMITTEE ON CANCER (AJCC) 8th EDITION (2017) TNM STAGING SYSTEM FOR THYROID CANCER

Papillary, Follicular, Poorly Differentiated, Hurthle Cell, and Anaplastic Thyroid Carcinoma

Primary Tumor (T)

TX		Primary tumor cannot be assessed
T0		No evidence of primary tumor
T1		Tumor ≤2 cm in greatest dimension limited to the thyroid
	T1a	Tumor ≤1 cm in greatest dimension limited to thyroid
	T1b	Tumor >1 cm but ≤2 cm in greatest dimension limited to the thyroid
T2		Tumor >2 cm but ≤4 cm in greatest dimension limited to the thyroid
T3		Tumor >4 cm limited to the thyroid, or gross extrathyroidal extension invading only strap muscles
	T3a	Tumor >4 cm limited to the thyroid
	T3b	Gross extrathyroidal extension invading only strap muscles (sternohyoid, sternothyroid, thyrohyoid, or omohyoid muscles) from a tumor of any size
T4		Includes gross extrathyroidal extension
	T4a	Gross extrathyroidal extension invading subcutaneous soft tissues, larynx, trachea, esophagus, or recurrent laryngeal nerve from a tumor of any size
	T4b	Gross extrathyroidal extension invading prevertebral fascia or encasing the carotid artery or mediastinal vessels from a tumor of any size

Regional Lymph Node (N)

NX		Regional lymph nodes cannot be assessed
N0		No evidence of locoregional lymph node metastasis
	N0a	One or more cytologically or histologically confirmed benign lymph nodes
	N0b	No radiologic or clinical evidence of locoregional lymph node metastasis
N1		Metastasis to regional nodes
	N1a	Metastasis to level VI or VII (pretracheal, paratracheal, or prelaryngeal/delphian, or upper mediastinal) lymph nodes. This can be unilateral or bilateral disease.
	N1b	Metastasis to unilateral, bilateral, or contralateral lateral neck lymph nodes (levels I, II, III, IV, or V) or retropharyngeal lymph nodes

Distant Metastasis (M)

M0	No distant metastasis
M1	Distant metastasis

Prognostic Stage Groups
Differentiated

When age at diagnosis is...	And T is...	And N is...	And M is...	Then, the stage group is...
<55 y	Any T	Any N	M0	I
	Any T	Any N	M1	II
≥55 y	T1	N0/NX	M0	I
	T1	N1	M0	II
	T2	N0/NX	M0	I
	T2	N1	M0	II
	T3a/T3b	Any N	M0	II
	T4a	Any N	M0	III
	T4b	Any N	M0	IVA
	Any T	Any N	M1	IVB

Anaplastic

When T is...	And N is...	And M is...	Then, the stage group is...
T1-T3a	N0/NX	M0	IVA
T1-T3a	N1	M0	IVB
T3b	Any N	M0	IVB
T4	Any N	M0	IVB
Any T	Any N	M1	IVC

From Amin MB, Edge SB, Greene FL, et al., eds. *AJCC cancer staging manual.* 8th ed. New York: Springer, 2017. Reproduced with permission of Springer International Publishing in the format Book via Copyright Clearance Center.

OUTCOME AND PROGNOSTIC FACTORS

The AJCC staging system documents the major prognostic factors that determine disease-specific survival after diagnosis of thyroid cancer (Table 53.4 and Figure 53.7). There are major differences in the staging system from prior versions and from the many prognostic models from other groups. The remainder of this subsection will discuss some of the issues that deserve additional explanation.

Recurrence Versus Survival

Many discussions of treatment for thyroid cancer are controversial. A major reason for disagreement is an inability to agree on the outcome endpoint. The major options are as follows: overall survival (an event is death from any cause), disease-specific survival (an event is death from thyroid cancer), relapse-free survival (an event is cancer recurrence), and locoregional control (an event is cancer recurrence in the thyroid bed or regional neck nodes).

Most types of thyroid cancer have an indolent growth rate such that patients live many years with uncontrolled tumor. An additional complicating factor is that DTC shares with prostate cancer the feature of exhibiting a highly specific serum marker of tumor activity. Serum thyroglobulin (Tg) level is to DTC what prostate-specific antigen is to prostate cancer. Therefore, with most forms of thyroid cancer, there is also the debate about biochemical versus clinical evidence of cancer control.

Most major studies of outcome of thyroid cancer use either overall or disease-specific survival as the outcome endpoint. The major limitation of these survival endpoints is that they do not reflect the morbidity from tumor recurrence that does not cause death. Psychological stress from living with recurrent cancer or uncertainty about cancer cure is substantial,[36,37] and there is physical morbidity that comes from additional diagnostic testing and salvage therapy. This limitation runs through almost every major debate about thyroid cancer treatment because the difference between recurrence and survival results is usually large. Figure 53.8 shows the key figure from a classic study demonstrating this concept.

In this chapter, we do not present specific studies related to a treatment recommendation in a specific situation. Summarizing specific studies would make this chapter unacceptably long and it would not end with definitive answers. For this reason, our approach is to list the major guideline references and to summarize their opinions in some of the

major treatment situations. These major guidelines contain a long list of references of the specific studies that inform the discussion topic.

Age

Age is a major prognostic variable in the AJCC staging systems. The current AJCC system dichotomizes staging based on age under 55 years versus 55 years and older. Age is a major

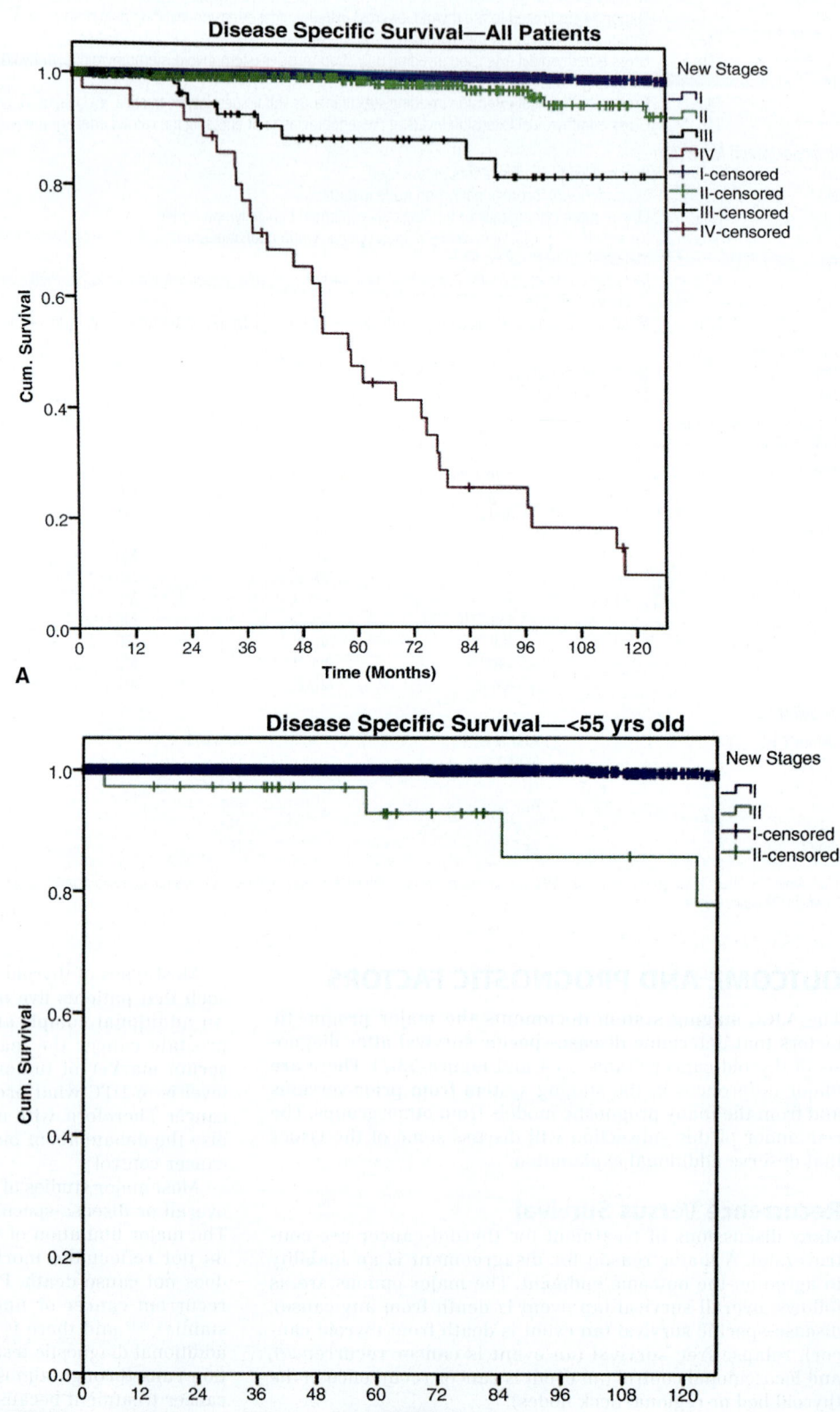

FIGURE 53.7. Disease-specific survival (death from thyroid cancer) using the 8th edition of the American Joint Committee on Cancer staging system for all patients **(A)**, patients age <55 years **(B)**, and patients age >55 years **(C)**.

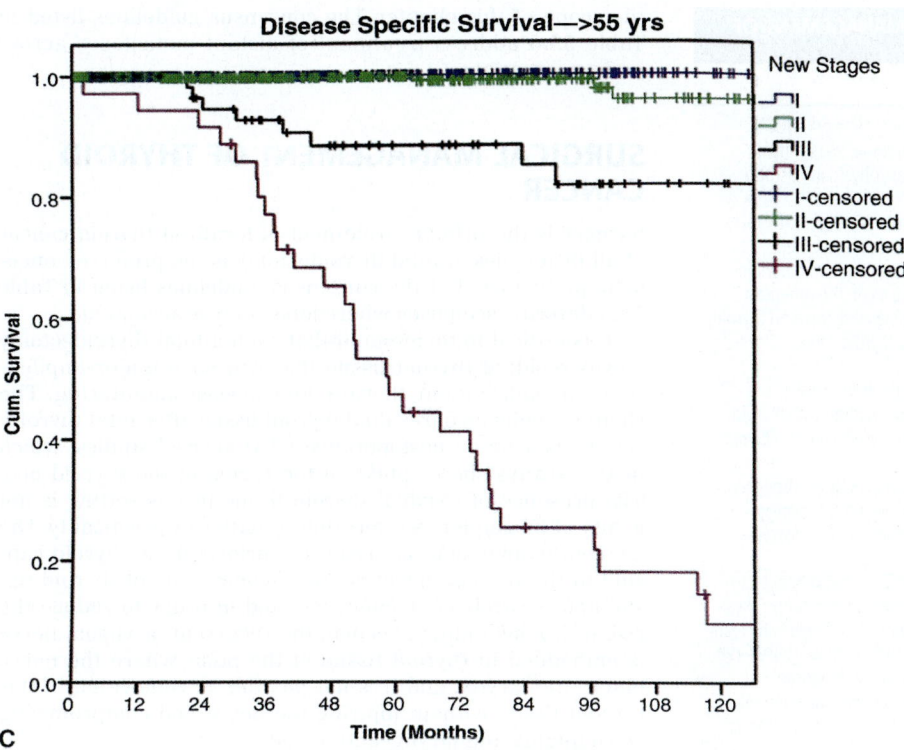

C

FIGURE 53.7. *(Continued)*

factor in all outcome studies because of the consistent finding that younger patients do better than older patients, especially those in the older adult age groups. Of course, the prognostic effect of age is really a continuous variable, but it is more useful for treatment decisions to force a dichotomous breakpoint. But, the major limitation of this approach to age is that it ignores the data that young children (<12 years old) do worse than young adults.[38] The explanation for this difference may be that young children present with more advanced-stage disease at diagnosis, frequently with distant metastases.[39,40]

Unfavorable Variants of Papillary Thyroid Cancer

The most important prognostic factor for disease recurrence and cancer mortality is the histologic classification. DTC, when diagnosed in an early stage, has a favorable prognosis.

FIGURE 53.8. Tumor recurrence and cancer deaths in 1,355 patients treated for follicular and papillary thyroid carcinoma. (Reprinted from Mazzaferri EL, Jhiang SM. Long-term impact of initial surgical and medical therapy on papillary and follicular thyroid cancer. *Am J Med* 1994;97[5]:418–428. Copyright © 1994 Elsevier. With permission.)

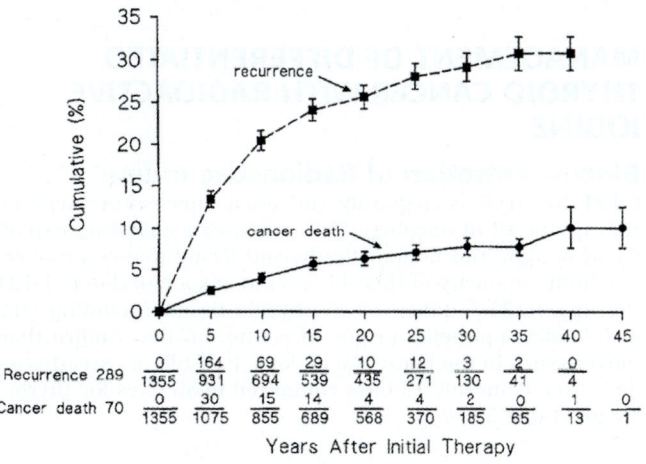

However, tall cell variant can have a 10-year mortality of up to 25%.[41] Columnar cell variant and diffuse sclerosing variants likewise carry a poor prognosis relative to other forms of DTC.[42] However, follicular-variant PTC and classic histology have the same prognoses, which is similar to that of follicular thyroid cancer.

Hurthle Cell Carcinoma

There is major disagreement about the prognosis of Hurthle cell carcinoma relative to other forms of DTC such that some authors recommend a separate staging system. A summary of this debate is beyond the scope of this chapter. A paper from our group summarizes the main issues and presents our data on the subject.[43]

Positive Surgical Margin

A positive surgical margin is an important prognostic factor in most cancer situations. But, microscopic margin status is not a factor in the American Thyroid Association (ATA) and National Comprehensive Cancer Network (NCCN) treatment guidelines (Table 53.5). Data on the independent significance of a microscopic positive margin in DTC are scarce. Some studies suggest that a positive margin warrants more aggressive treatment,[44] but the most respected study on this subject concludes that a positive margin does not affect the recurrence rate following standard treatment.[45] As with many other debates in thyroid cancer, the studies evaluate different endpoints. In the Memorial Sloan Kettering series, the endpoint is clinical recurrence (visible tumor recurrence) without discussion of biochemical recurrence data.[45] Our view is that a microscopically positive margin should be taken into account such that we are reluctant to recommend observation regardless of other factors (Table 53.7).

Number of Positive Lymph Nodes

The prognostic importance of positive neck nodes from DTC has been a major controversy for decades. The AJCC staging system reflects the conclusion that the distinction between no positive nodes and at least 1 positive node has some

TABLE 53.5 CONSENSUS GUIDELINES FOR MANAGEMENT OF THYROID CANCER

Organization	Reference
National Comprehensive Cancer Network: All Types	National Comprehensive Cancer Network. NCCN guidelines for thyroid carcinoma. 2011; https://www.nccn.org/professionals/physician_gls/pdf/thyroid.pdf
American Thyroid Association: DTC in Adults	Haugen BR, Alexander EK, Bible KC, et al. 2015 American Thyroid Association Management guidelines for adult patients with thyroid nodules and differentiated thyroid cancer: the American Thyroid Association guidelines task force on thyroid nodules and differentiated thyroid cancer. *Thyroid* 2016;26(1):1–133
American Thyroid Association: DTC in Children	Francis GL, Waguespack SG, Bauer AJ, et al. Management guidelines for children with thyroid nodules and differentiated thyroid cancer. *Thyroid* 2015;25(7):716–759
American Thyroid Association: Medullary Carcinoma	Wells SA Jr, Asa SL, Dralle H, et al. Revised American Thyroid Association guidelines for the management of medullary thyroid carcinoma. *Thyroid* 2015;25(6):567–610
American Head and Neck Society: EBRT for DTC	Kiess AP, Agrawal N, Brierley JD, et al. External beam radiotherapy for differentiated thyroid cancer local-regional control: a statement of the American Head and Neck Society. *Head Neck* 2016;38(4):493–498
American Thyroid Association: Anaplastic Carcinoma	Smallridge RC, Ain KB, Asa SL, et al. American Thyroid Association guidelines for management of patients with anaplastic thyroid cancer. *Thyroid* 2012;22(11):1104–1139

DTC, differentiated thyroid cancer; EBRT, external beam radiation therapy.

importance, but stage does not change based on the number of positive nodes (Table 53.4). Guidelines from the ATA and NCCN do take into account the number of positive nodes by specifying that patients with ≤5 central compartment nodes are still "low risk" (Table 53.5).

Our opinion is that these guidelines undervalue the significance of many positive nodes in predicting outcome and making treatment decisions. Multiple studies show that multiple positive nodes are a powerful negative prognostic factor. For example, in 2015, Adams and colleagues studied this question with the National Cancer Database and SEER database in young patients with an otherwise favorable prognosis.[46] They found that "increasing number of metastatic lymph nodes was associated with decreasing overall survival up to six metastatic nodes." We take the number of positive nodes into account when making treatment decisions (Table 53.7).

Extranodal Extension

Extranodal extension of metastatic tumor is an important prognostic factor in most types of cancer. In thyroid cancer, this factor is not included in the AJCC staging system nor in the factors that determine treatment in the ATA and NCCN guidelines (Tables 53.4 and 53.5). However, there is evidence that extranodal extension predicts a higher recurrence rate in patients with DTC.[47] We take extranodal extension into account when making treatment decisions (Table 53.7).

Distant Metastases

A unique feature of thyroid cancer is that patients with extensive distant metastases from DTC may be cured with I-131 therapy and most experience long-term survival.[48] Treatment of distant metastases depends on the specific situation, and the scenarios vary so greatly that further discussion is beyond

the scope of this chapter. The consensus guidelines listed in Table 53.5 address treatment of distant metastases across various situations.

SURGICAL MANAGEMENT OF THYROID CANCER

Surgery is the primary treatment of localized thyroid cancer of all histologies. A total thyroidectomy is the preferred oncologic procedure, but the consensus guidelines listed in Table 53.5 describe scenarios where lobectomy is acceptable.

It is critical to understand that even a total thyroidectomy leaves residual thyroid tissue that will have major implications for subsequent therapy and disease monitoring. The clearest evidence of residual thyroid tissue after total thyroidectomy is seen on postoperative I-131 thyroid studies, which nearly always show uptake in the region of the thyroid bed. The presence of residual thyroid tissue in this setting is not a sign of incomplete surgery, but a matter of practicality. The ligament connecting the posterior surface of the thyroid capsule to the trachea harbors microscopic nests of thyroid tissue and is rarely completely resected in order to reduce the risk of tracheal injury. Second, the recurrent laryngeal nerve is embedded in thyroid tissue at the point where the nerve enters the larynx, and it is not possible to remove all of this thyroid tissue without injuring the nerve and compromising voice quality and laryngeal function.

Several important complications can arise from thyroidectomy. The most common are recurrent laryngeal nerve injury (temporary 30% and permanent 2%) and hypoparathyroidism (temporary 5% and permanent 0.5%).[49]

Neck Dissection in Differentiated Thyroid Cancer

As with squamous cell carcinomas, a modified radical neck dissection is done for thyroid cancer when there is a visible or palpably positive node. However, elective neck dissection (removal of lymphatic regions at risk for subclinical disease) is generally not performed for DTC, unlike primary surgery for most other head and neck cancers. Despite a high incidence of subclinical lymph node involvement in even small DTCs, elective neck dissection is not included in the initial surgical approach because the results without neck dissection have been good.[50]

An ongoing controversy is the role of central (level 6) node dissection as part of the thyroidectomy procedure. The consensus guidelines listed in Table 53.5 summarize this controversy. In our opinion, thorough dissection of the central compartment is not necessary in the absence of clinically suspicious nodes at the time of surgery.

MANAGEMENT OF DIFFERENTIATED THYROID CANCER WITH RADIOACTIVE IODINE

Bioconcentration of Radioactive Iodine

I-131 for DTC is arguably the most successful targeted therapy in all of oncology. The iodine-concentrating capacity of benign and neoplastic thyroid tissue makes an overwhelming majority of thyroid carcinomas amenable to I-131 therapy. I-131 is taken up by thyroid tissue, including DTC of follicular epithelial origin, at a rate 6.6 times more than most tissues in the body. The biologic half-life in extrathyroidal tissue is merely 12 days compared to 80 days for thyroid tissue (Table 53.6).

TABLE 53.6 PHYSICAL, BIOLOGIC, AND EFFECTIVE HALF-LIVES (T½) OF I-131

Tissue	Physical T½	Biologic T½	Effective T½
Thyroid	8 d	80 d	7.3 d
Extrathyroidal	8 d	12 d	8 h

Radioactive Decay of Iodine-131

I-131 is produced from the fission of uranium atoms during the operation of nuclear reactors or in the detonation of nuclear bombs. I-131 decays by negatron emission (beta-minus decay) to xenon-131 (Xe-131). A neutron from the I-131 nucleus converts to a proton and an electron (beta particle) is emitted from the nucleus. This first transition results in a beta particle with a range of energies from 250 to 800 keV. These beta particles are core to I-131's ability to deliver targeted cytotoxicity. Because electrons of this energy range will deposit their energy within a millimeter, only the cells taking up the I-131 are affected. In the second decay step, unstable Xe-131 decays to stable xenon, releasing a photon with the energy of 364 keV. This product is therapeutically undesirable, because the photon will travel far from the source where iodine is concentrated. It contributes very little cytotoxicity to thyroid cancer cells and increases the total-body dose; however, it is this property that makes iodine useful for diagnostic imaging, forming the foundation for DxWBS and RxWBS.

Goals of Radioactive Iodine Therapy for Differentiated Thyroid Cancer

Broadly speaking, the two basic purposes of adjuvant I-131 are (a) thyroid remnant ablation and (b) adjuvant therapy for residual microscopic disease. First, I-131 provides potent cytotoxicity by targeting thyroid cancer cells remaining in the operative bed, occult lymph node metastases, and distant metastases. Second, RxWBS provides critical information including staging, prognosis, and determining which patients are likely to require additional treatments. Lastly, ablation of the remaining thyroid tissue facilitates the use of serum Tg as a very sensitive and specific marker for disease persistence after primary therapy. Serum Tg provides a powerful means of monitoring for early disease recurrences that are likely to be amenable to curative retreatment.

Dose of Radioactive Iodine (I-131) to Treat Differentiated Thyroid Cancer

There are two main approaches to selecting the dose of radioactive iodine, or I-131, for remnant ablation or treatment of known residual DTC: empiric and dosimetric. With the empiric method, all patients with the same disease risk factors get the same dose. With the dosimetric method, patients undergo tests of iodine metabolism to customize the dose based on individual physiology. It is beyond the scope of this chapter to discuss the many dosimetric approaches that have been described in the literature. The bottom line is that today most experts recommend empiric dosing in the absence of renal insufficiency or multiple prior I-131 treatments (Table 53.5).

Table 53.7 summarizes the indications and dose of I-131 that we currently use in our program. There are differences between these guidelines and those of the ATA and NCCN (Table 53.5).

TABLE 53.7 EMPIRIC I-131 DOSING FOR TREATMENT OF DIFFERENTIATED THYROID CANCER: UNIVERSITY OF FLORIDA DEPARTMENT OF RADIATION ONCOLOGY [a,b]

Adjuvant Treatment Soon after Total Thyroidectomy (No Prior I-131 Treatment and No Visible Tumor)

Observation[c] (No I-131 treatment)	**All must be present:** pT1-2, pN0-1a, M0 ≤3 positive nodes No extranodal extension Negative margin Postop Tg[d] < 1.0 ng/mL
30 mCi	All other scenarios
150 mCi	**If any are present:** pT3b ≥4 positive nodes ENE that is not extensive[e] Positive margin and postop Tg[d] ≥ 1.0 ng/mL
200 mCi	**If any are present:** pT4 Extensive ENE[e] M1 (with the exception of large-volume disease)

For Recurrent Tumor Based Only on Serum Thyroglobulin Level (No Visible Disease) Following At least One Prior I-131 Treatment

Observation without additional I-131 is always a reasonable option.

We recommend observation when life expectancy unrelated to thyroid cancer is <5 y or when the risk of additional I-131 treatment is high: renal insufficiency, peripheral blood count deficiency, or substantial dry eye from prior I-131 treatment.

Our usual dose when treating recurrent tumor based only on serum thyroglobulin level is 150 mCi.

Other Situations of Recurrent Tumor Following At least One Prior I-131 Treatment:

The range of scenarios in the category is wide: distant metastasis, small-volume unresectable disease in the neck, and gross total resection of neck disease with a high risk of recurrence based on pathologic findings, positive margin, soft tissue invasion, multiple positive nodes, extranodal extension.

We usually do not give I-131 treatment in this setting when the risk of I-131 treatment is high (major renal insufficiency, peripheral blood count deficiency, or dry eye problems).

When we treat with I-131 in this setting, our usual dose is 200 mCi.

[a]There are differences between these guidelines and those of the American Thyroid Association and National Comprehensive Cancer Network.
[b]8th Edition (2017) of the AJCC staging system.[1]
[c]Observation is always reasonable and we explain this as part of the discussion of treatment options.
[d]Serum thyroglobulin (Tg) value obtained ≥ 6 wk after thyroidectomy with any level of thyroid-stimulating hormone. The 1.0 ng/mL Tg threshold is only applicable in the absence of anti-thyroglobulin antibodies.
[e]ENE, extranodal extension of tumor beyond the node capsule. We do not have a definition of "extensive" in this setting.

Preparing Patients for Iodine-131 Treatment

Appropriate preparation for I-131 therapy is critical to obtaining the optimal desired effect of therapy, whether for remnant ablation or adjuvant therapy residual disease. There are many elements to consider when deciding how thorough to be. Table 53.8 summarizes how we prepare patients in our program. These factors are discussed in detail in the consensus guidelines from the ATA (Table 53.5).

Outpatient Management of Iodine-131

Grigsby et al.[51] described the pattern of radiation exposure in 65 household members of 30 patients treated with I-131. The mean dose to family members was well below regulatory standards at 0.24 mSv and the maximum dose was 1.11 mSv. The Nuclear Regulatory Commission (NRC) has issued guidance on the release of patients following I-131 treatment for thyroid cancer, and a copy of all material related to the issue can be found on the NRC Web site. Major recommendations were issued in 1997 (NRC Regulatory Guide 8.39) and have largely remained in place. Several minor subsequent recommendations have been issued, most recently in early 2011

TABLE 53.8 PREPARATION OF PATIENTS FOR I-131: GUIDELINES FROM THE UNIVERSITY OF FLORIDA DEPARTMENT OF RADIATION ONCOLOGY

Component	Description	Comments
Low-iodine diet	A diet that is low in iodine ($\leq$50 μg/d) for 2 wk before, and 2 d after, I-131 administration. Diet instructions are available at www.thyca.org.	The purpose of a low-iodine diet is to deplete the total-body iodine stores to a degree that maximizes the uptake of I-131 by thyroid tissue and thyroid cancer.[72,73]
Intravenous iodinated contrast exposure	Iodine contrast, as used with CT scans, results in a large amount of iodine stored in interstitial tissues.	In patients who have received intravenous iodinated contrast within 3 mo of the planned date of therapeutic I-131 administration, we measure the urine iodine level 1–2 wk before the planned date of administration (see below).
Urinary iodine measurement	Total-body iodine level is determined by the amount of iodine in the urine. The gold standard is a 24-h urine specimen, but we use a spot urine sample because it is more convenient for the patient.	Ideally, urine iodine is $\leq$ 50 μg/L before cancer treatment with I-131. When we suspect inadequate iodine depletion, we measure urine iodine 1–2 wk before the planned date of I-131 administration, on day $\geq$ 7 of a low-iodine diet. If the urine iodine is $\leq$150 μg/L, we administer I-131 as planned. If the level is higher, we delay administration, with the patient on a low-iodine diet for as long as we think it will take to adequately deplete total-body iodine stores. It is ideal to recheck the urine iodine concentration, but we do not do this when the initial value was <300 μg/L.
rhTSH instead of T$_4$ deprivation	rhTSH 0.9-mg intramuscular injection twice (2 d and 1 d) before I-131 administration	Compared to T$_4$ deprivation, rhTSH injections avoid the problems of hypothyroidism and result in less total-body radiation exposure but may decrease the potency of I-131 cancer treatment. Also, the cost of rhTSH may not be covered by the patient's insurance. We use rhTSH in all adults when the patient can afford the cost. We do not use rhTSH in children as it is not FDA approved in children and because children tolerate hypothyroidism better than adults do.
T$_4$ deprivation instead of rhTSH	Stop all thyroid hormone (usually levothyroxine, T$_4$) replacement for as long as it takes to raise the TSH level to $\geq$30 μU/mL by the day of I-131 administration. Ideally, pretreatment testing and the administration date should be scheduled well in advance. For this reason, our standard program is to stop thyroid hormone replacement 6 wk before the planned date of I-131 administration because TSH is almost always >30 μU/mL after ~5 wk of deprivation when we check it 5–10 d before the planned date of administration.	Compared to rhTSH, T$_4$ deprivation may make I-131 treatment more effective because hypothyroidism decreases urinary excretion of I-131 and thus increases biologic half-life. Another advantage of T$_4$ deprivation is that it does not have the cost of rhTSH injections. But, T$_4$ deprivation causes the physiologic problems of hypothyroidism and results in a higher total-body radiation dose. We use T$_4$ deprivation, instead of rhTSH, in adults that cannot afford rhTSH. We use T$_4$ deprivation in all children because rhTSH is not FDA approved in children and because children tolerate hypothyroidism better than adults do.
Lithium	The recommended dose of lithium carbonate is ~20 mg/kg/d (usually 300 mg 3 times a day) for 7 d, beginning 5 d before I-131 administration. At this dose, serum lithium concentration should be measured on day 4 and/or 5 (therapeutic range 0.6–1.2 mEq/L). We have found it difficult to get serum lithium results back in a timely fashion. For this reason, in standard-size patients, we often use an empiric dose of 300 mg twice a day and do not check serum levels.	Lithium increases radiation dose in target tissue by increasing iodine retention time preferentially in normal and malignant thyroid cells.[74,75] We use lithium in most patients that do not have a published contraindication, including psychiatric problems, dementia, seizure disorder, cardiac arrhythmia, renal insufficiency, hepatic impairment, hypo- or hypernatremia, and any of these medications: diuretic, antidepressant, nonsteroidal anti-inflammatory drugs, seizure medication, and calcium channel blockers. In patients who are at high risk for tumor recurrence, we often stop contraindicated medications for the week of lithium treatment or administer lithium without stopping the medication.
Stopping T$_4$ for 4 d with the rhTSH program	Discontinue thyroid hormone replacement 3 d prior to, and the day of, I-131 administration in patients prepared with rhTSH injections	Thyroid hormones contain iodine. Stopping thyroid hormone replacement for a short time before I-131 administration may increase the efficacy of treatment by augmenting the low-iodine diet.[76] We stop T$_4$ for 4 d in all patients prepared with rhTSH injections.
Scopolamine	Scopolamine transdermal patch of 0.33 mg/24 h. Apply patch behind your ear as soon as you get up in the morning on the day of I-131 administration. Remove patch 48–72 h later. Dispense 1 patch. No refills.	Scopolamine is an antimuscarinic that decreases stimulation of the salivary glands. Less salivary stimulation may decrease iodine uptake and thus decrease radiation dose to the salivary glands from I-131 therapy. We use scopolamine in all patients without major contraindications such as angle-closure glaucoma, pyloric obstruction, or serious dementia.
Sour candy	Do NOT eat sour candy for ~3 d after I-131 administration.	Some programs recommend sucking on sour candy during the first few days after I-131 administration. The idea behind sour candy is that stimulating salivary production "washes" iodine out of the saliva glands. One of the few studies on this issue suggested that sour candy INCREASES the radiation dose to the saliva glands.[77] For this reason, we give the patient instructions to NOT chew gum, suck on any type of candy, or eat spicy food for 3 d after I-131 administration.
T$_3$ during T$_4$ deprivation	Tri-iodothyronine (T$_3$, liothyronine sodium) 25 mcg orally twice a day starting the day of discontinuation of T$_4$ and stopping 2 wk before the day of I-131 administration.	T$_3$ has a much shorter half-life than T$_4$. The idea behind administering T$_3$ is to decrease the fatigue and other symptoms of T$_4$ deprivation. We do not use T$_3$ because a formal study failed to show a quality of life benefit.[78]
Diagnostic whole-body scan (DxWBS)	Total-body image ~3 d after administration of I-131 (1–3 mCi) or I-123 (1.5–3 mCi) with TSH $\geq$ 30 μU/mL.	Some experts use this study to determine the therapeutic dose of I-131. We do not perform this study.

CT, computed tomography; T$_3$, 3,5,3′ iodothyronine; T$_4$, 3,5,3′,5′ iodothyronine; TSH, thyroid-stimulating hormone.

TABLE 53.9 SIDE EFFECTS AND RISKS OF I-131 THERAPY: UNIVERSITY OF FLORIDA DEPARTMENT OF RADIATION ONCOLOGY CONSENT DOCUMENT LANGUAGE

The Most Common Temporary Side Effects from I-131 Treatment

Swelling of the saliva glands or neck: It is common to experience mild pain and swelling of the saliva glands that are located near the jawbone. This discomfort usually goes away in 3–5 d.

Taste change: It is common to experience a change in the way food tastes. Taste usually returns to normal within 3 wk after taking I-131.

Nausea: Some patients have nausea—possibly with vomiting—for 1–3 d after taking I-131. Take the nausea medication that we give you as often as you need it.

The Main Serious and Permanent Problems That May Occur after I-131 Treatment

Decrease in saliva and tears causing dry mouth, tooth decay (cavities), and dry eyes:

The risk of these problems depends mainly on I-131 dose and the status of your saliva and tear glands.

Bone marrow damage causing infection, bleeding, and problems from anemia:

The risk of these problems depends mainly on I-131 dose and the status of your bone marrow.

I-131 can cause cancer to develop in the future:

We will try to estimate the risk of cancer from I-131 in your situation.

A publication with a formula is Second primary malignancies in thyroid cancer patients.[79]

A Web site for cancer risk calculation is https://radiationcalculators.cancer.gov/radrat.

Damage to testicles or ovaries: I-131 therapy may cause early menopause if you are a woman and impotence and other problems if you are a man. The chance that you could get these problems depends on your age and dose of I-131.

I-131 therapy may decrease your fertility or ability to produce a normal baby. You should definitely not get pregnant if you are a woman, or get a woman pregnant if you are a man, for at least 6 mo after I-131 therapy.

To Decrease the Change of Problems, Do These Things

Do not wear contact lenses for 3 d after receiving I-131

Stay well hydrated for 3 d after taking I-131: Drink enough fluid so that you need to urinate every few hours. This will decrease radiation exposure to your saliva glands, bladder, and other organs.

Have at least one bowel movement each day for 3 d after taking I-131: Eat prunes or take a laxative, such as Dulcolax 15 mg, as needed.

Avoid things that stimulate saliva production for 3 d after taking I-131: Do not chew gum, use smokeless tobacco, or suck on candy.

under 10 CFR 35.75.[52] Overall, the recommendations are intended to keep the exposure to the public "as low as reasonably achievable (ALARA)."

Risks of I-131 Therapy

A therapeutic dose of I-131 exposes all tissues in the body to ionizing radiation. For this reason, I-131 may damage any tissue in the body and may cause the formation of all types of benign and malignant tumors. The risk of toxicity from I-131 treatment for thyroid cancer depends on the administered dose, the patient's physiology related to iodine metabolism, the sensitivity of the patient to ionizing radiation, the tumor burden, the tumor location, and the ability of tumor cells to concentrate iodine.

A discussion of all possible acute and late toxicities that have been reported following I-131 treatment will not be useful to most clinicians. Table 53.9 is a version of the consent document that we use to explain the main side effects and complications of I-131 therapy.

EXTERNAL BEAM RADIOTHERAPY FOR THYROID CANCER

Indications for External Beam Radiotherapy for Differentiated Thyroid Cancer

There are no randomized control trials defining the indications for external beam radiotherapy (EBRT) in thyroid cancer. The European Multicentre Study on Differentiated

Thyroid Cancer trial was planned as a prospective multicenter trial to evaluate the benefit of adjuvant EBRT in locally advanced DTC. Patients with pT4 disease with or without lymph node metastases and no known distant metastases who underwent total thyroidectomy, I-131, and TSH suppression were to be randomized to EBRT or observation. The trial closed prematurely, however, as only 16% of patients consented to be randomized to EBRT. The trial was converted to a prospective cohort study, and subsequent results failed to define the role of EBRT in this population.[53–55] Therefore, recommendations for EBRT are based on institutional retrospective experiences. Table 53.10 summarizes indications for EBRT from our department and the major consensus guideline publications.

External Beam Radiotherapy Technique

Techniques for treating metastatic disease will vary by site, tumor burden, and clinical circumstances; therefore, this chapter will only discuss the technique used for treating the primary site and nodal regions.

CT simulation is used for treatment planning with patients positioned supine with arms at their side and the neck extended such that the mandible is at 90 degrees with respect to the treatment couch. An Aquaplast (WFR/Aquaplast Corporation, Avondale, PA) mask, custom head holder, and shoulder straps are used to immobilize the head and neck and to depress the level of the shoulders. Bolus material should be applied over scars in the neck. Intravenous contrast may be helpful in defining target volumes and normal-tissue structures, but this is contraindicated if I-131 is being considered within the next 3 months. Axial CT images are acquired from above the skull base to the middle of the chest. Although not necessary, preoperative image sets may be fused to treatment planning CT scans to aid in target definitions. Historically, conventional anterior posterior/posterior anterior or lateral fields have been described to treat thyroid cancer, often requiring custom bolus materials to ensure homogenous dose distributions. Because the target volume straddles the level of the shoulder and, in nearly all cases, contains concavities with envaginated critical normal tissues, we treat all thyroid cancer cases with intensity-modulated radiotherapy (IMRT). We do not routinely bolus neck scars because the tangential beams in the IMRT plan deliver a high dose to the skin of the low neck.

External Beam Radiotherapy Dose and Target Guidelines

Table 53.11 lists the major publications from the modern era with dose and target volume information related to EBRT with curative intent for thyroid cancer. Table 53.10 summarizes the guidelines that we use.

Sequencing of External Beam Radiotherapy and I-131 Treatment

When there are indications for both EBRT and I-131 treatment, there is the question of sequencing. There is no high-quality study specific to this question. In the words of the American Head and Neck Society Consensus guidelines: "There is no consensus on the optimal sequence of EBRT and I-131."[56]

The argument for starting with EBRT is that it often minimizes delay to starting adjuvant treatment. The argument for starting with I-131 is concern that EBRT will "stun" cancer cells in a way that decreases uptake of I-131.

We individualize the decision based on projected delay to administering I-131 treatment and the likelihood that I-131 treatment will increase the chance of cure. In most cases, we deliver EBRT first.

TABLE 53.10 INDICATIONS FOR EXTERNAL BEAM RADIOTHERAPY FOR DIFFERENTIATED THYROID CANCER

Age	University of Florida	ATA Guidelines[62,80]	NCCN Guidelines v1.2017[41]	AHNS Guidelines[56]
Age ≤ 18 y	Painful metastases or impending normal tissue damage from a growing tumor not amenable to other treatment	No child-specific guidelines	No child-specific guidelines	No child-specific guidelines
Age > 18 y with visible, unresectable neck disease	Most situations where surgery is not able to remove all visible tumor with acceptable morbidity, but age is a factor. Because of the increased risk of complications from EBRT in young patients, we usually treat small-volume (<2 cm³), unresectable residual tumor in the neck in patients < 55 years old with I-131 without EBRT if the patient is I-131 naive. We do not use EBRT if I-131 may be curative, or elevated Tg is the only sign of disease.	Recommendation 71 [C22]: EBRT is considered for locoregional recurrence that is not surgically resectable, particularly in patients with no evidence of distant disease.	Consider EBRT for gross disease that is unresectable and/or threatening vital structures.	EBRT is recommended for patients with gross residual or unresectable locoregional disease, except for patients <45 years old with limited gross disease that is I-131-avid.
Age > 18 y: *Adjuvant treatment soon after thyroidectomy*	Most cases with stage T₄ primary tumor or nodal metastases with extensive extranodal extension, but age is a factor. We often do not give adjuvant EBRT in patients < 55 years old with risk factors for microscopic residual tumor. We do not use EBRT if I-131 may be curative, or elevated Tg is the only sign of disease.	There is no role for routine adjuvant EBRT to the neck in patients with DTC after initial complete surgical removal of the tumor.	No guidelines in the absence of unresectable disease	EBRT should not be used routinely as adjuvant therapy after complete resection of gross disease.
Age > 18 y: *After gross total resection of recurrence following initial therapy*	Same as for adjuvant EBRT after thyroidectomy	No guidelines in the absence of unresectable disease	No guidelines in the absence of unresectable disease	After complete resection, EBRT may be considered in select patients older than 45 y of age with a high likelihood of microscopic residual disease and a low likelihood of responding to I-131. This scenario may occur in the setting of gross extrathyroidal extension or with revision surgery for persistent or recurrent disease.

AHNS, American Head & Neck Society; ATA, American Thyroid Association; DTC, differentiated thyroid cancer; EBRT, external beam radiotherapy; NCCN, National Comprehensive Cancer Network.

TABLE 53.11 MAJOR PUBLICATIONS WITH DOSE AND TARGET INFORMATION FOR EXTERNAL BEAM RADIOTHERAPY OF THE NECK FOR DIFFERENTIATED THYROID CANCER

Organization	Reference
American Head and Neck Society	Kiess AP, Agrawal N, Brierley JD, et al. External-beam radiotherapy for differentiated thyroid cancer local-regional control: a statement of the American Head and Neck Society. *Head Neck* 2016;38(4):493–498
National Cancer Center, Korea	Lee EK, Lee YJ, Jung YS, et al. Postoperative simultaneous integrated boost-intensity modulated radiation therapy for patients with locoregionally advanced papillary thyroid carcinoma: preliminary results of a phase II trial and propensity score analysis. *J Clin Endocrinol Metab* 2015;100(3):1009–1017
Memorial Sloan Kettering Cancer Center	Romesser PB, Sherman EJ, Shaha AR, et al. External beam radiotherapy with or without concurrent chemotherapy in advanced or recurrent non-anaplastic non-medullary thyroid cancer. *J Surg Oncol* 2014;110(4):375–382
MD Anderson Cancer Center	Schwartz DL, Lobo MJ, Ang KK, et al. Postoperative external beam radiotherapy for differentiated thyroid cancer: outcomes and morbidity with conformal treatment. *Int J Radiat Oncol Biol Phys* 2009;74(4):1083–1091

THYROID-STIMULATING HORMONE SUPPRESSION FOR DIFFERENTIATED THYROID CANCER

A common practice in management of DTC is administration of supratherapeutic doses of T₄ in an effort to drive the TSH below detectable limits (<0.1 mIU/L), thereby decreasing stimulation of residual benign and malignant follicular-derived thyroid cells. There is *in vitro* evidence that TSH receptor stimulation

is sufficient to initiate thyroid tumorigenesis.[57] A large retrospective series of patients with DTC with 30 years of follow-up showed that, compared with no adjunctive therapy, treatment with TSH suppression with T₄ resulted in a 50% reduction in cancer deaths (6% vs. 12%).[58] Another study showed that the degree of TSH suppression (TSH ≤ 0.05 mIU/L vs. ≥1 mIU/L) was associated with improved relapse-free survival.[59]

A major limitation to TSH suppression is the associated toxicity as these patients experience subclinical and even overt thyrotoxicosis. As such, these patients are prone to bone demineralization and cardiac abnormalities, including tachyarrhythmia, conduction abnormalities, increased contractility, ventricular hypertrophy, systolic and diastolic dysfunction, and even cardiac death.[60] Nevertheless, a meta-analysis with over 4,000 patients with DTC demonstrated that the relative risk of major adverse clinical events was 0.73 (*P* < .05) favoring a "likely" or "questionable" benefit to TSH suppression in 15 of 17 trials.[61] The authors concluded that TSH suppression is justified following initial therapy for DTC. The authors recommend TSH suppression to just below 0.1 mU/L for high-risk thyroid cancer patients, while maintaining the TSH at or slightly below the lower limit of normal (0.1 to 0.5 mU/L) in patients at low risk of recurring.

CHEMOTHERAPY AND TARGETED AGENTS FOR DIFFERENTIATED THYROID CARCINOMA

There are two settings where chemotherapy or targeted systemic therapy is indicated: adjuvant treatment or treatment for recurrent or metastatic disease for which surgery, EBRT, or I-131 treatment is not a reasonable option.

The ATA's statement summarizes the view of most experts regarding the adjuvant situation: "RECOMMENDATION 61: There is no role for routine systemic adjuvant therapy in patients with DTC (beyond I-131 and/or TSH suppressive therapy using [levothyroxine])."[62]

There is no standard treatment for DTC that is not likely to respond to surgery or radiation therapy. Traditional systemic cytotoxic therapies have no significant role because of poor response rates.[63] Recent advances in targeted therapeutics have opened new doors for effective systemic therapy for recurrent or metastatic disease that is unresponsive to I-131. Most of the agents currently under investigation target specific pathways involved in cellular proliferation through inhibition of tyrosine kinase (TKI) receptors and angiogenesis through inhibition of vascular endothelial growth factor receptors (VEGFRs). This is a rapidly evolving area. Section C41 of the ATA guidelines summarizes the status of this issue as of late 2015.[62] The NCCN guidelines include a brief summary about the most common systemic programs.[41]

MANAGEMENT OF MEDULLARY THYROID CARCINOMA

All patients with MTC should be tested for *RET* mutations, including sporadic cases. Genetic screening and testing is also indicated. Similar to follicular epithelial–derived DTC, initial primary management of localized MTC is total thyroidectomy, which is the only completely effective therapy. Central neck dissection should be performed in all cases, and compartment-oriented lateral neck dissection is indicated when clinically involved. There is no role for adjuvant I-131 therapy. All patients should be followed with serum calcitonin levels as this presents a sensitive and specific marker for extent of residual disease.

MTC is uncommon and most of the time it behaves as an indolent disease where long survival with uncontrolled tumor is common. For these reasons, there are few studies on the role of EBRT. The American Head and Neck Society consensus document is currently the best summary of this issue.[64]

Traditional cytotoxic systemic therapies have been ineffective in the management of metastatic or recurrent MTC; however, recent advances in therapies targeting the *RET*–tyrosine kinase receptors have shown promising preclinical and early clinical results.[65-69]

MANAGEMENT OF ANAPLASTIC THYROID CARCINOMA

The ATA consensus guidelines explain the major issues and relevant literature related to diagnosis and treatment of ATC.[70]

Complete surgical excision should be the goal of initial therapy, when feasible. However, surgery should be avoided when complete excision is not possible as debulking does not improve outcomes. There is no therapeutic role for I-131.

The great majority of patients with ATC present with poor performance status and locally advanced disease such that gross total resection is not possible. For this reason, the goal of treatment in most ATC cases is palliation.

Patients with a good performance status and no evidence of distant metastases should be offered aggressive treatment with maximum safe resection and EBRT, with or without concurrent chemotherapy. There is no consensus on the EBRT fractionation program, but a recent study of the National Cancer Database showed that survival was better when the EBRT total dose was 60 to 75 Gy as compared to lower doses.[71] In our program, we usually use the 70/63/56 Gy program described in Table 53.12.

TABLE 53.12 UNIVERSITY OF FLORIDA EXTERNAL BEAM RADIOTHERAPY NECK TARGET VOLUME AND DOSE GUIDELINES FOR THYROID CANCER

Standard Fractionation with Moderate Risk of Recurrence: 60/54-Gy Prescriptions

We use this program when our indication for EBRT is met and there is NO evidence of visible residual tumor, extranodal extension of tumor, or surgical margin < 0.5 cm.

CTV 60 Gy at 2 Gy = Postoperative areas thought to be at high risk for recurrence. These include areas where recurrent tumor was resected plus a 1-cm margin edited for anatomic boundaries to tumor spread and dissected nodal stations with pathologically positive nodes.

CTV 54 Gy at 1.8 Gy = Undissected nodal stations that we judge to be at > 10% risk of recurrence

PTVs = CTV + 0.3 cm

Standard Fractionation with High Risk of Recurrence: 70/63/56-Gy Prescriptions

We use this program when our indication for EBRT is met and there is visible residual tumor, extranodal extension of tumor, or surgical margin < 0.5 cm

CTV 70 Gy at 2 Gy = Visible residual tumor and/or postoperative areas with close margin or extranodal extension, plus a 1-cm margin edited for anatomic boundaries to tumor spread.

CTV 63 Gy at 1.8 Gy = Dissected nodal stations with pathologically positive nodes

CTV 56 Gy at 1.6 Gy = Undissected nodal stations that we judge to be at > 10% risk of recurrence

PTVs = CTV + 0.3 cm

Stereotactic Body Radiation Therapy (SBRT)

We use neck SBRT for small-volume (<2 cm³) visible disease in situations where we judge the risk of treating a larger volume to be unacceptable. We do not have criteria for choosing the 50 vs. 35 Gy schedules

A single target volume: CTV = GTV, PTV = CTV + 0.2 cm

Dose to 95% of PTV = 50 Gy at 5 Gy (10 treatments) or 35 Gy at 7 Gy (5 treatments)

The most aggressive approach is to combine EBRT with chemotherapy involving a taxane, anthracycline, platin, or a combination. In our program, we rarely use chemotherapy with EBRT for ATC because of the high toxicity of combination therapy in this setting.

REFERENCES

1. Amin MB, Edge SB, Greene FL, et al. *AJCC cancer staging manual*. 8th ed. New York, NY: Springer, 2017.
2. Ghossein R. Update to the College of American Pathologists reporting on thyroid carcinomas. *Head Neck Pathol* 2009;3(1):86–93.
3. Hay ID. Papillary thyroid carcinoma. *Endocrinol Metab Clin North Am* 1990;19(3):545–576.
4. Pacini F, Elisei R, Capezzone M, et al. Contralateral papillary thyroid cancer is frequent at completion thyroidectomy with no difference in low- and high-risk patients. *Thyroid* 2001;11(9):877–881.
5. Kawaura M, Pathak I, Gullane PJ, et al. Multicentricity in papillary thyroid carcinoma: analysis of predictive factors. *J Otolaryngol* 2001;30(2):102–105.
6. Cannon J. The significance of hurthle cells in thyroid disease. *Oncologist* 2011;16(10):1380–1387.
7. Nagaiah G, Hossain A, Mooney CJ, et al. Anaplastic thyroid cancer: a review of epidemiology, pathogenesis, and treatment. *J Oncol* 2011;2011:542358.
8. Lim H, Devesa SS, Sosa JA, et al. Trends in thyroid cancer incidence and mortality in the United States, 1974–2013. *JAMA* 2017;317(13):1338–1348.
9. Wood JW, Tamagaki H, Neriishi S, et al. Thyroid carcinoma in atomic bomb survivors Hiroshima and Nagasaki. *Am J Epidemiol* 1969;89(1):4–14.
10. Parker LN, Belsky JL, Yamamoto T, et al. Thyroid carcinoma after exposure to atomic radiation. A continuing survey of a fixed population, Hiroshima and Nagasaki, 1958–1971. *Ann Intern Med* 1974;80(5):600–604.
11. Sampson RJ, Key CR, Buncher CR, et al. Thyroid carcinoma in Hiroshima and Nagasaki. I. Prevalence of thyroid carcinoma at autopsy. *JAMA* 1969;209(1):65–70.
12. Richardson DB. Exposure to ionizing radiation in adulthood and thyroid cancer incidence. *Epidemiology* 2009;20(2):181–187.
13. Preston DL, Ron E, Tokuoka S, et al. Solid cancer incidence in atomic bomb survivors: 1958–1998. *Radiat Res* 2007;168(1):1–64.
14. Cardis E, Hatch M. The Chernobyl accident--an epidemiological perspective. *Clin Oncol (R Coll Radiol)* 2011;23(4):251–260.
15. Cardis E, Krewski D, Boniol M, et al. Estimates of the cancer burden in Europe from radioactive fallout from the Chernobyl accident. *Int J Cancer* 2006;119(6):1224–1235.
16. Ron E, Lubin JH, Shore RE, et al. Thyroid cancer after exposure to external radiation: a pooled analysis of seven studies. *Radiat Res* 1995;141(3):259–277.
17. Tucker MA, Jones PH, Boice JD Jr, et al. Therapeutic radiation at a young age is linked to secondary thyroid cancer. The Late Effects Study Group. *Cancer Res* 1991;51(11):2885–2888.

Section III

18. Sadetzki S, Chetrit A, Lubina A, et al. Risk of thyroid cancer after childhood exposure to ionizing radiation for tinea capitis. *J Clin Endocrinol Metab* 2006;91(12):4798–4804.

19. Naing S, Collins BJ, Schneider AB. Clinical behavior of radiation-induced thyroid cancer: factors related to recurrence. *Thyroid* 2009;19(5):479–485.

20. Schneider AB, Sarne DH. Long-term risks for thyroid cancer and other neoplasms after exposure to radiation. *Nat Clin Pract Endocrinol Metab* 2005;1(2):82–91.

21. Acharya S, Sarafoglou K, LaQuaglia M, et al. Thyroid neoplasms after therapeutic radiation for malignancies during childhood or adolescence. *Cancer* 2003;97(10):2397–2403.

22. Tuttle RM, Vaisman F, Tronko MD. Clinical presentation and clinical outcomes in Chernobyl-related paediatric thyroid cancers: what do we know now? What can we expect in the future? *Clin Oncol (R Coll Radiol)* 2011;23(4):268–275.

23. Nose V. Familial thyroid cancer: a review. *Mod Pathol* 2011;24(Suppl 2):S19–S33.

24. Udelsman R, Zhang Y. The epidemic of thyroid cancer in the United States: the role of endocrinologists and ultrasounds. *Thyroid* 2014;24(3):472–479.

25. Franceschi S, Vaccarella S. Thyroid cancer: an epidemic of disease or an epidemic of diagnosis? *Int J Cancer* 2015;136(11):2738–2739.

26. Gomez NR, Kouniavsky G, Tsai HL, et al. Tumor size and presence of calcifications on ultrasonography are pre-operative predictors of lymph node metastases in patients with papillary thyroid cancer. *J Surg Oncol* 2011;104(6):613–616.

27. Mazzaferri EL. Neck Ultrasonography in patients with thyroid cancer. In: Amdur RJ, Mazzaferri EL, eds. *Essentials of thyroid cancer management (cancer treatment and research)*. New York, NY: Springer, 2005:101–120.

28. Gorges R, Eising EG, Fotescu D, et al. Diagnostic value of high-resolution B-mode and power-mode sonography in the follow-up of thyroid cancer. *Eur J Ultrasound* 2003;16(3):191–206.

29. Kouvaraki MA, Shapiro SE, Fornage BD, et al. Role of preoperative ultrasonography in the surgical management of patients with thyroid cancer. *Surgery* 2003;134(6):946–954; discussion 954–945.

30. Stulak JM, Grant CS, Farley DR, et al. Value of preoperative ultrasonography in the surgical management of initial and reoperative papillary thyroid cancer. *Arch Surg* 2006;141(5):489–494; discussion 494–486.

31. Mancuso AA, Mendenhall WM, Vaysberg M. Thyroid: nodules and malignant tumors. In: Mancuso AA, ed. *Head and neck radiology*. Philadelphia: Lippincott Williams & Wilkins; 2010:1457–1481.

32. Kwon SY, Choi EK, Kong EJ, et al. Prognostic value of preoperative 18F-FDG PET/CT in papillary thyroid cancer patients with a high metastatic lymph node ratio: a multicenter retrospective cohort study. *Nucl Med Commun* 2017;38(5):402–406.

33. Giraudet AL, Taieb D. PET imaging for thyroid cancers: current status and future directions. *Ann Endocrinol (Paris)* 2017;78(1):38–42.

34. Chin BB, Patel P, Cohade C, et al. Recombinant human thyrotropin stimulation of fluoro-D-glucose positron emission tomography uptake in well-differentiated thyroid carcinoma. *J Clin Endocrinol Metab* 2004;89(1):91–95.

35. Cooper DS, Doherty GM, Haugen BR, et al. Revised American Thyroid Association management guidelines for patients with thyroid nodules and differentiated thyroid cancer. *Thyroid* 2009;19(11):1167–1214.

36. Bresner L, Banach R, Rodin G, et al. Cancer-related worry in Canadian thyroid cancer survivors. *J Clin Endocrinol Metab* 2015;100(3):977–985.

37. Husson O, Nieuwlaat WA, Oranje WA, et al. Fatigue among short- and long-term thyroid cancer survivors: results from the population-based PROFILES registry. *Thyroid* 2013;23(10):1247–1255.

38. Mazzaferri EL, Kloos RT. Clinical review 128: current approaches to primary therapy for papillary and follicular thyroid cancer. *J Clin Endocrinol Metab* 2001;86(4):1447–1463.

39. Vaisman F, Corbo R, Vaisman M. Thyroid carcinoma in children and adolescents-systematic review of the literature. *J Thyroid Res* 2011;2011:845362.

40. Chow SM, Law SC, Mendenhall WM, et al. Differentiated thyroid carcinoma in childhood and adolescence-clinical course and role of radioiodine. *Pediatr Blood Cancer* 2004;42(2):176–183.

41. National Comprehensive Cancer Network. NCCN guidelines for thyroid carcinoma. 2017; https://www.nccn.org/professionals/physician_gls/pdf/thyroid.pdf. Accessed April 25, 2017.

42. Bongiovanni M, Mermod M, Canberk S, et al. Columnar cell variant of papillary thyroid carcinoma: cytomorphological characteristics of 11 cases with histological correlation and literature review. *Cancer* 2017;125(6):389–397.

43. Zavitsanos P, Amdur RJ, Drew PA, et al. Favorable outcome of hurthle cell carcinoma of the thyroid treated with total thyroidectomy, radioiodine, and selective use of external-beam radiotherapy. *Am J Clin Oncol* 2017;40(4):433–437.

44. Hong CM, Ahn BC, Park JY, et al. Prognostic implications of microscopic involvement of surgical resection margin in patients with differentiated papillary thyroid cancer after high-dose radioactive iodine ablation. *Ann Nucl Med* 2012;26(4):311–318.

45. Wang LY, Ghossein R, Palmer FL, et al. Microscopic positive margins in differentiated thyroid cancer is not an independent predictor of local failure. *Thyroid* 2015;25(9):993–998.

46. Adam MA, Pura J, Goffredo P, et al. Presence and number of lymph node metastases are associated with compromised survival for patients younger than age 45 years with papillary thyroid cancer. *J Clin Oncol* 2015;33(21):2370–2375.

47. Randolph GW, Duh QY, Heller KS, et al. The prognostic significance of nodal metastases from papillary thyroid carcinoma can be stratified based on the size and number of metastatic lymph nodes, as well as the presence of extranodal extension. *Thyroid* 2012;22(11):1144–1152.

48. Qiu ZL, Shen CT, Luo QY. Clinical management and outcomes in patients with hyperfunctioning distant metastases from differentiated thyroid cancer after total thyroidectomy and radioactive iodine therapy. *Thyroid* 2015;25(2):229–237.

49. Sosa JA, Udelsman R. Total thyroidectomy for differentiated thyroid cancer. *J Surg Oncol* 2006;94(8):701–707.

50. Villaret DB, Amdur RJ, Mazzaferri EL. Neck dissections to remove malignant lymph nodes. In: Amdur RJ, Mazzaferri EL, eds. *Essentials of thyroid cancer management (cancer treatment and research)*. New York, NY: Springer, 2005:131–140.

51. Grigsby PW, Siegel BA, Baker S, et al. Radiation exposure from outpatient radioactive iodine (131I) therapy for thyroid carcinoma. *JAMA* 2000;283(17):2272–2274.

52. NRC Regulatory Issue Summary 2011–01 NRC policy on release of iodine-131 therapy patients under 10 CFR 35.75 to locations other than private residences. 2011; https://www.nrc.gov/docs/ML1036/ML103620153.pdf. Accessed April 25, 2017.

53. Biermann M, Pixberg MK, Schuck A, et al. Multicenter study differentiated thyroid carcinoma (MSDS). Diminished acceptance of adjuvant external beam radiotherapy. *Nuklearmedizin* 2003;42(6):244–250.

54. Biermann M, Pixberg M, Riemann B, et al. Clinical outcomes of adjuvant external-beam radiotherapy for differentiated thyroid cancer—results after 874 patient-years of follow-up in the MSDS-trial. *Nuklearmedizin* 2009;48(3):89–98; quiz N15.

55. Powell C, Newbold K, Harrington KJ, et al. External beam radiotherapy for differentiated thyroid cancer. *Clin Oncol (R Coll Radiol)* 2010;22(6):456–463.

56. Kiess AP, Agrawal N, Brierley JD, et al. External-beam radiotherapy for differentiated thyroid cancer locoregional control: a statement of the American Head and Neck Society. *Head Neck* 2016;38(4):493–498.

57. Ludgate M, Gire V, Crisp M, et al. Contrasting effects of activating mutations of GalphaS and the thyrotropin receptor on proliferation and differentiation of thyroid follicular cells. *Oncogene* 1999;18(34):4798–4807.

58. Mazzaferri EL, Jhiang SM. Long-term impact of initial surgical and medical therapy on papillary and follicular thyroid cancer. *Am J Med* 1994;97(5):418–428.

59. Pujol P, Daures JP, Nsakala N, et al. Degree of thyrotropin suppression as a prognostic determinant in differentiated thyroid cancer. *J Clin Endocrinol Metab* 1996;81(12):4318–4323.

60. Suppression of TSH and the potential toxicity of I-131 therapy. In: Amdur RJ, Mazzaferri EL, eds. *Essentials of thyroid cancer management (cancer treatment and research)*. New York, NY: Springer, 2005:262.

61. McGriff NJ, Csako G, Gourgiotis L, et al. Effects of thyroid hormone suppression therapy on adverse clinical outcomes in thyroid cancer. *Ann Med* 2002;34(7–8):554–564.

62. Haugen BR, Alexander EK, Bible KC, et al. 2015 American Thyroid Association Management guidelines for adult patients with thyroid nodules and differentiated thyroid cancer: the American Thyroid Association guidelines task force on thyroid nodules and differentiated thyroid cancer. *Thyroid* 2016;26(1):1–133.

63. Haugen BR. Management of the patient with progressive radioiodine non-responsive disease. *Semin Surg Oncol* 1999;16(1):34–41.

64. Wells SA Jr, Asa SL, Dralle H, et al. Revised American Thyroid Association guidelines for the management of medullary thyroid carcinoma. *Thyroid* 2015;25(6):567–610.

65. Lam ET, Ringel MD, Kloos RT, et al. Phase II clinical trial of sorafenib in metastatic medullary thyroid cancer. *J Clin Oncol* 2010;28(14):2323–2330.

66. Wells SA Jr, Gosnell JE, Gagel RF, et al. Vandetanib for the treatment of patients with locally advanced or metastatic hereditary medullary thyroid cancer. *J Clin Oncol* 2010;28(5):767–772.

67. Ye L, Santarpia L, Gagel RF. Targeted therapy for endocrine cancer: the medullary thyroid carcinoma paradigm. *Endocr Pract* 2009;15(6):597–604.

68. Torino F, Paragliola RM, Barnabei A, et al. Medullary thyroid cancer: a promising model for targeted therapy. *Curr Mol Med* 2010;10(7):608–625.

69. Schlumberger MJ, Elisei R, Bastholt L, et al. Phase II study of safety and efficacy of motesanib in patients with progressive or symptomatic, advanced or metastatic medullary thyroid cancer. *J Clin Oncol* 2009;27(23):3794–3801.

70. Smallridge RC, Ain KB, Asa SL, et al. American Thyroid Association guidelines for management of patients with anaplastic thyroid cancer. *Thyroid* 2012;22(11):1104–1139.

71. Pezzi TA, Mohamed ASR, Sheu T, et al. Radiation therapy dose is associated with improved survival for unresected anaplastic thyroid carcinoma: outcomes from the National Cancer Data Base. *Cancer* 2017;123(9):1653–1661.

72. Maxon HR, Thomas SR, Boehringer A, et al. Low iodine diet in I-131 ablation of thyroid remnants. *Clin Nucl Med* 1983;8(3):123–126.

73. Sawka AM, Ibrahim-Zada I, Galacgac P, et al. Dietary iodine restriction in preparation for radioactive iodine treatment or scanning in well-differentiated thyroid cancer: a systematic review. *Thyroid* 2010;20(10):1129–1138.

74. Barbaro D, Grosso M, Boni G, et al. Recombinant human TSH and ablation of post-surgical thyroid remnants in differentiated thyroid cancer: the effect of pre-treatment with furosemide and furosemide plus lithium. *Eur J Nucl Med Mol Imaging* 2010;37(2):242–249.

75. Koong SS, Reynolds JC, Movius EG, et al. Lithium as a potential adjuvant to 131I therapy of metastatic, well differentiated thyroid carcinoma. *J Clin Endocrinol Metab* 1999;84(3):912–916.

76. Barbaro D, Boni G, Meucci G, et al. Radioiodine treatment with 30 mCi after recombinant human thyrotropin stimulation in thyroid cancer: effectiveness for postsurgical remnants ablation and possible role of iodine content in L-thyroxine in the outcome of ablation. *J Clin Endocrinol Metab* 2003;88(9):4110–4115.

77. Nakada K, Ishibashi T, Takei T, et al. Does lemon candy decrease salivary gland damage after radioiodine therapy for thyroid cancer? *J Nucl Med* 2005;46(2):261–266.

78. Regalbuto C, Maiorana R, Alagona C, et al. Effects of either LT4 monotherapy or LT4/LT3 combined therapy in patients totally thyroidectomized for thyroid cancer. *Thyroid* 2007;17(4):323–331.

79. Rubino C, de Vathaire F, Dottorini ME, et al. Second primary malignancies in thyroid cancer patients. *Br J Cancer* 2003;89(9):1638–1644.

80. Francis GL, Waguespack SG, Bauer AJ, et al. Management guidelines for children with thyroid nodules and differentiated thyroid cancer. *Thyroid* 2015;25(7):716–759.

PART D
Thorax

CHAPTER 54

Lung Cancer

Jing Zeng, Ramesh Rengan, Indrin J. Chetty, Roy H. Decker, Rafael Santana-Davila,
Corey J. Langer, William P. O'Meara, and Benjamin Movsas

EPIDEMIOLOGY

Throughout the world, lung cancer accounts for 13% (1.8 million) of the total cases of cancer and 18% (1.6 million) of the cancer-related deaths based on 2012 estimates.[1] Among males, lung cancer is the most commonly diagnosed cancer and leading cause of cancer death. Among females worldwide, it is the fourth most commonly diagnosed cancer and the second leading cause of cancer death.

In the United States, lung cancer is the second most common cancer and the most common cause of cancer-related death in both men and women. The American Cancer Society estimates 155,870 people in the United States died of lung cancer in 2017, including 84,590 men and 71,280 women.[2] More people in the United States die of lung cancer than from breast, prostate, and colorectal cancer combined. The overall 5-year survival rate for lung cancer is approximately 18%.[3]

The overall incidence and mortality rate for lung cancer rose steadily from the 1930s until peaking in the early 1990s. The incidence and mortality rates for men began to drop around 1990, and a slight drop in the incidence and mortality rates for women has only recently been measured. The lag in the trend of lung cancer rates in women compared with men reflects historical differences in cigarette smoking between the sexes; cigarette smoking in women peaked about 20 years later than in men. Gender and racial disparities exist in the incidence and mortality for lung cancer with rates highest in men, particularly those who are African American. In terms of socioeconomics, lung cancer demonstrates the largest disparity of all cancers, with the death rate in men five times higher for the least educated than for the most educated.[2]

Although the lung cancer numbers in the general population are startling, the main risk of lung cancer is based on exposures to carcinogens; most lung cancer cases are attributable to cigarette smoking. Voluntary or involuntary cigarette exposure accounts for 80% to 90% of all cases of lung cancer. Since the 1964 landmark report by US surgeon general citing smoking as a causal agent for the development of lung cancer, the prevalence of smoking in the United States has declined significantly. More recently, exposure to secondhand smoke has been considered a risk for lung cancer with up to a 30% increase in risk from secondhand smoke exposure associated with living with a smoker. Indoor radon exposure is now considered the second leading cause of lung cancer in the United States. Other known risk factors for lung cancer include exposure to occupational and environmental carcinogens such as asbestos, arsenic, and polycyclic aromatic hydrocarbons.

ANATOMY

In the past, a simplified and relatively superficial understanding of thoracic anatomy provided an acceptable framework for the radiation oncologist to design treatment fields in lung cancer patients utilizing conventional techniques with the carina and bony structures as landmarks. As the field of thoracic radiation oncology has moved toward more conformal therapy, however, a more detailed understanding of thoracic anatomy is essential for proper target delineation and treatment design.

The lungs are situated on each side of the mediastinum, which contains the heart, trachea, esophagus, and great vessels. The lungs are conical in shape with an apex projecting upward into the neck for approximately 2 to 3 cm above the clavicle, a base sitting on the diaphragm, a costal surface along the chest wall, and a mediastinal surface that is molded to the heart and other mediastinal structures. Visceral pleura cover the lungs, and parietal pleura cover the inside of the chest cavity. The lungs are freely suspended but are rooted to the mediastinum by the structures emerging from the hilum.

The lungs are divided into distinct lobes—three lobes to the right lung and two to the left. The right lung is divided into the upper, middle, and lower lobes by the oblique (major) and horizontal (minor) fissures. The oblique fissure runs forward and downward from approximately the level of the fifth thoracic vertebral body to the diaphragm, dividing the lungs into upper and lower lobes. The horizontal fissure separates the right middle from the right upper lobe, fanning out forward and laterally from the hilum. The middle lobe is thus a small, triangular lobe bounded by the horizontal and oblique fissures and actually rests on the diaphragm. The left lung is divided by only the oblique fissure into two lobes—the upper and lower lobes. The lingula, located in the left upper lobe, is homologous to the right middle lobe and also touches the diaphragm.

The bronchopulmonary segment is the functional unit of the lung and is defined by the segmental bronchi. The trachea bifurcates at the carina, which lies at the junction between the manubrium and body of the sternum, into the right and left main bronchi. Each main bronchus divides into lobar bronchi, each supplying a lobe of the lung. Although the lingula is located in the left upper lobe, the lingular bronchus is considered by many a lobar bronchus. Each lobar bronchus divides into smaller bronchi that form the bronchopulmonary segments. These segments are pyramidal in shape, with an apex toward the lung root and a base at the pleural surface.

Structures entering each bronchopulmonary segment (i.e., bronchus and artery) tend to lie centrally. Structures leaving the segment (i.e., veins and lymphatics) lie in the periphery of the segment within the connective tissue that separates the segments. Segmental bronchi divide into bronchioles, continue to branch, and eventually form the alveoli, where blood–gas exchange occurs.

The main lymphatic drainage for each bronchopulmonary segment follows the vasculature and airways toward the hilum, where it ultimately drains into the mediastinum. However, the rich network of lymphatics within the thorax leads to complex variability in drainage patterns.

The International Association for the Study of Lung Cancer (IASLC) developed a lymph node map that reconciles differences among older maps and provides precise anatomic definitions for all lymph node stations.[4] The IASLC lymph node map has been endorsed by the American Joint Committee on Cancer (AJCC) and incorporated into the staging manual. The IASLC lymph node map designates 14 lymph node levels compartmentalized into intrapulmonary, hilar, and mediastinal zones that have prognostic implications and are utilized in common clinical practice.

CLINICAL PRESENTATION AND PATTERNS OF SPREAD

Lung cancer spreads locally by direct extension of the primary tumor, regionally via involvement of the lymphatics, and distantly via invasion into vascular channels leading to hematogenous spread. In a Surveillance Epidemiology and End Results (SEER) analysis involving all lung cancer histologies, 15% of all cases of lung cancer were localized to the primary site at initial diagnosis; 22% had regional lymph node spread and 56% distant metastasis; and the remaining 7% were stage unknown.[3] In non–small cell lung cancer (NSCLC), half the patients present with localized or locally advanced disease and half with advanced disease. In small cell lung cancer (SCLC), 20% to 30% present with locally advanced disease, and 70% to 80% present with advanced disease. Table 54.1 shows the site of metastasis based on histologic type.[5] Signs and symptoms of lung cancer directly reflect the patient's local, regional, or distant pattern of spread.

Intrathoracic Spread

The intrathoracic spread of lung cancer involves direct extension of the primary tumor or lymphatic spread to regional lymph nodes involving the hilum or mediastinum. There is a wide range of symptoms owing to the intrathoracic effects of lung cancer; the most common include cough, dyspnea, hemoptysis, and chest pain.

The central etiology for many symptoms is owing to a growing tumor involving the airway. Cough is present in 50% to 75% of lung cancer patients at presentation and occurs most frequently in patients with squamous cell and small cell carcinomas because of their tendency to involve central airways. Tumor eroding into a blood vessel or bleeding from the neovasculature supplying the tumor may lead to hemoptysis, which is a presenting symptom in approximately 25% of patients. If tumor blocks airflow through a portion of the lung, shortness of breath may develop and is identified at presentation in approximately 25% of cases.[6] Dyspnea may also be due to the development of atelectasis, postobstructive pneumonia, or a pleural or pericardial effusion.

Chest pain is present in approximately 20% of patients presenting with lung cancer.[6] Pain may be attributed to direct extension to the mediastinum, parietal pleura, or chest wall. Pleuritic pain may also be the result of obstructive pneumonitis or a pulmonary embolus related to a hypercoagulable state. Pleural involvement can also manifest as pleural thickening or pleural effusion. During the course of lung cancer, 10% to 15% of all cases will eventually develop a malignant pleural effusion.

Direct extension of a central primary tumor or mediastinal lymph node involvement may lead to nerve involvement. Involvement of the recurrent laryngeal nerve along its course under the arch of the aorta can result in hoarseness. Irritation of the phrenic nerve may initially produce hiccups, and progressive damage can produce unilateral paralysis of the diaphragm with shortness of breath.

Obstruction of the superior vena cava (SVC) from primary tumor or mediastinal lymphadenopathy causes symptoms that commonly include a sensation of fullness in the head and dyspnea. Physical findings include jugular venous distension and occasionally swelling of the face and arms. SVC syndrome is more common in patients with SCLC than NSCLC. The pathophysiology and treatment options for the management of patients with SVC syndrome are discussed in more detail later.

Primary tumors arising within the superior sulcus may produce the classic Pancoast syndrome manifested by shoulder pain, Horner syndrome, and brachial plexopathy. Pancoast syndrome is most commonly caused by NSCLC and only rarely by SCLC. The treatment of patients with superior sulcus tumors (SSTs) will be discussed later.

Distant Extrathoracic Spread

Once vascular or lymphatic invasion occurs, metastatic dissemination to distant sites is common. Contralateral lung, liver, bone, adrenals, and brain are the most frequent sites of distant disease; however, lung cancer can spread to any part of the body (Table 54.1).

Asymptomatic liver metastases may be detected at presentation by liver enzyme abnormalities or on staging workup imaging. Pain in the back, chest, or extremity and elevated levels of serum alkaline phosphatase are usually present in patients with bone metastasis. The serum calcium may be elevated owing to extensive bone disease, although the majority of patients with elevated calcium have paraneoplastic parathyroid hormone (PTH)–like syndrome. Approximately 20% of patients with NSCLC and 30% to 40% of patients with SCLC have bone metastases at presentation. An osteolytic radiographic appearance is more frequent than an osteoblastic one, although a mixed picture is common. The most common sites of involvement are the vertebral bodies.

The adrenal glands are a frequent site of metastasis; however, such metastases are only rarely symptomatic. Concern about adrenal metastasis usually occurs when a unilateral mass is found by staging computed tomography (CT) in a patient with a known or suspected lung cancer. Most adrenal

TABLE 54.1 SITE OF METASTASIS CORRELATED WITH HISTOLOGIC SUBTYPE IN LUNG CANCER: NECROPSY FINDINGS IN CARCINOMA OF THE BRONCHUS IN 255 PATIENTS WITH METASTASES TO 431 SITES

Site of Metastasis	Squamous	Small Cell	Anaplastic	Adenocarcinoma
Lymph nodes	137 (54%)	163 (85%)	135 (76%)	42 (75%)
Liver	58 (23%)	122 (64%)	67 (38%)	26 (47%)
Adrenals	54 (21%)	84 (44%)	69 (39%)	17 (30%)
Bones	59 (23%)	75 (39%)	53 (30%)	23 (41%)
Brain	26 (17%)	45 (42%)	30 (24%)	13 (39%)
Kidney	39 (15%)	28 (15%)	24 (14%)	11 (20%)
Pancreas	9 (4%)	46 (24%)	25 (14%)	3 (5%)
Lung	31 (2%)	13 (7%)	15 (8%)	8 (14%)
Pleura	18 (7%)	21 (11%)	9 (5%)	3 (5%)
Total	**255**	**191**	**179**	**56**

Reprinted from Line DH, Deeley TJ. The necropsy findings in carcinoma of the bronchus. *Br J Dis Chest* 1971;65(4):238–242. Copyright © 1971 Elsevier. With permission.

masses detected on staging scans are benign. Conversely, a negative imaging study does not exclude adrenal metastases. The lack of specificity of an initial CT scan in identifying an adrenal mass creates a special problem in patients with an otherwise resectable lung cancer. In this situation, positron emission tomography (PET) may be particularly useful in distinguishing a benign from malignant adrenal mass. Other procedures that may be useful in excluding a metastasis include magnetic resonance imaging (MRI) consistent with a benign adenoma or a negative needle biopsy. Involvement of the adrenal glands is more frequent in patients with widely disseminated disease. In autopsy series, adrenal metastases were identified in about 40% of patients with lung cancer.[7] Patients with an isolated adrenal metastasis but otherwise limited thoracic disease seem to have a much better prognosis than other stage IV disease and may be considered for aggressive definitive management.

Symptoms from brain metastasis include headache, vomiting, visual field loss, hemiparesis, cranial nerve deficit, and seizures. In patients with NSCLC, the frequency of brain metastasis is greatest with adenocarcinoma and least with squamous cell carcinoma. The risk of brain metastasis increases with larger primary tumor size and regional node involvement. In patients with SCLC, metastasis to brain is present in approximately 20% to 30% of patients at presentation. An autopsy series of SCLC patients disclosed central nervous system (CNS) metastases in 80% of cases.[8]

Paraneoplastic Syndromes

A paraneoplastic syndrome is a disease or symptom that is the consequence of cancer cells in the body but is not attributable to the local presence of tumor. These phenomena are thought to be mediated by humoral factors secreted by tumor cells or by an immune response against the tumor. Treating the cancer, if successful, usually resolves the syndrome. Some of the more common paraneoplastic syndromes are described next.

Cushing Syndrome

Ectopic production of adrenocorticotropic hormone (ACTH) can cause Cushing syndrome. Patients typically present with muscle weakness, weight loss, hypertension, hirsutism, and osteoporosis. Hypokalemic alkalosis and hyperglycemia are usually present. Cushing syndrome is relatively common in patients with SCLC and with carcinoid tumors of the lung. SCLC patients with Cushing syndrome appear to have a worse prognosis than those without Cushing syndrome.

Syndrome of Inappropriate Antidiuretic Hormone Secretion

The syndrome of inappropriate antidiuretic hormone (SIADH) secretion is frequently caused by SCLC and results in hyponatremia. Approximately 10% of patients who have SCLC exhibit SIADH, and SCLC accounts for approximately 75% of all SIADH. Symptoms include headache, muscle cramps, anorexia, and decreased urine output. If left untreated, cerebral edema can develop, leading to mental status changes, coma, seizures, and respiratory arrest. Besides treating the underlying cancer, demeclocycline is the agent of choice.

Hypercalcemia

Hypercalcemia in patients with lung cancer may be attributable to the secretion of a parathyroid hormone–related protein (PTHrP), calcitriol, or other cytokines, including osteoclast-activating factors. In one study of 1,149 consecutive lung cancers, 6% of patients had hypercalcemia.[9] Among those with hypercalcemia, squamous cell carcinoma, adenocarcinoma, and SCLC were responsible in 51%, 22%, and 15% of cases, respectively. Symptoms of hypercalcemia include anorexia,

nausea, vomiting, constipation, lethargy, polyuria, polydipsia, and dehydration. Renal failure, confusion, and coma are late manifestations.

Lambert-Eaton Myasthenic Syndrome

Lambert-Eaton myasthenic syndrome (LEMS) is an autoimmune disorder characterized by muscle weakness of the limbs that improves with repeated testing, in contrast to myasthenia gravis, which worsens with repetition. Proximal muscles are predominantly affected, and patients complain of difficulty climbing stairs and rising from a sitting position. Approximately 3% of patients with SCLC exhibit LEMS, and SCLC accounts for approximately 60% of all LEMS.[10] The neurologic symptoms of LEMS precede the diagnosis of SCLC in >80% of cases, often by months or years.

Hypertrophic Osteoarthropathy

Hypertrophic pulmonary osteoarthropathy (HPO), most frequently associated with adenocarcinoma, is defined by clubbing and periosteal proliferation of the tubular bones. HPO is further characterized by a symmetrical, painful arthropathy that usually involves the ankles, knees, wrists, and elbows. A radiograph of the long bones shows characteristic periosteal new bone formation. A bone scan or PET typically demonstrates diffuse uptake by the long bones. In a series of 111 lung cancer patients, clubbing was present in 29%.[11]

SCREENING, DIAGNOSTIC STAGING, AND WORKUP

Screening for Lung Cancer

Given the high mortality rate of lung cancer and that the majority of patients are diagnosed at a late stage, lung cancer researchers have theorized that identifying lung cancer at an earlier stage might improve outcomes. Early screening trials involving chest x-rays and/or sputum failed to demonstrate a survival benefit. The role of screening has recently been reinvestigated with the advent of spiral CT scans. Early pilot trials of spiral CT in lung cancer screening looked promising with an increase in the identification of stage I detectable cancer. A subsequent international observational trial using spiral CT screening in a cohort of 31,000 high-risk individuals corroborated the findings, showing that annual spiral CT screening could detect lung cancer at an early, potentially more curable stage, suggesting that the stage I disease detection rate and 10-year survival rate could both exceed 80%.[12] This set the groundwork for the landmark National Lung Screening Trial (NLST).[13] From 2002 to 2004, 53,454 current or former heavy smokers at 33 US medical centers were randomly assigned to three annual screenings with either low-dose CT (26,722 participants) or standard chest x-ray (26,732). Eligible participants were between 55 and 74 years of age with a history of cigarette smoking of at least 30 pack-years and, if former smokers, had quit within the previous 15 years. Persons who had previously received a diagnosis of lung cancer, had undergone chest CT within 18 months before enrollment, had hemoptysis, or had an unexplained weight loss >6.8 kg (15 lb) in the preceding year were excluded. The findings revealed that participants who received low-dose helical CT scans had a 20% relative reduction in risk of death caused by lung cancer compared with the control radiography group ($P = .004$). Additionally, the all-cause mortality was reduced in the CT screening group by 6.7% when compared with the control group ($P = .02$). This is the first randomized trial to demonstrate a reduction in all-cause mortality with screening and has led to the development of lung cancer screening programs throughout the country.

Diagnostic Staging and Workup

When a patient presents with suspected lung cancer, testing is indicated to confirm the diagnosis, identify the histologic type, and determine the disease stage, all in an effort to guide management decisions. The process begins with a thorough history and physical examination to identify signs or symptoms suggestive of locally extensive or metastatic disease, assess pulmonary health status, identify significant comorbidities, and assess overall health status. Each impacts the therapeutic options in a more comprehensive manner than stage alone. A detailed history should also elicit tobacco use and past exposure to environmental carcinogens. Weight loss >5% from baseline has direct prognostic implications for survival in lung cancer.

Physical examination of the chest may detect signs of partial or complete obstruction of the airways, pneumonia, or pleural effusion. Examination of the neck can reveal evidence of supraclavicular lymphadenopathy. Abdominal examination may detect hepatomegaly. Neurologic examination can detect signs of brain metastasis.

Laboratory studies include complete blood count, liver function tests, and serum electrolytes including calcium. Renal function tests should be performed to assess whether the patient can tolerate intravenous contrast for CT examination or subsequent platinum-based therapy. Liver function test abnormalities could be owing to liver metastasis. Elevation of alkaline phosphatase could be due to liver or bone metastasis. Calcium elevation could be from bone metastasis or paraneoplastic syndrome. Anemia could be owing to metastatic disease.

Radiologic Examinations

Computed Tomography

All patients with suspected lung cancer, with or without an abnormal chest x-ray, should undergo a contrast-enhanced CT scan of the chest and upper abdomen to include the entire liver and adrenal glands. Intravenous contrast helps to distinguish vascular structures from mediastinal structures. This not only adds detail to the imaging characteristics of the primary tumor but also is critical to accurately identify suspicious lymph nodes in the mediastinum. CT assessment can establish T-stage by determining tumor size, presence of separate tumor nodules, presence of atelectasis or postobstructive pneumonia, invasion of adjacent structures, and proximal extent of the tumor.

Lymph node enlargement on CT presumes lymph node metastasis in the context of newly diagnosed lung cancer. Most normal mediastinal lymph nodes measure <1 cm, although normal nodes subcarinal lymph can reach a diameter 1.5 of cm. In a patient with known lung cancer, a lymph node is considered suspicious if it measures >1 cm in diameter on its short axis. Unfortunately, many subcentimeter regional lymph nodes may still harbor metastasis. In one study involving pathologic staging, up to 44% of nodes with metastatic deposits were <1 cm in diameter, and 18% of patients with pathologically involved mediastinal nodes did not have any nodes >1 cm.[14]

Positron Emission Tomography or Positron Emission Tomography–Computed Tomography

PET scanning has become standard in the staging workup of lung cancer patients. Although the primary tumor characteristics are usually clearly staged with a CT scan, PET can help distinguish atelectasis from tumor in certain cases. The largest benefit provided by PET is the identification of malignant disease in lymph nodes of normal size or distant metastasis not seen on CT scan. Kalff et al.[15] prospectively evaluated the utility of PET in patients with lung cancer, performing a PET scan on 105 consecutive clinically staged patients with a diagnosis of NSCLC. They found that PET correctly upstaged 26% of patients to palliative from curative intent therapy and appropriately downstaged 10 of 16 patients initially designated for palliative therapy. Integrated PET-CT scanners fuse images obtained in tandem from PET and CT, thus providing both anatomic and metabolic information simultaneously. This is superior to CT or PET alone and can detect malignancy in tumors as small as 0.5 cm.

Although PET has dramatically improved the noninvasive staging of lung cancer patients, it does have some key limitations. On meta-analysis, the sensitivity and specificity of CT for mediastinal nodal metastasis were estimated to be approximately 59% and 79%, respectively, and the sensitivity and specificity of PET were approximately 81% and 90%, respectively.[16] This same meta-analysis also found a difference in the accuracy of PET based on the CT size of a lymph node with a sensitivity of 91% for enlarged mediastinal nodes and 75% for nonenlarged nodes. Because false positives and false negatives are observed with PET, tissue sampling should be pursued to confirm the presence or absence of regional lymph node involvement before a treatment decision is made. A positive PET should not be considered proof of lymph node metastasis, especially if such a conclusion would otherwise exclude surgery.

With highly conformal radiation therapy for lung cancer becoming commonplace, PET is now being used to aid radiation oncologists in the target delineation process for involved-field radiotherapy (IFRT). Registration of PET with the planning CT scan at the contouring stage has been shown to enhance the accuracy of defining gross tumor volumes (GTVs). The clinician must be mindful that target volumes based solely on 18F-fluorodeoxyglucose (FDG)-PET positivity have their limitations, with the most notable being a false-negative rate of approximately 25% in mediastinal lymph nodes <1 cm in size.[16] Additionally, the optimal windowing algorithm for the purposes of contouring remains to be determined. Depending on the algorithm employed, the volume that is contoured can vary significantly. When benchmarked against the true pathologic volume, at present, the CT-derived contour appears to be more accurate than that derived from FDG-PET regardless of the algorithm employed.

Special Diagnostic Procedures

Percutaneous Fine Needle Aspiration

CT-guided fine needle aspiration (FNA) is an excellent method for establishing a tissue diagnosis from a suspicious peripheral pulmonary nodule that cannot be reached by bronchoscopy. The risk of a pneumothorax from this procedure is 25%. However, most of these are small and asymptomatic and resolve without intervention; only approximately 5% require a chest tube. The overall diagnostic yield is 80%. Indeterminate biopsies must be interpreted with caution. FNA cannot rule out malignancy unless another benign diagnosis can clearly be established. Abnormalities involving bone, liver, and adrenal glands can also be confirmed by CT-guided FNA. Frequently, biopsy of one of these suspected metastatic sites simultaneously establishes tissue diagnosis and stage of the disease. Increasingly, as we enter the modern era of molecularly guided therapy, core biopsies are displacing FNAs. This increases the risk but also increases the yield.

Bronchoscopy

Fiberoptic bronchoscopy enables visualization of the tracheobronchial tree to the second or third segmental divisions. Cytologic brushings or biopsy forceps specimens can be obtained from identified lesions. Even when no visible lesion is identified, the bronchus draining the area of suspicion can be lavaged for cytologic analysis. Navigational bronchoscopy is a real-time guidance system that combines fiberoptic bronchoscopy with special CT imaging techniques to guide the bronchoscope to specified locations within the bronchial tree. Using this approach, a virtual map of the bronchial tree is generated from a high-resolution CT scan of the chest, enabling the physician to monitor the location of the bronchoscope in real time through feedback from a positional sensor attached to the tip of the bronchoscope. This approach may significantly improve the diagnostic yield for peripheral lesions.

Endoscopic Ultrasound

Fiberoptic endoscopy techniques can also be combined with ultrasound to evaluate mediastinal and hilar lymph nodes. Endobronchial ultrasound-guided needle transbronchial aspiration (EBUS-TBNA) involves FNA sampling of ultrasound-suspicious lymph nodes, especially those located in the paratracheal (lymph node levels 2 and 4), subcarinal (level 7), or hilar lymph node stations (level 10). A prospective study comparing EBUS-TBNA with PET-CT scans revealed an accuracy of 98% and a sensitivity and specificity of 92% and 100%, respectively.[17] An esophageal approach known as transesophageal endoscopic ultrasound-guided fine needle aspiration (EUS-FNA) can perform the same function, especially the sampling of mediastinal nodes that are posterior or inferior, such as the retrotracheal (lymph node station 3p), subcarinal (level 7), paraesophageal (level 8), and pulmonary ligament lymph nodes (level 9).

Thoracentesis

Most pleural effusions in lung cancer patients are owing to tumor and should be evaluated with thoracentesis. In general, a diagnosis of cancer can be established in 70% to 80% of malignant effusions by thoracentesis. Even if cytology fails to identify cancer cells, repeat thoracenteses improve the diagnostic yield. If on multiple taps the fluid is consistently bloody or exudative, it should be considered malignant. Light criteria[18] can be used to help classify an effusion as exudative or transudative. As an alternative to repeat thoracentesis, thoracoscopy can be used to simultaneously collect pleural fluid for cytology, visualize the pleural space and biopsy suspicious lesions if present, and perform lymph node biopsies if indicated.

Mediastinoscopy and Mediastinotomy

Mediastinoscopy remains the most accurate technique to assess upper and lower paratracheal (lymph node stations 2 and 4), prevascular (station 3a), retrotracheal (station 3p), subcarinal (station 7), and hilar lymph nodes (station 7) in lung cancer patients. Lymph nodes within the aortopulmonary window (lymph node station 5) and along the ascending aorta (station 6) are not accessible by standard mediastinoscopy techniques; however, they can be evaluated by anterior mediastinotomy (also known as the Chamberlain procedure) or video-assisted thoracoscopic techniques. Although considered the gold standard, mediastinoscopy does have a false-negative rate of approximately 10%. Furthermore, the role of mediastinoscopy for lung cancer has evolved recently. Less invasive techniques such as EBUS-TBNA or EUS-FNA are frequently utilized instead to sample lymph nodes found to be clinically suspicious on imaging. Mediastinoscopy should still be considered in situations where less invasive techniques are nondiagnostic. It is reasonable to forgo invasive staging of the mediastinum in patients with clinical stage I peripheral disease, particularly those with PET-positive primary tumors but no mediastinal uptake and no obviously enlarged nodes on CT. Patients with more locally advanced disease being considered for surgery should undergo mediastinoscopy to rule out N3 disease and to identify those with N2 disease for whom induction therapy should be considered prior to surgery.

Thoracoscopy

Video-assisted thoracoscopy is frequently used for the diagnosis, staging, and resection of lung cancer. Peripheral nodules can be identified and excised using video-assisted, minimally invasive techniques. As discussed previously, this technique is also extremely valuable for evaluation of suspected pleural disease when thoracentesis has been nondiagnostic. Thoracoscopy can also be used to reach mediastinal nodes not accessible by standard mediastinoscopy, EBUS-TBNA, or EUS-FNA techniques.

STAGING

The eighth edition of the AJCC *Cancer Staging Manual* was published in late 2016 and will be enacted in January 2018. The IASLC established a Lung Cancer Staging Project in 1998 to bring together larger databases available worldwide. The IASLC lung cancer database is comprised of 94,708 cases available for analysis from 35 sources in more than 16 countries, diagnosed between 1999 and 2000, and treated by all therapeutic modalities.[19] The results of this project were accepted by the AJCC in their staging manual. Definitions of TNM for the eighth edition of the manual are shown in Table 54.2; the stage groupings are shown in Table 54.3. This

TABLE 54.2 AJCC STAGING OF LUNG CANCER, 8TH EDITION

Tx	Primary tumor cannot be assessed, or tumor proven by the presence of malignant cells in sputum or bronchial washings but not visualized by imaging or bronchoscopy
T0	No evidence of primary tumor
Tis	Carcinoma in situ
T1	Tumor 3 cm or less in greatest dimension, surrounded by lung or visceral pleura, without bronchoscopic evidence of invasion more proximal than the lobar bronchus (i.e., not in the main bronchus)
T1mi	Minimally invasive adenocarcinoma: adenocarcinoma ($\leq$3 cm in greatest dimension) with a predominantly lepidic pattern and $\leq$5 mm invasion in greatest dimension
T1a	**Tumor is $\leq$1 cm in greatest dimension**
T1b	**Tumor >1 cm but $\leq$2 cm in greatest dimension**
T1c	**Tumor >2 cm but $\leq$3 cm in greatest dimension**
T2	Tumor >3 cm **but $\leq$5 cm** or having any of the following features: **involves the main bronchus but without involvement of the carina**; invades the visceral pleura; or **associated with atelectasis or obstructive pneumonitis that extends to the hilar region, involving part or all of the lung**
T2a	**Tumor >3 cm but $\leq$4 cm in greatest dimension**
T2b	**Tumor >4 cm but $\leq$5 cm in greatest dimension**
T3	**Tumor >5 cm but $\leq$7 cm in greatest dimension** or directly invading any of the following: parietal pleura, chest wall (including superior sulcus tumors), phrenic nerve, parietal pericardium, or separate tumor nodule(s) in same lobe as the primary
T4	**Tumor >7 cm** or tumor of any size of that invades diaphragm, mediastinum, heart, great vessels, trachea, recurrent laryngeal nerve, esophagus, vertebral body, or carina; separate tumor nodule(s) in an ipsilateral lobe different from that of the primary
N0	No regional lymph node involvement
N1	Involvement of ipsilateral intrapulmonary, or peribronchial, hilar lymph nodes
N2	Involvement of mediastinal or subcarinal lymph nodes
N3	Involvement of contralateral mediastinal or hilar lymph nodes. Involvement of ipsilateral or contralateral scalene or supraclavicular nodes
M0	No distant metastasis
M1	Distant metastasis present
M1a	Separate tumor nodule(s) in a contralateral lobe; tumor with pleural or pericardial nodule(s) or malignant pleural or pericardial effusion.
M1b	**Single extrathoracic metastasis**
M1c	**Multiple extrathoracic metastases in one or several organs**

Note: Changes from the 7th edition are in bold.
Reprinted from Goldstraw P, Chansky K, Crowley J, et al. The IASLC Lung Cancer Staging Project: Proposals for the revision of the TNM stage groupings in the forthcoming (eighth) edition of the TNM of Classification for Lung Cancer. *J Thorac Oncol* 2016;11(1):39–51. Crown copyright © 2015 Elsevier. With permission.

TABLE 54.3 STAGE GROUPING: TNM SUBSETS, 8TH EDITION

Occult carcinoma	TX	N0	M0
Stage 0	Tis	N0	M0
Stage IA1	**T1(mi)**	**N0**	**M0**
	T1a	**N0**	**M0**
Stage IA2	**T1b**	**N0**	**M0**
Stage IA3	**T1c**	**N0**	**M0**
Stage IB	T2a	N0	M0
Stage IIA	T2b	N0	M0
Stage IIB	**T1a-c**	**N1**	**M0**
	T2a	**N1**	**M0**
	T2b	N1	M0
	T3	N0	M0
Stage IIIA	**T1a-c**	**N2**	**M0**
	T2a-b	N2	M0
	T3	N1	M0
	T4	N0	M0
	T4	N1	M0
Stage IIIB	**T1a-c**	**N3**	**M0**
	T2a-b	N3	M0
	T3	**N2**	**M0**
	T4	N2	M0
Stage IIIC	**T3**	**N3**	**M0**
	T4	**N3**	**M0**
Stage IVA	**Any T**	**Any N**	**M1a**
	Any T	Any N	M1b
Stage IVB	**Any T**	**Any N**	**M1c**

Note: Changes from the 7th edition are in bold.
Reprinted from Goldstraw P, Chansky K, Crowley J, et al. The IASLC Lung Cancer Staging Project: Proposals for the revision of the TNM stage groupings in the forthcoming (eighth) edition of the TNM of Classification for Lung Cancer. *J Thorac Oncol* 2016;11(1):39–51. Crown copyright © 2015 Elsevier. With permission.

new staging system more accurately expresses the prognostic significance of both the T and N stages in lung cancer outcome.

Given all of the various ways to assess lymph node status, accuracy in determining the nodal stage is essential. In accordance with IASLC recommendations adopted by the AJCC, when pathologic staging of lymph nodes is pursued, sampling of paratracheal (stations 2R and 4R), subcarinal (station 7), hilar (station 10R), and interlobar lymph nodes (station 11R) should be obtained for right-sided tumors, and aortopulmonary window (station 5), ascending aorta (station 6), subcarinal (station 7), hilar (station 10L), and interlobar (station 11L) lymph nodes for all left-sided tumors. Pulmonary ligament lymph nodes (station 9) should also be evaluated for lower lobe tumors. At least six lymph nodes (three from the mediastinum and three from the hilar region) should be examined. If all resected lymph nodes are negative but the number recommended is not met, the patient is still classified as pN0 in the AJCC staging system. For the radiation oncologist, proper staging of nodal disease has taken on increased importance as advances in conformal radiotherapy have resulted in elective mediastinal nodal irradiation being replaced by IFRT.

PATHOLOGIC CLASSIFICATION

The pathologic classification of lung cancer is undergoing significant transformation, driven primarily by recent therapeutic advancements in the management of advanced disease and the movement toward minimally invasive tissue acquisition procedures. The primary charge of the pathologist in the past had been to distinguish between non–small cell carcinoma and small cell carcinoma of the lung. However, since 2000, there are now important therapeutic implications for each of the four major classifications of lung cancer: (a) squamous cell carcinoma, (b) adenocarcinoma of the lung, (c) small cell carcinoma, and (d) large cell carcinoma. Histology is an important determinant in the selection of systemic therapy for advanced NSCLC. Bevacizumab, a monoclonal antibody (MAb) targeting VEGF, resulted in grade 4 and 5 pulmonary hemorrhage in patients with squamous cell histology; however, this agent in combination with standard chemotherapy has yielded a statistically significant survival advantage in patients with nonsquamous histology.[20] An association between nonsquamous histology (including adenocarcinoma and large cell carcinoma) and improved survival has been observed with pemetrexed in combination with platinum-based chemotherapy.[21] Adenocarcinoma histology is often associated with the presence of epidermal growth factor receptor (EGFR) mutations that confer heightened sensitivity to EGFR tyrosine kinase inhibitor (TKI) therapy and with echinoderm microtubule-associated protein-like 4 (EML4) and anaplastic lymphoma kinase (ALK) translocations that confer sensitivity to the mesenchymal-epithelial transition factor (MET)/ALK inhibitor crizotinib. All of these changes are being incorporated into the pathologic classification scheme for lung and have resulted in modifications to the 2015 World Health Organization (WHO) classification scheme for resected specimens.[22]

PROGNOSTIC AND PREDICTIVE FACTORS

The recent advancements in our understanding of tumor biology have underscored the fact that lung cancer is a heterogeneous cluster of illnesses rather than simply a dual (small cell, non–small cell) disease entity. Given the varied clinical outcomes and significant toxicity of treatment, there is an underlying need for robust prognostic and predictive factors in this disease. Prognostic factors, such as TNM stage, are those that predict clinical outcome independent of therapy, and predictive factors are those that predict response to a particular therapeutic regimen. In general, a discussion of prognostic and predictive factors is divided into two categories: tumor-related factors and patient-related factors. In the near future, these factors may be incorporated into a comprehensive approach to tailor therapy not simply by TNM stage but individualized to the patient and the biology of the patient's tumor.

Tumor-Related Prognostic and Predictive Factors

The past decade has seen significant advances in our understanding of tumor-related prognostic and predictive factors. Sensitizing mutations in EGFR have been demonstrated to be predictive for response to therapy with EGFR inhibitors, such as erlotinib or gefitinib. KRAS mutations are both prognostic of poor survival and predictive for lack of response to EGFR inhibitors. ALK and ROS1 rearrangements are predictive for response to agents such as crizotinib. Other targetable mutations such as RET gene arrangement, BRAF mutations, MET amplification or mutation, and HER2 have also been identified, and targeted agents have been approved for other malignancies but may be available in the near future or on a clinical trial.

Patient-Related Prognostic and Predictive Factors

Given the significant metabolic toll that lung cancer takes on patients, several patient-related factors have been identified as powerful prognostic indicators of clinical outcome. Performance status, as quantified by either the Karnofsky scale or the Eastern Cooperative Oncology Group (ECOG) scale, and weight loss in the 6 months preceding diagnosis have been shown in large trials to be among the factors most predictive of survival (along with TNM stage).[23] Additionally, age, gender, and marital status have been shown to be prognostic for survival in a number of studies. Movsas et al.[24] reported that baseline quality of life (QOL), as quantified by validated instruments, superseded performance status, age, gender, and other classic prognostic indicators for survival in a prospectively collected dataset in patients enrolled on a Radiation Therapy Oncology Group (RTOG) clinical trial, suggesting that QOL may be one of the most important predictors of long-term survival.[24]

GENERAL MANAGEMENT: NON–SMALL CELL LUNG CANCER

The management of NSCLC presents a formidable challenge. Oncologists not only must account for the stage and extent of disease spread at the time of diagnosis but also must carefully weigh the impact of baseline pulmonary functional status and comorbidities on the patient's ability to tolerate treatment. NSCLC is an aggressive tumor of a vital organ that is poorly functioning at baseline in the majority of patients. Therefore, the final therapeutic approach must be tailored to the individual. The treatment principles presented in this section should be viewed as guidelines and not as a cookbook for the management of this disease.

In general, the standard of care for operable patients with stage I and stage II disease is complete surgical resection with the possible addition of adjuvant chemotherapy. For medically inoperable patients, stereotactic body radiation therapy (SBRT), also known as stereotactic ablative radiotherapy (SABR), is an excellent treatment option. For stage III patients, a significant amount of controversy exists regarding optimal management. For select patients with stage IIIA disease at diagnosis who are candidates for surgical resection, neoadjuvant chemotherapy or chemoradiotherapy is often used. For patients with unresectable stage III disease, the standard approach is concurrent chemoradiotherapy for fit patients or sequential chemotherapy and radiotherapy for patients who cannot tolerate concurrent treatment. Approximately 50% of patients present with evidence of hematogenous dissemination at the time of diagnosis.[25] For stage IV patients without significant local presenting symptoms or need for urgent radiation, systemic therapy is the standard initial treatment approach. For stage IV patients with significant local presenting symptoms requiring urgent radiotherapy, such as SVC obstruction, hemoptysis, or cord compression, palliative radiotherapy followed by systemic therapy is the preferred treatment approach. For patients with stage IV disease, owing to the poor prognosis, a detailed discussion of the goals of care with consideration of early referral to hospice should be part of the initial treatment approach. Recent evidence suggests that early introduction of palliative care into the standard treatment paradigm in this setting not only improves QOL and reduces inappropriate hospitalization at the end of life but also may improve survival.[26]

Resectable Tumors

Preoperative Assessment

Patient selection is critical when an operative approach is being considered for the management of NSCLC. This includes an assessment by the pulmonologist and operating surgeon of the clinical extent of disease, the predicted postresection pulmonary reserve of the patient, and preoperative cardiac clearance for the intended surgical procedure. Although there are no strict guidelines for operability, traditionally, patients are considered to be suitable for resection if their predicted postoperative forced expiratory volume in 1 second (FEV1) is >60% and diffusing capacity of the lungs for carbon monoxide DLCO > 60%.[27] Patients who do not meet those criteria should undergo additional testing including exercise test or ventilation–perfusion imaging to determine the regional variance in pulmonary function, including the potential loss of functional lung tissue within the planned area of excision.

Stage I and Stage II Non–Small Cell Lung Cancer

The standard of care for a patient with stage I or II lung cancer is surgical resection through either a lobectomy or pneumonectomy with mediastinal lymph node dissection. The Lung Cancer Study Group performed a randomized trial of lobectomy versus limited surgical resection (either wedge resection or segmentectomy) in patients with T1N0 or T2N0 NSCLC. This trial randomized 276 patients and found a 17% risk of local recurrence with limited resection versus 6% with lobectomy ($P = .008$) and a trend toward an increase in all-cause and cancer-specific risk of death in patients randomized to limited resection (30% and 50% increased risk, respectively [$P = .09$], for both). Additionally, the report did not demonstrate any late functional advantages or decreased perioperative morbidity with limited resection.[28] This study firmly established lobectomy as the standard of care for early-stage lung cancer.

There have been several recent series comparing sublobar resection (SR) in appropriately selected early-stage NSCLC with lobectomy, showing comparable oncologic outcomes with the more limited resection. Okada et al.[29] performed a retrospective multi-institutional comparison of 567 patients undergoing either a sublobar ($N = 305$) or a lobar ($N = 262$) resection for cT1N0M0 (tumor size <2 cm) disease. With a median follow-up >5 years, they reported a 5-year overall survival (OS) of 89.6% for the SR group and 89.1% for the lobar resection group. The recurrence rate with SR was not inferior to those obtained with lobar resection, and postoperative lung function was significantly better in patients who underwent SR.[29] Results are still pending from Cancer and Leukemia Group B (CALGB) 140,503, a randomized trial of SR versus lobectomy in small, peripheral early-stage operable NSCLC. American College of Surgeons Oncology Group (ACOSOG) Z4032, a prospective randomized trial of sublobar resection (SR) with or without brachytherapy (SRB) for high-risk early-stage NSCLC, reported 224 patients were randomized.[30] Median (range) age was 71 (49 to 87) years; no differences were found in baseline characteristics between the two groups. Adverse events, previously reported, were not different between arms. Median follow-up was 4.38 (0.04, 5.59) years. There was no difference between arms in time to local recurrence, LR (hazard ratio [HR] 1.01; 95% confidence interval [CI] 0.51, 1.98; $P = .98$), or type of LR. In subgroups of patients with potentially compromised surgical margin (margin < 1cm; margin:tumor ratio <1; positive staple line cytology; wedge resection, nodule size >2 cm), SRB did not reduce LR, although trends favored the SRB arm, especially in the 14 patients with positive staple line cytology (HR 0.11, $P = .24$). Overall 3-year survival was similar for SR (71%) and SRB (71%) ($P = .97$). They concluded that there was no impact of brachytherapy on oncologic outcome in these patients.

There is also controversy regarding the role of mediastinal lymph node dissection in early-stage NSCLC. The American College of Surgeons Oncology Group (ACOSOG) Z0030 trial was a randomized trial of 1,111 patients with N0 or N1 (less than hilar) early-stage NSCLC to either mediastinal lymph node sampling or complete lymphadenectomy during pulmonary resection. The 5-year disease-free survival was 69% in the mediastinal lymph node sampling group and 68% in the mediastinal lymph node dissection group ($P = .92$). There was no difference in local ($P = .52$), regional ($P = .10$), or distant ($P = .76$) recurrence between the two groups, suggesting that complete lymphadenectomy does not improve survival in patients with early-stage NSCLC.

Based upon the favorable data with SBRT in medically inoperable patients, the possibility of this approach as a treatment option for a subset of resectable early-stage NSCLC patients has been raised. The RTOG (RTOG 0618) initiated a phase II study of SBRT in operable patients with early-stage NSCLC. Of 26 evaluable patients, 23 had T1 and 3 had T2 tumors. Four patients (16%) had SBRT-related grade 3 AEs, whereas 0 had grade 4 to 5 AEs. Median follow-up was 25 months. Two patients have been scored with in-field failure, INF (11.7 and 12.4 months post SBRT), and 1 with marginal failure, MF (32.5 months post SBRT), giving an estimated 2-year primary tumor failure rate of 7.7% (95% CI 0.0%, 18.1%). Two-year estimates of LF (primary tumor plus involved lobe failure), RF, and DF are 19.2% (95% CI 3.7%, 34.7%), 11.7% (95% CI 0.0%, 24.5%), and 15.4% (95% CI 1.2%, 29.6%), respectively. Only one patient was eligible for attempted surgical salvage and underwent lobectomy 1.2 years post SBRT complicated by a grade 4 cardiac arrhythmia. Two-year estimates of progression-free survival (PFS) and OS are 65.4% (95% CI 44.0%, 80.3%) and 84.4% (95% CI 63.7%, 93.9%), respectively. This study suggested that SBRT was associated with a high rate of tumor control, moderate treatment-related morbidity, and infrequent need for surgical salvage in operable early-stage lung cancer patients with peripheral lesions.[31]

As such, three separate prospective randomized trials comparing SBRT with sublobar or lobectomy in resectable early-stage NSCLC were launched, as described in refs[32,33] and [NCT00840749]. These trials have all failed to meet their primary end point because of lack of accrual and therefore are now closed. Two of these trials were retrospectively matched and compared for the primary end point of survival, the STARS and ROSEL trial. In the 2 studies, a total of 58 patients were enrolled and randomly assigned (31 to SABR and 27 to surgery). Median follow-up was 40.2 months for the SABR group and 35.4 months for the surgery group. Six patients in the surgery group died compared with one patient in the SABR group. Estimated OS at 3 years was 95% (95% CI 85 to 100) in the SABR group compared with 79% (64 to 97) in the surgery group (HR 0.14 [95% CI 0.017 to 1.190], log-rank P = .037). Recurrence-free survival at 3 years was 86% (95% CI 74 to 100) in the SABR group and 80% (65 to 97) in the surgery group (HR 0.69 [95% CI 0.21 to 2.29], log-rank P = .54). In the surgery group, one patient had regional nodal recurrence and two had distant metastases; in the SABR group, one patient had local recurrence, four had regional nodal recurrence, and one had distant metastases.[34] Although based on a small pooled randomized experience, these data suggest that SBRT may in the future become a viable noninvasive option for selected patients with early-stage operable NSCLC (e.g., who may be at increased risk from surgical resection).

Stage III Non–Small Cell Lung Cancer

Considerable controversy exists regarding the role of surgery in stage III NSCLC. In the 1960s and 1970s, patients with documented N2 disease were generally regarded as incurable and referred for nonoperative approaches. Martini et al.[35] reported the outcome of 1,598 patients who underwent surgical resection, 706 of whom had mediastinal nodal involvement. Of these, 151 patients underwent complete surgical resection with mediastinal node dissection. They reported an OS rate of 74% at 1 year, 43% at 3 years, and 29% at 5 years. Survival in patients with clinical stage I or II (pathologic N2) was favorable at 50% at 3 years. Survival in patients with obvious clinical N2 disease was extremely poor at 8% at 3 years. Martini et al.[35] stated: "Very few patients with gross mediastinal nodal involvement benefit from resection. We believe that this group of patients should not be considered for thoracotomy unless innovative forms of treatment can be offered." Beyond gross mediastinal nodal involvement, multistation N2 disease and subcarinal nodal involvement are also shown in multiple series to be protend to poor outcomes.[36,37]

Based, in part, on these and similar results with surgical resection alone in stage III disease, neoadjuvant approaches—either preoperative chemotherapy or chemoradiotherapy—were explored in an attempt to facilitate surgical resection. However, significant controversy still exists regarding the role of surgical resection in stage III disease. Van Meerbeeck et al.[38] reported the results of a European Organisation for Research and Treatment of Cancer (EORTC) phase III randomized trial of surgical resection versus radiotherapy after induction chemotherapy in patients with pathologically proven N2 disease. In this study, 579 eligible patients were enrolled and received three cycles of cisplatin-based induction chemotherapy. The 332 patients who responded to induction chemotherapy were then randomized to surgery (167 patients) or radiotherapy (165 patients). Median and 5-year OS for patients randomly assigned to resection versus radiotherapy were 16.4 versus 17.5 months and 15.7% versus 14%, respectively (HR 1.06, 95% CI 0.84 to 1.35). Rates of PFS were also similar in both groups. The authors concluded that radiotherapy is the preferred approach in these patients owing to lower rates of treatment-related morbidity and mortality.[38]

Neoadjuvant (Induction) Therapy

Preoperative Chemotherapy

The primary rationale for induction chemotherapy is similar to the rationale for preoperative radiotherapy: to facilitate complete surgical resection of disease. Additionally, induction chemotherapy may potentially sterilize micrometastatic disease beyond the thorax. Several early randomized trials compared preoperative chemotherapy versus surgical resection alone in stage III NSCLC and saw a significant survival benefit to the addition of neoadjuvant chemotherapy, causing trials to close early (Table 54.4).[39,41] The Neoadjuvant versus Adjuvant Taxol/Carbo Hope trial (NATCH) randomized 624 patients with stage IA (>2 cm), IB, II, or T3N1 to neoadjuvant versus adjuvant versus surgery alone.[42] Chemotherapy was three cycles of carboplatin–paclitaxel. Neoadjuvant arm had a trend toward better DFS than surgery alone arm, but results were not statistically significant (5-year DFS 38% vs. 34%, HR 0.92, P = .176). One possible explanation for the lack of benefit is due to the proportion of patients with early-stage disease in the trial (75% had clinical stage I disease). With subset analysis of only stage II-T3N1 patients, 5-year DFS was 36.6% in the neoadjuvant arm and 25% in the surgery arm (HR 0.81, P = .07). The adjuvant arm showed less benefit than the neoadjuvant arm, and more patients in the neoadjuvant arm were able to complete their planned chemotherapy (90.4% vs. 60.9% for neoadjuvant vs. adjuvant). Chemotherapy for Early Stages Trial assigned 270 patients with stages IB-IIIA NSCLC to surgery versus neoadjuvant cisplatin/gemcitabine for three cycles.[43] PFS and OS HRs were 0.70 (95% CI, 0.50 to 0.97; P = .003) and 0.63 (95% CI, 0.43 to 0.92; P = .02), respectively, both in favor of chemotherapy.

TABLE 54.4 SURGERY ALONE VERSUS NEOADJUVANT CHEMOTHERAPY FOLLOWED BY SURGERY IN STAGE III NON–SMALL CELL LUNG CANCER

Author	Patients	CT	Stages	Resection Rates PCT/Surgery (%)	OR Rates (%)	pCR	Operative Mortality PCT/Surgery (%)	Median PCT/Surgery Survival (Months)
Pass et al.[39]	27	E/P	IIIA N2	85 vs. 86	61	7.6	0	28.7 vs. 15.6 (P = .09)
Rosell et al.[40]	60	M/I/P	IIIA	85 vs. 90	53	3.3	6.6 vs. 6.6	26 vs. 8 (P = .001)
Roth et al.[41]	60	C/E/P	IIIA	61 vs. 66	35	3.6	3 vs. 6	21 vs. 14 (P = .056)
Felip et al.[42]	624 (3 arms)	B/X	IA-T3N1	91 vs. 95	53	10.5	5 vs. 5.5	5-yr OS 41.3% vs. 34.5%, P = .31)
Scagliotti et al.[43]	270	P/G	IB-IIIA	87 vs. 96	35.4	4	3 vs. 4	7.8 yrs vs. 4.8 yrs

B, carboplatin; C, cyclophosphamide; CT, chemotherapy; E, etoposide; G, gemcitabine; I, ifosfamide; M, mitomycin; OR, objective response; P, cisplatin; pCR, pathologic complete response rate; PCT, preoperative chemotherapy group; V, vinblastine; X, paclitaxel.
Reprinted from Depierre A, Westeel V, Jacoulet P. Preoperative chemotherapy for non-small cell lung cancer. *Cancer Treat Rev* 2001;27(2):119–127. Copyright © 2001 Elsevier. With permission.

When looking at just stage IIB/IIIA patients, a statistically significant impact of neoadjuvant chemotherapy was seen (3-year PFS rate: 36.1% vs. 55.4%; *P* = .002).

Preoperative Chemoradiotherapy

The rationale for preoperative chemoradiotherapy is that surgical resection after chemoradiotherapy will optimize local control, thereby improving clinical outcomes in locally advanced disease. A phase II trial by the Southwest Oncology Group (SWOG) of induction chemoradiotherapy followed by surgical resection in 126 patients with stage IIIA/IIIB disease showed a promising 3-year survival of 26%.[44] Motivated by these results, an intergroup randomized phase III trial was initiated to determine the value of adding surgery to chemoradiotherapy in stage III disease with a primary endpoint of OS. Patients with stage T1 to T3 pN2 M0 NSCLC were randomly assigned to concurrent induction platin-based chemotherapy plus radiotherapy (45 Gy). If no progression, patients either underwent resection or continued radiotherapy to 61 Gy.[45] A total of 202 patients were randomized to surgery and 194 to concurrent chemoradiotherapy. The median OS was 23.6 months in the trimodality arm and 22.2 months in the bimodality group (*P* = .24). For those with pN0 status at thoracotomy, the median OS was 34.4 months. PFS was better in the trimodality arm, median 12.8 months (5.3 to 42.2 months) versus 10.5 months (*P* = .017). An unplanned, exploratory analysis suggested that patients who underwent lobectomy in the trimodality arm had improved survival compared to matched patients receiving chemoradiotherapy; however, this result is hypothesis-generating only. One of the most important findings from this trial was the significant toxicity of right-sided pneumonectomy after induction chemoradiotherapy. Among the 29 patients who underwent a right pneumonectomy, there were

11 postoperative deaths (38%).[46] Overall, this trial did not demonstrate a survival benefit for the addition of surgery to chemoradiotherapy in patients with stage IIIA NSCLC.

The German Lung Cancer Cooperative Group (GLCCG) conducted a phase III trial with 558 patients comparing neoadjuvant chemotherapy with cisplatin and etoposide, followed by surgery and postoperative radiation, versus neoadjuvant chemotherapy with cisplatin and etoposide, and then twice-daily chemoradiation with carboplatin and vindesine, followed by surgery and a further radiation boost if positive margins.[47] Mediastinal downstaging (46% vs. 29%) and pathologic response (60% vs. 20%) favored the neoadjuvant chemoradiation arm, but PFS was no different (5-year PFS 16% vs. 14%, *P* = .87). Pneumonectomy after chemoradiation had a higher mortality rate than chemotherapy (14% vs. 6%).

In conclusion, the role of neoadjuvant chemoradiotherapy in stage III NSCLC remains unclear. Using a multidisciplinary approach, this strategy should be carefully tailored to the individual patient, accounting for his or her performance status, pulmonary function, extent of disease, extent of surgical resection required, and experience of the clinical team.

Adjuvant Therapy

Postoperative Radiotherapy

The predominant pattern of intrathoracic failure after surgical resection is along the surgical stump or in the mediastinal nodes (Fig. 54.1). Concern over locoregional failure led to the idea that postoperative radiotherapy (PORT) in completely resected stages II and IIIA NSCLC might be beneficial based on evidence that it reduced local recurrence.[48] However, the role of PORT was called into question in 1998 when the Medical Research Council published a meta-analysis of nine

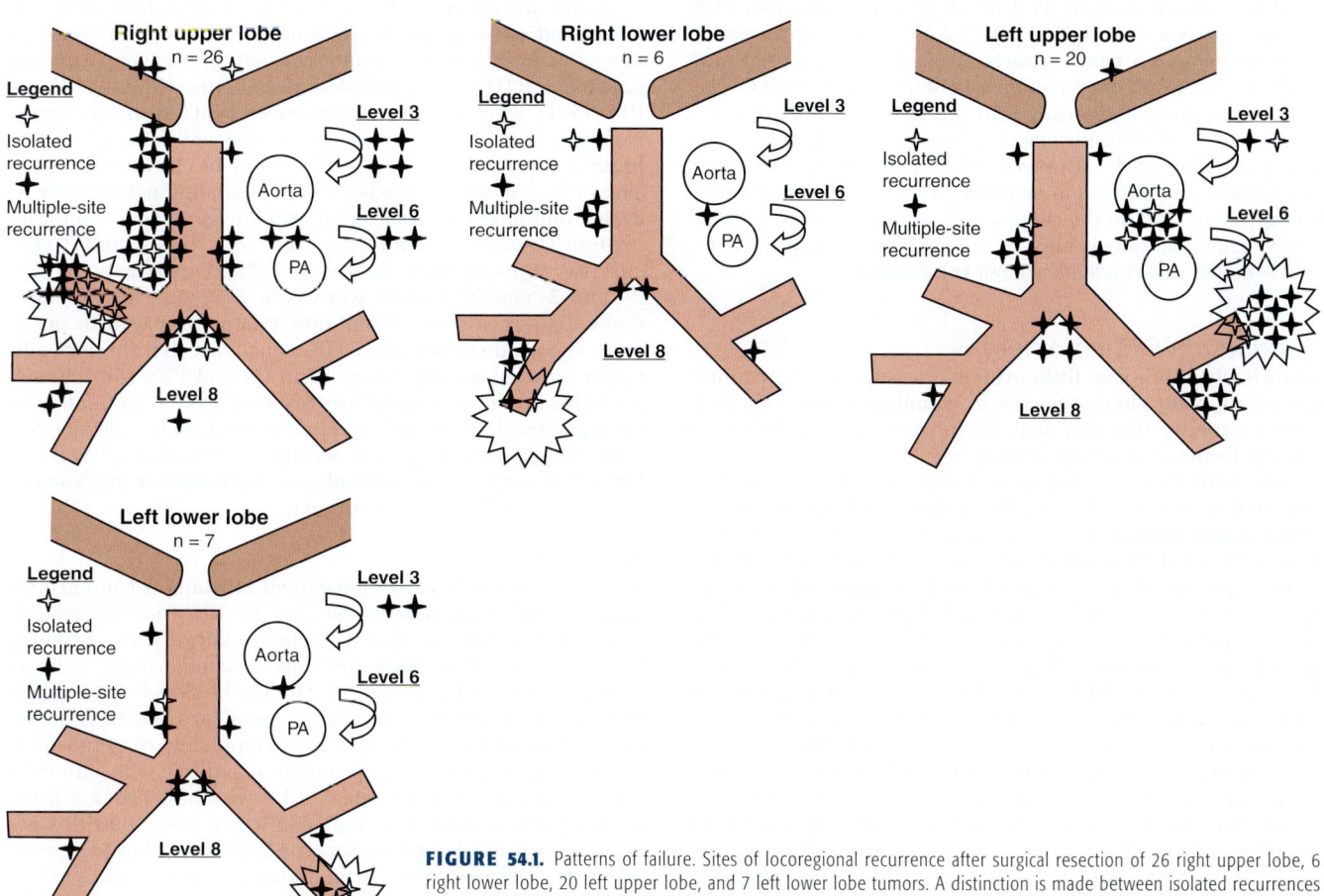

FIGURE 54.1. Patterns of failure. Sites of locoregional recurrence after surgical resection of 26 right upper lobe, 6 right lower lobe, 20 left upper lobe, and 7 left lower lobe tumors. A distinction is made between isolated recurrences (patients with a single recurrent site: *open stars*) and nonisolated recurrences (*filled stars*). (Reprinted from Kelsey CR, Light KL, Marks LB. Patterns of failure after resection of NSCLC. *Int J Radiat Oncol Biol Phys* 2006;65[4]:1097–1105. Copyright © 2006 Elsevier. With permission.)

randomized controlled trials assessing the effect of PORT after resection.[49] The PORT meta-analysis included information on 2,128 patients on and 1,368 deaths. PORT was associated with a decrease in survival for patients with pN1 disease. Given the theoretical benefit of radiotherapy on local control, the detriment in survival was attributed to excessive radiotherapy-induced morbidity exceeding any benefit. There was no survival difference for pN2 patients, although the incidence of locoregional recurrence was reduced in this group. This analysis has been criticized for many reasons. Twenty-five percent of the patients had pN0 tumors and did not need adjuvant therapy. There was no quality control in the radiotherapy arms, and the nature of the radiation was felt to be inferior to modern standards; many of the patients were treated to large volumes using older cobalt 60 equipment to fields designed under fluoroscopy. A subsequent SEER analysis provided insights to counter some of the findings from the PORT meta-analysis. In this study, over 7,400 patients with stage II/III resected NSCLC were evaluated. PORT showed an improved 5-year OS for pN2 patients (27% vs. 20%) but reduced OS for pN0 and pN1 patients.[50]

Additional support for the use of PORT in the modern era can be found in the Adjuvant Navelbine International Trialist Association (ANITA) trial.[51] This trial randomized 840 patients with stage IB through stage IIIA between 1994 and 2000 to adjuvant chemotherapy with vinorelbine and cisplatin or observation. The use of radiotherapy was not randomized; however, each center decided whether to use PORT before initiation of the study. Radiotherapy doses ranged from 45 to 60 Gy in 2 Gy fractions and were given after completion of chemotherapy. In patients with pN1 disease, PORT led to improved survival in the observation arm (median survival 25.9 vs. 50.2 months) but a detrimental effect in the chemotherapy group (median survival 93.6 months and 46.6 months). In contrast, in patients with pN2 disease, survival was improved both in the chemotherapy (median survival 23.8 vs. 47.4 months) and observation arm (median survival 12.7 vs. 22.7 months). The retrospective evaluation of the ANITA trial supports the findings from the SEER analysis that PORT may confer a benefit in pN2 NSCLC. The Lung Adjuvant Radiotherapy trial (Lung-ART), an intergroup collaborative effort in Europe, randomizes patients with completely resected locally advanced NSCLC with mediastinal nodal involvement to observation or PORT to 54Gy. Adjuvant chemotherapy is allowed on the control arm, and pre- and/or postoperative chemotherapy is allowed on the radiotherapy arm. The trial is ongoing, and results are not yet available.

Postoperative Chemotherapy

Historically, there was little evidence to support the routine use of adjuvant chemotherapy in completely resected lung cancer patients. However, benefits to chemotherapy began to emerge from various clinical trials.

The International Adjuvant Lung Cancer Trial (IALT) reported a statistically significant survival benefit for cisplatin-based adjuvant therapy in patients with completely resected stage I, II, or III NSCLC.[52] In this trial, 1,867 patients were randomized to cisplatin-based adjuvant chemotherapy or observation. With a median follow-up duration of 56 months, patients receiving chemotherapy had a significantly higher survival rate (44.5% vs. 40.4% at 5 years) and disease-free survival rate (39.4% vs. 34.3% at 5 years) compared with observation. However, after 7.5 years of follow-up, the survival curves started to converge and cross, the benefit of chemotherapy decreased over time, and there were more deaths in the chemotherapy group by 7.5 years ($P = .10$).[53]

The National Cancer Institute of Canada JBR.10 trial tested the effectiveness of adjuvant vinorelbine plus cisplatin versus observation in 482 patients with completely resected stage IB and II NSCLC.[54] Compared to observation, adjuvant chemotherapy significantly prolonged median OS (94 vs. 73 months) and median relapse-free survival (not reached in chemo arm vs. 46.7 months) compared to observation alone. Like the IALT trial, some of the benefit diminished with longer follow-up; however, unlike IALT, the survival difference remained statistically significant beyond 5 years. After 9 years of follow-up, adjuvant chemotherapy was found beneficial for stage II (median survival 6.8 vs. 3.6 years), although not for stage IB patients.[55]

In the ANITA trial, 840 patients with stage IB through stage IIIA NSCLC were randomized to adjuvant vinorelbine plus cisplatin or to observation.[56] Median survival was 65.7 months (95% CI 47.9 to 88.5) in the chemotherapy group and 43.7 (35.7 to 52.3) months in the observation group, and 5-year OS was improved by 8.6%, which was maintained at 7 years (8.4%). On subset analysis, this benefit was limited to node-positive patients (stage II through stage IIIA). The Lung Adjuvant Cisplatin Evaluation (LACE) meta-analysis showed similar results by pooling data from five large randomized trials enrolling 4,584 patients to examine the role of cisplatin-based adjuvant chemotherapy in completely resected patients. They demonstrated a statistically significant 5.4% absolute survival benefit favoring adjuvant cisplatin.[57]

Postoperative Chemoradiotherapy

With the positive early results from adjuvant chemotherapy trials and prior to the publication of the PORT meta-analysis, a few groups began to explore the role of chemoradiotherapy in the postoperative setting.

ECOG 3590 was one of the first multi-institutional randomized trials to investigate postoperative chemoradiotherapy. This trial randomized 488 patients with stage II and IIIA NSCLC and negative margins after surgery to either radiotherapy alone or radiotherapy plus four cycles of EP chemotherapy. Radiotherapy in both arms consisted of 50.4 Gy in 28 daily fractions. There was no difference in local recurrence or survival between the two arms.[58]

Before the results of ECOG 3590 were published, the RTOG embarked on a phase II combined modality study using a newer chemotherapy regimen consisting of carboplatin and paclitaxel. RTOG 9705 included 88 patients with stage II and IIIA NSCLC after surgery who received PORT with concurrent carboplatin and paclitaxel. Radiotherapy consisted of 50.4 Gy in 28 fractions with a boost of 10.8 Gy in extranodal extension or T3 lesions. The radiotherapy was administered during cycles one and two. At a median follow-up of 56.7 months, median OS time was 56.3 months, with 1-, 2-, and 3-year survival rates of 86%, 70%, and 61%, respectively. The 1-, 2-, and 3- year PFS rates were 70%, 57%, and 50%, respectively. Toxicities were acceptable. When compared to previously reported studies, the RTOG concluded that these results might portend an improvement in OS and PFS with chemoradiotherapy in postoperative resected NSCLC patients.[59] In current practice, concurrent chemoradiation is typically recommended in the adjuvant setting if gross disease was left behind at surgery and variably recommended if microscopic disease was left behind at surgery.

Summary

Adjuvant chemotherapy is accepted as standard of care for patients with node-positive (stages IIA, IIB, and IIIA) NSCLC. For patients with N2 disease prior to surgery, neoadjuvant therapy with either chemotherapy or chemoradiation is an option in selected patients. PORT may be beneficial in stage IIIA NSCLC, although it has never been "proven" in randomized testing and is not indicated in completely resected stage I and stage II NSCLC. In practice, a patient who clinically appears to have early-stage NSCLC who undergoes a gross total resection with pathology-confirmed clear margins but is unexpectedly found to have pN2 disease should receive adjuvant chemotherapy first (because of the known survival benefit) and may subsequently be considered for PORT (because of the reported local control benefit) on completion of chemotherapy.

The role of postoperative therapy for NSCLC patients at high risk for local recurrence has not been clearly established. If a patient who is clinically felt to have early-stage NSCLC undergoes surgery that results in a positive microscopic margin or residual macroscopic disease, radiation therapy should start earlier, as local recurrence is the most common cause of failure in this group of patients.[60] Chemoradiotherapy should be considered in this setting if the patient is medically fit.[59,61]

INOPERABLE TUMORS

Stage I/II Non–Small Cell Lung Cancer

The standard of care for a patient with operable early-stage lung cancer remains lobectomy or pneumonectomy with mediastinal lymph node dissection. However, a significant percentage of these patients cannot tolerate invasive procedures because of the comorbidities prevalent in patients with lung cancer, such as chronic obstructive pulmonary disease and poor cardiovascular health. Historically, the standard therapeutic approach for these patients has been conventionally fractionated definitive radiotherapy alone, with daily fractions delivered over a period of 6 to 8 weeks.[62] More recently, a hypofractionated approach with delivery of a small number of large fractions over a short period of time has gained acceptance. This approach has most commonly been referred to as stereotactic body radiation therapy (SBRT), although recently, there has been a move to rename this approach stereotactic ablative radiotherapy (SABR) to emphasize its distinct radiobiology.[63]

Conventionally Fractionated External Beam Radiotherapy

The RTOG performed a multi-institutional dose escalation study for inoperable NSCLC using three-dimensional conformal radiotherapy (3D-CRT). Patients with small, early-stage tumors were escalated to doses as high as 83.8Gy with acceptable toxicity. The 1-year local control rate for patients treated to this dose was 76%.[64] Hayman et al.[65] performed an adaptive dose escalation trial allowing safe delivery of doses up to 102.9 Gy to small peripheral tumors. However, the OS rates for patients with medically inoperable early-stage NSCLC remain poor when compared to surgery. The 5-year survival for patients treated with definitive radiotherapy range from 10% to 30% and are approximately one-half that reported in surgical series. Several possible explanations exist for this disparity in outcomes, including the poorer overall health of the medically inoperable patient and the fact that most of these patients are clinically, rather than surgically, staged. An additional limitation is the maximum dose that can be delivered to the tumor through conventionally fractionated external beam radiotherapy (EBRT) utilizing currently available techniques. Based on fundamental radiobiologic principles, Fletcher[66] predicted that using conventional fraction sizes of 1.8 to 2 Gy, doses of 100 Gy or higher might be required for the sterilization of most NSCLC tumors. These doses are not routinely achievable with conventionally fractionated radiotherapy in the medically inoperable patient without excessive toxicity.

Stereotactic Body Radiotherapy

SBRT refers to the delivery of large doses of radiation to a small treatment volume, usually employing multiple beams, using a small number of fractions (usually five fractions or less). It has been known for quite some time that this approach is remarkably effective at tumor sterilization, presumably because of greater radiobiologic efficacy.[67] This treatment approach was initially put to clinical use over a half-century ago by a Swedish neurosurgeon, Lars Leksell, for the treatment of intracranial metastases. However, unlike the cranial vault, the lung is a highly mobile structure. Thus, application of SBRT in lung cancer was impractical until advanced imaging treatment delivery techniques were developed (Fig. 54.2).

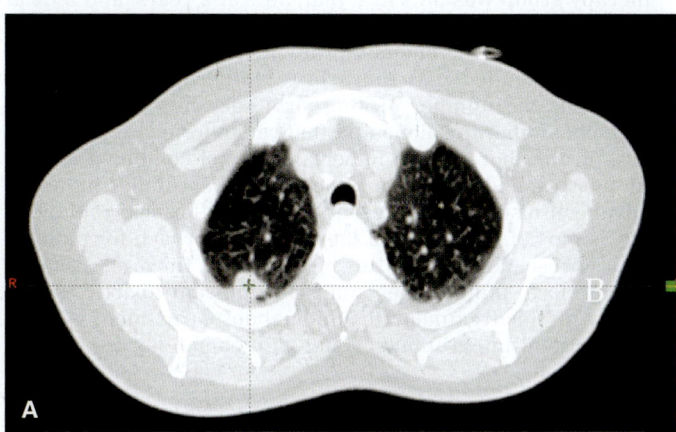

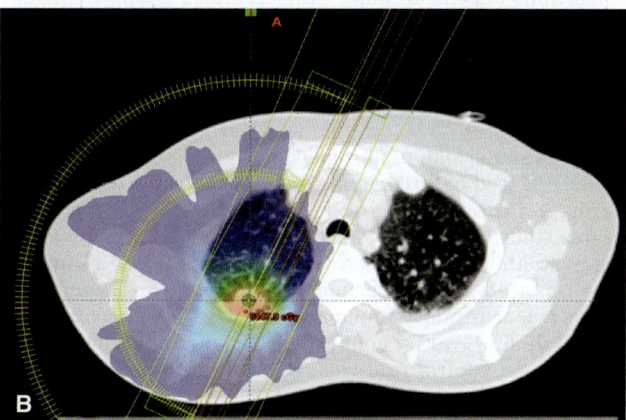

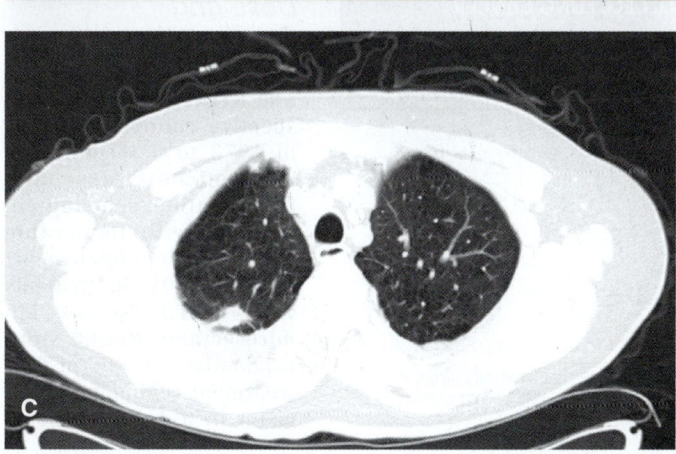

FIGURE 54.2. Stereotactic body radiation therapy (SBRT) in stage I non–small cell lung carcinoma (NSCLC). The patient was diagnosed as having T1N0M0 right upper lobe NSCLC and was treated with SBRT. **A:** Pretreatment tumor volume. **B:** Treatment plan with dose color wash. **C:** CT showing response 6 weeks after treatment.

A phase I dose escalation trial enrolled patients with T1-T2 N0 NSCLC, stratified into three-dose escalation groups based on T-stage and size (T1, T2 <5 cm, and T2 5 to 7 cm). This trial reported a maximally tolerated dose for T2 tumors >5 cm of 22 Gy × 3 and was not reached at 20 Gy × 3 for T1 tumors or at 22 Gy × 3 for T2 tumors <5 cm.[68] There was a loose association between total delivered dose and likelihood of local failure, with 9 of 10 local failures observed in patients treated to the lower-dose levels (<16 Gy × 3). Based on these results, this group moved forward with a phase II trial, utilizing the dose levels identified in the phase I trial. They were able to duplicate the excellent local control results in this expanded cohort of 70 patients. With a median follow-up of 17.5 months, the local control rate was 95%. However, with such large fraction sizes (of ~20 Gy), the group also identified an association between tumor location and toxicity, with severe toxicity occurring at a median of 10.5 months in 17% of those patients with peripheral lesions versus 46% with central lesions.[69] Data from other institutions suggest that early, central lesions can be treated safely and effectively using a lower dose per fraction (e.g., 10 to 12 Gy × 4 to 5 fractions).[70,71] The initial report from VUMC showed 63 patients with central tumors treated with >90% 3-year local control and no grade 4/5 toxicity, although 9 patients died of cardiopulmonary causes, which might be related to grade 5 toxicity. To further explore the treatment of central tumors, RTOG 0813 is a phase I/II trial for patients with centrally located, medically inoperable stage I (<5 cm) NSCLC. Preliminary results show that 120 patients were dose escalated starting at 10 Gy ×5 fraction, with 7.2% rate of dose-limiting toxicity at the highest dose level.[72,73] The maximum tolerated dose was the highest dose level allowed on the study, 12 Gy/fr × 5 fractions. Seventy-one patients were treated at the two highest dose levels (11.5 Gy and 12 Gy per fraction) with 2-year local control of 88% to 89%, PFS of 52% to 51%, and OS of 70% to 73%. Four patients with grade 5 toxicity were seen, one at 10.5 Gy per fraction, two at 11 Gy, and one at 12 Gy. Optimal dose/fraction and normal tissue constraints in central tumor SBRT remains a topic of ongoing investigation.

A variety of dose fractionation and prescription schemes have been published in SBRT for early (primarily peripheral) lung cancer (Table 54.5). Most studies report 80% to 100% local control, >40% 2- to 3-year survival, and 0% to 4% grade 3 toxicity Timmerman et al. reported the results of RTOG 0236, a phase II trial of SBRT in medically inoperable patients with T1 or T2 tumors treated to 54 Gy in three 18-Gy fractions.[76] In this study, 59 patients were enrolled, with 55 patients having evaluable disease. At a median follow-up of 34 months, they reported a 3-year primary tumor control rate of 97.6% and a 3-year primary tumor and involved lobe (local) control rate of 90.6%. Two patients experienced regional failure; the locoregional control rate was 87.2%. Eleven patients experienced distant recurrence with a 3-year rate of distant failure of 22.1%. The rates for disease-free survival and OS at 3 years were 48.3% and 55.8%, respectively. The median OS was 48.1 months. Protocol-specific treatment-related grade 3 adverse events were reported in seven patients; grade 4 adverse events were reported in two patients. No grade 5 adverse events were reported. Because of the 16% grade 3 and 4 protocol-specified toxicity in RTOG 0236 and an additional six patients with chest wall toxicity for a total of 25% overall toxicity rate, RTOG 0915 was launched to test two other fractionation regimens that have promising data, 34 Gy in one fraction (arm 1) versus 12 Gy times in four fractions (arm 2).[79] Ninety-four patients with T1-2N0M0 peripheral tumors were accrued and 84 were analyzable. With a median follow-up of 30 months, 4 patients on arm 1 (10.3%) and 6 patients on arm 2 (13.3%) had grade 3+ protocol-specified toxicity. Two-year OS was 61.3% and 77.7% for Arms 1 and 2, respectively. One-year primary control was 97% for arm 1 and 92.7% for arm 2. As results of these trials mature, chest wall toxicity is receiving more attention as patients present with late pain and fractures, with dose constraints for ribs, chest wall, and skin in the more recent trials.[76,79] SBRT, with its advantage of patient convenience and promising local control results, has largely replaced conventionally fractionated radiotherapy as the standard approach in the medically inoperable patient.

Stage III Non–Small Cell Lung Cancer

Definitive Radiotherapy

The majority of patients with inoperable locally advanced NSCLC will receive definitive thoracic radiotherapy as a part of their treatment strategy. The rationale for definitive radiotherapy in patients with inoperable NSCLC is to provide intrathoracic control of disease. Kubota et al.[80] performed a prospective randomized trial in 63 patients with stage III NSCLC comparing chemotherapy alone to chemotherapy plus thoracic radiotherapy. The survival rate in the thoracic radiotherapy group was 58% at 1 year, 36% at 2 years, and 29% at 3 years, compared with 66%, 9%, and 3% at 1, 2, and 3 years, respectively, in the chemotherapy-alone group. The investigators concluded that thoracic radiotherapy "significantly increases the number of long-term survivors as compared with chemotherapy alone and that radiotherapy to bulky disease in the thorax is an important part of combined modality therapy, and a necessary part of further studies in locally advanced disease." At present, definitive thoracic radiotherapy is part of the standard therapeutic approach for patients with unresectable locally advanced NSCLC. However, because of high local failure rates and the significant toxicity associated with this treatment, the optimal dose, treatment volume, and optimal integration scheme with chemotherapy remain to be defined.

TABLE 54.5 OUTCOME FOR PATIENTS WITH EARLY-STAGE NON–SMALL CELL LUNG CANCER RECEIVING STEREOTACTIC BODY RADIATION THERAPY

Authors (Reference)	Patient	Dose (Gy)	Stage	Local Control Years 3 (%)	Overall Survival Years 3 (%)
Prospective SBRT Trials					
Baumann et al.[74]	57	15 Gy × 3 to 67%	IA/B	92	60
Fakiris et al.[75]	70	T1: 20 Gy × 3	T1–T2N0M0	88	43
		T2: 22 Gy × 3			
Timmerman et al. (RTOG 0236)[76]	55	18 Gy × 3	T1–T2N0M0	98	56
Nagata et al.[77]	45	12 Gy × 4	IA/B	98 (30 m)	83
Retrospective SBRT Studies					
Onishi et al.[78]	257	4.4–35 Gy × 1–14	IA/B	84.2	56.8

SBRT, stereotactic body radiation therapy.
All studies are phase II.
Adapted from Onishi H, Shirato H, Nagata Y, et al. Hypofractionated stereotactic radiotherapy (HypoFXSRT) for stage I non-small cell lung cancer: updated results of 257 patients in a Japanese multi-institutional study. *J Thorac Oncol* 2007;2(7 Suppl 3):S94–S100. Copyright © 2007 International Association for the Study of Lung Cancer. With permission.

Dose and Fractionation with Radiotherapy Alone

The RTOG launched a prospective randomized trial in 1973 to determine the most effective dose and fractionation schedule in patients with inoperable NSCLC. In the initial report of RTOG 7301, 365 patients with T1-T3, N0-N2, M0 unresectable NSCLC were randomized to one of four treatment regimens: 40 Gy given in a split course of

20 Gy in five fractions in 1 week, a 2-week rest, and then an additional 20 Gy in 1 week or 40 Gy, 50 Gy, or 60 Gy given in 2 Gy per fraction continuous course 5 days/week. The split-course group had the poorest survival: 10% at 2 years.[81] The incidence of tumor recurrence in the irradiated volume was 58% for the patients receiving 40 Gy continuous course, 53% for those treated with 40 Gy split course, 49% with 50 Gy continuous irradiation, and 35% in the patients receiving 60 Gy.[82] There were no differences in 5-year survival rates between the four arms. However, based on the differences in local tumor control and short-term survival, this study established 60 Gy as the standard of care.

Motivated by these results, the RTOG moved to explore methods of escalating radiation dose while maintaining the therapeutic ratio through altered fractionation schedules or improved treatment delivery techniques. RTOG 8311 was a randomized phase I/II trial that delivered thoracic radiation at a dose of 1.2 Gy with twice-daily fractions escalating from a starting point of 60.0 to 79.2 Gy. A total of 848 patients were enrolled and analyzed for outcome. No significant differences in the risks of acute or late effects in normal tissues were found in the five arms. In a subset analysis of good performance status patients (stage III, Karnofsky performance scale [KPS] ≥70, <6% weight loss), there was a dose–response identified for survival with 69.6 Gy yielding improved survival over the lower-dose arms (P = .02). There were no differences in survival among the three high-dose arms; therefore, 69.6 Gy became the standard altered fractionation regimen for subsequent RTOG trials.[83]

The development of 3D-CRT in the early 1990s allowed radiation oncologists to increase the dose distribution to the tumor while restricting the dose to surrounding critical normal structures. Bradley et al.[84] examined 207 patients with inoperable NSCLC and demonstrated by multivariate analysis that GTV was strongly predictive of overall and cause-specific survival, suggesting that large-volume disease might require escalated doses of radiotherapy, if feasible without significantly increased toxicity risk. Rengan et al.[85] examined the value of dose escalation in patients with large-volume stage III disease and found that even in patients with large tumor volumes, local failure rates were significantly reduced when treated to ≥64 Gy.

Seventy-nine patients with NSCLC were enrolled and escalation of dose per fraction was performed according to patients' stratified risk for radiation pneumonitis with total RT doses ranging from 57 to 85.5 Gy in 25 daily fractions over 5 weeks using intensity-modulated radiotherapy. Based upon their protocol-defined criteria, investigators identified 63.25 Gy in 25 fractions (2.53 Gy per fraction) to be the maximally tolerated dose. This was due to late grade 4 to 5 toxicities that was attributable to damage to central and perihilar structures and correlated with dose to the proximal bronchial tree. Although the reported rates of pneumonitis were low, the late toxicities because of damage to the proximal bronchial tree highlights the sensitivity of these structures to hypofractionation. Taken together, these data suggest that dose escalation can be achieved safely in locally advanced NSCLC via novel hypofractionation and treatment delivery approaches. However, caution should be employed when considering hypofractionated regimens.[86]

Volume of Radiation with Definitive Radiotherapy: Involved-Field Versus Elective Nodal Irradiation in Inoperable Stage III Non–Small Cell Lung Cancer

In the era of two-dimensional (2D) radiation therapy for NSCLC, it was customary to include the elective nodal basin in the radiation portals for any patient receiving curative intent radiotherapy, regardless of stage. There is ample evidence

that the elective nodal basins can be safely omitted in stage I NSCLC, as there is low risk of nodal failure after IFRT either with conventionally fractionated radiotherapy or SBRT in this setting in patients who have undergone modern clinical staging.[76,84] Although [18]FDG-PET/CT has become an indispensible tool for noninvasive staging of the mediastinum, studies have shown that FDG-PET may carry up to a 25% false-negative rate in lymph nodes <1 cm in the short axis.[16] Therefore, some have argued that although IFRT may decrease toxicity or allow for dose escalation, this may come at the expense of clinical outcome in this disease.[87]

Motivated by this concern, several studies have examined the rate of elective nodal failure in patients treated with IFRT and have shown this to be a relatively rare event.[88] In a study of 524 inoperable patients treated with IFRT, Rosenzweig et al.[89] reported a 2-year elective nodal control rate of 92.4%. Kepka et al.[90] performed a comparative analysis of IFRT, limited elective nodal irradiation (ENI), and extended ENI and reported that substantial incidental radiation dose was delivered to the elective nodal basins even with IFRT; the median dose delivered to these areas ranged from 18 to 45 Gy, depending on the location of the primary tumor and involved nodes as well as the technique employed. Further, there was no significant difference in dose delivered to much of the elective nodal basin between extended and limited ENI. In the only prospective study of ENI versus IFRT, Yuan et al.[91] demonstrated an increase in local control with IFRT of 8% and 15% at 2 and 5 years, respectively. This increase, however, was only statistically significant at the 5-year time point. Additionally, Yuan et al. demonstrated an improved OS rate at 2 years with IFRT (39.4% vs. 25.6%, P = .048) and significantly higher pneumonitis rates in patients treated with ENI (29% vs. 17%, P = .044). Although interesting, this study has been criticized for the imbalances in several factors, including the radiation dose delivered (68 to 74 Gy for IFRT vs. 60 to 64 Gy for ENI) and V_{20} between the two arms, making attribution of the results observed solely to IFRT or ENI problematic. In a single-institution retrospective cohort comparison of patients receiving definitive 3D-CRT for locally advanced NSCLC, Fernandes et al.[92] analyzed 108 consecutive patients treated with either ENI or IFRT. The median follow-up time for survivors was 18.9 months. The median dose for patients treated with IFRT was 69.9 Gy versus 63.6 Gy for ENI. In a multivariable logistic regression analysis, patients treated with IFRT demonstrated a significantly lower risk of high-grade esophagitis (odds ratio 0.31, P = .036). There was a suggestion of improved 2-year local control with IFRT (59.6% IFRT vs. 39.2% ENI); however, this was not significant (P = .23). There were no significant differences in elective nodal control (84.3% vs. 84.3%), distant control (52.7 IFRT vs. 47.7% ENI), and OS (43.7% IFRT vs. 40.1% ENI) rates between ENI and IFRT. The authors concluded that IFRT had favorable therapeutic ratio compared with ENI owing to reduced to acute toxicity. Taken together, these data suggest that IFRT can be employed in patients with locally advanced NSCLC without risk of significant compromise in clinical outcome.

Combined Modality Therapy for Inoperable Stage III Non–Small Cell Lung Cancer

Sequential Chemoradiotherapy

Although dose escalation was achievable and appeared to be associated with improvements in local control in locally advanced NSCLC, the dominant pattern of failure in these patients was through distant dissemination in about 75% to 80% of patients.[82] To address the issue of systemic disease in locally advanced cases, the CALGB initiated a phase III randomized trial of 155 patients with unresectable stage III NSCLC with excellent performance status and minimal weight loss either to radiotherapy alone to 60 Gy or to induction chemotherapy with cisplatin and vinblastine followed by radiotherapy to 60 Gy. Median survival was improved with induction chemotherapy to 13.7 months versus 9.6 months with radiotherapy alone (*P* = .0066). The 5-year survival was improved from 6% to 17% with induction chemotherapy.[93] A subsequent intergroup trial was launched randomizing 490 patients with inoperable locally advanced NSCLC to one of the following regimens: (a) standard radiation therapy to 60 Gy, (b) induction chemotherapy followed by standard radiation therapy to 60 Gy, and (c) twice-daily radiation therapy to 69.6 Gy as 1.2 Gy given twice daily. Median survival was improved to 13.8 months with induction chemotherapy compared to 11.4 months with standard radiotherapy and 12.3 months with hyperfractionated radiotherapy (*P* = .03).[94] Overall, these trials established the role of chemotherapy, in addition to radiation, in the management of unresectable stage III NSCLC (Table 54.6).

Concurrent Chemoradiotherapy

The EORTC performed a phase III randomized trial comparing concurrent cisplatin-based chemoradiation to radiotherapy alone and demonstrated a clear survival benefit to this approach.[97] Of note, there was no difference in rate of distant metastases; thus, the authors concluded that the benefit in OS was attributable to an improvement in local control secondary to enhanced radiosensitization of the tumor by low-dose cisplatin. A meta-analysis performed in 2010 to examine the value of concurrent chemotherapy in definitive management of NSCLC by O'Rourke et al.[98] included 19 randomized studies with a total of 2,728 patients with NSCLC (stages I through III), who were randomized to receive either concurrent chemoradiotherapy or radiotherapy alone. Concurrent chemotherapy significantly reduced overall risk of death (HR 0.71) and improved overall PFS at any site (HR 0.69). However, this clinical benefit came at the expense of increased acute toxicity, especially severe esophagitis with concurrent treatment (RR 4.96).

Concurrent Versus Sequential Chemoradiotherapy

Initial phase II trials suggested that concurrent chemoradiotherapy might be an even more effective treatment than sequential chemoradiotherapy.[99] Therefore, Furuse et al.[99] performed a phase III randomized trial comparing concurrent chemoradiotherapy with mitomycin, vindesine, and cisplatin (MVP) given at systemic doses to sequential chemotherapy and radiation therapy. They demonstrated a statistically significant survival advantage to the concurrent approach (median survival of 16.5 months vs. 13.3 months and 5-year survival of 15.8% vs. 8.9%). RTOG 9410 compared two different concurrent regimens (cisplatin and vinblastine

with conventional radiotherapy, arm 1, or cisplatin and oral etoposide with hyperfractionated radiotherapy, arm 2) to a "standard" sequential regimen of cisplatin and vinblastine followed by conventional radiotherapy (arm 3). Comparing arm 1 to arm 3 (as per the study design), median survival times improved significantly (17 vs. 14.6 months), as did 5-year survival (15% vs. 10%) with an increase in acute grade 3 through grade 5 nonhematologic toxicities.[100,101] The survival in arm 2 was not significantly better than arm 1, although this intensive regimen was associated with much higher esophageal toxicity. A meta-analysis performed by Auperin et al.[102] evaluated data from six clinical trials involving 1,205 patients. The median follow-up was 6 years. Auperin et al. observed a significant benefit favoring concurrent over sequential chemotherapy and radiotherapy with respect to OS (HR 0.84, *P* = .004), with an absolute increase in survival of 5.7% (from 18.1% to 23.8%) at 3 years and 4.5% at 5 years. PFS was also improved with concurrent chemoradiotherapy (HR 0.90, *P* = .07). Concurrent chemoradiotherapy decreased locoregional progression (HR 0.77, *P* = .01), although not distant progression. Again, this improvement in locoregional control came at the expense of greater acute toxicity for patients receiving concurrent chemoradiotherapy, with an increase in acute esophageal toxicity (grades 3 and 4) from 4% to 18% with a relative risk of 4.9 (*P* <.001).

Because of the increased toxicity with concurrent chemoradiation, especially acute esophagitis, there are often treatment delays that are potentially detrimental in terms of radiobiologic efficacy. Cox et al.[103] examined the impact of prolonged treatment time in stage III NSCLC treated with radiotherapy alone and documented an association with decreased locoregional control and 5-year survival (15% vs. 0%). To determine whether treatment time had a similar impact in the setting of concurrent chemoradiation, Machtay et al.[104] performed a retrospective study of three prospective RTOG trials (RTOG 9106, 9204, and 9410), all of which included good performance status stage III NSCLC patients treated with cisplatin-based concurrent chemoradiotherapy. The authors defined "short" treatment time as finishing treatment within 5 days of the projected end date. They found that "long" treatment time was significantly associated with acute esophagitis. They also found a nonsignificant trend toward improved median survival for "short" (19.5 months) versus "long" treatment time (14.8 months). This study, although retrospective, indicated that even with concurrent chemoradiation, there could be a detrimental effect on survival with delayed treatment time.[104] Thus, appropriate patient selection and maneuvers to minimize toxicity are increasingly important to minimize the likelihood of treatment delays that can compromise the efficacy of concurrent therapy.

In summary, these prospective data strongly support concurrent chemoradiotherapy as the standard approach for patients

TABLE 54.6 SEQUENTIAL CHEMOTHERAPY VERSUS RADIATION THERAPY ALONE FOR LOCALLY ADVANCED NON–SMALL CELL LUNG CANCER

Author (Reference)	RT (Gy)	CT	Sequence	Number of Patients	Median Survival (Months)	Overall Survival (%)			
						1 Year	2 Year	3 Year	5 Year
Le Chevalier et al.[95]	65	–	–	177	10	41	14	4	–
	65	VCPC	CT → RT → CT	176	12	51	21	12	–
Sause et al.[94]	60	–	–	149	11.4	46	19	6	5
	60	PV	CT → RT–	151	13.2	60	32	15	8
	69.6	–	–152	12	51	24	13	6	
Dillman et al.[93]	60	–	–	77	9.7	40	13	11	7
	60	PV	CT → RT	79	13.8	55	26	23	19
NSCLC Collaborative Group meta-analysis[96]	32–65	Various	Neoadjuvant no CT; concurrent CT	3,033	–	41	15.7	6.7	2.7
						45	17.7	10.1	4.8

CT, chemotherapy; MACC, methotrexate, doxorubicin, cyclophosphamide, lomustine; NSCLC, non–small cell lung cancer; PV, cisplatin, vinblastine; RT, radiation therapy; VCPC, vindesine, cyclophosphamide, cisplatin, lomustine.

with good performance status and minimal weight loss. This therapeutic strategy results in improved OS, likely driven by an improvement in locoregional control in patients with locally advanced NSCLC. Of note, this comes at the expense of greater toxicity to the patient, especially esophagitis, and therefore, patient selection is critical when using this approach.

Cytotoxic Platforms for Concurrent Chemoradiotherapy in Locally Advanced Non–Small Cell Lung Cancer

Several chemotherapy regimens that pair cisplatin or carboplatin with etoposide, vinorelbine, mitomycin, vindesine, irinotecan, paclitaxel, docetaxel, and pemetrexed have each been studied; unfortunately, few head-to-head trials comparing these agents have been conducted. There is no single regimen that could be considered standard. In North America, the most common prescribed regimens are either cisplatin and etoposide (EP) at systemic doses or carboplatin and paclitaxel administered weekly during radiation therapy (XRT). Unlike limited SCLC, where cisplatin is dosed at 60 mg/m^2 every 3 weeks and etoposide at 80 to 120 mg/m^2 daily × 3 both during and after radiation,[105] an alternative dose and schedule is generally used. There are abundant data from the SWOG and RTOG for a schedule that was ultimately phase III tested in RTOG 9309 and later by the Hoosier Oncology Group: specifically, cisplatin 50 mg/m^2 days 1, 8, 29, and 36 and etoposide 50 mg/m^2 intravenously days 1 through 5 and days 19 through 33.[44,45,106] This schedule, while inconvenient, is tried and tested and generally safe. The carboplatin/paclitaxel regimen is administered weekly during radiation with a carboplatin dose of AUC of 2 and paclitaxel at 40 to 50 mg/m^2. After radiation is completed, two more cycles are usually administered 3 weeks apart using a higher (systemic) dosage of both agents (carboplatin AUC 6 and paclitaxel 200 mg/m^2). Summary of trials involving concurrent chemoradiation can be found in Table 54.7.

Some have argued that carboplatin-based therapy is inferior to cisplatin in the treatment of locally advanced NSCLC. However, data from Japan in a combined modality trial (West Japan Oncology Group Trial WJTOG 0105) evaluating various concurrent chemoradiation regimens failed to show superiority for cisplatin over carboplatin in the context of concurrent chemoradiation.[111] Investigators led by Nobuyuki Yamamoto compared their erstwhile standard of MVP to weekly carboplatin in combination with either irinotecan or paclitaxel during XRT; in each arm, those without disease progression or untoward toxicity went on to receive two cycles of full-dose chemotherapy during the "consolidation" period using the same agents administered during XRT. The paclitaxel/carboplatin regimen resulted in less toxicity, fewer dose reductions or omissions, and equivalent if not superior survival at 5 years: 19.5% versus 17.5% for MVP and 17.8% for irinotecan–carboplatin. In fairness, this study also compared second-generation to third-generation chemotherapy. A Chinese study compared the EP regimen with carboplatin and paclitaxel in a randomized study.[113] Although the 3-year OS was higher in the EP arm, the study failed to meet its primary end point of OS and median survival times were 23.3 months in the EP arm and 20.7 months in the PC arm (log-rank test $P = 0.095$, HR 0.76, 95% CI 0.55 to 1.05). Furthermore, the trial had some methodologic issues. The role of consolidation treatment as will be detailed below is controversial for patients who receive EP, but standard using carboplatin-based treatments; in this study, half the patients in the EP arm received consolidation treatment, whereas only 35% of patients in the carboplatin arm received it. Therefore, most patients in the carboplatin arm received incomplete treatment, which could potentially account for the decreased survival rate seen in this cohort. In a retrospective analysis of patients treated within the Veterans Health Administration, the outcomes of 499 patients treated with EP and 1,343 treated with CP were compared.[114] No difference in OS was noted between the two regimens, but EP was associated with an increased incidence of toxicities and more hospitalizations. This study has several limitations associated with the inherent biases of retrospective studies; however, it suggests that any difference in survival outcomes between the two regimens is likely to be small. One concern pertaining to paclitaxel-containing regimens is a potential increase in the incidence of radiation pneumonitis; this was raised after an individual patient meta-analysis identified that elderly patients receiving carboplatin/paclitaxel chemotherapy were at highest risk of developing this complication.[115]

Given its favorable toxicity profile and superiority to gemcitabine in combination with cisplatin in advanced

TABLE 54.7	CONCURRENT CHEMORADIOTHERAPY FOR STAGE III NON–SMALL CELL LUNG CANCER									
Trial (Reference)	Phase	Number of Patients	Additional Nonconcomitant Agents	Concomitant Chemotherapy	XRT Dose (Gy)	Median PFS (Months)	Median OS (Months)	2-Year OS	4-Year OS	5-Year OS
RTOG 9801[107]	III	243	± Amifostine	Carbo + Pac	69.6 bid	9	17.9	39%	21%	16%
CALGB 9431[108]	II	62	DDP + Gem	DDP + Gem	66	8.4	18.3	37%	17%	9%
		58	DDP + Pac	DDP + Pac	66	9.1	14.8	29		
		55	DDP + Vinorelbine	DDP + Vinorelbine	66	11.5	17.7	40%		
Hoosier[106]	III	203	± Docetaxel	DDP + VP-16	59.4	11	21.7	33%	20%	20%
CALGB 39801[109]	III	182	–	Carbo + Pac	66	7	12	29%	14%	11%
		184	Carbo + Pac	Carbo + Pac	66	8	14	31%	17%	14%
LAMP[110]	II	74	Carbo + Pac (induction)	Carbo + Pac	63	6.7	12.7	25%	NR	NR
		92	Carbo + Pac (adjuvant)	Carbo + Pac	63	8.7	16.3	31%	NR	NR
RTOG 9410[100]	III	≈198	DDP + Vinblastine	–	63	NR	14.6	31%	12%	10
		≈198	–	DDP + Vinblastine	63	NR	17.0	37%	21%	16
		≈198	–	VP-16 + DDP	69.6 bid	NR	15.2	32%	17%	13
West Japan[99]	III	156	–	MMC + Vindesine + DDP	56	10	15	35%	17%	15.8%
WJTOG0105[111]	III	153	DDP + Vindesine + MMC	DDP + Vindesine + MMC	60 split	8.2	20.5	45%	28%	17.5%
		152	Carbo + CPT-11	Carbo + CPT-11	60	8.0	19.8	40%	20%	17.8%
		156	Carbo + Pac	Carbo + Pac	60	9.5	22.0	45%	22%	19.5%
OLCSG 0007[112]	III	99		DDP + Docetaxel	60	13.4	26.8	60.3%	30%	23%
		101		MMC + Vindesine + DDP	60	10.5	23.7	48.1%	23%	16%

bid, twice daily; Carbo, carboplatin; CPT-11, irinotecan; DDP, cisplatin; Gem, gemcitabine; MMC, mitomycin C; NR, not reached; OS, overall survival; Pac, paclitaxel; PFS, progression-free survival; VP-16, etoposide; XRT, radiotherapy.

nonsquamous NSCLC, pemetrexed has been widely adopted in the metastatic setting. The PROCLAIM study randomized patients with stage III nonsquamous histologies either to EP or to cisplatin with pemetrexed during definitive thoracic XRT.[116] After 598 patients were enrolled, the study was stopped early because of futility; no difference were observed between the two arms with respect to OS (26.8 vs. 25 months, HR = 0.98 (95% CI: 0.79 to 1.20), P = .83), median progression-free survival (11.4 vs. 9.8 months HR, 0.86; 95% CI, 0.71 to 1.04; P = .13), and response rates (35.9% vs. 33% P = .45). The only clear toxicity difference was a higher incidence of neutropenia for patients treated with EP (54.8 vs. 44.5%, P = <.05).

Given the lack of evidence for a "best" or preferred regimen, clinicians and patients need to decide which chemotherapy to choose based on other considerations: these include histology (pemetrexed only useful for patients with nonsquamous histology), potential toxicities (e.g., kidney injury for cisplatin, neuropathy for paclitaxel), and cost (significantly higher for pemetrexed).

In patients with baseline V20s (percentage of normal lung that will receive >20 Gy) >35% or in those with borderline pulmonary function or other comorbidities, many clinicians consider administration of chemotherapy first for two or even three cycles, followed by radiation alone or concurrent chemoradiation if there has been sufficient tumor shrinkage to allow a more reasonable radiotherapy treatment field. In those with minimal or no tumor shrinkage using this approach, some investigators omit concurrent chemotherapy during XRT to avoid untoward toxicity, proceeding with XRT alone. These patients are often much more symptomatic than those with smaller-volume tumors, with postobstructive symptoms including wheezing, pneumonitis, and hypoxia, and often have compromised performance status. However, the one study to isolate the role of induction therapy prior to concurrent chemoradiation with paclitaxel and carboplatin failed to show a survival advantage compared to concurrent chemoradiation alone.[109]

Toxicity mitigation is another major challenge that has been inadequately addressed. Both acute esophagitis and long-term pneumonitis and pulmonary fibrosis are common complications of combined modality therapy. A recent meta-analysis by Auperin et al.[117] demonstrated a sixfold increase in short-term esophagitis, grade 3 or worse (18% vs. 3%) in those receiving concurrent chemoradiation as opposed to asynchronous or sequential chemotherapy and radiation. A phase III study evaluating amifostine as an esophageal protectant failed to show a significant reduction in esophagitis rates, as determined by objective measures, compared to a control arm that did not feature this agent[118]; however, a subsequent analysis based on patient-reported outcomes (PROs) suggested a modest benefit with reduction in pain and weight loss.[24,107] There is continued interest in evaluating mucosal protectants, including palifermin and other agents, although to date, no prospective randomized phase III trial has demonstrated a palliative benefit. Consequently, the approach to in-field toxicity has generally been reactive rather than pre-emptive. Newer technologies including proton beam may help to reduce the severity and duration of acute and late esophageal and pulmonary effects. This is currently under investigation.

Consolidative Chemotherapy
Consolidative chemotherapy remains highly controversial. A phase II SWOG trial using the EP/XRT regimen as a platform investigated the role of consolidation docetaxel in stage IIIB patients, yielding a 5-year survival rate of nearly 30%, which at the time, was virtually unprecedented in the realm of locally advanced NSCLC.[44] However, in a phase III randomized Hoosier Oncology Group trial, docetaxel consolidation failed to yield a survival advantage compared to standard "observation" in patients who had completed concurrent chemoradiation with EP, in part because the reference arm "outperformed" its historic controls.[106] These results were disappointing. However,

there was a borderline significant imbalance in baseline pulmonary function favoring the control arm: Nearly 60% of patients on the arm featuring no consolidation had an FEV1 ≥2 L, compared to slightly >40% in the investigational arm. Similarly, empiric use of gefitinib as maintenance therapy in a SWOG trial led to a paradoxical survival decrement compared to placebo after completion of docetaxel consolidation.[119] A more recent randomized trial in Asia tested consolidation chemotherapy with docetaxel and cisplatin after concurrent chemoradiation with the same agents (vs. no consolidation radiation) and found no difference in OS between the two arms (median OS 20.6 vs. 21.8 months in the observation vs. consolidation arms, HR 0.91, P = .44).[120] Hence, based on these trials, there is no proven role for consolidative chemotherapy in patients who have already received systemically dosed chemotherapy during thoracic XRT. In those who receive a radiosensitizing schedule of chemotherapy during XRT (mainly weekly carboplatin/paclitaxel), the general consensus favors at least two cycles of full-dose chemotherapy after chemoradiation is completed, although its role as consolidation has never been formally tested in phase III trials. Despite the disappointing data thus far, the role of consolidation or maintenance therapy after chemoradiation remains an open question.

Targeted Agents in Locally Advanced Disease
There are no data to support the empiric use of targeted agents such as EGFRs, TKIs, EGFR MAbs, ALK inhibitors, immunotherapy agents, or angiogenesis inhibitors either during or after chemoradiation. RTOG 0617 showed that the addition of cetuximab to standard chemoradiation in an unselected population provided no OS benefit.[121] As described in the previous section, a SWOG trial of adjuvant gefitinib or placebo after chemoradiation led to a paradoxical survival decrement compared to placebo.[119] RTOG 1306/Alliance 31101 is comparing standard chemoradiation versus induction erlotinib or crizotinib for 12 weeks followed by chemoradiation, for patients with EGFR and ALK mutations, respectively. Attempts to integrate bevacizumab into the combined modality approach have been unsuccessful, with adverse events including tracheoesophageal fistulas and pulmonary hemorrhages.[122,123] There is tremendous interest in integrating immunotherapy in the treatment of stage III NSCLC. The randomized START trial looked at whether the MUC1 antigen-specific cancer immunotherapy, tecemotide, improves survival in patients with stage III unresectable NSCLC when given as maintenance therapy after chemoradiation. Out of 1,513 patients randomized, 1,239 were analyzable with median OS of 25.6 months in the tecemotide arm versus 22.3 months in the placebo arm (HR 0.88, P = .123). On subset analysis with just patients who received concurrent chemoradiation (65% of patients) and not sequential (35%), median OS was 30.8 months versus 20.6 months in favor of the tecemotide arm (adjusted HR 0.78, P = .016).[124] The PACIFIC Trial (NCT 02125461) is looking at a randomization between MED14736, an antibody to PDL-1, and placebo as adjuvant therapy for a year after concurrent chemoradiation for unresectable stage III NSCLC. A Hoosier phase II trial (NCT 02343952) is looking at consolidation pembrolizumab following chemoradiation in patients with unresectable stage III NSCLC. More data on the clinical efficacy of these agents will be forthcoming in the next few years.

Dose Escalation with Concurrent Chemoradiotherapy
Although concurrent chemoradiotherapy has emerged as the standard therapeutic approach for fit patients with unresectable locally advanced disease, this has come at the cost of increased toxicity. It is therefore unclear whether dose escalation in the setting of concurrent chemotherapy will provide meaningful clinical benefit. Although phase II trials showed promise in dose escalation with concurrent chemotherapy,[125,126]

RTOG 0617 showed a detriment to 74 Gy compared with 60 Gy, and 60 Gy remains the standard dose in stage III NSCLC treatment. RTOG 0617 was a 2 × 2 phase III randomized trial to simultaneously examine the question of 60 Gy versus 74 Gy and concurrent chemoradiotherapy with or without cetuximab for patients with inoperable stage III NSCLC. A total of 544 patients were randomized to the four arms. Median follow-up for the radiotherapy comparison was 22.9 months (IQR 27.5 to 33.3). Median OS was 28.7 months (95% CI 24.1 to 36.9) for patients who received standard-dose radiotherapy and 20.3 months (17.7 to 25.0) for those who received high-dose radiotherapy (HR 1.38, 95% CI 1.09 to 1.76, P = .004). Median OS in patients who received cetuximab was 25.0 months (95% CI 20.2 to 30.5) compared with 24.0 months (19.8 to 28.6) in those who did not (HR 1.07, 95% CI 0.84 to 1.35, P = .29). Both the radiation dose and cetuximab results crossed protocol-specified futility boundaries. There were no statistical differences in grade 3 or worse toxic effects between radiotherapy groups. By contrast, the use of cetuximab was associated with a higher rate of grade 3 or worse toxic effects (205 [86%] of 237 vs. 160 [70%] of 228 patients; P < .0001). There were more treatment-related deaths in the high-dose chemoradiotherapy and cetuximab groups (radiotherapy comparison: eight vs. three patients; cetuximab comparison: ten vs. five patients). There were no differences in severe pulmonary events between treatment groups. A multivariate analysis with OS as an end point revealed that radiation dose (60 Gy), maximum esophagitis grade, planning target volume (PTV), and heart V_5 and V_{30} were all significantly associated with mortality. Emerging studies are testing novel approaches to radiation dose escalation, such as employing functional imaging to decrease the volume to be dose escalated using an adaptive radiation therapy (ART) approach.

Superior Sulcus Tumors and Pancoast Syndrome

SSTs were first described in 1838 and the characteristic accompanying neurologic symptoms in 1932 by Dr. Henry Pancoast. SSTs account for <5% of all lung cancer.[127]

Signs and Symptoms

The most common symptom among patients with SST is pain in the shoulder, which may radiate down the arm. This can be attributable to direct tumor invasion of the parietal pleura, vertebral body, ribs one through three, or the brachial plexus (Fig. 54.3). Pain radiating down the ulnar aspect of the arm past the elbow indicates involvement of the T1 nerve root, whereas extension to the fourth and fifth digits indicates involvement of the C8 nerve root or more distally the ulnar

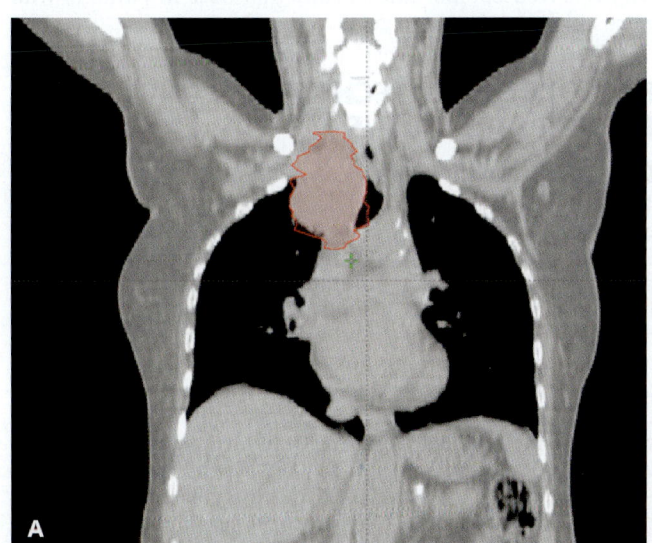

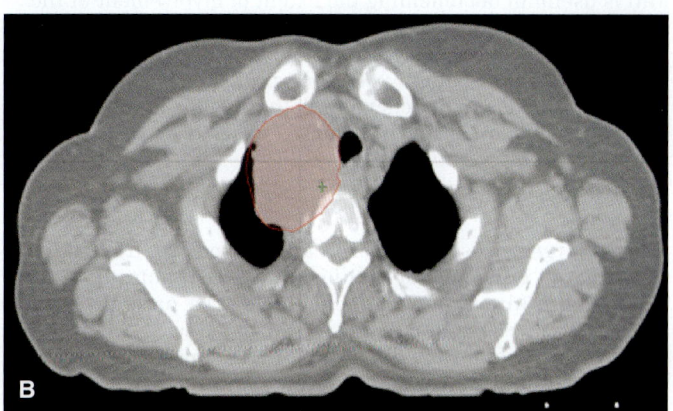

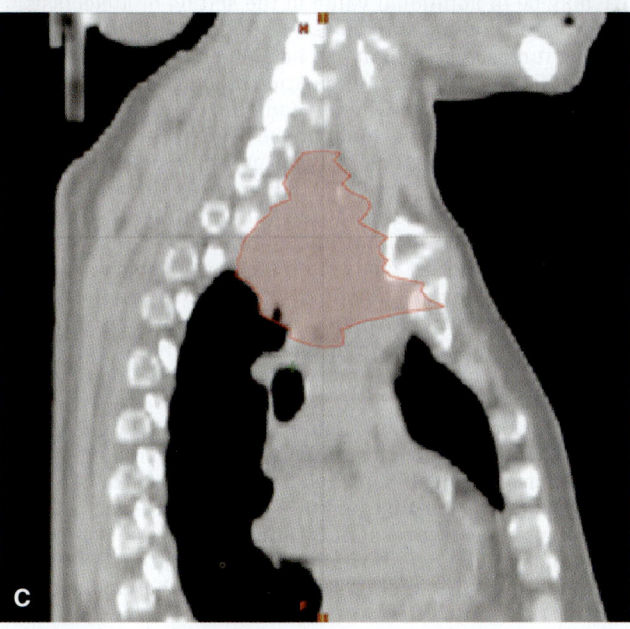

FIGURE 54.3. A 51-year-old former smoker presented with right shoulder pain and right-sided Horner syndrome and was found to have an adenocarcinoma in the right superior sulcus. **A:** Coronal view with gross tumor volume (GTV) contoured. **B:** An axial view with GTV contoured. A 4-cm tumor is seen invading the mediastinum with displacement of the trachea. He underwent a staging evaluation including mediastinoscopy and was staged as T4N0M0. **C:** Sagittal view with GTV contoured showing vertebral body impingement. The patient was treated with radiotherapy with concurrent cisplatin and etoposide to 50 Gy and underwent resection with negative margins.

nerve. There may be weakness or atrophy of the intrinsic muscles of the hand. SSTs that invade the neural foramina may cause spinal cord compression, which can ultimately occur in up to 25% of patients. Involvement of the stellate ganglion may manifest as Horner syndrome: the triad of ptosis, papillary miosis, and hemifacial anhidrosis. Irritation or compression of the adjacent sympathetic chain may cause ipsilateral flushing and sweating of the face or reflex sympathetic dystrophy, a regional syndrome of burning neuropathic pain. Pancoast syndrome is a constellation of signs and symptoms including shoulder/arm pain, Horner syndrome, and unilateral upper extremity weakness.

Diagnosis and Staging

SSTs are staged in the same way that SCLC and NSCLC are staged elsewhere in the thorax. For patients without metastatic disease, it is important to assess resectability. Surgery typically involves lobectomy with en bloc resection of the chest wall, which may be accompanied by resection of portions of the parasympathetic chain, stellate ganglion, lower trunks of the brachial plexus, subclavian artery, and portions of vertebral bodies.

Management

Determining the feasibility of resection is a critical decision point in the management of NSCLC SSTs. Because of the apical location of the tumor, invasion of the brachial plexus, vertebral bodies, and subclavian vessels are not uncommon and may preclude surgical resection as an option, depending on the extent of invasion. In addition to CT, PET, and bone scan, MRI is useful in documenting the extent of involvement of the brachial plexus, spinal nerve roots, vertebral bodies, and subclavian vessels and is more sensitive than CT for this purpose. Small cell SSTs in patient with good performance status are treated with concurrent chemoradiotherapy for limited-stage disease or chemotherapy for extensive-stage disease.

Multimodality Therapy for Superior Sulcus Tumors

Several large retrospective series and prospective trials have investigated outcomes of multimodality treatment of SSTs. SWOG 9416/Intergroup 0160 included 110 patients with T3-T4, N0-N1 SSTs. All patients were treated with two cycles of EP with radiotherapy (45 Gy in 25 fractions), followed by surgery within 3 to 5 weeks, and then two further cycles of chemotherapy.[128] The study included patients with apical tumors and Pancoast syndrome, or SSTs with chest wall invasion, or involvement of the vertebrae or subclavian vessels. In this study, 88 patients (80%) underwent surgery, and 83 (76%) had complete resection. The 5-year OS was 44%. As well, 61 resected patients (56%) had a pathologic complete response to induction therapy, and their 5-year survival was significantly better at 54%. A Japan Clinical Oncology Group (JCOG) study enrolled 76 patients and used induction MVP with 45 Gy in 27 fractions (split course) followed by surgery.[129] The study included patients with SSTs, staged T3 to 4, N0 to N1, and nonbulky N2 disease; 76% of patients underwent resection, and 68% had complete resection. The 5-year OS was 56%.

In patients who are resectable at diagnosis, surgery may be offered as initial therapy. A prospective trial at the University of Texas MD Anderson Cancer Center enrolled 32 patients with resectable or marginally resectable SSTs.[130] All patients underwent gross total resection initially; 28% had microscopic residual disease. Postoperatively, patients were treated with radiotherapy to 60 in Gy fractions (for 1.2-Gy negative margins) or 64.8 Gy in 1.2-Gy fractions (for positive margins) with concurrent EP. The 5-year locoregional control was 76%, and 5-year OS was 50%. The long-term results of this trial were

updated showing the 10-year locoregional control to remain excellent at 76% and the 10-year OS to be 45%.

Chemoradiotherapy

Retrospective evidence suggests that patients who undergo surgery have better local control and survival than those treated with radiation therapy, although such data are subject to significant selection bias.[131] Patients with unresectable localized SSTs and those with stage III disease and bulky N2 (or N3) lymph nodes should be treated with definitive chemotherapy and radiation. Early studies of radiotherapy alone for SSTs show acceptable local control and survival. In a series of 32 patients treated with definitive radiation, 91% of patients with pain reported relief, and 75% of patients with Horner syndrome had symptomatic improvement.[132] The addition of concurrent chemotherapy improves local control and survival in patients with stage III NSCLC—an observation that has led to the widespread use of concurrent therapy in SSTs. Small series in patients with SSTs appear to support this. A retrospective analysis from the Netherlands examined the outcome of patients treated with chemoradiotherapy.[133] In this study, 49 patients with stage II or III SST received 66 Gy with daily cisplatin (6 mg/m²); 19 patients had sufficient response to undergo resection, and in these patients, there was a 53% pathologic complete response rate. The 5-year OS was 18% in patients who received chemoradiotherapy and 33% in patients who were able to undergo surgery.

RADIOTHERAPY TECHNIQUES AND FUTURE DIRECTIONS

Gross Tumor Volume

The clinically macroscopic disease, as typically identified on any imaging modality, is defined as the GTV. The GTV in the lung cancer patient is usually derived from a treatment planning CT or PET-CT obtained during quiet respiration. Intravenous contrast is usually not required for identification of the primary tumor unless it is located adjacent to the hilum or mediastinum. Studies have shown that the size of the contoured GTV is highly sensitive to the windowing of the CT dataset.[134] Harris et al.[134] reported that measurements of pulmonary nodules using the standard "lung" windowing width of 850 Hounsfield units, with a windowing length of −750 Hounsfield units, resulted in highly accurate sizing of the parenchymal tumor. Therefore, lung windowing should be used for delineation of the primary tumor GTV. An FDG-PET may be of additional value in the setting of atelectasis.[135] However, the optimal standardized uptake value threshold for defining tumor edge remains to be defined.

Identification of the mediastinal nodal GTV may prove more challenging. Intravenous contrast may be valuable in identifying nodal disease and may be used if there are no contraindications such as allergy or renal insufficiency. Chapet et al.[136] at the University of Michigan developed an axial CT-based definition of the thoracic nodal stations for use in radiation treatment planning and nodal identification. On CT, a short-axis diameter ≥1 cm is often employed for identification of pathologically involved nodes. However, this cutoff is unsatisfactory, having a relatively poor accuracy of approximately 60% for correctly identifying the location and size of nodal disease. FDG-PET/CT can add significant value to CT alone in the identification of mediastinal nodal disease. Dwamena et al.[137] performed a meta-analysis of FDG-PET and CT for the identification of mediastinal nodal disease in lung cancer. They reported a mean sensitivity and specificity of 0.79 and 0.91, respectively, for PET and 0.60 and 0.77, respectively, for CT. Although this represents a significant improvement, the gold standard for identification of mediastinal nodal disease is through invasive staging. When feasible, the mediastinum should be pathologically staged through either cervical or mediastinoscopy endobronchial ultrasound with transbronchial needle aspiration; this information should be incorporated into delineating the nodal GTV.

Clinical Target Volume

The clinical target volume (CTV) represents a volumetric expansion of the GTV to encompass microscopic disease. For the primary tumor, pathologically derived correlative data have shown that a 9-mm margin would encompass all microscopic disease in approximately 90% of lung adenocarcinomas.[138] Others have advocated the use of a differential margin based on histology of 8 mm for adenocarcinoma and 6 mm for squamous cell carcinomas to account for 95% of the microscopic extension of disease.[139] For nodal disease, surgical series have shown that a 3-mm margin will encompass 95% of the microscopic extranodal extension of disease in lymph nodes <2 cm. However, larger margins may be required for lymph nodes >2 cm.[140]

Internal Target Volume

The internal target volume (ITV) is defined by International Commission on Radiation Units and Measurements (ICRU) 62 as an expansion of the CTV to account for tumor motion. However, as the CTV includes subclinical disease whose motion cannot be visualized, most clinicians will create an "IGTV," which represents the summation of the contoured GTV on all CT datasets obtained in a respiratory-correlated (or four-dimensional [4D]) CT using established methodologies for image acquisition and correlation.[141] In the absence of a 4D CT, a "slow" CT may be used with an extended image acquisition time to encompass a full breathing cycle.[142] The IGTV can then be expanded with a uniform volumetric margin to account for microscopic extension of disease and generation of a CTV.

Planning Target Volume

The PTV is a volumetric expansion of the CTV to account for setup variability. In the past, empiric margins have been used to account for daily variations in patient positioning. However, with the incorporation of image guidance to aid in patient positioning and daily setup, these margins can likely be reduced. Grills et al.[143] showed that calculated population setup margins were reduced from 9 to 13 mm for patients immobilized with a stereotactic body frame and positioned without cone-beam CT to 1 to 2 mm with cone-beam CT. Ideally, with greater integration of image guidance into lung cancer treatment delivery, patient-specific margins will be employed to account for tumor setup uncertainty.[143,144]

Dose Constraints

Normal tissue organs at risk (OARs) should be defined using guidelines outlined in prospective protocols, or using a consensus contouring atlas, so that consistent data can be collected and analyzed. The bilateral lungs excluding the GTV, esophagus, and spinal cord should be defined for all patients; and the heart, pericardium, and brachial plexus should be defined when clinically indicated. For all patients, OAR dose limits should be balanced against adequate coverage of the target volume. A multidisciplinary effort was undertaken—the Quantitative Analysis of Normal Tissue Effects in the Clinic (QUANTEC)—to summarize the published 3D dose–volume/toxicity data in the literature and provide practical guidance for the clinician.[145,146] For SBRT or intermediate hypofractionated schedules, there are less data to recommend dose–volume constraints for most relevant organs. American Association of Physicists in Medicine (AAPM) Task Group 101 provides suggested dose limits in one to five fractions for many parallel and serial organs.[147]

THREE-DIMENSIONAL CONFORMAL RADIOTHERAPY AND INTENSITY-MODULATED RADIOTHERAPY FOR LUNG CANCER PLANNING AND DELIVERY

Introduction

Accurate treatment planning and delivery of radiation for the treatment of lung cancer are confounded by several technical factors, including proper patient setup and localization, the mobility of lung tumors, and tissue inhomogeneity in the vicinity of the lung, as well as the physical and biologic dose implications of delivering dose in >30 fractions versus ≤5 fractions, as in the case of SBRT. To understand the effects of these factors on the accuracy of treatment, one must look more closely at each of the procedures involved in treatment planning and delivery, including treatment simulation, treatment planning, plan evaluation and quality assurance, and treatment delivery. Among other studies, comprehensive reviews of current techniques for lung cancer treatment planning and delivery have been presented.[148]

Treatment Simulation

The goal of treatment simulation is to acquire an image-based representation of the patient for the purposes of tumor and normal organ delineation for treatment planning. The imaging study is traditionally performed with CT. Serial CT images are acquired of the patient in the same treatment position, using the same immobilization devices as those used during radiation treatment. Slice thickness is typically ≤5 mm; smaller slice thicknesses allow for reconstruction of higher-resolution digitally reconstructed radiographs (DRRs),[148] which may improve localization accuracy during treatment. The anatomic region scanned should include both lungs and often extends from the level of the cricoid cartilage to the second lumbar vertebra. Immobilization refers to the process of "patient fixation" to ensure reproducible patient setup during treatment and between treatment fractions. Custom devices, composed of Styrofoam or other materials that mold to the patient surface, are often fabricated for immobilization. Examples include the Alpha Cradle (KGF Enterprises, Chesterfield, MI) and BodyFIX (Elekta Oncology Systems, Norcross, GA) immobilization systems. In the context of SBRT, the AAPM Task Group Report No. 101[147] recommends the use of 1- to 3-mm axial slice thickness during CT acquisition and the use of standard-of-care immobilization/fixation systems (including stereotactic body frames[149]) for reproducible treatment setup.

Management of Tumor Motion

Motion can result in significant distortion of axial or helical CT scans, manifested as artifacts in the vicinity of the tumor in the 3D image dataset.[150] Motion-related artifacts not only render it difficult to assess the full extent of motion but also confound the ability to contour the target accurately on the planning CT dataset. As a result of this, the AAPM Task Group Report No. 76 recommends that motion management strategies be considered when the range of tumor motion is >5 mm in any direction. The recommended 5-mm criterion may be reduced for techniques, such as SBRT, where tumor motion may become an accuracy-limiting factor. Several different techniques have been proposed to manage and mitigate the effects of tumor motion.[148] To assess the range of mobility of tumors in the coronal plane, investigators have employed fluoroscopy.[148] Information from fluoroscopy cannot be directly linked to the volumetric simulation CT scan and is also limited by visualization of the target, although the use of implanted markers may overcome this problem. Motion-encompassing methods are utilized to manage the effects of motion during the planning process. These include the generation of 4D CT scans, which contain spatial and temporal information during the CT acquisition process. 4D CT scans are typically reconstructed to generate multiple datasets at different phases of the respiratory cycle, ultimately generating an "envelope" of the moving tumor for treatment planning.[151] The use of "slow" CT scans (4 seconds per slice) acquired during quiet respiration has also been shown to capture reproducible target volumes for peripheral lung cancers.[142] Methods to limit motion, such as shallow breathing that is forced using abdominal compression devices, have shown to be effective in patients who can tolerate these devices. Techniques such as deep inspiration breath-hold, automatic breathing control, respiratory gating, and tumor tracking, although technically challenging to implement, can afford improvement in normal lung sparing, particularly in circumstances where the magnitude of motion is large.[152]

With regard to motion-encompassing approaches, automatic tools have been developed to improve efficiency in the contouring of GTVs on multiple datasets to form an ITV. The maximum intensity projection (MIP) represents the highest intensity value encountered along the viewing ray for each pixel in the volumetric dataset for the respective breathing phase. The summation of MIP images for each breathing phase therefore results in a composite view of the tumor incorporating all phases of motion. Other techniques, such as a color intensity projection (CIP) technique, in which the motion information from the cumulative 4D datasets are composited into a single color image, have also been proposed.[153] Figure 54.4 provides views of variance in GTV position in different phases of the breathing cycle.

Treatment Planning

The goal of treatment planning is to optimize the therapeutic ratio—that is, to maximize the dose to the target while minimizing dose to surrounding normal organs (Fig. 54.5). As described earlier, target and OAR volumes are defined based on imaging studies, primarily CT and PET. PET can be used to differentiate atelectasis from tumor and to determine nodal involvement for central disease. Respiratory-induced mobility of the tumor is accounted for using the internal margin, which represents the "envelope" encompassing tumor movement determined during the simulation 4D CT acquisition. The internal margin is expanded to form the PTV, which accounts

for geometric variation in the CTV owing to day-to-day (interfraction) uncertainties in the patient setup. According to ICRU Report No. 62,[154] a margin (planning risk volume [PRV]) should also be added to an OAR to account for interfraction variation in the OAR position. Margins for the PTV must be designed with an understanding of the random and systematic errors associated with patient setup. For advanced-stage NSCLC, typical margins for the PTV are on the order of 5 to 10 mm if an ITV is used for motion compensation and daily image-guided radiotherapy (IGRT) is employed during treatment. In the absence of motion compensation or IGRT, margins should typically be larger (10 to 20 mm) to minimize the chance of missing the target as a result of motion. Daily IGRT-based setup has been shown to significantly reduce residual errors and, consequently, planning margins.[155] For SBRT-based treatments, where motion management and IGRT are the recommended standard of care,[147] PTV margins can range from 3 to 6 mm.[149]

Beam arrangements for treatment planning can range from simple two-field, parallel-opposed fields (e.g., anterior–posterior, opposed, anterior–posterior/posterior–anterior [AP/PA]) for late-stage NSCLC to complex multiple gantry angle, modulated beams for more focal treatments. Beams are shaped with a multileaf collimator (MLC), which enables conformation of radiation to the target. Treatment plans should be designed to minimize dose to surrounding normal organs and thereby limit the risk of treatment toxicity, implying sharp gradients in the dose falloff outside the target.[147] AP/PA fields may be considered when disease is more extensive and located centrally. The goal in such cases is to produce a homogeneous dose distribution across the treated volume to encompass the extent of the disease. However, AP/PA beams can only be used for cumulative PTV doses in the range of 40 to 45 Gy (in 1.8 to 2 Gy per fraction) because of spinal cord tolerance. "Off-cord" fields are typically required beyond this dose. When treating large volumes of lung, it is especially important to design treatment plans that adhere to normal lung tolerance doses; dose indices, such as V_{20}, V_5, and MLD, must be closely observed to avoid possible treatment complications.[156] For treatment planning of localized disease, more conformal dose distributions employing multiple beam angles are warranted. Treatment plans can be developed using 3D CRT or IMRT techniques and should include beams from multiple gantry angles, particularly in the context of SBRT.

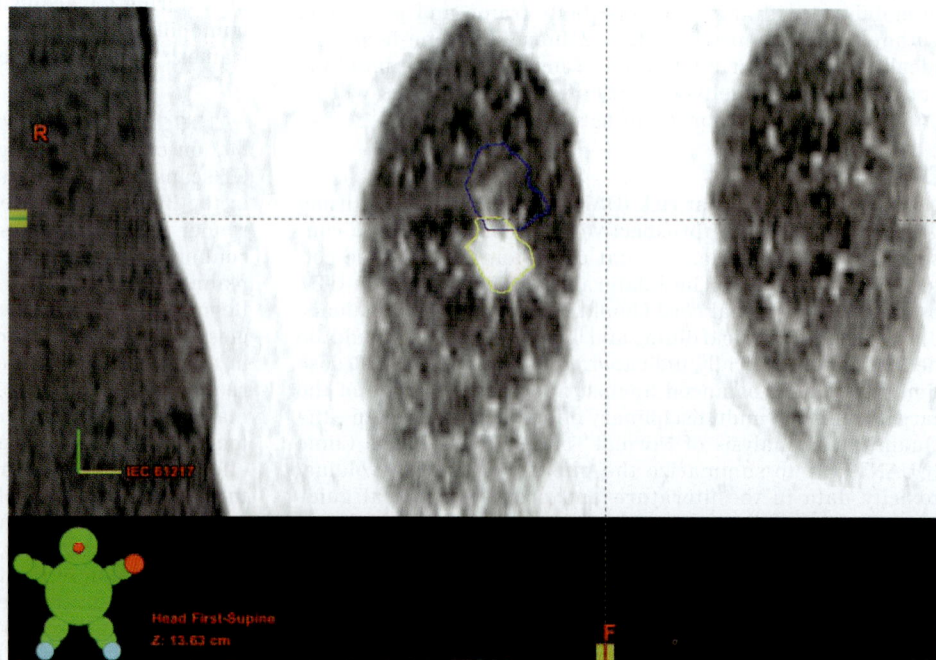

FIGURE 54.4. Tumor motion during a patient's normal respiratory cycle. The yellow wireframe shows the tumor position at full inspiration. The blue wireframe shows the tumor position at full expiration.

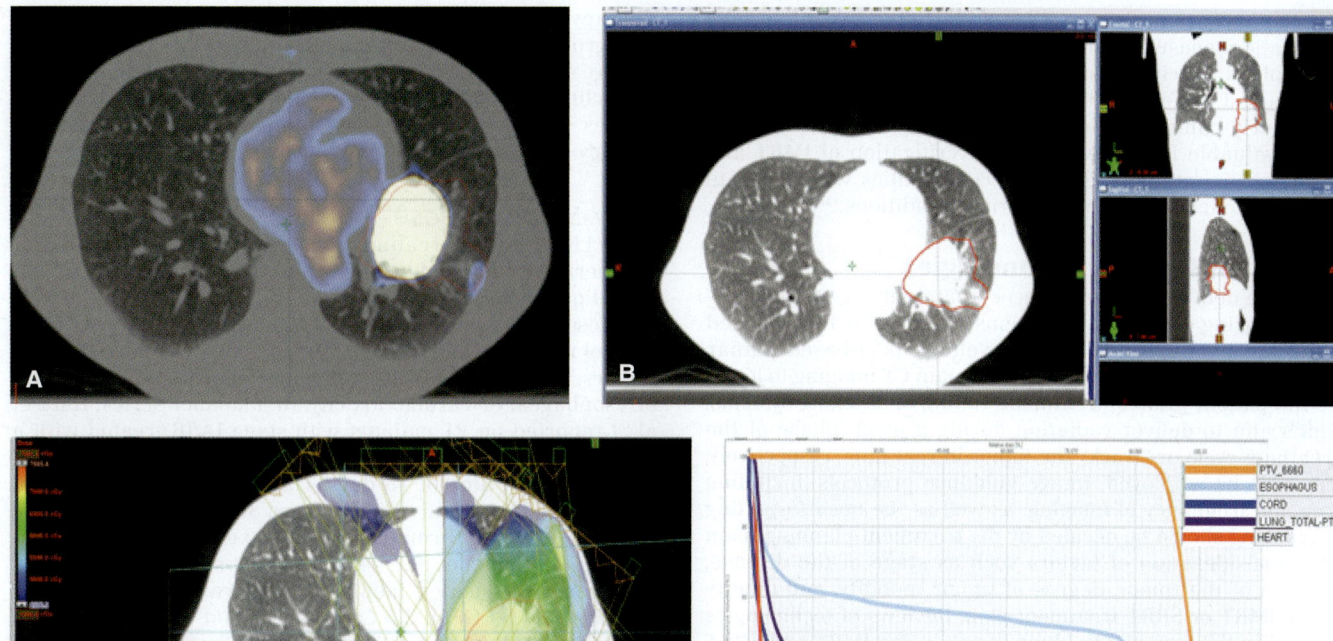

FIGURE 54.5. **A:** CT- and PET-fused image showing FDG-avid primary tumor. **B:** Axial, coronal, and sagittal views of GTV contour. **C:** Transverse CT image of field arrangement and dose color wash of treatment plan. **D:** Dose–volume histogram showing coverage of the planning target volume (*orange*) and dose to esophagus (*light blue*), spinal cord (*dark blue*), total lung (*purple*), and heart (*red*).

For IMRT-based planning, one must bear in mind the interplay effect, which describes the interplay between a given MLC position and instance of radiation delivery with the position of the tumor in the respiratory-induced motion cycle at the same instance.[157] The interplay effect has been shown to average out over the course of ≥30 treatment fractions.[157] However, in the SBRT setting, where 3 to 5 dose fractions are delivered, the interplay effect may compromise the planned dose distribution, suggesting that IMRT must be used cautiously for SBRT. Planning for SBRT must be done with an understanding of the dose gradients so as to develop dose distributions with sharp gradients. This is typically achieved using multiple non-overlapping and noncoplanar beams as necessary and a MLC with ≤5 mm leaf width.[147] The dose prescription line can be low (e.g., 80%) with much smaller margins for beam penumbra ("block edge") than conventional radiotherapy; the motivation is to produce a faster dose falloff and thereby improve sparing of surrounding healthy tissues. The AAPM Task Group No. 101 discourages the use of calculation grid sizes >3 mm for SBRT planning.

Low-density lung tissue in the vicinity of or surrounding thoracic tumors significantly confounds the radiation dose computation problem in lung cancer treatment planning. Conditions of loss of charged-particle equilibrium are produced when the field size is reduced such that the lateral ranges of the secondary electrons become comparable to (or greater than) the field size; such conditions occur for larger field sizes in lung than in water-equivalent tissues because of the increased electron range in lung. Under such circumstances, the dose to the target is determined primarily by the secondary electron interactions and dose deposition. Because conventional dose algorithms do not account explicitly for transport of secondary electrons, they can be severely limited in accuracy under nonequilibrium

conditions. Moreover, in low-density, lung-equivalent tissues, the range of the secondary electrons contributes to the dose "build-down" effect at the edges of the tumor (at the lung–tumor interface), an effect that increases with beam energy. The article by Reynaert et al. and AAPM Task Group No. 105[158] provide examples of numerous studies reporting on the inaccuracies associated with conventional algorithms for dose calculations in the lung. Therefore, for lung cancer treatment planning in general, and especially when dealing with smaller tumors, where the field sizes are <5 × 5 cm², more advanced dose algorithms such as convolution/superposition or the Monte Carlo method are necessary—the latter accounts explicitly for electron transport.[147] The AAPM TG Report No. 101[147] and other articles[159] recommend that pencil beam algorithms not be utilized for SBRT-based lung dose calculations.

Plan Evaluation and Quality Assurance

Plan evaluation of IMRT and SBRT treatment plans requires careful evaluation of DVHs and the entire 3D dose distributions.[147] The following items, among others, must be considered to properly evaluate a treatment plan prior to radiation delivery[147]: organ contours and dose–volume–based organ constraints; planning margins for targets and OARs; intrafraction motion and impact on margins; inhomogeneity corrections; dose uniformity and "hot" or "cold" spots in the target region; normal tissue tolerance doses; plan deliverability—that is, the presence of many low-intensity segments that could possibly be removed without compromising plan quality; and unusual beam orientations that might involve collision during gantry rotation. In accordance with national practice guidelines for IMRT[160] and SBRT[147], redundant verification of the patient-specific treatment plan monitor units and verification measurements of the planned isocenter and 2D dose distributions are necessary. When performing patient-specific verification measurements of highly modulated IMRT fields or SBRT plans, special consideration must be given to the detector size and performance under nonequilibrium conditions.[161] A properly commissioned Monte Carlo dose algorithm may prove valuable for patient-specific verification of IMRT and SBRT treatment plans, given the complexities with accurate measurements under nonequilibrium conditions.[147,161]

Treatment Delivery Technologies

Radiation delivery for lung cancer treatment is generally performed using IGRT-based systems, which can be acquired using megavoltage (MV)- or kilovoltage (kV)-based planar imaging, as well as volumetric, cone-beam CT imaging to localize the patient prior to treatment. Gating or tracking systems, which aim to deliver radiation during a given phase of the breathing cycle or "track" the tumor in real time, respectively, may also be employed. Image-guidance protocols, including type and frequency of imaging, as well as the need for gating or tracking should be decided by the treatment planning team after consideration of factors such as stage of the disease, location of the tumor, degree of tumor mobility, and quality of the IMRT or SBRT treatment plan. Reviews of technologies utilized in the treatment of lung cancer using IMRT and SBRT are provided elsewhere. More recently, volumetric modulated arc therapies (VMATs) have become available for treatment of lung cancers. In one study, an SBRT lung treatment plan performed with VMAT was compared with that of a conventional IMRT plan using the same optimization objective function and constraints.[143] The VMAT plan consisted of a single arc, with partial angles to spare the contralateral lung. The VMAT plan yielded improved target coverage and comparable normal tissue doses compared with the conventional IMRT plan while reducing treatment time by approximately 60%. The faster delivery of radiation with VMAT is likely to substantially mitigate patient movement on the treatment table as a result of discomfort during a long treatment procedure, thereby improving delivery quality. However, as with conventional IMRT, VMAT-based plans are also subject to the interplay effect, which must be considered depending on the mobility of the tumor and the degree of modulation of the MLC fields.

The emergence of linear accelerators with flattening filter free (FFF) beams, in addition to VMAT, has yield much larger gains in treatment efficiency.[162]. Vassiliev et al.,[163] in applying FFF beams to the treatment of early lung cancer patients with SBRT showed a significant improvement in treatment efficiency, with beam-on time being reduced over a factor of 2, from 25 to 11 seconds, on average. They found insignificant differences in target and normal organ doses with and without the use of FFF beams. They concluded that the increase in treatment efficiency afforded by FFF beams facilitates breath-hold and gated treatments. A recent meta-analysis by Dang et al.[164] comprising 210 studies from 2010 to 2015, involving the use of treatments with and without FFF beams, showed significant improvement in treatment efficiency without compromising target dose coverage or normal tissue sparing. A clinical meta-analysis by Prendergast et al. of 64 patients with early-stage NSCLC treated with SBRT using FFF beams showed minimal acute toxicity and reasonable rates of ≥ grade 2 late toxicity.[165]

Particle Beam Radiotherapy for Non–Small Cell Lung Cancer

Because of their physical properties and method of interaction with matter, particle beams, such as protons, neutrons, and heavy ions, have the potential to offer improved dose deposition profiles in tissue when compared with photon beam radiation. Although protons have a similar biologic potency to photons, neutrons and heavy ions such as carbon ions deliver a more biologically effective dose than either photons or protons. A consensus statement was recently issued by the Particle Therapy Co-operative Group (PTCOG) Thoracic Subcommittee task group on the role of proton therapy in NSCLC, reviewing passive scattering proton therapy, pencil beam scanning, available clinical data, and potential for improvement.[166] Further studies are emerging to assess the potential role of particle therapy in the management of lung cancer.

Early-Stage Disease

Loma Linda started treating early-stage lung cancer with proton therapy as detailed by Bush et al.,[167] beginning at 51 Cobalt Gray Equivalent (CGE) protons in 10 fractions and ultimately dose escalating to 70 CGE in 10 fractions. The 4-year local control rate was 96% in peripheral T1 tumors and 75% in T2 tumors. The treatment was well tolerated, with no cases of RP or esophageal or cardiac toxicity. In a smaller series, Hata et al.[168] reported on 21 patients with stage IA/IB treated with a total dose of 50 to 60 CGE at a dose per fraction of 5 to 6 CGE over a median time of 15 days. The 2-year local control and cause-specific survival were 95% and 86%, respectively. There were no grade 3 through grade 5 toxicities in this patient population. Chang et al.[169] reported on a series of 18 patients with centrally located medically inoperable stage I NSCLC treated to 87.5 CGE in 2.5 CGE per fraction with proton beam radiotherapy. With a median follow-up time of 16.3 months, no grade 4 or 5 toxicities were observed. The most common toxicities observed were dermatitis (grade 2, 67%; grade 3, 17%), followed by grade 2 fatigue (44%), grade 2 pneumonitis (11%), grade 2 esophagitis (6%), and grade 2 chest wall pain (6%). The crude local control in these 18 patients was 88.9%, with 11.1% experiencing regional lymph node failure and 27.8% experiencing distant metastasis. At the time of last follow-up, 12 patients (67%) were still alive with 5 patients dying of distant metastatic disease and 1 patient dying of a cardiopulmonary event unrelated to treatment. Miyamoto et al.[170] reported the results of a four-fraction phase II trial of carbon ion radiotherapy in early-stage NSCLC; 79 patients were enrolled and received either 52.8 cGE (stage IA) or 60 CGE (stage IB). The local control rate for all patients was 90% (T1: 98%, T2: 80%). The patients' 5-year lung cancer–specific survival rate was 68% (IA: 87%, IB: 42%). The OS was 45% (IA: 62%, IB: 25%). Half of the deaths were attributable to intercurrent disease. No toxic reactions in the lung greater than grade 3 were detected. Although these results are promising, whether particle beam therapy provides an advantage over photon-based SBRT is not known at this time.

Locally Advanced Disease

Because of the requirement of delivery of tumoricidal doses of radiation to the mediastinal nodes in locally advanced NSCLC, particle beam radiotherapy may be of particular value in this patient population. There are no prospective data to date examining carbon ion radiotherapy in locally advanced disease; however, there are emerging data with proton beam radiotherapy in this setting. Chang et al.[171] reported the results of the first 44 patients enrolled on a phase II trial of weekly concurrent carboplatin and paclitaxel with proton beam radiotherapy to 74 CGE in patients with inoperable stage IIIA/IIIB NSCLC. With a median follow-up of 19 months, they observed a promising median OS of 29.4 months in these patients. No patient experienced grade 4 or 5 proton-related adverse events. Although these results compare favorably to the 74 Gy arm of RTOG 0617, preliminary results from a phase 2 randomized study to compare passive scatter proton therapy with IMRT in stage III NSCLC treated with radiation therapy to 74 Gy with concurrent carboplatin and paclitaxel was reported in abstract form and found no difference between IMRT and proton therapy.[172] With 255 patients enrolled, patients in the proton group had larger target volumes ($P = 0.07$) and more patients received higher doses to the tumors than the IMRT group. Pneumonitis rates were 8.7% overall, 7.2% in IMRT, and 11% in proton therapy. Median time to local recurrence was 13 months in both groups.[166] RTOG 1308 is an ongoing randomized trial comparing IMRT with proton therapy in stage III NSCLC with survival as the primary end point.

In addition to conventionally fractionated radiation treatment, Gomez et al.[173] reported the results of a phase I hypofractionation trial for patients with locally advanced NSCLC who are unable to receive concurrent chemotherapy that demonstrated the feasibility of a 3-week regimen of hypofractionated proton beam radiotherapy in this patient population. More clinical trials are ongoing to explore hypofractionation with proton therapy in locally advanced lung cancer.

METASTATIC NON–SMALL CELL LUNG CANCER

Basic Therapeutic Precepts

The treatment of advanced NSCLC has evolved. By the early 1990s, it was clear that platinum-based chemotherapy could prolong survival, improve symptom control, and yield superior QOL compared with best supportive care.[174] In the 1990s, new agents emerged with enhanced therapeutic index. Carboplatin, although no more effective than cisplatin, was considerably safer with less nephrotoxicity, neurotoxicity, and gastrointestinal toxicity. In addition, several new agents, including paclitaxel, docetaxel, gemcitabine, vinorelbine, and irinotecan, were tested and proved compatible with either carboplatin or cisplatin. Phase III studies of these agents partnered with platinum demonstrated no clear preferred doublet.[175] In the early 2000s, histology became an important determinant in the selection of systemic therapy for advanced NSCLC. The antiangiogenic agent, bevacizumab, was proven to be an effective therapy in patients with nonsquamous lung cancer when coupled with carboplatin and paclitaxel.[20] Similarly, for patients with a nonsquamous histology, the combination of cisplatin and pemetrexed had an improved response and survival compared to cisplatin and gemcitabine, whereas the opposite was true for patients with a squamous histology.[21]

In terms of duration of chemotherapy, treatment with a platinum doublet beyond the initial four to six cycles is not a useful strategy as it is associated with an increase in adverse events, a decrease in QOL and a marginal effect on survival.[176] For patients with nonsquamous histologies who receive pemetrexed, continuation of this agent, also known as maintenance chemotherapy, has been demonstrated to achieve an OS advantage.[177]

Treatment of metastatic NSCLC is palliative and invariably patients treated with chemotherapy will acquire resistance to chemotherapy. Second-line treatment has also shown a survival advantage to best supportive care in phase III trials.[178] Prior to the immunotherapy era, docetaxel and pemetrexed became the standard second-line chemotherapy regimen depending on histology and prior chemotherapy use.[179]

Advent of Immunotherapy

Harnessing the immune system as a tool to treat cancer had long been pursued in a variety of malignancies but with largely disappointing results in the majority of them. The immune system is tightly regulated to avoid immune over activation that could result in harm to healthy tissues. These regulatory mechanisms are exploited by several cancers to escape from immune recognition. T cells, the major effector cell of the immune system, are regulated by a balance between costimulatory and inhibitory signals commonly referred as immune checkpoints. These checkpoints can be dysregulated by tumors as an important immune resistance mechanism.[180] Programmed death 1 (PD-1) receptor is a T-cell coinhibitory receptor that is activated upon its interaction with ligand PD-L1. Blocking this interaction with the use of antibodies against either of these receptors has been proven as successful strategy in a variety of cancers. In NSCLC, treatment with pembrolizumab or nivolumab, both

PD1 antagonists, as well as atezolizumab, a PDL1 antagonist, has been shown to improve response rates and OS compared to docetaxel in patients who have progressed through a platinum doublet. Therefore, immune checkpoint inhibition with anti-PD1 or anti-PDL1 agents has become the de facto standard second line for patients who are eligible to receive them.[181] Treatment with these medications have a distinct set of side effect compared to chemotherapy but they are generally better tolerated than cytotoxic agents. Given the success in the second-line setting, these agents have also been studied in patients who are treatment naive. However, in this setting the results have been more challenging to interpret. In patients who have a PDL1 expression in more than 50% of tumors cells, treatment with pembrolizumab is associated with an improvement in OS compared to a platinum doublet in NSCLC (HR 0.6, 95% CI 0.41 to 0.89),[182] establishing pembrolizumab as the new standard of care in this select population of roughly 23% to 28% of all advanced NSCLC patients.

The combination of these immune checkpoint inhibitors with chemotherapy is also being investigated. A phase 2 trials of pembrolizumab with carboplatin and pemetrexed compared to chemotherapy alone in patients with nonsquamous histology showed an increase in response rate (55% vs. 29%) and progression-free survival (13 vs. 8.9 months, HR 0.53, 95% CI 0.31 to 0.91, $P = 0.010$) in the investigational arm.[183] Overall survival appeared similar but one has to consider that this was not the primary end point and 74% of patients received immunotherapy at progression possibly diluting its effect. The combination arm was accompanied by more toxicities with an increase in the incidence of grade 3 or 4 AEs (40% vs. 25%). Phase III studies asking this question with pembrolizumab and other PD1/PDL1 blockers are underway.

In patients with melanoma, where a longer track record exists with the use of checkpoint inhibitors, 21% of patients are alive a decade after treatment.[184] More time is needed to establish if this is true for patients with NSCLC. Despite this excitement, it is important to remember that currently, only a minority of patients are helped by immunotherapy. Novel immunotherapy combinations with other checkpoint inhibitors and/or other modulators of immune activation such as vaccines or cytokines are being developed and the results of these studies are coming at a pace that we could only have dreamt of a few years ago.

Molecular Determinants of Therapy

Another major advance that dramatically improved the survival of a subset of patients with NSCLC in the last two decades is the discovery that a fraction of patients with mostly adenocarcinomas have a driver genetic abnormality. Pharmacologically inhibiting this abnormality with TKIs is now the standard of care for these patients.

Epidermal Growth Factor Receptor

The presence of EGFR-activating mutations in approximately 10% to 15% of lung cancer patients and their association with heightened sensitivity to EGFR TKIs were first recognized in 2004.[185] However, it is only since 2009 that the association between EGFR mutations and improved response rate and PFS have been confirmed in prospective phase III trials. The Iressa Pan-Asia Study (IPASS), a phase III, multicenter, randomized, study in patients with advanced adenocarcinoma of the lung,[186] randomized treatment-naive East Asian patients ($n = 1,217$), either nonsmokers or former light smokers, to gefitinib monotherapy 250 mg/day orally or to combination paclitaxel 200 mg/m^2 and carboplatin (AUC, 5 to 6 mg/mL/minute) every 3 weeks for up to six cycles. Among the overall study population, tumors from 437 patients (35.9%) were evaluable for mutation analysis; approximately 60% carried EGFR mutations. Of those with mutations randomized to gefitinib, the response rate exceeded 70%, whereas wild-type patients randomized to gefitinib had a response rate of roughly 1%. At 12 months, PFS was significantly longer in mutation-positive patients in the gefitinib group compared to patients in the chemotherapy group (HR 0.48, 95% CI 0.36 to 0.64, *P* <.001). Conversely, PFS was significantly shorter for gefitinib compared to chemotherapy in patients whose tumors did not harbor mutations (HR 2.85, 95% CI 2.05 to 3.98, *P* <.001). Final OS results for the gefitinib and chemotherapy groups were not significantly different, presumably because of crossover to an EGFR TKI in mutation-positive patients randomized to chemotherapy. Despite the absence of a survival benefit, this trial has irrevocably altered the therapeutic paradigm in advanced NSCLC and has laid the groundwork for subsequent phase III trials comparing EGFR TKIs to standard chemotherapy conducted exclusively in patients with an EGFR mutation.

Taken together, the results of these trials, particularly with respect to response rate and PFS, support the use of EGFR TKIs in the first-line setting in patients harboring EGFR-activating mutations. To date, however, largely because of crossover at the time of disease progression, this response rate and PFS benefit has not yet translated into an OS advantage. However, it appears that patients who harbor this mutation live longer than wild-type patients as long as they receive an oral EGFR TKI at some point in their disease course. The choice of which EGFR TKI to use, among those approved in the first-line setting, is a question of debate. Erlotinib, gefitinib and afatinib all have similar activity in this setting. Few studies have conducted head-to-head comparisons of these agents. Erlotinib and gefitinib have been compared in 2 Asian trials and both demonstrate similar response rates, progression free, and OS with similar toxicities.[187,188] Afatinib and gefitinib were compared in a phase IIB study. In a preliminary report, patients treated with afatinib had a slightly longer PFS (11 vs. 10.9 month, HR 0.73 95% CI, 0.57 to 0.95, *P* = 017) and no difference in OS (27.9 vs. 24.5 HR 0.86 95% CI, 0.66 to 1.12, *P* = 258).[189] The incidence and severity of adverse events were higher for patients treated with afatinib with grade 3/4 adverse events reported in 50 (31%) patients given afatinib and 28 (17%) patients given gefitinib, with diarrhea and rash being the most common.

Invariably, patients will acquire resistance to an initial TKI. The most common cause of resistance is the development of a new mutation (T790M) that results in a structural change in the EGFR protein and is present in 50% to 60% of cases.[190] Osimertinib is a third-generation EGFR TKI that still binds to the EGFR receptor despite a T790M mutation. When it was compared to carboplatin and pemetrexed in patients that had progressed after an initial TKI, it was associated with an increase in the response rate (71% vs. 31%) and an increase in median progression-free survival (10.1 vs. 4.4 months, HR 0.30; 95% CI, 0.23 to 0.41; *P* <0.001).[191] Overall survival has not been reported, but with a 60% crossover rate an advantage may not be apparent. Osimertinib is currently being evaluated in the treatment-naive patients with an EGFR mutation against gefitinib or erlotinib (NCT02296125).

ALK

ALK positivity defines a distinct molecular subset of NSCLC (3% to 7%). Here, the driver molecular abnormality arises because of an inversion in chromosome 2 that juxtaposes the 5′ end of the EML4 gene with the 3′ end of the ALK gene. Nearly all patients have adenocarcinomas, and they are more likely to be nonsmokers. Crizotinib, a selective inhibitor of the ALK and MET tyrosine kinases, was approved for this subset of patients after results of a phase I study in previously treated patients with NSCLC whose tumors expressed EML4-ALK showed remarkable activity.[192] When treatment with crizotinib was compared to a platinum-pemetrexed based regimen, crizotinib was associated with a higher response rate (74% vs. 45%) and longer progression-free survival (10.9 vs. 7 months, HR 0.45; 95% CI, 0.35 to 0.60; *P* <0.001). Similar to what is

seen in EGFR-positive cancers, with a crossover rate of about 70%, no difference in OS was noted (HR, 0.82; 95% CI, 0.54 to 1.26; *P* = 0.36).[193] The most common adverse events were mild to moderate and gastrointestinal in nature and included nausea (56%), diarrhea (61%), and vomiting (46%). Other adverse events included liver function test elevations and transient difficulty with light–dark visual accommodation (71%).

Invariably, either resistance to crizotinib develops or patients develop progressive disease within the CNS as crizotinib appears to have modest CNS activity. When resistance occurs, in contrast to the EGFR subset, there is no predominant molecular mechanism that accounts for it. Ceritinib and alectinib are second-generation ALK inhibitors that can overcome resistance to crizotinib and have good CNS activity. In the case of ceritinib, treatment with this agent in patients who had previously been treated with crizotinib resulted in a response rate of 57% (*n* = 92/163) including 3 complete response. In the same study, in 28 patients who had measurable CNS disease that developed while on crizotinib, the intracranial response rate was 36% (*n* = 10) with a median duration of response of 11.1 months.[194] Alectinib has been studied in two phase II trials of patients who developed resistance to crizotinib, and the response rates were 48 and 50% (in 87 and 138 patients) with progression-free survivals of 8.1 months (95% CI 6.2 to 12.6) and 8.9 months (95% CI, 5.6 to 11.3 months).[195,196] In those patients with measurable CNS disease in the first trial, the response rate was an impressive 75% (*n* = 12/16). In the second study of 35 patients with measurable lesions, the CNS response rate was 57%. The most common adverse events of alectinib reported have been constipation (33%), fatigue (26%), and peripheral edema (25%). Ceritinib and alectinib agents have not been compared head to head in a randomized setting and both have been approved for use after progression on crizotinib. Brigatinib and lorlatinib are other second-generation agents that are currently being evaluated. Brigatinib, alectinib, and lorlatinib are being evaluated in treatment-naive patients in randomized controlled trials comparting them against crizotinib in patients with ALK translocations (NCT02737501, NCT02604342, NCT03052608, respectively). The results of these ongoing studies may change the current standard of care in the near future.

ROS1

The translocation between *ROS1* and other genes, the most common of which is *CD74*, occurs in 1% to 2% of NSCLC.[197] These fusions lead to the constitutive activation of *ROS1*. This activation can be inhibited with crizotinib. In an open-label study of 50 patients treated with crizotinib, the objective response rate was 72 percent (3 complete and 33 partial responses) with a PFS of 19.2 months.[198] Crizotinib is currently approved for this indication. Little is known about the mechanisms of resistance is this setting and early phase trials are currently evaluating brigatinib and lorlatinib.

BRAFV600E

BRAF can also act as an oncogenic driver in the presence of an activating mutation, the most common one of which is V600E, observed in 1% to 2% of lung adenocarcinomas.[199] A BRAF inhibitor, dabrafenib, has been found to have activity in these patients with a response rate of 33% (*n* = 26/78) and a PFS of 5·5 months.[200] Vemurafenib, another BRAF inhibitor, also has activity with a response rate of 42% (*n* = 8/19) and a PFS of 7.3 months.[201] In patients with melanoma where the BRAFV600E mutation is more prevalent, studies using a MEK inhibitor along dabrafenib is synergistic. A phase II of the combination of dabrafenib and the MEK inhibitor, trametinib, reported that in 57 previously treated patients, the response rate was 63% with a PFS of 9.7 months (95% CI 6.9 to 19.6). The most common adverse events were pyrexia (44%), nausea (40%), vomiting (35%), and diarrhea (32%). These were typically mild and manageable; the most common grade 3/4 adverse events were neutropenia (9%) and hyponatremia (7%).[200] A study of this combination in previously treatment-naive patients is ongoing.

Role of Radiation in Oligometastatic/Oligoprogressive NSCLC

Although survival for patients with metastatic NSCLC remain poor with 5-year OS of <10%, there is a subset of patients who have better prognosis and may benefit from aggressive local therapy. The challenge has been to identify those patients. One subgroup that has consistently shown superior outcome is patients with limited systemic disease burden (oligometastatic disease), and this has been incorporated into the AJCC 8th edition staging system, with M1b being patients with a single site of extrathoracic metastasis.[19] The exact definition of oligometastatic is still evolving and varies based on studies. An international analysis of 757 NSCLC patients with 1 to 5 synchronous or metachronous metastases and a controlled primary (treated with curative intent local therapy including surgery, SBRT, curative dose radiation, or some combination) showed 5-year OS of 29.4% for the entire population, with 5-year OS of 47.8% for the best risk group on recursive partitioning analysis in patients with metachronous disease and 5-year OS of 13.8% in the worst risk group for patients with synchronous metastases and N1/N2 disease.[202] Beyond treating the primary lung tumor, aggressive radiation may also have a role in managing the oligometastatic sites. A multicenter, phase II trial randomized patients with metastatic NSCLC with 3 or fewer metastatic lesions after first-line systemic therapy to either local consolidative therapy to all sites of disease +/- maintenance treatment or to maintenance treatment alone.[203] Local consolidative therapy included surgery or radiation, and radiation was given with curative intent when possible. SBRT, hypofractionated radiotherapy (e.g., 15 fractions to the mediastinum), and concurrent chemoradiotherapy were allowed. The study was terminated early after randomization of 49 patients because of improved median PFS in the local consolidative therapy group (11·9 months (90% CI 5·7 to 20·9) versus 3·9 months (2·3 to 6·6) with HR 0·35 [90% CI 0·18 to 0·66], log-rank P = 0054). Adverse events were similar between groups, with no grade 4 adverse events or deaths because of treatment. A single arm, phase II study in 24 patients who progressed through platinum-based chemotherapy but were eligible to receive erlotinib and SBRT to 6 or less sites of extracranial disease showed it was possible to achieve median OS of 20.4 months with median PFS of 14.7 months, and most patients progressed in new distant sites, with only 3/47 measurable lesions recurring inside a prior SBRT field.[204] This was an unselected group of NSCLC from the standpoint of EGFR mutation status, with 0/13 tested patients positive for EGFR mutation.

As systemic therapies improve, there is also a category of patients with "oligoprogressive" disease, who may have many sites of metastasis that are all responding to systemic therapy (usually targeted agents), but one or a few sites of disease that are progressing. In this scenario, aggressive radiation therapy, such as with SBRT, to the sites of oligoprogressive disease can give patients more time on the targeted agent before having to switch systemic therapies. In published series of patients on erlotinib or crizotinib with four or fewer sites of extracranial progressive disease, ablative local therapy such as SBRT to the oligoprogressive sites can provide an additional 6 months or more of PFS on the same targeted agent.[205,206]

Conclusion

These are very exciting times for the treatment of metastatic NSCLC as significant advances have become available that are dramatically changing the paradigm of how we treat this disease. Chemotherapy remained the standard of care for several decades, and although it is still the predominant first-line treatment in the majority of patients, a growing subset of patients can be more effectively treated with either targeted therapy when an actionable molecular driver exists or with immunotherapy when they have a strong expression of PDL1. As systemic therapies improve, there may also be an increasing role for local therapy in providing durable disease control.

PALLIATIVE RADIOTHERAPY

Given the propensity of lung cancer for locoregional recurrence and/or distant metastatic disease, radiotherapy plays an important role in the palliation of symptomatic disease in many lung cancer patients. The most common sites of disease that require palliative radiotherapy include the thorax, bone, and brain. Intrathoracic disease and bone metastasis will be covered here. The reader is referred to the CNS section (see Chapter 94) for management of brain metastasis from lung cancer.

Palliation of Intrathoracic Disease

Symptoms from progression of intrathoracic lung cancer that may benefit from a course of palliative radiotherapy include cough, hemoptysis, chest wall pain, SVC syndrome, dyspnea from airway obstruction, and hoarseness from involvement of the recurrent laryngeal nerve. The rate of palliation of local symptoms is high for chest pain and hemoptysis at 60% to 80%, whereas cough and dyspnea are improved in only 50% to 70%.[207] For intrathoracic disease with an obstructive component, 30 to 45 Gy in 2.5- to 3-Gy fractions over 2 to 3 weeks is generally recommended. For patients with poor performance status or for whom daily radiotherapy over 2 to 3 weeks is logistically difficult, hypofractionated regimens (of one to two fractions) have been utilized with good palliative results. The use of concurrent chemotherapy in the palliative setting is not supported by the current medical literature.

Endobronchial brachytherapy provides relief for patients with endobronchial lesions causing obstruction or hemoptysis. The lesion to be treated should be visible by bronchoscopy and generally located in the trachea, main stem, or lower lobe bronchi. This procedure requires the combined efforts of an interventional pulmonologist and brachytherapist. The pulmonologist performs fiberoptic bronchoscopy, placing an afterloading catheter within the airway adjacent to the tumor under direct visualization. In a retrospective study from MD Anderson Cancer Center involving 175 patients with lung cancer who received high–dose rate brachytherapy for metastatic or locally recurrent lung cancer, 115 patients (66%) demonstrated symptomatic improvement.[208] Endobronchial brachytherapy is primarily indicated in patients with obstructive endobronchial lesions who have already received EBRT. It can also be combined with other interventions that can acutely relieve symptoms related to airway obstruction such as stenting or debulking procedures.

Superior Vena Cava Syndrome

Lung cancer is the most common cause of SVC syndrome and accounts for approximately 80% of cases at diagnosis. If the SVC becomes obstructed because of an extrinsic mass, blood returns to the heart through collateral vessels to the azygos vein or inferior vena cava. Venous collaterals dilate over weeks so that the upper body venous pressure and resulting edema of the arm and face decrease over time. The severity of the symptoms is therefore attributable not only to the degree of SVC narrowing but also to the rapidity with which it develops. The characteristic signs include cyanosis, plethora, distension of subcutaneous veins, and edema of the head, neck, and arm. Patients may report dyspnea or cough. Rarely, severe and acute obstruction can result in cerebral edema or laryngeal stridor. The clinical course may be exacerbated by the development of a thrombus or the simultaneous tumor mass effect on the bronchi or heart.

Traditionally, SVC syndrome was viewed as a medical emergency. Accumulating experience, however, demonstrates that the course of SVC is rarely life threatening.[209] In malignant SVC syndrome, immediate intervention is warranted when the symptoms are life threatening (e.g., cerebral edema leading to altered mental status, stridor, or clinically significant hemodynamic compromise). When urgent intervention is indicated, intravascular stenting provides the most immediate relief and can be accomplished even when there is complete obstruction. In the absence of life-threatening symptoms, the patient should be appropriately staged and biopsied and the underlying malignancy treated in a manner appropriate for its stage and presentation. The majority of patients with SVC syndrome attributed to SCLC will respond to systemic therapy, and patients with extensive-stage SCLC and SVC syndrome should start chemotherapy after a staging evaluation. Similarly, patients with limited-stage SCLC and SVC syndrome with bulky disease should respond rapidly to a cycle of chemotherapy, after which radiation can be added, treating the smaller, postchemotherapy volume to spare normal lung tissue. Patients with NSCLC and SVC syndrome are less likely to respond to chemotherapy, thus the threshold for starting radiation or placing an endovascular stent should be lower. In patients with metastatic NSCLC, palliative radiotherapy is commonly recommended as part of initial therapy.

SMALL CELL LUNG CARCINOMA

In the United States in 2011, approximately 28,000 patients were diagnosed with SCLC, constituting approximately 13% of all lung cancer diagnoses. Over the past several decades, the proportion of SCLC among all lung cancer histologies has been decreasing, perhaps because of smoking cessation and the proliferation of low-tar cigarettes. Although there has been a modest but statistically significant improvement in 2- and 5-year survival in both limited- and extensive-stage diseases in recent decades, the outcomes are still extremely poor, particularly because the majority (~60%) of patients present with extensive-stage disease with an expected 2-year survival of only 4%.

Pathology

The establishment of a firm pathologic diagnosis distinguishing SCLC from NSCLC variants such as carcinoma with neuroendocrine features and carcinoid is extremely important in this disease, as it can have a significant impact on management and clinical outcome. Histologically, SCLC is one of the small, round, blue cell tumors (along with neuroblastoma, rhabdomyosarcoma, Merkel cell carcinoma, etc.) with scant cytoplasm and indistinct nucleoli. Cells are often molded together, and crush artifact is commonly noted after needle biopsy but is not pathognomonic. Almost all SCLC samples are immunoreactive to keratin and epithelial membrane antigen, and approximately 80% express thyroid transcription factor-1 (TTF-1).[210] The majority of tumors will stain for neuroendocrine markers including synaptophysin, neuron-specific chromogranin A, enolase, and CD56. Immunohistochemistry alone, however, cannot distinguish SCLC from small cell cancer of nonthoracic origin or from NSCLC with neuroendocrine differentiation. The WHO recognizes that SCLC can occur in a pure type or mixed with NSCLC in up to 30% of cases.

Prognostic Factors in Small Cell Lung Cancer

The most clinically important prognostic factor in SCLC is stage (limited vs. extensive), with a median survival of approximately 23 months for patients with limited disease versus 8

to 9 months for those with extensive disease.[105] Other clinical factors consistently reported to correlate with improved survival include good performance status, female gender, and normal lactate dehydrogenase levels at baseline.[211]

Staging Workup

As in patients with NSCLC, patients with SCLC should undergo a timely and efficient history, physical exam, and laboratory and radiographic evaluation. The history and physical should be performed with particular attention to signs and symptoms of paraneoplastic syndromes, including SIADH and elevated ACTH. Laboratory evaluation should include a complete blood count and comprehensive chemistry panel. Radiographic studies should include a CT scan of the chest and abdomen with intravenous contrast, with PET/CT for suspected limited-stage disease. All patients with SCLC, regardless of stage, should undergo a brain MRI with gadolinium or a head CT with contrast to evaluate for brain metastases. A diagnostic thoracentesis should be performed for any identified pleural effusion to determine the presence of malignant cells. The TNM staging system adopted by the American Joint Commission for Cancer (AJCC) is applicable to both NSCLC and SCLC. Most historical studies and ongoing prospective trials, however, classify patients as having limited or extensive disease based on the 1973 Veteran's Administration Lung Group staging scheme.[212] In this system, limited stage is defined as disease confined to the ipsilateral hemithorax, which can be safely encompassed within a tolerable radiation portal. Virtually all studies in limited disease exclude malignant pleural effusions. From a practical standpoint, hemithoracic radiotherapy to encompass the entire ipsilateral pleura has little justification because it would confer a significant risk of pulmonary toxicity in a high-risk patient population with little chance of cure. As such, patients with malignant pleural effusions are classified as having extensive-stage disease.

Paraneoplastic Syndromes

Paraneoplastic syndromes are commonly encountered in lung cancer; however, the spectrum of paraneoplastic syndromes in SCLC is distinct from that observed in NSCLC. Neurologic paraneoplastic syndromes are more commonly encountered in SCLC and are thought to be primarily autoimmune in nature. LEMS is seen in 3% of all SCLC patients at presentation and is characterized by proximal muscle weakness that improves with continued activity. This syndrome occurs when autoantibodies are generated against voltage-gated calcium channel receptors on the presynaptic membrane, impeding release of acetylcholine into the neuromuscular junction and resulting in muscular weakness. A wide variety of other rare autoimmune neurologic paraneoplastic syndromes have been described in SCLC, including encephalomyelitis, cerebellar degeneration, and retinopathy. SCLC can also elaborate hormonally active peptides including ACTH and vasopressin leading to Cushing syndrome and SIADH, respectively. Although SCLC is the most common tumor associated with SIADH, only 10% of patients meet the clinical criteria for SIADH. Similarly, only 5% of SCLC patients present with Cushing syndrome. Despite the fact that paraneoplastic syndromes may lead to early identification and diagnosis of SCLC, some of these syndromes, such as Cushing's, have been associated with poorer survival.[213] Treatment of the cancer will often, although not always, ameliorate the paraneoplastic syndromes.

General Therapeutic Precepts

Early-stage (i.e., T1 to T2, N0) SCLC is diagnosed in <5% of incident cases. For these patients, definitive surgical resection is a potential therapeutic option. In a population-based study, lobectomy without adjuvant radiation was associated with an approximately 50% OS.[214] Given the propensity for early nodal dissemination with SCLC, invasive staging of the mediastinum should be performed prior to surgical resection. After surgical resection, the primary mode of failure for these patients is distant dissemination. Tsuchiya et al.[215] reported the results of JCOG9101, a JCOG Lung Cancer Study Group multi-institutional phase II prospective trial evaluating adjuvant EP after complete surgical resection of stage I through stage IIIA SCLC. The majority of patients enrolled had clinical stage I disease (44/62). Three-year survival was 61% overall, 68% in patients with clinical stage I disease, 56% in patients with stage II disease, and 13% in patients with stage IIIa disease. These data suggest a possible role for surgical resection in select patients with pathologically proven stage I or II SCLC.

The majority of patients present with evidence of nodal or distant dissemination at the time of diagnosis. Multiagent chemotherapy, usually a platinum-based combination, is an essential part of therapy for these patients. For patients with limited-stage disease, the addition of thoracic radiation significantly improves survival and therefore is an integral of part their treatment regimen. Two meta-analyses have demonstrated not only an improvement in thoracic control but also a significant increase in OS of about 5% (and relative improvement of about 50%) in patients with limited-stage disease treated with combined modality therapy compared to those with treated chemotherapy alone.[216,217] For select good performance status patients with extensive-stage disease who have complete resolution of their extrathoracic tumor burden, consolidative thoracic radiotherapy may be of benefit to reduce the risk of intrathoracic failure.[218,219] Patients with limited-stage disease selected (and with patients extensive-stage disease) who respond to initial therapy should be offered prophylactic cranial irradiation (PCI), as this has been shown to provide a significant improvement in absolute survival for these patients.[220,221]

Combining Radiation and Chemotherapy for Limited-Stage Disease

A randomized trial by the JCOG evaluated concurrent versus sequential chemotherapy and thoracic radiation in patients with limited-stage SCLC.[222] All patients received 45 Gy in 1.5-Gy fractions twice daily and were randomized to receive four cycles of cisplatin (80 mg/m² on day 1) and etoposide (100 mg/m² days 1, 2, and 3) every 4 weeks concurrent with radiotherapy (beginning day 2) or every 3 weeks sequentially before radiotherapy. Patients treated concurrently had longer median survival compared to patients treated sequentially: 27 months versus 20 months. A second randomized trial by the National Cancer Institute of Canada compared early with late concurrent chemoradiotherapy.[223] In this trial, 308 patients received cyclophosphamide, doxorubicin, and vincristine alternating with EP and were randomized to 40 Gy in 15 daily fractions given with either the first cycle of EP (week 3) or the last (week 15). The median survival improved to 21 months with radiotherapy early 16 versus months with treatment late ($P = .008$). These two trials were included in a meta-analysis by Fried et al.[224] that included >1,500 patients from seven randomized trials evaluating the timing of radiotherapy when given concurrently with multiagent chemotherapy. The use of early thoracic radiotherapy, with cycle one or two of chemotherapy, was associated with improved 2-year OS compared to delayed or sequential chemotherapy and radiation. The benefit was more pronounced when the radiotherapy was given with platinum-based chemotherapy. The chemotherapy most commonly prescribed in the curative setting is cisplatin and etoposide.

Dose and Fractionation

The optimal dose and fractionation scheme for concurrent chemoradiation for limited-stage small cell is an area of active investigation. SCLC is highly radiosensitive, suggesting that hyperfractionation could be employed to reduce late normal tissue toxicity. It also has a high proliferative rate, arguing for accelerated treatment to counteract repopulation. Between 1989 and 1992, 417 patients were enrolled in a randomized, intergroup trial of concurrent accelerated hyperfractionated radiotherapy versus standard daily radiotherapy in patients with limited-stage SCLC.[105] All patients received four cycles of cisplatin (60 mg/m² on day 1) and etoposide (120 mg/m² on days 1, 2, and 3), and radiotherapy began with cycle 1. In the once-daily arm, patients received 45 Gy in 1.8-Gy fractions over 5 weeks. In the twice-daily arm, patients received 45 Gy in 1.5-Gy fractions over 3 weeks. Patients who achieved a complete response were offered PCI. OS was significantly higher in the twice-daily arm, 26% versus 16% at 5 years, and local recurrence was significantly lower, 36% versus 52%. There was a significant increase in grade 3 acute esophagitis, 26% versus 11%, in the twice-daily arm, with no difference in late toxicity.

The high intrathoracic relapse rate observed in both arms of the Turrisi study highlights the inadequacy of these modest doses to achieve meaningful local control.[105] Dose escalation, either through an altered fractionation or conventionally fractionated approach, has been explored with a goal of improving intrathoracic control of disease. In 2005, the RTOG reported the results of a phase I dose escalation trial in which 64 patients were enrolled and dose escalated in a stepwise fashion from 50.4 Gy to 64.8 Gy in 1.8 Gy per fraction.[225] The lowest dose cohort received 1.8 Gy once daily for 20 fractions, followed by 1.8 Gy twice daily on the final 3 days. Dose escalation was achieved by the addition of a second daily fraction on the last 5, 7, 9, or 11 days, retaining the 5-week treatment duration. The maximum tolerated dose was determined to be 61.2 Gy in 5 weeks using this scheme. In a follow-up phase 2 study, RTOG 0239,[226] 72 patients were treated to 61.2 Gy in 5 weeks, with twice-daily radiotherapy for the last 9 treatment days. With 19 months median follow-up, 2-year OS was 37% and 2-year locoregional control was 80%.

Dose escalation has also been examined utilizing a daily fractionation scheme. Choi et al.[227] conducted a phase I dose escalation study with both twice-daily and once-daily arms. In the twice-daily arm, 45 Gy in 30 fractions over 3 weeks was the maximum tolerated dose. In the once-daily arm, the dose was escalated to the maximum of 70 Gy in 35 fractions over 7 weeks without dose-limiting toxicity. CALGB 39808 tested the feasibility of this approach with concurrent platinum and etoposide.[228] In this study, 63 patients were treated with two cycles of induction paclitaxel (175 mg/m² day 1) and topotecan (1 mg/m² days 1 through 5), followed by concurrent thoracic radiation with carboplatin (AUC 5) and etoposide (100 mg/m² days 1 through 3). Thoracic radiation consisted of 44 Gy to the mediastinum and primary tumor delivered in 2 Gy per fraction, followed by a cone down to encompass the involved nodes and primary tumor alone for an additional 26 Gy, totaling 70 Gy in 35 fractions over 7 weeks. The OS at 2 years was 48%. Results of the Concurrent Once-daily Versus Twice-daily Radiotherapy (CONVERT) trial were reported in 2016. This study enrolled 547 patients between 2008 and 2013 at 88 centers worldwide, randomizing patients with limited-stage disease to 45 Gy twice daily or 66 Gy once daily. The 2-year OS was not significantly different (56% for twice daily, 51% for once daily), and the rate of grade 3 or greater esophagitis was 19% in both arms. The authors concluded that once-daily radiation is an acceptable alternative to twice-daily radiation.[229]

An ongoing intergroup effort (CALGB 30610, RTOG 0538, NCT00632853) continues to compare 45 Gy in 30 fractions over 3 weeks versus 70 Gy in 35 fractions. A third arm was closed, which administered 61.2 Gy in 5 weeks per RTOG 0239. All patients receive concurrent EP, and radiotherapy begins with cycle 1 or cycle 2.

Radiotherapy Volume

Limited-stage SCLC is frequently bulky at presentation, requiring large treatment fields to encompass all sites of intrathoracic disease. Therefore, induction chemotherapy has been employed to achieve cytoreduction of disease prior to initiation of thoracic radiotherapy. This approach raises the concern of potentially increasing the risk of marginal treatment failure if the postchemotherapy volume alone is included in the radiation portal. To address this question, the SWOG conducted a randomized study, enrolling 191 patients who had a partial response or stable disease after 6 weeks of induction chemotherapy. They were randomized to receive radiotherapy (48 Gy split course) to either the preinduction or postinduction volume.[230] There was no difference in local recurrence rates: 32% in the preinduction versus 28% in the postinduction arm. Careful retrospective studies of patients treated with preinduction or postinduction thoracic radiotherapy show that local failure is not significantly higher if smaller fields are used. Furthermore, most intrathoracic failures occur in the smaller postchemotherapy radiation field, arguing, as in locally advanced NSCLC, against the use of ENI.[231,232]

Thoracic Radiotherapy for Extensive-Stage Disease

Systemic therapy is the essential element in the treatment of patients with extensive-stage SCLC with good performance status; however, thoracic radiotherapy may play a role in selected patients. Based on the observation that patients have high rates of thoracic relapse after systemic therapy alone, a single-institution prospective randomized trial was undertaken in Yugoslavia.[218] In this trial, 209 patients with extensive disease were enrolled and treated with three cycles of EP. Of those, 110 patients who had a partial response in the chest and a complete response outside the chest were randomized to receive thoracic radiation with concurrent carboplatin and etoposide, followed by two cycles of EP, versus four further cycles of EP alone. All eligible patients received PCI. The thoracic radiation was delivered in 54 Gy in 36 fractions over 12 days. At 5 years, the OS was higher in the arm that featured thoracic radiation: 9% versus 4%.

RTOG 0937 was a randomized phase II study in patients with metastatic SMLC with 1 to 4 extrathoracic sites of disease (excluding brain metastasis); patients were randomized to receive 45 Gy in 15 fractions to all sites of disease followed by PCI, versus PCI alone, after chemotherapy. The trial was closed for futility after an interim analysis of 86 patients.[233] With a median follow-up of 9 months, there was no significant difference in 1 year OS: 60% for PCI versus 51% for PCI and RT to thoracic and metastatic sites. Yet, the Chest Irradiation in Extensive Stage Small Cell Lung Cancer (CREST) trial, conducted by the Dutch Lung Cancer Study Group suggests a benefit of thoracic radiation in this setting. In this study, 498 patients with extensive-stage disease who responded to chemotherapy were randomized to thoracic radiotherapy (30 Gy in 10 fractions) and PCI versus PCI alone. The dose of thoracic RT was 30 Gy in 10 fractions. The primary end point was OS at 1 year, and there was no significant improvement at this time point (33% for TRT vs. 28%). At 2 years, however, there was a significant improvement in OS, 13% versus 3%, favoring TRT.[219] Overall, these results suggest that TRT may benefit a subset of patients with extensive disease after chemotherapy.

Prophylactic Cranial Irradiation

Brain metastases are present at diagnosis in approximately 20% of patients with SCLC. The brain is also a frequent site of failure after chemotherapy for extensive disease or chemoradiotherapy for limited-stage disease. Several randomized trials have addressed the value of PCI following a response to initial therapy and have consistently demonstrated a decrease

in the incidence of brain metastases. A meta-analysis reported the results of 987 patients treated in seven randomized trials enrolling between 1977 and 1995.[221] Here, 85% of these patients had limited stage and 15% extensive. All were randomized either to PCI or to observation following a complete response to initial therapy, although response was most commonly assessed by chest x-ray rather than CT scan. PCI regimens varied from 8 Gy in a single fraction to 40 Gy in 20 fractions. At 3 years, PCI was found to significantly decrease the incidence of brain metastases (59% vs. 33%) and significantly improve OS (21% vs. 15%). There was trend toward improved brain control when PCI was administered earlier and at higher dose. The publication of this study demonstrated the value of PCI in limited-stage SCLC.

PCI in extensive-stage SCLC was addressed separately in a randomized trial conducted by the EORTC.[220] In this study, 286 patients with extensive-stage SCLC were randomized to either PCI or observation after any response to four to six cycles of chemotherapy. Those assigned to the PCI arm were treated within 4 to 6 weeks of completing systemic therapy. Of note, this study did not require brain imaging prior to initiation of PCI. The 1-year cumulative incidence of brain metastases was significantly decreased in the PCI arm at 15% versus 40%, and 1-year OS was significantly increased in the PCI arm at 27% versus 13%. Six different PCI regimens were permitted, with biologically effective dose ranging from 25 to 39 Gy. A similar Japanese randomized trial did not replicate these results; the trial was terminated after enrollment of 163 patients when an interim futility analysis determined that no benefit was possible. Patients were randomized after any response to chemotherapy, but unlike the EORTC study, brain imaging was done before enrollment. The median OS was not significantly different between the two arms with a trend toward worse survival in the PCI arm: 11.6 months for patients who received PCI versus 13.7 months for those who did not (HR 1.27, CI 0.96 to 1.68, $P = 0.094$).[234] Thus, the role of PCI in extensive-stage SCLC remains an ongoing controversy.

Despite the survival benefit reported in the Auperin meta-analysis and the EORTC trial in extensive-stage disease, a variety of dose and fractionation schemes were employed to treat the patients enrolled in the trials. To help define the optimal dose and fractionation for PCI, a multi-institutional intergroup trial was launched to examine standard-dose PCI versus high-dose PCI. Patients with limited-stage SCLC who had achieved a complete response to chemoradiotherapy were randomized to receive PCI in standard dose, 25 Gy in 10 daily fractions, or high-dose, 36 Gy in either 18 daily fractions or 24 twice-daily fractions.[235] In this study, 720 patients were randomized; at 2 years, the cumulative incidence of brain metastases was not significantly different between the two arms: 29% in the standard-dose arm versus 23% for high dose. Surprisingly, there was poorer OS in the high-dose arm: 2-year survival was 42% in the standard-dose arm versus 36% for high dose. This was attributed to a higher cancer-related mortality in the high-dose arm. Patients enrolled in this trial participated in baseline and follow-up neuropsychologic test batteries along with QOL assessments. Wolfson et al.[236] recently reported the results of these assessments and observed an increased incidence of chronic neurotoxicity at 12 months after PCI in the 36-Gy cohort ($P = .02$). Taken together, these results establish 2.5 Gy in 10 fractions as the current preferred regimen to deliver PCI.

Extensive-Stage Disease

For patients with extensive-stage disease, treatment is largely palliative, and for patients with adequate performance status, systemic chemotherapy is the cornerstone of treatment. Given a more favorable toxicity profile, cisplatin is often substituted by carboplatin. A meta-analysis of four trials concluded that in the metastatic setting, there was no differences in efficacy between cisplatin and carboplatin.[237] Other drug partners aside from etoposide have been tested with no clear advantage. Recurrence is inevitable and few effective options exist at the time of progression. The only US Food and Drug Administration (FDA)–approved regimen in this setting is topotecan. Treatment with this agent in the second-line setting has been associated with a slower deterioration of QOL and better symptom control compared to best supportive care despite having a response rate of only 7%.[238]

After decades with no major advance in the treatment of patients with extensive-stage SCLC, two new developments provide hope that a breakthrough maybe in the horizon. On one hand, immunotherapy has gained considerable interest. In a phase 1/2 study, patients who have progressed after chemotherapy were treated with immune checkpoint inhibitors in different cohorts.[239] Nivolumab alone had an objective response rate of 10% in 98 patients. The combination of nivolumab and ipilimumab proved to be more efficacious with a response rate of 23% in the cohort using nivolumab 1 mg/kg plus ipilimumab 3 mg/kg (n = 14/61) and 19% (n = 10/54) in the nivolumab 3 mg/kg plus ipilimumab 1 mg/kg cohort. The use of combination immunotherapy was associated with increase toxicity, with an incidence of grade 3/4 adverse events of 24% versus 13% in monotherapy. Immunotherapy is currently being explored in several clinical trials in this setting.

The second exciting development is targeted therapy. The delta like 3 gene (*DLL3*) is highly expressed in neuroendocrine tumors, including approximately 80% of SCLC.[240] Rovalpituzumab tesirine is an antibody drug conjugate directed against *DLL3* that is linked to a pyrrolobenzodiazepine (PBD) dimer toxin. This agent was evaluated in a phase 1 study with 74 patients with previously treated metastatic SCLC. In patients who had an *DLL3* expression of >50% of neoplastic cells (n = 29), 10 (35%) had a confirmed objective response and 26 (90%) achieved disease control. The most common grade 3 or higher toxicities were serosal effusions (11%) and thrombocytopenia (11%). This agent is currently being evaluated in the relapsed setting in a single arm phase 2 trial (NCT02674568) and in a phase 3 trial.

NORMAL TISSUE TOXICITY

The risk and severity of radiation toxicity in normal tissue are related to the dose and volume irradiated, as well as the functional organization of the OAR. In serial tissue such as spinal cord, esophagus, and trachea and bronchi, injury of any one organ subunit may result in total organ dysfunction. Therefore, high dose to even small volumes can lead to significant toxicity. In parallel tissues, such as lung, dysfunction of any one organ subunit leads to partial organ dysfunction. In this case, the volume irradiated, even to lower doses, plays a larger role.

Emami et al.[241] published partial-volume organ tolerances for normal tissue that served for more than a decade as the standard source for radiation dose limits. Dose limits were defined for specific toxicity endpoints, using a 5% complication rate at 5 years (TD$_{5/5}$) or 50% complication rate at 5 years (TD$_{50/5}$). These parameters were based predominantly on clinical data from 2D radiotherapy planning. More recently, a multidisciplinary effort was undertaken, the QUANTEC, to summarize the published 3D dose–volume/toxicity data in the literature, review NTCP modeling, and provide practical guidance for the clinician[145,146] (Table 54.8).

Lung

Clinically significant pneumonitis occurs in 5% to 20% of patients receiving radiation for lung cancer and is one of the key dose-limiting factors in radiation planning for patients

TABLE 54.8 DOSE–VOLUME CONSTRAINTS FOR NORMAL TISSUES USING STANDARD FRACTIONATION TO TARGET VOLUME AND TRADITIONAL ESTIMATES OF NORMAL TISSUE TOLERANCE OF THERAPEUTIC IRRADIATION

Organ	Conventional RT Alone	SBRT[a] Number Fx	SBRT[a] Vol (mL)	SBRT[a] Vol Max (Gy)	SBRT[a] Point Max (Gy)	Chemo/RT	Chemo/RT, Then Surgery	TD$_{5/5}$ Volume[b] (Gy) 1/3	TD$_{5/5}$ Volume[b] (Gy) 2/3	TD$_{5/5}$ Volume[b] (Gy) 3/3	TD$_{50/5}$ Volume[b] (Gy) 1/3	TD$_{50/5}$ Volume[b] (Gy) 2/3	TD$_{50/5}$ Volume[b] (Gy) 3/3	Selected End TD Point
Brachial plexus	–	1	3	14.4	16	–	–	62	61	60	77	76	75	Clinical nerve damage
		3		7.5/fx	8/fx									
		5		6/fx	6.4/fx									
Cord[c]	50 Gy	1	0.25	10	14	45 Gy	45 Gy	50	50	47	70	70	–	Myelitis
		3		6/fx	7.5/fx									
		5		4.5/fx	6/fx									
Esophagus	D_{max} <75 Gy V_{60} <50%	1	5	14.5	19	D_{max} <75 Gy V_{55} <50%	D_{max} <75 Gy V_{55} <50%	60	58	55	72	70	68	Stricture/perforation/fistula
		3		7/fx	9/fx									
		5		5.5/fx	7/fx									
Heart	V_{40} <50%	1	15	16	22	Same as RT alone	Same as RT alone	60	45	40	70	55	50	Pericarditis
		3		8/fx	10/fx									
		5		6.4/fx	7.6/fx									
Kidney[d]	20 Gy[e]	1	<66% (200)[f]	10.6 (8.4)		Same as RT alone	Same as RT alone	50	30	23	–	40	28	Clinical nephritis
		3		6.2/fx (4.8/fx)										
		5		4.6/fx (3.5/fx)										
Liver	30 Gy (<40%)	1	700	9.1		Same as RT alone	Same as RT alone	50	35	30	55	45	40	Liver failure
		3		5.7/fx										
		5		4.2/fx										
Lung[g]	MLd <20 Gy V_{20} <40%	1	1,000	7.4		MLd <20 Gy V_{20} <35% V_{10} <45% V_5 <65%	MLd <20 Gy V_{20} <20% V_{10} <40% V_{40} <55%	45	30	17.5	65	40	24.5	Pneumonitis
		3		3.8/fx										
		5		2.7/fx										

Chemo, chemotherapy; Fx, fractions; Max, maximum; MLD, mean lung dose; RT, radiation therapy; SBRT, stereotactic body radiation therapy; TD, tolerance dose; Vol, volume.
[a]Hypofractionation dose constraints not validated by long-term follow-up.
[b]TD$_{5/5}$ and TD$_{50/5}$ represent the estimated dose for each organ volume or partial organ volume resulting in a 1% to 5% risk and a 50% risk, respectively, at 5 years.
[c]The chance of spinal cord damage is increased as treated volume is increased. Physicians should consider off cord earlier if a significant amount of spinal cord has received constraints dose. In general, spinal cord should not receive dose >60 Gy even in very limited volume. Higher fraction size of radiation or higher daily dose will decrease the tolerance. If the patient is treated with 3 Gy per fraction, the cord constraint should be around 40 Gy (based on biologic effective dose calculation).
[d]Consider a kidney scan if the large volume of one kidney will be treated to a high dose.
[e]Less than 50% of combined both kidneys, or <75% of one side of kidney if another kidney is not functional.
[f]First constraint applies to bilateral kidney hilum and vascular trunk. Second parenthetical constraint applies to bilateral kidney cortices.
[g]For patients receiving concurrent chemo/RT, V_{15} may also be an important parameter to be considered. V_{20} = effective lung volume (total lung volume – GTV) received ≥20 Gy.

with locally advanced disease. RP may occur during fractionated treatment or up to 18 months afterward, with a peak incidence at 2 to 6 months posttreatment. The most clinical common presentation includes a persistent nonproductive cough, dyspnea, low-grade fever, and fatigue. Chest x-ray or CT scan may be normal, or, depending on the time course, there may be ground-glass opacification (within 2 to 6 months), patchy consolidation (4 to 12 months), or fibrosis (10 months or more) that loosely corresponds to the radiation field. Pulmonary function testing shows reduced lung volumes, tidal volumes, and diffusion capacity.

A variety of dose–volume models have been evaluated as predictive metrics of RP, including threshold volumes (i.e., V_{dose}), MLD, and Lyman–Kutcher–Burman NTCP models. MLD and dose–volume threshold models are more widely used because of their simplicity, and MLD-based risk assessment for RP correlates closely to that calculated using NTCP modeling. A logistic regression of RP versus MLD and the cross-correlation of various V_{dose} parameters suggest a gradual increase in dose–response, with no safe threshold dose below which the risk of RP is zero.[242]

From collected data in the QUANTEC effort, the risk of RP is <20% when the MLD is less than approximately 20 Gy with conventional fractionation. With regard to V_{dose} threshold models, where the volume of lung outside of the GTV or PTV receiving a threshold dose is quantified, individual datasets have found different thresholds to be optimal, reflecting the interdependence of the dosimetric parameters as well as differences in technique and the specific clinical endpoint used. The risk of RP is <20% for V_{20Gy} <35% or V_5 <60% with conventional fractionation.

All models of conventional fractionation are extrapolated from datasets using standard, simple planning techniques and may have lower predictive power for IMRT, proton therapy, or hypofractionated radiotherapy. Caution is warranted when using IMRT and absolute dose–volume thresholds, because planning algorithms may meet strict dosimetric constraints at the cost of higher dose at other, unconstrained cut points. However, in an analysis of patients treated with IMRT for locally advanced NSCLC on the RTOG 0617, V20 remained the most accurate predictive metric of RP.[243]

RP occurs less commonly after SBRT in comparison to conventionally fractionated radiation.[69] The risk of symptomatic RP does seem to follow a similar relationship to dose and volume irradiated as seen in conventionally fractionated treatment, although specific dose thresholds corresponding to risk thresholds have not yet been fully elucidated. In one large series, the risk of grade 2 or greater RP was 17% when the MLD was >4 Gy versus 4% for lower values and 16% when the V_{20} was >4% versus 4% for lower values.[244] The AAPM Task Group 101 report included a first approximation of tissue dose tolerances for SBRT.[147] For bilateral lung, they recommended maximum dose to 10 and 15 cc of lung of 7.4 and 7 Gy for single-fraction SBRT, 12.4 and 11.6 Gy for three-fraction SBRT, and 13.5 and 12.5 Gy for five-fraction SBRT.

Radiotherapy-induced dyspnea may have several contributing causes, including not only RP but also radiotherapy to other thoracic OARs. Emerging evidence suggests an interaction between cardiac dose and RP,[245] or there may be additive dyspnea owing to pleural and pericardial effusions, restrictive pericarditis, cardiomyopathy, and bronchial stenosis or bronchiectasis. Bronchial toxicity has been reported with conventional radiotherapy after dose escalation,[246] and QUANTEC recommendations include the caution that doses >80 Gy to the major airways should be avoided.[242] For SBRT, the risk of bronchial stenosis is felt to be higher because of the higher biologically effective dose delivered, and this may be one cause of the reported higher risk of pulmonary toxicity when lesions near the proximal bronchi are being treated. The AAPM Task Group 101 recommends maximum doses to 4 cc and maximum point

doses to the proximal tracheobronchial tree of 10.5 and 20.2 Gy for single-fraction SBRT, 15 and 30 Gy for three-fraction SBRT, and 16.5 and 40 Gy for five-fraction SBRT.

Several patient- and treatment-related factors impact the risk of RP, independent of dose and volume. In a large dataset derived from patients treated on RTOG trials, the risk of RP was significantly higher for tumors in the lower lung fields.[247] Older age may increase the risk of RP, and patients who continue to smoke through their radiotherapy may be at decreased risk, although the benefits of smoking cessation far outweigh any potential benefit in terms of reduction of risk of RP.[242] Several chemotherapy agents that are commonly administered to lung cancer patients are associated with an increased risk of RP, including docetaxel, gemcitabine, and immune checkpoint inhibitors.

Glucocorticoids are commonly used to treat developing RP, although this has not been evaluated in a prospective fashion, and the starting dose and tapering schedule are undefined. A starting dose of approximately 60 mg or 1 mg/kg of prednisone may be given for 1 to 2 weeks, followed by a slow taper over 4 to 8 weeks. Symptoms may recur when steroids are discontinued, and although it is hoped that treatment may mitigate the development of lung fibrosis, this has not been established. Prophylactic antibiotics or anticoagulants do not appear to effect the development of RP. Pentoxifylline is a xanthine derivative that improves microvascular blood flow; it was used in a single randomized trial of 40 patients undergoing breast or lung irradiation.[248] The proportion of patients with grade 2 or 3 pulmonary toxicity was significantly lower in the patients who received pentoxifylline (20% vs. 50%), as was the measured diffusion capacity. Captopril is an angiotensin-converting enzyme inhibitor that has been shown to reduce the development of radiation-induced fibrosis in rats, although no such protective effect has been demonstrated in humans.[249]

Esophagus

Acute esophagitis is often the most prominent symptom during fractionated radiotherapy for thoracic malignancy, leading to inpatient admissions, dehydration, weight loss, and treatment interruption. Late esophageal toxicity may include stricture, perforation, or fistula formation. Grade 3 or greater acute esophagitis (symptoms requiring hospitalization, endoscopic intervention, surgery, or treatment breaks) occurs in 15% to 25% of patients during or shortly after chemoradiation. Acute esophagitis may coexist with, and be exacerbated by, comorbid conditions such as candidiasis or reflux disease. Severe late toxicity is less common, occurring in <5% of patients,[250] and manifests as stenosis or, more rarely, fistula formation.

Several dose–volume metrics have been evaluated as predictors of severe esophagitis. The maximum esophageal dose correlates with symptoms, as do multiple absolute dose and volume thresholds. These are highly cross-correlated, and no consensus has been reached regarding the optimum parameter for radiotherapy planning. Circumferential measures (i.e., limits to the length of entire esophageal circumference treated to threshold dose) have also been significantly correlated with symptoms, as has the mean esophageal dose.[251] QUANTEC analysis concludes that volumes treated above 40 to 50 Gy correlate with acute esophagitis and further suggests that no dose above prescription be allowed to even small volumes of esophagus, to reduce the risk of severe ulceration or fistula. This latter information is especially important for heterogeneous IMRT planning.

Esophageal toxicity is related to both dose and volume of irradiation, and the risk and severity are therefore also a function of the size, anatomic arrangement, and proximity of target structures. Other factors identified as increasing the risk or severity of acute esophagitis include the use of accelerated fractionation,[105] older patient age, and the use of concurrent chemotherapy.[93,99] Recently, an unexpectedly high risk of tracheoesophageal fistula formation was reported after radiotherapy with concurrent chemotherapy and bevacizumab.[122]

Treatment of acute esophagitis is primarily supportive care, frequently requiring topical agents, dietary changes, and narcotic pain medication. It is often prudent to evaluate patients for viral or candidal esophagitis. Patients may be treated empirically with antifungal agents or with proton pump inhibitors for comorbid reflux disease. When esophageal stricture develops, it is usually reversible with repeated dilations. An esophageal fistula can be life threatening, although stenting or surgical management may restore function.

Heart

The cardiotoxicity of radiotherapy has been primarily studied after treatment for breast cancer or mediastinal lymphoma. In these patients, the excess cardiac mortality manifests years after thoracic radiotherapy and depends on the dose, volume, and the patient's existing cardiac risk factors. More recently, analysis of the RTOG 0617 demonstrated that heart dose correlated with worse OS.[121] Acute toxicities include pericarditis, which uncommonly may progress to chronic pericardial fibrosis, effusion, or even more rarely a constrictive pericarditis. Ischemic changes in the cardiac muscle can manifest after a long latency and may lead to late cardiac events. Valvular abnormalities have been reported, presumably owing to late fibrotic changes.

Most of the data regarding dose and volume tolerances for the heart are derived from patients treated for breast cancer or lymphoma, typically with distinct beam arrangements that have limited application to 3D conformal or IMRT treatment of lung malignancies. The risk of pericardial toxicity has been correlated with treatment of >50% of the heart contour in 2D planning and to the volume receiving ≥30 Gy in 3D planning. NTCP modeling has been done using both breast and lymphoma patient data; the derived parameters differ, reflecting the significant differences in technique-related cardiac exposure and underlying patient risk factors. Recommendations made as part of the QUANTEC effort reflect a conservative interpretation of the existing literature: If the V_{25} is <10%, then the excess risk of cardiac mortality attributable to ischemic changes is <1% at 15 years. The risk of pericarditis can be minimized by keeping the mean pericardial dose <26 Gy or the pericardial V_{30} <46%. Heart and pericardial exposure should otherwise be minimized without compromise of target coverage.

Other clinical risk factors for cardiac mortality increasing the risk of radiotherapy-induced cardiac toxicity include hypertension, diabetes, obesity, and genetic predisposition. The risk of cardiac mortality from radiotherapy has been specifically demonstrated to be increased in patients >60 years old and by tobacco use.[252]

Brachial Plexus

Radiation brachial plexopathy is relatively poorly described with a low incidence. There are case reports of an early, transient plexopathy that occurs during or within weeks to months of radiation at relatively low dose and may resolve spontaneously.[253] Late radiation plexopathy is more clinically significant; it manifests years after radiation to the supraclavicular area with hypesthesia, paresthesia, and weakness of the affected arm and shoulder. It may progress to total paralysis of the affected arm and severe pain.

The dose tolerance of the brachial plexus is less defined than other thoracic organs, partly because of the difficulty in contouring and defining the OAR. A consensus contouring atlas has been created so that more robust clinical data can be collected.[254] Peripheral nerves respond as a serial organ; thus, it is thought that the maximum point dose should be predictive of plexopathy. Late plexopathy is rare in patients who have received ≤60 Gy. Proposed brachial plexus dose limits for standard, fractionated radiotherapy planning vary considerably; RTOG 0617 suggests a point maximum limit of 66 Gy.

For SBRT, brachial plexopathy has been reported after treatment of apical tumors. In a series of 37 apical tumors in 36 patients treated with SBRT at Indiana University, 7 patients developed plexopathy at a median of 7 months posttreatment.[255] The cumulative risk of grade 2 to 4 plexopathy was 46% when the plexus received >26 Gy versus 8% when the plexus received ≤26 Gy. AAPM Task Group 101 recommends maximum dose to 3 cc and maximum point dose of 14 and 17.5 Gy for single-fraction SBRT, 20.4 and 24 Gy for three-fraction SBRT, and 27 and 30.5 Gy for five-fraction SBRT.[147]

Reirradiation

As systemic therapy improves, more patients are presenting with locally recurrent lung cancer without systemic progression of disease, such as in stage III NSCLC previously treated with chemoradiation. This presents a challenge in management as local therapy is indicated, but surgery is usually not feasible, and we are still just beginning to understand normal tissue dose constraints in the setting of reirradiation. With conventional radiation techniques such as 3D conformal radiation, it is often not feasible to give a second, curative (i.e., >45 Gy) dose of radiation to the same thoracic region without exceeding dose constraints of nearby organ. Many small series have been published on using SBRT for reirradiation, both after prior SBRT as well as conventional radiation.[256] There is also increasing interest in using proton therapy in thoracic reirradiation because of the dosimetric advantages of proton therapy. There is a lot of variability in terms of efficacy, with median time to disease progression of typically 6 to 12 months with mean OS usually of about 18 months. Significant toxicity can be seen, including pneumonitis, esophagitis, fistulas, chest wall toxicity, and potentially fatal bleeding. Many studies do not publish detailed dosimetric analysis, which makes it difficult to apply the results clinically. A series of 102 patients from MD Anderson treated with proton therapy or IMRT for thoracic reirradiation reported acceptable toxicity rates with 7% grade 3+ esophageal toxicity and 10% grade 3+ pneumonitis.[257] Median initial dose was 70 EQD2Gy and median reirradiation dose was 60.48 EQD2Gy. At a median follow-up of 6.5 months, 41% had a local failure and 49% distant metastasis. Most local failures (88%) were within the original or reirradiation field or margins. Median OS was 14.7 months. Patients tended to have better OS with concurrent chemotherapy and higher EQD2, and worse OS with higher T-stage, poor performance status, squamous histology, and larger reirradiation volumes. Reirradiation appears feasible, but it is important to carefully select patients who are likely to benefit from this potentially high-risk treatment.

Patient-Reported Outcomes In Lung Cancer

A PRO is defined as any report of the status of a patient's health condition provided directly by the patient (such as QOL), without interpretation of the patient's response by others. Examples of validated QOL instruments that include both generic and site-specific lung modules are the Functional Assessment of Cancer Therapy-Lung (FACT-L) and the EORTC QOL Questionnaire Core-30 (QLQ-C30) and QLQ-LC13. The Lung Cancer Symptom Scale (LCSS) is a shorter (9-item) QOL instrument that is specific for lung cancer.

There are many compelling reasons to study PROs in lung cancer patients. When used to assess the impact of clinical regimens, PROs can often identify meaningful differences that may not have been anticipated.[258] For example, Temel et al.[26] assessed the impact of early palliative care on QOL (using FACT-L) among patients with newly diagnosed metastatic NSCLC randomized to early palliative care or to standard care. They found that patients in the early palliative care arm not only had significant improvement in QOL, with less depression or anxiety, but also had longer median survival ($P = .02$), despite receiving less therapy.

Another clinically relevant aspect of QOL is its ability to serve as an independent prognostic factor for survival. Movsas et al.[24] reported that the baseline QOL score independently predicted for 5-year survival in patients with stage III NSCLC treated with chemoradiation on RTOG 9801. Similarly, in RTOG 0617, every 10 points higher on the FACT-TOI instrument at baseline corresponded to a 10% decreased risk of death.[259] Moreover, although RTOG 0617 was not randomized by radiation technology, significantly fewer patients who received intensity-modulated radiation therapy (vs. 3D conformal radiation) had a clinically meaningful decline in QOL a full year after treatment ($P = 0.005$). Interestingly, studies are beginning to elucidate the biologic underpinnings supporting the relationship between QOL and outcomes.[260]

Studies have highlighted a critical "disconnect" between PROs and provider-reported observations.[261] In light of the above, a PRO measurement system has been developed by the NCI as a companion to the Common Terminology Criteria of Adverse Events (CTCAE), termed the PRO-CTCAE.[262] The PRO-CTCAE is novel in that it integrates the patient perspective directly into the toxicity reporting using a validated methodology that can guide future treatment recommendations. Indeed, randomized data have demonstrated that incorporating PROs into the clinical setting can improve physician–patient communication.[263] Ultimately, PROs should become a routine tool in the clinical care for our patients with lung cancer.

ACKNOWLEDGMENTS

The authors thank Mindy Langer for her exhaustive and critical review of the chapter. They also thank Eric Xanthopoulos for his input and assistance in the preparation of the figures and tables.

REFERENCES

1. Torre LA, Bray F, Siegel RL, et al. Global cancer statistics, 2012. *CA Cancer J Clin* 2015;65(2):87–108.
2. Siegel RL, Miller KD, Jemal A. Cancer statistics, 2017. *CA Cancer J Clin* 2017;67(1):7–30.
3. Howlader N, Noone AM, Krapcho M. *SEER stat fact sheets: lung and bronchus.* Bethesda, MD: National Cancer Institute, 2016.
4. Rusch VW, Asamura H, Watanabe H, et al. The IASLC lung cancer staging project: a proposal for a new international lymph node map in the forthcoming seventh edition of the TNM classification for lung cancer. *J Thorac Oncol* 2009;4(5):568–577.
5. Line DH, Deeley TJ. The necropsy findings in carcinoma of the bronchus. *Br J Dis Chest* 1971;65(4):238–242.
6. Kuo CW, Chen YM, Chao JY, et al. Non-small cell lung cancer in very young and very old patients. *Chest* 2000;117(2):354–357.
7. Stenbygaard LE, Sorensen JB, Olsen JE. Metastatic pattern at autopsy in non-resectable adenocarcinoma of the lung—a study from a cohort of 259 consecutive patients treated with chemotherapy. *Acta Oncol* 1997;36(3):301–306.
8. Nugent JL, Bunn PA Jr, Matthews MJ, et al. CNS metastases in small cell bronchogenic carcinoma: increasing frequency and changing pattern with lengthening survival. *Cancer* 1979;44(5):1885–1893.
9. Hiraki A, Ueoka H, Takata I, et al. Hypercalcemia-leukocytosis syndrome associated with lung cancer. *Lung Cancer* 2004;43(3):301–307.
10. Mareska M, Gutmann L. Lambert-Eaton myasthenic syndrome. *Semin Neurol* 2004;24(2):149–153.
11. Sridhar KS, Lobo CF, Altman RD. Digital clubbing and lung cancer. *Chest* 1998;114(6):1535–1537.
12. International Early Lung Cancer Action Program Investigators; Henschke CI, Yankelevitz DF, Libby DM, et al. Survival of patients with stage I lung cancer detected on CT screening. *N Engl J Med* 2006;355(17):1763–1771.
13. National Lung Screening Trial Research Team; Aberle DR, Adams AM, Berg CD, et al. Reduced lung-cancer mortality with low-dose computed tomographic screening. *N Engl J Med* 2011;365(5):395–409.
14. Arita T, Matsumoto T, Kuramitsu T, et al. Is it possible to differentiate malignant mediastinal nodes from benign nodes by size? Reevaluation by CT, transesophageal echocardiography, and nodal specimen. *Chest* 1996;110(4):1004–1008.

15. Kalff V, Hicks RJ, MacManus MP, et al. Clinical impact of (18)F fluorodeoxyglucose positron emission tomography in patients with non-small-cell lung cancer: a prospective study. *J Clin Oncol* 2001;19(1):111–118.
16. Gould MK, Kuschner WG, Rydzak CE, et al. Test performance of positron emission tomography and computed tomography for mediastinal staging in patients with non-small-cell lung cancer: a meta-analysis. *Ann Intern Med* 2003;139(11):879–892.
17. Yasufuku K, Nakajima T, Motoori K, et al. Comparison of endobronchial ultrasound, positron emission tomography, and CT for lymph node staging of lung cancer. *Chest* 2006;130(3):710–718.
18. Light RW. The undiagnosed pleural effusion. *Clin Chest Med* 2006;27(2):309–319.
19. Goldstraw P, Chansky K, Crowley J, et al. The IASLC Lung Cancer Staging Project: Proposals for Revision of the TNM Stage Groupings in the Forthcoming (Eighth) Edition of the TNM Classification for Lung Cancer. *J Thorac Oncol* 2016;11(1):39–51.
20. Sandler A, Gray R, Perry MC, et al. Paclitaxel-carboplatin alone or with bevacizumab for non-small-cell lung cancer. *N Engl J Med* 2006;355(24):2542–2550.
21. Scagliotti GV, Parikh P, von Pawel J, et al. Phase III study comparing cisplatin plus gemcitabine with cisplatin plus pemetrexed in chemotherapy-naive patients with advanced-stage non-small-cell lung cancer. *J Clin Oncol* 2008;26(21):3543–3551.
22. Travis WD, Brambilla E, Nicholson AG, et al. The 2015 World Health Organization Classification of Lung Tumors: Impact of Genetic, Clinical and Radiologic Advances Since the 2004 Classification. *J Thorac Oncol* 2015;10(9):1243–1260.
23. Stanley KE. Prognostic factors for survival in patients with inoperable lung cancer. *J Natl Cancer Inst* 1980;65(1):25–32.
24. Movsas B, Moughan J, Sarna L, et al. Quality of life supersedes the classic prognosticators for long-term survival in locally advanced non-small-cell lung cancer: an analysis of RTOG 9801. *J Clin Oncol* 2009;27(34):5816–5822.
25. Jemal A, Siegel R, Xu J, et al. Cancer statistics, 2010. *CA Cancer J Clin* 2010;60(5):277–300.
26. Temel JS, Greer JA, Muzikansky A, et al. Early palliative care for patients with metastatic non-small-cell lung cancer. *N Engl J Med* 2010;363(8):733–742.
27. Brunelli A, Kim AW, Berger KI, et al. Physiologic evaluation of the patient with lung cancer being considered for resectional surgery: diagnosis and management of lung cancer, 3rd ed: American College of Chest Physicians evidence-based clinical practice guidelines. *Chest* 2013;143(5 Suppl):e166S–e190S.
28. Ginsberg RJ, Rubinstein LV. Randomized trial of lobectomy versus limited resection for T1 N0 non-small cell lung cancer. Lung Cancer Study Group. *Ann Thorac Surg* 1995;60(3):615–622; discussion 622–613.
29. Okada M, Koike T, Higashiyama M, et al. Radical sublobar resection for small-sized non-small cell lung cancer: a multicenter study. *J Thorac Cardiovasc Surg* 2006;132(4):769–775.
30. Fernando HC, Landreneau RJ, Mandrekar SJ, et al. Impact of brachytherapy on local recurrence rates after sublobar resection: results from ACOSOG Z4032 (Alliance), a phase III randomized trial for high-risk operable non-small-cell lung cancer. *J Clin Oncol* 2014;32(23):2456–2462.
31. Timmerman RD, Paulas R, Pass HI, et al. RTOG 0618: stereotactic body radiation therapy (SBRT) to treat operable early-stage lung cancer patients. *J Clin Oncol* 2013;31(15 Suppl):7323.
32. Fernando HC, Timmerman R. American College of Surgeons Oncology Group Z4099/Radiation Therapy Oncology Group 1021: a randomized study of sublobar resection compared with stereotactic body radiotherapy for high-risk stage I non-small cell lung cancer. *J Thorac Cardiovasc Surg* 2012;144(3):S35–S38.
33. Hurkmans CW, Cuijpers JP, Lagerwaard FJ, et al. Recommendations for implementing stereotactic radiotherapy in peripheral stage IA non-small cell lung cancer: report from the Quality Assurance Working Party of the randomised phase III ROSEL study. *Radiat Oncol* 2009;4:1.
34. Chang JY, Senan S, Paul MA, et al. Stereotactic ablative radiotherapy versus lobectomy for operable stage I non-small-cell lung cancer: a pooled analysis of two randomised trials. *Lancet Oncol* 2015;16(6):630–637.
35. Martini N, Flehinger BJ, Zaman MB, et al. Results of resection in non-oat cell carcinoma of the lung with mediastinal lymph node metastases. *Ann Surg* 1983;198(3):386–397.
36. Iwasaki A, Shirakusa T, Miyoshi T, et al. Prognostic significance of subcarinal station in non-small cell lung cancer with T1-3 N2 disease. *Thorac Cardiovasc Surg* 2006;54(1):42–46.
37. Misthos P, Sepsas E, Kokotsakis J, et al. The significance of one-station N2 disease in the prognosis of patients with nonsmall-cell lung cancer. *Ann Thorac Surg* 2008;86(5):1626–1630.
38. van Meerbeeck JP, Kramer GW, Van Schil PE, et al. Randomized controlled trial of resection versus radiotherapy after induction chemotherapy in stage IIIA-N2 non-small-cell lung cancer. *J Natl Cancer Inst* 2007;99(6):442–450.
39. Pass HI, Pogrebniak HW, Steinberg SM, et al. Randomized trial of neoadjuvant therapy for lung cancer: interim analysis. *Ann Thorac Surg* 1992;53(6):992–998.
40. Rosell R, Gomez-Codina J, Camps C, et al. A randomized trial comparing preoperative chemotherapy plus surgery with surgery alone in patients with non-small-cell lung cancer. *N Engl J Med* 1994;330(3):153–158.
41. Roth JA, Fossella F, Komaki R, et al. A randomized trial comparing perioperative chemotherapy and surgery with surgery alone in resectable stage IIIA non-small-cell lung cancer. *J Natl Cancer Inst* 1994;86(9):673–680.
42. Felip E, Rosell R, Maestre JA, et al. Preoperative chemotherapy plus surgery versus surgery plus adjuvant chemotherapy versus surgery alone in early-stage non-small-cell lung cancer. *J Clin Oncol* 2010;28(19):3138–3145.
43. Scagliotti GV, Pastorino U, Vansteenkiste JF, et al. Randomized phase III study of surgery alone or surgery plus preoperative cisplatin and gemcitabine in stages IB to IIIA non-small-cell lung cancer. *J Clin Oncol* 2012;30(2):172–178.
44. Albain KS, Rusch VW, Crowley JJ, et al. Concurrent cisplatin/etoposide plus chest radiotherapy followed by surgery for stages IIIA (N2) and IIIB non-small-cell lung cancer: mature results of Southwest Oncology Group phase II study 8805. *J Clin Oncol* 1995;13(8):1880–1892.

45. Albain KS, Swann RS, Rusch VW, et al. Radiotherapy plus chemotherapy with or without surgical resection for stage III non-small-cell lung cancer: a phase III randomised controlled trial. *Lancet* 2009;374(9687):379–386.
46. Albain KS, Swann RS, Rusch VR, et al. Phase III study of concurrent chemotherapy and radiotherapy (CT/RT) vs CT/RT followed by surgical resection for stage IIIA(pN2) non-small cell lung cancer (NSCLC): outcomes update of North American Intergroup 0139 (RTOG 9309). *J Clin Oncol* 2005;23(16):624s.
47. Thomas M, Rube C, Hoffknecht P, et al. Effect of preoperative chemoradiation in addition to preoperative chemotherapy: a randomised trial in stage III non-small-cell lung cancer. *Lancet Oncol* 2008;9(7):636–648.
48. Logan DM, Lochrin CA, Darling G, et al. Adjuvant radiotherapy and chemotherapy for stage II or IIIA non-small-cell lung cancer after complete resection. Provincial Lung Cancer Disease Site Group. *Cancer Prev Control* 1997;1(5):366–378.
49. Postoperative radiotherapy in non-small-cell lung cancer: systematic review and meta-analysis of individual patient data from nine randomised controlled trials. PORT Meta-analysis Trialists Group. *Lancet* 1998;352(9124):257–263.
50. Lally BE, Zelterman D, Colasanto JM, et al. Postoperative radiotherapy for stage II or III non-small-cell lung cancer using the surveillance, epidemiology, and end results database. *J Clin Oncol* 2006;24(19):2998–3006.
51. Douillard JY, Rosell R, De Lena M, et al. Impact of postoperative radiation therapy on survival in patients with complete resection and stage I, II, or IIIA non-small-cell lung cancer treated with adjuvant chemotherapy: the adjuvant Navelbine International Trialist Association (ANITA) Randomized Trial. *Int J Radiat Oncol Biol Phys* 2008;72(3):695–701.
52. Arriagada R, Bergman B, Dunant A, et al. Cisplatin-based adjuvant chemotherapy in patients with completely resected non-small-cell lung cancer. *N Engl J Med* 2004;350(4):351–360.
53. Arriagada R, Dunant A, Pignon JP, et al. Long-term results of the international adjuvant lung cancer trial evaluating adjuvant Cisplatin-based chemotherapy in resected lung cancer. *J Clin Oncol* 2010;28(1):35–42.
54. Winton T, Livingston R, Johnson D, et al. Vinorelbine plus cisplatin vs. observation in resected non-small-cell lung cancer. *N Engl J Med* 2005;352(25):2589–2597.
55. Butts C, Murray N, Maksymiuk A, et al. Randomized phase IIB trial of BLP25 liposome vaccine in stage IIIB and IV non-small-cell lung cancer. *J Clin Oncol* 2005;23(27):6674–6681.
56. Douillard JY, Rosell R, De Lena M, et al. Adjuvant vinorelbine plus cisplatin versus observation in patients with completely resected stage IB-IIIA non-small-cell lung cancer (Adjuvant Navelbine International Trialist Association [ANITA]): a randomised controlled trial. *Lancet Oncol* 2006;7(9):719–727.
57. Pignon JP, Tribodet H, Scagliotti GV, et al. Lung adjuvant cisplatin evaluation: a pooled analysis by the LACE Collaborative Group. *J Clin Oncol* 2008;26(21):3552–3559.
58. Keller SM, Adak S, Wagner H, et al. A randomized trial of postoperative adjuvant therapy in patients with completely resected stage II or IIIA non-small-cell lung cancer. Eastern Cooperative Oncology Group. *N Engl J Med* 2000;343(17):1217–1222.
59. Bradley JD, Paulus R, Graham MV, et al. Phase II trial of postoperative adjuvant paclitaxel/carboplatin and thoracic radiotherapy in resected stage II and IIIA non-small-cell lung cancer: promising long-term results of the radiation therapy oncology group—RTOG 9705. *J Clin Oncol* 2005;23(15):3480–3487.
60. Jaklitsch MT, Herndon JE II, DeCamp MM Jr, et al. Nodal downstaging predicts survival following induction chemotherapy for stage IIIA (N2) non-small cell lung cancer in CALGB protocol #8935. *J Surg Oncol* 2006;94(7):599–606.
61. Feigenberg SJ, Hanlon AL, Langer C, et al. A phase II study of concurrent carboplatin and paclitaxel and thoracic radiotherapy for completely resected stage II and IIIA non-small cell lung cancer. *J Thorac Oncol* 2007;2(4):287–292.
62. Scott WJ, Howington J, Feigenberg S, et al. Treatment of non-small cell lung cancer stage I and stage II: ACCP evidence-based clinical practice guidelines (2nd edition). *Chest* 2007;132(3 Suppl):234S–242S.
63. Heinzerling JH, Kavanagh B, Timmerman RD. Stereotactic ablative radiation therapy for primary lung tumors. *Cancer J* 2011;17(1):28–32.
64. Bradley J, Graham MV, Winter K, et al. Toxicity and outcome results of RTOG 9311: a phase I-II dose-escalation study using three-dimensional conformal radiotherapy in patients with inoperable non-small-cell lung carcinoma. *Int J Radiat Oncol Biol Phys* 2005;61(2):318–328.
65. Hayman JA, Martel MK, Ten Haken RK, et al. Dose escalation in non-small-cell lung cancer using three-dimensional conformal radiation therapy: update of a phase I trial. *J Clin Oncol* 2001;19(1):127–136.
66. Fletcher GH. Clinical dose response curves of human malignant epithelial tumours. *Br J Radiol* 1973;46(542):151.
67. Hadziahmetovic M, Loo BW, Timmerman RD, et al. Stereotactic body radiation therapy (stereotactic ablative radiotherapy) for stage I non-small cell lung cancer—updates of radiobiology, techniques, and clinical outcomes. *Discov Med* 2010;9(48):411–417.
68. McGarry RC, Papiez L, Williams M, et al. Stereotactic body radiation therapy of early-stage non-small-cell lung carcinoma: phase I study. *Int J Radiat Oncol Biol Phys* 2005;63(4):1010–1015.
69. Timmerman R, McGarry R, Yiannoutsos C, et al. Excessive toxicity when treating central tumors in a phase II study of stereotactic body radiation therapy for medically inoperable early-stage lung cancer. *J Clin Oncol* 2006;24(30):4833–4839.
70. Haasbeek CJ, Lagerwaard FJ, Slotman BJ, et al. Outcomes of stereotactic ablative radiotherapy for centrally located early-stage lung cancer. *J Thorac Oncol* 2011;6(12):2036–2043.
71. Lagerwaard FJ, Haasbeek CJ, Smit EF, et al. Outcomes of risk-adapted fractionated stereotactic radiotherapy for stage I non-small-cell lung cancer. *Int J Radiat Oncol Biol Phys* 2008;70(3):685–692.
72. Bezjak A, Paulus R, Gaspar L, et al. Primary study endpoint analysis for NRG oncology/RTOG 0813 Trial of Stereotactic Body Radiation Therapy (SBRT) for Centrally Located Non-Small Cell Lung Cancer (NSCLC). *Int J Radiat Oncol Biol Phys* 2016;94(1):5–6.
73. Bezjak A, Paulus R, Gaspar L, et al. Efficacy and toxicity analysis of NRG oncology/RTOG 0813 Trial of Stereotactic Body Radiation Therapy (SBRT) for Centrally Located Non-Small Cell Lung Cancer (NSCLC). *Int J Radiat Oncol Biol Phys* 2016;96(2):S8.
74. Baumann P, Nyman J, Hoyer M, et al. Outcome in a prospective phase II trial of medically inoperable stage I non-small-cell lung cancer patients treated with stereotactic body radiotherapy. *J Clin Oncol* 2009;27(20):3290–3296.
75. Fakiris AJ, McGarry RC, Yiannoutsos CT, et al. Stereotactic body radiation therapy for early-stage non-small-cell lung carcinoma: four-year results of a prospective phase II study. *Int J Radiat Oncol Biol Phys* 2009;75(3):677–682.
76. Timmerman R, Paulus R, Galvin J, et al. Stereotactic body radiation therapy for inoperable early stage lung cancer. *JAMA* 2010;303(11):1070–1076.
77. Nagata Y, Takayama K, Matsuo Y, et al. Clinical outcomes of a phase I/II study of 48 Gy of stereotactic body radiotherapy in 4 fractions for primary lung cancer using a stereotactic body frame. *Int J Radiat Oncol Biol Phys* 2005;63(5):1427–1431.
78. Onishi H, Shirato H, Nagata Y, et al. Hypofractionated stereotactic radiotherapy (HypoFXSRT) for stage I non-small cell lung cancer: updated results of 257 patients in a Japanese multi-institutional study. *J Thorac Oncol* 2007;2(7 Suppl 3):S94–S100.
79. Videtic GM, Hu C, Singh AK, et al. A randomized phase 2 study comparing 2 stereotactic body radiation therapy schedules for medically inoperable patients with stage I peripheral non-small cell lung cancer: NRG Oncology RTOG 0915 (NCCTG N0927). *Int J Radiat Oncol Biol Phys* 2015;93(4):757–764.
80. Kubota K, Furuse K, Kawahara M, et al. Role of radiotherapy in combined modality treatment of locally advanced non-small-cell lung cancer. *J Clin Oncol* 1994;12(8):1547–1552.
81. Perez CA, Stanley K, Rubin P, et al. A prospective randomized study of various irradiation doses and fractionation schedules in the treatment of inoperable non-oat-cell carcinoma of the lung. Preliminary report by the Radiation Therapy Oncology Group. *Cancer* 1980;45(11):2744–2753.
82. Perez CA, Pajak TF, Rubin P, et al. Long-term observations of the patterns of failure in patients with unresectable non-oat cell carcinoma of the lung treated with definitive radiotherapy. Report by the Radiation Therapy Oncology Group. *Cancer* 1987;59(11):1874–1881.
83. Cox JD, Azarnia N, Byhardt RW, Shin KH, Emami B, Pajak TF. A randomized phase I/II trial of hyperfractionated radiation therapy with total doses of 60.0 Gy to 79.2 Gy: possible survival benefit with greater than or equal to 69.6 Gy in favorable patients with Radiation Therapy Oncology Group stage III non-small-cell lung carcinoma: Report of Radiation Therapy Oncology Group 83-11. *J Clin Oncol* 1990;8(9):1543–1555.
84. Bradley JD, Ieumwananonthachai N, Purdy JA, et al. Gross tumor volume, critical prognostic factor in patients treated with three-dimensional conformal radiation therapy for non-small-cell lung carcinoma. *Int J Radiat Oncol Biol Phys* 2002;52(1):49–57.
85. Rengan R, Rosenzweig KE, Venkatraman E, et al. Improved local control with higher doses of radiation in large-volume stage III non-small-cell lung cancer. *Int J Radiat Oncol Biol Phys* 2004;60(3):741–747.
86. Cannon DM, Mehta MP, Adkison JB, et al. Dose-limiting toxicity after hypofractionated dose-escalated radiotherapy in non-small-cell lung cancer. *J Clin Oncol* 2013;31(34):4343–4348.
87. Jeremic B. Low incidence of isolated nodal failures after involved-field radiation therapy for non-small-cell lung cancer: blinded by the light? *J Clin Oncol* 2007;25(35):5543–5545.
88. Senan S, Burgers S, Samson MJ, et al. Can elective nodal irradiation be omitted in stage III non-small-cell lung cancer? Analysis of recurrences in a phase II study of induction chemotherapy and involved-field radiotherapy. *Int J Radiat Oncol Biol Phys* 2002;54(4):999–1006.
89. Rosenzweig KE, Sura S, Jackson A, et al. Involved-field radiation therapy for inoperable non small-cell lung cancer. *J Clin Oncol* 2007;25(35):5557–5561.
90. Kepka L, Bujko K, Zolciak-Siwinska A, et al. Incidental irradiation of mediastinal and hilar lymph node stations during 3D-conformal radiotherapy for non-small cell lung cancer. *Acta Oncol* 2008;47(5):954–961.
91. Yuan S, Sun X, Li M, et al. A randomized study of involved-field irradiation versus elective nodal irradiation in combination with concurrent chemotherapy for inoperable stage III nonsmall cell lung cancer. *Am J Clin Oncol* 2007;30(3):239–244.
92. Fernandes AT, Shen J, Finlay J, et al. Elective nodal irradiation (ENI) vs. involved field radiotherapy (IFRT) for locally advanced non-small cell lung cancer (NSCLC): a comparative analysis of toxicities and clinical outcomes. *Radiother Oncol* 2010;95(2):178–184.
93. Dillman RO, Herndon J, Seagren SL, et al. Improved survival in stage III non-small-cell lung cancer: seven-year follow-up of cancer and leukemia group B (CALGB) 8433 trial. *J Natl Cancer Inst* 1996;88(17):1210–1215.
94. Sause W, Kolesar P, Taylor S, et al. Final results of phase III trial in regionally advanced unresectable non-small cell lung cancer—Radiation Therapy Oncology Group, Eastern Cooperative Oncology Group, and Southwest Oncology Group. *Chest* 2000;117(2):358–364.
95. Le Chevalier T, Arriagada R, Tarayre M, et al. Significant effect of adjuvant chemotherapy on survival in locally advanced non-small-cell lung carcinoma. *J Natl Cancer Inst* 1992;84(1):58.
96. Chemotherapy in non-small cell lung cancer: a meta-analysis using updated data on individual patients from 52 randomised clinical trials. Non-small Cell Lung Cancer Collaborative Group. *BMJ* 1995;311(7010):899–909.
97. Schaake-Koning C, van den Bogaert W, Dalesio O, et al. Effects of concomitant cisplatin and radiotherapy on inoperable non-small-cell lung cancer. *N Engl J Med* 1992;326(8):524–530.
98. O'Rourke N, Roque IFM, Farre Bernado N, et al. Concurrent chemoradiotherapy in non-small cell lung cancer. *Cochrane Database Syst Rev* 2010(6):CD002140.
99. Furuse K, Fukuoka M, Kawahara M, et al. Phase III study of concurrent versus sequential thoracic radiotherapy in combination with mitomycin, vindesine, and cisplatin in unresectable stage III non-small-cell lung cancer. *J Clin Oncol* 1999;17(9):2692–2699.

100. Curran WJ, Scott C, Langer CJ, et al. Long-term benefit is observed in a phase III comparison of sequential vs concurrent chemo-radiation for patients with unresected stage III NSCLC: RTOG 9410. *Proc Am Soc Clin Oncol* 2003;22:2499.

101. Curran W, Paulus R, Langer CJ, et al. Sequential vs. concurrent chemoradiation for stage III non-small cell lung cancer (NSCLC): randomized phase III trial RTOG 9410. *J Natl Cancer Inst* 2011;103(19):1452–1460.

102. Auperin A, Rolland E, Curran WJ, et al. Concomitant radio-chemotherapy (RT-CT) versus sequential RT-CT in locally advanced non-small cell lung cancer (NSCLC): a meta-analysis using individual patient data (IPD) from randomised clinical trials (RCTs). *J Thorac Oncol* 2007;2(8):S310.

103. Cox JD, Pajak TF, Asbell S, et al. Interruptions of high-dose radiation therapy decrease long-term survival of favorable patients with unresectable non-small cell carcinoma of the lung: analysis of 1244 cases from 3 Radiation Therapy Oncology Group (RTOG) trials. *Int J Radiat Oncol Biol Phys* 1993;27(3):493–498.

104. Machtay M, Hsu C, Komaki R, et al. Effect of overall treatment time on outcomes after concurrent chemoradiation for locally advanced non-small-cell lung carcinoma: analysis of the Radiation Therapy Oncology Group (RTOG) experience. *Int J Radiat Oncol Biol Phys* 2005;63(3):667–671.

105. Turrisi AT III, Kim K, Blum R, et al. Twice-daily compared with once-daily thoracic radiotherapy in limited small-cell lung cancer treated concurrently with cisplatin and etoposide. *N Engl J Med* 1999;340(4):265–271.

106. Hanna N, Neubauer M, Yiannoutsos C, et al. Phase III study of cisplatin, etoposide, and concurrent chest radiation with or without consolidation docetaxel in patients with inoperable stage III non-small-cell lung cancer: the Hoosier Oncology Group and U.S. Oncology. *J Clin Oncol* 2008;26(35):5755–5760.

107. Movsas B, Scott C, Langer C, et al. Randomized trial of amifostine in locally advanced non-small-cell lung cancer patients receiving chemotherapy and hyperfractionated radiation: radiation therapy oncology group trial 98-01. *J Clin Oncol* 2005;23(10):2145–2154.

108. Vokes EE, Herndon JE II, Crawford J, et al. Randomized phase II study of cisplatin with gemcitabine or paclitaxel or vinorelbine as induction chemotherapy followed by concomitant chemoradiotherapy for stage IIIB non-small-cell lung cancer: cancer and leukemia group B study 9431. *J Clin Oncol* 2002;20(20):4191–4198.

109. Vokes EE, Herndon JE II, Kelley MJ, et al. Induction chemotherapy followed by chemoradiotherapy compared with chemoradiotherapy alone for regionally advanced unresectable stage III non-small-cell lung cancer: Cancer and Leukemia Group B. *J Clin Oncol* 2007;25(13):1698–1704.

110. Belani CP, Choy H, Bonomi P, et al. Combined chemoradiotherapy regimens of paclitaxel and carboplatin for locally advanced non-small-cell lung cancer: a randomized phase II locally advanced multi-modality protocol. *J Clin Oncol* 2005;23(25):5883–5891.

111. Yamamoto N, Nakagawa K, Nishimura Y, et al. Phase III study comparing second- and third-generation regimens with concurrent thoracic radiotherapy in patients with unresectable stage III non-small-cell lung cancer: West Japan Thoracic Oncology Group WJTOG0105. *J Clin Oncol* 2010;28(23):3739–3745.

112. Segawa Y, Kiura K, Takigawa N, et al. Phase III trial comparing docetaxel and cisplatin combination chemotherapy with mitomycin, vindesine, and cisplatin combination chemotherapy with concurrent thoracic radiotherapy in locally advanced non-small-cell lung cancer: OLCSG 0007. *J Clin Oncol* 2010;28(20):3299–3306.

113. Liang J, Bi N, Wu S, et al. Etoposide and cisplatin vs paclitaxel and carboplatin with concurrent thoracic radiotherapy in unresectable stage III non-small cell lung cancer: a multicenter randomized phase III trial. *Ann Oncol* 2017;28(4):777–783.

114. Santana-Davila R, Devisetty K, Szabo A, et al. Cisplatin and etoposide versus carboplatin and paclitaxel with concurrent radiotherapy for stage III non-small-cell lung cancer: an analysis of Veterans Health Administration data. *J Clin Oncol* 2015;33(6):567–574.

115. Palma DA, Senan S, Tsujino K, et al. Predicting radiation pneumonitis after chemoradiation therapy for lung cancer: an international individual patient data meta-analysis. *Int J Radiat Oncol Biol Phys* 2013;85(2):444–450.

116. Senan S, Brade A, Wang LH, et al. PROCLAIM: randomized phase III trial of pemetrexed-cisplatin or etoposide-cisplatin plus thoracic radiation therapy followed by consolidation chemotherapy in locally advanced nonsquamous non-small-cell lung cancer. *J Clin Oncol* 2016;34(9):953–962.

117. Auperin A, Le Pechoux C, Rolland E, et al. Meta-analysis of concomitant versus sequential radiochemotherapy in locally advanced non-small-cell lung cancer. *J Clin Oncol* 2010;28(13):2181–2190.

118. Senzer N. A phase III randomized evaluation of amifostine in stage IIIA/IIIB non-small cell lung cancer patients receiving concurrent carboplatin, paclitaxel, and radiation therapy followed by gemcitabine and cisplatin intensification: preliminary findings. *Semin Oncol* 2002;29(6 Suppl 19):38–41.

119. Kelly K, Chansky K, Gaspar LE, et al. Phase III trial of maintenance gefitinib or placebo after concurrent chemoradiotherapy and docetaxel consolidation in inoperable stage III non-small-cell lung cancer: SWOG S0023. *J Clin Oncol* 2008;26(15):2450–2456.

120. Ahn JS, Ahn YC, Kim JH, et al. Multinational randomized phase III trial with or without consolidation chemotherapy using docetaxel and cisplatin after concurrent chemoradiation in inoperable stage III non-small-cell lung cancer: KCSG-LU05-04. *J Clin Oncol* 2015;33(24):2660–2666.

121. Bradley JD, Paulus R, Komaki R, et al. Standard-dose versus high-dose conformal radiotherapy with concurrent and consolidation carboplatin plus paclitaxel with or without cetuximab for patients with stage IIIA or IIIB non-small-cell lung cancer (RTOG 0617): a randomised, two-by-two factorial phase 3 study. *Lancet Oncol* 2015;16(2):187–199.

122. Spigel DR, Hainsworth JD, Yardley DA, et al. Tracheoesophageal fistula formation in patients with lung cancer treated with chemoradiation and bevacizumab. *J Clin Oncol* 2010;28(1):43–48.

123. Stinchcombe T, Socinski MA, Moore DT. Phase I/II trial of bevacizumab (B) and erlotinib (E) with induction (IND) and concurrent (CON) carboplatin (Cb)/paclitaxel (P) and 74 Gy of thoracic conformal radiotherapy (TCRT) in stage III non-small cell lung cancer (NSCLC). *J Clin Oncol* 2011;29:S7016.

124. Butts C, Socinski MA, Mitchell PL, et al. Tecemotide (L-BLP25) versus placebo after chemoradiotherapy for stage III non-small-cell lung cancer (START): a randomised, double-blind, phase 3 trial. *Lancet Oncol* 2014;15(1):59–68.

125. Bradley JD, Bae K, Graham MV, et al. Primary analysis of the phase II component of a phase I/II dose intensification study using three-dimensional conformal radiation therapy and concurrent chemotherapy for patients with inoperable non-small-cell lung cancer: RTOG 0117. *J Clin Oncol* 2010;28(14):2475–2480.

126. Socinski MA, Blackstock AW, Bogart JA, et al. Randomized phase II trial of induction chemotherapy followed by concurrent chemotherapy and dose-escalated thoracic conformal radiotherapy (74 Gy) in stage III non-small-cell lung cancer: CALGB 30105. *J Clin Oncol* 2008;26(15):2457–2463.

127. Arcasoy SM, Jett JR. Superior pulmonary sulcus tumors and Pancoast's syndrome. *N Engl J Med* 1997;337(19):1370–1376.

128. Rusch VW, Giroux DJ, Kraut MJ, et al. Induction chemoradiation and surgical resection for superior sulcus non-small-cell lung carcinomas: long-term results of Southwest Oncology Group Trial 9416 (Intergroup Trial 0160). *J Clin Oncol* 2007;25(3):313–318.

129. Kunitoh H, Kato H, Tsuboi M, et al. Phase II trial of preoperative chemoradiotherapy followed by surgical resection in patients with superior sulcus non-small-cell lung cancers: report of Japan Clinical Oncology Group trial 9806. *J Clin Oncol* 2008;26(4):644–649.

130. Gomez DR, Cox JD, Roth JA, et al. A prospective phase 2 study of surgery followed by chemotherapy and radiation for superior sulcus tumors. *Cancer* 2012;118(2):444–451.

131. Komaki R, Roth JA, Walsh GL, et al. Outcome predictors for 143 patients with superior sulcus tumors treated by multidisciplinary approach at the University of Texas M. D. Anderson Cancer Center. *Int J Radiat Oncol Biol Phys* 2000;48(2):347–354.

132. Komaki R, Roh J, Cox JD, et al. Superior sulcus tumors: results of irradiation of 36 patients. *Cancer* 1981;48(7):1563–1568.

133. Kappers I, Klomp HM, Koolen MG, et al. Concurrent high-dose radiotherapy with low-dose chemotherapy in patients with non-small cell lung cancer of the superior sulcus. *Radiother Oncol* 2011;101(2):278–283.

134. Harris KM, Adams H, Lloyd DC, et al. The effect on apparent size of simulated pulmonary nodules of using three standard CT window settings. *Clin Radiol* 1993;47(4):241–244.

135. Nestle U, Walter K, Schmidt S, et al. 18F-deoxyglucose positron emission tomography (FDG-PET) for the planning of radiotherapy in lung cancer: high impact in patients with atelectasis. *Int J Radiat Oncol Biol Phys* 1999;44(3):593–597.

136. Chapet O, Kong FM, Quint LE, et al. CT-based definition of thoracic lymph node stations: an atlas from the University of Michigan. *Int J Radiat Oncol Biol Phys* 2005;63(1):170–178.

137. Dwamena BA, Sonnad SS, Angobaldo JO, et al. Metastases from non-small cell lung cancer: mediastinal staging in the 1990s—meta-analytic comparison of PET and CT. *Radiology* 1999;213(2):530–536.

138. Grills IS, Fitch DL, Goldstein NS, et al. Clinicopathologic analysis of microscopic extension in lung adenocarcinoma: defining clinical target volume for radiotherapy. *Int J Radiat Oncol Biol Phys* 2007;69(2):334–341.

139. Giraud P, Antoine M, Larrouy A, et al. Evaluation of microscopic tumor extension in non-small-cell lung cancer for three-dimensional conformal radiotherapy planning. *Int J Radiat Oncol Biol Phys* 2000;48(4):1015–1024.

140. Yuan S, Meng X, Yu J, et al. Determining optimal clinical target volume margins on the basis of microscopic extracapsular extension of metastatic nodes in patients with non-small-cell lung cancer. *Int J Radiat Oncol Biol Phys* 2007;67(3):727–734.

141. Vedam SS, Keall PJ, Kini VR, et al. Acquiring a four-dimensional computed tomography dataset using an external respiratory signal. *Phys Med Biol* 2003;48(1):45–62.

142. Lagerwaard FJ, Van Sornsen de Koste JR, Nijssen-Visser MR, et al. Multiple "slow" CT scans for incorporating lung tumor mobility in radiotherapy planning. *Int J Radiat Oncol Biol Phys* 2001;51(4):932–937.

143. Grills IS, Hugo G, Kestin LL, et al. Image-guided radiotherapy via daily online cone-beam CT substantially reduces margin requirements for stereotactic lung radiotherapy. *Int J Radiat Oncol Biol Phys* 2008;70(4):1045–1056.

144. Hugo GD, Yan D, Liang J. Population and patient-specific target margins for 4D adaptive radiotherapy to account for intra- and inter-fraction variation in lung tumour position. *Phys Med Biol* 2007;52(1):257–274.

145. Marks LB, Ten Haken RK, Martel MK. Guest editor's introduction to QUANTEC: a users guide. *Int J Radiat Oncol Biol Phys* 2010;76(3 Suppl):S1–S2.

146. Bentzen SM, Constine LS, Deasy JO, et al. Quantitative Analyses of Normal Tissue Effects in the Clinic (QUANTEC): an introduction to the scientific issues. *Int J Radiat Oncol Biol Phys* 2010;76(3 Suppl):S3–S9.

147. Benedict SH, Yenice KM, Followill D, et al. Stereotactic body radiation therapy: the report of AAPM Task Group 101. *Med Phys* 2010;37(8):4078–4101.

148. Senan S, De Ruysscher D, Giraud P, et al. Literature-based recommendations for treatment planning and execution in high-dose radiotherapy for lung cancer. *Radiother Oncol* 2004;71(2):139–146.

149. Shah C, Grills IS, Kestin LL, et al. Intrafraction variation of mean tumor position during image-guided hypofractionated stereotactic body radiotherapy for lung cancer. *Int J Radiat Oncol Biol Phys* 2012;82(5):1636–1641.

150. Keall PJ, Mageras GS, Balter JM, et al. The management of respiratory motion in radiation oncology report of AAPM Task Group 76. *Med Phys* 2006;33(10):3874–3900.

151. Rietzel E, Liu AK, Doppke KP, et al. Design of 4D treatment planning target volumes. *Int J Radiat Oncol Biol Phys* 2006;66(1):287–295.

152. Korreman SS. Image-guided radiotherapy and motion management in lung cancer. *Br J Radiol* 2015;88(1051):20150100.

153. Lagerwaard FJ, Senan S. Lung cancer: intensity-modulated radiation therapy, four-dimensional imaging and mobility management. *Front Radiat Ther Oncol* 2007;40:239–252.

154. International Commission on Radiation Units and Measurements (ICRU). *Prescribing, recording and reporting photon beam therapy.* Bethesda, MD: ICRU, 1993.

155. Bissonnette J, Purdie T, Sharpe MB. Image-guided stereotactic lung radiation therapy. *Radiother Oncol* 2005;76(Suppl 1):S15–16.

156. Allen AM, Czerminska M, Janne PA, et al. Fatal pneumonitis associated with intensity-modulated radiation therapy for mesothelioma. *Int J Radiat Oncol Biol Phys* 2006;65(3):640–645.

157. Bortfeld T, Jokivarsi K, Goitein M, et al. Effects of intra-fraction motion on IMRT dose delivery: statistical analysis and simulation. *Phys Med Biol* 2002;47(13):2203–2220.

158. Sterpin E, Tomsej M, De Smedt B, et al. Monte carlo evaluation of the AAA treatment planning algorithm in a heterogeneous multilayer phantom and IMRT clinical treatments for an Elekta SL25 linear accelerator. *Med Phys* 2007;34(5):1665–1677.

159. Fragoso M, Wen N, Kumar S, et al. Dosimetric verification and clinical evaluation of a new commercially available Monte Carlo-based dose algorithm for application in stereotactic body radiation therapy (SBRT) treatment planning. *Phys Med Biol* 2010;55(16):4445–4464.

160. Moran JM, Dempsey M, Eisbruch A. Safety considerations for IMRT. *Pract Radiat Oncol* 2008;1(3):190–195.

161. Das IJ, Ding GX, Ahnesjo A. Small fields: nonequilibrium radiation dosimetry. *Med Phys* 2008;35(1):206–215.

162. Xiao Y, Kry SF, Popple R, et al. Flattening filter-free accelerators: a report from the AAPM Therapy Emerging Technology Assessment Work Group. *J Appl Clin Med Phys* 2015;16(3):5219.

163. Vassiliev ON, Kry SF, Chang JY, et al. Stereotactic radiotherapy for lung cancer using a flattening filter free Clinac. *J Appl Clin Med Phys* 2009;10(1):2880.

164. Dang TM, Peters MJ, Hickey B, et al. Efficacy of flattening-filter-free beam in stereotactic body radiation therapy planning and treatment: a systematic review with meta-analysis. *J Med Imaging Radiat Oncol* 2017;61(3):379–387.

165. Prendergast BM, Dobelbower MC, Bonner JA, et al. Stereotactic body radiation therapy (SBRT) for lung malignancies: preliminary toxicity results using a flattening filter-free linear accelerator operating at 2400 monitor units per minute. *Radiat Oncol* 2013;8:273.

166. Chang JY, Jabbour SK, De Ruysscher D, et al. Consensus statement on proton therapy in early-stage and locally advanced non-small cell lung cancer. *Int J Radiat Oncol Biol Phys* 2016;95(1):505–516.

167. Bush DA, Cheek G, Zaheer S, et al. High-dose hypofractionated proton beam radiation therapy is safe and effective for central and peripheral early-stage non-small cell lung cancer: results of a 12-year experience at Loma Linda University Medical Center. *Int J Radiat Oncol Biol Phys* 2013;86(5):964–968.

168. Hata M, Tokuuye K, Kagei K, et al. Hypofractionated high-dose proton beam therapy for stage I non-small-cell lung cancer: preliminary results of a phase I/II clinical study. *Int J Radiat Oncol Biol Phys* 2007;68(3):786–793.

169. Chang JY, Komaki R, Wen HY, et al. Toxicity and patterns of failure of adaptive/ablative proton therapy for early-stage, medically inoperable non-small cell lung cancer. *Int J Radiat Oncol Biol Phys* 2011;80(5):1350–1357.

170. Miyamoto T, Baba M, Sugane T, et al. Carbon ion radiotherapy for stage I non-small cell lung cancer using a regimen of four fractions during 1 week. *J Thorac Oncol* 2007;2(10):916–926.

171. Chang JY, Komaki R, Lu C, et al. Phase 2 study of high-dose proton therapy with concurrent chemotherapy for unresectable stage III nonsmall cell lung cancer. *Cancer* 2011;117(20):4707–4713.

172. Liao Z, Lee J, Komaki R, et al. Bayesian randomized trial comparing intensity-modulated radiation therapy vs. passively scattered proton therapy for locally advanced non-small cell lung carcinoma. *J Clin Oncol* 2016;34(Suppl):abstr 8500.

173. Gomez DR, Gillin M, Liao Z, et al. Phase 1 study of dose escalation in hypofractionated proton beam therapy for non-small cell lung cancer. *Int J Radiat Oncol Biol Phys* 2013;86(4):665–670.

174. Rapp E, Pater JL, Willan A, et al. Chemotherapy can prolong survival in patients with advanced non-small-cell lung cancer—report of a Canadian multicenter randomized trial. *J Clin Oncol* 1988;6(4):633–641.

175. Schiller JH, Harrington D, Belani CP, et al. Comparison of four chemotherapy regimens for advanced non-small-cell lung cancer. *N Engl J Med* 2002;346(2):92–98.

176. Soon YY, Stockler MR, Askie LM, et al. Duration of chemotherapy for advanced non-small-cell lung cancer: a systematic review and meta-analysis of randomized trials. *J Clin Oncol* 2009;27(20):3277–3283.

177. Paz-Ares LG, de Marinis F, Dediu M, et al. PARAMOUNT: final overall survival results of the phase III study of maintenance pemetrexed versus placebo immediately after induction treatment with pemetrexed plus cisplatin for advanced nonsquamous non-small-cell lung cancer. *J Clin Oncol* 2013;31(23):2895–2902.

178. Shepherd FA, Dancey J, Ramlau R, et al. Prospective randomized trial of docetaxel versus best supportive care in patients with non-small-cell lung cancer previously treated with platinum-based chemotherapy. *J Clin Oncol* 2000;18(10):2095–2103.

179. Hanna N, Shepherd FA, Fossella FV, et al. Randomized phase III trial of pemetrexed versus docetaxel in patients with non-small-cell lung cancer previously treated with chemotherapy. *J Clin Oncol* 2004;22(9):1589–1597.

180. Pardoll DM. The blockade of immune checkpoints in cancer immunotherapy. *Nat Rev Cancer* 2012;12(4):252–264.

181. Rafei H, El-Bahesh E, Finianos A, et al. Immune-based therapies for non-small cell lung cancer. *Anticancer Res* 2017;37(2):377–387.

182. Reck M, Rodriguez-Abreu D, Robinson AG, et al. Pembrolizumab versus chemotherapy for PD-L1-positive non-small-cell lung cancer. *N Engl J Med* 2016;375(19):1823–1833.

183. Langer CJ, Gadgeel SM, Borghaei H, et al. Carboplatin and pemetrexed with or without pembrolizumab for advanced, non-squamous non-small-cell lung cancer: a randomised, phase 2 cohort of the open-label KEYNOTE-021 study. *Lancet Oncol* 2016;17(11):1497–1508.

184. Schadendorf D, Hodi FS, Robert C, et al. Pooled analysis of long-term survival data from phase II and phase III trials of ipilimumab in unresectable or metastatic melanoma. *J Clin Oncol* 2015;33(17):1889–1894.

185. Lynch TJ, Bell DW, Sordella R, et al. Activating mutations in the epidermal growth factor receptor underlying responsiveness of non-small-cell lung cancer to gefitinib. *N Engl J Med* 2004;350(21):2129–2139.

186. Mok TS, Wu YL, Thongprasert S, et al. Gefitinib or carboplatin-paclitaxel in pulmonary adenocarcinoma. *N Engl J Med* 2009;361(10):947–957.

187. Urata Y, Katakami N, Morita S, et al. Randomized phase III study comparing gefitinib with erlotinib in patients with previously treated advanced lung adenocarcinoma: WJOG 5108L. *J Clin Oncol* 2016;34(27):3248–3257.

188. Yang JJ, Zhou Q, Yan HH, et al. A phase III randomised controlled trial of erlotinib vs gefitinib in advanced non-small cell lung cancer with EGFR mutations. *Br J Cancer* 2017;116(5):568–574.

189. Park K, Tan EH, O'Byrne K, et al. Afatinib versus gefitinib as first-line treatment of patients with EGFR mutation-positive non-small-cell lung cancer (LUX-Lung 7): a phase 2B, open-label, randomised controlled trial. *Lancet Oncol* 2016;17(5):577–589.

190. Sequist LV, Waltman BA, Dias-Santagata D, et al. Genotypic and histological evolution of lung cancers acquiring resistance to EGFR inhibitors. *Sci Transl Med* 2011;3(75):75ra26.

191. Mok TS, Wu YL, Ahn MJ, et al. Osimertinib or platinum-pemetrexed in EGFR T790M-positive lung cancer. *N Engl J Med* 2017;376(7):629–640.

192. Camidge DR, Theodoro M, Maxson DA, et al. Correlations between the percentage of tumor cells showing an anaplastic lymphoma kinase (ALK) gene rearrangement, ALK signal copy number, and response to crizotinib therapy in ALK fluorescence in situ hybridization-positive nonsmall cell lung cancer. *Cancer* 2012;118(18):4486–4494.

193. Solomon BJ, Mok T, Kim DW, et al. First-line crizotinib versus chemotherapy in ALK-positive lung cancer. *N Engl J Med* 2014;371(23):2167–2177.

194. Kim DW, Mehra R, Tan DS, et al. Activity and safety of ceritinib in patients with ALK-rearranged non-small-cell lung cancer (ASCEND-1): updated results from the multicentre, open-label, phase 1 trial. *Lancet Oncol* 2016;17(4):452–463.

195. Shaw AT, Spigel DR, Tan DS, et al. MINI01.01: whole body and intracranial efficacy of ceritinib in ALK-inhibitor naive patients with ALK+ NSCLC and brain metastases: results of ASCEND 1 and 3: topic: medical oncology. *J Thorac Oncol* 2016;11(11S):S256.

196. Ou SH, Sommers KR, Azada MC, et al. Alectinib induces a durable (>15 months) complete response in an ALK-positive non-small cell lung cancer patient who progressed on crizotinib with diffuse leptomeningeal carcinomatosis. *Oncologist* 2015;20(2):224–226.

197. Bergethon K, Shaw AT, Ou SH, et al. ROS1 rearrangements define a unique molecular class of lung cancers. *J Clin Oncol* 2012;30(8):863–870.

198. Shaw AT, Ou SH, Bang YJ, et al. Crizotinib in ROS1-rearranged non-small-cell lung cancer. *N Engl J Med* 2014;371(21):1963–1971.

199. Kris MG, Johnson BE, Berry LD, et al. Using multiplexed assays of oncogenic drivers in lung cancers to select targeted drugs. *JAMA* 2014;311(19):1998–2006.

200. Planchard D, Kim TM, Mazieres J, et al. Dabrafenib in patients with BRAF(V600E)-positive advanced non-small-cell lung cancer: a single-arm, multicentre, open-label, phase 2 trial. *Lancet Oncol* 2016;17(5):642–650.

201. Hyman DM, Puzanov I, Subbiah V, et al. Vemurafenib in multiple nonmelanoma cancers with BRAF V600 mutations. *N Engl J Med* 2015;373(8):726–736.

202. Ashworth AB, Senan S, Palma DA, et al. An individual patient data metaanalysis of outcomes and prognostic factors after treatment of oligometastatic non-small cell lung cancer. *Clin Lung Cancer* 2014;15(5):346–355.

203. Gomez DR, Blumenschein GR, Jr., Lee JJ, et al. Local consolidative therapy versus maintenance therapy or observation for patients with oligometastatic non-small-cell lung cancer without progression after first-line systemic therapy: a multicentre, randomised, controlled, phase 2 study. *Lancet Oncol* 2016;17(12):1672–1682.

204. Iyengar P, Kavanagh BD, Wardak Z, et al. Phase II trial of stereotactic body radiation therapy combined with erlotinib for patients with limited but progressive metastatic non-small-cell lung cancer. *J Clin Oncol* 2014;32(34):3824–3830.

205. Gan GN, Weickhardt AJ, Scheier B, et al. Stereotactic radiation therapy can safely and durably control sites of extra-central nervous system oligoprogressive disease in anaplastic lymphoma kinase-positive lung cancer patients receiving crizotinib. *Int J Radiat Oncol Biol Phys* 2014;88(4):892–898.

206. Weickhardt AJ, Scheier B, Burke JM, et al. Local ablative therapy of oligoprogressive disease prolongs disease control by tyrosine kinase inhibitors in oncogene-addicted non-small-cell lung cancer. *J Thorac Oncol* 2012;7(12):1807–1814.

207. Numico G, Russi E, Merlano M. Best supportive care in non-small cell lung cancer: is there a role for radiotherapy and chemotherapy? *Lung Cancer* 2001;32(3):213–226.

208. Kelly JF, Delclos ME, Morice RC, et al. High-dose-rate endobronchial brachytherapy effectively palliates symptoms due to airway tumors: the 10-year M. D. Anderson cancer center experience. *Int J Radiat Oncol Biol Phys* 2000;48(3):697–702.

209. Wilson LD, Detterbeck FC, Yahalom J. Clinical practice. Superior vena cava syndrome with malignant causes. *N Engl J Med* 2007;356(18):1862–1869.

210. Ordonez NG. Value of thyroid transcription factor-1 immunostaining in distinguishing small cell lung carcinomas from other small cell carcinomas. *Am J Surg Pathol* 2000;24(9):1217–1223.

211. Jackman DM, Johnson BE. Small-cell lung cancer. *Lancet* 2005;366(9494):1385–1396.

212. Zelen M. Keynote address on biostatistics and data retrieval. *Cancer Chemother Rep* 1973;4(2):31–42.

213. Shepherd FA, Laskey J, Evans WK, et al. Cushing's syndrome associated with ectopic corticotropin production and small-cell lung cancer. *J Clin Oncol* 1992;10(1):21–27.

214. Yu JB, Decker RH, Detterbeck FC, et al. Surveillance epidemiology and end results evaluation of the role of surgery for stage I small cell lung cancer. *J Thorac Oncol* 2010;5(2):215–219.

215. Tsuchiya R, Suzuki K, Ichinose Y, et al. Phase II trial of postoperative adjuvant cisplatin and etoposide in patients with completely resected stage I-IIIa small cell lung cancer: the Japan Clinical Oncology Lung Cancer Study Group Trial (JCOG9101). *J Thorac Cardiovasc Surg* 2005;129(5):977–983.

216. Warde P, Payne D. Does thoracic irradiation improve survival and local control in limited-stage small-cell carcinoma of the lung? A meta-analysis. *J Clin Oncol* 1992;10(6):890–895.

217. Arriagada R, Pignon JP, Ihde DC, et al. Effect of thoracic radiotherapy on mortality in limited small cell lung cancer. A meta-analysis of 13 randomized trials among 2,140 patients. *Anticancer Res* 1994;14(1B):333–335.

218. Jeremic B, Shibamoto Y, Nikolic N, et al. Role of radiation therapy in the combined-modality treatment of patients with extensive disease small-cell lung cancer: a randomized study. *J Clin Oncol* 1999;17(7):2092–2099.

219. Slotman BJ, van Tinteren H, Praag JO, et al. Use of thoracic radiotherapy for extensive stage small-cell lung cancer: a phase 3 randomised controlled trial. *Lancet* 2015;385(9962):36–42.

220. Slotman B, Faivre-Finn C, Kramer G, et al. Prophylactic cranial irradiation in extensive small-cell lung cancer. *N Engl J Med* 2007;357(7):664–672.

221. Auperin A, Arriagada R, Pignon JP, et al. Prophylactic cranial irradiation for patients with small-cell lung cancer in complete remission. Prophylactic Cranial Irradiation Overview Collaborative Group. *N Engl J Med* 1999;341(7):476–484.

222. Takada M, Fukuoka M, Kawahara M, et al. Phase III study of concurrent versus sequential thoracic radiotherapy in combination with cisplatin and etoposide for limited-stage small-cell lung cancer: results of the Japan Clinical Oncology Group Study 9104. *J Clin Oncol* 2002;20(14):3054–3060.

223. Murray N, Coy P, Pater JL, et al. Importance of timing for thoracic irradiation in the combined modality treatment of limited-stage small-cell lung cancer. The National Cancer Institute of Canada Clinical Trials Group. *J Clin Oncol* 1993;11(2):336–344.

224. Fried DB, Morris DE, Poole C, et al. Systematic review evaluating the timing of thoracic radiation therapy in combined modality therapy for limited-stage small-cell lung cancer. *J Clin Oncol* 2004;22(23):4837–4845.

225. Komaki R, Swann RS, Ettinger DS, et al. Phase I study of thoracic radiation dose escalation with concurrent chemotherapy for patients with limited small-cell lung cancer: Report of Radiation Therapy Oncology Group (RTOG) protocol 97-12. *Int J Radiat Oncol Biol Phys* 2005;62(2):342–350.

226. Komaki R, Paulus R, Ettinger D. Patterns of first failure in a phase ii study of accelerated high dose thoracic radiation therapy (TRT) with concurrent chemotherapy for limited small-cell lung cancer (LSCLC): Radiation Therapy Oncology Group (RTOG) 0239. *Int J Radiat Oncol Biol Phys* 2009; 75(3 Suppl):S34–S35.

227. Choi NC, Herndon JE, 2nd, Rosenman J, et al. Phase I study to determine the maximum-tolerated dose of radiation in standard daily and hyperfractionated-accelerated twice-daily radiation schedules with concurrent chemotherapy for limited-stage small-cell lung cancer. *J Clin Oncol* 1998;16(11):3528–3536.

228. Bogart JA, Herndon JE II, Lyss AP, et al. 70 Gy thoracic radiotherapy is feasible concurrent with chemotherapy for limited-stage small-cell lung cancer: analysis of Cancer and Leukemia Group B study 39808. *Int J Radiat Oncol Biol Phys* 2004;59(2):460–468.

229. Faivre-Finn C, Falk S, Ashcroft L, et al. Protocol for the CONVERT trial-Concurrent ONce-daily VErsus twice-daily Radiotherapy: an international 2-arm randomised controlled trial of concurrent chemoradiotherapy comparing twice-daily and once-daily radiotherapy schedules in patients with limited stage small cell lung cancer (LS-SCLC) and good performance status. *BMJ Open* 2016;6(1):e009849.

230. Kies MS, Mira JG, Crowley JJ, et al. Multimodal therapy for limited small-cell lung cancer: a randomized study of induction combination chemotherapy with or without thoracic radiation in complete responders; and with wide-field versus reduced-field radiation in partial responders: a Southwest Oncology Group Study. *J Clin Oncol* 1987;5(4):592–600.

231. Liengswangwong V, Bonner JA, Shaw EG, et al. Limited-stage small-cell lung cancer: patterns of intrathoracic recurrence and the implications for thoracic radiotherapy. *J Clin Oncol* 1994;12(3):496–502.

232. Arriagada R, Pellae-Cosset B, Ladron de Guevara JC, et al. Alternating radiotherapy and chemotherapy schedules in limited small cell lung cancer: analysis of local chest recurrences. *Radiother Oncol* 1991;20(2):91–98.

233. Gore EM, Hu C, Sun AY, et al. Randomized Phase II Study Comparing Prophylactic Cranial Irradiation Alone to Prophylactic Cranial Irradiation and Consolidative Extracranial Irradiation for Extensive-Disease Small Cell Lung Cancer (ED SCLC): NRG Oncology RTOG 0937. *J Thorac Oncol* 2017;12(10):1561–1570.

234. Takahashi T, Yamanaka T, Seto T, et al. Prophylactic cranial irradiation versus observation in patients with extensive-disease small-cell lung cancer: a multicentre, randomised, open-label, phase 3 trial. *Lancet Oncol* 2017;18(5):663–671.

235. Le Pechoux C, Dunant A, Senan S, et al. Standard-dose versus higher-dose prophylactic cranial irradiation (PCI) in patients with limited-stage small-cell lung cancer in complete remission after chemotherapy and thoracic radiotherapy (PCI 99-01, EORTC 22003-08004, RTOG 0212, and IFCT 99-01): a randomised clinical trial. *Lancet Oncol* 2009;10(5):467–474.

236. Wolfson AH, Bae K, Komaki R, et al. Primary analysis of a phase II randomized trial Radiation Therapy Oncology Group (RTOG) 0212: impact of different total doses and schedules of prophylactic cranial irradiation on chronic neurotoxicity and quality of life for patients with limited-disease small-cell lung cancer. *Int J Radiat Oncol Biol Phys* 2011;81(1):77–84.

237. Rossi A, Di Maio M, Chiodini P, et al. Carboplatin- or cisplatin-based chemotherapy in first-line treatment of small-cell lung cancer: the COCIS meta-analysis of individual patient data. *J Clin Oncol* 2012;30(14):1692–1698.

238. O'Brien ME, Ciuleanu TE, Tsekov H, et al. Phase III trial comparing supportive care alone with supportive care with oral topotecan in patients with relapsed small-cell lung cancer. *J Clin Oncol* 2006;24(34):5441–5447.

239. Antonia SJ, Lopez-Martin JA, Bendell J, et al. Nivolumab alone and nivolumab plus ipilimumab in recurrent small-cell lung cancer (CheckMate 032): a multicentre, open-label, phase 1/2 trial. *Lancet Oncol* 2016;17(7):883–895.

240. Rudin CM, Pietanza MC, Bauer TM, et al. Rovalpituzumab tesirine, a DLL3-targeted antibody-drug conjugate, in recurrent small-cell lung cancer: a first-in-human, first-in-class, open-label, phase 1 study. *Lancet Oncol* 2017;18(1):42–51.

241. Emami B, Lyman J, Brown A, et al. Tolerance of normal tissue to therapeutic irradiation. *Int J Radiat Oncol Biol Phys* 1991;21(1):109–122.

242. Marks LB, Bentzen SM, Deasy JO, et al. Radiation dose-volume effects in the lung. *Int J Radiat Oncol Biol Phys* 2010;76(3 Suppl):S70–S76.

243. Chun SG, Hu C, Choy H, et al. Impact of Intensity-Modulated Radiation Therapy Technique for Locally Advanced Non-Small-Cell Lung Cancer: a Secondary Analysis of the NRG Oncology RTOG 0617 Randomized Clinical Trial. *J Clin Oncol* 2017;35(1):56–62.

244. Barriger RB, Forquer JA, Brabham JG, et al. A dose-volume analysis of radiation pneumonitis in non-small cell lung cancer patients treated with stereotactic body radiation therapy. *Int J Radiat Oncol Biol Phys* 2012;82(1):457–462.

245. Huang EX, Hope AJ, Lindsay PE, et al. Heart irradiation as a risk factor for radiation pneumonitis. *Acta Oncol* 2011;50(1):51–60.

246. Miller ME, Bush D. Review of the Federal Child Labor Regulations: updating hazardous and prohibited occupations. *Am J Ind Med* 2004;45(2):218–221.

247. Bradley JD, Hope A, El Naqa I, et al. A nomogram to predict radiation pneumonitis, derived from a combined analysis of RTOG 9311 and institutional data. *Int J Radiat Oncol Biol Phys* 2007;69(4):985–992.

248. Ozturk B, Egehan I, Atavci S, et al. Pentoxifylline in prevention of radiation-induced lung toxicity in patients with breast and lung cancer: a double-blind randomized trial. *Int J Radiat Oncol Biol Phys* 2004;58(1):213–219.

249. Ward WF, Molteni A, Ts'ao CH. Radiation-induced endothelial dysfunction and fibrosis in rat lung: modification by the angiotensin converting enzyme inhibitor CL242817. *Radiat Res* 1989;117(2):342–350.

250. Qiao WB, Zhao YH, Zhao YB, et al. Clinical and dosimetric factors of radiation-induced esophageal injury: radiation-induced esophageal toxicity. *World J Gastroenterol* 2005;11(17):2626–2629.

251. Belderbos J, Heemsbergen W, Hoogeman M, et al. Acute esophageal toxicity in non-small cell lung cancer patients after high dose conformal radiotherapy. *Radiother Oncol* 2005;75(2):157–164.

252. Hooning MJ, Botma A, Aleman BM, et al. Long-term risk of cardiovascular disease in 10-year survivors of breast cancer. *J Natl Cancer Inst* 2007;99(5):365–375.

253. Churn M, Clough V, Slater A. Early onset of bilateral brachial plexopathy during mantle radiotherapy for Hodgkin's disease. *Clin Oncol* 2000;12(5):289–291.

254. Kong FM, Ritter T, Quint DJ, et al. Consideration of dose limits for organs at risk of thoracic radiotherapy: atlas for lung, proximal bronchial tree, esophagus, spinal cord, ribs, and brachial plexus. *Int J Radiat Oncol Biol Phys* 2011;81(5):1442–1457.

255. Forquer JA, Fakiris AJ, Timmerman RD, et al. Brachial plexopathy from stereotactic body radiotherapy in early-stage NSCLC: dose-limiting toxicity in apical tumor sites. *Radiother Oncol* 2009;93(3):408–413.

256. De Ruysscher D, Faivre-Finn C, Le Pechoux C, et al. High-dose re-irradiation following radical radiotherapy for non-small-cell lung cancer. *Lancet Oncol* 2014;15(13):e620–e624.

257. McAvoy S, Ciura K, Wei C, et al. Definitive reirradiation for locoregionally recurrent non-small cell lung cancer with proton beam therapy or intensity modulated radiation therapy: predictors of high-grade toxicity and survival outcomes. *Int J Radiat Oncol Biol Phys* 2014;90(4):819–827.

258. Siddiqui F, Liu AK, Watkins-Bruner D, et al. Patient-reported outcomes and survivorship in radiation oncology: overcoming the cons. *J Clin Oncol* 2014;32(26):2920–2927.

259. Movsas B, Hu C, Sloan J, et al. Quality of Life Analysis of a Radiation Dose-Escalation Study of Patients With Non-Small-Cell Lung Cancer: A Secondary Analysis of the Radiation Therapy Oncology Group 0617 Randomized Clinical Trial. *JAMA Oncol* 2016;2(3):359–367.

260. Sprangers MA, Sloan JA, Veenhoven R, et al. The establishment of the GENEQOL consortium to investigate the genetic disposition of patient-reported quality-of-life outcomes. *Twin Res Hum Genet* 2009;12(3):301–311.

261. Movsas B. PROceeding With the Patient-Reported Outcomes (PROs) Version of the Common Terminology Criteria for Adverse Events. *JAMA Oncol* 2015;1(8):1059–1060.

262. Dueck AC, Mendoza TR, Mitchell SA, et al. Validity and Reliability of the US National Cancer Institute's Patient-Reported Outcomes Version of the Common Terminology Criteria for Adverse Events (PRO-CTCAE). *JAMA Oncol* 2015;1(8):1051–1059.

263. Detmar SB, Muller MJ, Schornagel JH, et al. Health-related quality-of-life assessments and patient-physician communication: a randomized controlled trial. *JAMA* 2002;288(23):3027–3034.

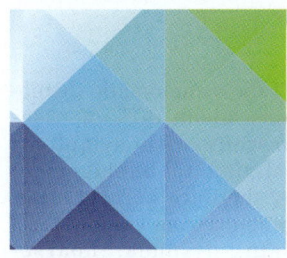

CHAPTER 55

Mediastinum and Trachea

Shervin M. Shirvani, Daniel R. Gomez, Clifton David Fuller, and Charles R. Thomas Jr.

MEDIASTINAL TUMORS

The mediastinum is a trapezoidal structure in the center of the thoracic cavity. It is bound by the sternum anteriorly, the vertebral column posteriorly, and the lungs and pleura laterally (Fig. 55.1). The diaphragm forms the floor of the mediastinum, whereas the thoracic outlet at the first thoracic vertebra, its rib, and the manubrium form the roof.[1] Conceptually, it is helpful to divide the mediastinum into anterior, middle, and posterior compartments, but no anatomic barriers specifically separate these regions.[2-4] The anterior mediastinum is the space anterior to the pericardium and great vessels and is occupied by the thymus, lymph nodes, and small vessels. The middle mediastinum is composed of the heart, proximal great vessels, central airway structures, and lymph nodes. The International Thymic Malignancy Interest Group (ITMIG) has codified these anatomic boundaries into a series of computed tomography (CT)-based radiographic standards for aiding clinical diagnosis and research.[5]

Tracheal anatomy is depicted in Figure 55.2. The posterior mediastinum is posterior to the heart and great vessels and contains the sympathetic chain ganglia, vagus nerve, thoracic duct, and esophagus. Given the number of structures within the mediastinum, it is not surprising that a heterogenous group of malignancies can arise in this location.

Thymic, neurogenic, germinal, and mesenchymal tissues may all give rise to neoplasms. The malignancies that occur within the various compartments in the mediastinum are listed in Table 55.1.

Incidence of Primary Mediastinal Tumors

Lymphomas represent the most common type of mediastinal tumor. The malignancies with the next highest incidence—tumors of thymic origin—are rare and represent about 0.2% to 1.5% of all malignancies.[6] Thymic carcinomas are especially rare and account for only 0.06% of all thymic neoplasms.[7] The frequency and prevalence of primary mediastinal tumors seem to be increasing over time.[8-11] Adults generally develop thymic tumors and lymphomas, but they can also develop germ cell tumors and carcinomas.[11,12] Neurogenic tumors are usually seen in children.[9,13,14]

THYMOMAS

The thymus gland is an irregular lobulated lymphoepithelial organ in the anterior mediastinum. Embryologically, the thymus is derived from the endoderm of the lower portion of the third pharyngeal pouch and involutes during adulthood, gradually being replaced by adipose tissue. Its blood supply is from the internal mammary arteries, and its venous return drains to the innominate and internal thoracic veins. Its lymphatics drain into the lower cervical, internal mammary, and hilar lymph nodes.

The vast majority of thymic tumors are thymomas, 90% of which are found in the anterosuperior mediastinum; other variants occur in the middle and posterior mediastinum or neck.[15] Thymomas are epithelial tumors associated with an exuberant lymphoid component composed of immature cortical thymocytes. Although lymphomas, carcinoid tumors, and germ cell tumors can all arise within the thymus, only thymomas, thymic carcinomas, and thymolipomas arise from true thymic elements.

FIGURE 55.1. Anatomy of the mediastinum.

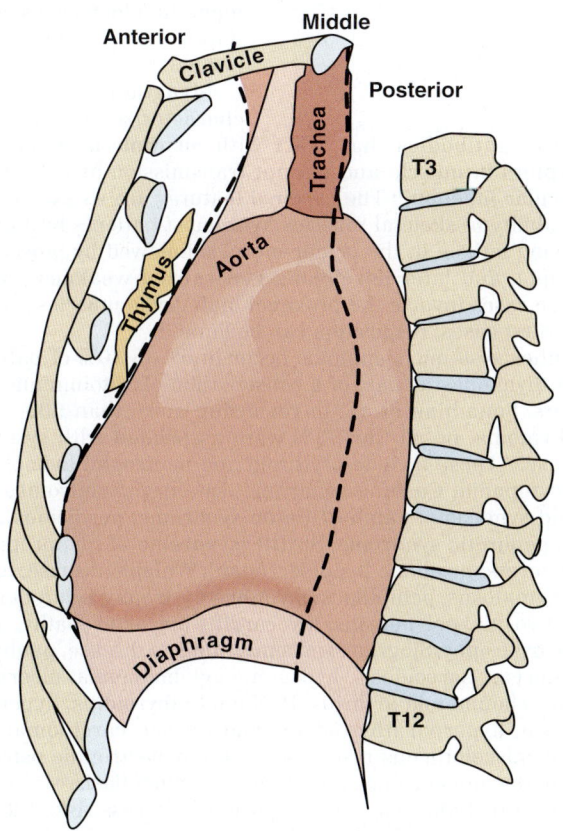

FIGURE 55.2. Representative schema of the trachea. Note the lateral longitudinal anastomotic artery running parallel to the organ and the intercartilaginous branches feeding each tracheal segment. The trachea resides in close proximity to the esophagus.

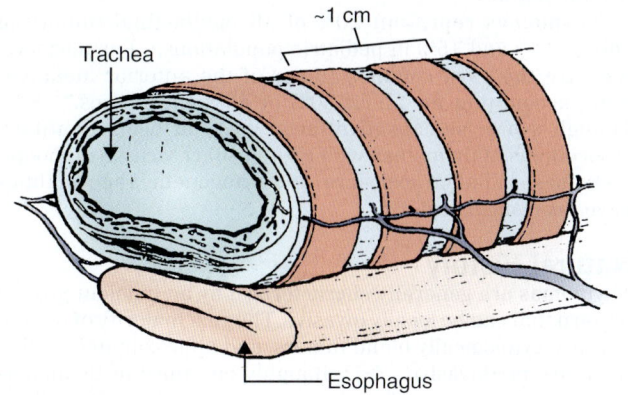

TABLE 55.1 HISTOLOGIES OF TUMORS APPEARING IN THE VARIOUS COMPARTMENTS OF THE MEDIASTINUM

Anterior (Anterosuperior)	Middle	Posterior
Thymic tumors	Lymphomas	Lymphomas
Thymomas	Cysts	Neurogenic tumors
Thymic carcinomas	Bronchogenic	Peripheral nerves
Thymic cysts	Foregut	Malignant peripheral nerve sheath tumors
Carcinoids	Pericardial	Schwannomas
Thymolipomas	Thoracic duct	Neurosarcomas
Lymphomas	Meningoceles	Sympathetic ganglia
Hodgkin disease	Mesenchymal tumors	Ganglioneuroblastomas
Non–Hodgkin lymphomas	Tracheal tumors	Ganglioneuromas
Undifferentiated	Carcinomas	Neuroblastomas
Germ cell tumors	Cardiac and pericardial tumors	Paraganglia
Seminomas	Hernias	Paragangliomas
Nonseminomas	Hiatal	Mesenchymal tumors
Embryonal carcinomas	Morgagni	Endocrine tumors
Choriocarcinomas	Vascular tumors	Esophageal tumors and cysts
Mixed germ cell tumors	Ascending aortic	Hiatal hernias
Teratomas (dermoid cysts)	Transverse arch	Lateral thoracic meningoceles
Endocrine tumors	Descending aortic	
Parathyroid adenomas	Great vessels	
Thyroid tumors	Lymphadenopathy	
Mesenchymal tumors	Inflammatory	
Amyloid tumors	Granulomatous	
Castleman disease	Sarcoidosis	
Chordomas		
Extramedullary hematopoiesis		
Fibromas, fibrosarcomas, malignant fibrous histiocytoma		
Hemangiomas, hemangioendotheliomas, hemangiopericytomas		
Intrathoracic meningioma		
Lipomas, liposarcomas		
Leiomyomas, leiomyosarcomas, leiomyoblastomas		
Lymphangiomas, lymphangiosarcoma, lymphangiomyomatosis		
Mesotheliomas		
Mesenchymomas		
Myxomas		
Rhabdomyosarcomas, rhabdomyomas		
Xanthogranulomas		
Morgagni hernias		

Epidemiology

Thymomas are exceedingly rare. The Surveillance, Epidemiology, and End Results (SEER) project reported the thymoma incidence to be 0.13 per 100,000 person-years.[16] For patients with associated myasthenia gravis, the peak age is in the 4th decade, whereas for patients without myasthenia gravis, the peak age is in the 7th decade or later.[17–22] According to the SEER data, the incidence of thymoma increases into the 8th decade of age and then decreases.[23] Thymomas are more common in men than in women (P = .007) and are most common among Asians/Pacific Islanders (0.49 per 100,000 person-years).

Thymomas represent 20% of all mediastinal tumors in adults[4,12,24,25] and 15% in pediatric populations.[15] Furthermore, they are the most common tumor of the anterior mediastinum, accounting for about 30% of all such masses.[9–11,15,26,27] Though a precise causative factor has not been identified, associations of thymomas with Epstein-Barr virus, lymphoepitheliomas, radiation exposure, and cytogenetic abnormalities have been suggested.[28–34]

Natural History

Thymomas are generally characterized by an indolent growth pattern that can be locally invasive. The vast majority of thymomas are cytologically bland tumors, and approximately half of them are noninvasive.[11,22,35–45] Roughly one-third of thymomas are asymptomatic and found incidentally on chest x-rays.[41,42,46]

Of the symptomatic thymomas, about 40% of cases present with symptoms relating to impingement by the intrathoracic mass, ranging from cough, chest pain, dyspnea, hoarseness, superior vena cava obstruction, and even tumor hemorrhage.[47] The remainder of symptomatic patients present with one of several parathymic syndromes, the most common of which are myasthenia gravis, benign cytopenias, hypogammaglobulinemia, and polymyositis.[17,20,48–51]

Myasthenia gravis has the highest incidence among the parathymic syndromes and occurs in approximately 45% of patients with thymomas, with the reported prevalence in studies involving more than 100 patients ranging from 10% to 67%.[18,19,21,22,52,53] Conversely, only 10% to 15% of patients with myasthenia gravis have a thymoma; 60% of myasthenia patients will have thymic lymphoid hyperplasia, and roughly 25% will have a normal thymus.[19,54–57] Thymectomy results in clinical improvement in most cases even when the thymus is normal.[58]

Myasthenia gravis is characterized by the presence of antibodies that react with nicotinic acetylcholine receptors in muscle and disrupt transmission at the neuromuscular junction.[54] The cardinal features are weakness and fatigability of skeletal muscles, with most patients first experiencing fatigue in the ocular muscles followed by ptosis and diplopia, and later developing generalized weakness. More severe cases involve the proximal limb girdle muscles and, in the worst cases, respiration can be limited.[59–61]

Other systemic symptoms occur in 5% to 10% of patients with thymomas as part of a constellation of autoimmune disorders. Souadjian et al., in reviewing more than 500 cases of thymoma, noted that 71% were associated with systemic disease.[51] These include erythroid and neutrophil hypoplasia, pancytopenia, Cushing syndrome, DiGeorge syndrome, carcinoid syndrome, Lambert-Eaton syndrome, pernicious anemia, nephrotic syndrome, SIADH [syndrome of inappropriate antidiuretic hormone hypersecretion], Whipple disease, lupus erythematosus, pemphigus, myotonic dystrophy, scleroderma, polymyositis, polyneuritis, myocarditis polyarthropathy, myotonic dystrophy, Sjogren syndrome, Addison disease, panhypopituitarism, sarcoidosis, hypogammaglobulinemia, ulcerative colitis, rheumatoid arthritis, Hashimoto thyroiditis, hyperthyroidism, hyperparathyroidism, and thyroid carcinoma.[15,62–65] Other miscellaneous diseases include hypertrophic osteoarthropathy and chronic mucocutaneous candidiasis.[64]

Several studies have also reported an excess risk of developing a second primary malignancy of approximately 15%

among thymoma patients.[48,49,51,66–68] An aberrant immune system is postulated to be a mechanism for the development of these metachronous malignancies.[69] The highest excess risk of subsequent malignancy appears to be for non-Hodgkin lymphoma, but thymoma patients are also at risk for digestive system malignancies and soft tissue sarcomas.[23] Patients with higher-grade and advanced stage tumors seem to have the highest risk of metachronous extrathymic malignancies.[69]

The vast majority of thymomas are indolent, but if the tumors spread, they most commonly implant on regional pleural surfaces (so-called drop metastases), which can progress to malignant pleural effusions.[17] Other mechanisms for metastases are uncommon for this histology. The rate of lymphogenous metastasis in a large database of 1093 patients with thymomas was 1.8%, with 90% of positive lymph nodes located in the anterior mediastinum.[70] Only rarely do thymomas spread hematogenously, though metastases have been reported in the liver, lung, and bone.[71]

Diagnosis

The radiographic presence of an anterior mediastinal mass is suggestive of a thymic tumor as these histologies account for the majority of masses in this location (see Table 55.1).[11] A clinical diagnosis of thymoma can sometimes be made based on the presence of an anterior mediastinal mass in conjunction with clear evidence of a parathymic syndrome such as myasthenia. The absence of symptoms suggestive of lymphoma (fevers, weight loss, adenopathy) or tell-tale radiographic findings for rare histologies such as teratoma are further clues suggestive of a thymic malignancy.

Nonetheless, histologic confirmation is usually required to establish a definitive diagnosis. Biopsy can be performed via a fine needle aspiration, bronchoscopy, mediastinoscopy, video-assisted thoracoscopy, or open biopsy. Historically, biopsies were assumed to be relatively contraindicated because of a concern for tumor spillage into the pleural space when the capsule was breached.[72,73] However, no cases of seeding of a needle tract or the biopsy site have been reported, and only three recurrences in thoracotomy scars have been reported.[74,75] In fact, multivariate analysis in one series of 136 patients being treated for thymomas showed better survival among patients who underwent biopsy before surgery ($P = .056$).[49] Therefore, many centers routinely obtain biopsy samples of anterior mediastinal tumors for histologic assessment.[19,48,74,76–79]

When thymoma is suspected or confirmed, the diagnostic workup begins with a careful evaluation for myasthenia gravis. Routine blood work for common associated syndromes should be done, with serum alpha-fetoprotein and beta-human chorionic gonadotropin in men to rule out a germ cell tumor.[80] In addition to laboratory studies, imaging is a hallmark of thymoma diagnosis and treatment planning.

Plain film chest x-rays were historically the main diagnostic modality for identifying and measuring thymic tumors. Thymomas tend to appear as ovoid, smooth, and unilateral masses occupying the space between the thoracic inlet and the cardiophrenic angle.[81] More advanced presentations may present an irregular border between the mediastinum and the lung, suggesting lung invasion, or elevation of the diaphragm if the phrenic nerve has been infiltrated.

CT is the most common technique for visualization of thymomas and other anterior mediastinal masses.[44,82–84] Magnetic resonance imaging (MRI) can provide more detail when needed, delineating the musculoskeletal anatomy and neurovascular structures of the mediastinum.[85–87] MRI may also improve sensitivity for defining the soft tissue extent of the mass in addition to providing information regarding tumor grade and invasiveness beyond that which can be gleaned from CT. Common features indicative of a high-grade tumor

include low T2-signal foci within the mass, the presence of mediastinal lymphadenopathy, an incomplete capsule, and inhomogeneous enhancement.[88,89]

The use of ^{18}F-fluorodeoxyglucose positron emission tomography (PET) is expanding for visualizing several types of malignancies, including thymoma. In the mediastinum, the results of PET can be confounded by the physiologic uptake of fluorodeoxyglucose by the thymus in children and young adults.[90–93] Nevertheless, this imaging modality has continued to show promise for disease detection and for evaluating prognosis. Recent studies have shown that PET not only can improve the sensitivity of diagnosis but also can be helpful for establishing the grade of the disease and for distinguishing thymoma from thymic carcinoma, which tends to have significantly higher metabolic activity.[94–98] In terms of distinguishing among lower- and higher-risk thymomas, maximum standardized uptake value may lack sensitivity, though some emerging data suggest that homogenously distributed uptake is more characteristic of lower-risk thymomas (types A, AB, and B1).[99]

In one provocative study in which 49 patients with thymic tumors underwent PET imaging, the rate of fluorodeoxyglucose uptake was compared with the expression of several biologic markers, including GLUT1, GLUT3, HIF-1α, vascular endothelial growth factor (VEGF), microvessel density, CD31 and CD34, p53, and bcl-2. The authors found a direct correlation between fluorodeoxyglucose uptake on PET and expression of GLUT1, HIF-1α, VEGF, and p53 as well as microvessel density, and several of these markers also correlated with tumor grade.[100] Predicting the presence of HIF-1α may also be germane to therapeutic strategies that seek to match radiation dose to the presence of hypoxia and its associated radioresistance in the tumor microenvironment.[99]

These findings are important because they imply that metabolic response may be a viable marker for measuring treatment efficacy. Figure 55.3 demonstrates PET findings from a patient with locally advanced thymoma treated with trimodality therapy. Indium 111-octreotide, carbon-11 methionine, and gallium-67 citrate, three other nuclear medicine agents, have also been reported to show some activity for thymic malignancies, but utilization of these modalities has been limited by their lack of sensitivity in distinguishing benign conditions such as thymic hyperplasia from frank neoplasia.[81,101]

Pathologic Classification

The varied appearances and the frequent absence of classic malignant features have made thymomas challenging to classify pathologically. Disagreements on the prognostic importance of certain pathologic features have led to multiple proposed classification systems (Table 55.2). Indeed, even simple terminology such as "invasive versus noninvasive" or "benign versus malignant" has not accurately captured clinical behavior. Recurrences and metastases after resection have been reported in all large series[18,19,102–104] regardless of disease stage or histologic subtype.[17–19,21,22,43,48,49,103–111] Ultimately, even bland-appearing, noninvasive thymomas have the fundamental characteristics of a malignant tumor in their ability to recur and metastasize.

A historical perspective of thymoma classification systems is illustrative of the challenges of pathologic classification for thymoma. The earliest system, proposed by Bernatz, identified four categories based on the predominant cell type: lymphocytic, epithelial, mixed, and spindle cell.[112] In practice, this classification system poorly correlated with clinical prognosis. Verley and Hollman later also identified four categories: spindle or oval, lymphocyte-rich, differentiated epithelial cell–rich, and undifferentiated epithelial.[103] The first three types are cytologically bland, whereas the fourth category includes pleomorphic tumors with high numbers of mitoses and atypia,

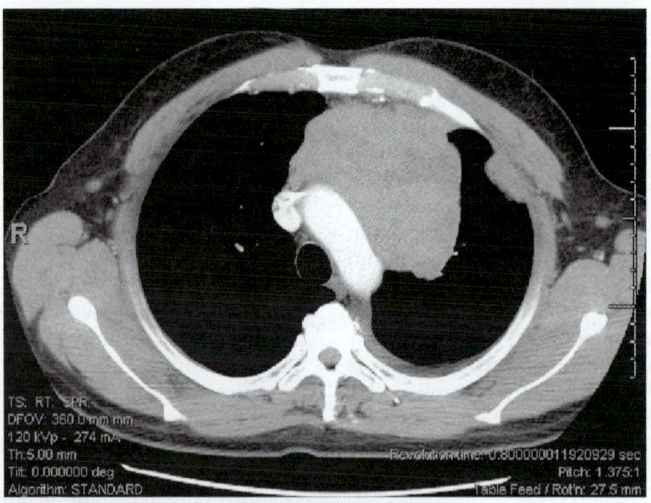

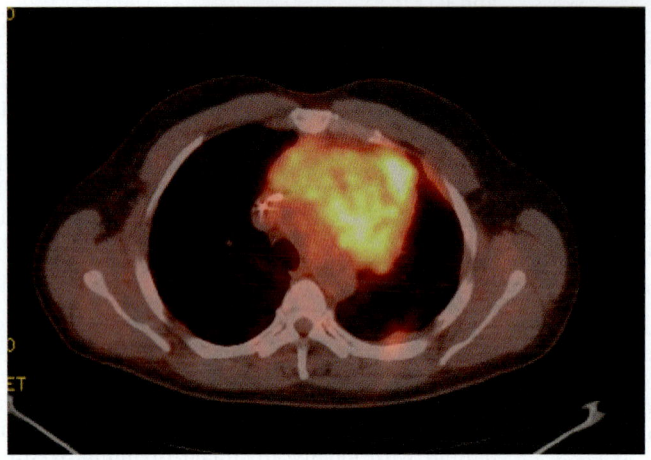
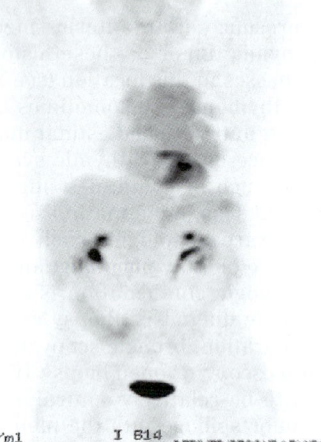

FIGURE 55.3. PET scanning in thymic malignancies. PET imaging has been shown to aid in delineating the extent of disease and assessing for metastases.

which are also considered thymic carcinoma. Unfortunately, this categorization also did not correlate well with prognosis.

A third classification system based on work by Müller-Hermelink et al. based classification on the different subsets of epithelial cells found in the thymus: cortical, medullary, mixed cortical and medullary, and well-differentiated.[113] Although this system was widely used, again a strong like between epithelial cell morphology and clinical prognosis has not been validated.[116] Although some associations have been found, such as cortical thymomas behaving more aggressively and being more often associated with myasthenia gravis, several multivariate analyses have shown that the Müller-Hermelink classification system is not an independent predictor of survival, casting doubt on the link between this histologic classification and prognosis.[17,20,76–78,103,107,116–120] Another confounder for these classification schemes is that they do not consistently correlate with other schemes.[116] Concordance rates for thymomas classified independently by a panel of pathologists were often as low as 35% within one system, although two small studies demonstrated 78% concordance when using the Müller-Hermelink classification system.[121,122] The poor correlation between the histopathology of thymomas and their potential for aggressive malignant behavior or systemic syndromes underlines the need for a consistent and predictive classification system.[44] The current system—the World Health Organization (WHO) classification—represents an important step in this direction though further refinement that perhaps includes a molecular component will likely be required.

The WHO classification, first proposed in 1999 and updated in 2004, is similar to the Müller-Hermelink system but recognizes six different types of thymic tumors (A, AB, B1, B2, B3, C; see Table 55.2).[115,123,124] Type A tumors are composed of neoplastic oval or spindle-shaped epithelial cells without atypia or lymphocytes. Type AB is similar to type A, but with foci of lymphocytes. Type B tumors consist of plump epithelioid cells that can be subdivided into three subtypes defined by increasing proportions of epithelial cells and increasing atypia. Type B1 tumors resemble normal thymic cortex with areas similar to thymic medulla. Type B2 have scattered neoplastic epithelial cells with vesicular nuclei and distinct nucleoli among a heavy population of lymphocytes; perivascular spaces are prominent and a palisading effect of tumor cells along the perivascular spaces may be present.

TABLE 55.2	THYMOMA CLASSIFICATION SYSTEMS		
Bernatz et al. (1961)[112]	Müller-Hermelink and Kirchner (1985)[113]	Suster and Moran (1999)[114]	WHO (1999)[115]
Spindle cell	Medullary	Thymoma, well-differentiated	Type A
–	Mixed		Type AB
–	Predominantly cortical		Type B1
Lymphocyte-rich Lymphoepithelial	Cortical		Type B2
Epithelial-rich	Well-differentiated thymic carcinoma	Atypical thymoma	Type B3
–	High-grade thymic carcinoma	Thymic carcinoma	Type C

TABLE 55.3 MASAOKA STAGING SYSTEM FOR THYMOMAS

Stage		Description
I		Macroscopically completely encapsulated, with no microscopic capsular invasion
II	a	Macroscopic invasion into surrounding mediastinal fatty tissue or mediastinal pleura
	b	Microscopic invasion into the capsule
III		Macroscopic invasion into surrounding organs
IV	a	Pleural or pericardial implants/dissemination
	b	Lymphogenous or hematogenous metastases

Adapted from Masaoka A, Monden Y, Nakahara K, et al. Follow-up study of thymomas with special reference to their clinical stages. *Cancer* 1981;48(11):2485–2492. Copyright © 1981 American Cancer Society. Reprinted by permission of John Wiley & Sons, Inc.

Type B3 is composed of predominantly round or polygonal epithelial cells exhibiting mild atypia admixed with a minor component of lymphocytes; thus, this type resembles what others have described as well-differentiated thymic carcinoma. Thymic carcinomas are designated type C tumors and have cytologic atypia and a cytoarchitecture resembling carcinoma that is distinctly unlike normal thymus tissue.[125]

Concordance rates among different pathologists using the WHO system were reported to be 90% and 95% in two independent studies.[126,127] The most clinically distinct subtypes are type B3, formerly known as well-differentiated thymic carcinoma, and type C, thymic carcinomas. The clinical characteristics associated with the other WHO subtypes still vary considerably, but the WHO system at least seems to correlate well with Masaoka stage (Table 55.3) in studies in which patients were analyzed with the WHO system.[125] The vast majority of type A and AB tumors are Masaoka stage I or II, and the B subtypes tend to resemble the higher Masaoka stages.[125]

With regard to prognosis, the WHO system has been found to have independent prognostic value for disease-specific survival, with only two small studies indicating that stage was the only prognostic variable.[125] Most of the prognostic value of the WHO classification is attributable to type C having distinctly worse survival,[128–130] but even studies that excluded type C could demonstrate WHO type as having independent prognostic value.[130,131]

More recent pathologic studies have provided intriguing insights on prognostic histologic features. In one such study by Shim et al. that involved assessing the effect of stromal lymphocytic infiltration in thymic carcinoma,[132] patients with low levels of CD4+ lymphocytes and CD20+ lymphocytes within the tumor stroma were found to have lower survival rates, and various combinations of CD4+, CD8+, and CD20+ cells were particularly predictive of worse survival outcomes. These authors concluded that these lymphocytes may work together to suppress cancer progression and that combinations of them may be useful for stratifying patients in terms of long-term prognosis.[132]

Molecular Characterization

During the past several years, pathologic classification systems for several thoracic malignancies have been refined by the incorporation of molecular markers. Likewise, there has been vast interest in clinical studies targeting these molecular markers with specific therapeutic agents. These innovations have been explored in thymomas as well, albeit at a smaller scale than non–small cell lung cancer (NSCLC).

Several studies have shown elevated expression of the epidermal growth factor receptor (EGFR) in large percentages of thymic malignancies, similar to what is observed among NSCLC and other epithelial cancers.[133–136] However, among thymic malignancies, the elevated EGFR levels have rarely been associated with accompanying mutations.[137–139] Therefore, targeted EGFR inhibitors have not shown consistent improvements in thymic tumor response or control rates.[140–142]

Other signaling pathways that often show overexpression are the VEGF,[143] IGF-1R,[144] and KIT pathways,[145,146] although again in most circumstances the overexpression takes place mainly in thymic carcinomas rather than thymomas.

More recent studies utilizing genomic, proteomic, and transcriptomic technologies have revealed new discoveries with regard to the molecular biology of thymomas. For instance, Radovich et al. used RNA sequencing to compare the transcriptomes of thymic malignancies to normal thymus tissue and found that large microRNA cluster on chromosome 19 is a hallmark of type A and AB thymoma; this cluster was associated with the PI3K pathway, suggesting a potential role for the use of PI3K inhibitors in this disease.[147] Similarly, Badve et al. conducted whole-genome expression of 34 thymoma patients and identified 4 clusters of thymic tumors that appeared to correlate with histologic classification.[148]

These efforts have recently culminated in a project by the Cancer Genome Atlas Project to molecularly subtype thymic epithelial tumors using a dataset of 120 patients using a robust approach that incorporated DNA mutational analysis, mRNA expression, and somatic copy number alterations.[149] This tour de force analysis identified four distinct subtypes. The first two were characterized, respectively, by general transcription factor II-I mutation or mRNA clusters associated with T-cell signaling expression. The next two subtypes were characterized by the presence or absence of chromosomal stability based upon somatic copy number. These subtypes were associated with disease-free and overall survival. As in other malignancies like breast cancer, the identification of molecular subtypes holds promise for testing of thymomas for their genetic type in the clinic and then selecting treatments or clinical trials based upon the result.[150]

Staging

The most commonly used staging system for thymomas was published by Masaoka et al. in 1981 (Table 55.3).[105] Staging is based on the extent of either macroscopic or microscopic invasion into structures including the thymoma capsule and surrounding mediastinal structures at the time of surgery. Other groups have tried to improve upon the Masaoka system. For example, the French Groupe d'Etudes des Tumeurs Thymiques (GETT) classification (Table 55.4) incorporates completeness of resection, which may be of prognostic value but does not allow patients to be compared independent of treatment factors.[151]

It is a testament to the robustness of Masaoka's classification system that it has persisted nearly unchanged for 30 years. But despite its popularity, areas of ambiguity have persisted, especially with regard to the Masaoka system's tendency to incorporate both clinical and pathologic data. For instance, some clinicians have questioned the precision with which one can assess that a "tumor is adherent to but not breaking through mediastinal pleura." After all, the mediastinal pleura is not typically in the pathologic specimen.[152] Therefore, a

TABLE 55.4 GROUPE D'ETUDES DES TUMEURS THYMIQUES (GETT) THYMOMA STAGING SYSTEM

Stage		Description
I	a	Encapsulated tumor, completely resected
	b	Macroscopically encapsulated tumor, completely resected
		Surgeon suspects mediastinal adhesions and potential capsular invasion
II		Invasive tumor, completely resected
III	a	Invasive tumor, subtotal resection
	b	Invasive tumor, biopsy only
IV	a	Distant pleural implants or supraclavicular metastasis
	b	Distant metastasis

From Gamondes JP, Balawi A, Greenland T, et al. Seventeen years of surgical treatment of thymoma: factors influencing survival. *Eur J Cardiothorac Surg* 1991;5(3):124–131. Reproduced by permission of European Journal of Cardio-Thoracic Surgery.

TABLE 55.5 OVERALL SURVIVAL RATES FOR PATIENTS WITH THYMOMAS AT 5 AND 10 YEARS

Study and Reference	Institution	Study Years	n	% R0	5–Year Survival				10–Year Survival			
					I	II	III	IV	I	II	III	IV
Kondo and Monden[52]	JACS	1990–1994	924	92	100	98	89	71	100	98	78	47
Regnard et al.[161]	ML, Paris	1955–1993	307	85	89	87	68	66	80	78	47	30
Maggi et al.[19]	Torino	Before 1991	241	88	89	71	72	59	87	60	64	40
Rena et al.[130]	Torino	1988–2000	175	84	100	100	100	100	100	100	85	–
Zhu et al.[162]	Fudan, Shanghai	1989–2002	175	89	100	96	78	57	–	–	–	–
Nakahara et al.[22]	Osaka	Before 1988	141	80	100	92	88	47	100	84	77	47
Wilkins et al.[49]	Johns Hopkins	1957–1997	136	68	84	66	63	40	75	50	44	40
Rea et al.[163]	Padua	1970–2001	132	82	93	93	60	36	84	82	51	0
Blumberg et al.[48]	MSKCC	1949–1993	118	73	95	70	50	100	86	54	26	0
Quintanilla-Martinez et al.[117]	MGH	Before 1994	116	94	100	100	70	70	100	100	60	0
Pan et al.[20]	Taipei	1961–1991	112	80	94	85	63	41	87	69	58	22
Elert et al.[164]	Wurzburg	1957–1988	102	–	83	90	46	–	–	–	–	–

JACS, Japanese Association for Chest Surgery; MGH, Massachusetts General Hospital; ML, Marie Lannelongue Hospital, Le Plessis-Robinson, France; MSKCC, Memorial Sloan-Kettering Cancer Center; R0, complete resection.

group headed by the ITMIG proposed a new staging classification in 2013 based upon TNM staging principles.[153] The T-stage—which still drives staging—has been more finely characterized as pathologically observed microscopic invasion into mediastinal fat (T1a), mediastinal pleura (T1b), pericardium (T2), "more resectable" organs (T3), and "less or unresectable" organs (T4).[154] Although it remains to be seen whether this staging system can provide better prognostic information above historical staging systems, at the very least it provides a standard template for communication among physicians and for the design of collaborative trials, an essential contribution by the staging system for the investigation of a rare disease like thymoma.

Prognostic Factors

The two factors that have consistently demonstrated prognostic value in multivariate analyses in large studies are tumor invasiveness (i.e., disease stage) and completeness of resection.[17,18,20,21,35-37,42,48,49,76,102,105,155-159] Disease stage has proven important for prognosis in every large study.[17-19,21,22,43,48,49,102,105,160] Mean overall survival rates at 15 years are 78% for those with stage I disease, 73% for stage II, 30% for stage III, and 8% for stage IV (Table 55.5).[18] At 10 years, mean disease-free survival rates are 92% for those with stage I disease, 87% for stage II, 60% for stage III, and 35% for stage IV (recurrence rates are summarized in Table 55.6).[18,21,102,117,159]

The extent of resection is the other major factor consistently identified as being prognostic in thymic malignancies.[18,48,49,166-168] Patients for whom complete (R0) resections can be done have significantly better survival than do those with R1 or R2 resections.[105,169] R0 resections are almost always possible for stage I tumors, but resectability rates decrease on average to 50% for stage III tumors.[19,22,43,105]

As mentioned previously, the WHO histology classification was found to be independently associated with prognosis. Major studies reporting analyses of stage, histology, and resection status as independent predictors of survival in thymic tumors are summarized in Table 55.7. Other potential prognostic factors are tumor size and the presence of symptoms.[17,48,107] Interestingly, although bulky tumor size was classically defined in terms of a 10-cm threshold, a more recent publication of 154 consecutive patients with thymic epithelial tumors treated in the modern era (2000–2014) demonstrated that a size >4 cm was associated with worse relapse-free survival, even among patients with stage I disease.[170] With regard to symptoms, older series reported that patients with parathymic syndromes such as myasthenia gravis and other autoimmune diseases fared worse than those without such syndromes,[45,48,159] but this finding has not been replicated in newer series.[18,21,22,49,77,78,105,107,157,171-173] Indeed, some studies have found survival to be better for patients with myasthenia gravis,[19,49,174] perhaps because of earlier detection of thymomas.[48,175-177] A study published in 2005 indicated that myasthenia gravis, present in 25% of 1,089 patients from Japan,[53] did not affect 5-year overall survival rates among patients with stage III disease. For patients with stage IV disease, 5-year overall survival rates were 85.1% for patients with myasthenia gravis versus 63.9% for patients without. R0 resection was accomplished in a significantly higher proportion of patients with myasthenia gravis (60%) than those without it (38%).

Another potential prognostic factor is patient age. Patients older than 30 to 40 years may have a better prognosis than younger patients.[17,76,159] Thymomas in children seem to follow a more malignant course than those in adults.[181] Fortunately, malignant thymomas in children are extremely rare.[182]

TABLE 55.6 RECURRENCE RATES OF THYMOMAS

Study and Reference	Study Years	Institution	n	% Receiving			5-Year Recurrence Rates by Stage			
				R0	Chemo	RT	I	II	III	IVa
Kondo and Monden[52]	1990–1994	JACS institutions	862	100	12	32	1	4	28	34
Regnard et al.[161]	1955–1993	ML, Paris	307	85	Few	Half	4	7	16	58
Maggi et al.[19]	Before 1991	Torino	241	88	7	12	2	13	30	25
Wright et al.[165]	1972–2003	MGH	179	90	–	–	0	0	22	41
Rena et al.[130]	1988–2000	Torino	178	84	13	43	1.6	8.6	28	40
Zhu et al.[162]	1989–2002	Fudan, Shanghai	175	80	14	97	4	2.4	43	57
Cowen et al.[26]	1979–1990	FNCLCC	149	42	100	50	0	7	23	25
Wilkins et al.[45]	1957–1997	Johns Hopkins	136	68	7	37	8	10	24	0
Blumberg et al.[48]	1949–1993	MSKCC	118	73	32	58	4	21	47	80
Ruffini et al.[104]	1974–1993	Torino	114	100	–	25	5	10	30	33

FNCLCC, Federation Nationale des Centres de Lutte Contre le Cancer; JACS, Japanese Association for Chest Surgery; MGH, Massachusetts General Hospital; ML, Marie Lannelongue Hospital, Le Plessis-Robinson, France; MSKCC, Memorial Sloan Kettering Cancer Center; R0, complete resection; RT, radiation therapy.

TABLE 55.7 RESULTS OF MULTIVARIATE ANALYSES OF FACTORS PREDICTING THYMOMA-SPECIFIC SURVIVAL

Study and Reference	Institution	Study Years	n	P Value		
				Histology	Stage	R₀
Okamura et al.[178]	Osaka	1957–2000	273	0.05	0.0001	NS
Rieker et al.[179]	Heidelberg	1967–1998	218	<0.0024	<0.001	–
Wright et al.[165]	MGH	1972–2003	179	0.004	0.002	NS
Rena et al.[130a]	Torino	1988–2000	178	0.014	0.012	0.0001
Park et al.[127b]	Yonsei	1992–2002	150	0.019	<0.001	0.947
Rea et al.[163b]	Padua	1970–2001	132	0.0001	0.003	NS
Kondo et al.[180b]	Tokushima	1973–2001	100	NS	0.04	<0.05

[a]Type C excluded.
[b]Overall survival instead of disease-free survival.
MGH, Massachusetts General Hospital; NS, not statistically significant; R₀, complete resection.

General Management

Treatment modalities that have shown activity for thymoma are numerous and include surgery, radiation, cytotoxic chemotherapy, and targeted agents. The optimal utilization and sequencing of these treatments is not well defined by randomized prospective trials. Therefore, treatment selection for these tumors can be daunting. The ITMIG advocates that patients with thymic epithelial tumors are best served in a setting in which multimodality consultation can occur prior to initiation of treatment.[183] The authors agree that multidisciplinary consultation is critical to achieve best outcomes.

Surgery

Surgical resection is the mainstay of treatment for thymomas. A complete en bloc surgical resection (R₀) remains the treatment of choice for all thymomas regardless of invasiveness, except in rare advanced cases with extensive intrathoracic or extrathoracic metastasis. Fortunately, the vast majority (90% to 95%) of thymomas are localized.[184] Operative mortality rates average 2.5% (range 0.7% to 4.9%).[17–19,22,43,48,102,164] Resectability rates for stage I thymomas should approximate 100%, but those rates vary widely for higher-stage thymomas: 43% to 100% (mean 85%) for stage II, 0% to 89% (mean 47%) for stage III, and 0% to 78% (mean 26%) for stage IV.[102]

Because the completeness of resection is such an important prognostic factor, an aggressive surgical approach is justified to remove as much of the lesion as possible at surgery. If residual microscopic disease is suspected of being present (an R₁ operation), metallic clips should be placed to help delineate the radiation field. Whether subtotal resections are beneficial is controversial, with some authors demonstrating better survival when debulking takes place before adjuvant radiation therapy[19,22,52,105,106,159] and others finding no benefit from debulking over biopsy alone.[18,19,22,48,76,151,159,174,185] One large study found significant differences in 5-year survival rates among patients undergoing subtotal resection versus biopsy only (64% vs. 36%) but little difference in 10-year survival rates, suggesting that any benefit may only be in intermediate-term survival.[52]

Traditional surgical techniques for patients with stage I thymic tumors produce 5-year survival rates in excess of 90%, with survival rates decreasing slightly at 10 years,[19,22,65] and with local recurrence rates of <5%. For stage II and III disease, recurrence rates after surgery alone range from 10% to 47%. In a study of more than 100 patients previously treated for thymoma, causes of death were as follows: 38% were related to thymoma (range 19% to 58%), 9% to postoperative causes (range 2% to 19%), 22% to myasthenia gravis (range 16% to 27%), 9% to other autoimmune diseases (range 2% to 19%), and 29% to unrelated causes (including other cancers) (range 8% to 47%).[17–19,21,43,49,103,106,117,159] Recurrence rates are summarized in Table 55.6.

Minimally invasive techniques including video-assisted thoracoscopic (VATS) thymectomy and robotic thymectomy have come to enter use over the last decade. Video-assisted techniques are generally accepted for benign conditions of the thymus, but their appropriateness in oncologic settings is a matter of active investigation. A Japanese center reported on using this procedure to treat 35 patients with clinical stage I thymoma from 1998 to 2009.[186] The authors reported the technique to be safe, with no perioperative deaths and three minor complications. Disease in 20 of the 35 patients was upstaged to Masaoka stage II or III at the time of surgery. At an average follow-up time of 65 months, one patient had experienced recurrence in the bilateral lung.[186] Similarly, a Polish group reported on 24 patients operated on for thymoma with VATS, which resulted in no operative mortality and one bleeding complication.[187] Finally, a Chinese center reported on comparative outcomes between 15 early-stage thymoma patients with myasthenia gravis treated with VATS and 18 patients treated with transsternal technique. The VATS patients achieved similar perioperative morbidity and significantly better oncologic outcomes, although the authors noted that selection bias may have influenced the latter finding as the open sternotomy patients had, on average, more advanced tumors.[188]

Despite this promising safety profile, it is an open question whether the oncologic outcomes will be the same as open procedures. Kimura et al. compared 45 early-stage thymoma patients who underwent VATS thymectomy with 29 patients who underwent open sternotomy.[189] They noted that all three cases of pleural recurrence occurred in the VATS group. Their conclusion was that VATS was oncologically feasible but that the technique should be favored for patients for whom en bloc resection is possible; special caution should be exercised for large or cystic tumors, for which the risk of capsular injury and tumor spillage is high.

Robotic surgical techniques have also become an accepted approach at specialized centers. The potential advantages of robotic techniques include increased rates of preserved pulmonary function, improved cosmesis, and higher rates of patient compliance because of the minimally invasive nature of the surgery.[190] The improved visualization and versatility of the robotic technique may allow for increased radicality of thymectomies by allowing surgeons to achieve resections in challenging anatomies such as patients with tumor located between the aorta and innominate vein or in those with encasement of the left phrenic nerve.[191]

Several institutions have explored the use of robotics in thymectomy, and a few studies have been published. Rückert et al. demonstrated the feasibility of this technique for patients undergoing thymectomy for myasthenia gravis.[192] That same group of investigators then published a retrospective cohort study comparing robotic and nonrobotic thoracoscopic thymectomy and found that rates of remission of myasthenia gravis were actually higher for patients who had received a robotic thymectomy; the authors attributed this finding to the potential for improved mediastinal dissection with the robotic technique.[193] A survey of the utilization of robotic techniques published in 2013 revealed that nearly 3,500 robotic thymectomy cases had been performed at approximately 100 centers worldwide.

Finally, surgeons have recently asked whether patients with early-stage thymoma and no evidence of myasthenia may be served by thymomectomy (removal of the tumor alone, akin to a wide local excision) rather than complete thymectomy. Tseng et al. reported on a cohort of 95 patients treated at a Taiwanese center between 2002 and 2011.[194] Forty-two patients underwent thymomectomy, whereas 53 underwent complete thymectomy. As expected, patients undergoing thymomectomy had lower morbidity and shorter hospitalizations. Intriguingly, after a median follow-up of 57 months, neither the rate of tumor recurrences nor myasthenia neurologic outcomes were significantly different in the two groups.

Section III

Because this was a nonrandomized retrospective study with limited patient numbers and length of follow-up, the results should be interpreted with caution. Nevertheless, minimizing not just surgical technique, but also the surgical target itself, is a compelling subject for further inquiry.

The appropriate use of these newer surgical techniques and surgical paradigms will clearly evolve as more evidence is collected on their safety and oncologic efficacy. Publication of long-term outcomes and development of clinical trials, whenever possible, will be critical for defining the role of these novel approaches in the spectrum of thymic malignancies.

Patterns of Failure After Surgical Resection

The pattern of failure in the overwhelming majority of thymomas is locoregional: 81% of recurrences are local, 9% are distant, and 11% are both.[17,18,43,48,103,104] Figure 55.4 demonstrates that, although recurrences in a radiation field are rare, a significant number of intrathoracic recurrences are observed along pleural surfaces.[195]

Most recurrences arise within 3 to 7 years,[17-19,48,49,104] but recurrence has been documented as late as 32 years after the initial resection.[43,55,172,196,197] Given the tendency for late recurrences, patients require at least 15 years of follow-up after potentially curative therapy.

If technically feasible, the traditional recommendation for recurrence has been surgery and adjuvant radiation.[75,104,198] Most recurrences (50% to 75%) are operable, and of those that are operable, the reported rates of a successful R₀ resection range from 45% to 71%.[48,75,102,104,199] Patients with a recurrence after an R₀ resection generally experience acceptable short-term and long-term results,[75,198] with 10-year actuarial survival rates ranging from 53% to 72%[75,102,104,200]; 10-year survival rates after an incomplete resection, by contrast, range from 0% to 35%.[18,75,102,104,200]

Despite the historical tendency to reresect operable recurrences, some emerging data suggest that this recommendation for reresection should be tempered by the high rate of additional recurrences. In one study from Memorial Sloan-Kettering Cancer Center, of 25 patients who experienced recurrent disease after initial resection, 11 (44%) had disease that was amenable to reresection. In that same study, 50% of patients undergoing surgery for recurrent disease had an R₀ resection, but 82% of these patients still experienced a second recurrence. The authors concluded that "despite the historical enthusiasm for re-resection...reoperation should be considered only in selected patients."[201]

When recurrent disease is unresectable, radiation and chemotherapy have been used with modest results: 5-year overall survival rates reportedly range from 25% to 50%, with poorer longer-term survival.[19,48,102,104,199,202]

Radiation Therapy

Adjuvant Radiation After Complete Resection

Recurrence rates for stage I thymomas after an R₀ resection are so low that radiation is considered unlikely to offer improvement. More commonly, radiation therapy is offered as an adjuvant treatment for patients with resected stage II and III thymomas or those with incompletely resected tumors. However, patterns of care studies demonstrate significant controversy even around these indications; some centers recommend adjuvant radiation for all patients,[22,106] others recommend adjuvant radiation for stage II and III thymomas,[18,65,79,151,159] and still others recommend radiation only after an incomplete resection.[52,151,159] The reason for this diversity of opinions is that the evidence regarding adjuvant radiation is retrospective, and, because of the rarity of thymoma, studies span many decades. Nonetheless, because disease stage and completeness of resection are such important prognostic factors, analyses of adjuvant radiation have tended to focus on these factors.

For completely resected stage II thymoma, studies have been mixed with regard to local control benefit of adjuvant radiotherapy, with some studies showing trends toward better local control after adjuvant radiation, others finding no difference in recurrence rates, and one series reporting worse results with adjuvant radiation.[52,104,195-198] A report by Chang et al. of patients with completely resected stage II or III thymoma demonstrated similar overall survival rates but improved disease-free survival rates with adjuvant radiation therapy (93% with radiation vs. 70% without).[203] In counterpoint, Berman et al. found that the local recurrence rate among 74 patients after complete resection for stage II disease was only 3% and was not affected by receipt of adjuvant radiation.[204] Utsumi et al. reported similar findings in a study of patients with stage I or II completely resected disease.[205] Finally, a SEER analysis of 901 patients showed no clear benefit from adjuvant radiation for patients with completely resected disease.[206] Some studies have sought to fine-tune the pathologic indications for adjuvant radiotherapy in stage II disease with additional high-risk features beyond capsular invasion. For instance, Haniuda et al. found that patients with fibrous adhesion to the mediastinal pleura without microscopic

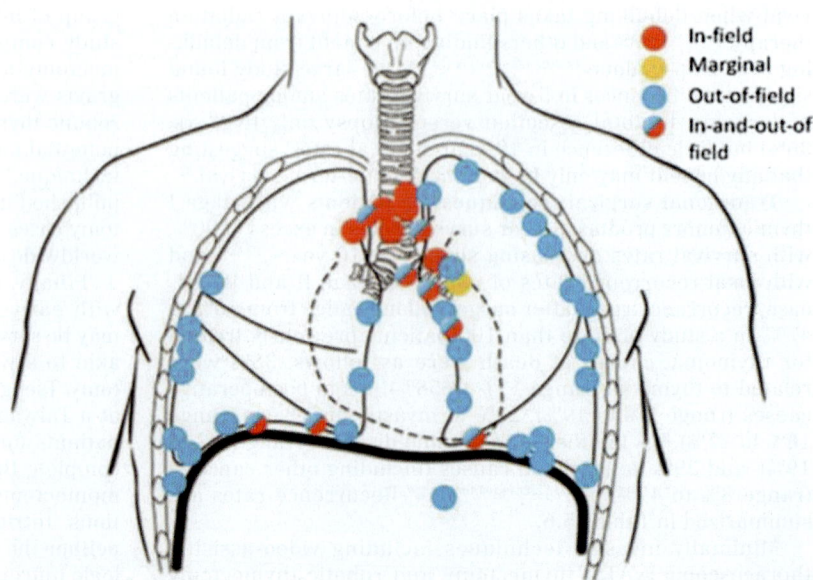

In-field
Marginal
Out-of-field
In-and-out-of field

FIGURE 55.4. Graphical illustration of failure patterns following radiotherapy for stage II to IV thymoma. (Reprinted from Rimner A, Gomez DR, Wu AJ, et al. Failure patterns relative to radiation treatment fields for stage II-IV thymoma. *J Thorac Oncol* 2014;9[3]:403–409. Copyright © 2014 International Association for the Study of Lung Cancer. With permission.)

invasion benefited the most from postoperative therapy[207]: Recurrence rates among patients with such adhesion were 36.4% versus 0% among those without adhesion.

Similar to the literature for stage II disease, there are mixed findings in the literature regarding the role of adjuvant radiation after R_0 resection for stage III thymoma. Traditionally, the literature has consisted of small retrospective studies showing excellent local control after radiation but unclear survival benefit with conflicting results. An illustrative example of a positive result in terms of local control is an early study by Urgesi et al., who reported no in-field recurrences and only 3 out-of-field recurrences among a cohort of 33 stage III and IVa patients treated with surgery and radiation.[157] Similarly, Ogawa reported on 103 patients with stage I to IV thymoma treated with postoperative radiation and found a 100% in-field control rate.[208] And yet, the impact of local control benefit on survival outcomes has not been borne out in some single-institution studies. For instance, Shen et al. reported on 83 patients with completely resected stage II and stage III thymic epithelial tumors and found no survival benefit to adjuvant radiation in these groups.[209]

More recently, large population-based databases have sought to answer the question of radiation's role, but just as in the preceding single-institution studies, these population-based studies have been inconsistent in their findings. The Japanese Association for Research on the Thymus Database Study published its findings on postoperative radiotherapy for stage II to III thymoma in 2015 using the records of 2,835 registered patients. In multivariate analysis comparing those who either did or did not receive adjuvant radiation, the study found no benefit to radiotherapy for either relapse-free survival or overall survival.[210] Furthermore, subgroup exploratory analysis failed to identify factors among the stage III patients that could reliably predict a benefit to adjuvant radiation.

In contrast to the Japanese study, three population-based analyses found an association with adjuvant radiation with improved outcomes. Weksler et al. reviewed the outcomes of 798 stage III thymoma patients in the SEER database. In multivariate analysis, postoperative radiation therapy after surgery was associated with improved disease-free survival but not overall survival.[211] Jackson et al. reported on a population cohort of 4,056 patients in the National Cancer Database with all stages of thymoma and found that adjuvant radiation was associated with improved overall survival after adjustment for other clinical factors. Subgroup analysis found that this benefit was most pronounced in patients with stage IIB to III disease and with positive margin.[212] Lastly, an analysis of 1,263 patients in the ITMIG database who had undergone complete resection of a stage II or III thymoma found a 7% improvement in the 10-year overall survival among those given postoperative radiotherapy (86% vs. 79%, P = .002).[213] Furthermore, the association of radiotherapy with overall survival was significant after multivariate adjustment.

The dose–response relationship is also a matter of controversy in the literature. Harnath et al. found that doses in excess of 50 Gy were associated with improved disease-free and overall survival among 27 patients diagnosed with thymic epithelial tumors and treated with adjuvant radiation. However, Fan et al. reviewed the cases of 53 patients who underwent complete resection of stage III thymoma followed by radiation (range 28 to 60 Gy) and found no clear dose–response relationship.[214]

Even if local control is achieved, it is not evident that distant or regional recurrences or overall survival are clearly impacted by adjuvant radiation.[48,52,215-217] Until a randomized controlled trial rigorously addresses the controversy around postoperative radiotherapy for completely resected tumors, we recommend that treatment for stage II or III disease should be made on an individual basis and should consider risk factors such as frank pleural or pericardial invasion, tumor grade, margin status, and comorbid conditions. We further strongly encourage that proposed treatment strategies be discussed in a multidisciplinary setting before the final recommendation is made.

In the scenario of an incomplete resection, radiotherapy is often considered to be an important adjunctive treatment for addressing residual disease. Although rigorous prospective evidence is unavailable for this clinical scenario, retrospective analyses have observed very low rates of mediastinal failure among patients with gross residual disease treated with adjuvant radiation.[38,157,218]

Radiation as Neoadjuvant Therapy

Radiation has been proposed as a neoadjuvant strategy to reduce tumor burden and improve resectability, especially for cases involving gross invasion of critical structures.[35,108,160,219-223] Response rates of up to 80% have been reported, and a theoretical decrease in the potential for tumor seeding during surgery has been proposed as well.[19,38,159,219] The rates of R_0 resections after neoadjuvant radiation for stage III thymoma can be as high as 53% to 75%,[108,223] which are favorable compared with the typical 50% rate of R_0 resections of stage III thymomas.[18,21,22,38,48,79,105,151] Ten-year survival rates do not seem to be better after preoperative radiation, but to date, the studies evaluating this approach have been small.[108,222,223]

Radiation as Definitive Therapy

Radiation therapy alone has been used for patients who cannot undergo surgery because of medical conditions, or those for whom surgical resection is not possible, with modest results. Arakawa et al. reported that 7 of 12 patients presenting with unresectable tumors treated with primary radiation therapy were still alive at follow-up times ranging from 1 to 5 years.[224] Ciernik et al. reported a 5-year survival rate of 87% for a small group of patients with stage III and IV disease who underwent radiation without resection,[218] and Jackson et al. found 10-year survival rates of 44% for patients who received radiation after biopsies or incomplete resections.[225] As for the use of radiation for recurrent disease, Urgesi and others reported outcomes of 21 patients given radiation alone after intrathoracic recurrences of thymoma.[199] The 7-year survival rate of 70% was similar for those treated with radiation alone and for those treated with surgery and adjuvant therapy. Although these results are informative, in the era of combined modality therapy, the use of preoperative and definitive radiation therapy in the absence of chemotherapy is rarely a primary recommendation in the management of inoperable thymomas.

Chemotherapy

Thymomas are quite sensitive to chemotherapy, with approximately two-thirds of patients showing a clinical response and one-third experiencing a complete response to systemic cytotoxic agents.[68,173,226-233] The duration of response ranges from 12 to 93 months. Whether chemotherapy influences long-term survival is more difficult to assess. In one retrospective analysis of 90 patients, chemotherapy reduced the rates of metastases to the lung, pleura, or other sites by half (17% vs. 38%, P < .05). All of those patients were high risk with stage III or IV tumors treated with radiation and partial or no resection.[159] Another study reported a nonsignificant trend toward better disease-free survival from the addition of chemotherapy.[185]

As is true for the literature on the effects of radiation, most of the series describing the use of chemotherapy are small and retrospective. Drugs commonly used in combination chemotherapy include cisplatin, doxorubicin, and cyclophosphamide. One prospective intergroup study reported disappointing results with combined etoposide, ifosfamide, and cisplatin.[227] A more recent study of patients with advanced disease showed that the combination of carboplatin and paclitaxel produced response rates of 43%, with a median survival time of 20 months. The authors of that report concluded that the clinical activity of that combination was less than that of anthracycline-based therapy.[234]

The most promising use of chemotherapy is in the neoadjuvant setting. Like preoperative radiation, chemotherapy seems to render tumors more suitable for complete resection. An early investigation suggested that neoadjuvant chemotherapy was associated with improved survival for patients with stage III or IVa thymomas.[177] This hypothesis was more rigorously tested in a phase II prospective trial by Park et al.: 27 patients with radiographic evidence of stage III or IV thymic malignancies were enrolled (9 had thymoma and 18 had thymic carcinoma).[235] After induction therapy with docetaxel/cisplatin, 19 of the 27 patients underwent surgery and 15 among the 19 achieved a complete resection, which represents 55.6% of the intent-to-treat population. Overall survival at 4 years was 92.9% and 62.2% among those who did and did not achieve complete resection, respectively, though statistical significance was not achieved (possibly as a result of the small numbers involved). This study serves as evidence that tumor resectability can potentially be improved with a course of systemic chemotherapy.

Aside from cytotoxic agents, somatostatin analogs (e.g., octreotide) and high-dose corticosteroids have shown promise in thymomas.[236,237] In one prospective study, two courses of glucocorticoid therapy before surgery led to a 47% response rate among 17 patients with resectable thymomas.[238] This therapy seems to work by exploiting the ability of corticosteroids to induce apoptosis in CD4+CD8+ immature thymocytes. Another prospective study by the Eastern Cooperative Oncology Group enrolled 42 patients with unresectable, advanced thymic malignancies for whom octreotide scans were positive. Patients were treated with octreotide with or without prednisone. Two patients had complete responses and ten had partial responses, which led the investigators to conclude that octreotide alone had modest activity and that prednisone improved the overall response rate.[239]

Targeted therapies, which seek to take advantage of aberrations in signaling pathways, have been investigated in small series for thymic malignancies. Early studies have focused on c-KIT, EGFR, IGF-1R, and VEGF angiogenesis and histone deacetylation pathways.[142,240,241] Phase I/II trials with agents targeting receptors in these pathways, like those with EGFR-targeted agents, have been largely disappointing,[242,243] although figitumumab, an anti–IGF-1R antibody, has shown efficacy in early clinical trials for advanced/refractory thymomas.[244,245] In addition, a phase II study evaluating the efficacy of the histone deacetylase inhibitor belinostat in patients with recurrent or refractory advanced thymic epithelial tumors showed that of 41 patients enrolled (25 with thymoma, 16 with thymic carcinoma), the response rate was 8%, with median times to progression and survival of 5.8 and 19.1 months, respectively. These investigators concluded that this agent had "modest" antitumor activity in this setting, but the prolonged duration of the response warranted further study.[246] mTOR inhibition

represents a newer line of investigation with promising early results reported in a phase I trial.[247]

Although steroid receptor expression has been thoroughly studied in other malignancies such as breast cancer, less research on this topic has been done in thymic malignancies. Glucocorticoid receptors are known to be expressed in epithelial cells, and the delivery of glucocorticoids can induce apoptosis in thymocytes.[248,249] A recent study evaluating the presence of glucocorticoid, estrogen, and progesterone receptors in thymomas and thymic carcinomas showed that glucocorticoid and estrogen receptors were overexpressed in 83% and 76% of thymic malignancies and progesterone receptors were overexpressed in <1%. Glucocorticoid receptor expression was also associated with better prognosis among patients who underwent resection.[250] Interestingly, these receptors may underpin the observation that prednisone is an active agent in this disease.

Other small investigations of agents that exploit molecular pathways—including agents such as imatinib, sorafenib, sunitinib, cetuximab, cixutumumab, and bevacizumab—have largely failed to demonstrate major activity for thymic malignancies although observations of modest response have been sporadically noted. The most compelling data for these agents comes from a phase 2 study of everolimus in a cohort of patients with advanced or recurrent thymoma or thymic carcinoma who failed cisplatinum. In this trial of 51 patients, 88% had a degree of disease control (mainly stable disease) and median survival was 25.7 months.[250a] Ultimately, better understanding of tumor biology coupled with studies involving larger numbers of patients is necessary to advance this approach.

Combined Modality Therapy

Some evidence exists to suggest that multimodality treatment can improve both resectability and long-term survival among patients with stage III or IV thymomas; typical combinations include neoadjuvant chemotherapy followed by surgery and postoperative radiation, chemotherapy, or both. Prospective trials of preoperative combination chemotherapy have been undertaken at several institutions[76,231,233,251]; the regimens in all cases included cisplatin with some combination of cyclophosphamide, doxorubicin, vincristine, prednisone, or epirubicin. Reported response rates to these regimens range from 77% to 100% (Table 55.8); R_0 resections were possible in 57% to 82% of cases; and pathologic complete response rates ranged from 4% to 31%. Overall survival rates at 5 years (57% to 95%) were quite favorable for unresectable stage III or IV thymoma.[76,231,233,251,252] In many of these studies, most if not all patients received postoperative radiation (Table 55.8), and the results seem superior to historical results from patients who underwent surgical resection alone. In summary, multimodality therapy consisting of preoperative combination cisplatin-based chemotherapy followed by surgery and postoperative radiation can produce excellent results.

Modest results have also been obtained from the combination of chemotherapy plus definitive radiation therapy for limited-stage, unresectable thymoma. A prospective intergroup study[210] reported a 5-year survival rate of 52%

TABLE 55.8   OUTCOMES AFTER COMBINED MODALITY THERAPY FOR THYMOMAS

Study and Reference	Institution	n	Preop Chemo	Adjuvant Therapy	% Response	% R₀	% pCR	% 5-Year Survival
Lucchi et al.[177]	Pisa	36	Cisplatin, vp, epi	RT and Chemo	67	78	6	65 (est)
Venuta et al.[76]	Rome	25	Cisplatin, vp, epi	RT and Chemo	–	80	4	80
Kim et al.[233]	MD Anderson	22	Cyclo, doxo, cisplatin, pred	RT and Chemo	77	82	18	95
Rea et al.[231]	Padua	16	Cyclo, doxo, cisplatin, vin	RT or Chemo	100	69	31	57
Yokoi et al.[253]	Tochigi	17	Cyclo, doxo, pred	RT and Chemo	93	12	7	81

Cyclo, cyclophosphamide; doxo, doxorubicin; epi, epirubicin; pCR, pathologic complete response; pred, prednisone; R₀, complete resection; vin, vincristine; vp, etoposide.

for 26 patients who were treated with cisplatin, doxorubicin, and cyclophosphamide followed by radiation therapy for patients with unresectable thymomas. The median survival time was 93 months.

Management of Myasthenia Gravis

Thymectomy has been used effectively to induce remission or reduce symptoms of myasthenia gravis. Removal of even normal-appearing thymuses improves symptoms in about half of patients with myasthenia gravis,[254–256] which may be related to the associated high acetylcholine receptor activity and the presence of antibodies to striated muscle within the thymus.[257]

In fact, the value of thymectomy in the management of nonthymomatous myasthenia was rigorously evaluated in the MGTX trial, which randomized 126 adult patients with myasthenia gravis in the absence of thymoma to extended transsternal thymectomy plus alternate-day prednisone with alternate-day prednisone alone. Patients who underwent thymectomy had improved symptomatology over a 3-year period, required lower prednisone doses, had fewer episodes requiring immunosuppression with azathioprine, and had fewer hospitalizations for myasthenia exacerbations (9% vs. 37%, $P < .001$).[258] The results of this trial put the use of thymectomy in the treatment of nonthymomatous myasthenia on unequivocal footing.[259,260]

The mortality rate associated with thymectomy, at centers with experience in the preoperative and postoperative management of myasthenia gravis, is essentially the same as that associated with general anesthesia.[54] An important consideration to optimize perioperative outcomes is to ensure that the anesthesiology team is experienced in compensating for the effects of myasthenia on diaphragmatic function, which may have implications for respiratory function while under anesthesia.

Interestingly, radiation therapy to the thymus has also been reported to be effective for treating myasthenia gravis, with symptom improvement or response noted in about 50% of patients.[261–263] However, radiation treatment alone for myasthenia gravis is mostly of historical interest given the advances in surgical expertise and perioperative management of this syndrome.

Radiation Therapy Dose

Radiation doses given for thymoma have ranged from 30 to 70 Gy, most often given in standard 1.8- to 2.0-Gy fractions. Typical postoperative doses are 45 to 50 Gy, with higher doses for positive surgical margins (54 Gy) or gross disease (60 to 70 Gy). Dose–response effects have been difficult to determine owing to the retrospective nature of most published studies; one study did not identify a dose response,[264] but two others did.[185,265]

Radiation Targets

As radiation planning techniques have evolved, the trend in treating thymic tumors, like NSCLC, has been toward use of involved-field techniques. Because thymomas do not routinely spread via the lymphatic system, the draining nodal distributions do not need to be included in the radiation fields.[104] In general, neoadjuvant or definitive radiation therapy delivered a clinical tumor volume consisting of the entire extent of gross disease as visualized on imaging with a further clinical tumor margin (1 to 2 cm) to account for microscopic infiltration. Extending the clinical tumor margin into the lung parenchyma is generally unnecessary.

When radiation is to be given as adjuvant therapy, the radiation treatment fields are designed to treat any residual gross disease and the surgical bed. This region is defined based on the pretreatment images, with the field generally encompassing the surgical field, which can be defined by the placement of surgical clips, and preoperative imaging that delineates the superior–inferior extent of disease before treatment. A clinical tumor margin is added to account for infiltration beyond the area previously occupied by gross tumor.

It is highly advisable to review the treatment volumes for adjuvant radiotherapy with the operating surgeon to ensure that all areas of concern for recurrence are addressed. Likewise, the surgeon can aid the radiation oncologist by placing radiopaque clips at the time of surgery to help define the tumor bed and other areas of interest. It is especially critical to mark in this way regions known to harbor an unresected positive margin based on frozen section or wherever there is a high expectation of margin positivity on permanent section.

There is evidence that these principles of delineation lead to good interobserver consensus; an investigation by Holliday et al. sought to measure interobserver variability by comparing contours among seven radiation oncologists given a pilot dataset for a preoperative and postoperative case.[266] Their results showed exceptional agreement in the preoperative contours although lower agreement was observed in the postoperative setting, further highlighting the benefit of multidisciplinary involvement that includes the surgeon for these cases.

In theory, hemithoracic radiation could be beneficial in thymic malignancies because of their tendency to recur along the pleural surfaces. This technique has been assessed in several studies. In one such study, Sugie et al.[267] reported findings from 60 patients with stage I to IV invasive thymoma, 48 of whom had been treated with fields limited to the mediastinum to a dose of 30 to 64 Gy and the other 12 given hemithoracic radiation therapy to a dose of 11.2 to 16 Gy. Although the toxicity of the extended-field (hemithoracic) radiation was acceptable and seemed to produce modest improvements in pleural dissemination rates, no differences were found in overall survival between the two techniques.[267] Other small studies have also tested hemithoracic radiation to doses of 15 to 20 Gy, and some have had promising results.[268–270] However, these studies were small and primarily retrospective. Ultimately, the dose that can be delivered safely in hemithoracic therapy is probably not sufficient for controlling microscopic disease, which typically requires 40 to 45 Gy. However, conformal techniques such as those noted below may allow further dose escalation in future investigations.

Radiation Modalities and Simulation Techniques

CT-based treatment planning is essential for targeting the tumor and for accurate dosimetry of critical structures. In the modern era, 4D techniques to manage respiratory are also helpful for ensuring coverage of the target as well as optimizing avoidance of organs at risk. As is true for all thoracic and mediastinal tumors, the major critical structures include the spinal cord, lung parenchyma, pericardium, heart, and esophagus. The guidelines to be followed to minimize dose to these structures are the same as those used in the treatment of lung cancer. Table 55.9 lists common dose constraints for radiation therapy, with or without chemotherapy, for mediastinal malignancies. These constraints were derived from a Quantitative Analysis of Normal Tissue Effects in the Clinic (QUANTEC) consensus analysis published in 2010.[271–274] Any deviations from these dose constraints should be reviewed in a radiation quality assurance setting and discussed with the patient before treatment is begun.

Major advances in radiation delivery over the past decade have led to great improvements in both conformality and therapeutic ratio of radiation for thoracic malignancies. Intensity-modulated radiation therapy (IMRT) has been shown to allow the dose to normal structures to be reduced relative to that from 3D conformal radiation and to allow accurate target localization.[275–281] Indeed, a recent study of 496 patients with

TABLE 55.9 STANDARD DOSE CONSTRAINTS USED IN RADIATION THERAPY FOR THORACIC MALIGNANCIES

Organ at Risk	RT Alone	Chemo and RT	Chemo and RT before Surgery
Spinal cord[1]	$D_{max} < 45$ Gy	$D_{max} < 45$ Gy	$D_{max} < 45$ Gy
Lung[2]	Mean dose ≤ 20 Gy	Mean dose ≤ 20 Gy	Mean dose ≤ 20 Gy
	$V_{20} \leq 40\%$	$V_{20} \leq 35\%$	$V_{20} \leq 30\%$
		$V_{10} \leq 45\%$	$V_{10} \leq 40\%$
		$V_5 \leq 65\%$	$V_5 \leq 55\%$
Heart	$V_{30} \leq 45\%$	$V_{30} \leq 45\%$	$V_{30} \leq 45\%$
	Mean dose < 26 Gy	Mean dose < 26 Gy	Mean dose < 26 Gy
Esophagus	$D_{max} \leq 80$ Gy	$D_{max} \leq 80$ Gy	$D_{max} \leq 80$ Gy
	$V_{70} < 20\%$	$V_{70} < 20\%$	$V_{70} < 20\%$
	$V_{50} < 50\%$	$V_{50} < 40\%$	$V_{50} < 40\%$
	Mean dose < 34 Gy	Mean dose < 34 Gy	Mean dose < 34 Gy
Kidney[5]	20 Gy $< 32\%$ of bilateral kidney	20 Gy $< 32\%$ of bilateral kidney	20 Gy $< 32\%$ of bilateral kidney
Liver	$V_{30} \leq 40\%$	$V_{30} \leq 40\%$	$V_{30} \leq 40\%$
	Mean dose < 30 Gy	Mean dose < 30 Gy	Mean dose < 30 Gy

D_{max}, maximum dose; V_x, percent volume of organ receiving x dose.
From Marks LB, Bentzen SM, Deasy JO, et al. Radiation dose-volume effects in the lung. *Int J Radiat Oncol Biol Phys* 2010;76(3 Suppl):S70–S76.

locally advanced, unresectable NSCLC demonstrated that the more advanced technique (4D CT with IMRT) led to lower rates of high-grade radiation pneumonitis and better overall survival compared with 3D simulation and 3D conformal therapy.[282] Although similar comparisons for thymic malignancies have not been done because of the rarity of this disease, the same principles would be expected to apply given the mediastinal location of these tumors and hence their close proximity to the lungs, heart, and esophagus.

Another treatment modality, proton beam therapy, has shown promise for reducing the dose to normal structures while maintaining adequate doses to the tumor target in NSCLC.[275,283–290] Indeed, the dose distribution properties of proton therapy, specifically the "Bragg peak" that minimizes dose distal to the tumor, are well suited for anteriorly located thymic tumors. Proton therapy has been shown to produce greatly reduced doses to critical structures in mediastinal lymphoma, which often presents in the same anterior location as thymic malignancies, compared with photon-based techniques.[291] Vogel et al. tested this hypothesis by comparing double-scattered proton beam plans to IMRT plans for 22 consecutive patients requiring treatment for thymic malignancies. They confirmed that proton beam therapy resulted in statistically significant reductions in dose to the heart, lungs, left ventricle, and spinal cord and that the baseline risk of major cardiac events was increased by 135% after IMRT and 74% after proton therapy ($P = .04$).[292] Further investigation via rigorous, prospective clinical trials will be essential in determining if the dosimetric benefits of proton beam therapy (Fig. 55.5) translate to clinical benefits.

Regardless of treatment modality, we recommend that all treatment simulations for patients with thymic tumors take place while the patients are supine, and well immobilized with their arms above their head, to maximize the number of potential beam arrangements. We recommend that 4D CT scans be obtained at the time of simulation to assess the motion of the tumor during respiration. If 4D CT scanning is not available, we recommend either a slow helical scan to encompass all phases of the breathing cycle or that CT images be obtained at full inspiration and expiration to assess the extremes of respiratory motion. Full descriptions of radiation techniques for thymic malignancies are available elsewhere.[293,294]

FIGURE 55.5. Axial, sagittal, and coronal views of a typical proton plan for postoperative treatment of thymoma. Surrounding structures including the lungs, heart, and esophagus have significantly diminished radiation exposure with this approach, as illustrated in the dose–volume histogram.

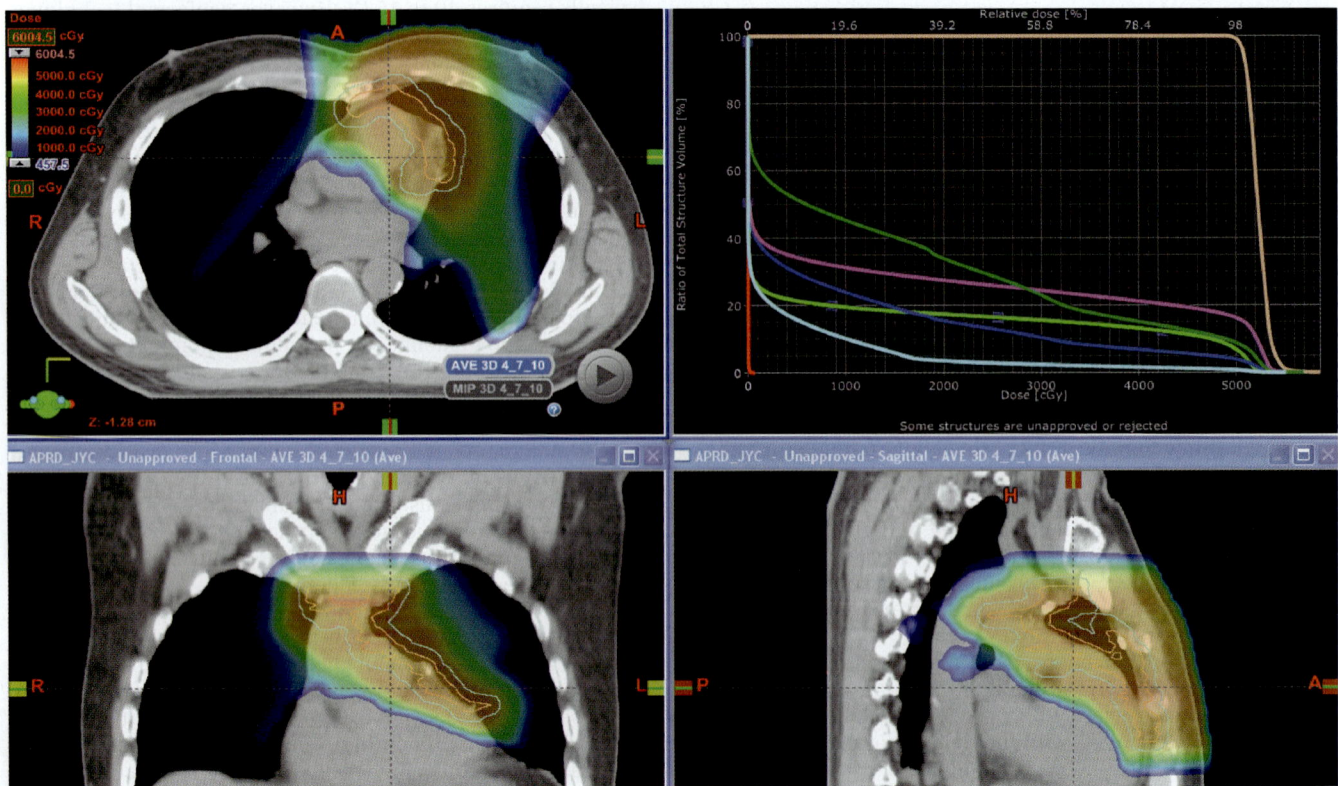

THYMIC CARCINOMA

Natural History and Diagnosis

Thymic carcinomas are considerably less common than thymomas. Like thymomas, thymic carcinomas are thought to arise from thymic epithelium and typically appear in the anterosuperior mediastinum. The clinical behavior of thymic carcinoma is quite different from that of thymoma; they are generally more aggressive and have a higher propensity for capsular invasion and metastatic proliferation. Because of these features, thymic carcinoma often presents as advanced disease and its 5-year survival rates are much poorer than for thymomas.[52,295,296]

Clinically, thymic carcinoma can present with cough, dyspnea, pleuritic chest pain, phrenic nerve palsy, or superior vena cava syndrome.[295,297,298] Associated paraneoplastic syndromes have been observed occasionally though these are less commonly seen compared to thymoma.[298-300] CT scans often demonstrate an irregular mass with necrotic, cystic, or calcified regions.[297,301-303] In about 80% of cases, thymic carcinoma shows radiographic evidence of invasion into adjacent structures in the mediastinum, and mediastinal lymphadenopathy is evident at presentation in about 40% of cases.[298,304-306] Distant metastases to regional lymphatics, bone, liver, kidney, and lung are also common clinical features.[298,307-309] Therefore, bone scanning, MRI, PET with ^{18}F-flourodeoxyglucose or ^{11}C-labeled methionine, and single photon emission computed tomography (SPECT) have been used for both staging and evaluation of response to therapy.[90,310-313]

Historically, thymic carcinomas have been classified as type C thymic tumors in the WHO classification, and disease staging is most often done with the Masaoka clinical staging system for thymomas.[105,314] Most thymic carcinomas are undifferentiated high-grade lesions with anaplasia and marked cellular atypia, lacking the histologic features of a normal thymus[315]; others may be of adenocarcinomatous, sarcomatous, squamous, basaloid, mucoepidermoid, or lymphoepithelial-like histology.[297,316,317] Some thymic carcinomas are associated with the multilocular thymic cysts, which are acquired lesions of the thymic gland associated with an inflammatory reaction. Recent studies have demonstrated the importance of thorough sampling of thymic cysts to rule out underlying carcinoma.[318]

Because histologic grade is one of the most significant indicators of prognosis, a revised histologic classification has been proposed that broadly divides thymic carcinomas into high-grade or low-grade lesions.[319] Tumors in the low-grade histologic group are characterized by a relatively favorable clinical course and a low incidence of local recurrence and metastasis.[320-322] High-grade variants of thymic carcinoma are more lethal, with frequent metastases to regional lymph nodes, bone, liver, and lung.[303,323]

The extent of surgical resection, Masaoka stage, TNM stage, and receipt of adjuvant therapy are also associated with improved survival[324-327]; interestingly, the specific histology of thymic carcinoma, just as in thymoma, does not appear to reliably confer an impact on survival. Stage IVb patients with lymph node–only metastases may have better outcomes than those with distant metastatic disease at presentation, a result which may be driven by the possibility of curative resection in some of these patients.[328]

General Management

Owing to the paucity of experience with this rare tumor, the ideal therapeutic regimen is unknown. Current management strategies borrow from the principles of treating non–small cell carcinoma of the lung. Thus, an aggressive multimodality approach is often employed, which includes the consideration of primary surgical resection, adjuvant cisplatin-based chemotherapy, and postoperative radiation therapy.

Although incomplete resection does not necessarily preclude long-term survival if multimodality platinum-based therapy is used,[329] complete resection is nevertheless the cornerstone of treatment.[324-327] Reflecting multiple other single-institution studies, Takeda et al. observed a median survival time of 57 months for patients with completely resected thymic carcinomas versus 13 incomplete resection.[330] A multi-institutional study of patients with thymic carcinoma showed that the 5-year survival rates of total resection, subtotal resection, and inoperable groups were 67%, 30%, and 24%, respectively.[52] Likewise, the largest modern series of 1,042 cases from the combined European Society of Thoracic Surgeons (ESTS) and ITMIG databases reported overall survival rates for R0, R1, and R2 groups were 70%, 55%, and 42%, respectively.[326] In light of this consistent finding in multiple datasets, complete resection of the primary tumor is a fundamental recommendation.

The routine addition of lymph node dissection is more controversial though it has merited attention because of the higher rate at which thymic carcinomas spread to regional lymph nodes in comparison to thymomas. Park et al. retrospectively reviewed 37 thymic carcinoma patients who were divided into 4 groups: No node dissection, N0 by limited dissection, N0 by extensive dissection, and N1 by dissection of any type.[331] Among the 29 patients who underwent node dissections, 6 (20.7%) were found to harbor nodal metastases. Furthermore, patients who underwent no dissection or node negative after limited dissection had outcomes that were inferior to those who were node negative after an extensive dissection. These results suggest that an extensive dissection may impart more accurate staging and better prognostic information. Though this study requires confirmation in larger investigations, it raises an intriguing hypothesis that routine lymph node dissection may improve outcomes either by the therapeutic effect of completely excising gross disease or by providing better guidance for necessary adjuvant therapies.

The role of radiotherapy for thymic carcinoma is not well defined, again owing to the rarity of the disease and the absence of prospective clinical trials. Although radiotherapy should be considered in all cases of thymic carcinoma, there is limited evidence that omission in completely resected, early-stage disease may be feasible. A small investigation of four patients fitting this characterization who were treated with radical surgery alone found that all four were alive and free from relapse at a median follow-up of 72 months (range 12 to 167 months).[332]

Most single-institution retrospective studies have reported on outcomes with adjuvant radiation therapy, typically to a dose of 40 to 70 Gy delivered in standard fractionation (1.8- to 2.0-Gy fractions).[264,321,330,333-336] In one such series of 26 patients treated with surgery and postoperative radiation without chemotherapy, Hsu et al. observed a 5-year overall survival rate of 77% for all patients,[336] 82% for patients with completely resected tumors, and 66% for those with subtotally resected tumors. The 5-year local control rate was 91% with a median radiation dose of 60 Gy. In another study of 40 patients given either surgery and adjuvant radiation or definitive radiation therapy with or without chemotherapy, Ogawa et al. reported no local recurrences among the cohort of patients with complete resection who had received adjuvant radiation of at last 50 Gy.[321] Kondo and Monden observed no survival benefit from adding adjuvant radiation to surgical resection in a retrospective multi-institutional study of 186 patients, although the authors did note that the retrospective nature of the study and its small subgroup sizes precluded any definitive conclusions.[52]

Investigators of the ESTS database reported on 229 patients treated with thymic carcinoma between 1999 and 2010. Compared to patients receiving surgery alone, a significant survival advantage was observed among patients receiving surgery and postoperative radiotherapy. Ahmad et al. went further to study the combined ESTS and ITMIG databases to create a cohort of 1,042 thymic carcinomas, 60% of whom received adjuvant radiotherapy. In their multivariable analysis, attaining R0 resection and administration of radiotherapy were the only variables associated with prolonged overall survival (hazard ratio for radiotherapy, 0.45).[326]

In aggregate, these studies seem to indicate that local control is improved with radiation and that a survival benefit may also accrue. The quality of the evidence, however, is limited by its retrospective nature and vulnerability to selection bias. As is true for all mediastinal tumors, better knowledge will depend on conducting randomized clinical trials. The formation of international collaborations such as the ESTS and the ITMIG is a reassuring development as they will likely underpin the design and completion of such trials.

With regard to systemic therapy, thymic carcinoma generally is less responsive to chemotherapy than thymoma,[337] and outcomes after chemotherapy alone are dismal. However, the use of adjuvant cisplatin-based chemotherapy has shown significantly beneficial effects in several studies.[226,338,339] In one such study, Nakamura et al. treated 10 patients with unresectable thymic carcinoma with platinum-based protocols, with or without radiation therapy, and observed a median survival time of 11 months.[339] Yoh and others reported excellent preliminary results (i.e., a 42% response rate) from the use of weekly cisplatin, vincristine, doxorubicin, and etoposide for the treatment of advanced tumors.[340] Other studies have shown favorable responses from various combinations of cisplatin, etoposide, ifosfamide, doxorubicin, nedaplatin, cyclophosphamide, and vincristine.[226,227,338–342] Finally, although data are limited, some centers advocate combined chemoradiation in select circumstances for thymic carcinoma, particularly after R1 or R2 resections.[343]

Finally, molecular pathways may provide a new avenue for treatment. Exploratory studies have shown the association of thymic carcinoma with certain mutations (VEGF,[143] IGF-1R,[144] and KIT pathways).[145,146,344] Validation of this approach, especially in combination with the other modalities, requires additional study.

Because of the rarity of thymic carcinoma, few treatment recommendations can be made; however, it seems clear that for patients with resectable disease, complete surgical resection is the preferred initial therapeutic intervention.[52,102,330,345,346] For patients with unresectable lesions, neoadjuvant chemotherapy, with or without thoracic radiotherapy, seems reasonable. Ultimately, after complete resection, the most important prognostic factors are initial disease stage and tumor grade. Five-year survival rates for patients with higher disease stage and higher-grade neoplasms range from 15% to 20%, whereas for patients with low-grade, localized disease, those rates can range from 80% to 90%.[319,323] The addition of adjuvant therapies for patients with poor prognostic factors should be made on an individual basis in the context of multidisciplinary review.

THYMIC CARCINOID

Thymic carcinoid (neuroendocrine) tumors of the thymus are very rare, accounting for <5% of all neoplasms of the anterior mediastinum. They originate from normal thymic Kulchitsky cells, which belong to the amine-precursor-uptake-and-decarboxylation group.[347] Thymic carcinoid tumors are often confused with thymomas because of similarities in their clinical behavior. Most patients with thymic carcinoid are men aged 30 to 50 years; the male-to-female ratio is 3 to 1.[348] Roughly half of thyroid carcinoids are associated with endocrine disorders such as MEN-1

[multiple endocrine neoplasia type 1] or secondary Cushing syndrome.[349–351]

Thymic carcinoids can present with symptoms related to compression of normal structures (chest pain, dyspnea, cough, hoarseness, superior vena cava syndrome)[347,352] or with no symptoms.[351] These tumors are best evaluated by CT or MRI for visualizing local invasion of the surrounding structures (pericardium, great vessels, pleura, sternum) and metastases within or outside the thorax. Most thymic carcinoids detected on radiographic studies are already advanced, commonly metastasizing to regional lymph nodes. Metastases are present in up to 40% to 70% of patients within 8 years of the initial diagnosis,[353,354] which may explain the poor prognosis associated with these tumors.

The Masaoka staging system for thymoma has been used for staging thymic carcinoids.[105,348] The WHO system classifies the pathology of thymic carcinoids into typical carcinoid, atypical carcinoid, large-cell neuroendocrine carcinoma, or small-cell carcinoma,[115,123] and a system proposed by Klemm and Moran classifies these tumors as well-differentiated (low grade), moderately differentiated (intermediate grade), or poorly differentiated (high grade).[355] Notably, neither grading nor other histologic variables have shown a consistent association with prognosis.[348]

Complete surgical resection is the preferred method of treatment, although recurrence is common. Incomplete resections followed by adjuvant radiation, chemotherapy, or both seem to provide some benefit without increasing morbidity or mortality.[351,353,356,357] Distant metastases to the bone, liver, or skin occur in 30% to 40% of cases.[358] Despite aggressive treatment, the prognosis in most cases is poor. According to one report, the overall 5-year survival rate was 31% and all 14 patients expired within 9 years.[352] A more recent analysis of 205 patients from the combined ESTS and ITMIG databases was more reassuring with a reported 5-year survival rate of 68%, although this result should be tempered by the observation that 39% of patients experienced recurrence in this time frame.[354] Similar to the other thymic malignancies, overall survival was influenced primarily by Masaoka stage and completeness of resection. Neither chemotherapy nor radiotherapy showed statistical significance with regard to overall survival benefit. Thymic carcinoids associated with MEN-1 are especially lethal; in one study, the 5-year survival rate for patients with thymic carcinoid without associated endocrinopathy was about 70% but was only 35% for those with an endocrinopathy.[351,352,359]

OTHER RARE TUMORS OF THE THYMUS

Thymoliposarcoma was first described by Havlicek and Rosai in 1984.[360] This rare and distinctive entity is considered the malignant counterpart of thymolipoma. Thymoliposarcomas have appeared in adults aged 36 to 77 years, with a slight female predominance. Unlike its thymolipoma counterpart, thymoliposarcoma is not associated with myasthenia gravis. It grows by expansion and has a relatively low risk of distant metastasis in the absence of histologic dedifferentiation. Complete surgical resection or subtotal resection with adjuvant radiation therapy has been used for local control.[360,361]

MALIGNANT MEDIASTINAL GERM CELL TUMORS

Epidemiology

Primary extragonadal germ cell tumors account for 2% to 5% of all germ cell tumors.[362] About two-thirds of these tumors occur in the mediastinum,[363–365] making the mediastinum the most common site of primary extragonadal germ cell tumors among young adults.[366] Germ cell tumors contribute about 10% of all malignant mediastinal tumors and about 2% of mediastinal neoplasms.[156,367] In a pooled analysis of 341 patients with mediastinal germ cell tumors treated at 11 cancer centers over a 20-year period, the median age of presentation was 33 years for seminomatous tumors and 28 years for nonseminomatous tumors.[368]

Primary extragonadal germ cell tumors have several unexplained associations. Klinefelter syndrome has been documented in patients with mediastinal germ cell tumors but not in patients with testicular germ cell tumors.[369–372] In one study, up to 20% of patients with mediastinal germ cell tumors were found to have the Klinefelter karyotype (47,XXY).[373,374] Several unusual malignant processes are associated with nonseminomatous germ cell tumors, including hematologic malignancies such as acute myeloid leukemia, acute nonlymphocytic leukemia, acute megakaryocytic leukemia, myelodysplastic syndrome, and malignant histiocytosis.[374–378] In another pooled analysis of primary extragonadal germ cell tumors, 1 in 17 patients with primary mediastinal nonseminomatous germ cell tumors developed a fatal hematologic disorder after the diagnosis of the germ cell tumor.[379]

Natural History

Primary extragonadal germ cell tumors arise along midline structures of the body extending from the pineal gland, through the mediastinum and retroperitoneum, to the presacral areas. The origin of these primary extragonadal germ cell tumors remains controversial,[380–382] but presumably they arise from germ cells that migrate along the urogenital ridge during embryonic development.[374,383] Because the embryologic urogenital ridge extends from C-6 to L-4, malignant transformation of displaced germ cells can give rise to primary germ cell tumors outside the gonads.

Because primary gonadal germ cell tumors can spread to the retroperitoneum and mediastinum,[364,374] the diagnostic workup must be thorough and meticulous to avoid overlooking an occult gonadal primary. Although primary mediastinal germ cell tumors have the same morphologic and histologic appearance as those of the testes, primary germ cell tumors of the mediastinum are more aggressive and have a poorer prognosis.[384–386] Like testicular germ cell tumors, mediastinal germ cell tumors can be seminomatous or nonseminomatous. Benign teratomas arise from germ cell elements, but they are not included in this discussion because they are not malignant and surgical resection is often curative.

Primary mediastinal seminomatous germ cell tumors are sensitive to radiation and chemotherapy, but nonseminomatous tumors are less vulnerable to treatment and are considered poor-risk disease in all staging systems.[386] Nonseminomatous tumors are often invasive at the time of diagnosis, and approximately half of such tumors will present with distant metastases, most often to the lung.[368]

Tumor markers can aid in the diagnosis of mediastinal germ cell tumors; serum alpha-fetoprotein levels are elevated in 75% of patients (median, 2,500 ng/mL) at diagnosis, and beta-human chorionic gonadotropin and lactate dehydrogenase levels are elevated in about 50% of patients at presentation.[368] Pure seminomatous histologies are less likely to be associated with biomarker elevation, although occasionally a modest rise in beta-human chorionic gonadotropin can be observed.

Clinical Presentation

As is true for the other mediastinal tumors, local symptoms are usually caused by tumor compression or invasion of adjacent structures. Primary extragonadal germ cell tumors present with clinical symptoms in 90% to 100% of cases,[387] with dyspnea (25%), chest pain (23%), cough (17%), fever (13%),

weight loss (11%), vena cava occlusion syndrome, and fatigue/weakness (6% each) being the most common.[368,388,389] Nevertheless, these tumors are asymptomatic in many cases, and a mass is found incidentally on chest x-ray.[390,391] Roughly one-third of seminomatous mediastinal germ cell tumors present with metastases at diagnosis. The cervical lymph nodes are enlarged in about 25% of such cases, but abdominal lymphadenopathy has also been observed. Distant metastases from nonseminomatous germ cell tumors are even more common, with rates of 85% to 90% at diagnosis in prior series and 50% in more recent series.[368,392–395]

Diagnostic Workup

Mediastinal germ cell tumors are usually readily detected on chest x-rays, with most masses noted in the anterosuperior mediastinum. CT scans of the chest, abdomen, and pelvis are essential to evaluate the mass and to screen for metastases and lymphadenopathy. A careful physical examination and testicular sonography should be performed to rule out an occult primary gonadal tumor. As mentioned above, levels of tumor markers such as alpha-fetoprotein, beta-human chorionic gonadotropin, and lactate dehydrogenase can be helpful for diagnosis, for evaluating treatment efficacy, and for monitoring recurrence.[11,396–398] Thus, the determination of baseline tumor marker levels both before treatment is begun and after treatment is completed is essential.

The initial diagnosis of mediastinal germ cell tumors is usually reached through a combination of findings from CT, radiography, sonography, and tumor marker measurements. Whether PET has a place in the management of these tumors is unclear. In some instances, the tumor marker findings are sufficient to classify the lesion as an extragonadal nonseminomatous germ cell tumor without histologic confirmation, but false-positive beta-human chorionic gonadotropin levels have been reported.[399,400] Histopathologic analysis can often be done easily via fine needle aspiration and cytologic staining for tumor markers. Biopsy samples should be obtained whenever possible because both choice of treatment and prognosis depend greatly on histology.[399,400]

Prognostic Factors

The most important prognostic factor for mediastinal germ cell tumors is histologic type. Seminomas are highly curable, but nonseminomatous germ cell tumors, despite advances in therapy, are associated with poor progression-free and overall survival. The presence of metastases with tumors of either histologic type is also associated with adverse progression-free and overall survival. In nonseminomatous tumors, elevated beta-human chorionic gonadotropin levels are associated with inferior overall survival.[368]

General Management

Seminomatous Tumors

Seminomas are quite sensitive to both radiation therapy and chemotherapy, and thus all patients with tumors of seminomatous histology should be treated with curative intent even in the presence of widely metastatic disease. The choice of treatment has evolved with the development of cisplatin-based chemotherapy regimens, and most patients should be initially treated with systemic chemotherapy.[401]

Historically, mediastinal seminomatous tumors (like all mediastinal tumors) were treated surgically.[374,402] Complete radical resection can be considered in some cases if it is technically feasible and if the patients do not want radiation or chemotherapy. Definitive radiation replaced surgical resection for localized mediastinal seminomatous germ cell tumors, with long-term survival rates of 60% to 80% achieved even for those with bulky tumors.[362,374,377,402] Before the advent of platinum-based chemotherapy, radiation therapy had the advantage of being more tolerable and less toxic, and relapses could be effectively treated with systemic chemotherapy.[362] However, cisplatin-based chemotherapy has eclipsed radiation; in an early application of this approach, Einhorn and Williams at the University of Indiana reported a complete response rate of 63% lasting a median duration of 18 months for 19 patients with disseminated seminoma treated with cisplatin-based chemotherapy.[403] In more modern series, the response to primary systemic chemotherapy is favorable for 92% of patients, and 5-year overall survival rates exceeding 90% are standard.[401]

Residual radiographic abnormalities after the completion of chemotherapy for bulky mediastinal seminomas are not uncommon, but the management strategy in such cases is still controversial. In the vast majority (80% to 90%) of such cases, the residual masses represent dense fibrosis with no viable tumor.[374,404-406] Some clinicians have advocated surgical resection or biopsy of all postchemotherapy masses larger than 3 cm,[85,405-407] and others recommend close follow-up in such cases, with early intervention if the mass enlarges on chest x-ray or CT scan and resection, radiation, or salvage chemotherapy reserved for progressive disease.[374,377,406,408] Whether ^{18}F-fluorodeoxyglucose PET is useful for predicting viable tumor is debatable and under investigation.[409,410] Even though seminomas are extremely sensitive to radiation therapy, radiation therapy delivered to residual masses after chemotherapy has not shown a significant benefit.

Circumstances in which radiation may be appropriate include patients who refuse chemotherapy, in whom chemotherapy is contraindicated, or who likely harbor viable residual disease after chemotherapy based upon highly suspicious imaging findings or pathologic confirmation. Radiation doses and treatment techniques for mediastinal seminomatous germ cell tumors have varied.[411-416] Doses as low as 30 Gy and as high as 50 Gy have been recommended.[367,413] Given the absence of unambiguous clinical trial guidance, radiation dose should be adjusted based on the size of the lesion, the history of chemotherapy exposure, and the clinical circumstance. Because the disease is infiltrative and susceptible to nodal involvement, the entire mediastinum was traditionally encompassed with anteroposterior–posteroanterior fields with CT guidance. In the prechemotherapy era, use of smaller portals was associated with marginal relapses,[412] and in fact, the clinical target volume for definitive radiation alone often electively covered the supraclavicular, cervical, and para-aortic lymph nodes.[397,411,414,417] Extrapolating from the experience with prophylactic treatment of para-aortic nodes in testicular seminomas, one could assume that the contiguous lymphatic drainage sites for a mediastinal primary could be treated effectively with 20 Gy with minimal morbidity.[418]

In conclusion, cisplatin-based combination chemotherapy can consistently produce 5-year overall survival rates in excess of 90% for mediastinal seminomas. However, for selected patients, definitive radiation therapy has produced local tumor control rates of 89% to 100% and long-term survival rates of 60% to 80%.[367,374,412,414,419]

Nonseminomatous Germ Cell Tumors

The primary treatment for nonseminomatous germ cell tumor is intensive cisplatin-based chemotherapy, but surgical resection of all residual masses after first-line chemotherapy is recommended whenever technically possible, either as a one-stage or as a sequential procedure.[420-423] Chemotherapy regimens should include either cisplatin and etoposide or cisplatin, etoposide, and bleomycin. Patients whose tumors respond well to initial chemotherapy followed by complete resection of any residual mass can have excellent outcomes, but the outcome for patients who do not respond to primary therapy is poor, as salvage therapy is rarely effective.[386]

The role of radiation therapy in nonseminomatous germ cell tumors is not clear. Radiation may be useful for unresectable residual masses given the relatively high rate of persistent viable tumor and the poor success rates of salvage therapy. Nonseminomatous germ cell tumors are in fact radiosensitive, but they require higher doses than seminomatous tumors. Akin to other solid tumors, doses of 60 Gy or more may be necessary to achieve disease control.[424]

Before the cisplatin-based chemotherapy era, fewer than 5% of patients with mediastinal nonseminomatous germ cell tumors survived.[397] Since that time, long-term disease-free survival rates have varied from 45% to 72% in studies using cisplatin-based combination chemotherapy followed by surgery.[368,386,425] Several salvage regimens have been used for disease that progresses during or after initial chemotherapy, but unfortunately, long-term survival rates for patients with relapsed mediastinal germ cell tumors are <10%.[368,386,427] Thus, surgical resection and even radiation therapy may be appropriate in select cases to augment chemotherapy or as an alternative treatment modality when no further chemotherapy is available.

MEDIASTINAL MESENCHYMAL TUMORS

Epidemiology

True mediastinal mesenchymal lesions are exceedingly rare tumors. Retrospective series suggest that 2% to 8% of all mediastinal lesions are primary mesenchymal tumors; extrapolation of these values puts the estimated incidence at approximately 0.1 to 0.2 per million.[11,428-430] Approximately three-quarters of mediastinal mesenchymal tumors are of lipomatous, lymphangitic, or vascular histology, with the rest composed of unusual histologic variants.[431] The age predilection depends on the specific histologic subtype.[48,391,428-430,432]

Clinical Presentation and Workup

Mesenchymal lesions can arise in any of the three mediastinal compartments. Mesenchymal tumors that present in children seem to be more malignant than those presenting in adults.[432,433]

Mediastinal mesenchymal lesions can reach impressively large sizes before detection, typically presenting with symptoms such as chest pain and dyspnea. At least one series suggests that symptomatic presentation is a harbinger of malignant character, with 80% of patients with malignant disease presenting with symptoms versus 44% of patients with benign masses.[11] An accurate histopathologic diagnosis is critical.[432] Tissue for these analyses can be obtained via mediastinoscopic biopsy, fine needle aspiration, or endoscopy. Disease can be staged according to the American Joint Committee on Cancer staging system for soft tissue tumors.

Tumors of Adipose Tissue

Mediastinal lipomas are the most common of the mediastinal mesenchymal lesions; they represent 1% to 5% of all lipomas.[431,434-436] Mediastinal lesions can occur in isolation or in multiples and may mimic cardiomegaly or pleural effusion on a chest x-ray. They are usually well circumscribed and encapsulated but can grow to 20 cm in diameter before detection.[437,438] Though these tumors can be quite large and cause significant compressive symptoms,[439-441] gross total resection is almost always curative.[13,442-445] Technically, lipomas are considered "benign" tumors, but those that are growing or causing symptoms should be referred for surgical resection.

In contrast to lipomas, liposarcomas consist of immature fat cells with malignant histology and behavior. Distinguishing lipomas from liposarcomas can be difficult histologically; liposarcomas are distinguished by size heterogeneity, hyperchromatic nuclei, and eosinophilic cytoplasm.[446] Primary mediastinal

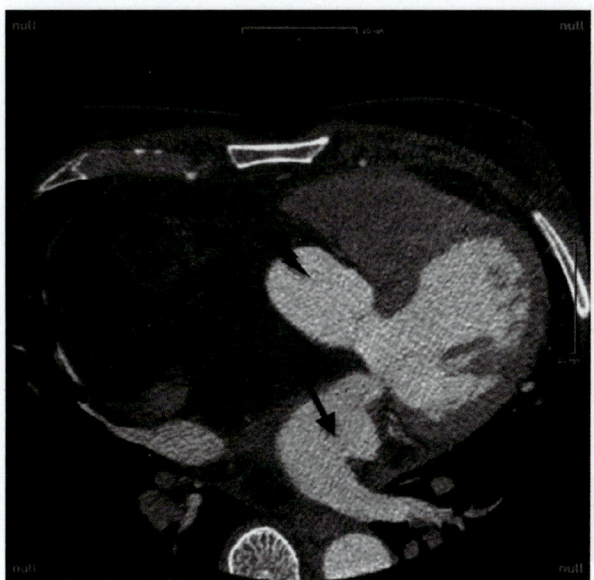
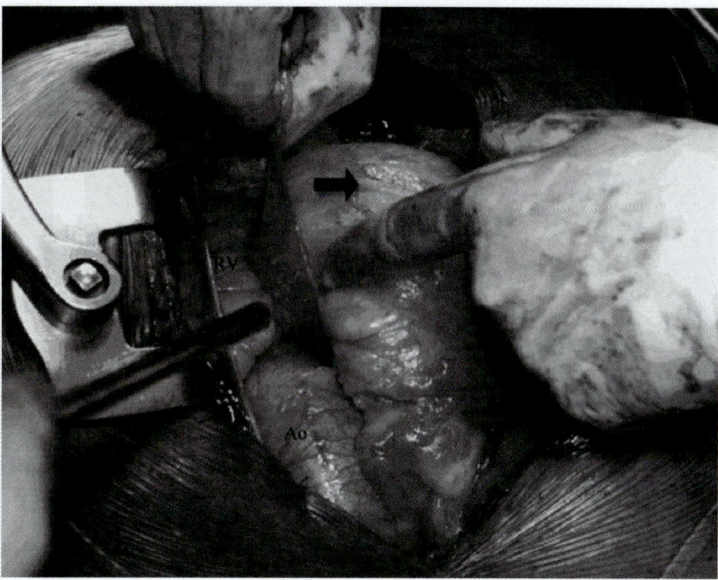

FIGURE 55.6. CT scan (*left*) and intraoperative photograph (*right*) of a primary mediastinal liposarcoma filling the right thoracic cavity. The recommended treatment for this malignancy is aggressive surgical resection with adjuvant radiation therapy and consideration of systemic therapy. (From Wiedemann D, Schistek R, Gassner E, et al. Mediastinal liposarcoma. *J Card Surg* 2011;26[2]:162–164. Copyright © 2010 Wiley Periodicals, Inc. Reprinted by permission of John Wiley & Sons, Inc.)

liposarcomas often appear in the posterior portion of the mediastinum. Anterior mediastinal liposarcomas are possible albeit rare.[447] Tumors often appear to be encapsulated and well-circumscribed, even when invasion is present (Fig. 55.6), giving rise to the term "pseudocapsule." In one historical review, survival times for patients with well-circumscribed lesions ranged from 3 to 17 years, whereas patients with grossly invasive tumors died within 2 years.[448] As is true for all sarcomas, the prognosis depends on the histologic grade.[449,450]

Like other sarcomas, optimal treatment consists of surgical resection and adjuvant radiation therapy.[451] Because well-differentiated tumors have little propensity for distant metastases, withholding adjuvant radiation for a trial of observation can be considered after an R₀ resection, but the significant local recurrence rates of 20% to 30% should be acknowledged during multidisciplinary discussion and with the patient.[449,450,452–455]

Tumors of Lymph Tissue

Tumors arising from the vascular or lymphatic components of the mediastinum make up the bulk of the remaining mediastinal mesenchymal lesions.[428–430] Lymphangiomas and hemangiomas are morphologically similar under light microscopy, and the presence of red blood cells or chyle within the tumor lumen often serves as a primary diagnostic aid.[442] Localized lymphangiomas are rare; more than 90% will have some degree of cervical extension.[456] A cystic lymphangioma is illustrated in Figure 55.7.[457] Lymphangiomatosis is usually seen in children and is characterized by synchronous widespread lymphangiomas.[458] Mediastinal or pulmonary involvement carries a poor prognosis.[442,459–467]

Lymphangiosarcoma seems to be a malignant variant of lymphangiomas and should probably be treated like other soft tissue sarcomas, with the optimal treatment being full extirpation.[468] In the largest reported retrospective series of 25 patients with mediastinal and cervicomediastinal lymphangiomas, survival rates were excellent after surgical resection alone, and only one patient died of a complication from lymphangioma.[469]

Adjuvant radiation has little role in most cases and may actually be detrimental for lymphangiomas. In one study, radiation was conjectured to transform a benign lymphangioma

into a malignant lymphangiosarcoma.[470–472] However, radiation may be helpful for controlling symptomatic unresectable disease; Johnson et al. described a young patient with surgically refractory chylothorax and lymphangioma who experienced prompt resolution after mediastinal radiation to 20 Gy in 10 fractions.[470] In another report, radiation produced complete local control of large, unresectable lymphangiomas in three patients, findings that are consistent with other anecdotal reports of lymphangiomyomatosis.[462,471]

Tumors of Vascular Tissue

Mediastinal mesenchymal lesions of endothelial origin include hemangiomas, hemangioendotheliomas, and hemangiopericytomas. Many of these tumors have an indolent course, but hemangiopericytomas are notable for high rates of metastasis at presentation.[473–476] Hemangiomas can be capillary or cavernous; cavernous hemangiomas (i.e., angiomyomas or hamartomas) are distinguished from capillary hemangiomas by the presence of smooth muscle. Hemangiomas and hemangioendotheliomas are typically well circumscribed. Hemangioendotheliomas contain the hallmark cytoplasmic Weibel-Palade bodies.[477,478]

Hemangiopericytomas arise from the capillary contractile pericytes of Zimmerman.[473] Although most are indolent, recurrence and metastases have been observed many years after resection.[479] Retrospective studies suggest that high mitotic rates and proliferative indices may portend malignant behavior.[480,481] Nevertheless, long-term survival is still possible with aggressive treatment of metastatic disease.[482] Surgery remains the mainstay of therapy and is often curative.[483] Because of their benign nature, hemangiomas or hemangioendotheliomas should not be treated with radiation.[483] An endoscopic approach has been proposed for several types of intrathoracic tumors including benign hemangiomas and should be explored further.[484] Radiation remains an option for incompletely resected hemangiopericytomas.

Miscellaneous Mediastinal Mesenchymal Lesions

A mélange of other mediastinal mesenchymal lesions have been occasionally encountered; usually of musculoskeletal

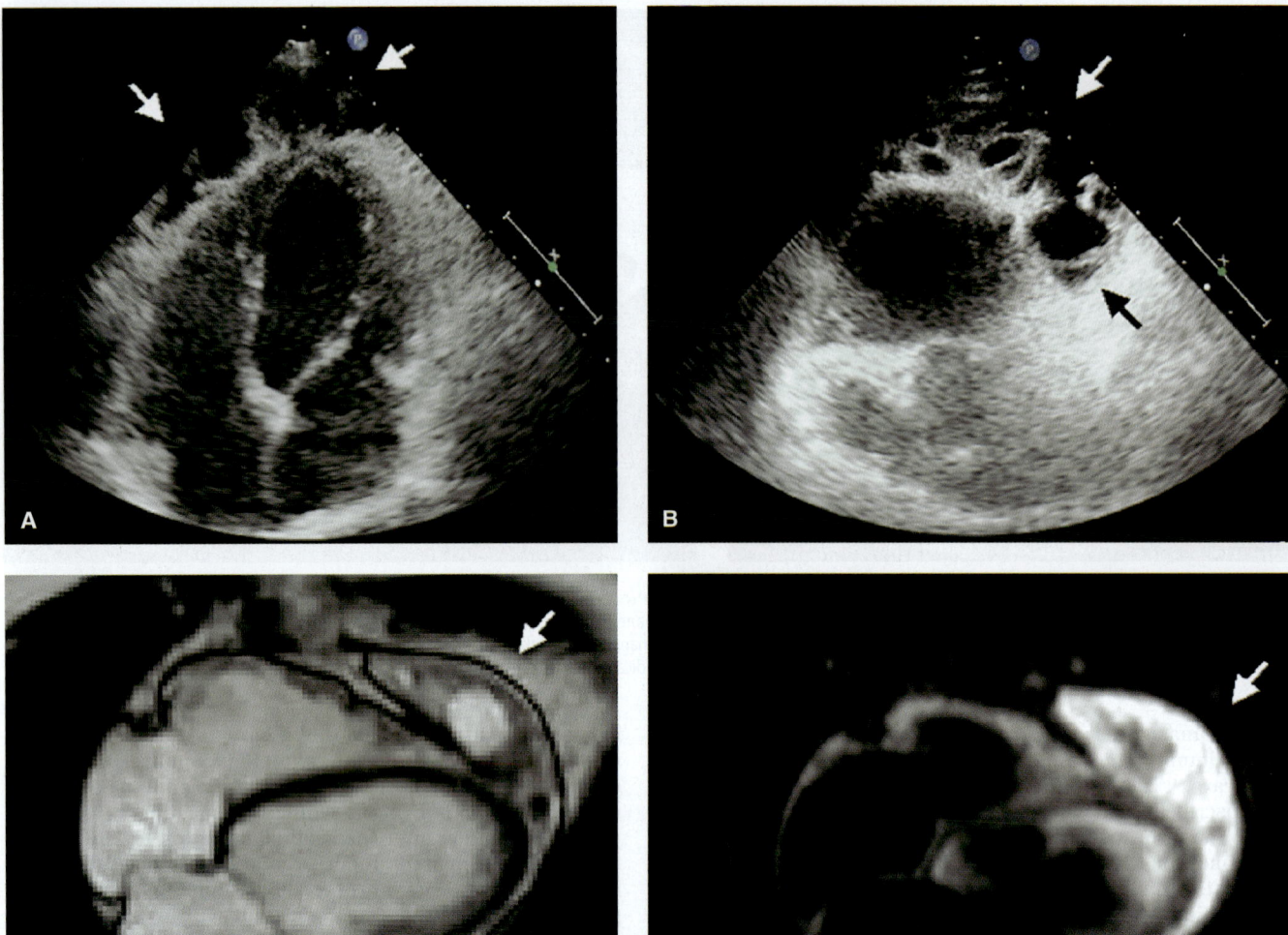

FIGURE 55.7. Echocardiographs **(A,B)** and cardiac magnetic resonance images **(C,D)** of mediastinal lymphangioma. The patient presented with palpitations and was found to have a cystic lymphangioma surrounding both ventricles from the apex to the left atrioventricular groove. (Reprinted from Conte G, Aldrovandi A, Reverberi C, et al. Mediastinal cystic lymphangioma. *J Am Coll Cardiol* 2011;57[16]:e207. Copyright © 2011 American College of Cardiology Foundation. With permission.)

or connective tissue origin, these lesions typically appear within the posterior mediastinum.[431] These lesions have been treated with surgical excision and occasionally postoperative radiation therapy, depending on the histology and clinical presentation.[428–431,485–489]

MEDIASTINAL NEUROGENIC TUMORS

Epidemiology

Neurogenic tumors of the thorax are generally classified by their neural cell of origin, including tumors of the nerve sheath (schwannomas and neurofibromas), autonomic ganglion (ganglioneuromas and neuroblastomas), and paraganglion (paragangliomas and pheochromocytomas). Most neurogenic lesions arise in the posterior mediastinum. Indeed, they are the most common cause of a posterior mediastinal mass and account for roughly one-quarter to one-third of all mediastinal neoplasms.[9,11,490,491]

Neurogenic neoplasms are rare, with an incidence of 0.5 per million in adults.[11] Neuroblastoma, an aggressive

variant of neurogenic tumors, occurs primarily in children[492] and appears in the mediastinum in about 20% of cases. Neuroblastomas are more common in male Caucasians, whereas other malignant neurogenic tumors occur at equal rates in both sexes.[493–495]

Paragangliomas are rare tumors that arise from extra-adrenal paraganglia and can be either functional (catecholamine-secreting) or nonfunctional.[496,497] Most of these tumors are benign and surgical resection is usually curative, but some studies have suggested that the risk of the tumor being malignant is >10%.[498,499]

The most common neurogenic tumors in adults are benign schwannomas and neurofibromas, often presenting in the setting of neurofibromatosis type 1 (NF-1), an autosomal dominant neurocutaneous disorder, with an estimated birth incidence of 1 in 2,500.[500] Individuals affected with NF-1 are at increased risk of developing both benign and malignant tumors. The most common benign tumor in individuals with NF-1 is neurofibroma, a heterogeneous benign peripheral nerve sheath tumor.[501,502] Neurofibromas can occur as discrete focal cutaneous or subcutaneous growths, as intraforaminal spinal tumors, or as plexiform tumors. Plexiform neurofibromas are composed of the same cell types as dermal neurofibromas but have an expanded extracellular matrix and a rich vascular supply.[502] In one study of 125 patients with NF-1, plexiform neurofibromas were clinically visible in 30%.[503] Schwannomas often originate from the intercostal or sympathetic nerves and can become quite large before being detected.[442] Surgery is the mainstay of treatment, but the possibility of achieving a R0 resection depends on the extent of locoregional disease. Long-term local control rates range from 90% to 100%.[491,493,504,505] In adults, most malignant mediastinal neurogenic tumors are malignant peripheral nerve sheath tumors (MPNSTs). Individuals with NF-1 carry heightened risk of developing MPNSTs, with a lifetime risk of almost 10%.[506,507] Because most NF-1–associated MPNSTs arise within pre-existing plexiform neurofibromas, individuals with NF-1 and plexiform neurofibromas warrant increased surveillance. In addition to their association with NF-1, MPNSTs have also been linked with prior radiation exposure.[508-511] In one series from the Mayo Clinic, almost 10% of the patients treated there over a 20-year period had a history of radiation exposure.[511]

With regard to anatomical origin, one single-institution experience reported that MPNSTs were located in the trunk in half of the patients studied.[495] The authors did not distinguish between mediastinal and retroperitoneal locations, but this distinction can be difficult given the lack of an anatomical barrier. Roughly, one-third of the patients in that study had NF-1. The median age at presentation of the MPNST was 37 years overall (27 years for patients with NF-1 and 40 for patients without).

Natural History and General Management

In up to 80% of cases, mediastinal neurogenic tumors present as an asymptomatic mass on a routine chest x-ray (Figs. 55.8 and 55.9). In some cases, these masses can grow slowly enough to involve nearly the entire hemithorax before detection.[494,512,513] Large or rapidly growing lesions can cause chest pain and nerve dysfunction (including Horner syndrome) from compression.[514] Proximal organs such as the vagus or phrenic nerves, esophagus, trachea, and cardiac chambers may be involved by direct extension or via the nerve sheath.[515-522] Local invasion and bony destruction are common.[523] Distant metastases are present in up to one-third of patients at diagnosis.[510] Because MPNSTs are difficult to detect before they infiltrate

nearby structures (making surgery difficult) and metastasize, they carry a poor prognosis.[524]

Management of malignant mediastinal neurogenic tumors entails a multidisciplinary approach similar to the management of adult soft tissue sarcomas. High-resolution CT (Fig. 55.10) is essential, as is MRI (Fig. 55.11), to evaluate the neural and spinal anatomy if involvement is suspected.[525] A definitive pathologic diagnosis is often reached after surgical intervention; examples of histologic slides of a schwannoma and a neurofibroma are shown in Figures 55.12 and 55.13. Histologic examination often reveals nuclear atypia, mitotic figures, cellularity, typical Antoni A and B areas, and tumor necrosis; these findings, in combination with positive immunohistochemical staining for S-100 protein and negative staining for smooth muscle markers such as desmin, are suggestive of a nerve sheath origin. Of these features, the factor most reliably correlated with malignancy is a mitotic figure of 5 or more in 50 high-power fields.

Surgical resection is the mainstay of therapy. An R0 resection should be attempted but is often difficult for mediastinal tumors because of impingement on surrounding structures and, in the case of neurofibromas, the risk of drastic neurologic deficits. Advances in surgical technique, including minimally invasive approaches such as video-assisted thoracoscopic surgery, are available but should be undertaken only by experienced thoracic surgeons.[526-528]

As is true for the treatment of soft tissue sarcomas, radiation appears to improve local control for MPNSTs when combined with surgery. The largest published series to date describes findings from 134 patients with NPNSTs treated at the Mayo Clinic between 1975 and 1993.[511] Only 25 of those patients had mediastinal tumors, and an R0 operation was possible for 70%, which was an improvement over a historical series showing an R0/R1 rate of only 55% for mediastinal MPNSTs.[529] About half of the patients received adjuvant radiation to a mean dose of 51 Gy using a variety of radiation techniques. At 10 years, the overall survival rate was 42% and local tumor control rate was 50% for the entire group of patients.

Prognostic factors for overall survival found to be significant in multivariate analyses were surgical margin status and history of radiation. Prognostic factors for local control were surgical margin status, radiation dose, and use of intraoperative radiation or brachytherapy. The use of adjuvant radiation nearly doubled local control rates from 40% to 73% at 3 years and from 34% to 65% at 5 years (*P* = .0004), but an apparent benefit in survival (43% vs. 58% at 5 years) was not statistically significant.

FIGURE 55.8. Posteroanterior chest radiographs of **(A)** a mediastinal schwannoma and **(B)** a mediastinal neurofibroma. (Courtesy of Steve Primack, MD.)

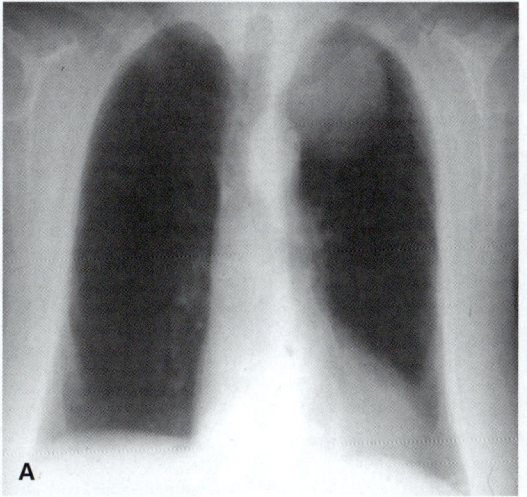
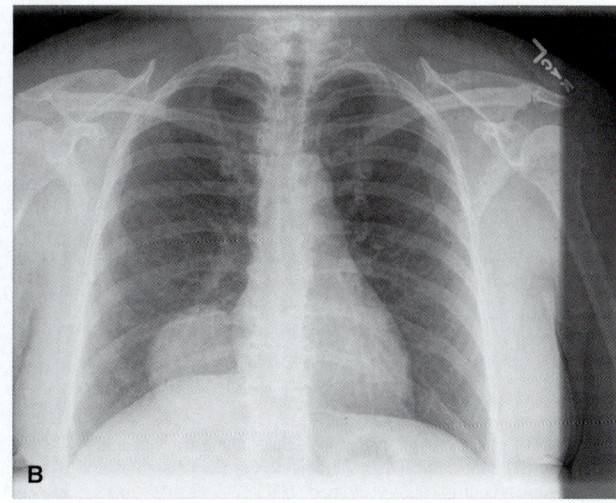

A

B

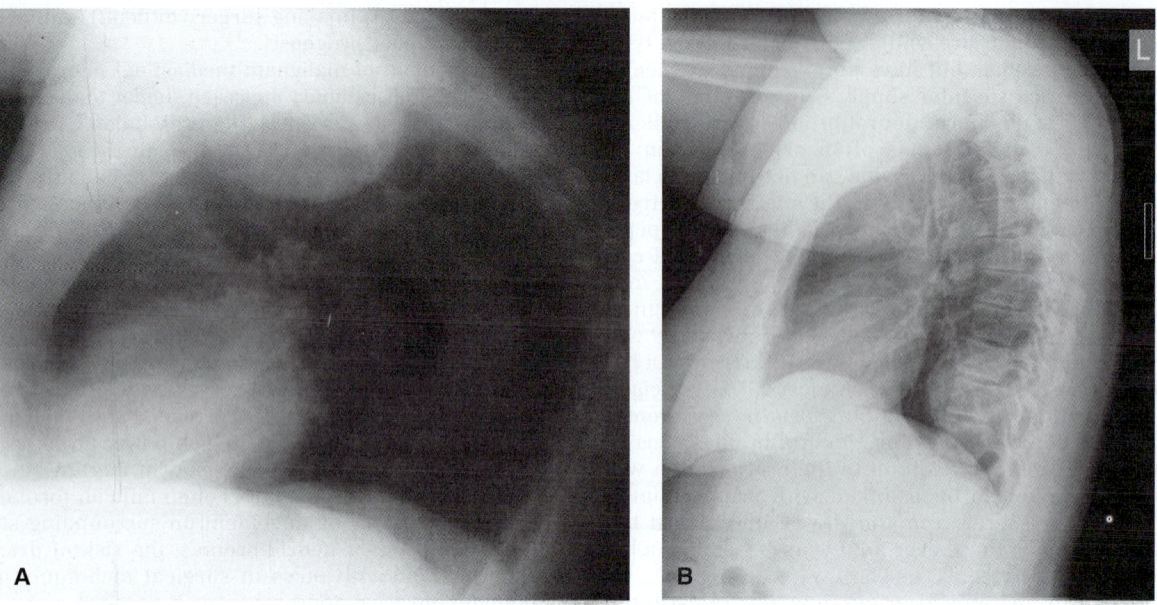

FIGURE 55.9. **A**, Lateral chest radiograph of a mediastinal schwannoma. (Courtesy of Steve Primack, MD.) **B**, Posteroanterior chest radiograph of a mediastinal neurofibroma. (Courtesy of Steve Primack, MD.)

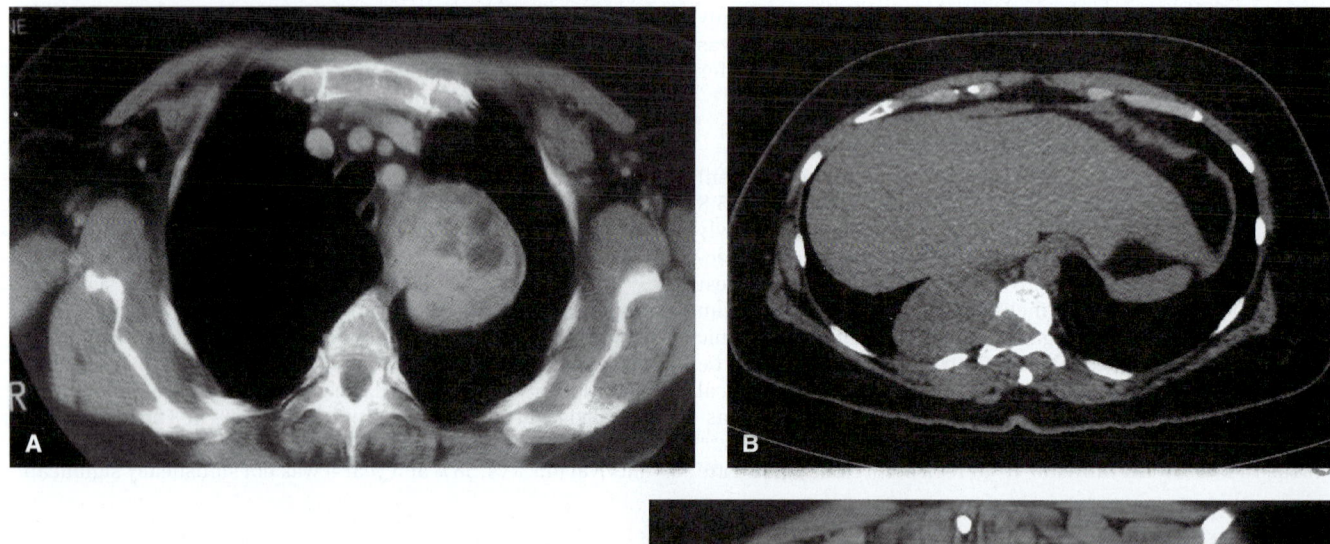

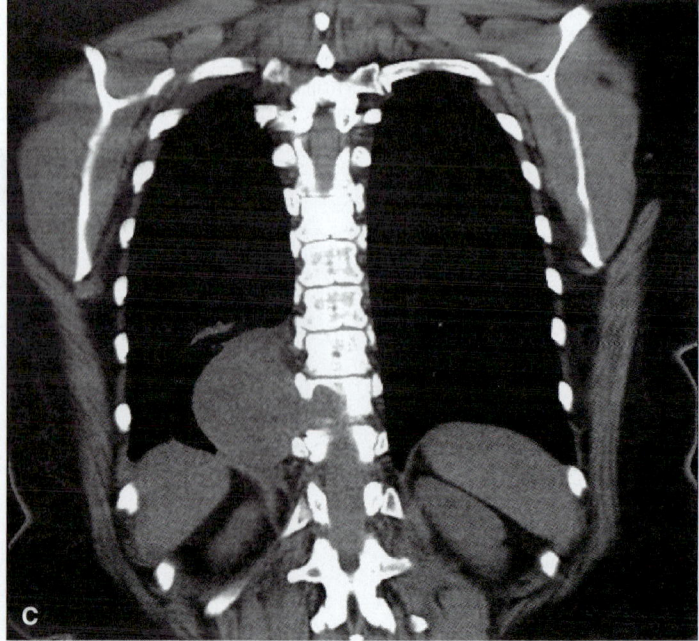

FIGURE 55.10. Axial CT scans of **(A)** a mediastinal schwannoma involving the sympathetic chain and **(B)** a mediastinal neurofibroma. **C**, Coronal CT scan of a mediastinal neurofibroma. (Courtesy of Steve Primack, MD.)

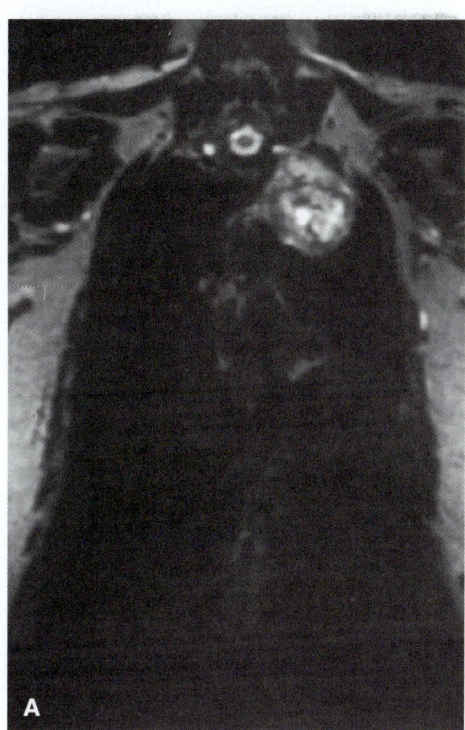 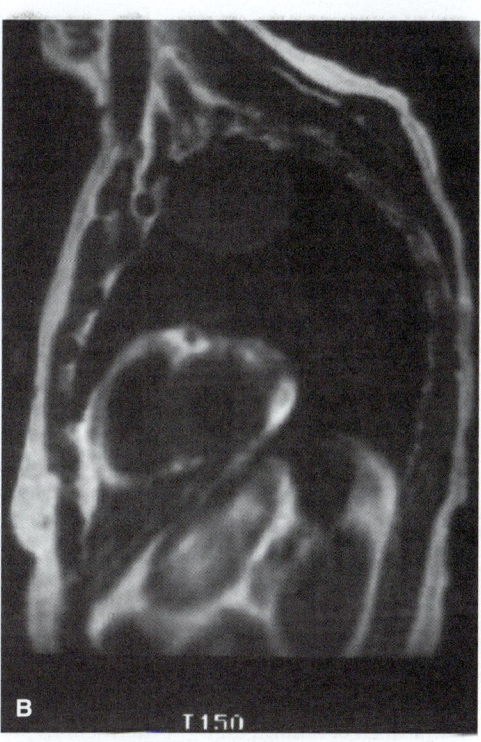

FIGURE 55.11. Coronal **(A)** and sagittal **(B)** magnetic resonance images of a mediastinal schwannoma involving the sympathetic chain. (Courtesy of Steve Primack, MD.)

Other evidence supporting the use of radiation after surgery for MPNSTs come from a review of 205 patients with localized MPNSTs at all body sites treated over a 25-year period at the Istituto Nazionale per lo Studio e la Cura dei Tumori in Milan, Italy.[495] That study reported a disease-specific mortality rate of 43% at 10 years in the context of only half of the patients receiving radiation therapy. Variables found to be significant in multivariate analyses for survival included tumor site, tumor size (>12 cm), surgical margin status, and the use of adjuvant radiation ($P = .016$). All of the same factors except for radiation were significantly associated with local control. Patients who received radiation seemed to have had fewer recurrences, but this was not statistically significant. About 30% of patients eventually developed distant metastases, the vast majority of which were pulmonary.

Planning and delivery of external beam radiation therapy for MPNSTs is facilitated with the use of modern approaches, including 3D conformal radiation, IMRT, and image-guided radiation using on-board imaging approaches. Patients with these tumors, which are complicated to manage, should be treated at centers with extensive multidisciplinary experience in thoracic and paraspinal neoplasms. Radiation treatment after surgery for microscopic disease should be given at a minimum dose of 60 Gy in 30 fractions, similar to the adjuvant dose given in other soft tissue sarcomas. Given the close proximity of the posterior mediastinum to the spinal cord, careful attention should be paid to immobilization and use of image guidance techniques. Although placing the patient in the prone position may reduce the distance from the localization points to the treatment volume, the patient must be able to rest comfortably in the same position throughout the

FIGURE 55.12. Hematoxylin-and-eosin–stained section of a schwannoma shows a circumscribed and encapsulated neoplasm composed of low-grade spindled and wavy Schwann cells with alternating palisaded cellular and stroma-rich areas (Verocay bodies) with nonpalisaded cellular foci (Antoni A areas) and hypocellular foci (Antoni B areas) (original magnification 100×). (Courtesy of David Sauer, MD.)

FIGURE 55.13. Hematoxylin-and-eosin–stained section of a neurofibroma shows a circumscribed and encapsulated neoplasm composed of a disorganized proliferation of low-grade spindled fibroblastic and Schwann cells within a myomatous and collagenous stroma (fibrils resembling shredded carrots). Scattered background mast cells and entrapped axons are also present (original magnification 100×). (Courtesy of David Sauer, MD.)

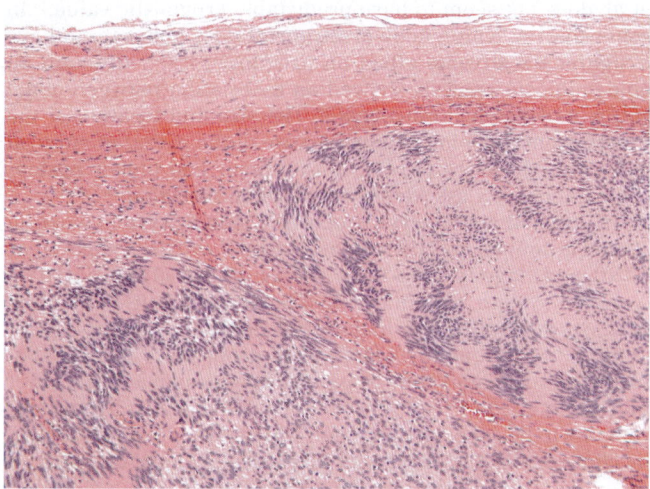 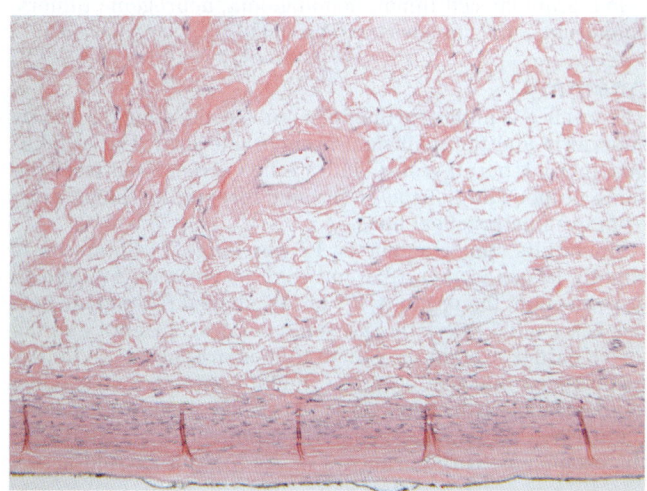

treatments. Daily on-board imaging with stereoscopic guidance can ensure daily accuracy. IMRT is often necessary to provide a concave dose distribution around the spinal cord. In cases of gross residual disease, higher doses may be beneficial but can be challenging to deliver given the constraints on exposure of normal tissues.

For patients with unresectable disease, radiation can be delivered either alone or with chemotherapeutic agents that are typically used for soft tissue sarcomas. Few agents are effective for MPNSTs, and treatment regimens usually include doxorubicin or ifosfamide.[530] Finally, significant progress has been made in recent years in elucidating the molecular genetics and biology of MPNSTs, especially in patients with NF-1. A variety of genetic alterations have been reported in MPNSTs, but it is yet unclear whether any of them are causally related to tumorigenesis or can be exploited for treatment effect.[531]

TRACHEAL CARCINOMAS

Tracheal neoplasms are quite rare, contributing to fewer than 0.5% of all tumors.[532] Most of the information available to date is derived from pooled population-based datasets or single-institution series involving a variety of treatment regimens. Review of the largely retrospective data has revealed several patterns: First, surgical resection is the cornerstone of therapy; second, local recurrence is a major pattern of failure; and third, adjuvant radiation seems to have some positive effect on outcomes.

Demographics

Primary tracheal malignancy is exceedingly uncommon, accounting for approximately 0.1% to 0.4% of all diagnosed malignancies.[533] Epidemiologic data from the SEER project estimate an incidence of 0.2 per 100,000 persons in the United States; the true incidence of tracheal carcinomas is likely even lower.[37] Traditionally, adenoid cystic carcinomas (formerly known as cylindromas) were considered the most common tracheal neoplasms, but recent reports suggest that the most prevalent histology worldwide is squamous cell carcinoma (60% to 90%).[534]

Tracheal cancer affects roughly twice as many men as women; estimates of incidence from SEER database are 0.2 per 100,000 for men and 0.1 per 100,000 for women.[535] The male-to-female ratio is 2 to 3:1 for squamous cancer but is closer to 1:1 for adenoid cystic carcinomas.[536] Use of tobacco is associated with squamous cell carcinoma of the trachea but generally not with adenoid cystic carcinoma.[490] Squamous cell variants typically present during the sixth decade of life, whereas adenoid cystic carcinomas seem to present at younger ages. Other histologies include carcinoid, carcinosarcoma, granular cell tumor, hemangioma, neurogenic tumors, chondroma, and chondrosarcoma.[537-583]

Anatomy

The trachea is a fibrocartilaginous tube connecting the larynx superiorly and the mainstem bronchi inferiorly. The esophagus, thyroid, parathyroids, and trachea are derived from the same outpouching of the embryonic foregut; the lungs arise from terminal tracheal buds.

In adults, the trachea is 12 cm long; its diameter is slightly larger in men (2.3 cm) than in women (2.0 cm). In cross-section, the organ is "C" or "U" shaped. The upper border lies around the sixth or seventh cervical vertebra and the lower border around the fourth (full expiration) or sixth (full inspiration) thoracic vertebra. Each centimeter of trachea contains about two cartilaginous rings. The posterior aspect of the trachea is membranous and is intimately associated with the esophagus. Three branches of the inferior thyroid artery

supply blood to the upper half of the trachea and connect to the superior thyroid artery, which contributes small vessels that run from the tracheal wall adjacent to the thyroid isthmus. The bronchial arteries supply blood to the lower trachea and carina. Arterial branches interdigitate between each cartilaginous ring (see Fig. 55.2).

Natural History

Tracheal carcinomas can present with a variety of symptoms, including cough, dyspnea, dysphagia, and hemoptysis.[565,584] Yang et al. reported cough to be the most common symptom (present in 72% of patients), followed by dyspnea (66%), stridor (39%), hemoptysis (39%), and dysphonia (31%).[585] Adenoid cystic carcinomas in particular are often first mistaken for asthma, which is often treated as such until "refractory" obstructive symptoms are evaluated with bronchoscopy, typically after numerous "normal" chest radiographs.[583,584,586-595] Hemoptysis is more likely to be the presenting symptom of squamous cell carcinoma,[585,596] and dysphagia is considered an ominous sign.[597] In one study of nonadenoid cystic/nonsquamous tracheal tumors, benign tumors presented with dyspnea, whereas malignant tumors were associated with hemoptysis.[540]

In 40% to 50% of cases, adenoid cystic carcinomas are diagnosed with metastases,[598] but survival is relatively long despite the presence of such metastases.[596,599-602] In one series, the median survival time for such patients was 37 months,[536] and median reported survival from the time of diagnosis was approximately 5 years.[534,585] When these tumors spread, they almost always do so in distant nodes rather than in the locoregional paratracheal lymph nodes. Local recurrence is the predominant form of treatment failure and can appear 10 or more years after treatment.[603-605]

Unlike adenoid cystic carcinoma, squamous cell carcinoma has a much more aggressive course, with reported median survival times of only 6 to 12 months depending on resectability.[18,596,600,601,606-610] The disease often presents with local extension via paratracheal lymph nodes (in ~30% of cases) and distant metastases.[611]

The clinical course and natural history of other pathologic variants of tracheal tumors are difficult to accurately characterize because of the scarcity of reported findings. Adenocarcinomas and sarcomas are thought to have poor prognoses.[540,576,578,582,612-625] Granular cell tumor, carcinoid, lymphoma, leiomyoma, and small cell carcinoma all have variable prognoses, yet they seem to be less aggressive than the squamous carcinomas, adenocarcinomas, or sarcomas.[540]

Staging and Prognostic Factors

No system for staging tracheal neoplasms has been universally accepted or adopted. One staging system proposed by Licht et al. does not seem to have predictable prognostic value.[46] In some studies, lymph node involvement does not seem to have a significant adverse effect on prognosis,[18,585,611] although an epidemiologic analysis showed an association between nodal status and survival outcomes.[626] The size and location of the tumor seem to be important because of the extent of surgical resection necessary to remove the tumor and higher postoperative mortality associated with carinal resection.[586,626,627]

In 2004, Bhattacharyya proposed a staging system wherein stage I is defined as T1N0 disease, stage II as T2N0, stage III as T3N0, and stage IV as T4N0 or any N1 disease (Table 55.10).[626] A similar system, with minor modifications, was used by Webb et al. in evaluating the experience at MD Anderson Cancer Center.[534] Subsequently, Macchiarini proposed a more elaborate staging model that draws from experience with other thoracic malignancies[532] (Table 55.10). However, at this time, it remains to be seen which system will be broadly implemented by clinicians or validated with large-scale clinical datasets.

TABLE 55.10 STAGING SYSTEMS FOR TRACHEAL CARCINOMA

Bhattacharyya Staging System[581]

Primary Tumor (T)

T1	Primary tumor confined to the trachea; size <2 cm
T2	Primary tumor confined to the trachea; size >2 cm
T3	Spread outside the trachea but not to adjacent organs or structures[a]
T4	Spread to adjacent organs or structures[a]
Tx	Unknown or cannot be assessed

Regional Lymph Nodes (N)

N0	No evidence of regional nodal disease
N1	Positive regional nodal disease
Nx	Unknown or cannot be assessed

[a]The MD Anderson system denotes "arising from but extending outside of trachea" as T3 disease and does not use T4.[490]

Anatomic Stage/Prognostic Groups

Stage

I	T1	N0
II	T2	N0
III	T3	N0
IV	Any	N1
IV	T4	Any

Macchiarini Staging System[487]

Primary Tumor (T)

Tx	Cannot be assessed
Tis	Any tumor without invasion
T1a	<3 cm limited to mucosa
T1b	≥3 cm limited to mucosa
T2*	Any tumor that invades cartilage or adventitia
T3	Any tumor that invades trachea or larynx
T4a	Any tumor that invades carina or main bronchus
T4b	Any tumor that invades neighboring structures

Regional Lymph Nodes (N)

Nx	Regional lymph nodes cannot be assessed
N0	No evidence of node metastasis
N1	Local nodes positive (N1a < 3 cm; N1b ≥ 3 cm)
Upper third	Highest mediastinal nodes; upper paratracheal nodes, prevascular and retrotracheal
Middle third	Upper paratracheal nodes; prevascular and retrotracheal; lower paratracheal nodes; para-aortic nodes (ascending aorta or phrenic)
Lower third	Upper paratracheal nodes; prevascular and retrotracheal; subaortic nodes (aortopulmonalis window)
N1A	1–3 positive nodes in upper third
N1B	>3 positive nodes in upper third
N2	Regional nodes positive
Upper third	Lower paratracheal nodes; subaortic nodes (aortopulmonalis window)
Middle third	Highest mediastinal nodes; subaortic nodes (aortopulmonalis window)
Lower third	Upper paratracheal nodes; pulmonary ligament

Distant Metastasis (M)

Mx	Distant metastasis cannot be assessed
M0	No distant metastasis
M1	Metastasis to nodes other than N1 and N2
M2	Distant metastasis (e.g., lung)

Anatomic Stage/Prognostic Groups

Stage

0	Tis	N0	M0
Ia	T1a	N0	M0
Ib	T1b–2	N0	M0
IIa	T1b–2	N1	M0
IIb	T1b–2	N2	M0
IIIa	T3	N0	M0
IIIb	T3	N1–2	M0
IVa	Any	N1–2	M1
IVb	Any	N1–2	M2

General Management

Bronchoscopy is essential for diagnosis of tracheal malignancies and for preoperative surgical planning.[584,628–630] In acute respiratory compromise, rigid bronchoscopy (see Fig. 55.2) may be indicated to "core out" the tracheal neoplasm.[586,631,632]

In one series of 56 patients reported by Mathisen and Grillo, rigid bronchoscopy led to improved airway symptoms in 90% of cases, with 5% experiencing mild, easily controlled bleeding.[633] Esophagoscopy is suggested for all patients to rule out esophageal invasion. A CT scan of the chest is indicated to aid in evaluation of tumor extension, resectability, involvement of lymph nodes, and pulmonary metastases,[565,584,630,634–638] and coronal reconstruction can be helpful to evaluate tracheal wall thickening and extraluminal extension.[639]

Treatment Approaches

Resectability is universally associated with lower mortality in reported series[18,601,628,640] and as such is the initial strategy for most tracheal primaries.[532,610,611,628,635,641–643] Resection rates vary, however, by institutional and national practice, from 10% to over 65% based on the above cited studies. Historic registry data from the Netherlands demonstrated a resection rate of 12%[606]; however, a recent update[644] suggests that 24% underwent resection in 2000 to 2005 (vs. 58% who received radiotherapy). Contraindications to resection depend in large part on the preference of the surgeon; for example, Pearson recommends tracheal resection for at least some patients with adenoid cystic carcinoma with low burden pulmonary metastases, yet many would consider such cases unresectable.[536,598,645] Regardless, many tracheal carcinomas are either improperly classified (e.g., nontracheal primaries with tracheal extension) or are systematically undertreated surgically.[644]

Most patients undergoing surgery have a median sternotomy and cervical collar excision, although extensive subglottic or high tracheal disease may require cervical exenteration with mediastinal tracheostomy.[598,604,611] Margins may of necessity be compromised to ensure a functioning airway. Technical advances in surgical procedures such as complete mobilization of the right hilar ligament, detachment/implantation of the left hilum, mobilization of the cervical trachea, and techniques for carinal resection/reconstruction and intrapericardial dissection have improved the likelihood of an R_0 resection.[338,627,640,646] Gaissert et al. reported improvements in both complete resection rates (from 68% to 82%) and in-hospital mortality (declining from 21% to 3%) with the increasing use of such techniques over a 40-year period.[600,641]

After resection, postoperative radiation is usually recommended.[534,600,601,628,629,632,641] Pathologic features such as completeness of resection, involvement of the thyroid gland, and lymphatic invasion have clearly been shown to have prognostic value,[647] and postoperative radiotherapy is routinely recommended for all patients at many institutions.[534,647] Preoperative radiotherapy has also been attempted, but fewer reports of this experience have been published. In aggregate, several small retrospective series seem to show a benefit for adjuvant radiation (Table 55.11). Chow et al. found that patients who underwent resection plus adjuvant radiation had a median survival time of 61 months versus 16 months for those who received only surgery.[648] Regnand and others found that 31 patients who had had a complete resection with adjuvant radiation had seemingly better 5-year survival rates than did 27 patients without adjuvant radiation (74% vs. 53%), but this apparent difference was not statistically significant.[18]

Postoperative radiation seems to be effective for incompletely resected disease as well, with 5-year survival rates of 45% for such patients versus 0% for patients who did not receive radiation ($P < .05$).[18] Webb et al., describing the experience at MD Anderson, demonstrated a statistically significant improvement in survival for patients given adjuvant radiotherapy rather than chemoradiation; however, no difference in survival was found between adjuvant radiotherapy and surgery alone.[534] The results of studies of definitive therapy for tracheal tumors are summarized in Table 55.12.

Section III

TABLE 55.11 RESULTS OF RESECTION WITH ADJUVANT IRRADIATION FOR PRIMARY TRACHEAL CARCINOMA

Study and Reference	Histology	Treatment	Median Survival Times or Rates
Grillo and Mathisen[601]	Squamous (n = 70)	Surgery ± RT[a]	34 mo
		RT	10 mo
	Adenoid cystic (n = 80)	Surgery ± RT[a]	118 mo
		RT	28 mo
Licht et al.[46]	–	Surgery alone (n = 6)	48% (5-year actuarial)
		RT alone (n = 35)	7%
		Laser/cautery ± RT (n = 24)	28%
		RT + chemo (n = 2)	0%
Chow et al.[648]	–	Surgery alone (n = 5)	16 mo
		RT alone (n = 12)	26 mo
		Surgery + RT (n = 5)	61 mo
Regnard et al.[18]	–	R_0 + RT (n = 31)	74% (5-y actuarial)
		R_0 (n = 27)	53% (P = NS)
		$R_{1,2}$ + RT (n = 15)	47%
		$R_{1,2}$ (n = 6)	0% (P < .05)
Maziak et al.[536]	Adenoid cystic (n = 35)	R_0 ± RT (n = 14)[a]	9.8 y
		$R_{1,2}$ + RT (n = 15)	7.5 y
		RT alone (n = 6)	6.2 y

[a]A minority of these patients received surgery alone.
R_0, complete resection; $R_{1,2}$, incomplete resection; RT, radiation therapy.

Radiation has also been used as monotherapy for unresectable tumors. Results are best when doses have exceeded 60 Gy.[607,650,652] Mornex et al. found that the 5-year survival rate decreased from 12% for those receiving at least 56 Gy to 5% for those receiving lower doses.[654] However, Chow et al. caution against giving doses higher than 60 Gy, as three of six patients in their study given doses in excess of 60 Gy had severe complications requiring surgical intervention, such as tracheoesophageal fistula, esophageal stricture, and severe tracheal crusting,[648] whereas none of the six patients treated with <60 Gy in that study had late side effects. Other authors have corroborated the concern of high doses contributing to the risk of complications.[655] Still, Chow et al. noted significantly better local control among patients who received >50 Gy as adjuvant therapy and >60 Gy as definitive therapy.[603] By way of comparison, Fuwa et al. reported reasonable results with a novel endoluminal-centering catheter; the median dose delivered to the group as a whole was 91 Gy (given as external beam radiation with low–dose rate ^{192}Ir brachytherapy). Only one treatment-related death was reported 1 year after therapy in a patient who had received a total dose of 113 Gy.[653] Harms et al., using median doses of 60 Gy delivered by external beam radiation plus 15- to 18-Gy brachytherapy boosts, reported minimal rates of severe (grade 3 to 4) toxicity (8% of 25 patients).[656] Exploratory studies of fast neutrons for locally advanced adenoid cystic carcinomas have been reported; in the University of Washington experience with endoluminal brachytherapy, fast neutrons were considered feasible with acceptable toxicity.[657] A summary of the experience with radiation as monotherapy for primary tracheal neoplasms is given in Table 55.11.

Combined chemoradiotherapy without resection has been attempted at some institutions, usually for nonsquamous tumors, with mixed results.[534,596,658,659] In general, patients with squamous cell carcinoma have fared poorly, and those with small cell carcinoma or lymphoma have done better.[46,534,585,660]

Radiation Techniques

No evidence is available to suggest that adjuvant radiation therapy is not beneficial in tracheal malignancies; however, any postoperative radiation should not be begun before 30 to 45 days after surgery to allow sufficient wound healing. Modern CT-based 3D conformal or intensity-modulated radiation techniques should be used. Aggressive treatment is warranted to prevent airway obstruction even when the intent is palliative.[654] External beam doses should be about 60 Gy for fully resected disease,[534] with a boost considered for squamous cell lesions with high-risk features.[647] An intraluminal boost technique allows the dose to be increased (and, theoretically, local control to be increased as well) with minimal added acute or late side effects.[609,648,656,661–663] Standard constraints on organs at risk should be observed in all cases.[271,272,274,664]

Intraluminal brachytherapy is also useful for palliative treatment. Skowronek et al., in a study of patients treated with 10 to 30 Gy in one to three fractions, found that high-dose brachytherapy as monotherapy led to prolonged survival and improved quality of life.[663] In patients with locally extensive disease, the gravest complication of radiation therapy is the development of a tracheoesophageal fistula, which can be difficult if not impossible to avoid. For patients with emergent airway obstruction, rigid bronchoscopy should be performed instead of urgent radiotherapy.

The role of elective nodal irradiation for tracheal carcinoma is uncertain. As mentioned earlier, nodal status does not seem to have prognostic significance; even cervical adenopathy was not associated with poorer outcome.[585] Given the low proclivity for lymphatic spread of adenoid cystic carcinomas, the choice to avoid elective nodal irradiation for this variant is certainly reasonable. Because local recurrence is the major factor influencing survival, nodal and regional failure patterns are not a main concern. Yet, if mediastinal or cervical nodes are seen on radiographic or pathologic examination, or if worrisome pathologic risk features[647] are discovered at surgery, radiation to these regions should be considered.

TABLE 55.12 RETROSPECTIVE SERIES EXAMINING RADIOTHERAPY ALONE FOR PRIMARY TRACHEAL CARCINOMA

Study and Reference	Histology	Treatment	Local Control	Survival
Schraube et al.[609]	Squamous (n = 11)	46–60 Gy RT + 15–20 Gy HDR	6/11	31 mo median
Cheung[649]	Squamous (n = 20)	40–60 Gy		5 mo median
	Adenoid cystic (n = 4)	40–60 Gy		12 mo median
Fields et al.[650]	Squamous (n = 17)	>60 Gy	5/6	25% at 5 y (n = 18)
		40–60 Gy	1/7	
		<40 Gy	0/4	
	Adenoid cystic (n = 1)	>60 Gy	1/1	
Rostom and Morgan[651]	Squamous (n = 28)	60–70 Gy	16/24	11% (4-y actuarial)
	Adenoid cystic (n = 3)	<60 Gy	0/4	67% at 4 y
		50–70 Gy		
Makarewick and Mross[652]		60 Gy RT + 6–12 Gy HDR (n = 8)	6/8	9.5 mo median (n = 23)
		40–60 Gy RT (n = 3)	1/3	
		<40 Gy (n = 12)	0/12	
Fuwa et al.[653]		RT + LDR (n = 4) (80–128 Gy)[a]	3/4	75% at 3 y

[a]One treatment-related death in patient receiving 60 Gy RT + 53 Gy LDR Ir-192.
HDR, high-dose rate brachytherapy; LDR, low-dose rate brachytherapy; RT, external beam radiotherapy.

CONCLUSION

Primary tracheal cancer is quite rare and, in most cases, is of squamous or adenoid cystic histology. The optimal management strategy for these tumors seems to be a combined modality approach incorporating surgical resection and postoperative radiation. For localized disease, the role of chemotherapy, either alone or concurrent with radiation, is unknown.

REFERENCES

1. Nagaishi C, Nagasawa N. *Functional anatomy and histology of the lung.* Tokyo, Japan: Igaku Shoin, 1972.
2. Burkell CC, Cross JM, Kent HP, et al. Mass lesions of the mediastinum. *Curr Probl Surg* 1969;6(6):2–57.
3. Fraser RS, Fraser RG, et al. The normal chest. In: Fraser RS, Fraser RG, et al., eds. *Synopsis of diseases of the chest.* 2nd ed. Philadelphia: W.B. Saunders, 1994.
4. Strollo DC, Rosado-de-Christenson ML, Jett JR. Primary mediastinal tumors: part II. Tumors of the middle and posterior mediastinum. *Chest* 1997;112(5):1344–1357.
5. Carter BW, Benveniste MF, Madan R, et al. ITMIG classification of mediastinal compartments and multidisciplinary approach to mediastinal masses. *Radiographics* 2017;37(2):413–436.
6. Fornasiero A, Daniele O, Ghiotto C, et al. Chemotherapy of invasive thymoma. *J Clin Oncol* 1990;8(8):1419–1423.
7. Greene MA, Malias MA. Aggressive multimodality treatment of invasive thymic carcinoma. *J Thorac Cardiovasc Surg* 2003;125(2):434–436.
8. Adkins RB Jr, Maples MD, Hainsworth JD. Primary malignant mediastinal tumors. *Ann Thorac Surg* 1984;38(6):648–659.
9. Azarow KS, Pearl RH, Zurcher R, et al. Primary mediastinal masses. A comparison of adult and pediatric populations. *J Thorac Cardiovasc Surg* 1993;106(1):67–72.
10. Cohen AJ, Thompson L, Edwards FH, et al. Primary cysts and tumors of the mediastinum. *Ann Thorac Surg* 1991;51(3):378–384; discussion 385–376.
11. Davis RD Jr, Oldham HN Jr, Sabiston DC Jr. Primary cysts and neoplasms of the mediastinum: recent changes in clinical presentation, methods of diagnosis, management, and results. *Ann Thorac Surg* 1987;44(3):229–237.
12. Whooley BP, Urschel JD, Antkowiak JG, et al. Primary tumors of the mediastinum. *J Surg Oncol* 1999;70(2):95–99.
13. Grosfeld JL. Primary tumors of the chest wall and mediastinum in children. *Semin Thorac Cardiovasc Surg* 1994;6(4):235–239.
14. Grosfeld JL, Weinberger M, Kilman JW, et al. Primary mediastinal neoplasms in infants and children. *Ann Thorac Surg* 1971;12(2):179–190.
15. Mullen B, Richardson JD. Primary anterior mediastinal tumors in children and adults. *Ann Thorac Surg* 1986;42(3):338–345.
16. Engels EA. Epidemiology of thymoma and associated malignancies. *J Thorac Oncol* 2010;5(10 Suppl 4):S260–S265.
17. Lewis JE, Wick MR, Scheithauer BW, et al. Thymoma. A clinicopathologic review. *Cancer* 1987;60(11):2727–2743.
18. Regnard JF, Fourquier P, Levasseur P. Results and prognostic factors in resections of primary tracheal tumors: a multicenter retrospective study. The French Society of Cardiovascular Surgery. *J Thorac Cardiovasc Surg* 1996;111(4):808–813; discussion 813–804.
19. Maggi G, Casadio C, Cavallo A, et al. Thymoma: results of 241 operated cases. *Ann Thorac Surg* 1991;51(1):152–156.
20. Pan CC, Wu HP, Yang CF, et al. The clinicopathological correlation of epithelial subtyping in thymoma: a study of 112 consecutive cases. *Hum Pathol* 1994;25(9):893–899.
21. Okumura M, Miyoshi S, Takeuchi Y, et al. Results of surgical treatment of thymomas with special reference to the involved organs. *J Thorac Cardiovasc Surg* 1999;117(3):605–613.
22. Nakahara K, Ohno K, Hashimoto J, et al. Thymoma: results with complete resection and adjuvant postoperative irradiation in 141 consecutive patients. *J Thorac Cardiovasc Surg* 1988;95(6):1041–1047.
23. Engels EA, Pfeiffer RM. Malignant thymoma in the United States: demographic patterns in incidence and associations with subsequent malignancies. *Int J Cancer* 2003;105(4):546–551.
24. Gonzales DG. The need for clinical studies in thymomas. *Radiother Oncol* 1991;21:75–76.
25. Lewis BD, Hurt RD, Payne WS, et al. Benign teratomas of the mediastinum. *J Thorac Cardiovasc Surg* 1983;86(5):727–731.
26. Cowen D, Hannoun-Levi JM, Resbeut M, et al. Natural history and treatment of malignant thymoma. *Oncology (Williston Park)* 1998;12(7):1001–1005; discussion 1006.
27. Thomas CR, Wright CD, Loehrer PJ. Thymoma: state of the art. *J Clin Oncol* 1999;17(7):2280–2289.
28. Dimery IW, Lee JS, Blick M, et al. Association of the Epstein-Barr virus with lymphoepithelioma of the thymus. *Cancer* 1988;61(12):2475–2480.
29. McGuire LJ, Huang DP, Teoh R, et al. Epstein-Barr virus genome in thymoma and thymic lymphoid hyperplasia. *Am J Pathol* 1988;131(3):385–390.
30. Teoh R, McGuire L, Wong K, et al. Increased incidence of thymoma in Chinese myasthenia gravis: possible relationship with Epstein-Barr virus. *Acta Neurol Scand* 1989;80(3):221–225.
31. Jensen MO, Antonenko D. Thyroid and thymic malignancy following childhood irradiation. *J Surg Oncol* 1992;50(3):206–208.
32. Lam WW, Chan FL, Lau YL, et al. Paediatric thymoma: unusual occurrence in two siblings. *Pediatr Radiol* 1993;23(2):124–126.
33. Matani A, Dritsas C. Familial occurrence of thymoma. *Arch Pathol* 1973;95(2):90–91.
34. Wick MR, Carney JA, Bernatz PE, et al. Primary mediastinal carcinoid tumors. *Am J Surg Pathol* 1982;6(3):195–205.
35. Batata MA, Martini N, Huvos AG, et al. Thymomas: clinicopathologic features, therapy, and prognosis. *Cancer* 1974;34(2):389–396.
36. Bergh NP, Gatzinsky P, Larsson S, et al. Tumors of the thymus and thymic region: I. Clinicopathological studies on thymomas. *Ann Thorac Surg* 1978;25(2):91–98.
37. Bernatz PE, Khonsari S, Harrison EG Jr, et al. Thymoma: factors influencing prognosis. *Surg Clin North Am* 1973;53(4):885–892.
38. Curran WJ Jr, Kornstein MJ, Brooks JJ, et al. Invasive thymoma: the role of mediastinal irradiation following complete or incomplete surgical resection. *J Clin Oncol* 1988;6(11):1722–1727.
39. Fujimura S, Kondo T, Handa M, et al. Results of surgical treatment for thymoma based on 66 patients. *J Thorac Cardiovasc Surg* 1987;93(5):708–714.
40. Kilman JW, Klassen KP. Thymoma. *Am J Surg* 1971;121(6):710–711.
41. Legg MA, Brady WJ. Pathology and clinical behavior of thymomas: a survey of 51 cases. *Cancer* 1965;18:1131–1144.
42. LeGolvan DP, Abell MR. Thymomas. *Cancer* 1977;39(5):2142–2157.
43. Maggi G, Giaccone G, Donadio M, et al. Thymomas. A review of 169 cases, with particular reference to results of surgical treatment. *Cancer* 1986;58(3):765–776.
44. Salyer WR, Eggleston JC. Thymoma: a clinical and pathological study of 65 cases. *Cancer* 1976;37(1):229–249.
45. Wilkins EW Jr, Castleman B. Thymoma: a continuing survey at the Massachusetts General Hospital. *Ann Thorac Surg* 1979;28(3):252–256.
46. Licht PB, Friis S, Pettersson G. Tracheal cancer in Denmark: a nationwide study. *Eur J Cardiothorac Surg* 2001;19(3):339–345.
47. Patterson GA. Thymomas. *Semin Thorac Cardiovasc Surg* 1992;4(1):39–44.
48. Blumberg D, Port JL, Weksler B, et al. Thymoma: a multivariate analysis of factors predicting survival. *Ann Thorac Surg* 1995;60(4):908–913; discussion 914.
49. Wilkins KB, Sheikh E, Green R, et al. Clinical and pathologic predictors of survival in patients with thymoma. *Ann Surg* 1999;230(4):562–572; discussion 572–564.
50. Rosenow EC III, Hurley BT. Disorders of the thymus. A review. *Arch Intern Med* 1984;144(4):763–770.
51. Souadjian JV, Enriquez P, Silverstein MN III. The spectrum of diseases associated with thymoma. Coincidence or syndrome? *Arch Intern Med* 1974;134(2):374–379.
52. Kondo K, Monden Y. Therapy for thymic epithelial tumors: a clinical study of 1,320 patients from Japan. *Ann Thorac Surg* 2003;76(3):878–884; discussion 884-875.
53. Kondo K, Monden Y. Thymoma and myasthenia gravis: a clinical study of 1,089 patients from Japan. *Ann Thorac Surg* 2005;79(1):219–224.
54. Drachman DB. Myasthenia gravis. *N Engl J Med* 1994;330(25):1797–1810.
55. Morgenthaler TI, Brown LR, Colby TV, et al. Thymoma. *Mayo Clin Proc* 1993;68(11):1110–1123.
56. Castleman B. The pathology of the thymus gland in myasthenia gravis. *Ann N Y Acad Sci* 1966;135(1):496–505.
57. Rosenberg J. Neoplasms of the mediastinum. In: DeVita VT Jr, Hellman S, Rosenberg SA, eds. *Cancer: Principles and Practice of Oncology.* 3rd ed. Philadelphia: Lippincott, 1989:706.
58. Buckingham JM, Howard FM Jr, Bernatz PE, et al. The value of thymectomy in myasthenia gravis: a computer-assisted matched study. *Ann Surg* 1976;184(4):453–458.
59. Drachman DB. Myasthenia gravis (first of two parts). *N Engl J Med* 1978;298(3):136–142.
60. Drachman DB. Myasthenia gravis (second of two parts). *N Engl J Med* 1978;298(4):186–193.
61. Vincent A, Palace J, Hilton-Jones D. Myasthenia gravis. *Lancet* 2001;357(9274):2122–2128.
62. Chahinian AP, Bhardwaj S, Meyer RJ, et al. Treatment of invasive or metastatic thymoma: report of eleven cases. *Cancer* 1981;47(7):1752–1761.
63. Cohen DJ, Ronnigen LD, Graeber GM, et al. Management of patients with malignant thymoma. *J Thorac Cardiovasc Surg* 1984;87(2):301–307.
64. Marchevsky AM, Kaneko M, Cohen BA. *Surgical pathology of the mediastinum.* New York: Raven, 1984.
65. Wilkens EW, Grillo HC, Scannell G. Role of staging in prognosis and management of thymoma. *Ann Thorac Surg* 1991;51:888–892.
66. Masaoka A, Yamakawa Y, Niwa H, et al. Thymectomy and malignancy. *Eur J Cardiothorac Surg* 1994;8(5):251–253.
67. Vessey MP, Doll R, Norman-Smith B, et al. Thymectomy and cancer: a further report. *Br J Cancer* 1979;39(2):193–195.
68. Loehrer PJ Sr, Kim K, Aisner SC, et al. Cisplatin plus doxorubicin plus cyclophosphamide in metastatic or recurrent thymoma: final results of an intergroup trial. The Eastern Cooperative Oncology Group, Southwest Oncology Group, and Southeastern Cancer Study Group. *J Clin Oncol* 1994;12(6):1164–1168.
69. Filosso PL, Galassi C, Ruffini E, et al. Thymoma and the increased risk of developing extrathymic malignancies: a multicentre study. *Eur J Cardiothorac Surg* 2013;44(2):219–224; discussion 224.
70. Kondo K, Monden Y. Lymphogenous and hematogenous metastasis of thymic epithelial tumors. *Ann Thorac Surg* 2003;76(6):1859–1864; discussion 1864–1855.
71. Jose B, Yu AT, Morgan TF, et al. Malignant thymoma with extrathoracic metastasis: a case report and review of literature. *J Surg Oncol* 1980;15(3):259–263.
72. Moran CA, Travis WD, Rosado-de-Christenson M, et al. Thymomas presenting as pleural tumors. Report of eight cases. *Am J Surg Pathol* 1992;16(2):138–144.
73. Shih DF, Wang JS, Tseng HH, et al. Primary pleural thymoma. *Arch Pathol Lab Med* 1997;121(1):79–82.
74. Shamji F, Pearson FG, Todd TR, et al. Results of surgical treatment for thymoma. *J Thorac Cardiovasc Surg* 1984;87(1):43–47.

Section III

75. Regnard JF, Zinzindohoue F, Magdeleinat P, et al. Results of re-resection for recurrent thymomas. *Ann Thorac Surg* 1997;64(6):1593–1598.

76. Venuta F, Rendina EA, Pescarmona EO, et al. Multimodality treatment of thymoma: a prospective study. *Ann Thorac Surg* 1997;64(6):1585–1591; discussion 1591–1582.

77. Lardinois D, Rechsteiner R, Lang RH, et al. Prognostic relevance of Masaoka and Muller-Hermelink classification in patients with thymic tumors. *Ann Thorac Surg* 2000;69(5):1550–1555.

78. Moore KH, McKenzie PR, Kennedy CW, et al. Thymoma: trends over time. *Ann Thorac Surg* 2001;72(1):203–207.

79. Kaiser LR, Martini N. Clinical management of thymomas: The Memorial Sloan-Kettering Cancer Center experience. In: Martini N, Vogt-Moykopf I, eds. *Thoracic surgery: frontiers and uncommon neoplasms.* vol. 5. Baltimore, MD: Mosby,1989:176–183.

80. Shields TW. Primary tumors and cysts of the mediastinum. In: Shields TW, ed. *General Thoracic Surgery.* Philadelphia: Lea & Febiger, 1983:927.

81. Marom EM. Advances in thymoma imaging. *J Thorac Imaging* 2013;28(2):69–80; quiz 81–63.

82. Baron RL, Lee JK, Sagel SS, et al. Computed tomography of the abnormal thymus. *Radiology* 1982;142(1):127–134.

83. Levitt RG, Husband JE, Glazer HS. CT of primary germ-cell tumors of the mediastinum. *AJR Am J Roentgenol* 1984;142(1):73–78.

84. Sagel SS, Aronberg DJ. Thoracic anatomy and mediastinum. In: Lee JKT, Sagel SS, Stanley RB, eds. *Computed Body Tomography.* New York: Raven Press, 1983.

85. Casamassima F, Villari N, Fargnoli R, et al. Magnetic resonance imaging and high-resolution computed tomography in tumors of the lung and the mediastinum. *Radiother Oncol* 1988;11(1):21–29.

86. Landwehr P, Schulte O, Lackner K. MR imaging of the chest: mediastinum and chest wall. *Eur Radiol* 1999;9(9):1737–1744.

87. Thompson BH, Stabford W. MR Imaging of pulmonary and mediastinal malignancies. *Magn Reson Imaging Clin N Am* 2000;8(4):729–739.

88. Inoue A, Tomiyama N, Fujimoto K, et al. MR imaging of thymic epithelial tumors: correlation with World Health Organization classification. *Radiat Med* 2006;24(3):171–181.

89. Sadohara J, Fujimoto K, Muller NL, et al. Thymic epithelial tumors: comparison of CT and MR imaging findings of low-risk thymomas, high-risk thymomas, and thymic carcinomas. *Eur J Radiol* 2006;60(1):70–79.

90. Kubota K, Yamada S, Kondo T, et al. PET imaging of primary mediastinal tumours. *Br J Cancer* 1996;73(7):882–886.

91. Liu RS, Yeh SH, Huang MH, et al. Use of fluorine-18 fluorodeoxyglucose positron emission tomography in the detection of thymoma: a preliminary report. *Eur J Nucl Med* 1995;22(12):1402–1407.

92. Ferdinand B, Gupta P, Kramer EL. Spectrum of thymic uptake at 18F-FDG PET. *Radiographics* 2004;24(6):1611–1616.

93. Otsuka H. The utility of FDG-PET in the diagnosis of thymic epithelial tumors. *J Med Invest* 2012;59(3–4):225–234.

94. El-Bawab H, Al-Sugair AA, Rafay M, et al. Role of flourine-18 fluorodeoxyglucose positron emission tomography in thymic pathology. *Eur J Cardiothorac Surg* 2007;31(4):731–736.

95. Endo M, Nakagawa K, Ohde Y, et al. Utility of 18FDG-PET for differentiating the grade of malignancy in thymic epithelial tumors. *Lung Cancer* 2008;61(3):350–355.

96. Kumar A, Regmi SK, Dutta R, et al. Characterization of thymic masses using (18)F-FDG PET-CT. *Ann Nucl Med* 2009;23(6):569–577.

97. Sung YM, Lee KS, Kim BT, et al. 18 F-FDG PET/CT of thymic epithelial tumors: usefulness for distinguishing and staging tumor subgroups. *J Nucl Med* 2006;47(10):1628–1634.

98. Fukumoto K,Taniguchi T,Ishikawa Y,et al.The utility of [18F]-fluorodeoxyglucose positron emission tomography-computed tomography in thymic epithelial tumours. *Eur J Cardiothorac Surg* 2012;42(6):e152–e156.

99. Toba H, Kondo K, Sadohara Y, et al. 18F-fluorodeoxyglucose positron emission tomography/computed tomography and the relationship between fluorodeoxyglucose uptake and the expression of hypoxia-inducible factor-1alpha, glucose transporter-1 and vascular endothelial growth factor in thymic epithelial tumours. *Eur J Cardiothorac Surg* 2013;44(2):e105–e112.

100. Kaira K, Endo M, Abe M, et al. Biologic correlation of 2-[18F]-fluoro-2-deoxy-D-glucose uptake on positron emission tomography in thymic epithelial tumors. *J Clin Oncol* 2010;28(23):3746–3753.

101. Lastoria S, Vergara E, Palmieri G, et al. In vivo detection of malignant thymic masses by indium-111-DTPA-D-Phe1-octreotide scintigraphy. *J Nucl Med* 1998;39(4):634–639.

102. Detterbeck FC, Parsons AM. Thymic tumors. *Ann Thorac Surg* 2004;77(5):1860–1869.

103. Verley JM, Hollmann KH. Thymoma. A comparative study of clinical stages, histologic features, and survival in 200 cases. *Cancer* 1985;55(5):1074–1086.

104. Ruffini E, Mancuso M, Oliaro A, et al. Recurrence of thymoma: analysis of clinicopathologic features, treatment, and outcome. *J Thorac Cardiovasc Surg* 1997;113(1):55–63.

105. Masaoka A, Monden Y, Nakahara K, et al. Follow-up study of thymomas with special reference to their clinical stages. *Cancer* 1981;48(11):2485–2492.

106. Monden Y, Nakahara K, Iioka S, et al. Recurrence of thymoma: clinicopathological features, therapy, and prognosis. *Ann Thorac Surg* 1985;39(2):165–169.

107. Pescarmona E, Rendina EA, Venuta F, et al. Analysis of prognostic factors and clinicopathological staging of thymoma. *Ann Thorac Surg* 1990;50(4):534–538.

108. Akaogi E, Ohara K, Mitsui K, et al. Preoperative radiotherapy and surgery for advanced thymoma with invasion to the great vessels. *J Surg Oncol* 1996;63(1):17–22.

109. Akwari OE, Payne WS, Onofrio BM, et al. Dumbbell neurogenic tumors of the mediastinum. Diagnosis and management. *Mayo Clin Proc* 1978;53(6):353–358.

110. Bader JL, Horowitz ME, Dewan R, et al. Intensive combined modality therapy of small round cell and undifferentiated sarcomas in children and young adults: local control and patterns of failure. *Radiother Oncol* 1989;16(3):189–201.

111. Benjamin SP, McCormack LJ, Effler DB, et al. Primary tumors of the mediastinum. *Chest* 1972;62(3):297–303.

112. Bernatz PE, Harrison EG, Clagett OT. Thymoma: a clinicopathologic study. *J West Soc Periodontol Periodontal Abstr* 1961;42:424–444.

113. Muller-Hermelink HK, Marino M, Palestro G, et al. Immunohistological evidences of cortical and medullary differentiation in thymoma. *Virchows Arch A Pathol Anat Histopathol* 1985;408(2–3):143–161.

114. Suster S, Moran CA. Primary thymic epithelial neoplasms: Spectrum of differentiation and histological features. *Semin Diagn Pathol* 1999;16(1):2.

115. Rosai J, Sobin LH. *Histological typing of tumours of the thymus.* Berlin, New York: Springer, 1999.

116. Kornstein MJ, Curran WJ Jr, Turrisi AT III, et al. Cortical versus medullary thymomas: a useful morphologic distinction? *Hum Pathol* 1988;19(11):1335–1339.

117. Quintanilla-Martinez L, Wilkins EW Jr, Choi N, et al. Thymoma. Histologic subclassification is an independent prognostic factor. *Cancer* 1994;74(2):606–617.

118. Ho FC, Fu KH, Lam SY, et al. Evaluation of a histogenetic classification for thymic epithelial tumours. *Histopathology* 1994;25(1):21–29.

119. Ricci C, Rendina EA, Pescarmona EO, et al. Correlations between histological type, clinical behaviour, and prognosis in thymoma. *Thorax* 1989;44(6):455–460.

120. Tan PH, Sng IT. Thymoma—a study of 60 cases in Singapore. *Histopathology* 1995;26(6):509–518.

121. Dawson A, Ibrahim NB, Gibbs AR. Observer variation in the histopathological classification of thymoma: correlation with prognosis. *J Clin Pathol* 1994;47(6):519–523.

122. Close PM, Kirchner T, Uys CJ, et al. Reproducibility of a histogenetic classification of thymic epithelial tumours. *Histopathology* 1995;26(4):339–343.

123. Travis WD; World Health Organization, International Agency for Research on Cancer, International Association for the Study of Lung Cancer, International Academy of Pathology. *Pathology and genetics of tumours of the lung, pleura, thymus and heart.* Lyon, Oxford: IARC Press Oxford University Press (distributor), 2004.

124. Strobel P, Marx A, Zettl A, et al. Thymoma and thymic carcinoma: an update of the WHO Classification 2004. *Surg Today* 2005;35(10):805–811.

125. Detterbeck FC. Clinical value of the WHO classification system of thymoma. *Ann Thorac Surg* 2006;81(6):2328–2334.

126. Chen G, Marx A, Wen-Hu C, et al. New WHO histologic classification predicts prognosis of thymic epithelial tumors: a clinicopathologic study of 200 thymoma cases from China. *Cancer* 2002;95(2):420–429.

127. Park MS, Chung KY, Kim KD, et al. Prognosis of thymic epithelial tumors according to the new World Health Organization histologic classification. *Ann Thorac Surg* 2004;78(3):992–997; discussion 997–998.

128. Kim DJ, Yang WI, Choi SS, et al. Prognostic and clinical relevance of the World Health Organization schema for the classification of thymic epithelial tumors: a clinicopathologic study of 108 patients and literature review. *Chest* 2005;127(3):755–761.

129. Okumura M, Ohta M, Miyoshi S, et al. Oncological significance of WHO histological thymoma classification. A clinical study based on 286 patients. *Jpn J Thorac Cardiovasc Surg* 2002;50(5):189–194.

130. Rena O, Papalia E, Maggi G, et al. World Health Organization histologic classification: an independent prognostic factor in resected thymomas. *Lung Cancer* 2005;50(1):59–66.

131. Zisis C, Rontogianni D, Tzavara C, et al. Prognostic factors in thymic epithelial tumors undergoing complete resection. *Ann Thorac Surg* 2005;80(3):1056–1062.

132. Shim HS, Byun CS, Bae MK, et al. Prognostic effect of stromal lymphocyte infiltration in thymic tumors. *Lung Cancer* 2011;74(2):338–343.

133. Gilhus NE, Jones M, Turley H, et al. Oncogene proteins and proliferation antigens in thymomas: increased expression of epidermal growth factor receptor and Ki67 antigen. *J Clin Pathol* 1995;48(5):447–455.

134. Henley JD, Koukoulis GK, Loehrer PJ Sr. Epidermal growth factor receptor expression in invasive thymoma. *J Cancer Res Clin Oncol* 2002;128(3):167–170.

135. Meister M, Schirmacher P, Dienemann H, et al. Mutational status of the epidermal growth factor receptor (EGFR) gene in thymomas and thymic carcinomas. *Cancer Lett* 2007;248(2):186–191.

136. Pescarmona E, Pisacane A, Pignatelli E, et al. Expression of epidermal and nerve growth factor receptors in human thymus and thymomas. *Histopathology* 1993;23(1):39–44.

137. Girard N, Shen R, Guo T, et al. Comprehensive genomic analysis reveals clinically relevant molecular distinctions between thymic carcinomas and thymomas. *Clin Cancer Res* 2009;15(22):6790–6799.

138. Yoh K, Nishiwaki Y, Ishii G, et al. Mutational status of EGFR and KIT in thymoma and thymic carcinoma. *Lung Cancer* 2008;62(3):316–320.

139. Mimae T, Tsuta K, Kondo T, et al. Protein expression and gene copy number changes of receptor tyrosine kinase in thymomas and thymic carcinomas. *Ann Oncol* 2012;23(12):3129–3137.

140. Christodoulou C, Murray S, Dahabreh J, et al. Response of malignant thymoma to erlotinib. *Ann Oncol* 2008;19(7):1361–1362.

141. Chuah C, Lim TH, Lim AS, et al. Dasatinib induces a response in malignant thymoma. *J Clin Oncol* 2006;24(34):e56–e58.

142. Farina G, Garassino MC, Gambacorta M, et al. Response of thymoma to cetuximab. *Lancet Oncol* 2007;8(5):449–450.

143. Cimpean AM, Raica M, Encica S, et al. Immunohistochemical expression of vascular endothelial growth factor A (VEGF), and its receptors (VEGFR1, 2) in normal and pathologic conditions of the human thymus. *Ann Anat* 2008;190(3):238–245.

144. Girard N, Teruya-Feldstein J, Payabyab EC, et al. Insulin-like growth factor-1 receptor expression in thymic malignancies. *J Thorac Oncol* 2010;5(9):1439–1446.

145. Nakagawa K, Matsuno Y, Kunitoh H, et al. Immunohistochemical KIT (CD117) expression in thymic epithelial tumors. *Chest* 2005;128(1):140–144.
146. Pan CC, Chen PC, Chiang H. KIT (CD117) is frequently overexpressed in thymic carcinomas but is absent in thymomas. *J Pathol* 2004;202(3):375–381.
147. Radovich M, Solzak JP, Hancock BA, et al. A large microRNA cluster on chromosome 19 is a transcriptional hallmark of WHO type A and AB thymomas. *Br J Cancer* 2016;114(4):477–484.
148. Badve S, Goswami C, Gokmen-Polar Y, et al. Molecular analysis of thymoma. *PLoS One* 2012;7(8):e42669.
149. Lee HS, Jang HJ, Shah R, et al. Genomic analysis of thymic epithelial tumors identifies novel subtypes associated with distinct clinical features. *Clin Cancer Res* 2017;23(16):4855–4864.
150. Kelly RJ. Thymoma versus thymic carcinoma: differences in biology impacting treatment. *J Natl Compr Canc Netw* 2013;11(5):577–583.
151. Gamondes JP, Balawi A, Greenland T, et al. Seventeen years of surgical treatment of thymoma: factors influencing survival. *Eur J Cardiothorac Surg* 1991;5(3):124–131.
152. Huang J. A new staging system for thymoma—will it improve outcomes? *J Thorac Cardiovasc Surg* 2016;151(1):20–22.
153. Detterbeck FC, Asamura H, Crowley J, et al. The IASLC/ITMIG thymic malignancies staging project: development of a stage classification for thymic malignancies. *J Thorac Oncol* 2013;8(12):1467–1473.
154. Nicholson AG, Detterbeck FC, Marino M, et al. The IASLC/ITMIG Thymic Epithelial Tumors Staging Project: proposals for the T Component for the forthcoming (8th) edition of the TNM classification of malignant tumors. *J Thorac Oncol* 2014;9(9 Suppl 2):S73–S80.
155. Cameron R, Loeher P, Thomas C. Neoplasms of the mediastinum. In: DeVita V, Lawrence T, Rosenberg S, eds. *Cancer: principles & practice of oncology*. 9th ed. Philadelphia: Lippincott-Raven, 2011:871–881.
156. Davis RD, Oldham HN, Sabiston DC. The mediastinum. In: Sabiston DC, Spencer FC, eds. *Surgery of the chest*. Philadelphia: W.B. Saunders, 1995.
157. Urgesi A, Monetti U, Rossi G, et al. Role of radiation therapy in locally advanced thymoma. *Radiother Oncol* 1990;19(3):273–280.
158. Okumura M, Miyoshi S, Fujii Y, et al. Clinical and functional significance of WHO classification on human thymic epithelial neoplasms: a study of 146 consecutive tumors. *Am J Surg Pathol* 2001;25(1):103–110.
159. Cowen D, Richaud P, Mornex F, et al. Thymoma: results of a multicentric retrospective series of 149 non-metastatic irradiated patients and review of the literature. FNCLCC trialists. Federation Nationale des Centres de Lutte Contre le Cancer. *Radiother Oncol* 1995;34(1):9–16.
160. Myojin M, Choi NC, Wright CD, et al. Stage III thymoma: pattern of failure after surgery and postoperative radiotherapy and its implication for future study. *Int J Radiat Oncol Biol Phys* 2000;46(4):927–933.
161. Regnard JF, Magdeleinat P, Dromer C, et al. Prognostic factors and long-term results after thymoma resection: a series of 307 patients. *J Thorac Cardiovasc Surg* 1996;112(2):376–384.
162. Zhu G, He S, Fu X, et al. Radiotherapy and prognostic factors for thymoma: a retrospective study of 175 patients. *Int J Radiat Oncol Biol Phys* 2004;60(4):1113–1119.
163. Rea F, Marulli G, Girardi R, et al. Long-term survival and prognostic factors in thymic epithelial tumours. *Eur J Cardiothorac Surg* 2004;26(2):412–418.
164. Elert O, Buchwald J, Wolf K. Epithelial thymus tumors—therapy and prognosis. *Thorac Cardiovasc Surg* 1988;36(2):109–113.
165. Wright CD, Wain JC, Wong DR, et al. Predictors of recurrence in thymic tumors: importance of invasion, World Health Organization histology, and size. *J Thorac Cardiovasc Surg* 2005;130(5):1413–1421.
166. Gawrychowski J, Rokicki M, Gabriel A, et al. Thymoma- the usefulness of some prognostic factors for diagnosis and surgical treatment. *Eur J Surg Oncol* 2000;26 203–208.
167. Thomas CR Jr, Bonomi PD. Mediastinal tumors. *Curr Opin Oncol* 1991;3(2):335–343.
168. Whooley BP, Urschel JD, Antkowiak JG, et al. A 25-year thymoma treatment review. *J Exp Clin Cancer Res* 2000;19(1):3–5.
169. Pollack A, Komaki R, Cox JD, et al. Thymoma: treatment and prognosis. *Int J Radiat Oncol Biol Phys* 1992;23(5):1037–1043.
170. Fukui T, Fukumoto K, Okasaka T, et al. Prognostic impact of tumour size in completely resected thymic epithelial tumours. *Eur J Cardiothorac Surg* 2016;50(6):1068–1074.
171. McCart JA, Gaspar L, Inculet R, et al. Predictors of survival following surgical resection of thymoma. *J Surg Oncol* 1993;54(4):233–238.
172. Murakawa T, Nakajima J, Kohno T, et al. Results from surgical treatment for thymoma: 43 years of experience. *Jpn J Thorac Cardiovasc Surg* 2000;48(2):89–95.
173. Park HS, Shin DM, Lee JS, et al. Thymoma. A retrospective study of 87 cases. *Cancer* 1994;73(10):2491–2498.
174. Wang LS, Huang MH, Lin TS, et al. Malignant thymoma. *Cancer* 1992;70(2):443–450.
175. Kohman LJ. Controversies in the management of malignant thymoma. *Chest* 1997;112(4 Suppl):296S–300S.
176. Verstandig AG, Epstein DM, Miller WT Jr, et al. Thymoma—report of 71 cases and a review. *Crit Rev Diagn Imaging* 1992;33(3):201–230.
177. Lucchi M, Ambrogi MC, Duranti L, et al. Advanced stage thymomas and thymic carcinomas: results of multimodality treatments. *Ann Thorac Surg* 2005;79(6):1840–1844.
178. Okumura M, Ohta M, Tateyama H, et al. The World Health Organization histologic classification system reflects the oncologic behavior of thymoma: a clinical study of 273 patients. *Cancer* 2002;94(3):624–632.
179. Rieker RJ, Hoegel J, Morresi-Hauf A, et al. Histologic classification of thymic epithelial tumors: comparison of established classification schemes. *Int J Cancer* 2002;98(6):900–906.
180. Kondo K, Yoshizawa K, Tsuyuguchi M, et al. WHO histologic classification is a prognostic indicator in thymoma. *Ann Thorac Surg* 2004;77(4):1183.
181. Welch KJ, Tapper D, Vawter GP. Surgical treatment of thymic cysts and neoplasms in children. *J Pediatr Surg* 1979;14(6):691–698.
182. Chatten J, Katz SM. Thymoma in a 12-year-old boy. *Cancer* 1976;37(2):953–957.
183. Shepherd A, Riely G, Detterbeck F, et al. Thymic carcinoma management patterns among International Thymic Malignancy Interest Group (ITMIG) Physicians with Consensus from the Thymic Carcinoma Working Group. *J Thorac Oncol* 2017;12(4):745–751.
184. Yamakawa Y, Masaoka A, Hashimoto T, et al. A tentative tumor-node-metastasis classification of thymoma. *Cancer* 1991;68(9):1984–1987.
185. Mornex F, Resbeut M, Richaud P, et al. Radiotherapy and chemotherapy for invasive thymomas: a multicentric retrospective review of 90 cases. The FNCLCC trialists. Federation Nationale des Centres de Lutte Contre le Cancer. *Int J Radiat Oncol Biol Phys* 1995;32(3):651–659.
186. Takeo S, Tsukamoto S, Kawano D, et al. Outcome of an original video-assisted thoracoscopic extended thymectomy for thymoma. *Ann Thorac Surg* 2011;92(6):2000–2005.
187. Zielinski M, Czajkowski W, Gwozdz P, et al. Resection of thymomas with use of the new minimally-invasive technique of extended thymectomy performed through the subxiphoid-right video-thoracoscopic approach with double elevation of the sternum. *Eur J Cardiothorac Surg* 2013;44(2):e113–e119; discussion e119.
188. He Z, Zhu Q, Wen W, et al. Surgical approaches for stage I and II thymoma-associated myasthenia gravis: feasibility of complete video-assisted thoracoscopic surgery (VATS) thymectomy in comparison with trans-sternal resection. *J Biomed Res* 2013;27(1):62–70.
189. Kimura T, Inoue M, Kadota Y, et al. The oncological feasibility and limitations of video-assisted thoracoscopic thymectomy for early-stage thymomas. *Eur J Cardiothorac Surg* 2013;44(3):e214–e218.
190. Rückert JC, Walter M, Muller JM. Pulmonary function after thoracoscopic thymectomy versus median sternotomy for myasthenia gravis. *Ann Thorac Surg* 2000;70(5):1656–1661.
191. Ismail M, Swierzy M, Rückert JC. State of the art of robotic thymectomy. *World J Surg* 2013;37(12):2740–2746.
192. Rückert JC, Ismail M, Swierzy M, et al. Thoracoscopic thymectomy with the da Vinci robotic system for myasthenia gravis. *Ann N Y Acad Sci* 2008;1132:329–335.
193. Rückert JC, Swierzy M, Ismail M. Comparison of robotic and nonrobotic thoracoscopic thymectomy: a cohort study. *J Thorac Cardiovasc Surg* 2011;141(3):673–677.
194. Tseng YC, Hsieh CC, Huang HY, et al. Is thymectomy necessary in nonmyasthenic patients with early thymoma? *J Thorac Oncol* 2013;8(7):952–958.
195. Rimner A, Gomez DR, Wu AJ, et al. Failure patterns relative to radiation treatment fields for stage II–IV thymoma. *J Thorac Oncol* 2014;9(3):403–409.
196. Awad WI, Symmans PJ, Dussek JE. Recurrence of stage I thymoma 32 years after total excision. *Ann Thorac Surg* 1998;66(6):2106–2108.
197. Schmidt R, Monig SP, Selzner M, et al. Surgical therapy of malignant thymoma. *J Cardiovasc Surg (Torino)* 1997;38(3):317–322.
198. Kirschner PA. Reoperation for thymoma: report of 23 cases. *Ann Thorac Surg* 1990;49(4):550.
199. Urgesi A, Monetti U, Rossi G, et al. Aggressive treatment of intrathoracic recurrences of thymoma. *Radiother Oncol* 1992;24(4):221–225.
200. Okumura M, Shiono H, Inoue M, et al. Outcome of surgical treatment for recurrent thymic epithelial tumors with reference to world health organization histologic classification system. *J Surg Oncol* 2007;95(1):40–44.
201. Bott MJ, Wang H, Travis W, et al. Management and outcomes of relapse after treatment for thymoma and thymic carcinoma. *Ann Thorac Surg* 2011;92(6):1984–1992.
202. Goldel N, Boning L, Fredrik A, et al. Chemotherapy of invasive thymoma. A retrospective study of 22 cases. *Cancer* 1989;63(8):1493–1500.
203. Chang JH, Kim HJ, Wu HG, et al. Postoperative Radiotherapy for completely resected stage II or III thymoma. *J Thorac Oncol* 2011;6(7):1282–1286.
204. Berman AT, Litzky L, Livolsi V, et al. Adjuvant radiotherapy for completely resected stage 2 thymoma. *Cancer* 2011;117(15):3502–3508.
205. Utsumi T, Shiono H, Kadota Y, et al. Postoperative radiation therapy after complete resection of thymoma has little impact on survival. *Cancer* 2009;115(23):5413–5420.
206. Forquer JA, Rong N, Fakiris AJ, et al. Postoperative radiotherapy after surgical resection of thymoma: differing roles in localized and regional disease. *Int J Radiat Oncol Biol Phys* 2010;76(2):440–445.
207. Haniuda M, Morimoto M, Nishimura H, et al. Adjuvant radiotherapy after complete resection of thymoma. *Ann Thorac Surg* 1992;54(2):311–315.
208. Ogawa K, Uno T, Toita T, et al. Postoperative radiotherapy for patients with completely resected thymoma: a multi-institutional, retrospective review of 103 patients. *Cancer* 2002;94(5):1405–1413.
209. Shen S, Ai X, Lu S. Long-term survival in thymic epithelial tumors: a single-center experience from China. *J Surg Oncol* 2013;107(2):167–172.
210. Omasa M, Date H, Sozu T, et al. Postoperative radiotherapy is effective for thymic carcinoma but not for thymoma in stage II and III thymic epithelial tumors: the Japanese Association for Research on the Thymus Database Study. *Cancer* 2015;121(7):1008–1016.
211. Weksler B, Shende M, Nason KS, et al. The role of adjuvant radiation therapy for resected stage III thymoma: a population-based study. *Ann Thorac Surg* 2012;93(6):1822–1828; discussion 1828–1829.
212. Jackson MW, Palma DA, Camidge DR, et al. The impact of postoperative radiotherapy for thymoma and thymic carcinoma. *J Thorac Oncol* 2017;12(4): 734–744.
213. Rimner A, Yao X, Huang J, et al. Postoperative radiation therapy is associated with longer overall survival in completely resected stage II and III thymoma—an analysis of the International Thymic Malignancies Interest Group Retrospective Database. *J Thorac Oncol* 2016;11(10):1785–1792.
214. Fan C, Feng Q, Chen Y, et al. Postoperative radiotherapy for completely resected Masaoka stage III thymoma: a retrospective study of 65 cases from a single institution. *Radiat Oncol* 2013;8:199.

215. Haniuda M, Miyazawa M, Yoshida K, et al. Is postoperative radiotherapy for thymoma effective? *Ann Surg* 1996;224(2):219–224.

216. Mangi AA, Wain JC, Donahue DM, et al. Adjuvant radiation of stage III thymoma: is it necessary? *Ann Thorac Surg* 2005;79(6):1834–1839.

217. Mangi AA, Wright CD, Allan JS, et al. Adjuvant radiation therapy for stage II thymoma. *Ann Thorac Surg* 2002;74(4):1033–1037.

218. Ciernik IF, Meier U, Lutolf UM. Prognostic factors and outcome of incompletely resected invasive thymoma following radiation therapy. *J Clin Oncol* 1994;12(7):1484–1490.

219. Ohara K, Okumura T, Sugahara S, et al. The role of preoperative radiotherapy for invasive thymoma. *Acta Oncol* 1990;29(4):425–429.

220. Sellors TH, Thackray AC, Thomson AD. Tumours of the thymus. A review of 88 operation cases. *Thorax* 1967;22(3):193–220.

221. Weissberg D, Goldberg M, Pearson FG. Thymoma. *Ann Thorac Surg* 1973;16(2):141–147.

222. Yagi K, Hirata T, Fukuse T, et al. Surgical treatment for invasive thymoma, especially when the superior vena cava is invaded. *Ann Thorac Surg* 1996;61(2):521–524.

223. Ribet M, Voisin C, Pruvot FR, et al. Lympho-epithelial thymomas. A retrospective study of 88 resections. *Eur J Cardiothorac Surg* 1988;2(4):261–264.

224. Arakawa A, Yasunaga T, Saitoh Y, et al. Radiation therapy of invasive thymoma. *Int J Radiat Oncol Biol Phys* 1990;18(3):529–534.

225. Jackson MA, Ball DL. Post-operative radiotherapy in invasive thymoma. *Radiother Oncol* 1991;21(2):77.

226. Loehrer PJ Sr, Chen M, Kim K, et al. Cisplatin, doxorubicin, and cyclophosphamide plus thoracic radiation therapy for limited-stage unresectable thymoma: an intergroup trial. *J Clin Oncol* 1997;15(9):3093–3099.

227. Loehrer PJ Sr, Jiroutek M, Aisner S, et al. Combined etoposide, ifosfamide, and cisplatin in the treatment of patients with advanced thymoma and thymic carcinoma: an intergroup trial. *Cancer* 2001;91(11):2010–2015.

228. Fornasiero A, Daniele O, Ghiotto C, et al. Chemotherapy for invasive thymoma. A 13-year experience. *Cancer* 1991;68(1):30–33.

229. Highley M, Underhill, CR Parnis, FX, et al. Treatment of invasive thymoma with single agent ifosfamide. *J Clin Oncol* 1999;17(9):2737–2744.

230. Bonomi PD, Finkelstein D, Aisner S, et al. EST 2582 phase II trial of cisplatin in metastatic or recurrent thymoma. *Am J Clin Oncol* 1993;16(4):342–345.

231. Rea F, Sartori F, Loy M, et al. Chemotherapy and operation for invasive thymoma. *J Thorac Cardiovasc Surg* 1993;106(3):543–549.

232. Giaccone G, Ardizzoni A, Kirkpatrick A, et al. Cisplatin and etoposide combination chemotherapy for locally advanced or metastatic thymoma. A phase II study of the European Organization for Research and Treatment of Cancer Lung Cancer Cooperative Group. *J Clin Oncol* 1996;14(3):814–820.

233. Kim ES, Putnam JB, Komaki R, et al. Phase II study of a multidisciplinary approach with induction chemotherapy, followed by surgical resection, radiation therapy, and consolidation chemotherapy for unresectable malignant thymomas: final report. *Lung Cancer* 2004;44(3):369–379.

234. Lemma GL, Lee JW, Aisner SC, et al. Phase II study of carboplatin and paclitaxel in advanced thymoma and thymic carcinoma. *J Clin Oncol* 2011;29(15):2060–2065.

235. Park S, Ahn MJ, Ahn JS, et al. A prospective phase II trial of induction chemotherapy with docetaxel/cisplatin for Masaoka stage III/IV thymic epithelial tumors. *J Thorac Oncol* 2013;8(7):959–966.

236. Palmieri G, Lastoria S, Colao A, et al. Successful treatment of a patient with a thymoma and pure red-cell aplasia with octreotide and prednisone. *N Engl J Med* 1997;336(4):263–265.

237. Palmieri G, Montella L, Martignetti A, et al. Somatostatin analogs and prednisone in advanced refractory thymic tumors. *Cancer* 2002;94(5):1414–1420.

238. Kobayashi Y, Fujii Y, Yano M, et al. Preoperative steroid pulse therapy for invasive thymoma: clinical experience and mechanism of action. *Cancer* 2006;106(9):1901–1907.

239. Loehrer PJ Sr, Wang W, Johnson DH, et al. Octreotide alone or with prednisone in patients with advanced thymoma and thymic carcinoma: an Eastern Cooperative Oncology Group Phase II Trial. *J Clin Oncol* 2004;22(2):293–299.

240. Lamarca A, Moreno V, Feliu J. Thymoma and thymic carcinoma in the target therapies era. *Cancer Treat Rev* 2013;39(5):413–420.

241. Rajan A, Giaccone G. Targeted therapy for advanced thymic tumors. *J Thorac Oncol* 2010;5(10 Suppl 4):S361–S364.

242. Giaccone G, Rajan A, Ruijter R, et al. Imatinib mesylate in patients with WHO B3 thymomas and thymic carcinomas. *J Thorac Oncol* 2009;4(10):1270–1273.

243. Girard N. Thymic tumors: relevant molecular data in the clinic. *J Thorac Oncol* 2010;5(10 Suppl 4):S291–S295.

244. Haluska P, Shaw HM, Batzel GN, et al. Phase I dose escalation study of the anti insulin-like growth factor-I receptor monoclonal antibody CP-751,871 in patients with refractory solid tumors. *Clin Cancer Res* 2007;13(19):5834–5840.

245. Karp DD, Paz-Ares LG, Novello S, et al. Phase II study of the anti-insulin-like growth factor type 1 receptor antibody CP-751,871 in combination with paclitaxel and carboplatin in previously untreated, locally advanced, or metastatic non-small-cell lung cancer. *J Clin Oncol* 2009;27(15):2516–2522.

246. Giaccone G, Rajan A, Berman A, et al. Phase II study of belinostat in patients with recurrent or refractory advanced thymic epithelial tumors. *J Clin Oncol* 2011;29(15):2052–2059.

247. Wheler J, Hong D, Swisher SG, et al. Thymoma patients treated in a phase I clinic at MD Anderson Cancer Center: responses to mTOR inhibitors and molecular analyses. *Oncotarget* 2013;4(6):890–898.

248. Funakoshi Y, Shiono H, Inoue M, et al. Glucocorticoids induce G1 cell cycle arrest in human neoplastic thymic epithelial cells. *J Cancer Res Clin Oncol* 2005;131(5):314–322.

249. Wyllie AH. Glucocorticoid-induced thymocyte apoptosis is associated with endogenous endonuclease activation. *Nature* 1980;284(5756):555–556.

250. Mimae T, Tsuta K, Takahashi F, et al. Steroid receptor expression in thymomas and thymic carcinomas. *Cancer* 2011;117(19):4396–4405.

250a. Zucali PA, De Pas T, Palmieri G, et al. Phase II study of everolimus in patients with thymoma and thymic carcinoma previously treated with cisplatin-based chemotherapy. *J Clin Oncol* 2018;36(4):342–349.

251. Macchiarini P, Chella A, Ducci F, et al. Neoadjuvant chemotherapy, surgery, and postoperative radiation therapy for invasive thymoma. *Cancer* 1991;68(4):706–713.

252. Rea F, Marulli G, Di Chiara F, et al. Multidisciplinary approach for advanced stage thymic tumors: long-term outcome. *Lung Cancer* 2011;72(1):68–72.

253. Yokoi K, Matsuguma H, Nakahara R, et al. Multidisciplinary treatment for advanced invasive thymoma with cisplatin, doxorubicin, and methylprednisolone. *Chest* 2005;128(4):145S-b-146.

254. Braitman H, Li W, Herrmann C Jr, et al. Surgery for thymic tumors. *Arch Surg* 1971;103(1):14–16.

255. Evoli A, Batocchi AP, Provenzano C, et al. Thymectomy in the treatment of myasthenia gravis: report of 247 patients. *J Neurol* 1988;235(5):272–276.

256. Jaretzki A III, Wolff M. "Maximal" thymectomy for myasthenia gravis. Surgical anatomy and operative technique. *J Thorac Cardiovasc Surg* 1988;96(5):711–716.

257. Williams CL, Hay JE, Huiatt TW, et al. Paraneoplastic IgG striational autoantibodies produced by clonal thymic B cells and in serum of patients with myasthenia gravis and thymoma react with titin. *Lab Invest* 1992;66(3):331–336.

258. Wolfe GI, Kaminski HJ, Aban IB, et al. Randomized trial of thymectomy in myasthenia gravis. *N Engl J Med* 2016;375(6):511–522.

259. Sonett JR, Magee MJ, Gorenstein L. Thymectomy and myasthenia gravis: a history of surgical passion and scientific excellence. *J Thorac Cardiovasc Surg* 2017;154(1):306–309.

260. Hsin MK. It's been a long time coming but It finally came. *J Thorac Cardiovasc Surg* 2017;154(1):310–311.

261. Phillips TL, Buschke F. The role of radiation therapy in myasthenia gravis. *Calif Med* 1967;106(4):282–289.

262. Schulz MD, Schwab RS. Results of thymic (mediastinal) irradiation in patients with myasthenia gravis. *Ann N Y Acad Sci* 1971;183:303–307.

263. Currier RD, Routh A, Hickman BT, et al. Thymus irradiation for myasthenia gravis. *Radiology* 1983;146(1):199–201.

264. Arriagada R, Bretel JJ, Caillaud JM, et al. Invasive carcinoma of the thymus. A multicenter retrospective review of 56 cases. *Eur J Cancer Clin Oncol* 1984;20(1):69–74.

265. Mayer R, Beham-Schmid C, Groell R, et al. Radiotherapy for invasive thymoma and thymic carcinoma. Clinicopathological review. *Strahlenther Onkol* 1999;175(6):271–278.

266. Holliday E, Fuller CD, Kalpathy-Cramer J, et al. Quantitative assessment of target delineation variability for thymic cancers: agreement evaluation of a prospective segmentation challenge. *J Radiat Oncol* 2016;5(1):55–61.

267. Sugie C, Shibamoto Y, Ikeya-Hashizume C, et al. Invasive thymoma: postoperative mediastinal irradiation, and low-dose entire hemithorax irradiation in patients with pleural dissemination. *J Thorac Oncol* 2008;3(1):75–81.

268. Kaseda S, Horinouchi H, Kato R, et al. Treatment of invasive thymoma using low dose and extended-field irradiation including hemi-thorax or whole-thorax. *Kyobu Geka* 1993;46(1):31–40.

269. Uematsu M, Yoshida H, Kondo M, et al. Entire hemithorax irradiation following complete resection in patients with stage II-III invasive thymoma. *Int J Radiat Oncol Biol Phys* 1996;35(2):357–360.

270. Yoshida H, Uematsu M, Itami J, et al. The role of low-dose hemithoracic radiotherapy for thoracic dissemination of thymoma. *Radiat Med* 1997;15(6):399–403.

271. Gagliardi G, Constine LS, Moiseenko V, et al. Radiation dose-volume effects in the heart. *Int J Radiat Oncol Biol Phys* 2010;76(3 Suppl):S77–S85.

272. Marks LB, Bentzen SM, Deasy JO, et al. Radiation dose-volume effects in the lung. *Int J Radiat Oncol Biol Phys* 2010;76(3 Suppl):S70–S76.

273. Marks LB, Yorke ED, Jackson A, et al. Use of normal tissue complication probability models in the clinic. *Int J Radiat Oncol Biol Phys* 2010;76(3 Suppl):S10–S19.

274. Werner-Wasik M, Yorke E, Deasy J, et al. Radiation dose-volume effects in the esophagus. *Int J Radiat Oncol Biol Phys* 2010;76(3 Suppl):S86–S93.

275. Grills IS, Yan D, Martinez AA, et al. Potential for reduced toxicity and dose escalation in the treatment of inoperable non-small-cell lung cancer: a comparison of intensity-modulated radiation therapy (IMRT), 3D conformal radiation, and elective nodal irradiation. *Int J Radiat Oncol Biol Phys* 2003;57(3):875–890.

276. Lievens Y, Nulens A, Gaber MA, et al. Intensity-modulated radiotherapy for locally advanced non-small-cell lung cancer: a dose-escalation planning study. *Int J Radiat Oncol Biol Phys* 2011;80(1):306–313.

277. Liu HH, Wang X, Dong L, et al. Feasibility of sparing lung and other thoracic structures with intensity-modulated radiotherapy for non-small-cell lung cancer. *Int J Radiat Oncol Biol Phys* 2004;58(4):1268–1279.

278. Munawar I, Yaremko BP, Craig J, et al. Intensity modulated radiotherapy of non-small-cell lung cancer incorporating SPECT ventilation imaging. *Med Phys* 2010;37(4):1863–1872.

279. Murshed H, Liu HH, Liao Z, et al. Dose and volume reduction for normal lung using intensity-modulated radiotherapy for advanced-stage non-small-cell lung cancer. *Int J Radiat Oncol Biol Phys* 2004;58(4):1258–1267.

280. Shi A, Zhu G, Wu H, et al. Analysis of clinical and dosimetric factors associated with severe acute radiation pneumonitis in patients with locally advanced non-small cell lung cancer treated with concurrent chemotherapy and intensity-modulated radiotherapy. *Radiat Oncol* 2010;5:35.

281. Videtic GM, Stephans K, Reddy C, et al. Intensity-modulated radiotherapy-based stereotactic body radiotherapy for medically inoperable early-stage lung cancer: excellent local control. *Int J Radiat Oncol Biol Phys* 2010;77(2):344–349.

282. Liao ZX, Komaki RR, Thames HD Jr, et al. Influence of technologic advances on outcomes in patients with unresectable, locally advanced non-small-cell lung cancer receiving concomitant chemoradiotherapy. *Int J Radiat Oncol Biol Phys* 2010;76(3):775–781.

283. Chang JY, Komaki R, Lu C, et al. Phase 2 study of high-dose proton therapy with concurrent chemotherapy for unresectable stage III nonsmall cell lung cancer. *Cancer* 2011;117(20):4707–4713.

284. Chang JY, Zhang X, Wang X, et al. Significant reduction of normal tissue dose by proton radiotherapy compared with three-dimensional conformal or intensity-modulated radiation therapy in Stage I or Stage III non-small-cell lung cancer. *Int J Radiat Oncol Biol Phys* 2006;65(4):1087–1096.

285. Macdonald OK, Kruse JJ, Miller JM, et al. Proton beam radiotherapy versus three-dimensional conformal stereotactic body radiotherapy in primary peripheral, early-stage non-small-cell lung carcinoma: a comparative dosimetric analysis. *Int J Radiat Oncol Biol Phys* 2009;75(3):950–958.

286. Nakayama H, Sugahara S, Tokita M, et al. Proton beam therapy for patients with medically inoperable stage I non-small-cell lung cancer at the university of tsukuba. *Int J Radiat Oncol Biol Phys* 2010;78(2):467–471.

287. Nichols RC, Huh SN, Henderson RH, et al. Proton radiation therapy offers reduced normal lung and bone marrow exposure for patients receiving dose-escalated radiation therapy for unresectable stage III non-small-cell lung cancer: a Dosimetric Study. *Clin Lung Cancer* 2011;12(4):252–257.

288. Sejpal S, Komaki R, Tsao A, et al. Early findings on toxicity of proton beam therapy with concurrent chemotherapy for nonsmall cell lung cancer. *Cancer* 2011;117(13):3004–3013.

289. Wang C, Nakayama H, Sugahara S, et al. Comparisons of dose-volume histograms for proton-beam versus 3-D conformal x-ray therapy in patients with stage I non-small cell lung cancer. *Strahlenther Onkol* 2009;185(4):231–234.

290. Zhang X, Li Y, Pan X, et al. Intensity-modulated proton therapy reduces the dose to normal tissue compared with intensity-modulated radiation therapy or passive scattering proton therapy and enables individualized radical radiotherapy for extensive stage IIIB non-small-cell lung cancer: a virtual clinical study. *Int J Radiat Oncol Biol Phys* 2010;77(2):357–366.

291. Li J, Dabaja B, Reed V, et al. Rationale for and preliminary results of proton beam therapy for mediastinal lymphoma. *Int J Radiat Oncol Biol Phys* 2011;81(1):167–174.

292. Vogel J, Lin L, Simone CB II, et al. Risk of major cardiac events following adjuvant proton versus photon radiation therapy for patients with thymic malignancies. *Acta Oncol* 2017;56(8):1060–1064.

293. Gomez D, Komaki R. Technical advances of radiation therapy for thymic malignancies. *J Thorac Oncol* 2010;5(10 Suppl 4):S336–S343.

294. Gomez D, Komaki R, Yu J, et al. Radiation therapy definitions and reporting guidelines for thymic malignancies. *J Thorac Oncol* 2011;6(7):S1743–S1748

295. Kondo K, Monden Y. Thymic carcinoma. *Kyobu Geka* 2002;55(8 Suppl):701–708.

296. Wick MR, Scheithauer BW, Weiland LH, et al. Primary thymic carcinomas. *Am J Surg Pathol* 1982;6(7):613–630.

297. Chalabreysse L, Etienne-Mastroianni B, Adeleine P, et al. Thymic carcinoma: a clinicopathological and immunohistological study of 19 cases. *Histopathology* 2004;44(4):367–374.

298. Jung KJ, Lee KS, Han J, et al. Malignant thymic epithelial tumors: CT-pathologic correlation. *AJR Am J Roentgenol* 2001;176(2):433–439.

299. Negron-Soto JM, Cascade PN. Squamous cell carcinoma of the thymus with paraneoplastic hypercalcemia. *Clin Imaging* 1995;19(2):122–124.

300. Suzuki K, Tanaka H, Shibusa T, et al. Parathyroid-hormone-related-protein-producing thymic carcinoma presenting as a giant extrathoracic mass. *Respiration* 1998;65(1):83–85.

301. Tomiyama N, Johkoh T, Mihara N, et al. Using the World Health Organization Classification of thymic epithelial neoplasms to describe CT findings. *AJR Am J Roentgenol* 2002;179(4):881–886.

302. Seto H, Kageyama M, Shimizu M, et al. Assessment of residual tumor viability in thymic carcinoma by sequential thallium-201 SPECT: comparison with CT and biopsy findings. *J Nucl Med* 1994;35(10):1659–1661.

303. Quagliano PV. Thymic carcinoma: case reports and review. *J Thorac Imaging* 1996;11(1):66–74.

304. Do YS, Im JG, Lee BH, et al. CT findings in malignant tumors of thymic epithelium. *J Comput Assist Tomogr* 1995;19(2):192–197.

305. Kushihashi T, Fujisawa H, Munechika H. Magnetic resonance imaging of thymic epithelial tumors. *Crit Rev Diagn Imaging* 1996;37(3):191–259.

306. Lee JD. CT findings in primary thymic carcinoma. *J Comput Assist Tomogr* 1991;15:429–433.

307. Zhang Z, Cui Y, Li B, et al. Thymic carcinoma (report of 14 cases). *Chin Med Sci J* 1997;12(4):252–255.

308. Chang HK, Wang CH, Liaw CC, et al. Prognosis of thymic carcinoma: analysis of 16 cases. *J Formos Med Assoc* 1992;91(8):764–769.

309. Shimosato Y, Kameya T, Nagai K, et al. Squamous cell carcinoma of the thymus. An analysis of eight cases. *Am J Surg Pathol* 1977;1(2):109–121.

310. Sakai S, Murayama S, Soeda H, et al. Differential diagnosis between thymoma and non-thymoma by dynamic MR imaging. *Acta Radiol* 2002;43(3):262–268.

311. Sasaki M, Kuwabara Y, Ichiya Y, et al. Differential diagnosis of thymic tumors using a combination of 11C-methionine PET and FDG PET. *J Nucl Med* 1999;40(10):1595–1601.

312. Adams S, Baum RP, Hertel A, et al. Metabolic (PET) and receptor (SPET) imaging of well- and less well-differentiated tumours: comparison with the expression of the Ki-67 antigen. *Nucl Med Commun* 1998;19(7):641–647.

313. Kageyama M, Seto H, Shimizu M, et al. Thallium-201 single photon emission computed tomography in the evaluation of thymic carcinoma. *Radiat Med* 1994;12(5):237–239.

314. Dadmanesh F, Sekihara T, Rosai J. Histologic typing of thymoma according to the new World Health Organization classification. *Chest Surg Clin N Am* 2001;11(2):407–420.

315. Snover DC, Levine GD, Rosai J. Thymic carcinoma. Five distinctive histological variants. *Am J Surg Pathol* 1982;6(5):451–470.

316. Nonaka D, Klimstra D, Rosai J. Thymic mucoepidermoid carcinomas: a clinicopathologic study of 10 cases and review of the literature. *Am J Surg Pathol* 2004;28(11):1526–1531.

317. Suster S. Thymic carcinoma: update of current diagnostic criteria and histologic types. *Semin Diagn Pathol* 2005;22(3):198–212.

318. Weissferdt A, Moran CA. Thymic carcinoma associated with multilocular thymic cyst: a clinicopathologic study of 7 cases. *Am J Surg Pathol* 2011;35(7):1074–1079.

319. Suster S, Rosai J. Thymic carcinoma. A clinicopathologic study of 60 cases. *Cancer* 1991;67(4):1025–1032.

320. Ritter JH, Wick MR. Primary carcinomas of the thymus gland. *Semin Diagn Pathol* 1999;16(1):18–31.

321. Ogawa K, Toita T, Uno T, et al. Treatment and prognosis of thymic carcinoma: a retrospective analysis of 40 cases. *Cancer* 2002;94(12):3115–3119.

322. Hartmann CA, Roth C, Minck C, et al. Thymic carcinoma. Report of five cases and review of the literature. *J Cancer Res Clin Oncol* 1990;116(1):69.

323. Suster S, Moran CA. Thymic carcinoma: spectrum of differentiation and histologic types. *Pathology* 1998;30(2):111–122.

324. Thomas de Montpreville V, Ghigna MR, Lacroix L, et al. Thymic carcinomas: clinicopathologic study of 37 cases from a single institution. *Virchows Arch* 2013;462(3):307–313.

325. Ruffini E, Detterbeck F, Van Raemdonck D, et al. Thymic carcinoma: a cohort study of patients from the European Society of Thoracic Surgeons database. *J Thorac Oncol* 2014;9(4):541–548.

326. Ahmad U, Yao X, Detterbeck F, et al. Thymic carcinoma outcomes and prognosis: results of an international analysis. *J Thorac Cardiovasc Surg* 2015;149(1):95–100, 101 e101–102.

327. Roden AC, Yi ES, Cassivi SD, et al. Clinicopathological features of thymic carcinomas and the impact of histopathological agreement on prognostical studies. *Eur J Cardiothorac Surg* 2013;43(6):1131–1139.

328. Litvak AM, Woo K, Hayes S, et al. Clinical characteristics and outcomes for patients with thymic carcinoma: evaluation of Masaoka staging. *J Thorac Oncol* 2014;9(12):1810–1815.

329. Hernandez-Ilizaliturri FJ, Tan D, Cipolla D, et al. Multimodality therapy for thymic carcinoma (TCA): results of a 30-year single-institution experience. *Am J Clin Oncol* 2004;27(1):68–72.

330. Takeda S, Sawabata N, Inoue M, et al. Thymic carcinoma. Clinical institutional experience with 15 patients. *Eur J Cardiothorac Surg* 2004;26(2):401–406.

331. Park IK, Kim YT, Jeon JH, et al. Importance of lymph node dissection in thymic carcinoma. *Ann Thorac Surg* 2013;96(3):1025–1032; discussion 1032.

332. Sakai M, Onuki T, Inagaki M, et al. Early-stage thymic carcinoma: is adjuvant therapy required? *J Thorac Dis* 2013;5(2):161–164.

333. Nonaka T, Tamaki Y, Higuchi K, et al. The role of radiotherapy for thymic carcinoma. *Jpn J Clin Oncol* 2004;34(12):722–726.

334. Lin JT, Wei-Shu W, Yen CC, et al. Stage IV thymic carcinoma: a study of 20 patients. *Am J Med Sci* 2005;330(4):172–175.

335. Eng TY, Fuller CD, Jagirdar J, et al. Thymic carcinoma: state of the art review. *Int J Radiat Oncol Biol Phys* 2004;59(3):654–664.

336. Hsu HC, Huang EY, Wang CJ, et al. Postoperative radiotherapy in thymic carcinoma: treatment results and prognostic factors. *Int J Radiat Oncol Biol Phys* 2002;52(3):801–805.

337. Chahinian AP. Chemotherapy of thymomas and thymic carcinomas. *Chest Surg Clin N Am* 2001;11(2):447–456.

338. Koizumi T, Takabayashi Y, Yamagishi S, et al. Chemotherapy for advanced thymic carcinoma: clinical response to cisplatin, doxorubicin, vincristine, and cyclophosphamide (ADOC chemotherapy). *Am J Clin Oncol* 2002;25(3):266–268.

339. Nakamura Y, Kunitoh H, Kubota K, et al. Platinum-based chemotherapy with or without thoracic radiation therapy in patients with unresectable thymic carcinoma. *Jpn J Clin Oncol* 2000;30(9):385–388.

340. Yoh K, Goto K, Ishii G, et al. Weekly chemotherapy with cisplatin, vincristine, doxorubicin, and etoposide is an effective treatment for advanced thymic carcinoma. *Cancer* 2003;98(5):926–931.

341. Kitami A, Suzuki T, Suzuki S, et al. Effective treatment of thymic carcinoma with operation and combination chemotherapy against acute monocyte leukemia: case report and review of the literature. *Jpn J Clin Oncol* 1998;28(9):555–558.

342. Lucchi M, Mussi A, Basolo F, et al. The multimodality treatment of thymic carcinoma. *Eur J Cardiothorac Surg* 2001;19(5):566–569.

343. Komaki R, Gomez DR. Radiotherapy for thymic carcinoma: adjuvant, inductive, and definitive. *Front Oncol* 2014;3:330.

344. Schirosi L, Nannini N, Nicoli D, et al. Activating c-KIT mutations in a subset of thymic carcinoma and response to different c-KIT inhibitors. *Ann Oncol* 2012;23(9):2409–2414.

345. Tseng YL, Wang ST, Wu MH, et al. Thymic carcinoma: involvement of great vessels indicates poor prognosis. *Ann Thorac Surg* 2003;76(4):1041–1045.

346. Kurup A, Loehrer PJ Sr. Thymoma and thymic carcinoma: therapeutic approaches. *Clin Lung Cancer* 2004;6(1):28–32.

347. Rosai J, Higa E. Mediastinal endocrine neoplasm, of probable thymic origin, related to carcinoid tumor. Clinicopathologic study of 8 cases. *Cancer* 1972;29(4):1061–1074.

348. Tiffet O, Nicholson AG, Ladas G, et al. A clinicopathologic study of 12 neuroendocrine tumors arising in the thymus. *Chest* 2003;124(1):141–146.

349. Lim LC, Tan MH, Eng C, et al. Thymic carcinoid in multiple endocrine neoplasia 1: genotype-phenotype correlation and prevention. *J Intern Med* 2006;259(4):428–432.

350. Wen Cc, Hsu YP, Sheu MH. Atypical carcinoid tumor of the thymus: a case report. *Chin J Radiol* 2003;28:317–321.

351. Lin FC, Lin CM, Hsieh CC, et al. Atypical thymic carcinoid and malignant somatostatinoma in type I multiple endocrine neoplasia syndrome: case report. *Am J Clin Oncol* 2003;26(3):270–272.

352. de Montpreville VT, Macchiarini P, Dulmet E. Thymic neuroendocrine carcinoma (carcinoid): a clinicopathologic study of fourteen cases. *J Thorac Cardiovasc Surg* 1996;111(1):134–141.

353. Asbun HJ, Calabria RP, Calmes S, et al. Thymic carcinoid. *Am Surg* 1991;57(7):442–445.

354. Filosso PL, Yao X, Ahmad U, et al. Outcome of primary neuroendocrine tumors of the thymus: a joint analysis of the International Thymic Malignancy Interest Group and the European Society of Thoracic Surgeons databases. *J Thorac Cardiovasc Surg* 2015;149(1):103–109 e102.

355. Klemm KM, Moran CA. Primary neuroendocrine carcinomas of the thymus. *Semin Diagn Pathol* 1999;16(1):32–41.

356. Economopoulos GC, Lewis JW Jr, Lee MW, et al. Carcinoid tumors of the thymus. *Ann Thorac Surg* 1990;50(1):58–61.

357. Wang DY, Chang DB, Kuo SH, et al. Carcinoid tumours of the thymus. *Thorax* 1994;49(4):357–360.

358. Wick MR, Rosai J. Neuroendocrine neoplasms of the mediastinum. *Semin Diagn Pathol* 1991;8(1):35–51.

359. Teh BT, Zedenius J, Kytola S, et al. Thymic carcinoids in multiple endocrine neoplasia type 1. *Ann Surg* 1998;228(1):99–105.

360. Havlicek F, Rosai J. A sarcoma of thymic stroma with features of liposarcoma. *Am J Clin Pathol* 1984;82(2):217–224.

361. Howling SJ, Flint JD, Muller NL. Thymoliposarcoma: CT and pathologic findings. *Clin Radiol* 1999;54(5):341.

362. Hainsworth JD, Greco FA. Extragonadal germ cell tumors and unrecognized germ cell tumors. *Semin Oncol* 1992;19(2):119–127.

363. Andac A, Mert B, Sevil B, et al. Adult primary extragonadal germ cell tumors: treatment results and long-term follow-up. *Med Pediatr Oncol* 2003;41(1):49–53.

364. Nichols CR, Fox EP. Extragonadal and pediatric germ cell tumors. *Hematol Oncol Clin North Am* 1991;5(6):1189–1209.

365. Kuhn MW, Weissbach L. Localization, incidence, diagnosis and treatment of extratesticular germ cell tumors. *Urol Int* 1985;40(3):166–172.

366. Weiland K, Conley J. A primary germ cell tumor of the anterior mediastinum: a case report and discussion. *S D J Med* 2000;53(10):441–444.

367. Cox J. Primary malignant germinal tumors of the mediastinum: a study of 24 patients. *Cancer* 1975;36:1162.

368. Bokemeyer C, Nichols CR, Droz JP, et al. Extragonadal germ cell tumors of the mediastinum and retroperitoneum: results from an international analysis. *J Clin Oncol* 2002;20(7):1864–1873.

369. Curry WA, McKay CE, Richardson RL, et al. Klinefelter's syndrome and mediastinal germ cell neoplasms. *J Urol* 1981;125(1):127–129.

370. Dexeus FH, Logothetis CJ, Chong C, et al. Genetic abnormalities in men with germ cell tumors. *J Urol* 1988;140(1):80–84.

371. Nichols CR, Heerema NA, Palmer C, et al. Klinefelter's syndrome associated with mediastinal germ cell neoplasms. *J Clin Oncol* 1987;5(8):1290–1294.

372. Turner AR, MacDonald RN, Gilbert JA, et al. Mediastinal germ cell cancers in Klinefelter's syndrome. *Ann Intern Med* 1981;94(2):279.

373. Aguirre D, Nieto K, Lazos M, et al. Extragonadal germ cell tumors are often associated with Klinefelter syndrome. *Hum Pathol* 2006;37(4):477–480.

374. Nichols CR. Mediastinal germ cell tumors. *Semin Thorac Cardiovasc Surg* 1992;4(1):45–50.

375. Nichols CR, Hoffman R, Einhorn LH, et al. Hematologic malignancies associated with primary mediastinal germ-cell tumors. *Ann Intern Med* 1985;102(5):603–609.

376. Nichols CR, Roth BJ, Heerema N, et al. Hematologic neoplasia associated with primary mediastinal germ-cell tumors. *N Engl J Med* 1990;322(20):1425–1429.

377. Hainsworth JD, Greco FA. Germ cell neoplasms and other malignancies of the mediastinum. *Cancer Treat Res* 2001;105:303–325.

378. Chariot P, Monnet I, Gaulard P, et al. Systemic mastocytosis following mediastinal germ cell tumor: an association confirmed. *Hum Pathol* 1993;24(1):111–112.

379. Hartmann JT, Nichols CR, Droz JP, et al. Hematologic disorders associated with primary mediastinal nonseminomatous germ cell tumors. *J Natl Cancer Inst* 2000;92(1):54–61.

380. Chaganti RS, Rodriguez E, Mathew S. Origin of adult male mediastinal germ-cell tumours. *Lancet* 1994;343(8906):1130–1132.

381. Friedman NB. The comparative morphogenesis of extragenital and gonadal teratoid tumors. *Cancer* 1951;4(2):265–276.

382. Hailemariam S, Engeler DS, Bannwart F, et al. Primary mediastinal germ cell tumor with intratubular germ cell neoplasia of the testis—further support for germ cell origin of these tumors: a case report. *Cancer* 1997;79(5):1031–1036.

383. Luna MA, Valenzuela-Tamariz J. Germ-cell tumors of the mediastinum, postmortem findings. *Am J Clin Pathol* 1976;65(4):450–454.

384. Aliotta PJ, Castillo J, Englander LS, et al. Primary mediastinal germ cell tumors. Histologic patterns of treatment failures at autopsy. *Cancer* 1988;62(5):982–984.

385. Kantoff P. Surgical and medical management of germ cell tumors of the chest. *Chest* 1993;103(4 Suppl):331S–333S.

386. Ganjoo KN, Rieger KM, Kesler KA, et al. Results of modern therapy for patients with mediastinal nonseminomatous germ cell tumors. *Cancer* 2000;88(5):1051–1056.

387. Knapp RH, Hurt RD, Payne WS, et al. Malignant germ cell tumors of the mediastinum. *J Thorac Cardiovasc Surg* 1985;89(1):82–89.

388. Lemarie E, Assouline PS, Diot P, et al. Primary mediastinal germ cell tumors. Results of a French retrospective study. *Chest* 1992;102(5):1477–1483.

389. Lemarie E, Lemarie E. Malignant germinal tumours of the mediastinum: diagnosis and treatment. *Rev Pneumol Clin* 2004;60(5 Pt 2):3S79–3S85.

390. Martini N, Golbey RB, Hajdu SI, et al. Primary mediastinal germ cell tumors. *Cancer* 1974;33(3):763–769.

391. Pachter MR, Lattes R. "Germinal" tumors of the mediastinum: a clinicopathologic study of adult teratomas, teratocarcinomas, choriocarcinomas and seminomas. *Dis Chest* 1964;45:301–310.

392. Logothetis CJ, Samuels ML, Selig DE, et al. Chemotherapy of extragonadal germ cell tumors. *J Clin Oncol* 1985;3(3):316–325.

393. Sickles EA, Belliveau RE, Wiernik PH. Primary mediastinal choriocarcinoma in the male. *Cancer* 1974;33(4):1196–1203.

394. Israel A, Bosl GJ, Golbey RB, et al. The results of chemotherapy for extragonadal germ-cell tumors in the cisplatin era: the Memorial Sloan-Kettering Cancer Center experience (1975 to 1982). *J Clin Oncol* 1985;3(8):1073–1078.

395. Hainsworth JD, Einhorn LH, Williams SD, et al. Advanced extragonadal germ-cell tumors. Successful treatment with combination chemotherapy. *Ann Intern Med* 1982;97(1):7–11.

396. Javadpour N. The value of biologic markers in diagnosis and treatment of testicular cancer. *Semin Oncol* 1979;6(1):37–47.

397. Economou JS, Trump DL, Holmes EC, et al. Management of primary germ cell tumors of the mediastinum. *J Thorac Cardiovasc Surg* 1982;83(5):643–649.

398. Burt ME, Javadpour N. Germ-cell tumors in patients with apparently normal testes. *Cancer* 1981;47(7):1911–1915.

399. Cole LA, Rinne KM, Shahabi S, et al. False-positive hCG assay results leading to unnecessary surgery and chemotherapy and needless occurrences of diabetes and coma. *Clin Chem* 1999;45(2):313–314.

400. Rotmensch S, Cole LA. False diagnosis and needless therapy of presumed malignant disease in women with false-positive human chorionic gonadotropin concentrations. *Lancet* 2000;355(9205):712–715.

401. Bokemeyer C, Droz JP, Horwich A, et al. Extragonadal seminoma: an international multicenter analysis of prognostic factors and long term treatment outcome. *Cancer* 2001;91(7):1394–1401.

402. Ginsberg RJ. Mediastinal germ cell tumors: the role of surgery. *Semin Thorac Cardiovasc Surg* 1992;4(1):51–54.

403. Einhorn LH, Williams SD. Chemotherapy of disseminated seminoma. *Cancer Clin Trials* 1980;3(4):307–313.

404. Motzer R, Bosl G, Heelan R, et al. Residual mass: an indication for further therapy in patients with advanced seminoma following systemic chemotherapy. *J Clin Oncol* 1987;5(7):1064–1070.

405. Puc HS, Heelan R, Mazumdar M, et al. Management of residual mass in advanced seminoma: results and recommendations from the Memorial Sloan-Kettering Cancer Center. *J Clin Oncol* 1996;14(2):454–460.

406. Schultz SM, Einhorn LH, Conces DJ Jr, et al. Management of postchemotherapy residual mass in patients with advanced seminoma: Indiana University experience. *J Clin Oncol* 1989;7(10):1497–1503.

407. Herr HW, Sheinfeld J, Puc HS, et al. Surgery for a post-chemotherapy residual mass in seminoma. *J Urol* 1997;157(3):860–862.

408. Hainsworth JD, Hainsworth JD. Diagnosis, staging, and clinical characteristics of the patient with mediastinal germ cell carcinoma. *Chest Surg Clin N Am* 2002;12(4):665–672.

409. Becherer A, De Santis M, Karanikas G, et al. FDG PET is superior to CT in the prediction of viable tumour in post-chemotherapy seminoma residuals. *Eur J Radiol* 2005;54(2):284–288.

410. Ganjoo KN, Chan RJ, Sharma M, et al. Positron emission tomography scans in the evaluation of postchemotherapy residual masses in patients with seminoma. *J Clin Oncol* 1999;17(11):3457–3460.

411. Hurt RD, Bruckman JE, Farrow GM, et al. Primary anterior mediastinal seminoma. *Cancer* 1982;49(8):1658–1663.

412. Uematsu M, Kondo M, Dokiya T, et al. The role of radiotherapy in the treatment of primary mediastinal seminoma. *Radiother Oncol* 1992;24(4):226–230.

413. Bagshaw MA, McLaughlin WT, Earle JD. Definitive radiotherapy of primary mediastinal seminoma. *Am J Roentgenol Radium Ther Nucl Med* 1969;105(1):86–94.

414. Bush SE, Martinez A, Bagshaw MA. Primary mediastinal seminoma. *Cancer* 1981;48(8):1877–1882.

415. Clamon GH. Management of primary mediastinal seminoma. *Chest* 1983;83(2):263–267.

416. Fizazi K, Culine S, Droz JP, et al. Initial management of primary mediastinal seminoma: radiotherapy or cisplatin-based chemotherapy? *Eur J Cancer* 1998;34(3):347–352.

417. Schantz A, Sewall W, Castleman B. Mediastinal germinoma. A study of 21 cases with an excellent prognosis. *Cancer* 1972;30(5):1189–1194.

418. Jones WG, Fossa SD, Mead GM, et al. Randomized trial of 30 versus 20 Gy in the adjuvant treatment of stage I testicular seminoma: a report on Medical Research Council Trial TE18, European Organisation for the Research and Treatment of Cancer Trial 30942 (ISRCTN18525328). *J Clin Oncol* 2005;23(6):1200–1208.

419. Aygun C, Slawson RG, Bajaj K, et al. Primary mediastinal seminoma. *Urology* 1984;23(2):109–117.

420. Nichols CR, Saxman S, Williams SD, et al. Primary mediastinal nonseminomatous germ cell tumors. A modern single institution experience. *Cancer* 1990;65(7):1641–1646.

421. Kay PH, Wells FC, Goldstraw P. A multidisciplinary approach to primary nonseminomatous germ cell tumors of the mediastinum. *Ann Thorac Surg* 1987;44(6):578–582.

422. Wright CD, Kesler KA, Nichols CR, et al. Primary mediastinal nonseminomatous germ cell tumors. Results of a multimodality approach. *J Thorac Cardiovasc Surg* 1990;99(2):210–217.

423. Hartmann JT, Schmoll HJ, Kuczyk MA, et al. Postchemotherapy resections of residual masses from metastatic non-seminomatous testicular germ cell tumors. *Ann Oncol* 1997;8(6):531–538.

424. Kersh CR, Eisert DR, Constable WC, et al. Primary malignant mediastinal germ-cell tumors and the contribution of radiotherapy: a southeastern multi-institutional study. *Am J Clin Oncol* 1987;10(4):302–306.

425. Walsh GL, Taylor GD, Nesbitt JC, et al. Intensive chemotherapy and radical resections for primary nonseminomatous mediastinal germ cell tumors. *Ann Thorac Surg* 2000;69(2):337–343; discussion 343–334.

426. Saxman SB, Nichols CR, Einhorn LH. Salvage chemotherapy in patients with extragonadal nonseminomatous germ cell tumors: the Indiana University experience. *J Clin Oncol* 1994;12(7):1390–1393.

427. Hidalgo M, Paz-Ares L, Rivera F, et al. Mediastinal non-seminomatous germ cell tumours (MNSGCT) treated with cisplatin-based combination chemotherapy. *Ann Oncol* 1997;8(6):555–559.

428. Pachter MR, Lattes R. Mesenchymal tumors of the mediastinum. I. Tumors of fibrous tissue, adipose tissue, smooth muscle, and striated muscle. *Cancer* 1963;16:74–94.

429. Pachter MR, Lattes R. Mesenchymal tumors of the mediastinum. III. Tumors of lymph vascular origin. *Cancer* 1963;16:108–117.

430. Pachter MR, Lattes R. Mesenchymal tumors of the mediastinum. II. Tumors of blood vascular origin. *Cancer* 1963;16:95–107.

431. Macchiarini P, Ostertag H. Uncommon primary mediastinal tumours. *Lancet Oncol* 2004;5(2):107–118.

432. Swanson PE. Soft tissue neoplasma of the mediastinum. *Semin Diagn Pathol* 1991;8(1):14–34.

433. Billmire DF. Germ cell, mesenchymal, and thymic tumors of the mediastinum. *Semin Pediatr Surg* 1999;8(2):85–91.

434. Alden JF, Bjornson RB, Sterner ER, et al. Mediastinal lipoma. *Dis Chest* 1957;32(5):580–581.

435. Blades B. Relative frequency and site of predilection of intrathoracic tumors. *Am J Surg* 1941;54:139–148.

436. Daniel RA Jr, Diveley WL, Edwards WH, et al. Mediastinal tumors. *Ann Surg* 1960;151:783–795.

437. Keeley JL, Gumbiner SH, Guzauskus AC, et al. Mediastinal lipoma; the successful removal of 1,700 gram mass; case report and review of recent literature of intrathoracic lipomas. *J Thorac Surg* 1953;25(3):316–323.

438. Keeley JL, Vana AJ. Lipomas of the mediastinum; 1940 to 1955. *Surg Gynecol Obstet* 1956;103(4):313–322.

439. Alar T, Ozcelik C, Kilnc N. Giant mediastinal mass: thymolipoma. *South Med J* 2011;104(5):353–354.

440. Minematsu N, Minato N, Kamohara K, et al. Complete removal of heart-compressing large mediastinal lipoma: a case report. *J Cardiothorac Surg* 2010;5:48.

441. Morris LM, Thurston RS. Massive thoracic lipoma: a case report. *J La State Med Soc* 2011;163(1):40–42.

442. Weiss SW, Goldblum JR, Enzinger FM. *Enzinger and Weiss's soft tissue tumors.* 4th ed. St. Louis, MO: Mosby, 2001.

443. Nomimura T, Takahashi T, Kato Y, et al. Mid mediastinal lipoma—a case report. *Nihon Kyobu Geka Gakkai Zasshi* 1996;44(4):580–584.

444. Grosfeld JL, Skinner MA, Rescorla FJ, et al. Mediastinal tumors in children: experience with 196 cases. *Ann Surg Oncol* 1994;1(2):121–127.

445. Takeo S, Fukuyama S. Video-assisted thoracoscopic resection of a giant anterior mediastinal tumor (lipoma) using an original sternum-lifting technique. *Jpn J Thorac Cardiovasc Surg* 2005;53(10):565–568.

446. Wiedemann D, Schistek R, Gassner E, et al. Mediastinal liposarcoma. *J Card Surg* 2011;26(2):162–164.

447. Barbetakis N, Asteriou C, Kleontas A, et al. Primary pleomorphic liposarcoma: a rare mediastinal tumor. *Interact Cardiovasc Thorac Surg* 2010;11(3):327.

448. Standerfer RJ, Armistead SH, Paneth M. Liposarcoma of the mediastinum: report of two cases and review of the literature. *Thorax* 1981;36(9):693–694.

449. Burt M, Ihde JK, Hajdu SI, et al. Primary sarcomas of the mediastinum: results of therapy. *J Thorac Cardiovasc Surg* 1998;115(3):671–680.

450. Klimstra DS, Moran CA, Perino G, et al. Liposarcoma of the anterior mediastinum and thymus. A clinicopathologic study of 28 cases. *Am J Surg Pathol* 1995;19(7):782–791.

451. Zagars GK, Goswitz MS, Pollack A. Liposarcoma: outcome and prognostic factors following conservation surgery and radiation therapy. *Int J Radiat Oncol Biol Phys* 1996;36(2):311–319.

452. Alho A, Eeg Larsen T. A case of multifocal liposarcoma? *Acta Orthop Scand* 1992;63(1):98–99.

453. Chung C, Lu CC, Chang SC, et al. Mediastinal liposarcoma with local recurrence: a case report. *Zhonghua Yi Xue Za Zhi (Taipei)* 1996;57(1):70–73.

454. Kara M, Ozkan M, Dizbay Sak S, et al. Successful removal of a giant recurrent mediastinal liposarcoma involving both hemithoraces. *Eur J Cardiothorac Surg* 2001;20(3):647–649.

455. Kendall SW, Williams EA, Hunt JB, et al. Recurrent primary liposarcoma of the pericardium: management by repeated resections. *Ann Thorac Surg* 1993;56(3):560–562.

456. Sumner TE, Volberg FM, Kiser PE, et al. Mediastinal cystic hygroma in children. *Pediatr Radiol* 1981;11(3):160–162.

457. Conte G, Aldrovandi A, Reverberi C, et al. Mediastinal cystic lymphangioma. *J Am Coll Cardiol* 2011;57(16):e207.

458. Oztunc F, Koca B, Adaletli I. Generalised lymphangiomatosis in an 8-year-old girl who presented with cardiomegaly. *Cardiol Young* 2011;21(4):465–467.

459. Alvarez OA, Kjellin I, Zuppan CW. Thoracic lymphangiomatosis in a child. *J Pediatr Hematol Oncol* 2004;26(2):136–141.

460. Bugaeva MI, Tararaev IA. Lymphangiomatosis complicated by chylothorax. *Sov Med* 1984;(7):112–113.

461. Chang JH, Newkirk J, Carlton G, et al. Generalized lymphangiomatosis with chylous ascites—treatment by peritoneo-venous shunting. *J Pediatr Surg* 1980;15(6):748–750.

462. Dajee H, Woodhouse R. Lymphangiomatosis of the mediastinum with chylothorax and chylopericardium: role of radiation treatment. *J Thorac Cardiovasc Surg* 1994;108(3):594–595.

463. Shahriari A, Odell JA. Cervical and thoracic components of multiorgan lymphangiomatosis managed surgically. *Ann Thorac Surg* 2001;71(2):694–696.

464. Swensen SJ, Hartman TE, Mayo JR, et al. Diffuse pulmonary lymphangiomatosis: CT findings. *J Comput Assist Tomogr* 1995;19(3):348–352.

465. Takahashi K, Takahashi H, Maeda K, et al. An adult case of lymphangiomatosis of the mediastinum, pulmonary interstitium and retroperitoneum complicated by chronic disseminated intravascular coagulation. *Eur Respir J* 1995;8(10):1799–1802.

466. Tamay Z, Saribeyoglu E, Ones U, et al. Diffuse thoracic lymphangiomatosis with disseminated intravascular coagulation in a child. *J Pediatr Hematol Oncol* 2005;27(12):685–687.

467. Watts MA, Gibbons JA, Aaron BL. Mediastinal and osseous lymphangiomatosis: case report and review. *Ann Thorac Surg* 1982;34(3):324–328.

468. Okubo T, Okayasu T, Osaka Y, et al. Surgical analysis of mediastinal lymphangioma—analysis of 7 cases. *Nihon Kyobu Geka Gakkai Zasshi* 1992;40(4):583–586.

469. Park JG, Aubry MC, Godfrey JA, et al. Mediastinal lymphangioma: Mayo Clinic experience of 25 cases. *Mayo Clin Proc* 2006;81(9):1197–1203.

470. Johnson DW, Klazynski PT, Gordon WH, et al. Mediastinal lymphangioma and chylothorax: the role of radiotherapy. *Ann Thorac Surg* 1986;41(3):325–328.

471. Kandil A, Rostom AY, Mourad WA, et al. Successful control of extensive thoracic lymphangiomatosis by irradiation. *Clin Oncol (R Coll Radiol)* 1997;9(6):407–411.

472. King DF, Hirose FM, Gurevitch AW, et al. Lymphangiosarcoma following radiation therapy. *J Am Acad Dermatol* 1986;14(4):684.

473. Chnaris A, Barbetakis N, Efstathiou A, et al. Primary mediastinal hemangiopericytoma. *World J Surg Oncol* 2006;4:23.

474. Hayashi A, Takamori S, Tayama K, et al. Primary hemangiopericytoma of the superior mediastinum: a case report. *Ann Thorac Cardiovasc Surg* 1998;4(5):283–285.

475. Osanai T, Kanazawa T, Nakamura K, et al. A case of primary cystic mediastinal hemangiopericytoma. *Arch Pathol Lab Med* 1994;118(5):575–577.

476. Backwinkel KD, Diddams JA. Hemangiopericytoma. Report of a case and comprehensive review of the literature. *Cancer* 1970;25(4):896–901.

477. Weidner N. Atypical tumor of the mediastinum: epithelioid hemangioendothelioma containing metaplastic bone and osteoclastlike giant cells. *Ultrastruct Pathol* 1991;15(4–5):481–488.

478. Llombart-Bosch A, Peydro-Olaya A, Paris-Romeu F. Fine structure of a malignant hemangioendothelioma of the esophagus. *Virchows Arch A Pathol Anat Histol* 1981;391(1):107–115.

479. Hiraki A, Murakami T, Aoe K, et al. Recurrent superior mediastinal primary hemangiopericytoma 23 years after the complete initial excision: a case report. *Acta Med Okayama* 2006;60(3):197–200.

480. Finn WG, Goolsby CL, Rao MS. DNA flow cytometric analysis of hemangiopericytoma. *Am J Clin Pathol* 1994;101(2):181–185.

481. McMaster MJ, Soule EH, Ivins JC. Hemangiopericytoma. A clinicopathologic study and long-term followup of 60 patients. *Cancer* 1975;36(6):2232–2244.

482. Dube VE, Paulson JF. Metastatic hemangiopericytoma cured by radiotherapy. a case report. *J Bone Joint Surg Am* 1974;56(4):833–835.

483. Cohen AJ, Sbaschnig RJ, Hochholzer L, et al. Mediastinal hemangiomas. *Ann Thorac Surg* 1987;43(6):656–659.

484. Ponce FA, Killory BD, Wait SD, et al. Endoscopic resection of intrathoracic tumors: experience with and long-term results for 26 patients. *J Neurosurg Spine* 2011;14(3):377–381.

485. Okubo K, Kuwabara M, Ito K, et al. A case of mediastinal fibrosarcoma. *Nihon Kyobu Geka Gakkai Zasshi* 1995;43(2):221–225.

486. Suster S, Moran CA. Malignant cartilaginous tumors of the mediastinum: clinicopathological study of six cases presenting as extraskeletal soft tissue masses. *Hum Pathol* 1997;28(5):588–594.

487. De Nictolis M, Goteri G, Campanati G, et al. Elastofibrolipoma of the mediastinum. A previously undescribed benign tumor containing abnormal elastic fibers. *Am J Surg Pathol* 1995;19(3):364–367.

488. Dikshtein EA, Sadovnik EE. Mesenchymoma of the mediastinum. *Arkh Patol* 1985;47(12):59–61.

489. Suster S, Moran CA. Chordomas of the mediastinum: clinicopathologic, immunohistochemical, and ultrastructural study of six cases presenting as posterior mediastinal masses. *Hum Pathol* 1995;26(12):1354–1362.

490. Chavez Espinosa JL CFJ, Hoyer OH, et al. Endothoracic neurogenic neoplasm (analysis of 30 cases). *Rev Interam Radiol* 1980;5(2):49–54.

491. Topcu S, Alper A, Gulhan E, et al. Neurogenic tumours of the mediastinum: a report of 60 cases. *Can Respir J* 2000;7(3):261–265.

492. Ohtaki Y, Ishii G, Hasegawa T, et al. Adult neuroblastoma arising in the superior mediastinum. *Interact Cardiovasc Thorac Surg* 2011;13(2):220–222.

493. Liu HP, Yim AP, Wan J, et al. Thoracoscopic removal of intrathoracic neurogenic tumors: a combined Chinese experience. *Ann Surg* 2000;232(2):187–190.

494. Reed JC, Hallet KK, Feigin DS. Neural tumors of the thorax: subject review from the AFIP. *Radiology* 1978;126(1):9–17.

495. Anghileri M, Miceli R, Fiore M, et al. Malignant peripheral nerve sheath tumors: prognostic factors and survival in a series of patients treated at a single institution. *Cancer* 2006;107(5):1065–1074.

496. Hayat J, Ahmed R, Alizai S, et al. Giant ganglioneuroma of the posterior mediastinum. *Interact Cardiovasc Thorac Surg* 2011;13(3):344–345.

497. Lin MW, Chang YL, Lee YC, et al. Non-functional paraganglioma of the posterior mediastinum. *Interact Cardiovasc Thorac Surg* 2009;9(3):540–542.

498. Dahia PL, Dahia PLM. Evolving concepts in pheochromocytoma and paraganglioma. *Curr Opin Oncol* 2006;18(1):1–8.

499. Elder EE, Elder G, Larsson C, et al. Pheochromocytoma and functional paraganglioma syndrome: no longer the 10% tumor. *J Surg Oncol* 2005;89(3):193–201.

500. Huson SM, Compston DA, Clark P, et al. A genetic study of von Recklinghausen neurofibromatosis in south east Wales. I. Prevalence, fitness, mutation rate, and effect of parental transmission on severity. *J Med Genet* 1989;26(11):704–711.

501. Harkin JC. Pathology of nerve sheath tumors. *Ann N Y Acad Sci* 1986; 486:147–154.

502. Ferner RE, Gutmann DH, Ferner RE, et al. International consensus statement on malignant peripheral nerve sheath tumors in neurofibromatosis. *Cancer Res* 2002;62(5):1573–1577.

503. Huson SM, Harper PS, Compston DA. Von Recklinghausen neurofibromatosis. A clinical and population study in south-east Wales. *Brain* 1988;111(Pt 6):1355–1381.

Section III

504. Netto MX, Almeida AW. Mediastinal tumors. *J Pneumol* 1984;10(1):15–24.

505. Paris P. Mediastinal neural tumors, a report of 27 cases. *Diss Abstr Int [C]* 1991;52(3):418.

506. Tucker T, Wolkenstein P, Revuz J, et al. Association between benign and malignant peripheral nerve sheath tumors in NF1. *Neurology* 2005;65(2):205–211.

507. McGaughran JM, Harris DI, Donnai D, et al. A clinical study of type 1 neurofibromatosis in north west England. *J Med Genet* 1999;36(3):197–203.

508. Bloechle C, Peiper M, Schwarz R, et al. Post-irradiation soft tissue sarcoma. *Eur J Cancer* 1995;31A(1):31–34.

509. Dini M, Caldarella A, Lo Russo G, et al. Malignant tumors of the peripheral nerve sheath (MPNST) after irradiation]. *Pathologica* 1997;89(4):441–445.

510. Storm FK, Eilber FR, Mirra J, et al. Neurofibrosarcoma. *Cancer* 1980;45(1):126–129.

511. Wong WW, Hirose T, Scheithauer BW, et al. Malignant peripheral nerve sheath tumor: analysis of treatment outcome. *Int J Radiat Oncol Biol Phys* 1998;42(2):351–360.

512. Gale AW, Jelihovsky T, Grant AF, et al. Neurogenic tumors of the mediastinum. *Ann Thorac Surg* 1974;17(5):434–443.

513. Kumar S, Rafiq MU, Ahamed I, et al. Asymptomatic giant thoracic schwannoma. *Ann Thorac Surg* 2006;82(3):e26.

514. Takeda S, Miyoshi S, Minami M, et al. Intrathoracic neurogenic tumors—50 years' experience in a Japanese institution. *Eur J Cardiothorac Surg* 2004;26(4):807–812.

515. Dutta R, Kumar A, Jindal T, et al. Concurrent benign schwannoma of oesophagus and posterior mediastinum. *Interact Cardiovasc Thorac Surg* 2009;9(6):1032–1034.

516. Eguchi T, Yoshida K, Kobayashi N, et al. Multiple schwannomas of the bilateral mediastinal vagus nerves. *Ann Thorac Surg* 2011;91(4):1280–1281.

517. Kaneko M, Matsumoto I, Oda M, et al. Multiple schwannoma of the intrathoracic vagal nerve; report of a case. *Kyobu Geka* 2008;61(9):820–823.

518. La Francesca S, Gregoric ID, Cohn WE, et al. Successful resection of a primary left ventricular schwannoma. *Ann Thorac Surg* 2007;83(5):1881–1882.

519. Mizuguchi S, Inoue K, Imagawa A, et al. Benign esophageal schwannoma compressing the trachea in pregnancy. *Ann Thorac Surg* 2008;85(2):660–662.

520. Rammos KS, Rammos SK, Foroulis CN, et al. Schwannoma of the vagus nerve, a rare middle mediastinal neurogenic tumor: case report. *J Cardiothorac Surg* 2009;4:68.

521. Smahi M, Lakranbi M, Ouadnouni Y, et al. Intrathoracic phrenic nerve neurofibroma. *Ann Thorac Surg* 2011;91(4):e57–e58.

522. Wang S, Zheng J, Ruan Z, et al. Long-term survival in a rare case of malignant esophageal schwannoma cured by surgical excision. *Ann Thorac Surg* 2011;92(1):357–358.

523. Lee JY, Lee KS, Han J, et al. Spectrum of neurogenic tumors in the thorax: CT and pathologic findings. *J Comput Assist Tomogr* 1999;23(3):399–406.

524. Ducatman BS, Scheithauer BW, Piepgras DG, et al. Malignant peripheral nerve sheath tumors. A clinicopathologic study of 120 cases. *Cancer* 1986;57(10):2006–2021.

525. Reeder LB. Neurogenic tumors of the mediastinum. *Semin Thorac Cardiovasc Surg* 2000;12(4):261–267.

526. Barrenechea IJ, Fukumoto R, Lesser JB, et al. Endoscopic resection of thoracic paravertebral and dumbbell tumors. *Neurosurgery* 2006;59(6):1195–1201; discussion 1201–1192.

527. Cardillo G, Carleo F, Khalil MW, et al. Surgical treatment of benign neurogenic tumours of the mediastinum: a single institution report. *Eur J Cardiothorac Surg* 2008;34(6):1210–1214.

528. Kan P, Schmidt MH. Minimally invasive thoracoscopic resection of paraspinal neurogenic tumors: technical case report. *Neurosurgery* 2008;63(1 Suppl 1):ONSE54; discussion ONSE54.

529. Kruger M, Uschinsky K, Engelmann C. Surgical treatment of malignant thoracic schwannomas. *Zentralbl Chir* 2001;126(3):223–228.

530. Santoro A, Tursz T, Mouridsen H, et al. Doxorubicin versus CYVADIC versus doxorubicin plus ifosfamide in first-line treatment of advanced soft tissue sarcomas: a randomized study of the European Organization for Research and Treatment of Cancer Soft Tissue and Bone Sarcoma Group. *J Clin Oncol* 1995;13(7):1537–1545.

531. Guha A, Lau N, Huvar I, et al. Ras-GTP levels are elevated in human NF1 peripheral nerve tumors. *Oncogene* 1996;12(3):507–513.

532. Macchiarini P. Primary tracheal tumours. *Lancet Oncol* 2006;7(1):83–91.

533. Houston HE, Payne WS, Harrison EG Jr, et al. Primary cancers of the trachea. *Arch Surg* 1969;99(2):132–140.

534. Webb BD, Walsh GL, Roberts DB, et al. Primary tracheal malignant neoplasms: the University of Texas MD Anderson Cancer Center experience. *J Am Coll Surg* 2006;202(2):237–246.

535. Hu J, Shen ZX, Sun GL, et al. Long-term survival and prognostic study in acute promyelocytic leukemia treated with all-trans-retinoic acid, chemotherapy, and As2O3: an experience of 120 patients at a single institution. *Int J Hematol* 1999;70(4):248–260.

536. Maziak DE, Todd TR, Keshavjee SH, et al. Adenoid cystic carcinoma of the airway: thirty-two-year experience. *J Thorac Cardiovasc Surg* 1996;112(6):1522–1531; discussion 1531–1522.

537. Amiraliev MA, Alekseev VI, Kolodiazhnyi AP, et al. Carcinoid of the trachea simulating bronchial asthma (1 case). *Vopr Onkol* 1985;31(6):107–108.

538. Briselli M, Mark GJ, Grillo HC. Tracheal carcinoids. *Cancer* 1978;42(6):2870–2879.

539. Chizh GI, Pichko RT. Malignant carcinoid tumor of the trachea. *Vestn Otorinolaringol* 1983;(3):84–85.

540. Gaissert HA, Grillo HC, Shadmehr MB, et al. Uncommon primary tracheal tumors. *Ann Thorac Surg* 2006;82(1):268–272; discussion 272–263.

541. Hulka GF, Rothschild MA, Warner BW, et al. Carcinoid tumor of the trachea in a pediatric patient. *Otolaryngol Head Neck Surg* 1996;114(6):822–825.

542. Koikkalainen K, Keskitalo E, Luosto R, et al. Carcinoid tumours and cylindromas of the tracheobronchial tree. *Ann Chir Gynaecol Fenn* 1974;63(4):332–341.

543. Kononov EP. Carcinoid of the trachea. *Zh Ushn Nos Gorl Bolezn* 1967;27(5):104.

544. Pant K, Bhagat R, Chawla R, et al. Primary carcinoid tumour of trachea. *Indian J Chest Dis Allied Sci* 1990;32(3):193–197.

545. Shi ML, Fan KH, Zhou CW, et al. X-ray features of primary non-squamous cell carcinoma and other malignant neoplasms in the trachea and main bronchi—analysis of 23 cases. *Zhonghua Zhong Liu Za Zhi* 1987;9(3):208–211.

546. Wang Y, Wang L, Zhang D. Carcinoid of trachea and bronchus: a report of 20 cases. *Zhonghua Zhong Liu Za Zhi* 2001;23(1):70–72.

547. Yamamoto K, Alarcon JP, Armengod EB, et al. Tracheal carcinoid during pregnancy. *J Cardiovasc Surg (Torino)* 2004;45(5):525.

548. Salm R. Primary carcinoma of the trachea: a review. *Br J Dis Chest* 1964;58:61–72.

549. Amar YG, Nguyen LH, Manoukian JJ, et al. Granular cell tumor of the trachea in a child. *Int J Pediatr Otorhinolaryngol* 2002;62(1):75–80.

550. Burton DM, Heffner DK, Patow CA. Granular cell tumors of the trachea. *Laryngoscope* 1992;102(7):807–813.

551. Desai DP, Maddalozzo J, Holinger LD. Granular cell tumor of the trachea. *Otolaryngol Head Neck Surg* 1999;120(4):595–598.

552. Ipakchi R, Zager WH, de Baca ME, et al. Granular cell tumor of the trachea in pregnancy: a case report and review of literature. *Laryngoscope* 2004;114(1):143–147.

553. Jobard P, Vandooren M, Baudouin J, et al. Granular cell tumor of the trachea. *Laval Med* 1966;37(5):602–604.

554. Kintanar EB, Giordano TJ, Thompson NW, et al. Granular-cell tumor of trachea masquerading as Hurthle-cell neoplasm on fine-needle aspirate: a case report. *Diagn Cytopathol* 2000;22(6):379–382.

555. Mikaelian DO, Cohn H, Israel H, et al. Granular cell tumor of the trachea. *Ann Otol Rhinol Laryngol* 1984;93(5 Pt 1):457–459.

556. Mulhollan TJ, Ro JY, el-Naggar AK, et al. Granular cell tumor of the biliary tree. *Am J Surg Pathol* 1992;16(2):204–206.

557. Raymond GS, Murray SK, Logan PM. Granular cell tumour of the trachea: case report. *Can Assoc Radiol J* 1997;48(1):48–50.

558. Spandow O, Lindholm CE. Granular cell tumour in a child's trachea—a diagnostic and therapeutic challenge. *Int J Pediatr Otorhinolaryngol* 1994; 30(2):159–166.

559. Stieglitz F, Kitz R, Schafers HJ, et al. Granular cell tumor of the trachea in a child. *Ann Thorac Surg* 2005;79(2):e15–e16.

560. van der Maten J, Blaauwgeers JL, Sutedja TG, et al. Granular cell tumors of the tracheobronchial tree. *J Thorac Cardiovasc Surg* 2003;126(3):740–743.

561. Littler ER. Asphyxia due to hemangioma in trachea. *J Thorac Cardiovasc Surg* 1963;45:552–558.

562. Madhumita K, Sreekumar KP, Malini H, et al. Tracheal haemangioma: case report. *J Laryngol Otol* 2004;118(8):655–658.

563. Maier HC. Hemangiomas of the subglottic region, trachea, and mediastinum in infancy and childhood. *Ann Thorac Surg* 1967;3(6):514–525.

564. Pogorzelski A, Zebrak J. Tracheal hemangioma. *Pediatr Pol* 1995;70(6):519–520.

565. Zimmer W, DeLuca SA. Primary tracheal neoplasms: recognition, diagnosis and evaluation. *Am Fam Physician* 1992;45(6):2651–2657.

566. Davies MJ, Hall DR, Ross BA. Rare tracheal tumours: two case reports of primary neurogenic tumours occurring in the trachea. *Respir Med* 1993;87(2):145–146.

567. Dincer SI, Demir A, Kara HV, et al. Primary tracheal schwannoma: a case report. *Acta Chir Belg* 2006;106(2):254–256.

568. Dorfman J, Jamison BM, Morin JE. Primary tracheal schwannoma. *Ann Thorac Surg* 2000;69(1):280–281.

569. Low SY, Eng P, Thirugnanam A. Primary endotracheal neurogenic tumors. *Surg Endosc* 2004;18(2):348.

570. Tiedemann R. Neurogenic tumors of the trachea. *HNO* 1992;40(2):41–43.

571. Brewster DC, MacMillan IK, Edwards FR. Chondroma of the trachea: report of a case and review of the literature. *Ann Thorac Surg* 1975;19(5):576–584.

572. Jortay AM, Bisschop P. Chondroma of the trachea. *Acta Otorhinolaryngol Belg* 1998;52(3):247–251.

573. Swain ME, Coblentz CL. Tracheal chondroma: CT appearance. *J Comput Assist Tomogr* 1988;12(6):1085–1086.

574. Zizmor J, Noyek AM, Lewis JS. Radiologic diagnosis of chondroma and chondrosarcoma of the larynx. *Arch Otolaryngol* 1975;101(4):232–234.

575. Arevalo M, Ordi J, Renedo G, et al. Chondrosarcoma of the trachea. Report of a case. *Respiration* 1986;49(2):147–151.

576. Fallahnejad M, Harrell D, Tucker J, et al. Chondrosarcoma of the trachea. Report of a case and five-year follow-up. *J Thorac Cardiovasc Surg* 1973;65(2):210–213.

577. Farrell ML, Gluckman JL, Biddinger P. Tracheal chondrosarcoma: a case report. *Head Neck* 1998;20(6):568–572.

578. Kiriyama M, Masaoka A, Yamakawa Y, et al. Chondrosarcoma originating from the trachea. *Ann Thorac Surg* 1997;63(6):1772–1773.

579. Maish M, Vaporciyan AA. Chondrosarcoma arising in the trachea: a case report and review of the literature. *J Thorac Cardiovasc Surg* 2003;126(6):2077–2080.

580. Matsuo T, Kinoshita S, Iwasaki K, et al. Chondrosarcoma of the trachea. A case report and literature review. *Acta Cytol* 1988;32(6):908–912.

581. Nakano Y, Asakura K, Himi T, et al. Chondrosarcoma of larynx: a case successfully reconstructed after total cricoidectomy. *Auris Nasus Larynx* 1999;26(2):207–211.

582. Slasky BS, Hardesty RL, Wilson S. Tracheal chondrosarcoma with an overview of other tumors of the trachea. *J Comput Tomogr* 1985;9(3):225–231.

583. Weber AL, Grillo HC. Tracheal tumor: radiological, clinical and pathological evaluation. *Adv Otorhinolaryngol* 1978;24:170–176.

584. Adachi MM, Pamies RJ. Carcinoma of the trachea: a hidden tumor. *Hosp Pract (Off Ed)* 1993;28(7):81–84.

585. Yang KY, Chen YM, Huang MH, et al. Revisit of primary malignant neoplasms of the trachea: clinical characteristics and survival analysis. *Jpn J Clin Oncol* 1997;27(5):305–309.

586. Allen MS. Malignant tracheal tumors. *Mayo Clin Proc* 1993;68(7):680–684.

587. Baydur A, Gottlieb LS. Adenoid cystic carcinoma (cylindroma) of the trachea masquerading as asthma. *JAMA* 1975;234(8):829–831.

588. Cleveland RH, Nice CM Jr, Ziskind J. Primary adenoid cystic carcinoma (cylindroma) of the trachea. *Radiology* 1977;122(3):597–600.

589. Filatova NM. Cancer of trachea presenting as bronchial asthma. *Vrach Delo* 1977;(5):58–59.

590. Leonova LA, Mel'nikova VG. Cancer of the trachea simulating bronchial asthma. *Vrach Delo* 1972;4:107–108.

591. Takami A, Okumura H, Maeda Y, et al. Primary tracheal lymphoma: case report and literature review. *Int J Hematol* 2005;82(4):338–342.

592. van Nostrand AW. Tracheal tumors—early diagnosis and treatment. *J Otolaryngol* 1977;6(1):74–84.

593. Janower ML, Grillo HC, MacMillan AS Jr, et al. The radiological appearance of carcinoma of the trachea. *Radiology* 1970;96(1):39–43.

594. Kallenbach J, Song E, Zwi S. Haemoptysis with no radiological evidence of tumour—the value of early bronchoscopy. *S Afr Med J* 1981;59(16):556–558.

595. McCarthy MJ, Rosado-de-Christenson ML. Tumors of the trachea. *J Thorac Imaging* 1995;10(3):180–198.

596. Thotathil ZS, Agarwal JP, Shrivastava SK, et al. Primary malignant tumors of the trachea—the Tata Memorial Hospital experience. *Med Princ Pract* 2004;13(2):69–73.

597. Lee CH, Lin HC. Descriptive study of prognostic factors influencing survival of patients with primary tracheal tumors. *Changgeng Yi Xue Za Zhi* 1995;18(3):224–230.

598. Pearson FG, Cooper JD. Experience with primary neoplasms of the trachea and carina. *Nihon Kyobu Geka Gakkai Zasshi* 1984;32(5):661–664.

599. Douglas JG, Laramore GE, Austin-Seymour M, et al. Treatment of locally advanced adenoid cystic carcinoma of the head and neck with neutron radiotherapy. *Int J Radiat Oncol Biol Phys* 2000;46(3):551–557.

600. Gaissert HA, Grillo HC, Shadmehr MB, et al. Long-term survival after resection of primary adenoid cystic and squamous cell carcinoma of the trachea and carina. *Ann Thorac Surg* 2004;78(6):1889–1896; discussion 1896–1887.

601. Grillo HC, Mathisen DJ. Primary tracheal tumors: treatment and results. *Ann Thorac Surg* 1990;49(1):69–77.

602. Kohno N, Tateno H, Kawaida M, et al. Primary adenoid cystic carcinoma of the trachea: a case report of a twelve year survivor. *Keio J Med* 1995;44(1):30–32.

603. Inoue H. Long-term prognosis of adenoid cystic carcinoma of the trachea. *Kyobu Geka* 1991;44(13):1121–1125.

604. Prommegger R, Salzer GM. Long-term results of surgery for adenoid cystic carcinoma of the trachea and bronchi. *Eur J Surg Oncol* 1998;24(5):440–444.

605. Ramsden D, Sheridan BF, Newton NC, et al. Adenoid cystic carcinoma of the head and neck: a report of 30 cases. *Aust N Z J Surg* 1973;43(2):102–108.

606. Honings J, van Dijck JA, Verhagen AF, et al. Incidence and treatment of tracheal cancer: a Nationwide Study in The Netherlands. *Ann Surg Oncol* 2007;14(2):968–976.

607. Jeremic B, Shibamoto Y, Acimovic L, et al. Radiotherapy for primary squamous cell carcinoma of the trachea. *Radiother Oncol* 1996;41(2):135–138.

608. Manninen MP, Pukander JS, Flander MK, et al. Treatment of primary tracheal carcinoma in Finland in 1967–1985. *Acta Oncol* 1993;32(3):277–282.

609. Schraube P, Latz D, Wannenmacher M. Treatment of primary squamous cell carcinoma of the trachea: the role of radiation therapy. *Radiother Oncol* 1994;33(3):254–258.

610. D'Cunha J, Maddaus MA. Surgical treatment of tracheal and carinal tumors. *Chest Surg Clin N Am* 2003;13(1):95–110, vi.

611. Grillo HC, Mathisen DJ. Cervical exenteration. *Ann Thorac Surg* 1990;49(3):401–408; discussion 408–409.

612. Harvey JC, Keen CW, Makowka L, et al. Adenocarcinoma of the trachea: palliative response to cobalt-60 irradiation. *Can J Surg* 1979;22(3):268–270.

613. Avilova OM, Vasilevskaia ZA. Sarcoma of the trachea. *Vrach Delo* 1974;5(0):34–36.

614. Chen JS, Chang YL, Shu HS, et al. Surgical treatment of a primary tracheal angiosarcoma. *J Thorac Cardiovasc Surg* 2003;125(1):191–193.

615. Cohen SR, Landing BH, Isaacs H. Fibrous histiocytoma of the trachea. *Ann Otol Rhinol Laryngol Suppl* 1978;87(5 Pt 2 Suppl 52):2–4.

616. Daniels AC, Conner GH, Straus FH. Primary chondrosarcoma of the tracheobronchial tree. Report of a unique case and brief review. *Arch Pathol* 1967;84(6):615–624.

617. Ho KL, Rassekh ZS. Rhabdomyosarcoma of the trachea: first reported case. *Hum Pathol* 1980;11(5 Suppl):572–574.

618. Larsson S, Lepore V, Cardillo G, et al. Primary tracheal rhabdomyosarcoma. Case report. *Scand J Thorac Cardiovasc Surg* 1989;23(3):293–295.

619. McKenzie GE, Rezek PR. Myosarcoma of trachea associated with Riedel struma. *AMA Arch Otolaryngol* 1953;57(1):22–39.

620. Outzen KE, Lunding J, Jakobsen J. Leiomyosarcoma of the trachea. *J Laryngol Otol* 1986;100(8):979–984.

621. Roncoroni AJ, Puy RJ, Goldman E, et al. Fibrosarcoma of the trachea with severe tracheal obstruction. *Thorax* 1973;28(6):777–781.

622. Saito H, Mizusawa A, Oketani N, et al. Suspected leiomyosarcoma of the trachea. *Nihon Kyobu Shikkan Gakkai Zasshi* 1997;35(4):420–425.

623. Sennaroglu L, Sozeri B, Ataman M, et al. Malignant fibrous histiocytoma of the trachea. Case report. *Acta Otorhinolaryngol Belg* 1996;50(2):147–149.

624. Smirnov NM. Sarcoma of the trachea. *Zh Ushn Nos Gorl Bolezn* 1979;(2):81–82.

625. Van Den Beukel JT, Wagenaar SJ, Vanderschueren R. Liposarcoma of the trachea. *Thorax* 1979;34(6):817–818.

626. Bhattacharyya N. Contemporary staging and prognosis for primary tracheal malignancies: a population-based analysis. *Otolaryngol Head Neck Surg* 2004;131(5):639–642.

627. Grillo HC. Primary tracheal tumours. *Thorax* 1993;48(7):681–682.

628. Grillo HC, Mathisen DJ, Wain JC. Management of tumors of the trachea. *Oncology (Williston Park)* 1992;6(2):61–67; discussion 68, 70, 72.

629. Mathisen DJ. Tracheal tumors. *Chest Surg Clin N Am* 1996;6(4):875–898.

630. Compeau CG, Keshavjee S. Management of tracheal neoplasms. *Oncologist* 1996;1(6):347–353.

631. Wood DE. Management of malignant tracheobronchial obstruction. *Surg Clin North Am* 2002;82(3):621–642.

632. Mathisen DJ. Primary tracheal tumor management. *Surg Oncol Clin N Am* 1999;8(2):307.

633. Mathisen DJ, Grillo HC. Endoscopic relief of malignant airway obstruction. *Ann Thorac Surg* 1989;48(4):469–473; discussion 473–465.

634. Aberle DR, Brown K, Young DA, et al. Imaging techniques in the evaluation of tracheobronchial neoplasms. *Chest* 1991;99(1):211–215.

635. Abudallo K, Romanoff H, Stern Z, et al. Primary tumors of the thoracic trachea with special emphasis on surgical management. *Int Surg* 1976;61(6–7):347–349.

636. Karlan MS, Livingston PA, Baker DC Jr. Diagnosis of tracheal tumors. *Ann Otol Rhinol Laryngol* 1973;82(6):790–799.

637. Gamsu G, Webb WR. Computed tomography of the trachea: normal and abnormal. *AJR Am J Roentgenol* 1982;139(2):321–326.

638. Rabkin I, Ovchinnikov VI, Iudin AL, et al. Diagnosis of tumors of the trachea and main bronchi by computerized tomography. *Vestn Rentgenol Radiol* 1993;(3):5–9.

639. Abbate G, Lancella A, Contini R, et al. A primary squamous cell carcinoma of the trachea: case report and review of the literature. *Acta Otorhinolaryngol Ital* 2010;30(4):209.

640. Grillo HC. Management of tracheal tumors. *Am J Surg* 1982;143(6):697–700.

641. Gaissert HA. Primary tracheal tumors. *Chest Surg Clin N Am* 2003;13(2):247–256.

642. Hetzel MR. Tracheal tumours: could treatment be better? *Clin Oncol (R Coll Radiol)* 1993;5(5):272–276.

643. Larsson S, Cardillo G, Lepore V. Surgical management of tracheal tumours. *Scand J Thorac Cardiovasc Surg* 1987;21(2):97–103.

644. Honings J, Gaissert HA, Verhagen AF, et al. Undertreatment of tracheal carcinoma: multidisciplinary audit of epidemiologic data. *Ann Surg Oncol* 2009;16(2):246–253.

645. Pearson FG, Thompson DW, Weissberg D, et al. Adenoid cystic carcinoma of the trachea. Experience with 16 patients managed by tracheal resection. *Ann Thorac Surg* 1974;18(1):16–29.

646. Grillo HC. New methods for the treatment of tracheal tumors. *GP* 1965;32(6):78–85.

647. Honings J, Gaissert HA, Ruangchira-Urai R, et al. Pathologic characteristics of resected squamous cell carcinoma of the trachea: prognostic factors based on an analysis of 59 cases. *Virchows Arch* 2009;455(5):423–429.

648. Chow DC, Komaki R, Libshitz HI, et al. Treatment of primary neoplasms of the trachea. The role of radiation therapy. *Cancer* 1993;71(10):2946–2952.

649. Cheung AY. Radiotherapy for primary carcinoma of the trachea. *Radiother Oncol* 1989;14(4):279–285.

650. Fields JN, Rigaud G, Emami BN. Primary tumors of the trachea. Results of radiation therapy. *Cancer* 1989;63(12):2429–2433.

651. Rostom AY, Morgan RL. Results of treating primary tumours of the trachea by irradiation. *Thorax* 1978;33(3):387–393.

652. Makarewicz R, Mross M. Radiation therapy alone in the treatment of tumours of the trachea. *Lung Cancer* 1998;20(3):169–174.

653. Fuwa N, Ito Y, Matsumoto A, et al. The treatment results of 40 patients with localized endobronchial cancer with external beam irradiation and intraluminal irradiation using low dose rate (192)Ir thin wires with a new catheter. *Radiother Oncol* 2000;56(2):189–195.

654. Mornex F, Coquard R, Danhier S, et al. Role of radiation therapy in the treatment of primary tracheal carcinoma. *Int J Radiat Oncol Biol Phys* 1998;41(2):299–305.

655. Green N, Kulber H, Landman M, et al. The experience with definitive irradiation of clinically limited squamous cell cancer of the trachea. *Int J Radiat Oncol Biol Phys* 1985;11(7):1401–1405.

656. Harms W, Latz D, Becker H, et al. Treatment of primary tracheal carcinoma. The role of external and endoluminal radiotherapy. *Strahlenther Onkol* 2000;176(1):22–27.

657. Bittner N, Koh WJ, Laramore GE, et al. Treatment of locally advanced adenoid cystic carcinoma of the trachea with neutron radiotherapy. *Int J Radiat Oncol Biol Phys* 2008;72(2):410–414.

658. Zhang HQ, Zhu ZJ, Peng DW, et al. Primary tracheal carcinoma—report of 5 patients. *Zhonghua Zhong Liu Za Zhi* 1988;10(1):45–47.

659. Videtic GM, Campbell C, Vincent MD. Primary chemoradiation as definitive treatment for unresectable cancer of the trachea. *Can Respir J* 2003;10(3):143–144.

660. Kobayashi H, Nemoto Y, Namiki K, et al. Primary malignant lymphoma of the trachea and subglottic region. *Intern Med* 1992;31(5):655–658.

661. Carvalho Hde A, Figueiredo V, Pedreira WL Jr, et al. High dose-rate brachytherapy as a treatment option in primary tracheal tumors. *Clinics* 2005;60(4):299–304.

662. Meyers BF, Mathisen DJ. Management of tracheal neoplasms. *Oncologist* 1997;2(4):245–253.

663. Skowronek J, Piotrowski T, Mlynarczyk W, et al. Advanced tracheal carcinoma—a therapeutic significance of HDR brachytherapy in palliative treatment. *Neoplasma* 2004;51(4):313–318.

664. Kirkpatrick JP, van der Kogel AJ, Schultheiss TE. Radiation dose-volume effects in the spinal cord. *Int J Radiat Oncol Biol Phys* 2010;76(3 Suppl):S42–S49.

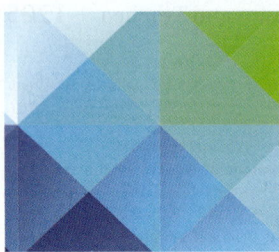

C H A P T E R   5 6

Esophageal Cancer

Brian G. Czito, Manisha Palta, and Christopher G. Willett

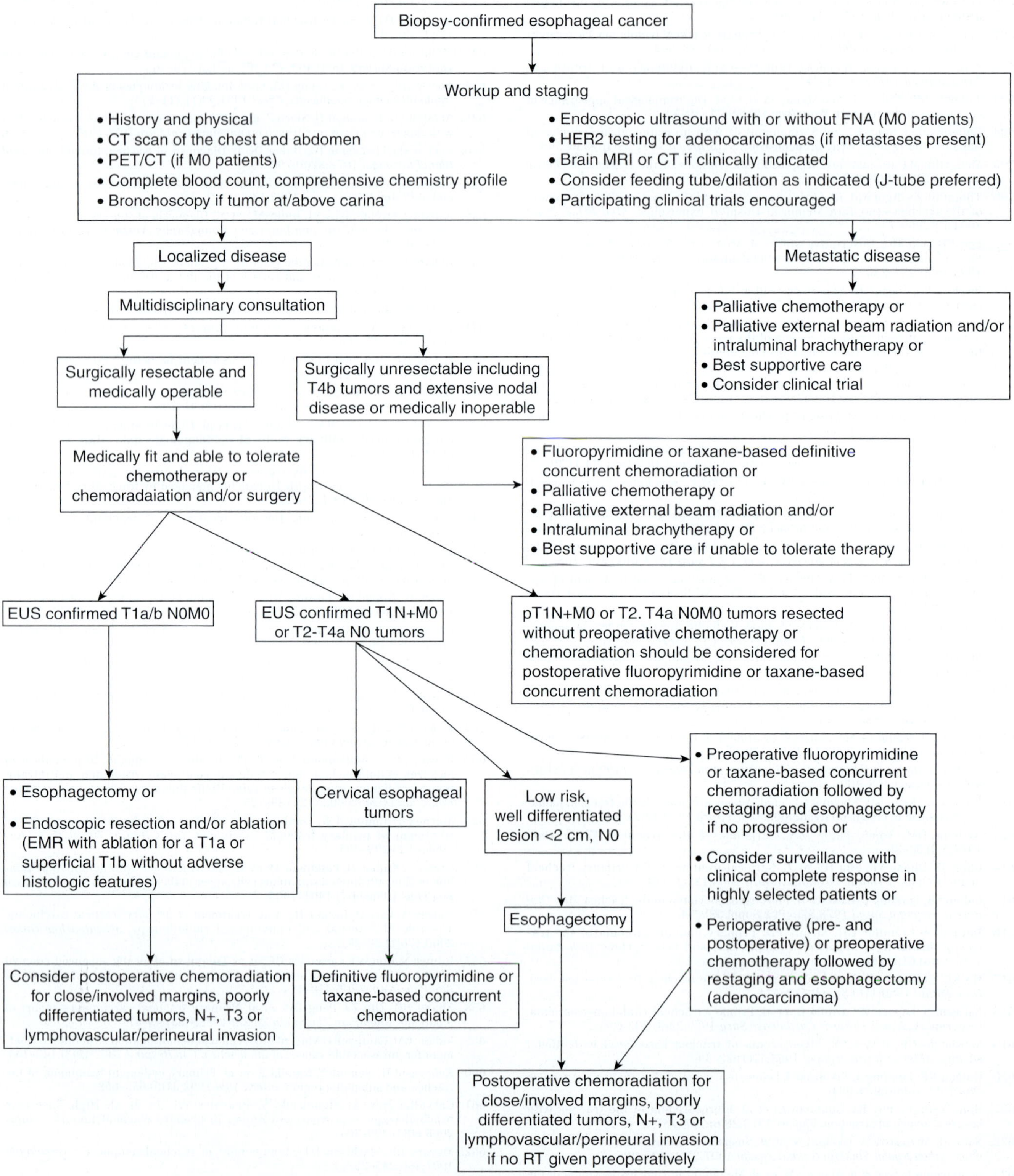

Biopsy-confirmed esophageal cancer

Workup and staging

- History and physical
- CT scan of the chest and abdomen
- PET/CT (if M0 patients)
- Complete blood count, comprehensive chemistry profile
- Bronchoscopy if tumor at/above carina

- Endoscopic ultrasound with or without FNA (M0 patients)
- HER2 testing for adenocarcinomas (if metastases present)
- Brain MRI or CT if clinically indicated
- Consider feeding tube/dilation as indicated (J-tube preferred)
- Participating clinical trials encouraged

Localized disease

Metastatic disease

- Palliative chemotherapy or
- Palliative external beam radiation and/or intraluminal brachytherapy or
- Best supportive care
- Consider clinical trial

Multidisciplinary consultation

Surgically resectable and medically operable

Surgically unresectable including T4b tumors and extensive nodal disease or medically inoperable

Medically fit and able to tolerate chemotherapy or chemoradaiation and/or surgery

- Fluoropyrimidine or taxane-based definitive concurrent chemoradiation or
- Palliative chemotherapy or
- Palliative external beam radiation and/or
- Intraluminal brachytherapy or
- Best supportive care if unable to tolerate therapy

EUS confirmed T1a/b N0M0

EUS confirmed T1N+M0 or T2-T4a N0 tumors

pT1N+M0 or T2. T4a N0M0 tumors resected without preoperative chemotherapy or chemoradiation should be considered for postoperative fluoropyrimidine or taxane-based concurrent chemoradiation

- Esophagectomy or
- Endoscopic resection and/or ablation (EMR with ablation for a T1a or superficial T1b without adverse histologic features)

Cervical esophageal tumors

Low risk, well differentiated lesion <2 cm, N0

- Preoperative fluoropyrimidine or taxane-based concurrent chemoradiation followed by restaging and esophagectomy if no progression or
- Consider surveillance with clinical complete response in highly selected patients or
- Perioperative (pre- and postoperative) or preoperative chemotherapy followed by restaging and esophagectomy (adenocarcinoma)

Esophagectomy

Consider postoperative chemoradiation for close/involved margins, poorly differentiated tumors, N+, T3 or lymphovascular/perineural invasion

Definitive fluoropyrimidine or taxane-based concurrent chemoradiation

Postoperative chemoradiation for close/involved margins, poorly differentiated tumors, N+, T3 or lymphovascular/perineural invasion if no RT given preoperatively

Treatment algorithm for newly diagnosed esophageal cancer. Treatment approaches are based in location and stage of the tumor, as well as surgical resectability and medical comorbidities of the patient. CT, computed tomography; EUS, endoscopic ultrasound; FNA, fine-needle aspiration; MRI magnetic resonance imaging; PET, positron emission tomography.

Less than 15% of patients diagnosed with esophageal cancer are cured, with approximately half of patients presenting with unresectable or metastatic disease. This chapter reviews the natural history and treatment of esophageal cancer, including anatomy, risk factors, patterns of spread and recurrence, staging, results of current therapeutic approaches, radiation planning techniques, toxicity data, and future treatment strategies.

ANATOMY

The esophagus is a thin-walled, hollow tube approximately 25 cm in length. It is lined with stratified keratinized squamous epithelium, extending from the cricopharyngeus muscle at the level of the cricoid cartilage superiorly to the gastroesophageal junction inferiorly. The lower one-third (5 to 10 cm) of the esophagus may contain glandular elements. Replacement of the stratified squamous epithelium with columnar epithelium is referred to as Barrett esophagus, often occurring in the lower one-third. The Z line refers to the endoscopically visible junction of the squamous and glandular epithelium. The esophageal wall is composed of three layers: the mucosa, submucosa, and muscularis propria (Fig. 56.1). The mucosal layer contains the epithelium,

lamina propria, and muscularis mucosae. The epithelium is separated from the lamina propria by a basement membrane. In the portion of the esophagus containing columnar-type epithelium, the muscularis mucosae may consist of two layers. The mucosa may be divided into distinct layers, including M1 (epithelium), M2 (lamina propria), and M3 (muscularis mucosae). Similarly, the submucosal layer may be divided into inner (SM1), middle (SM2), and outer (SM3) layers. The muscularis propria consists of a circular inner layer and longitudinal outer layer. The adventitia (periesophageal connective tissue) lies directly on the muscularis propria.[1] No serosa is present, facilitating extraesophageal spread of disease.

Although somewhat arbitrary, the esophagus is frequently divided into cervical and thoracic components. The most recent American Joint Committee on Cancer (AJCC) report divides the esophagus into four regions: cervical, upper thoracic, midthoracic, and lower thoracic (Fig. 56.2).[1] The cervical esophagus lies within the neck and begins at the cricopharyngeus muscle (approximately the C7 level or 15 cm from the incisors) and extends to the thoracic inlet (at approximately the T3 level or at ~20 cm from the incisors [the level of the suprasternal notch]). The thoracic esophagus extends from approximately the level of T3 (beginning at about 20 cm) to T10 or T11.[1,2] The upper

FIGURE 56.1. Diagram of esophageal wall. (CCF © 2016. The original source for this material is Rice TW, Ishwaran H, Ferguson MK, et al. Cancer of the esophagus and esophagogastric junction: an eighth edition staging primer. *J Thorac Oncol* 2017;12[1]:36–42. Copyright © 2016 International Association for the Study of Lung Cancer. With permission.)

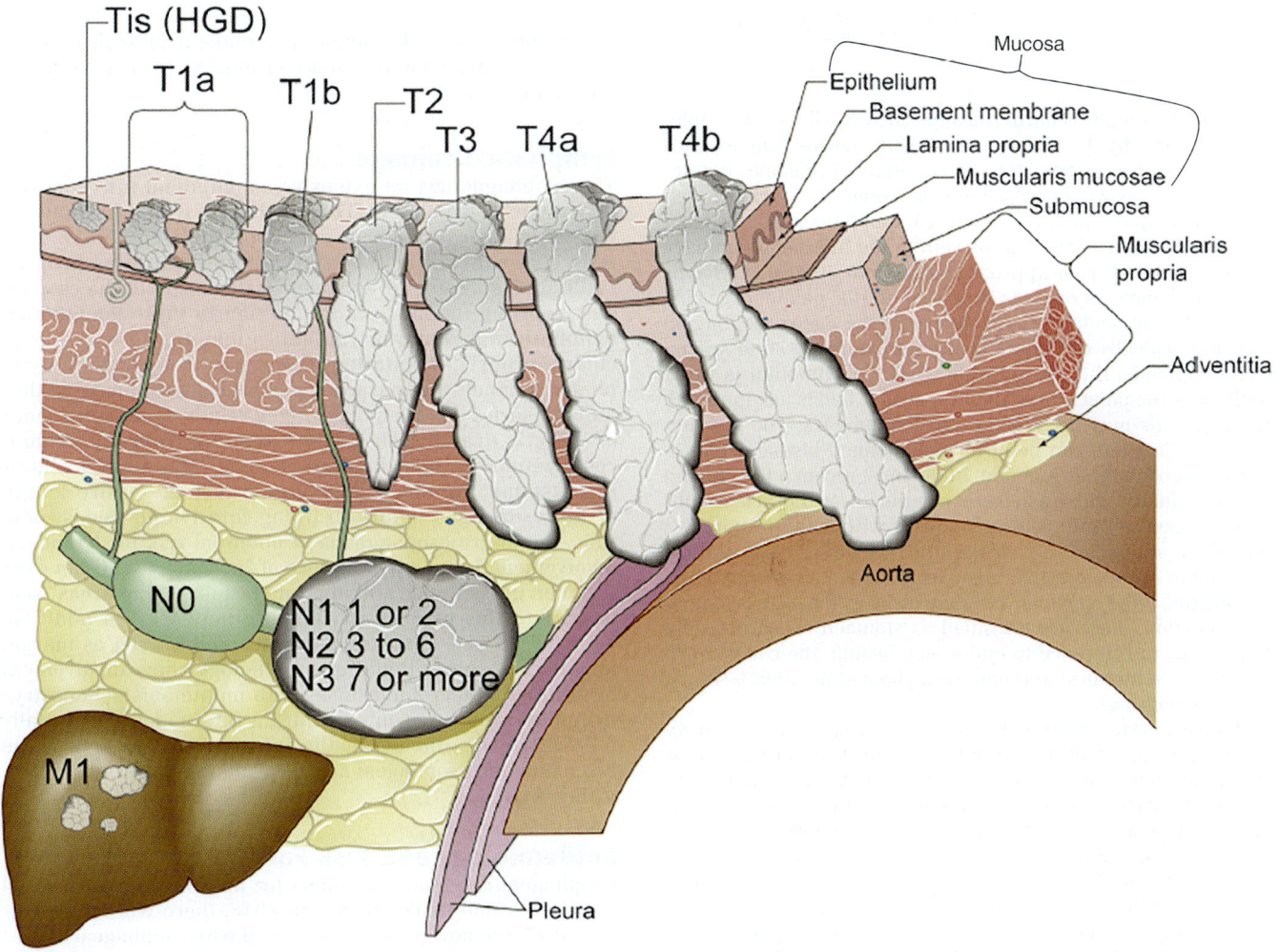

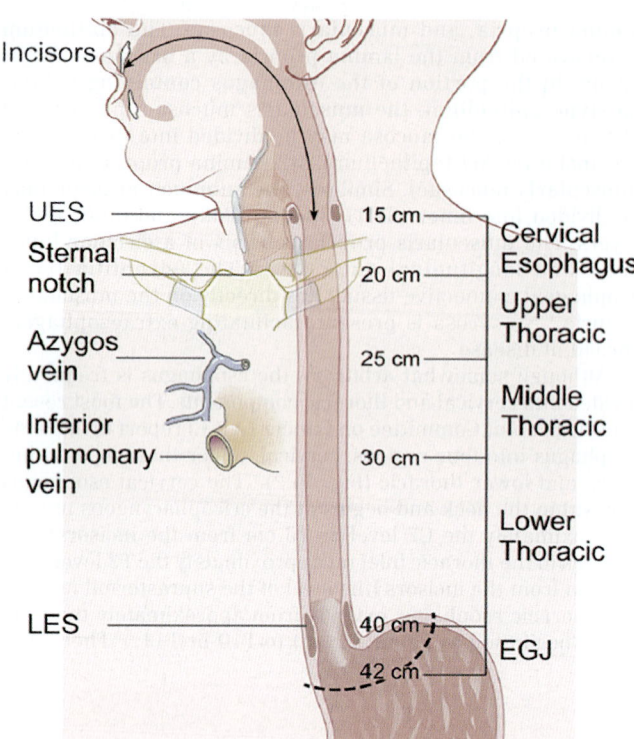

FIGURE 56.2. Anatomy of the esophagus. Note the lengths of various segments of the esophagus as measured from the upper central incisors. (CCF © 2016. The original source for this material is Rice TW, Ishwaran H, Ferguson MK et al. Cancer of the esophagus and esophagogastric junction: an eighth edition staging primer. *J Thorac Oncol* 2017;12[1]:36–42. Copyright © 2016 International Association for the Study of Lung Cancer. With permission.)

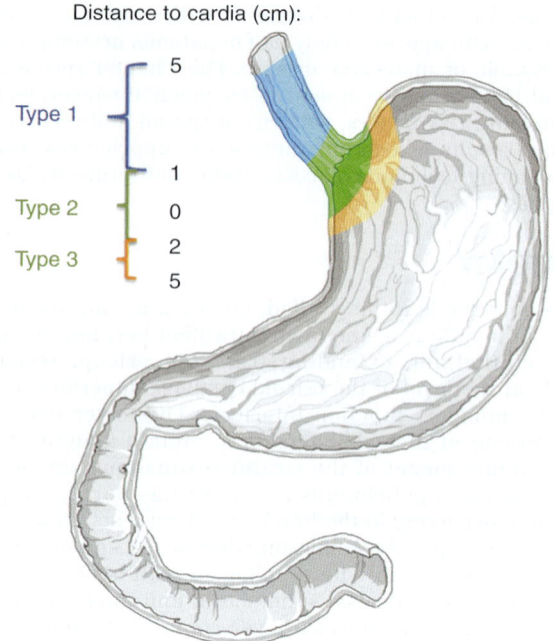

FIGURE 56.3. Siewert classification of the gastroesophageal junction cancers according to the location of the tumor. (Reprinted from Matzinger O, Gerber E, Bernstein Z, et al. EORTC-ROG expert opinion: radiotherapy volume and treatment guidelines for neoadjuvant radiation of adenocarcinomas of the gastroesophageal junction and the stomach. *Radiother Oncol* 2009;92[2]:164–175. Copyright © 2009 Elsevier Ireland Ltd. With permission.)

thoracic esophagus is bordered superiorly by the thoracic inlet and inferiorly by the lower border of the azygos vein, extending from approximately 20 to 25 cm. Radiographically, tumors in this location would be located between the sternal notch and azygos vein. The middle thoracic esophagus extends from the lower border of the azygos vein to the inferior pulmonary veins, extending from approximately 25 to 30 cm. The lower thoracic esophagus extends from the inferior pulmonary veins and to the stomach and is inclusive of the gastroesophageal junction, typically extending from approximately 30 to 40 cm. Endoscopically, the gastroesophageal (GE) junction is often defined as the point where the first gastric fold is encountered, although this may be a "theoretical" landmark. The location of the GE junction can be accurately defined histologically as the squamocolumnar junction. In the most recent AJCC staging system, cancers with an epicenter in the lower thoracic esophagus or gastroesophageal junction or within the proximal 2 cm of the stomach (i.e., cardia) and extending up to the GE junction or esophagus are staged as an adenocarcinoma of the esophagus. If the epicenter is >2 cm distal to the gastroesophageal junction, these are classified as stomach cancers. Useful landmarks in reference to endoscopy include the carina (~25 cm from the incisors) and gastroesophageal junction (~40 cm from the incisors).

Siewert et al.[3,4] characterized cancer *involving the gastroesophageal junction* according to the location of the tumor (Fig. 56.3). If the tumor center is located from >1 cm up to 5 cm above the gastroesophageal junction (Z line), the tumor is classified as a type I adenocarcinoma of the distal esophagus. If the tumor center is located within 1 cm cephalad to 2 cm caudad to the gastroesophageal junction, it is classified as type II. If the tumor center is located >2 cm below the gastroesophageal junction, the tumor is classified as type III. Only Siewert type I/II tumors would be staged as esophageal cancer in the most recent staging AJCC staging system. However,

locally advanced/bulky tumors can make it difficult to accurately distinguish where tumors originated in relationship to the GE junction.

Lymphatic Drainage

The esophagus has an extensive, longitudinal interconnecting system of lymphatics. The esophageal lymphatic network is primarily located within the submucosa (Fig. 56.1); however, channels are also present within the lamina propria, facilitating spread of even superficial cancers of the esophagus involving the mucosa. In addition to these longitudinal lymphatics, intramural lymphatics may traverse the muscularis propria, facilitating tumor spread to regional lymphatic channels and paraesophageal nodes. Supporting this, autopsy series have demonstrated a relatively high incidence of directly draining channels extending from the submucosa lymphatics into the thoracic duct (Fig. 56.1), facilitating systemic spread. Lymph can travel the entire length of the esophagus before draining into lymph nodes,[2] and thus, the entire esophagus is at potential risk for lymphatic involvement. Up to 8 cm or more of "normal" tissue can exist between gross tumor and micrometastases "skip areas" secondary to this extensive lymphatic network.[5] In addition, as many as 71% of frozen tissue sections scored as margin negative by conventional histopathology show involvement by lymphatic micrometastases with immunohistochemistry.[6] Lymphatics of the esophagus drain into nodes that usually follow arteries, including the inferior thyroid artery, the bronchial and esophageal arteries, and the left gastric artery (celiac axis).[7]

Epidemiology and Risk Factors

Esophageal carcinoma accounts for approximately 6% of all gastrointestinal malignancies. In 2018, there will be an estimated 17,290 new patients diagnosed with esophageal cancer in the United States and 15,850 deaths. Worldwide, in 2012, an estimated 455,800 esophageal cancer cases and 400,200 deaths occurred. Most cases occur in males, at a rate of 4:1 relative to females.[8–10]

The incidence of esophageal carcinoma varies according to geography. The highest incidence occurs in Linxian, China, Russia, and the Caspian region of Iran. The incidence in these regions is 100/100,000 persons. What is often referred to as the "esophageal cancer belt" extends from northern Iran through the Central Asian republics to north-central China. In areas such as northern France, Kazakhstan, and South Africa, incidence can be as high as 50 to 99/100,000. Although the reasons for the geographic discrepancy are unknown, some reports have linked the arid climate and alkaline soil with these high-risk areas, as well as the ingestion of nitrosamines, and inversely to the consumption of riboflavin, nicotinic acid, magnesium, and zinc.[11,12] In the United States, the incidence rate among males is <5/100,000. Over the last 20 years, there has been an increase in the incidence of adenocarcinoma at a rate of 5% to 10% per year.[13] In 1987, adenocarcinoma was reported to represent 34% and 12% of esophageal cancers in white men and women versus 3% and 1% for African American men and women, respectively.[13] As of 1998, esophageal adenocarcinoma accounted for almost 55% of all diagnosed cases in white men, and in the United States, the rates of adenocarcinoma now exceed those of squamous cell carcinoma. African American men are more frequently diagnosed with squamous cell carcinoma.[13–15]

In North America and Western Europe, alcohol use and tobacco use are the major risk factors for squamous cell carcinoma, accounting for 80% to 90% of cases.[16] Reports have described the relative risk of esophageal cancer by the amount of alcohol and tobacco consumed, including a relative risk of 155:1 when consuming >30 g/day of tobacco along with 121 g/day of alcohol.[17]

Diets low in fruits, vegetables, and animal products result in marginal deficiencies in vitamins and trace elements and are associated with development of squamous cell carcinoma.[18] Patients with Plummer-Vinson (Paterson-Kelly) syndrome, a condition characterized by iron deficiency anemia and low riboflavin levels, are at an increased risk for oral cavity, hypopharyngeal, and esophageal cancer. In addition, dietary intake of nitrosamines, nitrosamides, and *N*-nitroso compounds and exposure to polyaromatic hydrocarbons have been implicated in esophageal carcinoma. Examples of nitrate-rich foods include pickled vegetables, alcoholic beverages, cured meats, and fish. Betel quid chewing in Taiwan and India has been implicated as a potential cause as well.[19–21] Thermal irritation from consumption of hot beverages, soup, and food and physical irritation due to loss of teeth (poor oral hygiene) have been implicated in some studies. The role of HPV 16 and 18 has been linked to squamous cell carcinoma in some geographic areas although these results are inconsistent.[21]

Other risk factors associated with esophageal carcinoma include achalasia and tylosis. Achalasia of long duration (25 years) is associated with a 5% incidence of squamous cell carcinoma.[22,23] Patients with tylosis (hyperkeratosis of the palms and soles and papilloma of the esophagus) have a reported 38% risk in developing esophageal cancer at a mean age of 45 years.[24] In addition, carcinoma of the esophagus occurs in 2% to 4% of patients with head and neck cancer.

Risk factors leading to the development of adenocarcinoma of the esophagus are being increasingly understood. Most esophageal adenocarcinomas tend to arise from the metaplastic columnar-lined epithelium known as Barrett esophagus.[25] Severe and long-standing gastroesophageal reflux disease has clearly been shown to be a significant risk factor for Barrett esophagus, which may lead to adenocarcinoma. It has been estimated that patients with long-standing severe reflux have a 44-fold risk of developing adenocarcinoma.[26] Tobacco use is a more moderate risk factor for adenocarcinoma development. Smokers appear to have a two- to threefold greater risk for developing esophageal adenocarcinoma than do nonsmokers.[27,28] The relative risk of esophageal adenocarcinoma persists even after three decades following smoking cessation, in contrast to a significant decline in similar patients with squamous cell carcinoma.[29] Obesity has also been linked to a threefold to fourfold risk of adenocarcinoma, possibly because of an increased risk of reflux.[30] It has been estimated that a middle-aged patient with Barrett esophagus has a 10% to 15% risk of developing esophageal adenocarcinoma during his or her lifetime, although other reports have suggested this risk may be overstated.[31]

Although many risk factors are associated with esophageal carcinoma, few studies have demonstrated a causal relationship leading to pathogenesis. Montesano et al.[32] reported possible genetic abnormalities involved in the genesis of esophageal cancer. In addition, possible differences in mechanisms of pathogenesis for squamous cell carcinoma and adenocarcinoma were described. Genetic abnormalities in squamous cell carcinoma include p53 mutations and multiple allelic losses at 3p and 9q, with amplification of cyclin D1 and epidermal growth factor receptor (EGFR). These mutations lead to cell hyperplasia, low- and high-grade dysplasia, and, ultimately, squamous cell carcinoma. In contrast, genetic abnormalities in adenocarcinoma include overexpression of p53; multiple allelic losses at 17p, 5q, and 13q; and amplification and overexpression of EGFR and human epidermal growth factor receptor 2 (HER-2). These abnormalities may be involved in the stepwise development of Barrett esophagus, dysplasia, and, ultimately, adenocarcinoma. These differences suggest that squamous cell carcinoma and adenocarcinoma have different series of genetic mutations as etiologies, but these abnormalities occur in 23% to 94% of tumors studied. Whole exome sequencing has identified mutations in p53 and the cyclin-dependent kinase inhibitor CDKN2, as well as multiple other known tumor-associated genes, in both adenocarcinoma and squamous cell carcinoma.[33,34]

NATURAL HISTORY AND PATTERNS OF SPREAD

Squamous cell carcinoma is characterized by extensive local growth and proclivity to lymph node metastases. Because the esophagus has no covering serosa, direct invasion of contiguous structures may occur early. Lesions in the upper esophagus can impinge on or invade the recurrent laryngeal nerves, carotid arteries, and trachea. If extraesophageal extension occurs in the mediastinum, tracheoesophageal or bronchoesophageal fistula may occur. Tumors in the lower one-third of the esophagus can invade the aorta or pericardium, resulting in mediastinitis, massive hemorrhage, or empyema.

A review correlating the incidence of lymph node metastases with depth of penetration revealed that 18% of patients with spread to the submucosa had lymph node involvement.[35] For T1 lesions, the reported incidence of nodal spread is 10% to 21%, although this may be higher or lower depending on depth of involvement; for T2 lesions, this rises to 33% to 69%.[36–39] The location of involved lymph nodes is influenced by the origin of the primary tumor. At autopsy, lymph node metastases are found in approximately 70% of patients.[40–42] In patients with cervical lesions, lymph node metastases to the abdominal lymph nodes are rare. Distant metastasis can occur at almost any site (Table 56.1).[43]

A review of 1,077 patients with squamous cell carcinoma of the thoracic esophagus undergoing esophagectomy further

TABLE 56.1 DISTRIBUTION OF METASTASES BY ANATOMIC SITE

Site	(n = 79)	Percentage
Lymph nodes	58	73
Lung	41	52
Liver	37	47
Adrenals	16	20
Diaphragm	15	19
Bronchus	13	17
Pleura	13	17
Stomach	12	15
Bone	11	14
Kidneys	10	13
Trachea	10	13
Pericardium	9	11
Pancreas	9	11

From Anderson LL, Lad TE. Autopsy findings in squamous-cell carcinoma of the esophagus. *Cancer* 1982;50(8):1587–1590. Copyright © 1982 American Cancer Society. Reprinted by permission of John Wiley & Sons, Inc.

characterized patterns of nodal spread. Primary disease was located in the upper (5%), middle (63%), and lower (32%) thoracic esophagus. In total, 47% of patients had lymph node metastases. On multivariate analysis, T stage, tumoral length, and degree of differentiation significantly correlated with incidence of lymph node metastases. In approximately 6% of cases, skip metastasis (distant lymph node metastases without regional lymph node metastasis) occurred, usually in patients with poorly differentiated, large, and deeply invasive tumors. Of involved nodes, 37% were macroscopically involved versus 63% microscopically involved, indicating that most lymph node metastases would be below the resolution of detection using contemporary imaging tools. Lymph node involvement was grouped into five categories: cervical, thoracic upper mediastinum, thoracic middle mediastinum, thoracic lower mediastinum, and abdominal lymph nodes. Figure 56.4 shows the incidence of nodal metastases based on primary tumor location.[44] A similar study of 1,893 thoracic squamous cell carcinoma patients from China mapped patterns of lymph node metastases by primary tumor location, with similar patterns of spread. In this study, independent prognostic factors for lymph node metastases included tumor length, differentiation, and depth of invasion. The authors recommended treating nodal basins according to clinicopathologic factors, including enlargement of fields of patients of adverse histologic features, demonstrating similar rates of spread compared to the previously described series.[45]

For lower esophageal and gastroesophageal junctional adenocarcinomas, approximately 70% of patients will have nodal metastases at presentation. This is influenced by tumoral depth of penetration, with nearly all T3 and T4 lesions exhibiting metastases in surgical series. Pathologic resection data demonstrated rates of lymphatic involvement for lower esophageal and GE junctional tumors of 45%, 85%, and 100% for T2, T3, and T4 tumors, respectively (Fig. 56.5).[37] In patients with lower esophageal cancer, involvement of both mediastinal and abdominal lymph nodes is common (Fig. 56.6).[37] The primary direction for lymphatic flow for the lower esophagus is toward the abdomen. According to the classification by Siewert, nodal metastases are often seen in the mediastinum and abdomen for type I tumors, whereas type III tumors metastasize almost exclusively inferiorly, toward the celiac axis. Type II tumors are intermediate, preferentially spreading inferiorly and less frequently into the mediastinum. The primary value in the Siewert classification is to the guidance of appropriate type surgery (i.e., type I tumors are generally treated with esophagectomy and mediastinal lymph node resection, with types II and III approached through the abdomen), although it may be useful in radiation field design as well.[3] Generally speaking, the incidence of abdominal nodal involvement increases as one proceeds distally in the esophagus to the gastroesophageal junction. For patients with tumors arising from the gastroesophageal junction, mediastinal involvement is less common. Nodal metastases above the level of the carina are rare in lower esophageal and junctional tumors.[46] In addition, histologic analyses of lower esophagus and gastroesophageal junction adenocarcinoma specimens suggest that many patients without nodal involvement on conventional histopathology actually are involved when assessed by immunohistochemistry.[47]

Extensive nodal mapping has been performed by Japanese investigators, who have devised the Japanese Gastric Cancer Association Classification (Fig. 56.7).[48] Using this system of nodal classification, investigators from Erlangen evaluated 326 patients with esophagogastric junction carcinoma undergoing primary resection. Tumors were stratified as AEG type I (distal esophagus), II (gastric cardia), and III (subcardia). Note there was significant overlap in the majority of tumors for all stages, with an overall incidence of lymph node metastasis of 71%. In T1 patients, only 17% exhibited lymph node metastasis, whereas 78%, 86%, and 90% of T2, T3, and T4, respectively, had involved nodes. Figure 56.8 shows varying patterns of nodal spread based on T stage as well as AEG location. Additional generalizations from this study include the following: (a) lymph vascular invasion was highly predictive of nodal spread and (b) proximal extension of type II and III

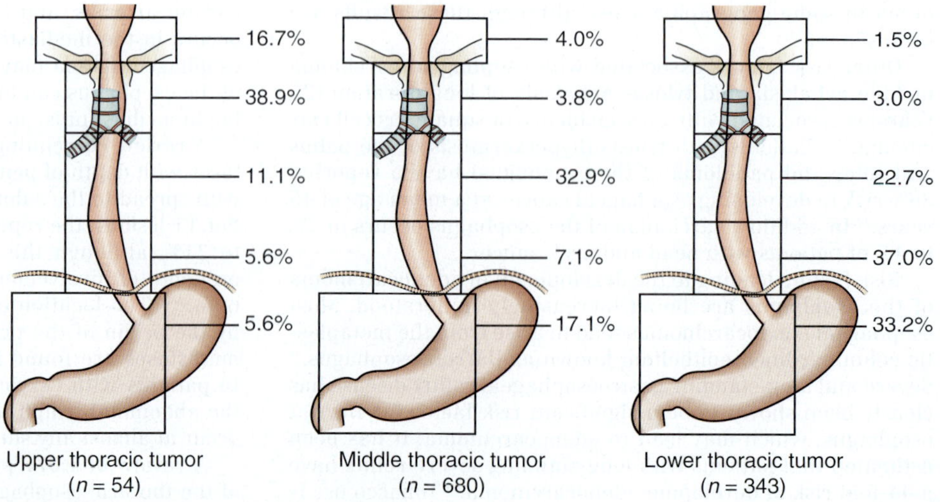

FIGURE 56.4. Positive lymph node distribution according to the location of the primary tumor, squamous cell carcinoma. (Reprinted from Huang W, Li B, Gong H, et al. Pattern of lymph node metastases and its implication in radiotherapeutic clinical target volume in patients with thoracic esophageal squamous cell carcinoma: a report of 1077 cases. *Radiother Oncol* 2010;95[2]:229–233. Copyright © 2010 Elsevier Ireland Ltd. With permission.)

Upper thoracic tumor (n = 54)

16.7%
38.9%
11.1%
5.6%
5.6%

Middle thoracic tumor (n = 680)

4.0%
3.8%
32.9%
7.1%
17.1%

Lower thoracic tumor (n = 343)

1.5%
3.0%
22.7%
37.0%
33.2%

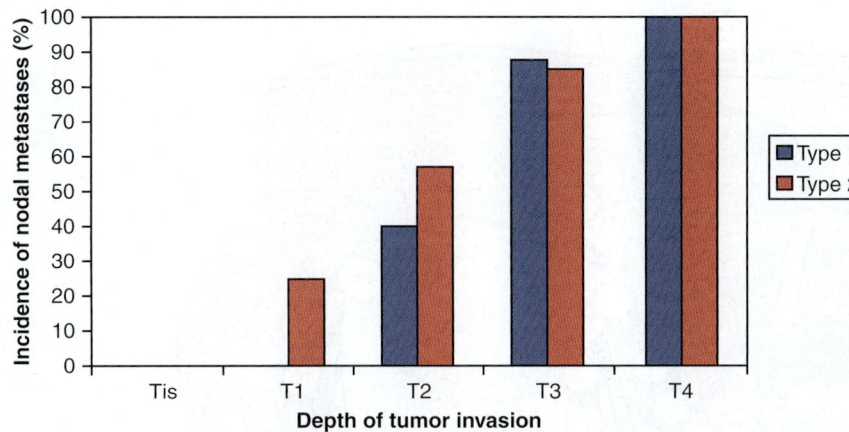

FIGURE 56.5. The incidence of nodal metastases related to depth of tumor invasion, adenocarcinoma. (Reprinted from Dresner SM, Lamb PJ, Bennett MK, et al. The pattern of metastatic lymph node dissemination from adenocarcinoma of the esophagogastric junction. *Surgery* 2001;129[1]:103–109. Copyright © 2001 Elsevier. With permission.)

tumors into the distal esophagus (particularly beyond the Z line) predicted an increasing incidence of paraesophageal lymph node involvement.[49]

LOCAL FAILURE

In an older series at the University of Pennsylvania and Fox Chase Cancer Center of patients with adenocarcinoma of the esophagus and gastroesophageal junction treated with surgery alone, the locoregional recurrence rate was 77%.[50] In contemporary randomized trials, local failure rates with surgery alone range from 29% to 45%.[51–54] Similarly, data from contemporary randomized trials of esophageal cancer using "definitive" chemoradiation also indicate that local failure is a major cause of failure, with approximately 50% of patients failing locally (Table 56.2). Similarly, in a study of 239 patients receiving definitive chemoradiotherapy, 50% presented with local failure, 48% distant failure, and 31% no failure. Of local failures, 90% were within the gross tumor volume (GTV), whereas clinical target volume (CTV) and planning target volume (PTV) failures were seen in only 23% and 12%,

respectively.[58] In many trials, patterns of failure are reported as first site of recurrence. This fact, along with infrequent post-therapy imaging and inability to detect subclinical recurrences, likely leads to underestimates of local recurrence rates. These data clearly emphasize the need for improvements in local treatment modalities.

CLINICAL PRESENTATION

Symptoms of esophageal cancer often start 3 to 4 months before diagnosis. Location of the primary tumor in the esophagus may influence presenting symptoms. Dysphagia is seen in >90% of patients regardless of location. Odynophagia is present in up to 50% of patients.[59] Weight loss is common, with 40% to 70% of patients reporting a loss of >5% of total body weight. This extent of weight loss has been associated with a worse prognosis. Less frequent symptoms may include vague chest pain, hoarseness, cough, and glossopharyngeal neuralgia.[60]

Advanced lesions can produce signs and symptoms from tumor invasion into local structures. Hematemesis,

FIGURE 56.6. Distribution of nodal metastases by frequency of site involved for adenocarcinoma. (Reprinted from Dresner SM, Lamb PJ, Bennett MK, et al. The pattern of metastatic lymph node dissemination from adenocarcinoma of the esophagogastric junction. *Surgery* 2001;129[1]:103–109. Copyright © 2001 Elsevier. With permission.)

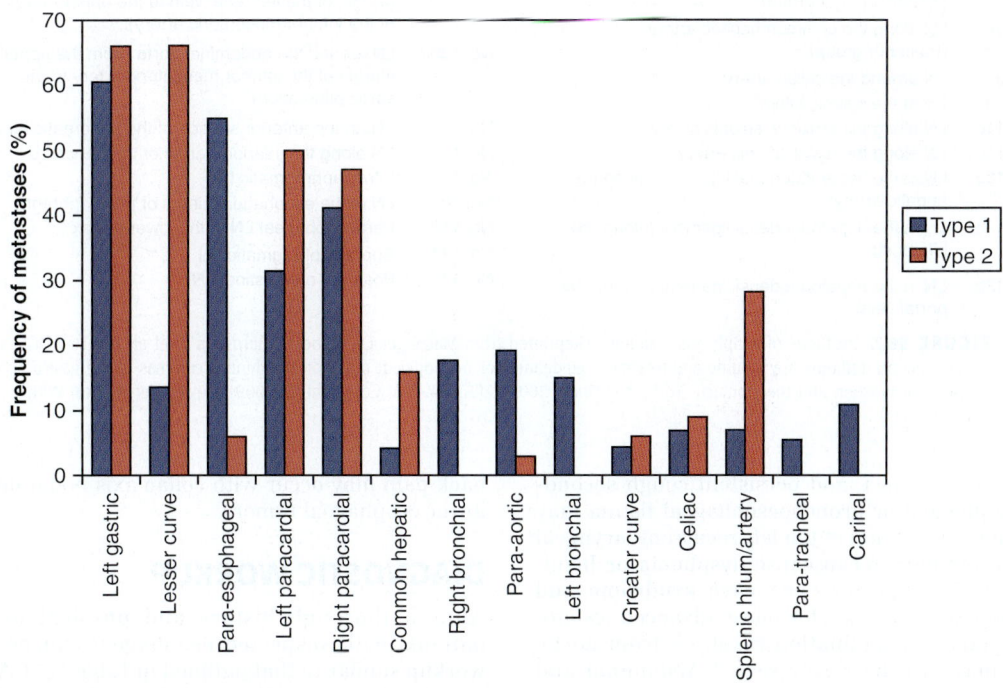

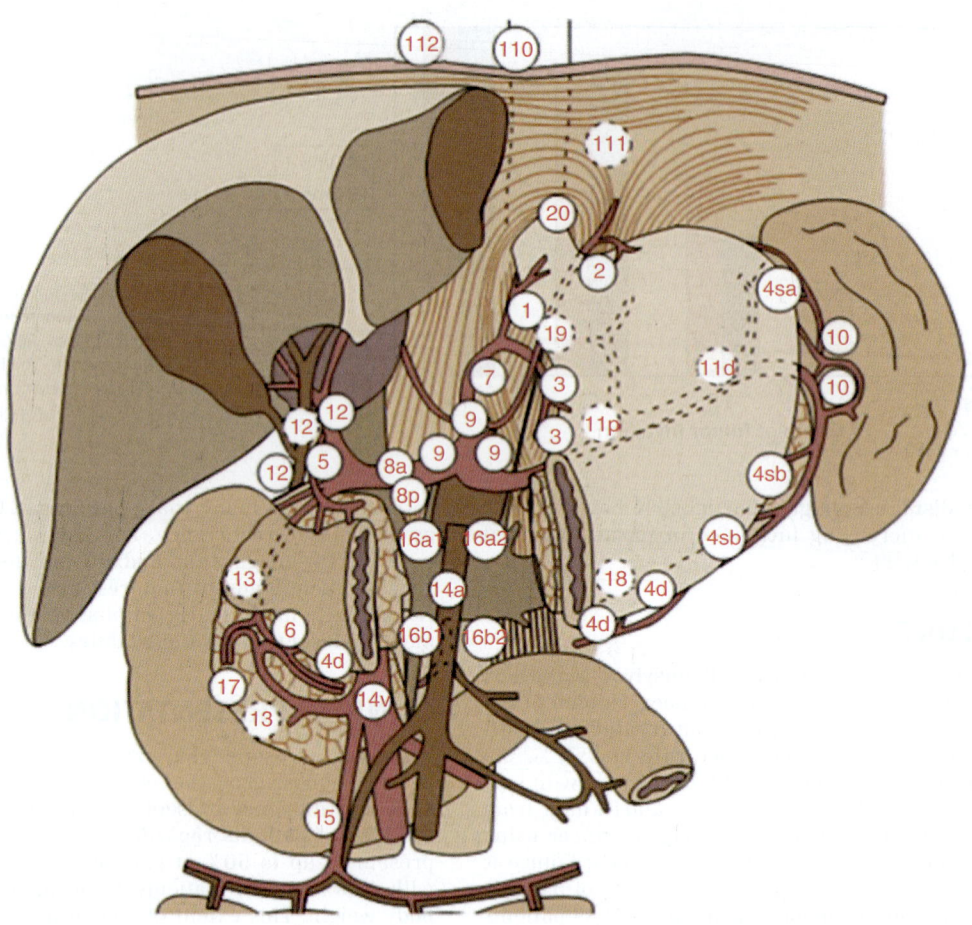

No. 1	Right paracardial LN
No. 2	Left paracardial LN
No. 3	LN along the lesser curvature
No. 4sa	LN along the short gastric vessels
No. 4sb	LN along the left gastroepiploic vessels
No. 4d	LN along the right gastroepiploic vessels
No. 5	Suprapyloric LN
No. 6	Infrapyloric LN
No. 7	LN along the left gastric artery
No. 8a	LN along the common hepatic artery (Anterosuperior group)
No. 8p	LN along the common hepatic artery (Posterior group)
No. 9	LN around the celiac artery
No. 10	LN at the splenic hilum
No. 11p	LN along the proximal splenic artery
No. 11d	LN along the distal splenic artery
No. 12a	LN in the hepatoduodenal ligament (along the hepatic artery)
No. 12b	LN in the hepatoduodenal ligament (along the bile duct)
No. 12p	LN in the hepatoduodenal ligament (behind the portal vein)

No. 13	LN on the posterior surface of the pancreatic head
No. 14v	LN along the superior mesenteric vein
No. 14a	LN along the superior mesenteric artery
No. 15	LN along the middle colic vessels
No. 16a1	LN in the aortic hiatus
No. 16a2	LN around the abdominal aorta (from the upper margin of the celiac trunk to the lower margin of the left renal vein)
No. 16b1	LN around the abdominal aorta (from the lower margin of the left renal vein to the upper margin of the inferior mesenteric artery)
No. 16b2	LN around the abdominal aorta (from the upper margin of the inferior mesenteric artery to the aortic bifurcation)
No. 17	LN on the anterior surface of the pancreatic head
No. 18	LN along the inferior margin of the pancreas
No. 19	Infradiaphragmatic LN
No. 20	LN in the esophageal hiatus of the diaphragm
No. 110	Paraesophageal LN in the lower thorax
No. 111	Supradiaphragmatic LN
No. 112	Posterior mediastinal LN

FIGURE 56.7. Locations of lymph node stations. (Reprinted from Matzinger O, Gerber E, Bernstein Z, et al. EORTC-ROG expert opinion: radiotherapy volume and treatment guidelines for neoadjuvant radiation of adenocarcinomas of the gastro-esophageal junction and the stomach. *Radiother Oncol* 2009;92[2]:164–175. Copyright © 2009 Elsevier Ireland Ltd. With permission.)

hemoptysis, melena, dyspnea, and persistent cough secondary to tracheoesophageal or bronchoesophageal fistula may occur. Compression or invasion of the left recurrent laryngeal nerve or the phrenic nerves can cause dysphonia or hemidiaphragm paralysis. Superior vena cava syndrome and Horner syndrome can also occur for more advanced lesions. Pleural effusion and exsanguination resulting from aortic communication may also be rarely seen.[59] Abdominal and back pain may occur with celiac axis nodal involvement with lower esophageal tumors.

DIAGNOSTIC WORKUP

After a thorough history and physical examination, all patients with suspected esophageal cancer should have a workup similar to that outlined in Table 56.3. Attention should

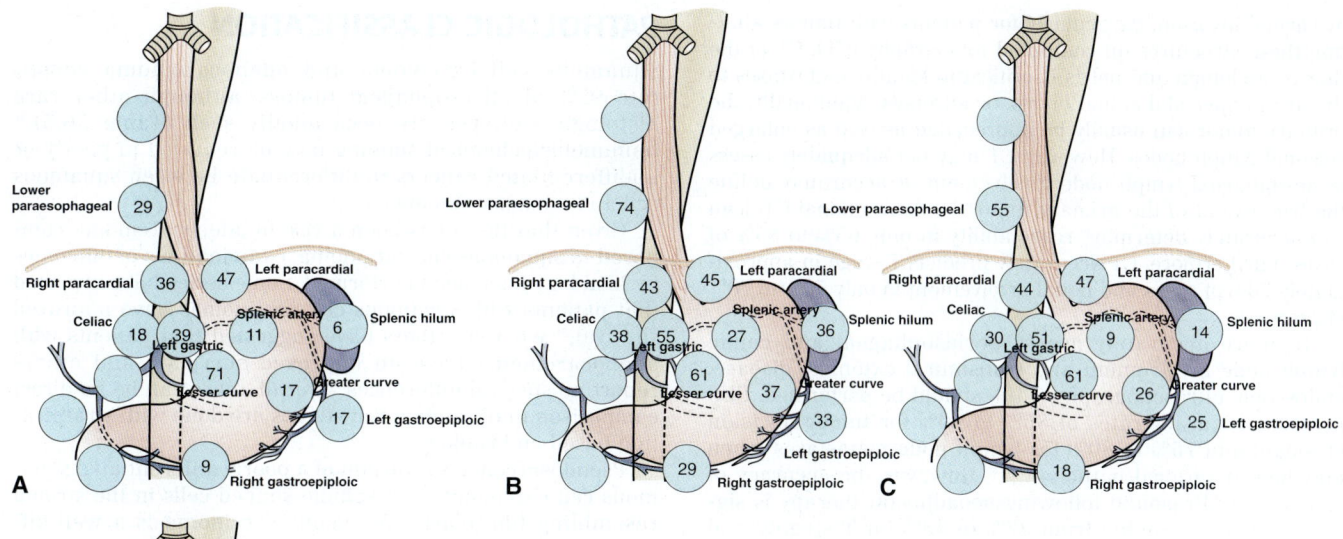

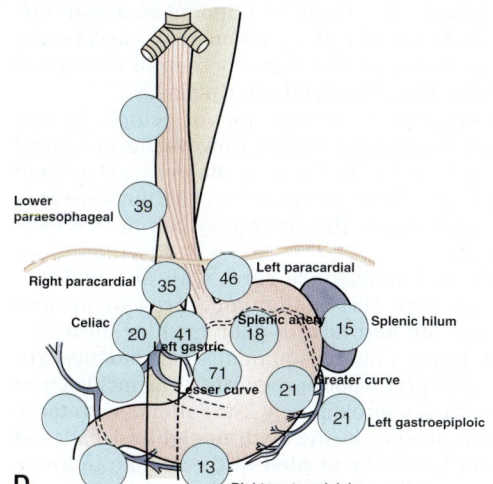

FIGURE 56.8. A: Frequency percent of nodal involvement for T2 tumors. **B:** Frequency percent of nodal involvement for T3-T4 tumors. **C:** Frequency percent of involvement for AEG type I tumors. **D:** Frequency percent of nodal involvement for AEG type II/III tumors. (Based on data from Meier I, Merkel S, Papadopoulos T, et al. Adenocarcinoma of the esophagogastric junction: the pattern of metastatic lymph node dissemination as a rationale for elective lymphatic target volume definition. *Int J Radiat Oncol Biol Phys* 2008;70:1408–1417.)

be paid to cervical and supraclavicular lymph nodes. Basic blood counts and a metabolic panel with liver function tests should be obtained.

Although the esophagogram may be used to define lesion extent, endoscopy is the best tool to diagnose and define the extent of the lesion. During flexible endoscopy, biopsies and brushings should be taken of the primary site and suspicious areas harboring satellites or submucosal spread. In addition, accurate endoscopic measurement and characterization of tumor and gastroesophageal junction in relation to the incisors facilitate radiation treatment planning as may strategic

placement of radioopaque fiducials at the superior and inferior extent of the primary lesion. Examination with panendoscopy of the oral cavity, pharynx, larynx, and tracheobronchial tree may also be performed at the time of esophagoscopy in patients with squamous cell carcinomas, given the high incidence of second tumors in the head and neck and upper airway.[2] In addition, bronchoscopy should generally be performed in patients with proximal malignancies to evaluate for the presence of tracheal

TABLE 56.2 LOCAL FAILURE RATES FROM RANDOMIZED TRIALS EVALUATING CHEMORADIATION ALONE IN ESOPHAGEAL CANCER

	Dose (Gy)	Local Failure (Crude) (%)	Local Failure (2-Year) (%)
RTOG 85-01[55]	50	45	47
INT 0123[56]	50	55	52
INT 0123[56]	64	50	56
German[57]	>60	51	58
SCOPE[183]	50	40	NS

INT, Intergroup; RTOG, Radiation Therapy Oncology Group.

TABLE 56.3 DIAGNOSTIC WORKUP FOR ESOPHAGEAL CANCER

Multidisciplinary evaluation (surgical, radiation, and medical oncology)
History and physical
Complete blood count and chemistry profile
Upper gastrointestinal endoscopy and biopsy
Chest, abdomen, and pelvic computed tomography (CT) with intravenous +/− oral contrast (combined positron emission tomography [PET]-CT optimal)
PET evaluation (combined PET-CT optimal)
Endoscopic ultrasound, with fine needle aspiration if indicated (if no evidence of distant metastases)
Bronchoscopy if tumor is located at or above the carina or there is suspected airway involvement
Nutritional assessment and consideration of feeding tube (nasogastric or feeding jejunostomy) in selected situations

or carinal invasion, particularly for patients with tumors abutting these structures on computed tomography (CT). CT of the thorax, abdomen and pelvis is critical to identify metastases to the liver, upper abdominal nodes, or adrenals; additionally, the primary tumor can usually be appreciated as well as enlarged regional lymph nodes. However, CT may not adequately assess periesophageal lymph node involvement or accurately define the true extent of the primary tumor.[61,62] Conventional CT scan can accurately determine resectability in only 65% to 85% of cases. Furthermore, CT accurately predicts T stage in approximately 70% of cases and nodal involvement in only 50% to 70% of cases.[63-65]

To more accurately assess periesophageal and celiac lymph node involvement and transmural extent of disease, endoscopic ultrasonography (EUS) should be performed. EUS provides accuracy rates of 85% to 90% for tumor invasion (T stage) and 75% to 80% for lymph node metastases when matched to surgical pathology.[66-69] However, the accuracy of endoscopic ultrasound following neoadjuvant therapy is significantly less, ranging from 27% to 48% for T staging and 38% to 71% for N staging. This is possibly due to the failure to discriminate tumor from postradiation inflammation and fibrosis.[70-72] Illustrating the potential limitations associated with contemporary staging techniques, in one series of 102 patients with clinically staged (by PET, EUS, and/or CT) T2-3 N0 tumors receiving induction chemotherapy alone, 60% of patients were found to have metastatic nodal disease.[73]

Surgical staging procedures, including thoracoscopy, mediastinoscopy, and laparoscopy, may provide additional staging information and are considered in selected patients at some institutions.[74] Laparoscopy would primarily be used for tumors at the gastroesophageal junction.

Patients with significant obstruction and inability to maintain their weight may require placement of a feeding tube. If surgery is planned, gastric tube placement is generally avoided, given that the stomach will ultimately serve as the "neoesophagus" following resection and a feeding jejunostomy tube may be placed.

Positron emission tomography (PET) has proven to be a valuable staging tool in esophageal cancer patients. The addition of PET to standard staging studies such as CT can improve the accuracy of detecting stage III and stage IV disease by 23% and 18%, respectively.[75,76] Overall, it is estimated that PET will detect distant metastatic disease in approximately 20% of patients who are considered to have locoregional disease only by CT. However, PET also appears to have a lower accuracy in detecting local nodal disease compared to CT alone or in combination with endoscopic ultrasound. Of importance, some series suggest that PET can be used to predict response to therapy, with PET "responders" experiencing significantly improved outcomes compared to "nonresponders."[77] In addition, PET has been used to predict response to treatment early during the treatment course. This has led to ongoing investigation of early treatment response as measured by PET as a surrogate for therapeutic efficacy and clinical outcomes, with potential subsequent therapy modification based on early repsonse.[78,79]

STAGING SYSTEMS

Esophageal staging can be based on pathologic or clinical criteria. Pathologic staging is performed after invasive procedures, including esophagectomy, mediastinotomy, or thoracotomy. Clinical staging is often employed with "definitive" and neoadjuvant chemoradiation approaches and is less accurate. With the combination of CT, PET, and EUS, clinical staging closely correlates with pathologic stage. Note that the most recent AJCC staging system takes into consideration tumor type and grade, as well as involved number of lymph nodes (Table 56.4).

PATHOLOGIC CLASSIFICATION

Squamous cell carcinoma and adenocarcinoma constitute 95% of all esophageal tumors, although other rare histologic subtypes are occasionally seen (Table 56.5).[80] Immunohistochemical staining may be required in poorly or undifferentiated cancers to differentiate between squamous cell and adenocarcinoma.

Given that there has been a rise in adenocarcinoma compared to squamous cell carcinoma, examinations of outcomes by histology have been performed. Some series have reported that patients with squamous cell carcinomas have improved survival,[81] whereas others have suggested that patients with adenocarcinoma have an improved survival[82] and others report no survival differences. Overall, there can be no direct comparison until randomized studies are done with stratification based on histology.

Pseudosarcoma is a variant of a poorly differentiated squamous cell carcinoma with spindle-shaped cells in the stroma resembling fibroblasts. Verrucous carcinoma is a well-differentiated, papillary variant of squamous cell carcinoma.[2] Squamous cell carcinoma *in situ* is rarely seen in the United States and should be distinguished from dysplasia.[83-85]

Adenocarcinoma may arise from foci of ectopic gastric mucosa or intrinsic esophageal glands. However, as described previously, it is believed that the vast majority arise from Barrett esophagus. If a focus of squamous cell metaplasia is found in an adenocarcinoma, the tumor may be referred to as an adenoacanthoma.[86]

Adenoid cystic carcinomas are rare, with an incidence of 0.75%. Patients with this malignancy present around the sixth decade of life and have a poor median survival.[87] Mucoepidermoid tumors (adenosquamous carcinomas) are more aggressive and carry a poor prognosis.[88] The incidence of small cell carcinoma is approximately 2%. Patients with these malignancies often present in the sixth to eighth decades of life, and the lesion is usually located in the middle to lower esophagus in males.[89,90] These are believed to originate in the argyrophilic cells in the esophagus and may produce paraneoplastic syndromes, such as antidiuretic hormone secretion and hypercalcemia.[91] The clinical course of small cell carcinoma is similar to that of small cell carcinoma of the lung and may be responsive to chemotherapy and radiation therapy.[88,90]

Nonepithelial tumors of the esophagus are rare. Among these, leiomyosarcomas are the most common. Twenty-five percent of patients with this tumor present with metastases.[92-94] Histologically, these tumors have interlacing bundles of spindle-shaped cells. Less aggressive forms have fewer mitotic figures and less anaplasia. Prognosis has been reported to be more favorable than that of squamous cell carcinoma.[88] In patients with Kaposi sarcoma, gastrointestinal involvement of the esophagus can be seen.[95]

Malignant melanoma is rare and can occur as a primary esophageal tumor or as a metastasis. These lesions are usually large and often covered by intact squamous mucosa with focal areas of ulceration. Spread is usually submucosal. Mean survival is approximately 7 months.[96,97] Lymphoma constitutes approximately 1% of esophageal malignancies. It is usually associated with direct extension from other organs, although primary esophageal lymphoma has been reported.[98]

PROGNOSTIC FACTORS

According to the Union Internationale Contre le Cancer/American Joint Cancer Committee seventh-edition staging system, R-status, age, and histologic subtype were independent prognostic factors of survival, whereas tumor grade and site were not.[99] It should be recalled that these data consider patients treated with surgery alone and as such do not apply to patients receiving chemotherapy or radiotherapy.

TABLE 56.4 AMERICAN JOINT COMMITTEE ON CANCER 2017 ESOPHAGEAL CANCER STAGING SYSTEM (EIGHTH EDITION)

Category	Criteria
T category	
TX	Tumor cannot be assessed.
T0	No evidence of primary tumor
Tis	High-grade dysplasia, defined as malignant cells confined by the basement membrane
T1	Tumor invades the lamina propria, muscularis mucosae, or submucosa
T1a[a]	Tumor invades the lamina propria or muscularis mucosae
T1b[a]	Tumor invades the submucosa
T2	Tumor invades the muscularis propria
T3	Tumor invades the adventitia
T4	Tumor invades adjacent structures
T4a[a]	Tumor invades the pleura, pericardium, azygos vein, diaphragm, or peritoneum
T4b[a]	Tumor invades other adjacent structures, such as the aorta, vertebral body, or trachea
N category	
NX	Regional lymph nodes cannot be assessed
N0	No regional lymph node metastasis
N1	Metastasis in 1–2 regional lymph nodes
N2	Metastasis in 3–6 regional lymph nodes
N3	Metastasis in ≥7 regional lymph nodes
M category	
M0	No distant metastasis
M1	Distant metastasis
Adenocarcinoma G category	
GX	Differentiation cannot be assessed
G1	Well differentiated, with >95% of the tumor composed of well-formed glands
G2	Moderately differentiated, with 50% 95% of the tumor showing gland formation
G3[b]	Poorly differentiated, with tumors composed of nest and sheets of cells with <50% of the tumor demonstrating glandular formation
Squamous cell carcinoma G category	
GX	Differentiation cannot be assessed
G1	Well-differentiated, with prominent keratinization with pearl formation and a minor component of nonkeratinizing basal-like cells, tumor cells arranged in sheets, and mitotic counts low
G2	Moderately differentiated, with variable histologic features ranging from parakeratotic to poorly keratinizing lesions and pearl formation generally absent
G3[c]	Poorly differentiated, consisting predominantly of basal-like cells forming large and small nests with frequent central necrosis and with the nests consisting of sheets or pavementlike arrangements of tumor cells that are occasionally punctuated by small numbers of parakeratotic or keratinizing cells
Squamous cell carcinoma L category[d]	
LX	Location unknown
Upper	Cervical esophagus to lower border of the azygos vein
Middle	Lower border of the azygos vein to lower border of the inferior pulmonary vein
Lower	Lower border of the inferior pulmonary vein to the stomach, including the esophagogastric junction

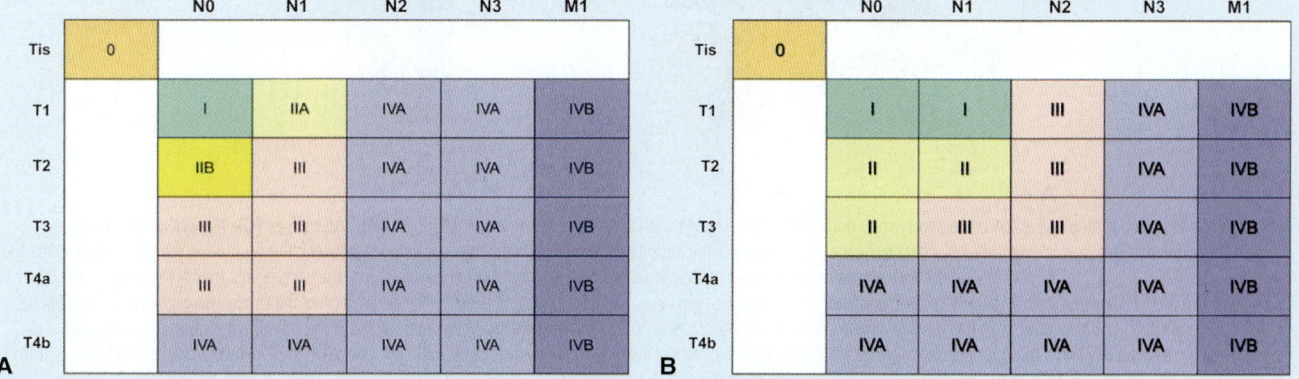

cTNM Adenocarcinoma

	N0	N1	N2	N3	M1
Tis	0				
T1		I	IIA	IVA	IVA	IVB
T2		IIB	III	IVA	IVA	IVB
T3		III	III	IVA	IVA	IVB
T4a		III	III	IVA	IVA	IVB
T4b		IVA	IVA	IVA	IVA	IVB

A

cTNM Squamous Cell Carcinoma

	N0	N1	N2	N3	M1
Tis	0				
T1		I	I	III	IVA	IVB
T2		II	II	III	IVA	IVB
T3		II	III	III	IVA	IVB
T4a		IVA	IVA	IVA	IVA	IVB
T4b		IVA	IVA	IVA	IVA	IVB

B

(A) Clinical stage groups (cTNM): adenocarcinoma. **(B)** Clinical stage groups (cTNM): squamous cell carcinoma.

(Continued)

pTNM Adenocarcinoma

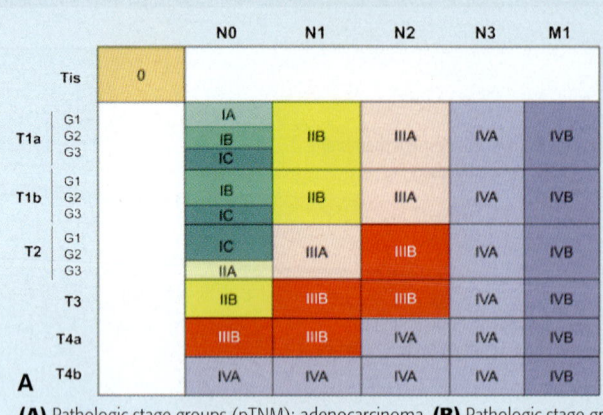

		N0	N1	N2	N3	M1
Tis		0				
T1a	G1	IA				
	G2	IB	IIB	IIIA	IVA	IVB
	G3	IC				
T1b	G1	IB				
	G2	IB	IIB	IIIA	IVA	IVB
	G3	IC				
T2	G1	IC	IIIA	IIIB	IVA	IVB
	G2					
	G3	IIA				
T3		IIB	IIIB	IIIB	IVA	IVB
T4a		IIIB	IIIB	IVA	IVA	IVB
T4b		IVA	IVA	IVA	IVA	IVB

pTNM Squamous Cell Carcinoma

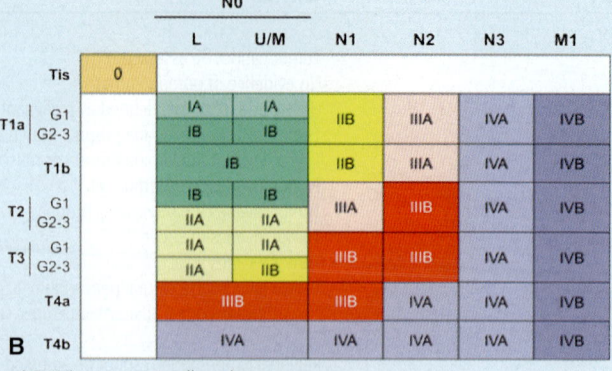

		N0 L	N0 U/M	N1	N2	N3	M1
Tis		0					
T1a	G1	IA	IA				
	G2-3	IB	IB	IIB	IIIA	IVA	IVB
T1b		IB	IB	IIB	IIIA	IVA	IVB
T2	G1	IB	IB	IIIA	IIIB	IVA	IVB
	G2-3	IIA	IIA				
T3	G1	IIA	IIA	IIIB	IIIB	IVA	IVB
	G2-3	IIA	IIB				
T4a		IIIB		IIIB	IVA	IVA	IVB
T4b		IVA		IVA	IVA	IVA	IVB

(A) Pathologic stage groups (pTNM): adenocarcinoma. **(B)** Pathologic stage groups (pTNM): squamous cell carcinoma.

ypTNM

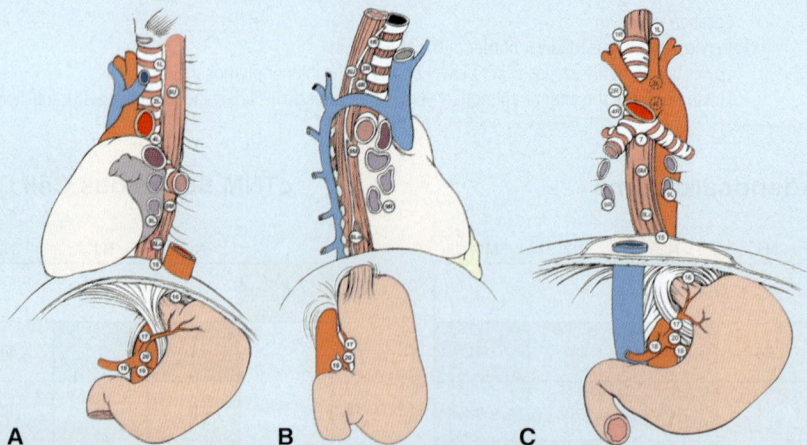

	N0	N1	N2	N3	M1
T0	I	IIIA	IIIB	IVA	IVB
Tis	I	IIIA	IIIB	IVA	IVB
T1	I	IIIA	IIIB	IVA	IVB
T2	I	IIIA	IIIB	IVA	IVB
T3	II	IIIB	IIIB	IVA	IVB
T4a	IIIB	IVA	IVA	IVA	IVB
T4b	IVA	IVA	IVA	IVA	IVB

Postneoadjuvant pathologic stage groups (ypTNM): adenocarcinoma and squamous cell carcinoma.

Lymph node maps for esophageal cancer. Regional lymph node stations for staging esophageal cancer from the left **(A)**, right **(B)**, and anterior **(C)**. 1R, right lower cervical paratracheal nodes, between the supraclavicular paratracheal space and apex of the lung; 1L, left lower cervical paratracheal nodes, between the supraclavicular paratracheal space and apex of the lung; 2R, right upper paratracheal nodes, between the intersection of the caudal margin of the brachiocephalic artery with the trachea and apex of the lung; 2L, left upper paratracheal nodes, between the top of the aortic arch and apex of the lung; 4R, right lower paratracheal nodes, between the intersection of the caudal margin of the brachiocephalic artery with the trachea and cephalic border of the azygos vein; 4L, left lower paratracheal nodes, between the top of the aortic arch and the carina; 7, subcarinal nodes, caudal to the carina of the trachea; 8U, upper thoracic paraesophageal lymph nodes, from the apex of the lung to the tracheal bifurcation; 8M, middle thoracic paraesophageal lymph nodes, from the tracheal bifurcation to the caudal margin of the inferior pulmonary vein; 8Lo, lower thoracic paraesophageal lymph nodes, from the caudal margin of the inferior pulmonary vein to the esophagogastric junction; 9R, pulmonary ligament nodes, within the right inferior pulmonary ligament; 9L, pulmonary ligament nodes, within the left inferior pulmonary ligament; 15, diaphragmatic nodes, lying on the dome of the diaphragm and adjacent to or behind its crura; 16, paracardial nodes, immediately adjacent to the gastroesophageal junction; 17, left gastric nodes, along the course of the left gastric artery; 18, common hepatic nodes, immediately on the proximal common hepatic artery; 19, splenic nodes, immediately on the proximal splenic artery; 20, celiac nodes, at the base of the celiac artery. Cervical periesophageal level VI and level VII lymph nodes are named as per the head and neck map.

[a]Subcategories.
[b]If further testing of "undifferentiated" cancers reveals a glandular component, categorize as adenocarcinoma G3.
[c]If further testing of "undifferentiated" cancers reveals squamous cell component or if after further testing they remain undifferentiated, categorize as squamous cell carcinoma G3.
[d]Location is defined by epicenter of esophageal tumor.

TABLE 56.5 PATHOLOGIC CLASSIFICATION OF MALIGNANT ESOPHAGEAL TUMORS

Epithelial Tumors
Squamous cell carcinoma
Variants of squamous cell carcinoma
Basaloid squamous cell carcinoma
Squamous cell carcinoma with sarcomatoid features
Undifferentiated carcinoma
Spindle cell carcinoma
Pseudosarcoma and carcinosarcoma
Verrucous carcinoma
In situ carcinoma
Adenocarcinoma
Adenoacanthoma
Adenoid cystic carcinoma (cylindroma)
Mucoepidermoid carcinoma
Adenosquamous carcinoma
Carcinoid
Small cell carcinoma

Nonepithelial Tumors
Sarcoma, 13 variants reported, most common is leiomyosarcoma.
Malignant melanoma
Myoblastoma
Choriocarcinoma
Lymphoma

A study published by Nomura et al.[100] evaluating 301 patients treated with chemoradiotherapy showed that T stage, M stage, and gender were prognostic factors in multivariate analysis. In addition to stage, other factors portend outcome. Tumor length/size may also impact outcome. In a study of 582 patients undergoing surgical resection as primary treatment, tumoral length adversely affected survival, with 5-year survival rates of 77%, 48%, 38%, and 23% for tumor lengths of 1, 2, 3, or >3 cm, respectively ($P < .001$).[101] Of note, length was not prognostic if patients were N+ or M+. Similarly, in adenocarcinoma patients, 5-year survival rates have been shown to be significantly higher for patients with tumors ≤2 cm compared to those >2 cm.[102] Another study of 1,553 patients with squamous cell carcinoma of the esophagus determined that tumor size, grade, lymphadenopathy, stage, and family history were prognostic following esophagectomy.[103]

In another large study from the Mayo Clinic, clinicopathologic factors that affected prognosis included T and N status, tumor grade, age > 76 years, extracapsular lymph node extension, and the absence of chemotherapy or radiotherapy; anatomic location did not influence survival.[104] In addition, weight loss and low overall performance status also indicate poor prognosis.[105] Deep ulceration of the tumor, sinus tract formation, and fistula formation are other poor prognostic factors.[59]

Obtaining uninvolved pathologic margins at resection is of significant importance with regard to long-term outcome. An Intergroup study (discussed later) evaluating chemotherapy preceding and following esophagectomy showed that outcomes were similar in patients undergoing R1 resection (positive microscopic margins) or R2 resection (gross residual disease) or patients not undergoing resection at all. Only patients undergoing R0 resection (uninvolved margins) had a substantial chance of long-term disease-free survival.[106] A meta-analysis of 17 studies found that major pathologic response following neoadjuvant therapy in gastroesophageal cancer patients was predictive of survival.[107] Another meta-analysis of 13 series showed that perineural invasion is an adverse prognostic biomarker in esophageal cancer, often associated with more advanced stage and poor differentiation.[108] A patterns-of-care survey examined the outcomes of patients with adenocarcinoma and squamous cell carcinoma of the esophagus between 1996 and 1999. Patients were treated with radiation therapy across 59 institutions. On multivariate analysis, significant improvements in survival were seen in patients treated at centers with ≥500 new cancer patients per year compared to centers seeing <500 (hazard ratio 1.32; $P = .03$).[109]

GENERAL MANAGEMENT

Treatment for esophageal carcinoma is characterized as either curative or palliative. According to one historical study,[110] only 20% patients present with cancer of the esophagus that is truly localized to the esophagus, indicating that at the time of diagnosis, approximately 80% patients have either locally advanced or distant disease.

Surgery with Curative Intent

Surgery of the thoracic esophagus usually requires a subtotal or total esophagectomy and is usually undertaken for lesions of the middle to lower one-third of the thoracic esophagus and gastroesophageal junction. Patients with stage I to III are often considered for potentially curative resection; however, aortic, tracheal, heart, or great vessel invasion may preclude resection. Esophagectomy may be accomplished by a number of techniques, including a transhiatal esophagectomy, right thoracotomy with laparotomy with intrathoracic anastomosis (Ivor Lewis esophagogastrectomy), right thoracotomy with laparotomy with cervical anastomosis (McKeown or "three-hole" esophagogastrectomy), and left thoracoabdominal, transhiatal, or radical esophagectomy via open or laparoscopic approaches. Each technique has its advantages and disadvantages. In general, advantages of the transthoracic approach include better visualization with access and resection of the upper two-thirds of the esophagus and mediastinal lymph nodes. One potential advantage of the McKeown approach is a cervical anastomosis, which may be easier management of anastomotic leaks. Alternatively, the transhiatal approach has less morbidity than does thoracotomy (including respiratory compromise) with easier access to anastomotic leaks. In any instance, achievement of negative margins at resection has been reported to be a significant prognostic factor and should be the goal of esophageal resection. Exemplifying this, in a study of 500 patients undergoing transthoracic resection, patients undergoing margin-negative resection had a 5-year survival rate of 29% versus no 5-year survivors in patients with involved margins.[111]

The Ivor Lewis procedure is the classic approach to expose midesophageal lesions. A left thoracotomy procedure exposes lesions of the gastroesophageal junction. Transhiatal esophagectomy is performed without a thoracotomy and is useful in lower esophageal lesions, although direct visualization and dissection of varying mediastinal lymph nodes cannot be achieved. An emerging treatment option in addition to the above techniques is the use of minimally invasive esophagectomy, which can include laparoscopic-assisted, thoracoscopic, or more limited thoracotomy. The optimal surgical approach is unknown and remains a topic of ongoing investigation.

Laparotomy or laparoscopy can be performed before neoadjuvant therapy or concurrently with esophagectomy to rule out peritoneal-based disease below the diaphragm, particularly in more advanced adenocarcinomas of the gastroesophageal junction. Multiple reconstruction options are available following definitive surgery; esophagogastrostomy is the most widely used, using the stomach as a conduit to replace the esophagus. Patients with significant obstruction and inability to maintain their weight often require placement of feeding jejunostomy. If possible surgery is planned, gastric tube placement is generally avoided, given that the stomach will ultimately serve as the "neoesophagus" following resection, with feeding jejunostomy often preferred. Colon interposition, preferably with the left colon, can also be used; however, this approach is generally reserved for patients who have previously undergone gastric surgery or other procedures that have devascularized the stomach. Similarly, jejunal interposition may be utilized.

Squamous cell carcinoma of the cervical esophagus presents a difficult management situation. Proximal esophageal

Section III

tumors <5 cm from the cricopharyngeus are generally treated with definitive chemoradiotherapy. If surgery is performed, resection of portions of the pharynx, the entire larynx, the thyroid gland, and the proximal esophagus is often required. Radical neck dissections are also carried out.[59] Because of the significant morbidity and loss of organ function with surgery, chemoradiation alone has been frequently employed. The survival probability with definitive chemoradiotherapy is similar, without the major functional impairments, morbidity, and mortality associated with surgery.[112] The optimum time to surgery following neoadjuvant therapy remains a topic of investigation, although delaying surgery from the traditional 4-6 weeks to greater than 12 weeks might improve tumor response to neoadjuvant therapy and thereby facilitate radical resection. This remains a topic of investigation.[112a]

Curative Combination Therapy

In the treatment of patients with esophageal cancer, an approach of radiation therapy with concurrent chemotherapy, with or without surgery, is frequently adopted. Multiagent chemotherapy with cisplatin and 5-fluorouracil (5-FU) has been used historically, although other combinations (e.g., paclitaxel and carboplatin; 5-FU with oxaliplatin) are now commonly utilized. Additional combinations of novel systemic agents (that also act as radiosensitizers) with radiation therapy are under investigation.

Palliative Treatment

Palliative treatment is frequently used for the relief of symptoms of esophageal carcinoma, especially dysphagia.[113] Surgical palliation involves resection and reconstruction, if possible, removing the bulk of the disease, potentially preventing abscess and fistula formation, as well as bleeding. Substernal bypass with the colon or entire stomach has also been carried out.[113] However, given the poor prognosis in patients with advanced disease and morbidity associated with resection, a surgical approach is rarely adopted and should be avoided in patients who can be managed with nonsurgical modalities.

Endoscopic dilatation is a reasonable alternative. When the lumen of the esophagus is dilated to 15 mm, dysphagia is often no longer experienced. Repeat dilatation is often required.[59] Esophageal stenting with either conventional plastic stents or metallic self-expanding stents can also be used to maintain patency.[114]

Palliative irradiation is frequently used to control the primary disease, as well as distant metastases. Resolution of symptoms, especially pain and dysphagia, can be accomplished in up to 87% of patients. Palliative treatment regimens range from 20 Gy over 1 week[60] to 50 Gy over 5 weeks. Laser ablation with or without intraluminal brachytherapy can be used. The addition of three fractions of 7 Gy each can improve the stenosis-free interval and prevent obstruction.[114]

RADIATION THERAPY TECHNIQUES

Simulation

When patients are simulated, the radiation oncologist should know the extent of disease based on imaging (barium swallow, CT, PET), as well as on endoscopy. CT simulation is appropriate for treatment planning. During simulation, the patient is positioned, straightened, and immobilized on the simulation table. An immobilization device (e.g., wing board, alpha cradle, body fix, or Vac-Lok on indexed wing board) is used to minimize variation in daily setup. Arms are generally placed overhead and knee support placed underneath the legs. Palpable neck disease should be marked with a radiopaque wire. The administration of oral contrast to delineate the esophagus is generally used and helps to define the extent of mucosal irregularity whereas small-bowel contrast can help identify any bowel in field. For GE junctional tumors (particularly with significant gastric

involvement), it may be advisable to have the patient come in with an empty stomach. Fasting prior to simulation and treatment each day may allow for greater reproducibility of treatment. In contrast, simulation without fasting and delivery of oral contrast may allow for planning in a "worst-case" scenario, with the patient is later instructed to fast prior to treatment delivery. For cervical and upper thoracic lesions, an immobilization mask may assist in creating a reproducible position. Some authors have also advocated that midesophageal primaries be simulated in prone position to maximize distance between the target volumes and spinal cord. The patient is placed on the CT simulator in the treatment position, and a scan of the entire area of interest with margin is obtained. At minimum, 3- to 5-mm slices should be used, allowing accurate tumor characterization, as well as improved quality of digitally reconstructed radiographs. If patients lose >10% of their body weight during therapy, consideration should be given to repeat CT planning. Arterial phase intravenous contrast is generally used to delineate mediastinal and abdominal vascular nodal basins, including the celiac axis and to allow the radiation oncologist to discern normal vasculature from other adjacent normal structures, and potential adenopathy. The tumor and vital structures are then outlined on each slice on the treatment planning system. The use of respiratory gating or breath-hold techniques may help to reduce target motion with respiration and, therefore, avoid normal-tissue irradiation associated with larger margins used in free-breathing approaches, particularly for lower esophageal cancers. Additional techniques to minimize physiologic motion include abdominal compression devices. Four-dimensional CT scan may be appropriate to assess tumoral motion, facilitating appropriate margin placement on the target volumes, particularly in lower esophageal tumors and/or disease involving the stomach.

Treatment Planning

Target Design

In the design of radiation fields for esophageal cancer, it is important to define varying target volumes, including gross disease as well as potential areas of subclinical involvement (i.e., the GTVs and CTVs, respectively). Definition of GTV is based on multiple studies, including endoscopic descriptions (from both esophagogastroduodenoscopy [EGD] and EUS). The proximal and distal aspects of the tumor should be standardly defined by the gastroenterologist based on distance from the incisors, as well as relationship to varying landmarks as measured from the incisors (e.g., the GE junction). The radiation oncologist is able to use these measurements to help correlate with disease extent visualized on planning CT scan, using varying anatomic landmarks (e.g., the GE junction, which is frequently located ~40 cm from the incisors in many patients), as well as carina (which is frequently located at ~25 cm in most patients) to help more accurately define the GTV. Additionally, endoscopists may place radioopaque fiducial markers at the superior and inferior extent of the primary tumor to help facilitate disease extent. Esophageal wall thickening correlating to the GTV can frequently be visualized on diagnostic and radiation planning CT. Similarly, EUS appears to be the most reliable test in detecting lymphadenopathy related to nodal spread. As in EGD, the endoscopist should be encouraged to accurately define not only the primary disease extent on EUS as measured by distances from the incisors but also depth of penetration and potential involvement of adjacent structures, which can also be used to help guide GTV delineation. Similarly, EUS may detect lymph nodes that may not be appreciated on CT or PET imaging, and the endoscopist should describe the size as well as the location (e.g., distance from incisors, relationship to adjacent mediastinal structures, etc.) of these, further facilitating accurate definition of potentially involved lymph nodes, either adjacent to or well removed from the primary tumor itself. In addition, radiographic areas of lymphadenopathy should similarly be included in the GTV.

Although the utility of PET in esophageal cancer staging primarily lies in its ability to detect distant metastases not fully appreciated on CT imaging (and thereby alter treatment approach of these patients),[115,116] diagnostic PET-CT has more recently been integrated into radiation planning of esophageal cancer patients and definition of GTV. Generally, gross disease as defined on PET is characterized by a standard uptake value of >2 to 2.5.[117] Generally speaking, PET-avid nodes should be included within the GTV volume. In a study from Fox Chase Cancer Center, the mean GTV length as determined by PET-CT closely correlated with endoscopy findings.[68] Another study from Australian investigators reported that CT-alone–based definition of GTV excluded PET-avid disease in a majority of patients, resulting in a potential geographic miss of disease in a significant minority of patients.[118] Similarly, the fusion of CT-PET has been shown to prompt GTV and PTV modification in a majority of patients.[119] Another analysis of PET-CT-based (as compared to CT alone) radiotherapy planning of esophageal cancer patients indicated a reduction of intraobserver and interobserver variability in GTV delineation.[120] However, another study compared the planning of patients with CT-alone treatment plans followed by adjustment based on PET findings. Although PET scan influenced GTV volume in half of patients, no locoregional recurrences were seen following CT-based radiotherapy that could have been prevented by the addition of PET.[121]

Finally, although the routine use of fluoroscopic barium swallow in esophageal cancer has decreased, this study may still be useful to the radiation oncologist for field design. A study by Chinese investigators suggested that, as compared to CT, endoscopy with barium swallow more accurately defines the true length of middle and lower esophageal tumors, although CT appeared to better determine this for tumors located at the GE junction.[122]

In summary, accurate definition of primary and nodal gross disease is paramount in radiation esophageal cancer planning. It is important to rely on all diagnostic studies, including barium swallow (when available), EGD, EUS, and CT, as well as PET scan.

The identification of potential direct and nodal pathways for spread of subclinical disease (i.e., CTV definition) in esophageal cancer is also of paramount importance. These areas vary significantly, depending on site of origin of disease, making esophageal cancer planning somewhat complex. In terms of direct disease extension along the esophagus itself, varying reports have assessed the histologic findings at primary esophagectomy to determine subclinical extent of disease. One prospective analysis of 66 resection specimens showed that placement of a 3-cm margin proximally and distally on the primary tumor would cover microscopic disease extension in 94% of squamous cell carcinomas. Similarly, in GE junctional carcinomas, a 3-cm proximal margin included subclinical disease extension in 100% of patients and 5 cm distally covered 94% of subclinical spread.[122]

As described previously, the esophagus is characterized by a rich submucosal network of lymphatics that facilitates early lymph node spread of disease, even for superficial esophageal cancers. The appropriate cranial and caudal margins remain a matter of debate in the treatment of esophageal cancer. Historically, very large fields were treated, encompassing potential pathways and lymphatic spread from the thoracic inlet down to the celiac axis region; however, such fields are potentially fraught with treatment-related toxicity and may be difficult for patients to tolerate, particularly in the context of concurrent chemotherapy delivery. Most contemporary radiation trials used margins of 3 to 5 cm cranially and caudally on the GTV, along with an approximate 2-cm radial margin. With disease located at or above the carina (or middle/upper one-third of the esophagus in some instances), many of these trials recommended fields inclusive of the supraclavicular lymph

node basins, whereas celiac axis nodal basin coverage was recommended for disease of the distal esophagus.[123] However, the appropriate field size for patients with esophageal cancer remains controversial, particularly the role of elective nodal irradiation.

Even the concept of what constitutes "involved-field" and "extended-field" can vary between series. Comparative series have yielded conflicting results to this effect, although recent reviews have suggested that elective nodal irradiation appears to prevent or delay regional nodal relapse. However, its impact on survival in these patients remains less clear, with a higher incidence of esophageal and lung toxicities in the latter.[124,125] This remains a topic of ongoing study and randomized studies are needed. Further description of lymph node basin coverage follows.

Field Design

Historically, the treatment of very proximal (cervical) esophageal cancers has been challenging. Because of the changing contour from the neck to the thoracic inlet, treatment of lesions in the upper one-third of the esophagus may present a difficult technical problem. Lesions in the upper cervical or postcricoid esophagus are often treated from the laryngopharynx to the carina, depending on extent of disease. Supraclavicular and superior mediastinal nodes are irradiated electively. Using older/conventional methods, this was achieved with lateral parallel opposed or oblique portals to the primary tumor and a single anterior field for the supraclavicular and superior mediastinal nodes.[105] Another historical technique treated lesions in this region by means of a four-field box approach, using a wax bolus to build up the lack of tissue above the shoulders, acting as a compensator. A high-energy beam (>15 MV) is used, and both sides of the neck are treated prophylactically. Other methods of treating lesions at the thoracic inlet include 140-degree arc rotations, anterior wedged pairs, and three- or four-field techniques using posterior oblique portals combined with a single anterior portal or anteroposterior–posteroanterior (AP/PA) fields.[105] Using three-dimensional (3D) approaches, varying techniques have been implemented, including treatment of the primary tumor and lymph nodes using an AP/PA approach to 39.6 to 41.4 Gy at 1.8 Gy/fraction, followed by a left or right opposed oblique pair to bring the total dose to 50.4 Gy, thereby limiting the spinal cord dose. This technique will generally exclude the supraclavicular fossa, and a separate electron field is often added, treating to a depth of 2 to 3 cm, depending upon individual anatomy. More recently, however, intensity-modulated radiation therapy (IMRT)-based planning has facilitated the treatment of upper esophageal lesions and is our preferred method for treating these tumors (Fig. 56.9) Strict normal-tissue constraints, including normal lung and spinal cord, are important considerations in using these techniques (discussed later).

Based on the previously described and other pathologic patterns of spread data in squamous cell carcinoma of the esophagus, general guidelines in terms of field design can be made as follows: For cervical and upper thoracic squamous cell carcinoma, the CTV should generally include nodal basins extending from the lower cervical and supraclavicular region superiorly to the subcarinal lymph node basin inferiorly, inclusive of the upper paraesophageal lymph nodes (Fig. 56.9). For lower esophageal squamous cell carcinomas, lymph node basins from the subcarinal region superiorly to the left gastric and common hepatic artery/celiac lymph nodal basins inferiorly should generally be included (described further later in this chapter). In a small series of patients without celiac radiation coverage, 6 (10%) had celiac nodal failure, portending a worse prognosis. The authors concluded that although overt celiac failure only occurred in 1 of

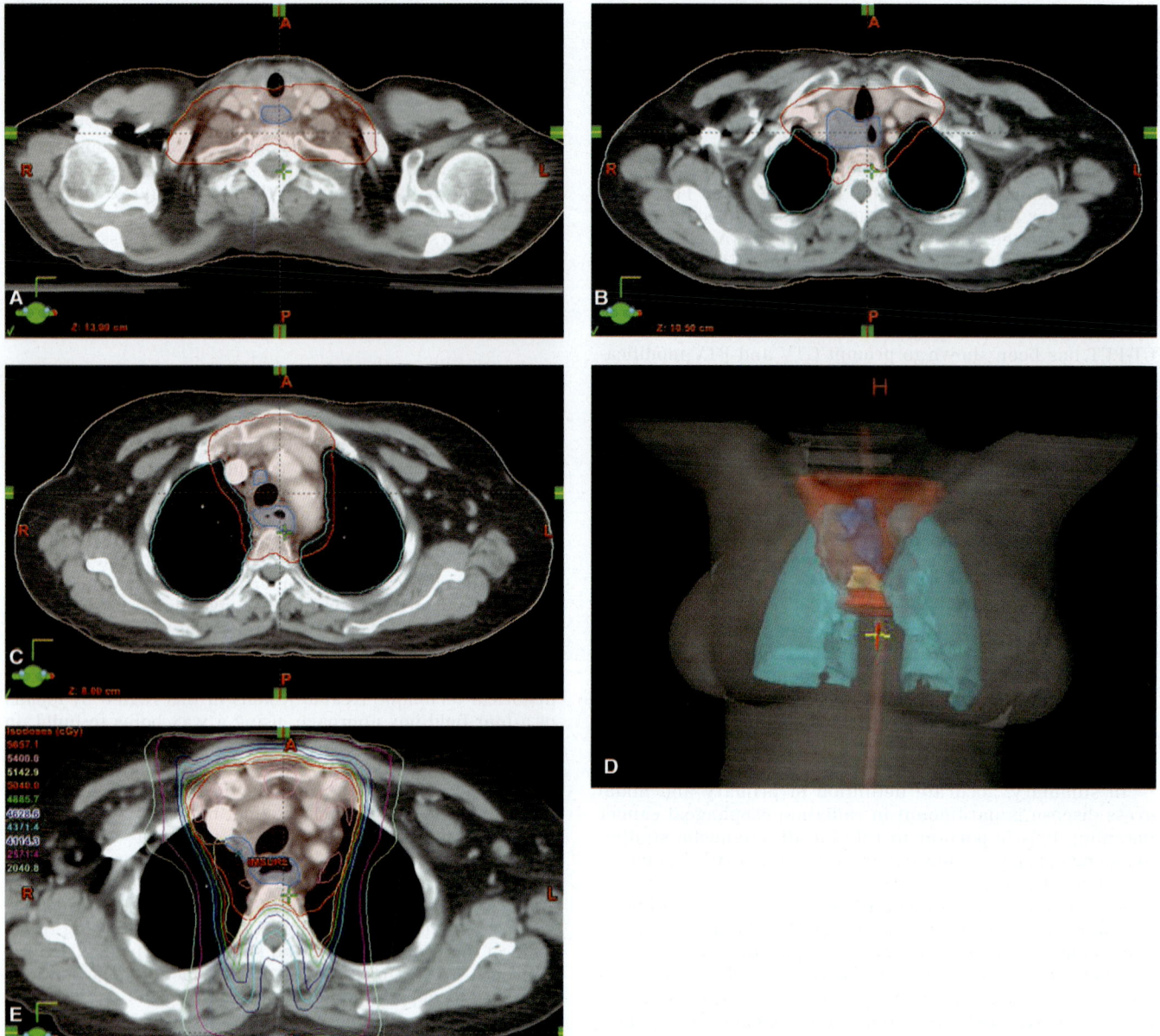

FIGURE 56.9.   A–C: Examples of planning target volume (PTV) in a 62-year-old woman with a cT3 N1 squamous cell carcinoma of cervical esophagus. Gross tumor volume (GTV), *blue* volume; PTV, *red* volume. **D:** Three-dimensional reconstruction of PTV from above the patient. Carina, *yellow*; GTV, *dark blue*; lungs, *light blue*; PTV, *red*; spinal cord, *brown*. **E:** Isodose curves of this patient treated with a nine-field intensity-modulated radiation therapy plan. Note that beams are primarily anteriorly oriented. (Courtesy of Rodney Hood, CMD.)

10 patients, the lack of effective salvage in treatments may justify treatment of this basin in distal esophageal cancer patients.[126] For tumors of the middle esophagus, we recommend individual field design according to clinical scenarios, with a more complete coverage of paraesophageal mediastinal lymph nodes, particularly in patients with a good performance status (Fig. 56.10).[43] These are general guidelines, and all plans should be individualized based on available imaging and endoscopic findings.

In field design, potential nodal involvement (and therefore target volumes) based on nodal size is problematic, given that some reports demonstrated that <15% of metastatic nodes are >1 cm and that average size differences between involved and uninvolved nodes are frequently not significantly different.[127] In addition, fluorodeoxyglucose-PET scanning has an estimated sensitivity of only 67% of detecting nodal metastases.[8] Even endoscopic ultrasound, generally considered the most

sensitive test for detecting lymph node metastases, is only able to detect such disease in approximately 75% of patients.[128] Therefore, it is not appropriate to rely exclusively on varying imaging modalities to define areas of subclinical spread for esophageal cancer, realizing that patterns-of-spread data are important in determining radiation field design.

The design of radiation fields for the treatment of adenocarcinoma of the esophagus is similar to that of lower thoracic squamous cell carcinomas but deserves special mention. Periesophageal lymph nodes are generally included in all patients. Given that lymph node involvement is clearly associated with depth of tumor penetration (T stage) and the fact that most patients in the United States and Europe presenting with GE junctional carcinoma will have more advanced disease, inclusion of celiac lymph basins for adenocarcinoma of the distal esophagus/GE junction is usually indicated, although remains an area of controversy. Based on the previously

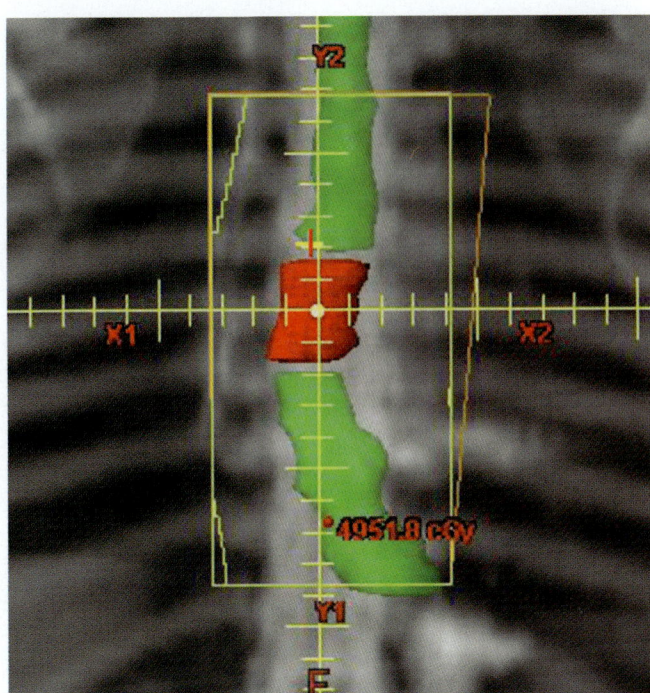

FIGURE 56.10. Example field for a midesophageal squamous cell carcinoma. Note that the field is inclusive of adjacent mediastinal/paraesophageal nodes, with approximately 5 cm margin superiorly on the gross tumor volume (GTV), as well as slightly larger margin on the inferior aspect of the GTV based on concern of previously unappreciated spread at the time of endoscopy.

described patterns of spread data from Erlangen and others, specific considerations include the following: Lymph vascular invasion is highly predictive of nodal spread. Proximal extension of tumors (particularly beyond the Z line into the distal esophagus for type II and III tumors) predicts an increasing incidence of paraesophageal lymph node involvement. Based on an estimated nodal incidence cutoff of 20% for inclusion, specific considerations include the following: (a) The lower paraesophageal, paracardial, lesser curvature, and left gastric artery nodes should be included in the CTV. (b) The presence of lymph vascular invasion predicts a nodal positivity rate of >20% in the left and right gastroepiploic, greater curvature, celiac trunk, and splenic hilar regions. (c) In T3/4 disease, the gastroepiploic, greater curvature, celiac trunk, splenic hilar, splenic artery, and common hepatic artery should be included. (d) High-grade tumors should also include the left gastroepiploic, greater curvature, and celiac trunk nodes in CT design. (e) Larger and more deeply penetrating tumors should also include the splenic artery and splenic hilar nodes, as well as those along the greater curvature. (f) Tumors extending above the diaphragm and those extending >1.5 cm beyond the Z line should include the mid paraesophageal nodes, treating up to the carina. Of note, significant involvement of the distal esophagus by GE junctional tumors (>1.5 cm beyond the Z line) should lead to inclusion of not only lower but also middle paraesophageal nodes based on patterns of spread. However, treating these more extensive fields must be weighed against potential side effects of increased normal-tissue irradiation. In summary, middle and lower paraesophageal nodes should be included in patients with T2-T4 type I and T2-T4 type II tumors extending >1.5 cm above the Z line and T3-T4 type II patients. The splenic hilar and artery nodes are considered "spareable" in T2 tumors, notably type I.[49]

Although, historically, two-dimensional–based radiation planning has been carried out primarily using anatomic landmarks such as bone and carina, as well as fluoroscopic barium swallow, to determine field borders, contemporary treatment planning using CT-based planning allows improved visualization of both target and nontarget structures, along with three-dimensional reconstruction and creation of a "beam's-eye" view of varying fields, allowing improved conformity around target structures and improvements in normal-tissue sparing. Because volumetric data can be obtained by CT scans, dose–volume histogram data can also be generated. A variety of three-dimensional techniques are being used and are described later.

Potential beam orientations for the treatment of thoracic esophageal and gastroesophageal junction tumors (again defined as tumors involving the gastroesophageal junction with an epicenter within 5 cm proximal or distal to the GE junction) include an initial AP/PA approach followed by AP/right posterior oblique (RPO)/left posterior oblique (LPO) fields with or without boost, an initial APPA approach followed by RAO/LPO fields with or without boost, and a three-field technique (AP/PA with left lateral or oblique field). One potential approach in lesions of the thoracic esophagus or GE junction is to use initial AP/PA/RAO/LPO fields, with boost fields using laterally oriented beams. The inferior margin of the initial fields includes the gastroesophageal junction and, for lower or middle one-third lesions, the celiac axis nodal basins (generally located at the level of T12 and identifiable on CT), as well as gastrohepatic ligament. Initial fields are often treated to a dose of 45 Gy, taking care to avoid as much of the heart as reasonably possible while continuing to minimize the kidney volume in the radiation field, inclusive of the above nodal basins. Reduced fields encompassing gross disease with an approximate 2-cm margin through oblique or lateral fields may then be used for an additional 5.4 Gy. Doses usually do not exceed 50 Gy, and lower doses (e.g., 41.4 Gy) may be appropriate (discussed later).

A margin of 5 cm above and below the GTV is generally recommended to cover subclinical submucosal/nodal disease, as well as an approximate 2.0- to 2.5-cm radial margin, although individual margins are case dependent. Because it is imperative to account for daily setup uncertainty as well as physiologic internal organ motion (secondary to respiration, peristalsis, cardiac motion, etc.), additional margin must be added to a CTV, particularly to the more mobile distal esophagus. The internal target volume (ITV) has been used to account for physiologic motion of the target volume, which is included in the PTV. Varying reports analyzing esophageal motion have shown average anterior and posterior motion ranges from 0.1 to 4 mm, lateral motion from 0.3 to 4.2 mm, and superior-to-inferior motion from 3.7 to 10 mm.[123] An analysis evaluating interfraction esophageal motion in the right–left and AP direction showed average right–left motion of 1.8 ± 5.1 mm (favoring leftward movement) and average AP motion of 0.6 ± 4.8 mm (favoring posterior movement), with an average absolute motion of 4.2 mm or less in the right–left and AP directions. The authors concluded that 12-mm left, 10-mm posterior, and 9-mm anterior margins are appropriate.[129] Some authors have recommended defining 1-cm radial, 1.5-cm distal, and 1-cm proximal margins from CTV to ITV if target motion data are not available. Image-guided radiation therapy, including cone beam CT, may also be useful in localizing tumor and establishing physiologic variability between daily treatments.

Figure 56.11 shows general recommendations for elective target nodal station coverage in a patient with a type I GE junctional tumor with an accompanying example field. Figure 56.12 shows general recommendations for elective target nodal station coverage in a patient with a type II GE junctional tumor. Nodal basins are similar to type I tumors with the exception of inclusion of nodal basins along the splenic artery course. Figure 56.13 shows general recommendations for elective target nodal station coverage in a patient with a type III GE junctional tumor with accompanying example fields. Note that in type III tumors, there is less emphasis

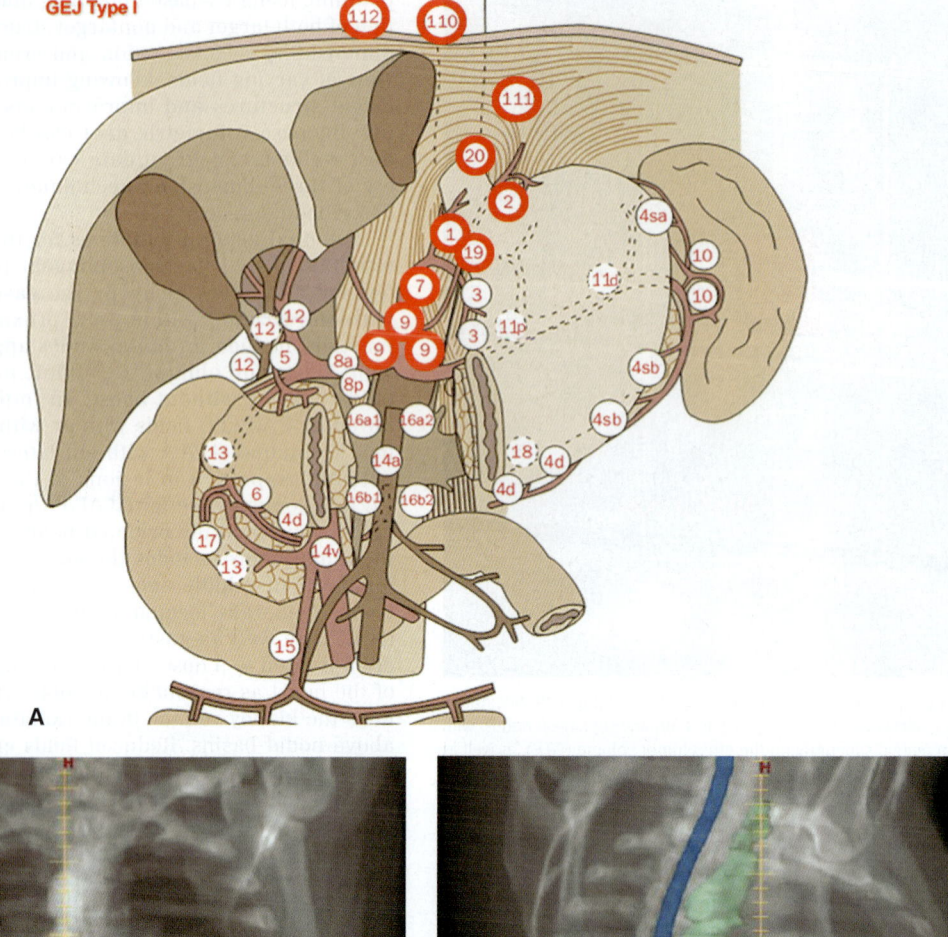

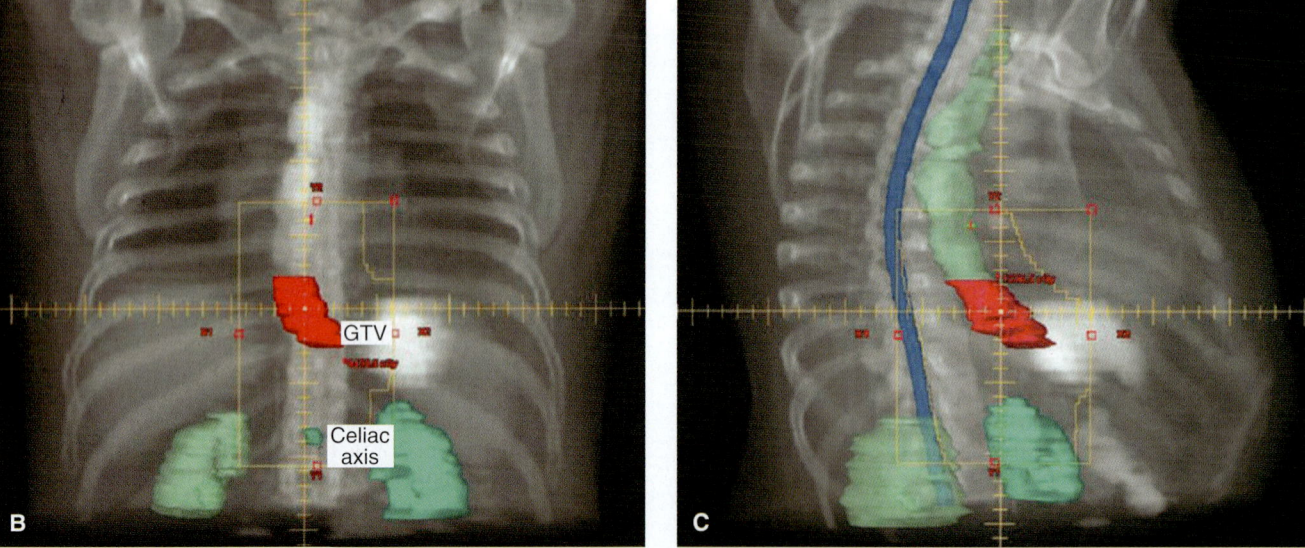

FIGURE 56.11.   A: Recommended nodal basins to be included for type I gastroesophageal (GE) junctional tumors based on Japanese Gastric Cancer Association lymph node stations. (Reprinted from Matzinger O, Gerber E, Bernstein Z, et al. EORTC-ROG expert opinion: radiotherapy volume and treatment guidelines for neoadjuvant radiation of adenocarcinomas of the gastroesophageal junction and the stomach. *Radiother Oncol* 2009;92[2]:164–175. Copyright © 2009 Elsevier Ireland Ltd. With permission.) **B:** Example field for a type I GE junctional adenocarcinoma. **C:** Example oblique field for a type I GE junctional tumor, inclusive of the above nodal basins.

on more proximal (lower mediastinal) nodes and more comprehensive coverage of the splenic artery course, including splenic hilum. Figure 56.14 shows examples of varying nodal locations on axial CT images.

Another potential treatment planning approach for thoracic esophageal cancer is the use of IMRT. IMRT also uses CT-based planning, again allowing 3D reconstruction of varying structures. However, IMRT differs from 3D planning through the delivery of radiation dose by partitioning a radiation field into multiple smaller fields of varying shapes and sizes, varying the dose intensity between each area. This is carried out with either dynamic IMRT (in which collimating

leaves move in and out of the radiation beam path during treatment) or "step-and-shoot" IMRT (in which the leaves change the radiation field shape while the beam is turned off). Either method is particularly effective at conforming radiation dose to the target structures while avoiding dose to normal tissue. Radiation oncologists must determine which structures are most critical and weight their importance during the treatment planning process. Of importance, the greater the number of "avoidance" normal structures, the more difficult it is to meet all dose constraints. IMRT uses "inverse planning," in which an intended prescription dose is placed on target volumes and dose constraints are placed on normal-tissue

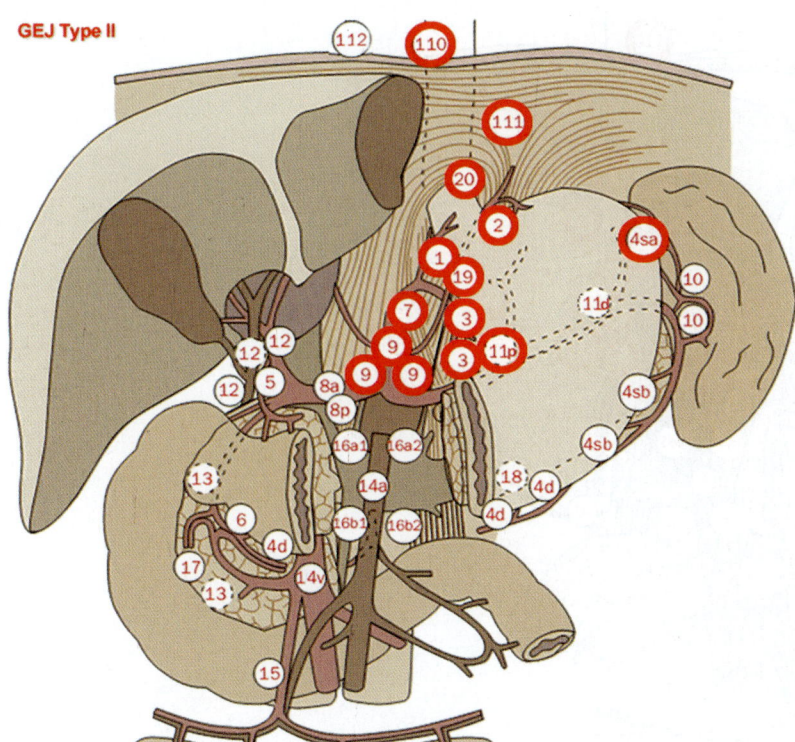

GEJ Type II

FIGURE 56.12. Recommended nodal basins to be included for type II gastroesophageal junctional tumors based on Japanese Gastric Cancer Association lymph node stations. (Reprinted from Matzinger O, Gerber E, Bernstein Z, et al. EORTC-ROG expert opinion: radiotherapy volume and treatment guidelines for neoadjuvant radiation of adenocarcinomas of the gastroesophageal junction and the stomach. *Radiother Oncol* 2009,92[2]:164–175. Copyright © 2009 Elsevier Ireland Ltd. With permission.)

structures. Thereafter, computer software algorithms allow design of unconventional treatment fields that would not otherwise be possible with standard planning methods. Radiation oncologists and medical physicists critically evaluate numerous plans until dose constraints are satisfactorily met. The result should be a series of radiation doses that closely conform to the target volumes while minimizing dose to normal tissues. Similarly, volumetric arc therapy (VMAT) also utilizes IMRT delivery, although doing so while the gantry is actively rotating during treatment. Dosimetric comparisons of IMRT versus 3D conformal therapy in cervical esophageal cancer have demonstrated superior target volume coverage and conformality with decreased normal-tissue dose.[130] A potential disadvantage of IMRT is the possibility of delivering low doses of radiation therapy to normal-tissue areas that might not normally be irradiated using 2D or 3D techniques. The influence of this on toxicity (e.g., low-dose pulmonary irradiation and development of postoperative pulmonary complications) remains uncertain. Another potential disadvantage of IMRT is possible dose inhomogeneity, leading to potential hot spots in normal organs. Because IMRT requires precise target definition, the potential for marginal miss increases and careful target delineation is of paramount importance. With setup uncertainty, physiologic organ motion must be considered to ensure accurate and reproducible setup, including the use of immobilization devices, possible respiratory gating/breath-hold techniques, etc. Generally, high-energy photons (4 to 18 MV) are recommended when using 3D conformal or IMRT therapy, potentially facilitating a reduction of the integral lung dose. A multi-institutional experience of 580 patients treated across three academic centers compared patients receiving 3D versus IMRT and proton beam therapy. Advanced treatment technologies (IMRT and proton beam) were associated with significantly reduced rate of postoperative complications and length of stay. The authors indicated prospective randomized data will be needed to validate these results.[131] Additionally, a registry-based study of patients >65 years old comparing 3D- versus IMRT-treated patients, IMRT was not associated with esophageal cancer–specific mortality or pulmonary mortality, but was with improved all-cause mortality, including

cardiac and other cause mortality.[132] Similarly, in analysis of the RTOG 0617 trial randomizing patients with non–small cell lung cancer to receive concurrent carboplatin and paclitaxel with or without cetuximab with a second randomization to 60 versus 74 Gy, no benefit was seen in terms of radiation dose escalation. On secondary analysis, however, IMRT was associated with less ≥ grade 3 pneumonitis (7.9 vs. 3.5%, P = .039), lower heart doses (P < .05), and lower heart V40 doses, with the heart V40 significantly associated with overall survival (P < .05). Additionally, the lung V20 dose was also associated with increased ≥ grade 3 pneumonitis risk on multivariable analysis (P = .026), with the authors concluding IMRT was associated with lower rates of severe pneumonitis and cardiac doses.[133]

More recently, an expert panel published contouring guidelines for esophageal and gastroesophageal junction CTV volumes for IMRT planning. Examples of consensus CTV are illustrated in Figure 56.15. Delineation of the proximal border of the CTV was described as 3 to 4 cm above the proximal edge of the GTV, or 1 cm above any grossly involved periesophageal nodes, oriented along the esophageal mucosa and not a simple geometric expansion. For proximal tumors, the upper border was not extended beyond the level of the cricoid cartilage unless disease presence precludes such. For proximal or midesophageal tumors, the distal border for CTV creation was described as 3 to 4 cm below the proximal edge of the GTV, again oriented along the esophagus. For lower tumors, what is described as at least a 2-cm margin along clinically involved gastric mucosa was recommended if treating definitively, or if treating to lower, preoperative-intent doses (≤45 Gy), a 4-cm or greater gastric margin was felt appropriate, particularly with significant gastric extension. CTV radial margin was described as at least 1 cm in all direction on GTV, with a 1-cm radial margin from the outer esophageal wall to encompass periesophageal lymph nodes, with a limit of 5 mm into cardiac tissue, including the pericardium. For more distal tumors involving or approaching the GE junction, the CTV was described as being extended inferiorly to the level of the celiac axis origin, bounded by the lateral aspect of the vertebral body on the right and 0.5 to 1 cm

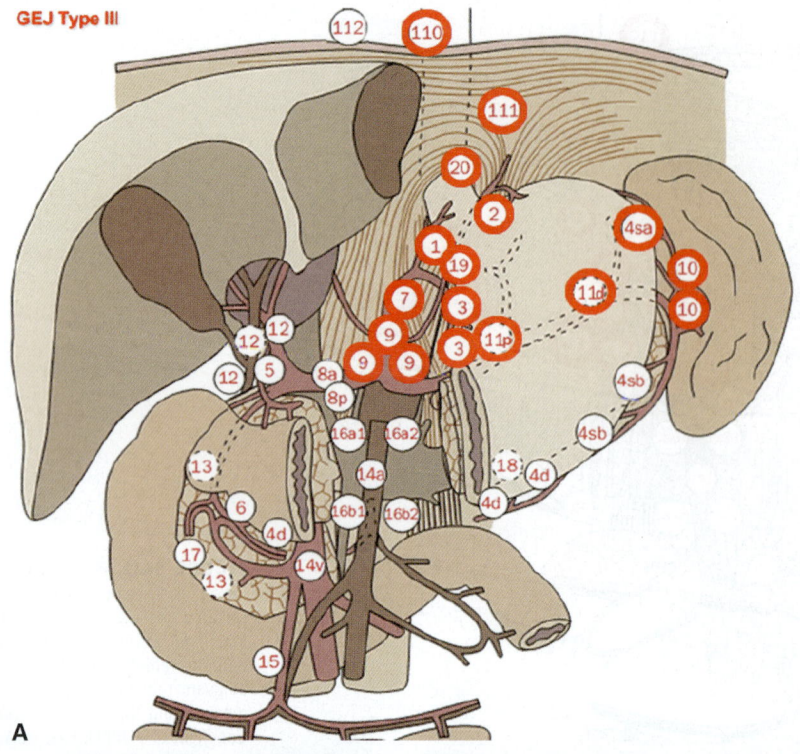

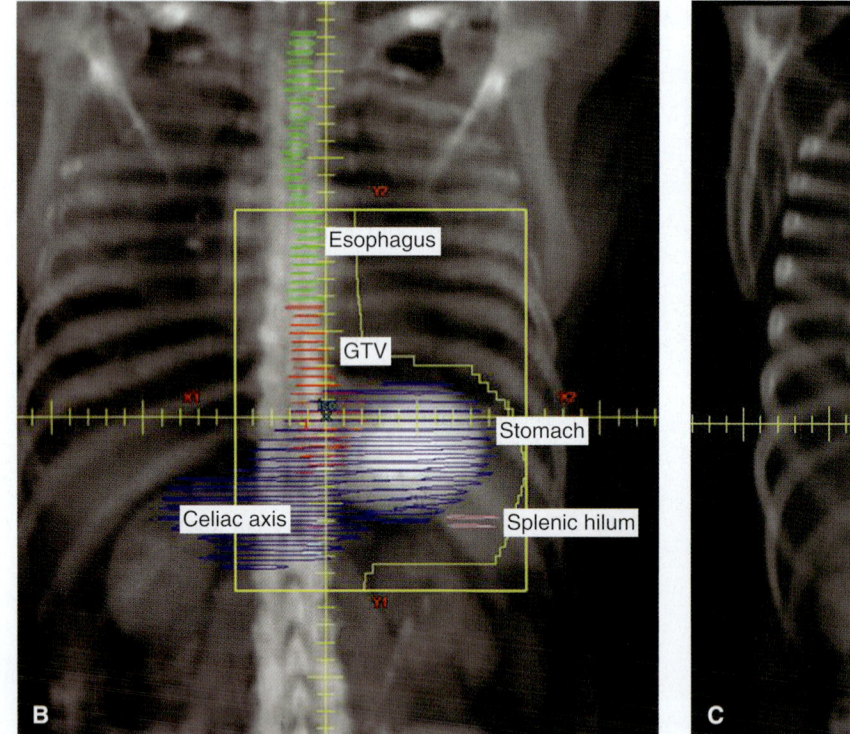

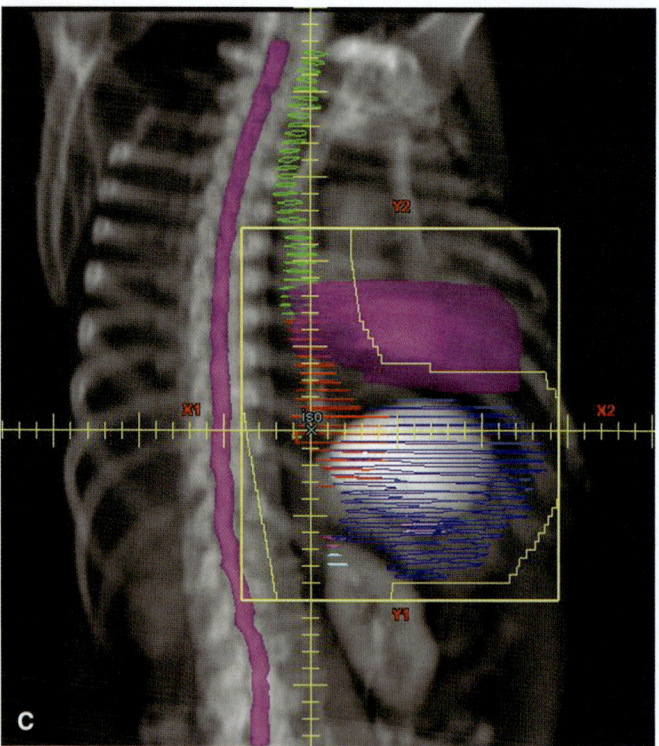

FIGURE 56.13. **A:** Recommended nodal basins to be included for type III gastroesophageal (GE) junctional tumors based on Japanese Gastric Cancer Association lymph node stations. (Reprinted from Matzinger O, Gerber E, Bernstein Z, et al. EORTC-ROG expert opinion: radiotherapy volume and treatment guidelines for neoadjuvant radiation of adenocarcinomas of the gastroesophageal junction and the stomach. *Radiother Oncol* 2009;92[2]:164–175. Copyright © 2009 Elsevier Ireland Ltd. With permission.) **B:** Example field for a type III gastroesophageal junctional adenocarcinoma. **C:** Example oblique field for a type III GE junctional tumor, inclusive of the above nodal basins.

beyond the lateral aspect of the aorta on the left, vertebral body posteriorly and pancreatic body anteriorly. Periaortic and gastrohepatic (sometimes classified as lesser curve or left gastric) lymph nodes were deemed appropriate for inclusion. Examples of CTVs are shown in Figures 56.16–56.18. Inclusion of some or all nodes in the splenic hilum and greater curvature region was felt potentially appropriate for Siewert type II gastroesophageal junction tumors depending on clinical and pathologic features. For tumors above the level of the carina, inclusion of the bilateral supraclavicular nodal basins was recommended. PTV delineation was created by adding 0.5 to 1 cm to the CTV in all directions (which is essentially

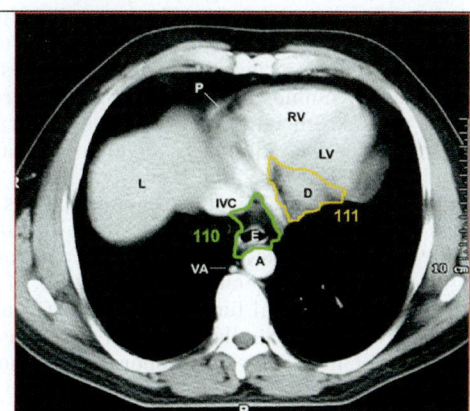

110 - Paraoesophageal LN
111 - Supradiaphragmatic LN

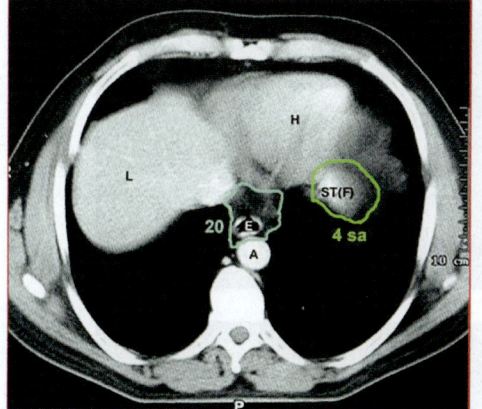

20 -   LN in the oesophageal hiatus of the diaphragm
4sa - LN along the short gastric vessels

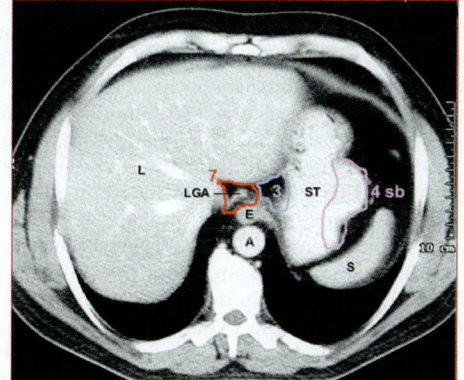

3 -   LN along the lesser curvature
4sb - LN along the left gastroepiploic vessels
7 -   LN along the left gastric artery

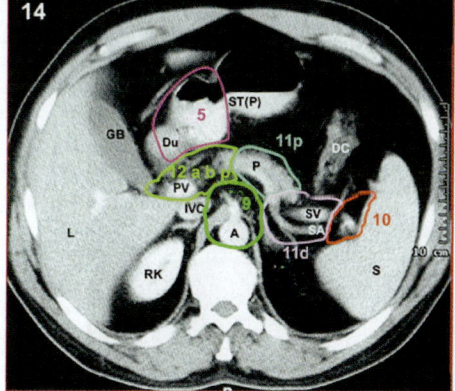

5 -   Suprapyloric LN,
9 -   LN around the celiac artery
10 -   LN at the splenic hilum
11p - LN along the proximal splenic artery
11d - LN along the distal splenic artery
12 a, b, p - LN in the hepatoduodenal ligament

LEGEND:
A – Aorta; AC – Ascending Colon; D - Diaphragma; DC – Descending Colon; Du – Duodenum; E - Oesophagus; GB – Gall Bladder; I – Ilium; H – Heart; J – Jejunum; IVC – Inferior Cava Vein; L – Liver; L-1 – First Lumbar Vertebra; LK – Left Kidney, LRV – Left Renal Vein; LV – Left Ventricle; P – Pancreas; PV – Portal Vein; RGA – Right Gastric Artery; RK – Right Kidney; RV – Right Ventricle; S – Spleen; SA – Splenic Artery; SMA&V – Superior Mesenteric Artery and Vein; SV – Splenic Vein; ST – Stomach; ST(F) – Stomach Fundus; ST(P) – Stomach Pylorus; TC - Transverse Colon; VA – Azygos Vein

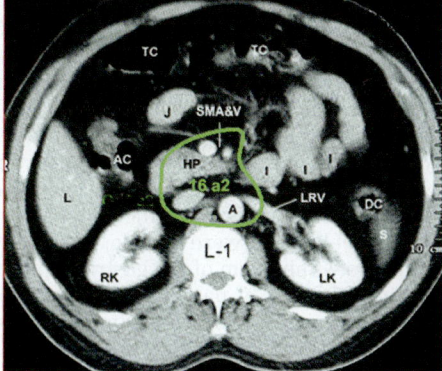

16 a2 LN around the abdominal aorta

FIGURE 56.14. Examples of lymph node stations on corresponding computed tomography slices. (Reprinted from Matzinger O, Gerber E, Bernstein Z, et al. EORTC-ROG expert opinion: radiotherapy volume and treatment guidelines for neoadjuvant radiation of adenocarcinomas of the gastroesophageal junction and the stomach. *Radiother Oncol* 2009;92[2]:164–175. Copyright © 2009 Elsevier Ireland Ltd. With permission.)

equivalent to the traditional practice of placing the field border 5 cm above and below the GTV).[134]

Dose Constraints

In radiation therapy planning of esophageal cancer, normal-tissue tolerance should always be considered. The spinal cord dose is generally limited to 45 Gy using 1.8-Gy fractions (and potentially less when delivered with novel systemic agents). Efforts to minimize radiation to the heart (in particular the left ventricle in lower esophageal/gastroesophageal junction lesions) should be made. Adopting an off-heart approach using oblique orientations (including right anterior and left

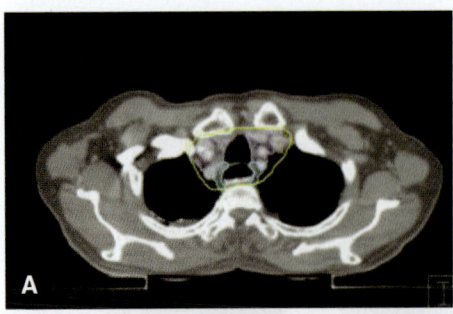

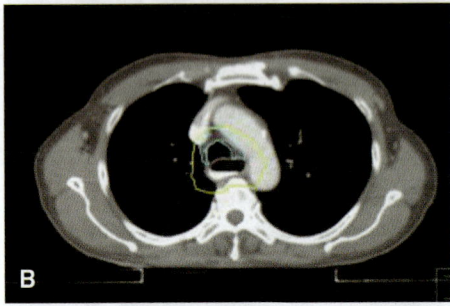

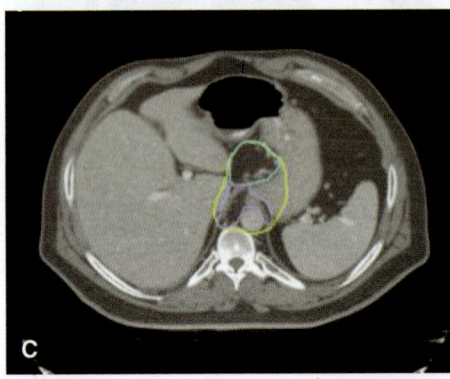

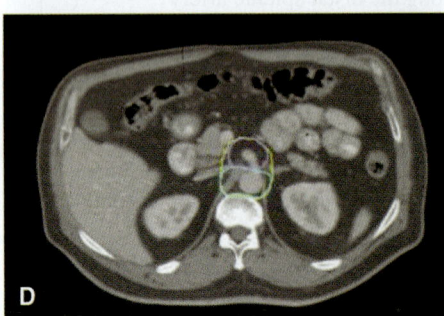

FIGURE 56.15. Examples of consensus contours encompassing defined nodal regions. **A:** CTV contour (*yellow*) encompasses level 3 retrotracheal (*blue*) and level 2 upper paratracheal (*purple*) nodes. **B:** CTV encompasses level 4 lower paratracheal (*blue*) and level 8 periesophageal nodes. **C:** CTV encompasses lesser curvature/gastrohepatic ligament (*blue*) and paracardial (*purple*) nodes. **D:** CTV encompasses para-aortic (*blue*) and celiac (*purple*) nodes. (Reprinted from Wu AJ, Bosch WR, Chang DT, et al. Expert consensus contouring guidelines for intensity modulated radiation therapy in esophageal and gastroesophageal junction cancer. *Int J Radiat Oncol Biol Phys* 2015;92(4);911–920. Copyright © 2015 Elsevier. With permission.)

posterior, described earlier) is one potential way of achieving this, although multiple approaches exist, including IMRT-based techniques. Similarly, efforts to minimize dose to normal pulmonary tissues should be made, based on data suggesting that the volume of irradiated lung may correspond to postoperative complications and worsened pulmonary function (described later). Frequently, the volume of irradiated lung can be minimized using a simple AP/PA approach. However,

this sometimes results in significant cardiac dose, particularly in lower esophagus and gastroesophageal junction tumors. Therefore, oblique orientations are sometimes used, resulting in increased volumes of normal lung being irradiated. When giving concurrent chemotherapy, we generally limit these fields to 13 to 15 Gy. Similarly, advanced radiation techniques including IMRT are frequently utilized.

Accurate delineation of adjacent organs, including the lungs, liver, kidneys, heart, and spinal cord, is important. Varying dose–volume normal-organ constraints have been suggested, including achieving a lung V_{20} of <20%, limiting >2,300 cm³ of normal lung tissue to <5 Gy, and using mean lung dose of <18 Gy. Similarly, a V_{10} of ≤60% has been proposed to reduce the incidence of postoperative pulmonary complications. Historically, heart dose constraints have included maintaining one-third, two-thirds, and total heart volumes of <45, 40, and 30 Gy, respectively. Recommended heart constraints include keeping <30% of the cardiac volume to a total dose of 40 Gy and <50% receiving 25 Gy, minimizing dose to the left ventricle. In the setting of potentially significant volumes of the heart in the radiation field, consideration of respiratory gating and/or breath-hold techniques can be made. For lower esophageal and gastroesophageal cancers, it is recommended that at least 70% of one physiologically functioning kidney receive a total dose of <20 Gy and that, collectively, no more than 50% of the combined functional renal volume should receive >20 Gy.[48] One should also consider the possibility of impaired kidney function in the context of varying comorbidities, using nuclear medicine renal studies to assess individual renal function in such situations or where significant volumes of kidneys are anticipated to be within the radiation field. Generally, 70% of the liver parenchyma should be kept to a dose of <30 Gy. Many of these constraints can be achieved with three-dimensional planning with appropriate and careful design of shielding blocks/multileaf collimation and dose–volume histogram analysis, with the use of IMRT in select cases. Examples of normal tissue constraints for esophageal cancer planning are seen in Table 56.6.

Doses of Radiation

Because locoregional failure is common after conventional chemoradiation, investigators have evaluated dose escalation techniques. Varying series using doses beyond 50 Gy have shown local control rates ranging from approximately 77% to 88%.[135,136] However, Minsky et al.[56,137] reported the results of a randomized trial in which 236 patients with clinical stage T1-4, N0/1, M0 squamous cell, or adenocarcinoma of the esophagus were selected for nonsurgical therapy. Patients were randomized to receive 64.8 versus 50.4 Gy, both with concurrent 5-fluorouracil and cisplatin chemotherapy. Patients with cervical, mid, or distal esophageal cancer were eligible, with the exception of those with tumors within 2 cm of the gastroesophageal junction, with approximately 85% of patients with squamous cell histology. This study was closed after interim analysis showed no probability of superiority in the high-dose arm. No significant difference in median survival (13 vs. 18.1 months), 2-year survival (31% vs. 40%), or locoregional failure/persistence of disease (56% vs. 52%) was seen between the high-dose and standard-dose arms. Eleven treatment-related deaths occurred in the high-dose arm compared with 2 in the standard-dose arm, with 7 of the 11 high-dose arm deaths occurring in patients who received 50.4 Gy or less. The authors performed a separate survival analysis including only patients receiving the assigned radiation dose. Despite this, no survival advantage was noted in the high-dose arm. These authors concluded that higher radiation doses did not increase survival or locoregional control and that the standard radiation dose for patients treated with concurrent 5-FU and cisplatin chemotherapy is 50.4 Gy. Based on these data, standard dose of radiation therapy for esophageal

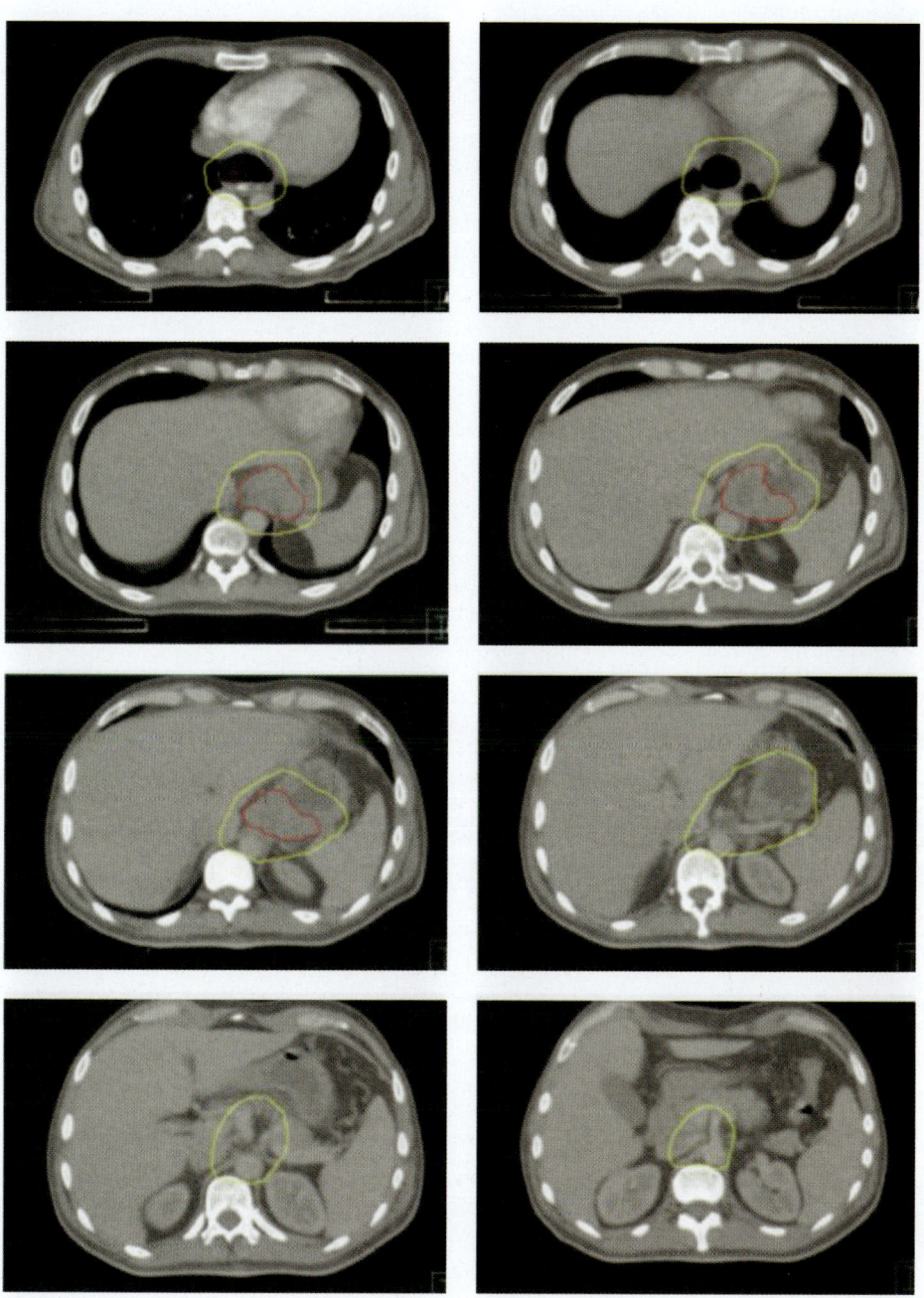

FIGURE 56.16. Consensus CTV contours for T3N0, Siewert II gastroesophageal junction cancer, gross tumor volume in *red*.

cancer is usually 50 to 50.4 Gy at 1.8 to 2 Gy per fraction, including delivery of similar doses in the definitive, adjuvant (45 to 50 Gy) or neoadjuvant (41.4 to 50 Gy) settings. Nonetheless, critics of this trial argue that older radiation techniques were utilized and that dose escalation should be evaluated using modern techniques. Randomized studies are ongoing to further evaluate this concept. The French Concorde trial is currently randomizing patients to receive 66 versus 50 Gy combined with FOLFOX for using IMRT/VMAT techniques in patients receiving definitive chemoradiotherapy with an elective nodal dose to 40 Gy.[138] Similarly, the Dutch ART deco trial is evaluating radiation dose escalation in nonoperable esophageal cancer patients (50.4 vs. 61 Gy with increasing dose per fraction concomitant boost) with concurrent carboplatin and paclitaxel. The United Kingdom SCOPE 2 study is a four-arm trial comparing carboplatin/paclitaxel versus cisplatin-/capecitabine-based chemoradiation, with a second randomization to standard versus high-dose radiation therapy (50 vs. 60 Gy, both in 25 fractions). Patients will receive a lead in of chemotherapy then be further randomized based on intratreatment PET analyses. Finally, a Chinese study is comparing a regimen of 50 Gy in 25

fractions with concurrent cisplatin and 5-FU versus a simultaneous integrated boost treatment to a total of 66 Gy in 30 fractions with concurrent cisplatin and 5-FU in nonoperable squamous cell carcinoma patients.

Brachytherapy

In addition to external beam radiation therapy (EBRT), intracavitary therapy can be used with curative or palliative intent. Brachytherapy has also been used as a dose escalation tool in addition to EBRT. The advantage of brachytherapy centers on exploitation of the inverse-square law and quick dose falloff, thus sparing surrounding tissues from radiation while providing focal dose escalation. The radioactive source of choice is usually [192]Ir. High–dose rate (HDR) techniques can deliver 100 to 400 Gy/hour, allowing treatment to be given in 5 to 10 minutes.

With brachytherapy, an afterloading catheter is introduced through the nose into the esophagus to the primary tumor site under fluoroscopic guidance. This is often performed with the patient on the simulation table. Contrast may be used to define the tumor site. CT scan can also be used to discern tumor location. After localization films are taken

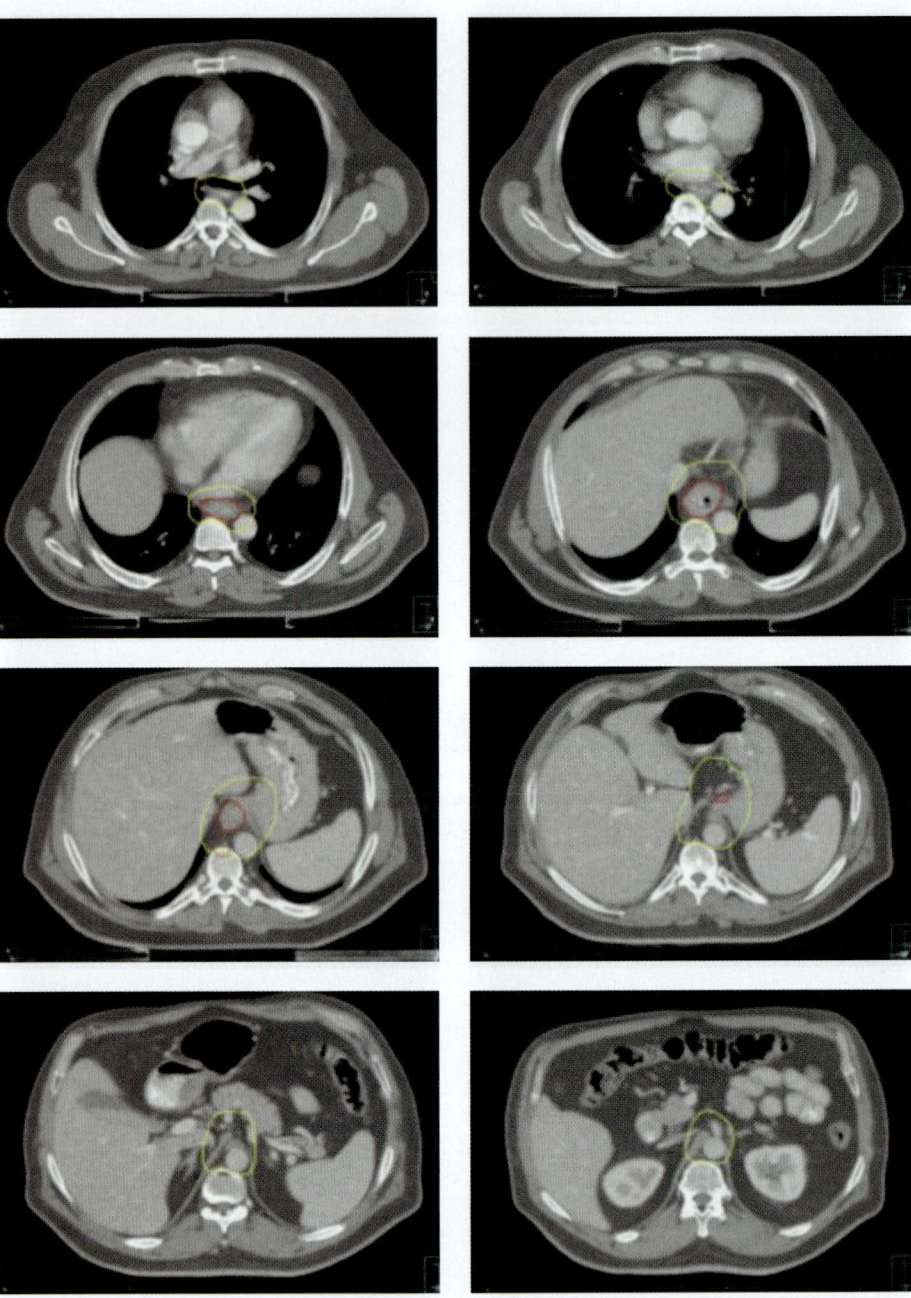

FIGURE 56.17. Consensus CTV contours for T3N1 distal esophageal cancer.

and dosimetry is generated, the catheter is then attached to a remote afterloader through a guide cable and the ^{192}Ir source inserted through remote control. Doses of 5 to 20 Gy are usually delivered to a depth of 1 cm from the center of the catheter. Dose can be shaped and modified through the use of dwell times.

RESULTS OF THERAPY

The best survival results have been reported in patients who have esophageal tumors that are truly localized. Survival rates range from 25% to >35% at 5 years, and these results have been attained using an array of treatment approaches. Problems arise in comparisons of various modalities, however, because of patient selection factors. A historical review of the Princess Margaret Hospital data[139] supported the concept that extent of tumor, rather than therapy, is the most important factor influencing survival. They found a significant correlation between T stage and response to treatment: T1 lesions showed a 100% response rate, whereas T2 and T3 lesions had response rates of 68% and 58%, respectively. Not unexpectedly,

they also found differences in survival according to T stage, M stage, and overall stage. Almost 20% of patients with stage I disease were alive at 3.5 years, whereas only 11% of stage II patients were alive after the same interval, and all patients with stage III died of disease by approximately 1.5 years following therapy.

Surgery Alone

Surgery remains a benchmark to which other modalities are compared. Surgery removes the tumor, a length of normal esophagus, and lymph nodes. Although multiple techniques exist for the resection of esophageal cancer, no one surgical approach has clearly been shown to be superior with regard to complications or outcomes. Proponents of more extended resection (including transthoracic approaches) have advocated that such procedures result in a superior nodal clearance and therefore offer a more complete "oncologic" resection. A trial from the Netherlands randomized 220 patients with esophageal adenocarcinoma to transhiatal esophagectomy alone or transthoracic esophagectomy with extended lymph node dissection. Patients undergoing transhiatal resection experienced

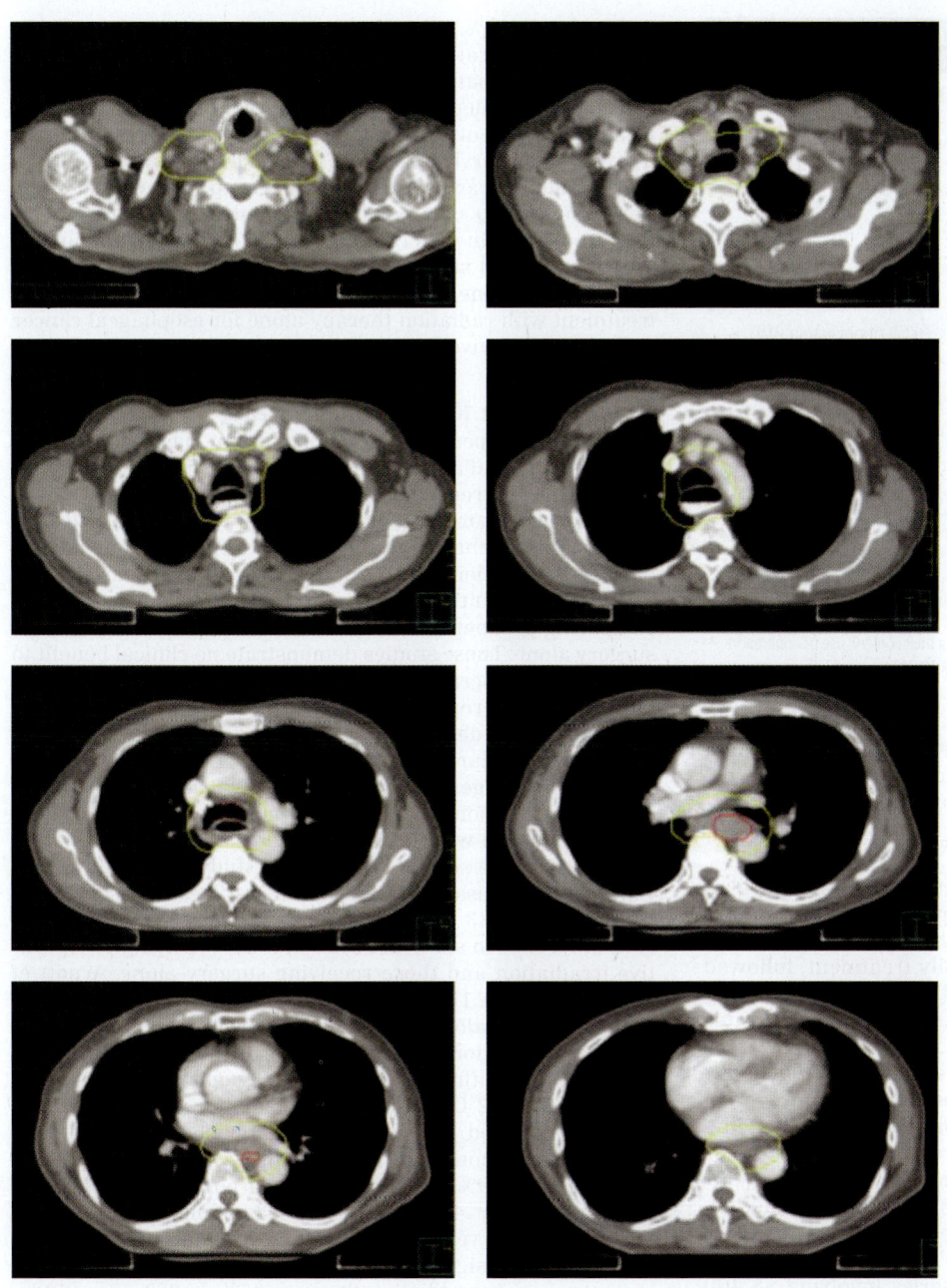

FIGURE 56.18. Consensus contours for T3N1 proximal esophageal cancer.

significantly fewer pulmonary complications and chylous leaks, as well as significantly reduced ventilator dependence and intensive care unit and hospital stays. At a median 4.7-year follow-up, no significant difference in locoregional recurrence was seen between the two groups (32% transhiatal vs. 31% transthoracic). Furthermore, no significant differences were seen in median disease-free survival (1.4 vs. 1.7 years; $P = .15$) or median overall survival (1.8 vs. 2.0 years; $P = .38$). However, there did appear to be a nonsignificant trend favoring the transthoracic approach in improved disease-free survival (5-year, 27% vs. 39%) and overall survival (5-year, 29% vs. 39%). The authors concluded that a transhiatal approach was associated with less morbidity relative to transthoracic surgery, with no apparent survival advantage with either technique, although a trend toward improved survival with a transthoracic approach was seen with longer follow-up.[51] Updated 5-year survival results were 34% versus 36%, respectively.[140] In contrast, a randomized trial from Japan comparing transhiatal to left thoracoabdominal approaches in patients with esophagogastric junction cancers. Both groups underwent total gastrectomy and splenectomy with extensive nodal dissection.

Ten-year survival was 37% for the transhiatal approach versus 24% for the thoracoabdominal approach ($P = .06$). The authors concluded left thoracoabdominal resection should be avoided in patients of the esophagogastric junction or gastric cardia.[141]

In summary, none of the surgical approaches to localized esophageal cancer has clearly been shown to be superior with regard to complications or outcomes, and no one standard surgical approach exists for esophageal cancer resection.

After resection alone, however, locoregional relapse is a common mode of failure. Contemporary randomized trials with surgery-alone arms have reported locoregional failure rates of 32% to 45%.[51,52,106,142] It should be remembered that patterns of failure reports often describe the first site of failure only and may include only patients undergoing R0 resection, potentially underreporting the true incidence of locoregional recurrence. These and other data suggest that even with modern surgical techniques, locoregional persistence of disease after resection remains a major problem. Prospective, randomized trials using surgery alone in the treatment of esophageal cancer have reported 3-year survival rates ranging from 6% to 48%, with more favorable rates likely reflecting inclusion of patients

TABLE 56.6 EXAMPLE OF NORMAL TISSUE DOSE CONSTRAINTS IN PLANNING OF ESOPHAGEAL CANCER

- Lung
  - $V_{40Gy} \leq 10\%$
  - $V_{30Gy} \leq 15\%$
  - $V_{20Gy} \leq 20\%$
  - $V_{10Gy} \leq 40\%$
  - $V_{05Gy} \leq 50\%$
  - Mean < 20 Gy
- Cord
  - Max ≤ 45 Gy
- Bowel
  - Max bowel dose < max PTV dose
  - $D_{05} \leq 45$ Gy
- Heart
  - $V_{30Gy} \leq 30\%$ (closer to 20% preferred)
  - Mean < 30 Gy
- Left Kidney, Right Kidney (evaluate each one separately):
  - No more than 33% of the volume can receive 18 Gy.
  - Mean dose < 18 Gy
- Liver
  - $V_{20Gy} \leq 30\%$
  - $V_{30Gy} \leq 20\%$
  - Mean < 25 Gy
- Stomach
  - Mean < 30 Gy (if not within PTV)
  - Max dose < 54 Gy

with earlier-stage disease[53,143–146] (Table 56.7). Given these high rates of relapse and poor long-term survival, the integration of adjuvant or neoadjuvant chemoradiation approaches into the treatment of esophageal cancer is rational and indicated.

Radiation Therapy Alone

A trial from China randomized 269 patients to either surgery alone or radiation therapy alone. Surgery entailed esophagectomy while radiation field varied by location of primary. Patients received 50 to 50.4 Gy of daily treatment, followed by reduced fields receiving 1.5 Gy BID to a cumulative dose of 68.4 to 71 Gy. The 1-, 3-, and 5-year overall survival rates in the surgery-alone group were 93%, 62%, and 37% versus 89%, 56%, and 35%, respectively. The authors concluded survival might be equivalent between these arms.[148] However, in most series, radiation therapy alone has been usually delivered when lesions are deemed inoperable because of tumor extent or medical contraindications and/or palliative treatment is indicated. In most series, patients receiving radiation as a sole treatment modality have a median survival of 6 to 12 months and 5-year survival of <10%.

A historical review analyzing 49 series involving >8,400 patients treated primarily with radiation therapy alone found overall survival rates at 1, 2, and 5 years to be 18%, 8%, and 6%, respectively.[149] Hancock and Glatstein[112] reviewed 9,511 patients and found only 5.8% were alive at 5 years. Okawa et al.[150] reported 5-year survival rates by stage. For patients with stage I disease, the 5-year survival rate was

20%; stage II, 10%; stage III, 3%; and stage IV, 0%. Overall, the 5-year survival rate was 9%. For cervical esophageal lesions treated with radiation alone, the cure rates were comparable with those in patients treated with surgery alone. Lederman[151] treated 263 patients with radiation therapy alone and reported 3- and 5-year survival rates of 11% and 7%, respectively. In a more contemporary series, an Intergroup randomized study (discussed later) comparing combined chemotherapy with 5-FU and cisplatin with radiotherapy (50 Gy) versus radiotherapy only (64 Gy) showed that 3-year actuarial survival with radiotherapy alone was 0%. These and other data suggest that treatment with radiation therapy alone for esophageal cancer patients is palliative in the vast majority of patients.

Preoperative Radiation Therapy

The use of preoperative radiation therapy has potential biologic and physical advantages, including increased resectability of tumors, increased tumor radioresponsiveness secondary to improved tumor oxygenation, a theoretical decreased likelihood of dissemination at the time of surgery, and avoidance of surgery in patients with rapidly progressive disease.

There are multiple, largely historical randomized studies comparing preoperative irradiation followed by surgery with surgery alone. These studies demonstrate no clinical benefit to the use of preoperative radiation therapy alone (Table 56.8). Launois et al.[152] reported delivering 40 Gy over 8 to 12 days with surgery 8 days later versus surgery alone. Resection rates were similar—70% and 58% for preoperative irradiation and for surgery alone, respectively. The 5-year survival rate after resection was 11.5% for those treated with surgery alone, compared with 9.5% for those treated with irradiation and surgery. The second randomized study, published by the European Organisation for Research and Treatment of Cancer (EORTC), used 33 Gy over 12 days.[153] There was no significant difference in survival between those receiving preoperative irradiation and those receiving surgery alone. Arnott et al.[154] reported on 176 patients, 86 of whom were treated with esophagectomy alone versus 90 who were treated with preoperative radiation therapy. Preoperative radiation therapy was delivered with 4-MV photons using opposed fields, delivering 20 Gy at 2 Gy/fraction. Resectability and local failure were not reported. Patients receiving low-dose radiation therapy did not demonstrate a benefit in 5-year overall survival rates (17% vs. 9% for surgery and preoperative radiation, respectively; $P = .4$). Wang et al.[155] randomized 206 patients to surgery alone versus 40 Gy in 2-Gy fractions delivered preoperatively. No significant survival advantage was seen for patients receiving radiation therapy (35% vs. 30%; $P > .05$).

A meta-analysis from the Oesophageal Cancer Collaborative Group updated data from five randomized trials of >1,100 patients comparing preoperative radiotherapy alone versus surgery alone. The majority of patients had squamous cell carcinoma. At a median follow-up of 9 years, the hazard ratio was 0.89, suggestive of an overall reduction in the risk of death of 11% and absolute survival benefit of 4% at 5 years with the use of preoperative radiotherapy. However, this was not statistically significant ($P = .06$). The authors concluded that there was no clear evidence that preoperative radiotherapy improves survival of patients with potentially resectable esophageal cancer.[4]

In general, there were no differences in resectability rates or survival in almost all of the individual studies. Interpretation of these varying studies is complicated by differences in radiation techniques, suboptimal radiation doses, and inadequate radiation volumes. Nonetheless, although preoperative radiation therapy alone may improve local control, there is no convincing data that it results in improved survival in esophageal cancer patients.

Postoperative Radiation Therapy

The main advantage of adjuvant versus neoadjuvant approaches is knowledge of the pathologic staging for

TABLE 56.7 COMPARISON OF SURGICAL ARMS IN RANDOMIZED STUDIES

Trial	Year	Patients (Total)	Patients (Surgical)	Median Survival (Months)	Two-Year Survival (%)	Three-Year Survival (%)
Walsh et al.[143]	1996	110	55	11	26	6
Urba et al.[52]	2001	100	50	18	NA	15
Bosset et al.[145]	1997	282	139	19	40	35
Kelsen et al.[106]	1998	440	227	16	37	23
MRC[144]	2002	802	402	13	34	NA
Burmeister[147]	2005	256	128	19	NA	31
van Hagen et al.[146]	2015	368	188	24	50	44
Mariette et al.[53]	2014	195	97	41	NA	34

MRC, Medical Research Council Oesophageal Cancer Working Group; NA, not applicable.

TABLE 56.8 RANDOMIZED TRIALS OF PREOPERATIVE RADIATION THERAPY FOR ESOPHAGEAL CANCER

Author	Patients	Dose (Gy)	Fraction (Gy)	Local Failure		Survival (5-Year)	
				Surgery	RT + Surgery	Surgery	RT + Surgery
Launois et al.[152]	109	40	NA	NA	NA	12	10
Gignoux et al.[153]	229	33	3.3	67	46	8	10
Arnott et al.[a154]	176	20	2	NA	NA	17	9
Wang et al.[155]	160	40	2	NA	NA	30	35

[a]Both squamous and adenocarcinoma.
NA, not applicable; RT, radiation therapy.

appropriately selected patients for therapy. Postoperative therapy may allow the radiation oncologist to treat areas at risk for recurrence while sparing otherwise normal radiosensitive structures, thereby decreasing toxicity. In addition, patients with pathologic T1, N0, and M0 or metastatic disease may be spared treatment. Postoperative irradiation has historically been delivered to patients with esophageal cancer who have bulky tumors with gross residual disease or histologically proven microscopic residual disease. Potential disadvantages of postoperative radiation include limited tolerance of normal tissues after gastric pull-up or intestinal interposition and irradiation of a devascularized tumor bed, potentially larger fields compared to a preoperative approach, and potential delays in adjuvant treatment delivery.

Three randomized trials have assessed surgery alone versus surgery followed by postoperative radiation therapy.[156–158] In a French trial, 221 patients with squamous cell carcinoma of the mid–lower esophagus undergoing esophagectomy were randomized to postoperative radiation therapy or no further treatment. Patients were stratified by extent of nodal involvement. Total dose was 45 to 55 Gy at 1.8 Gy/fraction, beginning within 3 months of surgery. Five-year survival in node-negative patients was 38% versus 7% with involved nodes. No significant survival difference was seen in patients receiving postoperative radiation versus surgery alone. Rates of locoregional recurrence were lower in patients receiving radiation therapy (85% vs. 70%; P = NS). However, in patients without nodal involvement, locoregional recurrence was significantly improved in patients receiving postoperative therapy (90% vs. 65%; P < .2). The authors concluded that postoperative radiation therapy did not improve survival after resection for squamous cell carcinoma.[156]

Investigators from the University of Hong Kong reported the results of a randomized trial of 130 patients treated with postoperative radiation therapy versus surgery alone. Patients who underwent either curative or palliative resections were included in this trial. Radiation therapy was delivered to a total dose of 49 Gy (curative patients) or 52.5 Gy (palliative patients) using 3.5-Gy fractions. Most patients had squamous cell histology. Local recurrence was noted in 15% of patients receiving radiation and 31% of patients with surgery only (P = .06). In patients with squamous cell carcinoma, the local recurrence rate was 15% with radiation therapy versus 36% with surgery alone (P = .02). Median survival in patients was worse in patients receiving postoperative radiotherapy versus control patients (8.7 vs. 15.2 months; P = .02). Ten patients undergoing surgery alone had tracheobronchial recurrence resulting in death versus three patients receiving adjuvant radiation therapy (P = .07). The authors concluded that postoperative radiation therapy was associated with increased morbidity and death caused by radiation injury, as well as with the early appearance of metastatic disease and a reduced overall survival, although patients receiving radiation therapy were less likely to have a tracheobronchial recurrence. However, it should be noted that the high rate of complications associated with radiation therapy in this study might possibly be related to the high dose per fraction and large total dose delivered.[157]

Last, a study conducted by Xiao et al.[158] randomized 549 patients to radical resection versus radical resection followed by radiation therapy. All patients had squamous cell carcinoma. The radiation dose delivered was 60 Gy in 6 weeks. Patients were classified into three groups: group 1, no lymph node involvement; group 2, one to two lymph nodes involved; and group 3, three or more lymph nodes involved. Results showed T stage, stage group, and the number of lymph nodes involved by tumor were highly predictive of survival. The 5-year survival rates for groups 1, 2, and 3 were 58.1%, 30.6%, and 14.4%, respectively. Local control and survival were improved in patients receiving postoperative irradiation. For patients with involved lymph nodes, 5-year survival rates for resection-only patients versus patients receiving resection and radiation therapy were 17.6% and 34.1%, respectively (P = .04).

In summary, postoperative radiation therapy may decrease local recurrence, particularly in the setting of involved margins, although the impact of this adjuvant treatment on overall survival remains less clear.

Postoperative Combined Chemoradiation

A large randomized Intergroup trial evaluating the role of adjuvant chemoradiation after surgery versus surgery alone for patients with adenocarcinoma of the stomach and GE junction was reported. In this study, patients with resected, margin-negative gastric or gastroesophageal junction adenocarcinoma were randomly assigned to surgery alone versus surgery with postoperative chemoradiotherapy. Approximately 20% of patients had lesions in the gastroesophageal junction. A significant survival advantage was seen in the adjuvantly treated group (median survival 27 vs. 36 months; p = .005). On subset analysis, this benefit was detected in patients with gastroesophageal cancer.[159] Long-term results at >10-year median follow-up continued to show significant improvement in overall and disease-free survival in the chemoradiation group, benefiting all T- and N-stage patients included in the trial.[160] Therefore, in patients with resected-stage group IB to IV, nonmetastatic GE junctional carcinoma, it is appropriate to advise adjuvant chemoradiotherapy in efforts to potentially improve upon local control and survival. In squamous cell carcinoma, no adjuvant randomized data exist, although institutional series suggests a potential survival benefit in lymph node–positive disease with adjuvant chemoradiation.[161,162]

Preoperative Chemotherapy

Five randomized trials showed conflicting results with the use of neoadjuvant chemotherapy alone in the treatment of esophageal cancer, with two of these trials also including gastric cancers. Kelsen et al.[106] reported the results of an Intergroup study randomizing 440 patients with squamous cell carcinoma and adenocarcinoma to receive either combined cisplatin or 5-FU chemotherapy for three cycles followed by resection, followed by a similar regimen of adjuvant chemotherapy, versus immediate resection with no chemotherapy. No apparent survival advantage (3-year survival of 23% vs. 26%) was seen in patients receiving chemotherapy. In addition, rates of local failure (32% vs. 31%) and distant metastasis development (41% vs. 50%) were not significantly different between the two groups. The authors concluded that neoadjuvant chemotherapy with cisplatin and 5-FU did not improve survival in patients with resectable esophageal cancer. Long-term results reported that only 59% and 63% of patients undergoing preoperative chemotherapy and surgery alone, respectively, underwent R0 resection, and patients undergoing less than R0 resection had an ominous prognosis, with only 5% of patients undergoing R1 resection surviving >5 years and no difference in median survival rates for patients with R1, R2, or no resection. In this follow-up study, patients with objective tumor regression after preoperative chemotherapy experienced improved survival. An important caveat from this study is that all long-term R1 survivors received adjuvant RT, and the authors concluded that after R1 resection, postoperative chemoradiotherapy offers the possibility of long-term disease-free survival to a small percentage of patients.[163]

In contrast to the Intergroup study, a similar trial from the Medical Research Council (MRC) randomized 802 patients with squamous cell carcinoma or adenocarcinoma of the esophagus to either two cycles of combined cisplatin/5-FU chemotherapy or surgery alone. Patients receiving neoadjuvant chemotherapy had a statistically improved 2-year survival (43% vs. 34%).[144] Follow-up analysis at a median follow-up of 6 years showed a persistent, significant survival benefit in the chemotherapy group (5-year survival 23% vs. 17%), with the effect maintained for both squamous cell carcinoma and adenocarcinoma patients.[164] The reason for outcomes differences between these trials is not clear. A follow-up trial from the MRC (OE05) randomized patients to neoadjuvant cisplatin/5-FU for 2 cycles versus 4 cycles of ECX (epirubicin, cisplatin, and capecitabine) for esophageal adenocarcinoma. No overall survival difference was seen between the arms. The authors concluded four cycles of neoadjuvant ECX compared with two cycles of CF did not increase survival, and cannot be considered standard of care.[164a]

A smaller trial of 169 patients with squamous cell carcinoma of the esophagus randomized patients to receive preoperative chemotherapy alone with two to four cycles of etoposide- and cisplatin-based chemotherapy versus surgery alone. Median and 5-year survival rates significantly favored the chemotherapy group at 16 versus 12 months and 26 versus 17%, respectively. The authors concluded that preoperative chemotherapy with a combination of etoposide and cisplatin improves survival in patients with squamous carcinoma of the esophagus.[165]

A more heterogeneous European study (the Medical Research Council Adjuvant Gastric Infusional Chemotherapy, or MAGIC, trial) randomly assigned patients with resectable adenocarcinoma of the stomach, gastroesophageal junction, or lower esophagus to preoperative and postoperative chemotherapy with epirubicin, cisplatin, and 5-FU versus surgery alone. Although originally designed to include patients with only tumors of the stomach, eligibility was later expanded to include tumors of the lower one-third of the esophagus. Approximately one-fourth of patients had adenocarcinoma involving the lower esophagus or gastroesophageal junction. No patient achieved pathologic complete response. However, patients receiving perioperative chemotherapy had a hazard ratio for death of 0.75, which was highly significant. Five-year survival in patients receiving chemotherapy was 36% versus 23% in patients undergoing surgery alone (P = .009). Subgroup analysis of patients with lower esophageal or gastroesophageal junction tumors showed benefit to the delivery of perioperative chemotherapy.[166]

A follow-up study to the MAGIC trial investigated the role of perioperative epirubicin, cisplatin, and capecitabine, with or without the addition of bevacizumab. One thousand sixty-three patients with esophagogastric adenocarcinoma were randomized. No survival benefit was seen in the bevacizumab arm, whereas wound healing complications were more prevalent with higher rates of postoperative anastomotic leak rates with bevacizumab, prompting discontinuation of recruitment of patients with lower esophageal or junctional tumors planned for esophagogastric resection.[167]

French investigators reported the results of a similar randomized trial of 224 patients assigned to perioperative chemotherapy (cisplatin and 5-FU) versus surgery alone. Although originally designed to include only patients with tumors of the lower one-third of the esophagus or gastroesophageal junction, eligibility was later expanded to include gastric cancers. Most patients (75%) had disease of the lower esophagus or gastroesophageal junction. Chemotherapy consisted of planned two or three preoperative and three or four postoperative cycles. This study was prematurely terminated because of low accrual. Patients receiving chemotherapy had improved overall survival (5-year, 38% vs. 24%; P = .02), disease-free survival (5-year, 34% vs. 19%, P = .003), and R0 resection rates (84% vs. 73%; P = .04). Only 50% of patients received postoperative chemotherapy. T0 disease (complete pathologic response at the primary site) was seen in 3% of neoadjuvantly treated patients. Total locoregional recurrence rates were 24% and 26%, respectively, in the chemotherapy versus surgery group, with distant recurrence rates of 42% versus 56%, respectively.[168] In addition to the foregoing studies, two meta-analyses suggested that neoadjuvant chemotherapy resulted in absolute 2- and 5-year survival benefit of 7% and 4%, respectively.[169,170]

Preoperative Chemoradiation Versus Surgery Alone

Walsh et al.[143] reported a randomized study to evaluate the role of concurrent preoperative chemoradiation combined with surgery. A total of 110 patients with adenocarcinoma of the esophagus were randomized to receive cisplatin, 5-FU, and concurrent radiation therapy followed by surgery versus surgery alone. Combined-modality patients received two courses of chemotherapy at weeks 1 and 6. Patients were treated using anteroposterior–posteroanterior fields (later changed to a three-field technique) to a total dose of 4,000 cGy in 15 fractions. Surgery was performed 4 to 6 weeks later, using five separate approaches. Median survival was 16 months with preoperative chemoradiation therapy compared to 11 months for the patients treated with surgery alone (P = .01). The 1-, 2-, and 3-year survival rates were 52%, 37%, and 32%, respectively, for patients who received multimodality therapy and 44%, 26%, and 6%, respectively, for those patients assigned to surgery. These results were significant at 3 years (P = .01). The authors concluded that neoadjuvant chemoradiation was superior to surgery alone in patients with resectable esophageal adenocarcinoma. A follow-up report of this study described two simultaneously conducted randomized trials in patients with (a) adenocarcinoma and (b) squamous cell carcinoma. Combined trial results suggest that neoadjuvant chemoradiotherapy conferred a significant survival advantage in both groups, with an associated 54% relative risk reduction in lymph node metastases (64% vs. 29%, P < .001). Pathologic complete response was seen in 25% and 31% of adenocarcinoma and squamous cell carcinoma patients, respectively. Patients receiving neoadjuvant therapy, achieving pathologic complete response, and those with lymph node–negative disease demonstrated superior survival.[171] This trial has been criticized for its poor surgery-alone results, short follow-up, and lack of prerandomization CT staging.

Urba et al.[52] reported the results of 100 patients with nonmetastatic esophageal carcinoma (squamous and adenocarcinoma histology) randomized to receive preoperative chemoradiation followed by surgery versus transhiatal esophagectomy alone. Chemotherapy consisted of cisplatin, 5-FU, and vinblastine. Only 69% of the patients were able to receive the intended chemotherapy dose. Radiation was delivered at 1.5 Gy twice daily for 3 weeks to a total dose of 4,500 cGy. No elective nodal irradiation was performed. Surgery was performed on day 42. Tumors >5 cm, patient age >70 years, and squamous cell histology were associated with inferior survival. At median follow-up of

8 years, no significant difference in survival was seen between treatment arms, with a median survival of 17 months. However, 3-year survival rate was 16% in the surgery-alone arm versus 30% in the combined modality arm (P = .15). A higher incidence of locoregional failure as first site of failure was seen in surgery-alone patients (42% vs. 19%, P = .02). In patients experiencing pathologic complete response, a median survival of 50 months and a 3-year survival rate of 64% were seen versus patients with residual tumor in the surgical specimen, where median survival was 12 months with a 3-year survival rate of 19% (P = .01). The investigators stated that "Although this is not statistically significant, this suggests a possible trend to the benefit of multimodality therapy, but the sample size was too small to detect a more subtle survival difference," and that surgery should be continued as a standard of care.

Bosset et al.[145] reported an EORTC trial randomizing 282 patients with squamous cell carcinoma of the esophagus to either immediate surgical resection or preoperative therapy using concurrent cisplatin chemotherapy with radiation therapy. Patients were treated with split-course radiotherapy with a 2-week interval, using 3.7 Gy/fraction to a total of 37 Gy. Postoperative mortality was significantly higher in patients receiving preoperative therapy (12% vs. 4%). Outcomes showed patients receiving neoadjuvant therapy experienced a significant improvement in disease-free survival, cancer-related mortality, margin-negative resection, and local control; however, no improvement in overall survival was seen versus patients undergoing surgery alone (median survival was 18.6 months for both groups). The authors concluded that neoadjuvant chemoradiation improved disease-free survival and local control in patients with squamous cell carcinoma of the esophagus but had no impact on overall survival. They judged that the increase in postoperative mortality in the combined group "could be due to deleterious effects of the high-dose of radiation per fraction," among other factors, and believed that the dose of 3.7 Gy/fraction "probably had a detrimental effect." This trial has also been criticized for the split-course treatment approach, as well as for potential delivery of suboptimal chemotherapy.

Burmeister et al.[147] reported an Australian study randomizing 257 patients with adenocarcinoma and squamous cell carcinoma of the esophagus to surgery alone versus neoadjuvant therapy using concomitant 5-FU and cisplatin. Patient received 2.33 Gy/fraction to a total dose of 35 Gy. Patients undergoing neoadjuvant therapy had a 16% pathologic complete response rate at resection. Patients receiving neoadjuvant therapy were more likely to undergo curative resection and have negative lymph nodes on histologic examination. However, no significant improvement in median survival was seen (19 vs. 22 months; hazard ratio 0.89; P = .57). On subset analysis, there appeared to be a trend toward improved survival in patients with squamous cell carcinoma undergoing neoadjuvant therapy versus surgery alone (progression-free survival hazard ratio, 0.47; P = .01; overall survival hazard ratio, 0.69; P = .16). The authors concluded that neoadjuvant chemoradiation as delivered in their study provided no obvious survival benefit in patients with esophageal cancer, although further study was warranted in patients with squamous cell carcinoma. Potential criticisms of this trial include delivery of a single chemotherapy cycle, as well as delivery of lower radiation doses.

Results of a Cancer and Leukemia Group B study described 56 patients (75% with adenocarcinoma) randomized to either surgery alone or neoadjuvant chemoradiation followed by surgical resection. Patients in the neoadjuvant therapy arm received cisplatin/5-FU–based chemotherapy and 50.4 Gy of EBRT at 1.8 Gy/fraction. This trial was closed prematurely because of poor accrual. In patients undergoing neoadjuvant therapy, pathologic complete response rate was 40%. A significant improvement in local control and survival was seen in patients receiving neoadjuvant combined-modality therapy (5-year survival, 39% vs. 16%). The authors concluded that neoadjuvant chemoradiation

in patients with esophageal cancer significantly improves progression-free and overall survival.[172]

Results of the largest randomized trial (the Chemoradiotherapy for Oesophageal Cancer Followed by Surgery Study, or CROSS trial) assessing neoadjuvant chemoradiotherapy in the treatment of esophageal cancer showed a significant survival benefit in patients receiving preoperative therapy, with the majority of patients included in this trial having locally advanced adenocarcinoma.[146] Patients with resectable T1N1 or T2-3 N0-1 tumors received preoperative chemoradiotherapy consisting of weekly paclitaxel and carboplatin with concurrent radiotherapy to a dose of 41.4 Gy versus surgery alone. R0 resection rates were 92% in patients receiving neoadjuvant chemoradiotherapy versus 69% for surgery alone, with a pathologic complete response rate of 29% in patients receiving preoperative therapy. No significant differences were seen in in-hospital mortality (4% vs. 4%). Median survival was 49 months in patients receiving chemoradiotherapy versus 24 months in surgery alone, with a significant improvement in 3-year survival (58% vs. 44%). An updated analysis of this trial showed that 95% of patients were able to complete the entire neoadjuvant chemoradiotherapy regimen. After a median follow-up of 84.1 months in surviving patients, median overall survival was 48.6 months in neoadjuvant arm versus 24 months with surgery alone. Most strikingly, median overall survival in squamous cell patients was 81.6 months versus 21.1 months (P = .008), whereas it was 43.2 months versus 27.1 months in adenocarcinoma patients (P = .038). Patients receiving neoadjuvant treatment had a significant decrease in both locoregional progression (22% vs. 38%) and distant progression (39% vs. 48%).[54] The authors concluded that weekly administration of carboplatin and paclitaxel with concurrent radiotherapy improves overall survival compared to surgery alone and that this regimen can be considered the standard of care for patients with resectable esophageal or esophagogastric junction cancer. A pattern of recurrence analysis of the CROSS study indicated that preoperative therapy reduced locoregional recurrence from 34% to 14% (P < .001) as well as reduction in peritoneal carcinomatosis (14% vs. 4%, P < .001) and hematogenous spread (35% vs. 29%, P = .025). Locoregional recurrence occurred in 5% of cases within the target volume, 2% at the field border, and 6% outside the radiation target volume, whereas only 1% had an isolated in-field recurrence.[173]

In contrast, a trial from France of 195 patients with clinically staged early-stage esophageal cancer randomized patients to receive preoperative chemoradiotherapy versus surgery alone. Study outcomes showed no significant difference in survival.[53] In this study, patients with early-stage disease (stage I to II) were randomized to receive surgery alone versus neoadjuvant chemoradiotherapy using concurrent 5-FU and cisplatin with 45 Gy. Postoperative mortality rates were 3.4% in the surgery-alone group versus 11.1% in the neoadjuvant group (P = .049). Three-year overall survival was 53.0% versus 47.5% (P = .749); however, despite the higher postoperative mortality rates, 5-year survival outcomes were 41% versus 34% in favor of the combined arm (NS). Additionally, patterns of failure analysis showed a significant improvement in local control in patients who were assigned to receive neoadjuvant therapy, nearly halving the rate of locoregional recurrence (29% vs. 15%). Disease recurrence rates were also significantly reduced in patients receiving neoadjuvant treatment. A follow-up report of surgery alone patients in this trial reported recurrent disease in 47% of patients undergoing surgery alone versus 31% neoadjuvant therapy (P = .03); locoregional recurrence was seen in 17% versus 30% (P = .047) and distant recurrence 23% versus 31% (P = .244) in the neoadjuvant and surgery arms, respectively.[174] The authors concluded that neoadjuvant chemoradiotherapy with cisplatin and 5-FU did not improve survival but increased postoperative mortality for patients with early-stage esophageal cancer. However, the lack of survival benefit with trimodality therapy in this study seems to be a result of increased

TABLE 56.9 RESULTS OF PREOPERATIVE COMBINED CHEMORADIATION VERSUS SURGERY ALONE—PHASE III TRIALS

Study	Median Follow-up (Year)	Pathology	Regimen	Number of Patients	Pathologic Complete Response	Three-Year Survival	Survival Difference
Urba et al.[52] (Michigan)	8.2	SCC + adeno	5-FU–CDDP–Vinb/45 Gy Surg	50 / 50	28 / –	CMT/Surg: 30% / Surg alone: 16%	$P = .15$
Bosset et al.[145] (EORTC)	4.6	SCC	CDDP/37 Gy Surg	143 / 138	20 / –	CMT/Surg: 33% / Surg alone: 36%	NS
Walsh et al.[143] (Ireland)	1.5	Adeno	5-FU–CDDP/40 Gy Surg	58 / 55	22 / –	CMT/Surg: 32% / Surg alone: 6%	$P = .01$
Burmeister et al.[147] (Australia)	5.4	SCC + adeno	5-FU–CDDP/35 Gy Surg	128 / 128	16 / –	CMT/Surg: 35% / Surg alone: 31%	NS
Tepper et al.[172] (USA)	6.0	SCC + adeno	5-FU–CDDP/50 Gy Surg	30 / 26	40 / –	CMT/Surg: 39% (5 y) / Surg alone: 16% (5 y)	$P = .008$
van Hagen et al.[54,146] (Netherlands)	7	SCC + adeno	Pac–Carbo/41.4 Gy Surg	180 / 188	29 / –	CMT/Surg: 58% / Surg alone: 44%	$P = .003$
Mariette et al.[53] (France)	7.8	SCC + adeno	5-FU–CDDP/45 Gy Surg	97 / 98	33 / –	CMT/Surg: 47.5% / Surg alone: 53%	NS

adeno, adenocarcinoma; Carbo, carboplatin; CDDP, cisplatin; CMT, combined modality therapy; EORTC, European Organisation for Research and Treatment of Cancer; 5-FU, 5-fluorouracil; med OS, median overall survival; Pac, paclitaxel; SCC, squamous cell carcinoma; Surg, surgery; Vinb, vinblastine.

postoperative mortality, which is likely multifactorial. A report from Chinese investigators of 451 patients with Stage IIb-III squamous cell carcinoma of the thoracic esophagus randomized patients to receive neoadjuvant vinorelbine/cisplatin with 40 Gy followed by resection versus resection alone. Pathologic complete response was seen in 43% of patients in the radiation containing arm. R0 resection (98% vs. 91%, p=0.002), and overall survival rates were significantly improved in the combined modality therapy arm (70% vs. 62% 3-year survival, p=0.035). The authors concluded neoadjuvant chemoradiotherapy plus surgery improved survival among patients with locally advanced esophageal squamous cell carcinoma.[174a]

Outcomes of these trials are shown in Table 56.9.

Given these conflicting results of contemporary trials, multiple meta-analyses have been performed. Two of the largest and most contemporary of these demonstrated an absolute 2- and 5-year overall survival benefit of 13% and 6.5% with the use of neoadjuvant chemoradiotherapy, respectively, when compared to surgery-alone approaches, also suggesting a larger benefit of preoperative chemoradiotherapy as compared to a chemotherapy alone.[169,170] It should be kept in mind that some of the included trials used sequential (vs. concurrent) chemotherapy, delivered what would be considered suboptimal doses of radiation therapy, used antiquated radiation therapy techniques, delivered (arguably) inadequate chemotherapy, and so on, potentially underestimating the effect of neoadjuvant combined modality therapy. That being said, an updated meta-analysis including a total of 24 randomized trials evaluating the role of neoadjuvant chemoradiotherapy, neoadjuvant chemotherapy, or comparison of the two in patients with resectable esophageal cancer was reported,[175] evaluating the outcomes of >4,000 patients. All-cause mortality for neoadjuvant chemoradiotherapy trials estimated an absolute survival benefit at 2 years of 8.7%, with survival benefits similar between squamous cell carcinoma and adenocarcinoma patients. By comparison, estimated absolute survival difference at 2 years was 5.1% in patients receiving neoadjuvant chemotherapy and was significant only for adenocarcinoma patients. The authors concluded that neoadjuvant chemoradiotherapy improves survival compared with surgery alone in operable patients, as does neoadjuvant chemotherapy, although the benefit of neoadjuvant chemotherapy was not as great as with neoadjuvant chemoradiotherapy. They also concluded that a clear advantage of one over the other is not established, and further randomized trials comparing these two strategies are warranted.

In summary, the above data suggest that neoadjuvant concurrent chemoradiation improves local control and overall survival versus surgery alone in patients with potentially resectable esophageal cancer.

Preoperative Chemoradiation Versus Preoperative Chemotherapy

A randomized trial comparing neoadjuvant chemotherapy alone versus neoadjuvant combined-modality therapy was conducted by German investigators (Preoperative Chemotherapy, or Radiochemotherapy in Esophagogastric Adenocarcinoma, or POET, trial).[176] Patients with advanced esophagogastric adenocarcinoma were randomized to receive (a) cisplatin-/5-FU–based chemotherapy alone versus (b) a similar induction chemotherapy, followed by concurrent cisplatin/etoposide with 30 Gy of radiation therapy. Both groups went on to receive surgery. Although this study was closed early because of poor accrual, patients receiving preoperative chemoradiotherapy had significantly higher N0 rates (37% vs. 64%; $P = .04$) and pathologic complete response rates (2% vs. 16%; $P = .03$), as well as significant trends toward improved local control (59% vs. 76%; $P = .06$) and overall survival (3-year survival, 28% vs. 47%; $P = .07$; hazard ratio, .67). The authors concluded that preoperative combined modality improves overall survival as compared to chemotherapy alone in patients with locally advanced esophagogastric adenocarcinoma.

A multicenter phase II Scandinavian trial randomised 181 patients with esophageal or gastroesophageal cancer to neoadjuvant chemotherapy with cisplatin/5-FU or the same chemotherapy concurrent with 40 Gy of radiotherapy. Primary trial end point of histologic complete response was higher in the radiation containing arm (28% vs. 9%, p=0.02), as was lymph node positivity rate (62% vs. 35%, p=0.001) and R0 resection rate (74% vs. 87%, p=0.04), although no significant survival difference was seen. The authors postulated that the lack of survival benefit may be due to increased deaths related to radiation therapy.[176a] A smaller phase II study from Australian investigators randomized 75 patients to receive either preoperative chemotherapy with cisplatin and infusional 5-FU or preoperative chemoradiotherapy with the same drugs with radiation therapy commencing day 21 of chemotherapy, delivering 35 Gy in 15 fractions.[177] Histopathologic response rate and noncurative resection rates were significantly improved in the radiation-containing arm (8% vs. 31% and 11% vs. 0%, respectively). However, median overall survival was not significantly different between the groups (29 vs. 32 months). The authors concluded that despite their being no difference in survival, the potential advantage of achieving negative margins made preoperative chemoradiotherapy a reasonable option for bulky, locally advanced resectable adenocarcinoma of the esophagus. A meta-analysis analyzing 5 randomized control trials (709 patients) demonstrated that neoadjuvant chemoradiotherapy significantly increased rates of pathologic complete response/R0 resection rates in both adenocarcinoma and squamous cell carcinoma patients compared to chemotherapy alone. A significant increase in 3-year survival was seen only in squamous cell carcinoma patients (56.8% vs. 42.8%, $P = .003$), whereas in adenocarcinoma patients, no significant difference was seen (46.3% vs. 41%, $P = .34$).[178]

Ongoing trials are evaluating the optimal approach in these patients. The European MAGIC versus CROSS (NeoAEGIS) trial is comparing neoadjuvant chemotherapy to chemoradiation in esophagogastric junctional adenocarcinomas. A Japanese three-arm randomized trial (the NExT trial) is comparing neoadjuvant cisplatin/5-FU versus docetaxel, cisplatin, and 5-FU versus radiotherapy with concurrent cisplatin/5-FU in patients with locally advanced esophageal cancer.

The Australian TOPGEAR study is currently randomizing patients to perioperative ECF versus preoperative chemoradiation plus perioperative ECF for resectable gastric cancer and resectable adenocarcinoma of the stomach and gastroesophageal junction. The ESOPEC trial from Germany is randomizing operable patients with esophageal adenocarcinoma to preoperative chemotherapy (FLOT: 5-FU, leucovorin, oxaliplatin, docetaxel) versus chemoradiation (CROSS regimen).

Radiation Therapy Alone Versus Chemoradiation

There are multiple randomized studies comparing radiation therapy alone with concurrent radiation and chemotherapy[55,179,180] as definitive therapy. However, small patient numbers, substandard chemotherapy delivery, and the use of suboptimal radiotherapy techniques handicap many of these studies. This makes treatment results difficult to interpret. The landmark trial establishing the superiority of concurrent chemoradiation to radiation therapy alone was Radiation Therapy Oncology Group (RTOG) 85-01. Herskovic et al.[181] reported results of this two-arm trial that treated 60 control patients with radiation alone to a total dose of 64 Gy versus 61 patients with 50 Gy of radiation therapy with concurrent 5-FU and cisplatin. The chemotherapy protocol consisted of four planned courses of infusional 5-FU and cisplatin. Although less radiation was delivered in the concurrent-therapy arm, the results demonstrated a significant advantage of the combined modality arm over the radiation-alone arm. The median survival in patients treated by radiation alone was 8.9 months compared with 12.5 months for those treated with combined therapy, with 2-year survival rate 10% versus 38%; the incidence of local recurrence decreased from 24% to 16%, and the 2-year distant metastasis rate decreased from 26% to 12%. Because of this highly significant survival difference, the randomization was stopped, and 69 additional patients were treated on the chemoradiation arm. Updated trial results[55,182] showed that at 5 years, survival rates were 26% and 0%, respectively, for chemoradiation and radiation therapy alone. Local recurrence rates were also decreased with the use of combined modality therapy versus radiation alone (45% vs. 69%), and distant metastases were more frequent in the radiation-alone arm at 40% versus 12% for the combined-modality group. The incidence of acute toxicity, however, was higher for the combined-modality arm versus the radiation-alone arm (44% vs. 25%). Similarly, the incidence of life-threatening side effects, including hematologic toxicity and fistula formation, was increased from 3% to 20%. In conclusion, this study demonstrated a significant improvement in local control, median and overall survival, and distant metastasis development with the addition of chemotherapy, at the cost of increased side effects.

Comparison of outcomes data from "definitive" chemoradiation approaches suggests that survival with combined chemoradiation is similar to that achieved by surgery alone. In previously discussed studies, median survivals of 14 to 20 months and 5-year survival rates of 20% to 30% were achieved with chemoradiation alone; in comparison, in the MRC trial and Intergroup trial evaluating surgery alone, median survivals were 13 to 16 months, with 5-year survivals of approximately 20%. In addition, local failure rates appear similar. For example, in the RTOG/ Intergroup studies using chemoradiation therapy alone, local failure rates as a first site of failure range from 39% to 45%. In comparison, local failure rate for the Intergroup study evaluating surgery alone was 31%. However, this analysis was limited to patients undergoing R0 resection only (59% of patients).[163] This would undoubtedly be higher if all patients were considered. Therefore, local failure and survival rates appear similar between "definitive" chemoradiation and surgical approaches.

Novel Chemoradiation Approaches

In attempts to improve outcomes in patients with nonoperable esophageal cancer, the SCOPE-1 trial was initiated in the United Kingdom. Patients were randomized to receive neoadjuvant cisplatin and capecitabine for 2 cycles, followed by initiation of radiation therapy cycles 3 and 4 (50 Gy in 25 fractions), with or without concurrent cetuximab. Two hundred fifty-eight patients were recruited (73% squamous cell). Median overall survival was 34.5 months in the non-cetuximab arm versus 24.7 months in the cetuximab-containing arm ($P = .137$), and 3-year overall survival 47% vs. 38%.[183] Similarly, a trial conducted through the RTOG (0436) randomized 344 patients with nonoperable esophageal cancer to weekly cisplatin, paclitaxel, and radiation therapy (50.4 Gy), with or without the addition of weekly cetuximab. Based on interim analyses, the study stopped accrual of adenocarcinoma patients and later squamous cell carcinoma patients. The 12- and 24-month survival rates for the cetuximab-containing arm were 64% and 44%, respectively, versus 65% and 42%, respectively ($P = .70$). Additionally, no difference in outcomes was seen when stratifying by histology. The authors concluded the addition of cetuximab to concurrent chemoradiation did not improve overall survival.[184]

The French PRODIGE5/ACCORD17 phase III trial compared 5-FU/cisplatin with FOLFOX4-based chemoradiotherapy. After a median follow-up of 25 months, progression-free survival was 9.4 and 9.7 months, respectively, with no significant differences observed in terms of high-grade toxicities between the two arms.[185]

Based on an overall survival advantage seen in metastatic esophagogastric patients with the addition of trastuzumab (a monoclonal antibody against HER2 receptors) to fluoropyrimidine-/cisplatin-based chemotherapy,[186] the RTOG is currently conducting a trial (RTOG 1010) randomizing patients with locally advanced esophageal adenocarcinoma to receive 50.4 Gy with weekly carboplatin and paclitaxel versus the same regimen with concurrent and maintenance trastuzumab (HER-2–overexpressing patients). The PROTECT from France is comparing preoperative chemoradiation with paclitaxel/ carboplatin versus a FOLFOX-based regimen in resectable esophageal and gastroesophageal junction tumors.

Chemoradiation Versus Chemoradiation Followed by Surgery

Two randomized trials examined whether surgery is necessary after combined-modality therapy. A report from French investigators randomized 445 patients with clinically resectable squamous cell or adenocarcinoma of the esophagus.[187] All patients received concurrent 5-fluorouracil and cisplatin-based chemoradiation. Patients were treated with one of two radiation regimens: 46 Gy over 4.5 weeks (continuous) or 30 Gy at 15 Gy/ week (split course). Two hundred fifty-nine patients who had at least a partial response were then randomized to either surgery or additional combined-modality therapy of 5-FU and cisplatin delivered concurrent with radiation (either an additional 20 Gy at 2 Gy/day or a split course of 15 Gy). No significant difference in 2-year survival (34% vs. 40%; $P = .56$) or median survival (18 vs. 19 months) was seen between the groups, although 2-year local control results favored the surgical arm (66% vs. 57%). The death rate at 3 months following treatment was 9% in the surgery group versus 1% in the combined-modality therapy–alone group. In addition, patients undergoing surgery were found to have a worse quality of life. However, the rate of stent and dilatation requirement was higher in the nonsurgical arm. Additionally, in a separate analysis, patients who were not randomized in this trial (i.e., nonresponders) were found to have a survival benefit with surgical resection.[188] The results of this trial suggest that surgery after chemoradiation in responding patients does not further enhance survival.

In another study, from Germany, patients with potentially resectable squamous cell carcinoma of the esophagus received induction chemotherapy with 5-FU, leucovorin, etoposide, and cisplatin for three cycles, followed by concurrent etoposide and cisplatin with 40 Gy of EBRT.[57] Patients were then randomized to receive surgery versus continuing with combined chemoradiation (total radiation dose increased to 60 to 65 Gy, with or without brachytherapy). Local control was significantly improved in patients undergoing surgery (2-year local control, 64% vs. 41%; P < .05). Despite this, no significant difference in survival was seen (median survival, 16 vs. 15 months; 3-year survival; 31% vs. 24%; P = NS). The "severe" postoperative complication rate (including infection, leak) was 70%, and the hospital mortality rate was 11%. Overall, treatment-related mortality was significantly higher in patients undergoing surgery (13% vs. 3.5%). In patients who did not respond to induction chemotherapy, 3-year survival was improved in patients undergoing surgery (18% vs. 9%). On regression analysis, only tumor response to induction chemotherapy was found to be a significant prognostic factor. An important caveat to this trial was that only approximately two-thirds of patients in the surgery arm actually had surgery. The authors concluded that (a) surgery after combined-modality therapy improves local control but had no impact on overall survival and (b) nonresponders to induction chemotherapy may benefit from surgery, and it may be appropriate to individualize therapy based on response to induction treatment. Although it has not been well studied, retrospective experience suggested that definitive chemoradiation in patients with adenocarcinoma of the esophagus results in median survival of 21 months and 2-, 3-, and 5-year survival rates of 44%, 33%, and 20% respectively.[189]

A large, multicenter study was conducted to assess the impact of salvage esophagectomy following definitive chemoradiotherapy on clinical outcome. Comparisons were performed between patients undergoing salvage (n = 308) versus planned (n = 540) esophagectomy. Additionally, patients were analyzed in the salvage arm by persistent versus recurrent disease. In-hospital mortality was similar in both salvage and planned resections (8.4 vs. 9.3%). Anastomotic leak rates (17.2 vs. 10.7%) and surgical site infection were both more frequent in the salvage group. Overall and disease-free survival rates were similar between the cohorts. In the salvage group, overall survival was worse in the persistent group. Of note is that doses higher than 55 Gy were linked with increased postoperative morbidity and mortality in this analysis. The authors concluded that salvage esophagectomy can offer acceptable short- and long-term outcomes in selected patients at experienced centers and that persistent cancer following chemoradiotherapy may be more aggressive and associated with a poor survival.[190] Similarly, RTOG 0246 was a single-arm trial in which patients received induction chemotherapy with fluorouracil, cisplatin, and paclitaxel followed by concurrent chemoradiation with 5-FU/cisplatin to 50.4 Gy. In follow-up evaluation, if there was clinical suspicion of residual disease, patients were taken immediately to surgery; however, clinical completely responding patients were followed with serial endoscopy and imaging. Of 41 patients entered, 21 (52%) were deemed to have persistent disease with 17 taken immediately to surgery, all with residual disease noted. Of 15 clinical complete responders, 3 (20%) developed recurrent locoregional disease without distant metastases and underwent salvage resection at 3 to 8 months following treatment completion. Overall, 5-year survival was 37%, and 20/41 patients (49%) did not require esophagectomy. The authors concluded that selective salvage

esophagectomy is a viable option in patients who are at higher risk of resection or refuse to undergo surgery.[191]

The role of salvage (versus upfront) esophagectomy following chemoradiotherapy remains a topic of investigation. The French ESOSTRATE trial is currently randomizing patients with operable esophageal cancer achieving clinical complete response following neoadjuvant chemoradiotherapy between systematic surgery and surveillance with selective salvage surgery. The nonrandomized preSANO trial from the Netherlands is investigating the feasibility of salvage surgery with endoscopic ultrasound, biopsies, and PET-CT as response assessment diagnostics, with surgical resection offered only to those patients in whom a locoregional recurrence is highly suspected or proven.

In summary, although surgery after combined chemoradiation for esophageal cancer appears to improve local control, its effect on ultimate survival remains unclear.

Brachytherapy

Gaspar et al.[192,193] reported the results of a prospective trial evaluating intraluminal brachytherapy in patients with nonoperable esophageal cancer. Patients initially received 50 Gy of external irradiation with concurrent chemotherapy, followed by a 2-week break and brachytherapy administration. Patients received either 15 Gy using HDR techniques over three consecutive weeks (5 Gy/fraction) or a single administration of 20 Gy using low–dose rate (LDR) techniques. Dose was prescribed to 1 cm from the source axis. Treatments were accomplished by placement of a 10- to 12-French applicator inserted transnasally or transorally. The target length was defined as the pretreatment tumor length with 1-cm margin proximally and distally as determined by CT, barium swallow, and endoscopy. Both external irradiation and brachytherapy were given concurrently with 5-FU chemotherapy. After the development of fistulas in six patients, the HDR dose was reduced to 10 Gy in two fractions, and the LDR arm was ultimately closed because of poor accrual. Results showed a median survival of 11 months in all patients. Local disease persistence/recurrence was observed in 63% of 49 eligible patients receiving HDR therapy. Six patients developed esophageal fistulas, resulting in three deaths. These fistulas were deemed treatment related. The 1-year actuarial fistula development rate was 18%. The investigators concluded that esophageal brachytherapy, particularly in conjunction with chemotherapy, should be approached with caution. Chinese investigators randomized 160 patients to receive either a stent loaded with I-125 seeds or conventional stenting. Median overall survival was 177 days in the irradiation group versus 147 days in the control group (P = .0046). Major complications included severe chest pain (23 vs. 20%) and fistula formation (8 vs. 7%).[194] Review of other combined brachytherapy/EBRT series suggests that fistula formation rates range from 0% to 12%, with a possible trend toward a higher incidence in patients receiving concurrent chemotherapy with brachytherapy. The incidence of brachytherapy-related mortality varies from 0% to 8%, with most series reporting rates of 4% or less.[195] A meta-analysis of prospective studies of brachytherapy encompassing 623 patients concluded that brachytherapy was a highly effective and relatively safe treatment option that was currently underused. However, the severe adverse event rate was 23% (stenosis 12%, fistula development 8%).[196]

Other studies have suggested that HDR brachytherapy is effective for palliation of dysphagia in up to 90% of patients.[195] Danish investigators reported the results of a randomized trial of 209 patients with dysphagia due to inoperable esophageal or gastroesophageal junctional tumors.[197] Patients were randomized to either endoscopic stent placement or single-dose HDR brachytherapy. Patient exclusion criteria included tumors >12 cm, tumors within 3 cm of the upper esophageal sphincter, deeply ulcerated tumors, tracheoesophageal fistula/tracheal involvement, presence of a pacemaker, and previous radiation treatment or stent placement. Brachytherapy was delivered through a flexible 1-cm applicator delivering a dose of 12 Gy prescribed to 1 cm from the source axis. The treatment length was defined as gross disease plus 2 cm proximally and distally. Although trial results showed a more rapid improvement in dysphagia after stent insertion, long-term dysphagia relief was significantly improved in the group receiving brachytherapy. Patients undergoing brachytherapy experienced more days with low-grade or no dysphagia versus patients with stent placement. Complication rates were higher following stent placement (33% vs. 21%), primarily because of an increased incidence of late hemorrhage in the stent group. The authors concluded that single-dose brachytherapy is preferable to stent placement as the initial treatment for patients with progressive dysphagia due to inoperable esophageal or gastroesophageal junction carcinoma. A trial from the International Atomic Energy Agency randomized 219 palliatively approached patients to HDR brachytherapy (8 Gy × 2), with or without the addition of 30 Gy of EBRT in 10 fractions. Dysphagia relief was significantly improved in the combined approach, with an absolute benefit of 18% at 200 days from randomization (P = .019).[198] In a smaller trial, 65 patients with advanced cancer of the esophagus or gastroesophageal junction were randomized to either expandable stent or HDR endoluminal brachytherapy (7 Gy × 3) delivered over 2 to 4 weeks. Although the stent-alone patients reported significantly better dysphagia scores at 1 month, other health-related quality of life scores were worse relative to brachytherapy, and at 3 months, dysphagia-related scores were improved with brachytherapy.[199]

For patients treated with curative intent (unifocal thoracic tumors <10 cm, no distant metastases, no airway involvement or cervical esophageal location), the American Brachytherapy Society recommends a brachytherapy dose of 10 Gy in two weekly fractions of 5 Gy each (HDR) or 20 Gy in a single course at 0.4 to 1 Gy/hour (LDR). The dose is prescribed to 1 cm from midsource and delivered through a 6- to 10-mm applicator. The recommended active length is the visible mucosal tumor with a 1- to 2-cm proximal and distal margin. Ideally, brachytherapy is started 2 to 3 weeks after completion of concurrent external irradiation/chemotherapy to allow mucositis resolution. Concurrent chemotherapy with brachytherapy is not recommended. In palliative cases, a similar approach is recommended, with delivery of 10 to 14 Gy in one or two fractions (HDR) or 20 to 25 Gy in a single course (LDR). In previously untreated patients with a short life expectancy (<3 months), a dose of 15 to 20 Gy in two to four fractions (HDR) or of 25 to 40 Gy (LDR) without external irradiation is recommended (Tables 56.10–56.12).[200] In summary, the use of brachytherapy in the curative approach to esophageal cancer does not appear to significantly improve results achieved with combined EBRT with chemotherapy alone. However, in the palliative setting, brachytherapy has shown good efficacy in the relief of dysphagia.

Palliative Treatment

Although treatment advances have occurred in esophageal cancer over the last 20 years, the majority of patients diagnosed with esophageal cancer will die of their malignancy. Therefore, palliation remains an important goal. Dysphagia is a common

presenting symptom and may significantly impair patient's quality of life. Many studies report a 60% to >80% rate of relief from dysphagia with radiation.[201] Coia et al.[201] reported that nearly half of patients with baseline dysphagia experienced an improvement in swallowing within 2 weeks of treatment initiation. By the completion of the 6th week, >80% experienced improvement. A median time to maximal improvement was approximately 1 month. In another series of 148 patients receiving palliative radiation therapy (most received a dose of 20 Gy in five fractions), 75% experienced an improvement in dysphagia, with 26% of these patients requiring stent placement subsequently.[202] Given the superior outcomes of patients receiving concurrent chemotherapy with radiation therapy in nonmetastatic disease, palliative chemoradiation may be preferable to radiation alone for patients with advanced-stage esophageal carcinoma who have a good performance status. However, Trans-Tasman Radiation Oncology Group (TROG) 03.01/National Cancer Institute of Canada (NCIC) CTG (ES.2) investigators enrolled 220 patients with advanced/metastatic esophageal cancer and randomized them to receive 35 Gy in 15 fractions (or alternatively 30 Gy in 10 fractions) with or without the addition of concurrent cisplatin and fluorouracil. 45% of patients in the chemoradiotherapy group and 35% in the radiotherapy group obtained dysphagia relief (p=0.13). Median dysphagia progression-free survival was 4.1 months versus 3.4 months in the chemoradiotherapy and radiotherapy groups, respectively (p=0.58), and median overall survival was 6.9 months versus 6.7 months, respectively (p=0.88). Grade 3-4 acute toxicity occurred in 36% of patients in the chemoradiotherapy group and in 16% patients in the radiotherapy group (p=0.0017). The authors concluded that a palliative chemoradiotherapy showed a modest, but not statistically significant, increase in dysphagia relief compared with radiotherapy alone, with minimal improvement in dysphagia progression-free survival and overall survival with chemoradiotherapy but at a cost of increased toxicity, and that a short course of radiotherapy

---

TABLE 56.11 SUGGESTED SCHEMA FOR DEFINITIVE EXTERNAL BEAM RADIATION AND ESOPHAGEAL BRACHYTHERAPY

External Beam Radiation
From 45 to 50 Gy in 1.8- to 2.0-Gy fractions, 5 fractions/wk, wk 1 to 5

Brachytherapy
High dose rate: total dose of 10 Gy, 5 Gy/fraction, 1 fraction/wk, starting 2 to 3 wk after completion of external beam
Low dose rate: total dose of 20 Gy, single course, 0.4 to 1.0 Gy/h, starting 2 to 3 wk from completion of external beam

All doses are specified 1 cm from the midsource or mid-dwell position.

TABLE 56.12 SUGGESTED SCHEMA FOR EXTERNAL BEAM RADIATION AND BRACHYTHERAPY IN THE PALLIATIVE TREATMENT OF ESOPHAGEAL CANCER

1. Recurrent after external beam radiation and short life expectancy
   Brachytherapy:
   HDR: total dose of 10 to 14 Gy, one or two fractions
   LDR: total dose of 20 to 40 Gy, one or two fractions, 0.4 to 1.0 Gy/h
2. No previous external beam radiation
   External beam radiation:
   From 30 to 40 Gy in 2- to 3-Gy fractions
   Brachytherapy
   HDR: 10 to 14 Gy, one or two fractions
   LDR: total dose of 20 to 25 Gy, single course, 0.4 to 1.0 Gy/h
3. No previous external beam radiation, life expectancy >6 mo
   External beam radiation:
   From 45 to 50 Gy in 1.8- to 2.0-Gy fractions, 5 fractions/wk, wk 1 to 5
   Brachytherapy
   HDR: total dose of 10 Gy, 5 Gy/fraction, 1 fraction/wk, starting 2 to 3 wk after completion of external beam
   LDR: total dose of 20 Gy, single course, 0.4 to 1.0 Gy/h, starting 2 to 3 wk after completion of external beam

All doses are specified 1 cm from the midsource or mid-dwell position.
HDR, high dose rate; LDR, low dose rate.

TABLE 56.10 SELECTION CRITERIA FOR BRACHYTHERAPY IN THE TREATMENT OF ESOPHAGEAL CANCER

Good Candidates	Poor Candidates	Contraindications
Primary tumor ≤10 cm length	Extraesophageal extension	Esophageal fistula
Tumor confined to the esophageal wall	Tumor >10 cm in length	Cervical esophageal location
Thoracic esophagus location	Regional lymphadenopathy	Stenosis that cannot be bypassed
No regional lymph node or systemic metastases	Tumor involving gastro-esophageal junction or cardia	

alone should be considered a safe and well tolerated treatment for malignant dysphagia in the palliative setting.[203] As described earlier, intraluminal brachytherapy has also been used for palliation of dysphagia. The previously described randomized trial from the Netherlands comparing intraluminal brachytherapy to stent placement showed that although patients undergoing stenting experienced a more rapid improvement in dysphagia, long-term palliation was significantly improved in patients treated with brachytherapy.[197]

The palliative management of patients with tracheoesophageal fistula presents a clinical dilemma. Fistulazation usually precludes surgery. These patients are often treated effectively with the placement of silicone-covered, self-expanding metal stents, often obviating palliative surgery. In addition, placement of feeding gastrostomy or jejunostomy may be appropriate. Although considered a "relative" contraindication to radiation therapy, limited data from a Mayo Clinic series suggest that radiation therapy may not increase fistula severity and can be administered safely in this setting; however, the presence of fistula is a poor prognostic factor.[204]

REIRRADIATION

Although local control rates with trimodality therapy are high, the incidence of local recurrence remains common in nonoperative patients. Varying investigators have evaluated the role of reirradiation in clinical practice. In one report of 54 patients (21 previously irradiated), radiation was associated with an improvement in dysphagia in 68% and median survival of 1 year. Dose range was 30 to 68 Gy with a median of 45. No grade 5 toxicities were seen, with 1 of 21 patients previously irradiated developing a late esophageal stenosis. The authors indicated that if reirradiation of esophageal carcinoma is contemplated, three-dimensional conformal techniques and a minimum total dose of 45 Gy are recommended.[205] In a smaller series of 10 patients who were reirradiated, the total dose of primary radiotherapy was a median of 50.4 Gy (range, 50.4 to 63.0 Gy). The total dose of reirradiation was a median of 46.5 Gy (range, 44.0 to 50.4 Gy). Three patients developed a grade 5 tracheoesophageal fistula, and five experienced progressive disease 3 months following treatment. The authors concluded that reirradiation of recurrent esophageal cancer after primary radiotherapy can cause severe toxicity.[206] A small, prospective trial of 14 patients with history of prior thoracic radiation with newly diagnosed or locally recurrent esophageal cancer explored the use of proton beam treatment. Median reirradiation prescription dose was 54 Gy and median cumulative prescription dose was 110 Gy. Four of ten symptomatic patients had complete resolution of symptoms and four decreased or stable symptoms. One grade 5 toxicity of esophageal pleural fistula was seen, possibly related to tumor progression. Median time to local failure was 10 months and median survival 14 months. The authors conclude that reirradiation is feasible with encouraging symptom control rate and with a modest toxicity profile.[207]

TREATMENT SEQUELAE

Advances in surgical technique, as well as improved preoperative and postoperative management, have decreased treatment-related mortality. Contemporary operative mortality rates are generally <10%.[54,57,208] Complication rates can exceed 75%, including pulmonary and cardiac complications, anastomotic leak, and recurrent laryngeal nerve paralysis. Stricture formation can occur in 14% to 27% of patients. The addition of preoperative radiation therapy and chemotherapy may enhance surgical complication rates, although this remains a subject of debate.[53,54]

More than 75% of patients receiving radiation experience transient esophagitis and dysphagia, sometimes requiring nutritional support. Chemotherapy-related leukopenia and thrombocytopenia are common, although this may be less common with contemporary chemotherapy regimens.[146] Additional acute toxicities of radiation therapy include esophagitis, dermatitis, fatigue, and weight loss in most patients. Nausea and vomiting are relatively common, particularly in patients with lower esophageal and gastroesophageal junction tumors. Many symptoms resolve within 1 to 2 weeks of treatment completion. A perforated esophagus is life threatening and can be characterized by substernal chest pain, a high pulse rate, fever, and hemorrhage.[105] The addition of chemotherapy can significantly increase acute complications. Moderate-to-severe and even life-threatening toxicities have been reported in 50% to 66% of patients.[82,181,209] In the previously discussed RTOG study of chemoradiation alone, patients treated with combined therapy had a higher incidence of acute grade 3 (44% vs. 25%) and grade 4 toxicity (20% vs. 3%) compared to patients receiving radiation therapy alone.[55] Chemoradiation treatment–related mortality rates range from 0% to 3%.[57,82,143,147,181]

The most common late effects following radiation therapy are esophageal stenosis and stricture formation. Stenosis can occur in >60% of patients. Symptomatic stricture requiring dilation has been reported to occur at least 15% to 20% of the time. Dysphagia may be relieved with two to three dilations.[82] Long-term results from the RTOG study showed that late grade 3 or greater toxicity was similar in the combined versus radiation-alone arms (29% vs. 23%). However, grade 4 or greater toxicity was higher in patients receiving combined modality therapy (10% vs. 2%).[182] Other complications include clinically apparent damage to organs within the radiation therapy volume, although this is uncommon. Chemotherapy may further increase the risk of late treatment-related toxicities.

The effects of radiation on pulmonary and cardiac function deserve special mention. Pulmonary complications associated with either the definitive or neoadjuvant treatment of esophageal cancer patients can be broadly broken up into symptomatic pneumonitis following treatment completion and postoperative pulmonary complications in patients undergoing resection. Although they are still relatively ill-defined, various institutional series have described predictive factors for these complications (which are not mutually exclusive), and are described in the following.

Radiation pneumonitis is a relatively common complication in the treatment of thoracic (lung) malignancies, which can range from minimally symptomatic to fatal. Common symptoms include nonproductive cough, dyspnea, and, uncommonly, respiratory distress. Generally, this occurs 2 to 6 months after radiation therapy completion. The ability to predict radiation pneumonitis has been a significant topic of investigation. However, most data come from patients with lung cancer, who may have more underlying intrinsic pulmonary/smoking-related disease. A variety of predictive parameters have been suggested, including V_{20} of >25% to 30%, mean lung dose of >15 to 20 Gy, V_5 of >42%, and absolute V_5 of >3,000 cm.[123]

In nonoperative patients, an analysis of esophageal cancer patients from Japan treated definitively to a dose of 60 Gy with concurrent 5-FU and cisplatin showed a radiation pneumonitis incidence of 27%.[210] The authors concluded that an optimal V_{20} threshold to predict symptomatic pneumonitis was approximately 30%. In a study of 101 both operative and nonoperative patients (88% distal esophagus/GE junction) from the MD Anderson Cancer Center undergoing a mix of 3D and IMRT radiation therapy, 59%, 5%, and 1% of patients experienced grade 2, 3, and 5 radiation pneumonitis, respectively.[211] An analysis from Japan using fields inclusive of supraclavicular, mediastinal, and celiac regions up to a dose of 60 Gy with concurrent cisplatin and 5-FU showed a 2-year cumulative incidence of late, high-grade cardiopulmonary toxicities for patients ≥75 years of 29% versus 3% in younger patients. They concluded that older patients might not tolerate extensive radiation fields.[212] Other studies have shown that significant declines in diffusion capacity and total lung capacity may occur in patients irradiated for esophageal cancer.[213] The current RTOG 1010 study recommends maintaining a V10 ≤ 40%, mean lung dose of <20 Gy, V20 ≤ 30% (ideally < 25%), and V30 ≤ 20%. For IMRT, interval dose is limited to 60% of the lungs receiving 5 Gy or less.

In operative patients, a study of 110 patients treated with preoperative chemoradiotherapy followed by resection at the MD Anderson Cancer Center showed that mean lung dose, effective dose, and absolute lung dose receiving ≤5 Gy were predictors of development of postoperative pulmonary complications.[214] In a report on patients from the same institution describing complications in patients receiving neoadjuvant combined modality therapy,[215] 18% experienced pulmonary complications, with higher rates when the V_{10} was ≥40% (35% vs. 8%) and V_{15} was ≥30% (33% vs. 10%), leading the authors to conclude that minimization of lung volume irradiation was important in the preoperative planning of these patients. This increase in postoperative pulmonary complications (pneumonia, acute respiratory distress syndrome) when the V_{10} was >40% suggests that the volume of remaining/undamaged functional lung may determine postoperative pulmonary function, that is, patients with a small lung volume initially may be at higher risk of experiencing pulmonary complications, even if the relative V_5 is low, and that patients with small lung volume with less functional reserve may be more susceptible to postoperative pulmonary complications. Therefore, it is important to consider not only the dose–volume histogram of the lung but also the total lung volume.

A study from China evaluating patients receiving chemoradiotherapy followed by resection showed that the volume of lung spared from doses of ≥5 Gy was the only independent dosimetric factor on multivariate analysis in predicting postoperative pulmonary complications.[216] Wang et al.[217] similarly described that the relative V_5 and all spared volumes from 5 to 35 Gy significantly correlated with the incidence of postoperative pulmonary complications, although on multivariate analysis, V_5 was the only significant independent predictive factor, indicating that the volume of "unexposed" lung during induction therapy was predictive. Of note in this study was that the majority of patients were treated with induction chemotherapy alone initially (most paclitaxel), which has been shown to increase rates of pneumonitis in other disease sites. A significant association of induction chemotherapy alone prior to concurrent chemoradiotherapy was seen as a predictor of grade 2 or greater pneumonitis (49% vs. 14%; P = .003), leading the authors to conclude that induction chemotherapy alone may sensitize lung tissue to radiation damage. In contrast to the foregoing studies, however, another analysis of 98 patients receiving preoperative chemoradiotherapy with 5-FU and cisplatin showed no difference in pulmonary complications versus patients undergoing surgery alone, with no correlation of any lung dose–volume histogram findings with development of postoperative pulmonary complications seen, leading the authors to conclude that neoadjuvant chemoradiotherapy had no detrimental impact on postoperative course.[218] An analysis from Taiwan of neoadjuvantly, IMRT-treated esophageal cancer patients undergoing resection suggested that preoperative (not prechemoradiation) forced expiratory volume in 1 second was an independent factor associated with postoperative pulmonary complications and that reducing the absolute volume of the right lung irradiated might decrease the risk of postoperative pulmonary complications.[219] Finally, a review from Fox Chase Cancer Center of 139 patients with esophageal cancer receiving taxane-based trimodality therapy showed that 14% of patients experienced grade 2+ radiation pneumonitis. The V5, V10, V20, and V30 were associated with an increased risk of clinically significant grade 2 pneumonitis. Multivariable analysis showed that V5 and V20 remained associated with this, with V5 of ≤65% and V20 of ≤25% optimal thresholds.[220]

Radiation-induced cardiac toxicity is a broad term describing potential radiation injury to a number of cardiac structures, including the pericardium (as manifested by effusion, pericarditis), coronary arteries, the heart muscle itself/cardiomyopathy, and cardiac valves, as well as nerve/conduction injury. Radiation injury primarily consists of fibrosis and/or small-vessel injury. "Classic" radiation tolerance (TD5/5) of the heart is about 60 Gy when 25% or less of the heart is irradiated and 45 Gy if 65% of the heart is irradiated, assuming 2 Gy/fraction. The mechanism of radiation-induced cardiac injury is relatively poorly defined, particularly in the context of esophageal cancer. Historical data from the treatment of Hodgkin disease patients suggest that a dose of >40 Gy may increase the risk of cardiac death, as well as of pericarditis.[221,222] Several studies of cardiac toxicity and esophageal cancer patient demonstrated that a V_{30} of >46% predicted a significant increase in pericardial effusion, and increasing fraction size (particularly ≥3.5 Gy) also predicted the same. In addition, some authors have shown a possible trend for decrease in ejection fraction in patients with increasing V_{20} of the left ventricle.[123] In a study of 150 esophageal cancer patients receiving chemoradiotherapy (49 neoadjuvantly), the incidence of pericardial effusion was 28%, usually developing within 15 months of radiation therapy, with median onset time of approximately 5 months. The risk of pericardial effusion was associated with mean pericardial doses over an array of dose–volume points to the pericardium from 5 to 45 Gy. A matched-pair analysis of nonradiation patients receiving surgery versus those treated neoadjuvantly was performed, with 42% of patients in the radiation group demonstrating ischemia/scarring on single-photon emission CT images versus 4% in the surgical group, with a median onset to abnormality of 3 months.[223] In a Japanese study, long-term analysis of 139 patients treated with definitive chemoradiotherapy (cisplatin/5-FU with 60 Gy EBRT) for squamous cell carcinoma revealed grade 2, 3, and 4 late pericarditis occurring in 6%, 5%, and 1% of patients, respectively; grade 4 heart failure in 2 patients; grade 2, 3, and 4 pleural effusion development in 5%, 6%, and 0% of patients, respectively; and grade 2, 3, and 4 radiation pneumonitis development in 1%, 2%, and 0% of patients, respectively.[224] A more recent retrospective review of 343 esophageal cancer patients demonstrated the rate of symptomatic cardiac disease at 5 years was 14%. Multivariable analysis revealed this increase with increasing heart dose with the lowest significant cutoff values of V45, V50, and V55 of 15%, 10%, and 5%, respectively.[225] As described previously, an analysis of esophageal cancer patients showed no difference in disease-specific or pulmonary mortality in patients treated with either conformal therapy or IMRT, but did show an improvement in all-cause cardiac mortality with IMRT.[132] In a literature search concerning cardiac toxicity in esophageal cancer patients treated with radiotherapy, with or without chemotherapy, the overall accrued incidence of symptomatic cardiac toxicity was as high as 10.8%, corresponding with several dose–volume parameters of the heart. The most frequent complications were pericardial effusion, ischemic heart disease, and heart failure. Most events occurred within 2 years following treatment. The authors concluded that normal tissue complication probability models for esophageal cancer were not available at present.[226]

FUTURE CONSIDERATIONS

Although modest improvements in survival have been achieved by combining neoadjuvant chemoradiation and surgery, patients treated with chemoradiation alone or with surgery have unacceptably high locoregional relapse rates and mortality rates. Ultimately, approximately 75% of patients succumb to metastatic disease. As described previously, efforts at radiation dose escalation have not resulted in significant gains for this disease, although newer efforts are now underway to further define optimal dose. Current clinical trials are also evaluating new and potentially more effective chemotherapeutic agents with radiation therapy, attempting to optimize combined regimens and integrate novel systemic agents in combination with radiation.

SUMMARY

The prognosis for patients with carcinoma of the esophagus remains poor despite recent advances in combined-modality therapies. No firm recommendation can be made for managing locally advanced disease. The data suggest that neoadjuvant chemoradiation improves outcomes in patients who are candidates for surgery. Alternatively, randomized trials have also suggested that perioperative chemotherapy improves outcomes in these patients. However, many patients are not able to tolerate surgery, and combined chemoradiation may be more appropriate in selected patients because definitive chemoradiation has resulted in survival rates comparable to those from surgery alone. Locoregional failure remains a significant pattern of relapse in nonoperable patients. For patients with stage IV disease, palliation with single-modality therapy or several modalities should be used and tailored to the patient's specific symptoms. Current unresolved issues include the following:

1. Which subsets of patients are more likely to benefit from the addition of surgery than others? Is a response-based surgical approach following chemoradiation appropriate for widespread use?
2. Which subsets of patients are more likely to benefit from the addition of neoadjuvant and/or perioperative therapies? Is there a superiority of a neoadjuvant chemoradiation versus a perioperative chemotherapy approach, and will some patients benefit from one particular treatment approach?
3. Can introduction of newer chemotherapy/targeted agents in the neoadjuvant or concurrent setting improve the results over "standard" chemoradiation with cisplatin/5-FU or carboplatin/paclitaxel? What is the optimal "standard" regimen in combination patients?
4. Will new technologies such as PET-based planning, IMRT, proton therapy, and image-guided radiation therapy decrease complication rates and influence cure rates? Is it appropriate to reduce radiation treatment volumes to "involved-field" given the high propensity for distant metastases development?
5. Will PET scan allow early prediction of both response to treatment and ultimate outcomes and potentially allow avoidance of delivery of ineffective treatments early on during the course of therapy?
6. Will the identification of molecular prognostic markers allow "individualization" of treatments among patients?
7. Will further studies of dose escalation improve local control rates in patients treated with "definitive" chemoradiation?

REFERENCES

1. Rice TW, Ishwaran H, Ferguson MK et al. Cancer of the esophagus and esophagogastric junction: an eighth edition staging primer. *J Thorac Oncol* 2017;12(1):36–42.
2. Rosenberg JC, Franklin R, Steiger Z. Squamous cell carcinoma of the thoracic esophagus: an interdisciplinary approach. *Curr Probl Cancer* 1981;5:1–52.
3. Rudiger Siewert J, Feith M, Werner M, et al. Adenocarcinoma of the esophagogastric junction: results of surgical therapy based on anatomical/topographic classification in 1,002 consecutive patients. *Ann Surg* 2000;232:353–361.
4. Arnott SJ, Duncan W, Gignoux M, et al. Preoperative radiotherapy for esophageal carcinoma. *Cochrane Database Syst Rev* 2005;(4):CD001799.
5. Goodner JT, Miller TP, Pack GT, et al. Torek esophagectomy; the case against segmental resection for esophageal cancer. *J Thorac Surg* 1956;32:347–359.
6. Hosch SB, Stoecklein NH, Pichlmeier U, et al. Esophageal cancer: the mode of lymphatic tumor cell spread and its prognostic significance. *J Clin Oncol* 2001;19:1970–1975.
7. Sharpiro A, Robillard G. The esophageal arteries. *Ann Surg* 1950;131:171.
8. Ott K, Weber W, Siewert JR. The importance of PET in the diagnosis and response evaluation of esophageal cancer. *Dis Esophagus* 2006;19:433–442.
9. Siegel RL, Miller KD, Jemal A. Cancer statistics, 2018. *CA Cancer J Clin* 2018;68(1):7–30.
10. Ferlay J, Soerjomataram I, Ervik M, et al. GLOBOCAN 2012 v1.0, Cancer Incidence and Mortality Worldwide: IARC CancerBase No. 11 [Internet]. [cited 2015 July 30]. Available from: http://globocan.iarc.fr
11. Cheng KK. The etiology of esophageal cancer in Chinese. *Semin Oncol* 1994;21:411–415.
12. Mahboubi M, Kmet J, Cook P. Esophageal cancer studies in the Caspian littoral of Iran: the Caspian Cancer Registry. *Br J Cancer* 1973;28:196.
13. Blot WJ, McLaughlin JK. The changing epidemiology of esophageal cancer. *Semin Oncol* 1999;26:2–8.
14. Denham JW, Burmeister BH, Lamb DS, et al. Factors influencing outcome following radio-chemotherapy for oesophageal cancer. The Trans Tasman Radiation Oncology Group (TROG). *Radiother Oncol* 1996;40:31–43.
15. Pohl H, Welch HG. The role of overdiagnosis and reclassification in the marked increase of esophageal adenocarcinoma incidence. *J Natl Cancer Inst* 2005;97:142–146.
16. Schottenfeld D. Epidemiology of cancer of the esophagus. *Semin Oncol* 1984;11:92–100.
17. Blot WJ. Alcohol and cancer. *Cancer Res* 1992;52:2119s–2123s.
18. van Rensburg SJ. Epidemiologic and dietary evidence for a specific nutritional predisposition to esophageal cancer. *J Natl Cancer Inst* 1981;67:243–251.
19. Lijinsky W. *Current concepts in the toxicology of nitrates, nitrites and nitrosamines.* Washington, DC: Hemisphere, 1979.
20. Miao C, Guo F, Zhang J. The relationship between fungi and nitrosamines and their precursors: II. The action of fungi isolated from grains in Linxian Med Ref. *Med Ref* 1978;2:46.
21. Yang CS, Chen X, Tu S. Etiology and Prevention of Esophageal Cancer. *Gastrointest Tumors* 2016;3(1):3–16.
22. Appelqvist P, Salmo M. Lye corrosion carcinoma of the esophagus: a review of 63 cases. *Cancer* 1980;45:2655–2658.
23. Hopkins RA, Postlethwait RW. Caustic burns and carcinoma of the esophagus. *Ann Surg* 1981;194:146–148.
24. Harper PS, Harper RM, Howel-Evans AW. Carcinoma of the oesophagus with tylosis. *Q J Med* 1970;39:317–333.
25. Spechler SJ. Barrett's esophagus. *Gastroenterologist* 1994;2:273–284.
26. Lagergren J, Bergstrom R, Lindgren A, et al. Symptomatic gastroesophageal reflux as a risk factor for esophageal adenocarcinoma. *N Engl J Med* 1999;340:825–831.
27. Devesa SS, Blot WJ, Fraumeni JF Jr. Changing patterns in the incidence of esophageal and gastric carcinoma in the United States. *Cancer* 1998;83:2049–2053.
28. Zhang ZF, Kurtz RC, Sun M, et al. Adenocarcinomas of the esophagus and gastric cardia: medical conditions, tobacco, alcohol, and socioeconomic factors. *Cancer Epidemiol Biomarkers Prev* 1996;5:761–768.
29. Heath EI, Limburg PJ, Hawk ET, et al. Adenocarcinoma of the esophagus: risk factors and prevention. *Oncology (Williston Park)* 2000;14:507–514; discussion 518–520, 522–503.
30. Brown LM, Swanson CA, Gridley G, et al. Adenocarcinoma of the esophagus: role of obesity and diet. *J Natl Cancer Inst* 1995;87:104–109.
31. DeMeester TR. Clinical biology of the Barrett's metaplasia, dysplasia to carcinoma sequence. *Surg Oncol* 2001;10:91–102.
32. Montesano R, Hollstein M, Hainaut P. Genetic alterations in esophageal cancer and their relevance to etiology and pathogenesis: a review. *Int J Cancer* 1996;69:225–235.
33. Dulak AM, Stojanov P, Peng S, et al. Exome and whole-genome sequencing of esophageal adenocarcinoma identifies recurrent driver events and mutational complexity. *Nat Genet* 2013;45(5):478–486.
34. Song Y, Li L, Ou Y, et al. Identification of genomic alterations in oesophageal squamous cell cancer. *Nature* 2014;509(7498):91.
35. Holdscher A, Bollschweiller E, Bumm R, et al. Prognostic factors of resected adenocarcinoma of the esophagus. *Surgery* 1995;118:845–855.
36. Collard JM, Otte JB, Fiasse R, et al. Skeletonizing en bloc esophagectomy for cancer. *Ann Surg* 2001;234:25–32.
37. Dresner SM, Lamb PJ, Bennett MK, et al. The pattern of metastatic lymph node dissemination from adenocarcinoma of the esophagogastric junction. *Surgery* 2001;129:103–109.
38. Siewert JR, Stein HJ, Feith M, et al. Histologic tumor type is an independent prognostic parameter in esophageal cancer: lessons from more than 1,000 consecutive resections at a single center in the Western world. *Ann Surg* 2001;234:360–367.
39. Rice TW, Zuccaro G Jr, Adelstein DJ, et al. Esophageal carcinoma: depth of tumor invasion is predictive of regional lymph node status. *Ann Thorac Surg* 1998;65:787–792.
40. Akiyama H, Tsurumaru M, Kawamura T, et al. Principles of surgical treatment for carcinoma of the esophagus: analysis of lymph node involvement. *Ann Surg* 1981;194:438–446.
41. Bloedorn F, Kasdorf H. *Radiotherapy in squamous cell carcinoma of the esophagus.* Chicago, IL: Year Book Medical, 1971.
42. Dormans E. Das Oesophaguscarcinoma: Ergebnisse der unter Mitarbet von 29 patholgischem Instituten Deutschlands Durgefuhrten Erhebung uber das Oesophaguscarcinomon (1925–1933). *Z Krebforsch* 1939;49:86.
43. Anderson LL, Lad TE. Autopsy findings in squamous-cell carcinoma of the esophagus. *Cancer* 1982;50:1587–1590.
44. Huang W, Li B, Gong H, et al. Pattern of lymph node metastases and its implication in radiotherapeutic clinical target volume in patients with thoracic esophageal squamous cell carcinoma: a report of 1077 cases. *Radiother Oncol* 2010;95:229–233.
45. Cheng J, Kong L, Huang W. Explore the radiotherapeutic clinical target volume delineation for thoracic esophageal squamous cell carcinoma from the pattern of lymphatic metastases. *J Thorac Oncol* 2013;8:359–365.
46. Monig SP, Baldus SE, Zirbes TK, et al. Topographical distribution of lymph node metastasis in adenocarcinoma of the gastroesophageal junction. *Hepatogastroenterology* 2002;49:419–422.
47. Schurr PG, Yekebas EF, Kaifi JT, et al. Lymphatic spread and microinvolvement in adenocarcinoma of the esophago-gastric junction. *J Surg Oncol* 2006;94:307–315.

48. Matzinger O, Gerber E, Bernstein Z, et al. EORTC-ROG expert opinion: radiotherapy volume and treatment guidelines for neoadjuvant radiation of adenocarcinomas of the gastroesophageal junction and the stomach. *Radiother Oncol* 2009;92:164–175.

49. Meier I, Merkel S, Papadopoulos T, et al. Adenocarcinoma of the esophagogastric junction: the pattern of metastatic lymph node dissemination as a rationale for elective lymphatic target volume definition. *Int J Radiat Oncol Biol Phys* 2008;70:1408–1417.

50. Whittington R, Coia LR, Haller DG, et al. Adenocarcinoma of the esophagus and esophago-gastric junction: the effects of single and combined modalities on the survival and patterns of failure following treatment. *Int J Radiat Oncol Biol Phys* 1990;19:593–603.

51. Hulscher JB, van Sandick JW, de Boer AG, et al. Extended transthoracic resection compared with limited transhiatal resection for adenocarcinoma of the esophagus. *N Engl J Med* 2002;347:1662–1669.

52. Urba SG, Orringer MB, Turrisi A, et al. Randomized trial of preoperative chemoradiation versus surgery alone in patients with locoregional esophageal carcinoma. *J Clin Oncol* 2001;19:305–313.

53. Mariette C, Dahan L, Mornex F, et al. Surgery alone versus chemoradiotherapy followed by surgery for stage I and II esophageal cancer: final results of a randomized controlled phase III trial FFCD 9901. *J Clin Oncol* 2014;32(23):2416–2422.

54. Shapiro J, van Lanschot J, Hulshof MC, et al. Neoadjuvant chemoradiotherapy plus surgery versus surgery alone for oesophageal or junctional cancer (CROSS): long-term results of a randomised controlled trial. *Lancet Oncol* 2015;16(9):1090–1098.

55. al-Sarraf M, Martz K, Herskovic A, et al. Progress report of combined chemoradiotherapy versus radiotherapy alone in patients with esophageal cancer: an intergroup study. *J Clin Oncol* 1997;15:277–284.

56. Minsky BD, Neuberg D, Kelsen DP, et al. Final report of Intergroup Trial 0122 (ECOG PE-289, RTOG 90-12): phase II trial of neoadjuvant chemotherapy plus concurrent chemotherapy and high-dose radiation for squamous cell carcinoma of the esophagus. *Int J Radiat Oncol Biol Phys* 1999;43:517–523.

57. Stahl M, Stuschke M, Lehmann N, et al. Chemoradiation with and without surgery in patients with locally advanced squamous cell carcinoma of the esophagus. *J Clin Oncol* 2005;23:2310–2317.

58. Welsh J, Settle S, Amini A, et al. Failure patterns in patients with esophageal cancer treated with definitive chemoradiation. *Cancer* 2012;118:2632–2640.

59. Rosenberg J, Lichter A, Leichman L. *Cancer of the esophagus*. Philadelphia: JB Lippincott, 1989.

60. Moertel C. *The esophagus*. Philadelphia: Lea & Febiger, 1982.

61. Lea JWt, Prager RL, Bender HW Jr. The questionable role of computed tomography in preoperative staging of esophageal cancer. *Ann Thorac Surg* 1984;38:479–481.

62. Picus D, Balfe DM, Koehler RE, et al. Computed tomography in the staging of esophageal carcinoma. *Radiology* 1983;146:433–438.

63. Griffith JF, Chan AC, Chow LT, et al. Assessing chemotherapy response of squamous cell oesophageal carcinoma with spiral CT. *Br J Radiol* 1999;72:678–684.

64. Rankin SC, Taylor H, Cook GJ, et al. Computed tomography and positron emission tomography in the pre-operative staging of oesophageal carcinoma. *Clin Radiol* 1998;53:659–665.

65. Kole AC, Plukker JT, Nieweg OE, et al. Positron emission tomography for staging of oesophageal and gastroesophageal malignancy. *Br J Cancer* 1998;78:521–527.

66. Earlam R, Cunha-Melo JR. Oesophageal squamous cell carcinomas: II. A critical view of radiotherapy. *Br J Surg* 1980;67:457–461.

67. Kelly S, Harris KM, Berry E, et al. A systematic review of the staging performance of endoscopic ultrasound in gastro-oesophageal carcinoma. *Gut* 2001;49:534–539.

68. Konski A, Doss M, Milestone B, et al. The integration of 18–fluoro-deoxy-glucose positron emission tomography and endoscopic ultrasound in the treatment-planning process for esophageal carcinoma. *Int J Radiat Oncol Biol Phys* 2005;61:1123–1128.

69. Rosch T. Endosonographic staging of esophageal cancer: a review of literature results. *Gastrointest Endosc Clin N Am* 1995;5:537–547.

70. Beseth BD, Bedford R, Isacoff WH, et al. Endoscopic ultrasound does not accurately assess pathologic stage of esophageal cancer after neoadjuvant chemoradiotherapy. *Am Surg* 2000;66:827–831.

71. Laterza E, de Manzoni G, Guglielmi A, et al. Endoscopic ultrasonography in the staging of esophageal carcinoma after preoperative radiotherapy and chemotherapy. *Ann Thorac Surg* 1999;67:1466–1469.

72. Zeccaro G, Rice T, Goldbloom J, et al. Endoscopic ultrasound can not determine suitability for esophagectomy after aggressive chemoradiotherapy for esophageal cancer. *Am J Gastroenterol* 1999;94:906–912.

73. Stiles B, Mirza F, Coppolino A, et al. Clinical T2-T3N0M0 esophageal cancer: the risk of node positive disease. *Ann Thorac Surg* 2011;92(2):491–498.

74. Jaklitsch MT, Harpole DH Jr, Healey EA, et al. Current issues in the staging of esophageal cancer. *Semin Radiat Oncol* 1994;4:135–145.

75. Blackstock AW, Farmer MR, Lovato J, et al. A prospective evaluation of the impact of 18-F-fluoro-deoxy-D-glucose positron emission tomography staging on survival for patients with locally advanced esophageal cancer. *Int J Radiat Oncol Biol Phys* 2006;64:455–460.

76. Flamen P, Lerut A, Van Cutsem E, et al. Utility of positron emission tomography for the staging of patients with potentially operable esophageal carcinoma. *J Clin Oncol* 2000;18:3202–3210.

77. Monjazeb AM, Riedlinger G, Aklilu M, et al. Outcomes of patients with esophageal cancer staged with [¹⁸F]fluorodeoxyglucose positron emission tomography (FDG-PET): can postchemoradiotherapy FDG-PET predict the utility of resection? *J Clin Oncol* 2010;28:4714–4721.

78. Weber WA, Ott K. Imaging of esophageal and gastric cancer. *Semin Oncol* 2004;31:530–541.

79. Schmidt T, Lordick F, Herrmann K, et al. Value of functional imaging by PET in esophageal cancer. *J Natl Compr Canc Netw* 2015;13(2):239–247.

80. Oota K, Shin L. *Histological typing of gastric and oesophageal tumors*. Geneva, Switzerland: World Health Organization, 1977.

81. Gill PG, Denham JW, Jamieson GG, et al. Patterns of treatment failure and prognostic factors associated with the treatment of esophageal carcinoma with chemotherapy and radiotherapy either as sole treatment or followed by surgery. *J Clin Oncol* 1992;10:1037–1043.

82. Coia LR, Engstrom PF, Paul AR, et al. Long-term results of infusional 5-FU, mitomycin-C and radiation as primary management of esophageal carcinoma. *Int J Radiat Oncol Biol Phys* 1991;20:29–36.

83. Burke EL, Sturm J, Williamson D. The diagnosis of microscopic carcinoma of the esophagus. *Am J Dig Dis* 1978;23:148–151.

84. Maimon HN, Dreskin RB, Cocco AE. Positive esophageal cytology without detectable neoplasm. *Gastrointest Endosc* 1974;20:156–159.

85. Smoron GL, O'Brien CA, Sullivan CA. Tumor localization and treatment technique for cancer of the esophagus. *Radiology* 1974;111:735–736.

86. Thompson WM. Esophageal cancer. *Int J Radiat Oncol Biol Phys* 1983;9:1533–1565.

87. Epstein JI, Sears DL, Tucker RS, et al. Carcinoma of the esophagus with adenoid cystic differentiation. *Cancer* 1984;53:1131–1136.

88. Turnbull AD, Rosen P, Goodner JT, et al. Primary malignant tumors of the esophagus other than typical epidermoid carcinoma. *Ann Thorac Surg* 1973;15:463–473.

89. Briggs JC, Ibrahim NB. Oat cell carcinomas of the oesophagus: a clinico-pathological study of 23 cases. *Histopathology* 1983;7:261–277.

90. Imai T, Sannohe Y, Okano H. Oat cell carcinoma (apudoma) of the esophagus: a case report. *Cancer* 1978;41:358–364.

91. Doherty MA, McIntyre M, Arnott SJ. Oat cell carcinoma of esophagus: a report of six British patients with a review of the literature. *Int J Radiat Oncol Biol Phys* 1984;10:147–152.

92. Gaede JT, Postlethwait RW, Shelburne JD, et al. Leiomyosarcoma of the esophagus: report of two cases, one with associated squamous cell carcinoma. *J Thorac Cardiovasc Surg* 1978;75:740–746.

93. Partyka EK, Sanowski RA, Kozarek RA. Endoscopic diagnosis of a giant esophageal leiomyosarcoma. *Am J Gastroenterol* 1981;75:132–134.

94. Postlethwait R, Sealy W. *Surgery of the esophagus*. New York: Appleton-Century-Crofts, 1979.

95. Gelb A, Miller S. AIDS and gastroenterology. *Am J Gastroenterol* 1986;81:619–622.

96. Ludwig ME, Shaw R, de Suto-Nagy G. Primary malignant melanoma of the esophagus. *Cancer* 1981;48:2528–2534.

97. Son YH. Primary mucosal malignant melanoma. Appraisal of role of radiation therapy. *Acta Radiol Oncol* 1980;19:177–181.

98. Orvidas LJ, McCaffrey TV, Lewis JE, et al. Lymphoma involving the esophagus. *Ann Otol Rhinol Laryngol* 1994;103:843–848.

99. Gertler R, Stein HJ, Langer R, et al. Long-term outcome of 2920 patients with cancers of the esophagus and esophagogastric junction: evaluation of the New Union Internationale Contre le Cancer/American Joint Cancer Committee staging system. *Ann Surg* 2011;253:689–698.

100. Nomura M, Shitara K, Kodaira T, et al. Prognostic impact of the 6th and 7th American Joint Committee on Cancer TNM staging systems on esophageal cancer patients treated with chemoradiotherapy. *Int J Radiat Oncol Biol Phys* 2012;82:946–952.

101. Wang BY, Goan YG, Hsu PK, et al. Tumor length as a prognostic factor in esophageal squamous cell carcinoma. *Ann Thorac Surg* 2011;91:887–893.

102. Gaur P, Sepesi B, Hofstetter WL, et al. Endoscopic esophageal tumor length: a prognostic factor for patients with esophageal cancer *Cancer* 2011;117.63–69.

103. Yueguan J, Shifeng C, Bing Z. Prognostic factors and family history for survival of esophageal squamous cell carcinoma patients after surgery. *Ann Thorac Surg* 2010;90(3):908–913.

104. Yoon HH, Khan M, Shi Q, et al. The prognostic value of clinical and pathologic factors in esophageal adenocarcinoma: a Mayo cohort of 796 patients with extended follow-up after surgical resection. *Mayo Clin Proc* 2010;85:1080–1089.

105. Hussey D, Barakley T, Bloedorn F. *Carcinoma of the esophagus*. Philadelphia: Lea & Febiger, 1980.

106. Kelsen DP, Ginsberg R, Pajak TF, et al. Chemotherapy followed by surgery compared with surgery alone for localized esophageal cancer. *N Engl J Med* 1998;339:1979–1984.

107. Tomasello G, Petrelli F, Ghidini M, et al. Tumor regression grade and survival after neoadjuvant treatment in gastro-esophageal cancer: a meta-analysis of 17 published studies. *Eur J Surg Oncol* 2017;43(9):1607–1616.

108. Gao A, Wang L, Lei J, et al. Prognostic value of perineural invasion in esophageal and esophagogastric junction carcinoma: a meta-analysis. *Dis Markers* 2016;2016:7340180.

109. Suntharalingam M, Moughan J, Coia LR, et al. Outcome results of the 1996–1999 patterns of care survey of the national practice for patients receiving radiation therapy for carcinoma of the esophagus. *J Clin Oncol* 2005;23:2325–2331.

110. Pearson JG. The present status and future potential of radiotherapy in the management of esophageal cancer. *Cancer* 1977;39:882–890.

111. Ellis FH Jr. Standard resection for cancer of the esophagus and cardia. *Surg Oncol Clin N Am* 1999;8:279–294.

112. Hancock SL, Glatstein E. Radiation therapy of esophageal cancer. *Semin Oncol* 1984;11:144–158.

112a. Haisley K, Laird A, Nabavizadeh N, et al. Association of intervals between neoadjuvant chemoradiation and surgical resection with pathologic complete response and survival in patients with esophageal cancer. *JAMA Surg* 2016;151:E162743.

113. Skinner DB. En bloc resection for neoplasms of the esophagus and cardia. *J Thorac Cardiovasc Surg* 1983;85:59–71.

114. Sander R, Hagenmueller F, Sander C, et al. Laser versus laser plus afterloading with iridium-192 in the palliative treatment of malignant stenosis of the esophagus: a prospective, randomized, and controlled study. *Gastrointest Endosc* 1991;37:433–440.
115. Luketich JD, Friedman DM, Weigel TL, et al. Evaluation of distant metastases in esophageal cancer:100 consecutive positron emission tomography scans. *Ann Thorac Surg* 1999;68:1133–1136; discussion 1136–1137.
116. van Westreenen HL, Westerterp M, Bossuyt PM, et al. Systematic review of the staging performance of 18 F-fluorodeoxyglucose positron emission tomography in esophageal cancer. *J Clin Oncol* 2004;22:3805–3812.
117. Zhong X, Yu J, Zhang B, et al. Optimal SUV threshold of gross tumor volume delineation validated by pathologic examination in patients with esophageal cancer. *Int J Radiat Oncol Biol Phys* 2007;69:108–109.
118. Leong T, Everitt K, Yuen K, et al. A prospective study to evaluate the impact of coregistered PET-CT images in radiotherapy treatment planning for esophageal cancer. *Int J Radiat Oncol Biol Phys* 2004;60:S139–S140.
119. Zobotto L, Toubouol E, Lerouge D, et al. Impact of Ct and 18F-deoxyglucose positron emission tomography image fusion for conformal radiotherapy in esophageal carcinoma. *Int J Radiat Oncol Biol Phys* 2005;63:340.
120. Vesprini D, Ung Y, Kamra J, et al. The addition of 18-fluoodeoxglucose positron emission tomography (FDG-PET) to CT based radiotherapy planning of carcinoma of the esophagus decreases both the intra- and interobserver variability of GTV delineation. *Int J Radiat Oncol Biol Phys* 2006;66:S299–S300.
121. Muijs C, Beukema J, Woutersen D, et al. Clinical validation of FDG-PET/CT in the radiation treatment planning for patients with oesophageal cancer. *Radiother Oncol* 2014;113(2):188–192.
122. Gao XS, Qiao X, Wu F, et al. Pathological analysis of clinical target volume margin for radiotherapy in patients with esophageal and gastroesophageal junction carcinoma. *Int J Radiat Oncol Biol Phys* 2007;67:389–396.
123. Hazard L, Yang G, McAleer M, et al. Principles and techniques of radiation therapy for esophageal and gastroesophageal junction cancers. *J Natl Compr Canc Netw* 2008;6:870–878.
124. Li, M, Zhang X, Zhao F, et al. Involved-field radiotherapy for esophageal squamous cell carcinoma: theory and practice. *Radiat Oncol* 2016;11:18.
125. Wang X, Miao C, Chen Z, et al. Can involved-field irradiation replace elective nodal irradiation in chemoradiotherapy for esophageal cancer? A systematic review and meta-analysis. *Onco Targets Ther* 2017;10:2087–2095.
126. Amini A, Xiao L, Allen P, et al. Celiac node failure patterns after definitive chemoradiation for esophageal cancer in the modern era. *Int J Radiat Oncol Biol Phys* 2012;83:E231–E239.
127. Schroder W, Baldus SE, Monig SP, et al. Lymph node staging of esophageal squamous cell carcinoma in patients with and without neoadjuvant radiochemotherapy: histomorphologic analysis. *World J Surg* 2002;26:584–587.
128. Lightdale CJ, Kulkarni KG. Role of endoscopic ultrasonography in the staging and follow-up of esophageal cancer. *J Clin Oncol* 2005;23:4483–4489.
129. Cohen RJ, Paskalev K, Litwin S, et al. Esophageal motion during radiotherapy: quantification and margin implications. *Dis Esophagus* 2010;23:473–479.
130. Fenkell L, Kaminsky I, Breen S, et al. Dosimetric comparison of IMRT vs. 3D conformal radiotherapy in the treatment of cancer of the cervical esophagus. *Radiother Oncol* 2008;89:287–291.
131. Lin SH, Merrell KW, Shen J, et al. Multi-institutional analysis of radiation modality use and postoperative outcomes of neoadjuvant chemoradiation for esophageal cancer. *Radiother Oncol* 2017;123(3):376–381.
132. Lin S, Zhang N, Godby J, et al. Radiation modality use and cardiopulmonary mortality risk in elderly patients with esophageal cancer. *Cancer* 2016;122(6):917–928.
133. Chun S, Hu C, Choy H, et al. Impact of intensity-modulated radiation therapy technique for locally advanced non-small-cell lung cancer: a secondary analysis of the NRG oncology RTOG 0617 randomized clinical trial. *J Clin Oncol* 2017;35(1):56–62.
134. Wu AJ, Bosch WR, Chang DT, et al. Expert consensus contouring guidelines for intensity modulated radiation therapy in esophageal and gastroesophageal junction cancer. *Int J Radiat Oncol Biol Phys* 2015;92:911–920.
135. Burmeister BH, Dickie G, Smithers BM, et al. Thirty-four patients with carcinoma of the cervical esophagus treated with chemoradiation therapy. *Arch Otolaryngol Head Neck Surg* 2000;126:205–208.
136. Murakami M, Kuroda Y, Okamoto Y, et al. Neoadjuvant concurrent chemoradiotherapy followed by definitive high-dose radiotherapy or surgery for operable thoracic esophageal carcinoma. *Int J Radiat Oncol Biol Phys* 1998;40:1049–1059.
137. Minsky BD, Pajak TF, Ginsberg RJ, et al. INT 0123 (Radiation Therapy Oncology Group 94-05) phase III trial of combined-modality therapy for esophageal cancer: high-dose versus standard-dose radiation therapy. *J Clin Oncol* 2002;20:1167–1174.
138. Crehange G, Bonnetain F, Peiffert D, et al. Phase II/III randomized trial of exclusive chemoradiotherapy with or without dose escalation in locally advanced esophageal carcinoma: The CONCORDE study (PRODIGA 26). *J Clin Oncol* 2016;34:Abstract TPS190.
139. Beatty JD, DeBoer G, Rider WD. Carcinoma of the esophagus: pretreatment assessment, correlation of radiation treatment parameters with survival, and identification and management of radiation treatment failure. *Cancer* 1979;43:2254–2267.
140. Omlooj Lagarde S, Hulscher J, et al. Extended transthoracic resection compared with limited transhiatal resection for adenocarcinoma of the mid/distal esophagus: five-year survival of a randomized clinical trial. *Ann Surg* 2007;246(6):992–1000.
141. Kurokawa Y, Sasako M, Sano T, et al. Ten-year follow-up results of a randomized clinical trial comparing left thoracoabdominal and abdominal transhiatal approaches to total gastrectomy for adenocarcinoma of the oesophagogastric junction or gastric cardia. *Br J Surg* 2015;102(4):341–348.
142. Law SY, Fok M, Wong J. Pattern of recurrence after oesophageal resection for cancer: clinical implications. *Br J Surg* 1996;83:107–111.
143. Walsh TN, Noonan N, Hollywood D, et al. A comparison of multimodal therapy and surgery for esophageal adenocarcinoma. *N Engl J Med* 1996;335:462–467.
144. Medical Research Council Oesophageal Cancer Working Group. Surgical resection with or without preoperative chemotherapy in oesophageal cancer: a randomized controlled trial. *Lancet Oncol* 2002;359:1727–1733.
145. Bosset JF, Gignoux M, Triboulet JP, et al. Chemoradiotherapy followed by surgery compared with surgery alone in squamous-cell cancer of the esophagus. *N Engl J Med* 1997;337:161–167.
146. van Hagen P, Hulshof M, van Lanschot JJB, et al. Preoperative Chemoradiotherapy for Esophageal or Junctional Cancer. *N Engl J Med* 2012;366:2074–2084.
147. Burmeister BH, Smithers BM, Gebski V, et al. Surgery alone versus chemoradiotherapy followed by surgery for resectable cancer of the oesophagus: a randomised controlled phase III trial. *Lancet Oncol* 2005;6:659–668.
148. Sun X, Yu J, Fan X, et al. Randomized clinical study of surgery versus radiotherapy alone in the treatment of resectable esophageal cancer in the chest. *Zhonghua Zhong Liu Za Zhi* 2006;28(10):784–787.
149. Earlam R, Cunha-Melo JR. Oesophageal squamous cell carcinoma: I. A critical review of surgery. *Br J Surg* 1980;67:381–390.
150. Okawa T, Kita M, Tanaka M, et al. Results of radiotherapy for inoperable locally advanced esophageal cancer. *Int J Radiat Oncol Biol Phys* 1989;17:49–54.
151. Lederman M. Carcinoma of the oesophagus with special reference to the upper third: part I. Clinical considerations. *Br J Cancer* 1982;39:193.
152. Launois B, Delarue D, Campion JP, et al. Preoperative radiotherapy for carcinoma of the esophagus. *Surg Gynecol Obstet* 1981;153:690–692.
153. Gignoux M, Roussel A, Paillot B, et al. The value of preoperative radiotherapy in esophageal cancer: results of a study of the E.O.R.T.C. *World J Surg* 1987;11:426–432.
154. Arnott SJ, Duncan W, Kerr GR, et al. Low dose preoperative radiotherapy for carcinoma of the oesophagus: results of a randomized clinical trial. *Radiother Oncol* 1992;24:108–113.
155. Wang M, Gu XZ, Yin WB, et al. Randomized clinical trial on the combination of preoperative irradiation and surgery in the treatment of esophageal carcinoma: report on 206 patients. *Int J Radiat Oncol Biol Phys* 1989;16:325–327.
156. Teniere P, Hay JM, Fingerhut A, et al. Postoperative radiation therapy does not increase survival after curative resection for squamous cell carcinoma of the middle and lower esophagus as shown by a multicenter controlled trial. French University Association for Surgical Research. *Surg Gynecol Obstet* 1991;173:123–130.
157. Fok M, Sham JS, Choy D, et al. Postoperative radiotherapy for carcinoma of the esophagus: a prospective, randomized controlled study. *Surgery* 1993;113:138–147.
158. Xiao ZF, Yang ZY, Miao YJ, et al. Influence of number of metastatic lymph nodes on survival of curative resected thoracic esophageal cancer patients and value of radiotherapy: report of 549 cases. *Int J Radiat Oncol Biol Phys* 2005;62:82–90.
159. Macdonald JS, Smalley SR, Benedetti J, et al. Chemoradiotherapy after surgery compared with surgery alone for adenocarcinoma of the stomach or gastroesophageal junction. *N Engl J Med* 2001;345:725–730.
160. Smalley SR, Benedetti J, Haller DG, et al. Updated analysis of SWOG-directed intergroup study 0116: a phase III trial of adjuvant radiochemotherapy versus observation after curative gastric cancer resection. *J Clin Oncol* 2012;30:2327.
161. Hsu P, Huang C, Wang BY, et al. Survival benefits of postoperative chemoradiation for lymph node-positive esophageal squamous cell carcinoma. *Ann Thorac Surg* 2014;97:1734–1741.
162. Bedard E, Inculet R, Malthaner R, et al. The role of surgery and postoperative chemoradiation therapy in patients with lymph node positive esophageal carcinoma. *Cancer* 2001;91:2423–2430.
163. Kelsen DP, Winter KA, Gunderson LL, et al. Long-term results of RTOG trial 8911 (USA Intergroup 113): a random assignment trial comparison of chemotherapy followed by surgery compared with surgery alone for esophageal cancer. *J Clin Oncol* 2007;25:3719–3725.
164. Allum WH, Stenning SP, Bancewicz J, et al. Long-term results of a randomized trial of surgery with or without preoperative chemotherapy in esophageal cancer. *J Clin Oncol* 2009;27:5062–5067.
164a. Alderson D, Cunningham D, Nankivell M, et al. Neoadjuvant cisplatin and fluorouracil versus epirubicin, cisplatin, and capecitabine followed by resection in patients with oesophageal adenocarcinoma (UK MRC OE05): an open-label, randomised phase 3 trial. *Lancet Oncol* 2017;18(9):1249–1260.
165. Boonstra JJ, Kok TC, Wijnhoven BP, et al. Chemotherapy followed by surgery versus surgery alone in patients with resectable oesophageal squamous cell carcinoma: long-term results of a randomized controlled trial. *BMC Cancer* 2011;11:181.
166. Cunningham D, Allum WH, Stenning SP, et al. Perioperative chemotherapy versus surgery alone for resectable gastroesophageal cancer. *N Engl J Med* 2006;355:11–20.
167. Cunningham D, Stenning S, Smyth E, et al. Peri-operative chemotherapy with or without bevacizumab in operable oesophagogastric adenocarcinoma (UK Medical Research Council ST03); primary analysis results of a multicentre, open-label, randomised phase 2-3 trial. *Lancet Oncol* 2017;18(3):357–370.
168. Ychou M, Boige V, Pignon JP, et al. Perioperative chemotherapy compared with surgery alone for resectable gastroesophageal adenocarcinoma: an FNCLCC and FFCD multicenter phase III trial. *J Clin Oncol* 2011;29:1715–1721.
169. Gebski V, Burmeister B, Smithers BM, et al. Survival benefits from neoadjuvant chemoradiotherapy or chemotherapy in oesophageal carcinoma: a meta-analysis. *Lancet Oncol* 2007;8:226–234.
170. Thirion P, Michiels S, Le Maitre A, et al. Individual patient data-based meta-analysis assessing pre-operative chemotherapy in resectable oesophageal carcinoma. *J Clin Oncol* 2007;25:200s.
171. Bass G, Furlong H, O'Sullivan K, et al. Chemoradiotherapy, with adjuvant surgery for local control, confers a durable survival advantage in adenocarcinoma and squamous cell carcinoma of the oesophagus. *Eur J Cancer* 2014;50(6):1065–1075.
172. Tepper J, Krasna MJ, Niedzwiecki D, et al. Phase III trial of trimodality therapy with cisplatin, fluorouracil, radiotherapy, and surgery compared with surgery alone for esophageal cancer: CALGB 9781. *J Clin Oncol* 2008;26:1086–1092.

173. Oppedijk V, van der Gaast A, Van Lanschot J, et al. Patterns of recurrence after surgery alone versus preoperative chemoradiotherapy and surgery in the CROSS trials. *J Clin Oncol* 2014;32(5):385–391.

174. Robb W, Messager M, Dahan L, et al. Patterns of recurrence in early-stage oesophageal cancer after chemoradiotherapy and surgery compared with surgery alone. *Br J Surg* 2016;103(1):117–125.

174a. Yang H, Fu J, Liu M, et al. A phase III clinical trial of neoadjuvant chemoradiotherapy followed by surgery versus surgery alone for locally advanced squamous cell carcinoma of the esophagus. *Annals of Oncology* 2016;27(suppl_6):6110.

175. Sjoquist KM, Burmeister BH, Smithers BM, et al. Survival after neoadjuvant chemotherapy or chemoradiotherapy for resectable oesophageal carcinoma: an updated meta-analysis. *Lancet Oncol* 2011;12:681–692.

176. Stahl M, Walz MK, Stuschke M, et al. Phase III comparison of preoperative chemotherapy compared with chemoradiotherapy in patients with locally advanced adenocarcinoma of the esophagogastric junction. *J Clin Oncol* 2009;27:851–856.

176a. Klevebro F, Von Dobeln A, Wang N, et al. A randomized clinical trial of neoadjuvant chemotherapy versus neoadjuvant chemoradiotherapy for cancer of the oesophagus or gastro-oesophageal junction. *Ann Oncol* 2016;27(4):660–667.

177. Burmeister BH, Thomas JM, Burmeister EA, et al. Is concurrent radiation therapy required in patients receiving preoperative chemotherapy for adenocarcinoma of the oesophagus? A randomised phase II trial. *Eur J Cancer* 2011;47:354–360.

178. Deng H, Wang W, Wang Y, et al. Neoadjuvant chemoradiotherapy or chemotherapy? A comprehensive systematic review and meta-analysis of the options for neoadjuvant therapy for treating oesophageal cancer. *Eur J Cardiothorac Surg* 2017;51(3):421–431.

179. Araujo CM, Souhami L, Gil RA, et al. A randomized trial comparing radiation therapy versus concomitant radiation therapy and chemotherapy in carcinoma of the thoracic esophagus. *Cancer* 1991;67:2258–2261.

180. Roussell A, Jacob J, Haegele P, et al. Controlled clinical trial for the treatment of patients with inoperable esophageal carcinoma: a study of EORTC Gastrointestinal Tract Cancer Cooperative Group. *Recent Results Cancer Res* 1988;110:21–29.

181. Herskovic A, Martz K, al-Sarraf M, et al. Combined chemotherapy and radiotherapy compared with radiotherapy alone in patients with cancer of the esophagus. *N Engl J Med* 1992;326:1593–1598.

182. Cooper JS, Guo MD, Herskovic A, et al. Chemoradiotherapy of locally advanced esophageal cancer: long-term follow-up of a prospective randomized trial (RTOG 85-01). Radiation Therapy Oncology Group. *JAMA* 1999;281:1623–1627.

183. Crosby T, Hurt C, Falk S, et al. Long-term results and recurrence patterns from SCOPE-1: a phase II/III randomised trial of definitive chemoradiotherapy +/− cetuximab in oesophageal cancer. *Br J Cancer* 2017;116(6):709–716.

184. Suntharalingam M, Winter K, Ilson D, et al. The initial report of RTOG 0436: a phase III trial evaluating the addition of cetuximab to paclitaxel, cisplatin and radiation for patients with esophageal cancer treated without surgery. *J Clin Oncol* 2014;32(Suppl 3):abstr LBA6.

185. Conroy T, Galais M, Raoul J, et al. Definitive chemoradiotherapy with FOLFOX vs fluorouracil and cisplatin in patients with oesophageal cancer (PRODIGE5/ACCORD17): Final results of a randomised, phase 2/3 trial. *Lancet Oncol* 2014;15(3):305–314.

186. Bang Y, Van Cutsem E, Feyereislova A, et al. Trastuzumab in combination with chemotherapy versus chemotherapy alone for treatment of HER2-positive advanced gastric or gastro-oesophageal junctional cancer (ToGA): a phase 3, open-label, randomised controlled trial. *Lancet* 2010;376(9742):687–697.

187. Bedenne L, Michel P, Bouche O, et al. Chemoradiation followed by surgery compared with chemoradiation alone in squamous cancer of the esophagus: FFCD 9102. *J Clin Oncol* 2007;25:1160–1168.

188. Jouve J, Michel P, Mariette C, et al. Outcome of the nonrandomized patients in the FFCD 9102 trial: Chemoradiation followed by surgery compared with chemoradiation alone in squamous cancer of the esophagus. *J Clin Oncol* 2008;26(20s):4555.

189. Gwynne S, Hurt C, Evans M, et al. Definitive chemoradiation for oesophageal cancer—a standard of care in patients with non-metastatic oesophageal cancer. *Clin Oncol (R Coll Radiol)* 2011;23:182–188.

190. Markar S, Gronnier C, Duhamel A, et al. Salvage surgery after chemoradiotherapy in the management of esophageal cancer: is it a viable therapeutic option? *J Clin Oncol* 2015;33(33):3866–3873.

191. Swisher S, Moughan J, Komaki R, et al. Final results of NRG Oncology RTOG 0246: an organ-preserving selective resection strategy in esophageal cancer patients treated with definitive chemoradiation. *J Thorac Oncol* 2017;12:368–374.

192. Gaspar L, Winter K, Kocha W, et al. Swallowing function and weight change observed in a phase I/II study of external-beam radiation, brachytherapy and concurrent chemotherapy in localized cancer of the esophagus (RTOG 9207). *Cancer J* 2001;7(5):388–394.

193. Gaspar LE, Winter K, Kocha WI, et al. A phase I/II study of external beam radiation, brachytherapy, and concurrent chemotherapy for patients with localized carcinoma of the esophagus (Radiation Therapy Oncology Group Study 9207): final report. *Cancer* 2000;88:988–995.

194. Zhu H, Guo J, Mao A, et al. Conventional stents versus stents loaded with (125) iodine seeds for the treatment of unresectable oesophageal cancer: a multicentre, randomised phase 3 trial. *Lancet Oncol* 2014;15(6):612–619.

195. Vuong T, Szego P, David M, et al. The safety and usefulness of high-dose-rate endoluminal brachytherapy as a boost in the treatment of patients with esophageal cancer with external beam radiation with or without chemotherapy. *Int J Radiat Oncol Biol Phys* 2005;63:758–764.

196. Fuccio L, Mandolesi D, Farioli A, et al. Brachytherapy for the palliation of dysphagia owing to esophageal cancer: A systematic review and meta-analysis of prospective studies. *Radiother Oncol* 2017;122(3):332–339.

197. Homs MY, Steyerberg EW, Eijkenboom WM, et al. Single-dose brachytherapy versus metal stent placement for the palliation of dysphagia from oesophageal cancer: multicentre randomised trial. *Lancet* 2004;364:1497–1504.

198. Rosenblatt E, Jones G, Sur R, et al. Adding external beam to intra-luminal brachytherapy improves palliation in obstructive squamous cell oesophageal carcinoma: a prospective multi-centre randomized trial of the International Atomic Energy Agency. *Radiother Oncol* 2010;97(3):488–494.

199. Berquist H, Wenger U, Johnsson E, et al. Stent insertion or endoluminal brachytherapy as palliation of patients with advanced cancer of the esophagus and gastroesophageal junction: results of a randomized, controlled clinical trial. *Dis Esophagus* 2005;18(3):131–139.

200. Gaspar LE, Nag S, Herskovic A, et al. American Brachytherapy Society (ABS) consensus guidelines for brachytherapy of esophageal cancer. Clinical Research Committee, American Brachytherapy Society, Philadelphia, PA. *Int J Radiat Oncol Biol Phys* 1997;38:127–132.

201. Coia LR, Soffen EM, Schultheiss TE, et al. Swallowing function in patients with esophageal cancer treated with concurrent radiation and chemotherapy. *Cancer* 1993;71:281–286.

202. Murray L, Din O, Kumar V, et al. Palliative radiotherapy in patients with esophageal carcinoma: a retrospective review. *Pract Radiat Oncol* 2012;2(4):257–264.

203. Penniment MG, De Ieso PB, Harvey JA, et al. Palliative chemoradiotherapy versus radiotherapy alone for dysphagia in advanced oesophageal cancer: a multicentre randomised controlled trial (TROG 03.01). *Lancet Gastroenterol Hepatol* 2018;3(2):114–124.

204. Gschossmann JM, Bonner JA, Foote RL, et al. Malignant tracheoesophageal fistula in patients with esophageal cancer. *Cancer* 1993;72:1513–1521.

205. Fakhrian K, Gamisch N, Schuster T, et al. Salvage radiotherapy in patients with recurrent esophageal carcinoma. *Strahlenther Onkol* 2012;188(2):136–142.

206. Kim YS, Lee C, Kim K, et al. Re-irradiation of recurrent esophageal cancer after primary definitive radiotherapy. *Radiat Oncol J* 2012;30(4):182–188.

207. Fernandes A, Berman A, Mick R, et al. A Prospective Study of Proton Beam Reirradiation for Esophageal Cancer. *Int J Radiat Oncol Biol Phys* 2016;95(1):43–47.

208. Tsutsui S, Moriguchi S, Morita M, et al. Multivariate analysis of postoperative complications after esophageal resection. *Ann Thorac Surg* 1992;53:1052–1056.

209. Baquet CR, Commiskey P, Mack K, et al. Esophageal cancer epidemiology in blacks and whites: racial and gender disparities in incidence, mortality, survival rates and histology. *J Natl Med Assoc* 2005;97:1471–1478.

210. Asakura H, Hashimoto T, Zenda S, et al. Analysis of dose-volume histogram parameters for radiation pneumonitis after definitive concurrent chemoradiotherapy for esophageal cancer. *Radiother Oncol* 2010;95:240–244.

211. Hart JP, McCurdy MR, Ezhil M, et al. Radiation pneumonitis: correlation of toxicity with pulmonary metabolic radiation response. *Int J Radiat Oncol Biol Phys* 2008;71:967–971.

212. Morota M, Gomi K, Kozuka T, et al. Late toxicity after definitive concurrent chemoradiotherapy for thoracic esophageal carcinoma. *Int J Radiat Oncol Biol Phys* 2009;75:122–128.

213. Gergel TJ, Leichman L, Nava HR, et al. Effect of concurrent radiation therapy and chemotherapy on pulmonary function in patients with esophageal cancer: dose-volume histogram analysis. *Cancer J* 2002;8:451–460.

214. Tucker SL, Liu HH, Wang S, et al. Dose-volume modeling of the risk of postoperative pulmonary complications among esophageal cancer patients treated with concurrent chemoradiotherapy followed by surgery. *Int J Radiat Oncol Biol Phys* 2006;66:754–761.

215. Lee HK, Vaporciyan AA, Cox JD, et al. Postoperative pulmonary complications after preoperative chemoradiation for esophageal carcinoma: correlation with pulmonary dose-volume histogram parameters. *Int J Radiat Oncol Biol Phys* 2003;57:1317–1322.

216. Wang SL, Liao Z, Vaporciyan AA, et al. Investigation of clinical and dosimetric factors associated with postoperative pulmonary complications in esophageal cancer patients treated with concurrent chemoradiotherapy followed by surgery. *Int J Radiat Oncol Biol Phys* 2006;64:692–699.

217. Wang S, Liao Z, Wei X, et al. Association between systemic chemotherapy before chemoradiation and increased risk of treatment-related pneumonitis in esophageal cancer patients treated with definitive chemoradiotherapy. *J Thorac Oncol* 2008;3:277–282.

218. Dahn D, Martell J, Vorwerk H, et al. Influence of irradiated lung volumes on perioperative morbidity and mortality in patients after neoadjuvant radiochemotherapy for esophageal cancer. *Int J Radiat Oncol Biol Phys* 2010;77:44–52.

219. Hsu FM, Lee YC, Lee JM, et al. Association of clinical and dosimetric factors with postoperative pulmonary complications in esophageal cancer patients receiving intensity-modulated radiation therapy and concurrent chemotherapy followed by thoracic esophagectomy. *Ann Surg Oncol* 2009;16:1669–1677.

220. Shaikh T, Churilla T, Monpara P, et al. Risk of radiation pneumonitis in patients receiving taxane-based trimodality therapy for locally advanced esophageal cancer. *Pract Radiat Oncol* 2016;6(6):388–394.

221. Cosset JM, Henry-Amar M, Pellae-Cosset B, et al. Pericarditis and myocardial infarctions after Hodgkin's disease therapy. *Int J Radiat Oncol Biol Phys* 1991;21:447–449.

222. Hancock SL, Donaldson SS, Hoppe RT. Cardiac disease following treatment of Hodgkin's disease in children and adolescents. *J Clin Oncol* 1993;11:1208–1215.

223. Gayed IW, Liu H, Yusuf SW, et al. The prevalence of myocardial ischemia after concurrent chemoradiation therapy as detected by gated myocardial perfusion imaging in patients with esophageal cancer. *J Nucl Med* 2006;47:1756–1762.

224. Ishikura S, Nihei K, Ohtsu A, et al. Long-term toxicity after definitive chemoradiotherapy for squamous cell carcinoma of the thoracic esophagus. *J Clin Oncol* 2003;21:2697–2702.

225. Ogino I, Watanabe S, Iwahashi N, et al. Symptomatic radiation-induced cardiac disease in long-term survivors of esophageal cancer. *Strahlenther Onkol* 2016;192(6):359–367.

226. Beukema J, van Luijk P, Widder J, et al. Is cardiac toxicity a relevant issue in the radiation treatment of esophageal cancer? *Radiother Oncol* 2015;114:85–90.

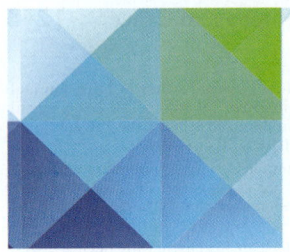

CHAPTER 57

Tumors of the Heart, Pericardium, and Great Vessels

Gregory M.M. Videtic and Roger M. Macklis

ANATOMY

The heart is a hollow, conical (MB1) organ with muscular walls. In the adult, it measures approximately 12 cm in length, 8 to 9 cm in width, and 6 cm in thickness. It is located in the inferior aspect of the middle mediastinum, with two-thirds lying to the left of midline and one-third to the right. The heart lies posterior to the sternum and rib cage, and anatomic landmarks on the chest wall may be used to approximate its position. The apex is located roughly 8 cm to the left of midline in the fifth intercostal space, and the base is at the level of the third costal cartilage. It rests on the diaphragm inferiorly. The heart receives its blood supply from the coronary arteries, which are located in the space between the myocardium and epicardium. The pericardial fat provides a smooth contour and is also located in this space. The heart has four chambers: two ventricles with thick muscular walls and two atria with thin muscular walls. Although the heart is not attached to surrounding organs, it is held in position by its association with the great vessels (GVs) and the pericardium. The GVs include the aorta, superior and inferior vena cava (IVC), pulmonary artery, and pulmonary veins, which arise from (or terminate in) the left ventricle, right atrium, right ventricle, and left atrium, respectively. The roots of the GVs, along with the heart, are encompassed by the parietal pericardium. In combination with the epicardium, this fibrous layer provides a smooth cavity in which the heart can pump freely. Externally, the pericardium is adherent to, but separate from, the mediastinal pleura, creating a potential space through which the phrenic nerve traverses.[1]

INCIDENCE AND EPIDEMIOLOGY

Tumors of the heart, GVs, and pericardium are rare and include a range of disease presentations: primary neoplasms; secondary metastases from a known malignancy; or direct tumor invasion into the structures, which is seen in certain cancers such as Hodgkin or non-Hodgkin lymphoma, lung cancer, or malignant thymoma. The focus of this chapter will be to review the epidemiology, diagnosis, natural history, and management of primary tumors arising from the heart, pericardium, and GVs as well as metastatic disease to these sites.

The first described case of a primary cardiac tumor was by Albers in 1835.[2] Reynen[3] performed a compilation of autopsy series consisting of over 700,000 cases and found 157 primary cardiac tumors. The overall incidence of primary tumors is 0.021%, with a range from 0% to 0.19%. Approximately 75% of primary tumors of the heart are benign, and about half of those are atrial myxomas arising from the interatrial septum.[4–6] Lipomas, papillary fibroelastomas, and rhabdomyomas each account for approximately 10% of cases. Fibromas, hemangiomas, and teratomas are less common benign cardiac tumors.[7] Cystic atrioventricular node tumors are extremely rare but may lead to sudden death, despite their small size.[8] There is an increased incidence of cardiac myxomas among females and in patients with Carney complex, an inherited autosomal dominant disorder that also shows hyperpigmented lentigines, blue nevi, schwannomas, endocrine tumors, and endocrinopathies.[9,10] The syndrome is most commonly caused by an inactivating germ-line mutation of the *PRKAR1 A* tumor-suppressor gene on chromosome 17q23-q24.[9,11,12] Variants include the LAMB (*l*entigines, *a*trial myxoma, *m*ucocutaneous myxoma, and *b*lue nevi) and NAME (*n*evi, *a*trial myxoma, *m*yxoid neurofibroma, and *e*phelides) syndromes.[8] Myxomas in patients with Carney complex account for 7% of all cardiac myxomas, are typically found at a younger age, and may have higher recurrence rates.[4,13] Hamartomas, rhabdomyomas, and fibromas are diagnosed almost exclusively in children.[14] Rhabdomyomas are the most common pediatric cardiac tumor and are associated with tuberous sclerosis.

Malignant primary tumors constitute the remaining 25% of cardiac neoplasms. Primary malignancies of the myocardium constitute the bulk of the remaining cases, of which sarcomas account for the vast majority. Malignant fibrous histiocytoma, angiosarcoma, fibrosarcoma, and rhabdomyosarcoma are among the more common histologic types.[15] Table 57.1 summarizes the relative frequency of specific subtypes of sarcoma that may be diagnosed. The median age at diagnosis is 30 to 40 years, slightly younger than that for benign tumors, and there is no sex predilection as seen in myxoma.[15] Lymphomas account for only about 2% of primary cardiac tumors, but the incidence appears to be increasing.[19] Melanoma and carcinoma may also occur infrequently.

Primary malignant tumors of the pericardium are exceedingly rare and include mesothelioma, fibrosarcoma, angiosarcoma, and malignant teratoma.[20] An American Medical Association survey of nearly 500,000 autopsies revealed a 0.0022% incidence of primary malignant pericardial neoplasms.[21] It appears that malignant mesothelioma is the most common primary malignancy of the pericardium, accounting for 50% of primary pericardial tumors. Asbestos has well-established associations with pleural and peritoneal mesothelioma, and there appears to be some correlation in pericardial mesothelioma.[22] Unfortunately, because of the low incidence, this association has been inconsistent, and no other risk factors have been identified.[23–25] There have been very few cases reported since 1994, when 140 cases had been reported in the literature.[20,21,23–29] Fibrosarcoma, angiosarcoma, synovial sarcoma, and teratoma of the pericardium have also been documented.[20,24,29]

TABLE 57.1 DISTRIBUTION OF HISTOLOGIC SUBTYPES OF CARDIAC SARCOMA

Subtype of Sarcoma	Number of Cases	Percentage of Cases
Angiosarcoma	105	28
Rhabdomyosarcoma	43	12
Undifferentiated/NOS	43	12
Fibrosarcoma	39	10
Malignant fibrous histiocytoma	33	9
Leiomyosarcoma	26	7
Liposarcoma	20	5
Other	64	17
Total	373	100

NOS, not otherwise specified.
Data compiled from references 7 and 15–18.

With advances in echocardiography, computed tomography (CT), and magnetic resonance imaging (MRI), the postmortem diagnosis of cardiac tumors is becoming less common. Surgical series seem to demonstrate an increase in the ratio of benign to malignant tumors, with malignant tumors accounting for only 10% of cases in a narrow range of 6% to 20%.[14,16,30–34] This is likely the result of surgical management of benign myxoma, which accounts for over 80% of patients in some series, combined with changes in patient selection.[16,30,33]

The majority of primary cardiac tumors arise in adults with a median age of 45 to 55 years, but they can be seen at any age.[14,16,30–34] Among 533 cases in the database of the Armed Forces Institute of Pathology, McAllister and Fenoglio[7] noted that 83% of patients were adults. Infants (<1 year of age) constituted 9% of the patients, and in this group, 96% of tumors were benign and only 4% were malignant. In a review of the data from the National Cancer Institute Surveillance, Epidemiology, and End Results from 1973 to 1987, Mack[15] reported no sex predilection for the incidence of sarcoma of the mediastinum and heart.

Metastatic disease to the heart and pericardium occurs at a frequency much greater than that of primary tumors.[35–41] In a review of more than 12,000 autopsies in Hong Kong, Lam et al.[39] noted that cardiac metastases were over 20 times more common than primary tumors and may be present in up to 20% of patients dying of disease. The majority of cases have involvement of the pericardium, whereas myocardial involvement is uncommon. In a review of autopsy series of patients with a known malignancy, Hanfling[37] noted the rate of reported cardiac involvement increased steadily from 1.5% in the late 1800s to 18.3% in 1960. Contemporary series indicate the rate of cardiac metastases in patients dying of cancer may be as high as 20%.[7,37–40,42,43]

The sites of origin of cardiac metastases from solid tumors are summarized in Table 57.2. Lung cancer is the most common cause of cardiac metastases and accounts for nearly one-half of all cases. Upper gastrointestinal malignancies and breast cancer are also common causes of cardiac metastases, accounting for one-fourth of all cases. The remaining one-fourth of cases arise from a wide variety of other malignancies.[35–40] Melanoma is purported to have the highest propensity for metastatic spread to the heart and tends to involve the endocardium or myocardium, with some series showing its incidence of cardiac metastases rivaling or exceeding that of lung cancers.[2,43] Cardiac metastases may also originate from lymphoma or leukemia. In 1960, Hanfling[37] reported that the proportion of cardiac metastases arising from these malignancies rivals that arising from solid tumors. However, multiple medical advances in both chemotherapy and diagnosis have occurred since then, and modern series consistently report that these histologies account for approximately 17% of cardiac metastases.[35,36,38,39]

Tumors of the GVs are extremely rare. The literature on these consists mainly of case reports, and approximately 130 cases have been documented. As a whole, tumors of the GVs are about as common as primary malignant pericardial mesothelioma. The largest series has been reported by Burke and

Virmani.[44] They evaluated 45 tumors on the files of the Armed Forces Institute of Pathology and found that all of the tumors were sarcomas, including intimal (undifferentiated) sarcoma, angiosarcoma, leiomyosarcoma, and synovial sarcoma. There appeared to be no sex predilection for tumors of the aorta or pulmonary artery, although the female-to-male ratio was 3 to 1 among patients with tumors of the IVC.

NATURAL HISTORY

Tumors of the Myocardium

Myxomas, as discussed previously, are the most common benign tumors of the heart, are seen in women twice as frequently as men, and are diagnosed at a mean age of 45 to 55 years but have been documented in infants and octogenarians.[16,30–34,45] Benign myxomas tend to be slow growing and are minimally invasive and as such may have a long duration of symptoms before diagnosis. Typically, these tumors arise from the interatrial septum and grow into the adjacent chamber. The left atrium is the most common site of involvement for myxoma, and this is six to seven times more common than myxoma of the right atrium. The tumor may also be located in the ventricles or the valves and can be bilateral. Although they are considered benign, the tumor can elicit dramatic symptoms from valvular insufficiency, congestive heart failure, and embolic phenomena. Surgical excision is the treatment of choice, with local recurrence rates ranging from 0% to 5.4%.[8]

Primary malignant tumors of the myocardium, most commonly sarcomas, do not show a predilection for developing in any particular part of the heart, except for angiosarcomas, which tend to occur more frequently in the right atrium, and often present late with advanced disease and lung metastases.[14,16,30,32,33] The duration of symptoms is on the order of months, and survival is poor. Even after attempts at curative resection, recurrences are common, and the median survival ranges from 6 to 18 months.[14,16–18,30–34] The cause of death is most often complications of locally recurrent disease with invasion of adjacent chambers, valves, or pericardium. Tamponade, hemopericardium, and distant metastases are common.[18] About 30% of primary cardiac sarcomas have distant metastases at the time of diagnosis.[2] The high incidence of hematogenous dissemination of a cardiac sarcoma may be explained by the high rate of blood flow through the heart.[46]

Tumors of the Pericardium

Mesothelioma is the most common pericardial neoplasm and may either be confined to the pericardial sac at diagnosis or extend beyond it, involving the myocardium or mediastinal structures.[23–25] Of 140 primary malignant pericardial mesotheliomas reported in the literature, only 28% of cases were diagnosed antemortem.[24] These tumors have been documented to metastasize by lymphatic and hematogenous routes to involve regional lymph nodes, lung, liver, brain, bone, and adrenal glands.[20,21,23–28] Despite the metastatic potential, pericardial tumors are more often fatal because of local complications, such as restrictive pericarditis with resultant cardiac tamponade, arrhythmia due to myocardial invasion, or vena caval obstruction. Even if the tumor can be diagnosed antemortem, survival is poor. Typically, the onset of symptoms does not occur until the tumor is well advanced, and from that time, the median survival is <6 months, with only a handful of patients surviving beyond 1 year.[26–28]

Tumors of the Great Vessels

The median age at presentation for tumors of the GVs is between 40 and 60 years.[44] The natural history and clinical presentation depend on the exact location of the primary tumor. Depending on the location, symptoms may include dyspnea, cough, hemoptysis, pain, and thromboembolic

TABLE 57.2 SITE OF ORIGIN FOR CARDIAC METASTASES		
Primary Tumor	**Number of Patients**	**Percentage of Cases**
Lung	271	47
Upper gastrointestinal[a]	107	19
Breast	42	7
Genitourinary (nonprostate)	37	6
Melanoma	28	5
Other	93	16
Total	578	100

[a]Includes esophagus, stomach, small bowel, pancreas, and hepatobiliary primary tumors.
Data compiled from references 35–40.

Section III

phenomena, including pulseless extremities, stroke, peripheral edema, and superior vena cava (SVC) syndrome. In the series by Burke and Virmani,[44] they found that in contrast to the tumors of the aorta and pulmonary artery that were aggressive sarcomas arising from the vessel lumen, tumors of the IVC were mostly low-grade leiomyosarcomas originating from the medial layer of smooth muscle in the vessel wall.

DIAGNOSIS

Tumors of the heart have been referred to as the "great imitators" of the cardiovascular system, and although there are no pathognomonic signs or symptoms, cardiac tumors can often be detected through careful attention to both cardiac and extracardiac manifestations of the disease.[47,48] It is not surprising that tumors of the heart are often asymptomatic until they become advanced enough to affect blood flow or cardiac function.[37] As the tumor enlarges, disturbances in normal heart function produce different signs and symptoms depending on the location of the tumor. The scope of clinical presentation is summarized in Table 57.3. Tumors involving the right heart may result in pulmonary emboli, pulmonary hypertension, tricuspid valve disease, or SVC or IVC obstruction. Left-sided tumors can cause mitral valve disease, thromboembolic phenomena, and rapidly progressive congestive heart failure, which may be refractory to treatment. A characteristic auscultation finding referred to as a tumor plop may be heard during early diastole in 30% of patients.[49] Arrhythmias are very common and are predominantly supraventricular tachycardia or nonspecific conduction anomalies.[48] Specific presenting complaints are equally varied. Dyspnea is the most common presenting complaint and is noted in 59% to 88% of patients.[17,35,50,51] Palpitations or syncope is also seen frequently and may be positional, and if the tumor obstructs a valve orifice, sudden death may result. Chest pain can be anginal, resulting from direct myocardial invasion or obstruction of the main coronary ostia. It can also be sharp, due to invasion of the pericardium, with resulting pericarditis. Constitutional symptoms also occur, with fever, malaise, anemia, and weight loss.[17,35,37,48,50,51] Tumors of the pericardium and GVs show a similarly variable constellation of symptoms, and as such, they pose the same diagnostic difficulties as tumors of the myocardium.

Physical examination may reveal tachycardia, murmur (which may be positional), pericardial rub, gallops, peripheral edema, jugular venous distention, rales, and stigmata of thromboembolic disease. Electrocardiography (ECG) most often reveals nonspecific ST- and T-wave changes, although low-voltage ECG, supraventricular tachycardia, bundle-branch block, or second-degree (type II) or third-degree atrioventricular node block may also be noted. Laboratory studies may reveal anemia, erythrocytosis, thrombocytosis, thrombocytopenia, leukocytosis, and elevated erythroid sedimentation rate.[17,48,51,52]

DIAGNOSTIC WORKUP

Before the advent of echocardiography and angiography, 66% of tumors were diagnosed intraoperatively during exploration for suspected valvular disease. With current techniques, the diagnosis can be made reliably in the preoperative setting in almost 90% of cases.[16] The diagnostic evaluation of patients with suspected cardiac tumors is presented in Table 57.4.

Physical examination and ECG findings have been described above. The imaging techniques used in the diagnosis and evaluation of cardiac tumors include chest radiography, CT, MRI, echocardiography, radionuclide scintigraphy, and cardiac catheterization. Although there is considerable overlap among these studies, each modality is unique and complements the others in evaluating the tumor. Chest radiography shows abnormalities in over 80% of patients. Unfortunately, abnormalities are usually nonspecific and therefore of limited usefulness. Findings include cardiomegaly, an abnormal cardiac contour, mediastinal widening, or evidence of congestive heart failure.[48,53,54] Calcifications are present in up to 20% of cases, perhaps relating to the presence of valvular or pericardial disease.[53,55] Calcifications on imaging may also suggest the presence of a fibroma. In the setting of a malignant tumor, chest radiography may also reveal hilar nodal, pulmonary, or osseous metastatic disease.

Echocardiography, M-mode and two-dimensional, is the diagnostic procedure of choice among patients with suspected cardiac tumors. Either transthoracic (TTE) or transesophageal (TEE) techniques can be performed, yielding valuable information regarding size, shape, location, mobility, and areas of attachment.[48] In a review of 533 primary cardiac tumors, Blondeau[16] found echocardiography provided a 98% diagnostic accuracy rate among the 437 patients for whom it was used. Bogren et al.[54] found that echocardiography detected abnormalities in 63 of 65 (97%) patients with primary cardiac tumors. With this high level of diagnostic yield, and because the use of TTE has no known side effects, it

TABLE 57.3 SCOPE OF CLINICAL MANIFESTATIONS OF CARDIAC TUMORS

Cardiovascular Manifestations	Extracardiac Manifestations
Electrocardiogram findings	Pulmonary
Low voltage	Rales
Atrial fibrillation or flutter	Dyspnea
Supraventricular tachycardia	Hemoptysis
Conduction anomalies	Pulmonary hypertension
Bundle branch block	Upper digestive tract
Atrioventricular block (2nd or 3rd degree)	Hematemesis
Ventricular tachycardia	Dysphagia
Ventricular fibrillation	Embolic phenomena
Pericardial signs	Right-sided tumors
Friction rub	Pulmonary emboli
Pericarditis	Left-sided tumors
Effusion	Stroke
Tamponade	Splinter hemorrhages
Congestive heart failure	Peripheral arterial occlusion
Peripheral edema	Raynaud phenomenon
Jugular venous distention	Peripheral findings
Valvular insufficiency	Clubbing
Chest pain	Ascites
Palpitations	Constitutional symptoms
Syncope	Anemia
Sudden death	Fatigue
Superior or inferior vena caval obstruction	Fever
Myalgia	Weight loss
	Arthralgia

TABLE 57.4 DIAGNOSTIC EVALUATION FOR A SUSPECTED OR KNOWN CARDIAC TUMOR

Required Studies	Optional Studies
History	Cardiac catheterization, right or left sided
Physical examination	Pressure and output measurements
Blood work	Coronary angiography
Complete blood count	Endomyocardial biopsy
Liver function tests	Transesophageal echocardiography
Renal profile	ECG-gated MRI
Electrolytes	Radionuclide scintigraphy, including PET
ECG	Pericardiocentesis
Imaging	Staging for malignant tumors
Chest radiography	CT of the abdomen, pelvis, and brain
Transthoracic echocardiography	Bone scan
Contrast-enhanced dynamic CT	

CT, computed tomography; ECG, electrocardiography; MRI, magnetic resonance imaging; PET, positron emission tomography.

should be performed for all patients. TEE is a complementary procedure to TTE. It is a more invasive procedure and is not required in all patients, but it may be used for guidance during endomyocardial biopsy and may also provide better evaluation of the left atrial appendage and right-sided tumors.[56–58]

Cross-sectional imaging has also become indispensable in the evaluation of nonmyxomatous cardiac tumors. With the development of contrast-enhanced dynamic CT (Fig. 57.1B) and ECG-gated MRI (Fig. 57.1A and C), real-time imaging of the heart provides fine details of the tumor, with delineation of intraluminal, intramyocardial, and extracardiac extension.[48,59–62] The findings may be used to plan the surgical approach and, should adjuvant therapy be required, could also be used for radiotherapy treatment planning. Compared to chest radiographs, both CT and MRI are more sensitive in detecting metastatic disease. If these studies are positive, tissue diagnosis may be made without the need for endomyocardial biopsy or thoracotomy. If they have not been performed before surgery, CT of the brain, chest, and upper abdomen and a bone scan are recommended in the staging of malignant cardiac tumors.

Radionuclide imaging has been used in the evaluation of cardiac tumors. Gated cardiac blood pool scintigraphy has limited resolution, but it may be able to detect tumors when other modalities have failed. Gallium-67 and thallium-201 scans may reveal intramyocardial invasion.[48,54] Positron emission tomography (PET), with or without CT fusion (PET-CT) (Fig. 57.1D), is rapidly gaining favor in the staging of many

FIGURE 57.1. Axial contrast-enhanced fat-saturated T1 magnetic resonance image (MRI) of a primary cardiac neoplasm arising from the left atrium **(A)**; corresponding axial contrast-enhanced computed tomography (CT) **(B)**, coronal contrast-enhanced fat-saturated T1 MRI **(C)**, and coronal fluorodeoxyglucose positron emission tomography CT **(D)** images. Tumor indicated by *white arrows*.

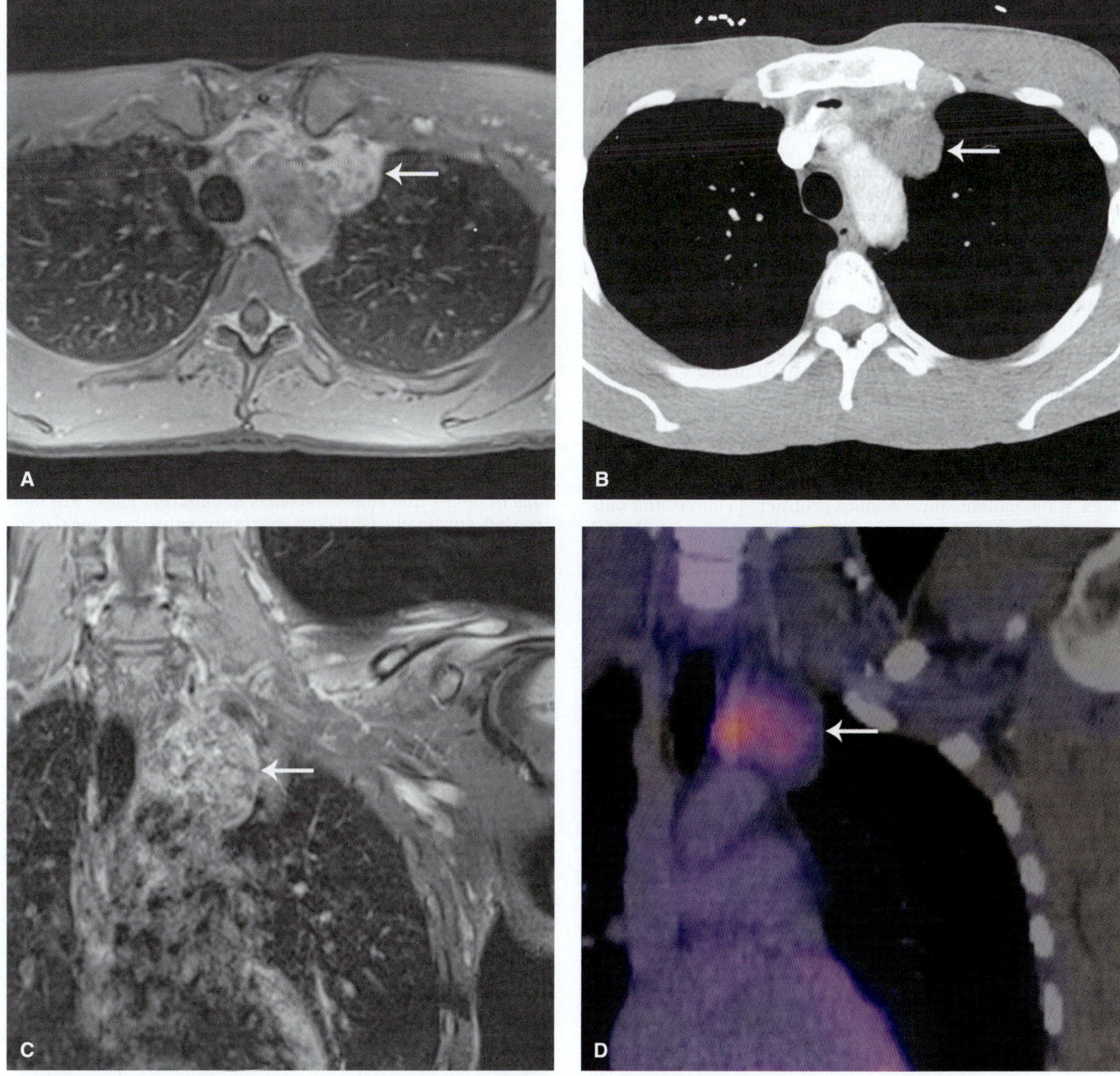

cancers, and there are scattered case reports on its usefulness in evaluating cardiac tumors.[63,64]

Cardiac catheterization was heavily utilized in the past, but its usefulness has diminished with the emergence of the noninvasive techniques noted previously. Catheterization may reveal wall structural or motion abnormalities, intracavitary filling defects, or evidence of neovascularization of the tumor.[48,54] If a malignant tumor is suspected, endocardial biopsy may provide tissue for pathologic diagnosis. For patients who may undergo surgical resection of their tumor, catheterization is still recommended for the detection of coronary artery disease and pulmonary hypertension.

STAGING SYSTEM AND PATHOLOGIC CLASSIFICATION

There is no accepted staging system available for cardiac tumors. With respect to pathologic classification, tumors of the heart and pericardium may be classified as primary (originating from the heart) or metastatic (originating from malignancies of other organs). Primary cardiac tumors can be further subclassified by the site of origin and by malignant potential (Table 57.5).

PROGNOSTIC FACTORS

In general, the prognosis for patients with either primary or secondary malignant tumors of the heart is poor. The median survival of patients with malignant primary tumors is approximately 1 year, and both local and distant relapses are common. Blondeau[16] reported that angiosarcoma had a median survival of 2.14 years, compared with only 0.75 years for fibrosarcoma. Llombart-Cussac et al.,[65] on the other hand, noted a worse survival for angiosarcomas due to their propensity to present late with advanced disease. The series from Burke et al.[17] and Putnam et al.[18] indicate that the histologic subtype does not appear to have prognostic value, although the microscopic finding of more than 10 mitoses per high-power field does portend a worse prognosis. Tazelaar et al.[66] also noted a worse outcome for tumors with high mitotic activity and necrosis. Conversely, the ability to resect all gross tumor and a left atrial site of origin predict for longer survival.[17,18] Although the duration of symptoms is typically short, some patients have a more protracted course, and outcome may be better in those with symptoms for more than 3 months before diagnosis.[67] The use of adjuvant radiotherapy has been associated with longer median survival (22.7 vs. 9.6 months), whereas adjuvant chemotherapy has provided mixed results.[17,67] Given the retrospective nature of these studies, patient selection may be a source of bias. If a controlled,

prospective study could be completed, it is unclear if it would confirm an improved prognosis with either type of adjuvant therapy.

The discovery and diagnosis of metastatic disease in the myocardium is rare in the antemortem setting, and hence prognostic factors have not been elucidated. Malignant pericardial effusion, on the other hand, is more easily diagnosed in life and can be appropriately palliated with pericardiocentesis, pericardiotomy, or pericardial sclerosis. Among patients with metastases from a solid tumor, the median survival after the procedure is approximately 3 to 4 months, and it appears to be improved with better performance status.[68,69]

MANAGEMENT

Primary Pericardial Tumors

Fewer than 200 primary pericardial malignant tumors have been reported in the literature to date, and less than one-third of these were diagnosed during life.[20,21,23–28,70–73] Among those diagnosed before autopsy, locally advanced or metastatic disease is common, and palliative treatment may be the most appropriate option. Relief of pericardial tamponade can be achieved rapidly through pericardiocentesis. Palliative surgical approaches include pericardiectomy or pericardial sclerosis to alleviate the symptoms of effusion and potentially prevent its recurrence. In keeping with the contemporary data supporting the use of radiotherapy in cases of primary pleural mesothelioma, it is appropriate to consider its use in the setting of primary pericardial mesothelioma, although there are few clinical data defining its use.[74] Both external-beam radiotherapy and instillation of radiopharmaceuticals (phosphorus-32, gold-198) have been reported in the palliative setting for this disease.[6,20]

Surgical resection of all gross disease is the treatment of choice in the definitive setting. As with pleural mesothelioma, a high rate of local recurrence should be expected without adjuvant therapy, and postoperative radiotherapy and chemotherapy should be considered. The radiation treatment volume should include the entire pericardial surface and likely should include the mediastinal lymph nodes.

Benign Cardiac Tumors

The most common benign cardiac tumors are atrial myxomas in adults and rhabdomyomas in children. These are both treated surgically with low mortality rates and local control rates in excess of 95%.[14,16,30–33,50,67] Endo et al.[31] reported a 5-year overall survival rate of 86% after resection of atrial myxoma. Bogren et al.[54] found the 5-year survival rate was 87% for patients with myxoma and 76% for all patients treated for a benign cardiac tumor. Blondeau[16] reported 444 patients had resection of a myxoma with a 4% 30-day surgical mortality rate, a 1% late tumor- or treatment-related mortality rate, and only a 2% risk of local relapse. Given the high rate of cure, with an acceptable rate of morbidity, surgical resection without adjuvant chemotherapy or radiotherapy is generally appropriate for benign primary cardiac neoplasms. Some rhabdomyomas may even regress spontaneously without the need for aggressive resection.[75]

Malignant Primary Cardiac Tumors

Surgical resection is the primary treatment of choice for patients with primary malignant cardiac tumors. Unfortunately, local resection is often incomplete because of the extent and invasiveness of the tumor and lack of experience with extended cardiac resection and partly because of uncertainty of diagnosis at the time of initial surgery.[76] In experienced hands, even tumors requiring complete reconstruction of the entire right and left atria and up to 30% of the right ventricle may be resectable and still retain

TABLE 57.5 PATHOLOGIC CLASSIFICATION OF CARDIAC TUMORS	
Pericardial Tumors	**Myocardial Tumors**
Benign Subtypes	**Benign Subtypes**
Teratoma	Myxoma
Pericardial cysts	Lipoma
Fibroma	Papillary fibroelastoma
Angioma	Rhabdomyoma
Lipoma	Fibroma
Malignant Subtypes	Hamartoma
Mesothelioma	Hemangioma
Angiosarcoma	Teratoma
Fibrosarcoma	**Malignant Subtypes**
Malignant teratoma	Sarcoma
	Lymphoma
	Malignant teratoma
	Melanoma
	Carcinoma

adequate cardiac function.[76] Even in the presence of a complete excision, local relapse is common and accounts for as much as one-third of deaths. Sarcomas account for almost all primary malignant cardiac neoplasms, and the treatment principles should be similar to those for soft tissue sarcoma arising from other areas of the body.[77] After complete or incomplete resection of the tumor, adjuvant radiotherapy and chemotherapy may be used in an attempt to gain control of local and distant disease, respectively. There are conflicting reports on the effectiveness of chemotherapy, and given the small sample sizes, it is difficult to draw conclusions, but it seems to be less beneficial if patients are not able to obtain a complete resection.[17,18,76] Combination chemotherapy appears to have greater efficacy than single-agent therapy, with different combinations of agents such as cyclophosphamide, ifosfamide, doxorubicin, and paclitaxel in use.[18,78–81]

Anecdotal cases of orthotopic heart transplantation for patients with malignant neoplasms of the heart were first described in 1981 by Jamieson et al.[82] and in several reports in the literature since then, with some promising results in selected cases.[83–92] Although this technique should ideally achieve a complete tumor resection, the results have been mixed. There have been some case reports of long-term survivors, whereas many other patients have developed distant metastases and subsequent death within months of transplant. Some have attempted cardiac explantation, tumor removal, and autotransplantation.[81] Although orthotopic heart transplantation has promise, theoretical dangers exist, including the potential protumor effect of immune suppression and a decreased ability to tolerate adjuvant radiotherapy or chemotherapy.

Metastatic Tumors of the Heart and Pericardium

There is no known curative therapy for patients with metastatic disease to the heart. Appropriate management of the primary metastatic tumor with systemic therapy may be indicated as a first-line approach for cardiac, pericardial, or GV metastases. Surgery may have a role in both diagnosis and palliation for patients with malignant pericardial disease.[68,69] Emergency pericardiocentesis or pericardiotomy can alleviate cardiac tamponade and yield the diagnosis, and the instillation of a sclerosing agent, such as tetracycline, can often effectively prevent the reaccumulation of the pericardial effusion. Palliative radiotherapy may be used to relieve symptoms of life-threatening outflow obstruction or pericardial disease.

Tumors of the Great Vessels

Resection of the tumor with graft reconstruction of the vessel is the treatment of choice. As with sarcomas of the heart, sarcomas of the GVs are treated based on the same philosophy as used for treatment of soft tissue sarcoma.[77] Postoperative radiotherapy should be considered for all patients, even those with low-grade tumors, because local recurrence would likely not be amenable to salvage surgical resection.[17,33,44]

RADIOTHERAPY

In general, the most common indication for radiotherapy is in the postoperative setting, for example, as adjuvant therapy after resection of a primary malignant cardiac tumor. Less common is the use of radiotherapy in the definitive setting for a tumor that is not technically resectable. There are rare reports of preoperative radiotherapy being used to render a technically unresectable cardiac tumors appropriate

for surgery. Lastly, palliative radiotherapy may be considered when metastatic tumors to the heart cause clinically significant symptoms causing interference with cardiac function.

Decisions on radiation dose and target definitions for cardiac tumors will be determined by the tumor type and the particular clinical indication for treatment. Given that sarcomas are the most common primary malignant cardiac tumors, the radiotherapy model used in their management has been extrapolated from the approach used for soft tissues sarcomas arising at extracardiac sites. Thus, for completely resected tumors with negative margins, postoperative doses of 45 to 50 Gy at 1.8 to 2 Gy/fraction are recommended.[77] The initial target should include all areas known to harbor tumor before surgery, with a margin of about 2 cm. This target should be derived from diagnostic imaging and other investigations and also by the operative description of the surgeon. In the setting of incomplete resection (i.e., involved microscopic margins or gross residual disease), an additional 10 to 20 Gy boost should be added to initial dose and target the postoperative volume at risk. In definitive cases, the goal is to achieve a total dose of at least 70 Gy delivered to the unresected primary tumor, but normal tissues may impose limitations in achieving this. For GV tumors, the target volume will vary depending on the tumor origin but, as with cardiac primaries, should include a minimum expansion of 2 cm around the preoperative mass. Doses from 45 to 50 Gy are suggested for microscopic residual disease and 60 to 70 Gy for gross residual or unresectable disease, allowing for accepted normal tissue tolerances.[93–96] For patients with pericardial mesothelioma, the entire pericardium needs to be included in the initial target volume, but the total dose deliverable will be limited by the tolerance of the myocardium itself and may only be as high as 40 Gy if the whole heart is treated. Focal involvement of the pericardium may be treated to doses as high as 64 Gy.[97] For tumors with a high propensity for nodal involvement (i.e., mesothelioma, angiosarcoma, rhabdomyosarcoma, carcinoma, or lymphoma), coverage of the mediastinal lymph nodes is also recommended. With respect to altered fractionation approaches for cardiac tumors, there are few reports on dose variations to improve the efficacy of conventional radiotherapy. A rare example is a case report on the use of hyperfractionation for a cardiac sarcoma treated to a dose of 70.5 Gy at 1.5 Gy/fraction delivered twice daily with a radiosensitizer, iododeoxyuridine.[46] Regarding palliative radiotherapy, dose schedules should reflect the clinical urgency and the patient's performance status. The origin of the primary tumor may also have a bearing on dose schedules. A survey of palliative case reports showed wide ranges in dose/fractionation schedules with the most common ones being short-course accelerated hypofractionated approaches such as 20 to 30 Gy in 5 to 10 fractions.[98]

With respect to radiation delivery, historic practice has involved two-dimensional planning and static beam arrangements, such as anteroposterior parallel-opposed (APPA) techniques to cover the desired initial target volume. Contemporary radiotherapy should now be planned using a three-dimensional (3D) conformal approach, with careful delineation of gross tumor volumes, clinical target volumes, and planning target volumes as defined by the nature of the primary tumor, its expected natural history, and the management approach (definitive or adjuvant). When planning radiotherapy, normal tissue constraints should be observed for each case, with an emphasis on cardiac, lung, spinal cord, and esophageal tolerances. If required, advanced techniques such as intensity-modulated radiotherapy (IMRT) may be of use in the delivery of desired doses to target volumes while highly limiting dose to normal structures. IMRT techniques allow for the selective intensification or reduction of dose to areas of specific concern and may allow for greater sparing of normal tissues without sacrificing tumor coverage or dosing. A recent innovation in radiotherapy highly relevant to cardiac tumors is the use of four-dimensional (4D) CT scanning at the time of patient simulation. 4DCT allows an understanding of the effect of breathing motion on the target and normal structures within the chest. For each structure, 4DCT can generate volumetric datasets representing the various phases of the respiratory cycle. By more clearly understanding tumor motion, relevant normal structures at risk can be optimally spared by restricting treatment margins.

One of the more important advances in the field of radiotherapy has been developing technology that can deliver extremely high-dose focused radiation. Stereotactic body radiotherapy (SBRT), also known as stereotactic ablative radiotherapy-(SABR) involves the precise delivery of very high (ablative) doses of radiation to discrete targets over a small number of treatment sessions (usually five or less) by treating the target with high degree of conformality and employing rigorous pretreatment set-up verification. Given the complexity of heart tumors by virtue of their location and their relationships to a number of organs-at-risk, SBRT has proved to be of particular interest in their management. Soltys et al.[99] treated a recurrent pulmonary artery sarcoma with 33 Gy in 3 fractions. Bonomo et al. used SBRT for recurrent and metastatic cardiac tumors with doses ranging from 24 to 36 Gy in 3 to 5 fractions.[100,101] Although the total doses used for cardiac tumors reported so far have been less than the curative doses seen in the early-stage lung cancer SBRT literature, clinicians treating heart tumors have nonetheless employed the critical organ dose constraints used in lung SBRT planning.[102-104] Mindful of the limited reported use of such high-dose, highly conformal techniques for heart tumors, it is conceivable that they may offer a means to safely escalate doses to those which would theoretically be optimal for tumor control. This is attractive given the poor outcomes seen with current nonsurgical therapies.[99] Patients who may be the best candidates for using such novel approaches may also be those who have received prior radiotherapy and suffer an isolated in-field recurrence. Because using conventional radiotherapy techniques would likely exceed critical structure dose constraints, SBRT may make high-dose therapy feasible in the setting where otherwise anything other than palliative doses might not have been possible.

Particle-based therapies are also increasingly being investigated in the management of cancers because of their physical properties, which might provide better sparing of normal tissues. A clinical report from Japan (see further below in "Results") is an example of this modality for a heart malignancy, describing the use of carbon-ion radiotherapy for a case of cardiac sarcomas that employed 64 Gy in 16 fractions over 4 weeks.[105]

Advanced technologies must be used with caution, however, because cardiac and respiratory motions introduce considerable uncertainty in tumor localization and predictability of dose delivery. In the setting of SBRT, normal tissue and tumor motion must be therefore be effectively evaluated using 4D CT techniques. Image guidance (image-guided radiotherapy [IGRT]) at the time of delivery to further ensure targeting accuracy is also critical. Alternative delivery approaches such as gating procedures may be considered to decrease positioning uncertainty and thus decrease the necessary target expansions for daily set-up variations.[106] As a demonstration of different planning result, representative isodose distributions, and their corresponding dose–volume histogram (DVH) data, for two primary cardiac tumors are shown in Figure 57.2 for a 3D conformal radiotherapy plan and in Figure 57.3 for an SBRT plan.

As noted above, the total dose deliverable to any given cardiac tumor is primarily limited by heart and lung tolerance. Much of the available evidence on tolerance of the heart is based on patients previously treated for malignancies such as Hodgkin lymphoma or breast cancer. In general, radiation-induced heart disease (RIHD) may manifest as pericarditis, myocarditis, conduction defects, or coronary vascular disease.[107,108] Damage to the pericardium is most often observed clinically. Risk factors for developing RIHD include total dose, dose per fraction, irradiated volume, radiation technique, age at exposure, and use of concurrent or anthracycline-based chemotherapy. Emami et al.[93] estimated the tolerance dose for the heart to be 40 Gy for the whole heart and 60 Gy for one-third of the heart based on a 5% complication rate of developing pericarditis within 5 years of treatment (TD5/5). However, current estimates of normal tissue tolerances tend to be more accurate, and administration of chemotherapeutic agents must also be taken into account as enhancing risk.[109] Most recently, Gagliardi et al.[94] reviewed all the available data on cardiac toxicities and concluded that the whole-organ dose at which toxicity occurs in 50% of cases (TD50) is on the order of 48 to 50.6 Gy, but that side-effect profiles must be considered in relation to the probability of tumor control for the specific patient. Certainly, in aggressive tumors with poor outcomes, recurrence is equally or more morbid than the potential treatment-related toxicities, and this must be balanced and discussed with the individual patient. With respect to other normal structures relevant to 3D-target planning for cardiac or GV tumors, Werner-Wasik et al.[96] have reported that doses as high as 74 Gy with concurrent chemotherapy can be delivered safely to segments of the esophagus, but that no single best threshold is identifiable for limiting esophageal toxicity. In a comprehensive literature review on lung tolerances performed by Marks et al.,[95] the authors recommended limiting the volume of lung receiving 20 Gy (V20) to ≤30% to 35%, and the mean lung dose to ≤20 to 23 Gy in order to minimize lung toxicity. All of these values are for patients receiving conventionally fractionated radiotherapy because as noted earlier, SBRT-based approaches employ a different set of normal tissue constraints.

RESULTS

Case reports and small retrospective series have been the primary means of understanding outcomes for this rare class of tumors. A classic example is the 1964 report by Sagerman et al.,[110] which included one of the earliest descriptions of adjuvant radiotherapy for attempted cure. The patient was a 55-year-old woman with a primary cardiac fibromyxosarcoma. After incomplete resection, she underwent external-beam radiotherapy to a dose up to 75 Gy to the primary site, with proper shielding of the spinal cord. As a result of the use of lateral fields, the left lung received 35 Gy to a large volume. The patient was treated with prophylactic steroids to prevent radiation pneumonitis and fibrosis. She died 8 months later with brain and lung metastases. Autopsy revealed complete sterilization of the primary tumor.

Despite the use of aggressive treatment regimens including surgical resection, postoperative radiotherapy, and chemotherapy, the overall survival for patients with primary malignant cardiac tumors is poor, and this is true even in light of more recent reports that have suggested better outcomes with contemporary adjuvant radiotherapy or chemoradiotherapy.[17,78,79,81] Operative mortality is relatively common, at 8% to 9%, and is twice as high compared to that following resection of benign tumors.[76,111] The median survival in most surgical series is in the range of 9 to 12 months,[14,16,18,30,32,65,78,111,112]

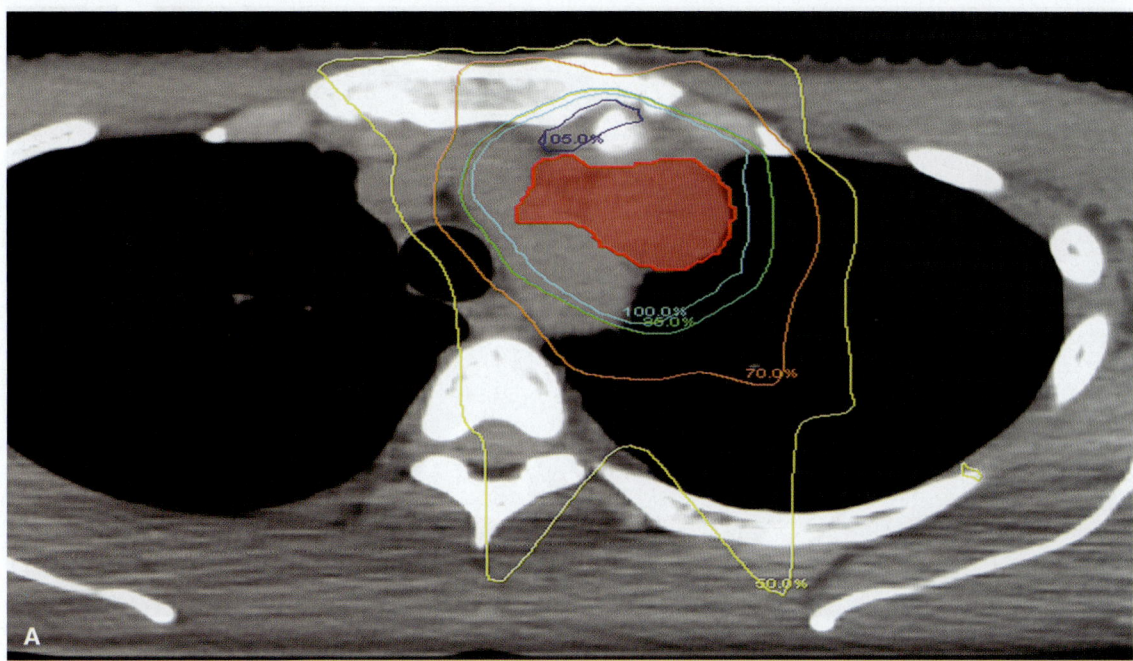

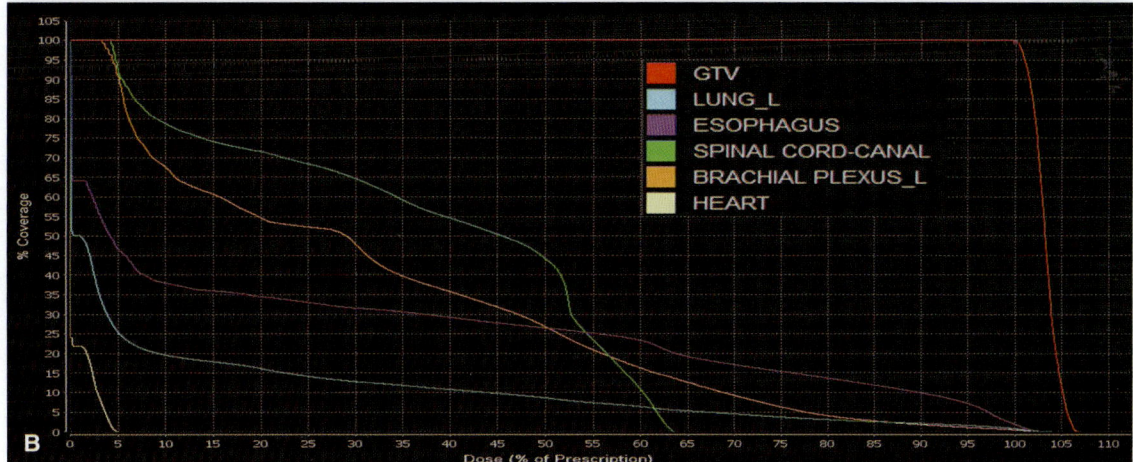

FIGURE 57.2. Sample three-dimensional conformal plan developed for a patient with an unresectable epithelioid hemangioendothelioma of the aortic arch **(A)** and corresponding dose–volume histogram data **(B)**. GTV, gross tumor volume.

with outliers as low as 6 months[17,33,113] and as high as 23.5 months among patients who survived surgery in one of the most recent reports.[76] Putnam et al.[18] reported a median survival of 11 months and a 2-year overall survival rate of only 14%. In this series, the authors also noted the importance of complete resection. For patients in whom complete resection was possible, the median survival was 24 months, compared with only 10 months for those with incomplete resection. Llombart-Cussac et al.[65] also noted improved survival with complete resection (22 vs. 7 months). Burke et al.[17] reported significantly improved median survival of 12 months among patients who underwent adjuvant radiotherapy, chemotherapy, or both, compared with 3 months in those who did not have adjuvant therapy.

With respect to the use of definitive carbon-ion radiotherapy in the treatment of a patient with cardiac angiosarcoma,[105] the tumor volume reduced by 86% following treatment and became negative on PET scan. After 18 months, the primary tumor remained controlled, but the

patient had developed bilateral lung metastases 4 months after treatment.

Selected patients who develop recurrence after undergoing combined modality therapy may still benefit from aggressive management of their disease, with one author reporting an improvement in median survival from 25 months with no treatment to 47 months with resection, radiofrequency ablation, or radiotherapy.[76] Others have shown similar benefits to this approach at the time of recurrences.[81]

The median survival for patients with metastatic disease to the heart is approximately 3 to 4 months, but rare cases of long-term survival, some as long as 3 years, have been documented and may be related to primary tumor histologic type and performance status.[68,69,114] Pericardiotomy or pericardial sclerosis appears to offer at least temporary control of tamponade and effusion in up to 90% of cases.[68,69] Palliative treatment with radiation is well tolerated and is effective in controlling cardiac tamponade in approximately 60% of patients. Cham et al.[115] reported the results

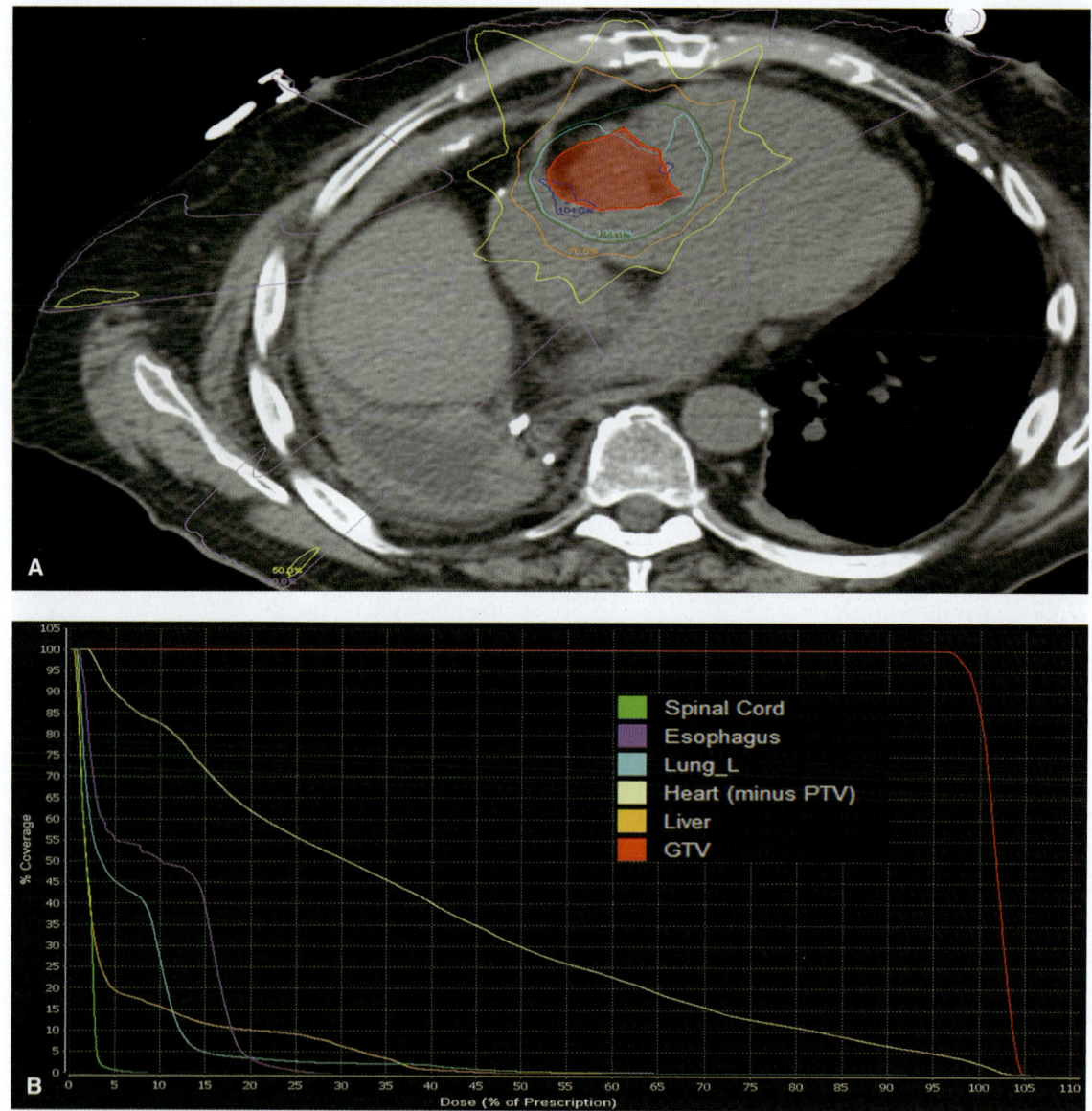

FIGURE 57.3. Sample stereotactic body radiotherapy plan developed for a patient with a local recurrence of a pleomorphic sarcoma of the pulmonary artery **(A)** and corresponding dose–volume histogram data **(B)**. GTV, gross tumor volume.

of radiotherapeutic palliation for 38 patients with secondary tumors of the heart and pericardium. Thirty-seven patients were noted to have pericardial involvement, nine also had invasion of the myocardium, and one had only endocardial involvement. The radiation dose was 25 to 30 Gy in 3 to 4 weeks for 32 patients. The dose was 15 to 20 Gy in 1.5 to 2 weeks for the remaining six patients, all of whom had lymphoreticular tumors. The overall response rate was 61%, with a median duration of response of 3 to 4 months. Lymphoreticular tumors had the best response rate (6 of 7 cases) followed by breast cancer (11 of 16 cases). Only 6 of the remaining 15 cases showed a response. Although the median survival among patients with metastases to the heart and pericardium is short, palliative efforts are not in vain because tamponade appears to be effectively controlled with these measures.

Among patients treated for GV tumors, median survival depends on the location, resectability, and grade of the primary tumor. Burke and Virmani[44] reported the median

survival was 5 months for aortic sarcoma, 23 months for sarcoma of the pulmonary artery, and 37 months for sarcoma of the IVC. Two patients with sarcoma of the SVC were alive and without disease 10 and 72 months after treatment. Local relapse was documented in two patients, although metastatic disease occurred in 19 of 45 patients. The sites most commonly involved by metastases were the lung, liver, and bone. Involvement of the peritoneum, adrenals, kidneys, skin, and lymph nodes was also noted.

Treatment Sequelae

Late radiation-induced cardiac or pulmonary sequelae after the definitive treatment of cardiac tumors have not been well documented, probably as a result of the poor overall survival for these malignancies. In a recent report of 17 patients treated for different cardiac malignancies, with follow-ups ranging from 5 to 137 months, Lestuzzi et al. described late toxicities from cardiac radiotherapy in six of these cases.[116] Three patients developed recurring atrial fibrillation, two segmental hypokinesis and one constrictive pericarditis. The cardiotoxic effects of doxorubicin have been well documented, and there is evidence for increased risk when it is given in conjunction with radiotherapy[109]; therefore, concurrent therapy should be avoided to the degree possible.

ACKNOWLEDGMENTS

The authors gratefully acknowledge the critical contribution played by Dr. Lawrence Sheplan Olsen as the primary author on the last edition of this chapter.

REFERENCES

1. Gray H, Clemente CD. *Anatomy of the human body*. 30th American ed. Philadelphia: Lea & Febiger, 1985.
2. Burke AP, Virmani R. *Tumors of the heart and great vessels. Atlas of tumor pathology*. 3rd series. Vol. 16. Washington, DC: Armed Forces Institute of Pathology, 1996.
3. Reynen K. Frequency of primary tumors of the heart. *Am J Cardiol* 1996;77(1):107.
4. Reynen K. Cardiac myxomas. *N Engl J Med* 1995;333(24):1610–1617.
5. Sarjeant JM, Butany J, Cusimano RJ. Cancer of the heart: epidemiology and management of primary tumors and metastases. *Am J Cardiovasc Drugs* 2003;3(6):407–421.
6. Lokich JJ. The management of malignant pericardial effusions. *JAMA* 1973;224(10):1401–1404.
7. McAllister HA, Fenoglio JJ. *Tumors of the cardiovascular system. Atlas of tumor pathology*. Washington, DC: Armed Forces Institute of Pathology, 1978.
8. Butany J, Nair V, Naseemuddin A, et al. Cardiac tumours: diagnosis and management. *Lancet Oncol* 2005;6(4):219–228.
9. Carney JA, Hruska LS, Beauchamp GD, et al. Dominant inheritance of the complex of myxomas, spotty pigmentation, and endocrine overactivity. *Mayo Clin Proc* 1986;61(3):165–172.
10. Nwokoro NA, Korytkowski MT, Rose S, et al. Spectrum of malignancy and premalignancy in Carney syndrome. *Am J Med Genet* 1997;73(4):369–377.
11. Wilkes D, McDermott DA, Basson CT. Clinical phenotypes and molecular genetic mechanisms of Carney complex. *Lancet Oncol* 2005;6(7):501–508.
12. Kirschner LS, Sandrini F, Monbo J, et al. Genetic heterogeneity and spectrum of mutations of the PRKAR1A gene in patients with the carney complex. *Hum Mol Genet* 2000;9(20):3037–3046.
13. Vidaillet HJ Jr, Seward JB, Fyke FE III, et al. "Syndrome myxoma": a subset of patients with cardiac myxoma associated with pigmented skin lesions and peripheral and endocrine neoplasms. *Br Heart J* 1987;57(3):247–255.
14. Murphy MC, Sweeney MS, Putnam JB Jr, et al. Surgical treatment of cardiac tumors: a 25-year experience. *Ann Thorac Surg* 1990;49(4):612–618.
15. Mack TM. Sarcomas and other malignancies of soft tissue, retroperitoneum, peritoneum, pleura, heart, mediastinum, and spleen. *Cancer* 1995;75(1 Suppl):211–244.
16. Blondeau P. Primary cardiac tumors—French studies of 533 cases. *Thorac Cardiovasc Surg* 1990;38(Suppl 2):192–195.
17. Burke AP, Cowan D, Virmani R. Primary sarcomas of the heart. *Cancer* 1992;69(2):387–395.
18. Putnam JB Jr, Sweeney MS, Colon R, et al. Primary cardiac sarcomas. *Ann Thorac Surg* 1991;51(6):906–910.
19. Petrich A, Cho SI, Billett H. Primary cardiac lymphoma: an analysis of presentation, treatment, and outcome patterns. *Cancer* 2011;117(3):581–589.
20. Kralstein J, Frishman W. Malignant pericardial diseases: diagnosis and treatment. *Am Heart J* 1987;113(3):785–790.
21. Strauss R, Merliss R. Primary tumor of the heart. *Arch Pathol* 1945;39:74–78.
22. Mensi C, Giacomini S, Sieno C, et al. Pericardial mesothelioma and asbestos exposure. *Int J Hyg Environ Health* 2011;214(3):276–279.
23. Aggarwal P, Wali JP, Agarwal J. Pericardial mesothelioma presenting as a mediastinal mass. *Singapore Med J* 1991;32(3):185–186.
24. Kaul TK, Fields BL, Kahn DR. Primary malignant pericardial mesothelioma: a case report and review. *J Cardiovasc Surg (Torino)* 1994;35(3):261–267.
25. Thomason R, Schlegel W, Lucca M, et al. Primary malignant mesothelioma of the pericardium. Case report and literature review. *Tex Heart Inst J* 1994;21(2):170–174.
26. Norman MG. Primary mesothelioma of the pericardium. *Can Med Assoc J* 1965;92:129–133.
27. Sytman AL, MacAlpin RN. Primary pericardial mesothelioma: report of two cases and review of the literature. *Am Heart J* 1971;81(6):760–769.
28. Andersen JA, MacAlpin RN. Primary pericardial mesothelioma. *Dan Med Bull* 1974;21(5):195–200.
29. Yokouchi Y, Hiruta N, Oharaseki T, et al. Primary cardiac synovial sarcoma: a case report and literature review. *Pathol Int* 2011;61(3):150–155.
30. Centofanti P, Di Rosa E, Deorsola L, et al. Primary cardiac tumors: early and late results of surgical treatment in 91 patients. *Ann Thorac Surg* 1999;68(4):1236–1241.
31. Endo A, Ohtahara A, Kinugawa T, et al. Characteristics of 161 patients with cardiac tumors diagnosed during 1993 and 1994 in Japan. *Am J Cardiol* 1997;79(12):1708–1711.
32. Miralles A, Bracamonte L, Soncul H, et al. Cardiac tumors: clinical experience and surgical results in 74 patients. *Ann Thorac Surg* 1991;52(4):886–895.
33. Molina JE, Edwards JE, Ward HB. Primary cardiac tumors: experience at the University of Minnesota. *Thorac Cardiovasc Surg* 1990;38(Suppl 2):183–191.
34. Perchinsky MJ, Lichtenstein SV, Tyers GF. Primary cardiac tumors: forty years' experience with 71 patients. *Cancer* 1997;79(9):1809–1815.
35. Adenle AD, Edwards JE. Clinical and pathologic features of metastatic neoplasms of the pericardium. *Chest* 1982;81(2):166–169.
36. Fabian JT, Rose AG. Tumours of the heart. A study of 89 cases. *S Afr Med J* 1982;61(3):71–77.
37. Hanfling SM. Metastatic cancer to the heart. Review of the literature and report of 127 cases. *Circulation* 1960;22:474–483.
38. Klatt EC, Heitz DR. Cardiac metastases. *Cancer* 1990;65(6):1456–1459.
39. Lam KY, Dickens P, Chan AC. A 20-year experience with a review of 12,485 consecutive autopsies. *Arch Pathol Lab Med* 1993;117(10):1027–1031.
40. Lockwood WB, Broghamer WL Jr. The changing prevalence of secondary cardiac neoplasms as related to cancer therapy. *Cancer* 1980;45(10):2659–2662.
41. Reynen K, Kockeritz U, Strasser RH. Metastases to the heart. *Ann Oncol* 2004;15(3):375–381.
42. Salcedo EE, Cohen GI, White RD, et al. Cardiac tumors: diagnosis and management. *Curr Probl Cardiol* 1992;17(2):73–137.
43. Silvestri F, Bussani R, Pavletic N, et al. Metastases of the heart and pericardium. *G Ital Cardiol* 1997;27(12):1252–1255.
44. Burke AP, Virmani R. Sarcomas of the great vessels. A clinicopathologic study. *Cancer* 1993;71(5):1761–1773.
45. St John Sutton MG, Mercier LA, Giuliani ER, et al. Atrial myxomas. a review of clinical experience in 40 patients. *Mayo Clin Proc* 1980;55(6):371–376.
46. Movsas B, Teruya-Feldstein J, Smith J, et al. Primary cardiac sarcoma: a novel treatment approach. *Chest* 1998;114(2):648–652.
47. Goodwin JF. The spectrum of cardiac tumors. *Am J Cardiol* 1968;21(3):307–314.
48. Thomas CR Jr, Johnson GW Jr, Stoddard MF, et al. Primary malignant cardiac tumors: update 1992. *Med Pediatr Oncol* 1992;20(6):519–531.
49. Keren A, Chenzbruna A, Schuger L, et al. The etiology of tumor plop in a patient with huge right atrial myxoma. *Chest* 1989;95(5):1147–1149.
50. Livi U, Bortolotti U, Milano A, et al. Cardiac myxomas: results of 14 years' experience. *Thorac Cardiovasc Surg* 1984;32(3):143–147.
51. Peters MN, Hall RJ, Cooley DA, et al. The clinical syndrome of atrial myxoma. *JAMA* 1974;230(5):695–701.
52. Becker RC, Hobbs RE, Ratliff NB. Cardiac rhabdomyosarcoma: case report with review of clinical and pathologic features. *Cleve Clin Q* 1984;51(1):83–88.
53. Abrams HL, Adams DF, Grant HA. The radiology of tumors of the heart. *Radiol Clin North Am* 1971;9(2):299–326.
54. Bogren HG, DeMaria AN, Mason DT. Imaging procedures in the detection of cardiac tumors, with emphasis on echocardiography: a review. *Cardiovasc Intervent Radiol* 1980;3(3):107–125.
55. Steiner RE. Radiologic aspects of cardiac tumors. *Am J Cardiol* 1968;21(3):344–356.
56. Mugge A, Daniel WG, Haverich A, et al. Diagnosis of noninfective cardiac mass lesions by two-dimensional echocardiography. Comparison of the transthoracic and transesophageal approaches. *Circulation* 1991;83(1):70–78.
57. Lynch M, Clements SD, Shanewise JS, et al. Right-sided cardiac tumors detected by transesophageal echocardiography and its usefulness in differentiating the benign from the malignant ones. *Am J Cardiol* 1997;79(6):781–784.
58. Fye WB, Molina JE. Right atrial angiosarcoma: echocardiographic diagnosis and surgical correlation. *Johns Hopkins Med J* 1980;147(3):111–116.
59. Freedberg RS, Kronzon I, Rumancik WM, et al. The contribution of magnetic resonance imaging to the evaluation of intracardiac tumors diagnosed by echocardiography. *Circulation* 1988;77(1):96–103.
60. Lipton MJ, Brundage BH, Higgins CB, et al. Clinical applications of dynamic computed tomography. *Prog Cardiovasc Dis* 1986;28(5):349–366.
61. Lund JT, Ehman RL, Julsrud PR, et al. Cardiac masses: assessment by MR imaging. *AJR Am J Roentgenol* 1989;152(3):469–473.
62. Restrepo CS, Largoza A, Lemos DF, et al. CT and MR imaging findings of malignant cardiac tumors. *Curr Probl Diagn Radiol* 2005;34(1):1–11.
63. Lee JC, Platts DG, Huang YT, et al. Positron emission tomography combined with computed tomography as an integral component in evaluation of primary cardiac lymphoma. *Clin Cardiol* 2010;33(6):E106–E108.
64. Probst S, Seltzer A, Spieler B, et al. The appearance of cardiac metastasis from squamous cell carcinoma of the lung on F-18 FDG PET/CT and post hoc PET/MRI. *Clin Nucl Med* 2011;36(4):311–312.
65. Llombart-Cussac A, Pivot X, Contesso G, et al. Adjuvant chemotherapy for primary cardiac sarcomas: the IGR experience. *Br J Cancer* 1998;78(12):1624–1628.
66. Tazelaar HD, Locke TJ, McGregor CG. Pathology of surgically excised primary cardiac tumors. *Mayo Clin Proc* 1992;67(10):957–965.

Section III

67. Poole GV Jr, Breyer RH, Holliday RH, et al. Tumors of the heart: surgical considerations. *J Cardiovasc Surg (Torino)* 1984;25(1):5–11.

68. Davis S, Rambotti P, Grignani F. Intrapericardial tetracycline sclerosis in the treatment of malignant pericardial effusion: an analysis of thirty-three cases. *J Clin Oncol* 1984;2(6):631–636.

69. Appelqvist P, Maamies T, Grohn P. Emergency pericardiotomy as primary diagnostic and therapeutic procedure in malignant pericardial tamponade: report of three cases and review of the literature. *J Surg Oncol* 1982;21(1):18–22.

70. Lee MJ, Kim DH, Kwan J, et al. A case of malignant pericardial mesothelioma with constrictive pericarditis physiology misdiagnosed as pericardial metastatic cancer. *Korean Circ J* 2011;41(6):338–341.

71. Morita S, Goto A, Sakatani T, et al. Multicystic mesothelioma of the pericardium. *Pathol Int* 2011;61(5):319–321.

72. Terada T. Primary sarcomatoid malignant mesothelioma of the pericardium. *Med Oncol* 2012;29(2):1345–1346.

73. Marinaccio A, Binazzi A, Di Marzio D, et al. Incidence of extrapleural malignant mesothelioma and asbestos exposure, from the Italian national register. *Occup Environ Med* 2010;67(11):760–765.

74. Raja S, Murthy SC, Mason DP. Malignant pleural mesothelioma. *Curr Oncol Rep* 2011;13(4):259–264.

75. Nir A, Tajik AJ, Freeman WK, et al. Tuberous sclerosis and cardiac rhabdomyoma. *Am J Cardiol* 1995;76(5):419–421.

76. Bakaeen FG, Jaroszewski DE, Rice DC, et al. Outcomes after surgical resection of cardiac sarcoma in the multimodality treatment era. *J Thorac Cardiovasc Surg* 2009;137(6):1454–1460.

77. O'Sullivan B, Davis AM, Turcotte R, et al. Preoperative versus postoperative radiotherapy in soft-tissue sarcoma of the limbs: a randomised trial. *Lancet* 2002;359(9325):2235–2241.

78. Pessotto R, Samet H, Ohana M, et al. Primary cardiac leiomyosarcoma: seven-year survival with combined surgical and adjuvant therapy. *Int J Cardiol* 1997;60(1):91–94.

79. Antunes MJ, Vanderdonck KM, Andrade CM, et al. Primary cardiac leiomyosarcomas. *Ann Thorac Surg* 1991;51(6):999–1001.

80. Loffler H, Grille W. Classification of malignant cardiac tumors with respect to oncological treatment. *Thorac Cardiovasc Surg* 1990;38(Suppl 2):173–175.

81. Mery GM, Reardon MJ, Haas J, et al. A combined modality approach to recurrent cardiac sarcoma resulting in a prolonged remission: a case report. *Chest* 2003;15(6):1766–1768.

82. Jamieson SW, Gaudiani VA, Reitz BA, et al. Operative treatment of an unresectable tumor of the left ventricle. *J Thorac Cardiovasc Surg* 1981;81(5):797–799.

83. Coelho PN, Banazol NG, Soares RJ, et al. Long-term survival with heart transplantation for fibrosarcoma of the heart. *Ann Thorac Surg* 2010;90(2):635–636.

84. Armitage JM, Kormos RL, Griffith BP, et al. Heart transplantation in patients with malignant disease. *J Heart Transplant* 1990;9(6):627–630.

85. Aufiero TX, Pae WE Jr, Clemson BS, et al. Heart transplantation for tumor. *Ann Thorac Surg* 1993;56(5):1174–1176.

86. Crespo MG, Pulpón LA, Pradas G, et al. Heart transplantation for cardiac angiosarcoma: should its indication be questioned? *J Heart Lung Transplant* 1993;12(3):527–530.

87. Goldstein DJ, Oz MC, Rose EA, et al. Experience with heart transplantation for cardiac tumors. *J Heart Lung Transplant* 1995;14(2):382–386.

88. Grandmougin D, Fayad G, Decoene C, et al. Total orthotopic heart transplantation for primary cardiac rhabdomyosarcoma: factors influencing long-term survival. *Ann Thorac Surg* 2001;71(5):1438–1441.

89. Michler RE, Goldstein DJ. Treatment of cardiac tumors by orthotopic cardiac transplantation. *Semin Oncol* 1997;24(5):534–539.

90. Siebenmann R, Jenni R, Makek M, et al. Primary synovial sarcoma of the heart treated by heart transplantation. *J Thorac Cardiovasc Surg* 1990;99(3):567–568.

91. Talbot SM, Taub RN, Keohan ML, et al. Combined heart and lung transplantation for unresectable primary cardiac sarcoma. *J Thorac Cardiovasc Surg* 2002;124(6):1145–1148.

92. Uberfuhr P, Meiser B, Fuchs A, et al. Heart transplantation: an approach to treating primary cardiac sarcoma? *J Heart Lung Transplant* 2002;21(10):1135–1139.

93. Emami B, Lyman J, Brown A, et al. Tolerance of normal tissue to therapeutic irradiation. *Int J Radiat Oncol Biol Phys* 1991;21(1):109–122.

94. Gagliardi G, Constine LS, Moiseenko V, et al. Radiation dose-volume effects in the heart. *Int J Radiat Oncol Biol Phys* 2010;76(3 Suppl):S77–S85.

95. Marks LB, Bentzen SM, Deasy JO, et al. Radiation dose-volume effects in the lung. *Int J Radiat Oncol Biol Phys* 2010;76(3 Suppl):S70–S76.

96. Werner-Wasik M, Yorke E, Deasy J, et al. Radiation dose-volume effects in the esophagus. *Int J Radiat Oncol Biol Phys* 2010;76(3 Suppl):S86–S93.

97. Reardon KA, Reardon MA, Moskaluk CA, et al. Primary pericardial malignant mesothelioma and response to radiation therapy. *Rare Tumors* 2010;2(3):e51.

98. Fotouhi Ghiam A, Dawson LA, Abuzeid W, et al. Role of palliative radiotherapy in the management of mural cardiac metastases: who, when and how to treat? A case series of 10 patients. *Cancer Med* 2016;5(6):989–996.

99. Soltys SG, Kalani MY, Cheshier SH, et al. Stereotactic radiosurgery for a cardiac sarcoma: a case report. *Technol Cancer Res Treat* 2008;7(5):363–368.

100. Bonomo P, Cipressi S, Desideri I, et al. Stereotactic body radiotherapy with CyberKnife for cardiac malignancies. *Tumori* 2015;101(3):294–297.

101. Bonomo P, Livi L, Rampini A, et al. Stereotactic body radiotherapy for cardiac and paracardiac metastases: University of Florence experience. *Radiol Med* 2013;118(6):1055–1065.

102. Timmerman R, Paulus R, Galvin J, et al. Stereotactic body radiation therapy for inoperable early stage lung cancer. *JAMA* 2010;303(11):1070–1076.

103. Timmerman R, Papiez L, McGarry R, et al. Extracranial stereotactic radioablation: results of a phase I study in medically inoperable stage I non-small cell lung cancer. *Chest* 2003;124(5):1946–1955.

104. Timmerman R, McGarry R, Yiannoutsos C, et al. Excessive toxicity when treating central tumors in a phase II study of stereotactic body radiation therapy for medically inoperable early-stage lung cancer. *J Clin Oncol* 2006;24(30):4833–4839.

105. Bezjak A. *RTOG 0831: Seamless phase i/ii study of stereotactic lung radiotherapy (SBRT) for early stage, centrally located, non-small cell lung cancer (NSCLC) in medically inoperable patients.* 2011. Available at: http://www.rtog.org/ClinicalTrials/ProtocolTable/StudyDetails.aspx?study=0813

106. Aoka Y, Kamada T, Kawana M, et al. Primary cardiac angiosarcoma treated with carbon-ion radiotherapy. *Lancet Oncol* 2004;5(10):636–638.

107. Li G, Citrin D, Camphausen K, et al. Advances in 4D medical imaging and 4D radiation therapy. *Technol Cancer Res Treat* 2008;7(1):67–81.

108. Gaya AM, Ashford RF. Cardiac complications of radiation therapy. *Clin Oncol (R Coll Radiol)* 2005;17(3):153–159.

109. Prosnitz RG, Bristow MR, Glatstein E, et al. Cardiac toxicity following thoracic radiation. *Semin Oncol* 2005;32(2 Suppl 3):S71–S80.

110. Sagerman RH, Hurley E, Bagshaw MA. Successful sterilization of a primary cardiac sarcoma by supervoltage radiation therapy. *Am J Roentgenol Radium Ther Nucl Med* 1964;92:942–946.

111. Billingham ME, Bristow MR, Glatstein E, et al. Adriamycin cardiotoxicity: endomyocardial biopsy evidence of enhancement by irradiation. *Am J Surg Pathol* 1977;1(1):17–23.

112. Bakaeen FG, Reardon MJ, Coselli JS, et al. Surgical outcome in 85 patients with primary cardiac tumors. *Am J Surg* 2003;186(6):641–647.

113. Bear PA, Moodie DS. Malignant primary cardiac tumors. The Cleveland Clinic experience, 1956 to 1986. *Chest* 1987;92(5):860–862.

114. Herrmann MA, Shankerman RA, Edwards WD, et al. Primary cardiac angiosarcoma: a clinicopathologic study of six cases. *J Thorac Cardiovasc Surg* 1992;103(4):655–664.

115. Cham WC, Freiman AH, Carstens PH, et al. Radiation therapy of cardiac and pericardial metastases. *Radiology* 1975;114(3):701–704.

116. Lestuzzi C, et al. Malignant cardiac tumors: diagnosis and treatment. *Future Cardiol* 2015;11(4):485–500.

PART E
Breast

CHAPTER 58

Breast Cancer: Stage TIS

Alfredo I. Urdaneta, Todd Adams, David E. Wazer, and Douglas W. Arthur

INTRODUCTION

Noninvasive carcinoma of the breast (stage Tis) includes Paget disease of the nipple and two histopathologic entities that are distinct in both their clinical presentation and biologic potential: lobular carcinoma *in situ* (LCIS) and ductal carcinoma *in situ* (DCIS). As a result of the increase in the use of mammography, these three histopathologic entities comprise a larger percentage of all breast cancer cases seen today. There remains considerable controversy regarding the optimal treatment approach and, as a consequence, treatment recommendations range from observation to breast-conservation therapy to mastectomy. It is, therefore, important to understand the distinguishing pathologic appearances, biologic characteristics, and natural history of these three noninvasive breast disease entities to appropriately formulate coherent treatment recommendations.

LOBULAR CARCINOMA *IN SITU*

LCIS is characterized by multicentric breast involvement and consists of loose, discohesive epithelial cells that are large in size, variable in shape, and contain a normal cytoplasm to nucleus ratio.[1] The extent of involvement of the lobular lumen ranges from simple filling to moderate to severe distention with extension into the adjacent extralobular ducts.[2] As such, the lines of histologic delineation can become blurred between atypical ductal hyperplasia, LCIS, and, when ductal extension is seen, DCIS. This overlap of histologic morphology may complicate the interpretation of studies from different institutions.[1-4]

LCIS has been reported to present with a multicentric distribution in up to 90% of mastectomy specimens, with bilateral involvement in 35% to 59%.[5-7] LCIS cells are commonly estrogen receptor positive, although overexpression of c-erbB-2 and p53 are uncommon.[4,8-10] The loss of E-cadherin is often observed,[8,11,12] and the absence of this adhesion molecule may explain the growth pattern seen with LCIS.

LCIS represents <15% of all noninvasive breast cancer.[13-15] The majority of women are premenopausal at diagnosis, with an average age of 45 years.[1,3,16] Risk factors for the development of LCIS correspond to those identified for invasive carcinoma.[17] Because the male breast lacks lobular elements, this entity has not been described in men.[3] As there are no clinical or mammographic indicators that are characteristic of LCIS, it is often detected as an incidental biopsy finding.[1,4] In a minority of cases, LCIS can be detected with mammographic calcifications; however, more commonly, calcifications are in adjacent tissue and are not histologically associated with LCIS.[18-20] In excisional biopsy specimens, DCIS or invasive carcinoma are frequently identified even when LCIS is the sole histologic entity seen on core biopsy.[21-23]

LCIS is considered a marker of increased risk for the subsequent development of invasive (usually ductal) carcinoma[3,13,14,16] that may be greatest for high-grade or more extensive lesions.[1,24] This risk appears to be nearly equal for both breasts.[25]

The question as to whether LCIS can serve as a direct precursor lesion to the subsequent development of invasive lobular carcinoma is unresolved. Some studies have suggested a clonal link of synchronously detected LCIS and invasive lobular carcinoma,[26] whereas others have not.[27] In an analysis of 182 patients with LCIS who were inadvertently enrolled on the National Surgical Adjuvant Breast and Bowel Project (NSABP) B-17 trial for DCIS and treated with lumpectomy only, there was a 14.4% in-breast tumor recurrence (IBTR) rate and a 7.8% contralateral breast tumor recurrence rate after a median follow-up of 12 years.[28] Nine IBTRs (5% of the total cohort) were invasive carcinoma, and 17 (9% of total cohort) were DCIS. Although the frequency of contralateral breast tumor recurrence rate was less than that of IBTR, the frequency of invasive contralateral breast tumor recurrence rate (5.6% of total cohort) was similar to invasive IBTR (5% of total cohort). Of note, all of the IBTR were documented to be at the site of the index lesion except for one, characterized as pure LCIS, that was found at a remote site.

The evidence associating LCIS with the subsequent development of invasive disease raises the question as to whether magnetic resonance imaging (MRI) would be a useful screening tool. Limited data exist to formulate a firm recommendation. In 2007, the American Cancer Society stated there were insufficient data; however, in 2009, the National Comprehensive Cancer Network published guidelines reflecting a panel consensus opinion that annual breast MRI should be considered in patients with LCIS. Several studies have been published evaluating the role of MRI in patients with LCIS.[29-32] Each document revealed a small but defined 3.3% to 4.5% breast cancer detection rate and a positive predictive value of 31% based on biopsies performed supporting consideration for an annual MRI in this subset of patients. Management for LCIS depends on whether it is associated with another malignancy (DCIS or invasive carcinoma) or if LCIS is the sole histologic diagnosis. Approximately 10% of early-stage breast cancers have an associated component of LCIS.[33-35] The effect that LCIS has on the outcome of conservative management of early-stage breast cancer has been evaluated. Limited studies suggest that the presence of LCIS should influence treatment approach[36]; however, the most widely accepted treatment approach is to manage the breast according to the dominant malignant histology (DCIS or invasive carcinoma) and disregard the LCIS. In such circumstances, it is not necessary to pursue additional surgery to obtain clear margins for LCIS.[27,33,34,37,38]

If LCIS is the sole histologic diagnosis, treatment recommendations range from conservative to radical. When first described as an entity, the significance of LCIS was unknown and mastectomy was often performed.[39] The high frequency of contralateral breast involvement was subsequently used to justify contralateral biopsy and even bilateral mastectomy.[16,39] Observational studies after wide local excision alone have led to a better understanding of the natural history of this condition, and a more conservative approach is now commonly practiced.[3,13,14] In patients with LCIS as the sole histologic diagnosis, the most widely accepted clinical practice is close observation with regular physical examination and mammographic surveillance.[3,13-15,28] There is no role for radiotherapy in the management of LCIS. The fact that LCIS commonly involves both breasts makes treatment with unilateral mastectomy both inadequate and illogic. Bilateral prophylactic mastectomy is likely excessive in all but those patients believed to be at highest risk: young age, diffuse high-grade lesion, and significant family history. A less radical prophylactic approach in high-risk patients is to consider the use of tamoxifen. Tamoxifen has demonstrated efficacy in the prevention of invasive carcinoma and, in the context of LCIS, has been shown to reduce risk by 56%.[40,41]

PAGET DISEASE

The clinical presentation of crusting and eczematous changes of the nipple–areola complex were first described in 1856. However, it was not until 1874 that the association with an underlying breast cancer was reported by Sir James Paget.[42] Paget disease of the nipple is characterized by the presence of Paget cells that are located throughout the epidermis.[43] Paget cells are large and have hyperchromatic, round to oval nuclei with abundant amphophilic to clear cytoplasm. Mitoses are commonly seen, and the cells can be found in clusters or individually in the basal layers. The fact that Paget disease is associated with an underlying malignancy in >95% of cases has generated discussion regarding the origin of these malignant cells. The epidermotropic theory appears to be the prevailing opinion, with the belief that the disease originates from the underlying *in situ* or invasive disease. This is supported by histologic evidence of intraepithelial extension, immunohistochemical studies, and evidence suggesting that the epidermal keratinocytes release a motility factor, heregulin-α, that results in the chemotaxis of Paget cells that migrate to the overlying nipple epidermis.[44,45]

Paget disease is a rare entity representing <5% of all breast cancer cases[46,47] and is typically diagnosed in the fifth or sixth decade of life. Synchronous bilateral Paget disease and male Paget disease have been reported.[44,48,49]

Patients with Paget disease describe itching and burning of the nipple and areola. There is a slow progression toward a crusting eczematoid appearance that can extend to the periareolar skin. If neglected, bleeding, pain, and ulceration can occur.[47,50] Alternatively, Paget disease can be asymptomatic and present as a pathologic finding after incidental surgical removal of the nipple–areolar complex.[51] The differential diagnosis includes superficial spreading melanoma,

pagetoid squamous cell carcinoma *in situ*, and clear cells of Toker.[43,52] A palpable mass is detected in approximately 50% of patients at diagnosis; in >90% of cases, this will be an invasive carcinoma. In contrast, if no palpable mass is detected, 66% to 86% will have an underlying DCIS. These associated malignancies are usually located centrally, although they can occur elsewhere in the breast.[44,47,53] Mammographic findings are frequent in the presence of a palpable mass; however, normal mammograms are reported in as many as 50% of cases.[47,54]

At presentation, clinical evaluation includes bilateral breast examination, mammography, and biopsy to confirm the diagnosis of Paget disease and to fully evaluate the extent of the associated malignancy. The prognosis does not depend on the diagnosis of Paget disease but rather on the associated malignancy. Therefore, local treatment, as well as systemic and regional nodal disease risk management, should be based on the associated disease.

Management of Paget disease continues to evolve. Mastectomy was employed in the past, although this has been increasingly supplanted by breast-conserving treatment.[55-58] The infrequent occurrence of this disease entity, the range of disease presentations (nipple involvement with or without an underlying mass and association with invasive vs. noninvasive disease), and the variable extent of surgical resection has made the evaluation of treatment options difficult. Small series have described results with various forms of breast-conserving treatment, including wide local surgical resection alone, radiotherapy alone, and wide excision followed by whole-breast radiotherapy. Conservative surgery alone for Paget disease appears to be inadequate, with reported local recurrence rates of 25% to 40%.[5,59-63] The use of radiotherapy alone has been reported as achieving an 85% local control rate in a small series of patients with Paget disease of the nipple who presented without an associated palpable mass.[64] However, this approach has not been widely adopted because of the undefined histologic type and extent of the underlying disease leading to uncertainty in field design and total radiation dose.

The combination of limited surgical resection and postoperative radiotherapy appears to be the most practical breast-conserving approach. Two studies have evaluated the combined use of surgery and radiotherapy in Paget disease of the nipple. The European Organization for Research and Treatment of Cancer (EORTC) Study 10873 was a multiinstitutional registry trial that reported a 5-year local recurrence rate of 5.2%.[65] In this study, a complete excision with tumor-free margins of the nipple–areolar complex and underlying breast tissue was followed by whole-breast radiotherapy. The median follow-up was 6.4 years, and the majority of these patients were found to have an underlying DCIS without a palpable mass. A separate study consisted of a seven-institution collaborative review of 36 patients with Paget disease without a palpable mass or mammographic density.[66,67] Patient follow-up was a median of 9.4 years. The extent of surgical resection varied as patients underwent complete (69%) or partial (25%) excision of the nipple–areolar complex and underlying breast tissue, with 6% reported as biopsy only. The final margin status was documented as negative in 56%, positive in 6%, and unknown in 39%. All received whole-breast irradiation, and most received an additional boost dose to the tumor bed. The actuarial rate of local failure as the only site of first recurrence was 9% at 5 years and 13% at both 10 and 15 years. Two additional patients recurred in the treated breast simultaneously with regional and distant metastasis at 69 and 122 months. Despite the differences in clinical, pathologic, and treatment factors, statistical evaluation did not identify any factors that significantly predicted for risk of local recurrence.

Current data suggest that a combined modality approach that conserves the breast is an appropriate alternative to mastectomy in properly selected patients with underlying noninvasive or invasive carcinoma of limited extent. As with any breast-conserving approach, patients with multicentric disease extension should be excluded. Surgical resection should include the nipple–areolar complex with microscopically clear margins surrounding both the Paget disease and the associated malignancy. Whole-breast radiotherapy is delivered with standard techniques. Management of regional nodes and the risk of systemic disease are dictated by the associated malignancy.

DUCTAL CARCINOMA *IN SITU*

Clinical Presentation and Epidemiology

DCIS is a neoplastic process that is confined to the ductal system of the breast and lacks histologic evidence of invasion. These cells neither disrupt the basement membrane nor involve the surrounding breast stroma. This entity lacks the ability to metastasize and is confined to the breast.[68-71] Axillary node involvement is rare (0% to 5%) and most likely is associated with an undetected focus of invasive carcinoma.[72] Risk factors for the development of DCIS are the same as those identified for invasive carcinoma,[17] including family history, reproductive events such as delayed age of first live birth and nulliparity, history of benign breast biopsy, and dietary factors such as alcohol consumption. Before the use of screening mammography, DCIS typically presented as a palpable mass or nipple discharge. An invasive component commonly was found, and pure DCIS rarely was encountered. The widespread use of mammography now routinely detects DCIS <1 cm in diameter and results in breast cancer–free survival rates that approach 100%.[72]

With the increased use of mammography and as pathologists began to recognize DCIS as a pathologic entity, the incidence of DCIS has markedly increased.[73-75] The incidence of DCIS in the United States rose from 4,800 cases in 1983 to >50,000 cases in 2004, representing a 10-fold increase in only 20 years.[76] Of the more than 250,000 new breast cancers that occur annually, approximately 63,000 are anticipated to be noninvasive, of which 85% will be DCIS.[77] Of these, 90% are expected to be nonpalpable.[45] Studies have shown that the rate of screen-detected DCIS increases with age despite that it accounts for a progressively smaller proportion of the total breast cancers detected.[78] The rate of DCIS detection has been reported to increase from 0.56 per 1,000 mammograms among women aged 40 to 49 years to 1.07 per 1,000 mammograms among women aged 70 to 84 years.[78]

Imaging

Ninety-five percent of new cases of DCIS present with mammographic abnormalities, of which microcalcifications are most typical.[79] Noncalcified mammographic abnormalities make up the remaining findings, with asymmetric densities identified in 10%, dominant masses in 8%, and abnormal galactograms (performed for evaluation of nipple discharge) in 6%. Amorphous, coarse, fine pleomorphic, and fine linear are all forms of calcifications that can be related to DCIS. Linear and segmental calcifications are considered suspicious distribution and can be associated with DCIS in up to 80% of cases.[80] Linear and branching calcifications frequently are associated with high-grade DCIS and necrosis, whereas fine and granular calcifications are associated more commonly with low-grade DCIS[81-84] (Fig. 58.1A and B).

Initial evaluation should include magnification views that allow for complete characterization of mammographic findings and determination of the need for biopsy. The extent of the lesion as determined mammographically may be used as a guide for excision; however, the size typically is underestimated by 1 to 2 cm when compared with pathologic measurements.[82,85,86] Prior to 2000, MRI was not considered a useful imaging modality for DCIS. However, change in MRI imaging acquisition and an improved understanding of non–mass-like malignant lesion imaging characteristics now has MRI considered a valuable imaging tool for DCIS.[87] MRI now presents as the imaging modality with the highest sensitivity to detect DCIS, particularly high-grade DCIS. MRI has additionally been shown to better establish the extent of DCIS, thus aiding treatment planning.[88] In cases that present with nipple discharge and a negative mammogram, galactography may be helpful in determining the likelihood of underlying DCIS versus papilloma[89] (Fig. 58.1C).

Pathology and Biology

The histologic diversity of DCIS can lead to difficulty in distinguishing it from other pathologic entities.[70,71] The spectrum of DCIS extends from noncomedo, low-grade DCIS that can be similar in appearance to atypical ductal hyperplasia to comedo, high-grade DCIS. In addition, DCIS can extend into lobules, making it difficult to distinguish from LCIS.[90] Traditionally, classification of DCIS has followed its architectural or morphologic appearance. The five subtypes of DCIS are comedo, solid, cribriform, micropapillary, and papillary,[70,71,91] and it is common to encounter a mixture of subtypes within the same specimen.[89] The characteristic features of each type are shown in Figure 58.2. Less common subtypes have been described and include apocrine, neuroendocrine, signet-cell cystic hypersecretory carcinoma, and clinging DCIS.[92]

In 1997, a consensus conference committee was convened to reach an agreement on the pathologic classification of DCIS and the identification of specific features that may convey prognostic significance.[69] Methods of processing and evaluating the pathologic specimen were also addressed. Rather than endorsing any specific classification system, the committee recommended and described features that should be documented for each case of DCIS, thus separating out important pathologic components and providing a comprehensive evaluation of the pathologic findings. These features include nuclear grade, presence of necrosis, polarization, and architectural pattern(s). The committee extended its recommendations to include margin status, lesion size, extent of microcalcifications, and correlation between specimen x-ray and mammographic findings. The DCIS Working Party of the EORTC arrived at similar conclusions and emphasized the importance of cytonuclear and architectural differentiation.[93]

Three-dimensional examination and reconstruction techniques have resulted in a better understanding of the enormously complex structure of the mammary duct–lobular system and the patterns by which DCIS can spread within the breast[6,85,94] (Fig. 58.3). Knowledge of the anatomy and distribution of DCIS within the mammary ductal tree can be useful in selecting patients for breast conservation and assuring maximal surgical clearance of the lesion while preserving an acceptable cosmetic result. For example, Ohtake et al.[6,85] studied the duct–lobular system with computer graphic reconstruction and found that the breast consists of 16 to 24 duct–lobular systems, each culminating in a corresponding collecting duct at the nipple. They also identified ductal anastomoses that established a connection between the various ductal–lobular units and provided a potential pathway for tumor extension and subsequent diffuse involvement.[6,85] Their proposed model for the development of widespread

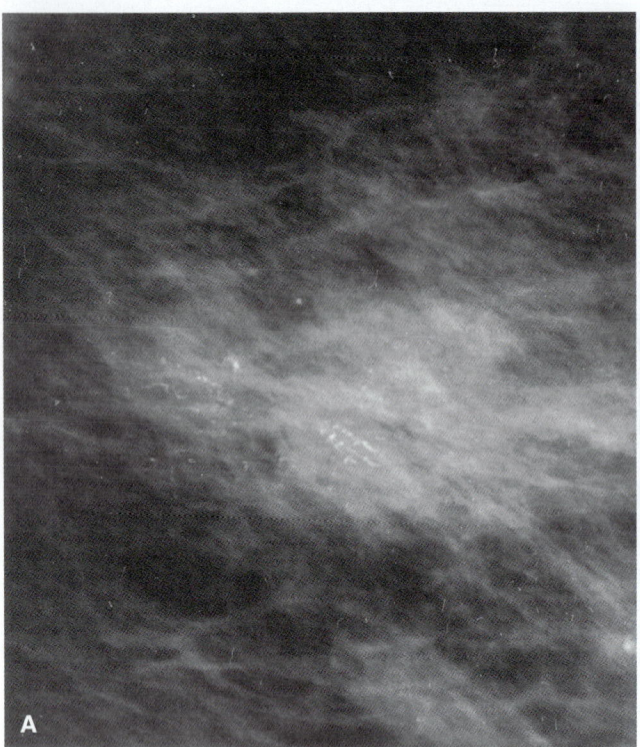

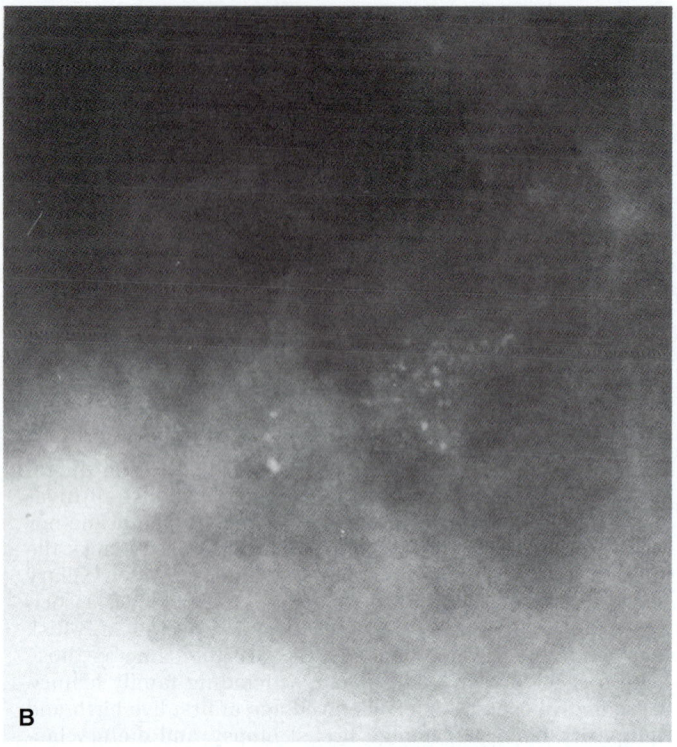

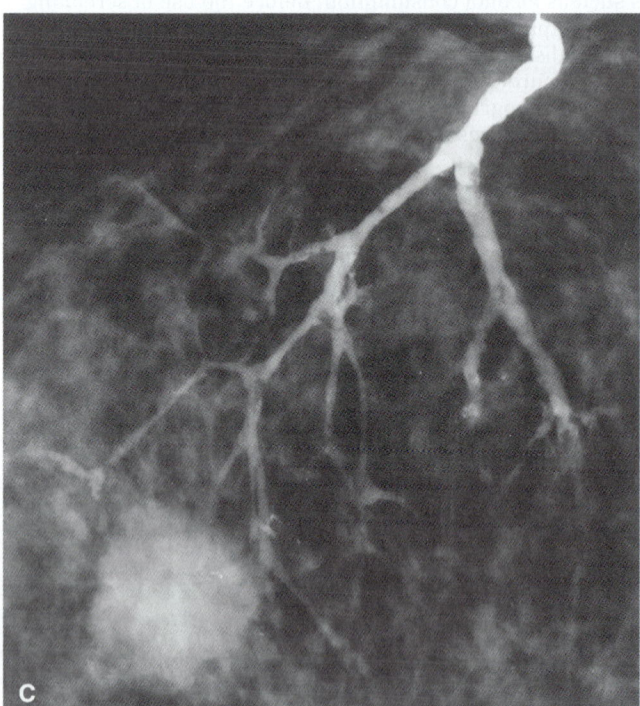

FIGURE 58.1. A: Linear and branching calcifications frequently associated with high-grade ductal carcinoma *in situ* (DCIS). **B:** Fine and granular calcifications commonly associated with low-grade DCIS. **C:** Galactogram with the multiple filling defects associated with DCIS.

intraductal tumor extension within the breast is seen in Figure 58.4.

Faverly et al.[95] have described the DCIS growth pattern within the ductal tree and the implications for surgical excision. The growth patterns documented include unicentric (one area only), multicentric (two distinct areas separated by >4 cm), continuous (extension along ductal system without gaps), and discontinuous or multifocal (two or more areas separated by <4 cm). They found that in mammographically detected DCIS, a multicentric growth pattern was rare (<2%), with most cases showing an even distribution between discontinuous and continuous growth patterns. Of cases with a discontinuous growth pattern, 63% had foci separated by gaps that measured <5 mm, 83% had foci separated by <10 mm, and only 8% had foci separated by >10 mm. There was a correlation between differentiation and growth pattern such that 90% of poorly differentiated DCIS showed a continuous growth pattern, whereas 70% of well-differentiated DCIS had a discontinuous growth pattern. Based on these findings, the authors concluded that a 1-cm margin of normal tissue around the lesion would lead to complete surgical clearance of histologically evident DCIS in 90% of cases. DCIS is a precursor lesion to invasive ductal carcinoma and exists along an evolutionary continuum that starts with benign breast tissue and ends with an invasive breast

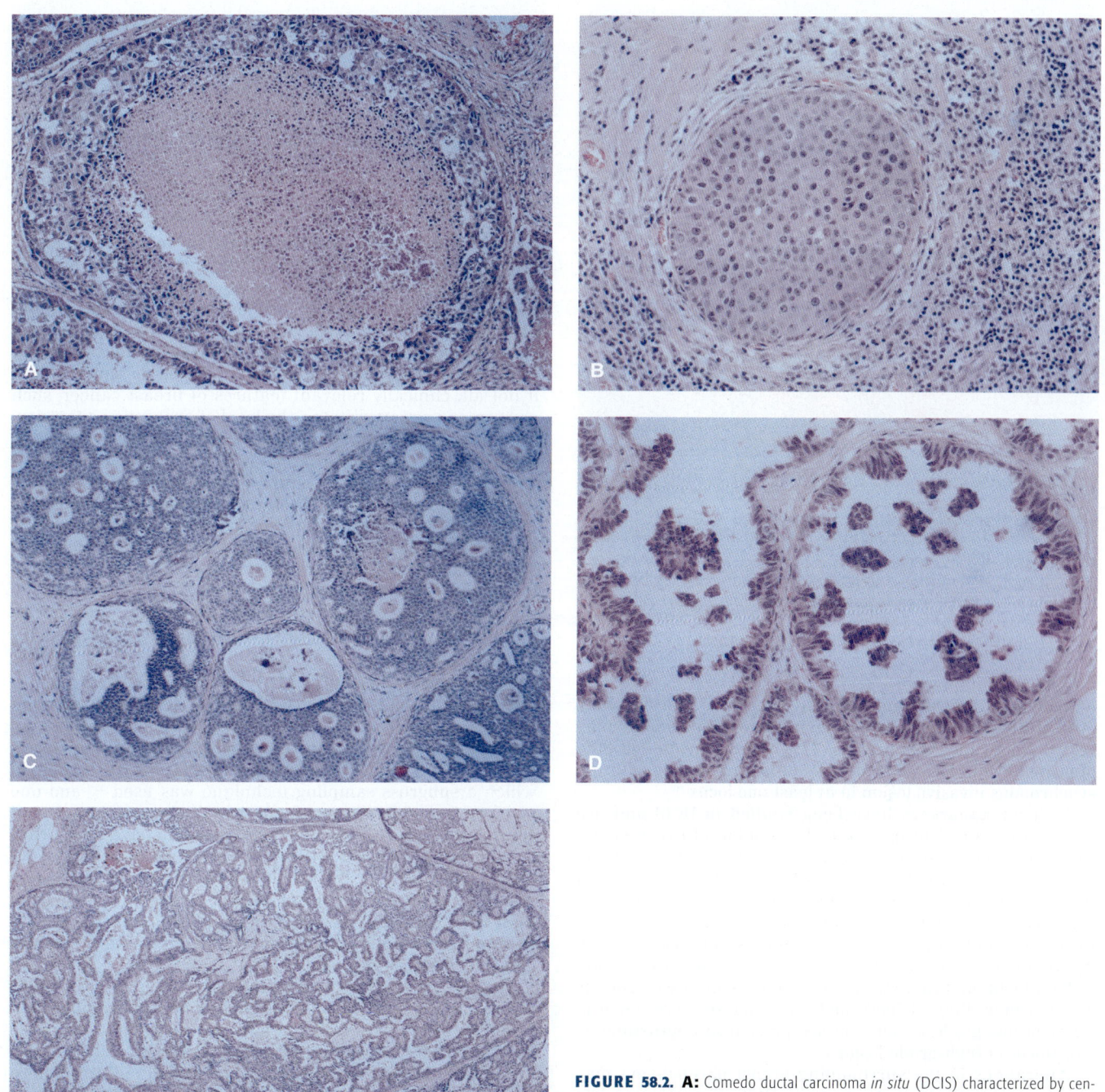

FIGURE 58.2. A: Comedo ductal carcinoma *in situ* (DCIS) characterized by central necrosis, large cells, and poorly differentiated nuclei. **B:** Solid DCIS characterized by ductal spaces filled with neoplastic cells with limited necrosis. **C:** Cribriform DCIS characterized by microlumens and fenestrations. **D:** Micropapillary DCIS characterized by intraluminal projections with no fibrovascular core. **E:** Papillary DCIS characterized by intraluminal projections with a fibrovascular core.

carcinoma.[96] This concept has been validated in several ways. For years, pathologists have recognized and documented confirmation of a histologic progression from benign breast cells to invasive breast cancer. The evolutionary concept is supported by the recognized association between the presence of DCIS and the subsequent increased risk of developing an invasive breast cancer.[76,97,98] In some series, a 10-fold risk of developing an invasive lesion has been reported. At the biologic and molecular level, many studies have demonstrated that DCIS and invasive breast cancer are highly similar at the cellular and molecular levels.[96,99–103] These similarities have now been shown to extend to global gene expression profiles as DCIS has been classified under luminal, basal, and erbB2 intrinsic

molecular subtypes.[99,104] Additionally, these shared identical genetic abnormalities between DCIS and synchronous invasive breast cancer demonstrate a clonal relationship of biologic progression.[76,97,98,105] The biologic evolution from benign breast cells to invasive breast cancer occurs through highly diverse genetic mechanisms.

Genetic and molecular differences have been documented that differentiate DCIS from normal breast tissue. Genetic alterations have been evaluated with an analysis of loss of heterozygosity that has demonstrated gain or loss of multiple loci.[97,98,105–107] Loss of heterozygosity is not seen in normal breast tissue. The frequency of loss of heterozygosity correlates with histologic progression of breast tissue from benign

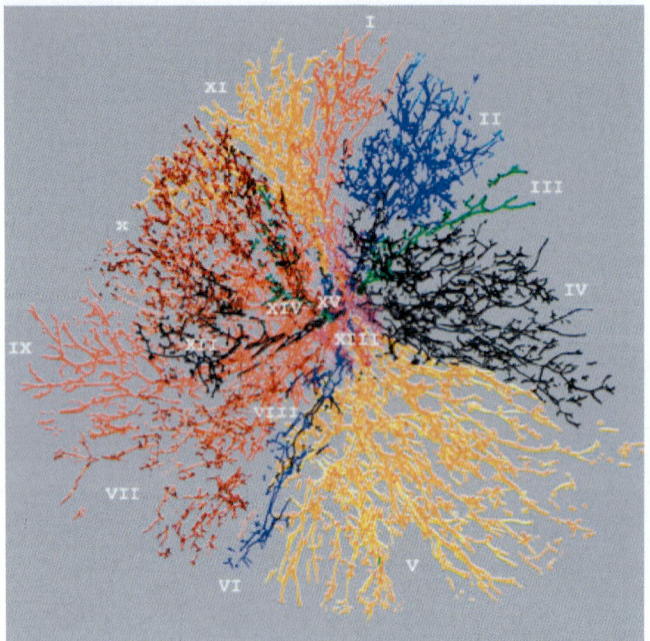

FIGURE 58.3. All ducts and their branches in an autopsy breast, viewed *en face*. Each Roman numeral refers to a different independent duct system. (From Going JJ, Moffat DF. Escaping from flatland: clinical and biological aspects of human mammary duct anatomy in three dimensions. *J Pathol* 2004;203[1]:538–544. Copyright © 2004 Pathological Society of Great Britain and Ireland. Reprinted by permission of John Wiley & Sons, Inc.)

and angiogenesis in the surrounding stromal tissues.[109,110] Whether these stromal changes reflect important steps that facilitate primary tumor transformation or secondary alterations in response to ductal epithelium that is being transformed is unknown. Quantitative changes in the expression of genes related to cell motility, adhesion, and extracellular matrix composition—all of which may be related to the acquisition of invasiveness—occur as DCIS evolves into invasive carcinoma.[111]

Data suggest that DCIS represents a stage in the development of breast cancer in which most of the molecular changes that characterize invasive breast cancer are already present, although the lesion has not yet assumed a fully malignant phenotype. A final set of events, which probably includes gain of function by malignant cells and loss of function and integrity by surrounding normal tissues, is associated with the transition from a preinvasive DCIS lesion to invasive cancer. Most, if not all, clinically relevant features of breast cancer, such as hormone receptor status, the level of oncogene expression, and histologic grade, are probably determined by the time that DCIS has evolved.[112–115]

An occult microinvasive tumor (one that does not exceed 0.1 cm in diameter) may be seen with some cases of DCIS. Such cases are classified as *microinvasive breast cancer*[116] and are generally treated according to the guidelines for invasive disease. Occult microinvasive tumors are most common in patients with DCIS lesions that are >2.5 cm in diameter,[117] those presenting with palpable masses or nipple discharge, and those with high-grade DCIS or comedonecrosis.[89,118]

Natural History of Ductal Carcinoma *In Situ*

The overall incidence of DCIS in the general population is unclear. In an attempt to address this incidence, a small number of autopsy studies have been reported. One series examined 185 randomly selected breasts from 101 women in which a subgross sampling technique was used [119] and one or more foci of DCIS were found in 6% of cases. A review of seven autopsy series of women not known to have breast cancer during life showed a median prevalence of DCIS of 8.9% (range, 0% to 14.7%).[120] The fact that some autopsy series document a greater incidence of DCIS in asymptomatic women than most clinical series suggests either the possibility that DCIS is either underdiagnosed or that many cases are not clinically significant.

A primary consideration in the natural history of DCIS is the risk of progression to invasive carcinoma. The published evidence on the clinical course of untreated DCIS is sparse because it has been recognized as a distinct entity for only a relatively brief period, having been considered rare before the widespread use of mammography and having been treated most frequently by mastectomy. Those cases for which long-term follow-up data are available were grossly palpable DCIS—a form that may not be equivalent to the

to malignant. Loss of heterozygosity is seen in approximately 50% of atypical ductal hyperplasia. Among specimens harvested from cancerous breasts, 77% of noncomedo and 80% of comedo DCIS lesions share loss of heterozygosity with the synchronous invasive lesion in at least one locus.[105]

Molecular markers have been studied in DCIS and are found to have a heterogeneous distribution of expression.[76] The estrogen receptor is present in 70% of DCIS; however, the rate of expression is higher in low-grade lesions (90%) than in high-grade lesions (25%). This association with histologic grade is reversed for the rate of overexpression of HER2/neu protooncogene and the p53 tumor suppression gene. Approximately 50% of all DCIS lesions have overexpression of HER2/neu, and in 25%, the p53 tumor suppressor gene is also detected. Both of these molecular markers are noted in <20% of low-grade lesions but are present in approximately two-thirds of high-grade lesions.

Alterations in the surrounding breast parenchyma may also be seen with DCIS. High-grade DCIS, in particular, has been associated with the breakdown of the myoepithelial cell layer and basement membrane surrounding the ductal lumen,[108] proliferation of fibroblasts, lymphocyte infiltration,

FIGURE 58.4. Models for the formation of widespread intraductal tumor extension over multiple mammary duct–lobular systems. *Blue lines,* normal mammary duct–lobular systems; *red lines,* intraductal tumor extension; *closed circle,* invasive tumor foci. **Left:** Multicentric development. **Middle:** Unicentric development with continuous intraductal tumor extension. **Right:** Unicentric development with continuous intraductal tumor extension through ductal anastomoses connecting adjacent duct–lobular systems. (From Ohtake T, Abe R, Kimijima I, et al. Intraductal extension of primary invasive breast carcinoma treated by breast-conservation surgery. *Cancer* 1995;76[1]:32–45. Copyright © 1995 American Cancer Society. Reprinted by permission of John Wiley & Sons, Inc.)

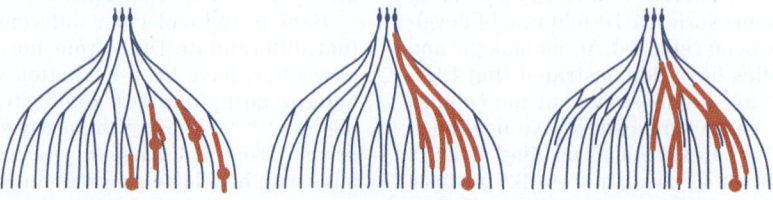

mammographic DCIS that is seen more commonly today. The few published long-term follow-up studies of DCIS after only biopsy document an overall incidence of subsequent invasive carcinoma of >36%.[7,121–123] Most of these subsequent malignancies occur within 10 years, although as many as one-third may develop after 15 years.[7,121]

Women with DCIS in one breast are at risk for a second tumor (either invasive or *in situ*) in the contralateral breast [124]; the rate at which such tumors develop is similar to that among women with primary invasive breast cancer at approximately 0.5% to 1% per year.

DCIS is a part of the breast/ovarian cancer syndromes defined by BRCA1 and BRCA2, with mutation rates similar to those found for invasive breast cancer.[125] These findings suggest that patients with DCIS with an appropriate personal or family history of breast and/or ovarian cancer should be screened and followed according to the same high-risk protocols as developed for invasive breast cancer.

Treatment Options for Ductal Carcinoma In Situ

Prognostic Factors and Their Interpretation

The goal of treatment with DCIS is prevention of local recurrence, with particular emphasis on the prevention of invasive breast cancer. Treatment decisions are largely based on information provided by mammography and, most especially, pathologic evaluation of the biopsy specimen. As such, in the consideration of treatment options, it is important for the clinician to be aware of some of the technical limitations associated with the clinical and histopathologic assessment of DCIS.

Studies performed during the past two decades clearly have suggested that DCIS is not a single disease. Rather, DCIS encompasses a diverse group of lesions that differ with regard to their clinical presentation, mammographic features, extent and distribution within the breast, histologic characteristics, and biologic markers. Moreover, clinical follow-up studies have indicated that these lesions vary in their propensity to recur or progress to invasive breast cancer. As a consequence, a significant proportion of patients diagnosed with DCIS can be treated adequately with breast-conserving therapy (i.e., excision with or without radiation therapy). Which patients with DCIS can be treated safely with excision alone and which patients require radiation therapy after excision are pressing clinical questions. Attempts to resolve this issue have focused on the identification of risk factors for local recurrence after breast conservation therapy for DCIS. Through multiple retrospective studies, several factors have been identified that may be important in defining local failure risk. These include symptomatic presentation,[126–128] lesion size,[128,129] histopathologic subtype,[126] nuclear/cytologic grade,[127,128,130] central necrosis,[127,128,130] margin status,[128,131,132] and patient age.[126,132–134]

The relative importance of any histopathologic factor in predicting the probability of local recurrence and in turn selecting the appropriate therapeutic option for a given patient is unclear. This is partly the result of the inherent difficulty associated with the establishment of standardized and reproducible systems of pathologic classification, including such apparently straightforward assessments of grade, margin width, and lesion size.

Efforts to classify DCIS have been based primarily on the nuclear grade of the lesion and/or the presence or absence of necrosis. Several studies have shown that there is an association between high nuclear grade and/or necrosis and the risk of local recurrence and progression to invasion.[127,128,130] Although the criteria for histologic grading systems have been published, there are limited data regarding the ability of pathologists to apply them in a reproducible manner.

Several studies have shown that the status of the microscopic margins appears to be important in predicting the

likelihood of recurrence in the breast for patients with both invasive breast cancer and DCIS treated with breast-conserving therapy.[128,131,132] In 2016, a consensus guideline was published from the Society of Surgical Oncology, the American Society for Radiation Oncology, and the American Society of Clinical Oncology on appropriate margins for breast-conserving surgery with whole breast radiation in DCIS.[135] The consensus panel recommended a 2-mm margin as the standard adequate margin and clinical judgment be used to determine the need for further surgery in patients with negative margins <2 mm. However, there are numerous technical problems in the evaluation of margins of breast excision specimens. First, if a specimen is removed in more than one fragment, the margins cannot be evaluated. Second, there is no standardized method for sampling or reporting margins, and this process is subject to sampling error. Finally, it is often difficult to provide an accurate assessment of the margin width for patients who undergo a reexcision because the initial biopsy site can be eccentrically located in the surgical specimen.

Most DCIS lesions present as a nonpalpable, grossly inapparent mammographic abnormality, which can make accurate determination of the size or extent of the lesion difficult (Fig. 58.5). The modalities available to assess the size of the lesion are mammography, MRI, and pathologic examination. Mammography frequently will underestimate the pathologic extent of DCIS, particularly for well-differentiated lesions in which substantial areas of the tumor may not contain microcalcifications. MRI has been demonstrated to more accurately estimate the disease extent; however, it should be recognized that pathologic assessment of lesion size can be difficult. Macroscopic examination of a specimen containing DCIS rarely reveals a grossly evident tumor that can be measured. Therefore, the assessment of the size of the lesion must be estimated from histologic sections.

Mastectomy for Ductal Carcinoma In Situ

Mastectomy was the standard treatment of DCIS through the first four decades of its recognition as a distinct histopathologic entity. Mastectomy is a highly effective treatment for DCIS, with a locoregional control rate of 96% to 100% and cancer-specific mortality rates of ≤4%.[136] No randomized study has compared mastectomy with breast-conservation

FIGURE 58.5. Extensive ductal carcinoma *in situ* (DCIS) in a mastectomy breast sectioned in the coronal plane. Every parenchymal structure (duct or lobule) within the marked perimeter is colonized by DCIS; outside that boundary there is none. (From Going JJ, Moffat DF. Escaping from flatland: clinical and biological aspects of human mammary duct anatomy in three dimensions. *J Pathol* 2004;203[1]:538–544. Copyright © 2004 Pathological Society of Great Britain and Ireland. Reprinted by permission of John Wiley & Sons, Inc.)

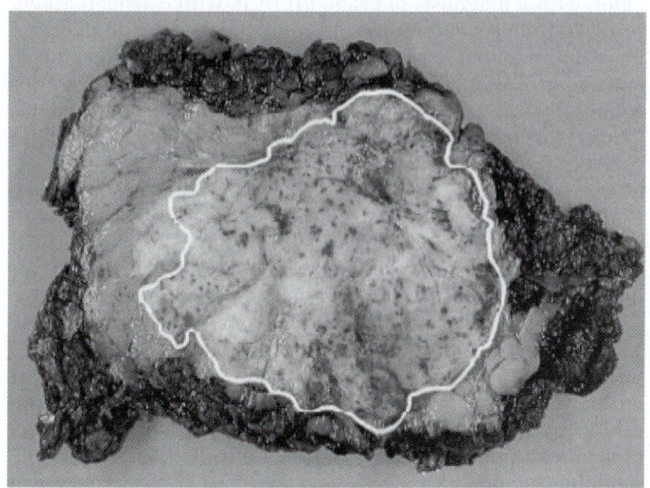

Section III

treatment for DCIS. Therefore, the relative outcomes for mastectomy and breast-conservation treatment can be estimated only by reviewing nonrandomized, retrospective studies. Local treatment failure after mastectomy[136] may occur because of unrecognized invasive carcinoma that results in local recurrence or distant metastasis, or it may be the result of incomplete removal of breast tissue with the subsequent formation of a new primary tumor.

Data from some surgical trials[137] and large treatment registries[138] suggest that the rates of local or regional recurrence are significantly lower after mastectomy than after breast-conserving surgery, although there have been no significant differences in overall survival. Metastatic breast cancer can follow the recurrence of an invasive tumor or the development of invasive cancer in the contralateral breast. However, death related to breast cancer within 10 years after the diagnosis of DCIS occurs in only 1% to 2% of all patients, irrespective of whether mastectomy or breast-conserving surgery was performed.[138]

The role of postmastectomy chest wall radiation following mastectomy or skin-sparing mastectomy and close pathologic margins has been debated in the literature but is not presently considered the standard of care. Some studies show an increased risk of chest wall failure in selected cases of high-grade DCIS undergoing mastectomy with pathologic margins <1 mm, leading to a routine recommendation of postmastectomy radiation in these cases.[139] The empiric use of a close or positive margins as a trigger for postmastectomy radiation has been challenged, providing a strong argument against postmastectomy radiation.[140] This retrospective review evaluated the risk of chest wall recurrence following mastectomy, specifically looking at skin-sparing mastectomy and high-risk features of high-grade and close margins. In this series, the overall risk of chest wall recurrence was rare at 1.7% and only 3.3% for high-grade DCIS. Margins <5 mm were not at increased risk. It was concluded that the chest wall failure rate was sufficiently low that a routine recommendation of postmastectomy radiation DCIS with high-risk features was not warranted. Furthermore, a population-based analysis using the Ontario Cancer Registry identified >1,500 women with DCIS who underwent mastectomy without radiotherapy. With a median follow-up of 10 years, the overall rate of chest wall recurrence was 2.3% with no significant difference seen between positive, close (2 mm or less), or negative margins. Univariate and multivariate analysis failed to show a significant effect of age, nuclear grade, necrosis, or multifocality.[141]

Recent interest has surged regarding active surveillance in women with low-risk DCIS. The COMET trial is comparing guideline concordant care which includes surgery +/− radiation therapy and choice of endocrine therapy vs active surveillance with choice of endocrine therapy in women 40 years or older, with a diagnosis of grade I/II DCIS with estrogen and/or progesterone receptors present and lack of comedo necrosis. Primary end point is rate of ipsilateral invasive disease development at 2 years. Two additional trials, LORIS, of the United Kingdom, and LORD sponsored by the EORTC have recently opened for accrual with similar randomizations.

Breast Conservation for Ductal Carcinoma In Situ

Four prospective randomized studies of excision only versus excision plus breast irradiation for DCIS have been performed with reported results, and all have shown that the rate of local recurrence was reduced with the addition of radiation (Table 58.1). The NSABP B-17 trial[142,143] consisted of 813 patients who were stratified by age (≤49 vs. >49 years), DCIS versus DCIS plus LCIS, method of detection, and whether an axillary dissection was performed. Tumor size was determined by mammogram, gross pathologic measurement, or clinical examination. Of the patients enrolled, 83% had nonpalpable tumors. The 17.5-year rate of local recurrence was

TABLE 58.1 LUMPECTOMY VERSUS LUMPECTOMY AND WHOLE-BREAST RADIOTHERAPY: RANDOMIZED CLINICAL TRIALS FOR DUCTAL CARCINOMA *IN SITU*

Trial Group	Number of Patients	Follow-Up	Local Recurrence (Cumulative %) DCIS + Invasive Carcinoma		
			L	L + XRT	P Value
NSABP B-17	818	12-y actuarial	31.7	15.7	<.000005
		17.25-y median	35.0	19.8	—
EORTC 10853	1,010	15.7-y median	31.0	18.0	<.0001
UK/ANZ	1,030	12.7-y median	19.4	7.1	<.00001
SweDCIS	1,046	17-y mean	32	20	—

DCIS, ductal carcinoma *in situ*; EORTC, European Organisation for Research and Treatment of Cancer; L, lumpectomy; L + XRT, lumpectomy and postoperative radiotherapy; NSABP, National Surgical Adjuvant Bowel and Breast Project; SweDCIS, Swedish Breast Cancer Group DCIS study; UK/ANZ, United Kingdom, Australia, and New Zealand.

19.8% with radiation and 35.9% without radiation. The average annual incidence rates of ipsilateral noninvasive recurrences and ipsilateral invasive recurrences were reduced with breast irradiation by 47% and 52%, respectively.[144] An analysis of clinical variables showed that microcalcifications extending beyond a maximum dimension >1 cm were associated with an elevated risk of breast recurrence. A central pathology review was performed, including a multivariate analysis of histopathologic variables (Table 58.2). Comedonecrosis in patients treated on NSABP B-24 did not correlate with an increased risk of IBTR; however, comedonecrosis did relate to the risk of DCIS-IBTR. The prognostic value of margin status (free vs. unknown/involved) depended on the treatment group and was greater among those treated with lumpectomy and radiotherapy alone as compared to those that also received tamoxifen.[133,143,144]

The EORTC 10853 trial[145,146] randomly allocated 1,010 patients with ≤5 cm DCIS and negative margins to excision versus excision plus breast irradiation. Lesions were nonpalpable in 79% of patients, and the mean maximal tumor diameter was approximately 2 cm. The 15-year rate of local recurrence was 18% for patients treated with radiation, as compared with 31% for patients treated without radiation (P <.0001). At a median follow-up of 15.7 years, radiation therapy resulted in risk reduction for both invasive and noninvasive breast relapse of 48%. As with the NSABP B-17 study, a central pathology review was performed.[126,145,146] In a multivariate analysis, factors associated with an increased risk of local recurrence were ≤40 years of age, clinically symptomatic presentation (nipple discharge or palpable mass), intermediate or poorly differentiated DCIS, solid/comedo and cribriform histologic growth pattern, involved or uncertain margins, and treatment by local excision alone. The risk of DCIS recurrence

TABLE 58.2 HAZARD RATIOS FOR INVASIVE IPSILATERAL BREAST TUMOR (I-IBTR) RECURRENCE OR DUCTAL CARCINOMA *IN SITU* (DCIS-IBTR) BASED ON COMEDONECROSIS AND MARGIN STATUS ADAPTED FROM NSABP B-17 AND B-24

Histopathologic Variable	I-IBTR HR (95% CI)	DCIS-IBTR HR (95% CI)
Comedonecrosis		
Absent	1.00	1.00
Present	0.87 (0.62–1.21) P = .41	2.21 (1.52–3.2) P = <.001
Margin status		
LRT, margin-free	1.00	1.00
LRT, involved/uncertain	2.61 (1.68–4.05) P = <.001	1.65 (1.00–2.73) P = .05
LRT + TAM, margin free	1.00	1.00
LRT + TAM, involved/uncertain	1.27 (0.73–2.20) P = .40	1.32 (0.77–2.28) P = .31

CI, confidence interval; DCIS-IBTR, ductal carcinoma *in situ* in-breast tumor recurrence; HR, hazard ratio; I-IBTR, ipsilateral in-breast tumor recurrence; LRT, lumpectomy + radiotherapy; NSABP, National Surgical Adjuvant Breast and Bowel Project; TAM, tamoxifen.

was documented to be less following treatment of clinging/ micropapillary DCIS; however, in this group, breast irradiation reduced the rate of invasive recurrence in over 50%. Although early publications suggested a relationship between histologic type and risk of distant metastasis and death, with additional follow-up, no statistically significant relationship is now appreciated.

The EORTC 10853 trial did not allow the identification of an appropriate margin width for treatment with or without radiotherapy because the eligibility criteria did not require reporting of the margin status. Nonetheless, the central review of cases did provide some information regarding the relative importance of surgical margin as related to local failure risk. A recurrence rate of 24% at 4 years was observed in cases with close/involved margins after excision alone. Radiotherapy was not adequate to compensate for involved margins because even with the application of irradiation, the recurrence rate was 20% in this group[147]. These data and others[128,129,131,132] are strongly suggestive that obtaining a microscopic complete excision is essential for optimal local control in breast-conserving therapy for DCIS. Of further note, even in the group of DCIS cases for which margins could be considered optimal (i.e., those patients who underwent a surgical reexcision in which no residual DCIS was found), a 4-year local recurrence rate of 18% was observed when these patients were treated with surgery alone.[126]

The United Kingdom, Australia, and New Zealand (UK/ANZ) DCIS trial was a randomized trial investigating the role of adjuvant radiotherapy.[148,149] With a 2 × 2 factorial protocol design, the aim of this study was to compare excision alone versus excision plus tamoxifen versus excision plus radiotherapy versus excision plus radiotherapy and tamoxifen. Tamoxifen was prescribed at 20 mg per day, and radiotherapy was delivered through whole-breast tangential fields to a total dose of 50 Gy. A boost was not recommended, and elective decision to withhold or provide one of the treatments was permitted. Data have been reported with a median follow-up of 12.7 years. The addition of radiotherapy was demonstrated to reduce the risk of IBTR. Of the 1,030 patients randomized between no radiotherapy versus radiotherapy, ipsilateral IBTR was 19.4% versus 7.1%, respectively ($P < .0001$). The addition of tamoxifen offered no benefit toward overall ipsilateral local control when administered in addition to radiotherapy; however, tamoxifen reduced the ipsilateral recurrence rate of DCIS (but not invasive carcinoma) in the absence of radiotherapy.[148,149]

The Swedish Breast Cancer Group SweDCIS study was a randomized trial that enrolled 1,067 patients from 1987 to 1999, with 1,046 of these patients followed for a median of 17 years. Patients were randomized between lumpectomy followed by radiotherapy and lumpectomy only for treatment of DCIS.[150] Following sector resection, microscopically clear resection margins were not required, and 50 Gy in 25 fractions to the whole breast was delivered in the majority of patients. A split course, 54 Gy in 2 Gy fractions, delivered in two treatment series separated by a 2-week break was allowed. No boost dose was delivered. The in-breast failure risk reduction for the addition of radiotherapy was 12% at 20 years (95% confidence interval [CI] 6.5% to 17.7%) with a relative risk reduction of 37.5% (95% CI 0.30 to 0.54). Detailed analysis did not identify any patient or tumor characteristic subgroups, which did not benefit from the addition of postoperative radiotherapy. Additionally, despite combining factors entailing a low risk of recurrence without radiotherapy, a low-risk group without significant benefit from the addition of radiotherapy could not be identified.

A meta-analysis was completed utilizing the individual patient data from each of the four randomized trials discussed above, and an overview of results was reported by the Early Breast Cancer Trialists' Collaborative Group (EBCTCG).[151] With a total of 3,729 women eligible for analysis, it was demonstrated that radiotherapy reduced the absolute 10-year risk of any ipsilateral breast event (recurrent DCIS or invasive disease) by 15.2% (standard error [SE] 1.6%, 12.9% vs. 28.1%, $2 P < .00001$). This analysis further establishes strong and consistent evidence that the addition of radiotherapy following breast-conserving surgery for DCIS approximately reduces the risk of IBTR by 50%. Subgroup analyses from these randomized trials have demonstrated that the absolute benefit of radiotherapy is greater in women at increased risk for tumor recurrence, such as women with involved surgical margins (identified on retrospective pathologic review), younger women, and those with tumors that have high-grade or comedonecrotic features.[126,142,143,145,151] However, this meta-analysis confirmed that no matter what the underlying rate of ipsilateral IBTR was within subgroups evaluated, the risk reduction of approximately 50% remained. This was demonstrated across categories defined by patient age, type of excision, use of tamoxifen, method of detection, margin status, tumor focality, and histologic or nuclear grade. There was little impact of radiotherapy on contralateral or distant events, and a difference in the risk of death from breast cancer was not appreciated.

Patient age is an important prognostic variable for local recurrence after breast conservation for DCIS.[126,132-134] In younger patients, DCIS more frequently contains adverse pathologic features and extends over a greater distance in the breast than in older patients.[134] In series with adequate follow-up, younger patients treated with lumpectomy and radiation therapy had a significantly higher rate of local recurrence than older patients, especially invasive local recurrences.[134] Some studies have suggested that careful attention to margin status and excising larger volumes of tissue can reduce this difference substantially.[132,134] No available data show that younger patients have better long-term cancer-free survival rates if treated by mastectomy rather than lumpectomy and radiation therapy. Successful treatment of younger patients with DCIS with lumpectomy and radiation therapy requires careful attention to patient evaluation, selection, and surgical technique. When this is done, age at diagnosis should not be a contraindication to breast-conserving therapy.

The randomized trials discussed were designed and conducted over a decade ago. Since then, imaging technology, surgical techniques, and pathologic evaluation have continued to advance, suggesting that the patients encountered with DCIS presently may represent a group a patients with smaller, less extensive disease that is better surgically cleared as compared to those included in the randomized trials. As a result, the value of adjuvant radiotherapy has been hypothesized to be lower than indicated in previous trials. However, it should be noted that the tumor characteristics of those included in the randomized trials represented limited and mammographically detected disease. Despite this, several recent studies have attempted to identify and treat patients with highly selected favorable tumor characteristics with excision alone (i.e., without whole-breast irradiation) and report 10-year local failure rates of 3% to 25%.[131,136] One of these studies[129] has proposed a scoring system using histopathologic features including tumor size, grade, and margin width in an attempt to stratify patients according to local failure risk after excision plus or minus whole-breast irradiation. Each variable was assigned a score of 1 to 3, and the sum total defined the Van Nuys Prognostic Index. Although appealingly simple, this schema[129] is drawn from the retrospective analysis of a patient cohort in which there existed several methodologic shortcomings, and it has not been independently validated.[152]

The Radiation Oncology Group (RTOG) published the results of a prospective randomized trial of 585 women who were defined as having good-risk DCIS (low or intermediate grade, <2.5 cm size primary, and ≥ 3 mm margins) treated with adjuvant whole breast irradiation (50.4 Gy in 28 fractions and later amended to allow 42.5Gy in 16 fractions without a boost) or observation. The use of tamoxifen was optional. The study was closed early because of low accrual (expected accrual 1,790). With a median follow up of >7 years, the rate of local failure was 6.7% and 0.9% for the observation and radiation groups, respectively. Grade 1 to 2 acute toxicity was higher in the XRT arm, 76% versus 30%, with no difference in grade 3 to 4 toxicity in either arm. Despite the lower than expected accrual in this good-risk population, adjuvant XRT improved local failure. Additional follow up is needed to determine long term benefits.[153]

Wong et al.[154] performed a prospective study that attempted to identify patients with "low-risk" DCIS who can be spared whole-breast radiation therapy. This trial enrolled 158 patients with lesions that were mostly grade 1 or 2 and with a mammographic extent of ≤2.5 cm who were treated with wide excision, with final margins ≥1 cm or a re-excision without residual DCIS. Tamoxifen was not permitted. The median age was 51 years. The most recent data, with a median follow-up of 11 years,[155] reported an estimated annual local recurrence percentage rate of 1.9%. Of those with an IBTR, 68% had a DCIS recurrence and 32% experienced recurrence with invasive carcinoma. This data provides prospective evidence that despite margins of >1 cm, the local recurrence rate is substantial even in patients with small grade 1 or 2 DCIS following treatment with wide excision alone.

In an intergroup trial run by the Eastern Cooperative Oncology Group and North Central Cancer Treatment Group, wide excision only in a population of conservatively selected patients with DCIS was evaluated.[156,157] Eligibility included patients with low- or intermediate-grade DCIS measuring ≤2.5 cm (cohort 1, n = 561) or high-grade DCIS measuring ≤1 cm (cohort 2, n = 104). Microscopic margin width was required to be ≥3 mm with no residual calcifications on postoperative mammograms. The majority of these patients had a more favorable profile than that reflected by the eligibility criteria with median lesion size of 6 mm and 7 mm for cohorts 1 and 2, respectively, and the majority having margins >5 mm. The use of tamoxifen was optional after the year 2000, potentially impacting recurrence rates and/or time to recurrence intervals (30% and 24% for cohorts 1 and 2 respectively). With a median follow-up of 12.3 years, the 12-year rates of ipsilateral in-breast failure and invasive in-breast failure were 14.4% and 7.5%, respectively, for the low-inermediate group and 24.6% and 13.4%, respectively, for the high grade group. Whether this identifies the low-intermediate grade group as a group that could avoid radiotherapy remains to be demonstrated, as this may represent a group with a delayed IBTR pattern, as no plateau was identified. The NSABP and Radiation Therapy Oncology Group have jointly launched a phase III accelerated partial-breast irradiation trial which randomly allocates patients between standard whole-breast irradiation following lumpectomy versus accelerated partial-breast irradiation to determine if in-breast control rates are comparable. As the in-breast failure patterns for DCIS suggest that treatment directed to the primary lesion plus a 2-cm margin should achieve local control rates that equate to whole-breast treatment approaches, patients with pure DCIS or DCIS and LCIS are eligible for stratified randomization. This trial is now closed and results are pending.

Follow-Up and Management of Recurrence

Ipsilateral tumor recurrences in patients with DCIS are usually detected on surveillance mammography, although one-quarter may be detected on the basis of changes on physical examination of the breast or chest wall.[158,159] For this reason, patients should be scheduled for a baseline mammogram 6 to 12 months after initial therapy and at least annually thereafter. Distant breast cancer metastases in the absence of regional recurrence are unusual. Local recurrences after

breast-conserving surgery and radiotherapy are generally treated with mastectomy. Selected patients with local recurrences who have not previously received radiotherapy may be candidates for local excision and radiotherapy. The clinical outcome of ipsilateral tumor recurrence is governed by the nature of the recurrence. Patients with recurrent DCIS have an excellent prognosis, with <1% risk of further recurrence after salvage mastectomy. Patients with invasive recurrence after breast-conserving surgery for DCIS have a prognosis similar to those with early-stage breast cancer, with a 15% to 20% risk of metastatic recurrence at 8 years.[159]

The Role of Tamoxifen and Aromatase Inhibitors for Ductal Carcinoma In Situ

The use of tamoxifen in the treatment of DCIS has been studied; however, results have been conflicting. Therefore, its role is not yet clearly defined. The role ofHer2Neu targeted treatment is presently being investigated in the NSABP B-43 trial. In this prospective randomized trial, patients with Her2Neu-positive DCIS are treated with postlumpectomy radiotherapy and randomized between Herceptin or observation. The NSABP B-24 trial[133,144] compared excision plus radiotherapy to excision, radiotherapy, and tamoxifen. Patients who received tamoxifen had a decreased incidence of breast cancer events (invasive or noninvasive ipsilateral or contralateral breast cancer) compared with patients who did not receive tamoxifen. With a median follow-up of 163 months, the addition of tamoxifen translated into a significant 32% reduction in invasive IBTR (9.0% vs. 6.6%, P = .025), a nonsignificant 16% reduction in DCIS-IBTR (7.6% vs. 6.7%, P = .33), and a 32% reduction in contralateral breast cancer (8.1% vs. 4.9%, P = .023); however, no survival benefit was found (Table 58.3). Positive tumor margins were significantly associated with breast recurrence. The 15-year cumulative incidence of invasive IBTR was reduced from 17.4% in patients with positive margins to 11.5% with the addition of tamoxifen. In those with tumor-free margins, tamoxifen did not improve in-breast disease control with a 7.4% and 7.5% incidence of invasive IBTR with and without tamoxifen, respectively.

In contrast to the findings of the NSABP B-24 trial, the UK/ANZ DCIS trial found that tamoxifen had no effect in reducing local recurrence rate when combined with whole-breast radiation therapy (Table 58.3). When used as single agent without radiation therapy after lumpectomy, tamoxifen had no effect on the incidence of invasive recurrence but did show a statistically significant reduction in the risk of DCIS recurrence (10.4% vs. 7.4%, P = .04).[148,149] As such, the role of tamoxifen for DCIS in the absence of whole-breast radiotherapy remains to be defined.

The role of tamoxifen versus anastrazole (an aromatase inhibitor) in the management of DCIS has been evaluated in the NSABP B-35 trial. Eligibility included postmenopausal women with DCIS, with or without associated LCIS with estrogen or progesterone positive receptors who underwent lumpectomy with clear margins and adjuvant whole breast radiation therapy. Patients were stratified by age <60 versus ≥60 years. A total of 3,104 women were enrolled with 3,084 women having a median follow up of 9 years. Breast cancer-free interval

TABLE 58.3 TAMOXIFEN VERSUS NO TAMOXIFEN: RANDOMIZED CLINICAL TRIALS FOR DUCTAL CARCINOMA *IN SITU*

Trial Group	Number of Patients	Follow-Up	Local Recurrence (Cumulative %) DCIS + Invasive Carcinoma		
			– Tam	+ Tam	P Value
NSABP B-24	1,798	13.6-y median	16.6	13.2	–
UK/ANZ	1,053	12.7-y median	17.0	13.2	.04
No radiotherapy Radiotherapy	523		2.6	2.4	.8

DCIS, ductal carcinoma *in situ*; NSABP, National Surgical Adjuvant Bowel and Breast Project; Tam, tamoxifen; UK/ANZ, United Kingdom, Australia, and New Zealand.

improved with the use of anastrazole, 7.8% versus 5.7%, with no significant difference in regard to the rates of in-breast recurrence, contralateral breast cancer, or distant disease. Improvement in disease-free survival was reported in women under the age of 60 years with the use of anastrazole compared to the tamoxifen arm, 89.8% versus 85.7%. Except for higher rates of thrombosis in the tamoxifen arm, no significant difference with regard to toxicity or treatment adherence was seen.[160] Because DCIS is a precursor to invasive breast cancer and shares many biologic features of invasive carcinoma, it is increasingly recognized as a target for preventive measures. In the largest trials of the prevention of primary breast cancer among women at high risk for breast cancer by virtue of age, family history, or prior benign breast disease, tamoxifen reduced the risk of DCIS by 50% to 70%.[40,161]

A Decision Tree for Ductal Carcinoma *In Situ*

The management of DCIS requires the coordinated, multidisciplinary interaction of radiologists, surgeons, pathologists, and oncologists. Patients are first assessed to determine if they are candidates for breast-conserving surgery. Women with multicentric DCIS, as defined by the presence of two or more tumors in separate quadrants of the breast, and those with extensive or diffuse DCIS or suspicious-appearing microcalcifications throughout the breast are candidates for mastectomy, as are women in whom negative margins or acceptable cosmesis cannot be achieved with the use of breast-conserving surgery. Some women may prefer mastectomy to breast conservation to minimize the chance of ipsilateral recurrence or for other reasons.

Patients deemed to be appropriate candidates for breast conservation require complete surgical excision of the affected area. The extent of DCIS in the breast and the existing margin determine the likelihood of identifying residual disease on re-excision. Nearly half of patients with margins <1 mm have residual DCIS on re-excision.[38]

Neither dissection of axillary lymph nodes nor mapping of sentinel lymph nodes is routinely warranted in patients with DCIS because of the very low incidence of axillary metastases.[162] Three to 13% of patients with DCIS, and a slightly greater percentage with DCIS and microinvasion, have isolated tumor cells in sentinel axillary lymph nodes.[163] The prognostic significance of these cells is not clear. Clinical experience suggests that patients have a much better outcome than would be predicted by such rates of nodal metastases, and in most instances these represent micrometastases of unclear metastatic potential. However, sentinel lymph node mapping may be used in selected patients with a higher likelihood of occult invasive cancer—those with extensive, high-grade DCIS or palpable masses—and those undergoing mastectomy as sentinel node mapping cannot be performed afterward if an invasive tumor is identified.[164]

After breast-conserving surgery, radiotherapy is administered using tangential fields to the whole breast with a standard dose of 45 to 50 Gy delivered in daily fractions of 180 to 200 cGy. On the basis of extrapolation from data on the treatment of invasive breast cancer,[165] a radiation boost to the tumor bed may be added to whole-breast treatment, particularly for women with close surgical margins, although the benefit of a boost in the management of DCIS is not established. There is no role for postmastectomy or nodal irradiation in the treatment of DCIS.

It is not yet possible to prospectively identify women who are at sufficiently low risk that radiotherapy may not be of some clinical advantage in preventing recurrences. After discussing the various options, patients may elect not to receive radiation treatment; however, they must understand and accept the increased risk of recurrence that this choice probably entails.[166]

In summary, despite considerable advances in our clinical knowledge base, the answer to the question "when should radiotherapy be used for DCIS?" remains complex and surrounded by considerable controversy. Two fundamental considerations must be emphasized:

1. A primary goal of breast-conserving therapy for DCIS is to achieve the best possible cosmetic outcome. Attempts to obtain wide surgical margins through deforming, large-volume breast excisions represent cosmetic failures and defeat the purpose of breast conservation.
2. Breast irradiation reduces the risk of subsequent invasive or noninvasive carcinoma in the treated breast and thus reduces the risk of the ultimate cosmetic failure—mastectomy.

According to prospectively randomized trials of breast-conserving therapy for DCIS, radiotherapy reduces subsequent breast recurrence in all patient groups irrespective of prognostic risk factors. That is not to say, however, that radiotherapy must be used for all patients with DCIS. In all cases, a realistic and balanced discussion of the relative risks and benefits of treatment options should be presented to the patient. Reasonable estimates of breast recurrence during the ensuing decade with or without radiotherapy are available based on level I evidence from prospective clinical trials.

Section III

REFERENCES

1. Page DL, Kidd TE, Dupont WD, et al. Lobular neoplasia of the breast: higher risk for subsequent invasive cancer predicted by more extensive disease. *Hum Pathol* 1991;22:1232–1239.
2. Tavassoli FA. Lobular neoplasia. In: Tavassoli FA. *Pathology of the breast*. 2nd ed. New York: Elsevier, 1999:373–400.
3. Frykberg ER, Bland KI. In situ breast carcinoma. *Adv Surg* 1993;26:29–72.
4. Schnitt SJ, Morrow M. Lobular carcinoma in situ: current concepts and controversies. *Semin Diagn Pathol* 1999;16:209–223.
5. Lagios MD, Westdahl PR, Marye RR, et al. Paget's disease of the nipple. *Cancer* 1984;54:545–551.
6. Ohtake T, Abe R, Kimijima I, et al. Intraductal extension of primary invasive breast carcinoma treated by breast—conservation surgery. *Cancer* 1995;76:32–45.
7. Sanders ME, Schuyler PA, Dupont WD, et al. The natural history of low-grade ductal carcinoma in situ of the breast in women treated by biopsy only revealed over 30 years of long-term follow-up. *Cancer* 2005;103:2481–2484.
8. Acs G, Lawton TJ, Rebbeck TR, et al. Differential expression of E-cadherin in lobular and ductal neoplasms of the breast and its biologic and diagnostic implications. *Am J Clin Pathol* 2001;115:85–98.
9. Albonico G, Querzoli P, Ferretti S, et al. Biological profile of in situ breast cancer investigated by immunohistochemical technique. *Cancer Detect Prev* 1998;22:313–318.
10. Bur ME, Zimarowski MJ, Schmitt SJ, et al. Estrogen receptor immunohistochemistry in carcinoma in situ of the breast. *Cancer* 1992;69:1174–1181.
11. Jacobs TW, Pliss N, Kouria G. Carcinomas in situ of the breast with indeterminate features. *Am J Surg Pathol* 2001;25:229–236.
12. Vos CB, Cleton-Jansen AM, Verx G, et al. E-cadherin inactivation in lobular carcinoma in situ of the breast: an early event in tumorigenesis. *Br J Cancer* 1997;76:1131–1133.
13. Andersen JA. Lobular carcinoma in situ of the breast—an approach to rational treatment. *Cancer* 1977;39:2597–2602.
14. Haagensen CD, Bodian C, Haagensen DE. *Lobular neoplasia (lobular carcinoma in situ). Breast carcinoma: risk and detection.* Philadelphia: WB Saunders, 1981:238–292.
15. Wheeler JE, Enterline HT, Roseman JM, et al. Lobular carcinoma in situ of the breast—long term follow-up. *Cancer* 1974;34:554–563.
16. Rosen PP, Kosloff C, Lieberman PH, et al. Lobular carcinoma in situ of the breast. Detailed analysis of 99 patients with average follow-up of 24 years. *Am J Surg Pathol* 1978;2:225–251.
17. Trentham-Dietz A, Newcomb PA, Storer BE, et al. Risk factors for carcinoma in situ of the breast. *Cancer Epidemiol Biomarkers Prev* 2000;9:697–703.
18. Georgian-Smith D, Lawton TJ. Calcifications of lobular carcinoma in situ of the breast: radiologic-pathologic correlation. *AJR Am J Roentgenol* 2001;176:1255–1259.
19. Sapino A, Frigerio A, Peterse JL, et al. Mammographically detected in situ lobular carcinomas of the breast. *Virchows Arch* 2000;436:421–430.
20. Sonnenfeld MR, Frenna TH, Weidner N, et al. Lobular carcinoma in situ: mammographic-pathologic correlation of results of needle-directed biopsy. *Radiology* 1991;181:363–367.
21. Cohen MA. Cancer upgrades at excisional biopsy after diagnosis of atypical lobular hyperplasia or lobular carcinoma in situ core-needle biopsy: some reasons why. *Radiology* 2004;231:617–621.
22. Foster MC, Helvie MA, Gregory NE, et al. Lobular carcinoma in situ or atypical lobular hyperplasia at core-needle biopsy: is excisional biopsy necessary? *Radiology* 2004;231:813–819.
23. Liberman L, Sama M, Susnik B, et al. Lobular carcinoma in situ at percutaneous breast biopsy: surgical biopsy findings. *AJR Am J Roentgenol* 1999;173:219–299.
24. Ottesen GL, Graversen HP, Blichert-Toft M, et al. Carcinoma in situ of the female breast. 10 year follow-up results of a prospective nationwide study. *Breast Cancer Res Treat* 2000;62:197–210.
25. Chuba PJ, Hamre MR, Yap J, et al. Bilateral risk for subsequent breast cancer after lobular carcinoma-in-situ: analysis of surveillance, epidemiology, and end results data. *J Clin Oncol* 2005;23:5534–5541.

26. Hwang ES, Nyante SJ, Chen YY, et al. Clonality of lobular carcinoma in situ and synchronous invasive lobular carcinoma. *Cancer* 2004;100:2562–2572.

27. Ben-David MA, Kleer CG, Paramagul C, et al. Is lobular carcinoma in situ as a component of breast carcinoma a risk factor for local failure after breast-conserving therapy? *Cancer* 2006;106:28–34.

28. Fisher ER, Land SR, Fisher B, et al. Pathologic findings from the National Surgical Adjuvant Breast and Bowel Project—twelve-year observations concerning lobular carcinoma in situ. *Cancer* 2004;100:238–244.

29. Friedlander LC, Roth SO, Gavenonis SC. Results of MR imaging screening for breast cancer in high-risk patients with lobular carcinoma in situ. *Radiology* 2011;261(2):421–427.

30. Port ER, Park A, Borgen PI, et al. Results of MRI screening for breast cancer in high risk patients with LCIS and atypical hyperplasia. *Ann Surg Oncol* 2007;14:1051–1057.

31. Sung JS, Malak SF, Bajaj P, et al. Screening breast MR imaging in women with a history of lobular carcinoma in situ. *Radiology* 2011;261(2):414–420.

32. Ehsani S, Strigel RM, Pettke E, et al. Screening magnetic resonance imaging recommendations and outcomes in patients at high risk for breast cancer. *Breast J* 2015;3:246–253.

33. Abner AL, Connolly JL, Recht A, et al. The relationship between the presence and extent of lobular carcinoma in situ and the risk of local recurrence for patients with infiltrating carcinoma of the breast treated with conservative surgery and radiation therapy. *Cancer* 2000;88:1072–1077.

34. Moran M, Haffty B. Lobular carcinoma in situ as a component of breast cancer: the long-term outcome in patients treated with breast-conservation therapy. *Int J Radiat Oncol Biol Phys* 1998;40:353–358.

35. Sasson AR, Fowble B, Hanlon AL, et al. Lobular carcinoma in situ increases the risk of local recurrence in selected patients with stages I and II breast carcinoma treated with conservative surgery and radiation. *Cancer* 2001;91:1862–1869.

36. Jolly S, Kestin LL, Goldstein NS, et al. The impact of lobular carcinoma in situ in association with invasive breast cancer on the rate of local recurrence in patients with early-stage breast cancer treated with breast-conserving therapy. *Int J Radiat Oncol Biol Phys* 2006;66:365–371.

37. Ciocca RM, Li T, Freedman GM, et al. Presence of lobular carcinoma in situ does not increase local recurrence in patients treated with breast-conserving therapy. *Ann Surg Oncol* 2008;15:2263–2271.

38. Neuschatz AC, DiPetrillo T, Steinhoff M, et al. The value of breast lumpectomy margin assessment as a predictor of residual tumor burden in ductal carcinoma in situ of the breast. *Cancer* 2002;94:1917–1924.

39. Foote FW, Stewart FW. Lobular carcinoma in situ—a rare form of mammary cancer. *Am J Pathol* 1941;17:491–495.

40. Fisher B, Costantino J, Wickerham DL, et al. Tamoxifen for prevention of breast cancer: report of the National Surgical Adjuvant Breast and Bowel Project P-1 study. *J Natl Cancer Inst* 1998;90:1371–1388.

41. Vogel VG, Costantino JP, Wickerham DL, et al. National Surgical Adjuvant Breast and Bowel Project update: prevention trials and endocrine therapy of ductal carcinoma in situ. *Clin Cancer Res* 2003;9:495S–501S.

42. Paget J. On the disease of the mammary areola preceding cancer of the mammary gland. *St Bartholomew Hosp Rep* 1874;10:87–89.

43. Lloyd J, Flanagan AM. Mammary and extramammary Paget's disease. *J Clin Pathol* 2000;53:742–749.

44. Desai DC, Brennan EJ, Carp NZ. Paget's disease of the male breast. *Am Surg* 1996;62:1068–1072.

45. Ernster VL, Barclay J, Kerlikowske K, et al. Incidence of and treatment for ductal carcinoma in situ of the breast. *JAMA* 1996;275:913–918.

46. Jamali FR, Ricci A, Deckers PJ. Paget's disease of the nipple-areola complex. *Surg Clin North Am* 1996;76:365–381.

47. Sakorafas GH, Blanchard K, Sarr MG, et al. Paget's disease of the breast. *Cancer Treat Rev* 2001;27:9–18.

48. Adams SJ, Kanthan R. Paget's disease of the male breast in the 21st century: a systematic review. *Breast* 2016;29:14–23.

49. Markpoulos CH, Gogas H, Sampalis F, et al. Bilateral Paget's disease of the breast. *Eur J Gynaecol Oncol* 1997;18:495–496.

50. Ward KA, Burton JL. Dermatological diseases of the breast in young women. *Clin Dermatol* 1997;15:45–52.

51. Inwang ER, Fentiman IS. Paget's disease of the nipple. *Br J Hosp Med* 1990;44:392–395.

52. Kohler S, Rouse RV, Smoller BR. The differential diagnosis of pagetoid cells in the epidermis. *Mod Pathol* 1998;11:79–92.

53. Chaudary MA, Millis RR, Lane B, et al. Paget's disease of the nipple: a ten year review including clinical, pathological, and immunohistochemical findings. *Breast Cancer Res Treat* 1986;8:139–146.

54. Ikeda DM, Helvie MA, Frank TS, et al. Paget disease of the nipple: radiologic-pathologic correlation. *Radiology* 1993;189:89–94.

55. Ashikari R, Park K, Huvos AG, et al. Paget's disease of the breast. *Cancer* 1970;26:680–685.

56. Kawase K, DiMaio DJ, Tucker SL, et al. Pagets disease of the breast: there is a role for breast conserving therapy. *Ann Surg Oncol* 2005;12:1–7.

57. Paone JF, Baker RR. Pathogenesis and treatment of Paget's disease of the breast. *Cancer* 1981;48:825–829.

58. Yim JH, Wick MR, Philpott GW, et al. Underlying pathology in mammary Paget's disease. *Ann Surg Oncol* 1997;4:287–292.

59. Dixon AR, Galea RR. Pathogenesis and treatment of Paget's disease of the breast. *Cancer* 1981;48:825–829.

60. Fischer B, Anderson S, Bryant J, et al. Twenty-year follow-up of a randomized trial comparing total mastectomy, lumpectomy, and lumpectomy plus irradiation for the treatment of invasive breast cancer. *N Engl J Med* 2002;347:1233–1241.

61. Fourquet A, Campana F, Vielh P, et al. Paget's disease of the nipple without detectable breast tumor: conservative management with radiation therapy. *Int J Radiat Oncol Biol Phys* 1987;13:1463–1465.

62. Polgar C, Orosz Z, Kovacs T, et al. Breast-conserving therapy for Paget disease of the nipple. *Cancer* 2002;94:1904–1905.

63. Veronesi U, Cascinelli N, Mariani L, et al. Twenty-year follow-up of randomized study comparing breast-conserving surgery with radical (Halstead) mastectomy for early breast cancer. *N Engl J Med* 2002;347:1227–1232.

64. Stockdale AD, Brierly JD, White WF, et al. Radiotherapy for Paget's disease of the nipple: a conservative alternative. *Lancet* 1989;2:664–666.

65. Bijker N, Rutgers EJT, Duchateau L, et al. Breast-conserving therapy for Paget disease of the nipple. *Cancer* 2001;91:472–477.

66. Marshall JK, Griffith KA, Haffty BG, et al. Conservative management of Paget disease of the breast with radiotherapy. *Cancer* 2003;97:2142–2149.

67. Pierce LJ, Haffty BG, Solin LJ, et al. The conservative management of Paget's disease of the breast with radiotherapy. *Cancer* 1997;80:1065–1072.

68. Catzavelos C. Part III. The pathobiology of ductal carcinoma in situ. *Curr Probl Cancer* 2000;24:125–140.

69. Consensus conference on the classification of ductal carcinoma in situ. The Consensus Conference Committee. *Cancer* 1997;80:1798–1802.

70. Page DL, Anderson TJ. *Diagnostic histopathology of the breast*. Edinburgh, Scotland: Churchill Livingstone, 1987.

71. Rosen PP. *Rosen's breast pathology*. Philadelphia: Lippincott Raven, 1997:237–245.

72. Silverstein MJ. Current management of noninvasive (in situ) breast cancer. *Adv Surg* 2000;34:17–41.

73. Lenhard RE. Cancer statistics, a measure of progress. *CA Cancer J Clin* 1996;46:3–7.

74. Simon MS, Lemanne D, Schwartz AG, et al. Recent trends in the incidence of in situ and invasive breast cancer in the Detroit Metropolitan area (1975–1988). *Cancer* 1993;71:769–774.

75. Simon MS, Schwartz AG, Martino S, et al. Trends in the diagnosis of in situ breast cancer in the Detroit Metropolitan area, 1973 to 1987. *Cancer* 1992;69:466–469.

76. Burstein HJ, Polyak K, Wong JS, et al. Ductal carcinoma in situ of the breast. *N Engl J Med* 2004;350:1430–1441.

77. American Cancer Society. *Cancer facts and figures*. Atlanta, GA: American Cancer Society, 2017.

78. Ernster VL, Ballard-Barbash R, Barlow WE, et al. Detection of ductal carcinoma in situ in women undergoing screening mammography. *J Natl Cancer Inst* 2002;94:1546–1554.

79. Tabar L, Gad A, Parsons WC, et al. Mammographic appearances of in situ carcinomas. In: Silverstein MJ, ed. *Ductal carcinoma in situ of the breast*. Baltimore, MD: Williams & Wilkins, 1997:413–420.

80. D'Orsi CJ. Imaging for the diagnosis and management of ductal carcinoma in situ. *J Natl Cancer Inst Monogr* 2010;2010(4):214–217.

81. Dinkel H-P, Gassel AM, Tschammler A. Is the appearance of microcalcifications on mammography useful in predicting histological grade of malignancy in ductal cancer in situ? *Br J Radiol* 2000;73:938–944.

82. Holland R, Hendriks J, Verbeek A, et al. Extent, distribution and mammographic/histological correlations of breast ductal carcinoma in situ. *Lancet* 1990;335:519–522.

83. Recht A, Rutgers EJ, Fentiman IS, et al. The fourth EORTC DCIS consensus meeting (Chateau Marguette, Heemskerk, The Netherlands 23–24 January 1998)—conference report. *Eur J Cancer* 1998;34:1664–1669.

84. Wright B, Shumak R. Part II. Medical imaging of ductal carcinoma in situ. *Curr Probl Cancer* 2000;24:112–124.

85. Ohtake T, Kimijima I, Fukushima T, et al. Computer-assisted complete three-dimensional reconstruction of the mammary ductal/lobular systems. *Cancer* 2001;91:2263–2272.

86. Satake H, Shimamoto K, Sawaki A, et al. Role of ultrasonography in the detection of intraductal spread of breast cancer: correlation with pathologic findings, mammography and MR imaging. *Eur Radiol* 2000;10:1726–1732.

87. Lehman CD. Magnetic resonance imaging in the evaluation of ductal carcinoma in situ. *J Natl Cancer Inst Monogr* 2010;(4):214–217.

88. Berg WA, Gutierrez L, Nessairer MS, et al. Diagnositic accuracy of mammography, US, and MR imaging in preoperative assessment of breast cancer. *Radiology* 2004;133:830–849.

89. Patchefsky AS, Schwartz GF, Finkelstein SD, et al. Heterogeneity of intraductal carcinoma of the breast. *Cancer* 1989;63:731–741.

90. Fechner RE. Epithelial alterations in the extralobular ducts of breasts with lobular carcinoma. *Arch Pathol* 1972;93:164–171.

91. Azzopardi JG. *Problems in breast pathology*. Philadelphia: WB Saunders, 1983.

92. Lagios MD. Ductal carcinoma in situ: controversies in diagnosis, biology, and treatment. *Breast J* 1995;1:68–78.

93. Recht A, van Dongen JA, Fentimen IS, et al. Third meeting of the DCIS Working Party of the EORTC (Fondazione Cini, Isola s. Giorgio, Venezia, 28 February 1994)—conference report. *Eur J Cancer* 1994;30A:1895–1901.

94. Going JJ, Moffat DF. Escaping from Flatland: clinical and biological aspects of human mammary duct anatomy in three dimensions. *J Pathol* 2004;203:538–544.

95. Faverly DRG, Burgers L, Bult P, et al. Three dimensional imaging of mammary ductal carcinoma in situ; clinical implications. *Semin Diagn Pathol* 1994;11:193–198.

96. Allred DC, Mohsin SK, Fuqua SAW. Histological and biological evolution of human premalignant breast disease. *Endocr Relat Cancer* 2001;8:47–61.

97. Radford DM, Phillips NHJ, Fair KL, et al. Allelic loss and the progression of breast cancer. *Cancer Res* 1995;55:5180–5183.

98. Stratton MR, Collins N, Lakhani SR, et al. Loss of heterozygosity in ductal carcinoma in situ of the breast. *J Pathol* 1995;175:195–201.

99. Allred DC. Ductal carcinoma in situ: terminology, classification and natural history. *J Natl Cancer Inst Monogr* 2010;2010(41):134–138.

100. Hannemann J, Velds A, Halfwerk JB, et al. Classification of ductal carcinoma in situ by gene expression profiling. *Breast Cancer Res* 2006;8(5):R61.

101. Kuerer HM, Albarracin CT, Yang WT, et al. Ductal carcinoma in situ: state of the science and roadmap to advance the field. *J Clin Oncol* 2009;27:279–288.

102. Ma XJ, Salunga R, Tuggle JT, et al. Gene expression profiles of human breast cancer progression. *Proc Natl Acad Sci U S A* 2003;100(10):5974–5979.

103. Porter D, Lahti-Domenici J, Keshaviah A, et al. Molecular markers in ductal carcinoma in situ of the breast. *Mol Cancer Res* 2003;1(5):362–375.
104. Allred DC, Wu Y, Mao S, et al. Ductal carcinoma in situ and the emergence of diversity during breast cancer evolution. *Clin Cancer Res* 2008;14:370–378.
105. O'Connell P, Pekkel V, Fuqua SA, et al. Analysis of loss of heterozygosity in 399 premalignant breast lesions at 15 genetic loci. *J Natl Cancer Inst* 1998;90:697–703.
106. Aubele MM, Cummings MC, Mattis AE, et al. Accumulation of chromosomal imbalances from intraductal proliferative lesions to adjacent in situ and invasive ductal breast cancer. *Diagn Mol Pathol* 2000;9:14–19.
107. Farabegoli F, Champeme MH, Bieche I, et al. Genetic pathways in the evolution of breast ductal carcinoma in situ. *J Pathol* 2002;196:280–286.
108. Damiani S, Ludvikova M, Tomasic G, et al. Myoepithelial cells and basal lamina in poorly differentiated in situ duct carcinoma of the breast: an immunocytochemical study. *Virchows Arch* 1999;434:227–234.
109. Guidi AJ, Fischer L, Harris JR, et al. Microvessel density and distribution of ductal carcinoma in situ of the breast. *J Natl Cancer Inst* 1994;86:614–619.
110. Guidi AJ, Schnitt SJ, Fischer L, et al. Vascular permeability factor (vascular endothelial growth factor) expression and angiogenesis in patients with ductal carcinoma in situ of the breast. *Cancer* 1997;80:1945–1953.
111. Allred DC, Wu Y, Tsimelzon A, et al. The progression of DCIS to IBC: a cDNA expression microarray study [abstract]. *Breast Cancer Res Treat* 2002;76(Suppl 1):S81.
112. Buerger H, Otterbach F, Simon R, et al. Different genetic pathways in the evolution of invasive breast cancer are associated with distinct morphological subtypes. *J Pathol* 1999;189:521–526.
113. Gupta SK, Douglas-Jones AG, Fenn N, et al. The clinical behavior of breast carcinoma is probably determined at the preinvasive stage (ductal carcinoma in situ). *Cancer* 1997;80:1740–1745.
114. Lampejo OT, Barnes DM, Smith P, et al. Evaluation of infiltrating ductal carcinomas with a DCIS component: correlation of the histologic type of the in situ component with grade of the infiltrating component. *Semin Diagn Pathol* 1994;11:215–222.
115. Warnberg F, Nordgren H, Bergkvist L, et al. Tumour markers in breast carcinoma correlate with grade rather than with invasiveness. *Br J Cancer* 2001;85:869–874.
116. Singletary SE, Allred C, Ashley P, et al. Revision of the American Joint Committee on Cancer staging system for breast cancer. *J Clin Oncol* 2002;20:3628–3636.
117. Lagios MD, Margolin FR, Westdahl PR, et al. Mammographically detected duct carcinoma in situ: frequency of local recurrence following tylectomy and prognostic effect of nuclear grade on local recurrence. *Cancer* 1989;63:618–624.
118. Silver SA, Tavassoli FA. Mammary ductal carcinoma in situ with microinvasion. *Cancer* 1998;82:2382–2390.
119. Alpers C, Wellings S. The prevalence of carcinoma in situ in normal and cancer associated breast. *Hum Pathol* 1985;16:796.
120. Welch HG, Black WC. Using autopsy series to estimate the disease "reservoir" for ductal carcinoma in situ of the breast: how much more breast cancer can we find? *Ann Intern Med* 1997;11:1023–1028.
121. Betsill WL, Rosen PP, Lieberman PH, et al. Intraductal carcinoma: long-term follow-up after treatment by biopsy alone. *JAMA* 1978;239:1863–1867.
122. Collins LC, Tamimi RM, Baer HJ, et al. Outcome of patients with ductal carcinoma in situ untreated after diagnostic biopsy: results from the Nurses' Health Study. *Cancer* 2005;103:1778–1784.
123. Millis RR, Thynne GSJ. In situ intraduct carcinoma of the breast: a long-term follow-up study. *Br J Surg* 1975;62:957–962.
124. Habel LA, Moe RE, Daling JR, et al. Risk of contralateral breast cancer among women with carcinoma in situ of the breast. *Ann Surg* 1997;225:69–75.
125. Claus EB, Petruzella S, Matloff E, et al. Prevalence of BRCA1 and BRCA2 mutations in women diagnosed with ductal carcinoma in situ. *JAMA* 2005;293:553–554.
126. Bijker N, Peterse JL, Duchateau L, et al. Risk factors for recurrence and metastasis after breast-conserving therapy for ductal carcinoma-in-situ: analysis of European Organization for Research and Treatment of Cancer Trial 10853. *J Clin Oncol* 2001;19:2263–2271.
127. Ottesen GL, Graversen HP, Blichert-Toft M, et al. Ductal carcinoma in situ of the female breast: short-term results of a prospective nationwide study—the Danish Breast Cancer Cooperative Group. *Am J Surg Pathol* 1992;16:1183–1196.
128. Sneige N, McNeese MD, Atkinson EN, et al. Ductal carcinoma in situ treated with lumpectomy and irradiation: histopathological analysis of 49 specimens with emphasis on risk factors and long term results. *Hum Pathol* 1995;26:642–649.
129. Silverstein MJ, Lagios MD, Craig PH, et al. A prognostic index for ductal carcinoma in situ of the breast. *Cancer* 1996;77:2267–2274.
130. Solin LJ, Yeh IT, Kurtz J, et al. Ductal carcinoma in situ (intraductal carcinoma) of the breast treated with breast-conserving surgery and definitive irradiation: correlation of pathologic parameters with outcome of treatment. *Cancer* 1993;71:2532–2542.
131. Silverstein MJ, Lagios MD, Groshen S, et al. The influence of margin width on local control of ductal carcinoma in situ of the breast. *N Engl J Med* 1999;340:1455–1461.
132. Solin LJ, Fourquet A, Vicini FA, et al. Long-term outcome after breast-conservation treatment with radiation for mammographically detected ductal carcinoma in situ of the breast. *Cancer* 2005;103:1137–1146.
133. Fisher B, Dignam J, Wolmark N, et al. Tamoxifen in treatment of intraductal breast cancer: National Surgical Adjuvant Breast and Bowel Project B-24 randomised controlled trial. *Lancet* 1999;353:1993–2000.
134. Vicini FA, Recht A. Age at diagnosis and outcome for women with ductal carcinoma-in-situ of the breast: a critical review of the literature. *J Clin Oncol* 2002;20:2736–2744.
135. Morrow M, Van Zee KJ, Solin LJ, et al. Society of surgical oncology-american society for radiation oncology-american society of clinical oncology consensus guideline on margins for breast-conserving surgery with whole-breast irradiation in ductal carcinoma in situ. *Pract Radiat Oncol* 2016;6:287–95.
136. Silverstein MJ. Van Nuys experience by treatment. In: Silverstein MJ, Lagios MD, Poller DN, et al, eds. *Ductal carcinoma in situ of the breast*. Philadelphia: Williams & Wilkins, 1997:443–447.
137. Fisher ER, Leeming R, Anderson S, et al. Conservative management of intraductal carcinoma (DCIS) of the breast. *J Surg Oncol* 1991;47:139–147.
138. Ernster VL, Barclay J, Kerlikowske K, et al. Mortality among women with ductal carcinoma in situ of the breast in the population-based Surveillance, Epidemiology and End Results program. *Arch Intern Med* 2000;160:953–958.
139. Carlson G, Page A, Johnson E, et al. Local recurrence of ductal carcinoma in situ after skin-sparing mastectomy. *J Am Coll Surg* 2007;204:1074–1078.
140. Chan LW, Rabban JR, Hwang ES, et al. Is radiation indicated in patients with ductal carcinoma in situ and close or positive mastectomy margins. *Int J Radiat Oncol Biol Phys* 2011;80:25–30.
141. Klein J, Kong I, Paszat L, et al. Close or positive resection margins are not associated with an increase risk of chest wall recurrence in women with DCIS treated by mastectomy: a population-based analysis. *Springerplus* 2015;4:335.
142. Fisher B, Dignam J, Wolmark N, et al. Lumpectomy and radiation therapy for the treatment of intraductal breast cancer: findings from National Surgical Adjuvant Breast and Bowel Project B-17. *J Clin Oncol* 1998;16:441–452.
143. Fisher B, Land S, Mamounas E, et al. Prevention of invasive breast cancer in women with ductal carcinoma in situ: an update of the National Surgical Adjuvant Breast and Bowel Project experience. *Semin Oncol* 2001;28:400–418.
144. Wapnir IL, Dignam JJ, Fisher B, et al. Long-term outcomes of invasive ipsilateral breast tumor recurrences after lumpectomy in NSABP B-17 and B-24 randomized clinical trials for DCIS. *J Natl Cancer Inst* 2011;103:478–488.
145. Bijker N, Meijnen PH, Bogaerts J, et al. Radiotherapy in breast-conserving treatment for ductal carcinoma in situ (DCIS): ten-year results of European organization for research and treatment of cancer (EORTC) randomized trial 10853. *J Clin Oncol* 2006;24:3381–3387.
146. Donker M, Litiere GW, Julien J-P, et al. Breast-conserving treatment with or without radiotherapy in ductal carcinoma in situ: 15-year recurrence rates and outcomes after a recurrence, from the EORTC 10853 randomized phase III trial. *J Clin Oncol* 2013;31:4054–4059.
147. Julien JP, Bijker N, Fentiman IS, et al. Radiotherapy in breast-conserving treatment for ductal carcinoma in situ: first results of the EORTC randomised phase III trial 10853. EORTC Breast Cancer Cooperative Group and EORTC Radiotherapy Group. *Lancet* 2000;355:528–533.
148. Cusck J, Sestak I, Pinder SE, et al. Effect of tamoxifen and radiotherapy in women with locally excised ductal carcinoma in situ: long-term resulrs from the UK/ANZ DCIS trial. *Lancet Oncol* 2011;12:21–29
149. Houghton J, George WD, Cuzick J, et al. Radiotherapy and tamoxifen in women with completely excised ductal carcinoma in situ of the breast in the UK, Australia, and New Zealand: randomized controlled trial. *Lancet* 2003;362:95–102.
150. Warnberg F, Garmo H, Emdin S, et al. Effect of radiotherapy after breas-conserving surgery for ductal carcinoma in situ: 20 years follow-up in the randomized SweDCIS trial. *J Clin Oncol* 2014;32:3613–3618.
151. Early Breast Cancer Trialists' Collaborative Group, Correa C, McGale P, Taylor C, et al. Overview of the randomized trials of radiotherapy in dictal carcinoma in situ of the breast. *J Natl Cancer Inst Monogr* 2010;(41):162–167.
152. De Mascarel I, Bonichon F, MacGrogan G, et al. Application of the Van Nuys Prognostic Index in a retrospective series of 367 ductal carcinomas in situ of the breast examined by serial macroscopic sectioning: practical considerations. *Breast Cancer Res Treat* 2000;61:151–159.
153. Wong JS, Kaelin CM, Troyan SL, et al. Prospective study of wide excision alone for ductal carcinoma in situ of the breast. *J Clin Oncol* 2006;24:1031–1036.
154. McCormick B, Winter K, Hudis C, et al. RTOG 904: a prospective randomized trial for good-risk ductal carcinoma in situ comparing radiotherapy with observation. *J Clin Oncol* 2015;33:709–715.
155. Wong JS, ChenY-H, Gadd MA, et al. Eight-year update of a prospective study of wide excision alone for a small low- or intermediate-grade ductal carcinoma in situ. *Breast Cancer Res Treat* 2014;143:343–350.
156. Hughes LL, Wang M, Page DL, et al. Local excision alone without irradiation for ductal carcinoma in situ of the breast: a trial of the Eastern Cooperative Oncology Group. *J Clin Oncol* 2009;27:5319–5324.
157. Solin LJ, Gray R, Hughes LL, et al. Surgical excision without radiation for ductal carcinoma in situ of the breast: 12-year results from the ECOG-ACRIN E5194 study. *J Clin Oncol* 2015;33:3938–3944.
158. Liberman L, Van Zee KJ, Dershaw DD, et al. Mammographic features of local recurrence in women who have undergone breast-conserving therapy for ductal carcinoma in situ. *AJR Am J Roentgenol* 1997;168:489–493.
159. Solin LJ, Fourquet A, Vicini FA, et al. Salvage treatment for local recurrence after breast-conserving surgery and radiation as initial treatment for mammographically detected ductal carcinoma in situ of the breast. *Cancer* 2001;91:1090–1097.
160. Margolese RG, Cecchini RS, Julian TB, et al. Anastrazole versus tamoxifen in postmenopausal women with ductal carcinoma in situ undergoing lumpectomy plus radiotherapy (NSABP B-35): a randomized, double-blind, phase 3 clinical trial. *Lancet* 2016;387:849–856.
161. Cuzick J, Forbes J, Edwards R, et al. First results from the International Breast Cancer Intervention Study (IBIS-I): a randomised prevention trial. *Lancet* 2002;360:817–824.
162. Silverstein MJ, Rosser RJ, Gierson ED, et al. Axillary lymph node dissection for intraductal breast carcinoma—is it indicated? *Cancer* 1987;59:1819–1824.
163. Intra M, Veronesi P, Mazzarol G, et al. Axillary sentinel lymph node biopsy in patients with pure ductal carcinoma in situ of the breast. *Arch Surg* 2003;138:309–313.
164. McMasters KM, Chao C, Wong SL, et al. Sentinel lymph node biopsy in patients with ductal carcinoma in situ: a proposal. *Cancer* 2002;95:15–20.
165. Bartelink H, Horiot J-C, Poortmans P, et al. Recurrence rates after treatment of breast cancer with standard radiotherapy with or without additional radiation. *N Engl J Med* 2001;345:1378–1387.
166. Schwartz GF, Solin LJ, Olivotto IA, et al. Consensus conference on the treatment of in situ ductal carcinoma of the breast, April 22–25, 1999. *Cancer* 2000;88:946–954.

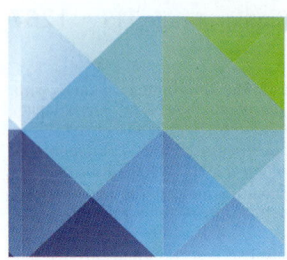

CHAPTER 59

Breast Cancer: Early Stage

Sharad Goyal, Thomas Buchholz, and Bruce G. Haffty

Radiation therapy (RT) plays an essential and critical role in the management of breast cancer. In a general radiation oncology practice, breast cancer typically constitutes approximately 25% of total patient caseload. This chapter will provide an overview of general concepts in breast cancer and will then focus on management of early-stage invasive disease. The management of early-stage disease by breast conservation is a major focus of this chapter. Postmastectomy radiation, as well as advanced invasive disease and locoregional recurrence, will be covered in the advanced disease chapter that follows. Management of ductal carcinoma *in situ* (DCIS) and lobular carcinoma *in situ* (LCIS) are the focus of the previous chapter.

ANATOMY

The female breast lies on the anterior chest wall superficial to the pectoralis major muscle.[1] The breast can extend from the midline to near the midaxillary line and cranial caudally from the second anterior rib to the sixth anterior rib. The upper outer quadrant of the breast extends into the region of the low axilla and is frequently referred to as the axillary tail of Spence. This anatomical feature results in the upper outer quadrant of the breast containing a greater percentage of total breast tissue compared with the other quadrants, and, therefore, a greater percentage of breast cancers occur in this anatomical location.

The breast is made up of the mammary gland, fat, blood vessels, nerves, and lymphatics[2] (Fig. 59.1). The surface of the breast has deep attachments of fibrous septa, called Cooper ligaments, which run between the superficial fascia (attached to the skin) and the deep fascia (covering the pectoralis major and other muscles of the chest wall). Skin dimpling may be caused by tumors affecting these supporting structures. It is important to realize, from a staging perspective, that the chest wall includes the ribs, intercostal muscles, and the serratus anterior muscle, but not the pectoral muscles.

The breast parenchyma is composed of lobules and ducts. The function of the lobules is to produce milk, and the function of the ducts is to transport lactation products to the nipple. The peripheral ducts converge into major lactiferous ducts, which then communicate with the nipple–areola complex. Most breast cancers develop at the interface between the ductal system and the lobules, a region called the terminal ductal lobular unit.

The breast parenchyma is intermixed with connective tissue, which has a rich vascular and lymphatic network.

FIGURE 59.1. Anatomy of the breast and lymphatic drainage. (From Osborne MP. Breast development and anatomy. In: Harris JR, Hellman S, Henderson IC, et al., eds. *Breast diseases*. Philadelphia, PA: JB Lippincott, 1987:1–14. With permission.)

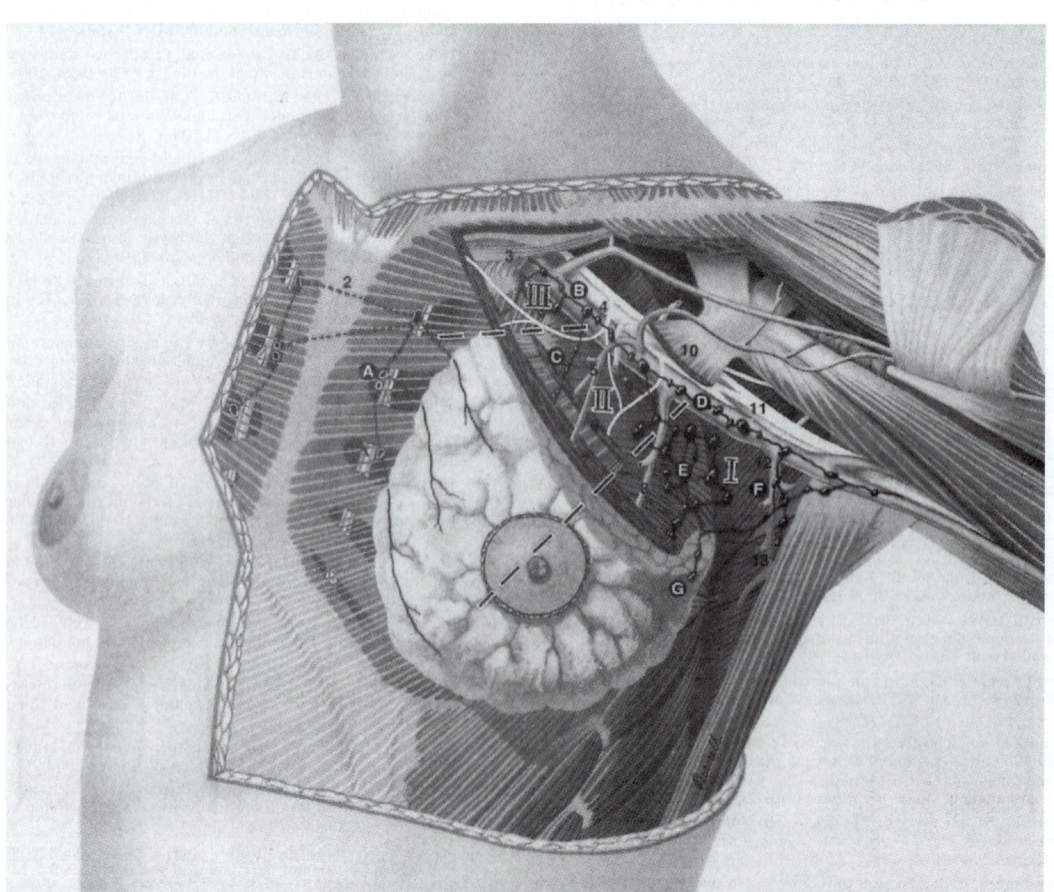

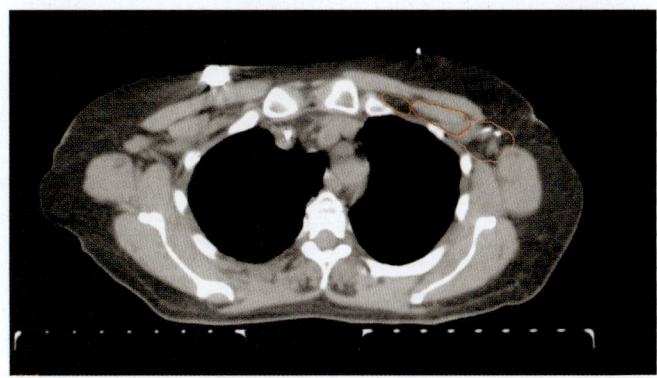

FIGURE 59.2. Location of the three levels of axillary lymph nodes (Level 1 – *pink*; Level 2 – *red*; Level 3 – *orange*).

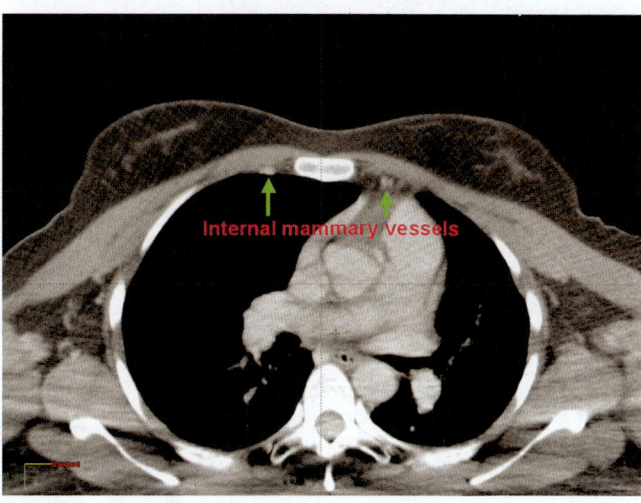

FIGURE 59.3. Treatment planning CT scan of the chest demonstrating the location of the internal mammary vessels, which are typically located approximately 3 to 4 cm lateral to midline and approximately 3 cm deep to the surface. The IMNs are in close proximity to the vessels, with the most critical nodes being located in the first three intercostal spaces.

Mammary gland lymphatics begin in the interlobular or prelobular spaces, follow the ducts, and end in the subareolar network of lymphatics of the skin. The predominant lymphatic drainage of the breast is to axillary lymph nodes, which is commonly described in three levels, based on the relation of the lymph node regions to the pectoralis minor muscle (Fig. 59.2). The level I axilla is caudal and lateral to the muscle, level II is beneath the muscle, and level III (also known as the infraclavicular region) is cranial and medial to the muscle. A standard axillary lymph node dissection (ALND) resects the tissue and lymph nodes within levels I and II. It is very unusual to have involvement of level III of the axilla without disease in level I or II. The axillary lymph nodes continue underneath the clavicle to become the supraclavicular lymph nodes, which can be involved in locally advanced breast cancers.

Lymphatics can also drain directly into the internal mammary lymph node chain (IMC), which are intrathoracic structures located in the parasternal space. Although these nodes are not usually visualized on computed tomography (CT), the anatomical region of the IMC can be determined by the internal mammary artery and vein, which are easily visualized by CT (Fig. 59.3) and usually lie 3 to 4 cm lateral to midline. When breast cancer involves the IMC, the majority of patients will have disease that is limited to lymph nodes in the first three interspaces. Regardless of location in the breast, the axilla is the most common site of lymphatic involvement. However, breast cancers that develop in the medial, central, or lower breast more commonly drain to the IMC (in addition to the axilla) than do those occurring in the lateral and upper quadrants.

The use of lymphoscintigraphy, by injecting technetium-99 radiocolloid into the peritumoral region followed by scintillation scanning, is used now for sentinel lymph node imaging. This technique has helped to delineate primary lymphatic drainage patterns of breast cancer. The distribution of axillary and internal mammary drainage is summarized in Figure 59.4.[3] Even in inner quadrant lesions, axillary drainage is more common than internal mammary drainage. However, internal mammary drainage was present in over 50% of lower inner quadrant lesions.

EPIDEMIOLOGY

Breast cancer is the most frequently diagnosed cancer in women, and it is estimated that there will be 252,710 new cases of invasive breast cancer and 63,410 new cases of *in situ* breast cancers among women in the United States in 2017[4]. Primarily because of increased utilization of screening mammography, breast cancer incidence rates increased rapidly in the 1980s, and breast cancer alone is expected to account for 30% of all new cancer diagnoses in women. It is estimated that 40,610 breast cancer deaths will occur in 2017, with breast cancer ranking second among cancer deaths in women, after lung cancer. In contrast to the significant number of breast cancer cases in women, it is expected that 2,470 cases of breast cancer will be diagnosed in men in 2017, with approximately 460 breast cancer deaths in men.

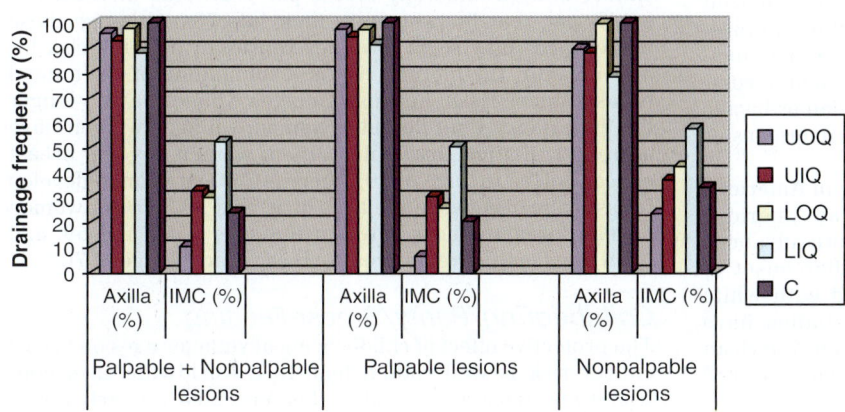

FIGURE 59.4. Distribution of lymphatic drainage of the breast to axillary and internal mammary chains according to the location within the breast. (Data extracted from study of 700 patients undergoing sentinel lymph node mapping by Estourgie SH, Nieweg OE, Olmos RA, et al. Lymphatic drainage patterns from the breast. *Ann Surg* 2004;239[2]:232–237.)

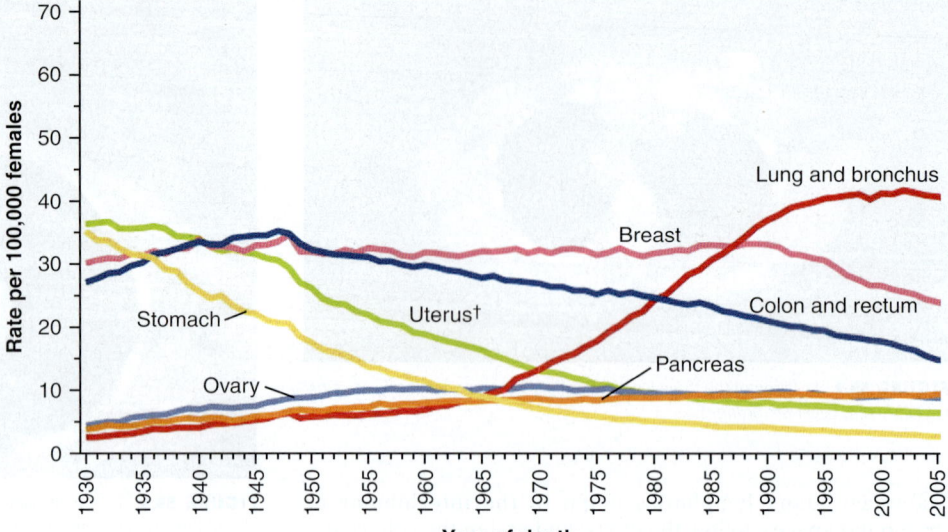

FIGURE 59.5. Age-adjusted cancer death rates for women. Statistics show a recent decrease in breast cancer mortality due to an increase in screening-detected malignancies and improvements in treatment. (From Jemal A, Siegel R, Xu J, et al. Cancer statistics, 2010. *CA Cancer J Clin* 2010;60[5]:277–300. Copyright © 2010 American Cancer Society, Inc. Reprinted by permission of John Wiley & Sons, Inc.)

Because of a combination of early detection, increased awareness, and improvements in therapy, death rates from breast cancer actually declined 38% from 1989 to 2014 for female breast cancer. The decrease in breast cancer mortality is demonstrated in Figure 59.5.

There is considerable geographic, ethnic, and racial variability in breast cancer incidence. Ethnicity and national origin rank highly as predictors of risk for breast cancer, with up to a 10-fold variation throughout the world.[5] Compared with other well-established risk factors such as age of menarche and menopause, age at first childbirth, and family history, geographic and ethnic variability is quite significant. It is likely that a complex interaction of multiple factors, including genetic, environmental, and socioeconomic, contribute to the wide variability in age-adjusted incidence across populations.

The potential contribution of environmental factors and lifestyle is clearly demonstrated in the increasing incidence of breast cancers among Japanese American women and in trends of increasing incidence of breast cancer in Japan with recent changes in lifestyle. It is well recognized that the relatively low incidence of breast cancer in Asian immigrants to the United States has gradually increased as these immigrants have adapted to Western lifestyles.[6] In Japan, incidence rates have more than doubled from 1960 to 1990. This is likely a result of adaptation of Western lifestyles, including fewer children, later marriage, increasing rates of obesity, and possibly dietary influences.[7]

In the United States, the incidence of breast cancer in white women is higher than in all other populations. Recent data from the National Cancer Institute's Surveillance, Epidemiology, and End Results (SEER) program report incidence rates of 128.3 cases per 100,000 white women, compared with 125.1 in African American, 89.3 in Asian or Pacific Islanders, 91.7 in Hispanics, and 98.1 in Native Americans or Alaskan Natives[4].

Although incidence is slightly lower in African American women, the age of onset is younger and African American women are more likely to be diagnosed at a more advanced stage. Several studies have reported an earlier onset of breast cancer in African American, compared with white women, by approximately 10 years; other studies have indicated that after correcting for stage, African American women have more aggressive biology and a poorer overall prognosis.[8,9]

Risk Factors

Table 59.1 summarizes the major risk factors associated with development of breast cancer. With the exception of female gender, increasing age is the most consistent and significant risk factor, with most populations demonstrating increasing incidence rates with age. Other risk factors include personal history and family history of breast cancer, nulliparity or late age at first childbirth, early menarche and late menopause, prior breast biopsy with hyperplasia or atypical hyperplasia, high breast tissue density, radiation exposure at a young age, alcohol consumption, and use of postmenopausal hormone therapy. Some of the national origin or ethnicity variability discussed above may be explained in part by differences in established risk factors, such as age of menarche, parity, and age at first childbirth. However, these factors explain only part of the variability observed in national origin, indicating underlying genetic, environmental, and dietary factors are likely to contribute to the differences in the worldwide incidence of breast cancer.[10] Breast-feeding, physical activity, and maintaining a healthy body weight have been demonstrated in various studies to be associated with a lower risk of breast cancer.[10]

Age

The risk of breast cancer increases exponentially up to the age of menopause, at which time the rate of increase in the risk slows significantly. After the age of 80, the incidence of breast cancer begins to show a slight decline. For women in their late 30s, the annual increase in risk of developing breast cancer is approximately 0.07% per year. This increases to 0.44% per year for women in their late 70s. Although these percentages may seem low, they represent only the risk for a given year; the lifetime risk is a summation of the annual breast cancer risks. Because younger women have a longer life expectancy than do older women, younger women have a greater lifetime risk. Only 1.9% of women develop breast cancer before the age of 50, whereas 2.3% of women develop breast cancer between the ages of 50 and 59, 3.5% of women develop breast cancer between the ages of 60 and 69, and 6.8% of women develop breast cancer over the age of 70.[11]

Childbearing/Parity/Breast-Feeding

The protective effect of childbearing at younger ages on breast cancer risk is well established. In a worldwide case–control study, MacMahon et al.[5,12] demonstrated a nearly linear

TABLE 59.1 RISK FACTORS FOR BREAST CANCER IN WOMEN

Risk Factors	Category at Risk	Comparison Category
Established Risk Factors		
Older age	Older than 50	Younger than 50
Country of residence	North America or Northern Europe	Asia or Africa
Germline mutation	With *BRCA1* or *BRCA2* mutations	Without *BRCA1* or *BRCA2* mutations
Personal history of breast cancer	With history of invasive breast carcinoma	No history of invasive breast carcinoma
High radiation exposure to chest area	With high radiation exposure to chest	Without radiation exposure
Atypical hyperplasia in breast biopsy	With atypical hyperplasia	Without hyperplasia
Cytologic findings (fine needle aspiration; nipple aspiration fluid)	Proliferation with atypia	No abnormality detected
Family history of breast cancer	With one or more close relatives with breast cancer	No close relatives with breast cancer
Early menarche	Menarche before age 12	Menarche after age 14
Late menopause	Menopause after age 55	Menopause before age 55
Older age at 1st full-term birth	Older than 30 years when first child was born	Younger than 20 years when first child was born
Not having children	Without children	With one or more children
Using menopausal hormone therapy	With hormone treatment after menopause	Without hormone treatment after menopause
Obesity after menopause	Obese after menopause	Not obese after menopause
Other Reported Risk Factors		
Using birth control pills	Current use	None
Tall height	Taller than 5 ft 9 inches	Shorter than 5 ft 3 inches
Regular alcohol consumption	Regularly consume alcoholic beverages	No alcoholic beverages consumption
Breast-feeding	None	Longer than 1 year
Postmenopausal body mass index (BMI)	Higher BMI	Lower BMI
Jewish heritage	Yes	No
Possible Risk		
High-density breasts on mammograms	With high-density mammograms	With low-density mammograms
High socioeconomic position	Have high socioeconomic position	Have low socioeconomic position
Physical activity	Lower	>3 h/wk
Dietary factors	High fat, low fiber	Low fat, high fiber

relation between relative risk (RR) of breast cancer and age at first birth, with women aged 20 to 25 having nearly a 50% reduction in the RR of breast cancer compared with nulliparous women. Interestingly, for women whose first childbirth occurred over age 35, the risk appears greater than that for nulliparous women. Data on the effect of breast-feeding are not as strong as the data on age at first childbirth, but they do suggest a protective effect. The Oxford Collaborative Group conducted an analysis of 47 studies evaluating breast-feeding and breast cancer risk and reported a decrease in RR of breast cancer by 4.3% for each 12 months of breast-feeding.[13]

Ovarian Function

The relation between ovarian function and breast cancer risk has long been recognized, with long menstrual history (early menarche and late menopause) contributing significantly to breast cancer risk. In experimental models and observational studies, removal of the ovaries reduces the risk of breast cancer.[5] Women with surgically induced menopause have been shown to have significantly reduced risks of breast cancer compared with women whose menopause occurred naturally. In comparison with women whose menopause occurs between the ages of 45 and 54 (RR = 1), women with early menopause before age 45 have a RR of breast cancer of 0.73 and women with late menopause at age 55 or older have a RR of 1.48. The data on early onset of menses and its association with breast cancer risk are also well established.[5]

Exogenous Hormone

The risk of breast cancer associated with hormonal therapy has been controversial. A collaborative meta-analysis from 51 epidemiologic studies of over 150,000 women did show an increased RR of 1.35 for current or recent users of hormonal replacement therapy.[14] The authors reported that postmenopausal hormone replacement therapy increased the annual RR of developing breast cancer by 2.3% for each year of hormonal therapy. A randomized trial of postmenopausal

hormone therapy from the Women's Health Initiative Study comparing estrogen and progestin with placebo was closed prematurely, demonstrating a 24% increase in breast cancer, coronary heart disease, stroke, and pulmonary emboli. This study of 46,000 women reported that the combined use of estrogen and progesterone increased the RR of breast cancer 8% compared with the risk in nonusers, whereas the use of estrogen alone increased the RR only 1%.[15] After publication of this study, a dramatic decrease of almost 7% between 2002 and 2003 was primarily attributed to the reduction in the use of hormone replacement therapy. Since then, breast cancer incidence rates have been generally stable.[16] Other studies have also demonstrated increased risks of breast cancer with long-term use of hormonal replacement therapy.[17] However, short-term use of hormonal replacement, particularly in women with severe menopausal symptoms, has not been consistently associated with breast cancer risk. For women who have undergone hysterectomy, it seems that hormone replacement therapy with estrogen alone rather than estrogen and progesterone has a minimal effect on breast cancer risk. For women who have not undergone hysterectomy and who elect to be treated with hormone replacement therapy, combined estrogen and progesterone remains the standard for hormone replacement therapy to avoid the risk of endometrial cancer that is associated with unopposed estrogen replacement.[17]

The use of oral contraceptives has not been consistently shown to increase the risk of breast cancer. There is some evidence that use of oral contraceptives for more than 4 years prior to first pregnancy increases the risk of breast cancer. Other studies, however, have not demonstrated increased risks of breast cancer, even with long-term exposures of more than 15 years.[18,19]

Family History

The increased risk of breast cancer as a function of family history is well established. For women with a second-degree relative (aunt, grandmother) with breast cancer, the risk is about 1.5, and for women with a history in first-degree relatives (mother or sister), the risk is 1.7 to 2.5.[20] This may be explained in part by inheritance of a genetic condition that predisposes an individual to breast cancer development (e.g., mutations in BRCA1 or BRCA2); shared lifestyle; and inheritance of genes that affect risk factors, such as body habitus and age at menarche. Between 20% and 25% of women diagnosed with breast cancer have a positive family history of the disease, and approximately 10% of women with breast cancer are from families who display an autosomal dominant pattern of breast cancer inheritance.[21] The actual risk that family history conveys depends on the number of relatives affected and their age at diagnosis (having a first-degree relative with premenopausal breast cancer conveys a greater risk than does having a first-degree relative with postmenopausal cancer). Women with one first-degree relative affected by the disease have an increased RR of developing breast cancer two to three times that of women with no family history. Women with two or more first-degree relatives with a diagnosis of breast cancer have a still greater risk, four to six times that of women with no family history.[20]

Women with a strong family history, particularly those with multiple first- and second-degree relatives diagnosed with breast cancer in the premenopausal years, are at risk for carrying mutations in the breast cancer susceptibility genes, BRCA1 or BRCA2. Although these mutations are present in <1% of the population and account for approximately 5% to 10% of all breast cancer cases, women carrying these mutations have a lifetime risk of developing breast cancer of up to 70% to 80%.[21] Genetic counseling or testing should be considered in women at risk for carrying these mutations. Recently, the National Comprehensive Cancer Network (NCCN) published guidelines for genetic testing.[22] In the context of pre- and posttest counseling, the NCCN recommends that genetic testing be offered when:

1. The individual has a family history of a known BRCA1/BRCA2 mutation
2. Personal history of breast cancer plus one of the following:
   a. Diagnosed age 45 years or younger
   b. Diagnosed age ≤50 years with one or more close blood relatives with breast cancer at any age, one or more close blood relatives with pancreatic cancer, one or more close blood relatives with prostate cancer, or an unknown or limited family history. Diagnosed age ≤60 years with a triple negative (TN) breast cancer. Diagnosed at any age with two or more close blood relatives with breast, pancreatic, or prostate cancer at any age, ≥1 close blood relative with breast cancer ≥50 years, ≥1 close blood relative with ovarian cancer, close male blood relative with breast cancer or an individual of ethnicity associated with higher mutation frequency (e.g., Ashkenazi Jewish).
3. Personal history of epithelial ovarian/fallopian tube/primary peritoneal cancer, or
4. Personal history of male breast cancer

Personal History of Breast Cancer and History of "Benign" Breast Biopsy

Women with a prior history of breast cancer are at an elevated risk to develop a second contralateral breast cancer.[1] Studies with long-term follow-up have demonstrated a risk of breast cancer in the contralateral breast of approximately 10% to 15%, depending on the patient population and length of follow-up.[23] Patients treated for invasive breast cancer or DCIS have similar risks of developing a contralateral breast cancer, which does not appear to be effected by the type of local therapy for the initial lesion. A recent analysis of the SEER database demonstrated that 4.2% of localized invasive or intraductal **breast cancer** patients surviving at least

3 months developed contralateral breast cancer with the 10- and 20-year actuarial rate of CBC being 6.1% and 12%.[24] The risk of contralateral breast cancer as a function of prior radiation treatment is discussed in detail later.

Although women with a history of fibrocystic changes have been reported to have an elevated risk of breast cancer, recent evidence suggests that the majority of the elevated risk is due to the smaller proportion of women whose biopsy reveals atypical hyperplasia. Results from the Breast Cancer Detection Demonstration Project, which included over 280,000 women in 29 centers, demonstrated that women with atypical hyperplasia had 4.3 times the breast cancer risk of women without proliferative disease (95% confidence interval [CI], 1.7 to 11.0). In women with proliferative disease lacking atypical hyperplasia, the RR was 1.3 (95% CI, 0.77 to 2.2). In that study, the joint occurrence of family history and atypical hyperplasia had a strong synergistic effect on breast cancer risk.[25]

Radiation Exposure

Exposure to ionizing radiation during or after puberty increases the risk for development of carcinoma of the breast. Land et al.[26,27] reviewed reports on three populations of patients exposed to ionizing radiation by atomic bombings, multiple fluoroscopic examinations for tuberculosis, and multiple examinations for mastitis. They concluded that the risk of radiation-induced cancer of the breast increased approximately linearly with increasing dose and was heavily dependent on age at exposure.

In a study of 31,710 women who had tuberculosis and were examined with repeated fluoroscopic studies, a substantial proportion (26.4%) received doses to the breast of ≥0.1 Gy; the breast cancer risk was greatest among women who had radiation exposure between the ages of 10 and 14 years (RR 4.5 per 0.01 Gy and an additive risk of 6.1 per 104 person-years per 0.01 Gy); there was substantially less excess risk with increasing age at first exposure.[28]

A high risk of solid tumors, especially breast cancer, has been described in women treated with RT at a young age for Hodgkin lymphoma. In a recent study, RRs of breast cancer were defined by radiation dose to the chest (0, 20 ≤40 Gy, or ≥40 Gy). Estimates were from this case–control study conducted within an international population-based cohort of 3,817 female survivors of Hodgkin lymphoma diagnosed at age 30 years or younger. For a survivor who was treated at age 25 years with a chest radiation dose of at least 40 Gy without alkylating agents, estimated cumulative absolute risks of breast cancer by age 35, 45, and 55 years were 1.4% (95% CI, 0.9% to 2.1%), 11.1% (95% CI, 7.4% to 16.3%), and 29.0% (95% CI, 20.2% to 40.1%), respectively.[29] A reduced volume of radiation fields has also been shown to reduce the breast cancer risk associated with treatment of Hodgkin lymphoma. The current practice of limiting radiation fields to involved nodal regions may help to further reduce the risk of radiation-related breast cancers in Hodgkin's survivors.[30]

Body Mass Index, Physical Activity, and Dietary Factors

The inherent complex interaction between body mass, physical activity, and diet complicates interpretation of epidemiologic studies correlating these factors with breast cancer risk. Body mass index (BMI) has been clearly associated with breast cancer risk in a number of studies, but it appears to influence breast cancer risk predominantly in postmenopausal women. In premenopausal women, most studies have not observed a strong relation between BMI and breast cancer risk. In postmenopausal women, a pooled analysis of prospective studies demonstrated the risk of breast cancer to be 30% higher in postmenopausal women with a BMI over 31 kg/m^2 compared with women with a BMI of 20 kg/m^2.[31] The higher risk of breast cancer with increased BMI in postmenopausal women is likely due to higher estradiol levels associated with increased adipose tissue and increased aromatase, which is involved in the conversion of androgens to estradiol. In postmenopausal women, this is the primary source of estradiol, whereas in premenopausal women, estradiol is predominantly from the ovaries so there is little association with BMI and estradiol levels.

Physical activity can have a significant impact on BMI, so it is sometimes difficult to separate these two effects in interpreting breast cancer risk. A majority of studies, however, have observed a lower risk of breast cancer among women who are more physically active compared with women who are sedentary.

Although it has been suggested that obesity and high intake of meat, dairy products, and fat may increase risk and fiber, fruits and vegetables, and phytoestrogens (soy products) may reduce risk, strong links between diet and breast cancer risk have not been clearly established.[32] Accurate data regarding nutritional factors are difficult to evaluate in most epidemiologic studies. A pooled analysis of eight prospective studies did not conclude a relation between dietary fat intake and breast cancer risk. Similarly, large prospective studies have failed to demonstrate an association between dietary fiber intake and breast cancer risk.[33] Phytoestrogens found in soy products and many cereals, tea, and vegetables may reduce the effects of estrogens. Given the lower incidence of breast cancer in Asian countries with high soy intake, one might hypothesize a relation between this dietary factor and breast cancer risk. Although animal studies suggest that high soy intake is protective, human studies have not been as conclusive.

Alcohol Consumption

In an analysis by the Oxford Group of 53 epidemiologic studies, including 58,515 women with breast cancer and 95,067 women without breast cancer, women with daily consumption of four or more drinks a day had a 50% higher breast cancer risk.[34] The average consumption of alcohol reported was 6.0 g/day (about half a unit or drink of alcohol per day). Compared with women who reported drinking no alcohol, the RR of breast cancer was 1.32 (1.19 to 1.45, $P < .00001$) for an intake of 35 to 44 g/day alcohol and 1.46 (1.33 to 1.61; $P < .00001$) for ≥45 g/day or more of alcohol. The RR of breast cancer increased by 7.1% (95% CI, 5.5 to 8.7%; $P < .00001$) for each additional drink of alcohol consumed on a daily basis. Chen et al.[35] reported on a prospective observational study of 105,986 women enrolled in the Nurses' Health Study between 1980 and 2008. With 2.4 million person-years of follow-up, 7,690 cases of invasive breast cancer were diagnosed. They found that increasing alcohol consumption was associated with increased breast cancer risk that was statistically significant at levels as low as 3 to 6 drinks per week (RR 1.15; 95% CI, 1.06 to 1.24). Moreover, binge drinking, but not frequency of drinking, was associated with breast cancer risk after controlling for cumulative alcohol intake. They concluded that low levels of alcohol consumption were associated with a small increase in breast cancer risk, with the most consistent measure being cumulative alcohol intake throughout adult life.

Although the relation among physical activity, BMI, and dietary factors may be difficult to separate, it is apparent that maintaining a sound, varied diet; limiting alcohol intake; avoiding obesity, and moderate physical activity are modifiable behaviors that can impact breast cancer risk (as well as other health-related issues) and should be encouraged.

Mammographic Density

There is a large body of evidence suggesting a correlation between mammographic breast density and breast cancer risk.[36–40] The risk of breast cancer associated with the highest category of density has been estimated to be two to six times greater than in the lowest category. Although the causal link between mammographic density remains poorly understood, breast density is in part attributable to genetic factors.

Determining an Individual's Risk

It is important to consider the combination of risk factors when a generalized risk profile is determined. Gail et al.[41] have used these epidemiologic risk factors to derive a model for predicting an individual's annual and lifetime risks of breast cancer. In the Gail model, an individual's annual risk of breast cancer is based on her present age, number of first-degree relatives with breast cancer, age at first birth, age at menarche, number of breast biopsies, and history of atypical ductal hyperplasia. The use of exogenous hormones is not considered in this model, and many of the other risk factors discussed above are not incorporated into this specific model.

PREVENTION AND GENETIC SCREENING

Approximately 10% of breast cancer patients have familial breast cancer, typically defined as breast cancer showing an autosomal dominant inheritance pattern.[21] During the 1990s, germline mutations in three important tumor suppressor genes—*p53*, *BRCA1*, and *BRCA2*—were discovered in family members of individuals with familial breast cancer.[42–44] All three genes have been shown unequivocally to predispose to breast cancer. A number of genetic conditions associated with increased risk of breast cancer are summarized in Table 59.2.

Mutations in *p53*

Germline mutations in the *p53* gene are very rare and result in Li-Fraumeni syndrome, named after two investigators who made significant contributions to the understanding of this condition.[44] The *p53* gene is one of the most important tumor suppressor genes and has been called the "guardian of the genome" because of its critical role in cellular pathways that recognize and direct a response to DNA injury. One consequence of a germline mutation in *p53* is an increased risk for a variety of cancers, including childhood sarcomas, gynecologic tumors, and breast cancer. Breast cancer is the most common malignancy in patients with Li-Fraumeni syndrome; the lifetime risk is estimated to be 90%.[44]

Mutations in *BRCA1* and *BRCA2*

Studies of patients with familial breast cancer led to the discovery of *BRCA1* in 1995 and *BRCA2* in 1996. Similar to *p53*, both *BRCA1* and *BRCA2* are tumor suppressor genes that contribute to the stability of the genome by mediating

TABLE 59.2 GENES ASSOCIATED WITH HEREDITARY BREAST CANCER

Gene/Syndrome	Approximate Relative Breast Cancer Risk
BRCA1/BRCA2	10–20 times relative risk
P53-Li-Fraumeni	2–6 times relative risk
PTEN Cowden	2–4 times risk
STK11 Peutz-Jeghers	10–15 times risk
ATM (ataxia–telangiectasia)	3–4 times risk
CHEK2	2 times risk
BRIP1-Fanconi anemia	2 times risk
PALB2	2–3 times risk

the effects of the cellular response to DNA injury. Individuals with a germline mutation in *BRCA1* have a lifetime risk of breast cancer of 65% to 85%. In addition, these individuals have an elevated lifetime risk of ovarian cancer, which may approach 50%. Other types of cancer that develop more frequently in *BRCA1* carriers include colon and prostate cancers. The lifetime risk of breast cancer for women with germline *BRCA2* mutations mirrors that for women with *BRCA1* mutations. *BRCA2* mutation carriers are also at increased risk for ovarian cancer compared with the general population, but their risk is much less than the risk in women with *BRCA1* mutations. *BRCA2* is also associated with male breast cancer and pancreatic cancer. Genetic screening for germline mutations in *BRCA1* and *BRCA2* is now possible. Testing should be performed in centers equipped with genetic counseling programs designed to properly inform individuals of the social, economic, and legal consequences associated with genetic testing. Germline mutations in *BRCA1* and *BRCA2* are rare, occurring in fewer than 7% of patients with breast cancer. Thus, only a minority of breast cancer patients with a family history of the disease would be predicted to carry a mutation in one of these genes. Table 59.3 contains data concerning the probability of carrying a *BRCA1* mutation based on an individual's age at cancer diagnosis, personal cancer history, and family cancer history and whether the individual is of Ashkenazi Jewish descent.[45]

No definitive data exist on which to base screening recommendations for individuals with a proven germline mutation in a gene predisposing to the development of breast cancer. The NCCN has published a guideline recommending that individuals with a genetic predisposition undergo breast awareness starting at age 18, annual clinical and self-breast examination starting at age 25, and annual mammography or magnetic resonance imaging (MRI) and semiannual clinical and self-breast examination after age 25.[22] In addition, annual pelvic examinations with transvaginal sonography, color Doppler examinations of the ovaries, and measurement of serum cancer antigen (CA-125) levels can be considered beginning at age 35 to 35 years. For those women aged 35 to 40, a risk-reducing bilateral salpingo-oophorectomy is recommended, with possible short-term hormone replacement therapy.

Breast Cancer Prevention Strategies

Tamoxifen

Understanding of the role of estrogens and progesterones in breast cancer development has led to the development of pharmacologic strategies that could significantly decrease the incidence of breast cancer over the next two decades.

Several pharmaceuticals that affect the estrogenic pathways have been studied as chemopreventive agents, but the only agent for which mature data from clinical trials are available is tamoxifen.[46–51] Interest in tamoxifen as a chemopreventive agent arose after a number of randomized trials designed to test the efficacy of hormonal therapy for invasive breast cancer reported that tamoxifen reduced the incidence of contralateral breast cancer. On the basis of these data, in 1992, the National Surgical Adjuvant Breast and Bowel Project (NSABP) began a randomized, placebo-controlled study (the P-1 trial) to test the efficacy of 5 years of tamoxifen in the prevention of breast cancer.[51] Between 1992 and 1997, 13,388 women with a 1.67% or greater predicted risk of developing breast cancer within 5 years were enrolled in this trial. Risk was assessed using a modification of the Gail model, which permitted enrollment of any woman older than 60 years of age and selected women younger than 60 years with additional risk factors that increased their annual risk to at least that of a 60-year-old. In addition, women with a history of LCIS were included. Women were not allowed to use estrogen replacement therapy during their participation in the trial. The results of the NSABP P-1 trial indicated that tamoxifen reduced the rates of invasive and noninvasive breast cancer by 49% and 50%, respectively. The benefit of tamoxifen was seen in all age groups (≤49 years, 50 to 59 years, ≥60 years). In addition, women with a history of atypical ductal hyperplasia had an 86% risk reduction, and women with a history of LCIS had a 56% risk reduction. Finally, the benefit was seen across all subgroups specified according to family history of breast cancer. Tamoxifen selectively reduced the incidence of estrogen receptor–positive tumors; estrogen receptor–negative tumors developed at an equal rate in the tamoxifen and placebo groups. No evidence was shown of a cardioprotective effect of tamoxifen in this trial, but the number of osteoporosis-related fractures was reduced in the tamoxifen-treated cohort. Tamoxifen increased the risk of developing stage I endometrial cancer (risk ratio of 2.53).

Subsequently, a landmark study was published that compared tamoxifen to raloxifene as a preventative agent in postmenopausal women with breast cancer. Raloxifene, a drug that is primarily used in prevention of osteoporosis, had been shown in prior studies to decrease the incidence of breast cancers. The NSABP study of tamoxifen and raloxifene was a prospective, double-blind, randomized clinical trial.[52] There were 19,747 postmenopausal women of mean age 58.5 years with increased 5-year breast cancer risk. Patients were randomized to oral tamoxifen (20 mg/day) or raloxifene (60 mg/day) for 5 years. There were 163 cases of invasive breast cancer in women assigned to tamoxifen and 168 in those assigned to raloxifene, which was not significantly different between the two arms. The main benefit of raloxifene was in toxicity. There were 36 cases of uterine cancer with tamoxifen and 23 with raloxifene. No differences were found for other invasive cancer sites, for ischemic heart disease events, or for stroke. Thromboembolic events also occurred less often in the raloxifene group. The number of osteoporotic fractures in the groups was similar, and there were fewer cataract surgeries with raloxifene. There was no difference in the total number of deaths (101 vs. 96 for tamoxifen vs. raloxifene) or in causes of death. It appears from this study that raloxifene is as effective as tamoxifen in reducing the risk of invasive breast cancer and has a lower risk of thromboembolic events. Of note, there were slightly more noninvasive cancers in the raloxifene group, but that was not statistically significant.

TABLE 59.3 PROBABILITY OF *BRCA1* GERMLINE MUTATIONS IN VARIOUS CLINICAL SCENARIOS

Scenario	Probability
Mother or father proven carrier	50%
40-year-old with breast cancer and a first-degree relative with breast cancer	
Ashkenazi	20%
Non-Ashkenazi	5%
60-year-old with bilateral breast cancer and a first-degree relative with breast cancer	
Ashkenazi	20%
Non-Ashkenazi	5%
30-year-old with breast cancer and a first-degree relative with ovarian cancer	
Ashkenazi	50%
Non-Ashkenazi	20%

Data from Shattuck-Eidens D, Oliphant A, McClure M, et al. *BRCA1* sequence analysis in women at high risk for susceptibility mutations. Risk factor analysis and implications for genetic testing. *JAMA* 1997;278:1242–1250.

TABLE 59.4 RESULTS OF CHEMOPREVENTION TRIALS

	Royal Marsden (Tamoxifen vs. Placebo)[55]	NSABP-P1 (Tamoxifen vs. Placebo)[51]	Italian (Tamoxifen vs. Placebo)[54]	IBIS-1 (Tamoxifen vs. Placebo)[48]	MORE (Raloxifene vs. Placebo)[47]	STARR (Tamoxifen vs. Raloxifene)[52]
Entry dates	1986–1996	1992–1997	1992–1997	1992–2001	1994–1999	1999–2005
Number randomized	2,494 (1,238 vs. 1,233)	6,681 vs. 6,707	2,700 vs. 2,708	3,573 vs. 3,566	2,557 + 2,572 vs. 2,576	9,726 vs. 9,745
Age (yr)	30–70	≥35	35–70	35–70	66.5 (median)	≥35
Agent dose	Tamoxifen 20 mg	Tamoxifen 20 mg	Tamoxifen 20 mg	Tamoxifen 20 mg	Raloxifene 60 mg or 120 mg	Tamoxifen 20 mg, raloxifene 60 mg
Planned length (yr) of treatment	5–8	5	5	5	4	5
Breast Cancers						
Total	62 vs. 75	124 vs. 244	34 vs. 45	69 vs. 101	31/2 vs. 43	220 vs. 248
Invasive	54 vs. 64	89 vs. 175	28 vs. 40	64 vs. 85	22/2 vs. 39	163 vs. 168
Noninvasive	7 vs. 7	35 vs. 69	5 vs. 4	5 vs. 16	9/2 vs. 4	57 vs. 80
Unknown	1 vs. 4	–	1 vs. 1	–	–	–
ER Status (Invasive Only)						
Positive	31 vs. 44	41 vs. 130	–	44 vs. 63	10/2 vs. 31	115 vs. 109
Negative	17 vs. 10	38 vs. 31	–	19 vs. 19	9/2 vs. 4	44 vs. 51

Section III

A comparison of the tamoxifen P-1, P-2, and other tamoxifen prevention trials is outlined in Table 59.4.[46–50,53,54]

Prophylactic Surgery

An alternative strategy used to prevent breast cancer development is prophylactic surgical intervention. Hartmann et al.[55] analyzed outcomes in women with a family history of breast cancer who underwent bilateral prophylactic mastectomy at the Mayo Clinic between 1960 and 1993. With a median follow-up time of 14 years, only 4 of the 639 treated patients developed breast cancer. According to the Gail model, 37.4 cases of breast cancer would have been expected to develop in this population, so the prophylactic surgery resulted in an 89.5% risk reduction ($P < .001$).[55]

Breast cancer prevention strategies will continue to be a dynamic area of preclinical and clinical research.

NATURAL HISTORY AND ORIGINS

All forms of breast cancer are believed to develop as a consequence of unregulated cell growth and the development of phenotypic changes such as the ability to invade, recruit a new blood supply, and metastasize. These changes in phenotypes are secondary to the development of aberrations in genetic pathways. Some of these aberrations are inherited (germline mutations), whereas others develop during the life of a breast cell (somatic mutations). It is currently believed that most breast cancer is a consequence of a series of somatic mutations. As previously noted, only 20% to 25% of breast cancer patients have a history of breast cancer in a first-degree relative. However, it is possible that some women without a first-degree relative with breast cancer still inherit a genetic background that predisposes to breast cancer. These mutations may be insufficient to cause breast cancer unless accompanied by other mutations and, therefore, would be predicted to have a low penetrance. Historically, it has been much more difficult to discover low-penetrance mutations than to discover germline mutations that result in an autosomal dominant pattern of breast cancer development. However, with newer molecular techniques, such as DNA-array assays, the identification of low-penetrance predisposing mutations may be more feasible.

Left untreated, breast cancer can have a variable clinical course. A classic article by Bloom et al.[56] outlined the natural history of breast cancer patients, seen between 1805 and 1933, not treated by surgery or irradiation, 250 of whom had a pathologic diagnosis of cancer. There were no patients with stage I disease, 2.4% with stage II, 23% with stage III, and 74% with stage IV. Survival in the untreated group was 3.6% compared with an overall survival of 34% in patients treated with radical or modified radical mastectomy with or without radiation.

Concepts regarding the natural history of breast cancer have undergone great evolution over the past 100 years, with a profound impact on the management of these patients. The Halsted[57] model was based on an orderly progression to the regional lymph nodes and from there to distant metastatic sites. Later, Keynes[58] and Crile et al.[59] suggested that breast cancer is a systemic disease and that extensive surgery to achieve local tumor control was not as important as originally believed. This alternative hypothesis was fully demonstrated in both laboratory and clinical studies by Fisher,[60] who advanced the concept that breast cancer, as a systemic process involving host–tumor interactions, would not show substantial effects on survival with variations in locoregional treatment. A third hypothesis put forward by Hellman[61] considers breast cancer as a heterogeneous disease with a spectrum extending from a tumor that remains localized throughout its course to one that disseminates systemically, even when detected as a small lesion, suggesting that metastases are a function of tumor growth and progression factors.

The most common site of origin of breast cancer is the upper outer quadrant (38.5%), followed by the central area (29%), the upper inner quadrant (14.2%), the lower outer quadrant (8.8%), and the lower inner quadrant (5%).[62] These rates correlate with the amount of breast tissue in the various quadrants. Cancer is somewhat more common in the left than in the right breast and may appear in both breasts simultaneously (1% to 2%). As noted above, women with a history of breast cancer have a 10% to 15% risk of developing a new primary in the contralateral breast.

As the cancer grows, it travels along the ducts, eventually breaking through the basement membrane of the duct, invading adjacent lobules, ducts, fascial strands, and the mammary fat, spreading through the breast lymphatics and into the peripheral lymphatics. The tumor can grow through the wall of blood vessels, spread into the deep lymphatics of the dermis, and eventually produce edema of the skin (*peau d'orange*), which usually indicates that the superficial as well as the deep lymphatics are involved. Skin dimpling can be caused by involvement of Cooper ligament. Ulceration and infiltration of overlying skin, which may develop late in the course of the disease, are usually preceded by fixation and localized redness of the skin over the tumor and are less frequently seen because of the current emphasis on screening and early diagnosis.[62]

Axillary Spread

A common route of spread of breast carcinoma is first through the axillary lymph nodes, with the incidence increasing with larger tumors. Depending on mode of detection, tumor size, histology, and other clinical or pathologic factors, between 10% and 40% of newly diagnosed stage T1 and T2 breast cancers have pathologic evidence of axillary nodal metastases. Voogd et al.[63] assessed 7,680 patients with documented invasive breast cancer; of 5,125 patients known to have clinically negative lymph nodes who underwent axillary dissection, 1,748 (34%) had positive lymph nodes at pathologic examination. Univariate analysis showed that lymph node metastases were associated with tumors larger than 1 cm (P = .001), moderate or poorly differentiated nuclear grade (P = .005), high fraction of cells in the growth phase (S phase) of the cell cycle (P = .041), presence of lymphatic vascular invasion (P < .001), and age younger than 60 years (P = .01).

Multiple studies have shown a strong relation between primary tumor size and axillary nodal involvement.[64–68] Even patients with T1a and T1b disease have significant nodal involvement. Mustafa et al.[69] noted an overall frequency of axillary lymph node metastases in T1a and T1b lesions of 16%; integrating age, tumor size, and grade predicted the frequency of nodal metastases. Overall, patients with all three poor prognostic indicators had a 34% incidence of nodal involvement, and those with no poor prognostic factors had a ≤7% probability of nodal metastases. Gann et al.[70] reviewed 18,025 patients with a diagnosis of breast carcinoma from the American College of Surgeons database. On multivariate analysis, the following factors were independently associated with a greater likelihood of one or more positive lymph nodes: larger tumor size, young age, African American or Hispanic race, outer-half tumor location, poor or moderate differentiation, aneuploidy, and infiltrating ductal histologic type.

Although up to 30% to 40% of T1 or T2 clinically node-negative breast cancers may have pathologically involved lymph nodes, data from NSABP-04 suggest that less than half of clinically negative but pathologically positive axilla will experience a clinical relapse in the axilla.[71] In this study, operable breast cancer patients, who were primarily diagnosed with palpable breast tumors in the premammography era, were randomized to one of three arms: simple mastectomy without axillary dissection, simple mastectomy with axillary dissection, or simple mastectomy with comprehensive chest wall and regional nodal irradiation (RNI).

In the arm undergoing axillary dissection, nodal positivity was approximately 40%. Nodal control was excellent (>97%) in this arm as well as in the arm treated with radiation. In the simple mastectomy arm, where no nodal treatment by radiation or dissection was administered, the axillary failure rate was approximately 20%. Assuming equal distribution among the arms, it is presumed the pathologic involvement was approximately 40%, indicating that less than half of those with pathologic involvement eventually failed clinically.

Internal Mammary Spread

Metastases to the internal mammary nodes (IMNs) are correlated with tumor size, are more frequent from medial half and central lesions, and occur more frequently when there is axillary node involvement (Table 59.5).[72] Veronesi et al.[73] found that, among women with tumors larger than 2 cm who were younger than 40 years of age and had positive axillary nodes, there was a 41% risk of having positive IMNs on IMN dissection; the corresponding risk for patients of that age with negative nodes was 16%. Sugg et al.[74] reviewed 286 patients with breast cancer who underwent IMN dissection. Positive IMNs were associated with primary tumor size (P < .0001) and the number of positive axillary nodes (P < .0001) but not with age or primary tumor location. Patients who had positive IMNs (25% of all patients) had a significantly worse overall 20-year disease-free survival rate than did patients with negative IMNs (P < .0001). Clinical failure of the IMNs is extremely rare, despite the evidence of pathologic involvement from these studies. Most studies looking at nodal failure patterns report failure in the internal mammary region of <1%.[75–79]

Supraclavicular Spread

Spread to supraclavicular lymph nodes usually follows involvement in the high axillary lymph nodes or IMNs depending on the location of the primary lesion. Chen et al.[80] reviewed 2,658 patients with invasive breast cancer who underwent surgery and adjuvant therapy. With a median follow-up period of 39 months, supraclavicular lymph node metastasis developed in 113 (4.3%). Young age (≤40 years), tumor size >3 cm, angiolymphatic invasion, negative estrogen-receptor status, and DNA synthetic phase fraction >4% were significant for predicting supraclavicular metastasis on univariate analysis. Three predictive factors were significant after multivariate analysis: high histologic grade, more than four positive nodes, and axillary level II or III involved nodes. In patients with axillary level I involved nodes and four or fewer positive nodes, the incidence of supraclavicular lymph node metastasis was 4.4%, but if axillary level III was involved, it increased to 15.1%.

TABLE 59.5 INTERNAL MAMMARY NODE INVOLVEMENT RELATED TO LOCATION OF PRIMARY TUMOR AND TO AXILLARY NODE INVOLVEMENT[a]

| | Location of Primary Tumor | | | | |
Axillary Involvement	Upper Inner Quadrant (%)	Lower Inner Quadrant (%)	Central (%)	Upper Outer Quadrant (%)	Lower Outer Quadrant (%)
Axilla not involved	20/143 (14)	2/36 (6)	5/76 (7)	7/170 (4)	2/40 (5)
Axilla involved	47/105 (45)	18/25 (72)	65/140 (46)	47/212 (22)	10/53 (19)
Total	67/248 (27)	20/61 (33)	70/216 (32)	54/382 (14)	12/93 (13)

[a]Number of patients with internal mammary node involvement/total number of patients.
Reproduced with permission of The Royal College of Surgeons of England from Handley RS. Carcinoma of the breast. *Ann R Coll Surg Engl* 1975;57(2):59–66. Copyright ©1975 The Royal College of Surgeons of England; permission conveyed through Copyright Clearance Center, Inc.

Clinical failure in the supraclavicular fossa is relatively rare in patients with early-stage breast cancer and is dependent on the degree of axillary involvement. For patients with no or minimal nodal involvement (less than three involved axillary nodes), supraclavicular failure is extremely rare. In an analysis of 691 patients with zero to three nodes involved undergoing breast-conserving surgery and RT to tangential fields only without RNI, Galper et al.[76] reported failure in the supraclavicular fossa in 1.3% of patients.

Several studies have demonstrated that the failure rate in supraclavicular nodes, left untreated, may be as high as 20% in patients with advanced disease or more than four lymph nodes involved.[81–85] In a cohort of 1,031 patients with operable breast cancer treated with mastectomy and level I or II node dissection plus adriamycin-based chemotherapy, but no radiation, Strom et al.[85] reported failure in the supraclavicular fossa was 8% at 10 years. Predictors of supraclavicular failure included four or more involved nodes and gross extranodal extension. In these subgroups, supraclavicular failure ranged from 14% to 19%. Radiation to the supraclavicular fossa in these higher-risk patients results in high local control rates, with isolated supraclavicular failures occurring in <1% of prophylactically treated nodes.

Systemic Spread

Using monoclonal antibodies to epithelial cytokeratins or tumor-associated cell membrane glycoproteins, carcinoma cells can be detected on cytologic bone marrow (or lymph node) preparations. Braun et al.[86] combined patient data from nine studies involving 4,703 patients with stage I, II, or III breast cancer. Micrometastasis was detected in 30.6% of the patients. With a median follow-up of 5.2 years, patients with bone marrow micrometastasis had larger tumors and tumors with a higher histologic grade and more often had lymph node metastases and hormone receptor–negative tumors, compared with those without bone marrow micrometastasis. The presence of micrometastasis was a significant prognostic factor for poorer overall survival (RR 2.15; $P < .001$), breast cancer–specific survival (RR 2.44; $P < .001$), disease-free survival (RR 2.13), and distant disease-free survival (RR 2.33; $P < .001$ for all outcomes measures). In multivariable analysis, micrometastasis was an independent predictor of a poor outcome.

Local Control and Systemic Metastasis

Patients treated for breast cancer are at risk for locoregional failure, as well as systemic metastasis. It is evident from the available literature that optimizing local control can impact systemic metastasis and survival, and similarly, systemic therapy can impact local control.[87–90] Integration of systemic therapy with radiation will be discussed in detail later, but numerous studies have clearly demonstrated a significant improvement in local control with the use of RT and systemic therapy (both cytotoxic and hormonal) compared with RT without the use of systemic therapy.[90–95] Appropriate integration of both local and systemic treatments through a multidisciplinary approach is thus essential to optimize outcome. Although there is some overlap, prognostic factors for locoregional control and systemic metastasis often differ.

For patients with early-stage invasive breast cancer, even with appropriate systemic therapy, development of metastasis can vary from <5% in women with T1a disease and favorable histology to >40% for women with T2 tumors and pathologically involved lymph nodes. Similarly, locoregional failure rates can vary from <5% to over 40% depending on local treatment and prognostic factors for local failure.[91–94,96–100]

The impact of local control on systemic metastasis in breast cancer as well as other malignancies has been the subject of considerable debate and controversy. Although the benefits of local control with respect to cosmesis and quality of life are apparent, the independent effect of local control on systemic disease and survival has been questioned. Several studies have identified local control as an independent predictor of disease-free or overall survival.[9,10,12–15,17–21,23,25–97,97–100,100–109] Fisher et al.,[106] in an analysis of patients treated in NSABP protocol B-06, concluded that ipsilateral breast tumor recurrence (IBTR) was a harbinger, but not a cause, of distant metastases. Although mastectomy or breast irradiation after lumpectomy prevented expression of the marker (breast relapse), neither lowered the risk of distant metastases, which was determined by a host of prognostic factors.

More recent meta-analyses, however, have demonstrated a small but significant impact of local control on systemic metastasis and overall survival.[87,88] A meta-analysis of randomized trials by Vinh-Hung and Verschraegen[88] comparing breast-conserving surgery without radiation to breast-conserving surgery with radiation confirms an approximate threefold reduction in local relapse with RT and an 8.6% improvement in mortality in the radiated cohorts.

One of the most convincing and authoritative studies related to this subject is the recent analysis of the Early Breast Cancer Trialists' Collaborative Group (EBCTCG).[87] In this analysis, over 42,000 women were enrolled in 78 randomized trials that compared 24 types of local treatment (radiotherapy vs. no radiotherapy, more vs. less surgery, or more surgery vs. radiotherapy). The EBCTCG attempted to relate the effect on local control to breast cancer mortality by grouping studies into whether the 5-year local relapse risk difference between the two comparisons of local therapy exceeded 10%. In those comparisons in which the difference in 5-year local recurrence risk was <10%, there was no impact on 15-year breast cancer mortality. However, there were 25,000 women enrolled in trials in whom the comparisons involved >10% differences in local control. In those studies, the difference in local recurrence risks at 5 years were 7% versus 26%, and the 15-year mortality risks were 44.6% versus 49.5% ($P < .00001$). Figure 59.6 summarizes the results of this meta-analysis with respect to the impact of radiation on breast cancer mortality both in breast conservation and following mastectomy. An update from the EBCTCG focused on 10,801 women enrolled in 17 randomized trials of radiotherapy versus no radiotherapy after breast-conserving surgery and relates the absolute reduction in 15-year risk of breast cancer death to the absolute reduction in 10-year recurrence risk.[110] Overall, radiotherapy reduced the 10-year risk of any first recurrence from 35.0% to 19.3% ($P < 00001$) and reduced the 15-year risk of breast cancer death from 25.2% to 21.4% ($P < 0001$). In women with pN+ disease ($n = 1,050$), radiotherapy reduced the 10-year recurrence risk from 63.7% to 42.5% ($P < 00001$) and the 15-year risk of breast cancer death from 51.3% to 42.8% ($P = 01$). Overall, about one breast cancer death was avoided by year 15 for every four recurrences avoided by year 10.

CLINICAL PRESENTATION

The majority of patients with T1 or T2 breast cancers present with a painless or slightly tender breast mass or have an abnormal screening mammogram. Patients with more advanced tumors may have breast tenderness, skin changes, bloody nipple discharge, or occasionally change in the shape and size of the breast. Rarely, patients may present

RT after BCS, generally with AC: 7,311 women, 17% with node-positive disease

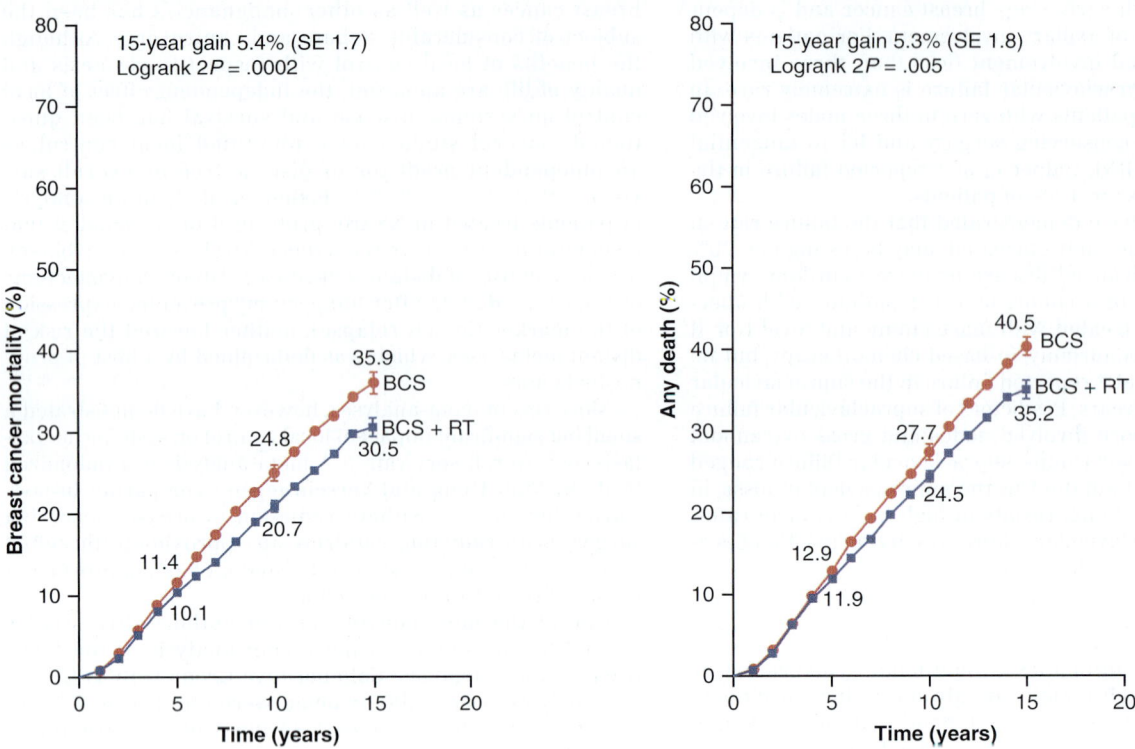

RT after mastectomy with AC: 8,505 women with node-positive disease

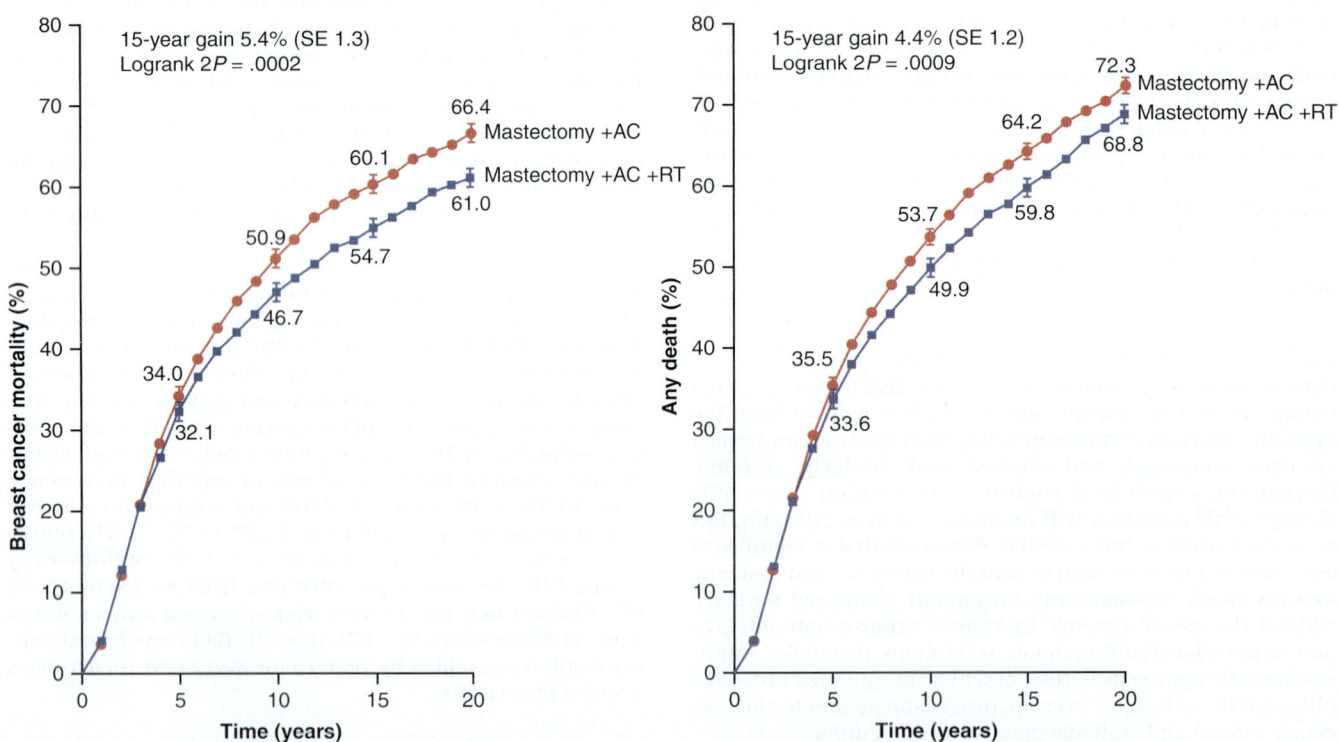

FIGURE 59.6. Effect of radiotherapy on breast cancer mortality and on all-cause mortality after breast conservation surgery or after mastectomy with axillary clearance: 15-year or 20-year probabilities. (Reprinted from Clarke M, Collins R, Darby S, et al. Effects of radiotherapy and of differences in the extent of surgery for early breast cancer on local recurrence and 15-year survival: an overview of the randomised trials. *Lancet* 2005;366[9503]:2087–2106. Copyright © 2005 Elsevier. With permission.)

with axillary lymphadenopathy or even distant metastasis. As noted previously, however, depending on tumor size, method of detection, and pathologic factors associated with the primary tumor, up to 30% to 40% of women with a clinically

negative axilla may harbor subclinical pathologically involved axillary nodes.

The impact of delays in evaluation or treatment on the survival of patients with breast cancer is controversial. Richards

TABLE 59.6 BREAST CANCER SCREENING GUIDELINES

Age Group	Developed by the ACS and Endorsed by the ACR, SBI
20–39	BSE optional; CBE every 3 y
40–44	Women should have the opportunity to begin annual screening between the ages of 40 and 44 y (qualified recommendation)
45-54	Women should be screened annually (qualified recommendation)
55+	Women 55 y and older should transition to biennial screening or have the opportunity to continue screening annually (qualified recommendation)
At increased risk	Consult with their doctors about the benefits and limitations of starting mammography screening earlier, having additional tests (i.e., breast ultrasound and MRI), or having more frequent exams

ACR, American College of Radiology; ACS, American College of Surgeons; BSE, breast self-examination; CBE, clinical breast examination; SBI, Society of Breast Imagers; MRI, magnetic resonance imaging.

et al.,[111] in a review of 2,964 patients, found 942 (32%) who had symptoms for 12 or more weeks before their first hospital visit. Locally advanced or metastatic disease was detected in 32% of patients with delays compared with 10% of patients with intervals of <12 weeks between the onset of symptoms and hospital referral (*P* < .0001). Olivotto et al.[112] found that delays in diagnosis of 6 to 12 months led to increased risk of larger tumor size and more lymph node metastases compared with patients diagnosed within 4 to 12 weeks of an abnormal screening mammogram result.

SCREENING IN BREAST CANCER

Mammography

Screening mammography has resulted in a shift in both the incidence and stage of patients presenting with breast cancer. In a simplified model described by Harris et al.,[113] for every 1,000 screening mammograms, 80 women (8%) will be recalled for additional diagnostic imaging, 10 (1%) will require tissue diagnosis, and of those undergoing biopsy only 3 (0.3%) will have a malignancy.

There is a large body of evidence that early detection by mammography, followed by appropriate local, regional, and systemic treatment, is associated with reduced breast cancer mortality rates for women 50 years of age and older.[114–117] Although it remains an active area of debate, several authors agree that screening mammography in women 40 to 49 years of age may reduce mortality from breast cancer,[25,115–121] and mammographic screening beginning at age 40 is encouraged in the majority of published guidelines (Table 59.6). The reader is referred elsewhere for an extensive discussion of

screening mammography studies.[115–117] Selected series will be briefly discussed here, and a summary of the classic screening mammography trials is summarized in Table 59.7.[68,123–131] Collectively, these studies demonstrate a decrease in mortality and migration of patients from later stages of disease to earlier stages of disease with the use of screening mammography.[25,115–121,123,130,131]

Sixteen-year results are available from the Health Insurance Plan study, which involved two systematically selected, randomly sampled groups of approximately 31,000 women aged 40 to 64 years who were offered screening examinations.[122,132] Compared with the control group, which was observed and monitored, the mortality rate was reduced by approximately one-third in screened women 50 to 59 years of age. The survival difference between mammography-only and clinical examination–only cases appeared in years 7 to 10 after diagnosis. Although the greatest difference in mortality between screened and control group was detected in women 50 to 59 years of age when they entered the study, the differences are in favor of the study group at all ages.

Tabár et al.[124,130,131] demonstrated the benefit from mammography screening in two Swedish counties. In the group of women 20 to 69 years of age, there were 6,807 diagnosed with breast carcinoma over a 29-year period and 1,863 breast carcinoma deaths. The mortality rate from breast carcinoma diagnosed in women 40 to 69 years of age who were screened during the screening period (1988–1996) declined by 63% (RR 0.37) compared with the breast carcinoma mortality rate during the period when no screening was available (1968–1977). The reduction in mortality rate observed during the service-screening period, adjusted for selection bias, was 48%. No significant change in breast carcinoma mortality rate

TABLE 59.7 RANDOMIZED CONTROLLED TRIALS OF BREAST CANCER SCREENING

Trial (Reference)	Screening Protocol		Population			Follow-Up (Years)	Relative Risk (95% Confidence Interval)
	Approach	Frequency	Age Group	Invited	Control		
HIP, 1963–1969[122]	2 VMM 1 CBE	24 mo 4 rounds	40–49	14,432	14,701	18	0.77 (0.53–1.11)
			50–64	16,568	16,299	18	0.80 (0.59–1.08)
Malmo, 1976–1990[123]	1 or 2 VMM	18–24 mo 5 rounds	45–49	13,528	12,242	12.7	0.64 (0.45–0.89)
			50–69	17,134	17,165	9	0.86 (0.64–1.16)
Kopparberg, 1977–1985[124]	1 VMM	24 mo 4 rounds	40–49	9,650	5,009	20	0.76 (0.42–1.40)
			50–74	28,939	13,551	20	1.06 (0.65–1.76)
Ostergotland, 1977–1985[124]	1 VMM	24 mo 4 rounds	40–49	10,240	10,441	20	0.52 (0.39–0.70)
			50–74	28,229	26,830	20	0.81 (0.64–1.03)
Edinburgh, 1979–1988[125]	1 or 2 VMM CBE (initial)	24 mo 4 rounds	45–49	11,755	10,641	14	0.83 (0.54–1.27)
			50–64	11,245	12,359	10	0.85 (0.62–1.15)
CNBSS-1, 1980–1987[126]	2 VMM CBE	12 mo 4–5 rounds	40–49	25,214	25,216	11–16	1.07 (0.75–1.52)
CNBSS-2, 1980–1987[127]	2 VMM CBE	12 mo 4–5 rounds	50–59	19,711	19,694	13	1.02 (0.78–1.33)
Stockholm, 1981–1985[128]	1 VMM	28 mo 2 rounds	40–49	14,185	7,985	11.4	1.01 (0.51–2.02)
			50–64	25,815	12,015	7	0.65 (0.4–1.08)
Gothenburg[129]	2 VMM	18 mo 5 rounds	39–49	11,724	14,217	12	0.56 (0.32–0.98)
			50–59	9,276	16,394	13	0.91 (0.61–1.36)

CBE, clinical breast examination; 1 VMM, one-view mammography of each breast; 2 VMM, two-view mammography of each breast.

was observed over the three periods in women who did not undergo screening. In a recent long-term update, there has remained a highly significant reduction in breast cancer mortality in women invited to screening (RR 0.69; 95% CI: 0.56 to 0.84; $P = .001$). At 29 years of follow-up, there was a reduction in 1 death for every 414 women undergoing screening for 7 years. They conclude that the group invited to screening resulted in a highly significant decrease in breast cancer specific mortality.[133]

In contrast to the above, a Canadian study revealed that in women aged 50 to 59 years, the addition of annual mammography screening to physical examination had no effect on breast cancer mortality. Miller et al.[127] reported a study of 39,405 women (aged 50 to 59 years) randomly assigned to one of two study groups. By December 31, 1993, 622 invasive and 71 *in situ* breast cancers were observed in the mammography plus physical examination group, compared with 610 and 16, respectively, in the physical examination–only group. At 13-year follow-up, the number of deaths from breast cancer was 107 in the mammography plus physical examination group and 105 in the physical examination–only group. The results of the Canadian study may be due to the unbalanced allocation of women with advanced cancers (large tumors, four or more positive nodes) to the screened group, the poor quality of the mammography in the trial, and an insufficient sample size.[119,134]

Screening in Women under Age 50

Although the majority of studies clearly support the impact of screening mammography on mortality in women over 50 years of age, data on screening younger women are more conflicting. Frisell and Lidbrink[128] presented updated data on breast cancer mortality for women younger than age 50 years from the Stockholm Mammographic Screening Trial. Approximately 40,000 women aged 40 to 64 years (14,842 aged 40 to 49 years) were randomized to a trial of breast cancer screening by single-view mammography alone; 20,000 women (7,103 aged 40 to 49) were randomized to a control group. In the 40- to 49-year age group, 24 and 12 breast cancer deaths were found in the study and control groups, respectively, after 11.4 years of follow-up. The RR of breast cancer death in screened versus nonscreened women was 1.08 (95% CI, 0.54 to 2.17).

A large trial was conducted in the United Kingdom involving 45,841 women aged 45 to 64 years who were offered annual screening by clinical examination and mammography; 63,636 were taught breast self-examination, and 127,117, for whom no extra services were provided, constituted a control population.[135] After 16 years of follow-up, the breast cancer mortality rate was 27% lower in the two screening centers combined than in the four comparison centers. A 35% decrease in mortality rate was observed in mammographically screened women in all cohorts aged 45 to 64 years at entry. There was no evidence of less benefit in women aged 45 to 49 years at initial screening compared with a reduction of 25% in women aged 50 to 74 years.[136]

In a Swedish study evaluating women in the 40- to 49-year age group, Hellquist et al.[137] reported 803 breast cancer deaths in a screening study group compared with 1,238 deaths in a control group after 16 years of follow-up. The estimated RR for women screened in this younger population was 0.74 (95% CI, 0.66 to 0.83), concluding that screening mammography reduced the breast cancer mortality rate in this younger population.

In the United States, screening mammography beginning at age 40 years is recommended for the general population.[138] For some women at high risk for development of breast cancer, annual screening may be started at an earlier age. These women include those with a personal history of breast cancer, those who have had therapeutic radiation to the breast area especially for Hodgkin lymphoma, *BRCA*-positive women, women with a family history of a first-degree relative with breast cancer at a young age, and women with a biopsy diagnosis of LCIS or atypical ductal hyperplasia.

Despite some conflicting data in the large randomized trials and meta-analyses summarized above, there is general agreement that screening mammography can have a significant impact on stage of presentation of disease and breast cancer mortality. Given the incidence of breast cancer, promotion of screening for breast cancer is a major public health issue. The American Cancer Society, the American College of Radiology (ACR), and Society of Breast Imaging (SBI) recommend that women with an average risk of breast cancer should undergo regular screening mammography starting at age 45 years (strong recommendation). Women aged 45 to 54 years should be screened annually (qualified recommendation). Women 55 years and older should transition to biennial screening or have the opportunity to continue screening annually (qualified recommendation). Women should have the opportunity to begin annual screening between the ages of 40 and 44 years (qualified recommendation). Women should continue screening mammography as long as their overall health is good and they have a life expectancy of 10 years or longer (qualified recommend[139]. The US Preventive Services Task Force (USPSTF) published a controversial recommendation statement on screening breast cancer in the general population.[140] For women before the age of 50 years, the decision to start regular, biennial screening mammography should be an individual one and take patient context into account, including the patient's values regarding specific benefits and harms. They recommended biennial screening mammography for women between the ages of 50 and 74 years. The group felt there was insufficient evidence to assess the additional benefits and harms of screening mammography in women 75 years or older.

This issue continues to be controversial. Even though the guidelines still differ in their recommendations on key issues, they have become more consistent. In addition, the inconsistencies that exist may be secondary to differences in guideline member composition and evidence grading systems between the ACS and the USPSTF, as well as differences in what evidence is considered and what constitutes a favorable benefit-to-harm ratio for recommending screening.

Digital Versus Screen Film Mammography

There has been increased utilization of digital mammography for screening. This technology utilizes a special detector capable of transforming x-ray images into electronic digital image. Advantages include no film processing, faster image acquisition, and less callbacks due to the ability to manipulate the image digitally. Results of a large-scale American College of Radiology Imaging Network (ACRIN) trial of 49,000 women revealed that digital mammography overall was at least as good as screen film mammography but was superior in younger women and women with dense breasts.[141] Given the potential efficiencies and advantages of digital mammography, most centers are moving in this direction.

Magnetic Resonance Imaging Screening

The role of MRI screening is rapidly evolving. MRI is unlikely to replace mammography for screening of the general population and is not recommended by the USPSTF in their statement on breast cancer screening.[140,142,143] However, its use in screening high-risk populations has recently been supported in several studies. For women at high risk for breast cancer due to strong family history or positive *BRCA1/BRCA2* status, the standard screening techniques of breast self-examination, clinical breast examination, and mammography may be suboptimal. Nearly half of the cancers in this population are detected by physical examination between routine radiographic surveillance. In this population, increased breast density and rapid proliferative rates likely contribute to the relative insensitivity of mammography. Although MRI has not yet been shown to impact mortality, the sensitivity of MRI over mammography, clinical examination, and ultrasound in this high-risk population has been demonstrated in several prospective, nonrandomized studies[144–149].

Despite substantial differences in patient population (age, risk, etc.) and MRI technique, all reported significantly higher sensitivity for MRI compared with mammography (or any of the other modalities). All studies that included more than one round of screening reported interval cancer rates below 10%. Participants in each of these studies had either a documented *BRCA1* or *BRCA2* mutation or a very strong family history of breast cancer. Some of the studies included women with a prior personal history of breast cancer. Overall, studies have found high sensitivity for MRI, ranging from 71% to 100% versus 16% to 40% for mammography in these high-risk populations. Three studies included ultrasound, which had sensitivity similar to mammography.

In a landmark study by Kriege et al.,[150] 1,909 eligible women (cumulative lifetime risk of breast cancer of 15% or more) at high risk for familial breast cancer, including 358 carriers of germline mutations, were screened with an annual MRI and mammography. Within a median follow-up period of 2.9 years, the screening program yielded 51 tumors. The sensitivity of clinical breast examination, mammography, and MRI for detecting invasive breast cancer was 17.9%, 33.3%, and 79.5%, respectively, and the specificity was 98.1%, 95.0%, and 89.8%, respectively. The overall discriminating capacity of MRI was significantly better than that of mammography ($P < .05$). From this study, it appears that MRI is more sensitive than mammography in detecting tumors in women at high risk for familial breast cancer.

Ultrasound Screening

Ultrasound is a complementary tool to mammography for the diagnosis of breast cancer. As with MRI, it is unlikely to replace mammography for screening the general population. The NCCN recommends ultrasound for those women presenting with a dominant mass or asymmetric thickening or nodularity.[105,151] In a randomized trial of ultrasound and mammography of 2,809 women with dense breasts from ACRIN, adding a single screening ultrasound yielded an additional 1.1 to 7.2 additional cancers found in high-risk women but substantially increased the number of false positives.[152] The role of screening ultrasound and selection of patients remains controversial and will likely continue to evolve over the next decade.

Screening by Physical Examination

Two studies have evaluated the effectiveness of screening by breast self-examination alone, the UK and the Canadian trials. Using Breast Cancer Registry data, Costanza and Foster[153,154] found fewer deaths from breast cancer (14% vs. 26%) and improved estimated 5-year survival rates (75% vs. 59%) among women who reported performing breast self-examination compared with those who did not. In the Breast Cancer Detection Demonstration Project, the estimated overall sensitivity of breast self-examination in detecting breast cancer was 26%, compared with 75% for the combination of clinical breast examination and mammography.[155]

Clinical breast examination and self-examination may be complementary to mammography, perhaps detecting interval cancers in the 10% to 12% of cancers not visualized by mammography. Although it is evident that clinical screening is not as sensitive as mammography, the combination of clinical examination and mammography appears to yield optimal results in early detection.

TABLE 59.8 DIAGNOSTIC WORKUP FOR CARCINOMA OF THE BREAST, STAGES T1 AND T2

General
History with emphasis on presenting symptoms, menstrual status, parity, family history of cancer, other risk factors
Physical examination with emphasis on breast, axilla, supraclavicular area, abdomen

Special Tests
Biopsy (core biopsy directed by physical examination, ultrasound, or mammography as indicated, or needle localization)

Radiologic Studies
Before biopsy
Bilateral diagnostic mammography/ultrasonography
Chest radiographs
Magnetic resonance imaging of breast (selected cases)
After positive biopsy
Bone scan (when clinically indicated, for stage II or III disease or elevated serum alkaline phosphatase levels)
Computed tomography of the chest, abdomen, and pelvis for stage II or III disease and/or abnormal liver function tests

Laboratory Studies
Complete blood cell count,
Comprehensive metabolic panel, including liver function tests and alkaline phosphatase

Other Studies
Hormone receptor status (ER, PR)*HER2/neu* status
Consider genetic counseling/*BRCA* testing in high-risk patients
Counseling for fertility if premenopausal
Assess for distress

DIAGNOSIS AND WORKUP

The workup of a patient with a breast mass, including complete clinical and family history, is summarized in Table 59.8. The patient should be examined both sitting up and lying down (to confirm masses felt on the sitting-up examination and to detect lesions deeper in the breast or against the chest wall). Careful inspection of both breasts should be made, including size, form, and symmetry; changes in pigmentation; scaling or discharge from the nipple, and dilated veins or edema of the skin in a nonpregnant patient. The location, size, consistency, tenderness, and mobility of the palpable tumor should be recorded. It is useful to draw and photograph the projection of any suspect or palpable masses on the skin of the breast or nodal areas.

In addition to examination of the breast, careful evaluation of the axilla and supraclavicular node areas is mandatory. The number, consistency, tenderness, mobility or fixation, and size of lymph nodes should be noted. Clinically node-negative patients have pathologic involvement in 10% to 40% of cases (depending on primary tumor size), whereas no pathologic evidence of tumor is found in 25% to 30% of patients with clinically palpable axillary nodes.

Examination of the abdomen for liver enlargement and evaluation for bony pain are also essential. Finally, a complete pelvic examination should be part of the overall evaluation of the patient, if not recently performed by the patient's other physicians.

Laboratory studies include a complete blood count and chemistry profile, including liver function tests (e.g., aspartate aminotransferase, alanine aminotransferase, lactate dehydrogenase, bilirubin).

Imaging in Breast Cancer Diagnosis and Workup

Routine radiographic studies include chest radiography and bilateral mammograms. As clinically indicated, these may be supplemented by CT scanning, MRI, or positron emission tomography (PET) scans, bone scans, and plain radiographs of *symptomatic* bones, if clinically warranted.

TABLE 59.9 AMERICAN COLLEGE OF RADIOLOGY BIRADS ASSESSMENT CATEGORIES: MAMMOGRAPHY

Complete Final Assessment Categories

Category 1 Negative	There is nothing to comment on. The breasts are symmetric, and no masses, architectural disturbances, or suspect calcifications are present.
Category 2 Benign finding	This is also a negative mammogram, but the interpreter may wish to describe a finding. Involuting, calcified fibroadenomas, multiple secretory calcifications, fat-containing lesions such as oil cysts, lipomas, galactoceles, and mixed-density hamartomas all have characteristic appearances and may be labeled with confidence. The interpreter might wish to describe intramammary lymph nodes, implants, and the like while still concluding that there is no mammographic evidence of malignancy.
Category 3 Probably benign finding—short-interval follow-up suggested	A finding placed in this category should have a very high probability of being benign. It is not expected to change over the follow-up interval, but the radiologist would prefer to establish its stability. Data are becoming available that shed light on the efficacy of short-interval follow-up. At present, most approaches are intuitive. These will likely undergo future modification as more data accrue as to the validity of an approach, the interval required, and the type of findings that should be followed.
Category 4 Suspicious abnormality—biopsy should be considered	These are lesions that do not have the characteristic morphologies of breast cancer but have a definite probability of being malignant. The radiologist has sufficient concern to urge a biopsy. If possible, the relevant probabilities should be cited so that the patient and her physician can make the decision on the ultimate course of action.
Category 5 Highly suggestive of malignancy—appropriate action should be taken	These lesions have a high probability of being cancer.
Category 0 Need additional imaging evaluation	Finding for which additional imaging evaluation is needed. This is almost always used in a screening situation and should rarely be used after a full imaging workup. A recommendation for additional imaging evaluation includes the use of spot compression, magnification, special mammographic views, ultrasound, and so forth.

From ACR Bi-RADS® Assessment Categories: Mammography, Bi-RADS® and Digital Mammo QC, 3rd ed., 1998. Reprinted with permission of the American College of Radiology. No other representation of this material is authorized without expressed, written permission from the American College of Radiology.

Mammography

Mammography remains the most critical component of diagnostic imaging in breast cancer patients, and bilateral mammograms should be performed routinely in the workup of the breast cancer patient. The BIRADS (Breast Imaging Reporting and Data System) classification system, outlined in Table 59.9, has been widely adopted in classifying mammograms with respect to appropriate follow-up and intervention.[156]

The radiation oncologist should be familiar with the difference between diagnostic and screening mammography, because a majority of conservatively treated breast cancer patients will have undergone diagnostic mammography prior to treatment, as well as in follow-up. Screening mammography refers to routine mammographic images in asymptomatic women and consists of two views: craniocaudal and mediolateral oblique of each breast. Diagnostic mammography is used to characterize abnormalities detected at screening or in women with palpable masses, employs additional magnification views, and is generally done with the radiologist present to determine the need for additional views or follow-up studies. Following breast conservation, most patients will undergo diagnostic mammograms, as additional images are often needed to rule out suspicious findings in the previously radiated breast. Some mammographers recommend reverting to screening studies after several years of stable mammography in the conservatively managed breast cancer patient.

Classically, breast carcinoma is seen as an ill-defined mass that may have spiculated margins (Fig. 59.7), although rarely cancers may also be seen with a knobby, lobulated, or even a smooth contour (ultrasonography may distinguish them from cystic masses). Architectural distortion of the breast tissue may be present. The appearance of linear, radiated, or spiculated changes around a central focus should always be considered suspect for carcinoma. The tumor may be hidden by dense parenchyma; review of previous mammogram compression views and sometimes ultrasonograms is very important in detecting subtle interval changes in the appearance of the breast.[113]

Calcifications can be associated with either benign or malignant conditions of the breast. However, calcifications associated with malignant tumors are typically 100 to 300 μm in size and are rodlike, tubular, branching, or punctate. Clusters of microcalcifications (more than five) are suggestive of intraductal disease, and in nonpalpable lesions, needle localization aids in the diagnosis (Fig. 59.8). For patients undergoing biopsy of a suspicious mass or calcifications, about 30% will yield a diagnosis of malignancy.[113] The average sensitivity of mammography is approximately 90% (60% to 95%), and the specificity is 94% (50% to 98%). The positive predictive value is approximately 8% to 14% for screened patients but is significantly higher for patients with symptoms or palpable masses.[157] If microcalcifications were initially present, radiographs of the surgical specimen and postlumpectomy mammography are important to rule out residual disease for patients considering breast conservation therapy.[158]

Ultrasound

Ultrasound can be a useful tool to complement physical examination and mammography in the diagnosis and treatment of breast cancer. Its use as a screening tool is limited and is the focus of ongoing investigations, as previously noted. Ultrasonography has a reported sensitivity of 73% and specificity of 95%. It is very helpful in differentiating cysts from solid tumors, and its primary use is the identification and characterization of palpable and nonpalpable abnormalities of the breast detected by physical examination or mammography.[113,159] In the evaluation of a palpable mass in 420 patients, if both mammography and ultrasound are negative, Soo et al.[160] reported the negative predictive value to be >99%. This was confirmed in a larger study of 3,516 patients from the Netherlands reported by Flobbe et al.[161]

In addition to complementing physical examination and mammography in diagnosis, ultrasound is often used as a guide for interventional procedures. Ultrasound-guided core biopsies are routinely performed in the diagnosis of breast cancer and have been shown to be more cost-effective than stereotactic biopsy. Ultrasound can also be used for fine needle aspiration biopsies, cyst aspirations, presurgical localizations, and evaluation of breast tissue surrounding implants.

Magnetic Resonance Imaging

Although controversial for routine use, the use of MRI to supplement mammography in breast cancer diagnosis and treatment is rapidly increasing (see Fig. 59.7). In a review of MRI

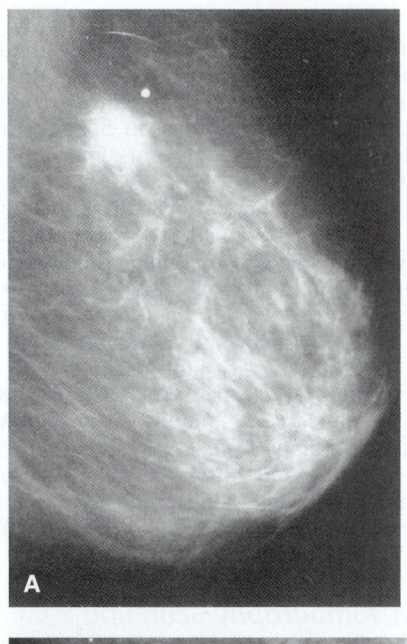

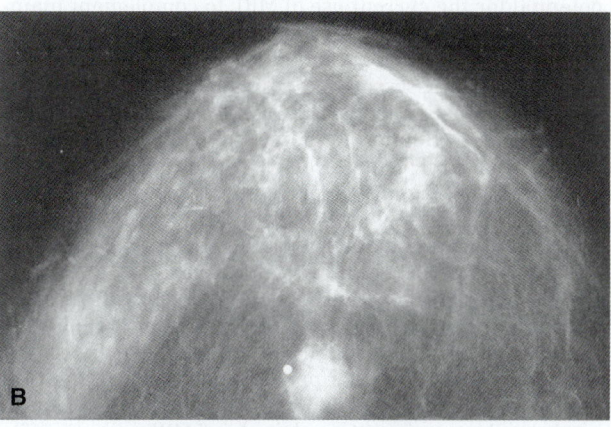

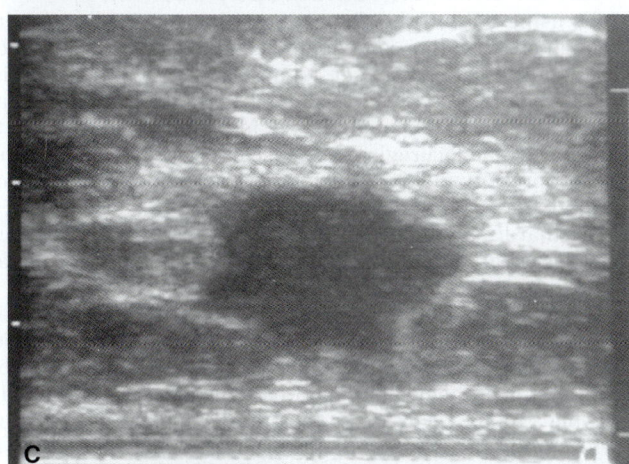

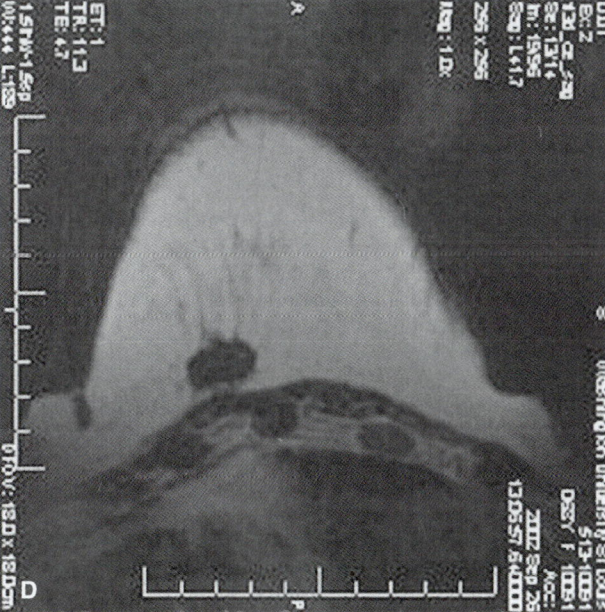

FIGURE 59.7. Mediolateral **(A)** and cephalocaudal **(B)** views of mammogram depicting a 1-cm mass with stellate margins deeply located in the upper quadrant of the left breast, histologically proven to be an IDC. Example of ultrasonogram of the breast showing a hypoechoic mass with "shadowing" deeper to the lesion, characteristic of invasive carcinoma **(C)**. T1-weighted magnetic resonance image of the breast demonstrating a mass that proved to be an invasive carcinoma **(D)**.

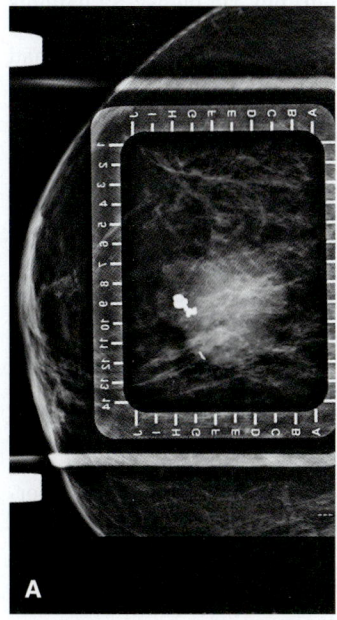

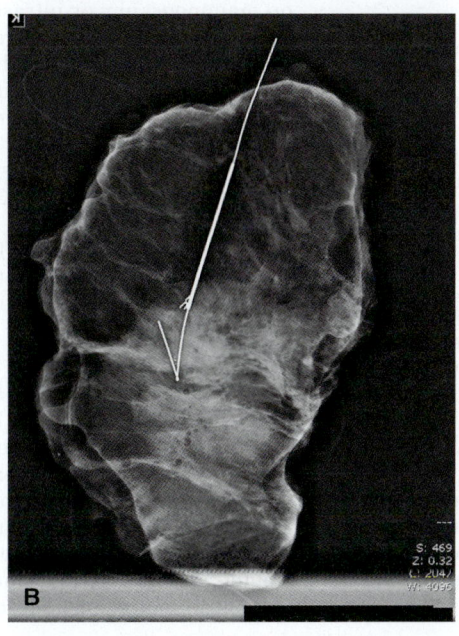

FIGURE 59.8. A: Mammogram demonstrating microcalcifications in the central portion of the breast with needle localization in place. **B:** Radiograph showing microcalcifications in the central portion of the wide excisional biopsy specimen. Pathologic diagnosis was intraductal carcinoma. Postlumpectomy mammogram showed no residual calcifications in the breast. The patient was treated with breast conservation surgery and irradiation years ago and remains tumor free.

in the management of breast cancer, Hylton[162] summarized the potential for the current use of MRI, to complement mammography in screening; for differential diagnosis of questionable findings on physical examination, mammography, and ultrasound; and for assessment of response in the neoadjuvant treatment of breast cancers. The NCCN recommends breast MRI for staging evaluation to define the extent of cancer or presence of multifocal or multicentric cancer in the ipsilateral breast or as screening of the contralateral breast at the time of initial diagnosis. They also indicate MRI would be useful for evaluation before and after neoadjuvant chemotherapy, to identify the primary cancer in women with axillary nodal carcinoma or occult primary cancer, or in patients with invasive lobular carcinoma (ILC) poorly defined on mammography[163].

In a retrospective study of MRI in the management of 441 women with breast cancer, Upponi and Warren[164] reported the indications for MRI studies were diagnostic in 176, monitoring chemotherapy in 126, and study of MRI screening for breast cancer in 139. MRI results were confusing or incorrect in 6% of the diagnostic group, 13% of the chemotherapy group, and 9% of the screening group. The authors report that MRI resulted in an increase in confidence or change in clinical plan in 46% of the diagnostic group, 72% of the chemotherapy group, and 80% of the screening group. In 44 of 283 of these, MRI caused a beneficial change in the clinical plan based on conventional radiology.

Esserman et al.[165] reported that MRI successfully detected cancer in 55 of 58 cases. There were two false-positive and two false-negative results, including a nonsignificant enhancement of one lesion. The anatomic extent of disease was correctly identified in 98% of cases by MRI but in only 55% by mammography.

MRI has a clear role in the evaluation of patients who present with axillary metastasis with no evidence of a primary tumor in the breast by physical examination or mammography. Buchanan et al.[166] reported on 55 patients who presented with axillary adenopathy without evidence of distant disease. MRI revealed suspicious lesions in 76% (42 of 55). In 62% (26 of 42), the MRI finding proved to be the occult primary tumor, of whom 58% (15 of 26) were candidates for breast conservation. MRI did not identify the primary tumor in 25 women. Of these 25, 12 underwent mastectomy, and cancer was found in 4 of these 12. The authors concluded that breast MRI detects mammographically occult cancer in half of women with axillary metastases and is a valuable tool for patients with occult primary breast cancer.

Computed Tomography

There is no established role for CT scans in routine staging of patients with early-stage breast cancer. The need for iodine contrast material to differentiate benign from malignant conditions, high radiation dose, cost per study, and inability to detect small lesions precludes the use of CT for initial evaluation, except under special circumstances. Most patients with node-negative breast cancer do not need to undergo routine CT scans for staging, because the yield is exceeding low. A small percentage of women with very high-risk node-negative disease or with node-positive disease may be upstaged by routine CT scans and, although the yield is low, it is common practice to CT stage high-risk node-negative and node-positive breast cancer patients. At present, the NCCN guidelines on breast cancer recommend an abdomino-pelvic CT if abnormal lab values on physical examination are present or if the patient is deemed as a stage IIIA (T3N1M0) or greater[163].

Many women undergoing breast-conserving surgery and radiation do have CT scans as part of RT treatment planning. Without the use of contrast and specific diagnostic imaging protocols, these scans should not be considered as part of a staging procedure.

Bone Scans

Routine bone scan at the time of initial treatment of stage I and II breast cancer is of limited value and should be reserved for patients with bone pain.[167] In patients with stage I disease, the incidence of abnormalities on bone scan is approximately 2%, but a greater incidence of abnormalities is found in stages II (10%) and III (>20%).[168] In a group of 7,604 patients who had bone scans, of over 20,000 women operated for breast cancer in Denmark, approximately 5% had abnormal study results.[169] The incidence of abnormal scan results was greater in patients older than 60 years (8%) than in the younger group (3%), most likely because of the many benign bone and joint disorders frequently seen in older women.

Koizumi et al.[170] reviewed records from 5,538 patients with breast cancer. The overall incidence of metastasis to bone was 2.13% (0% in patients with stage 0, 0.08% in stage I, 1.09% in stage II, 9.96% in stage III, and 34.04% in stage IV). Bone scans are more commonly recommended in patients with stage II larger tumors (>3 cm), aggressive histopathologic features, and in stage III or IV cancer.

Positron Emission Tomography Scanning

PET using ^{18}F-labeled fluorodeoxyglucose (FDG) scanning, though not a routine component of staging, is being used more frequently in breast cancer. Its application in patients on initial presentation with early-stage disease has not been established. However, its potential role in patients with metastatic, advanced, and locoregional relapse of disease is rapidly evolving. At present, the NCCN guidelines recommend against routine PET scans in patients with stage 0 to IIIA disease but do state that it may be useful for patients with locally advanced disease or in situations where standard imaging results are equivocal or suspicious.[105,171,172]

In an analysis of PET scanning in 165 patients from British Columbia, Weir et al.[173] concluded that there are two clinical situations in which PET appears to be particularly valuable. The first is in the evaluation of patients who are suspected of having a tumor recurrence. The other is in identifying patients with multifocal or distant sites of malignancy who otherwise appear to have an isolated, potentially curable, locoregional recurrence.

Schirrmeister et al.[174] also evaluated FDG-PET scanning and compared it prospectively with standard staging procedures within 2 weeks before surgery in 117 women who had palpable breast tumors or lesions suggestive of cancer on mammography or ultrasonography. On biopsy, 89 patients were determined to have breast cancer and 28 benign tumors. For interpreting results as being breast cancer, FDG-PET had a sensitivity of 93%, a specificity of 78%, an accuracy of 89%, a positive predictive value of 92%, and a negative predictive value of 96%. In detecting multifocal lesions, FDG-PET was twice as sensitive (63%) as the combination of mammography and ultrasonography (32%). Distant metastases in three patients were missed with the standard staging procedures but detected with FDG-PET. Because FDG-PET had a false-negative rate of 20% for detection of lymph node metastases, this imaging method cannot replace histologic evaluation of axillary nodes.

Summary of Imaging for Breast Cancer

All women should undergo history and physical examination, with mammography and liver function tests. Ultrasound or MRI may be useful in selected cases to complement mammography. For women who have operable disease with normal liver function tests, surgical staging of the breast and node sampling is performed. For low-risk patients, no further staging is required. For women with more advanced disease and those being considered for neoadjuvant chemotherapy, preoperative staging would routinely include a bone scan, chest x-ray and CT, or abdominal ultrasound. PET scanning may be considered in selected cases.

Pathologic Studies

Histopathologic diagnosis may be obtained by fine needle aspiration of cystic or solid masses or biopsies of solid masses; any fluid aspirated from the breast should be examined for malignant cells. Fine needle aspiration of the breast is a simple, low-cost, accurate diagnostic technique that has been used for many years in Europe and is gaining increasing acceptance in the United States.[175,176] A potential limitation of fine needle aspiration is that it provides cytology and no tissue architecture. Therefore, while the presence of malignant cells can be detected, cytology from fine needle aspiration cannot conclusively differentiate invasive from noninvasive disease. However, for lesions that are palpable or easily visualized on ultrasound, this method results in rapid and efficient diagnosis.

Stereotactic core needle biopsy is increasingly used to obtain a histologic diagnosis with high accuracy, particularly in small breast lesions.[177] In 6,152 lesions sampled at multiple institutions, 817 (13.3%) showed infiltrating breast cancer, 167 (2.7%) showed intermediate or high-grade DCIS, and 213 (3.5%) showed atypical hyperplasia or low-grade DCIS. Complete agreement between the core biopsy and subsequent histologic sections was reached in 89.7% of lesions and partial agreement in 9.2%. Clinically significant complications occurred in only 6 of 3,765 cases (0.2%) for which follow-up was available.

Breast biopsy of any suspicious mass is mandatory. The biopsy usually can be done using local anesthesia; the patient should be informed of the nature of the lesion to allow for her greater participation in therapeutic decisions. There has been no evidence that delay in treatment up to 2 weeks after biopsy worsens prognosis.[178]

In nonpalpable lesions, needle localization and radiographic techniques are necessary to identify the tissue to be removed. Failure to remove the mammographic abnormality has been reported in 2% to 8% of patients undergoing needle localization.[179] The localizing wires should be left in place in the specimen and a radiograph obtained to ensure that the area of abnormality has been adequately excised. If the specimen radiograph does not document complete tumor removal, an immediate re-excision of the area at the tip of the wire should be carried out. However, specimen mammography may be of questionable benefit in the management or outcome of most patients undergoing image-guided, needle-localized breast biopsies. Bimston et al.[180] reviewed 164 patients who underwent 165 needle/dye-localized breast biopsies for suspect mammographic abnormalities. In only three (1.8%) cases did the patient clearly benefit from specimen mammography; in no patient was a malignant neoplasm missed.

If there is any question, particularly in patients with microcalcifications, a postbiopsy mammogram should be obtained to determine the completeness of tumor excision.[113] The surgeon should prepare (orient) the specimen accordingly, and the margins of the resected breast tissue should be identified and inked before processing. The pathologist should be made aware of the nature of the lesion for appropriate processing of the specimen.[181] Radiation oncologists should be familiar with the implications of the diagnostic procedures for carcinoma of the breast as active participants in a breast preservation therapeutic approach.

In the United States, estrogen-receptor (ER) and progesterone-receptor (PR) assays are routinely done for patients with breast cancer; these parameters are correlated with prognosis and tumor response to chemotherapeutic and hormonal agents.[182,183] Immunohistochemical techniques are commonly employed and correlate well with other hormonal-receptor assays. Cellular assays measure the growth fraction (S-phase fraction [SPF]) of tumors, either by thymidine-labeling index (TLI) or flow cytometry methods, and other tumor markers have prognostic implications, sometimes independent of tumor stage and hormone-receptor status.[184,185] HER-2/neu assay is being done routinely because overexpression is associated with poor prognosis, and these patients are currently being offered adjuvant therapy directed at HER2/neu.[186,187] HER2/neu analysis by fluorescent in situ hybridization (FISH) techniques has evolved as the standard for determining response to therapy directed at the HER2/neu oncogene.[186,187]

Staging

Two staging systems are widely used for breast cancer: the American Joint Committee on Cancer (AJCC) (Table 59.10) and the Union Internationale Contre le Cancer systems.[188,189] Major changes made in the eighth edition of the *AJCC Cancer Staging Manual* include the following[190]:

- The inclusion of 2 stage grouping systems: The anatomic stage group table is based solely on anatomic extent of cancer as defined by the T, N, and M categories. The prognostic stage group table is based on populations of persons with breast cancer that have been offered—and mostly treated with appropriate endocrine and/or systemic chemotherapy, which includes anatomic T, N, and M plus tumor grade and the status of the biomarkers human epidermal growth factor receptor 2 (HER2), estrogen receptor (ER), and progesterone receptor (PR).
- LCIS is removed as a pathologic tumor *in situ* (pTis) category for T categorization. LCIS is a benign entity and is removed from TNM staging.
- The general rules for rounding to the nearest millimeter do not apply for tumors between 1.0 and 1.5 mm, so that these cancers are not classified as microinvasive (T1mi) carcinomas (defined as invasive tumor foci 1.0 mm or smaller). Tumors > 1 mm and < 2 mm should be reported rounding to 2 mm.

The T categorization of multiple synchronous tumors is identified clinically and/or by macroscopic pathologic examination, and their presence is documented using the (m) modifier for the T category. The Columbia staging system is important both historically and because it clearly identifies prognostic factors affecting operability.[62] Figure 59.9 depicts the various clinical stages according to tumor and nodal characteristics.

Pathologic Classification

The World Health Organization (WHO) has classified proliferative conditions and tumors of the breast into the following categories: benign mammary dysplasias, benign or apparently benign tumors, carcinoma, sarcoma, carcinosarcoma, and unclassified tumors.[191] The AJCC has adopted the WHO classification of tumors as shown in Table 59.11.[188]

Numerous detailed reports and monographs describe the pathologic features and clinical implications of carcinoma of the breast, which are reviewed elsewhere.[113,192–195] The radiation oncologist should be familiar with the histologic characteristics of breast cancer because many of them affect prognosis and may have important therapeutic implications. Brief descriptions of several types of carcinoma of the breast follow.

Microinvasive carcinoma is defined as "the extension of cancer cells beyond the basement membrane into the adjacent tissues with no focus more than 0.1 cm in greatest dimension."

TABLE 59.10 AMERICAN JOINT COMMITTEE ON CANCER STAGING OF BREAST CANCER

Primary Tumor (T)

Definitions for classifying the primary tumor (T) are the same for clinical and for pathologic classification. If the measurement is made by physical examination, the examiner will use the major headings (T1, T2, or T3). If other measurements, such as mammographic or pathologic measurements, are used, the subsets of T1 can be used. Tumors should be measured to the nearest 0.1-cm increment.

TX	Primary tumor cannot be assessed
T0	No evidence of primary tumor
Tis	Carcinoma *in situ*
Tis (DCIS)	Ductal carcinoma *in situ*
Tis (Paget's)	Paget disease of the nipple with no tumor

Note: Paget disease associated with a tumor is classified according to the size of the tumor.

T1	Tumor ≤20 mm in greatest dimension
T1mic	Tumor ≤1 mm in greatest dimension
T1a	Tumor >1 mm but ≤5 mm in greatest dimension
T1b	Tumor >5 mm but ≤10 mm in greatest dimension
T1c	Tumor >10 mm but ≤20 mm in greatest dimension
T2	Tumor >20 mm but ≤50 mm in greatest dimension
T3	Tumor >50 mm in greatest dimension
T4	Tumor of any size with direct extension to the chest wall and/or to the skin (ulceration or macroscopic nodules); invasion of the dermis alone does not qualify as T4
T4a	Extension to the chest wall; invasion or adherence to pectoralis muscle in the absence of invasion of chest wall structures does not qualify as T4
T4b	Ulceration and/or ipsilateral macroscopic satellite nodules and/or edema (including peau d'orange) of the skin that does not meet the criteria for inflammatory carcinoma
T4c	Both (T4a and T4b)
T4d	Inflammatory carcinoma

Regional Lymph Nodes (N)

NX	Regional lymph nodes cannot be assessed (e.g., previously removed)
N0	No regional lymph node metastasis
N1	Metastasis to movable ipsilateral axillary lymph node(s)
N2	Metastasis to ipsilateral axillary lymph node(s) fixed or matted or in clinically apparent[a] ipsilateral internal mammary nodes in the absence of clinically evident axillary lymph node metastasis
N2a	Metastasis in ipsilateral axillary lymph nodes fixed to one another (matted) or to other structures
N2b	Metastasis only in clinically apparent[a] ipsilateral internal mammary nodes and in the absence of clinically evident axillary lymph node metastasis
N3	Metastasis to ipsilateral mammary lymph node(s) with or without axillary lymph node involvement or in clinically apparent[a] ipsilateral internal mammary lymph node(s) and in the presence of clinically evident axillary lymph node metastasis; or metastasis in ipsilateral supraclavicular lymph node(s) with or without axillary or internal mammary lymph node involvement
N3a	Metastasis in ipsilateral infraclavicular lymph node(s)
N3b	Metastasis in ipsilateral internal mammary lymph node(s) and axillary lymph node(s)
N3c	Metastasis in ipsilateral supraclavicular lymph node(s)

Pathologic Classification (*p*N)

*p*NX	Regional lymph nodes cannot be assessed (e.g., previously removed or not removed for pathologic study)
*P*N0	No regional lymph node metastasis histologically, no additional examination for isolated tumor cells (ITC)

Note: ITC are defined as single tumor cells or small cell clusters not >0.2 mm, usually detected only by immunohistochemical (IHC) or molecular methods but which may be verified on hematoxylin and eosin stains. ITCs do not usually show evidence of malignant activity (e.g., proliferation or stromal reaction).

p N0(i−)	No regional lymph node metastasis histologically, negative IHC
p N0(i+)	No regional lymph node metastasis histologically, positive IHC, IHC cluster no >0.2 mm
p N0(mol−)	No regional lymph node metastasis histologically, negative molecular findings [reverse transcriptase polymerase chain reaction (RT-PCR)]
p N0(mol+)	No regional lymph node metastasis histologically, positive molecular findings (RT-PCR)
p N1	Metastasis in 1 to 3 axillary lymph nodes and/or in internal mammary nodes with microscopic disease detected by sentinel lymph node dissection but not clinically apparent[b]
p N1mi	Micrometastasis (approximately 200 cells, >0.2 mm, none larger than 2.0 mm)
p N1a	Metastasis in 1 to 3 axillary lymph nodes, one larger than 2.0 mm
p N1b	Metastasis in internal mammary nodes with microscopic disease detected by sentinel node dissection but not clinically apparent[c]
p N1c	pN1a and pN1b combined
p N2	Metastasis in 4–9 axillary lymph nodes or in clinically apparent[b] internal mammary lymph nodes in the absence of axillary lymph node metastasis
p N2a	Metastasis in 4 to 9 axillary lymph nodes (at least one tumor deposit >2.0 mm)
p N2b	Metastasis in clinically apparent[b] internal mammary lymph nodes in the absence of axillary lymph node metastasis
p N3	Metastasis in 10 or more axillary lymph nodes, or in infraclavicular lymph nodes, or in clinically apparent[b] ipsilateral internal mammary lymph nodes in the presence of 1 or more positive axillary lymph nodes; or in more than 3 axillary lymph nodes with clinically negative microscopic metastasis in internal mammary lymph nodes or in ipsilateral supraclavicular lymph nodes
p N3a	Metastasis in 10 or more axillary lymph nodes (at least one tumor deposit >2.0 mm) or metastasis to the infraclavicular lymph nodes
p N3b	Metastasis in clinically apparent[b] ipsilateral internal mammary lymph nodes in the presence of 1 or more positive axillary lymph nodes or in more than 3 axillary lymph nodes and in internal mammary lymph nodes with microscopic disease detected by sentinel lymph node dissection but not clinically apparent[c]
p N3c	Metastasis in ipsilateral supraclavicular lymph nodes

Distant Metastasis (M)

M0	No distant metastasis
cM0(i+)	No clinical or radiographic evidence of distant metastases in the presence of tumor cells or and no deposits no >0.2 mm detected microscopically or by using molecular techniques in circulating blood, bone marrow, or other nonregional lymph node tissue in a patient without symptoms or signs of metastases
M1	Distant metastases detected by clinical and radiographic means (cM) and/or histologically proven metastases larger than 0.2 mm (pM)

[a]Clinically apparent is defined as detected by imaging studies (excluding lymphoscintigraphy) or by clinical examination or grossly visible pathologically.
[b]Clinically apparent is defined as detected by imaging studies (excluding lymphoscintigraphy) or by clinical examination.
[c]Not clinically apparent is defined as not detected by imaging studies (excluding lymphoscintigraphy) or by clinical breast.

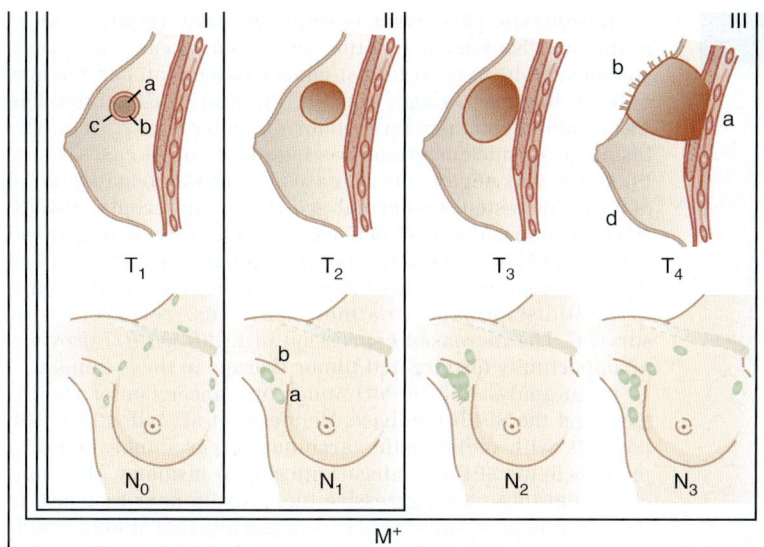

FIGURE 59.9. Clinical staging of carcinoma of the breast. Stages, in part, reflect curability by locoregional treatment modalities prognostically (surgery and radiation therapy). The equivalence of T and N categories are as follows: T2 = N1, T3 = N2, T4 = N3. The American Joint Committee on Cancer and Union Internationale Contre le Cancer classification systems use similar categories and stages. (Reprinted from Langmuir VK, Poulter CA, Qazi R, et al. Breast cancer. In: Rubin P, ed. *Clinical oncology: a multidisciplinary approach for physicians and students.* 7th ed. Philadelphia, PA: WB Saunders, 1993. Copyright © 1993 Elsevier. With permission.)

Lesions that fulfill this definition are staged as T1mic, a subset of T1 breast cancer. The AJCC staging manual further states that "when there are multiple foci of microinvasion, the size of only the largest focus is used to classify the microinvasion" and that the sizes of the individual foci should not be added together. They also state that "the prognosis of microinvasive carcinoma is generally thought to be quite favorable, although the clinical impact of multifocal microinvasive disease is not well understood at this time." Widely varying definitions of microinvasion have been used, and some differ substantially from that offered here.[188]

Invasive (infiltrating) ductal carcinoma is the most common type of breast cancer, constituting more than 50% of all cases. It appears as solid cords or groups of ductal tumor cells varying in size and cytoplasmic content and degree of differentiation.[196] Necrosis is rare, but lymphatic invasion may be present. An associated *in situ* component is frequently seen.

Tubular carcinoma is composed of tubular structures typically lined by a single layer of well-differentiated epithelium. The tubular cells simulate those of normal ducts or ductules, are arranged in multiglandular cribriform or adenocystic configurations, and are frequently associated with other *in situ* carcinomas of the breast.[197] Tubular carcinomas have a nonaggressive growth pattern, with an excellent prognosis. A meta-analysis of 680 women showed an overall frequency of nodal metastasis of 13.8%.[198] In view of the low incidence of axillary node metastases at presentation (7%) in low-risk tubular carcinoma of the breast (≤1 cm), some have advocated that axillary dissection may be omitted. In a retrospective review of 73 cases of tubular carcinoma, Sullivan et al.[199] reported treatment with conservative surgery (CS) plus radiation therapy (RT) in 67%, CS without RT in 18%, and mastectomy in 15%. The published literature of 529 conservatively treated tubular carcinomas was reviewed along with the 62 conservative cases from their series. No patients developed distant metastasis or died from disease. Local failure occurred in three (4%) of the cases. The literature review showed that adjuvant RT reduces local failure following CS for tubular carcinoma.

Medullary carcinoma is composed of cords and masses of large cells with reticular pleomorphic nuclei containing prominent nucleoli. There is a scant fibrous stroma, but lymphoid infiltrate is prominent. These tumors are microscopically and grossly well circumscribed. Prognosis, in general, is better than for other tumors. These tumors are more frequently seen in younger women and are commonly associated with patients with *BRCA1* mutations.[200]

Lobular invasive carcinoma may be interspersed with; the cells appear singly or in small clusters in a targetoid or single-file pattern. Some scirrhous carcinomas probably are invasive lobular lesions; these tumors tend to be aggressive and multicentric and are prone to development of distant metastases. Du Toit et al.[201] reported five subtypes of lobular carcinomas in 171 cases and observed a 12-year actuarial survival rate of 100% for the tubulolobular subtype but only 47% for the solid variant. Two other characteristics of ILC is that it is often "mammographically silent," meaning its detection or the full appreciation of extent of disease is often not visualized mammographically. Invasive lobular cancers are much more commonly ER positive than is invasive ductal carcinoma (IDC). Infiltrating pleomorphic lobular carcinoma, an aggressive variant of ILC, was described in 38 cases; 29% of the specimens demonstrated signet ring cells.[202]

Mucinous carcinoma, also called mucoid or colloid carcinoma, has been observed in older women with relatively long duration of symptoms.[203] It is more likely to be devoid of a cellular reaction; necrosis and lymphatic invasion are very rare. It is slowly growing with a pushing border and has a low frequency of axillary lymph node metastasis. Survival is appreciably better than with IDC.[204] Anan et al.[205] evaluated 76 patients with mucinous carcinoma (52 pure type and 24 mixed type). The incidence of lymphatic vessel invasion (4%) and nodal involvement (4%) was lower in pure mucinous carcinoma than in mixed carcinoma ($P < .05$). No nodal involvement occurred in patients with pure mucinous carcinoma <3 cm in diameter.

Adenocystic carcinoma is rarely found in the breast. Histologic features and clinical behavior are similar to its counterpart in the salivary gland and the upper respiratory tract.[206] In 28 patients, only 1 had axillary node metastases; 22 were treated with mastectomy and 6 with local excision (with breast irradiation in 5). With a median follow-up of 7 years, there were no local recurrences; the 5-year disease-free survival rate was 95%.[207]

Invasive micropapillary carcinoma of the breast is characterized by growth of tumor cell clusters in prominent clear spaces resembling dilated angiolymphatic vessels. Nassar et al.[208] reported on 83 invasive micropapillary carcinomas; the mean tumor size was 4 cm, 22% invaded skin, 58% were poorly differentiated, and 71% were ER positive. Axillary node metastases were present in 77% of cases and were typically multiple (51% had three or more positive). Forty-six percent of the patients died from their disease (mean interval to death, 36 months). Skin involvement and nodal status were the only parameters predictive of poor survival ($P = .01$).

Section III

TABLE 59.11 AMERICAN JOINT COMMITTEE ON CANCER HISTOPATHOLOGIC CLASSIFICATION OF BREAST TUMORS

Type

Precursor lesions
  Ductal carcinoma *in situ*
  Lobular neoplasia
    Lobular carcinoma *in situ*
      Classic lobular carcinoma *in situ*
      Pleomorphic lobular carcinoma *in situ*
    Atypical lobular hyperplasia
Intraductal proliferative lesions
  Usual ductal hyperplasia
  Columnar cell lesions including flat epithelial atypia
  Atypical ductal hyperplasia
Papillary lesions
  Intraductal papilloma
    Intraductal papilloma with atypical hyperplasia
    Intraductal papilloma with ductal carcinoma *in situ*
    Intraductal papilloma with lobular carcinoma *in situ*
  Intraductal papillary carcinoma
  Encapsulated papillary carcinoma
    Encapsulated papillary carcinoma with invasion
  Solid papillary carcinoma
    In situ
    Invasive
Invasive carcinoma of no special type (NST)
  Pleomorphic carcinoma
  Carcinoma with osteoclast-like stromal giant cells
  Carcinoma with choriocarcinomatous features
  Carcinoma with melanotic features
Invasive lobular carcinoma
  Classic lobular carcinoma
  Solid lobular carcinoma
  Alveolar lobular carcinoma
  Pleomorphic lobular carcinoma
  Tubulolobular carcinoma
  Mixed lobular carcinoma
Tubular carcinoma
Cribriform carcinoma
Mucinous carcinoma
Carcinoma with medullary features
  Medullary carcinoma
  Atypical medullary carcinoma
  Invasive carcinoma NST with medullary features
Carcinoma with apocrine differentiation
Carcinoma with signet-ring-cell differentiation
Invasive micropapillary carcinoma
Metaplastic carcinoma of no special type
  Low-grade adenosquamous carcinoma
  Fibromatosis-like metaplastic carcinoma
  Squamous cell carcinoma
  Spindle cell carcinoma
  Metaplastic carcinoma with mesenchymal
    differentiation
      Chondroid differentiation
      Osseous differentiation
      Other types of mesenchymal differentiation
  Mixed metaplastic carcinoma
  Myoepithelial carcinoma
Epithelial–myoepithelial tumors
Adenomyoepithelioma with carcinoma
Adenoid cystic carcinoma
Rare types
Carcinoma with neuroendocrine features
  Neuroendocrine tumor, well differentiated
  Neuroendocrine carcinoma poorly differentiated (small cell carcinoma)
  Carcinoma with neuroendocrine differentiation
Secretory carcinoma
Invasive papillary carcinoma
Acinic cell carcinoma
Mucoepidermoid carcinoma
Polymorphous carcinoma
Oncocytic carcinoma
Lipid-rich carcinoma
Glycogen-rich clear cell carcinoma
Sebaceous carcinoma

From Amin MB, Edge SB, Greene FL, et al., eds. *AJCC cancer staging manual.* 8th ed. New York: Springer, 2017. Reproduced with permission of Springer International Publishing in the format Book via Copyright Clearance Center.

Metaplastic carcinoma is relatively rare. Beatty et al.,[209] of the Swedish Cancer Institute, identified 24 cases that were compared with typical breast cancer cases matched for age; date of diagnosis; stage; and ER, PR, and *HER2* status. The mean metaplastic primary tumor diameter was 2.5 cm. The histologic or nuclear grade was high in 21 of 24 cases. ER or PR status was negative in all cases. *HER2* was negative in 10 of 11 cases tested. Epidermal growth factor receptor (EGFR; *HER1*) was positive in 7 of 7 cases tested. Five-year survival was 83% (95% CI, 66% to 100%). Comparison with matched typical breast cancer cases revealed no significant difference in multidisciplinary treatment patterns, recurrence, or survival. The increased expression of EGFR (*HER1*) provides an opportunity for targeted tumor therapy in these tumors.

In an analysis of the MD Anderson Cancer Center experience and the SEER database, Hennessy et al.[210] identified 100 patients with metaplastic sarcomatoid carcinoma and 213 patients in the SEER database with similar histology. They conclude that these are aggressive tumors with poor response to therapy and poor outcomes, also suggesting that studies evaluating novel targeted therapy are needed for these patients.

Spindle cell carcinoma of the breast, a variant of metaplastic carcinoma, includes a wide spectrum of lesions with mildly atypical features that may resemble fasciitis, fibromatosis, or myofibroblastic tumors. Unlike spindle cell carcinomas in general, they have no propensity for distant metastasis and should be termed *tumors* rather than *carcinomas*. Sneige et al.[211] studied 24 cases of fibromatosis-like spindle cell breast carcinoma. Treatment consisted of local excision (7 cases) or modified radical mastectomy (13 cases) and was not specified in 4 cases. In patients who underwent axillary nodal dissection, no lymph node metastases were found. Local recurrences developed in two of the six patients who underwent local excision only.

Primary neuroendocrine small cell carcinoma is uncommon. Francois et al.[212] reported seven cases, and Shin et al.[213] described nine cases. Immunohistochemical analysis showed consistent staining for cytokeratin markers but variable staining with neuroendocrine markers. The histologic type and prognosis are identical to those of lung cancer. It is important to distinguish these lesions from metastatic lung tumors or direct invasion of breast by Merkel cell carcinoma, lymphoma, or carcinoid tumor. It is reasonable to treat these patients with aggressive multiagent chemotherapy, excision of the primary tumor, and breast irradiation, although no data are available on the outcome of this approach.

Paget disease describes involvement of the nipple by tumor. Most investigators agree that it represents extension of neoplasms from subjacent ducts in the nipple or metastases from an underlying carcinoma.[1] The tumor seems to travel linearly down the ducts and may appear to be multicentric. There may be an associated subareolar tumor. Breast-conserving surgery followed by radiation is effective in this disease.[214,215]

Cystosarcoma phyllodes is usually a benign lesion; in broad, fibrous beads that look "leaflike" are cystic clefts lined by a single layer of cells. These tumors are large; usually, they are encapsulated, without invasion of the adjacent breast.[62] The lesions frequently develop from preexisting fibromas and have a long initial period of slow growth followed by a sudden, rapid increase in size. The grade (mitotic rate), surgical margins, and proliferative index have prognostic importance.[216]

Primary mammary lymphomas are rare and constitute approximately 0.5% of breast malignancies and approximately 1% of all non-Hodgkin lymphomas (NHL). Diffuse large B-cell lymphoma (DLBCL) is the most common histologic subtype of PBL (50% to 80%). The indolent histologic subtypes of marginal zone lymphoma (10% to 30%) and follicular lymphoma (10% to 20%) are the next most frequent. Burkitt lymphoma (typically in pregnancy or lactation) constitutes approximately 5%, with the recently described entity of breast implant–associated anaplastic large cell lymphoma (BIA-ALCL) making up an increasing proportion of the remaining cases.[217]

Sarcoma

Primary breast sarcomas are occasionally seen. McGowan et al.[218] described 78 cases of primary breast sarcoma without metastatic disease (76 women, 2 men); 32 patients had malignant cystosarcoma phyllodes, and the others had stromal sarcomas (14 patients), angiosarcomas (8 patients), fibrosarcomas (7 patients), carcinosarcomas (5 patients), liposarcomas (4 patients), or other lesions (8 patients). The cause-specific survival rate was 48%, the relapse-free rate was 42%, and the local relapse-free rate was 75% at 10 years. No statistically significant difference in outcome was noted between those treated with conservation surgery and those undergoing mastectomy. Patients with negative margins had a significantly better local relapse-free rate than did those with positive margins (80% vs. 33%; P = .009).

PROGNOSTIC FACTORS FOR SURVIVAL AND METASTASIS

Carcinoma of the breast represents a wide spectrum of tumors with a variety of clinical, biologic, and genetic characteristics resulting in a considerable variation in prognosis. It is important to understand, particularly from the radiation oncologists' perspective, that prognostic factors for systemic relapses and prognostic factors for local relapse differ significantly. Furthermore, prognostic factors for local relapse after mastectomy differ substantially from prognostic factors for local relapse after lumpectomy and radiation.[219] For example, tumor size and nodal status are clearly among the strongest predictors of overall survival and metastasis and are also strong predictors of postmastectomy chest wall relapse when radiation is not used.[113,220,221] However, these factors have not been consistently reported to be prognostic for an in-breast relapse after cancer surgery. On the other hand, margin status is a strong predictor of relapse in the conservatively treated breast but is not strongly correlated with distant metastasis.[222–224] Young age is also a very strong predictor of local relapse after breast-conserving therapy, and although it has been shown to be predictive of systemic metastasis, the effect of young age on distant metastasis as an independent factor is clearly not as significant as it is for local relapse in the conservatively managed patient.[225] Patients, as well as clinicians, often become confused regarding these issues, resulting in misconceptions regarding appropriate decision-making and treatment. Below, prognostic factors for systemic relapse (i.e., distant metastasis and disease-free and overall survival) are discussed. A more in-depth discussion of prognostic factors for local relapse following lumpectomy and radiation is included later in the section on selection factors for the conservative management of breast cancer. Prognostic factors related to postmastectomy chest wall recurrence for patients with early-stage disease are discussed in Chapter 57.

Tumor Size

The size of the primary tumor ranks among the strongest predictors of distant metastasis and disease-free and overall survival. Although tumor size correlates strongly with the presence and number of involved axillary lymph nodes, it is clearly an independent prognostic factor. Among patients with documented node-negative disease, tumor size remains a strong and independent predictor of disease-free and overall survival. In a classic study with over 20 years of follow-up, Rosen et al.[192] reported a recurrence-free survival of 88% for tumors <1 cm, 72% for tumors 1.1 to 3.0 cm, and 59% for tumors 3.1 to 5.0 cm. In an analysis of 826 women with node-negative breast cancer treated by mastectomy at the University of Chicago with a median follow-up of 13.5 years, Quiet et al.[226] reported a 20-year disease-free survival of 79% for patients with tumors <2 cm, compared with 64% with

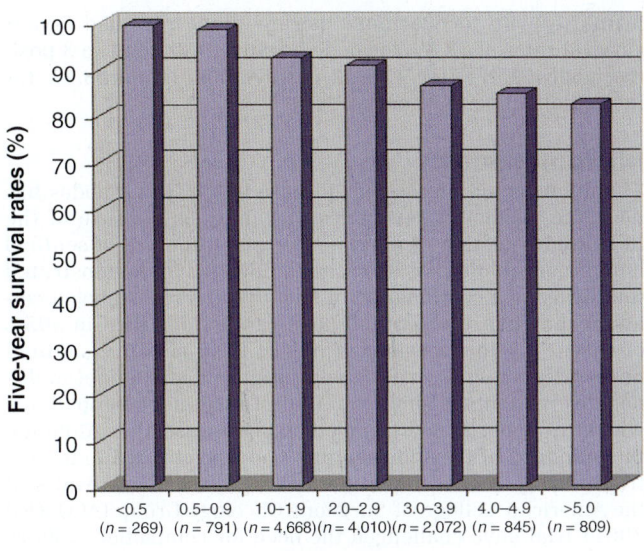

FIGURE 59.10. Five-year survival according to tumor size in node-negative breast cancers. (Data adapted from Carter CL, Allen C, Henson DE. Relation of tumor size, lymph node status and survival in 24,740 breast cancer cases. *Cancer* 1989;63:181–187.)

tumors >2 cm. In multivariate analysis, the strongest predictor of outcome and time to relapse was pathologic tumor size. Survival as a function of primary tumor size in node-negative breast cancer patients is illustrated in Figure 59.10.

Axillary Nodal Status

Of all prognostic factors, nodal status continues to be the strongest predictor of disease-free and overall survival and is the primary factor that governs breast cancer staging (Fig. 59.11).[188] Although there is a direct relation between the number of axillary nodes involved and the risk of distant metastasis, the most commonly employed schema is to group patients into four prognostic categories (node negative, 1 to 3 involved nodes, 4 to 9 involved nodes, and more than 10 involved nodes). These nodal prognostic categories are employed in the N staging of the current AJCC staging system. Although outcomes will continually improve as systemic therapies advance, data from previous NSABP trials treated

FIGURE 59.11. Five-year survival according to tumor size and nodal status. (Data adapted from Carter CL, Allen C, Henson DE. Relation of tumor size, lymph node status and survival in 24,740 breast cancer cases. *Cancer* 1989;63:181–187.)

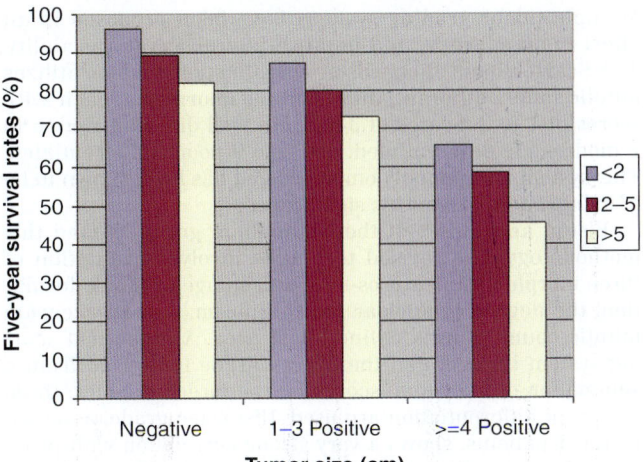

primarily with locoregional therapy alone revealed 5-year survival rates of 82.8% for node negative, 73% for 1 to 3 positive nodes, 45.7% for 4 to 12 positive nodes, and 28.4% for more than 13 positive nodes.[71,178,227–229]

Micrometastasis

The influence of microscopic disease in the lymph nodes has been the subject of several recent analyses because of the increased detection of micrometastasis in the era of sentinel lymph node biopsy. Most recent studies have demonstrated that by using a combination of blue dye and radiolabeled colloid techniques, the sentinel node can be identified in >95% of cases.[230–232] In experienced hands, false-negative sentinel node rates are low (<10%), and prognosis of sentinel node–negative patients is similar to that of node-negative patients who have undergone a complete axillary dissection. Although the standard of care for sentinel node–positive patients has traditionally been completion axillary dissection, results of the American College of Surgeons Oncology Group (ACOSOG) Z0011 trial have challenged the need for completion axillary dissection in selected sentinel node–positive patients.[233] The need for axillary dissection in node-positive patients will likely continue to be highly individualized and will be further evaluated in ongoing clinical trials.[234]

Hansen et al.[235] evaluated the sentinel node in 696 women by hematoxylin and eosin staining and immunohistochemistry. With a median follow-up of 38 months, the size of the sentinel node metastasis (<2 mm or >2 mm) was a significant prognostic factor. There was no difference in disease-free or overall survival, however, between true node-negative and immunohistochemistry-only–positive cases. Additional data from large databases will continue to emerge in the coming years to further refine the prognostic significance of micrometastasis and immunohistochemistry-only positive lymph node metastasis in breast cancer patients.

Tumor Type

The histologic subtype of invasive cancer has been shown to be of prognostic value in several studies. The tubular, mucinous, and medullary subtypes have been shown to have a more favorable prognosis, compared with invasive ductal.[192,199,236,237] Invasive lobular tumors appear to have a prognosis similar to invasive ductal tumors.[238] Poor prognostic categories include metaplastic, undifferentiated, and other rarer subtypes.[113,193] In a classic analysis of 293 T2N0 breast cancers with over 20 years of follow-up treated by mastectomy, Rosen et al.[192] reported more favorable relapse rates in medullary, mucinous, tubular, and papillary subtypes compared with invasive ductal and invasive lobular tumors.

Tumor Grade

Multiple tumor grading systems have been proposed in an effort to standardize and improve interobserver variability. The Scarff-Bloom-Richardson classification system utilizes mitotic index, differentiation, and pleomorphism, each with scores of 1 to 3. Scores of 3 to 5 are well differentiated, 6 to 7 moderately differentiated, and 8 to 9 poorly differentiated. This system is commonly employed and has been shown to be of independent prognostic significance.[239]

Elston and Ellis[240] of the Nottingham group refined this methodology. The revised technique involves evaluation of three morphologic features—the percentage of tubule formation, the degree of nuclear pleomorphism, and an accurate mitotic count using a defined field area. A numerical scoring system is used, and the overall grade is derived from a summation of individual scores for the three variables: three grades of differentiation are used. Histologic grade, assessed in 1,831 patients, shows a very strong correlation with prognosis; patients with grade I tumors have a significantly better

survival than do those with grade II and III tumors ($P < .0001$). If the protocol is followed, reproducible and consistent results regarding prognosis can be obtained.

Estrogen and Progesterone Hormonal Receptors in Tumor Cells

Several studies have indicated that patients with hormonal receptors have a significantly higher survival rate.[241,242] Crowe et al.[243] studied 1,392 patients with carcinoma of the breast treated with modified radical mastectomy. ER-positive tumors (≥3 fmol/mg cytosol protein) were found in 1,063 patients (76.4%). Their 10-year overall survival rate of 65.9% was significantly better than the 56% rate in 329 patients with ER-negative tumors ($P = .0001$). However, this correlation is not consistent, with conflicting reports regarding the prognostic significance of hormonal receptor status.[244] The apparent discrepancy in some of these reports may be explained by technical nuances. Esteban et al.[245] noted that quantitative immunohistochemistry of ERs provides results with better predictive value than the biochemically procured ones.[246]

Tumors that express both ER and PR have the greatest benefit from hormonal therapy, but those containing only ER or PR still have significant responses. Two types of ERs—ER-α and ER-β—have been identified. PR also exists in two forms, PRA and PRB.[247] Patients with tumors negative for hormonal receptors have only a small probability of responding to hormonal therapy.[183,247]

Lymphatic and Vascular Invasion

Lymphatic and vascular invasion (LVI) in the peritumoral region has been clearly demonstrated to be of independent prognostic significance in several studies.[248–252] In the study by Rosen et al.,[192] recurrence rate for LVI-positive stage I patients was 38% compared with 22% for LVI-negative patients.

Proliferative Indices, S-Phase, and Thymidine Labeling Index

Various techniques for evaluating the proliferative rate of a tumor have been shown to correlate with distant metastasis and survival. The most common are the fraction of cells in SPF, TLI, mitotic index, or antibodies directed against proliferative markers such as Ki-67 and proliferating cell nuclear antigen.

Thymidine labeling represents the fraction of cells in S phase of the cell cycle and is based on the active incorporation of labeled thymidine into DNA; the TLI of primary breast cancers appears closely related to steroid receptor status and generally unrelated to pathologic stage. Retrospective analyses have shown that TLI is a prognostic indicator, independent of tumor size, steroid receptors, and p53, and Bcl-2 protein expression. Together with patient age and tumor size, TLI is able to identify patients at different levels of risk for locoregional or distant metastases.[253]

Wenger and Clark[254] concluded that despite different techniques and cut points, a higher SPF is in general associated with worse tumor grade, absence of steroid receptors, larger tumors, and positive axillary lymph nodes. Higher SPF is usually associated with worse disease-free and overall survival rates in both univariate and multivariate analyses.

Bryant et al.,[255] in over 4,000 patients from NSABP protocol B-14 who had ER-positive tumors and no axillary lymph node involvement, found a strong association between SPF and disease-free and overall survival rate.

DNA Ploidy Index

Chromosome instability (CIN) is gaining increasing interest as a central process in cancer. CIN, either past or present, is indicated whenever tumour cells harbor an abnormal quantity of DNA, termed "aneuploidy".[256] At present, the most widely used approach to detecting aneuploidy is DNA cytometry—a method that involves staining of DNA in the nuclei of cells from a tissue sample, followed by analysis using quantitative flow cytometry or microscopic imaging. Most breast cancers exhibit a bimodal distribution of DNA values. DNA ploidy as measured by flow cytometry correlates with nuclear grade, with low-grade tumors being diploid and high-grade tumors being aneuploid.[257] Ploidy was found to be associated with histologic type, tumor grade, and SPF values, but not with patient age, menopausal status, tumor size, axillary nodal status, ER status, or PR status.[258] Diploid tumors tend to be ER positive, whereas aneuploid tumors are frequently ER negative. Older patients are more likely to have hyperdiploid tumors.[259] Diploid tumors tend to have a better prognosis than do those with an aneuploid DNA distribution.[260,261] Toikkanen et al.,[262] in 351 patients monitored for a minimum of 22 years, observed a 25-year survival rate of 28% for patients with nondiploid tumors, in contrast to 48% for those with a diploid DNA pattern. In a European Organisation for Research on Treatment of Cancer (EORTC) trial evaluation of DNA, proliferative compartment was the most important predicting factor for overall survival and metastasis-free survival in 281 premenopausal, lymph node–negative patients with invasive carcinoma of the breast.[263]

Studies by Ewers et al.[264] and Fallenius et al.[265] also confirm the prognostic significance of DNA ploidy. Keyhani-Rofagha et al.[266] and Witzig et al.[267] reported no statistically significant prognostic significance of DNA ploidy.

HER2/neu

The *HER2/neu* proto-oncogene (also called *c-erbB-2*) located on chromosome 17 codes for a transmembrane glycoprotein, p185, which has tyrosine kinase activity and is homologous to the EGFR.[268] It is amplified or overexpressed in up to 30% of human breast carcinomas. Overexpression of the protein is associated with tumor aggressiveness and decreased disease-free survival in node-positive patients, with variable prognostic significance among node-negative patients. The conflicting reports regarding the prognostic significance of *HER2/neu* may be related to interobserver variability in interpretation of staining and uncertainty regarding the significance of intermediate staining.[186,187,268] Staining for overexpression of *HER2/neu* is interpreted on a 0 to 3+ scale. The available data suggest that the majority of 0 to 1 staining is clearly negative and 3+ is clearly positive, while the classification of those patients with 2+ staining remains uncertain. Amplification of the oncogene identified using FISH techniques has been found to be of more prognostic value.[186,187,268,269]

Variability in the prognostic value of *HER2/neu* may be related to variability in interpretation of protein expression levels. Birner et al.[270] correlated results of the HercepTest with *HER-2/neu* oncogene gene amplification assessed by FISH in 303 patients with lymph node–positive breast cancer.[270] Results were compared with FISH analysis performed in all 2+ and 3+ specimens (103 cases) and 104 *HER-2/neu*-negative specimens; 3+ carcinomas were found in 8.9% to 15.7% of specimens. FISH revealed that almost exclusively 3+ positive cases had *HER-2/neu* gene amplification.

More critical than its prognostic significance, however, is its predictive value with respect to response to therapy and its value in identifying patients who may benefit from adjuvant targeted therapy directed at the protein.[271] Several studies have demonstrated that *HER-2/neu* status may be predictive of response to hormonal therapy, resistance to alkylating agent–based chemotherapy, and response to taxanes.[272,273]

p53 Gene

The *p53* tumor suppressor gene encodes a nuclear phosphoprotein that is thought to be important to cell cycle regulation and DNA repair and that also may regulate induction of apoptosis by ionizing radiation.[274,275] The *p53* gene is most frequently mutated in sporadic breast cancer; alterations of this gene were identified in 43 of 192 tumors (22%).[275] Mutations of *p53* were found more often in tumors of younger women ($P = .002$) and African American women ($P = .04$) and in tumors lacking ER ($P = .03$), PR ($P = .04$), or both ($P = .06$). In 843 cases of breast cancer, *p53* mutations were not found in low-grade carcinomas (tubular, mucinous, papillary, and invasive cribriform types) but were observed in 4.2% of ILCs (6 of 140 cases), 15.5% of high-grade IDCs (99 of 640 cases), and 50% of pure medullary carcinomas (5 of 10 cases).[276] The overall survival rates were not significantly different in patients with mutant or wild-type *p53* tumors. In another study of 156 patients with primary invasive breast cancer, overexpression of p53 protein emerged as a reliable and independent predictor for disease recurrence and reduced survival.[277] Jansen et al.,[278] in a study of 345 patients with breast cancer with a median follow-up of more than 10 years, noted that *Bcl-2* expression was not a prognostic factor, but *p53* was an independent prognostic factor for overall survival ($P = .005$) and postrelapse survival ($P = .006$). However, *p53* status was important only in the *Bcl-2*–positive subgroup.

Genetic Profiling

Recent developments in DNA microarray technologies allow for extensive profiling of tumors based on their gene expression signatures.[279] Using this technology, investigators from the Netherlands Cancer Institute screened thousands of genes to develop a 70-gene prognostic signature that in 295 women demonstrated a 10-year disease-free survival of 50.6% in 180 poor prognosis signature patients compared with 85.2% in 115 women with a favorable signature. In a recent validation study, the profiling outperformed classic prognostic criteria, but the magnitude of the prognostic value was not as strong.[280–282]

Gene expression profiling has had a marked impact on our understanding of the biology of breast cancers and is routinely used in clinical decision-making. Categorizing breast cancer into distinct clinical subtypes of luminal A, luminal B, *HER2/neu*, and basal-like has significant prognostic value and impacts on decisions regarding systemic therapy options.[283,284] Although gene profiling forms the basis of this subtyping, most clinicians rely on common molecular markers of ER, PR, *HER2/neu*, Ki-67, and others as a surrogate to classify patients into these intrinsic subtypes of breast cancer for clinical decision making.[285]

An assay using gene profiling on paraffin-embedded specimens has been developed by Genomics Health Inc. (Redwood City, CA, USA). The Oncotype DX Breast Recurrence Score Assay measures RNA expression levels of 21 genes (16 cancer-related and 5 reference genes) using quantitative real-time reverse transcriptase polymerase chain reaction (qRT-PCR) on formalin-fixed, paraffin-embedded (FFPE) tissue samples to compute a recurrence score (RS) (0 to 100), which is used to estimate the odds of relapse over 10 years. Specimens from patients in NSABP trials with ER-positive HER2-negative tumors treated with tamoxifen alone were used to validate this scheme in which patients were categorized as low risk (<18 score), intermediate risk,[19–21,23,25–29,101–104] or high risk.[30–98,105] As shown in Figure 59.12, the likelihood of distant metastasis is low in those patients with favorable scores treated with tamoxifen alone.[286] These data can be used to determine which patients with ER-positive tumors and otherwise favorable factors may avoid chemotherapy and aid the clinician and patient in clinical decision-making. For intermediate Recurrence Score patients where chemotherapy benefit remains unclear, two phase III clinical trials (one in the node-negative and the other in the node-positive setting) are ongoing to determine whether endocrine treatment alone is noninferior to chemoendocrine treatment in this patient group[287].

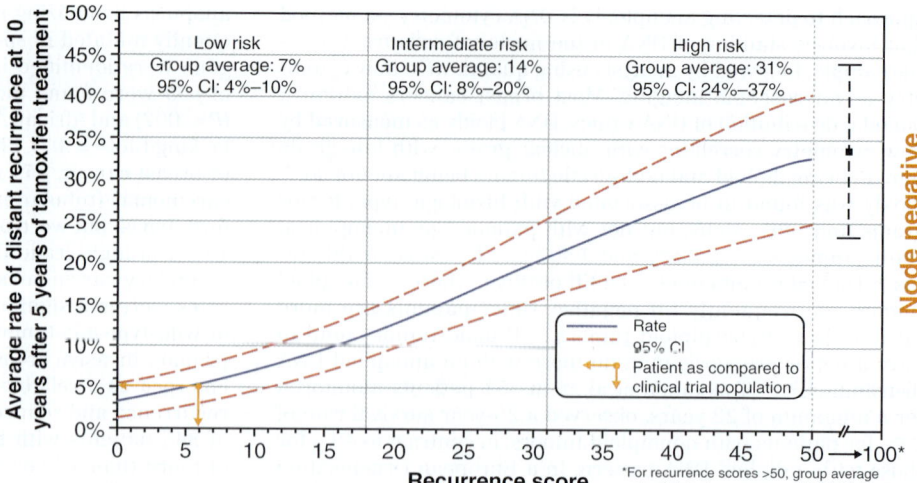

FIGURE 59.12. Risk stratification in patients with receptor positive tumors treated with hormonal therapy broken as a function of recurrence score using the Oncotype DX gene profiling scheme.

Age

Although young age has consistently been shown to be a predictor of local relapse following breast-conserving surgery, there are conflicting data regarding its prognostic significance for distant metastasis and overall survival.[11,219,225,288–291] The available data are confounded by the fact that younger women often present with palpable disease and have larger tumors with a higher percentage of positive nodes. Several studies, however, have shown that when corrected for stage, young age remains a significant prognostic factor for distant metastasis. In an analysis of 1,751 patients with nonmetastatic breast cancer, Vanlemmens et al.[292] demonstrated that younger women had a higher proportion of patients with ER-negative and high-grade tumors and lower disease-free and breast cancer–specific survival. In multivariate analysis, young age at diagnosis was an independent poor prognostic factor. Kollias et al.,[293] however, in an analysis of 2,879 patients younger than 70 years old with operable disease in the Nottingham database, demonstrated that the association of young age at diagnosis with a worse prognosis was explained by a higher proportion of poorly differentiated cancers in young women and that young age itself had no influence on the prognosis of the individual. Although clearly not as valid as tumor size and nodal status, young age may be considered in combination with other prognostic factors in clinical decision-making as a potential negative prognostic factor.

Race

African American women are commonly diagnosed with more advanced stages of breast cancer than are white women.[11] Simon and Severson,[294] in a review of 10,502 women diagnosed with breast cancer (82% white and 18% African American), observed that African American women were more likely to present with regional or distant disease (45%) than were white women (37%). White women had a better survival rate than did African American women during the first 4 years after diagnosis (P < .0001), but there were no significant differences in survival by race in women who lived longer than 4 years (P = .64). Black women are more likely than are whites to report that they have not had a mammogram within 3 years before diagnosis. However, history of mammographic screening accounted for <10% of the observed differences in stage at diagnosis.[295]

In 75 black and 615 white women with stage I and II breast cancer treated with breast conservation therapy and CMF (cyclophosphamide, methotrexate, and fluorouracil), with or without prednisone and tamoxifen, the 5-year actuarial local-only first failure rates were 5% for black women and 6% for white women (P = .53); regional-only failure, 9% and 1% (P = .002); and regional recurrence as any component of first failure, 16% and 4%, respectively (P = .001).[296] The 5-year overall survival rate for the black patients was 82% versus 91% for the white patients (P = .01); the disease-free survival rates were 64% and 83%, respectively (P = .0002).

Eley et al.[297] reported on a study of 612 black and 518 white women aged 20 to 79 years with primary invasive breast cancer. After controlling for geographic site and age, the risk of dying was 2.2 times greater for blacks than whites. Adjustment for stage reduced risk from 2.2 to 1.7; further adjustment for sociodemographic variables had no effect. They concluded that approximately 75% of the racial difference in survival was explained by prognostic factors. Other studies have also indicated that black women more commonly develop breast cancers that are high grade and negative for ER, PR, and *HER2/neu*.[298,299]

Obesity and Body Mass Index

In a study of 923 women treated by mastectomy and axillary dissection, those who were obese (25% or more over optimal weight for height) at the time of primary breast cancer treatment 10 years after diagnosis were at significantly greater risk for recurrence (42%), compared with nonobese patients (32%; P < .01).[300] On multivariate analysis, obesity remained a statistically significant prognostic factor after controlling for tumor size, number of positive axillary lymph nodes, age at diagnosis, and adjuvant chemotherapy. Recurrent disease developed in 32% of obese patients compared with 19% of nonobese women.

Daling et al.,[301] in a study of 1,177 women 45 years of age and younger who had invasive ductal breast carcinoma, found that women with breast carcinoma who were in the highest quartile of BMI were 2.5 times more likely to die of their disease within 5 years of diagnosis compared with women in the lowest quartile of BMI.[301]

Smoking

High plasma levels of estrogens are associated with increased breast cancer risk. Manjer et al.[302] in an analysis of 792 women in a mammographic screening trial with a mean follow-up of 12.1 years observed that 145 patients died of breast cancer. The RRs for smokers and ex-smokers, compared with those who had never smoked, were 1.44 and 1.13, respectively. The association with smoking remained significant after adjustment for age and stage at diagnosis and other potential confounders.

Pregnancy

Kroman et al.[303] investigated the prognostic effect of age at first birth and total parity in 10,703 women with primary breast cancer. After adjusting for age and stage of tumor, the number of full-term pregnancies had no prognostic value. However, women with primary childbirth between 20 and 29 years experienced a significantly reduced risk of death compared with women with primary childbirth before the age of 20 years (20 to 24 years, RR 0.88; 25 to 29 years, RR 0.80). Psyrri and Burtness[304] reviewed 117 articles and three abstracts referring to breast cancer in pregnancy. They concluded the prognosis of the pregnant breast cancer patient is similar to her stage-matched nonpregnant counterparts in most series. Management of breast cancer during and after pregnancy is discussed in detail later.

Although in the past it was thought that pregnancy after the diagnosis of breast cancer was associated with a worse prognosis, recent evidence suggests the opposite.[305] Women with a history of breast cancer should be reassured that there is not strong evidence to suggest that subsequent pregnancy will increase the risk of recurrence.

Tumor Location

There is some evidence that medially located tumors have a poorer prognosis than do laterally located tumors. An analysis of 45,880 patients from the SEER database by Gaffney et al.[306] demonstrated that the hazard ratio (HR) for inner quadrant location compared with outer quadrant was 1.27 for breast cancer–specific survival and 1.11 for overall survival. Both were significant on multivariate analysis. Lohrisch et al.,[307] in an analysis of 6,781 patients, also demonstrated a twofold risk of relapse and breast cancer death associated with high-risk medial breast tumors compared with lateral tumors. They postulate that this may be due to occult spread to IMNs.

Selected Other Prognostic Factors

A wide variety of other prognostic factors have been extensively evaluated. Although some of these have been promising in initial reports, they have not been applied in routine clinical decision-making. However, these markers may help to supplement information obtained with more established prognostic factors. Furthermore, with additional testing and validation, some of these markers may serve as targets for therapeutic interventions. Extensively evaluated and reported potentially useful prognostic factors include cathepsin-D, vascular endothelial growth factor, EGF, *Bcl-2*, carcinoembryonic antigen, prostate-specific antigen, E-cadherin, and others. The reader is referred elsewhere for an extensive review of molecular prognostic factors in breast cancer.[308,309]

MANAGEMENT OF BREAST CANCER

Management of invasive breast cancer should be based on the clinical extent and pathologic characteristics of the tumor, in addition to the age of the patient (menopausal status), some biologic prognostic factors, and the preference and psychological profile of the individual patient, optimally in a multidisciplinary setting. Although surgical, medical, and radiation oncology remain the primary therapeutic disciplines in the management of breast cancer, the patients management often is dependent on input from diagnostic radiology and pathology, the primary physician involved, and support services such as genetic counseling, social work, nursing, and others.

Surgical Management of Breast Cancer

The surgical management of patients with early-stage operable breast cancer addresses both the primary tumor and regional lymphatics. The primary tumor may be managed by mastectomy or lumpectomy, and the nodal regions may be surgically addressed by lymph node dissection or sentinel node biopsy. The radiation oncologist should be aware of the various surgical procedures, as it may influence the radiotherapeutic management. Procedures that remove the bulk of parenchymal breast tissue include the radical mastectomy, extended radical mastectomy, modified radical mastectomy, simple mastectomy (also referred to as total mastectomy), skin-sparing mastectomy, and nipple-sparing mastectomy. Partial mastectomy, lumpectomy, tylectomy, and quadrantectomy are collectively referred to as breast-conserving surgery.

Breast-conserving approaches, as well as the skin-sparing and nipple-sparing mastectomy, used in early-stage breast cancers, are briefly discussed here as they are often used in early-stage disease. Details of the mastectomy procedures are summarized in Chapter 57.

Skin-Sparing Mastectomy

Skin-sparing mastectomy is a standard mastectomy, with minimal skin sacrifice at the mastectomy site.[113] This is often performed when immediate reconstruction is planned. This technique attempts to remove all breast tissue, but the preservation of skin provides cosmetic and reconstructive advantages. The procedure is oncologically sound, and patients undergoing skin-sparing mastectomy do not require postmastectomy radiation unless they have risk factors that place them at higher risk (i.e., positive nodes, positive margins, large primary tumors), as discussed in Chapter 57.

Nipple-Sparing Mastectomy

The nipple-sparing mastectomy is distinct from the skin-sparing mastectomy in that the nipple and/or nipple areola complex are conserved. This procedure is more controversial and is not routinely employed in cancer patients. However, there have been recent studies employing this technique in combination with intraoperative electrons in patients with operable breast cancer.[310]

Lumpectomy

Another treatment of breast cancer, initially described by Keynes in 1929 and 1937, combined breast-conserving surgery by wide local excision of the tumor followed by definitive irradiation to the intact breast.[58,311–313] Various terms have been used to describe the surgical approach, including lumpectomy, wide local excision, breast-conserving surgery, tylectomy, tumorectomy, segmental mastectomy, partial mastectomy, and quadrantectomy. This approach is extensively discussed in this chapter. The NSABP recommends specific types of incisions depending on the location of the tumor (Fig. 59.13). The radiation oncologist may play an

FIGURE 59.13. National Surgical Adjuvant Breast Project recommendations for the direction of incisions used for tumorectomy **(A)** and for axillary node dissection **(B)**. (Courtesy of Bernard Fisher, MD, Chairman, National Surgical Adjuvant Breast Project. From Bedwinek JM. Treatment of stage I and II adenocarcinoma of the breast by tumor excision and irradiation. *Int J Radiat Oncol Biol Phys* 1981;7[11]:1553–1559. Copyright © 1981 Elsevier. With permission.)

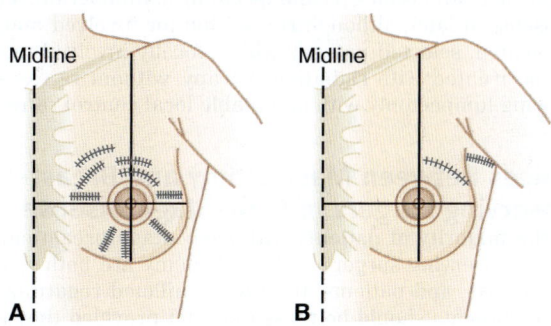

advisory role, as in many cases the patient may be evaluated by both the surgeon and the radiation oncologist before the definitive operation.

The optimal extent of breast resection for treatment of T1 and T2 breast cancer has not been defined. Increasing the size of the resection may lower the risk of local recurrence but also has an adverse impact on the cosmetic outcome. Because cosmesis is a critical reason for performing tumor excision and irradiation instead of mastectomy, wide local excision with microscopically negative margins is preferable to segmental mastectomy or quadrantectomy.

Surgical removal of additional breast tissue surrounding the original excision site is indicated when margins are positive and there is a substantial probability that the tumor cell burden exceeds what can be controlled by the usual doses of radiation. The percentage of patients with residual tumor at the time of re-excision varies widely (32% to 62%), depending on the criteria used for taking a patient back to the operating room for more breast surgery. If the initial margins of resection are positive, 55% to 69% of re-excision specimens contain cancer cells, compared with 49% in cases with unknown margins.[314-317] Tumor size alone is not usually considered an indication for re-excision in the absence of other factors.

Some authors have advocated re-excision of the primary site if the biopsy was performed at an outside hospital and margins of resection were unknown. Of 210 patients having surgery at the MD Anderson Cancer Center, 67 underwent re-excision after biopsies performed at other institutions, and invasive carcinoma was identified in 57%.[315] An 8.2% incidence of breast recurrence (12 of 135 patients) was noted when the tumor excision was performed before referral to the MD Anderson Cancer Center, but only 2% (4 of 210) when it was performed at that institution.

Other factors that may have an impact on the rate of positive re-excisions include extensive intraductal carcinoma (EIC) and residual calcifications on a postlumpectomy preirradiation mammogram. At Harvard University, when EIC was detected on the initial biopsy, 88% of the re-excisions were positive, compared with 48% when EIC was absent.[316] At the University of Pennsylvania, when a posttylectomy mammogram detected residual microcalcifications, 86% of the re-excisions contained tumor.[317] In a series from Yale, reported by Lally et al.,[318] of 34 patients with a postlumpectomy mammogram that showed suspicious residual calcification who underwent re-excision, 20 (59%) were found to have residual disease. Patients whose initial tumor was associated with calcifications with questionable, close, or positive margins should be evaluated with a prelumpectomy mammogram with guided re-excision if suspicious residual calcifications are present.

Based on these findings, the authors recommend re-excision at the primary tumor site (a) when the surgical procedure was less than a complete lumpectomy, such as an initial incisional biopsy or core biopsy, (b) when pathologic margins on the initial excisional biopsy are shown to be involved by tumor, and (c) when there are residual suspicious microcalcifications on a postlumpectomy mammogram. As will be discussed later, although re-excision for involved margins is indicated, selected patients with a focally involved margin may be treated with radiation therapy, without re-excision, following lumpectomy with acceptable local control rates.

Choices Between Mastectomy and Breast-Conserving Surgery in Early-Stage Disease

For the majority of patients with early-stage breast cancer, breast-conserving surgery and mastectomy are both reasonable options, and patients are often conflicted regarding the choice. Patients should be reassured that provided they meet the criteria for breast-conserving surgery, all of the available medical evidence demonstrates equivalent long-term survival rates with both modalities.

A modified radical mastectomy may be preferable for some patients who wish to avoid radiation, for those in whom removal of clinical and radiographically apparent disease will result in a suboptimal cosmetic result, for those with diffusely positive margins which cannot be cleared with re-excision, and those with diffuse suspicious microcalcifications. Even patients who are ideally suited for breast-conserving therapy may have a personal preference for mastectomy, based on a number of factors.

Whelan et al.[319] reported on the decision-making process in 82 consecutive node-negative patients presented with a decision board of therapeutic choices. Overall, 95% of women chose lumpectomy and breast irradiation. Kelemen et al.[320] evaluated the choice between breast-conserving surgery and modified radical mastectomy in 7,815 women with early-stage breast cancer. There was a progressive increase from 16% to 47% in the use of breast-conserving therapy to treat tumors of all sizes over the 11 years of the study ($P < .0001$), and it was more frequently used for ≤2 cm tumors with an odds ratio (OR) of 2.46. Breast-conserving therapy was used at a slightly higher rate in medical centers than in community hospitals (31% vs. 28%; $P < .0001$); its use varied among geographic regions from a low of 24% in the southwestern United States to 36% in the northeast and 40% in hospitals outside the continental United States ($P < .0001$). Local availability of radiation therapy did not influence choice of treatment.

In response to a questionnaire mailed to 2,405 oncologists from all three disciplines and 60 oncology nurses in the United States, Tannock and Belanger[321] noted that more than 60% thought that modified radical mastectomy and conservation surgery plus irradiation were equivalent options for patients with stage T1 and T2 carcinoma of the breast; 31% of the surgical oncologists favored the former and 35% of the radiation oncologists favored the latter approach. Medical oncologists were equally divided between the two procedures (14% and 18%, respectively).

In an analysis from Canada, Temple et al.[322] prospectively evaluated participants with a first diagnosis of localized unilateral breast cancer who were candidates for breast-conserving therapy or mastectomy. Of 157 patients between 1992 and 1995, 71.3% anticipated having breast-conserving surgery and 28.7% anticipated modified radical mastectomy. The patient, physician, and significant other were perceived to play a role in the decision process. The two top-ranked items perceived to have influenced treatment choice were doctor's advice and possibility of complete cure. The authors concluded that both patient and surgeon factors are important predictors of type of planned surgery, but there is a gap between women's preferences and actual experiences with regard to information provided.

Some patients with early-stage breast cancer will choose mastectomy to avoid the course of radiation, either because of the logistics of 6 weeks of therapy or because of fears of radiation therapy. It is likely that accelerated partial breast irradiation (APBI) may further impact the choice between mastectomy and breast-conserving surgery for those women in whom the time commitment of treatment is an issue.

Patients selecting mastectomy should also be made aware that this procedure does not totally eliminate the need for radiation treatment. For patients with early-stage operable breast cancer treated by modified radical mastectomy, postoperative irradiation of the chest wall and peripheral lymphatics may be indicated in selected patients with high-risk characteristics, positive nodes, or positive resection margins. Indications for postmastectomy radiation are discussed in Chapter 54.

Surgical Management of Axillary Lymph Nodes

An axillary node dissection or sentinel node biopsy are a standard component of the staging process for a majority of women with early-stage invasive breast cancer.[188] Although the role of complete axillary dissection is evolving, there is compelling evidence that ALND is not necessary in most women with early-stage breast cancer who have only one or two sentinel lymph node metastases and who will receive whole-breast irradiation as part of breast-conserving therapy. If, however, whole-breast irradiation is not planned, then ALND is indicated for such patients. Clearly the procedure is most important for women in whom axillary nodal status will influence subsequent management with respect to adjuvant systemic therapy. Two randomized trials, the ACOSOG Z-0011 trial and the International Breast Cancer Study Group 23-01 (IBCSG 23-01) trial (discussed later), demonstrated that many of these patients with one or two metastatic sentinel nodes can safely avoid a completion axillary node dissection. It is not uncommon for clinicians to avoid axillary staging if it is not going to influence management.[66,323,324] This is relevant in elderly women with receptor-positive tumors who will receive hormonal therapy, regardless of nodal status, and who are not thought to be candidates for cytotoxic chemotherapy. The decision to omit SLNB in older women should be discussed in a multidisciplinary setting with input from the treating oncologists to ensure all providers are in agreement as to whether or not axillary staging information is important for adjuvant-therapy decisions. As will be discussed later, axillary radiation, as with axillary dissection, results in a high rate of regional control.[66,323,324]

Axillary Node Dissection

The axillary contents are divided into three levels: level I represents tissue between the axillary vein and the latissimus dorsi muscle and the lateral border of the pectoralis minor muscle; level II is located between the lateral and medial borders of the pectoralis minor muscle; and level III is between the medial border of the pectoralis minor and Halsted ligament (the apex of the axilla).[1] Thorough dissection of levels I and II has traditionally been the most common axillary surgical procedure in patients with clinically node-negative breast cancer. Complete axillary dissection, including level III, may be performed in patients with clinically positive lymph nodes. A higher incidence of breast and arm edema has been noted with level III axillary node dissection, and the benefit of dissecting the level III lymph nodes has not been demonstrated.[325] Pigott et al.[326] reported on 146 patients treated with radical mastectomy (either modified or Halsted) for invasive ductal or lobular carcinoma of the breast. Eighty patients (55%) had histologically proven axillary lymph node metastases. If only the low (level I) axillary lymph nodes had been removed, 18 patients (25%) would have had metastases confined to levels II and III that would have gone undetected. However, only 1.4% of patients showed positive level III lymph nodes if levels I and II were negative.

Approximately 20% to 40% of patients with carcinoma of the breast and clinically negative lymph nodes have pathologic evidence of lymph node metastases.[1,113,229,327,328] Yet, in patients with stage I or II breast cancer and clinically negative axillary lymph nodes, if an axillary dissection is not performed, axillary recurrence develops in only approximately 20%.[71] In patients with clinically positive axilla, 20% to 30% have no histologic evidence of nodal metastatic disease.[71]

The necessity of axillary dissection has been questioned in selected patients with a low probability of nodal involvement by Silverstein et al.,[66] who reported positive axillary lymph nodes in only 3 (3%) of 96 patients with tumors ≤5 mm in diameter and in 27 (17%) of 156 patients with

tumors 6 to 10 mm in diameter. Iwasaki et al.,[329] in a group of 823 patients with T1N0M0 invasive breast cancer, also identified a subgroup of patients who may not need to undergo ALND. Certain tumor types (medullary, mucinous, and tubular carcinoma) had lower positive rates for lymph node involvement. With regard to the histologic grade, lymph node positivity increased significantly with high-grade tumors.

In a randomized trial, evaluating the necessity of axillary dissection in older women, Martelli et al.[330] reported on 219 women, 65 to 80 years of age, with early breast cancer and clinically negative axillary nodes who were randomized to conservative breast surgery with or without axillary dissection. Tamoxifen was prescribed to all patients for 5 years. With a follow-up of 60 months, there were no significant differences in overall or breast cancer mortality or crude cumulative incidence of breast events between the two groups. Only two patients in the no axillary dissection arm (8 and 40 months after surgery) developed overt axillary involvement during follow-up. They conclude that older patients with T1N0 breast cancer can be treated by conservative breast surgery and no axillary dissection without adversely affecting breast cancer mortality or overall survival.

In light of the increased use of primary tumor-related factors, including molecular profiling, for decision-making regarding systemic therapy, combined with sentinel node procedures and low rates of regional relapse with radiation therapy or observation in selected patients, axillary dissection has been less frequently employed in the management of early-stage breast cancer patients.

Sentinel Lymph Node Biopsies

In recent years, there has been a substantial increase in the use of sentinel lymph node biopsies to stage patients with breast cancer. Patients are injected around the tumor with technetium-99m (^{99m}Tc) sulfur colloid and vital blue dye, and a handheld γ-probe is used to identify areas of highest radioisotope uptake in the lymphatic system. The lymph nodes underlying this area (sentinel lymph nodes) are removed.[231,331–333] The sentinel node procedure has been widely embraced as an acceptable standard for women with breast cancer and has a high degree of sensitivity and specificity.[334]

Recently, the standard of care that mandated performing an ALND in node-positive patients was reexamined after the publication of IBCSG 23-01 and the ACOSOG Z11 studies[335,336]. The IBCSG 23-01 study randomized 931 patients with micrometastatic (<2 mm) deposit in the SLNB to ALND or no additional surgery[337]. The majority of the patients (97%) received adjuvant RT without RNI. In the ALND arm, additional axillary nodal involvement was detected in 13% of the patients. There was no difference in the overall survival or disease-free survival between the two study arms. Although the study closed before meeting target accrual, the authors concluded that breast cancer patients with limited SLN involvement could be spared the morbidity of an ALND.

In contrast to the previous study, the ACOSOG Z11 study was a prospective trial examining survival of patients with sentinel node metastases detected by standard hematoxylin and eosin staining, who were randomized to undergo ALND after sentinel lymph node dissection (SLND) versus SLND alone; all patients received whole-breast irradiation. There were 446 patients randomized to SLND alone and 445 to SLND plus ALND. Patients were equally stratified according to multiple factors; those randomized to SLND plus ALND had a median of 17 axillary nodes removed compared with a median of only 2 sentinel nodes removed with SLND alone ($P < .001$). At a median follow-up time of 6.3 years, there were no statistically significant differences in local recurrence ($P = .11$) or regional recurrence ($P = .45$) between the two groups. Interestingly, ALND also removed more positive lymph nodes ($P < .001$) in 27% of the patients in this group. The

TABLE 59.12 SUGGESTED APPROACH FOR RADIATION FIELD DESIGN IN SENTINEL NODE–POSITIVE PATIENTS NOT UNDERGOING AXILLARY LYMPH NODE DISSECTION

Clinical Scenario	Sentinel Nodes +/Total Sentinel Nodes Sampled	Probability of Additional Nodes MSKCC[338] (%)	Probability of Additional Nodes MDACC[339] (%)	Probability of Four or More Nodes Involved[340] (%)	Field Design
IDC, 1.0 cm, ER+, LVI–	1 (IHC only)/3	3	8	<1	Tangents only
IDC, 1.8 cm, G3, ER+, LVI–, Unifocal	1 (macro)/2	27	24	2	High tangents
IDC, 2.0 cm, ER–, LVI+	2 (macro)/2	63	55	30	High tangents/consider full nodal treatment
ILC, 4.0 cm ER+, multifocal, LVI–	2 (macro)/2	77	64	40	High tangents/consider full nodal treatment
IDC, 3 cm, ER–, LVI+, multifocal	3 (macro with ENE)/3	78	95	80	Full nodal treatment

ENE, extranodal extension; ER, estrogen receptor; G, grade; IDC, infiltrating ductal carcinoma; IHC, immunohistochemistry; ILC, infiltrating lobular carcinoma; LVI, lymphovascular invasion; macro, macroscopic.

patients in this trial all had whole-breast irradiation, but RNI was not allowed; however, there was no radiotherapy quality assurance and field design was not uniform. The reason for the low regional relapse rates is likely a combination of factors, including a favorable subset of patients with a low likelihood of a high residual axillary burden of disease, the use of systemic therapy, and incidental radiation to the residual nodes in level I or II from the tangential breast irradiation.

Several studies describe an approach to radiation field design based on probability of additional axillary nodal involvement in patients with positive sentinel nodes (Table 59.12).[234,338–341]

The ALMANAC (Axillary Lymphatic Mapping Against Nodal Axillary Clearance) trial is a multicenter randomized trial of 1,031 patients randomly assigned to sentinel node biopsy (n = 515) or standard axillary dissection (n = 516).[332] Mansel et al.[332] reported the primary outcome measures, which were arm and shoulder morbidity and quality of life. Drain usage, length of hospital stay, and resumption of normal activities after surgery were all highly significantly better in the sentinel lymph node group. In addition, patient recorded quality of life and arm functioning scores were also significantly better, with no increase in anxiety levels in the sentinel node group. The authors conclude that sentinel node biopsy is the treatment of choice for patients who have early-stage breast cancer and clinically negative nodes.

Veronesi et al.[342] also reported on a randomized trial of 516 patients with T1 tumors, randomized to either sentinel node biopsy or total axillary dissection. Axillary dissection was performed in the sentinel node group if the sentinel node contained metastases. In the axillary dissection group, the overall accuracy of the sentinel node status was 96.9%, the sensitivity 91.2%, and the specificity 100%. There was less pain and better arm mobility in the patients who underwent sentinel node biopsy only than in those who also underwent axillary dissection. There were 15 events associated with breast cancer in the axillary dissection group and 10 such events in the sentinel node group. Among the 167 patients who did not undergo axillary dissection, there were no cases of overt axillary metastasis during follow-up.

Weaver et al.[343] evaluated 443 patients with breast cancer. After sentinel node biopsies, a complete ALND was performed. Original pathologic material was reviewed for 431 patients enrolled in this study and for 214 patients with node-negative disease. Metastases were detected in 16% of the sentinel lymph nodes and in 4% of the nonsentinel nodes (OR 4.3; P < .001). Occult metastases were detected in 4% of the sentinel lymph nodes and in 0.3% of the nonsentinel nodes. The probability of detecting metastases in nonsentinel nodes was more than 13 times greater in patients with positive sentinel lymph nodes than in patients with negative sentinel lymph nodes (P < .001).

The role of sentinel lymph node procedures in patients undergoing neoadjuvant chemotherapy is covered in Chapter 57.

SYSTEMIC MANAGEMENT OF BREAST CANCER

Systemic therapy is an essential component of both early-stage node-negative breast cancer and advanced-stage disease. Hormonal therapy, cytotoxic chemotherapy, and the more recently introduced biologic therapies are routinely employed in the vast majority of patients with early-stage breast cancer. For patients with all stages of breast cancer, systemic therapy has been shown to decrease the RR of relapse and mortality. However, there are subsets of patients with a very favorable prognosis and extremely low rate of relapse, in whom the risk reduction results in only a very small absolute benefit. It is beyond the scope of this chapter to discuss all of the issues related to systemic management of breast cancer, and the reader is referred to comprehensive reviews on the use of chemotherapy, endocrine therapies, and biologic therapies in the systemic management of breast cancer. These issues are also discussed in more detail in Chapter 57.[344–346]

In the recent 2011 St. Galen consensus meeting, the panel adopted the approach that systemic therapy should be made based on recognition of intrinsic subtypes and that for practical reasons these intrinsic subtypes could be approximated based on more conventional parameters of estrogen receptor, progesterone receptor, HER2/neu, and Ki-67. Endocrine therapy alone is generally adequate for luminal A-type cancers, while chemotherapy is typically indicated for luminal B and TN cancers, and trastuzumab is generally added for HER2-positive disease.[347]

RADIATION THERAPY IN THE MANAGEMENT OF EARLY-STAGE INVASIVE BREAST CANCER

The radiation oncologist plays a critical role in the management of early-stage breast cancer. As noted previously, the role of radiation therapy in postmastectomy radiation and in the neoadjuvant treatment of advanced breast cancers will be discussed in Chapter 57. The remainder of this chapter will primarily be focused on the role of radiation therapy in the conservative management of early-stage invasive breast cancer.

This will include an extensive discussion of the studies establishing breast-conserving surgery and radiation as the preferred standard of care for the majority of women with early-stage invasive disease and studies evaluating the avoidance of radiation therapy in selected patients. Integration of radiation therapy with systemic therapy will be discussed, as will selection of patients for breast-conserving therapy. Risk factors for local relapse and controversies in the management of patients with special circumstances will be discussed. Technical issues in the delivery of radiation therapy for early-stage breast cancer, including dosing and fractionation, matching techniques, and newer technical approaches, will be presented. The rapidly evolving area of partial breast irradiation will also be discussed. Follow-up of the breast cancer patient and sequelae of treatment will be presented. Management of local relapse in the conservatively treated breast and postmastectomy will be covered in Chapter 57. The role of radiation therapy in the management of DCIS and LCIS was discussed Chapter 55.

Breast-Conserving Therapy and Patient Selection

Breast-conserving surgery followed by radiation therapy to the intact breast is now clearly established as the most acceptable standard of care for the majority of women with early-stage invasive breast cancer. Recommended techniques for breast conservation treatment are wide local excision of the primary tumor, preferably with clear margins, ALND, and breast irradiation (45 to 50 Gy), usually with a boost (10 to 20 Gy, depending on tumor size and status of the surgical margins). As will be discussed in detail under prognostic factors, while widely negative margins are desirable, patients with focally involved margins can be treated with radiation with excellent local control rates.

In addition to tumor control and survival, conservation of the breast with optimal cosmetic results is a crucial goal of this therapy, which is associated with improved psychoemotional adjustment of the patient to the diagnosis and treatment of carcinoma of the breast. It also enhances the acceptance by women of mammographic screening for early detection of this disease.

The widespread embracement of breast-conserving surgery followed by radiation therapy is based on numerous mature and well-documented studies, both prospectively designed randomized trials and large retrospective series of appropriately selected patients treated with breast conservation followed by radiation therapy.

It is important to select appropriate patients and tumors for breast conservation therapy, with close consultation between the surgeon, medical oncologist, and the radiation oncologist and after thorough discussion of therapeutic alternatives with the patient. Risks and benefits of breast-conserving therapy compared with mastectomy should be discussed. Despite the clear evidence of equivalence, some patients will still prefer mastectomy, which remains an acceptable standard of care for all women with operable breast cancers. Although avoidance of radiation may be a primary rationale for some patients in choosing mastectomy, patients should realize that even with early-stage operable disease postmastectomy radiation may be indicated based on the pathologic findings at mastectomy. It is likely that over the next several years, long-term results and selection factors for APBI will become available and may further influence patient choices regarding breast-conserving surgery with more rapid radiation compared with mastectomy.[348–350]

Ideally, patients electing breast-conserving surgery and radiation will have unicentric primary tumors that are <4 to 5 cm in diameter, as cosmesis is affected by the amount of tissue that must be removed in relation to the size of the breast.[351] For patients in whom the size of the tumor, compared with the size of the breast, will result in an unacceptable cosmetic outcome, neoadjuvant chemotherapy followed by lumpectomy and radiation has been demonstrated to result excellent breast conservation rates.[352–354] This was discussed in detail in Chapter 54.

With careful attention to surgical margins, radiation technique, and the appropriate use of systemic therapy, local relapse rates in the majority of conservatively managed patients are low, and only a minority of patients with early-stage invasive breast cancer are not suitable for breast-conserving therapy. There are several perceived relative "contraindications" to breast-conserving therapy, including patients with collagen vascular disease, patients with germline mutations that predispose to breast cancer development, and those with positive margins, more advanced disease, multicentric disease, pregnancy, or who have had prior radiation. Although many of these factors require careful consideration and discussion between the treating physicians and the patient, as will be discussed in the section on special circumstances, selected patients faced with breast cancer in the setting of these controversial circumstances can be offered breast-conserving therapy with acceptable outcomes. Although some clinicians believe that patients at higher risk for development of local recurrence should not be treated with conservation surgery, there are relatively few absolute contraindications.

Perhaps with the exception of the patients with persistently positive diffuse margins or gross multicentric disease, where removal of clinically and radiographically apparent disease would result in an unacceptable cosmetic outcome, breast-conserving therapy followed by radiation can be offered to most women with early-stage breast cancer and may be offered to a high percentage of women with advanced cancers following neoadjuvant chemo- or hormonal therapy. The decision regarding breast-conserving therapy compared with mastectomy is often based on personal preference as the available medical and scientific evidence suggests equivalent overall and disease-free survival in all subsets of patients.

Early Reports of Breast-Conserving Therapy

In 1937, Keynes[58] stated that "widespread operations based upon the permeation theory of lymphatics and fascial planes have no real justification and the idea of conservative treatment of cancer of the breast may become less repugnant to us [surgeons]." He treated 325 patients with local removal of the breast tumor and radium implantation at the site of local incision as well as in the axilla. In 250 patients, the 5-year survival rate was 71% for group 1 (disease confined to the breast), 29% for group 2 (disease apparently confined to breast and axilla), and 23.6% for group 3 (advanced disease or inoperable cancer). At the time, the results were comparable with those achieved with radical mastectomy. Other early reports[312,355–358] paved the way for the development of randomized trials that have now clearly established breast-conserving surgery followed by radiation therapy as an accepted standard of care.

Randomized Studies Comparing Breast-Conserving Surgery Plus Radiation Therapy to Mastectomy

There have been numerous randomized trials that have now clearly established breast-conserving surgery followed by radiation therapy as equivalent to mastectomy for appropriately selected patients with early-stage breast cancer. Table 59.13 summarizes these randomized trials. In all of these trials, local tumor excision (tylectomy, lumpectomy), segmental mastectomy, or quadrantectomy combined with irradiation to the breast yielded survival and tumor control rates similar to those achieved with modified or classic radical mastectomy.[91,99,100,361–365] Each of these randomized trials, as well as meta-analyses of the trials, clearly demonstrates equivalent mortality rates in conservatively treated patients compared with mastectomy.[366–368]

The earliest prospective, randomized trial comparing breast conservation with radical mastectomy was conducted at Guy's Hospital in London. Three hundred and seventy women with stage I or II breast cancer were randomly assigned to receive either standard radical mastectomy or wide local excision plus irradiation.[369] Although the rates of survival and distant metastasis were not significantly different for stage I disease, in stage II, the recurrence rates in the breast and axilla were higher in the group treated with local excision and irradiation, and survival was significantly lower because of a higher rate of distant metastasis. Major weaknesses of this study were the low doses of irradiation used

TABLE 59.13 PROSPECTIVE RANDOMIZED TRIALS COMPARING CONSERVATIVE SURGERY AND RADIATION WITH MASTECTOMY FOR EARLY-STAGE BREAST CANCER

	Institut Gustave-Roussy (1972–84)[359]	Milan (1973–80)[100]	NSABP B-06 (1976–84)[91]	NCI (1979–87)[360]	EORTC (1980–86)[361]	Danish (1983–89)[362]
Number of patients	179	701	1219	237	874	904
Stage	1	1	1 and 2	1 and 2	1 and 2	1, 2, 3
Surgery	2-cm gross margin	Quadrantectomy	Lumpectomy	Gross excision	1-cm gross margin	Wide excision
Follow-up (yr)	15	20	20	18	10	6
Overall Survival						
CS+RT (%)	73	42	46	59	65	79
Mastectomy (%)	65	41	47	58	66	82
Local Recurrence						
CS+RT (%)	9	9	14	22	20	3
Mastectomy (%)	14	2	10	6	12	4

CS+RT, conservative therapy; EORTC, European Organisation for Research and Treatment of Cancer; NCI, National Cancer Institute; NSABP, National Surgical Adjuvant Breast and Bowel Project; RT, Radiation therapy.

(35 to 38 Gy to the breast and 25 to 27 Gy to the axilla), probably patient selection, and surgical techniques.

Veronesi et al.[365] reported on 701 patients with tumors <2 cm in diameter and without palpable axillary nodes of whom 352 were randomly assigned to treatment with either quadrantectomy and axillary dissection plus irradiation (50 Gy in 5 weeks to the breast and 10-Gy boost) and 349 to radical (Halsted) mastectomy. Women with positive axillary lymph nodes also received 12 cycles of adjuvant chemotherapy with CMF. Actuarial 20-year overall and disease-free survival rates were comparable in the two groups (58%). The death rates from breast cancer were 26.1% and 24.3%. The incidence of local failure was 2.3% with mastectomy and 8.8% with quadrantectomy and irradiation. There was no difference in the incidence of contralateral breast cancer (10.2% and 8.7%, respectively).[100]

Fisher et al.[91,363] updated the results of the NSABP protocol B-06 in 1,843 women with clinical stage I or II carcinoma of the breast <4 cm in diameter. Patients were randomly assigned to be treated with total mastectomy or lumpectomy (segmental mastectomy), with or without irradiation. Irradiated patients received 50 Gy to the breast through tangential fields irradiation and a boost to the operative site was not given. With 20-year follow-up, there was no significant difference in survival among patients treated with mastectomy, lumpectomy alone, or lumpectomy combined with irradiation (Fig. 59.14). For the patients treated with lumpectomy alone, the ipsilateral breast relapse rates were approximately 40% if the nodes were negative and 50% if they were positive. For patients treated with lumpectomy and irradiation, the corresponding rates were 10% for all patients and those with negative nodes and 5% for those with positive nodes, illustrating the interaction of irradiation and adjuvant chemotherapy in local tumor control. Cumulate incidence of ipsilateral breast tumor relapse in the lumpectomy alone compared with the lumpectomy and radiation arm is shown in Figure 59.15.

The Institut Gustave-Roussy conducted a prospective, randomized trial comparing mastectomy with local excision plus irradiation for women with cancers measuring ≤2 cm.[359,370] The 15-year disease-free survival rate was 55% for the tumorectomy group and 45% for the mastectomy group (P = .23). The 15-year local recurrence rate was 9% in the conservation surgery and irradiation group and 14% in the mastectomy group.

The EORTC Breast Cancer Cooperative Group conducted a randomized trial of women with stage I or II breast cancer comparing modified radical mastectomy (420 patients) with breast conservation therapy (448 patients).[361] The actuarial 8-year local tumor control rate was similar in both arms, 91% in the mastectomy group, and 87% in the breast conservation therapy group. There was one axillary recurrence in the mastectomy group and three in the conservation therapy group.

FIGURE 59.14. Life-table analysis showing disease-free survival among patients in the three cohorts who were treated by total mastectomy, lumpectomy, or lumpectomy and breast irradiation. The number of events includes those that occurred after the 20-year follow-up period. (From Fisher B, Anderson S, Bryant J, et al. Twenty-year follow-up of a randomized trial comparing total mastectomy, lumpectomy, and lumpectomy plus irradiation for the treatment of invasive breast cancer. *N Engl J Med* 2002;347[16]:1233–1241. Copyright © 2002 Massachusetts Medical Society. Reprinted with permission from Massachusetts Medical Society.)

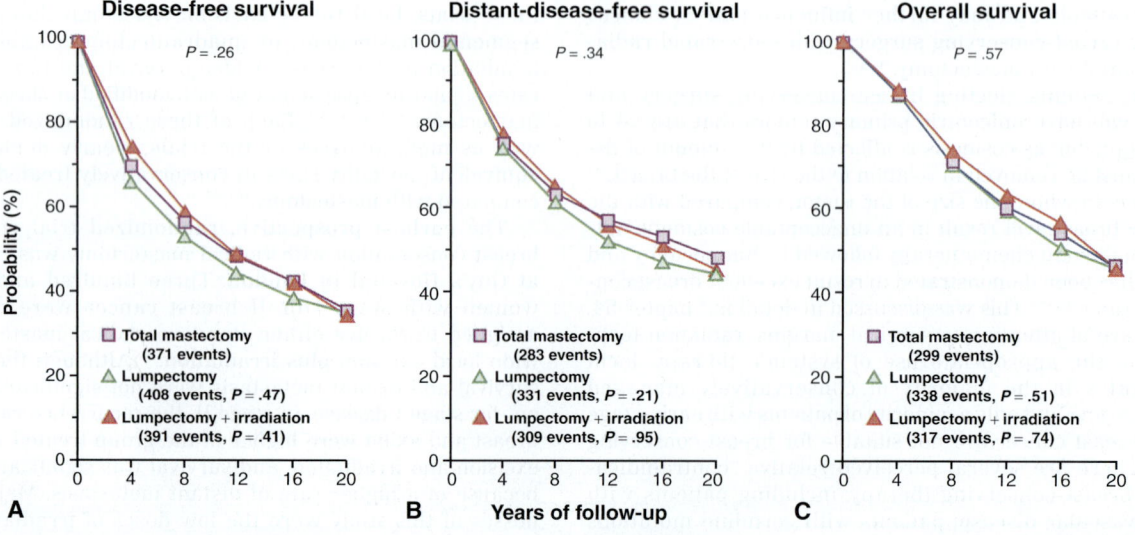

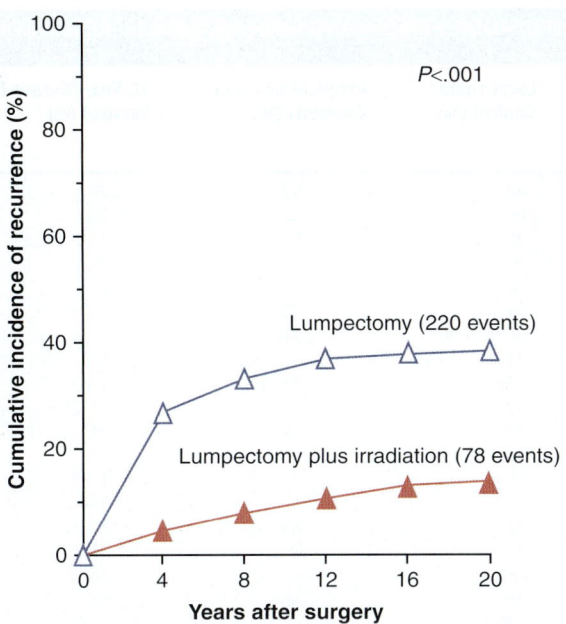

FIGURE 59.15. Cumulative incidence of IBR after lumpectomy (*open triangle*) or lumpectomy plus breast irradiation (*solid triangle*) in 1,137 patients in the current-update cohort (cohort B) who had either negative or positive nodes and tumor-negative specimen margins. (From Fisher B, Anderson S, Bryant J, et al. Twenty-year follow-up of a randomized trial comparing total mastectomy, lumpectomy, and lumpectomy plus irradiation for the treatment of invasive breast cancer. *N Engl J Med* 2002;347[16]:1233–1241. Copyright © 2002 Massachusetts Medical Society. Reprinted with permission from Massachusetts Medical Society.)

A Danish Cooperative Study carried out a similar randomized trial in 905 women (another 248 patients were treated with mastectomy or breast conservation therapy according to preference without randomization).[371] High-risk patients (tumor >5 cm, invasion to skin or deep fascia, metastatic axillary lymph nodes) who were treated with breast conservation therapy received radiation therapy to the regional lymph nodes. Those who were treated with mastectomy also received irradiation of the same target volume and all high-risk patients received adjuvant CMF. At 6 years, the recurrence-free survival rate in 430 patients treated with breast conservation therapy was 70%, compared with 66% in 429 patients treated with mastectomy. Overall survival rates were 79% and 82%, respectively. There were 12 breast relapses in the former group (3%) and 19 chest wall recurrences in the latter group (4%). In the breast conservation therapy group, 31% of patients had excellent and 41% had satisfactory cosmesis.

The US National Cancer Institute reported results of a randomized study in which 122 patients with T1-2N0M0 disease were treated with modified radical mastectomy and 125 with breast conservation therapy (45 to 50 Gy to breast plus 15- to 20-Gy boost).[372] Recently updated by Poggi et al.[360] with a median follow-up of 18.4 years, there was no detectable difference with regard to overall survival between patients treated with mastectomy and those treated with breast-conserving therapy (58% vs. 54%; *P* = .67 overall). Twenty-seven women in the breast-conserving therapy arm (22%) experienced an in-breast event. After censoring in-breast events in the breast-conserving therapy arm that were salvaged successfully by mastectomy, disease-free survival also was found to be statistically similar (67% in the mastectomy arm vs. 63% in the breast-conserving therapy arm; *P* = .64 overall). There was no statistically significant difference in the incidence of contralateral breast carcinoma between the two treatment groups.

Van Dongen et al.[99,361] reported on an EORTC trial comparing modified radical mastectomy with breast-conserving therapy (lumpectomy, axillary clearance, and irradiation to the breast, 50 Gy in 5 weeks and a 25-Gy boost with iridium implant) in 168 patients with stage I and 734 with stage II disease. Patients with microscopically incomplete excision of the tumor were included. Updated analysis from this trial with a median follow-up period of 13.4 years revealed that locoregional recurrence (LRR) rates were higher in the breast conservation therapy group (10-year rate, 19.7%) than in the mastectomy group (10-year rate, 12.2%, *P* = .0097). The overall survival rate at 10 years was 66.1% for patients undergoing mastectomies and 65.2% for patients undergoing breast conservation therapy (*P* = .11).

Additional Experiences with Breast-Conserving Surgery Plus Radiation Therapy

Although the acceptance of breast-conserving surgery plus radiation therapy as an alternative to mastectomy has been established based on the numerous randomized trials outlined above, large retrospective experiences with long-term follow-up have provided additional data regarding the selection of patients for breast-conserving therapy and radiation, prognostic factors for locoregional end points, impact of various treatment policies and techniques, complications, cosmesis, and long-term outcomes.

Mature Retrospective Series of Breast-Conserving Surgery Plus Radiation Therapy

There have been numerous reports of breast-conserving therapy and radiation, now with follow-up exceeding 10 to 15 years. These studies have provided valuable data regarding technical issues related to treatment and have provided additional data regarding outcomes in subsets of patients, prognostic factors for local control, cosmesis, and other sequelae. Lessons learned from these retrospective series have yielded valuable insight into the conservative management of breast cancer and provide the basis for further prospective studies. Selected publications are highlighted below and in the section on prognostic factors for local control. Long-term outcome from some of these experiences are summarized in Table 59.14.[97,107,296,313,355,370,373–390] Collectively, these studies clearly show long-term outcomes that are consistent with the randomized trials noted above. Local failure rates will depend on follow-up, selection factors, and treatment, as discussed later, but in general are expected to range between 0.5% and 1% per year.

PROGNOSTIC FACTORS FOR LOCAL RELAPSE FOLLOWING BREAST-CONSERVING SURGERY PLUS RADIATION THERAPY

The retrospective experiences outlined above together with the prospective randomized trials have provided additional data confirming acceptable long-term local control, cosmesis, and toxicities and have identified prognostic factors that lead to higher local relapse rates and impact treatment policies.

Local relapse in the conservatively managed breast is an active area of investigation, with numerous studies dedicated to the evaluation of factors that identify patients at increased risk for local relapse following lumpectomy and radiation therapy. Although prognostic factors for local relapse are not as well evaluated as they have been for systemic relapse, there have been numerous studies demonstrating the prognostic value of molecular and genetic markers for local relapse. Local relapse following breast-conserving surgery and radiation can be governed by a complex array of host, primary tumor, and treatment factors.

Given the complex interaction of these factors, it is sometimes difficult to separate out the independent significance of any one factor. There have, however, been several factors that have been consistently reported in

TABLE 59.14 CONSERVATION SURGERY AND IRRADIATION: NONRANDOMIZED STUDIES STAGE I AND II BREAST CANCER: RESULTS OF SELECTED STUDIES

Study (Reference)	Number of Patients	Stage	Dose (Gy) Breast	Dose (Gy) Boost	Local Tumor Control (%)	Excellent or Good Cosmesis (%)	10-Year Disease-Free Survival (%)
Amalric et al.[355]	1,440	I, II	60	15–20	80	90	74
Barr et al.[373]	411	I, II, III	48.4	20	88	NS	NS
Bartelink et al.[574]	585	T1,T2	50	25	98	NS	T1,92[a] T2,85
Calle et al.[375]	411	I, II	50	10	89	88	78
Clark et al.[376]	1,504	T1–2N0	40/3 wk	5–15	86	NS	70
Clarke et al.[577]	436	T1,T2	45	15	90	NS	–
Delouche et al.[778]	410	T1,T2	50–60	Yes	T1,94 T2,86	93	62.5
Dewar et al.[379]	757	T0–2	45	15	92	–	69
Dubois et al.[380]	231	I	45	10–15	1,91	90	1–84
	161	II			84		11–75
Fagundes et al.[381]	425	T1,T2	50	10–15	92	77	74[b]
Fourquet et al.[382]	518	T1,T2	57–62	5–12	90	NS	NS
Fowble et al.[107]	697	I, II	50	10–15	91	93	1–79
							II-67
Gage et al.[383]	1,870	I, II	45–50	10–20	87	NS	NS
Haffty et al.[97]	433	I, II	48	10–20	92	NS	81
Kurtz et al.[296]	1,593	I, II	50–60	20	89	–	86
Leborgne et al.[384]	796	I, II	50	10–20	87[b]	NS	82[c]
Osborne et al.[385]	263	T1,T2	45	10	I, 85	–	I, 54
					11,81		II, 29
Pierquin et al.[386]	245	I, II	50	10–20	90	82	75[c]
Recht et al.[387]	366	I, II	50	10	I, 96	–	–
					II, 90		
Sarrazin et al.[370]	179	T1smT2	45	15	95	92	85[b]
Solin et al.[388]	217	T1	45–50	10–15	95	90	T1, 80[b]
	166	T2	45–50	10–15	92	90	T2, 69[b]
van Limbergen et al.[389]	235	T1,T2(3)	40–65	8–20	90	–	T1,75.4
							T2, 61.9
Vicini et al.[390]	1,396	I, II	50	10	92	87	NS
Vilcoq et al.[313]	314	T1,T2	50–55	10–20	90	–	84[b]

[a]Six-year disease-free survival.
[b]Five-year disease-free survival.
[c]Fifteen-year disease-free survival.
NS, not stated.

TABLE 59.15 SUMMARY OF RISK FACTORS FOR LOCAL RELAPSE

Prognostic Factor	Effect	Strength of Data	Comment
Age	Young age increases local relapse	Multiple studies. Upheld in multivariate analysis. Few conflicting reports	Remains among the strongest factors
Margins	Positive margins increase local relapse	Multiple studies. Upheld in multivariate analysis. Few conflicting reports	Remains among the strongest factors. Data on "close" margins are less consistent.
Systemic therapy	Systemic therapy (chemo and hormonal) lowers risk of local relapse	Multiple studies support. Some conflicting reports	May delay rather than counteract risk
Radiation dose	Higher doses decrease local relapse	Multiple studies support. Confirmed in randomized trials (boost vs. no boost). Some conflicting data regarding doses above 50 Gy	Interaction with margins and age. Necessity of "boost" in women over 50 and with widely negative margins unclear
Extensive intraductal component (EIC)	EIC positive tumors have higher rates of local relapse	Initial studies supportive. Some confirmatory studies. Some conflicting studies	Recent data suggest that negative margin status eliminates this as a risk factor
LCIS as a component	LCIS as a component increases risk of local relapse	Conflicting data with no clear consensus	Patients with LCIS are suitable candidates for BCS. Debate remains regarding need for clear LCIS margins.
Lobular histology	Lobular histology has higher local relapse rates	Conflicting data with no clear consensus	Should be treated similar to invasive ductal cancers
BRCA1/2	Higher late local relapses in BRCA1/2 patients	Several confirmatory studies. Some conflicting data	Higher relapse rates related to late "new primaries." This may be minimized by prophylactic hormonal manipulation
Tumor size	Larger tumors result in higher local relapses	Some confirmatory studies. Several conflicting studies	Data are confounded by more frequent use of systemic therapy in larger tumors
Nodal status	Higher local relapse rates in node-positive patients	Several conflicting studies	As with tumor size, data are confounded by more frequent use of systemic therapy in node-positive patients
Receptor status	Higher local relapse rates in triple-negative and HER2-positive patients	Some confirmatory studies. Few conflicting studies. Under active investigation	Would offer these patients conventional whole-breast irradiation

BCS, breast-conserving surgery; LCIS, lobular carcinoma in situ.

TABLE 59.16 IPSILATERAL BREAST RECURRENCE RATES BY AGE

Study (Reference)	Follow-Up (Year)	≤35 Year		>35 Year	
		Number of Patients	**Recurrence**	**Number of Patients**	**Recurrence**
Clarke and Martinez[391]	5 (mean)	32	3 (9%)	424	21 (5%)
Fowble et al.[291]	8 (actuarial)	64	15 (24%)	916	119 (13%)
Haffty et al.[90]	8.2 (median)	34	5 (15%)	349	38 (11%)
Halverson et al.[392]	7 (actuarial)	37	3 (9%)	474	57 (12%)
Kini et al.[393]	10 (median)		24%		7%
Kurtz et al.[394]	11 (mean)	91	15 (16%)	1,291	129 (10%)
Matthews et al.[395]	≥2	72	11 (15%)	306	15 (5%)
Nixon et al.[396]	8.3 (median)	107	15 (14%)	1,026	92 (9%)
Veronesi et al.[397]	6 (median)	95	9 (9%)	1,137	45 (4%)
Vicini et al.[390]	5 (actuarial)	65	14 (21%)	721	65 (9%)

influencing local relapse in the conservatively managed breast cancer patient. Table 59.15 summarizes some of the more commonly reported prognostic factors for local relapse. The factors that most consistently have been reported to influence local relapse, namely, young age, margin status, and the use of systemic therapy, are discussed first, followed by other commonly evaluated prognostic factors.

Age

Young age has been shown in numerous studies to be a risk factor for breast recurrence in conservation surgery and irradiation. These are summarized in Table 59.16.[90,291,391–400]

Different investigators have used various age cutoffs, such as 40, 35, and 30 years. Vilcoq et al.[313] found an LRR rate of 35% versus 4% in women younger or older than 30 years.

Kurtz et al.[399] reported a 19% incidence of local recurrence in 210 women younger than 40 years of age, compared with 9% in 1,172 older women. This observation correlated with EIC, high tumor grade, and a major mononuclear cell reaction. The Harvard Joint Center's inferior results in younger women also correlated with the presence of EIC.[401] These findings have also been reported by other authors.[378,389,402]

One of the most significant and powerful studies correlating young age with local relapse was the large EORTC boost versus no-boost trial.[403] Overall in this study, young patient age was a significant predictor of local relapse. As shown in Figure 59.16, the use of a boost, as will be discussed later, was most effective in younger women, although the more recent update found an advantage to the boost in all age groups.[404] In a review of 3,602 women who underwent

FIGURE 59.16. Cumulative incidence of recurrence of tumor in the ipsilateral breast after whole-breast irradiation at 50 Gy, with or without an additional dose to the tumor bed as a function of age group. (From Bartelink H, Horiot JC, Poortmans PM, et al. Impact of a higher radiation dose on local control and survival in breast-conserving therapy of early breast cancer: 10-year results of the randomized boost versus no boost EORTC 22881–10882 trial. *J Clin Oncol* 2007;25[22]:3259–3265. Reprinted with permission. Copyright © 2007 American Society of Clinical Oncology. All rights reserved.)

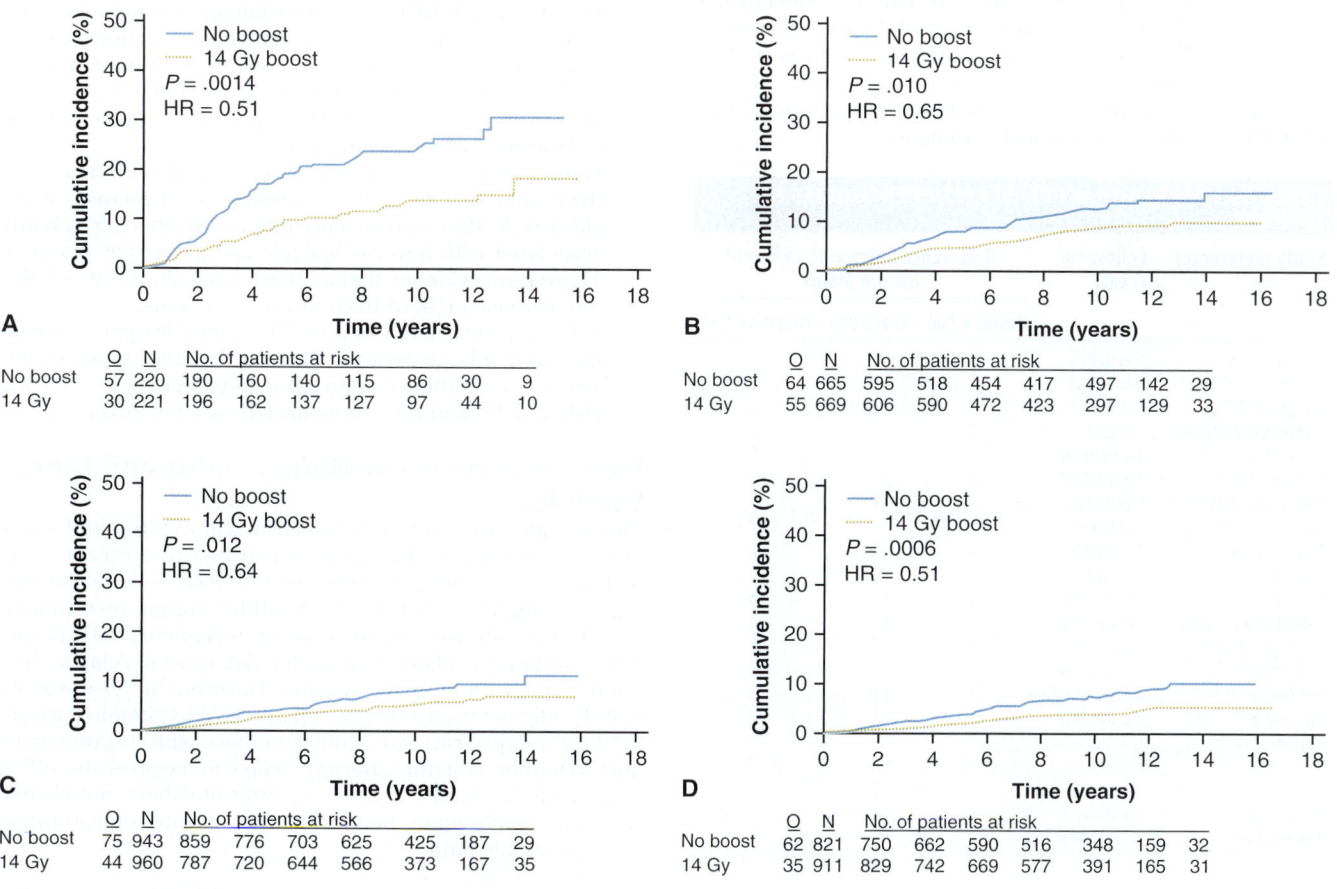

surgery (breast conservation, 55%, or mastectomy, 45%) for early breast cancer and were rolled in EORTC studies, de Bock et al.[405] clearly demonstrated the impact of young age on local relapse. The results of multivariate analysis showed that younger age and breast conservation were risk factors for isolated LRR (breast cancer under 35 years of age vs. over 50 years of age: HR 2.80; 95% CI, 1.41 to 5.60; breast cancer age 35 to 50 years vs. over 50 years: HR 1.72; 95% CI, 1.17 to 2.54; breast conservation: HR 1.82; 95% CI, 1.17 to 2.86). After perioperative chemotherapy, less isolated LRRs were observed (HR 0.63; 95% CI, 0.44 to 0.91). It is concluded that young age and breast-conserving therapy are both independent predictors for isolated LRR. The authors note that as an isolated LRR is a potentially curable condition, women treated with breast conservation or diagnosed with breast cancer at a young age should be monitored closely to detect local recurrence at an early stage.

Numerous other studies have confirmed in univariate and multivariate analyses a significant correlation between younger age and local relapse rates. Although there is no apparent cutoff age where relapse rates significantly change, most of the studies have selected 35 years of age or 40 years of age to demonstrate the differences.[288,290,291,396,398,406,407] However, one study that compared the outcome of breast conservation in patients under 40 found that those under 35 had a higher risk of recurrence compared with those aged 36 to 40.[408]

Margin Status

Positive margin status has been one of the most consistently reported factors associated with higher local relapse rates. Selected studies are summarized in Table 59.17.[222,223,374,379,391,409-415,417-420,422-426] Because of the varying definitions of margin status and the complex interaction between margin status and use of systemic therapy, radiation dose, and patient age, there are conflicting conclusions regarding the influence of margin status on local relapse.

Definition of a negative margin is variable between institutions and in national studies. Although some consider no tumor cells seen on the inked margin definitive, as defined by the NSABP, others consider negative as margins of 1 or 2 mm beyond invasive cancer; of note, many of the studies evaluating margin status utilized pathologic reports without a central re-review of the original pathology.

The degree of margin involvement (i.e., whether it is focally involved or more diffusely involved) is also a critical issue in determining the significance of margin involvement and how it should influence management. Although there are clearly conflicting reports, it is evident that obtaining a wide negative margin is desirable. However, a focally involved margin, particularly when re-excision is not technically feasible, as may be the case with a focally involved deep margin at the pectoralis facia, is not a contraindication to breast-conserving therapy.

Recently, a multidisciplinary panel of breast experts from the Society of Surgical Oncology-American Society for Radiation Oncology examined the relationship between margin width and IBTR and developed a guideline for defining adequate margins in the setting of breast-conserving surgery and adjuvant radiation therapy[427]. The meta-analysis was based on 33 eligible studies published between 1965 and 2013 and included 28,162 patients, of whom 1,506 had an IBTR (5.3%). The median follow-up was 79.2 months. Their conclusions and recommendations are as follows:

1. A positive margin, defined as ink on invasive cancer or DCIS, is associated with at least a twofold increase in IBTR. This increased risk in IBTR is not nullified by (a) delivery of a boost dose of radiation, (b) delivery of systemic therapy (endocrine therapy, chemotherapy, or biologic therapy), or (c) favorable biology.
2. Negative margins (no ink on tumor) minimize the risk of IBTR. Wider margin widths do not significantly lower this risk. The routine practice to obtain negative margin widths wider than no ink on tumor is not indicated.
3. The rates of IBTR are reduced with the use of systemic therapy. In the uncommon circumstance of a patient not receiving adjuvant systemic therapy, there is no evidence suggesting that margins wider than no ink on tumor are needed.
4. Margins wider than no ink on tumor are not indicated based on biologic subtype.
5. The choice of WBRT delivery technique, fractionation, and boost dose should not be dependent on margin width.
6. Wider negative margins than no ink on tumor are not indicated for ILC. Classic LCIS at the margin is not an indication for re-excision. The significance of pleomorphic LCIS at the margin is uncertain.
7. Young age (≤40 years) is associated with both increased IBTR after BCT as well as increased local relapse on the chest wall after mastectomy and is also more frequently associated with adverse biologic and pathologic features. There is no evidence that increased margin width nullifies the increased risk of IBTR in young patients.
8. A lobular carcinoma in situ (EIC) identifies patients who may have a large residual DCIS burden after lumpectomy. There is no evidence of an association between increased risk of IBTR and EIC when margins are negative.

Interaction between Margin Status and Other Variables

The complex interaction between margin status and other treatment-related factors is demonstrated in a recent study by Park et al.[418] They demonstrated that local relapse was significantly higher in patients with diffuse margin involvement than in patients with negative margins. Patients with focally involved margins also had a higher risk of local relapse than did patients with negative margins. However, in those women with focally involved margins who received systemic therapy, the local relapse rate was similar to those with negative margins. Whether systemic therapy delays or negates the effect of a focally involved margin is a matter of debate, but clearly, there are confounding factors that complicate interpretation of the available data.

TABLE 59.17 IPSILATERAL BREAST RECURRENCE RATES BY MARGINS

Study (Reference)	Follow-Up (Year)	Recurrence Rates with Different Margin Status		
		Positive (%)	Close (%)	Negative (%)
Anscher et al.[409]	5 actuarial	10	–	2
Bartelink et al.[374]	6 actuarial	7	–	2
Borger et al.[410]	5 actuarial	16	–	2
Clarke and Martinez[391]	5 mean	9	–	4
Dewar et al.[379]	10 actuarial	14	–	6
DiBiase et al.[411]	10 actuarial	33	–	12
Freedman et al.[412]	5 actuarial	12	14	7
Ghossein et al.[413]	7 median	10	–	12
Hartsell et al.[414]	3.4 median	11	–	2
Heimann et al.[415]	5 actuarial	11	–	2
Jobsen et al.[416]	10 actuarial	12	–	5
Obedian and Haffty[222]	10 actuarial	17	2	2
Peterson et al.[417]	8 actuarial	10	17	8
Park et al.[418]	8 crude rate	18	7	7
Pittinger et al.[419]	4.5 crude rate	25	2.9	3
Ryoo et al.[420]	3.5 median	–	13	8
Schnitt et al.[421]	6.2 median	13	4	2
Smitt et al.[223]	–	9	16	2
Solin et al.[422]	5 actuarial	2	11	7
Vicini et al.[423]	12 actuarial	30	18-24	9
Wazer et al.[424]	12 actuarial	17	9	5

Freedman et al.[412] studied 1,262 patients with clinical stage I or II breast cancer treated by breast-conserving surgery, axillary node dissection, and radiation therapy. The final margins were negative in 77%, positive in 12%, and close (≤2 mm) in 11%. The 5-year incidence of IBTR was not significantly different among patients with negative (4%), positive (5%), or close (7%) margins. However, by 10 years, a significant difference in IBTR became apparent (negative 7%, positive 12%, close 14%; P = .04). The 5-year cumulative IBTR rate in patients with close or positive margins was 1% with adjuvant systemic therapy and 13% with no adjuvant therapy. However, by 10 years, the IBTR rate was similar (18% vs. 14%), because of more late failures in the patients who received adjuvant systemic therapy.

A study by Jobsen et al.[416] demonstrates some of the difficulties associated with interpretation of studies related to margin status and local relapse as it relates to other prognostic factors. In a study of 1,752 patients with known margin status and a median follow-up of 78 months, the 10-year local relapse rate was 5.6% and 12.2% for negative and positive margins, respectively. An interaction between age category and margin status was noted in relation to local relapse-free survival. The 5-year local relapse rate for women younger than 40 years of age was 8.4% for negative margins and 36.9% for positive margins (P = .005). On the other hand, the 5-year local relapse rate for women over 40 years old was 2.6% for negative and 2.2% for positive margins.

Although it is clear that margin status is a significant risk factor for local relapse, and negative margins are desirable, the available data suggest that patients with a focally involved margin are suitable candidates for breast-conserving therapy followed by radiation therapy to the intact breast.

Effect of Systemic Therapy on Local Control

The use of systemic therapy, in the form of adjuvant tamoxifen or adjuvant chemotherapy, has been clearly shown to impact local control in numerous retrospective and prospective randomized trials. Although it has been clearly demonstrated in randomized trials that chemotherapy and tamoxifen are not appropriate substitutes for radiation therapy, in patients who are treated with radiation therapy, the use of systemic therapy improves local control.[91,92,95,428] As with the other critical prognostic factors, the degree to which systemic therapy influences local control is confounded by other factors.

In the NSABP B-06 trial, patients with lymph node–positive disease who were treated with radiation therapy and chemotherapy had an 8-year local recurrence rate of 5% compared with a local recurrence rate of 12% in lymph node–negative patients treated with surgery and radiation therapy alone.[363] In the NSABP B-21 trial, tamoxifen similarly improved local control rates in patients with lymph node–negative breast tumors smaller than 1 cm. The crude rate of breast tumor recurrence was only 3% in women randomly assigned to undergo lumpectomy, radiation therapy, and tamoxifen compared with 7% in women treated with lumpectomy and radiation therapy alone.[93] A retrospective analysis from the MD Anderson Cancer Center investigating the impact of systemic therapy on local control after breast-conserving therapy in patients with lymph node–negative breast cancer further confirmed these data.[95] In this study, 277 patients treated with systemic therapy had improved 5-year (97.5% vs. 89.8%) and 10-year (95.6% vs. 85.2%) local control rates compared with 207 patients who received no systemic treatment. No statistically significant difference was evident in local control between patients treated with chemotherapy and those treated with tamoxifen alone (P = .219). In a Cox regression analysis, the use of systemic therapy was the most powerful clinical, pathologic, or treatment predictor of local control, producing a 3.3-fold reduction in the risk of local recurrence. Similar results have been reported in series from Yale as well

TABLE 59.18 IPSILATERAL BREAST RECURRENCE RATES BY SYSTEMIC TREATMENT (SYSTX)

Study (Reference)	Number of Patients	Follow-Up (Year)	SysTx	Local Relapse		
				With SysTx	Without SysTx	P
NSABP-13[430]	760	8	CTX	2.6%	13%	.001
NSABP-14[451]	1,400	10	Tam	3.4%	10.3%	.001
Buchholz[95]	484	8	CTX+Tam	4.4%	14.8%	.004
Haffty et al.[90]	548	7	CTX+Tam	6%	12%	.02
Park et al. (positive margin)[418]	45	8	CTX	7%	18%	.05
Van der Leest[428]	758	8.5	CTX	5%	12%	.002

CTX, chemotherapy; Tam, tamoxifen.

as the Netherlands, where the risk of local relapse was lower among patients treated by breast-conserving surgery and radiation with adjuvant chemotherapy or adjuvant tamoxifen, compared with patients treated without adjuvant systemic therapy.[428,429] Table 59.18 summarizes several of these studies that have evaluated local control as a function of systemic therapy. It is evident that both hormonal therapy as well as cytotoxic chemotherapy influence local relapse rates.[430–432]

Trastuzumab (Herceptin) is a humanized monoclonal antibody against the human EGFR-2 (HER2), which is amplified or overexpressed in about 15% to 20% of invasive breast cancers; these tumors are known to be more aggressive and more susceptible to recurrence than HER2-negative tumors. Romond et al.[271] reported on a combine analysis from two large cooperative group studies investigating the utility of trastuzumab in HER2-positive patients with operable breast cancer and found that trastuzumab improved disease-free survival by an absolute value of 12% at 3 years and was associated with a 33% reduction in the risk of death (P = .015). Interestingly, they also reported that IBTR as a site of first failure was reduced from 57 patients to 27 patients with the use of trastuzumab. Recently, Kiess et al.[433] reported on a series of 197 women with early-stage breast cancer; 70 women did not receive trastuzumab while 102 did receive trastuzumab. They found that the 3-year LRR-free survival rate was 90% without trastuzumab and 99% with trastuzumab. Moreover, LRRs were reduced from 7 to 1 with the use of trastuzumab. These data lend support to the notion that systemic therapy has an impact on local control.

Tumor Size

Although tumor size is clearly a strong predictor of systemic relapse and overall survival, its prognostic value in local relapse has not been consistently reported (Table 59.19).[96,365,373–375,378,380,386,388,389,391,434–438] Differences are probably related to the treatment techniques used (e.g., completeness of tumor excision, use of irradiation boost) and the complex interaction of other prognostic factors, as noted above.

Tumor Location

Location of the primary tumor within the breast is not known to be a contraindication to breast-conserving surgery, and any specific location is not associated with a higher local relapse rate. Haffty et al.,[439] in a review of 1,014 patients with early breast cancer treated with breast conservation therapy, identified 98 patients who had a central or subareolar tumor. Ten of 98 patients had the nipple–areola complex sacrificed at the time of surgery, whereas the remaining 88 patients had the entire area included in the boost cone–down field. The 10-year actuarial breast recurrence-free survival rate was 84%, the distant disease-free survival rate was 88%, and the overall survival rate was 79%, similar to patients with

TABLE 59.19 CONSERVATION SURGERY AND IRRADIATION IN BREAST CANCER: LOCAL RECURRENCE AT 5 YEARS CORRELATED WITH INITIAL TUMOR STAGE

Study (Reference)	Percent Local Recurrence (Total Number of Patients in Study)			
	Stage T1 or I		Stage T2 or II	
Barr et al.[373]	12	(101)	12	(255)
Bartelink et al.[374]	2	(360)	2	(197)
Calle et al.[375]	7	(190)	11	(113)
Clarke et al.[391]	6	(305)	3	(95)
Delouche et al.[378]	6	(220)	14	(190)
Dubois et al.[380]	10.8	(231)	16.1	(161)
Eberlein et al.[434]	13	–	12	–
Fisher et al.[435]	7	(306)	12	(257)
Fowble et al.[107]	8		8	
Leung et al.[436]	7.4	(150)	12.8	(335)
Perez et al.[437]	5	(1039)	10	(308)
Pierquin et al.[386]	8	–	12	–
Solin et al.[388]	5	(217)	8	(166)
Stotter et al.[438]	10	(249)	12	(241)
van Limbergen et al.[389]	5	(57)	11.5	(104)

TABLE 59.20 INCIDENCE OF BREAST RELAPSE CORRELATED WITH EXTENSIVE INTRADUCTAL CARCINOMA COMPONENT IN PRIMARY BREAST TUMOR ADJACENT BREAST

Study (Reference)	Percent Breast Recurrence at 5 Years (Total Number of Patients in Study)			
	EIC Present		EIC Absent	
Bartelink et al.[374]	9	(79)	2	(208)
Boyages et al.[444]	24	(166)	6	(418)
Eberlein et al.[434]	27	(166)	7	(418)
Fisher et al.[194]	11	(56)	9	(366)
Fowble et al.[96]	22	(23)	4	(252)
Kurtz et al.[296]	18	(106)	8	(390)
Schnitt et al.[445]	15	(133)	1	(98)
Veronesi et al.[397]				
Quadrantectomy	10	(22)	4	(338)
Tumorectomy	30	(38)	8	(307)
Zafrani et al.[196]	11	(63)	6	(361)

EIC, extensive intraductal carcinoma.

tumors in other locations. The nipple–areola complex could be preserved in most patients, and there were no significant complications. Thus, a subareolar breast cancer presentation was not a contraindication to breast-conserving therapy in early-stage disease.

However, Gajdos et al.[440] reported on 95 women with tumors located within 2 cm of the border of the areola, considered to be subareolar carcinomas; 62 were treated with breast-conserving surgery and 33 with mastectomies. Radiation therapy was given to 87% of the breast-conserving surgery group and to 13% of the mastectomy group. The nipple–areola complex was removed in 11 women in the breast-conserving group. On univariate analysis, variables significantly related to pathologic involvement of the nipple–areola complex were clinical involvement of the nipple–areola complex (P = .001), mammographic calcifications or Paget disease (P < .001), pathologic tumor size (P = .019), and the presence of an EIC (P = .098). When radiation therapy was accounted for in multivariate analysis, the only variable significantly related to local recurrence in patients undergoing breast-conserving surgery was clinical involvement of the nipple–areola complex.

Extensive Intraductal Carcinoma

According to the Harvard definition of EIC, 25% or more of the primary tumor is intraductal carcinoma, and intraductal carcinoma is seen outside (adjacent to) the infiltrating tumor border.[441] Fourquet et al.[382] reported a 20% incidence of EIC in 185 women younger than 45 years of age compared with 10.4% in 279 older women. EIC involving the primary tumor and adjacent tissues has been reported by some groups, particularly Harvard University and Marseilles, to be associated with a higher incidence of breast recurrences.[399,442,443] In contrast, others have found no significant impact on local tumor control with EIC.[194,228,377,389] This difference may be related to the definition of EIC, adequacy of tumor excision, doses of irradiation delivered to the boost volume, as well as interactions with other factors. It has been reported by some that a somewhat higher breast relapse rate in EIC-positive patients was seen only in women younger than 40 years of age. Table 59.20 summarizes reports of breast relapse correlated with presence of EIC in selected studies.[96,194,196,374,397,401,434,443–445]

Holland et al.[446] stated that an EIC component is associated with subsequent breast recurrence because of the presence of residual intraductal carcinoma in these patients. In a series of 214 women who underwent mastectomy, 71% of those with EIC had residual intraductal carcinoma, compared with 28%

of those without that pathologic feature. In particular, 44% of the EIC-positive patients had prominent residual tumor compared with 3% of those who were EIC negative (P < .00001).

The impact of EIC on local relapse, however, appears to be minimized if negative margins are achieved. Although negative margins are desirable in all patients undergoing breast-conserving surgery, attention to margins in patients with EIC is particularly relevant, as a negative margin may decrease or eliminate the significance of EIC with respect to local failure. In a study from the Harvard group, Gage et al.[447] evaluated clinical stage I or II breast carcinoma treated with radiation therapy as part of breast-conserving therapy, of whom 343 had invasive ductal histology evaluable for an extensive intraductal component, had inked margins that were evaluable for an review of their pathology slides, and received ≥60 Gy to the tumor bed. The 5-year rate of ipsilateral breast recurrence (IBR) for patients with negative margins was 2%; for patients with positive margins, the rate was 16%. Among patients with negative margins, the 5-year rate of IBR was 2% for all patients with close margins (negative ≤1 mm) and 3% for those with negative margins >1 mm. For patients with close margins, the rates were 2% and 0% for EIC-negative and EIC-positive tumors, respectively; the corresponding rates for patients with negative margins >1 mm were 1% and 14%. The 5-year rate of IBR for patients with focally positive margins was 9% (9% for EIC-negative and 7% for EIC-positive patients). The 5-year crude rate of IBR for patients with greater than focally positive margins was 28% (19% for EIC-negative and 42% for EIC-positive patients). The authors conclude that patients with negative margins of excision have a low rate of recurrence in the treated breast, whether the margin is >1 mm or ≤1 mm and whether the carcinoma is EIC negative or EIC positive. It appears from this study that although EIC may be a poor prognostic factor for local relapse, achievement of a negative margin eliminates EIC as a risk factor.

From a group of 885 patients treated for clinical stage I or II invasive breast cancer, Schnitt et al.[421] limited their study to 181 patients with IDC who received a radiation dose to the surgical site of 60 Gy or greater, whose final microscopic margins of resection were evaluable, and who had at least 5 years of follow-up. In 157 patients (87%), the tumor was evaluable for the presence or absence of EIC. The 5-year rates of recurrence among patients with negative, close, focally positive, and more than focally positive margins were 0%, 4%, 6%, and 21%, respectively. Among the 127 patients with EIC-negative tumors, the 5-year recurrence rate was <10% in all margin groups. Among the 30 patients with EIC-positive tumors, the 5-year recurrence rate was 0% when margins

TABLE 59.21 LOBULAR CARCINOMA TREATED WITH BREAST-CONSERVING SURGERY AND RADIATION (SELECTED SERIES WITH 10-YEAR FOLLOW-UP)

Study (Reference)	Number Lobular/ Number Ductal	Local Relapse Lobular/ Ductal	Contralateral Lobular/ Ductal	Overall Survival Lobular/Ductal
Santiago et al.[449]	55/1,093	18% vs. 12% (NS)	12% vs. 8% (NS)	85% vs. 79% (NS)
Vo et al.[450]	84/1,126	4% vs. 9% (NS)	11.3% vs. 11.9% (NS)	81% vs. 85% (NS)
Moran et al.[453]	142/1,760	20% vs. 13% (NS)	26% vs. 12% (P = .006)	68% v. 78% (P = .08)
Salvadori et al.[452]	286/1,903	8% vs. 8% (NS)	NR	NR
Peiro et al.[451]	93/1,089	15% vs. 13% (NS)	4% vs. 6% (NS)	NR

NR, no results; NS, not significant.

were negative or close but 50% when margins were more than focally positive. These results provide support for the use of breast-conserving therapy (including an irradiation boost to the primary site) for patients with EIC-positive tumors and negative margins.

Histology

In general, studies that have evaluated local relapse in relation to histologic subtypes of breast cancer have not demonstrated higher relapse rates associated with specific histologic patterns. Weiss et al.[236] reported on 879 patients with stage I and II breast cancer treated with conservation surgery and irradiation. The patients were divided into 7 groups based on histologic subtype: 368 patients with infiltrating and intraductal ductal carcinoma, 389 with IDC, 41 with ILC, 23 with combined infiltrating ductal and lobular carcinoma, 28 with medullary carcinoma, 12 with colloid carcinoma, and 18 with tubular carcinoma. There were no significant differences in 5-year actuarial overall survival, cause-specific survival, or relapse-free survival rates among the histologic categories. There was, however, a difference among the seven groups in distant metastasis only at first failure, with IDCs having the highest rate.

Thurman et al.,[237] in an analysis of the Harvard series, identified twenty clinical stage I and II patients with mucinous carcinoma, 27 with medullary carcinoma, 28 with tubular carcinoma, and 1,055 with IDC. No significant difference was seen in the site of first failure among the four histologic types within the first 10 years after treatment. Local failure was significantly associated with age <50 years (P = .04), positive surgical margins (P = .007), lymphovascular invasion (P = .04), and presence of an extensive intraductal component (P < .001).

An analysis of medullary carcinomas treated conservatively was performed by the Yale group, who identified 46 cases of conservatively treated patients with medullary histology who were compared with 1,444 patients with infiltrating ductal carcinoma.[200] The medullary cohort presented at a younger age with a higher percentage of patients in the 35 years or younger age group (26.1% vs. 6.6%; P < .00001). Twelve patients with medullary histology underwent genetic screening, and six patients were identified with deleterious mutations. This group showed greater association with *BRCA1/2* mutations compared with screened patients in the control group (50.0% vs. 15.8%; P = .0035). The medullary

cohort was also significantly associated with greater T stage and tumor size (37.0% vs. 17.2%; T2 mean size 3.2 vs. 2.5 cm; P = .00097) as well as negative ER (84.9% vs. 37.6%; P < .00001) and PR (87.5% vs. 48.1%; P = .00001) status. Breast relapse-free rates were not significantly different from the invasive ductal cancers (76.7% vs. 85.2%); however, 10-year distant relapse-free survival in the medullary cohort was significantly better than in the control group (94.9% vs. 77.5%; P = .028).

Tubular carcinomas treated with CS and radiation were reviewed by Sullivan et al.[199] They reviewed 62 of their own cases from the Massachusetts General as well as 529 cases from the literature. They conclude that tubular carcinoma is associated with an excellent prognosis, but long-term follow-up is essential for detecting local failures. Adjuvant RT reduces the incidence of local failure following CS for tubular carcinoma. However, elderly women treated by CS may have a very low risk of local recurrence without adjuvant RT.

Infiltrating Lobular Carcinoma

A review of the literature strongly supports local tumor resection and breast irradiation as appropriate therapy for invasive lobular breast cancer, following the same guidelines used for invasive ductal tumors. Breast tumor control and survival after breast-conserving therapy are equivalent in patients with invasive ductal or lobular carcinoma. Because of the presumed multicentric nature of lobular carcinomas, several groups have attempted to assess whether these subtypes are more prone to local failure with breast-conserving approaches.[238,448-453] Table 59.21 summarizes results of several selected series of patients treated with breast-conserving surgery and radiation comparing outcomes in lobular carcinoma to IDCs. Although some of the studies show higher contralateral rates in lobular carcinomas, local relapse, disease-free, and overall survival appear to be comparable to IDCs. The majority of studies show locoregional control, disease-free, and overall survival rates in lobular carcinomas that are comparable to patients with IDCs.

Lobular Carcinoma *in Situ* as a Component of Invasive Cancers

Several groups have evaluated whether patients with LCIS as a component of invasive cancer or DCIS were associated with higher local relapse rates. Conflicting results from these studies,

TABLE 59.22 STUDIES EVALUATING LCIS AS A COMPONENT OF BREAST CANCER LOCAL RELAPSE IN BREAST-CONSERVING THERAPY PLUS RADIATION THERAPY

Study (Reference)	Number of Patients and Controls		Follow-Up (Median, Year)	Local Relapse		P
	With LCIS	Without LCIS		With LCIS (%)	Without LCIS (%)	
Moran and Haffty[454]	51	1,045	10.6	5	7	NS
Abner et al.[455]	119	1,062	13.4	13	12	NS
Ben-David et al.[456]	64	121	3.9	100	99.1	NS
Jolly et al.[457]	46	551	8.7	14	7	.04
Sasson et al.[458]	65	1,209	6.3	15	5	.001
Ciocca et al.[459]	290	2,604	6.0	4.5	3.8	NS

LCIS, lobular carcinoma *in situ*; NS, not significant.

Section III

as outlined in Table 59.22, preclude firm conclusions.[454-458] Sasson et al.[458] noted that LCIS was present in 65 of 1,274 patients (5%) with stage I or II breast cancer. LCIS was more likely to be associated with an ILC (30 of 59 patients; 51%) than with IDC (26 of 1,125 patients; 2%). The 10-year cumulative incidence rate of IBTR was 6% in women without LCIS compared with 29% in women with LCIS (P = .0003). In both groups, the majority of recurrences were invasive. The 10-year cumulative incidence rate of IBTR in patients who received tamoxifen was 8% when LCIS was present compared with 6% when LCIS was absent (P = .46). In a series of 56 patients with an LCIS component, Jolly et al.[457] reported a higher risk of local relapse at 10 years (14%) compared with a rate of 7% in cases without an LCIS component. In multivariate analysis, a component of LCIS was associated with a higher risk of local relapse.

However, studies from Yale, Harvard, and Michigan and a more recent study from Fox Chase failed to show a higher local relapse rate in patients with a component of LCIS. Abner et al.[455] reviewed 1,181 patients with stage I or II infiltrating ductal, infiltrating lobular, or infiltrating carcinoma with mixed features who had received at least 60 Gy to the tumor bed and had a minimum follow-up of 8 years. Of the 1,181 patients, 137 had detectable LCIS in or adjacent to the tumor. The 8-year local recurrence rate was not significantly increased for patients with LCIS overall or for the subgroup of patients with LCIS in or adjacent to the tumor. The risk of contralateral disease and of distant treatment failure also was unaffected by the presence or extent of LCIS (5% to 10% in all groups). Similar results were reported by Moran and Haffty[454] in an analysis of the Yale series where there was no statistically significant difference between patients with or without a component of LCIS in the 10-year overall survival (67% vs. 72%), distant disease-free survival (62% vs. 79%), or IBTR-free survival (77% LCIS vs. 84% control). Ben-David et al.[456] reported the results on 64 cases treated at the University of Michigan and also found no association between local failure and presence of LCIS. The presence of LCIS at the margins and the size and presence of multifocal LCIS did not alter the rate of local control. Ciocca et al.,[459] in an analysis of 290 patients with LCIS as a component compared with 2,604 without LCIS as a component, showed no difference in local control, even if LCIS was present at the final margin.

Other Histologic Features

Clemente et al.,[460] in 506 cases of infiltrating ductal carcinoma (T1-2N0M0), described peritumoral lymphatic infiltration in 6.9% of routinely evaluated specimens, whereas in a randomly selected group of 234 cases, the frequency was 20%. Patients with peritumoral lymphatic infiltration had worse disease-free and total survival rates than did those without this feature (P = .0001 for each), as well as more local recurrences (P = .0001) and a higher incidence of distant metastases (P = .0576).

Wong et al.,[461] in a study of 234 patients with clinical T1N0 breast cancer treated with breast conservation surgery and radiation therapy, scored 180 patients as lymphatic vessel invasion negative and 54 as invasion positive (23 focal and 31 extensive). The local first failure rates were 14% and 22%, respectively. The percentages of regional distant failure (without local failure) were 12% and 21%, respectively. At 10 years, 60% of the lymphatic vessel invasion–negative patients remained free of any failure, compared with 50% of the lymphatic vessel invasion–positive patients.

Nodal Status

Although nodal status is the strongest predictor of distant metastasis and overall survival, most studies have not clearly demonstrated an effect of nodal status on local control in the conservatively managed breast cancer patient. This may be because a majority of node-positive patients receive chemotherapy or hormonal therapy, which may counteract any adverse effects on local relapse. There are some data, however, that suggest an effect of nodal status on local relapse in conservatively managed patients. The Primary Therapy of Breast Cancer Study Group and others noted lower survival and a greater incidence of local recurrences in patients with positive axillary nodes after partial mastectomy.[229,462-464] At the Institut Gustave-Roussy, among 356 patients, local recurrence was noted in 26% of those with and 6.5% of those without nodal involvement; the greater the number of nodes involved, the more likely the occurrence of local failure and the lower the survival rate.[238,465] Increased incidence of breast relapse was also observed by van Limbergen et al.[389] in patients with N1b metastasis (8 of 42 patients, or 19%) and in those in whom three or more lymph nodes (4 of 14 patients, or 28.6%) compared with patients with N0 or N1a lymph nodes (14 of 187; 7.5%). However, more recent reports by several investigators noted lower survival rates but fewer breast relapses after breast conservation therapy in patients with positive nodes. Again, this is likely a result of the interaction of irradiation to the breast with adjuvant chemotherapy. Because most node-positive patients receive chemotherapy, which is synergistic with radiation in lowering the local relapse rate, any potential adverse effect of positive nodes on local relapse may be lost.

Molecular Factors and Local Relapse

In comparison with an explosion of data regarding molecular markers as risk factors for overall survival and distant metastasis in breast cancer, there are relatively few data relating molecular markers to local relapse in the conservatively managed breast. There have been several studies, however, that demonstrate the potential application of molecular markers in predicting locoregional relapse in breast cancer patients.[466-468] Particularly exciting is the potential not only to use these markers to identify patients at risk for relapse but also to consider the molecular markers as potential targets for therapeutic intervention and increasing radiation sensitivity. Several molecular markers have been shown in bench studies to be associated with radiation resistance, including p53, HER2/neu, insulin-like growth factor-1 receptor, and other markers associated with hypoxia.[467-490] In general, molecular subtypes of breast cancer may be organized into the following general categories: luminal A (ER positive or PR positive and Ki-67 <14%), luminal B (ER positive or PR positive and Ki-67 ≥14%), luminal-HER2 (ER positive or PR positive and HER2 positive), HER2 enriched (ER negative, PR negative, and HER2 positive), and basal-like (ER negative, PR negative, HER2 negative, and EFGR positive or CK5/6 positive).

Haffty et al.[491] examined patients treated with breast-conserving therapy plus radiation and identified 482 patients with ER, PR, and HER2 available for analysis. Patients were then stratified into TN and non-TN status. They found that at 5 years, the TN cohort had a poorer distant metastasis-free rate compared with the other subtypes (67% vs. 82%, respectively; P = .002). TN subtype was an independent predictor of distant metastasis (HR 2.14; 95% CI, 1.31 to 3.53; P = .002) and cause-specific survival (HR 1.79; 95% CI, 1.03 to 3.22; P = .047). However, there was no significant difference in local control between the TN and other subtypes (83% vs. 83%, respectively). The authors concluded that although patients classified as TN have a poor prognosis, there was no evidence that these patients are at higher risk for local relapse after CS and radiation.

Nguyen et al.[492] reported on 793 patients with invasive breast cancer who received breast-conserving therapy and radiation. With a median follow-up of 70 months, the 5-year rate of local recurrence was 1.8%; 0.8% (0.3, 2.2) for luminal A, 1.5% (0.2, 10) for luminal B, 8.4% (2.2, 30) for HER2, and 7.1% (3.0, 16) for basal. In addition, on multivariate analysis, HER2 and basal subtypes were associated with increased local recurrence as compared with luminal A (P < .01). Luminal B and basal subtypes were associated with increased distant metastases as compared with luminal A (P < .04).

Voduc et al.[493] investigated the rate of local and regional relapse in 2,985 patients stratified by molecular subtype. With a median follow-up of 12 years, they found that after breast-conserving therapy and radiation, patients with luminal A tumors had the most favorable prognosis, with local relapse and regional relapse rates of only 8% and 3% at 10 years, respectively. HER2-enriched and basal-like groups exhibited the highest rates of LR (21% and 14%, respectively) and regional relapse (16% and 14%, respectively). After mastectomy, patients with luminal A tumors again had the best prognosis, with rates of local relapse and regional relapse (8% and 4%, respectively, at 10 years). All non–luminal A subtypes exhibited a greater risk of local relapse and regional relapse.

A recent analysis of TN breast cancers from a large Canadian database revealed an interesting observation. Abdulkarim et al.[494] reported a higher rate of local relapse among T1/T2 node-negative mastectomy patients treated without radiation who had TN disease compared with a similar node-negative cohort treated with breast-conserving surgery and radiation. These results emphasize the point that TN breast cancers do not necessarily fare better with mastectomy, possibly because of the incidental irradiation of lymphatics in the low axilla.[495] Wang et al. conducted a prospective trial where patients with stage I to II TN breast cancer were treated with mastectomy and randomized to chemotherapy +/− PMRT. With 86.5 months' follow-up, the 5-year DFS rates were 88.3% and 74.6% for adjuvant chemotherapy plus radiation and adjuvant chemotherapy alone, respectively (P = 0.02). The 5-year OS was significantly improved in adjuvant chemotherapy plus radiation group compared with chemotherapy alone (90.4% and 78.7%, P = 0.03)[496].

Mamounas et al.[497] investigated the risk of LRR in patients with early-stage, node-negative ER-positive breast cancer treated on the NSABP B14 and B20 based on the Oncotype DX recurrence score (RS). The RS was available in 355 placebo-treated patients (B14), 424 chemotherapy plus tamoxifen patients (B20), and 895 tamoxifen patients (B14 and B20). In the tamoxifen-treated patients, the risk of LRR was 4.3% for patients with low RS (<18), 7.2% for those with intermediate RS (18 to 30) and 15.8% for those with high RS (>30). In placebo-treated patients, the risk of LRR was 10.8% for patients with low RS, 20.0% for those with intermediate RS, and 18.4% for those with high RS. In chemotherapy-treated patients, the risk of LRR was 1.6% for patients with low RS, 2.7% for those with intermediate RS, and 7.8% for those with high RS. The authors concluded that the Oncotype DX recurrence score was a significant predictor of LRR.

These analyses, while showing a consistent trend, should be considered exploratory and are not significant enough to base clinical decision-making on. This is clearly an area that is an active area of investigation, ideally with molecular studies linked to large clinical trials, to help identify molecular markers predictive of locoregional outcomes and hopefully identify potential targets for improving outcomes. Table 59.23 summarizes selected studies evaluating molecular markers for locoregional relapse in conservatively managed breast cancers.[490,498,499]

TABLE 59.23 MOLECULAR MARKERS IN THE LOCAL MANAGEMENT OF EARLY BREAST CANCER TREATED WITH BREAST CONSERVATION SURGERY PLUS RADIATION THERAPY

Markers	Study (Reference)	Patient Population	Local Relapse
ER/PR	Silvestrini, 1995[485]	970 node negative	No correlation for either ER or PR
	Elkhuizen et al., 1999[472]	195 case–control IBC	Higher frequency of PR-negative tumors in locally recurrent population (75% vs. 60%; P = .03)
	Vrieling et al., 2003[498]	5,569 cases	Higher recurrence rate was observed in ER-negative or PR-negative tumors
	Grills et al., 2003[499]	1,500 IBC	Regional nodal failure was associated with ER status on univariate analysis
	Choi et al., 2005[483]	103 IBC	Neither ER nor PR correlated with local relapse rate. PR negativity was related with distant metastasis
	Santiago et al., 2004[477]	937 IBC	Negative PR status was related to local relapse rate
HER2/neu	Haffty et al., 1996[469]	20 case–control IBC	Higher expression of HER2/neu in patients experiencing local relapse (19% vs. 10%; P = .10)
	Pierce et al., 1994[474]	137 IBC	HER2/neu correlated with extensive intraductal component but did not correlate to local relapse.
	Kim et al., 2003[484]	611 IBC	HER2/neu correlated with overall survival but not local relapse
	Choi et al., 2005[483]	103 IBC	HER2/neu was not related with local or distant failure
	Harris et al., 2006[488]	356 IBC	HER2/neu was not related to local failure
Triple negative (TN)	Haffty et al., 2006[491]	482 IDC	TN was not related to local control
	Nguyen et al., 2008[492]	793 IDC	Increased local failure with TN or HER2+ subtypes
	Voduc et al., 2010[493]	2,985 IDC	Increased local failure with TN or HER2+ subtypes
	Mamounas et al., 2010[497]	1,674 IDC	Increased local failure with higher Oncotype DX score
p53	Silvestrini et al., 1997[482]	496 IBC	No correlation with p53 and local relapse
	Turner et al., 2000[470]	94 IBC	p53 overexpression more common in locally recurrent group compared to locally controlled group (26% vs. 9%; P = .02)
	Elkhuizen et al., 1999[472]	195 case–control IBC	p53 expression similar in locally recurrent and locally controlled group (21% vs. 23%; P = .61)
	Amornmarn et al., 2000[487]	112 IBC	p53 expression associated with all local recurrence cases (only four local relapses in series)
	Choi et al., 2005[483]	103 IBC	p53 was not related with local or distant failure
Proliferative markers	Choi et al., 2005[483]	103 IBC	Ki-67 positivity was related with distant but not local failure
	Silvestrini et al., 1997[481]	496 IBC	Thymidine-labeling index was not related with local failure
ATM mutation	Meyer et al., 2004[489]	135 IBC	ATM gene alterations were not related to patient outcomes

ATM, ataxia telangiectasis mutations; ER, estrogen receptor; IBC, inflammatory breast cancer; IDC, invasive ductal carcinoma; PR, progesterone receptor.

BREAST-CONSERVING SURGERY WITHOUT RADIATION

Based on the mature data from the well-conducted randomized trials outlined above and on long-term follow-up from the several large retrospective series, it is apparent that breast-conserving surgery followed by radiation therapy is a safe and effective modality for the majority of women with early-stage invasive breast cancer.[113] Whether subsets of patients can be treated with breast-conserving surgery alone without irradiation has been the subject of considerable debate and several randomized trials. With the possible exception of selected elderly women, which will be discussed in a later section, subsets of patients in whom radiation therapy can be safely avoided have yet to be clearly identified. Collectively, the randomized studies to date consistently demonstrate an approximately threefold greater local relapse rate in the unirradiated cohorts.[88] Although the majority of these trials did not demonstrate an impact on survival, recent pooled analysis of these randomized trials demonstrates a small but statistically significant impact on mortality as a result of the omission of radiation.

Vinh-Hung and Verschraegen[88] conducted a pooled analysis of published randomized clinical trials that compared radiotherapy versus no radiotherapy after breast-conserving surgery. The outcomes studied were IBTR and patient death from any cause. A search of the literature identified 15 trials with a pooled total of 9,422 patients available for analysis. The RR of ipsilateral breast tumor recurrence after breast-conserving surgery, comparing patients treated with no radiotherapy or radiotherapy, was 3.00 (95% CI, 2.65 to 3.40). Mortality data were available for 13 trials with a pooled total of 8,206 patients. The RR of mortality was 1.086 (95% CI, 1.003 to 1.175), corresponding to an estimated 8.6% (95% CI, 0.3% to 17.5%) relative excess mortality if radiotherapy was omitted (Fig. 59.17A and B).

In an analysis from the EBCTCG, similar conclusions were reached evaluating various forms of local therapy.[87,110] Within this meta-analysis were 10,801 women treated with breast-conserving surgery in trials randomizing patients to radiation therapy versus no radiation therapy. The majority included patients with axillary clearance of node-negative disease and generally were treated with radiation to the conserved breast alone. The reduction in local recurrence (mainly in the conserved breast) in patients treated with radiotherapy was highly significant ($P < .00001$) in every separate trial. As seen in Figure 59.18, the recurrence rate ratio, comparing those allocated radiotherapy with those not, is about 0.3 in

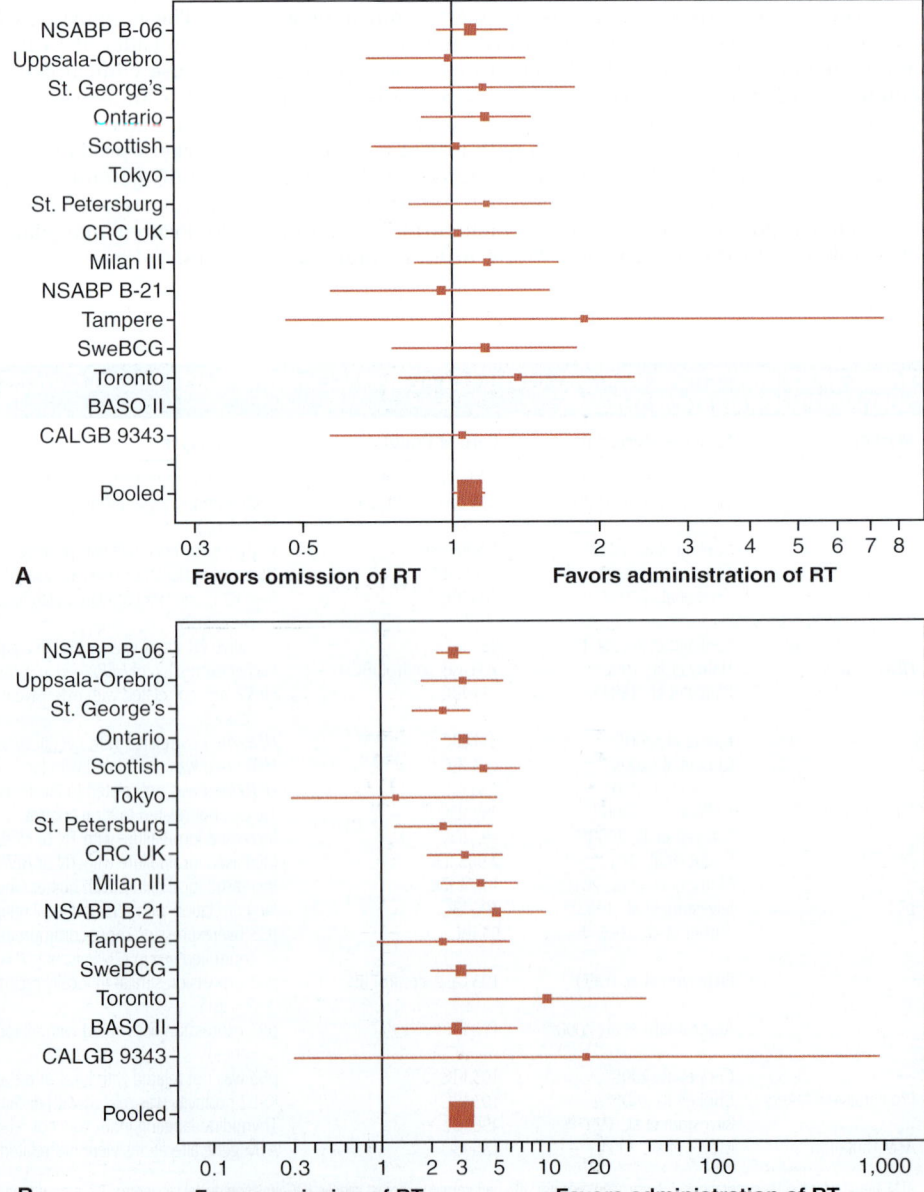

FIGURE 59.17. Meta-analysis of survival **(A)** and local control **(B)** in randomized trials comparing breast-conserving surgery with or without radiation. This meta-analysis demonstrated a threefold reduction in local relapse and a small but significant increase in survival with the use of radiation therapy following lumpectomy. (From Vinh-Hung V, Verschraegen C. Breast-conserving surgery with or without radiotherapy: pooled-analysis for risks of ipsilateral breast tumor recurrence and mortality. *J Natl Cancer Inst* 2004;96[2]:115–121. Reproduced by permission of Oxford University Press.)

Isolated local recurrence (events/woman-years)

Year started and study name	RT sites	Events/woman-years		BCS+RT events		Ratio of annual event rates
		Allocated BCS + RT	Allocated BCS	Logrank O–E	Variance of O–E	BCS + RT : BCS

(a) Radiotherapy only to conserved breast: 14% node positive

1976 NSABP B-06	BW*	125/6,862	285/4,991	−93.3	84.8	
1981 Uppsala-Örebro	BW	10/1,636	43/1,511	−17.7	12.7	
1982 St. George's London	BW*	12/1,202	31/1,047	−11.5	9.6	
1984 Ontario COG	BW + S	53/3,543	155/2,754	−58.2	48.2	
1987 INT Milan 3	BW + S*	19/2,478	60/2,005	−25.1	18.2	
1989 NSABP B-21	BW + S*	6/1,810	40/1,729	−17.3	11.2	
1991 Swedish BCCG	BW	33/3,718	92/3,429	−30.8	30.5	
(a) Subtotal		258/ 21,249	706/ 17.466	−254.0	215.3	0.31 (SE 0.04), 2P <.00001
5-year risk		7.2%	25.6%			

(b) Radiotherapy to conserved breast and other sites: 24% node positive

1982 St. George's London	BW + AF*	14/620	30/380	−10.9	9.7	
1985 Scottish	BW + S + (AF) + IMC	16/2,598	83/2,260	−33.0	22.5	
1985 West Midlands, UK	BW + S + AF + IMC	42/2,398	104/1,929	−36.8	34.2	
1986 CRC, UK	Various	33/1,604	77/1,454	−24.3	25.7	
(b) Subtotal		105/ 7,220	294/ 6,023	−105.0	92.1	0.32 (SE 0.06), 2P <.00001
5-year risk		7.7%	26.7%			
Total (a + b)		363/ 20,409	1000/ 23,489	−359.0	307.4	0.31 (SE 0.03), 2P <.00001
5-year risk		7.3%	25.9%			

Heterogeneity between 11 strata: $\chi^2_{10} = 7.8$; $P = .6$

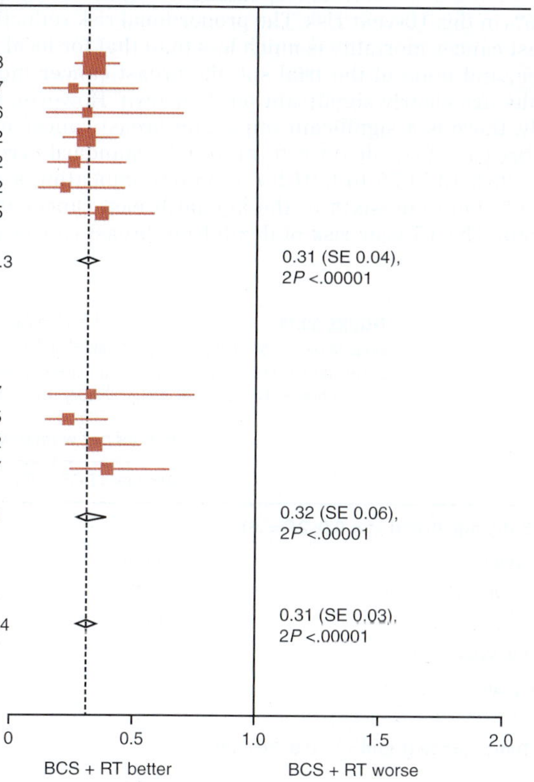

BCS + RT better   BCS + RT worse

Isolated local recurrence (events/woman-years)

Year started and study name	RT sites	Events/woman-years		BCS + RT deaths		Ratio of annual death rates
		Allocated BCS + RT	Allocated BCS	Logrank O–E	Variance of O–E	BCS + RT : BCS

(a) Radiotherapy only to conserved breast: 14% node positive

1976 NSABP B-06	BW*	267/731	305/719	−19.7	135.0	
1981 Uppsala Örebro	BW	37/184	34/197	2.3	16.8	
1982 St. George's London	BW*	24/128	25/122	−2.5	10.9	
1984 Ontario COG	BW + S	91/416	123/421	−16.4	51.5	
1987 INT Milan 3	BW + S*	40/294	51/273	−6.2	21.3	
1989 NSABP B-21	BW + S*	8/337	8/336	0.5	3.9	
1991 Swedish BCCG	BW	32/593	41/594	−3.9	18.0	
(a) Subtotal		499/ 2,683	587/ 2,662	−45.8	257.4	0.84 (SE 0.06), 2P = .004
15-year risk		28.0%	33.2%			

(b) Radiotherapy to conserved breast and other sites: 24% node positive

1982 St. George's London	BW + AF*	31/80	28/70	−2.1	12.2	
1985 Scottish	BW + S + (AF) + IMC	59/293	78/296	−5.0	30.2	
1985 West Midlands, UK	BW + S + AF + IMC	88/358	107/349	−11.4	45.3	
1986 CRC, UK	Various	76/259	89/261	−8.3	37.6	
(b) Subtotal		254/ 990	302/ 976	−26.9	125.3	0.81 (SE 0.08), 2P = .02
10-year risk		28.2%	35.1%			
Total (a + b)		753/ 3,673	889/ 3,638	−72.7	382.7	0.83 (SE 0.05), 2P = .0002
15-year risk		30.5%	35.9%			

Heterogeneity between 11 strata: $\chi^2_{10} = 3.8$; $P = .96$

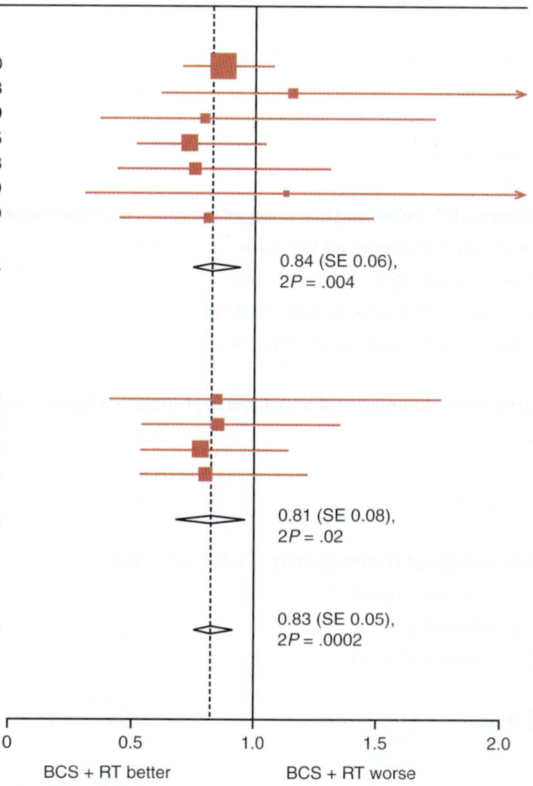

BCS + RT better   BCS + RT worse

FIGURE 59.18. Meta-analysis of local control and survival from the Early Breast Cancer Trialists Collaborative Group demonstrating the impact of radiation therapy on both local control and survival in the management of breast cancer. (Reprinted from Clarke M, Collins R, Darby S, et al. Effects of radiotherapy and of differences in the extent of surgery for early breast cancer on local recurrence and 15-year survival: an overview of the randomised trials. *Lancet* 2005;366[9503]:2087–2106. Copyright © 2005 Elsevier. With permission.)

Section III

every trial, corresponding to a proportional reduction of 70%. Considering all 17 trials together, the 10-year risk of local recurrence is 19% among those allocated radiotherapy and 35% among those not, corresponding to an absolute reduction of 16% in this 10-year risk. The proportional risk reduction for breast cancer mortality is much less than that for local recurrence, and none of the trial-specific breast cancer mortality results are clearly significant on their own. However, collectively, there is a significant impact on breast cancer mortality (breast cancer death rate ratio 0.83, standard error [SE] 0.05; 95% CI, 0.75 to 0.912; $P = .0002$), indicating a reduction of about one-sixth in the annual breast cancer mortality rate. The 15-year risk of death from breast cancer (in the hypothetical absence of other causes) is 30·5% among those allocated post–breast-conserving surgery radiotherapy and 35.9% among those not (corresponding to an absolute reduction of 5.4%; SE 1.7). Figure 59.19 highlights a recent update of the EBCTCG, demonstrating the impact of radiation therapy on outcome in early-stage breast cancer.[110]

Randomized Trials

Selected trials comparing breast-conserving surgery alone to breast-conserving surgery with radiation are summarized in Table 59.24.[91,93,500-503] The Uppsala-Orebro Breast Cancer Study group reported on a trial in which women with stage I breast carcinoma were randomly assigned to be treated with either

FIGURE 59.19. Updated meta-analysis from the Early Breast Cancer Trialists Collaborative Group comparing breast-conserving surgery alone to breast-conserving surgery with radiation therapy. (Reprinted from Darby S, McGale P, Correa C, et al. Effect of radiotherapy after breast-conserving surgery on 10-year recurrence and 15-year breast cancer death: meta-analysis of individual patient data for 10,801 women in 17 randomised trials. *Lancet* 2011;378[9804]:1707–1716. Copyright © 2011 Elsevier. With permission.)

	Events per woman-year during years 0–9		Ratio of annual event rates BCS + RT vs. BCS (CI)*
	Allocated BCS + RT	Allocated BCS	
(a) Entry age (trend $\chi_1^2 = 0.0$; $2P = .9$)			
<40 years	5.9%	11.5%	0.49 (0.32–0.76)
40–49 years	2.7%	6.1%	0.44 (0.33–0.58)
50–59 years	1.9%	4.0%	0.47 (0.36–0.61)
60–69 years	1.6%	3.6%	0.45 (0.35–0.59)
70+ years	1.0%	2.1%	0.45 (0.28–0.72)
(b) Tumor grade (trend $\chi_1^2 = 0.0$; $2P = .9$)			
Low	1.0%	2.5%	0.43 (0.29–0.65)
Intermediate	2.2%	4.4%	0.47 (0.35–0.63)
High	4.1%	9.8%	0.43 (0.32–0.58)
Grade unknown	1.8%	3.6%	0.48 (0.39–0.59)
(c) Tumor size (trend $\chi_1^2 = 1.7$; $2P = .2$)			
T1 (1–20 mm)	1.5%	3.5%	0.42 (0.36–0.50)
T2 (21–50 mm)	4.5%	8.9%	0.50 (0.37–0.66)
Various/unknown	2.9%	4.2%	0.74 (0.43–1.27)
(d) Surgery, ER status, and trial policy of tamoxifen use† (heterogeneity $\chi_3^2 = 11.4$; $2P = .01$)			
Lumpectomy, ER-positive no tamoxifen	3.3%	8.0%	0.41 (0.33–0.52)
Lumpectomy, ER-poor	5.2%	8.5%	0.65 (0.46–0.94)
>Lumpectomy, ER-positive no tamoxifen/ER-poor	1.6%	3.2%	0.51 (0.39–0.67)
Lumpectomy, ER-positive with tamoxifen	0.9%	2.4%	0.38 (0.29–0.51)
(e) Trial policy of using additional therapy† (heterogeneity $\chi_1^2 = 0.0$; $2P = 1.0$)			
Yes	2.0%	4.1%	0.46 (0.38–0.56)
No	2.0%	4.2%	0.46 (0.37–0.56)
Some/unknown	2.4%	3.8%	0.69 (0.24–2.01)
(f) Trial category‡ (heterogeneity $\chi_2^2 = 9.4$; $2P = .009$)			
(A) Lumpectomy: original	3.7%	7.7%	0.49 (0.41–0.59)
(B) >Lumpectomy	1.6%	3.2%	0.51 (0.39–0.67)
(C) Lumpectomy: low risk	0.6%	2.0%	0.32 (0.22–0.45)
Total	**2.0%**	**4.2%**	**0.46 (0.41–0.51)**
			2P<.00001

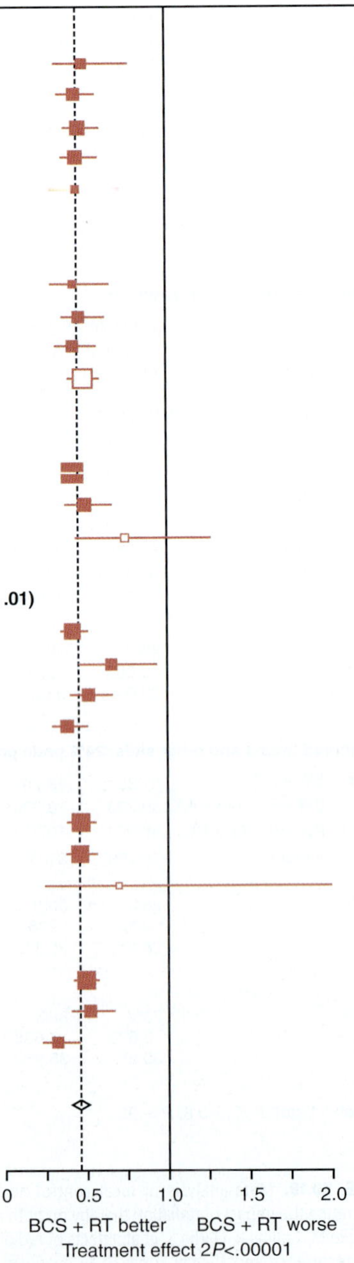

0   0.5   1.0   1.5   2.0
BCS + RT better   BCS + RT worse
Treatment effect 2P<.00001

*■ 99% CI or ◁▷ 95% CI

TABLE 59.24 RESULTS OF SELECTED RANDOMIZED TRIALS OF BREAST-CONSERVING SURGERY WITH OR WITHOUT RADIATION

Study (Reference)	Criteria for Eligibility	Number of Patients	Follow-Up (Years)	Radiation Therapy		
				With (%)	Without (%)	P
Fisher et al. B-06[91]	<4 cm node positive/negative	930	10	12.4	40.9	<.001
Liljegren et al.[500]	<2 cm node negative	381	10	8.5	24.0	.0001
Veronesi et al.[501]	<2.5 cm	579	10	5.8	23.5	<.001
Clark et al.[502]	<2 cm node negative	837	3	5.5	25.7	<.001
Fisher et al. B-21[93]	<2 cm node negative	1,009	8	2.8	16.5	<.001
Winzer et al.[503]	<2 cm node negative	347	5.9	3.2	27.8	.001

sector resection and axillary dissection plus 54 Gy breast irradiation (184 patients) or the same surgical procedure alone (197 patients).[500] The actuarial local recurrence rates after a median follow-up of 63 to 65 months were 2.3% in the irradiated group and 18.4% with surgery only. The 5-year disease-free survival rates were 91% and 87%, and the 5-year overall survival rates were 91% and 90%, respectively.

Whelan et al.[504] reported on a randomized study of women with stage I or II node-negative breast cancer; 403 had lumpectomy, axillary dissection, and breast irradiation, and 396 had the same surgical procedure without irradiation. A dose of 40 Gy was given in 16 fractions to the whole breast, followed by a boost of 12.5 Gy in 5 fractions to the primary site. No patient received adjuvant systemic therapy. The 5-year ipsilateral breast relapse rate was 8% in patients receiving irradiation and 30% in the surgery-alone group (P < .0001). Survival rates at 5 years were 88% and 86%, respectively. Ipsilateral breast relapse correlated with increased incidence of distant metastases and greater mortality from cancer.

Clark et al.[502] reported on a randomized study of 421 patients with tumors 4 cm or smaller and negative nodes who were treated with wide local excision and axillary dissection alone and 416 patients who were treated with the same surgery plus breast irradiation (40 Gy in 3 weeks, 16 fractions, and 12.5-Gy boost in 5 fractions). With 7.6 years' median follow-up, breast recurrences were seen in 148 (35%) of the nonirradiated patients and in 147 (11%) of the irradiated patients (P < .0001); 99 patients (24%) in the former group and 87 (21%) in the latter group died during the study period.

Forrest et al.,[505] after local excision of breast tumors <4 cm in diameter and axillary dissection, randomly assigned 291 patients to receive irradiation of 50 Gy to the breast plus a 10- to 15-Gy boost and 294 to receive no irradiation. Patients received either tamoxifen or 6 cycles of CMF. Overall survival was equivalent in the two groups. The rates of locoregional relapse were 6.1% (18 patients) in the irradiated group and 28.6% (84 patients) in the excision-alone group.

Renton et al.[506] analyzed 418 patients treated by wide local excision and adjuvant chemotherapy (tamoxifen if ER positive and CMF chemotherapy if ER negative) who were randomized to have radiation therapy to the breast or not. At a minimum 5-year follow-up, the local recurrence rate in patients receiving irradiation was 13% compared with 35% in those not so treated. When histologically local excision was incomplete and patients received radiation therapy, the local recurrence rate was 17%.

One of the most significant trials addressing the issue of local relapse following lumpectomy alone was from the NSABP-06.[91] This trial included three arms—modified radical mastectomy, lumpectomy with radiation, and lumpectomy without radiation—and included both node-positive and node-negative patients. In this trial, breast irradiation decreased the likelihood of a recurrence in the ipsilateral breast in the group of 1,137 lumpectomy-treated women whose surgical specimens had tumor-free margins. The cumulative incidence of a recurrence in the ipsilateral breast 20 years after surgery was 14.3% among the women who underwent irradiation after lumpectomy and 39.2% among those who underwent lumpectomy without irradiation (P < .001). The benefit of radiation therapy was independent of the nodal status. Among the women with negative nodes, 36.2% of those who did not receive radiation therapy and 17.0% of those who did had a recurrence in the ipsilateral breast within 20 years (P < .001). Among the women with positive nodes, 44.2% of those who did not undergo irradiation and 8.8% of those who did had a recurrence in the ipsilateral breast (P < .001). Among the lumpectomy-treated women whose surgical specimens had tumor-free margins, the HR for death among the women who underwent postoperative breast irradiation, as compared with those who did not, was 0.91 (95% CI, 0.77 to 1.06; P = .23). Radiation therapy was associated with a marginally significant decrease in deaths due to breast cancer. This decrease was partially offset by an increase in deaths from other causes.

Because of continued uncertainty regarding the need for radiation in more favorable tumors, the NSABP continued to investigate this issue of elimination of irradiation. In the B-21 trial, 1,009 women treated by lumpectomy were randomly assigned to tamoxifen (n = 336), radiation therapy and placebo (n = 336), or radiation therapy and tamoxifen (n = 337).[92] Endpoints were divided rates of breast relapse, distant recurrence, and contralateral breast cancer. Radiation and placebo resulted in a 49% lower hazard rate of local relapse as opposed to tamoxifen alone; radiation and tamoxifen resulted in a 63% lower rate as opposed to radiation and placebo. When compared with tamoxifen alone, radiation plus tamoxifen resulted in an 81% reduction in hazard rate of IBTR. Cumulative incidences of local relapse through 8 years were 16.5% with tamoxifen, 9.3% with radiation and placebo, and 2.8% with radiation and tamoxifen. The authors concluded that in women with tumors ≤1 cm, local relapse occurs with enough frequency after lumpectomy to justify considering radiation therapy regardless of ER status.

In another landmark trial, Veronesi et al.[397,501] randomly assigned 567 women with small cancers of the breast (<2.5 cm in diameter) to quadrantectomy followed by radiation therapy or to quadrantectomy alone. All patients underwent total axillary dissection. The number of IBTRs was significantly higher in patients treated with surgery alone (59 cases of 273; 10-year crude cumulative incidence of 23.5%) than in patients treated with surgery plus radiotherapy (16 cases of 294; 10-year crude cumulative incidence of 5.8%). The difference in IBTR frequency between the two treatments was high in women up to 45 years of age, tending to decrease with increasing age up to no apparent difference in women older than 65 years. Overall survival curves for the two groups did not differ significantly (P = .326). However, a limited survival advantage was evident after radiotherapy for node-positive women.

Other Nonrandomized Studies of Lumpectomy Alone

Lim et al.[507] recently updated a prospective single-arm trial addressing omission of radiation for highly selected favorable patients from the Harvard group. Eighty-seven (of 90 planned) patients enrolled from 1986 until closure in 1992, when a predefined stopping boundary was crossed. Patients were required to have a unicentric, T1, pathologic node-negative invasive ductal, mucinous, or tubular carcinoma without an extensive intraductal component or lymphatic vessel invasion. Surgery included local excision with margins of at least 1 cm or a negative re-excision. No RT or systemic therapy was given. Nineteen patients (23%) had local recurrence as a first site of failure (average annual local recurrence: 3.5 per 100 patient-years of follow-up). The authors concluded that even in this highly selected cohort, a substantial risk of local recurrence occurred after breast-conserving therapy alone with margins of ≥1.0 cm.

McCready et al.[508] reported on a postmenopausal group of 244 patients with breast cancer treated with lumpectomy alone. With a median follow-up of 9.1 years, the overall breast relapse rate was 24% (59 of 244). On univariate analysis, smaller tumor size, negative nodes, positive ER status, and no lymphovascular or perineural invasion were associated with significantly lower relapse rates ($P < .05$). On multivariate analyses, lymphovascular or perineural invasion, age, and amount of DCIS were all significantly associated with greater risk of local relapse. The authors defined a low-risk subgroup (node negative, younger than 65 years of age, no comedo, ER positive, no emboli) with a crude 10-year local recurrence rate of 9%.

Conservative Surgery Alone in Elderly Women

The available evidence clearly establishes lumpectomy followed by radiation as the standard of care for the majority of women with early-stage invasive breast cancer. As noted in the numerous randomized trials reported above, lumpectomy alone results in a threefold increase in local relapse and compromised breast cancer–related survival to a lesser degree.[88] Given the lower reported local relapse rates in elderly women, however, the absolute benefit of radiation therapy following breast-conserving surgery, however, may be less. The question of whether radiation can be eliminated following breast-conserving therapy has been addressed in both retrospective and, more recently, carefully designed prospective randomized trials.

There is evidence from several retrospective and prospective series that elderly women may be spared radiation. Cooke et al.[509] identified 44 women treated with partial mastectomy, breast irradiation, and tamoxifen and compared them with 53 women treated in a similar fashion but without breast irradiation. At 39 months, the breast tumor recurrence rate was 5% with breast irradiation and 21% when irradiation was omitted. Of those not receiving irradiation, no breast relapses were seen in 22 patients older than 70 years of age at diagnosis, in contrast to 8 breast recurrences in 31 patients younger than 70 years.

In the trial of quadrantectomy versus quadrantectomy plus radiation reported by Veronesi et al.,[501] although there was a clear benefit in local control overall, the benefit was significant and apparent only in younger women; for patients over age 65, there was no significant benefit.

Gajdos et al.[510] noted that reported rates of local and distant recurrence for elderly patients were comparable with those for younger patients after both mastectomy and breast conservation. Ninety-eight of 920 patients older than 70 years of age were undertreated by conventional criteria. Undertreated elderly patients were significantly older (78 vs. 76 years; $P = .003$), were diagnosed with excisional biopsy

more often (69% vs. 57%; $P = .069$) and had fine needle aspiration less frequently (22% vs. 38%; $P = .069$), and were more likely to have breast conservation therapy (90% vs. 73%; $P = .004$). Local and distant disease-free survival rates for both groups were comparable. Tamoxifen treatment significantly reduced the chances for development of distant metastasis in node-negative elderly patients with invasive tumors ($P = .028$). Omission of chemotherapy had no impact on disease control in the elderly. Therefore, elderly women with favorable prognostic factors may be candidates for treatment with tumor resection and tamoxifen without irradiation or chemotherapy and with close follow-up.

Given the apparent biologic differences in breast cancers in the elderly, as well as the logistic issues in daily radiation treatment, two randomized trials have addressed the issue of the need for radiation therapy in elderly women with early-stage breast cancer.[173,511] The first trial from the Cancer and Leukemia Group B (CALGB), published by Hughes et al.,[511] randomly assigned 636 women with clinical stage I, ER-positive breast carcinoma treated by lumpectomy to receive tamoxifen plus radiation therapy (317 women) or tamoxifen alone (319 women). The only significant difference between the two groups was the rate of local or regional recurrence at 5 years (1% in the group given tamoxifen plus irradiation and 4% in the group given tamoxifen alone; $P < .001$). There were no significant differences between the two groups with regard to the rates of mastectomy for local recurrence, distant metastases, or 5-year rates of overall survival. The authors concluded that lumpectomy plus adjuvant therapy with tamoxifen alone is a reasonable choice for the treatment of women 70 years of age or older who have early, ER-positive breast cancer. An update of this trial revealed that at 10 years, 98% of patients receiving tamoxifen plus irradiation compared with 90% of those receiving tamoxifen alone were free from local and regional recurrences. There were no significant differences in mastectomy rates, distant metastases, or 10-year rates of OS[512].

The second trial was a Canadian study published by Fyles et al.[513] of women 50 years of age or older who had T1 or T2 node-negative breast cancer. In this trial, 769 women with early breast cancer with a tumor diameter of ≤5 cm were randomly assigned to receive breast irradiation plus tamoxifen (386 women) or tamoxifen alone (383 women). With a median follow-up of 5.6 years, the rate of local relapse at 5 years was 7.7% in the tamoxifen group and 0.6% in the group given tamoxifen plus irradiation (HR 8.3; 95% CI, 3.3 to 21.2; $P < .001$). The corresponding 5-year disease-free survival rates were 84% and 91% ($P = .004$). A subgroup analysis of 611 women with T1, receptor-positive tumors, similar to the CALGB cohorts, also indicated a benefit from radiotherapy, with the 5-year rates of local relapse of 0.4% with tamoxifen plus radiotherapy and 5.9% with tamoxifen alone ($P < .001$). There was also a significant difference in the rate of axillary relapse at 5 years (2.5% in the tamoxifen group and 0.5% in the group given tamoxifen plus irradiation; $P = .049$), but there were no significant difference in the rates of distant relapse or overall survival. In both of these trials, women were not required to have surgical staging of the axilla, but they did have clinically negative axilla in both, and follow-up remains relatively short. Both studies show that even this favorable subgroup benefits from radiation with respect to local control, but the absolute benefit is small.

As a follow-up to the CALGB study, Smith et al.[513] conducted a detailed analysis of women over age 70 from the SEER-Medicare database. They identified 8,724 women aged 70 years or older treated with CS for small, lymph node-negative, ER-positive (or unknown receptor status) breast cancer. Using a proportional hazards model, they tested whether radiation therapy was associated with a lower risk of a combined outcome, defined as a second ipsilateral breast cancer reported by SEER, or a subsequent mastectomy reported by

Medicare claims. The results, summarized in Figure 59.20, were similar to those reported by the randomized studies above in that radiation therapy, compared with no radiation therapy, was associated with a lower risk of the combined outcome (HR 0.19; 95% CI, 0.14 to 0.28). Radiation therapy was associated with an absolute risk reduction of 4.0 events per 100 women at 5 years (from 5.1 events without radiation therapy to 1.1 with radiation therapy) and 5.7 events per 100 women at 8 years (from 8.0 events without radiation therapy to 2.3 with radiation therapy; $P < .001$).

Using a comorbidity analysis, radiation therapy was most likely to benefit those aged 70 to 79 years without comorbidity

(number needed to treat to prevent one event, 21 to 22 patients) and was least likely to benefit those aged 80 years or older with moderate to severe comorbidity (number needed to treat, 61 to 125 patients). The authors conclude that for older women with early breast cancer, radiation therapy was associated with a lower risk of a second ipsilateral breast cancer and subsequent mastectomy. Patients aged 70 to 79 years with minimal comorbidity were the most likely to benefit and older patients with substantial comorbidity were least likely to benefit.

Collectively, these studies indicate that the benefit of radiation therapy for elderly women is significant in terms of local control, but this absolute benefit is relatively small and must

FIGURE 59.20. Association of radiation therapy with outcomes in elderly women. Patients were at risk for all outcomes beginning 9 months after diagnosis. **A:** Second ipsilateral breast cancer reported by Surveillance, Epidemiology, and End Results (SEER). This outcome was defined as a second ipsilateral, pathologically confirmed, invasive breast cancer. **B:** Subsequent mastectomy reported by Medicare claims. **C:** Second breast cancer event defined as a second ipsilateral, pathologically confirmed, invasive breast cancer reported by SEER data or as a subsequent mastectomy reported by Medicare claims. **D:** Repeat breast-conserving surgery as reported by Medicare claims. RT, radiation therapy. Error bars equal 95% CIs. *P* values were calculated from a two-sided logrank test. (From Smith BD, Gross CP, Smith GL, et al. Effectiveness of radiation therapy for older women with early breast cancer. *J Natl Cancer Inst* 2006;98[10]:681–690. Reproduced by permission of Oxford University Press.)

Section III

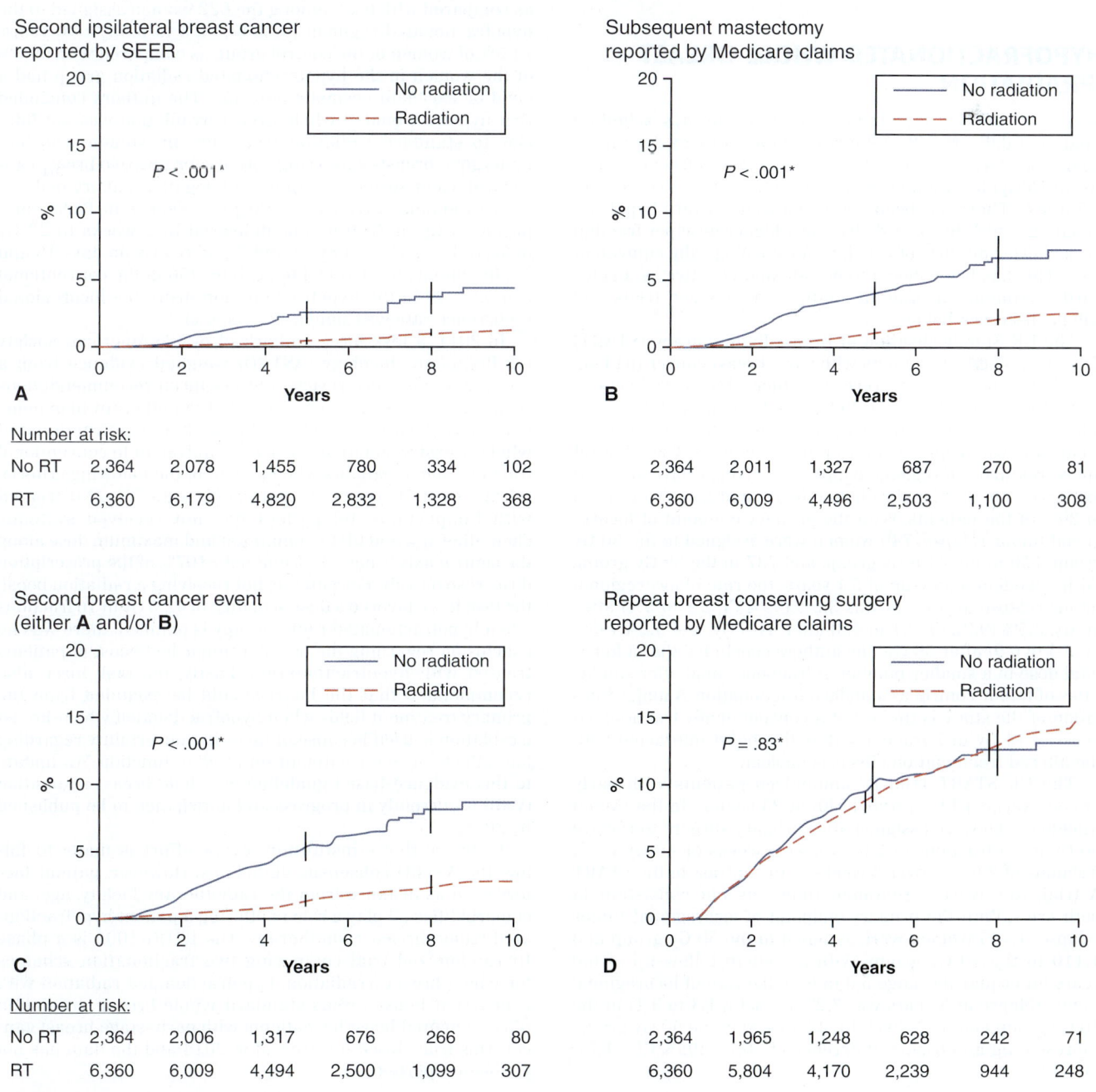

Second ipsilateral breast cancer reported by SEER

Number at risk:

No RT	2,364	2,078	1,455	780	334	102
RT	6,360	6,179	4,820	2,832	1,328	368

Subsequent mastectomy reported by Medicare claims

	2,364	2,011	1,327	687	270	81
	6,360	6,009	4,496	2,503	1,100	308

Second breast cancer event (either **A** and/or **B**)

Number at risk:

No RT	2,364	2,006	1,317	676	266	80
RT	6,360	6,009	4,494	2,500	1,099	307

Repeat breast conserving surgery reported by Medicare claims

	2,364	1,965	1,248	628	242	71
	6,360	5,804	4,170	2,239	944	248

TABLE 59.25 FIVE-YEAR OUTCOME OF BREAST-CONSERVING SURGERY WITH OR WITHOUT RADIOTHERAPY IN ELDERLY WOMEN WITH BREAST CANCER

Study (Reference)	Age (Year)	Number of Patients		Follow-Up	Ipsilateral Relapse			Axillary Relapse			Distant Relapse		
		CS	CS+RT		CS (%)	CS+RT (%)	P	CS (%)	CS+RT (%)	P	CS (%)	CS+RT (%)	P
Fyles et al.[513]	≥50	383	386	5.6 (median)	7.7	0.6	<.001	2.5	0.5	.049	4.0	4.5	.69
Hughes et al.[511]	≥70	319	317	>8	4.1	0.6	<.01	0.6	0	.08	1.9	2.2	.77
Smith et al.[514]	≥70	2364	6360	5.0 (median)	5.1	1.1	<.001	–	–	–	–	–	–

be weighed against comorbidities and other competing risks. The two randomized trials and the SEER-Medicare analysis are summarized in Table 59.25. For women with favorable T1N0 receptor-positive breast cancers, tamoxifen alone is a reasonable option that should be discussed. For patients with multiple comorbidities and shorter life expectancies, this option is often chosen. The author's own preference in patients with low comorbidity and long life expectancy is to offer radiation, even in those over age 70 with ER-positive tumors.

HYPOFRACTIONATED WHOLE-BREAST IRRADIATION

In breast cancer, the standard radiation therapy schedule treatment delivers 1.8 to 2.0 Gy/day for 25 to 28 days for a total dose of 45 to 50.4 Gy followed by a 5 to 8 fraction boost (10 to 16 Gy) for a total dose of 60 to 66 Gy delivered for 6 to 7.5 weeks. There has been a growing trend toward hypofractionation, which involves delivering a higher dose per fraction for a shorter number of fractions for a biologically equivalent dose. This has been shown to be safe and effective as a standard treatment schedule in multiple randomized trials and will be discussed below.

The UK Standardisation of Breast Radiotherapy (START) Trial A randomized patients with early breast cancer (pT1-3a pN0-1 M0); these patients received either 50 Gy in 25 fractions of 2.0 Gy versus 41.6 Gy or 39 Gy in 13 fractions of 3.2 Gy or 3.0 Gy over 5 weeks after surgery.[515] Thus, the overall treatment time was kept constant in all three arms. The trial did allow treatment of regional lymph nodes (supraclavicular and axillary) with additional radiation fields, and these were used in 20% of the patients. With the primary endpoint of locoregional tumor relapse, 749 women were assigned to the 50 Gy group, 750 to the 41.6 Gy group, and 737 to the 39 Gy group. With a median follow-up of 5.1 years, the rate of locoregional tumor relapse at 5 years was 3.6% (95% CI, 2.2 to 5.1) after 50 Gy, 3.5% (95% CI, 2.1 to 4.3) after 41.6 Gy, and 5.2% (95% CI, 3.5 to 6.9) after 39 Gy. The authors concluded that a lower total dose in a smaller number of fractions could offer similar rates of tumor control as standard fractionation. A major limitation of the study is the use of a conventionally fractionated boost of 14 Gy in 7 fractions. How this boost interacted with the altered fractionation effects is unclear.

The UK START Trial B randomized patients with early breast cancer (pT1-3a pN0-1 M0) at 23 centers in the United Kingdom who were assigned after primary surgery to receive 50 Gy in 25 fractions of 2.0 Gy over 5 weeks or 40 Gy in 15 fractions of 2.67 Gy over 3 weeks.[516] In contrast to the START A trial, the overall treatment time was not consistent in both arms. With the primary endpoint of locoregional tumor relapse, 1,105 women were assigned to the 50 Gy group and 1,110 to the 40 Gy group. With a median follow-up of 6.0 years (interquartile range 5.0 to 6.2), the rate of locoregional tumor relapse at 5 years was 2.2% (95% CI, 1.3 to 3.1) in the 40 Gy group and 3.3% (95% CI, 2.2 to 4.5) in the 50 Gy group, representing an absolute difference of –0.7% (95% CI, –1.7% to 0.9%).

Whelan et al.[517] reported on a study of women with invasive breast cancer who had undergone breast-conserving surgery and were randomized to whole-breast irradiation either at a standard dose of 50.0 Gy in 25 fractions over a period of 35 days (the control group) or at a dose of 42.5 Gy in 16 fractions over a period of 22 days (the hypofractionated radiation group). Notably, women with breast separations >25 cm were excluded. The risk of local recurrence at 10 years was 6.7% among the 612 women assigned to standard irradiation as compared with 6.2% among the 622 women assigned to the hypofractionated regimen (95% CI, –2.5 to 3.5). At 10 years, 71.3% of women in the control group as compared with 69.8% of the women in the hypofractionated radiation group had a good or excellent cosmetic outcome. The authors concluded that hypofractionated whole-breast irradiation was not inferior to standard radiation treatment in women who had undergone breast-conserving surgery for invasive breast cancer with clear surgical margins and negative axillary nodes.

A randomized trial from Hospital Necker in Paris compared 45 Gy in 25 fractions delivered in 5 weeks to 23 Gy delivered as 5 Gy on days 1 and 3 and 6.5 Gy on days 15 and 17. In patients treated by lumpectomy (56 in the conventional arm and 45 in the hypofractionation arm), the locoregional recurrence rate was similar (7% vs. 4%).[518]

In 2011, a task force authorized by the American Society for Radiation Oncology (ASTRO) weighed evidence from a systematic literature review and produced recommendations regarding the use of hypofractionated radiotherapy in patients with breast cancer.[519] They stated that hypofractionated whole-breast irradiation was likely equivalent to conventional fractionation in patients who meet all of the following criteria: (a) age over 50 years, (b) pathologic state T1–2N0 treated with lumpectomy, (c) patient has not received systemic chemotherapy, and (d) the minimum and maximum dose along the central axis is not <93% and not >107% of the prescription dose, respectively. For patients not receiving a radiation boost, the task force favored a dose schedule of 42.5 Gy in 16 fractions when hypofractionated radiotherapy is planned; there was no conclusion regarding the use of a tumor bed boost in patients treated with hypofractionation. Lastly, the task force also recommended that the heart should be excluded from the primary treatment fields when hypofractionated whole-breast irradiation is used because of lingering uncertainty regarding late effects of this treatment on cardiac function. An update to this evidence-based guideline on whole-breast irradiation (WBI) is currently in progress and anticipated to be published by 2018.

In the author's institution, every effort is made to follow the ASTRO consensus guidelines. However, patient factors such as distance from the radiotherapy facility, age, and comorbidities all play a role in offering a patient hypofractionated whole-breast radiotherapy. The RTOG-1005 is a phase III randomized trial comparing two fractionation schemes for whole-breast irradiation: hypofractionated radiation with concurrent boost versus standard whole-breast irradiation plus sequential boost for patients with early-stage breast cancer. This trial closed for accrual in 2014 and the data has not yet been reported.

TABLE 59.26 TREATMENT POLICY FOR CONSERVATIVE MANAGEMENT OF EARLY-STAGE INVASIVE BREAST CANCER

Treatment Volume	Indication	Fraction Size/Technique	Total Dose	Comment
Whole breast	Routinely following BCS	2 (prefer) or 1.8 Gy/ tangents with wedges or dynamic wedges to optimize homogeneity	45–50.4 Gy	Consider omission of RT in elderly with stage I disease and comorbidities
Boost	Routinely following whole breast	2 or 1.8 Gy (prefer 2 Gy)/*en face* electrons	10–16 Gy to bring total dose to >60 Gy	Consider no boost for widely negative margins in women over 60
Accelerated whole breast	On protocol or ASTRO consensus guidelines	2.66 Gy tangents with no nodal fields/no boost	42.5 Gy	
Accelerated partial breast	On protocol or ASTRO consensus guidelines	3.4–3.8 Gy/external beam conformal, interstitial, or MammoSite	34–38.5 Gy	

ASTRO, American Society for Radiation Oncology; BCS, breast-conserving surgery; RT, radiation therapy.

RADIATION MANAGEMENT OF THE REGIONAL LYMPHATICS

Radiation therapy of the regional lymphatics remains one of the most variable aspects of breast-conserving therapy.[324,520,521] The role of radiation therapy in management of the regional lymphatics is influenced by the risk of subclinical microscopic disease in regional nodal basins and patterns of failure. This risk is in part determined by disease characteristics and in part determined by the extent of surgical evaluation of the axilla, which has become increasingly relevant as a result of increased use of sentinel node, and whether completion axillary dissections are performed for those patients with sentinel node–positive disease. Furthermore, clinicians differ significantly regarding their philosophy with respect to the treatment of subclinical microscopic disease, particularly as it relates to the internal mammary chain.

The issue of whether one treats the "axilla" in conservatively managed patients is further complicated by both uncertainty and misconceptions about the degree to which the axilla receives radiation from a standard tangential field. Although this will vary considerably, as will be discussed in the section on radiation techniques, tangential radiation ports will likely treat most level I nodes and a portion of level II nodes.[522]

All of this uncertainty, debate, and controversy is well founded as there are little in the way of randomized data to establish a clear standard. Studies are under way randomizing high-risk node-negative and node-positive patients to treatment to the breast or chest wall only compared with the breast or chest wall and regional lymphatics. In the interim, reliance on available retrospective data, calculated risks of subclinical disease, and patterns of failure form the basis for various treatment policies. Current treatment policies and guidelines at the authors institutions are outlined in Tables 59.26 and 59.27.

Although in the earlier years of breast conservation therapy, node-negative as well as node-positive patients often received regional nodal treatment, most authors currently agree that it is not necessary to irradiate the regional lymphatics if the nodes are pathologically negative and an adequate axillary dissection has been performed.[77,324,523] This general practice has now been extended to those patients with a negative sentinel node, because available studies have demonstrated a low rate of pathologically involved nodes after a negative sentinel node procedure performed by an experienced surgeon.[230,332,524] However, several recently published studies have swung the pendulum toward treating the regional nodes, even in node-negative patients. They demonstrated a survival benefit to chest wall or WBI with RNI by addressing postsurgical axillary residual microscopic disease subclinical disease in the supraclavicular (SCV) and internal mammary nodes (IMN) not accessible to surgery.[525,526]

However, as noted previously, the clinically negative axilla harbors subclinical microscopic disease in up to 40% of patients with early-stage operable breast cancer,[328] and both axillary dissection and axillary radiation result in high rates of regional nodal control.[77,113,324,328,523]

Radiation Compared with Axillary Surgery

Sentinel node sampling, with or without full axillary dissection, is now the most common method of axillary management in women with early-stage breast cancer. For patients in whom full axillary staging will not affect subsequent systemic management, who have not undergone any axillary staging procedure, or who have a positive sentinel node and did not undergo further axillary staging, axillary radiation has

TABLE 59.27 TREATMENT POLICY FOR REGIONAL NODES

Treatment Volume	Indication	Fraction Size/Technique	Total Dose	Comment
Supraclav	• Clinical N2 or N3 disease • >4 +LN after axillary dissection • 1–3 + LN with high-risk features • Node + sentinel lymph node with no dissection unless risk of additional axillary disease is very small • High risk[a] no dissection	1.8–2.0 Gy (prefer 200)/AP or AP-PA	45–50.4 Gy	May omit with 1–3 positive nodes in select cases
Axilla	• N+ with extensive ECE • SN+ with no dissection • Inadequate axillary dissection • High risk[a] with no dissection	1.8–2.0 Gy/AP—Consider posterior axillary boost if suboptimal coverage with AP only	45–50.4 Gy	Axilla may be intentionally included with use of high tangents.
Internal mammary	Individualized but consider for: • Positive axillary nodes • Central and medial lesions with high risk[a] • Stage III breast cancer • +SLN in the IM chain • +SLN in axilla with drainage to IM on lymphosintigraphy	1.8–2.0 Gy/Partially wide tangents or separate IM electron/photon	45–50.4 Gy	

[a]High risk is defined as estimated probability of nodal involvement >10% to 15%.
AP, anterior–posterior; ECE, extracapsular extension; IM, internal mammary; LN, lymph node; PA, posterior–anterior; +, positive; SN, sentinel node; SLN, sentinel lymph node.

TABLE 59.28 AXILLARY RECURRENCE AFTER AXILLARY LYMPH NODE DISSECTIONOR AXILLARY RADIATION IN CONSERVATIVELY MANAGED PATIENTS

Study (Reference)	Number of Patients		RT Dose (Gy)	Follow-Up (Year)	Axillary Failure/Number of Failures (% Failure)	
	N0	N1 (Clinical)			N0	N1
Royal Marsden[385]	211	52	50/25	120 (min)	3 (1)	15 (29)
Institut Curie[528]	332	–	50/25	54 (ave)	7 (2)	–
Santiago[529]	171	–	50/25	62 (med)	4 (2)	–
Charlebourg[378]	281	–	50–70	60 (min)	4 (1)	–
Henri Mondor[436]	446	47	69/33	120 (ave)	0 (0)	3 (6)
Groupe European[530]	1,040	181	45–70	>60 (med)	19 (2)	7 (4)
Tufts[531]	73	–	45/25	54	1 (1)	–
JCRT[79]	335	35	44–55/22–30	73 (med)	3 (1)	1 (3)
Yale University[77]	590	–	46	>120	18 (2)	–
JCRT[532]	292	126[a]	64–68	96	3 (1)	3 (2)

[a]All the patients received limited axillary dissection; RT dose, radiotherapy dose to axilla, given as total dose in Gy/number of fractions. RT, radiation therapy.

been shown to result in high rates of regional nodal control.[77,113,324,523,527] Selected series demonstrating nodal control rates with radiation therapy in breast-conserving therapy are summarized in Table 59.28.[79,378,385,436,528–532] Table 59.29 summarizes results of randomized trials comparing axillary surgery to radiation or observation.[71,330,533–542]

Retrospective Experiences

Haffty et al.[77] reported actuarial nodal control rates of 97% and 96% at 10 years for two groups of patients, 245 receiving irradiation alone without axillary dissection and 187 treated with irradiation to the supraclavicular lymph nodes and IMNs after axillary dissection. Minimal morbidity was associated with this treatment policy. Recently Pejavar et al.[543] updated the Yale experience, demonstrating a 98% 5-year regional nodal control rate in 582 patients with invasive breast cancer treated by RNI without dissection compared with 98% 5-year nodal control rate in 1,440 patients treated by axillary dissection. Within this experience were 16 patients with positive sentinel nodes who did not undergo completion axillary dissection and were treated with radiation therapy. None of those sentinel node–positive patients recurred.

Galper et al.[532] estimated the efficacy of axillary radiation therapy after a positive sentinel node biopsy and evaluated the risk of regional nodal failure for patients with clinical stage I or II, clinically node-negative invasive breast cancer treated with either no dissection or a limited dissection (removal of five nodes or less) followed by axillary radiation therapy. Two hundred ninety-two patients had axillary radiation therapy instead of axillary dissection; 126 underwent axillary radiation therapy

following limited node dissection. The median dose to the axilla was 46 Gy and to the supraclavicular fossa 45 Gy. Among patients found to have positive nodes on limited dissection, adjuvant chemotherapy and tamoxifen were administered to 81% and 7% of subjects, respectively. All patients had an 8-year follow-up. Six of the 418 patients (1.4%) had regional nodal failure within 8 years; four had simultaneous regional and distant recurrences; and two had isolated axillary failures. Three of the 292 patients (1%) with no axillary dissection, 0 of 84 patients with pathologically negative nodes, and 3 of 42 patients (7%) with pathologically involved nodes had regional node failure as a first site of failure.

A group of 511 patients with 519 stage I and II breast cancers treated with lumpectomy, with or without axillary dissection, and irradiation were reviewed by Halverson et al.[544] Management of the axilla consisted of irradiation after axillary dissection in 74, irradiation alone in 75, and observation in 21 patients; the extent of nodal irradiation was at the discretion of the attending radiation oncologist. Overall, axillary recurrence was uncommon (1.2%) but was slightly more frequent after irradiation alone (2.7%) than after surgery alone (0.3%; P = .14). There was no benefit for supplemental axillary irradiation after an axillary dissection yielding negative nodes or one to three positive nodes. Among the 21 patients in whom the axilla was not treated, axillary recurrence was not observed. Supraclavicular failures were rare in women with negative or one to three positive axillary lymph nodes (0.5%) and were not significantly affected by elective irradiation. IMN recurrence was seen in only one patient and was not influenced by elective internal mammary irradiation.

TABLE 59.29 AXILLARY FAILURE RATES IN PATIENTS IN RANDOMIZED TRIALS COMPARING AXILLARY TREATMENTS

Trials (Reference)	Study Design	Number of Patients	Follow-Up (Month)	Positive LNs (%)	Axillary Failure Rates		
					AxD (%)	AxRT(%)	OBS (%)
NSABP B-04[328]	M (AxD vs. AxRT vs OBS)	1079	126 (ave)	40	1	3	19
Institut Curie[533]	CS (AxD vs. AxRT)	658	180 (med)	18	1	3	NA
Edinburgh[534]	M (AxD vs. AxRT)	275	72 (min)	30	1	14	NA
Guy's I[535]	M vs. CS (AxD vs. AxRT)	232	180 (min)	25	1	19	NA
Guy's II[535]	M vs. CS (AxD vs. AxRT)	258	120 (min)	31	1	13	NA
Manchester I[536]	M (AxRT vs. OBS)	714	60 (min)	NA	NA	19	37
Manchester II[537]	CS (AxRT vs. OBS)	708	65 (med)	NA	NA	10	23
International Breast Cancer Study Group[538]	M or CS (AxD vs. OBS)	454	79 (med)	14	0.4	NA	1.3
Italian Oncological Senology Group[539]	CS	435	63 (med)	NA	NA	0.5	1.5
Milan[330]	CS	219	60	23	1	NA	1.8

ave, average length of follow-up; AxRT, axillary radiotherapy; CS, breast-conserving surgery; M, simple or radical mastectomy; med, median length of follow-up; min, minimum length of follow-up; NA, not applicable; OBS, observation; Positive LNs, incidence of pathologically involved lymph nodes in patients undergoing axillary lymph node dissection.

Randomized Studies

Randomized studies evaluating axillary treatment (dissection vs. observation vs. radiation) are summarized in Table 59.29. One of the largest and earliest comparisons of axillary surgery to radiation was the NSABP-04 study, in which operable clinically node-negative patients were randomly assigned to radical mastectomy, simple mastectomy, or simple mastectomy with radiation to the chest wall and regional lymphatics.[71] The nodal relapse rate approached 20% in those assigned to simple mastectomy without radiation. The nodal control rates in the radical mastectomy arm and simple mastectomy plus radiation arm were comparable, with <3% relapse rate in each of these arms.

A direct comparison of axillary treatment by dissection compared with radiation was recently reported by Louis-Sylvestre et al.,[533] in which 658 patients with a breast carcinoma <3 cm in diameter and clinically uninvolved lymph nodes were randomly assigned to axillary dissection or axillary radiotherapy after breast-conserving surgery with radiation to the breast. Of the group undergoing dissection, 21% of the patients in the axillary dissection group were node positive. At 10 and 15 years, survival rates were identical in both groups (73.8% vs. 75.5% at 15 years). Recurrences in the axilla were less frequent in the axillary dissection group at 15 years (1% vs. 3%; P = .04). There was no difference in recurrence rates in the breast or supraclavicular region or distant metastases between the two groups.

Veronesi et al.[539] carried out a study in which women older than 45 years of age with breast cancer up to 1.2 cm were randomized, 214 of whom were treated with breast conservation surgery and irradiation without axillary treatment and 221 with conservation surgery plus breast and axillary radiation therapy (50 Gy in 5 weeks). After a median follow-up of 63 months, overt axillary metastases were fewer than expected: three cases in the no axillary treatment group (1.5%) and one in the RT group (0.5%). This study suggests that occult axillary metastases might never become clinically overt and axillary dissection might be avoided in patients with small carcinomas and a clinically negative axilla. Axillary RT seems to protect the patients from axillary recurrence almost completely. It is possible that systemic therapy, the undamaged immunocompetent tissue in the axillary lymph nodes, and axillary irradiation may all be factors contributing to the low incidence of axillary failures in these patients. Also, in the patients receiving no axillary irradiation, it is highly likely that the level I lymph nodes were included in the standard tangential fields.[324,522,545]

Irradiation of Lymphatics in Patients with Positive Axillary Lymph Nodes

Although there is general consensus that radiation to the regional lymph nodes is not necessary in patients with pathologically node-negative disease, there is considerable variability in radiation to the regional lymphatics in patients with pathologically node-positive disease.[75–77,324,527,546] Many radiation oncologists favor irradiation of the regional lymphatics in addition to the breast in node-positive women, while others favor no nodal irradiation, particularly in women with one to three positive nodes. Based on the potential disease-free and overall survival advantage, as well as the risk of failure in the supraclavicular region, most radiation oncologists favor at least supraclavicular nodal irradiation in patients with four or more nodes. The recent presentation of preliminary results of the National Cancer Institute of Canada's MA.20 trial demonstrates a distant metastasis, disease-free survival, and potential survival advantage to regional nodal irradiaton.[547] The majority of patients in this trial had one to three positive nodes and were randomized after breast-conserving surgery to tangential breast irradiation alone or breast irradiation with RNI to the supraclavicular and internal mammary regions. Full publication of this trial is eagerly awaited. A similar trial of the EORTC, randomizing high-risk node-negative and node-positive patients to treatment to the breast or chest wall alone or breast or chest wall and regional lymphatics, may help to further clarify this important issue.

The Canadian MA.20 intergroup study showed the benefit for RNI in node-positive or high-risk node-negative disease[525]. One thousand eight hundred thirty-two women were randomized after lumpectomy, ALND, and adjuvant therapy (91% of patients received adjuvant chemotherapy and 71% received hormonal therapy) to either WBI with or without regional nodal coverage (axillary, SCV, and ipsilateral IMN in the upper 3 intercostal spaces). Eighty-five percent of patients had 1 to 3 positive nodes. RNI improved 10-year DFS (82% vs. 77%, HR 0.76, P = .01), distant DFS (86.3% vs. 82.4%, HR 0.76, P = .03), and isolated locoregional DFS (95.2% vs. 92.2%, HR .59, P = .009). Certain high-risk patient population on subgroup analysis (especially those with negative estrogen and progesterone receptor statuses) benefited from RNI. Overall survival was not significant.

Similarly, the EORTC 22922/10925 study randomized 4004 node-positive or node-negative breast cancer with central or medial tumors after lumpectomy or mastectomy and adjuvant therapy (85% of patients received either chemotherapy, hormonal therapy, or both) to either RNI or observation[526]. At a median follow-up of 11 years, RNI improved DFS (72.1% vs. 69.1%, HR 0.89, P = .04), distant DFS (78% vs. 75%, HR 0.86, P = .02), and breast cancer mortality (12.5% vs. 14.4%, HR 0.82, P = .02).

The relative reduction of 24% of distant metastasis seen in the MA.20 study was substantiated in the EORTC study and is probably due to the reduction in regional nodal recurrence and subclinical regional nodal disease[548,549]. Interestingly, OS was nonsignificant in either study. However, a meta-analysis of both studies showed a significant improvement of OS (HR 0.88, CI 0.78–0.99) with absolute benefits at 10 years of 1% in the MA.20 trial and 1.6% in the EORTC trial[550]. Subgroup analysis suggests that patients with N0 disease and a complete ALND (>10 nodes) have a larger OS advantage from RNI than do those with N1-N3 disease or an incomplete ALND. Further investigation remains necessary to identify patients who benefit the most from RNI.

The European After Mapping of the Axilla Radiation or Surgery (AMAROS) Trial randomized patients after positive sentinel nodes to axillary dissection or axillary radiation and will help to address issues of locoregional control, survival, and morbidity using these two approaches.[551] Between 2001 and 2010, 4,806 patients were enrolled in this phase III non-inferiority trial and randomized for their axillary treatment if their sentinel node biopsy was positive (n = 1,425). Of these patients, ALND was performed in 744 patients and axillary radiotherapy in 681 patients. With a median follow-up of 6.1 years, the 5-year axillary recurrence rate was 0.54% after ALND and 1.03% after axillary radiotherapy (P = NS). There was no difference in DFS or OS. Interestingly, lymphedema occurred more often following ALND (40% at 1 year and 28% at 5 year) than after axillary radiotherapy (22% at 1 year and 14% at 5 years (P < .0001)). There was a nonsignificant trend toward more impairment of shoulder movement in the first year after axillary radiotherapy.

Acknowledging the lack of definitive data and clear consensus and allowing for flexibility depending on patient and physician preferences, the guidelines that the authors advocate are summarized in Tables 59.26 and 59.27. In general, the authors favor treatment of the supraclavicular fossa in patients with positive nodes. Treatment of the axilla and internal mammary will vary, with attention to the indications outlined in the table.

Sarrazin et al.[359] carried out a randomized study comparing 88 patients treated with tumorectomy and irradiation and 91 patients treated with mastectomy. In a second randomization in the study, the patients with positive axillary lymph nodes in the first randomization were randomly assigned to receive or not receive nodal irradiation. There was no significant difference in overall survival between the two groups. Nevertheless, Yarnold[523] advised elective irradiation of the axilla and the supraclavicular fossa in selected patients, such as those with four or more metastatic axillary lymph nodes, involvement of the apex of the axilla, or gross extracapsular tumor extension, even if the patients are to receive adjuvant chemotherapy. These recommendations are supported by reports that document the benefit of postmastectomy irradiation in patients receiving chemotherapy, which are reviewed in more detail in Chapter 54.

Treatment of the axilla varies significantly in patients with positive nodes. For those patients with negative nodes or with one to three positive nodes without extracapsular extension (ECE) who undergo adequate axillary dissection, there does not appear to be a benefit to targeting the full axilla.[75-78,324,544] There is considerable variability regarding treatment of the full axilla, even in patients with multiple positive nodes.[75,79,522,546] The risk of axillary recurrence after full dissection is low in patients with ECE, even without axillary lymph node irradiation. Whether to treat the full axilla following dissection for patients with multiple positive nodes or ECE generally includes consideration of the extent of dissection, the degree of nodal involvement and ECE, and the degree to which the patient and physician are willing to accept some increased risk of lymphedema with full axillary radiation following dissection.[113,324]

Hetelekidis et al.[251] evaluated 368 patients with T1 or T2 breast cancer and pathologically positive lymph nodes treated with breast-conserving therapy. The median number of sampled lymph nodes was 10. Twenty percent of the patients were treated with supraclavicular radiation therapy, and 64% received both axillary and supraclavicular radiation therapy (45 Gy). One hundred twenty-two patients (33%) had ECE. There was no significant correlation of either disease-free or overall survival or local, regional nodal, or distant failure rates in patients with ECE compared with those without it.

Pierce et al.,[552] in a review of 72 women with breast cancer treated with conservation surgery and irradiation, identified 27 patients (37.5%) who had evidence of ECE in the axilla. With a median follow-up of 14 months, 1 of 27 (4%) patients with ECE experienced an axillary failure, compared with 0 of 45 patients without ECE. Several authors concluded that ECE is associated with decreased survival but not with increased axillary failures and that radiation therapy may be omitted in a dissected axilla if the sole indication is extracapsular disease.

Internal Mammary Node Irradiation

The role of internal mammary nodal irradiation in node-positive breast cancer patients remains a controversial issue. Although, recently reported trials from the National Cancer Institute of Canada and EORTC help to address this, currently, there is no clear consensus on the role of internal mammary irradiation.[520,521,553-555] The EORTC 22922-10925 randomized patients with an involved axilla and/or medial primary tumor to WBI +/− internal mammary and medial supraclavicular LN (IM-MS) after lumpectomy and ALND. After enrolling over 4,000 women with a follow-up of 10.9 years, it was reported that IM-MS irradiation improved overall, disease-free and metastases-free survival without an increase in non–breast cancer–related mortality[526]. Similarly, the NCIC MA-20 randomized 1832 women with high-risk node-negative or node-positive breast cancer to WBI +/− RNI (internal

mammary, supraclavicular, and high axillary lymph nodes) and lumpectomy and ALND[548,549]. With a median follow-up of 9.5 years, the authors reported that RNI offered women a statistically significant benefit in terms of locoregional DFS and distant DFS but not OS with acceptable rates of toxicities. These studies lend credence to the notion of RNI in patients with a positive axilla.

Recently, a prospective Danish study reported the results 3,089 early-stage breast cancer patients treated according national guidelines that directed RNI (including IM nodes) of all right-sided disease but RNI (excluding IM nodes) of all left-sided disease[556]. RT was given 48 Gy in 24 fractions regardless of cancer laterality. With a median follow up of 8.9 years, the overall survival rates (75.9% vs. 72.2%, HR 0.82, $P = .005$), breast cancer mortality (20.9% vs. 23.4%, HR 0.85, $P = .03$), and risk of distant recurrence (27.4% vs. 29.7%, HR 0.89, $P = .07$) all favored internal mammary irradiation. Subgroup analysis suggested that tumor size ≥51 mm and ≥4 axillary nodes positive (especially if the primary cancer was in the lateral quadrants) predicted an overall survival benefit for internal mammary irradiation.

The Danish study suggested that the effect of treating the IMNs depended on risk of IM node metastasis. In contrast, a French randomized trial of patients with node-positive breast cancer treated with postmastectomy radiation, randomized to internal mammary radiation or no internal mammary radiation, with two-dimensional radiotherapy techniques[557]. After a median follow-up of 11.3 years among the survivors, no benefit of IMN irradiation on the overall survival was demonstrated. In addition, an older study examining the dissection of IMNs in T1-T3, N0-N1 invasive breast cancer patients who underwent either Halsted mastectomy or extended mastectomy with regional node dissection without postoperative RT showed that in 30 years, the dissection of IMNs does not improve the survival of patients. However, the prognostic value of axillary and internal mammary nodal positivity is high as it impacts overall survival. Annual death rates were 0.163 with both sites positive, 0.077 with axillary LNs positive, 0.055 with IMNs positive, and 0.031 with neither site positive for disease[558].

Several surgical series comparing extended radical mastectomy and radical mastectomy, without adjuvant systemic therapy, have shown that extended radical mastectomy was associated with improved survival rates in patients with medial T1 or T2 tumors and positive axillary nodes.[559,560] These surgical series and selected series evaluating internal mammary irradiation are summarized in Table 59.30.[553-555,559,560] The majority of randomized trials evaluating postoperative radiation therapy did include radiation to the internal mammary chain. However, it is difficult to distinguish whether the benefit derived from such treatment related specifically to radiation of the internal mammary chain or to the breast or chest wall, supraclavicular, or axillary treatment administered.

Freedman et al.[561] examined data regarding patterns of failure after elective IMN treatment. Although controversial, data from the prospective, randomized trials of IMN treatment did not seem to support elective dissection or irradiation. IMN irradiation did not contribute to survival, yet it raised the risk of cardiac toxic effects. Sentinel lymph node mapping provided an opportunity to examine the IMN chain in early breast cancer. It is possible that biopsy of the "hot" nodes could be used to select patients who are most likely to benefit from additional regional therapy to these nodes.

Fowble et al.[553] compared the outcome in 1,383 women with stage I or II breast cancer who underwent wide excision, axillary node dissection with 10 or more nodes removed, and breast irradiation. A total of 114 women had radiation to the IMNs with deep tangents and 1,269 did not. All axillary

TABLE 59.30 STUDIES EVALUATING IMPACT OF INTERNAL MAMMARY TREATMENT (SURGERY OR RADIATION) ON 10-YEAR SURVIVAL

Study (Reference)	Type of IMN Treatment	Number of Patients		Follow-Up (Year)	Overall Survival			Distant Metastasis-Free Survival			Disease-Free Survival		
		With IMN Treatment	Without IMN Treatment		With IMN Treatment (%)	Without IMN Treatment (%)	P	Without IMN Treatment (%)	With IMN Treatment (%)	P	Without IMN Treatment (%)	With IMN Treatment (%)	P
Meier et al.[560]	dissection	56	56	10	73.6	60.4	.130	–	–	–	–	–	–
Lacour et al.[559]	dissection	750	703	10	56	53	.40	44	49	NS	–	–	–
Fowble et al.[553]	radiation	114	1,269	6	80	81	0.87	–	–	–	82	87	.38
Obedian and Haffty[554]	radiation	535	411	13	72	84	NS	77	87	NS	–	–	–
Stemmer et al.[a][555]	radiation	67	33	6.4	78	64	.08	–	–	–	73	52	.02
Poortmans[526]	radiation	2,002	2,002	10	82.3	80.7	0.06	78	75	0.02	72.1	69.1	0.04
Whelan[525]	radiation	916	916	9.5	82.8	81.8	0.35	86.3	82.4	0.03	82	77	0.01
Thorsen[556]	radiation	1,492	1,597	8.9	75.9	72.2	0.005	72.6	70.3	0.06	–	–	–
Romestaing[557]	radiation	1,200 Total		11.3	62.6	59.6	.87	–	–	–	–	–	–

[a]Survival data documented at the end point of follow-up.
IMN, internal mammary lymph nodes; NS, not significant.

node-positive women received adjuvant chemotherapy or tamoxifen or both. There were no significant differences in IBTR, regional node recurrence, and initial or total distant metastases for the two groups. No IMN failures were observed among the 114 patients whose IMNs were treated, and only 4 IMN failures were found in the 1,269 other patients (2 of whom had distant metastases). Similarly, 5- and 10-year actuarial overall and cause-specific survival rates were not significantly different.

In a series from Yale, Obedian and Haffty[554] found no difference in the 10-year disease-free survival rate after breast irradiation and excision, regardless of whether IMNs were irradiated. Of 984 patients with invasive breast cancer who were treated with CS and radiotherapy, patients were divided into two groups: those treated by intentionally targeting the IMNs (n = 535) and without intentionally targeting the IMNs (n = 411). The decision not to use a separate internal mammary field was a result of a change in treatment policy over time and generally not based on number of nodes or tumor location. There were no significant differences between the groups with respect to age, ER or PR status, or use of adjuvant chemotherapy or hormone therapy. There were more patients with T2 tumors, positive nodes, medial lesions, indeterminate margins, and slightly longer follow-up in the group treated to the internal mammary chain. There were no significant differences between the groups with respect to overall survival or distant metastasis-free survival.

In a study by Stemmer et al.[555] of 100 node-positive patients scheduled to receive radiation to the internal mammary chain, 67 received the radiation and 33 did not because of technical difficulties. At a median follow-up of 77 months, disease-free survival was significantly prolonged in patients receiving internal mammary radiation compared with those without internal mammary radiation (73% vs. 52%; P = .02). A trend was seen for overall survival (78% vs. 64%; P = .08). Cox regression multivariate analysis found IMN radiotherapy to be significant both for disease-free and overall survival. There was no treatment-related mortality.

It is evident that data are conflicting, and opinions regarding the role of internal mammary radiation remain unresolved. Until more definitive data become available, it is likely that patient and physician biases will dictate practice. The authors' approach is summarized in Tables 59.26 and 59.27, acknowledging that uncertainties in the available data allow for substantial flexibility. The radiation oncologist, however, must be familiar with the various techniques to treat IMNs, which are summarized later in the section on techniques.

SEQUENCING CHEMOTHERAPY AND HORMONAL THERAPY

Sequencing Chemoradiation in the Conservative Management of Breast Cancer

With the increasing use of systemic therapy in patients with early-stage breast cancer, the integration of this treatment with surgery and radiation therapy has become an important clinical question. Initial retrospective series evaluating treatment sequencing suggested that a delay in the onset of radiation therapy to permit delivery of chemotherapy increased local recurrence rates.[89,562,563] These data are summarized in a pooled analysis by Huang et al.[89] Ten retrospective studies involving 7,401 patients investigated the association between delay in initiating postoperative RT and local control in breast cancer (after lumpectomy in nine studies and lumpectomy or mastectomy in one study). Eight of these studies compared local control between patients who were treated more than 8 weeks after surgery and those treated within 8 weeks of surgery. The pooled random-effects OR from the combined analysis was 1.62 (95% CI, 1.21 to 2.16), corresponding to an increase in the 5-year LRR from 5.8% in those patients treated within 8 weeks to 9.1% in those patients treated between 9 and 16 weeks after surgery. In a separate analysis exploring the optimum sequencing of adjuvant RT and systemic chemotherapy after surgery for breast cancer from 11 retrospective series, the pooled random-effects OR in these 11 studies was 2.28 (95% CI, 1.45 to 3.57), corresponding to an increase in the 5-year LRR from 6.0% in the RT-first group to 16.0% in the chemotherapy-first group (Fig. 59.21).

Most of these data are subject to criticism because of their retrospective nature, the fact that patients were treated in an earlier era with different surgical techniques and lack of attention to margins, and inclusion of heterogenous groups of patients with these caveats, but there appears to be a trend toward higher local relapse rates with delays in radiation therapy, which appears to have been an appropriate concern with respect to integration of radiation therapy and chemotherapy in the conservatively managed patients.

Initial data regarding these concerns related to the delay in radiation while chemotherapy was being delivered led the Harvard group at Joint Center for Radiation Therapy (JCRT) to investigate the sequencing of radiation therapy and chemotherapy in a randomized prospective clinical trial.[562,563] In this trial, women treated with breast-conserving surgery were randomly assigned to 4 cycles of doxorubicin-based combination chemotherapy, followed by radiation therapy or radiation

Section III

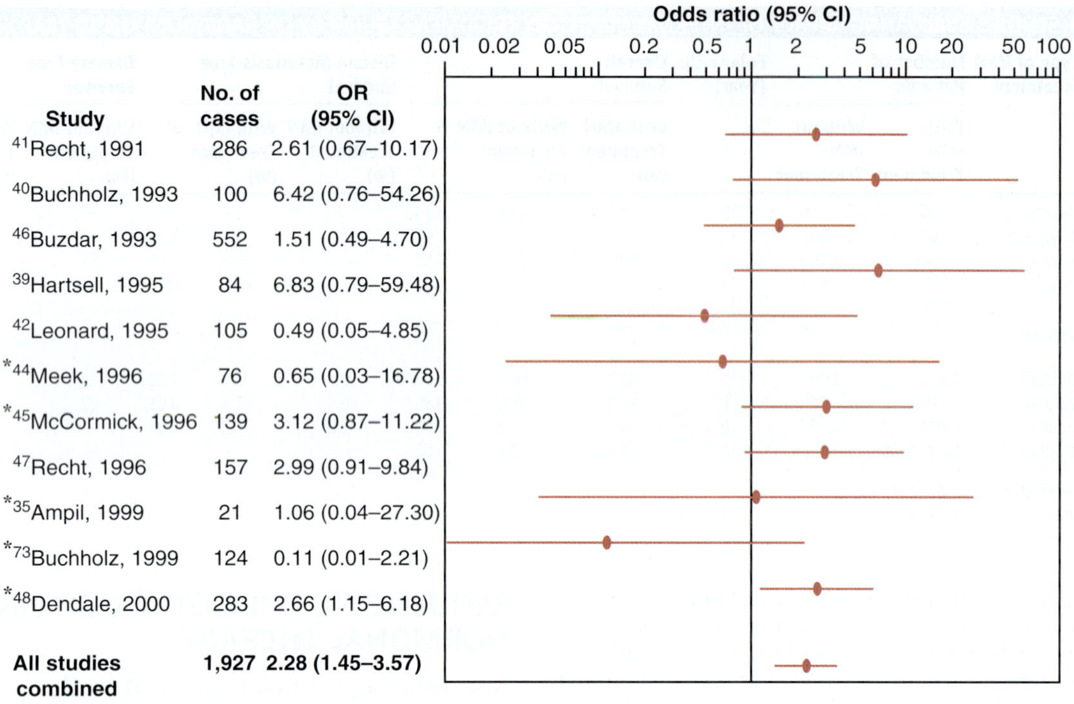

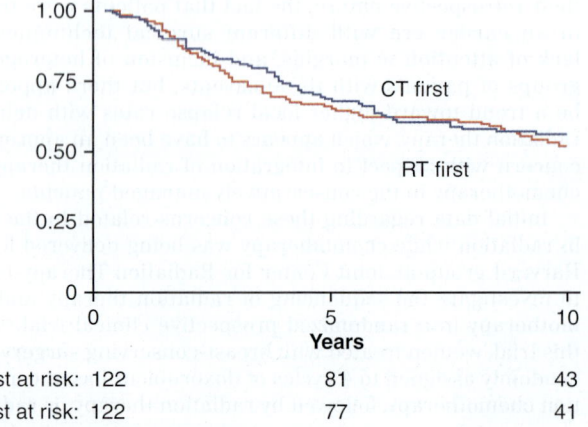

Odds ratio (95% CI)
0.01 0.02 0.05 0.2 0.5 1 2 5 10 20 50 100
Study
No. of cases
OR (95% CI)
41Recht, 1991 286 2.61 (0.67–10.17)
40Buchholz, 1993 100 6.42 (0.76–54.26)
46Buzdar, 1993 552 1.51 (0.49–4.70)
39Hartsell, 1995 84 6.83 (0.79–59.48)
42Leonard, 1995 105 0.49 (0.05–4.85)
*44Meek, 1996 76 0.65 (0.03–16.78)
*45McCormick, 1996 139 3.12 (0.87–11.22)
47Recht, 1996 157 2.99 (0.91–9.84)
*35Ampil, 1999 21 1.06 (0.04–27.30)
*73Buchholz, 1999 124 0.11 (0.01–2.21)
*48Dendale, 2000 283 2.66 (1.15–6.18)
All studies combined 1,927 2.28 (1.45–3.57)

FIGURE 59.21. Associations between delay in postoperative radiotherapy (RT) and local recurrence rates (LRRs) in studies of the sequencing of adjuvant RT and chemotherapy for breast cancer. LRRs in patients who received delayed RT following initial chemotherapy are compared with the rates observed in those patients who received early RT by chemotherapy. Low-quality studies are indicated by an asterisk. (From Huang J, Barbera L, Brouwers M, et al. Does delay in starting treatment affect the outcomes of radiotherapy? A systematic review. *J Clin Oncol* 2003;21[3]:555–563. Reprinted with permission. Copyright © 2003 American Society of Clinical Oncology. All rights reserved.)

therapy followed by 4 cycles of the same chemotherapy. In an update of this trial, Bellon et al.[564] reported no statistically significant treatment difference in the rates of freedom from any event, including breast cancer recurrence, contralateral breast cancer, second malignancy, or death (Fig. 59.22). The 10-year rate of any event was 46% for patients in the chemotherapy-first arm compared with 51% in the radiation-first arm. The 10-year rates of distant metastasis were 35% and 36% in the two arms, respectively, and the 10-year rates of death were 28% and 33%, respectively. For the 123 patients with negative margins, the crude local recurrence rates for

FIGURE 59.22. Event-free survival (including breast cancer recurrence, contralateral breast cancer, second malignancy, or death) by sequencing of chemotherapy and radiation following breast-conserving therapy, from the Harvard randomized trial. (From Bellon JR, Come SE, Gelman RS, et al. Sequencing of chemotherapy and radiation therapy in early-stage breast cancer: updated results of a prospective randomized trial. *J Clin Oncol* 2005;23[9]:1934–1940. Reprinted with permission. Copyright © 2005 American Society of Clinical Oncology. All rights reserved.)

1.00
0.75
0.50
0.25
0
CT first
RT first
0
5
10
Years
CT first at risk: 122 81 43
RT first at risk: 122 77 41

chemotherapy-first and radiation-first patients were 6% and 13%, respectively. Corresponding rates of distant and regional recurrences were 18% and 26%. Among women with close margins (n = 47), crude local recurrence rates were 32% and 4%, respectively; distant or regional recurrences were 37% and 43%. In the group with positive margins (n = 51), local recurrences occurred in 23% of chemotherapy-first and 20% of radiation-first patients.

Although the JCRT study provided important data concerning treatment sequencing, this study predominantly focused on patients with lymph node–positive disease. Investigators from the MD Anderson Cancer Center performed a retrospective analysis of sequencing of chemotherapy and radiation in 124 patients with lymph node–negative disease treated with breast-conserving therapy.[565] In this series, 79% of the patients had negative margins. The 5-year actuarial rates of local control were 100% for the chemotherapy-first group (most commonly 6 cycles of doxorubicin-based chemotherapy) and 94% for the radiation-first group (P = .351). The 5-year recurrence-free survival rates for the chemotherapy-first and radiation-first groups were 92% and 77% (P = .083), respectively. These data again support an adjuvant-therapy schedule in which chemotherapy is delivered first. The median delays in radiation delivery were 6.7 months in the MD Anderson Cancer Center series and 16 weeks in the JCRT series.

More recently, with the addition of taxane-based chemotherapy to adriamycin-based regimens, concerns have arisen regarding the additional delays in initiating radiation therapy in conservatively managed patients. This was addressed in a study by Sartor et al.[566] In this randomized CALGB study evaluating adriamycin and cytoxan versus adriamycin and cytoxan, followed by taxane, there were 345 conservatively managed patients. Although the sequencing of radiation was not randomized, patients in the adriamycin plus taxane arm had radiation delayed by an additional 84 days (4 21-day cycles of taxol). Despite this added delay, locoregional relapses were lower in the adriamycin plus taxane compared with the adriamycin arm (9.7% vs. 3.7%; *P* = .04). (The majority of patients in this randomized trial presumably had negative surgical margins.)

For the majority of patients undergoing breast-conserving surgery with negative margins, these data collectively indicate that administration of chemotherapy prior to radiation therapy does not result in excessive rates of local relapse, provided all modalities are given in a timely fashion without excessive delays. Whether patients with positive or close margins or other risk factors for local relapse would benefit from earlier administration of radiation remains an unresolved issue.

Concurrent Chemoradiation in Breast-Conserving Therapy

Although the concurrent use of chemoradiation therapy in conservatively managed breast cancer has fallen out of favor, there are data that suggest a high rate of local control in patients treated concurrently. These studies are summarized in Table 59.31.[567–570,572] The chemotherapy regimens used in these studies are no longer routinely employed because they are less effective.

A randomized trial of concurrent versus sequential CMF chemotherapy was reported by Arcangeli et al.[572] A total of 206 patients who had quadrantectomy and axillary dissection for breast cancer and were planned to receive adjuvant CMF chemotherapy were randomized to concurrent or sequential radiotherapy. Radiotherapy was delivered only to the whole breast through tangential fields to a dose of 50 Gy in 20 fractions over 4 weeks, followed by an electron boost of 10 to 15 Gy in 4 to 6 fractions to the tumor bed. No differences in 5-year breast recurrence-free, metastasis-free, disease-free, and overall survival were observed in the two treatment groups. All patients completed the planned radiotherapy. No evidence of an increased risk of toxicity was observed between the two arms. No difference in radiotherapy and in the chemotherapy dose intensity was observed in the two groups. The authors concluded that in patients with negative surgical margins receiving adjuvant chemotherapy, radiotherapy can be delayed for up to 7 months. However, concurrent administration of CMF chemotherapy and radiotherapy was safe, and the authors suggest that such an approach might be reserved for patients at high risk of local recurrence.

Another randomized study of concurrent versus sequential radiation therapy was reported by Rouesse et al.[570] This study supports the concept that concurrent use of chemotherapy with radiation therapy improves local control in breast cancer. This trial compared concurrent chemoradiotherapy with FNC (5-fluorouracil [5-FU] 500 mg/m², mitoxantrone 12 mg/m², and cyclophosphamide 500 mg/m² to sequential FEC (5-fluorouracil 500 mg/m², epirubicin 60 mg/m², and cyclophosphamide 500 mg/m² followed by radiation in node-positive breast cancer in 650 women with operable breast cancer. All patients had node-positive disease and were randomized to sequential or concurrent chemoradiotherapy. Although there were no differences in disease-free or overall survival, local recurrences were significantly lower with concurrent therapy (3% vs. 7%). Of patients undergoing breast conservation, there were 6 locoregional relapses in the concurrent arm compared with 18 locoregional relapses in the sequential arm (*P* = .01). In multivariate Cox analysis, the sequential group had an increased risk of locoregional relapse compared with those in the concurrent group (RR 2.8; 95% CI, 1.1 to 7.2).

Toledano et al.[571] recently reported the results of the ARCOSEIN sequential versus concurrent adjuvant chemotherapy with radiation therapy after breast-conserving surgery. After breast-conserving surgery, patients were treated either with sequential treatment with chemotherapy first followed by RT (arm A) or chemotherapy administered concurrently with RT (arm B). In all patients, the chemotherapy regimen consisted of mitoxantrone (12 mg/m²), 5-FU (500 mg/m²), and cyclophosphamide (500 mg/m², 6 cycles [day 1 to day 21]). Among the 214 evaluable patients, 107 were treated in each arm. Although local control was slightly superior in the concurrent arm, subcutaneous fibrosis, telangiectasia, skin pigmentation, and breast atrophy were significantly increased in arm B. No statistical difference was observed between the two arms of the study concerning grade 2 or greater pain, breast edema, or lymphedema.

Another randomized trial recently reported by Calais et al.,[573] which is similar to the Rouesse et al.[570] study, compared concurrent radiotherapy with mitoxantrone, 5-FU, and cyclophosphamide to the same regimen followed by radiation therapy. Although toxicities were higher in the concurrent group, those patients with positive nodes had a significantly lower local relapse rate in the concurrent arm.

The concurrent use of chemotherapy and radiation following breast-conserving therapy has been reported in several nonrandomized studies. A prospective single-arm study by Bellon et al.[568] also demonstrated favorable local control in a high-risk group of patients treated with concurrent CMF chemotherapy and reduced-dose radiation. Several other retrospective series, including one conducted from Yale, have demonstrated favorable local control rates and acceptable

TABLE 59.31 SELECTED STUDIES EVALUATING CONCURRENT CHEMORADIATION IN BREAST-CONSERVING SURGERY WITH RADIATION

Study (Reference)	Number of Patients		Follow-Up (Median, Year)	Type of Chemo	Local Control		*P*	Toxicity with CON-CRT
	CON-CRT	Non-CON-CRT			CON-CRT (%)	Non-CON-CRT (%)		
Haffty et al.[567]	109	426	8.8	CMF (mainly)	92	83	<.001	Cosmetic results, toxicities, and long-term complications acceptable
Bellon et al.[568]	112	–	7.8	CMF (prospective)	96	–	–	
Markiewicz et al.[569]	210	–	5.2 for node negative; 7.6 for node positive	CF during radiation therapy flowed by further CMF	87 (10 y)	–	–	Cosmesis and complications acceptable
Rouesse et al.[570]	210	206	5.25	FNC for CON-CRT, FEC for sequential RT	97	91	.01	Febrile neutropenia and grade 3–4 leukopenia significantly more frequent
Toledano et al.[571]	107	107	6.7	CNF	–	–	–	Increased incidence of grade 2 or greater late side effects.
Arcangeli et al.[572]	106	100	5.4	CMF	97	96	NS	Late toxicity and cosmesis not available yet

CF, oral cyclophosphamide/intravenous 5-fluorouracil; CMF, cyclophosphamide/methotrexate/5-fluofouracil; CNF, cyclophosphamide/mitoxantrone/5-fluorouracil; CON-CRT, concurrent chemotherapy; NS, not significant.

toxicity in patients at high risk for local relapse using concurrent chemoradiotherapy.[429] In the Yale retrospective series, which compared 109 patients treated with concurrent chemoradiation to 426 patients treated with sequential chemoradiation, the concurrent group had a lower rate of local relapse, despite overall poorer prognostic factors for local control. However, the majority of these studies did not employ the most commonly used current chemotherapy agents such as adriamycin and taxanes. Therefore, it is difficult to extrapolate these results to current practice.

More recently, monoclonal antibodies such as trastuzumab and bevacizumab (Avastin) are being used commonly in the management of breast cancer patients. Romond et al.[271] reported on a combine analysis from two large cooperative group studies investigating the utility of trastuzumab in HER2-positive patients with operable breast cancer and found that trastuzumab improved patient outcomes. There was no difference in acute locoregional toxicities, but it should be noted that the use of trastuzumab was associated with an increased risk of congestive heart failure or death from cardiac causes (4.1% vs. 0.8%). Goyal et al.[574] reported on a series of 14 patients receiving bevacizumab in combination with whole-breast irradiation who were then matched to a group of patients who received whole-breast irradiation alone. No patient receiving bevacizumab plus RT experienced grade 3 or higher toxicity; however, three matched control patients experienced a grade 3 skin reaction. Five patients (35%) developed reduction in ejection fraction in the bevacizumab arm: two with right-sided and three with left-sided treatment. Patients with left-sided treatment experienced a persistent reduction in ejection fraction compared with those receiving right-sided treatment. Thus, when treating patients with left-sided breast cancer, exclusion of the heart from the beam's eye view should be undertaken such that no unnecessary radiation dose is delivered to the heart. One challenge moving forward is determining the toxicities of these novel therapies in combination with conventionally fractionated and hypofractionated radiotherapy regimens.

The critical issue that arises with conservatively managed breast cancer is whether the modest gain in local control outweighs the added toxicities and risks of concurrent chemoradiotherapy, using currently available agents. The benefit in locoregional control obtained in the Rouesse et al.[570] study was statistically significant, but it remains debatable whether the added toxicity of the concurrent program is worth the added risk. Potential issues with concurrent chemoradiation, as pointed out in a study by Burstein et al.,[575] include high rates of radiation pneumonitis in patients treated with radiation given in combination with weekly paclitaxel. Although they observed more favorable results with less frequent dosing,

this study highlights the importance of prospective evaluation of radiation in combination with newer chemotherapeutic agents. Furthermore, this study highlights the importance of the dosing and scheduling of the chemotherapy agents given in combination with radiation.

The challenge over the next few years will be to identify those patients, who when treated by the traditional approach of surgery followed by chemotherapy followed by radiation therapy remain at elevated risk of local relapse. Also at risk may be subsets of patients treated with neoadjuvant chemotherapy followed by surgery followed by radiation. Those patients who, when treated by these traditional sequencing approaches, are at high risk of local relapse are ideally suited for prospective evaluation of novel approaches using concurrent chemoradiation strategies. From such trials, we can hopefully minimize locoregional relapse and optimize disease-free and overall survival, with acceptable treatment-related morbidity.

Sequencing Tamoxifen/Hormonal Therapy and Radiation Therapy in Conservatively Managed Patients

The question of optimal scheduling of hormonal therapy and radiation has been raised because of theoretical concerns that tamoxifen may decrease the radiation sensitivity of tumors. In cell culture studies, tamoxifen causes arrest of breast cancer cells in culture in the relatively radioresistant G_0/G_1 phases of the cell cycle. Although there are conflicting data, suggesting both no effect and increased radiation sensitivity, clinicians and patients have been in a quandary as to whether it is reasonable to begin tamoxifen during radiation. In addition, clinical studies have suggested increased pulmonary and breast fibrosis, possibly related to increased concentrations of transforming growth factor-β with the concurrent use of tamoxifen.[576] In a retrospective case series, Wazer et al.[577] reported a trend for an adverse cosmetic outcome associated with breast fibrosis in patients treated with tamoxifen and breast irradiation given either concurrently or sequentially ($P = .06$), although this was not confirmed in other series.[578-580]

A series of three separate retrospective series, however, performed independently but published simultaneously, reached similar conclusions that sequential or concurrent use of tamoxifen were both acceptable.[578-581] These studies are summarized in Table 59.32. The largest study by Ahn et al.[578] from the Yale group compared 254 patients treated with concurrent tamoxifen and radiation therapy to 241 treated by radiation therapy followed by tamoxifen ($n = 241$). There were no significant differences in the risk of IBTR, disease-free survival, or overall survival. The HR for ipsilateral breast tumor

TABLE 59.32 OUTCOMES OF CONCURRENT OR SEQUENTIAL TAMOXIFEN WITH RADIATION THERAPY IN EARLY-STAGE BREAST CANCER

Study (Reference)	Number of Patients CON-TAM	Number of Patients SEQ-TAM	Follow-Up (Median, Year)	Total Local Relapse CON-TAM (%)	Total Local Relapse SEQ-TAM (%)	P	Distant Metastasis CON-TAM (%)	Distant Metastasis SEQ-TAM (%)	P	Secondary Malignancy CON-TAM (%)	Secondary Malignancy SEQ-TAM (%)	P	Complications
Ahn et al.[578]	254	241	10.0	5.9	7.5	.59	8.3	12.0	.16	17.3	15.8	.16	
Harris et al.[579]	174	104	8.6	4.0	4.8	.76	—	—	—	—	—	—	No significant difference between the two groups for arm edema, pneumonitis, and rib fracture
Pierce et al.[581]	202	107	10.3	15.8	14.0	.67	—	—	—	—	—	—	No significant differences between two groups for grade 3 or 4 toxicity; one grade 3 pulmonary toxicity observed in CON-TAM group

CON-TAM, concurrent tamoxifen; SEQ-TAM, sequential tamoxifen.

recurrence comparing sequential with concurrent tamoxifen and radiation therapy was 0.93 (95% CI, 0.42 to 2.05; *P* = .86). In this study, morbidity outcomes were not reported.

The second study, by Harris et al.,[579] from the group at the University of Pennsylvania compared 174 patients treated with concurrent tamoxifen and radiation therapy with 104 patients treated with radiation therapy followed sequentially by tamoxifen. Similar to the Yale study, patients were accrued throughout a long period between 1980 and 1995, and again no significant differences in IBTR, disease-free survival, or overall survival were observed between groups. The HR for ipsilateral breast tumor recurrence (sequential vs. concurrent) was 1.23 (95% CI, 0.33 to 4.49; *P* = .78). In this study, breast edema and arm edema as well as cosmetic outcome and pneumonitis were analyzed and no significant differences were observed.

The third study, by Pierce et al.,[581] evaluated results from a randomized trial, in which patients were randomly assigned to cyclophosphamide, doxorubicin, and fluorouracil (CAF) followed by tamoxifen, CMF, or CMF followed by tamoxifen. Although the sequencing of tamoxifen was not randomized, 202 patients received concurrent tamoxifen and radiation therapy and 107 received radiation therapy followed sequentially by tamoxifen. In this study, no differences were noted in the risk of IBTR, disease-free survival, or survival between radiation therapy followed sequentially by tamoxifen and concurrent tamoxifen and radiation therapy group. Patients who received concurrent tamoxifen and radiation therapy were more likely to receive radiation after chemotherapy, with less delay. The HR for risk of IBTR (radiation therapy followed sequentially by tamoxifen vs. concurrent tamoxifen and radiation therapy) was 0.73 (95% CI, 0.26 to 2.04; *P* = .54).

Although these studies are limited by their retrospective design, they do offer some reassurance that the concurrent use of hormonal therapy with radiation therapy does not result in excessive rates of local relapse. Although a large randomized trial would be the appropriate next step in addressing this issue, it is unclear whether this issue will be addressed by such a trial in the near future. Given the lack of more definitive data, it appears that either the concurrent or the sequential use of tamoxifen is acceptable in the conservatively managed breast cancer patient. The majority of available data on the use of hormonal therapy and radiation are with tamoxifen. In a prospective phase II randomized trial evaluating concurrent or sequential letrozole, Azria et al.[582] reported no difference in local relapse (one in each arm) at 26 months of follow-up. In addition, only two patients in each group had grade 2 or worse late effects. These authors conclude that letrozole can be safely delivered concomitantly with radiation, but longer follow-up is awaited from this trial.

BREAST-CONSERVING THERAPY: CONTROVERSIES AND SPECIAL CIRCUMSTANCES

The available evidence from all of the retrospective and prospective trials above suggests that although there are clearly cohorts of patients who are at increased risk of local relapse, there are relatively few contraindications to breast-conserving therapy and there is little evidence that treatment of patients at higher risk for local relapse with breast-conserving therapy compromises overall survival. Careful attention to patient selection, surgical technique, and radiation technique, with the appropriate integration of systemic therapy, should minimize the probability of local relapse. There are several areas of controversy and special circumstances in the selection of patients for breast-conserving therapy that warrant specific discussion.

Breast-Conserving Surgery and Radiation in Familial Breast Cancer and Carriers of *BRCA1/2* Mutations

There is considerable controversy and uncertainty regarding the role of breast-conserving surgery and radiation in carriers of *BRCA1/2* mutations.[466,583,584] It has been just over two decades since these two major breast cancer predisposition genes were identified. Genetic linkage studies from families at high risk for predisposing germline mutations have led to the identification of the *BRCA1/2* genes, and these two genes are thought to account for 5% to 10% of breast cancers.[21,43,585-588] Patients with either mutation have up to an 80% lifetime risk of developing breast cancer depending on variable penetrance of the gene. Inherited mutation of *BRCA1* also confers a 20% to 40% lifetime risk of ovarian cancer. Typical patient characteristics of *BRCA*-associated breast cancer include young age at onset and bilateral involvement. The median age at breast cancer diagnosis is 40 for *BRCA1* carriers and 45 for *BRCA2* carriers.[21,585-588] Tumor characteristics of *BRCA1* carriers have been well described. Histopathologic features are often more aggressive, with high nuclear grade, aneuploidy, and high proliferation indices; tumors with a medullary component are more common. Estrogen and progesterone receptors are more likely to be negative when compared with *BRCA2* or sporadic counterparts. Although there are some conflicting data, *BRCA1/2* carriers with breast cancer appear to have equivalent survival when compared with age and staged matched patients with sporadic disease.[21,43,589-591]

The loci for *BRCA1* and *BRCA2* are chromosome 17q21 and chromosome 13q12-13, respectively.[21,585-588] Both function as tumor suppressor genes and are involved in DNA double-strand break repair. The role of *BRCA1/2* in DNA repair suggests the possibility of hypersensitivity to radiation, as well as the potential for radiation-induced complications including second cancers. DNA double-strand breaks caused by ionizing radiation in *BRCA1/2* carriers could theoretically result in increased cell kill secondary to deficient repair mechanisms.[21,45,592-594]

The risk of both contralateral primary breast cancer and ovarian cancer is substantially higher in patients with *BRCA1/2* mutations than sporadic counterparts. An early publication by the Breast Cancer Linkage Consortium estimated a 64% risk of contralateral breast cancer by the age of 70 years in patients who have had *BRCA1*-associated breast cancer.[43,595] The cumulative risk of ovarian cancer in these patients was 44% by age 70 years. Women with *BRCA2* mutations have a risk of breast cancer similar to patients with *BRCA1* mutations. There is a lesser risk of ovarian cancer, with a cumulative risk of <10% by age 70 years. These results have been interpreted with caution, as linkage studies are likely to overestimate the cancer risk associated with *BRCA1/2* mutations. Several studies of known germline *BRCA1/2* carriers have demonstrated a less pronounced increase in the rate of contralateral breast cancer compared with sporadic controls.[21,43,595]

Early study of familiar breast cancer used positive family history as a surrogate for genetic predisposition. Many of the patients included likely did not harbor germline mutations of the *BRCA1/2* genes. Seynaeve et al.[591] for the Dutch Cancer Society investigated local recurrence after breast conservation therapy in patients with *three or more* first-degree relatives with breast or ovarian cancer or *BRCA1/2* families. Local recurrence rates were initially similar, but with longer follow-up, there was a higher rate of recurrence in the hereditary group when compared with age-matched sporadic patients. Other studies of breast conservation therapy in patients with a family history of breast cancer have not shown an increase in IBR.[406,407,596] Disparate results are expected, as family history is not the sole factor in genetic predisposition.

TABLE 59.33 RATE OF IPSILATERAL BREAST TUMOR RELAPSE IN *BRCA* MUTATION CARRIERS COMPARED TO SPORADIC CONTROLS

Study (Reference)	Number of Patients Genetic	Number of Patients Sporadic	Follow-Up (Year)	IBTR Sporadic (%)	IBTR Genetic (%)	P	Notes
Seynaeve et al.[591]	87	174	10	16	30	.05	More recurrences elsewhere? in cancers
Robson et al.[607]	28	277	10	6.9	22	.25	Only tested for founder mutations in Ashkenazi women
Robson et al.[590]	56	440	9.6	7	13	.68	As above
Haffty et al.[598]	23	135	12	21	46	.007	No oophorectomy or Tamoxifen in *BRCA* group
Pierce et al.[601]	160	445	7.9	17	24	.19	HR for IBTR was significant in those carriers who did not undergo prophylactic oophorectomy
Kirova et al.[599]	29	107	13	19	24	.47	
Garcia-Etienne et al.[597]	54	162	5	4	15	.03	

HR, hazard ratio; IBTR, ipsilateral breast tumor recurrence.

The risk of local and contralateral breast cancers as a function of *BRCA1* and *BRCA2* status has been evaluated by numerous groups over the past 10 years.[285,584,590,591,597-608] These are summarized in Table 59.33.

Robson et al.[584] studied breast conservation therapy in Ashkenazi women with the *BRCA* gene founder mutations (*BRCA1* 185delAG, *BRCA1* 5382insC, and *BRCA2* 617delT). Archival tissue samples were retrieved from 305 women, and 28 *BRCA* gene founder mutations were detected. *BRCA1/2* carriers had a nonsignificant trend toward increased ipsilateral breast cancer recurrence and decreased overall survival at 5 and 10 years. This trend may be related to the greater likelihood of young age and axillary lymph node involvement in women with *BRCA* founder mutations. On univariate analysis, age but not *BRCA* mutation status was associated with IBTR. The significance of age was maintained on multivariate analysis, with a RR of 2.5. The risk of contralateral breast cancer at 5 and 10 years was 14.8% and 27.0%, respectively.

This series from Memorial Hospital was later combined with data from McGill University, yielding a total of 56 women with founder mutations. Again, *BRCA1/2* carriers had an increased risk of contralateral breast cancer at a median follow-up of 9.7 years (27% vs. 8%; P < .001). Ipsilateral breast cancer recurrence for *BRCA1/2* carriers was similar to noncarriers, and age <50 at diagnosis was the only significant

predictor of metachronous ipsilateral disease (P = .002).[590] *BRCA1* mutations were an independent predictor of breast cancer mortality on multivariate analysis but only for women who did not receive chemotherapy. *BRCA2* mutations had no impact on breast cancer-specific survival.

Haffty et al.[598] studied breast conservation therapy in germline carriers with early-onset breast cancer. One hundred and twenty-seven women diagnosed with breast cancer at age 42 years or younger agreed to undergo genetic testing, and 22 were found to have *BRCA1/2* mutations. Adjuvant tamoxifen or oophorectomy was not used in any of the carriers of *BRCA1/2* mutations. Patients in the genetic group were younger than sporadic patients, and this difference was significant on multivariate analysis. Treatment outcomes were compared with results from patients with sporadic disease. With a median follow-up of 12.7 years, the genetic group had a higher rate of ipsilateral (49% vs. 21%; P = .007) and contralateral breast events (42% vs. 9%; P = .001). Nine of the 11 IBRs were classified as second primary tumors, based on a difference in tumor location (n = 7) or histology (n = 8). The rate of ipsilateral and contralateral events was much higher than those reported in earlier series and may be attributable to both the young age of the patients at diagnosis and longer duration of follow-up. The proportion of relapse-free *BRCA1/2* carriers was similar to noncarriers at 5 years and then progressively declined with time (Fig. 59.23). It is

FIGURE 59.23. Risk of ipsilateral **(A)** and contralateral breast tumor relapse **(B)** as a function of *BRCA1/BRCA2* mutation status in a cohort of conservatively managed breast cancer patients. (Reprinted from Haffty BG, Harrold E, Khan AJ, et al. Outcome of conservatively managed early-onset breast cancer by BRCA1/2 status. *Lancet* 2002;359[9316]:1471–1477. Copyright © 2002 Elsevier. With permission.)

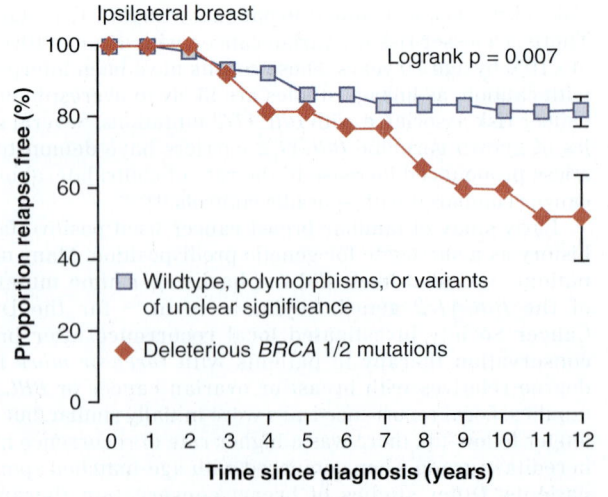

Ipsilateral breast

Logrank p = 0.007

☐ Wildtype, polymorphisms, or variants of unclear significance

◆ Deleterious *BRCA* 1/2 mutations

Number at risk

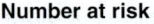

Sporadic	105	105	103	96	93	84	79	67	62	58	54	48	39
Genetic	22	22	22	19	17	16	16	14	11	10	8	6	6

A

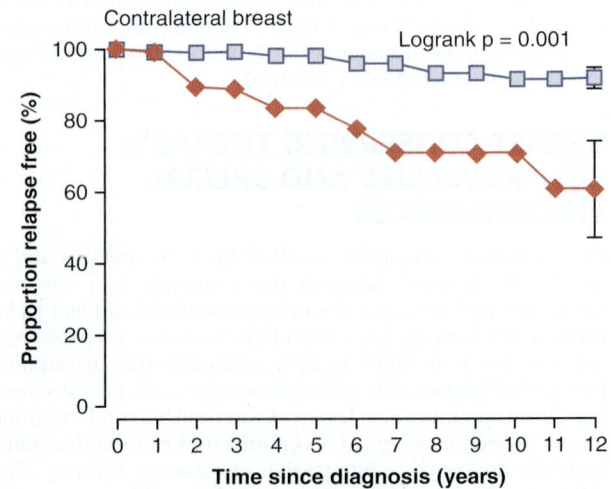

Contralateral breast

Logrank p = 0.001

Number at risk

Sporadic	105	99	98	97	97	93	88	85	74	67	62	57	51
Genetic	22	18	16	15	14	14	12	10	10	10	6	5	5

B

promising that all of the second events in *BRCA1/2* carriers were successfully salvaged and remained disease-free. Steinmann et al.[609] confirmed the increased risk of developing ipsilateral second primaries in *BRCA1/2* carriers and extended this concern to patients with bilateral breast cancer. Although the high rate of local relapses and contralateral events in these studies might be considered unacceptable, it is likely that the use of risk reduction strategies, such as tamoxifen or oophorectomy, would reduce these events to an acceptable level. Recent similar case–control-type studies were undertaken by and Garcia-Etienne et al.[597] and Kirova et al.[599] The study by Kirova et al. did not show a statistically higher local relapse rate in *BRCA1/2* carriers. However, the study by Garcia-Etienne et al., comparing 54 genetic cases to 162 sporadic cases, reported a 15% local relapse rate in the genetic group compared with a 4% local relapse rate in the sporadic group (*P* = .03).

Although the data presented above have some apparent conflicting conclusions, a study by Pierce et al.[601] helps to resolve some of these issues. In a large collaborative study, these authors evaluated a total of 160 *BRCA1/2* mutation carriers with breast cancer matched to 445 controls with sporadic breast cancer (Fig. 59.24). Median follow-up was 7.9 years for mutation carriers and 6.7 years for controls. Although there was no significant difference in IBTR overall between carriers and controls (15-year estimates were 24% for carriers and 17% for controls; HR 1.37; *P* = .19), a subset analysis revealed higher rates of local relapse in those carriers who had not undergone prophylactic oophorectomy. Multivariate analyses for IBTR found *BRCA1/2* mutation status to be an independent predictor of IBTR when carriers who had undergone oophorectomy were removed from analysis (HR 1.99; *P* = .04); the incidence of IBTR in carriers who had undergone oophorectomy was not significantly different from that in sporadic controls (*P* = .37). Contralateral breast cancers were significantly more frequent in carriers versus controls, with 10- and 15-year estimates of 26% and 39% for carriers and 3% and 7% for controls, respectively (HR 10.43; *P* < .0001). Tamoxifen use significantly reduced the risk of contralateral breast cancers in mutation carriers (HR 0.31; *P* = .05). Thus, it appears that this study confirms the findings of Haffty et al.[598]

that *BRCA1/2* carriers have a high rate of both contralateral and ipsilateral breast events if they do not undergo specific measures to reduce the risk of subsequent breast cancers by undergoing oophorectomy or tamoxifen. Prophylactic mastectomy has been shown to significantly reduce the incidence of breast cancer in women with a family history of breast cancer and specifically women with *BRCA1/2* mutations.[55] This risk reduction strategy has complex emotional and psychological implications, and there are no data to suggest an improvement in survival when compared with close surveillance. Most preventative strategies have focused on primary prevention, but prophylactic strategies should also be considered at the time of breast cancer diagnosis. Oophorectomy and tamoxifen offer similar risk reduction for breast cancer patients with germline mutations. These agents have not been widely used in studies of conservatively managed breast cancer patients with *BRCA1/2* mutations. Their potential benefits must be weighed against the possible complications of premature menopause following oophorectomy and the side effects of tamoxifen.

In a study of 655 women with *BRCA1/2* mutations diagnosed with breast cancer and treated with breast-conserving therapy (*n* = 302) or mastectomy (*n* = 353) from a multicenter collaborative group, Pierce et al.[605] reported on local failure, as first failure was significantly more likely in those treated with breast conservation (23.5% vs. 5.5%, respectively), at 15 years (*P* < .0001). Of note, the in-breast relapse rate appeared to be reduced in the breast conservation group by chemotherapy, whereas the 15-year estimate in carriers treated with breast-conserving therapy and chemotherapy was 11.9% and did not significantly differ from those treated with mastectomy. There were no differences seen in regional or systemic recurrences between the breast-conserving therapy and mastectomy groups and no difference in overall survival, but contralateral breast cancers were common in both cohorts.

Women with *BRCA1/2* mutations who underwent prophylactic oophorectomy to reduce the risk of ovarian cancer were found to have a decreased incidence of breast cancer. Rebbeck[610] studied the risk of breast cancer in 43 *BRCA1* carriers with no history of breast or ovarian cancer who

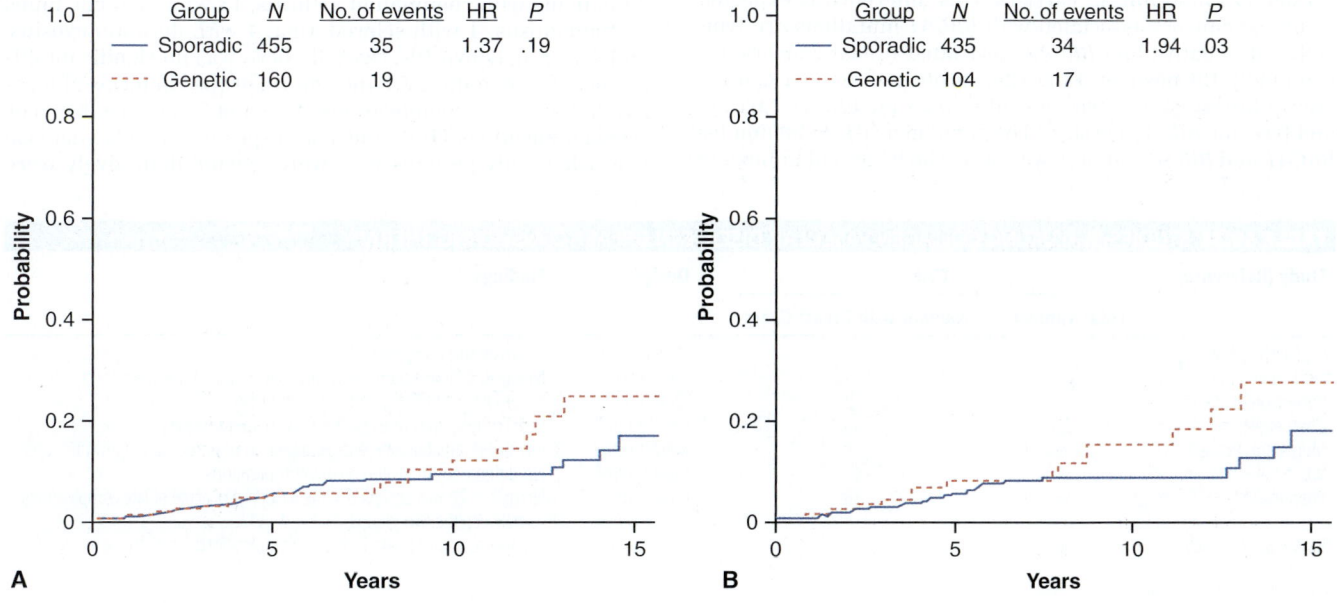

FIGURE 59.24. A: Risk of ipsilateral breast tumor relapse in *BRCA* carriers as a function of whether carriers had undergone prophylactic oophorectomy. In *BRCA* carriers who did not undergo oophorectomy **(B)**, the risk of late local relapses was significantly greater than in sporadic controls. (From Pierce L, Levin AM, Rebbeck TR, et al. Ten-year multi-institutional results of breast-conserving surgery and radiotherapy in BRCA1/2-associated stage I/II breast cancer. *J Clin Oncol* 2006;24[16]:2437–2443. Reprinted with permission. Copyright © 2006 American Society of Clinical Oncology. All rights reserved.)

underwent prophylactic bilateral oophorectomy. When these patients were compared with *BRCA1* controls who did not undergo oophorectomy, there was a significant reduction in breast cancer risk (HR 0.53). A follow-up report from this author identified 551 women with *BRCA1/2* germline mutations and reported the incidence of ovarian and breast cancer in women who had undergone prophylactic oophorectomy and matched controls.[611,612] Six women who underwent prophylactic oophorectomy were diagnosed with stage I ovarian cancer at the time of the procedure. With a median follow-up of 8 years, two women developed papillary serous peritoneal carcinoma after oophorectomy and 58 controls were diagnosed with ovarian cancer. After the exclusion of women who were diagnosed with cancer at surgery, oophorectomy reduced the risk of ovarian cancer by 96%. Oophorectomy also reduced the incidence of breast cancer in the subgroup of 241 women with no history of breast cancer or prophylactic mastectomy. Twenty-one of the 99 (21.2%) women who underwent prophylactic oophorectomy developed breast cancer versus 60 of the 142 (42.3%) women in the control group (HR 0.47).

Kauff et al.[613] conducted a prospective study of the risk of gynecologic cancer and breast cancer in 170 *BRCA1/2* carriers who chose to undergo surveillance or prophylactic oophorectomy. In the 98 women who chose prophylactic oophorectomy, 3 were later diagnosed with breast cancer and peritoneal cancer was diagnosed in 1 patient. The surveillance group of 72 patients yielded 8 breast cancers, 4 ovarian cancers, and 1 peritoneal cancer. With a median follow-up of only 24 months, this prospective study supports an early reduction in breast and ovarian cancer risk with prophylactic oophorectomy.

In prospective trials, tamoxifen has been shown to reduce both the risk of breast cancer in high-risk women and the risk of contralateral breast cancer in patients with breast cancer.[51,614] An analysis of the NSABP-P1 data from the tamoxifen versus placebo prevention trial identified 19 *BRCA1/2* mutations in the 288 women who developed breast cancer.[94] Five of the 8 women with *BRCA1* mutations had taken tamoxifen versus 3 of 11 women with *BRCA2* mutations. This represented a 62% reduction in breast cancer incidence for *BRCA2* carriers, but no benefit for tamoxifen in *BRCA1* carriers. The dataset was small, however, with low power to detect a protective effect.

Narod et al.[594] studied tamoxifen and the risk of contralateral breast cancer in *BRCA1/2* carriers. This collaborative effort compared women with bilateral breast cancer and women with unilateral breast cancer in a case–control study. Sixty-four (13%) *BRCA1* mutation carriers used tamoxifen versus 39 (33%) *BRCA2* carriers. This difference is expected as breast cancers associated with *BRCA1* mutations are typically ER-negative and *BRCA2*-associated breast cancers are commonly ER positive. Tamoxifen protected against contralateral breast cancer, with an OR of 0.38 for *BRCA1* carriers and 0.63 for *BRCA2* carriers. The combined risk reduction for *BRCA1* and *BRCA2* carriers was 50%. The benefit of tamoxifen

in *BRCA1* carriers was possibly detected because of the larger sample size. This study also noted a reduction in contralateral breast cancer in patients who received oophorectomy. The OR was 0.42, which is similar to the reduction in contralateral breast cancer noted with tamoxifen.

Although the conservative management of breast cancer in patients with *BRCA1/2* germline mutations warrants further study, the available evidence indicates that breast-conserving therapy followed by radiation therapy is an appropriate alternative to bilateral mastectomy in early-stage breast cancer in these women. Theoretical concerns for radiation-induced complications have not been demonstrated.[615] Although development of second primary tumors in the ipsilateral and contralateral breast remains a concern, prophylactic oophorectomy and tamoxifen appear to significantly reduce the probability of these secondary events.[21,594,601,610] Prophylactic oophorectomy is even more critical in the risk-reduction strategy for the development of primary tumors of the ovary. For those women considering breast-conserving surgery and radiation therapy, strategies to reduce secondary events, including prophylactic oophorectomy as soon as childbearing issues have been addressed and resolved, with or without tamoxifen or other hormonal agents as indicated, appear to be rational and viable options. Despite some evidence that tamoxifen reduces the risk of secondary breast cancers in patients who are carriers of *BRCA1/2* mutations, the use of tamoxifen in *BRCA1* breast cancer patients who are ER-negative remains unresolved and controversial.

Collagen Vascular Disease

Increased acute and late effects of irradiation have been reported in patients with pre-existing collagen vascular disease (CVD). Selected studies addressing this issue are summarized in Table 59.34.[616–623]

Fleck et al.[617] reported on five women in whom CVD developed 3 months to 10 years after radiation therapy and who had no complications. However, in three of four women with pre-existing CVD, severe complications developed, characterized by persistent moist desquamation, paresthesias in the ipsilateral arm, chest wall necrosis requiring surgical resection, and osteonecrosis of the clavicle, sternum, and rib cage. These authors concluded that a history of active CVD appeared to be a contraindication to breast conservation surgery and irradiation.

On the other hand, Ross et al.[621] evaluated a group of 61 patients with CVD who were compared with a matched control group of 61 patients without CVD. The CVD group included 39 patients with rheumatoid arthritis, 13 with systemic lupus erythematosus, 4 with scleroderma, 4 with dermatomyositis, and 4 with polymyositis. Overall, there was no significant difference between the CVD and control groups in terms of postirradiation acute complications (11% and 7%, respectively) or late complications (10% and 7%, respectively). This was also true when only patients who were treated definitively were

TABLE 59.34 STUDIES EVALUATING COLLAGEN VASCULAR DISEASE IN BREAST-CONSERVING THERAPY

Study (Reference)	CVD		Design	Findings
	Total Number	Number with Breast Cancer		
De Naeyer et al.[616]	3	1	Case report	Necrosis and progressive fibrosis
Fleck et al.[617]	9	4	Case report	Necrosis, brachial plexopathy, and severe moist desquamation
Robertson et al.[618]	2	2	Case report	Severe breast fibrosis, erythema, and pain
Chen et al.[619]	36	36	Case control	Late complication rates higher only in scleroderma
Morris and Powell[620]	209	19	Retrospective	Increased radiation late effects appear in nonrheumatoid arthritis cases
Ross et al.[621]	61	61	Case control	No differences in acute/chronic complications
Phan et al.[622]	38	38	Case control	No difference was observed in the incidence of acute or late complications between the two groups
Rakfal and Deutsch[623]	6	4	Case report	No severe acute or late radiation complications

CVD, collagen vascular disease.

considered. Three patients in the CVD group had fatal complications, compared with none in the control group. Rheumatoid arthritis was associated with a slight increase in late complications in definitively treated patients, whereas systemic lupus erythematosus was associated with a slight increase in acute reactions. No significant acute or late reactions were observed in the patients with scleroderma, dermatomyositis, or polymyositis.

Morris and Powell[620] treated 96 patients with documented CVD with breast conservation therapy (127 sites irradiated). Grade 3 or higher acute complications were seen in 15 of the 127 (11.8%) sites, and the actuarial rate of significant late complications was 24% at 10 years. There was a single in-field sarcoma. Patients with rheumatoid arthritis had less severe late effects than did those with other CVD (6% vs. 37% at 5 years; $P = .0001$).

In a study specifically evaluating conservatively treated breast cancer patients, Chen et al.[619] from the Yale group identified 36 patients with documented CVD conservatively treated for early-stage breast cancer between 1975 and 1998. All of these patients were treated with conventional radiation therapy to a median total dose of 64 Gy. Seventeen had rheumatoid arthritis; four, scleroderma; four, Raynaud phenomenon; five, lupus erythematosus; two, Sjögren disease; and four, polymyositis. Each of these patients was matched to two control patients without a history of CVD. Acute and late complications were assessed using a six-point scale from the toxicity criteria of the RTOG and the EORTC. No significant difference was detected between the CVD and control groups with respect to acute complications (14% vs. 8%). With respect to late complications, a significant difference was observed (17% vs. 3%) between the two groups. However, when patients in the CVD group were analyzed by specific disease, this significance disappeared in all but the scleroderma group.

Collectively, these data suggest that with the exception of patients with scleroderma, there does not appear to be a significantly greater late complication rate associated with CVD. Nevertheless, when patients with CVD are irradiated, it is prudent to limit the whole-breast dose to 45 Gy with 1.8-Gy fractions, use 6-MV photons, optimize homogeneity of dose distribution, avoid concurrent chemoirradiation, and discuss with patients the potential increased risks of radiation sequelae. There are small, limited case series of treating breast cancer in patients with CVD with hypofractioned whole-breast or partial-breast radiotherapy.

Pregnancy

Breast Cancer during Pregnancy

Breast cancer is the most common cancer diagnosed during pregnancy and represents a significant therapeutic challenge. Recently, an expert international panel met and published general recommendations for breast cancer developing during pregnancy.[624] The panel noted that the goal for the pregnant women with breast cancer is the same as that of the nonpregnant women: local control of disease and prevention of systemic metastasis. However, because of adverse effects on the fetus, certain treatment modalities, including radiation, must be avoided.

The incidence of breast cancer associated with pregnancy is estimated to be 1.5 to 2 in 10,000 pregnancies. Albrektsen et al.,[625] in a study of 802,457 women from the Cancer Registry of Norway, observed a RR of 1.24 for breast cancer in the 3 to 4 years immediately after a pregnancy, followed by a decreased risk thereafter.

The prognosis of patients developing breast cancer during pregnancy, stage for stage, appears to be similar to age-matched controls, although delays in diagnosis may result in higher stages in pregnant women. Several studies have stated that poorer prognosis in breast cancer associated with pregnancy may be related to delay in diagnosis because pregnancy impedes early detection and possibly to the biology of the tumor.[626] Zemlickis et al.[627] compared 118 women with breast cancer (119 pregnancies) with 269 nonpregnant control patients. The distribution of breast cancer stages among the 118 pregnant women was compared with that among 5,115 cases of breast cancer in nonpregnant women of reproductive age. Women having breast cancer in pregnancy were 2.5 times more likely to have metastatic disease (95% CI, 1.1 to 5.3) and had a significantly lower chance of having stage I disease ($P = .015$). However, stage for stage survival of pregnant women did not differ from that of the control patients. A number of authors have commented on the high percentage of pregnant patients with lymph node involvement, compared with nonpregnant patients. Others have also suggested that the poorer outcome relates to the young age of the patient and not necessarily to the pregnancy.[304,628,629] A single-institution retrospective chart review was performed on 99 patients identified with pregnancy-associated breast cancer (PABC), where non-PABC controls were matched 2 to 1 to PABC cases by year of diagnosis and age.[630] They found that PABC cases were more likely than controls to be negative for estrogen receptor (59% vs. 31%; $P < .0001$) and negative for progesterone receptor (72% vs. 40%; $P < .0001$). Cases were also more likely to have advanced T class ($P = .03$) and N class ($P = .01$) and higher grade tumors ($P = .0115$). With a median follow-up of 6.3 years for cases and 4.7 years for controls, overall survival did not differ between cases and controls ($P = .08$).

As will be discussed below, selected chemotherapy agents can be administered during the second and third trimesters. Although therapeutic abortion is not necessary, women with high-risk disease may find this preferable. They also note that in women with known deleterious mutations in *BRCA1/2*, early pregnancy is not known to decrease subsequent breast cancer risk. In addition, the available evidence suggests that in women with a history of breast cancer, subsequent pregnancy does not increase the risk of recurrence.

In addition to requiring close coordination among multidisciplinary cancer care givers, management of breast cancer during pregnancy also benefits from having obstetricians and pediatricians closely involved in therapeutic decision making. It is likely that as pregnancy in Western society is delayed to older ages, the incidence of breast cancer developing during pregnancy will increase.

Breast cancers during pregnancy are almost universally diagnosed after an abnormal physical examination finding.[304] There frequently may be a delay in diagnosis because the breast mass is thought to represent obstructed milk ducts and inflammatory changes of the breast may be misdiagnosed as cellulitis. For patients who present with a breast mass, a careful history and physical examination should be performed. The overall goal of managing breast cancer during pregnancy requires attention to both the mother and the fetus. Certain diagnostic and therapeutic interventions are known to be teratogenic and therefore are best avoided. Although theoretically a chest radiograph may be safely performed because the maximum dose to the fetus is <0.005 Gy, radiographic and scintigraphic imaging for staging should be minimized or deferred.[290] Mammography is somewhat controversial, although the irradiation dose to the fetus is minimal (<0.5 mrem).[631] Ultrasound evaluations of the breast and lymph nodes can provide diagnostic information and serve as a method of guidance for core biopsy. Pathology of breast cancer during pregnancy is most frequently invasive ductal with high nuclear grade and lower rates of ER and PR positivity.[304]

The management of the patient and the risks of certain interventions are also highly dependent on the week of gestation. In general, potentially harmful interventions carry the greatest risk during the period of organogenesis (first trimester) and are safest during the final trimester. For patients with operable disease, data suggest that surgery can be safely performed after the 12th week of pregnancy. The type of surgical procedure is dependent on the extent of disease and the trimester of the pregnancy.[304,625,627,628] Few data exist concerning the safety and efficacy of sentinel lymph node biopsy. Although the blue dye used in sentinel lymph node surgery is not approved for use in pregnant patients, the estimated radiation dose to the fetus from the radiocolloid tracer is low. Except for radiation, treatment should not be altered or delayed because of pregnancy. Either a modified radical mastectomy or lumpectomy with axillary dissection is acceptable local treatment. Immediate breast reconstruction should not be performed.

Systemic chemotherapy with FAC (5-fluorouracil, doxorubicin, cyclophosphamide) has been used in pregnancy. Investigators from MD Anderson Cancer Center reported a prospective series of 57 pregnant breast cancer patients who were treated on a single-arm, multidisciplinary, protocol with FAC in the adjuvant ($n = 32$) or neoadjuvant ($n = 25$) setting.[632] Parents and guardians were surveyed by mail or telephone regarding outcomes of children exposed to chemotherapy *in utero*. All women who delivered had live births. One child has Down syndrome and two have congenital anomalies (club foot; congenital bilateral ureteral reflux). They conclude that breast cancer can be treated with FAC chemotherapy during the second and third trimesters without significant short-term complications for the majority of children exposed to chemotherapy *in utero*. Longer follow-up of the children is needed to evaluate possible late side effects such as impaired cardiac function and fertility. Administration of chemotherapy in the first trimester is associated with a high risk of birth defects (17%, 24 of 139), in terms of probability of intrauterine growth retardation, prematurity, fetal malformation, or death; this risk is less in the second and third trimesters (1.3%, 2 of 150).[633]

As a general principle, hormonal therapy and radiation therapy should be avoided until after delivery. In one study, the estimated dose to the fetus from breast or chest wall radiation to a dose of 0.5 Gy is 0.02 Gy in the first trimester, 0.022 to 0.246 Gy during the second trimester, and 0.02 to 0.586 Gy during the third trimester. Dose to the fetus in the range of 0.1 to 0.9 Gy during the first trimester have been associated with mental retardation.[634]

When the patient chooses breast-conserving therapy, irradiation should be deferred until the fetus is delivered because 50 Gy delivered to the breast, even with external shielding, exposes the fetus to 0.1 to 0.15 Gy if it is small and contained in the true pelvis. During later gestation, when the fetus is larger and high in the abdomen, some fetal areas may receive as much as 2 Gy.[634] In another study using a phantom (film dosimetry), doses to the pelvis ranged from 0.043 Gy with 4-MV x-rays to 0.158 Gy with cobalt-60 (^{60}Co) to the midpelvis.[635]

Although there is some question whether there is any safe dose of irradiation to the fetus, Brent,[636] in an extensive review of the literature, defined 0.05 Gy as a relatively safe upper limit of fetal exposure. Hall[637] suggested that 0.1 Gy *in utero* exposure be used as a dose beyond which a therapeutic abortion should be considered.

Some authors have suggested therapeutic abortion based on a study by Adair,[638] who reported in the early 1950s a better outcome in patients who terminated their pregnancies. However, in 63 patients treated at Mayo Clinic, the 5-year survival rate was 59% in the women who carried to term and 43% in those who underwent a therapeutic abortion. The latter group had more advanced tumors.[639] Petrek[626] also noted that therapeutic abortion does not alter the outcome in patients with breast cancer. Contrary to popular belief, pregnancy does not appear to stimulate the growth of breast cancer. Therefore, no justification exists for therapeutic abortion,

which may be relevant only in the patient who has rapidly progressing disease, such as inflammatory breast cancer (IBC) or metastatic disease.

Pregnancy after Breast Cancer

Almost one-third of women of reproductive age in whom breast cancer later develops have one or more pregnancies, and 70% of these occur within 5 years of treatment.[640] No data are available to suggest that subsequent pregnancy hastens or induces breast cancer recurrence. When matched by age and stage with nonpregnant patients, pregnant women with breast cancer do not have a worse outcome than nonpregnant patients with comparable stages. However, in patients receiving adjuvant chemotherapy, a minimum of 12 months between treatment and conception is advised. Breast-feeding is contraindicated in patients receiving chemotherapy because antineoplastic agents are excreted in the milk.[304,626,628]

Sutton et al.[641] reviewed 227 women 35 years of age or younger at diagnosis who became pregnant after treatment with CAF adjuvant chemotherapy. Twenty-five patients had 33 pregnancies. The median interval between completion of chemotherapy and pregnancy was 12 months (range, 0 to 87 months). Ten pregnancies were terminated, 2 ended in spontaneous abortion, 2 patients were still pregnant at the time of the report, and 19 produced normal full-term infants. The incidence of recurrence was 46% in patients without pregnancy, compared with 28% in those who had subsequent pregnancies. Similarly, 38% of patients without subsequent pregnancy were dead at the time of the report, compared with 12% of patients who became pregnant after chemotherapy treatment for breast cancer.

A population-based matched survival study assessed the risk of death for patients with breast cancer in relation to whether they delivered a live child subsequent to their cancer diagnosis.[642] Among 2,548 women younger than 40 years of age diagnosed with carcinoma of the breast, 91 experienced subsequent deliveries (10 months or longer after the diagnosis) and 471 control patients were matched for stage, age, and year of breast cancer diagnosis. The control subjects had to survive at least the interval between the cancer diagnosis and the delivery of their matched counterparts. The control subjects had a 4.8-fold greater risk of death compared with those who delivered after the diagnosis of breast cancer. These authors' interpretation of this result was that there was a "healthy mother effect" (only women who felt healthy gave birth, and those who were affected by the disease did not). Nevertheless, 6 of 8 deaths among the 91 patients who did give birth were related to breast cancer.

It may be helpful to suggest a waiting time (2 to 3 years) for the patient to regain health before attempting the physical stress of pregnancy and deferral of childbearing until after the period of greatest risk of recurrence of the tumor.[640] The individual woman's prognosis, well-being, desire for children, support from spouse or significant other, and other sociodemographic factors must be carefully considered in this difficult decision-making process.

Lactation after Breast Conservation Therapy

Successful breast-feeding, from the untreated as well as the treated breast, is possible after conservation surgery and irradiation. Higgins and Haffty[643] reviewed the records of 890 patients treated with radiation therapy for early-stage (stage I or II) breast cancer. This series was recently updated by Moran et al.[644] Of over 3,000 patients treated from 1965 to 2003, a cohort of 21 premenopausal women who underwent breast-conserving therapy and subsequently sustained full-term pregnancies were identified. Lactation outcome parameters (breast swelling, ability to lactate, and volume of lactation in the treated and untreated breasts) were the main outcome measures. There were 28 pregnancies in 21 patients. One patient underwent bilateral breast treatment; therefore, a total of 22 breasts were irradiated. All patients interviewed reported little or no swelling of the treated breast during pregnancy. Of the patients studied, 4 (18.2%) elected pharmacologic suppression of lactation. Of the remaining 18 breasts, lactation occurred in 10 (55.6%), did not occur in 7 (38.9%), and was unknown for 1 (5.5%). The volume was reported as significantly diminished in 80% of breasts treated. Lactation in the contralateral breast occurred in all patients who did not undergo pharmacologic suppression. The authors confirm that successful lactation in the contralateral, untreated breast after breast-conserving therapy is expressed. In the treated breast, functional lactation is possible but is significantly diminished in the majority of patients. Tralins[645] reported results of a survey describing 53 women who became pregnant after conservation therapy and breast irradiation. Eighteen exhibited some lactation and 13 (24.5%) were able to breast-feed from the involved breast. Pregnancy or lactation had no impact on prognosis; with a 5.4-year mean follow-up, the tumor-free survival rate was 82%.

Breast Irradiation in Patients Previously Irradiated for Hodgkin Lymphoma

There is an increased incidence of breast cancer in female patients who have previously undergone mantle irradiation for Hodgkin lymphoma. Numerous studies have demonstrated a significantly increased RR of breast cancer in women treated for Hodgkin lymphoma, with the risk significantly increasing with decreasing age of exposure. Table 59.35 summarizes the findings of several series.[29,104,646-664]

Travis et al.[29] estimated that for a female Hodgkin lymphoma survivor who was treated at age 25 years with a chest radiation dose of at least 40 Gy without alkylating agents, the cumulative absolute risks of breast cancer by age 35, 45, and 55 years were 1.4% (95% CI, 0.9% to 2.1%), 11.1% (95% CI, 7.4% to 16.3%), and 29.0% (95% CI, 20.2% to

40.1%), respectively. In addition to radiation dose, treatment volumes may also play a role in determining a woman's risk of developing breast cancer after radiotherapy for Hodgkin lymphoma. A study by De Bruin et al.[665] reported on a cohort of 1,122 female patients with Hodgkin lymphoma treated between 1965 and 1995. The overall cumulative incidence 30 years after treatment was 19%; for those treated before age 21 years, it was 26%. Moreover, mantle field irradiation was associated with a 2.7-fold increased risk in developing breast cancer compared with similarly dosed (36 to 44 Gy) mediastinal irradiation alone.

Mastectomy has been recommended as the preferred treatment option in these women. Lumpectomy followed by breast irradiation has been considered by some to be contraindicated because of the cumulative radiation dose to the breast. However, in selected patients using careful breast irradiation techniques that avoid significant overlap with the previous mantle port, anecdotal and retrospective reports in small numbers of patients suggest that it is possible to offer breast conservation therapy. Therapeutic options and the potential increased risk of reirradiation sequelae should be thoroughly discussed with the patient. A second issue that should also be considered is the risk of the development of new primary. Similar to patients with *BRCA* mutations, patients who have a history of breast cancer development after irradiation for Hodgkin lymphoma are at risk in the development of subsequent new primaries and may benefit from prevention strategies such as mastectomy.

Elkin et al.[666] reported on a retrospective multicenter, cohort study of 253 patients treated for Hodgkin lymphoma with radiation therapy who developed breast cancer and matched 3 to 1 with 741 patients with sporadic breast cancer. They found that patients had a median time from diagnosis of Hodgkin's to breast cancer of 18 years, with a median age at breast cancer diagnosis of 42 years. Breast cancer after RT for Hodgkin lymphoma was more likely to be detected by screening, was more likely to be diagnosed at an earlier stage, and was more likely to be bilateral at diagnosis. Hodgkin

TABLE 59.35 RISK OF SECONDARY BREAST CANCER DEVELOPMENT AFTER MANTLE RADIOTHERAPY FOR HODGKIN LYMPHOMA

Study (Reference)	Population			Treatment	Average Follow-Up (Year)	Interval to Breast Cancer Detection	Breast Cancer Cases		Relative Risk (95% CI)
	Number	Sex	Age (Year)				Number	Age Range (Year)	
Aisenberg et al.[641]	111	F		RT ± CT	18	8.5–25	14	23–49	
			≤19						56 (23.3–107)
			20–29						7.0 (2.3–16.4)
			≥30						0.9 (0–5.3)
Chung et al.[646]	136	F	–	RT ± CT	14.8	6–22	11	30–63	AR = 55.1 cases/10,000 patient-years
Carey et al.[647]	164	F	–	RT	–	11–17	4	37.3	5.45
Guibout et al.[648]	1,258	F	≥17	RT ± CT	16	16–28	4	30–34	7.01 (22–164)[a]
Hoppe[649]	2,498	F and M	–	RT ± CT	–	–	25	–	4.1
Tinger et al.[650]	152	F	–	RT ± CT	>5	4–23	10	27–64	2.2
Bhatia et al.[104]	483	F	<16	RT ± CT	11.4	–	17	16–42	75.3
Mauch et al.[651]	349	F	3–69	RT ± CT	10.7	–	13	–	6.5 (3.5–11.2)
Salloum et al.[652]	144	F	–	RT ± CT	13.5	13.9–14	2	39–41	2 (0.6–7.4)
Hancock et al.[653]	885	F	–	RT ± CT	10	4.5–23	25	22–75	4.1 (2.6–5.9)
Prior and Pope[654]	777	F	–	RT ± CT	6.7	10–19	9	–	2.2
Tucker et al.[655]	1,507	F and M	–	RT ± CT	6.2	8	3	–	12 (2.3–35)
Kaldor et al.[656]	11,491	F	–	RT ± CT	1–20+	–	62	–	1.4
Travis et al.[657]	3,817	F	≤30	RT ± CT	–	7–30	105	27–57	3.2 (1.4–8.2)
Metayer et al.[658]	2,725	F	≤21	RT ± CT	10.5	–	52	–	4.9
Swerdlow et al.[659]	2,085	F	–	RT ± CT	1–15	–	19	–	14.4 (5.7–29.3)[b]
Van Leeuwen et al.[660]	544	F	<40	RT ± CT	14.1	1–20+	27	–	5.2 (3.4–7.6)
Gervais-Fagnou et al.[661]	427	F	≤30	RT ± CT	12.3	9–25	15	30–52	10.6 (5.8–17)
Hudson et al.[662]	165	F	–	RT ± CT	15.1	3.6–24.9	6	–	33 (12–72)[a]
Wolden et al.[663]	207	F	<21	RT ± CT	13.1	8.5–27.9	16	–	26 (15–42)

[a]Standardized incidence ratio.
[b]For treated at ages younger than 25 years.
AR, absolute risk; CT, chemotherapy; CI, confidence interval; F, female; M, male; RT, radiation therapy.

lymphoma survivors had an increased risk of metachronous contralateral breast cancer (HR 4.3; 95% CI, 1.7 to 11.0) and death as a result of any cause (HR 1.9; 95% CI, 1.1 to 3.3).

Cutuli et al.[667] reported on a retrospective multicenter analysis in which 117 women and 2 men treated for Hodgkin lymphoma subsequently developed 133 breast cancers. Hodgkin lymphoma treatment was radiation therapy alone in 74 patients and combined modality with chemotherapy in 43 patients. Breast cancer occurred after a median interval of 16 years. Tumors were treated by mastectomy without ($n = 67$) or with ($n = 10$) irradiation. Forty-four tumors were treated with lumpectomy without ($n = 12$) or with ($n = 32$) radiation therapy. Sixteen patients had isolated breast relapses, 39 had metastases, and 34 died. Young women treated for Hodgkin lymphoma should be carefully monitored in the long term by clinical examination, mammography, and ultrasonography. The authors suggested that a baseline mammography be performed 5 to 8 years after supradiaphragmatic irradiation (complete mantle or involved field) in patients treated before 30 years of age. Subsequently, mammography should be performed every 2 years or each year, depending on the characteristics of the breast tissue (e.g., density) and especially in the case of an association with other breast cancer risk factors.

Wolden et al.[668] described 71 cases of breast cancer in 65 survivors of Hodgkin lymphoma. Median age at diagnosis was 24.6 years for Hodgkin lymphoma and 42.6 years for breast cancer; the RR for invasive breast cancer after Hodgkin lymphoma was 4.7 compared with an age-matched cohort. Cancers were detected by self-examination in 63%, by mammography in 30%, and by physical examination alone in 7%. The majority were of invasive ductal histology and 27% had positive axillary nodes. The tumor was ER positive in 63% of the cases, and 25% of patients had an associated family history. The majority of tumors were smaller than 4 cm. Ninety-five percent of cases were managed by mastectomy because of prior irradiation, and two women underwent excisional biopsy with breast irradiation. One of these patients had tissue necrosis in the region of overlap with the prior mantle field. The incidence of bilateral breast cancer was 10%. The 10-year disease-specific survival rate for DCIS was 100%; stage I, 88%; stage II, 55%; stage III, 60%; and stage IV, 0%.

One of the largest series using breast-conserving therapy plus radiation in patients previously treated for Hodgkin lymphoma is from Deutsch et al.[669] In this retrospective review, 12 women treated with radiotherapy with or without chemotherapy for Hodgkin lymphoma (11 patients) and non-Hodgkin lymphoma (1 patient) in whom breast cancer developed 10 to 29 years later were treated with lumpectomy and breast irradiation. Patients were treated with whole-breast daily irradiation with a fractionation of 2 Gy to 50 Gy with boost to the operative area. Six also received adjuvant chemotherapy for breast cancer. Breast irradiation was well tolerated without any unusual acute or chronic sequelae. They conclude that this may be an option for previously radiated Hodgkin's survivors who develop early-stage breast cancer.

This controversial area will continue to evolve. Given the development of partial breast irradiation programs over the past several years, it is likely that data regarding reirradiation with partial breast irradiation or proton therapy will be reported.[670,671] Clearly, however, Hodgkin's survivors and others who receive radiotherapy to breast at a young age are at high risk for developing breast cancers and should be carefully monitored. Women who develop breast cancer should be advised that mastectomy remains the treatment of choice. However, for patients highly motivated for breast preservation, anecdotal experiences using a variety of approaches have revealed acceptable toxicity and cosmesis.

Patients with More than One Invasive Carcinoma (Multicentric Disease)

Multicentricity of breast cancer has been considered by some a contraindication to breast-conserving surgery and suggest mastectomy as the preferred option.[672] Conservation surgery and breast radiation therapy as an alternative to mastectomy is controversial in patients with two or more lesions in the same breast. Several studies have addressed this issue, and it appears that the risk of relapse in the conservatively treated patient is slightly higher than if there is one lesion, but the risk may be acceptable in patients with two or perhaps three lesions provided these lesions are surgically excised with negative margins and there are no residual areas of suspicion on physical examination, mammogram, or imaging studies. Selected studies evaluating the conservative management of breast cancer in patients with multicentric disease are summarized in Table 59.36.[673–677]

Kurtz et al.,[677] in an analysis of 586 patients with unilateral stage I or II breast cancer treated with breast-conserving surgery and irradiation, found 61 patients who had two or more microscopic tumor nodules. After a median follow-up of 71 months, 15 patients (25%) had a recurrence in the treated breast, compared with 56 of 525 (11%) patients with single tumors ($P < .005$). Recurrence was noted more often in patients with multiple tumors diagnosed clinically or mammographically (8 of 22, 36%) than when multicentricity was apparent only on pathologic examination (7 of 39, 18%).

TABLE 59.36 CONSERVATIVE SURGERY AND RADIATION IN THE TREATMENT OF MULTICENTRIC BREAST CANCER

Study (Reference)	Patients		Follow-Up (Year)		Local Relapse Rate			Comment
	Number of SIBC	Controls	SIBC	Controls	SIBC (%)	Controls (%)	P	
Yale[673]	13	1,047	6	6	25	12	.403	Local recurrence rate in SIBC is greater than seen in patients with single lesions.
JCRT[674]	10	707	5.3 (median)	6.3 (median)	40	11	.019	The presence of two or more primary tumors in the breast is associated with a high likelihood of local recurrence.
St Luke's[675]	36	19[a]	5	5	3	0	.54	No significant differences in the local or distant disease-free survival between the group treated with breast conservation and the group treated with mastectomy.
Rush[676]	27		4.4 (median)		3.7	–	–	
France[677]	61	525	5.9 (median)	5.9 (median)	25	11	<.005	Macroscopically multiple breast cancers are at higher local failure risk, especially if multiplicity is clinically apparent, or if three or more gross nodules are seen on pathologic examination.

[a]All are SIBC treated with mastectomy.
SIBC, synchronous ipsilateral breast cancer.

Wilson et al.[673] reviewed their experience in 1,060 patients treated with conservation surgery and breast irradiation of whom 13 (1.2%) presented with synchronous multicentric ipsilateral breast cancer. With a median follow-up of 71 months, 3 of the 13 (23%) had an IBR (72-month actuarial rate of 25%) compared with 12% in the single-lesion population. The use of conservation therapy in patients with more than one primary lesion should be considered with caution, and patients should be forewarned of the need for more extensive resections and the increased risk of breast relapse. Because resection of a larger volume of breast is required, cosmetic results may be compromised, and expectations may not be met. In such instances, a mastectomy may be the preferred approach.

Conservation Surgery and Irradiation after Breast Augmentation

A growing number of breast cancers occur in women with prior augmentation mammoplasty. The stage of breast cancer at diagnosis in women who have undergone augmentation mammoplasty has been examined with conflicting results. In a retrospective review, Clark et al.[678] reported that 24% of 33 patients with augmented breasts and 42% of 1,735 patients with nonaugmented breasts had mammographically detected cancers (P = not significant). The incidence of DCIS in the two groups was similar (18% vs. 15%, respectively). Sizes of the mammographically detected tumors in the two groups were comparable. However, palpable tumors in the augmented group were significantly smaller than those in the nonaugmented group. Axillary lymph node involvement was detected in 19% of the augmented group and 41% of the nonaugmented group. Among those with mammographically detected tumors, there was no significant difference in axillary lymph node metastases between patients with augmented versus nonaugmented breasts (13% vs. 15%, respectively).

Patients with augmentations who have breast cancer are currently being treated with conservation therapy, but no study has investigated the complications and cosmetic results of radiation therapy specifically in this group of women.

Breast conservation therapy in 17 augmented patients with breast cancer was reported by Handel et al.,[679] where 15 patients were available for follow-up. In 10 patients (67%), significant capsular contracture occurred in the irradiated breast an average of 12 weeks after completion of treatment. Four patients underwent revision surgery to correct symptoms arising from contracture. These authors concluded that irradiation of the breast for cancer in augmented women results in a high incidence of scar tissue contracture and poor cosmetic results.

In contrast, Guenther et al.[680] evaluated 20 women in whom breast cancer developed after augmentation mammoplasty (14 subcutaneous implants and 6 retromuscular implants). Patients were treated with wide local tumor excision and level I and II ALND. Irradiation was delivered to the breast (45 to 50 Gy), and a boost (14 to 21 Gy) was given to the tumor excision site with either photons, electrons, or iridium-192 (^{192}Ir) implant. With a median follow-up of 3.8 years (range, 6 months to 9.3 years), there were no local recurrences, although distant metastases developed in two patients. Seventeen patients (85%) had good or excellent cosmetic results.

Breast Conservation and Mammoplasty

Women with large, pendulous breasts have been documented to have poorer cosmetic outcomes when undergoing irradiation after breast conservation surgery (thought to be caused by dose inhomogeneity) compared with women who have small or medium-size breasts. Smith et al.[681] evaluated 10 women who had undergone bilateral reduction mammoplasty for breast malignancy followed by radiation therapy. A variety of reduction techniques were used to include the malignant

lesions. Patients received 50 Gy in 25 fractions in 5 weeks after surgery. Radiation therapy was usually initiated within 4 weeks after surgery. With a follow-up of 37 months, no patients have had complications from the surgery or radiation therapy. No local recurrent malignancies have been detected. Cosmesis has been good to excellent in all patients.

Bilateral Carcinoma of the Breast

Among factors reported to be associated with an increased risk of bilateral breast carcinoma are younger age, family history of breast cancer, lobular carcinoma, multicentric disease, histologic differentiation of the primary tumor, parity, and PR-positive status.[682-687] The appearance may be synchronous (1% to 2%) or metachronous (5% to 8%). Synchronous breast carcinoma was defined as a contralateral cancer diagnosed within 1 year of initial diagnosis.

Patients with bilateral carcinoma have been treated with total or modified radical mastectomy. However, the available evidence clearly supports lumpectomy followed by breast irradiation as an acceptable alternative for appropriately selected women. Solin et al.[688] reported on 30 treated with breast conservation therapy (11 with concurrent and 19 with metachronous carcinoma). A dose of 45 to 50 Gy was delivered to both breasts with tangential fields, in addition to a boost of 10 to 15 Gy with either iridium implant or electrons. The tangential fields were matched in the midline in 17 patients and overlapped by up to 3 cm in 10 patients. In the 60 treated breasts, the 5-year actuarial local failure rate was 6%. In 25 treated breasts with a minimum of 2 years of follow-up, 68% had excellent and 24% had good cosmetic results. The incidence of arm edema was 6%, similar to that reported in patients with unilateral disease.

Hungness et al.[689] reviewed their experience with 51 patients with bilateral synchronous breast cancer (2.1% of 2,382 treated for breast cancer during the same period). The first cancer was detected by palpation in 81% and by mammography in 14%. The corresponding figures for the contralateral cancer were 24% and 54%, respectively. The histologic type of cancer was identical in the two breasts in 29 patients (57%) and was different in 22 patients (43%). The overall 10-year survival rate was 66%.

Heron et al.[690] compared the outcomes in 1,315 patients (89.9%) with unilateral, 103 (7.1%) with metachronous, and 47 (3.0%) with synchronous breast carcinoma treated with either mastectomy or breast conservation therapy. Patients with synchronous and metachronous bilateral carcinoma had a worse 8-year disease-free survival rate compared with patients who had unilateral breast carcinoma, as well as increased risk of distant metastasis. In multivariate analysis, differences in local tumor control and overall survival were not statistically significant for patients who had bilateral or metachronous cancer compared with those who had unilateral disease.

Kollias et al.,[691] in 3,210 women age 70 years or younger treated for primary operable breast cancer, identified 106 who had bilateral breast cancer; in 26 (0.8%), the disease was synchronous, and in 80 (24%), a contralateral breast cancer developed after treatment for an initial primary breast cancer. There was a significant difference in survival between women with unilateral breast cancer, synchronous bilateral breast cancers, and metachronous contralateral breast cancer, with survival rates at 16 years of 53.8%, 42.4%, and 60.1%, respectively (P < .0001), from the date of the diagnosis of the first primary tumor. There was no difference in survival among the three groups from the date of diagnosis of the second primary in cases of metachronous contralateral breast cancer (P = .31).

Ninety-five patients with bilateral carcinoma of the breast treated with mastectomy (60 patients), conservation of the breast (17 patients), or both (18 patients) were studied by

Gustafsson et al.[692] Cumulative 5-year local tumor control rates were 94% for the 138 mastectomy patients and 90% for the 52 patients treated with breast conservation therapy. Twenty-eight percent of the first carcinomas were stage I, compared with 43% of second carcinomas ($P < .05$), probably reflecting the close follow-up after initial treatment. The 5-year distant disease-free survival rate from treatment for the second carcinoma was 74%. The 5-year distant recurrence-free survival rate when second carcinomas were diagnosed within 5 years was 58%, compared with 95% for patients diagnosed more than 5 years after the first carcinoma.

de la Rochefordiere et al.[693] reported on 149 patients with simultaneous bilateral breast cancer (diagnosed within 6 months). Of 298 tumors, 40% were T0 or T1, 45% were T2, and 15% were T3 or T4. The majority (83%) were clinically node negative. Treatments were bilateral mastectomy in 43%, irradiation in 16%, and both in 41% of the patients. Fifty-one patients had bilateral breast-conserving therapy and 24 were treated exclusively with irradiation. The 5-year disease-free survival rates were 70% to 86%, respectively, similar to those observed at the same institution in patients with unilateral tumors. Cosmesis was assessed in 48 patients and was acceptable in 37 (77%). These authors advised special attention should be paid to any possible overlap of the supraclavicular and internal mammary fields over the spinal cord; in one patient, spinal cord myelopathy developed at T6.

Freedman et al.[596] reviewed records of 116 patients with bilateral breast cancer and a breast cancer family history. The primary treatment was a breast-conserving procedure in 55 and a mastectomy in 61. LRRs occurred in 4 of 46 cases treated with breast-conserving therapy, resulting in a 10-year actuarial locoregional tumor control rate of 83%. Of nine patients who did not receive radiation as a component of their breast-conserving therapy, LRRs developed in four patients (10-year locoregional control rate of 49%). The 10-year actuarial rates of locoregional control after mastectomy with and without radiation were 91% and 89%, respectively.

Fung et al.[694] reported on 55 women with stage 0, I, or II concurrent ($n = 12$) or sequential ($n = 43$) bilateral breast cancers treated with irradiation after breast-conserving surgery. The tangential fields were matched with no overlap in 40 patients (73%); there was overlap on skin of up to 4 cm in 14 patients (25%). For the 110 treated breast cancers, the 10-year actuarial local failure rate was 15%. Complications included breast edema (28%), arm edema (8%), pneumonitis (4%), cellulitis (3%), rib fracture (1%), and brachial plexopathy (1%). No patient had match line fibrosis. For patients with

a minimum of 3 years of relapse-free follow-up, the rate of excellent or good cosmetic outcome for 104 treated breasts was 85%.

TECHNICAL ISSUES IN RADIATION MANAGEMENT OF EARLY-STAGE DISEASE

Treatment Position

Most patients are treated in the supine position, with the arm abducted (90 degrees or greater). Commercially available or custom-made breast tilt boards with armrests that maintain the patient's daily position with the slope of the chest wall parallel to the table, often in combination with immobilization devices (e.g., Alpha cradle, plastic molds), are typically used to reproduce daily positioning and minimize day-to-day setup errors (Fig. 59.25).

Other treatment positions have been used to improve the dosimetry in patients with large, pendulous breasts. A lateral decubitus position has been suggested by investigators at the Institut Curie.[695,696]

Irradiation in the prone position has been proposed by Merchant and McCormick,[697] with reduction of dose in the high-dose region to 102% to 103% of the dose to the irradiated breast, as well as reduction of volume and dose to the underlying lung and heart and reduction of scattered dose to the contralateral breast. This technique is being increasingly employed and follow-up data appear to be promising with respect to toxicity and early outcomes.[698] Patient positioning and a corresponding CT image are shown in Figures 59.26 and 59.27.

Treatment Volume

The entire breast and chest wall are included in the irradiated volume as shown in Figures 59.28 and 59.29. Radiopaque surgical clips placed at the margin of the tumor bed may assist in defining the target volume.[699] The upper margin of the portals should be placed at the head of the clavicle to include the entire breast. The medial margin, if no internal mammary portal is used, should be at or 1 cm over the midline. If an internal mammary field is used, the medial tangential portal is located at the lateral margin of the internal mammary field. (See discussion later on regional nodal irradiation.) The lateral–posterior margin should be placed 2 cm beyond all palpable breast tissue, which is usually near the midaxillary line. The inferior margin is drawn 2 to 3 cm below the inframammary fold. The RTOG published their consensus definitions

FIGURE 59.25. Patient immobilized for breast irradiation on a slant board with custom mold to minimize day-to-day positioning errors.

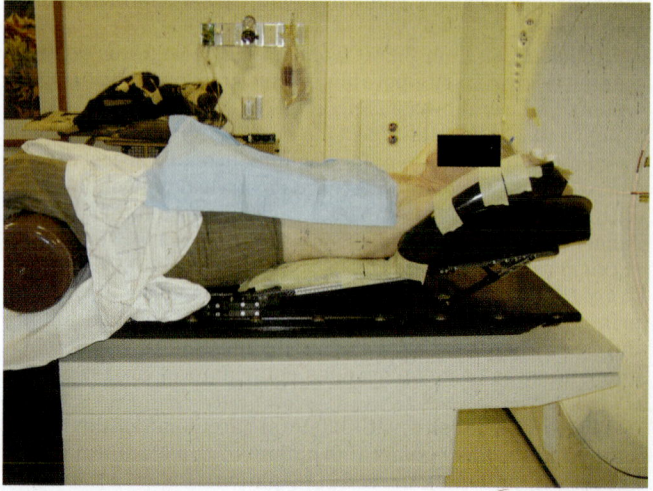

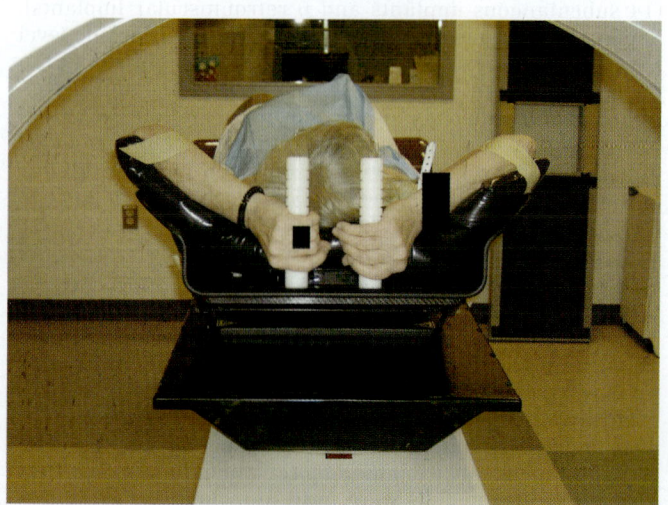

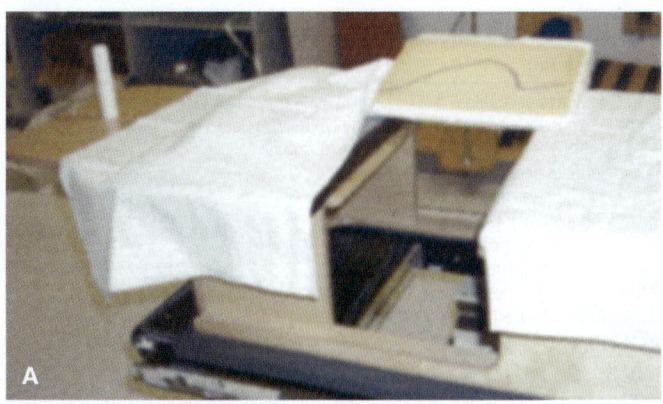

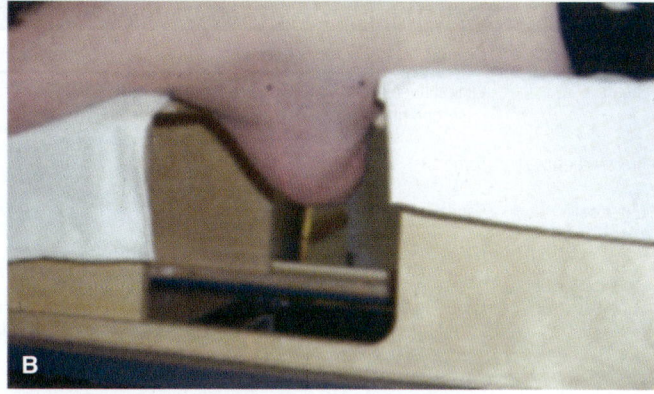

FIGURE 59.26. Prone breast board. **A:** Customized prone breast board with adjustable aperture and wedge for contralateral breast. **B:** Ipsilateral breast and anterior chest wall hang in dependent fashion away from thorax with ipsilateral arm placed above head. (Reprinted from Goodman K, Hong L, Wagman R, et al. Dosimetric analysis of a simplified intensity modulation technique for prone breast radiotherapy. *Int J Radiat Oncol Biol Phys* 2004;60[1]:95–102. Copyright © 2004 Elsevier. With permission.)

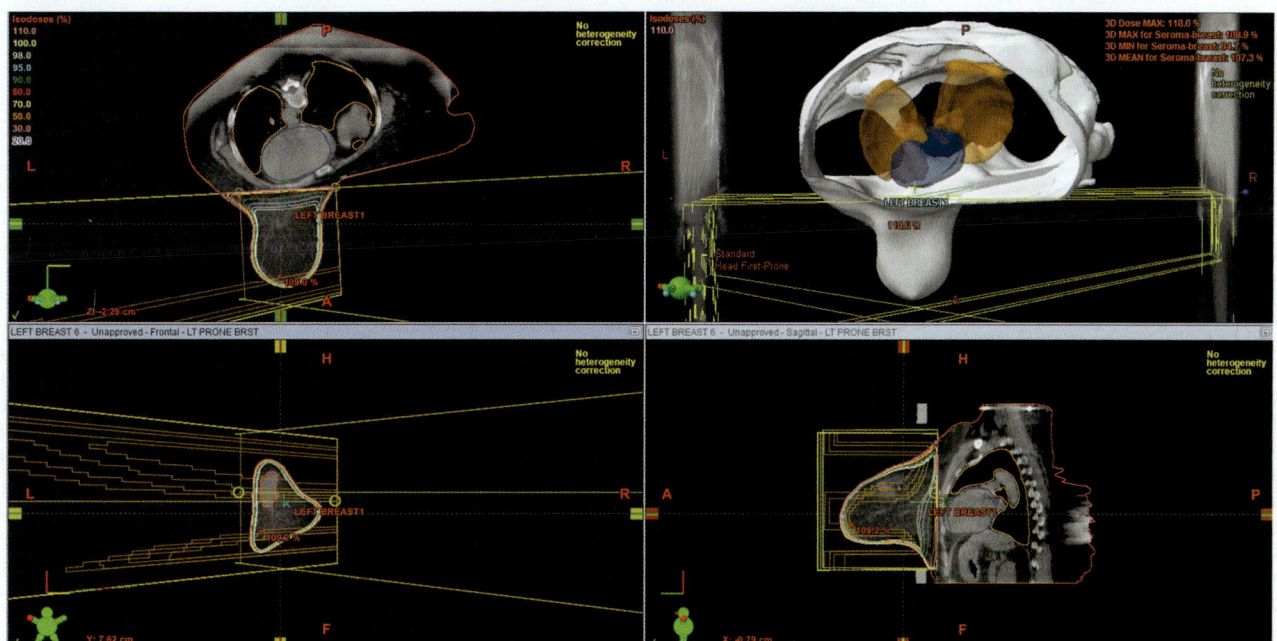

FIGURE 59.27. Computed tomography simulation images used to determine arrangement of tangent beams in prone breast irradiation. (Reprinted from Goodman K, Hong L, Wagman R, et al. Dosimetric analysis of a simplified intensity modulation technique for prone breast radiotherapy. *Int J Radiat Oncol Biol Phys* 2004;60[1]:95–102. Copyright © 2004 Elsevier. With permission.)

FIGURE 59.28. Axial treatment planning CT cut with contours of the level I, II, and III nodes.

FIGURE 59.29. A tangential breast radiation field, demonstrating projection of tangential field on simulation film and patient surface.

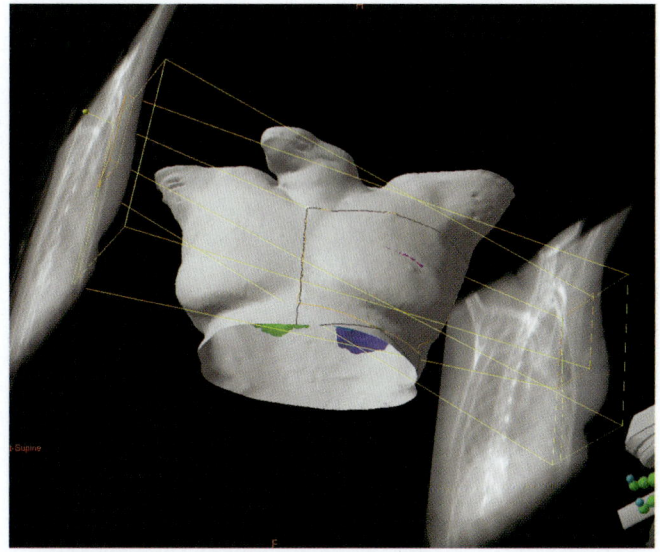

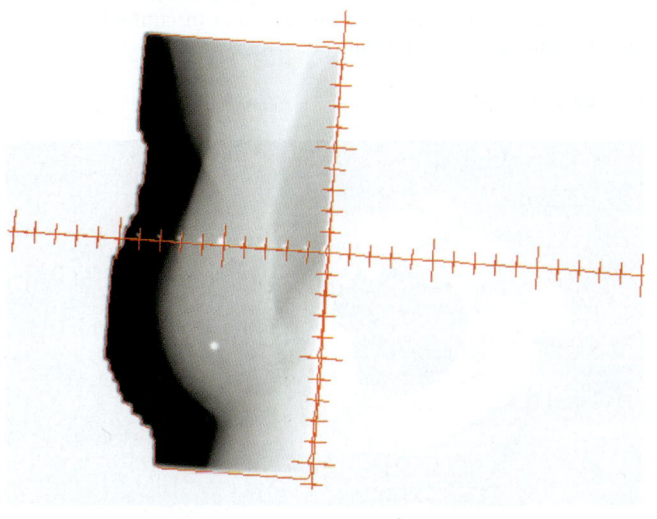

TABLE 59.37 RADIATION THERAPY ONCOLOGY GROUP CONSENSUS DEFINITIONS FOR BREAST CANCER RADIATION THERAPY PLANNING

	Cranial	Caudal	Anterior	Posterior	Lateral	Medial
Breast	Clinical reference + second rib insertion	Clinical reference + loss of CT apparent breast	Skin	Excludes pectoralis muscles, chest wall muscles, ribs	Clinical reference/midaxillary line typically, excludes lattissimus dorsi	Sternal–rib junction
Breast+chest wall	Same	Same	Same	Includes pectoralis muscles, chest wall muscles, ribs	Same	Same
Chest wall	Caudal border of the clavicle head	Clinical reference + loss of CT apparent contralateral breast	Skin	Rib–pleural interface. (includes pectoralis muscles, chest wall muscles, ribs)	Same	Same
Supraclavicular	Caudal to the cricoid cartilage	Junction of brachioceph.–axillary vns./caudal edge clavicle head	Sternocleidomastoid (SCM) muscle	Anterior aspect of the scalene m.	Cranial: lateral edge of SCM m. Caudal: junction 1st rib–clavicle	Excludes thyroid and trachea
Axilla: Level I	Axillary vessels cross lateral edge of pec. minor m.	Pec. major muscle insert into ribs	Plane defined by: anterior surface of pec. maj. m. and lat. dorsi m.	Anterior surface of subscapular is m.	Medial border of lat. dorsi m.	Lateral border of pec. minor m.
Axilla: Level II	Axillary vessels cross medial edge of pec. minor m.	Axillary vessels cross lateral edge of pec. minor m.	Anterior surface pec. minor m.	Ribs and intercostal muscles	Lateral border of pec. minor m.	Medial border of pec. minor m.
Axilla: Level III	Pec. minor m. insert on cricoid	Axillary vessels cross medial edge of pec. minor m.	Posterior surface pec. major m.	Ribs and intercostal muscles	Medial border of pec. minor m.	Thoracic inlet
Internal mammary	Superior aspect of the medial 1st rib.	Cranial aspect of the 4th rib				

Brachioceph.–axillary vns, brachiocephalic–axillary veins; CT, computed tomography; lat. dorsi m., latissimus dorsi muscle; pec. minor m., pectoralis minor muscle; pec. major m., pectoralis major muscle.

for breast cancer radiation therapy planning, which are listed in Table 59.37. An illustration of nodal volumes drawn on an axial planning CT scan is shown in Figure 59.30.

In patients treated with 6-MV or lower-energy photons with wide tangential fields in whom separation is >22 cm, there may be significant dose inhomogeneity in the breast; this may correlate with less satisfactory cosmetic results.[351,700] This problem can be minimized by using higher-energy photons (10 to 18 MV) to deliver a portion of the breast radiation (approximately 50%) as determined with treatment planning to maintain the inhomogeneity throughout the entire breast to between 93% and 105%. If desired, the buildup of the beam may be modified with a "degrader." "Simple intensity-modulated radiation therapy" techniques such as field-in-field or dynamic multileaf collimators (MLCs) to achieve electronic tissue compensation may be utilized to reduce dose inhomogeneity as well. Bolus should be avoided in conservatively managed patients. A variety of immobilizing devices or molds may be constructed to support the breast in the treatment position (Fig. 59.31). A polyvinyl chloride, ring-shaped device, held by a strap, has been used around the breast to aid in positioning of patients with large, pendulous or flaccid breasts. Skin reactions where material is in contact with the skin should be closely monitored.[701]

Alignment of the Tangential Beam with the Chest Wall Contour

The anterior chest wall slopes downward from the midchest to the neck. To make the posterior edge of the tangential beam follow this downward-sloping contour, the collimator of the tangential beam may be rotated, or the patient may be placed on a slant so that the slope of the chest wall is parallel to the table. An alternative is to make the deep posterior edge of the tangential beam follow the chest wall contour by means of a rotating beam splitter mounted on a tray without rotation of the collimator or using multileaf collimation. In this way, the superior edge of the tangential beam remains in the true vertical and matches perfectly the vertical inferior edge of the supraclavicular field if used.

Usually up to 2 to 3 cm of underlying lung may be included in the tangential portals. The amount of lung included in the irradiated volume is greatly influenced by the portals used. Bornstein et al.[702] determined the amount of lung irradiated in 40 patients with breast cancer using CT scans for treatment planning in the treatment position. Parameters measured from simulator films included the perpendicular distance

FIGURE 59.30. Nodal volumes drawn on axial planning CT scan.

FIGURE 59.31. Immobilization material placed over breast tissue to help maintain day-to-day positioning of the breast.

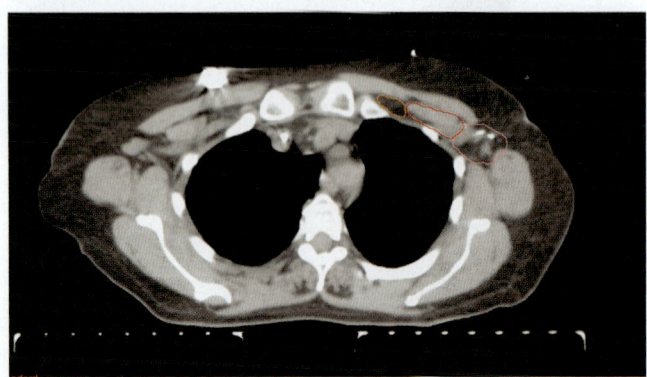

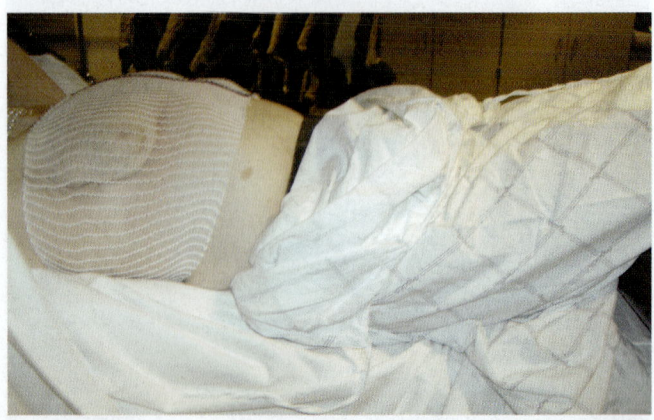

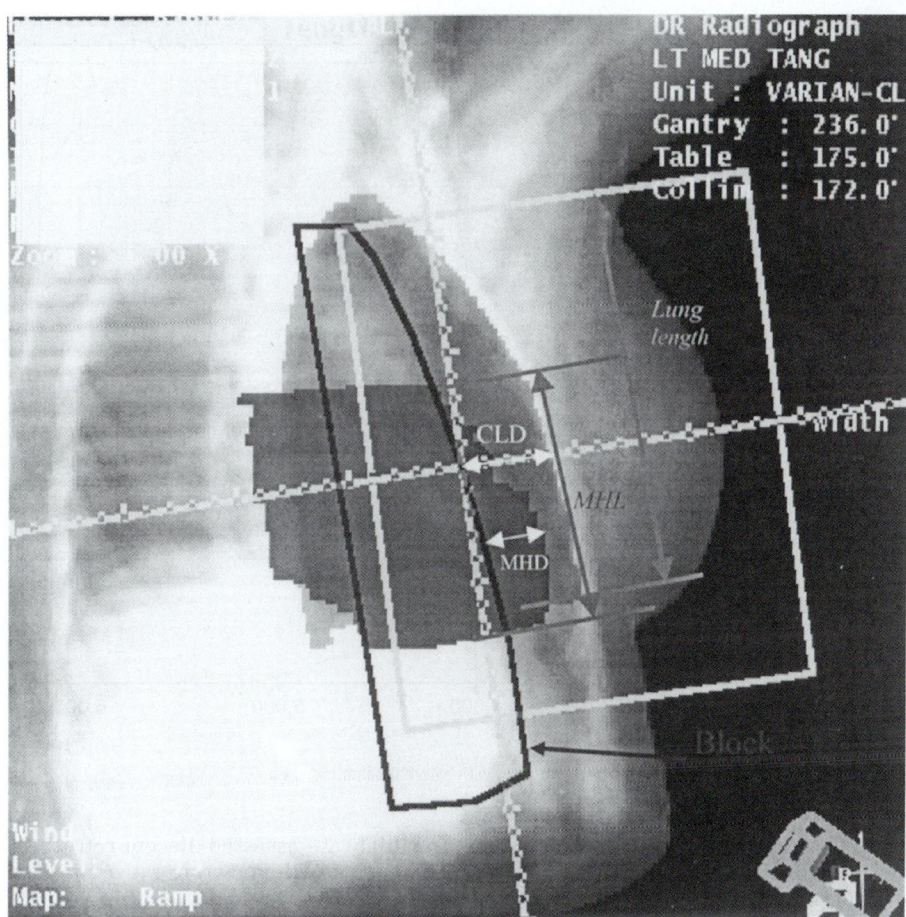

FIGURE 59.32. Measurement of the radiographic parameters using virtual simulator. The contoured heart is shown in *black*, the lung in *gray*. The central lung distance (CLD) is the lung distance in the projection of the tangential fields at the level of the central axis. Lung length is the vertical lung distance included in the radiation port. The maximal heart distance (MHD) is the width of heart in the tangent fields at its maximal level, whereas the maximal heart length (MHL) is the maximal length in tangential fields referring to the heart contour in a digitally reconstructed radiograph (DRR). (Reprinted from Kong F-M, Klein EE, Bradley JD, et al. The impact of central lung distance, maximal heart distance, and radiation technique on the volumetric dose of the lung and heart for intact breast radiation. *Int J Radiat Oncol Biol Phys* 2002;54[3]:963–971. Copyright © 2002 Elsevier. With permission.)

from the posterior tangential field edge to the posterior part of the anterior chest wall at the center of the field (central lung distance [CLD]), the maximum perpendicular distance from the posterior tangential field edge to the posterior part of the anterior chest wall (maximum lung distance [MLD]), and the length of lung as measured at the posterior tangential field edge on the simulator film (Fig. 59.32). The best predictor of the percentage of ipsilateral lung volume treated by the tangential fields was the CLD. A CLD of 1.5 cm predicted that approximately 6% of the ipsilateral lung would be included in the tangential field; a CLD of 2.5 cm, approximately 16%; and a CLD of 3.5 cm, approximately 26% of the ipsilateral lung. A typical acceptable dose–volume histogram of a left-sided breast cancer treated with external beam radiation is given in Figure 59.33.

When the CLD is >3 cm, in treatment of the left breast, a significant volume of heart will also be irradiated. To avoid this, a medial tangential breast port (3- to 5-cm wide), somewhat similar to an internal mammary port, may be designed. The beam is angled 10 to 15 degrees laterally to conform to the angle of the medial breast port. The dose is prescribed to the posterior border of the chest wall as determined by CT scanning.

Special attention should be paid to minimizing the volume of heart irradiated.[703] As will be discussed later in the section on cardiac sequelae, even small amounts of heart in the field can affect cardiac function. Marks et al.[704] have suggested the use of a cardiac block if the heart is in the tangential field, which can be supplemented by an electron field as shown in Figure 59.34. Use of short (10- to 15-second) treatments while the patient holds her breath is also feasible as a way of reducing cardiac radiation during left-sided breast cancer treatment.[705]

Doses of Radiation and Fractionation

Whole-Breast Dose
With whole-breast irradiation, tumor doses of approximately 45 to 50 Gy are delivered to the entire breast over 5 to 6 weeks (1.8- to 2-Gy tumor dose daily, 5 weekly fractions). Some authors have suggested daily fractions of 1.8 Gy for patients with large, pendulous breasts or when irradiation is combined with chemotherapy.[308,369,706] The authors' preference is to use 2 Gy fractions to 50 Gy because this is the scheme used in the vast majority of randomized trials using whole-breast radiation therapy following CS.

Alternative fractionation schemes have been employed and have been shown to be acceptable. These are discussed in greater detail in the hypofractionation section.

Radiation Beams
X-ray energies of 4 to 6 MV are preferred to treat the breast. Photon energies >6 MV underdose superficial tissues beneath the skin surface, but higher-energy photons may be helpful in large breasts to decrease the integral breast dose. In these patients, the high-energy photon beam may be "degraded" to bring the maximum dose to more superficial tissues. It is not necessary to apply bolus to the breast because the skin is usually not at risk for recurrence after complete excision of a T1 or T2 lesion, as is the skin of the chest wall after a mastectomy. Use of bolus results in impaired cosmetic results.[351]

Wedges or compensating filters must be used for a portion of the treatment to achieve a uniform dose distribution in the breast (5% to 8% dose variance from the chest wall to the apex). Although conventional wedges improve dose homogeneity at the central axis of the breast, significant inhomogeneity can occur in the superior and inferior portions

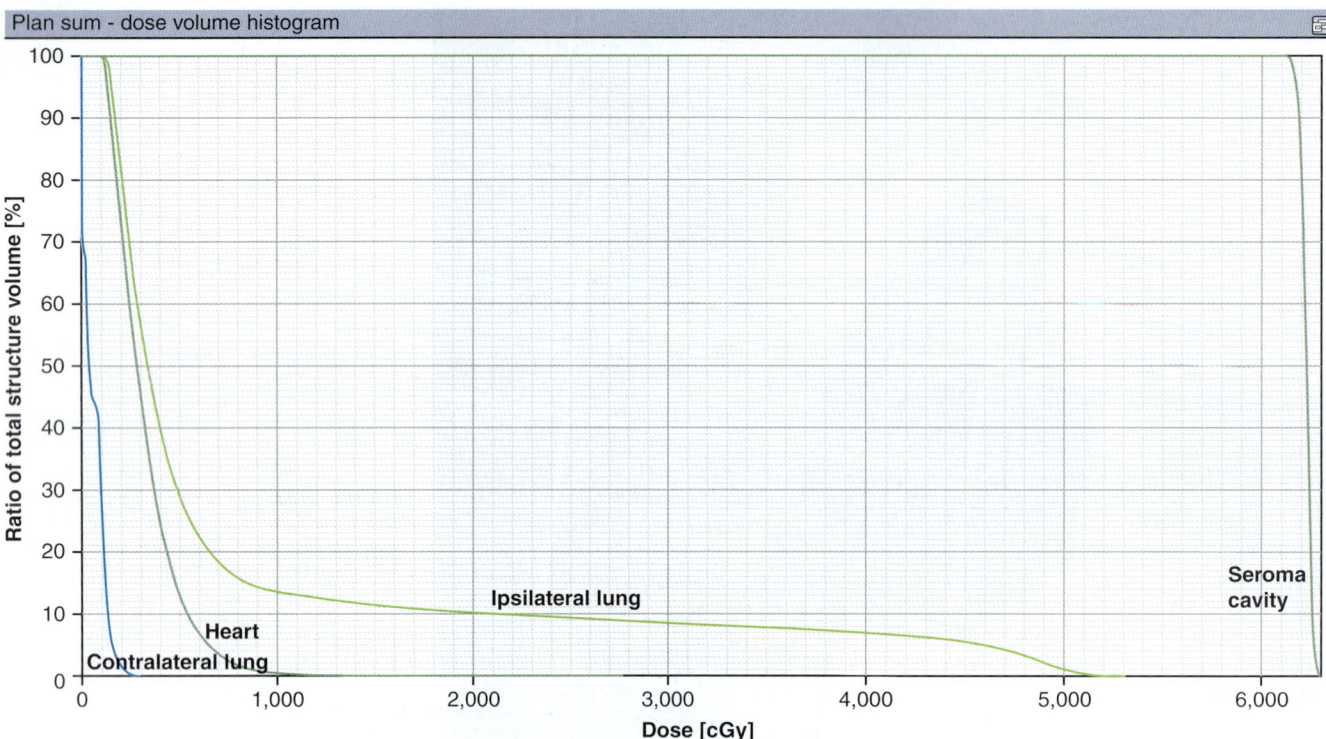

FIGURE 59.33. Dose–volume histogram of left-sided breast cancer treated with external beam radiation.

of the breast. Currently, with the use of MLCs and more sophisticated treatment planning techniques, optimization of homogeneity throughout the breast can be achieved through the use of a variety of techniques. Dose homogeneity in a breast plan uncompensated (without wedges), with standard wedges, and with electronic dynamic wedge technique to improve homogeneity in the superior–inferior plane is outlined in Figure 59.35. These techniques are discussed in more detail later.

Boost to Tumor Site

The need for a boost to the tumor bed following lumpectomy and whole-breast radiation remains an area of debate. In the earlier years of breast-conserving surgery, status of the surgical margins was not always assessed. Recent retrospective data suggest that patients with known negative margins have high local control rates with no boost following whole-breast irradiation.[707] Fisher et al.[708] have all raised the question of the need for a radiation dose boost at the excision site.

Most authors report that 65% to 80% of breast recurrences after conservation surgery and irradiation occur around the primary tumor site.[107,109,194,296,375,387,679–711] These data provide a strong rationale for a tumor bed boost. Various series suggest that patients treated with higher doses have a greater probability of tumor control. Clark et al.[376] noted in 1,504 patients a greater incidence of failures at 10 years of 17% in those to whom no boost was delivered, compared with 11% in those who received doses of 5 to 15 Gy at the primary excision site

FIGURE 59.34. A and **B:** Left tangential breast field with heart block to shield left ventricle from radiation port. Projection of heart block on breast shields minimal amount of breast tissue. If necessary, a shadow electron field may be added to cover the portion of breast tissue shielded by heart block.

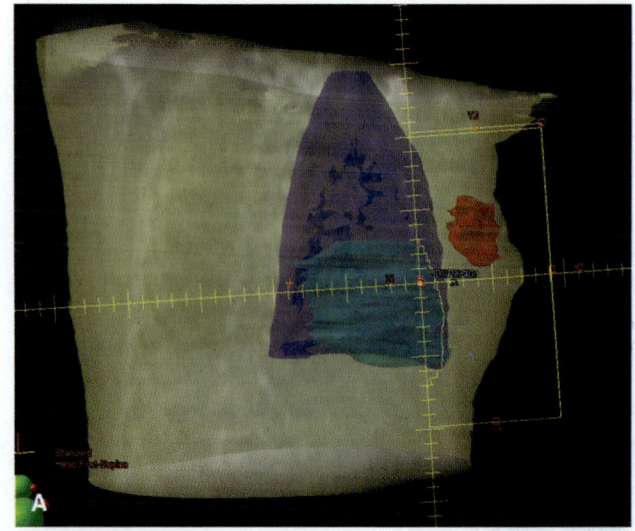
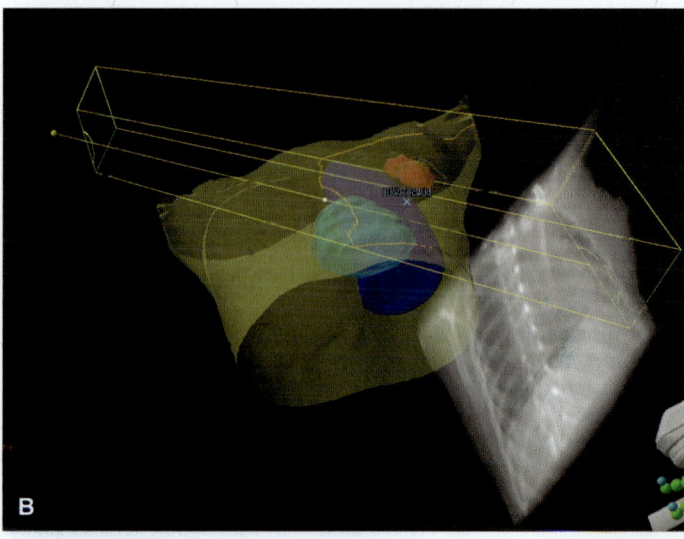

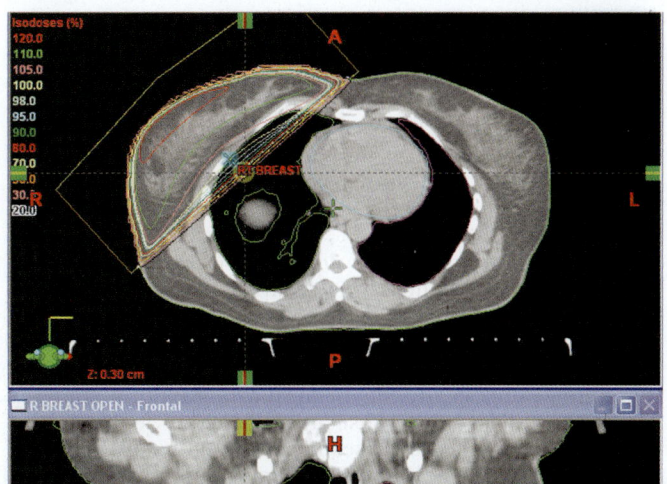

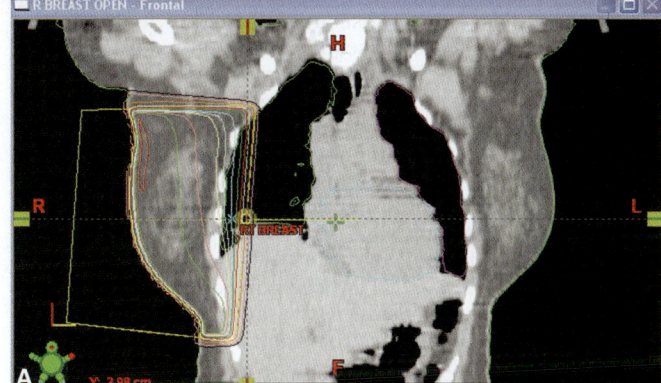

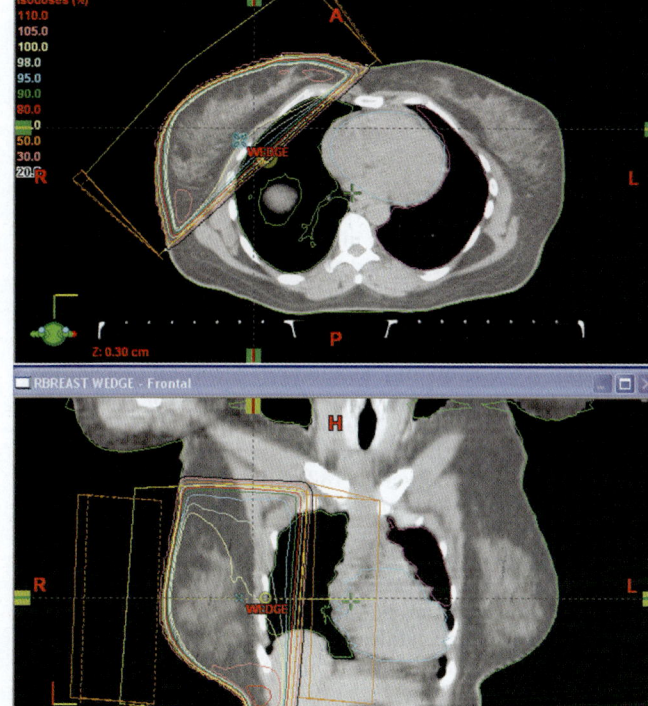

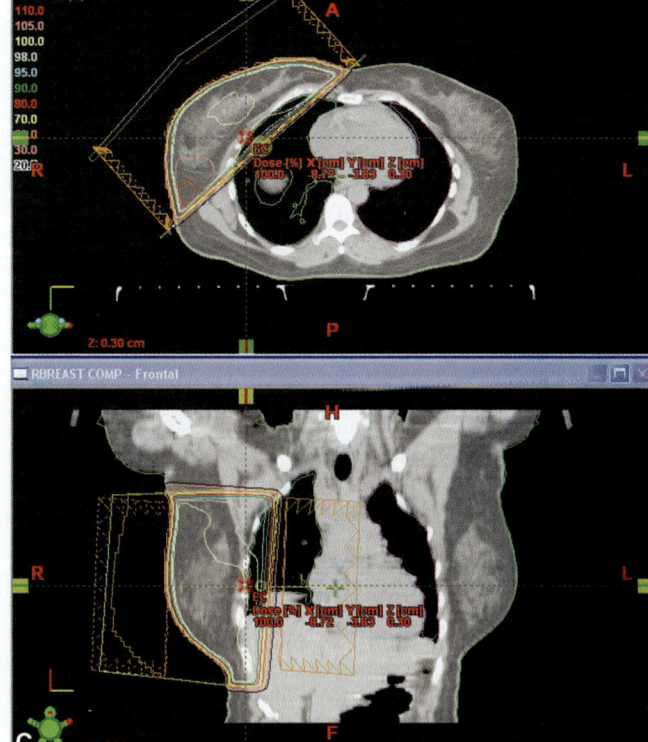

FIGURE 59.35. Isodose distributions from three breast plans. **A:** Open fields demonstrating inhomogeneity. **B:** Standard wedges demonstrating improvement in central axis, but with a hot spot in the superior inferior plane. **C:** Dynamic wedge plan showing improved homogeneity in both the central axis as well as the superior–inferior plane.

($P = .03$). In other series of patients with unknown surgical margins, patients receiving a boost had roughly half the breast failure rate (6% to 11%) compared with those with no boost (9% to 20%).[113,387,403,712]

Others have advocated tailoring the need for a boost depending on margins. Arthur et al.[707] reported on 205 patients who underwent re-excision prior to radiation. All patients in this cohort had no tumor on re-excision and were treated

with whole-breast irradiation to a dose of 50 Gy without a boost. Five failures were documented, resulting in a 15-year local control rate of 92.4%. The authors advocate selective avoidance of the boost in these patients.

Randomized Data

The Lyon Breast Cancer Trial conducted a randomized study to assess the role of the boost in breast-conserving therapy in patients with stage I and II breast cancer (≤3 cm) who were treated with complete local tumor excision, axillary dissection, and 50 Gy to the breast in 20 fractions over 5 weeks and randomly assigned to receive or not a boost of 10 Gy with electrons to the tumor bed.[713] With a median follow-up of 3.3 years, at 5 years 10 of 521 women who received a boost (3.6%) and 20 of 503 (4.5%) who received no further treatment experienced a local breast relapse (P = .044). Time to local recurrence is shown in Figure 59.52, with more patients failing after 7 years in the no-boost arm.

Bartelink et al.[403] reported the results of the EORTC trial in which, after complete lumpectomy and axillary dissection, patients with stage I or II breast cancer received 50 Gy of radiation to the whole breast in 2-Gy fractions over a 5-week period and were randomly assigned to receive either no further local treatment (2,657 patients) or a boost of 16 Gy, usually given in 8 fractions by electron beam (2,661 patients). In the initial report, with a median follow-up of 5.1 years, local recurrences were observed in 182 of the 2,657 patients in the standard-treatment group and 109 of the 2,661 patients in the additional-radiation group. The 5-year actuarial rates of local recurrence were 7.3% and 4.3%, respectively (P < .001). Patients 40 years of age or younger benefited most; at 5 years, their rate of local recurrence was 19.5% with standard treatment and 10.2% with additional radiation (RR 0.46; 99% CI, 0.23 to 0.89; P = .002). In an update of this study published in 2007, with a median follow-up of 10.8 years, a significant benefit to the boost was noted in all age groups, with an overall HR of 0.59 in favor of the boost[404] (see Fig. 59.16).

If a decision is made not to use a boost, careful assessment of lumpectomy margins is critical, as discussed in the following section.

Electron Versus Interstitial Boosts

Before the widespread availability of electron beam therapy, interstitial brachytherapy or cone-down photon boost was popular. Experiences with interstitial boosts have been reported by several groups, using both high-dose rate after loading and low–dose rate temporary implants.[714–723] The reader is referred to these studies and the chapter on brachytherapy for a more extensive discussion of techniques related to interstitial tumor bed boosts. Currently, most institutions prefer electron beam boost because of its relative ease in setup, outpatient setting, lower cost, decreased time demands on the physician, and excellent results compared with ^{192}Ir implants. The introduction of single lumen or multilumen balloon catheters, used primarily in partial breast irradiation, can also be considered an interstitial boost technique. Cosmetic results with either boost technique at various institutions are summarized in Table 59.38.

Electron Boosts

The patient is positioned with the arm toward the head to flatten the breast contour and may be rolled so the tumor bed is parallel to the table and the accelerator head can point straight down onto the target volume. An electron energy is

selected that covers the target volume depth (usual range is 9 to 16 MeV electrons), based on review of the physical examination, mammogram, ultrasound, CT, or other imaging used to ascertain the location and depth of the tumor or metallic surgical clips. The 90% prescription isodose line is limited to the chest wall to decrease dose to the lung. The clinical setup for electron boost involves marking the projection of the post-lumpectomy volume on the skin and adding 2 to 3 cm in all directions.

Accurate target volume definition is critical with any boost technique. Methods vary from simple and unsophisticated (as described in the previous paragraph) to complex and expensive, such as ultrasound and CT definition of the target volume.[724,725] The accuracy of using the scar to define the lumpectomy cavity has been questioned. In a study by Oh et al.,[724] 30 women consecutively treated for 31 breast cancers had simulation CT scans performed before and after whole-breast irradiation. CT breast volumes were delineated using clinically defined borders, and excision cavity volumes were contoured based on surgical clips, the presence of a hematoma, or other surgical changes. Hypothetical electron boost plans were generated using the surgical scar with a 3-cm margin and analyzed for coverage. The volume reduction (R) in the excision cavity was inversely correlated with time elapsed since surgery (R = 0.46; P < .01) and body weight (R = 0.50; P < .01). The scar-guided hypothetical plans failed to cover the excision cavity adequately in 62% and 53.8% of cases using the pretreatment and postradiation CTs, respectively.

Surgical clips are ideal for the localization of the tumor bed.[699,725,726] The surgical clip method requires the cooperation of the surgical team. Despite the fact that it would theoretically take an infinite number of clips to define every extension of a typical tylectomy cavity, in practice six clips suffice (superficial, deep, medial, lateral, cephalad, and caudal). In a study reported by Denham et al.,[727] surgical hemoclips were left *in situ* in 27 patients to demarcate the limits of the excision cavity. The position of these clips varied widely in relation to the patient's recollection of the position of the original lump, the surgical notes, and the surgical scar. Incomplete coverage of the excision cavity in the "coronal" (*en face*) plane using an electron field could have occurred in an estimated 10 of 24 (42%) cases had surgical clips not been left *in situ*. Depth of the surgical clips below the skin surface also varied markedly; in 19 of 26 (73%) cases, the clips were observed to be ≥3 cm below the skin surface, whereas in only 5 of 26 (19.2%) cases were the clips found to be ≤2 cm deep to the surface. Had a 9-MeV electron beam been used to treat all of the patients, a major underdose of the excision cavity would have been likely in 21 of 26 (81%) evaluable cases. Coverage would have improved to 11 of the 26 (42%) had a 12-MeV beam been used.

Fein et al.[726] described a study in patients with stage I or II breast cancer treated with breast conservation therapy; surgical clips were placed in the excision cavity in 556 patients, and no clips were placed in 808. After breast irradiation with tangential fields, the primary tumor incision site was boosted with electron beam (14 to 20 Gy). The actuarial breast recurrence rates at 10 years were 11% in patients with clips and 5% in patients without clips (P = .01). Increased rates of breast recurrence were noted for patients with clips who had some of the following: no adjuvant treatment, unknown surgical margins, no re-excision, pathologic negative nodes, and outer location of primary tumor. The higher incidence of breast relapse may be related to a specific surgeon who had a breast recurrence rate of 21%, compared with 6% for the remainder of the surgeons (P = .01); the status of the margins was unknown in 48% of these patients, compared with 10% overall (P = .001). The authors concluded that failure to ink the surgical specimen and inadequate assessment of margins cannot

TABLE 59.38 EXCELLENT OR GOOD COSMETIC RESULTS WITH ELECTRON BEAM OR INTERSTITIAL BRACHYTHERAPY BOOST IN BREAST CONSERVATION THERAPY

Study (Reference)	Electron Beam	Brachytherapy	Follow-Up
Fourquet et al.[718]	39/52 (75%)	48/68 (71%)	3–7.3 yr
Mansfield et al.[712]	357/376 (95%)	575/629 (91%)	1 mo to 12 yr
Olivotto et al.[719]	36/36 (100%)	298/497 (60%)	5 yr
Perez et al.[720]	366/449 (81%)	97/129 (75%)	3–20 yr
Ray and Fish[721]	97/107 (91%)	12/23 (52%)	6–120 mo
Touboul et al.[715]	104/126 (82%)	91/148 (61%)	29–1 39 mo
Vicini et al.[716]	(90%)	(88%)	59.3 mo (median)

be compensated by placement of surgical clips or treatment planning using CT to delineate the surgical bed. On the other hand, this study failed to show any benefit from use of surgical clips at the tumor excision margins to design the boost volume.

Ultrasonography can provide the depth of the biopsy cavity, as well as the other dimensions, for use in designing electron portal borders and selection of electron energy.[725,728] Ultrasonography was used in 30 patients to measure breast thickness for determination of the most appropriate electron beam energy for the boost. In most patients, the depth was ≤4 cm, but in eight patients (32%), energy higher than 12 MeV should have been used to cover adequately the depth of the target volume.

CT-guided portal design should be done in the treatment position. This technique gives good definition of the depth of the chest wall and has been shown to be similar to ultrasound in delineating the lumpectomy cavity.[725,728] Delineation of the biopsy cavity becomes more difficult with increased interval from surgery. The combination of surgical clips with a treatment planning CT scan to define the lumpectomy site for electron boost is most ideal. In the absence of surgical clips, the CT scan evaluation of the biopsy cavity or postsurgical changes, in combination with clinical information including mammography findings, scar location, operative reports, and patient input, will provide accurate information regarding placement of the field and energy of the electron boost.

A recent multi-institutional study reported interobserver variabilities in the delineation of the seroma cavity and organs at risk in breast cancer patients undergoing breast-conserving surgery and whole-breast irradiation.[729] Nine radiation oncologists specializing in breast radiotherapy from eight institutions independently delineated target volumes on the same three breast cancer patients. They concluded that "variations in delineating the targets and OARs [organs at risk] for breast RT by well-experienced observers from different institutions are substantial for all relevant structures."

To reduce these variations, guidelines for contouring the seroma cavity have been established; the Seroma Clarity Scale (SCS), developed by the British Columbia Cancer Agency and the Cavity Visualization Score (CVS), developed by a Stanford group.[725,730] Both scoring systems are remarkably similar with the distinction being the SCS is a scale from 0 to 5, with 0 being no visible seroma cavity and 1 being a scar or shadow; the CVS is a scale from 1 to 5, with 1 being no visible seroma cavity, and omits the presence of a scar or shadow on the scale. The scores of 2 to 5 are relatively consistent between the two classification methods.

It is pertinent to note that each of these classification systems was developed without noting the presence of surgical clips or fiducial markers with respect to the seroma cavity. However, the authors, along with other investigators, have previously published that the presence of surgical clips or fiducial markers in the surgical bed improve the interphysician accuracy in the delineation of the seroma cavity in early-stage breast cancer patients.[731,732] In a study by Shaikh et al.,[733] the presence of fiducial markers improved the mean CVS score (from 2.5 to 3.5) and accuracy of physician contours compared with patients without fiducial markers. The use of titanium clips in patients treated with APBI is a focus of the United Kingdom IMPORT LOW (Intensity Modulated and Partial Organ Radiotherapy) trial.[734] An audit of the trial was performed to determine inter- and intraphysician variation for tumor bed localization for radiotherapy planning. Although no control group was used, clips were essential for the localization of the surgical cavity in 22 of 30 (73%) patients and led to modifications in radiotherapy field borders in 18 of 30 (60%) patients. A recent study by Dzhugashvili et al.[732] found that the visualization of the lumpectomy cavity was greatly improved in treatment-planning CT scans when clips were present; this was found to be even more pronounced in patients with very dense mammary glands, regardless of the physician reading the CT image.

Irradiation of Regional Lymphatics

Radiation therapy to the breast or chest wall and regional lymphatics can be technically challenging and, as previously discussed, remains one of the more variable and controversial aspects in management. A wide variety of available techniques, in combination with difficulties associated with matching fields, anatomic variability between patients, and lack of clear evidence regarding the superiority of any single approach, has resulted in a lack of consensus in regional nodal management.

Anatomic variation was highlighted in a study by Mansur et al.[735] They reported on 65 patients with breast cancer who had volumetric CT scanning in the treatment position. The IMNs and axillary lymph node regions were delineated according to a cross-sectional nodal atlas. The variable depths of IMNs at different intercostal spaces result in dose variations if the internal mammary port is treated with a single or inadequate electron beam energy. Axillary lymph nodes frequently overlapped the head of the humerus anteriorly when the arm was angled more than 90 degrees, but did not when the arm was angled 90 degrees or less. The larger the angle, the less head of the humerus could be spared in the supraclavicular port.

Arthur et al.[736] evaluated treatment techniques for coverage of the intact breast and ipsilateral lymph node regions. Anatomic outlines were obtained from five randomly selected patients with CT scanning in treatment position (three with cancer of the left breast and two of the right). Three techniques used to treat ipsilateral breast and internal mammary and supraclavicular nodes (extended tangents, five-field, partially wide tangents) were configured and compared with a supraclavicular field matched to standard tangential fields. All of the treatment techniques covering IMNs included at least 10% more lung and heart volume than that covered by standard tangential fields. Because of increased chest wall thickness and depth of IMNs superiorly, complete coverage was not achieved with any technique if the IMN target extended superiorly into the medial supraclavicular field.

Goodman et al.[737] examined the relation between tangential, anterior, and posterior radiation fields and regional lymph nodes, including level I to III axillary and supraclavicular lymph nodes in 55 patients who underwent CT scanning in the supine position. The mean depths of the level I to III axillary nodes were 4.6, 5.1, and 3.6 cm, respectively. The mean depth of the supraclavicular nodes was 3.9 cm. With the treatment using two tangential fields, level I axillary nodes appeared in the tangential portals in nine of nine patients, either alone or with other lymph node groups. In the three-field group, level I axillary nodes were in 16 of 16 tangential fields either alone or with level II nodes (8 patients). In eight patients, level III and the supraclavicular nodes were included in the anterior field, and in the other eight, levels II and III and the supraclavicular nodes were in the anterior field. There was considerable variation in the depth of supraclavicular and axillary lymph nodes in the fields in which these nodal groups appear and in the nodal group present in the posterior axillary boost field. To be certain that nodal groups to be treated are actually treated, as well as to minimize tissue irradiated, these authors recommended that before the placement of radiation fields, the nodal groups be outlined on a CT scan. From a practical standpoint, whether this results in better tumor control than standard techniques has not been demonstrated.

Supraclavicular Lymph Nodes

The inferior border of the supraclavicular field is matched to the tangential field usually just below the clavicular head. The medial border is 1 cm across the midline, extending upward, following the medial border of the sternocleidomastoid muscle to the thyrocricoid groove. The lateral border is a vertical line at the level of the coracoid process, just medial to the humeral head. This field is angled approximately 10 to 15 degrees laterally to spare the cervical spine (Fig. 59.36). The typical width of the supraclavicular field is 7 to 9 cm. The supraclavicular field is extended laterally to treat the full axilla, as clinically indicated. Figure 59.36 demonstrates a supraclavicular field with the supraclavicular and level I, II, and III nodes outlined. Level I as well as a portion of level II nodes will often be included in the tangential field; level III and supraclavicular nodes are covered in the supraclavicular field.

The total dose delivered to the supraclavicular field is 46 to 50.4 Gy at 1.8 to 2 Gy/day (calculated at a depth of 3 cm) in 5 fractions per week. For obese patients, an assessment of the depth of lymph nodes with ultrasound or CT treatment planning is useful to ensure adequate dose is delivered to the target. For patients in whom the target is deeper than 3 cm, higher-energy photons should be considered.

Axillary Lymph Nodes

When the axilla is treated in patients with positive nodes, or in patients with inadequate or undissected axillae, the supraclavicular field is extended laterally to cover at least two-thirds of the humeral head, as demonstrated in Figure 59.36. The dose to the midplane of the axilla from the supraclavicular field is calculated at a point approximately 2 cm inferior to the midportion of the clavicle. Depending on the dose distribution and patient's anatomy, a posterior axillary boost may be considered or anterior axillary boost, as suggested by Wang et al.,[738] may be considered.

Posterior Axillary Boost

There is considerable debate regarding the necessity of a posterior axillary boost. Bentel et al.[739] questioned its necessity in a majority of patients. In 49 patients undergoing treatment-planning CT scanning in the treatment position, the maximum depth of the supraclavicular and axillary lymph nodes was measured on CT images, and the relation between the supraclavicular and axillary lymph node depth and patient diameter was determined. For an anterior field, the relative dose to the supraclavicular and axillary lymph nodes were calculated for a 6-MV photon beam. If an anterior 6-MV beam only is used to treat both supraclavicular and axillary lymph nodes, the dose to the axilla is within ±5% of the supraclavicular dose in 53% (26 of 49) patients and is 90% or more of the dose delivered to the supraclavicular nodes in 90% (44 of 49) of patients. These authors concluded that higher-energy

beams or anterior–posterior/posterior–anterior supraclavicular axillary fields may be reasonable when the axillary and supraclavicular nodes are deep.

The posterior axillary boost has been employed to supplement axillary dose. At the end of the treatments to the supraclavicular field, the dose to the midplane of the axilla may be supplemented by a posterior axillary field, as shown in Figure 59.37. Alternatively, the axilla should be contoured in CT-treatment planning as variation of the depth of the axilla from the anterior-posterior skin surface varies from patient to patient and the supplement prescription point can be adjusted accordingly. If the dose is determined to be inadequate, a posterior boost or anterior boost, as suggested by Wang et al.,[738] may be employed. When a posterior axillary boost is used, the borders are as follows: medially, the border is drawn to allow 1.5 to 2 cm of lung to show on the portal film; inferiorly, the border is at the same level as the inferior border of the supraclavicular field; laterally, the border just blocks fall-off across the posterior axillary fold; lastly, the superior border splits the clavicle and the superolateral border shields or splits the humeral head. Additional dose to the axilla midplane is usually administered to complete 46 to 50 Gy (2 Gy daily). When indicated, a boost of 10 to 15 Gy is delivered with reduced portals.

If the supraclavicular nodes are not felt to be at risk, a separate axillary field may not always be necessary to treat the axilla. In a study of 39 women with surgical clips in the axilla, Schlembach et al.[522] demonstrated that with tangential fields, placing the caudal border of the field within 2 cm of the humeral head and 2 cm deep to the chest wall–lung interface includes the majority of level I and level II lymph nodes (Fig. 59.38).

Internal Mammary Lymph Nodes

The benefit of irradiation of the IMNs is an unresolved issue because clinical failures at this site are very rare and the majority of patients at risk receive adjuvant therapy.[554,561] However, the IMNs are difficult to treat because their exact location is often uncertain and the radiation fields that include them irradiate more normal tissue.[740,741] Several techniques are used, the most common of which is a direct anterior field matched to tangential fields, which was developed for postmastectomy radiation therapy and increases the volume of heart and lung tissue in the field. With this technique, the rising contour of the intact breast interferes with dosimetry, which may affect the traditional dose prescription point at depths of 4 to 5 cm and may prevent an easy match to the breast tangential fields. Including the IMNs in the tangential fields (wide or deep tangents) may significantly increase the

FIGURE 59.36. Supraclavicular and axillary field and field borders. Level I, II, and III nodes are demonstrated on the film. Note that level I nodes are included primarily in the tangential field in this case.

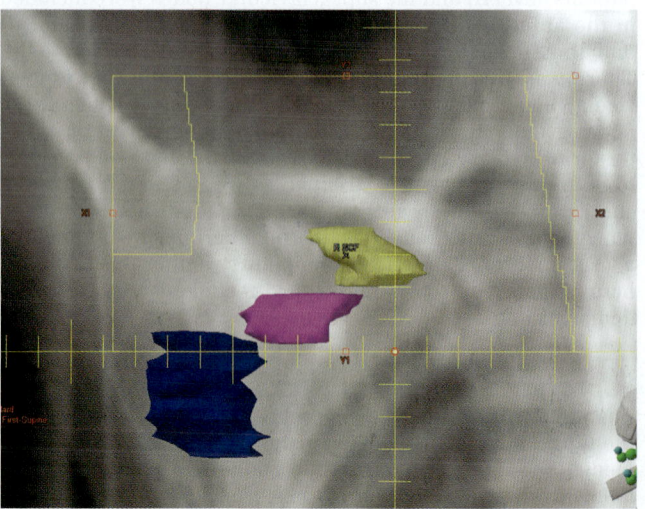

FIGURE 59.37. Posterior axillary field used to supplement the dose at midplane of the axilla. Note the small amount of lung included and the shielding of the humeral head (whenever possible).

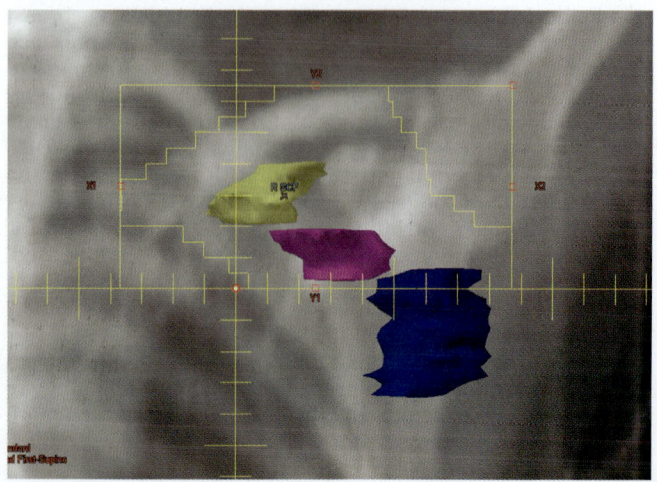

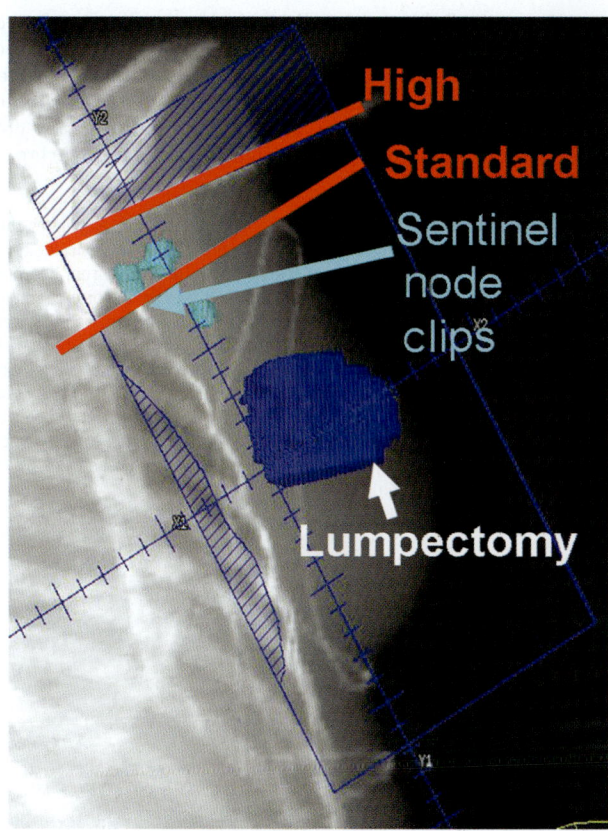

FIGURE 59.38. "High" tangential field shown coverage of level I and portion of level II nodes. With caudal edge of the field within 2 cm of the humeral head and leading edge approximately 2 cm from lung–chest wall interface, the majority of nodes in level I and level II will be covered by this technique.

volume of irradiated lung and heart tissue and often includes a portion of the contralateral breast as well.

The medial border of the IMN field is the midline. The lateral border is usually 5 to 6 cm lateral to the midline. The superior border abuts the inferior border of the supraclavicular field and the inferior border is at the xiphoid or higher. If only the IMNs are to be treated, the superior border of the field is at the first intercostal space (superior border of the head of the clavicle). The field is set, as described previously, with an oblique incidence to match the medial tangential portal (Fig. 59.39).

The dose to the IMN field (45 to 50 Gy at 1.8 to 2 Gy/day) is calculated at a point 4 to 5 cm beneath the skin surface (depending on the thickness of anterior chest wall and ideally based on CT localization). Careful individualized planning and use of electrons of appropriate energy for all or a major portion of the IMN irradiation are necessary to minimize dose to the lung. To spare underlying lung, mediastinum, and spinal cord, electrons in the range of 12 to 16 MeV are preferred for a portion of the treatment, for example, 14.4 to 16.2 Gy delivered with 4- to 6-MV photons and 30.6 to 32.4 Gy with electrons.

A solution that avoids matching of fields is the use of partially wide tangential fields to treat the internal mammary chain.[742] Although IMNs can be imaged more clearly by radionuclide techniques, the nodes are typically located by identification of the internal mammary vessels, which can be seen on the CT simulator. The nodes in the first three intercostal spaces are thought to be most clinically significant. The medial border of the tangential field is moved 3 to 5 cm across the midline to cover the IMNs in the first three intercostal spaces. To minimize lung and cardiac exposure, a block is drawn in, as demonstrated in Figure 59.40, to block the inferior mediastinal nodes. The portal films should be inspected carefully to ensure that an excessive amount of lung or heart is not being irradiated. It is important to verify on the clinical setup that targeted breast tissue is not covered by the block.

FIGURE 59.39. Irradiation of the breast: field configurations and isodose lines for 6-MV photons. **A:** "Standard tangents" technique. **B:** Deep tangents technique. **C:** *En face* internal mammary field (IMF) technique. **D:** Twenty-degree IMF technique. (Reprinted from Roberson PL, Lichter AS, Bodner A, et al. Dose to lung in primary breast irradiation. *Int J Radiat Oncol Biol Phys* 1982;9[1]:97–102. Copyright © 1982 Elsevier. With permission.)

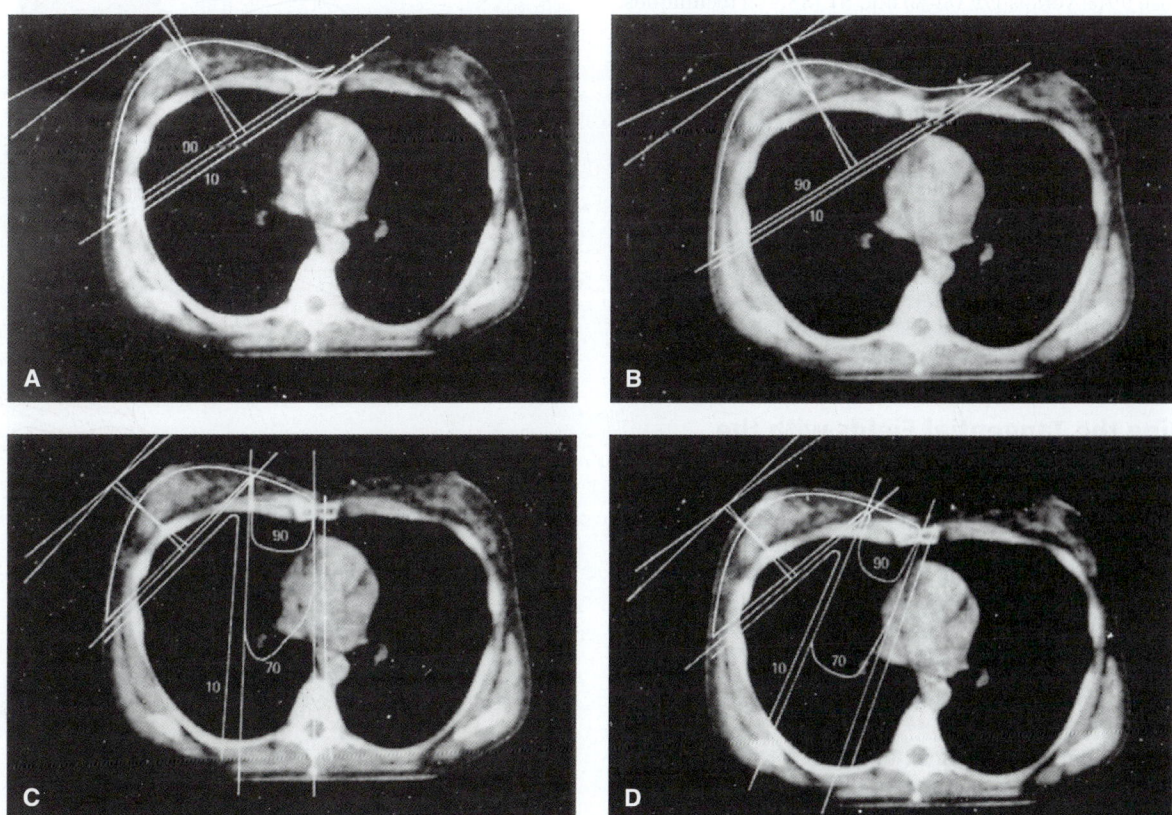

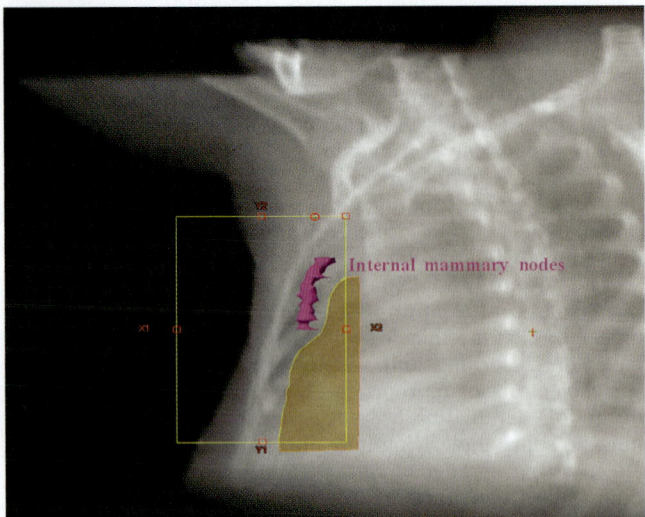

FIGURE 59.40. Partially wide tangential field covering internal mammary chain. The medial border of the tangential field is set 2 to 3 cm to the contralateral side to include the internal mammary chain. Below the fourth intercostal space, the field is blocked to minimize dose to the lungs and heart. Projection of the field on the patient's surface demonstrates adequate coverage of the involved breast–chest wall with this technique. With this technique, there may be a small amount of overlap onto the superior contralateral breast.

Severin et al.[742] compared the partially wide tangent technique (PWT) of breast and internal mammary chain irradiation with photon/electron (P/E) and standard tangent (ST) techniques in terms of dose homogeneity within the breast and the dose to critical structures such as the heart and lung in 16 patients who underwent CT simulation for left-sided breast cancers. The mean dose to the left breast with the ST, P/E, and PWT techniques was 94.7%, 98.4%, and 96.5%, respectively ($P = .029$). The left lung received the lowest mean dose with the ST technique (13.9%) compared with PWT (22.8%) and P/E (24.3%). The internal mammary chain volume was most consistently treated with the PWT (mean dose 99%) versus P/E (86%) and ST (38.4%) techniques, although this technique was associated with the greatest amount of contralateral breast (mean dose 5.8%) versus ST (3.2%) versus P/E (2.8%). The heart received the least dose with ST (mean dose 6.7%) versus PWT (10.3%) and P/E (19%). Pierce et al.,[741] evaluating seven techniques of treating postmastectomy chest wall and lymphatics, also reported that the PWT technique was the most appropriate balance of target coverage and normal tissue sparing when irradiating the chest wall and internal mammary chain.

CT treatment planning is useful for irradiation of the IMN. Although the lymph nodes are most often not visible, the internal mammary vessels can be clearly seen and contoured on axial CT slices. This anatomic region can then be visualized in treatment field design and in dosimetry planning.

Matching the Tangential Fields with the Supraclavicular Field

A hot spot caused by divergence of the tangential beams into the supraclavicular field and of the supraclavicular beam into the tangential fields can exist just beneath the skin surface at the junction of the inferior border of the supraclavicular field and the superior border of the tangential fields.[743] The sharp beam of a linear accelerator and the "horns" at the edge of this beam produce a marked increase in dose beneath the match line if these divergences are not corrected. This increased dose may result in severe match line fibrosis or even rib fracture.

There are numerous methods to adjust for divergence of the beams and minimize match line fibrosis. The divergence

of the tangential fields can be eliminated by angling the foot of the treatment couch away from the radiation source to direct the tangential beams inferiorly so that the superior edges of these beams line up perfectly with the inferior border of the supraclavicular field (Fig. 59.41).[744] In addition, the collimator may be rotated to geometrically eliminate overlap at

FIGURE 59.41. A: Inferior angulation of the tangential beams eliminates their divergence into the supraclavicular field. **B:** Splitting the supraclavicular beam eliminates its divergence down into the tangential field. (**A** and **B** from Bedwinek JM. Treatment of stage I and II adenocarcinoma of the breast by tumor excision and irradiation. *Int J Radiat Oncol Biol Phys* 1981;7:1553, with permission from Elsevier.) **C:** Three-field treatment beam geometry in irradiation of the intact breast and supraclavicular fields illustrated in coronal, cross-sectional, and sagittal projections. The supraclavicular and tangential field blocks are shaded. (**C** from Svensson GK, Chin LM, Siddon RL, et al. Breast treatment techniques at the Joint Center for Radiation Therapy. In: Harris JR, Hellman S, Silen W, eds. *Conservative management of breast cancer: new surgical and radiotherapeutic techniques.* Philadelphia, PA: JB Lippincott, 1983. With permission.)

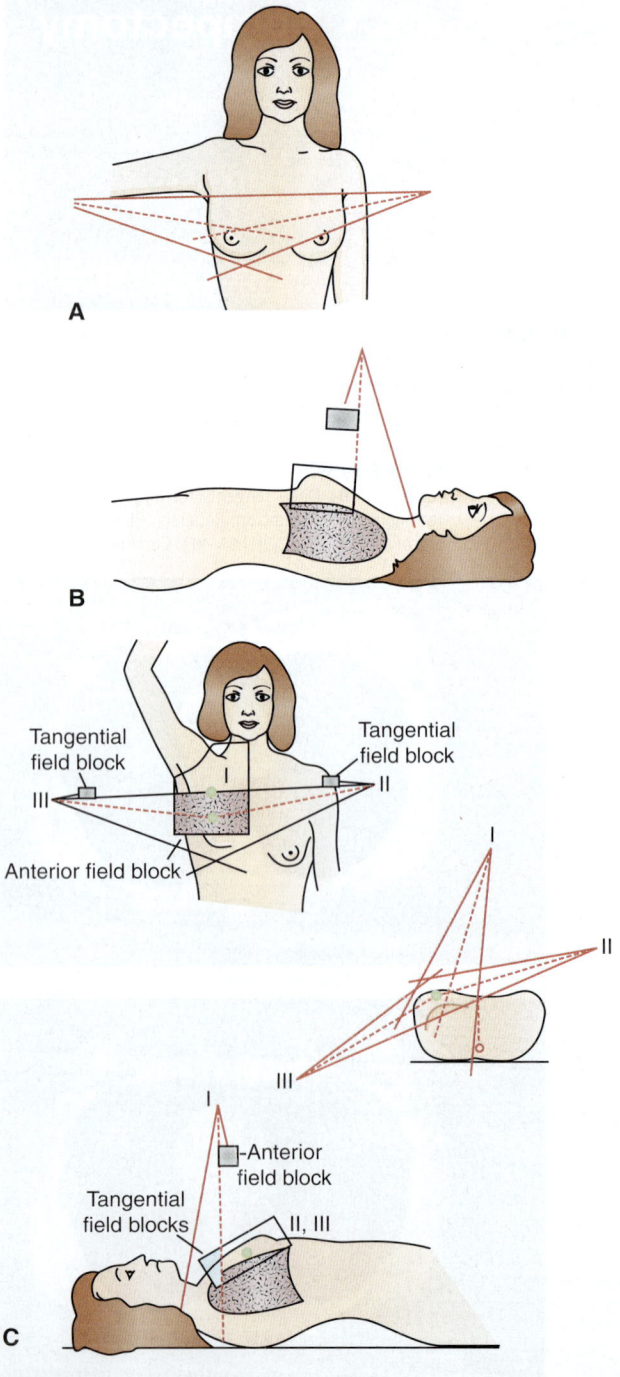

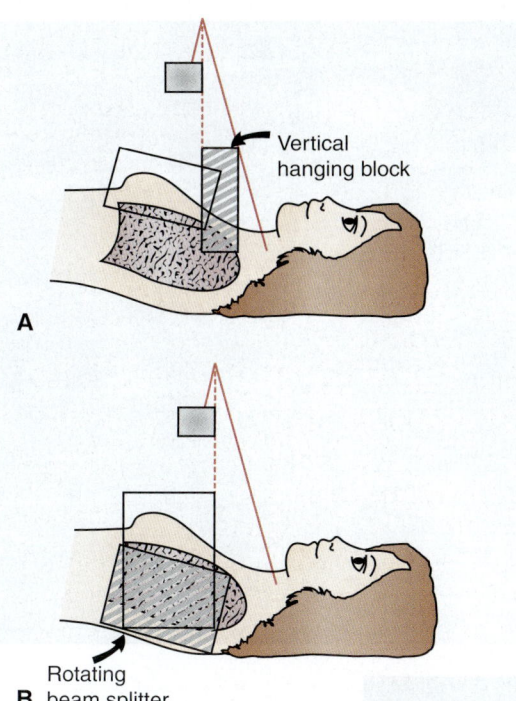

FIGURE 59.42. The superior edge of the tangential beams can be made perfectly vertical by means of the "hanging block" technique **(A)** or by avoiding collimator rotation with the use of a rotating beam splitter **(R)**. (Reprinted from Bedwinek JM. Treatment of stage I and II adenocarcinoma of the breast by tumor excision and irradiation. *Int J Radiat Oncol Biol Phys* 1981;7[11]:1553–1559. Copyright © 1981 Elsevier. With permission.)

this junction. Alternatively, the "hanging block" technique, in which a vertical block is affixed to the superior portion of the collimator to block off the nonvertical portion of the tangential beam, can be used (Fig. 59.42).

The inferior divergence of the supraclavicular beam can be eliminated by blocking the inferior half of the beam. This can be accomplished with a beam splitter or with multileaf collimation so that the central, nondiverging portion of the beam becomes the inferior border of this field (see Fig. 59.43B). The combination of the half-beam block supraclavicular field and the couch kick technique for the tangential field results in minimal overlap and has essentially eliminated the problem of match line fibrosis.

The Single Isocenter Technique for Matching Supraclavicular and Tangential Fields

An alternative and attractive method for minimizing field matching problems between the supraclavicular and tangential fields is to use a technique that employs a single isocenter placed at the junction of the supraclavicular and tangential fields, as demonstrated in Figure 59.44. This single isocenter serves as the isocenter for both the supraclavicular/axillary axillary field and the tangential field, such that the nondivergent central axis single isocenter results in a perfect match of the supraclavicular and tangential fields.[745] As demonstrated, when treating the supraclavicular field, the beam below the isocenter is completely blocked. The supraclavicular field is typically angled 5% to 10% away from the spinal cord. Without moving the isocenter or patient, the tangential field is treated by closing the field above the isocenter and angling the beam to treat the tangential fields. Using this technique, there is not an option for rotating the collimator. If the patient's anatomy and positioning is ideal, the tangential field is closed down to the central axis, an acceptable amount of lung is exposed (<3 cm), and no block may be required. In some cases, the tangential field needs to be opened up beyond the central axis and a block drawn to minimize lung exposure while maintaining coverage of the breast. Because much of the setup is performed on the CT simulator, it is critical when using this technique to clinically view the medial and lateral setups on the patient to ensure that the entire breast is covered, the medial border is not extending to the contralateral breast, and the blocks are not covering any of the targeted breast tissue.

Matching the Tangential Fields with the Internal Mammary Field

When an internal mammary field is required, the match between it and the medial tangential field can be a problem if there is a significant amount of breast tissue beneath the match line. In this situation, a cold spot can exist (Fig. 59.43). The effect may be negligible if the breast tissue beneath this match line is thin (see Fig. 59.43B), or it can be avoided by including the IMNs in the tangential field, as described above (see Fig. 59.43C). Woudstra and van der Werf[746] described a technique using an oblique incidence of the internal mammary portal to match the orientation of the adjacent medial tangential portal; this results in a more homogeneous

FIGURE 59.43. Diagrams showing several relationships between internal mammary and tangential fields. **A:** A significant cold region exists if the internal mammary (IM) tangential matchline overlies a large amount of breast tissue. **B:** The cold area may be negligible if the breast tissue beneath the matchline is thin. **C:** The lack of a separate IM field can result in irradiation of an excessive volume of lung, particularly in large-chested patients. (Reprinted from Bedwinek JM. Treatment of stage I and II adenocarcinoma of the breast by tumor excision and irradiation. *Int J Radiat Oncol Biol Phys* 1981;7[11]:1553–1559. Copyright © 1981 Elsevier. With permission.)

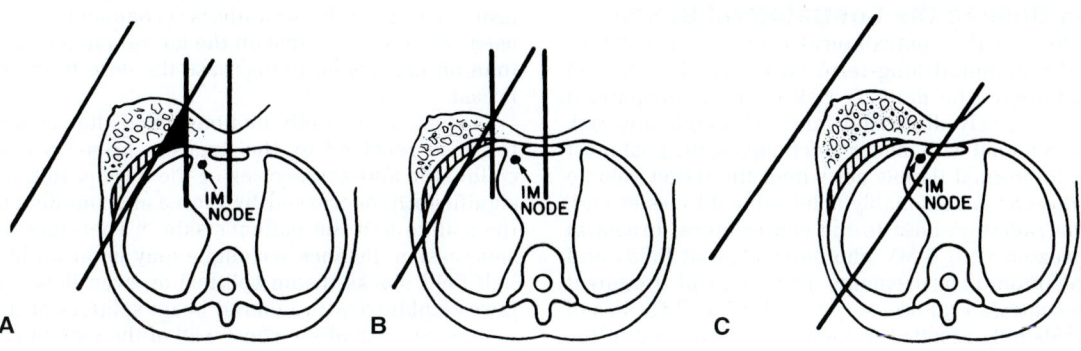

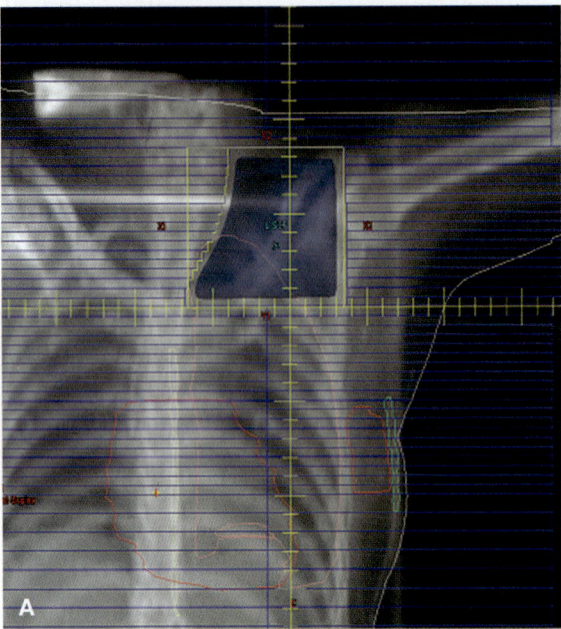
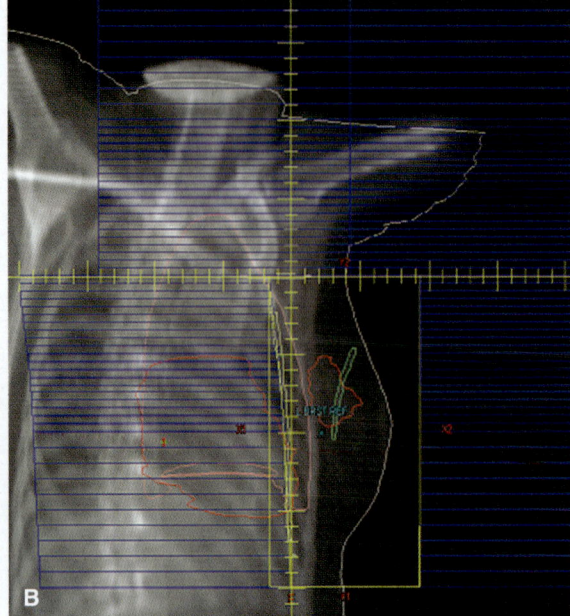
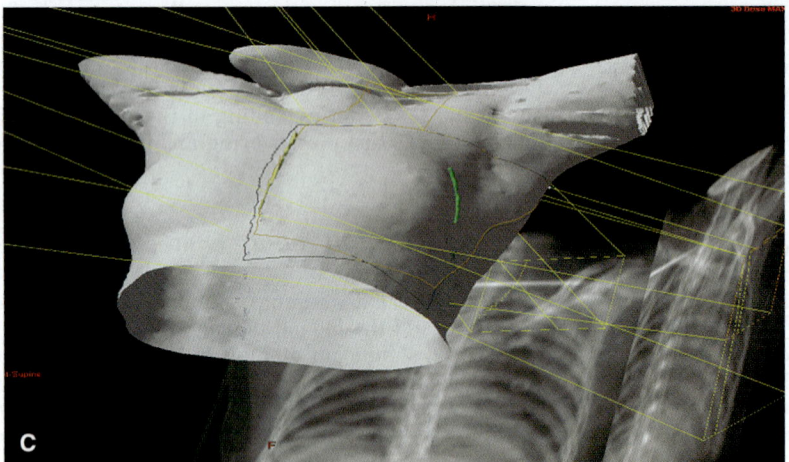

FIGURE 59.44. A–C: Monoisocentric matching technique. Single isocenter is set at the match between the supraclavicular and tangential fields. The inferior portion of the beam is blocked for the supraclavicular treatment and the superior blocked for the tangential field, with no movement of the isocenter, resulting in an ideal match. Blocks are drawn as indicated to shield lung and heart. The field should be viewed clinically to ensure that the blocks drawn to shield the heart and lungs to not block target tissue on the breast–chest wall. Projection of fields onto patient surface demonstrates perfect match of the supraclavicular and tangential fields.

dose distribution at the junction of the two fields (Fig. 59.45). One potential advantage of the partially wide tangential field in the conservatively managed patient is that it avoids the problem of matching over breast tissue.

Irradiation Dose to the Contralateral Breast

Irradiation dose to the contralateral breast is of concern because of the potential long-term carcinogenic effect of scattered radiation. The data on risk of the contralateral breast are extensively discussed later. Although this risk appears to be minimal with modern techniques, the goal must be to expose all normal tissues not within the target volume to as low a dose as is reasonably achievable. Fraass et al.[747] measured the radiation dose to the contralateral breast in 16 women treated with 6-MV photon tangential fields and performed phantom measurements. For a typical treatment of 50 Gy, the contralateral breast received 0.5 to 2 Gy. Use of tangential fields only resulted in more dose delivered to the surface of the opposite breast, whereas use of the internal

mammary field in addition to the tangential portals gave more dose deeper in the breast. Use of a 2.5-cm-thick lead shield over the contralateral breast during treatment with a medial tangential field reduced the dose to 35% of its original value. Similar shields used on the lateral tangential field had no protective effect. These authors recommended that wedges be used whenever possible on the lateral tangential fields rather than on the medial to decrease the dose to the contralateral breast.

A dosimetric study demonstrated that most of the scatter dose received by the opposite breast originates in the collimator and accessories of the accelerator, and it can be significantly decreased by increasing the distance between the source and the patient's skin.[748] Therefore, an isocentric source–skin distance technique may be desirable. The use of half-field blocks (beam splitter) or, even better, independent jaws combined with tailored beam splitters or a MLC following the contour of the chest wall of the patient is very helpful in decreasing the dose to the contralateral breast.

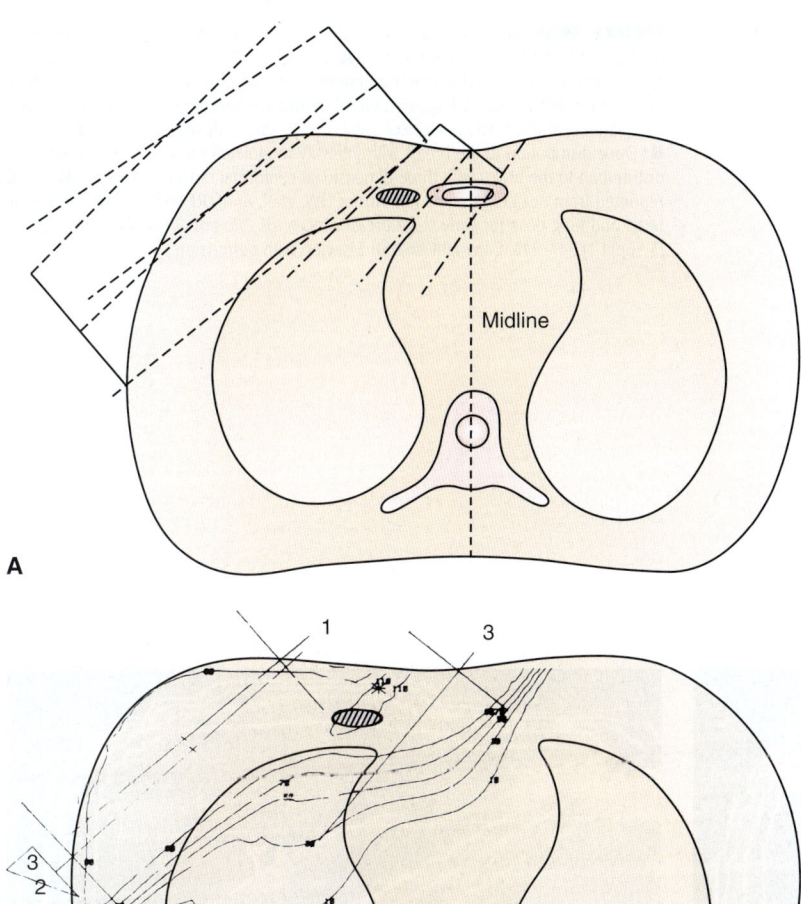

Midline

A

B

Section
III

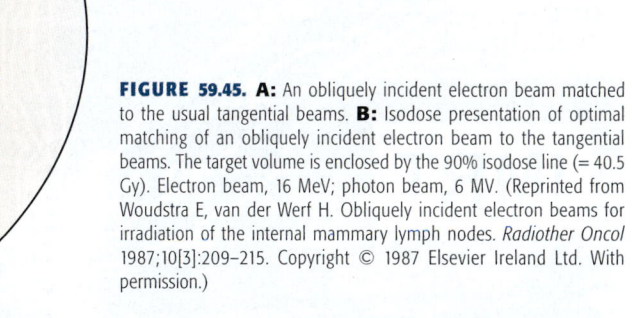

FIGURE 59.45. A: An obliquely incident electron beam matched to the usual tangential beams. **B:** Isodose presentation of optimal matching of an obliquely incident electron beam to the tangential beams. The target volume is enclosed by the 90% isodose line (= 40.5 Gy). Electron beam, 16 MeV; photon beam, 6 MV. (Reprinted from Woudstra E, van der Werf H. Obliquely incident electron beams for irradiation of the internal mammary lymph nodes. *Radiother Oncol* 1987;10[3]:209–215. Copyright © 1987 Elsevier Ireland Ltd. With permission.)

Kelly et al.[749] reviewed the dose to the contralateral breast from breast irradiation with tangential fields using four different techniques. The highest dose was delivered with the use of Cerrobend half-beam blocks (regardless of the proportion of wedge used). Remaining techniques gave similar dose ranges, with the lowest total dose produced by the asymmetric jaw with no medial wedge.

The clinical significance of this inadvertent radiation dose to the opposite breast is uncertain, as various investigators have shown no increased risk of contralateral breast malignancy after treatment of the original breast by radiation therapy.[23,91,686,750]

Three-Dimensional Conformal or Intensity-Modulated Radiation Therapy

Standard opposed tangential fields with appropriate use of wedges to optimize dose homogeneity remains the most commonly employed method for delivery of whole-breast irradiation. A number of publications have explored the potential advantages of three-dimensional conformal radiation therapy (3D-CRT) or intensity-modulated radiation therapy (IMRT) to treat patients with breast cancer. Theoretically, 3D-CRT involves a reduction in the volume of normal tissues receiving a high dose, with an increase in dose to the target volume that includes the tumor and a limited amount of normal tissue. IMRT potentially can further improve the dose distribution between the target and nontarget tissue but may also increase the volume of tissue exposed to lower doses of radiation. As suggested in a review by Hall and Wuu,[637] this may increase the risk of second malignancies; the potential gains and limitations of advanced planning techniques must be weighed carefully.

Solin et al.[751] devised 38 3D treatment plans in two patients using multiple CT scan sections and compared various dose distributions. Breast inhomogeneity doses ranged from 5% to 10%. Cobalt-60 produced greater inhomogeneities than did 6-MV photons, with minimal improvement in tumor dose coverage. In contrast, 15-MV photons had significantly worse tumor coverage at shallow depths, although there was a slight reduction in hot spots. These authors were unable to identify any beam arrangement that improved dose distributions compared with standard tangential fields.

Vicini et al.[752] reported on 281 patients treated with whole-breast IMRT using multiple static MLC segments. Figure 59.46 shows a representative dose distribution. The median volume of breast receiving 105% of the prescribed dose was 11% (range, 0% to 67.6%). The median breast volume receiving 110% of the prescribed dose was 0% (range, 0% to 39%), and the median breast volume receiving 115% of the prescribed dose was also 0%. Only three (1%) experienced grade III toxicity. The cosmetic results at 12 months (95 patients analyzable) were rated as excellent or good in 94 patients (99%). No skin telangiectasias, significant

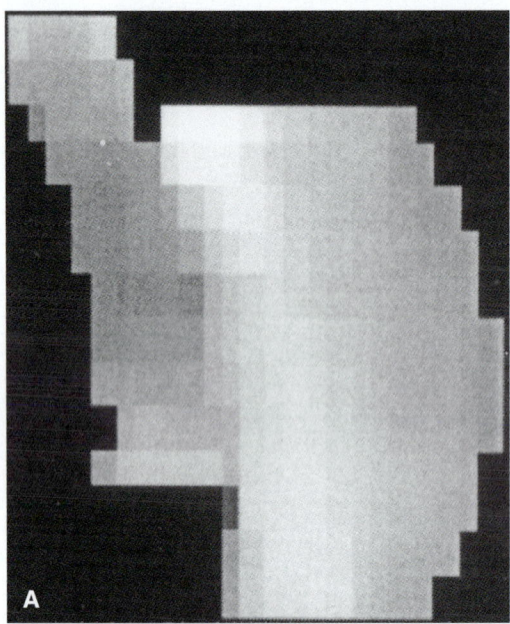

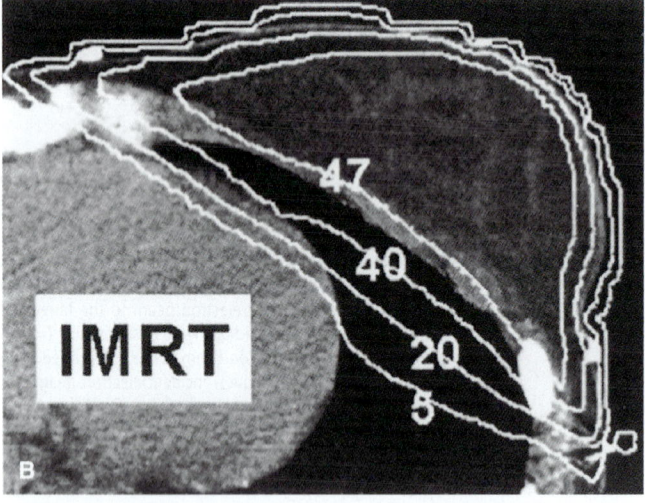

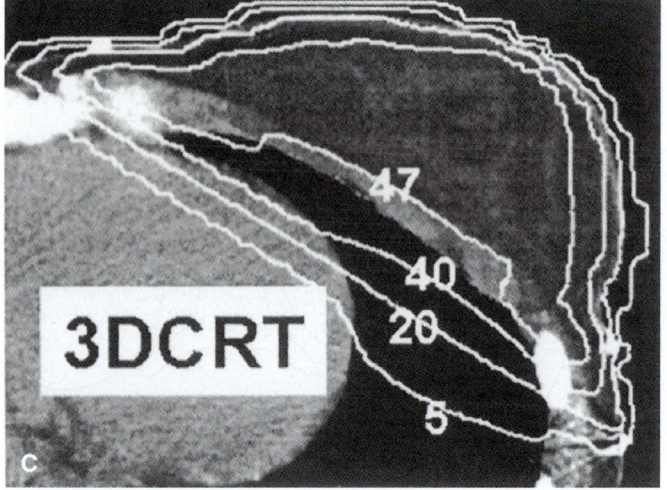

fibrosis, or persistent breast pain was noted. These authors concluded that the use of intensity modulation with a static MLC technique for tangential whole-breast RT is an efficient method for achieving a uniform and standardized dose throughout the whole breast, and widespread implementation of this technology can be achieved with minimal imposition on clinic resources and time constraints. As demonstrated in Figure 59.47, Dunst et al.[753] compared optimized IMRT with 3D-CRT and reported a small

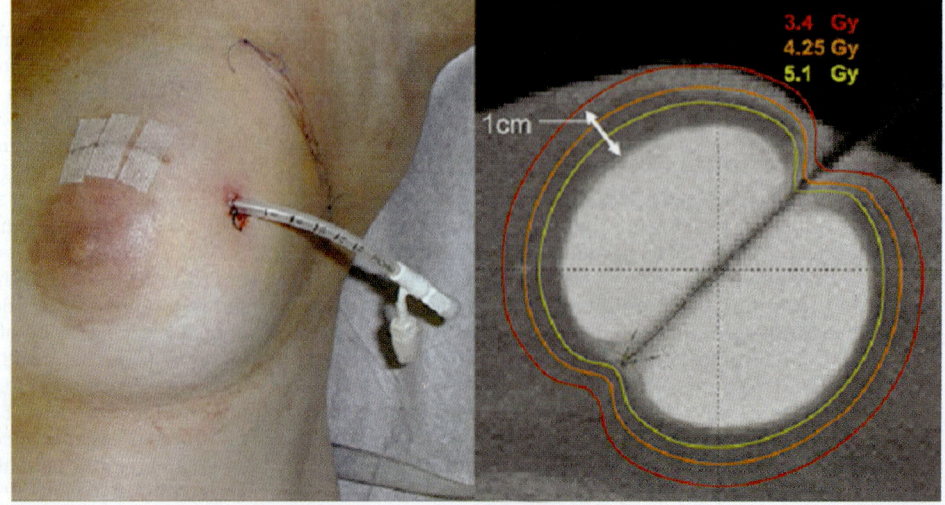

FIGURE 59.47. Partial breast irradiation demonstrating the MammoSite breast brachytherapy device. (From Arthur DW, Vicini FA. Accelerated partial breast irradiation as a part of breast conservation therapy. *J Clin Oncol* 2005;23[8]:1726–1735. Reprinted with permission. Copyright © 2005 American Society of Clinical Oncology. All rights reserved.)

reduction in does to the heart, lungs, and contralateral breast with IMRT.

In a trial of patients undergoing breast-conserving therapy, 358 patients undergoing whole-breast irradiation were randomized to radiation to the breast with standard wedges or with IMRT. Those randomized to IMRT experienced significantly lower degrees of moist desquamation due to the improved homogeneity with the IMRT techniques employed.[754,755] In another randomized trial of IMRT in breast cancer, 306 women were randomized to standard treatment with tangential fields with wedge compensators compared with IMRT. The standard control patients were 1.7 times more likely to have a change in photographic appearance compared with those in the IMRT arm.[756] Further follow-up and additional studies relating to the technical delivery of radiation therapy in early-stage breast cancer will evolve rapidly in the next several years because of the rapid advances in technology.

It is important to recognize that the term IMRT has been used in various ways to describe breast cancer treatment. In some studies, IMRT is described as a method of 3D dose compensation without a change in the gantry angles of pre-designed tangential fields. In such instances, dose distribution has been improved but the fields are not more conformal. Accordingly, low dose to other organs is not an issue. For others, IMRT attempts to improve conformality of the high-dose region by using multiple field angles that increase the volume of normal tissues that receive low radiation doses.

ACCELERATED PARTIAL BREAST IRRADIATION

The current standard of care for women with invasive breast cancer remains whole-breast irradiation following breast-conserving surgery.[757] With the notable exception of selected elderly women, omission of radiation therapy has now been proven in numerous randomized trials and meta-analysis to compromise local control and to a lesser extent breast cancer–related mortality. For some women, the 6-week course of daily radiation with its associated time and travel issues is not feasible. In response to this, a wide variety of accelerated forms of treatment have been developed and have been proven safe and effective in short-term studies.[671] These approaches include multicatheter interstitial implants placed around the excision cavity, a single balloon catheter that can be after loaded with a central radiation source (MammoSite) that is placed into the excision cavity, external beam conformal partial breast irradiation, and intraoperative single-dose

irradiation. Although these techniques vary considerably, they share the common strategy of delivering the radiation to a smaller volume of breast tissue around the lumpectomy site, using fewer larger fractions delivered over a shorter time. The rationale behind this approach is that the majority of breast relapses occur at or near the lumpectomy site. Pathologic studies from mastectomy specimens have demonstrated a lower probability of subclinical microscopic disease with increasing distance from the primary tumor.[100,106,219,296,390,671,758–760] Although the early results clearly demonstrate the feasibility and acceptable toxicity of APBI, this approach has not yet been demonstrated in a randomized trial to be equivalent to whole-breast irradiation. There are several randomized ongoing trials that will attempt to answer the question of whether this approach is equivalent to whole-breast irradiation for selected patients. The current NSABP-39/RTOG-0413 is well under way with high enrollment.[761] Although the mature results of this trial will not be available for several years, it should help to identify appropriate patients for this approach. Ongoing randomized trials investigating partial breast irradiation are summarized in Table 59.39. The NSABP-RTOG trial randomized 4,300 women with early-stage breast cancer (including DCIS) to whole-breast versus APBI. This trial allows for any one of the three techniques of partial breast irradiation, namely, interstitial brachytherapy, MammoSite, or 3D-CRT.[671] The techniques were selected based on physician or patient preference prior to randomization. Fraction size is slightly higher for the external beam conformal (3.85 Gy vs. 3.4 Gy), but all three employ twice daily radiation for a total of 10 treatments for a total dose of 38.5 or 34 Gy, respectively, over 5 days. Each of the various techniques of partial breast irradiation is discussed below.

Multicatheter Interstitial Techniques

Experience is greatest with the multicatherter interstitial technique, as it was initially developed (and is still employed) as a boost technique following whole-breast irradiation.[762–764] As demonstrated in Figure 59.48, multiple catheters are generally position at 1.0- to 1.5-cm intervals, with the total number of catheters and planes employed dependent on the size, extent, and shape of the target. With refinements in image-guided techniques, this approach is generally quite adaptable to most cavities and locations within the breast. Because of its complexity, user dependence, and logistics, however, the use of this technique has been less widely embraced, compared with the MammoSite (described below) and external beam techniques.

TABLE 59.39 RANDOMIZED TRIALS OF ACCELERATED PARTIAL BREAST IRRADIATION			
Institution/Trial	**Number of Cases**	**Control Arm**	**Experimental Arm**
NSABP B 39 RTOG 0413	3,000	50–50.4 Gy WB +/– 10–16 Gy boost	1. Interstitial Brachytx 2. MammoSite 3. 3D conformal EBRT
National Institute of Oncology Budapest, Hungary	570	50 Gy WB	1. Interstitial Brachytx (5.2 Gy × 7) or 2. Electrons (50 Gy)
European Brachytherapy GEC-ESTRO Working Group	1,170	50–50.4 Gy WB + 10 Gy boost	Brachytherapy only 32.0 Gy 8 fractions HDR 30.3 Gy 7 fractions HDR 50 Gy PDR
European Institute of Oncology(ELIOT)	824	50 Gy WB + 10 Gy boost	Intraoperative Single-fraction EBRT 21 Gy × 1
University College of London (TARGIT)	1,600	WBRT (per center) + boost	Intraoperative Single-fraction EBRT 5 Gy × 1
Canadian Trial (RAPID)	2,128	WBRT 42.5 in 16 or 50 in 25	3 CRT 38.5 Gy in 10
Medical Research Council-UK Import Low	1,935	WB 2.67 Gy × 15	PBI 2.67 Gy × 15

CRT, conformal radiation therapy; EBRT, external beam radiation therapy; HDR, high-dose rate; PBI, partial breast irradiation; PDR, pulsed-dose rate; WB, whole breast.

Section III

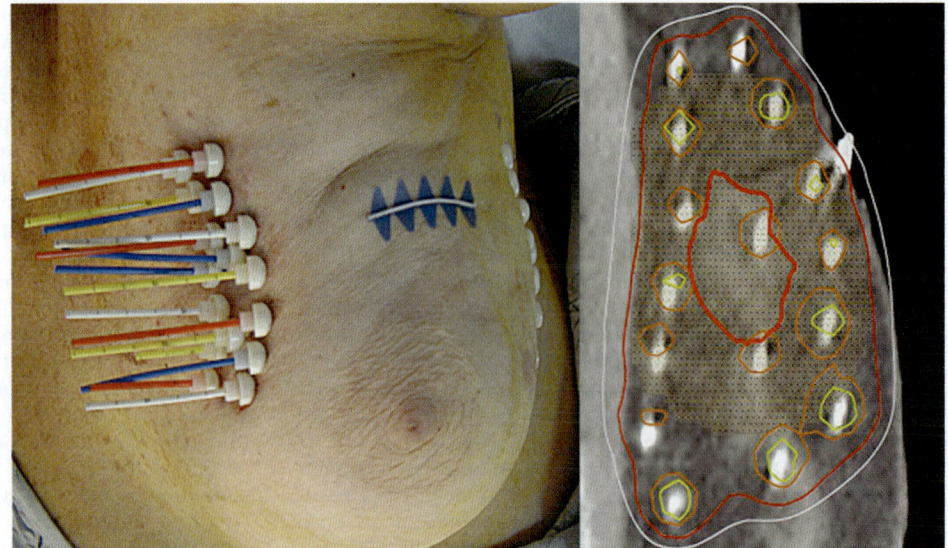

FIGURE 59.48. Partial breast irradiation demonstrating the multiplane interstitial implant technique. (From Arthur DW, Vicini FA. Accelerated partial breast irradiation as a part of breast conservation therapy. *J Clin Oncol* 2005;23[8]:1726–1735. Reprinted with permission. Copyright © 2005 American Society of Clinical Oncology. All rights reserved.)

Kuske et al.[765] recently reported the results of RTOG-95-17, a phase I and II study employing APBI using multiplane interstitial catheters in 99 women with early-stage breast cancer. The inclusion criteria for this study included invasive non-lobular tumors ≤3 cm after lumpectomy with negative surgical margins and axillary dissection with zero to three positive axillary nodes without ECE. The patients were treated with either low-dose-rate (LDR) APBI (45 Gy in 3.5 to 5 days) or high-dose-rate (HDR) APBI (34 Gy in 10 twice-daily fractions within 5 days). Chemotherapy and/or tamoxifen was administered at the discretion of the treating physicians. Of the 99 women, 33 were treated with LDR and 66 with HDR APBI. Of the 66 patients treated with HDR APBI, 2 (3%) had grade 3 or 4 toxicity. Of the 33 patients treated with LDR, 3 (9%) had grade 3 or 4 toxicity during brachytherapy. No patient experienced late grade 4 toxicity; the rate of grade 3 toxicity was 18% for the LDR and 4% for the HDR groups.

Vicini et al.[224] reported on 133 cases of early-stage breast cancer managed with lumpectomy and ALND followed by interstitial implant alone (99 cases using LDR and 34 with HDR implant) to the tumor bed, matched to a control group treated with external beam from the same institution. The number of catheters per patient ranged from 11 to 18 (median, 16). Tumor size ranged from 0.1 to 3 cm (median, 1.1 cm), with margins of excision >2 mm. Patients treated with LDR implants received 50 Gy over 96 hours as an inpatient procedure and those treated with HDR implants received 32 Gy in 8 fractions over 4 days (twice daily) as an outpatient procedure. The median follow-up for the external beam radiation therapy group was 5.7 years versus 3.2 years for brachytherapy. No local or regional failures have been detected and only one patient failed distantly in the HDR group. No significant adverse sequelae were noted, and cosmetic results were judged to be good or excellent in 98% of patients. No statistically significant differences were noted in the 5-year actuarial rates of ipsilateral breast (3% vs. 0%; *P* = .17) or locoregional failure (4% vs. 0%; *P* = .37) between patients treated with external beam radiation therapy and those treated with brachytherapy alone. In a recent update of this study with 12 years follow-up, there was no difference in the rate of local recurrence (3.8% vs. 5.0%; *P* = .40), regional recurrence (0% vs. 1.1%; *P* = .15), disease-free survival (87% vs. 91%; *P* = .30), cause-specific survival (93% vs. 95%; *P* = .28), or overall survival (78% vs. 71%; *P* = .06) between the WBI and APBI groups, respectively.[766]

Arthur et al.[767] used HDR brachytherapy (34 Gy in 10 fractions twice a day over 5 days) in 26 patients or LDR (45 Gy given at a dose rate of 0.45 to 0.50 Gy/hour) in 18 patients. After a median follow-up of 31 months (range, 11 to 61 months), all patients remain locally controlled. Among patients receiving doxorubicin after brachytherapy, at a median follow-up of 12 months, recall reactions involving the skin overlying the implant site were observed in 42% of patients (6 of 14). On multivariate analysis, a recall reaction (*P* = .0007) and LDR brachytherapy (*P* = .04) were significant predictors of fibrosis and telangiectasis.

Wazer et al.[768] reported the results of APBI using high-dose-rate interstitial brachytherapy in a phase I or II single multi-institutional study in 33 women with early-stage breast cancer. Eligible patients included those with T1, T2, N0, N1 (≤3 nodes positive), and M0 tumors of nonlobular histologic features with negative surgical margins, no extracapsular lymph node extension, and a negative postexcision mammogram. High-activity ^{192}Ir (3 to 10 Ci) was used to deliver 3.4 Gy per fraction, 2 fractions per day, for 5 consecutive days, to a total dose of 34 Gy to the target volume. The mean tumor size was 1.3 cm, and 55% had an extensive intraductal component. Three patients had positive axillary nodes. The RTOG late radiation morbidity scoring scheme was applied. Clinically evident fat necrosis occurred in eight patients at a median of 7.5 months after HDR brachytherapy completion. The only variables significantly associated with grade 3 or 4 toxicity were the number of source dwell positions and the volume of tissue encompassed by the prescription isodose shell. The global cosmetic scores after a minimum of 18 months' follow-up were 0 cases with poor, 4 with fair, 5 with good, and 24 with excellent scores. One case of IBTR was diagnosed.

MAMMOSITE

MammoSite as an alternative method of delivering APBI has been widely embraced because of its simplicity and less dependence on user experience.[350,671,769,770] The technique employs a single balloon catheter introduced into the lumpectomy site either at the time of lumpectomy or percutaneously after the procedure. In the current NSABP/RTOG clinical trial, patients cannot be randomized until after the lumpectomy procedure when final margins and nodal status are known, and hence, the device must be placed after the lumpectomy procedure. As shown in Figure 59.48, the catheter is located centrally within a distal balloon, which is inflated once the catheter is placed in the lumpectomy cavity. Adequacy of placement requires symmetry of the balloon, conformance of the balloon surface to the lumpectomy cavity, and a minimum distance between the surface of the balloon and skin of >5 mm (ideally >7 mm). Treatment is delivered via a HDR remote afterloading system to a circumferential 1-cm distance from the balloon surface. This technique is one of the three methods employed in the ongoing randomized trial, with a dose prescription of 3.4 Gy delivered at 1 cm twice daily to a total dose of 34 Gy over 5 days.

Although early experiences with this technique are promising, the results of the ongoing randomized trial will help to identify suitable patients. The most extensive experience with this technique has been reported by the American Society of Breast Surgeons MammoSite Registry Trial, which included 1,419 patients treated in 87 institutions.[350,771,772] This was a nonrandomized single-arm registration trial in which data were collected prospectively on clinical use of the MammoSite breast brachytherapy catheter for delivering breast irradiation. They reported on 1,237 patients (87% of enrolled patients) who received APBI (34 Gy to 1.0 cm in 10 fractions; 91% of the patients with invasive carcinoma (977 of 1,068 patients) had negative lymph node status, and 99% of all patients had negative margins. The median patient age was 65 years. Five hundred fifty-four catheters (45%) were placed with an open cavity at the time of lumpectomy, and 683 catheters (55%) were placed after lumpectomy. Skin spacing ranged from 2 to 75 mm (median, 10 mm). At 5 years, 37 cases (2.6%) developed an IBTR, for a 5-year actuarial rate of 3.80% (3.86% for IBC and 3.39% for DCIS). Negative ER status ($P = .0011$) was the only clinical, pathologic, or treatment-related variable associated with IBTR for patients with IBC and young age (<50 years; $P = .0096$) and positive margin status ($P = .0126$) in those with DCIS. The percentage of breasts with good or excellent cosmetic results at 60 months ($n = 371$) was 90.6%. The authors concluded that treatment efficacy, cosmesis, and toxicity 5 years after treatment with APBI using the MammoSite device are good and similar to those reported with other forms of APBI with similar follow-up.

External Beam Conformal Radiation

Although external beam conformal radiation has been developed only recently, it is the one that is most widely employed in the ongoing randomized trial.[214,773,774] Recent data suggest that over 70% of patients in the randomized trial are opting for the 3D-CRT. Its widespread acceptance is likely because it is totally noninvasive and delivers a homogenous dose distribution. Although the ongoing trial mandates supine position, some authors have advocated prone accelerated breast irradiation.[214,773,774]

Three-dimensional-CRT, as shown in Figure 59.49, generally employs multiple conformal fields, although plans as simple as two opposing small conformal fields may be adequate. Challenges with this technique include daily positioning of the target, movement with breathing, and delivery of higher doses to surrounding normal breast tissue than with the brachytherapy. Nonetheless, this approach has been widely embraced and has been shown to be reproducible. In the phase I and II RTOG-0319 trial of external beam conformal radiation, Vicini et al.[774] examined the use of 3D-CRT to deliver APBI. Reproducibility, as measured by technical feasibility, was the primary endpoint. This study was designed such that if fewer than 5 cases in the first 42 patients evaluable were scored as unacceptable, the treatment would be considered reproducible. Patients received 38.5 Gy in 3.85 Gy per fraction delivered twice daily. The clinical target volume included the lumpectomy cavity plus a 10- to 15-mm margin bounded by 5 mm within the skin surface and the lung–chest wall interface. The planning target volume included the clinical target volume plus a 10-mm margin. A total of 58 patients were enrolled on this study over an 8-month period, 5 of whom were ineligible or did not receive protocol treatment. There were 4 cases with major variations and a total of 32 cases with minor variations in treatment plans. Based on this analysis, the authors concluded that APBI using 3D conformal external beam radiation therapy was technically feasible and reproducible in a multi-institutional trial using exceptionally strict dosimetric criteria. An update of this study found that the ipsilateral breast failure rate was 6%, in-field failure rate was 2%, and contralateral breast failure rate was 0%.[775] Only two (4%) grade 3 toxicities were observed. There have, however, been some reports of increased toxicity with external beam radiation using the fractionation schedule of 3.85 Gy per fraction, twice daily for 10 fractions.[776,777] Longer follow-up and detailed outcomes from the NSABP/RTOG randomized trial will help to shed further light on this issue.

Olivotto et al. published a report of the RAPID (Randomized Trial of Accelerated Partial Breast Irradiation Using Three-Dimensional Conformal External Beam Radiation Therapy) trial where 2,135 women age >40 years with invasive or *in situ* breast cancer ≤3 cm were randomly assigned after breast-conserving surgery to 3D-CRT APBI (38.5 Gy in 10 fractions twice daily) or WBI (42.5 Gy in 16 or 50 Gy in 25 daily fractions ± boost irradiation)[778]. With a secondary endpoint of cosmesis, they reported adverse cosmesis at 3 years was increased among those treated with APBI compared with WBI as assessed by trained nurses (29% vs. 17%; $P < .001$), by patients (26% vs. 18%; $P = .0022$), and by physicians reviewing digital photographs (35% vs. 17%; $P < .001$). They found that

FIGURE 59.49. A and **B:** Partial breast irradiation demonstrating the external beam conformal radiation technique.

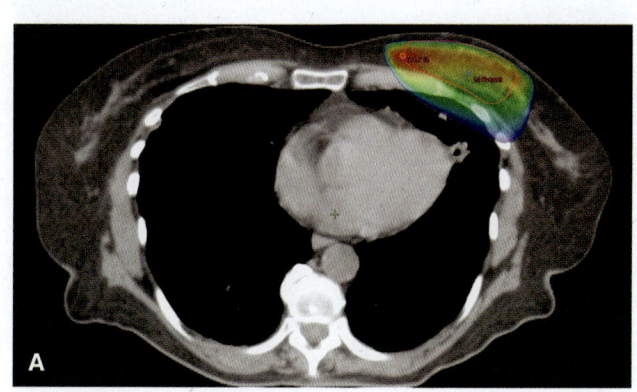

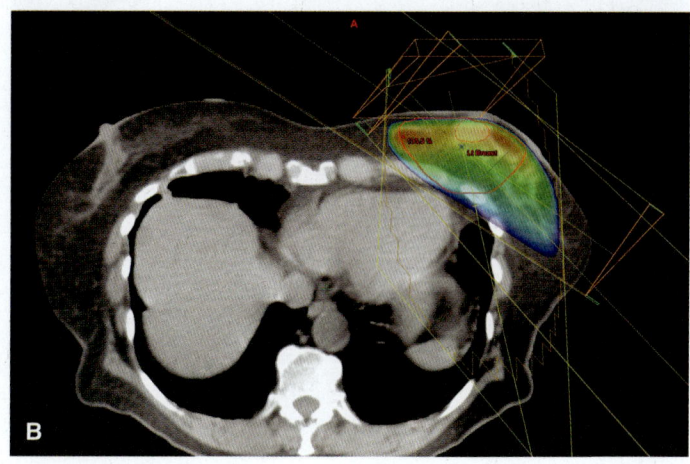

there was an adverse effect of the fractionation from APBI and boost irradiation from WBI on cosmesis.

Again, the NSABP/RTOG randomized trial will help to further define acceptability and reproducibility of 3D conformal external beam radiation as an option for women with early-stage invasive breast cancer.

Intraoperative Accelerated Partial Breast Irradiation

APBI using intraoperative therapy has been most widely employed outside of the United States.[779,780] The radiation is delivered in a single intraoperative dose to the lumpectomy site at the time of surgery, using intraoperative electrons or intraoperative photons (Fig. 59.50). Vaidya et al.[781] describe a preliminary report using a 50 kV spherical source to deliver a dose of 20 Gy at a depth of 1 cm, with acceptable toxicity. This group recently published the results of a phase III study that randomized 3,451 women to either targeted intraoperative radiation therapy (IORT) or whole-breast irradiation.[782] The 5-year risks for local recurrence in the conserved breast for IORT versus EBRT were 3·3% (95% CI 2.1–5.1) versus 1·3% (0.7–2.5; $P = 0·042$). Veronesi et al.[779] developed an IORT technique for a breast quadrant after the removal of the primary carcinoma using a mobile linear accelerator with a robotic arm to deliver electron beams with energies from 3 to 9 MeV.

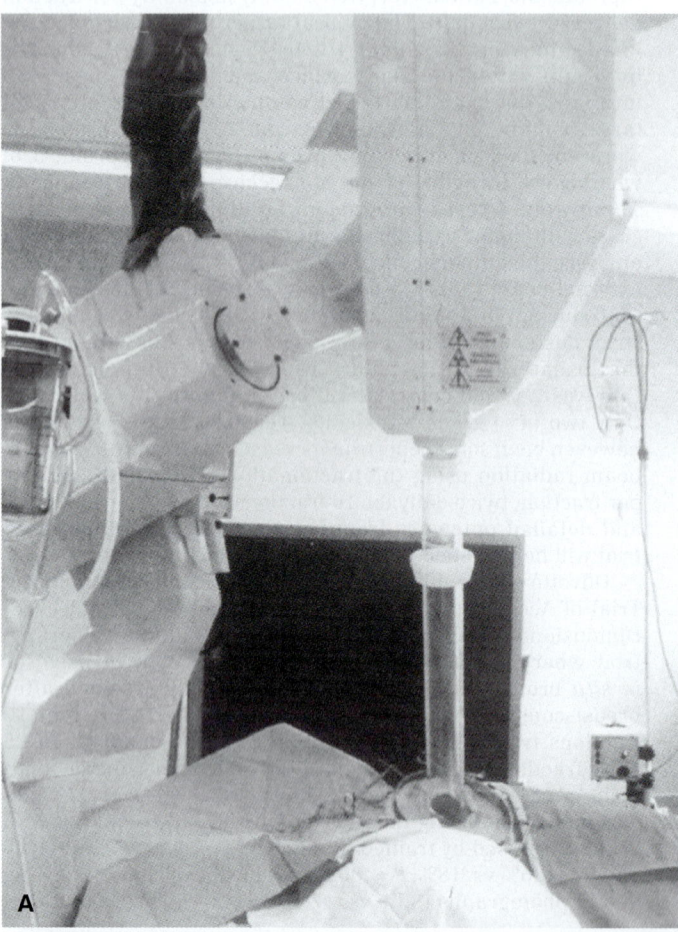

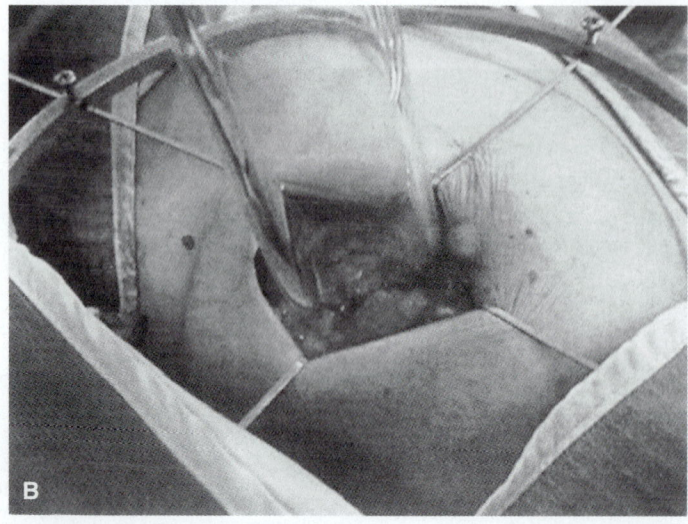

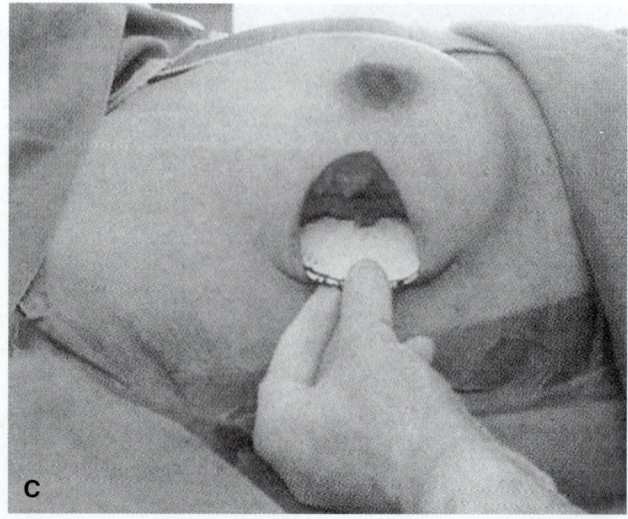

FIGURE 59.50. A: Linear electron beam accelerator in operating room during intraoperative radiation therapy. **B:** Proper placement of applicator in the breast. **C:** Before intraoperative radiation therapy delivery, an aluminum-lead disc (4 mm Al and 5 mm Pb thick) is placed between the deep face of residual breast and pectoralis muscle. (Reprinted from Veronesi U, Oreechia R, Luini A, et al. A preliminary report on intraoperative radiotherapy (IORT) in limited-stage breast cancers that are conservatively treated. *Eur J Cancer* 2001;37[17]:2178–2183. Copyright © 2001 Elsevier. With permission.)

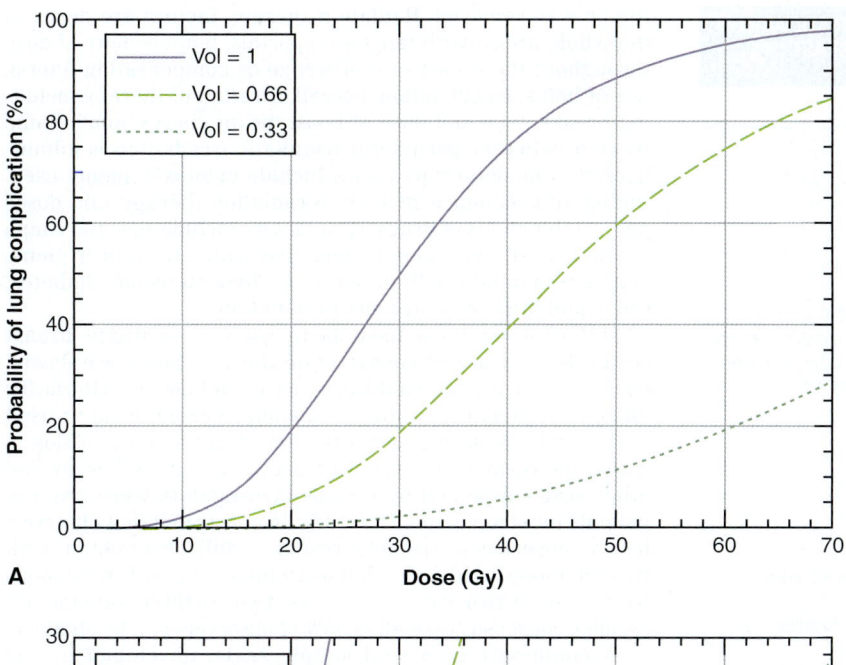

A

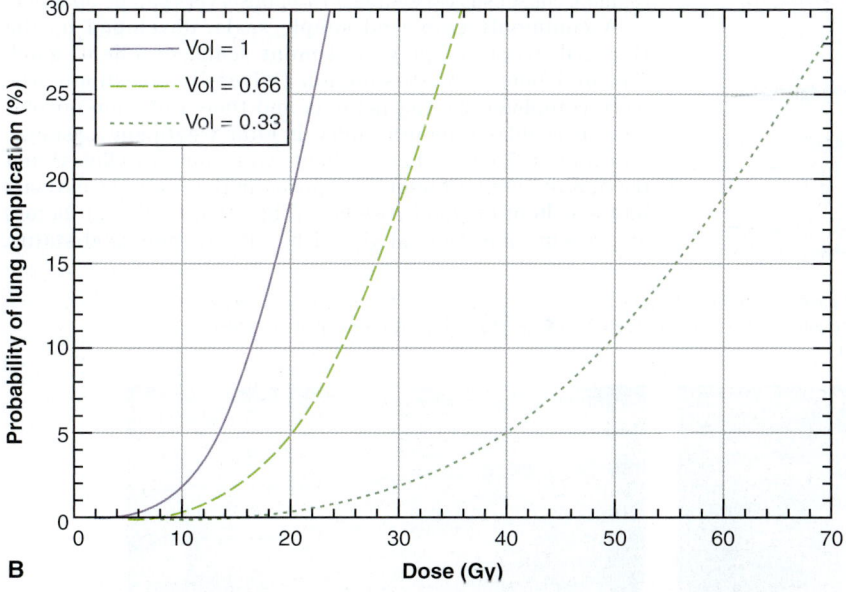

B

FIGURE 59.51. Probability of radiation pneumonitis versus dose. The relative lung volumes are 100%, 66%, and 33%. The curve parameters are $D_{50} = 30$ Gy, $\gamma = 1.01$, $s = 0.01$. The curve covers the probability range up to 100% **(A)**, and up to 30% (i.e., within the interval of the clinical data) **(B)**. (Reprinted from Gagliardi G, Bjohle J, Lax I, et al. Radiation pneumonitis after breast cancer irradiation: analysis of the complication probability using the relative seriality model. *Int J Radiat Oncol Biol Phys* 2000;46[2]:373–381. Copyright © 2000 Elsevier. With permission.)

Through a Perspex applicator, the radiation is delivered directly to the mammary gland, and to spare the skin from radiation, the skin margins are stretched out of the radiation field (Fig. 59.51A and B). To protect the thoracic wall, an aluminum–lead disc is placed between the gland and the pectoralis muscle (see Fig. 59.50C). Different dose levels were tested from 10 to 21 Gy without important side effects. They estimated that a single fraction of 21 Gy is equivalent to 60 Gy delivered in 30 fractions at 2 Gy per fraction. Seventeen patients received an IORT dose of 10 to 15 Gy as a boost to external radiation therapy, whereas 86 patients received 17, 19, or 21 Gy intraoperatively as their whole treatment. The follow-up time of the 101 patients ranged from 1 to 17 months (mean, 8 months). The IORT treatment was very well accepted by all patients. The authors believe that single-dose IORT after breast resection for small mammary carcinomas may be an excellent alternative to the traditional postoperative radiation therapy. Based on these data, the European Institute of Oncology has conducted a randomized trial comparing this option to whole-breast irradiation for selected patients, and results of this trial are eagerly awaited.[780]

In 2009, a task force of experts in the field of breast cancer developed a consensus statement on behalf of ASTRO on the use of APBI. These guidelines have since been updated in 2016. They reported their recommendations on the suitability of patients receiving APBI outside the context of a clinical trial and divided patients into three categories: suitable, cautionary, and unsuitable (Table 59.40).[783–785] In general, patients ≥50 years, with node-negative, invasive ductal or DCIS tumors ≤2 cm and with negative margins, ER positivity, and no lymphovascular space involvement were deemed suitable for use of APBI off trial. The task force hoped their recommendations would provide guidance regarding the use of APBI outside a clinical trial and serve as a framework to promote additional research into the optimal role of APBI in the treatment of breast cancer.

COSMETIC OUTCOMES AND SEQUELAE

Cosmesis

Surgical, radiotherapeutic, chemotherapeutic, and host factors may influence cosmetic outcome.[351] Surgical factors to be considered include extent of surgical resection, re-excision, orientation and length of the scar, closure or not of the tylectomy cavity, separate or continuous axilla–tylectomy scars, extent of the axillary dissection, and whether an ellipse of skin over the

TABLE 59.40 ASTRO CONSENSUS GUIDELINES FOR SUITABILITY OF PATIENTS TO RECEIVE ACCELERATED PARTIAL BREAST IRRADIATION (APBI) OFF TRIAL

Patient Group	Risk Factor	Factor
Suitability	Age	≥50 y
	Margins	Negative by at least 2 mm
	T stage	Tis or T1
	DCIS	If all of the below:
		Screen-detected
		• Low to intermediate nuclear grade
		• Size ≤2.5 cm
		• Resected with margins negative at ≥3 mm
Cautionary	Age	• 40–49 y if all other criteria for "suitable" are met
		• ≥50 y if patient has at least 1 of the pathologic factors below and does not have any "unsuitable" factors
		• *Pathologic factors:*
		• Size 2.1–3.0 cm[a]
		• T2
		• Close margins (<2 mm)
		• Limited/focal LVSI
		• ER(-)
		• Clinically unifocal with total size 2.1-3.0 cm[b]
		• Invasive lobular histology
		• Pure DCIS ≤3 cm if criteria for "suitable" not fully met
		• EIC ≤3 cm
	Margins	Close (<2 mm)
	DCIS	≤3 cm and does not meet criteria for "suitable"
Unsuitable	Age	• <40 y
		• 40–49 y and do not meet the criteria for cautionary
	Margins	Positive
	DCIS	>3 cm

APBI, accelerated partial breast irradiation; DCIS, ductal carcinoma *in situ*; EIC, extensive intraductal carcinoma; ER, estrogen receptor; LVSI, lymphovascular space involvement; T, tumor stage.

tumor was removed. Radiation therapy factors are doses to the whole breast with tangential portals, homogeneity of dose throughout the breast (use of wedge or compensating filters), use of bolus, fractionation, overall duration of therapy including breaks, type and dose of boost, beam energy, and volume treated (whether peripheral lymphatic irradiation is administered). Chemotherapy issues include cytotoxic agents used, timing and sequence relative to radiation therapy, and doses and combinations of drugs. Host factors include size and shape of the breast, age, race, compliance with care and hygiene, concurrent medical illnesses (e.g., hypertension, diabetes, CVD), and intrinsic sensitivity to radiation.

Different methods have been used to evaluate breast cosmesis after breast conservation therapy. Some are flawed because they do not establish strict guidelines or criteria for objectively judging cosmetic outcome. Pezner et al.[786] used scales and standard procedures for obtaining color slides to assess the cosmetic results of breast conservation therapy and other scales designed by various investigators were given to patients for comparison. The study demonstrated that observer-based consensus of cosmetic results is difficult to obtain with two commonly used scales, but by changing the scale gradations from four to two (zero to one vs. two to three satisfactory results), consensus exceeding 85% of observers can be obtained.

A commonly employed simple scale, developed by the Harvard group, employs a 4-point scale: excellent, good, fair, and poor.[787] At Washington University, questionnaires were completed by 458 patients and their radiation oncologists at regular 6-month intervals after treatment. Cosmetic outcome analysis of these patients was done for clinical and treatment-related factors.[351] Approximately 80% of patients had excellent or good cosmesis (Fig. 59.52). Clinical factors at presentation were analyzed by age, menopausal status,

FIGURE 59.52. A–D: Photographs of patients showing excellent cosmetic results obtained with conservation surgery and irradiation for patients with T1 and T2 carcinomas of the breast. The patient in **C** has minimal telangiectasia in the area treated with a boost (upper region of left breast).

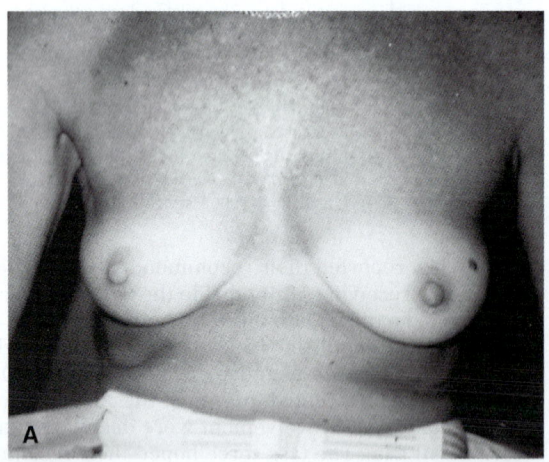

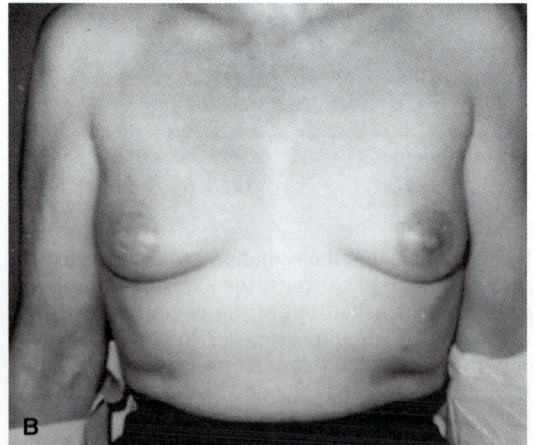

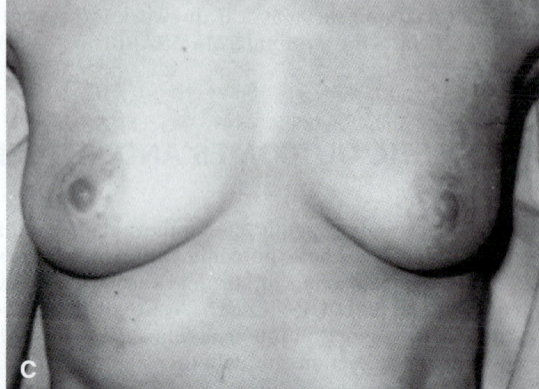

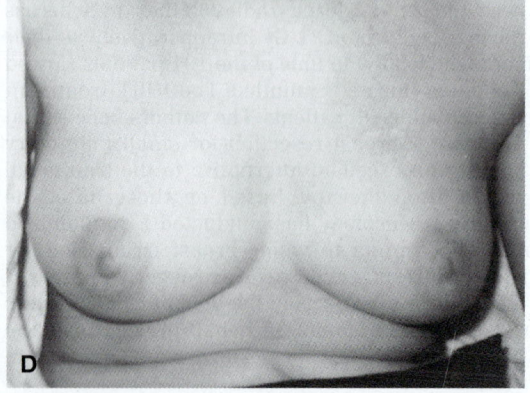

race, and tumor-related parameters of size, palpable status, and location. Patients older than 60 years of age had lower excellent cosmetic scores compared with patients 60 years of age or younger. Tumor size significantly influenced cosmetic outcome, most likely related to the volume of breast removed and perhaps boost dose. Cosmetic outcome by race indicated 40% of whites had an excellent cosmetic rating, compared with only 18% for African Americans. Thirty percent of African American patients received concurrent chemotherapy or hormonal therapy with irradiation, compared with 23% of white patients. Of African American patients, 14% were obese, 17% were hypertensive, 25% had both obesity and hypertension, and 4% had diabetes.

Poorer cosmetic outcomes in African American women have also been reported by Pierce et al.[490] and Tuomokumo and Haffty.[299] In the study by Tuomokomo and Haffty,[299] a detailed cosmetic analysis was performed on a subset of 20 African American patients and 20 white patients from the Yale database. The two groups were intentionally matched by age, follow-up, adjuvant therapy, and breast size and were asked to participate in a detailed cosmetic evaluation. With respect to overall cosmetic outcome and all specific cosmetic measures (edema, fibrosis, and pigmentation), African American patients fared more poorly than did white patients. Overall cosmesis was good to excellent in 55% of African Americans, compared with 90% of whites.

Cosmesis may be affected by multiple breast and axillary surgical factors.[351] The type of breast surgery is important, with patients undergoing excisional biopsy having the highest rate of excellent cosmesis (56%) compared with wide excision (35%) or quadrantectomy (13%; $P = .0001$). Scar orientation compliance with NSABP guidelines was a significant factor, with a 44% excellent cosmetic rating compared with 27% for patients with noncompliant scar orientations ($P = .0034$). Re-excision of the primary site also resulted in a lower rate of excellent cosmesis ($P = .0002$). Breast tissue resection of >100 cm^3 was associated with lower rates of excellent or good cosmesis, independent of breast size ($P = .0001$). Similarly, a resected skin area of >20 cm^2 was correlated with a lower excellent cosmetic result ($P = .045$). Extent of axillary surgery did not significantly affect breast cosmesis.

Radiation factors affecting cosmesis included treatment volume (tangential breast fields only vs. three fields or more; $P = .034$), whole-breast dose >50 Gy ($P = .024$), total dose to the tumor site >65 Gy ($P = .06$), and optimum dose distribution created with use of compensating filters. Daily fraction size of 1.8 Gy versus 2 Gy, boost versus no boost, type of boost (brachytherapy vs. electrons), total irradiation dose, and use of bolus were not significant factors. Vrieling et al.[486] published a report of the randomized EORTC trial in which 5,318 women with early-stage breast cancer after tumorectomy were randomized to a boost of 16 Gy to the tumor bed or no further treatment. Patients with microscopically incomplete excision were randomized to receive a boost of 10 Gy or 25 or 26 Gy with interstitial implant or external beam radiation. Cosmetic results at 3 years were assessed in 731 women (364 with boost, 367 without boost) using digitizer measurements, and displacement of the nipple cosmesis in the boost group was excellent in 33%, good in 38%, fair in 26%, and poor in 3%. In the no-boost group, the results were 42%, 44%, 13%, and 1%, respectively. The position of the nipple was the only moderately representative parameter of the overall cosmetic outcome. Other measurements had no significant correlation with cosmesis. A global assessment of the appearance of the breast was thought to be a reliable method to assess cosmetic results. Factors associated with worse cosmesis were inferior tumor location, large excision volume, presence of postoperative complications, and radiation therapy boost.

TABLE 59.41 IMPACT OF ADJUVANT CHEMOTHERAPY ON COSMESIS IN BREAST CONSERVATION THERAPY

Institution (Reference)	Chemotherapy	Good to Excellent Cosmesis (%)	
		Radiation Therapy without Chemotherapy	Radiation Therapy with Chemotherapy
Harvard University[788]	CMF, A	92	67
Palo Alto[325]	CMF	88	73
National Cancer Institute[789]	AC	80	70
University of Pennsylvania[569]	CMF ± P	89	81
Washington University[351]	CMF	81	78

A, doxorubicin; AC, doxorubicin, cyclophosphamide; CMF, cyclophosphamide, methotrexate, 5-fluorouracil; P, prednisone.

Impact of Adjuvant Chemotherapy on Cosmesis

Adjuvant chemotherapy may have a deleterious influence on excellent to good cosmetic results (Table 59.41).[325,351,787,788,790] In several studies, the main effect was a switch from "excellent" results to the "good" category. In particular, concomitant administration of chemotherapy and irradiation appears to have a more pronounced affect on cosmesis. The majority of studies using concurrent chemotherapy, however, employed agents that are no longer routinely employed.

Rose et al.[787] reported on the Harvard cosmesis data and found that 68% of women not receiving chemotherapy had an excellent result at 3 years, compared with 37% who did receive chemotherapy. Conversely, 9% of patients who did not receive chemotherapy were judged to have fair or poor cosmetic results, compared with 24% of those who received chemotherapy. These differences were mostly the result of an increase in breast retraction and, to a lesser extent, development of telangiectasia.

Taylor et al.[351] also reported impaired cosmetic outcome with concurrent administration of chemoirradiation. Excellent cosmetic outcome was observed in 43% of patients receiving sequential chemotherapy, in 25% receiving concomitant chemoirradiation, and in 41% receiving no adjuvant therapy ($P = .02$). The specific effect of methotrexate on cosmetic outcome was evaluated, and the proportion of excellent cosmetic outcomes with methotrexate omitted was 41% versus 16% with methotrexate included. Good results were obtained in 23% versus 58%, fair results in 23% versus 26%, and poor results in 12% versus 0%, respectively ($P = .14$). Similarly, studies by Markiewicz et al.[569,790] and Danoff et al.[789] report no compromise of cosmesis in patients receiving concurrent chemoradiation if methotrexate was held during the radiation.

In a randomized trial of concurrent versus sequential radiation therapy, using fluorouracil, Cytoxan, and mitoxantrone, Rouesse et al.[570] also reported comparable and acceptable cosmetic outcomes, whether patients were treated with sequential or concurrent chemotherapy.

Breast Cosmetic Surgery after Irradiation

Breast deformities after conservation therapy may represent difficult reconstructive problems.[791] Correction of a locally damaged breast is a surgical challenge that can result in a fully restored breast if selection of the surgical procedure is properly carried out. In 37 patients who underwent correction of deformities after breast conservation surgery, which included simple submuscular placement of traditional or expandable implants, breast reshaping, transposition of a latissimus dorsi muscle or musculocutaneous flap, transverse rectus abdominis muscle flap, and reverse abdominoplasty, aesthetic outcome was judged to be good or excellent in 78% of patients.

When partial mastectomy, a term that encompasses a diversity of excisional techniques, follows radiation therapy, breast defects characterized by parenchymal loss, nipple–areola complex distortion, and cutaneous abnormalities can occur. Slavin et al.[792] reported on eight patients who had reconstructive correction of an irradiated partial mastectomy deformity. Mammograms were obtained before and after the myocutaneous flap procedure. Six patients had reconstructions with latissimus dorsi flaps and two with rectus flaps. No patient underwent reconstruction sooner than 1 year after completion of radiation therapy for the entire group; a mean of 2.6 years elapsed from completion of radiation therapy to flap reconstruction of the breast. An aesthetic improvement of the partial mastectomy deformity was achieved in all eight patients. Complications consisted only of seroma formation in two patients after latissimus flap reconstruction. Mammographic evaluation revealed degeneration of the soft tissues of both types of flaps, a change that occurs as early as 6 months after operation and appears as a radiolucent area.

In a review of the MD Anderson Cancer Center experience, Kronowitz et al.[793] evaluated results of 69 patients who underwent repair of a partial mastectomy defect after radiation. They concluded that immediate repair of partial mastectomy defects with local tissues results in a lower risk of complications and better aesthetic outcomes than does immediate repair of partial mastectomy defects with a latissimus dorsi flap.

Follow-Up of Patients Treated with Breast Conservation Surgery and Irradiation

It is important to closely monitor patients treated with conservation surgery and irradiation because early detection of a local recurrence may allow for another wide local excision or a total mastectomy, without significantly compromising the overall survival of the patient.[106,219,758,794-797] Although the optimal interval for follow-up mammography has not been determined, a postradiation bilateral diagnostic mammogram should be obtained within the first year following radiation therapy.[158,798-800]

A careful history and physical examination are indicated every 3 to 6 months for 3 years and every 6 months for the following 2 years and annually thereafter. In patients who underwent breast conservation therapy, a diagnostic mammogram within 3 to 6 months postradiation therapy and then annually thereafter is sufficient unless the radiologist recommends more frequent examinations.[158,799,800] Monthly breast self-examination should be emphasized to every patient, including demonstration of the examination in the upright and supine positions. At least yearly evaluation is mandatory even 10 years after therapy because of the possibility of late breast relapses and occasional distant metastases. According to the American Society of Clinical Oncology's surveillance guidelines, intensive follow-up should be limited to high-risk patients with breast cancer, especially those who enter randomized clinical trials.[801]

If there is strong evidence of suspect microcalcifications, masses, or architectural distortions of the breast after conservation surgery and irradiation, a biopsy should be obtained to rule out a recurrence. At times, these patients are difficult to evaluate. Posttreatment hematomas, fat necrosis, seromas, cysts, and scar tissue pose frequent dilemmas. Consultation with an experienced mammographer is essential.

Kollias et al.[802] in the United Kingdom evaluated 5,102 contralateral screening mammograms performed biennially on 2,511 women aged ≤70 years after treatment for primary operable breast cancer. Sixty-five metachronous contralateral breast cancers were identified: 21 (32%) at routine clinical examination, 24 (37%) at mammography, and 20 (31%) by patients between routine follow-up appointments. The prognostic features of metachronous cancers were better than or similar to those of the first cancer in 59 of 65 (91%)

cases. Mammography may have contributed to the long-term survival of 16 of 26 women in whom the histologic characteristics of the first cancer predicted a good prognosis. The cancer detection rate with mammography for these women was 6.5 per 1,000 contralateral mammograms at a cost of 3,852 pounds sterling (6,108 dollars) per cancer detected, suggesting that surveillance mammography of the contralateral breast is of value in women whose first cancer predicted a favorable prognosis.

Kramer et al.[803] assessed the efficacy of contrast-enhanced dynamic MRI compared with palpation, mammography, and ultrasonography in 33 patients after breast conservation therapy. The sensitivities for the diagnosis of local recurrences were 51% for palpation, 67% for mammography, 85% for ultrasonography, and 91% for MRI. All multicentric local recurrences were diagnosed by MRI. Mammography did not diagnose 11 local recurrences in radiodense breast, and ultrasonography was able to diagnose 8 of the 11, whereas MRI diagnosed 10 of the 11 recurrences. MRI may be useful as a complement to mammography and ultrasonography in the radiodense breast.[799]

It is important to define the cost–benefit ratio of follow-up procedures. In a controlled trial in Italy, 655 women were randomly assigned to be monitored with an intensive surveillance program including physician visits, bone scan, liver ultrasonography, chest radiography, and laboratory tests after initial treatment for breast cancer.[804] A control group of 665 women was monitored by their physicians with physical examination and only the clinically indicated tests. Both groups received a yearly mammogram. Compliance in both protocols was more than 80%. With a median follow-up of 71 months, there was no difference in overall survival between the two groups. There were 132 deaths (20%) in the intensive surveillance group and 122 deaths (18%) in the control group. Time to detection of recurrence and parameters related to quality of life were similar in both groups. Therefore, unnecessary tests are discouraged in the follow-up of patients treated for breast cancer.

Radiographic Findings after Breast Conservation Therapy

Dershaw[158] summarized the most frequent mammographic findings: parenchymal distortion and fibrosis at the tumor excision site (secondary to surgical scar and irradiation); skin thickening, seen in 90% of patients, which may be diffuse or more prominent at the surgical excision site; and calcifications, due to fat necrosis, which are coarse and round and have radiolucent centers. Dershaw et al.[800] retrospectively reviewed the mammograms of 22 patients with local tumor recurrence that were usually associated with 10 or more calcifications (17 patients, 77%). Recurrences commonly contained very suspect patterns of calcification, with linear forms in 15 cases (68%) and pleomorphic forms in 17 cases (77%). The distribution of calcifications was usually clustered (73%, 16 of 22) or segmental (18%, 4 of 22). Recurrences were characterized as obviously malignant in 77% of cases. The remainder were indeterminate, requiring biopsy. Therefore, women without worrisome mammographic patterns need not undergo breast biopsy. If the findings are stable, mammographic follow-up is sufficient. However, a change in number or characteristic pattern warrants a biopsy to rule out recurrent tumor. Mammographic findings were correlated with clinical observations in several studies.[387,709,712,758,796,799,805-807] Most changes are observed in the first 12 months after therapy, with stabilization achieved at 12 to 36 months after completion of therapy. Breast edema is mammographically present in virtually all patients at completion of therapy, with a steady increase over 36 months and stabilization by 42 months.

Tian et al. longitudinally compare the incidence of common mammographic sequelae seen after breast-conserving surgery and RT in patients treated with APBI, hypofractionated whole-breast irradiation (HWBI), and conventionally fractionated WBI[808]. In their cohort of 89 patients, 29 had received APBI, 30 had received HWBI, and 30 had received WBI. A total of 605 mammograms were evaluated, with a median follow-up of 48 months. The fractionation scheme did not affect the severity of architectural distortion when the groups were evaluated longitudinally. The likelihood of finding skin thickening decreased with increasing follow-up duration (OR 0.6; $P < .001$) adjusted for fractionation schemes. No differences were seen with respect to changes in skin thickening, fluid collections, or calcifications among the treatment groups, after adjustment for the follow-up time. The clinical characteristics, including age, race, T stage, and chemotherapy use, were not linked to the likelihood of finding several mammographic phenomena over time. The authors concluded that fractionation did not alter the relative incidence or severity of architectural distortion, skin thickening, fluid collections, or calcifications.

Pretreatment and posttreatment mammograms were reviewed in 103 patients undergoing conservation therapy.[809] The main posttreatment findings were a diffuse increase in parenchymal density with coarse stromal pattern, some parenchymal distortion, and thickening of the skin. Changes reached a peak at 9 months and slowly resolved over the next 2 years. At 31 to 33 months, 3 of 15 patients still had dense parenchyma and 6 had skin thickening. Sixty-nine patients had fibroadenosis. Scar with retraction in the surgical area was observed on the mammograms of 71 patients. Fat necrosis was noted in two patients. During the 3-year follow-up, recurrent cancer was noted in two treated breasts, and contralateral breast cancer developed in three women.

Orel et al.[810] reported on 1,145 women with early breast cancer treated with lumpectomy and irradiation. One hundred two women with various mammographic and clinical findings later required biopsy at the treated site, and 58 had two sets of mammograms available for review (one within 3 months of the biopsy). Recurring cancer was documented in 38 (66%) of 58 patients. Thirteen (34%) of the recurrences were detected solely with mammography, and eight others were detected both mammographically and clinically. The positive predictive value for mammographic abnormalities was 72% (76% for soft tissue microcalcifications and 62% for other findings). Twenty-one recurrences (55%) were within the lumpectomy quadrant. Within the lumpectomy site, sensitivity was substantially better for physical examination (71%) than for mammography (43%). In the remaining breast outside the lumpectomy quadrant, mammography had a significantly higher sensitivity (71%) and positive predictive value (86%). The most common posttreatment findings reported by Orel et al.[810,811] and Stomper et al.[812] were calcifications alone (48%) or with a mass (29%), distortion of the breast parenchyma (20%), and inflammatory thickening of the breast skin.

Stomper et al.[812] reported on 50 of 1,600 patients with stage I or II invasive breast cancer treated with conservation surgery and irradiation on whom biopsies were performed within 4 months of a mammogram for suspected recurrence in the irradiated breast. The tumor was suspected based on mammography in only eight patients (35%), on physical examination in nine (39%), and on both in six (26%). The most common radiographic findings were calcifications with or without a mass. Histologic evidence of recurrent cancer was found in 23 of 45 (51%) biopsy specimens. Sixty-five percent of patients had recurrences at the primary site and 22% in other sites; 13% were multifocal.

MRI is increasingly used in the evaluation of patients with equivocal mammographic findings. Viehweg et al.[813] followed 207 patients with breast cancer treated with breast conservation therapy; 40 patients were examined 0 to 12 months and 167 patients later than 12 months after radiation therapy. Suspect or indeterminate findings were suggested by clinical examination or conventional imaging in 80 studies. In 127 women, MRI was performed in breast tissue that was difficult to assess because of scarring or dense breast tissue. Recurrent carcinoma was confirmed in 27 patients by surgical biopsy. All 27 carcinomas, except for one with a slow signal increase, demonstrated early rise of signal intensity on dynamic T1-weighted, contrast-enhanced images. During the first year after therapy, the diagnostic accuracy was not improved by additional use of contrast-enhanced MRI because of strong and sometimes early and ill-circumscribed enhancement. Later than 12 months after therapy, enhancement decreased significantly and the false-positive calls could be reduced from 49 (conventional imaging) to 12 (conventional imaging plus MRI). A total of 12 of 26 recurrences and multifocality in four of five cases were diagnosed by MRI alone at this time.

Dao et al.[814] evaluated 35 women with breast carcinoma treated with conservation therapy who underwent posttreatment MRI. Nine patients had recurrent tumors, and 26 had a benign fibrotic mass confirmed at biopsy. In all cases, a localized hypointense area was present on plain spin-echo T1-weighted images. In all recurrent tumors, dynamic gadolinium-enhanced T1-weighted images demonstrated early increased signal intensity of the lesion within 3 minutes after bolus injection.

Drew et al.[815] also investigated MRI for screening for local recurrence after breast-conserving therapy. One hundred five patients were recruited for the study. Sixteen biopsies were performed and nine recurrences were confirmed histologically. The sensitivity for clinical examination, mammography, examination combined with mammography, and MRI alone for the detection of recurrent cancer were 89%, 67%, 100%, and 100%, respectively, and the specificity was 76%, 85%, 67%, and 93%. The authors concluded that when combined, clinical examination and mammography are as sensitive as MRI of the breast for the detection of LRR, but MRI has greater specificity.

SEQUELAE OF IRRADIATION IN BREAST CANCER

The most frequent complications associated with conservation surgery plus irradiation are arm or breast edema, breast fibrosis, painful mastitis or myositis, pneumonitis, and rib fracture. Apical pulmonary fibrosis is occasionally noted when the regional lymph nodes are irradiated.[1,113,314,351,816,817]

Lymphedema and Breast Edema

Complications from axillary surgery, regardless of breast surgical procedure, have been reported by several authors. It should be emphasized that before the treatment of arm lymphedema after breast carcinoma, it is mandatory to differentiate between treatment-associated complications and tumor recurrence in the regional lymphatics.

An extensive review of the literature related to arm edema following breast surgery was conducted by Erickson et al.[818] They found that arm edema is a common complication of breast cancer therapy that can result in substantial functional impairment and psychological morbidity. The risk of arm edema increases when axillary dissection and axillary radiation therapy are used. Preventive measures have not been well studied. Nonpharmacologic treatments, such as massage and exercise, have been shown to be effective therapies for lymphedema, but the effect of pharmacologic interventions remains uncertain. They conclude that as arm edema becomes more prevalent with the increasing survival of breast cancer patients, further research is needed to evaluate the efficacy of preventive strategies and therapeutic interventions.[43]

Maunsell et al.[819] evaluated frequency of upper extremity problems from axillary surgery in 223 patients. At 3 months after surgery, 82% of patients reported at least one arm problem: swelling (24%), weakness (26%), some limitation in range of movement (32%), stiffness (40%), pain (55%), and numbness (58%). The severity of these problems changed little 15 months later. Regardless of the type of mastectomy, women who underwent axillary dissection had more problems.

Clarke et al.[402] observed breast edema in approximately 20% of patients not undergoing axillary dissection, compared with 80% of those in whom this procedure was performed. The extent of the axillary dissection (medial or lateral to the tendon of the pectoralis minor) influences the incidence of breast or arm edema, with this complication being more frequent when more extensive axillary dissections are carried out (beyond level II—middle). On the other hand, Dewar et al.[820] reported a greater incidence of upper limb sequelae in patients undergoing axillary surgery and irradiation (33.7%) or irradiation alone (26%) than in patients treated with axillary dissection only (7.2%). The most frequently noted complications were edema, impaired shoulder mobility, pain on movement, sensory or motor deficit, and pectoral muscle fibrosis.

Pain and discomfort after ALND were significantly related to quality of life. Hack et al.,[821] in 220 women with breast cancer who had undergone ALND, noted that 73% had sensation of pain or discomfort or the point of maximum arm–shoulder movement was different between the affected and nonaffected side. Although more than half of the patients experienced pain-related discomfort and disability, patients in general reported a good quality of life and mental health. Younger women had significantly greater pain than did older women. Patients with more than 13 lymph nodes dissected and patients receiving chemotherapy reported more pain.

Sentinel node sampling appears to be associated with a much lower degree of lymphedema.[332] Sener et al.[822] reported that 9 of 303 patients (3%) who underwent only sentinel lymphadenectomy had lymphedema, compared with 20 of 117 patients (17%) who underwent sentinel lymphadenectomy combined with axillary dissection ($P < .0001$). Among 303 patients who underwent sentinel lymphadenectomy only, lymphedema developed in 8 of 155 patients (5%) who had tumors in the upper outer quadrant and in 1 of 148 patients (0.7%) whose tumors were in other locations. The ALMANAC randomized trial also confirms lower morbidity and improved quality of life following sentinel node biopsy compared with axillary dissection.[332]

Various treatment regimens have been used to treat lymphedema.[823] The compression pump, along with skin care, exercise, and compression garments, is one. A second treatment is known as *complex decongestive physiotherapy* or *complex physical therapy*. Arm care, therapeutic exercises, manual lymph node drainage, and compression bandages or garments constitute this treatment regimen. Decreases in lymphedema are noted if women are compliant with the prescribed treatment program.

Brorson et al.[824] reported on 20 patients with arm lymphedema after breast cancer treatment who underwent liposuction combined with controlled compression therapy or controlled compression therapy alone. Liposuction combined with controlled compression therapy reduced arm edema volume by (median) 115% (range, 92% to 179%), whereas controlled compression therapy alone decreased arm edema volume by only 54% (range, 7% to 81%; $P = .008$).

In general, the incidence of breast or arm edema after conservation therapy varies, and it is related to performance and technique of axillary dissection, whether the axillary lymph nodes were irradiated, and the dose of radiation delivered.

Skin and Breast Complications

A wide variety of symptoms may occur following radiation treatment to the conservatively treated breast. McCormick et al.[314] showed that breast swelling was the most frequently noted symptom (31% of patients), followed by muscle pain (on motion), incision site pain, and general breast discomfort (approximately 20%). Rib pain was noted by 13%. Forty-eight percent of patients reported more breast discomfort in the treated breast compared with the untreated breast during sexual activity (64 sexually active patients).

In addition to host factors such as such as CVS and diabetes, underlying genetic factors may play a role in radiation complications. Iannuzzi et al.[825] evaluated 46 patients with early-stage breast carcinoma who underwent limited surgery and breast irradiation. DNA was isolated from blood lymphocytes. Nine ataxia telangiectasis mutations were identified in six patients (eight novel and one rare). The median follow-up was 3.2 years (range, 1.3 to 19.3 years). All three of the patients (100%) who manifested grade 3 or 4 subcutaneous late sequelae possessed ataxia telangiectasis mutations, whereas only 3 of the 43 patients (7%) who did not have this form of severe toxicity harbored an ataxia telangiectasis mutation ($P = .001$).

Skin effects after postlumpectomy radiation therapy may be affected more significantly by the increase in the dose of radiation per fraction than by the total dose. Gorodetsky et al.[826] studied 110 women with breast cancer who had been treated with lumpectomies and radiation therapy and normal controls using a viscoelasticity skin analyzer. With increasing age, the viscoelasticity of the skin decreased and anisotropy increased significantly. A small but significant increase in skin stiffness was noted with radiation therapy in the range of 45 to 50 Gy given in fractions of 1.8 Gy. A dose of 50 Gy given in fractions of 2.5 Gy produced a more pronounced effect.

Pseudosclerodermatosus panniculitis is an unusual variant of panniculitis seen as a complication of radiation therapy. Carrasco et al.[827] described four women in whom this unusual entity developed on the anterior chest and abdominal skin after they received radiation therapy for either breast carcinoma or painful bone metastases from breast carcinoma. Histopathologically, the epidermis and dermis of the involved area showed little or no evidence of radiodermatitis. The main findings were in subcutaneous tissue and consisted of thickened sclerotic septa, composed of both thick and thin collagen bundles, and a lobular panniculitis characterized by lipophagic granulomas and scattered lymphocytes and plasma cells. This sequela should be distinguished from subcutaneous metastatic disease, cellulitis, or connective tissue diseases involving the subcutaneous fat.

Rayan et al.[828] reported on a randomized clinical trial of breast-conserving surgery and tamoxifen with or without radiation therapy in women 50 years of age and older treated for stage T1 or T2, node-negative breast cancer. A companion study to assess breast pain was carried out during the past 2 years of accrual to the trial, in which 86 patients participated. Forty-one received radiation therapy and tamoxifen and 45 tamoxifen alone. The median age was 70 years. Baseline pain and quality-of-life scores were similar for the two groups. At 3 months, patients receiving radiation therapy experienced more breast pain compared with those receiving tamoxifen alone, but this did not reach statistical significance. At 3 months, the pain scores for the radiation therapy and tamoxifen and tamoxifen alone groups were 2.39 and 1.83, respectively ($P = .47$). At 12 months, pain scores were lower and fairly similar in both groups, with a difference of 0.20 ($P = .71$).

Tamoxifen has been shown to induce secretion of tumor growth factor-β, which has been implicated in pathogenesis of radiation fibrosis. Li et al.[729] in a study of 91 patients with T1 or T2 breast cancer, noted that tumor growth factor-β and the receptor–ligand complex appeared to be of clinical value in identifying patients at risk for development of postirradiation fibrosis of the breast. Wazer et al.[577] showed a trend toward decreased cosmesis in patients receiving tamoxifen. In a randomized study, pulmonary fibrosis developed in 15 of 24 (63%) women treated with 36.6 Gy in 12 fractions and tamoxifen, compared with 10 of 30 (33%) receiving irradiation alone. Also, 5 of 14 (36%) women treated with 40.9 Gy in 22 fractions and tamoxifen had lung fibrosis, compared with 2 of 16 (13%) receiving irradiation alone.[576] In contrast, Fowble et al.[829] observed no difference in cosmetic results or complications in 154 patients who received tamoxifen in combination with breast conservation therapy compared with 337 patients who did not receive tamoxifen. The incidences of radiation pneumonitis were 0.2% and 0.3%, respectively. The sequence of tamoxifen, given concurrently or following radiation, has not been clearly shown to correlate with complications or cosmesis.[578–580]

Markiewicz et al.[790] analyzed complications in 1,053 women with stage I or II breast cancer treated with breast-conserving therapy. Of this group, 206 received chemotherapy alone, 141 had hormonal therapy alone, 94 had both, and 612 received no adjuvant therapy. The incidence of grade 4 or 5 arm edema (≥ 2 cm difference in arm circumference) was 2% without chemotherapy and 8% with chemotherapy ($P - .00002$). However, the incidence of arm edema was not affected by sequencing or type of chemotherapy; it occurred in 10% and 7% of patients with sequential or concurrent treatment, respectively, and in 8% and 18% of patients treated with CMF or CAF, respectively. The incidence of clinical pneumonitis and rib fracture was not influenced by use of chemotherapy, sequencing of drugs, or use of hormonal therapy. These authors concluded that some chemotherapy could be given concurrently with radiation therapy to the breast without significant compromise of cosmetic results or sequelae of treatment.

Hyperbaric oxygen therapy has been shown to be effective in the treatment of some late radiation sequelae. Carl et al.[830] reported on 44 patients with persistent local symptoms after breast-conserving therapy. Hyperbaric oxygen therapy (100% oxygen at 240 kPa for 90-minute sessions) was administered to 32 patients for a median of 25 sessions (range, 7 to 60 sessions). The remaining 12 patients declined hyperbaric treatment and acted as control subjects. The patients given hyperbaric oxygen therapy demonstrated a significant reduction in pain, edema, and erythema scores compared with untreated control subjects ($P < .001$). Seven of the 32 women who were treated with hyperbaric oxygen therapy were free of symptoms after treatment, whereas all 12 patients in the control group had persistent complaints. However, hyperbaric oxygen therapy did not have a significant effect on fibrosis and telangiectasia in the irradiated breast.

Brachial Plexopathy

Brachial plexus dysfunction is a possible complication of regional nodal radiation therapy. In a review of 1,624 patients, brachial plexus sequelae were observed in 1.8% of patients.[831] Pierce et al.[831] found that the incidence of brachial plexopathy was significantly higher when the axillary dose was >50 Gy ($P = .004$). However, dose alone did not determine whether radiation damage would develop in a given patient. Treatment technique (two vs. three fields; $P = .0009$) and concomitant chemotherapy were also risk factors. Other investigators have found the incidence of this complication to be $\leq 1\%$.[96,378] It is very important but difficult to distinguish between metastatic and radiation-induced brachial plexopathy.

Treatment for radiation brachial plexopathy consists of transdermal electrical nerve stimulation, dorsal column stimulators, neurolysis, and neurolysis with omentoplasty. Physical therapy, tricyclics, antiarrhythmics, anticonvulsives, nonsteroidal anti-inflammatory drugs, and steroids are helpful in therapy of both radiation-induced and metastatic brachial plexopathies.[832]

Pritchard et al.[833] used hyperbaric oxygen in 34 volunteers with radiation-induced brachial plexopathy who were randomized to hyperbaric oxygen or a control group. The hyperbaric oxygen group breathed 100% oxygen for 100 minutes in a hyperbaric chamber (30 sessions over 6 weeks). The control group breathed a gas mixture equivalent to breathing 100% oxygen at surface pressure. Normalization of the warm sensory threshold was seen in two of the patients receiving hyperbaric oxygen therapy. Two cases with marked chronic arm lymphedema reported major improvement in arm volume. These authors concluded that there is no reliable evidence to support hyperbaric oxygen therapy to slow or reverse radiation-induced brachial plexopathy, although improvements in warm sensory threshold suggest a therapeutic effect improvement in long-standing arm lymphedema and justify further investigation.

Pulmonary Sequelae

Symptomatic pneumonitis is infrequent. This clinical syndrome is noted one to several months after irradiation.[834] Patients present with dry cough (88%), shortness of breath (35%), or fever (53%), and on radiographic studies, a pulmonary infiltrate is observed in the irradiated volume.[816] The risk for development of radiation pneumonitis may be related to the volume of lung irradiated.[816,835]

The addition of regional nodal radiation therapy to breast irradiation significantly increase the incidence of symptomatic pneumonitis (1% without and 4% with regional node radiation therapy; $P < .001$). Combined axillary dissection and nodal irradiation result in a significantly higher incidence of arm edema compared with either alone (9.5% with axillary dissection, 6.1% with radiation therapy to the axilla and supraclavicular fossa, and 31% with combined modality therapy; $P < .001$).[835]

Lingos et al.[816] reported on radiation pneumonitis in a retrospective review of 1,624 patients treated with conservation surgery and irradiation. Overall, pneumonitis developed in 1% of patients. No patient had late or persisting pulmonary symptoms. The incidence of radiation pneumonitis was correlated with the combined use of chemotherapy and a supraclavicular field ($P = .0001$). Fourteen of 17 patients who had radiation pneumonitis also had IMNs treated. When patients treated with the three-field technique received chemotherapy concurrently with irradiation, the incidence of radiation pneumonitis was 8.8% (8 of 92) compared with 1.3% (3 of 236) for those who received sequential chemotherapy and irradiation to the breast only and 0.5% (6 of 1,296) for those treated with irradiation to the breast only without chemotherapy ($P = .002$). In this study, the volume of lung irradiated did not correlate with the risk for development of radiation pneumonitis.

Taghian et al.,[836] in 41 patients treated with radiation therapy and paclitaxel (21 concurrent, 20 sequential), also described a higher incidence of pneumonitis (14.6%) compared with control patients irradiated and not receiving chemotherapy (1.1%; $P < .0001$). Burstein et al.[575] also recently reported that the concurrent use of weekly paclitaxel with radiation result in high rates of pneumonitis. However, an analysis of patients treated with radiation as a component of a randomized trial, in which 50% of the patients were treated with paclitaxel and 50% were treated with a nontaxane regimen, found that the rates of pneumonitis were very low and not significantly different between the two arms.[837]

The effect of tangential field technique on pulmonary function was reported by Lund et al.[838] in 25 patients treated with conservation surgery and irradiation. Dynamic and static lung volumes, distribution of ventilation, and gas transfer were measured before irradiation and at varying intervals up to 1 year after completion of therapy. There was a small but statistically significant decrease in the forced vital capacity and forced expired volume in 1 second 3 months after irradiation ($P < .05$). These changes normalized within 1 year. The reduction in total lung capacity after 3 months almost achieved statistical significance ($P = .06$). These slight restrictive ventilatory changes are reversible and have no clinical importance.

Radiation pneumonitis was retrospectively assessed on the basis of clinical symptoms and radiologic findings using a serial organ model by Gagliardi et al.[839] As demonstrated in Figure 59.52, a lung volume effect was relevant in the description of radiation pneumonitis. Lind et al.[840] measured pulmonary function 5 months after radiation therapy in 144 patients with node-positive stage II breast cancer. No deterioration of pulmonary function was detected among the patients who were treated with local radiation therapy. Patients undergoing locoregional radiation therapy showed a 5% mean reduction in diffusion capacity ($P < .001$) and a 3% mean reduction in vital capacity ($P = .001$).

Cardiac Sequelae

The potential for excess cardiac morbidity associated with the use of radiation therapy in breast cancer has been extensively evaluated. It has been clearly demonstrated, based on data from randomized trials, overview, and meta-analyses, that when using older techniques, excess cardiac mortality from radiation offsets some of the benefits that radiation therapy clearly produced with respect to breast cancer mortality.[68,366,841] Although the evidence from more modern trials, using techniques that minimize exposure to the normal cardiac and pulmonary structures, have reduced cardiac toxicity, the radiation oncologist must be cognizant of the potential for adverse cardiac effects of incidental irradiation, particularly in the setting of left-sided breast cancers in patients receiving other cardiotoxic therapies, including adriamycin, epirubicin, and trastuzumab.[842,843]

Earlier techniques of radiation therapy from large pools of randomized data have clearly been implicated in excess cardiac mortality. In an analysis of over 90,000 Swedish women, comparing left- to right-sided cancers, Darby et al.[844] from the Oxford group reported excess ischemic heart disease mortality more than 10 years after initial treatment in the left-sided cancer group (HR 1.13; 95% CI, 1.03 to 1.25; $P = .01$). The majority of cardiovascular deaths were from earlier studies using techniques that are no longer used. However, for patients treated after 1980, although the ratio was still 1.11, the CIs were much larger (0.95 to 1.29), so the hazard remains uncertain for the more modern techniques.

In a separate report, Darby et al. conducted a population-based case–control study of major coronary events (i.e., myocardial infarction, coronary revascularization, or death from ischemic heart disease) in 2168 women who underwent radiotherapy for breast cancer between 1958 and 2001 in Sweden and Denmark[845]. They found that rates of major coronary events increased linearly with the mean dose to the heart by 7.4% per gray (95% CI, 2.9 to 14.5; $P < .001$), with no apparent threshold. The increase started within the first 5 years after radiotherapy and continued into the third decade after radiotherapy.

Gyenes et al.[846] reported on the incidence of ischemic heart disease 15 to 20 years after adjuvant radiation therapy in 960 patients with breast cancer enrolled in the Stockholm Breast Cancer Trial. Of 37 long-term survivors, 20 received left-sided therapy and 17 received right-sided therapy or no

therapy. Radiation therapy consisted of tangential fields for preoperative treatment and electron beam portals, which included the IMNs, for postoperative therapy (45 to 50 Gy). Evaluation consisted of echocardiography, exercise stress tests with ^{99m}Tc myocardial perfusion scan, and careful history for cardiac risk factors. Results showed that 5 of 20 (25%) patients treated with left-sided radiation had defects on ^{99m}Tc scan, compared with 0 of 17 control patients ($P = .05$).

Paszat et al.[847] conducted a study of 25,570 cases of invasive female breast cancer that were linked to radiation therapy records from Ontario cancer centers. Postlumpectomy radiation therapy was administered to 1,555 patients on the left side and to 1,451 on the right side. Two percent of women with left-sided radiation therapy had a fatal myocardial infarction compared with 1% of women with right-sided radiation therapy ($P = .02$). Adjusting for age at diagnosis, the RR for fatal myocardial infarction with left-sided postlumpectomy radiation therapy was 2.10.

Rutqvist et al.[848] followed 684 patients with breast cancer treated with breast-conserving surgery and radiation therapy using tangential photon fields (48 to 52 Gy in 4.5 to 5.5 weeks). The median follow-up was 9 years. In 88% of patients, the target volume involved the breast only; in the remaining patients, regional nodes were irradiated. A control group included 4,996 patients with breast cancer who underwent mastectomies without postoperative radiation therapy. Twelve patients (1.8%) in the irradiated group had myocardial infarctions and five patients (0.7%) died as a result of myocardial infarctions. The RR for a myocardial infarction between the irradiated group and the control group was 0.6, and the RR for death was 0.4. The study presents no evidence that the risk for myocardial infarction is increased with radiation therapy after breast-conserving surgery regardless of which side the tumor was located. However, because the number of myocardial infarctions in the study was small, there is no way to rule out the possibility of cardiac problems in patients with left breast carcinomas.

Shapiro et al.[842] assessed the cardiac effects in 299 patients with breast cancer prospectively randomized to receive either 5 cycles or 10 cycles of cyclophosphamide and a doxorubicin intravenous bolus every 21 days. Of the 299 patients, 122 received radiation therapy. The risk of major cardiac events (congestive heart failure, acute myocardial infarction) was assessable in 276 patients, with a median follow-up of 6 years (range, 0.5 to 19.4 years). The estimated risk of cardiac events per 100 patient-years was significantly higher for 10 cycles than for 5 cycles of chemotherapy (1.7 vs. 0.5; $P = .02$). The risk of cardiac events in the 5-cycle patients, regardless of the cardiac radiation therapy dose volume, did not differ significantly from rates of cardiac events predicted for a general female population. For patients receiving 10 cycles, the incidence of cardiac events was significantly increased (RR 3.6; $P < .00003$) compared with the general population, particularly in groups that also received moderate- and high–dose-volume cardiac radiation therapy.

Cuzick et al.[841] updated cardiac toxicity data from eight randomized trials initiated before 1975 in which radiotherapy was the randomized option and surgery was the same for both treatment arms. An initial analysis of these trials demonstrated an increased all-cause mortality rate in 10-year survivors associated with radiation, but in the update this was no longer present. The initial increase in mortality in the radiation arms was strongly influenced by the earliest trials, and more recent trials have found a nonsignificant net benefit in overall mortality associated with radiation therapy. However, an excess of cardiac deaths was apparent in both early and more recent trials ($P < .001$), but this was offset by a reduced number of deaths due to breast cancer, especially in more recent trials. Based on this, it is clearly prudent to use techniques that minimize cardiac dose.

Although clinical evidence of cardiac morbidity has decreased with modern techniques, care should be taken to exclude heart from the tangential radiation field. In an analysis of 114 patients, Marks et al.[704] assessed RT-induced left ventricular perfusion defects and whether these perfusion defects are related to changes in cardiac wall motion or alterations in ejection fraction. Patients were imaged 30 to 60 minutes after injection of [99mTc] sestamibi or tetrofosmin. Post-RT perfusion scans were compared with the pre-RT studies to assess for RT-induced perfusion defects as well as functional changes in wall motion and ejection fraction. The incidence of new perfusion defects 6, 12, 18, and 24 months after RT was 27%, 29%, 38%, and 42%, respectively. New defects occurred in approximately 10% to 20% and 50% to 60% of patients with <5% and >5% of their left ventricle included within the RT fields, respectively. The rates of wall motion abnormalities in patients with and without perfusion defects were 12% to 40% versus 0% to 9%. These authors note that RT causes volume-dependent perfusion defects in approximately 40% of patients within 2 years of RT, and that these perfusion defects are associated with corresponding wall-motion abnormalities. However, additional study is necessary to determine if these defects are associated with functional consequences.

Given these findings, the authors suggest the use of a heart block if needed to reduce or eliminate cardiac irradiation. CT-based 3D treatment planning is used to design such cardiac blocks and select the optimal gantry angle to minimize the need for a heart block. There may be a small amount of breast tissue underdosed if the block overlies the medial inferior breast, but this tissue is typically <5%. In situations where the heart block may underdose the high-risk volume of the breast or chest wall, an "electron patch" can be used to treat the target tissue in the shadow of the heart block. A tangential field with a heart block is demonstrated in Figure 59.33.

Although it is clearly prudent to minimize exposure of the heart during radiation therapy, using modern techniques, the available evidence does not suggest a higher incidence of cardiac mortality in left-sided radiation therapy.

Analysis of the randomized postmastectomy Danish trials, with over 10 years of follow-up, showed no excess cardiac mortality with the use of postmastectomy radiation. Hojris et al.[274] reported that the relative hazard of morbidity from ischemic heart disease among patients in the radiotherapy compared with the no-radiotherapy group was 0.86 (95% CI, 0.6 to 1.3), and that for death from ischemic heart disease was 0.84 (0.4 to 1.8). The hazard rate of morbidity from ischemic heart disease in the radiotherapy group compared with the no-radiotherapy group did not increase with time from treatment.

Patt et al.[849] analyzed data from the SEER-Medicare database for women who were diagnosed with nonmetastatic breast cancer from 1986 to 1993, had known disease laterality, underwent breast surgery, and received adjuvant radiotherapy; 8,363 patients had left-sided breast cancer and 7,907 had right-sided breast cancer. With a mean follow-up of 9.5 years (range, 0 to 15 years), there were no significant differences in patients with left- versus right-sided cancers for hospitalization for ischemic heart disease (9.9% vs. 9.7%), valvular heart disease (2.9% vs. 2.8%), conduction abnormalities (9.7% vs. 9.6%), or heart failure (9.7% vs. 9.7%). The adjusted HR for left- versus right-sided breast cancer was 1.05 (95% CI, 0.94 to 1.16) for ischemic heart disease, 1.07 (95% CI, 0.89 to 1.30) for valvular heart disease, 1.07 (95% CI, 0.96 to 1.19) for conduction abnormalities, and 1.05 (95% CI, 0.95 to 1.17) for heart failure.

Similar conclusions were reached by Nixon et al.[850] who reviewed 365 patients with 12-year follow-up who received irradiation to the left breast and 380 who received irradiation to the right breast as part of conservation therapy. Equivalent proportions from each group died of non–breast cancer causes (11%), including nine patients (2%) from each group who died from cardiac causes. Also, Vallis et al.,[851] in a retrospective review of 2,128 women treated with lumpectomy and breast irradiation with a median follow-up of 10.2 years, noted that the incidence of myocardial infarction in the study cohort was comparable with that in an age-matched general population of women in Ontario.

The potential for cardiac vessel injury from radiation was recently explored in an elegant study by Nilsson et al.[852] who analyzed radiation fields and subsequent coronary angiograms in a Swedish breast cancer cohort study. For right-sided compared with left-sided breast cancers, the OR for grade 3 to 5 stenosis in arteries likely to be within the tangential radiation port was 4.38 (95% CI, 1.64 to 11.7) and was 7.22 (95% CI, 1.64 to 31.8) for grade 4 or 5 stenosis. They conclude there is an increased risk and direct link between radiation and the location of the coronary stenosis. In a related editorial Zagar and Marks[853] emphasize the potential effects of radiation on the heart but point out that improved radiation techniques, including custom blocking of the heart and other techniques to manipulate the radiation dose, are likely to minimize these risks and improve the therapeutic ratio.

Collectively, these data suggest that although there may be excess cardiac morbidity using tangential fields to treat left-sided breast cancers, these effects can be minimized through careful treatment planning. It remains prudent to minimize cardiac exposure in all patients and particularly in those receiving left-sided radiation in combination with other potentially cardiotoxic drugs.

Risk of Stroke with Supraclavicular Radiation

For patients with node-positive disease undergoing supraclavicular radiation, there is a theoretical concern regarding the potential for development of accelerated carotid artery stenosis. In a study by Jagsi et al.,[854] rates of stroke in 820 eligible early-stage breast cancer patients treated with radiation therapy were compared with expected rates. The relation between potential risk factors and actuarial rate of first stroke was analyzed. On multivariate analysis, only age ($P < .001$) and hypertension ($P = .003$) remained significant predictors of cardiovascular accident or transient ischemic attack. Age was the only significant predictor of cardiovascular accident alone ($P < .001$). This study found no significant association between supraclavicular RT and stroke after controlling for other factors. This study is in agreement with the findings of the EBCTCG who reported the causes of nonbreast cancer death in 32,800 patients treated in trials of surgery with and without RT. Although the incidence of heart disease was found to be significantly greater in those women who received RT, no significant excess mortality from RT was observed because of stroke. However, a recent nested case–control study by Nilsson et al.[855] showed a significant increase in stroke (OR 1.8; 95% CI, 1.1 to 2.8) when comparing patients treated to the supraclavicular and internal mammary regions with those not treated to these regions. In addition, a study by Woodward et al.[856] of the SEER database comparing 5,281 women presumably without supraclavicular radiation with negative nodes to 482 women presumably treated to the supraclavicular region with more than four nodes did not find any increased rate of hospitalization for stroke in the treated population.

Contralateral Breast Cancer and Irradiation

Although all patients with a diagnosis of breast cancer are at increased risk for developing a contralateral breast cancer, the additional risk contributed by radiation treatment appears to be minimal, particularly when one uses modern techniques and maintains a dose to the contralateral breast that is as low as is reasonably achievable. Although this issue is often a concern raised by patients, the available data using modern radiation techniques do not suggest a significant increase of risk for contralateral breast cancers in breast cancer patients who have been irradiated, in comparison to similar cohorts of breast cancer patients who have not undergone radiation.[1,23,91,113,686,750,857-860] Although there is some evidence suggesting a slight excess risk in women who are irradiated at a relatively young age (i.e., <45 years at diagnosis), the risk is extremely small and may be related to use of older techniques, and most experts would agree that the benefit of radiation far outweighs the risk.[857] Nonetheless, it appears prudent to be aware of these potential risks and employ techniques that minimize scattered dose to the contralateral breast. As demonstrated in Table 59.42, the reported incidence of contralateral cancer in the majority of these studies of patients treated with CS and radiation do not appear to be elevated compared with those treated by mastectomy without radiation.

However, the EBCTCG overview analysis does suggest an elevated incidence of contralateral breast cancer in patients receiving radiation compared with those who did not receive radiation.[87] This overview analysis of all randomized trials comparing radiation to surgery demonstrated an increased RR of contralateral breast cancers of 1.18 (=.002). Although the excess risk appears to be driven primarily by older trials using antiquated techniques, these data do demonstrate the potential long-term effects of radiation-related secondary cancers and highlight the need to maintain dose to the contralateral breast as low as possible.

A report by Hankey et al.,[862] involving 27,175 women treated for breast cancer between 1960 and 1975, disclosed a RR of 1.2 to 1.4 for development of cancer in the contralateral breast in irradiated patients compared with those who did not receive irradiation. These authors, however, concluded that the data did not indicate a pattern of RR consistent with an increased incidence of carcinoma in the opposite breast.

Boice et al.[857] evaluated the risk of second cancers associated with radiation therapy to the breast in 41,109 women with breast cancer who were registered in the Connecticut Tumor Registry between 1935 and 1982. They reviewed the records of 655 women in whom a second breast cancer developed 5 years or longer after initial treatment

and compared the radiation exposure in these patients with the exposure in 1,189 matched control patients who did not have a second cancer. The average dose to the contralateral breast in women exposed to radiation was 2.82 Gy. The RR for development of a second breast cancer was 1.9 in the women who received radiation therapy, and among patients who survived for 10 years or longer, the RR was 1.33. Women <45 years of age had a RR of 1.59 for development of a second breast cancer, compared with 1.01 for older women. According to these authors, younger patients should be informed that, based on the results of this study, after 10 years the risk for development of a second cancer increases from 14% if they do not receive irradiation to 22% if they choose treatment involving irradiation.

On the other hand, Levitt and Mandell[863] estimated the dose delivered to the contralateral breast to be between 1 and 4 Gy. Assuming that 20,000 women undergo radiation therapy after conservation surgery and using data on the risk for development of breast cancer after various doses of ionizing radiation, they concluded that fewer than one additional case of breast cancer would occur after 10 years. Storm et al.,[864] in a case-controlled study of a registry-based cohort of patients with breast cancer in Denmark, also concluded there was little, if any, risk of radiation-induced breast cancer associated with exposure of adult breast tissue to low-dose irradiation.

Obedian et al.[23] compared 1,029 breast cancer patients treated with CS and radiation to a cohort of 1,387 breast cancer patients who underwent surgical treatment by mastectomy and who did not receive postoperative radiation during the same time period. The median follow-up was 14.6 years for the conservatively treated group and 16 years for the mastectomy group. The 15-year risk of any second malignancy was nearly identical for both cohorts (17.5% vs. 19%, respectively). The second breast malignancy rate at 15 years was 10% for both groups. In the subset of patients ≤45 years of age at the time of treatment, the second breast and nonbreast malignancy rates at 15 years were 10% and 5% for patients undergoing breast-conserving therapy versus 7% and 4%, respectively, for patients undergoing mastectomy (probability not statistically significant).

To address whether the radiation administered may influence the development of breast cancers on the contralateral side, Khan and Haffty[865] evaluated the location of contralateral breast cancers developing after radiation. There was not a preponderance of medial lesions developing in the contralateral group (where radiation dose would be higher), suggesting that there was no cause–effect relation with respect to the prior radiation. In a study by Hill-Kayser et al.[861] the 20-year risk of contralateral breast cancer in 1,801 patients treated with breast-conserving surgery and radiation was 15.4%. They also demonstrated that the distribution of location of the contralateral tumors did not appear to be influenced by the prior irradiation.

In a recent update of the Danish randomized trials of postmastectomy radiation, Nielsen et al.[750] also reported no excess risk of second malignancies in the contralateral breast in patients randomized to receive radiation. In this long-term follow-up performed among the 3,083 patients from the Danish Breast Cancer Cooperative Group 82B and 82C, randomized to postmastectomy radiation or not, there was no significant difference in the risk of contralateral breast cancers (6% RT vs. 5% no RT) between the two groups.

Hooning et al.,[859] in a study from Amsterdam of over 7,000 predominantly young women treated with or without radiation, did note an increase in contralateral breast cancer with decreasing age with tangential breast irradiation, particularly in young women with a strong family history. Of note, patients treated with mastectomy and chest wall electrons, where scattered dose to the contralateral breast was less, did not experience an increased contralateral breast cancer risk. The

TABLE 59.42 INCIDENCE OF CONTRALATERAL BREAST CANCER IN CARCINOMA OF THE BREAST TREATED WITH CONSERVATION SURGERY AND IRRADIATION OR MASTECTOMY

Study (Reference)	Conservation Therapy	Mastectomy
Arriagada et al.[858a]	88 (14%)	91 (11%)
Broët et al.[744]	1,819 (3.8%)	1,815 (3.9%)
Clark et al.[376]	1,504 (3%)	–
Dewar et al.[379]	757 (6%)[b]	–
Hill-Kayser et al.[861]	1,801 (15.4%)[c]	–
Montague[315]	316 (1.9%)[d]	576 (5.2%)
Nielsen et al.[860]	–	No RT 1,545 (4%)
		RT 1,538 (5%)
Obedian et al.[23]	1,029 (10%)[e]	1,387, (10%)[e]
Recht et al.[387]	366 (9%)[f]	–
Rosen et al.[195]	–	RT, 76 (10.7%)
	–	No RT, 47 (9.4%)
Sarrazin et al.[359]	88 (9%)	91 (9%)
Veronesi et al.[100]	349 (5%)[g]	352 (5%)[g]
Hooning et al.[859]	RR 1.5[h]	RR 1.0

[a]Risk at 15 years (update of Sarrazin data [Feigenberg SJ, Mendenhall NP, Reith JD, et al. Angiosarcoma after breast-conserving therapy: experience with hyperfractionated radiotherapy. *Int J Radiat Oncol Biol Phys* 2002;52(3):620–626.].
[b]Actuarial relapse at 10 years.
[c]Actuarial risk at 20 years.
[d]Excludes simultaneous bilateral cancer.
[e]Actuarial risk at 15 years
[f]Actuarial risk at 5 years.
[g]Actuarial risk at 12 years.
[h]Relative risk of tangential fields increased compared to mastectomy with electron fields.
RT, radiation therapy.

joint effects of tangential breast irradiation following lumpectomy and strong family history on contralateral breast cancer resulted in a HR of 3.52 (95% CI, 2.07 to 6.02; P = .043).

With modern technology scattered dose to the contralateral breast is lower and should minimize this issue, but care should be taken, particularly in younger women, to ensure that the dose to the contralateral breast is as low as possible.

Incidence of Other Second Malignancies

The incidence of secondary malignancies, as with the issue of contralateral breast cancer, appears to be very low, and it is evident that the appropriate use of radiation therapy far outweighs the risk of radiation-induced malignancy. Nonetheless, there is some evidence, with very long-term follow-up, of higher rates of secondary cancers. Although this may be more prevalent with older techniques, it is an important component of treatment planning to minimize dose to nontarget normal tissues. In addition to the excess risk of contralateral breast cancers discussed previously, the EBCTCG overview analysis did demonstrate an excess risk of secondary cancers of the lung and esophagus as well as leukemia and sarcoma in all randomized trials of breast cancer that compared patients treated with and without radiation. The increased RR for each of these secondary malignancies as a function of radiation treatment for breast cancer was lung cancer, 1.61 (±0.18; P = .007); esophageal cancer, 2.06 (±0.53; P = .05); leukemia, 1.71 (±0.36; P = .03); and sarcoma, 2.34 (±0.62; P = .03). The total RR for all secondary nonbreast malignancies was 1.20 (±0.06; P = .001). Although the increased risk of secondary malignancies may be driven primarily by trials using older techniques, they highlight the importance of limiting dose to nontarget tissues.

Huang and Mackillop,[866] in an analysis of 194,798 women from the SEER database who were diagnosed with invasive breast carcinoma (exclusive of those with distant metastasis) between 1973 and 1995, identified 54 women in a radiation therapy cohort and 81 women in a non–radiation therapy cohort in whom soft tissue sarcoma subsequently developed. In the radiation therapy cohort, the standardized incidence ratio was 26.2 for angiosarcoma and 2.5 for other sarcomas; in the non–radiation therapy cohort, the standardized incidence ratios were 2.1 and 1.3 (95% CI, 1.0 to 1.7), respectively. The largest increase was observed in the chest wall breast. The elevated RR was significant even within 5 years of radiation therapy, but it reached a maximum between 5 and 10 years.

Karlsson et al.[867] quantified the risk of posttreatment sarcoma in 122,991 women with breast cancer in the Swedish Cancer Register. One-hundred and sixteen cases were found, giving a standardized incidence ratio of 1.9 per 10^4 women. The absolute risk was 1.3 per 10^4 person-years. There were 40 angiosarcomas and 76 sarcomas of other types. The sarcomas were located in the breast region or on the ipsilateral arm in 63% (67 of 106). In a case–control study, angiosarcoma correlated significantly with lymphedema of the arm (OR 0.5), but no correlation with previous irradiation was observed. However, for other histologic types of sarcomas, the risk increased linearly with the integral dose to 150 to 200 J and stabilized at higher energies. The risk was 2.4 for an energy of 50 J, approximately corresponding to the radiation of the breast after breast-conserving surgery.

More contemporary retrospective series have not reported an excess risk of secondary malignancies. However, interpretation of these series is limited by follow-up periods of <20 years, which may not be adequate. A study by Fowble et al.[868] evaluated nonbreast malignancies with approximately 9 years of follow-up and reported the 10-year risk of second malignancy was 16% for all cancers, 7% for contralateral breast cancer, and 8% for all second non–breast cancer malignancies. Obedian et al.[23] also reported no increased

risk of second non-breast malignancies in patients treated with CS and radiation compared with a cohort treated with mastectomy without radiation during the same time interval. The 15-year risk of a second nonbreast malignancy was 11% for the radiation group and 10% for the mastectomy group.

Galper et al.[869] analyzed the risk for development of second nonbreast malignancies in 1,884 patients with clinical stage I or II breast cancer treated with excision and radiation therapy. By 8 years of follow-up, 147 (8%) had a second nonbreast malignancy compared with the 127.7 expected from SEER. This corresponds to an absolute excess of 1% of the study population and a relative increase of 15% greater than expected from SEER (P = .05). Lung as a second nonbreast malignancy was observed in 33 women, 50% more than the 21.67 predicted by SEER (P = .01), although most of the lung malignancies occurred <5 years after treatment. Of seven sarcomas, three developed in the radiation field. Second nonbreast malignancies occurred in a substantial minority (8%) of patients treated with conservation surgery and radiation therapy. However, the absolute excess risk compared with the general population was very small (1%) and only evident after 5 years.

Ahsan and Neugut[870] reviewed SEER data in 220,806 women in whom breast cancer was diagnosed between January 1, 1973 and December 31, 1993. In women who had received radiation therapy for breast cancer, the RR for esophageal squamous cell carcinoma increased to 5.42 and the RR for esophageal adenocarcinoma increased to 4.22 10 years or more after radiation therapy. No increased risk was seen for either type of carcinoma among patients with breast cancer who did not receive radiation therapy.

The available evidence of the risk of lung cancer in patients undergoing radiation suggests that smoking and radiation may be synergistic in contributing to the risk of lung cancer. Ford et al.[871] analyzed smoking, radiation, and both exposures on lung carcinoma development in women who were treated previously for breast carcinoma in a case–control study of 280 female patients with a diagnosis of breast cancer prior to lung cancer. Smoking increased the odds of lung carcinoma in women without radiation (OR 6.0; 95% CI, 3.6 to 10.1), but radiation did not increase lung carcinoma risk in nonsmoking women (OR 0.5; 95% CI, 0.3 to 1.1). Overall, the OR for both radiation and smoking, compared with no radiation or smoking, was 9.0 (95% CI, 5.1 to 15.9). The authors conclude that smoking is a significant independent risk factor for lung carcinoma after breast carcinoma, but radiation alone was not. Smoking and radiation combined enhanced the effect of either alone.

Deutsch et al.[872] in a long-term analysis of the NSABP-04 and NSABP-06 trials, suggest an excess risk of lung cancers associated with the extent of radiation. The records of all patients who developed a recurrence in the lung or a new primary lung tumor were reviewed to determine the incidence and laterality of confirmed and probable primary lung carcinoma. For the NSABP-04 trial, which employed more comprehensive radiation with larger lung volumes, there were a total of 23 subsequent confirmed and probable ipsilateral or contralateral primary lung carcinomas. In those patients who had received comprehensive postmastectomy radiotherapy, there was a statistically significant increase in the incidence of these new primary tumors (P = .029). With regard to the development of confirmed new primary ipsilateral lung carcinoma alone, the incidence was statistically significantly increased (P = .013) in those patients who had received radiotherapy as part of their treatment, and when confirmed and probable ipsilateral lung carcinomas were analyzed, there was a strong trend toward a statistically significant increase in those patients who had received radiotherapy (P = .066). For the NSABP-06 (mean follow-up of 19.0 years), there was a total of 30 second primary lung carcinomas but no increase in either ipsilateral or contralateral primary tumors of the lung in those patients who had received radiotherapy. They conclude that extensive postmastectomy irradiation of the chest wall and regional lymphatic node areas, with consequent exposure of a greater volume of lung to higher doses as administered in the NSABP-04 trial, compared with post-lumpectomy breast irradiation in the NSABP-06 trial, was associated with an increased incidence of subsequent primary lung tumors, both ipsilateral and contralateral. Unfortunately, data regarding smoking were not available in this analysis.

Postirradiation Angiosarcoma of the Breast

Special attention should be paid to uncommon skin changes of the treated breast because clinical suspicion is the main clue to the diagnosis of postirradiation angiosarcoma. The primary therapy is simple mastectomy if wide tumor-free margins can be achieved. At this time, there is no clear indication for standard adjuvant chemotherapy or irradiation. Angiosarcomas arising in the field of radiation therapy are rare. Unlike other radiation-induced sarcomas, cutaneous angiosarcoma often occurs within a short time after irradiation. It is important to differentiate atypical vascular lesions from angiosarcoma, but currently, there is no evidence that they represent a precursor to radiation-induced angiosarcoma. Deutsch and Rosenstein[873] reported an angiosarcoma arising in the breast more than 7 years after lumpectomy and breast irradiation. The initial appearance was very similar to late radiation dermatitis, and the true nature of the malignant lesion was not known for 23 months. Fineberg and Rosen[874] studied three patients with cutaneous angiosarcoma and four patients with atypical vascular lesions. All had breast-conserving surgery and ALND, and six patients received conventional high-energy postoperative doses of external beam radiation to the breast. Angiosarcoma was diagnosed 3.5, 3.7, and 5.25 years after radiation therapy. The three angiosarcomas were multifocal or diffuse and high grade, with solid cellular foci located mainly in the dermis. Two patients with angiosarcoma underwent mastectomy; one died 10 months after diagnosis with recurrent local angiosarcoma, and the other was alive and tumor free 2 months after diagnosis.

Feigenberg et al.[875] reported results of hyperfractionated radiation therapy in conjunction with surgery for angiosarcoma occurring after breast-conserving therapy in three patients. All three patients were treated initially with radical surgery for the angiosarcoma, but extensive recurrences were noted within 1 to 2 months of surgery. Because of the extremely rapid growth before and after surgery, hyperfractionated radiation therapy was used. Two of the patients underwent resection of the recurrence after radiation therapy, and neither specimen demonstrated any evidence of high-grade angiosarcoma. All three patients were alive without any recurrent disease 22, 38, and 39 months, respectively, after treatment. For previously untreated angiosarcoma, the authors recommend hyperfractionated radiation therapy followed by surgery to enhance disease control and, in recurring tumors, removing as much reirradiated tissue as possible.

Thirty-six cases of angiosarcoma after irradiation had been reported in the literature, and Edeiken et al.[876] presented two additional patients treated with breast-conserving treatment in whom angiosarcoma developed in the field of prior irradiation. Seven cases of angiosarcoma after radiation therapy for breast-conserving treatment of breast carcinoma had been reported, and the average time between the administration of radiation therapy and development of angiosarcoma was 8.6 years.

Marchal et al.[877] reported on nine breast angiosarcomas identified in a review of 18,115 patients who underwent breast-conserving treatment for carcinomas at 11 French cancer centers over a 20-year period ending in 1997. The estimated prevalence of angiosarcomas after breast-conserving

therapy for carcinomas was 5 per 10,000, which is approximately the same as for primary angiosarcomas in healthy breasts. The patients had a mean age of 62.5 years when the primary breast cancer was treated and 69 years when the angiosarcoma was diagnosed. Most angiosarcomas were stage T1N0M0 and were treated with radical mastectomy; two patients underwent reirradiation, and two patients were given adjuvant chemotherapy. The median time to the median survival after diagnosis of an angiosarcoma was 15.5 months. One patient was alive without progression of disease 32 months after a salvage mastectomy and the rest had died.

In a series of 3,295 patients treated with CS and irradiation for breast cancer, Zucali et al.[878] observed three cases of soft tissue sarcoma in irradiated breasts. It appears from these collective experiences that the risk of a second primary tumor in the irradiated breast is too low to justify modification of current policies of conservation therapy of breast cancer.

A rare complication after radical mastectomy is development of lymphangiosarcoma. It is associated with the development of lymphedema in the affected extremity and occurs in approximately 5 of 1,000 patients who had radical mastectomy and survived 5 years.[879]

Cost Versus Benefit in Breast Cancer Treatment

Barlow et al.[880] compared the total medical care costs from a regional nonprofit health management organization of breast conservation therapy versus a mastectomy 5 years after diagnosis in 1,675 women with early-stage breast cancer who had initial diagnoses between 1990 and 1997 and were 35 years of age or older. These women were classified into four groups according to treatment: mastectomy only (group 1, $n = 183$), mastectomy plus adjuvant therapy (group 2, $n = 417$), breast conservation therapy plus radiation therapy (group 3, $n = 405$), and breast conservation therapy plus radiation therapy and adjuvant therapy (group 4, $n = 670$). At 6 months, the costs of the treatments differed significantly ($P < .001$). Breast conservation therapy was more expensive than mastectomy. At 1 year, costs still differed significantly ($P < .001$) but were influenced more by the use of adjuvant therapy. By 5 years, the overall cost for breast conservation therapy was lower than for a mastectomy, presumably because of costs of reconstruction or complications of mastectomy.

Warren et al.[881] linked data of women with breast cancer from the SEER cancer registries with their Medicare claims from 1990 through 1998. Initial care costs for the 6 months after diagnosis for women who underwent breast conservation therapy and irradiation were approximately $450 per month higher than for women with modified radical mastectomy in the continuing-care phase; costs for women undergoing breast-conserving surgery with radiation therapy were significantly less than for modified radical mastectomy cases. The two groups had similar costs in the terminal-care phase. Long-term costs for women undergoing breast-conserving therapy with radiation therapy were not statistically different from those for women undergoing modified radical mastectomy.

Liljegren et al.[882] evaluated the cost-effectiveness of radiation therapy in a prospective, randomized trial of 381 women treated with sector resection plus axillary dissection with or without radiation therapy in stage I breast cancer. After a median follow-up of 5 years, 43 local recurrences, 6 of them in the radiation therapy group, had occurred ($P < .0001$). No differences in regional and distant metastases or survival rate were observed. Direct medical costs as well as indirect costs, in terms of production lost during the treatment period and travel expenses, were estimated from data in the medical records and the Swedish National Insurance Registry of each patient. Taking into account the cost of primary treatment, follow-up, cost of treatment of a local recurrence, travel expenses, and indirect costs (production lost) and excluding costs for treatment of regional and distant recurrence, the cost per avoided local recurrence at 5 years was $44,438. Adjustment of quality of life showed a cost for every gained quality-adjusted life-year (QALY) to be approximately $210,526. These results stress the importance of identifying risk factors for local recurrence, a better understanding of the impact on quality of life of a local recurrence, and adding cost evaluations to clinical trials in early breast cancer.

Hayman et al.[883] performed a cost-utility analysis of electron beam boost using a Markov model. From a societal perspective, outcomes were measured in QALYs. On the basis of the Lyon trial, the electron-beam boost was assumed to reduce local recurrences by approximately 2% at 10 years but to have no impact on survival. Direct medical, time, and travel costs were considered. The electron-beam boost led to an additional cost of $2,008, an increase of 0.0065 QALY, and an incremental cost-effectiveness ratio of over $300,000 QALY. Even if patients do value a small cancer risk reduction, the mean cost-effectiveness ratio remains high, at $70,859 QALY, which is well above the commonly cited threshold for cost-effectiveness care ($50,000 QALY). The electron beam boost is cost-effective only if patients place an unexpectedly high value on the small absolute reduction in local tumor recurrences achievable with it.

The usage of hypofractionation, with its associated reduced number of treatments, has recently been evaluated with respect to its costs by Bekelman et al.[884] in a retrospective, observational cohort study, using administrative claims data from 14 commercial health care plans covering 7.4% of US adult women. They classified patients with incident early-stage breast cancer treated with lumpectomy and WBI into 2 cohorts: (a) the hypofractionation-endorsed cohort (n = 8,924) included patients aged 50 years or older without prior chemotherapy or axillary lymph node involvement and (b) the hypofractionation-permitted cohort (n = 6,719) included patients younger than 50 years or those with prior chemotherapy or axillary lymph node involvement. They published that hypofractionated WBI increased from 10.6% in 2008 to 34.5% in the hypofractionation-endorsed cohort and from 8.1% in 2008 to 21.2% in the hypofractionation-permitted cohort. Adjusted mean total health care expenditures in the 1 year after diagnosis were $28 747 for hypofractionated and $31 641 for conventional WBI in the hypofractionation-endorsed cohort. Hypofractionated WBI was associated with savings of 9.1% and 11.8% in the hypofractionation-endorsed cohort and hypofractionation-permitted cohort, respectively. The adjusted mean total 1-year patient out-of-pocket expenses were not significantly different between hypofractionated vs conventional WBI in either cohort.

Psychoemotional Aspects and Quality of Life in Patients with Breast Cancer

Approximately 25% to 35% of patients diagnosed with breast cancer have significant psychosocial distress manifested by anxiety or depression and some level of sexual dysfunction. These disruptive consequences of treatment remain bothersome for at least 2 years after initial therapy. Jensen,[885] in a review of the literature studying psychosocial factors and their relation to breast cancer, revealed major methodologic problems in evaluation of the data, including small sample size, retrospective design, lack of cross-referencing for other important factors, cross-referencing studies instead of longitudinal studies, and insufficient statistical analysis. Regarding psychosocial factors, some of the most valid studies indicate that the risk of getting breast cancer may be connected with difficulties in expressing feelings, especially ones of aggression-coping strategy, amount of stress, and

level of activity, which seem to be of possible influence on the prognosis. A possible connection between psyche and the immunologic system has been proposed, but there have been few data to support it.

The specific types, magnitude, and duration of emotional dysfunction of women undergoing breast conservation therapy compared with those treated with mastectomy are highly variable, and although somewhat different, they require the attention and psychotherapeutic support of the treating physicians.[886,887] Radical surgery produces more psychoemotional disruption in terms of feelings about body image, physical attractiveness, and sexuality, whereas lumpectomy and irradiation may interfere temporarily with the patient's lifestyle and may cause worries about cancer and the perceived adverse effects of irradiation. However, at present, this assumption is not supported by research findings; the fear of recurrence has been reported to be similar in women undergoing mastectomy or breast conservation therapy.

A clinical decision analysis on the quality-adjusted life expectancy of patients with breast cancer, comparing a group treated with mastectomy and one treated with breast conservation therapy, showed that breast conservation therapy yields better quality-adjusted life expectancy than mastectomy. However, there are selected subgroups of patients who should preferably undergo mastectomy.[888] Lasry and Margolese,[889] in a comparison of psychological effects on some patients randomly assigned to NSABP protocol B-06, noted that patients who underwent more radical surgery did not express less fear of cancer recurrence than those treated with lumpectomy. The expected tradeoff between breast conservation and increased fear of cancer recurrence did not occur.

Body image, as a component of self-concept, was compared through mailed questionnaires sent to 257 patients treated with mastectomy, mastectomy with delayed reconstruction, mastectomy with immediate reconstruction, or conservation therapy.[890] When analysis of covariance with age was used, body image in the conservation therapy group was significantly more positive than in either the mastectomy group or the mastectomy with immediate reconstruction group. No differences in self-concept were evident among the four groups.

The advantage of breast conservation therapy is psychological because preservation of the configuration of the body maintains the sensation of female identity and body image to a better extent than mastectomy.[371] Breast conservation therapy does not, however, reduce the high frequency of anxiety phenomena, mental instability, and depression. Psychosocial adjustment, body image, and sexual function were retrospectively assessed in 72 women who had partial and 147 women who had total mastectomy and immediate breast reconstruction.[891,892] Questionnaires completed at a mean of 4 years after surgery (44% of questionnaires returned) showed that fewer than 20% of women reported good adjustment in the areas measured. There was no significant difference between the two groups with regard to body image, sexual attractiveness, or marital happiness. Of 184 women who answered the question, 109 (59%) believed that cancer had brought them closer to their partner, 44 (24%) saw no significant impact, and 31 (17%) believed that cancer had interfered with their relationships. There was no significant differences between the two surgery groups with regard to frequency of sexual expression, desire for sex, or actual sexual activity. Pleasure with breast caressing had decreased since cancer treatment for 44% of women with partial mastectomy and for 83% of those with mastectomy and breast reconstruction. With regard to satisfaction with appearance of the breast, there was no significant difference between the surgical groups.

Schain et al.[887] prospectively studied 142 women participating in clinical trials who were randomly assigned to undergo mastectomy or lumpectomy and radiation therapy. Baseline assessments were made before randomization and at 6, 12, and 24 months after treatment. At 6 months, patients receiving mastectomy reported significantly less control of events in their lives ($P = .003$) and more problems with sexual relations ($P = .021$) than did their conservatively treated counterparts. In addition, there were marked differences between patients receiving mastectomy and those undergoing lumpectomy or irradiation in the degree of distress over body image ($P = .059$ at 24 months). This study concluded that breast conservation therapy protects a woman's perception of her body but does not, over time, contribute to more positive sexual adjustment.

Despite numerous studies of partial mastectomy and psychological morbidity in the first 24 months after surgery, little is known about the long-term psychosocial repercussions. Dorval et al.[893] assessed the effect of the type of mastectomy on psychological adjustment in 124 breast carcinoma survivors, 47 of whom underwent partial mastectomy and 77 total mastectomy, 8 years after initial treatment. Interviews were also conducted 3 and 18 months after surgery. Psychological distress was assessed using the Psychiatric Symptom Index. No statistically significant differences between partial and total mastectomy were observed with respect to long-term quality of life. Among women younger than 50 years of age, partial mastectomy appeared to be protective against distress compared with total mastectomy ($P = .04$). In contrast, among women 50 years of age or older, partial mastectomy was associated with higher psychological distress.

With the increasing use of adjuvant chemotherapy in younger women with early-stage breast cancer, the long-term impact on quality of life, effects of premature menopause, and changes in perceived sexual attractiveness must be given a high priority for research to improve posttreatment adjustment and satisfaction in these patients.[891,894,895] Women who received chemotherapy were more likely to worry about breast cancer recurrence ($P = .001$), had sex less frequently ($P = .013$), tended to desire sex less frequently ($P = .032$), and had more vaginal dryness ($P < .001$) and dyspareunia ($P < .001$). Their ability to reach orgasm through intercourse tended to be reduced ($P = .043$), and their sexual satisfaction was significantly poorer ($P = .001$). The ability to have orgasm through noncoital caressing did not differ from that of other women. There was a significant correlation between the age of the patient and the frequency of sexual desire and activity.

In two large-scale clinical trials in Switzerland, adjuvant chemotherapy had a measurable effect on health-related quality of life, but this effect was transient and minor compared with the effect of patients' adjustment and coping after diagnosis and surgery.[896]

Ganz et al.[894] conducted a survey of 864 breast cancer survivors. RAND Health Survey scores were as good or better than those of healthy, age-matched women, and the frequency of depression was similar to general population samples. Marital or partner adjustment was similar to that in normal healthy samples, and sexual functioning mirrored that of healthy, age-matched postmenopausal women. However, these breast cancer survivors reported higher rates of physical symptom (e.g., joint pains, headaches, and hot flashes) than healthy women. Sexual dysfunction occurred more frequently in women who had received chemotherapy (all ages) and in younger women who were no longer menstruating. In women 50 years of age and older, tamoxifen therapy was unrelated to sexual functioning. Clinicians should inquire about common symptoms to provide symptomatic management or counseling for these women.

Ganz et al.[895] also surveyed 1,096 women diagnosed with early-stage breast cancer between 1 and 5 years earlier in two large metropolitan centers in the United States; 356 had received tamoxifen alone, 180 chemotherapy alone, 395 chemotherapy and tamoxifen, and 265 received no adjuvant therapy. No significant differences in global quality-of-life or in depression scores were observed among the four treatment groups. The group receiving no adjuvant therapy had a

physical functioning composite score that was at the mean for a normal population of healthy women, whereas those in the adjuvant treatment groups scored slightly lower. The mental health score was not significantly different among the four treatment groups and approximated scores from the normal population of healthy women. Overall, breast cancer survivors function at a high level, similar to healthy women without cancer. However, compared with survivors with no adjuvant therapy, those who received chemotherapy have significantly more sexual problems, and those treated with tamoxifen experience more vasomotor symptoms.

Nissen et al.[897] carried out a quality-of-life study in women 30 to 85 years of age with newly diagnosed breast carcinoma who underwent breast-conserving surgery ($n = 103$), mastectomy alone ($n = 55$), or mastectomy with reconstruction ($n = 40$). Quality of life was assessed after diagnosis (baseline) and at 1, 3, 6, 12, 18, and 24 months. Women who underwent mastectomy with reconstruction had greater mood disturbance ($P = .002$) and poorer well-being ($P = .002$) after baseline than women who had mastectomy alone, and these differences remained 18 months after surgery. The breast-conserving surgery and mastectomy-only groups did not differ significantly regarding well-being.

CONCLUSION

Radiation therapy plays an essential and critical role in the management of breast cancer, the most common cancer diagnosed in women. Early detection by mammography, followed by appropriate oncologic therapy, may be associated with reduced breast cancer mortality rates for women aged 50 years and older. After breast-conserving surgery, WBI improves local control and survival rates in appropriately selected patients and therefore should be considered for all patients. The development of molecular signatures predictive for LRR may revolutionize how we select patients for radiotherapy; significant progress has been made in this area with systemic therapy but similar work is needed with regard to locoregional therapies. Accelerated forms of treatment including HWBI and APBI may increase the utilization rate of radiotherapy after breast-conserving surgery. Ongoing research will help to further define the safety and acceptability of these techniques in women with early-stage breast cancer.

REFERENCES

1. Wallgren A, Bernier J, Gelber RD, et al. Timing of radiotherapy and chemotherapy following breast-conserving surgery for patients with node-positive breast cancer. International Breast Cancer Study Group. *Int J Radiat Oncol Biol Phys* 1996;35(4):649–659.
2. Weinstein SP, Orel SG, Heller R, et al. MR imaging of the breast in patients with invasive lobular carcinoma. *AJR Am J Roentgenol* 2001;176(2):399–406.
3. Estourgie SH, Nieweg OE, Olmos RA, et al. Lymphatic drainage patterns from the breast. *Ann Surg* 2004;239(2):232–237.
4. Siegel RL, Miller KD, Jemal A. Cancer Statistics, 2017. *CA Cancer J Clin* 2017;67(1):7–30.
5. MacMahon B. Epidemiology and the causes of breast cancer. *Int J Cancer* 2006;118(10):2373–2378.
6. Deapen D, Liu L, Perkins C, et al. Rapidly rising breast cancer incidence rates among Asian-American women. *Int J Cancer* 2002;99(5):747–750.
7. Chlebowski RT, Chen Z, Anderson GL, et al. Ethnicity and breast cancer: factors influencing differences in incidence and outcome. *J Natl Cancer Inst* 2005;97(6):439–448.
8. Blaszyk H, Vaughn CB, Hartmann A, et al. Novel pattern of p53 gene mutations in an American black cohort with high mortality from breast cancer. *Lancet* 1994;343(8907):1195–1197.
9. Joslyn SA, West MM. Racial differences in breast carcinoma survival. *Cancer* 2000;88(1):114–123.
10. Colditz GA. Epidemiology and prevention of breast cancer. *Cancer Epidemiol Biomarkers Prev* 2005;14(4):768–772.
11. Jemal A, Siegel R, Ward E, et al. Cancer statistics, 2006. *CA Cancer J Clin* 2006;56(2):106–130.
12. MacMahon B, Purde M, Cramer D, et al. Association of breast cancer risk with age at first and subsequent births: a study in the population of the Estonian Republic. *J Natl Cancer Inst* 1982;69(5):1035–1038.

13. Bonadonna G, Veronesi U, Brambilla C, et al. Primary chemotherapy for resectable breast cancer. *Recent Results Cancer Res* 1993;127:113–117.
14. Breast cancer and hormone replacement therapy: collaborative reanalysis of data from 51 epidemiological studies of 52,705 women with breast cancer and 108,411 women without breast cancer. Collaborative Group on Hormonal Factors in Breast Cancer. *Lancet* 1997;350(9084):1047–1059.
15. Rossouw JE, Anderson GL, Prentice RL, et al. Risks and benefits of estrogen plus progestin in healthy postmenopausal women: principal results from the Women's Health Initiative Randomized Controlled Trial. *JAMA* 2002;288(3):321–333.
16. Jemal A, Siegel R, Xu J, et al. Cancer statistics, 2010. *CA Cancer J Clin* 2010; 60(5):277–300.
17. Schairer C, Lubin J, Troisi R, et al. Menopausal estrogen and estrogen-progestin replacement therapy and breast cancer risk. *JAMA* 2000;283(4):485–491.
18. Grabrick DM, Hartmann LC, Cerhan JR, et al. Risk of breast cancer with oral contraceptive use in women with a family history of breast cancer. *JAMA* 2000;284(14):1791–1798.
19. Van Hoften C, Burger H, Peeters PH, et al. Long-term oral contraceptive use increases breast cancer risk in women over 55 years of age: the DOM cohort. *Int J Cancer* 2000;87(4):591–594.
20. Burke W, Daly M, Garber J, et al. Recommendations for follow-up care of individuals with an inherited predisposition to cancer. II. BRCA1 and BRCA2. Cancer Genetics Studies Consortium. *JAMA* 1997;277(12):997–1003.
21. Robson ME, Boyd J, Borgen PI, et al. Hereditary breast cancer. *Curr Probl Surg* 2001;38(6):387–480.
22. Daly MB, Pilarski R, Berry M, et al. NCCN Guidelines Insights: Genetic/Familial High-Risk Assessment: Breast and Ovarian, Version 2.2017. *J Natl Compr Canc Netw* 2017;15(1):9–20
23. Obedian E, Fischer DB, Haffty BG. Second malignancies after treatment of early-stage breast cancer: lumpectomy and radiation therapy versus mastectomy. *J Clin Oncol* 2000;18(12):2406–2412.
24. Gao X, Fisher SG, Emami B. Risk of second primary cancer in the contralateral breast in women treated for early-stage breast cancer: a population-based study. *Int J Radiat Oncol Biol Phys* 2003;56(4):1038–1045.
25. Smart CR, Byrne C, Smith RA, et al. Twenty-year follow-up of the breast cancers diagnosed during the Breast Cancer Detection Demonstration Project. *CA Cancer J Clin* 1997;47(3):134–149.
26. Land CE, Boice JD Jr, Shore RE, et al. Breast cancer risk from low-dose exposures to ionizing radiation: results of parallel analysis of three exposed populations of women. *J Natl Cancer Inst* 1980;65(2):353–376.
27. Land CE. Studies of cancer and radiation dose among atomic bomb survivors. The example of breast cancer. *JAMA* 1995;274(5):402–407.
28. Miller AB, Howe GR, Sherman GJ, et al. Mortality from breast cancer after irradiation during fluoroscopic examinations in patients being treated for tuberculosis. *N Engl J Med* 1989;321(19):1285–1289.
29. Travis LB, Hill D, Dores GM, et al. Cumulative absolute breast cancer risk for young women treated for Hodgkin lymphoma. *J Natl Cancer Inst* 2005;97(19):1428–1437.
30. De Bruin ML, Sparidans J, van't Veer MB, et al. Breast cancer risk in female survivors of Hodgkin's lymphoma: lower risk after smaller radiation volumes. *J Clin Oncol* 2009;27(26):4239–4246.
31. van den Brandt PA, Spiegelman D, Yaun SS, et al. Pooled analysis of prospective cohort studies on height, weight, and breast cancer risk. *Am J Epidemiol* 2000;152(6):514–527.
32. Wu AH, Pike MC, Stram DO. Meta-analysis: dietary fat intake, serum estrogen levels, and the risk of breast cancer. *J Natl Cancer Inst* 1999;91(6):529–534.
33. Hunter DJ, Spiegelman D, Adami HO, et al. Non-dietary factors as risk factors for breast cancer, and as effect modifiers of the association of fat intake and risk of breast cancer. *Cancer Causes Control* 1997;8(1):49–56.
34. Hamajima N, Hirose K, Tajima K, et al. Alcohol, tobacco and breast cancer—collaborative reanalysis of individual data from 53 epidemiological studies, including 58,515 women with breast cancer and 95,067 women without the disease. *Br J Cancer* 2002;87(11):1234–1245.
35. Chen WY, Rosner B, Hankinson SE, et al. Moderate alcohol consumption during adult life, drinking patterns, and breast cancer risk. *JAMA* 2011;306(17):1884–1890.
36. Boyd NF, Dite GS, Stone J, et al. Heritability of mammographic density, a risk factor for breast cancer. *N Engl J Med* 2002;347(12):886–894.
37. Boyd NF, Stone J, Vogt KN, et al. Dietary fat and breast cancer risk revisited: a meta-analysis of the published literature. *Br J Cancer* 2003;89(9):1672–1685.
38. Yaffe M, Boyd N. Mammographic breast density and cancer risk: the radiological view. *Gynecol Endocrinol* 2005;21(Suppl 1):6–11.
39. Boyd NF, Lockwood GA, Byng JW, et al. Mammographic densities and breast cancer risk. *Cancer Epidemiol Biomarkers Prev* 1998;7(12):1133–1144.
40. Byrne C, Schairer C, Wolfe J, et al. Mammographic features and breast cancer risk: effects with time, age, and menopause status. *J Natl Cancer Inst* 1995;87(21):1622–1629.
41. Gail MH, Brinton LA, Byar DP, et al. Projecting individualized probabilities of developing breast cancer for white females who are being examined annually. *J Natl Cancer Inst* 1989;81(24):1879–1886.
42. Malkin D, Li FP, Strong LC, et al. Germline p53 mutations in a familial syndrome of breast cancer, sarcomas, and other neoplasms. *Science* 1990;250(4985):1233–1238.
43. The Breast Cancer Linkage Consortium. Cancer risks in BRCA2 mutation carriers. *J Natl Cancer Inst* 1999;91(15):1310–1316.
44. Hollstein M, Soussi T, Thomas G, et al. P53 gene alterations in human tumors: perspectives for cancer control. *Recent Results Cancer Res* 1997;143:369–389.
45. Shattuck-Eidens D, Oliphant A, McClure M, et al. BRCA1 sequence analysis in women at high risk for susceptibility mutations. Risk factor analysis and implications for genetic testing. *JAMA* 1997;278(15):1242–1250.
46. Barrett-Connor E, Mosca L, Collins P, et al. Effects of raloxifene on cardiovascular events and breast cancer in postmenopausal women. *N Engl J Med* 2006;355(2):125–137.
47. Cummings SR, Eckert S, Krueger KA, et al. The effect of raloxifene on risk of breast cancer in postmenopausal women: results from the MORE randomized trial. Multiple Outcomes of Raloxifene Evaluation. *JAMA* 1999;281(23):2189–2197.
48. Cuzick J, Forbes J, Edwards R, et al. First results from the International Breast Cancer Intervention Study (IBIS-I): a randomised prevention trial. *Lancet* 2002;360(9336):817–824.
49. Cuzick J, Powles T, Veronesi U, et al. Overview of the main outcomes in breast-cancer prevention trials. *Lancet* 2003;361(9354):296–300.
50. Veronesi U, Maisonneuve P, Rotmensz N, et al. Italian randomized trial among women with hysterectomy: tamoxifen and hormone-dependent breast cancer in high-risk women. *J Natl Cancer Inst* 2003;95(2):160–165.
51. Fisher B, Costantino JP, Wickerham DL, et al. Tamoxifen for prevention of breast cancer: report of the National Surgical Adjuvant Breast and Bowel Project P-1 study. *J Natl Cancer Inst* 1998;90(18):1371–1388.
52. Vogel VG, Costantino JP, Wickerham DL, et al. Effects of tamoxifen vs raloxifene on the risk of developing invasive breast cancer and other disease outcomes: the NSABP Study of Tamoxifen and Raloxifene (STAR) P-2 trial. *JAMA* 2006;295(23):2727–2741.
53. Powles T, Eeles R, Ashley S, et al. Interim analysis of the incidence of breast cancer in the Royal Marsden Hospital tamoxifen randomised chemoprevention trial. *Lancet* 1998;352(9122):98–101.
54. Veronesi U, Maisonneuve P, Sacchini V, et al. Tamoxifen for breast cancer among hysterectomised women. *Lancet* 2002;359(9312):1122–1124.
55. Hartmann LC, Schaid DJ, Woods JE, et al. Efficacy of bilateral prophylactic mastectomy in women with a family history of breast cancer. *N Engl J Med* 1999;340(2):77–84.
56. Bloom HJ, Richardson WW, Harries EJ. Natural history of untreated breast cancer (1805–1933). Comparison of untreated and treated cases according to histological grade of malignancy. *Br Med J* 1962;5299:213–221.
57. Halsted WS. The results of operations for the cure of cancer of the breast performed at Johns Hopkins Hospital from June 1889 to January 1894. *Johns Hopkins Hosp Bull* 1894;4:297.
58. Keynes G. Carcinoma of the breast, the unorthodox view. *Proc Cardiff Med Soc* 1954;40.
59. Crile G Jr, Cooperman A, Esselstyn CB Jr, et al. Results of partial mastectomy in 173 patients followed for from five to ten years. *Surg Gynecol Obstet* 1980;150(4):563–566.
60. Fisher B. Laboratory and clinical research in breast cancer, a personal adventure. The David A Karnovsky Memorial Lecture. *Cancer Res* 1980;40:3863–3874.
61. Hellman S. Karnofsky Memorial Lecture. Natural history of small breast cancers. *J Clin Oncol* 1994;12(10):2229–2234.
62. Haagenson C. *Diseases of the breast*. Philadelphia, PA: WB Saunders, 1986.
63. Voogd AC, Coebergh JW, Repelaer van Driel OJ, et al. The risk of nodal metastases in breast cancer patients with clinically negative lymph nodes: a population-based analysis. *Breast Cancer Res Treat* 2000;62(1):63–69.
64. Greco M, Crippa F, Agresti R, et al. Axillary lymph node staging in breast cancer by 2-fluoro-2-deoxy-D-glucose-positron emission tomography: clinical evaluation and alternative management. *J Natl Cancer Inst* 2001;93(8):630–635.
65. Kambouris AA. Axillary node metastases in relation to size and location of breast cancers: analysis of 147 patients. *Am Surg* 1996;62(7):519–524.
66. Silverstein MJ, Gierson ED, Waisman JR, et al. Axillary lymph node dissection for T1a breast carcinoma. Is it indicated? *Cancer* 1994;73(3):664–667.
67. Tinnemans JG, Wobbes T, Holland R, et al. Treatment and survival of female patients with nonpalpable breast carcinoma. *Ann Surg* 1989;209(2):249–253.
68. Fein DA, Fowble BL, Hanlon AL, et al. Identification of women with T1–T2 breast cancer at low risk of positive axillary nodes. *J Surg Oncol* 1997;65(1):34–39.
69. Mustafa IA, Cole B, Wanebo HJ, et al. Prognostic analysis of survival in small breast cancers. *J Am Coll Surg* 1998;186(5):562–569.
70. Gann PH, Colilla SA, Gapstur SM, et al. Factors associated with axillary lymph node metastasis from breast carcinoma: descriptive and predictive analyses. *Cancer* 1999;86(8):1511–1519.
71. Fisher B, Montague E, Redmond C, et al. Findings from NSABP protocol no. B-04-comparison of radical mastectomy with alternative treatments for primary breast cancer. I. Radiation compliance and its relation to treatment outcome. *Cancer* 1980;46(1):1–13.
72. Handley RS. Carcinoma of the breast. *Ann R Coll Surg Engl* 1975;57(2):59–66.
73. Veronesi U, Cascinelli N, Bufalino R, et al. Risk of internal mammary lymph node metastases and its relevance on prognosis of breast cancer patients. *Ann Surg* 1983;198(6):681–684.
74. Sugg SL, Ferguson DJ, Posner MC, et al. Should internal mammary nodes be sampled in the sentinel lymph node era? *Ann Surg Oncol* 2000;7(3):188–192.
75. Fowble B, Solin LJ, Schultz DJ, et al. Frequency, sites of relapse, and outcome of regional node failures following conservative surgery and radiation for early breast cancer. *Int J Radiat Oncol Biol Phys* 1989;17(4):703–710.
76. Galper S, Recht A, Silver B, et al. Factors associated with regional nodal failure in patients with early stage breast cancer with 0-3 positive axillary nodes following tangential irradiation alone. *Int J Radiat Oncol Biol Phys* 1999;45(5):1157–1166.
77. Haffty BG, Fischer D, Fischer JJ. Regional nodal irradiation in the conservative treatment of breast cancer. *Int J Radiat Oncol Biol Phys* 1990;19(4):859–865.
78. Halverson KJ, Taylor ME, Perez CA, et al. Regional nodal management and patterns of failure following conservative surgery and radiation therapy for stage I and II breast cancer. *Int J Radiat Oncol Biol Phys* 1993;26(4):593–599.
79. Recht A, Pierce SM, Abner A, et al. Regional nodal failure after conservative surgery and radiotherapy for early-stage breast carcinoma. *J Clin Oncol* 1991;9(6):988–996.

80. Chen SC, Chen MF, Hwang TL, et al. Prediction of supraclavicular lymph node metastasis in breast carcinoma. *Int J Radiat Oncol Biol Phys* 2002;52(3):614–619.

81. Fisher B, Bauer M, Wickerham DL, et al. Relation of number of positive axillary nodes to the prognosis of patients with primary breast cancer. An NSABP update. *Cancer* 1983;52(9):1551–1557.

82. Fisher BJ, Perera FE, Cooke AL, et al. Extracapsular axillary node extension in patients receiving adjuvant systemic therapy: an indication for radiotherapy?. *Int J Radiat Oncol Biol Phys* 1997;38(3):551–559.

83. Fisher BJ, Perera FE, Cooke AL, et al. Long-term follow-up of axillary node-positive breast cancer patients receiving adjuvant systemic therapy alone: patterns of recurrence. *Int J Radiat Oncol Biol Phys* 1997;38(3):541–550.

84. Vicini FA, Horwitz EM, Lacerna MD, et al. The role of regional nodal irradiation in the management of patients with early-stage breast cancer treated with breast-conserving therapy. *Int J Radiat Oncol Biol Phys* 1997;39(5):1069–1076.

85. Strom EA, Woodward WA, Katz A, et al. Clinical investigation: regional nodal failure patterns in breast cancer patients treated with mastectomy without radiotherapy. *Int J Radiat Oncol Biol Phys* 2005;63(5):1508–1513.

86. Braun S, Vogl FD, Naume B, et al. A pooled analysis of bone marrow micrometastasis in breast cancer. *N Engl J Med* 2005;353(8):793–802.

87. Clarke M, Collins R, Darby S, et al. Effects of radiotherapy and of differences in the extent of surgery for early breast cancer on local recurrence and 15-year survival: an overview of the randomised trials. *Lancet* 2005;366(9503):2087–2106.

88. Vinh-Hung V, Verschraegen C. Breast-conserving surgery with or without radiotherapy: pooled-analysis for risks of ipsilateral breast tumor recurrence and mortality. *J Natl Cancer Inst* 2004;96(2):115–121.

89. Huang J, Barbera L, Brouwers M, et al. Does delay in starting treatment affect the outcomes of radiotherapy? A systematic review. *J Clin Oncol* 2003;21(3):555–563.

90. Haffty BG, Fischer D, Rose M, et al. Prognostic factors for local recurrence in the conservatively treated breast cancer patient: a cautious interpretation of the data. *J Clin Oncol* 1991;9(6):997–1003.

91. Fisher B, Anderson S, Bryant J, et al. Twenty-year follow-up of a randomized trial comparing total mastectomy, lumpectomy, and lumpectomy plus irradiation for the treatment of invasive breast cancer. *N Engl J Med* 2002;347(16):1233–1241.

92. Fisher B, Anderson S, Tan-Chiu E, et al. Tamoxifen and chemotherapy for axillary node-negative, estrogen receptor-negative breast cancer: findings from National Surgical Adjuvant Breast and Bowel Project B-23. *J Clin Oncol* 2001;19(4):931–942.

93. Fisher B, Bryant J, Dignam JJ, et al. Tamoxifen, radiation therapy, or both for prevention of ipsilateral breast tumor recurrence after lumpectomy in women with invasive breast cancers of one centimeter or less. *J Clin Oncol* 2002;20(20):4141–4149.

94. King MC, Wieand S, Hale K, et al. Tamoxifen and breast cancer incidence among women with inherited mutations in BRCA1 and BRCA2: National Surgical Adjuvant Breast and Bowel Project (NSABP-P1) Breast Cancer Prevention Trial. *JAMA* 2001;286(18):2251–2256.

95. Buchholz TA, Tucker SL, Erwin J, et al. Impact of systemic treatment on local control for patients with lymph node-negative breast cancer treated with breast-conservation therapy. *J Clin Oncol* 2001;19(8):2240–2246.

96. Fowble BL, Solin LJ, Schultz DJ, et al. Ten year results of conservative surgery and irradiation for stage I and II breast cancer. *Int J Radiat Oncol Biol Phys* 1991;21(2):269–277.

97. Haffty BG, Goldberg NB, Fischer D, et al. Conservative surgery and radiation therapy in breast carcinoma: local recurrence and prognostic implications. *Int J Radiat Oncol Biol Phys* 1989;17(4):727–732.

98. Recht A. Selection of patients with early stage invasive breast cancer for treatment with conservative surgery and radiation therapy. *Semin Oncol* 1996;23(1 Suppl 2):19–30.

99. van Dongen JA, Voogd AC, Fentiman IS, et al. Long-term results of a randomized trial comparing breast-conserving therapy with mastectomy: European Organization for Research and Treatment of Cancer 10801 trial. *J Natl Cancer Inst* 2000;92(14):1143–1150.

100. Veronesi U, Cascinelli N, Mariani L, et al. Twenty-year follow-up of a randomized study comparing breast-conserving surgery with radical mastectomy for early breast cancer. *N Engl J Med* 2002;347(16):1227–1232.

101. Ready K, Arun B. Clinical assessment of breast cancer risk based on family history. *J Natl Compr Canc Netw* 2010;8(10):1148–1155.

102. Ready K, Gutierrez-Barrera AM, Amos C, et al. Cancer risk management decisions of women with BRCA1 or BRCA2 variants of uncertain significance. *Breast J* 2011;17(2):210–212.

103. Claus EB, Stowe M, Carter D, et al. The risk of a contralateral breast cancer among women diagnosed with ductal and lobular breast carcinoma in situ: data from the Connecticut Tumor Registry. *Breast* 2003;12(6):451–456.

104. Bhatia S, Robison LL, Oberlin O, et al. Breast cancer and other second neoplasms after childhood Hodgkin's disease. *N Engl J Med* 1996;334(12):745–751.

105. Bevers TB, Anderson BO, Bonaccio E, et al. NCCN clinical practice guidelines in oncology: breast cancer screening and diagnosis. *J Natl Compr Canc Netw* 2009;7(10):1060–1096.

106. Fisher B, Anderson S, Fisher ER, et al. Significance of ipsilateral breast tumour recurrence after lumpectomy. *Lancet* 1991;338(8763):327–331.

107. Fowble B, Solin LJ, Schultz DJ, et al. Breast recurrence following conservative surgery and radiation: patterns of failure, prognosis, and pathologic findings from mastectomy specimens with implications for treatment. *Int J Radiat Oncol Biol Phys* 1990;19(4):833–842.

108. Haffty BG, Reiss M, Beinfield M, et al. Ipsilateral breast tumor recurrence as a predictor of distant disease: implications for systemic therapy at the time of local relapse. *J Clin Oncol* 1996;14(1):52–57.

109. Cheng JC, Chen CM, Liu MC, et al. Locoregional failure of postmastectomy patients with 1–3 positive axillary lymph nodes without adjuvant radiotherapy. *Int J Radiat Oncol Biol Phys* 2002;52(4):980–988.

110. Darby S, McGale P, Correa C, et al. Effect of radiotherapy after breast-conserving surgery on 10-year recurrence and 15-year breast cancer death: meta-analysis of individual patient data for 10,801 women in 17 randomised trials. *Lancet* 2011;378(9804):1707–1716.

111. Richards MA, Smith P, Ramirez AJ, et al. The influence on survival of delay in the presentation and treatment of symptomatic breast cancer. *Br J Cancer* 1999;79(5–6):858–864.

112. Olivotto IA, Gomi A, Bancej C, et al. Influence of delay to diagnosis on prognostic indicators of screen-detected breast carcinoma. *Cancer* 2002;94(8):2143–2150.

113. Harris J, Lippman M, Morrow M, et al. *Diseases of the breast.* 3rd. ed. Philadelphia, PA: Lippincott Williams & Wilkins, 2004.

114. O'Malley MS, Fletcher SW. US Preventive Services Task Force. Screening for breast cancer with breast self-examination. A critical review. *JAMA* 1987;257(16):2196–2203.

115. Elmore JG, Armstrong K, Lehman CD, et al. Screening for breast cancer. *JAMA* 2005;293(10):1245–1256.

116. Elmore JG, Reisch LM, Barton MB, et al. Efficacy of breast cancer screening in the community according to risk level. *J Natl Cancer Inst* 2005;97(14):1035–1043.

117. Fenton JJ, Barton MB, Geiger AM, et al. Screening clinical breast examination: how often does it miss lethal breast cancer?. *J Natl Cancer Inst Monogr* 2005(35):67–71.

118. Kopans DB. An overview of the breast cancer screening controversy. *J Natl Cancer Inst Monogr* 1997(22):1–3.

119. Kopans DB, Feig SA. The Canadian National Breast Screening Study: a critical review. *AJR Am J Roentgenol* 1993;161(4):755–760.

120. Smart CR, Hendrick RE, Rutledge JH III, et al. Benefit of mammography screening in women ages 40 to 49 years. Current evidence from randomized controlled trials. *Cancer* 1995;75(7):1619–1626.

121. Tabar L, Vitak B, Chen HH, et al. Beyond randomized controlled trials: organized mammographic screening substantially reduces breast carcinoma mortality. *Cancer* 2001;91(9):1724–1731.

122. Shapiro S, Venet W, Strax P, et al. Selection, follow-up, and analysis in the Health Insurance Plan Study: a randomized trial with breast cancer screening. *Natl Cancer Inst Monogr* 1985;67:65–74.

123. Andersson I, Aspegren K, Janzon L, et al. Mammographic screening and mortality from breast cancer: the Malmo mammographic screening trial. *BMJ* 1988;297(6654):943–948.

124. Tabár L, Vitak B, Chen HH, et al. The Swedish Two-County Trial twenty years later. Updated mortality results and new insights from long-term follow-up. *Radiol Clin North Am* 2000;38(4):625–651.

125. Alexander FE, Anderson TJ, Brown HK, et al. 14 years of follow-up from the Edinburgh randomised trial of breast-cancer screening. *Lancet* 1999;353(9168):1903–1908.

126. Miller AB, To T, Baines CJ, et al. The Canadian National Breast Screening Study: update on breast cancer mortality. *J Natl Cancer Inst Monogr* 1997(22):37–41.

127. Miller AB, To T, Baines CJ, et al. Canadian National Breast Screening Study 2: 13-year results of a randomized trial in women aged 50–59 years. *J Natl Cancer Inst* 2000;92(18):1490–1499.

128. Frisell J, Lidbrink E. The Stockholm Mammographic Screening Trial: risks and benefits in age group 40–49 years. *J Natl Cancer Inst Monogr* 1997(22):49–51.

129. Bjurstam N, Bjorneld L, Warwick J, et al. The Gothenburg Breast Screening Trial. *Cancer* 2003;97(10):2387–2396.

130. Tabár L, Duffy SW, Burhenne LW. New Swedish breast cancer detection results for women aged 40–49. *Cancer* 1993;72(4 Suppl):1437–1448.

131. Tabár L, Duffy SW, Vitak B, et al. The natural history of breast carcinoma: what have we learned from screening?. *Cancer* 1999;86(3):449–462.

132. Shapiro S, Venet W, Strax P, et al. Ten- to fourteen-year effect of screening on breast cancer mortality. *J Natl Cancer Inst* 1982;69(2):349–355.

133. Tabar L, Vitak B, Chen TH, et al. Swedish two-county trial: impact of mammographic screening on breast cancer mortality during 3 decades. *Radiology* 2011;260(3):658–663.

134. Tarone RE. The excess of patients with advanced breast cancer in young women screened with mammography in the Canadian National Breast Screening Study. *Cancer* 1995;75(4):997–1003.

135. UK Trial Group. 16-year mortality from breast cancer in the UK Trial of Early Detection of Breast Cancer. *Lancet* 1999;353(9168):1909–1914.

136. Wald NJ, Hackshaw A, Chamberlain J. The efficacy and safety of periodic mammographic breast cancer screening: summary of report of the European Society of Mastology. *Clin Radiol* 1994;49(9):592–593.

137. Hellquist BN, Duffy SW, Abdsaleh S, et al. Effectiveness of population-based service screening with mammography for women ages 40 to 49 years: evaluation of the Swedish Mammography Screening in Young Women (SCRY) cohort. *Cancer* 2011;117(4):714–722.

138. American Cancer Society. *Cancer facts & figures 2002.* Atlanta, GA: American Cancer Society, 2002.

139. Oeffinger KC, Fontham ET, Etzioni R et al. Breast cancer screening for women at average risk: 2015 guideline update from the American Cancer Society. *JAMA* 2015;314(15):1599–1614.

140. Nelson HD, Tyne K, Naik A, et al. Screening for breast cancer: an update for the U.S. Preventive Services Task Force. *Ann Intern Med* 2009;151(10):727–737.

141. Pisano ED, Gatsonis C, Hendrick E, et al. Diagnostic performance of digital versus film mammography for breast-cancer screening. *N Engl J Med* 2005;353(17):1773–1783.

142. U.S. Preventive Services Task Force. Screening for breast cancer: U.S. Preventive Services Task Force recommendation statement. *Ann Intern Med* 2009;151(10):716–726, W-236.

143. Summaries for patients. Screening for breast cancer: U.S. Preventive Services Task Force recommendations. *Ann Intern Med* 2009;151(10):I44.

144. Kriege M, Brekelmans CT, Boetes C et al. Efficacy of MRI and mammography for breast-cancer screening in women with a familial or genetic predisposition. *N Engl J Med* 2004;351(5):427–437.
145. Kuhl CK, Schrading S, Leutner CC, et al. Mammography, breast ultrasound, and magnetic resonance imaging for surveillance of women at high familial risk for breast cancer. *J Clin Oncol* 2005;23(33):8469–8476.
146. Leach MO, Boggis CR, Dixon AK, et al. Screening with magnetic resonance imaging and mammography of a UK population at high familial risk of breast cancer: a prospective multicentre cohort study (MARIBS). *Lancet* 2005;365(9473):1769–1778.
147. Lehman CD, Blume JD, Weatherall P, et al. Screening women at high risk for breast cancer with mammography and magnetic resonance imaging. *Cancer* 2005;103(9):1898–1905.
148. Sardanelli F, Podo F. Breast MR imaging in women at high-risk of breast cancer. Is something changing in early breast cancer detection? *Eur Radiol* 2007;17(4):873–887.
149. Warner E, Plewes DB, Hill KA et al: Surveillance of BRCA1 and BRCA2 mutation carriers with magnetic resonance imaging, ultrasound, mammography, and clinical breast examination. *JAMA* 2004;292(11):1317–1325.
150. Kriege M, Brekelmans CT, Boetes C, et al. Efficacy of MRI and mammography for breast-cancer screening in women with a familial or genetic predisposition. *N Engl J Med* 2004;351(5):427–437.
151. Bevers TB. Ultrasound for the screening of breast cancer. *Curr Oncol Rep* 2008;10(6):527–528.
152. Berg WA, Blume JD, Cormack JB, et al. Combined screening with ultrasound and mammography vs mammography alone in women at elevated risk of breast cancer. *JAMA* 2008;299(18):2151–2163.
153. Costanza MC, Foster RS Jr. Relationship between breast self-examination and death from breast cancer by age groups. *Cancer Detect Prev* 1984;7(2):103–108.
154. Foster RS Jr, Costanza MC. Breast self-examination practices and breast cancer survival. *Cancer* 1984;53(4):999–1005.
155. Seidman H, Gelb SK, Silverberg E, et al. Survival experience in the Breast Cancer Detection Demonstration Project. *CA Cancer J Clin* 1987;37(5):258–290.
156. Orel SG, Kay N, Reynolds C, et al. BI-RADS categorization as a predictor of malignancy. *Radiology* 1999;211(3):845–850.
157. Kopans DB, Meyer JE, Sadowsky N. Breast imaging. *N Engl J Med* 1984;310(15):960–967.
158. Dershaw DD. Mammography in patients with breast cancer treated by breast conservation (lumpectomy with or without radiation). *AJR Am J Roentgenol* 1995;164(2):309–316.
159. Smallwood JA, Guyer P, Dewbury K, et al. The accuracy of ultrasound in the diagnosis of breast disease. *Ann R Coll Surg Engl* 1986;68(1):19–22.
160. Soo MS, Rosen EL, Baker JA, et al. Negative predictive value of sonography with mammography in patients with palpable breast lesions. *AJR Am J Roentgenol* 2001;177(5):1167–1170.
161. Flobbe K, Bosch AM, Kessels AG, et al. The additional diagnostic value of ultrasonography in the diagnosis of breast cancer. *Arch Intern Med* 2003;163(10):1194–1199.
162. Hylton N. Magnetic resonance imaging of the breast: opportunities to improve breast cancer management. *J Clin Oncol* 2005;23(8):1678–1684.
163. Gradishar WJ, Anderson BO, Balassanian R, et al. NCCN Guidelines Insights: Breast Cancer, Version 1.2017. *J Natl Compr Canc Netw* 2017;15(4):433–451.
164. Upponi SS, Warren RM. The diagnostic impact of contrast-enhanced MRI in management of breast disease. *Breast* 2006;15(6):736–743.
165. Esserman L, Hylton N, Yassa L, et al. Utility of magnetic resonance imaging in the management of breast cancer: evidence for improved preoperative staging. *J Clin Oncol* 1999;17(1):110–119.
166. Buchanan CL, Morris EA, Dorn PL, et al. Utility of breast magnetic resonance imaging in patients with occult primary breast cancer. *Ann Surg Oncol* 2005;12(12):1045–1053.
167. Thomsen HS, Lund JO, Munck O, et al. The value of pre-scheduled bone scintigraphies in breast cancer. *Acta Oncol* 1988;27(6A):617–619.
168. Butzelaar RM, van Dongen JA, van der Schoot JB, et al. Evaluation of routine pre-operative bone scintigraphy in patients with breast cancer. *Eur J Cancer* 1977;13(1):19–21.
169. Thomsen HS, Lund JO, Munck O, et al. Experience with 7,604 bone scintigraphies at time of operation for breast cancer 1977–1987. *Dan Med Bull* 1989;36(5):481–483.
170. Koizumi M, Yoshimoto M, Kasumi F, et al. What do breast cancer patients benefit from staging bone scintigraphy?. *Jpn J Clin Oncol* 2001;31(6):263–269.
171. Carlson RW, Allred DC, Anderson BO, et al. Invasive breast cancer. *J Natl Compr Canc Netw* 2011;9(2):136–222.
172. Carlson RW, Allred DC, Anderson BO, et al. Breast cancer. Clinical practice guidelines in oncology. *J Natl Compr Canc Netw* 2009;7(2):122–192.
173. Weir L, Worsley D, Bernstein V. The value of FDG positron emission tomography in the management of patients with breast cancer. *Breast J* 2005;11(3):204–209.
174. Schirrmeister H, Kuhn T, Guhlmann A, et al. Fluorine-18 2-deoxy-2-fluoro-D-glucose PET in the preoperative staging of breast cancer: comparison with the standard staging procedures. *Eur J Nucl Med* 2001;28(3):351–358.
175. Winchester D, Bernstein J, Paige M. *The early detection and diagnosis of breast cancer*. Atlanta, GA: American Cancer Society, 1988.
176. Zajdela A, Ghossein NA, Pilleron JP, et al. The value of aspiration cytology in the diagnosis of breast cancer: experience at the Fondation Curie. *Cancer* 1975;35(2):499–506.
177. Parker SH, Burbank F, Jackman RJ, et al. Percutaneous large-core breast biopsy: a multi-institutional study. *Radiology* 1994;193(2):359–364.
178. Fisher B. *Some thoughts concerning the primary therapy of breast cancer*. Berlin, Germany: Springer-Verlag, 1976.
179. Landercasper J, Gundersen SB Jr, Gundersen AL, et al. Needle localization and biopsy of nonpalpable lesions of the breast. *Surg Gynecol Obstet* 1987;164(5):399–403.
180. Bimston DN, Bebb GG, Wagman LD. Is specimen mammography beneficial?. *Arch Surg* 2000;135(9):1083–1089.
181. Schnitt SJ, Connolly JL. Processing and evaluation of breast excision specimens. A clinically oriented approach. *Am J Clin Pathol* 1992;98(1):125–137.
182. Lippman ME, Allegra JC. Current concepts in cancer. Receptors in breast cancer. *N Engl J Med* 1978;299(17):930–933.
183. Wittliff JL. Steroid-hormone receptors in breast cancer. *Cancer* 1984;53(3 Suppl):630–643.
184. Meyer JS, Friedman E, McCrate MM, et al. Prediction of early course of breast carcinoma by thymidine labeling. *Cancer* 1983;51(10):1879–1886.
185. Meyer JS, Province MA. S-phase fraction and nuclear size in long term prognosis of patients with breast cancer. *Cancer* 1994;74(8):2287–2299.
186. Perez EA, Roche PC, Jenkins RB, et al. HER2 testing in patients with breast cancer: poor correlation between weak positivity by immunohistochemistry and gene amplification by fluorescence in situ hybridization. *Mayo Clin Proc* 2002;77(2):148–154.
187. Perez EA, Suman VJ, Davidson NE, et al. HER2 testing by local, central, and reference laboratories in specimens from the North Central Cancer Treatment Group N9831 intergroup adjuvant trial. *J Clin Oncol* 2006;24(19):3032–3038.
188. American Joint Committee on Cancer. *AJCC cancer staging manual*, 7th ed. New York: Springer Science and Business Media LLC, 2010.
189. *Union Internationale Contre le Cancer*. Berlin, Germany: Springer-Verlag; 1982.
190. Giuliano AE, Connolly JL, Edge SB, et al: Breast Cancer-Major changes in the American Joint Committee on Cancer eighth edition cancer staging manual. *CA Cancer J Clin* 2017;67(4):290–303.
191. Ambrosone CB, Freudenheim JL, Sinha R, et al. Breast cancer risk, meat consumption and N-acetyltransferase (NAT2) genetic polymorphisms. *Int J Cancer* 1998;75(6):825–830.
192. Rosen PR, Groshen S, Saigo PE, et al. A long-term follow-up study of survival in stage I (T1N0M0) and stage II (T1N1M0) breast carcinoma. *J Clin Oncol* 1989;7(3):355–366.
193. Fisher ER, Gregorio RM, Fisher B, et al. The pathology of invasive breast cancer. A syllabus derived from findings of the National Surgical Adjuvant Breast Project (protocol no. 4). *Cancer* 1975;36(1):1–85.
194. Fisher ER, Sass R, Fisher B, et al. Pathologic findings from the National Surgical Adjuvant Breast Project (protocol 6). II. Relation of local breast recurrence to multicentricity. *Cancer* 1986;57(9):1717–1724.
195. Rosen PP, Groshen S, Kinne DW, et al. Contralateral breast carcinoma: an assessment of risk and prognosis in stage I (T1N0M0) and stage II (T1N1M0) patients with 20-year follow-up. *Surgery* 1989;106(5):904–910.
196. Zafrani B, Vielh P, Fourquet A, et al. Conservative treatment of early breast cancer: prognostic value of the ductal in situ component and other pathological variables on local control and survival. Long-term results. *Eur J Cancer Clin Oncol* 1989;25(11):1645–1650.
197. McDivitt RW, Stone KR, Craig RB, et al. A proposed classification of breast cancer based on kinetic information: derived from a comparison of risk factors in 168 primary operable breast cancers. *Cancer* 1986;57(2):269–276.
198. Papadatos G, Rangan AM, Psarianos T, et al. Probability of axillary node involvement in patients with tubular carcinoma of the breast. *Br J Surg* 2001;88(6):860–864.
199. Sullivan T, Raad RA, Goldberg S, et al. Tubular carcinoma of the breast: a retrospective analysis and review of the literature. *Breast Cancer Res Treat* 2005;93(3):199–205.
200. Vu-Nishino H, Tavassoli FA, Ahrens WA, et al. Clinicopathologic features and long-term outcome of patients with medullary breast carcinoma managed with breast-conserving therapy (BCT). *Int J Radiat Oncol Biol Phys* 2005;62(4):1040–1047.
201. du Toit RS, Locker AP, Ellis IO, et al. Invasive lobular carcinomas of the breast—the prognosis of histopathological subtypes. *Br J Cancer* 1989;60(4):605–609.
202. Middleton LP, Palacios DM, Bryant BR, et al. Pleomorphic lobular carcinoma: morphology, immunohistochemistry, and molecular analysis. *Am J Surg Pathol* 2000;24(12):1650–1656.
203. Silverberg SG, Kay S, Chitale AR, et al. Colloid carcinoma of the breast. *Am J Clin Pathol* 1971;55(3):355–363.
204. Norris HJ, Taylor HB. Prognosis of mucinous (gelatinous) carcinoma of the breast. *Cancer* 1965;18:879–885.
205. Anan K, Mitsuyama S, Tamae K, et al. Pathological features of mucinous carcinoma of the breast are favourable for breast-conserving therapy. *Eur J Surg Oncol* 2001;27(5):459–463.
206. Santamaria G, Velasco M, Zanon G, et al. Adenoid cystic carcinoma of the breast: mammographic appearance and pathologic correlation. *AJR Am J Roentgenol* 1998;171(6):1679–1683.
207. Arpino G, Clark GM, Mohsin S, et al. Adenoid cystic carcinoma of the breast: molecular markers, treatment, and clinical outcome. *Cancer* 2002;94(8):2119–2127.
208. Nassar H, Wallis T, Andea A, et al. Clinicopathologic analysis of invasive micropapillary differentiation in breast carcinoma. *Mod Pathol* 2001;14(9):836–841.
209. Beatty JD, Atwood M, Tickman R, et al. Metaplastic breast cancer: clinical significance. *Am J Surg* 2006;191(5):657–664.
210. Hennessy BT, Giordano S, Broglio K, et al. Biphasic metaplastic sarcomatoid carcinoma of the breast. *Ann Oncol* 2006;17(4):605–613.
211. Sneige N, Yaziji H, Mandavilli SR, et al. Low-grade (fibromatosis-like) spindle cell carcinoma of the breast. *Am J Surg Pathol* 2001;25(8):1009–1016.
212. Francois A, Chatikhine VA, Chevallier B, et al. Neuroendocrine primary small cell carcinoma of the breast. Report of a case and review of the literature. *Am J Clin Oncol* 1995;18(2):133–138.
213. Shin SJ, DeLellis RA, Ying L, et al. Small cell carcinoma of the breast: a clinicopathologic and immunohistochemical study of nine patients. *Am J Surg Pathol* 2000;24(9):1231–1238.
214. Marshall JK, Griffith KA, Haffty BG, et al. Conservative management of Paget disease of the breast with radiotherapy: 10- and 15-year results. *Cancer* 2003;97(9):2142–2149.

215. Bijker N, Rutgers EJ, Duchateau L, et al. Breast-conserving therapy for Paget disease of the nipple: a prospective European Organization for Research and Treatment of Cancer study of 61 patients. *Cancer* 2001;91(3):472–477.

216. el-Naggar AK, Ro JY, McLemore D, et al. DNA content and proliferative activity of cystosarcoma phyllodes of the breast. Potential prognostic significance. *Am J Clin Pathol* 1990;93(4):480–485.

217. Blombery P, Prince HM, Seymour JF. Primary breast lymphoma-population-level insights into an infrequent but increasingly recognized subtype of lymphoma. *J Natl Cancer Inst* 2017;109(6).

218. McGowan TS, Cummings BJ, O'Sullivan B, et al. An analysis of 78 breast sarcoma patients without distant metastases at presentation. *Int J Radiat Oncol Biol Phys* 2000;46(2):383–390.

219. Veronesi U, Marubini E, Del Vecchio M, et al. Local recurrences and distant metastases after conservative breast cancer treatments: partly independent events. *J Natl Cancer Inst* 1995;87(1):19–27.

220. Wilson LD, Haffty BG. National Residency Matching Program (NRMP) results for radiation oncology, 2004 update. *Int J Radiat Oncol Biol Phys* 2004;60(2):689–690.

221. Recht A, Edge SB, Solin LJ, et al. Postmastectomy radiotherapy: clinical practice guidelines of the American Society of Clinical Oncology. *J Clin Oncol* 2001;19(5):1539–1569.

222. Obedian E, Haffty BG. Negative margin status improves local control in conservatively managed breast cancer patients. *Cancer J Sci Am* 2000;6(1):28–33.

223. Smitt MC, Nowels KW, Zdeblick MJ, et al. The importance of the lumpectomy surgical margin status in long-term results of breast conservation. *Cancer* 1995;76(2):259–267.

224. Vicini FA, Baglan KL, Kestin LL, et al. Accelerated treatment of breast cancer. *J Clin Oncol* 2001;19(7):1993–2001.

225. Zhou P, Gautam S, Recht A. Factors affecting outcome for young women with early stage invasive breast cancer treated with breast-conserving therapy. *Breast Cancer Res Treat* 2007;10(1):51–57.

226. Quiet CA, Ferguson DJ, Weichselbaum RR, et al. Natural history of node-negative breast cancer: a study of 826 patients with long-term follow-up. *J Clin Oncol* 1995;13(5):1144–1151.

227. Fisher B. Laboratory and clinical research in breast cancer—a personal adventure: the David A. Karnofsky memorial lecture. *Cancer Res* 1980;40(11):3863–3874.

228. Fisher B, Anderson S. Conservative surgery for the management of invasive and noninvasive carcinoma of the breast: NSABP trials. National Surgical Adjuvant Breast and Bowel Project. *World J Surg* 1994;18(1):63–69.

229. Fisher B, Redmond C, Fisher ER. The contribution of recent NSABP clinical trials of primary breast cancer therapy to an understanding of tumor biology—an overview of findings. *Cancer* 1980;46(4 Suppl):1009–1025.

230. Krag D, Harlow S, Julian T. Breast cancer and the NSABP-B32 sentinel node trial. *Breast Cancer* 2004;11(3):221–226.

231. Krag DN, Harlow S, Weaver D, et al. Radiolabeled sentinel node biopsy: collaborative trial with the National Cancer Institute. *World J Surg* 2001;25(6):823–828.

232. Krag DN, Julian TB, Harlow SP, et al. NSABP-32: phase III, randomized trial comparing axillary resection with sentinel lymph node dissection: a description of the trial. *Ann Surg Oncol* 2004;11(3 Suppl):208S–210S.

233. Giuliano AE, Hunt KK, Ballman KV, et al. Axillary dissection vs no axillary dissection in women with invasive breast cancer and sentinel node metastasis: a randomized clinical trial. *JAMA* 2011;305(6):569–575.

234. Haffty BG, Hunt KK, Harris JR, et al. Positive sentinel nodes without axillary dissection: implications for the radiation oncologist. *J Clin Oncol* 2011;29(34):4479–4481.

235. Hansen NM, Ye X, Grube BJ, et al. Manipulation of the primary breast tumor and the incidence of sentinel node metastases from invasive breast cancer. *Arch Surg* 2004;139(6):634–640.

236. Weiss MC, Fowble BL, Solin LJ, et al. Outcome of conservative therapy for invasive breast cancer by histologic subtype. *Int J Radiat Oncol Biol Phys* 1992;23(5):941–947.

237. Thurman SA, Schnitt SJ, Connolly JL, et al. Outcome after breast-conserving therapy for patients with stage I or II mucinous, medullary, or tubular breast carcinoma. *Int J Radiat Oncol Biol Phys* 2004;59(1):152–159.

238. Sastre-Garau X, Jouve M, Asselain B, et al. Infiltrating lobular carcinoma of the breast. Clinicopathologic analysis of 975 cases with reference to data on conservative therapy and metastatic patterns. *Cancer* 1996;77(1):113–120.

239. Bloom HJ, Richardson WW. Histological grading and prognosis in breast cancer; a study of 1409 cases of which 359 have been followed for 15 years. *Br J Cancer* 1957;11(3):359–377.

240. Elston CW, Ellis IO. Pathological prognostic factors in breast cancer. I. The value of histological grade in breast cancer: experience from a large study with long-term follow-up. *Histopathology* 1991;19(5):403–410.

241. McGuire WL, Clark GM. Prognostic factors and treatment decisions in axillary-node-negative breast cancer. *N Engl J Med* 1992;326(26):1756–1761.

242. McGuire WL, Tandon AK, Allred DC, et al. How to use prognostic factors in axillary node-negative breast cancer patients. *J Natl Cancer Inst* 1990;82(12):1006–1015.

243. Crowe JP Jr, Gordon NH, Hubay CA, et al. Estrogen receptor determination and long term survival of patients with carcinoma of the breast. *Surg Gynecol Obstet* 1991;173(4):273–278.

244. Tsangaris TN, Knox SM, Cheek JH. Tumor hormone receptor status and recurrences in premenopausal patients with node-negative breast carcinoma. *Cancer* 1992;69(4):984–987.

245. Esteban JM, Felder B, Ahn C, et al. Prognostic relevance of carcinoembryonic antigen and estrogen receptor status in breast cancer patients. *Cancer* 1994;74(5):1575–1583.

246. Gaffney EV, Halpin DP, Blakemore WS. Relationship between low estrogen receptor values and other prognostic factors in primary breast tumors. *Surgery* 1995;117(3):241–246.

247. Osborne CK. Steroid hormone receptors in breast cancer management. *Breast Cancer Res Treat* 1998;51(3):227–238.

248. Epstein AH, Connolly JL, Gelman R, et al. The predictors of distant relapse following conservative surgery and radiotherapy for early breast cancer are similar to those following mastectomy. *Int J Radiat Oncol Biol Phys* 1989;17(4):755–760.

249. Gruber G, Berclaz G, Altermatt HJ, et al. Can the addition of regional radiotherapy counterbalance important risk factors in breast cancer patients with extracapsular invasion of axillary lymph node metastases?. *Strahlenther Onkol* 2003;179(10):661–666.

250. Hanrahan EO, Valero V, Gonzalez-Angulo AM, et al. Prognosis and management of patients with node-negative invasive breast carcinoma that is 1 cm or smaller in size (stage 1; T1a,bN0M0): a review of the literature. *J Clin Oncol* 2006;24(13):2113–2122.

251. Hetelekidis S, Schnitt SJ, Silver B, et al. The significance of extracapsular extension of axillary lymph node metastases in early-stage breast cancer. *Int J Radiat Oncol Biol Phys* 2000;46(1):31–34.

252. Truong PT, Yong CM, Abnousi F, et al. Lymphovascular invasion is associated with reduced locoregional control and survival in women with node-negative breast cancer treated with mastectomy and systemic therapy. *J Am Coll Surg* 2005;200(6):912–921.

253. Amadori D, Silvestrini R. Prognostic and predictive value of thymidine labelling index in breast cancer. *Breast Cancer Res Treat* 1998;51(3):267–281.

254. Wenger CR, Clark GM. S-phase fraction and breast cancer—a decade of experience. *Breast Cancer Res Treat* 1998;51(3):255–265.

255. Bryant J, Fisher B, Gunduz N, et al. S-phase fraction combined with other patient and tumor characteristics for the prognosis of node-negative, estrogen-receptor-positive breast cancer. *Breast Cancer Res Treat* 1998;51(3):239–253.

256. Danielsen HE, Pradhan M, Novelli M. Revisiting tumour aneuploidy - the place of ploidy assessment in the molecular era. *Nat Rev Clin Oncol* 2016, 13(5):291–304.

257. Patek E, Johannisson E, Krauer F, et al. Microfluorometric grading of mammary tumors. A pilot study. *Anal Quant Cytol* 1980;2(4):264–271.

258. Frierson HF Jr. Ploidy analysis and S-phase fraction determination by flow cytometry of invasive adenocarcinomas of the breast. *Am J Surg Pathol* 1991;15(4):358–367.

259. Taylor IW, Musgrove EA, Friedlander ML, et al. The influence of age on the DNA ploidy levels of breast tumours. *Eur J Cancer Clin Oncol* 1983;19(5):623–628.

260. Ellis CN, Frey ES, Burnette JJ, et al. The content of tumor DNA as an indicator of prognosis in patients with T1N0M0 and T2N0M0 carcinoma of the breast. *Surgery* 1989;106(2):133–138.

261. Kallioniemi OP, Blanco G, Alavaikko M, et al. Tumour DNA ploidy as an independent prognostic factor in breast cancer. *Br J Cancer* 1987;56(5):637–642.

262. Toikkanen S, Joensuu H, Klemi P. The prognostic significance of nuclear DNA content in invasive breast cancer—a study with long-term follow-up. *Br J Cancer* 1989;60(5):693–700.

263. Mandard AM, Denoux Y, Herlin P, et al. Prognostic value of DNA cytometry in 281 premenopausal patients with lymph node negative breast carcinoma randomized in a control trial: multivariate analysis with Ki-67 index, mitotic count, and microvessel density. *Cancer* 2000;89(8):1748–1757.

264. Ewers SB, Langstrom E, Baldetorp B, et al. Flow-cytometric DNA analysis in primary breast carcinomas and clinicopathological correlations. *Cytometry* 1984;5(4):408–419.

265. Fallenius AG, Franzen SA, Auer GU. Predictive value of nuclear DNA content in breast cancer in relation to clinical and morphologic factors. A retrospective study of 227 consecutive cases. *Cancer* 1988;62(3):521–530.

266. Keyhani-Rofagha S, O'Toole RV, Farrar WB, et al. Is DNA ploidy an independent prognostic indicator in infiltrative node-negative breast adenocarcinoma?. *Cancer* 1990;65(7):1577–1582.

267. Witzig TE, Ingle JN, Cha SS, et al. DNA ploidy and the percentage of cells in S-phase as prognostic factors for women with lymph node negative breast cancer. *Cancer* 1994;74(6):1752–1761.

268. Slamon DJ, Clark GM, Wong SG, et al. Human breast cancer: correlation of relapse and survival with amplification of the HER-2/neu oncogene. *Science* 1987;235(4785):177–182.

269. Hoang MP, Sahin AA, Ordonez NG, et al. HER-2/neu gene amplification compared with HER-2/neu protein overexpression and interobserver reproducibility in invasive breast carcinoma. *Am J Clin Pathol* 2000;113(6):852–859.

270. Birner P, Oberhuber G, Stani J, et al. Evaluation of the United States Food and Drug Administration-approved scoring and test system of HER-2 protein expression in breast cancer. *Clin Cancer Res* 2001;7(6):1669–1675.

271. Romond EH, Perez EA, Bryant J, et al. Trastuzumab plus adjuvant chemotherapy for operable HER2-positive breast cancer. *N Engl J Med* 2005;353(16):1673–1684.

272. Menard S, Valagussa P, Pilotti S, et al. Response to cyclophosphamide, methotrexate, and fluorouracil in lymph node-positive breast cancer according to HER2 overexpression and other tumor biologic variables. *J Clin Oncol* 2001;19(2):329–335.

273. Slamon DJ, Romond EH, Perez EA. Advances in adjuvant therapy for breast cancer. *Clin Adv Hematol Oncol* 2006;4(3 Suppl 1):4–9.

274. Hojris I, Andersen J, Overgaard M, et al. Late treatment-related morbidity in breast cancer patients randomized to postmastectomy radiotherapy and systemic treatment versus systemic treatment alone. *Acta Oncol* 2000;39(3):355–372.

275. Caleffi M, Teague MW, Jensen RA, et al. p53 gene mutations and steroid receptor status in breast cancer. Clinicopathologic correlations and prognostic assessment. *Cancer* 1994;73(8):2147–2156.

276. Martinazzi M, Crivelli F, Zampatti C, et al. Relationship between p53 expression and other prognostic factors in human breast carcinoma. An immunohistochemical study. *Am J Clin Pathol* 1993;100(3):213–217.

277. Friedrichs K, Gluba S, Eidtmann H, et al. Overexpression of p53 and prognosis in breast cancer. *Cancer* 1993;72(12):3641–3647.

278. Jansen RL, Joosten-Achjanie SR, Volovics A, et al. Relevance of the expression of bcl-2 in combination with p53 as a prognostic factor in breast cancer. *Anticancer Res* 1998;18(6A):4455–4462.

279. Hayes DF. Prognostic and predictive factors revisited. *Breast* 2005;14(6):493–499.

280. Buyse M, Loi S, van't Veer L, et al. Validation and clinical utility of a 70-gene prognostic signature for women with node-negative breast cancer. *J Natl Cancer Inst* 2006;98(17):1183–1192.

281. van't Veer LJ, Paik S, Hayes DF. Gene expression profiling of breast cancer: a new tumor marker. *J Clin Oncol* 2005;23(8):1631–1635.

282. van de Vijver MJ, He YD, van't Veer LJ, et al. A gene-expression signature as a predictor of survival in breast cancer. *N Engl J Med* 2002;347(25):1999–2009.

283. Perou CM, Sorlie T, Eisen MB, et al. Molecular portraits of human breast tumours. *Nature* 2000;406(6797):747–752.

284. Sorlie T, Perou CM, Tibshirani R, et al. Gene expression patterns of breast carcinomas distinguish tumor subclasses with clinical implications. *Proc Natl Acad Sci U S A* 2001;98(19):10869–10874.

285. Morris SR, Carey LA. Molecular profiling in breast cancer. *Rev Endocr Metab Disord* 2007;8(3):185–198.

286. Paik S, Shak S, Tang G, et al. A multigene assay to predict recurrence of tamoxifen-treated, node-negative breast cancer. *N Engl J Med* 2004;351(27):2817–2826.

287. Curtit E, Mansi L, Maisonnette-Escot Y, et al. Prognostic and predictive indicators in early-stage breast cancer and the role of genomic profiling: Focus on the Oncotype DX(R) Breast Recurrence Score Assay. *Eur J Surg Oncol* 2017, 43(5):921–930.

288. Chabner E, Nixon A, Gelman R, et al. Family history and treatment outcome in young women after breast-conserving surgery and radiation therapy for early-stage breast cancer. *J Clin Oncol* 1998;16(6):2045–2051.

289. Chung M, Chang HR, Bland KI, et al. Younger women with breast carcinoma have a poorer prognosis than older women. *Cancer* 1996;77(1):97–103.

290. de la Rochefordiere A, Asselain B, Campana F, et al. Age as prognostic factor in premenopausal breast carcinoma. *Lancet* 1993;341(8852):1039–1043.

291. Fowble BL, Schultz DJ, Overmoyer B, et al. The influence of young age on outcome in early stage breast cancer. *Int J Radiat Oncol Biol Phys* 1994;30(1):23–33.

292. Vanlemmens L, Hebbar M, Peyrat JP, et al. Age as a prognostic factor in breast cancer. *Anticancer Res* 1998;18(3B):1891–1896.

293. Kollias J, Murphy CA, Elston CW, et al. The prognosis of small primary breast cancers. *Eur J Cancer* 1999;35(6):908–912.

294. Simon MS, Severson RK. Racial differences in survival of female breast cancer in the Detroit metropolitan area. *Cancer* 1996;77(2):308–314.

295. Jones BA, Kasl SV, Curnen MG, et al. Can mammography screening explain the race difference in stage at diagnosis of breast cancer?. *Cancer* 1995;75(8):2103–2113.

296. Kurtz JM, Amalric R, Brandone H, et al. Local recurrence after breast-conserving surgery and radiotherapy. Frequency, time course, and prognosis. *Cancer* 1989;63(10):1912–1917.

297. Eley JW, Hill HA, Chen VW, et al. Racial differences in survival from breast cancer. Results of the National Cancer Institute Black/White Cancer Survival Study. *JAMA* 1994;272(12):947–954.

298. Jones BA, Kasl SV, Howe CL, et al. African-American/white differences in breast carcinoma: p53 alterations and other tumor characteristics. *Cancer* 2004;101(6):1293–1301.

299. Tuamokumo NL, Haffty BG. Clinical outcome and cosmesis in African-American patients treated with conservative surgery and radiation therapy. *Cancer J* 2003;9(4):313–320.

300. Senie RT, Rosen PP, Rhodes P, et al. Obesity at diagnosis of breast carcinoma influences duration of disease-free survival. *Ann Intern Med* 1992;116(1):26–32.

301. Daling JR, Malone KE, Doody DR, et al. Relation of body mass index to tumor markers and survival among young women with invasive ductal breast carcinoma. *Cancer* 2001;92(4):720–729.

302. Manjer J, Berglund G, Bondesson L, et al. Breast cancer incidence in relation to smoking cessation. *Breast Cancer Res Treat* 2000;61(2):121–129.

303. Kroman N, Wohlfahrt J, Andersen KW, et al. Parity, age at first childbirth and the prognosis of primary breast cancer. *Br J Cancer* 1998;78(11):1529–1533.

304. Psyrri A, Burtness B. Pregnancy-associated breast cancer. *Cancer J* 2005;11(2):83–95.

305. Hornstein E, Skornick Y, Rozin R. The management of breast carcinoma in pregnancy and lactation. *J Surg Oncol* 1982;21(3):179–182.

306. Gaffney DK, Tsodikov A, Wiggins CL. Diminished survival in patients with inner versus outer quadrant breast cancers. *J Clin Oncol* 2003;21(3):467–472.

307. Lohrisch C, Jackson J, Jones A, et al. Relationship between tumor location and relapse in 6,781 women with early invasive breast cancer. *J Clin Oncol* 2000;18(15):2828–2835.

308. Ross JS, Linette GP, Stec J, et al. Breast cancer biomarkers and molecular medicine. *Expert Rev Mol Diagn* 2003;3(5):573–585.

309. Ross JS, Linette GP, Stec J, et al. Breast cancer biomarkers and molecular medicine: part II. *Expert Rev Mol Diagn* 2004;4(2):169–188.

310. Petit JY, Veronesi U, Orecchia R, et al. Nipple-sparing mastectomy in association with intra operative radiotherapy (ELIOT): a new type of mastectomy for breast cancer treatment. *Breast Cancer Res Treat* 2006;96(1):47–51.

311. Calle R, Pilleron JP, Schlienger P, et al. Conservative management of operable breast cancer: ten years experience at the Foundation Curie. *Cancer* 1978;42(4):2045–2053.

312. Peters MV. Wedge resection with or without radiation in early breast cancer. *Int J Radiat Oncol Biol Phys* 1977;2(11–12):1151–1156.

313. Vilcoq JR, Calle R, Stacey P, et al. The outcome of treatment by tumorectomy and radiotherapy of patients with operable breast cancer. *Int J Radiat Oncol Biol Phys* 1981;7(10):1327–1332.

314. McCormick B, Yahalom J, Cox L, et al. The patients perception of her breast following radiation and limited surgery. *Int J Radiat Oncol Biol Phys* 1989;17(6):1299–1302.

315. Montague ED. Conservation surgery and radiation therapy in the treatment of operable breast cancer. *Cancer* 1984;53(3 Suppl):700–704.

316. Schnitt SJ, Connolly JL, Khettry U, et al. Pathologic findings on re-excision of the primary site in breast cancer patients considered for treatment by primary radiation therapy. *Cancer* 1987;59(4):675–681.

317. Solin LJ, Fowble B, Martz K, et al. Results of re-excisional biopsy of the primary tumor in preparation for definitive irradiation of patients with early stage breast cancer. *Int J Radiat Oncol Biol Phys* 1986;12(5):721–725.

318. Lally BE, Haffty BG, Moran MS, et al. Management of suspicious or indeterminate calcifications and impact on local control. *Cancer* 2005;103(11):2236–2240.

319. Whelan TJ, Levine MN, Gafni A, et al. Breast irradiation postlumpectomy: development and evaluation of a decision instrument. *J Clin Oncol* 1995;13(4):847–853.

320. Kelemen JJ III, Poulton T, Swartz MT, et al. Surgical treatment of early-stage breast cancer in the Department of Defense Healthcare System. *J Am Coll Surg* 2001;192(3):293–297.

321. Tannock IF, Belanger D. Use of a physician-directed questionnaire to define a consensus about management of breast cancer: implications for assessing costs and benefits of treatment. *J Natl Cancer Inst Monogr* 1992(11):137–142.

322. Temple WJ, Russell ML, Parsons LL, et al. Conservation surgery for breast cancer as the preferred choice: a prospective analysis. *J Clin Oncol* 2006;24(21):3367–3373.

323. Haffty BG, McKhann C, Beinfield M, et al. Breast conservation therapy without axillary dissection. A rational treatment strategy in selected patients. *Arch Surg* 1993;128(12):1315–1319.

324. Recht A, Houlihan MJ. Axillary lymph nodes and breast cancer: a review. *Cancer* 1995;76(9):1491–1512.

325. Ray GR, Fish VJ, Marmor JB, et al. Impact of adjuvant chemotherapy on cosmesis and complications in stages I and II carcinoma of the breast treated by biopsy and radiation therapy. *Int J Radiat Oncol Biol Phys* 1984;10(6):837–841.

326. Pigott J, Nichols R, Maddox WA, et al. Metastases to the upper levels of the axillary nodes in carcinoma of the breast and its implications for nodal sampling procedures. *Surg Gynecol Obstet* 1984;158(3):255–259.

327. Danforth DN Jr, Findlay PA, McDonald HD, et al. Complete axillary lymph node dissection for stage I–II carcinoma of the breast. *J Clin Oncol* 1986;4(5):655–662.

328. Fisher B, Jeong JH, Anderson S, et al. Twenty-five-year follow-up of a randomized trial comparing radical mastectomy, total mastectomy, and total mastectomy followed by irradiation. *N Engl J Med* 2002;347(8):567–575.

329. Iwasaki Y, Fukutomi T, Akashi-Tanaka S, et al. Axillary node metastasis from T1N0M0 breast cancer: possible avoidance of dissection in a subgroup. *Jpn J Clin Oncol* 1998;28(10):601–603.

330. Martelli G, Boracchi P, De Palo M, et al. A randomized trial comparing axillary dissection to no axillary dissection in older patients with T1N0 breast cancer: results after 5 years of follow-up. *Ann Surg* 2005;242(1):1–9.

331. Clarke D, Khonji NI, Mansel RE. Sentinel node biopsy in breast cancer: ALMANAC trial. *World J Surg* 2001;25(6):819–822.

332. Mansel RE, Fallowfield L, Kissin M, et al. Randomized multicenter trial of sentinel node biopsy versus standard axillary treatment in operable breast cancer: the ALMANAC Trial. *J Natl Cancer Inst* 2006;98(9):599–609.

333. Mansel RE, Goyal A, Newcombe RG. Internal mammary node drainage and its role in sentinel lymph node biopsy: the initial ALMANAC experience. *Clin Breast Cancer* 2004;5(4):279–286.

334. Krag D, Weaver D, Ashikaga T, et al. The sentinel node in breast cancer—a multicenter validation study. *N Engl J Med* 1998;339(14):941–946.

335. Lyman GH, Giuliano AE, Somerfield MR et al. American Society of Clinical Oncology guideline recommendations for sentinel lymph node biopsy in early-stage breast cancer. *J Clin Oncol* 2005, 23(30):7703–7720.

336. Lyman GH, Somerfield MR, Bosserman LD, et al. Sentinel lymph node biopsy for patients with early-stage breast cancer: American Society of Clinical Oncology Clinical Practice Guideline Update. *J Clin Oncol* 2013;54:1177.

337. Galimberti V, Cole BF, Zurrida S et al. Axillary dissection versus no axillary dissection in patients with sentinel-node micrometastases (IBCSG 23-01): a phase 3 randomised controlled trial. *Lancet Oncol* 2013;14(4):297–305.

338. Van Zee KJ, Kattan MW. Validating a predictive model for presence of additional disease in the non-sentinel lymph nodes of a woman with sentinel node positive breast cancer. *Ann Surg Oncol* 2007;14(8):2177–2178.

339. Lambert LA, Ayers GD, Hwang RF, et al. Validation of a breast cancer nomogram for predicting nonsentinel lymph node metastases after a positive sentinel node biopsy. *Ann Surg Oncol* 2006;13(3):310–320.

340. Katz A, Smith BL, Golshan M, et al. Nomogram for the prediction of having four or more involved nodes for sentinel lymph node-positive breast cancer. *J Clin Oncol* 2008;26(13):2093–2098.

341. Van Zee KJ, Manasseh DM, Bevilacqua JL, et al. A nomogram for predicting the likelihood of additional nodal metastases in breast cancer patients with a positive sentinel node biopsy. *Ann Surg Oncol* 2003;10(10):1140–1151.

342. Veronesi U, Paganelli G, Viale G, et al. A randomized comparison of sentinel-node biopsy with routine axillary dissection in breast cancer. *N Engl J Med* 2003;349(6):546–553.

343. Weaver DL, Krag DN, Ashikaga T, et al. Pathologic analysis of sentinel and nonsentinel lymph nodes in breast carcinoma: a multicenter study. *Cancer* 2000;88(5):1099–1107.

344. Hortobagyi GN, Buzdar AU. Current status of adjuvant systemic therapy for primary breast cancer: progress and controversy. *CA Cancer J Clin* 1995;45(4):199–226.

345. Hudis CA, Gianni L. Triple-negative breast cancer: an unmet medical need. *Oncologist* 2011;16(Suppl 1):1–11.

346. Arteaga CL, Sliwkowski MX, Osborne CK, et al. Treatment of HER2-positive breast cancer: current status and future perspectives. *Nat Rev Clin Oncol* 2011;9(1):16–32.

347. Goldhirsch A, Wood WC, Coates AS, et al. Strategies for subtypes—dealing with the diversity of breast cancer: highlights of the St. Gallen International Expert Consensus on the Primary Therapy of Early Breast Cancer 2011. *Ann Oncol* 2011;22(8):1736–1747.

348. Arthur DW, Vicini FA, Kuske RR, et al. Accelerated partial breast irradiation: an updated report from the American Brachytherapy Society. *Brachytherapy* 2003;2(2):124–130.

349. Haffty BG. Accelerated partial breast irradiation: where do we go from here?. *Breast J* 2005;11(5):303–305.

350. Vicini FA, Beitsch PD, Quiet CA, et al. First analysis of patient demographics, technical reproducibility, cosmesis, and early toxicity: results of the American Society of Breast Surgeons MammoSite breast brachytherapy trial. *Cancer* 2005;104(6):1138–1148.

351. Taylor ME, Perez CA, Halverson KJ, et al. Factors influencing cosmetic results after conservation therapy for breast cancer. *Int J Radiat Oncol Biol Phys* 1995;31(4):753–764.

352. Buchholz TA, Tu X, Ang KK, et al. Epidermal growth factor receptor expression correlates with poor survival in patients who have breast carcinoma treated with doxorubicin-based neoadjuvant chemotherapy. *Cancer* 2005;104(4):676–681.

353. Chen AM, Meric-Bernstam F, Hunt KK, et al. Breast conservation after neoadjuvant chemotherapy: the MD Anderson cancer center experience. *J Clin Oncol* 2004;22(12):2303–2312.

354. Chen AM, Meric-Bernstam F, Hunt KK, et al. Breast conservation after neoadjuvant chemotherapy. *Cancer* 2005;103(4):689–695.

355. Amalric R, Santamaria F, Robert F, et al. Radiation therapy with or without primary limited surgery for operable breast cancer: a 20-year experience at the Marseilles Cancer Institute. *Cancer* 1982;49(1):30–34.

356. Janjan NA, Murray KJ, Conway P, et al. Prognosis for breast cancer surgery and radiation therapy compared with mastectomy alone. A retrospective analysis of 759 patients with stage I/II breast cancer. *Cancer* 1992;69(11):2842–2848.

357. Montague ED, Paulus DD, Schell SR. Selection and follow-up of patients for conservation surgery and irradiation. *Front Radiat Ther Oncol* 1983;17:124–130.

358. Rissanen PM. A comparison of conservative and radical surgery combined with radiotherapy in the treatment of stage I carcinoma of the breast. *Br J Radiol* 1969;42(498):423–426.

359. Sarrazin D, Le MG, Arriagada R, et al. Ten-year results of a randomized trial comparing a conservative treatment to mastectomy in early breast cancer. *Radiother Oncol* 1989;14(3):177–184.

360. Poggi MM, Danforth DN, Sciuto LC, et al. Eighteen-year results in the treatment of early breast carcinoma with mastectomy versus breast conservation therapy: the National Cancer Institute Randomized Trial. *Cancer* 2003;98(4):697–702.

361. van Dongen JA, Bartelink H, Fentiman IS, et al. Randomized clinical trial to assess the value of breast-conserving therapy in stage I and II breast cancer, EORTC 10801 trial. *J Natl Cancer Inst Monogr* 1992(11):15–18.

362. Blichert-Toft M, Rose C, Andersen JA, et al. Danish randomized trial comparing breast conservation therapy with mastectomy: six years of life-table analysis. Danish Breast Cancer Cooperative Group. *J Natl Cancer Inst Monogr* 1992(11):19–25.

363. Fisher B, Anderson S, Redmond CK, et al. Reanalysis and results after 12 years of follow-up in a randomized clinical trial comparing total mastectomy with lumpectomy with or without irradiation in the treatment of breast cancer. *N Engl J Med* 1995;333(22):1456–1461.

364. Lichter AS, Fraass BA, Yanke B. Treatment techniques in the conservative management of breast cancer. *Semin Radiat Oncol* 1992;2(2):94–106.

365. Veronesi U, Zucali R, Luini A. Local control and survival in early breast cancer: the Milan trial. *Int J Radiat Oncol Biol Phys* 1986;12(5):717–720.

366. Fowble B. Postmastectomy radiation in patients with one to three positive axillary nodes receiving adjuvant chemotherapy: an unresolved issue. *Semin Radiat Oncol* 1999;9(3):230–240.

367. Jatoi I, Proschan MA. Randomized trials of breast-conserving therapy versus mastectomy for primary breast cancer: a pooled analysis of updated results. *Am J Clin Oncol* 2005;28(3):289–294.

368. Morris AD, Morris RD, Wilson JF, et al. Breast-conserving therapy vs mastectomy in early-stage breast cancer: a meta-analysis of 10-year survival. *Cancer J Sci Am* 1997;3(1):6–12.

369. Atkins H, Hayward JL, Klugman DJ, et al. Treatment of early breast cancer: a report after ten years of a clinical trial. *Br Med J* 1972;2(811):423–429.

370. Sarrazin D, Le M, Rouesse J, et al. Conservative treatment versus mastectomy in breast cancer tumors with macroscopic diameter of 20 millimeters or less. The experience of the Institut Gustave-Roussy. *Cancer* 1984;53(5): 1209–1213.

371. Blichert-Toft M. Breast-conserving therapy for mammary carcinoma: psychosocial aspects, indications and limitations. *Ann Med* 1992;24(6):445–451.

372. Jacobson JA, Danforth DN, Cowan KH, et al. Ten-year results of a comparison of conservation with mastectomy in the treatment of stage I and II breast cancer. *N Engl J Med* 1995;332(14):907–911.

373. Barr LC, Brunt AM, Goodman AG, et al. Uncontrolled local recurrence after treatment of breast cancer with breast conservation. *Cancer* 1989;64(6):1203–1207.

374. Bartelink H, Borger JH, van Dongen JA, et al. The impact of tumor size and histology on local control after breast-conserving therapy. *Radiother Oncol* 1988;11(4):297–303.

375. Calle R, Vilcoq JR, Zafrani B, et al. Local control and survival of breast cancer treated by limited surgery followed by irradiation. *Int J Radiat Oncol Biol Phys* 1986;12(6):873–878.

376. Clark RM, Wilkinson RH, Miceli PN, et al. Breast cancer. Experiences with conservation therapy. *Am J Clin Oncol* 1987;10(6):461–468.

377. Clarke DH, Le MG, Sarrazin D, et al. Analysis of local-regional relapses in patients with early breast cancers treated by excision and radiotherapy: experience of the Institut Gustave-Roussy. *Int J Radiat Oncol Biol Phys* 1985;11(1):137–145.

378. Delouche G, Bachelot F, Premont M, et al. Conservation treatment of early breast cancer: long term results and complications. *Int J Radiat Oncol Biol Phys* 1987;13(1):29–34.

379. Dewar JA, Arriagada R, Benhamou S, et al. Local relapse and contralateral tumor rates in patients with breast cancer treated with conservative surgery and radiotherapy (Institut Gustave Roussy 1970–1982). IGR Breast Cancer Group. *Cancer* 1995;76(11):2260–2265.

380. Dubois JB, Gary-Bobo J, Pourquier H, et al. Tumorectomy and radiotherapy in early breast cancer: a report on 392 patients. *Int J Radiat Oncol Biol Phys* 1988;15(6):1275–1282.

381. Fagundes MA, Fagundes HM, Brito CS, et al. Breast-conserving surgery and definitive radiation: a comparison between quadrantectomy and local excision with special focus on local-regional control and cosmesis. *Int J Radiat Oncol Biol Phys* 1993;27(3):553–560.

382. Fourquet A, Campana F, Zafrani B, et al. Prognostic factors of breast recurrence in the conservative management of early breast cancer: a 25-year follow-up. *Int J Radiat Oncol Biol Phys* 1989;17(4):719–725.

383. Gage I, Recht A, Gelman R, et al. Long-term outcome following breast-conserving surgery and radiation therapy. *Int J Radiat Oncol Biol Phys* 1995;33(2):245–251.

384. Leborgne F, Leborgne JH, Ortega B, et al. Breast conservation treatment of early stage breast cancer: patterns of failure. *Int J Radiat Oncol Biol Phys* 1995;31(4):765–775.

385. Osborne MP, Ormiston N, Harmer CL, et al. Breast conservation in the treatment of early breast cancer. A 20-year follow-up. *Cancer* 1984;53(2):349–355.

386. Pierquin B, Huart J, Raynal M, et al. Conservative treatment for breast cancer: long-term results (15 years). *Radiother Oncol* 1991;20(1):16–23.

387. Recht A, Silen W, Schnitt SJ, et al. Time-course of local recurrence following conservative surgery and radiotherapy for early stage breast cancer. *Int J Radiat Oncol Biol Phys* 1988;15(2):255–261.

388. Solin LJ, Fowble B, Martz KL, et al. Definitive irradiation for early stage breast cancer: the University of Pennsylvania experience. *Int J Radiat Oncol Biol Phys* 1988;14(2):235–242.

389. van Limbergen E, van den Bogaert W, van der Schueren E, et al. Tumor excision and radiotherapy as primary treatment of breast cancer. Analysis of patient and treatment parameters and local control. *Radiother Oncol* 1987;8(1):1–9.

390. Vicini FA, Recht A, Abner A, et al. Recurrence in the breast following conservative surgery and radiation therapy for early-stage breast cancer. *J Natl Cancer Inst Monogr* 1992(11):33–39.

391. Clarke DH, Martinez AA. Identification of patients who are at high risk for locoregional breast cancer recurrence after conservative surgery and radiotherapy: a review article for surgeons, pathologists, and radiation and medical oncologists. *J Clin Oncol* 1992;10(3):474–483.

392. Halverson KJ, Perez CA, Taylor ME, et al. Age as a prognostic factor for breast and regional nodal recurrence following breast conserving surgery and irradiation in stage I and II breast cancer. *Int J Radiat Oncol Biol Phys* 1993;27(5):1045–1050.

393. Kini VR, White JR, Horwitz EM, et al. Long term results with breast-conserving therapy for patients with early stage breast carcinoma in a community hospital setting. *Cancer* 1998;82(1):127–133.

394. Kurtz JM, Jacquemier J, Amalric R, et al. Why are local recurrences after breast-conserving therapy more frequent in younger patients?. *J Clin Oncol* 1990;8(4):591–598.

395. Matthews RH, McNeese MD, Montague ED, et al. Prognostic implications of age in breast cancer patients treated with tumorectomy and irradiation or with mastectomy. *Int J Radiat Oncol Biol Phys* 1988;14(4):659–663.

396. Nixon AJ, Neuberg D, Hayes DF, et al. Relationship of patient age to pathologic features of the tumor and prognosis for patients with stage I or II breast cancer. *J Clin Oncol* 1994;12(5):888–894.

397. Veronesi U, Salvadori B, Luini A, et al. Conservative treatment of early breast cancer. Long-term results of 1232 cases treated with quadrantectomy, axillary dissection, and radiotherapy. *Ann Surg* 1990;211(3):250–259.

398. Kini VR, Vicini FA, Frazier R, et al. Mammographic, pathologic, and treatment-related factors associated with local recurrence in patients with early-stage breast cancer treated with breast conserving therapy. *Int J Radiat Oncol Biol Phys* 1999;43(2):341–346.

399. Kurtz JM, Spitalier JM, Amalric R, et al. Mammary recurrences in women younger than forty. *Int J Radiat Oncol Biol Phys* 1988;15(2):271–276.

400. Curtis RE, Boice JD Jr, Stovall M, et al. Risk of leukemia after chemotherapy and radiation treatment for breast cancer. *N Engl J Med* 1992;326(26): 1745–1751.

401. Recht A, Connolly JL, Schnitt SJ, et al. The effect of young age on tumor recurrence in the treated breast after conservative surgery and radiotherapy. *Int J Radiat Oncol Biol Phys* 1988;14(1):3–10.

402. Clarke D, Martinez A, Cox RS, et al. Breast edema following staging axillary node dissection in patients with breast carcinoma treated by radical radiotherapy. *Cancer* 1982;49(11):2295–2299.

403. Bartelink H, Horiot JC, Poortmans P, et al. Recurrence rates after treatment of breast cancer with standard radiotherapy with or without additional radiation. *N Engl J Med* 2001;345(19):1378–1387.

404. Bartelink H, Horiot JC, Poortmans PM, et al. Impact of a higher radiation dose on local control and survival in breast-conserving therapy of early breast cancer: 10-year results of the randomized boost versus no boost EORTC 22881-10882 trial. *J Clin Oncol* 2007;25(22):3259–3265.

405. de Bock GH, van der Hage JA, Putter H, et al. Isolated loco-regional recurrence of breast cancer is more common in young patients and following breast conserving therapy: long-term results of European Organisation for Research and Treatment of Cancer studies. *Eur J Cancer* 2006;42(3):351–356.

406. Haas JA, Schultz DJ, Peterson ME, et al. An analysis of age and family history on outcome after breast-conservation treatment: the University of Pennsylvania experience. *Cancer J Sci Am* 1998;4(5):308–315.

407. Harrold EV, Turner BC, Matloff ET, et al. Local recurrence in the conservatively treated breast cancer patient: a correlation with age and family history. *Cancer J Sci Am* 1998;4(5):302–307.

408. Oh JL, Bonnen M, Outlaw ED, et al. The impact of young age on locoregional recurrence after doxorubicin-based breast conservation therapy in patients 40 years old or younger: how young is "young"?. *Int J Radiat Oncol Biol Phys* 2006;65(5):1345–1352.

409. Anscher MS, Jones P, Prosnitz LR, et al. Local failure and margin status in early-stage breast carcinoma treated with conservation surgery and radiation therapy. *Ann Surg* 1993;218(1):22–28.

410. Borger J, Kemperman H, Hart A, et al. Risk factors in breast-conservation therapy. *J Clin Oncol* 1994;12(4):653–660.

411. DiBiase SJ, Komarnicky LT, Heron DE, et al. Influence of radiation dose on positive surgical margins in women undergoing breast conservation therapy. *Int J Radiat Oncol Biol Phys* 2002;53(3):680–686.

412. Freedman G, Fowble B, Hanlon A, et al. Patients with early stage invasive cancer with close or positive margins treated with conservative surgery and radiation have an increased risk of breast recurrence that is delayed by adjuvant systemic therapy. *Int J Radiat Oncol Biol Phys* 1999;44(5):1005–1015.

413. Ghossein NA, Vilcoq J, Stacey P, et al. Is it necessary to irradiate the breast after conservative surgery for localized cancer?. *Arch Surg* 1987;122(8):913–917.

414. Hartsell WF, Recine DC, Griem KL, et al. Delaying the initiation of intact breast irradiation for patients with lymph node positive breast cancer increases the risk of local recurrence. *Cancer* 1995;76(12):2497–2503.

415. Heimann R, Powers C, Halpem HJ, et al. Breast preservation in stage I and II carcinoma of the breast. The University of Chicago experience. *Cancer* 1996;78(8):1722–1730.

416. Jobsen JJ, van der Palen J, Ong F, et al. The value of a positive margin for invasive carcinoma in breast-conservative treatment in relation to local recurrence is limited to young women only. *Int J Radiat Oncol Biol Phys* 2003;57(3):724–731.

417. Peterson ME, Schultz DJ, Reynolds C, et al. Outcomes in breast cancer patients relative to margin status after treatment with breast-conserving surgery and radiation therapy: the University of Pennsylvania experience. *Int J Radiat Oncol Biol Phys* 1999;43(5):1029–1035.

418. Park CC, Mitsumori M, Nixon A, et al. Outcome at 8 years after breast-conserving surgery and radiation therapy for invasive breast cancer: influence of margin status and systemic therapy on local recurrence. *J Clin Oncol* 2000;18(8):1668–1675.

419. Pittinger TP, Maronian NC, Poulter CA, et al. Importance of margin status in outcome of breast conserving surgery for carcinoma. *Surgery* 1994;116(4):605–609.

420. Ryoo MC, Kagan AR, Wollin M, et al. Prognostic factors for recurrence and cosmesis in 393 patients after radiation therapy for early mammary carcinoma. *Radiology* 1989;172(2):555–559.

421. Schnitt SJ, Abner A, Gelman R, et al. The relationship between microscopic margins of resection and the risk of local recurrence in patients with breast cancer treated with breast-conserving surgery and radiation therapy. *Cancer* 1994;74(6):1746–1751.

422. Solin LJ, Fowble BL, Schultz DJ, et al. The significance of the pathology margins of the tumor excision on the outcome of patients treated with definitive irradiation for early stage breast cancer. *Int J Radiat Oncol Biol Phys* 1991;21(2):279–287.

423. Vicini FA, Goldstein NS, Pass H, et al. Use of pathologic factors to assist in establishing adequacy of excision before radiotherapy in patients treated with breast-conserving therapy. *Int J Radiat Oncol Biol Phys* 2004;60(1):86–94.

424. Wazer DE, Jabro G, Ruthazer R, et al. Extent of margin positivity as a predictor for local recurrence after breast conserving irradiation. *Radiat Oncol Investig* 1999;7(2):111–117.

425. Abner AL, Recht A, Eberlein T, et al. Prognosis following salvage mastectomy for recurrence in the breast after conservative surgery and radiation therapy for early-stage breast cancer. *J Clin Oncol* 1993;11(1):44–48.

426. Slotman BJ, Meyer OW, Njo KH, et al. Importance of timing of radiotherapy in breast conserving treatment for early stage breast cancer. *Radiother Oncol* 1994;30(3):206–212.

427. Moran MS, Schnitt SJ, Giuliano AE, et al: Society of Surgical Oncology-American Society for Radiation Oncology consensus guideline on margins for breast-conserving surgery with whole-breast irradiation in stages I and II invasive breast cancer. *Int J Radiat Oncol Biol Phys* 2014;88(3):553–564.

428. van der Leest M, Evers L, van der Sangen MJ, et al. The safety of breast-conserving therapy in patients with breast cancer aged < or = 40 years. *Cancer* 2007;109(10):1957–1964.

429. Haffty BG, Wilmarth L, Wilson L, et al. Adjuvant systemic chemotherapy and hormonal therapy. Effect on local recurrence in the conservatively treated breast cancer patient. *Cancer* 1994;73(10):2543–2548.

430. Fisher B, Redmond C, Dimitrov NV, et al. A randomized clinical trial evaluating sequential methotrexate and fluorouracil in the treatment of patients with node-negative breast cancer who have estrogen-receptor-negative tumors. *N Engl J Med* 1989;320(8):473–478.

431. Fisher B, Dignam J, Wolmark N, et al. Tamoxifen and chemotherapy for lymph node-negative, estrogen receptor-positive breast cancer. *J Natl Cancer Inst* 1997;89(22):1673–1682.

432. Fisher B, Costantino J, Redmond C, et al. A randomized clinical trial evaluating tamoxifen in the treatment of patients with node-negative breast cancer who have estrogen-receptor-positive tumors. *N Engl J Med* 1989;320(8):479–484.

433. Kiess AP, McArthur HL, Mahoney K, et al. Adjuvant trastuzumab reduces locoregional recurrence in women who receive breast-conservation therapy for lymph node-negative, human epidermal growth factor receptor 2-positive breast cancer. *Cancer* 2012;118(8):1982–1988.

434. Eberlein TJ, Connolly JL, Schnitt SJ, et al. Predictors of local recurrence following conservative breast surgery and radiation therapy. The influence of tumor size. *Arch Surg* 1990;125(6):771–777.

435. Fisher B, Wickerham DL, Deutsch M, et al. Breast tumor recurrence following lumpectomy with and without breast irradiation: an overview of recent NSABP findings. *Semin Surg Oncol* 1992;8(3):153–160.

436. Leung S, Otmezguine Y, Calitchi E, et al. Locoregional recurrences following radical external beam irradiation and interstitial implantation for operable breast cancer—a twenty three year experience. *Radiother Oncol* 1986;5(1):1–10.

437. Perez CA, Garcia DM, Kuske RR, et al. Organ preservation therapy in stage T1 and T2 carcinoma of the breast. *Front Radiat Ther Oncol* 1993;27:62–88.

438. Stotter AT, McNeese MD, Ames FC, et al. Predicting the rate and extent of locoregional failure after breast conservation therapy for early breast cancer. *Cancer* 1989;64(11):2217–2225.

439. Haffty BG, Wilson LD, Smith R, et al. Subareolar breast cancer: long-term results with conservative surgery and radiation therapy. *Int J Radiat Oncol Biol Phys* 1995;33(1):53–57.

440. Gajdos C, Tartter PI, Bleiweiss IJ. Subareolar breast cancers. *Am J Surg* 2000;180(3):167–170.

441. Harris JR, Connolly JL, Schnitt SJ, et al. The use of pathologic features in selecting the extent of surgical resection necessary for breast cancer patients treated by primary radiation therapy. *Ann Surg* 1985;201(2):164–169.

442. Harris JR, Botnick L, Bloomer WD, et al. Primary radiation therapy for early breast cancer: the experience at the Joint Center for Radiation Therapy. *Int J Radiat Oncol Biol Phys* 1981;7(11):1549–1552.

443. Kurtz JM, Jacquemier J, Amalric R, et al. Risk factors for breast recurrence in premenopausal and postmenopausal patients with ductal cancers treated by conservation therapy. *Cancer* 1990;65(8):1867–1878.

444. Boyages J, Recht A, Connolly J, et al. Factors associated with local recurrence as a first site of failure following the conservative treatment of early breast cancer. *Recent Results Cancer Res* 1989;115:92–102.

445. Schnitt SJ, Connolly JL, Harris JR, et al. Pathologic predictors of early local recurrence in stage I and II breast cancer treated by primary radiation therapy. *Cancer* 1984;53(5):1049–1057.

446. Holland R, Connolly JL, Gelman R, et al. The presence of an extensive intraductal component following a limited excision correlates with prominent residual disease in the remainder of the breast. *J Clin Oncol* 1990;8(1):113–118.

447. Gage I, Schnitt SJ, Nixon AJ, et al. Pathologic margin involvement and the risk of recurrence in patients treated with breast-conserving therapy. *Cancer* 1996;78(9):1921–1928.

448. Schnitt SJ, Connolly JL, Recht A, et al. Influence of infiltrating lobular histology on local tumor control in breast cancer patients treated with conservative surgery and radiotherapy. *Cancer* 1989;64(2):448–454.

449. Santiago RJ, Harris EE, Qin L, et al. Similar long-term results of breast-conservation treatment for stage I and II invasive lobular carcinoma compared with invasive ductal carcinoma of the breast: the University of Pennsylvania experience. *Cancer* 2005;103(12):2447–2454.

450. Vo TN, Meric-Bernstam F, Yi M, et al. Outcomes of breast-conservation therapy for invasive lobular carcinoma are equivalent to those for invasive ductal carcinoma. *Am J Surg* 2006;192(4):552–555.

451. Peiro G, Bornstein BA, Connolly JL, et al. The influence of infiltrating lobular carcinoma on the outcome of patients treated with breast-conserving surgery and radiation therapy. *Breast Cancer Res Treat* 2000;59(1):49–54.

452. Salvadori B, Biganzoli E, Veronesi P, et al. Conservative surgery for infiltrating lobular breast carcinoma. *Br J Surg* 1997;84(1):106–109.

453. Moran MS, Yang Q, Haffty BG. The Yale University experience of early-stage invasive lobular carcinoma (ILC) and invasive ductal carcinoma (IDC) treated with breast conservation treatment (BCT): analysis of clinical-pathologic features, long-term outcomes, and molecular expression of COX-2, Bcl-2, and p53 as a function of histology. *Breast J* 2009;15(6):571–578.

454. Moran M, Haffty BG. Lobular carcinoma in situ as a component of breast cancer: the long-term outcome in patients treated with breast-conservation therapy. *Int J Radiat Oncol Biol Phys* 1998;40(2):353–358.

455. Abner AL, Connolly JL, Recht A, et al. The relation between the presence and extent of lobular carcinoma in situ and the risk of local recurrence for patients with infiltrating carcinoma of the breast treated with conservative surgery and radiation therapy. *Cancer* 2000;88(5):1072–1077.

456. Ben-David MA, Kleer CG, Paramagul C, et al. Is lobular carcinoma in situ as a component of breast carcinoma a risk factor for local failure after breast-conserving therapy? Results of a matched pair analysis. *Cancer* 2006;106(1):28–34.

457. Jolly S, Kestin LL, Goldstein NS, et al. The impact of lobular carcinoma in situ in association with invasive breast cancer on the rate of local recurrence in patients with early-stage breast cancer treated with breast-conserving therapy. *Int J Radiat Oncol Biol Phys* 2006;66(2):365–371.

458. Sasson AR, Fowble B, Hanlon AL, et al. Lobular carcinoma in situ increases the risk of local recurrence in selected patients with stages I and II breast carcinoma treated with conservative surgery and radiation. *Cancer* 2001;91(10):1862–1869.

459. Ciocca RM, Li T, Freedman GM, et al. Presence of lobular carcinoma in situ does not increase local recurrence in patients treated with breast-conserving therapy. *Ann Surg Oncol* 2008;15(8):2263–2271.

460. Clemente CG, Boracchi P, Andreola S, et al. Peritumoral lymphatic invasion in patients with node-negative mammary duct carcinoma. *Cancer* 1992;69(6):1396–1403.

461. Wong JS, O'Neill A, Recht A, et al. The relationship between lymphatic vessel invasion, tumor size, and pathologic nodal status: can we predict who can avoid a third field in the absence of axillary dissection?. *Int J Radiat Oncol Biol Phys* 2000;48(1):133–137.

462. Lash TL, Silliman RA, Guadagnoli E, et al. The effect of less than definitive care on breast carcinoma recurrence and mortality. *Cancer* 2000;89(8):1739–1747.

463. Identification of breast cancer patients with high risk of early recurrence after radical mastectomy. II. Clinical and pathological correlations. A report of the Primary Therapy of Breast Cancer Study Group. *Cancer* 1978;42(6):2809–2826.

464. Ege GN, Clark RM. Internal mammary lymphoscintigraphy in the conservative management of breast carcinoma: an update and recommendations for a new TNM staging. *Clin Radiol* 1985;36(5):469–472.

465. Donegan WL, Perez-Mesa CM, Watson FR. A biostatistical study of locally recurrent breast carcinoma. *Surg Gynecol Obstet* 1966;122(3):529–540.

466. Haffty BG. Molecular and genetic markers in the local-regional management of breast cancer. *Semin Radiat Oncol* 2002;12(4):329–340.

467. Moran MS, Haffty BG. Local-regional breast cancer recurrence: prognostic groups based on patterns of failure. *Breast J* 2002;8(2):81–87.

468. Haffty BG, Glazer PM. Molecular markers in clinical radiation oncology. *Oncogene* 2003;22(37):5915–5925.

469. Haffty BG, Brown F, Carter D, et al. Evaluation of HER-2 neu oncoprotein expression as a prognostic indicator of local recurrence in conservatively treated breast cancer: a case-control study. *Int J Radiat Oncol Biol Phys* 1996;35(4):751–757.

470. Turner BC, Gumbs AA, Carbone CJ, et al. Mutant p53 protein overexpression in women with ipsilateral breast tumor recurrence following lumpectomy and radiation therapy. *Cancer* 2000;88(5):1091–1098.

471. Elkhuizen PH, Hermans J, Leer JW, et al. Isolated late local recurrences with high mitotic count and early local recurrences following breast-conserving therapy are associated with increased risk on distant metastasis. *Int J Radiat Oncol Biol Phys* 2001;50(2):387–396.

472. Elkhuizen PH, Voogd AC, van den Broek LC, et al. Risk factors for local recurrence after breast-conserving therapy for invasive carcinomas: a case-control study of histological factors and alterations in oncogene expression. *Int J Radiat Oncol Biol Phys* 1999;45(1):73–83.

473. Linderholm B, Tavelin B, Grankvist K, et al. Does vascular endothelial growth factor (VEGF) predict local relapse and survival in radiotherapy-treated node-negative breast cancer?. *Br J Cancer* 1999;81(4):727–732.

474. Pierce LJ, Merino MJ, D'Angelo T, et al. Is c-erb B-2 a predictor for recurrent disease in early stage breast cancer?. *Int J Radiat Oncol Biol Phys* 1994;28(2):395–403.

475. Ringberg A, Anagnostaki L, Anderson H, et al. Cell biological factors in ductal carcinoma in situ (DCIS) of the breast-relationship to ipsilateral local recurrence and histopathological characteristics. *Eur J Cancer* 2001;37(12):1514–1522.

476. Ringberg A, Idvall I, Ferno M, et al. Ipsilateral local recurrence in relation to therapy and morphological characteristics in patients with ductal carcinoma in situ of the breast. *Eur J Surg Oncol* 2000;26(5):444–451.

477. Santiago RJ, Wu L, Harris E, et al. Fifteen-year results of breast-conserving surgery and definitive irradiation for stage I and II breast carcinoma: the University of Pennsylvania experience. *Int J Radiat Oncol Biol Phys* 2004;58(1):233–240.

478. Silvestrini R, Benini E, Veneroni S, et al. p53 and bcl-2 expression correlates with clinical outcome in a series of node-positive breast cancer patients. *J Clin Oncol* 1996;14(5):1604–1610.

479. Stal O, Sullivan S, Wingren S, et al. c-erbB-2 expression and benefit from adjuvant chemotherapy and radiotherapy of breast cancer. *Eur J Cancer* 1995;31A(13–14):2185–2190.

480. Zellars RC, Hilsenbeck SG, Clark GM, et al. Prognostic value of p53 for local failure in mastectomy-treated breast cancer patients. *J Clin Oncol* 2000;18(9):1906–1913.

481. Silvestrini R, Daidone MG, Luisi A, et al. Cell proliferation in 3,800 node-negative breast cancers: consistency over time of biological and clinical information provided by 3H-thymidine labeling index. *Int J Cancer* 1997;74(1):122–127.

482. Silvestrini R, Veneroni S, Benini E, et al. Expression of p53, glutathione S-transferase-pi, and Bcl-2 proteins and benefit from adjuvant radiotherapy in breast cancer. *J Natl Cancer Inst* 1997;89(9):639–645.

483. Choi DH, Kim S, Rimm DL, et al. Immunohistochemical biomarkers in patients with early-onset breast carcinoma by tissue microarray. *Cancer J* 2005;11(5):404–411.

484. Kim S, Rimm D, Carter D, et al. BRCA status, molecular markers, and clinical variables in early, conservatively managed breast cancer. *Breast J* 2003;9(3):167–174.

485. Silvestrini R, Daidone MG, Luisi A, et al. Biologic and clinicopathologic factors as indicators of specific relapse types in node-negative breast cancer. *J Clin Oncol* 1995;13(3):697–704.

486. Vrieling C, Collette L, Fourquet A, et al. The influence of patient, tumor and treatment factors on the cosmetic results after breast-conserving therapy in the EORTC "boost vs. no boost" trial. EORTC Radiotherapy and Breast Cancer Cooperative Groups. *Radiother Oncol* 2000;55(3):219–232.

487. Amornmarn R, Bui MM, Prempree TB, et al. Molecular predictive factors for local recurrence and distant metastasis of breast cancer after lumpectomy with postoperative radiation therapy. *Ann Clin Lab Sci* 2000;30(1):33–40.

488. Harris EE, Hwang WT, Lee EA, et al. The impact of HER-2 status on local recurrence in women with stage I–II breast cancer treated with breast-conserving therapy. *Breast J* 2006;12(5):431–436.

489. Meyer A, John E, Dork T, et al. Breast cancer in female carriers of ATM gene alterations: outcome of adjuvant radiotherapy. *Radiother Oncol* 2004;72(3):319–323.

490. Pierce L, Fowble B, Solin LJ, et al. Conservative surgery and radiation therapy in black women with early stage breast cancer. Patterns of failure and analysis of outcome. *Cancer* 1992;69(11):2831–2841.

491. Haffty BG, Yang Q, Reiss M, et al. Locoregional relapse and distant metastasis in conservatively managed triple negative early-stage breast cancer. *J Clin Oncol* 2006;24(36):5652–5657.

492. Nguyen PL, Taghian AG, Katz MS, et al. Breast cancer subtype approximated by estrogen receptor, progesterone receptor, and HER-2 is associated with local and distant recurrence after breast-conserving therapy. *J Clin Oncol* 2008;26(14):2373–2378.

493. Voduc KD, Cheang MC, Tyldesley S, et al. Breast cancer subtypes and the risk of local and regional relapse. *J Clin Oncol* 2010;28(10):1684–1691.

494. Abdulkarim BS, Cuartero J, Hanson J, et al. Increased risk of locoregional recurrence for women with T1-2N0 triple-negative breast cancer treated with modified radical mastectomy without adjuvant radiation therapy compared with breast-conserving therapy. *J Clin Oncol* 2011;29(21):2852–2858.

495. Pignol JP, Rakovitch E, Olivotto IA. Is breast conservation therapy superior to mastectomy for women with triple-negative breast cancers?. *J Clin Oncol* 2011;29(21):2841–2843.

496. Wang J, Shi M, Ling R, et al. Adjuvant chemotherapy and radiotherapy in triple-negative breast carcinoma: a prospective randomized controlled multi-center trial. *Radiother Oncol* 2011;100(2):200–204.

497. Mamounas EP, Tang G, Fisher B, et al. Association between the 21-gene recurrence score assay and risk of locoregional recurrence in node-negative, estrogen receptor-positive breast cancer: results from NSABP B-14 and NSABP B-20. *J Clin Oncol* 2010;28(10):1677–1683.

498. Vrieling C, Collette L, Fourquet A, et al. Can patient-, treatment- and pathology-related characteristics explain the high local recurrence rate following breast-conserving therapy in young patients?. *Eur J Cancer* 2003;39(7):932–944.

499. Grills IS, Kestin LL, Goldstein N, et al. Risk factors for regional nodal failure after breast-conserving therapy: regional nodal irradiation reduces rate of axillary failure in patients with four or more positive lymph nodes. *Int J Radiat Oncol Biol Phys* 2003;56(3):658–670.

500. Liljegren G, Holmberg L, Adami HO, et al. Sector resection with or without postoperative radiotherapy for stage I breast cancer: five-year results of a randomized trial. Uppsala-Orebro Breast Cancer Study Group. *J Natl Cancer Inst* 1994;86(9):717–722.

501. Veronesi U, Marubini E, Mariani L, et al. Radiotherapy after breast-conserving surgery in small breast carcinoma: long-term results of a randomized trial. *Ann Oncol* 2001;12(7):997–1003.

502. Clark RM, Whelan T, Levine M, et al. Randomized clinical trial of breast irradiation following lumpectomy and axillary dissection for node-negative breast cancer: an update. Ontario Clinical Oncology Group. *J Natl Cancer Inst* 1996;88(22):1659–1664.

503. Winzer KJ, Sauer R, Sauerbrei W, et al. Radiation therapy after breast-conserving surgery; first results of a randomised clinical trial in patients with low risk of recurrence. *Eur J Cancer* 2004;40(7):998–1005.

504. Whelan T, Clark R, Roberts R, et al. Ipsilateral breast tumor recurrence post-lumpectomy is predictive of subsequent mortality: results from a randomized trial. Investigators of the Ontario Clinical Oncology Group. *Int J Radiat Oncol Biol Phys* 1994;30(1):11–16.

505. Forrest AP, Stewart HJ, Everington D, et al. Randomised controlled trial of conservation therapy for breast cancer: 6-year analysis of the Scottish trial. Scottish Cancer Trials Breast Group. *Lancet* 1996;348(9029):708–713.

506. Renton SC, Gazet JC, Ford HT, et al. The importance of the resection margin in conservative surgery for breast cancer. *Eur J Surg Oncol* 1996;22(1):17–22.

507. Lim M, Bellon JR, Gelman R, et al. A prospective study of conservative surgery without radiation therapy in select patients with stage I breast cancer. *Int J Radiat Oncol Biol Phys* 2006;65(4):1149–1154.

508. McCready DR, Chapman JA, Hanna WM, et al. Factors associated with local breast cancer recurrence after lumpectomy alone: postmenopausal patients. *Ann Surg Oncol* 2000;7(8):562–567.

509. Cooke AL, Perera F, Fisher B, et al. Tamoxifen with and without radiation after partial mastectomy in patients with involved nodes. *Int J Radiat Oncol Biol Phys* 1995;31(4):777–781.

510. Gajdos C, Tartter PI, Bleiweiss IJ, et al. The consequence of undertreating breast cancer in the elderly. *J Am Coll Surg* 2001;192(6):698–707.

511. Hughes KS, Schnaper LA, Berry D, et al. Lumpectomy plus tamoxifen with or without irradiation in women 70 years of age or older with early breast cancer. *N Engl J Med* 2004;351(10):971–977.

512. Hughes KS, Schnaper LA, Bellon JR, et al: Lumpectomy plus tamoxifen with or without irradiation in women age 70 years or older with early breast cancer: long-term follow-up of CALGB 9343. *J Clin Oncol* 2013, 31(19):2382–2387.

513. Fyles AW, McCready DR, Manchul LA, et al. Tamoxifen with or without breast irradiation in women 50 years of age or older with early breast cancer. *N Engl J Med* 2004;351(10):963–970.

514. Smith BD, Gross CP, Smith GL, et al. Effectiveness of radiation therapy for older women with early breast cancer. *J Natl Cancer Inst* 2006;98(10):681–690.

515. Bentzen SM, Agrawal RK, Aird EG, et al. The UK Standardisation of Breast Radiotherapy (START) Trial A of radiotherapy hypofractionation for treatment of early breast cancer: a randomised trial. *Lancet Oncol* 2008;9(4):331–341.

516. Bentzen SM, Agrawal RK, Aird EG, et al. The UK Standardisation of Breast Radiotherapy (START) Trial B of radiotherapy hypofractionation for treatment of early breast cancer: a randomised trial. *Lancet* 2008;371(9618):1098–1107.

517. Whelan TJ, Pignol JP, Levine MN, et al. Long-term results of hypofractionated radiation therapy for breast cancer. *N Engl J Med* 2010;362(6):513–520.

518. Jacquillat C, Weil M, Baillet F, et al. Results of neoadjuvant chemotherapy and radiation therapy in the breast-conserving treatment of 250 patients with all stages of infiltrative breast cancer. *Cancer* 1990;66(1):119–129.

519. Smith BD, Bentzen S, Correa C, et al. Fractionation for whole breast irradiation: an American Society for Radiation Oncology (ASTRO) evidence-based guideline. *Int J Radiat Oncol Biol Phys* 2011;81(1):59–68.

520. Ceilley E, Jagsi R, Goldberg S, et al. Radiotherapy for invasive breast cancer in North America and Europe: results of a survey. *Int J Radiat Oncol Biol Phys* 2005;61(2):365–373.

521. Jagsi R, Makris A, Goldberg S, et al. Intra-European differences in the radiotherapeutic management of breast cancer: a survey study. *Clin Oncol (R Coll Radiol)* 2006;18(5):369–375.

522. Schlembach PJ, Buchholz TA, Ross MI, et al. Relationship of sentinel and axillary level I–II lymph nodes to tangential fields used in breast irradiation. *Int J Radiat Oncol Biol Phys* 2001;51(3):671–678.

523. Yarnold JR. Selective avoidance of lymphatic irradiation in the conservative management of breast cancer. *Radiother Oncol* 1984;2(2):79–92.

524. Giuliano AE, Haigh PI, Brennan MB, et al. Prospective observational study of sentinel lymphadenectomy without further axillary dissection in patients with sentinel node-negative breast cancer. *J Clin Oncol* 2000;18(13):2553–2559.

525. Whelan TJ, Olivotto IA, Parulekar WR et al. Regional nodal irradiation in early-stage breast cancer. *N Engl J Med* 2015;373(4):307–316.

526. Poortmans PM, Collette S, Kirkove C, et al. Internal mammary and medial supra-clavicular irradiation in breast cancer. *N Engl J Med* 2015; 373(4):317–327.

527. Recht A. Should irradiation replace dissection for patients with breast cancer with clinically negative axillary lymph nodes?. *J Surg Oncol* 1999;72(4):184–192.

528. Cabanes PA, Salmon RJ, Vilcoq JR, et al. Value of axillary dissection in addition to lumpectomy and radiotherapy in early breast cancer. The Breast Carcinoma Collaborative Group of the Institut Curie. *Lancet* 1992;339(8804):1245–1248.

529. Baeza MR, Sole J, Leon A, et al. Conservative treatment of early breast cancer. *Int J Radiat Oncol Biol Phys* 1988;14(4):669–676.

530. Pierquin B, Mazeron JJ, Glaubiger D. Conservative treatment of breast cancer in Europe: report of the Groupe Europeen de Curietherapie. *Radiother Oncol* 1986;6(3):187–198.

531. Wazer DE, Erban JK, Robert NJ, et al. Breast conservation in elderly women for clinically negative axillary lymph nodes without axillary dissection. *Cancer* 1994;74(3):878–883.

532. Galper S, Recht A, Silver B, et al. Is radiation alone adequate treatment to the axilla for patients with limited axillary surgery? Implications for treatment after a positive sentinel node biopsy. *Int J Radiat Oncol Biol Phys* 2000;48(1):125–132.

533. Louis-Sylvestre C, Clough K, Asselain B, et al. Axillary treatment in conservative management of operable breast cancer: dissection or radiotherapy? Results of a randomized study with 15 years of follow-up. *J Clin Oncol* 2004;22(1):97–101.

534. Langlands AO, Prescott RJ, Hamilton T. A clinical trial in the management of operable cancer of the breast. *Br J Surg* 1980;67(3):170–174.

535. Hayward J, Caleffi M. The significance of local control in the primary treatment of breast cancer. Lucy Wortham James Clinical Research Award. *Arch Surg* 1987;122(11):1244–1247.

536. Lythgoe JP, Palmer MK. Manchester regional breast study—5 and 10 year results. *Br J Surg* 1982;69(12):693–696.

537. Ribeiro GG, Magee B, Swindell R, et al. The Christie Hospital breast conservation trial: an update at 8 years from inception. *Clin Oncol (R Coll Radiol)* 1993;5(5):278–283.

538. Rudenstam CM, Zahrieh D, Forbes JF, et al. Randomized trial comparing axillary clearance versus no axillary clearance in older patients with breast cancer: first results of International Breast Cancer Study Group Trial 10–93. *J Clin Oncol* 2006;24(3):337–344.

539. Veronesi U, Orecchia R, Zurrida S, et al. Avoiding axillary dissection in breast cancer surgery: a randomized trial to assess the role of axillary radiotherapy. *Ann Oncol* 2005;16(3):383–388.

540. Hamilton T, Langlands AO, Prescott RJ. The treatment of operable cancer of the breast: a clinical trial in the South-East region of Scotland. *Br J Surg* 1974;61(10):758–761.

541. Sanuki-Fujimoto N. Benefits of axillary radiotherapy unclear in women with early stage breast cancer undergoing conservative breast surgery without axillary dissection. *Cancer Treat Rev* 2005;31(6):496–500.

542. Zurrida S, Orecchia R, Galimberti V, et al. Axillary radiotherapy instead of axillary dissection: a randomized trial. Italian Oncological Senology Group. *Ann Surg Oncol* 2002;9(2):156–160.

543. Pejavar S, Wilson LD, Haffty BG. Regional nodal recurrence in breast cancer patients treated with conservative surgery and radiation therapy (BCS+RT). *Int J Radiat Oncol Biol Phys* 2006;66(5):1320–1327.

544. Halverson KJ, Taylor ME, Perez CA, et al. Management of the axilla in patients with breast cancers one centimeter or smaller. *Am J Clin Oncol* 1994;17(6):461–466.

545. Wong JS, Recht A, Beard CJ, et al. Treatment outcome after tangential radiation therapy without axillary dissection in patients with early-stage breast cancer and clinically negative axillary nodes. *Int J Radiat Oncol Biol Phys* 1997;39(4):915–920.

546. Mehta K, Haffty BG. Long-term outcome in patients with four or more positive lymph nodes treated with conservative surgery and radiation therapy. *Int J Radiat Oncol Biol Phys* 1996;35(4):679–685.

547. Whelan T. NCIC CTG MA.20: an intergroup trial of regional nodal irradiation in early breast cancer. *J Clin Oncol* 2011;9(Suppl):(abstr LBA1003).

548. Huang O, Wang L, Shen K, et al. Breast cancer subpopulation with high risk of internal mammary lymph nodes metastasis: analysis of 2,269 Chinese breast cancer patients treated with extended radical mastectomy. *Breast Cancer Res Treat* 2008, 107(3):379–387.

549. Veronesi U, Arnone P, Veronesi P, et al. The value of radiotherapy on metastatic internal mammary nodes in breast cancer. Results on a large series. *Ann Oncol* 2008;19(9):1553–1560.

550. Budach W, Kammers K, Boelke E, et al. Adjuvant radiotherapy of regional lymph nodes in breast cancer—a meta-analysis of randomized trials. *Radiat Oncol* 2013;8:267.

551. Straver ME, Meijnen P, van Tienhoven G, et al. Sentinel node identification rate and nodal involvement in the EORTC 10981–22023 AMAROS trial. *Ann Surg Oncol* 2010;17(7):1854–1861.

552. Pierce LJ, Oberman HA, Strawderman MH, et al. Microscopic extracapsular extension in the axilla: is this an indication for axillary radiotherapy?. *Int J Radiat Oncol Biol Phys* 1995;33(2):253–259.

553. Fowble B, Hanlon A, Freedman G, et al. Internal mammary node irradiation neither decreases distant metastases nor improves survival in stage I and II breast cancer. *Int J Radiat Oncol Biol Phys* 2000;47(4):883–894.

554. Obedian E, Haffty BG. Internal mammary nodal irradiation in conservatively-managed breast cancer patients: is there a benefit?. *Int J Radiat Oncol Biol Phys* 1999;44(5):997–1003.

555. Stemmer SM, Rizel S, Hardan I, et al. The role of irradiation of the internal mammary lymph nodes in high-risk stage II to IIIA breast cancer patients after high-dose chemotherapy: a prospective sequential nonrandomized study. *J Clin Oncol* 2003;21(14):2713–2718.

556. Thorsen LB, Offersen BV, Dano H, et al. DBCG-IMN: a population-based cohort study on the effect of internal mammary node irradiation in early node-positive breast cancer. *J Clin Oncol* 2016;34(4):314–320.

557. Hennequin C, Bossard N, Servagi-Vernat S et al. Ten-year survival results of a randomized trial of irradiation of internal mammary nodes after mastectomy. *Int J Radiat Oncol Biol Phys* 2013;86(5):860–866.

558. Veronesi U, Marubini E, Mariani L, et al. The dissection of internal mammary nodes does not improve the survival of breast cancer patients. 30-year results of a randomised trial. *Eur J Cancer* 1999;35(9):1320–1325.

559. Lacour J, Bucalossi P, Cacers E, et al. Radical mastectomy versus radical mastectomy plus internal mammary dissection. Five-year results of an international cooperative study. *Cancer* 1976;37(1):206–214.

560. Meier P, Ferguson DJ, Karrison T. A controlled trial of extended radical versus radical mastectomy. Ten-year results. *Cancer* 1989;63(1):188–195.

561. Freedman GM, Fowble BL, Nicolaou N, et al. Should internal mammary lymph nodes in breast cancer be a target for the radiation oncologist?. *Int J Radiat Oncol Biol Phys* 2000;46(4):805–814.

562. Recht A. Integration of systemic therapy and radiation therapy for patients with early-stage breast cancer treated with conservative surgery. *Clin Breast Cancer* 2003;4(2):104–113.

563. Recht A, Come SE, Henderson IC, et al. The sequencing of chemotherapy and radiation therapy after conservative surgery for early-stage breast cancer. *N Engl J Med* 1996;334(21):1356–1361.

564. Bellon JR, Come SE, Gelman RS, et al. Sequencing of chemotherapy and radiation therapy in early-stage breast cancer: updated results of a prospective randomized trial. *J Clin Oncol* 2005;23(9):1934–1940.

565. Buchholz TA, Hunt KK, Amosson CM, et al. Sequencing of chemotherapy and radiation in lymph node-negative breast cancer. *Cancer J Sci Am* 1999;5(3):159–164.

566. Sartor CI, Peterson BL, Woolf S, et al. Effect of addition of adjuvant paclitaxel on radiotherapy delivery and locoregional control of node-positive breast cancer: cancer and leukemia group B 9344. *J Clin Oncol* 2005;23(1):30–40.

567. Haffty BG, Kim JH, Yang Q, et al. Concurrent chemo-radiation in the conservative management of breast cancer. *Int J Radiat Oncol Biol Phys* 2006;66(5):1306–1312.

568. Bellon JR, Shulman LN, Come SE, et al. A prospective study of concurrent cyclophosphamide/methotrexate/5-fluorouracil and reduced-dose radiotherapy in patients with early-stage breast carcinoma. *Cancer* 2004;100(7):1358–1364.

569. Markiewicz DA, Fox KR, Schultz DJ, et al. Concurrent chemotherapy and radiation for breast conservation treatment of early-stage breast cancer. *Cancer J Sci Am* 1998;4(3):185–193.

570. Rouesse J, de la Lande B, Bertheault-Cvitkovic F, et al. A phase III randomized trial comparing adjuvant concomitant chemoradiotherapy versus standard adjuvant chemotherapy followed by radiotherapy in operable node-positive breast cancer: final results. *Int J Radiat Oncol Biol Phys* 2006;64(4):1072–1080.

571. Toledano A, Garaud P, Serin D, et al. Concurrent administration of adjuvant chemotherapy and radiotherapy after breast-conserving surgery enhances late toxicities: long-term results of the ARCOSEIN multicenter randomized study. *Int J Radiat Oncol Biol Phys* 2006;65(2):324–332.

572. Arcangeli G, Pinnaro P, Rambone R, et al. A phase III randomized study on the sequencing of radiotherapy and chemotherapy in the conservative management of early-stage breast cancer. *Int J Radiat Oncol Biol Phys* 2006;64(1):161–167.

573. Calais G, Berger C, Descamps P, et al. Conservative treatment feasibility with induction chemotherapy, surgery, and radiotherapy for patients with breast carcinoma larger than 3 cm. *Cancer* 1994;74(4):1283–1288.

574. Goyal S, Rao MS, Khan A, et al. Evaluation of acute locoregional toxicity in patients with breast cancer treated with adjuvant radiotherapy in combination with bevacizumab. *Int J Radiat Oncol Biol Phys* 2011;79(2):408–413.

575. Burstein HJ, Bellon JR, Galper S, et al. Prospective evaluation of concurrent paclitaxel and radiation therapy after adjuvant doxorubicin and cyclophosphamide chemotherapy for stage II or III breast cancer. *Int J Radiat Oncol Biol Phys* 2006;64(2):496–504.

576. Bentzen SM, Skoczylas JZ, Overgaard M, et al. Radiotherapy-related lung fibrosis enhanced by tamoxifen. *J Natl Cancer Inst* 1996;88(13):918–922.

577. Wazer DE, DiPetrillo T, Schmidt-Ullrich R, et al. Factors influencing cosmetic outcome and complication risk after conservative surgery and radiotherapy for early-stage breast carcinoma. *J Clin Oncol* 1992;10(3):356–363.

578. Ahn PH, Vu HT, Lannin D, et al. Sequence of radiotherapy with tamoxifen in conservatively managed breast cancer does not affect local relapse rates. *J Clin Oncol* 2005;23(1):17–23.

579. Harris EE, Christensen VJ, Hwang WT, et al. Impact of concurrent versus sequential tamoxifen with radiation therapy in early-stage breast cancer patients undergoing breast conservation treatment. *J Clin Oncol* 2005;23(1):11–16.

580. Suh WW, Pierce LJ, Vicini FA, et al. A cost comparison analysis of partial versus whole-breast irradiation after breast-conserving surgery for early-stage breast cancer. *Int J Radiat Oncol Biol Phys* 2005;62(3):790–796.

581. Pierce LJ, Hutchins LF, Green SR, et al. Sequencing of tamoxifen and radiotherapy after breast-conserving surgery in early-stage breast cancer. *J Clin Oncol* 2005;23(1):24–29.

582. Azria D, Belkacemi Y, Romieu G, et al. Concurrent or sequential adjuvant letrozole and radiotherapy after conservative surgery for early-stage breast cancer (CO-HO-RT): a phase 2 randomised trial. *Lancet Oncol* 2010;11(3):258–265.

583. Alpert TE, Haffty BG. Conservative management of breast cancer in BRCA1/2 mutation carriers. *Clin Breast Cancer* 2004;5(1):37–42.

584. Robson M, Svahn T, McCormick B, et al. Appropriateness of breast-conserving treatment of breast carcinoma in women with germline mutations in BRCA1 or BRCA2: a clinic-based series. *Cancer* 2005;103(1):44–51.

585. Easton DF. How many more breast cancer predisposition genes are there?. *Breast Cancer Res* 1999;1(1):14–17.

586. Easton DF, Steele L, Fields P, et al. Cancer risks in two large breast cancer families linked to BRCA2 on chromosome 13q12-13. *Am J Hum Genet* 1997;61(1):120–128.

587. Ford D, Easton DF, Peto J. Estimates of the gene frequency of BRCA1 and its contribution to breast and ovarian cancer incidence. *Am J Hum Genet* 1995;57(6):1457–1462.

588. Ford D, Easton DF, Stratton M, et al. Genetic heterogeneity and penetrance analysis of the BRCA1 and BRCA2 genes in breast cancer families. The Breast Cancer Linkage Consortium. *Am J Hum Genet* 1998;62(3):676–689.

589. Ansquer Y, Gautier C, Fourquet A, et al. Survival in early-onset BRCA1 breast-cancer patients. Institut Curie Breast Cancer Group. *Lancet* 1998;352(9127):541.

590. Robson ME, Chappuis PO, Satagopan J, et al. A combined analysis of outcome following breast cancer: differences in survival based on BRCA1/BRCA2 mutation status and administration of adjuvant treatment. *Breast Cancer Res* 2004;6(1):R8–R17.

591. Seynaeve C, Verhoog LC, Van De Bosch LM, et al. Ipsilateral breast tumour recurrence in hereditary breast cancer following breast-conserving therapy. *Eur J Cancer* 2004;40(8):1150–1158.

592. Moynahan ME, Pierce AJ, Jasin M. BRCA2 is required for homology-directed repair of chromosomal breaks. *Mol Cell* 2001;7(2):263–272.

593. Noguchi S, Kasugai T, Miki Y, et al. Clinicopathologic analysis of BRCA1- or BRCA2-associated hereditary breast carcinoma in Japanese women. *Cancer* 1999;85(10):2200–2205.

594. Narod SA, Brunet JS, Ghadirian P, et al. Tamoxifen and risk of contralateral breast cancer in BRCA1 and BRCA2 mutation carriers: a case-control study. Hereditary Breast Cancer Clinical Study Group. *Lancet* 2000;356(9245):1876–1881.

595. Prevalence and penetrance of BRCA1 and BRCA2 mutations in a population-based series of breast cancer cases. Anglian Breast Cancer Study Group. *Br J Cancer* 2000;83(10):1301–1308.

596. Freedman LM, Buchholz TA, Thames HD, et al. Local-regional control in breast cancer patients with a possible genetic predisposition. *Int J Radiat Oncol Biol Phys* 2000;48(4):951–957.

597. Garcia-Etienne CA, Barile M, Gentilini OD, et al. Breast-conserving surgery in BRCA1/2 mutation carriers: are we approaching an answer?. *Ann Surg Oncol* 2009;16(12):3380–3387.

598. Haffty BG, Harrold E, Khan AJ, et al. Outcome of conservatively managed early-onset breast cancer by BRCA1/2 status. *Lancet* 2002;359(9316):1471–1477.

599. Kirova YM, Savignoni A, Sigal-Zafrani B, et al. Is the breast-conserving treatment with radiotherapy appropriate in BRCA1/2 mutation carriers? Long-term results and review of the literature. *Breast Cancer Res Treat* 2010;120(1):119–126.

600. Kirova YM, Stoppa-Lyonnet D, Savignoni A, et al. Risk of breast cancer recurrence and contralateral breast cancer in relation to BRCA1 and BRCA2 mutation status following breast-conserving surgery and radiotherapy. *Eur J Cancer* 2005;41(15):2304–2311.

601. Pierce LJ, Levin AM, Rebbeck TR, et al. Ten-year multi-institutional results of breast-conserving surgery and radiotherapy in BRCA1/2-associated stage I/II breast cancer. *J Clin Oncol* 2006;24(16):2437–2443.

602. Pierce LJ, Phillips KA, Griffith KA, et al. Local therapy in BRCA1 and BRCA2 mutation carriers with operable breast cancer: comparison of breast conservation and mastectomy. *Breast Cancer Res Treat* 2010;121(2):389–398.

603. Turner BC, Harrold E, Matloff E, et al. BRCA1/BRCA2 germline mutations in locally recurrent breast cancer patients after lumpectomy and radiation therapy: implications for breast-conserving management in patients with BRCA1/BRCA2 mutations. *J Clin Oncol* 1999;17(10):3017–3024.

604. Pierce LJ, Haffty BG. Radiotherapy in the treatment of hereditary breast cancer. *Semin Radiat Oncol* 2011;21(1):43–50.

605. Pierce LJ, Phillips KA, Griffith KA, et al. Local therapy in BRCA1 and BRCA2 mutation carriers with operable breast cancer: comparison of breast conservation and mastectomy. *Breast Cancer Res Treat* 2010;121(2):389–398.

606. Robson M. Are BRCA1- and BRCA2-associated breast cancers different? Prognosis of BRCA1-associated breast cancer. *J Clin Oncol* 2000;18(21 Suppl):113S–118S.

607. Robson M, Levin D, Federici M, et al. Breast conservation therapy for invasive breast cancer in Ashkenazi women with BRCA gene founder mutations. *J Natl Cancer Inst* 1999;91(24):2112–2117.

608. Pierce LJ. Postmastectomy radiotherapy: future directions. *Semin Radiat Oncol* 1999;9(3):300–304.

609. Steinmann D, Bremer M, Rades D, et al. Mutations of the BRCA1 and BRCA2 genes in patients with bilateral breast cancer. *Br J Cancer* 2001;85(6):850–858.

610. Rebbeck TR. Prophylactic oophorectomy in BRCA1 and BRCA2 mutation carriers. *J Clin Oncol* 2000;18(21 Suppl):100S–103S.

611. Rebbeck TR, Friebel T, Lynch HT, et al. Bilateral prophylactic mastectomy reduces breast cancer risk in BRCA1 and BRCA2 mutation carriers: the PROSE Study Group. *J Clin Oncol* 2004;22(6):1055–1062.

612. Rebbeck TR, Friebel T, Wagner T, et al. Effect of short-term hormone replacement therapy on breast cancer risk reduction after bilateral prophylactic oophorectomy in BRCA1 and BRCA2 mutation carriers: the PROSE Study Group. *J Clin Oncol* 2005;23(31):7804–7810.

613. Kauff ND, Satagopan JM, Robson ME, et al. Risk-reducing salpingo-oophorectomy in women with a BRCA1 or BRCA2 mutation. *N Engl J Med* 2002;346(21):1609–1615.

614. Fowble B, Hanlon AL, Patchefsky A, et al. The presence of proliferative breast disease with atypia does not significantly influence outcome in early-stage invasive breast cancer treated with conservative surgery and radiation. *Int J Radiat Oncol Biol Phys* 1998;42(1):105–115.

615. Pierce LJ, Strawderman M, Narod SA, et al. Effect of radiotherapy after breast-conserving treatment in women with breast cancer and germline BRCA1/2 mutations. *J Clin Oncol* 2000;18(19):3360–3369.

616. De Naeyer B, De Meerleer G, Braems S, et al. Collagen vascular diseases and radiation therapy: a critical review. *Int J Radiat Oncol Biol Phys* 1999;44(5):975–980.

617. Fleck R, McNeese MD, Ellerbroek NA, et al. Consequences of breast irradiation in patients with pre-existing collagen vascular diseases. *Int J Radiat Oncol Biol Phys* 1989;17(4):829–833.

618. Robertson JM, Clarke DH, Pevzner MM, et al. Breast conservation therapy. Severe breast fibrosis after radiation therapy in patients with collagen vascular disease. *Cancer* 1991;68(3):502–508.

619. Chen AM, Obedian E, Haffty BG. Breast-conserving therapy in the setting of collagen vascular disease. *Cancer J* 2001;7(6):480–491.

620. Morris MM, Powell SN. Irradiation in the setting of collagen vascular disease: acute and late complications. *J Clin Oncol* 1997;15(7):2728–2735.

621. Ross JG, Hussey DH, Mayr NA, et al. Acute and late reactions to radiation therapy in patients with collagen vascular diseases. *Cancer* 1993;71(11):3744–3752.

622. Phan C, Mindrum M, Silverman C, et al. Matched-control retrospective study of the acute and late complications in patients with collagen vascular diseases treated with radiation therapy. *Cancer J* 2003;9(6):461–466.

623. Rakfal SM, Deutsch M. Radiotherapy for malignancies associated with lupus: case reports of acute and late reactions. *Am J Clin Oncol* 1998;21(1):54–57.

624. Loibl S, von Minckwitz G, Gwyn K, et al. Breast carcinoma during pregnancy. International recommendations from an expert meeting. *Cancer* 2006;106(2):237–246.

625. Albrektsen G, Heuch I, Kvale G. The short-term and long-term effect of a pregnancy on breast cancer risk: a prospective study of 802,457 parous Norwegian women. *Br J Cancer* 1995;72(2):480–484.

626. Petrek JA. Breast cancer during pregnancy. *Cancer* 1994;74(1 Suppl):518–527.

627. Zemlickis D, Lishner M, Degendorfer P, et al. Maternal and fetal outcome after breast cancer in pregnancy. *Am J Obstet Gynecol* 1992;166(3):781–787.

628. Nugent P, O'Connell TX. Breast cancer and pregnancy. *Arch Surg* 1985;120(11):1221–1224.

629. Adami HO, Malker B, Holmberg L, et al. The relation between survival and age at diagnosis in breast cancer. *N Engl J Med* 1986;315(9):559–563.

630. Murphy CG, Mallam D, Stein S, et al. Current or recent pregnancy is associated with adverse pathologic features but not impaired survival in early breast cancer. *Cancer* 2012;118(13):2354–2359.

631. Liberman L, Giess CS, Dershaw DD, et al. Imaging of pregnancy-associated breast cancer. *Radiology* 1994;191(1):245–248.

632. Hahn KM, Johnson PH, Gordon N, et al. Treatment of pregnant breast cancer patients and outcomes of children exposed to chemotherapy in utero. *Cancer* 2006;107(6):1219–1226.

633. Doll DC, Ringenberg QS, Yarbro JW. Antineoplastic agents and pregnancy. *Semin Oncol* 1989;16(5):337–346.

634. Wolmark N, Dunn BK. The role of tamoxifen in breast cancer prevention: issues sparked by the NSABP Breast Cancer Prevention Trial (P-1). *Ann NY Acad Sci* 2001;949:99–108.

635. Diallo I, Lamon A, Shamsaldin A, et al. Estimation of the radiation dose delivered to any point outside the target volume per patient treated with external beam radiotherapy. *Radiother Oncol* 1996;38(3):269–271.

636. Brent RL. The effect of embryonic and fetal exposure to x-ray, microwaves, and ultrasound: counseling the pregnant and nonpregnant patient about these risks. *Semin Oncol* 1989;16(5):347–368.

637. Hall EJ, Wuu CS. Radiation-induced second cancers: the impact of 3D-CRT and IMRT. *Int J Radiat Oncol Biol Phys* 2003;56(1):83–88.

638. Adair FE. Cancer of the breast. *Surg Clin North Am* 1953:313–327.

639. King RM, Welch JS, Martin JK Jr, et al. Carcinoma of the breast associated with pregnancy. *Surg Gynecol Obstet* 1985;160(3):228–232.

640. Danforth DN Jr. How subsequent pregnancy affects outcome in women with a prior breast cancer. *Oncology (Williston Park)* 1991;5(11):23–31, 35.

641. Sutton R, Buzdar AU, Hortobagyi GN. Pregnancy and offspring after adjuvant chemotherapy in breast cancer patients. *Cancer* 1990;65(4):847–850.

642. Sankila R, Heinavaara S, Hakulinen T. Survival of breast cancer patients after subsequent term pregnancy: "healthy mother effect." *Am J Obstet Gynecol* 1994;170(3):818–823.

643. Higgins S, Haffty BG. Pregnancy and lactation after breast-conserving therapy for early stage breast cancer. *Cancer* 1994;73(8):2175–2180.

644. Moran MS, Colasanto JM, Haffty BG, et al. Effects of breast-conserving therapy on lactation after pregnancy. *Cancer J* 2005;11(5):399–403.

645. Tralins AH. Lactation after conservative breast surgery combined with radiation therapy. *Am J Clin Oncol* 1995;18(1):40–43.

646. Chung CT, Bogart JA, Adams JF, et al. Increased risk of breast cancer in splenectomized patients undergoing radiation therapy for Hodgkin's disease. *Int J Radiat Oncol Biol Phys* 1997;37(2):405–409.

647. Carey RW, Linggood RM, Wood W, et al. Breast cancer developing in four women cured of Hodgkin's disease. *Cancer* 1984;54(10):2234–2236.

648. Guibout C, Adjadj E, Rubino C, et al. Malignant breast tumors after radiotherapy for a first cancer during childhood. *J Clin Oncol* 2005;23(1):197–204.

649. Hoppe RT. Hodgkin's disease: complications of therapy and excess mortality. *Ann Oncol* 1997;8(Suppl 1):115–118.

650. Tinger A, Wasserman TH, Klein EE, et al. The incidence of breast cancer following mantle field radiation therapy as a function of dose and technique. *Int J Radiat Oncol Biol Phys* 1997;37(4):865–870.

651. Mauch PM, Kalish LA, Marcus KC, et al. Second malignancies after treatment for laparotomy staged IA-IIIB Hodgkin's disease: long-term analysis of risk factors and outcome. *Blood* 1996;87(9):3625–3632.

652. Salloum E, Doria R, Schubert W, et al. Second solid tumors in patients with Hodgkin's disease cured after radiation or chemotherapy plus adjuvant low-dose radiation. *J Clin Oncol* 1996;14(9):2435–2443.

653. Hancock SL, Tucker MA, Hoppe RT. Breast cancer after treatment of Hodgkin's disease. *J Natl Cancer Inst* 1993;85(1):25–31.

654. Prior P, Pope DJ. Hodgkin's disease: subsequent primary cancers in relation to treatment. *Br J Cancer* 1988;58(4):512–517.

655. Tucker MA, Coleman CN, Cox RS, et al. Risk of second cancers after treatment for Hodgkin's disease. *N Engl J Med* 1988;318(2):76–81.

656. Kaldor JM, Day NE, Band P, et al. Second malignancies following testicular cancer, ovarian cancer and Hodgkin's disease: an international collaborative study among cancer registries. *Int J Cancer* 1987;39(5):571–585.

657. Travis LB, Hill DA, Dores GM, et al. Breast cancer following radiotherapy and chemotherapy among young women with Hodgkin disease. *JAMA* 2003;290(4):465–475.

658. Metayer C, Lynch CF, Clarke EA, et al. Second cancers among long-term survivors of Hodgkin's disease diagnosed in childhood and adolescence. *J Clin Oncol* 2000;18(12):2435–2443.

659. Swerdlow AJ, Barber JA, Hudson GV, et al. Risk of second malignancy after Hodgkin's disease in a collaborative British cohort: the relation to age at treatment. *J Clin Oncol* 2000;18(3):498–509.

660. van Leeuwen FE, Klokman WJ, Veer MB, et al. Long-term risk of second malignancy in survivors of Hodgkin's disease treated during adolescence or young adulthood. *J Clin Oncol* 2000;18(3):487–497.

661. Gervais-Fagnou DD, Girouard C, Laperriere N, et al. Breast cancer in women following supradiaphragmatic irradiation for Hodgkin's disease. *Oncology* 1999;57(3):224–231.

662. Hudson MM, Poquette CA, Lee J, et al. Increased mortality after successful treatment for Hodgkin's disease. *J Clin Oncol* 1998;16(11):3592–3600.

663. Wolden SL, Lamborn KR, Cleary SF, et al. Second cancers following pediatric Hodgkin's disease. *J Clin Oncol* 1998;16(2):536–544.

664. Aisenberg AC, Finkelstein DM, Doppke KP, et al. High risk of breast carcinoma after irradiation of young women with Hodgkin's disease. *Cancer* 1997;79(6):1203–1210.

665. De Bruin ML, Sparidans J, van't Veer MB, et al. Breast cancer risk in female survivors of Hodgkin's lymphoma: lower risk after smaller radiation volumes. *J Clin Oncol* 2009;27(26):4239–4246.

666. Elkin EB, Klem ML, Gonzales AM, et al. Characteristics and outcomes of breast cancer in women with and without a history of radiation for Hodgkin's lymphoma: a multi-institutional, matched cohort study. *J Clin Oncol* 2011;29(18):2466–2473.

667. Cutuli B, Borel C, Dhermain F, et al. Breast cancer occurred after treatment for Hodgkin's disease: analysis of 133 cases. *Radiother Oncol* 2001;59(3):247–255.

668. Wolden SL, Hancock SL, Carlson RW, et al. Management of breast cancer after Hodgkin's disease. *J Clin Oncol* 2000;18(4):765–772.

669. Deutsch M, Gerszten K, Bloomer WD, et al. Lumpectomy and breast irradiation for breast cancer arising after previous radiotherapy for Hodgkin's disease or lymphoma. *Am J Clin Oncol* 2001;24(1):33–34.

670. Alpert TE, Kuerer HM, Arthur DW, et al. Ipsilateral breast tumor recurrence after breast conservation therapy: outcomes of salvage mastectomy vs. salvage breast-conserving surgery and prognostic factors for salvage breast preservation. *Int J Radiat Oncol Biol Phys* 2005;63(3):845–851.

671. Arthur DW, Vicini FA. Accelerated partial breast irradiation as a part of breast conservation therapy. *J Clin Oncol* 2005;23(8):1726–1735.

672. Morgenstern L, Kaufman PA, Friedman NB. The case against tylectomy for carcinoma of the breast. The factor of multicentricity. *Am J Surg* 1975;130(2):251–258.

673. Wilson LD, Beinfield M, McKhann CF, et al. Conservative surgery and radiation in the treatment of synchronous ipsilateral breast cancers. *Cancer* 1993;72(1):137–142.

674. Leopold KA, Recht A, Schnitt SJ, et al. Results of conservative surgery and radiation therapy for multiple synchronous cancers of one breast. *Int J Radiat Oncol Biol Phys* 1989;16(1):11–16.

675. Kaplan J, Giron G, Tartter PI, et al. Breast conservation in patients with multiple ipsilateral synchronous cancers. *J Am Coll Surg* 2003;197(5):726–729.

676. Hartsell WF, Recine DC, Griem KL, et al. Should multicentric disease be an absolute contraindication to the use of breast-conserving therapy?. *Int J Radiat Oncol Biol Phys* 1994;30(1):49–53.

677. Kurtz JM, Jacquemier J, Amalric R, et al. Breast-conserving therapy for macroscopically multiple cancers. *Ann Surg* 1990;212(1):38–44.

678. Clark CP III, Peters GN, O'Brien KM. Cancer in the augmented breast. Diagnosis and prognosis. *Cancer* 1993;72(7):2170–2174.

679. Handel N, Lewinsky B, Silverstein MJ, et al. Conservation therapy for breast cancer following augmentation mammaplasty. *Plast Reconstr Surg* 1991;87(5):873–878.

680. Guenther JM, Tokita KM, Giuliano AE. Breast-conserving surgery and radiation after augmentation mammoplasty. *Cancer* 1994;73(10):2613–2618.

681. Smith ML, Evans GR, Gurlek A, et al. Reduction mammaplasty: its role in breast conservation surgery for early-stage breast cancer. *Ann Plast Surg* 1998;41(3):234–239.

682. Horn PL, Thompson WD. Risk of contralateral breast cancer. Associations with histologic, clinical, and therapeutic factors. *Cancer* 1988;62(2):412–424.

683. Recht A. Radiotherapy and surgery in early breast cancer. *N Engl J Med* 1996;334(15):989.

684. Hislop TG, Elwood JM, Coldman AJ, et al. Second primary cancers of the breast: incidence and risk factors. *Br J Cancer* 1984;49(1):79–85.

685. Lewis TR, Casey J, Buerk CA, et al. Incidence of lobular carcinoma in bilateral breast cancer. *Am J Surg* 1982;144(6):635–638.

686. Nielsen M, Christensen L, Andersen J. Contralateral cancerous breast lesions in women with clinical invasive breast carcinoma. *Cancer* 1986;57(5):897–903.

687. Sears HF, Janus C, McDermott A, et al. Bilateral breast carcinoma: prospective evaluation of factors assisting diagnosis. *J Surg Oncol* 1986;32(4):203–207.

688. Solin LJ, Fowble BL, Schultz DJ, et al. Bilateral breast carcinoma treated with definitive irradiation. *Int J Radiat Oncol Biol Phys* 1989;17(2):263–271.

689. Hungness ES, Safa M, Shaughnessy EA, et al. Bilateral synchronous breast cancer: mode of detection and comparison of histologic features between the 2 breasts. *Surgery* 2000;128(4):702–707.

690. Heron DE, Komarnicky LT, Hyslop T, et al. Bilateral breast carcinoma: risk factors and outcomes for patients with synchronous and metachronous disease. *Cancer* 2000;88(12):2739–2750.

691. Kollias J, Evans AJ, Wilson AR, et al. Value of contralateral surveillance mammography for primary breast cancer follow-up. *World J Surg* 2000;24(8):983–989.

692. Gustafsson A, Tartter PI, Brower ST, et al. Prognosis of patients with bilateral carcinoma of the breast. *J Am Coll Surg* 1994;178(2):111–116.

693. de la Rochefordiere A, Asselain B, Scholl S, et al. Simultaneous bilateral breast carcinomas: a retrospective review of 149 cases. *Int J Radiat Oncol Biol Phys* 1994;30(1):35–41.

694. Fung MC, Schultz DJ, Solin LJ. Early-stage bilateral breast cancer treated with breast-conserving surgery and definitive irradiation: the University of Pennsylvania experience. *Int J Radiat Oncol Biol Phys* 1997;38(5):959–967.

695. Fourquet A, Campana F, Rosenwald JC, et al. Breast irradiation in the lateral decubitus position: technique of the Institut Curie. *Radiother Oncol* 1991;22(4):261–265.

696. Cross MA, Elson HR, Aron BS. Breast conservation radiation therapy technique for women with large breasts. *Int J Radiat Oncol Biol Phys* 1989;17(1):199–203.

697. Merchant TE, McCormick B. Prone position breast irradiation. *Int J Radiat Oncol Biol Phys* 1994;30(1):197–203.

698. Stegman LD, Beal KP, Hunt MA, et al. Long-term clinical outcomes of whole-breast irradiation delivered in the prone position. *Int J Radiat Oncol Biol Phys* 2007;68(1):73–81.

699. Solin LJ, Danoff BF, Schwartz GF, et al. A practical technique for the localization of the tumor volume in definitive irradiation of the breast. *Int J Radiat Oncol Biol Phys* 1985;11(6):1215–1220.

700. Moody AM, Mayles WP, Bliss JM, et al. The influence of breast size on late radiation effects and association with radiotherapy dose inhomogeneity. *Radiother Oncol* 1994;33(2):106–112.

701. Bentel GC, Marks LB. A simple device to position large/flaccid breasts during tangential breast irradiation. *Int J Radiat Oncol Biol Phys* 1994;29(4):879–882.

702. Bornstein BA, Cheng CW, Rhodes LM, et al. Can simulation measurements be used to predict the irradiated lung volume in the tangential fields in patients treated for breast cancer?. *Int J Radiat Oncol Biol Phys* 1990;18(1):181–187.

703. Kong FM, Klein EE, Bradley JD, et al. The impact of central lung distance, maximal heart distance, and radiation technique on the volumetric dose of the lung and heart for intact breast radiation. *Int J Radiat Oncol Biol Phys* 2002;54(3):963–971.

704. Marks LB, Yu X, Prosnitz RG, et al. The incidence and functional consequences of RT-associated cardiac perfusion defects. *Int J Radiat Oncol Biol Phys* 2005;63(1):214–223.

705. Lu HM, Cash E, Chen MH, et al. Reduction of cardiac volume in left-breast treatment fields by respiratory maneuvers: a CT study. *Int J Radiat Oncol Biol Phys* 2000;47(4):895–904.

706. Recht A, Come SE, Gelman RS, et al. Integration of conservative surgery, radiotherapy, and chemotherapy for the treatment of early-stage, node-positive breast cancer: sequencing, timing, and outcome. *J Clin Oncol* 1991;9(9):1662–1667.

707. Arthur DW, Cuttino LW, Neuschatz AC, et al. Tumor bed boost omission after negative re-excision in breast-conservation treatment. *Ann Surg Oncol* 2006;13(6):794–801.

708. Fisher B, Bauer M, Margolese R, et al. Five-year results of a randomized clinical trial comparing total mastectomy and segmental mastectomy with or without radiation in the treatment of breast cancer. *N Engl J Med* 1985;312(11):665–673.

709. Haffty BG, Fischer D, Beinfield M, et al. Prognosis following local recurrence in the conservatively treated breast cancer patient. *Int J Radiat Oncol Biol Phys* 1991;21(2):293–298.

710. Harris JR, Recht A, Amalric R, et al. Time course and prognosis of local recurrence following primary radiation therapy for early breast cancer. *J Clin Oncol* 1984;2(1):37–41.

711. Smith TE, Lee D, Turner BC, et al. True recurrence vs. new primary ipsilateral breast tumor relapse: an analysis of clinical and pathologic differences and their implications in natural history, prognoses, and therapeutic management. *Int J Radiat Oncol Biol Phys* 2000;48(5):1281–1289.

712. Recht A, Silver B, Schnitt S, et al. Breast relapse following primary radiation therapy for early breast cancer. I. Classification, frequency and salvage. *Int J Radiat Oncol Biol Phys* 1985;11(7):1271–1276.

713. Romestaing P, Lehingue Y, Carrie C, et al. Role of a 10-Gy boost in the conservative treatment of early breast cancer: results of a randomized clinical trial in Lyon, France. *J Clin Oncol* 1997;15(3):963–968.

714. Mansfield CM, Komarnicky LT, Schwartz GF, et al. Perioperative implantation of iridium-192 as the best technique for stage I and II breast cancer: results of a 10-year study of 655 patients. *Radiology* 1994;192(1):33–36.

715. Mansfield CM, Komarnicky LT, Schwartz GF, et al. Ten-year results in 1070 patients with stages I and II breast cancer treated by conservative surgery and radiation therapy. *Cancer* 1995;75(9):2328–2336.

716. Mariani L, Salvadori B, Marubini E, et al. Ten year results of a randomised trial comparing two conservative treatment strategies for small size breast cancer. *Eur J Cancer* 1998;34(8):1156–1162.

717. Touboul E, Belkacemi Y, Lefranc JP, et al. Early breast cancer: influence of type of boost (electrons vs iridium-192 implant) on local control and cosmesis after conservative surgery and radiation therapy. *Radiother Oncol* 1995;34(2):105–113.

718. Vicini F, White J, Gustafson G, et al. The use of iodine-125 seeds as a substitute for iridium-192 seeds in temporary interstitial breast implants. *Int J Radiat Oncol Biol Phys* 1993;27(3):561–566.

Section
III

719. Vicini FA, Kestin LL, Edmundson GK, et al. Dose-volume analysis for quality assurance of interstitial brachytherapy for breast cancer. *Int J Radiat Oncol Biol Phys* 1999;45(3):803–810.

720. Fourquet A, Campana F, Mosseri V, et al. Iridium-192 versus cobalt-60 boost in 3–7 cm breast cancer treated by irradiation alone: final results of a randomized trial. *Radiother Oncol* 1995;34(2):114–120.

721. Olivotto IA, Rose MA, Osteen RT, et al. Late cosmetic outcome after conservative surgery and radiotherapy: analysis of causes of cosmetic failure. *Int J Radiat Oncol Biol Phys* 1989;17(4):747–753.

722. Perez CA, Taylor ME, Halverson K, et al. Brachytherapy or electron beam boost in conservation therapy of carcinoma of the breast: a nonrandomized comparison. *Int J Radiat Oncol Biol Phys* 1996;34(5):995–1007.

723. Ray GR, Fish VJ. Biopsy and definitive radiation therapy in stage I and II adenocarcinoma of the female breast: analysis of cosmesis and the role of electron beam supplementation. *Int J Radiat Oncol Biol Phys* 1983;9(6):813–818.

724. Oh KS, Kong FM, Griffith KA, et al. Planning the breast tumor bed boost: changes in the excision cavity volume and surgical scar location after breast-conserving surgery and whole-breast irradiation. *Int J Radiat Oncol Biol Phys* 2006;66(3):680–686.

725. Smitt MC, Birdwell RL, Goffinet DR. Breast electron boost planning: comparison of CT and US. *Radiology* 2001;219(1):203–206.

726. Fein DA, Fowble BL, Hanlon AL, et al. Does the placement of surgical clips within the excision cavity influence local control for patients treated with breast-conserving surgery and irradiation. *Int J Radiat Oncol Biol Phys* 1996;34(5):1009–1017.

727. Denham JW, Sillar RW, Clarke D. Boost dosage to the excision site following conservative surgery for breast cancer: it's easy to miss! *Clin Oncol (R Coll Radiol)* 1991;3(5):257–261.

728. Ringash J, Whelan T, Elliott E, et al. Accuracy of ultrasound in localization of breast boost field. *Radiother Oncol* 2004;72(1):61–66.

729. Li XA, Tai A, Arthur DW, et al. Variability of target and normal structure delineation for breast cancer radiotherapy: an RTOG multi-institutional and multiobserver study. *Int J Radiat Oncol Biol Phys* 2009;73(3):944–951.

730. Petersen RP, Truong PT, Kader HA, et al. Target volume delineation for partial breast radiotherapy planning: clinical characteristics associated with low interobserver concordance. *Int J Radiat Oncol Biol Phys* 2007;69(1):41–48.

731. Coles CE, Wishart G, et al. The IMPORT Gold Seed Study: evaluation of tumour bed localisation and image-guided radiotherapy for breast cancer. *Clin Oncol (R Coll Radiol)* 2007;19(3 Suppl):S26–S27.

732. Dzhugashvili M, Pichenot C, Dunant A, et al. Surgical clips assist in the visualization of the lumpectomy cavity in three-dimensional conformal accelerated partial-breast irradiation. *Int J Radiat Oncol Biol Phys* 2010;76(5):1320–1324.

733. Shaikh T, Chen T, Khan A, et al. Improvement in interobserver accuracy in delineation of the lumpectomy cavity using fiducial markers. *Int J Radiat Oncol Biol Phys* 2010;78(4):1127–1134.

734. Coles CE, Wilson CB, Cumming J, et al. Titanium clip placement to allow accurate tumour bed localisation following breast conserving surgery: audit on behalf of the IMPORT Trial Management Group. *Eur J Surg Oncol* 2009;35(6):578–582.

735. Mansur DB, El Naqa I, Kong F, et al. Localization of internal mammary lymph nodes by CT simulation: implications for breast radiation therapy planning. *Radiother Oncol* 2004;73(3):355–357.

736. Arthur DW, Arnfield MR, Warwicke LA, et al. Internal mammary node coverage: an investigation of presently accepted techniques. *Int J Radiat Oncol Biol Phys* 2000;48(1):139–146.

737. Goodman RL, Grann A, Saracco P, et al. The relationship between radiation fields and regional lymph nodes in carcinoma of the breast. *Int J Radiat Oncol Biol Phys* 2001;50(1):99–105.

738. Wang X, Yu TK, Salehpour M, et al. Breast cancer regional radiation fields for supraclavicular and axillary lymph node treatment: is a posterior axillary boost field technique optimal?. *Int J Radiat Oncol Biol Phys* 2009;74(1):86–91.

739. Bentel GC, Marks LB, Hardenbergh PH, et al. Variability of the depth of supraclavicular and axillary lymph nodes in patients with breast cancer: is a posterior axillary boost field necessary?. *Int J Radiat Oncol Biol Phys* 2000;47(3):755–758.

740. Bentel G, Marks LB, Hardenbergh P, et al. Variability of the location of internal mammary vessels and glandular breast tissue in breast cancer patients undergoing routine CT-based treatment planning. *Int J Radiat Oncol Biol Phys* 1999;44(5):1017–1025.

741. Pierce LJ, Butler JB, Martel MK, et al. Postmastectomy radiotherapy of the chest wall: dosimetric comparison of common techniques. *Int J Radiat Oncol Biol Phys* 2002;52(5):1220–1230.

742. Severin D, Connors S, Thompson H, et al. Breast radiotherapy with inclusion of internal mammary nodes: a comparison of techniques with three-dimensional planning. *Int J Radiat Oncol Biol Phys* 2003;55(3):633–644.

743. Bedwinek JM, Brady L, Perez CA, et al. Irradiation as the primary management of stage I and II adenocarcinoma of the breast: analysis of the RTOG breast registry. *Cancer Clin Trials* 1980;3(1):11–18.

744. Broët P, de la Rochefordiere A, Scholl SM, et al. Contralateral breast cancer: annual incidence and risk parameters. *J Clin Oncol* 1995;13(7):1578–1583.

745. Hartsell WF, Kelly CA, Schneider L, et al. A single isocenter three-field breast irradiation technique using an empiric simulation and asymmetric collimator. *Med Dosim* 1994;19(3):169–173.

746. Woudstra E, van der Werf H. Obliquely incident electron beams for irradiation of the internal mammary lymph nodes. *Radiother Oncol* 1987;10(3):209–215.

747. Fraass BA, Roberson PL, Lichter AS. Dose to the contralateral breast due to primary breast irradiation. *Int J Radiat Oncol Biol Phys* 1985;11(3):485–497.

748. Muller-Runkel R, Kalokhe UP. Scatter dose from tangential breast irradiation to the uninvolved breast. *Radiology* 1990;175(3):873–876.

749. Kelly CA, Wang XY, Chu JC, et al. Dose to contralateral breast: a comparison of four primary breast irradiation techniques. *Int J Radiat Oncol Biol Phys* 1996;34(3):727–732.

750. Nielsen HM, Overgaard M, Grau C, et al. Study of failure pattern among high-risk breast cancer patients with or without postmastectomy radiotherapy in addition to adjuvant systemic therapy: long-term results from the Danish Breast Cancer Cooperative Group DBCG 82 B and C randomized studies. *J Clin Oncol* 2006;24(15):2268–2275.

751. Solin LJ, Chu JC, Sontag MR, et al. Three-dimensional photon treatment planning of the intact breast. *Int J Radiat Oncol Biol Phys* 1991;21(1):193–203.

752. Vicini FA, Sharpe M, Kestin L, et al. Optimizing breast cancer treatment efficacy with intensity-modulated radiotherapy. *Int J Radiat Oncol Biol Phys* 2002;54(5):1336–1344.

753. Dunst J, Steil B, Furch S, et al. Prognostic significance of local recurrence in breast cancer after postmastectomy radiotherapy. *Strahlenther Onkol* 2001;177(10):504–510.

754. Pignol J. A multicentre randomized trial of breast IMRT to reduce acute radiation dermatitis. *J Clin Oncol* 2008;26(13):2085–2092.

755. Pignol J, Olivotto I, Rakovitch E, et al. Phase III randomized study of intensity modulated radiation therapy versus standard wedging technique for adjuvant breast radiotherapy. Paper presented at Proceedings of the ASTRO 48th annual meeting 2006; Philadelphia, *PA*

756. Donovan E, Bleakley N, Denholm E, et al. Randomised trial of standard 2D radiotherapy (RT) versus intensity modulated radiotherapy (IMRT) in patients prescribed breast radiotherapy. *Radiother Oncol* 2007;82(3):254–264.

757. National Institutes of Health Consensus Development Conference Statement: Adjuvant therapy for breast cancer, November 1–3, 2000. *J Natl Cancer Inst Monogr* 2001;2001(30):5–15.

758. Fowble B. Ipsilateral breast tumor recurrence following breast-conserving surgery for early-stage invasive cancer. *Acta Oncol* 1999;38(Suppl 13):9–17.

759. Freedman GM, Anderson PR, Hanlon AL, et al. Pattern of local recurrence after conservative surgery and whole-breast irradiation. *Int J Radiat Oncol Biol Phys* 2005;61(5):1328–1336.

760. Haffty BG, Carter D, Flynn SD, et al. Local recurrence versus new primary: clinical analysis of 82 breast relapses and potential applications for genetic fingerprinting. *Int J Radiat Oncol Biol Phys* 1993;27(3):575–583.

761. NSABP-B39, RTOG-0413. A randomized phase III study of conventional whole breast irradiation versus partial breast irradiation for women with stage 0, I, or II breast cancer. Available at: http://www.rtog.org/members/protocols/0413/0413.pdf.

762. Kuske RR Jr. Breast brachytherapy. *Hematol Oncol Clin North Am* 1999;13(3):543–558, vi–vii.

763. Vicini FA, Arthur DW. Breast brachytherapy: North American experience. *Semin Radiat Oncol* 2005;15(2):108–115.

764. Wazer DE, Lowther D, Boyle T, et al. Clinically evident fat necrosis in women treated with high-dose-rate brachytherapy alone for early-stage breast cancer. *Int J Radiat Oncol Biol Phys* 2001;50(1):107–111.

765. Kuske RR, Winter K, Arthur DW, et al. Phase II trial of brachytherapy alone after lumpectomy for select breast cancer: toxicity analysis of RTOG 95–17. *Int J Radiat Oncol Biol Phys* 2006;65(1):45–51.

766. Shah C, Antonucci JV, Wilkinson JB, et al. Twelve-year clinical outcomes and patterns of failure with accelerated partial breast irradiation versus whole-breast irradiation: results of a matched-pair analysis. *Radiother Oncol* 2011;100(2):210–214.

767. Arthur DW, Koo D, Zwicker RD, et al. Partial breast brachytherapy after lumpectomy: low-dose-rate and high-dose-rate experience. *Int J Radiat Oncol Biol Phys* 2003;56(3):681–689.

768. Wazer DE, Berle L, Graham R, et al. Preliminary results of a phase I/II study of HDR brachytherapy alone for T1/T2 breast cancer. *Int J Radiat Oncol Biol Phys* 2002;53(4):889–897.

769. Arthur DW, Vicini FA. MammoSite RTS: the reporting of initial experiences and how to interpret. *Ann Surg Oncol* 2004;11(8):723–724.

770. Keisch M, Vicini F, Kuske RR, et al. Initial clinical experience with the MammoSite breast brachytherapy applicator in women with early-stage breast cancer treated with breast-conserving therapy. *Int J Radiat Oncol Biol Phys* 2003;55(2):289–293.

771. Vicini F, Beitsch P, Quiet C, et al. Five-year analysis of treatment efficacy and cosmesis by the American Society of Breast Surgeons MammoSite Breast Brachytherapy Registry Trial in patients treated with accelerated partial breast irradiation. *Int J Radiat Oncol Biol Phys* 2011;79(3):808–817.

772. Vicini F, Beitsch PD, Quiet CA, et al. Three-year analysis of treatment efficacy, cosmesis, and toxicity by the American Society of Breast Surgeons MammoSite Breast Brachytherapy Registry Trial in patients treated with accelerated partial breast irradiation (APBI). *Cancer* 2008;112(4):758–766.

773. Formenti SC. External-beam partial-breast irradiation. *Semin Radiat Oncol* 2005;15(2):92–99.

774. Vicini F, Winter K, Straube W, et al. A phase I/II trial to evaluate three-dimensional conformal radiation therapy confined to the region of the lumpectomy cavity for stage I/II breast carcinoma: initial report of feasibility and reproducibility of Radiation Therapy Oncology Group (RTOG) Study 0319. *Int J Radiat Oncol Biol Phys* 2005;63(5):1531–1537.

775. Vicini F, Winter K, Wong J, et al. Initial efficacy results of RTOG 0319: three-dimensional conformal radiation therapy (3D-CRT) confined to the region of the lumpectomy cavity for stage I/II breast carcinoma. *Int J Radiat Oncol Biol Phys* 2010;77(4):1120–1127.

776. Jagsi R, Ben-David MA, Moran JM, et al. Unacceptable cosmesis in a protocol investigating intensity-modulated radiotherapy with active breathing control for accelerated partial-breast irradiation. *Int J Radiat Oncol Biol Phys* 2010;76(1):71–78.

777. Hepel JT, Tokita M, MacAusland SG, et al. Toxicity of three-dimensional conformal radiotherapy for accelerated partial breast irradiation. *Int J Radiat Oncol Biol Phys* 2009;75(5):1290–1296.

778. Olivotto IA, Whelan TJ, Parpia S, et al. Interim cosmetic and toxicity results from RAPID: a randomized trial of accelerated partial breast irradiation using three-dimensional conformal external beam radiation therapy. *J Clin Oncol* 2013;31(32):4038–4045.

779. Veronesi U, Gatti G, Luini A, et al. Full-dose intraoperative radiotherapy with electrons during breast-conserving surgery. *Arch Surg* 2003;138(11):1253–1256.

780. Orecchia R, Veronesi U. Intraoperative electrons. *Semin Radiat Oncol* 2005;15(2):76–83.

781. Vaidya JS, Baum M, Tobias JS, et al. The novel technique of delivering targeted intraoperative radiotherapy (Targit) for early breast cancer. *Eur J Surg Oncol* 2002;28(4):447–454.

782. Vaidya JS, Joseph DJ, Tobias JS, et al. Targeted intraoperative radiotherapy versus whole breast radiotherapy for breast cancer (TARGIT-A trial): an international, prospective, randomised, non-inferiority phase 3 trial. *Lancet* 2010;376(9735):91–102.

783. Smith BD, Arthur DW, Buchholz TA, et al. Accelerated partial breast irradiation consensus statement from the American Society for Radiation Oncology (ASTRO). *J Am Coll Surg* 2009;209(2):269–277.

784. Smith BD, Arthur DW, Buchholz TA, et al. Accelerated partial breast irradiation consensus statement from the American Society for Radiation Oncology (ASTRO). *Int J Radiat Oncol Biol Phys* 2009;74(4):987–1001.

785. Correa C, Harris EE, Leonardi MC, et al. Accelerated partial breast irradiation: executive summary for the update of an ASTRO Evidence-Based Consensus Statement. *Pract Radiat Oncol* 2017;7(2):73–79.

786. Pezner RD, Lipsett JA, Vora NL, et al. Limited usefulness of observer-based cosmesis scales employed to evaluate patients treated conservatively for breast cancer. *Int J Radiat Oncol Biol Phys* 1985;11(6):1117–1119.

787. Rose MA, Olivotto I, Cady B, et al. Conservative surgery and radiation therapy for early breast cancer. Long-term cosmetic results. *Arch Surg* 1989;124(2):153–157.

788. Beadle GF, Come S, Henderson IC, et al. The effect of adjuvant chemotherapy on the cosmetic results after primary radiation treatment for early stage breast cancer. *Int J Radiat Oncol Biol Phys* 1984;10(11):2131–2137.

789. Danoff BF, Goodman RL, Glick JH, et al. The effect of adjuvant chemotherapy on cosmesis and complications in patients with breast cancer treated by definitive irradiation. *Int J Radiat Oncol Biol Phys* 1983;9(11):1625–1630.

790. Markiewicz DA, Schultz DJ, Haas JA, et al. The effects of sequence and type of chemotherapy and radiation therapy on cosmesis and complications after breast conservation therapy. *Int J Radiat Oncol Biol Phys* 1996;35(4):661–668.

791. Berrino P, Campora E, Leone S, et al. Correction of type II breast deformities following conservative cancer surgery. *Plast Reconstr Surg* 1992;90(5):846–853.

792. Slavin SA, Love SM, Sadowsky NL. Reconstruction of the radiated partial mastectomy defect with autogenous tissues. *Plast Reconstr Surg* 1992;90(5):854–869.

793. Kronowitz SJ, Feledy JA, Hunt KK, et al. Determining the optimal approach to breast reconstruction after partial mastectomy. *Plast Reconstr Surg* 2006;117(1):1–14.

794. Veronesi U. NIH consensus meeting on early breast cancer. *Eur J Cancer* 1990;26(7):843–844.

795. Freedman GM, Fowble BL. Local recurrence after mastectomy or breast-conserving surgery and radiation. *Oncology (Williston Park)* 2000;14(11):1561–1584.

796. Haffty BG. Follow-up and salvage therapy for the conservatively treated breast cancer patient. *Semin Radiat Oncol* 1992;2(2):132–139.

797. Veronesi U, Banfi A, Salvadori B, et al. Breast conservation is the treatment of choice in small breast cancer: long-term results of a randomized trial. *Eur J Cancer* 1990;26(6):668–670.

798. Weight SC, Windle R, Stotter AT. Optimizing surveillance mammography following breast conservation surgery. *Eur J Surg Oncol* 2002;28(1):11–13.

799. Dershaw DD. Breast imaging and the conservative treatment of breast cancer. *Radiol Clin North Am* 2002;40(3):501–516.

800. Dershaw DD, Giess CS, McCormick B, et al. Patterns of mammographically detected calcifications after breast-conserving therapy associated with tumor recurrence. *Cancer* 1997;79(7):1355–1361.

801. American Society of Clinical Oncology. Recommended breast cancer surveillance guidelines. *J Clin Oncol* 1997;15:2149–2156.

802. Kollias J, Ellis IO, Elston CW, et al. Prognostic significance of synchronous and metachronous bilateral breast cancer. *World J Surg* 2001;25(9):1117–1124.

803. Kramer S, Schulz-Wendtland R, Hagedorn K, et al. Magnetic resonance imaging in the diagnosis of local recurrences in breast cancer. *Anticancer Res* 1998;18(3C):2159–2161.

804. Verhoog LC, Brekelmans CT, Seynaeve C, et al. Survival and tumour characteristics of breast-cancer patients with germline mutations of BRCA1. *Lancet* 1998;351(9099):316–321.

805. Mendelson EB. Evaluation of the postoperative breast. *Radiol Clin North Am* 1992;30(1):107–138.

806. Solin LJ, Fowble BL, Troupin RH, et al. Biopsy results of new calcifications in the postirradiated breast. *Cancer* 1989;63(10):1956–1961.

807. Samuels JR, Haffty BG, Lee CH, et al. Breast conservation therapy in patients with mammographically undetected breast cancer. *Radiology* 1992;185(2):425–427.

808. Tian S, Paster LF, Kim S, et al. Comparison of mammographic changes across three different fractionation schedules for early-stage breast cancer. *Int J Radiat Oncol Biol Phys* 2016;95(2):597–604.

809. Braw M, Erlandsson I, Ewers SB, et al. Mammographic follow-up after breast conserving surgery and postoperative radiotherapy without boost irradiation for mammary carcinoma. *Acta Radiol* 1991;32(5):398–402.

810. Orel SG, Fowble BL, Solin LJ, et al. Breast cancer recurrence after lumpectomy and radiation therapy for early-stage disease: prognostic significance of detection method. *Radiology* 1993;188(1):189–194.

811. Orel SG, Troupin RH, Patterson EA, et al. Breast cancer recurrence after lumpectomy and irradiation: role of mammography in detection. *Radiology* 1992;183(1):201–206.

812. Stomper PC, Recht A, Berenberg AL, et al. Mammographic detection of recurrent cancer in the irradiated breast. *AJR Am J Roentgenol* 1987;148(1):39–43.

813. Viehweg P, Heinig A, Lampe D, et al. Retrospective analysis for evaluation of the value of contrast-enhanced MRI in patients treated with breast conservative therapy. *MAGMA* 1998;7(3):141–152.

814. Dao TH, Rahmouni A, Campana F, et al. Tumor recurrence versus fibrosis in the irradiated breast: differentiation with dynamic gadolinium-enhanced MR imaging. *Radiology* 1993;187(3):751–755.

815. Drew PJ, Kerin MJ, Turnbull LW, et al. Routine screening for local recurrence following breast-conserving therapy for cancer with dynamic contrast-enhanced magnetic resonance imaging of the breast. *Ann Surg Oncol* 1998;5(3):265–270.

816. Lingos TI, Recht A, Vicini F, et al. Radiation pneumonitis in breast cancer patients treated with conservative surgery and radiation therapy. *Int J Radiat Oncol Biol Phys* 1991;21(2):355–360.

817. Taylor PJ, Cooper GG, Sarkar TK. Upper-limb arterial disease in women treated for breast cancer. *Br J Surg* 1995;82(8):1089–1091.

818. Erickson VS, Pearson ML, Ganz PA, et al. Arm edema in breast cancer patients. *J Natl Cancer Inst* 2001;93(2):96–111.

819. Maunsell E, Brisson J, Deschenes L. Arm problems and psychological distress after surgery for breast cancer. *Can J Surg* 1993;36(4):315–320.

820. Dewar JA, Sarrazin D, Benhamou E, et al. Management of the axilla in conservatively treated breast cancer: 592 patients treated at Institut Gustave-Roussy. *Int J Radiat Oncol Biol Phys* 1987;13(4):475–481.

821. Hack TF, Cohen L, Katz J, et al. Physical and psychological morbidity after axillary lymph node dissection for breast cancer. *J Clin Oncol* 1999;17(1):143–149.

822. Sener SF, Winchester DJ, Martz CH, et al. Lymphedema after sentinel lymphadenectomy for breast carcinoma. *Cancer* 2001;92(4):748–752.

823. Morrell RM, Halyard MY, Schild SE, et al. Breast cancer-related lymphedema. *Mayo Clin Proc* 2005;80(11):1480–1484.

824. Brorson H, Svensson H, Norrgren K, et al. Liposuction reduces arm lymphedema without significantly altering the already impaired lymph transport. *Lymphology* 1998;31(4):156–172.

825. Iannuzzi CM, Atencio DP, Green S, et al. ATM mutations in female breast cancer patients predict for an increase in radiation-induced late effects. *Int J Radiat Oncol Biol Phys* 2002;52(3):606–613.

826. Gorodetsky R, Lotan C, Piggot K, et al. Late effects of dose fractionation on the mechanical properties of breast skin following post-lumpectomy radiotherapy. *Int J Radiat Oncol Biol Phys* 1999;45(4):893–900.

827. Carrasco L, Moreno C, Pastor MA, et al. Postirradiation pseudosclerodermatous panniculitis. *Am J Dermatopathol* 2001;23(4):283–287.

828. Rayan G, Dawson LA, Bezjak A, et al. Prospective comparison of breast pain in patients participating in a randomized trial of breast-conserving surgery and tamoxifen with or without radiotherapy. *Int J Radiat Oncol Biol Phys* 2003;55(1):154–161.

829. Fowble B, Fein DA, Hanlon AL, et al. The impact of tamoxifen on breast recurrence, cosmesis, complications, and survival in estrogen receptor-positive early-stage breast cancer. *Int J Radiat Oncol Biol Phys* 1996;35(4):669–677.

830. Carl UM, Feldmeier JJ, Schmitt G, et al. Hyperbaric oxygen therapy for late sequelae in women receiving radiation after breast-conserving surgery. *Int J Radiat Oncol Biol Phys* 2001;49(4):1029–1031.

831. Pierce SM, Recht A, Lingos TI, et al. Long-term radiation complications following conservative surgery (CS) and radiation therapy (RT) in patients with early stage breast cancer. *Int J Radiat Oncol Biol Phys* 1992;23(5):915–923.

832. Kori SH. Diagnosis and management of brachial plexus lesions in cancer patients. *Oncology (Williston Park)* 1995;9(8):756–760; discussion 765.

833. Pritchard J, Anand P, Broome J, et al. Double-blind randomized phase II study of hyperbaric oxygen in patients with radiation-induced brachial plexopathy. *Radiother Oncol* 2001;58(3):279–286.

834. Kaufman J, Gunn W, Hartz AJ, et al. The pathophysiologic and roentgenologic effects of chest irradiation in breast carcinoma. *Int J Radiat Oncol Biol Phys* 1986;12(6):887–893.

835. Rothwell RI, Kelly SA, Joslin CA. Radiation pneumonitis in patients treated for breast cancer. *Radiother Oncol* 1985;4(1):9–14.

836. Taghian AG, Assaad SI, Niemierko A, et al. Risk of pneumonitis in breast cancer patients treated with radiation therapy and combination chemotherapy with paclitaxel. *J Natl Cancer Inst* 2001;93(23):1806–1811.

837. Yu TK, Whitman GJ, Thames HD, et al. Clinically relevant pneumonitis after sequential paclitaxel-based chemotherapy and radiotherapy in breast cancer patients. *J Natl Cancer Inst* 2004;96(22):1676–1681.

838. Lund MB, Myhre KI, Melsom H, et al. The effect on pulmonary function of tangential field technique in radiotherapy for carcinoma of the breast. *Br J Radiol* 1991;64(762):520–523.

839. Gagliardi G, Bjohle J, Lax I, et al. Radiation pneumonitis after breast cancer irradiation: analysis of the complication probability using the relative seriality model. *Int J Radiat Oncol Biol Phys* 2000;46(2):373–381.

840. Lind PA, Rosfors S, Wennberg B, et al. Pulmonary function following adjuvant chemotherapy and radiotherapy for breast cancer and the issue of three-dimensional treatment planning. *Radiother Oncol* 1998;49(3):245–254.

841. Cuzick J, Stewart H, Peto R, et al. Overview of randomized trials of postoperative adjuvant radiotherapy in breast cancer. *Cancer Treat Rep* 1987;71(1):15–29.

842. Shapiro CL, Hardenbergh PH, Gelman R, et al. Cardiac effects of adjuvant doxorubicin and radiation therapy in breast cancer patients. *J Clin Oncol* 1998;16(11):3493–3501.

843. Shapiro CL, Recht A. Side effects of adjuvant treatment of breast cancer. *N Engl J Med* 2001;344(26):1997–2008.

844. Darby SC, McGale P, Taylor CW, et al. Long-term mortality from heart disease and lung cancer after radiotherapy for early breast cancer: prospective cohort study of about 300,000 women in US SEER cancer registries. *Lancet Oncol* 2005;6(8):557–565.

845. Darby SC, Ewertz M, McGale P, et al. Risk of ischemic heart disease in women after radiotherapy for breast cancer. *N Engl J Med* 2013, 368(11):987–998.

846. Gyenes G, Fornander T, Carlens P, et al. Morbidity of ischemic heart disease in early breast cancer 15–20 years after adjuvant radiotherapy. *Int J Radiat Oncol Biol Phys* 1994;28(5):1235–1241.

847. Paszat LF, Mackillop WJ, Groome PA, et al. Mortality from myocardial infarction following postlumpectomy radiotherapy for breast cancer: a population-based study in Ontario, Canada. *Int J Radiat Oncol Biol Phys* 1999;43(4):755–762.

848. Rutqvist LE, Liedberg A, Hammar N, et al. Myocardial infarction among women with early-stage breast cancer treated with conservative surgery and breast irradiation. *Int J Radiat Oncol Biol Phys* 1998;40(2):359–363.

849. Patt DA, Goodwin JS, Kuo YF, et al. Cardiac morbidity of adjuvant radiotherapy for breast cancer. *J Clin Oncol* 2005;23(30):7475–7482.

850. Nixon AJ, Manola J, Gelman R, et al. No long-term increase in cardiac-related mortality after breast-conserving surgery and radiation therapy using modern techniques. *J Clin Oncol* 1998;16(4):1374–1379.

851. Vallis KA, Pintilie M, Chong N, et al. Assessment of coronary heart disease morbidity and mortality after radiation therapy for early breast cancer. *J Clin Oncol* 2002;20(4):1036–1042.

852. Nilsson G, Holmberg L, Garmo H, et al. Distribution of coronary artery stenosis after radiation for breast cancer. *J Clin Oncol* 2012;30(4):380–386.

853. Zagar TM, Marks LB. Breast cancer radiotherapy and coronary artery stenosis: location, location, location. *J Clin Oncol* 2012;30(4):350–352.

854. Jagsi R, Griffith KA, Koelling T, et al. Stroke rates and risk factors in patients treated with radiation therapy for early-stage breast cancer. *J Clin Oncol* 2006;24(18):2779–2785.

855. Nilsson G, Holmberg L, Garmo H, et al. Radiation to supraclavicular and internal mammary lymph nodes in breast cancer increases the risk of stroke. *Br J Cancer* 2009;100(5):811–816.

856. Woodward WA, Giordano SH, Duan Z, et al. Supraclavicular radiation for breast cancer does not increase the 10-year risk of stroke. *Cancer* 2006;106(12):2556–2562.

857. Boice JD Jr, Harvey EB, Blettner M, et al. Cancer in the contralateral breast after radiotherapy for breast cancer. *N Engl J Med* 1992;326(12):781–785.

858. Arriagada R, Le MG, Rochard F, et al. Conservative treatment versus mastectomy in early breast cancer: patterns of failure with 15 years of follow-up data. Institut Gustave-Roussy Breast Cancer Group. *J Clin Oncol* 1996;14(5):1558–1564.

859. Hooning MJ, Aleman BM, Hauptmann M, et al. Roles of radiotherapy and chemotherapy in the development of contralateral breast cancer. *J Clin Oncol* 2008;26(34):5561–5568.

860. Nielsen HM, Overgaard M, Grau C, et al. Loco-regional recurrence after mastectomy in high-risk breast cancer—risk and prognosis. An analysis of patients from the DBCG 82 B& C randomization trials. *Radiother Oncol* 2006;79(2):147–155.

861. Hill-Kayser CE, Harris EE, Hwang WT, et al. Twenty-year incidence and patterns of contralateral breast cancer after breast conservation treatment with radiation. *Int J Radiat Oncol Biol Phys* 2006;66(5):1313–1319.

862. Hankey BF, Curtis RE, Naughton MD, et al. A retrospective cohort analysis of second breast cancer risk for primary breast cancer patients with an assessment of the effect of radiation therapy. *J Natl Cancer Inst* 1983;70(5):797–804.

863. Levitt SH, Mandel J. Benefits versus risks in conservation surgery with irradiation for breast cancer. *Am J Med* 1984;77(1):93–100.

864. Storm HH, Andersson M, Boice JD Jr, et al. Adjuvant radiotherapy and risk of contralateral breast cancer. *J Natl Cancer Inst* 1992;84(16):1245–1250.

865. Khan AJ, Haffty BG. The location of contralateral breast cancers after radiation therapy. *Breast* 2001;7(5):331–336.

866. Huang J, Mackillop WJ. Increased risk of soft tissue sarcoma after radiotherapy in women with breast carcinoma. *Cancer* 2001;92(1):172–180.

867. Karlsson P, Holmberg E, Samuelsson A, et al. Soft tissue sarcoma after treatment for breast cancer—a Swedish population-based study. *Eur J Cancer* 1998;34(13):2068–2075.

868. Fowble B, Hanlon A, Freedman G, et al. Second cancers after conservative surgery and radiation for stages I–II breast cancer: identifying a subset of women at increased risk. *Int J Radiat Oncol Biol Phys* 2001;51(3):679–690.

869. Galper S, Gelman R, Recht A, et al. Second nonbreast malignancies after conservative surgery and radiation therapy for early-stage breast cancer. *Int J Radiat Oncol Biol Phys* 2002;52(2):406–414.

870. Ahsan H, Neugut AI. Radiation therapy for breast cancer and increased risk of esophageal carcinoma. *Ann Intern Med* 1998;128(2):114–117.

871. Ford MB, Sigurdson AJ, Petrulis ES, et al. Effects of smoking and radiotherapy on lung carcinoma in breast carcinoma survivors. *Cancer* 2003;98(7):1457–1464.

872. Deutsch M, Land SR, Begovic M, et al. The incidence of lung carcinoma after surgery for breast carcinoma with and without postoperative radiotherapy. Results of National Surgical Adjuvant Breast and Bowel Project (NSABP) clinical trials B-04 and B-06. *Cancer* 2003;98(7):1362–1368.

873. Deutsch M, Rosenstein MM. Angiosarcoma of the breast mimicking radiation dermatitis arising after lumpectomy and breast irradiation: a case report. *Am J Clin Oncol* 1998;21(6):608–609.

874. Fineberg S, Rosen PP. Cutaneous angiosarcoma and atypical vascular lesions of the skin and breast after radiation therapy for breast carcinoma. *Am J Clin Pathol* 1994;102(6):757–763.

875. Feigenberg SJ, Mendenhall NP, Reith JD, et al. Angiosarcoma after breast-conserving therapy: experience with hyperfractionated radiotherapy. *Int J Radiat Oncol Biol Phys* 2002;52(3):620–626.

876. Edeiken S, Russo DP, Knecht J, et al. Angiosarcoma after tylectomy and radiation therapy for carcinoma of the breast. *Cancer* 1992;70(3):644–647.

877. Marchal C, Weber B, de Lafontan B, et al. Nine breast angiosarcomas after conservative treatment for breast carcinoma: a survey from French comprehensive Cancer Centers. *Int J Radiat Oncol Biol Phys* 1999;44(1):113–119.

878. Zucali R, Merson M, Placucci M, et al. Soft tissue sarcoma of the breast after conservative surgery and irradiation for early mammary cancer. *Radiother Oncol* 1994;30(3):271–273.

879. Martin MB, Kon ND, Kawamoto EH, et al. Postmastectomy angiosarcoma. *Am Surg* 1984;50(10):541–545.

880. Barlow WE, Taplin SH, Yoshida CK, et al. Cost comparison of mastectomy versus breast-conserving therapy for early-stage breast cancer. *J Natl Cancer Inst* 2001;93(6):447–455.

881. Warren JL, Brown ML, Fay MP, et al. Costs of treatment for elderly women with early-stage breast cancer in fee-for-service settings. *J Clin Oncol* 2002;20(1):307–316.

882. Liljegren G, Karlsson G, Bergh J, et al. The cost-effectiveness of routine postoperative radiotherapy after sector resection and axillary dissection for breast cancer stage I. Results from a randomized trial. *Ann Oncol* 1997;8(8):757–763.

883. Hayman JA, Hillner BE, Harris JR, et al. Cost-effectiveness of adding an electron-beam boost to tangential radiation therapy in patients with negative margins after conservative surgery for early-stage breast cancer. *J Clin Oncol* 2000;18(2):287–295.

884. Bekelman JE, Sylwestrzak G, Barron J, et al. Uptake and costs of hypofractionated vs conventional whole breast irradiation after breast conserving surgery in the United States, 2008-2013. *JAMA* 2014;312(23):2542–2550.

885. Jensen AB. Psychosocial factors in breast cancer and their possible impact upon prognosis. *Cancer Treat Rev* 1991;18(3):191–210.

886. Schain W, Edwards BK, Gorrell CR, et al. Psychosocial and physical outcomes of primary breast cancer therapy: mastectomy vs excisional biopsy and irradiation. *Breast Cancer Res Treat* 1983;3(4):377–382.

887. Schain WS, d'Angelo TM, Dunn ME, et al. Mastectomy versus conservative surgery and radiation therapy. Psychosocial consequences. *Cancer* 1994;73(4):1221–1228.

888. Verhoef LC, Stalpers LJ, Verbeek AL, et al. Breast-conserving treatment or mastectomy in early breast cancer: a clinical decision analysis with special reference to the risk of local recurrence. *Eur J Cancer* 1991;27(9):1132–1137.

889. Lasry JC, Margolese RG. Fear of recurrence, breast-conserving surgery, and the trade-off hypothesis. *Cancer* 1992;69(8):2111–2115.

890. Mock V. Body image in women treated for breast cancer. *Nurs Res* 1993;42(3):153–157.

891. Schover LR. Sexuality and body image in younger women with breast cancer. *J Natl Cancer Inst Monogr* 1994(16):177–182.

892. Schover LR, Yetman RJ, Tuason LJ, et al. Partial mastectomy and breast reconstruction. A comparison of their effects on psychosocial adjustment, body image, and sexuality. *Cancer* 1995;75(1):54–64.

893. Dorval M, Maunsell E, Deschenes L, et al. Type of mastectomy and quality of life for long term breast carcinoma survivors. *Cancer* 1998;83(10):2130–2138.

894. Ganz PA, Rowland JH, Desmond K, et al. Life after breast cancer: understanding women's health-related quality of life and sexual functioning. *J Clin Oncol* 1998;16(2):501–514.

895. Ganz PA, Rowland JH, Meyerowitz BE, et al. Impact of different adjuvant therapy strategies on quality of life in breast cancer survivors. *Recent Results Cancer Res* 1998;152:396–411.

896. Hurny C, Bernhard J, Coates A. Quality of life assessment in the International Breast Cancer Study Group: past, present, and future. *Recent Results Cancer Res* 1998;152:390–395.

897. Nissen MJ, Swenson KK, Ritz LJ, et al. Quality of life after breast carcinoma surgery: a comparison of three surgical procedures. *Cancer* 2001;91(7):1238–1246.

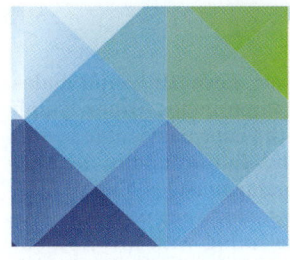

CHAPTER 60

Breast Cancer: Locally Advanced, Part 1

Ron Y. Shiloh, Brandon A. Mahal, Serena Wong, Atif J. Khan, and
Jennifer R. Bellon

BACKGROUND

This chapter focuses on the management of locally advanced breast cancer as well as locally recurrent breast cancer and selected unusual presentations of breast cancer. The emphasis is on locoregional control and radiation therapy, though systemic treatments are also reviewed.

Locally advanced breast cancer is not clearly defined, though it commonly refers to stage III disease, which includes advanced primary or nodal disease without evidence of systemic metastases. Patients who present with locally advanced breast cancer require care from a multidisciplinary team that includes radiologists, pathologists, surgical oncologists, medical oncologists, and radiation oncologists. Incorporating and coordinating the input of each specialty is of utmost importance in the management of patients with locally advanced disease, as these patients are at high risk of disease recurrence and require complex decision-making.

Fortunately, the outcome for patients who present with locally advanced breast cancer has improved substantially in recent decades. Prior to the routine use of chemotherapy, patients treated with mastectomy, radiation, or both had high rates of distant metastases and death.[1-3] Chemotherapy and hormone therapy regimens in both the neoadjuvant and adjuvant settings have significantly improved the prognosis. By decreasing the burden of distant metastases, modern chemotherapy and biologic therapies have also resulted in increased importance of local disease control.

EPIDEMIOLOGY

Between 1980 and 1987, the incidence of breast cancer increased by approximately 4% each year, due in large part to the increase in the use of screening mammography.[4] Between 1987 and 1994, the incidence remained constant and then increased again at a 1.6% rate from 1994 to 1999. Since 1999, there has been a steady decrease in incidence by 2% a year. There was a particularly sharp drop of 7% between 2002 and 2003, likely because of the decreased use of menopausal hormones after the 2002 publication of clinical trial results that demonstrated an association between hormone replacement and increased rates of breast cancer and cardiovascular disease.[4] Between 1988 and 2000, there was a steady increase in tumors diagnosed at a size of 2.0 cm or less, but since 2000, this incidence rate has decreased by 3.3% per year, and the rate of tumors of >5.0 cm has increased by 2% per year since 1992.[4] A few reasons have likely contributed to the decline in the percentage of cases of locally advanced disease at diagnosis during the late 1980s. First, mammographic screening resulted in a larger proportion of patients being diagnosed with breast cancer at earlier stages. Second, an increase in women's health initiatives and public education efforts prompted women to seek medical care at the first sign of a breast mass. Finally, the medical community has become better educated about appropriate standards for evaluating a breast mass.

An estimated 252,710 new cases of breast cancer will be diagnosed in women in 2017, and an estimated 40,610 breast cancer deaths will occur, according to the American Cancer Society.[4] As illustrated in Figure 60.1, the incidence of breast cancer is highest in the non-Hispanic White population and lowest in the Asian/Pacific Islander population. However, mortality is highest in the non-Hispanic Black population; it is 1.4 times higher than mortality in the non-Hispanic White population and 2.7 times higher than mortality in the Asian/Pacific Islander population, the population with the lowest mortality.

This significant difference in mortality has been attributed to both biologic and socioeconomic factors. Black women have been noted to be diagnosed more frequently with breast

FIGURE 60.1. Female breast cancer incidence and mortality rates per 100,000 by race and ethnicity in the United States in 2008 to 2012. (From Copeland G, Lake A, Firth R, et al., eds. *Cancer in North America: 2008–2012. Volume one: combined cancer incidence for the United States, Canada and North America.* Springfield, IL: North American Association of Central Cancer Registries, Inc., 2012).

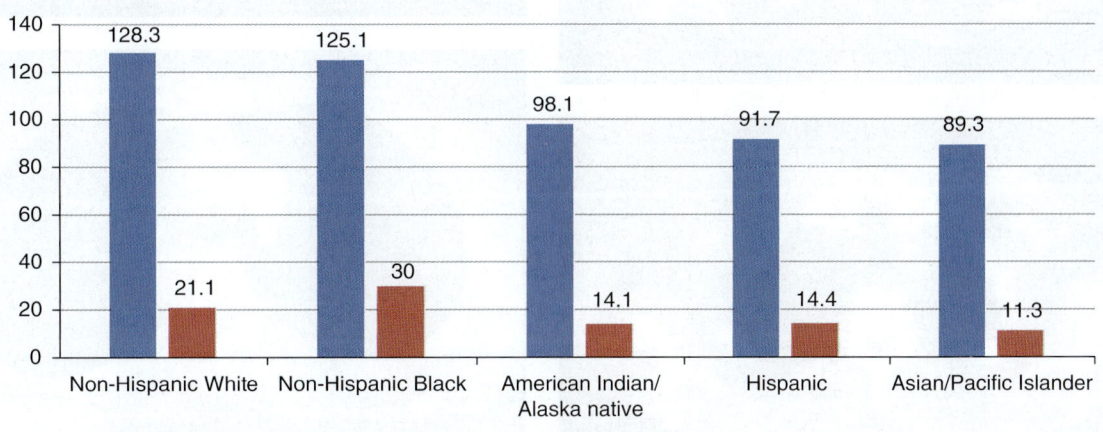

cancers of higher nuclear grade and estrogen receptor–negative disease compared with white women. Differences in access to medical care and screening mammography have also contributed to this disparity.[5,6]

NATURAL HISTORY

Prior to recent decades, a diagnosis with locally advanced breast cancer portended a poor prognosis. However, treatment advances have allowed many individuals with locally advanced disease to be cured. The clinical course of locally advanced breast cancer may vary based on several factors, including the specific disease characteristics at presentation, the biologic features of the cancer, and the treatment given.

Locally, as disease grows within the breast, the tumor may infiltrate or invade the dermis or chest wall. Invasion of Cooper ligaments may lead to skin retraction; this can also occur in early-stage disease but is more likely as the tumor grows. When lymphatic drainage of the breast or skin occurs, edema may occur, leading to dilated dermal hair follicles appearing like the skin of an orange; this peau d'orange appearance is sometimes associated with inflammatory breast cancer (IBC).

Because of the propensity of larger tumors to invade the lymphatic system, most advanced primary tumors have spread to the axillary lymph nodes at the time of diagnosis. The axillary lymph node region is divided into three levels, each defined in relationship to the pectoralis minor muscle. Level I lymph nodes are inferolateral to the muscle, level II lymph nodes are beneath the muscle, and level III lymph

nodes are superomedial to the muscle. Level III lymph nodes are also known as infraclavicular lymph nodes. Other lymph nodes that may be involved include the supraclavicular nodes, internal mammary (IM) nodes, and Rotter nodes, located between the pectoralis minor and major muscles. Figure 60.2 shows computed tomography (CT) scans from patients with locally advanced breast cancer presenting with involvement of the level II axilla (Fig. 60.2A), an infraclavicular lymph node (Fig. 60.2B), a Rotter lymph node (Fig. 60.2C), and an IM lymph node (Fig. 60.2D).

Local disease progression can lead to ulceration of the breast skin, pain, bleeding, and infection. In addition to these sequelae, arm edema, brachial plexopathy, and obstruction and thrombosis of the brachial vasculature may also occur due to progression of regional lymphatic disease. Primary tumor growth also increases the risk of spread through the lymphatic system to regional lymph nodes or hematogenous spread to distant sites like the liver, lung, bone, and brain. Without treatment, almost all locally advanced breast cancers will metastasize to visceral organs and eventually become life threatening.[1,2]

Survival rates for women with locally advanced breast cancer have improved due to treatment advances. Before the use of systemic treatment became a standard of care, individuals with advanced disease treated with mastectomy, radiation therapy, or both had 5-year survival rates of only 25% to 45%.[1–3] After the introduction of combined modality treatments including surgery, radiation therapy, and chemotherapy, the 5-year survival rates have approached 80% for patients with stage IIA disease and 45% for patients with stage

FIGURE 60.2. CT images of patients with lymph node involvement at the time of diagnosis. **A:** Image from a patient with involvement of axillary lymph nodes in the level II axilla. The *white arrows* show the involved lymph nodes, which are just beneath the pectoralis minor muscle. **B:** An involved level III axillary lymph node (*white arrow*) that extends superomedially to the pectoralis minor muscle. **C:** An involved Rotter lymph node (*white arrow*), which is anterior to the pectoralis minor and beneath the pectoralis major muscle. **D:** Image from a patient with an involved IM lymph node (*white arrow*).

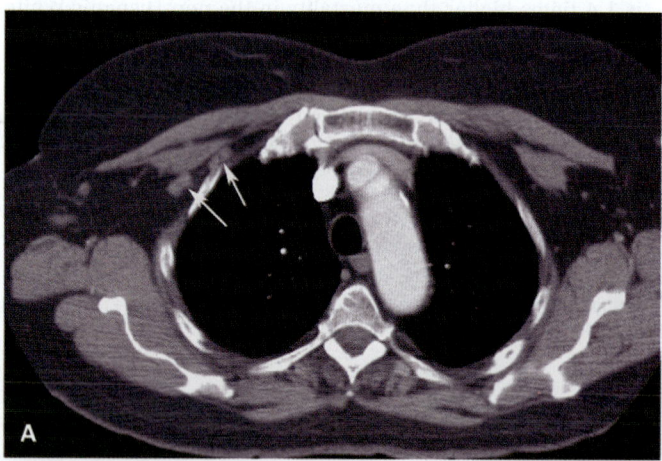
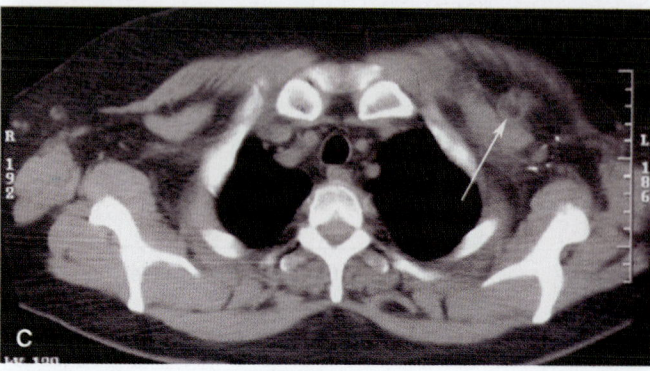
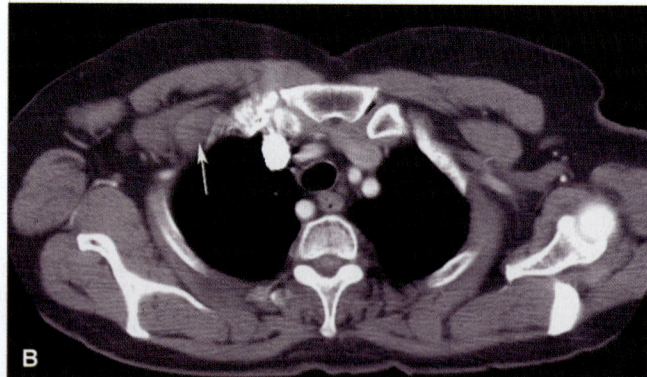
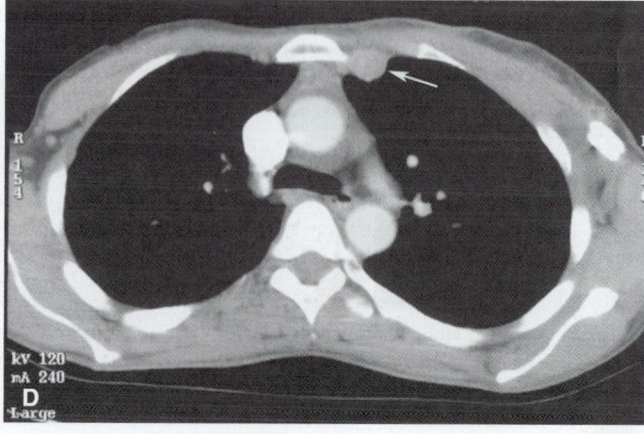

IIIB disease.[7] Continued improvement has been observed with the addition of even more effective systemic regimens.

Although treatment advances may be credited for much of the improvement in prognosis for individuals with stage III disease in recent decades, it is important to recognize how stage migration has affected the statistics as well. Diagnostic imaging has improved over the same time period, increasing the likelihood of detecting metastatic disease. As a result, some cases that would have been classified as stage III historically may now be classified as stage IV. The reclassification of patients with a relatively low burden of metastatic disease from stage III to stage IV may improve the outcome statistics for both stage III and stage IV diseases. A similar effect was introduced by the 2003 change in the American Joint Committee on Cancer (AJCC) breast cancer staging system, which incorporated the number of positive lymph nodes in the pathologic disease stage. Specifically, many patients with four or more positive lymph nodes in the past would have had stage II disease but are classified as having stage III disease in the 2003 staging system. Indeed, a study that compared the stage-specific survival of 1,350 patients staged according to the 1988 AJCC staging system to the stage-specific survival of the same patients restaged according to the 2003 AJCC system found that the 10-year overall survival (OS) rates were significantly higher when the 2003 system was used, both for patients with stage II disease (76% [2003] vs. 65% [1988], $P < .0001$) and for those with stage IIIA disease (59% [2003] vs. 45% [1988], $P < .0001$).[8] The reason for the better stage-specific outcome was that restaging into the 2003 system led to most of the patients with four or more positive lymph nodes being moved from stage II to the stage III category.

PATHOLOGY AND BIOLOGY OF LOCALLY ADVANCED BREAST CANCER

The histopathology of locally advanced disease is similar to that of early-stage disease. Both of the most common subtypes, infiltrating ductal carcinoma and lobular carcinoma, can present as early-stage or locally advanced disease. However, those subtypes considered to behave less aggressively (e.g., tubular carcinoma, mucinous carcinoma, and medullary carcinoma) are unlikely to present at advanced clinical stages unless the breast mass has been present for a long time.

The term "locally advanced breast cancer" encompasses a biologic spectrum of diseases. Locally advanced disease that has developed between annual interval screening mammograms is most often ER-negative with a high nuclear grade and a high proliferative index. These cancers may be of the luminal B, nonluminal Her-2–positive, or triple-negative subtypes. In contrast, patients who present with extensive locoregional disease after years of medical neglect more often are found to have ER-positive disease with a low nuclear grade and a low proliferative index (luminal A subtype). IBC also has biologic characteristics that differ from those of non-IBC; these will be discussed further in the section on IBC later in this chapter.

CLINICAL PRESENTATION OF LOCALLY ADVANCED BREAST CANCER

Locally advanced breast cancer most commonly is diagnosed after a palpable mass is detected within the breast. Advanced disease can cause symptoms such as local or regional pain, bleeding, paresthesia, and paresis. As previously indicated, it is critically important to determine the onset of symptoms and the rate of disease progression to reach an accurate diagnosis as to whether an advanced breast cancer should more accurately be designated an inflammatory carcinoma.

Diagnostic Workup

For patients with locally advanced breast cancer, the workup should start with a careful history and physical examination. The breast examination should include note of the breast symmetry, as well as careful inspection for involvement or edema of the skin. Peau d'orange and skin erythema can sometimes be subtle, particularly in non-Caucasian women; comparison with the contralateral side can often be helpful.

Other times, physical examination findings are more obvious. Figure 60.3 shows a photograph of a patient with a neglected locally advanced breast cancer presenting with peau d'orange, breast retraction and involution, and effacement of the nipple–areola complex. Medical photographs are highly helpful to document the extent of visible abnormalities before treatment is begun and can also be used to assess disease response.

The extent of palpable disease should also be measured and documented. Fixation of a breast mass to the pectoralis muscle or chest wall should be determined by assessing the mobility of the mass with the pectoralis muscle relaxed and contracted. Regional lymph nodes should be thoroughly evaluated by careful clinical examination with the patient in both supine and sitting positions. Clinical nodal evaluation may be supplemented with ultrasonographic imaging coupled with fine needle aspiration of suspicious lymph nodes.[9]

All cases of locally advanced disease require complete staging before initiation of therapy. Laboratory studies should include a complete blood cell count and serum chemistry profile with liver function tests. Radiographic studies should include a CT scan of the chest, abdomen, and pelvis, a bone scan, and plain radiographs of symptomatic regions or areas of increased uptake on bone scans. If any neurologic symptoms suggestive of cerebral metastases are present, a contrast-enhanced CT scan or gadolinium-enhanced magnetic resonance imaging (MRI) scan of the brain should be obtained. Gadolinium-enhanced MRI is the preferred imaging technique if leptomeningeal carcinomatosis is suspected. There are early data suggesting that subsets of women with breast cancer may have a higher risk of brain disease and may be appropriately screened with MRI. These include women with HER2-positive and triple-negative subtypes who present with extracranial metastatic disease[10] and women with IBC who present with extracranial metastases.[11]

There is increasing interest in the use of [18F]fluorodeoxyglucose positron emission tomography (PET)/CT for disease staging of patients with locally advanced breast cancer, particularly those with IBC. Several small retrospective studies have shown that PET/CT increases detection of both previously

FIGURE 60.3. Photograph of a patient with a neglected locally advanced breast cancer presenting with peau d'orange, breast retraction and involution, and effacement of the nipple–areola complex.

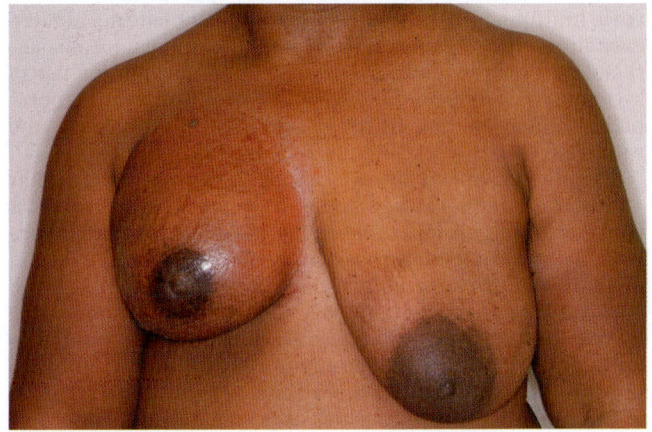

unsuspected sites of metastatic disease as well as additional sites of extra-axillary nodal disease when compared to conventional imaging.[12,13] Researchers from MD Anderson showed that the addition of PET/CT in the staging of 41 women with IBC not only detected new sites of disease in 44% of patients when compared to standard imaging but also resulted in a change in radiation doses or fields in 18%.[14]

Staging of Locally Advanced Breast Cancer

A comprehensive discussion of disease staging systems for breast cancer is provided in the previous chapter. Some staging considerations are particularly relevant to patients with stage III disease. Stage III breast cancer can represent either T3 disease (tumors >5.0 cm) with involved lymph nodes, N2 or N3 disease, or T4 disease.[15]

Specific aspects of both primary tumor and nodal staging in locally advanced breast cancer warrant additional consideration. Specifically, T4 disease may represent invasion into the chest wall (T4a), tumors associated with breast edema or skin ulceration or satellite nodules (T4b), both invasion and T4b characteristics (T4c), or IBC (T4d). Invasion of disease into the pectoralis major muscle without chest wall invasion and dimpling or fixation of the overlying skin does not qualify as T4 disease. Both clinical and pathologic staging systems have been established for N2 and N3 disease. Clinical N2 disease signifies either involved axillary lymph nodes that are fixed to one another or to surrounding structures (N2a) or involved IM lymph nodes without concurrent disease in the axilla (N2b), as determined by physical examination or imaging studies. Clinical N3 disease is a disease that involves the infraclavicular region (N3a), both the axilla and IM lymph nodes (N3b), or the supraclavicular region (N3c). Pathologic N2 disease represents involvement of 4 to 9 axillary lymph nodes with at least 1 focus measuring >2.0 mm (N2a) or clinical involvement of IM lymph nodes with pathologically negative axillary lymph nodes (N2b). Pathologic N3 disease represents involvement of an infraclavicular lymph node or 10 or more involved lymph nodes with at least 1 focus measuring >2.0 mm (N3a), clinical involvement of IM lymph nodes with 1 to 9 axillary lymph nodes involved, pathologic involvement of a sentinel IM lymph node with 4 or more axillary lymph nodes involved (N3b), or a metastasis in the supraclavicular region (N3c).[15]

Neoadjuvant chemotherapy is recommended for most patients with locally advanced breast cancer. The initial extent of disease is an important factor for later locoregional treatment decisions and for future research. It is therefore imperative that disease in all patients be carefully assigned a clinical stage before any treatment is begun.

OVERVIEW OF TREATMENT

Combined Modality Therapy

Locally advanced breast cancer is most appropriately treated with multimodality therapy aimed at eradicating all disease in the locoregional area and preventing distant disease recurrence. These goals are best achieved through the use of systemic therapy (generally chemotherapy and, when appropriate, endocrine and HER2-directed therapy), surgery, and radiation.

Locally advanced breast cancer can present as either operable or inoperable disease. In general, the disease is considered to be inoperable if an initial surgical procedure is unlikely to completely resect all gross disease with achievement of negative surgical margins. Most patients with T4 disease and all patients with IBC are considered to be inoperable at presentation. Inoperable disease requires the administration of upfront systemic therapy to reduce tumor volume in order to facilitate definitive local therapy. Neoadjuvant therapy (also known as preoperative or primary systemic therapy)

usually takes the form of chemotherapy, although, in certain situations as discussed later on, endocrine therapy may also be an option. In addition to downstaging the tumor, systemic therapy also reduces the risk of recurrence and breast cancer mortality by eradicating occult micrometastatic disease and aiding radiation in obtaining long-term local control.

Patients who have operable disease at the time of presentation have the option of either receiving neoadjuvant chemotherapy or proceeding directly with definitive surgery followed by adjuvant systemic therapy at a later date. Multiple studies have demonstrated equivalent survival and distant disease recurrence rates between the two approaches,[16,17] and each approach has its own merits.

Neoadjuvant Chemotherapy

The landmark NSABP B-18 trial randomized 1,523 patients with operable breast cancer to receive neoadjuvant doxorubicin and cyclophosphamide (AC) for 4 cycles followed by surgery versus surgery followed by 4 cycles of AC. Although this trial included only patients with operable breast cancer, the results demonstrated the feasibility of preoperative chemotherapy. The planned surgical approach was determined prior to randomization, with approximately two-thirds of patients in each group deemed initially eligible for lumpectomy. There was no difference in OS or disease-free survival (DFS) between the two groups, but a larger proportion of patients who received neoadjuvant chemotherapy were able to undergo breast-conserving surgery (BCS) compared to those who received adjuvant chemotherapy (68% vs. 60%).[18,19] This increase was largely due to a higher percentage of patients with T3 disease being offered breast conservation after responding to neoadjuvant chemotherapy. The percentage of patients with pathologically negative nodes was also higher in the neoadjuvant group compared to the adjuvant group (59% vs. 43%, $P < .001$). Results from another pivotal neoadjuvant trial EORTC 10902 also demonstrated an increase in the percentage of patients eligible for BCS, with 23% of patients initially requiring mastectomy being able to undergo lumpectomy after the receipt of chemotherapy. OS and recurrence rates were equivalent between the preoperative and postoperative chemotherapy groups.[20]

Patients with locally advanced breast cancer who have complete clinical resolution of skin changes and chest wall involvement may also be offered breast conservation therapy. This has been demonstrated in a study reviewing outcomes of 340 patients treated with neoadjuvant chemotherapy followed by BCS and radiation therapy. In that study, patients with T3 or T4 disease were found to have acceptably low rates of locoregional recurrence and ipsilateral breast tumor recurrence. Those with T4 disease and those with N2–N3 disease had a 5-year IBTR-free survival rate of 92% and 89%, respectively, and both had a 5-year LRR-free survival rate of 84%.[21]

A key finding that emerged from the early neoadjuvant trials was the correlation between response to therapy and long-term outcome. In B-18, patients who achieved a pathologic complete response (pCR) in the breast after neoadjuvant chemotherapy had improved DFS (hazard ratio [HR] 0.47, $P = .0001$) and OS (HR 0.32, $P = .0001$) compared to those who did not.[22] This finding has been replicated in several other studies, though the definition of pCR varied, with some studies using the definition of absence of invasive tumor in the breast and nodes and others the absence of invasive disease in the breast. The currently accepted definition of pCR is the lack of residual invasive cancer in the breast and nodes. Patients who achieve a pCR consistently demonstrate improved long-term outcomes compared to those with significant residual disease.[23,24]

In addition to downstaging the tumor to improve surgical outcomes and providing valuable prognostic information, neoadjuvant chemotherapy also allows an *in vivo* assessment of the tumor's response to chemotherapy. Patients whose tumors demonstrate resistance to initial therapy should be offered a non–cross-resistant regimen or proceed directly to local therapy. It should be noted, however, that the benefit of transitioning to an alternate chemotherapy regimen in nonresponding patients is unclear. In the GeparTrio trial, patients who did not respond to two cycles of docetaxel/doxorubicin/cyclophosphamide (TAC) were randomized to four additional cycles of the same regimen or to four cycles of vinorelbine/capecitabine (NX). pCR rates were similarly low in both groups of these nonresponders (5.3% in the TAC group vs. 6.0% in the NX group). In contrast, patients who responded initially achieved a pCR rate of 21% after 6 additional cycles of TAC and 23.5% after 8 additional cycles.[25] It appears that tumors that are resistant to one chemotherapy regimen tend to be broadly chemoresistant, posing a significant management challenge.

For patients with locally advanced but operable disease at presentation, primary surgery followed by adjuvant therapy may be a consideration. A potential advantage of this approach is a shorter time interval between diagnosis and effective treatment for patients with disease that is resistant to chemotherapy. Primary surgery also allows for more accurate pathologic staging of the tumor and axillary nodes, which is important to guide prognosis and selection of appropriate adjuvant treatment. However, the amount of residual disease after neoadjuvant chemotherapy may ultimately provide a more individualized assessment of prognosis. Furthermore, tumor biology has become a driving force in the selection of appropriate systemic therapy, and appropriate treatment decisions can often be made at the time of diagnosis based on the clinical stage and molecular subtype of the tumor. Given equivalent DFS and OS between the two approaches, there has been a paradigm shift in the treatment of locally advanced breast cancer, with increased use of neoadjuvant chemotherapy.

As discussed above, pathologic evaluation of the tumor bed and lymph nodes after neoadjuvant chemotherapy provides important prognostic information. However, the value of pCR as a prognostic tool is highly dependent on the molecular subtype of the tumor. Tumors that are highly proliferative (luminal B, nonluminal/HER2-positive, and triple-negative) tend to demonstrate increased chemosensitivity and are associated with higher rates of pCR compared to low proliferative subtypes with high expression of hormone receptors (luminal A).[26] pCR appears to be most predictive of DFS and OS in nonluminal/HER2-positive (treated with trastuzumab) and triple-negative subtypes, with those achieving a pCR having an excellent prognosis and those with significant residual disease having a high risk of recurrence and overall worse survival. pCR in patients with luminal A tumors does not appear to be a good predictor of long-term outcome, whereas the utility of pCR as a predictive tool in patients with luminal B (HER2-negative or HER2-positive) tumors seems to be better than for luminal A tumors but worse than for nonluminal/Her2-positive or triple-negative tumors.[24,26]

Neoadjuvant Endocrine Therapy

Given the lower response rates to neoadjuvant chemotherapy in patients with tumors having high hormone receptor expression, there has been interest in evaluating the role of neoadjuvant endocrine therapy in this population. The IMPACT trial randomized 330 postmenopausal patients with clinical stage II or III HR+ breast cancer to receive tamoxifen versus anastrozole versus tamoxifen plus anastrozole for 12 weeks. There was no difference in clinical and radiographic response rates among the three groups, but a higher percentage of women receiving anastrozole were eligible for BCS compared with those receiving tamoxifen (44% vs. 22%, P = .022). The authors also found that higher expression of ER was associated with increased response rates.[27] P024 compared the efficacy of letrozole to tamoxifen in the neoadjuvant setting in 324 postmenopausal women with hormone receptor–positive breast cancer. After 16 weeks, treatment with letrozole resulted in improved clinical response rates compared to treatment with tamoxifen.[28]

Neoadjuvant endocrine therapy may therefore be considered for postmenopausal patients whose tumors are of low- to intermediate-grade and express high levels of ER. Treatment with an aromatase inhibitor appears to be superior to tamoxifen, and the recommended duration is at least 4 to 6 months. The choice of aromatase inhibitor is a matter of personal preference, as all 3 third-generation aromatase inhibitors have demonstrated similar response rates, reductions in Ki67 levels, and rates of conversion to BCS when compared head-to-head.[29] The use of neoadjuvant endocrine therapy in the premenopausal population has not been established.

Choice of Systemic Agents in the Neoadjuvant Setting

Neoadjuvant Chemotherapy for HER2-Negative Disease

The optimal neoadjuvant chemotherapy regimen for patients with HER2-negative disease has not been established, but it is generally accepted that regimens with proven effectiveness in the adjuvant setting may also be used in the neoadjuvant setting. Because patients with locally advanced breast cancer are considered to have high-risk disease, a regimen containing an anthracycline and taxane is generally preferred.

These recommendations are based on results from the Early Breast Cancer Trialists' Collaborative Group meta-analyses, which demonstrated that adjuvant polychemotherapy reduced the risk of recurrence and breast cancer mortality in patients with node-positive and node-negative disease.[30] Anthracycline-based regimens were found to be superior to CMF (cyclophosphamide, methotrexate, fluorouracil) regimens, and the addition of taxanes to anthracyclines further improved outcomes.[31] Overall, taxane-plus-anthracycline–based regimens reduced 10-year breast cancer mortality by one-third.

NSABP B-27 established the role of adding a taxane after an anthracycline-based regimen in the neoadjuvant setting. In this study, 2,411 patients were randomized to one of three groups: 4 cycles of AC followed by surgery versus AC followed by 4 cycles of docetaxel followed by surgery versus AC followed by surgery and then 4 cycles of docetaxel in the postoperative setting. The addition of docetaxel to AC prior to surgery resulted in a doubling of pCR rate (26% vs. 13%; P < .001). There was no significant improvement in DFS or OS with either preoperative or postoperative docetaxel for the overall study population. However, achievement of pCR was a significant predictor of OS regardless of treatment (HR 0.33; 95% CI, 0.23 to 0.47; P = .0001).[32] In a subset analysis, patients who achieved a clinical partial response after AC had improved DFS with preoperative, but not postoperative, docetaxel (HR 0.71; 95% CI, 0.55 to 0.91; P = .007). Based on these findings, outside of a clinical trial, it is preferable to administer the entire chemotherapy regimen prior to surgery if possible.

For patients with contraindications to anthracyclines or taxanes, alternate regimens are available (Table 60.1). A non–anthracycline-containing regimen may be preferred in patients who have cardiac disease or who have other risk factors for anthracycline-associated congestive heart failure such as hypertension, diabetes, or advanced age. For patients with a hypersensitivity reaction to solvent-based paclitaxel, nanoparticle albumin–bound paclitaxel (nab-paclitaxel) may be used. In GeparSepto, patients were randomized to 12 weeks of weekly paclitaxel (80 mg/m²) versus weekly nab-paclitaxel (initially 150 mg/m² but later reduced

Preferred Regimens

Dose-dense AC (every 2 wk with filgrastim support) × 4 followed by dose-dense paclitaxel (every 2 wk with filgrastim support) × 4

Dose-dense AC × 4 followed by weekly paclitaxel × 12 wk

TC every 3 wk × 4

Other Regimens

Dose-dense AC × 4

AC every 3 wk × 4

CMF every 28 d × 6

AC × 4 followed by docetaxel every 3 wk × 4

AC followed by weekly paclitaxel

EC every 3 wk × 8

TAC every 3 wk × 6

AC, doxorubicin/cyclophosphamide; CMF, cyclophosphamide/methotrexate/fluorouracil; EC, epirubicin/cyclophosphamide; TAC, docetaxel/doxorubicin/cyclophosphamide; TC, docetaxel/cyclophosphamide.

to 125 mg/m^2 because of toxicities) and followed by epirubicin plus cyclophosphamide in the neoadjuvant setting. There was a higher pCR rate in the group receiving nab-paclitaxel (38% vs. 29%, $P = .00065$), but there was also a higher rate of grade 3 to 4 sensory neuropathy and anemia. It is not yet known whether the improvement in pCR will translate into a survival benefit.[33]

Several studies have examined the role of adding additional cytotoxic agents such as capecitabine and gemcitabine to anthracycline-plus-taxane–based regimens. However, incorporation of these agents has been associated with added toxicities without improvements in pCR or survival.[34,35] Some studies have demonstrated an improvement in pCR rates in subsets of patients with the addition of the angiogenesis inhibitor bevacizumab, but use of the drug has also been associated with increased toxicities (hypertension, bleeding, thromboembolic events, surgical complications), and it remains unclear which patients are most likely to derive benefit. Furthermore, studies in the adjuvant setting have not demonstrated an improvement in survival with bevacizumab. Given the above, antiangiogenic agents should not be routinely used outside of a clinical trial setting.

The role of adding carboplatin in the treatment of triple-negative breast cancer has garnered particular interest. Results from two randomized trials demonstrated significantly higher pCR rates with the incorporation of platinum to an anthracycline-plus-taxane–based regimen in this population. In CALGB 40603, every-3-week carboplatin added to weekly paclitaxel followed by dose-dense AC-x 4 resulted in an increased pCR rate in the breast and axilla (54% vs. 41%; $P = .0029$) but did not result in an improved 3-year EFS or OS.[36,37] Patients who achieved a pCR had significantly lower event rates and mortality, but these improved outcomes were not specifically associated with receipt of carboplatin. On the other hand, in GeparSixto, patients were randomized to weekly paclitaxel and liposomal doxorubicin, with or without weekly carboplatin. In the subset of patients with TNBC, pCR rates improved from 37% to 53% ($P = .005$) with the addition of carboplatin. In addition, a significant improvement in DFS in these patients was also observed (85.8% vs. 76.1%, HR 0.56, $P = .035$).[38,39] Given the conflicting results from these two trials and the added toxicities associated with carboplatin, the routine incorporation of carboplatin in the neoadjuvant setting is not generally recommended. It can, however, be considered in patients who need a rapid response or greater cytoreduction for optimal locoregional management.

Neoadjuvant Chemotherapy for HER2-Positive Disease

One of the most significant advances in breast cancer treatment has been the introduction of trastuzumab, a monoclonal antibody directed against the HER2 protein, into the adjuvant treatment for patients with HER2-overexpressing cancer. Several prospective randomized trials have demonstrated that the addition of trastuzumab to chemotherapy in the adjuvant setting confers an approximate 50% improvement in DFS and 35% improvement in OS in this population.[40,41] Subsequent studies in the neoadjuvant setting have confirmed an important role for trastuzumab in the neoadjuvant setting as well, although there are few data comparing different chemotherapy regimens.

In the phase II NOAH trial, the addition of trastuzumab to a neoadjuvant anthracycline- and taxane-containing regimen resulted in a pCR rate of 38% compared to 19% with chemotherapy alone. More women in the trastuzumab arm were able to undergo BCS (23% vs. 13%), and EFS was also improved (58% vs. 43%).[42] In a meta-analysis, the addition of trastuzumab to neoadjuvant chemotherapy resulted in an improvement in pCR rate from 23% to 40% in women with HER2+ breast cancer. pCR was also found to be a predictor of EFS (HR 0.39; 95% CI, 0.31 to 0.50) and OS (HR 0.34; 95% CI, 0.24 to 0.47).[24]

More recently, the development of pertuzumab, a monoclonal antibody that binds to the HER2 protein at the site of HER2/HER3 dimerization, has led to even further improvements in pCR rates when added to trastuzumab and chemotherapy. NeoSphere was a phase 2 study of 417 patients with HER2+ breast cancer who were randomized to receive neoadjuvant therapy with 4 cycles of docetaxel/trastuzumab versus docetaxel/trastuzumab/pertuzumab versus trastuzumab/pertuzumab versus docetaxel/pertuzumab. Following surgery, all patients received an anthracycline in the adjuvant setting. pCR rates were 29%, 46%, 17%, and 24%, respectively.[43]

The benefit of adding pertuzumab to chemotherapy and trastuzumab was corroborated by results from the phase II TRYPHAENA trial, which yielded a pCR rate of 56% in patients receiving neoadjuvant FEC (fluorouracil, epirubicin, cyclophosphamide)-THP (docetaxel, trastuzumab, pertuzumab) and 64% for TCHP (docetaxel, carboplatin, trastuzumab, pertuzumab).[44] Based on the results of these two studies and the improvement in DFS that was subsequently demonstrated when pertuzumab was added to trastuzumab and chemotherapy in the adjuvant setting,[45] the FDA granted approval for the use of pertuzumab in the neoadjuvant treatment of patients with HER2-positive, locally advanced, inflammatory, or early stage breast cancer (either greater than 2 cm in diameter or node positive).

Table 60.2 lists recommended regimens for treatment of HER2-positive breast cancer.

Preferred Regimens[a]

AC × 4 followed by paclitaxel + trastuzumab ± pertuzumab (various schedules)

TCH ± pertuzumab

Paclitaxel + trastuzumab (for low-risk stage I disease)

Other Regimens[a]

AC × 4 followed by docetaxel + trastuzumab ± pertuzumab various schedules

TC × 4 + trastuzumab

[a]Following completion of chemotherapy, trastuzumab should be continued in the adjuvant setting to complete 1-y total of anti-HER2 therapy.

AC, doxorubicin/cyclophosphamide; FEC, fluorouracil/epirubicin/cyclophosphamide; TC, docetaxel/cyclophosphamide; TCH, docetaxel/carboplatin/trastuzumab.

Selection of Patients for Breast-Conserving Surgery

The decision to offer BCS is dependent on the extent of tumor present after completion of neoadjuvant therapy and the breast size relative to residual tumor size. Clinical and radiographic assessments are used to determine eligibility for BCS. In those patients who undergo BCS after neoadjuvant chemotherapy, advanced nodal involvement at diagnosis, residual tumor larger than 2 cm, multifocal residual disease, and lymphovascular space invasion predict higher rates of LRR and IBTR.[21] Although the presence of these features should not preclude BCS, they are relevant prognostic factors, and mastectomy may be considered in patients who possess multiple risk factors after neoadjuvant chemotherapy. It is important to note that a complete clinical or radiographic response may still be associated with residual disease on pathologic examination of the final surgical specimen. The discrepancy may be due to persistence of scattered areas of invasive cancer in a background of tumor that has been partially eradicated in a fragmented fashion, or of intraductal cancer, which is not affected by chemotherapy.

All areas containing cancer must be resected to provide optimal breast cancer outcomes. In a meta-analysis of 9 randomized trials, a higher rate of BCS was seen in patients who had received neoadjuvant chemotherapy compared to those who had received adjuvant therapy. Although there was no difference in OS and distant disease recurrence between the two groups, there was an increased risk of locoregional recurrence in the group that received neoadjuvant chemotherapy. However, these results were confounded by the inclusion of three trials in which patients who achieved a clinical complete response (CR) received radiation but were not required to undergo surgery.[16] After excluding these trials, locoregional recurrence rates were similar between neoadjuvant and adjuvant groups.[17] These results underscore the importance of performing definitive surgery in all patients undergoing neoadjuvant therapy even if a clinical CR is achieved.

Systemic Therapy After Surgery

A full discussion of adjuvant systemic therapies is beyond the scope of this chapter. However, the following section will highlight the salient points of adjuvant therapy as they pertain to patients with locally advanced breast cancer who have completed neoadjuvant chemotherapy.

Chemotherapy

Until recently, there were no data to support the use of additional chemotherapy in the postoperative setting if the full intended course of neoadjuvant chemotherapy was administered. The CREATE-X trial, however, was the first to demonstrate a potential benefit of adding capecitabine in patients with residual disease found at the time of surgery. In this study conducted in Japan, 910 women with HER2-negative breast cancer who had residual disease after neoadjuvant therapy with an anthracycline and/or taxane were randomized after surgery to either standard therapy (endocrine therapy for patients with hormone receptor–positive disease or no systemic therapy for hormone receptor–negative disease) or to standard therapy plus capecitabine for 8 cycles. At 5 years, DFS was 74% for the capecitabine arm compared to 68% for the control arm (HR 0.70, P = .01). OS was also improved (89% vs. 84%, HR = 0.59, P = .01). In the triple-negative subgroup, DFS was 70% vs 56% (HR 0.58) and OS was 79% vs 70% for the capecitabine and controls groups, respectively. These results have been practice changing and offer the opportunity to improve long-term outcomes in a population with high-risk disease.[45] Other ongoing clinical trials are evaluating the role of platinum chemotherapy versus capecitabine, as well as the role of the immune checkpoint inhibitor pembrolizumab, in the postoperative setting in patients with residual triple-negative breast cancer following neoadjuvant chemotherapy.

Adjuvant Endocrine Therapy

Patients with HR+ breast cancer should receive adjuvant endocrine therapy to reduce the risk of recurrence and breast cancer–specific mortality. The choice of therapy is influenced by menopausal status. Although tamoxifen remains a standard for both pre- and postmenopausal women, the use of aromatase inhibitors is limited to women who are postmenopausal, though there are now data supporting the use of aromatase inhibitors when given concurrently with ovarian function suppression in the premenopausal setting.

The EBCTCG meta-analysis demonstrated that 5 years of adjuvant tamoxifen was associated with a one-third proportional reduction in breast cancer mortality at 15 years in patients with estrogen receptor–positive disease, irrespective of age, nodal status, or receipt of chemotherapy. Subsequent data from the ATLAS trial demonstrated a further reduction in recurrence risk and breast cancer mortality with 10 years of tamoxifen compared to 5 years, suggesting that compared to no endocrine therapy, 10 years of tamoxifen was associated with an almost 50% reduction in disease-specific mortality.[46]

For postmenopausal women with HR+ breast cancer, use of an aromatase inhibitor is recommended in the adjuvant setting, either as upfront therapy or following tamoxifen. Support for this recommendation comes from multiple studies demonstrating improvement in recurrence rates and breast cancer mortality with the use of an aromatase inhibitor compared to tamoxifen. In a recent meta-analysis conducted by the EBCTCG, 5 years of aromatase inhibitor therapy was associated with a 15% reduction in 10-year breast cancer mortality compared with 5 years of tamoxifen.[47]

Recent data from the SOFT and TEXT trials have demonstrated a role for ovarian function suppression plus either tamoxifen or aromatase inhibition in select premenopausal women with HR+ breast cancer. Although the addition of ovarian suppression did not confer benefit over tamoxifen alone for the overall population of premenopausal women with HR+ disease, there was an improvement in DFS when ovarian suppression was administered with tamoxifen or an aromatase inhibitor in the subset of women who were younger than 35 years or whose disease was considered to be of sufficiently high risk to warrant the administration of chemotherapy. Given that women with locally advanced breast cancer comprise a high-risk group, those who are premenopausal should be offered this strategy in the adjuvant setting.[48,49]

Adjuvant HER2-Directed Therapy

For patients with HER2-positive breast cancer, trastuzumab should be continued in the adjuvant setting to complete 1-year total of HER2-directed therapy. This recommendation is based on studies demonstrating improved DFS and OS with the addition of 1 year of trastuzumab.[40,41] More recently, results from the APHINITY trial demonstrated that the addition of 1 year of pertuzumab to trastuzumab in the adjuvant setting led to a small but statistically significant improvement in DFS (94% in the pertuzumab group vs. 93% in the placebo group, HR 0.81, P = .045).[45] The KATHERINE trial is comparing trastuzumab emtansine (TDM-1), a novel antibody–drug conjugate approved in the metastatic setting, versus trastuzumab as adjuvant therapy in patients with HER2-positive breast cancer with residual disease after neoadjuvant therapy.

Treatment Results for Locally Advanced Breast Cancer

As noted earlier in this chapter, stage III breast cancer historically has been associated with a very poor prognosis, with high rates of locoregional recurrence, distant metastases, and death. However, advances in all of the disciplines involved in breast cancer treatment have improved the outcome of such patients. With modern treatment strategies that include systemic therapy with taxanes and anthracyclines, appropriate surgical intervention, and locoregional irradiation, outcomes have significantly improved. A reasonable estimate of 10-year survival rates for patients given modern treatments for stage III breast cancer is approximately 50%.[7]

Patients with supraclavicular lymph node (SCV) disease at diagnosis have a poorer outcome than do other patients with stage III disease. However, because some studies of patients treated with chemotherapy have reported 10-year survival rates of 25%, the AJCC recategorized this stage of disease from stage IV to stage IIIC.[50] One study investigating the outcome of 71 patients with supraclavicular disease who were treated with neoadjuvant chemotherapy, surgery, and radiation reported a 5-year locoregional control rate of 77% and a 5-year OS rate of 47%.[51] Patients in whom the supraclavicular disease showed a clinical CR to neoadjuvant chemotherapy had better outcomes than did those with persistent disease after chemotherapy.

IM nodal involvement at presentation also confers a poor prognosis, although the incidence of IM involvement is difficult to assess in modern series as extended radical mastectomies are not typically performed. Older series, prior to the use of routine screening mammography, have shown that IM involvement is a risk factor for poor OS independent of axillary nodal status.[52] A more modern series from the European Institute of Oncology included 107 patients with either IM or SCV involvement between 1997 and 2009.[53] Nodal involvement was determined by a combination of clinical examination, surgical biopsy, FDG-PET, and ultrasound. Five-year outcomes were better in those with IM compared to SCV disease (DFS 84% vs. 39%, respectively). Patients with both IM and SCV involvement have a particularly high risk of distant disease. A study from Korea found a 33% 5-year DFS among 18 patients with disease involving both nodal sites.[54]

Patients presenting with SCV or IM disease should receive treatment similar to other patients with stage III disease. Typically, this includes preoperative systemic therapy and breast and axillary surgery, followed by comprehensive adjuvant radiation therapy. As neither SCV nor IM sites are typically operated on, these areas should be included in the radiation fields. There are insufficient data to guide radiation dose selection in this setting, but consideration should be given to a cone down to the area of clinical involvement. Dose is typically limited in this site because of the adjacent brachial plexus (SCV) and heart and/or lung (IM).

INFLAMMATORY BREAST CANCER

Epidemiology of Inflammatory Breast Cancer
IBC is an important subcategory of locally advanced breast cancer that is notable for both its similarities to and differences from noninflammatory locally advanced breast cancer. IBC is not common and accounts for 0.5% to 2% of all invasive breast cancers diagnosed in the United States but is disproportionately lethal, accounting for about 10% of breast cancer deaths.[55] In a study of 9 SEER registries (Surveillance, Epidemiology, and End Results), the incidence of IBC was found to have increased slightly during the 1990s, even while the incidence of locally advanced breast cancer (LABC) and non-T4 breast cancer decreased.[56] The rates of IBC, and mortality from IBC, were higher in black women than in white women. IBC tends to occur in younger patients than non-IBC. Women with IBC are more likely to have positive axillary lymph nodes, higher tumor grade, and negative hormone receptors.[55–57] Distant metastases at diagnosis are also more common with IBC. Risk factors for IBC, including menstrual/reproductive factors, obesity, smoking, alcohol, and exposure

to the mouse mammary tumor virus (MMTV), have been evaluated, but results are not consistent.[57] The strongest epidemiologic associations of IBC are with black race, young age, and high body mass index (BMI).[58]

Natural History of Inflammatory Breast Cancer
Inflammatory breast cancer, as defined by the AJCC, is a composite clinical–pathologic entity characterized by diffuse edema and erythema of the breast with acute/subacute onset and pathologic demonstration of invasive breast cancer. The erythema and skin changes must involve at least one-third of the breast, and duration of symptoms must be <6 months. A critical and determinative feature of IBC is the rapid onset of clinical findings including skin erythema, peau d'orange, brawny breast induration, warmth, and asymmetric enlargement (Fig. 60.4).

One hallmark of IBC is extensive lymphovascular invasion of the superficial plexus of vessels in the papillary and high reticular dermis by tumor emboli. These emboli can be demonstrated with skin punch biopsies directed to areas of erythema in up to 75% of cases.[58] However, the presence of invasive cells in the dermal lymphatics alone is neither sufficient nor necessary for the diagnosis.

It is important to distinguish IBCs from locally advanced breast cancer with secondary lymphatic congestion. Neglected primary tumors can also lead to breast erythema, edema, warmth, and asymmetric enlargement, particularly when bulky axillary adenopathy impedes the normal lymphatic flow from the breast. However, the former has a history of rapid onset, whereas the latter tends to have a long interval between the first symptom and the presentation for medical treatment.

Despite the natural history of IBC being one of rapid disease progression and early distant dissemination, in the United States, approximately 70% of patients with IBC have only evidence of locoregional disease at the time of diagnosis.[55] Patients with IBC typically have a worse clinical outcome than do other patients with T4 disease, suggesting that IBC is a distinct biologic entity.[59] However, the prognosis for patients with IBC has improved with combined (or

FIGURE 60.4. Photograph of a patient with erythema and peau d'orange consistent with IBC.

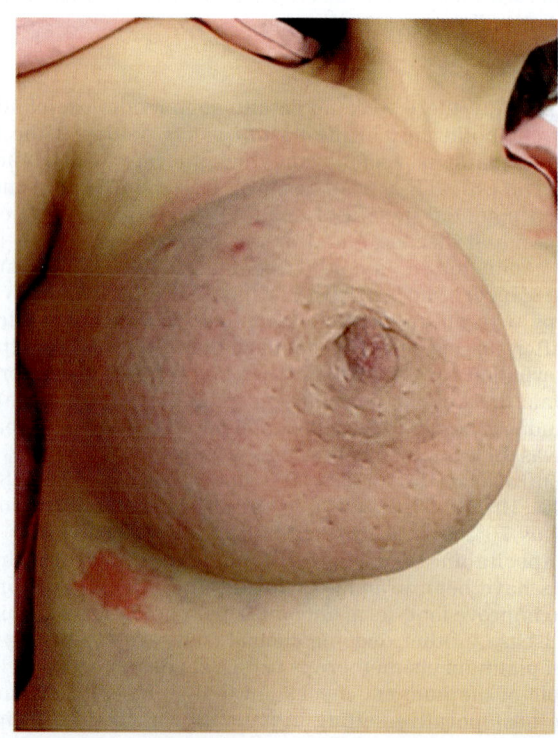

tri-) modality therapy including neoadjuvant chemotherapy, mastectomy, and postmastectomy radiation therapy (PMRT). Before the availability of combination chemotherapy, IBC was almost uniformly fatal. Fewer than 5% of patients treated with surgery, radiation therapy, or both survived past 5 years, and the expected median survival time for such patients was <15 months.[60] Local recurrence rates after surgery or radiation therapy were also high at approximately 50%.[61,62] The introduction of doxorubicin-based chemotherapy was the first step toward improved outcomes.[63,64] An evaluation of the outcome of patients with IBC registered in the SEER Program found that breast cancer–specific survival rates for patients with IBC improved continuously throughout the 1990s.[55] Currently, local control rates for patients treated with chemotherapy, mastectomy, and postmastectomy radiation approach 80% to 95%, and 5-year survival rates are approximately 40% to 60%.[65-69]

Diagnostic Workup

Although mammograms are considered a routine part of imaging workup for unspecified breast cancer, they are often of limited value for IBC. Over 90% of women with IBC have dense breasts[70] (a finding that has contributed to the "soil hypothesis" of IBC pathogenesis,[71] which may also obscure skin changes, masses, and nodules. The diagnosis of IBC is often made without a clinically detectable mass. There are no specific IBC findings on mammography, but skin and trabecular thickening are the most frequent findings. MRI, with dynamic contrast enhancement studies, is the most accurate test for identifying primary breast lesions in IBC. MRI abnormalities on MRI can include asymmetric non–mass-like enhancement, multifocality/centricity, and postcontrast peak signal intensity higher than that for other presentations of LABC. As discussed earlier in the chapter, there is increasing interest in the use of [18F]fluorodeoxyglucose PET-CT for disease staging of patients with locally advanced breast cancer, particularly those with IBC.

Pathology and Biology of Inflammatory Cancer

IBC cells appear similar to high-grade ductal breast cancer cells from noninflammatory breast carcinoma. Molecular subtypes of non-IBC, including the basal subtypes, all exist in IBC. However, inflammatory cancer is more commonly high histologic grade and shows high percentages of cells in S phase and aneuploidy. IBC is also more likely to lack expression of ER/PR and more likely to express high levels of p53 and epidermal growth factor.[72] Most strikingly, HER2/neu amplification/overexpression is more frequent in IBC (36% to 60%) than in non-IBC. Other more recently discovered markers include the propensity of inflammatory tumors to overexpress RhoC GTPase and to not express the tumor suppressor gene WIPS3.[73,74] Finally, others have described that IBCs with loss of MUC-1 may be associated with poorer survival than tumors that express MUC-1. More recently, investigators have noted that overexpression of E-cadherin may play an important role in the tumor emboli formation that is typically noted in the dermal lymphatics, and preclinical work suggests that targeting E-cadherin may decrease invasiveness.[75,76] As such, there are several important areas of research that may further characterize IBC and lead to the development of novel therapeutics.

General Management and Treatment Results for Inflammatory Breast Cancer

Because IBC is relatively uncommon, no data from randomized studies are available regarding the optimal therapeutic approach for this disease. From the aggregate of data reporting on IBC, it is quite clear that the best reported outcomes are with trimodality therapy, with a general sequence of

neoadjuvant chemotherapy, mastectomy, and PMRT. Clearly, management of IBC requires integrated care by a multidisciplinary team. Ideally, such patients should be evaluated in a multidisciplinary center by all specialists at the time of presentation to confirm the diagnosis of inflammatory disease, document the extent of disease (including photographs of areas of the involved skin), and agree on a treatment plan.

Chemotherapy for Inflammatory Breast Cancer

IBC is considered inoperable at presentation and should be treated initially with neoadjuvant chemotherapy (with consideration of trastuzumab if the tumor is HER2/neu-positive). Patients should be carefully monitored for response, and after achievement of the maximal clinical response, patients should be reevaluated for mastectomy. About 80% of patients with IBC will achieve a clinical response, and their disease will become operable.[77]

The optimal chemotherapy regimen for patients with IBC includes both anthracyclines and taxanes. The introduction of anthracycline chemotherapy, when combined with locoregional treatments, provided the first evidence of treatment efficacy in this disease. Investigators at MD Anderson conducted a series of single-group prospective trials for patients with IBC and found that neoadjuvant chemotherapy with FAC followed by locoregional therapy led to a 5-year survival rate of 25%. Subsequently, these investigators introduced sequential FAC or FEC followed by weekly paclitaxel and reported that the addition of taxanes improved the progression-free and OS of patients with inflammatory disease.[77]

IBC outcome is also affected by biologic subtype, as determined by ER, PR, and HER2/neu status. An update of the MD Anderson IBC experience analyzed 316 patients with non-metastatic IBC treated with curative intent between 1974 and 2008 who had known ER, PR, and HER2/neu status.[78] The 5-year rate of locoregional recurrence in patients with triple-negative disease was much higher than that for other subtypes—39% despite aggressive locoregional treatments—and the 5-year rate of distant metastasis was 57%. New therapeutic targets are needed in such patients, and recent research has identified potential biologic roles of NF-κB, RhoC GTPase, WISP3, and E-cadherin.[58]

Surgery for Inflammatory Breast Cancer

Locoregional treatment is an essential component of therapy for inflammatory disease. Before the routine use of chemotherapy, mastectomy, with or without postmastectomy radiation, was associated with a dismal prognosis, and so many physicians abandoned mastectomy in favor of radiation-only treatments. Outcomes after radiation therapy as the sole treatment modality were equally poor. After neoadjuvant chemotherapy became routine, combinations of surgery and radiation have been reevaluated.

De Boer et al.[79] reported on 54 patients with IBC treated after neoadjuvant chemotherapy with either radiation only (n = 35) or mastectomy plus radiation (n = 19). For the patients treated with radiation only, the median progression-free survival time was only 16 months, and the local recurrence rate was 34%. These results were not statistically different from the patients treated with mastectomy, and the authors concluded that surgery provided no clinical advantage over chemotherapy and radiation alone. In contrast, Perez et al.[80] found that the addition of mastectomy to local treatment significantly improved the outcome of IBC treatment. Patients given neoadjuvant chemotherapy, mastectomy, and postmastectomy radiation had a local control rate of 79% and a 5-year DFS of 40%. This was among the earliest demonstration of the efficacy of trimodality therapy. These data were supported by the report from Panades et al.,[81] who evaluated 308 patients given chemotherapy as a component of their treatment and found that the 10-year local recurrence–free survival rates were significantly better for patients who underwent mastectomy than for those who did not (about 60% vs. 34%, respectively; P = .0001), as were the 10-year breast cancer–specific survival rates (about 34% with mastectomy vs. 23% without, P = .005). A multivariate analysis that considered other potential prognostic factors found that the use of mastectomy remained a significant factor for improved local recurrence–free survival (P = .04). Results from an MD Anderson study also confirmed these results, with multivariate analysis revealing that a complete or partial response to neoadjuvant chemotherapy, the use of radiotherapy, and the addition of mastectomy to the therapeutic regimen all significantly improved disease-specific survival.[82]

A related question is whether breast conservation is appropriate and safe for patients who achieve a CR to neoadjuvant chemotherapy.[83–85] The enthusiasm for breast conservation has been limited due to the diffuse nature of IBC coupled with its predilection for skin involvement. One report from Arthur et al. challenges this conventional wisdom.[83] In that study, 52 patients treated for IBC at Virginia Commonwealth University hospitals and Tufts-New England Medical Center were treated on a prospective study of breast conservation, accelerated "suprafractionated" radiotherapy (1.5 bid to the entire breast and nodes and boost of 18 to 21 Gy for total of dose of 63 to 66 Gy to all initially involved areas). Mastectomy was reserved for nonresponders. With a median follow-up of 24 months, the breast preservation rate was 74%. In contrast, Swain reported a local recurrence rate of 30% despite their patients having achieved a clinical CR to neoadjuvant chemotherapy and multiple negative biopsies before irradiation.[86] Low and colleagues also reported a 40% local recurrence rate in 15 patients with IBC treated with radiation therapy alone after a biopsy-proven CR.[84] Finally, Brun et al.[85] reported a 54% local failure rate with attempts at breast conservation, and Chevallier et al.[87] reported a 61% local failure rate in patients treated with breast conservation after they had achieved a CR to neoadjuvant chemotherapy. In summary, mastectomy appears to be the prudent surgical choice based on current data.

Radiation therapy for IBC: Radiation therapy also has an important role in the management of IBC. The randomized data supporting PMRT for LABC have been discussed elsewhere and will not be reviewed. Although IBC was not represented in those trials, the lessons are still germane to a discussion on IBC. Furthermore, the best reported outcomes in IBC have all employed trimodality therapy and had aggressively designed and dosed radiation therapy. Because IBC has a rapid doubling time, investigators from MD Anderson investigated an accelerated hyperfractionated radiation delivery schedule in which 51 Gy is delivered to the chest wall and draining lymphatic fields by giving 1.5 Gy twice a day.[88] Subsequently, the chest wall was boosted to an additional 15 Gy, given in ten 1.5-Gy fractions twice daily. This approach was found to significantly improve locoregional disease control compared with a group treated with only 60 Gy, but also with a twice daily schedule. Respective 10-year locoregional control rates were 77% versus 58% (P = .04). Statistically significant improvements were also seen in 5- and 10-year OS rates between these two groups (P = .03), and a trend toward improvement in 5- and 10-year DFS rates was noted as well (P = .06). In a more recent update from these investigators in which the outcome of 192 patients treated with neoadjuvant chemotherapy, mastectomy, and postmastectomy radiation was evaluated, the authors reported a 5-year locoregional control rate of 84%.[69] Factors associated with higher rates of locoregional control included partial response to chemotherapy, negative margins, three or fewer positive lymph nodes, and the use of taxane chemotherapy. Similarly good outcomes have also been reported from centers that used once-daily RT

with high doses or daily use of bolus. Nonetheless, a recent report from Loveland-Jones et al.[89] demonstrated distressing underutilization of any PMRT in the National Cancer Database and identified several parameters associated with underutilization.

In summary, all patients with IBC require management by a multidisciplinary team. After initial staging and careful documentation of the extent of disease, patients should receive initial chemotherapy. The chemotherapy course should include both an anthracycline and a taxane, which can be given either concurrently or sequentially. Anti-HER2 therapy (trastuzumab) should be given with chemotherapy for patients with HER2/neu–positive disease. The majority of patients who exhibit a disease response and become operable should then undergo a modified radical mastectomy. Comprehensive and aggressive postmastectomy radiation treatments to the chest wall and draining lymphatics should be given as adjuvant therapy. This approach was recently endorsed by a consensus panel of IBC experts.[69] The dose of radiation to the initial fields should be 50 Gy in 25 fractions given once a day or 51 Gy in 1.5-Gy fractions given twice a day. Subsequently, the chest wall and any areas of gross disease that has not been resected should be boosted to 60 to 66 Gy. Attention should be paid to skin dose, and many institutions use tissue equivalent bolus material to ensure full dose to the skin of the chest wall. Patients with ER-positive disease should also receive hormonal therapy.

Some patients will continue to have inoperable disease after neoadjuvant chemotherapy. In a retrospective review of 38 patients with IBC who were inoperable after neoadjuvant chemotherapy, 32 (84%) of the 38 patients were able to undergo mastectomy after radiotherapy.[90] Preoperative radiation doses of 54 Gy or higher were significantly associated with the development of complications that required surgical treatment. Therefore, these patients should receive either preoperative radiation to the breast and draining lymphatics to a dose of 50 to 51 Gy, or, if the disease is unlikely to become resectable, high dose (72 Gy) definitive radiation is indicated using a reduced-field technique.

Clearly, great strides have been made over the last two decades in the management of IBC, and patients whose disease is managed with trimodality therapy can have locoregional control rates >80% and 5-year survival rates of ≥40% to 60% or more. Improvements in systemic therapy will, it is hoped, further augment these results.

GENERAL MANAGEMENT AND TREATMENT RESULTS FOR LOCALLY OR REGIONALLY RECURRENT BREAST CANCER

Women who receive initial potentially curative therapy for invasive cancer with either breast conservation therapy or mastectomy are at risk of developing locoregional recurrence. Locoregional recurrences are relatively uncommon with recurrence rates at approximately 5% to 10% and 10% to 15% after mastectomy and breast conservation therapy, respectively.[91] Most patients present clinically with a palpable mass or with findings on post–conserving therapy surveillance imaging.[92] Although still potentially curable, the development of a locoregional recurrence after primary treatment of an invasive breast cancer portends a high risk for distant metastases and death because of breast cancer. Accordingly, patients should undergo disease restaging at the time of recurrence to rule out metastatic disease and should have a biopsy for histopathologic confirmation and reevaluation of hormone receptor and HER2 status. Given that locoregional recurrences are relatively uncommon and are heterogeneous in presentation and prior treatment, treatment strategies must be tailored to individual cases.

Recurrence in the Breast After Breast Conservation Therapy

Local recurrences after breast conservation therapy are classified and can sometimes be distinguished from second primary cancers based on location, appearance on imaging, histologic subtype, and HER2 status. It is important to try to identify true relapses, as there are data showing that compared with patients with new primaries, patients with true relapses have poorer 10-year OS (55% vs. 75%; $P < .0001$) and distant DFS (41% vs. 85%; $P < .0001$).[93] Risk factors for developing local recurrence after an initial breast-conserving approach are dictated mostly by margin status and receipt of radiotherapy; other known poor prognostic factors include greater T-stage, younger age, higher-grade histology, receptor-negative disease, and LVI.[94,95]

Appropriate management for locoregional recurrence after breast-conserving therapy depends on initial disease presentation and management. However, mastectomy remains the standard salvage treatment and is associated with a 50% to 95% local control rate depending on other prognostic factors of the disease.[96–98] There is no high-level evidence to support the use of postmastectomy radiotherapy after mastectomy for locoregional recurrence after initial breast-conserving therapy; however, this may be considered in patients with positive nodes (who did not receive initial regional nodal irradiation as a part of initial therapy), tumors larger than 5 cm, or multiple adverse risk factors, particularly in patients in whom their initial radiation was many years prior to the recurrence.

Given most patients treated with initial lumpectomy are also treated with breast irradiation, mastectomy remains the standard of care at the time of recurrence. However, some single-institutional studies investigated additional BCS with or without radiation. Salvadori et al.[99] compared the outcome of 134 patients treated with mastectomy for a localized breast recurrence to 54 highly selected patients treated with a second BCS alone. They found that a second breast recurrence was more common at 5 years in the reexcision group (19% vs. 4%); however, there was no difference in disease-specific survival between the two groups at 5 years. Komoike et al.[100] also reported a relatively high rate (30%) of a second breast relapse after local surgery only for recurrent disease. Gentilini et al.[101] examined outcomes for BCS alone after recurrence by predictive factors and found that repeating conserving therapy alone was associated with a 15.2% 5-year risk of local recurrence in patients with a tumor 2 cm or smaller and time to recurrence >2 years, whereas small tumors with early recurrence had a 31.2% 5-year local recurrence risk, and tumors >2 cm were associated with a 71.2% risk of 5-year local recurrence. This suggests that the best candidates for second BCS may be those with small tumors and late recurrence.

Experience with giving a second course of radiation therapy following local resection of a breast recurrence has also been limited, with most approaches being limited to a partial breast reirradiation strategy because of concerns for the morbidity of reirradiation to the whole breast. Deutsch et al.[102] treated 39 women with 50 Gy to the operative area using electrons after a repeat lumpectomy for an intact breast recurrence but reported a rate of second recurrence of 23%, whereas Wahl et al.[103] found a 53% recurrence rate at 1 year after repeat external beam radiotherapy. Resch et al.[104] treated 17 ipsilateral breast tumor recurrence patients with pulsed–dose rate brachytherapy following repeat lumpectomy and noted a second breast recurrence in 5, whereas Guix et al.[105] treated 36 patients with small low-risk local recurrences with excision and high dose rate brachytherapy and noted a local control rate of 89.4% at 10 years. Furthermore, Hannoun-Levi et al.[106] treated 69 highly selected patients with interstitial brachytherapy after a second lumpectomy

for an intact breast recurrence and after a median follow-up of 50 months reported that 11 (16%) developed a second recurrence. Grade 2 to 3 late complications developed in 0% to 32% of the patients, depending on the radiation dose. In RTOG 1014, a phase II trial of 55 patients who received accelerated partial breast irradiation following repeat lumpectomy for in-breast recurrence, there was only one grade 3 or higher toxicity (grade 3 fibrosis of deep connective tissue) at 1 year; however, long-term toxicity data are not yet available.[107]

There are limited data on reirradiation of the whole breast. In a small retrospective study of 47 women who received reirradiation for locally recurrent refractory breast cancer, investigators from the University of Toronto reported that the mean 2-Gy equivalent dose (EQD2) to the whole breast and tumor cavity was 99.8 Gy and 109.2 Gy, respectively. Two-year local control and OS were 50% and 67%, respectively, with acceptable short- and long-term toxicity (five cases of grade 3 to 4 acute radiation dermatitis and four cases of grade 3 fibrosis).[108]

Patients with recurrence in the breast are also at risk of axillary metastases. No high-level evidence or consensus exists for the management of the axilla in this setting. Rates of positive nodes in the recurrent setting in older series where axillary dissection was standardly employed at initial diagnosis report rates of lymph node involvement at the time of recurrence at approximately 25% but are as high as 50%.[109] In patients who have already had an axillary dissection at initial presentation, radiographic staging followed by surgical resection of gross axillary disease should be attempted if technically feasible. For patients who initially underwent sentinel lymph node surgery, restaging with repeat sentinel node evaluation may be feasible, but its diagnostic accuracy and prognostic significance are unknown.[110]

Although there are no high-level data regarding radiation of the regional nodes in the setting of nodal relapse, radiation of the axillary and supraclavicular nodes may provide durable local control. In this setting, maximal debulking with either surgical resection of disease or systemic chemotherapy is recommended to maximize local control.

The use of chemotherapy in the recurrent setting was studied in the phase III Chemotherapy for Isolated Locoregional Recurrence of Breast Cancer (CALOR) trial where 162 patients with locoregional recurrence after mastectomy or breast-conserving therapy were randomized to chemotherapy versus no chemotherapy.[111] Compared to the control group, chemotherapy was associated with significant improvements in OS (HR 0.41, 88% vs. 76%) and DFS (HR 0.59, 69% vs. 57%), with a larger benefit ($P_{interaction} = .046$) noted among women with ER-negative disease (67% vs. 35%) compared to ER-positive disease (70% vs. 69%). Although these data support the use of chemotherapy in the locoregionally recurrent setting especially for ER-negative disease, this trial was limited by small size and poor accrual and thus poor generalizability. The use of systemic therapy after breast recurrence should be decided on an individual basis according to the risk of metastatic disease, the previous systemic treatments used, and the hormone receptor status.

Several investigators have examined prognostic factors associated with outcome for patients with breast recurrence after treatment for an invasive breast cancer. A consistent finding in these studies is the finding that patients with an interval to development of recurrence of ≤2 years have a worse outcome than those who develop recurrent disease many years after treatment. In part, this may be explained by the hypothesis that early breast recurrences develop from repopulation of persistent microscopic disease, whereas some late breast recurrences represent a new primary tumor. Investigators from Yale University were among the first to provide insights into the prognostic importance of this distinction. These authors evaluated a series of 136 such patients and used clinical criteria to classify recurrences as either true recurrences or new primary tumors.[93] New primary tumors were defined by one of the following: location in the breast remote from the original tumor bed site, a change in histology, or a change from aneuploid to diploid status. Subsequently, a retrospective series from MDACC of 126 patients suggested that patients with a new primary tumor had significantly better 10-year survival (77% vs. 46%, P = .0002), cancer-specific survival (83% vs. 49%, P = .0001), and distant DFS (77% vs. 26%, P < .0001).[112] Both studies found that patients considered to have new primary tumors had significantly longer intervals between their initial primary tumor and the recurrence and had significantly lower rates of distant metastasis and death after the recurrence. These data were later validated in a study of 447 patients.[113] Furthermore, a retrospective study from Harvard suggests that estrogen receptor–negative status is associated with poorer DFS compared to patients with estrogen receptor–positive disease.[114] These findings may be valuable in decisions regarding management of recurrent disease.

Reconstructive surgery should be considered for patients treated with mastectomy, although previous history of breast radiation may limit the success of implant-based procedures. Forman et al.[115] reported significant complications in 6 of the 10 patients in whom a tissue expander and implant were attempted after mastectomy in the setting of an ipsilateral breast recurrent treatment. Autologous tissue reconstruction may provide better outcomes. Moran et al.[116] reported on 14 patients who underwent free TRAM flaps with anastomosis to the thoracodorsal vessels in patients being treated for a breast recurrence. The complication rate was only 14%, and the aesthetic result was rated as excellent. Determination of reconstructive approach should be made based on institutional experience for the best chances at successful outcome.

Locoregional Recurrence After Mastectomy

Recurrences after mastectomy tend to occur earlier and are more likely to be diagnosed on exam when compared to recurrence after breast-conserving therapy. The major risk factors for recurrence after mastectomy as initial therapy are the number of axillary lymph nodes positive at surgery in addition to other poor prognostic factors including younger age, higher-grade histology, receptor-negative disease, and LVI.[30,117]

Patients with recurrent disease after initial mastectomy may have a worse prognosis than those with recurrent disease after initial breast conservation therapy. In the Canadian and the Danish postmastectomy radiation randomized control trials, patients who developed locoregional recurrence had very high rates of subsequently developing metastatic disease.[118,119] In the Vancouver trial, of the 39 patients who developed a locoregional recurrence, 37 eventually developed metastatic disease.[118] In the Danish trial, the 5-year rate of distant metastatic disease development after an isolated locoregional recurrence was 73%. This rate was no different for those in whom disease recurred after mastectomy only versus those with recurrent disease after mastectomy and radiation,[119] though the ability to use radiation for salvage therapy, especially in isolated chest wall recurrences, may influence outcome, as discussed below.[120]

The general management strategy for an isolated locoregional recurrence after mastectomy requires input from a multidisciplinary team, but whenever possible should be wide local excision. The initial evaluation should define the sites of disease involvement and determine whether the patient is able to undergo resection of all gross disease with negative surgical margins. Surgical therapy is recommended for patients with resectable disease, provided surgery can be done with acceptable morbidity. If the patient had not previously been given radiation therapy, a standard approach would be comprehensive locoregional radiation with similar techniques used for newly diagnosed disease. A study from Washington University found that patients who had radiation therapy to the chest wall and regional lymphatics had better outcomes than those in whom radiation fields were limited to the site of the recurrent disease.[121] Finally, because patients with recurrent disease after mastectomy are at high risk of developing distant metastatic disease, those who have not been previously treated with chemotherapy (or trastuzumab if the tumor is HER2/neu-positive) should strongly consider treatment with these agents.[111,122] Patients with ER-positive disease should receive appropriate second-line endocrine therapy. A retrospective series of 115 patients with recurrence after mastectomy suggest that patients who receive combined modality therapy with wide local excision and radiotherapy in addition to systemic therapy have better DFS (52% vs. 39%) and OS (63% vs. 50%) compared to patients who get more limited treatment.[123] Patients presenting with bulky unresectable disease or who are poor surgical candidates should be considered for neoadjuvant chemotherapy if active systemic agents are available. If the disease responds favorably, some of these patients may become candidates for surgical resection, which then can be consolidated with comprehensive radiation. The prognosis for those with persistent gross disease is very poor, and radiation treatments alone are unlikely to render such patients free of disease. Nevertheless, aggressive locoregional radiation is often used to help stabilize the disease and to avoid the significant adverse consequences of uncontrolled growth of locoregional disease. The dose of radiation depends on the presence or absence of gross disease and whether patients have previously undergone radiation therapy. For patients who have not had prior radiation therapy and do not have residual gross disease, we recommend comprehensive treatment to the chest wall and draining lymphatics to a dose of 50 Gy followed by a boost to the sites of prior disease to 60 to 66 Gy. Hyperfractionated chest wall irradiation does not seem to provide any benefit over that of conventional therapy given once daily.[124] Investigators from Duke University have had modest success with combining a second course of radiation with chemotherapy and hyperthermia.[125]

Few data are available to quantify the benefits of systemic therapy for patients with locoregional recurrence. As discussed under management for recurrent disease of conservation therapy, the use of chemotherapy was studied in the CALOR trial where, compared to the control group, chemotherapy was associated with significant improvements in OS. A randomized trial that investigated tamoxifen use versus no systemic therapy after salvage local therapy for patients with recurrent disease after mastectomy found improvement in 5-year DFS from 36% to 59% (P = .007),[126] supporting the use of endocrine treatments in the management of patients with recurrent disease. Finally, investigators from MD Anderson conducted a series of four prospective single-group protocols evaluating systemic therapies for patients with either locoregional recurrence or metastatic disease that was converted to "no evidence of disease" after surgery, radiation, or both.[127] The findings suggest that for patients with anthracycline-naïve disease, the introduction of doxorubicin at the time of recurrence may be associated with improved survival. More recently, the use of docetaxel also seemed to lead to favorable outcome for patients who had previously had anthracycline treatment. The 3-year DFS rate for such patients was 58%.[127] The use of systemic therapy after breast recurrence should be decided on an individual basis according to the risk of metastatic disease, the previous systemic treatments used, and the hormone receptor status.

Several publications have provided insight into the factors of prognostic significance for patients with locoregional recurrence after mastectomy. One of the largest series was an analysis of the 535 patients who developed a postmastectomy recurrence after treatment in the Danish 82b and 82c randomized trials.[119] In multivariable analyses, the investigators found the following factors to be associated with a poorer outcome at recurrence: large initial primary tumor and high number of positive lymph nodes, extracapsular extension, recurrence in the infraclavicular or supraclavicular regions, and a disease-free interval of <2 years. Other series have reported similar findings. In general, patients who present with an isolated chest wall recurrence, particularly those who have resectable disease and have not undergone radiation, may have a greater probability of disease control and improved outcome compared to patients with other locoregional recurrences. Investigators from MD Anderson found that initial nodal status, time to recurrence, and ability to use radiation to treat the recurrence were all independent predictors of outcome for patients with a chest wall recurrence.[120] The 19 patients in whom these three factors were favorable had a 5-year OS of 86% (median survival time, 141 months). The 5-year survival rate for the 89 patients who had one or two unfavorable features was 48% (median survival time, 54 months), and all 22 of the patients who had all three unfavorable factors died within 5 years of the recurrence (median survival, 16 months). Outcome for patients with T1/T2 disease with one to three positive lymph nodes was as poor after a locoregional recurrence as was the outcome for patients with four or more positive lymph nodes.[128] In contrast, patients with initial lymph node–negative disease had a significantly better outcome.

Axillary Metastases with Unknown Primary

The presentation of metastatic disease within axillary lymph nodes without an identifiable primary source is unusual, accounting for <1% of newly diagnosed breast cancer cases.[129-131] The initial workup for patients who present with axillary disease and an occult primary is typically directed toward establishing the source, that is, a regional metastasis from breast cancer or a distant metastasis from a different site. As such, the initial evaluation should include a history and physical examination, routine serum studies, bilateral mammography, chest radiography, liver imaging, and bone scan. If no primary disease is detected with mammography, ultrasound and MRI scan of the breast are indicated. Although literature in this area is quite scant to begin with, most of it predates the widespread availability of MRI. Contrast-enhanced MRIs can detect occult lesions in about 80% of patients with "occult" primary and a negative mammogram. As such, true "occult" presentations will likely become even more uncommon in the current era. Cytologic confirmation of disease within axillary lymph nodes can be obtained with ultrasound-guided fine needle aspiration. Tumor markers, including ER, PR, and HER2/neu, can and should be performed on the cytologic specimens. In the absence of evidence for a remote, nonbreast primary, and a negative mammogram/ultrasound, a patient can be assumed to have an occult or unknown breast primary, and treated as such, particularly if the nodal biopsy results support a breast primary (i.e., based on markers). Most individuals present with advanced nodal disease at presentation and are clinically staged as having T0 N2 to 3 disease.

Modified radical mastectomy and postmastectomy radiation have been the historical locoregional treatments for patients with occult breast primary and axillary metastases. Studies vary significantly with respect to the frequency with which a primary is found within the breast during pathologic examination. Again, most of these studies predate the use of MRI screening or other improvements in diagnostic imaging. In general, however, approximately two-thirds of the patients are found to have an invasive breast cancer on pathologic examination of a mastectomy specimen.[129] Many patients with inoperable nodal disease (LABC) at presentation may receive neoadjuvant chemotherapy, and the probability of finding pathologic evidence of disease within the breast is likely lower in the current era.

A few investigators have investigated and reported on the safety of breast conservation therapy for patients with occult primary disease. One reported strategy for such patients includes neoadjuvant chemotherapy, reimaging of the breast to evaluate for calcifications resulting from tumor cell death, axillary dissection, and irradiation of the breast and draining lymphatics. Early attempts at breast conservation without breast irradiation resulted in high subsequent breast recurrence rates.[132,133] More recent studies that incorporate breast irradiation have yielded better results. In one of the largest series, investigators from MD Anderson evaluated 45 patients treated over a 47-year period and compared the outcome of those treated with mastectomy ($n = 13$) to those treated with breast conservation ($n = 32$).[131] These authors found equivalent rates of locoregional control, DFS, and OS between the mastectomy and breast conservation cohorts. With a median follow-up of 7 years, only 2 of the 25 breast conservation patients who received breast irradiation developed a local recurrence. Similar results have been reported from The Royal Marsden Hospital. In a series of 48 patients, they found a 14% locoregional recurrence rate after breast radiation and an unacceptable rate of 80% if breast radiation was omitted.[134] These data suggest that microscopic/undetectable primary lesions can successfully be sterilized with the combination of systemic therapy and radiation therapy. One can feel particularly reassured with this strategy for lesions treated in the MRI age (i.e., for lesions below the threshold for MRI detectability). Patients presenting with an occult breast primary and axillary disease should receive regional nodal RT, whether as a part of PMRT or breast conservation therapy.[135,136]

Male Breast Cancer

Breast cancer developing in males is uncommon and accounts for <1% of total new breast cancer cases in the United States.[4] The American Cancer Society estimated that in 2017, there would be approximately 2,470 new cases of male breast cancer and 460 deaths because of male breast cancer in the United States. The incidence of male breast cancer is positively correlated with age, and the highest rates occur in black males (2.7 per 100,000) and white males (1.9 per 100,000).[4]

The presenting symptom for male breast cancer patients is typically a breast mass or axillary adenopathy, and most male breast cancer patients present with locally advanced disease. The ratio of the number of deaths to new cases is 19% for males, compared to a ratio of 16% for females, with a 5-year OS of 84% in men compared to 90% in women.[4] Retrospective national database evidence suggests differences in cancer-specific mortality may be attributable to stage migration, as there are no gender-specific differences when comparing outcome within stage II or stage III.[137]

The known risk factors for male breast cancer, similar to those in postmenopausal female breast cancer, include family history, age, conditions that affect testosterone and estrogen levels, BRCA2 mutations, and prior history of radiotherapy.[138] Germ-line mutations in the BRCA2 gene have been reported in 4% to 16% of men with breast cancer and, unlike female breast cancer, are more common than germ-line mutations in BRCA1.[139,140] Nevertheless, most male breast cancers present without an identifiable risk factor.

Section III

Males have a similar histopathologic spectrum of breast cancers to females with the exception of lower rates of invasive lobular carcinoma given the lack of acini and lobules in normal breast tissue. Specifically, <2% of invasive male breast carcinomas are lobular, as compared to approximately 15% in female cancers.[141] In addition, male breast cancers more frequently are ER-positive (estimated rate of 90%) and HER2/neu-negative compared to female breast cancer.[137] Diagnostic workup and staging are similar to that for female breast cancer and should include bilateral mammography, biopsy, and staging workup. Treatment decisions are also similar to those used in women.

Mastectomy with or without postmastectomy radiation is the most common locoregional treatment approach, with increasing attention being placed on postmastectomy reconstruction and potential psychological distress related to cosmetic outcomes. Investigators at MD Anderson reviewed 142 patients treated with mastectomy without radiation therapy and found that, similar to female patients, margin status, number of positive nodes, and tumor size predicted locoregional failure.[142] Accordingly, decisions concerning postmastectomy radiation should be based on the same criteria used in the treatment of female breast cancer.

Similarly, systemic treatments are indicated for male breast cancer patients who have a clinically relevant risk of distant metastases, and treatment decisions should follow those for female breast cancers. Level 1 data supporting the use of particular chemotherapy regimens specifically in men are lacking, given the rarity of the disease. In addition to chemotherapy, because most male breast cancers are receptor positive, tamoxifen is indicated for the majority of cases. Retrospective series have suggested that tamoxifen can reduce the risk of recurrence and death.[143] The role of aromatase inhibitors in males is unclear, but retrospective data support the adjuvant use of tamoxifen rather than aromatase inhibitors.[144]

REFERENCES

1. Haagensen CD, Cooley E. Radical mastectomy for mammary carcinoma. *Ann Surg* 1969;170:884.
2. Haagensen CD, Stout AP. Carcinoma of the breast: criteria of inoperability. *Ann Surg* 1943;118:859–870.
3. Fracchia AA, Evans JF, Eisenberg BC. Stage III carcinoma of the breast—a detailed analysis. *Ann Surg* 1980;192:705.
4. American Cancer Society. *Cancer facts and figures 2017*. Atlanta, GA: American Cancer Society, 2017:1–76.
5. Li CL, Malone KE, Daling JR. Differences in breast cancer hormone receptor status and histology among women 50 years of age and older. *Cancer Epidemiol Biomarkers Prev* 2002;11:601–607.
6. Elledge RM, et al. Tumor biologic factors and breast cancer prognosis among white, Hispanic, and black women in the United States. *J Natl Cancer Inst* 1994;86:705–712.
7. Hortobagyi GN, Singletary SE, Buchholz TA. Locally advanced breast cancer. In: Singletary SE, Robb GL, Hortobagyi GN, eds. *Advanced therapy of breast disease*. 2nd ed. Hamilton, Canada: BC Decker, Inc., 2004:498–508.
8. Woodward WA, et al. Changes in the 2003 American Joint Committee on Cancer staging for breast cancer dramatically affect stage-specific survival. *J Clin Oncol* 2003;21(17):3244–3248.
9. Krishnamurthy S, Sneige N, Bedi DG, et al. Role of ultrasound-guided fine-needle aspiration of indeterminate and suspicious axillary lymph nodes in the initial staging of breast carcinoma. *Cancer* 2002;95(5):982–988.
10. Martin AM, Cagney DN, Catalano PJ, et al. Brain metastases in newly diagnosed breast cancer: a population-based study. *JAMA Oncol* 2017;3(8):1069–1077.
11. Warren LE, Guo H, Regan MM, et al. Inflammatory breast cancer and development of brain metastases: risk factors and outcomes. *Breast Cancer Res Treat* 2015;151(1):225–232.
12. Alberini JL, Lerebours F, Wartski M, et al. 18 F-fluorodeoxyglucose positron emission tomography/computed tomography (FDG-PET/CT) imaging in the staging and prognosis of inflammatory breast cancer. *Cancer* 2009;115(21):5038–5047.
13. Groheux D, Giacchetti S, Delord M, et al. 18 F-FDG PET/CT in staging patients with locally advanced or inflammatory breast cancer: comparison to conventional staging. *J Nucl Med* 2013;54(1):5–11.
14. Walker GV, Niikura N, Yang W, et al. Pretreatment staging positron emission tomography/computed tomography in patients with inflammatory breast cancer influences radiation treatment field designs. *Int J Radiat Oncol Biol Phys* 2012;83(5):1381–1386.
15. Singletary SE, Greene FL. Revision of breast cancer staging: the 6th edition of the TNM classification. *Semin Surg Oncol* 2003;21(1):53–59.
16. Mauri D, Pavlidis N, Ioannidis JP. Neoadjuvant versus adjuvant systemic treatment in breast cancer: a meta-analysis. *J Natl Cancer Inst* 2005;97:188–194.
17. Mieog JS, van der Hage JA, van de Velde CJ. Neoadjuvant chemotherapy for operable breast cancer. *Br J Surg* 2007;94:1189–1200.
18. Fisher B, Brown A, Mamounas E, et al. Effect of preoperative chemotherapy on local-regional disease in women with operable breast cancer: findings from National Surgical Adjuvant Breast and Bowel Project B-18. *J Clin Oncol* 1997;15:2483–2493.
19. Fisher B, Bryant J, Wolmark N, et al. Effect of preoperative chemotherapy on the outcome of women with operable breast cancer. *J Clin Oncol* 1998;16:2672–2685.
20. van der Hage JA, van de Velde CJ, Julien JP, et al. Preoperative chemotherapy in primary operable breast cancer: results from the European Organization for Research and Treatment of Cancer trial 10902. *J Clin Oncol* 2001;19:4224–4237.
21. Chen AM, Meric-Bernstam F, Hunt KK, et al. Breast conservation after neoadjuvant chemotherapy: the M.D. Anderson Cancer Center Experience. *J Clin Oncol* 2004;22:2303–2312.
22. Rastogi P, Anderson SJ, Bear HD, et al. Preoperative chemotherapy: updates of National Surgical Adjuvant Breast and Bowel Project Protocols B-18 and B-27. *J Clin Oncol* 2008;26:778–785.
23. Guarneri V, Broglio K, Kau SW, et al. Prognostic value of pathologic complete response after primary chemotherapy in relation to hormone receptor status and other factors. *J Clin Oncol* 2006;24:1037–1044.
24. Cortazar P, Zhang L, Untch M, et al. Pathological complete response and long-term clinical benefit in breast cancer: the CTNeoBC pooled analysis. *Lancet* 2014;384:164–172.
25. von Minckwitz G, Kümmel S, Vogel P, et al. Neoadjuvant vinorelbine-capecitabine versus docetaxel-doxorubicin-cyclophosphamide in early nonresponsive breast cancer: phase III randomized GeparTrio trial. *J Natl Cancer Inst* 2008;100:542–551.
26. von Minckwitz G, Untch M, Blohmer JU, et al. Definition and impact of pathologic complete response on prognosis after neoadjuvant chemotherapy in various intrinsic breast cancer subtypes. *J Clin Oncol* 2012;30:1796–1804.
27. Smith IE, Dowsett M, Ebbs SR, et al. Neoadjuvant treatment of postmenopausal breast cancer with anastrozole, tamoxifen, or both in combination: the Immediate Preoperative Anastrozole, Tamoxifen, or Combined with Tamoxifen (IMPACT) multicenter double-blind randomized trial. *J Clin Oncol* 2005;23:5108–5116.
28. Eiermann W, Paepke S, Appfelstaedt J, et al. Preoperative treatment of postmenopausal breast cancer patients with letrozole: a randomized double-blind multicenter study. *Ann Oncol* 2001;12:1527–1532.
29. Ellis MJ, Suman VJ, Hoog J, et al. Randomized phase II neoadjuvant comparison between letrozole, anastrozole, and exemestane for postmenopausal women with estrogen receptor-rich stage 2 to 3 breast cancer: clinical and biomarker outcomes and predictive value of the baseline PAM50-based intrinsic subtype—ACOSOG Z1031. *J Clin Oncol* 2011;29:2342–2349.
30. Early Breast Cancer Trialists' Collaborative Group (EBCTCG). Effects of chemotherapy and hormonal therapy for early breast cancer on recurrence and 15-year survival: an overview of the randomised trials. *Lancet* 2005;365:1687–1717.
31. Peto R, Davies C, Godwin J, et al. Comparisons between different polychemotherapy regimens for early breast cancer: meta-analyses of long-term outcome among 100,000 women in 123 randomised trials. *Lancet* 2012;379:432–444.
32. Bear HD, Anderson S, Smith RE, et al. Sequential preoperative or postoperative docetaxel added to preoperative doxorubicin plus cyclophosphamide for operable breast cancer: National Surgical Adjuvant Breast and Bowel Project Protocol B-27. *J Clin Oncol* 2006;24:2019–2027.
33. Untch M, Jackisch C, Schneeweiss A, et al. Nab-paclitaxel versus solvent-based paclitaxel in neoadjuvant chemotherapy for early breast cancer (GeparSepto-GBG 69): a randomised, phase 3 trial. *Lancet Oncol* 2016;17:345–356.
34. von Minckwitz G, Rezai M, Loibl S, et al. Capecitabine in addition to anthracycline- and taxane-based neoadjuvant treatment in patients with primary breast cancer: phase III GeparQuattro study. *J Clin Oncol* 2010;28:2015–2023.
35. Bear HD, Tang G, Rastogi P, et al. Neoadjuvant plus adjuvant bevacizumab in early breast cancer (NSABP B-40 [NRG Oncology]): secondary outcomes of a phase 3, randomised controlled trial. *Lancet Oncol* 2015;16:1037–1048.
36. Sikov WM, Berry DA, Perou CM, et al. Impact of the addition of carboplatin and/or bevacizumab to neoadjuvant once-per-week paclitaxel followed by dose-dense doxorubicin and cyclophosphamide on pathologic complete response rates in stage II to III triple-negative breast cancer: CALGB 40603 (Alliance). *J Clin Oncol* 2015;33:13–21.
37. Sikov W, Berry D, Perou C. Event-free and overall survival following neoadjuvant weekly paclitaxel and dose-dense AC ± carboplatin and/or bevacizumab in triple-negative breast cancer: outcomes from CALGB 40603 (Alliance). 2015 San Antonio Breast Cancer Symposium. Abstract S2-05. Presented December 9, 2015.
38. von Minckwitz G, Schneeweiss A, Loibl S, et al. Neoadjuvant carboplatin in patients with triple-negative and HER2-positive early breast cancer (GeparSixto; GBG 66): a randomised phase 2 trial. *Lancet Oncol* 2014;15:747–756.
39. von Minckwitz G, Loibl S, Schneeweiss A, et al. Early survival analysis of the randomized phase II trial investigating the addition of carboplatin to neoadjuvant therapy for triple-negative and HER2-positive early breast cancer (GeparSixto). 2015 San Antonio Breast Cancer Symposium. Abstract S2-04. Presented December 9, 2015.

40. Piccart-Gebhart MJ, Procter M, Leyland-Jones B, et al. Trastuzumab after adjuvant chemotherapy in HER2-positive breast cancer. *N Engl J Med* 2005;353:1659–1672.

41. Romond EH, Perez EA, Bryant J, et al. Trastuzumab plus adjuvant chemotherapy for operable HER2-positive breast cancer. *N Engl J Med* 2005;353:1673–1684.

42. Semiglazov V, Eiermann W, Zambetti M, et al. Surgery following neoadjuvant therapy in patients with HER2-positive locally advanced or inflammatory breast cancer participating in the NeOAdjuvant Herceptin (NOAH) study. *Eur J Surg Oncol* 2011;37:856–863.

43. Gianni L, Pienkowski T, Im YH, et al. Efficacy and safety of neoadjuvant pertuzumab and trastuzumab in women with locally advanced, inflammatory, or early HER2-positive breast cancer (NeoSphere): a randomised multicentre, open-label, phase 2 trial. *Lancet Oncol* 2012;13:25–32.

44. Schneeweiss A, Chia S, Hickish T, et al. Pertuzumab plus trastuzumab in combination with standard neoadjuvant anthracycline-containing and anthracycline-free chemotherapy regimens in patients with HER2-positive early breast cancer: a randomized phase II cardiac safety study (TRYPHAENA). *Ann Oncol* 2013;24:2278–2284.

45. Masuda N, Lee S-J, Ohtani S, et al. Adjuvant capecitabine for breast cancer after preoperative chemotherapy. *N Engl J Med* 2017;376:2147–2159.

46. Davies C, Pan H, Godwin J, et al. Long-term effects of continuing adjuvant tamoxifen to 10 years versus stopping at 5 years after diagnosis of oestrogen receptor-positive breast cancer: ATLAS, a randomised trial. *Lancet* 2013;381:805–816.

47. Dowsett M, Forbes JF, Bradley R, et al. Aromatase inhibitors versus tamoxifen in early breast cancer: patient-level meta-analysis of the randomised trials. *Lancet* 2015;386:1341–1352.

48. Pagani O, Regan MM, Walley BA, et al. Adjuvant exemestane with ovarian suppression in premenopausal breast cancer. *N Engl J Med* 2014;371:107–118.

49. Francis PA, Regan MM, Fleming GF. Adjuvant ovarian suppression in premenopausal breast cancer. *N Engl J Med* 2015;372:1673.

50. Brito RA, Valero V, Buzdar AU, et al. Long-term results of combined-modality therapy for locally advanced breast cancer with ipsilateral supraclavicular metastases: the University of Texas M.D. Anderson Cancer Center experience. *J Clin Oncol* 2001;19(3):628–633.

51. Huang EH, Tucker SL, Strom EA, et al. Postmastectomy radiation improves local-regional control and survival for selected patients with locally advanced breast cancer treated with neoadjuvant chemotherapy and mastectomy. *J Clin Oncol* 2004;22(3):4691–4699.

52. Livingston SF, Arlen M. The extended extrapleural radical mastectomy: its role in the treatment of carcinoma of the breast. *Ann Surg* 1974;179:260–265.

53. Dellapasqua S, Bagnardi V, Balduzzi A, et al. Outcomes of patients who present with ipsilateral supraclavicular or internal mammary lymph node metastases. *Clin Breast Cancer* 2014;14(1):53–60.

54. Noh JM, Kim KH, Park W, et al. Prognostic significance of nodal involvement region in clinical stage IIIc breast cancer patients who received primary systemic treatment, surgery, and radiotherapy. *Breast* 2015;24(5):637–641.

55. Wingo PA, Jamison PM, Young JL, et al. Population-based statistics for women diagnosed with inflammatory breast cancer (United States). *Cancer Causes Control* 2004;15:321–328.

56. Hance KW, Anderson WF, Devesa SS, et al. Trends in inflammatory breast carcinoma incidence and survival: the surveillance, epidemiology, and end results program at the National Cancer Institute. *J Natl Cancer Inst* 2005;97:966–975.

57. Anderson WF, Schairer C, Chen BE, et al. Epidemiology of inflammatory breast cancer (IBC). *Breast Dis* 2005;22:9–23.

58. Robertson FM, Bondy M, Yang W, et al. Inflammatory breast cancer: the disease, the biology, the treatment. *CA Cancer J Clin* 2010;60:351–375.

59. Dawood S, Ueno NT, Valero V, et al. Differences in survival among women with stage III inflammatory and noninflammatory locally advanced breast cancer appear early: a large population-based study. *Cancer* 2011;117:1819–1826.

60. Bozzetti F, Saccozzi R, De Lena M, et al. Inflammatory cancer of the breast: analysis of 114 cases. *J Surg Oncol* 1981;18:355–361.

61. Barker JL, Nelson AJ, Montague ED. Inflammatory carcinoma of the breast. *Radiology* 1976;121:173–176.

62. Zucali R, Uslenghi C, Kenda R, et al. Natural history and survival of inoperable breast cancer treated with radiotherapy and radiotherapy followed by radical mastectomy. *Cancer* 1976;37:1422–1431.

63. Fields JN, Perez CA, Kuske RR, et al. Inflammatory carcinoma of the breast: treatment results on 107 patients. *Int J Radiat Oncol Biol Phys* 1989;17:249–255.

64. Krutchik AN, Buzdar AU, Blumenschein GR, et al. Combined chemoimmunotherapy and radiation therapy of inflammatory breast carcinoma. *J Surg Oncol* 1979;11:325–332.

65. Brown L, Harmsen W, Blanchard M, et al. Once-daily radiation therapy for inflammatory breast cancer. *Int J Radiat Oncol Biol Phys* 2014;89:997–1003.

66. Rehman S, Reddy CA, Tendulkar RD. Modern outcomes of inflammatory breast cancer. *Int J Radiat Oncol Biol Phys* 2012;84:619–624.

67. Damast S, Ho AY, Montgomery L, et al. Locoregional outcomes of inflammatory breast cancer patients treated with standard fractionation radiation and daily skin bolus in the taxane era. *Int J Radiat Oncol Biol Phys* 2010;77:1105–1112.

68. Abramowitz MC, Li T, Morrow M, et al. Dermal lymphatic invasion and inflammatory breast cancer are independent predictors of outcome after postmastectomy radiation. *Am J Clin Oncol* 2009;32:30–33.

69. Bristol IJ, Woodward WA, Strom EA, et al. Locoregional treatment outcomes after multimodality management of inflammatory breast cancer. *Int J Radiat Oncol Biol Phys* 2008;72:474–484.

70. Yang WT, Le-Petross HT, Macapinlac H, et al. Inflammatory breast cancer: PET/CT, MRI, mammography, and sonography findings. *Breast Cancer Res Treat* 2008;109:417–426.

71. Woodward WA. Inflammatory breast cancer: unique biological and therapeutic considerations. *Lancet Oncol* 2015;16:e568–e576.

72. Guerin M, Gabillot M, Mathieu MC, et al. Structure and expression of c-erbB-2 and EGF receptor genes in inflammatory and non-inflammatory breast cancer: prognostic significance. *Int J Cancer* 1989;43:201–208.

73. van Golen KL, Davies S, Wu ZF, et al. A novel putative low-affinity insulin-like growth factor-binding protein, LIBC (lost in inflammatory breast cancer), and RhoC GTPase correlate with the inflammatory breast cancer phenotype. *Clin Cancer Res* 1999;5:2511–2519.

74. Kleer CG, Zhang Y, Pan Q, et al. WISP3 and RhoC guanosine triphosphatase cooperate in the development of inflammatory breast cancer. *Breast Cancer Res* 2004;6:R110–R115.

75. Dong HM, Liu G, Hou YF, et al. Dominant-negative E-cadherin inhibits the invasiveness of inflammatory breast cancer cells in vitro. *J Cancer Res Clin Oncol* 2007;133:83–92.

76. Tomlinson JS, Alpaugh ML, Barsky SH. An intact overexpressed E-cadherin/alpha,beta-catenin axis characterizes the lymphovascular emboli of inflammatory breast carcinoma. *Cancer Res* 2001;61:5231–5241.

77. Cristofanilli M, Gonzalez-Angulo AM, Buzdar AU, et al. Paclitaxel improves the prognosis in estrogen receptor negative inflammatory breast cancer: the M. D. Anderson Cancer Center experience. *Clin Breast Cancer* 2004;4:415–419.

78. Li J, Gonzalez-Angulo AM, Allen PK, et al. Triple-negative subtype predicts poor overall survival and high locoregional relapse in inflammatory breast cancer. *Oncologist* 2011;16:1675–1683.

79. De Boer RH, Allum WH, Ebbs SR, et al. Multimodality therapy in inflammatory breast cancer: is there a place for surgery? *Ann Oncol* 2000;11:1147–1153.

80. Perez CA, Fields JN, Fracasso PM, et al. Management of locally advanced carcinoma of the breast. II. Inflammatory carcinoma. *Cancer* 1994;74:466–476.

81. Panades M, Olivotto IA, Speers CH, et al. Evolving treatment strategies for inflammatory breast cancer: a population-based survival analysis. *J Clin Oncol* 2005;23:1941–1950.

82. Fleming RY, Asmar L, Buzdar AU, et al. Effectiveness of mastectomy by response to induction chemotherapy for control in inflammatory breast carcinoma. *Ann Surg Oncol* 1997;4:452–461.

83. Arthur DW, Schmidt-Ullrich RK, Friedman RB, et al. Accelerated superfractionated radiotherapy for inflammatory breast carcinoma: complete response predicts outcome and allows for breast conservation. *Int J Radiat Oncol Biol Phys* 1999;44:289–296.

84. Low JA, Berman AW, Steinberg SM, et al. Long-term follow-up for locally advanced and inflammatory breast cancer patients treated with multimodality therapy. *J Clin Oncol* 2004;22:4067–4074.

85. Brun B, Otmezguine Y, Feuilhade F, et al. Treatment of inflammatory breast cancer with combination chemotherapy and mastectomy versus breast conservation. *Cancer* 1988;61:1096–1103.

86. Swain SM, Lippman ME. Treatment of patients with inflammatory breast cancer. *Important Adv Oncol* 1989:129–150.

87. Chevallier B, Asselain B, Kunlin A, et al. Inflammatory breast cancer. Determination of prognostic factors by univariate and multivariate analysis. *Cancer* 1987;60:897–902.

88. Liao Z, Strom EA, Buzdar AU, et al. Locoregional irradiation for inflammatory breast cancer: effectiveness of dose escalation in decreasing recurrence. *Int J Radiat Oncol Biol Phys* 2000;47:1191–1200.

89. Loveland-Jones C, Lin H, Shen Y, et al. Disparities in the use of postmastectomy radiation therapy for inflammatory breast cancer. *Int J Radiat Oncol Biol Phys* 2016;95:1218–1225.

90. Huang E, McNeese MD, Strom EA, et al. Locoregional treatment outcomes for inoperable anthracycline-resistant breast cancer. *Int J Radiat Oncol Biol Phys* 2002;53:1225–1233.

91. Yang SH, Yang KH, Li YP, et al. Breast conservation therapy for stage I or stage II breast cancer: a meta-analysis of randomized controlled trials. *Ann Oncol* 2008;19:1039.

92. Montgomery DA, Krupa K, Jack WJ, et al. Changing pattern of the detection of locoregional relapse in breast cancer: the Edinburgh experience. *Br J Cancer* 2007;96:1802.

93. Smith TE, Lee D, Turner BC, et al. True recurrence vs. new primary ipsilateral breast tumor relapse: an analysis of clinical and pathologic differences and their implications in natural history, prognoses, and therapeutic management. *Int J Radiat Oncol Biol Phys* 2000;48:1281–1289.

94. Houssami N, Macaskill P, Marinovich ML, et al. Meta-analysis of the impact of surgical margins on local recurrence in women with early-stage invasive breast cancer treated with breast-conserving therapy. *Eur J Cancer* 2010;46:3219.

95. Botteri E, Bagnardi V, Rotmensz N, et al. Analysis of local and regional recurrences in breast cancer after conservative surgery. *Ann Oncol* 2010;21:723.

96. Galper S, Blood E, Gelman R, et al. Prognosis after local recurrence after conservative surgery and radiation for early-stage breast cancer. *Int J Radiat Oncol Biol Phys* 2005;61:348.

97. Doyle T, Schultz DJ, Peters C, et al. Long-term results of local recurrence after breast conservation treatment for invasive breast cancer. *Int J Radiat Oncol Biol Phys* 2001;51:74.

98. Shen J, Hunt KK, Mirza NQ, et al. Predictors of systemic recurrence and disease-specific survival after ipsilateral breast tumor recurrence. *Cancer* 2005;104:479.

99. Salvadori B, Marubini E, Miceli R, et al. Reoperation for locally recurrent breast cancer in patients previously treated with conservative surgery. *Br J Surg* 1999;86(1):84–87.

100. Komoike Y, Motomura K, Inaji H, et al. Repeat lumpectomy for patients with ipsilateral breast tumor recurrence after breast-conserving surgery. Preliminary results. *Oncology* 2003;64(1):1–6.

101. Gentilini O, Botteri E, Veronesi P, et al. Repeating conservative surgery after ipsilateral breast tumor reappearance: criteria for selecting the best candidates. *Ann Surg Oncol* 2012;19:3771.

102. Deutsch M. Repeat high-dose external beam irradiation for in-breast tumor recurrence after previous lumpectomy and whole breast irradiation. *Int J Radiat Oncol Biol Phys* 2002;53(3):687–691.

103. Wahl AO, Rademaker A, Kiel KD, et al. Multi-institutional review of repeat irradiation of chest wall and breast for recurrent breast cancer. *Int J Radiat Oncol Biol Phys* 2008;70:477.

104. Resch A, Fellner C, Mock U, et al. Locally recurrent breast cancer: pulse dose rate brachytherapy for repeat irradiation following lumpectomy—a second chance to preserve the breast. *Radiology* 2002;225(3):713–718.

105. Guix B, Lejárcegui JA, Tello JI, et al. Exeresis and brachytherapy as salvage treatment for local recurrence after conservative treatment for breast cancer: results of a ten-year pilot study. *Int J Radiat Oncol Biol Phys* 2010; 78:804.

106. Hannoun-Levi JM, Houvenaeghel G, Ellis S, et al. Partial breast irradiation as second conservative treatment for local breast cancer recurrence. *Int J Radiat Oncol Biol Phys* 2004;60(5):1385–1392.

107. Arthur DW, Winter K, Kuerer HM, et al. NRG Oncology/RTOG 1014: 1-Year Toxicity Report From a Phase II Study of Repeat Breast Preserving Surgery and 3D Conformal Partial-Breast Reirradiation (PBrI) for In-Breast Recurrence. ASTRO 2015, San Antonio.

108. Merino T, Tran WT, Czarnota GJ. Re-irradiation for locally recurrent refractory breast cancer. *Oncotarget* 2015;6(33):35051–35062.

109. Hsi RA, Antell A, Schultz DJ, et al. Radiation therapy for chest wall recurrence of breast cancer after mastectomy in a favorable subgroup of patients. *Int J Radiat Oncol Biol Phys* 1998;42:495.

110. Vugts G, Maaskant-Braat AJ, Voogd AC. Repeat sentinel node biopsy should be considered in patients with locally recurrent breast cancer. *Breast Cancer Res Treat* 2015;153(3):549–556.

111. Aebi S, Gelber S, Anderson SJ, et al. Chemotherapy for isolated locoregional recurrence of breast cancer (CALOR): a randomised trial. *Lancet Oncol* 2014;15:156.

112. Huang E, Buchholz TA, Meric F, et al. Classifying local disease recurrences after breast conservation therapy based on location and histology: new primary tumors have more favorable outcomes than true local disease recurrences. *Cancer* 2002;95(10):2059–2067.

113. Yi M, Buchholz TA, Meric-Bernstam F, et al. Classification of ipsilateral breast tumor recurrences after breast conservation therapy can predict patient prognosis and facilitate treatment planning. *Ann Surg* 2011;253(3): 572–579.

114. Braunstein LZ, Niemierko A, Shenouda MN, et al. Outcome following local-regional recurrence in women with early-stage breast cancer: impact of biologic subtype. *Breast J* 2015;21(2):161–167.

115. Forman DL, Chiu J, Restifo RJ, et al. Breast reconstruction in previously irradiated patients using tissue expanders and implants: a potentially unfavorable result. *Ann Plast Surg* 1998;40(4):360–363; discussion 363–364.

116. Moran SL, Serletti JM, Fox I. Immediate free TRAM reconstruction in lumpectomy and radiation failure patients. *Plast Reconstr Surg* 2000;106(7):1527–1531.

117. Katz A, Strom EA, Buchholz TA, et al. Locoregional recurrence patterns after mastectomy and doxorubicin-based chemotherapy: implications for postoperative irradiation. *J Clin Oncol* 2000;18:2817.

118. Ragaz J, Olivotto IA, Spinelli JJ, et al. Locoregional radiation therapy in patients with high-risk breast cancer receiving adjuvant chemotherapy: 20-year results of the British Columbia randomized trial. *J Natl Cancer Inst* 2005;97(2):116–126.

119. Nielsen HM, Overgaard M, Grau C, et al. Loco-regional recurrence after mastectomy in high-risk breast cancer–risk and prognosis. An analysis of patients from the DBCG 82 b& c randomization trials. *Radiother Oncol* 2006;79(2):147–155.

120. Chagpar A, Meric-Bernstam F, Hunt KK, et al. Chest wall recurrence after mastectomy does not always portend a dismal outcome. *Ann Surg Oncol* 2003;10(6):628–634.

121. Halverson KJ, Perez CA, Kuske RR, et al. Isolated local-regional recurrence of breast cancer following mastectomy: radiotherapeutic management. *Int J Radiat Oncol Biol Phys* 1990;19(4):851–858.

122. Haylock BJ, Coppin CM, Jackson J, et al. Locoregional first recurrence after mastectomy: prospective cohort studies with and without immediate chemotherapy. *Int J Radiat Oncol Biol Phys* 2000;46(2):355–362.

123. Kuo SH, Huang CS, Kuo WH, et al. Comprehensive locoregional treatment and systemic therapy for postmastectomy isolated locoregional recurrence. *Int J Radiat Oncol Biol Phys* 2008;72:1456.

124. Ballo MT, Strom EA, Prost H, et al. Local-regional control of recurrent breast carcinoma after mastectomy: does hyperfractionated accelerated radiotherapy improve local control?. *Int J Radiat Oncol Biol Phys* 1999;44(1): 105–112.

125. Zagar TM, Higgins KA, Miles EF, et al. Durable palliation of breast cancer chest wall recurrence with radiation therapy, hyperthermia, and chemotherapy. *Radiother Oncol* 2010;97(3):535–540.

126. Borner M, Bacchi M, Goldhirsch A, et al. First isolated locoregional recurrence following mastectomy for breast cancer: results of a phase III multicenter study comparing systemic treatment with observation after excision and radiation. Swiss Group for Clinical Cancer Research. *J Clin Oncol* 1994;12(10): 2071–2077.

127. Hanrahan EO, Broglio ER, Buzdar AU, et al. Combined-modality treatment for isolated recurrences of breast carcinoma: update on 30 years of experience at the University of Texas M.D. Anderson Cancer Center and assessment of prognostic factors. *Cancer* 2005;104(6):1158–1171.

128. Chagpar A, Kuerer HM, Hunt KK, et al. Outcome of treatment for breast cancer patients with chest wall recurrence according to initial stage: implications for post-mastectomy radiation therapy. *Int J Radiat Oncol Biol Phys* 2003;57(1):128–135.

129. Knapper WH. Management of occult breast cancer presenting as an axillary metastasis. *Semin Surg Oncol* 1991;7:311–313.

130. Vezzoni P, Balestrazzi A, Bignami P, et al. Axillary lymph node metastases from occult carcinoma of the breast. *Tumori* 1979;65:87–91.

131. Vlastos G, Jean ME, Mirza AN, et al. Feasibility of breast preservation in the treatment of occult primary carcinoma presenting with axillary metastases. *Ann Surg Oncol* 2001;8:425–431.

132. Bhatia SK, Saclarides TJ, Witt TR, et al. Hormone receptor studies in axillary metastases from occult breast cancers. *Cancer* 1987;59:1170–1172.

133. Ellerbroek N, Holmes F, Singletary E, et al. Treatment of patients with isolated axillary nodal metastases from an occult primary carcinoma consistent with breast origin. *Cancer* 1990;66:1461–1467.

134. Barton SR, Smith IE, Kirby AM, et al. The role of ipsilateral breast radiotherapy in management of occult primary breast cancer presenting as axillary lymphadenopathy. *Eur J Cancer* 2011;47:2099–2106.

135. Whelan TJ, Olivotto IA, Levine MN. Regional nodal irradiation in early-stage breast cancer. *N Engl J Med* 2015;373:1878–1879.

136. Poortmans PM, Collette S, Kirkove C, et al. Internal mammary and medial supraclavicular irradiation in breast cancer. *N Engl J Med* 2015;373: 317–327.

137. Gnerlich JL, Deshpande AD, Jeffe DB, et al. Poorer survival outcomes for male breast cancer compared with female breast cancer may be attributable to in-stage migration. *Ann Surg Oncol* 2011;18(7):1837–1844.

138. Ruddy KJ, Winer EP. Male breast cancer: risk factors, biology, diagnosis, treatment, and survivorship. *Ann Oncol* 2013;24(6):1434–1443.

139. Ferzoco RM, Ruddy KJ. The epidemiology of male breast cancer. *Curr Oncol Rep* 2016;18(1):1.

140. Ottini L, Masala G, D'Amico C, et al. BRCA1 and BRCA2 mutation status and tumor characteristics in male breast cancer: a population-based study in Italy. *Cancer Res* 2003;63(2):342–347.

141. Giordano SH, Cohen DS, Buzdar AU, et al. Breast carcinoma in men: a population-based study. *Cancer* 2004;101(1):51.

142. Buchholz TA, Katz A, Strom EA, et al. Pathologic tumor size and lymph node status predict for different rates of locoregional recurrence after mastectomy for breast cancer patients treated with neoadjuvant versus adjuvant chemotherapy. *Int J Radiat Oncol Biol Phys* 2002;53(4):880–888.

143. Ribeiro G, Swindell R. Adjuvant tamoxifen for male breast cancer (MBC). *Br J Cancer* 1992;65(2):252–254.

144. Eggemann H, Ignatov A, Smith BJ, et al. Adjuvant therapy with tamoxifen compared to aromatase inhibitors for 257 male breast cancer patients. *Breast Cancer Res Treat* 2013;137(2):465–470.

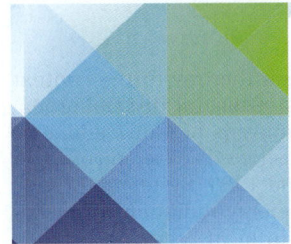

CHAPTER 61

Breast Cancer: Locally Advanced, Part 2

Meena S. Moran and Pauline Truong

INTRODUCTION

Locally advanced breast cancer (LABC) is a heterogeneous entity in the spectrum of malignant breast diseases. Definitions of LABC vary but generally encompass stage III A, B, and C (TNM stage T3 to T4 or N2 to N3) and may include stage IIB (T3N0 or T2N1) disease, as defined by the *AJCC Cancer Staging Manual*, 6th edition.[1] It is well established that women with stage III breast cancer have high risks of locoregional and distant recurrence compromising survival. Corresponding recurrence risks in women with stage IIB cancer are lower but may still be substantial. Breast cancer management is evolving toward an era of personalized medicine with advances in pathologic processing, molecular profiling, sentinel nodal staging, chemotherapy and targeted drug therapies, and conformal radiation treatment techniques. Although these advances are shifting paradigms and increasing complexities in prognostication and therapeutic decisions, the shared goals among multidisciplinary cancer care professionals treating patients with LABC remain focused on improving survival and disease control, minimizing treatment-related toxicity, and providing optimal function and cosmesis. In this context, communication between radiation oncologists with allied radiation medicine professionals, surgical and medical oncologists, plastic surgeons, radiologists, and pathologists is essential to achieve coordinated, individualized care plans for each patient with LABC.

An overview of the general management strategies for LABC has been provided in the previous chapter. The current chapter will focus on the role of radiation therapy, including regional nodal irradiation (RNI), as an adjunct to mastectomy or breast-conserving surgery in the setting of stage IIB and III disease. Data from meta-analyses and prospective randomized trials conducted in the past three decades providing valuable data to define the role of locoregional radiation therapy in contemporary practice will be reviewed. Locoregional recurrence (LRR) risks after mastectomy and systemic therapy will be examined. With the expanded use of neoadjuvant chemotherapy (NCT) not only in the setting of inoperable LABC but also in less advanced cases, radiation therapy decisions taking into consideration pretreatment disease extent, and response after NCT will be discussed.

In contemporary practice, the goal of safe and effective implementation of locoregional radiation therapy for women with LABC has been advanced by technological innovations in treatment planning and delivery. We will review and provide illustrative examples of locoregional radiation therapy techniques, with an emphasis on standardized contouring methods and rigorous adherence to dose–volume constraints. Dosimetric considerations to achieve conformal targeting and dose homogeneity to the breast/chest wall and regional nodes will be discussed. We will examine the effects of radiation therapy on critical organs at risk (OAR), particularly the cardiovascular structures, along with modern techniques including three-dimensional conformal planning and gating or active breath hold techniques to minimize cardiac exposure. Finally, issues regarding the complex interdisciplinary integration of radiation therapy with mastectomy and breast reconstruction will be discussed.

LOCOREGIONAL RADIATION THERAPY AFTER MASTECTOMY OR BREAST-CONSERVING SURGERY

Meta-Analyses of Prospective Trials

The foundation of radiation therapy as an integral component of locoregional treatment for patients with stage IIB and stage III breast cancer was built upon decades of clinical trials dating back to the 1960s, when mastectomy was considered standard of care. Accordingly, the available data from meta-analyses of adjuvant locoregional radiation therapy were predominantly derived from postmastectomy radiation therapy (PMRT) trials, which enrolled patients with operable breast and nodal disease, a proportion of whom had stage IIB or III breast cancer. In comparison, prospective trials and meta-analyses of patients with inoperable LABC and of patients with LABC managed with breast-conserving therapy are much fewer.

In an early meta-analysis published in 1987 of 7,941 patients enrolled in eight PMRT trials initiated before 1975, Cuzick et al.[2] reported no difference in survival in the first 10 years of follow-up; but beyond 10 years, an excess of deaths among radiated patients was observed. Radiation therapy was associated with reduced breast cancer–specific mortality, but this was counterbalanced by an increased risk of cardiovascular death, a risk related to radiation treatment techniques that would be considered substandard today, such as large photon fields that exposed substantial volumes of the cardiovascular and pulmonary structures to high radiation doses.[3] Although these trials were conducted in an era that predated effective systemic therapies and many of the surgical and radiation practices used are no longer applied in modern practice, the work by Cuzick et al. provided relevant early lessons in the association between locoregional control and improved breast cancer–specific survival and the importance of using heart-sparing radiation techniques to mitigate the risks of cardiac injury and cardiac death.

In 1985, the Early Breast Cancer Trialists' Collaborative Group (EBCTCG) formed an international collaborative organization with the mandate of generating and regularly updating meta-analyses using individual patient data from randomized trials of breast cancer treatment. The group defined early breast cancer as disease "in which all clinically apparent disease can be removed surgically."[4] As such, the trials analyzed in the EBCTCG overview may include LABC cases with stage IIB and III disease. As large systematic overviews using individual patient data provide the highest level evidence to address issues that may not be readily addressed by smaller trials,[5,6] the EBCTCG has, over time, contributed important data which provide the basis for current treatment guidelines and which continue to inform contemporary practice.

The first cycle of the EBCTCG meta-analysis, published in 1995, included 36 randomized trials comparing surgery alone versus surgery plus radiation therapy. Among 17,273 women enrolled in these trials, the use of radiation therapy after surgery was associated with a threefold reduced rate of local recurrence compared with surgery alone.[4]

In 2000, the group reported the 10- and 20-year results from 40 randomized trials of radiation therapy enrolling 20,000 women, half of whom had node-positive disease.[7] In these trials, adjuvant radiation therapy generally included not only the breast or chest wall, but also the axillary, supraclavicular, and internal mammary nodes (IMN). Across the trials, radiation therapy was associated with a decrease in LRR by approximately two-thirds (8.8% vs. 27.2% at 10 years), a decrease in breast cancer mortality ($2P = .0001$) but an increase in cardiovascular mortality ($2P = .0003$), and no significant difference in overall survival at 20 years ($2P = .06$).[7]

In 2005, the EBCTCG published an influential analysis reporting that, among 8,340 subjects with node-positive breast cancer treated with mastectomy and axillary dissection, PMRT to the chest wall and regional lymphatics reduced 5-year LRR by 17% from 22.8% to 5.8%.[8] By 15 years, breast cancer mortality was reduced by 5.4% (54.7% vs. 60.1%, $2P = .0002$) and overall mortality was reduced by 4.4% (64.2% vs. 59.8%, $2P = .0009$), suggesting the concept that for every four local recurrences prevented at 5 years by radiation therapy, one breast cancer death may be spared at 15 years. Importantly, radiation therapy produced similar reductions in the relative risk of LRR across trials and across subjects, irrespective of age, stage, and tumor characteristics. Although the relative risk in LRR was consistently decreased by two-thirds, the absolute risk reduction in individual subjects varied, depending on the baseline (or control) risk without therapy. As such, women with baseline LRR risks >10% would have larger absolute reductions in LRR with radiation therapy, compared to women with low risks <10%.

In the breast-conservation therapy setting, the EBCTCG investigators have contributed data in women with node-negative and node-positive breast cancer treated with breast-conserving surgery with versus without adjuvant radiation therapy.[9] Among 1,050 women with node-positive disease, radiation therapy conferred an absolute 10-year recurrence reduction of 21.2% (42.5% vs. 63.7%; 95% confidence interval [CI], 14.5 to 27.9; $2P < .00001$) and a 15-year absolute reduction in breast cancer death of 8.5% (42.8% vs. 51.3%; 95% CI, 1.8 to 15.2; $2P = .01$).

Although the EBCTCG meta-analyses provided valuable insight into the long-term effects of radiation therapy on recurrence and survival, there were limitations. Many trials included in these analyses were conducted in the 1960s and 1970s, time periods in which systemic therapy was not used and the available radiation techniques were suboptimal. Generalizability of results from such trials to the modern setting is hence limited. To address these concerns, several investigators have performed meta-analyses of trials selected based on study time period and treatment quality.

In a reanalysis of trials included in the EBCTCG meta-analysis, but with exclusion of trials initiated prior to 1970, trials with small samples, and trials that employed suboptimal radiation techniques and dose prescriptions, Van de Steene et al.[10] found significant survival benefits with radiation therapy, highlighting the need for techniques that limit radiation exposure to the cardiopulmonary structures and other normal tissues. Similarly, Gebski et al.[11] reanalyzed data from the EBCTCG 2000 meta-analysis using predefined categories of radiation therapy, classified as "optimal: doses ranging between 40 and 60 Gray (Gy) in 2 Gy fractions or a biologically equivalent dose to the chest wall, axilla, and supraclavicular fossa with or without the IMN," "inadequate or excessive: doses <40 Gy or >60 Gy in 2-Gy fractions," and "incomplete tissue coverage: target volume covered less than the chest wall and regional nodes." Local control, breast cancer–specific survival, and overall survival were all significantly improved in the "optimal" radiation group, whereas there were no survival benefits with radiation in the other groups.

To address the effect of radiation therapy in the context of systemic therapy reducing risks of distant dissemination, Whelan et al. conducted a meta-analysis of 6,367 subjects, the majority of whom had node-positive disease, enrolled in 18 trials of PMRT between 1967 and 1999. Systemic therapy was used in all subjects. Postmastectomy radiation was associated with significant reductions in local recurrence (odds ratio [OR] 0.25; 95% CI, 0.19 to 0.34) and overall mortality (OR 0.83; 95% CI, 0.74 to 0.94).[12]

In the most recent fifth update of the EBCTCG meta-analysis, published in 2014, 8,135 patients in 22 PMRT trials from 1964 to 1986 were analyzed. In this version of the overview, disease recurrence and survival outcomes were examined with stratification by pathologic nodal status. The 20-year breast cancer mortality reduction associated with PMRT was statistically significant for all patients with node-positive disease, including those with 1 to 3 and 4 or more positive nodes.[13] Among 3,786 women who underwent axillary dissection, 700 had node-negative disease, 1,214 had 1 to 3 positive nodes, and 1,772 had 4 or more positive nodes. Distinct from women with node-negative disease in whom radiation therapy had no significant effect on LRR or breast cancer mortality, women with 1 to 3 positive nodes treated with radiation experienced significantly reduced rates of LRR ($2P < .00001$), overall recurrence (relative risk [RR] 0.68; 95% CI, 0.57 to 0.82; $2P = .00006$), and breast cancer mortality (RR 0.80; 95% CI, 0.67 to 0.95; $2P = .01$). These improved outcomes were also observed among 1,133 women with 1 to 3 positive nodes who received systemic therapy with cyclophosphamide, methotrexate, and fluorouracil (CMF) or tamoxifen. In these women, PMRT was associated with significantly lower rates of 10-year isolated LRR (4.3% vs. 21.0%, $P < .00001$), overall recurrence (33.8% vs. 45.5%, $P < .00001$), and 20-year breast cancer mortality (41.5% vs. 49.4%, $P = .01$). Among 1,677 women with 4 or more positive nodes treated with systemic therapy, PMRT similarly reduced LRR (13.6% vs. 31.5%, $P < .00001$), overall recurrence (RR 0.79; 95% CI, 0.69 to 0.90; $2P = .0003$), and 20-year breast cancer mortality (70.0% vs. 78.0%, $P = .08$).

Compared to the previous 2005 EBCTCG report, which suggested a 4 to 1 relationship between recurrences and breast cancer death avoided, the 2014 EBCTCG postmastectomy analysis included women with more advanced cancer treated with more extensive radiation therapy. For these women, the 2014 meta-analysis suggested that for every 1.5 recurrences of any type avoided during the first 10 years after radiation therapy, 1 breast cancer death would be avoided at 20 years.[13]

Phase III Randomized Trials—Postmastectomy Radiation Therapy

In 1982, the Eastern Cooperative Oncology Group (ECOG) initiated a trial of PMRT, which enrolled 426 patients with operable LABC, including pathologic T3 disease with positive nodes, T4a to T4c disease (excluding T4d), N2 disease, or primary tumors fixed to underlying muscle.[14] Subjects underwent mastectomy and axillary dissection, followed by chemotherapy and hormone therapy, then restaging. The 332 patients without disease progression were randomized to PMRT versus observation with radiation reserved at time of progression. Of these, 312 patients were eligible for analysis for both time to relapse and death. After a median follow-up of 9 years, there were no significant differences in these endpoints between the two treatment arms. Patients who received radiotherapy had significantly lower LRRs (15% vs. 24%, P value not reported), but higher rates of distant progression (50% vs. 35%, $P = .003$). The trial, while well designed to address a relevant clinical issue, was ultimately limited by high proportions of noncompliance with study treatment allocation, and the numbers of patients analyzed were likely insufficient to detect a small but clinically meaningful survival difference.

In 1995, Arriagada et al.[15] reported results of a randomized trial with 960 patients treated with mastectomy without adjuvant systemic therapy randomized to receive preoperative radiotherapy, postoperative radiotherapy, or no adjuvant therapy. In this trial, PMRT use in patients with node-positive disease was associated with significantly reduced distant metastasis and overall mortality compared to unirradiated patients. These results were among the earliest data illustrating the concept that effective locoregional disease control can reduce distant dissemination and improve survival.

Danish Breast Cancer Cooperative Group and British Columbia Trials

The Danish Breast Cancer Cooperative Group (DBCG) 82b and 82c trials and the British Columbia, Canada, trials, published in 1997 and 1999, demonstrated that PMRT was associated with not only improved locoregional control but also improved overall survival.[16–18] These landmark trials, which employed protocol-defined radiation techniques treating the chest wall, IMN, supraclavicular, and axillary nodes in women treated with adjuvant systemic therapy, contributed important prospective data that defined the role of PMRT in contemporary practice.

The DBCG 82b trial enrolled 1,708 premenopausal subjects with high-risk pathologic stage II or III breast cancer, accrued between 1982 and 1989.[16] In this trial, high-risk status was defined as one or more of the following features: involvement of axillary nodes, primary tumors more than 5 cm, or invasion of the skin or pectoral fascia. After mastectomy and level I to II axillary surgery removing a median of 7 nodes, women were randomized to systemic therapy with 9 cycles of CMF chemotherapy without radiation therapy versus 8 cycles of CMF plus radiation therapy, 50 Gy in 25 fractions or 48 Gy in 22 fractions using megavoltage equipment. At a median follow-up time of 9.5 years, compared to the control group, women who received PMRT had significantly lower LRR (9% vs. 32%, $P < .001$), improved disease-free survival (48% vs. 34%, $P < .001$), and improved overall survival (54% vs. 45%, $P < .001$).

The DBCG 82c trial evaluated 1,375 postmenopausal women, accrued between 1982 and 1990, randomized to mastectomy plus 1 year of tamoxifen versus mastectomy, tamoxifen, and radiation therapy.[17] Similar to the DBCG 82b results, PMRT was associated with reduced 10-year LRR (8% vs. 35%, $P < .001$), improved disease-free survival (36% vs. 24%, $P < .001$), and improved overall survival (45% vs. 36%, $P = .03$).

In the updated analysis of both DBCG 82b and 82c trials with 15-year follow-up, which also analyzed outcomes stratified by nodal subgroups (1 to 3 vs. ≥4 positive nodes), PMRT significantly reduced LRR from 51% to 10% in patients with ≥4 positive nodes and from 27% to 4% in patients with 1 to 3 positive nodes.[19] Overall survival improvement with PMRT use was demonstrated in both subgroups with 1 to 3 positive nodes (57% vs. 48%, $P = .03$) and with ≥4 positive nodes (21% vs. 12%, $P = .03$). Chest wall failures were the most common type of LRR, representing 55% of all LRR events in the no-PMRT group and 70% of all LRR events in the PMRT group. Axillary failures were more common in the no-PMRT group, representing 43% of all LRR events in the no-PMRT group and 24% of all LRR events in the PMRT group.[20]

In an important analysis examining relationships between locoregional control and survival in three subgroups classified as good, intermediate, or poor based on tumor size, nodal status, grade, and biomarkers, Kyndi et al. reported that the magnitude of overall survival improvement with PMRT use was highest in patients with favorable-risk disease (tumors <2 cm, fewer than 3 positive nodes, grade 1, hormone receptors positive, Her2-negative disease).[21] In contrast, the high-risk subgroup (>3 positive nodes, tumors >5 cm, grade 3) had larger improvements in locoregional control, but no overall survival advantage. These findings suggest that improved locoregional control may exert a greater impact on survival in patients with favorable-risk disease with low competing risks of distant metastasis. Accordingly, these patients may gain larger survival improvements with radiation therapy optimizing locoregional control, compared to counterparts with high LRR risk and concomitant high distant progression risk.

The DBCG trials also contributed useful subset analyses documenting the risks of radiation-related late toxicities.[22–24] As older trials and meta-analyses have raised concerns regarding cardiovascular morbidity and mortality in radiated subjects, Højris et al. retrospectively analyzed data from both DBCG trials, which employed PMRT techniques that avoided cardiac exposure. At 10-year median follow-up, the rates of ischemic heart disease, acute myocardial infarction (MI), and cardiac death were similar between women treated with or without PMRT.[22] In a subset of 84 patients without evidence of disease, women who received PMRT had higher rates of lymphedema (14% vs. 3%, $P = $ ns) and impaired shoulder function (17% vs. 2%, $P = .001$).[23] Disabling brachial plexopathy was present in 5% of radiated patients.[24]

The British Columbia trial was a smaller study that randomly assigned 318 premenopausal women with node-positive disease after mastectomy and CMF chemotherapy to PMRT or no additional treatment.[18] In this trial, PMRT employed hypofractionated prescriptions of 37.5 Gy in 16 fractions to the chest wall and IMN and 35 Gy in 16 fractions to the midaxilla. In the 20-year update, women treated with PMRT were confirmed to have significantly reduced rates of LRR (10% vs. 26%, $P = .002$) and improved distant relapse-free survival (31% vs. 48%, $P = .004$) and overall survival (47% vs. 37%, $P = .03$).[25] The rates of cardiac death were 1.8% in the PMRT group and 0.6% in the control group ($P = .62$). Women treated with PMRT had higher rates of lymphedema (9% vs. 3%, $P = .035$).

In summary, the Danish and British Columbia PMRT trials reported consistent outcomes. Women with high-risk breast cancer treated with PMRT and systemic therapy had significantly reduced risks of LRR. These improvements led to improved disease-free survival and overall survival at 15- and 20-year follow-up.[19,25] These trials, taken together with the EBCTCG meta-analyses, supported the principle that by reducing LRR in the setting of effective systemic therapies, radiation therapy contributed to improved overall survival. As systemic treatment lowered the competing risk of distant metastasis, the effect of optimal locoregional control on improved survival became evident.

Phase III Randomized Trials—Regional Nodal Irradiation after Breast-Conserving Surgery or Mastectomy

In the setting of LABC, particularly in patients presenting with large T3 tumors or T4 disease, including inflammatory breast cancer, standard surgical treatment remains modified radical mastectomy. The use of breast-conserving surgery for patients with LABC, while more controversial, is being increasingly considered. Breast-conservation therapy may be applied to patients with T2 tumors with positive nodes, selected patients with operable T3 tumors with clinically node-negative disease or limited N1 involvement, and may be considered on an individualized basis with multidisciplinary review for patients with LABC with excellent response to neoadjuvant systemic therapy.

In patients with operable stage II to III breast cancer who are candidates for breast-conservation therapy, prospective trial results have emerged evaluating the role of RNI as a component of adjuvant management. The characteristics and results of these trials are summarized in Table 61.1.

TABLE 61.1 SUMMARY OF RESULTS OF THE MA20, EORTC, AND FRENCH IMN TRIALS EVALUATING REGIONAL NODAL IRRADIATION

	MA20[26]	EORTC 22922[27]	French IMN[28]
Number of subjects	1,832	4,004	1,334
	N+ or high-risk N0	N+ or medial/central tumor	N+ or medial/central tumor
Accrual period	2000–2007	1996–2004	1991–1997
Breast surgery	All BCS	75% BCS	All mastectomy
Randomization	Breast alone vs. breast + IMN/SCN/level III ± level I–II	Breast/chest wall alone vs. breast/chest wall + IMN/SCN	IMN vs. no IMN
Node positive	90% (85% 1–3N+)	56%	75%
Chemotherapy	91%	55%	61%
Outcomes (RNI vs. control)	LRRFS 95.2% vs. 92.2%, P = .009	LRRFS not reported	LRRFS not reported
	DMFS 86.3% vs. 82.4%, P = .03	DMFS 78.0% vs. 75.0%, P = .02	DMFS not reported
	DFS 82% vs. 77%, P = .01	DFS 72.1% vs. 69.1%, P = .04	DFS 53.2% vs. 49.9%, P = .35
	OS 82.8% vs. 81.8%, P = .38	OS 82.3% vs. 80.7%, p = .06	OS 62.6% vs. 59.3%, P = .8

BCS, breast-conserving surgery; DFS, disease-free survival; DMFS, distant metastasis-free survival; IMN, internal mammary nodes; LRRFS, locoregional recurrence-free survival; N+, node positive; OS, overall survival; RNI, regional nodal irradiation; SC, supraclavicular nodes.

National Cancer Institute of Canada Clinical Trial Group MA20 Trial

In 2015, the National Cancer Institute of Canada Clinical Trial Group (NCIC-CTG) MA20 trial was published after a median follow-up time of 9.5 years.[26] In this multicenter trial, 1,832 patients who underwent breast-conserving surgery and systemic therapy were randomized to receive radiation therapy to the whole breast alone (50 Gy in 25 fractions) versus radiation therapy to the whole breast (50 Gy in 25 fractions) plus regional nodes (45 Gy in 25 fractions). Axillary dissection was performed in 96% of subjects. Overall, 85% had 1 to 3 positive nodes, 5% had 4 or more positive nodes, and 10% had high-risk node-negative disease, defined as tumors >2 cm with ≤10 nodes removed, plus one or more of the following features: grade 3 histology, lymphovascular invasion, or estrogen receptor (ER)-negative disease. LABC, defined as stage IIB to III disease, was represented by 45% of subjects. RNI included the ipsilateral IMN in the first 3 intercostal spaces and the supraclavicular and level III axillary nodes. For patients with fewer than 10 nodes removed or 4 or more positive nodes, the target volume also included level I and II axillary nodes.

At 10 years, RNI was associated with improved locoregional disease-free survival (95.2% vs. 92.2%, P = .009) and distant disease-free survival (86.3% vs. 82.4%, P = .03), but no difference in overall survival (82.8% and 81.8%, P = .38). In a planned subset analysis, women with ER-negative disease randomized to RNI had improved disease-free survival and overall survival compared to no RNI. The majority of regional recurrences occurred in the axilla (63% of patients) or the supraclavicular nodes (27%). The rate of lymphedema was higher in the RNI group (8.4% vs. 4.5%, P = .001). The rates of grade 2 or higher cardiac and pulmonary toxicities were low (<1%) and were similar in the two study groups.

European Organisation for Research and Treatment of Cancer 22922 Trial

The European Organisation for Research and Treatment of Cancer (EORTC) 22922 trial evaluated elective radiation to the IMN and medial supraclavicular fossa in conjunction with whole-breast radiation after breast-conserving surgery or chest wall radiation after mastectomy.[27] Between 1996 and 2004, 4,004 patients with stage I to III breast cancer with a central or inner quadrant tumor with node-negative or node-positive disease or an outer quadrant tumor with node-positive disease were enrolled after breast-conserving surgery (76%) or mastectomy (24%). In this trial, the majority of patients had early-stage breast cancer (34% stage I and 32% stage IIA disease). 33% of subjects had LABC, including 19% stage IIB and 14% stage III disease. Systemic therapy was used in 99% of node-positive and 66% of node-negative subjects. Subjects were randomized to radiation to the IMN and supraclavicular

nodes: 50 Gy in 25 fractions, 26 Gy with photons (ranging from Co60 to 10 MV photons), and 24 Gy with electrons or no IMN–supraclavicular radiation. Radiation was delivered to the IMN in the first three intercostal spaces, up to and including the first five intercostal spaces in patients with lower inner quadrant tumors. Among subjects who underwent mastectomy, 76% had chest wall radiation in conjunction with RNI. The axillary nodes were included in the target volume in 8.3% of the IMN–supraclavicular radiation group and 7.4% in the control (no IMN–supraclavicular radiation) group. At 10 years, the RNI group had lower rate of any first recurrence (19.4% vs. 22.9%, P = .02) and higher rates of distant disease-free survival (78% vs. 72%, P = .02). Overall survival was 82.3% in the RNI group and 80.7% in the control groups (P = .06). As in the MA20 trial, the EORTC trial demonstrated that RNI was beneficial for women with node-positive disease with respect to breast cancer–specific outcomes, but the difference in overall survival at 10 years was small and did not reach statistical significance. The rate of lung fibrosis was higher in the RNI group (4.4% vs. 1.7%, P < .001), whereas the rate of cardiac disease was comparable in the two groups (6.5% vs. 5.6%, P = .25).

French Trial of Internal Mammary Nodal Irradiation

The MA20 and EORTC trials both reported improved recurrence and disease-free survival with RNI including the IMN and supraclavicular nodes, but their studies were not designed to address the question of which specific nodal basin coverage contributed to the observed improvements in outcomes. A French multicenter prospective trial attempted to evaluate the impact of specific IMN targeting in patients undergoing total mastectomy and axillary dissection.[28] From 1991 to 1997, 1,334 patients with stage I to III disease were enrolled, approximately 35% of whom had LABC. All subjects received radiation with two-dimensional planning to the chest wall, supraclavicular, and apical axillary nodes, with randomization to radiation to the IMN in the first five intercostal spaces versus no IMN inclusion. Ten-year overall survival rates were 62.6% in the IMN-treated group and 59.3% in the control group, but this difference was not statistically significant (P = .8).

Although the trial attempted to address an important question, its design was unfortunately limited. The sample size was calculated to detect a 10% difference in 10-year overall survival, an expectation inconsistent with the finding from the EBCTCG meta-analysis that the survival benefit with PMRT was approximately 4% to 5%.[8] The trial was hence underpowered to detect a small survival difference. Other limitations include the use of two-dimensional planning and a lack of rigorous methods to capture cardiac toxicity events, further limiting the trial's applicability to modern practice.

Budach et al. Meta-Analysis

After publication of the MA20, EORTC, and French IMN trials, Budach et al.[29] performed a meta-analysis of these three trials. RNI of the IMN and supraclavicular nodes as delivered in the MA20 and EORTC trials was associated with significant improvement in disease-free survival (HR 0.86; 95% CI, 0.78 to 0.95), distant disease-free survival (HR 0.84; 95 % CI, 0.75 to 0.94), and overall survival (HR 0.88; 95% CI, 0.78 to 0.99). Adding results of the French trial using a random effects model to take into account the different design of the French trial, the effect of RNI on overall survival remained significant (HR 0.90; 95% CI, 0.82 to 0.99).

In summary, the meta-analyses and randomized PMRT trials with 15- to 20-year follow-up and the more recent trials of RNI after breast-conserving surgery or mastectomy with 10-year follow-up have advanced our insight into the role of radiation therapy in the management of patients with operable LABC. Although LABC is a heterogeneous entity, consistent improvements in the recurrence and survival outcomes reported across these trials support the use of locoregional RT as an essential component of management for women with LABC, a population with high to extreme risks of locoregional and distant recurrence. When used in conjunction with systemic therapy, radiation therapy can optimize locoregional and distant disease control, reduce the morbidity of uncontrolled cancer progression, and provide incremental improvements in survival.

ADJUVANT REGIONAL NODAL IRRADIATION CONSIDERATIONS

Indications in Stage IIB and IIIC Disease

The EBCTCG meta-analyses and randomized trials of locoregional radiation therapy after mastectomy or breast-conserving surgery have provided valuable data for the development of clinical practice guidelines and consensus statements from national and international expert panels.[30–39] Across the available guidelines, there is clear consensus that locoregional radiation therapy encompassing the breast/chest wall plus regional nodes is indicated for patients with advanced primary T3 and T4 tumors, N2 to N3 disease, and inflammatory breast cancer because of their high risk of LRR in excess of 30% to 40%.[40–46] The role of locoregional radiation therapy for patients with stage IIB disease with 1 to 3 positive nodes or T3N0 disease requires multidisciplinary, individualized consideration.

Target Volume Considerations

As the randomized trials of locoregional radiation therapy employed comprehensive targeting of the IMN and supraclavicular/apical level III axillary nodes and, in some cases, level I and II axilla, data regarding the individual effects of targeting specific nodal basins are lacking. Recognizing this caveat, decision-making regarding when to treat the regional nodes and which nodal basins to target may still be informed by available prospective trials and studies of patterns of relapse.

After mastectomy without radiation therapy, the most common site of locoregional relapse is the chest wall, occurring in more than 50% of patients who experienced LRR.[20,43–46] Another common site of LRR is the supraclavicular nodes and axillary apex, representing 20% to 40% of all LRR events.[43–46] Based on these relapse patterns, for women with stage IIB to III disease who are candidates for locoregional radiation therapy, the target volume should encompass at a minimum the entire chest wall, supraclavicular nodes, and axillary apex.

As LABC represents a wide spectrum of nodal recurrence risk, the use of full axillary nodal irradiation should be individualized. In an analysis of regional nodal failure patterns

in 1,031 patients treated with mastectomy including level I to II axillary dissection and enrolled in five trials doxorubicin-based chemotherapy with no PMRT at the MD Anderson Cancer Center (MDACC), Strom et al.[45] reported that the 10-year rates of recurrence were 3% within the low-mid axilla. The risk of failure in the low-mid axilla was not significantly higher for patients with increasing numbers of involved nodes, percentage of involved nodes, nodal size, or gross extranodal extension. These findings suggest that radiation targeting the dissected axilla may not be warranted for most patients, when balanced against increased risks of lymphedema and arm morbidity. This benefit versus risk balance, however, is changing as nodal staging standards have shifted from routine axillary dissection to sentinel node biopsy.[47–51] As in all therapeutic decision-making for locoregional RT, the estimated risks of regional nodal recurrence and estimated benefits that axillary RT may provide should be carefully balanced against risks of adverse effects including lymphedema, chronic arm morbidity, and brachial plexopathy.

IMN Irradiation

Indications for the specific targeting of the IMN remain controversial.[52–54] Historically, studies of extended radical mastectomy have identified IMN metastases in large proportions of patients with LABC, particularly in association with extensive nodal disease and central or medial tumor location.[55] Patients with clinically or pathologically detected IMN disease clearly warrant radiation therapy targeting the disease. In patients without IMN involvement, the relative benefits of treating the IMN are unclear and hence difficult to balance against potential risks of increasing heart and lung exposure with IMN inclusion. It is noted that in all of the randomized trials that demonstrated benefits with RNI, the IMNs were routinely included in the target volume. Although the benefits observed with RNI in these trials may be attributed to the principle of radiation eradicating subclinical disease that may be a source for distant metastasis, it is not possible to assess how much of the benefits observed may be specifically attributed to IMN treatment.

In this context, additional insight into the effect of IMN radiation may be gained from the DBCG IMN study, a prospective population-based cohort study with 3,089 patients with node-positive breast cancer.[56] In this study, patients with right-sided disease were treated with IMN irradiation and patients with left-sided disease were followed without IMN treatment. At a median follow-up of 8.9 years, statistically significant improvements in breast cancer–specific survival and overall survival were observed with IMN irradiation. In an exploratory subset analysis, the benefit of IMN irradiation was more pronounced in patients at high risk of IMN involvement, specifically those with node-positive medial/central tumors and those with 4 or more positive nodes irrespective of tumor location. The rate of death from ischemic heart disease was not elevated in the IMN-treated group. These data, while interesting, should be interpreted with caution. The study was nonrandomized, and the use of systemic therapy was lower than today's standards. It is also noteworthy that in this analysis, IMN irradiation was not observed to be associated with improved survival in women with lateral tumors and 1 to 3 positive nodes, a group of women likely with lower risk compared to central/medial tumors or more advanced nodal disease.

Based on the available data discussed, decisions regarding IMN inclusion in the target volume require caution and careful consideration of the uncertainty regarding its relative benefit and the potential for increased cardiopulmonary exposure. IMN treatment is justified for women with clinical or pathologically IMN involvement. As a component of adjuvant locoregional treatment, in light of randomized controlled data demonstrating benefits with comprehensive nodal treatment, IMN inclusion may be considered, particularly for women with advanced primary (T3/T4) or nodal disease (N2/N3), and women with node-positive medial/central tumors. When the decision is made to include the IMN as a component of PMRT or RNI, careful treatment planning using conformal techniques is essential to ensure that dose constraints to the heart and lungs are safely met.

RISKS OF LOCOREGIONAL RECURRENCE AFTER MASTECTOMY AND SYSTEMIC TREATMENT

Stage III

Estimates of the risks of LRR after mastectomy and systemic treatment may be derived from meta-analyses of prospective trials comparing cohorts treated with versus without radiation therapy. The 2014 EBCTCG meta-analysis suggested that for every 1.5 recurrences of any type avoided during the first 10 years after radiation, 1 breast cancer death would be avoided at 20 years.[13] It is thus important to note that, with the exception of patients with node-negative cancer treated with axillary dissection who have low LRR risk <10%, all other subgroups, the majority of whom had node-positive disease treated with mastectomy and axillary dissection without RT, had LRR risks in the 20% to 30% range. At this risk magnitude, adjuvant locoregional radiation may reasonably be considered for the potential benefits in reductions of recurrence and breast mortality risk previously discussed.

Corroborating data from randomized trials and meta-analyses, multiple institutional studies have reported that patients with advanced primary T3 or T4 tumors or ≥4 positive lymph nodes have high LRR risks >30% following mastectomy and chemotherapy.[57-62] As modern randomized trials have demonstrated that PMRT improved the 15- and 20-year overall survival outcomes of breast cancer patients with LRR risks of this magnitude, international consensus statements and guidelines have clearly endorsed recommendations for PMRT in these high-risk subgroups.[31-40]

Stage IIB T2N1

Distinct from patients with advanced primary tumors or extensive nodal burden, LRR risk estimates and locoregional management in patients with T1 to T2 breast cancer with 1 to 3 positive axillary nodes have long been more controversial. A paradigm shift, however, may be occurring as we now have data from the 2014 EBCTCG meta-analysis providing evidence that PMRT significantly improves overall survival in all patient subsets with node-positive breast cancer, including women with 1 to 3 positive nodes, irrespective of axillary surgery extent or systemic therapy use.[13] We also now have consistent data from the MA20 trial (which included predominantly women with 1 to 3 positive nodes) and the EORTC trial that RNI significantly reduced not only LRR but also distant relapse and breast cancer mortality.[27,28] The DBCG PMRT subset analysis showed that the magnitude of overall survival improvement was greatest not in women with the highest LRR risk but in women with more favorable risk in whom the competing risk of distant metastasis was lower.[23] These data, interpreted in light of the concept from the EBCTCG 2014 meta-analysis that for every 1.5 recurrences avoided, 1 breast cancer death could be spared,[13] support considerations for using RNI for women with 1 to 3 positive nodes after mastectomy and breast-conserving surgery.

The long-standing controversy in the setting of 1 to 3 positive nodes centered on observed discrepancies between the magnitudes of LRR risks reported in the PMRT trials compared to large institutional series of patients treated with mastectomy and systemic therapy. In the Danish trials, the 10-year LRR rate without PMRT was approximately 30%[16,17] and the 18-year rate was 37%,[20] substantially higher than the LRR rates observed in the British Columbia trial (16% at 10 years and 21% at 20 years)[18,21] and in numerous institutional studies of patients treated with mastectomy and adjuvant systemic therapy without radiation (LRR ~10% to 15% at 10 years).[58-80] Variations in surgical staging and axillary clearance have been implicated as the source of discrepancy in these observed risks. The disproportionately greater rates of LRR in the DBCG trials have been attributed to limited axillary surgery potentially compromising staging accuracy and locoregional disease control. The DBCG investigators have addressed this by reanalyzing their data evaluating specifically subjects with eight or more nodes resected.[19] Among patients with 1 to 3 positive nodes, PMRT was still associated with significant reduced LRR (4% vs. 27%) and improved overall survival (57% vs. 48%).

In the EBCTCG 2014 meta-analysis, 10-year LRR rates among patients with 1 to 3 positive nodes treated with mastectomy and systemic therapy were 21% without PMRT and 4.3% with PMRT ($P < .0001$).[13] The 10-year LRR rates reported in institutional studies in women with 1 to 3 positive nodes treated with mastectomy and systemic therapy without PMRT were lower by comparison, approximating 10% to 15%.[58-80] Notably, the more recent series reported rates even lower LRR rates of <10%.[74-76] These trends in declining LRR rates over time may be attributable to earlier diagnosis, less advanced stage at presentation, improved surgical techniques, and availability of more effective systemic therapies.

Numerous groups have examined prognostic factors for high LRR risk among patients with 1 to 3 positive nodes treated with mastectomy and systemic therapy without radiation therapy. Factors that have been identified to be associated with LRR risk include age, tumor size, tumor location, grade, lymphovascular invasion, surgical margins, number of positive nodes, nodal ratio, extranodal extension, biomarker status, and systemic therapy use. Prognostic models have been proposed[62-66] using combinations of such factors to estimate LRR risk, but these models require validation before they can be applied to routine practice. Molecular subtyping[81-83] has also emerged as a promising tool to improve prognostication and treatment selection, but further studies are still needed.

A joint ASCO/ASTRO/SSO expert panel recently convened to formulate a focused PMRT guideline update in response to the publication of the 2014 EBCTCG meta-analysis.[37] Although the panel unanimously accepted that the available evidence supported the findings that PMRT reduced the risks of recurrence and mortality in patients with T1 to T2 breast cancer with 1 to 3 positive nodes, concerns remained that the results of EBCTCG meta-analysis based on older trials may not be generalizable to the advances available in modern practice. Concerns also remained that there may still be some patient subsets with such low LRR risks that the absolute benefit of radiation therapy may be offset by potential toxicities. The panel hence agreed that clinicians should consider factors that may be associated with decreased risks of LRR when balancing benefits versus risks of PMRT. Although there are no current validated methods to identify node-positive, low-risk subsets, the panel suggested that these factors may include patient characteristics such as age, life expectancy, and comorbid conditions; pathologic findings such as T1 tumors, no lymphovascular invasion, single positive node, and/or small size of nodal metastasis; substantial response to neoadjuvant systemic therapy; and favorable intrinsic characteristics such as low-grade disease and strongly positive hormone receptors.

Until such low-risk subsets can be clearly identified, decision-making in patients with 1 to 3 positive nodes should continue to be multidisciplinary, taking into consideration the results of the randomized trials and meta-analyses demonstrating that radiation therapy reduces LRR, distant recurrence, and breast cancer mortality not only in patients with high LRR risks but also in those with more favorable-risk disease. The benefits in reducing recurrence and improving survival should be balanced against potential risks and should be carefully communicated, taking into consideration the individual patient's therapeutic goals and personal preferences.

Prospective randomized trials are needed to provide evidence-based data for prognostication and locoregional treatment decisions in women with 1 to 3 positive nodes. The United Kingdom *Selective Use of Postoperative Radiotherapy AftEr MastectOmy* (SUPREMO) randomized trial is designed to evaluate the role of postmastectomy radiation to the chest wall in women with intermediate-risk stage II disease.[84] The trial has enrolled 1,688 patients between 2006 and 2013. Although the trial is not generalizable to the vast majority of patients with LABC and does not address ongoing questions regarding nodal irradiation, it will provide valuable data regarding the role of chest wall irradiation, patterns of relapse, and survival outcomes for patients with intermediate-risk breast cancer.

Another highly pertinent trial is the Canadian Cancer Trials Group MA39 Tailor RT trial, currently in planning stages. In this multi-institutional phase III trial, molecular analysis will be performed to identify women with favorable-risk subtype with 1 to 2 positive nodes after sentinel node staging or 1 to 3 positive nodes after axillary dissection. Eligible subjects treated with breast-conserving surgery will be randomized to radiation therapy to the breast alone versus breast and regional nodes, whereas subjects treated with mastectomy will be randomized to PMRT versus observation. The trial, which will be conducted internationally during the modern era of sentinel node staging, 3D conformal RT planning, and effective targeted systemic therapy, will provide essential data to advance our efforts to optimize therapy for women with 1 to 3 positive nodes.

Stage IIB T3N0

Women with pT3N0 breast cancer, as defined by the AJCC Cancer Staging Manual, 6th edition, as stage IIB breast cancer with primary tumor >5 cm without direct extension to the chest wall or skin, and no nodal metastasis,[1] comprise another group of patients in whom LRR risk estimate is controversial. Prospective randomized trials included very few pT3N0 cases.[16–18,26–28] The relative rarity of pT3N0 breast cancer is likely related to the fact that the majority of patients with large tumors >5 cm will be found to have nodal involvement at surgery, including those deemed clinically node-negative. As with other uncommon clinical scenarios, risk estimates in pT3N0 disease are challenging because of limited data available.

The DBCG 82b and 82c trials performed subgroup analysis on high-risk node-negative disease, comprising 8% to 10% of subjects enrolled. This subgroup included pT3 and pT4 disease with involvement of chest wall and skin.[16,17] In the DBCG82b trial of premenopausal women treated with CMF, PMRT in this subgroup was associated with reduced 10-year LRR from 17% to 3% and improved overall survival from 70% to 82%.[16] However, in the DBCG82c trial of postmenopausal women treated with tamoxifen, PMRT reduced 10-year LRR from 23% to 6%, but there was no difference in overall survival (56% with PMRT vs. 55% without PMRT).[17]

In the absence of consistent prospective data on LRR risk and the effect of PMRT in pT3N0 breast cancer, investigators have used other data sources to address the controversy. Floyd and Taghian[85] highlighted a wide range in reported LRR from 7.1% to 60% among patients with T3N0 disease. In a multi-institutional analysis that combined pT2 = 5 cm N0 and pT3 > 5 cm N0 cases treated without PMRT yielding 70 cases, the 5-year cumulative LRR rate was 7.6%.[86] Similarly,

in a pooled analysis of five National Surgical Adjuvant Breast Project (NSABP) randomized trials of systemic therapy with 313 cases, Taghian et al.[87] reported a 10-year isolated LRR of 7%. Although neither study included a comparison cohort treated with PMRT, the low LRR rates observed raised questions regarding whether PMRT should be routinely used in these subjects.

Several retrospective studies have reported LRR rates in women with T3N0 breast cancer treated with and without PMRT. Mignano et al.[88] reported on 101 cases with T3N0 breast cancer treated with mastectomy without radiation. At a median follow-up of 93 months, the rate of LRR was 11%. Helinto et al.[89] compared 33 patients with pT3N0 breast cancer treated with PMRT with 5 patients treated without PMRT. LRR was significantly lower in the PMRT compared to the no-PMRT group, 9% versus 40%. In analysis from the British Columbia Cancer Agency with 100 node-negative cases with tumors ≥5 cm, 44 of whom received PMRT, Goulart et al.[90] reported that the 10-year LRR rates in women treated with PMRT was 2.3%, compared to 8.9% without PMRT. These series, however, were limited by very small samples and selection biases inherent in their retrospective design.

The effect of PMRT on disease-specific survival and overall survival has also been examined in retrospective, registry-based analyses with variable results. Using the Surveillance Epidemiology and End Results (SEER) database, McCammon et al.[91] analyzed a cohort of 1865 women with T3N0 tumors treated with mastectomy from 1988 to 2002, in which one-third of patients received PMRT. No significant difference in 10-year breast cancer–specific survival was found between the subgroups treated with or without PMRT. In contrast, in a more contemporary SEER analysis, Johnson et al.[92] examined 2,525 women with T3N0 disease treated with mastectomy from 2000 to 2010, 1,063 of whom received PMRT. At a median follow-up of 56 months, PMRT was found to be associated with significant improvements in both breasts cancer–specific survival and overall survival. Similarly, Cassidy et al.[93] analyzed 3,437 patients with T3N0 breast cancer treated with mastectomy between 2003 and 2011 identified in the National Cancer Database (NCDB). PMRT was found to be associated with improved overall survival, regardless of surgical margin status, tumor size, and systemic therapy use. Francis et al. reported comparable results in another NCDB analysis of 4291 T3N0 patients treated between 2004 and 2012, 47% of whom underwent PMRT.[94] After propensity score matching analysis to address potential confounders, PMRT use was found to be associated with improved overall survival at 5 years and 10 years.

Acknowledging the limitations of available data, in the 2001 ASCO guidelines, PMRT was "suggested" for patients with pT3, node-positive and operable stage III breast cancer.[36] Similarly, the 2017 NCCN Guidelines advised clinicians to "consider" radiation therapy after mastectomy for patients with pT3N0 disease.[34]

LOCOREGIONAL RADIATION THERAPY AFTER NEOADJUVANT CHEMOTHERAPY

In the multimodality management of patients with LABC, NCT is now standard of care. As an initial treatment, NCT has the potential to simultaneously reduce tumor bulk in the breast and regional nodes and reduce the risk of distant dissemination. In recent years, NCT use has expanded beyond the setting of inoperable disease to also include patients with operable tumors who may experience disease downstaging and gain opportunities to be considered for breast-conserving therapy or less extensive and morbid axillary surgery. As NCT use increases, knowledge on its impact on subsequent locoregional treatment decisions continues to evolve. Data to guide radiation therapy decision-making after NCT are limited. A systematic review by Fowble et al. included 24 studies, 23 of which were single institution retrospective analyses plus one combined analysis of the NSAPBP B18 and B27 trials of NCT providing the sole source of prospective, multi-institutional data.[95]

Retrospective Data of LRR Risk after NAC and Mastectomy with Versus without PMRT

The MDACC has contributed several retrospective analyses documenting recurrence risks in patients with predominantly stage II to III disease treated with NCT followed by mastectomy with or without PMRT. In these series, when used, locoregional radiation therapy encompassed the chest wall, IMN, and undissected lymphatics in the supraclavicular and axillary regions. Among 150 patients with LABC treated with NAC followed by mastectomy without radiation therapy, Buchholz et al.[96] documented that the 10-year rate of LRR was 27%. On multivariable analysis, clinical IIIB or more advanced disease, pathologic involvement of 4 or more axillary nodes, and lack of tamoxifen use were significantly associated with higher LRR.

In another series also from MDACC, Huang et al. compared 542 patients treated with NAC and mastectomy with PMRT to 134 patients treated with NAC and mastectomy without PMRT.[97,98] At 10 years, PMRT was associated with reduced LRR (11% vs. 22%, $P = .0001$). Patients with clinical stage III to IV disease and pathologic complete response (pCR) who received PMRT had lower rates of LRR at 10 years compared to counterparts who did not receive PMRT (3% vs. 33%, $P = .006$).

McGuire et al. reported a series of 226 patients treated at MDACC who achieved pCR after NAC and mastectomy. Patients with stage I to II disease with pCR who were treated with PMRT did not experience LRR. The 10-year LRR rates among patients with stage III disease who had pCR treated with PMRT was 7.3%, compared to 33% without PMRT ($P = .04$).[99] Finally, Garg et al.[100] reported on 132 patients with clinical stage I to II disease treated with NAC and mastectomy without PMRT. Factors associated with increased LRR were young age, stage T3N0 disease, 4 or more positive nodes, and lack of tamoxifen use.

Despite selection biases inherent in retrospective studies, these contributions from the MDACC were instructive in highlighting the finding that patients with locally advanced or T3N0 disease, despite having pCR to NAC, still have high LRR risk when PMRT was not used and that patients with early-stage (I to II) disease with pCR had low rates of LRR, irrespective of PMRT use.

NSAPBP B18 and B27 Combined Analysis of Recurrence Patterns after NCT and Mastectomy

The NSABP B18 and B27 randomized trials were trials of NAC with doxorubicin and cyclophosphamide alone or followed by neoadjuvant/adjuvant docetaxel.[101] These trials did not permit the use of chest wall/RNI after mastectomy or RNI after breast-conserving surgery as during that study era (accrual between 1988 and 1993 for B18 and between 1995 and 2000 for B27), it was not yet known that radiation can improve survival. Trial participants had operable cT1-3N0-1 breast cancer, diagnosed by fine needle aspiration or core biopsy. Patients with LABC with T4 or N2/3 disease were not included. In the combined analysis with 3,088 patients (1,947 mastectomy and 1,100 breast-conserving surgery), the 10-year cumulative incidence of LRR after mastectomy was 12.3% (8.9% local and 3.4% regional) and 10.3% after breast-conserving therapy (8.1% local and 2.2% regional). The 10-year LRR risks after NAC and mastectomy according to pre-NAC clinical stage and post-NAC pathologic response

TABLE 61.2 SUMMARY OF RESULTS OF THE NSABP B18 AND B27 COMBINED ANALYSIS OF 10-YEAR LRR RISK AFTER NCT IN PATIENTS TREATED WITH MASTECTOMY

	ypN0; Breast pCR		ypN0; No Breast pCR		ypN+; Any Breast Response	
	N	10-year LRR	N	10-year LRR	N	10-year LRR
≤5 cm; cN0	46	6.5%	178	6.3%	184	11.2%
>5 cm; cN0	16	6.2%	95	11.8%	179	14.6%
≤5 cm; cN+	21	0%	37	10.8%	143	17.0%
>5 cm; cN+	11	0%	33	9.2%	128	22.5%

cN0 or cN+, clinical node-negative or node-positive before NAC; NAC, neoadjuvant chemotherapy; pCR, pathologic complete response; ypN0 or ypN+, pathologic node-negative or node-positive after NAC.

are summarized in Table 61.2. Among patients treated with mastectomy with pathologic node-positive disease after NAC, LRR risks ranged between 11.2% and 22.5%, a risk magnitude at which locoregional RT should be considered. Patients who presented with either clinical node-negative or node-positive disease who were found to have no pathologic nodal disease after NAC had LRR risks ranging from 6% to 12%. Finally, in patients with clinically node-positive disease before NAC but who achieved pCR at mastectomy, the LRR rate was 0% at 10 years, suggesting that this may be a favorable-risk subset in whom PMRT avoidance may be studied in a clinical trial setting. In patients treated with breast-conserving therapy, the risk of regional nodal recurrence was approximately 7% to 9% in patients with clinical or pathologic node-positive disease, supporting consideration for RNI.

On multivariable analysis, clinical node-positive disease before NAC and no breast or nodal pCR after NAC were predictors of increased LRR after mastectomy or breast-conserving therapy. Additional risk factors for LRR were clinical tumor size >5 cm in patients treated with mastectomy and age <50 in patients treated with breast-conserving therapy. Although the NASBP combined analysis provided useful data from a large patient cohort documenting the 10-year LRR risks without adjuvant PMRT or post–breast-conserving surgery (BCS) RNI after NAC, interpretation of these results in the modern context is limited as the study lacked information on hormone receptors and Her2 status at presentation and was conducted before the era of more effective chemotherapy and targeted anti-Her2 therapy.

Until additional data from more modern prospective trials become available, the outcomes derived from available institutional series and the NSABP B18 and B27 combined analysis support the position that PMRT should be recommended after NAC and mastectomy for patients presenting with stage III disease as these patients, including those with pCR, have high LRR risks. Patients with pathologically positive nodes after NAC constitute another group with high LRR risk warranting PMRT consideration. These recommendations are consistent with a National Cancer Institute statement that supports the use of PMRT to the chest wall and regional nodes for patients with clinical stage III disease or patients with residual histologically positive nodes after NAC.[102]

In contrast, the role of PMRT in patients with stage I to II disease is less clear as these patients have intermediate LRR risks. The ASCO/ASTRO/SSO panel stated that, on the basis of available data, stage I to II patients with persistently involved nodes on axillary dissection after NAC have sufficiently high risks of LRR to warrant PMRT recommendations.[37] Rates of LRR in patients with residual invasive cancer in the breast but pathologically negative nodes after NAC were inconsistent across different reports. Although stage I to II patients with pCR may have low rates of LRR, there remain insufficient data to exclude the possibility that some subgroups may still benefit from PMRT. Hence, the panel was not able to provide recommendations for or against PMRT use in these patients at this time.

Since the publication of the combined analysis of the NSABP B18 and B27 trials, other investigators have examined the impact of PMRT or post-BCS RNI in patients with clinically node-positive disease treated with NAC. In an analysis of 15,315 patients identified in the National Cancer Database (NCDB) with cT1-3cN1 disease, stratified into four subgroups by type of surgery and pathologic nodal status after NAC (ypN0 vs. ypN+), the use of PMRT was associated with improved overall survival for all pathologic nodal subgroups, whereas the addition of post-BCS RNI to breast RT was not associated with overall survival differences.[103] Interesting reports have also emerged suggesting that molecular subtype[104,105] and novel strategies to combine clinical and pathologic staging variables[106] may be used to improve prognostication of LRR risk after NAC.

Finally, in a study of practice patterns, Haffty et al.[107] evaluated participants of the American College of Surgeons Oncology Group Z1071 trial, a prospective study designed to evaluate the false-negative rate of sentinel node surgery after NAC. In this trial, RT decisions were at the discretion of the treating radiation oncologists. Although the majority of patients with clinically node-positive cancer treated with NAC received PMRT, the use of PMRT was less common in patients undergoing reconstruction and that there were wide variations in PMRT field design. These practices were not consistent with expert recommendations, highlighting the need for improved uniformity in RT following NAC.

Ultimately, prospective trial data are needed to address the role of locoregional RT after NAC and surgery. Two North American multicenter trials are underway for patients with biopsy-proven node-positive disease before NAC. The NRG Oncology Group 9353 trial, initiated in 2013, randomizes patients with clinical T1 to T3, N1 breast cancer (after fine needle aspiration cytology or core biopsy confirmation of positive nodes) who undergo NAC followed by mastectomy or BCS and have pathologically negative nodes, to either no radiation or PMRT to the chest wall or reconstructed breast and regional nodes or radiation to the breast or breast plus RNI (ClinicalTrials.gov identifier NCT01872975). The Alliance for Clinical Trials in Oncology A011202 trial will randomize patients with a positive sentinel node biopsy after NAC to axillary dissection versus axillary radiation therapy without axillary surgery (ClinicalTrials.gov identifier NCT01901094). These trials will provide valuable data to improve our understanding of the role of locoregional radiation after NCT for patients with LABC.

TREATMENT TECHNIQUES AFTER MASTECTOMY OR BCT WITH REGIONAL NODAL IRRADIATION

Though external beam radiation can be delivered using cobalt machines or linear accelerators (LINACs), the techniques for radiation treatment to the breast and chest wall have evolved significantly since their initial use in the 1940s. Compared with cobalt machines, which deliver photon energies of 1.2 and 1.3 MV and only have the ability to adequately penetrate superficial depths, modern radiation delivery techniques utilize LINACs with multiple beam energies up to 20 MV, and three-dimensional treatment planning and delivery are facilitated by tools such as multislice computed tomography (CT) simulators, computerized treatment planning software, and on-board imaging systems. It is now widely recognized that the techniques utilized in the early breast-conservation therapy and PMRT trials using cobalt machines and older radiation delivery techniques subjected patients unintentionally to excessive doses to normal tissues such as the heart, lung, and contralateral breast. Over time and with longer follow-up, we have learned that this exposure to normal tissue increases

risks of cardiovascular, pulmonary, and soft tissue complications including cardiac-related deaths (in left-sided treatment) and secondary malignancies (contralateral breast, lung cancer).[2-4,7,8]

With improvements in treatment planning and delivery, the benefits of radiation for locoregional and disease-free outcomes for breast cancer after breast-conserving surgery and after mastectomy have resulted in a small but significant survival benefit.[7-13] Though it is unlikely that these modern radiation advances have improved the *absolute* magnitude of the benefits in locoregional control, these technologic improvements have resulted in more precise and conformal treatment delivery that spares normal tissue. In this context, improved techniques have the potential to significantly affect survival outcomes, by shifting the proportions in the risks to benefits to ultimately achieve an improvement in the therapeutic ratio. This section will examine the traditional tangential and more conformal radiation techniques for breast, chest wall, and regional nodal radiation. We will discuss considerations in target volume delineation, dose prescriptions, optimal dosimetry to optimize homogeneity to target tissues and meet normal tissue constraints, and methods of delivery to maximize locoregional control and minimize toxicity.

Simulation

At the time of simulation, a virtual simulation with CT simulator is preferable for treatment planning purposes, though a fluoroscopic simulator may be used for two-dimensional treatment planning when CT technology or modern treatment planning software and linear accelerators are not available. Patients are initially immobilized in the treatment position, with immobilization devices ranging from commonly utilized commercial supine breast boards or prone boards to customized VacLok, Alpha Cradle, and lateral decubitus positioning devices.[108] Typically, one or both arms may be positioned above the head when in the supine or prone position but may be adjusted as needed for patient comfort but ensuring that the arm(s) do not intercept with treatment beams. The supine position is most common, with the ipsilateral arm abducted to 90 to 120 degrees and externally rotated. In assessing arm position, it is important to have the soft tissues of the arm cranial to the junction of the tangent and supraclavicular fossa field. In addition, skin folds within the supraclavicular fossa should be avoided if possible. Patients are placed on a 10- to 15-degree angle board to flatten the slope of the chest wall in the region of the sternum. The face should be turned to the contralateral side to displace the mandible from the supraclavicular field.

At simulation, patients should be clinically assessed with palpation of the areas at risk and delineation of the clinical borders of the breast/chest wall and surgical scars with radio-opaque wire markers. Thus, the clinical target volume (CTV) may be visualized on the planning CT together with the anatomic landmarks, allowing for conformal treatment beam design. The volumes to be wired should include all breast tissue, and in the case of mastectomy, the entire chest wall and mastectomy scar. The traditional clinical borders were typically defined at the inferior portion of the clavicular head superiorly; the midaxillary line laterally; the midsternum medially; 2 cm below the inframammary fold (using the contralateral inframammary fold as a reference, in patients treated with mastectomy), clearing air by 2 to 3 cm over the chest wall/breast tissue anteriorly; and 1 to 3 cm of the lung posteriorly to the edge of the tangential field edge.[109] For PMRT, the entire chest wall and mastectomy scar should be encompassed. Although these clinical borders solely define the treatment borders with fluoroscopic simulation, they also provide a general guide in the case of three-dimensional CT planning and therefore should be considered at the time of CT simulation.

Section III

Typically, CT slice thicknesses of 2 to 3 mm should be used. Because the anatomic structures are reconstructed from these slices with a certain thickness from the planning CT, a maximum slice thickness exceeding 3 mm is generally not recommended, in order to minimize enlargement of the field borders, as during the planning process, the clinical treatment volume (CTV) is typically enlarged by 1 slice thickness in the craniocaudal direction to compensate for partial volume effect.[110]

Target Delineation

In the era of 3D treatment planning, consistent delineation of the breast, chest wall, regional lymph nodes, and OAR is critical for accurate assessment of the dose distributions prior to approving a treatment plan. Inadequate delineation of target tissues and OARs can result in the misinterpretation of dose–volume histograms (DVHs) and ultimately influence treatment plan evaluation. The OARs include the heart, ipsilateral/contralateral lung, contralateral breast, brachial plexus, esophagus, thyroid, and spinal cord.

Significant variations have been reported in contoured volumes among radiation oncologists.[111,112] To reduce these inconsistencies, several contouring proposals and guidelines have been published, with the goal of reducing multi-institutional and interobserver variability in target delineation.[110,113–115] These include institution-based studies with proposals for anatomic delineation and professional organizations, which have developed definitions from data systematically quantified and collected from experts in breast radiation oncology. For example, the Radiation Therapy Oncology Group (RTOG) has established a breast cancer atlas based on target delineation of 3 illustrative patient cases performed by 9 breast radiation oncologists and describes the general principles of contouring for CTVs of the breast, chest wall, and nodal regions, which include the axilla, supraclavicular fossa, and IMN (Table 61.3).[113,116] Similarly, the European Society

TABLE 61.4 EXAMPLE OF DOSE–VOLUME CONSTRAINTS AS RECOMMENDED BY DANISH BREAST CANCER COOPERATIVE GROUP[114]

Organ at Risk	Danish Guideline Dosimetric Parameter
Heart	LAD $V_{20\ Gy}$ = 0%
	$V_{20\ Gy}$ = 10%
	$V_{40\ Gy}$ = 5%
Ipsilateral lung	$V_{20\ Gy}$ = 25% (no SCNI)
	$V_{20\ Gy}$ = 35% (with SCNI)
Spinal cord	Max 45 Gy
Brachial plexus	Max 54 Gy
CTV	$CTV_{max}\ V_{107\%}$ = 53.5 Gy
PTV	Max dose outside PTV = 54 Gy

From Nielsen MH, Berg M, Pedersen AN, et al. Delineation of target volumes and organs at risk in adjuvant radiotherapy of early breast cancer: national guidelines and contouring atlas by the Danish Breast Cancer Cooperative Group. *Acta Oncol* 2013;52(4):703–710. Copyright © Acta Oncologica Foundation, reprinted by permission of Taylor & Francis Ltd, www.tandfonline.com on behalf of Acta Oncologica Foundation.

Therapeutic Radiation Oncology (ESTRO) has developed a breast-contouring consensus for delineation of the CTV for the breast, chest wall, and regional lymph node basins, which additionally includes the interpectoral (Rotter) nodes, and describes planning target volumes (PTV).[110] Finally, the Danish Breast Cancer Cooperative Group has published a national guideline and contouring atlas, which additionally provides recommended dose–volume constraints (Table 61.4).[114]

Typically, in early-stage patients, the pectoralis muscle, chest wall muscles, and ribs may be excluded when contouring the breast; but for locally advanced cases, the chest wall and ribs should be included irrespective of the breast conservation or mastectomy setting.[113] In the case of advanced breast cancer, it is important to note that the abovementioned guidelines can be used as a starting point for contouring but require individual adaptation based on the extent of the primary tumor and the lymph node involvement, with the

TABLE 61.3 RTOG CONSENSUS DEFINITIONS FOR BREAST CANCER TREATMENT PLANNING

	Breast/Chest Wall	Axilla I	Axilla II	Axilla III	Supraclavicular Fossa	Internal Mammary Nodes
Cranial	Clinical reference + second rib insertion	Axillary vessels cross lateral edge of pectoralis minor muscle	Axillary vessels cross medial edge of pectoralis minor muscle	Pectoralis minor muscle insert on cricoid	Caudal to the cricoid cartilage	Superior aspect of the medial first rib
Caudal	Clinical reference + loss of CT apparent breast	Pectoralis major muscle insert into ribs	Axillary vessels cross lateral edge of pectoralis minor muscle	Axillary vessels cross medial edge of pectoralis minor muscle	Junction of brachioceph.–axillary veins/caudal edge clavicle head	Cranial aspect of the fourth rib
Lateral	Clinical reference/mid Axillary line, excludes latissimus dorsi muscle	Medial border of latissimus dorsi muscle	Lateral border of pectoralis minor muscle	Medial border of pectoralis minor muscle	Caudal: junction first rib, clavicle Cranial: lateral edge of SCM muscle	Encompass the IM/thoracic vessels
Medial	Sternal–rib junction	Lateral border of pectoralis minor muscle	Medial border of pectoralis minor muscle	Thoracic inlet	Excludes thyroid and trachea	Encompass the IM/thoracic vessels
Posterior	Br: Excludes pectoralis muscles, chest wall muscles, ribs CW: Includes ribs, pectoralis muscles, pleural interface. ribs, chest muscles	Anterior surface of subscapularis muscle	Ribs and intercostal muscles	Ribs and intercostal muscles	Anterior aspect of the scalene muscle	Encompass the IM/thoracic vessels
Anterior	Skin	Plane defined by anterior surface of pectoralis major muscle and lateral dorsi muscle	Anterior surface pectoralis minor muscle	Posterior surface of the pectoralis major muscle	Sternocleidomastoid muscle	Encompass the IM/thoracic vessels

Table adapted from online version of the 'Breast Cancer Atlas for Therapy Planning: Consensus Definitions" https://www.rtog.org/LinkClick.aspx?fileticket=vzJFhPaBipE%3d&tabid=236. Reproduced with permission of RTOG for the Radiation Therapy Oncology Group.

obvious need for coverage of any gross disease with an added margin to the CTV to obtain a PTV for planning purposes.

Ultimately, there remain significant variations in philosophies regarding the target volumes requiring irradiation and the contouring of these volumes for LABC. Often, they are based on specific clinical/pathologic details of an individual case but can be influenced also by the treating physician's opinions regarding these issues and policies of the treating institution.[6] These variations in RNI patterns of practice have been highlighted in an international survey of radiation oncologists.[117,118]

Treatment Techniques

Various methods to incorporate the regional nodes in the locoregional treatment volume have been described. Two-dimensional tangential techniques in the breast-conserving therapy and PMRT settings have used bony and soft tissue landmarks to treat the entire breast or chest wall (with mastectomy scar) and typically only assess the dose at the level of the isocenter. In contrast, three-dimensional treatment planning uses CT imaging to delineate the volume to be radiated and can use "wedges" to attenuate the beam depending on the slope and thickness of the breast or chest wall to achieve a more uniform distribution and match anatomic contour using wedge-shaped pieces of metal in the head of the machine. When electron beams are used, such as for IMN treatment or delivery of a "boost" to the tumor bed after breast-conserving surgery or, in selected cases, the mastectomy scar, physical blocks are placed in the path of beam in the machine head to deliver a more conformal electron beam dose.

In contrast, 3D/IMRT techniques are based on the volumes delineated on planning CT and permits dosimetric and volumetric assessment at all levels above and below the central axis. As described earlier in this chapter, there are variations in the definitions for anatomic volumes and in physician judgment regarding which nodal basins require treatment (i.e., supraclavicular, internal mammary [IM], axilla).[15] Nevertheless, the vast majority of patients with locally advanced disease treated with either breast-conservation therapy or mastectomy have node-positive disease with high LRR risk, and therefore, the ipsilateral supraclavicular (SC) fossa and axillary apex (level III axilla) are generally included in the treatment volume. The intentional inclusion of the dissected axilla and IM nodes is significantly more variable and decisions regarding their inclusion require individualized consideration.[117,118] Typically, the volume for the IM vessels is within the first three intercostal interspaces, though the depth of the supraclavicular fossa and level III axilla varies greatly depending on individual anatomy and patient habitus. Inclusion of the intended nodal volumes in the CTV will ensure that these targets are adequately covered within the desired isodose volumes.

Various forward and inverse planning solutions have been described to generate 3D/IMRT plans that have been shown to significantly improve dose distribution over the standard wedge pair.[119,120] Additionally, methods using a combination of both forward and inverse planning have been described and are termed hybrid plans.[121,122] Unlike other disease sites such as head and neck and prostate cancer where intensity-modulated radiation therapy (IMRT), by definition, is inverse planned, for breast treatment planning, the modulation of the tangential beams can be achieved with forward planning, inverse planning, or a combination of both. For this reason, the exact definitions of breast IMRT versus three-dimensional treatment in breast cancer radiation treatment remain broad.[109] In this chapter, these modulated treatment plans will be termed 3D/IMRT.

Several forward-planned, "field-within-field" techniques have been described to deliver a more conformal dose by shaping the radiation beam and modulating high-dose regions.[123] Initially, the diverging posterior edges of the medial

and lateral borders of the tangential beams are adjusted to be nondivergent and the fields are weighted and optimized with adjustments to the beam depth, gantry angles, and collimator angles to minimize irradiation to OAR and ensure full coverage of the treatment volume. Unlike a standard 3D treatment plan with wedges, forward-planned 3D/IMRT has additional sub-fields with manually created apertures that are used to block specific hot spots in the original tangential fields. The dose distribution for these tangential fields is typically equally weighted, with open medial and lateral fields, and the normalization point defined at approximately mid-depth and 1 to 1.5 cm superficial to the deep edge of the chest wall in the plane of the central axis of the beams. Next, the highest dose cloud of the >115% isodose curve volume is projected in the beam's eye view of the treatment fields. A new segment is created using MLCs onto the medial/lateral tangent fields to account for 15% of the dose. This process can then be repeated for the 110% dose cloud, the 107% dose cloud, and so on, typically requiring 2 to 6 additional subfields to optimize dose homogeneity, as shown in Figure 61.1.[109,122] When using forward planning techniques, modifications to the weighting of the subfields and mixing of 4 to 6 MV with higher-energy photons should be manually adjusted to enhance dose homogeneity, particularly when the patient separation is large.[124] The criteria used for choosing the numbers of additional subfields is generally based on reducing maximum isodose volumes by approximately 3% per subfield down to a goal of 107% of the prescription dose or until PTV starts to break up.

With inverse treatment planning, multisegment fields are created using inverse planning software that makes use of computer-generated intensity-modulated fields by adding dose to particular areas of the breast or chest wall using supplementary individually shaped beam portals (segments) that are coplanar to the tangential fields. The inverse-planned IMRT technique uses optimization algorithms to create fluence maps to shape dose distributions with the number of segments varying based on the different types of planning and optimization tools used to plan each case[125] and can be performed using a linear accelerator with either dynamic or static MLCs, arc therapy, or tomotherapy.[126,127] Typically, the same beam orientations and angles used for forward planning are used with inverse planning when the intent is to deliver a more homogeneous plan, although non-coplanar beams are often necessary to generate a more conformal treatment plan. The PTV is the same used for the 3D plans plus an extension into the air anteriorly of the chest of 1.5 cm to ensure appropriate opening of the multileaf collimator. The dose is prescribed to the PTV, and initial dose–volume constraints are provided. These automated priority-based computer algorithms deliver the prescribed dose to the predefined PTV volume while taking into consideration the relative prioritized dose constraints for normal tissues. Although the use of automated inverse software provides excellent homogeneity and normal tissue sparing, particularly for anatomically challenging cases, a more conformal plan typically requires rotational IMRT techniques or fixed-gantry IMRT techniques using multiple angles and non-coplanar beams, which result in larger volumes of normal tissue structures being exposed to low-dose radiation.[128]

Overall, no one breast modulation method (forward or inverse) has been shown to have a clear dosimetric or clinical advantage over another[120,129] and the method for developing the modulated plan is often based on institutional preferences and practices or determined based on anatomic specifics of an individual patient. Nevertheless, inverse planning typically results in a reduced treatment planning time with the trade-off of increasing monitor units to the patient compared to forward planning.[121] Unless necessary for particularly anatomically challenging cases, the routine use of multiple-angle rotational IMRT techniques and non-coplanar beams is

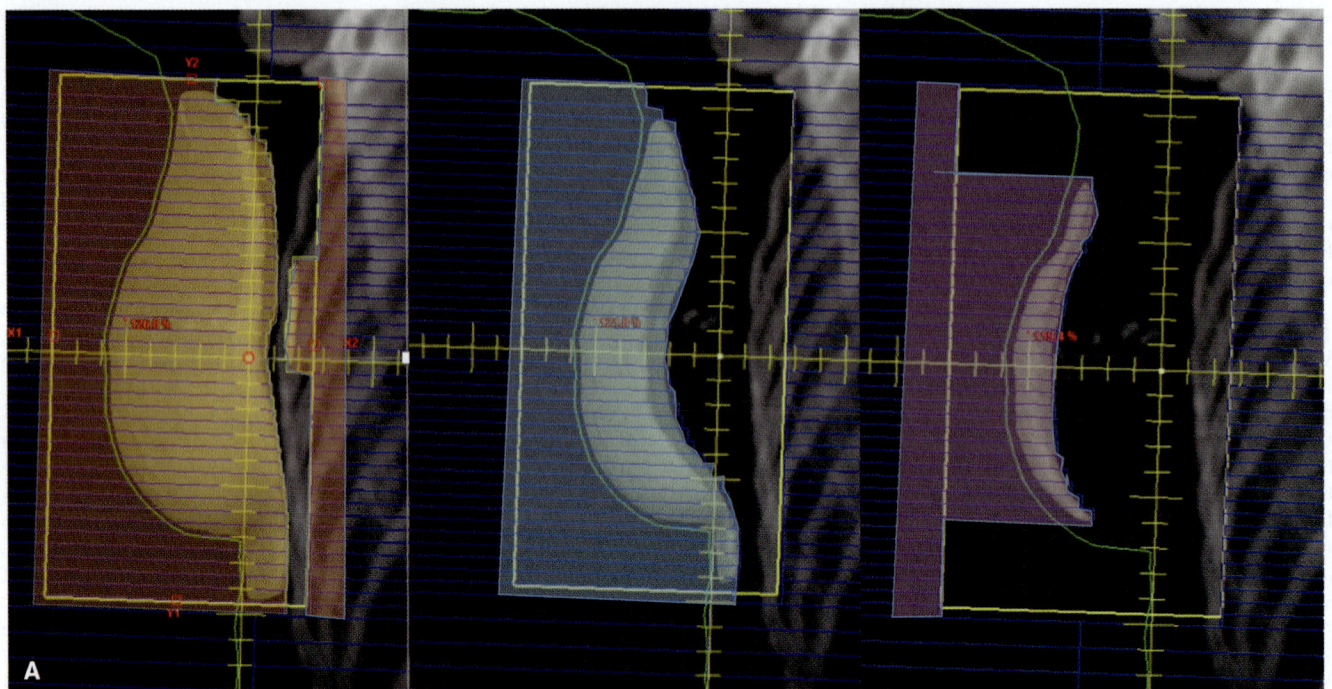

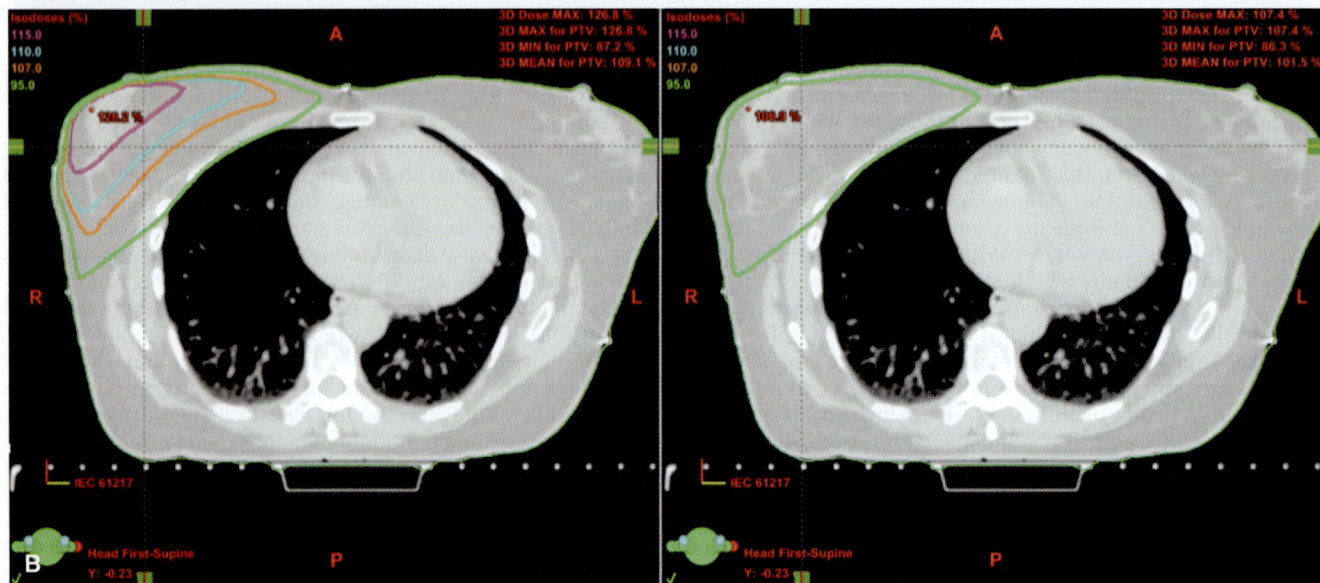

FIGURE 61.1. Field-in-field technique. **A:** Each segment is created as a subfield of the medial/lateral tangent fields blocking >115%, then >110%, then >107% dose cloud, etc. Typically, 2 to 6 additional subfields are used to optimize dose homogeneity. **B:** Treatment plan showing improvement in dose homogeneity with the addition of subfields. (Courtesy of Gifty Arthur, BS, CMD, Yale New Haven Hospital, Madison, CT.)

discouraged, because of the potential for long-term sequelae from the exposure of low-dose radiation to a significantly higher volume of normal tissue (Fig. 61.2).[128,129]

Coverage of SC/Axilla/IMN

Whether using 2-D treatment planning using bony landmarks or 3-D treatment planning with regional nodal basins contoured to guide field design, the inclusion of SC/axilla may require the addition of a third anterior–posterior field to deliver a dose to a depth that will adequately cover the SC and axillary regions. This anterior field is typically angled 10 to 20 degrees to avoid the spinal cord and esophagus.

In all cases, it is important that the inferior border of the supraclavicular (with or without axilla) field be nondivergent to avoid overlap with the tangents. This can be accomplished using either independent collimator jaws or a half-beam block. A commonly used method is the single isocenter technique, in which the isocenter is identified on the axis conjoining the tangential fields and AP supraclavicular field with a gantry angle of zero, and shielding and wedges are typically used because table and collimator angles would result in asymmetric exit dose. When the depth of the axillary nodes exceeds approximately 5 cm and may not be adequately covered with the AP field using 4- to 6-MV photons, the use of higher photon energy or anterior–medial/posterior–lateral beam arrangement may be considered. The additional posterior–anterior (PA) supplemental field, traditionally referred to as the posterior axillary boost (PAB), allows delivery of additional dose to the midaxillary depth.

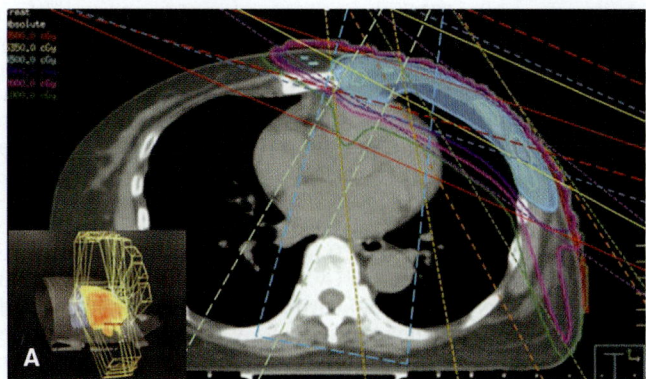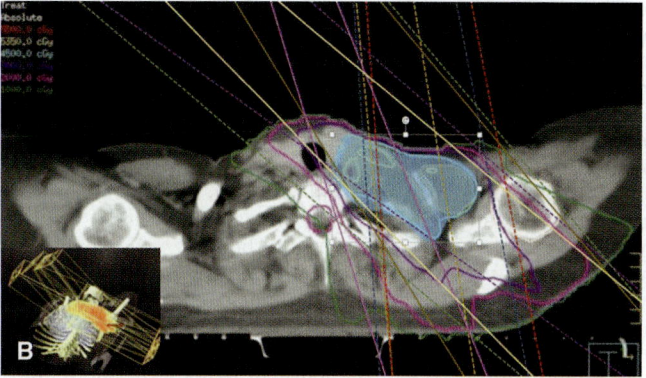

FIGURE 61.2. Inverse-planned IMRT plan of postmastectomy and comprehensive regional nodal radiation. As depicted in *blue*, the prescribed dose is very conformal to the PTV, but multiple beams and beam angles are required, resulting in a greater volume of low-dose radiation to normal tissue structures. *Inset* depicts the multiple coplanar beams, resulting in exposure to contralateral and posterior normal tissue. **A:** Chest wall and IM chain inverse IMRT plan. **B:** Supraclavicular, high axilla inverse IMRT plan.

More challenging is the coverage of the IMN, particularly in patients with left-sided disease, because the heart is located directly below the IMN and inevitably will receive more radiation than when the IMN are not covered. Several commonly described methods for IMN inclusion are described below.

Wide Tangents/Partially Wide Tangents

This is particularly useful when deep inspiration breath hold (DIBH) techniques are available (see below). Three photon beams are used including the supraclavicular, wide medial and wide lateral tangential fields, with the isocenter at the inferior border of the supraclavicular photon beam. Overlapping the inferior supraclavicular field with the tangents is assured without divergence using half-beam blocking and prohibiting collimator rotation. The medial border is extended onto the opposite breast/chest wall, to ensure that the ipsilateral IMNs are covered. When the wide tangents are to be split inferiorly with a heart block and computer-optimized wedge angles to minimize dose to heart and lung, this technique is termed partially wide tangents. This technique avoids the issue of matching fields and, depending on the patient's anatomy, offers an attractive alternative to a separate IMN field in selected patients. Care must be taken to ensure complete coverage of all target tissue and the entire chest wall and mastectomy scar in the inferior portion of the field, in the region of the block, if a partially wide tangent is used, and should be adjusted to follow the chest wall at the rib cage so that the IMN, breast, and chest wall receive adequate dose while sparing normal lungs.

Photon/Electron Matching Techniques

These techniques may be considered when attempts to encompass the IMN in the wide tangential fields result in excessive heart and lung exposure and when DIBH techniques are not available or successful. The supraclavicular and tangential photon fields are created using the standard single isocenter, 3-field technique described above. An IMN field using electron beams is matched on the skin to the medial tangential field, with the medial tangential border moved laterally so that it does not include the IMC. Traditionally, IMN portals have been 5 to 6 cm in width, extending from midline medially, just below the clavicular head superiorly to include the first 3 intercostal spaces, with the inferior border at the fourth interspace, but should be tailored three-dimensionally based on the CT contour.[109] The electrons may be a combination of two electron beam energies, a higher energy superiorly to provide full coverage to the IM regions at risk, whereas lower-energy electron beams are used at the inferior portion to encompass the breast/chest wall. The electron IM field can be

treated with electrons alone or a combination of low-energy photons and electrons, with a maximum of 50% of the dose being delivered by photons to minimize the dose to underlying heart and lung tissue. A popular technique is to tilt the gantry angle of the electron field 5 degrees to 15 degrees less than the medial tangent, minimizing the cold triangle just below the skin match of the 2 fields, and to feather this junction 1 to 3 times during the treatment course.

IMRT Inverse-Planned IMN Treatment

Using the contoured volumes to define the PTV, the inverse planning software uses a set of procedural guidelines to include specifications of the clinical planning goals to fulfill. Dose constraints for the OARs are prioritized and the software program automatically generates an optimized treatment plan, using optimization algorithms to create fluence maps to shape dose distributions. Intended dose distributions for targets are achieved while reducing OAR doses with the use of MLCs (dynamic or static), arc therapy,[127] tomotherapy, or topotherapy.[126] Although the development of a plan that will meet heart and lung dose constraints is achievable with inverse-planned IMRT, this typically comes at the cost of spreading low dose radiation to larger volumes of normal healthy tissue (Fig. 61.2).[128]

Dosimetry and Dose

For treatment planning purposes, the breast/CTV volume is defined as clinically demarcated tissue at CT simulation, and the volume may be adjusted to include all glandular breast tissue visualized by CT. In patients with early-stage disease, the breast CTV is typically limited anteriorly to within 5 mm from the skin and excludes the chest wall. In patient with LABC, it is particularly important to contour volumes that correlate with the clinical presentation, pathology, and residual disease, if present when planning treatment. As mentioned above, for advanced breast cancer and recurrent disease, it is important to remember that the target delineation guidelines can only be used as a starting point for contouring, but individual adaptation is essential to ensure coverage of all gross disease and tissues at risk.

The recommended dose prescriptions for whole-breast irradiation are 46 to 50 Gy in 23 to 25 fractions or 40 to 42.5 Gy in 15 to 16 fractions (in appropriately selected patients),[130] delivered 5 days per week, with a boost to the tumor bed with 10 to 16 Gy in 4 to 8 fractions for higher-risk patients.[131] In the postmastectomy setting, the target includes the ipsilateral chest wall, mastectomy scar, and drain sites when indicated. The typical prescribed dose to the PTV (chest wall with or without reconstruction and regional nodes) is 46 to 50 Gy in 23 to 25 or 40 Gy in 16 fractions. The use of a boost to the mastectomy scar is controversial. When the decision is made to boost, a typical prescription of 2 Gy per fraction to a total dose of approximately 60 Gy is reasonable.

The use of tissue-equivalent bolus in the PMRT setting to increase the dose to skin[131,132] is also controversial.[133] Although bolus use is known to increase acute skin toxicity,[134] its specific contribution to improve local control is unknown. Reports have emerged suggesting that postmastectomy local recurrence rates are low in the absence of bolus.[135,136] For patients with inflammatory breast cancer or advanced primary tumors with high risks of skin recurrence, the use of bolus is justified. For other situations such as patients with low-risk disease and patients undergoing reconstruction, the bolus may be reasonably omitted. When the decision is made to use bolus, tissue-equivalent material of 0.5 to 1.0 cm is typically incorporated into the treatment plan and may be applied every day to every other day on the entire chest wall skin surface or, alternatively, may be applied during the initial portion of the radiation and removed for the second half, depending on the clinical scenario and physician and institutional preference.[132]

Although routine use of inverse planning and noncoplanar beam techniques may be appealing to generate homogenous plans requiring less treatment planning time compared with manual planning, many centers continue to routinely use forward planning techniques because of the disadvantages of inverse planning, which, as described previously, result in higher radiation monitor units, longer daily treatment time, increased low-dose exposure to larger volumes of normal tissue (which is associated with concerns for potential long-term toxicity such as secondary malignancies), and the inevitable association with higher health care costs. For this reason, 3D/IMRT with inverse-planned, non-coplanar techniques should be reserved for select cases where acceptable dose constraints cannot be met using 3D conformal RT (3D-CRT) methods.

Although standards for dose homogeneity have yet to be consistently adopted, most 3D/IMRT planning techniques typically achieve no more than 110% of the prescribed dose to the intact breast. In the case of PMRT, achieving this inhomogeneity can sometimes be more challenging depending on patient anatomy. DVHs of the PTV and OAR of the 3D/IMRT plans should be generated and compared. All attempts should be made to observe dose constraints for OAR, though these parameters vary depending on the volumes targeted and varying protocols. For example, the Danish Breast Cancer Guideline/Atlas suggests that the heart $V_{20\,Gy}$ should be <10%, heart $V_{40\,Gy}$ should be <5%, and the ipsilateral lung $V_{20\,Gy}$ should be <25% using tangents only and <35% when a third supraclavicular/axillary field is included.[114] These dose constraints typically pertain to early-stage disease, and occasionally, despite the use of contemporary techniques in the PMRT setting, left-sided PMRT heart dose constraints may be difficult to meet. One study evaluated 3 different modern PMRT planning techniques, which included (a) forward-planned FIF 3D/IMRT, (b) inverse-planned 3D/IMRT (using 5 beams consisting of 2 opposed tangential beams with the same gantry angles as the forward planning technique, 2 anterior beams with a 10-degree angle from the tangential ones, and a supraclavicular beam, and segments with 166 control points), and (c) a VMAT 3D/IMRT plan consisting of two optimized coplanar partial arcs. This study demonstrated that the heart $V_{20\,Gy}$ was 12.48% ± 6.36, 10.54% ± 5.17, and 19.48% ± 8.84, respectively, for each of the techniques.[137] Another dosimetric evaluation of forward versus inverse-planned 3D/IMRT in the PMRT setting described mean heart doses of 877 and 704 cGy, respectively.[138]

Comparison of homogeneity and conformality across treatment plans can be quantitatively assessed using parameters such as the homogeneity index (HI), calculated as the fraction of the PTV with a dose between 95% and 105% of the prescribed dose ($V_{95\%}$ to $V_{105\%}$) and the conformity index (CI), defined as the fraction of the PTV surrounded by the reference dose ($V_{95\%}$) multiplied by the fraction of the total body volume covered by the reference PTV dose ([$PTV_{95\%}$/PTV] × [$PTV_{95\%}$/$V_{95\%}$]).[138]

When using inverse planning to generate a 3D/IMRT plan, various optimization algorithms and techniques have been described and are often institution based. For example, one described optimization process starts with dose–volume constraints of as follows: 90% of PTV to receive 50 Gy/25 fractions; ipsilateral mean lung dose ≤20 Gy and ≤30% of the ipsilateral lung to receive ≤20 Gy; ≤5% of the heart to receive ≤30 Gy, mean heart dose ≤8 Gy for left-sided lesions, and ≤10 Gy if IMN is included; spinal cord maximum dose ≤45 Gy; and contralateral breast mean dose ≤1.5 Gy. Priority is high for the PTV, heart and lung constraints relative to other structures, and optimization proceeds with these settings until no further improvement are seen. Priority is then increased for other structures until a balance is reached between PTV coverage and normal tissues sparing. Once PTV and normal tissue dose constraints are met, the dosimetrist expands the anterior border of chest wall field 1.5 to 2 cm beyond the skin surface to ensure coverage of the chest wall (and bolus, if used).[139,140]

BREAST RADIOTHERAPY AND THE HEART

Cardiac Toxicity with Breast XRT

It has been well documented that standard tangential radiotherapy fields used for breast cancer consequentially result in irradiation of cardiac tissues, particularly in women receiving left-sided radiotherapy, who have been demonstrated to have more cardiac exposure when comparing right- versus left-sided breast cancer patients receive radiotherapy.[141] As a direct result of older techniques, this increase in cardiac exposure historically mitigated some of the benefits of adjuvant radiation, though more recently, with improvements in technology and treatment planning to sparing normal tissue, more recent meta-analyses in both the breast conservation and mastectomy setting demonstrate the ultimate benefits of radiation in reducing breast cancer–specific mortality.[8,9]

It is now established that incidental dose to the heart results in coronary events such as pericarditis, pericardial fibrosis, diffuse myocardial fibrosis, coronary artery disease (CAD), and, in more rare cases, valvular disease.[142] Although breast cancer–related cardiac toxicity typically takes a decade or more years to manifest, there is a dose gradient such that high-dose exposure above 30 Gy results in cardiac complications that become apparent within a year or two of exposure, with the risk of cardiac complications increasing with younger age of exposure and the presence of conventional risk factors.[142]

Cardiac Injury Pathogenesis

Radiation exposure to the heart results in an increase in micro- and macrovascular injury. The cardiac damage that results from radiation typically can be characterized into four major categories: pericardial fibrosis, myocardial fibrosis, pericarditis, and CAD.[142] The development of fibrosis consists of the deposition of collagen in either the parietal pericardium or the myocardial, which over time replaces normal tissue, and inhibits normal function. With pericardial fibrosis, the normal peripheral adipose layer (typically measuring <0.5 mm) is replaced with a thick fibrous layer, increasing the thickness of pericardium to as much as 8 mm and resulting in a rigid, constricted pericardial sac that is often accompanied by effusion. When collagen is deposited in the myocardium, which classically occurs in patches on the anterior wall of the left ventricle, this results in damage to the endothelium of the myocardial blood capillaries and can lead to transient ischemia and myocardial fibrosis, which, if extensive, can result in congestive heart failure.[143]

Alternatively, when a variable amount of protein-rich exudate accumulates within the pericardial sac resulting in a pericardial effusion, this accumulation of fluid result in pericarditis or cause potentially fatal cardiac tamponade.[143] Atherosclerosis and the resultant CAD resulting from radiation exposure occurs with the same pathogenesis as normal physiologic atherosclerosis from other causes. The reduction in the arterial lumen is a result of intimal proliferation of myofibroblasts, with lipid-containing macrophages forming plaques that can fracture and cause thrombosis and can clinically manifest in symptoms of ischemic heart disease such as stable and unstable angina pectoris, MI, and chronic ischemic heart disease.[144]

Cardiac Toxicity Dose–Volume Data

Though QUANTEC recommends restricting the volume of the heart receiving at least 25 Gy (V_{25}) to <10% to keep the risk of cardiac mortality under 1%, much of the data supporting this recommendation come from a combination of both lymphoma and breast cancer patients.[145,146] Unlike studies that have evaluated radiation-related cardiac toxicity from diseases like Hodgkin disease where the degree of the cardiac exposure has been significantly larger, RT in breast cancer patients has resulted in cardiac complications of smaller magnitude, which have been much more difficult to elucidate. Much of data were derived from women enrolled in prospective, phase III trials in which half of the women were randomized to receive adjuvant radiotherapy. Earlier analysis of these randomized trials demonstrated that long-term survival beyond 10 years was significantly worse in women receiving radiation[2,3] and, ultimately, that mortality from heart disease was significantly increased by 27% in patients receiving RT.[8] Most of the increase was due to CAD. It has been elucidated that delivery techniques utilized in the earlier trials, including tangential field placement in close proximity to the heart, large daily fraction size and high total doses, use of anterior–posterior (AP) fields, inclusion of IMN, and use of orthovoltage and cobalt radiation, all may have contributed to these earlier results.[147] Updated analyses of these trials provide clear evidence demonstrating the larger mean cardiac RT doses with the risk of death from heart disease. The EBCTCG assessed the risk of death from RT-related heart disease, though notably not estimated from individual patient treatment plans, to be approximately increased by 3% per Gy mean cardiac heart dose,[148] whereas Darby et al.[149] estimated major coronary events in population-based case–control study of patients treated in Sweden and Denmark between 1958 and 2001 to be estimated at 7.4% per Gy. Although they attempted to estimate this risk correcting for differences in doses and fractionation schedules using the linear-quadratic model to convert all treatments to an equivalent dose in 2-Gy fractions, and estimated cardiac volumes and doses of these pre-CT era patients with reconstruction using one standard representative CT scan, the validity of individual variability and correcting for these dosing differences brings to question the applicability of their findings to current clinical practice.[149] Nevertheless, since the time of this publication, cardiac dose constraints for the whole heart in breast cancer of a mean heart dose <4 Gy have generally been considered an achievable standard.

Outside the context of a randomized trial, comparisons of mortality after various different treatment regimens are often misleading because the prognosis of patients given different treatments will vary.[141] Radiation-induced heart disease is generally regarded a classical "deterministic" radiation effect, which is only expected to occur if the radiation dose exceeds a well-defined threshold. Cardiac dose–volume data from studies among atomic bomb survivors in the Hiroshima-Nagasaki Life Span Study, with mortality from heart disease after radiation exposure, suggest that although it remains unclear if there is any increased cardiac mortality risk when mean heart dose is below 0.5 Gy, at some undefined point in this range, there begins to be a clear association with level of exposure and the increased cardiac death risk is estimated at 14% per Gy.[150] Specifically, there is a significant quadratic dose–response relationships for MI among survivors exposed at <40 years of age ($P = .049$).[151]

This difference in the estimates of cardiac mortality risk of 14% in atomic bomb survivors versus 7.4% to 3% per Gy mean heart dose from women treated for breast cancer has been suggested to be unlikely because of confounding factors such as predisposing cardiac risk factors, because of the minimal presence of confounders such as obesity, diabetes, alcohol use, and smoking in the atomic bomb cohort. More likely, this difference in risk-per-Gy has been postulated to be secondary to the fractionated exposure and substantially less homogeneous cardiac radiation exposure in breast cancer patients or differences in age at exposure.[152]

The first study to assess cardiac toxicity outcomes in a population treated uniformly with RT using three-dimensional, CT-based simulation and assess this risk with consideration for the individual's cardiac risk factors (including hypertension, smoking history, and body mass index [BMI], diabetes, etc.) reported a risk of acute coronary events to be 16.5% (95% CI, 0.6 to 35.0) per Gy of radiation to the whole heart in the first 9 years after treatment, similar to that reported by Darby et al. at 15.5% between 5 and 9 years after RT. Additionally, the authors describe that the normal tissue complication probability (NTCP) model could be improved by using left ventricular V_5 instead of mean heart dose.[153]

Cardiac Avoidance Techniques

In the contemporary era where the vast majority of breast cancer patients receive some form of systemic treatment, efforts to spare the heart are even more crucial, because of increased cardiovascular risks associated with modern systemic agents, such as trastuzumab and anthracyclines and long-term use of aromatase inhibitors. More contemporary data support the decrease in incidental cardiac exposure to radiation for left-sided breast cancers with the use of modern techniques. Nevertheless, there will be significant variability in cardiac exposure based on individual patient factors, which include anatomy, history of smoking, and preexisting comorbidities. Several techniques for reducing the radiation exposure to the heart and lung have demonstrated significant impact in decreasing incidental dose to these OAR.

This section reviews some of the common techniques utilized to effectively decrease heart (and lung) exposure.[154,155]

Heart Blocks

A heart block is one of the oldest and possibly the simplest methods for minimizing heart dose, though it is only technically possible in certain patients in whom the lumpectomy cavity is readily identifiable to be remote from the heart block. The relationship between the tumor(s) to the chest wall is particularly important in the setting of oncoplastic reduction or any situation in which the lumpectomy cavity is ambiguous, to avoid placing the heart block in a location even remotely close to the original tumor(s). With selective and appropriate use of the heart block, the dose to the PTV has been shown to be reduced by only 2.8% and has been demonstrated to have no effect on compromising local control in appropriately selected patients (Fig. 61.3).[156]

Patient Positioning Using Prone Breast Board

In certain patients requiring left-sided breast cancer treatment, and occasionally for right-sided patients with large, pendulous breasts, those in whom the lung dose needs to be further minimized, or those with challenging anatomy such as pectus excavatum, positioning using a prone breast board at the time of simulation for treatment planning can

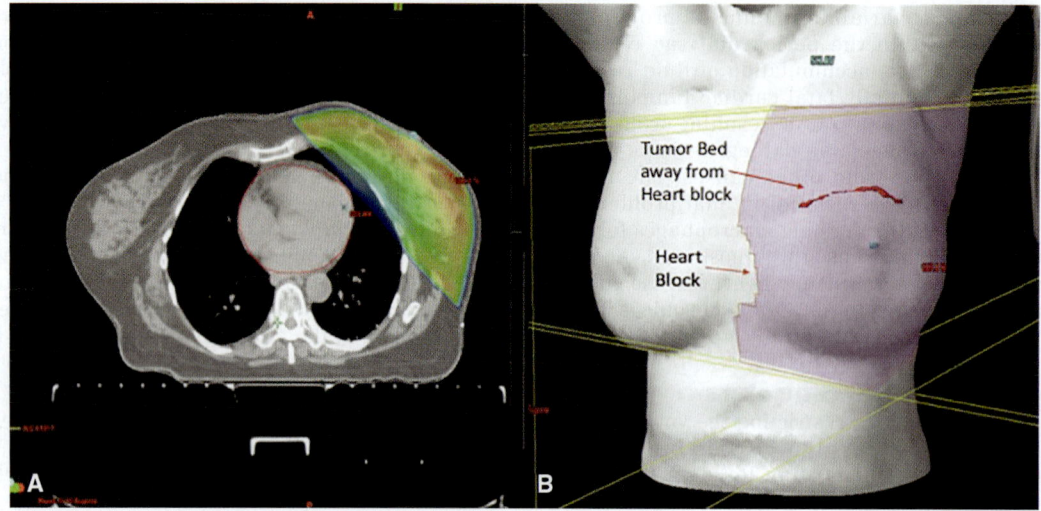

FIGURE 61.3. Heart block placement allows for Mean$_{\text{heart dose}}$ = 193 cGy. Multileaf collimators are added to the cardiac silhouette on the digital reconstruction and should be confirmed clinically on the patient and on the skin rendition to verify its placement away from the tumor bed. **A:** Axial dose distribution at the level of the heart. **B:** Skin rendition showing that the heart block placement not compromise coverage when limited to the cardiac silhouette and tumor bed is remote from the heart block.

significantly reduce heart and lung doses. The traditional immobilization is the supine breast board, which allows for variable incline but nevertheless results in flattening of the breast across the chest wall so that larger volumes of chest wall receive incidental radiation when covering the PTV. With the prone board, gravity facilitates the anterior displacement of the breast tissue, allowing for significantly less inclusion of tissues deep to the chest wall (and hence underlying normal tissue).[157,158] In a dosimetric analysis comparing women simulated with both prone and supine positioning, prone positioning decreases lung exposure in 100% of patients and heart exposure in 85% of patients with left breast cancer, irrespective of breast size (Fig. 61.4).[159] Furthermore, cosmetic assessment using photographs of patients treated in the prone versus supine position suggests more favorable cosmesis with lower rates of hyperpigmentation and cosmetic deterioration among patients treated in the prone position.[160] No difference in 5-year local recurrence was observed in patients treated in the prone position.[158] There are a variety of commercially

available prone breast boards, each with advantages and disadvantages, with the limitations of each prone board including the learning curve for daily positioning and reproducibility. Furthermore, prone boards can only be utilized for patients who are able to lie relatively comfortably on their abdomen with the head turned away at a >45 degree angle. Lastly, most current commercially available boards are intended to treat tangential breast plans and therefore are not used to treat 3-field breast plans to include a matched supraclavicular/axillary field. However, data are emerging reporting feasibility of locoregional treatment in the prone position, creating a potential for expansion of prone applications for patients with more advanced-stage disease.[161]

Deep Inspiration Breath Hold/Respiratory Gating Methods

There are several commercially available devices for delivering radiation in breast cancer patients, which synchronize the

FIGURE 61.4. Supine versus prone positioning. **A:** Axial image depicting the tangential beams in the supine position at the level of the heart; Mean$_{\text{heart dose}}$ = 450 cGy. **B:** Axial image depicting the tangential beams in the prone position at the level of the heart; Mean$_{\text{heart dose}}$ = 173 cGy.

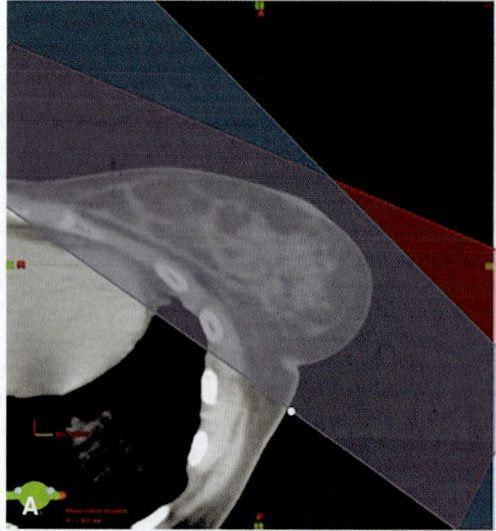
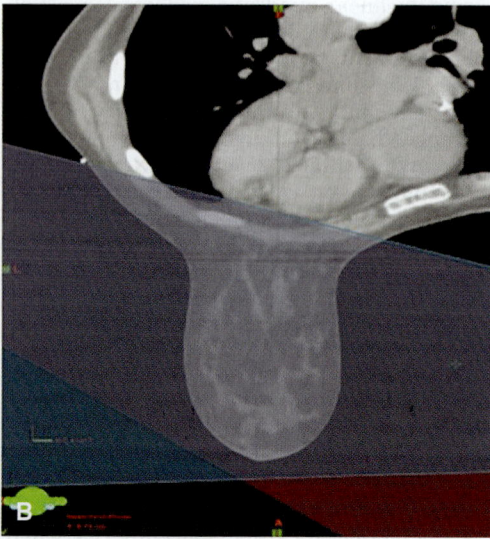

delivery of radiation with the respiratory cycle. This concept makes use of the normal physiologic inferior and posterior–medial movement of the heart when a patient takes (and holds) a deep breath and only delivers radiation when the patient is in specified portions of the breath (or breath hold) cycle. This, in turn, reduces the irradiated volume and dose to the heart.

There are two major methods that make use of the respiratory cycle. The first is an active-breathing control (ABC) device used for regulation of respiratory inspiratory volume; the second relies on patient coaching for voluntary DIBH that is verified with either surface anatomy verification or direct volume measurement. For this, the patient is trained to hold a deep breath, typically for 20 to 30 seconds. At the time of simulation, each patient undergoes two CT simulation scans, one with free breathing, which is obtained as a reference for treatment setups, and the second in the deep breath hold position, which is used for the actual treatment plan. Use of this method has resulted in significant lowering of cardiac dose and volumes in both the breast conservation and postmastectomy settings (Fig. 61.5).

CT-based studies have demonstrated the magnitude in the benefit of DIBH to approximate *complete* removal of the heart from the radiated field in nearly half of the patients and an approximately 80% reduction in cardiac volumes overall.[162]

In one study, moderate DIBH with ABC resulted in a significant decrease in mean heart dose in 88% of the patients studied (mean heart dose $_{ABC}$ = 254 cGy vs. mean heart dose $_{free\ breathing}$ = 423 cGy, $P < .001$).[163] Although the reductions in cardiac exposure are considerable in most patients with left-sided breast

FIGURE 61.5. The use of DIBH significantly reduces cardiac volume irradiated. **A:** Free breathing scan showing tangential beams with a substantial portion of the left ventricle in the radiated field. **B:** DIBH scan—heart moves away from the chest wall with expansion of the diaphragm. **C:** Using the same clinical borders, the dose–volume histogram (DVH) showing Mean$_{heart\ dose}$ = 377 cGy with free breathing and Mean$_{heart\ dose}$ = 195 cGy with DIBH.

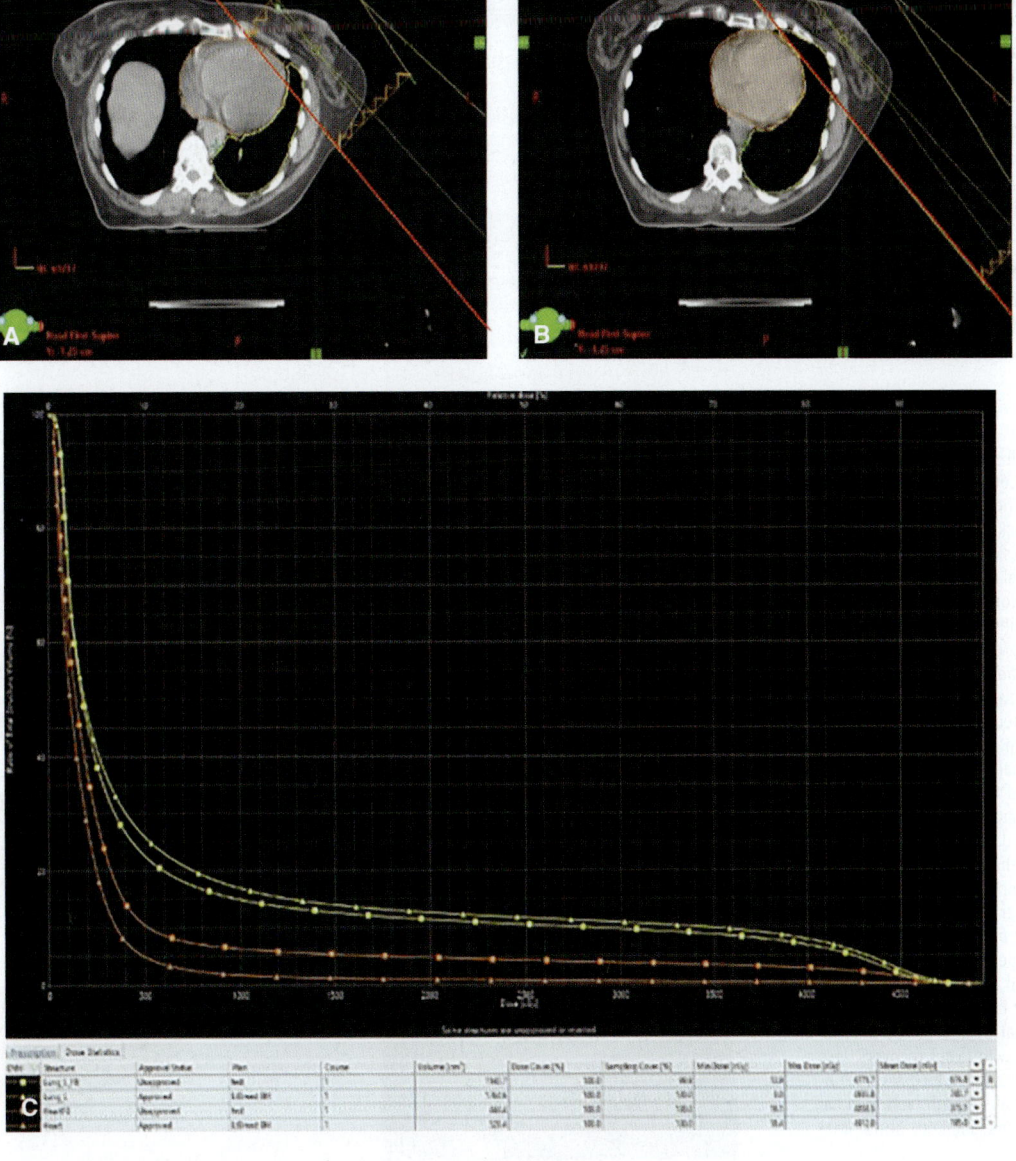

cancers, it is particularly notable that the benefits in decreasing cardiac dose with DIBH appear to be of greater magnitude in patients receiving PMRT, for which treatment planning to minimize cardiac dose can be more challenging because of the need to treat the much larger surgical bed including scars, compared to whole-breast irradiation following BCS.[164]

BREAST RECONSTRUCTION

The benefits of reconstruction after mastectomy are well described in the literature and include improvements in cosmetic outcomes, psychological health, self-esteem, body image, postdiagnosis sexuality, and overall satisfaction scores.[165,166] Although the benefits of PMRT have been described in detail elsewhere, in brief, for patients undergoing mastectomy with high-risk features such as node-positive disease, positive margins, large tumors, or recurrent disease, the adjuvant use of PMRT results in a decrease in LRRs and, in selected patients, has long-term survival benefits.

Although an increasing proportion of patients are opting to undergo reconstruction after mastectomy, the timing of when to incorporate reconstruction with adjuvant radiation remains challenging. It is well documented that the use of radiation and reconstruction results in increased complications, such as a higher risk of fibrosis and soft tissue shrinkage, capsular contractions around prosthesis, increased need for revision surgeries, and increased autologous reconstruction failures.[167–169] Ultimately, the complications associated with PMRT and reconstruction have the potential to significantly affect the quality of life and cosmetic outcomes of these women. Unfortunately, the data regarding patient-centered outcomes with regard to types of reconstruction and timing of reconstruction relative to PMRT are largely retrospective series or population-based analysis, and published prospective data are limited.

Types of Breast Reconstruction

There are two major categories of postmastectomy breast reconstruction. The most common has traditionally been an implant-based reconstruction, which can be performed as a one- or two-step procedure. With the one-step procedure, the implant of choice (saline or silicone) is placed immediately after the mastectomy and PMRT is delivered thereafter. With the two-step procedure, an expander is placed at the time of mastectomy and optimally expanded prior to the delivery of PMRT. The benefits of a two-step procedure include the ability to revise any radiation effects and allow for correction of PMRT-related asymmetry. Furthermore, with a two-step procedure, it is not mandated that the patient decide on implant-based or autologous reconstruction prior to the mastectomy, as this can be determined at the time of tissue expander removal and, if needed, allows for patient flexibility in changing their decision from one reconstruction approach to another. Options for autologous reconstruction include immediate reconstruction versus a delayed one-step or possibly a delayed two-step operative approach. The method of delayed autologous or two-step delayed-immediate autologous reconstruction has been reported to be utilized to decrease the soft tissue effects of PMRT.[170] With delayed-immediate reconstruction, patients who do not require radiation therapy can achieve aesthetic outcomes similar to those undergoing immediate reconstruction, and patients whose need for postoperative PMRT becomes apparent after review of the permanent pathologic sections after mastectomy, as it can avoid delivery of radiation to the permanent reconstruction.

Although patients with locally advanced disease historically have not been eligible for implant-based reconstruction because of the absence of a breast skin envelope following mastectomy and PMRT, which resulted in a fibrotic chest wall that was difficult to expand and made delayed breast reconstruction extremely challenging, the use of delayed-immediate reconstruction has resulted in a paradigm shift in allowing patients with locally advanced disease to have reconstruction options by allowing immediate expander placement so that the breast skin envelope can be preserved for subsequent delayed reconstruction after PMRT.[171]

The 2 most common form of autologous reconstruction methods currently used are the TRAM and DIEP flaps (Fig. 61.6). The traditional autologous implant for many years was the TRAM flap, which was classically performed in one of three ways. The initial TRAM approach was the pedicled

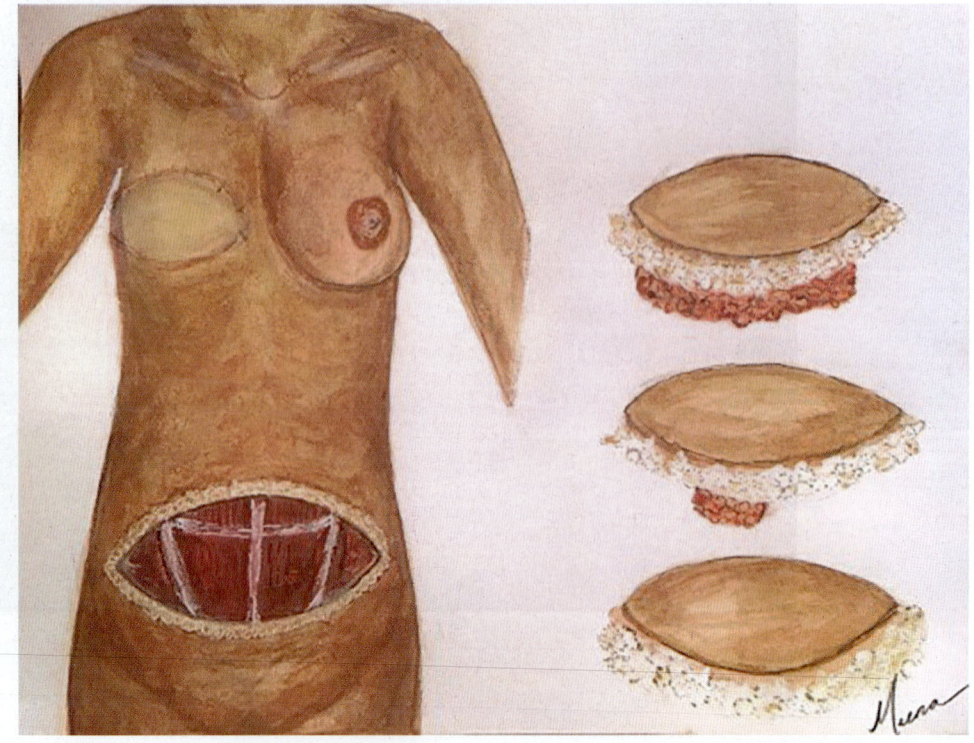

FIGURE 61.6. Illustration of TRAM and DIEP autologous reconstructions by Meena S. Moran. *Right top*: The traditional TRAM flap-A pedicled, full-thickness flap of the lower abdominal tissue (skin, fat and ipsilateral, full rectus abdominal muscle). Disadvantages include loss of abdominal muscle strength, and risks of "tunneling" of the flap under the skin around the rib cage area and abdominal hernia. *Right middle*: A "muscle-sparing free TRAM" uses only a small portion of the rectus muscle dissected from the anterior rectus sheath, which is completely detached from the abdominal wall and microsurgically reanastomosed to the blood supply on the chest wall. Advantages of this technique include a better blood supply than the pedicled flap, no "tunneling," less risk of healing and fat necrosis complications, and increased preservation of lower abdominal motor–sensory function. *Right bottom*: The DIEP (deep inferior epigastric perforator) flap uses the patient's abdominal skin and fat to reconstruct a natural, soft breast after mastectomy, but without removal of any rectus muscle, which is associated with faster recovery, less associated postsurgical pain, long-term maintenance of abdominal strength, and minimal risk of complications such as abdominal bulging and hernia.

TRAM, which requires an incision from hip to hip after which the lower abdominal tissue (including skin, fat and ipsilateral, full-thickness rectus abdominal muscle) below the navel is tunneled under the upper abdominal skin to the ipsilateral chest wall to reconstruct the new breast (Fig. 61.6, right top). With this procedure, the surgery is generally difficult and long, and the patient experiences clinically significant loss of abdominal muscle strength, and there is also some degree of "tunneling" under the skin with an upper abdominal bulge around the rib cage area.

The free-TRAM flap uses the same tissue as the pedicled TRAM but in this case is completely detached from the abdominal wall, transplanted to the chest, with the blood supply reestablished with microsurgery. The main advantage of the free TRAM over the pedicled TRAM is a better blood supply and therefore less risk of healing problems and fat necrosis, and no "tunneling." Most recently, the technique for muscle-sparing free TRAM was developed, which requires dissection of the anterior rectus sheath with procurement of only a small portion of the rectus muscle as part of the flap (Fig. 61.6, right middle). This approach has the benefit of preservation of an increased amount of rectus abdominis muscle to improve the integrity of the abdominal wall and preserve lateral intercostal nerve innervations, which are reported to be important to the strength of the abdominal wall than the muscles themselves.[172,173]

The most advanced autologous reconstruction to date is the DIEP (deep inferior epigastric perforator), which is increasingly replacing the TRAM techniques. Similar to the muscle-sparing free TRAM, the DIEP uses the patient's abdominal skin and fat to reconstruct a natural, soft breast after mastectomy, but without removal of any rectus muscle (Fig. 61.6, right bottom). Sometimes described as the "tummy tuck" reconstruction, it is associated with a faster recovery, with less associated pain after surgery, long-term maintenance of abdominal strength, and minimal risk of complications such as abdominal bulging and hernia.

Sequencing of PMRT and Reconstruction

The timing of breast reconstruction is of critical importance in the decision-making process and needs to be discussed early with any patient considering mastectomy. The expanding indications for PMRT have added to the complexity of the reconstruction decision-making process, and therefore, a multidisciplinary approach is required to discern the likelihood of requiring PMRT based on the preoperative risk assessment. Whether or not a patient has a likelihood to require PMRT is a critical factor in the decision-making process when discussing reconstruction options and timing of (possible) radiation. Currently, the typical approach is to do immediate (permanent) reconstruction if the patient is considered low risk for requiring PMRT RT, as this generally results in better cosmesis.[171] Alternatively, if the patient is considered intermediate to high risk for requiring PMRT, delaying the definitive (flap or implant placement) with initial placement of a tissue expander to preserve and expand the breast skin envelope for a skin preservation and then delayed placement of the permanent reconstruction after PMRT is typically the preferred course.[174] Currently, the vast majority of reconstructions currently performed in the United States in the setting of PMRT consist of delayed reconstruction,[175] which is not necessarily supported by the published literature but may be related to risk aversion and medical–legal implications for radiating a permanent implant.

Timing for Implant-Based Reconstruction

There are numerous publications describing and attempting to discern the best algorithm for reconstruction to minimize the effects of PMRT. The vast majority of the existing literature assesses absolute risk of complications such as contractures,

revision surgeries, and reconstruction failures (and not patient-centered outcomes). Although there is significant controversy about the optimal approach regarding strategies for timing of reconstruction with PMRT to the tissue expander versus the permanent implant, the published data to date are difficult to interpret because of differences in outcomes measured.

Although delivering radiation therapy to a temporary tissue expander is feasible, there are challenges. Large expanders can make radiation treatment planning more challenging, creating steep sloping contours particularly at the medial chest wall that can increase normal tissue exposure and compromise dose distribution. In a survey study, 66% of radiation oncologists agreed that tissue expander volume affects radiation dose distribution and render planning more difficult[176] and 47% will ask plastic surgeons to adjust expander volume to 150 to 250 cc, with the most common reason for this request being to minimize dose to the heart and lungs. With few data to guide radiation oncologists regarding whether an expander should be deflated or inflated during PMRT, decision-making must be individualized taking into consideration the patient's anatomy and may require an initial planning CT for assessment prior to deciding whether adjustments in the volume of fluid in the implant is needed.

For example, the data are consistent in demonstrating higher rates of reconstructive failures in patients receiving PMRT to the tissue expander compared with permanent implants.[177–179] Yet conflicting these results, the risk of GIII/IV capsular contractures is reported to be worse when irradiating the permanent implant.[180,181] Confounding these findings further, very few patient-centered studies assessing irradiation to permanent implant versus tissue expander have been published. An institutional experience of nearly 300 patients with either expanders or permanent implants from Memorial Sloan Kettering reported that although tissue expanders had a higher risk of reconstructive failure, permanent implants were associated with worse aesthetic results and capsular contracture. Though the patient-reported outcomes did not differ across the 2 cohorts, these authors concluded that any sequence of radiotherapy in two-stage prosthetic reconstruction negatively impacts the final aesthetic outcome and survival of the implant.[180] From the same institution, these group of authors reported on outcomes of a cohort of 151 stage II or III patients that underwent a 2-step immediate expander placement, followed by initiation of systemic chemotherapy and expansion of expander and exchange of expander for permanent implant at the completion of chemotherapy prior PMRT. They reported the 7-year permanent implant failure to be 29%, with the most common causes for failure reported as severe capsular contractures and infection.[182] More recently, these data were updated to report an overall success rate of 94% when the permanent implant was in place prior to PMRT versus 60% when the exchange occurred after radiation.[183]

Nevertheless, the traditional and most common preferred method for implant-based reconstruction has been to wait until after the completion of radiation therapy to perform the exchange procedure to the permanent implant. This practice pattern has likely been more popular because of concerns regarding potential delays in initiating PMRT, the opportunity to release capsular contractures around the expander after PMRT, and capacity to revise any radiation effects and allow for correction of PMRT-related asymmetry. However, there are increasing body of data, including meta-analysis, to suggest that exchanging the expander for the permanent implant prior to starting PMRT is associated with decreased complications and improved cosmetic outcomes.[180,181,183–190]

For example, one meta-analysis of studies of reconstruction published reported on results from 37 combined studies and found that for the cohort undergoing implant-based reconstruction, there were more complications and a higher revision rate if the permanent implant reconstruction was performed after radiotherapy.[185] Ultimately, the use of variable endpoints across studies makes it difficult to draw definitive conclusions from these data, and patients undergoing mastectomy should have risks and benefits presented to them prior to their definitive surgery, with the integration of reconstruction and PMRT addressed in a multidisciplinary setting.

Timing for Autologous Reconstructions

The literature regarding the timing of autologous reconstruction, similar to implant-based reconstruction, continues to be conflicting and remains a topic of debate. Options when discussing PMRT with patients intending on mastectomy and autologous reconstruction include immediate autologous reconstruction prior to PMRT, a delayed autologous procedure performed 6 or more months after PMRT, or the delayed-immediate (2-step) approach discussed above. To date, the studies evaluating these approaches and the best cosmetic outcomes and satisfaction scores have reported conflicting results. There are several studies that have suggested that the outcomes of aesthetics and satisfaction are better with immediate reconstruction,[186-189] though these studies are limited in their small cohort size and use of non-validated outcomes measures.

A meta-analysis of studies of reconstruction published in 2014 reported on results from 37 combined studies. They found that, for the cohort undergoing autologous reconstruction, though the incidence of fibrosis was higher if autologous reconstruction was done prior to PMRT, they were not able to demonstrate any significant differences in total complication rate before or after PMRT, ultimately concluding that in the setting of autologous implants, the data do not support sequencing of PMRT and autologous reconstruction has any impact on severe complication rates.[181] Currently, most plastic surgeons opt for immediate versus delayed versus two-step based on their own clinical experience and institutional preferences rather than data- or patient-driven timing decisions. Other factors that may play a role when considering sequencing of PMRT and autologous reconstruction include the technical and economic benefits of immediate reconstruction, which include performing a technically less challenging procedure when performed prior to PMRT, the decrease in cost associated with one versus two separate surgeries and hospitalizations for the patient, and data suggesting an association with patient-reported improvements in measures of quality of life when autologous implants are performed immediately compared with delayed.[190-193]

Comparison of Implant Versus Autologous Reconstruction in the Setting of PMRT

Generally, much of the existing literature suggests that autologous reconstruction has a better complication and PMRT-related toxicity profile compared with implant-based reconstruction. Furthermore, autologous reconstruction has been demonstrated to result in superior patient-centered cosmetic outcomes in settings where PMRT is delivered.[192,194]

The effects of PMRT and systemic chemotherapy with either autologous or implant-based reconstructions were comprehensively assessed in a meta-analysis that analyzed 62 published manuscripts and over 6,000 reconstructed patients. Pooled analysis of the PMRT cohort revealed significantly higher-weighted incidences of reoperation ($P <$ .0001), total complications ($P < .0001$), and reconstructive failure ($P < .0001$) in prosthetic compared to autologous reconstructions. The use of postoperative chemotherapy did not appear to affect the overall outcomes of the reconstruction.[175] Though together, the body of data to date suggest that autologous reconstruction results in a better complication profile and success rate than implant-based reconstruction when PMRT is needed,[175,192-194] there are many significant factors to consider when counseling a patient regarding reconstruction and PMRT, which include but are not limited to patient preferences, comorbidities, technical feasibility, clinical–

pathologic features and ultimate breast cancer-related prognosis (i.e., reconstruction in an inflammatory breast cancer patient with 14/14+ axillary lymph nodes in comparison to a patient undergoing mastectomy for a T1, N1 breast cancer).

CONCLUSIONS

Indications for radiation therapy have expanded with contemporary prospective trials and meta-analyses providing evidence-based data that radiation therapy reduces not only LRR but also distant recurrence and improves survival for women with breast cancer. In the setting of women with node-positive breast cancer, including LABC, locoregional treatment decision-making is complex and requires multidisciplinary assessment to generate individualized recommendations. A meticulous approach should include interdisciplinary input to coordinate systemic therapy, radiation therapy, surgery, and potentially reconstruction. Modern technologic advances in radiation planning and delivery, using CT-based three-dimensional treatment planning to minimize radiation to OAR and deliver a homogenous treatment plan using techniques described in this chapter, will increase the potential for radiation oncologists to improve the therapeutic ratio for patients with breast cancer.

REFERENCES

1. American Joint Committee on Cancer; Greene FL, Page DL, Fleming ID, et al., eds. *AJCC cancer staging manual.* 6th ed. New York: Springer, 2002.
2. Cuzick J, et al. Overview of randomized trials of postoperative adjuvant radiotherapy in breast cancer. *Cancer Treat Rep* 1987;71(1):15–29.
3. Cuzick J, et al. Cause-specific mortality in long-term survivors of breast cancer who participated in trials of radiotherapy. *J Clin Oncol* 1994;12(3):447–453.
4. Early Breast Cancer Trialists' Collaborative Group. Effects of radiotherapy and surgery in early breast cancer. An overview of the randomized trials. *N Engl J Med* 1995;333(22):1444–1455.
5. Simmonds MC, Higgins JP, Stewart LA, et al. Meta-analysis of individual patient data from randomized trials: a review of methods used in practice. *Clin Trials* 2005;2(3):209–217.
6. Stewart LA, Parmar MK. Meta-analysis of the literature or of individual patient data: is there a difference? *Lancet* 1993;341(8842):418–422.
7. Early Breast Cancer Trialists' Collaborative Group. Favourable and unfavourable effects on long-term survival of radiotherapy for early breast cancer: an overview of the randomised trials. *Lancet* 2000;355(9217):1757–1770.
8. Early Breast Cancer Trialists' Collaborative Group. Effects of radiotherapy and of differences in the extent of surgery for early breast cancer on local recurrence and 15-year survival: an overview of the randomised trials. *Lancet* 2005;366(9503):2087–2106.
9. Early Breast Cancer Trialists' Collaborative Group. Effect of radiotherapy after breast-conserving surgery on 10-year recurrence and 15-year breast cancer death: meta-analysis of individual patient data for 10,801 women in 17 randomised trials. *Lancet* 2011;378(9804):1707–1716.
10. Van de Steene J, Soete G, Storme G. Adjuvant radiotherapy for breast cancer significantly improves overall survival: the missing link. *Radiother Oncol* 2000;55(3):263–272.
11. Gebski V, Lagleva M, Keech A, et al. Survival effects of postmastectomy adjuvant radiation therapy using biologically equivalent doses: a clinical perspective. *J Natl Cancer Inst* 2006;98(1):26–38. Erratum in: *J Natl Cancer Inst* 2006;98(12):876.
12. Whelan TJ, Julian J, Wright J, et al. Does locoregional radiation therapy improve survival in breast cancer? A meta-analysis *J Clin Oncol* 2000;18(6):1220–1229.
13. Early Breast Cancer Trialists' Collaborative Group. Effect of radiotherapy after mastectomy and axillary surgery on 10-year recurrence and 20-year breast cancer mortality: meta-analysis of individual patient data for 8135 women in 22 randomised trials. *Lancet* 2014;383(9935):2127–2135.
14. Olson JE, Neuberg D, Pandya KJ, et al. The role of radiotherapy in the management of operable locally advanced breast carcinoma: results of a randomized trial by the eastern cooperative oncology group. *Cancer* 1997;79(6):1138–1149.
15. Arriagada R, Rutqvist LE, Mattsson A, et al. Adequate locoregional treatment for early breast cancer may prevent secondary dissemination. *J Clin Oncol* 1995;13:2869–2878.
16. Overgaard M, Hansen PS, Overgaard J, et al. Postoperative radiotherapy in high-risk premenopausal women with breast cancer who receive adjuvant chemotherapy. *N Engl J Med* 1997;337:949–955.
17. Overgaard M, et al. Randomized trial evaluating postoperative radiotherapy in high risk postmenopausal breast cancer patients given adjuvant tamoxifen: results from the DBCG 82c trial. *Lancet* 1999;353:1641–1648.
18. Ragaz J, Jackson SM, Le N, et al. Adjuvant radiotherapy and chemotherapy in node-positive premenopausal women with breast cancer. *N Engl J Med* 1997;337(14):956–962.
19. Overgaard M, Nielsen HM, Overgaard J. Is the benefit of postmastectomy irradiation limited to patients with four or more positive nodes, as recommended in international consensus reports? A subgroup analysis of the DBCG 82 b&c randomized trials. *Radiother Oncol* 2007;82(3):247–253.

20. Nielsen HM, Overgaard M, Grau C, et al. Study of failure pattern among high-risk breast cancer patients with or without postmastectomy radiotherapy in addition to adjuvant systemic therapy: long-term results from the Danish Breast Cancer Cooperative Group DBCG 82b and c randomized studies. *J Clin Oncol* 2006;24(15):2268–2275.

21. Kyndi M, et al. High local recurrence risk is not associated with large survival reduction after postmastectomy radiotherapy in high-risk breast cancer: a subgroup analysis of DBCG 82 b& c. *Radiother Oncol* 2009;90(1):74–79.

22. Højris I, Overgaard M, Christensen JJ, et al. Morbidity and mortality of ischaemic heart disease in high-risk breast-cancer patients after adjuvant postmastectomy systemic treatment with or without radiotherapy: analysis of DBCG 82b and 82c randomised trials. *Lancet* 1999;354(9188):1425–1430.

23. Højris I, Andersen J, Overgaard M, et al. Late treatment-related morbidity in breast cancer patients randomized to postmastectomy radiotherapy and systemic treatment versus systemic treatment alone. *Acta Oncol* 2000;39(3):355–372.

24. Olsen N, Pfeiffer P, Johanssen L, et al. Radiation-induced brachial plexopathy, neurological follow-up in 161 recurrence-free breast cancer patients. *Int J Radiat Oncol Biol Phys* 1993;26:43–49.

25. Ragaz J, et al. Locoregional radiation therapy in patients with high-risk breast cancer receiving adjuvant chemotherapy: 20-year results of the British Columbia randomized trial. *J Natl Cancer Inst* 2005;97(2):116–126.

26. Whelan T, Olivotto IA, Parulekar WR, et al. Regional nodal irradiation in early breast cancer. *N Engl J Med* 2015;373(4):307–316.

27. Poortmans P, Colette L, Kirkove C, et al. Internal mammary and medial supraclavicular irradiation in breast cancer. *N Engl J Med* 2015;373:317–327.

28. Hennequin C, Bossard N, Servagi-Vernat S, et al. Ten-year survival results of a randomized trial of irradiation of internal mammary nodes after mastectomy. *Int J Radiat Oncol Biol Phys* 2013;86:860–866.

29. Budach W, Bolke E, Kammers K, et al. Adjuvant radiation therapy of regional lymph nodes in breast cancer—a meta-analysis of randomized trials—an update. *Radiat Oncol* 2015;10:258.

30. Macdonald SM, Harris EE, Arthur DW, et al. *American College of Radiology ACR appropriateness criteria: locally advanced breast cancer.* Reston, VA: American College of Radiology, 2011. Accessed at: http://www.acr.org/a2c

31. Shenkier T, Weir L, Levine M, et al. Clinical practice guidelines for the care and treatment of breast cancer: 15. Treatment for women with stage III or locally advanced breast cancer. *CMAJ* 2004;170(6):983–994.

32. Sautter-Bihl ML, Souchon R, Budach W, et al. DEGRO practical guidelines for radiotherapy of breast cancer II. Postmastectomy radiotherapy, irradiation of regional lymphatics, and treatment of locally advanced disease. *Strahlenther Onkol* 2008;184(7):347–353.

33. Brackstone M, Fletcher GG, Dayes IS, et al. Locoregional therapy of locally advanced breast cancer: a clinical practice guideline. *Curr Oncol* 2015;22(Suppl 1):S54–S66.

34. Gradishar WJ, Anderson BO, Blair SL, et al. NCCN clinical practice guidelines in oncology (NCCN guidelines) breast cancer. Version 2.2017. *National Comprehensive Cancer Network*; Accessed at: https://www.nccn.org/professionals/physician_gls/pdf/breast.pdf

35. Harris JR, et al. Consensus statement on postmastectomy radiation therapy. *Int J Radiat Oncol Biol Phys* 1999;44(5):989–990.

36. Recht A, Edge SB, Solin LJ, et al. Postmastectomy radiotherapy: clinical practice guidelines of the American Society of Clinical Oncology. *J Clin Oncol* 2001;19(5):1539–1569.

37. Recht A, Comen EA, Fine RE, et al. Postmastectomy radiotherapy: an American Society of Clinical Oncology, American Society for Radiation Oncology, and Society of Surgical Oncology focused guideline update. *J Clin Oncol* 2016;34(36):4431–4442.

38. Truong PT, Olivotto IA, Whelan TJ, et al.; Steering Committee on Clinical Practice Guidelines for the Care and Treatment of Breast Cancer. Clinical practice guidelines for the care and treatment of breast cancer: 16. Locoregional post-mastectomy radiotherapy. *CMAJ* 2004;170(8):1263–1273.

39. Belkacemi Y, Fourquet A, Cutuli B, et al. Radiotherapy for invasive breast cancer: guidelines for clinical practice from the French expert review board of Nice/Saint-Paul de Vence. *Crit Rev Oncol Hematol* 2011;79(2):91–102.

40. Hortobagyi GN, Ames FC, Buzdar AU, et al. Management of stage III primary breast cancer with primary chemotherapy, surgery and radiation therapy. *Cancer* 1988;62:2507–2516.

41. Buchholz TA, Tucker SL, Masullo L, et al. Predictors of local-regional recurrence after neoadjuvant chemotherapy and mastectomy without radiation. *J Clin Oncol.* 2002;20(1):17–23.

42. Panades M, Olivotto IA, Speers CH. Evolving treatment strategies for inflammatory breast cancer: a population-based survival analysis. *J Clin Oncol* 2005;23(9):1941–1950.

43. Recht A, Gray R, Davidson NE, et al. Locoregional failure ten years after mastectomy and adjuvant chemotherapy with or without tamoxifen without irradiation: experience of the Eastern Cooperative Oncology Group. *J Clin Oncol* 1999;17:1689–1700.

44. Katz A, Strom EA, Buchholz TA, et al. Loco-regional recurrence patterns following mastectomy and doxorubicin-based chemotherapy: implications for postoperative irradiation. *J Clin Oncol* 2000;18(15):2817–2827.

45. Strom EA, Woodward WA, Katz A, et al. Clinical investigation: regional nodal failure patterns in breast cancer patients treated with mastectomy without radiotherapy. *Int J Radiat Oncol Biol Phys* 2005;63(5):1508–1513.

46. Pisansky TM, Ingle JN, Schaid DJ, et al. Patterns of tumor relapse following mastectomy and adjuvant systemic therapy in patients with axillary lymph node-positive breast cancer. Impact of clinical, histopathologic, and flow cytometric factors. *Cancer* 1993;72(4):1247–1260.

47. Belkacemi Y, Truong PT, Khan AJ, et al. Adjuvant nodal radiotherapy in the era of sentinel node biopsy staging of breast cancer: a review of published guidelines and prospective trials and their implications on clinical practice. *Crit Rev Oncol Hematol* 2017;112:171–178.

48. Giuliano AE, McCall L, Beitsch P, et al. Locoregional recurrence after sentinel lymph node dissection with or without axillary dissection in patients with sentinel lymph node metastases: the American College of Surgeons Oncology Group Z0011 randomized trial. *Ann Surg* 2010;252(3):426–432.

49. Krag DN, Anderson SJ, Julian TB, et al. Sentinel lymph-node resection compared with conventional axillary-lymph-node dissection in clinically node-negative patients with breast cancer: overall survival findings from the NSABP B-32 randomized phase 3 trial. *Lancet Oncol* 2010;11:927–933.

50. Galimberti V, Cole BF, Zurrida S, et al. Axillary dissection versus no axillary dissection in patients with sentinel-node micrometastases (IBCSG 23–01): a phase 3 randomised controlled trial. *Lancet Oncol* 2013;14(4):297–305.

51. Donker M, van Tienhoven G, Straver ME, et al. Radiotherapy or surgery of the axilla after a positive sentinel node in breast cancer (EORTC 10981–22023 AMAROS): a randomised, multicentre, open-label, phase 3 non-inferiority trial. *Lancet Oncol* 2014;15:1303–1310.

52. Buchholz T. Internal mammary lymph nodes: to treat or not to treat. *Int J Rad Oncol Biol Phys* 2000;46:801–803.

53. Freedman G, Fowble BL, Nicolaou N, et al. Should internal mammary lymph nodes in breast cancer be a target for the radiation oncologist? *Int J Rad Oncol Biol Phys* 2000;46:805–814.

54. Jagsi R, Pierce L. Radiation therapy to the internal mammary nodal region in breast cancer: the debate continues. *Int J Radiat Oncol Biol Phys* 2013;86:813–815.

55. Lacour J, Bucalossi P, Caceres E, et al. Radical mastectomy versus radical mastectomy plus internal mammary dissection: five-year results of an international cooperative study. *Cancer* 1976;37:206–214.

56. Thorsen LB, Offersen BV, Danø H, et al. DBCG-IMN: a population-based cohort study on the effect of internal mammary node irradiation in early node-positive breast cancer. *J Clin Oncol* 2016;34(4):314–320.

57. Katz A, Strom EA, Buchholz TA, et al. The influence of pathologic tumor characteristics on locoregional recurrence rates following mastectomy. *Int J Radiat Oncol Biol Phys* 2001;50(3):735–742.

58. Katz A, Buchholz TA, Thames HD, et al. Recursive partitioning analysis of locoregional recurrence following mastectomy and doxorubicin-based chemotherapy: implications for postoperative irradiation. *Int J Radiat Oncol Biol Phys* 2001;50(2):397–403.

59. Wallgren A, et al. Risk factors for locoregional recurrence among breast cancer patients: results from International Breast Cancer Study Group Trials I through VII. *J Clin Oncol* 2003;21(7):1205–1213.

60. Taghian A, et al. Patterns of locoregional failure in patients with operable breast cancer treated by mastectomy and adjuvant chemotherapy with or without tamoxifen and without radiotherapy: results from five National Surgical Adjuvant Breast and Bowel Project randomized clinical trials. *J Clin Oncol* 2004;22(21):4247–4254.

61. Truong PT, Woodward W, Buchholz TA. Optimizing locoregional control and survival for women with breast cancer: a review of current developments in postmastectomy radiotherapy. *Expert Rev Anticancer Ther* 2006;6(2):205–216.

62. Truong PT, Olivotto IA, Kader HA, et al. Selecting breast cancer patients with T1-T2 tumors and one to three positive axillary nodes at high postmastectomy locoregional recurrence risk for adjuvant radiotherapy. *Int J Radiat Oncol Biol Phys* 2005;61:1337–1347.

63. Yildirim E, Berberoglu U. Local recurrence in breast carcinoma patients with T(1,2) and 1–3 positive nodes: indications for radiotherapy. *Eur J Surg Oncol* 2007;33:28–32.

64. Moo TA, McMillan R, Lee M, et al. Selection criteria for postmastectomy radiotherapy in t1-t2 tumors with 1 to 3 positive lymph nodes. *Ann Surg Oncol* 2013;20:3169–3174.

65. Tam MM, Wu SP, Perez C, et al. The effect of post-mastectomy radiation in women with one to three positive nodes enrolled on the control arm of BCIRG-005 at ten year follow-up. *Radiother Oncol* 2017;123(1):10–14.

66. Macdonald SM, Abi-Raad RF, Alm El-Din MA, et al. Chest wall radiotherapy: middle ground for treatment of patients with one to three positive lymph nodes after mastectomy. *Int J Radiat Oncol Biol Phys* 2009;75:1297–1303.

67. Hamamoto Y, Ohsumi S, Aogi K, et al. Are there high-risk subgroups for isolated locoregional failure in patients who had T1/2 breast cancer with one to three positive lymph nodes and received mastectomy without radiotherapy? *Breast Cancer* 2014;21:177–182.

68. Truong PT, Berthelet E, Lee J, et al. The prognostic significance of the percentage of positive/dissected axillary lymph nodes in breast cancer recurrence and survival in patients with one to three positive axillary lymph nodes. *Cancer* 2005;103:2006–2014.

69. Huang CJ, Hou MF, Chuang HY, et al. Comparison of clinical outcome of breast cancer patients with T1-2 tumor and one to three positive nodes with or without postmastectomy radiation therapy. *Jpn J Clin Oncol* 2012;42:711–720.

70. Kim SI, Park S, Park HS, et al. Comparison of treatment outcome between breast-conservation surgery with radiation and total mastectomy without radiation in patients with one to three positive axillary lymph nodes. *Int J Radiat Oncol Biol Phys* 2011;80:1446–1452.

71. Sartor CI, Peterson BL, Woolf S, et al. Effect of addition of adjuvant paclitaxel on radiotherapy delivery and locoregional control of node-positive breast cancer: cancer and leukemia group B 9344. *J Clin Oncol* 2005;23:30–40.

72. Harris EE, Freilich J, Lin HY, et al. The impact of the size of nodal metastases on recurrence risk in breast cancer patients with 1–3 positive axillary nodes after mastectomy. *Int J Radiat Oncol Biol Phys* 2013;85:609–614.

73. Botteri E, Gentilini O, Rotmensz N, et al. Mastectomy without radiotherapy: outcome analysis after 10 years of follow-up in a single institution. *Breast Cancer Res Treat* 2012;134:1221–1228.

74. Sharma R, Bedrosian I, Lucci A, et al. Present-day locoregional control in patients with t1 or t2 breast cancer with 0 and 1 to 3 positive lymph nodes after mastectomy without radiotherapy. *Ann Surg Oncol* 2010;17:2899–2908.

75. McBride A, Allen P, Woodward W, et al. Locoregional recurrence risk for patients with T1,2 breast cancer with 1–3 positive lymph nodes treated

with mastectomy and systemic treatment. *Int J Radiat Oncol Biol Phys* 2014;89:392–398.

76. Tendulkar RD, Rehman S, Shukla ME, et al. Impact of postmastectomy radiation on locoregional recurrence in breast cancer patients with 1–3 positive lymph nodes treated with modern systemic therapy. *Int J Radiat Oncol Biol Phys* 2012;83:e577–e581.
77. Cheng JC, et al. Locoregional failure of postmastectomy patients with 1–3 positive axillary lymph nodes without adjuvant radiotherapy. *Int J Radiat Oncol Biol Phys* 2002;52(4):980–988.
78. Lin J, Li C, Zhang C, et al. Postmastectomy radiation therapy for breast cancer patients with one to three positive lymph nodes: a propensity score matching analysis. *Future Oncol* 2017;13(16):1395–1404. doi: 10.2217/fon-2017-0099.
79. Lai SF, Chen YH, Kuo WH, et al. Locoregional recurrence risk for postmastectomy breast cancer patients with T1-2 and one to three positive lymph nodes receiving modern systemic treatment without radiotherapy. *Ann Surg Oncol* 2016;23(12):3860–3869.
80. Li Y, Moran MS, Huo Q, et al. Post-mastectomy radiotherapy for breast cancer patients with t1-t2 and 1–3 positive lymph nodes: a meta-analysis. *PLoS One* 2013;8(12):e81765.
81. Mamounas EP, Tang G, Fisher B, et al. Association between the 21-gene recurrence score assay and risk of locoregional recurrence in node-negative, estrogen receptor-positive breast cancer: results from NSABP B-14 and NSABP B-20. *J Clin Oncol* 2010;28:1677–1683.
82. Wen G, Zhang JS, Zhang YJ, et al. Predictive value of molecular subtyping for locoregional recurrence in early-stage breast cancer with N1 without postmastectomy radiotherapy. *J Breast Cancer* 2016;19(2):176–184.
83. Moo TA, McMillan R, Lee M, et al. Impact of molecular subtype on locoregional recurrence in mastectomy patients with T1-T2 breast cancer and 1–3 positive lymph nodes. *Ann Surg Oncol* 2014;21(5):1569–1574.
84. Kunkler IH, Canney P, van Tienhoven G, et al. Elucidating the role of chest wall irradiation in 'intermediate-risk' breast cancer: the MRC/EORTC SUPREMO trial. *Clin Oncol (R Coll Radiol)* 2008;20:31–34.
85. Floyd SR, Taghian AG. Post-mastectomy radiation in large node-negative breast tumors: does size really matter? *Radiother Oncol* 2009;9(1):33–37.
86. Floyd SR, Buchholz TA, Haffty BG, et al. Low local recurrence rate without postmastectomy radiation in node-negative breast cancer patients with tumors 5 cm and larger. *Int J Radiat Oncol Biol Phys* 2006;66:358–364.
87. Taghian AG, Jeong JH, Mamounas EP, et al. Low locoregional recurrence rate among node-negative breast cancer patients with tumors 5 cm or larger treated by mastectomy, with or without adjuvant systemic therapy and without radiotherapy: results from five national surgical adjuvant breast and bowel project randomized clinical trials. *J Clin Oncol* 2006;24:3927–3932.
88. Mignano JE, Gage I, Piantadosi S, et al. Local recurrence after mastectomy in patients with T3pN0 breast carcinoma treated without postoperative radiation therapy. *Am J Clin Oncol* 2007;30:466–472.
89. Helinto M, Blomqvist C, Heikkila P, et al. Post-mastectomy radiotherapy in pT3N0M0 breast cancer: is it needed? *Radiother Oncol* 1999;52:213–217.
90. Goulart J, Truong P, Woods R, et al. Outcomes of node-negative breast cancer 5 centimeters and larger treated with and without postmastectomy radiotherapy. *Int J Radiat Oncol Biol Phys* 2011;80:758–764.
91. McCammon R, Finlayson C, Schwer A, et al. Impact of postmastectomy radiotherapy in T3N0 invasive carcinoma of the breast: a surveillance, epidemiology, and end results database analysis. *Cancer* 2008;113:683–689.
92. Johnson ME, Handorf EA, Martin JM, et al. Postmastectomy radiation therapy for T3N0: a SEER analysis. *Cancer* 2014;120(22):3569–3574.
93. Cassidy RJ, Liu Y, Kahn ST, et al. The role of postmastectomy radiotherapy in women with pathologic T3N0M0 breast cancer. *Cancer* 2017;123(15):2829–2839. doi: 10.1002/cncr.30675.
94. Francis SR, Frandsen J, Kokeny KE. Outcomes and utilization of postmastectomy radiotherapy for T3N0 breast cancers. *Breast* 2017;32:156–161.
95. Fowble BL, Einck JP, Kim DN, et al. Role of postmastectomy radiation after neoadjuvant chemotherapy in stage II-III breast cancer. *Int J Radiat Oncol Biol Phys* 2012;83(2):494–503.
96. Buchholz TA, Katz A, Strom EA, et al. Pathologic tumor size and lymph node status predict for different rates of locoregional recurrence after mastectomy for breast cancer patients treated with neoadjuvant versus adjuvant chemotherapy. *Int J Radiat Oncol Biol Phys* 2002;53(4):880–888.
97. Huang EH, Tucker SL, Strom EA, et al. Postmastectomy radiation improves local-regional control and survival for selected patients with locally advanced breast cancer treated with neoadjuvant chemotherapy and mastectomy. *J Clin Oncol* 2004;22(23):4691–4699.
98. Huang EH, Tucker SL, Strom EA, et al. Predictors of locoregional recurrence in patients with locally advanced breast cancer treated with neoadjuvant chemotherapy, mastectomy, and radiotherapy. *Int J Radiat Oncol Biol Phys* 2005;62(2):351–357.
99. McGuire SE, Gonzalez-Angulo AM, Huang EH, et al. Postmastectomy radiation improves the outcome of patients with locally advanced breast cancer who achieve a pathologic complete response to neoadjuvant chemotherapy. *Int J Radiat Oncol Biol Phys* 2007;68(4):1004–1009.
100. Garg AK, Strom EA, McNeese MD, et al. T3 disease at presentation or pathologic involvement of four or more lymph nodes predict for locoregional recurrence in stage II breast cancer treated with neoadjuvant chemotherapy and mastectomy without radiotherapy. *Int J Radiat Oncol Biol Phys* 2004;59(1):138–145.
101. Mamounas EP, Anderson SJ, Dignam JJ, et al. Predictors of locoregional recurrence after neoadjuvant chemotherapy: results from combined analysis of National Surgical Adjuvant Breast and Bowel Project B-18 and B-27. *J Clin Oncol* 2012;30(32):3960–3966.
102. Buchholz TA, Lehman CD, Harris JR, et al. Statement of the science concerning locoregional treatments after preoperative chemotherapy for breast cancer: a National Cancer Institute conference. *J Clin Oncol* 2008;26:791–797.
103. Rusthoven CG, Rabinovitch RA, Jones BL, et al. The impact of postmastectomy and regional nodal radiation after neoadjuvant chemotherapy for clinically lymph node-positive breast cancer: a National Cancer Database (NCDB) analysis. *Ann Oncol* 2016;27(5):818–827.
104. Yang TJ, Morrow M, Modi S, et al. The effect of molecular subtype and Residual disease on locoregional recurrence in breast cancer patients treated with neoadjuvant chemotherapy and postmastectomy radiation. *Ann Surg Oncol* 2015;22(Suppl 3):S495–S501.
105. Swisher SK, Vila J, Tucker SL, et al. Locoregional control according to breast cancer subtype and response to neoadjuvant chemotherapy in breast cancer patients undergoing breast-conserving therapy. *Ann Surg Oncol* 2016;23(3):749–756.
106. Vila J, Teshome M, Tucker SL, et al. Combining clinical and pathologic staging variables has prognostic value in predicting local-regional recurrence following neoadjuvant chemotherapy for breast cancer. *Ann Surg* 2017;265(3):574–580.
107. Haffty BG, McCall LM, Ballman KV, et al. Patterns of local-regional management following neoadjuvant chemotherapy in breast cancer: results from ACOSOG Z1071 (Alliance). *Int J Radiat Oncol Biol Phys* 2016;94(3):493–502.
108. Fourquet A, Campana F, Rosenwald JC, et al. Breast irradiation in the lateral decubitus position: technique of the Institut Curie. *Radiother Oncol* 1991;22(4):261–265.
109. Moran MS, Haffty BG. Radiation techniques and toxicities for locally advanced breast cancer. *Semin Radiat Oncol* 2009;19(4):244–255.
110. Offersen BV, Boersma LJ, Kirkove C, et al. ESTRO consensus guideline on target volume delineation for elective radiation therapy of early stage breast cancer. *Radiother Oncol* 2016;114(1):3–10.
111. Landis DM, Luo W, Song J, et al. Variability among breast radiation oncologists in delineation of the postsurgical lumpectomy cavity. *Int J Radiat Oncol Biol Phys* 2007;67(5):1299–1308.
112. Hurkmans CW, Borger JH, Pieters BR, et al. Variability in target volume delineation on CT scans of the breast. *Int J Radiat Oncol Biol Phys* 2001;50(5):1366–1372.
113. White J, Tai A, Arthur D, et al. *RTOG Breast Atlas* https://wwwrtogorg/LinkClickaspx?fileticket=vzJFhPaBipE%3d&tabid=236. Accessed on March 1, 2018.
114. Nielsen MH, Berg M, Pedersen AN, et al. Delineation of target volumes and organs at risk in adjuvant radiotherapy of early breast cancer: national guidelines and contouring atlas by the Danish Breast Cancer Cooperative Group. *Acta Oncol* 2013;52(4):703–710.
115. Castro Pena P, Kirova YM, Campana F, et al. Anatomical, clinical and radiological delineation of target volumes in breast cancer radiotherapy planning: individual variability, questions and answers. *Br J Radiol* 2009;82:595–599.
116. Li XA, Tai A, Arthur DW, et al. Variability of target and normal structure delineation for breast cancer radiotherapy: an RTOG Multi-Institutional and Multiobserver Study. *Int J Radiat Oncol Biol Phys* 2009;73(3):944–951.
117. Taghian A, Jagsi R, Makris A, et al. Results of a survey regarding irradiation of internal mammary chain in patients with breast cancer: practice is culture driven rather than evidence based. *Int J Radiat Oncol Biol Phys* 2004;60(3):706–714.
118. Belkacemi Y, Kaidar-Person O, Poortmans P, et al. Patterns of practice of regional nodal irradiation in breast cancer: results of the European Organization for Research and Treatment of Cancer (EORTC) NOdal Radiotherapy (NORA) survey. *Ann Oncol* 2015;26(3):529–535.
119. Kestin LL, Sharpe MB, Frazier RC, et al. Intensity modulation to improve dose uniformity with tangential breast radiotherapy: initial clinical experience. *Int J Radiat Oncol Biol Phys* 2000;48(5):1559–1568.
120. Donovan EM, Yarnold JR, Adams EJ, et al. An investigation into methods of IMRT planning applied to breast radiotherapy. *Br J Radiol* 2008;81(964):311–322.
121. Smith W, Menon G, Wolfe N, et al. IMRT for the breast: a comparison of tangential planning techniques. *Phys Med Biol* 2010;55(4):1231–1241.
122. Descovich M, Fowble B, Bevan A, et al. Comparison between hybrid direct aperture optimized intensity-modulated radiotherapy and forward planning intensity-modulated radiotherapy for whole breast irradiation. *Int J Radiat Oncol Biol Phys* 2010;76(1):91–99.
123. Vicini FA, Sharpe M, Kestin L, et al. Optimizing breast cancer treatment efficacy with intensity-modulated radiotherapy. *Int J Radiat Oncol Biol Phys* 2002;54(5):1336–1344.
124. Buchholtz TA. Breast cancer. In: Chao C, Apisrathanarax S, Ozyigit G, eds. *Practical essentials of intensity modulated radiation therapy.* Philadelphia: Lippincott Williams & Wilkins, 2005:248.
125. Fraass BA, Kessler ML, McShan DL, et al. Optimization and clinical use of multisegment intensity-modulated radiation therapy for high-dose conformal therapy. *Semin Radiat Oncol* 1999;9(1):60–77.
126. Caudrelier JM, Morgan SC, Montgomery L, et al. Helical tomotherapy for locoregional irradiation including the internal mammary chain in left-sided breast cancer: dosimetric evaluation. *Radiat Oncol* 2009;9(1):99–105.
127. Giorgia N, Antonella F, Alessandro C, et al. Planning strategies in volumetric modulated arc therapy for breast. *Med Phys* 2011;38(7):4025–4031.
128. Hall EJ, Wuu CS. Radiation-induced second cancers: the impact of 3D-CRT and IMRT. *Int J Radiat Oncol Biol Phys* 2003;56(1):83–88.
129. Schubert LK, Gondi V, Sengbusch E, et al. Dosimetric comparison of left-sided whole breast irradiation with 3DCRT, forward-planned IMRT, inverse-planned IMRT, helical tomotherapy, and topotherapy. *Radiother Oncol* 2011;100(2):241–246.
130. Smith BD, Bentzen SM, Correa CR, et al. Fractionation for whole breast irradiation: an American Society for Radiation Oncology (ASTRO) evidence-based guideline. *Int J Radiat Oncol Biol Phys* 2011;81(1):59–68.
131. Gradishar WJ, Anderson BO, Balassanian R, et al. NCCN guidelines insights: breast cancer, Version 1.2017. *J Natl Compr Canc Netw* 2017;15(4):433–451.
132. Gradishar WJ, Anderson BO, Balassanian R, et al. Invasive breast cancer version 1.2016, NCCN clinical practice guidelines in oncology. *J Natl Compr Canc Netw* 2016;14(3):324–354.
133. Vu TT, Pignol JP, Rakovitch E, et al. Variability in radiation oncologists' opinion on the indication of a bolus in post-mastectomy radiotherapy: an international survey. *Clin Oncol (R Coll Radiol)* 2007;19(2):115–119.

134. Pignol JP, Vu TT, Mitera G, et al. Prospective evaluation of severe skin toxicity and pain during postmastectomy radiation therapy. *Int J Radiat Oncol Biol Phys* 2015;91(1):157–164. doi: 10.1016/j.ijrobp.2014.09.022. Erratum in: *Int J Radiat Oncol Biol Phys* 2015;92(3):702.

135. Nakamura N, Arahira S, Zenda S, et al. Post-mastectomy radiation therapy without usage of a bolus may be a reasonable option. *J Radiat Res* 2017;58(1):66–70.

136. Abel S, Renz P, Trombetta M, et al. Local failure and acute radiodermatological toxicity in patients undergoing radiation therapy with and without postmastectomy chest wall bolus: is bolus ever necessary? *Pract Radiat Oncol* 2017;7(3):167–172. pii: S1879-8500(16)30245-4.

137. Ma C, Zhang W, Lu J, et al. Dosimetric comparison and evaluation of three radiotherapy techniques for use after modified radical mastectomy for locally advanced left-sided breast cancer. *Sci Rep* 2015;5:12274.

138. Rudat V, Aziz Alaradi A, Mohamed A, et al. Tangential beam IMRT versus tangential beam 3D-CRT of the chest wall in postmastectomy breast cancer patients: a dosimetric comparison. *Radiat Oncol* 2011;6(1):26.

139. Cho BCJ, Schwarz M, Mijnheer BJ, et al. Simplified intensity-modulated radiotherapy using pre-defined segments to reduce cardiac complications in left-sided breast cancer. *Radiother Oncol* 2004;70(3):231–241.

140. Ma J, Li J, Xie J, et al. Post mastectomy linac IMRT irradiation of chest wall and regional nodes: dosimetry data and acute toxicities. *Radiat Oncol* 2013;8(1):81.

141. Taylor CW, Bronnum D, Darby SC, et al. Cardiac dose estimates from Danish and Swedish breast cancer radiotherapy during 1977–2001. *Radiother Oncol* 2011;100(2):176–183.

142. Darby SC, Cutter DJ, Boerma M, et al. Radiation-related heart disease: current knowledge and future prospects. *Int J Radiat Oncol Biol Phys* 2010;76(3):656–665.

143. Fajardo LF, Stewart JR. Pathogenesis of radiation-induced myocardial fibrosis. *Lab Invest* 1973;29:244–257.

144. Fajardo LF. The pathology of ionizing radiation as defined by morphologic patterns. Keynote lecture, 5th Nordic Conference on Radiation Oncology, Bergen, Norway. *Acta Oncol* 2005;44:13–22.

145. Moiseenko V, Einck J, Murphy J, et al. Clinical evaluation of QUANTEC guidelines to predict the risk of cardiac mortality in breast cancer patients. *Acta Oncol* 2016;55(12):1506–1510.

146. Gagliardi G, Constine LS, Moiseenko V, et al. Radiation dose-volume effects in the heart. *Int J Radiat Oncol Biol Phys* 2010;76(3 Suppl):S77–S85.

147. Taylor CW, Nisbet A, McGale P, et al. Cardiac exposures in breast cancer radiotherapy: 1950s-1990s. *Int J Radiat Oncol Biol Phys* 2007;69(5):1484–1495.

148. EBCTCG. Long term toxicity of radiation therapy. In: *2006 Update of the Early Breast Cancer Trialists' Collaborative group overview of radiation therapy for early breast cancer. American Society of Clinical Oncology Annual Meeting, June 1–5, 2007, Chicago*. 2007.

149. Darby SC, Ewertz M, McGale P, et al. Risk of ischemic heart disease in women after radiotherapy for breast cancer. *N Engl J Med* 2013;368(11):987–998.

150. Preston DL, Shimizu Y, Pierce DA, et al. Studies of mortality of atomic bomb survivors. Report 13: solid cancer and noncancer disease mortality: 1950–1997. *Radiat Res* 2003;160:381–407.

151. Yamada M, Wong FL, Fujiwara S, et al. Noncancer disease incidence in atomic bomb survivors, 1958–1998. *Radiat Res* 2004;161(6):622–632.

152. Schultz-Hector S, Trott KR. Radiation-induced cardiovascular diseases: is the epidemiologic evidence compatible with the radiobiologic data? *Int J Radiat Oncol Biol Phys* 2007;67(1):10–18.

153. van den Bogaard VA, Ta BD, van der Schaaf A, et al. Validation and modification of a prediction model for acute cardiac events in patients with breast cancer treated with radiotherapy based on three-dimensional dose distributions to cardiac substructures. *J Clin Oncol* 2017;35(11):1171–1178.

154. Amir E, Seruga B, Niraula S, et al. Toxicity of adjuvant endocrine therapy in postmenopausal breast cancer patients: a systematic review and meta-analysis. *J Natl Cancer Inst* 2011;103(17):1299–1309.

155. Alarid-Escudero F, Blaes AH, Kuntz KM. Trade-offs between efficacy and cardiac toxicity of adjuvant chemotherapy in early-stage breast cancer patients: do competing risks matter? *Breast J* 2017;23(4):401–409. doi: 10.1111/tbj.12757

156. Raj KA, Evans ES, Prosnitz RG, et al. Is there an increased risk of local recurrence under the heart block in patients with left-sided breast cancer? *Cancer J* 2006;12:309–317.

157. Varga Z, Hideghety K, Mezo T, et al. Individual positioning: a comparative study of adjuvant breast radiotherapy in the prone versus supine position. *Int J Radiat Oncol Biol Phys* 2009;75(1):94–100.

158. Stegman LD, Beal KP, Hunt MA, et al. Long-term clinical outcomes of whole-breast irradiation delivered in the prone position. *Int J Radiat Oncol Biol Phys* 2007;68(1):73–81.

159. Formenti SC, DeWyngaert JK, Jozsef G, et al. Prone vs supine positioning for breast cancer radiotherapy. *JAMA* 2012;308(9):861–863.

160. Veldeman L, Schiettecatte K, De Sutter C, et al. The 2-year cosmetic outcome of a randomized trial comparing prone and supine whole-breast irradiation in large-breasted women. *Int J Radiat Oncol Biol Phys* 2016;95(4):1210–1217.

161. Shin SM, No HS, Vega RM, et al. Breast, chest wall, and nodal irradiation with prone set-up: results of a hypofractionated trial with a median follow-up of 35 months. *Pract Radiat Oncol* 2016;6(4):e81–e88.

162. Lu HM, Cash E, Chen MH, et al. Reduction of cardiac volume in left-breast treatment fields by respiratory maneuvers: a CT study. *Int J Radiat Oncol Biol Phys* 2000;47(4):895–904.

163. Swanson T, Grills IS, Ye H, et al. Six-year experience routinely using moderate deep inspiration breath-hold for the reduction of cardiac dose in left-sided breast irradiation for patients with early-stage or locally advanced breast cancer. *Am J Clin Oncol* 2013;36(1):24–30.

164. Lin A, Sharieff W, Juhasz J, et al. The benefit of deep inspiration breath hold: evaluating cardiac radiation exposure in patients after mastectomy and after breast-conserving surgery. *Breast Cancer* 2017;24(1):86–91.

165. Alderman AK, Wilkins EG, Lowery JC, et al. Determinants of patient satisfaction in postmastectomy breast reconstruction. *Plast ReconstrSurg* 2000;106(4):769–776.

166. Wilkins EG, Cederna PS, Lowery JC, et al. Prospective analysis of psychosocial outcomes in breast reconstruction: one-year postoperative results from the Michigan Breast Reconstruction Outcome Study. *Plast Reconstr Surg* 2000;106(5):1014–1025; discussion 26–27.

167. Spear SL, Ducic I, Low M, et al. The effect of radiation on pedicled TRAM flap breast reconstruction: outcomes and implications. *Plast Reconstr Surg* 2005;115(1):84–95.

168. Hirsch EM, Seth AK, Dumanian GA, et al. Outcomes of immediate tissue expander breast reconstruction followed by reconstruction of choice in the setting of postmastectomy radiation therapy. *Ann Plast Surg* 2014;72(3): 274–278.

169. Hirsch EM, Seth AK, Kim JY, et al. Analysis of risk factors for complications in expander/implant breast reconstruction by stage of reconstruction. *Plast Reconstr Surg* 2014;134(5):692e–699e.

170. Tran N, Chang D, Gupta A, et al. Comparison of immediate and delayed free TRAM flap breast reconstruction in patients receiving postmastectomy radiation therapy. *Plast Reconstr Surg* 2001;108:78–82.

171. Kronowitz SJ. State of the art and science in postmastectomy breast reconstruction. *Plast Reconstr Surg* 2015;135(4):755e–771e.

172. Nahabedian MY, Dooley W, Singh N, et al. Contour abnormalities of the abdomen after breast reconstruction with abdominal flaps: the role of muscle preservation. *Plast Reconstr Surg* 2002;109(1):91–101.

173. Nahabedian MY, Manson PN. Contour abnormalities of the abdomen after transverse rectus abdominis muscle flap breast reconstruction: a multifactorial analysis. *Plast Reconstr Surg* 2002;109(1):81–87; discussion 8–90.

174. Kronowitz SJ. Delayed-immediate breast reconstruction: technical and timing considerations. *Plast Reconstr Surg* 2010;125(2):463–474.

175. Gurunluoglu R, Gurunluoglu A, Williams SA, et al. Current trends in breast reconstruction: survey of American Society of Plastic Surgeons 2010. *Ann Plast Surg* 2013;70(1):103–110.

176. Chen SA, Hiley C, Nickleach D, et al. Breast reconstruction and post-mastectomy radiation practice. *Radiat Oncol* 2013;8:45.

177. Anderson P, Freedman G, Nicolaou N, et al. Postmastectomy chest wall radiation to a temporary tissue expander or permanent breast implant—is there a difference in complication rates? *Int J Radiat Oncol Biol Phys* 2009;74: 81–85.

178. El-Sabawi B, Sosin M, Carey JN, et al. Breast reconstruction and adjuvant therapy: a systematic review of surgical outcomes. *J Surg Oncol* 2015;112(5):458–464.

179. Collier P, Williams J, Edhayan G, et al. The effect of timing of postmastectomy radiation on implant-based breast reconstruction: a retrospective comparison of complication outcomes. *Am J Surg* 2014;207:408–411.

180. Cordeiro P, Albornoz C, Mccormick B, et al. What is the optimum timing of post-mastectomy radiotherapy in two-stage prosthetic reconstruction: radiation to the tissue expander or permanent implant? *Plast Reconstr Surg* 2015;135:1509–1517.

181. Nava M, Pennati A, Lozza L, et al. Outcome of different timings of radiotherapy in implant-based breast re- constructions. *Plast Reconstr Surg* 2011;128:353–359.

182. Ho A, Cordeiro P, Disa J, et al. Long-term outcomes in breast cancer patients undergoing immediate 2-stage expander/implant reconstruction and postmastectomy radiation. *Cancer* 2012;118(9):2552–2559.

183. Cordeiro PG, McCarthy CM. A single surgeon's 12-year experience with tissue expander/implant breast reconstruction: part II. An analysis of long-term complications, aesthetic outcomes, and patient satisfaction. *Plast Reconstr Surg* 2006;118(4):832–839.

184. Lam TC, Hsieh F, Boyages J. The effects of postmastectomy adjuvant radiotherapy on immediate two-stage prosthetic breast reconstruction: a systematic review. *Plast Reconstr Surg* 2013;132(3):511–518.

185. Berbers J, van Baardwijk A, Houben R, et al. 'Reconstruction: before or after postmastectomy radiotherapy?' A systematic review of the literature. *Eur J Cancer* 2014;50(16):2752–2762.

186. Lee BT, A Adesiyun T, Colakoglu S, et al. Postmastectomy radiation therapy and breast reconstruction: an analysis of complications and patient satisfaction. *Ann Plast Surg* 2010;64(5):679–683.

187. Kim SH, Kim JM, Park SH, et al. Analysis of the effects of breast reconstruction in breast cancer patients receiving radiotherapy after mastectomy. *Arch Plast Surg* 2012;39(3):222–226.

188. Albino FP, Patel KM, Smith JR, et al. Delayed versus delayed-immediate autologous breast reconstruction: a blinded evaluation of aesthetic outcomes. *Arch Plast Surg* 2014;41(3):264–270.

189. Carlson GW, Page AL, Peters K, et al. Effects of radiation therapy on pedicled transverse rectus abdominis myocutaneous flap breast reconstruction. *Ann Plast Surg* 2008;60(5):568–572.

190. Veronesi P, Ballardini B, De Lorenzi F, et al. Immediate breast reconstruction after mastectomy. *Breast* 2011;20(Suppl 3):S104–S107.

191. Al-Ghazal SK, Sully L, Fallowfield L, et al. The psychological impact of immediate rather than delayed breast reconstruction. *Eur J Surg Oncol* 2000;26(1):17–19.

192. Jagsi R, Li Y, Morrow M, et al. Patient-reported quality of life and satisfaction with cosmetic outcomes after breast conservation and mastectomy with and without reconstruction: results of a survey of breast cancer survivors. *Ann Surg* 2015;261(6):1198–1206.

193. Jhaveri JD, Rush SC, Kostroff K, et al. Clinical outcomes of postmastectomy radiation therapy after immediate breast reconstruction. *Int J Radiat Oncol Biol Phys* 2008;72(3):859–865.

194. Kronowitz S, Robb G. Radiation therapy and breast reconstruction: a critical review of the literature. *Plast Reconstr Surg* 2009;124:395–408.

CHAPTER 62
Stomach Cancer

Brian G. Czito, Manisha Palta, and Christopher G. Willett

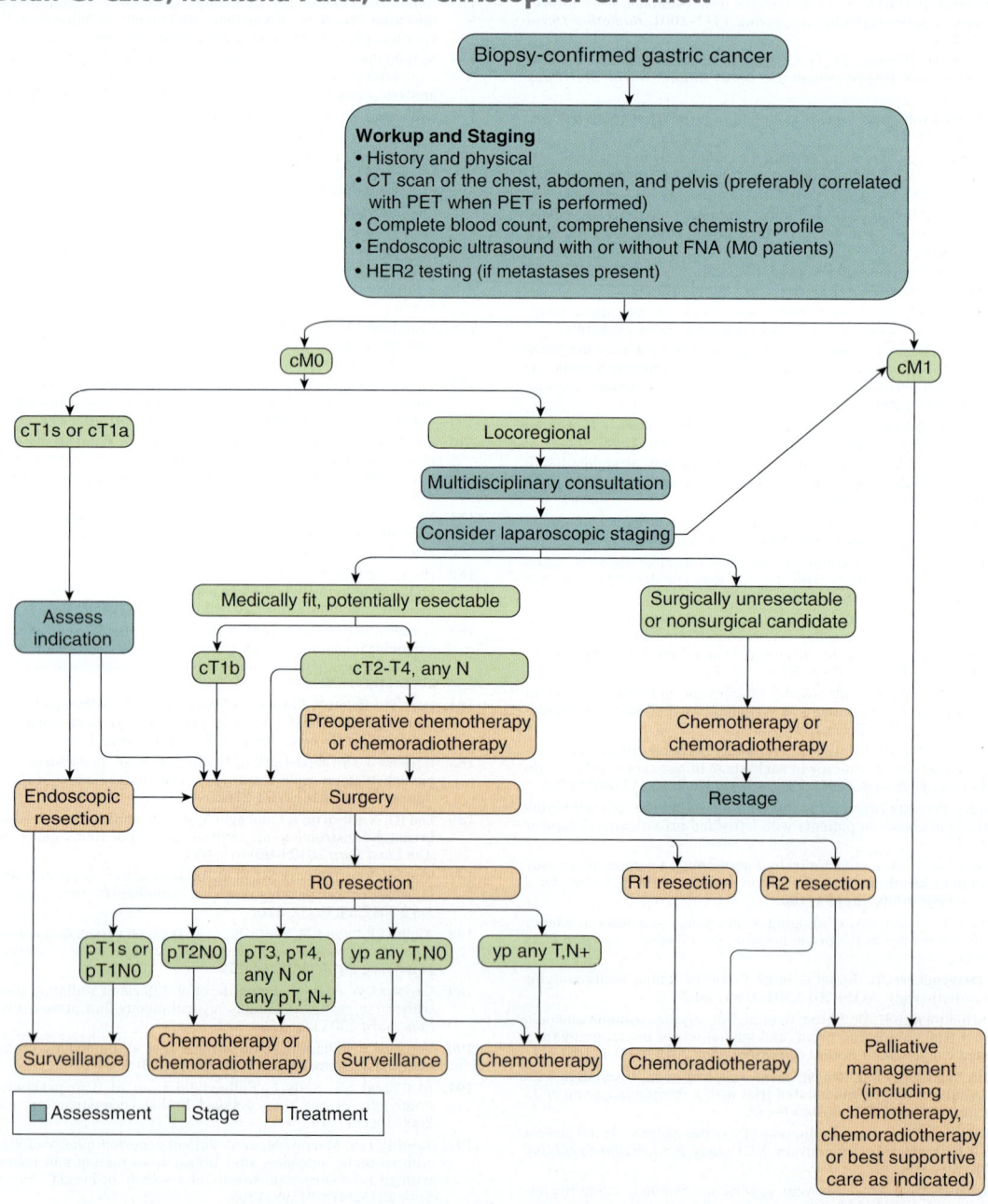

Treatment algorithm for newly diagnosed gastric cancer. Treatment approaches are based in location and stage of the tumor, as well as surgical resectability and medical comorbidities of the patient. CT, computed tomography; EUS, endoscopic ultrasound; FNA, fine-needle aspiration; PET, positron emission tomography. Reprinted by permission from Nature: Ajani JA, Lee J, Sano T, et al. Gastric adenocarcinoma. Nat Rev Dis Primers 2017;3:17036. Copyright © 2017 Springer Nature.

ANATOMY

The stomach begins at the gastroesophageal (GE) junction and ends at the pylorus. The stomach is generally divided into anatomic regions, including the gastric cardia (the region surrounding the superior opening of the stomach where it connects with the GE junction/level of the lower esophageal sphincter), the fundus (situated superiorly, a rounded portion superior to the body and to the left of the cardia), the body (a large, central portion of the stomach), and the pyloric canal (distally, connecting to the duodenum). The pylorus is composed of two parts: the pyloric antrum, which connects to the body of the stomach, and the pyloric canal, which empties into the duodenum (Fig. 62.1). The pylorus communicates with the duodenum of the small intestine via the pyloric sphincter (valve). This valve regulates the passage of chyme from the stomach to the duodenum and prevents backflow from the duodenum to the stomach. A plane passing through the incisura angularis on the lesser curvature divides the stomach into the body and the pyloric portion (antrum). The anterior surface of the stomach is covered with the peritoneum of the greater sac. At the left and cranially, it abuts the diaphragm.

FIGURE 62.1. Gastric anatomy. (Republished with permission of John Wiley & Sons, Inc. from Tortora GJ, Grabowski SR. *Principles of anatomy and physiology*. 9th ed. New York: John Wiley & Sons, Inc. Copyright © 2000 Biological Sciences Textbooks, Inc. and Sandra Reynolds Grabowski; permission conveyed through Copyright Clearance Center, Inc.)

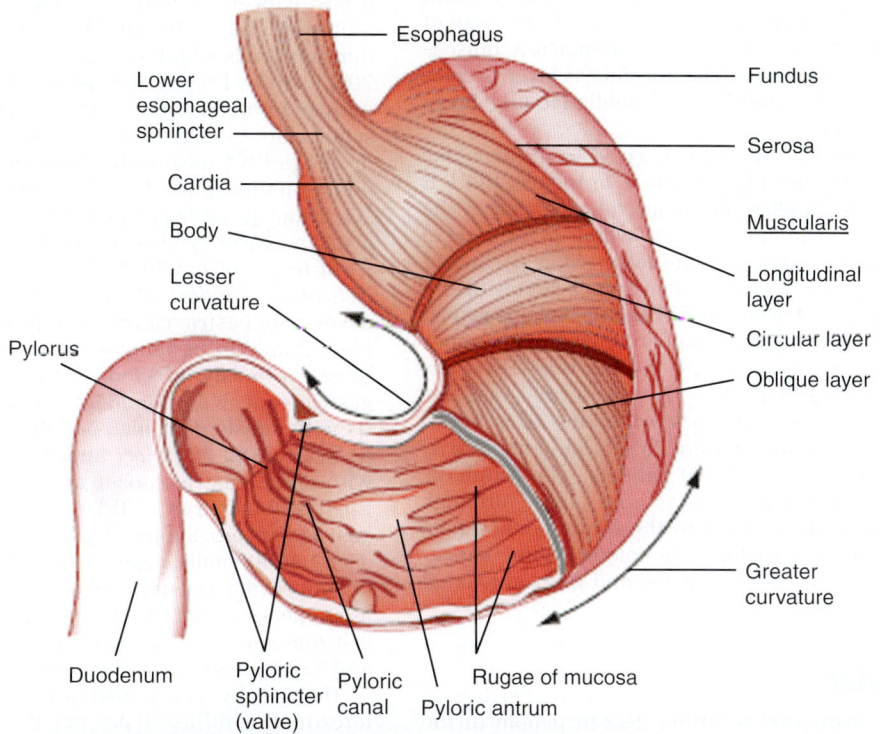

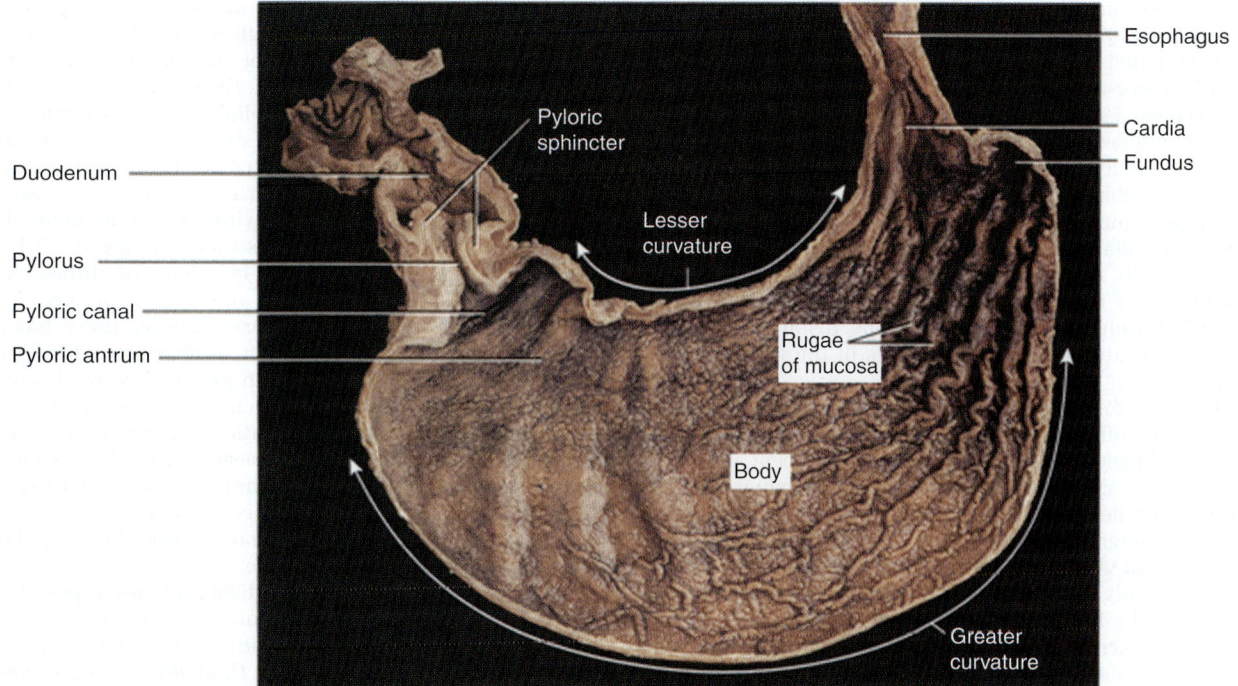

Section
III

In view of the increasing incidence of gastric cancer at the GE junction, it is important to note that there is either no or variable visceral peritoneal covering at the most proximal portion of the GE junction.[1] Positive radial margins at this site are often "true" positive margins, whereas many other positive margins in the stomach are free serosal margins unless the tumor is adherent to an adjacent organ or structure. The right portion of the anterior gastric surface is adjacent to the left lobe of the liver and the anterior abdominal wall. Posteriorly, the stomach is covered with peritoneum of the lesser sac or omental bursa. The stomach contacts many visceral structures; from superior to inferior, it is adjacent to the spleen, left adrenal gland, superior portion of the left kidney, ventral portion of the pancreas, and transverse colon. The hepatogastric ligament or lesser omentum is attached to the lesser curvature and contains the left gastric artery and the right gastric branch of the hepatic artery. Histologically, the wall of the stomach has five layers: the mucosa, submucosa, muscular layer, subserosa, and serosa. The muscularis layer is composed of an outer longitudinal layer, a middle circular layer, and inner oblique layer.

The stomach's vascular supply is derived from the celiac axis. The celiac artery usually has three branches: the left gastric artery, which supplies the upper right portion of the stomach; the common hepatic artery, which gives rise to the right gastric artery supplying the lower right portion of the stomach and the right gastroepiploic branch supplying the lower portion of the greater curvature; and the splenic artery, which gives rise to the left gastroepiploic supplying the upper portion of the greater curvature and the short gastric arteries supplying the fundus. Variations in this normal vascular supply are common. The celiac axis originates at or below the pedicle of T12 in approximately 75% of patients and at or above the pedicle of L1 in 25% of patients.[2] The lymphatic drainage of the stomach follows the arterial supply. Although most lymphatics ultimately drain to the celiac nodal basin, lymph drainage sites can include the splenic hilum, suprapancreatic nodal groups, porta hepatis, and gastroduodenal areas.

EPIDEMIOLOGY

Gastric cancer is estimated to afflict 26,240 people in the United States in 2018 and result in 10,800 deaths.[3] Worldwide, gastric cancer remains a significant cause of cancer-related mortality, with approximately 1,313,000 new cases annually and an estimated 819,000 deaths, making it the third-leading cause of cancer-related deaths.[4] During the past 70 years, there has been a significant decline in the incidence of gastric cancer in both sexes in Western countries. The causes of this decline are unknown.[4-6] Although the overall decrease in gastric cancer incidence is encouraging, there has been a steady and dramatic increase in the incidence of proximal lesser curvature, cardia, and GE junction tumors over the past 20 years, especially in white males.[7] In contrast to the increasing incidence of more proximal gastric cancers seen in the Western Hemisphere and parts of Europe, distal tumors continue to constitute most gastric cancers in the Far East and other parts of the world.

Risk factors for gastric cancer can be classified as modifiable or nonmodifiable (Table 62.1). Race or ethnicity, specifically being of East Asian or Pacific Islanders descent, portends increased risk. Although potentially related to environment, this incidence persists following immigration and into offspring when migrating to the West. Age is also an important risk factor, with 90% of cases occurring in patients older than 45 years. Family history similarly contributes to risk, with studies from the East and West demonstrating a first-degree relative likely increases an individual's risk from two- to fourfold. Similarly, male sex portends a two- to fivefold increased

TABLE 62.1 RISK FACTORS FOR GASTRIC CANCER DEVELOPMENT

Modifiable	Intrinsic
H. pylori infection	Ethnicity (East Asian or Pacific Islander)
Tobacco smoking	Male gender
Obesity	Age
High-salt diet; low-fruit or -vegetable diet	Family history

risk, possibly accounted for by protective effects of estrogen in females. Approximately 10% of gastric cancers are linked to genetic syndromes, with the most common being hereditary diffuse gastric cancer (HDGC), which is characterized by an autosomal dominant inheritance, portending a 60% to 80% increase risk of gastric cancer and 40% to 50% increase in breast cancer. Some of these cases are believed to be due to mutations in E-cadherin (CDH1). The presence of CDH1 mutations portends a lifetime risk of gastric cancer development of 70% to 80%.[8] Prophylactic gastrectomy is often recommended once patients are >20 years of age in these patients. Other syndromes associated with increased risk include Lynch syndrome (a DNA mismatch repair gene mutation), familial adenomatous polyposis (an APC gene mutation), Peutz-Jeghers syndrome, juvenile polyposis syndrome, hereditary breast and ovarian cancer syndrome, and Li-Fraumeni syndrome.[9]

In terms of modifiable risk factors, the most common is *Helicobacter pylori* (*H. pylori*) infection. Although the risk of developing gastric cancer is approximately 1% once present, more than 90% of patients with gastric cancer diagnosis have been previously infected. *H. pylori* appears to contribute to gastric cancer development through development of gastritis with subsequent histopathologic changes. The increased association of *H. pylori* appears to be confined to patients with distal gastric cancer and intestinal-type histology. The Epstein-Barr virus (EBV) has been found in 5% to 16% of gastric cancers, supporting its possible role in the genesis of such.[8] Additionally, cigarette use appears to increase the risk of both cardia and noncardia cancers, whereas obesity (BMI > 30) appears to increase the risk of noncardia cancers. A high-salt diet seems to increase risk, whereas diets high in fruit and vegetables seem to be protective.[5,9-11]

Historically, gastric adenocarcinomas have been labeled as intestinal or diffuse types per the Lauren classification system. Intestinal types are more prevalent in high-incidence areas and responsible for much of the observed global ethnic variation of disease, although the incidence is believed to be decreasing.[12] Intestinal-type carcinomas are primarily well to moderately differentiated. Histologically, these tumors generally show malignant epithelial cells in hyperchromatic, irregular, angulated glands with cohesiveness and glandular differentiation infiltrating the stroma. These tumors can be polypoid with a wide base, ulcerated with sharp/heaped-up margins, and ulcerated disease without obvious limits. These are generally seen more in males than females in a 2:1 ratio. In contrast, the incidence of the less common diffuse gastric cancer appears to be increasing and is fairly uniform among geographic regions or race. More recently, there has been an emergence of another distinct subtype—proximal gastric (cardia) cancers. These are often grouped with GE junction and distal esophageal adenocarcinomas, with a rapidly rising incidence in industrialized nations. Gastric cardia cancers are associated with reflux and obesity, resembling esophageal adenocarcinomas. These malignancies are generally more aggressive and carry a worse prognosis than do noncardia tumors. These tumors are associated with white populations with a strong male predominance.

The risks factors for these individual types appear to vary significantly. Risk factors for intestinal, noncardia gastric cancers appear to center around inflammatory causes and environmental factors, primarily *H. pylori*, as well as chronic gastritis, tobacco, high salt intake, and alcohol consumption. The less common diffuse gastric cancer subtype appears to be distinct, with E-cadherin mutations/silencing thought to be a common precursor event with this histology. HDGC is a genetic syndrome in which there is loss of function/mutation in the E-cadherin gene. In proximal gastric cancer (and in contrast to intestinal types), *H. pylori* infection has been found to be potentially protective in several randomized trials, possibly through associated atrophic gastritis and reduced acid production with subsequent reduction in gastroesophageal reflux disease (GERD), although this remains controversial.[13] As opposed to intestinal types, there is often no precancerous lesion seen, and histologically, cells generally lack cohesion and invade independently or in smaller clusters. Diffuse carcinomas are poorly differentiated. These are often more diffusely infiltrating and nonulcerated and can present as a "signet-ring" carcinoma, which is a variant with cytoplasmic mucin that displaces the cell nucleus peripherally. The presence of signet-ring (or poorly differentiated) phenotype has been associated with therapy resistance and poor prognosis[13] (Fig. 62.2). However, a large database analysis indicated patients with signet-ring gastric cancer, when compared to adenocarcinoma patients, tended to present at a younger age and less often in men. Additionally, despite more advanced stage, median survival was not different relative to "traditional" adenocarcinoma patients.[12,14,15]

An alternative gastric cancer classification from the World Health Organization is based predominantly on histologic cancer patterns (tubular, papillary, mucinous, poorly cohesive, and rare variants). The tubular and papillary subtypes roughly correspond to the Lauren intestinal type and poorly cohesive to the diffuse type. More recently, the Cancer Genome Atlas Research Network published the results of genomic profiling of 295 primary gastric adenocarcinomas. Four tumor subtypes were identified: (a) Epstein-Barr virus (9%), (b) microsatellite-unstable tumors (22%), (c) genomically stable tumors (20%), and (d) chromosomally unstable tumors (50%). This classification has the potential to determine prognosis and help individualize treatment in the future.[14]

PATTERNS OF SPREAD

Cancer of the stomach may extend directly into the omentum, pancreas, diaphragm, transverse colon or mesocolon, and duodenum. Peritoneal contamination with carcinomatosis is possible after a lesion extends beyond the gastric wall to a free peritoneal (serosal) surface.[16]

Microscopic or subclinical spread beyond the visible gross lesion occurs frequently because of the abundant lymphatic channels within the submucosal and subserosal layers of the gastric wall. The submucosal plexus in the esophagus and subserosal plexus in the duodenum allow proximal and distal spread.

It is difficult to perform a complete node dissection because of the numerous pathways of lymphatic drainage from the stomach (Fig. 62.3). Initial drainage is to lymph nodes along the lesser and greater curvatures (i.e., gastric and gastroepiploic nodes) but also includes the celiac axis, porta hepatis, splenic, suprapancreatic, pancreaticoduodenal, adjacent para-aortics, and distal paraesophageal system. The relative risks for nodal involvement in gastric cancer depend on the location of the primary tumor as well as extent of gastric wall involvement.

Gastric venous drainage is primarily to the liver by the portal system. Liver involvement is found in as many as 30% of patients at initial exploration, and it can occur as a result of venous metastasis, peritoneal-based spread, and direct extension (Fig. 62.4).

CLINICAL PRESENTATION

The most common presenting symptoms of stomach cancer are anorexia, early satiety, abdominal discomfort, unintentional weight loss, dysphagia (notably if GE junction or proximal stomach involvement), anemia-related weakness, nausea and vomiting, and tarry stools. Duration of symptoms is <3 months in almost 40% of patients and >1 year in 20%. Physical examination can reveal advanced disease, for which the presentation may include an abdominal mass (epigastric or liver mass as well as a periumbilical node [i.e., Sister Mary Joseph node]), palpable left supraclavicular nodes (i.e., Virchow node), an enlarged left axillary lymph node (Irish node), or a rectal shelf (representing peritoneal seeding [i.e., Blumer shelf]).

DIAGNOSTIC WORKUP

Many patients with early-stage gastric cancer are asymptomatic, and therefore patients are often diagnosed with a more advanced stage. Diagnosis is usually confirmed by

FIGURE 62.2. A: Hematoxylin and eosin–stained slide of Lauren classification diffuse-type gastric adenocarcinoma (GAC) with many cancer cells isolated from other cells. *Arrows* point to signet-ring cells, in which the nucleus is pushed out to the periphery of the cytoplasm. **B:** Hematoxylin and eosin–stained slide of Lauren classification intestinal-type GAC. *Arrows* are pointing to gland formation by tumor cells. (Reprinted by permission from Nature: Ajani JA, Lee J, Sano T, et al. Gastric adenocarcinoma. *Nat Rev Dis Primers* 2017;3:17036. Copyright © 2017 Springer Nature.)

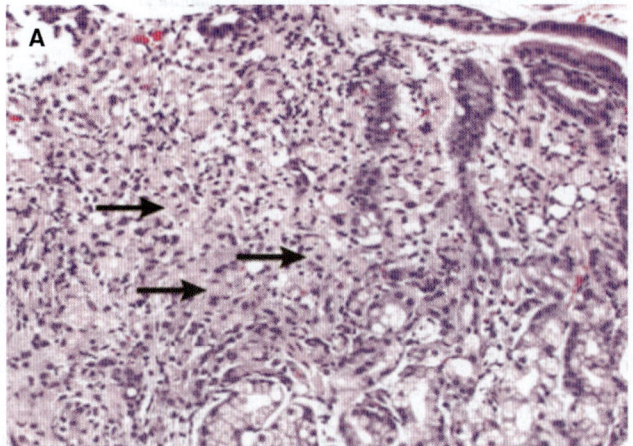

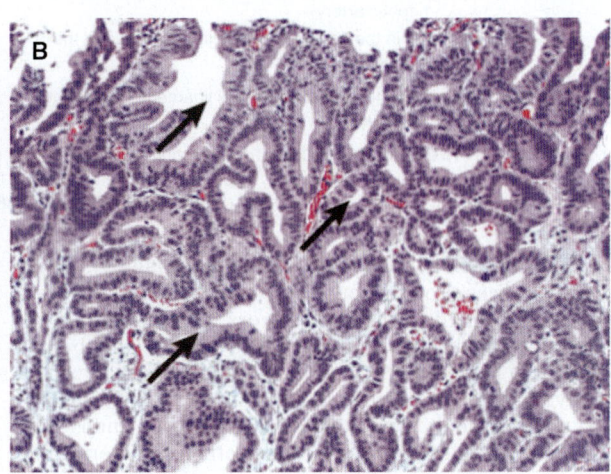

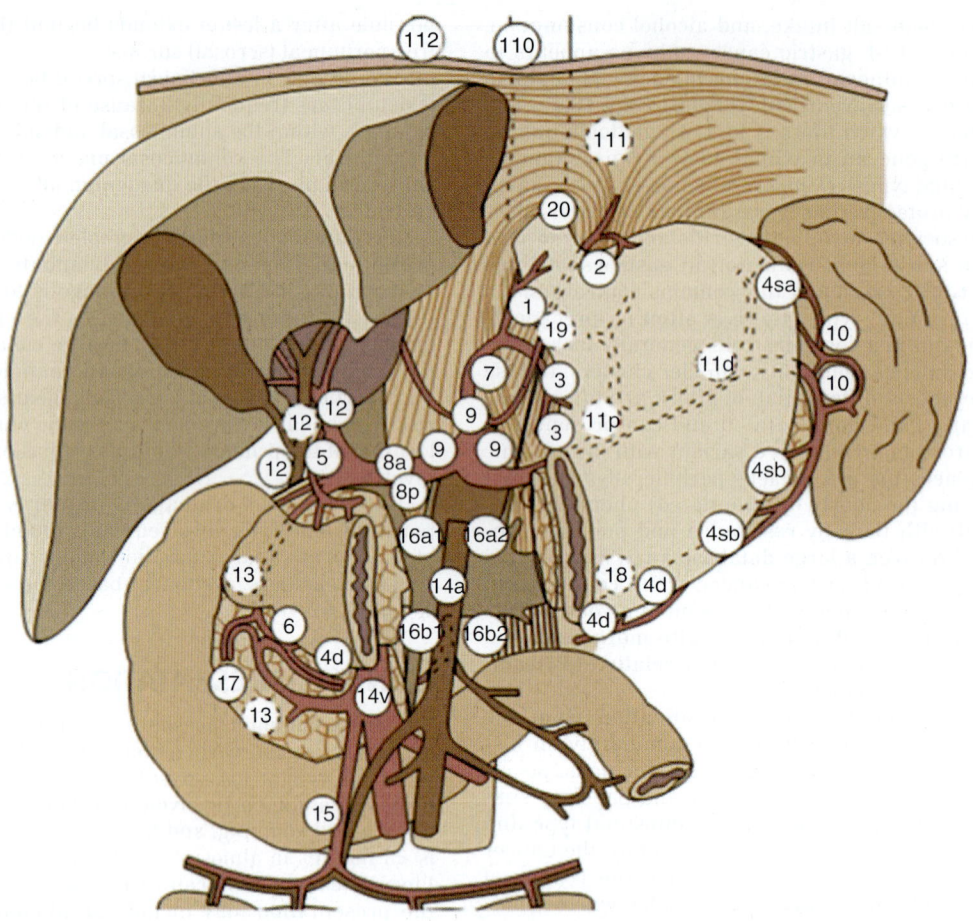

No. 1	Right paracardial LN
No. 2	Left paracardial LN
No. 3	LN along the lesser curvature
No. 4sa	LN along the short gastric vessels
No. 4sb	LN along the left gastroepiploic vessels
No. 4d	LN along the right gastroepiploic vessels
No. 5	Suprapyloric LN
No. 6	Infrapyloric LN
No. 7	LN along the left gastric artery
No. 8a	LN along the common hepatic artery (Anterosuperior group)
No. 8p	LN along the common hepatic artery (Posterior group)
No. 9	LN around the celiac artery
No. 10	LN at the splenic hilum
No. 11p	LN along the proximal splenic artery
No. 11d	LN along the distal splenic artery
No. 12a	LN in the hepatoduodenal ligament (along the hepatic artery)
No. 12b	LN in the hepatoduodenal ligament (along the bile duct)
No. 12p	LN in the hepatoduodenal ligament (behind the portal vein)

No. 13	LN on the posterior surface of the pancreatic head
No. 14v	LN along the superior mesenteric vein
No. 14a	LN along the superior mesenteric artery
No. 15	LN along the middle colic vessels
No. 16a1	LN in the aortic hiatus
No. 16a2	LN around the abdominal aorta (from the upper margin of the celiac trunk to the lower margin of the left renal vein)
No. 16b1	LN around the abdominal aorta (from the lower margin of the left renal vein to the upper margin of the inferior mesenteric artery)
No. 16b2	LN around the abdominal aorta (from the upper margin of the inferior mesenteric artery to the aortic bifurcation)
No. 17	LN on the anterior surface of the pancreatic head
No. 18	LN along the inferior margin of the pancreas
No. 19	Infradiaphragmatic LN
No. 20	LN in the esophageal hiatus of the diaphragm
No. 110	Paraesophageal LN in the lower thorax
No. 111	Supradiaphragmatic LN
No. 112	Posterior mediastinal LN

FIGURE 62.3. Locations of gastric lymph node stations. (Reprinted from Matzinger O, Gerber E, Bernstein Z, et al. EORTC-ROG expert opinion: radiotherapy volume and treatment guidelines for neoadjuvant radiation of adenocarcinomas of the gastroesophageal junction and the stomach. *Radiother Oncol* 2009;92[2]:164–175. Copyright © 2009 Elsevier Ireland Ltd. With permission.)

upper gastrointestinal endoscopy as well as imaging studies in some instances. Double-contrast x-ray studies may reveal small lesions limited to the inner layers of the gastric wall. Endoscopy with direct visualization, cytology, and biopsy yields the diagnosis in ≥90% of exophytic lesions; however, infiltrative (linitis plastica), small (<3 cm), or cardia lesions may be more difficult to diagnose endoscopically. Endoscopic ultrasonography is the most accurate method of determining depth of tumor invasion (intramural vs. extramural extension) prior to resection but is less accurate in detecting regional nodal metastases.[17,18] In some instances, needle biopsies of suspicious nodes are performed at the time of endoscopic ultrasound.

One principle goal of staging computed tomography (CT) is the identification of distant metastases, although it can also provide T- and N-stage data. Abdominal CT is useful in

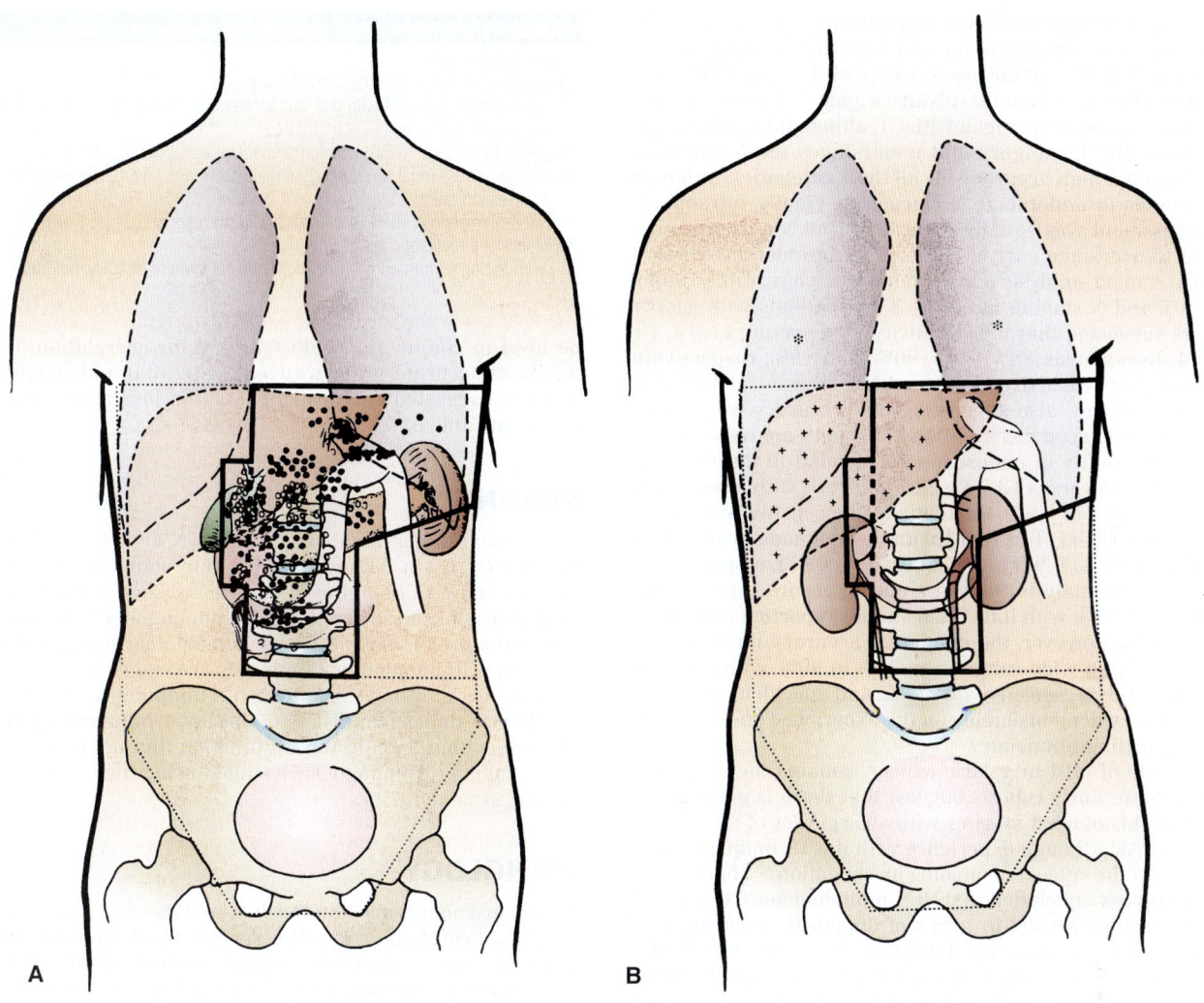

FIGURE 62.4. Patterns of failure in 82 evaluable patients in the University of Minnesota Reoperation series. **A:** *Large bold circles* indicate local failures in surrounding organs or tissues; *large open circles* indicate lymph node failures. **B:** *Asterisk* (*) indicates lung metastasis; *plus* (+) indicates liver metastasis. Superimposed irradiation portals encompass postsurgical gastric remnant, anastomoses, duodenal stump, gastric bed structures, and primary and secondary areas of lymph node drainage; *broken lines* represent upper and total abdomen fields. (Reprinted from Gunderson LL, Sosin H. Adenocarcinoma of the stomach: areas of failure in a reoperation series [second or symptomatic looks]. Clinicopathologic correlation and implications for adjuvant therapy. *Int J Radiat Oncol Biol Phys* 1982;8[1]:1–11. Copyright © 1982 Elsevier. With permission.)

determining the abdominal extent of disease and may help to determine which lesions extend to surgically unresectable structures but are of lesser value in detecting small lymph node metastases or peritoneal spread. Distant metastases should be ruled out with contrast-enhanced CT of the chest, abdomen, and pelvis. CT may provide valuable tumor localization information if radiation is indicated. If a proximal gastric cancer extends to involve the esophagus, CT of the chest will help to rule out involvement of mediastinal nodes or the lung parenchyma. A meta-analysis suggested that CT accuracy in terms of T stage was 72% although there was an indication that multidetector (4 or more) scanners demonstrated an overall accuracy of 80%.[19] However, multidetector status did not seem to influence nodal or distant metastatic assessment. In the same study, CT accuracy, compared to histologic findings, was 66% in terms of N stage.

The value of laparoscopy in the staging of gastric cancer remains a subject of study. The primary value of laparoscopy lies in the detection of occult metastatic deposits. A large series from Memorial Sloan Kettering Cancer Center of >600 patients with potentially resectable gastric adenocarcinoma by conventional imaging underwent laparoscopic staging, resulting in distant metastases being detected in 31% of patients.[20]

A systematic review on the role of diagnostic laparoscopy showed that change in patient management occurred in 9% to 60% of patients initially deemed resectable by preoperative imaging, with 9% to 44% avoiding laparotomy, predominantly through the identification of patients with metastatic disease who would not benefit from either laparotomy or neoadjuvant therapy, thereby avoiding unnecessary interventions. This is primarily related to patients with advanced (T3, T4) gastric cancer, with relatively minimal benefit in early-stage patients, prompting the authors to recommend diagnostic laparoscopy for patients with locally advanced-stage disease.[21,22] In addition, peritoneal fluid can be sampled for cytology at laparoscopy by direct aspiration of ascitic fluid or peritoneal lavage. If positive, this is a poor prognostic indicator, and although the bearing on treatment approach remains somewhat controversial, the patient should be considered as having M1 disease.

Overall treatment planning in gastric cancer may be improved by accurate preoperative classification of key prognostic factors, namely, depth of invasion (T category) and lymph node involvement (N category). A prospective study in 108 patients evaluated endogastric ultrasonography (EUS), CT, and intraoperative surgical assessment for T and N classification.[23] T staging was accurately characterized by CT in 43% of the cases, EUS in 86% of cases, and intraoperative assessment in 56% of cases. Staging of N1 and N2 lymph nodes was correct with CT in 51% of the cases, 74% with EUS, and 54% with intraoperative assessment. Advanced gastric tumors tended to be more accurately staged with CT, although CT, in general, overstages the T category and understages the N category. EUS showed a high accuracy for all the T categories, although it also tends to understage N categories. Finally, intraoperative assessment was equally accurate for all N categories but tended to overstage early T stages and to understage N categories. A meta-analysis and systematic review of the role of EUS in T and N staging in nearly 2,000 patients with gastric cancers suggested that the sensitivity for detecting T1, T2, T3, and T4 disease was 88%, 82%, 90%, and 99%, respectively. Nodal staging sensitivity for N1 and N2 disease was 58% and 65%, respectively, also suggesting that accuracy was higher with more advanced disease.[24] Another meta-analysis demonstrated the ability of endoscopic ultrasound to discriminate between T1-T2 versus T3-T4 gastric cancers, with a sensitivity of 0.86 (CI 0.81 to 0.90); additionally, the sensitivity for diagnosis of superficial (T1a vs. T1b) and lymph node involvement was 0.87 (0.81 to 0.92) and 0.83 (0.79 to 0.87), respectively.[25] Another meta-analysis showed a pooled accuracy for T-stage diagnosis of 75%, with individual studies reporting rates from 57% to 88%. However, the diagnostic accuracy for N staging was less, with a wide range from 30% to 90%, with a pooled accuracy of 64%, sensitivity of 74%, and specificity of 80%.[26] EUS accuracy depends highly on the experience and expertise of the operating physician.

The role of MRI in gastric cancer remains the subject of investigation. Early reports suggest that there is good agreement with histologic T staging, with an accuracy of 83% (range 77% to 87%), although experience with this technique is more limited and the subject of ongoing investigation.[22] Another systematic review concluded that EUS, multidetector CT, and MRI achieve similar results in terms of diagnostic accuracy of T staging and assessing serosal involvement.[27] Presently, MRI is primarily used in further characterization of indeterminate liver lesions seen on other staging investigations in gastric cancer patients.

Positron emission tomography (PET) scan has a lower detection rate in some cases of gastric cancers owing to the low fluorine-18 fluorodeoxyglucose (FDG) accumulation in patients with diffuse or mucinous/signet-ring tumors.[28] Approximately 40% of gastric carcinomas, notably the above histologies, may not be detected with PET scan.[29] PET alone has been described as displaying a lower sensitivity when compared to CT in detecting nodal involvement, although specificity is improved.[30] Because of its low-resolution images, the value of PET-CT primarily lies in its ability to detect metastatic disease, with a relatively low T-stage sensitivity for T1-T2 tumors, with improvement for more advanced disease. Estimated sensitivity for N stage is 40%, although specificity has been reported as high as 98%. As above, the accuracy in identifying distant metastases was 88% and higher than CT alone, and PET has been reported to detect occult metastases in operable patients in 10% and changing patient management in 15%. Additionally, PET response to neoadjuvant therapy, including treatment modification in poor responders as well as a potential indicator of prognosis in these patients, remains an active area of investigation.[22] The ongoing Alliance A021302 study is comparing overall survival of patients with locally advanced gastric cancer classified as PET nonresponders following one cycle of preoperative chemotherapy, with nonresponding patients receiving either salvage chemotherapy before and after surgery or immediate surgery followed by fluorouracil-sensitized radiotherapy. Given the above, PET alone is likely not an adequate diagnostic procedure for evaluation of gastric cancer and generally should

TABLE 62.2 DIAGNOSTIC WORKUP FOR GASTRIC CANCER
History and physical
Upper gastrointestinal endoscopy and biopsy
Chest, abdomen, pelvic CT with oral and intravenous contrast (preferably correlated with PET when PET is performed)
Complete blood count (CBC) and comprehensive metabolic panel
Endoscopic ultrasound if no evidence of metastases with fine-needle aspiration (FNA) as indicated
Biopsy confirmation of suspected metastatic gastric cancer
HER2 testing if metastatic
H. pylori testing performed and treatment delivered where clinically indicated

be used in conjunction with CT scan for correlation, allowing more accurate preoperative staging than either modality alone. A suggested diagnostic evaluation for gastric cancer is shown in Table 62.2.

STAGING

The current tumor–node–metastasis (TNM) system is depicted in Table 62.3.[31] In the most recent American Joint Committee on Cancer (AJCC) staging of gastric cancers, cancers whose midpoint is in the lower thoracic esophagus, GE junction, or within the proximal 2 cm of the stomach (cardia) *and* extending to the GE junction or esophagus are staged as esophageal neoplasms. All other cancers with a midpoint in the stomach lying more than 2 cm distal to and involving the GE junction or those within 2 cm of the GE junction (but not involving the GE junction or esophagus) are staged using the gastric cancer staging system.

PATHOLOGY

Adenocarcinomas account for 90% to 95% of all gastric malignancies. Lymphomas are the second most common malignancies. Rarely, gastrointestinal stromal tumors (GISTs), carcinoid (neuroendocrine) tumors, adenoacanthomas (1%), and squamous cell carcinomas (1%) occur.

The site of origin of gastric cancers within the stomach has changed in the United States over recent decades, and proximal lesions are being diagnosed and treated more frequently. Although the highest frequency is still in the antrum/distal stomach (~40%), the lowest frequency is now in the body (~25%) rather than the proximal portion of the stomach, with intermediate frequency in the proximal stomach and GE junction (~35%). Several investigators have reported an increased frequency of cardia lesions. As described previously, cardia lesions appear to have different epidemiologic factors, exhibit different tumor biology, and have an inferior prognosis relative to lesions in the other sites.[32-36] Gastric cancers have historically been categorized according to Borrmann's five types. Type I tumors are polypoid or fungating; type II are ulcerating lesions surrounded by elevated borders; type III have ulceration with invasion of the gastric wall; type IV are diffusely infiltrating (linitis plastica); and type V are unclassifiable.[37]

PROGNOSTIC FACTORS

The most important prognostic indicators reflect tumor extent. If hematogenous or transperitoneal spread is present, the outcome is, essentially, uniformly fatal. Survival rates decrease with progressive tumor extension within or beyond the gastric wall.[32,38-40] The number of involved lymph nodes also has a significant impact on survival. Lymph node involvement is important, as are the number and locations of nodes affected.[32,40-42] Minimal nodal involvement adjacent to the primary lesion only moderately affects prognosis.[38,42,43] The finding of either

TABLE 62.3 AMERICAN JOINT COMMITTEE ON CANCER 8TH EDITION GASTRIC CANCER STAGING

T Category	T Criteria
TX	Primary tumor cannot be assessed
T0	No evidence of primary tumor
Tis	Carcinoma *in situ*: intraepithelial tumor without invasice of the lamina propria, high grade dysplasia
T1	Tumor invades the lamina propria, muscularis mucosae or submocosa
T1a	Tumor invades the lamina propria or muscularis mucosae
T1b	Tumor invades the submocosa
T2	Tumor invades the muscularis propria[a]
T3	Tumor penetrates the subserosal connective tissue without invasion of the visceral peritoneum or adjacent structures[b,c]
T4	Tumor invades the serosa (visceral peritoneum) or adjacent structures[b,c]
T4a	Tumor invades the serosa (visceral peritoneum)
T4b	Tumor invades the adjacent structures/organs

Definition of Distant Lymph Node (M)

N Category	N Criteria
NX	Regional lymph node(s) cannot be assessed
N0	No regional lymph node metastasis
N1	Metastasis in 1 or 2 regional lymph nodes
N2	Metastasis in 3 to 6 regional lymph nodes
N3	Metastasis in 7 or more regional lymph nodes
N3a	Metastasis in 7 to 15 regional lymph nodes
N3b	Metastasis in 16 or more regional lymph nodes

Definition of Distant Metastasis (M)

M Category	M Criteria
M0	No distant metastasis
M1	Distant metastasis

AJCC PROGNOSTIC STAGE GROUPS

Clinical (cTNM)

When T is...	And N is...	And M is...	Then stage group is...
Tis	N0	M0	0
T1	N0	M0	I
T2	N0	M0	I
T1	N1, N2, or N3	M0	IIA
T2	N1, N2, or N3	M0	IIA
T3	N0	M0	IIB
T4a	N0	M0	IIB
T3	N1, N2, or N3	M0	III
T4a	N1, N2, or N3	M0	III
T4b	Any N	M0	IVA
Any T	Any N	M1	IVB

Pathological (pTNM)

When T is...	And N is...	And M is...	Then stage group is...
Tis	N0	M0	0
T1	N0	M0	IA
T1	N1	M0	IB
T2	N0	M0	IB
T1	N2	M0	IIA
T2	N1	M0	IIA
T3	N0	M0	IIA
T1	N3a	M0	IIB
T2	N2	M0	IIB
T3	N1	M0	IIB
T4a	N0	M0	IIB
T2	N3a	M0	IIIA
T3	N2	M0	IIIA
T4a	N1	M0	IIIA
T4a	N2	M0	IIIA
T4b	N0	M0	IIIA
T1	N3b	M0	IIIB
T2	N3b	M0	IIIB
T3	N3a	M0	IIIB
T4a	N3a	M0	IIIB
T4b	N1	M0	IIIB
T4b	N2	M0	IIIB
T3	N3b	M0	IIIC
T4a	N3b	M0	IIIC
T4b	N3a	M0	IIIC
T4b	N3b	M0	IIIC
Any T	Any N	M1	IV

(Continued)

TABLE 62.3 AMERICAN JOINT COMMITTEE ON CANCER 8TH EDITION GASTRIC CANCER STAGING (*Continued*)

Post-Neoadjuvant Therapy (ypTNM)

When T is...	And N is...	And M is...	Then stage group is...
T1	N0	M0	I
T2	N0	M0	I
T1	N1	M0	I
T3	N0	M0	II
T2	N1	M0	II
T1	N2	M0	II
T4a	N0	M0	II
T3	N1	M0	II
T2	N2	M0	II
T1	N3	M0	II
T4a	N1	M0	III
T3	N2	M0	III
T2	N3	M0	III
T4b	N0	M0	III
T4b	N1	M0	III
T4a	N2	M0	III
T3	N3	M0	III
T4b	N2	M0	III
T4b	N3	M0	III
T4a	N3	M0	III
Any T	Any N	M1	IV

The specific regional nodal areas are as follows.
- Perigastric along the greater curvature (including greater curvature, greater omental)
- Perigastric along the lesser curvature (including lesser curvature, lesser omental)
- Right and left paracardial (cardioesophageal)
- Suprapyloric (including gastroduodenal)
- Infrapyloric (including gastroepiploic)
- Left gastric artery
- Celiac artery
- Common hepatic artery
- Hepatoduodenal (along the proper hepatic artery, including portal)
- Splenic artery
- Splenic hilum

[a]A tumor may penetrate the muscularis propria with extension into the gastrocolic or gastrohepatic ligaments, or into the greater or lesser omentum, without perforation of the visceral peritoneum covering these structures. In this case, the tumor is classified as T3. If there is perforation of the visceral peritoneum covering the gastric ligaments or the omentum, the tumor should be classified as T4.
[b]The adjacent structures of the stomach include the spleen, transverse colon, liver, diaphragm, pancreas, abdominal wall, adrenal gland, kidney, small intestine, and retroperitoneum.
[c]Intramural extension to the duodenum or esophagus is not considered invasion of an adjacent structure, but is classified using the depth of the greatest invasion in any of these sites.
From Amin MB, Edge SB, Greene FL, et al., eds. *AJCC Cancer Staging Manual*. 8th ed. New York: Springer, 2017. Reproduced with permission of Springer International Publishing in the format Book via Copyright Clearance Center.

involved lymph nodes or complete wall penetration is usually not as ominous as the presence of both[38,40,42,44] Additional prognostic indicators include a poor performance status, elevated alkaline phosphatase levels, and ethnicity.[45] In one study, Asian Pacific Islanders born in the United States were compared to those born abroad, finding that only foreign-born Asian Pacific Islanders had a more favorable survival compared to indigenous Caucasians.[46] Proposed hypothesis to explain disparities in survival outcomes between Western and Asian populations include early detection in the latter, leading to stage migration, differences in treatment policy, as well as potential differences in tumor biology.

Flow cytometry may also be prognostically valuable; aneuploidy is associated with unfavorable tumor location, lymph node metastasis, and primary tumor invasion.[47–49] Unfavorable DNA flow cytometry correlates with a poor prognosis.[47] The prognosis is worse for cardia lesions, and flow cytometry reveals a greater incidence of aneuploidy.[49] The gross pathologic appearance of the primary lesion also reveals prognostic information, although it is not known whether this factor is independent of tumor stage. Patients with Borrmann type I and II tumors have relatively favorable 5-year survival rates, although patients with type IV (linitis plastica) fare poorly.[43,50–52]

The molecular biology of gastric cancer reflects the heterogeneity of its causes and its histologic subtypes. A detailed discussion of the molecular biology of gastric cancer is beyond the scope of this chapter and is well detailed elsewhere.[13] However, identification of the genetic and phenotypic variables existing among gastric cancers may lead to more directed therapeutic approaches and a more accurate prediction of clinical outcome. Changes that may affect the behavior of gastric tumor cells involve four major types of alterations. Loss of tumor suppressor gene function, especially inactivation of the p53 gene, appears to play a critical role. The p53 gene is located on the short arm of chromosome 17 and plays a key role in tumor suppression and cell cycle regulation.[53] The p53 gene halts DNA replication and triggers programmed cell death in response to DNA damage.[54] Loss of p53 function allows malignancy to develop, affects the effectiveness of chemotherapy and irradiation, and predisposes cells to genetic instability.[55,56] The latter is particularly important because p53 mutations occur early in tumorogenesis.[57]

A second major aberration affecting gastric epithelial cells is the impact of alterations in mismatch repair genes. Two such genes, hMSH3 and hMLH1, on chromosomes 2 and 3, respectively, account for replication errors throughout the genome. Mutations in these genes are implicated in cancer family syndromes and hereditary nonpolyposis colorectal cancer, which is a disease associated with an increased tendency for the development of gastric tumors.[58] Mutations in these genes generate genetic instability and have the potential to lead to further alterations in oncogenes.

Two proto-oncogenes, c-met and k-sam, are associated with scirrhous carcinoma of the stomach. The former encodes hepatocyte growth factor, which is a potent endogenous promoter of gastric epithelial cell growth.[59] Its overexpression correlates with tumor progression and metastasis.[60] The latter encodes a tyrosine kinase receptor family.[60] In scirrhous carcinoma, c-met and k-sam amplification may occur independently. There is a tendency for k-sam to be activated in women <40 years of age and c-met to be amplified in men >50 years of age.[57,61]

Peptide receptors, including estrogen receptors and epidermal growth factor receptors, are associated with adverse prognoses.[62,63] Epidermal growth factor receptors and levels correlate with higher rates of primary tumor infiltration, poorer histologic differentiation, and linitis plastica.[64] The pathophysiologic relation between these peptide receptors and their association with poor prognoses is not well understood.

Modern molecular biology observations confirm the heterogeneity of human gastric cancer. Genetic alterations detected and potentially associated with a worse prognosis include CD44 expression; telomerase reactivation; p53 gene inactivation; dysfunction of repair genes such as hMSH3 and hMLH1; overexpression of proto-oncogenes such as erb-B2, bcl-2, c-met, and k-sam; estrogenic receptor expression; and presence of viral genomes.[65] Gastric cancers with class II major histocompatibility complex antigen expression have a better prognosis; however, the loss of expression is not an independent prognostic factor.[64] Illustrating the importance of understanding and potential exploitation of these genetic alterations, a randomized study was conducted in patients with HER2 overexpression. Patients with locally advanced or metastatic gastric or GE cancer (the ToGA trial) were randomized to determine whether trastuzumab (an antibody against the HER2 gene product/receptor) enhanced treatment efficacy when added to cisplatin and 5-fluorouracil (5-FU)/capecitabine therapy. This study demonstrated that the addition of trastuzumab achieved a significant improvement in overall and progression-free survival.[66] These and other data have led to the ongoing Radiation Therapy Oncology Group (RTOG) 1010 trial, which is randomizing patients with esophageal/GE junction tumors to receive preoperative radiation therapy concurrent with paclitaxel/carboplatin, with or without trastuzumab, followed by resection.

GENERAL MANAGEMENT

Surgical Management

Complete tumor and regional lymph node resection remains the primary curative modality for gastric adenocarcinoma and may require total or distal gastrectomy. Operative attempts are highly successful if disease is limited to the mucosa; however, the incidence of such early lesions at diagnosis is <5% in most US series. In Japan, the incidence of lesions initially confined to the mucosa or submucosa was only 3.8% in 1955 and 1956, although by 1966, as a result of screening procedures, this figure had increased to 34.5%, with corresponding survival rates of 90.9%.[67] For very early gastric cancer (Tis and T1a), endoscopic mucosal dissection and endoscopic submucosal dissection have been successfully used as less radical alternatives to standard surgery. Appropriateness of endoscopic resection is based on the tumor depth, tumor diameter, histologic grade, and ulcerative component. As in other endoscopic procedures, outcomes are operator dependent. Endoscopic laser surgery has been applied successfully to patients with very early gastric cancer whose tumors are inoperable because of complicating medical illness. Small lesions that are pedunculated, noninvasive, and well differentiated have lymph node metastasis in <5% of cases and can be completely removed endoscopically in 75% of cases.[67] Radiation therapy with chemotherapy may be considered as adjuvant therapy in selected situations. These approaches in early gastric cancer (uncommonly seen in Western society) require meticulous patient selection and remain a topic of investigation.

Curative or palliative surgical resection is possible for 50% to 60% of patients at the time of initial disease presentation. However, only approximately 25% to 40% are eligible for potentially curative resection. Generally, patients with evidence of peritoneal involvement, distant metastases, or locally advanced disease (including encasement of unresectable/major blood vessels) are generally considered to have unresectable disease. Palliative resection is usually reserved for rare cases, including symptomatic palliation of bleeding uncontrolled by other methods, and is generally considered a last resort in patients with locally unresectable or metastatic disease. A recent randomized trial from Asia (the REGATTA trial) enrolled 175 gastric cancer patients. Patients were randomized to receive either chemotherapy (oral S1 + cisplatin) or palliative D1 gastrectomy followed by the same regimen. At interim analysis, no significant difference was seen in 2-year survival between the arms. The authors concluded that palliative gastrectomy could not be justified even in the setting of a solitary metastasis.[68] In some instances, unresectable tumors may be debulked successfully, with sites of minimal residual disease marked judiciously with clips. This may palliate and permit accurate delivery of postoperative radiation therapy. In patients with gastric outlet obstruction, gastrojejunostomy may be performed as an alternative to endoscopic placement of a stent in patients with expected longer survival.

No prospective randomized trials have definitively established optimal surgical therapy.[69,70] Generally, it is recommended that gastric cancer surgery be performed by experienced surgeons in high-volume centers, entailing removal of the perigastric lymph nodes (D1) as well as those along the main vessels of the celiac trunk (D2), with the goal of examining ≥16 lymph nodes (discussed later).[7] Total gastrectomy is generally necessary in most cases of proximal and midgastric carcinomas, although proximal gastrectomy may be appropriate depending on extent of disease. However, for more distal lesions, distal gastrectomy is preferred if adequate margins can be obtained. Generally, the distal margin in subtotal gastrectomy needs to be approximately 2 cm. This operation removes approximately 80% of the stomach along with the node-bearing tissue, the gastrohepatic and gastrocolic omenta, and the first portion of the duodenum. Larger lesions may require total gastrectomy. Total gastrectomy is not recommended where 4- to 6-cm margins can be achieved with partial gastrectomy given improved safety and long-term functional outcome improvements in the latter.[71] Patients treated with total gastrectomy characteristically have 5-year survival rates of 10% to 15%, and those undergoing radical subtotal gastrectomy have 5-year survival rates of 25% to 45%.[41,70,72] The inferior survivorship of patients undergoing total gastrectomy reflects larger tumors and unfavorable proximal lesions that prompt such a procedure. The value of splenectomy has not been addressed in prospective randomized trials; however, retrospective Japanese data do not support a survival benefit.[73] Because routine splenectomy has not shown significant improved outcomes and potentially increases complication rates, complete removal of splenic nodes is not commonly performed by Western surgeons. Roux-en-Y reconstruction may be used to avoid bile reflux gastritis/esophagitis. Vitamin B supplementation is generally required following total gastrectomy because of lack of intrinsic factor production from the stomach.

Minimally invasive gastrectomy (including laparoscopic or robot-assisted resection) is being increasingly utilized, although these approaches remain a subject of investigation. These approaches carry potential advantages, including less intraoperative blood loss, faster recovery times, reduced pain, and decreased hospital length of stay. Multiple trials have indicated that minimally invasive techniques provide equivalent surgical and oncologic outcomes to open approaches.[74] However, patient selection is important. In patients who undergo adjuvant chemoradiotherapy, it may be prudent to place feeding jejunostomy at the time of resection.

The propensity for gastric carcinoma to spread via the submucosal lymphatics suggests that a 5-cm margin of normal tissue proximally and distally may be optimal. It may be necessary to include a portion of the esophagus or duodenum to achieve adequate margins. Frozen section pathologic evaluation of surgical margins has been advocated to confirm their adequacy.[41] The importance of careful evaluation of longitudinal margins is emphasized in multiple series with documented positive pathologic margins in approximately one-quarter of "curatively" resected specimens.[75-82] The approximate 25% positive longitudinal margin correlates almost precisely with the incidence of locoregional recurrence in the anastomosis or stump, as discussed later.

Although R0 resection with adequate lymph node sampling is a primary goal for gastric cancer surgery, many patients end up with involved margins. Even though the longitudinal margin is routinely evaluated, equally important but frequently not assessed are the radial or circumferential margins. The incidence of radial margin positivity is not well reported in the literature. The rising incidence of T3 and T4 GE tumors will likely result in an increasing rate of microscopically positive radial margins. Because the perigastric tissue surrounding the GE junction and distal esophagus has no serosa, lesions that extend to the pathologic radial margin likely represent a true positive margin in a large percentage of cases.

The extent of lymph node dissection remains an ongoing area of controversy. The Japanese Research Society for gastric cancer categorizes draining stomach lymph nodes into 16 stations, 6 perigastric and 10 regional along major vessels and adjacent to the pancreas (Fig. 62.3). A D1 dissection only includes perigastric nodes (stations 1 to 6); a D2 dissection includes those along the common hepatic, left gastric, celiac, and splenic arteries (stations 7 to 11); a D3 dissection includes additional nodes with any of the porta hepatis and adjacent to the aorta (stations 12 to 16).[71] According to the most recent AJCC Cancer staging manual, accurate nodal staging demands evaluation of at least 16 lymph nodes. This may reduce stage migration. In a D0 dissection, there is generally incomplete removal of the lymph nodes along the greater and lesser curvature. In series with rigorous pathologic evaluation of these nodes,[83] the likelihood of discovering lymph node metastasis increases markedly in both D1 and D2 procedures. There appears to be a small subset of patients who have limited metastasis in the celiac axis, superior pancreatic, or retroduodenal chains and may be cured by a D2 lymph node resection.[84,85] Data from the Surveillance Epidemiology and End Results (SEER) database show that the number of nodes examined correlated with overall survival, potentially reflecting improved staging in these patients.[86] Japanese researchers advocate complete lymph node removal to improve the rates of local control and survival. Several nonrandomized clinical trials suggested that extended lymphadenectomy may improve survival.[87-90] Others[91] reported that increasingly radical lymphadenectomies failed to improve survival or reduce the risk of locoregional failure. Multiple prospective randomized trials of lymphadenectomies have been reported[84,92-96] and show no survival advantage with more extensive lymph node dissection. A more recent update of a Dutch randomized trial showed D2 dissections to be associated with improved disease-specific survival versus D1 at a median follow-up of 15 years.[97] However, morbidity and mortality rates have been significantly higher for patients undergoing more extensive nodal dissection. Despite the mixed evidence of randomized trials, it is generally recommend that spleen-sparing D2 lymphadenectomy be performed by experienced surgeons in high-volume centers. An even more extensive lymph node dissection may entail para-aortic nodal dissection. However, a Japanese trial comparing D2 lymphadenectomy versus the same with para-aortic (D3) nodal dissection did not show any differences in overall or relapse-free survival between the groups, indicating the latter approach should not be used in

TABLE 62.4 PATTERNS OF FAILURE AFTER "CURATIVE" RESECTION OF GASTRIC CANCER

Pattern of Failure	Incidence in Total Patient Group (%)		
	Clinical[103]	University of Minnesota Reoperation[a39]	Autopsy[1,100,101,104]
Locoregional[b]	38	67	80–93
Peritoneal seeding	28	41	30–43
Localized	–	19	–
Diffuse	–	22	–
Distant metastases	52	22	49

[a]107 patients at risk.
[b]Local or regional failure based on direct extension of tumor, lymphatic spread, or operative wound implant; one or more distant metastases on hematologic basis; abdominal involvement on the basis of peritoneal seeding or peritoneal lymphatics.

patients with curable gastric cancer.[98] However, other important principles of lymph node dissection have been elucidated through these trials. The first is that as more lymph node areas are dissected and as pathologic lymph node evaluation is more rigorous, considerable stage migration occurs. This stage migration produces an apparent improvement in stage-specific survival without improvement in survival in the group overall.

Failure Patterns after Surgical Resection

Local failures in the tumor bed and/or regional lymph nodes and distant failures by hematogenous or peritoneal routes are common mechanisms of failure after "curative" resection in clinical, reoperative, and autopsy series[44,99-102] (Tables 62.4 and 62.5). For GE junction lesions, the liver and lungs are common sites of distant metastases. With gastric lesions that do not extend to the esophagus, the initial site of distant metastasis is usually the liver, and many failures could be prevented if an effective abdominal treatment could be combined with treatment to the primary site. In the series of Landry et al.,[103] 50 of 88 (57%) failing patients had disease progression within the abdomen only. Abdominal treatment also could address peritoneal seeding, which occurs in 23% to 43% of postgastrectomy patients.[99-107]

Locoregional failures occur commonly in organs and structures of the gastric bed and in lymph nodes and an established mode of failure (Table 62.5). Clinically detectable locoregional recurrence following surgical resection alone generally exceeds 25%. As an example, in long-term follow-up of the previously described Dutch Gastric Cancer Trial, even with D2 dissection, locoregional recurrence rates were 25%, and 41% following D1 surgery.[97] However, reoperation and autopsy series have suggested that these rates are much higher.[44,99-102,105] Failures in the anastomoses, gastric remnant, or duodenal stump also are frequent, as suggested by the incidence of positive longitudinal resection margins (Table 62.5). As is true for most sites, clinical series underestimate the true incidence of locoregional failure when compared with reoperative or autopsy series (Table 62.4). Progressive extension of the operative procedure to include routine splenectomy, omentectomy, and radical lymph node dissection neither

TABLE 62.5 PATTERNS OF LOCOREGIONAL FAILURE AFTER RESECTION OF GASTRIC CANCER

Failure Area	Incidence (%)		
	Clinical[a105]	Reoperation[b39]	Autopsy[c106]
Gastric bed	21	54	52–68
Anastomosis or stumps	25	26	54–60
Abdominal or stab wound	–	5	–
Lymph node(s)	8	42	52

[a]130 patients at risk.
[b]107 patients at risk.
[c]92 patients at risk and 28 patients at risk.

improved survival nor decreased the incidence of locoregional failures in the University of Minnesota series.[44] Subsequent failure in areas of initial node dissection occurred frequently, even with radical lymph node dissections[44] (Fig. 62.4). The high rate of regional node relapse (including para-aortic basins) provides a partial explanation for the lack of survival benefit with a D2 (extended lymphadenectomy) versus D1 (limited lymphadenectomy) node dissection in the phase III surgical trials discussed previously. A more contemporary analysis of 382 patients with stage III (N3) disease undergoing D2 resection receiving adjuvant chemotherapy alone demonstrated that first site of recurrence (some patients had multiple) was local in 7% (most at anastomosis and few in gastric bed), regional failure as any component of first recurrence occurred in 24% of patients (isolated in 12.8% of patients), and peritoneal based in 33%. Most commonly involved lymph node groups were 16, 12, 14, 13, and 9 (primarily outside of the D2 nodal basin).[108] A further analysis of this trial of nodal CT recurrences suggested that vessel-based delineations of these volumes on CT may assist in target design.[109] (Fig. 62.5A). A pattern of failure analysis of the ARTIST trial (discussed below) evaluating patterns of recurrence suggested a significant decrease in regional recurrence with the addition of radiation therapy in node-positive patients. Specifically, patients in the nonradiation arm had significantly higher likelihood of failure in the retroperito-neal lymph node basins, emphasizing the importance of covering this area in gastric cancer patients, whereas as true local recurrence rates did not differ significantly between the two arms (Fig. 62.5B).[110]

Indications for Radiation Therapy

The results of the U.S. Gastrointestinal Intergroup Gastric Adjuvant Trial changed the standard of care in the United States to the use of both chemotherapy and radiation therapy in the postoperative setting for patients with disease extension through the gastric wall and/or with lymph nodes positive for tumor (discussed later).[111] Postoperative irradiation plus concurrent and maintenance fluoropyrimidine-based chemotherapy is recommended for patients with stage IB-IV and M0 gastric cancer.[111] Quality control of irradiation field design was conducted during the cycle of chemotherapy given before the start of concurrent chemoradiation. The up-front quality control provided the mechanism to correct most of the major or minor deviations (35% incidence) in irradiation field design before the start of treatment and resulted in only a 6.5% final major deviation rate.

Radiation therapy, usually administered with concomitant fluoropyrimidine-based chemotherapy, is also indicated for locally confined gastric cancer that either is not technically resectable or occurs in medically inoperable patients. In this setting, therapy can be administered with curative or palliative

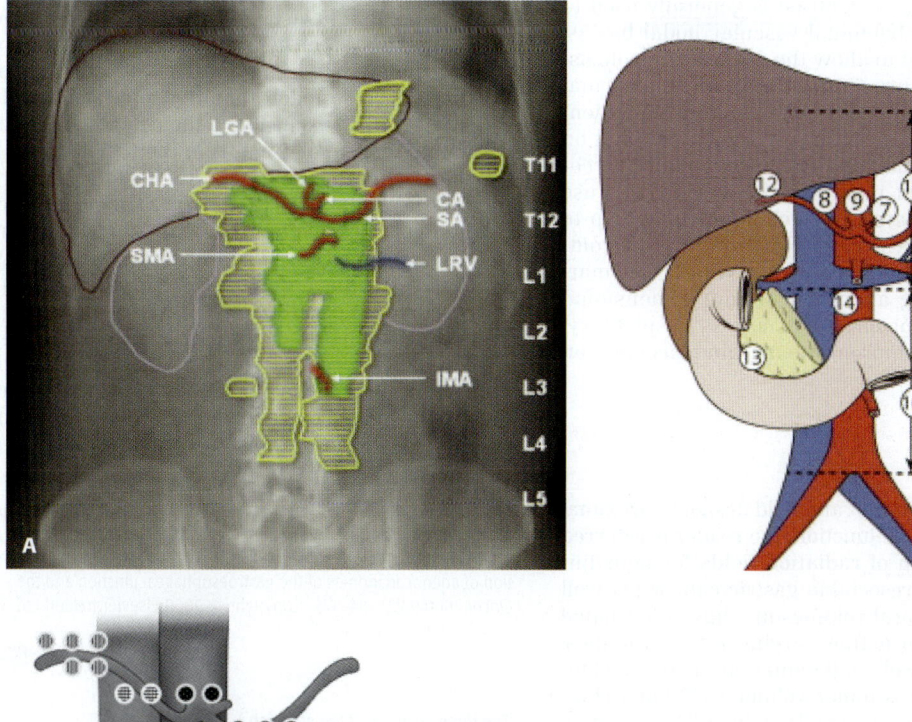

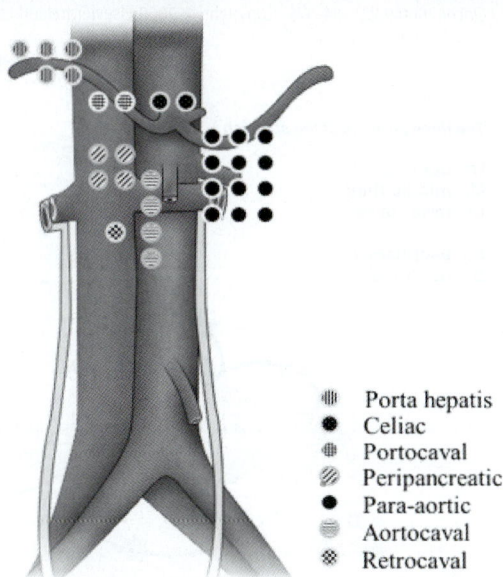

⫴	Porta hepatis
●	Celiac
⊕	Portocaval
▨	Peripancreatic
●	Para-aortic
⊜	Aortocaval
❊	Retrocaval

FIGURE 62.5. A: Common nodal recurrent regions (*green*) overlapped by more than five recurrent nodal gross tumor volumes depicted on a digitally reconstructed radiograph image. The volume of total GTVs (*yellow*), liver (*cobalt purple*), and both kidneys (*violet*) are also seen. Common hepatic artery (CHA), splenic artery (SA), left gastric artery (LGA), celiac artery (CA), superior mesenteric artery (SMA), inferior mesenteric artery (IMA), and left renal vein (LRV) are shown in *solid lines*. **B:** Retroperitoneal patterns of failure in the nonradiation arm of the ARTIST trial.

intent, depending on the clinical situation. Those who undergo gastric resection with incomplete tumor resection or have truly positive margins of resection are also managed appropriately by combined modality postoperative therapy.

RADIATION THERAPY TECHNIQUES

Simulation

When gastric cancer patients are simulated, the radiation oncologist should know the extent of disease based on imaging (barium swallow, CT, PET) as well as endoscopic procedures. CT simulation is appropriate for treatment planning. Some authors have recommended fasting for >2 hours before simulation as well as at treatment.[112] During simulation, the patient is positioned, straightened, and immobilized on the simulation table. An immobilization device is used to minimize variation in daily setup. Arms are generally placed. The administration of oral contrast to delineate the stomach is generally used and may help define the extent of mucosal irregularity (if the patient is surgically naïve). The patient is placed on the CT simulator in the treatment position, and a scan of the entire area of interest with margin is obtained. At minimum, 3- to 5-mm slices should be used, allowing accurate tumor characterization as well as improved quality of digitally reconstructed radiographs. If patients lose >10% of their body weight during therapy, consideration should be given to repeat CT planning. IV contrast is generally used to delineate mediastinal and abdominal vascular nodal basins, including the celiac axis, and to allow the radiation oncologist to discern normal vasculature from other adjacent normal structures and potential adenopathy. The tumor (if the patient is surgically naïve) and vital structures are then outlined on each slice on the treatment planning system, enabling a three-dimensional (3-D) treatment plan to be generated. The use of respiratory gating or breath hold techniques may help to reduce target motion with respiration and, therefore, avoidance of normal tissue irradiation associated with larger margins used in free-breathing approaches. Four-dimensional (4-D) CT scan may be appropriate to assess respiratory/tumoral motion, facilitating appropriate margin placement on the target volumes.

Treatment Planning

Target Design

For a detailed description of target and field design in proximal gastric cancer involving the GE junction, the reader is referred to Chapter 56. In the design of radiation fields for neoadjuvantly treated or locally unresectable gastric cancer (as well as in the re-creation of tumoral volumes in adjuvantly treated patients), it is important to define varying target volumes, including gross disease as well as potential areas of subclinical involvement (i.e., the gross tumor volume [GTV] and clinical target volume [CTV], respectively). Defining GTV (including re-creation of volumes in the adjuvant setting) is based on multiple studies, including endoscopic descriptions (from both esophagogastroduodenoscopy and endoscopic ultrasound) as well as cross-sectional imaging. Gastric wall thickening correlating to the GTV can frequently be visualized on diagnostic and radiation planning CT. Similarly, EUS appears to be the most reliable test in detecting lymphadenopathy related to nodal spread. The endoscopist should be encouraged to accurately define not only the primary disease extent on EGD but also depth of penetration and potential involvement of adjacent structures on EUS, which can also be used to help guide GTV delineation. Similarly, EUS may allow detection of lymph nodes that may not be appreciated on CT or PET imaging, and the endoscopist should be encouraged to describe the size as well as location (e.g., relationship to tumor or adjacent structures). Additionally, radiographic areas of lymphadenopathy

should similarly be included in the GTV. In GTV design, basing potential nodal involvement (and therefore target volumes) on nodal size is problematic given that metastatic nodes may frequently be below the resolution of conventional imaging. Therefore, it is not appropriate to rely exclusively on imaging modalities to define areas of subclinical spread for gastric cancer, realizing established pathologic patterns of spread data are important in determining radiation field design.

The identification of potential direct and nodal pathways for spread of subclinical disease (i.e., CTV definition) in gastric cancer is of paramount importance. These areas vary significantly depending on site of origin of disease, making gastric cancer planning somewhat complex. As described previously, the stomach is characterized by a rich network of lymphatics that facilitates early lymph node spread of disease. Some authors have recommended dividing the stomach into three equal lengths (upper/proximal, middle, and distal), with tumors classified by location of the bulk of their masses in these respective sites. Therefore, practically speaking, the stomach can be divided into proximal (remembering that in the AJCC eighth edition staging system, involvement of the GE junction by very proximal third tumors would be classified as an esophageal tumor), middle, or distal segments (Fig. 62.6).

Primarily based on extensive analysis of patterns of nodal spread from surgical series, Japanese investigators have developed lymph node station classifications (the Japanese classification of gastric carcinoma of the Japanese Gastric Cancer Association) that have been validated in other series (Fig. 62.3). Based on this system, general recommendations for CTV definition for tumors in varying parts of the stomach are as follows. Proximal third stomach tumors should include the contour of the stomach with exclusion of the pylorus and antrum (keeping a minimal margin of 5 cm from the GTV). Middle third tumors should include the contour of the stomach from the cardia to the pylorus. Distal third tumor CTVs should include the stomach except for the cardia/fundus, again keeping a minimal margin of 5 cm from the GTV. However, some authors have noted that surgical series have demonstrated that <5% of patients have microscopic mucosal extension >3 cm beyond gross disease, suggesting smaller margins may be feasible.[112] If pyloric/duodenal invasion is present, the CTV would be expanded along the duodenum with a margin of 3 cm from the tumor. Nodal volumes to be included are further described later, and it has been recommended that the CTV consist of a 5-mm margin around

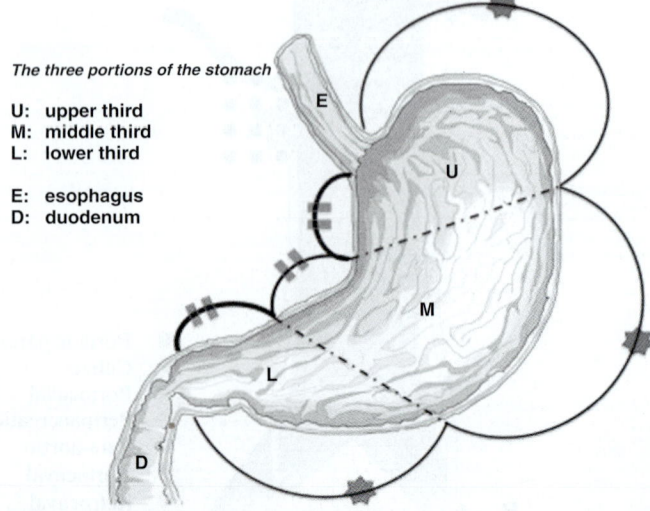

FIGURE 62.6. Subdivision of the stomach into equal lengths along greater and lesser curves. (Reprinted from Matzinger O, Gerber E, Bernstein Z, et al. EORTC-ROG expert opinion: radiotherapy volume and treatment guidelines for neoadjuvant radiation of adenocarcinomas of the gastroesophageal junction and the stomach. *Radiother Oncol* 2009;92[2]:164–175. Copyright © 2009 Elsevier Ireland Ltd. With permission.)

The three portions of the stomach

U: upper third
M: middle third
L: lower third

E: esophagus
D: duodenum

corresponding vessels. An internal target volume (ITV) may be created based on 4-D imaging, with PTV expansion variable, although this typically ranges from 5 to 15 mm depending on immobilization technique and use of image guidance. If target motion is not accounted for, the minimal recommended 3-D margins to the CTV to obtain the ITV are 1.5 cm in all directions, taking into account physiologic organ motion, particularly respiratory motion. The PTV can then be defined as the ITV volume plus a 3-D margin of 5 mm.[113]

Field Design

Field design is based on established patterns of nodal involvement following gastrectomy and lymph node dissection as well as patterns of disease recurrence (Table 62.5). This is also dependent on tumor location within the stomach, stage of disease, as well as extent of lymph node dissection. In resected patients, the gastric/tumor bed, anastomosis and gastric remnant, and pertinent regional lymphatics should be included in most patients.[44,102,106,107,111,113] Major nodal chains at risk include the lesser and greater curvature, celiac axis, pancreaticoduodenal, splenic, suprapancreatic, porta hepatis, and, in many, para-aortics to the level of mid-L3. However, included basins are frequently modified based on margin status, type of surgery (i.e., D0, D1, D2), location within the stomach, as well as stage.

The relative risk of nodal metastases at a specific nodal location depends on both the site of origin of the primary tumor[113-115] and other factors including width and depth of invasion of the gastric wall. On the basis of previously described patterns of failure data, general guidelines in terms of field design can be made as illustrated in Figures 62.7 through 62.9 and are discussed below. These are general guidelines, and all plans should be individualized according to available imaging and endoscopic data, and generalized portals based on patterns of failure data frequently need to be modified on the basis of the individual patient's initial extent of disease.[113-115] As seen in Figures 62.7 to 62.9, gastric tumors (i.e., without GE junction

involvement) that originate in the proximal portion of the stomach have a higher propensity of spread to nodes in the paracardial region but a lower likelihood of involvement of nodes in the region of the gastric antrum, periduodenal area, and porta hepatis. In patients with proximal gastric cancers (gastric cardia and GE junction) undergoing esophagogastrectomy with intrathoracic anastomosis, the CTV typically includes 3 to 4 cm of the mucosa of the esophagus and distal stomach, tumor bed (typically determined by preoperative imaging and including the medial two-thirds of the left hemidiaphragm), as well as lymph node stations 1 to 4, 7, and 9 to 11 with some authors recommending inclusion of stations 12 to 13.[112]; if the GE junction is involved, stations 20 and 110 to 111 are also included, and if the tumor extended to the middle stomach, stations 5, 6, and 8 frequently are included.[112] Tumors that originate in the body of the stomach can spread to all nodal sites but have the highest likelihood of spreading to nodes along the greater and lesser curvature near the location of the primary tumor mass. Nodal basins are similar to upper third tumors with the exception of inclusion of nodal basins along the pyloric region, common hepatic artery, and additional coverage along the greater curvature. For middle third patients undergoing total gastrectomy with Roux-en-Y esophagojejunal anastomosis, the CTV typically includes 3 to 4 cm of mucosa of the esophagus and jejunum, tumor bed delineated as above, as well as lymph node stations 3 to 11, with some authors advocating inclusions of stations 12 to 13,[112] as well as considerations of 1 to 2 if there is proximal third stomach involvement. Tumors that originate in the distal stomach, in the region of the gastric antrum, have a high likelihood of spread to the periduodenal, peripancreatic, and porta hepatis nodes, whereas they have a lower likelihood of spread to the nodes near the cardia of the stomach, the periesophageal and mediastinal nodes, or to the splenic hilar nodes—that is, there is less emphasis placed on more proximal nodes (including coverage of the splenic artery course,

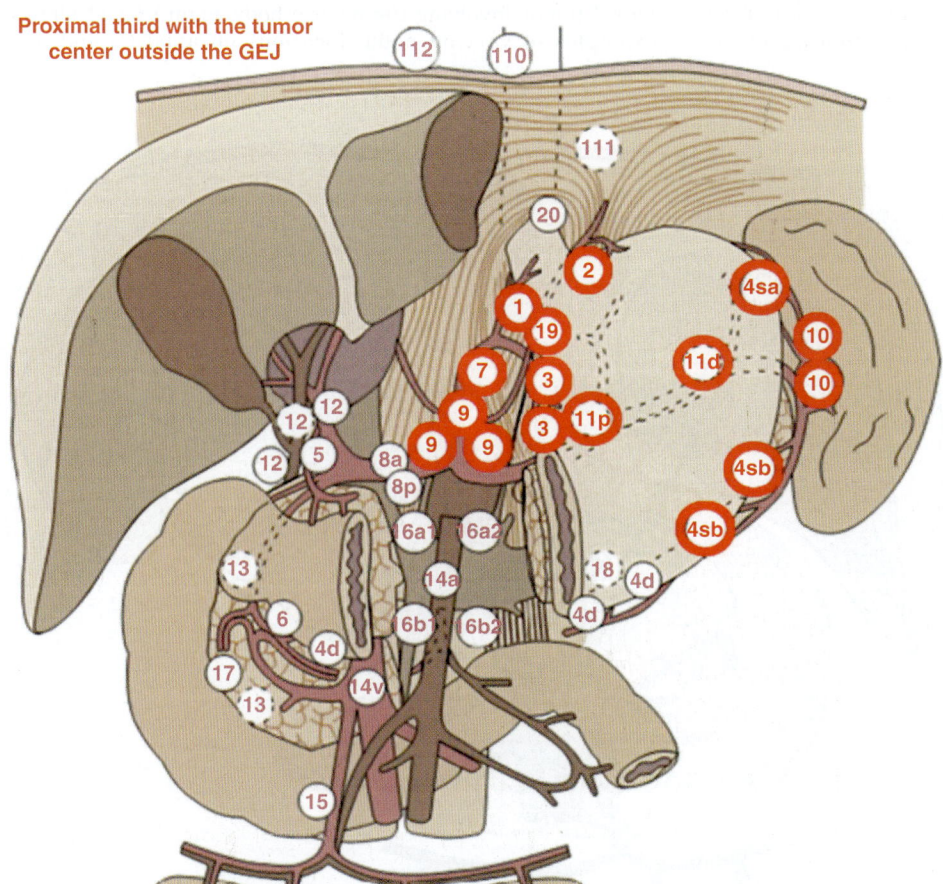

Proximal third with the tumor center outside the GEJ

FIGURE 62.7. Suggested lymph node station coverage for tumors of the proximal third of the stomach without involvement of the GE junction. (Reprinted from Matzinger O, Gerber E, Bernstein Z, et al. EORTC-ROG expert opinion: radiotherapy volume and treatment guidelines for neoadjuvant radiation of adenocarcinomas of the gastroesophageal junction and the stomach. *Radiother Oncol* 2009;92[2]:164–175. Copyright © 2009 Elsevier Ireland Ltd. With permission.)

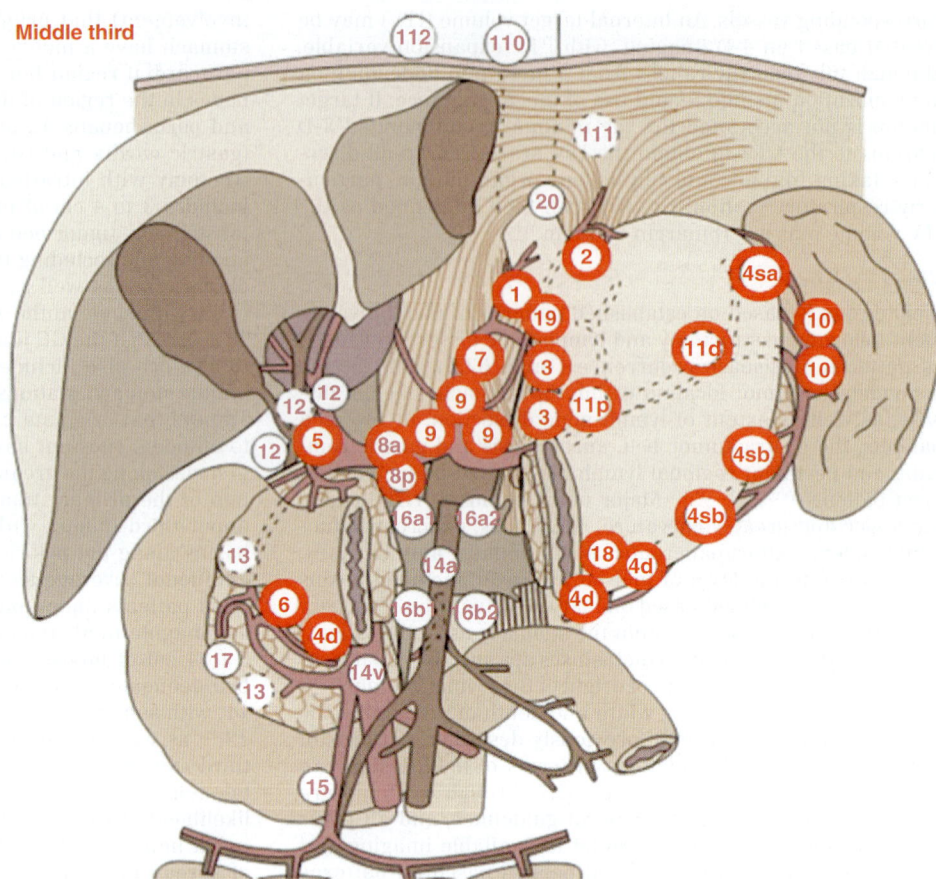

FIGURE 62.8. Suggested lymph node nodal coverage of patients with middle third gastric carcinomas. (Reprinted from Matzinger O, Gerber E, Bernstein Z, et al. EORTC-ROG expert opinion: radiotherapy volume and treatment guidelines for neoadjuvant radiation of adenocarcinomas of the gastroesophageal junction and the stomach. *Radiother Oncol* 2009;92[2]:164–175. Copyright © 2009 Elsevier Ireland Ltd. With permission.)

including splenic hilum) and more comprehensive coverage of pancreaticoduodenal nodal basins. For distal third tumors undergoing distal gastrectomy with gastrojejunal anastomosis, the CTV typically includes 3 to 4 cm of the mucosa of the proximal stomach and jejunum as well as 3 to 4 cm of the duodenal stump, tumor bed as delineated using preoperative imaging as above, and lymph node stations 3 to 9 and 11 to 13.[112] Figure 62.10 shows an example of 3-D fields for a T3N1 antral tumor involving the gastric body. Figure 62.11 shows examples of varying nodal locations on axial CT images.

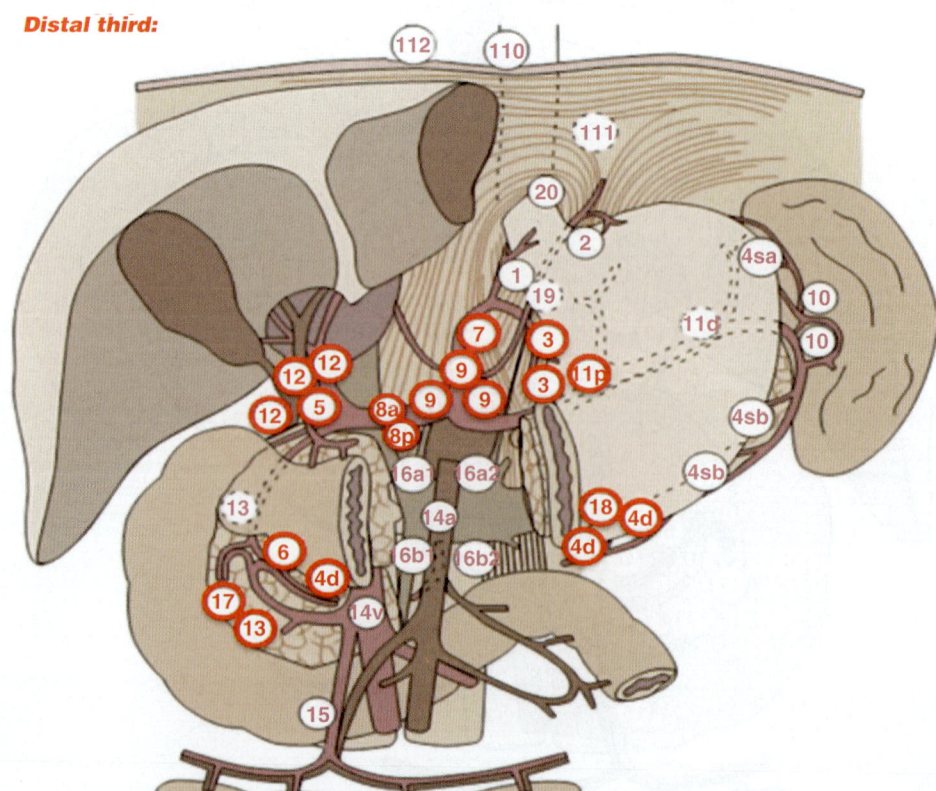

FIGURE 62.9. Suggested nodal coverage for primary gastric cancers of the distal third of the stomach. (Reprinted from Matzinger O, Gerber E, Bernstein Z, et al. EORTC-ROG expert opinion: radiotherapy volume and treatment guidelines for neoadjuvant radiation of adenocarcinomas of the gastroesophageal junction and the stomach. *Radiother Oncol* 2009;92[2]:164–175. Copyright © 2009 Elsevier Ireland Ltd. With permission.)

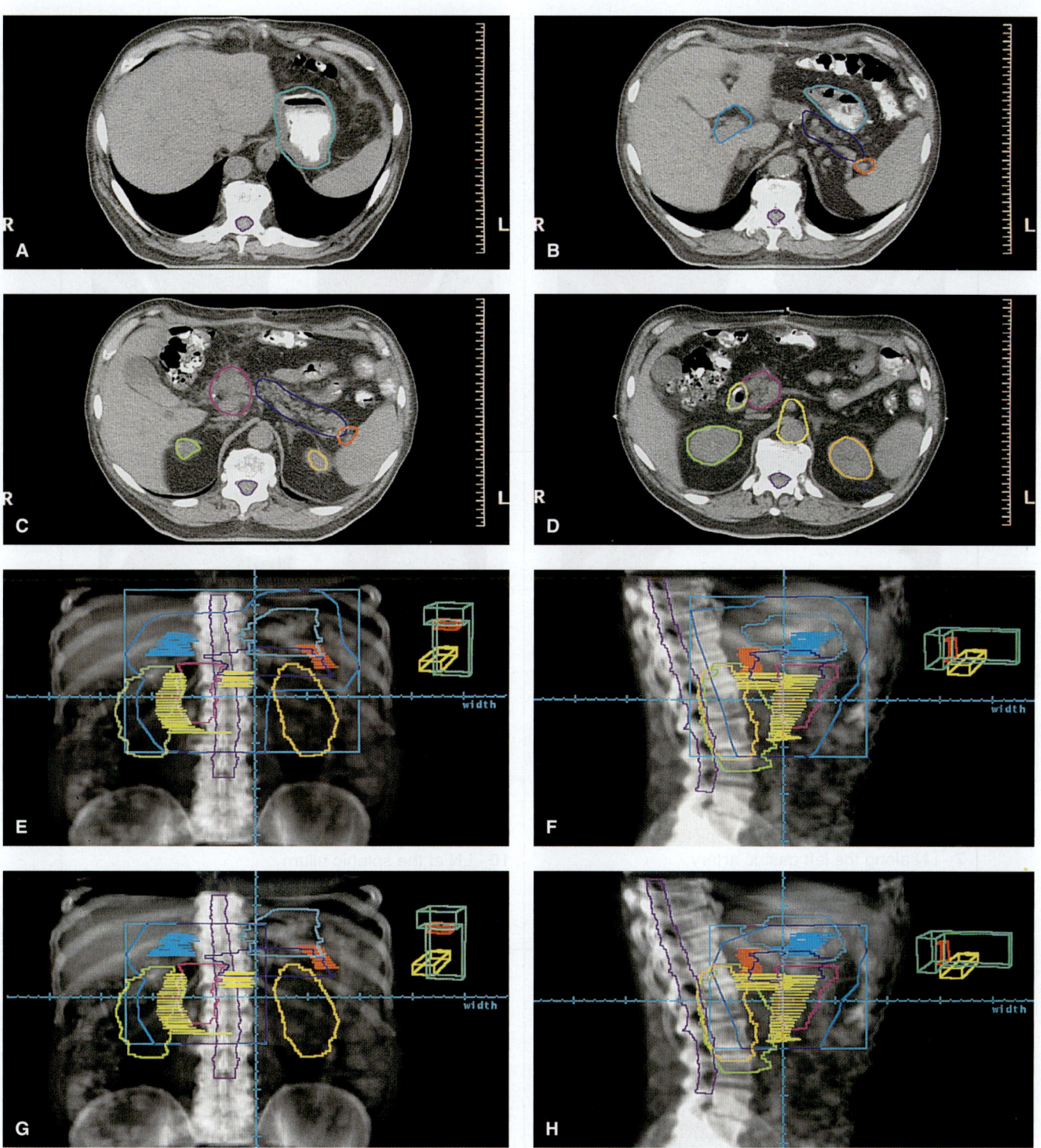

FIGURE 62.10. Optimized postoperative irradiation fields for patient with T3N1 antral primary. Structures of interest were delineated at the time of computed tomography simulation **(A–D)**, and irradiation fields were designed with the aid of digitally reconstructed radiographs **(E–H)**. **A:** Gastric remnant (*teal*). **B:** Gastric remnant plus body/tail of the pancreas (*dark blue*), splenic hilum (*salmon*), and porta hepatis (*medium blue*). **C:** Head of the pancreas (*magenta*) and kidneys (*left, orange; right, light green*) are delineated in addition to body/tail of the pancreas and splenic hilum. **D:** Celiac artery (*yellow*) and duodenum (*yellow–green*) are shown together with head of pancreas and kidneys. A four-field technique of AP (antero-posterior), PA (posteroanterior), and paired laterals was designed to include the gastric remnant (*teal*), tumor bed (head of the pancreas [*magenta*], first and second part of the duodenum [*yellow–green cross hatched*]), pertinent nodal volumes (perigastric, pancreaticoduodenal, porta hepatic [*medium blue cross hatched*], celiac [*yellow cross hatched*], and suprapancreatic), and the optional nodal volume of splenic hilum (*salmon cross hatched*). **E:** Initial AP field (field margins as shown in medium blue exclude approximately two-thirds of the left kidney while including about 50% of the right kidney). Exclusion of the optional splenic hilar nodes would have allowed additional but minimal sparing of the left kidney in view of the adjacency of gastric antrum and splenic hilum. **F:** Initial right lateral field demonstrated exclusion of the spinal cord. **G:** Reduced AP field with exclusion of splenic hilar nodes and most of the gastric remnant. **H:** Reduced right lateral field.

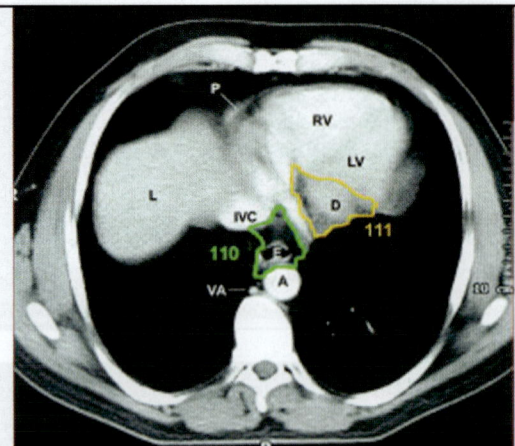

110 - Paraoesophageal LN
111 - Supradiaphragmatic LN

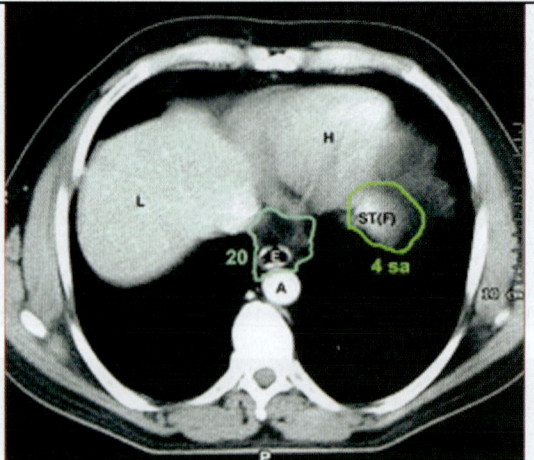

20 - LN in the oesophageal hiatus of the diaphragm
4sa - LN along the short gastric vessels

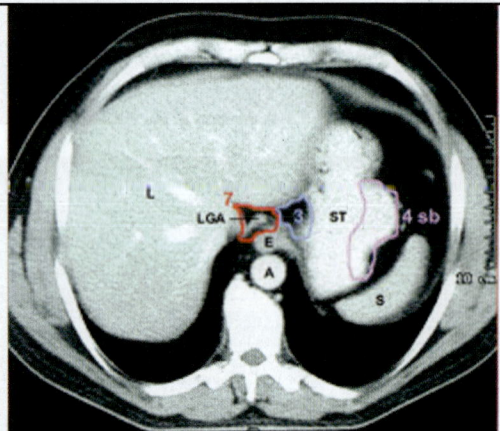

3 - LN along the lesser curvature
4sb - LN along the left gastroepiploic vessels
7 - LN along the left gastric artery

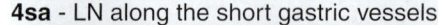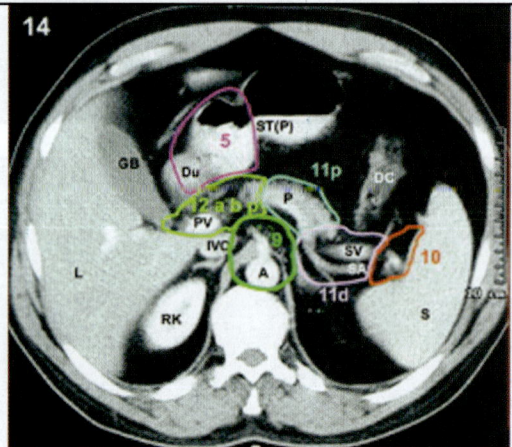

5 - Suprapyloric LN,
9 - LN around the celiac artery
10 - LN at the splenic hilum
11p - LN along the proximal splenic artery
11d - LN along the distal splenic artery
12a, b, p - LN in the hepatoduodenal ligament

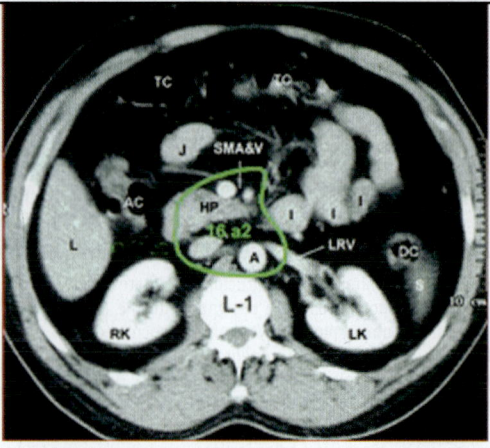

16 a2 LN around the abdominal aorta

LEGEND:
A, Aorta; AC, Ascending colon; D, Diaphragma;
DC, Descending colon; Du, Duodenum;
E, Oesophagus; GB, Gall bladder; I, Ilium; H, Heart;
J, Jejunum; IVC, Inferior cava vein; L, Liver;
L-1, First lumbar vertebra; LK, Left kidney,
LRV, Left renal vein; LV, Left ventricle; P, Pancreas;
PV, Portal vein; RGA, Right gastric artery;
RK, Right kidney; RV, Right ventricle; S, Spleen;
SA, Splenic artery; SMA&V, Superior mesenteric
artery and vein; SV, Splenic vein; ST, Stomach;
ST(F), Stomach fundus; ST(P), Stomach pylorus;
TC, Transverse colon; VA, Azygos vein

FIGURE 62.11. Examples of locations of varying nodal stations and anatomic structures on axial CT slices. (Reprinted from Matzinger O, Gerber E, Bernstein Z, et al. EORTC-ROG expert opinion: radiotherapy volume and treatment guidelines for neoadjuvant radiation of adenocarcinomas of the gastroesophageal junction and the stomach. *Radiother Oncol* 2009;92[2]: 164–175. Copyright © 2009 Elsevier Ireland Ltd. With permission.)

TABLE 62.6 GENERAL GUIDELINES OF IMPACT OF T AND N STAGE ON INCLUSION OF REMAINING STOMACH, TUMOR BED, AND NODAL SITES WITHIN IRRADIATION FIELDS

TN Stage	Remaining Stomach[a]	Tumor Bed	Nodes
T1–T2 (not into subserosa) N0	N	N	N
T2N0 (into subserosa)[b]	Variable	Y	N
T3N0	Variable	Y	N
T4N0	Variable	Y	Variable
T1-2N+	Y	N	Y
T3-4N+	Y	Y	Y

[a]Inclusion of the remaining stomach is preferable in most patients if two-thirds of one kidney can be excluded. This depends on the extent of surgical resection and uninvolved margins (in centimeters).

[b]Posterior wall T2N0 lesions, or those that extend beyond the muscularis propria, especially tumors located in the proximal or distal stomach, are at risk for local relapse. In addition, patients with low-stage disease with close or positive surgical margins should be considered for treatment to the tumor bed.

N, no; Y, yes.

Reprinted from Tepper JE, Gunderson LL. Radiation treatment parameters in the adjuvant postoperative therapy of gastric cancer. *Semin Radiat Oncol* 2002;12(2):187–195. Copyright © 2002 Elsevier. With permission.

Any tumor originating in the stomach has a high propensity of spread to nodes along the greater and lesser curvature, although they are most likely to spread to those sites in close anatomic proximity to the primary tumor mass.

Additional guidelines for defining the CTV for postoperative irradiation fields have been developed based on location and extent of the primary tumor (T stage) and location and extent of known nodal involvement (N stage).[114] Table 62.6 presents general guidelines on the impact of T and N stages on inclusion of the remaining stomach (gastric remnant), tumor bed, and nodal sites, whereas Tables 62.7 to 62.9 present treatment guidelines based on TN stage within each of three primary sites (proximal, mid, and distal stomach). With proximal gastric lesions or lesions at the GE junction, a 3- to 5-cm margin of distal esophagus should be included; if the lesion extends through the entire gastric wall, a major portion of the left hemidiaphragm should be included. In these circumstances, blocking can decrease the volume of irradiated heart. For unresectable lesions with moderate periesophageal

extension, it may not be possible to exclude an adequate amount of the heart with anteroposterior/posteroanterior (AP/PA) fields, and the use of lateral or oblique fields for a portion of treatment, as well as adopting intensity-modulated radiation therapy (IMRT) techniques, is likely indicated (Fig. 62.12; discussed below). In general, for patients with node-positive disease, there should be wide coverage of tumor bed, remaining stomach, resection margins, and nodal drainage regions. For node-negative disease, if there is a good surgical resection with pathologic evaluation of at least 16 nodes, and there are wide surgical margins on the primary tumor (at least 5 cm), treatment for the nodal beds may be optional. However, it is the authors' opinion that in most cases (particularly node positive) that the celiac basins/associated branches as well as periaortic nodes should be similarly covered (see above patterns of failure discussion). Treatment for the remaining stomach should depend on a balance of the likely normal tissue morbidity and the perceived risk of local relapse in the residual stomach.

Although parallel-opposed AP/PA fields are a practical arrangement for tumor bed and nodal irradiation, multifield techniques should be used if they can improve long-term tolerance of normal tissues. Tightly contoured AP/PA fields should be designed to spare as much normal tissue as possible (Figs. 62.13 and 62.14). In institutional series, the average irradiation field measured 15 cm × 15 cm.[39,115,116] More routine use of multifield techniques should be implemented when preoperative imaging exists to allow accurate reconstruction of target volumes. Single-institution data suggest that multifield arrangements may produce less toxicity. Although AP/PA fields can be weighted anteriorly to keep the spinal cord dose at acceptable levels, a four-field technique, if feasible, can spare spinal cord with improved dose homogeneity. Depending on the posterior extent of the gastric fundus, either obliqued or more routine lateral portals can be used to deliver a 10- to 20-Gy component of irradiation to spare spinal cord or kidney. When lateral fields are used, liver and kidney tolerance limits the use of lateral fields to ≤20 Gy. Patients should be treated with high-energy photons when possible. With the wide availability of 3D treatment planning systems, it may be possible

TABLE 62.7 IMPACT OF SITE OF PRIMARY GASTRIC LESION AND TN STAGE ON IRRADIATION VOLUMES: CARDIA/PROXIMAL ONE-THIRD OF THE STOMACH (GENERAL GUIDELINES)

Site of Primary and TN Stage	Remaining Stomach	Tumor Bed Volumes[a]	Nodal Volumes	Tolerance Organ Structures
Cardia/proximal one-third of the stomach	Preferred, but spare two-thirds of one kidney (usually right)	T-stage dependent	N-stage dependent	Kidneys, spinal cord, liver, heart, lung
T2N0 with invasion of subserosa	Variable dependent on surg–path findings[b]	Medial left hemidiaphragm, adjacent body of the pancreas (± tail)	None or perigastric[c]	
T3N0	Variable dependent on surg–path findings[b]	Medial left hemidiaphragm, adjacent body of the pancreas (± tail)	None or perigastric; optional: periesophageal, mediastinal, celiac[c]	
T4N0	Variable dependent on surg–path findings[b]	As for T3N0 plus site(s) of adherence with 3–5-cm margin	Nodes related to site of adherence, ± perigastric, periesophageal, mediastinal, celiac	
T1-2N+	Preferable	Not indicated for T1, as above for T2 into subserosa	Perigastric, celiac, splenic, suprapancreatic ± periesophageal, mediastinal, pancreaticoduodenal, porta hepatis[d]	
T3-4N+	Preferable	As for T3, T4N0	As for T1-2N+ and T4N0	

[a]Use preoperative imaging (computed tomography [CT], barium swallow), surgical clips, and postoperative imaging (CT, barium swallow).

[b]For tumors with wide (>5 cm) surgical margins confirmed pathologically, treatment of residual stomach may not be necessary, especially if this would result in substantial increased normal tissue morbidity.

[c]Optional node inclusion for T2-3N0 lesions if adequate surgical node dissection (D2 dissection) and at least 10 to 15 nodes are examined pathologically.

[d]Pancreaticoduodenal and porta hepatis nodes are at low risk if nodal positivity is minimal (i.e., 1 to 2 positive nodes with 10 to 15 nodes examined), and this region may not need to be irradiated. Periesophageal and mediastinal nodes are at risk if there is esophageal extension.

Surg–path, surgical–pathologic.

Reprinted from Tepper JE, Gunderson LL. Radiation treatment parameters in the adjuvant postoperative therapy of gastric cancer. *Semin Radiat Oncol* 2002;12(2):187–195. Copyright © 2002 Elsevier. With permission.

TABLE 62.8 IMPACT OF SITE OF PRIMARY GASTRIC LESION AND TN STAGE ON IRRADIATION VOLUMES: BODY/MIDDLE ONE-THIRD OF THE STOMACH (GENERAL GUIDELINES)

Site of Primary and TN Stage	Remaining Stomach	Tumor Bed Volumes[a]	Nodal Volumes	Tolerance Organ Structures
Body/middle one-third of the stomach	Yes—but spare two-thirds of one kidney	T-stage dependent	N-stage dependent—spare two-thirds of one kidney	Kidneys, spinal cord, liver
T2N0 with invasion of subserosa, especially post wall	Yes	Body of the pancreas (± tail)	None or perigastric; optional: celiac, splenic, suprapancreatic, pancreaticoduodenal, porta hepatis[b]	
T3N0	Yes	Body of the pancreas (± tail)	None or perigastric; optional: celiac, splenic, suprapancreatic, pancreaticoduodenal, porta hepatis[b]	
T4N0	Yes	As for T3N0 plus site(s) of adherence with 3–5-cm margin	Nodes related to site of adherence ± perigastric, celiac, splenic, suprapancreatic, pancreaticoduodenal, porta hepatis	
T1-2N+	Yes	Not indicated for T1; as for T2N0 with invasion of subserosa	Perigastric, celiac, splenic, suprapancreatic pancreaticoduodenal, porta hepatis	
T3-4N+	Yes	As for T3, T4N0	As for T1-2N+ and T4N0	

[a]Use preoperative imaging (computed tomography [CT], barium swallow), surgical clips, and postoperative imaging (CT, barium swallow).
[b]Optional node inclusion for T2-3N0 lesions if adequate surgical node dissection (D2 dissection) and at least 10 to 15 nodes examined pathologically.
Reprinted from Tepper JE, Gunderson LL. Radiation treatment parameters in the adjuvant postoperative therapy of gastric cancer. *Semin Radiat Oncol* 2002;12(2):187–195. Copyright © 2002 Elsevier. With permission.

to more accurately target the high-risk volume and to use unconventional field arrangements to produce superior dose distributions. To accomplish this without marginal misses, it will be necessary to both carefully define and encompass the various target volumes because the use of oblique or noncoplanar beams could exclude target volumes that would be included in AP/PA fields or nonoblique four-field techniques (AP/PA and laterals). Although, historically, two-dimensional (2D)-based radiation planning has been carried out primarily using anatomic landmarks as well as fluoroscopic barium swallow to determine field borders (Figs. 62.13 and 62.14), contemporary treatment planning using CT-based planning allows improved visualization of both target and nontarget structures, along with 3D reconstruction and creation of a "beam's eye" view of varying fields, allowing improved conformality around target structures and improvements in normal

tissue sparing. Because volumetric data can be obtained by CT scans, dose–volume histogram data can also be generated. A variety of 3D techniques are presently used and described later. Similarly, with the implementation of IMRT, utilization of this approach should be considered where meeting dose constraints with 3D techniques proves challenging.

Because it is important to account for daily setup uncertainty as well as physiologic internal organ motion (secondary to respiration, peristalsis, cardiac motion, etc.), an additional margin must be added to a CTV. Interfraction variability in stomach location occurs, often owing to variations in gastric filling. Intrafraction changes in target shape and location may be attributable to respiratory motion, which, particularly in the superior to inferior direction, may exceed 1 to 1.5 cm. In effort to reduce this, kilovoltage radiographic matching can be used with particular emphasis on matching of surgical clips.

TABLE 62.9 IMPACT OF SITE OF PRIMARY GASTRIC LESION AND TN STAGE ON IRRADIATION VOLUMES: ANTRUM/PYLORUS/DISTAL ONE-THIRD OF THE STOMACH (GENERAL GUIDELINES)

Site of Primary and TN Stage	Remaining Stomach	Tumor Bed Volumes[a]	Nodal Volumes	Tolerance Organ Structures
Antrum/pylorus/distal one-third of the stomach	Yes—but spare two-thirds of one kidney, usually left	T-stage dependent	N-stage dependent	Kidneys, liver, spinal cord
T2N0 with invasion of subserosa	Variable dependent on surg–path findings[b]	Head of the pancreas (± body), first and second part of the duodenum	None or perigastric; optional: pancreaticoduodenal, porta hepatis, celiac, suprapancreatic[c]	
T3N0	Variable dependent on surg–path findings[b]	Head of the pancreas (± body), first and second part of the duodenum	None or perigastric; optional: pancreaticoduodenal, porta hepatis, celiac, suprapancreatic[c]	
T4N0	Preferable but dependent on surg–path findings[b]	As for T3N0 plus site(s) of adherence with 3–5-cm margin	Nodes related to site(s) of adherence ± perigastric, pancreaticoduodenal, porta hepatis, celiac, suprapancreatic	
T1-2N+	Preferable	Not indicated for T1; as for T2N0 with invasion of subserosa	Perigastric, pancreaticoduodenal, porta hepatis, celiac, suprapancreatic, optional—splenic hilum	
T3-4N+	Preferable	As for T3, T4N0	As for T1-2N+ and T4N0	

[a]Use preoperative imaging (computed tomography [CT], barium swallow), surgical clips, and postoperative imaging (CT, barium swallow).
[b]For tumors with wide (>5 cm) surgical margins confirmed pathologically, treatment of residual stomach is optional if this would result in substantial increased normal tissue morbidity.
[c]Optional node inclusion for T2-3N0 lesions if adequate surgical node dissection (D2 dissection) and at least 10 to 15 nodes examined pathologically.
Surg–path, surgical–pathologic.
Reprinted from Tepper JE, Gunderson LL. Radiation treatment parameters in the adjuvant postoperative therapy of gastric cancer. *Semin Radiat Oncol* 2002;12(2):187–195. Copyright © 2002 Elsevier. With permission.

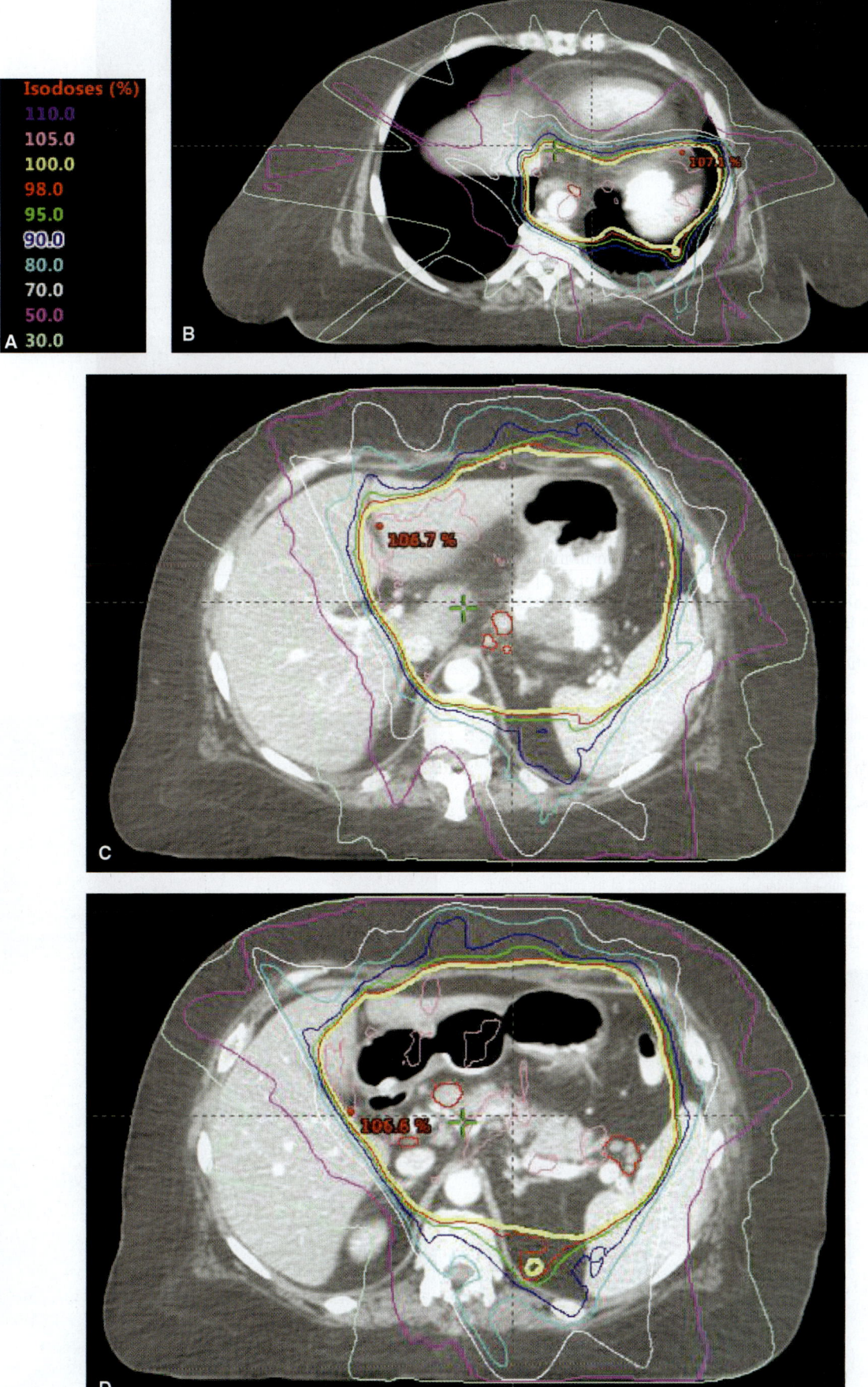

FIGURE 62.12. A 50-year-old female with a gastric body adenocarcinoma with multiple suspicious nodes noted on CT scan (delineated in *red*), including lower paraesophageal, perigastric, gastrohepatic, porta, and splenic hilum. IMRT was utilized to minimize adjacent normal tissue including the heart, liver, kidneys, and spinal cord.

(Continued)

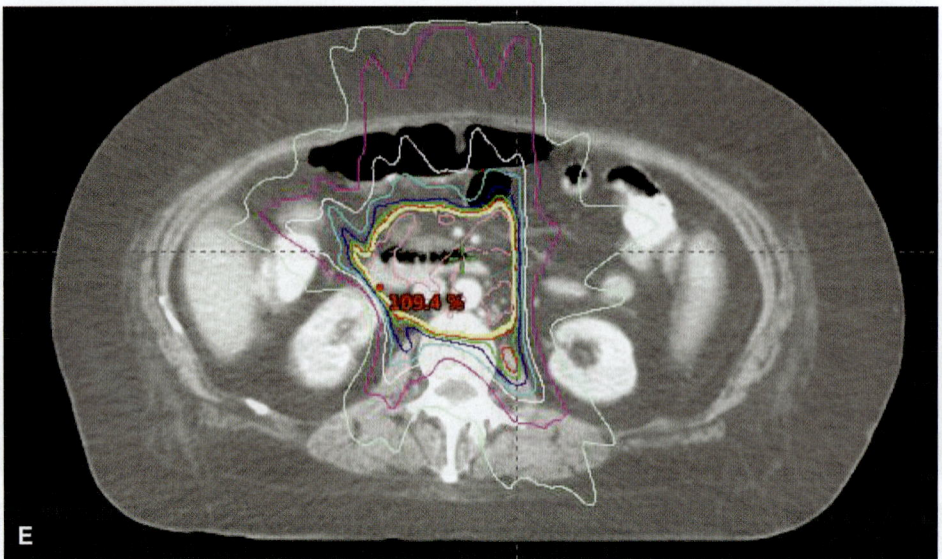

FIGURE 62.12. *(Continued)*

An additional technique that may improve treatment accuracy is cone-beam CT, which allows direct target matching within a given fraction. Movement related to respiratory motion can be assessed using 4D CT, which images the patient in all phases of respiration (similar to what is performed fluoroscopically but using CT). Similarly, respiratory gating techniques may allow reduction in the target volume/smaller margins, allowing for treatment during a more stationary phase of the respiratory cycle (either in expiration or breath hold).

FIGURE 62.13. Simulation film for T3 antral tumor with two of five peritumoral lymph nodes metastatically involved (radical subtotal gastrectomy with D1 node dissection). Simulation film identifies areas at risk for recurrence, including preoperative gastric/tumor bed (defined by preoperative computed tomography [CT] scan), anastomotic sites and gastric stump (staple line seen on precontrast simulation films and marked on postintravenous pyelogram/postcontrast film), and regional lymphatics (celiac, porta hepatis, superior mesenteric artery, and splenic nodes identified on CT and pancreaticoduodenal nodes lie in C-loop of the duodenum identified by preoperative CT). The right kidney is spared for approximately three-fourths of its volume, whereas the left kidney has about one-third of its volume blocked. (Reprinted from Smalley SS, Gunderson L, Tepper J, et al. Gastric surgical adjuvant radiotherapy consensus report: rationale and treatment implementation. *Int J Radiat Oncol Biol Phys* 2002;52[2]:283–293. Copyright © 2002 Elsevier. With permission)

FIGURE 62.14. Simulation film for a T4 (diaphragm invasion) gastroesophageal junction tumor with 4 of 15 involved lymph nodes (total gastrectomy with modified R3 node dissection). Areas at risk for recurrence include preoperative gastric/tumor bed (defined by preoperative upper gastrointestinal radiographs and hemoclips placed at the time of resection to mark tumor bed and diaphragm invasion), anastomotic sites and stump (anastomosis visualized at the juncture of residual distal esophagus and jejunum), and regional lymphatics (including the celiac, porta hepatis, and pancreaticoduodenal areas as well as the distal paraesophageal nodes). (Reprinted from Smalley SS, Gunderson L, Tepper J, et al. Gastric surgical adjuvant radiotherapy consensus report: rationale and treatment implementation. *Int J Radiat Oncol Biol Phys* 2002;52[2]:283–293. Copyright © 2002 Elsevier. With permission.)

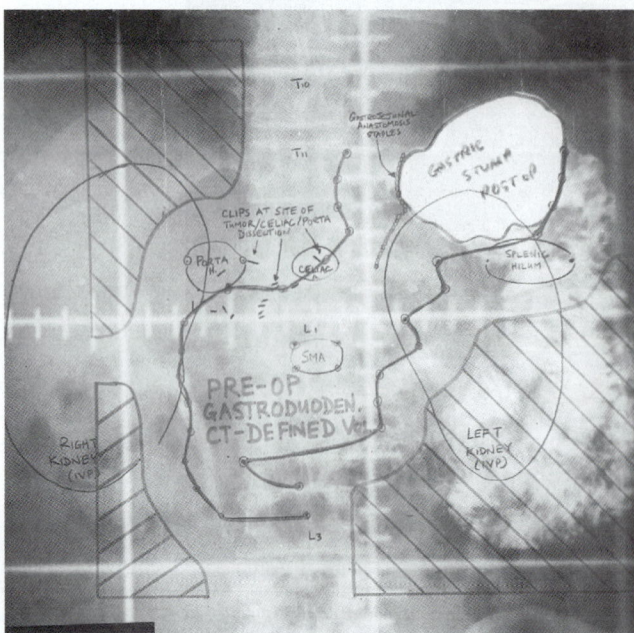

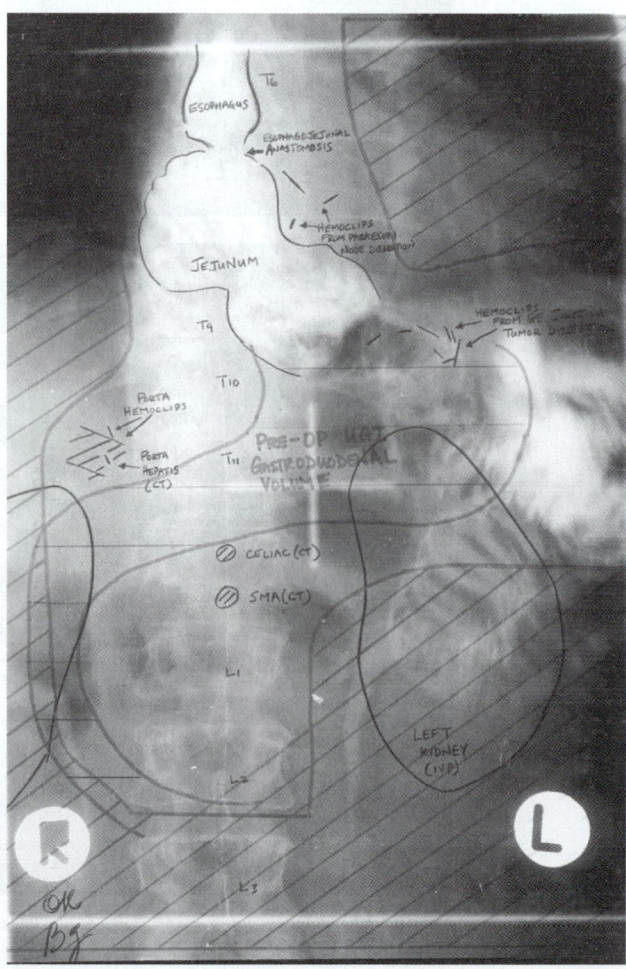

Another potential approach in the treatment for gastric cancer is the use of IMRT. IMRT also uses CT-based planning, again allowing 3D reconstruction of varying structures. However, IMRT differs from 3D planning through the delivery of radiation dose by partitioning a radiation field into multiple smaller fields of various shapes and sizes, varying the dose intensity between each area. This is carried out with either dynamic IMRT (where collimating leaves move in and out of the radiation beam path during treatment) or "step-and-shoot" IMRT (where the leaves change the radiation field shape while the beam is turned off). Either method is particularly effective at conforming radiation dose to the target structures while avoiding dose to normal tissue. Radiation oncologists must determine which structures are most critical and weight their importance during the treatment planning process. Importantly, the greater the number of "avoidance" normal structures, the more difficult it is to meet all dose constraints. IMRT utilizes "inverse planning," where an intended prescription dose is placed on target volumes and dose constraints are placed on normal tissue structures. Thereafter, computer software algorithms allow design of unconventional treatment fields that would not otherwise be possible with standard planning methods. Radiation oncologists and medical physicists critically evaluate numerous plans until dose constraints are satisfactorily met. The result should be a series of radiation doses that closely conform to the target volumes while minimizing dose to normal tissues. IMRT may be appropriate in selected cases to reduce doses to normal structures, including the heart, liver, and kidneys. A potential disadvantage of IMRT is the possibility of delivering low doses of radiation therapy to normal tissue areas that might not normally be irradiated using 2D or 3D techniques. Another potential disadvantage to IMRT is possible dose inhomogeneity, leading to potential "hot spots" in normal organs. Because IMRT requires precise target definition, the potential for "marginal miss" increases and careful, accurate target delineation is of paramount importance.

With setup uncertainty and physiologic organ motion, care must be taken to ensure accurate and reproducible setup, including with the use of immobilization devices as well as possible respiratory gating/breath-hold techniques. Block margins may be minimized with efforts to reduce intrafractional position variability, including breath-hold techniques. Generally, high-energy photons (10 to 18 MV) are recommended when using 3D conformal or IMRT therapy, potentially facilitating a reduction in the integral dose. When using more advanced radiation planning techniques, daily image guidance is generally recommended, with consideration of frequent cone-beam CT imaging and adaptive planning pending anatomic changes.[112]

Multiple dosimetric studies comparing IMRT to two-field and 3D conformal radiation therapy plans have shown significant reductions in kidney, liver, heart, lung, and spinal cord dose with the former. Although IMRT may result in improved normal tissue sparing, many of the acute toxicities encountered during radiation may persist given that many symptoms arise from radiation of the target, including gastric mucosa. The value of IMRT may lie primarily in normal organ sparing with potential reductions in long-term toxicity in surviving patients. There is ongoing investigation into further enhancements of this technique using volumetric modulated arc therapy, helical TomoTherapy, as well as proton therapy. This may also become important with the integration of newer/novel systemic agents, in conjunction with radiation therapy, of which many act as potent tumoral (as well as normal organ) radiation sensitizers and may reduce treatment-related toxicities as well as avoidance of treatment interruptions.

Dose Constraints

In radiation therapy planning of gastric cancer, normal tissue tolerance should always be considered. The spinal cord dose is generally limited to 45 Gy using 1.8-Gy fractions (and potentially less when delivered with novel systemic agents).

Accurate delineation of adjacent organs including lungs, liver, kidneys, heart, and spinal cord is important. Varying dose–volume normal organ constraints have been suggested. Historically, heart dose constraints have included maintaining one-third, two-thirds, and total heart volumes <45, 40, and 30 Gy, respectively. Recommended heart constraints include keeping <30% of the cardiac volume to a total dose of 40 Gy and <50% receiving 25 Gy, minimizing dose to the left ventricle. In a recent secondary analysis of the NRG Oncology RTOG 0617 Randomized Clinical Trial in which lung cancer patients received concurrent chemotherapy of carboplatin and paclitaxel with or without cetuximab, and 60- versus 74-Gy radiation doses, IMRT produced lower heart doses ($P < .05$), and the volume of heart receiving 40 Gy (V40) was significantly associated with OS on adjusted analysis ($P < .05$).[117] In the setting of potentially significant volumes of the heart in the radiation field, consideration of 4D CT and/or respiratory motion management can be made. It is recommended that at least 70% of one physiologically functioning kidney receive a total dose <20 Gy and that collectively ≤50% of the combined functional renal volume should receive >20 Gy.[113] In some patients, a portion of both kidneys will fall within the treatment field; however, at least two-thirds to three-fourths of one kidney should be excluded beyond a dose of 20 Gy. For proximal gastric lesions, ≥50% of the left kidney is commonly within the irradiation portal, and the right kidney must be appropriately spared. For distal lesions with narrow or positive duodenal margins, a similar amount of right kidney often is included, and every effort must be taken to spare enough left kidney to maintain function. Late renal sequelae have not generally been encountered with these techniques.[39,79,118] One should also consider the possibility of impaired kidney function in the context of varying comorbidities, using nuclear medicine renal studies to assess individual renal function in such situations or where significant volumes of kidneys are anticipated to be within the radiation field. Generally, 70% of the liver parenchyma should be kept to a dose <30 Gy. Many of these constraints can be achieved through the use of 3D planning with appropriate and careful design of shielding blocks/multileaf collimation and dose–volume histogram analysis, with the use of IMRT in appropriate cases. Table 62.10 shows examples of recommended normal tissue constraints.

Doses of Radiation

Generally, doses in the range of 45 to 50.4 Gy should be delivered at 1.8 Gy per fraction. Although primarily limited by normal tissue constraints in the upper abdomen, several series have reported improved locoregional control with radiation dose escalation in the adjuvant setting. A report from Mayo Clinic investigators reported high locoregional control rates with radiation doses >54 Gy.[118] Similarly, a report from Italian investigators treating patients adjuvantly with hyperfractionated radiation therapy to a dose of 55 Gy, with concurrent 5-FU, showed an in-field recurrence rate of only 7.5% and survival rate of 52% with a median follow-up >5 years.[119] With regimens using single daily fractions, the usual dose is 45 delivered in

TABLE 62.10 EXAMPLE NORMAL TISSUE CONSTRAINTS

	EORTC[113]	National Comprehensive Cancer Network[a]
Spinal Cord	<45 Gy	≤45 Gy
Lungs	V20 < 20%	V20 ≤ 30%; mean ≤20 Gy
Heart	V40 < 30%, V25 < 50%	V30 ≤ 30% (closer to 20% preferred); mean 30 Gy
Kidneys	Total V20 < 50%; at least one with V20 < 30%	(evaluate each separately): V20 ≤ 33%; mean <18 Gy
Liver	V30 < 30%	V30 ≤ 33%; mean < 25 Gy
Bowel	—	V45 < 195 cm³

*a*NCCN Clinical Practice Guidelines in Oncology (NCCN Guidelines)—Gastric Cancer Version 2.2017.2017. Accessed August 21, 2017.

1.8- to 2-Gy fractions over 5 weeks, with a field reduction after 45 Gy in patients receiving boost-field treatments. Reduced boost fields to small areas of residual disease and a small volume of stomach or small intestine sometimes can be cautiously carried to doses of 55 to 60 Gy with multifield techniques. In such instances, informed consent should include a discussion of an increased risk of grade 3 to 4 gastrointestinal toxicity.

RESULTS OF THERAPY

Locally Advanced Unresectable or Subtotally Resected Gastric Cancer

For patients with locally advanced unresectable or subtotally resected gastric carcinoma, radiotherapeutic approaches both with and without chemotherapy have been used because these tumors appear localized without clinically detectable metastases. Combined treatment with radiation therapy and chemotherapy appears to prolong survival but rarely results in long-term cure.[120] Although only a modest effect on survival is seen, these studies have established, importantly, the foundation of contemporary combined modality therapy and have served as a stimulus to further clinical investigation in gastric cancer as well as other gastrointestinal disease sites. The results of these phase III studies have had a significant impact on clinical trial development in gastrointestinal malignancies (Table 62.11).

In a historical trial from 1969, Moertel et al.[120] reported the results of a prospective, controlled double-blind study of patients with locally advanced unresectable gastric cancer. In this study, 48 patients were randomized to 35 to 40 Gy of radiation therapy over 4 weeks with and without 5-FU. Mean survival was 13 months in patients receiving radiation therapy and 5-FU versus 5.9 months for the radiation therapy patients ($P < .01$). These results demonstrated for the first time the clinical benefit of combining concurrent 5-FU with radiation therapy and encouraged further investigation of combination therapy in gastric cancer and other gastrointestinal disease sites (esophageal, pancreatic, rectal, and anal carcinomas).

As a follow-up to this study, the Gastrointestinal Tumor Study Group (GITSG) examined the combination of 5-FU/ MeCCNU, or 1-(2-chloroethyl)-3-(4-methylcyclohexyl)-1 nitrosourea, and radiotherapy (RT; 50 Gy/split course/8 weeks) versus the same chemotherapy alone in locally advanced gastric cancer.[121] Patients were eligible if the tumor involved regional lymph nodes or adjacent structures that could be completely resected en bloc. Of the 90 patients entered, 66 patients had a resection of the primary tumor. Of these, 23 patients had gross residual disease, 36 patients had microscopic residual, and 7 patients had no documented residual disease. The study was closed prematurely because of an excess of early deaths in the combined chemotherapy–RT arm. The excessive early mortality of the combined-modality arm was attributed to early tumor progression and poor tolerance of the combined-modality regimen. However, further follow-up beyond 3 years indicated continuing mortality among the chemotherapy-alone arm, whereas the combined chemoradiotherapy arm exhibited a plateau with 18% of patients surviving 5 years. Thus, despite an excess of early mortality, the combined-modality arm exhibited an overall superiority in 5-year survival. It is important to note that patients who had had their primary tumor resected experienced superior survival to those without resection. All of the survival benefit in patients receiving combined modality was in patients whose primary tumor had been resected. This trial showed that combined chemoradiation therapy is capable of rendering a substantial percentage of patients with microscopic residual gastric cancer free from disease. It furthermore supported the rationale of exploring chemoradiation adjuvant trials in completely resected patients at high risk for locoregional relapse, and that chemoradiation was able to control microscopic disease and lead to long-term survival in a significant number of these patients.

A more recent multicenter phase II trial from China treated patients with medically inoperable or unresectable gastric cancer with pre- and postradiation docetaxel, cisplatin, and 5-fluorouracil (DCF), in combination with chemoradiation with concurrent cisplatin in between. Clinical complete response rate was 36%, overall response rate 83%, median survival 26 months, and 2-year survival 52%. Medically inoperable patients had a better prognosis than patients with frankly unresectable disease.[122]

Resectable Gastric Cancer

The recognition of the high rates of local and regional failure following surgery in patterns of failure analyses has served as the basis for clinical trials assessing the value of radiation therapy both with and without chemotherapy as an adjuvant treatment (Table 62.4). Although these studies have all addressed the important question of whether clinical outcome is enhanced by adjuvant radiation therapy, there has been marked variability in radiation dose and schedule, sequence with surgery (preoperatively, intraoperatively, or postoperatively), and the use of concurrent and maintenance chemotherapy (Table 62.12). These differences in study design and included patients may explain in part the conflicting results observed in phase III studies.

Adjuvant Radiation Therapy

Two randomized phase III studies have studied the use of external beam radiation therapy (EBRT) alone with surgery.[76,123] Although both studies used similar radiation dose and schedule, sequence with surgery differed. In the British Stomach Cancer Group study, 436 patients were randomized to surgery alone, postoperative radiation therapy (45 to 50 Gy in 25 to 28 fractions), or cytotoxic chemotherapy with mitomycin, doxorubicin, and fluorouracil (FAM).[76,123] The 5-year survival for surgery alone was 20%, for surgery plus radiation therapy 12%, and for surgery plus chemotherapy 19%. In this study, no survival advantage was observed for patients who received postoperative EBRT, although there was an apparent improvement in local control, demonstrating that local disease could be affected by adjuvant radiation therapy. Locoregional failure was documented in only 15 of 153 patients (10%) in the irradiation arm versus 39 of 145 patients (27%) in the surgery-alone arm and 26 of 138 patients (19%) in the FAM group. Interpretation of the results is complicated by the inclusion of 171 patients undergoing resection with gross or microscopic residual carcinoma. These patients would not be candidates for contemporary gastric surgical adjuvant trials in the United States. In addition, approximately one-third of patients randomized to receive

TABLE 62.11	UNRESECTABLE OR RESIDUAL GASTRIC CANCER: TREATMENT RESULTS OF RANDOMIZED TRIALS				
Group or Institution	Treatment Arms	Number of Patients	EBRT Dose	Chemotherapy	Survival Results
Mayo Clinic[120]	EBRT + ChT vs. EBRT	48	35–40 Gy	5-FU	Increased survival for EBRT + 5-FU with mean survival 13 vs. 5.9 mo and 3/25 (12%) vs. 0/23 5-y survival
GITSG[121]	EBRT + ChT vs. ChT	90	50-Gy split course	5-FU + MeCCNU	Advantage in long-term survival with EBRT + ChT at 18% vs. 7% ($P < .05$)

ChT, chemotherapy; EBRT, external beam radiation therapy; 5-FU, 5-fluorouracil; GITSG, Gastrointestinal Tumor Study Group; MeCCNU, 1-(2-chloroethyl)-3-(4-methylcyclohexyl)-1 nitrosourea.

TABLE 62.12 ADJUVANT/NEOADJUVANT IRRADIATION FOR RESECTED GASTRIC CANCER: TREATMENT RESULTS OF RANDOMIZED TRIALS

Series/Treatment Method	Patients	Median Survival (Months)	Survival			Locoregional Relapse	
			Long Term[a] (%)	P Value	N	%	P Value
1. Mayo Clinic[107]							
a. Surgery alone	23	15	4	—	—	54	—
b. Postop EBRT + 5-FU	39	24	23	.05	—	39	—
2. British Stomach Group[123]							
a. Surgery alone	145	—	20	—	39	27 (3 y)	—
b. Postop ChT	138	—	19	—	26	19 (3 y)	—
c. Postop EBRT	153	—	12	—	15	10 (3 y)	—
3. China–Beijing[124]							
a. Surgery alone	199	—	20	—	—	52	—
b. Preop EBRT	171	—	30	.009	—	39	<.025
4. Intergroup 0116[111]						Disease-free survival (3 y)	
a. Surgery alone	275	27	41	—	—	31	—
b. Postop EBRT + ChT	281	36	50	.005	—	48	<.001
5. ARTIST Trial[125,126]							
a. Postop ChT	228	—	73	—	—	13	—
b. Postop EBRT + ChT → Postop EBRT + ChT	230	—	75	.484	—	7[b]	.0033
6. CRITICS Trial[133]							
a. Preop ChT → Surgery → Postop ChT	393	43	42	.90	—	—	—
b. Preop ChT → Surgery → Postop EBRT + ChT	395	37	40				

[a]Long-term survival is 5-year data for Mayo Clinic, ARTIST, CRITICS, and Beijing series, and 3-year data are for British and Intergroup 0116.
[b]In node-positive patients, 3-year disease-free survival 72% vs. 76%, P = .04; 83% vs. 94% in intestinal-type tumors.
ChT, chemotherapy; EBRT, external beam radiation therapy; N, patient number; preop, preoperative; postop, postoperative; 5-FU, 5-fluorouracil.

adjuvant treatment did not receive the assigned therapy. Of 153 patients randomized to the irradiation arm, only 104 (68%) received a dose ≥40.5 Gy, and 36 (24%) received none.

Neoadjuvant Radiation Therapy
In contrast, the results of a phase III study from Beijing demonstrated a survival benefit for patients with gastric cardia carcinoma receiving preoperative irradiation and surgery versus surgery only.[124] In this study, 370 patients with gastric cardia carcinoma were randomized to 40 Gy in 20 fractions over 4 weeks of preoperative irradiation and surgery or surgery only. The 5-year survival rates of preoperative irradiation and surgery and the surgery-alone group were 30% and 20%, respectively (10-year, 20% and 13%, respectively). These differences were statistically significant (P = .009). Further, local and regional nodal control was improved in patients undergoing preoperative irradiation and surgery (61% and 61%) versus surgery (48% and 45%) only. Morbidity and mortality rates were not increased in patients receiving preoperative irradiation and surgery.

Intraoperative Radiation Therapy
An alternative approach to postoperative or preoperative irradiation is intraoperative radiation therapy (IORT).[127,128] The advantage of this technique is the ability to deliver a single large fraction (10 to 35 Gy) of radiation to the tumor or tumor bed while excluding or protecting surrounding normal tissue from the high-dose field. This approach permits high-dose irradiation with minimal normal tissue treatment. Two randomized trials have examined the efficacy of IORT in combination with surgery for patients with gastric carcinoma. Abe et al.[127] from Kyoto University performed a randomized trial of 211 patients with gastric cancer comparing surgery alone with surgery and intraoperative radiation (28 to 35 Gy). Patients were randomized based on hospital day of admission for surgery. For patients with tumor confined to the gastric wall, 5-year survival rates were similar for IORT and for resection alone. However, patients with Japanese stages II to IV disease who received IORT in conjunction with resection showed improved survival over patients who underwent resection without irradiation. Among patients with stage IV disease (who usually had local residual disease after maximal resection), there were no 5-year survivors in patients who received surgery alone; however, 15% of the patients who received IORT were alive at

5 years. The experience with IORT in gastric cancer at Kyoto University suggested that IORT may be beneficial in the treatment for locally advanced malignancies of the stomach.

To further evaluate this approach, Sindelar et al.[128] at the National Cancer Institute conducted a prospectively randomized controlled trial comparing surgical resection and IORT with conventional therapy in gastric carcinoma. Patients in the experimental group underwent gastrectomy, and IORT was administered to the gastric bed (20 Gy). Patients in the control group underwent resection and postoperative EBRT to the upper abdomen (50 Gy in 25 fractions) in advanced-stage lesions extending beyond the gastric wall. Of the 100 patients screened for the study, 60 patients were randomized and underwent exploratory surgery. Nineteen patients were excluded intraoperatively because of unresectability or metastases, leaving 41 patients in the study. The median survival for patients with tumors of all stages was 25 months for the IORT group and 21 months for the control group (P = not significant [NS]). Locoregional disease relapse occurred in 7 of 16 IORT patients (44%) and in 23 of 25 control patients (92%) (P < .001). Complication rates were similar between IORT and control patients. Although IORT failed to afford a significant advantage over conventional therapy in overall survival, it significantly improved control of locoregional disease. The use of IORT in gastric cancer remains a topic of investigation.

Adjuvant Chemoradiation Therapy
Because of the promising results in the early studies of combined-modality therapy for locally advanced unresectable or subtotally resected gastric cancer, investigators also have studied this combination in resectable gastric carcinoma. A small study from South Africa randomized 66 patients with resected gastric cancer (T1 to T3, N1 or N2, M0) to low-dose postoperative irradiation (20 Gy in eight fractions over 10 days) and 5-FU or no further therapy.[96] No difference in survival was observed between the patients undergoing surgery and adjuvant therapy and those undergoing surgery alone. Given the subtherapeutic doses of radiation used in this study, it is difficult to draw any conclusions as to the efficacy of adjuvant radiation therapy and 5-FU.

In 1984, Moertel et al.[107] reported the results of a prospective randomized trial conducted at the Mayo Clinic of 62 patients with poor prognosis but completely resected gastric cancers who were randomized to either surgery alone or surgery followed by irradiation (37.5 Gy in 24 fractions over 4 to 5 weeks) with concurrent 5-FU. A nonstratified, prerandomization scheme was used with a 2:3 ratio favoring treatment. Informed consent was requested of only the 39 patients randomized to treatment. Ten of the 39 patients refused further therapy and were observed. When analyzed by intent to treat, the adjuvant arm had statistically significant improvement in both relapse-free and overall survival (overall 5-year survival 23% vs. 4%, $P < .05$). When patient outcome was compared with actual treatment received (29 adjuvant treatment, 33 surgery alone), 5-year survival still favored the adjuvant group (20% vs. 12%), although the differences were not statistically significant in view of the small patient numbers. The 10 patients who refused assignment to adjuvant treatment had more favorable prognostic findings than the other two groups of patients. When the two groups with equally poor prognostic factors were compared, the 5-year overall survival was 20% versus 4%, with an advantage to those receiving adjuvant treatment. When analyzed by treatment delivered, locoregional relapse was decreased with adjuvant treatments (54% incidence with surgery alone vs. 39% with irradiation and 5-FU).

Because of these conflicting results and the fact locoregional failure remained an established source of recurrence, an Intergroup trial (INT 0116) was initiated to evaluate postoperative combined 5-FU–based chemotherapy and irradiation to the gastric bed and regional nodes versus surgery only following resection of gastric cancer.[111] Eligibility included patients with pathologic stage group IB through IV nonmetastatic adenocarcinoma of the stomach or GE junction. After an en bloc resection (patients underwent D0-D1 dissection), 556 patients were randomized to either observation alone or postoperative 5-FU/leucovorin for one cycle followed by combined-modality therapy consisting of 45 Gy in 25 fractions plus concurrent 5-FU and leucovorin (4 days in week 1, 3 days in week 5) followed by two monthly 5-day cycles of 5-FU and leucovorin. Minor or major errors in field design were seen in 35% during preirradiation quality assurance review, allowing most deviations to be corrected prior to radiation therapy initiation, resulting in a 6.5% final major deviation rate. Nodal metastases were present in 85% of the cases. With 5 years of median follow-up, 3-year relapse-free survival was 48% for adjuvant treatment and 31% for observation ($P = .001$); 3-year overall survival was 50% for treatment and 41% for observation ($P = .005$). The median overall survival in the surgery-only group was 27 months, compared with 36 months in the chemoradiotherapy group; the HR for death was 1.35 (95% CI 1.09 to 1.66, $P = .005$). The HR for relapse in the surgery-only group as compared with the chemoradiotherapy group was 1.52 (95% CI 1.23 to 1.86, $P < .001$). The median duration of relapse-free survival was 30 months in the chemoradiotherapy group and 19 months in the surgery-only group. Patterns of failure were based on the site of first relapse only and were categorized as local, regional, or distant. Local recurrence occurred in 29% of patients who relapsed in the surgery-only group and 19% of those who relapsed in the chemoradiotherapy group. Regional relapse—typically abdominal carcinomatosis—was reported in 72% of those who relapsed in the surgery-only group and 65% of those who relapsed in the chemoradiotherapy group. Extra-abdominal distant metastases were diagnosed in 18% of those who relapsed in the surgery-only group and 33% of those who relapsed in the chemoradiotherapy group. Treatment was tolerable, with three (1%) toxic deaths. Grades 3 and 4 toxicity occurred in 41% and 32% of cases, respectively, and 17% of patients assigned to the chemoradiotherapy group stopped treatment owing to toxicity from therapy. Long-term results at >10-year median follow-up continued to show significant improvement in overall and disease-free survival in the chemoradiation group, benefiting all T- and N-stage patients included in the trial.[129] The results of this large study demonstrate a

clear survival advantage for the use of postoperative chemoradiation and strongly support its integration into the routine care of patients with curatively resected high-risk carcinoma of the stomach and GE junction.[129]

The follow-up Intergroup trial CALGB 80101 randomized 546 patients with resected gastric or GE junction adenocarcinoma to receive either (a) one cycle of 5-FU/leucovorin, followed by 45 Gy with concurrent continuous infusion 5-FU, followed by two additional cycles of 5-FU/leucovorin, or (b) one cycle of ECF (epirubicin, cisplatin, 5-FU), followed by 45 Gy with concurrent, continuous infusional 5-FU, followed by two additional cycles of reduced dose ECF. With a median follow-up duration of 6.5 years, 5-year overall survival rates were 44% in the FU plus LV arm and 44% in the ECF arm ($P = .69$; hazard ratio, 0.98; 95% CI, 0.78 to 1.24 comparing ECF with FU plus LV). Five-year disease-free survival rates were 39% in the FU plus LV arm and 37% in the ECF arm ($P = .94$; hazard ratio, 0.96; 95% CI, 0.77 to 1.20). The authors concluded that following curative resection of gastric or GE junction adenocarcinoma, postoperative chemoradiotherapy using ECF before and after 5-FU–based radiation does not improve survival compared to bolus 5-FU/leucovorin given in the same manner.[130]

A large retrospective study from Korea evaluated the role of adjuvant chemoradiation in patients undergoing D2 gastric cancer resection, a group that was not adequately represented in the aforementioned Intergroup trial. In the Korean study, 544 patients treated with D2 dissection and postoperative chemoradiation therapy were compared to 446 patients with similar characteristics treated with D2 dissection alone. Overall survival was significantly higher in patients treated with adjuvant chemoradiation (median survival 95 vs. 63 months, $P = .02$) as well as significant improvement in relapse-free survival.[91] Additionally, a collective review of nine randomized trials incorporating radiation therapy approaches with surgery alone also demonstrated a significant 5-year survival benefit with the addition of radiation therapy in resectable gastric cancer patients.[131]

A Korean phase III trial (the Adjuvant Chemoradiation Therapy in Stomach Cancer [ARTIST] study) compared the effects of adjuvant chemoradiation (capecitabine/cisplatin [XP] + RT) to adjuvant chemotherapy alone (capecitabine/cisplatin) following D2 resection of gastric cancer in 458 patients.[125] Treatment was completed as planned by 75.4% of patients (172 of 228) in the XP arm and 81.7% (188 of 230) in the XP/RT/XP arm. The addition of radiation to XP chemotherapy did not significantly prolong disease-free survival ($P = .086$). However, in the subgroup of patients with pathologic lymph node metastasis at the time of surgery ($n = 396$), patients randomly assigned to the XP/RT/XP arm experienced superior disease-free survival when compared with those who received XP alone ($P = .0365$), and the statistical significance was retained at multivariate analysis (estimated HR 0.69, $P = .047$). The authors concluded that the addition of RT to XP chemotherapy did not significantly reduce recurrence after curative resection and D2 lymph node dissection in gastric cancer. Of note is there was a relatively high proportion of early-stage disease in both trial arms, with approximately 60% of patients exhibiting stage Ib-II gastric cancer, as well as >60% demonstrating diffuse-type histology (vs. 39% in the Intergroup 0116 trial). A report of long-term outcomes of the ARTIST trial with 7-year follow-up showed disease-free survival remains similar between the treatment arms (hazard ratio 0.74, CI 0.52 to 1.05, $P = .09$), with similar overall survival rates. In this analysis, the effect of the addition of radiation therapy in disease-free and overall survival differed by Lauren classification and lymph node ratio. Subgroup analysis showed that chemoradiotherapy significantly improved disease-free survival in node-positive disease and intestinal-type gastric cancers with a similar trend for disease-free and overall survival by stage of disease[126]; a subsequent trial by this group (ARTIST-II) in patients with lymph node–positive/stage

II-III gastric cancer undergoing D2 resection stage II-III gastric cancer is randomizing patients to receive (a) adjuvant S1 for 1 year versus (b) adjuvant S1/oxaliplatin for 6 months versus (c) two cycles of S1/oxaliplatin, followed by concurrent S1/radiotherapy, followed by four additional cycles of S1/oxaliplatin with stage IB- IVA resectable gastric or gastro-oesophageal adenocarcinoma. Interpretation of these trial results are challenging given the high noncompliance rates, given that only 62%o f patients assigned to the radiation arm initiated radiation, with only 50% received the intended 5 weeks of therapy.

Chinese investigators randomized 380 patients undergoing D2 lymph node dissection to either radiation therapy using IMRT (45 Gy) with concurrent 5-FU and leucovorin or 5-FU and leucovorin alone. Five-year local recurrence rate in the radiation arm was 15.6% versus 24.2% without radiation (P = .042), although 5-year overall survival was not significantly different (48.4% vs. 41.8%, P = .122). However, median relapse-free survival (50 vs. 32 months, P = .029) was higher in the radiation group, and rates of all grade adverse events were similar between the two groups.[132]

Finally, a study by the Dutch Colorectal Cancer Group (the Chemoradiotherapy after Induction Chemotherapy in Cancer of the Stomach [CRITICS] trial) randomized 788 patients to receive preoperative chemotherapy (epirubicin, cisplatin, capecitabine or, alternatively, epirubicin, oxaliplatin, and capecitabine) for three cycles followed by D1+ resection, followed by a similar postoperative chemotherapy regimen, with or without radiotherapy concurrent with cisplatin/capecitabine. After preoperative chemotherapy, 372 (95%) of 393 patients in the chemotherapy group and 369 (93%) of 395 patients in the chemoradiotherapy group proceeded to surgery, with a potentially curative resection acheived in 310 (79%) of 393 patients in the chemotherapy group and 326 (83%) of 395 in the chemoradiotherapy group. Postoperatively, 233 (59%) of 393 patients started chemotherapy and 245 (62%) of 395 started chemoradiotherapy. At a median follow-up of 61·4 months, median overall survival was 43 months in the chemotherapy group and 37 months in the chemoradiotherapy group (p=0·90). After preoperative chemotherapy, in the total safety population of 781 patients (assessed together), there were 368 (47%) grade 3 adverse events; 130 (17%) grade 4 adverse events, and 13 (2%) deaths. During postoperative treatment, grade 3 and 4 adverse events occurred in 113 (48%) and 22 (9%) of 233 patients in the chemotherapy group, respectively, and in 101 (41%) and ten (4%) of 245 patients in the chemoradiotherapy group, respectively. The authors concluded postoperative chemoradiotherapy did not improve overall survival compared with postoperative chemotherapy in patients with resectable gastric cancer treated with adequate preoperative chemotherapy and surgery, although given the poor postoperative patient compliance in both treatment groups, future studies should focus on optimizing preoperative treatment strategies.[133]

Preoperative Chemoradiation Therapy

Because preoperative radiation therapy and chemotherapy have improved the surgical and disease-related outcomes in patients with rectal and esophageal cancer, this treatment is a logical approach to explore in gastric cancer as well. In the context of established limitations of perioperative and adjuvant strategies, potential advantages of preoperative therapy include improved tolerance relative to adjuvant treatments, potential downstaging with associated improvement in R0 resection rates, better target definition, better vascularization for optimal chemotherapy and radiosensitizing oxygen delivery, and allowing biologic stratification of patients for surgery, notably given that the presence of micrometastases is at initial diagnosis. Although no completed phase III trials have tested the value of preoperative radiation plus chemotherapy for patients with gastric cancer to date, two phase III trials for patients with esophagus cancer have included

either lesions of the gastric cardia[134] or the esophagogastric junction.[135] In both trials, the trimodality arm demonstrated an improvement in survival when compared with the control arm of surgery alone. The series by Walsh et al.[134] (adenocarcinoma of the esophagus or gastric cardia) demonstrated a median survival of 16 versus 11 months and 3-year survival of 32% versus 6% (P = .01), with the advantage to trimodality treatment. The U.S. Gastrointestinal Intergroup phase III trial (adenocarcinoma or squamous cell of the esophagus or GE junction), which closed prematurely owing to low accrual, resulted in a median survival of 54 versus 21.6 months and 5-year survival of 39% versus 16% (P = .008), with an advantage to the trimodality arm.[135]

Preoperative chemoradiation data for patients with gastric cancer are primarily limited to phase II studies from single institutions and cooperative groups. MD Anderson Cancer Center investigators reported a study in which 33 patients completed a preoperative protocol that started with induction chemotherapy of 5-FU, leucovorin, and cisplatin, followed by 45 Gy of radiation therapy in 25 fractions over 5 weeks. Infusional 5-FU was administered concurrently with radiation therapy. In 28 patients (85%), a gastrectomy was performed and D2 lymph node dissection was attempted. Pathologic complete and partial response was found in 64% of all operated patients. These patients showed a significantly longer median survival of 64 months in comparison with 13 months in patients with tumors not pathologically responding.[136] In a study from the same institution, 41 patients with operable gastric cancer received two cycles of continuous 5-FU, paclitaxel, and cisplatin followed by 45 Gy of radiation therapy with concurrent 5-FU and paclitaxel. An R0 resection was achieved in 78% of patients, pathologic complete response in 25%, and pathologic partial response in 15%. Pathologic response, R0 resection, and postoperative T and N stage were correlated with overall and disease-free survival.[137] The RTOG reported the results of a phase II study of 49 patients undergoing induction 5-FU, leucovorin, and cisplatin followed by concurrent radiation therapy and infusional 5-FU and paclitaxel.[138] Resection was attempted 5 to 6 weeks after radiation therapy and chemotherapy. The pathologic complete response and R0 resection rates were 26% and 77%, respectively. At 1 year, more patients with tumors exhibiting a pathologic complete response (89%) were living than patients with tumors exhibiting a less favorable response (66%). Grade 4 toxicity occurred in 21% of patients. These data appear to support a randomized phase III study evaluating preoperative versus postoperative radiation therapy and chemotherapy.[138] Although some concerns exist regarding potential for neoadjuvant radiation to increase perioperative morbidity, a national database analysis showed no differences in overall complications or 30-day mortality relative to up-front surgery alone with this approach.[139]

Preoperative Chemoradiation Versus Preoperative Chemotherapy

A randomized trial comparing neoadjuvant chemotherapy alone versus neoadjuvant combined modality therapy was conducted by German investigators (the Preoperative Chemotherapy or Radiochemotherapy in Esophago-gastric Adenocarcinoma Trial [POET]).[140] Patients with advanced esophagogastric adenocarcinoma were randomized to receive (a) cisplatin/5-FU–based chemotherapy alone versus (b) a similar induction chemotherapy followed by concurrent cisplatin/etoposide with 30 Gy of radiation therapy. Both groups went on to receive surgery. Although this study closed early owing to poor accrual, patients receiving preoperative chemoradiotherapy had significantly higher N0 rates (37% vs. 64%, P = .04) and pathologic complete response rates (2% vs. 16%, P = .03), as well as statistical trends toward improved local control (59% vs. 76%, P = .06) and overall survival (3-year survival 28% vs. 47%, P = .07, HR 0.67). The authors concluded that preoperative combined modality improves overall survival as compared to chemotherapy alone in patients with locally advanced esophagogastric adenocarcinoma.[140] Long-term follow up of this study showed local progression-free survival after tumour resection was significantly improved by CRT (hazard ratio 0.37; 0.16-0.85, p = value 0.01) and 20 versus 12 patients were free of local tumour progression at 5 years (p = 0.03). Although the rate of postoperative in-hospital mortality was somewhat higher with CRT (10.2% versus 3.8%, p = 0.26), more patients were alive at 3 and 5 years after CRT (46.7% and 39.5%) compared with chemotherapy (26.1% and 24.4%). Thus, overall survival showed a trend in favour of preoperative CRT (HR 0.65, 95% confidence interval [CI] 0.42-1.01, p = 0.055).[140a] Along these lines, an Australian randomized phase II/III trial (the TOPGEAR study) was initiated, randomizing resectable gastric and GE junction cancer patients to (a) preoperative chemotherapy alone (ECF) versus (b) the same regimen followed by concurrent 5-FU–based chemoradiotherapy, with both arms followed by adjuvant ECF. Interim analysis of the first 120 patients from this study demonstrated that preoperative chemoradiation could be safely delivered to the vast majority of patients without a significant increase in treatment toxicity or surgical morbidity. Specifically, 92% of patients allocated to preoperative chemoradiation received the specified treatment, which is much higher than the 50% compliance rate seen in the previously described CRITICS trial; greater than or equal to grade III gastrointestinal toxicity occurred in 30% of combined modality patients versus 32% in the chemotherapy-alone arm.[141] Similarly, a follow-up Dutch phase II trial (the CRITICS-II trial) is planning on examining the role of preoperative chemoradiotherapy using three preoperative strategies: chemotherapy (docetaxel , oxaliplatin, capecitabine), chemoradiotherapy (45 Gy, carboplatin, paclitaxel), and a combination of both in these patients.

Adjuvant Chemotherapy

The use of adjuvant chemotherapy has been explored in >30 randomized trials, most of which showed no benefit in survival compared to surgery alone. A randomized trial from Japan evaluated 579 patients undergoing resection to receive adjuvant chemotherapy alone versus observation alone. Primarily early T-stage patients in the treatment group received a combination of mitomycin and fluorouracil twice weekly for 3 weeks following surgery, followed by delivery of UFT (uracil + tegafur [an oral 5-FU prodrug]). No survival benefit was seen with adjuvant chemotherapy.[142] However, a more recent study from Japan (the ACTS-GC trial) evaluated the efficacy of adjuvant chemotherapy in patients with stage II/III gastric cancer undergoing R0, D2 dissection (excluding T1 patients). This study randomized 1,059 patients to surgery alone versus treatment with S1, an oral fluoropyrimidine combining tegafur and oxonic acid. Three- and five-year survival was significantly improved in patients receiving adjuvant chemotherapy (80% vs. 70%; 72% vs. 61%, respectively) in favor of the chemotherapy arm (hazard ratio of 0.669).[143,144] Whether the impact of S1 in the Asian population can be extrapolated to Western patients remains less clear and the subject of investigation, including potential biologic differences among populations regarding how this drug is metabolized.

A follow-up Japanese trial (the SAMIT trial) randomized patients with T4a/b gastric cancer following D2 dissection to (a) adjuvant UFT alone, (b) S1 alone, or (c) intermittent weekly paclitaxel, followed by either (a) UFT or (b) S1. The authors concluded that sequential treatment did not improve disease-free survival and UFT was not noninferior to S1 (and S1 was superior to UFT). The authors recommended S1 monotherapy should remain the standard adjuvant treatment for locally advanced gastric cancer in Japan.[145]

Another Asian study, the CLASSIC (capecitabine and oxaliplatin adjuvant study in stomach cancer) was conducted in South Korea, China, and Taiwan. A total of 1,035 patients with pathologic stage II-IIIB gastric cancer were randomized to a surgery-alone arm versus surgery plus adjuvant capecitabine/oxaliplatin for 6 months. Again, all patients underwent D2 gastrectomy. At a median follow-up of 62 months, the adjuvant chemotherapy group had a significant improvement in disease-free survival compared to the surgery-alone group (68% vs. 53%, P < .0001).[146]

A meta-analysis of 17 randomized controlled trials using individual patient data comparing surgery alone to surgery with adjuvant chemotherapy in patients with resectable gastric cancer was performed. In this study, adjuvant chemotherapy was associated with a significant survival benefit in terms of overall survival (hazard ratio [HR] 0.82, confidence interval [CI] 0.76 to 0.90, P < .001) and disease-free survival. Estimated 5-year overall survival was increased from approximately 50% to 55% with the use of chemotherapy. The authors[147] concluded that adjuvant chemotherapy with fluorouracil-containing regimens reduce the risk of death in gastric cancer compared to surgery alone. As discussed previously, how these varying studies apply to Western patients remains unclear.

Perioperative Chemotherapy

Various combinations of active drugs have been reported to improve the response rate among patients with metastatic or locally unresectable gastric carcinoma.[11] A combination of FAM (fluorouracil, doxorubicin, and methotrexate) has been associated with a 30% to 40% response rate and was the most widely prescribed regimen for patients with advanced disease in the 1980s.[11] Despite an initial response rate of 64% when a combination of etoposide, doxorubicin, and cisplatin (EAP) was used by German investigators, in subsequent trials, this regimen was considerably less effective and deemed extremely toxic.[148-150] A combination of fluorouracil, doxorubicin, and high-dose methotrexate (FAMTX) was associated with a significant improvement in response rate compared with either EAP or FAM. As a result of these studies, FAMTX became standard therapy for metastatic disease.

In a British study of patients with unresectable or metastatic gastric and esophageal adenocarcinoma, 274 patients were randomized to either 5-FU, doxorubicin, and methotrexate (FAMTX) or epirubicin, cisplatin, and continuous infusion 5-FU (ECF).[151,152] ECF was associated with a superior response rate (45% vs. 21%, P = .0002), median survival (8.7 vs. 5.7 months, P = .0006 vs. .006), and 1-year survival (36% vs. 21%). Moreover, ECF was associated with a superior quality of life and less toxicity.

The Medical Research Council (MRC) subsequently initiated a trial (the Medical Research Council Adjuvant Gastric Infusional Chemotherapy [MAGIC] trial) to address the question of perioperative chemotherapy (pre- and post-) in operable gastric cancer patients. Patients with resectable adenocarcinoma of the stomach, GE junction, or lower esophagus were randomized to preoperative and postoperative chemotherapy with epirubicin, cisplatin, and 5-FU (ECF) versus surgery alone. Although originally designed to include patients with only tumors of the stomach, eligibility was later expanded to include tumors of the lower third of the esophagus, with approximately one-fourth of patients having adenocarcinoma involving the lower esophagus or GE junction. Of note is that there were more patients with T1/T2 disease (52% vs. 37%, P = .002) as well as more N0/N1 patients (84% vs. 71%, P = .01) in the chemotherapy group. Additionally, a significantly higher percentage of gastric cancer patients receiving perioperative chemotherapy underwent surgery (79% vs. 70%, P = .03). Nonetheless, the resected tumors were significantly smaller and less advanced in the perioperative chemotherapy group. With a median follow-up of 4 years, 149 patients in the perioperative chemotherapy group and 170 patients in the surgery group had died. As compared with the surgery group, the perioperative chemotherapy group had statistically improved progression-free and overall survival rates. No patient achieved pathologic complete response. However, patients receiving perioperative chemotherapy had a HR for death of 0.75, which was highly significant, with 5-year survival in patients receiving chemotherapy 36% versus 23% in patients undergoing surgery alone (P = .009).[153] A follow-up MRC study (the ST03 trial) randomized 1,063 patients with perioperative resectable esophagogastric adenocarcinoma (36% gastric cancer, an additional 20% Siewert type III esophagogastric cancers) to epirubicin, cisplatin, and capecitabine (ECX) versus the same regimen plus bevacizumab. Three-year survival was 50.3% versus 48.1% (NS), with a higher rate of wound healing complications and anastomotic leaks in the bevacizumab group. The authors concluded their results did not provide evidence for the use of bevacizumab in combination with ECX in resectable esophagogastric patients.[154]

French investigators reported the results of a similar randomized trial of 224 patients assigned to perioperative chemotherapy (cisplatin and 5-FU only) versus surgery alone. Although originally designed to include only patients with tumors of the lower third of the esophagus or GE junction, eligibility was later expanded to include gastric cancers, although most (75%) of patients had disease of the lower esophagus or GE junction. Chemotherapy consisted of a planned two to three preoperative and three to four postoperative cycles. This study was prematurely terminated because of low accrual. Nonetheless, patients receiving chemotherapy had improved overall survival (5-year 38% vs. 24%, P = .02), disease-free survival (5-year 34% vs. 19%, P = .003), and R0 resection rates (84% vs. 73%, P = .04). Only 50% of patients received postoperative chemotherapy. T0 disease (complete pathologic response at the primary site) was seen in 3% of neoadjuvantly treated patients. Total locoregional recurrence rates were 24% and 26%, respectively, in the chemotherapy versus surgery group, with distant recurrence rates of 42% versus 56%, respectively.[155]

An EORTC study enrolling patients with locally advanced adenocarcinoma of the stomach or GE junction randomized patients to receive either cisplatin, leucovorin, and infusional 5-FU followed by surgery or surgery alone. Although only accruing 144 of 360 planned patients, neoadjuvantly treated patients had higher R0 resection rates (82% vs. 67%, P = .036); however, at a median follow-up of 4.4 years, no significant difference in overall survival was seen (P = .466).[156]

A meta-analysis of these along with other small trials was performed, revealing that neoadjuvant chemotherapy was associated with a significant improvement in overall survival and progression-free survival and improved R0 resection rates.[157] Given the above, some authors have suggested that in terms of patient selection, a perioperative chemotherapy strategy may be most appropriate for patients with bulky primary tumors or bulky adenopathy in which there is a significant risk of micrometastatic disease as well as incomplete resection.[158]

A preliminary report from Dutch investigators described a study randomizing patients with resectable gastric or GE junction patients to 5-FU, leucovorin, oxaliplatin, and docetaxel (FLOT) versus epirubicin, cisplatin, and 5-FU or capecitabine (ECF or ECX) given in a perioperative fashion. At a median of 43 months, median overall survival was 35 months in the ECF/ECX arm and 50 months with FLOT (hazard ratio 0.77, P = .012). Corresponding 3-year survivals were 48 and 57%, respectively.[159] Additionally, an ongoing French study (FFCD1103) is randomizing resectable signet-ring gastric cancer patients to receive neoadjuvant chemotherapy using perioperative ECF versus initial surgery followed by adjuvant ECF.

Palliative Radiation Therapy

Radiation therapy is capable of providing substantial palliation of local gastric cancer symptoms.[160-165] It appears that 50% to 75% of patients can expect improvement of symptoms such as gastric outlet obstruction, pain from local tumor extension, bleeding, or biliary obstruction.[163] The likelihood of benefit may increase with concomitant 5-FU administration, with less tumor bulk, and if the patient's performance score is better before therapy.[118,161,166,167] The median duration of palliation varies from 4 to 18 months in reports addressing this issue.[161,166,167] A systematic review of the use of palliative radiotherapy in gastric cancer showed large variations in radiation dose and fractionation. The pooled overall response rates for bleeding, pain, and obstruction were 74%, 67%, and 68%, respectively. No difference in bleeding response rates was seen with a BED of ≥39 versus lower doses. Grade III/IV toxicities occurred in up to 15% of patients treated with radiation alone versus up to 25% with combined modality therapy. The authors concluded that more than two-thirds of patients receiving radiation therapy would derive clinical benefit.[168]

SEQUELAE OF THERAPY

Anorexia, nausea, and fatigue are very common complaints during gastric radiation therapy; these symptoms can lead to potentially detrimental treatment breaks, with a National Cancer Data Base analysis evaluating overall adjuvant radiation therapy treatment time suggesting prolonged breaks were associated with inferior survival and that efforts to minimize cumulative interruptions to <7 days should be considered.[169] However, the understanding of these side effects is somewhat limited.[170-173] Although visceral afferents may play some role in the acute emetogenic effects of radiation, other unknown factors, possibly chemical in nature and mediated by the chemoreceptor trigger zone, appear to be more important. Although selective serotonin (5-HT$_3$) antagonists effectively treat radiation-induced emesis, it is not clear whether the mechanism of action is directed at the 5-HT$_3$ receptor alone or has an effect on inhibition of serotonin release.[174] Additionally, the use of low-dose corticosteroids may be beneficial in patients with refractory nausea. Other compounding factors may include the altered gastric motility and prolonged gastric emptying time observed in animal experiments as a response to irradiation.[104,170,171,175] Chemotherapy-related leukopenia and thrombocytopenia may occur. If chemotherapy is used with irradiation, blood counts are generally obtained once to twice weekly. Additional acute toxicities of radiation therapy include esophagitis, epidermitis, fatigue, and weight loss in most patients. Nausea, vomiting, dehydration, and anorexia are relatively common, particularly in patients with lower esophageal and GE junction tumors. During therapy, patient tolerance, weight, and blood counts are checked at least weekly. Many symptoms resolve within 1 to 2 weeks of treatment completion. Because of potential toxicities in the treatment for gastric cancer patients (dehydration, weight loss, anorexia, etc.), aggressive supportive measurements and symptom management are indicated in efforts to avoid treatment-related interruptions, hospitalizations, or failure to complete the intended treatment course. Varying antiemetics should be used liberally, including on a prophylactic basis. Antacids including proton pump inhibitors are frequently implemented, and antidiarrheal medications may be appropriate. Additionally, nutritional supportive measurements are paramount and, when appropriate, the use of enteral methods is implemented. In selected cases, the use of feeding jejunostomy may be appropriate. Patients may require intermittent hydration both during and shortly following the treatment course. Postoperatively, B$_{12}$, iron, and calcium levels should be monitored and supplemented as appropriate.

Nutritional complications of treatment and myelosuppression, if concurrent chemotherapy is used during irradiation, can carry substantial morbidity and even occasional mortality from therapy. The historical GITSG reported a minimum 13% treatment-related mortality from nutritional problems or septic events on their concurrent chemoradiation arm,[120] and almost 20% of the patients of Caudry et al.[176] were unable to complete therapy because of nutritional problems. However, others reported no severe or life-threatening nutritional compromise with aggressive chemoradiation.[116,118,177] Toxic gastrointestinal effects usually are managed with careful nutritional support and antiemetic therapy. It may be prudent to proactively prescribe antiemetics at the initiation of therapy in patients undergoing aggressive upper abdominal irradiation.

Myelosuppression causing serious or, rarely, lethal toxicity is also reported in many of the combined-modality trials.[116,118,177,178] If blood counts are monitored weekly during combined-modality therapy, serious problems with sepsis or bleeding should be uncommon.[177,178]

Moderate doses of 16 to 36 Gy reduce secretion of pepsin and hydrochloric acid.[1,104,179] For this reason, radiation therapy was once a common and successful therapy for peptic ulcer disease. Most of the gastric ulcers healed, although they recurred in approximately 40% of patients.[1,104,179] Gastric acid secretion decreased in almost all cases, with achlorhydria in 25% to 40%. The gastric acid decrease usually persisted from 1 to 6 months; however, 25% showed persistent decrease in acid production for 1 to 5 years or more.

Gastric late effects were categorized by the Walter Reed Group as dyspepsia, radiation gastritis, uncomplicated gastric ulcer, or gastric ulcer with perforation or obstruction.[180–182] The associations between dose and these late effects are described in Table 62.13. These data suggest a 20% to 30% incidence of ulceration with doses of 45 to 59 Gy, with complications of these ulcers in 30% to 50% of the treated patients. Some caution is necessary in interpreting this experience because the Walter Reed cohort was treated with 200-keV photons or 1-MV photons using a 70-cm target-skin distance, usually using only one field each day with daily fraction sizes of 3 Gy to midline, which sometimes produced daily given doses of 4 to 6 Gy.[181,182]

Most data suggest that gastric late effects are rare with doses of 40 to 52 Gy using conventional fractionation of 1.8 to 2 Gy. The relatively low risk of gastric late effects with doses <50 Gy is corroborated by many series using radiation therapy with or without chemotherapy for locally advanced gastric cancer.[42,48,62,73,81,134] However, doses in the range of 50 to 55 Gy may produce variable gastric late effects, which have been reported to reach 9% in some series. Doses of 60 Gy carried a 5% to 15% risk of gastric late effects.[1–3,52,62,69,90,118,134,152,161,167,172,174–177,179–184] The ability of histamine (H_2) blockers, proton pump inhibitors, and sucralfate to prevent the later development of radiation-induced gastric ulcerations is unproven. It may be reasonable to administer H_2 blockers or proton pump inhibitors prophylactically to patients receiving >45 Gy to any significant volume of the stomach or proximal duodenum.

Several series have described a gradual decline in renal function occurring ≥18 to 24 months following postoperative radiation therapy for gastric cancer. However, it is unclear that this is of clinical significance, and long-term renal function among gastric cancer survivors has not been reliably reported. One recent report described a dose-dependent nephrotoxicity as manifested by hypertension in gastric cancer patients,

which may take years to manifest.[185] Similarly, another study indicated that mean creatinine clearance as well as changes in renal parenchymal volume occurred primarily within the first 4 years following radiation therapy with a clear relationship between these changes and DVH parameters.[186] Nonetheless, advanced techniques may enhance renal sparing and also allow potential dose escalation as well as integration of novel (and potentially nephrotoxic) systemic agents.[187]

Radiation-induced cardiac toxicity is a broad term describing potential radiation injury to a number of cardiac structures, including the pericardium (as manifested by effusion, pericarditis), coronary arteries, the heart muscle itself, and cardiac valves as well as nerve/conduction injury. Radiation injury primarily consists of fibrosis and/or small-vessel injury. The mechanism of radiation-induced cardiac injury is relatively poorly defined, particularly in the context of gastric cancer. Historical data from the treatment for Hodgkin disease patients have suggested that dose >40 Gy may increase the risk of cardiac death as well as pericarditis.[188,189] Several studies of cardiac toxicity and esophageal cancer patients have demonstrated that an increasing V_{30} predicted for a significant increase in pericardial effusion and increasing fraction size (particularly ≥3.5 Gy) also predicted for the same. Additionally, some authors have shown a possible trend for decrease in ejection fraction in patients with increasing V_{20} of the left ventricle.[190] A more detailed discussion on potential long-term cardiac sequelae of radiation therapy can be found in Chapter 56.

CONCLUSIONS AND RECOMMENDATIONS

Radiation therapy, usually administered with concomitant fluoropyrimidine-based chemotherapy, is indicated for locally confined gastric cancer that either is not technically resectable or occurs in medically inoperable patients. In this setting, therapy can be administered with curative or palliative intent, depending on the clinical situation. Those who undergo gastric resection with incomplete tumor resection or have truly positive margins of resection are also appropriately managed by combined-modality therapy. Preferably, patients with locally advanced disease that is unresectable with negative margins would be identified preoperatively with endoscopic ultrasonography and CT staging. Preoperative chemoradiation then could precede an attempt at gross total resection, alone or in combination with IORT, and maintenance chemotherapy.

The results of the U.S. Gastrointestinal Intergroup Gastric Adjuvant Trial established a standard of care in the United States to the use of both chemotherapy and radiation therapy in the postoperative setting for patients with disease extension through the gastric wall and/or with nodes positive for tumor. Postoperative irradiation and concurrent and maintenance fluoropyrimidine-based chemotherapy are generally recommended for patients with stage IB, II, IIIA, IIIB, or IV and M0 gastric cancer. The role of postoperative chemoradiation in patients with T2N0 tumors remains more controversial. In patients with high-risk features (i.e., poorly differentiated or higher-grade cancers, lymph vascular invasion, perineural invasion, age <50 years, or suboptimal resection including lymph node resection), postoperative chemoradiotherapy may also be indicated.

Because extended node dissections were not commonly performed as a component of surgery in the Intergroup trial, some have questioned whether postoperative chemoradiation would give added benefit following a D2 nodal resection. Similarly, given the survival benefit from the use of perioperative chemotherapy alone in European esophagogastric patients, ongoing trials are examining the role of adjuvant chemoradiation in both the settings of perioperative chemotherapy and D2 lymph node dissection, including attempts to better stratify which patients might be most appropriate for adjuvant combined modality therapy. Additionally, further trials are investigating new systemic agents with radiation

TABLE 62.13 RADIATION DOSE COMPARED WITH LATE EFFECTS IN THE WALTER REED EXPERIENCE

Dose (Gy)	Number of Patients[b]	Radiation Late Effects (%)[a]			
		Dyspepsia	Gastritis	Ulcer	Complicated Ulcer[c]
<40	111	5	2	3	0
40–44.99	23	0	22	0	0
45–49.99	27	4	19	11	11
50–54.99	34	0	24	18	12
55–59.99	14	0	50	14	7
>60	8	0	0	13	38

[a]Results reported as number of patients with injury/total number of patients treated with this dose.
[b]Total number of patients treated at this dose.
[c]Ulcers complicated by obstruction or perforation.

therapy to establish efficacy compared with 5-FU and leucovorin. Given the poor prognosis with patients receiving either perioperative chemotherapy or adjuvant chemoradiotherapy, integration of the approaches has the potential to improve disease-related outcomes compared to either alone. Similarly, on the basis of encouraging outcomes with phase II preoperative chemoradiation trials in patients with gastric cancer and phase III esophagus (and other gastrointestinal) cancer trials, ongoing evaluation of this approach in patients with potentially resectable lesions is occurring in phase III trials and will likely help guide future treatment approaches.

The irradiation field design from the phase III U.S. Gastrointestinal Intergroup trial was based on optimized field design related to both site of the primary lesion and T and N stage of disease.[114] With the wide availability of 3-D conformal treatment planning systems, it may be possible to more accurately target the high-risk volume and to use unconventional field arrangements and/or IMRT to produce superior dose distributions. To accomplish this without marginal misses, however, it will be necessary to both carefully define and encompass the various target volumes (tumor bed, nodal sites at risk) given target volumes that would be included using older approaches may be missed with more contemporary planning approaches.

REFERENCES

1. Goss CM. *Anatomy of the human body.* Philadelphia, PA: Lea & Febiger, 1973.
2. Kao GD, Whittington R, Cola L. Anatomy of the celiac axis and superior mesenteric artery and its significance in radiation therapy. *Int J Radiat Oncol Biol Phys* 1993;25:131–134.
3. Siegel R, Miller K, Jemal A. Cancer statistics, 2018. *CA Cancer J Clin* 2018;68(1):7–30.
4. Global Burden of Disease Cancer Collaboration; Fitzmaurice C, Allen C, Barber RM, et al. Global, regional, and national cancer incidence, mortality, years of life lost, years lived with disability, and disability-adjusted life-years for 32 cancer groups, 1990 to 2015: a systematic analysis for the global burden of disease study. *JAMA Oncol* 2017;3(4):524–548.
5. Howson CP, Hiyama T, Wynder EL. The decline in gastric cancer: epidemiology of an unplanned triumph. *Epidemiol Rev* 1986;8:1–27.
6. Silverberg E, Boring CC, Squires TS. Cancer statistics, 1990. *CA Cancer J Clin* 1990;40:9–26.
7. Ajani JA, Barthel JS, Bekaii-Saab T, et al. Gastric cancer. *J Natl Compr Canc Netw* 2010;8:378–409.
8. Marques-Lespier J, Gonzalez-Pons M, Cruz-Correa M. Current perspectives on gastric cancer. *Gastro Enterol Clin North AM* 2016;45(3):413–428.
9. Zakko L, Lutzke L, Wang K. Screening and preventive strategies in esophagogastric cancer. *Surg Oncol Clin NA* 2017;26:163–178.
10. Coggon D, Barker DJ, Cole RB, et al. Stomach cancer and food storage. *J Natl Cancer Inst* 1989;81:1178–1182.
11. Fuchs CS, Mayer RJ. Gastric carcinoma. *N Engl J Med* 1995;333:32–41.
12. Shah MA, Kelsen DP. Gastric cancer: a primer on the epidemiology and biology of the disease and an overview of the medical management of advanced disease. *J Natl Compr Canc Netw* 2010;8:437–447.
13. Ajani J, Lee J, Sano T, et al. Gastric adenocarcinoma. *Nat Rev Dis Primers* 2017;3:17036.
14. Van Cutsem E, Sagaert X, Topal B, et al. Gastric Cancer. *Lancet* 2016;388: 2654–2664.
15. Taghavi S, Jayarajan S, Davey A, et al. Prognostic significance of signet ring gastric cancer. *J Clin Oncol* 2012;30(28):3493–3498.
16. Nakajima T, Harashima S, Hirata M, et al. Prognostic and therapeutic values of peritoneal cytology in gastric cancer. *Acta Cytol* 1978;22:225–229.
17. Caletti G, Ferrari A, Brocchi E, et al. Accuracy of endoscopic ultrasonography in the diagnosis and staging of gastric cancer and lymphoma. *Surgery* 1993;113:14–27.
18. Saito N, Takeshita K, Habu H, et al. The use of endoscopic ultrasound in determining the depth of cancer invasion in patients with gastric cancer. *Surg Endosc* 1991;5:14–19.
19. Seevaratnam R, Cardoso R, McGregor C, et al. How useful is preoperative imaging for tumor, node, metastasis (TNM) staging with gastric cancer? A meta-analysis. *Gastric Cancer* 2012;15:S3–S18.
20. Sarela AI, Lefkowitz R, Brennan MF, et al. Selection of patients with gastric adenocarcinoma for laparoscopic staging. *Am J Surg* 2006;191:134–138.
21. Leake PA, Cardoso R, Seevaratnam R, et al. A systematic review of the accuracy and indications for diagnostic laparoscopy prior to curative-intent resection of gastric cancer. *Gastric Cancer* 2012;15(Suppl 1):S38–S47.
22. Hayes T, Smyth E, Riddell A, et al. Staging in esophageal and gastric cancers. *Hematol Oncol Clin North AM* 2017;30(3):427–440.
23. Ziegler K, Sanft C, Zimmer T, et al. Comparison of computed tomography, endosonography, and intraoperative assessment in TN staging of gastric carcinoma. *Gut* 1993;34:604–610.
24. Puli SR, Batapati Krishna Reddy J, Bechtold ML, et al. How good is endoscopic ultrasound for TNM staging of gastric cancers? A meta-analysis and systematic review. *World J Gastroenterol* 2008;14:4011–4019.
25. Mocellin S, Pasquali S. Diagnostic accuracy of endoscopic ultrasonography (EUS) for the preoperative locoregional staging of primary gastric cancer. *Cochrane Database Syst Rev* 2015;2:CD009944
26. Cardoso R, Coburn N, Seevaratnam R, et al. A systemic review and meta-analysis of the utility of EUS for preoperative staging for gastric cancer. *Gastr Canc* 2012;15:19–26.
27. Kwee RM, Kwee TC. Imaging in local staging of gastric cancer: a systematic review. *J Clin Oncol* 2007;25:2107–2116.
28. Stahl A, Ott K, Weber WA, et al. FDG PET imaging of locally advanced gastric carcinomas: correlation with endoscopic and histopathological findings. *Eur J Nucl Med Mol Imaging* 2003;30:288–295.
29. Das P, Jiang Y, Lee JH, et al. Multimodality approaches to localized gastric cancer. *J Natl Compr Canc Netw* 2010;8:417–425.
30. Chen J, Cheong JH, Yun MJ, et al. Improvement in preoperative staging of gastric adenocarcinoma with positron emission tomography. *Cancer* 2005;103:2383–2390.
31. Edge S, Byrd D, Compton C, et al. *Stomach. AJCC cancer staging manual.* 8th ed. New York: Springer, 2017:203–220.
32. Hartley LC, Evans E, Windsor CJ. Factors influencing prognosis in gastric cancer. *Aust N Z J Surg* 1987;57:5–9.
33. Kalish RJ, Clancy PE, Orringer MB, et al. Clinical, epidemiologic, and morphologic comparison between adenocarcinomas arising in Barrett's esophageal mucosa and in the gastric cardia. *Gastroenterology* 1984;86:461–467.
34. MacDonald J, Cohn I, Gunderson LL. *Carcinoma of the stomach.* Philadelphia, PA: JB Lippincott, 1985.
35. Meyers WC, Damiano RJ Jr, Rotolo FS, et al. Adenocarcinoma of the stomach. Changing patterns over the last 4 decades. *Ann Surg* 1987;205:1–8.
36. Yamada Y, Kato Y. Greater tendency for submucosal invasion in fundic area gastric carcinomas than those arising in the pyloric area. *Cancer* 1989;63:1757–1760.
37. Borrmann R. *Geschwulste des magens und duodenums.* Berlin, Germany: Julius Springer, 1926.
38. Dockerty MB. *Pathologic aspects of primary malignant neoplasms of the stomach.* Philadelphia, PA: WB Saunders, 1964.
39. Gunderson LL, Sosin H. Adenocarcinoma of the stomach: areas of failure in a re-operation series (second or symptomatic look) clinicopathologic correlation and implications for adjuvant therapy. *Int J Radiat Oncol Biol Phys* 1982;8:1–11.
40. Kennedy BJ. T N M classification for stomach cancer. *Cancer* 1970;26:971–983.
41. Douglass HO Jr, Nava HR. Gastric adenocarcinoma—management of the primary disease. *Semin Oncol* 1985;12:32–45.
42. Nagatomo T, Murakami E, Kondo K. Histologic criteria of serosal rupture and prognosis in gastric carcinoma. *Cancer* 1972;29:180–190.
43. Maruta K, Shida H. Some factors which influence prognosis after surgery for advanced gastric cancer. *Ann Surg* 1968;167:313–318.
44. Gunderson LL. Gastric cancer—patterns of relapse after surgical resection. *Semin Radiat Oncol* 2002;12:150–161.
45. Chau I, Norman AR, Cunningham D, et al. Multivariate prognostic factor analysis in locally advanced and metastatic esophago-gastric cancer—pooled analysis from three multicenter, randomized, controlled trials using individual patient data. *J Clin Oncol* 2004;22:2395–2403.
46. Byfield SA, Earle CC, Ayanian JZ, et al. Treatment and outcomes of gastric cancer among United States-born and foreign-born Asians and Pacific Islanders. *Cancer* 2009;115:4595–4605.
47. Baba H, Korenaga D, Okamura T, et al. Prognostic significance of DNA content with special reference to age in gastric cancer. *Cancer* 1989;63:1768–1772.
48. Korenaga D, Okamura T, Saito A, et al. DNA ploidy is closely linked to tumor invasion, lymph node metastasis, and prognosis in clinical gastric cancer. *Cancer* 1988;62:309–313.
49. Nanus DM, Kelsen DP, Niedzwiecki D, et al. Flow cytometry as a predictive indicator in patients with operable gastric cancer. *J Clin Oncol* 1989;7:1105–1112.
50. Asakawa H, Otawa H, Yamada S, et al. Combination therapy of gastric carcinoma with radiation and chemotherapy. *Tohoku J Exp Med* 1982;137: 445–452.
51. Asakawa H, Takeda T. High energy x-ray therapy of gastric carcinoma. *Nihon Gan Chiryo Gakkai Shi* 1973;8:362–371.
52. Tsukiyama I, Akine Y, Kajiura Y, et al. Radiation therapy for advanced gastric cancer. *Int J Radiat Oncol Biol Phys* 1988;15:123–127.
53. Finlay CA, Hinds PW, Levine AJ. The p53 proto-oncogene can act as a suppressor of transformation. *Cell* 1989;57:1083–1093.
54. Lane DP. Worrying about p53. *Curr Biol* 1992;2:581–583.
55. Kastan MB, Onyekwere O, Sidransky D, et al. Participation of p53 protein in the cellular response to DNA damage. *Cancer Res* 1991;51:6304–6311.
56. O'Connor PM, Jackman J, Jondle D, et al. Role of the p53 tumor suppressor gene in cell cycle arrest and radiosensitivity of Burkitt's lymphoma cell lines. *Cancer Res* 1993;53:4776–4780.
57. Fenoglio-Preiser C. The effect of oncogenes on biology and prognosis of surgically resected gastric cancer. *ASCO Educational Book.* 1997:275–277.
58. Lynch HT, Smyrk TC, Watson P, et al. Genetics, natural history, tumor spectrum, and pathology of hereditary nonpolyposis colorectal cancer: an updated review. *Gastroenterology* 1993;104:1535–1549.
59. Takahashi M, Ota S, Shimada T, et al. Hepatocyte growth factor is the most potent endogenous stimulant of rabbit gastric epithelial cell proliferation and migration in primary culture. *J Clin Invest* 1995;95:1994–2003.
60. Tahara E, Yokozaki H, Yasui W. *Growth factors in gastric cancer.* Tokyo, Japan: Springer-Verlag, 1993.
61. Tahara E, Semba S, Tahara H. Molecular biological observations in gastric cancer. *Semin Oncol* 1996;23:307–315.
62. Harrison JD, Morris DL, Ellis IO, et al. The effect of tamoxifen and estrogen receptor status on survival in gastric carcinoma. *Cancer* 1989;64:1007–1010.

Section III

63. Tahara E. Molecular mechanism of stomach carcinogenesis. *J Cancer Res Clin Oncol* 1993;119:265–272.

64. Yonemura Y, Ninomiya I, Ohoyama S, et al. Expression of c-erbB-2 oncoprotein in gastric carcinoma. Immunoreactivity for c-erbB-2 protein is an independent indicator of poor short-term prognosis in patients with gastric carcinoma. *Cancer* 1991;67:2914–2918.

65. Hilton DA, West KP. An evaluation of the prognostic significance of HLA-DR expression in gastric carcinoma. *Cancer* 1990;66:1154–1157.

66. Bang YJ, Van Cutsem E, Feyereislova A, et al. Trastuzumab in combination with chemotherapy versus chemotherapy alone for treatment of HER2-positive advanced gastric or gastro-oesophageal junction cancer (ToGA): a phase 3, open-label, randomised controlled trial. *Lancet* 2010;376(9742):687–697. Erratum in: *Lancet* 2010;376(9749):1302.

67. Prolla JC, Kobayashi S, Kirsner JB. Gastric cancer. Some recent improvements in diagnosis based upon the Japanese experience. *Arch Intern Med* 1969;124:238–246.

68. Fujitani K, Yang H, Mizusawa J, et al. Gastrectomy plus chemotherapy versus chemotherapy alone for advanced gastric cancer with a single non-curable factor (REGATTA): a phase 3, randomised controlled trial. *Lancet Oncol* 2016;17(3):309–318.

69. Fukutomi H, Nakahara A. Endoscopic therapy of gastrointestinal cancer and its curability. *Gan To Kagaku Ryoho* 1988;15:1132–1136.

70. Kern KA. Gastric cancer: a neoplastic enigma. *J Surg Oncol* 1989;(Suppl 1):34–39.

71. Makris E, Poultsides G. Surgical considerations in the management of gastric adenocarcinoma. *Surg Clin North Am* 2017;97(2):295–316.

72. ReMine W, Priestley J, Berkson J. *Cancer of the stomach*. Philadelphia, PA: WB Saunders, 1964.

73. Serlin O, Keehn RJ, Higgins GA Jr, et al. Factors related to survival following resection for gastric carcinoma: analysis of 903 cases. *Cancer* 1977;40:1318–1329.

74. Gholami S, Cassidy M, Strong V. Minimally invasive surgical approaches to gastric resection. *Surg Clin North Am.* 2017;97(2):249–264.

75. Fenoglio-Preiser CM, Noffsinger AE, Belli J, et al. Pathologic and phenotypic features of gastric cancer. *Semin Oncol* 1996;23:292–306.

76. Allum WH, Hallissey MT, Ward LC, et al. A controlled, prospective, randomised trial of adjuvant chemotherapy or radiotherapy in resectable gastric cancer: interim report. British Stomach Cancer Group. *Br J Cancer* 1989;60:739–744.

77. Bleiberg H, Goffin JC, Dalesio O, et al. Adjuvant radiotherapy and chemotherapy in resectable gastric cancer. A randomized trial of the gastro-intestinal tract cancer cooperative group of the EORTC. *Eur J Surg Oncol* 1989;15:535–543.

78. Gez E, Sulkes A, Yablonsky-Peretz T, et al. Combined 5-fluorouracil (5-FU) and radiation therapy following resection of locally advanced gastric carcinoma. *J Surg Oncol* 1986;31:139–142.

79. Gill PG, Jamieson GG, Denham J, et al. Treatment of adenocarcinoma of the cardia with synchronous chemotherapy and radiotherapy. *Br J Surg* 1990;77:1020–1023.

80. Regine WF, Mohiuddin M. Impact of adjuvant therapy on locally advanced adenocarcinoma of the stomach. *Int J Radiat Oncol Biol Phys* 1992;24:921–927.

81. Siewert JR, Lange J, Bottcher K, et al. [Stomach cancer—the current situation from the surgical viewpoint]. *Dtsch Med Wochenschr* 1987;112:622–628.

82. Slot A, Meerwaldt JH, van Putten WL, et al. Adjuvant postoperative radiotherapy for gastric carcinoma with poor prognostic signs. *Radiother Oncol* 1989;16:269–274.

83. Whittington R, Coia LR, Haller DG, et al. Adenocarcinoma of the esophagus and esophago-gastric junction: the effects of single and combined modalities on the survival and patterns of failure following treatment. *Int J Radiat Oncol Biol Phys* 1990;19:593–603.

84. Bunt AM, Hogendoorn PC, van de Velde CJ, et al. Lymph node staging standards in gastric cancer. *J Clin Oncol* 1995;13:2309–2316.

85. Douglass HO, Clark JL, Barcewicz P, et al. Importance of the R₂ lymph node dissection in the surgical treatment of gastric cancer. *Proc Am Soc Clin Oncol* 1989;8:101.

86. Smith DD, Schwarz RR, Schwarz RE. Impact of total lymph node count on staging and survival after gastrectomy for gastric cancer: data from a large US-population database. *J Clin Oncol* 2005;23:7114–7124.

87. Soga J, Ohyama S, Miyashita K, et al. A statistical evaluation of advancement in gastric cancer surgery with special reference to the significance of lymphadenectomy for cure. *World J Surg* 1988;12:398–405.

88. Dupont JB Jr, Lee JR, Burton GR, et al. Adenocarcinoma of the stomach: review of 1,497 cases. *Cancer* 1978;41:941–947.

89. Potish R, Adcock L, Jones T Jr, et al. The morbidity and utility of periaortic radiotherapy in cervical carcinoma. *Gynecol Oncol* 1983;15:1–9.

90. Potish RA, Twiggs LB, Adcock LL, et al. Paraaortic lymph node radiotherapy in cancer of the uterine corpus. *Obstet Gynecol* 1985;65:251–256.

91. Kim S, Lim DH, Lee J, et al. An observational study suggesting clinical benefit for adjuvant postoperative chemoradiation in a population of over 500 cases after gastric resection with D2 nodal dissection for adenocarcinoma of the stomach. *Int J Radiat Oncol Biol Phys* 2005;63:1279–1285.

92. Bonenkamp JJ, Hermans J, Sasako M, et al. Extended lymph-node dissection for gastric cancer. *N Engl J Med* 1999;340:908–914.

93. Bonenkamp JJ, Songun I, Hermans J, et al. Randomised comparison of morbidity after D1 and D2 dissection for gastric cancer in 996 Dutch patients. *Lancet* 1995;345:745–748.

94. Bunt AM, Hermans J, Smit VT, et al. Surgical/pathologic-stage migration confounds comparisons of gastric cancer survival rates between Japan and Western countries. *J Clin Oncol* 1995;13:19–25.

95. Cuschieri A, Weeden S, Fielding J, et al. Patient survival after D1 and D2 resections for gastric cancer: long-term results of the MRC randomized surgical trial. Surgical Co-operative Group. *Br J Cancer* 1999;79:1522–1530.

96. Dent DM, Werner ID, Novis B, et al. Prospective randomized trial of combined oncological therapy for gastric carcinoma. *Cancer* 1979;44(2):385–391.

97. Songun I, Putter H, Kranenbarg E, et al. Surgical treatment of gastric cancer: 15-year follow-up results of the randomised nationwide Dutch D1D2 trial. *Lancet Oncol* 2010;11(5):439–449.

98. Sasako M, Sano T, Yamamoto S, et al. D2 lymphadenectomy alone or with para-aortic nodal dissection for gastric cancer. *N Engl J Med* 2008;359:453–462.

99. Gunderson LL, Hoskins RB, Cohen AC, et al. Combined modality treatment of gastric cancer. *Int J Radiat Oncol Biol Phys* 1983;9:965–975.

100. Gunderson LL, Willett C, Harrison LB, et al. *Intraoperative irradiation: techniques and results*. Totowa, NJ: Humana Press, 1999.

101. Horn RC Jr. Carcinoma of the stomach; autopsy findings in untreated cases. *Gastroenterology* 1955;29:515–523; discussion 523–515.

102. Papachristou DN, Fortner JG. Local recurrence of gastric adenocarcinomas after gastrectomy. *J Surg Oncol* 1981;18:47–53.

103. Landry J, Tepper JE, Wood WC, et al. Patterns of failure following curative resection of gastric carcinoma. *Int J Radiat Oncol Biol Phys* 1990;19:1357–1362.

104. Stout AP. Pathology of carcinoma of the stomach. *Arch Surg* 1943;46:807.

105. McNeer G, Vandenberg H, Donn F, et al. A critical evaluation of subtotal gastrectomy for the cure of cancer of the stomach. *Ann Surg* 1957;134:2.

106. Gilbertsen VA. Results of treatment of stomach cancer. An appraisal of efforts for more extensive surgery and a report of 1,983 cases. *Cancer* 1969;23:1305–1308.

107. Moertel CG, Childs DS, O'Fallon JR, et al. Combined 5-fluorouracil and radiation therapy as a surgical adjuvant for poor prognosis gastric carcinoma. *J Clin Oncol* 1984;2:1249–1254.

108. Chang J, Lim J, Noh S, et al. Patterns of regional recurrence after curative D2 resection for stage III (N3) gastric cancer: implications for postoperative radiotherapy. *Radiother Oncol* 2012;104(3):367–373.

109. Yoon H, Chang J, Lim J, et al. Defining the target volume for post-operative radiotherapy after D2 dissection in gastric cancer by CT-based vessel-guided delineation. *Radiother Oncol* 2013;108(1):72–77.

110. Yu J, Lim D, Ahn Y, et al. Effects of adjuvant radiotherapy on completely resected gastric cancer: A radiation oncologist's view of the ARTIST randomized phase III trial. *Radiother Oncol* 2015;117(1):171–177.

111. MacDonald JS, Smalley SR, Benedetti J, et al. Chemoradiotherapy after surgery compared with surgery alone for adenocarcinoma of the stomach or gastroesophageal junction. *N Engl J Med* 2001;345:725–730.

112. Hallemeier C, Haddock M, et al. Gastric cancer: radiation therapy planning. In: Hong T, Das P, eds. *Radiation therapy for gastrointestinal cancers*. Cham, Switzerland: Springer, 2017:59–71.

113. Matzinger O, Gerber E, Bernstein Z, et al. EORTC-ROG expert opinion: radiotherapy volume and treatment guidelines for neoadjuvant radiation of adenocarcinomas of the gastroesophageal junction and the stomach. *Radiother Oncol* 2009;92:164–175.

114. Smalley SR, Gunderson L, Tepper J, et al. Gastric surgical adjuvant radiotherapy consensus report: rationale and treatment implementation. *Int J Radiat Oncol Biol Phys* 2002;52:283–293.

115. Tepper JE, Gunderson LL. Radiation treatment parameters in the adjuvant postoperative therapy of gastric cancer. *Semin Radiat Oncol* 2002;12:187–195.

116. Thirlwell M, Keable H, Kost K, et al. Combination of 5-fluorouracil (5-FU) plus semustine (MECCNU) with and without radiotherapy (RT) in advanced gastric and pancreatic carcinoma. *Proc Am Soc Clin Oncol* 1981;22:449.

117. Chun S, Hu C, Choy H, et al. Impact of intensity-modulated radiation therapy technique for locally advanced non-small-cell lung cancer: a secondary analysis of the NRG oncology RTOG 0617 randomized clinical trial. *J Clin Oncol* 2017;35(1):56–62.

118. Henning GT, Schild SE, Stafford SL, et al. Results of irradiation or chemoirradiation following resection of gastric adenocarcinoma. *Int J Radiat Oncol Biol Phys* 2000;46:589–598.

119. Arcangeli G, Saracino B, Angelini F, et al. Postoperative adjuvant chemoradiation in completely resected locally advanced gastric cancer. *Int J Radiat Oncol Biol Phys* 2002;54:1069–1075.

120. Moertel CG, Childs DS, Reitemeier R, et al. Combined 5 fluorouracil and supervoltage radiation therapy of locally unresectable gastrointestinal cancer. *Lancet* 1969;865:867.

121. A comparison of combination chemotherapy and combined modality therapy for locally advanced gastric carcinoma. Gastrointestinal Tumor Study Group. *Cancer* 1982;49:1771–1777.

122. Liu Y, Zhao G, Xu Y, et al. Multicenter phase 2 study of peri-irradiation chemotherapy plus intensity modulated radiation therapy with concurrent weekly docetaxel for inoperable or medically unresectable nonmetastatic gastric cancer. *Int J Radiat Oncol Biol Phys* 2017;98(5):1096–1105.

123. Hallissey MT, Dunn JA, Ward LC, et al. The second British Stomach Cancer Group trial of adjuvant radiotherapy or chemotherapy in resectable gastric cancer: five-year follow-up. *Lancet* 1994;343:1309–1312.

124. Zhang ZX, Gu XZ, Yin WB, et al. Randomized clinical trial on the combination of preoperative irradiation and surgery in the treatment of adenocarcinoma of gastric cardia (AGC)—report on 370 patients. *Int J Radiat Oncol Biol Phys* 1998;42:929–934.

125. Lee J, Lim DH, Kim S, et al. Phase III trial comparing capecitabine plus cisplatin versus capecitabine plus cisplatin with concurrent capecitabine radiotherapy in completely resected gastric cancer with D2 lymph node dissection: the ARTIST trial. *J Clin Oncol* 2012;30(3):268–273.

126. Park S, Sohn T, Lee J, et al. Phase III trial to compare adjuvant chemotherapy with capecitabine and cisplatin versus concurrent chemoradiotherapy in gastric cancer: final report of the adjuvant chemoradiotherapy in stomach tumors trial, including survival and subset analyses. *J Clin Oncol* 2015;33(28):3130–3136.

127. Abe M, Takahashi M, Ono K, et al. Japan gastric trials in intraoperative radiation therapy. *Int J Radiat Oncol Biol Phys* 1988;15:1431–1433.

128. Sindelar WF, Kinsella TJ, Tepper JE, et al. Randomized trial of intraoperative radiotherapy in carcinoma of the stomach. *Am J Surg* 1993;165:178–186; discussion 186–177.

129. Macdonald JS, Benedetti J, Smalley SR, et al. Chemoradiation of resected gastric cancer: a 10-year follow-up of the phase III trial INT0116 (SWOG 9008). *J Clin Oncol* 2009;27:15S.

130. Fuchs CS, Niedzwiecki D, Mamon HJ, et al. Adjuvant chemoradiotherapy with epirubicin, cisplatin, and fluorouracil compared with adjuvant chemoradio-

therapy with fluorouracil and leucovorin after curative resection of gastric cancer: results from CALGB 80101 (Alliance). *J Clin Oncol* 2017;35(32):3671–3677.

131. Valentini V, Cellini F, Minsky BD, et al. Survival after radiotherapy in gastric cancer: systematic review and meta-analysis. *Radiother Oncol* 2009;92:176–183.

132. Zhu W, Xua D, Pu J, et al. A randomized, controlled, multicenter study comparing intensity-modulated radiotherapy plus concurrent chemotherapy with chemotherapy alone in gastric cancer patients with D2 resection. *Radiother Oncol* 2012;104:361–366.

133. Cats A, Jansen E, van Grieken N, et al. Chemotherapy versus chemoradiotherapy after surgery and preoperative chemotherapy for resectable gastric cancer (CRITICS): an international, open-label, randomised phase 3 trial. *Lancet Oncol* 2018;19(5):616–628.

134. Walsh TN, Noonan N, Hollywood D, et al. A comparison of multimodal therapy and surgery for esophageal adenocarcinoma. *N Engl J Med* 1996;335:462–467.

135. Krasna M, Tepper J, Niedzwiecki D, et al. Trimodality therapy is superior to surgery alone in esophageal cancer: results of CALGB 9871. ASCO Gastrointestinal Cancer Symposium, January 26–28, 2006, San Francisco, CA.

136. Ajani J, Mansfield P, Janjan N, et al. Multiinstitutional trial of preoperative chemoradiotherapy in patients with potentially resectable gastric carcinoma. *J Clin Oncol* 2004;22:2774–2780.

137. Ajani J, Mansfield P, Crane C, et al. Paclitaxel-based chemoradiotherapy in localized gastric carcinoma: degree of pathologic response and not clinical parameters dictated patient outcome. *J Clin Oncol* 2005;23:1237–1244.

138. Ajani J, Winter K, Okawara A, et al. Phase II trial of preoperative chemoradiation in patients with localized gastric adenocarcinoma (RTOG 9904): quality of combined modality therapy and pathologic response. *J Clin Oncol* 2006;24:3953–3958.

139. Sun Z, Nussbaum D, Speicher P, et al. Neoadjuvant radiation therapy does not increase perioperative morbidity among patients undergoing gastrectomy for gastric cancer. *J Surg Oncol* 2015;112(1):46–50.

140. Stahl M, Walz MK, Stuschke M, et al. Phase III comparison of preoperative chemotherapy compared with chemoradiotherapy in patients with locally advanced adenocarcinoma of the esophagogastric junction. *J Clin Oncol* 2009;27:851–856.

140a. Stahl M, Walz M, Riera-Knorrenschild J, et al. Preoperative chemotherapy versus chemoradiotherapy in locally advanced adenocarcinomas of the oesophagogastric junction (POET): long-term results of a controlled randomised trial. *Eur J Cancer* 2017;81:183–190.

141. Leong T, Smithers B, Haustermans K, et al. TOPGEAR: a randomised phase III trial of perioperative ECF chemotherapy with or without preoperative chemoradiation for resectable gastric cancer: interim results from an international, intergroup trial of the AGITG/TROG/EORTC/NCICCTG. *Ann Surg Oncol* 2017;24(8):2252–2258.

142. Nakajima T, Nashimoto A, Kitamura M, et al. Adjuvant mitomycin and fluorouracil followed by oral uracil plus tegafur in serosa-negative gastric cancer: a randomised trial. Gastric Cancer Surgical Study Group. *Lancet* 1999;354:273–277.

143. Sakuramoto S, Sasako M, Yamaguchi T, et al. Adjuvant chemotherapy for gastric cancer with S-1, an oral fluoropyrimidine. *N Engl J Med* 2007;357:1810–1820.

144. Sasako M, Sakuramoto S, Katai H, et al. Five-year outcomes of a randomized phase III trial compared adjuvant chemotherapy with S-1 versus surgery alone in stage II or III gastric cancer. *J Clin Oncol* 2011;29(33):4387–4393.

145. Tsuburaya A, Yoshida K, Kobayashi M, et al. Sequential paclitaxel followed by tegafur and uracil (UFT) or S-1 versus UFT or S-1 monotherapy as adjuvant chemotherapy for T4a/b gastric cancer (SAMIT): a phase 3 factorial randomised controlled trial. *Lancet Oncol* 2014;15(8):886–893.

146. Noh S, Park S, Yang H, et al. Adjuvant capecitabine plus oxaliplatin for gastric cancer after D2 gastrectomy (CLASSIC): 5-year follow-up of an open-label randomised phase 3 trial. *Lancet Oncol* 2014;15(12):1389–1396.

147. Paoletti X, Oba K, Burzykowski T, et al. Benefit of adjuvant chemotherapy for resectable gastric cancer: a meta-analysis. *JAMA* 2010;303:1729–1737.

148. Kelsen D, Atiq OT, Saltz L, et al. FAMTX versus etoposide, doxorubicin, and cisplatin: a random assignment trial in gastric cancer. *J Clin Oncol* 1992;10:541–548.

149. Lerner A, Gonin R, Steele GD Jr, et al. Etoposide, doxorubicin, and cisplatin chemotherapy for advanced gastric adenocarcinoma: results of a phase II trial. *J Clin Oncol* 1992;10:536–540.

150. Preusser P, Wilke H, Achterrath W, et al. Phase II study with the combination etoposide, doxorubicin, and cisplatin in advanced measurable gastric cancer. *J Clin Oncol* 1989;7:1310–1317.

151. Waters JS, Norman A, Cunningham D, et al. Long-term survival after epirubicin, cisplatin and fluorouracil for gastric cancer: results of a randomized trial. *Br J Cancer* 1999;80:269–272.

152. Webb A, Cunningham D, Scarffe JH, et al. Randomized trial comparing epirubicin, cisplatin, and fluorouracil versus fluorouracil, doxorubicin, and methotrexate in advanced esophagogastric cancer. *J Clin Oncol* 1997;15:261–267.

153. Cunningham D, Allum WH, Stenning SP, et al. Perioperative chemotherapy versus surgery alone for resectable gastroesophageal cancer. *N Engl J Med* 2006;355:11–20.

154. Cunningham D, Stenning S, Smyth E, et al. Peri-operative chemotherapy with or without bevacizumab in operable oesophagogastric adenocarcinoma (UK Medical Research Council ST03): primary analysis results of a multicentre, open-label, randomised phase 2–3 trial. *Lancet Oncol* 2017;18(3):357–370.

155. Ychou M, Boige V, Pignon JP, et al. Perioperative chemotherapy compared with surgery alone for resectable gastroesophageal adenocarcinoma: an FNCLCC and FFCD multicenter phase III trial. *J Clin Oncol* 2011;29:1715–1721.

156. Schumacher C, Gretschel S, Lordick F, et al. Neoadjuvant Chemotherapy Compared With Surgery Alone For Locally Advanced Cancer Of The Stomach And Cardia: European Organisation for Research and Treatment of Cancer Randomized Trial 40954. *J Clin Oncol* 2010;28(35):5210–5218.

157. Xiong B, Cheng Y, Ma L, et al. An updated meta-analysis of randomized controlled trial assessing the effect of neoadjuvant chemotherapy in advanced gastric cancer. *Cancer Invest* 2014;32(6):272–284.

158. Speigel D, Palta M, Uronis H. Role of chemotherapy and radiation therapy in the management of gastric adenocarcinoma. *Surg Clin North Am* 2017;97:421–435.

159. Al-Batran S, Homann N, Schmalenberg H, et al. Perioperative chemotherapy with docetaxel, oxaliplatin, and fluorouracil/leucovorin (FLOT) versus epirubicin, cisplatin, and fluorouracil or capecitabine (ECF/ECX) for resectable gastric or gastroesophageal junction (GEJ) adenocarcinoma (FLOT4-AIO): a multicenter, randomized phase 3 trial. *J Clin Oncol* 2017;35(Suppl):Abstract 4004

160. Buffet C, Turner K, Pelletier G, et al. Palliative radiotherapy (Letter to editor). *Br J Surg* 1983;70:131.

161. Falkson G, van Eden EB. A controlled clinical trial of fluorouracil plus imidazole carboxamide dimethyl triazeno plus vincristine plus bis-chloroethyl nitrosourea plus radiotherapy in stomach cancer. *Med Pediatr Oncol* 1976;2:111–117.

162. Freid JR, Goldberg H, Tenzel W, et al. Cobalt 60 beam therapy: three years experience at Montefiore Hospital (New York). *Radiology* 1956;67:200–209.

163. Klaassen DJ, MacIntyre JM, Catton GE, et al. Treatment of locally unresectable cancer of the stomach and pancreas: a randomized comparison of 5-fluorouracil alone with radiation plus concurrent and maintenance 5-fluorouracil—an Eastern Cooperative Oncology Group study. *J Clin Oncol* 1985;3:373–378.

164. Maus JH, McCormick NA. Three years' clinical experience with rotation therapy with the theratron. *Am J Roentgenol Radium Ther Nucl Med* 1958;79:382–386.

165. Moertel CG, Rubin J, O'Connell MJ, et al. A phase II study of combined 5-fluorouracil, doxorubicin, and cisplatin in the treatment of advanced upper gastrointestinal adenocarcinomas. *J Clin Oncol* 1986;4:1053–1057.

166. Falkson G. Halogenated pyrimidines as radiopotentiators in the treatment of stomach cancer. *Prog Biochem Pharmacol* 1965;1:695.

167. Nordman E. Value of megavolt therapy in gastric carcinoma. *Bull Cancer* 1976;63:217–222.

168. Tey J, Soon Y, Koh W, et al. Palliative radiotherapy for gastric cancer: a systematic review and meta-analysis. *Onco Target* 2017;8(15):25797–25805.

169. McMillan M, Ojerholm E, Roses R, et al. Adjuvant radiation therapy treatment time impacts overall survival in gastric cancer. *Int J Radiat Oncol Biol Phys* 2015;93(2):326–336.

170. Brecher G, Cronkite EP, Conard RA, et al. Gastric lesions in experimental animals following single exposures to ionizing radiations. *Am J Pathol* 1958;34:105–119.

171. Dickson HM. Effect of x-irradiation on glucose absorption. *Am J Physiol* 1955;182:477–478.

172. Fletcher GH, Lindberg RD, Caderao JB, et al. Hyperbaric oxygen as a radiotherapeutic adjuvant in advanced cancer of the uterine cervix: preliminary results of a randomized trial. *Cancer* 1977;39:617–623.

173. Smalley S, Evans R. *Radiation morbidity to the gastrointestinal tract and liver*. London: Butterworth, 1989.

174. Scarantino CW, Ornitz RD, Hoffman LG, et al. On the mechanism of radiation-induced emesis: the role of serotonin. *Int J Radiat Oncol Biol Phys* 1994;30:825–830.

175. Fenton PF, Dickson HM. Changes in some gastrointestinal functions following x-irradiation. *Am J Physiol* 1954;177:528–530.

176. Caudry M, Escarmant P, Maire JP, et al. Radiotherapy of gastric cancer with a three field combination: feasibility, tolerance, and survival. *Int J Radiat Oncol Biol Phys* 1987;13:1821–1827.

177. Schein P, Smith F, Dritschillo A, et al. Phase I-II trial of combined modality FAM plus split-course radiation (FAM-RT-FAM) for locally advanced gastric and pancreatic cancer: a Mid-Atlantic Oncology Program study. *Proc Am Soc Clin Oncol* 1983;2:126.

178. Haas CD, Mansfield CM, Leichman LP, et al. Combined nonsimultaneous radiation therapy and chemotherapy with 5-FU, doxorubicin, and mitomycin for residual localized gastric adenocarcinoma: a Southwest Oncology Group pilot study. *Cancer Treat Rep* 1983;67:421–424.

179. Carpender JW, Levin E, Clayman CB, et al. Radiation in the therapy of peptic ulcer. *Am J Roentgenol Radium Ther Nucl Med* 1956;75:374–379.

180. Amory HI, Brick IB. Irradiation damage of the intestines following 1,000-kv Roentgen therapy; evaluation of tolerance dose. *Radiology* 1951;56:49–57.

181. Brick IB. Effects of million volt irradiation on the gastrointestinal tract. *AMA Arch Intern Med* 1955;96:26–31.

182. Friedman M. Calculated risks of radiation injury of normal tissue in the treatment of cancer of the testis. In: *Proceedings of the second national cancer conference*. Cincinnati, OH: American Cancer Society, Inc., National Cancer Institute of the U.S. Public Health Service and American Association for Cancer Research, 1952:390–400.

183. Jolles CJ, Freedman RS, Hamberger AD, et al. Complications of extended-field therapy for cervical carcinoma without prior surgery. *Int J Radiat Oncol Biol Phys* 1986;12:179–183.

184. Rubin P, Casarett G. *Clinical radiation pathology*. Philadelphia, PA: WB Saunders, 1968.

185. Trip A, Nijkamp J, van Tinteren H, et al. IMRT limits nephrotoxicity after chemoradiotherapy for gastric cancer. *Radiother Oncol* 2014;112(2):289–294.

186. Inaba K, Okamoto H, Wakita A, et al. Long-term observations of radiation-induced creatinine clearance reduction and renal parenchymal volume atrophy. *Radiother Oncol* 2016;120(1):145–149.

187. Callister MD, Gunderson LL. Advancements in radiation techniques for gastric cancer. *J Natl Compr Canc Netw* 2010;8:428–435; quiz 436.

188. Cosset JM, Henry-Amar M, Pellae-Cosset B, et al. Pericarditis and myocardial infarctions after Hodgkin's disease therapy. *Int J Radiat Oncol Biol Phys* 1991;21:447–449.

189. Hancock SL, Donaldson SS, Hoppe RT. Cardiac disease following treatment of Hodgkin's disease in children and adolescents. *J Clin Oncol* 1993;11:1208–1215.

190. Hazard L, Yang G, McAleer M, et al. Principles and techniques of radiation therapy for esophageal and gastroesophageal junction cancers. *J Natl Compr Cancer Netw* 2008;6:870–878.

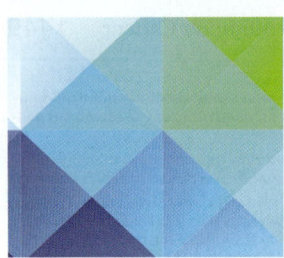

CHAPTER 63

Pancreatic Cancer

Manisha Palta, Christopher G. Willett, and Brian G. Czito

ANATOMY AND PATHWAYS OF SPREAD

The pancreas lies in the retroperitoneal space of the upper abdomen at about the level of the first two lumbar vertebrae. It is divided into head (including the uncinate process), neck, body, and tail (Fig. 63.1). It has intimate contact with surrounding organs, including stomach, duodenum, jejunum, kidneys, spleen, and major vessels, which can be involved by direct tumor extension. Tumors in the pancreatic head often invade or compress the common bile duct, causing jaundice and dilatation of the bile and pancreatic ducts and gallbladder.

The rich lymphatic drainage of the pancreas is interconnected with duodenal lymphatics. Regional drainage of the pancreatic head is to the peripancreatic, pancreaticoduodenal, porta hepatis, celiac, and superior mesenteric lymph nodes. The pancreatic body and tail drains to splenic artery, peripancreatic, celiac, superior mesenteric, and paraaortic nodal basins.[1] With posterior, retroperitoneal tumor extension, paraaortic nodes are at risk. The main venous channels drain via the portal system to the liver. The lungs and pleura may be involved with posterior tumor extension into tissues with venous drainage by the vena cava or its tributaries. Generalized peritoneal involvement is more common with carcinoma of the body and tail than with carcinoma of the head of the pancreas.

EPIDEMIOLOGY AND RISK FACTORS

In 2017, an estimated 53,670 new cases of pancreatic cancer will be diagnosed in the United States, with 43,090 estimated deaths from the disease, making pancreatic cancer the fourth leading cause of cancer-related death in the United States.[2] At present, surgery offers the only means of cure. Unfortunately, only 10% to 20% of patients present with tumors amenable to resection. Even among patients who present with localized disease, the 5-year overall survival (OS) is approximately 20%.[3] Contemporary survival rates have reported improved results, particularly in patients with complete surgical resection (R0) and node-negative (N0) disease.[4–6] Patients who present with locally advanced, unresectable pancreatic cancer have a median survival of approximately 8 to 14 months, with rare long-term survival. Up to 60% of patients present with metastatic disease, which carries a shorter median survival of 4 to 12 months.[7]

The incidence of pancreatic cancer rises sharply after age 45, with higher rates in males than in females (1.3:1) and in black males compared with the general population (14.8/100,000:8.8/100,000).[8] Familial aggregation of pancreatic cancer is estimated in 5% to 10% of newly diagnosed cases. It is associated with *BRCA1/2* and PALB2 mutations, familial atypical multiple mole melanoma syndrome, Peutz-Jeghers syndrome, familial adenomatous polyposis, hereditary nonpolyposis colorectal cancer, hereditary pancreatitis, ataxia telangiectasia, and Li-Fraumeni syndrome, with lifetime risk ranging from 5% to 40%.[9,10] Described risk factors for pancreatic cancer include chronic pancreatitis, smoking, alcohol consumption, *Helicobacter pylori* infection, and factors associated with metabolic syndrome such as obesity and glucose intolerance.[11,12]

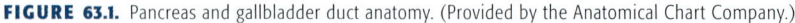

FIGURE 63.1. Pancreas and gallbladder duct anatomy. (Provided by the Anatomical Chart Company.)

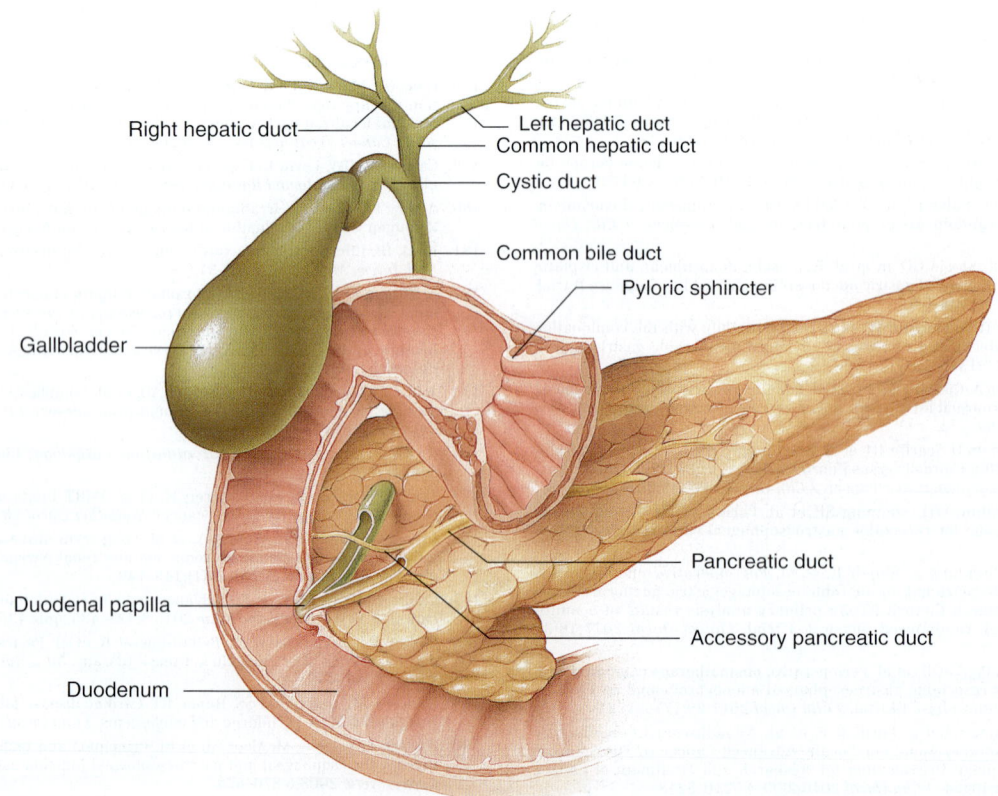

Right hepatic duct

Left hepatic duct
Common hepatic duct

Cystic duct

Common bile duct

Pyloric sphincter

Gallbladder

Pancreatic duct

Duodenal papilla

Accessory pancreatic duct

Duodenum

CLINICAL PRESENTATION

Most patients with pancreatic cancer experience pain, weight loss, or jaundice. Classically, pain from pancreatic cancer is characterized by radiation to the back, given the retroperitoneal location of the pancreas. Jaundice, due to biliary obstruction, is often accompanied by pruritus, acholic stools, and dark urine color. The initial presentation varies according to tumor location. Patients with tumors in the pancreatic body or tail usually present with pain and weight loss, whereas those in the head of the gland typically present with jaundice, steatorrhea, weight loss, and pain. Recent onset of atypical or exacerbation of preexisting diabetes mellitus, unexplained thrombophlebitis, or history of pancreatitis is often noted. Patients with pancreatic cancer frequently present with unresectable or metastatic disease, in part due to these nonspecific presenting symptoms and the tendency for local and distant spread. No effective screening method to detect disease at the localized stage has been identified. Positive physical findings, if any, generally reflect incurable disease. These may include a palpable abdominal mass (i.e., pancreas, liver, or gallbladder due to biliary obstruction), ascites, supraclavicular nodes, or palpable rectal shelf (i.e., peritoneal seeding).

EVALUATION

Significant advances have been achieved in the imaging and staging of pancreatic cancer.[13] Currently, the principal diagnostic tools are multiphasic, helical computed tomography (CT) scan; endoscopic ultrasound (EUS); and laparoscopy. Magnetic resonance imaging (MRI) and positron emission tomography (PET) imaging techniques may be used in initial evaluation of pancreatic malignancies. These tools have facilitated the characterization of the primary tumor (resectable or borderline resectable vs. unresectable) as well as the identification of metastatic disease so patients can be appropriately and reliably triaged to operative and nonoperative therapies.

CT scan is the most commonly used staging modality. Newer generation, multidetector, high-speed helical CT coupled with and thin section imaging allows high-resolution images of the pancreas and its surrounding structures to be obtained at varying phases of enhancement. This allows for adequate imaging of the pancreas and assessment of metastatic deposits in other intra-abdominal organs such as the liver.[14] Over 90% of patients deemed unresectable because of vascular involvement by CT are truly inoperable at time of surgery.[15] Although CT staging is limited in detection of nodal involvement and peritoneal disease, it is useful in evaluating for metastatic disease.

Another tool for local tumor staging and diagnosis is EUS. In this procedure, an endoscope with an ultrasound transducer at its tip is passed into the stomach and duodenum, where it provides high-resolution images of the pancreas and surrounding vessels. EUS facilitates FNA without exposing the peritoneum to potential tumor seeding, as may occur with CT-guided biopsy. Sensitivity for EUS is at least comparable to CT, with tumor detection reported as high as 97%.[16] An advantage of EUS over CT is the ability to detect small or isoattenuating lesions, which might not be well visualized on cross-sectional imaging.[17] Interpretation of EUS is highly operator dependent. Frequently, EUS is performed in conjunction with endoscopic retrograde cholangiopancreatography.[18] This combined diagnostic approach allows for staging, therapeutic stenting of the common bile duct when indicated, and diagnostic FNA simultaneously.

A limitation of current imaging techniques is the inability to visualize small (1 to 2 mm) liver and peritoneal implants. Staging laparoscopy has been used preoperatively to assess for intraperitoneal metastases. One meta-analysis demonstrated that the adoption of staging laparoscopy and laparoscopic ultrasound will prevent up to 50% of patients from undergoing unnecessary laparotomy.[19] Patients with locally advanced disease and involved peritoneal washings or positive peritoneal biopsies have the same prognosis as do those with metastatic disease.[20]

Advances in MRI, including high-resolution imaging, faster acquisition time, three-dimensional (3D) reconstruction, functional imaging, and MR cholangiopancreatography, have led to an improved ability of MRI to diagnose and stage pancreatic cancer.[14] This modality can be used in patients with poor renal function to assess the primary tumor and determine resectability; however, studies suggest that MRI is not as sensitive as EUS or CT in tumor detection.[21] A potential advantage of MRI is identification of small foci of hepatic metastatic disease difficult to appreciate by CT or to further characterize ill-defined lesions seen on CT.[22]

Initial studies showed that PET has a higher sensitivity, specificity, and accuracy than does CT in diagnosing pancreatic carcinomas.[23-25] Integrated PET-CT had a higher sensitivity for malignancy detection than did either PET or CT alone (96% vs. 84% vs. 77%) but did not improve specificity (64%). PET may also be a useful adjunct in the identification of benign versus malignant lesions and presence of metastatic disease. Although PET-CT may be useful in initial diagnosis, its role in determining resectability has been questioned as coregistration is often performed with lesser resolution CT images and high metabolism can obscure peripancreatic planes.[26]

High-resolution pancreatic CT and EUS remain the current standard for diagnosis and staging of pancreatic malignancies. Staging laparoscopy is useful in assessing for intraperitoneal and liver disease. MRI and PET-CT are technologies that may also be useful. All imaging modalities are inadequate to stage lymph node involvement, and further advances may improve the ability to diagnose, stage, and appropriately select further therapies.

TUMOR STAGING

Staging is rarely used in published series, and tumors are instead characterized as resectable, borderline resectable, unresectable, or metastatic.

The current American Joint Committee on Cancer 2010 tumor, node, and metastasis staging system is described in Table 63.1. Common criteria of resectability are outlined in Table 63.2.

PATHOLOGIC CLASSIFICATION

Approximately 85% to 90% of pancreatic cancers are adenocarcinomas. Other neoplasm histologic cell types include intraductal papillary mucinous neoplasm, mucinous cystic, solid pseudopapillary, acinar cell, pancreaticoblastoma, neuroendocrine, squamous cell, serous cystadenocarcinoma, and lymphoma. Management and treatment sections will focus on pancreatic adenocarcinomas, given this is the predominate histologic subtype. The histopathology of lesions in the periampullary region of the head of the pancreas is of particular importance as different types of adenocarcinomas, originating from the pancreas, bile duct, ampullary region, or duodenum, respectively, portend different prognoses.[27]

Pancreatic adenocarcinomas evolve from noninvasive pancreatic intraepithelial neoplasias, acquiring various genetic and epigenetic mutations. Several molecular abnormalities have been implicated in contributing to the development of pancreatic cancer. The most frequent genetic alterations are activation of the oncogene *KRAS* and inactivation of tumor suppressor genes including *TP53*, p16 (*CDKN2*), *DPC4 (SMAD4)*, and *BRCA2*, with reported incidences ranging from 50% to 95% in pancreatic tumors.[28] These molecular changes have the potential to identify precursor lesions with a high likelihood of progressing into carcinomas, characterizing pathologically ambiguous lesions, and useful in development of screening regimens.

TABLE 63.1 AMERICAN JOINT COMMITTEE ON CANCER STAGING 2010 CLASSIFICATION FOR PANCREATIC CANCER

American Joint Committee on Cancer (AJCC)

TNM Staging of Pancreatic Cancer (2010)

Because only a few patients with pancreatic cancer undergo surgical resection of the pancreas (and adjacent lymph nodes), a single TNM classification must apply to both clinical and pathologic staging.

Primary Tumor (T)

TX Primary tumor cannot be assessed

T0 No evidence of primary tumor

Tis Carcinoma *in situ**

T1 Tumor limited to the pancreas, 2 cm or less in greatest dimension

T2 Tumor limited to the pancreas, more than 2 cm in greatest

T3 Tumor extends beyond the pancreas but without involvement of the celiac axis or the superior mesenteric artery

T4 Tumor involves the celiac axis or the superior mesenteric artery (unresectable primary tumor)

* This also includes the "PanIn III" classification

Regional Lymph Nodes (N)

NX Regional lymph nodes cannot be assessed

N0 No regional lymph node metastasis

N1 Regional lymph node metastasis

Distant Metastasis (M)

M0 No distant metastasis

M1 Distant metastasis

Stage Grouping

Stage 0	Tis	N0	M0
Stage IA	T1	N0	M0
Stage IB	T2	N0	M0
Stage IIA	T3	N0	M0
Stage IIB	T1	N1	M0
	T2	N1	M0
	T3	N1	M0
Stage III	T4	Any N	M0
Stage IV	Any T	Any N	M1

From Edge SB, Byrd DR, Compton CC, et al., eds. *AJCC cancer staging manual.* 7th ed. New York: Springer, 2010. Copyright © 2010 American Joint Committee on Cancer. Reproduced with permission of Springer in the format Book via Copyright Clearance Center.

TABLE 63.2 CRITERIA DEFINING RESECTABILITY STATUS

Resectable (head, body, and tail)

No distant metastases

No arterial tumor contact (celiac axis [CA], superior mesenteric artery [SMA], or common hepatic artery [CHA])

No tumor contact with the superior mesenteric vein (SMV) or portal vein (PV) or ≤180-degree contact without vein contour irregularity

Borderline Resectable (head/uncinate)

Solid tumor contact with CHA without extension to celiac axis or hepatic artery bifurcation allowing for safe and complete resection and reconstruction

Solid tumor contact with the SMA of ≤180 degrees

Solid tumor contact with variant arterial anatomy (ex: accessory right hepatic, replaced right hepatic artery, replaced CHA, and the origin of replaced or accessory artery and the presence and degree of tumor contact should be noted if present as it may affect surgical planning

Solid tumor contact with the SMV or PV >180 degrees, contact of ≤180 degrees with contour irregularity of the vein or thrombosis of the vein but with suitable vessel proximal and distal to the site of involvement allowing for safe and complete resection and vein reconstruction

Solid tumor contact with the inferior vena cava (IVC)

Borderline Resectable (body/tail)

Solid tumor contact with the CA of ≤180 degrees

Solid tumor contact with the CA of >180 degrees without involvement of the aorta and with intact and uninvolved gastroduodenal artery thereby permitting a modified Appleby procedure

Unresectable

Distant metastases

Unresectable (head/uncinate)

Solid tumor contact with SMA >180 degrees

Solid tumor contact with the CA >180 degrees

Solid tumor contact with the first jejunal SMA branch

Unreconstructible SMV/PV due to tumor involvement or occlusion (can be due to tumor or bland thrombus)

Contact with most proximal draining jejunal branch into SMV

Unresectable (body/tail)

Solid tumor contact of >180 degrees with SMA or CA

Solid tumor contact with the CA and aortic involvement

Unreconstructible SMV/PV due to tumor involvement or occlusion (can be due to tumor or bland thrombus)

Modified from the NCCN Clinical Practice Guidelines in Oncology (NCCN Guidelines®) for Pancreatic Adenocarcinoma (V.2.2017).

GENERAL MANAGEMENT

Operative Considerations

Surgery, as part of a multimodality treatment approach for patients with resectable pancreatic cancer, represents the only potentially curative treatment strategy.[29] More than 80% of patients present with advanced disease that is not amenable to curative resection, with roughly two-thirds presenting in the pancreatic head. The standard surgical treatment for pancreatic cancer of the head or uncinate is pancreaticoduodenectomy, first described by Whipple et al.[30] in 1935. For pancreatic tail lesions, distal pancreatectomy is employed, frequently with splenectomy. Initially, high operative morbidity and mortality rates led to technical modifications of the operation that, combined with improvements in anesthesia and critical care, have resulted in current perioperative mortality rates of ≤2% at high-volume centers.[31–33] With reduced morbidity from the Whipple procedure, there is no age limitation, and selected patients, even at ages >80 years, may undergo pancreaticoduodenectomy.[34–36]

Several studies report low postoperative mortality rates and appropriate patient selection at high-volume institutions, highlighting the importance of performing such procedures at institutions with extensive experience.[37–40] In addition, the definition of resectable lesions has broadened with the ability to perform venous reconstructions with minimal increase in morbidity or mortality.[41,42]

The prognosis, even among resectable patients, remains poor, with 5-year survival rates of 10% to 25%. The number of nodes harvested appears to impact outcomes; data suggest that 12 to 15 lymph nodes constitute an adequate assessment, although impact on outcomes may simply reflect accurate staging.[43,44] Although appropriate lymph node dissection is desirable, trials of extended lymphadenectomy conveyed no survival benefit and compromised quality of life.[45,46] Pathologic assessment provides important prognostic information, including margin status, tumor grade, tumor size, lymphovascular invasion, and lymph node involvement. The presence of positive operative margins, poor histologic grade, larger tumor size, lymphovascular invasion, and lymph node involvement portends a poorer prognosis.[47–51] Similarly, patients with elevated pre- and postoperative carbohydrate antigen 19–9 (CA19-9) have inferior disease-free survival (DFS) and OS rates.[51–54]

In an effort to minimize surgical morbidity, pyloruspreserving pancreaticoduodenectomy and laparoscopic resection techniques have developed. Pylorus-sparing pancreaticoduodenectomy potentially improves gastrointestinal function without compromising oncologic management.[55,56] Laparoscopic pancreatic resection was first explored in the late 1990s, and its use has increased dramatically.[57,58] Although most experiences are small, retrospective, single-institution series, laparoscopic resection, in experienced hands, appears a reasonable option for distal pancreatic resections.[59–62] The data on laparoscopic pancreaticoduodenectomy are more limited; the difficulty with this procedure arises from more complex dissection and the need for reconstruction.[42,58] Data suggest, however, that despite prolonged operative times and potential increase in postoperative fistula formation, laparoscopic resection offers shortened hospitalization and equivalent oncologic results.[58,63–65]

Cause of Death and Patterns of Failure

For patients with locally unresectable tumors or metastatic disease, death usually results from hepatic failure secondary to biliary obstruction by local tumor extension or hepatic replacement by metastases. For the 10% to 20% of patients undergoing a potentially curative pancreaticoduodenectomy, three major

TABLE 63.3 PATTERNS OF FAILURE AFTER RESECTION OF PANCREATIC CANCER WITHOUT ADJUVANT RADIATION THERAPY OR CHEMOTHERAPY

Author (Reference)	Number of Patients	Local (%)	Incidence of Failure (%)	
			Peritoneal	Liver
Patterns of Failure after Surgery				
Tepper et al.[66]	26	13 (50)	NA	NA
Griffin et al.[67]	36[a]	19 (53)	11 (31)	16 (44)
Whittington et al.[68]	29	22 (85)	6 (23)	6 (23)
Ozaki[69]	14	12 (86)	5 (36)	11 (79)
Westerdahl et al.[70]	74	64 (86)	NA	68 (92)
Patterns of Failure with Surgery and Adjuvant Therapy				
Foo et al.[71]	29	3 (10)	12 (41)	12 (41)
Abrams et al.[72]b	29	10 (34)	4 (14)	9 (31)
Paulino and Latona[73]	38	– (25)	– (33)	– (80)
Hattangadi et al.[74]	86	– (31)	– (55)	– (53)
Regine[75]b				
Gemcitabine CRT	184	56 (30)	138 (75)[c]	
5-FU CRT	197	70 (36)	140 (71)[c]	

[a]Ten patients received external beam irradiation.
[b]First site of failure only.
[c]Distant failure.
CRT, chemoradiation; NA, not available; 5-FU, 5-fluorouracil.

sites of disease relapse dominate: locoregional, peritoneal cavity, and liver (Table 63.3). High local recurrence rates of 50% to 86% occur despite resection because of frequent lymphatic and perineural involvement and cancer invasion into the retroperitoneal soft tissues, with an inability to achieve wide retroperitoneal soft tissue margins due to anatomic constraints (SMA and SMV, portal vein, and inferior vena cava).[50,76,77] The incidence of microscopic residual disease after careful evaluation of the posterior peripancreatic soft tissue margin is as high as 40%.[77] Therefore, tumor stage, grade, and resection margin status are the best predictors of survival after surgery.[76,77] The use of adjuvant therapy after surgery can reduce the incidence of local failure, but distant disease recurrence rates remain high.

RADIATION THERAPY TECHNIQUES

Dose-Limiting Tissues

The dose-limiting organs for irradiation of upper abdominal malignancies include the small bowel, stomach, liver, kidneys, and spinal cord. Various techniques, such as 3D conformal radiotherapy (3DCRT) and intensity-modulated radiotherapy (IMRT), can spare these organs. Given long-term survival is low, the actual number of patients at risk for late complications is small. Late small bowel and gastric effects may also be decreased through reduction of the volume of these organs within the high-dose field.

Treatment Volumes, Fields, and Doses

In patients undergoing surgery, clips should be placed to mark the extent of the lesion for postoperative irradiation. The patient should be positioned supine during simulation and treatment. 3DCRT radiotherapy allows visualization of internal organs and target delineation. CT-based treatment planning allows the construction of normal tissue dose–volume histograms and the generation of treatment plans that optimize radiation dose delivery to tumor while sparing critical normal tissues. Multiple field, fractionated, external beam techniques utilizing high-energy photons to deliver 45 to 50 Gy in 1.8 Gy fractions to tumor bed, unresected or residual tumor, and lymph node–bearing areas at risk. After the primary fields, a boost field can be designed to include unresected or gross residual disease, as defined by CT scans and clips, while excluding most of the stomach and small bowel.

With lesions in the head of the pancreas, major node groups include the pancreaticoduodenal and peripancreatic (resected at the time of Whipple) and porta hepatis and paraaortic regions. Approximately two-thirds of the left kidney must be excluded from the AP/PA field because the right kidney is often in the field because of duodenal (bed) inclusion. The superior field extent is often at the middle or upper portion of the T11 vertebral body for adequate margins on the celiac vessels (T12, L1) and the inferior limit at the level L2–L3 to include the superior mesenteric lymph nodes and third portion of the duodenum. The upper field extent is sometimes more superior with body lesions to obtain adequate margin on the primary lesion. With lateral fields, the anterior field margin is 1.5 to 2.0 cm beyond initial gross disease. The posterior margin is often 1.5 cm behind the anterior portion of the vertebral body to allow adequate margins on paraaortic nodes, which are at risk with posterior tumor extension in head or body lesions. The lateral contribution usually is limited to 15 to 18 Gy because a moderate volume of kidney or liver may be in the irradiated volume (Fig. 63.2).

FIGURE 63.2. External beam four-field technique for pancreatic head lesion. **A:** The anteroposterior/posteroanterior (AP/PA) field, which includes gross tumor (*red*), duodenal loop (*pink*) (plus approximately 50% of the right kidney [*light green*]), liver (*brown*), and nodal areas at risk (porta hepatis: *orange*, superior mesenteric arteries: *green*, celiac: *magenta*). Most of the left kidney (*blue*) is excluded from the AP/PA field. **B:** The right lateral field with an anterior margin beyond gross disease and a posterior margin behind front edge of vertebral body. The liver contour (*brown*) has been removed from lateral field for visualization of other structures.

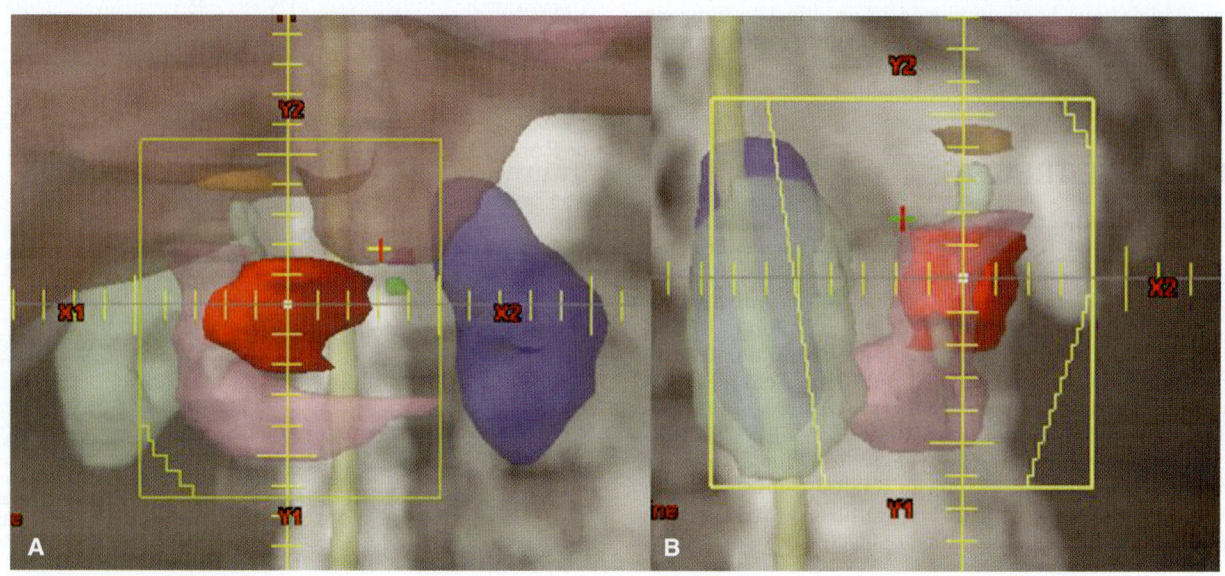

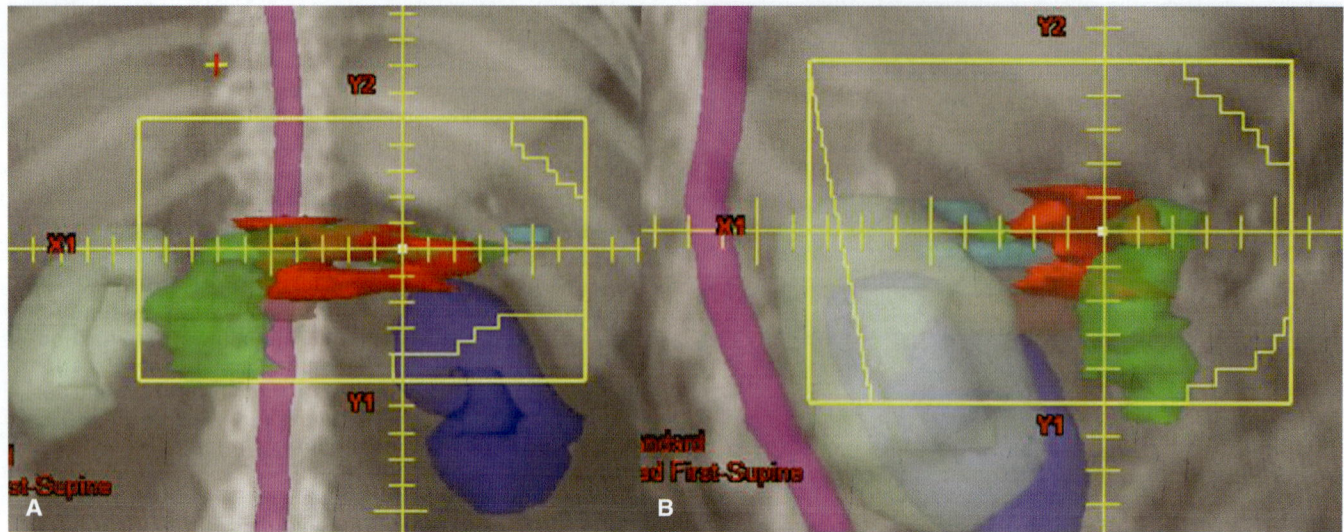

FIGURE 63.3. External beam four-field technique for unresectable tail of pancreas lesion. **A:** The anteroposterior/posteroanterior (AP/PA) field showing lesion (*red*) and head of pancreas (*green*). The field is extended to the patient's left to include coverage of the splenic hilum (*cyan*). Much of the right kidney (*light green*) is excluded from the field and multileaf collimators block most of the left kidney (*blue*). **B:** The right lateral field with an anterior margin beyond gross disease and a posterior margin at least 1.5 cm behind front edge of vertebral body.

With pancreatic body or tail lesions, at least 50% of the left kidney may be included to achieve adequate margins on node groups at risk (i.e., lateral suprapancreatic, splenic artery, and splenic hilum nodes). Inclusion of the pancreaticoduodenal nodes is often not indicated with body or tail lesions, and at least two-thirds of the right kidney can be preserved (Fig. 63.3).

After resection, AP/PA and lateral fields are often designed on the basis of preoperative CT primary tumor volumes, preoperative duodenal loop location, operative clip placement, and postoperative CT nodal volumes (Radiation Therapy Oncology Group [RTOG] contouring atlas accessible on their website). The anterior border is determined by vascular or nodal boundaries (porta hepatis, superior mesenteric, and celiac), as demonstrated on CT, as well as preoperative tumor location.[78]

RADIATION THERAPY RESULTS

Resectable Tumors: Adjuvant Therapy

After surgical resection of pancreatic cancer, local recurrence rates range from 50% to 86% and distant recurrence rates from 40% to 90%, most commonly to the liver or peritoneum.[50,66,67,69,70,77,79] This provides the rationale for adjuvant therapy, which have been employed in an effort to improve patient outcomes (Table 63.4). Despite multiple randomized trials, a definitive role for adjuvant radiotherapy for resected pancreatic cancer has not been established.

PROSPECTIVE TRIALS

Historical Prospective Studies

The Gastrointestinal Tumor Study Group (GITSG) conducted the first multicenter prospective trial of adjuvant CRT for patients with resected pancreatic cancer and negative surgical margins, laying the foundation for the adoption of CRT in the United States. Forty-three patients were randomized to observation or CRT to 40 Gy delivered in split-course fashion with concurrent 5-fluorouracil (5-FU) (500 mg/m²) as an intravenous bolus on the first 3 and last 3 days of radiation, followed by maintenance weekly 5-FU for 2 years or until disease progression. At interim analysis, improvements in median DFS and OS with CRT were observed: 11 versus 9 months and 20 versus 11 months, respectively. Two-year OS

was 42% in the CRT group versus 15% in the surgery-alone arm.[80] An additional 30 patients were later enrolled to receive adjuvant CRT. These additional patients confirmed the survival outcomes seen in the original trial, with median survival of 18 months and a 2-year survival of 46%.[81]

TABLE 63.4 PROSPECTIVE, RANDOMIZED TRIALS FOR ADJUVANT THERAPY FOR PANCREATIC CANCER

Series (Reference)	Number of Patients	Median Survival (Month)	2-Year Survival (%)	5-Year Survival (%)
GITSG[80]				
Chemoradiation	21	20.0	42	15
Observation	22	10.9	15	5
Chemoradiation (expanded cohort)[81]	30	18.0	46	17
EORTC[82,83]				
Chemoradiation	110	21.6	51	25
Observation	108	19.2	41	22
ESPAC-1 Pooled data[84]				
Chemotherapy	238	19.7	NA	NA
No chemotherapy	235	14.0	NA	NA
Chemoradiation	175	15.5	NA	NA
No chemoradiation	178	16.1	NA	NA
ESPAC-1 2X2 analysis[85]				
Chemotherapy	147	20.1	40	21
No chemotherapy	142	15.5	30	8
Chemoradiation	145	15.9	29	10
No chemoradiation	144	17.9	41	20
CONKO[86,87]				
Gemcitabine	186	23	30.5	21
Observation	182	20	14.5	9
ESPAC-3[88]				
5-FU	551	23	48	NA
Gemcitabine	537	23.6	49	NA
ESPAC-4[93]				
Gemcitabine	366	25.5	52.1	16.3
Gemcitabine and capecitabine	364	28	53.8	28.8
RTOG-9704 (pancreatic head)[75,89,90]				
Gemcitabine, then chemoradiation	187	20.5	31 (3 y)	22
5-FU, then chemoradiation	201	17.2	22 (3 y)	18

CONKO, Charite Onkologie; EORTC, European Organisation for Research and Treatment of Cancer; ESPAC, European Study Group for Pancreatic Cancer; GITSG, Gastrointestinal Tumor Study Group; NA, not available; RTOG, Radiation Therapy Oncology Group; 5-FU, 5-fluorouracil.

The GITSG trial has been criticized for a number of reasons. The trial closed prematurely following enrollment of 43 of an intended 100 patients because of slow accrual over the 8-year enrollment period. The EBRT approach in this trial was considered low dose and antiquated by contemporary standards because of a split-course technique and use of large treatment fields, which encompassed the entire pancreas or pancreatic bed and the celiac, pancreaticosplenic, peripancreatic, and retroperitoneal regional lymph nodes. Additionally, the inclusion of both CRT and adjuvant chemotherapy after surgery evaluated two treatment variables, making it difficult to discern the true effect of either treatment alone. In the CRT arm, there were issues of compliance, with 32% of patients assigned to CRT receiving inappropriate radiation and 25% of patients failing to initiate treatment within 10 weeks postsurgery, the protocol-specified time limit. Only 9% of patients completed the planned 2-year maintenance chemotherapy course. In addition, survival in the control arm was low compared to historical studies. Despite these limitations and the failure to reach the desired patient accrual, the GITSG trial demonstrated a benefit for CRT, which became standard adjuvant therapy, particularly in the United States.

A second study sponsored by the European Organisation for Research and Treatment of Cancer (EORTC) sought to confirm the findings of the original GITSG study. Two hundred eighteen patients with resected pancreas ($n = 114$) or periampullary cancers ($n = 104$) were randomly assigned to observation or CRT to 40 Gy in a split-dose fashion with concurrent continuous infusional 5-FU (25 mg/kg) without further adjuvant chemotherapy. This study showed no significant improvement ($P = .208$) in median survival (19 months [observation] vs. 24.5 months [CRT]) or 2-year survival (41% [observation] vs. 51% [CRT]).[82] Long-term follow-up of the EORTC trial demonstrated no difference in 5-year OS with CRT use: 22% (surgery alone) versus 25% (CRT). *Post hoc* analysis of pancreatic head lesions failed to demonstrate a benefit with CRT, with a median OS of 1.3 years for CRT versus 1 year for surgery alone.[83]

This trial has been criticized for its heterogeneous patient population, which included patients with both pancreatic and periampullary primary tumors. Periampullary carcinomas have a significantly better prognosis compared with pancreatic cancer; the two entities thus represent truly different diseases and potentially dilute any evidence of benefit for adjuvant CRT.[91] Similar to the GITSG trial, older EBRT techniques—split course and low total dose—were used. Also, >20% of patients in the CRT arm did not receive the intended treatment because of postoperative complications or patient refusal. The trial did not include maintenance chemotherapy in the treatment arm. Finally, although a small subset, patients undergoing noncurative resection and patients with positive surgical margins were still eligible for enrollment. The discordant results of the EORTC and GITSG trials have led some investigators to attribute the OS benefit seen in the GITSG trial to maintenance chemotherapy administration rather than to EBRT.

An additional European trial conducted by the European Study Group for Pancreatic Cancer (ESPAC) aimed to further explore the question of appropriate adjuvant therapy for "macroscopically" resected pancreatic cancers. Treating physicians were allowed to enroll patients into one of three parallel randomized studies:

1. Chemoradiation versus no chemoradiation ($n = 68$), consisting of 20 Gy over 2 weeks with 5-FU (500 mg/m^2) on days 1 through 3, then repeated after a 2-week break;
2. Chemotherapy versus no chemotherapy ($n = 188$), consisting of bolus 5-FU (425 mg/m^2) and leucovorin (20 mg/m^2) given for 5 days every 28 days for 6 cycles; or
3. A 2-by-2 factorial design of 285 patients enrolled on chemoradiotherapy ($n = 70$), chemotherapy ($n = 74$), chemoradiotherapy with maintenance chemotherapy ($n = 72$), or observation ($n = 69$).

The data from the treatment groups from all three parallel trials were then pooled for analysis. There was no survival difference between the 175 patients who received adjuvant chemoradiation and the 178 patients who did not receive therapy (median survival, 15.5 vs. 16.1 months; $P = .24$). In the chemotherapy arm, however, a 35% reduction in death was seen in the group who received adjuvant chemotherapy ($n = 238$) compared with those who received no chemotherapy ($n = 235$), with a difference in median survival of 19.7 versus 14 months ($P = .0005$).[84] On further follow-up of patients randomized using the 2-by-2 factorial design, the 5-year survival rate for the patients who received chemotherapy was 21% versus 8% for those who did not. Additionally, adjuvant CRT was associated with a deleterious effect on survival.[85]

A number of problems are associated with the interpretation of these data. First, the complex trial design has the potential for bias, because patients or physicians could select randomization for one treatment variable. Also, as in the aforementioned trials, the EBRT technique used was, by contemporary standards, considered outdated, using split course and low total dose. No details of EBRT delivery or central quality assurance for EBRT, surgery, or pathology are available. In addition, many treatment violations occurred, as only 62% of patients received full CRT treatment and only 42% of patients in the chemotherapy arms completed the predefined regimen. Although many have attempted to draw conclusions from the updated publication, the 2-by-2 factorial cohort of the study was not powered to detect OS differences. Additionally, patients receiving CRT in the ESPAC trial experienced poorer survival outcomes compared with those in other reported CRT series. Also, patients who had received prior "background" chemotherapy or radiation therapy were still eligible for enrollment. As in the EORTC trial, no maintenance chemotherapy was administered. Despite these critiques, some have speculated that the detriment seen in the CRT group may have resulted from delayed administration of systemic therapy shown to improve survival in the ESPAC trial.

A common critique of the aforementioned trials of adjuvant therapy is the lack of restaging to evaluate for the presence of persistent or metastatic disease after surgical resection and prior to the initiation of adjuvant therapy. The time between initial staging and the commencement of adjuvant treatment can be as long as 3 to 4 months, during which a significant number of patients would be expected to develop radiographically apparent metastases. Without interval restaging, these patients may inappropriately receive CRT. Although these three trials formed the foundation for adjuvant treatment approaches to resectable pancreatic cancer, perhaps because each trial was fraught with flaws, there continues to be little consensus regarding the "most appropriate" treatment. A relative dichotomy in adjuvant treatment approaches for resectable pancreatic cancer has emerged between the United States and parts of Europe, with adjuvant CRT frequently implemented in the United States and adjuvant chemotherapy alone administered in parts of Europe.

Modern Studies: Adjuvant Systemic Therapy

Building from the data showing potential benefit to adjuvant chemotherapy, investigators in Europe conducted a randomized phase III trial of observation versus adjuvant gemcitabine in patients with resected pancreatic cancer. Three hundred sixty-eight patients were enrolled on the Charite Onkologie (CONKO) trial and randomized to observation or adjuvant gemcitabine (1,000 mg/m^2 intravenous days 1, 8, and 15 every 4 weeks for 6 months).[86] The primary end point was DFS, and patients treated with gemcitabine achieved a statistically significantly longer DFS (14.2 vs. 7.5 months) than those observed after surgery. This improvement was seen in both the R0 and R1 subgroups. At initial publication, there was no difference in OS. With longer follow-up, median and 5-year

OS were both improved in patients receiving gemcitabine (23 vs. 20 months, and 21% vs. 9%, respectively).[87] These findings were supported by a smaller randomized study from Japan, which again demonstrated a DFS benefit for gemcitabine compared to surgery alone.[92]

At the same time the CONKO trial was enrolling patients, ESPAC-3, the largest randomized controlled trial in pancreatic cancer to date, enrolled 1,088 patients with pancreatic adenocarcinoma who underwent R0 or R1 resection. Patients were randomly assigned to 6 cycles of adjuvant gemcitabine (3 weekly infusions of 1,000 mg/m²) or 6 cycles of bolus 5-FU (425 mg/m²)/leucovorin (LV) (20 mg/m²). Patients receiving 5-FU/LV experienced significantly higher rates of grade 3 or 4 gastrointestinal toxicity (stomatitis and diarrhea), whereas patients receiving gemcitabine experienced significantly higher rates of grade 3 or 4 hematologic toxicity. At a median follow-up of 34.2 months, there was no difference between the two groups in the primary end point of OS.[88]

The recently completed ESPAC-4 trial randomized patients with resected pancreatic cancer to gemcitabine alone versus gemcitabine/capecitabine. Seven hundred and thirty patients with R0/R1 resection were evaluable for the primary end point of overall survival. The median survival for patients receiving adjuvant gemcitabine and capecitabine was 28 months compared to 25.5 months in the gemcitabine-alone arm. Estimated overall survival was 80.5% (95% CI 76.0 to 84.3) at 12 months and 52.1% (46.7 to 57.2) at 24 months in the gemcitabine group and 84.1% (79.9 to 87.5) at 12 months and 53.8% (48.4 to 58.8) at 24 months in the gemcitabine plus capecitabine group. Although clinically significant toxicities were low in both arms, the rates of grade 3 to 4 diarrhea, infection, neutropenia, and hand–foot syndrome were statistically higher in the combined chemotherapy arm. These data suggest that adjuvant gemcitabine and capecitabine may be a reasonable alternative to single-agent gemcitabine. The focus of future European adjuvant therapies for resectable pancreatic cancer has centered on finding the ideal combination of systemic agents.[93]

Modern Studies: Adjuvant Chemoradiation

In the United States, the GITSG trial laid the foundation for CRT as the predominant adjuvant treatment modality. The RTOG/Gastrointestinal Intergroup trial 9704 was a phase III randomized study comparing adjuvant 5-FU–based chemotherapy to gemcitabine-based chemotherapy, with both regimens followed by CRT. Four hundred fifty-one patients with resected pancreatic cancer were randomized to continuous infusion 5-FU (250 mg/m²/d) or gemcitabine (1,000 mg/m² weekly) for 3 weeks prior to CRT and 12 weeks after CRT. CRT in both groups consisted of 50.4 Gy delivered with continuous infusion 5-FU (250 mg/m²/d).[75] Prospective quality assurance of all radiation therapy plans was required. This trial was powered to demonstrate a survival benefit for the entire cohort and for the subgroup of patients with pancreatic head lesions. On initial analysis of the pancreatic head subgroup (n = 388), a nonsignificant trend toward improved median and 3-year OS was seen in the gemcitabine arm: 20.5 versus 16.9 months and 31% versus 22%, respectively. However, a higher incidence of grade 3 or higher hematologic toxicity was also seen in the gemcitabine group, with no significant differences seen in severe nonhematologic toxicities.

An update of this trial reported median and 5-year OS rates in patients with pancreatic head tumors of 20.5 months and 22% in those who received gemcitabine, compared with 17.2 months and 18% in those who received 5-FU. On multivariate analysis, in the subgroup of patients with pancreatic head lesions who received gemcitabine, there was a nonsignificant trend toward improved OS (P = .08).[89,90]

A secondary aim of RTOG-9704 was to assess the ability of postresection CA19-9 levels to predict survival. When CA19-9 levels were analyzed in a cohort of 385 patients as a

dichotomized variable (<180 IU/mL vs. ≥180 IU/mL, ≤90 IU/mL vs. >90 IU/mL), there was a significant survival difference favoring patients with CA19-9 levels of <180 IU/mL. This corresponded to a 72% reduction in the risk of death.[52] Unlike preceding randomized CRT studies, a major strength of the RTOG study was the rigorous, centralized quality control of radiation therapy techniques and delivery. A recent analysis demonstrated that patients treated per study guidelines had a significant survival advantage, indicating the importance of centralized review and treatment technique in this disease.[72]

The high rates of local failure and need for more efficacious systemic therapy, as well as controversy surrounding the role of CRT is resected patients, led to the design of the current RTOG-0848/EORTC trial. This trial randomly assigns patients with resected pancreatic head adenocarcinoma (stratified based on CA19-9 level, nodal involvement, and margin status) to receive treatment with gemcitabine alone for 5 cycles. If no progression is seen on restaging following the completion of systemic therapy, patients are further randomized either to receive an additional cycle of chemotherapy (for a total of 6 cycles) or to receive CRT (50.4 Gy with concurrent capecitabine or 5-FU) using modern techniques and central radiation therapy quality assurance. This trial seeks to evaluate the role of CRT in the era of modern chemotherapy, particularly in patients who do not experience early disease progression. (https://clinicaltrials.gov/ct2/show/NCT01013649)

Neoadjuvant Therapy

Even after undergoing curative resection for pancreatic cancer, 80% to 85% of patients will recur. In addition, positive margins or nodal disease increases this rate of recurrence to approximately 90%.[77,94] The use of neoadjuvant therapy offers an alternative approach to improve on these figures for several reasons:

1. Approximately one-third of patients experience a significant delay or do not receive adjuvant therapy following resection.[49,95,96]
2. Twenty percent to 40% of patients will be spared the morbidity of resection as their metastatic disease becomes clinically apparent during course of neoadjuvant therapy.[97–99]
3. Preoperative therapy could theoretically be less toxic and more effective as the chemotherapy and radiation would be given without the postsurgical issues of small bowel in the radiation field, decreased oxygenation and decreased drug delivery to the remaining tumor bed.[100,101]
4. Patients with local, borderline, and unresectable lesions may be able to be downstaged to allow for surgical resection and sterilization of the operative region, which potentially facilitates R0 resection and reduces the risk of spread during surgical manipulation.

Neoadjuvant Chemoradiation

Unlike with adjuvant therapy, no phase III randomized trials of neoadjuvant CRT in resectable pancreatic lesions have been conducted, and the vast majority of data come from phase II and retrospective studies.[102] At the MD Anderson Cancer Center, multiple trials of neoadjuvant CRT with a variety of radiosensitizers have been performed.[103–107]

A review of the Surveillance, Epidemiology, and End Results (SEER) database supports the use of neoadjuvant treatment. This analysis included 3,885 patients treated for resectable pancreatic cancer: 70 patients (2%) received neoadjuvant EBRT, 1,478 (38%) received adjuvant EBRT, and 2,337 (60%) were treated with surgery alone. Given that the SEER database does not provide information on administration of chemotherapy, this variable could not be assessed. Median OS was 23 months in patients receiving neoadjuvant EBRT, 17 months with adjuvant EBRT, and 12 months in the surgery-alone cohort.[108]

Despite the potential advantages and encouraging results using a neoadjuvant CRT approach, no randomized trial results exist comparing neoadjuvant to adjuvant therapy, and its role continues to be investigational. Therefore, in the future, the design of a trial with neoadjuvant radiotherapy might include induction chemotherapy in analogy to the current treatment strategies for LAPC as distant progression during neoadjuvant therapy is a more substantial problem.[109] With respect to chemoradiation, the first RCT phase II study comparing immediate surgery (arm A) with surgery after neoadjuvant chemoradiotherapy (arm B) for (potentially) resectable tumors was reported. Of note, the experimental arm started with chemoradiotherapy without induction chemotherapy. Simultaneous chemotherapy was gemcitabine 300 mg/m² and cisplatin 30 mg/m² weekly in weeks 1, 2, 4, and 5 of radiotherapy. Conventionally fractionated, 3DCRT included a tightly restricted elective nodal volume to a dose of 50.4 Gy and 55.8 Gy to the tumor. The trial under-recruited (73/254 planned patients) with considerable impact on statistical power. However, an important finding is that neoadjuvant therapy was well tolerated with only 7% grade 4 leukopenia and 3% grade 4 thrombocytopenia. No grade 4 gastrointestinal toxicity was observed but grade 3 nausea and vomiting was seen in 35% which was attributed to cisplatin. Resections were R0 in 67% versus 90% in arm A versus arm B. Postoperative complications were not more frequent after chemoradiotherapy compared to immediate surgery. At intention-to-treat analysis, OS was not different; at per-protocol analysis, mOS was 18 versus 25 months in arm A versus arm B (*P* >.05). After chemoradiotherapy, a trend for fewer local recurrences as the first site of progression was observed. Four versus eight patients (Arm A vs. B) had distant metastasis between randomization and laparotomy.[109]

Neoadjuvant Chemotherapy

With recent data demonstrating efficacy of combination chemotherapy in the metastatic setting, there has been growing interest to assess these agents in less advanced disease. The ongoing Southwest Oncology Group (SWOG) phase II study is comparing neoadjuvant gemcitabine and nab-paclitaxel to modified 5-FU, leucovorin, and irinotecan (m-FOLFIRNOX) for resectable pancreatic adenocarcinoma. The goal of this study is to identify the superior arm to test in a larger randomized trial. (https://clinicaltrials.gov/show/NCT02562716)

Therapy for Locally Advanced Carcinoma

Approximately 30% of patients present with locally advanced carcinoma of the pancreas, comprising a group of patients with an intermediate prognosis between resectable and metastatic disease. These patients have pancreatic tumors that are defined as surgically unresectable but have no evidence of distant metastases. A tumor is usually considered to be unresectable if it has one of the following features:

1. Distant metastases
2. Encasement or occlusion of the SMV or SMV/portal or vein confluence that is not amenable to reconstruction, contact with the most proximal draining jejunal branch into the SMV
3. ≥180 degree involvement of the SMA, celiac axis, first jejunal SMA branch, or aorta or celiac axis involvement with a body or tail lesion

Recent advances in surgical technique allow for resection of selected patients with tumors involving the SMV.[41,110] Treatment with radiation and chemotherapy increases median survival for patients with locally advanced cancers to approximately 8 to 14 months but rarely results in long-term survival. The therapeutic options of patients with locally advanced pancreatic cancer include chemotherapy alone,

CRT, intraoperative radiotherapy (IORT), and stereotactic body radiation therapy (SBRT). In evaluating the results of these various therapies, it is useful to remember that a median survival of 3 to 6 months has been reported for this subset of patients undergoing palliative gastric or biliary bypass only.[111]

PROSPECTIVE TRIALS

Prospective trials have evaluated the role of EBRT versus CRT, variations in CRT regimens, and CRT versus chemotherapy alone (Table 63.5). The Mayo Clinic undertook an early randomized trial in the 1960s in which 64 patients with locally unresectable, nonmetastatic stomach, large bowel, and pancreas adenocarcinoma received 35 to 40 Gy of EBRT alone or with concurrent bolus 5-FU (45 mg/kg). A significant survival advantage was seen for patients receiving EBRT with 5-FU versus EBRT only (10.4 vs. 6.3 months).[112]

The GITSG followed with a similar study comparing EBRT alone to EBRT with concurrent and maintenance 5-FU. One hundred and ninety-four eligible patients with surgically confirmed unresectable and nonmetastatic pancreatic adenocarcinoma were randomized to receive 60-Gy split-course EBRT alone, 40-Gy split-course EBRT with 2 to 3 cycles of concurrent bolus 5-FU chemotherapy (500 mg/m²), or 60-Gy split-course EBRT using a similar chemotherapy regimen. Patients in the latter groups received 2 years' maintenance 5-FU (500 mg/m²) after EBRT completion. The EBRT-alone arm was closed early as a result of an inferior survival rate. The 1-year survival rate in the two combined modality therapy arms was roughly 40% (with no statistical difference between CRT arms) versus 11% in the EBRT-alone arm.[113]

The Eastern Oncology Group's trial ECOG-8282 randomized 114 patients to EBRT alone (59.4 Gy) with or without continuous infusion 5-FU (1,000 mg/m²/d) on days 2 to 5 and 28 to 31 and mitomycin-C (10 mg/m²) on day 2. There was no difference in response rates, DFS, or OS with the addition of concurrent chemotherapy. Higher rates of toxicity, primarily hematologic, were noted in the CRT group.[114]

Further studies sought to determine a more efficacious CRT regimen. A second GITSG trial randomized 157 and analyzed results for 143 eligible patients with unresectable disease to 60-Gy split-course EBRT with concurrent and maintenance 5-FU (500 mg/m²) (as in the prior GITSG trial) or 40-Gy continuous course radiation with weekly, concurrent doxorubicin chemotherapy (10 mg/m²), followed by maintenance doxorubicin and 5-FU. A significant increase in treatment-related toxicity was seen in the doxorubicin arm, with no survival difference observed between the two groups (median survival 8.5 vs. 7.6 months). No clinical benefit was seen in substituting doxorubicin for 5-FU.[115]

As studies emerged demonstrating significant survival advantages with gemcitabine-based chemotherapy in the metastatic setting, it was incorporated into the locally advanced setting. A trial from Taipei randomized 34 patients to EBRT with concurrent 5-FU (500 mg/m²) or gemcitabine (600 mg/m²). Patients received 50.4- to 61.2-Gy EBRT and maintenance gemcitabine (1,000 mg/m²) at the completion of CRT. Median OS and time to progression were prolonged in the gemcitabine arm: 14.5 months and 7.1 months (gemcitabine) versus 6.7 months and 2.7 months (5-FU). There were no observed differences in grade 3 or 4 toxicity or hospitalization days between the two arms. Study criticisms include the small number of patients and relatively poor outcomes in the 5-FU arm compared with historical controls.[116]

A number of trials have compared CRT with chemotherapy alone. A subsequent GITSG trial compared combination streptozocin, mitomycin-C, and 5-FU (SMF) chemotherapy to chemoradiation with 5-FU. Forty-three patients were randomized to

TABLE 63.5 PROSPECTIVE RANDOMIZED TRIALS FOR LOCALLY ADVANCED, UNRESECTABLE PANCREATIC CANCER

Series (Reference)	Number of Patients	Median Survival (Month)	Local Progression (%)	1-Year (%)	18-Month (est %)
EBRT Versus CRT					
Mayo Clinic[112]					
EBRT (35–40 Gy/3–4 weeks) alone	32	6.3	NA	6	6
EBRT (35–40 Gy/3–4 weeks) + 5-FU	32	10.4	NA	22	13
GITSG[113]					
EBRT (60 Gy/10 weeks) alone	25	5.3	24	10	5
EBRT (40 Gy/6 weeks) + 5-FU	83	9.7	26	35	20
EBRT (60 Gy/10 weeks) + 5-FU	86	9.3	27	46	20
ECOG[114]					
EBRT (59.4 Gy) alone	49	7.1	NA	NA	NA
EBRT (59.5 Gy) + 5-FU/MMC	55	8.4	NA	NA	NA
Variations in CRT Regimen					
GITSG[115]					
EBRT (60 Gy/10 weeks) + 5-FU	73	8.5	58 (first site)	33	15
EBRT (40 Gy/4 weeks) + doxorubicin	70	7.6	51 (first site)	27	17
Taipei[116]					
EBRT (50.4–61.2 Gy) + 5-FU	16	6.7	56	31	0 (2 y)
EBRT (50.4–61.2 Gy) + gemcitabine	18	14.5	34	56	15 (2 y)
CRT versus Chemotherapy					
GITSG[117,118]					
EBRT (54 Gy/6 weeks) + 5-FU and SMF	22	9.7	45 (first site)	41	18
SMF alone	21	7.4	48 (first site)	19	0
ECOG[119]					
EBRT (40 Gy/4 weeks) + 5-FU	47	8.3	32	26	11
5-FU alone	44	8.2	32	32	21
FFCD/SFRO[120]					
EBRT (60 Gy) + 5-FU/CDDP	59	8.6	NA	32	NA
Gemcitabine alone	60	13	NA	53	NA
ECOG[121]					
EBRT (50.4 Gy) + gemcitabine	34	11.1	12 (first site)	50	29
Gemcitabine alone	37	9.2	30 (first site)	32	11
LAP07[122]					
Chemotherapy	136	16.5	46		
Chemotherapy then EBRT+ capecitabine	133	15.2	32		

CCDP, neoadjuvant cisplatin; CRT, chemoradiation; EBRT, external beam radiation therapy; ECOG, Eastern Cooperative Oncology Group; FFCD/SFRO, Fédération Francophone de Cancérologie Digestive/Société Francophone de Radiothérapie Oncologique; GITSG, Gastrointestinal Tumor Study Group; LAP, Locally advanced pancreas; MMC, mitomycin-C; NA, not available; SMF, streptozocin, mitomycin-C, and 5-flurouracil; 5-FU, 5-flurouracil.

receive SMF chemotherapy or 54 Gy of EBRT with 2 cycles of concurrent bolus 5-FU chemotherapy followed by adjuvant SMF chemotherapy. The chemoradiation arm demonstrated a significant survival advantage over the chemotherapy-alone arm (1-year survival 41% vs. 19%, respectively).[117]

In contrast, the ECOG reported no benefit to chemoradiation versus chemotherapy only. In this study, 191 patients with unresectable, nonmetastatic pancreatic or gastric adenocarcinoma were randomized to receive either 5-FU chemotherapy (600 mg/m^2) alone or 40-Gy EBRT with concurrent bolus 5-FU during week 1 (600 mg/m^2) followed by maintenance chemotherapy. Patients with locally recurrent disease as well as patients undergoing surgery with residual disease were eligible for this trial. In the 91 analyzable pancreatic patients, no survival difference was observed between the two groups (median survival 8.2 vs. 8.3 months).[119]

The FFCD/SFRO trial randomized 119 patients to CRT consisting of 60-Gy EBRT with continuous infusion 5-FU (300 mg/m^2/d) on days 1 to 5 for 6 weeks and intermittent CDDP (20 mg/m^2/d) on days 1 to 5 in weeks 1 and 5 with maintenance gemcitabine (1,000 mg/m^2) versus gemcitabine alone (1,000 mg/m^2). Survival was inferior in the CRT arm at 8.6 months compared with 13 months with gemcitabine alone. Higher grade 3 or 4 toxicity rates were observed in the CRT arm during CRT (36% vs. 22%) and maintenance chemotherapy phases (32% vs. 18%). This trial closed early because of poor accrual. Many criticize the inferior survival in the CRT arm, which is similar to early GITSG trials, despite use of continuous infusion chemotherapy and modern EBRT techniques.[120]

The ECOG published results from a randomized trial of CRT (50.4 Gy with concurrent gemcitabine: 600 mg/m^2/wk, weeks 1 to 5) versus gemcitabine alone (1,000 mg/m^2/wk). The trial closed early because of poor accrual. Analysis of the eligible, randomized 71 patients demonstrated no difference in progression-free survival; however, a survival benefit was seen in the CRT arm: 11.1 versus 9.2 months. This benefit came at the expense of higher grade 4 or 5 toxicity rates in the CRT arm (mainly hematologic) but with no difference in quality of life.[121]

A multicenter phase II study, the SCALOP trial, evaluated the role of gemcitabine-based or capecitabine-based CRT. All patients received 12 weeks of induction gemcitabine and capecitabine chemotherapy. Seventy-four patients were randomized and median OS in the capecitabine group was 15.2 months compared with 13.4 months in the gemcitabine arm ($P = .012$). More patients in the gemcitabine group than in the capecitabine group had grade 3 to 4 hematologic toxicity and grade 3 to 4 nonhematologic toxicity during CRT. These data suggest that concurrent capecitabine-based CRT may be preferable to gemcitabine-based CRT.[123]

More recently, the Locally Advanced Pancreas Cancer 07 (LAP07) trial was published. In this 2 × 2 randomization, all patients were initially randomized to gemcitabine or gemcitabine and erlotinib for 4 months. A second randomization was performed in patients with no evidence of progression to continuation of chemotherapy for an additional 2 months or chemoradiation. The primary study end point was overall survival. A total of 442 patients underwent the first randomization and 269 patients underwent the second randomization.

Interim analysis was performed after 221 patients died and early stopping rule for futility were reached. The median overall survival was 16.5 months for patient receiving systemic therapy and 15.2 months in the cohort receiving chemoradiation. Chemoradiation was associated with decreased local progression from 46% to 32% (P = .03)[122] and median delay to treatment reintroduction was 6.1 months (95% CI, 4.8 to 7.0 months) for the chemoradiotherapy group, significantly longer than the 3.7 months (95% CI, 3.0 to 4.6) for the chemotherapy group (P = .02). Some authors have critiqued the older chemotherapy regimen of gemcitabine alone, which has now largely been replaced with combination systemic therapies such as gemcitabine/nab-paclitaxel and m-FOLFIRINOX. In addition, quality of life analyses were not performed, which could have demonstrated a clinically meaningful difference between the arms.

With the recent publication of LAP07, many consider upfront chemotherapy with subsequent response assessment and directed CRT to facilitate selection of patients most likely to benefit from locoregional therapy as the current standard of care.

Borderline Resectable Disease

As surgery of the primary tumor remains the only potentially curative treatment for pancreatic cancer, neoadjuvant therapy has been evaluated to assess its ability to convert locally unresectable pancreatic cancer to resectable disease. Although the definition of borderline resectable disease is contentious, the National Comprehensive Cancer Network definition is accepted by many institutions (Table 63.2). Approximately 30% of patients with borderline resectable disease become resectable after neoadjuvant therapy.[124,125] Similarly, there appears to be higher rates of local control, R0 resection, and N0 disease in this patient subset after neoadjuvant therapy.[126–129]

A number of single-institution retrospective studies have evaluated this patient subset. An early study from the MD Anderson Cancer Center assessed 160 patients with borderline resectable disease. Patients received 50.4 Gy in 28 fractions or 30 Gy in 10 fractions with concurrent 5-FU, paclitaxel, gemcitabine, or capecitabine at radiosensitizing doses. Forty-one percent underwent pancreatectomy with margin-negative resection in 94%. Median survival in the 66 patients who completed preoperative therapy and surgery was 44 months, comparable to patients with initially resectable disease.[127]

A review from Fox Chase Cancer Center evaluated 109 patients who underwent resection of pancreatic adenocarcinoma with varying involvement of the portal vein or superior mesenteric vein as determined by CT. Patients received 5-FU or gemcitabine-based CRT. Median survival in the 74 patients who received preoperative therapy was 23 months compared with 15 months in the cohort undergoing upfront surgery. Preoperative CRT was associated with a higher rate of R0 resection and N0 disease.[128]

A smaller series from the University of Virginia reviewed the outcomes of 40 patients with borderline resectable disease. Patients received 50.4 Gy in 28 fractions or 50 Gy in 20 fractions with concurrent capecitabine. Forty-six percent of patients underwent surgery, with 75% undergoing an R0 resection. Patients undergoing surgery after neoadjuvant treatment had similar median survival rates as patients undergoing upfront surgery.[129]

The ECOG initiated a randomized phase II study of two neoadjuvant gemcitabine-containing regimens in patients with potentially resectable cancer. Patients received 50.4-Gy EBRT with weekly gemcitabine (500 mg/m²) or induction chemotherapy with gemcitabine (175 mg/m²), CDDP (20 mg/m²), and 5-FU (600 mg/m²) prior to CRT with 5-FU (225 mg/m²). All patients received adjuvant gemcitabine (1,000 mg/m²). This trial, the only randomized trial of borderline resectable pancreatic cancer, closed early because of poor accrual with 21 patients.[130] Although the subject of ongoing study, an approach utilizing neoadjuvant

chemoradiotherapy in patients with borderline resectable disease, in efforts to facilitate R0 resection, seems appropriate.

A systematic review and meta-analysis was performed of 18 studies with neoadjuvant chemotherapy or CRT with a total of 959 patients evaluating posttreatment response rates. The following response rates were achieved: CR, PR, SD, and PD were observed in 2.8%, 28.7%, 45.9%, and 16.9%, respectively. The weighted frequency of resected patients was 65.3% who achieved a median OS of 25.9 months. In contrast, patients without resection had a median OS of 11.9 months and the total group of 17.9 months.[131]

Dose Escalation

Given the limited tolerance of normal tissue in the upper abdomen (liver, kidney, spinal cord, and bowel) to EBRT, total doses of only 45 to 54 Gy in 25 to 30 Gy fractions have traditionally been administered. For an unresectable tumor, this dose of radiation is inadequate, as demonstrated by the high rates of local tumor progression and poor survival seen in both prospective and retrospective studies. Local progression as first site of failure occurred in 58% of patients treated to 60 Gy with concurrent 5-FU in the second GITSG trial.[115] Similarly, the Mayo Clinic reported a local recurrence rate of 72% for 122 patients with unresectable pancreatic cancer treated with an EBRT dose of 40 to 60 Gy.[132] Attempts have been made to evaluate whether increasing dose of radiation may improve outcomes through 3DCRT, IORT, IMRT, and stereotactic body radiotherapy (SBRT).

In a report from Thomas Jefferson University Hospital, 46 evaluable patients with unresectable disease by laparotomy were treated with 63- to 70-Gy EBRT with or without chemotherapy. Despite high-dose EBRT, the local recurrence rate was 78%.[133]

IORT is an alternative method to deliver higher radiation doses. This technique allows for administration of a single high dose of radiotherapy with the advantage of enabling healthy tissues to be displaced and shielded from radiation. IORT has been utilized postoperatively and in treatment of locally advanced disease. Institutional reports and a randomized trial have shown that surgery followed by IORT yields lower rates of locoregional recurrence; however, no significant difference in survival has been seen.[134–137] IORT has also been evaluated in patients with unresectable disease.[138,139] A study from investigators at Massachusetts General Hospital reported the results of 150 patients with unresectable pancreatic cancer treated with IORT, EBRT, and chemotherapy. Although the study spanned nearly 25 years, it demonstrated that long-term survival is possible for patients with unresectable pancreatic cancer. Furthermore, this study shows that postoperative and late treatment-related toxicity rates were acceptable.[139,140] A lower incidence of local recurrence in most series and improved median survival in some have been reported with these techniques when compared with conventional external beam irradiation, but it is uncertain whether this is due to treatment superiority or case selection.[132]

Advances in radiation technique and delivery, such as IMRT and SBRT, also enable dose escalation and potential sparing of normal tissues. IMRT is a technique that breaks up a typical radiation treatment field into smaller beamlets. It is implemented either as dynamic IMRT (collimating leaves move in and out of the radiation beam path during treatment) or as "step-and-shoot" IMRT (leaves change field shape while the machine is off). The cumulative effect is that the prescription dose conforms around delineated target volumes, significantly reducing doses to adjacent normal tissues. This technology has increasingly been used in a number of gastrointestinal malignancies, including pancreatic cancer. Early clinical data support both the feasibility of this technique and its potential for reducing acute gastrointestinal toxicity.[141–143]

An analysis from the University of Maryland evaluated 46 patients treated with IMRT and concurrent 5-FU–based chemotherapy. Acute toxicities in these patients were compared with those in a control group enrolled in RTOG-9704 who received conventional 3D treatment. There was a statistically significant reduction in acute grade 3 or 4 gastrointestinal toxicity in the patients who received radiotherapy via IMRT compared with those who received 3DCRT.[143] IMRT can also result in a significant reduction of dose to normal structures, including the liver, kidneys, stomach, and small bowel.[142] This may allow alternate novel systemic agents to be administered with radiotherapy.[141]

Although IMRT can reduce the dose to surrounding normal tissues, it also allows the opportunity for dose escalation. A phase I/II study by Ben Josef et al attempted to define the maximum tolerated radiation dose via IMRT in combination with gemcitabine for unresectable pancreas cancer. Fifty patients were accrued and dose-limiting toxicity was seen at 55Gy. Median survival was 14.8 months and 12 patients subsequently underwent resection.[144]

Another technique for dose escalation in the treatment of pancreatic cancers is SBRT, which involves the delivery of high dose per fraction radiation treatments over a small number of fractions (generally 1 to 5 treatments), utilizing techniques that allow very highly conformal dose delivery of external beam radiotherapy. The postulated advantage of SBRT is potentially improving local control through the delivery of ablative doses of radiation, while minimizing associated side effects. Early experience and data using this technique are in the setting of locally advanced disease.[145,146] Stanford University has implemented an institutional protocol for the treatment of locally advanced pancreatic cancer using a 25-Gy single fraction with systemic therapy. This single, high dose of radiation has been estimated to result in delivery of a higher biologically equivalent dose compared with a more standard, protracted course of radiation therapy, albeit at the potential for increased risk of normal tissue injury. A report from these investigators described 77 patients who were treated with SBRT and found that freedom from local progression was 91% at 6 months and 84% at 12 months. No patients experienced grade 3 acute toxicity, and 9% had grade 3 or higher late toxicity.[146]

Based on these data, a prospective, multi-institutional phase II study was conducted utilizing 5 fraction SBRT with primary end point to achieve a lower rate of late grade 2+ toxicity than with single-fraction SBRT. Forty-nine patient received up to 3 doses of gemcitabine followed by 33 Gy in 5 fractions. The rate of grade 2+ late toxicity was 11% and 1-year freedom from local progression was 78%. Four patients (8%) subsequently underwent a margin-negative resection.[147]

A meta-analysis of 19 studies encompassing over 1,000 patients treated with SBRT demonstrated a 1-year local control rate of 72%. The rate of acute grade 3+ toxicity ranged from 0% to 36% and the rate of late grade 3+ toxicity did not exceed 11%.[148] Select series have demonstrated high rates of margin-negative resection in patients with borderline and unresectable pancreas cancer who ultimately underwent surgical resection.[149,150]

Ultimately, the role of IMRT and SBRT as well as integration with systemic therapy are ongoing areas of active investigation.

Chemoradiation Effects on Quality of Life

Pain, anorexia, fatigue, and cachexia are relatively common symptoms, which significantly impact a patient's quality of life. When using EBRT with or without chemotherapy, approximately 35% to 65% of patients will experience pain resolution as well as some improvement in cachexia and obstructive symptoms.[115,151,152] Definite but less dramatic improvements in performance status and anorexia may be observed as well.[151,152] Patient-reported quality of life (QOL) with SBRT in unresectable pancreas cancer demonstrates no change in QOL at pretreatment compared to 1-month follow-up but statistical and clinical improvements in pancreatic pain and body image at 1 month.[153] Palliation from therapy can take many weeks for maximal effect, and alternative treatments, such as biliary and duodenal stents, may provide more rapid relief of obstructive symptoms. Given the high mortality rate associated with pancreatic cancer, QOL should be a study end point in trials for these patients.

TARGETED THERAPIES AND FUTURE DIRECTIONS

There is much room for improvement in the diagnosis and treatment of pancreatic cancer. Screening of high-risk individuals may allow for detection of disease in earlier disease stages by means of novel imaging methods or assessment of serum biomarkers.[154,155] As the biologic basis of cancer is better understood, the successful use of cancer-specific targeted therapies in other cancers supports the need to identify new targets and better predictors of response to therapy in pancreatic cancer.

There is evidence of additive or synergistic effects for several targeted agents (such as antibodies against EGFR and vascular endothelial growth factor [VEGF] receptor) with both chemotherapy and radiation therapy, making these topics of investigation. These targeted agents have been studied most extensively in the metastatic setting prior to evaluation in locally advanced and resectable disease. Currently, the only targeted agent that has shown a modest statistically significant survival benefit in the metastatic setting compared to chemotherapy alone is erlotinib, an anti-EGFR tyrosine kinase inhibitor. However, the survival benefit with addition of erlotinib is small, with median survival increased from 5.9 to 6.2 months and 1-year survival improvement from 17% to 24%.[156] The clinical significance of this difference has been questioned by investigators and treating physicians.

Another EGFR/*HER-1* inhibitor, cetuximab, initially showed promising phase II results in the metastatic setting. Efficacy was initially seen with the combination of cetuximab and EBRT in the treatment of locally advanced squamous cell carcinoma of the head and neck and subsequently tested in a phase III trial.[157] However, in pancreatic cancer, a phase III randomized study of gemcitabine plus cetuximab versus gemcitabine plus placebo (Southwest Oncology Group S0205) as first-line therapy in locally advanced, unresectable, or metastatic disease enrolled over 700 patients from the United States and Canada. No survival improvement was seen with the addition of cetuximab to gemcitabine (6.3 months gemcitabine plus cetuximab vs. 5.9 months gemcitabine alone). Even among patients tested for EGFR expression (90% specimens positive for expression), no benefit to cetuximab was seen in this patient subgroup.[158] An additional phase II study evaluated the efficacy and safety of multiagent chemotherapy in combination with cetuximab. Sixty-nine patients with locally advanced pancreatic cancer received cetuximab, gemcitabine, and oxaliplatin followed by cetuximab, capecitabine, and radiotherapy. Diagnostic cytology specimens were stained for Smad4 (Dpc4) expression. Median overall survival was 19.2 months, and the pattern of failure for patients with Smad4 (Dpc4) expression was primarily local, rather than distant, disease failure.[159] The addition of EGFR inhibitors in localized disease is currently being evaluated in phase I and phase II trials.

VEGF inhibitors bind to receptors involved in tumor growth via vasculogenesis and angiogenesis pathways. Preclinical data have shown that inhibition of VEGF has radiosensitizing effects. Initially, promising results in the metastatic setting, however, have ultimately not shown a benefit from the addition of an anti-VEGF antibody to chemotherapy. A phase II trial of the combination of gemcitabine and bevacizumab in 52 treated patients with advanced pancreatic cancer showed a response rate of 21%, a median progression-free survival of 5.4 months, and median overall survival of 8.8 months.[160] In response to these positive results, a phase III randomized study of gemcitabine plus bevacizumab versus placebo (Cancer and Leukemia Group B CALGB-80303) was initiated. No significant difference was observed in OS or PFS.[161] Bevacizumab has also been evaluated in combination with radiotherapy. An initial phase I study of radiotherapy, capecitabine, and bevacizumab led to incorporation in the phase II setting in patients with locally advanced pancreatic cancer (RTOG-0411).[162] Eighty-two patients were treated with radiotherapy to the gross tumor, capecitabine (825 mg/m²), and bevacizumab (5 mg/kg on days 1, 15, 29) followed by adjuvant gemcitabine (1,000 mg/m²). The median and 1-year survival rates were 11.9 months and 47%, respectively. These results were similar to prior RTOG trials of locally advanced pancreatic cancer.[163] An additional phase II trial assessed the efficacy of full-dose gemcitabine (1000 mg/m²), bevacizumab (10 mg/kg), and radiotherapy to 36 Gy (in 2.4 Gy fractions) with maintenance gemcitabine and bevacizumab in patients with unresected tumors with no evidence of disease progression. Median progression-free and overall survival were 9.9 and 11.8 months, respectively.[164] The incorporation of bevacizumab with radiotherapy has not led to profound improvements in treatment outcomes compared to 5-FU–based CRT.

Although improvements with targeted agents have been modest, other pathways are being evaluated. Pancreatic cells deficient in *BRCA* repair pathways are sensitive to poly-adenosine diphosphate-ribose polymerase (PARP) inhibitors. PARP inhibitors have been evaluated in ovarian and breast cancer, with response rates of 40%; clinical trials of PARP inhibitors in treatment of pancreatic cancer are under way.[7] Other therapeutic agents under evaluation include hedgehog pathway inhibitors, multikinase inhibitors (sorafenib), and agents targeting v-src sarcoma, γ-secretase, stem cell factor receptor (c-kit), secreted protein acidic and rich in cysteine, mitogen-activated protein kinase, mesothelin, *RAS*, prostate stem cell antigen, tumor necrosis factor-α, mucin-1, mammalian target of rapamycin, tumor necrosis factor superfamily member 10, and type 1 insulin-like growth factor receptor.[7,165]

There is growing interest in immunotherapies to target the heterogeneous pancreas tumor and immunosuppressive microenvironment. A number of clinical trials in pancreas cancer alone or advanced solid tumors have been completed or ongoing evaluating the role of immune checkpoint monotherapy, dual checkpoint blockade, immune checkpoint in combination with vaccine therapy, and in combination with cytotoxic and other systemic therapies.[166,167]

Summary

Treatment of pancreatic cancer remains a challenge in oncology. Despite advances in many aspects of oncologic evaluation and management, including preoperative evaluation, surgical techniques, perioperative care, systemic therapy, and radiotherapy, the 5-year OS rate for patients with resectable pancreatic cancer remains around 20%. Local tumor control has been improved by the use of specialized radiation techniques, allowing safe dose escalation. Even with these techniques, it is not clear that a survival benefit is achieved given the proclivity of metastases in this malignancy. Similarly, even in patients with metastatic disease, morbidity and mortality associated with locoregional progression remains a major cause of morbidity and mortality. Further advances in systemic therapies, study of the optimal sequencing of therapies, earlier detection of disease, and development of new and novel therapeutic options are urgently needed in the treatment of this formidable disease. Quality of life should be considered a paramount end point in the care and protocol design of clinical trials for these patients. Significant improvements in long-term survival will likely be achieved through ongoing attempts at exploitation of the malignancy's basic biologic anomalies.

REFERENCES

1. American Joint Committee on Cancer. *AJCC cancer staging manual*. New York: Springer-Verlag, 2010.
2. Siegel R, Naishadham D, Jemal A. Cancer statistics, 2017. *CA Cancer J Clin* 2017;67(1):7–30.
3. Geer RJ, Brennan MF. Prognostic indicators for survival after resection of pancreatic adenocarcinoma. *Am J Surg* 1993;165(1):68–73.
4. Yeo CJ, et al. Pancreaticoduodenectomy for cancer of the head of the pancreas. 201 patients. *Ann Surg* 1995;221(6):721–733.
5. Wagner M, et al. Curative resection is the single most important factor determining outcome in patients with pancreatic adenocarcinoma. *Br J Surg* 2004; 91(5):586–594.
6. Lim JE, Chien MW, Earle CC. Prognostic factors following curative resection for pancreatic adenocarcinoma: a population-based, linked database analysis of 396 patients. *Ann Surg* 2003;237(1):74–85.
7. Ryan DP, et al. Pancreatic adenocarcinoma. *N Engl J Med* 2014;371:1039–1049.
8. Ries LA, et al. The annual report to the nation on the status of cancer, 1973–1997, with a special section on colorectal cancer. *Cancer* 2000;88(10): 2398–2424.
9. Brentnall TA. Management strategies for patients with hereditary pancreatic cancer. *Curr Treat Options Oncol* 2005;6(5):437–445.
10. Klein AP, et al. Familial pancreatic cancer. *Cancer J* 2001;7(4):266–273.
11. Maisonneuve P, Lowenfels AB. Epidemiology of pancreatic cancer: an update. *Dig Dis* 2010;28(4–5):645–656.
12. Lowenfels AB, et al. Pancreatitis and the risk of pancreatic cancer. International Pancreatitis Study Group. *N Engl J Med* 1993;328(20):1433–1437.
13. Willett CG, et al. Locally advanced pancreatic cancer. *J Clin Oncol* 2005;23(20):4538–4544.
14. Kinney T. Evidence-based imaging of pancreatic malignancies. *Surg Clin North Am* 2010;90(2):235–249.
15. Karmazanovsky G, et al. Pancreatic head cancer: accuracy of CT in determination of resectability. *Abdom Imaging* 2005;30(4):488–500.
16. Hunt GC, Faigel DO. Assessment of EUS for diagnosing, staging, and determining resectability of pancreatic cancer: a review. *Gastrointest Endosc* 2002;55(2):232–237.
17. Rosch T, et al. Endoscopic ultrasound in pancreatic tumor diagnosis. *Gastrointest Endosc* 1991;37(3):347–352.
18. Brugge WR, Van Dam J. Pancreatic and biliary endoscopy. *N Engl J Med* 1999;341(24):1808–1816.
19. Hariharan D, et al. The role of laparoscopy and laparoscopic ultrasound in the preoperative staging of pancreatico-biliary cancers—a meta-analysis. *Eur J Surg Oncol* 2010;36(10):941–948.
20. Fernandez-del Castillo C, Rattner DW, Warshaw AL. Further experience with laparoscopy and peritoneal cytology in the staging of pancreatic cancer. *Br J Surg* 1995;82(8):1127–1129.
21. Bipat S, et al. Ultrasonography, computed tomography and magnetic resonance imaging for diagnosis and determining resectability of pancreatic adenocarcinoma: a meta-analysis. *J Comput Assist Tomogr* 2005;29(4):438–445.
22. Sica GT, Ji H, Ros PR. Computed tomography and magnetic resonance imaging of hepatic metastases. *Clin Liver Dis* 2002;6(1):165–179.
23. Lemke AJ, et al. Retrospective digital image fusion of multidetector CT and 18F-FDG PET: clinical value in pancreatic lesions—a prospective study with 104 patients. *J Nucl Med* 2004;45(8):1279–1286.
24. Sachelarie I, et al. Integrated PET-CT: evidence-based review of oncology indications. *Oncology (Williston Park)* 2005;19(4):481–490; discussion 490–492, 495–496.
25. Rose DM, et al. 18Fluorodeoxyglucose-positron emission tomography in the management of patients with suspected pancreatic cancer. *Ann Surg* 1999;229(5):729–738.
26. Grassetto G, Rubello D. Role of FDG-PET/CT in diagnosis, staging, response to treatment, and prognosis of pancreatic cancer. *Am J Clin Oncol* 2011;34(2):111–114.
27. Michelassi F, et al. Experience with 647 consecutive tumors of the duodenum, ampulla, head of the pancreas, and distal common bile duct. *Ann Surg* 1989;210(4):544–556.
28. Rozenblum E, et al. Tumor-suppressive pathways in pancreatic carcinoma. *Cancer Res* 1997;57(9):1731–1734.
29. Shaib Y, et al. The impact of curative intent surgery on the survival of pancreatic cancer patients: a U.S. Population-based study. *Am J Gastroenterol* 2007;102(7):1377–1382.
30. Whipple AO, Parsons WB, Mullins CR. Treatment of carcinoma of the ampulla of Vater. *Ann Surg* 1935;102(4):763–779.
31. Pellegrini CA, et al. An analysis of the reduced morbidity and mortality rates after pancreaticoduodenectomy. *Arch Surg* 1989;124(7):778–781.
32. Trede M, Schwall G, Saeger HD. Survival after pancreatoduodenectomy. 118 consecutive resections without an operative mortality. *Ann Surg* 1990; 211(4):447–458.
33. Cameron JL, et al. One thousand consecutive pancreaticoduodenectomies. *Ann Surg* 2006;244(1):10–15.
34. Brozzetti S, et al. Surgical treatment of pancreatic head carcinoma in elderly patients. *Arch Surg* 2006;141(2):137–142.
35. Sohn TA, et al. Should pancreaticoduodenectomy be performed in octogenarians? *J Gastrointest Surg* 1998;2(3):207–216.
36. Hodul P, et al. Age is not a contraindication to pancreaticoduodenectomy. *Am Surg* 2001;67(3):270–276.
37. Bilimoria KY, et al. National failure to operate on early stage pancreatic cancer. *Ann Surg* 2007;246(2):173–180.
38. Bilimoria KY, et al. Multimodality therapy for pancreatic cancer in the U.S.: utilization, outcomes, and the effect of hospital volume. *Cancer* 2007;110(6):1227–1234.
39. Bilimoria KY, et al. Assessment of pancreatic cancer care in the United States based on formally developed quality indicators. *J Natl Cancer Inst* 2009;101(12):848–859.
40. Sosa JA, et al. Importance of hospital volume in the overall management of pancreatic cancer. *Ann Surg* 1998;228(3):429–438.

41. Tseng JF, et al. Venous resection in pancreatic cancer surgery. *Best Pract Res Clin Gastroenterol* 2006;20(2):349–364.

42. Martin RC II, et al. Arterial and venous resection for pancreatic adenocarcinoma: operative and long-term outcomes. *Arch Surg* 2009;144(2):154–159.

43. Slidell MB, et al. Impact of total lymph node count and lymph node ratio on staging and survival after pancreatectomy for pancreatic adenocarcinoma: a large, population-based analysis. *Ann Surg Oncol* 2008;15(1):165–174.

44. Tomlinson JS, et al. Accuracy of staging node-negative pancreas cancer: a potential quality measure. *Arch Surg* 2007;142(8):767–724.

45. Yeo CJ, et al. Pancreaticoduodenectomy with or without distal gastrectomy and extended retroperitoneal lymphadenectomy for periampullary adenocarcinoma, part 2: randomized controlled trial evaluating survival, morbidity, and mortality. *Ann Surg* 2002;236(3):355–368.

46. Farnell MB, et al. A prospective randomized trial comparing standard pancreatoduodenectomy with pancreatoduodenectomy with extended lymphadenectomy in resectable pancreatic head adenocarcinoma. *Surgery* 2005;138(4):618–630.

47. Chang DK, et al. Margin clearance and outcome in resected pancreatic cancer. *J Clin Oncol* 2009;27(17):2855–2862.

48. Helm J, et al. Histologic characteristics enhance predictive value of American Joint Committee on Cancer staging in resectable pancreas cancer. *Cancer* 2009;115(18):4080–4089.

49. Sohn TA, et al. Resected adenocarcinoma of the pancreas—616 patients: results, outcomes, and prognostic indicators. *J Gastrointest Surg* 2000;4(6):567–579.

50. Raut CP, et al. Impact of resection status on pattern of failure and survival after pancreaticoduodenectomy for pancreatic adenocarcinoma. *Ann Surg* 2007;246(1):52–60.

51. Kinsella TJ, et al. The impact of resection margin status and postoperative CA19-9 levels on survival and patterns of recurrence after postoperative high-dose radiotherapy with 5-FU-based concurrent chemotherapy for resectable pancreatic cancer. *Am J Clin Oncol* 2008;31(5):446–453.

52. Berger AC, et al. Postresection CA19-9 predicts overall survival in patients with pancreatic cancer treated with adjuvant chemoradiation: a prospective validation by RTOG 9704. *J Clin Oncol* 2008;26(36):5918–5922.

53. Ferrone CR, et al. Perioperative CA19-9 levels can predict stage and survival in patients with resectable pancreatic adenocarcinoma. *J Clin Oncol* 2006;24(18):2897–2902.

54. Hernandez JM, et al. CA19-9 velocity predicts disease-free survival and overall survival after pancreatectomy of curative intent. *J Gastrointest Surg* 2009;13(2):349–353.

55. Iqbal N, et al. A comparison of pancreaticoduodenectomy with pylorus preserving pancreaticoduodenectomy: a meta-analysis of 2822 patients. *Eur J Surg Oncol* 2008;34(11):1237–1245.

56. Diener MK, et al. Pylorus-preserving pancreaticoduodenectomy (pp Whipple) versus pancreaticoduodenectomy (classic Whipple) for surgical treatment of periampullary and pancreatic carcinoma. *Cochrane Database Syst Rev* 2011;5:CD006053.

57. Sussman LA, Christie R, Whittle DE. Laparoscopic excision of distal pancreas including insulinoma. *Aust N Z J Surg* 1996;66(6):414–416.

58. Kooby DA, Chu CK. Laparoscopic management of pancreatic malignancies. *Surg Clin North Am* 2010;90(2):427–446.

59. Kooby DA, et al. A multicenter analysis of distal pancreatectomy for adenocarcinoma: is laparoscopic resection appropriate? *J Am Coll Surg* 2010;210(5):779–787.

60. Kooby DA, et al. Left-sided pancreatectomy: a multicenter comparison of laparoscopic and open approaches. *Ann Surg* 2008;248(3):438–446.

61. Mabrut JY, et al. Laparoscopic pancreatic resection: results of a multicenter European study of 127 patients. *Surgery* 2005;137(6):597–605.

62. Fernandez-Cruz L, et al. Curative laparoscopic resection for pancreatic neoplasms: a critical analysis from a single institution. *J Gastrointest Surg* 2007;11(12):1607–1622.

63. Gumbs AA, et al. Laparoscopic pancreatoduodenectomy: a review of 285 published cases. *Ann Surg Oncol* 2011;18(5):1335–1341.

64. Zureikat AH, et al. Robotic-assisted major pancreatic resection and reconstruction. *Arch Surg* 2011;146(3):256–261.

65. Kendrick ML, Cusati D. Total laparoscopic pancreaticoduodenectomy: feasibility and outcome in an early experience. *Arch Surg* 2010;145(1):19–23.

66. Tepper J, Nardi G, Sutt H. Carcinoma of the pancreas: review of MGH experience from 1963 to 1973. Analysis of surgical failure and implications for radiation therapy. *Cancer* 1976;37(3):1519–1524.

67. Griffin JF, et al. Patterns of failure after curative resection of pancreatic carcinoma. *Cancer* 1990;66(1):56–61.

68. Whittington R, et al. Adjuvant therapy of resected adenocarcinoma of the pancreas. *Int J Radiat Oncol Biol Phys* 1991;21(5):1137–1143.

69. Ozaki H. Improvement of pancreatic cancer treatment from the Japanese experience in the 1980s. *Int J Pancreatol* 1992;12(1):5–9.

70. Westerdahl J, Andren-Sandberg A, Ihse I. Recurrence of exocrine pancreatic cancer—local or hepatic? *Hepatogastroenterology* 1993;40(4):384–387.

71. Foo ML, et al. Patterns of failure in grossly resected pancreatic ductal adenocarcinoma treated with adjuvant irradiation ± 5 fluorouracil. *Int J Radiat Oncol Biol Phys* 1993;26(3):483–489.

72. Abrams RA, et al. Failure to adhere to protocol specified radiation therapy guidelines was associated with decreased survival in RTOG 9704-A phase III trial of adjuvant chemotherapy and chemoradiotherapy for patients with resected adenocarcinoma of the pancreas. *Int J Radiat Oncol Biol Phys* 2012;82(2):809–816.

73. Paulino AC, Latona C. Unresectable adenocarcinoma of the pancreas: patterns of failure and treatment results. *Cancer Invest* 2000;18(4):309–313.

74. Hattangadi JA, et al. Results and patterns of failure in patients treated with adjuvant combined chemoradiation therapy for resected pancreatic adenocarcinoma. *Cancer* 2009;115(16):3640–3650.

75. Regine WF, et al. Fluorouracil vs gemcitabine chemotherapy before and after fluorouracil-based chemoradiation following resection of pancreatic adenocarcinoma: a randomized controlled trial. *JAMA* 2008;299(9):1019–1026.

76. Allema JH, et al. Prognostic factors for survival after pancreaticoduodenectomy for patients with carcinoma of the pancreatic head region. *Cancer* 1995;75(8):2069–2076.

77. Willett CG, et al. Resection margins in carcinoma of the head of the pancreas. Implications for radiation therapy. *Ann Surg* 1993;217(2):144–148.

78. Goodman KA, Regine WF, Dawson LA, et al. Radiation Therapy Oncology Group consensus panel guidelines for the delineation of the clinical target volume in the postoperative treatment of pancreatic head cancer. *Int J Radiat Oncol Biol Phys* 2012;83(3):901–908. doi:10.1016/j.ijrobp.2012.01.022.

79. Allema JH, et al. Results of pancreaticoduodenectomy for ampullary carcinoma and analysis of prognostic factors for survival. *Surgery* 1995;117(3):247–253.

80. Kalser MH, Ellenberg SS. Pancreatic cancer. Adjuvant combined radiation and chemotherapy following curative resection. *Arch Surg* 1985;120(8):899–903.

81. Further evidence of effective adjuvant combined radiation and chemotherapy following curative resection of pancreatic cancer. Gastrointestinal Tumor Study Group. *Cancer* 1987;59(12):2006–2010.

82. Klinkenbijl JH, et al. Adjuvant radiotherapy and 5-fluorouracil after curative resection of cancer of the pancreas and periampullary region: phase III trial of the EORTC gastrointestinal tract cancer cooperative group. *Ann Surg* 1999;230(6):776–784.

83. Smeenk HG, et al. Long-term survival and metastatic pattern of pancreatic and periampullary cancer after adjuvant chemoradiation or observation: long-term results of EORTC trial 40891. *Ann Surg* 2007;246(5):734–740.

84. Neoptolemos JP, et al. Adjuvant chemoradiotherapy and chemotherapy in resectable pancreatic cancer: a randomised controlled trial. *Lancet* 2001;358(9293):1576–1585.

85. Neoptolemos JP, et al. A randomized trial of chemoradiotherapy and chemotherapy after resection of pancreatic cancer. *N Engl J Med* 2004;350(12):1200–1210.

86. Oettle H, et al. Adjuvant chemotherapy with gemcitabine vs observation in patients undergoing curative-intent resection of pancreatic cancer: a randomized controlled trial. *JAMA* 2007;297(3):267–277.

87. Neuhaus P, et al. CONKO-001: final results of the randomized, prospective, multicenter phase III trial of adjuvant chemotherapy with gemcitabine versus observation in patients with resected pancreatic cancer (PC). *J Clin Oncol* 2008;26:(abstr LBA4504).

88. Neoptolemos JP, et al. Adjuvant chemotherapy with fluorouracil plus folinic acid vs gemcitabine following pancreatic cancer resection: a randomized controlled trial. *JAMA* 2010;304(10):1073–1081.

89. Regine WF. Five-year results of the phase III intergroup trial (RTOG 97–04) of adjuvant pre- and postchemoradiation (CRT) 5-FU vs. gemcitabine (G) for resected pancreatic adenocarcinoma: implications for future international trial design. *Int J Radiat Oncol Biol Phys* 2009;75(3):S55–S56.

90. Regine WF, Winter KA, Abrams R. Fluorouracil-based chemoradiation with either gemcitabine or fluorouracil chemotherapy after resection of pancreatic adenocarcinoma: 5-year analysis of the U.S. Intergroup/RTOG 9704 phase III trial. *Ann Surg Oncol* 2011;18:1319–1326.

91. Mehta V, Fisher GA, Ford JM, et al. Adjuvant chemoradiotherapy for "unfavorable" carcinoma of the ampulla of Vater. *Arch Surg* 2001;136:65–69.

92. Ueno H, et al. A randomised phase III trial comparing gemcitabine with surgery-only in patients with resected pancreatic cancer: Japanese Study Group of Adjuvant Therapy for Pancreatic Cancer. *Br J Cancer* 2009;101(6):908–915.

93. Neoptolemos JP, Palmer DH, Ghaneh P, et al. Comparison of adjuvant gemcitabine and capecitabine with gemcitabine monotherapy in patients with resected pancreatic cancer (ESPAC-4): a multicentre, open-label, randomised, phase 3 trial. *Lancet* 2017;389:1011–1024.

94. Cameron JL, et al. Factors influencing survival after pancreaticoduodenectomy for pancreatic cancer. *Am J Surg* 1991;161(1):120–125.

95. Spitz FR, et al. Preoperative and postoperative chemoradiation strategies in patients treated with pancreaticoduodenectomy for adenocarcinoma of the pancreas. *J Clin Oncol* 1997;15(3):928–937.

96. Aloia TA, et al. Delayed recovery after pancreaticoduodenectomy: a major factor impairing the delivery of adjuvant therapy? *J Am Coll Surg* 2007;204(3):347–355.

97. Evans DB, et al. Preoperative chemoradiation strategies for localized adenocarcinoma of the pancreas. *J Hepatobiliary Pancreat Surg* 1998;5(3):242–250.

98. Raut CP, et al. Neoadjuvant therapy for resectable pancreatic cancer. *Surg Oncol Clin N Am* 2004;13(4):639–661.

99. Wayne JD, et al. Localized adenocarcinoma of the pancreas: the rationale for preoperative chemoradiation. *Oncologist* 2002;7(1):34–45.

100. White RR, Tyler DS. Neoadjuvant therapy for pancreatic cancer: the Duke experience. *Surg Oncol Clin N Am* 2004;13(4):675–684.

101. Cheng TY, et al. Effect of neoadjuvant chemoradiation on operative mortality and morbidity for pancreaticoduodenectomy. *Ann Surg Oncol* 2006;13(1):66–74.

102. Le Scodan R, et al. Preoperative chemoradiation in potentially resectable pancreatic adenocarcinoma: feasibility, treatment effect evaluation and prognostic factors, analysis of the SFRO-FFCD 9704 trial and literature review. *Ann Oncol* 2009;20(8):1387–1396.

103. Evans DB, et al. Preoperative chemoradiation and pancreaticoduodenectomy for adenocarcinoma of the pancreas. *Arch Surg* 1992;127(11):1335–1339.

104. Pisters PW, et al. Rapid-fractionation preoperative chemoradiation, pancreaticoduodenectomy, and intraoperative radiation therapy for resectable pancreatic adenocarcinoma. *J Clin Oncol* 1998;16(12):3843–3850.

105. Pisters PW, et al. Preoperative paclitaxel and concurrent rapid-fractionation radiation for resectable pancreatic adenocarcinoma: toxicities, histologic response rates, and event-free outcome. *J Clin Oncol* 2002;20(10):2537–2544.

106. Evans DB, et al. Preoperative gemcitabine-based chemoradiation for patients with resectable adenocarcinoma of the pancreatic head. *J Clin Oncol* 2008;26(21):3496–3502.

107. Varadhachary GR, et al. Preoperative gemcitabine and cisplatin followed by gemcitabine-based chemoradiation for resectable adenocarcinoma of the pancreatic head. *J Clin Oncol* 2008;26(21):3487–3495.

108. Stessin AM, Meyer JE, Sherr DL. Neoadjuvant radiation is associated with improved survival in patients with resectable pancreatic cancer: an analysis of data from the surveillance, epidemiology, and end results (SEER) registry. *Int J Radiat Oncol Biol Phys* 2008;72(4):1128–1133.

109. Golcher H, Brunner TB, Witzigmann H, et al. Neoadjuvant chemoradiation therapy with gemcitabine/cisplatin and surgery versus immediate surgery in resectable pancreatic cancer: results of the first prospective randomized phase II trial. *Strahlenther Onkol* 2015;191(1):7e16.

110. Leach SD, et al. Survival following pancreaticoduodenectomy with resection of the superior mesenteric-portal vein confluence for adenocarcinoma of the pancreatic head. *Br J Surg* 1998;85(5):611–617.

111. Gunderson LL, et al. Future role of radiotherapy as a component of treatment in biliopancreatic cancers. *Ann Oncol* 1999;10(Suppl 4):291–295.

112. Moertel CG, et al. Combined 5-fluorouracil and supervoltage radiation therapy of locally unresectable gastrointestinal cancer. *Lancet* 1969;2(7626):865–867.

113. Moertel CG, et al. Therapy of locally unresectable pancreatic carcinoma: a randomized comparison of high dose (6000 rads) radiation alone, moderate dose radiation (4000 rads + 5-fluorouracil), and high dose radiation +5-fluorouracil: the Gastrointestinal Tumor Study Group. *Cancer* 1981;48(8):1705–1710.

114. Cohen SJ, et al. A randomized phase III study of radiotherapy alone or with 5-fluorouracil and mitomycin-C in patients with locally advanced adenocarcinoma of the pancreas: Eastern Cooperative Oncology Group study E8282. *Int J Radiat Oncol Biol Phys* 2005;62(5):1345–1350.

115. Radiation therapy combined with Adriamycin or 5-fluorouracil for the treatment of locally unresectable pancreatic carcinoma. Gastrointestinal Tumor Study Group. *Cancer* 1985;56(11):2563–2568.

116. Li CP, et al. Concurrent chemoradiotherapy treatment of locally advanced pancreatic cancer: gemcitabine versus 5-fluorouracil, a randomized controlled study. *Int J Radiat Oncol Biol Phys* 2003;57(1):98–104.

117. Treatment of locally unresectable carcinoma of the pancreas: comparison of combined-modality therapy (chemotherapy plus radiotherapy) to chemotherapy alone. Gastrointestinal Tumor Study Group. *J Natl Cancer Inst* 1988;80(10):751–755.

118. Phase II studies of drug combinations in advanced pancreatic carcinoma. fluorouracil plus doxorubicin plus mitomycin C and two regimens of streptozotocin plus mitomycin C plus fluorouracil. The Gastrointestinal Tumor Study Group. *J Clin Oncol* 1986;4(12):1794–1798.

119. Klaassen DJ, et al. Treatment of locally unresectable cancer of the stomach and pancreas: a randomized comparison of 5-fluorouracil alone with radiation plus concurrent and maintenance 5-fluorouracil—an Eastern Cooperative Oncology Group study. *J Clin Oncol* 1985;3(3):373–378.

120. Chauffert B, et al. Phase III trial comparing intensive induction chemoradiotherapy (60 Gy, infusional 5-FU and intermittent cisplatin) followed by maintenance gemcitabine with gemcitabine alone for locally advanced unresectable pancreatic cancer. Definitive results of the 2000–01 FFCD/SFRO study. *Ann Oncol* 2008;19(9):1592–1599.

121. Loehrer PJ Sr, et al. Gemcitabine alone versus gemcitabine plus radiotherapy in patients with locally advanced pancreatic cancer: an eastern cooperative oncology group trial. *J Clin Oncol* 2011;29(31):4105–4112.

122. Hammel P, Huguet F, van Laethem JL, et al. Effect of chemoradiotherapy vs chemotherapy on survival in patients with locally advanced pancreatic cancer controlled after 4 months of gemcitabine with or without erlotinib: the LAP07 randomized clinical trial. *JAMA* 2016;315:1844–1853.

123. Mukherjee S, Hurt CN, Bridgewater J, et al. Gemcitabine-based or capecitabine-based chemoradiotherapy for locally advanced pancreatic cancer (SCALOP): a multicentre, randomised, phase 2 trial. *Lancet Oncol* 2013;14(4):317–326.

124. Gillen S, et al. Preoperative/neoadjuvant therapy in pancreatic cancer: a systematic review and meta-analysis of response and resection percentages. *PLoS Med* 2010;7(4):e1000267.

125. Massucco P, et al. Pancreatic resections after chemoradiotherapy for locally advanced ductal adenocarcinoma: analysis of perioperative outcome and survival. *Ann Surg Oncol* 2006;13(9):1201–1208.

126. Greer SE, et al. Effect of neoadjuvant therapy on local recurrence after resection of pancreatic adenocarcinoma. *J Am Coll Surg* 2008;206(3):451–457.

127. Katz MH, et al. Borderline resectable pancreatic cancer: the importance of this emerging stage of disease. *J Am Coll Surg* 2008;206(5):833–848.

128. Chun YS, et al. Defining venous involvement in borderline resectable pancreatic cancer. *Ann Surg Oncol* 2010;17(11):2832–2838.

129. Stokes JB, et al. Preoperative capecitabine and concurrent radiation for borderline resectable pancreatic cancer. *Ann Surg Oncol* 2011;18(3):619–627.

130. Landry J, et al. Randomized phase II study of gemcitabine plus radiotherapy versus gemcitabine, 5-fluorouracil, and cisplatin followed by radiotherapy and 5-fluorouracil for patients with locally advanced, potentially resectable pancreatic adenocarcinoma. *J Surg Oncol* 2010;101(7):587–592.

131. Tang K, Lu W, Qin W, et al. Neoadjuvant therapy for patients with borderline resectable pancreatic cancer: a systematic review and meta-analysis of response and resection percentages. *Pancreatology* 2016;16(1):28–37.

132. Roldan GE, et al. External beam versus intraoperative and external beam irradiation for locally advanced pancreatic cancer. *Cancer* 1988;61(6):1110–1116.

133. Whittington R, et al. Multimodality therapy of localized unresectable pancreatic adenocarcinoma. *Cancer* 1984;54(9):1991–1998.

134. Hiraoka T, et al. Intraoperative irradiation combined with radical resection for cancer of the head of the pancreas. *World J Surg* 1984;8(5):766–771.

135. Sindelar WF, Kinsella TJ. Studies of intraoperative radiotherapy in carcinoma of the pancreas. *Ann Oncol* 1999;10(Suppl 4):226–230.

136. Showalter TN, et al. Does intraoperative radiation therapy improve local tumor control in patients undergoing pancreaticoduodenectomy for pancreatic adenocarcinoma? A propensity score analysis. *Ann Surg Oncol* 2009;16(8):2116–2122.

137. Ogawa K, et al. Intraoperative radiotherapy for resected pancreatic cancer: a multi-institutional retrospective analysis of 210 patients. *Int J Radiat Oncol Biol Phys* 2010;77(3):734–742.

138. Ogawa K, et al. Intraoperative radiotherapy for unresectable pancreatic cancer: a multi-institutional retrospective analysis of 144 patients. *Int J Radiat Oncol Biol Phys* 2011;80(1):111–118.

139. Willett CG, et al. Long-term results of intraoperative electron beam irradiation (IOERT) for patients with unresectable pancreatic cancer. *Ann Surg* 2005;241(2):295–299.

140. Cai S, Hong TS, Goldberg SI, et al. Updated long-term outcomes and prognostic factors for patients with unresectable locally advanced pancreatic cancer treated with intraoperative radiotherapy at the Massachusetts General Hospital, 1978 to 2010. *Cancer* 2013;119(23):4196–204. doi:10.1002/cncr.28329.

141. Ben-Josef E, et al. Intensity-modulated radiotherapy (IMRT) and concurrent capecitabine for pancreatic cancer. *Int J Radiat Oncol Biol Phys* 2004;59(2):454–459.

142. Milano MT, et al. Intensity-modulated radiotherapy in treatment of pancreatic and bile duct malignancies: toxicity and clinical outcome. *Int J Radiat Oncol Biol Phys* 2004;59(2):445–453.

143. Yovino S, et al. Intensity-modulated radiation therapy significantly improves acute gastrointestinal toxicity in pancreatic and ampullary cancers. *Int J Radiat Oncol Biol Phys* 2011;79(1):158–162.

144. Ben-Josef E, Schipper M, Francis IR, et al. A phase I/II trial of intensity modulated radiation (IMRT) dose escalation with concurrent fixed-dose rate gemcitabine (FDR-G) in patients with unresectable pancreatic cancer. *Int J Radiat Oncol Biol Phys* 2012;84:1166–1171.

145. Rwigema JC, et al. Stereotactic body radiotherapy in the treatment of advanced adenocarcinoma of the pancreas. *Am J Clin Oncol* 2011;34(1):63–69.

146. Chang DT, et al. Stereotactic radiotherapy for unresectable adenocarcinoma of the pancreas. *Cancer* 2009;115(3):665–672.

147. Herman JM, Chang DT, Goodman KA, et al. Phase 2 multi-institutional trial evaluating gemcitabine and stereotactic body radiotherapy for patients with locally advanced unresectable pancreatic adenocarcinoma. *Cancer* 2015;121:1128–1137.

148. Petrelli F, Comito T, Ghidini A, et al. Stereotactic body radiation therapy for locally advanced pancreatic cancer: a systematic review and pooled analysis of 19 trials. *Int J Radiat Oncol Biol Phys* 2017;97:313–322.

149. Moningi S, Dholakia AS, Raman SP, et al. The role of stereotactic body radiation therapy for pancreatic cancer: a single-institution experience. *Ann Surg Oncol* 2015;22:2352–2358.

150. Mellon EA, Hoffe SE, Springett GM, et al. Long-term outcomes of induction chemotherapy and neoadjuvant stereotactic body radiotherapy for borderline resectable and locally advanced pancreatic adenocarcinoma. *Acta Oncol* 2015;54:979–985.

151. Dobelbower RR Jr, et al. Precision radiotherapy for cancer of the pancreas: technique and results. *Int J Radiat Oncol Biol Phys* 1980;6(9):1127–1133.

152. Haslam JB, Cavanaugh PJ, Stroup SL. Radiation therapy in the treatment of irresectable adenocarcinoma of the pancreas. *Cancer* 1973;32(6):1341–1345.

153. Rao AD, Sugar EA, Chang DT, et al. Patient-reported outcomes of a multicenter phase 2 study investigating gemcitabine and stereotactic body radiation therapy in locally advanced pancreatic cancer. *Pract Radiat Oncol* 2016;6:417–424.

154. Larghi A, et al. Screening for pancreatic cancer in high-risk individuals: a call for endoscopic ultrasound. *Clin Cancer Res* 2009;15(6):1907–1914.

155. Greenhalf W, et al. Screening of high-risk families for pancreatic cancer. *Pancreatology* 2009;9(3):215–222.

156. Moore MJ, et al. Erlotinib plus gemcitabine compared with gemcitabine alone in patients with advanced pancreatic cancer: a phase III trial of the National Cancer Institute of Canada Clinical Trials group. *J Clin Oncol* 2007;25(15):1960–1966.

157. Bonner JA, et al. Radiotherapy plus cetuximab for locoregionally advanced head and neck cancer: 5-year survival data from a phase 3 randomised trial, and relation between cetuximab-induced rash and survival. *Lancet Oncol* 2010;11(1):21–28.

158. Philip PA, et al. Phase III study comparing gemcitabine plus cetuximab versus gemcitabine in patients with advanced pancreatic adenocarcinoma: Southwest Oncology Group–directed intergroup trial S0205. *J Clin Oncol* 2010;28(22):3605–3610.

159. Crane CH, et al. Phase II trial of cetuximab, gemcitabine, and oxaliplatin followed by chemoradiation with cetuximab for locally advanced (T4) pancreatic adenocarcinoma: correlation of Smad4(Dpc4) immunostaining with pattern of disease progression. *J Clin Oncol* 2011;29(22):3037–3043.

160. Kindler HL, et al. Phase II trial of bevacizumab plus gemcitabine in patients with advanced pancreatic cancer. *J Clin Oncol* 2005;23(31):8033–8040.

161. Kindler HL, et al. Gemcitabine plus bevacizumab compared with gemcitabine plus placebo in patients with advanced pancreatic cancer: phase III trial of the Cancer and Leukemia Group B (CALGB 80303). *J Clin Oncol* 2010;28(22):36173622.

162. Crane CH, et al. Phase I trial evaluating the safety of bevacizumab with concurrent radiotherapy and capecitabine in locally advanced pancreatic cancer. *J Clin Oncol* 2006;24(7):1145–1151.

163. Crane CH, et al. Phase II study of bevacizumab with concurrent capecitabine and radiation followed by maintenance gemcitabine and bevacizumab for locally advanced pancreatic cancer: Radiation Therapy Oncology Group RTOG 0411. *J Clin Oncol* 2009;27(25):4096–4102.

164. Small W Jr, et al. Phase II trial of full-dose gemcitabine and bevacizumab in combination with attenuated three-dimensional conformal radiotherapy in patients with localized pancreatic cancer. *Int J Radiat Oncol Biol Phys* 2011;80(2):476–482.

165. Hidalgo M. Pancreatic cancer. *N Engl J Med* 2010;362(17):1605–1617.

166. Kotteas E, Saif MW, Syrigos K. Immunotherapy for pancreatic cancer. *J Cancer Res Clin Oncol* 2016;142:1795–1805.

167. Wang J, Reiss KA, Khatri R, et al. Immune therapy in GI malignancies: a review. *J Clin Oncol* 2015;33:1745–1753.

Section III

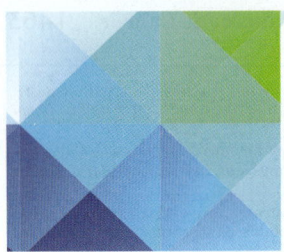

CHAPTER 64

Cancer of the Liver and Hepatobiliary Tract

Mirrorer Ming-Jiung Liu, Tsun-I Cheng, Skye Hung-Chun Cheng, and Andrew T. Huang

LIVER CANCER

Hepatobiliary malignancies include hepatocellular carcinoma (HCC), gallbladder cancer, intrahepatic cholangiocarcinoma (ICC), extrahepatic cholangiocarcinoma, and rare neoplasms such as sarcoma and hepatoblastoma.[1] Worldwide, there were estimated 792,000 patients with liver cancer in 2013. The male-to-female incidence ratio was about 2.5.[2] People living in developing countries, such as eastern Asia and middle and western Africa, have higher incidence of liver cancer than those live in the developed countries.[3] Age-standardized incidence rates per 100,000 population for liver cancer were higher in developing versus developed countries (16:7) for both genders in 2013.[2]

Patients with liver cancer usually are asymptomatic except for symptoms related to chronic liver disease. Disease-related symptoms, however, are associated with advanced disease. The overall prognosis is dismal, with a 5-year survival rates ranging from 0% to 10%. Only about one of five affected patients was amenable to curative resection[4,5] before the implementation of screening programs using α-fetoprotein (AFP) and ultrasonography. In recent years, improvements in surgical techniques have brought resection rates up to 30% to 50%.[6,7] The advent of liver transplantation in the recent decades contributes to the curability of the disease. Surgical resection remains to be the primary curative treatment for hepatobiliary malignancies, as the majority of patients have inoperable or unresectable disease at diagnosis. For patients with unresectable intrahepatic disease, treatment modalities such as transplantation, transcatheter arterial chemoembolization (TACE), local radiofrequency ablation (RFA), systemic chemotherapy, radiotherapy, molecular target therapy, and the use of current form of immunotherapy are treatment options.

HEPATOCELLULAR CARCINOMA

Topographic Anatomy

The liver is the largest solid organ of humans. Traditionally, it is divided into left and right lobes separated by the falciform ligament. Surgeons interested in hepatic resection need to understand the spatial relationship of a tumor to the hepatic vascular system preoperatively to determine resectability. Fortunately, progress in imaging modalities has made segmental division of the liver based on the anatomy of portal and hepatic veins feasible. The most common segmentation scheme proposed by Couinaud divides the liver parenchyma into right and left lobe with four segments each (Fig. 64.1). The left lobe of the liver consists of caudate lobe (segment I), lateral segment (segments II and III), and medial segment (segment IV). The anatomic landmark between the medial segment and lateral segment is drawn between the gallbladder and inferior vena cava (the falciform ligament). The right lobe of the liver consists of anterior segments (segments V and VIII) and posterior segments (segments VI and VII). The anatomic landmark that separates the anterior from posterior segment is the right hepatic vein; the anatomic landmark that divides the anterior segment from the left medial segment is the middle hepatic vein. No good anatomic landmarks exist that further divide the anterior and posterior segments into superior and inferior subsegments.[8] Dynamic computerized tomography is useful in distinctly defining segmental anatomy because the portal vein, hepatic vein, and inferior vena cava can be opacified at the same time.[9,10] Details of the anatomic information is available in the Web site: http://www.radiologyassistant.nl/en/p4375bb8dc241d.

Epidemiology

HCC is the most frequent primary cancer of the liver and ranks as the fifth most common cancer in the world and the third most common cause of cancer mortality.[11] The age-standardized incidence rate of liver cancer in 1990 worldwide was 14.7 per 100,000 men and 4.9 per 100,000 women.[12] The male-to-female ratio was 3:1. High-risk regions are eastern and southeast Asia and middle Africa.[11] The highest incidence rate is seen in the male population of South Korea, North Korea, Thailand, China, Gambia, and Senegal (28.5 to 48.8 per 100,000 populations).[11] In low-risk areas, such as Canada, Columbia, and United Kingdom, HCC occurs in only 1 to 3 per 100,000 population.[11] But the incidence rates of primary liver cancer have recently declined in Chinese population in Hong Kong, Shanghai, Taiwan, and Singapore.[11] On the contrary, the incidence rates in some low-rate areas such as United States, United Kingdom, and Australia have increased. The incidence of HCC tripled between 1975–1976 (1.4 per 100,000) and 2005–2007 (4.8 per 100,000) in the United States.[13,14] The most likely reason for this rise is related to higher prevalence of hepatitis C infection.[14]

Risk Factors

HCC is clearly associated with hepatitis B (HBV) and hepatitis C (HCV) viral infections and chronic liver disease. With persistent HBV infection, the relative risk of incidence of HCC is 223-fold higher than the uninfected population.[15] The risk of HCC is even higher in patients who are HBeAg positive compared with those who are HBeAg negative.[16] Similar to HBV, the relative risk of HCC among individuals with chronic HCV infection and cirrhosis is also approximately 100 times the risk of uninfected persons.[17] There also exists a synergistic interaction in patients having HBV and HCV combined infection toward the development of HCC.[18]

Other chronic liver cell injury is also associated with the development of HCC. Chemical injury induced by ethanol, nitrites, hydrocarbons, solvents, organochlorine pesticides, primary metals, and polychlorinated biphenyls has been implicated.[19,20] Ethanol is the most common culpable chemical agent and is thought to produce HCC through the development of liver cirrhosis or to play the role of a cocarcinogen. Chronic alcohol use of >80 g/day for more than 10 years increases the risk for HCC by approximately fivefold. In patients with HCV, alcohol use doubles the risk of HCC.[21] Environmental toxins including aflatoxin, contaminated drinking water, and betel nut chewing may also be associated with the pathogenesis of HCC. Aflatoxins, a well-known group of hepatotoxic agent, produced by the fungi, *Aspergillus flavus* and *Aspergillus parasiticus*, are associated with HCC. Aflatoxins could contaminate

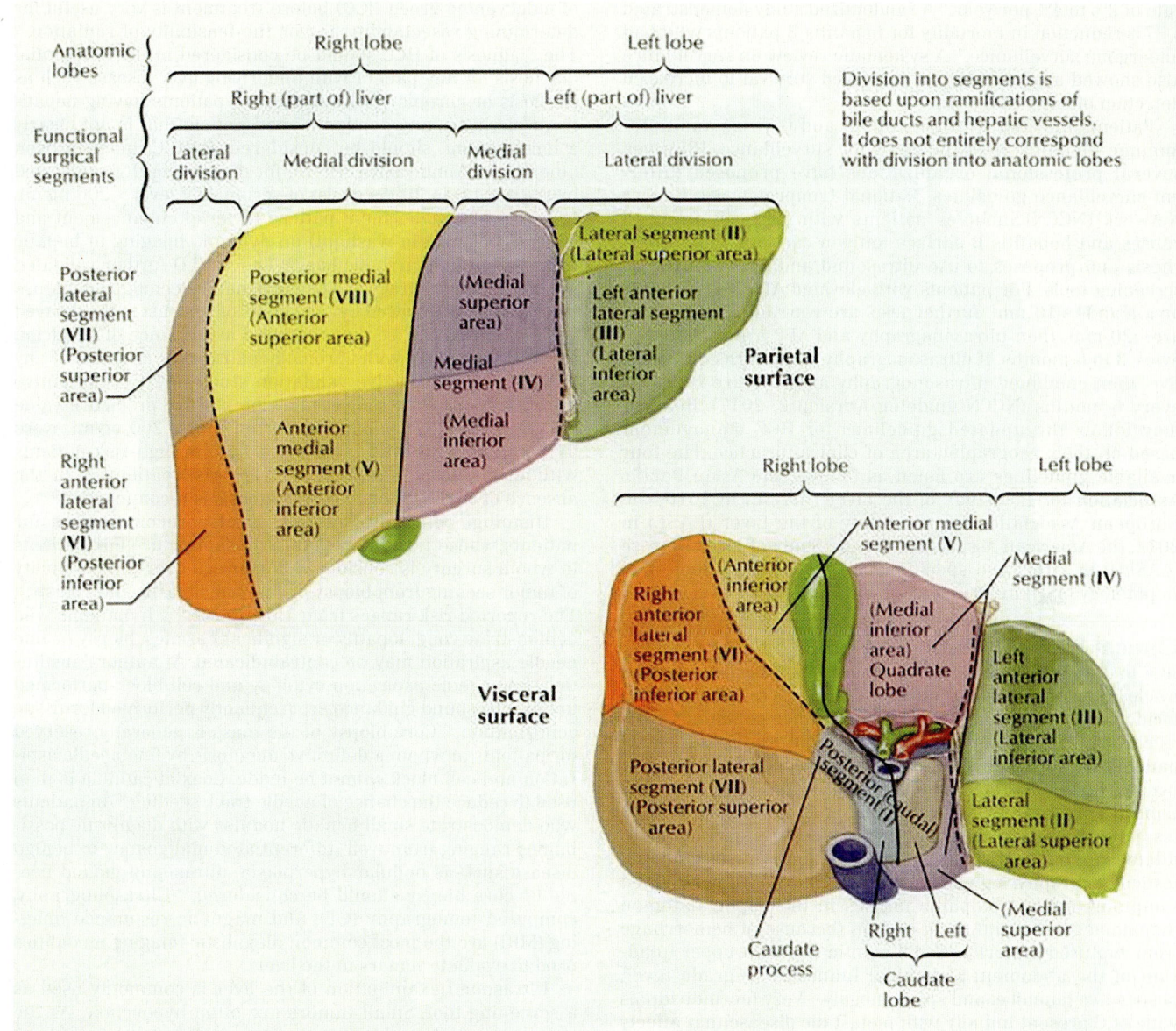

FIGURE 64.1. Segmentation schemes of the liver based on Couinaud proposal.

corn, soybeans, and peanuts. High dietary aflatoxin intake is known to be related to the development of HCC.[22,23] There is a synergistic interaction between chronic HBV infection and aflatoxin exposure on the risk of developing HCC.[18] Patients with hereditary liver disease, such as hemochromatosis, Wilson disease, hereditary tyrosinemia, and type I glycogen storage disease, are also at higher risk of developing HCC.[18,24] The common mechanism in these incidences of HCC may be related to chronic injury and inflammation of the liver.

Prevention

Because HCC is causally related to viral hepatitis and chemical injuries, public health measures against viral infection and avoidance of chemical exposure are essential for the prevention of HCC. The HBV vaccine has been available for decades. Universal HBV vaccination in many countries such as Taiwan has shown significant decrease in the incidence of HCC, from 0.70 to 0.36 per 100,000 children at the age of 6 to 14.[25] In patients with evidence of HBV or HCV infection, oral antiviral agents should be chosen to effectively control the progression of infection. Antiviral therapy has also been shown to reduce recurrence and improve survival for HBV-related HCC.[26]

When patients with HCC are treated with radiotherapy, HBV carriers or individuals with Child-Pugh B cirrhosis exhibit significantly greater susceptibility to radiation-induced liver disease.[27] Caution should be taken to survey and follow patients with HCC from hepatitis B endemic areas and patients with compromised liver reserve when radiotherapy is being considered. Prophylactic use of antiviral agents is recommended in this instance.

Vaccination against HCV is currently unavailable. Strategies of prevention of HCV infection include blood screening, the use of disposable needles and syringes, adoption of universal precaution for health care workers, and timely treatment of chronic HCV infection with currently available anti-HCV agents.[28] Recent advances in interferon-free anti-HCV treatment have achieved highly effective control of HCV in infected individuals. Readers are referred to the recent reports by van der Meer et al. and Morgan et al.[29,30]

Surveillance

The goal of surveillance is to detect HCC at its early stage by serial screening tests when curative treatment can be applied. Patients with cirrhosis developed HCC with an approximate rate of 2% to 4% per year.[31] A randomized study demonstrated a 37% reduction in mortality for hepatitis B patients who had undergone surveillance.[32] A systematic review on surveillance also showed a relationship of improved survival to increased detection of early-stage HCC.[33]

Patients infected with hepatitis B and C virus, and auto-immune hepatitis are candidates for surveillance. However, several professional organizations have proposed different surveillance guidelines. National Comprehensive Cancer Network (NCCN) includes patients with cirrhosis from all causes and hepatitis B surface antigen carriers without cirrhosis and proposes to use ultrasound and optional AFP as screening tools. For patients with elevated AFP > 100 ng/mL or a nodule >10 mm, further tests are warranted. If nodules are <20 mm, then ultrasonography and AFP are repeated in every 3 to 6 months. If ultrasonography alone turns out negative, then combined ultrasonography and AFP are repeated every 6 months (NCCN guideline version 2, 2017). Readers may follow the updated guidelines for HCC management based on their geographic area of clinical practice. The four available guidelines are listed as follows: the Asian Pacific Association for the Study of the Liver (APASL) in 2010, the European Association for the Study of the Liver (EASL) in 2012, the American Association for the Study of Liver Disease (AASLD) in 2017, and specific country: Japanese Society of Hepatology (JSH) in 2014, etc.

Clinical Presentation

HCC in the early stage is asymptomatic; it is generally detected by elevation of AFP and/or ultrasonography screening or as an incidental finding in the evaluation of other conditions such as chronic liver disease.[34] Even in the advanced stages, some patients are still asymptomatic. Symptoms in HCC patients are usually related to their chronic hepatitis and liver cirrhosis. Clinical symptoms include general fatigue, poor appetite, ascites, jaundice, upper gastrointestinal bleeding, splenomegaly, dilated abdominal veins, palmar erythema, gynecomastia, testicular atrophy, leg edema, and weight loss. Tumor-related symptoms include palpable masses in the upper abdomen (hepatomegaly), acute onset of pain (because of hemorrhage from ruptured tumor) and dull pain in the right upper quadrant of the abdomen, abdominal fullness, low-grade fever, obstructive jaundice, and splenomegaly.[35] Very few individuals with HCC present initially with metastatic disease that affects extrahepatic organs such as lungs, bones, adrenal glands, pancreas, and neck lymph nodes.[31,36]

Diagnostic Workup

In a patient in whom HCC is suspected, the clinical history frequently includes a history of hepatitis, jaundice, blood transfusion, use of intravenous drugs, or exposure to aflatoxins. A family history of hepatitis or hemochromatosis is also an important risk factor.[31] Details concerning alcohol abuse and industrial exposure to potential carcinogens are also helpful. The physical examination should include a search for signs of underlying liver disease such as jaundice, ascites, ankle edema, spider angiomata on the anterior chest wall, palmar erythema, splenomegaly, increasing abdominal girth, and weight loss. Evaluation of the abdomen for liver size, existence of tumor masses, tenderness, and abdominal bruits should also be included.

Blood tests should include serology for HBV and HCV and AFP. If HBV or HCV serology is positive, quantitative HBV DNA or HCV RNA should be obtained.[37] Evaluation of hepatic functional reserve includes prothrombin time, activated partial thromboplastin time, and serum albumin. Platelet, red cell, and white blood cell counts should also be obtained to look for simultaneous existence of portal hypertension and hypersplenism from liver cirrhosis. Fifteen-minute retention rate

of indocyanine green (ICG) before treatment is very useful for determining resectability and/or the feasibility of radiation.[38] The diagnosis of HCC should be considered in the differential diagnosis for any patient with underlying liver disease such as cirrhosis or chronic viral hepatitis. In patients having hepatitis or cirrhosis, any dominant solid nodule that is not clearly a hemangioma should be considered as HCC unless proven otherwise.[39] Noninvasive criteria for diagnosing HCC suggested by the AASLD in 2005 consist of serum AFP level > 200 ng/mL or a typical enhancement pattern (arterial enhancement and delayed portal vein washout) on dynamic imaging of hepatic mass >2 cm in a cirrhotic liver.[40] The AASLD further validated the diagnostic accuracy of a single dynamic technique if intense arterial uptake followed by "washout" of contrast in the delayed venous phases can be demonstrated as evidence of suspicion for HCC in patients with chronic hepatitis B or cirrhosis of any etiology.[41] A prospective validation study in 206 consecutive patients from Korea showed that the positive predictive value (PPV) of typical CT findings or serum AFP > 200 ng/mL were 97.8% in patients with cirrhosis, 89.6% in high-risk patients without cirrhosis, and 82.4% in low-risk patients.[42] In the absence of cirrhosis, histologic diagnosis is recommended.

Histologic diagnosis of HCC is also recommended for patients whose treatment plan is nonsurgical.[43] For patients in whom surgery is considered, a concern over the possibility of tumor seeding from biopsy or fine needle aspiration exists.[43] The reported risk ranges from 1.6% to 5%.[44-46] In patients who demonstrate coagulopathy or significant ascites, biopsy or fine needle aspiration may be contraindicated. At authors' institution, fine needle aspiration cytology and cell block performed under ultrasound guidance are frequently performed for tissue confirmation.[45] Core biopsy of the mass is generally reserved for patients in whom a definitive diagnosis by fine needle aspiration and cell block cannot be made. Coaxial cannula is then used to reduce the chance of needle track seeding.[47] In patients who demonstrate small hepatic nodules with diagnostic possibilities ranging from well-differentiated malignancy to benign disease such as nodular hyperplasia, ultrasound-guided needle or core biopsy should be considered.[48] Ultrasonography, computed tomography (CT), and magnetic resonance imaging (MRI) are the most common diagnostic imaging modalities used to evaluate tumors in the liver.

Ultrasound examination of the liver is commonly used as a screening tool. Small tumors are often hypoechoic. As the tumor grows, the echo pattern tends to become isoechoic or hyperechoic, and HCC can be difficult to distinguish from the surrounding liver.[49] Nodules <1 cm should be followed with ultrasonography again at intervals of 3 months. Nodules over 1 cm in a cirrhotic liver should be investigated further with four-phase dynamic CT scan. If the four-phase dynamic CT scan cannot confirm the diagnosis of HCC, contrast-enhanced MRI or biopsy is the next step. Another option is to use ultrasonography with carbon dioxide (CO_2) microbubbles or the like as ultrasound contrast agent given intra-arterially, which can overcome limitations of conventional B-mode and Doppler ultrasound techniques for studies of the focal lesion in the cirrhotic liver.[41] Extrahepatic metastases are not common at presentation; however, they occur mainly in patients with T4, multicentric disease, or in earlier stage disease following treatment. The most common sites of metastasis are lung, abdominal lymph nodes, and bone.[50] Routine metastatic survey in patients with early-stage HCC is not recommended unless transplantation is being considered.

Staging

HCC carries a generally poorer prognosis compared to other cancers because the underlying liver disease can negatively affect prognosis. Several factors have been identified as being important determinants of survival: the severity of underlying

TABLE 64.1 BCLC STAGING SYSTEM FOR HEPATOCELLULAR CARCINOMA

BCLC Stage	ECOG Performance Status	Tumor Features	Liver Function
0	0	Single nodule < 2 cm	Child-Pugh A
A	0	Single or 3 nodules < 3 cm	Child-Pugh A–B
B	0	Multinodular	Child-Pugh A–B
C	1–2	Portal invasion, N1, M1	Child-Pugh A–B
D	3–4		Child-Pugh C

N, node classification; M, metastasis classification.

TABLE 64.2 GRADING SYSTEM FOR CIRRHOSIS: THE CHILD-PUGH SCORE

Score	Bilirubin (mg/dL)	Albumin (g/dL)	Prothrombin Time (s)	Hepatic Encephalopathy (Grade)	Ascites
1	<2	>3.5	<4	None	None
2	2–3	2.8–3.5	4–6	1–2	Mild (detectable)
3	>3	<2.8	>6	3–4	Severe (tense)

Child class: A, 5 to 6; B, 7 to 9; C, >9.
From Pugh RN, Murray-Lyon IM, Dawson JL, et al. Transection of the oesophagus for bleeding oesophageal varices. *Br J Surg* 1973;60(8):646–649. Copyright © 1973 British Journal of Surgery Society Ltd. Reprinted by permission of John Wiley & Sons, Inc.

Section III

liver disease, the size and number of the tumor, vascular invasion, regional lymph node metastasis, and the presence of distant disease. There is no worldwide consensus on the use of any given HCC staging system. However, most major trials of HCC therapy have chosen the Barcelona clinic liver cancer (BCLC) staging system (Table 64.1), making it the *de facto* reference staging system.[41] Other systems such as the American Joint Committee on Cancer TNM staging system,[51] Okuda staging systems,[52] and the Cancer of the Liver Italian Program (CLIP) scoring system[48] are also in common use.

Pathologic Classification

Histologic classification of malignant tumors of the liver includes HCC (conventional type), HCC (fibrolamellar variant), cholangiocarcinoma (intrahepatic bile duct carcinoma), mixed hepatocellular cholangiocarcinoma, undifferentiated carcinoma, and hepatoblastoma. The fibrolamellar variant of HCC has a relatively better prognosis. It occurs more frequently in adolescents or young adults and has a more indolent clinical course than conventional HCC.[53] Hepatoblastoma occurs most commonly in young children (median age, 13 to 16 months) and usually presents in an advanced stage.[54,55]

General Management

HCC is often multicentric when it is associated with HCV infection. The incidence of multicentric disease in HCV-associated HCC (53.3%) is significantly higher (*P* < .05) than in the non–HCV-related HCC (7.7%).[56] The risk of multicentric occurrence increases with the progression of chronic liver disease and cirrhosis.[57,58] Although multiple tumors occur less often in HBV-associated HCC, the incidence of intrahepatic recurrence of HCC is significantly higher in patients with a sustained HBeAg positivity and high serum concentration of HBV DNA.[59] Despite these observations, the mainstay of therapy is surgical resection. The majority of patients, however, are not eligible for surgery because of the extent of tumor involvement or underlying liver dysfunction. Several other treatment modalities can be considered, including liver transplantation, RFA, percutaneous ethanol or acetic acid injection, TACE, cryoablation, radiation therapy, systemic chemotherapy, and immunotherapy, which is being tested for its efficacy currently.

Surgical Resection

Surgical resection is a reliable method to obtain long-term disease control. The main limiting factors for resection are poor liver function above all and size, location, and number of tumor. In virus-related HCC, the extent of surgical resection of hepatic tumor depends on the functional reserve of the residual liver after surgery. Previously, the selection of patients for resection has been based on the Child-Pugh functional classification (Table 64.2), but this method is known to be inconsistent with the outcome. Many Japanese and other Asian investigators rely on the ICG retention test.[59] In Europe and the United States, selection of optimal candidates for resection is usually based on the assessment of the presence of portal hypertension, which is assessed clinically or by hepatic vein

catheterization.[60] Clinically significant portal hypertension is suspected when the platelet count is below 100,000/μL associated with significant splenomegaly. The goal of surgery is to remove gross tumor with a margin of 1 to 2 cm of normal liver. Today, however, the 5-year survival after resection has improved by careful preoperative assessments as stated above and can exceed 50%.

Liver Transplantation

Many patients are not candidates for definitive surgery because of underlying liver dysfunction. The increasing availability of liver transplantation has made this procedure a viable alternative to tumor resection for selected patients. Based on the Milan study and others, liver transplantation is an effective option for HCC patients.[61] Milan criteria are still today's benchmark for patient selection. The major selection criteria are solitary tumor 5 cm or up to three tumors of smaller than 3 cm. Elevated AFP concentration adds prognostic information and may be used for decision-making in combination with imaging criteria.[62] When these selection criteria are strictly applied, excellent overall 3- to 4-year actuarial (75% to 85%) and recurrence-free survival rates (83% to 92%) can be achieved.[61,63,64] Risk factors of recurrence after transplantation include tumor size, number of tumors, vascular invasion, and persistence of HBV infection.[64–66] A major disadvantage with orthotopic liver transplantation is the unpredictable, potentially long waiting time for donor organs.[66] Living donor transplantation can be offered for HCC if the waiting time would likely be long.[62] Local treatment such as TACE or RFA could downstage HCC for transplantation purposes. Downstaging could increase the opportunity for transplantation and improve survival. Besides, local treatment could also be a bridging therapy for patients on the waiting list to keep them away from progression of disease diminishing the chance of transplantation.

Percutaneous Ablation

For patients with early-stage HCC who are not suitable for resection or transplantation, percutaneous ablation could be a treatment option.[67,68] Other methods by destroying tumor cells can also be achieved by the injection of chemical substances (using ethanol or acetic acid) or by modifying the temperature (with radiofrequency, microwave, laser, or cryotherapy). Percutaneous ethanol injection is highly effective for small HCC. It achieves necrosis rate of 90% to 100% of the HCC <2 cm in size, but the necrosis rate is reduced to 50% if HCC is >3 cm.[69–71]

RFA involves the local application of radiofrequency thermal energy to the lesion. RFA is a reasonable option for patients who do not meet resectability criteria for HCC and yet are candidates for a liver-directed procedure based on the presence of liver-only disease. The best outcomes are in patients with a single tumor >2 and <4 cm in diameter.

Randomized control trials comparing RFA and ethanol injection have shown that RFA provides superior local disease control that could result in an improved survival.[72-75]

Transcatheter Arterial Chemoembolization

HCC is a highly vascular tumor supplied mostly by the hepatic or adjoining arteries and has strong neoangiogenic activity during its progression. This character provides the theoretical basis for the radiological diagnosis of the disease. It is also the rationale in support of arterial embolization as a treatment option. TACE combines selective injection of chemotherapeutic agents through arteries feeding the tumor followed by intra-arterial embolization of tumor-feeding arteries with lipiodol, an iodized oily contrast agent, Gelfoam, or plastic particles such as Ivalon. Despite two prospective randomized studies failed to show significant survival benefit over conservative management in patients with unresectable HCC,[76,77] more recent systematic review of randomized prospective studies has shown TACE to have a positive impact on survival.[78] TACE has currently been accepted as the standard treatment for unresectable disease or inoperable patients such as with multicentric disease or repeated relapses, and it can be used selectively for tumors of different organ location and can be repeated if necessary.[1,79]

Conventional Radiotherapy

HCC is a radiosensitive tumor.[38] The major drawback is the poor radiation tolerance of adjacent normal liver and the difficulty of tumor localization.[80,81] Recent technological and conceptual developments in the field of radiation therapy, such as intensity-modulated radiation therapy, image-guided radiation therapy, respiratory gating, and stereotactic body radiation therapy (SBRT), raised the potential and feasibility of radiation treatment. By conforming the delivery of radiation dose distribution closer to the tumor or target volume outlined more accurately, radiotherapy can result in sparing more normal liver tissue from high-dose radiation.[82,83] For patients with liver-confined disease treated with conformal radiotherapy with or without TACE, local control response rates ranged from 40% to 90%, and the median survival ranged from 10 to 25 months.[84] Indications for conformal radiotherapy include larger unresectable HCC, relieving portal vein tumor–induced thrombosis, obstructive jaundice, failure of prior TACE to control disease progression and as component of a combined modality treatment with TACE, or percutaneous ablation therapy.[38,85,86] However, the combination of TACE and conformal radiotherapy in large unresectable HCC has not been shown to have added efficacy in randomized trial.

Radiation Doses

The tumor response to radiotherapy and survival of patients with HCC are related to the dose delivered.[85,87] Before the era of conformal radiotherapy, the dose of radiation treatment was limited to <30 to 40 Gy for the hepatic toxicity, as a result, partial response usually was <30%.[88,89] Seong et al.[90] reported an objective tumor-specific response rate of 67% after a mean dose of 51.8 ± 7.9 Gy for patients who failed TACE and were treated with conformal radiotherapy. Dawson et al.[87] escalated radiation doses for unresectable hepatobiliary cancer and observed that patients who received radiation doses >70 Gy had better median survival (>16.4 months). It appears that the higher the radiation doses given, the better the tumor response seen (Table 64.3). However, caution should be given in HBV-related HCC, and local radiotherapy may cause deterioration of liver function by radiation-induced liver disease (RILD), portal hypertension, and HBV reactivation. To fend off HBV reactivation, prophylactic anti-HBV treatment should be considered.

TABLE 64.3 RADIOTHERAPY WITH AND WITHOUT CHEMOTHERAPY FOR UNRESECTABLE HEPATOCELLULAR CARCINOMA

Series	Patient Number	Radiation Dose (Gy)	Chemotherapy	Response Rate (%)
Stillwagon et al.[89] (RTOG)	135	21, 3 q.d.	Concurrent ADR, 5-FU	22
Order et al.[88] (RTOG)	105	21, 3 q.d. + I[131] 10–12 × 2 courses	Concurrent ADR and 5-FU	48
Seong et al.[90]	27	51.8 (mean), 1.8 q.d.	None	67
Dawson et al.[87]	25	58.5 (median), 1.5 b.i.d.	Concurrent HAI fluorodeoxyuridine	68

RTOG, Radiation Therapy Oncology Group; q.d., every day; ADR, doxorubicin; 5-FU, 5-fluorouracil; b.i.d., twice daily; HAI, hepatic arterial infusion.

Treatment Volumes

Although higher radiation doses have been shown to produce higher treatment response, unfortunately, patients with HCC are often accompanied by liver cirrhosis and dysfunction, which forbids higher doses of radiation. Published reports on three-dimensional conformal radiotherapy (3DCRT) with photon beam suggest that tumor-affected portions of the liver can be treated with higher doses with acceptable side effects. Lawrence et al. developed a normal tissue complication probability (NTCP) model of radiotherapy for intrahepatic malignancy. Based on this model, authors have designed a protocol in which each patient receive maximum tolerated doses of radiation with no more than 10% risk of radiation-induced liver disease.[94] Thus, the mean doses that can be delivered according to this protocol are 56.6 ± 2.31 Gy (range, 40.5 to 81 Gy). Using this dosing range, they observed a reduction of radiation injury to 4.8% (95% confidence interval, 0% to 23.8%). This model, however, was derived using patients with relatively normal liver function, and only 4 of 21 of their study population had HCC.[94] The NTCP model for patients with impaired liver function still requires further evaluation.[95] For patients with cirrhosis but within Child-Pugh grade A functional classification, the mean dose of hepatic radiation tolerated for normal liver is 23 Gy.[96] The authors suggested a dose–volume histogram for irradiation to normal liver that the irradiated hepatic volume over 10, 20, 30, and 40 Gy should be <68%, 49%, 28%, and 20%, respectively. Multivariate analyses demonstrated that the severity of hepatic cirrhosis was the only independent predictor for radiation-induced liver disease.

ICG retention test can guide the treatment volume of HCC.[97] We propose a treatment guideline using ICG test for conformal radiotherapy for patients with impaired liver function (Table 64.4). We advise no radiation treatment for patients with Child-Pugh class C liver cirrhosis or prolonged ICG retention unless only a very small portion of the liver is included in the radiation treatment fields.[38]

TABLE 64.4 RADIATION TREATMENT GUIDELINES FOR HEPATOCELLULAR CARCINOMA

Nontumor Part of Liver	ICG (Gy)		
	≤10%	10.1%–20%	20.1%–30%
<1/3	40 (Gy)	No RT	No RT
1/3–1/2	50 (Gy)	40 (Gy)	No RT
>1/2	60 (Gy)	50 (Gy)	40 (Gy)

ICG, indocyanine green; RT, radiation therapy.
From Cheng SH, Lin YM, Chuang VP, et al. A pilot study of three-dimensional conformal radiotherapy in unresectable hepatocellular carcinoma. J Gastroenterol Hepatol 1999;14(10):1025–1033. Copyright © 1999 Blackwell Science Asia Pty Ltd. Reprinted by permission of John Wiley & Sons, Inc.

Stereotactic Body Radiotherapy

Stereotactic body radiotherapy (SBRT) to the intrahepatic lesion has emerged recently as a novel option of treatment following the advent of improved planning system using more current models of linear accelerators. For patients with unresectable tumors or medical conditions denying surgery, SBRT could be an alternative treatment. Stereotactic technique could deliver higher biologic equivalent doses (BED) to local tumor with similar or reduced normal tissue damages. There is a wider variety of dosing and fractionation schedules of SBRT for HCC, ranging from 24 to 60 Gy in 3 to 10 fractions. The local tumor control rate in the past 2 to 3 years ranged from 70% to 90%,[98–101] but the complete response rate measured with CT images is generally <20% by current size-based criteria, this discrepancy with local tumor control requires functional imaging assessment.[102] The progression-free survival and overall survival rates are still disappointing because of out-of-field progression after SBRT.

Simulation

Simulation for SBRT is best done with the four-dimensional (4D) CT to minimize the treatment volume to decrease normal tissue damage. The 4D CT with gating can generate 10-phase images to detect the tumor motion during respiratory cycle.[103] In addition, small bowel contrast and intravenous contrast should be done to allow tumor, stomach and intestine being clearly demarcated. Abdominal compression belt and breath-holding technique can minimize inter- and intrafraction motion during radiation treatment.[104]

Tumor Contouring

The tumor target is often difficult to delineate with images of 4D. We prefer patients to have TACE using Lipiodol as landmarks before SBRT. If possible, contrast MRI can be obtained to provide complimentary information to aid the target delineating process as MRI often offer high soft tissue contrast resolution. Deformable registration of image technique can be used to fuse the diagnostic CT scan and MRI.[105]

Planning and Prescription

The goal of conformal radiotherapy is to precisely target the tumor(s) and to reduce injury to the surrounding normal tissue. Respiratory organ motion induces the largest "intrafraction" organ motion during treatment. Aruga et al.[106] studied organ motions involving the use of CT images obtained during both the static exhalation phase and the static inhalation phase for upper abdomen irradiation. They found that the tumor shifted between the two respiratory phases. The variation ranged from 0.4 to 5.9 mm in the lateral direction, 2.2 to 24.5 mm in the longitudinal direction, and 0.2 to 11.7 mm in the vertical direction with the patient in supine position. As mentioned in previous section, breath-gating or breath-holding techniques may help overcome the problem of respiratory movement during radiotherapy to a certain degree.[107] In general, the radiation field margin to the target in the lateral direction could be within 6 to 9 mm, vertical direction 9 to 12 mm, superior (subphrenic) direction 10 mm, and inferior direction 19 to 21 mm.[108,109] To preserve more liver function, the radiation field margins can be set only 5 mm and patient receives radiation treatment in the expiratory or inspiratory phase, the beam-on time will occupy about 30% to 40% of the whole respiratory cycle. The exact radiation delivery interval is generally set based on the observation of tumor motion on 4D CT images.

Dose and Organs at Risk

The SBRT dose is dependent on the tolerance of surrounding organs (liver, stomach, duodenum, kidney, and spinal cord). The large fraction size with SBRT still makes tolerance of surrounding tissues difficult. Son et al.[110] reported that at least 800 mL of normal liver should receive no more than 18 Gy to reduce the risk of deterioration of hepatic function. For patients with Child-Pugh score B, a 5-fraction regimen is recommended.[111] The dose to one-third of the uninvolved liver should be restricted to ≤18 Gy (3.6 Gy per fraction), and ≥500 cc of uninvolved liver should receive <12 Gy (2.4 Gy per fraction). For patients with a Child-Pugh score of ≥B and score ≥ 8, the risk of radiation-induced liver disease will be much higher and SBRT may not be safe unless the patients are already on the list for liver transplantation soon enough. For lesions adjacent to the duodenum or stomach, Mahadevan et al.[112] reported that 24 to 36 Gy in 3 fractions was associated with acceptable side effects. Bujold et al.[113] suggested the maximal dose of 32 to 34 Gy in 6 fractions to the stomach, duodenum, and small bowel and 12 Gy to the kidney in SBRT to HCC were acceptable.

Acute and Late Complications

The dose-limiting tissue injuries in radiation treatment for HCC include the liver, stomach, duodenum, bowels, and kidneys. Acute complications include general fatigue, transient elevation of liver function test, and nausea and vomiting (mainly for tumors in the left lobe of the liver), fever, and pancytopenia.[38,90] Subacute and late complications include hepatic failure, radiation pneumonitis, and gastrointestinal bleeding (caution should especially be given in tumor located in the inferior portion of the right lobe of the liver where the duodenum and jejunum are nearby and radiation doses plan to give more than 50 Gy).[38,114] Hepatic failure can be avoided by limiting the radiation dose to the organs at risk as mentioned above.

Combined TACE and Local Radiation Therapy

TACE alone rarely produces complete pathologic remission for HCC > 5 cm, especially in the peripheral zone of the tumor.[115,116] Additional therapy is required to eradicate the residual disease or produce longer-term control of HCC. The combination of TACE and conformal radiotherapy shows promising results in large HCC (Table 64.5). Guo and Yu[120] reported 107 patients with large unresectable HCC treated with TACE followed by external beam irradiation. The largest dimension of the tumors ranged from 5 to 18 cm. After a median follow-up interval of 24 months, the cumulative survival rates at 3 and 5 years were 28.4% and 15.8%, respectively, with a median survival of 18 months. Cheng et al.[38] reported 17 patients with unresectable HCC treated with TACE and conformal radiotherapy. The mean tumor size was 8.6 cm (range, 3.7 to 18 cm). The overall survival rate at

TABLE 64.5 COMBINATION TACE AND LOCAL RADIOTHERAPY IN UNRESECTABLE HEPATOCELLULAR CARCINOMA

Series	Patient Number	Mean Tumor Size (cm)	Treatment	Overall Survival (3 y) (%)	Median Survival (mo)
Guo and Yu[120]	107	10.2	TACE–RT	28	18
Cheng et al.[38]	17	8.6	TACE–RT–TACE	58 (2 y)	>24
Yasuda et al.[120a]	44	Range 3–8	TAE–RT	81	Not available
Seong et al.[114]	50	8.3	TACE–RT	43%	17
Wu et al.[121]	94	10.7	TACE–RT	26	25

TACE, transcatheter arterial chemoembolization; RT, radiation therapy.

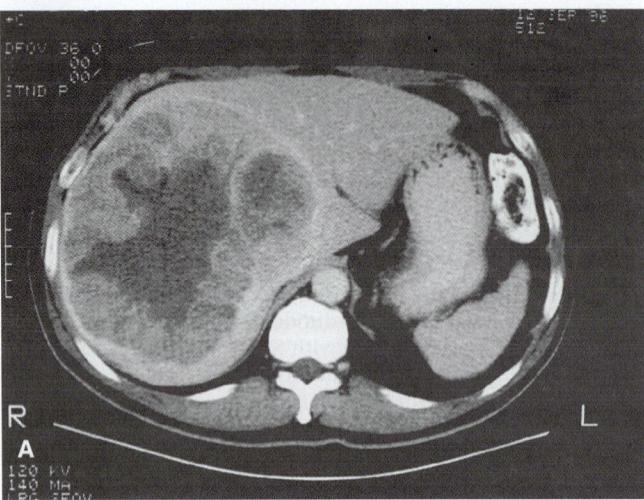

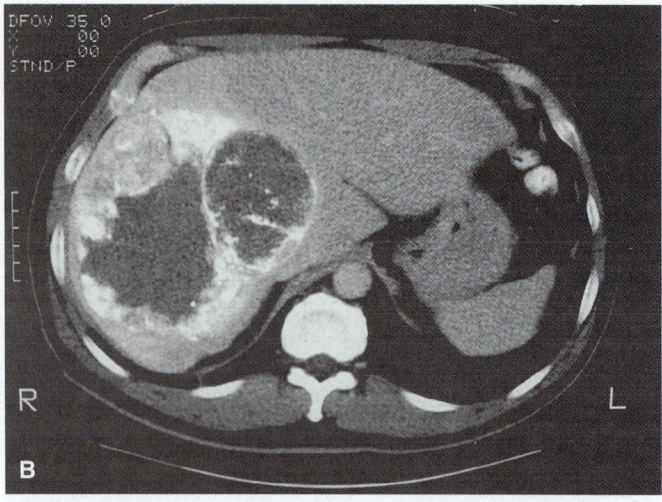

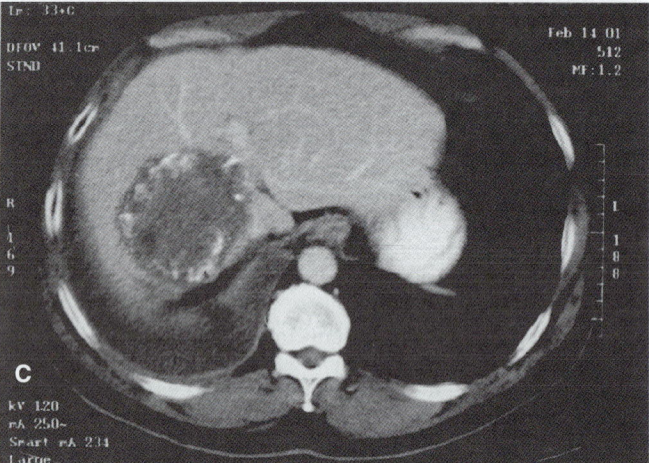

FIGURE 64.2. A: A 55-year-old man with hepatitis B virus infection developed a large hepatocellular carcinoma in the right lobe of the liver. The tumor measured 12 × 15 × 15 cm. Alpha-fetoprotein (AFP) was 901 ng/mL. **B:** After a first course of transcatheter arterial chemoembolization (TACE), his AFP dropped to 150 ng/mL. It rose again to 440 ng/mL 3 months later. Immediately thereafter, he had a second TACE followed by three-dimensional conformal radiotherapy. This image was taken after the second TACE but before conformal radiotherapy, revealing viable tumors in the peripheral zone of the main mass. **C:** Four years and 4 months after the first treatment, computed tomography revealed a nonenhancing tumor in the right lobe of the liver suggesting an effective control of the disease. His AFP remained <10 ng/mL after completion of radiotherapy.

2 years was 58%, and local progression-free tumor control was 83%. After 24 months of median follow-up, the median survival had not been reached, and 4 of 17 patients remained progression free (Fig. 64.2). Another study that combined TACE and local radiotherapy in 50 unresectable HCC patients reported a partial response rate of 66% and survival rates at 3 years of 43%.[114] Wu et al.[121] reported 94 patients with HCC who received 3DCRT combined with TACE. The response rate was 90.5%. The overall survival rates at 1, 2, and 3 years were 93.6%, 53.8%, and 26.0%, respectively, with the median survival of 25 months. Patients with branch portal vein thrombosis may benefit from combined treatments. Tazawa et al.[122] reported 19 patients with thrombus, presumably caused by the tumor, in the first branch of portal vein received 3DCRT with TACE. Eleven patients (58%) had an objective response, and 1-year survival rate was 41% (8 patients). Although we do not know yet whether combined TACE and conformal radiotherapy is a superior to TACE alone, the result of these studies suggests that in patients with large unresectable HCC, combined treatment can be a promising alternative treatment modality and is worthy of further investigation.

Chemotherapy

Systemic chemotherapy for HCC has limited value in clinical practice because only a small portion of patients obtain significant benefit at the price of remarkable toxicity.[123] In general, cytotoxic therapy should be reserved for medically appropriate patients with adequate hepatic functional reserve, preferably administered within the context of a clinical trial. The side effect profile of any chemotherapy regimen is substantial,

and its use should be carefully assessed in patients having advanced liver disease and a short life expectancy.

Several new drugs have been tested recently. One of the more promising of these drugs is gemcitabine. It has a lower toxicity profile, but its antitumor activity in patients with advanced HCC is marginal: the response rate is no more than 18%, and the response duration is about 35 weeks.[124] Combination chemotherapy regimens have shown better responses. Leung et al.[125] reported 50 patients treated with intravenous chemotherapy PIAF (cisplatin, doxorubicin, 5-fluorouracil, and interferon-α). The partial response was 26% (13/50), and 4 patients achieved pathologic complete remission.[125] Louafi et al.[126] reported 34 patients of advanced HCC treated with gemcitabine and oxaliplatin. The disease control rate was 76%. Median progression-free and overall survival times were 6.3 months and 11.5 months, respectively.

Molecular Targeted Therapy

Recent advances in molecular biology have uncovered the structures and/or functions of many cytokines thought to have a strong relationship with the mechanisms of the antitumor effect of biologic therapies. Thalidomide, a sedative with anti-angiogenesis potential previously associated with severe fetal malformations but highly effective for myeloma, has limited value in the treatment of HCC.[127,128] Molecular targeted therapy to the epidermal growth factor receptor and vascular endothelial growth factor has exhibited potential of inhibiting tumor growth of HCC.[129] The randomized trial of sorafenib, a tyrosine protein kinase inhibitor, has shown statistically significant tumor suppression with a median overall survival of

10.7 versus 7.9 months without sorafenib and longer median time to radiological progression (5.5 vs. 2.8 months).[130] Some clinical studies showed benefit in local control by combining sorafenib with conventional irradiation.[131] But hepatic toxicity and out-of-field progression remains the key factor affecting survival. Concurrent treatment of sorafenib with SBRT awaits further investigation.[132] However, the combination of sorafenib with radiation should be given cautiously; a single 8 Gy irradiation to lumbar spine has been reported associated with a complication of bowel perforation.[133] We recommend stopping antiangiogenic agent during radiotherapy. Combination of sorafenib or regorafenib with immunotherapy is also under active investigation.

Immunotherapy

HCC is most frequently a virally associated disease. Immune tolerance and imbalance are thought to be one of the mechanisms leading to the development of cancer.[134] There is evidence that immunotherapy may play a role in treating HCC. A phase I/II study including 48 patients demonstrated that the PD-1 inhibitor, nivolumab, is safe and effective in advanced HCC, and the overall response rate was 15%. The preliminary overall 1-year survival was 62%. Dose-limiting toxicity was hepatic decompensation. The most common adverse effects are skin rash, pruritus, and elevation of AST, ALT, lipase, and amylase.[135] Combination of immunotherapy and radiotherapy is in active clinical trial.

Areas of Failure and Cause of Death

Survival of HCC with various treatments depends largely on the clinical stage and liver function. Five-year survival in resectable HCC after partial hepatectomy is 50% to 73% in stage I patients, 30% to 56% in stage II patients, 10% to 29% in stage III patients, and approximately 10% in stage IV patients.[136,137] The 5-year survival for patients with unresectable HCC is usually <10%.[138] The major cause of failure after resection is tumor recurrence within the liver. Extrahepatic metastasis in advanced HCC has become more frequently encountered in recent years, probably related to improvements in the survival from intrahepatic disease.[139,140]

Future Study

The outcome in HCC from various treatments is generally unsatisfactory. The main cause of failure is intrahepatic recurrence. Future efforts should be directed more toward prevention of HBV via vaccination and HCV infection through screening of blood products and universal needle precaution in endemic regions. Antivirals including the recent advent of anti-HCV agents have been effective in the control of infected individuals. Treatment of HCC unfortunately relies mainly on surgical resection for limited stage disease at this moment in time. Investigation for newer target agents or novel immunotherapy is only in the early stage of development.

BILIARY TRACT CANCER

Biliary tract cancers consist of cancer of the gallbladder, the bile ducts, and the ampulla of Vater. They are clinically highly aggressive tumors and are usually discovered in locally advanced stage of disease at diagnosis. Gallbladder cancer is the most common cancer of the biliary tract and accounts for two-thirds of these cancers, whereas bile duct cancer accounts for the remaining one-third.[141] Biliary tract cancer can appear in small intrahepatic bile ducts, as well as large intrahepatic and extrahepatic bile ducts. The term cholangiocarcinoma is used to describe cancers arising from the epithelial cells of the bile ducts. At present, surgical excision of all resectable biliary tract cancers is associated with a good long-term survival, whereas for unresectable tumors, the treatment is usually palliative aiming to relieve obstructive jaundice with drainage of bile and management of biliary tract infection, pain, and ascites.

CHOLANGIOCARCINOMA

Topographic Anatomy

The bile ducts originate within the liver, with the left and right hepatic ducts joining to form the common hepatic duct. At the origin of the cystic duct, it becomes the common bile duct. The cystic duct drains bile from the gallbladder into the common bile duct. The gallbladder is adjacent to the undersurface of the liver.

There is a rich lymphatic network along the submucosa of bile ducts. The primary lymphatic drainage of the biliary tract is to the lymph nodes in the pericholedochal area, periportal region, hepatoduodenal ligament, common hepatic artery, and pancreaticoduodenal groups.[83,142,143]

Epidemiology and Risk Factors

Cholangiocarcinoma is a rare tumor in developed countries; there are approximately 2,000 to 3,000 cases per year in the United States. However, it is one of the most common cancers in endemic areas of developing countries, with incidences as high as 87 per 100,000 people in northeast Thailand.[144] Cholangiocarcinoma accounts for about 15% of the primary liver cancer worldwide. But the proportion differs regionally: 20% in Western countries, <10% in Asian nations, and as high as 90% in northern Thailand.[67,145]

A number of risk factors have been identified as important in the development of cholangiocarcinoma, most of which share a history of long-standing inflammation and chronic injury of the biliary epithelium.[146] The major risk factor in Western countries is primary sclerosing cholangitis, which is closely associated with chronic inflammatory bowel disease, particularly ulcerative colitis.[147] The risk of developing cholangiocarcinoma is higher in patients with primary sclerosing cholangitis, ulcerative colitis with colonic neoplasm than in patients with primary sclerosing cholangitis, and ulcerative colitis without colonic neoplasm.[148] Studies in Japan and the United states also showed that chronic hepatitis C infection elevates the incidence of ICC with the odds ratio between 4 and 17.[149,150] In Asia, chronic infections of the biliary tract related to the infestation by certain liver flukes, such as *Clonorchis sinensis* and *Opisthorchis viverrini*, are associated with cholangiocarcinoma and hepatolithiasis.[144] Hepatolithiasis itself is also a risk factor for cholangiocarcinoma. Five to ten percent of patients with intrahepatic stones develop this complication.[151,152] Moreover, the combination of liver fluke infestation and nitrosamine exposure may explain the very high incidence of cholangiocarcinoma in northeast Thailand.[153] Other risk factors, although rare, include congenital fibropolycystic disease of the biliary system such as choledochal cysts and Caroli disease (cystic dilatation of intrahepatic bile ducts).[154] The observed incidence and mortality of ICC has increased in the past three decades in Japan, the United States, and the United Kingdom.[14,155,156] However, the incidence of extrahepatic cholangiocarcinoma is almost the same.[157] In the United States, the age-adjusted mortality rate has increased from 0.07 per 100,000 in 1973 to 0.69 per 100,000 in 1997. The estimated annual percent increase of mortality rate was 9.44% during this period. Between 1973 and 2012, the incidence of ICC increased from 0.44 to 1.18 cases per 100,000, representing an annual percentage increase of 2.30%; this trend has accelerated during the past decades to an annual percent increase of 4.36%.[157] Better case ascertainment and diagnosis from improved imaging, use of image-guided biopsies, or increased use of endoscopic retrograde cholangiopancreatography (ERCP) cannot fully explain this observation.[156,158]

Diagnosis

The most common presenting symptoms of biliary tract cancer are caused by obstruction of the bile duct. Those include painless jaundice, clay-colored stools, tea-colored urine, and pruritus. Other signs and symptoms include abdominal pain, fever, general malaise, abdominal distention, fullness, anorexia, and weight loss. The spectrum of cholangiocarcinoma can be classified into three broad groups: (a) intrahepatic, (b) perihilar, and (c) distal tumors. The age of onset is similar among the three groups and ranges from 60 to 65 years.[159] Patients with extrahepatic tumor usually present with jaundice, acholic stools, and tea-colored urine. Patients with intrahepatic tumors are less likely to be jaundiced and more likely to present with abdominal symptoms and more advanced disease.

There are no reliable screening methods; early diagnosis is almost impossible even in patients with high-risk situations such as primary sclerosing cholangitis, parasitic infestation, and hepatolithiasis.[160] Some patients are diagnosed when screening blood work demonstrates elevation of alkaline phosphatase and γ-glutamyl transferase. Ultrasonography and CT are the initial primary tools to evaluate biliary tract tumor (Table 64.6). Further tests include percutaneous transhepatic cholangiography, ERCP with brushing cytology, serum carbohydrate antigen 19-9 (CA 19-9) levels, radiologic imaging with dynamic CT scan, MRI, or both, and angiography.

A serum CA 19-9 value >100 U/mL has a sensitivity of approximately 75% and a specificity of approximately 80%.[161] The optimal cutoff value for serum CA 19-9 that best discriminates between benign or malignant biliary tract diseases is influenced by the presence of cholangitis. Thus, in patients with symptoms of acute cholangitis, serum CA 19-9 concentrations should ideally be reevaluated after recovery. The sensitivity of serum carcinoembryonic antigen (CEA) is low, helpful only in one-third of the patients.[162] Biliary CEA levels increase significantly in patients with cholangiocarcinoma and also in patients with intrahepatic cholelithiasis (average, 50.2 to 57.4 ng/mL) compared with patients with benign strictures (average, 10.1 ng/mL) and patients with sclerosing cholangitis and choledochal cysts (average, 20.0 to 21.6 ng/mL).[161] Serum AFP may increase in some cases of cholangiocarcinoma, and this would suggest a diagnosis of mixed HCC and cholangiocarcinoma.[163]

Pathology

Cholangiocarcinomas arise from the epithelium of the biliary tract. There are two main histologic subtypes: bile ductular type (mixed), arising from small intrahepatic bile ducts, and bile duct type (mucinous), arising from large intrahepatic and extrahepatic bile ducts. Pathologic classification of ICC is based on a new concept.[164] Histologic diversity in cholangiocellular carcinoma reflects the different cholangiocyte phenotypes.[165] The majority of these cancers are adenocarcinomas (more than 90%). Squamous cell carcinoma is the second most common histologic type. Rare histologies include mucoepidermoid carcinoma, cystadenocarcinoma, and carcinoid tumor.

Adenocarcinomas are divided into three types: sclerosing, nodular, and papillary. Sclerosing tumors are characterized by an intense desmoplastic reaction. This type of tumor tends to invade the bile duct wall early and, as a result, is associated with low resectability and cure rates. Most cholangiocarcinomas are of this type.[159] The nodular cholangiocarcinomas are also highly invasive tumors. Most patients have advanced disease at diagnosis. The resection and cure rates are both very low. In contrast, papillary type tumors usually present as masses in the lumen of bile ducts causing biliary obstruction early in the course of disease. Therefore, these tumors have the more favorable prognosis.[166] Microscopically, cholangiocarcinoma is classically well differentiated to undifferentiated. Cells tend to be cuboidal or low columnar and resemble biliary epithelium; mucin is always demonstrable in the cytoplasm. Readers should be aware that bile duct obstruction can be associated with reactive hyperplasia of subepithelial mucous glands in the presence or absence of cholangiocarcinoma.[167] Cholangiocarcinomas frequently invade lymphatic, perineural, and periductal spaces, and portal tracts. Spreading along the lumen of large bile ducts can also be seen, especially in perihilar cholangiocarcinoma.[168]

The differential diagnosis of cholangiocarcinoma from HCC can be further affirmed by positive association with CEA, CA 19-9, and immunohistochemical stain with cytokeratin-19.[169] Mutations in p53 tumor suppressor gene and K-RAS protooncogene have been identified in cholangiocarcinoma.[92,170,171] p53 overexpression and K-RAS mutations are associated with a shortened survival.[170] Recent marker analysis of cholangiocarcinoma from the Cancer Genome Atlas revealed a distinct subtype enriched for isocitrate dehydrogenase (IDH) mutants.[172] IDH mutations block normal cellular differentiation and promote tumorigenesis via the abnormal production of the oncometabolite D-2-hydroxyglutarate (2-HG). Mutant IDH could be the potential future target for developing inhibitors of tumor growth.[173]

Pathways of Tumor Spread

Bile duct cancers commonly spread by direct extension through the biliary tract and the abundant lymphatic network in the submucosa layer. These tumors also commonly involve the surrounding structures by direct invasion. Lymph node metastases in the porta hepatis and celiac axis are common. The lymph nodes in porta hepatis are more frequently involved with tumors in the intrahepatic duct and proximal extrahepatic bile duct, and the pancreaticoduodenal nodes are more often involved with tumors in the distal bile duct.[168,174]

The incidence of lymph node metastasis in ICC ranges from 50% to 60%.[175,176] ICCs, irrespective of their intrahepatic location, mainly spread to the nodes in the hepatoduodenal ligament, then to the paraaortic nodes, retropancreatic nodes, or common hepatic artery node group. In addition, the left peripheral type or hilar type of cholangiocarcinoma tends to spread along the left gastric nodes through the lesser curvature.[176] Lymph node metastasis in perihilar cholangiocarcinoma is common, which occurs in about half of the patients, with the frequency of 43% in pericholedochal nodes, 31% in the periportal nodes, 27% in the common hepatic nodes, and 15% in the posterior pancreaticoduodenal nodes. The celiac and superior mesenteric nodes are rarely involved.[168]

Lymph node metastasis in distal duct cancer is commonly observed near the duodenopancreatic regions. Yoshida et al.[174]

TABLE 64.6 DIAGNOSTIC WORKUP FOR CARCINOMA OF THE BILE DUCT

General
  History
  Physical examination
Laboratory studies
  Complete blood cell counts
  Blood chemistry profile to include liver function studies
  Tumor markers: CA 19–9, CEA
Radiographic studies
Standard
  Computed tomography scan
  Ultrasonography
  Transhepatic cholangiography
  Endoscopic retrograde cholangiopancreatography
Optional
  Endoscopic ultrasound
  Magnetic resonance cholangiopancreatography
  Dynamic computed tomography scan
  Arteriography

Modified from Gunderson LL, Willett CG. Pancreas and hepatobiliary tract. In: Perez CA, Brady LW, eds. *Principles and practice of radiation oncology.* 3rd ed. New York: Lippincott-Raven Publishers, 2009.

examined 20 consecutive patients with distal bile duct cancer who underwent pancreaticoduodenectomy with extended lymph node dissection. Histologic evidence of lymph node metastasis was seen in 55% of the patients. The areas with frequent metastases were the posterior pancreaticoduodenal lymph nodes (35%), the nodes around the hepatoduodenal ligament (35%), and those around the common hepatic artery (30%). Paraaortic lymph node involvement occurred in 25% of patients and was significantly associated with pancreatic parenchymal invasion.

Staging for Cholangiocarcinoma

The American Joint Committee on Cancer TNM classifications (8th edition) for ICC are shown below:

T category:
T1: solitary tumor without vascular invasion
   T1a: solitary tumor ≤ 5 cm
   T1b: solitary tumor >5 cm
T2: solitary tumor with intrahepatic vascular invasion or multiple tumors, with or without vascular invasion
T3: tumor perforating the visceral peritoneum
T4: tumor involving local extrahepatic structures by direct invasion
N category:
N0: no regional lymph node metastasis
N1: regional lymph node metastasis present
M category:
M0: no distant metastasis
M1: distant metastasis present

The complete stage groups are listed in Table 64.7. The American Joint Committee on Cancer TNM staging for both perihilar and distal cholangiocarcinoma has been revised in 2017 (Table 64.7). The N category is classified based on the number of positive nodes (N1: one to three positive nodes; N2: four or more positive nodes). The T category of perihilar cholangiocarcinoma is as follows: T1 is tumor confined to the bile duct, T2 is tumor invaded beyond the bile duct wall, T3 is tumor invaded unilateral branches of portal vein or hepatic artery, and T4 is tumor invaded the main portal vein or its branches bilaterally. The T category in distal bile duct cancer is classified based on the depth of invasion (T1: <5 mm; T2: 5–12 mm; T3: >12 mm).

TABLE 64.7 AJCC STAGE GROUPS BY TNM CLASSIFICATION (8TH EDITION)

Intrahepatic Cholangiocarcinoma
Stage IA: T1aN0M0
Stage IB: T1bN0M0
Stage II: T2N0M0
Stage IIIA: T3N0M0
Stage IIIB: T4N0M0, or any T, N1M0
Stage IV: any T, any N, M1

Perihilar Cholangiocarcinoma
Stage I: T1N0M0
Stage II: T2a-bN0M0
Stage IIIA: T3N0M0
Stage IIIB: T4N0M0
Stage IIIC: any T, N1M0
Stage IVA: any T, N2M0
Stage IVB: any T, any N, M1

Distal Cholangiocarcinoma
Stage I: T1N0M0
Stage IIA: T2N0M0, T1N1M0
Stage IIB: T2-T3N1M0
Stage IIIA: T1-T3N2M0
Stage IIIB: T4, N1-N2, M0
Stage IV: any T, any N, M1

The most important prognostic factors for cholangiocarcinoma are resectability, regional lymph node metastasis, and distant metastasis. Multivariate analysis using Cox proportional hazards model demonstrated that multifocality, extrahepatic extension, grade, node positivity, and age >60 years (MEGNA) are independently associated with worse overall survival. This MEGNA prognostic score is an improvement of the discriminatory power of prognostication over AJCC 7th staging system.[177]

General Management

Surgical resection provides the only possibility of cure, but the resection rates for intrahepatic, perihilar, and distal lesions are 60%, 56%, and 91%, respectively, in one large series.[159] The 5-year survival rates after resection range from 10% to 40%, depending on the location of the primary tumor.[159] Patients with unresectable cholangiocarcinoma generally have a very poor prognosis; chemotherapy and radiotherapy have been used, but the results are disappointing.[178]

Intrahepatic Cholangiocarcinoma

ICC accounts for 5% to 10% of all biliary tract cancers and constitutes 10% to 20% of primary liver malignancies. The resectability rate in all patients is only 30% to 50%.[179,180] The outcomes after surgery for patients with lymph node metastasis are poor regardless of the site of nodal metastasis; the 5-year survival rate in patients with lymph node metastasis is lower than that in patients without lymph node metastasis (0% vs. 51%; $P < .0001$).[176]

Factors that affect tumor recurrence include lymph node metastasis, presence of satellite nodules, positive resection margin, tumor size, and bilobar distribution.[176,181-183] The patterns of failure after resection of ICC are primarily in the liver (56%), regional lymph node (20%), and peritoneal seeding (24%).[184]

The role of postoperative adjuvant radiotherapy with or without chemotherapy in the management of ICC is controversial. The typical reports in the literature are retrospective with small numbers of patients and marked variations in radiation fields and doses.[185] A delineation of radiation fields based on patterns of failure analysis and lymph node spread of the disease will be necessary to rationally define the role of radiotherapy in any proposed phase III study. For unresectable cholangiocarcinoma, the purpose of treatment is palliative; however, some long-term survivals (a 4-year rate of 20%) have been observed in unresectable cholangiocarcinoma treated with conformal radiotherapy and intra-arterial infusion of fluorodeoxyuridine.[186] SBRT is another treatment option. With a median follow-up of 5.4 years of 26 patients, the median progression-free survival and overall survival were 6.7 and 10.6 months, respectively.[187] Others have reported similar results in perihilar cholangiocarcinoma (Klatskin tumors) treated with SBRT.[188]

Total hepatectomy with orthotopic liver transplantation also can be considered in cholangiocarcinoma. One systematic review combining all studies that included a minimum of 10 patients reported a median survival of 11.8 months, the 5-year overall survival of 22%, and the 5-year disease-free survival of 13%.[189] Because of the high rate of recurrence and lack of selection criteria for good prognostic patient, transplantation should seldom be used as a treatment for cholangiocarcinoma.[190]

Perihilar Cholangiocarcinoma

Perihilar cholangiocarcinoma is the most common biliary tract carcinoma and accounts for 65% to 70% of tumors of the biliary tract.[159] Perihilar tumor involving bifurcation of the hepatic duct is also called Klatskin tumors.[191] These tumors are further classified by Bismuth et al.[192] as tumors below the confluence of the left and right hepatic ducts (type I), tumors reaching the confluence (type II), tumors occluding the common hepatic duct and the right or the left hepatic duct (types IIIa and IIIb, respectively), and tumors that are multicentric or that involve the confluence and both the right and left hepatic ducts (type IV).

Only 25% to 79% of patients are amenable to surgical resection. Definitive surgery may involve combined bile duct and liver resection with caudate lobe lobectomy.[193] The 3-year survival rate was 55% for patients without nodal involvement, 32% for patients with regional node metastasis, and 12% for patients with paraaortic node metastasis.[168] In multivariate prognostic analysis, only lymph node metastases and curative resection have proven to be of independent prognostic significance.[168]

The role of postoperative radiotherapy with or without chemotherapy in patients with completely resected cholangiocarcinoma remains unproven. A retrospective analysis from Johns Hopkins suggests that postoperative adjuvant radiation therapy does not improve survival.[194] However, postoperative radiotherapy or chemoradiotherapy reduces the rate of local recurrence in patients with incomplete resection.[195,196] In addition, many retrospective series and small phase II studies suggest superior outcomes for resected patients who receive external beam radiation therapy with or without concomitant chemotherapy.[68,197-199] For patients with microscopic residual disease after resection, a retrospective analysis from 63 patients with stage IV Klatskin tumor revealed that postoperative radiotherapy (with or without intraoperative radiotherapy) yielded significantly higher 5-year survival rates than in the resection-alone group (33.9% vs. 13.5%).[196]

An updated report from Mayo Clinic revealed that the 5-year survival in transplant patients of unresectable hilar cholangiocarcinoma after induction chemoradiotherapy was 80%, and in resection-only patients, it was 21%.[200] Others also have reported similar promising results in these unresectable cholangiocarcinoma treated with induction chemoradiotherapy followed by liver transplant.[201,202]

In general, patients with inoperable perihilar cholangiocarcinoma usually have obstructive jaundice and should be treated with endoscopic or percutaneous drainage and/or stent placement initially. External beam radiotherapy alone rarely controls advanced disease. Combinations of external beam radiotherapy, chemotherapy, and intraluminal brachytherapy may relieve pain and contribute to biliary decompression. Sometimes such approach achieves long-term survival. The most active chemotherapy agents include 5-FU, gemcitabine, docetaxel, and oxaliplatin.[203,204] The median survivals range from 17 to 21 months. In some cases, combined chemotherapy and radiotherapy could delay progression of cholangiocarcinomas while awaiting availability of liver transplant.[118,197]

Distal Bile Duct Carcinoma

Primary distal bile duct adenocarcinoma, which includes carcinoma of the ampulla of Vater, accounts for 25% to 30% of biliary tract carcinomas.[159] Patients with distal duct carcinoma have the highest rate of curative resection as compared to proximal duct carcinomas. In an analysis of 171 patients who underwent surgical exploration at Mayo Clinic for extrahepatic cholangiocarcinoma from 1976 to 1985, the rate of curative resection (achieving negative margins) by site of the primary tumor was 15% for proximal, 33% for middle, and 56% for distal duct lesions.[93] The prognosis of patients with distal duct carcinoma is clearly better than those with proximal duct carcinoma.[148]

The role of postoperative radiotherapy is uncertain. Investigators at Thomas Jefferson University found that postoperative radiotherapy did not improve survival in distal duct carcinoma after complete resection.[205] However, studies of concurrent chemotherapy and radiotherapy show more promising results. Mehta et al.[206] from Stanford University treated 12 patients having unfavorable (mainly lymph node metastasis) ampullary carcinoma with concurrent radiotherapy and protracted venous infusion of 5-FU. Actuarial overall survival at 2 years was 89%, and median survival

was 34 months. Another study conducted by the Eastern Cooperative Oncology Group revealed that unresectable pancreaticobiliary carcinoma treated with concomitant radiotherapy and protracted intravenous infusion of 5-FU achieved a 2-year survival of 19%.[199]

Systemic Chemotherapy

Although some retrospective reports showed benefit of postoperative chemotherapy,[207,208] a multi-institutional randomized trial from Japan showed only a trend toward better 5-year survival following a potential curative resection in patients who received postoperative chemotherapy.[195] But it was not a statistically significant difference. According to multiple retrospective studies, multivariate analysis, and expert consensus, adjuvant chemotherapy with fluoropyrimidine or gemcitabine-based chemotherapy is nonetheless recommended in margin-negative patients. Adjuvant chemoradiotherapy is also recommended for margin-positive patients.[195,209]

For treatment of advanced and metastatic cholangiocarcinoma, no single chemotherapy agent or combination regimen consistently leads to objective tumor shrinkage, although a small randomized trial showed a survival benefit with 5-FU–based chemotherapy comparing with best supportive care alone (median survival 6 vs. 2.5 months, respectively).[210] The most frequently used agents include 5-FU, gemcitabine, cisplatin, and oxaliplatin. Another phase III study enrolled 410 patients with locally advanced or metastatic cholangiocarcinoma, gallbladder cancer, or ampullary cancer. As compared with gemcitabine alone, cisplatin plus gemcitabine was associated with a significant survival advantage (11.7 vs. 8.1 months) without substantial toxicity. Cisplatin plus gemcitabine is an option for the treatment of patients with advanced biliary tract cancer.[211] In summary, for unresectable or metastatic cholangiocarcinoma, gemcitabine combined with cisplatin or gemcitabine alone is first-line treatment of choice for this patient group. If gemcitabine and cisplatin fail, no established regimens in the second-line setting are currently available. Enrolling such patients into newer clinical trial is recommended.

Target Therapy

Existing data demonstrate no or only very modest survival benefits with the target agents tested. EGFR inhibitors (cetuximab, erlotinib, panitumumab), anti-VEGF (bevacizumab, cediranib, vandetanib), ERB2, MEK (selumetinib, trametinib), multityrosine kinase inhibitors (such as dasatinib, imatinib, pazopanib, regorafenib, sorafenib, sunitinib), and c-MET–VEGF have been tested in ongoing or completed clinical trials. These agents can be used alone or in combination with chemotherapy.[212]

Radiation Therapy

The role of radiotherapy (with or without chemotherapy) in unresectable or recurrent cholangiocarcinoma is to relieve pain and biliary obstruction. At 1 year following conventional radiotherapy, 60% to 75% of patients have locoregional failure, and the median survival ranges only 7 to 12 months.[213,214] Local failure remains the first site of disease progression.[213] To enhance treatment effect, radiotherapy given with 5-FU–based chemotherapy is generally recommended.[198,206]

The development of novel technique in radiation in the past few years has made SBRT for biliary cancer more promising. Mahadevan et al.[215] reported a series of 34 patients with 42 lesions. With a median follow-up interval of 38 months, the 1-year local control rate with doses of 24 to 45 Gy in 3 to 5 fractions was 88% and the 4-year control rate was 79%. Another report included 27 patients with unresectable cholangiocarcinoma who underwent SBRT (45 Gy in 3 fractions). The local control was 84% in 1 year.[216] The major complications were severe duodenal/pyloric ulceration and bleeding, duodenal stenosis, and biliary stenosis. Radiotherapy technique for ICC is similar to the treatment for HCC. Tumor moves with respiratory excursion during radiation treatment. Oral contrast to delineate the duodenum, 4D CT, breath-holding, and abdominal compression are the techniques used to reduce the movement of the organ and the tumor and to avoid unnecessary exposure of normal adjacent organs. The surrounding organs to be protected from SBRT include the liver, duodenum, stomach, and spinal cord.

Treatment Volumes

The extent of the tumor within the bile duct can be defined by percutaneous cholangiography, ERCP, and MRCP. However, the extraductal disease is difficult to define by any noninvasive procedure. Clip placement at the time of surgery is useful in delineating the extrahepatic portion of ductal lesions and helps define the primary tumor bed. With the incorporation of CT in radiation treatment planning, and to reduce errors

to a minimum, we advocate placing patients in treatment position when performing pretreatment CT, using 1 to 3 mm per slice, and contrast medium to reconstruct the anatomy of bile ducts and gross tumor volume (GTV) (Fig. 64.3). The GTV is defined as any visible tumor by CT and/or MRI. Clinical target volume (CTV) is defined as 1.5-cm margin beyond the GTV, especially along the bile duct and potential lymphatic drainage areas, which include nodes along the porta hepatis, pancreaticoduodenal system, and celiac axis.[174,176,217,218] The planning target volume is defined by adding a margin of 0.5 to 1 cm to the CTV.[91]

Radiation Doses

Initial setup of radiation fields is to include GTV and CTV; the radiation fields can be coplanar or noncoplanar. The planning target volume is treated to 45 to 50 Gy in 1.8 to 2 Gy fractions given 5 days a week, using blocks to exclude the stomach,

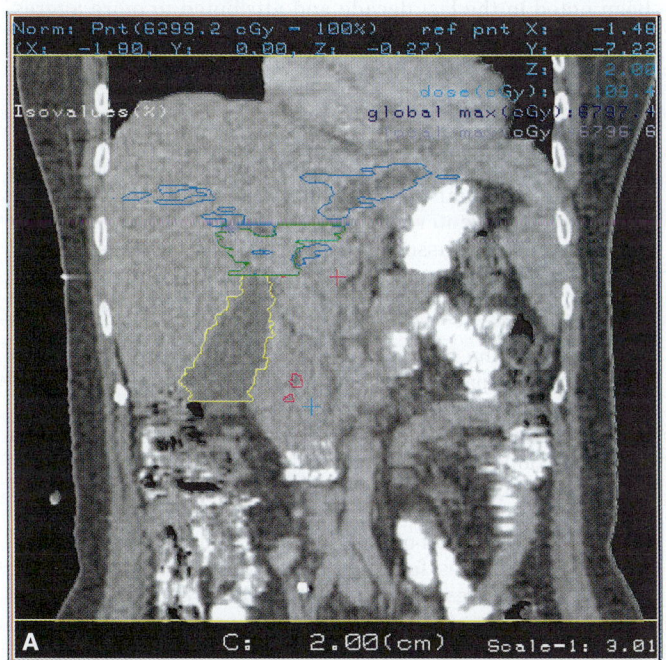

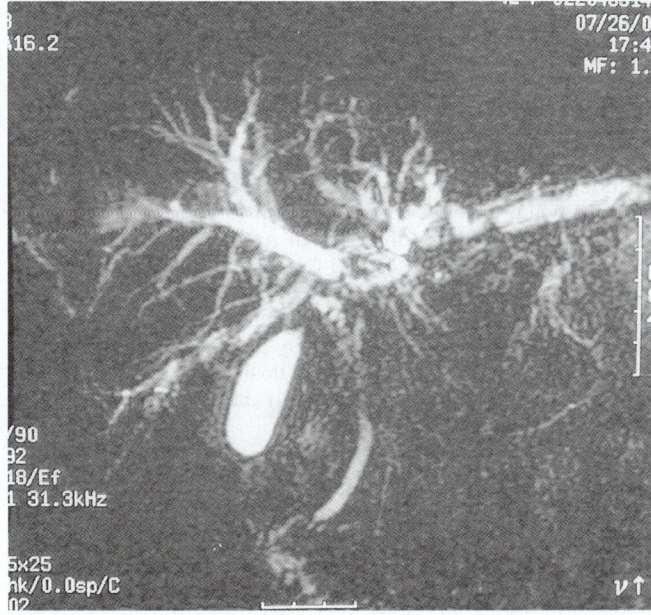

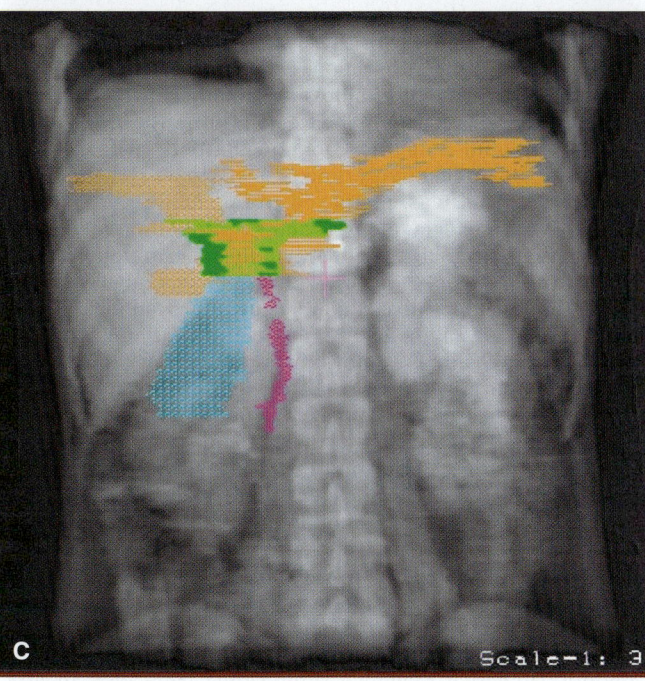

FIGURE 64.3. **A:** Computed tomography was performed in a 39-year-old woman who had cholangiocarcinoma of perihilar area. This image was reconstructed from a CT, at 2-mm slice interval. The tumor involved right and left hepatic ducts (*green line*). **B:** Magnetic resonance cholangiopancreatography affirmed the extent of tumor involvement. **C:** Digital reconstruction radiography revealed the gross tumor volume (*green*) and clinical target volume (*purple*).

small intestine, kidney, and liver.[192,219] Higher radiation doses are used only to treat the GTV with the application of 3DCRT.[87] If boost-dose irradiation is feasible with brachytherapy techniques, the GTV is carried to 45 to 50 Gy with external beam techniques or 20 to 30 Gy delivered via an intraluminal catheter.[82] The most commonly employed brachytherapy technique for the biliary tract begins with the placement, by an interventional diagnostic radiologist, of a percutaneous drainage catheter through the area of tumor. The radiation oncologist then threads a catheter inside the drainage system catheter. When a low-dose-rate system is employed, a wire with Ir-192 is then placed at the desired location inside the catheter.[220] If a remote high-dose-rate afterloading system is employed, then the appropriate dwell time and position are selected and programmed. It is a matter of some debate as to where the brachytherapy prescription point should be placed. Some physicians select the tumor's peripheral edge, away from the catheter, as determined by CT or MRI. Other practitioners prefer a point 0.5 or 1 cm away from the catheter. It is important to be familiar with the valves used to direct bile flow in the drainage system lest; during the administration of brachytherapy, bile leaks onto the patient's skin and dressings. If the drainage system remains in place for a long period of time (i.e., a month), enteric bacterial colonization and biliary tract infection are common. The combination of external beam irradiation and brachytherapy employed at Thomas Jefferson University resulted in 2 years and median survival rate to increase by twofold when doses were brought up to >55 Gy.[220] However, investigators at the University of Amsterdam reported no improved survival at doses >55 Gy.[221] The role of radiotherapy and its optimal dosage remains to be determined.

As for SBRT, the daily dose is similar to the treatment of HCC, and it ranges from 8 to 15 Gy per fraction with a total fraction number of 3 to 5. The daily dose to the duodenum and stomach should be limited to 400 cGy daily.

Acute and Late Complications

Acute complications of external beam and intraluminal radiotherapy include nausea, vomiting, and transient elevation of transaminases. These effects are usually mild and tolerable.[36]

Late complications are associated with radiation doses to surrounding organs. The most common complications are gastrointestinal bleeding, biliary bleeding, and duodenal stenosis.[36,220,221] With external beam doses of <55 Gy to the duodenum or stomach, the risk of severe gastrointestinal complications varies from 5% to 10%. At doses >55 Gy, one-third of the patients develop severe radiation-related complications.

Future Directions

There is a paucity of phase III studies for cholangiocarcinoma. We must rely on retrospective studies or prospective phase I–II trials. Further advances in treatment could potentially be made by: (a) defining when to use radiation and chemotherapy for high-risk patients after curative resection, (b) investigating the use of higher doses of conformal radiotherapy and chemotherapy in unresectable cholangiocarcinoma, and (c) identifying novel chemotherapeutic or novel pathway inhibitory agents. Patients with unresectable cholangiocarcinoma should be considered in the setting of investigative clinical trials.

ADENOCARCINOMA OF GALLBLADDER

Gallbladder carcinoma is the fifth most common cancer of the gastrointestinal tract. The incidence indicates a large geographic variation. The American Cancer Society's estimates for cancer of the gallbladder and nearby large bile ducts in the United States for 2017 are about 11,740 new cases diagnosed: 5,320 in men and 6,420 in women.[222] Cholelithiasis, anomalous junction of pancreaticobiliary ducts, and porcelain gallbladder are factors that predispose to gallbladder cancer.[223] Cigarette

smoking, alcohol consumption, and obesity may also contribute to the risk. Patients with polyps >10 mm in diameter may be at increased risk for gallbladder cancer.[224,225] Chronic infection with *Salmonella typhi* and *Helicobacter bilis* is also associated with the risk of developing carcinoma of the gallbladder.[226,227]

The most common clinical presentation is pain, followed by anorexia, nausea, or vomiting. Patients with early invasive gallbladder carcinoma are most often asymptomatic, or they have nonspecific symptoms that mimic or are due to cholelithiasis or cholecystitis. In general, patients having gallbladder carcinoma manifest symptoms such as jaundice, anorexia, and weight loss and are associated with more advanced disease, which accounts for the poor prognosis.[154] A French study of 724 patients revealed that only 4% of the patients had Tis lesions, 11% had T1 to T2 lesions, and 85% had T3 to T4 lesions.[228] Five-year survival rates according to more than 10,000 patients reported in the U.S. National Cancer Data Base were stage 0, 80%; stage I, 50%; stage II, 28%; and stage III, 7% to 8%.[222] However, improved outcomes have been noted in the last decade and attributed to more aggressive surgery and the use of postoperative adjuvant therapy.[229] Studies from Japan report a 5-year survival rate in stage I patients of 100%, stage II at 50% to 78%, stage III at 0% to 69%, and stage IV at 0% to 11%.[230,231]

Lymphatic metastasis initially is to cystic and pericholedochal nodes and then to the pancreaticoduodenal system, with later potential spread to the rest of the celiac axis or the superior mesenteric or aortic nodes.[230,232] The lymph node metastasis rate is associated with primary tumor stage: 0% to 2.5% in pT1a disease (involvement limited to the mucosa), 15% in T1b disease, 62% in pT2 disease, and 81% in pT3/pT4 disease.[230,233,234]

Surgery is the only potentially curative therapy, but only one-quarter of patients are eligible for resection.[235] The standard surgical procedure is removal of the gallbladder, resection of various amounts of liver surrounding the gallbladder bed, resection of the extrahepatic bile duct, and dissection of the regional lymph nodes. Patients with jaundice should be considered for preoperative percutaneous transhepatic biliary drainage for relief of biliary obstruction. Overall, the curative resection rates for gallbladder carcinoma range from 10% to 30% in Western countries.[236] The prognosis is related to the possibility of curative resection, primary tumor extension, and regional lymph node metastasis.

Patients with T1a disease often are cured after simple cholecystectomy and require no further adjuvant treatment.[234] However, for patients with ≥T2 disease, many reports support the benefit of radical resection.[229,233,237] In more advanced disease (≥T2), the benefit of adjuvant radiotherapy is uncertain. After "curative" resection, locoregional relapse in the tumor bed or regional nodes is common. Patients who received radiation postoperatively had a median survival of over 16 months. This was compared to <6 months for patients treated with surgery alone. Factors predicting recurrence are positive surgical margins, lymph node metastasis, and perineural invasion.[238] Several retrospective analyses demonstrate that postoperative radiotherapy improved local control and survival.[239–241] Benefits are also seen in patients who have microscopic residual tumors.[241] Combination radiotherapy and chemotherapy with 5-FU also reveal similar benefits.[242–244] However, there is a lack of phase III studies. Whether combination treatment is better than single modality is still unknown.

Patients with stage III and IV disease are at high risk for distant metastasis. The most frequent sites of involvement are the liver, peritoneum, and lung, with less frequent spread to ovaries, spleen, bones, and other organs.[91,243] In general, patients who are locally unresectable should be referred for chemoradiotherapy. Median survival is improved in several retrospective studies.[119,245] Systemic chemotherapy has limited success in the treatment of advanced gallbladder carcinoma. Objective response rates range from 25% to 50%.

Active agents include infusion of 5-FU in combination with agents such as leucovorin modulation, capecitabine, cisplatin, oxaliplatin, gemcitabine, and docetaxel, and 5-FU combined with recombinant IFN α-2b.[246–251] Currently, the standard of care for systemic chemotherapy is cisplatin and gemcitabine as mentioned in the section of Cholangiocarcinoma.[211]

OTHER RARE NEOPLASMS

Primary sarcomas of the liver are extremely rare in adults and represent only 1% to 2% of primary liver cancers.[252] Leiomyosarcoma is the most common histologic type, followed by malignant fibrous histiocytoma, epithelioid hemangioendothelioma, and angiosarcoma.[117] Some patients with angiosarcoma have a history of occupational exposure to vinyl chloride monomer.[253] Severity of histologic grade determines overall patient survival. Complete resection offers a chance of long-term survival.[117]

Hemangioma is a benign lesion and generally is asymptomatic. For symptomatic hemangioma, treatments include steroids, interferon-α, arterial embolization, and surgery.[254] If patients fail above treatments, radiotherapy may play a role. Long symptom-free duration has been obtained with doses as low as 13 to 30 Gy in 2.5 to 4 weeks to involved area.[255]

Hepatoblastoma is the most common malignant liver tumor of childhood. Children who have familial adenomatous polyposis of the colon and rectum are high risk for hepatoblastoma. The risk of hepatoblastoma in these children is 700 to 7,500 times higher than in the general population.[256,257] Surgery combined with chemotherapy has resulted in dramatic improvements in prognosis.[258] With the combination of chemotherapy and surgery, 75% to 80% of patients may be cured.[54] Preoperative chemotherapy often converts unresectable tumors to resectable and may reduce blood loss and technical complications.[259]

REFERENCES

1. Cance WG, Stewart AK, Menck HR. The National Cancer Data Base Report on treatment patterns for hepatocellular carcinomas: improved survival of surgically resected patients, 1985–1996. *Cancer* 2000;88:912–920.
2. Global Burden of Disease Cancer Collaboration. The global burden of cancer 2013. *JAMA Oncol* 2015;1(4):505–527.
3. Bosch FX, Ribes J, Díaz M, et al. Primary liver cancer: worldwide incidence and trends. *Gastroenterology* 2004;127:S5–S16.
4. Lin TY, Lee CS, Chen KM, et al. Role of surgery in the treatment of primary carcinoma of the liver: a 31-year experience. *Br J Surg* 1987;74:839–842.
5. Tsuzuki T, Sugioka A, Ueda M, et al. Hepatic resection for hepatocellular carcinoma. *Surgery* 1990;107:511–520.
6. Sasaki Y, Imaoka S, Nakano H, et al. Indications for hepatectomy for hepatocellular carcinoma: what stage of the disease is the best indication for surgery? *J Hepatobiliary Pancreat Surg* 1998;5:14–17.
7. Sotiropoulos GC, Lang H, Frilling A, et al. Resectability of hepatocellular carcinoma: evaluation of 333 consecutive cases at a single hepatobiliary specialty center and systematic review of the literature. *Hepatogastroenterology* 2006;53:322–329.
8. Dusenbery D, Ferris JV, Thaete FL, et al. Percutaneous ultrasound-guided needle biopsy of hepatic mass lesions using a cytohistologic approach. Comparison of two needle types. *Am J Clin Pathol* 1995;104:583–587.
9. Takayasu K, Okuda K. *Imaging in liver disease*. 1st ed. New York: Oxford University Press; 1997.
10. Hori M, Murakami T, Kim T, et al. Sensitivity of double-phase helical CT during arterial portography for detection of hypervascular hepatocellular carcinoma. *J Comput Assist Tomogr* 1998;22:861–867.
11. Kim T, Murakami T, Takahashi S, et al. Optimal phases of dynamic CT for detecting hepatocellular carcinoma: evaluation of unenhanced and triple-phase images. *Abdom Imaging* 1999;24:473–480.
12. El-Serag HB, Rudolph KL. Hepatocellular carcinoma: epidemiology and molecular carcinogenesis. *Gastroenterology* 2007;132:2557.
13. Devila JA, El-Serag H. The rising incidence of hepatocellular carcinoma in the United States: an update. *Gastroenterology* 2012;142(Suppl 1):S914–S914.
14. McGlynn KA, Tarone RE, El-Serag HB. A comparison of trends in the incidence of hepatocellular carcinoma and intrahepatic cholangiocarcinoma in the United States. *Cancer Epidemiol Biomarkers Prev* 2006;15:1198–1203.
15. Beasley RP, Lin CC, Hwang LY, et al. Hepatocellular carcinoma and hepatitis B virus: a prospective study of 22 707 men in Taiwan. *Lancet* 1981;318:1129.
16. Yang HI, Lu SN, Liaw YF, et al. Hepatitis B e antigen and the risk of hepatocellular carcinoma. *N Engl J Med* 2002;347:168–174.
17. Heintges T, Wands JR. Hepatitis C virus: epidemiology and transmission. *Hepatology* 1997;26:521–526.
18. Chen CJ, Yu MW, Liaw YF. Epidemiological characteristics and risk factors of hepatocellular carcinoma. *J Gastroenterol Hepatol* 1997;12:S294–S308.
19. Deuffic S, Poynard T, Buffat L, et al. Trends in primary liver cancer. *Lancet* 1998;351:214–215.
20. Haverkos HW. Viruses, chemicals and co-carcinogenesis. *Oncogene* 2004;23:6492–6499.
21. Morgan TR, Mandayam S, Jamal MM. Alcohol and hepatocellular carcinoma. *Gastroenterology* 2004;127:S87–S96.
22. Jackson PE, Groopman JD. Aflatoxin and liver cancer. *Baillieres Best Pract Res Clin Gastroenterol* 1999;13:545–555.
23. Yu SZ. Primary prevention of hepatocellular carcinoma. *J Gastroenterol Hepatol* 1995;10:674–682.
24. Fracanzani AL, Conte D, Fraquelli M, et al. Increased cancer risk in a cohort of 230 patients with hereditary hemochromatosis in comparison to matched control patients with non-iron-related chronic liver disease. *Hepatology* 2001;33:647–651.
25. Chang MH, Chen CJ, Lai MS, et al. Universal hepatitis B vaccination in Taiwan and the incidence of hepatocellular carcinoma in children. Taiwan Childhood Hepatoma Study Group. *N Engl J Med* 1997;336:1855–1859.
26. Ishikawa T. Anti-viral therapy to reduce recurrence and improve survival in hepatitis B virus-related hepatocellular carcinoma. *World J Gastroenterol* 2013;19:8861–8866.
27. Cheng JCH, Wu JK, Lee PCT, et al. Biologic susceptibility of hepatocellular carcinoma patients treated with radiotherapy to radiation-induced liver disease. *Int J Radiation Oncol Biol Phys* 2004;60:1502–1509.
28. Benvegnu L, Alberti A. Risk factors and prevention of hepatocellular carcinoma in HCV infection. *Dig Dis Sci* 1996;41:49S–55S.
29. van der Meer AJ, Veldt BJ, Feld JJ, et al. Association between sustained virological response and all-cause mortality among patients with chronic hepatitis C and advanced hepatic fibrosis. *JAMA* 2012;308:2584.
30. Morgan RL, Baack B, Smith BD, et al. Eradication of hepatitis C virus infection and the development of hepatocellular carcinoma: a meta-analysis of observational studies. *Ann Intern Med* 2013;158:329.
31. El-Serag HB. Hepatocellular carcinoma. *N Engl J Med* 2011;365:1118–1127.
32. Zhang BH, Yang BH, Tang ZY. Randomized controlled trial of screening for hepatocellular carcinoma. *J Cancer Res Clin Oncol* 2004;130:417–422.
33. Singal AG, Pillai A, Tiro J. Early detection, curative treatment, and survival rates for hepatocellular carcinoma surveillance in patients with cirrhosis: a meta-analysis. *PLoS Med* 2014;11(4):e1001624.
34. Yuen MF, Cheng CC, Lauder IJ, et al. Early detection of hepatocellular carcinoma increases the chance of treatment: Hong Kong experience. *Hepatology* 2000;31:330–335.
35. Lee CS, Sung JL, Hwang LY, et al. Surgical treatment of 109 patients with symptomatic and asymptomatic hepatocellular carcinoma. *Surgery* 1986;99:481–490.
36. Vallis KA, Benjamin IS, Munro AJ, et al. External beam and intraluminal radiotherapy for locally advanced bile duct cancer: role and tolerability. *Radiother Oncol* 1996;41:61–66.
37. Buti M, Sanchez F, Cotrina M, et al. Quantitative hepatitis B virus DNA testing for the early prediction of the maintenance of response during lamivudine therapy in patients with chronic hepatitis B. *J Infect Dis* 2001;183:1277–1280.
38. Cheng SH, Lin YM, Chuang VP, et al. A pilot study of three-dimensional conformal radiotherapy in unresectable hepatocellular carcinoma. *J Gastroenterol Hepatol* 1999;14:1025–1033.
39. Gogel BM, Goldstein RM, Kuhn JA, et al. Diagnostic evaluation of hepatocellular carcinoma in a cirrhotic liver. *Oncology (Williston Park)* 2000;14:15–20.
40. Bruix J, Sherman M. Management of hepatocellular carcinoma. *Hepatology* 2005;42:1208–1236.
41. Serra C, Righi S, Molo CD, et al. Current role of contrast-enhanced ultrasound in the diagnosis of hepatocellular carcinoma. *J Hepatol Gastroint Dis* 2015;1:102. doi:10.4172/2475-3181.1000102
42. Kim SE, Lee HC, Shim JH, et al. Noninvasive diagnostic criteria for hepatocellular carcinoma in hepatic masses >2 cm in a hepatitis B virus-endemic area. *Liver International* 2011;31:1468–1476.
43. Takamori R, Wong LL, Dang C, et al. Needle-tract implantation from hepatocellular cancer: is needle biopsy of the liver always necessary? *Liver Transpl* 2000;6:67–72.
44. Durand F, Regimbeau JM, Belghiti J, et al. Assessment of the benefits and risks of percutaneous biopsy before surgical resection of hepatocellular carcinoma. *J Hepatol* 2001;35:254–258.
45. Huang GT, Sheu JC, Yang PM, et al. Ultrasound-guided cutting biopsy for the diagnosis of hepatocellular carcinoma—a study based on 420 patients. *J Hepatol* 1996;25:334–338.
46. Kim SH, Lim HK, Lee WJ, et al. Needle-tract implantation in hepatocellular carcinoma: frequency and CT findings after biopsy with a 19.5-gauge automated biopsy gun. *Abdom Imaging* 2000;25:246–250.
47. Maturen KE, Nghiem HV, Marrero JA, et al. Lack of tumor seeding of hepatocellular carcinoma after percutaneous needle biopsy using coaxial cutting needle technique. *AJR Am J Roentgenol* 2006;187:1184–1187.
48. Kanematsu M, Hoshi H, Yamada T, et al. Small hepatic nodules in cirrhosis: ultrasonographic, CT, and MR imaging findings. *Abdom Imaging* 1999;24:47–55.
49. Ishiguchi T, Shimamoto K, Fukatsu H, et al. Radiologic diagnosis of hepatocellular carcinoma. *Semin Surg Oncol* 1996;12:164–169.
50. Katyal S, Oliver JH III, Peterson MS, et al. Extrahepatic metastases of hepatocellular carcinoma. *Radiology* 2000;216:698–703.
51. Amin MB, Edge S, Greene F, et al. *AJCC cancer staging manual*. New York: Springer, 2017.
52. Okuda K, Ohtsuki T, Obata H, et al. Natural history of hepatocellular carcinoma and prognosis in relation to treatment. Study of 850 patients. *Cancer* 1985;56:918–928.
53. Pinna AD, Iwatsuki S, Lee RG, et al. Treatment of fibrolamellar hepatoma with subtotal hepatectomy or transplantation. *Hepatology* 1997;26:877–883.

Section III

54. Carceller A, Blanchard H, Champagne J, et al. Surgical resection and chemotherapy improve survival rate for patients with hepatoblastoma. *J Pediatr Surg* 2001;36:755–759.
55. Jung SE, Kim KH, Kim MY, et al. Clinical characteristics and prognosis of patients with hepatoblastoma. *World J Surg* 2001;25:126–130.
56. Hanazaki K, Wakabayashi M, Sodeyama H, et al. Surgical outcome in cirrhotic patients with hepatitis C-related hepatocellular carcinoma. *Hepatogastroenterology* 2000;47:204–210.
57. Kubo S, Nishiguchi S, Hirohashi K, et al. Clinicopathological criteria for multicentricity of hepatocellular carcinoma and risk factors for such carcinogenesis. *Jpn J Cancer Res* 1998;89:419–426.
58. Poon RT, Fan ST, Ng IO, et al. Different risk factors and prognosis for early and late intrahepatic recurrence after resection of hepatocellular carcinoma. *Cancer* 2000;89:500–507.
59. Kubo S, Hirohashi K, Tanaka H, et al. Virologic and biochemical changes and prognosis after liver resection for hepatitis B virus-related hepatocellular carcinoma. *Dig Surg* 2001;18:26–33.
60. Bruix J, Castells A, Bosch J, et al. Surgical resection of hepatocellular carcinoma in cirrhotic patients: prognostic value of preoperative portal pressure. *Gastroenterology* 1996;111:1018–1022.
61. Yamamoto J, Iwatsuki S, Kosuge T, et al. Should hepatomas be treated with hepatic resection or transplantation? *Cancer* 1999;86:1151–1158.
62. Clavien PA, Lesurtel M, Bossuyt MM, et al. Recommendations for liver transplantation for hepatocellular carcinoma: an international consensus conference report. *Lancet Oncol* 2012;13(1):e11–e22.
63. Mazzaferro V, Regalia E, Doci R, et al. Liver transplantation for the treatment of small hepatocellular carcinomas in patients with cirrhosis. *N Engl J Med* 1996;334:693–699.
64. Michel J, Suc B, Montpeyroux F, et al. Liver resection or transplantation for hepatocellular carcinoma? Retrospective analysis of 215 patients with cirrhosis. *J Hepatol* 1997;26:1274–1280.
65. Bismuth H, Chiche L, Adam R, et al. Liver resection versus transplantation for hepatocellular carcinoma in cirrhotic patients. *Ann Surg* 1993;218:145–151.
66. Philosophe B, Greig PD, Hemming AW, et al. Surgical management of hepatocellular carcinoma: resection or transplantation? *J Gastrointest Surg* 1998;2:21–27.
67. Chapman RW. Risk factors for biliary tract carcinogenesis. *Ann Oncol* 1999;10(Suppl 4):308–311.
68. Gerhards MF, van Gulik TM, Gonzalez Gonzalez D, et al. Results of postoperative radiotherapy for resectable hilar cholangiocarcinoma. *World J Surg* 2003;27:173–179.
69. Ferrari FS, Stella A, Gambacorta D, et al. Treatment of large hepatocellular carcinoma: comparison between techniques and long term results. *Radiol Med (Torino)* 2004;108:356–371.
70. Lin SM, Lin CJ, Lin CC, et al. Randomised controlled trial comparing percutaneous radiofrequency thermal ablation, percutaneous ethanol injection, and percutaneous acetic acid injection to treat hepatocellular carcinoma of 3 cm or less. *Gut* 2005;54:1151–1156.
71. Meloni F, Lazzaroni S, Livraghi T. Percutaneous ethanol injection: single session treatment. *Eur J Ultrasound* 2001;13:107–115.
72. Lencioni RA, Allgaier HP, Cioni D, et al. Small hepatocellular carcinoma in cirrhosis: randomized comparison of radio-frequency thermal ablation versus percutaneous ethanol injection. *Radiology* 2003;228:235–240.
73. Lin SM, Lin CJ, Lin CC, et al. Radiofrequency ablation improves prognosis compared with ethanol injection for hepatocellular carcinoma < or = 4 cm. *Gastroenterology* 2004;127:1714–1723.
74. Livraghi T, Lazzaroni S, Meloni F. Radiofrequency thermal ablation of hepatocellular carcinoma. *Eur J Ultrasound* 2001;13:159–166.
75. Shiina S, Teratani T, Obi S, et al. A randomized controlled trial of radiofrequency ablation with ethanol injection for small hepatocellular carcinoma. *Gastroenterology* 2005;129:122–130.
76. Groupe d'Etude et de Traitement du Carcinome Hepatocellulaire. GA comparison of lipiodol chemoembolization and conservative treatment for unresectable hepatocellular carcinoma. *N Engl J Med* 1995;332:1256–1261.
77. Pelletier G, Roche A, Ink O, et al. A randomized trial of hepatic arterial chemoembolization in patients with unresectable hepatocellular carcinoma. *J Hepatol* 1990;11:181–184.
78. Llovet JM, Bruix J. Systematic review of randomized trials for unresectable hepatocellular carcinoma: chemoembolization improves survival. *Hepatology* 2003;37:429–442.
79. Chuang VP, Wallace S. Chemoembolization: transcatheter management of neoplasms. *JAMA* 1981;245:1151–1152.
80. Dhir V, Swaroop VS, Mohandas KM, et al. Combination chemotherapy and radiation for palliation of hepatocellular carcinoma. *Am J Clin Oncol* 1992;15:304–307.
81. Friedman MA, Volberding PA, Cassidy MJ, et al. Therapy for hepatocellular cancer with intrahepatic arterial adriamycin and 5-fluorouracil combined with whole-liver irradiation: a Northern California Oncology Group Study. *Cancer Treat Rep* 1979;63:1885–1888.
82. Gunderson LL, Haddock MG, Foo ML, et al. Conformal irradiation for hepatobiliary malignancies. *Ann Oncol* 1999;10(Suppl 4):221–225.
83. Shirato H, Seppenwoolde Y, Kitamura K, et al. Intrafractional tumor motion: lung and liver. *Semin Radiat Oncol* 2004;14:10–18.
84. Hawkins MA, Dawson LA. Radiation therapy for hepatocellular carcinoma: from palliation to cure. *Cancer* 2006;106:1653–1663.
85. Lin CS, Jen YM, Chiu SY, et al. Treatment of portal vein tumor thrombosis of hepatoma patients with either stereotactic radiotherapy or three-dimensional conformal radiotherapy. *Jpn J Clin Oncol* 2006;36:212–217.
86. Yamada K, Soejima T, Sugimoto K, et al. Pilot study of local radiotherapy for portal vein tumor thrombus in patients with unresectable hepatocellular carcinoma. *Jpn J Clin Oncol* 2001;31:147–152.
87. Dawson LA, McGinn CJ, Normolle D, et al. Escalated focal liver radiation and concurrent hepatic artery fluorodeoxyuridine for unresectable intrahepatic malignancies. *J Clin Oncol* 2000;18:2210–2218.
88. Order SE, Stillwagon GB, Klein JL, et al. Iodine 131 antiferritin, a new treatment modality in hepatoma: a Radiation Therapy Oncology Group study. *J Clin Oncol* 1985;3:1573–1582.
89. Stillwagon GB, Order SE, Guse C, et al. 194 Hepatocellular cancers treated by radiation and chemotherapy combinations: toxicity and response: a Radiation Therapy Oncology Group Study. *Int J Radiat Oncol Biol Phys* 1989;17:1223–1229.
90. Seong J, Park HC, Han KH, et al. Local radiotherapy for unresectable hepatocellular carcinoma patients who failed with transcatheter arterial chemoembolization. *Int J Radiat Oncol Biol Phys* 2000;47:1331–1335.
91. Kondo S, Nimura Y, Kamiya J, et al. Factors influencing postoperative hospital mortality and long-term survival after radical resection for stage IV gallbladder carcinoma. *World J Surg* 2003;27:272–277.
92. Sturm PD, Baas IO, Clement MJ, et al. Alterations of the p53 tumor-suppressor gene and K-RAS oncogene in perihilar cholangiocarcinomas from a high-incidence area. *Int J Cancer* 1998;78:695–698.
93. Nagorney DM, Donohue JH, Farnell MB, et al. Outcomes after curative resections of cholangiocarcinoma. *Arch Surg* 1993;128:871–879.
94. McGinn CJ, Ten Haken RK, Ensminger WD, et al. Treatment of intrahepatic cancers with radiation doses based on a normal tissue complication probability model. *J Clin Oncol* 1998;16:2246–2252.
95. Cheng JC, Wu JK, Huang CM, et al. Radiation-induced liver disease after three-dimensional conformal radiotherapy for patients with hepatocellular carcinoma: dosimetric analysis and implication. *Int J Radiat Oncol Biol Phys* 2002;54:156–162.
96. Liang SX, Zhu XD, Xu ZY, et al. Radiation-induced liver disease in three-dimensional conformal radiation therapy for primary liver carcinoma: the risk factors and hepatic radiation tolerance. *Int J Radiat Oncol Biol Phys* 2006;65:426–434.
97. Kawasaki S, Makuuchi M, Miyagawa S, et al. Results of hepatic resection for hepatocellular carcinoma. *World J Surg* 1995;19:31–34.
98. Kwon JH, Bae SH, Kim JY, et al. Long-term effect of stereotactic body radiation therapy for primary hepatocellular carcinoma ineligible for local ablation therapy or surgical resection. Stereotactic radiotherapy for liver cancer. *BMC Cancer* 2010;10:475.
99. Kang JK, Kim MS, Cho CK, et al. Stereotactic body radiation therapy for inoperable hepatocellular carcinoma as a local salvage treatment after incomplete transarterial chemoembolization. *Cancer* 2012;118:5424.
100. Sanuki N, Takeda A, Oku Y, et al. Stereotactic body radiotherapy for small hepatocellular carcinoma: a retrospective outcome analysis in 185 patients. *Acta Oncol* 2014;53:399.
101. Jang WI, Kim MS, Bae SH, et al. High-dose stereotactic body radiotherapy correlates increased local control and overall survival in patients with inoperable hepatocellular carcinoma. *Radiat Oncol* 2013;8:250.
102. Gonzalez-Guindalini FD, Botelho MPF, Harmath CB, et al. Assessment of liver tumor response to therapy: role of quantitative imaging. *Radiographics* 2013;33:1781–1800.
103. Deshpande S. To study tumor motion and planning target volume margins using four dimensional computed tomography for cancer of the thorax and abdomen regions. *J Med Phys* 2011;36:35–39.
104. Eccles CL, Dawson LA, Moseley JL, et al. Interfraction liver shape variability and impact on GTV position during liver stereotactic radiotherapy using abdominal compression. *Int J Radiation Oncol Biol Phys* 2011;80:938–946.
105. Yu JI, Kim JS, Park HC, et al. Evaluation of anatomical landmark position differences between respiration-gated MRI and four-dimensional CT for radiation therapy in patients with hepatocellular carcinoma. *Br J Radiol* 2013;86:20120221.
106. Aruga T, Itami J, Aruga M, et al. Target volume definition for upper abdominal irradiation using CT scans obtained during inhale and exhale phases. *Int J Radiat Oncol Biol Phys* 2000;48:465–469.
107. Ohara K, Okumura T, Akisada M, et al. Irradiation synchronized with respiration gate. *Int J Radiat Oncol Biol Phys* 1989;17:853–857.
108. Balter JM, Lam KL, McGinn CJ, et al. Improvement of CT-based treatment-planning models of abdominal targets using static exhale imaging. *Int J Radiat Oncol Biol Phys* 1998;41:939–943.
109. Shimizu S, Shirato H, Xo B, et al. Three-dimensional movement of a liver tumor detected by high-speed magnetic resonance imaging. *Radiother Oncol* 1999;50:367–370.
110. Son SH, Choi BO, Ryu MR, et al. Stereotactic body radiotherapy for patients with unresectable primary hepatocellular carcinoma: dose-volume parameters predicting the hepatic complication. *Int J Radiat Oncol Biol Phys* 2010;78:1073–1080.
111. Tarita O, Thomas TO, Shaakir Hasan S, et al. The tolerance of gastrointestinal organs to stereotactic body radiation therapy: what do we know so far? *J Gastrointest Oncol* 2014;5(3):236.
112. Mahadevan A, Jain S, Goldstein M, et al. Stereotactic body radiotherapy and gemcitabine for locally advanced pancreatic cancer. *Int J Radiat Oncol Biol Phys* 2010;78:735–742.
113. Bujold A, Massey CA, Kim JJ, et al. Sequential phase I and II trials of stereotactic body radiotherapy for locally advanced hepatocellular carcinoma. *J Clin Oncol* 2013;31(13):1631.
114. Seong J, Park HC, Han KH, et al. Clinical results of 3-dimensional conformal radiotherapy combined with transarterial chemoembolization for hepatocellular carcinoma in the cirrhotic patients. *Hepatol Res* 2003;27:30–35.
115. Adachi E, Matsumata T, Nishizaki T, et al. Effects of preoperative transcatheter hepatic arterial chemoembolization for hepatocellular carcinoma. The relationship between postoperative course and tumor necrosis. *Cancer* 1993;72:3593–5598.
116. Higuchi T, Kikuchi M, Okazaki M. Hepatocellular carcinoma after transcatheter hepatic arterial embolization. A histopathologic study of 84 resected cases. *Cancer* 1994;73:2259–2267.
117. Poggio JL, Nagorney DM, Nascimento AG, et al. Surgical treatment of adult primary hepatic sarcoma. *Br J Surg* 2000;87:1500–1505.
118. Minsky BD, Kemeny N, Armstrong JG, et al. Extrahepatic biliary system cancer: an update of a combined modality approach. *Am J Clin Oncol* 1991;14:433–437.
119. Czito BG, Hurwitz HI, Clough RW, et al. Adjuvant external-beam radiotherapy with concurrent chemotherapy after resection of primary gallbladder carcinoma: a 23-year experience. *Int J Radiat Oncol Biol Phys* 2005;62:1030–1034.

120. Guo WJ, Yu EX. Evaluation of combined therapy with chemoembolization and irradiation for large hepatocellular carcinoma. *Br J Radiol* 2000;73:1091–1097.

120a. Yasuda S, Ito H, Yoshikawa M, et al. Radiotherapy for large hepatocellular carcinoma combined with transcatheter arterial embolization and percutaneous ethanol injection therapy. *Int J Oncol* 1999;15:467–473.

121. Wu DH, Liu L, Chen LH. Therapeutic effects and prognostic factors in three-dimensional conformal radiotherapy combined with transcatheter arterial chemoembolization for hepatocellular carcinoma. *World J Gastroenterol* 2004;10:2184–2189.

122. Tazawa J, Maeda M, Sakai Y, et al. Radiation therapy in combination with transcatheter arterial chemoembolization for hepatocellular carcinoma with extensive portal vein involvement. *J Gastroenterol Hepatol* 2001;16:660.

123. Nagahama H, Okada S, Okusaka T, et al. Predictive factors for tumor response to systemic chemotherapy in patients with hepatocellular carcinoma. *Jpn J Clin Oncol* 1997;27:321–324.

124. Yang TS, Lin YC, Chen JS, et al. Phase II study of gemcitabine in patients with advanced hepatocellular carcinoma. *Cancer* 2000;89:750–756.

125. Leung TW, Patt YZ, Lau WY, et al. Complete pathological remission is possible with systemic combination chemotherapy for inoperable hepatocellular carcinoma. *Clin Cancer Res* 1999;5:1676–1681.

126. Louafi S, Boige V, Ducreux M, et al. Gemcitabine plus oxaliplatin (GEMOX) in patients with advanced hepatocellular carcinoma (HCC). *Cancer* 2007;109:1384.

127. Patt YZ, Hassan MM, Lozano RD, et al. Durable clinical response of refractory hepatocellular carcinoma to orally administered thalidomide. *Am J Clin Oncol* 2000;23:319–321.

128. Patt YZ, Hassan MM, Lozano RD, et al. Thalidomide in the treatment of patients with hepatocellular carcinoma: a phase II trial. *Cancer* 2005;103:749–755.

129. Zhu AX. Development of sorafenib and other molecularly targeted agents in hepatocellular carcinoma. *Cancer* 2008;112:250.

130. Llovet JM, Ricci S, Mazzaferro V, et al. Sorafenib in advanced hepatocellular carcinoma. *N Engl J Med* 2008;359:378.

131. Chen AW, Lin LC, Kuo YC, et al. Phase 2 study of combined sorafenib and radiation therapy in patients with advanced hepatocellular carcinoma. *Int J Radiation Oncol Biol Phys* 2014;88(5):1041–1047.

132. Dawson LA, Brade A, Cho C, et al. Phase I study of sorafenib and SBRT for advanced hepatocellular carcinoma. *Int J Radiation Oncol Biol Phys* 2014;84(3):S10–S11.

133. Peters N, Richel D, Verhoeff J, et al. Bowel perforation after radiotherapy in a patient receiving sorafenib. *J Clin Oncol* 2008;26(14):2405–2410.

134. Feun LG, Li YY, Wangpaichitr M, et al. Immunotherapy for hepatocellular carcinoma: the force awakens in HCC? *Hepatoma Res* 2017;3:43–51.

135. El-Khoueiry AB, Sangro B, Yau T, et al. Nivolumab in patients with advanced hepatocellular carcinoma (CheckMate 040): an open-label, non-comparative, phase 1/2 dose escalation and expansion trial. *Lancet* 2017;389:2492–2502.

136. Dohmen K, Shirahama M, Onohara S, et al. Differences in survival based on the type of follow-up for the detection of hepatocellular carcinoma: an analysis of 547 patients. *Hepatol Res* 2000;18:110–121.

137. Poon RT, Ng IO, Fan ST, et al. Clinicopathologic features of long-term survivors and disease-free survivors after resection of hepatocellular carcinoma: a study of a prospective cohort. *J Clin Oncol* 2001;19:3037–3044.

138. Nakamura H, Mitani T, Murakami T, et al. Five-year survival after transcatheter chemoembolization for hepatocellular carcinoma. *Cancer Chemother Pharmacol* 1994;33(Suppl):S89–S92.

139. Cheng JC, Chuang VP, Cheng SH, et al. Local radiotherapy with or without transcatheter arterial chemoembolization for patients with unresectable hepatocellular carcinoma. *Int J Radiat Oncol Biol Phys* 2000;47:435–442.

140. Seong J, Keum KC, Han KH, et al. Combined transcatheter arterial chemoembolization and local radiotherapy of unresectable hepatocellular carcinoma. *Int J Radiat Oncol Biol Phys* 1999;43:393–397.

141. Landis SH, Murray T, Bolden S, et al. Cancer statistics, 1998. *CA Cancer J Clin* 1998;48:6–29.

142. Duda SH, Huppert PE, Schott U, et al. Percutaneous transhepatic intraductal biliary sonography for lymph node staging at 12.5 MHz in malignant bile duct obstruction: work in progress. *Cardiovasc Intervent Radiol* 1997;20:133–138.

143. Shirabe K, Shimada M, Harimoto N, et al. Intrahepatic cholangiocarcinoma: its mode of spreading and therapeutic modalities. *Surgery* 2002;131:S159–S164.

144. Shin HR, Oh JK, Masuyer E, et al. Epidemiology of cholangiocarcinoma: an update focusing on risk factors. *Cancer Sci* 2010;101:579.

145. Shin HR, Lee CU, Park HJ, et al. Hepatitis B and C virus, *Clonorchis sinensis* for the risk of liver cancer: a case-control study in Pusan, Korea. *Int J Epidemiol* 1996;25:933–940.

146. Vatanasapt V, Martin N, Sriplung H, et al. Cancer incidence in Thailand, 1988–1991. *Cancer Epidemiol Biomarkers Prev* 1995;4:475–483.

147. Gores GJ. Early detection and treatment of cholangiocarcinoma. *Liver Transpl* 2000;6:S30–S34.

148. Bortolasi L, Burgart LJ, Tsiotos GG, et al. Adenocarcinoma of the distal bile duct. A clinicopathologic outcome analysis after curative resection. *Dig Surg* 2000;17:36–41.

149. Yamamoto S, Kubo S, Hai S, et al. Hepatitis C virus infection as a likely etiology of intrahepatic cholangiocarcinoma. *Cancer Sci* 2004;95:592–595.

150. Welzel TM, Graubard BI, El-Serag HB, et al. Risk factors for intra- and extrahepatic cholangiocarcinoma in the United States: a population based case-control study. *Clin Gastroenterol Hepatol* 2007;5:1221–1228.

151. Chijiiwa K, Ichimiya H, Kuroki S, et al. Late development of cholangiocarcinoma after the treatment of hepatolithiasis. *Surg Gynecol Obstet* 1993;177:279–282.

152. Kubo S, Kinoshita H, Hirohashi K, et al. Hepatolithiasis associated with cholangiocarcinoma. *World J Surg* 1995;19:637–641.

153. Parkin DM, Srivatanakul P, Khlat M, et al. Liver cancer in Thailand. I. A case-control study of cholangiocarcinoma. *Int J Cancer* 1991;48:323–328.

154. Chao TC, Greager JA. Primary carcinoma of the gallbladder. *J Surg Oncol* 1991;46:215–221.

155. Parkin DM, Pisani P, Ferlay J. Estimates of the worldwide incidence of 25 major cancers in 1990. *Int J Cancer* 1999;80:827–841.

156. Patel T. Increasing incidence and mortality of primary intrahepatic cholangiocarcinoma in the United States. *Hepatology* 2001;33:1353–1357.

157. Supriya K. Saha SK, Zhu AX, et al. Forty-year trends in cholangiocarcinoma incidence in the U.S.: intrahepatic disease on the rise. *The Oncologist* 2016;21:594–599.

158. Taylor-Robinson SD, Foster GR, Arora S, et al. Increase in primary liver cancer in the UK, 1979–94. *Lancet* 1997;350:1142–1143.

159. Nakeeb A, Pitt HA, Sohn TA, et al. Cholangiocarcinoma. A spectrum of intrahepatic, perihilar, and distal tumors. *Ann Surg* 1996;224:463–475.

160. Hultcrantz R, Olsson R, Danielsson A, et al. A 3-year prospective study on serum tumor markers used for detecting cholangiocarcinoma in patients with primary sclerosing cholangitis. *J Hepatol* 1999;30:669–673.

161. Nakeeb A, Lipsett PA, Lillemoe KD, et al. Biliary carcinoembryonic antigen levels are a marker for cholangiocarcinoma. *Am J Surg* 1996;171:147–153.

162. Bjornsson E, Kilander A, Olsson R. CA 19-9 and CEA are unreliable markers for cholangiocarcinoma in patients with primary sclerosing cholangitis. *Liver* 1999;19:501–508.

163. Nakamura S, Suzuki S, Sakaguchi T, et al. Surgical treatment of patients with mixed hepatocellular carcinoma and cholangiocarcinoma. *Cancer* 1996;78:1671–1676.

164. Nakanuma Y, Sato Y, Harada K, et al. Pathological classification of intrahepatic cholangiocarcinoma based on a new concept. *World J Hepatol* 2010;2:419–427.

165. Komuta M, Govaere O, Vandecaveye V, et al. Histological diversity in cholangiocellular carcinoma reflects the different cholangiocyte phenotypes. *Hepatology* 2012;55:1876–1888.

166. Jarnagin WR, Bowne W, Klimstra DS, et al. Papillary phenotype confers improved survival after resection of hilar cholangiocarcinoma. *Ann Surg* 2005;241:703–714.

167. Weinbren K, Mutum SS. Pathological aspects of cholangiocarcinoma. *J Pathol* 1983;139:217–238.

168. Klempnauer J, Ridder GJ, von Wasielewski R, et al. Resectional surgery of hilar cholangiocarcinoma: a multivariate analysis of prognostic factors. *J Clin Oncol* 1997;15:947–954.

169. Tsuji M, Kashihara T, Terada N, et al. An immunohistochemical study of hepatic atypical adenomatous hyperplasia, hepatocellular carcinoma, and cholangiocarcinoma with alpha-fetoprotein, carcinoembryonic antigen, CA19-9, epithelial membrane antigen, and cytokeratins 18 and 19. *Pathol Int* 1999;49:310–317.

170. Ahrendt SA, Rashid A, Chow JT, et al. p53 overexpression and K-RAS gene mutations in primary sclerosing cholangitis-associated biliary tract cancer. *J Hepatobiliary Pancreat Surg* 2000;7:426–431.

171. Ohashi K, Nakajima Y, Kanehiro H, et al. Ki-ras mutations and p53 protein expressions in intrahepatic cholangiocarcinomas: relation to gross tumor morphology. *Gastroenterology* 1995;109:1612–1617.

172. Farshidfar F, Zheng S, Gingras MC, et al. Integrative genomic analysis of cholangiocarcinoma identifies distinct IDH-mutant molecular Profiles. *Cell Reports* 2017;18:2780–2794.

173. Fujii T, Khawaja MR, DiNardo CD, et al. Targeting isocitrate dehydrogenase (IDH) in cancer. *Discov Med* 2016;21:373–380.

174. Yoshida T, Aramaki M, Bandoh T, et al. Para-aortic lymph node metastasis in carcinoma of the distal bile duct. *Hepatogastroenterology* 1998;45:2388–2391.

175. Tsuji T, Hiraoka T, Kanemitsu K, et al. Lymphatic spreading pattern of intrahepatic cholangiocarcinoma. *Surgery* 2001;129:401–407.

176. Yamamoto M, Takasaki K, Yoshikawa T. Lymph node metastasis in intrahepatic cholangiocarcinoma. *Jpn J Clin Oncol* 1999;29:147–150.

177. Raoof M, Dumitra S, Ituarte PHG, et al. Development and validation of a prognostic score for intrahepatic cholangiocarcinoma. *JAMA Surg* 2017;152(5):e170117.

178. Garner PD, Hall LD, Johnstone PA. Palliation of unresectable hilar cholangiocarcinoma. *J Surg Oncol* 2000;75:95–97.

179. Chen MF, Jan YY, Jeng LB, et al. Intrahepatic cholangiocarcinoma in Taiwan. *J Hepatobiliary Pancreat Surg* 1999;6:136–141.

180. Chu KM, Fan ST. Intrahepatic cholangiocarcinoma in Hong Kong. *J Hepatobiliary Pancreat Surg* 1999;6:149–153.

181. El Rassi ZE, Partensky C, Scoazec JY, et al. Peripheral cholangiocarcinoma: presentation, diagnosis, pathology and management. *Eur J Surg Oncol* 1999;25:375–380.

182. Roayaie S, Guarrera JV, Ye MQ, et al. Aggressive surgical treatment of intrahepatic cholangiocarcinoma: predictors of outcomes. *J Am Coll Surg* 1998;187:365–372.

183. Valverde A, Bonhomme N, Farges O, et al. Resection of intrahepatic cholangiocarcinoma: a Western experience. *J Hepatobiliary Pancreat Surg* 1999;6:122–127.

184. Yamamoto M, Takasaki K, Otsubo T, et al. Recurrence after surgical resection of intrahepatic cholangiocarcinoma. *J Hepatobiliary Pancreat Surg* 2001;8:154–157.

185. Yeo CJ, Pitt HA, Cameron JL. Cholangiocarcinoma. *Surg Clin North Am* 1990;70:1429–1447.

186. Robertson JM, Lawrence TS, Andrews JC, et al. Long-term results of hepatic artery fluorodeoxyuridine and conformal radiation therapy for primary hepatobiliary cancers. *Int J Radiat Oncol Biol Phys* 1997;37:325–330.

187. Kopek N, Holt MI, Hansen AT, et al. Stereotactic body radiotherapy for unresectable cholangiocarcinoma. *Radiother Oncol* 2010;94:47–52.

188. Momm F, Schubert E, Henne K, et al. Stereotactic fractionated radiotherapy for Klatskin tumours. *Radiother Oncol* 2010;95:99–102.

189. Beavers KL, Bonis PAL, Lau J. Liver transplantation for patients with hepatobiliary malignancies other than hepatocellular carcinoma. Available online at https://www.cms.gov/medicare-coverage-database/. Accessed on August 13, 2017.

190. Meyer CG, Penn I, James L. Liver transplantation for cholangiocarcinoma: results in 207 patients. *Transplantation* 2000;69:1633–1637.

191. Klatskin G. Adenocarcinoma of the hepatic duct at its bifurcation within the porta hepatis. An unusual tumor with distinctive clinical and pathological features. *Am J Med* 1965;38:241–256.

192. Bismuth H, Nakache R, Diamond T. Management strategies in resection for hilar cholangiocarcinoma. *Ann Surg* 1992;215:31–38.
193. Tsao JI, Nimura Y, Kamiya J, et al. Management of hilar cholangiocarcinoma: comparison of an American and a Japanese experience. *Ann Surg* 2000;232:166–174.
194. Pitt HA, Nakeeb A, Abrams RA, et al. Perihilar cholangiocarcinoma. Postoperative radiotherapy does not improve survival. *Ann Surg* 1995;221:788–798.
195. Takada T, Amano H, Yasuda H, et al. Is postoperative adjuvant chemotherapy useful for gallbladder carcinoma? A phase III multicenter prospective randomized controlled trial in patients with resected pancreaticobiliary carcinoma. *Cancer* 2002;95:1685–1695.
196. Todoroki T, Ohara K, Kawamoto T, et al. Benefits of adjuvant radiotherapy after radical resection of locally advanced main hepatic duct carcinoma. *Int J Radiat Oncol Biol Phys* 2000;46:581–587.
197. Morganti AG, Trodella L, Valentini V, et al. Combined modality treatment in unresectable extrahepatic biliary carcinoma. *Int J Radiat Oncol Biol Phys* 2000;46:913–919.
198. Verbeek PC, Van Leeuwen DJ, Van Der Heyde MN, et al. Does additive radiotherapy after hilar resection improve survival of cholangiocarcinoma? An analysis in sixty-four patients. *Ann Chir* 1991;45:350–354.
199. Whittington R, Neuberg D, Tester WJ, et al. Protracted intravenous fluorouracil infusion with radiation therapy in the management of localized pancreaticobiliary carcinoma: a phase I Eastern Cooperative Oncology Group Trial. *J Clin Oncol* 1995;13:227–232.
200. Rea DJ, Heimbach JK, Rosen CB, et al. Liver transplantation with neoadjuvant chemoradiation is more effective than resection for hilar cholangiocarcinoma. *Ann Surg* 2005;242:451–461.
201. Heimbach JK, Gores GJ, Haddock MG, et al. Liver transplantation for unresectable perihilar cholangiocarcinoma. *Semin Liver Dis* 2004;24:201–207.
202. Sudan D, DeRoover A, Chinnakotla S, et al. Radiochemotherapy and transplantation allow long-term survival for nonresectable hilar cholangiocarcinoma. *Am J Transplant* 2002;2:774–779.
203. Alberts SR, Al-Khatib H, Mahoney MR, et al. Gemcitabine, 5-fluorouracil, and leucovorin in advanced biliary tract and gallbladder carcinoma: a North Central Cancer Treatment Group phase II trial. *Cancer* 2005;103:111–118.
204. Verderame F, Russo A, Di Leo R, et al. Gemcitabine and oxaliplatin combination chemotherapy in advanced biliary tract cancers. *Ann Oncol* 2006;17:vii68–vii72.
205. Alden ME, Waterman FM, Topham AK, et al. Cholangiocarcinoma: clinical significance of tumor location along the extrahepatic bile duct. *Radiology* 1995;197:511–516.
206. Mehta VK, Fisher GA, Ford JM, et al. Adjuvant chemoradiotherapy for "unfavorable" carcinoma of the ampulla of Vater: preliminary report. *Arch Surg* 2001;136:65–69.
207. Murakami Y, Uemu K, Sudo T, et al. Gemcitabine-based adjuvant chemotherapy improves survival after aggressive surgery for hilar cholangiocarcinoma. *J Gastrointest Surg* 2009;13:1470.
208. Liu YB, Fang CH, Jian ZX, et al. Surgical management and prognostic factors of hilar cholangiocarcinoma: experience with 115 cases in China. *Ann Surg Oncol* 2008;15:2113–2119.
209. Horgan AM, Amir E, Walter T, et al. Adjuvant therapy in the treatment of biliary tract cancer: a systematic review and meta-analysis. *J Clin Oncol* 2012;30:1934–1940.
210. Glimelius B, Hoffman K, Sjoden PO, et al. Chemotherapy improves survival and quality of life in advanced pancreatic and biliary cancer. *Ann Oncol* 1996;7:593.
211. Valle J, Wasan H, Palmer DH, et al. Cisplatin plus gemcitabine versus gemcitabine for biliary tract cancer. *N Engl J Med* 2010;362:1273–1281.
212. Banales JM, Cardinale V, Carpino G, et al. Expert consensus document: cholangiocarcinoma: current knowledge and future perspectives consensus statement from the European Network for the Study of Cholangiocarcinoma. *Nat Rev Gastroenterol Hepatol* 2016;13:261–280.
213. Crane CH, MacDonald KO, Vauthey JN, et al. Limitations of conventional doses of chemoradiation for unresectable biliary cancer. *Int J Radiat Oncol Biol Phys* 2002;53:969–974.
214. Ben-David MA, Griffith KA, Abu-Isa E, et al. External-beam radiotherapy for localized extrahepatic cholangiocarcinoma. *Int J Radiat Oncol Biol Phys* 2006;66:772–779.
215. Mahadevan A, Dagoglu N, Mancias J, et al. Stereotactic body radiotherapy (SBRT) for intrahepatic and hilar cholangiocarcinoma. *J Cancer* 2015;6:1099–1104.
216. Kopek N, Holt MI, Hansen AT, et al. Stereotactic body radiotherapy for unresectable cholangiocarcinoma. *Radiothera Oncol* 2010;94:47–52.
217. Kitagawa Y, Nagino M, Kamiya J, et al. Lymph node metastasis from hilar cholangiocarcinoma: audit of 110 patients who underwent regional and paraaortic node dissection. *Ann Surg* 2001;233:385–392.
218. Yamaguchi K, Chijiiwa K, Saiki S, et al. Carcinoma of the extrahepatic bile duct: mode of spread and its prognostic implications. *Hepatogastroenterology* 1997;44:1256–1261.
219. Urego M, Flickinger JC, Carr BI. Radiotherapy and multimodality management of cholangiocarcinoma. *Int J Radiat Oncol Biol Phys* 1999;44:121–126.
220. Alden ME, Mohiuddin M. The impact of radiation dose in combined external beam and intraluminal Ir-192 brachytherapy for bile duct cancer. *Int J Radiat Oncol Biol Phys* 1994;28:945–951.
221. Gonzalez Gonzalez D, Gouma DJ, Rauws EA, et al. Role of radiotherapy, in particular intraluminal brachytherapy, in the treatment of proximal bile duct carcinoma. *Ann Oncol* 1999;10(Suppl 4):215–220.
222. The American Cancer Society medical and editorial content team: What are the key statistics about gallbladder cancer? Available online at https://www.cancer.org/cancer/gallbladder-cancer/about/key-statistics.htm. Accessed on August 13, 2017.
223. Sheth S, Bedford A, Chopra S. Primary gallbladder cancer: recognition of risk factors and the role of prophylactic cholecystectomy. *Am J Gastroenterol* 2000;95:1402–1410.
224. Moerman CJ, Bueno-de-Mesquita HB. The epidemiology of gallbladder cancer: lifestyle related risk factors and limited surgical possibilities for prevention. *Hepatogastroenterology* 1999;46:1533–1539.
225. Okamoto M, Okamoto H, Kitahara F, et al. Ultrasonographic evidence of association of polyps and stones with gallbladder cancer. *Am J Gastroenterol* 1999;94:446–450.
226. Dutta U, Garg PK, Kumar R, et al. Typhoid carriers among patients with gallstones are at increased risk for carcinoma of the gallbladder. *Am J Gastroenterol* 2000;95:784–787.
227. Matsukura N, Yokomuro S, Yamada S, et al. Association between *Helicobacter bilis* in bile and biliary tract malignancies: *H. bilis* in bile from Japanese and Thai patients with benign and malignant diseases in the biliary tract. *Jpn J Cancer Res* 2002;93:842–847.
228. Cubertafond P, Mathonnet M, Gainant A, et al. Radical surgery for gallbladder cancer. Results of the French Surgical Association survey. *Hepatogastroenterology* 1999;46:1567–1571.
229. Nakeeb A, Tran KQ, Black MJ, et al. Improved survival in resected biliary malignancies. *Surgery* 2002;132:555–564.
230. Shimada H, Endo I, Togo S, et al. The role of lymph node dissection in the treatment of gallbladder carcinoma. *Cancer* 1997;79:892–899.
231. Todoroki T, Kawamoto T, Takahashi H, et al. Treatment of gallbladder cancer by radical resection. *Br J Surg* 1999;86:622–627.
232. Tsukada K, Kurosaki I, Uchida K, et al. Lymph node spread from carcinoma of the gallbladder. *Cancer* 1997;80:661–667.
233. Shirai Y, Yoshida K, Tsukada K, et al. Inapparent carcinoma of the gallbladder. An appraisal of a radical second operation after simple cholecystectomy. *Ann Surg* 1992;215:326–331.
234. Wakai T, Shirai Y, Yokoyama N, et al. Early gallbladder carcinoma does not warrant radical resection. *Br J Surg* 2001;88:675–678.
235. Ruckert JC, Ruckert RI, Gellert K, et al. Surgery for carcinoma of the gallbladder. *Hepatogastroenterology* 1996;43:527–533.
236. Levin B. Gallbladder carcinoma. *Ann Oncol* 1999;10(Suppl 4):129–130.
237. Tashiro S, Konno T, Mochinaga M, et al. Treatment of carcinoma of the gallbladder in Japan. *Jpn J Surg* 1982;12:98–104.
238. Chijiiwa K, Nakano K, Ueda J, et al. Surgical treatment of patients with T2 gallbladder carcinoma invading the subserosal layer. *J Am Coll Surg* 2001;192:600–607.
239. Houry S, Haccart V, Huguier M, et al. Gallbladder cancer: role of radiation therapy. *Hepatogastroenterology* 1999;46:1578–1584.
240. Nadler LH, McSherry CK. Carcinoma of the gallbladder: review of the literature and report on 56 cases at the Beth Israel Medical Center. *Mt Sinai J Med* 1992;59:47–52.
241. Todoroki T, Kawamoto T, Otsuka M, et al. Benefits of combining radiotherapy with aggressive resection for stage IV gallbladder cancer. *Hepatogastroenterology* 1999;46:1585–1591.
242. de Aretxabala X, Roa I, Burgos L, et al. Preoperative chemoradiotherapy in the treatment of gallbladder cancer. *Am Surg* 1999;65:241–246.
243. Frezza EE, Mezghebe H. Gallbladder carcinoma: a 28 year experience. *Int Surg* 1997;82:295–300.
244. Kresl JJ, Schild SE, Henning GT, et al. Adjuvant external beam radiation therapy with concurrent chemotherapy in the management of gallbladder carcinoma. *Int J Radiat Oncol Biol Phys* 2002;52:167–175.
245. Hejna M, Zielinski CC. Nonsurgical management of gallbladder cancer: cytotoxic treatment and radiotherapy. *Expert Rev Anticancer Ther* 2001;1:291–300.
246. Gebbia V, Majello E, Testa A, et al. Treatment of advanced adenocarcinomas of the exocrine pancreas and the gallbladder with 5-fluorouracil, high dose levofolinic acid and oral hydroxyurea on a weekly schedule. Results of a multicenter study of the Southern Italy Oncology Group (G.O.I.M.). *Cancer* 1996;78:1300–1307.
247. Papakostas P, Kouroussis C, Androulakis N, et al. First-line chemotherapy with docetaxel for unresectable or metastatic carcinoma of the biliary tract. A multicentre phase II study. *Eur J Cancer* 2001;37:1833–1838.
248. Patt YZ, Hassan MM, Aguayo A, et al. Oral capecitabine for the treatment of hepatocellular carcinoma, cholangiocarcinoma, and gallbladder carcinoma. *Cancer* 2004;101:578–586.
249. Patt YZ, Jones DV Jr, Hoque A, et al. Phase II trial of intravenous fluorouracil and subcutaneous interferon alfa-2b for biliary tract cancer. *J Clin Oncol* 1996;14:2311–2315.
250. Penz M, Kornek GV, Raderer M, et al. Phase II trial of two-weekly gemcitabine in patients with advanced biliary tract cancer. *Ann Oncol* 2001;12:183–186.
251. Shirai Y, Ohtani T, Tsukada K, et al. Lymph node recurrence of gallbladder carcinoma successfully managed by systemic chemotherapy with 5-fluorouracil and mitomycin C: report of a 5-year survivor. *Eur J Surg Oncol* 1997;23:457–458.
252. Cioffi U, Quattrone P, De Simone M, et al. Primary multiple epithelioid leiomyosarcoma of the liver. *Hepatogastroenterology* 1996;43:1603–1605.
253. Hozo I, Miric D, Bojic L, et al. Liver angiosarcoma and hemangiopericytoma after occupational exposure to vinyl chloride monomer. *Environ Health Perspect* 2000;108:793–795.
254. Iyer CP, Stanley P, Mahour GH. Hepatic hemangiomas in infants and children: a review of 30 cases. *Am Surg* 1996;62:356–360.
255. Park WC, Rhillips R. The role of radiation therapy in the management of hemangiomas of the liver. *JAMA* 1970;212:1496–1498.
256. Aretz S, Koch A, Uhlhaas S, et al. Should children at risk for familial adenomatous polyposis be screened for hepatoblastoma and children with apparently sporadic hepatoblastoma be screened for APC germline mutations? *Pediatr Blood Cancer* 2006;47:811–818.
257. Giardiello FM, Offerhaus GJ, Krush AJ, et al. Risk of hepatoblastoma in familial adenomatous polyposis. *J Pediatr* 1991;119:766–768.
258. Douglass EC. Hepatic malignancies in childhood and adolescence (hepatoblastoma, hepatocellular carcinoma, and embryonal sarcoma). *Cancer Treat Res* 1997;92:201–212.
259. Seo T, Ando H, Watanabe Y, et al. Treatment of hepatoblastoma: less extensive hepatectomy after effective preoperative chemotherapy with cisplatin and Adriamycin. *Surgery* 1998;123:407–414.

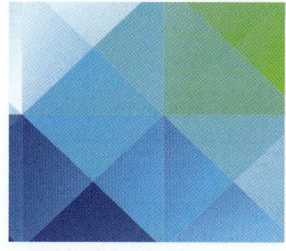

CHAPTER 65

Cancer of the Colon and Rectum

Manisha Palta, Brian G. Czito, and Christopher G. Willett

ANATOMY

The colorectum consists of the cecum, ascending colon, hepatic flexure, transverse colon, splenic flexure, descending colon, sigmoid colon, and rectum. Variability in the peritoneal investment, bowel mobility, and lymph node drainage of the colon and rectum presents unique therapeutic issues.[1]

The posterior and lateral surfaces of the ascending and descending colon are in direct contact with the retroperitoneum, whereas the anterior surface is draped with peritoneum.[1] These posterior attachments can prevent significant mobility, increasing the difficulty of surgical resection. In contrast, the transverse colon is completely surrounded with peritoneum and supported on a long mesentery. As the sigmoid colon evolves distally into the rectum, the peritoneal coverage recedes. The rectum, approximately 12 to 15 cm in length, extends from the rectosigmoid junction to the puborectalis ring. The upper one-third of the rectum is draped with peritoneum anteriorly and on both sides. As the middle one-third of the rectum moves deeper into the pelvis, only the anterior surface is covered with peritoneum, which forms the posterior border of the rectouterine pouch or rectovesical space. The lowest one-third of the rectum is devoid of peritoneal covering and in close proximity to adjacent structures, including the bony pelvis (Fig. 65.1). Distal rectal tumors have no serosal barrier to invasion of adjacent structures and are more difficult to resect, given the close confines of the deep pelvis.

Colonic nodal drainage consists of pericolic nodes and nodes in association with the vascular supply to the colon (i.e., mesenteric nodes). Because of the mobile and extensive nature of the colonic mesentery, complete regional lymph node coverage with external beam radiotherapy (EBRT) is challenging but is usually well treated surgically. In contrast, the major regional groups for rectal nodal drainage can be covered within a reasonable EBRT field and include the perirectal, presacral, and internal iliac nodes.

EPIDEMIOLOGY AND RISK FACTORS

Colorectal cancer (CRC) remains a major worldwide health problem. In the United States alone, it was estimated that there would be 135,430 patients diagnosed with CRC and 50,260 deaths in 2017.[2] Worldwide, approximately 1.2 million new cases per year are diagnosed, with 600,000 deaths.[3] In the United States, incidence of CRC over the last two decades declined by 2% to 3% annually; this is largely attributed to improvements in cancer prevention, early detection, and treatment.[4]

Genetic and environmental factors can increase the likelihood of developing CRC. A number of hereditary CRC syndromes exist, including familial adenomatous polyposis (FAP), MUTYH-associated polyposis, and Lynch syndrome (hereditary nonpolyposis colorectal cancer [HNPCC]). Factors shown to increase the risk of developing CRC include the following: increasing age; male sex; family history of CRC; inflammatory bowel disease; increasing height; increasing body mass index; consumption of processed meat, refined grains, starches, and sugars; excessive alcohol intake and smoking; and low folate consumption.[5,6] Of these risk factors, only increasing age, male sex, and excessive alcohol use have been associated with rectal cancer.[7] Age is a major risk factor for the development of CRC, with median age of diagnosis in the seventh decade. Incidence rates increase dramatically between ages 40 and 50 years and each subsequent decade thereafter (data from Surveillance, Epidemiology, and End Results Program accessible online at www.seer.cancer.gov).

Although CRC may be linked to chemical carcinogens within the bowel lumen, it is not established whether these are ingested, the result of chemical activation of substances in the fecal stream, or a bacterial by-product.[8,9] The value of consumption of fruits and vegetables in the prevention of CRC remains controversial, although recent studies suggested that these associations might have been overstated.[10] Contemporary prospective and randomized data do not support a high-fiber

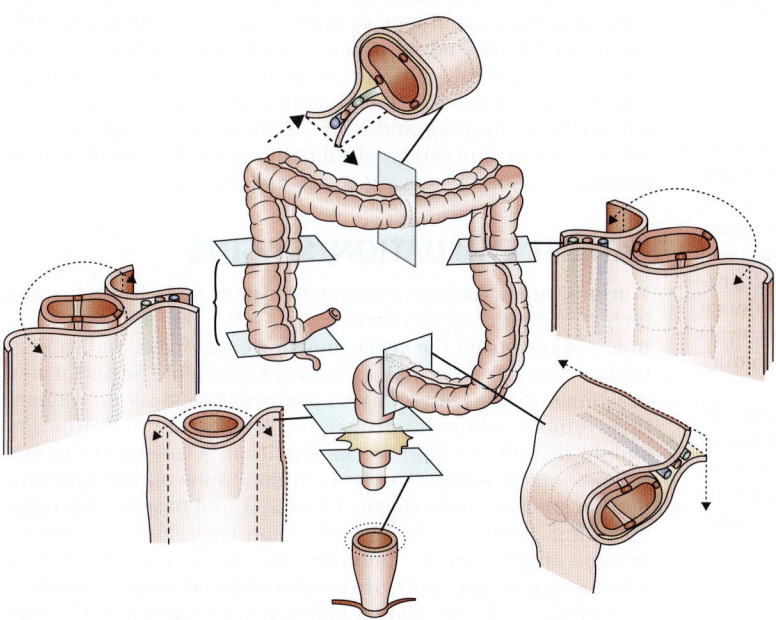

FIGURE 65.1. Idealized depiction of peritoneal relationships in the colon and rectum. The transverse and sigmoid colon are intraperitoneal, with a complete peritoneal covering (serosa) and mesentery. The ascending and descending colon are retroperitoneal, lack a true mesentery, and usually do not have a peritoneal covering posteriorly or laterally. The upper rectum begins above the peritoneal reflection and has peritoneum anteriorly and laterally. The lower one-half to two-thirds of the rectum is below the peritoneal reflection (infraperitoneal). (From Gunderson LL, O'Connell MJ. The postoperative chemotherapy/irradiation adjuvant strategy. In: Cohen AF, Winawer SJ, Friedman MA, et al., eds. *Cancer of the colon, rectum, and anus.* New York: McGraw-Hill, 1995;631–645. Copyright © 1995 McGraw-Hill, Inc. All rights reserved.)

diet in the prevention of CRC.[11] Other studies suggested that nonsteroidal anti-inflammatory drugs may serve in reducing recurrent adenomas and CRC, but long-term therapy must be weighed against potential side effects. The role of chemopreventive agents (carotenoids, aspirin, and other nonsteroidal anti-inflammatory drugs) in CRC remains an area of active investigation. A detailed discussion of the biologic and genetic pathways of development of CRC is beyond the scope of this chapter. In brief, it has been established that the development of colon cancer is a multifactorial process, involving genomic instability, mutational inactivation of tumor suppressor genes, and activation of oncogene pathways. Microsatellites are mutated short-repeat DNA sequences, usually consisting of one to five nucleotides. The majority of patients with HNPCC, as well as a minority of sporadic CRCs, harbor microsatellite instability. It has been shown that this instability occurs in patients with mutations in genes encoding enzymes that repair DNA replication errors. These defects in mismatch repair lead to high-frequency microsatellite and hence genomic instability.[12] Studies suggested that patients with tumors possessing a high frequency of microsatellite instability have more favorable outcomes and lower likelihood of developing metastatic disease.[13] CRC appears to arise through inactivation of the tumor suppressor genes adenomatous polyposis coli (APC), P53, and TGF-β, as well as activation of the RAS, BRAF, and PI3 K proto-oncogenes.[12] Further elucidation of the genetic pathways in the development of CRC remains an active area of investigation and may ultimately affect therapy of this disease.

CLINICAL PRESENTATION

CRC often produces minimal or no symptoms, emphasizing the need for screening programs in the general population. Patients with symptomatic CRC most commonly experience abdominal pain, change in bowel habits, hematochezia/melena, weakness, iron deficiency anemia, and weight loss.[14,15] Less commonly, patients present with nausea, vomiting, or abdominal distension, which may be signs of tumor-related obstruction.

The clinical presentation of CRC is determined largely by site of the tumor. Cancers of the right colon are often exophytic and commonly associated with iron deficiency anemia due to occult blood loss, resulting in delayed diagnosis. During the last 20 years, the incidence of cancer of the right colon appears to have increased and accounts for one-third of large-bowel cancers.[16] Cancers of the left colon and sigmoid colon are often deeply invasive and annular ("apple core lesions") and accompanied by obstruction, rectal bleeding, and alteration in bowel habits.

SCREENING

Neoplastic polyps, including tubular adenomas, villous adenomas, and tubulovillous adenomas, are precursors of colon cancers.[8,17] Most CRC arise from preexisting polyps. As the cumulative lifetime risk of developing CRC in the United States is about 6%, screening programs for the general population have been initiated. The goal of screening is to detect preinvasive polyps or early invasive cancer. Mounting evidence supports that screening of asymptomatic, average-risk individuals can detect CRC at early, curable stage, thereby reducing CRC mortality.[18-20]

Given the data in favor of screening, health organizations such as the American Cancer Society (ACS), the United States Preventive Services Task Force, and the American College of Radiology recommend screening in average-risk individuals starting at age 50. The ACS advocates for tests that detect adenomatous polyps and cancer as follows:

1. Flexible sigmoidoscopy every 5 years.
2. Double-contrast barium enema every 5 years.
3. Computed tomography (CT) colonography every 5 years.

4. Colonoscopy every 10 years.[19]
5. Guaiac-based fecal occult blood, fecal immunohistochemical, and stool DNA tests may be performed for CRC, but not polyp, detection.[21]

In high-risk patients (patients with adenomatous polyps, history of CRC, first-degree relative diagnosed with CRC or adenomas, inflammatory bowel disease, or high risk due to family history or genetic testing), more intensive surveillance is recommended. Individuals with FAP initiate annual sigmoidoscopy or colonoscopy beginning at age 10 to 12 years until age 35 to 40 years if negative. Patients with HNPCC initiate annual screening at age 20 to 25 years or 10 years prior to earliest familial CRC diagnosis.[22,23] Patients with inflammatory bowel disease should initiate screening with colonoscopy 8 to 10 years after initial diagnosis.[21] The American College of Gastroenterology recommends the following for high-risk individuals based on family history[24]:

1. Colonoscopy screening.
2. If single, first-degree relative diagnosed with CRC, or advanced adenoma at age 60+ years, screening every 10 years beginning at age 50 years.
3. If single, first-degree relative diagnosed with CRC, or advanced adenoma at age <60 years or two or more first-degree relatives with CRC or advanced adenoma at any age, screening beginning at age 40 years or 10 years before the youngest relative's diagnosis. Screening should be performed every 5 years.

Although screening methods can detect CRC at an early stage, <40% of patients are diagnosed with early disease, likely reflecting low rates of disease awareness, as well as the infrequency of screening in eligible candidates.[25] Approximately 50% to 60% of eligible adults aged 50 to 75 years underwent CRC screening in 2008.[26,27] Lower rates of screening are seen in younger patients, Hispanics, individuals of lower socioeconomic status, and individuals without health insurance.[27] Although all screening tests have potential drawbacks, patients should be educated regarding relative risks and benefits of screening modalities, including potential benefits in reducing risk of CRC.

PATHOLOGY AND PATHWAYS OF SPREAD

Tumors of the colorectum arise in the mucosa and virtually all (>90%) are adenocarcinomas.[8] Other histologic types include squamous cell carcinoma, melanoma, small cell carcinoma, carcinoid, sarcoma, and lymphoma. Most grading systems classify adenocarcinoma as well, moderately or poorly differentiated. Large-bowel tumors invade from mucosa through the bowel wall and beyond, with involvement of lymphatic channels and lymph nodes. Hematogenous spread can occur, primarily to the lung and liver. There is little propensity for colon cancer to spread longitudinally within the bowel wall, in contrast to esophageal or gastric cancers.

PATIENT EVALUATION/STAGING

Workup should include a complete history and physical exam, including digital rectal examination (DRE). On DRE, size, location, distance from the verge, mobile versus fixed, and sphincter function should be noted. Pelvic exam should be performed in women diagnosed with rectal cancer to assess for vaginal involvement where appropriate. Pretreatment evaluation should include pathologic confirmation of adenocarcinoma, colonoscopy to evaluate extent of tumor and rule out synchronous primaries (occurring in 1% to 5%), and baseline lab tests, including blood counts, liver function tests, and carcinoembryonic antigen levels.[9] India ink may be used at the time of colonoscopy to mark the proximal and distal disease extent.

Patients with CRC should undergo abdominopelvic CT scan and chest x-ray or chest CT to evaluate extent of locoregional disease, as well as the presence or absence of distant metastases. Efforts to improve the clinical assessment of rectal cancers have been enhanced considerably with the evolution of new imaging modalities. CT appears to be more useful in identifying enlarged pelvic lymph nodes and metastasis outside the pelvis than the extent or stage of the primary tumor.[28] Standard CT does not permit the visualization of the layers of the rectal wall, and therefore its utility in the assessment of smaller primary cancers is limited.[29] The sensitivity of CT scan is reported as 50% to 80% accurate, with a 30% to 80% specificity (65% to 75% accurate for tumor staging and 55% to 65% accurate in mesorectal lymph node staging).[30] The ability of CT scans for detecting distant metastasis (DM), including pelvic and para-aortic lymph nodes, is higher than for detecting perirectal nodal involvement (75% to 87% vs. 45%).[31,32] Any lymphadenopathy near the rectum seen on a CT scan should be considered abnormal.

For rectal malignancies, endoscopic ultrasound (EUS) or pelvic magnetic resonance imaging (MRI) can assess primary disease and, with less sensitivity, evaluate nodal extent. Transrectal EUS techniques have been more helpful in efforts to clinically stage rectal cancers. EUS is 80% to 95% accurate in tumor staging and 70% to 75% accurate in mesorectal lymph node staging.[33,34] Transrectal ultrasound is able to visualize layers of the rectal wall, including the mucosa, muscularis mucosa, submucosa, and muscularis propria.[35,36] Its use is more limited in tumors of the upper rectum or for stenosing tumors. EUS can also identify enlarged perirectal lymph nodes but is not effective outside of the perirectum.[37] One situation in which EUS can be very useful is in determining extension of disease into the anal canal, which is an area that is poorly visualized on CT but of critical importance for planning sphincter-preserving surgical procedures.[38]

More recently, MRI techniques have been found to be of high accuracy in defining the extent of rectal cancer extension into the mesorectum and in determining the location and stage of tumor.[39,40] Different approaches to MRI have been explored, including the use of body coils, endorectal MRI, and phased-array techniques. Although MRI appears to have high levels of accuracy, it requires a significant learning curve but is becoming a greater part of the standard presurgical workup for rectal cancer. Body-coil MRI, which first became available in the mid-1980s, has had an accuracy of 54% to 66% for T staging, but this has improved with the use of endorectal coil MRI, with reported accuracy rates of 80% to 95%.[16,41] A significant advantage of both endorectal and surface coil MRI is that it is less operator dependent and permits a larger field of view than does EUS. It also allows assessment for proximal tumors and stenotic lesions where EUS is not possible. Another advantage of MRI is that it can detect involved lymph nodes on the basis of characteristics other than size. MRI can also be helpful in determining the extent of lateral extension of disease, which is critical in predicting the adequacy of circumferential margins for surgical excision.[17] Several studies using phased-array MRI reported accuracy rates of 80% to 97% in predicting lateral disease extent and correlated the likelihood of tumor-free resection margin by visualizing tumor involvement of the mesorectal fascia.[42]

Positron emission tomography (PET) scan, although less accurate in assessment of primary disease, is useful in evaluating patients with oligometastatic disease who may be appropriate candidates for resection of metastatic sites with curative intent.[43] Liver MRI is considered the test of choice in assessment of hepatic metastases in patients with CRC.[44] All of these imaging techniques have advantages and limitations and should be considered complementary to physical examination. They are all less accurate in predicting response after neoadjuvant therapy, with high rates of false positivity, and should be interpreted with caution in this setting.[45,46] Prognostic factors influencing survival in CRC patients include the depth of tumor invasion into and beyond the bowel wall, the number of involved regional lymph nodes, and the

TABLE 65.1 AMERICAN JOINT COMMITTEE ON CANCER 2010 TNM STAGING OF COLORECTAL CANCER

Primary Tumor (T)

TX	Primary tumor cannot be assessed
T0	No evidence of primary tumor
Tis	Carcinoma *in situ*: intraepithelial or invasion of lamina propria
T1	Tumor invades submucosa
T2	Tumor invades muscularis propria
T3	Tumor invades through the muscularis propria into the subserosa or into pericolorectal tissues
T4a	Tumor penetrates to the surface of the visceral peritoneum[a]
T4b	Tumor directly invades or is adherent to other organs or structures[a,b]

Regional Lymph Nodes (N)

NX	Regional lymph nodes cannot be assessed
N0	No regional lymph node metastasis
N1	Metastasis in one to three regional lymph nodes
N1a	Metastasis in one regional lymph node
N1b	Metastasis in two to three lymph nodes
N1c	Tumor deposit(s) in the subserosa, mesentery, or nonperitonealized pericolorectal tissues without regional nodal metastasis
N2	Metastasis in four or more regional lymph nodes
N2a	Metastasis in four to six regional lymph nodes
N2b	Metastasis in seven or more regional lymph nodes

Distant Metastasis (M)

MX	Distant metastasis cannot be assessed
M0	No distant metastasis
M1	Distant metastasis
M1a	Metastasis confined to one organ or site
M1b	Metastasis in more than one organ/site or peritoneum

[a]Direct invasion in T4 includes invasion of other organs or other segments of the colorectum as a result of direct extension through the serosa, as confirmed on microscopic examination (e.g., invasion of the sigmoid colon by a carcinoma of the cecum) or, for cancers in a retroperitoneal or subperitoneal location, direct invasion of other organs or structures by virtue of extension beyond the muscularis propria (i.e., respectively, a tumor on the posterior wall of the descending colon invading the left kidney or lateral abdominal wall or a mid or distal rectal cancer with invasion of prostate, seminal vesicles, cervix, or vagina).
[b]Tumor that is adherent to other organs or structures grossly is classified cT4b. However, if no tumor is present in the adhesion microscopically, the classification should be pT1-4a, depending on the anatomic depth of wall invasion. The V and L classifications should be used to identify the presence or absence of vascular or lymphatic invasion, whereas the PN site-specific factor should be used for perineural invasion. Data from Edge SB, Byrd DR, Compton CC, et al., eds. *AJCC cancer staging handbook*. 7th ed. New York: Springer, 2010. Copyright © 2010 American Joint Committee on Cancer. Reproduced with permission of Springer International Publishing in the format Book via Copyright Clearance Center.

presence or absence of distant metastases. The tumor, node, metastasis (TNM) system of the American Joint Committee on Cancer can be used as a clinical (preoperative) or postoperative staging system (Tables 65.1 and 65.2).

TABLE 65.2 STAGING OF COLON AND RECTUM CANCER

Stage	American Joint Committee on Cancer[a]			Dukes[b]	MAC[c]
	T	N	M		
0	Tis	N0	M0	–	–
I	T1	N0	M0	A	A
	T2	N0	M0	A	B1
IIA	T3	N0	M0	B	B2
IIB	T4a	N0	M0	B	B2
IIC	T4b	N0	M0	B	B3
IIIA	T1-T2	N1/N1c	M0	C	C1
	T1	N2a	M0	C	C1
IIIB	T3-T4a	N1/N1c	M0	C	C2
	T2-T3	N2a	M0	C	C1/C2
	T1-T2	N2b	M0	C	C1
IIIC	T4a	N2a	M0	C	C2
	T3-T4a	N2b	M0	C	C2
	T4b	N1-N2	M0	C	C3
IVA	Any T	Any N	M1a	–	D
IVB	Any T	Any N	M1b		
IVC	Any T	Any N	M1c		

[a]Data from Edge SB, Greene FL, Byrd DR, et al., eds. Colon and rectum. In: American Joint Committee on Cancer Staging Manual. 8th ed. New York: Springer, 2017.
[b]Dukes B is a composite of better (T3 N0 M0) and worse (T4 N0 M0) prognostic groups, as is Dukes C (any TN1 M0 and Any T N2 M0).
[c]MAC, modified Astler-Coller classification.
M, metastasis; N, node; T, tumor.

TREATMENT OF COLON CANCER

Surgery

Surgery is the primary treatment modality for patients with colonic tumors. Resection with curative intent is possible in approximately 75% of patients.[9] Surgery of primary colon cancer is based on the anatomy and mechanisms by which this disease spreads. Adenocarcinomas of the colon may grow by direct extension into the lymphatics of the submucosa and bowel wall. To avoid cutting across tumor intramural lymphatics, sufficient lengths of bowel must be resected proximal and distal to the primary cancer. Colon cancer often extends through the serosa into mesenteric lymphatics that run along the blood vessels draining into the portal watershed at the root of the mesentery. Resection includes removal of the major lymphatic drainage system in the mesentery. Because anatomic resections are designed to include named blood vessels and draining lymphatics, the boundaries for resecting large-bowel cancer are relatively uniform. Right hemicolectomy, transverse colectomy, left hemicolectomy, and sigmoid resection are performed by adherence to surgical oncologic principles without major sacrifice of large-bowel function. Consensus guidelines recommend that a minimum of 12 lymph nodes should be excised for appropriate staging.[47–49] As with other gastrointestinal and pelvic malignancies, the use of laparoscopic techniques has increased. Data suggest no difference in recurrence or survival outcomes with open versus laparoscopic resection.[50–53]

Resection results in excellent cure rates for lesions limited to the bowel wall with negative nodes (average 5-year survival, 97% for T1 N0; 85% to 90% for T2 N0). With a single high-risk feature of extension beyond the colonic wall (T3-4 N0) or involved nodes (T0-2 N+), 5-year survival with surgery falls to 65% to 75%, and adjuvant treatment is often indicated. When both high-risk features are present (T3-4 N+), 5-year survival with surgery alone drops to approximately 50% (T3 N+) and 35% (T4 N+), and adjuvant treatment is recommended.

Adjuvant Chemotherapy

The benefit of adjuvant chemotherapy has been clearly demonstrated in stage III patients, whereas benefit in stage II patients is more controversial. Prospective randomized trials have shown that the addition of 5-flourouracil (5-FU) and leucovorin (LV) improves survival for resected stage III patients.[54,55] More recently, newer agents have been investigated and have shown potential benefit. Capecitabine, an oral 5-FU prodrug, demonstrated similar overall survival (OS) and disease-free survival (DFS) rates to 5-FU/LV in patients with resected stage III colon cancer.[56,57] Oxaliplatin has also been investigated in the adjuvant treatment of resected colon cancer. A randomized study comparing 5-FU/LV with 5-FU/LV/oxaliplatin (FOLFOX) in resected stage II or III colon cancer patients showed improved DFS and OS in stage III patients treated with oxaliplatin-containing regimens.[58,59] These results were validated in the National Surgical Adjuvant Breast and Bowel Project (NSABP) C-07 trial, demonstrating an improvement in DFS with addition of oxaliplatin.[60,61] A Cancer and Leukemia Group B (CALGB) trial examined 5-FU/LV with and without the addition of irinotecan in resected stage III colon patients. No benefit was seen in DFS or OS.[45] These data helped to establish FOLFOX or capecitabine and oxaliplatin (XELOX) as new standard chemotherapeutic regimens in the adjuvant treatment of completely resected, high-risk colon cancer. The use of monoclonal antibodies, such as bevacizumab and cetuximab, although potentially efficacious in the metastatic setting, has not yielded similar results in the adjuvant setting.[62–65]

Adjuvant Irradiation with or without Concurrent Chemotherapy

Given the documented efficacy of adjuvant chemotherapy, as well as the perception by many oncologists that colonic (as opposed to rectal) cancer is much more likely to relapse distantly than locally, there has been little evaluation of the efficacy of postoperative irradiation with chemotherapy. The potential indications for adjuvant radiation therapy in colon cancer are based on analyses of patterns of failure following resection (Table 65.3).[66,67] Advanced stage predicts for local failure in both colon and rectal cancers; however, local failure in colon cancer also depends on anatomic origin. The ascending and descending colon are considered "anatomically immobile," and their close proximity to the retroperitoneal tissues often limits wide surgical resection (Fig. 65.1). Limitations in achieving satisfactory circumferential margins increase the risk of residual disease and consequently local failure. In contrast, the midsigmoid and midtransverse colon are relatively "mobile," with a wide mesentery, permitting the surgeon to obtain wide margins regardless of extent of disease invasion into the mesentery. Unless there is adjacent organ adherence/invasion by tumor, local failure at these sites is uncommon. Local failure rates for cecal, hepatic/splenic flexure, and proximal/distal sigmoid tumors are variable, depending on the amount of mesentery present, tumor extension, and the adequacy of radial margins. When colon cancers adhere to or invade adjacent structures, local failure rates exceed 30% following surgery alone. In summary, local failure occurs in patients with colonic tumors where there are anatomic constraints on radial resection margins, including tumors adherent to or invading adjacent structures.

Data evaluating the use of adjuvant radiation therapy in high-risk colon cancer patients have largely been limited to single-institution retrospective analyses.[38,68–70] To summarize, these studies have suggested that operative bed failures in high-risk patients undergoing resection alone are at least 30% and that the risk of local failure is reduced by the administration of adjuvant radiation therapy. These are discussed in detail in what follows.

A report from the Massachusetts General Hospital (MGH) evaluated outcomes in high-risk patients undergoing resection followed by adjuvant radiation therapy and compared these to a similar cohort of patients treated over the same period undergoing surgery only.[70] Irradiated patients included those with T4 N0/N+, T3 N+ disease (excluding midsigmoid and midtransverse colon) and T3 N0 patients with margins of <1 cm. A total of 171 patients received postoperative radiation, with 63 patients receiving concurrent chemotherapy, usually with bolus 5-FU (500 mg/m^2/d) for 3 consecutive days during the first and last weeks of radiation therapy. Radiation treatment was administered through parallel-opposed or other multifield techniques to treat the

TABLE 65.3 FIVE-YEAR ACTUARIAL LOCAL CONTROL AND RELAPSE-FREE SURVIVAL AFTER SURGERY PLUS POSTOPERATIVE RADIOTHERAPY VERSUS SURGERY ALONE, ACCORDING TO STAGE, FROM THE MASSACHUSETTS GENERAL HOSPITAL

TNM Stage	Surgery Alone			Surgery Plus Postoperative Radiation		
	Number of Patients	LC (%)	RFS (%)	Number of Patients	LC (%)	RFS (%)
T3 N0	163	90	78	23	91	72
T4 N0	83	69	63	54	93	79[a]
T3 N+	100	64	48	55	70	47
T4 N+	49	47	38	39	72	53[a]

[a]P < .05.

LC, local control; RFS, relapse-free survival; TNM, tumor, node, metastasis.

tumor bed with an approximate 3- to 5-cm margin to a total dose of 45 Gy, followed by reduced fields to a total dose of 50.4 to 54 Gy. Draining nodes were included if they were believed to be at high risk for involvement. This cohort was compared to 395 patients with T3-4 N0/N+ tumors undergoing surgery alone during the same time period. Table 65.3 shows 5-year actuarial local control (LC) and relapse-free survival (RFS) in the adjuvant group compared to patients undergoing surgery alone. LC rates in T4 N0 and T4 N+ patients treated with radiation therapy were 93% and 72%, respectively, versus 69% and 47%, respectively, in patients undergoing surgery alone. Similarly, RFS rates were 79% and 53%, respectively, in T4 N0/T4 N+ patients undergoing adjuvant radiation versus 63% and 38%, respectively, in those undergoing surgery alone. No significant outcome differences were observed in patients with T3 N0 and T3 N+ lesions; however, there may be an element of selection bias, given that most patients were referred out of concerns of adequacy of LC following surgery alone. A trend toward improved LC in patients receiving 5-FU was seen (Table 65.4). The rate of acute enteritis in patients receiving irradiation and 5-FU was 16% versus 4% in patients undergoing irradiation only. This rate of enteritis is similar to data from studies of concurrent 5-FU and radiation therapy in rectal cancer. Late bowel complication rates were not increased by concomitant 5-FU administration. The conclusion was that patients with T4 tumors, abscess/fistula formation, or margin-positive resection may benefit from postoperative radiation. In an updated analysis from MGH, 152 patients with T4 tumors received adjuvant irradiation.[70] On pathologic examination, 42 patients had tumors with positive margins. For patients with negative margins, the 10-year actuarial LC in T4 N0 and T4 N+ patients was 78% and 48%, respectively. In patients with node-negative tumors, the 10-year actuarial LC and RFS rates were 87% and 58%, respectively, compared to 65% and 33%, respectively, in patients with node-positive tumors. For patients with one involved lymph node, LC and RFS rates were similar to those without nodal involvement; however, with increasing numbers of nodes involved, survival steadily decreased.

A report from the Mayo Clinic evaluated outcomes of 103 patients receiving radiation therapy following surgery for locally advanced colon cancer.[71] Microscopic and gross residual disease was present in 18 and 35 patients, respectively. Greater than 90% of patients had T4 N0/N+ disease. A median dose of 50.4 Gy was delivered through multifield techniques, and most patients received concurrent 5-FU–based chemotherapy. Eleven patients received an intraoperative radiotherapy (IORT) boost of 10 to 20 Gy. Five-year actuarial LC was 40%. Patients with margin-negative tumors had a 5-year local LC of 90%, compared to 46% for patients with microscopic residual tumor and 21% for those with gross residual tumor. In patients with residual disease, LC rates in patients undergoing intraoperative boost were 89%,

compared to 18% in those undergoing external irradiation alone. Similarly, 5-year OS rates were improved in patients undergoing margin-negative resection (66%) compared to those with microscopic residual (47%) or gross residual (23%) disease. In addition, patients undergoing intraoperative boost demonstrated improved survival (76% vs. 26%).

A study from the University of Florida of patients with locally advanced but completely resected colon cancers receiving adjuvant radiation reported a LC rate of 88%, similar to the 90% reported from the Mayo Clinic series.[68] In addition, there appeared to be a dose–response relationship to LC. The 5-year rate of LC was 96% for patients receiving 50 to 55 Gy versus 76% for patients receiving <50 Gy ($P = .0095$).

These retrospective studies laid the foundation for further testing in a phase III trial. To assess whether the addition of radiation therapy to adjuvant chemotherapy would result in superior OS and LC rates in resected, high-risk colon cancer patients, the U.S. Intergroup initiated a randomized, prospective trial in 1992.[72] In this trial, patients with resected colon cancer were randomized to postoperative irradiation with 5-FU and levamisole or 5-FU and levamisole alone. Eligibility criteria included margin-negative tumors with adherence to or invasion of surrounding structures (i.e., T4 N0 or N+ disease, excluding peritoneal invasion) or tumors arising in the ascending or descending colon with metastatic regional nodes (T3 N+). Patients were randomized to receive (a) weekly 5-FU combined with levamisole for 12 months or (b) 5-FU and levamisole for 12 months with combined radiation therapy and chemotherapy beginning 1 month after the first 5-FU administration. The recommended total radiation dose was 45 Gy in 25 fractions over 5 weeks, with an optional 5.4-Gy boost.

The initial trial accrual goal was 700 patients; however, the study was closed in 1996 because of poor accrual (222 patients; 189 evaluable). Total accrual was less than one-third of the initial goal, and there was reduced statistical power to detect differences between the groups. No difference in OS or DFS was seen between the two groups. Five-year OS of patients receiving chemotherapy only was 62% versus 58% for patients randomized to chemoirradiation ($P > .50$). LR rates were identical in both arms (18 patients each). Grade III or IV hematologic toxicity was higher in patients receiving radiation therapy. Interpretation of study results was handicapped by decreased statistical power, high ineligibility rates, and lack of surgical clips or preoperative imaging to assist in the definition of appropriate radiotherapy fields in a high percentage of patients. Therefore, no definitive conclusions can be made regarding the efficacy of postoperative irradiation with 5-FU and levamisole based on this underpowered study with many flaws; however, this study provides no data supporting its routine use.

A recent study has examined the role of adjuvant radiation therapy in locally advanced colon cancer in the era of modern chemotherapy.[73] The investigators reported the outcome of 62 patients with T4 colonic cancer treated with surgery only, surgery followed by adjuvant chemotherapy only, or 13 patients adjuvant chemoradiation. A multivariate analysis demonstrated that treatment with adjuvant chemoradiation (vs. adjuvant chemotherapy alone) enhanced locoregional control and disease-free survival. The investigators concluded that adjuvant radiation therapy may be appropriate in select patients, specifically those with T4b lesions and/or residual disease following resection.

Neoadjuvant Treatment

Neoadjuvant chemotherapy or chemoradiation therapy can be considered for locally advanced or unresectable colon cancer. The FOxTROT pilot study showed that neoadjuvant chemotherapy for large T3 or T4 tumors was feasible with acceptable

TABLE 65.4 FIVE-YEAR ACTUARIAL LOCAL CONTROL AND RELAPSE-FREE SURVIVAL OF ADJUVANTLY IRRADIATED PATIENTS BASED ON 5-FLUOROURACIL ADMINISTRATION— MASSACHUSETTS GENERAL HOSPITAL

TNM Stage	Without 5-Fluorouracil			With 5-Fluorouracil		
	Number of Patients	LC (%)	RFS (%)	Number of Patients	LC (%)	RFS (%)
T3 N0	16	87	69	7	100	80
T4 N0	37	94	78	16	100	83
T3 N+	41	69	48	14	70	43
T4 N+	24	67	53	15	79	52

LC, local control; RFS, relapse-free survival; TNM, tumor, node, metastasis.

toxicity rates[74]; this study group has moved forward with a phase 3 trial. Although neoadjuvant chemoradiation has been shown in randomized trials to improve LC/DFS in rectal cancer patients,[75,76] there is no high-level evidence demonstrating its effectiveness in colon cancer patients. For locally advanced colon cancer patients receiving neoadjuvant chemoradiation, high rates of R0 resection and LC with low toxicity rates have been reported in retrospective studies.[77]

Locally Advanced Disease and Palliation

Patients with unresectable tumors or metastatic disease at presentation are usually treated with systemic therapy. An irinotecan-based (e.g., FOLFIRI: irinotecan–fluorouracil–leucovorin)[78] or oxaliplatin-based (e.g., FOLFOX: oxaliplatin–fluorouracil–leucovorin) regimen with the addition of bevacizumab[79] or an epidermal growth factor receptor (EGFR) inhibitor (e.g., panitumumab or cetuximab)[80] (KRAS/NRAS wild-type tumors) can prolong progression-free survival and potentially OS. Patients with refractory disease may be treated with EGFR inhibitors containing regimens (KRAS/NRAS wild-type tumors), PD-1 inhibitors like pembrolizumab[81] (MMR-deficient tumors), oral multikinase inhibitors like regorafenib, or tipiracil/trifluridine. Additional targeted and immunotherapy agents are under evaluation.

Patients with near colonic obstruction may benefit from a diverting ostomy or stenting. Nonsurgical candidates may benefit from palliative radiation to shrink a painful, near-obstructing or bleeding mass.

Techniques of Irradiation

Treatment field design in colon cancer is based on patterns of failure data. As is true in the treatment of rectal carcinoma, great care must be taken in the design of postoperative treatment of adenocarcinoma of the colon. Field arrangement will vary, depending on the site of the primary disease, as well as on areas judged to be at high risk for local recurrence (LR).[82] Patient positioning (supine, prone, decubitus) should be considered in planning. The small bowel is often a dose-limiting structure in this therapy, and it may be advantageous to position patients in the right or left decubitus position for at least a portion of their treatment, allowing displacement of the small bowel away from the treatment field. Immobilization devices may improve reproducibility. Small-bowel contrast aids in delineation of small-bowel volume within the treatment field. It may be useful to compare films in both the decubitus and supine positions to determine the actual amount of small-bowel displacement. CT-based planning may facilitate defining the tumor bed, determining beam orientation, and estimating the volume of small bowel included within the treatment fields. As in other abdominal malignancies, a portion of one kidney may be irradiated. Unilateral renal irradiation results in minimal long-term clinical sequelae, assuming that baseline function in the contralateral kidney is normal.[83]

The total radiation dose used in the adjuvant treatment of colon carcinoma depends on the amount of suspected residual disease and tolerance constraints of surrounding normal tissue. Generally, an initial dose of 45 Gy in 25 fractions at 1.8 Gy/fraction is delivered through larger fields to the primary tumor and at-risk tissues. Reduced fields may be treated to 50 Gy if only a small portion of small bowel is included. For patients with T4 tumors, the general goal is to treat the tumor bed to a total dose of up to 54 to 60 Gy. Surgical clips may aid in the identification of high-risk areas (i.e., positive margins) to assist in target delineation. Any treatment beyond 50 Gy generally mandates exclusion of all small bowel from the field to minimize late toxicity. Spinal cord dose should generally be limited to 45 Gy. In addition, at least two-thirds of one functional kidney should receive no more than 18 to 20 Gy, and at least two-thirds of the total liver volume should not receive >30 Gy. In a Mayo Clinic

analysis, small-bowel obstruction rates were lower when more than two treatment fields were used, and attempts should be made to implement multifield techniques, which may be aided by CT-based planning.[84]

Generally, the primary tumor site should be covered with a 4- to 5-cm margin proximally and distally and with a 3- to 4-cm margin medially and laterally to cover areas of potential residual disease. The nodal basins in the mesentery beyond surgical margins are usually not treated, as satisfactory margin clearance is often obtained in these sites. An exception to this may be right colon tumors, for which both small bowel and right colon are supplied by ileocolic vessels, limiting the extent of resection. In some instances, treatment of the para-aortic nodes may be indicated, particularly with extensive retroperitoneal involvement by tumor. Treatment of proximal mesenteric nodes may be appropriate if nodes adjacent to the surgical or resection margin are involved. Figures 65.2 and 65.3 show idealized radiation fields for varying colonic sites, including cecum, descending, and sigmoid cancer. In many situations, it may be appropriate to exclude treatment of para-aortic nodal basins, based on operative and pathologic findings.

Endorectal brachytherapy is an alternative or adjunct to EBRT where a high dose of radiation is delivered to the tumor. This technique of contact therapy was first described by Jean Papillon who pioneered this approach at the University of Lyon in the mid-1940s. In addition to contact therapy, radiotherapy may be delivered via high dose rate endoluminal brachytherapy or interstitial rectal brachytherapy implant. These techniques are primarily delivered as a boost in an effort to escalate dose and achieve higher rates of clinical complete response (cCR), which may allow for nonoperative management (NOM). The use of rectal brachytherapy is an area of ongoing investigation.

CONCLUSION

Subsets of patients with colon cancer have LR rates similar to patients with rectal cancer if surgery only is undertaken. Encouraging results from single-institution series utilizing postoperative irradiation with or without 5-FU for patients with resected high-risk colon cancers and the positive results of 5-FU and levamisole in high-risk adjuvant colon cancer prompted an Intergroup randomized trial. Patients with high risk of LR following surgery were randomized to 5-FU and levamisole or 5-FU and levamisole with tumor bed irradiation. There was no benefit in survival in patients receiving adjuvant radiation therapy; however, interpretation of these results is impaired by inadequate accrual and significant flaws, as previously discussed.

The value of adjuvant postoperative irradiation combined with systemic therapy for patients at high risk for LR is unlikely to ever be addressed in a definitive randomized trial. Treatment recommendations should be made on a case-by-case basis with existing data in the setting of an informed consent. Adjuvant tumor bed irradiation with concurrent 5-FU–based chemotherapy should be considered for patients (a) with tumors invading adjoining structures, (b) with tumors complicated by perforation or fistula, and (c) with tumors where incomplete resection is performed.

The use of IORT as a supplement to EBRT in certain T4 tumors (i.e., those with uncertain margins) may also be appropriate. For patients with tumors adherent to or invading adjacent structures, one preferred treatment sequence would be preoperative EBRT plus 5-FU–based chemotherapy, followed by resection with or without IORT and postoperative systemic therapy, based on excellent results in preliminary IORT reports from both US and European institutions.[71,85,86] A similar approach would be reasonable for patients with locally recurrent cancers or with regional nodal relapse.[87,88]

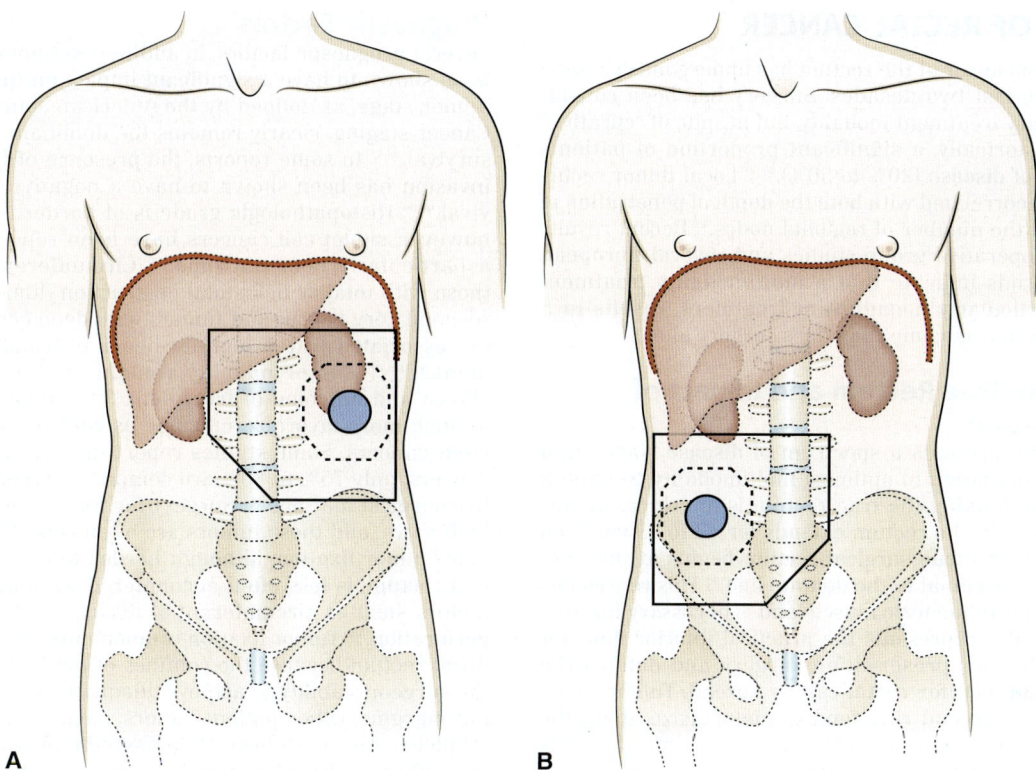

A   B

FIGURE 65.2. Idealized postoperative anteroposterior/posteroanterior irradiation fields of extrapelvic colon cancer (tumor bed and nodal regions). If treated preoperatively, lateral fields could be added based on imaging with computed tomography of the abdomen and colon radiograph. **A:** Para-aortic nodes may be at risk, in addition to tumor bed, because of tumor adherence to posterior abdominal wall with descending colon cancer. **B:** External and common iliac nodes may be at risk, in addition to tumor bed, from a proximal cecal/ascending colon cancer. (From Gunderson LL, Martenson JA, Smalley SR, et al. Lower gastrointestinal cancer: rationale, results, and techniques of treatment. *Front Radiat Ther Oncol* 1994;28:140 154. Copyright © 1994 Karger Publishers, Basel, Switzerland. Reprinted by permission.)

FIGURE 65.3. Idealized multiple-field preoperative or postoperative irradiation technique for a sigmoid colon cancer adherent to the bladder. Solid lines, large field; interrupted lines, boost field. **A:** Anteroposterior/posteroanterior. **B:** Paired laterals. (From Gunderson LL, Martenson JA, Smalley SR, et al. Lower gastrointestinal cancer: rationale, results, and techniques of treatment. *Front Radiat Ther Oncol* 1994;28:140–154. Copyright © 1994 Karger Publishers, Basel, Switzerland. Reprinted by permission.)

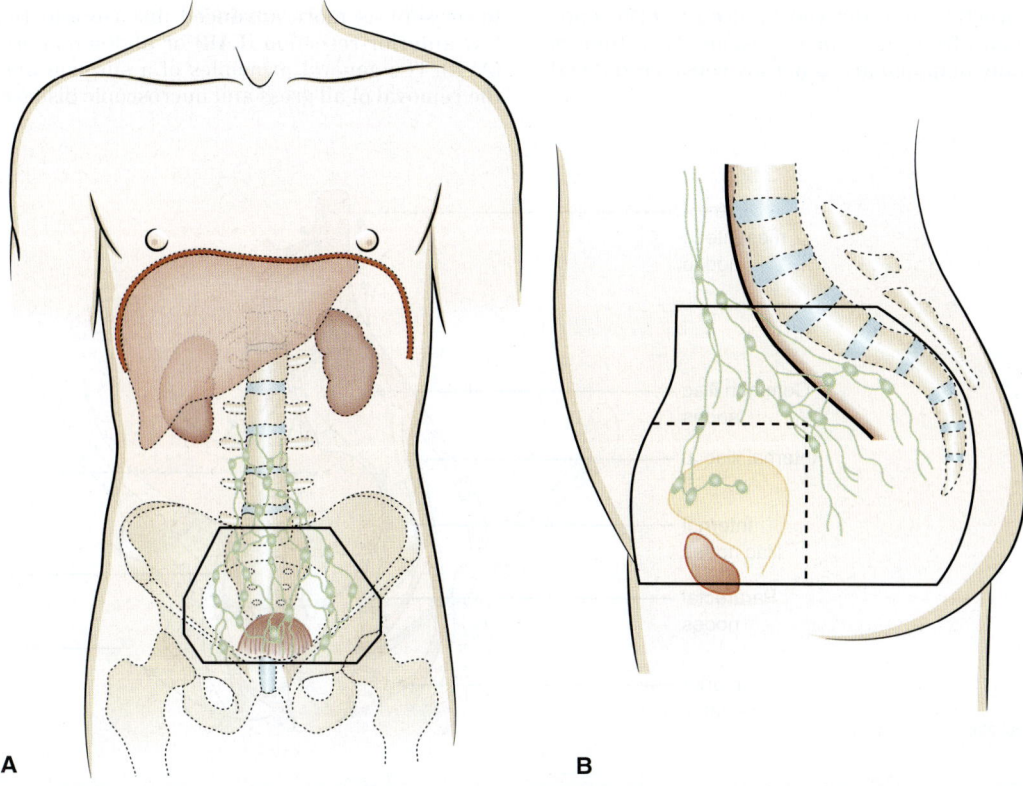

A   B

THERAPY OF RECTAL CANCER

Management of cancer of the rectum has undergone dramatic changes in the last two decades. Surgery has been considered the primary treatment modality, but in spite of "curative" resections, historically, a significant proportion of patients developed LR of disease (20% to 50%).[89,90] Local tumor recurrence is highly correlated with both the depth of penetration of the tumor and the number of regional nodes.[43] Recent results of national cooperative group studies and several European randomized trials indicate that a multimodality treatment approach, particularly neoadjuvant treatment, results in a significantly better outcome than does surgery alone.

Defining the True Rectum and Impact of Tumor Location

Rectal cancer represents a spectrum of disease stages that needs careful definition to optimize multimodality treatment strategies, and defining the true rectum is of critical importance. Traditionally, the rectum extends for 12 to 15 cm from the anal verge. The true surgical rectum begins at the anorectal ring, just proximal to the dentate line.[35] This represents the internal anal sphincteric muscle and is necessary for anal continence. It also represents the practical inferior limit for functional sphincter preservation surgery and defines the lymphatic watershed for rectal cancer spread. Tumors arising above the anorectal ring tend to metastasize along the distribution of the middle rectal vessels to the internal iliac lymph nodes, as compared to tumors that may extend into the anal canal, which may spread via nodes along the inferior rectal and external iliac pathways (Fig. 65.4).[91] Cancers that arise in the anal canal may metastasize to the lungs (caval drainage) rather than the liver (portal drainage), as is common with most true rectal cancers. The prognosis of patients worsens with more distal location of cancer, and these differences persist even with the addition of adjunctive therapy.[92–94] The proximal rectum has historically been defined by the level at which the peritoneum is reflected along the anterior surface of the rectum (usually at the level of S3).[95] This is a surgical observation and may be difficult to define in an intact patient. The middle valve of Houston is a useful landmark that can often be identified endoscopically (usually about 6 cm from the anorectal ring) and can be used to differentiate proximal tumors from more distal lesions. Most tumors that can be digitally palpated are generally considered distal cancers.

Prognostic Factors

Several prognostic factors, in addition to tumor location, have been shown to have a significant impact on tumor behavior.[92] Tumor stage, as defined by the American Joint Committee on Cancer staging, clearly remains the dominant determinant of survival.[96,97] In some reports, the presence of lymphovascular invasion has been shown to have a negative impact on survival.[98,99] Histopathologic grade is of borderline significance; however, signet cell cancers have been reported to portend a particularly poor outcome.[100] Circumferential tumors or those with total or near-total obstruction (lumen, <1 cm) may respond very poorly, and tumors with deep central ulceration are associated with a high incidence of lymph node involvement.[98,101,102] Tumor mobility remains a key factor in both choice and outcome of treatment.[103,104] Mobile cancers have a much more favorable outcome as compared to tethered or fixed cancers. Some studies report that even among mobile cancers, only 75% to 80% are completely resected with negative surgical margins.[105] Surgery for fixed cancers has proven ineffective, and these tumors are often classified as unresectable. Tumor fixation, although harder to assess in the proximal rectum, is less often encountered without other adverse factors such as circumferential disease with obstruction or perforation.[106] Tumor fixation is much more problematic in the distal rectum because the confines of the bony pelvis inhibits the surgeon's ability to achieve adequate lateral/circumferential margins. Other patient factors, such as age, gender, and ethnicity, appear to have little association with outcome but may affect choice of therapy.[107–109] As neoadjuvant therapy has emerged as the standard of care, degree of tumor regression has become an important prognostic factor.[110,111] Pathologic assessment of tumors after neoadjuvant therapy receives a special designation of ypTNM classification.

Treatment

Surgery

Surgery remains the mainstay of curative treatment for carcinoma of the rectum. Surgical management depends on the stage and location of a tumor within the rectum. Early cancers can be managed with limited surgery (i.e., local excision) in selected situations; however, the majority of tumors tend to present as more advanced disease and require either a low anterior resection (LAR) or abdominoperineal resection (APR). The general principles of a surgical approach remain the removal of all gross and microscopic disease with negative

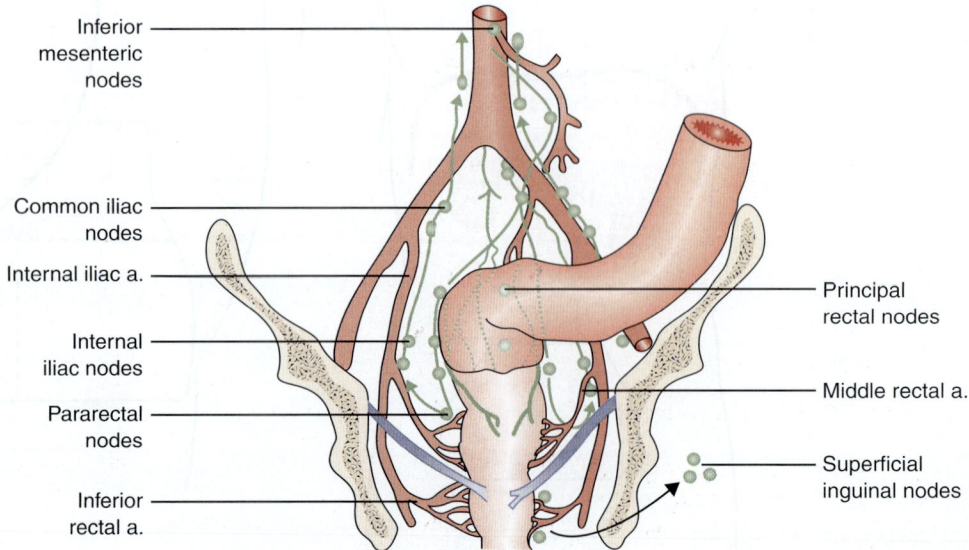

FIGURE 65.4. Lymphatics of the rectum.

proximal, distal, and circumferential margins. In the case of radical resection, this means removal of the adjacent mesorectal tissue (total mesorectal excision [TME]), containing the regional lymphatics and potential tumor deposits. Several studies have shown that the surgeon's experience with resection of CRC is an independent variable in the outcome of treatment.[112] The Intergroup 0114 trial found that for stage II and III rectal cancers, not only were APR rates higher in hospitals performing low-volume procedures (46% vs. 32%), but more patients had positive resection margins.[113]

Historically, the distal and proximal resection margins were considered important determinants in outcome, and a 5-cm distal margin of normal rectum was considered necessary for adequate surgical resection.[114-116] However, several retrospective studies have shown that distal intramural spread of tumor is rare beyond 1.5 cm, and, therefore, a 2-cm distal margin is generally considered acceptable, except in lesions that are poorly differentiated or widely metastatic.[117-119] The reduced requirement of 2-cm distal margin for adequate resection has led to a significant increase in the likelihood of sphincter preservation procedures in this disease.[120]

Laparoscopic surgery has emerged offering potential advantages of reduced blood loss/perioperative morbidity and shorter hospitalizations. In the hands of an experienced surgeon, outcomes from laparoscopic surgery appear no different than those from open resection in a number of randomized trials, although this remains a subject of ongoing investigation.[121-123]

Local Excision

Early rectal cancer may be resected with local excision techniques, avoiding major surgery and a colostomy, but patients should be carefully selected for these procedures. Transanal excision, transsphincteric excision (York-Mason), and a posterior parasacral approach (Kraske) permit removal of the tumor and adjoining rectum in one uninterrupted specimen. A transanal approach is usually associated with the least morbidity, but to be amenable for local excision, tumors generally need to be located <8 cm from the anal verge. An anal sphincter–splitting approach can be used for tumors close to the anorectal junction, and occasionally a presacral Kraske approach can be used to access more proximal tumors, although this is now generally considered a historical procedure. An adequate resection requires full thickness (into the fat), with the tumor being removed in one uninterrupted specimen with at least a 1-cm margin so that careful pathologic assessment can be performed. A primary closure of the rectal defect may then be performed, although this is variable. The inability to sample perirectal and mesenteric lymph nodes can result in underestimation of cancer stage. Lymph node metastases have been observed in 5% to 10% of patients with T1 lesions and 20% to 35% of patients with T2 lesions.[124] Given the potential risk of lymph node spread, it is necessary to restrict local excision to patients with low-risk tumors where the risk of recurrence is <10% (i.e., very favorable T1 cancers). Properly selected T1 lesions have excellent results with local excision alone, with 5-year LC ranging from 82% to 97% and OS rates of 90% or better.[125,126] The risk of perirectal nodal metastasis and high incidence of reported LR rates for T2 cancers following local excision alone indicate the need for further adjuvant therapy.[127]

Radiation Therapy Oncology Group (RTOG) 89-02 examined the efficacy of local excision in a study of 65 patients with distal rectal cancers. Tumors had to be grade 1 or 2 and have margins ≥3 mm, no lymphovascular invasion (LVI), and no regional lymph node ≥2 cm by CT scan to be eligible for observation. T2 tumors with margins ≤3 mm received 59.4 to 65 Gy. Fourteen patients with T1 tumors were observed after surgery, whereas 13 patients with T1 tumors, 25 patients with T2 tumors, and 13 patients with T3 tumors received local excision with postoperative radiation of 50 to 65 Gy with 5-FU (1,000 mg/m^2 on days 1 to 3 and 29 to 31). None of the T1 tumors receiving postoperative treatment relapsed, compared to one DM and one LR in the T1 observation arm. Five patients in the T2 group relapsed (2 local, 1 distant, 2 both), and 4 patients in the T3 group had recurrence (1 distant, 3 both). Therefore, 20% of T2 and 23% of T3 tumors experienced LR after local excision plus chemoradiation (CRT).[128] Therefore, although it is possible that highly selected T2 and limited T3 tumors may be treated with local excision and postoperative adjuvant therapy, the high rate of LR makes this a potentially inferior approach.

The CALGB 8984 study provides some support for postoperative CRT after local excision for appropriately selected early stage rectal cancers.[129] Fifty-nine patients with T1 disease were treated with local excision alone, and 51 patients with T2 disease received adjuvant therapy with 54 Gy and 5-FU (500 mg/m^2 on days 1 to 3 and 29 to 31). At 10 years, LR, DFS, and OS were 8%, 75%, and 84%, respectively, in T1 tumors. For T2 tumors LR, DFS, and OS were 18%, 64%, and 66%, respectively. Detailed information regarding salvage APR was not published in the updated study. In initial publication, one of two T1 local failures and four of five T2 local failures were salvaged by APR. Of note, 25% of the clinical T1 and T2 tumors were actually pathologic T3, highlighting the potential inaccuracy of preoperative staging.[130] The 20% recurrence rate and DFS of 64% for T2 cancers are considerably inferior to the results of radical surgery with TME alone or neoadjuvant therapy followed by surgery. This study supports the possibility of conservative sphincter-sparing surgery for well-selected T1 lesions, but for T2 tumors, the high rate of LR despite CRT warrants caution.

The American College of Surgeons Oncology Group conducted a multi-institutional, single-arm, open-label, non-randomized, phase 2 trial of patients with clinically staged T2N0 distal rectal cancer treated with neoadjuvant chemoradiotherapy.[131] Patients with clinical T2N0 rectal adenocarcinoma staged by endorectal ultrasound or endorectal coil MRI, measuring <4 cm in greatest diameter, involving <40% of the circumference of the rectum, located within 8 cm of the anal verge, were treated with neoadjuvant chemoradiotherapy consisted of capecitabine (original dose 825 mg/m^2 twice daily on days 1 to 14 and 22 to 35), oxaliplatin (50 mg/m^2 on weeks 1, 2, 4, and 5), and radiation (5 days a week at 1·8 Gy/day for 5 weeks to a dose of 45 Gy, followed by a boost of 9 Gy, for a total dose of 54 Gy) followed by local excision. Because of adverse events during chemoradiotherapy, the dose of capecitabine was reduced to 725 mg/m^2 twice daily, 5 days/week, for 5 weeks, and the boost of radiation was reduced to 5.4 Gy, for a total dose of 50.4 Gy. Seventy-nine eligible patients were recruited to the trial and started neoadjuvant chemoradiotherapy. Two patients had no surgery and one had a TME. Four additional patients completed protocol treatment, but one had a positive margin, and three had ypT3 tumors. Thus, the per-protocol population consisted of 72 patients. Median follow-up was 56 months (IQR 46 to 63) for all patients. The estimated 3-year DFS for the intention-to-treat group was 88.2% (95% CI, 81.3 to 95.8) and for the per-protocol group was 86.9% (79.3 to 95.3). Of 79 eligible patients, 23 (29%) had grade 3 gastrointestinal adverse events, 12 (15%) had grade 3 to 4 pain, and 12 (15%) had grade 3 to 4 hematologic adverse events during chemoradiation. Of the 77 patients who had surgery, six (8%) had grade 3 pain, three (4%) had grade 3 to 4 hemorrhage, and three (4%) had gastrointestinal adverse events. Although the observed 3-year DFS was not as high as anticipated, the investigators suggested that neoadjuvant chemoradiotherapy followed by local excision might be considered as an organ-preserving alternative in carefully selected patients with clinically staged T2N0 tumors who refuse or are not candidates for transabdominal resection.

Based on the available data, local excision should generally be limited to tumors that are small (<4 cm), clinically T1 (or favorable T2 patients in selected situations), and well to moderately differentiated and involve <40% of the circumference of the rectum. These tumors are usually mobile, polypoid, and not ulcerated and have favorable pathology, including no LVI.[132–134]

Low Anterior Resection

The availability of circular stapling devices has expanded the role of sphincter preservation surgical options in rectal cancers, and LAR is now being performed not just for cancers of the upper one-third of the rectum, but also for middle and lower one-third cancers.[135] Preserving adequate anorectal function becomes increasingly difficult the more distal the level of anorectal anastomosis.[136] Patients should have good anal sphincter continence prior to considering sphincter-preserving options. Patient age, pelvic anatomy, gender, and body habitus can affect suitability for sphincter preservation. A 2-cm distal margin of preserved normal rectum is considered optimal for preservation of adequate bowel function. In carefully selected patients, a functional coloanal anastomosis can be achieved with significantly reduced margins for more distal cancers, particularly after neoadjuvant therapy. If LAR is planned following neoadjuvant radiation therapy, it is necessary to mobilize the splenic flexure to allow an unirradiated segment of the bowel to be used for the anastomosis. The latter can be performed with several techniques—an end-to-end, a side-to-end, or a colonic J-pouch technique to maximize preservation of sphincter function.[137,138] Several studies comparing results of LAR to APR generally reported similar outcomes for local and distant recurrence rates and survival as long as surgical margins are negative.[139,140] The absence of a colostomy, although offering a better quality of life with LAR, can be compromised with bowel urgency, frequency, or poor sphincter control.[141]

Abdominoperineal Resection

APR has been considered the gold standard for surgical resection of distal rectal cancer and requires removal of the primary tumor along with a complete proctectomy, leading to a permanent colostomy. Recent data suggest a decline in the APR rate.[142] APR is associated with a slightly higher morbidity and mortality than LAR and a worse quality of life related to changes in body image and depression due to the presence of a colostomy.[140,142,143] There is also a higher risk of positive margins with APR because the mesorectum is thin in the distal segment of the rectum and margins are often restricted by the proximity of the prostate or vagina. The confines of the bony pelvis, particularly in males, can also restrict surgical access.[144]

Total Mesorectal Excision

The high LR of disease following standard APR or LAR (15% to 30% or more) has been believed by some to be due to blunt dissection that violates the planes of the mesorectal circumference.[145] Lateral spread of disease has been shown to occur not only at the level of the tumor but also distally within the mesorectum.[146] Heald et al.[147,148] recommended en bloc removal of the tumor within the envelope of the endopelvic fascia as necessary to obtain adequate lateral clearance of disease and reduced likelihood of LR. TME, as they described, has become the established standard for all radical rectal cancer resections and requires sharp dissection along the plane that separates the visceral from the parietal pelvic fascia with complete en bloc removal of the rectum so that all of the rectal mesentery remains within the envelope of the specimen.[149]

On gross pathology, an adequate TME specimen will have a bilobed, encapsulated appearance, with the surface looking smooth and unbroken, like a lipoma (Fig. 65.5). On pathologic

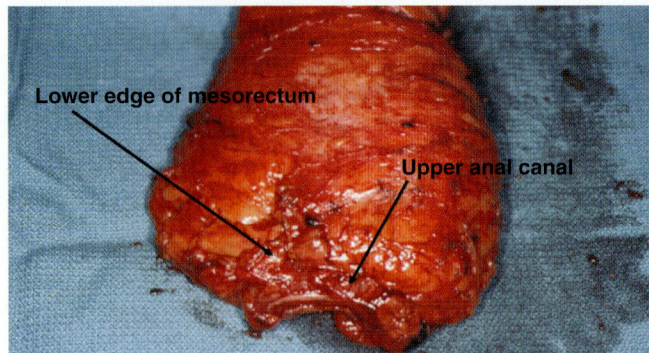

FIGURE 65.5. Total mesorectal excision specimen with designation of the lower mesorectum and upper anal canal.

review, an appropriate dissection should include a minimum of 12 to 15 perirectal and pelvic lymph nodes.[150–154] TME, although more difficult with APR than LAR, may be associated with a somewhat higher anastomotic leak rate, especially for low rectal lesions (15% to 17%).[105,149,155] Multiple series using TME surgery have reported low rates of LR (ranging from 5% to 10%) and an improvement in OS approaching 80% to 85% for stage II and 65% to 70% for stage III disease.[101,145,156–158]

Radial Margin

The National Institute of Health Consensus Conference on Rectal Cancer indicated that the principal reason for LR in resected rectal cancer appears to be related to the anatomic constraints in obtaining wide radial margins, despite adequate proximal and distal margins.[159] Using whole-mount specimens, Quirke et al. found that 27% (14 of 52) of patients showed spread to the lateral radial margin, even though the margins appeared negative with standard pathologic assessment. Eighty-six percent of those with positive radial margins developed LR of disease, as compared to only 3% without lateral resection margin involvement.[160] In addition, pathologic assessment in a large randomized trial found that the plane of surgery—mesorectal, intramesorectal, or muscularis propria plane—predicted for LR. Three-year LR was 4% in patients undergoing complete mesorectal excision, compared with 7% and 13% in the intramesorectal and muscularis propria groups, respectively.[101] A positive radial margin is a predictor not only of LR but also of inferior survival.[98] The mean surgical margin of resection has been shown to decrease with increasing stage of disease, ranging from 14 mm for T1 cancers to 3 mm for T4 cancers, with a corresponding increase in LR from 0% to 75%.[161]

Adjuvant Therapy

Postoperative

The problem of unacceptably high LR after surgery has led to many studies exploring the potential benefit of postoperative adjuvant therapy. One of the advantages of postoperative radiation is the ability to selectively treat patients at high risk of LF on the basis of pathologic criteria. Disadvantages include a potentially hypoxic postsurgical bed, making radiation and chemotherapy less effective, and potentially higher complications due to increased small bowel in the radiation field. Postoperative treatments tend to require larger treatment volumes, particularly in patients undergoing an APR where the perineal scar may need to be covered. A number of trials assessed the role of adjuvant radiotherapy compared to surgery alone. These trials showed reduced LF with radiotherapy; however, no improvement in DFS, DM, or OS was seen.[162] Given this, the role of adjuvant CRT was evaluated in an effort to improve treatment outcomes. In general, surgery alone resulted in a 25% LF rate and 40% to 50% OS for T3 or

T4 or node-positive patients, whereas CRT yielded a lower LF rate of 10% to 15% and higher OS of 50% to 60%.

The NSABP R-02 study enrolled 694 stage B and C patients and asked two questions in its study design: (a) Does the addition of radiation to chemotherapy improve outcome? (b) Are 5-FU, semustine, and vincristine superior to 5-FU/LV in men?[163] There were four treatment arms for male patients and two treatment arms for female patients. Five cycles of MOF were compared to six cycles of 5-FU/LV with or without radiation in male patients. For women, 5-FU/LV was compared against a similar regimen with radiation. The radiation dose was 50.4 Gy. At 5 years, the locoregional failure was 13% for the chemotherapy-only arm as compared to 8% with the addition of radiation to chemotherapy. 5-FU/LV demonstrated better RFS and DFS, but not OS, as compared to MOF chemotherapy. Although postoperative radiation treatment did not appear to improve OS, there was an improvement in LC.

Two trials of CRT demonstrating an improvement in OS were the Gastrointestinal Tumor Study Group (GITSG) and North Central Cancer Treatment Group (NCCTG) studies. The GITSG study was a four-arm trial of 227 patients with stage B2 and C rectal cancer who, after R0 resection, were randomized to (a) surgery alone, (b) postoperative chemotherapy of bolus 5-FU (500 mg/m^2 in weeks 1 and 5 and methyl-CCNU [semustine] given day 1), (c) postoperative radiation treatment of 40- to 48-Gy split course, or (d) postoperative CRT of 40 to 44 Gy plus bolus 5-FU.[34] The severe acute toxicity was 61% in the combined modality treatment arm, as compared to 31% with chemotherapy only and 18% with radiation only. This trial was terminated early, given the significant benefit seen with CRT. In a subsequent update, postoperative CRT improved 10-year OS, 45% versus 27%, compared with observation after surgery.[164] There was a prolonged time to recurrence and a decreased recurrence rate of 33% versus 55% with CRT. LF rate was decreased to 10% versus 25% with surgery alone. Therefore, this trial concluded that there was a significant OS advantage (near doubling of survival) for patients who had CRT after surgical resection.

The Mayo–NCCTG study compared postoperative radiation therapy against postoperative CRT.[165] Two hundred four patients with T3/T4 or node-positive tumors received one cycle of 5-FU and semustine before randomization. The radiation dose was 45 to 50.4 Gy to tumor bed and adjacent lymph node regions. Bolus 5-FU (500 mg/m^2) was administered concurrently with radiotherapy. The 5-year locoregional failure was higher in the radiation-only arm, 25% versus 13%, and the 5-year OS was 40% versus 55% (in favor of CRT). Postoperative CRT reduced recurrence by 47%, LR by 46%, and DM by 37%. Cancer deaths were reduced by 36%, and overall deaths were reduced by 29%.

Given the potential benefits seen with CRT, subsequent trials attempted to refine the type and delivery of chemotherapy to maximize benefit with lower toxicity. The NCCTG 86-47-51 study compared chemotherapy regimens to be added to postoperative radiation therapy.[166] Six hundred sixty stage II or III patients were randomized 2 × 2 to systemic chemotherapy (5-FU vs. 5-FU + semustine) and the method of delivery (bolus vs. continuous infusion [CI] 5-FU). Nine weeks of chemotherapy were given, followed by the experimental chemotherapy concurrently with 50.4- to 54-Gy radiation therapy and additional chemotherapy thereafter. The bolus 5-FU dose was 500 mg/m^2 on day 1 to 5 during weeks 1 and 5, and the CI 5-FU was 225 mg/m^2/d. With a median follow-up of 46 months, there was a 27% improvement in RFS of 63% versus 53% in favor of CI 5-FU. The 4-year OS was 70% versus 60% in favor of CI. The time to relapse and the DM rate (31% vs. 40%) were also lower. There was no difference in LR. Bolus 5-FU had a higher rate of leukopenia, whereas CI had more acute severe diarrhea, which did not persist after conclusion of CRT. Semustine was of no additional benefit beyond 5-FU chemotherapy.[167]

The Intergroup 0114 study compared different chemotherapy regimens with radiation treatment in 1,695 patients.[168] Patients were randomized to one of four arms: (a) bolus 5-FU alone, (b) 5-FU and LV, (c) 5-FU plus levamisole, and (d) 5-FU, LV, and levamisole. Levamisole was not given during the radiation treatment. The radiation treatment dose was 45 Gy with a 5.4- to 9-Gy boost to a total of 50.4 to 54 Gy. With a median follow-up of 7.4 years, there was no difference in OS or DFS among the four groups. Patients randomized to the three-drug regimen experienced greater toxicity. The addition of levamisole and/or LV did not appear to add any benefit to the 5-FU.

Favorable T3 N0

Several studies have shown that there may be a subset of tumors that might not need adjuvant therapy, given the low risk of recurrence with surgery alone. Memorial Sloan Kettering Cancer Center evaluated 95 patients with T3 N0 rectal cancer treated by surgery alone.[169] Seventy-nine patients underwent LAR and 16 patients underwent APR, both with sharp mesorectal excision. With 53.3-month follow-up, 6% had LR, 13% had DM, and 3% had both LR and DM. LVI was the only histologic factor that was important for LR. This study suggests that sharp mesorectal excision with LAR or APR for T3 N0 rectal cancers results in low LRs of <10% without the use of adjuvant therapy.

In a retrospective review of 117 patients with T3 N0 rectal cancer treated at MGH, perirectal tumor invasion ≥2 mm, LVI, and poorly differentiated histology were independent factors for increased risk of DM and worse RFS.[170] Only depth of invasion was significant for LC. Of the 25 patients with favorable histologic features (well differentiated/moderately differentiated, invading <2 mm into the perirectal fat, no LVI), the 10-year actuarial LC and RFS were 95% and 87%, respectively, as compared to 71% and 55% in the unfavorable group.

A pooled analysis of five randomized, controlled trial assessed survival and relapse rates by T and N stage.[97] In patients with T3 N0 disease, 5-year survival of patients undergoing surgery and adjuvant chemotherapy alone was 84% and compared favorably to the 74% to 80% survival in patients undergoing surgery and adjuvant CRT. DFS in the T3 N0 subgroup was 69%. Since many of these trials, EUS and/or pelvic MRI has become standard in staging rectal cancers. One issue for the T3 N0 subset is the concern of understaging despite these technologies. A report from Memorial Sloan Kettering evaluated the pathologic complete response (pCR) and mesorectal lymph node involvement rate in 188 patients with either EUS or MRI staging undergoing radical resection after CRT.[171] Twenty-two percent of patients had mesorectal lymph node involvement. Although overstaging and overtreatment are possible with preoperative treatment, a larger number of patients would be understaged and require postoperative therapy. Thus, there is likely a limited subset of patients with T3 N0 rectal cancer who might have an excellent outcome with surgery alone, but there are no randomized data to support the omission of (neo) adjuvant therapy for this group of patients at the present time.

Neoadjuvant

Neoadjuvant Radiotherapy

Although both preoperative and postoperative adjuvant therapies can be effective, neoadjuvant treatment has emerged as the standard of care. Neoadjuvant therapy is associated with tumor downstaging, improved resectability and tolerance (both acute and chronic), and potential for expanded sphincter preservation options in the distal rectum. Studies from Europe have demonstrated that appropriate neoadjuvant preoperative radiation results in improvement of both LC and OS, and these results have had a significant impact on the current management of this disease.[156,172]

The Swedish Rectal Cancer Trial included 1,168 patients accrued from 1987 to 1990 with resectable, Dukes A to C rectal cancer.[173] Patients were randomized to 25 Gy in five fractions in 1 week followed by surgery 1 week later versus surgery alone. The surgery was rated as curative if margins were negative. The 5-year LR (11% vs. 27%) and OS (58% vs. 48%) were superior with preoperative radiation treatment compared to surgery alone. The LR and OS benefit persisted with long-term follow-up. At a median of 13 years, LR was 9% versus 26% and OS was 38% versus 30%, both in favor of preoperative radiotherapy, with all stages benefiting.[172]

One caveat of this study is that the surgery-alone arm did not use TME, which may have resulted in an unacceptably high 5-year LF rate of 27%. Late effects suggested more bowel movement frequency, incontinence, urgency, and soiling in the preoperative radiation treatment arm, although overall quality of life was rated good.[174] A higher rate of small-bowel obstruction was also seen in the preoperative radiotherapy arm.[175] This trial set the standard of care in many European centers, but the dose of 5 Gy times five fractions may potentially contribute to late toxicity, and the short interval between radiation and surgery may not have allowed sufficient time for tumor regression (downstaging) for improved sphincter preservation.

Justification for a longer interval after preoperative radiation treatment before surgery was demonstrated in a French trial, Lyon 90-01, which delivered 39 Gy as 3 Gy/fraction (no preoperative chemotherapy).[176] Two hundred one patients were randomized to surgery within 2 weeks versus 6 to 8 weeks of radiotherapy. The LC and OS after a median follow-up of 33 months were the same in both arms of the study. However, the pCR was 7% versus 14% (P = NSS [not statistically significant]), and the pathologic downstaging was 10% versus 26% (P = .007) in favor of the longer interval before surgery.

The TME experience by Heald et al.[147] suggested that TME alone may be sufficient for achieving low LR rates. A Dutch (CKVO 95-04) multicenter, phase III study of 1,861 patients was undertaken to evaluate the role of short-course preoperative radiation with TME. Patients were randomized to TME alone versus 25 Gy in five fractions followed by TME surgery. No fixed tumors were included in the study, and approximately half of the patients had T1 or T2 disease. The 2-year OS was 82% in both arms of the study; however, the 2-year LR was 8.2% in the TME-only arm as compared to 2.4% in the preoperative arm. This highlighted the value of radiation treatment, despite the use of TME. The sphincter preservation rate was the same in both arms, and there was no clear evidence of any downstaging effect. The perineal complication rate was slightly higher in the preoperative radiation arm of 26% versus 18% in the TME arm.[105,177] Ten-year follow-up indicates persistent benefit in LR of 5% (RT) versus 11% (TME alone).[156] Updated toxicity analysis indicates a higher incidence of sexual dysfunction and slower recovery of bowel function, more fecal incontinence, and generally poorer quality of life with short-course preoperative radiation.[178,179]

Two meta-analyses of approximately 6,000 patients each were carried out to explore the benefit of preoperative radiation treatment. One analysis included 14 randomized, controlled trials and reported that neoadjuvant radiation treatment was associated with significantly fewer LRs, improved specific survival, and an OS benefit. The second meta-analysis, provided by the Colorectal Cancer Collaborative Group, also reported on 14 randomized, controlled trials.[162] They noted a significant reduction in the risk of LR and death from rectal cancer with preoperative radiotherapy.

Neoadjuvant Chemoradiation

The improvement in outcomes with CRT in the postoperative setting led to adoption of this approach in the treatment of this disease. In the United States, neoadjuvant CRT has become widely accepted, but in other parts of the world, several groups have undertaken studies to examine the potential benefit from neoadjuvant CRT compared to radiation alone.

Preoperative radiation therapy was compared with combined preoperative CRT in a French study (Fédération Francophone de la Canérologie Digestive 9203).[180] Seven hundred thirty-three patients with resectable T3 and T4 tumors accessible by DRE were randomized to 45 Gy of radiation alone versus radiation with concurrent bolus 5-FU (350 mg/m²) plus LV on days 1 to 5 during weeks 1 and 5. After surgery, four cycles of adjuvant chemotherapy were given. The primary endpoint was OS. Although there was no difference in 5-year OS between the two arms, pCR rates (11.4% vs. 3.6%) were higher and LR rates (8.1% vs. 16.5%) were lower with CRT. Grade 3/4 acute toxicity was more frequent in patients receiving CRT, at 14.6% versus 2.7%.

A similar study undertaken by the European Organization for Research and Treatment of Cancer (EORTC 22921)[181] randomized >1,000 patients to four arms (2 × 2 design): 45 Gy alone versus 45 Gy plus 5-FU (350 mg/m²) LV followed by surgery, with patients further randomized to adjuvant therapy with 5-FU/LV or no adjuvant therapy. Results of the study were similar to those of the French study, with increased tumor downstaging (14% vs. 5.3%; P = .0001) and lower rates of LR (9% vs. 17%) but no difference in 5-year OS (65% in both arms). This information suggests that although there are lower rates of recurrence, there is no conclusive evidence that combined treatment offers a survival benefit compared to radiation alone in the neoadjuvant setting. There is, however, a higher incidence of acute toxicity associated with combined CRT.

A subsequent meta-analysis pooled four trials and compared results of preoperative radiotherapy with preoperative CRT in patients with resectable stage II or III rectal cancer.[182] The addition of chemotherapy significantly increased rates of grade 3/4 acute toxicity (odds ratio [OR], 1.68 to 10) and higher rates of pCR (OR, 2.52 to 5.27) and lowered the incidence of LR (OR, 0.39 to 0.72). No difference was seen in 5-year DFS or OS. Although the aforementioned studies and meta-analysis do not show a DFS or OS benefit with the addition of chemotherapy to neoadjuvant RT, given higher pCR as well as improved LC, neoadjuvant CRT represents a reasonable standard of care.

Long-Course Neoadjuvant Chemoradiotherapy Versus Short-Course Neoadjuvant Radiotherapy

In parts of Europe where a hypofractionated preoperative radiotherapy regimen is preferred, a study to determine whether a short-course approach (5 Gy for five fractions) to neoadjuvant therapy is better than a protracted approach (50.4 Gy using 1.8- to 2-Gy fractions with concomitant bolus 5-FU/LV given during weeks 1 and 5) was undertaken by the Polish rectal cancer group.[183] Although a higher pCR rate was seen with CRT (16% vs. 1%) along with fewer positive radial margins (4% vs. 13%) and considerable size reduction of the tumor (by ~1.9 cm), no difference in the rate of sphincter preservation, LC, or OS was seen. In a follow-up study from the Polish rectal cancer group, patients with fixed cT3 or cT4 cancer were randomized either to 5 × 5 Gy and three cycles of FOLFOX4 (group A) or to 50.4 Gy in 28 fractions combined with two 5-day cycles of bolus 5-FU 325 mg/m²/d and LV 20 mg/m²/d during the first and fifth week of irradiation along with five infusions of oxaliplatin 50 mg/m² once weekly (group B).[241] The protocol was amended in 2012 to allow oxaliplatin to be then foregone in both groups. Of 541 entered patients, 515 were eligible for analysis: 261 in group A and 254 in group B. Preoperative treatment acute toxicity was lower in group A than group B (P = .006), any toxicity being, respectively, 75% versus 83%, grade III to IV 23% versus 21%, and toxic deaths 1% versus 3%. R0 resection rates (primary endpoint) and pathologic complete response rates in groups A and B were, respectively, 77% versus 71% ($P = .07$) and 16% versus 12% ($P = .17$). The median follow-up was 35 months. At 3 years, the rates of OS and DFS in groups A and B were, respectively, 73% versus 65% ($P = .046$) and 53% versus 52% ($P = .85$) together with the cumulative incidence of local failure and distant metastases being, respectively, 22% versus 21% ($P = .82$) and 30% versus 27% ($P = .26$). Postoperative and late complication rates in groups A and group B were, respectively, 29% versus 25% ($P = .18$) and 20% versus 22% ($P = .54$). No differences were observed in local efficacy between 5×5 Gy with consolidation chemotherapy and long-course chemoradiation. The investigators concluded that an improved OS and lower acute toxicity favored the 5×5-Gy schedule with consolidation chemotherapy.[3]

In the Australian Intergroup Trial, three hundred twenty-six patients with cT3NxM0 rectal cancer within 12 cm of the anal verge were randomized to short-course RT (25 Gy in 5 fractions) with surgery within 1 week or long-course CRT (50.4 Gy in 28 fractions with continuous infusion 5-FU 225 mg/m²) with surgery 4 to 6 weeks following completion of CRT.[184] Both regimens were followed by adjuvant 5-FU–based chemotherapy. The primary endpoint of this study was to compare LR rates at 3 years. Over 90% of patients were clinically staged with pelvic MRI or EUS. With a median follow-up of 5.9 years, there was no difference in 3-year LR (7.5% short course vs. 4.4% CRT), 5-year OS (74% short course vs. 70% CRT) or late toxicity. Despite tumor downstaging, there was no difference in rates of sphincter-sparing surgery. The optimal neoadjuvant approach for resectable rectal cancer remains far from clear. Both short-course RT (25 Gy in 5 fractions) and long-course CRT (50.4 Gy in 28 fractions) with concurrent 5-FU–based chemotherapy represent reasonable therapeutic options. Many await long-term data from these randomized trials to assess for differences in late toxicities, which, as seen in the Swedish and Dutch experiences, can take many years to emerge.

The more recently published Stockholm III trial evaluated both fractionation and timing after radiation therapy to surgery. Patients with resectable rectal cancer were randomized to 1 of the following: (1) 5 Gy × 5 followed by surgery within 1 week, (2) 5 Gy × 5 followed by surgery after 4 to 8 weeks, and (3) 50 Gy in 25 fractions followed by surgery after 4 to 8 weeks. The primary endpoint was time to LR. Outcomes were similar between all three treatment arms. Although there was noted to be an increase in radiation-related toxicities in the short-course RT arm with delay to surgery, there was a significant decrease in postoperative complications in these patients. The authors suggest that short-course RT with delay may be an alternative to conventional short-course RT followed by immediate surgery.[185]

Alternative Chemotherapy Regimens with Neoadjuvant Radiotherapy

There is considerable variability in the administration of chemotherapy in many of the trials undertaken and those that are ongoing. 5-FU has been used concurrent with radiation because of its well-established potentiating effect with radiation. However, several studies have used bolus 5-FU, whereas others have administered LV-modulated 5-FU during the first and last weeks of radiation. The results of the Intergroup study demonstrating a superiority of low-dose continuous-infusion (CI)-FU were extrapolated to the neoadjuvant setting, and it appears to be a preferred approach to treatment.[167] New drugs, including oral fluoropyrimidines (capecitabine), oxaliplatin, and irinotecan, have been shown to be effective in the treatment of metastatic CRC. Oral fluoropyrimidines, as part of a CRT regimen, are commonly replacing infusional

5-FU. The incorporation of oxaliplatin and irinotecan into the neoadjuvant regimen has been less promising.

Capecitabine is an oral fluoropyrimidine prodrug that is readily absorbed in the gastrointestinal tract and mimics the efficacy of CI 5-FU while avoiding the risk of side effects and complications due to a central line for CI 5-FU.[186] Capecitabine requires the presence of thymidine phosphorylase (TP) for conversion to the active form of 5-FU within the cells. TP is present in higher concentration in tumor cells, particularly CRC, than in normal tissues, and this potentially creates a therapeutic advantage for capecitabine as compared to intravenous 5-FU.[187] Capecitabine is generally given in two divided doses twice a day during the course of radiation treatment.

Two reports from randomized control trials indicate promising results for the use of capecitabine. A German trial compared capecitabine to infusional 5-FU, initially in the adjuvant setting and then later neoadjuvantly. Initially, patients in the capecitabine group were scheduled to receive two cycles of capecitabine (2,500 mg/m² days 1 to 14, repeated day 22), followed by chemoradiotherapy (50.4 Gy plus capecitabine 1,650 mg/m² days 1 to 38), and then three cycles of capecitabine. Patients in the fluorouracil group received two cycles of bolus fluorouracil (500 mg/m² days 1 to 5, repeated day 29), followed by chemoradiotherapy (50.4 Gy plus infusional fluorouracil 225 mg/m² daily), and then two cycles of bolus fluorouracil. The protocol was later amended to allow a neoadjuvant cohort in which patients in the capecitabine group received chemoradiotherapy (50.4 Gy plus capecitabine 1,650 mg/m² daily) followed by radical surgery and five cycles of capecitabine (2,500 mg/m²/d for 14 days) and patients in the fluorouracil group received chemoradiotherapy (50.4 Gy plus infusional fluorouracil 1,000 mg/m² days 1 to 5 and 29 to 33) followed by radical surgery and four cycles of bolus fluorouracil. Five-year OS in the capecitabine group was noninferior to that in the fluorouracil group (76% [95% CI 67 to 2] vs. 67% [58 to 74]; $P = .0004$; post hoc test for superiority $P = .05$). Three-year DFS was 75% (95% CI 68 to 81) in the capecitabine group and 67% (59 to 73) in the fluorouracil group ($P = .07$). Similar numbers of patients had LRs in each group (6% in the capecitabine group vs. 7% in the fluorouracil group, $P = .67$), but fewer patients developed distant metastases in the capecitabine group (19% vs. 28%; $P = .04$). Diarrhea was the most common adverse event in both groups (any grade, 53% patients in the capecitabine group vs. 44% in the fluorouracil group; grade 3 to 4, 9% vs. 2%). Patients in the capecitabine group had more hand–foot skin reaction, fatigue, and proctitis than did those in the fluorouracil group, whereas leukopenia was more frequent with fluorouracil arm.[188]

A second study, the NSABP R-04, compared the efficacy of four chemotherapy regimens. More than 1,600 patients were randomized to 5-FU (225 mg/m², 5 days/week) or capecitabine (825 mg/m², twice a day, 5 days/week) with radiation therapy with subsequent randomization to ±oxaliplatin (50 mg/m²/week ×5).[189] For patients who received 5-FU versus capecitabine, there were comparable rates of tumor downstaging, pCR, and sphincter preservation.

Several other options for neoadjuvant therapy that have been investigated include the addition of irinotecan or oxaliplatin to 5-FU–based CRT. Early data from phase I and II trials suggested that an oxaliplatin dose of 60 mg/m² can be combined safely with CI 5-FU and standard radiation approaches with acceptable grade 3 toxicity and promising rates of pathologic downstaging, with pCR rates of 20% to 30%.[190-193] These have not been confirmed in phase III testing, as reports from four randomized, control trials all demonstrate higher toxicity with oxaliplatin-containing regimens and no proven benefit. The STAR-01 trial randomized approximately 750 patients to CI 5-FU (225 mg/m²/d) ± oxaliplatin (60 mg/

m²).[194] With the addition of oxaliplatin, there was no difference in pCR rate (16% in both arms), pN+ disease, or rates of positive circumferential radial margin, although higher rates of acute toxicity were seen. The ACCORD 12 study randomized approximately 600 patients with resectable T2 to T4 rectal cancer to CRT (45 Gy) with capecitabine (800 mg/m² twice daily) versus capecitabine and oxaliplatin (50 mg/m² weekly) delivered with 50-Gy radiation.[195] Similar to results of the STAR-01 trial, the addition of oxaliplatin increased grade 3+ acute toxicity (25% vs. 11%) and did not significantly improve pCR or sphincter preservation rates. A follow-up report showed that pCR (the primary endpoint) was achieved in 13.9% versus 19.2% of patients, respectively (P = .09).[196] Clinical results showed that at 3 years, there was no significant difference between the arms (cumulative incidence of LR, 6.1% vs. 4.4%; OS, 87.6% vs. 88.3%; DFS, 67.9% vs. 72.7%). Grade 3 to 4 toxicity was reported in four patients in the capecitabine-alone group and in two patients in the oxaliplatin-containing group. Bowel continence, erectile dysfunction, and social life disturbance were not different between groups. In multivariate analysis, the sterilization rate (Dworak score) of the operative specimen was the main significant prognostic factor (hazard ratio [HR], 0.32; 95% CI, 0.21 to 0.50). The authors concluded that no significant difference in clinical outcome was achieved with the intensified oxaliplatin regimen and that when compared with other recent randomized trials, these results indicate that concurrent administration of oxaliplatin and RT is not recommended.[196] The results of the NSABP R-04 trial also suggest higher rates of toxicity with minimal or no improvement in outcomes.[189] However, the German CAO/ARO/AIO-04 trial randomized patients with clinically staged T3-4 or any node-positive disease to a control group receiving standard fluorouracil-based combined modality treatment, consisting of preoperative radiotherapy of 50.4 Gy plus infusional fluorouracil (1,000 mg/m² days 1 to 5 and 29 to 33), followed by surgery and four cycles of bolus fluorouracil (500 mg/m² days 1 to 5 and 29; fluorouracil group) versus an experimental group receiving preoperative radiotherapy of 50·4 Gy plus infusional fluorouracil (250 mg/m² days 1 to 14 and 22 to 35) and oxaliplatin (50 mg/m² days 1, 8, 22, and 29), followed by surgery and eight cycles of adjuvant chemotherapy with oxaliplatin (100 mg/m² days 1 and 15), LV (400 mg/m² days 1 and 15), and infusional fluorouracil (2,400 mg/m² days 1 to 2 and 15 to 16; fluorouracil plus oxaliplatin group). Of the 1,265 patients initially enrolled, 1,236 were assessable (613 in the investigational group and 623 in the control group). With a median follow-up of 50 months (IQR 38 to 61), DFS at 3 years was 75.9% (95% CI, 72.4 to 79.5) in the investigational group and 71.2% (95% CI 67.6 to 74.9) in the control group (HR, 0.79; 95% CI, 0.64 to 0.98; P = .03). Preoperative grade 3 to 4 toxic effects occurred in 144 (24%) of 607 patients who actually received fluorouracil and oxaliplatin during chemoradiotherapy and in 128 (20%) of 625 patients who actually received fluorouracil chemoradiotherapy. Of 445 patients who actually received adjuvant fluorouracil and LV and oxaliplatin, 158 (36%) had grade 3 to 4 toxic effects, as did 170 (36%) of 470 patients who actually received adjuvant fluorouracil. Late grade 3 to 4 adverse events in patients who received protocol-specified preoperative and postoperative treatment occurred in 112 (25%) of 445 patients in the investigational group and in 100 (21%) of 470 patients in the control group. The investigators concluded that adding oxaliplatin to fluorouracil-based neoadjuvant chemoradiotherapy and adjuvant chemotherapy (at the doses and intensities used in this trial) significantly improved DFS of patients with clinically staged cT3-4 or cN1-2 rectal cancer compared with our former fluorouracil-based combined modality regimen (based on CAO/ARO/AIO-94).[197]

The addition of irinotecan to 5-FU–based chemotherapy has also been investigated. Toxicity of irinotecan with a dose of 50 mg/m² weekly with CI 5-FU–based CRT is somewhat higher but appears to be tolerable and also has yielded high response rates, with pCR of 25% to 30%.[198] A number of retrospective studies suggest a benefit with the addition of irinotecan to neoadjuvant CRT.[199-201] The RTOG conducted a randomized, phase II study of neoadjuvant CRT for distal rectal cancer.[202] One hundred three patients with T3 or T4 distal rectal cancer (<9 cm from the dentate line) were randomized to CI 5-FU plus hyperfractionated radiation treatment of 55.2 to 60 Gy (1.2 Gy twice a day) versus CI 5-FU and irinotecan with conventional fractionation radiation of 50 to 54 Gy (1.8 Gy/fraction). The response rate between the two arms was similar, with a pCR of 28%. Other groups attempted to incorporate biologic agents into the neoadjuvant regimen. Although reports of the addition of bevacizumab and cetuximab to conventional preoperative regimens appear tolerable, the benefit remains unclear, and no phase III evaluation of these agents has been performed.[203-209]

Preoperative Versus Postoperative Therapy

A number of phase III trials have compared preoperative versus postoperative CRT treatment strategies. The first trial was an RTOG 94-01/Intergroup 0417 trial that accrued 53 patients but closed early because of poor accrual. The NSABP R-03 study was scheduled to accrue 900 patients but also closed, after accruing 267 patients.[75] In this study, individuals with operable adenocarcinoma of the rectum were randomized (and stratified based on age and sex) to surgery followed by one cycle of 5-FU/LV and then concurrent bolus (weeks 1 and 5) 5-FU/LV with radiation treatment versus 5-FU/LV for one cycle and then concurrent CRT treatment followed by surgery. All patients received adjuvant 5-FU and LV for four cycles. Although the study was underpowered, 5-year DFS was superior in the preoperative therapy group: 64.7% versus 53.4%. There was a trend, although not statistically significant, of improved 5-year OS with preoperative therapy: 74.5% versus 65.6%. A pCR was seen in 15% of patients undergoing preoperative therapy.

A Korean trial randomized 240 patients with locally advanced (cT3/T4 or N+) rectal cancer to preoperative or postoperative CRT.[210] CRT consisted of 50 Gy in 25 fractions with concurrent capecitabine (1,650 mg/m²/d). Standard surgical procedure was TME. Patients received four cycles of adjuvant chemotherapy with either capecitabine (2,500 mg/m²/d for 14 days followed by a 1-week break) or bolus 5-FU (375 mg/m²/d)/LV (for 5 days every 4 weeks). The 5-year DFS, OS, and LR rates were no different between the two arms. Patients with low-lying rectal tumors (<5 cm from the anal verge) had higher rates of sphincter preservation in the preoperative arm (68% vs. 42%).

The definitive phase III study in favor of preoperative radiation therapy was the CAO/ARO/AIO-94 study performed by the German Rectal Cancer Group.[211] Eight hundred twenty-three clinically staged T3/T4 or node-positive rectal cancers were randomized to preoperative CRT followed by TME 6 weeks later or TME followed by postoperative CRT. The radiation dose was 50.4 Gy in 28 fractions in all patients, with a 5.4-Gy small-volume boost in the postoperative arm. 5-FU (1 g/m²/d) was administered during the weeks 1 and 5 of radiotherapy as a 120-hour CI. Both arms received four additional cycles of 5-FU (500 mg/m²/d for 5 days every 4 weeks). All surgeons were trained in the use of TME and were asked, prior to treatment, to evaluate the possibility of sphincter preservation. The 5-year results revealed a pelvic recurrence rate of 6% versus 13% (P = .02) in favor of the preoperative arm. The distant recurrence rate was 36% versus 38% (P = NSS), DFS was 68% versus 65% (P = NSS), and OS was 76% versus 74% (P = NSS) for preoperative radiation versus postoperative, respectively.

There was significant tumor downstaging after preoperative CRT, with an 8% pCR. Nodal positivity was 25% in the preoperative versus 40% in the postoperative arm. The sphincter preservation rate in 188 patients with low-lying tumors (declared by the surgeon prior to randomization to require an APR) revealed that 39% versus 19% had a sphincter-preserving LAR (P = .004) in the preoperative versus the postoperative arm. There were fewer acute (27% vs. 40%) and late toxicities (14% vs. 24%) in preoperative treatment group. Thus, preoperative CRT resulted in half the LF and doubled the sphincter preservation rate compared to postoperative therapy. In addition, compliance rates were significantly improved in the preoperative arm. Of importance, there was no difference in OS or DFS between the two arms. An update, with a median follow-up of 11 years, continues to demonstrate an improvement in LC but no difference in DFS or OS with preoperative therapy.[76]

In the era of improved surgical technique, staging, and histologic assessment, the MRC CR07 trial reevaluated the role of radiotherapy.[212] A total of 1,350 patients were randomized to preoperative radiotherapy (25 Gy in five fractions) or up-front resection with selective postoperative chemoradiotherapy (45 Gy in 25 fractions with concurrent 5-FU) in patients with a ≤1-mm circumferential resection margin. At median follow-up of 4 years, the LR was significantly lower in the preoperative radiotherapy group (4.4% vs. 10.6%). Although 3-year DFS was improved in the preoperative therapy group (77.5% vs. 71.5%), there was no difference in OS. Attempts to identify patients at high risk of recurrence after resection (≤1-mm circumferential resection margin) and administration of selective CRT were inferior to up-front preoperative radiotherapy. Both the MRC CR07 and German rectal trial established preoperative therapy, either short-course (25 Gy in five fractions) or long-course chemoradiotherapy (50 Gy in 1.8-Gy fractions with concurrent 5-FU–based chemotherapy), as the current standard of care.

Locally Advanced Rectal Cancer

The definition of locally advanced rectal cancer is variable. One definition of locally advanced disease encompasses tumors that cannot be resected without high likelihood of residual gross or microscopic disease secondary to tumor fixation or adherence to adjacent structures. A preoperative therapy approach is recommended to potentially facilitate curative resections.

The superiority of preoperative CRT over radiotherapy alone was shown in a phase III, randomized control trial.[213] Two hundred seven patients with locally unresectable T4 primary rectal carcinoma or locally recurrent rectal cancer were randomized to CRT (50 Gy with 5-FU/LV) and further adjuvant systemic therapy for 16 weeks after surgery versus radiotherapy alone (50 Gy). Higher rates of R0 resections were seen in the CRT arm: 84% versus 68%. Results for LC (82% vs. 67%), time to treatment failure (63% vs. 44%), and cancer-specific survival (72% vs. 55%) all favored the CRT arm. Similarly, there was a nonsignificant trend to improved OS with CRT. As would be anticipated, patients receiving concurrent chemotherapy experienced higher grade 3/4 acute toxicity with no difference in late toxicity.

Despite preoperative CRT and complete surgical resection, LR rates in this subgroup remain high. In situations in which the margin of resection is compromised, IORT offers the possibility of improved LC. The IORT experience at MGH was reviewed by Nakfoor et al.[214] Preoperative CI 5-FU plus 50.4 to 54 Gy of radiation was given, followed by a 4- to 6-week break and surgery. No IORT was given if metastases were present at surgical exploration, if there were adequate margins >1 cm, or if there was less than T4 disease. 10 to 12.5 Gy was given for complete resection, 12.5 to 15 Gy for microscopic residual disease, and 17.5 to 20 Gy for gross residual disease.

The 5-year LC was 90%, 65%, and 55%, and the disease-specific survival at 5 years was 65%, 45%, and 15%, for these three dose levels, respectively. However, the 5-year actuarial risk of complications was 15%. The risk of peripheral neuropathy was 20% for doses >15 Gy. IORT appeared to improve LC, especially with a gross total resection, but not OS for locally advanced rectal cancers.

A series from the Mayo Clinic evaluated outcomes in 146 patients with primary locally advanced CRC.[215] Patients received conventionally fractionated EBRT (45 to 50 Gy) with chemotherapy, surgery, and IORT (10 to 20 Gy). The rates of 5-year freedom from LR and DFS were 86% and 43%, respectively. Late complications occurred in 77 patients (53%) and included peripheral neuropathy (19%), bowel obstruction (14%), and ureteral obstruction (12%). In summary, IORT is a valuable tool in an effort to improve LC in situations in which the risk of microscopic residual disease following resection remains high, albeit with potential risks for late toxicity.

Neoadjuvant Chemotherapy Only

The PROSPECT trial evaluates the efficacy of neoadjuvant chemotherapy utilizing contemporary chemotherapy regimens in hopes of permitting more selective use of RT. Patients with cT2N1, T3N0, or T3N1 disease located in the upper or middle thirds of the rectum, who are without evidence of mesorectal fascial involvement, are eligible.[216] In the experimental arm, patients receive six cycles of FOLFOX with subsequent assessment of treatment response. If the tumor has decreased in size by at least 20%, patients proceed directly to TME followed by six cycles of adjuvant FOLFOX. If the tumor has not decreased by at least 20%, patients receive neoadjuvant CRT (with 5-FU or capecitabine), TME, and then two cycles of adjuvant FOLFOX. This is being compared to standard long-course CRT (with 5-FU or capecitabine) followed by TME and eight cycles of adjuvant FOLFOX. Primary endpoints include rate of pelvic R0 resection and time to LR.

Neoadjuvant Chemotherapy and Radiation Therapy

The role of induction chemotherapy in patients with rectal cancer was examined in a phase II trial from Spain (GCR-3). Patients with clinical stage T3/4 tumors or node-positive disease with lesions in the distal or middle third of the rectum were randomized to neoadjuvant CRT followed by surgery and adjuvant CAPOX or four cycles of induction CAPOX followed by chemoradiation and then surgery. Clinical endpoints (LR, DM, DFS, and OS) were similar between the two groups at 5 years. There was improvement in compliance and lower rates of acute toxicity in patients undergoing induction chemotherapy. The authors advocated that this regimen deserves further evaluation in a phase III setting.[217]

A more recent prospective phase II trial has reported pCR rates following additional cycles of mFOLFOX6 after neoadjuvant chemoradiation and prior to surgery. All patients received CRT followed by TME 6 to 8 weeks later compared to 2, 4, or 6 cycles of mFOLFOX6 followed by TME. Increasing cycles of mFOLFOX6 improved the rate of pCR and this approach is currently being evaluated in a phase III setting.[218] However, extending the time after chemoradiation to surgery in this trial may also have contributed to improvement in pCR.

An ongoing phase II multicenter trial (NCI 13-213) evaluates 3-year DFS in patients with locally advanced rectal cancer randomizing patients to either induction or consolidation chemotherapy (FOLFOX or CapeOX) in conjunction with neoadjuvant CRT (5-FU or capecitabine). Patients then undergo restaging with clinical exam, endoscopy, and MRI. Those with significant clinical response will be managed nonoperatively. Those with inadequate clinical response will undergo TME.[219]

Section III

Nonoperative Management

Despite the oncologic benefits of TME in patients with rectal cancer, there are potentially serious complications associated with this procedure including vascular injury, infection, wound complications, ureteral injury, and sexual dysfunction.[220-225] Long-term complications include chronic bowel dysfunction, urinary incontinence, and small-bowel obstruction.[4,5] Despite these risks, most patients with rectal cancer undergo surgery. However, there has been increasing interest in NOM, especially in patients with distal rectal cancers requiring APR, in elderly patients, or those with significant medical comorbidities. Additionally, many patients experience significant impact on their quality of life following either LAR or APR procedures. Another potential rationale for NOM management comes from the rate of pCR observed in patients undergoing neoadjuvant therapy, particularly those who undergo long-course CRT.

Investigators from the University of São Paulo School of Medicine evaluated NOM for patients with potentially resectable rectal cancer. The study included patients with T2-4 and N0-1 disease, who received neoadjuvant CRT to 50.4 Gy with concurrent 5-FU. Patients were reevaluated 8 weeks postoperatively. Response was assessed radiographically and pathologically via endoscopic biopsies. Patients with an incomplete response were sent immediately for resection. Those with cCR were followed closely with monthly physical exams, frequent proctoscopy with biopsies of any suspicious areas, serial CEA monitoring, and abdominopelvic CT scans every 6 months for the first year. Patients without evidence of disease for 1 year were considered to have a cCR.[226] Updated results have also been published with a larger cohort of patients.[227] The most recent report indicates that 31% of patients with an initial cCR went on to develop a LR, the majority of which occurred in the first 12 months. Only 7% of these patients were not amenable to salvage surgery. Five-year cause-specific OS and DFS were 91% and 68%, respectively, with 14% of patients failing distantly.[228]

In a retrospective analysis, Lim and colleagues reported on the outcomes of medically inoperable patients or patients refusing surgery treated with chemoradiation or radiation therapy only from six Australian centers. The majority of patients had distal T3 lesions and underwent CRT. Patients were followed clinically. Those patients who achieved a cCR had significantly longer PFS.[229]

Maas and colleagues attempted to build upon the results of the São Paulo group by employing modern MRI staging techniques. In this study, there was a noticeably lower rate of cCR, likely the result of the strict imaging criteria that was used.[230] Memorial Sloan Kettering investigators compared the outcomes of 32 patients who had a cCR with NOM to a comparable group who had achieved a pCR with surgical resection. The LR rate for patients undergoing NOM was 21% versus 0% in the pCR group after 28 months; however, all patients that failed locally were successfully salvaged with surgery. The clinical outcomes were otherwise similar between the groups.[231] This series has since been updated with OS and DFS remaining similar between the NOM and pCR groups.[232]

More recently, a prospective trial from Denmark evaluated patients with resectable T2-3 primaries and N0-1 disease who were treated with high-dose radiation to 60 Gy in 30 fractions with a 5-Gy endorectal brachytherapy[240] boost and oral tegafur–uracil. Response was assessed via endoscopy and MRI/CT. If patients achieved a cCR, they were followed closely with exams, endoscopy, and PET scans. Only 26% of patients had LR failure by 2 years and all patients were surgically salvaged.[233]

Radiotherapy Treatment Technique

External beam treatment fields for rectal carcinoma should encompass potential sites at greatest risk for harboring disease, including the presacral space, primary tumor site, and (for post-APR cases) the perineum. Other areas at risk include the internal iliac and distal common iliac nodes. Generally, the risk of disease involvement of the para-aortic region is sufficiently low, and the morbidity from treatment is sufficiently high, to exclude this region from radiation fields. The external iliac nodes may be covered for lesions involving the anterior structures, including the bladder, prostate, and vagina.

In general, patients with rectal carcinoma should be treated in the prone position to reduce the volume of small bowel within the pelvis. Maneuvers to reduce the volume of small bowel include treatment with a full bladder and the use of bowel displacement techniques such as a bellyboard (a device with a false tabletop to allow the upper abdominal contents to fall anteriorly).[234] The use of shaped lateral fields reduces the dose to small bowel located in the anterior and superior aspects of the pelvis. A marker is generally placed at the anal verge, and intravenous, rectal, and small-bowel contrast is often administered at the time of simulation for accurate target and normal tissue delineation.

Generally, a four-field (anteroposterior/posteroanterior [AP/PA]/right/left [R/L] lateral) or three-field (PA/R/L lateral) technique is used. The superior field edge is placed at the L5/S1 interspace. The distal field edge depends on tumor location and should be roughly 3 to 5 cm below palpable tumor for patients receiving preoperative treatment. For postoperative cases, the distal field edge is about 5 cm below the best estimate of the preoperative tumor bed and (if an APR has been performed) below the perineum. AP/PA fields should have at least a 1.5-cm margin on the pelvic brim.

On lateral treatment fields, the superior and inferior borders remain the same as for AP/PA fields. Lateral fields should encompass the entire sacrum posteriorly to ensure adequate coverage of the presacral space. The anterior margin should be roughly 4 cm anterior to the rectum (ensuring adequate coverage of the mesorectum). If the tumor has considerable extrarectal extension, these guidelines should be modified to make certain that all disease is encompassed with appropriate margin.

The usual dose given to initial pelvic fields is 45 Gy in 25 fractions of 1.8 Gy each. An additional tumor boost may be administered, usually through opposed lateral fields, to an additional 5.4 to 9 Gy. Small bowel should be excluded from the boost volume after about 50 Gy in an effort to minimize acute and late toxicity (Fig. 65.6).

Management of Recurrent Rectal Cancer

Recurrent rectal cancer is often approached in the same way as T4 disease, often with an aggressive treatment plan of CRT, surgery, and adjuvant chemotherapy. At the time of surgery, IORT may be considered. Up to 10% of patients with T1 and T2 N0 disease will fail locally after surgery, usually because of an inadequate lymph node/mesorectal dissection. Recurrences may occur along the pelvic sidewall or in nonpelvic sidewall areas such as the uterus, prostate, or vagina. The 5-year OS is approximately 20% for all cases. LC is roughly 40% in patients with no prior radiation and 10% to 20% in patients with prior radiotherapy.[235] Given the difficulty of surgical resection of pelvic sidewall recurrences, these tend to fare worse.

In patients with no prior history of radiation, neoadjuvant CRT followed by surgical resection is a reasonable treatment approach. In one series, 123 patients with locally recurrent CRC received a course of EBRT (45 to 54 Gy) either before or

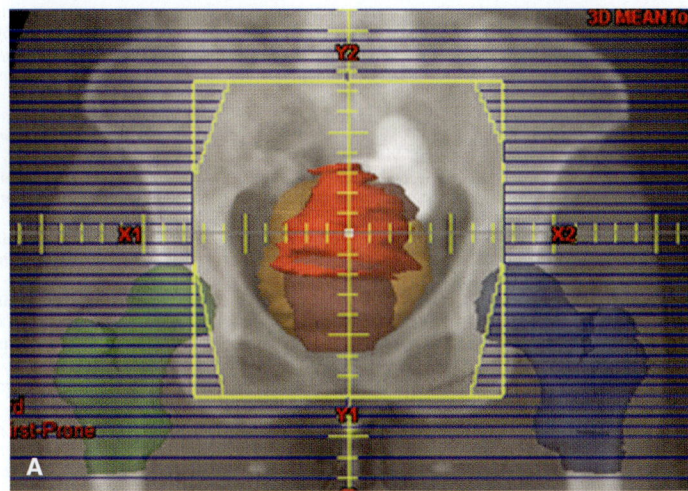
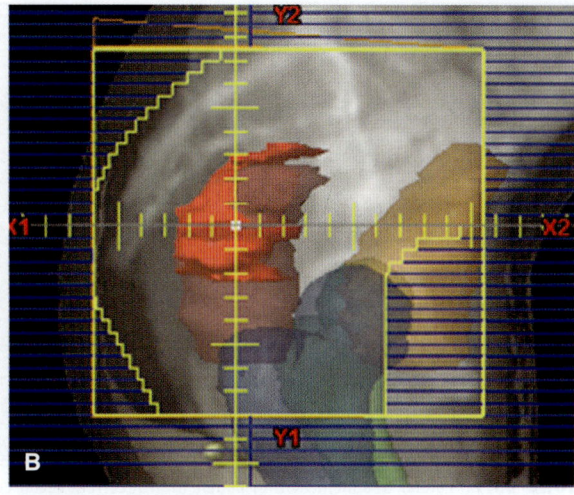

FIGURE 65.6.   A: Posteroanterior treatment field of patient with T3 N1 rectal cancer. **B:** Lateral treatment field of a patient with T3 N1 rectal cancer. *Red*, gross tumor volume; *brown*, rectum; *orange*, bladder; *green/blue*, femoral heads.

after surgical resection and IORT.[87,88] Five-year OS in patients undergoing gross total resection was 24%, compared to 18% in patients with gross residual disease. A second series using a similar treatment approach of neoadjuvant therapy, surgical resection, and IORT achieved 5-year LC and OS rates of 54% and 32%, respectively. The 5-year LC and OS rates in patients undergoing radical resection were 69% and 42%, respectively. A series of 35 patients with recurrent rectal cancer not amenable to up-front surgical resection was treated with a course of preoperative CRT (50.4 to 59.4 Gy with 5-FU chemotherapy).[236] Eighty percent underwent curative resection, and 60% achieved negative surgical margins. Three-year OS rate in patients with complete resection was 82%.

One randomized control trial compared outcomes of preoperative CRT or radiotherapy alone prior to surgical resection in patients with locally advanced or recurrent rectal cancer who had not received prior radiotherapy.[213] This series included 25 patients with recurrent disease. Higher rates of R0 resection, LC, time to treatment failure, and cancer-specific survival were seen in the chemoradiation arm (see section Locally Advanced Rectal Cancer). Five-year OS rate in patients with recurrent rectal cancer was 37%.

In patients with prior history of radiation, reirradiation is possible in carefully selected situations. Forty-seven patients in an Italian retrospective study were treated with preoperative CRT.[237] Patients who did not have prior radiation treatment received 45 Gy with CI 5-FU and mitomycin C, followed by surgery and IORT of 10 to 15 Gy. LV and 5-FU were given for six to nine cycles adjuvantly. If patients had prior radiation treatment, they received 23.4 Gy. The 5-year OS rate was 20% for all patients, 60% for resected tumors, 0% for unresected tumors, and 40% for patients treated by external beam, surgery, and IORT. The 5-year LC rate was 30% for all patients, 70% for completely resected tumors, 0% for unresectable tumors, and 80% for EBRT, surgery, and IORT. Eighty-five percent of patients had palliation of pain, with an average duration of 12 months.

Another retrospective series included 147 patients with locally recurrent rectal cancer, with the majority (127 patients) undergoing preoperative CRT.[86] Fifty-seven had received prior radiation and were reirradiated to a dose of 30.6 Gy. Preoperative treatment was followed by surgical resection and IORT. Five-year OS for the entire group was 32% and was 48% in patients with an R0 resection. Radical

resection correlated significantly with improved OS, DFS, and LC rates. There was no difference in late toxicity in patients who received reirradiation.

Long-term results of reirradiation for patients with recurrent rectal carcinoma were also reported by Mohiuddin et al.[238] One hundred three patients who developed LR after surgery with preoperative or postoperative radiation treatment (median dose, 50.4 Gy) were reirradiated with concurrent CI 5-FU. Patients were treated with opposed laterals or three-field technique (PA/L lateral/R lateral) to the presacral area and gross tumor volume with 2- to 4-cm margin. Patients received 30 Gy (1.2 Gy twice a day) or 30.6 Gy (1.8 Gy every day), followed by a boost of 6 to 20 Gy to gross tumor volume (2-cm margin). Forty-one patients were surgically explored after treatment and 34 underwent resection, with 6 patients undergoing sphincter-sparing surgery. With a median follow-up of 2 years, the 5-year OS rate was 19%. Patients who underwent resection had a higher survival rate, with tolerable acute and late toxicity. Twenty-two patients experienced late toxicity, including severe, persistent diarrhea (18 patients), small-bowel obstruction (15 patients), fistula formation (4 patients), and stricture (2 patients). Palliation of bleeding was achieved in 100% of patients.

Hyperfractionated radiotherapy may be an alternative in an effort to reduce late toxicity. A retrospective series from MD Anderson Cancer Center evaluated reirradiation outcomes in 50 patients with prior history of pelvic radiotherapy.[239] Patients were treated in 1.5-Gy fractions twice daily to a total dose of 30 to 39 Gy (depending on the time interval between radiotherapy treatment courses). Concurrent chemotherapy was administered to the majority of patients. The 3-year freedom rate from local progression and OS rate in the entire cohort were 33% and 39%, respectively. Three-year OS rate was 66% in patients undergoing surgery, and the 3-year rate of grade 3/4 late toxicity was 35%.

Patients with recurrent rectal cancer and no prior history of EBRT are generally treated with a course of concurrent, preoperative CRT (50 to 54 Gy with 5-FU–based chemotherapy) followed by surgical resection (and consideration of IORT). Patients with prior history of radiotherapy may receive reirradiation to doses of 30 to 39 Gy but have the potential to experience significant late toxicity; therefore, efforts should be made to avoid small bowel within treatment fields (Fig. 65.7).

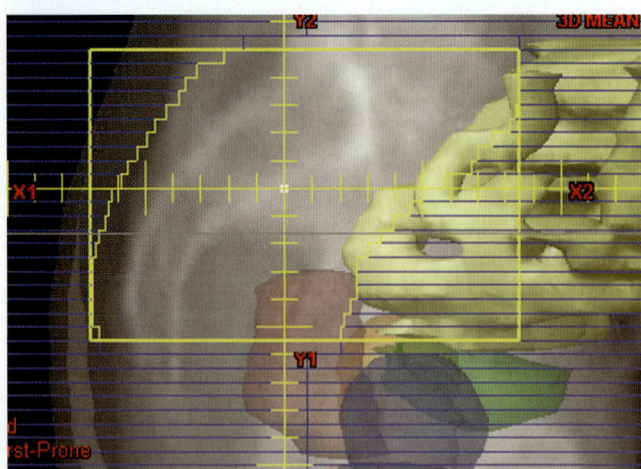

FIGURE 65.7. Lateral treatment field of patient with recurrent rectal cancer (with prior history of radiation) along presacral space. *Brown*, rectum; *yellow*, small bowel; *green*, bladder; *orange/blue*, femoral heads.

REFERENCES

1. Horton J, Tepper JE. Colorectal cancer. In: Haffty B, Wilson L, eds. *Handbook of radiation oncology: basic principles and clinical protocols.* Burlington, MA: Jones and Bartlett, 2006.
2. Siegel R, Miller K, Jemal A. Cancer statistics, 2017. *CA Cancer J Clin* 2017;67(1):7–30.
3. Heinrich S, et al. Adjuvant gemcitabine versus NEOadjuvant gemcitabine/oxaliplatin plus adjuvant gemcitabine in resectable pancreatic cancer: a randomized multicenter phase III study (NEOPAC study). *BMC Cancer* 2011;11:346.
4. Kohler BA, et al. Annual report to the nation on the status of cancer, 1975–2007, featuring tumors of the brain and other nervous system. *J Natl Cancer Inst* 2011;103(9):714–736.
5. Chan AT, Giovannucci EL. Primary prevention of colorectal cancer. *Gastroenterology* 2010;138(6):2029–2043e10.
6. Ekbom A, et al. Ulcerative colitis and colorectal cancer. A population-based study. *N Engl J Med* 1990;323(18):1228–1233.
7. Wei EK, et al. Comparison of risk factors for colon and rectal cancer. *Int J Cancer* 2004;108(3):433–442.
8. Czito BWC. Colon cancer. In: Tepper GA, ed. *Clinical radiation oncology.* Edinburgh, UK: Churchill Livingstone, 2007:1101–1111.
9. Steele GMR, Podolsky DK, et al. Cancer of the colon, rectum, and anus. In: *Cancer manual.* Framingham, MA: American Cancer Society, Massachusetts Division, 1996.
10. Michels KB, et al. Prospective study of fruit and vegetable consumption and incidence of colon and rectal cancers. *J Natl Cancer Inst* 2000;92(21):1740–1752.
11. Gustin DM, Brenner DE. Chemoprevention of colon cancer: current status and future prospects. *Cancer Metastasis Rev* 2002;21(3–4):323–348.
12. Markowitz SD, Bertagnolli MM. Molecular origins of cancer: molecular basis of colorectal cancer. *N Engl J Med* 2009;361(25):2449–2460.
13. Gryfe R, et al. Tumor microsatellite instability and clinical outcome in young patients with colorectal cancer. *N Engl J Med* 2000;342(2):69–77.
14. Speights VO, et al. Colorectal cancer: current trends in initial clinical manifestations. *South Med J* 1991;84(5):575–578.
15. Steinberg SM, et al. Prognostic indicators of colon tumors. The Gastrointestinal Tumor Study Group experience. *Cancer* 1986;57(9):1866–1870.
16. Beets-Tan RG, Beets GL, Bortslap AC, et al. Preoperative assessment of local tumor extent in advanced rectal cancer: CT or high resolution MRI? *Abdom Imaging* 2000;25:533.
17. Beets-Tan RG, Beets GL, Vliegen RF, et al. Accuracy of magnetic resonance imaging in prediction of tumour-free resection margin in rectal cancer surgery. *Lancet* 2001;357:497.
18. Screening for colorectal cancer: U.S. Preventive Services Task Force recommendation statement. *Ann Intern Med* 2008;149(9):627–637.
19. Levin B, et al. Screening and surveillance for the early detection of colorectal cancer and adenomatous polyps, 2008: a joint guideline from the American Cancer Society, the US Multi-Society Task Force on Colorectal Cancer, and the American College of Radiology. *CA Cancer J Clin* 2008;58(3):130–160.
20. Whitlock EP, et al. Screening for colorectal cancer: a targeted, updated systematic review for the U.S. Preventive Services Task Force. *Ann Intern Med* 2008;149(9):638–658.
21. Lieberman DA. Clinical practice. Screening for colorectal cancer. *N Engl J Med* 2009;361(12):1179–1187.
22. Engel C, et al. Efficacy of annual colonoscopic surveillance in individuals with hereditary nonpolyposis colorectal cancer. *Clin Gastroenterol Hepatol* 2010;8(2):174–182.
23. Burke W, et al. Recommendations for follow-up care of individuals with an inherited predisposition to cancer. I. Hereditary nonpolyposis colon cancer. Cancer Genetics Studies Consortium. *JAMA* 1997;277(11):915–919.
24. Rex DK, et al. American College of Gastroenterology guidelines for colorectal cancer screening 2009 [corrected]. *Am J Gastroenterol* 2009;104(3):739–750.
25. Smith RA, Cokkinides V, Eyre HJ. American Cancer Society guidelines for the early detection of cancer, 2006. *CA Cancer J Clin* 2006;56(1):11–25; quiz 49–50.
26. Steinwachs D, et al. National Institutes of Health state-of-the-science conference statement: Enhancing use and quality of colorectal cancer screening. *Ann Intern Med* 2010;152(10):663–667.
27. Centers for Disease Control and Prevention. Vital signs: colorectal cancer screening among adults aged 50–75 years—United States, 2008. *MMWR Morb Mortal Wkly Rep* 2010;59(26):808–812.
28. Farouk R, et al. Accuracy of computed tomography in determining resectability for locally advanced primary or recurrent colorectal cancers. *Am J Surg* 1998;175(4):283–287.
29. Isbister WH, al-Sanea O. The utility of pre-operative abdominal computerized tomography scanning in colorectal surgery. *J R Coll Surg Edinb* 1996;41(4):232–234.
30. Adalsteinsson B, et al. Computed tomography in staging of rectal carcinoma. *Acta Radiol Diagn (Stockh)* 1985;26(1):45–55.
31. Balthazar EJ, et al. Carcinoma of the colon: detection and preoperative staging by CT. *AJR Am J Roentgenol* 1988;150(2):301–306.
32. McAndrew MR, Saba AK. Efficacy of routine preoperative computed tomography scans in colon cancer. *Am Surg* 1999;65(3):205–208.
33. Beynon J, Foy DM, Roe AM, et al. Endoluminal ultrasound in the assessment of local invasion in rectal cancer. *Br J Surg* 1986;73:474.
34. Solomon MJ, McLeod RS. Endoluminal transrectal ultrasonography: accuracy, reliability, and validity. *Dis Colon Rectum* 1993;36:200.
35. Hulsmans FJH, Tio TL, Fockens P, et al. Assessment of tumor infiltration depth in rectal cancer with transrectal sonography. Caution is necessary. *Radiology* 1994;190:715.
36. Orrom WJ, Wong WD, Rothenberger DA, et al. Endorectal ultrasound in the preoperative staging of rectal tumors: a learning experience. *Dis Colon Rectum* 1990;33:654.
37. Hildebrandt U, Feifel G. Preoperative staging of rectal cancer by intrarectal ultrasound. *Dis Colon Rectum* 1985;28:42.
38. Gualdi GF, Casciani E, Guadalaxara A, et al. Local staging of rectal cancer with transrectal ultrasound and endorectal magnetic resonance imaging: comparison with histologic findings. *Dis Colon Rectum* 2000;43:338.
39. Blomqvist L, Machado M, Rubio C, et al. Rectal tumour staging: MR imaging using pelvic phased-array and endorectal coils vs endoscopic ultrasonography. *Eur Radiol* 2000;10:653.
40. Brown G, Richards CJ, Bourne MW, et al. Morphologic predictors of lymph node status in rectal cancer with use of high-spatial-resolution MR imaging with histopathologic comparison. *Radiology* 2003;227:371.
41. Kim NK, Kim MJ, Yun SH, et al. Comparative study of transrectal ultrasonography, pelvic computerized tomography, and magnetic resonance imaging in preoperative staging of rectal cancer. *Dis Colon Rectum* 1999;42:770.
42. Meyenberger C, et al. Endoscopic ultrasound and endorectal magnetic resonance imaging: a prospective, comparative study for preoperative staging and follow-up of rectal cancer. *Endoscopy* 1995;27(7):469–479.
43. Dukes CE. The surgical pathology of rectal cancer. *Proc R Soc Med* 1943;37:131.
44. Nahas CS, Akhurst T, Yeung H, et al. Positron emission tomography detection of distant metastatic or synchronous disease in patients with locally advanced rectal cancer receiving preoperative chemoradiation. *Ann Surg Oncol* 2008;15(3):704–711.
45. Saltz LB, et al. Irinotecan fluorouracil plus leucovorin is not superior to fluorouracil plus leucovorin alone as adjuvant treatment for stage III colon cancer: results of CALGB 89803. *J Clin Oncol* 2007;25(23):3456–3461.
46. Freeny PC, Marks WM, Ryan JA, et al. Colorectal carcinoma evaluation with CT: Preoperative staging and detection of postoperative recurrence. *Radiology* 1986;158:347.
47. Otchy D, et al. Practice parameters for colon cancer. *Dis Colon Rectum* 2004;47(8):1269–1284.
48. McGory ML, Shekelle PG, Ko CY. Development of quality indicators for patients undergoing colorectal cancer surgery. *J Natl Cancer Inst* 2006;98(22):1623–1633.
49. Benson AB III, et al. American Society of Clinical Oncology recommendations on adjuvant chemotherapy for stage II colon cancer. *J Clin Oncol* 2004;22(16):3408–3419.
50. The Clinical Outcomes of Surgical Therapy Study Group. A comparison of laparoscopically assisted and open colectomy for colon cancer. *N Engl J Med* 2004;350(20):2050–2059.
51. Fleshman J, et al. Laparoscopic colectomy for cancer is not inferior to open surgery based on 5-year data from the COST Study Group trial. *Ann Surg* 2007;246(4):655–662; discussion 662–664.
52. Bonjer HJ, et al. Laparoscopically assisted vs open colectomy for colon cancer: a meta-analysis. *Arch Surg* 2007;142(3):298–303.
53. Jackson TD, et al. Laparoscopic versus open resection for colorectal cancer: a metaanalysis of oncologic outcomes. *J Am Coll Surg* 2007;204(3):439–446.
54. Moertel CG, et al. Levamisole and fluorouracil for adjuvant therapy of resected colon carcinoma. *N Engl J Med* 1990;322(6):352–358.
55. O'Connell MJ, et al. Controlled trial of fluorouracil and low-dose leucovorin given for 6 months as postoperative adjuvant therapy for colon cancer. *J Clin Oncol* 1997;15(1):246–250.
56. Cassidy J, et al. First-line oral capecitabine therapy in metastatic colorectal cancer: a favorable safety profile compared with intravenous 5-fluorouracil/leucovorin. *Ann Oncol* 2002;13(4):566–575.
57. Twelves C, et al. Capecitabine versus 5-fluorouracil/folinic acid as adjuvant therapy for stage III colon cancer: final results from the X-ACT trial with analysis by age and preliminary evidence of a pharmacodynamic marker of efficacy. *Ann Oncol* 2012;23(5):1190–1197.
58. Andre T, et al. Oxaliplatin, fluorouracil, and leucovorin as adjuvant treatment for colon cancer. *N Engl J Med* 2004;350(23):2343–2351.

59. Andre T, et al. Improved overall survival with oxaliplatin, fluorouracil, and leucovorin as adjuvant treatment in stage II or III colon cancer in the MOSAIC trial. *J Clin Oncol* 2009;27(19):3109–3116.

60. Kuebler JP, et al. Oxaliplatin combined with weekly bolus fluorouracil and leucovorin as surgical adjuvant chemotherapy for stage II and III colon cancer: results from NSABP C-07. *J Clin Oncol* 2007;25(16):2198–2204.

61. Yothers G, et al. Oxaliplatin as adjuvant therapy for colon cancer: updated results of NSABP C-07 trial, including survival and subset analyses. *J Clin Oncol* 2011;29(28):3768–3774.

62. Allegra CJ, et al. Phase III trial assessing bevacizumab in stages II and III carcinoma of the colon: results of NSABP protocol C-08. *J Clin Oncol* 2011;29(1):11–16.

63. Alberts SR Sargent DJ, Smyrk TC, et al. Adjuvant mFOLFOX6 with and without cetuximab (Cmab) in KRAS wild-type (WT) patients with resected stage III colon cancer: results from NCCTG Intergroup Phase III Trial N0147. *Clin Oncol* 2010;28:959s.

64. Goldberg RM, Sargent D, Thibodeau SN, et al. Adjuvant mFOLFOX6 plus or minus cetuximab in patients with KRAS-mutant resected stage III colon cancer: NCCTG Intergroup Phase III Trial N0147 (abstract 3508). *J Clin Oncol* 2010;28:262s.

65. De Gramont A, van Cutsem E, Tabernero J, et al. AVANT: Results from a randomized, three-arm multinational phase III study to investigate bevacizumab with either XELOX or FOLFOX4 versus FOLFOX4 alone as adjuvant treatment for colon cancer. *J Clin Oncol* 2011;29(Suppl 4):362.

66. Gunderson LL, Sosin H, Levitt S. Extrapelvic colon–areas of failure in a reoperation series: implications for adjuvant therapy. *Int J Radiat Oncol Biol Phys* 1985;11(4):731–741.

67. Willett CG, et al. Failure patterns following curative resection of colonic carcinoma. *Ann Surg* 1984;200(6):685–690.

68. Amos EH, et al. Postoperative radiotherapy for locally advanced colon cancer. *Ann Surg Oncol* 1996;3(5):431–436.

69. Gunderson LL, et al. Locally advanced primary colorectal cancer: intraoperative electron and external beam irradiation +/– 5-FU. *Int J Radiat Oncol Biol Phys* 1997;37(3):601–614.

70. Willett CG, et al. Postoperative radiation therapy for high-risk colon carcinoma. *J Clin Oncol* 1993;11(6):1112–1117.

71. Gunderson LL, Nelson H, Martenson JA, et al. Intraoperative electron and external beam irradiation with or without 5-fluorouracil and maximum surgical resection for previously unirradiated, locally recurrent colorectal cancer. *Dis Colon Rectum* 1996;39(12):1379–1395.

72. Martenson JA Jr, et al. Phase III study of adjuvant chemotherapy and radiation therapy compared with chemotherapy alone in the surgical adjuvant treatment of colon cancer: results of intergroup protocol 0130. *J Clin Oncol* 2004;22(16):3277–3283.

73. Ludmir E, Arya R, Wu Y, et al. Role of adjuvant radiotherapy in locally advanced colonic carcinoma in the modern chemotherapy era. *Ann Surg Oncol* 2016;23:856–862.

74. Foxtrot Collaborative Group. Feasibility of preoperative chemotherapy for locally advanced, operable colon cancer: the pilot phase of a randomised controlled trial. *Lancet Oncol* 2012;13:1152–1160.

75. Roh MS, Colangelo LH, O'Connell MJ, et al. Preoperative multimodality therapy improves disease-free survival in patients with carcinoma of the rectum: NSABP R-03. *J Clin Oncol* 2009;27:5124–5130.

76. Sauer R, Liersch T, Merkel S, et al. Preoperative versus postoperative chemoradiotherapy for locally advanced rectal cancer: results of the German CAO/ARO/AIO-94 randomized phase III trial after a median follow-up of 11 years. *J Clin Oncol* 2012;30:1926–1933.

77. Cukier M, Soliman H, Smith A, et al. Neoadjuvant chemoradiotherapy and multivisceral resection for primary locally advanced adherent colon cancer. *J Clin Oncol* 2011;29:3544.

78. Hurwitz H, Fehrenbacher L, Novotny W, et al. Bevacizumab plus irinotecan, fluorouracil, and leucovorin for metastatic colorectal cancer. *N Engl J Med* 2004;350:2335–2342.

79. Kohne CH, Hofheinz R, Mineur L, et al. First-line panitumumab plus irinotecan/5-fluorouracil/leucovorin treatment in patients with metastatic colorectal cancer. *J Cancer Res Clin Oncol* 2012;138:65–72.

80. Cunningham D, Humblet Y, Siena S, et al. Cetuximab monotherapy and cetuximab plus irinotecan in irinotecan-refractory metastatic colorectal cancer. *N Engl J Med* 2004;351:337–345.

81. Le DT, Uram JN, Wang H, et al. PD-1 blockade in tumors with mismatch-repair deficiency. *N Engl J Med* 2015;372:2509–2520.

82. Gunderson LL, et al. Lower gastrointestinal cancers: rationale, results, and techniques of treatment. *Front Radiat Ther Oncol* 1994;28:140–154.

83. Willett CG, et al. Renal complications secondary to radiation treatment of upper abdominal malignancies. *Int J Radiat Oncol Biol Phys* 1986;12(9):1601–1604.

84. Schild SE, et al. The treatment of locally advanced colon cancer. *Int J Radiat Oncol Biol Phys* 1997;37(1):51–58.

85. Willett CG, et al. Intraoperative electron beam radiation therapy for primary locally advanced rectal and rectosigmoid carcinoma. *J Clin Oncol* 1991;9(5):843–849.

86. Dresen RC, et al. Radical resection after IORT-containing multimodality treatment is the most important determinant for outcome in patients treated for locally recurrent rectal cancer. *Ann Surg Oncol* 2008;15(7):1937–1947.

87. Haddock MG, et al. Intraoperative electron radiotherapy as a component of salvage therapy for patients with colorectal cancer and advanced nodal metastases. *Int J Radiat Oncol Biol Phys* 2003;56(4):966–973.

88. Haddock MG, et al. Intraoperative irradiation for locally recurrent colorectal cancer in previously irradiated patients. *Int J Radiat Oncol Biol Phys* 2001;49(5):1267–1274.

89. Pilipshen SJ, et al. Patterns of pelvic recurrence following definitive resections of rectal cancer. *Cancer* 1984;53(6):1354–1362.

90. Rich T, et al. Patterns of recurrence of rectal cancer after potentially curative surgery. *Cancer* 1983;52(7):1317–1329.

91. Aldridge MC, et al. Influence of tumour site on presentation, management and subsequent outcome in large bowel cancer. *Br J Surg* 1986;73(8):663–670.

92. Lingareddy V, Ahmad NR, Mohiuddin M. Palliative reirradiation for recurrent rectal cancer. *Int J Radiat Oncol Biol Phys* 1997;38(4):785–790.

93. Clinico-pathological features of prognostic significance in operable rectal cancer in 17 centres in the U.K. (Third report of the M.R.C. Trial, on behalf of the Working Party). *Br J Cancer* 1984;50(4):435–442.

94. Law WL, Chu KW. Abdominoperineal resection is associated with poor oncological outcome. *Br J Surg* 2004;91(11):1493–1499.

95. Kirklin JW, Dockerty MB, Waugh JM. The role of the peritoneal reflection in the prognosis of carcinoma of the rectum and sigmoid colon. *Surg Gynecol Obstet* 1949;88(3):326–331.

96. Edge SB, Greene FL, Byrd DR, et al., eds. Colon and rectum. In: American Joint Committee on Cancer Staging Manual. 8th ed. New York: Springer, 2017.

97. Gunderson LL, et al. Impact of T and N stage and treatment on survival and relapse in adjuvant rectal cancer: a pooled analysis. *J Clin Oncol* 2004;22(10):1785–1796.

98. Chapuis PH, et al. A multivariate analysis of clinical and pathological variables in prognosis after resection of large bowel cancer. *Br J Surg* 1985;72(9):698–702.

99. Crucitti F, et al. Prognostic factors in colorectal cancer: current status and new trends. *J Surg Oncol Suppl* 1991;2:76–82.

100. Sasaki O, Atkin WS, Jass JR. Mucinous carcinoma of the rectum. *Histopathology* 1987;11(3):259–272.

101. Quirke P, et al. Effect of the plane of surgery achieved on local recurrence in patients with operable rectal cancer: a prospective study using data from the MRC CR07 and NCIC-CTG CO16 randomised clinical trial. *Lancet* 2009;373(9666):821–828.

102. Nagtegaal ID, Quirke P. What is the role for the circumferential margin in the modern treatment of rectal cancer? *J Clin Oncol* 2008;26(2):303–312.

103. Habib NA, et al. Does fixity affect prognosis in colorectal tumours? *Br J Surg* 1983;70(7):423–424.

104. Mohiuddin M, Regine WF, Marks G. Prognostic significance of tumor fixation of rectal carcinoma. Implications for adjunctive radiation therapy. *Cancer* 1996;78(4):717–722.

105. Kapiteijn E, et al. Preoperative radiotherapy combined with total mesorectal excision for resectable rectal cancer. *N Engl J Med* 2001;345(9):638–646.

106. Carraro PG, et al. Obstructing colonic cancer: failure and survival patterns over a ten-year follow-up after one-stage curative surgery. *Dis Colon Rectum* 2001;44(2):243–250.

107. Beahrs OH, Sanfelippo PM. Factors in prognosis of colon and rectal cancer. *Cancer* 1971;28(1):213–218.

108. Copeland EM, Miller LD, Jones RS. Prognostic factors in carcinoma of the colon and rectum. *Am J Surg* 1968;116(6):875–881.

109. Rankin FW, Broders AC. Factors influencing prognosis in carcinoma of the rectum. *Surg Gynecol Obstet* 1928;46:660–667.

110. Rodel C, et al. Prognostic significance of tumor regression after preoperative chemoradiotherapy for rectal cancer. *J Clin Oncol* 2005;23(34):8688–8696.

111. Ryan R, et al. Pathological response following long-course neoadjuvant chemoradiotherapy for locally advanced rectal cancer. *Histopathology* 2005;47(2):141–146.

112. McArdle CS, Hole D. Impact of variability among surgeons on postoperative morbidity and mortality and ultimate survival. *BMJ* 1991;302(6791):1501–1505.

113. Meyerhardt JA, et al. Impact of hospital procedure volume on surgical operation and long-term outcomes in high-risk curatively resected rectal cancer: findings from the Intergroup 0114 Study. *J Clin Oncol* 2004;22(1):166–174.

114. Black WA, Waugh JM. The intramural extension of carcinoma of the descending colon, sigmoid, and rectosigmoid; a pathologic study. *Surg Gynecol Obstet* 1948;87(4):457–464.

115. Grinnell RS. Distal intramural spread of carcinoma of the rectum and rectosigmoid. *Surg Gynecol Obstet* 1954;99(4):421–430.

116. Quer EA, Dahlin DC, Mayo CW. Retrograde intramural spread of carcinoma of the rectum and rectosigmoid; a microscopic study. *Surg Gynecol Obstet* 1953;96(1):24–30.

117. Pollett WG, Nicholls RJ. The relationship between the extent of distal clearance and survival and local recurrence rates after curative anterior resection for carcinoma of the rectum. *Ann Surg* 1983;198(2):159–163.

118. Vernava AM III, et al. A prospective evaluation of distal margins in carcinoma of the rectum. *Surg Gynecol Obstet* 1992;175(4):333–336.

119. Williams NS, Dixon MF, Johnston D. Reappraisal of the 5 centimetre rule of distal excision for carcinoma of the rectum: a study of distal intramural spread and of patients' survival. *Br J Surg* 1983;70(3):150–154.

120. Wolmark N, Fisher B. An analysis of survival and treatment failure following abdominoperineal and sphincter-saving resection in Dukes' B and C rectal carcinoma. A report of the NSABP clinical trials. National Surgical Adjuvant Breast and Bowel Project. *Ann Surg* 1986;204(4):480–489.

121. Kang SB, et al. Open versus laparoscopic surgery for mid or low rectal cancer after neoadjuvant chemoradiotherapy (COREAN trial): short-term outcomes of an open-label randomised controlled trial. *Lancet Oncol* 2010;11(7):637–645.

122. Lujan J, et al. Randomized clinical trial comparing laparoscopic and open surgery in patients with rectal cancer. *Br J Surg* 2009;96(9):982–989.

123. Ng SS, et al. Long-term morbidity and oncologic outcomes of laparoscopic-assisted anterior resection for upper rectal cancer: ten-year results of a prospective, randomized trial. *Dis Colon Rectum* 2009;52(4):558–566.

124. Brodsky JT, et al. Variables correlated with the risk of lymph node metastasis in early rectal cancer. *Cancer* 1992;69(2):322–326.

125. Gall FP, Hermanek P. Cancer of the rectum–local excision. *Surg Clin North Am* 1988;68(6):1353–1365.

Section III

126. Nascimbeni R, et al. Risk of lymph node metastasis in T1 carcinoma of the colon and rectum. *Dis Colon Rectum* 2002;45(2):200–206.

127. Mellgren A, et al. Is local excision adequate therapy for early rectal cancer? *Dis Colon Rectum* 2000;43(8):1064–1071; discussion 1071–1074.

128. Russell AH, et al. Anal sphincter conservation for patients with adenocarcinoma of the distal rectum: long-term results of radiation therapy oncology group protocol 89-02. *Int J Radiat Oncol Biol Phys* 2000;46(2):313–322.

129. Greenberg JA, et al. Local excision of distal rectal cancer: an update of cancer and leukemia group B 8984. *Dis Colon Rectum* 2008;51(8):1185–1191; discussion 1191–1194.

130. Steele GD Jr, et al. Sphincter-sparing treatment for distal rectal adenocarcinoma. *Ann Surg Oncol* 1999;6(5):433–441.

131. Garcia-Aguilar J, et al. Organ preservation for clinical T2N0 distal rectal cancer using neoadjuvant chemoradiotherapy and local excision (ACOSOGZ6041): results of an open-label, single-arm, multi-institutional, phase 2 trial. *Lancet Oncol* 2015;16:1537–1546.

132. Minsky BD, et al. Selection criteria for local excision with or without adjuvant radiation therapy for rectal cancer. *Cancer* 1989;63(7):1421–1429.

133. You YN. Local excision: is it an adequate substitute for radical resection in T1/T2 patients? *Semin Radiat Oncol* 2011;21(3):178–184.

134. Blackstock W, et al. ACR appropriateness criteria: local excision in early-stage rectal cancer. *Curr Probl Cancer* 2010;34(3):193–200.

135. Lavery IC, et al. Chances of cure are not compromised with sphincter-saving procedures for cancer of the lower third of the rectum. *Surgery* 1997;122(4):779–784; discussion 784–785.

136. Zaheer S, et al. Surgical treatment of adenocarcinoma of the rectum. *Ann Surg* 1998;227(6):800–811.

137. Machado M, et al. Similar outcome after colonic pouch and side-to-end anastomosis in low anterior resection for rectal cancer: a prospective randomized trial. *Ann Surg* 2003;238(2):214–220.

138. Paty PB, et al. Long-term functional results of coloanal anastomosis for rectal cancer. *Am J Surg* 1994;167(1):90–94; discussion 94–95.

139. Nakagoe T, et al. Survival and recurrence after a sphincter-saving resection and abdominoperineal resection for adenocarcinoma of the rectum at or below the peritoneal reflection: a multivariate analysis. *Surg Today* 2004;34(1):32–39.

140. Williams NS, Durdey P, Johnston D. The outcome following sphincter-saving resection and abdominoperineal resection for low rectal cancer. *Br J Surg* 1985;72(8):595–598.

141. Ortiz H, Armendariz P. Anterior resection: do the patients perceive any clinical benefit? *Int J Colorectal Dis* 1996;11(4):191–195.

142. Jessup JM, Stewart AK, Menck HR. The National Cancer Data Base report on patterns of care for adenocarcinoma of the rectum, 1985–95. *Cancer* 1998;83(11):2408–2418.

143. Grumann MM, et al. Comparison of quality of life in patients undergoing abdominoperineal extirpation or anterior resection for rectal cancer. *Ann Surg* 2001;233(2):149–156.

144. Matzel KE, et al. Continence after colorectal reconstruction following resection: impact of level of anastomosis. *Int J Colorectal Dis* 1997;12(2):82–87.

145. Enker WE, et al. Total mesorectal excision in the operative treatment of carcinoma of the rectum. *J Am Coll Surg* 1995;181(4):335–346.

146. Cawthorn SJ, et al. Extent of mesorectal spread and involvement of lateral resection margin as prognostic factors after surgery for rectal cancer. *Lancet* 1990;335(8697):1055–1059.

147. Heald RJ, Husband EM, Ryall RD. The mesorectum in rectal cancer surgery—the clue to pelvic recurrence? *Br J Surg* 1982;69(10):613–616.

148. Heald RJ, et al. Rectal cancer: the Basingstoke experience of total mesorectal excision, 1978–1997. *Arch Surg* 1998;133(8):894–899.

149. MacFarlane JK, Ryall RD, Heald RJ. Mesorectal excision for rectal cancer. *Lancet* 1993;341(8843):457–460.

150. Baxter NN, et al. Lymph node evaluation in colorectal cancer patients: a population-based study. *J Natl Cancer Inst* 2005;97(3):219–225.

151. Havenga K, et al. Improved survival and local control after total mesorectal excision or D3 lymphadenectomy in the treatment of primary rectal cancer: an international analysis of 1411 patients. *Eur J Surg Oncol* 1999;25(4):368–374.

152. Tepper JE, et al. Impact of number of nodes retrieved on outcome in patients with rectal cancer. *J Clin Oncol* 2001;19(1):157–163.

153. Rajput A, et al. Meeting the 12 lymph node (LN) benchmark in colon cancer. *J Surg Oncol* 2010;102(1):3–9.

154. Compton CC, et al. Prognostic factors in colorectal cancer. College of American Pathologists Consensus Statement 1999. *Arch Pathol Lab Med* 2000;124(7):979–994.

155. Karanjia ND, et al. Leakage from stapled low anastomosis after total mesorectal excision for carcinoma of the rectum. *Br J Surg* 1994;81(8):1224–1226.

156. van Gijn W, et al. Preoperative radiotherapy combined with total mesorectal excision for resectable rectal cancer: 12-year follow-up of the multicentre, randomised controlled TME trial. *Lancet Oncol* 2011;12(6):575–582.

157. Arbman G, et al. Local recurrence following total mesorectal excision for rectal cancer. *Br J Surg* 1996;83(3):375–379.

158. Bolognese A, et al. Total mesorectal excision for surgical treatment of rectal cancer. *J Surg Oncol* 2000;74(1):21–23.

159. Nelson H, et al. Guidelines 2000 for colon and rectal cancer surgery. *J Natl Cancer Inst* 2001;93(8):583–596.

160. Quirke P, et al. Local recurrence of rectal adenocarcinoma due to inadequate surgical resection. Histopathological study of lateral tumour spread and surgical excision. *Lancet* 1986;2(8514):996–999.

161. Ng IO, et al. Surgical lateral clearance in resected rectal carcinomas. A multivariate analysis of clinicopathologic features. *Cancer* 1993;71(6):1972–1976.

162. Colorectal Cancer Collaborative Group. Adjuvant radiotherapy for rectal cancer: a systematic overview of 8,507 patients from 22 randomised trials. *Lancet* 2001;358(9290):1291–1304.

163. Wolmark N, et al. Randomized trial of postoperative adjuvant chemotherapy with or without radiotherapy for carcinoma of the rectum: National Surgical Adjuvant Breast and Bowel Project Protocol R-02. *J Natl Cancer Inst* 2000;92(5):388–396.

164. Thomas PR, Lindblad AS. Adjuvant postoperative radiotherapy and chemotherapy in rectal carcinoma: a review of the Gastrointestinal Tumor Study Group experience. *Radiother Oncol* 1988;13(4):245–252.

165. Krook JE, et al. Effective surgical adjuvant therapy for high-risk rectal carcinoma. *N Engl J Med* 1991;324(11):709–715.

166. Miller RC, et al. Acute diarrhea during adjuvant therapy for rectal cancer: a detailed analysis from a randomized intergroup trial. *Int J Radiat Oncol Biol Phys* 2002;54(2):409–413.

167. O'Connell MJ, et al. Improving adjuvant therapy for rectal cancer by combining protracted-infusion fluorouracil with radiation therapy after curative surgery. *N Engl J Med* 1994;331(8):502–507.

168. Tepper JE, et al. Adjuvant postoperative fluorouracil-modulated chemotherapy combined with pelvic radiation therapy for rectal cancer: initial results of intergroup 0114. *J Clin Oncol* 1997;15(5):2030–2039.

169. Merchant NB, et al. T3N0 rectal cancer: results following sharp mesorectal excision and no adjuvant therapy. *J Gastrointest Surg* 1999;3(6):642–647.

170. Willett CG, et al. Prognostic factors in stage T3N0 rectal cancer: do all patients require postoperative pelvic irradiation and chemotherapy. *Dis Colon Rectum* 1999;42:167–173.

171. Guillem JG, et al. cT3N0 rectal cancer: potential overtreatment with preoperative chemoradiotherapy is warranted. *J Clin Oncol* 2008;26(3):368–373.

172. Folkesson J, et al. Swedish Rectal Cancer Trial: long lasting benefits from radiotherapy on survival and local recurrence rate. *J Clin Oncol* 2005;23(24):5644–5650.

173. Swedish Rectal Cancer Trial. Improved survival with preoperative radiotherapy in resectable rectal cancer. *N Engl J Med* 1997;336(14):980–987.

174. Birgisson H, et al. Adverse effects of preoperative radiation therapy for rectal cancer: long-term follow-up of the Swedish Rectal Cancer Trial. *J Clin Oncol* 2005;23(34):8697–8705.

175. Birgisson H, et al. Late gastrointestinal disorders after rectal cancer surgery with and without preoperative radiation therapy. *Br J Surg* 2008;95(2):206–213.

176. Francois Y, et al. Influence of the interval between preoperative radiation therapy and surgery on downstaging and on the rate of sphincter-sparing surgery for rectal cancer: the Lyon R90-01 randomized trial. *J Clin Oncol* 1999;17(8):2396.

177. Marijnen CA, et al. Acute side effects and complications after short-term preoperative radiotherapy combined with total mesorectal excision in primary rectal cancer: report of a multicenter randomized trial. *J Clin Oncol* 2002;20(3):817–825.

178. Peeters KC, et al. Late side effects of short-course preoperative radiotherapy combined with total mesorectal excision for rectal cancer: increased bowel dysfunction in irradiated patients—a Dutch colorectal cancer group study. *J Clin Oncol* 2005;23(25):6199–6206.

179. Marijnen CA, et al. Impact of short-term preoperative radiotherapy on health-related quality of life and sexual functioning in primary rectal cancer: report of a multicenter randomized trial. *J Clin Oncol* 2005;23(9):1847–1858.

180. Gerard JP, et al. Preoperative radiotherapy with or without concurrent fluorouracil and leucovorin in T3-4 rectal cancers: results of FFCD 9203. *J Clin Oncol* 2006;24(28):4620–4625.

181. Bosset JF. Chemotherapy with preoperative radiotherapy in rectal cancer. *N Engl J Med* 2006;355(11):1114–1123.

182. Ceelen WP, Van Nieuwenhove Y, Fierens K. Preoperative chemoradiation versus radiation alone for stage II and III resectable rectal cancer. *Cochrane Database Syst Rev* 2009;(1):CD006041.

183. Bujko K, et al. Long-term results of a randomized trial comparing preoperative short-course radiotherapy with preoperative conventionally fractionated chemoradiation for rectal cancer. *Br J Surg* 2006;93(10):1215–1223.

184. Ngan SY, Burmeister B, Fisher RJ, et al. Randomized trial of short-course radiotherapy versus long-course chemoradiation comparing rates of local recurrence in patients with t3 rectal cancer: trans-tasman radiation oncology group trial 01.04. *J Clin Oncol* 2012;30(31):3827–3833.

185. Erlandsson J, Holm T, Pettersson D, et al. Optimal fractionation of preoperative radiotherapy and timing to surgery for rectal cancer (Stockholm III): a multicentre, randomised, non-blinded, phase 3, non-inferiority trial. *Lancet Oncol* 2017;18(3):336–346.

186. Di Costanzo F, Sdrobolini A, Gasperoni S. Capecitabine, a new oral fluoropyrimidine for the treatment of colorectal cancer. *Crit Rev Oncol Hematol* 2000;35(2):101–108.

187. Schuller J, et al. Preferential activation of capecitabine in tumor following oral administration to colorectal cancer patients. *Cancer Chemother Pharmacol* 2000;45(4):291–297.

188. Hofheinz ED, Wenz F, Post S, et al. Chemoradiotherapy with capecitabine versus fluorouracil for locally advanced rectal cancer: a randomised, multicentre, non-inferiority, phase 3 trial. *Lancet Oncol* 2012;13:579–588.

189. O'Connell MJ, Colangelo LH, Beart RW, et al. Capecitabine and oxaliplatin in the preoperative multimodality treatment of rectal cancer: surgical end points from National Surgical Adjuvant Breast and Bowel Project trial R-04. *J Clin Oncol* 2014;32(18):1927–1934.

190. Aschele C, et al. A phase I-II study of weekly oxaliplatin, 5-fluorouracil continuous infusion and preoperative radiotherapy in locally advanced rectal cancer. *Ann Oncol* 2005;16(7):1140–1146.

191. Machiels JP, et al. Phase II study of preoperative oxaliplatin, capecitabine and external beam radiotherapy in patients with rectal cancer: the RadiOxCape study. *Ann Oncol* 2005;16(12):1898–1905.

192. Rodel C, et al. Phase I/II trial of capecitabine, oxaliplatin, and radiation for rectal cancer. *J Clin Oncol* 2003;21(16):3098–3104.

193. Rosenthal DI, et al. Phase I study of preoperative radiation therapy with concurrent infusional 5-fluorouracil and oxaliplatin followed by surgery and postoperative 5-fluorouracil plus leucovorin for T3/T4 rectal adenocarcinoma: ECOG E1297. *Int J Radiat Oncol Biol Phys* 2008;72(1):108–113.

194. Aschele C, et al. Primary tumor response to preoperative chemoradiation with or without oxaliplatin in locally advanced rectal cancer: pathologic results of the STAR-01 randomized phase III trial. *J Clin Oncol* 2011;29(20):2773–2780.

195. Gerard JP, et al. Comparison of two neoadjuvant chemoradiotherapy regimens for locally advanced rectal cancer: results of the phase III trial ACCORD 12/0405-Prodige 2. *J Clin Oncol* 2010;28(10):1638–1644.

196. Gérard JP, Azria D, Gourgou-Bourgade S, et al. Clinical outcome of the ACCORD 12/0405 PRODIGE 2 randomized trial in rectal cancer. *J Clin Oncol* 2012;30(36):4558–4565.

197. Rodel C, Graeven U, Fietkau R, et al. Oxaliplatin added to fluorouracil-based preoperative chemoradiotherapy and postoperative chemotherapy of locally advanced rectal cancer (the German CAO/ARO/AIO-04 study): final results of the multicentre, open-label, randomised, phase 3 trial. *Lancet Oncol* 2015;16(8):979–989.

198. Mitchell EP, Anne P, Fry R, et al. Chemoradiation with CPT-11, 5-FU in neoadjuvant treatment of locally advanced or recurrent adenocarcinoma of the rectum: a phase I/II study update. *Proc Am Soc Clin Oncol* 2003;22(abstr 1052):262.

199. Gollins S, et al. Preoperative chemoradiotherapy using concurrent capecitabine and irinotecan in magnetic resonance imaging-defined locally advanced rectal cancer: impact on long-term clinical outcomes. *J Clin Oncol* 2011;29(8):1042–1049.

200. Navarro M, et al. A phase II study of preoperative radiotherapy and concomitant weekly irinotecan in combination with protracted venous infusion 5-fluorouracil, for resectable locally advanced rectal cancer. *Int J Radiat Oncol Biol Phys* 2006;66(1):201–205.

201. Willeke F, et al. A phase II study of capecitabine and irinotecan in combination with concurrent pelvic radiotherapy (CapIri-RT) as neoadjuvant treatment of locally advanced rectal cancer. *Br J Cancer* 2007;96(6):912–917.

202. Mohiuddin M, et al. Randomized phase II study of neoadjuvant combined-modality chemoradiation for distal rectal cancer: Radiation Therapy Oncology Group Trial 0012. *J Clin Oncol* 2006;24(4):650–655.

203. Willett CG, et al. A safety and survival analysis of neoadjuvant bevacizumab with standard chemoradiation in a phase I/II study compared with standard chemoradiation in locally advanced rectal cancer. *Oncologist* 2010;15(8):845–851.

204. Czito BG, et al. Bevacizumab, oxaliplatin, and capecitabine with radiation therapy in rectal cancer: phase I trial results. *Int J Radiat Oncol Biol Phys* 2007;68(2):472–478.

205. Crane CH, et al. Phase II trial of neoadjuvant bevacizumab, capecitabine, and radiotherapy for locally advanced rectal cancer. *Int J Radiat Oncol Biol Phys* 2010;76(3):824–830.

206. Willett CG, et al. Efficacy, safety, and biomarkers of neoadjuvant bevacizumab, radiation therapy, and fluorouracil in rectal cancer: a multidisciplinary phase II study. *J Clin Oncol* 2009;27(18):3020–3026.

207. Horisberger K, et al. Cetuximab in combination with capecitabine, irinotecan, and radiotherapy for patients with locally advanced rectal cancer: results of a Phase II MARGIT trial. *Int J Radiat Oncol Biol Phys* 2009;74(5):1487–1493.

208. Velenik V, et al. A phase II study of cetuximab, capecitabine and radiotherapy in neoadjuvant treatment of patients with locally advanced resectable rectal cancer. *Eur J Surg Oncol* 2010;36(3):244–250.

209. Debucquoy A, et al. Molecular response to cetuximab and efficacy of preoperative cetuximab-based chemoradiation in rectal cancer. *J Clin Oncol* 2009;27(17): 2751–2757.

210. Park JH, et al. Randomized phase 3 trial comparing preoperative and postoperative chemoradiotherapy with capecitabine for locally advanced rectal cancer. *Cancer* 2011;117(16):3703–3712.

211. Sauer R, et al. Preoperative versus postoperative chemoradiotherapy for rectal cancer. *N Engl J Med* 2004;351(17):1731–1740.

212. Sebag-Montefiore D, et al. Preoperative radiotherapy versus selective postoperative chemoradiotherapy in patients with rectal cancer (MRC CR07 and NCIC-CTG C016): a multicentre, randomised trial. *Lancet* 2009;373(9666):811–820.

213. Braendengen M, et al. Randomized phase III study comparing preoperative radiotherapy with chemoradiotherapy in nonresectable rectal cancer. *J Clin Oncol* 2008;26(22):3687–3694.

214. Nakfoor BM, et al. The impact of 5-fluorouracil and intraoperative electron beam radiation therapy on the outcome of patients with locally advanced primary rectal and rectosigmoid cancer. *Ann Surg* 1998;228(2):194–200.

215. Mathis KL, et al. Unresectable colorectal cancer can be cured with multimodality therapy. *Ann Surg* 2008;248(4):592–598.

216. Available: https://clinicaltrials.gov/ct2/show/NCT01515787

217. Fernandez-Martos C, Garcia-Albeniz X, Pericay C, et al. Chemoradiation, surgery and adjuvant chemotherapy versus induction chemotherapy followed by chemoradiation and surgery: long-term results of the Spanish GCR-3 phase II randomized trialdagger. *Ann Oncol* 2015;26(8):1722–1728.

218. Garcia-Aguilar J, Chow OS, Smith DD, et al. Effect of adding mFOLFOX6 after neoadjuvant chemoradiation in locally advanced rectal cancer: a multicentre, phase 2 trial. *Lancet Oncol* 2015;16(8):957–966.

219. Available: https://clinicaltrials.gov/ct2/show/NCT02008656, Accessed February 2017.

220. D'Ambra L, Berti S, Bonfante P, et al. Hemostatic step-by-step procedure to control presacral bleeding during laparoscopic total mesorectal excision. *World J Surg* 2009;33(4):812–815.

221. Halabi WJ, Jafari MD, Nguyen VQ, et al. Ureteral injuries in colorectal surgery: an analysis of trends, outcomes, and risk factors over a 10-year period in the United States. *Dis Colon Rectum* 2014;57(2):179–186.

222. Tekkis PP, Cornish JA, Remzi FH, et al. Measuring sexual and urinary outcomes in women after rectal cancer excision. *Dis Colon Rectum* 2009;52(1):46–54.

223. Ho VP, Lee Y, Stein SL, et al. Sexual function after treatment for rectal cancer: a review. *Dis Colon Rectum* 2011;54(1):113–125.

224. Pollack J, Holm T, Cedermark B, et al. Late adverse effects of short-course preoperative radiotherapy in rectal cancer. *Br J Surg* 2006;93(12):1519–1525.

225. Holm T, Singnomklao T, Rutqvist LE, et al. Adjuvant preoperative radiotherapy in patients with rectal carcinoma. Adverse effects during long term follow-up of two randomized trials. *Cancer* 1996;78(5):968–976.

226. Habr-Gama A, Perez RO, Nadalin W, et al. Operative versus nonoperative treatment for stage 0 distal rectal cancer following chemoradiation therapy: long-term results. *Ann Surg* 2004;240(4):711–717; discussion 717–718.

227. Habr-Gama A, Perez RO, Proscurshim I, et al. Patterns of failure and survival for nonoperative treatment of stage c0 distal rectal cancer following neoadjuvant chemoradiation therapy. *J Gastrointest Surg* 2006;10(10):1319–1328; discussion 1328–1319.

228. Habr-Gama A, Gama-Rodrigues J, Sao Juliao GP, et al. Local recurrence after complete clinical response and watch and wait in rectal cancer after neoadjuvant chemoradiation: impact of salvage therapy on local disease control. *Int J Radiat Oncol Biol Phys* 2014;88(4):822–828.

229. Lim L, Chao M, Shapiro J, et al. Long-term outcomes of patients with localized rectal cancer treated with chemoradiation or radiotherapy alone because of medical inoperability or patient refusal. *Dis Colon Rectum* 2007;50(12):2032–2039.

230. Maas M, Beets-Tan RG, Lambregts DM, et al. Wait-and-see policy for clinical complete responders after chemoradiation for rectal cancer. *J Clin Oncol* 2011;29(35):4633–4640.

231. Smith JD, Ruby JA, Goodman KA, et al. Nonoperative management of rectal cancer with complete clinical response after neoadjuvant therapy. *Ann Surg* 2012;256(6):965–972.

232. Smith JJ, Chow OS, Gollub MJ, et al. Organ preservation in rectal adenocarcinoma: a phase II randomized controlled trial evaluating 3-year disease-free survival in patients with locally advanced rectal cancer treated with chemoradiation plus induction or consolidation chemotherapy, and total mesorectal excision or nonoperative management. *BMC Cancer* 2015;15:767.

233. Appelt AL, Ploen J, Harling H, et al. High-dose chemoradiotherapy and watchful waiting for distal rectal cancer: a prospective observational study. *Lancet Oncol* 2015;16(8):919–927.

234. Gallagher MJ, et al. A prospective study of treatment techniques to minimize the volume of pelvic small bowel with reduction of acute and late effects associated with pelvic irradiation. *Int J Radiat Oncol Biol Phys* 1986;12(9):1565–1573.

235. Wanebo HJ, et al. Pelvic resection of recurrent rectal cancer: technical considerations and outcomes. *Dis Colon Rectum* 1999;42(11):1438–1448.

236. Rodel C, et al. Extensive surgery after high-dose preoperative chemoradiotherapy for locally advanced recurrent rectal cancer. *Dis Colon Rectum* 2000;43(3):312–319.

237. Valentini V, et al. Preoperative hyperfractionated chemoradiation for locally recurrent rectal cancer in patients previously irradiated to the pelvis: a multicentric phase II study. *Int J Radiat Oncol Biol Phys* 2006;64(4):1129–1139.

238. Mohiuddin M, Marks G, Marks J. Long-term results of reirradiation for patients with recurrent rectal carcinoma. *Cancer* 2002;95(5):1144–1150.

239. Das P, et al. Hyperfractionated accelerated radiotherapy for rectal cancer in patients with prior pelvic irradiation. *Int J Radiat Oncol Biol Phys* 2010;77(1):60–65.

240. Myint AS. Novel radiation techniques for rectal cancer. *J Gastrointest Oncol* 2014;5: 212–217.

241. Bujko K, Wyrwicz L, Rutkowski A, et al. Long-course oxaliplatin-based preoperative chemoradiation versus 5 × 5 Gy and consolidation chemotherapy for cT4 or fixed cT3 rectal cancer: results of a randomized phase III study. *Ann Oncol* 2016;27: 834–842.

Section
III

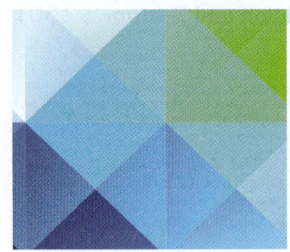

CHAPTER 66

Anal Cancer

James D. Murphy

INTRODUCTION

The standard treatment for primary squamous cell cancers of the anal canal is chemoradiation, using concurrent radiation therapy (RT), 5-fluorouracil (5-FU), and mitomycin C (MMC), with surgery reserved for residual cancer. This combination, developed empirically as preoperative adjuvant therapy in the 1970s,[1] has evolved to become the standard of care. Trials of other chemotherapy agents in combination with radiation have so far not improved results. Currently, about 65% of those with cancer confined to the pelvis will survive 5 years or more and about 75% will retain anorectal function.

In this chapter, the emphasis is on the management of squamous cell cancer of the anal canal. Note is also made of the role of RT in the treatment of squamous cell cancers of the perianal skin and of adenocarcinomas of the anal region.

ANATOMY

The anal canal is 3 to 4 cm in length, the posterior wall being longer than the anterior. The canal ends superiorly at the palpable upper border of the anal sphincter and puborectalis muscle of the anorectal ring. The distal end at the anal verge is the level at which the walls of the anal canal come in contact in their normal resting state; it approximates the palpable groove between the lower edge of the internal sphincter and the subcutaneous part of the external sphincter and the junction with true skin. The American Joint Committee on Cancer Clinical Staging (AJCC)[2] and the International Union Against Cancer (UICC)[3] recommend this definition rather than a convention used by some centers under which carcinomas that are above or exactly astride the dentate line are classified as anal canal tumors and those lying mainly or entirely below that line are called anal margin tumors (Fig. 66.1). The terms *anal margin* and *perianal skin* are now generally used interchangeably. Perianal carcinomas are arbitrarily considered to be cancers arising from the skin within a 5-cm radius of the anal verge.

Four different types of epithelium are found within the anal region.[4] The perianal skin is similar to hair-bearing skin elsewhere. At the anal verge, the skin blends with a pale-colored zone, sometimes called the pecten, lined by modified squamous epithelium that lacks hair or glandular structures. This squamous zone merges just below the dentate or pectinate

line, which marks the mucosal folds of the anal valves, with a transitional epithelium that incorporates features of rectal, urothelial, and squamous epithelium. The purplish red–colored transitional zone extends proximally for about 2 cm until the pinker glandular mucosa of the rectum becomes dominant.

The major lymphatic pathways flow to three lymph node systems. The perianal skin, the anal verge, and the canal distal to the dentate line drain predominantly to the superficial inguinal nodes, with some communication to the femoral nodes and to the external iliac systems. Lymphatics from around and above the dentate line flow with those from the distal rectum to the internal pudendal, hypogastric, and obturator nodes of the internal iliac systems. The proximal canal drains to the perirectal and superior hemorrhoidal nodes of the inferior mesenteric system. There are numerous lymphatic connections between the various levels of the anal canal, and an intramural system links the lymphatics of the canal with those of the rectum.[5]

The veins of the anal canal connect with both the systemic and the portal venous systems. Venous plexuses, which lie in and surround the mucosal and muscular structures of the anal wall, anastomose around the junction of the anal verge and distal canal. The veins draining the inferior parts of these plexuses communicate with the systemic venous system via the internal pudendal and internal iliac veins, and those from the superior canal flow predominately to the inferior mesenteric vein and then to the portal system.[5]

Anorectal continence is mediated by both cerebrospinal nerves and the autonomic system. The smooth muscle of the internal sphincter is supplied by parasympathetic fibers from the second, third, and fourth sacral segments as well as sympathetic fibers from the hypogastric plexus. The upper canal has selective sensitivity for intraluminal differences in pressure, and the autonomic nerves mediate both the inhibitor and facilitator reflexes of the internal sphincter. The striated muscle of the external sphincter is under voluntary control and innervated by the internal rectal nerve, a branch of the pudendal nerve arising from the second, third, and fourth sacral nerves. The internal rectal nerve also transmits pain, touch, and other sensations from the anal lining below the dentate line and from the perianal skin.[5]

PATHOLOGIC CLASSIFICATION

The most recent revision of the World Health Organization (WHO) classification of anal tumors, published in 2010, describes intraepithelial and invasive neoplasms.[6] The term *anal intraepithelial neoplasia* (AIN) is applied to precancerous changes in the epithelium of the anal canal and perianal skin.[7]

For invasive cancers, the term *squamous cell carcinoma* is applied to all the various subtypes: squamous; large-cell keratinizing and nonkeratinizing; and basaloid, cloacogenic, and transitional, all of which were considered separate entities in the previous classification.[6] Clinicians have for some years grouped these various subtypes as epidermoid cancers because of their similar natural history; the term epidermoid is not used in the WHO classification. About 85% to 90% of primary anal canal cancers are squamous cell type. The remaining 10% to 15% are predominantly adenocarcinomas, most of which arise from anal glands or within anal fistulae. Adenocarcinomas from the rectal-type mucosa in

FIGURE 66.1. Anatomy of the anal region.

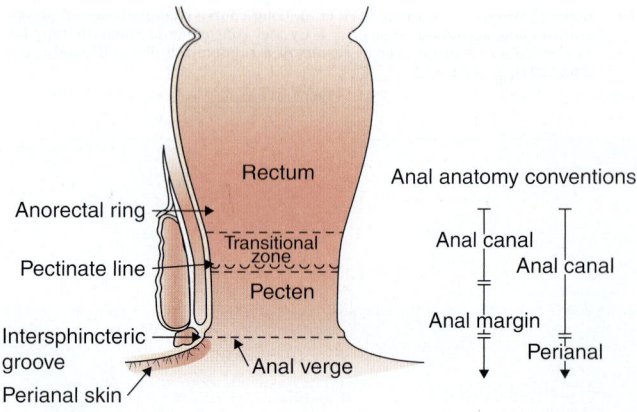

the upper canal are classified as primary rectal cancers. The WHO system retains as separate entities rare variants such as squamous cell carcinoma with mucous microcysts, small cell, and undifferentiated cancers.

Primary cancers of the perianal skin are similar to cancers of the skin in other sites. Most are squamous cell cancers, with occasional basal cell cancers and skin adnexal adenocarcinomas.

EPIDEMIOLOGY

Anal cancers are about one-tenth as common as cancers of the rectum. Cancers arise in the canal with three to four times the frequency of perianal cancers. In North America and Europe, anal canal cancers are more common in women than in men, although this difference is decreasing[8]; perianal cancers occur with about equal frequency in both sexes. The annual age-adjusted rates per 100,000 for squamous cell cancers of the anus, anal canal, and anorectum in the U.S. Surveillance, Epidemiology, and End Results (SEER) registry for 2010 to 2014 were 1.5 for males and 2.1 for females.[8] The incidence varies widely in different parts of the world but has been increasing in North America and Europe over the past 40 years.[8] The annual incidence of invasive and intraepithelial neoplasia almost doubled in men and rose by about half in women between the periods 1973 to 1979 and 1994 to 2000.[9] The risk of anal cancer increases with age; the median age at diagnosis is 61 years.

RISK FACTORS

The most significant risk factors so far identified are sexually transmissible viruses, immunosuppression, and tobacco smoking. The role of sexual practices and sexually transmissible agents has been investigated intensively. Several mucosotropic types of human papillomavirus (HPV) are linked to cancer and precancerous lesions in the anogenital epithelium.[10-12] Subtypes of HPV with a high risk of association with cancer are type 16 in particular and, to a lesser extent, types 18, 31, 33, 35, and others.[10-12] These high-risk HPV types have been found in about 85% of anal squamous cancers in many series,[10,11] more commonly in cancer of the canal than of the perianal skin.[11,13] Some geographic variation was noted in the types of high-risk HPV identified.[11,14] Case–control studies suggest that a history of multiple sexual partners in homosexual or heterosexual relationships or of unprotected anal intercourse in males and in females is predictive of an increased risk of AIN and invasive anal cancer.[15] Compared to the overall annual incidence of anal cancer in white males in the United States of approximately 0.7 per 100,000 in the early 1980s, the estimated incidence in the male homosexual population, prior to the human immunodeficiency virus (HIV) epidemic, ranged from about 12 to 37 per 100,000.[16] This rate increased to about 70 per 100,000 among HIV-positive male homosexuals.[17]

Compromise of cell-mediated immunity reduces the body's ability to prevent or eliminate infection by viruses such as HPV. An increased risk of anal cancer is associated with at least two situations in which cell-mediated immunity is significantly altered: infection with HIV and iatrogenic suppression of immunity in organ transplant patients. Interactions between HPV and HIV are complex. Although anal cancer has not been designated an acquired immunodeficiency syndrome (AIDS)-defining condition, data from the U.S. AIDS Cancer Registry linkage study showed that the rate of HPV-associated cancers and precursors was increased in HIV-infected persons for all anogenital sites compared with the general population. The relative risk for anal cancers was 6.8 in women and 37.9 in men.[18] A national cohort study in Sweden of 5,931 patients who had undergone organ transplantation showed a 10-fold excess risk of developing anal cancer.[19] Whatever

the cause of suppression of cell-mediated immunity, those affected have increased rates of HPV infection, higher progression rates from normal epithelium to AIN and from lower- to higher-grade AIN, and lower rates of clearance of HPV and regression from abnormal to normal epithelium.[20,21]

The increasing effectiveness of antiretroviral therapy has led to longer survival of HIV-infected patients and an increased number with anal cancer.[22,23] There was a threefold increase in incidence in the HIV-positive population from the period prior to the introduction of highly active antiretroviral therapy (HAART) in about 1996 and the later HAART era.[23] Although there was a decrease in the incidence of Kaposi sarcoma and lymphoma by a few years after HAART became available, at the time of the review, there had been no significant reduction in the incidence of less common malignancies such as anogenital cancers.[24] Early success of prophylactic vaccines against HPV in both men and women suggests that the incidence of anal cancer can be reduced in the future.[25,26]

Tobacco smoking is associated with up to a fourfold increase in risk in several case–control studies. Current smokers are at greater risk than are past smokers.[15,27] Benign conditions such as fistulae, fissures, and hemorrhoids do not appear to predispose to cancer.[28] Chronic anal inflammation due to inflammatory bowel disease has also been discounted as a risk factor.[29]

NATURAL HISTORY

Most squamous cell cancers of the anal region, especially the canal, are believed to be preceded by high-grade AIN.[7] However, it has been estimated that no more than 1% of cases with AIN develop invasive cancer per year,[30] a rate lower than that described for cervical intraepithelial neoplasia. Anal dysplasia recurs frequently despite excision, laser ablation, or topical therapies, presumably because of incomplete treatment or persistence of the HPV infection with which dysplasia is associated.[22] The natural history of AIN coexisting with anal cancers exposed to radiation, with or without chemotherapy, is unknown.

Squamous cancers of the anal canal spread most commonly by direct extension and lymphatic pathways. Hematogenous metastases are less common. Direct invasion from the anal mucosa into the sphincter muscles and perianal connective tissue spaces occurs early; in a series of 137 cases, cancers were confined to the mucosa and submucosa at diagnosis in only 12%, and to the sphincter muscles, without regional lymph node involvement, in only 34%.[31] In about half the cases, anal cancers extend into the rectum or perianal skin. Invasion of the vaginal septum and vaginal mucosa is more common than invasion of the prostate gland, but anovaginal fistulas occur in fewer than 5% of women. Extensive tumors may infiltrate the pelvic walls.

Lymphatic invasion occurs relatively early. The overall risk of regional nodal involvement at diagnosis is about 25%.[32,33] Pelvic lymph node metastases were found in as many as 30% of patients treated by abdominoperineal resection.[31,34,35] In an illustrative series, metastases were present in the superior hemorrhoidal nodes in 25% (15 of 61); in the external iliac, obturator, or hypogastric nodes in 30% (8 of 27); and in the inguinal nodes in 16% (12 of 74) of patients.[35] Inguinal metastases were detected clinically in up to approximately 20% of patients at initial diagnosis and were present subclinically in a further 10% to 20%.[31,35-37] Nodal metastases were associated with 30% of cancers confined to the sphincter muscles, and 60% of those that had extended through the sphincters or were more poorly differentiated.[34] Lymphatic metastases increase in frequency with progressive enlargement of the primary cancer.[34,38]

Extrapelvic metastases are identified at the time of first presentation in <10% of patients. They are found most frequently in the liver, lungs, and para-aortic nodes. Relapse after initial treatment is more common in the area of the primary tumor and the pelvic lymph nodes than in extrapelvic organs. Locoregional relapse rates of up to about 30% are common. Failure outside the pelvis occurs in up to about 20%.[31,39-41]

Perianal cancers tend to grow locally and may extend into the anal canal. When the site of origin is in doubt, it is conventional to classify the cancer as arising in the anal canal. The ipsilateral inguinal nodes are the most common site of metastasis and are involved in from 5% to 20% of cases. Extrapelvic metastases are uncommon except in locally advanced cancer or those with nodal metastases.

CLINICAL PRESENTATION

The symptoms of anal cancer are nonspecific, contributing to delay in presentation by the patient and in diagnosis by the physician of more than 6 months in a third of patients.[42,43] Bleeding and anal discomfort are the most common symptoms and are reported by about half the patients.[44] Less common complaints include awareness of an anal mass, pruritus, and anal discharge. Pain is uncommon but may be severe. In patients with tumors in the proximal canal, there may be an alteration in bowel habits, but this is uncommon with distal cancers.[44] Occasionally, asymptomatic tumors are found during physical examination or in the course of investigation of an enlarged inguinal node. Unsuspected microinvasive carcinoma is sometimes found in mucosa removed at hemorrhoidectomy.[45]

Small carcinomas are often nodular or plaque-like, but larger tumors are more typically ulcerated and infiltrative. Coexisting benign conditions such as anogenital warts, hemorrhoids, and anal fissures may be present. Anal sphincter tone is usually preserved and may be increased by painful spasm. Gross fecal incontinence resulting from sphincter destruction occurs in <5% of patients, although some fecal soiling is often reported. Similarly, vaginal fistulas are uncommon. Rarely, extrapelvic metastases may be the only symptomatic feature or finding.

DIAGNOSTIC WORKUP

The history and physical examination should stress features that delineate the extent of the primary tumor, including anal sphincter competence and possible invasion of adjacent organs. A biopsy of the primary tumor is necessary to establish the diagnosis and the histologic type. General anesthesia may be needed to permit detailed pelvic and anorectal examination, which should include proctoscopy. Sigmoidoscopy and colonoscopy, although often performed, infrequently disclose colonic pathology.[46] Physical examination should include detailed examination of the genital region, especially in patients who give a history of previous anogenital area dysplasia or cancer, genital warts, or anal-receptive intercourse or are HIV positive.

Only the inguinal and low perirectal lymph nodes are accessible to clinical examination. Because lymph node enlargement may be caused by reactive hyperplasia in as many as half of those with palpable inguinal nodes, clinically suspicious nodes should be assessed histologically by needle biopsy or simple excision.[44] Metastases in the internal iliac and superior hemorrhoidal node chains, about half of which are <0.5 cm in diameter,[47] cannot be identified reliably by current techniques of lymphangiography, pelvic lymphoscintigraphy, computed tomography (CT), magnetic resonance imaging (MRI), or transanorectal ultrasonography. MRI is considered the most accurate method for assessing the primary cancer and pelvic nodes.[48] Both fluorodeoxyglucose (FDG) positron emission tomography (PET) with CT and inguinal sentinel lymph node biopsy (ISLN) have been used to identify inguinal node metastases and to refine RT plans.[49-51] However, a comparison of FDG-PET-CT and ISLN biopsy in 27 patients found

several false-positive PET studies (4 of 7).[52] Also, late inguinal node metastases have been reported after a previous negative ISLN biopsy.[53] A meta-analysis of twelve studies found that FDG-PET resulted in a change in nodal staging in 28% of anal cancer patients. Guidelines from the National Comprehensive Cancer Network recommend considering a PET-CT for radiation planning as part of the workup for anal cancer patients.

Thoracic, abdominal, and pelvic CT and pelvic MRI identify liver or lung metastases or enlarged nodes. If the diagnosis is uncertain, image-guided biopsy should be considered. Skeletal studies are not indicated in the absence of focal symptoms.

Examination of blood and serum should include full blood count, renal and liver function tests, and, if any risk factors are present, assessment of HIV antibody status.

STAGING

The staging systems for anal canal and perianal cancers most commonly used are those proposed by the UICC[3] and the AJCC[2] (Tables 66.1 and 66.2). Most authors continue to report results by T (tumor) category or N (node) category rather than by composite TNM (tumor, node, metastasis) stages. Under the UICC and AJCC systems, the regional lymph nodes for anal canal cancer are the perirectal, internal iliac, and inguinal nodes. Spread to all other pelvic node groups, including the external iliac, common iliac, and sigmoid nodes, is classified as metastasis (M1). For perianal cancers, the only regional nodes are the ipsilateral inguinal nodes. The 8th edition of the AJCC staging manual for anal cancer includes changes to nodal classification and stage groupings.

In a review of 19,199 patients with squamous cell carcinoma of the anal canal, diagnosed between 1985 and 2000 and recorded in the U.S. National Cancer Database (NCDB), the stage distribution per AJCC 7th edition was stage I, 25.3%; II, 51.8%; III, 17.1%; and IV, 5.7%. Tumors were >5 cm in size (T3) in at least 20.6% (tumor size in T4 category not available). Nodal involvement was present in 21.8% of those for whom information on nodal status was recorded.[33]

TABLE 66.1 ANAL CANAL TNM CLASSIFICATION—8TH EDITION

Primary Tumor (T)

Tis	High-grade squamous intraepithelial lesion
T1	Tumor 2 cm or less in greatest dimension
T2	Tumor more than 2 cm but not more than 5 cm in greatest dimension
T3	Tumor more than 5 cm in greatest dimension
T4	Tumor of any size invades adjacent organ(s) (e.g., vagina, urethra, bladder) (invasion of the rectal wall, perirectal skin, subcutaneous tissue, or sphincter muscle is not included as T4).

Regional Lymph Nodes (N)

N0	No regional lymph node metastases
N1a	Inguinal, mesorectal, or internal iliac lymph nodes
N1b	External iliac nodes
N1c	External iliac nodes *plus* any node in the N1a group

Distant Metastases (M)

M0	No distant metastasis
M1	Distant metastasis

Stage Grouping

Stage 0	Tis	N0	M0
Stage I	T1	N0	M0
Stage II	T2	N0	M0
	T3	N0	M0
Stage IIIA	T1	N1	M0
	T2	N1	M0
Stage IIIB	T4	N0	M0
Stage IIIC	T3	N1	M0
	T4	N1	M0
Stage IV	Any T	Any N	M1

From Amin MB, Edge SB, Greene FL, et al., eds. *AJCC cancer staging manual*. 8th ed. New York: Springer, 2017. Reproduced with permission of Springer International Publishing in the format Book via Copyright Clearance Center.

TABLE 66.2 PERIANAL SKIN TNM CLASSIFICATION

Primary Tumor (T)

TX	Primary tumor (T)
T0	No evidence of primary tumor
Tis	Carcinoma *in situ*
T1	Tumor 2 cm or less in greatest dimension
T2	Tumor more than 2 cm but not more than 5 cm in greatest dimension
T3	Tumor more than 5 cm in greatest dimension
T4	Tumor invades deep extradermal structures (i.e., cartilage, skeletal muscle, or bone)

Regional Lymph Nodes (N)

NX	Regional lymph nodes cannot be assessed
N0	No regional lymph node metastasis
N1	Regional lymph node metastasis

Distant Metastasis (M)

MX	Distant metastasis cannot be assessed
M0	No distant metastasis
M1	Distant metastasis

Stage Grouping

Stage 0	Tis	N0	M0
Stage I	T1	N0	M0
Stage II	T2, T3	N0	M0
Stage III	T4	N0	M0
	Any T	N1	M0
Stage IV	Any T	Any N	M1

From Sobin LH, Gospodarowicz M, Wittekind C. *TNM classification of malignant tumours*. 7th ed. Hoboken, NJ: Wiley-Blackwell, 2009. Copyright © 2010 Blackwell Publishing Ltd. Reprinted by permission of John Wiley & Sons, Inc.

PROGNOSTIC FACTORS

Tumor Factors

Features related to the anatomic extent of disease generally provide the most prognostic value.[54] The most adverse factor for survival is the presence of extrapelvic metastasis.[55–57] When anal cancer is confined to the pelvis, the size of the primary tumor is the most useful predictor for local control and preservation of anorectal function and survival.[39,58,59] Involvement of regional lymph nodes is an adverse factor for survival but, in most series, not for control of the primary tumor.[39,59]

Among the 19,199 patients recorded in the NCDB between 1985 and 2000, the overall 5-year survival was 58%.[33] Patients with distant metastases had a 5-year survival of 18.7% versus 59.4% for those without metastases. Patients with regional node metastases had a 5-year survival of 37.4% versus 62.9% in node-negative patients. Five-year survival rates by T category were T1, 68.5%; T2, 58.9%; T3, 43.1%; and T4, 34.3%. The survival rates by AJCC stage are shown in Figure 66.2.

FIGURE 66.2. Five-year survival rates by American Joint Committee on Cancer Clinical Staging and the International Union Against Cancer stages, for 19,199 patients recorded in the U.S. National Cancer Database between 1985 and 2000. (Reprinted from Bilimoria KY, Bentrem DJ, Rock CE, et al. Outcomes and prognostic factors for squamous cell carcinoma of the anal canal: analysis of patients from the National Cancer Data Base. *Dis Colon Rectum* 2009;52[4]:624–631. With permission.)

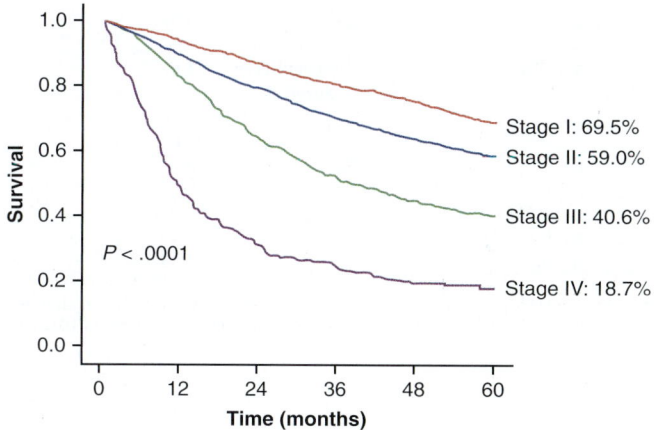

TABLE 66.3 PROGNOSTIC GROUPS: BASED ON DATA FROM RTOG TRIAL 9811

End Points (3 Y)	Group 1 T ≤5 cm, N-ve (n = 365)	Group 2 T >5 cm, N-ve (n = 112)	Group 3 T ≤5 cm, N+ve (n = 107)	Group 4 T >5 cm, N+ve (n = 60)
Disease-free survival (actuarial) (%)	74	65	48	30
Colostomy rate (crude) (%)	11	17	9	24
Overall survival (actuarial) (%)	86	75	75	63

N, any regional node; RTOG, Radiation Therapy Oncology Group; T, primary tumor.
Data from pooled trial groups treated by radiation therapy (RT), 5-fluorouracil, and mitomycin C or RT, 5-FU, and cisplatin (CDDP). Median follow-up 2.2 years. Most events occurred by 2 years.
From Ajani JA, Winter KA, Gunderson LL, et al. US Intergroup Anal Carcinoma Trial: tumor diameter predicts for colostomy. *J Clin Oncol* 2009;27:1116–1121; Ajani JA, Winter KA, Gunderson LL, et al. Prognostic factors derived from a prospective database dictate clinical biology of anal cancer. The Intergroup Trial (RTOG 98–11). *Cancer* 2010;116:4007–4013.

In detailed analyses of data collected prospectively for Radiation Therapy Oncology Group trial RTOG-9811,[59,60] tumor diameter >5 cm correlated with an increased likelihood of colostomy (hazard ratio [HR] 1.8; P = .008)[59] (Table 66.3). A tumor size >5 cm and clinically positive nodes were each associated with significantly poorer 5-year disease-free and overall survival.[60] These findings were combined into prognostic groups.[60] These groups are shown in Figure 66.3, with additional data drawn from the analyses by Ajani et al.[59,60] These groupings have not been verified prospectively.

Patient Factors

Patient-related factors are not consistent between series. Age, performance status, gender, baseline hemoglobin level, and race have all been considered prognostic in one or more series. Patients who continue to smoke tobacco may be at greater risk of local relapse.[61] In some series of HIV-positive patients, high viral load, low lymphocyte CD4-positive

FIGURE 66.3. Example of radiation fields used to cover pelvic nodes and primary cancer. Upper border generally lowered from lumbosacral junction to lower border of sacroiliac joints part way through course. Fields are later reduced further to give higher dose to primary tumor. Separate anterior fields are applied to cover lateral inguinal nodes.

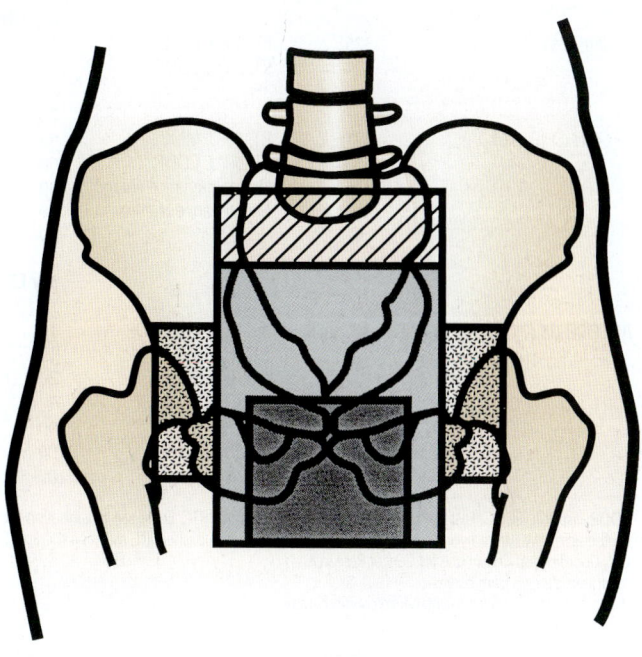

Section III

counts, and AIDS have been prognostic of poor local tumor control and survival and, in some series, of impaired tolerance of RT and chemotherapy.[62–64]

Biochemical and Molecular Factors

A survey of nearly 50 reports on cytogenetic, flow cytometric, immunohistochemical, and other factors considered that these studies offered some insights on pathogenesis but did not help with selection of treatment or provide guidance on prognosis.[65] Recent studies suggested that biomarkers such as p53,[66] Ki 67, nuclear factor kappa B, 5HH, and Gli-1[67] may be associated with locoregional control or disease-free survival. High levels of MCM7 protein detected in gene expression analysis were associated with improved cancer survival in one series.[68] None of these suggested markers has yet been validated in prospective studies. Recent studies suggest that HPV-positive anal squamous cell carcinoma may confer an overall survival advantage over HPV-negative anal cancer patients.

Treatment Factors

Early response and the extent of response to chemoradiation were correlated with survival in several multivariate analyses.[54,69,70] An association with total radiation dose or with treatment duration, although expected, has not been demonstrated consistently for either locoregional control or survival. A daily fraction size of 2.5 Gy appeared to be associated with increased acute and late toxicity, compared with 2-Gy fractions.[39]

TREATMENT OF ANAL CANCER

Although squamous cell cancer of the anal canal is a relatively uncommon malignancy, several multicenter randomized trials have been completed successfully. These have established RT, 5-FU, and MMC, with surgery reserved for failure, as the standard against which other treatments should be compared. These trials are outlined here and in Table 66.4.[41,71–78] The original references should be consulted for full details of patient

TABLE 66.4 SELECTED RESULTS OF PHASE III TRIALS

Trial (Reference)	N	Treatment	Local (LF) or Locoregional (LRF) Failure (%)	Colostomy Rate (CR) or Colostomy-Free Survival (CFS) (%)	Disease-Free Survival (%)	Overall Survival (%)
			3-y LRF	**3-y CR**	**3 y**	**3 y**
UKCCCR (ACT I) (41)	292	RT, 5-FU, MMC	39	24	np	65
	285	RT	61	40	np	58
	RR		0.54	np	np	0.86
	P		<.0001	np	np	.25
			10-y LRF	**10-y CFS**	**10 y**	**10 y**
Update (71)	292	RT, 5-FU, MMC	34	36	36	42
	285	RT	59	26	24	36
	HR		0.46	np	0.70	0.86
	P		<.001	sig	<.001	.12
			5-y LRF	**5-y CFS**	**5 y**	**5 y**
EORTC (72)	51	RT, 5-FU, MMC	32[a]	72[a]	np	58[a]
	52	RT	48[a]	40[a]	np	53[a]
	P		.02	.002	np	.17
			4-y LF	**4-y CR**	**4 y**	**4 y**
RTOG 8704/ECOG 1289 (73)	146	RT, 5-FU, MMC	16	9	73	76
	145	RT, 5-FU	34	22	51	67
	P		.0008	.002	.0003	.31
			5-y LRF	**3-y CR**	**3 y**	**3 y**
RTOG 9811 (74)	324	RT, 5-FU, MMC	25	10	60	75
	320	RT, 5-FU, CDDP	33	19	54	70
	HR		1.32	1.68	1.20	1.28
	P		.07	.02	.17	.10
			5-y LRF	**5-y CR**	**5 y**	**5 y**
Update (75)	325	RT, 5-FU, MMC	20	12	68	78
	324	RT, 5-FU, CDDP	27	17	58	71
	P		.089	.075	.004	.021
			3 y	**3-y CR**	**3 y**[b]	**3 y**[b]
UKCR (ACT II) (76)	471	RT, 5-FU, MMC	np	14	np	np
	469	RT, 5-FU, CDDP	np	11	np	np
	446	No maintenance chemo	np	np	75	85
	448	Maintenance chemo	np	np	75	84
	HR		np	11	0.89	0.79
	P			.26	.42	.19
			3-y LF	**3-y CFS**	**3-y Event-Free Survival**	**3 y**
ACCORD-03 (77,78)	307 total	Std RT, 5-FU, CDDP	10	86	67	np
		HD RT, 5-FU, CDDP	13	80	68	np
		Ind CT + Std RTCT	20	83	70	np
		Ind CT + HD RTCT	4	85	78	np
		Ind CT arms	np	84 vs. 83		
		HD RTCT arms	np	84 vs. 83		
	P		not sig	not sig	not sig	not sig

CDDP, cisplatin; ECOG, Eastern Cooperative Oncology Group; EORTC, European Organisation for Research on Treatment of Cancer; 5-FU, 5-fluorouracil; HD RT, high-dose radiation; Ind CT, induction chemotherapy; MMC, mitomycin C; not sig, not significant; np, not published; RT, radiation therapy; RTCT, chemoradiation; RTOG, Radiation Therapy Oncology Group; sig, significant; Std, standard; UKCCCR, U.K. Coordination Committee for Cancer Research.
[a]Numbers derived from curves.
[b]In patients who received maintenance chemotherapy.

eligibility, treatment regimens, outcomes, and statistical analyses. There have also been more than 100 nonrandomized studies, many of which provided hypotheses subsequently tested in the randomized studies, or information that guided the development of technical aspects of radiation treatment.[79]

It is of note that the combination of RT and chemotherapy has supplanted surgery as the preferred treatment for anal canal squamous cell cancer without formal comparison in a randomized trial. Nonrandomized comparisons of radical resection with this combination of RT, 5-FU, and MMC[32] or with RT alone[80] have shown the ability of radiation-based regimens to produce survival rates at least equal to those of surgical series while allowing preservation of anorectal function in the majority of patients.

COMBINED RADIATION AND CHEMOTHERAPY

Radiation, 5-Fluorouracil, and Mitomycin C Versus Radiation Alone

In both the United Kingdom and Europe in the 1970s, more so than in North America, there was already some acceptance of RT as the primary treatment for anal cancer[81]; this facilitated the development of the first multi-institutional randomized trials in which RT alone was compared with RT plus chemotherapy. The randomized trials conducted by the U.K. Coordination Committee for Cancer Research (UKCCCR)[41] and the European Organisation for Research and Treatment of Cancer (EORTC)[72] both demonstrated significant improvement in control of the primary cancer and regional nodes and in colostomy rate or colostomy-free survival in patients who received RT, 5-FU, and MMC. Overall survival rates were not improved significantly in the initial reports. However, in a later report of the UKCCCR trial after a median of 13 years' follow-up, locoregional control, colostomy-free survival, disease-free survival, and deaths due to anal cancer all significantly favored chemoradiation.[71] The absolute difference in risk of dying from all causes was 5.1% lower in the chemoradiation group at 5 years and 5.6% lower at 12 years from randomization. This difference approached statistical significance (HR 0.86; 95% confidence interval [CI], 0.70 to 1.04; $P = .12$).[71]

The UKCCCR trial included 577 patients with all stages (UICC staging system, 1987 edition) of squamous cell cancer of the anal canal (75% of patients) or anal margin (23%).[41] The radiation dose was 45 Gy in 20 to 25 fractions in 4 to 5 weeks. Those randomized to chemotherapy received 5-FU (1,000 mg/m²/d for 4 days or 750 mg/m²/d for 5 days) by continuous peripheral intravenous infusion in the first and final weeks of radiation treatment, plus MMC (12 mg/m²) by bolus intravenous injection on day 1 of the first course of chemotherapy. If the primary tumor had not regressed by at least 50% by 6 weeks after treatment (as occurred in 10% in each group), surgery was recommended; otherwise, the patients received an additional 15 Gy in 6 fractions by a perineal field or 25 Gy over 2 to 3 days by iridium-192 implant. The locoregional recurrence rates at 3 years were 61% after RT and 39% after RT, 5-FU, and MMC ($P < .0001$). The overall survival rates at 3 years were 58% and 65% ($P = .25$), respectively. There were six (2%) deaths due to treatment in the combined-modality arm and two (0.7%) in the irradiation-alone arm. Acute toxicity, other than hematologic, was considered comparable in each group. In the first few years after treatment, surgery that included colostomy was necessary for management of toxicity in 10 patients (3.5%) in each group.[41] Late toxicity events (severity was not graded) after a median of 13 years' follow-up were similar in each treatment group.[71]

In the EORTC study, 103 patients with advanced cancers of the anal canal were randomized in a trial of similar design.[72] The radiation dose was 45 Gy in 25 fractions over 5 weeks. Chemotherapy included 5-FU (750 mg/m²/d for 5 days) in weeks 1 and 5 of radiation, and a single dose of MMC (15 mg/m²) by bolus intravenous injection on day 1 of the first course of 5-FU only. After 6 weeks, boost irradiation of 15 Gy (if complete clinical response to previous treatment had occurred) or 20 Gy (after partial response) was given by external-beam or interstitial irradiation. The 5-year locoregional recurrence rate was 48% after RT and 32% after RT, 5-FU, and MMC ($P = .02$). The difference between overall survival rates (53% and 58%, respectively) was not significant. One of 51 patients who received combined modality treatment died of toxicity. Otherwise, acute and late toxicity rates did not differ markedly. These two trials established RT, 5-FU, and MMC as the standard first-line treatment.

Radiation, 5-Fluorouracil, and Mitomycin C Versus Radiation and 5-Fluorouracil

The RTOG and Eastern Cooperative Oncology Group (ECOG) established in a randomized trial that the combination of MMC with 5-FU and RT is more effective than is 5-FU alone with RT.[73] This study was undertaken to determine whether MMC was a necessary component of the protocol and whether the hematologic toxicity of that drug could be avoided. Two hundred and ninety-one patients with cancers of the anal canal of any T and N category (RTOG staging system) who did not have evidence of extrapelvic metastases received 45 Gy to 50.4 Gy in 25 to 28 fractions over 5 weeks, plus 2 courses of 5-FU (1,000 mg/m²/d by continuous peripheral intravenous infusion) over 4 days, with or without MMC (10 mg/m² by bolus intravenous injection) on the first day of each course of chemotherapy. Chemotherapy was administered in weeks 1 and 5 of RT. All patients underwent biopsy of the primary tumor site 6 weeks after treatment. Biopsies were positive in 15% of those who received 5-FU only and in 8% of those who received both MMC and 5-FU ($P = .14$). Patients with positive biopsies had the option of receiving an additional 9 Gy in 5 treatments concurrently with a 4-day infusion of 5-FU (1,000 mg/m²/d) and a single injection of cisplatin (CDDP) (100 mg/m²) if it was thought that anal function might still be salvaged. At 4 years, the rates of local failure (16% vs. 34%; $P = .0008$) and of colostomy (9% vs. 22%; $P = .002$), significantly favored treatment with radiation, 5-FU, and MMC. There was no significant difference in overall survival rates (76% with RT, 5-FU, and MMC vs. 67%); however, the disease-free survival rate (73% vs. 51%; $P = .0003$) was improved by the three-agent combination. Acute hematologic toxicity was more common in the patients who received MMC, but the rates of other acute and late toxic effects were similar in each treatment group. Four of 146 (2.7%) patients who received both 5-FU and MMC suffered fatal toxicity as did 1 of 145 treated with RT and 5-FU alone. On the evidence from this trial, MMC was retained in combination with RT and 5-FU.

Radiation, 5-Fluorouracil, and Mitomycin C Versus Radiation, 5-Fluorouracil, and Cisplatin

Several pilot studies suggested high tumor response rates to concurrent, induction, or induction plus concurrent 5-FU and CDDP with RT.[82–88] Cisplatin was known to be effective against squamous cell cancers in several other sites and to be associated with stronger laboratory evidence as a radiosensitizer than MMC.

The RTOG elected to evaluate a strategy of CDDP-based induction chemotherapy intended to downsize the primary tumor and nodal metastases prior to concurrent chemoradiation. This trial included a higher total radiation dose than the earlier RTOG randomized trial,[73] based on analysis of non-randomized studies that suggested a radiation dose–control relationship[89,90] and on pilot studies, which had demonstrated that a proportion of patients could tolerate uninterrupted radiation schedules of up to 59.4 Gy over 6.5 weeks with either concurrent MMC with 5-FU[91,92] or CDDP with 5-FU.[83]

In RTOG-9811,[74] one patient group received 59 Gy in 6.5 weeks (45 Gy in 1.8-Gy fractions, followed without interruption by 14 Gy in 2-Gy fractions), together with concurrent 5-FU (1,000 mg/m^2/d) by continuous infusion on days 1 to 4 and 29 to 32 plus MMC 10 mg/m^2 intravenous bolus on days 1 and 29; the other group received 5-FU (1,000 mg/m^2/d) days 1 to 4, 29 to 32, 57 to 60, and 85 to 88 plus CDDP (75 mg/m^2 bolus injection on days 1, 29, 57, and 85) with the same 59-Gy radiation schedule (start day 57). Acute grade 3 or 4 nonhematologic toxicity rates were 75% in each arm, but hematologic toxicity was higher in the MMC group (67% vs. 47%). No treatment-related deaths were reported. The rate of severe long-term toxicity was similar in each group (11% MMC vs. 10% CDDP). The first report of this trial (after median patient follow-up of 2.5 years) described a significantly higher rate of colostomy at 3 years in those who received CDDP rather than MMC plus 5-FU and RT. There were no significant differences in disease-free or overall survival rates.

After longer follow-up, the 5-year colostomy rates and locoregional failure rates showed trends in favor of 5-FU, MMC- and RT but were not significant. However, the 5-year disease-free (68% vs. 58%; $P = .004$) and overall survival rates (78% vs. 71%; $P = .021$) significantly favored RT, 5-FU, and MMC.[75] The investigators concluded that RT, 5-FU, and MMC should remain the standard approach.

The second U.K. Anal Cancer Trial (ACT II) also has not identified a role for CDDP in addition to or in place of MMC. This trial has so far been reported in abstract only.[76] The trial incorporates a double randomization, either to 5-FU and MMC or to 5-FU and CDDP concurrently with RT and to 2 courses of adjuvant (or maintenance) 5-FU and CDDP or to no additional chemotherapy following concurrent chemoradiation. The primary endpoints were improvements in complete tumor response rates and disease-free survival rates. Complete tumor response rates at 6 months were similar: 94% (MMC arm) and 95% (CDDP arm). Three-year disease-free and overall survival rates were not improved in those who received adjuvant 5-FU and CDDP. MMC-treated patients had more severe hematologic toxicity, but rates of neutropenic sepsis were similar (about 3%).

A French intergroup conducted a factorial-designed four-arm trial (ACCORD 03) that evaluated the addition of induction 5-FU and CDDP and of a higher dose of boost RT (20 Gy to 25 Gy vs. standard 15 Gy). The baseline standard RT schedule was 45 Gy in 25 fractions in 5 weeks. The outcome has been reported in abstract only.[77,78] The actuarial 3-year colostomy-free survival rate (the primary study endpoint) ranged from 80% to 85% in the four arms, with no significant advantages for either experimental treatment. Local control, event-free survival, and overall survival rates were similar in each arm.

Other Drug–Radiation Combinations

In an effort to develop a simplified schedule, the U.K. National Cancer Research Institute Anal Subgroup conducted a phase II trial of RT (50.4 Gy in 28 fractions in 5.5 weeks), a single intravenous injection of MMC (12 mg/m^2 on day 1) and oral capecitabine (825 mg/m^2 twice daily on each RT treatment day).[93] The schedule was described as well tolerated with acceptable compliance (although only 58% received the full planned doses). The overall tumor response rate after treatment was 90% (complete in 24 of 31 and partial in 4 of 31). Although this use of oral capecitabine is promising and removes the need for continuous intravenous infusions of 5-FU, at this time, delivery of both 5-FU and MMC intravenously remains standard.

The EORTC conducted a randomized phase II trial in which RT (36 Gy + 2-week gap + 23.4 Gy) was combined with either MMC and 5-FU or MMC and CDDP. The overall response rates at 8 weeks were 92% (34 of 37) to RT, MMC, and CDDP versus 80% (31 of 39) to RT, 5-FU, and MMC, although greater compliance to the full regimen was seen with RT, 5-FU, and MMC.[94] It is not known whether this group has proceeded with a planned phase III trial.[95]

Because epidermal growth factor receptor (EGFR) is known to be overexpressed in many epithelial cancers, including squamous cell cancer of the anal canal,[96] EGFR blockers are being evaluated. The ECOG is conducting a phase II study of RT, 5-FU, CDDP, and cetuximab in HIV-negative patients.[95] The AIDS Malignancy Clinical Trials Consortium is performing a similar study in HIV-positive patients.[95] Other anti-EGFR agents under study include nimotuzumab and panitumumab.[95] Initial laboratory studies suggest that EGFR and *K-RAS* mutation analysis are not likely to be useful as a screening test for sensitivity to anti-EGFR therapy in anal canal cancer.[96]

In Sweden, bleomycin was given concurrently with RT in nonrandomized studies, but no benefit was apparent.[97-99] A pilot study in the United Kingdom in which all three of the major drugs investigated, 5FU, MMC, and CDDP, were combined with RT was not pursued further because of excessive toxicity.[100]

CONCLUSION

Much remains to be learned about the mechanisms of interaction between radiation and chemotherapy in the treatment of cancer. The synergistic interactions of various combinations of RT, 5-FU, MMC, and CDDP observed in some laboratory studies are difficult to evaluate clinically, and no trials designed to study such interactions have been performed. Also, there have not been formal comparisons of more prolonged, but less daily dose-intense, infusions of 5-FU with the 96-hour to 120-hour infusions generally favored, nor of bolus injections with continuous infusions of 5-FU or CDDP. In most series, the timing of delivery of chemotherapy each day relative to irradiation was not tightly controlled, and the importance of scheduling is not known.

The current standard chemoradiation combination is RT with two concurrent 96-hour or 120-hour continuous intravenous infusions of 5-FU and one or two bolus injections of MMC. The most effective doses have not been established. When patients are to be managed outside a clinical trial, it is suggested that a schedule used in one of the prospective randomized trials, for which there are data on efficacy and toxicity, be adopted.

RADIATION THERAPY

The use of RT alone, either brachytherapy or external beam, has been greatly reduced since the confirmation of improved outcome of combined modality therapy. Radiation alone is now recommended mainly to patients who are unable to undergo RT plus chemotherapy or for the treatment of smaller cancers up to about 3 to 4 cm in size where the physician does not wish to add chemotherapy. As with combined RT and chemotherapy, primary tumor control is better with small tumors. Selected results, mainly from the period prior to the adoption of chemoradiation, are shown in Table 66.5.

TABLE 66.5 SELECTED STUDIES OF THREE-DIMENSIONAL CONFORMAL RADIATION AND INTENSITY-MODULATED RADIATION THERAPY

Study (Reference)	RTOG 9811 MMC arm (74)	Boston (159)	RTOG 0529 (158)	Toronto (139)
No. of patients	324	43	51	58
Radiation technique	3-D conformal	IMRT	IMRT	IMRT
Acute grade 3 or 4 toxicity				
Hematologic (%)	61	49	NP	38
Skin (%)	48	7	20	46
GI (%)	36	7	22 (GI/GU)	9
GU (%)	4	5	22 (GI/GU)	0
Treatment breaks	61	40	49	55
2-y results				
Locoregional control (%)	77	95 (local)	80	85
Colostomy-free survival (%)	84	94	86	87
Disease-free survival (%)	71	NP	77	75

3-D, three-dimensional; GI, gastrointestinal; GU, genitourinary; IMRT, intensity-modulated radiation therapy; MMC, mitomycin C; NP, not published; RTOG, Radiation Therapy Oncology Group.

SURGERY

For Residual and Recurrent Cancer

Random biopsies from the site of the primary tumor, or abnormal nodes, shortly after chemoradiation have been advocated by some but are not necessary. Elective biopsies at predetermined times do not appear to lead to better results than can be achieved by biopsies directed only to areas suspected clinically of harboring residual or recurrent cancer. A negative biopsy does not exclude the possibility of cancer regrowth.[101,102] Residual masses at the site of the original anal cancer may take several months to resolve fully after chemoradiation or RT alone.[39,102] A post hoc analysis of the ACT II study evaluated the optimal timepoint to assess clinical complete response. Patients in the ACT II study had assessments after chemoradiotherapy at 11 weeks, 18 weeks, and 26 weeks. The investigators found that among patients who did not have a clinical complete response by 11 weeks, 151 of 209 (72%) would ultimately achieve a clinical complete response by 26 weeks. Together, these findings highlight the potentially slow primary anal tumor response to chemoradiotherapy, and most authors now recommend biopsy only when persistent cancer is suspected clinically.

Suspected residual or recurrent cancer at the primary site or in regional nodes should be confirmed histologically if possible. Full restaging imaging is recommended. FDG-PET scans may disclose otherwise unidentified cancer.[103] Abdominoperineal resection or multivisceral pelvic resection is usually required. Survival rates are poor when R0 resection cannot be achieved.[104,105] Locoregional recurrence is common, despite apparent R0 resection.[104,106] Five-year survival rates following salvage surgery range from 30% to 50%, reflecting the varying criteria applied when selecting patients for surgery.[104–107]

Salvage for inguinal node metastases is usually by radical or selective inguinofemoral lymphadenectomy. Pelvic sidewall node metastases may not be resectable because of invasion of muscle or bone or neurovascular structures.

For Primary Cancer

Surgery is the principal treatment for AIN[108] but retains only a limited place in the initial management of primary invasive anal cancer. A few patients (<5% in most series) are incontinent for solid stool at presentation. This is usually due to extensive tumors that have destroyed the competence of the anal sphincters or fistulized into the vagina. Eradication of cancer by RT, with or without chemotherapy, does not restore continence in such patients, likely because the cancer is replaced by fibrous tissue rather than the specialized muscle of the anal sphincters. One approach is to perform colostomy before preoperative RT and chemotherapy using doses of 45 to 50 Gy over 5 weeks, followed by immediate or delayed resection. An alternative is initial abdominoperineal resection with postoperative RT and chemotherapy. There are insufficient data to compare the outcomes of these approaches.

Local excision, preserving anorectal function, is possible in some patients, although this is now usually restricted to small well-differentiated squamous cell cancers that have not invaded the sphincter muscles and are located distal to the dentate line.[109–111] This approach is based on the finding in surgical series that pararectal or superior hemorrhoidal system lymph node metastases were associated with <5% of well-differentiated squamous cell cancers <2 cm in size.[31,34] Local excision of small cancers of the distal canal or perianal skin is generally more expedient and associated with less morbidity than radiation-based treatments. However, if resection margins are positive or considered inadequate, and further local excision is not possible, the patient should receive chemoradiation or RT alone. There is no evidence that elective management by limited tumor excision and postoperative radiation-based protocols improves local control.[112]

The role of surgery in the management of inguinal node metastases detected at initial diagnosis has not been well defined. Although nodal metastases are generally treated successfully by the same doses of RT and chemotherapy effective against the primary cancer, there is no consensus on whether control of the nodal region involved is improved by limited node dissection prior to RT and chemotherapy and on how such an approach affects morbidity such as late limb edema.[36,38–40] After local excision of gross node metastases, the dose to the groin can usually be limited to 50 to 54 Gy over 5 to 6 weeks, provided imaging does not show residual metastases. The combination of local surgery and RT and chemotherapy has resulted in regional control rates in the groin of 80% or better.[38,39] However, 5-year survival rates are usually –20% less than in those who do not present with inguinal node metastases.

Extrapelvic Metastases

Deaths from extrapelvic metastases alone are relatively infrequent. Extrapelvic metastases are identified in about 10% to 20% of patients. Among 77 patients in the UKCCCR ACT I trial who died of anal cancer after treatment with RT, 5-FU, and MMC, 38 of 77 (49% of the cancer deaths) had cancer in the pelvis only and 21 of 77 (27%) had extrapelvic metastases only. In that trial, the overall crude rate of metastasis in those who received RT and chemotherapy was 10%, compared with 17% in those treated by RT alone.[41] In the EORTC trial, 17% of those treated by RT and chemotherapy developed metastases, as did 21% of those treated by RT only.[72] In RTOG-9811, the rates of distant metastases at 5 years were 13% in those who received RT, 5-FU, and MMC and 18% after RT, 5-FU, and CDDP.[75] In the U.K. ACT II trial, there was no suggestion in the 3-year disease-free and overall survival rates of benefit from the addition of 2 courses of adjuvant 5-FU and CDDP.[76] The rates of metastases in patients treated by chemoradiation are similar to those reported following management of the primary cancer and regional nodes by surgery or RT only. There is still considerable uncertainty regarding the effects on subclinical metastases outside the pelvis from the chemotherapy given concurrently with RT and as short-term induction or adjuvant treatment.

The median survival time after diagnosis of extrapelvic metastases ranges from 8 to about 24 months.[55,56,113] These metastases have been relatively resistant so far to all chemotherapy, RT, or combined modality protocols.[113] The most active combination is 5-FU and CDDP, although complete or durable responses are uncommon.

Many recently developed drugs and molecular targeted agents have not yet been evaluated, but the possibility of new approaches is illustrated by preliminary reports of responses to cetuximab and irinotecan.[114] A recently reported phase II trial evaluated the anti–PD-1 antibody nivolumab in patients with treatment of refractory metastatic anal squamous cell carcinoma. Among the 37 patients treated with nivolumab, two had complete responses and seven had partial responses for an overall response rate of 24%. Radiation alone may provide useful palliation, especially for painful metastases. Stereotactic body RT or metastasectomy may be offered to selected patients, but metastases are commonly multiple.

TREATMENT OF PERIANAL CANCER

The most common histologic type of invasive cancer of the perianal skin is squamous cell carcinoma, usually keratinizing. Basal cell cancers and adenocarcinomas can also occur.

Wide local excision with a 1-cm margin is recommended for all histologic types, provided anal continence can be preserved.[111] Radiation alone or in combination with chemotherapy is also effective against squamous cell cancers.[40,69,115-119] Radiation-based protocols identical to those for anal canal cancer are preferred when anal continence would be impaired by surgery. In the UKCCCR ACT I trial, one of four patients had a cancer that arose in the perianal skin (anal margin). Results by site of cancer origin were not reported, but local control and cause-specific survival rates favored combined modality therapy.[41,71] The UK investigators also included perianal cancers in their subsequent trial.[76] In institution-based series, locoregional control rates ranged from 60% to 90%, sphincter preservation rates from 65% to 85%, and 5-year overall survival from 55% to 80%.[40,69,115-119] Local necrosis was seen as a complication more frequently when brachytherapy was used, although in general, the rates of serious complications were <5%.

The regional nodes for the perianal skin are the ipsilateral inguinal nodes. Perirectal and pelvic node metastases are uncommon unless the cancer involves the anal canal extensively. The risk of inguinal node metastases is about 10%, principally with category T3 or T4 tumors or poorly differentiated cancers. Elective bilateral inguinal nodal irradiation may be considered when these larger tumors are treated, although some advocate elective inguinal RT for all perianal cancers.[119] The lower pelvic nodes should be included if the anal canal is invaded. The management of abnormal inguinal nodes is similar to that for anal canal cancer.

The principles of management for the uncommon basal cell and adenocarcinomas of the perianal skin are similar to those for these histologic types elsewhere on the skin.

PATIENTS WITH HUMAN IMMUNODEFICIENCY VIRUS/ACQUIRED IMMUNODEFICIENCY SYNDROME

The numbers of HIV-infected patients with anal squamous cell cancer are increasing.[23] The median age at diagnosis is in the fourth decade, about 20 years earlier than in non–HIV-infected patients. There is a marked preponderance of male patients.[23]

HIV-infected patients were not eligible for any of the randomized trials described earlier. Anal cancers in HIV-infected patients have been treated by combined modality therapy or RT alone.[62-64,120-124] HIV-infected patients are at increased risk of toxicity, particularly in the perineal skin, anorectal mucosa, and hematologic system when treated with RT with or without chemotherapy. The mechanisms for this increased toxicity are not known.[125] Most recent reports indicate that it is not necessary to electively modify standard protocols of RT (with respect to dose, fractionation, or volume) and chemotherapy (either 5-FU and MMC or 5-FU and CDDP), but modifications should be based on the severity of side effects in each individual patient.[62,120] Two factors may predict for heightened acute normal tissue toxicity or poor cancer control: a CD4 count <200/μL at the start of treatment or the presence of AIDS.[63,126] But these findings are not inevitably associated with poor tolerance. Concurrent antiretroviral therapy does not reliably reduce the severity or incidence of toxicity of RT and chemotherapy.[30]

Locoregional control rates of about 65% or better were described in some series, similar to those in HIV-negative patients. However, some investigators reported lower rates of local control and sphincter preservation in HIV-positive patients, despite earlier-stage disease and good initial tumor response.[64,124] In a study of 40 HIV-positive patients, the 5-year overall survival rate was similar to that in 81 HIV-negative patients, but the major cause of death in HIV-positive patients was anal cancer, in contradistinction to the HIV-negative patients in whom causes other than cancer predominated.[64]

ADENOCARCINOMAS

Most adenocarcinomas involving the anal canal arise from rectal-type mucosa that extends below the upper muscular boundary of the canal. They are generally treated similarly to those that arise in the rectum. The uncommon adenocarcinomas that develop from anal glands or in fistulae are more aggressive than squamous cancers and often metastasize early.[127] They have usually been managed by abdominoperineal resection. Five-year survival rates following surgery alone are commonly below 50%, with local recurrence rates of about 25%.[32,111,127-130] Any advantage from adjuvant radiation and chemotherapy is unknown, although, by analogy, protocols used for primary rectal cancers are sometimes applied. A few centers have treated some anal adenocarcinomas by chemoradiation protocols developed for squamous cell cancers or rectal adenocarcinomas and have deferred surgery. Experience is limited, but anorectal function has been retained, and apparent cures have been reported, particularly in patients with smaller cancers, following treatment with RT alone or with RT and chemotherapy.[127-133]

SMALL CELL CARCINOMAS

Small cell carcinomas are rare cancers characterized by early metastases and have a poor prognosis.[31] The primary tumor may be managed by surgery or radiation. Systemic chemotherapy similar to that used for small cell cancers that arise elsewhere may be combined with radiation for the primary tumor and used to treat metastases, but responses are generally limited.

RADIATION THERAPY: TECHNIQUES AND DOSES

Anal Canal Cancer

Current radiation treatment strategies have been developed through better understanding of the natural history of anal cancer and correlation of sites of treatment failure with the treatment plan.[134-136] Most failures were at the site of the primary tumor, followed by the regional and other pelvic node groups.

The treatment volumes of interest are also influenced by the philosophy adopted with regard to which lymph node groups should be treated electively. Only well-differentiated squamous cell cancers ≤2 cm in size situated in the distal canal appear to have a risk of nodal metastases <5%.[31,34] The finding in surgical series of histopathologically verified metastases in the pararectal and internal iliac nodes in up to 30%, and in the inguinal nodes in up to 20%, has encouraged most radiation oncologists to irradiate these node groups electively. Retrospective and prospective studies have shown the advantages of elective nodal irradiation (ENI).[38,39] Following ENI to a total dose of 40 to 50 Gy (1.8 to 2 Gy fractions), investigators from France reported 5-year cumulative rates of inguinal recurrence of 2% in those who received ENI ($n = 75$) versus 16% in those who did not ($n = 106$). In the no-ENI group, recurrence rates were 12% from T1 to T2 and 30% from T3 to T4 tumors.[38] In a prospective study in Australasia in which patients with T1 or T2 tumors up to 4 cm in diameter did not receive inguinal ENI, inguinal node failure occurred in 9 of 40 (23%), in 5 as first site of failure.[137] Treatment of larger cancers by interstitial brachytherapy alone resulted in failure in pelvic nodes above the treated volume in 16% (14 of 88).[138] Control of most subclinical pelvic node metastases by pelvic ENI and chemotherapy can be inferred from the low failure rates reported in pelvic node sites.[134-136] The minimum effective dose for ENI is not known. Doses as low as 24 Gy in 12 fractions in 2.5 weeks appeared effective in one series,[39] but most centers give from 30.6 Gy in 17 fractions in 3.5 weeks to 50 Gy in 25 fractions in 5 weeks.[38,73,74]

The randomized trials described earlier all used radiation plans generated by two- or three-dimensional (2-D or 3-D) planning techniques and, for the most part, employed predominantly anteroposterior opposed field techniques for a substantial part of the schedule. Most radiation oncologists prefer to treat the primary tumor, the regional internal iliac, and perirectal nodes and inguinal nodes and other pelvic node groups such as the external iliac and presacral nodes in continuity. If the patient is prone, the anus can be visualized readily and bolus placed selectively over any perianal tumor extension. However, it is difficult to boost the inguinal area when the patient is prone if a 2-D or 3-D treatment technique is used. Alternatively, the patient may be treated supine. This facilitates boosts to the inguinal areas and reduces some of the inhomogeneities produced by the natural curvatures of the pelvic soft tissues. In that position, it is difficult to ensure that bolus placed over the anal area remains in place.

In the discussion that follows, the radiation doses described are typical of those prescribed when RT is combined with 5-FU and MMC. When an anteroposterior opposed pair of fields is used, the upper border of the fields is placed at the lumbosacral junction if the intent is to include the common iliac, upper presacral, and lower rectosigmoid nodes, in addition to the regional nodes. This border is commonly moved down during treatment to the lower end of the sacroiliac joints (typically after 30.6 Gy in 17 fractions to 36 Gy in 20 fractions), thus encompassing in the reduced volume only the perirectal, lower presacral, and internal iliac nodes (and, if the fields are sufficiently wide, the lower external iliac nodes), in order to reduce the risk of radiation enteritis (Fig. 66.3). A further field reduction is made at 45 Gy, following which a final phase of treatment of 9 Gy in 5 fractions or 14.4 Gy in 8 fractions is delivered to the primary tumor. It is advisable to add a CTV margin of 2 to 3 cm around the primary tumor for this boost phase. If the primary tumor cannot be identified on

the planning CT, the anal sphincter complex is often used as a surrogate target, adjusted for any known tumor extension beyond the anal canal. The overall total dose to the primary tumor is 54 Gy in 30 fractions in 6 weeks to 59.4 Gy in 33 fractions in 6.5 weeks when all RT is delivered by external-beam radiation. If there are metastatic nodes, these are treated by appropriate fields to the same total dose as the primary tumor. It may not be possible to deliver more than about 45 to 50.4 Gy to abnormal nodes in the pelvis if these lie adjacent to small bowel; in many cases, these doses are enough to achieve control. In the absence of abnormal nodes in the lower pelvis, some consider elective treatment of radiologically normal nodes above the lower border of the sacroiliac joints unnecessary.[39,139,140]

The inferior field border is placed 3 cm distal to the lower most extension of the primary tumor, which should be indicated by a radio-opaque marker during simulation.

The position of the lateral borders depends on the philosophy adopted with respect to the desirability of treating a continuous homogeneous volume, without multiple fields and field junctions, and minimizing irradiation of the femoral head and neck. Options include anterior and posterior fields of equal size encompassing the inguinal nodes; anterior and posterior fields of equal size, but restricted to include the medial borders of the pelvis only, the inguinal nodes being treated by anterior electron beams matched to the photon fields; asymmetric photon fields, with a larger anterior field to cover the primary tumor and pelvic and inguinal nodes in continuity; and a posterior beam restricted to the primary tumor and pelvic nodes. In this latter arrangement, an anterior electron beam may be used to supplement the dose to the inguinal nodes to the desired level. The location and depth of the inguinal nodes should be obtained by axial imaging.[141] Another popular alternative, if 30.6 to 36 Gy in 3.5 to 4 weeks is felt to be sufficient dose for ENI for radiologically normal nodes, is to treat the primary and pelvic and inguinal nodes with the AP:PA fields and then to use a three-field arrangement (posterior and two lateral fields) to encompass the primary tumor to 45 to 59.4 Gy total dose, according to the size of the primary cancer and local practice. Other field arrangements, such as oblique fields[142] and a direct perineal field coupled with a posterior partial arc beam,[138] have been described. When asymmetric or matched fields are used, there is potential for both over- and underdosage.[143]

The final phase of treatment, beyond which includes both lymph nodes and primary cancer, typically delivers from 9 to 20 Gy to a reduced volume encompassing the primary tumor only. This phase may be delivered by brachytherapy. Brachytherapy is used more commonly in Europe than in North America, where external-beam treatment is favored. There are a number of reports of effective brachytherapy, including low–dose rate (LDR),[69,144,145] pulsed dose rate (PDR),[146-148] and high–dose rate (HDR) techniques.[149,150] Brachytherapy has usually been given 2 to 8 weeks after external beam therapy, although one schedule introduced HDR in the interval during split-course external beam therapy.[149] There is no agreement on whether the treatment volume should include the full extent of the initial primary cancer[69,138,147,149] or only the tumor remaining at the time of implant.[151] The brachytherapy dose depends on the composite dose of the total radiation prescription. Occasionally, significant toxicity has been encountered.

The introduction of intensity-modulated radiation therapy (IMRT) offers the possibility of further reducing the dose to normal tissues beyond that achievable with 3-D conformal techniques. Several initial studies of IMRT and similar highly conformal techniques described improvements in radiation dose distributions.[135,152-157] However, it is apparent from the

TABLE 66.6 SELECTED RESULTS OF RADIATION THERAPY ALONE

Author (Reference)	Radiation	Primary Tumor Control			Serious Complications—Colostomy	5-Year Survival
		T1	T2	T3 T4		
Newman et al. (178)	50 Gy/20/4 wk	8/9 (≤2 cm)	42/52 (81%) (≤5 cm)	13/20 (65%) (>5 cm or T4)	2	66%
Cummings et al. (139)	50 Gy/20/4 wk (some EB-l/l)	6/6 (≤2 cm)	19/29 (66%) (≤5 cm)	13/28 (46%) (>5 cm or T4)	6	61%
Martenson and Gunderson (179)	45–50 Gy/25–28/5–6 wk Plus boost to 55–67 Gy	9/9 (≤2 cm)	17/17 (100%) (≤5 cm)	—	2 temp	94%, actuarial
Otim-Oyet et al. (180)	60–65 Gy/30–33/6–7 wk (Some with boost)	2/2 (≤2 cm)	16/22 (73%) (≤4 cm)	8/17 (47%) (>4 cm)	1	56% Cause-specific
Papillon and Montbarbon (80)	42 Gy/10/2.5 wk Plus I 20 Gy at 8 wk	NS	29/39 (74%) (≤4 cm)	27/64 (42%) (>4 cm)	6	60%

EB, external beam; I, interstitial brachytherapy; NS, not stated; temp, temporary.

selected results in Table 66.6 that a wide range of severe acute toxicities was seen and that about half the patients treated by IMRT had breaks in treatment. Comparisons of the different case series and interpretation are difficult because most studies used differing RT techniques and doses and practices for recording toxicities. There are no high-quality data as yet on long-term toxicity following IMRT for anal cancer.

Highly conformal IMRT and related techniques require considerable attention to identifying gross target volumes (GTV) and relevant elective clinical target volumes (CTV). In a trial conducted by RTOG to test the reproducibility of IMRT in multiple centers, 79% of 51 cases were found on pretreatment review to not comply with the protocol treatment volumes, particularly those for nodal regions to be irradiated electively.[156] The RTOG study found that IMRT had similar rates of grade 2+ acute gastrointestinal/genitourinary toxicity (primary study endpoint) compared to historic RTOG controls treated with conformal radiation, though the IMRT patients had decreased rates of grade 2+ hematologic toxicity (73% vs. 85%), grade 3+ gastrointestinal toxicity (21% vs. 36%), and grade 3+ skin toxicity (23% vs. 49%) compared to historic controls. The RTOG subsequently published an atlas of elective CTV templates developed by a consensus panel for use in planning IMRT for anal and rectal cancers.[158] When IMRT techniques are to be used, particular attention to patient positioning and immobilization is necessary. If possible, the accuracy of setup should be verified frequently, for example, by image-guided radiation treatment.

The results of IMRT appear similar to those achieved with 3-D conformal RT, though we lack long-term clinical outcomes with IMRT. Despite this lack of data, current guidelines endorse IMRT as the preferred option over 3-D conformal RT.

There has been increasing attention to radiation dose–time factors. Recent protocols have sought to improve local control rates, particularly for larger tumors, by intensifying RT or chemotherapy or both. Primary tumor control rates (excluding salvage treatment) in most studies of RT, 5-FU, and MMC are about 90% to 100% for tumors up to 2 cm (T1), 65% to 75% for tumors from 2 to 5 cm (T2), and 40% to 55% for those >5 cm and for most deeply invasive cancers (T3 or T4); the primary tumor control rate is about 60% overall.[39,57,102,145,159–162]

Increases in total radiation doses have been advocated. When combined with 5-FU and MMC, radiation doses of as little as 30 Gy in 15 fractions over 3 weeks have been shown to eradicate up to about 90% of cancers ≤3 cm in size. Higher doses, from 45 Gy in 25 fractions in 5 weeks to 54 Gy in 30 fractions in 6 weeks, sometimes supplemented with additional radiation after an interval of 6 to 8

weeks to a total of 60 to 65 Gy over a total time of about 12 weeks, have controlled from 65% to 75% of primary tumors >4 cm.[39,57,102,159–162] Recent trials in North America used up to 59 Gy in 32 fractions over 6.5 weeks for large or node-positive cancers[74,83,91,92]; the effectiveness and long-term tolerability of these increased doses have not yet been reported in detail. Analysis of the UKCCCR ACT I trial suggested that delivery of boost radiation of 15 to 25 Gy 6 weeks after the initial 45 Gy in 4 to 5 weeks did not improve local control but was associated with an increased risk of necrosis (8% vs. 0% if no boost was given).[163] Many centers are developing graduated dose schedules according to the size of the primary tumor and lymph node metastases.[74,134,153,157]

A potential advantage frequently proposed for IMRT is the ability to selectively increase the radiation dose to the cancer. It is not known whether this will be possible as a strategy to increase control rates for larger anal tumors because of the limited tolerances of the distal rectum, anal canal, and perianal skin.[164,165] The introduction of single-phase IMRT plans has led to the use of nonstandard dose fractionation, particularly for lymph node regions treated electively. For example, if all target volumes are to be treated to 30 fractions and the primary tumor is to receive 54 Gy at 1.8 Gy/fraction, elective treatment of uninvolved nodes to 36 Gy would be delivered at 1.2 Gy/fraction and to 45 Gy at 1.5 Gy/fraction. Some authors have also introduced biologically effective dose corrections to allow for different fractional doses or alterations in time over which the lower doses are delivered.[153,157] The long-term effectiveness of these nonstandard doses has not been determined.

In the era of 2-D treatment planning, and later with 3-D conformal planning, interruptions in external-beam treatment, generally of no more than 2 weeks but of up to 4 weeks in some series, were introduced into many combined modality protocols, either as elective breaks after about 3 weeks' treatment or as required by individual patients, to reduce the severity of acute anoproctitis and perineal dermatitis. Longer intervals of 6 to 8 weeks were part of some schedules to allow time for tumor regression, particularly where further RT was to be prescribed based on the extent of the clinical or histopathologic response to the first phase of treatment.[41,72,73,138] The possible adverse effects of split-course irradiation on the control of anal cancer have not been studied formally, but the limited data available on the potential tumor doubling time of anal cancer suggest that it is relatively rapid and of the order of 4 days (range 1 to 30 days; $n = 26$),[166] so some adverse effect may be expected from unnecessarily prolonged treatment. Recent analyses of treatment duration indicate that the overall treatment time (OTT), including time for induction chemotherapy if given and for prolonged intervals prior to boost RT, may have more influence on outcome than the duration of radiation (RTT). Review of the UKCCCR ACT I trial did not identify an association between OTT and locoregional failure.[163] Analysis of two RTOG trials[73,74] showed a trend toward an association between longer OTT and colostomy failure and a statistically significant association with local failure. RTT and OTT were not correlated with overall or colostomy-free survival rates.[167] There are many potentially confounding factors in these retrospective comparisons, and the optimum duration of overall treatment or RT is not known. The introduction of IMRT techniques does not appear to have led to a consistent reduction in interruptions in RT. The general principle recommended is to avoid, or minimize the length of, all interruptions in the delivery of radiation.

Radiation Alone

If external-beam irradiation is given without concurrent chemotherapy, it is usual, as in other cancers, to prescribe doses close to the tolerance of the normal tissues. There have been no studies to establish the optimum dose–time factors. A dose to the primary tumor of 60 to 65 Gy over 6 to 7 weeks, in 1.8- to 2-Gy fractions, is commonly prescribed, with doses to lymph nodes to be treated electively in the range of 36 Gy in 4 weeks to 50.4 Gy in 5.5 weeks. Brachytherapy may be used for part of the treatment. As with chemoradiation, interruptions in treatment should be minimized.

Perianal Cancer

If small (<4 cm) perianal cancers with low risk of regional node metastases are treated by radiation, a dose of 60 to 66 Gy in 2-Gy fractions over 6 weeks may be used. A direct perineal field is preferred as this minimizes the area of skin irradiated. Orthovoltage equipment may suffice, although electrons or low-energy megavoltage photons (with bolus) are used more commonly. Care should be taken to flatten the perineum as much as possible to avoid areas of over- or underdosage. Larger perianal cancers, or cancers invading the anal canal, are usually treated by the techniques and schedules of radiation and chemotherapy used for anal canal cancers, based on the results of the UKCCCR ACT I trial.[41] Elective nodal irradiation is given to the inguinal and lower external iliac nodes and to the lower perirectal and internal iliac nodes if the tumor extends into the anal canal. The upper border of the fields is usually placed at the lower end of the sacroiliac joints. The final phase of radiation may be given by direct perineal photon or electron therapy. Although brachytherapy may be used for the final phase, full treatment of perianal cancers by brachytherapy was associated with high rates of necrosis in some series.

SEQUELAE OF THERAPY

Surveys of published studies suggest that the delivery of chemotherapy concurrently with RT is associated more with increases in acute rather than late normal tissue toxicity, beyond that expected with RT alone. Some nonrandomized series have described higher acute and late toxicity rates from combined modality therapy than those reported in the multicenter randomized trials. This probably results from use of different criteria for recording and reporting toxicity.

In programs that combined RT, 96-hour to 120-hour infusions of 5-FU (750 to 1,000 mg/m²/24 h) and bolus injections of MMC (10 to 15 mg/m²), moderate leukopenia, thrombocytopenia, anoproctitis, and perineal dermatitis were recorded in about 30% of patients after doses of 25 to 30 Gy in 2.5 to 3 weeks.[39,168] More profound proctitis and dermatitis occurred in up to 55% of those who received

from 50 Gy in 4 to 5 weeks[39,102] to 59.4 Gy in 6.5 weeks.[91] When CDDP was substituted for MMC, marrow toxicity was less, but at radiation doses of 59.4 Gy in 6.5 weeks, acute soft tissue toxicity rates were similar.[74,83] Most large studies of RT, 5-FU, and MMC or CDDP reported some mortality (<2% overall) associated with acute toxicity, usually as a result of neutropenia with sepsis. This risk can be reduced with prophylactic antibiotics[41] and aggressive supportive care.

Serious late toxicity has not been reported after doses of 30 Gy in 3 weeks with 5-FU and MMC, but significant complications, often requiring surgery, were recorded in about 5% to 10% of those receiving higher radiation doses. A review of anal cancer management in Denmark from 1995 to 2003 found 5-year cumulative incidences of tumor-related and treatment-related colostomy of 26% (95% CI, 21% to 32%) and 8% (95% CI, 5% to 12%), respectively.[169] In the randomized RTOG-9811 trial, in those who received RT, 5-FU, and MMC, only 10 of the 30 colostomy procedures performed by about 3 years were for treatment-related problems, a crude rate of about 3%.[59] It is probable that some reports, many of which were retrospective, also overlooked some treatment-related toxicity. For example, a large cohort study of 556 women aged ≥65 who developed anal cancer showed a higher risk of pelvic fracture, principally of the hip, in those who received radiation (n = 399) compared to those not irradiated (n = 157). The cumulative 5-year fracture rate was 14% versus 7.5% (P < .01).[170] One of the objectives of current 3-D conformal and IMRT techniques is to reduce RT dose to the proximal femurs.

There are two additional areas of possible toxicity that need further study. Pelvic RT increases the risk of secondary malignancies,[171] and some of the chemotherapy agents used to treat anal cancer also are associated with a raised risk; these risks have not been quantified in detail for patients treated for anal cancer. Second, in the only report so far of long-term follow-up of patients in a randomized trial, it was found that there were more deaths due to causes other than cancer, particularly cardiovascular related, in the first 10 years following treatment with RT, 5-FU, and MMC.[71] This difference reached +9% at 5 years, but the effect almost disappeared by 10 years. The magnitude of this difference was less than the reduction in deaths from anal cancer. Information from other randomized trials is needed to determine whether this observation was a chance phenomenon or a risk that should be addressed by further research.

Although preservation of anorectal anatomy is an advantage of treatment by chemoradiation, late anorectal function is often abnormal. Side effects of treatment are very common and may cause patients considerable discomfort and social disability, although they are often graded as only level 1 or 2 toxicity.[172–175] These effects include changes in anorectal function such as urgency and frequency of defecation, bleeding from anorectal telangiectasia, perineal dermatitis, pelvic fibrosis, dyspareunia, and impotence. They are usually managed medically with varying success. Systematic and prospective evaluations of the function of the anorectum and of other organs potentially affected by treatment are now being reported, as are formal quality-of-life studies.[135,176] There is often dissociation between a patient's and his or her physician's assessment of anal and rectal function and continence and physiologic measurements of anorectal function. The few studies in this area have been inconclusive.[174,177] Prospective studies of pelvic organ function can be expected to assist the development of radiation treatment protocols by facilitating correlation of function with radiation–chemotherapy interactions, radiation techniques and dose distributions, and time–dose factors.

REFERENCES

1. Nigro ND, Vaitkevicius VK, Considine B. Combined therapy for cancer of the anal canal: a preliminary report. *Dis Colon Rectum* 1974;17:354–356.

2. Edge SB, Byrd DR, Compton CC, et al., eds. *AJCC cancer staging manual.* 7th ed. New York: Springer, 2010.

3. Sobin L, Gospodarowicz M, Wittekind C, eds. *International Union Against Cancer (UICC). TNM classification of malignant tumours.* 7th ed. New York: Wiley-Blackwell, 2009.

4. Fenger C. Histology of the anal canal. *Am J Surg Pathol* 1988;12:41–55.

5. Godlewski G, Prudhomme M. Embryology and anatomy of the anorectum. *Surg Clin North Am* 2000;80:319–343.

6. Fenger C, Frisch M, Marti MC, et al. Tumours of the anal canal. In: Hamilton SR, Aaltonen LA, eds. *Pathology and genetics of tumours of the digestive system.* Lyon, France: IARC Press, 2000:145–155.

7. Shepherd NA. Anal intraepithelial neoplasia and other neoplastic precursor lesions of the anal canal and perianal region. *Gastroenterol Clin North Am* 2007;36:969–987.

8. Cook MB, Dawsey SM, Freedman ND, et al. Sex disparities in cancer incidence by period and age. *Cancer Epidemiol Biomarkers Prev* 2009;18:1174–1182.

9. Johnson LG, Madeleine MM, Newcomer LM, et al. Anal cancer incidence and survival: the Surveillance, Epidemiology, and End Results experience, 1973–2000. *Cancer* 2004;101:281–288.

10. IARC Cancer Monograph Working Group. A review of human carcinogens—Part B: biologic agents. *Lancet Oncol* 2009;10:321–322.

11. Hoots BE, Palefsky JM, Pimenta JM, et al. Human papillomavirus type distribution in anal cancer and anal intraepithelial lesions. *Int J Cancer* 2009;124:2375–2383.

12. De Vuyst H, Clifford GM, Nascimento MC, et al. Prevalence and type distribution of human papillomavirus in carcinoma and intraepithelial neoplasia of the vulva, vagina, and anus: a meta-analysis. *Int J Cancer* 2009;124:1626–1636.

13. Frisch M, Fenger C, van den Brule AJ, et al. Variants of squamous cell carcinoma of the anal canal and perianal skin and their relation to human papillomavirus. *Cancer Res* 1999;59:753–757.

14. Scholefield JH, Kerr IB, Shepherd NA, et al. Human papillomavirus type 16 DNA in anal cancers from six different countries. *Gut* 1991;32:674–676.

15. Frisch M. On the etiology of anal squamous carcinoma. *Dan Med Bull* 2002;49:194–209.

16. Daling JR, Weiss NS, Klopfenstein LL, et al. Correlates of homosexual behavior and the incidence of anal cancer. *JAMA* 1982;247:1988–1990.

17. Daling JR, Weiss NS, Hislop TG, et al. Sexual practices, sexually transmitted diseases, and the incidence of anal cancer. *N Engl J Med* 1987;317:973–977.

18. Frisch M, Biggar RJ, Engels EA, et al. Association of cancer with AIDS-related immunosuppression in adults. *JAMA* 2001;285:1736–1745.

19. Adami J, Gabel H, Lindelof B, et al. Cancer risk following organ transplantation: a nationwide cohort study in Sweden. *Br J Cancer* 2003;89:1221–1227.

20. Critchlow CW, Surawicz CM, Holmes KK, et al. Prospective study of high grade and intraepithelial neoplasia in a cohort of homosexual men: influence of HIV infection, immunosuppression and human papillomavirus infection. *AIDS* 1995;9:1255–1262.

21. Palefsky JM, Holly EA, Hogeboom CJ, et al. Virologic, immunologic, and clinical parameters in the incidence and progression of anal squamous intraepithelial lesions in HIV-positive and HIV-negative homosexual men. *J Acquir Immune Defic Syndr Hum Retrovirol* 1998;17:314–319.

22. Palefsky JM. Anal squamous intraepithelial lesions: relation to HIV and human papillomavirus infection. *J Acquir Immune Defic Syndr* 1999;21:542–548.

23. Simard EP, Pfeiffer RM, Engels EA. Spectrum of cancer risk late after AIDS onset in the United States. *Arch Intern Med* 2010;170:1337–1345.

24. International Collaboration on HIV and Cancer. Highly active antiretroviral therapy and incidence of cancer in human immunodeficiency virus-infected adults. *J Natl Cancer Inst* 2000;92:1823–1830.

25. Palefsky JM, Giuliano AR, Goldstone S, et al. HPV vaccine against anal HPV infection and anal intraepithelial neoplasia. *N Engl J Med* 2011;365:1576–1585.

26. Rambout L, Hopkins L, Hutton B, et al. Prophylactic vaccination against human papillomavirus infection and disease in women: a systematic review of randomized controlled trials. *CMAJ* 2007;177:469–479.

27. Daling JR, Sherman KJ, Hislop TG, et al. Cigarette smoking and the risk of anogenital cancer. *Am J Epidemiol* 1992;135:180–189.

28. Frisch M, Olsen JH, Bautz A, et al. Benign anal lesions and the risk of anal cancer. *N Engl J Med* 1994;331:300–302.

29. Frisch M, Johansen C. Anal carcinoma in inflammatory bowel disease. *Br J Cancer* 2000;83:89–90.

30. Klencke BJ, Palefsky JM. Anal cancer: an HIV-associated cancer. *Hematol Oncol Clin North Am* 2003;17:859–872.

31. Boman BM, Moertel CG, O'Connell M, et al. Carcinoma of the anal canal: a clinical and pathological study of 188 cases. *Cancer* 1984;54:114–125.

32. Myerson RJ, Karnell LH, Menck HR. The National Cancer Data Base report on carcinoma of the anus. *Cancer* 1997;80:805–815.

33. Bilimoria KY, Bentrem DJ, Rock CE, et al. Outcomes and prognostic factors for squamous cell carcinoma of the anal canal: analysis of patients from the National Cancer Data Base. *Dis Colon Rectum* 2009;52:624–631.

34. Frost DB, Richards PC, Montague ED, et al. Epidermoid cancer of the anorectum. *Cancer* 1984;53:1285.

35. Stearns MW, Urmacher C, Sternberg SS, et al. Cancer of the anal canal. *Curr Probl Cancer* 1980;4:1–44.

36. Gerard JP, Chapet O, Samiei F, et al. Management of inguinal lymph node metastases in patients with carcinoma of the anal canal. Experience in a

37. Salmon RJ, Fenton J, Asselain B, et al. Treatment of epidermoid anal canal cancer. *Am J Surg* 1984;147:43–48.

38. Ortholan C, Resbeut M, Hannoun-Levi JM, et al. Anal canal cancer: management of inguinal nodes and benefit of prophylactic inguinal irradiation (CORS-03 study). *Int J Radiat Oncol Biol Phys* 2012;82(5):1988–1995.

39. Cummings BJ, Keane TJ, O'Sullivan B, et al. Epidermoid anal cancer: treatment by radiation and 5-fluorouracil with and without mitomycin C. *Int J Radiat Oncol Biol Phys* 1991;21:1115–1125.

40. Touboul E, Schlienger M, Buffat L, et al. Epidermoid carcinoma of the anal canal. *Cancer* 1994;73:1569–1579.

41. UKCCCR Anal Canal Cancer Trial Working Party. Epidermoid anal cancer: results from the UKCCCR randomized trial of radiotherapy alone versus radiotherapy, 5-fluorouracil and mitomycin C. *Lancet* 1996;348:1049–1054.

42. Edwards AT, Morus LC, Goster ME, et al. Anal cancer: the case for earlier diagnosis. *J R Soc Med* 1991;84:395–397.

43. Tanum G, Tveit K, Karlsen KO. Diagnosis of anal carcinoma—doctor's finger still the best? *Oncology* 1991;48:383–386.

44. Wolfe HR, Bussey HJ. Squamous cell carcinoma of the anus. *Br J Surg* 1968;55:295–301.

45. Cataldo PA, MacKeigan JM. The necessity of routine pathologic evaluation of hemorrhoidectomy specimens. *Surg Gynecol Obstet* 1992;174:302–304.

46. Wasvary HJ, Barkel DC, Klein SN. Is total colonic evaluation for anal cancer necessary? *Am Surg* 2000;66:592–594.

47. Wade DS, Herrera L, Castillo NB, et al. Metastases to the lymph nodes in epidermoid carcinoma of the anal canal studied by a clearing technique. *Surg Gynecol Obstet* 1989;169:238–242.

48. Goh V, Gollub FK, Liaw J, et al. Magnetic resonance imaging assessment of squamous cell carcinoma of the anal canal before and after chemoradiation: can MRI predict for eventual clinical outcome? *Int J Radiat Oncol Biol Phys* 2010;78:715–721.

49. Cotter SE, Grigsby PW, Siegal BA, et al. FDG-PET/CT in the evaluation of anal carcinoma. *Int J Radiat Oncol Biol Phys* 2006;65:720–725.

50. Krengli M, Milia ME, Turri L, et al. FDG-PET/CT imaging for staging and target volume delineation in conformal radiotherapy of anal carcinoma. *Radiat Oncol* 2010;5:10.

51. Mai SK, Welzel G, Hermann B, Wenz F, Haberkorn U, Dinter DJ. Can the radiation dose to CT enlarged but FDG-PET-negative inguinal lymph node in anal cancer be reduced? *Strahlenther Onkol* 2009;185:254–259.

52. Mistrangelo M, Pelosi E, Bello M, et al. Comparison of positron emission tomography scanning and sentinel node biopsy in the detection of inguinal node metastases in patients with anal cancer. *Int J Radiat Oncol Biol Phys* 2010;77:73–78.

53. de Jong JS, Beukema JC, Van Dam GM, et al. Limited value of staging squamous cell carcinoma of the margin and canal using the sentinel lymph node procedure: a prospective study with long-term follow-up. *Ann Surg Oncol* 2010;17:2656–2662.

54. Cummings BJ. Anal cancer. In: Gospodarowicz MK, O'Sullivan B, Sobin LH, eds. *Prognostic factors in cancer.* 3rd ed. Hoboken, NJ: Wiley, 2006:139–142.

55. Greenall MJ, Quan SHQ, Decosse JJ. Epidermoid cancer of the anus. *Br J Surg* 1985;72(Suppl):S97.

56. Tanum G. Treatment of relapsing anal carcinoma. *Acta Oncol* 1993;32:33–35.

57. Tanum G, Tveit K, Karlsen KO, et al. Chemotherapy and radiation therapy for anal carcinoma: survival and late morbidity. *Cancer* 1991;67:2462–2466.

58. Goldman S, Auer G, Erhardt K, et al. Prognostic significance of clinical stage, histologic grade, and nuclear DNA content in squamous cell carcinoma of the anus. *Dis Colon Rectum* 1987;30:444–448.

59. Ajani JA, Winter KA, Gunderson LL, et al. US Intergroup Anal Carcinoma Trial: tumor diameter predicts for colostomy. *J Clin Oncol* 2009;27:1116–1121.

60. Ajani JA, Winter KA, Gunderson LL, et al. Prognostic factors derived from a prospective database dictate clinical biology of anal cancer. The Intergroup Trial (RTOG 98–11). *Cancer* 2010;116:4007–4013.

61. Ramamoorthy S, Luo L, Luo E, et al. Tobacco smoking and risk of recurrence for squamous cell cancer of the anus. *Cancer Detect Prev* 2008;32:116–120.

62. Hoffman R, Welton ML, Klenche B, et al. The significance of pretreatment CD4 count on the outcome and treatment tolerance of HIV-positive patients with anal cancer. *Int J Radiat Oncol Biol Phys* 1999;44:127–131.

63. Place RJ, Gregorcyk SG, Huber PJ, et al. Outcome analysis of HIV-positive patients with anal squamous cell carcinoma. *Dis Colon Rectum* 2001;44:506–512.

64. Oehler-Janne C, Huguet F, Provender S, et al. HIV-specific differences in outcome of squamous cell carcinoma of the anal canal: a multicentric cohort study of HIV-positive patients receiving highly active antiretroviral therapy. *J Clin Oncol* 2008;26:2550–2557.

65. Fenger C. Prognostic factors in anal carcinoma. *Pathology* 2002;34:573–578.

66. Mawdsley S, Meadows HH, Royston P. Role of molecular markers in the clinical outcome and prediction of response to treatment in squamous anal cancer. *Proc ASCO* 2003;22:3566.

67. Ajani JA, Wang X, Izzo JG, et al. Molecular biomarkers correlate with disease-free survival in patients with anal canal carcinoma treated with chemoradiation. *Dig Dis Sci* 2010;55:1098–1105.

68. Bruland O, Fluge O, Immervoll H, et al. Gene expression reveals 2 distinct groups of anal carcinomas with clinical implications. *Br J Cancer* 2008;98:1264–1273.

69. Peiffert D, Bey P, Pernot M, et al. Conservative treatment by irradiation of epidermoid cancers of the anal canal: prognostic factors of tumoral control and complications. *Int J Radiat Oncol Biol Phys* 1997;37:313–324.

series of 270 patients treated in Lyon and review of the literature. *Cancer* 2001;92:77–84.

70. Chapet O, Gerard JP, Riche B, et al. Prognostic value of tumor regression evaluated after first course of radiotherapy for anal canal cancer. *Int J Radiat Oncol Biol Phys* 2005;63:1316–1324.
71. Northover J, Glynne-Jones R, Sebag-Montefiore D, et al. Chemoradiation for the treatment of epidermoid anal cancer: 13-year follow-up of the first randomized UKCCCR Anal Cancer Trial (ACT I). *Br J Cancer* 2010;102:1123–1128.
72. Bartelink H, Roelofsen F, Eschwege F, et al. Concomitant radiotherapy and chemotherapy is superior to radiotherapy alone in the treatment of locally advanced anal cancer: results of a phase III randomized trial of the European Organization for Research and Treatment of Cancer Radiotherapy and Gastrointestinal Cooperative Groups. *J Clin Oncol* 1997;15:2040–2049.
73. Flam M, John M, Pajak TF, et al. The role of mitomycin C in combination with 5-fluorouracil and radiotherapy, and of salvage chemoradiation in the definitive nonsurgical treatment of epidermoid carcinoma of the anal canal: results of a phase III randomized Intergroup study. *J Clin Oncol* 1996;14:2527–2539.
74. Ajani JA, Winter KA, Gunderson LL, et al. Fluorouracil, mitomycin, and radiotherapy vs fluorouracil, cisplatin and radiotherapy for carcinoma of the anal canal; a randomized controlled trial. *JAMA* 2008;299:1914–1921.
75. Gunderson LL, Winter KA, Ajani JA, et al. Long-term update of US GI Intergroup RTOG 98–11 phase III trial for anal carcinoma: disease-free and overall survival with RT + 5FU – mitomycin versus RT + 5FU-cisplatin. *J Clin Oncol* 2011; 29(Suppl):4005.
76. James R, Wan S, Sebag-Montefiore D, et al. A randomized trial of chemoradiation using mitomycin or cisplatin, with or without maintenance cisplatin/5FU in squamous cell carcinoma of the anus (ACT II). *J Clin Oncol* 2009;27(Suppl):LBA4009.
77. Conroy T, Ducreux M, Lemanski C, et al. Treatment intensification by induction chemotherapy (ICT) and radiation dose escalation in locally advanced squamous cell anal canal carcinoma (LAAC): definitive analysis of the intergroup ACCORD 03 trial. *J Clin Oncol* 2009;27(Suppl):4033.
78. Peiffert D, Gerard JP, Ducreux M, et al. Induction chemotherapy (ICT) and dose intensification of the radiation boost in locally advanced anal canal carcinoma (LAACC): definitive analysis of the Intergroup ACCORD 03 trial (Federation Nationale des Centres de Lutte Contre le Cancer, Fondation Francaise de Cancerologie Digestive). *Radiother Oncol* 2008;88(Suppl 2):S20.
79. Lim F, Glynne-Jones R. Chemotherapy/chemoradiation in anal cancer: a systematic review. *Cancer Treat Rev* 2011;37:520–532.
80. Papillon J, Montbarbon JF. Epidermoid carcinoma of the anal canal: a series of 276 cases. *Dis Colon Rectum* 1987;30:324–333.
81. Cummings BJ. The place of radiation therapy in the treatment of carcinoma of the anal canal. *Cancer Treat Rev* 1982;9:125–147.
82. Gerard JP, Ayzac L, Hun D, et al. Treatment of anal canal carcinoma with high dose radiation therapy and concomitant fluorouracil-cisplatinum. Long term results in 95 patients. *Radiother Oncol* 1998;46:249–256.
83. Martenson JA, Lipsitz SR, Wagner H, et al. Initial results of a phase II trial of radiation therapy, 5-fluorouracil and cisplatin for patients with anal cancer. *Int J Radiat Oncol Biol Phys* 1996;35:745–749.
84. Doci R, Zucali R, La Monica G, et al. Primary chemoradiation therapy with fluorouracil and cisplatin for cancer of the anus: results in 35 consecutive patients. *J Clin Oncol* 1996;14:3121–3125.
85. Hung A, Crane C, Delclos M, et al. Cisplatin-based combined modality therapy for anal carcinoma: a wider therapeutic index. *Cancer* 2003;97:1195–1202.
86. Peiffert D, Giovanni M, Ducreux M, et al. High dose radiation therapy and neoadjuvant plus concomitant chemotherapy with 5 fluorouracil and cisplatin in patients with locally advanced squamous cell anal canal cancer: final results of a phase II study. *Ann Oncol* 2001;12:397–404.
87. Brunet R, Becouarn Y, Pigneux J, et al. Cisplatin et fluorouracile en chimiothérapie neoadjuvante des carcinomas épidermoides du canal anal. *Lyon Chir* 1990;87:77–79.
88. Roca E, De Simone G, Barugel M, et al. A phase II study of alternating chemoradiotherapy including cisplatin in anal canal carcinoma. *Proc Am Soc Clin Oncol* 1990;9:128(abstr).
89. Constantinou EC, Daly W, Fung CY, et al. Time-dose considerations with treatment of anal cancer. *Int J Radiat Oncol Biol Phys* 1997;39:651–657.
90. Rich TA, Ajani JA, Morrison WH, et al. Chemoradiation therapy for anal cancer: radiation plus continuous infusion of 5-fluorouracil with or without cisplatin. *Radiother Oncol* 1993;27:209–215.
91. John M, Pajak T, Flam M, et al. Dose acceleration in chemoradiation for anal cancer: preliminary results of RTOG 9208. *Cancer J Sci Am* 1996;2:205–207.
92. John M, Pajak T, Krieg R, et al. Dose escalation without split-course chemoradiation for anal cancer: results of a phase II RTOG study. *Int J Radiat Oncol Biol Phys* 1997;39(Suppl 2):203 (abstr).
93. Glynne-Jones R, Meadows H, Wan S, et al. EXTRA—A multicentre phase II study using a 5-day per week oral regimen of capecitabine and intravenous mitomycin C in anal cancer. *Int J Radiat Oncol Biol Phys* 2008;72:119–126.
94. Matzinger O, Roelofsen F, Mineur L, et al. Mitomycin C with continuous fluorouracil or with cisplatin in combination with radiotherapy for locally advanced anal cancer (European Organization for Research and Treatment of Cancer phase II study 22011–40014). *Eur J Cancer* 2009;45:2782–2791.
95. NIH Clinical Trials Registry. Available at: http://clinicaltrials.gov/
96. Van Damme N, Deron P, Van Roy N, et al. Epidermal growth factor receptor and K-RAS status in two cohorts of squamous cell cancers. *BMC Cancer* 2010;10:189.
97. Friberg B, Svensson C, Goldman S, et al. The Swedish National Care Programme for anal carcinoma. Implementation and overall results. *Acta Oncol* 1998;37:25–32.
98. Goldman S, Glimelius B, Glas U, et al. Management of anal epidermoid carcinoma: an evaluation of treatment results in two population-based series. *Int J Colorectal Dis* 1989;4:234–243.
99. Nilsson PJ, Svensson C, Goldman S, et al. Epidermoid anal cancer: a review of a population-based series of 308 consecutive patients treated according to prospective protocols. *Int J Radiat Oncol Biol Phys* 2005;61:92–102.
100. James RD, David C, Neville D, et al. Chemoradiation and maintenance chemotherapy for patients with anal carcinoma: a phase II study of the UK Coordinating Committee for Cancer Research (UKCCCR) Anal Cancer Trial Working Party. *Proc Am Soc Clin Oncol* 2000;19:268a(abstr).
101. Nigro ND. An evaluation of combined therapy for squamous cell cancer of the anal canal. *Dis Colon Rectum* 1984;27:763–766.
102. Tanum G, Tveit K, Karlsen KO, et al. Chemoradiotherapy of anal carcinoma: tumour response and acute toxicity. *Oncology* 1993;50:14–17.
103. Schwarz JK, Siegal BA, Dehdashti F, et al. Tumor response and survival predicted by post-therapy FDG-PET/CT in anal cancer. *Int J Radiat Oncol Biol Phys* 2008;71:180–186.
104. Akbari RP, Paty PB, Guillem JG, et al. Oncologic outcomes of salvage surgery of epidermoid carcinoma of the anus initially managed by combined modality therapy. *Dis Colon Rectum* 2004;47:1134–1144.
105. Renehan AG, Sanders MP, Schofield PF, et al. Patterns of local disease failure and outcome after salvage surgery in patients with anal cancer. *Br J Surg* 2005;92:605–614.
106. Schiller DE, Cummings BJ, Rai S, et al. Outcomes of salvage surgery for squamous cell carcinoma of the anal canal. *Ann Surg Oncol* 2007;14:2780–2789.
107. Ghouti L, Houvenaeghel G, Moutardier V, et al. Salvage abdominoperineal resection after failure of conservative treatment in anal epidermoid cancer. *Dis Colon Rectum* 2005;48:16–22.
108. Scholefield JH, Ogunbiji OA, Smith JH, et al. Treatment of anal intraepithelial neoplasia. *Br J Surg* 1994;81:1238–1240.
109. Greenall MJ, Quan SHQ, Stearns MW, et al. Epidermoid cancer of the anal margin. *Am J Surg* 1985;149:95–101.
110. Greenall MJ, Quan SHQ, Urmacher C, et al. Treatment of epidermoid carcinoma of the anal canal. *Surg Gynecol Obstet* 1985;161:509–517.
111. Klas JV, Rothenberger DA, Wong WD, et al. Malignant tumors of the anal canal. The spectrum of disease, treatment and outcomes. *Cancer* 1999;85:1686–1693.
112. Ortholan C, Ramaioli A, Peiffert D, et al. Anal canal carcinoma: early stage tumors ≤10 mm (T1 or Tis): therapeutic options and original pattern of local failure after radiotherapy. *Int J Radiat Oncol Biol Phys* 2005;62:479–485.
113. Eng C, Pathak P. Treatment options in metastatic squamous cell carcinoma of the anal canal. *Curr Treat Options Oncol* 2008;9:400–407.
114. Lukan N, Strobel P, Willer A, et al. Cetuximab-based treatment of metastatic anal cancer: correlation of response with KRAS mutational status. *Oncology* 2009;77:293–299.
115. Bieri S, Allal AS, Kurtz JM. Sphincter-conserving treatment of carcinomas of the anal margin. *Acta Oncol* 2001;40:29–33.
116. Newlin HE, Zlotecki RA, Morris CG, et al. Squamous cell carcinoma of the anal margin. *J Surg Oncol* 2004;86:55–62.
117. Chapet O, Gerard JP, Mornex F, et al. Prognostic factors of squamous cell carcinoma of the anal margin treated by radiotherapy: the Lyon experience. *Int J Colorectal Dis* 2007;22:191–199.
118. Papillon J, Chassard JL. Respective roles of radiotherapy and surgery in the management of epidermoid cancer of the anal margin. *Dis Colon Rectum* 1992;35:422–429.
119. Khanfir K, Ozsahin M, Bieri S, et al. Patterns of failure and outcome in patients with carcinoma of the anal margin. *Ann Surg Oncol* 2008;15:1092–1098.
120. Cleator S, Fife K, Nelson M, et al. Treatment of HIV-associated invasive anal cancer with combined chemoradiation. *Eur J Cancer* 2000;36:754–758.
121. Edelman S, Johnstone PA. Combined modality therapy for HIV-infected patients with squamous cell carcinoma of the anus: outcomes and toxicities. *Int J Radiat Oncol Biol Phys* 2006;66:206–211.
122. Peddada AV, Smith DE, Rao AR, et al. Chemotherapy and low-dose radiotherapy in the treatment of HIV-infected patients with carcinoma of the anal canal. *Int J Radiat Oncol Biol Phys* 1997;37:1101–1105.
123. Hammad N, Heilbrun LK, Gupta S, et al. Squamous cell cancer of the anal canal in HIV-infected patients receiving highly active antiretroviral therapy. *Am J Clin Oncol* 2011;34:135–139.
124. Chiao EY, Giordano TP, Richardson P, et al. Human immunodeficiency virus-associated squamous cell cancer of the anus: epidemiology and outcomes in the highly active antiretroviral therapy era. *J Clin Oncol* 2008;299:1914–1921.
125. Formenti SC, Chak L, Gill P, et al. Increased radiosensitivity of normal tissue fibroblasts in patients with acquired immunodeficiency syndrome (AIDS) and with Kaposi's sarcoma. *Int J Radiat Biol* 1995;68:411–412.
126. Holland JM, Swift PS. Tolerance of patients with human immunodeficiency virus and anal carcinoma to treatment with combined chemotherapy and radiation therapy. *Radiology* 1994;193:251–254.
127. Kounalakis N, Artinyan A, Smith D, et al. Abdominal perineal resection improves survival for nonmetastatic adenocarcinoma of the anal canal. *Ann Surg Oncol* 2009;16:1310–1315.
128. Belkacemi Y, Berger C, Poortmans P, et al. Management of anal canal adenocarcinoma: a large retrospective study from the Rare Cancer Network. *Int J Radiat Oncol Biol Phys* 2003;56:1274–1283.
129. Tarazi R, Nelson RL. Anal adenocarcinoma: a comprehensive review. *Semin Surg Oncol* 1994;10:235–240.
130. Chang GJ, Gonzalez RJ, Skibbar JM, et al. A twenty-year experience with adenocarcinoma of the anal canal. *Dis Colon Rectum* 2009;52:1375–1380.
131. Joon DL, Chao MW, Ngan SY, et al. Primary adenocarcinoma of the anus: a retrospective analysis. *Int J Radiat Oncol Biol Phys* 1999;45:1199–1205.
132. Lee J, Corman M. Recurrence of anal adenocarcinoma after local excision and adjuvant chemoradiation therapy: report of a case and review of the literature. *J Gastrointest Surg* 2009;13:150–154.

133. Papagikos M, Crane CH, Skibber J, et al. Chemoradiation for adenocarcinoma of the anus. *Int J Radiat Oncol Biol Phys* 2003;55:669–678.

134. Wright JL, Patil SM, Temple LK, et al. Squamous cell carcinoma of the anal canal: patterns and predictors of failure and implications for intensity-modulated radiation treatment and planning. *Int J Radiat Oncol Biol Phys* 2010;78:1064–1072.

135. Han K, Craig T, Skliarenko J, et al. Prospective evaluation of IMRT for anal and perianal cancer: early patterns of failure. *Int J Radiat Oncol Biol Phys* 2011;81(2 Suppl):S125–S126.

136. Das P, Bhatia S, Eng C, et al. Predictions and patterns of recurrence after definitive chemoradiation for anal cancer. *Int J Radiat Oncol Biol Phys* 2007;68:794–800.

137. Matthews JH, Burmeister BH, Borg M, et al. T1-T2 anal carcinoma requires elective inguinal radiation treatment—the results of Trans-Tasman Radiation Oncology Group Study TROG 99.02. *Radiother Oncol* 2011;98:93–98.

138. Papillon J. *Rectal and anal cancers: conservative treatment by irradiation. an alternative to radical surgery.* Berlin, Germany: Springer-Verlag, 1982.

139. Cummings BJ, Keane TJ, Thomas GM, et al. Results and toxicity of the treatment of anal canal carcinoma by radiation therapy or radiation therapy and chemotherapy. *Cancer* 1984;54:2062–2068.

140. Melcher AA, Sebag-Montefiore D. Concurrent chemoradiotherapy for squamous cell carcinoma of the anus using shrinking field radiotherapy technique without a boost. *Br J Cancer* 2003;88:1352–1357.

141. Koh WJ, Chiu M, Stelzer KJ, et al. Femoral vessel depth and the implications for groin node radiation. *Int J Radiat Oncol Biol Phys* 1993;27:969–974.

142. Vuong T, Devic S, Belliveau P, et al. Contribution of conformal therapy in the treatment of anal canal carcinoma with combined chemotherapy and radiotherapy: results of a phase II study. *Int J Radiat Oncol Biol Phys* 2003;56:823–831.

143. Chen YJ, Liu A, Tsai PT, et al. Organ sparing by conformal avoidance intensity-modulated radiation therapy for anal cancer: dosimetric evaluation of coverage of pelvis and inguinal/femoral nodes. *Int J Radiat Oncol Biol Phys* 2005;63:274–281.

144. Papillon J, Montbarbon JF, Gerard JP, et al. Interstitial curietherapy in the conservative treatment of anal and rectal cancers. *Int J Radiat Oncol Biol Phys* 1989;17:1161–1169.

145. Wagner JP, Mahe MA, Romestaing P, et al. Radiation therapy in the conservative treatment of epidermoid carcinoma of the anal canal. *Int J Radiat Oncol Biol Phys* 1994;29:17–23.

146. Gerard JP, Mauro F, Thomas L, et al. Treatment of squamous cell anal canal carcinoma with pulse dose rate brachytherapy. Feasibility study of a French Cooperative Group. *Radiother Oncol* 1999;51:129–131.

147. Roed H, Engelholm SA, Svendsen LB, et al. Pulsed dose rate (PDR) brachytherapy of anal carcinoma. *Radiother Oncol* 1996;41:131–134.

148. Peiffert D. Comment on pulsed dose rate (PDR) brachytherapy of anal carcinoma by Roed et al. [letter]. *Radiother Oncol* 1997;44:296–297.

149. Kapp KS, Geyer E, Gebhart FH, et al. Experience with split-course external beam irradiation +/− chemotherapy and integrated Ir-192 high–dose-rate brachytherapy in the treatment of primary carcinomas of the anal canal. *Int J Radiat Oncol Biol Phys* 2001;49:997–1005.

150. Vordermark D, Flentje M, Sailer M, et al. Intracavitary after-loading boost in anal canal carcinoma. Results, function and quality of life. *Strahlenther Onkol* 2001;177:252–258.

151. Doniec JM, Schniewind B, Kovacs G, et al. Multimodal therapy of anal cancer aided by new endosonographic-guided brachytherapy. *Surg Endosc* 2006;20:673–678.

152. Joseph KJ, Syme A, Small C, et al. A treatment planning study comparing helical tomotherapy with intensity-modulated radiotherapy for the treatment of anal cancer. *Radiother Oncol* 2010;94:60–66.

153. Vieillot S, Azria D, Lemanski C, et al. Plan comparison of volumetric-modulated arc therapy (RapidArc) and conventional intensity-modulated radiation therapy (IMRT) in anal canal cancer. *Radiat Oncol* 2010;5:92.

154. Salama JK, Mell LK, Schomas DA, et al. Concurrent chemotherapy and intensity-modulated radiation therapy for anal cancer patients: a multi-center experience. *J Clin Oncol* 2007;25:4581–4586.

155. Clivio A, Fogliata A, Franzetti-Pellanda A, et al. Volumetric-modulated arc radiotherapy for carcinoma of the anal canal: a treatment planning comparison with fixed field IMRT. *Radiother Oncol* 2009;92:118–124.

156. Kachnic L, Winter K, Myerson R, et al. RTOG 0529: a phase II evaluation of dose-painted IMRT in combination with 5-fluorouracil and mitomycin-C for reduction of acute morbidity in carcinoma of the anal canal. *Int J Radiat Oncol Biol Phys* 2009;75(Suppl):S5.

157. Kachnic LA, Tsai HK, Coen JJ, et al. Dose-painted intensity-modulated radiation therapy for anal cancer; a multi-institutional report of acute toxicity and response to therapy. *Int J Radiat Oncol Biol Phys* 2010;78(Suppl 3):S55.

158. Myerson RJ, Garofolo MC, El Naqa I, et al. Elective clinical target volumes for conformal therapy in anorectal cancer: a Radiation Therapy Oncology Group consensus panel contouring atlas. *Int J Radiat Oncol Biol Phys* 2009;74:824–830.

159. Hu K, Minsky BD, Cohen AM, et al. 30 Gy may be an adequate dose in patients with anal cancer treated with excisional biopsy followed by combined-modality therapy. *J Surg Oncol* 1999;70:71–77.

160. Leichman L, Nigro N, Vaitkevicius VK, et al. Cancer of the anal canal: model for preoperative adjuvant combined modality therapy. *Am J Med* 1985;78:211–215.

161. Doci R, Zucali R, Bombelli L, et al. Combined chemoradiation therapy for anal cancer. *Ann Surg* 1992;215:150–156.

162. Schneider IHF, Grabenbauer GG, Reck T, et al. Combined radiation and chemotherapy for epidermoid carcinoma of the anal canal. *Int J Colorectal Dis* 1992;7:192–196.

163. Glynne-Jones R, Sebag-Montefiore D, Adams R, et al. "Mind the gap"—the impact of variations in the duration of the treatment gap and overall treatment time in the first UK anal cancer trial (ACT I). *Int J Radiat Oncol Biol Phys* 2011;81:1488–1494.

164. Cummings BJ. Is there a limit to dose escalation for rectal cancer? *Clin Oncol* 2007;19:730–737.

165. Heemsbergen WD, Hoogeman MS, Hart GA, et al. Gastrointestinal toxicity and its relation to dose distributions in the anorectal region of prostate cancer patients treated with radiotherapy. *Int J Radiat Oncol Biol Phys* 2005;61:1101–1018.

166. Wong CS, Tsang RW, Cummings BJ, et al. Proliferation parameters in epidermoid carcinomas of the anal canal. *Radiother Oncol* 2000;56:349–353.

167. Ben-Josef E, Moughan J, Ajani JA, et al. Impact of overall treatment time on survival and local control in patients with anal cancer; a pooled data analysis of Radiation Therapy Oncology Group trials 87–04 and 98–11. *J Clin Oncol* 2010;28:5061–5066.

168. Sischy N, Doggett RL, Krall JM, et al. Definitive irradiation and chemotherapy for radiosensitization in management of anal carcinoma: interim report on Radiation Therapy Oncology Group Study no. 8314. *J Natl Cancer Inst* 1989;81:850–856.

169. Sunesen KG, Norgaard M, Lundby L, et al. Cause-specific colostomy rates after radiotherapy for anal cancer: a Danish multicentre cohort study. *J Clin Oncol* 2011;29:3535–3540.

170. Baxter NN, Habermann EB, Tepper JE, et al. Risk of pelvic fractures in older women following pelvic irradiation. *JAMA* 2005;294:2587–2593.

171. Wright JD, St Clair CM, Deutsch I, et al. Pelvic radiotherapy and the risk of secondary leukemia and multiple myeloma. *Cancer* 2010;116:2486–2492.

172. Allal AS, Sprangers MA, Laurencet F, et al. Assessment of long-term quality of life in patients with anal carcinomas treated by radiotherapy with or without chemotherapy. *Br J Cancer* 1999;80:1588–1594.

173. Jephcott CR, Pattiel C, Hay J. Quality of life after non-surgical treatment of anal carcinoma: a case control study of long-term survivors. *Clin Oncol* 2004;16:530–535.

174. Vordermark D, Sailer M, Flentje M, et al. Curative intent radiation therapy in anal carcinoma: quality of life and sphincter function. *Radiother Oncol* 1999;52:239–243.

175. Das P, Cantor SB, Parker CL, et al. Long-term quality of life after radiotherapy for the treatment of anal cancer. *Cancer* 2010;116:822–829.

176. Tournier-Rangeard L, Mercier M, Peiffert D, et al. Radiochemotherapy of locally advanced anal canal carcinoma: prospective assessment of early impact on the quality of life (randomized trial ACCORD 03). *Radiother Oncol* 2008;87:391–397.

177. Broens P, Van Limbergen E, Penninckx F, et al. Clinical and manometric effects of combined external beam irradiation and brachytherapy for anal cancer. *Int J Colorectal Dis* 1998;13:68–72.

178. Newman G, Calverley DC, Acker BD, et al. The management of carcinoma of the anal canal by external beam radiotherapy: experience in Vancouver 1971–1988. *Radiother Oncol* 1992;25:196–202.

179. Martenson JA, Gunderson LL. External radiation therapy without chemotherapy in the management of anal cancer. *Cancer* 1993;71:1736–1740.

180. Otim-Oyet D, Ford H, Fisher C, et al. Radical radiotherapy for carcinoma of the anal canal. *Clin Oncol* 1990;2:84–89.

CHAPTER 67

Cancer of the Kidney, Renal Pelvis, and Ureter

Hiram A. Gay and Jeff M. Michalski

ANATOMY

The kidneys are retroperitoneal structures located at the level between the 11th rib and the transverse process of the 3rd lumbar vertebral body. Usually, the right kidney is inferior to the right hepatic lobe and slightly more inferior than the left kidney. The renal axis runs parallel to the lateral margin of the psoas muscle. Each kidney is approximately 11 to 12 cm in length. The kidney is encased by a fibrous capsule and surrounded by perinephric fat, which is enveloped by Gerota fascia. At the renal hilus are the pelvis, ureter, renal artery, and vein. The organs adjacent to the right kidney include the liver superiorly, the duodenum and the vertebral bodies medially, and the transverse colon and small bowel anteriorly. On the left, the kidney abuts the spleen laterally; the stomach, pancreas, and vertebral bodies medially; and the small bowel and colon anteriorly.

The kidney consists of the cortex (glomeruli, convoluted tubules) and the medulla (Henle loops, collecting ducts, and pyramids of converging tubules). Each papilla opens in the minor calices, which unite in the major calices and drain into the renal pelvis. The caliceal collecting systems lie on the anteromedial surface of each kidney. The ureteropelvic junction is variable in position but serves as the landmark to separate the renal pelvis and the ureter. The ureters course posteriorly and inferiorly, paralleling the lateral border of the psoas muscle until they curve anteriorly to join the bladder at the trigone. The mucosal surfaces of the renal collecting tubules, calyces, renal pelvis, ureter, bladder, and urethra all have the same embryologic origin. The renal pelvis and ureter have the following layers: epithelium, subepithelial connective tissue, and muscularis, which is continuous with a connective tissue adventitial layer.

The lymphatics of the kidney and renal pelvis drain along the renal vessels. The right kidney drains predominantly into the paracaval and interaortocaval lymph nodes, and the left kidney drains exclusively to the para-aortic lymph nodes.[1] The lymphatic drainage of the ureter is segmented and diffuse and may involve any of the renal hilar, abdominal para-aortic, paracaval, common iliac, internal iliac, or external iliac lymph nodes.

EPIDEMIOLOGY AND RISK FACTORS

The lesions discussed in this chapter are limited to adult renal cell carcinoma (RCC) and urothelial carcinoma of the renal pelvis and ureter. Lymphomas, Wilms tumor, neuroblastoma, and primary retroperitoneal sarcomas, including rhabdomyosarcoma, are discussed in Chapters 79, 81, 82, 89, 90, and 91, respectively. Approximately 88% of solid renal masses are malignant, and the probability of malignancy is proportional to the size of the lesion.[2] RCCs comprise 80% to 85% of primary kidney tumors, whereas urothelial (transitional cell) carcinomas of the renal pelvis account for 7% of kidney tumors.

Renal Cell Carcinoma

Globally in 2012, the male kidney cancer incidence and mortality age-standardized rate per 100,000 (ASR) was 12.6 and 4.2 in more developed areas and 3.4 and 1.7 in less developed areas, respectively. The estimated new kidney cancer cases in males in developed countries were 125,400, with 47,900 deaths. In contrast, the female kidney cancer incidence and mortality ASR was 6.2 and 1.7 in more developed areas and 1.8 and 0.9 in less developed areas, respectively. The estimated new kidney cancer cases in females in developed countries were 47,900.[3]

In the United States in 2017, the estimated number of new cases of kidney and renal pelvis cancer was 64,990, with 14,400 deaths. Men are twice as likely as women to be diagnosed with kidney cancer. These figures represent approximately 4% of all new cancers and 2% of cancer-related deaths. Incidence rates of kidney cancers increased over the past decades from incidental diagnoses during abdominal imaging, but appear to have stabilized in recent years. Since 2002, kidney cancer death rates have decreased approximately 1% per year.[4]

The median age of RCC diagnosis is 65 years. Few large epidemiologic studies have demonstrated a significant link between occupational exposure and RCC. Danish workers exposed to trichloroethylene, an industrial solvent used as a metal degreaser, had an 8-fold higher incidence of kidney cancer.[5] Occupations associated with a higher risk of RCC are employment in the blast-furnace, coke-oven, or the iron and steel industry and exposure to asbestos, cadmium, drycleaning solvents, gasoline, and other petroleum products.[6] A number of other environmental (e.g., exposure to thorium dioxide), hormonal (e.g., diethylstilbestrol), dietary (e.g., high total energy intake and fried meats increase the risk, whereas vegetables, fruits, and alcohol are protective), cellular, and genetic factors have been associated with the development of RCC.[7–9]

Long-term cigarette smoking is associated with an increased risk of developing RCC. Obesity, diabetes, hepatitis C, and hypertension are also associated with a higher relative risk for development of these tumors.[10–12] Cytotoxic chemotherapy may predispose childhood cancer survivors to translocation RCC, bearing TFE3 or TFEB gene fusions.[13]

Acquired cystic kidney disease (ACKD), which occurs in up to 50% of patients on dialysis for more than 3 years, increases 50-fold the risk of developing RCC.[14,15] The ACKD-associated RCC is seen mostly in males, occurs approximately 20 years earlier than in the general population, and is frequently bilateral (9%) and multicentric (50%).[15]

Several inherited cancer syndromes affect the kidney: von Hippel-Lindau (VHL) disease, hereditary papillary renal cancer (HPRC), hereditary leiomyomatosis renal cell carcinoma (HLRCC), Birt-Hogg-Dubé (BHD) syndrome, and constitutional chromosome 3 translocation. VHL is autosomal dominant and is caused by germ-line mutations of the VHL tumor suppressor gene, located on chromosome 3p25–26. The VHL protein is involved in cell cycle regulation and angiogenesis. In patients with VHL disease, loss of the sole functioning VHL allele in somatic tissues causes a situation similar to hypoxia, with elevated levels of HIF-1-α, despite the presence of normal oxygen tension.[16] The renal manifestations of VHL are kidney cysts and clear cell RCC. The mean age onset for VHL-associated clear cell RCC is 37 years, and periodic screening with MRI should start after the age of 10 years.[17]

HPRC is autosomal dominant with high penetrance and is characterized by multiple, bilateral, late-onset papillary RCCs. HLRCC is autosomal dominant with a predisposition to papillary type 2 RCC. BHD is autosomal dominant with incomplete penetrance and is associated with multiple chromophobe and clear cell RCCs, papillary RCCs, and oncocytomas. Constitutional chromosome 3 translocation is associated with multiple, bilateral clear cell RCCs.[18] Autosomal dominant polycystic kidney disease does not appear to increase the incidence of RCC, but the tumors are more often multicentric (28% vs. 6%), bilateral (12% vs. 1% to 5%), and sarcomatoid in type (33% vs. 1% to 5%) than in the general population.[19]

Renal Pelvis and Ureter Carcinoma

Urothelial carcinoma of the upper urinary tract accounts for 7% of all kidney tumors and 5% of all urothelial malignancies.[20] The incidence of bilateral upper urinary tract tumors is 1.5% to 2% for synchronous and 6 to 8% for asynchronous presentations.[21] Renal pelvis tumors are found two to three times more commonly in men than in women, and the peak incidence is in the fifth and sixth decades of life. Because the mucosal surfaces of the renal pelvis, ureter, and bladder have the same embryologic origin, many of the etiologic factors in renal pelvis and ureter tumors also apply to tumors of the urinary bladder. Urothelial carcinomas of the upper urinary tract tend to be multifocal because of "field cancerization," which may be caused by exposure of the urothelium to potential carcinogens. Urothelial tumors can also spread to urothelial structures that are either distal or proximal to the primary tumor and are referred to as "drop metastases." About 40% to 50% of patients with upper urinary tract tumors will have a synchronous or metachronous bladder cancer.[22,23]

Cigarette smoking is the most important factor contributing to the overall incidence of urothelial cancer in Western countries. Patients with Lynch syndrome, an autosomal dominant genetic condition because of inherited mutations that impair DNA mismatch repair, have an increased risk of developing urinary tract cancer.[24]

Exposure to aristolochic acid has been associated with acute, near–end-stage renal disease. Aristolochic acid is commonly found in the Aristolochiaceae family of plants commonly used in Chinese herbal medicine. A high incidence of cellular atypia and urothelial carcinoma of the renal pelvis, ureter, and bladder has been associated with aristolochic acid nephropathy.[25] Arsenic-contaminated water has been associated with a high incidence of upper urinary tract urothelial carcinoma in Taiwan.[26] Prolonged heavy phenacetin-containing analgesic use can lead to urothelial carcinomas of the renal pelvis, ureter, and bladder (which may be multiple and bilateral).[27]

Balkan endemic nephropathy (BEN) is a chronic tubulointerstitial disease of unknown etiology most commonly reported in southeastern Europe. A high frequency of urothelial atypia, occasionally progressing to tumors of the renal pelvis and urethra, but also involving the bladder, is associated with BEN.[27]

NATURAL HISTORY

Renal Cell Carcinoma

Primary renal cell tumors may spread by local infiltration through the renal capsule to involve the perinephric fat and Gerota fascia. The tumor may grow directly along the venous channels to the renal vein or vena cava. Lymph node metastases occur with an incidence of 9% to 27%, and most often involve the renal hilar, para-aortic, and paracaval lymph nodes.[28,29] The renal vein is invaded by tumor in 21% of cases, and the inferior vena cava is invaded in as many as 4% of cases.[30]

Approximately 45% of patients with RCC have localized disease, 25% have regional disease, and about 30% have evidence of distant metastases at the time of diagnosis.[29,31] Of patients with metastases, about 1% to 3% have solitary lesions.[32] About half of the patients with RCC eventually develop metastatic disease.[33]

Among patients presenting with metastatic RCC, the sites of distribution include the lung, bone, brain, liver, adrenal gland, and distant lymph nodes. RCC can metastasize to unusual sites like nasal sinuses, skin, penis, etc. Patients with metastatic disease at diagnosis have an extremely poor prognosis, with an expected survival of <5 years regardless of the site of metastasis.[29,31]

Renal Pelvis and Ureter Carcinoma

Upper urinary tract carcinoma is frequently a multifocal process. Patients with cancer at one site in the upper urinary tract are at significant risk for development of tumors elsewhere along the urothelium. The probability of multifocal occurrence is greatest in patients with large tumors and those with carcinoma *in situ*. Ureteral tumors tend to occur in the distal third of the ureter.

Urothelial carcinoma of the upper urothelial tract may spread both by direct extension and by hematogenous and lymphatic metastases. Implantation of tumor cells in the bladder has been demonstrated, especially in previously traumatized areas. The incidence of lymph node metastasis is highly dependent on the grade of the primary tumor. Low-grade tumors have a very low metastatic propensity. In a series of 94 patients, none of 43 low-grade tumors had lymph node metastasis, compared with 3 of 22 grade 3 or 4 tumors.[34] Lymph node metastases were reported in 9 of 26 patients selected to receive adjuvant radiotherapy.[35]

CLINICAL PRESENTATION

Renal Cell Carcinoma

Patients with RCC may present with an occult primary tumor or with signs and symptoms attributable to a local mass or systemic paraneoplastic syndromes. Gross hematuria, palpable flank mass, and pain describe a classic triad that occurs only in 5% to 10% of patients.[36,37] Indeed, a finding of the classic triad often suggests advanced disease with a poor prognosis. The most frequent symptom associated with RCC is hematuria, either gross or microscopic, when there is invasion of the collecting system.[38] Scrotal varicoceles, mostly left-sided, are observed in as many as 11% of men with RCC.[39] Other symptoms include anemia, hepatic dysfunction in the absence of liver metastases (called Stauffer syndrome and because of a paraneoplastic elevation in alkaline phosphatase), secondary (AA) amyloidosis, fever, hypercalcemia, cachexia, erythrocytosis, thrombocytosis, and a syndrome resembling polymyalgia rheumatica.[39-45] RCC presenting as an incidental mass on a diagnostic imaging study ordered for other purposes accounts for 61% of all diagnoses.[46]

A wide range of paraneoplastic syndromes has been associated with RCC. Parathyroid-like hormones, erythropoietin, renin, gonadotropins, placental lactogen, prolactin, enteroglucagon, insulin-like hormones, adrenocorticotropic hormone, and prostaglandins have been identified in patients with RCC.[47,48]

Renal Pelvis and Ureter Carcinoma

Gross or microscopic hematuria occurs in 70% to 95% of patients with renal pelvis or ureter tumors.[20] The other less common symptoms include pain (8% to 40%), bladder irritation (5% to 10%), or other constitutional symptoms (5%). About 10% to 20% of patients may present with a flank mass secondary to tumor or hydronephrosis.

DIAGNOSTIC WORKUP

Renal Cell Carcinoma

Renal masses are not uncommon, and most of them are benign. A central renal mass may suggest the presence of urothelial carcinoma; if so, urine cytology, ureteroscopy, and biopsy should be considered. Renal masses are frequently diagnosed as an incidental finding during abdominal imaging for metastatic evaluation for an unrelated malignancy or other disease. An algorithm for the workup of renal masses has been proposed.[49] Most contrast-enhancing masses tend to be malignant, and the odds ratio of malignancy increases with increasing size.[50] If computed tomography (CT) or ultrasound clearly identifies the mass as a cyst, no further workup is necessary. If a solid lesion is identified, then tumor removal by nephrectomy should be considered. In the case of small lesions, a follow-up CT scan to evaluate potential growth of the mass may raise the suspicion of malignancy. The diagnostic and staging workup for RCC is given in Table 67.1. The diagnosis of RCC is established clinically and radiographically in most cases. Pathologic confirmation often is made at the time of nephrectomy.

Once a radiographic diagnosis is made, a staging evaluation should be undertaken, which should include a complete history and physical examination, complete blood count, and liver and kidney function tests. A metastatic workup should include a chest CT and an abdominal–pelvic CT or abdominal magnetic resonance imaging (MRI) scan of the abdomen. Patients with symptoms suggestive of bone metastases and those with an elevated alkaline phosphatase level should undergo a bone scan. If metastatic lesions are detected, histologic confirmation should be made by biopsy of either the metastatic focus or the primary tumor. MRI can be valuable when evaluating the extent of involvement of the collecting system or inferior vena cava, or radiographic contrast cannot be administered. Renal arteriography is sometimes helpful in planning surgery.

TABLE 67.1 DIAGNOSTIC WORKUP FOR RENAL CELL CARCINOMA

General
History and physical examination
If ≤46 years, refer to a hereditary cancer clinic for further evaluation[159]
Avoid biopsy if resection is being considered. Consider needle biopsy, if clinically indicated, for small lesions to confirm diagnosis or guide surveillance, cryosurgery, or radio-frequency ablation strategies

Radiographic Studies
Abdominal ± pelvic CT (preferred because it shows calcification and better visualization of other body parts) or abdominal MRI with or without contrast depending on renal function. MRI is superior to CT when evaluating the inferior vena cava and right atrium for tumor involvement
Consider CT urography, which allows imaging of both the renal parenchyma and the collecting system
As clinically indicated to rule out metastases:
   Chest CT or chest x-ray
   Bone scan, if patient has bone pain or has an elevated alkaline phosphatase
   Brain MRI with or without contrast depending on renal function, if clinical signs, presentation, and symptoms are suggestive of brain metastases

Laboratory Studies
Urinalysis
Complete blood cell count (CBC)
Comprehensive metabolic panel (including LDH, serum corrected calcium, liver function tests, blood urea nitrogen, and serum creatinine)

CT, computed tomography; MRI, magnetic resonance imaging.

TABLE 67.2 DIAGNOSTIC WORKUP FOR RENAL PELVIS AND URETER CARCINOMA

General
History and physical examination

Radiographic Studies
CT of the abdomen and pelvis or MRI urogram
Multidetector CT urography (CTU)
Chest CT or chest radiograph
Bone scan, if patient has bone pain or has an elevated alkaline phosphatase
Brain MRI, if suspecting brain metastases

Special Tests
Cystoscopy, the entire urinary tract has to be evaluated due to the high incidence of multiple tumors
Ureteroscopic visualization of the tumor is desirable, and tissue biopsy through a ureteroscope may be performed if feasible
Urine cytology may help determine tumor grade if tissue is not available. False-negative rate can be high in upper tract and low-grade tumors

Laboratory Studies
Complete blood cell count
Comprehensive metabolic panel (including liver function tests, blood urea nitrogen, and serum creatinine)
Urinalysis

CT, computed tomography.

Renal Pelvis and Ureter Carcinoma

The diagnostic workup for renal pelvis and ureter carcinoma is listed in Table 67.2. Staging includes a complete history and physical examination, complete blood count, and liver and kidney function tests. CT urography is now used to evaluate patients with renal pelvis carcinoma. CT or MRI of the abdomen and pelvis before and after contrast administration gives useful information regarding the possible extension of tumor outside the collecting system. Ureteroscopic visualization of the tumor is desirable, and tissue biopsy through a ureteroscope should be performed if feasible. Cystoscopy is very important because of the high incidence of multiple tumors. Urine cytology may help determine tumor grade if tissue is not available, but false-negative rates can be high for upper tract and low-grade tumors.

STAGING

Renal Cell Carcinoma

The American Joint Committee on Cancer (AJCC) system is currently being utilized to stage patients with RCC (Table 67.3).[50] T1 and T2 cancers are limited to the kidney. T3 tumors extend into major veins or perinephric tissues, but not into the ipsilateral adrenal gland and not beyond Gerota fascia. T4 tumors invade beyond Gerota fascia (including contiguous extension into the ipsilateral adrenal gland). Regional lymph node metastases may involve spread to the renal hilar, caval, and aortic drainage sites. Metastasis in regional lymph node(s) is classified as N1. This staging system underwent some modifications for the 8th edition: For T3a disease, the word "grossly" was eliminated from the description of renal vein involvement, "muscle containing" was eliminated, and "invasion of the pelvicalyceal system" was added.[50]

Renal Pelvis and Ureter Carcinoma

Tumors of the renal pelvis and ureter have a natural history that is not too dissimilar from that of other urothelial malignancies originating in the bladder. Their prognoses are dependent on tumor invasiveness and pathologic grade. The 2017 AJCC 8th edition staging classification for renal pelvis and ureter carcinoma is shown in Table 67.4.[51] This staging system underwent one modification for the 8th edition: The N3 category of a metastasis in a single lymph node larger than 5 cm in greatest dimension was collapsed into the N2 category.

TABLE 67.3 2017 KIDNEY CANCER TNM STAGING AJCC UICC

Primary Tumor (T)

TX	Primary tumor cannot be assessed
T0	No evidence of primary tumor
T1	Tumor ≤7 cm in greatest dimension, limited to the kidney
T1a	Tumor ≤4 cm in greatest dimension, limited to the kidney
T1b	Tumor >4 cm but ≤7 cm in greatest dimension limited to the kidney
T2	Tumor >7 cm in greatest dimension, limited to the kidney
T2a	Tumor >7 cm but ≤10 cm in greatest dimension, limited to the kidney
T2b	Tumor >10 cm, limited to the kidney
T3	Tumor extends into major veins or perinephric tissues, but not into the ipsilateral adrenal gland and not beyond Gerota fascia
T3a	Tumor extends into the renal vein or its segmental branches, or tumor invades the **pelvicalyceal system** or invades perirenal and/or renal sinus fat but not beyond Gerota fascia
T3b	Tumor extends into the vena cava below the diaphragm
T3c	Tumor extends into the vena cava above the diaphragm or invades the wall of the vena cava
T4	Tumor invades beyond Gerota fascia (including contiguous extension into the ipsilateral adrenal gland)

Regional Lymph Nodes (N)[a]

NX	Regional lymph nodes cannot be assessed
N0	No regional lymph node metastasis
N1	Metastasis in regional lymph node(s)

Distant Metastasis (M)

M0	No distant metastasis
M1	Distant metastasis

Stage Grouping

Stage I	T1	N0	M0
Stage II	T2	N0	M0
Stage III	T1 or T2	N1	M0
	T3	N0, N1	M0
Stage IV	T4	Any N	M0
	Any T	Any N	M1

Histopathologic Grade

GX	Grade cannot be assessed
G1	Nucleoli absent or inconspicuous and basophilic at 400× magnification
G2	Nucleoli conspicuous and eosinophilic at 400× magnification, visible but not prominent at 100× magnification
G3	Nucleoli conspicuous and eosinophilic at 100× magnification
G4	Marked nuclear pleomorphism and/or multinucleate giant cells and/or rhabdoid and/or sarcomatoid differentiation

[a]The regional lymph nodes are as follows: renal hilar, caval (precaval, interaortocaval, paracaval, and retrocaval), and aortic (preaortic, para-aortic, and retroaortic).
From AJCC: Kidney. In: Amin MB, Edge SB, Greene FL, et al., eds. *AJCC cancer staging manual.* 8th ed. New York: Springer, 2017:739–747. Reproduced with permission of Springer International Publishing in the format Book via Copyright Clearance Center.

TABLE 67.4 2017 TUMORS OF THE RENAL PELVIS AND URETER TNM STAGING AJCC UICC

Primary Tumor (T)

TX	Primary tumor cannot be assessed
T0	No evidence of primary tumor
Ta	Papillary noninvasive carcinoma
Tis	Carcinoma *in situ*
T1	Tumor invades subepithelial connective tissue
T2	Tumor invades muscularis
T3	For renal pelvis only: Tumor invades beyond the muscularis into peripelvic fat or into the renal parenchyma. For ureter only: Tumor invades beyond the muscularis into the periureteric fat
T4	Tumor invades adjacent organs, or through the kidney into the perinephric fat

Regional Lymph Nodes (N)[a]

NX	Regional lymph nodes cannot be assessed
N0	No regional lymph node metastasis
N1	Metastasis in a single lymph node, ≤2 cm in greatest dimension
N2	Metastasis in a single lymph node, >2 cm; or multiple lymph nodes

Distant Metastasis (M)

M0	No distant metastasis
M1	Distant metastasis

Stage Grouping

Stage 0a	Ta	N0	M0
Stage 0is	Tis	N0	M0
Stage I	T1	N0	M0
Stage II	T2	N0	M0
Stage III	T3	N0	M0
Stage IV	T4	N0	M0
	Any T	N1 or N2	M0
	Any T	Any N	M1

Histopathologic Grade

WHO/ISUP recommended grading for urothelial histologies:

LG	Low grade
HG	High grade

For squamous cell carcinoma and adenocarcinoma:

GX	Grade cannot be assessed
G1	Well differentiated
G2	Moderately differentiated
G3	Poorly differentiated
G4	Undifferentiated

[a]The regional lymph nodes for the renal pelvis are renal, hilar, paracaval, aortic, and retroperitoneal, NOS. The regional lymph nodes for the ureter are as follows: renal hilar, iliac (common, internal [hypogastric], external), paracaval, periureteral, and pelvic, NOS.
ISUP, International Society of Urologic Pathology; WHO, World Health Organization.
From AJCC: Renal Pelvis and Ureter. In: Amin MB, Edge SB, Greene FL, et al., eds. *AJCC cancer staging manual.* 8th ed. New York: Springer, 2017:749–755. Reproduced with permission of Springer International Publishing in the format Book via Copyright Clearance Center.

PATHOLOGIC CLASSIFICATION

Renal Cell Carcinoma

RCC is a group of malignancies arising from the epithelium of the renal tubules and comprises 90% of all malignancies in the kidney.[18] The World Health Organization (WHO) classifies renal cell tumors as clear cell RCC, multilocular cystic renal neoplasm of low malignant potential, papillary RCC, HLRCC-associated RCC, chromophobe RCC, collecting duct RCC, renal medullary carcinoma, MiT family translocation RCC, succinate dehydrogenase (SDH)-deficient RCC, mucinous tubular and spindle cell carcinoma, tubulocystic RCC, acquired cystic disease–associated RCC, clear cell papillary RCC, and unclassified RCC.[52]

Clear cell RCC is the most common (80% to 90% of tumors), followed papillary RCC (10% to 15%) and chromophobe RCC (4% to 5%). Papillary RCC can be subdivided into type 1, which tends to be low-grade and have a better prognosis, and type 2, which is the opposite, each biologically distinct. Renal medullary carcinoma is very aggressive malignancy mostly associated with young black patients with sickle cell trait and, less commonly, sickle cell disease.[53]

Renal Pelvis and Ureter Carcinoma

More than 90% of malignant tumors arising from the renal pelvis and ureter are urothelial (also called transitional cell) carcinomas. The WHO classifies urothelial tumors as infiltrating urothelial carcinoma or infiltrating urothelial carcinoma with the following variants: with squamous differentiation, with glandular differentiation, and with trophoblastic differentiation, nested, microcystic, micropapillary, lymphoepithelioma-like, plasmacytoid, sarcomatoid, giant cell, and undifferentiated.[52]

PROGNOSTIC FACTORS

Renal Cell Carcinoma

The 5-year survival rate of patients with kidney cancer has doubled over the last 50 years, from 34% in 1954 to 70.9% in 2007.[54,55] The stage at initial presentation remains the most important prognostic factor for RCC survival. Prognostic features for RCC are tumor, patient, and laboratory related. Tumor-related prognostic factors include stage, tumor size, tumor grade, histologic type, tumor necrosis, sarcomatoid transformation, and ≥2 sites of organ metastases. Patient-related factors include asymptomatic versus local symptoms versus systemic symptoms, weight loss, paraneoplastic syndromes, and an interval of less than a year from original diagnosis to start of systemic therapy. Laboratory prognostic factors include thrombocytosis, and elevated ESR or CRP.[50,56]

For patients with metastatic RCC, the following factors were predictive of survival in a retrospective study of 670 patients: low Karnofsky performance status (<80), high LDH (>1.5 times upper limit of normal), low hemoglobin (less than lower limit of normal), high "corrected" serum calcium (>10 mg/dL or 2.5 mmol/L), and absence of prior nephrectomy.[57]

Lymph node metastases are associated with increased rates of local recurrence and distant metastasis.[36,58–60] Nuclear grade, sarcomatoid component, tumor size, stage, and the presence of tumor necrosis increase the likelihood of lymph node involvement.[61] The overall risk of lymph node metastases is 20%.[62,63] Patients with lymph node metastases in radical nephrectomy specimens have a local failure rate of 21%, compared with only 4% in patients without lymph node metastases ($P = .0002$).[60] A select group of patients with solitary metastases may have a 5-year survival rate of 25% to 35%.[64,65]

Nuclear grade, after stage, is the most important prognostic feature of clear cell carcinoma. Fuhrman developed a four-tier grading system that is based upon nuclear and nucleolar size, shape, and content.[66] Fuhrman grade is the most widely used grading system. Grade is also an independent prognostic factor for papillary RCC and chromophobe RCC especially when using standardized criteria.[67] Worsening pathologic grade is associated with a poor 5-year disease-free survival.[31,36]

Papillary RCC has a 5-year survival rate that approaches 90% and metastasizes less frequently than clear cell RCC. The spindle cell or sarcomatoid variants of RCC are associated with statistically significant inferior 5-year survival rates, compared with pure clear or clear and granular histologic variants.[31,36]

Nuclear morphology is a strong predictor of tumor stage and prognosis.[66] High nuclear grade is associated with an increased incidence of advanced tumor stage, lymph node involvement, distant metastases, renal vein involvement, tumor size, and perirenal fat involvement. In a series of 190 patients reported by Bretheau and colleagues,[68] the 5-year actuarial survival rates of patients with grade I, II, III, and IV tumors were 76%, 72%, 51%, and 35%, respectively. Sarcomatoid differentiation carries a significantly poorer prognosis than the clear cell or granular cell subtypes. Almost half of patients with sarcomatoid RCC have bone metastases at presentation. The median survival time of patients with sarcomatoid renal cell cancer is only 6.6 months, compared with 19 months for other histologic types.[69]

Nomograms and algorithms have been described to facilitate the determination of cancer-free survival in patients with RCC. Based on 601 patients treated at Memorial Sloan Kettering Cancer Center with radical nephrectomy, Kattan used variables including patient symptoms (incidental, local, or systemic), histology (chromophobe, papillary, or conventional), tumor size, and pathologic stage to predict risk of recurrence after surgery (note: uses older 1997 staging and is available at the Memorial Sloan Kettering Cancer Center website https://www.mskcc.org/nomograms/renal/post-op).[70] Frank et al.[71] from the Mayo Clinic developed a predictive algorithm based upon 1,801 patients treated with radical nephrectomy. This system combines stage, size, grade, and necrosis (SSIGN) to predict patient survival. Finally, Zisman et al.[72] from UCLA have developed an algorithm that utilizes AJCC TNM stage, Fuhrman grade, and Eastern Cooperative Oncology Group (ECOG) performance status to divide patients into low-risk, intermediate-risk, and high-risk groups. This model is also known as the UISS or the UCLA integrated staging system.

A number of molecular markers are being explored for their prognostic significance including lack of B7H1 expression,[73] immunohistochemical detection of carbonic anhydrase IX (CAIX),[74] the proliferative marker Ki67,[74] immunohistochemical expression of IMP3,[75] and others.

Renal Pelvis and Ureter Carcinoma

The major prognostic factors in patients with renal pelvis or ureter carcinoma are initial stage and grade of the tumor. There is no significant difference in prognosis between urothelial carcinomas originating in the ureter compared to those arising in the renal pelvis.[76]

High-grade tumors are associated with a higher incidence of metastases and worse survival. Corrado et al.[77] reported 5-year survival rates of 83%, 75%, 52%, and 0% for grades 1 through 4, respectively. These results are comparable to those described by Heney and colleagues,[78] who reported 100% survival for grade 1, 81% for grade 2, and 0% for grade 3. Local recurrence was identified in three of 24 patients with grade 3 tumors. No survival differences were seen for patients with papillary versus solid tumors. In the series of Charbit et al.,[23] lymph node metastases were seen exclusively in patients with high-grade tumors. Of tumor-related deaths, 90% were in patients with high-grade tumors. Hall et al.[79] reported a retrospective series of 252 patients treated surgically for upper urinary tract urothelial cancers. Significant factors for recurrence included high tumor grade and advanced clinical stage. Older patients and patients treated with parenchymal-sparing surgical procedures had higher rates of recurrence. In their series of 77 patients, Akdogan et al.[80] reported from a multivariate analysis that higher recurrence rates were associated with tumor location, higher grade, and advanced T-stage. Tumors in the ureters were more likely to recur than tumors involving the renal pelvis. In a series of 86 patients, Park et al. also reported a higher rate of recurrence in ureteral tumors, compared to those arising in the renal pelvis.[81]

A prior history of bladder cancer has been reported to worsen the prognosis of patients with second urothelial cancers involving the upper tracts.[80,82] From the Memorial Sloan Kettering Cancer Center series of 129 patients, a multivariate analysis demonstrated that patients with advanced primary tumors and a prior history of bladder cancer were associated with worse disease-free survival.[82]

Flow cytometry may aid in estimating long-term prognosis. In a multivariate analysis, Corrado et al.[77] demonstrated that, although stage and grade were the most important prognostic indices, DNA pattern (diploid vs. nondiploid) and the number of lesions (unifocal vs. multifocal) identified at initial diagnosis also determined prognosis. Patients with diploid tumors had a 79% survival rate, compared with only 46% in patients with nondiploid tumors ($P = .0003$). Recent data suggest that hypermethylation of the promoter region of patients with urothelial cancers of the urothelium is associated with a worse prognosis. Tumors of the renal pelvis and ureters demonstrate hypermethylation in 94% of cases compared to 76% of similar appearing tumors in the bladder, $P < .0001$. Hypermethylation was also associated with higher tumor stage, tumor progression, and mortality.[83]

GENERAL MANAGEMENT

Renal Cell Carcinoma

Surgery is the therapeutic foundation for the management of kidney cancer. Radiotherapy has an important and growing role in the palliative management of RCC. Although RCC is traditionally considered to be radioresistant, it has a clear dose response to radiation.[84,85] As long as sufficient radiation dose is delivered to the tumor while respecting normal tissue dose constraints, RCC "radioresistance" can be overcome with modern techniques. The kidney cancer NCCN guidelines (version 2.2017) offer the following surgical options depending on the stage[86]:

- Stage I (pT1a): partial (preferred) or radical nephrectomy (if partial not feasible or central location), active surveillance, or ablative techniques in selected patients

- Stage I (pT1b): partial or radical nephrectomy
- Stage II and III: radical nephrectomy or partial nephrectomy if clinically indicated
- Stage IV: nephrectomy and surgical metastasectomy if potentially resectable primary with solitary metastatic site, followed by systemic first-line therapy; cytoreductive nephrectomy if potentially resectable primary with solitary metastatic site, followed by systemic first-line therapy; or systemic first-line therapy if surgically unresectable

Elderly patients and those with small renal masses and other comorbidities often have a low RCC-specific mortality.[87]

Surgery

A radical nephrectomy includes a perifascial resection of the kidney, perirenal fat, regional lymph nodes, and ipsilateral adrenal gland. It is the preferred treatment if the tumor extends into the inferior vena cava and usually requires the assistance of a cardiovascular surgeon if there is a caval or atrial thrombus. Adrenalectomy is not indicated when imaging shows a normal adrenal gland or if the tumor is not high-risk.[88] An experienced team should be involved in the context of thrombus, as treatment-related mortality can reach 10%.[86] Open, robotic, and laparoscopic techniques may be used to perform a radical nephrectomy. Improved preoperative assessment with CT can identify patients who have no significant risk of adrenal gland involvement.[89] In 76% of cases, the adrenal gland can be spared at the time of surgery. The EORTC conducted a randomized trial of radical nephrectomy with or without an elective lymph node dissection, and there was no survival advantage between the two study groups. The incidence of unsuspected lymph node metastases was low (4%).[90] Nevertheless, the lymph node dissection does provide valuable prognostic information.

Radical nephrectomies should be avoided if nephron-sparing surgery is feasible for T1a and T1b renal tumors. In this setting, nephron-sparing surgery has shown equivalent outcomes to radical nephrectomy.[91,92] Radical nephrectomy-induced chronic renal insufficiency is associated with an increased risk of cardiovascular death and death from any cause.[93] For this reason, nephron-sparing surgery is preferred in T1a and T1b tumors. Nephron-sparing surgery is also preferred in patients with hereditary RCC to preserve renal function and decrease the risk of cardiovascular events.[94] In a matched-pair analysis of 164 patients undergoing nephron-sparing surgery at the Mayo Clinic, the disease-free survival was 79%, which compared favorably to 77% in patients undergoing radical nephrectomy.[95] In 117 patients with renal tumors 4 cm or less undergoing partial nephrectomy at the Memorial Sloan Kettering Cancer Center, the 5-year freedom from recurrence was 98.6% compared to 96.4% in a similar group of 173 patients undergoing radical nephrectomy. Compared to patients undergoing partial nephrectomy, those undergoing radical nephrectomy were at a higher risk of chronic renal insufficiency.[96] There is some risk that sparing of the renal parenchyma may leave microscopic residual tumor or inadequately treat multifocal cancers.[97-99] Bilateral RCC occurs in 2% to 3% of patients. In these patients, nephron-sparing surgery is an attractive option because bilateral radical nephrectomy sentences the patient to a lifetime of renal dialysis or the need for a renal transplant.

Following surgery, 20% to 30% of patients with localized tumors relapse, with a median time to relapse of 1 to 2 years, and most occurring within 3 years.[86] Although at present there is no role for adjuvant therapy after surgery, a number of recent trials are exploring the role of targeted therapy.

Patients who have local symptoms, such as hematuria, pain, hypertension, or other paraneoplastic syndromes, may benefit from a palliative nephrectomy. Spontaneous regression of metastatic renal cell cancer after nephrectomy has been reported. In an extensive literature review, the incidence of regression of metastatic foci induced by nephrectomy was 0.8% (4 of 474 patients).[33] Cytoreductive surgery performed to prolong or increase the response of metastatic disease in response to systemic therapy may be beneficial.[100-102]

Thermal Ablation

Recently, the minimally invasive ablative technologies of cryoablation and radio-frequency ablation (RFA) have emerged as potential treatment options for clinically localized RCC, especially in the elderly, or patients with a solitary kidney or comorbidities impeding surgery. Long-term oncologic efficacy for these modalities remains to be established. The most favorable lesions for this approach are <4 cm and in the periphery of the kidney. Relative contraindications for RFA and cryoablation include distant metastases, tumors > 5 cm, tumors in the hilum or central collecting system, and life expectancy less than a year. A meta-analysis comparing cryoablation and RFA suggested that cryoablation results in fewer retreatments and improved local tumor control and that cryoablation may be associated with a lower risk of metastatic progression compared with RFA.[103]

Systemic Therapy in the Treatment for Relapsed, Metastatic, or Unresectable Renal Cell Carcinoma

Until 2005, systemic treatment for RCC was mostly limited to cytokine therapy. The NCCN guidelines list the following first-line systemic therapies for clear cell histology: pazopanib (Category 1, preferred), sunitinib (Category 1, preferred), bevacizumab + interferon (Category 1), temsirolimus (Category 1 for poor-prognosis patients and Category 2B for selected patients of other groups), axitinib, high-dose IL-2 for selected patients, and sorafenib for selected patients. Subsequent therapy includes cabozantinib (Category 1, preferred), nivolumab (Category 1, preferred), axitinib (Category 1), everolimus, pazopanib, sorafenib, sunitinib, bevacizumab (Category 2B), high-dose IL-2 for selected patients, or temsirolimus (Category 2B).[86]

For non–clear cell histology, the NCCN guidelines list the following first-line systemic therapies: sunitinib, axitinib, bevacizumab, cabozantinib, erlotinib, everolimus, lenvatinib + everolimus, nivolumab, pazopanib, sorafenib, and temsirolimus (Category 1 for poor-prognosis patients and Category 2A for other risk groups).[86]

Pazopanib is a multikinase inhibitor targeting c-KIT, FGFR, PDGFR, and VEGFR. Sunitinib is a multikinase inhibitor targeting c-KIT, FGFR, FLT-3, CSF-1R, PDGFR, VEGFR, and RET. Bevacizumab is a recombinant monoclonal antibody that binds VEGF-A. Temsirolimus and everolimus are mTOR inhibitors. Axitinib is a small molecule tyrosine kinase inhibitor targeting VEGF, c-KIT, and PDGFR. Sorafenib is a small inhibitor of several tyrosine protein kinases, such as VEGFR, PDGFR, and Raf family kinases. Cabozantinib is a small molecule inhibitor of the tyrosine kinases c-Met and VEGFR2. Nivolumab is an antibody that selectively blocks the interaction between PD-1 and its ligands. Erlotinib is a receptor tyrosine kinase inhibitor of EGFR. Lenvatinib is a multikinase inhibitor targeting VEGFR, FGFR, PDGFR, c-KIT, and RET.

Chemotherapy has limited use in RCC because it is one of the most chemotherapy-resistant solid tumors. Gemcitabine in combination with doxorubicin or sunitinib has shown some benefit in patients with sarcomatoid features (Category 2B).

Metastasectomy

Patients with a solitary metastatic lesion have a 5-year survival rate of 24% (compared with 4% for those with more than one metastatic focus), and they may benefit from aggressive therapy.[104] The resection of one or a limited number of metastases in combination with nephrectomy or at relapse has been associated with a 13% to 50% 5-year survival in small series of selected patients.[105-107] Selected lung, bone, brain, liver, and even pancreatic metastases, among other sites, have been treated using this approach.

Radiation Therapy (RT) Trends

A study of the National Cancer Database in the United States observed a decrease in the use of RT for patients with RCC from 1998 to 2010. Patients with more aggressive disease characteristics were more likely to receive RT. Of 233,572 patients diagnosed with nonmetastatic RCC between 1998 and 2010, 0.9% were treated using radiotherapy. Overall, there was a decreasing trend in the utilization of RT (1.5% in 1998 to 0.6% in 2010; $P < .001$). Of 45,855 patients diagnosed with metastatic RCC, 30% received radiotherapy. Overall, there was a decreasing trend in the utilization of RT from 1998 to 2010 (33.3% to 28.5%; $P < .001$).[108] Nevertheless, there is an increased interest in dose escalation using single fractions and other hypofractionated regimens for the primary treatment of kidney lesions and palliation of cranial and extracranial metastases.

Neoadjuvant (Preoperative) Radiation Therapy

Neoadjuvant radiotherapy is not recommended in patients with resectable RCC. Two European studies were undertaken to test the efficacy of neoadjuvant/preoperative RT in RCC (Table 67.5). A prospective randomized study of neoadjuvant RT and nephrectomy versus nephrectomy alone was conducted in Rotterdam. No advantage was demonstrated in patients receiving 30 Gy RT in 2 Gy fractions with respect to overall survival or survival free of distant metastasis. Neoadjuvant radiotherapy did appear to increase the rate of complete resectability in patients with locally advanced tumors.[109] Subsequent patients received 40 Gy in 2 Gy fractions. No benefit was demonstrated at the higher radiation dose.[110] In Sweden, a second prospective randomized clinical trial was also unable to demonstrate an advantage for neoadjuvant radiotherapy. In this trial, patients were randomly assigned to receive neoadjuvant RT to 33 Gy in 15 fractions administered to the flank with a betatron unit followed by nephrectomy or nephrectomy alone. Patients receiving neoadjuvant RT had a 5-year survival rate of 47%, compared with 63% for patients undergoing surgery alone.[111]

Adjuvant (Postoperative) Radiotherapy

Adjuvant radiation therapy is not recommended in RCC after complete resection. Two prospective randomized studies testing the value of adjuvant radiation therapy did not demonstrate an advantage to patients receiving RT after surgery (Table 67.6). The first study from New Castle, United Kingdom, demonstrated an inferior survival for patients receiving adjuvant RT compared with those treated by surgery alone.[112] Local tumor recurrence rates were not affected by adjuvant RT. Four patients died of fatal hepatotoxicity after RT to a right-sided nephrectomy bed. Patients in this study received 55 Gy in 2.04-Gy daily fractions.[7] A second randomized study conducted by the Copenhagen Renal Cancer Study Group

compared patients with stage II or III renal cell cancer treated with nephrectomy alone with patients who received nephrectomy and adjuvant RT to 50 Gy in 20 fractions to the kidney bed and regional ipsilateral and contralateral lymph nodes. No difference in the relapse rate was found between the two study groups. There were significant complications involving the stomach, duodenum, and liver in 44% of patients receiving adjuvant RT. Specifically, 19% of deaths in the RT group were attributed to RT-induced complications.[113]

Aref et al. analyzed the patterns of failure in 116 patients undergoing nephrectomy for RCC. They observed that locoregional failure is rare following nephrectomy and that distant metastases is the main pattern of failure. Consequently, their data did not support the role of adjuvant radiation in RCC.[114] Moreover, a retrospective study of 1,344 patients who underwent 1,390 partial nephrectomies for kidney cancer found that positive surgical margins were not associated with an increased risk of local tumor recurrence or metastatic disease.[115] A SEER-based study of adjuvant RT in sarcomatoid RCC did not show an overall survival benefit.[116]

In contrast, a meta-analysis including the two prospective randomized trials previously mentioned and five retrospective trials with a total of 735 patients observed a significant reduction in locoregional failure with adjuvant RT ($P < .0001$). The patient accrual for all the studies combined spanned from 1968 to 1999. There was no difference in overall survival or disease-free survival. The authors proposed a prospective randomized trial using modern RT techniques for high-risk patients with tumor size > 5 cm, positive margins or gross residual disease, perinephric fat invasion, capsule invasion, renal vein/inferior vena cava invasion, positive lymph nodes, or high-grade histology.[117]

Stereotactic Body Radiation Therapy (SBRT) for Primary Treatment

A number of small phase I and II trials are exploring the role of SBRT in the primary treatment of renal tumors. The largest of these studies included 40 patients, 11 with transitional cell cancer and 29 with RCC. All tumors were treated with a single 25-Gy fraction to the 70% isodose. The local tumor control rate 9 months after SBRT was 98% (95% CI 89 to 99). There was a measurable size reduction in 38 lesions, including complete remission in 19.[118]

Whole-Brain Radiation Therapy for Brain Metastases

A retrospective study of 60 patients receiving whole-brain radiotherapy (WBRT) for RCC brain metastases showed that local control (LC) at 6 months was 21% after 3 Gy × 10 and 57% after higher doses of 2 Gy × 20 or 3 Gy × 15 ($P = .013$). The LC at 12 months was 7% and 35%, respectively. The overall survival (OS) at 6 months was 29% after 3 Gy × 10 and 52% after higher doses ($P = .003$). The OS at 12 months was 13% and 47%, respectively. The authors concluded that escalating the WBRT dose beyond 3 Gy × 10 could improve the outcomes in RCC patients with brain metastases.[119]

TABLE 67.5 SURVIVAL AFTER NEPHRECTOMY OR NEOADJUVANT RADIOTHERAPY AND NEPHRECTOMY FOR RENAL CELL CARCINOMA, PROSPECTIVE RANDOMIZED TRIALS

Study	No. of Patients	Radiation Dose/ Fraction Size (Gy)	Treatment	5-Yr Survival Rate (%)	Comments
van der Werf-Messing et al.[109,110]	85	–	N	50	No significant survival difference
	89	30–40/2	N + NART		
Juusela et al., 1977[111]	50	–	N	63	No significant survival difference
	38	33/2.2	N + NART	47	

N, nephrectomy; NART, neoadjuvant radiotherapy.

TABLE 67.6 SURVIVAL AFTER NEPHRECTOMY OR NEPHRECTOMY AND ADJUVANT RADIATION THERAPY FOR RENAL CELL CARCINOMA, PROSPECTIVE RANDOMIZED TRIALS

Study	Stage	No. of Patients	Radiation Dose/ Fraction Size (Gy)	Treatment	5-Yr Survival Rate (%)	Local Recurrence (%)	RT-related Mortality (%)	RT Complications (%)
Fugitt, 1973[112]	NS	48	–	N	47 (17/35)	7	18	>20
		52	55/2.04	N + ART	36 (14/39)	7		
Kjaer et al., 1987[64]	II, III	33	–	N	63[a]	1	19	44
		32	55/2.5	N + ART	38[a]	0		

[a]Interpolated from graph; number at risk not known.
ART, adjuvant radiotherapy; N, nephrectomy; NS, not stated.

Stereotactic Radiosurgery (SRS) for Brain Metastases

A retrospective study of 280 consecutive patients with metastatic brain tumors (of which 80 were RCC) treated with gamma knife radiosurgery (GKS) observed that to control symptomatic peritumoral edema, a higher marginal dose of 25 Gy or more was necessary. The authors developed an algorithm for the management of RCC metastases where lesions ≥ 3 cm undergo resection; lesions > 2 cm with symptomatic peritumoral edema undergo resection (because a 25 Gy was not considered safe for tumors > 2 cm) and those without it GKS; and lesions ≤ 2 cm receive GKS.[120] Another retrospective study of 46 patients and 99 RCC brain lesions treated with radiosurgery observed that the good-response group (as assessed by MRI) survived significantly longer than the poor-response group (median survival times of 18.0 and 9.0 months, respectively; $P = .025$).[121]

Kano et al. reported 158 consecutive RCC patients (531 lesions) who underwent stereotactic radiosurgery. The overall survival after SRS was 60%, 38%, and 19% at 6, 12, and 24 months, respectively, with a median survival of 8.2 months. Median survival for patients with <2 brain metastases, higher KPS (>90), and no prior WBRT was 12 months after SRS. Sustained local tumor control was achieved in 92% of patients. Symptomatic adverse radiation effects occurred in 7%. Overall, 70% of patients improved or remained neurologically stable.[122]

A retrospective study of 61 patients with RCC treated with GKS, median dose 20 Gy, showed that the use of targeted agents (tyrosine kinase inhibitors, mammalian target rapamycin inhibitors, and bevacizumab) was the only factor that predicted for improved survival. The median survival for patients receiving targeted agents ($n = 24$) was 16.6 months compared with 7.2 months ($n = 37$) for those not receiving targeted therapy ($P = .04$).[123]

A systematic review including 16 publications of cranial RCC showed that the weighted local control was 92%, overall survival ranged from 6.7 to 25.6 months, grade 3 to 4 toxicity ranged from 0% to 6%, and the weighted rate of treatment-related mortality was 0.6% secondary to intratumoral hemorrhage.[124]

Conventional Radiation Therapy for Extracranial Metastases

Palliative radiotherapy is effective at relieving symptoms from metastatic renal cell cancer.[125–128] A patient with a solitary bone metastasis may have a long survival time, and a sufficient radiation dose should be administered to allow durable pain relief. If surgery is used to remove a metastatic lesion, postoperative radiotherapy is indicated to prevent its recurrence. In a prospective phase II study using validated quality of life questionnaires, Lee and colleagues from the Princess Margaret Hospital demonstrated that 83% of patients treated for pain had experienced significant pain relief with 30-Gy radiation delivered in 10 fractions.[127] DiBiase et al. observed a dose response in the palliative treatment of 107 patients with RCC. A biologically effective dose (BED) > 50 Gy_{10} (α/β ratio of 10) was associated with a statistically significant increased rate of response: 59% versus 39% ($P = .001$).[84]

Figure 67.1 illustrates a painful RCC cutaneous metastasis that had a complete response after 375 cGy × 13

FIGURE 67.1. Patient with RCC who received 375 cGy × 13 fractions over 5 weeks to a painful, fixed, and pulsatile cutaneous RCC metastasis. Appearance after **(A)** 3 fractions and **(B)** complete response 6 months after the completion of treatment. The patient had durable pain palliation without local recurrence until death. (From Gay HA, Cavalieri R, Allison RR, et al. Complete response in a cutaneous facial metastatic nodule from renal cell carcinoma after hypofractionated radiotherapy. *Dermatol Online J* 2007;13[4]:6; © 2007 Dermatology Online Journal. Reprinted with permission of Dr. Hiram A. Gay.)

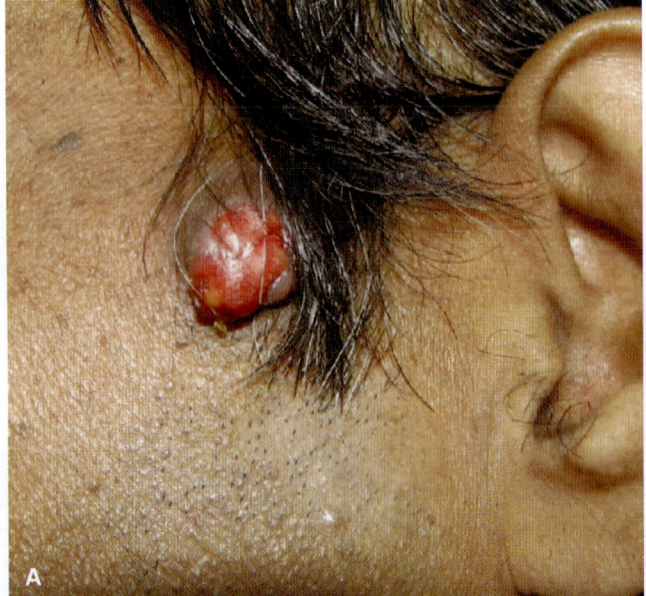

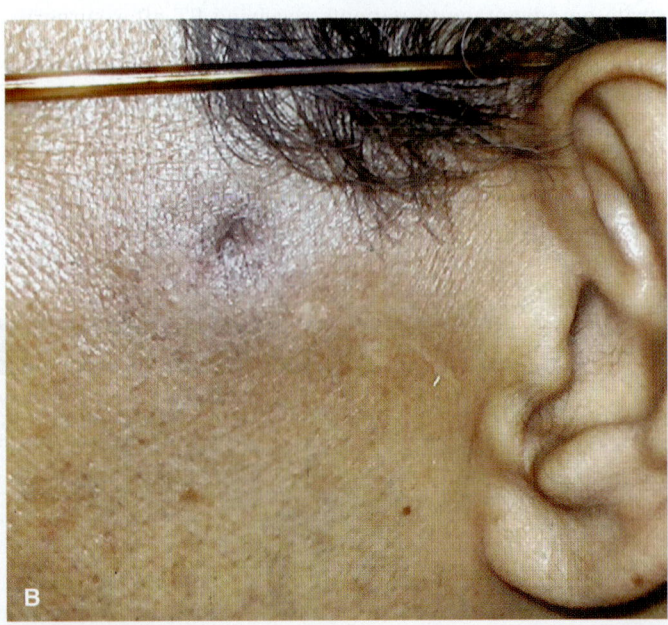

fractions (BED = 67 Gy$_{10}$) over 5 weeks. The lesion was treated with electrons, a custom bolus, and 2-cm peripheral margin.[129]

Stereotactic Body Radiation Therapy for Extracranial Metastases

A systematic review including 10 publications of extracranial RCC showed that the weighted local tumor control was 89%, overall survival ranged from 11.7 to 22 months, grade 3 to 4 toxicity ranged from 0% to 4%, and the weighted rate of treatment-related mortality was 0.5%.[124]

Zelefsky et al. reported 105 RCC lesions treated with either single-dose, image-guided, intensity-modulated radiotherapy (IMRT) to a prescription dose of 18 to 24 Gy (median, 24) or hypofractionation (3 or 5 fractions) with a prescription dose of 20 to 30 Gy. The 3-year local progression-free survival for those who received a high single-dose (24 Gy; n = 45), a low single-dose (<24 Gy; n = 14), or hypofractionation regimens (n = 46) was 88%, 21%, and 17%, respectively. Multivariate analysis showed that significant predictors of improved local progression-free survival were 24 Gy versus a lower dose (P = .009) and a single dose versus hypofractionation (P = .008).[130]

In a series of 50 patients with metastatic RCC, Wersäll et al. reported that stereotactically delivered radiation to sites including the lung, liver, and adrenal resulted in complete regression in 30% of cases and either partial regression or stabilization of the lesions in 60%.[131] Of 162 treated tumors, only 3 recurred. Dose and fractionation ranged from 8 Gy × 4, 10 Gy × 4, and 15 Gy × 3 all delivered in 1 week.

Spine

In a study of 48 patients (55 lesions) with metastatic RCC to the spine, patients received 24 Gy × 1, 9 Gy × 3, or 6 Gy × 5 fractions. The actuarial 1-year spine tumor progression-free survival was 82.1%. At pretreatment baseline, 23% patients were pain-free; at 1 and 12 months post-SBRT, 44% and 52% patients were pain-free, respectively. No grade 3 to 4 neurologic toxicity was observed.[132] A prospectively collected study of 71 spinal segments treated with SBRT showed that the 1-year overall survival and LC rates were 64% and 83%, respectively. The 1-year vertebral compression fracture (VCF)-free probability rate was 82%. Multivariate analysis identified single-fraction SBRT (18 to 24 Gy) and baseline VCF as significant predictors of SBRT-induced VCF (P = .028 and P = .012, respectively).[133] A retrospective study of 57 patients with RCC metastases to the spine who received single-fraction SBRT to 88 treatment sites showed that the median time to radiographic failure and unadjusted pain progression were 26.5 and 26.0 months, respectively. The median time to pain relief from simulation and duration of pain relief from treatment were 0.9 months (range 0.1 to 4.4 months) and 5.4 months (range 0.1 to 37.4 months), respectively. Multivariate analyses demonstrated that multilevel disease and neural foramen involvement were correlated with radiographic failure; multilevel disease and vertebral fracture were correlated with unadjusted pain progression. Twelve treatment sites (14%) were complicated by subsequent vertebral fractures.[134]

Bone

A study was conducted on 46 consecutive RCC patients with 95 lesions who were treated as follows: 50 SBRT and 45 conventional fractionation (CF) RT. A biologically effective dose ≥ 80 Gy (α/β = 7) was predictive of clinical local control. Median time to symptom control between SBRT and CFRT was

2 (range, 0 to 6 weeks) and 4 weeks (range, 0 to 7 weeks), respectively. Toxicity rates were low and equivalent in both groups, with no grade 4 or 5 toxicity reported.[135]

A potential added benefit of extracranial stereotactic radiotherapy is what is called the abscopal effect, in which there is tumor response at a distance from the irradiated volume. Wersäll and colleagues observed an abscopal effect in 4 out of 28 RCC patients with treated and untreated metastatic lesions. In these 4 patients, nonirradiated metastases regressed either temporarily or seemingly permanently after treatment with SBRT of either the primary tumor or other metastatic lesions. The authors' findings argued for a more active and liberal use of SBRT in metastatic RCC. They suggested that further studies were necessary to define the underlying mechanisms behind such responses or to combine SBRT with immunomodulating agents.[136]

Intraoperative Radiation Therapy for Advanced or Recurrent RCC

A retrospective study of 98 patients who received intraoperative radiation therapy (IORT) for advanced or locally recurrent RCC at 9 institutions showed a 5-year overall survival of 37% for advanced disease and 55% for locally recurrent disease. The respective 5-year disease-free survival was 39% and 52%. IORT was delivered during nephrectomy for advanced disease (28%) or during resection of locally recurrent RCC in the renal fossa (72%). Preoperative or postoperative external beam radiation therapy was administered to 27% and 35% of patients, respectively. Initial nodal involvement, presence of sarcomatoid features, and higher IORT dose were statistically significantly associated with decreased survival. The outcomes for patients receiving IORT in the setting of local recurrence compared favorably to similar cohorts treated by local resection alone.[137]

Ongoing Phase III Clinical Trials

There are numerous clinical trials taking place in advanced RCC. Many of these trials are employing antiangiogenesis agents, thymidine kinase inhibitors, tyrosine kinase inhibitors, mTOR inhibitors, anti–PD-1 monoclonal antibodies, and other immunologic therapies alone or in combination.

Renal Pelvis and Ureter Carcinoma

Surgery is the therapeutic foundation for the management of renal pelvis and ureter carcinoma. The bladder cancer NCCN guidelines (version 2.2017) recommend the following treatment options for renal pelvis low-grade tumors: nephroureterectomy with a cuff of bladder or endoscopic resection ± postsurgical intrapelvic chemotherapy or BCG.[138] High-grade renal pelvis tumors, large tumors, or tumors that invade the renal parenchyma have the following management options: nephroureterectomy with a cuff of bladder and regional lymphadenectomy, with consideration of neoadjuvant chemotherapy in selected patients.

The management of ureter tumors depends on the location of the tumor, upper, mid, or distal location, and on disease extent. Neoadjuvant chemotherapy may be considered in selected patients.[139]

For both renal pelvis and ureter tumors, once the pathologic staging is obtained, patients with pathologic stage pT2, pT3, pT4, or N+ should be considered for adjuvant chemotherapy with or without radiotherapy.

Surgery

Radical nephroureterectomy is the only potentially curative treatment for most patients with urothelial carcinoma of the renal pelvis or ureter. This operation includes removal of the contents of Gerota fascia, including the ipsilateral ureter with a cuff of bladder at its distal extent. Less radical surgeries have been plagued by high local or regional recurrence rates, sometimes approaching 30%.[140] Hall et al.[79] reported an increase rate of recurrence when parenchymal-sparing procedures were performed. Conservative surgical excision should be considered only in patients with low-grade, low-stage, solitary tumors in whom radical nephrectomy is not indicated because of poor kidney function or an absent contralateral kidney. Conservative surgical options in selected cases include laparoscopic nephroureterectomy, nephrectomy and partial ureterectomy, endoscopic resection, and fulguration. The role of lymph node dissection in this disease is unclear. Patients who have the highest risk of lymph node metastases also have a high risk of systemic disease.

Adjuvant Radiation Therapy

There are no randomized trials on the role of postoperative RT in patients who have had a complete resection of an upper urinary tract cancer. Tumors of the renal pelvis and ureter have a significantly high local recurrence rate after nephroureterectomy, particularly in patients with high-grade tumors or deep invasion.[141] Retrospective studies suggest that adjuvant RT may diminish the likelihood of local tumor recurrence, but it does not appear to have an impact on overall survival or reducing future distant metastases.[34,142]

Cozad et al. reported a retrospective study of 94 patients with urothelial carcinoma of the renal pelvis, of which 77 had resections without residual. On multivariate analysis, adjuvant RT had a significant effect on local control ($P = .02$). In terms of survival, the use of adjuvant radiation therapy was of borderline significance ($P = .07$). Of the 27 patients that were excluded from local failure and survival analysis, 19 had unresectable local disease and of these 11 received radiation therapy. Two long-term disease-free survivors in this group received 45 and 50.4 Gy. The authors recommended consideration of adjuvant radiotherapy in patients with high grade or stage, close surgical margins, or positive lymph nodes to improve local control.[34]

In another retrospective study of 133 patients with urothelial carcinoma of the renal pelvis, 67 patients received external beam RT following surgery (RT group) and 66 patients received intravesical chemotherapy (non-RT group). The clinical target volume included the renal fossa, the course of the ureter to the entire bladder, and the paracaval and para-aortic lymph nodes (Fig. 67.2). The tumor bed or residual tumor was targeted in 14 patients. The median radiation dose administered was 50 Gy. There was a significant difference between the survival rates for these groups based on patients with T3/T4 stage cancer. A significant difference was observed in the bladder tumor relapse rate between the irradiated and nonirradiated bladder groups ($P = .004$). The authors concluded that radiation therapy may improve the overall survival for patients with T3/T4 cancer of the renal pelvis or ureter and delay bladder tumor recurrences.[143]

The patterns of failure were described in 252 patients undergoing surgery at the University of Texas Southwest Medical Center for urothelial carcinoma of the upper urinary tract.[79] Local recurrence occurred only 9% of the time, whereas new invasive urothelial tumors or distant metastases occurred in 69% and 22% of cases, respectively. Isolated local recurrences were rare. Another series from the Princess Margaret Hospital confirms the high rate of distant metastases. Although local failure occurred in 35% of patients with locally advanced disease, most patients also experienced distant metastases as well.[144]

Systemic Chemotherapy

The pathologic similarity of urothelial carcinoma of the renal pelvis and ureter to bladder cancer has encouraged medical oncologists to use similar chemotherapeutic regimens in the management of upper tract urothelial carcinomas. Dose-dense methotrexate, vinblastine, doxorubicin, and cisplatin (ddMVAC) for 3 or 4 cycles and gemcitabine and cisplatin for 4 cycles are considered standard neoadjuvant or adjuvant regimens. Standard MVAC is no longer used because it is less efficacious and more toxic ddMVAC.[145] Radiosensitizing chemotherapeutic agents include cisplatin, taxanes (docetaxel or paclitaxel) (Category 2B), 5-FU (Category 2B), 5-FU and mitomycin (Category 2B), capecitabine (Category 3), and low-dose gemcitabine (Category 2B).[138]

Ongoing Phase III Clinical Trials

There are various clinical trials enrolling patients with renal pelvis and ureter carcinoma. Some of these trials are employing tyrosine kinase inhibitors, ATR kinase inhibitors, anti–PD-1 monoclonal antibodies, and other immunologic therapies alone or in combination with chemotherapy.

RADIATION THERAPY TECHNIQUES

Normal Tissue Dose Constraints

A number of organs at risk have to be taken into consideration when palliating an unresected kidney tumor or a kidney tumor bed recurrence. These organs include the spinal cord, liver, spleen, stomach, duodenum, small bowel, any normal contralateral or ipsilateral kidney, and normal adrenal gland(s).

There are no established dose constraints for sparing the remaining kidney after nephrectomy or in the palliative setting when both kidneys are present. In the context of two normal kidneys, the QUANTEC kidney panel recommended a mean bilateral kidney dose of <15 to 18 Gy and a bilateral kidney DVH with a $V_{12} < 55\%$, $V_{20} < 32\%$, $V_{23} < 30\%$, and $V_{28} < 20\%$.[146] The dose to the stomach should be kept below 45 Gy and the small bowel $V_{45} < 195$ cc when it is contoured as a bowel bag (Fig. 67.3).[147] The male and female RTOG normal pelvis atlases illustrate how to contour the bowel bag and are accessible at http://www.rtog.org/CoreLab/ContouringAtlases.aspx. The mean liver dose should be kept below 30 to 32 Gy, excluding patients with pre-existing liver disease or hepatocellular carcinoma who have a lower tolerance. Sparing at least 700 cc of the liver from radiation is another potential strategy to avoid complications.[148] There are no recognized splenic or adrenal dose constraints. Nevertheless, based on the spleen's exquisite radiosensitivity and experience with palliative radiotherapy for myeloproliferative disorders,[149] it seems prudent to limit the spleen to a total of 5 to 10 Gy. The spinal dose should be limited to an absolute maximum of 45 Gy.

Renal Cell Carcinoma

Neoadjuvant or adjuvant radiotherapy is not routinely recommended for patients with RCC. However, there may be special cases where the clinician may consider neoadjuvant radiotherapy to improve respectability or adjuvant radiotherapy if there are clinical tumor features suggestive of a high risk of local recurrence. Careful planning is paramount because ignoring any of the critical structures surrounding the kidney or nephrectomy bed could result in serious, even fatal, patient toxicity.

Patients receiving radiation therapy to the kidney may be simulated supine, arms up, using a wing board or alpha cradle, a wire on the surgical scar, and a planning CT scan.

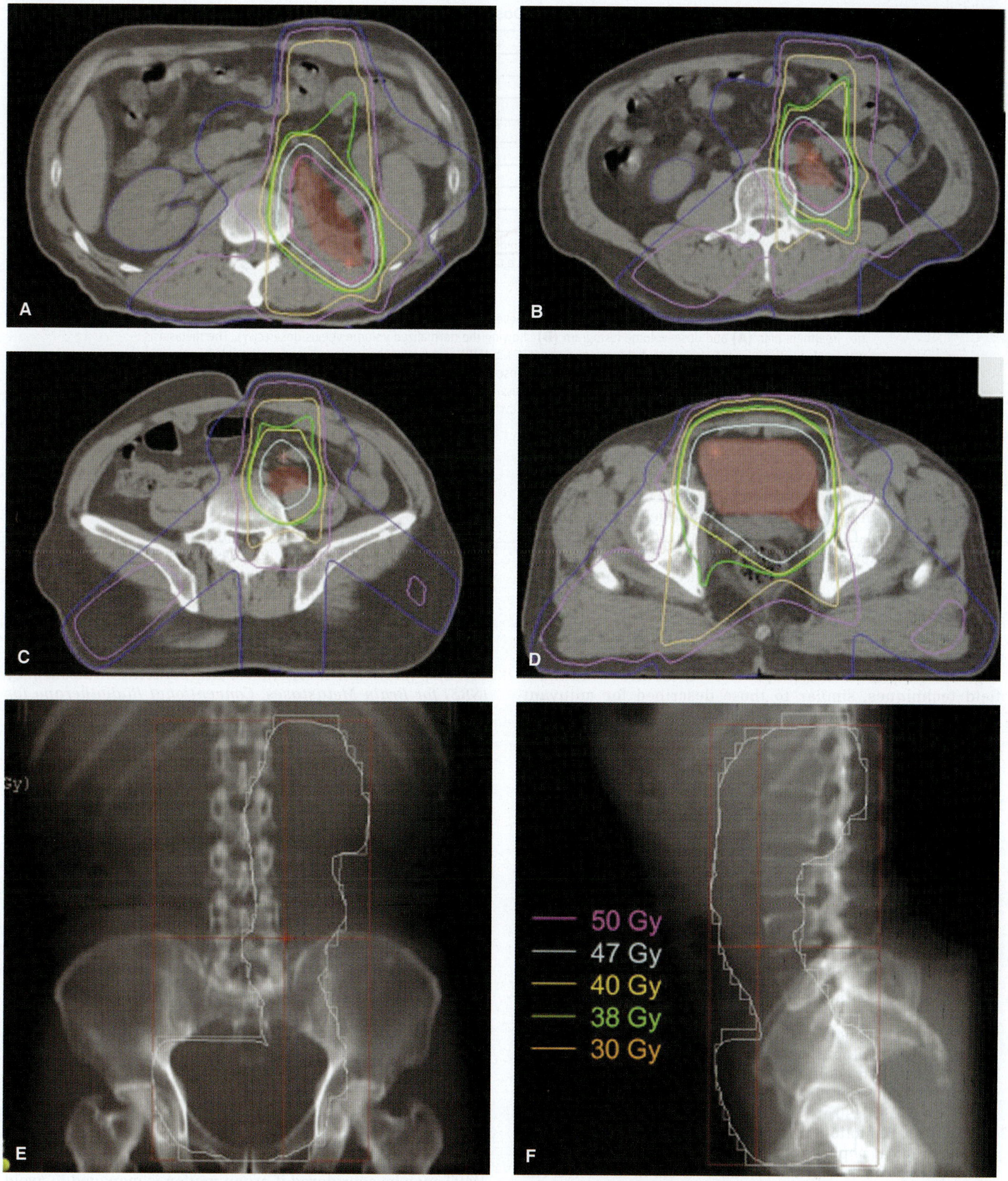

FIGURE 67.2. Dose distribution of a patient with renal pelvis cancer and beam arrangements of 0°, 129°, and 229° gantry: **(A)** renal fossa; **(B, C)** course of ureter; and **(D)** bladder. Digitally reconstructed radiograph for views of **(E)** 0° gantry and **(F)** 90° gantry. Internal *pink* and *yellow* lines represent the CTV$_{50}$ and CTV$_{40}$, respectively. (From Chen B, Zeng ZC, Wang GM, et al. Radiotherapy may improve overall survival of patients with T3/T4 transitional cell carcinoma of the renal pelvis or ureter and delay bladder tumour relapse. *BMC Cancer* 2011;11:297; © 2011 Chen et al; licensee BioMed Central Ltd.)

The kidneys are mobile organs and move vertically within the retroperitoneum an average of 0.9 to 1.3 cm and as much as 4 cm during normal respiration.[150–152] In going from the supine to upright position, the kidneys can shift inferiorly between 0.5 and 7.5 cm with an average of 3.6 cm.[153] This finding, although critical for total-body irradiation treatments, further highlights the mobility of the kidneys.

The high complication rates reported in the prospective trials of postoperative RT have taught radiation oncologists an important lesson regarding radiation therapy planning,

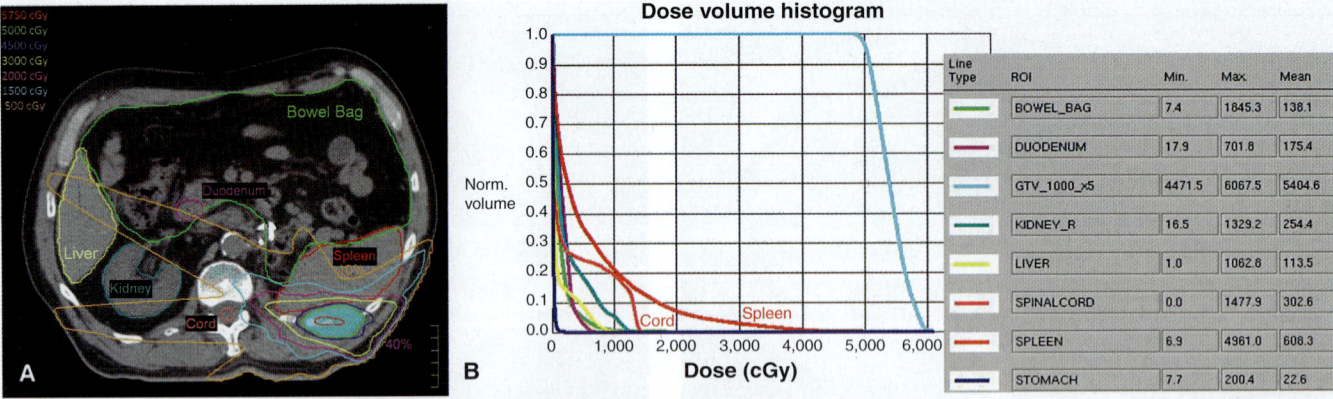

FIGURE 67.3. Patient with metastatic clear cell RCC who developed a painful, destructive, 55-cc metastasis in the left 12th rib. Treatment plan **(A)** and dose–volume histogram **(B)** showing the normalized volume versus dose (cGy). The metastasis was treated with 10 Gy × 5 using a six-field step-and-shoot, 6-MV IMRT technique. The isodose-based methodology was used to evaluate the plan.[155] The skin was limited to the 40% isodose (400 cGy × 5), the spinal cord to the 30% isodose (300 cGy × 5), and the spleen to the 10% isodose (100 cGy × 5) or less as feasible. The cyan-filled contour is the GTV. Doses to the bowel, liver, remaining kidney, and duodenum were well below tolerance.

patient selection, and the tolerance of the upper abdominal viscera. IMRT may be a reasonable consideration because of the sensitivity of adjacent surrounding structures. If IMRT is considered, a plan to manage the uncertainties in target localization such as 4-DCT treatment planning, IGRT, abdominal immobilization devices, gating, or breathing control needs to be considered. Renal function scans may assist in the treatment planning or patient selection process, but this has not been formally studied.

In unresectable lesions, 40 to 50 Gy neoadjuvant radiation therapy (1.8 to 2 Gy/fraction) directed to the kidney tumor and regional lymphatics may improve resectability.[110] Multiple-field techniques, similar to those described for adjuvant radiation therapy, should be considered in patients receiving preoperative treatment.

CT-based treatment planning contributes to good local control with minimal morbidity. Careful definition of the target volume to encompass the nephrectomy bed, lymph node drainage sites, and surgical clips on the planning CT scan is important. Exclusive use of anterior- and posterior-field arrangements, particularly on the right side, is likely to result in irradiation of large volumes of bowel and liver beyond tolerance. The use of multiple beams is paramount for protecting the surrounding normal structures. Total radiation doses of 45 to 50 Gy (1.8 to 2 Gy/fraction) to the nephrectomy bed and regional lymph nodes with a boost to small volumes of microscopic or gross residual disease of 10 to 15 Gy (total dose 50 to 60 Gy) are appropriate. Stein and coworkers[154] reported two scar recurrences and recommended that the incision site be included in the target volume. If the scar cannot be covered without increasing the amount of normal tissue irradiated, an additional electron-beam field to treat the scar may be considered.

Figure 67.3 illustrates a patient with metastatic clear cell RCC, with sarcomatoid and rhabdoid differentiation, status post left radical nephrectomy, pT3aN1M1. The kidney tumor was Fuhrman nuclear grade IV and 15.5 cm in diameter. The patient was treated with temsirolimus, pazopanib, bevacizumab, and finally adriamycin plus gemcitabine with some objective response. The patient developed a painful, destructive, 55-cc metastasis in the left 12th rib. The metastasis was treated with 10 Gy × 5 using a six-field (RPO 210, LAO 60, LT LAT 90, LPO 120, LPO 150, PA) step-and-shoot, 6-MV IMRT technique. The isodose-based methodology was used to evaluate the plan and is explained in detail in the reference.[155] The skin was limited to the 40% isodose (400 cGy × 5), the spinal cord to the 30% isodose (300 cGy × 5), and the spleen to the 10% isodose (100 cGy × 5) or less as feasible. Doses to

the bowel, liver, remaining kidney, and duodenum were well below tolerance (Fig. 67.3A). Daily imaging with 2D:2D match and cone-beam CT was used prior to the delivery of the 5 fractions over 3 weeks.

Because of the possibility of long survival even in the presence of distant metastases, aggressive treatment for palliation should be considered in patients who have limited metastatic disease with good performance status. Treatment fields should encompass metastatic foci with adequate (2 to 3 cm) margins. See previous sections on *Stereotactic Body Radiosurgery (SBRS) for Primary Treatment, Whole-Brain Radiation therapy for Brain Metastases, Stereotactic Radiosurgery (SRS) for Brain Metastases, Conventional Radiotherapy for Extracranial Metastases, and Stereotactic Body Radiation Therapy for Extracranial Metastases.*

Renal Pelvis and Ureter Carcinoma

Adjuvant radiation therapy has been used in the management of renal pelvis and ureter cancers. For elective radiotherapy, the clinical target volume should include the renal fossa, the course of the ureter to the bladder, the entire bladder, and the paracaval and para-aortic lymph nodes (Fig. 67.3).[143] As in RCC, CT-based planning may facilitate dosimetric coverage of the regions at risk while minimizing dose to normal tissues. Radiation doses of 45 to 50 Gy at 1.8 to 2 Gy per day are appropriate to treat subclinical and microscopic disease. For more extensive disease (e.g., multiple positive nodes), R1 (microscopic positive margins) or R2 (macroscopic residual margins) resections, a boost of 5 to 10 Gy should be considered. For unresectable or gross residual disease, higher doses may be necessary. In this event, multiple-field arrangements including oblique and lateral fields with field reductions are important to minimize toxicity to surrounding normal structures (Fig. 67.2). CT-based simulation, three-dimensional treatment planning, and contrast-enhanced radiographs are helpful in defining the radiation therapy target volume. IMRT may be considered if organ motion is managed to avoid underdosing the planning target volume. Chemotherapy may allow a lower radiation dose for gross disease.

FOLLOW-UP

Renal Cell Carcinoma

The NCCN Kidney Cancer Panel recommends patients be seen every 6 months for the first 2 years after surgery and then annually up to 5 years after diagnosis. Each visit should include a history and physical examination and comprehensive metabolic panel.[86] The NCCN recommends a baseline abdominal CT, MRI or ultrasound within 3 to 12 months of surgery, and chest imaging with its frequency depending on the initial stage. The UCLA UISS (described in *Prognostic Factors* section) uses the older 1997 TNM staging and also provides surveillance recommendations according to risk category.[156] The greatest risk of recurrence following surgery for RCC is in the first 1 to 2 years, with most relapses occurring within 3 years, but recurrences can occur more than a decade later. Early diagnosis of metastatic disease could identify patients who may be candidates for metastasectomy and potentially result in long-term survival.

Renal Pelvis and Ureter Carcinoma

Because patients with urothelial carcinoma of the upper urinary tract are at a high risk of urothelial tumors of the bladder, monitoring with cystoscopy at periodic intervals is necessary. For patients who underwent a renal-sparing procedure, imaging with CT or MRI and/or ureteroscopy may be necessary. The NCCN Bladder Cancer Panel recommends a cystoscopy every 3 months for 1 year and then at increasing intervals. For endoscopic procedures, imaging (IVP, CT urography, retrograde pyelogram, ureteroscopy, or MRI urogram) of the upper tract collecting system at 3- to 12-month intervals is recommended. Imaging to exclude metastatic disease such as a chest radiograph or chest CT or abdominal/pelvic CT or MRI should be considered.

SEQUELAE OF RADIATION THERAPY

The side effects and complications from radiation therapy for cancer of the kidney, renal pelvis, and ureters are similar to those expected from irradiation of the upper abdomen and pelvis. These side effects include nausea, vomiting, diarrhea, and abdominal cramping. Patients with right-sided tumors may have significant portions of the liver irradiated, and radiation-induced liver damage is possible. The Copenhagen Renal Cancer Study Group reported that 12 (44%) of 27 patients developed significant complications: Three had biochemical changes indicating radiation hepatitis, three had duodenum and small-bowel stenosis, and six had duodenum and small-bowel bleeding.[113] Surgery was performed on four of nine patients with bowel-related radiation therapy complications, and five patients died of treatment-related complications. The total radiation dose in this study was 50 Gy given in 2.5-Gy fractions per day—a fractionation schedule that may account for the high rate of complications. Fugitt also reported four cases of "liver" failure among 52 patients who received postoperative irradiation.[112]

The complication rate after radiation therapy for tumors of the kidney and upper urinary tract is related to the irradiated volume, total dose, fraction size, and technique of irradiation. CT-based simulation and 3-D treatment planning may decrease the risk of complications after elective radiotherapy in patients with upper urinary tract malignancies. In a prospective clinical trial, patients received single-fraction renal stereotactic ablative body RT (SABRT) (26 Gy) for tumors < 5 cm or fractionated SABR (3 × 14 Gy) for tumors ≥5 cm. For every 10 Gy of physical dose delivered, an exponential decline in affected kidney GFR was observed at 39% for 26 Gy in 1 fraction and 25% for 42 Gy in 3 fractions. When normalized to BED_{3Gy}, the dose–response relationship for each treatment prescription was similar with a plateau beyond 100 Gy. The authors concluded that sparing the functional kidney from high-dose regions (>50% isodoses) may help reduce risk of functional loss.[157] Another study of 14 patients receiving SBRT for RCC (50, 60,

or 70 Gy in 10 fractions) showed significant renal atrophic change. The dose distribution of SBRT at 20 to 30 Gy had a strong correlation with renal atrophy when using these 10 fraction regimens.[158]

ACKNOWLEDGMENTS

Thanks to Michael Watts, M.S., CMD, for masterfully planning the case in Figure 67.3 and obtaining the screen captures of the plan.

REFERENCES

1. Marshall FF Powell KC. Lymphadenectomy for renal cell carcinoma: anatomical and therapeutic considerations. *J Urol* 1982;128:677–681.
2. Thompson RH, et al. Tumor size is associated with malignant potential in renal cell carcinoma cases. *J Urol* 2009;181:2033–2036.
3. Torre LA, et al. Global cancer statistics, 2012. *CA Cancer J Clin* 2015;65:87–108.
4. American Cancer Society. *Cancer facts and figures 2017*, vol. 2017. Atlanta, GA: American Cancer Society, 2017.
5. Henschler D, et al. Increased incidence of renal cell tumors in a cohort of cardboard workers exposed to trichloroethene. *Arch Toxicol* 1995;69:291–299.
6. Mandel JS, et al. International renal-cell cancer study. IV. Occupation. *Int J Cancer* 1995;61:601–605.
7. Lai PP. Kidney, renal pelvis, and ureter. In: Perez CA, Brady LW, eds. *Principles and practice of radiation oncology*, 2nd ed. Philadelphia, PA: JB Lippincott, 1992.
8. Wolk A, et al. International renal cancer study. VII. Role of diet. *Int J Cancer* 1996;65:67–73.
9. Lew JQ, et al. Alcohol consumption and risk of renal cell cancer: the NIH-AARP diet and health study. *Br J Cancer* 2011;104:537–541.
10. Muscat JE, Hoffmann D, Wynder EL. The epidemiology of renal cell carcinoma. A second look. *Cancer* 1995;75:2552–2557.
11. Lindblad P, et al. The role of diabetes mellitus in the aetiology of renal cell cancer. *Diabetologia* 1999;42:107–112.
12. Gordon SC, et al. Risk for renal cell carcinoma in chronic hepatitis C infection. *Cancer Epidemiol Biomarkers Prev* 2010;19:1066–1073.
13. Argani P, et al. Translocation carcinomas of the kidney after chemotherapy in childhood. *J Clin Oncol* 2006;24:1529–1534.
14. Brennan JF, et al. Acquired renal cystic disease: implications for the urologist. *Br J Urol* 1991;67:342–348.
15. Truong LD, et al. Renal neoplasm in acquired cystic kidney disease. *Am J Kidney Dis* 1995;26:1–12.
16. Kim WY Kaelin WG. Role of vhl gene mutation in human cancer. *J Clin Oncol* 2004;22:4991–5004.
17. Pavlovich CP, Schmidt LS Phillips JL. The genetic basis of renal cell carcinoma. *Urol Clin North Am* 2003;30:437–454, vii.
18. *Pathology and genetics of tumours of the urinary system and male genital organs*. Lyon, France: IARC Press, 2004.
19. Keith DS, et al. Renal cell carcinoma in autosomal dominant polycystic kidney disease. *J Am Soc Nephrol* 1994;4:1661–1669.
20. Reitelman C, et al. Prognostic variables in patients with transitional cell carcinoma of the renal pelvis and proximal ureter. *J Urol* 1987;138:1144–1145.
21. Huben RP, Mounzer AM Murphy GP. Tumor grade and stage as prognostic variables in upper tract urothelial tumors. *Cancer* 1988;62:2016–2020.
22. Olgac S, et al. Urothelial carcinoma of the renal pelvis: a clinicopathologic study of 130 cases. *Am J Surg Pathol* 2004;28:1545–1552.
23. Charbit L, et al. Tumors of the upper urinary tract: 10 years of experience. *J Urol* 1991;146:1243–1246.
24. Gylling AH, et al. Differential cancer predisposition in lynch syndrome: insights from molecular analysis of brain and urinary tract tumors. *Carcinogenesis* 2008;29:1351–1359.
25. Nortier JL, et al. Urothelial carcinoma associated with the use of a Chinese herb (*Aristolochia fangchi*). *N Engl J Med* 2000;342:1686–1692.
26. Yang MH, et al. Unusually high incidence of upper urinary tract urothelial carcinoma in Taiwan. *Urology* 2002;59:681–687.
27. Blohme I Johansson S. Renal pelvic neoplasms and atypical urothelium in patients with end-stage analgesic nephropathy. *Kidney Int* 1981;20:671–675.
28. Flocks RH Kadesky MC. Malignant neoplasms of the kidney; an analysis of 353 patients followed five years or more. *J Urol* 1958;79:196–201.
29. Giuliani L, et al. Radical extensive surgery for renal cell carcinoma: long-term results and prognostic factors. *J Urol* 1990;143:468–473; discussion 473–474.
30. Waters WB Richie JP. Aggressive surgical approach to renal cell carcinoma: review of 130 cases. *J Urol* 1979;122:306–309.
31. Selli C, et al. Stratification of risk factors in renal cell carcinoma. *Cancer* 1983;52:899–903.
32. Tolia BM Whitmore WF Jr. Solitary metastasis from renal cell carcinoma. *J Urol* 1975;114:836–838.
33. Montie JE, et al. The role of adjunctive nephrectomy in patients with metastatic renal cell carcinoma. *J Urol* 1977;117:272–275.

Section III

34. Cozad SC, et al. Transitional cell carcinoma of the renal pelvis or ureter: patterns of failure. *Urology* 1995;46:796–800.

35. Maulard-Durdux C, et al. Postoperative radiation therapy in 26 patients with invasive transitional cell carcinoma of the upper urinary tract: no impact on survival? *J Urol* 1996;155:115–117.

36. Skinner DG, et al. Diagnosis and management of renal cell carcinoma. A clinical and pathologic study of 309 cases. *Cancer* 1971;28:1165–1177.

37. Smith RB, et al. Bilateral renal cell carcinoma and renal cell carcinoma in the solitary kidney. *J Urol* 1984;132:450–454.

38. Gibbons RP, et al. Manifestations of renal cell carcinoma. *Urology* 1976;8:201–206.

39. Pinals RS Krane SM. Medical aspects of renal carcinoma. *Postgrad Med J* 1962;38:507–519.

40. Gold PJ, Fefer A Thompson JA. Paraneoplastic manifestations of renal cell carcinoma. *Semin Urol Oncol* 1996;14:216–222.

41. Da Silva JL, et al. Tumor cells are the site of erythropoietin synthesis in human renal cancers associated with polycythemia. *Blood* 1990;75:577–582.

42. O'Keefe SC, et al. Thrombocytosis is associated with a significant increase in the cancer specific death rate after radical nephrectomy. *J Urol* 2002;168:1378–1380.

43. Pras M, et al. Amyloidosis associated with renal cell carcinoma of the aa type. *Am J Med* 1982;73:426–428.

44. Symbas NP, et al. Poor prognosis associated with thrombocytosis in patients with renal cell carcinoma. *BJU Int* 2000;86:203–207.

45. Sidhom OA, Basalaev M Sigal LH. Renal cell carcinoma presenting as polymyalgia rheumatica. Resolution after nephrectomy. *Arch Intern Med* 1993;153:2043–2045.

46. Jayson M Sanders H. Increased incidence of serendipitously discovered renal cell carcinoma. *Urology* 1998;51:203–205.

47. Da Silva JL, et al. Tumor cells are the site of erythropoietin synthesis in human renal cancers associated with polycythemia. *Blood* 1990;75:577–582.

48. Sufrin G, et al. Hormones in renal cancer. *J Urol* 1977;117:433–438.

49. McClennan BL. Oncologic imaging. Staging and follow-up of renal and adrenal carcinoma. *Cancer* 1991;67:1199–1208.

50. Kidney. In: Amin MB, Edge S, Greene F, et al., eds. *AJCC cancer staging manual.* New York: Springer-Verlag, 2017.

51. Renal pelvis and ureter. In: Amin MB, Edge S, Greene F, et al., eds. *AJCC cancer staging manual.* New York: Springer-Verlag, 2017.

52. Cancer IAfRo. *WHO classification of tumours of the urinary system and male genital organs.* World Health Organization, 2016.

53. Bruno D, et al. Genitourinary complications of sickle cell disease. *J Urol* 2001;166:803–811.

54. Howlader N, Noone AM, Krapcho M, et al., eds. *SEER cancer statistics review, 1975–2008, based on November 2010 SEER data submission, posted to the SEER web site 2011,* vol. 2011. Bethesda, MD: National Cancer Institute, 2011.

55. Pantuck AJ, Zisman A Belldegrun AS. The changing natural history of renal cell carcinoma. *J Urol* 2001;166:1611–1623.

56. Hudes G, et al. Temsirolimus, interferon alfa, or both for advanced renal-cell carcinoma. *N Engl J Med* 2007;356:2271–2281.

57. Motzer RJ, et al. Survival and prognostic stratification of 670 patients with advanced renal cell carcinoma. *J Clin Oncol* 1999;17:2530–2540.

58. Bassil B, Dosoretz DE, Prout GR Jr. Validation of the tumor, nodes and metastasis classification of renal cell carcinoma. *J Urol* 1985;134:450–454.

59. Golimbu M, et al. Renal cell carcinoma: survival and prognostic factors. *Urology* 1986;27:291–301.

60. Rabinovitch RA, et al. Patterns of failure following surgical resection of renal cell carcinoma: implications for adjuvant local and systemic therapy. *J Clin Oncol* 1994;12:206–212.

61. Blute ML, et al. A protocol for performing extended lymph node dissection using primary tumor pathological features for patients treated with radical nephrectomy for clear cell renal cell carcinoma. *J Urol* 2004;172:465–469.

62. Pantuck AJ, et al. Renal cell carcinoma with retroperitoneal lymph nodes. Impact on survival and benefits of immunotherapy. *Cancer* 2003;97:2995–3002.

63. Vasselli JR, et al. Lack of retroperitoneal lymphadenopathy predicts survival of patients with metastatic renal cell carcinoma. *J Urol* 2001;166:68–72.

64. Kjaer M. The treatment and prognosis of patients with renal adenocarcinoma with solitary metastasis. 10 year survival results. *Int J Radiat Oncol Biol Phys.* 1987;13:619–621.

65. Thrasher JB Paulson DF. Prognostic factors in renal cancer. *Urol Clin North Am* 1993;20:247–262.

66. Fuhrman SA, Lasky LC Limas C. Prognostic significance of morphologic parameters in renal cell carcinoma. *Am J Surg Pathol* 1982;6:655–663.

67. Lohse CM, et al. Comparison of standardized and nonstandardized nuclear grade of renal cell carcinoma to predict outcome among 2,042 patients. *Am J Clin Pathol* 2002;118:877–886.

68. Bretheau D, et al. Prognostic value of nuclear grade of renal cell carcinoma. *Cancer* 1995;76:2543–2549.

69. Sella A, et al. Sarcomatoid renal cell carcinoma. A treatable entity. *Cancer* 1987;60:1313–1318.

70. Kattan MW, et al. A postoperative prognostic nomogram for renal cell carcinoma. *J Urol* 2001;166:63–67.

71. Frank I, et al. An outcome prediction model for patients with clear cell renal cell carcinoma treated with radical nephrectomy based on tumor stage, size, grade and necrosis: the SSIGN score. *J Urol* 2002;168:2395–2400.

72. Zisman A, et al. Improved prognostication of renal cell carcinoma using an integrated staging system. *J Clin Oncol* 2001;19:1649–1657.

73. Thompson RH Kwon ED. Significance of b7-h1 overexpression in kidney cancer. *Clin Genitourin Cancer* 2006;5:206–211.

74. Bui MH, et al. Prognostic value of carbonic anhydrase IX and Ki67 as predictors of survival for renal clear cell carcinoma. *J Urol* 2004;171:2461–2466.

75. Jiang Z, et al. Analysis of RNA-binding protein IMP3 to predict metastasis and prognosis of renal-cell carcinoma: a retrospective study. *Lancet Oncol* 2006;7:556–564.

76. Raman JD, et al. Impact of tumor location on prognosis for patients with upper tract urothelial carcinoma managed by radical nephroureterectomy. *Eur Urol* 2010;57:1072–1079.

77. Corrado F, et al. Transitional cell carcinoma of the upper urinary tract: evaluation of prognostic factors by histopathology and flow cytometric analysis. *J Urol* 1991;145:1159–1163.

78. Heney NM, et al. Prognostic factors in carcinoma of the ureter. *J Urol* 1981;125:632–636.

79. Hall MC, et al. Prognostic factors, recurrence, and survival in transitional cell carcinoma of the upper urinary tract: a 30-year experience in 252 patients. *Urology* 1998;52:594–601.

80. Akdogan B, et al. Prognostic significance of bladder tumor history and tumor location in upper tract transitional cell carcinoma. *J Urol* 2006;176:48–52.

81. Park S, et al. The impact of tumor location on prognosis of transitional cell carcinoma of the upper urinary tract. *J Urol* 2004;171:621–625.

82. Mullerad M, et al. Bladder cancer as a prognostic factor for upper tract transitional cell carcinoma. *J Urol* 2004;172:2177–2181.

83. Catto JW, et al. Promoter hypermethylation is associated with tumor location, stage, and subsequent progression in transitional cell carcinoma. *J Clin Oncol* 2005;23:2903–2910.

84. DiBiase SJ, et al. Palliative irradiation for focally symptomatic metastatic renal cell carcinoma: support for dose escalation based on a biological model. *J Urol* 1997;158:746–749.

85. Zelefsky MJ, et al. Tumor control outcomes after hypofractionated and single-dose stereotactic image-guided intensity-modulated radiotherapy for extracranial metastases from renal cell carcinoma. *Int J Radiat Oncol Biol Phys* 2012;82:1744–1748.

86. Motzer RJ, Jonasch E, Agarwal N, et al. *Kidney cancer NCCN Clinical Practice Guidelines in Oncology, vol. 2017, ed. Version 2.2017.* National Comprehensive Cancer Network, 2016.

87. Lane BR, et al. Active treatment of localized renal tumors may not impact overall survival in patients aged 75 years or older. *Cancer* 2010;116:3119–3126.

88. Lane BR, et al. Management of the adrenal gland during partial nephrectomy. *J Urol* 2009;181:2430–2436; discussion 2436–2437.

89. Gill IS, et al. Adrenal involvement from renal cell carcinoma: predictive value of computerized tomography. *J Urol* 1994;152:1082–1085.

90. Blom JH, et al. Radical nephrectomy with and without lymph-node dissection: final results of European Organization for Research and Treatment of Cancer (EORTC) randomized phase 3 trial 30881. *Eur Urol* 2009;55:28–34.

91. Hollingsworth JM, et al. Surgical management of low-stage renal cell carcinoma: technology does not supersede biology. *Urology* 2006;67:1175–1180.

92. Leibovich BC, et al. Nephron sparing surgery for appropriately selected renal cell carcinoma between 4 and 7 cm results in outcome similar to radical nephrectomy. *J Urol* 2004;171:1066–1070.

93. Weight CJ, et al. Nephrectomy induced chronic renal insufficiency is associated with increased risk of cardiovascular death and death from any cause in patients with localized ct1b renal masses. *J Urol* 2010;183:1317–1323.

94. Weight CJ, et al. Partial nephrectomy is associated with improved overall survival compared to radical nephrectomy in patients with unanticipated benign renal tumours. *Eur Urol* 2010;58:293–298.

95. Lau WK, et al. Matched comparison of radical nephrectomy vs nephron-sparing surgery in patients with unilateral renal cell carcinoma and a normal contralateral kidney. *Mayo Clin Proc* 2000;75:1236–1242.

96. McKiernan J, et al. Natural history of chronic renal insufficiency after partial and radical nephrectomy. *Urology* 2002;59:816–820.

97. Nissenkorn I Bernheim J. Multicentricity in renal cell carcinoma. *J Urol* 1995;153:620–622.

98. Oya M, et al. Intrarenal satellites of renal cell carcinoma: histopathologic manifestation and clinical implication. *Urology* 1995;46:161–164.

99. Whang M, et al. The incidence of multifocal renal cell carcinoma in patients who are candidates for partial nephrectomy. *J Urol* 1995;154:968–970; discussion 970–971.

100. Bennett RT, et al. Cytoreductive surgery for stage iv renal cell carcinoma. *J Urol* 1995;154:32–34.

101. Flanigan RC, et al. Nephrectomy followed by interferon alfa-2b compared with interferon alfa-2b alone for metastatic renal-cell cancer. *N Engl J Med* 2001;345:1655–1659.

102. Mickisch GH, et al. Radical nephrectomy plus interferon-alfa-based immunotherapy compared with interferon alfa alone in metastatic renal-cell carcinoma: a randomised trial. *Lancet* 2001;358:966–970.

103. Kunkle DA Uzzo RG. Cryoablation or radiofrequency ablation of the small renal mass: a meta-analysis. *Cancer* 2008;113:2671–2680.

104. Frank W, et al. Stage iv renal cell carcinoma. *J Urol* 1994;152:1998–1999.

105. Kavolius JP, et al. Resection of metastatic renal cell carcinoma. *J Clin Oncol* 1998;16:2261–2266.

106. Piltz S, et al. Long-term results after pulmonary resection of renal cell carcinoma metastases. *Ann Thorac Surg* 2002;73:1082–1087.

107. Zerbi A, et al. Pancreatic metastasis from renal cell carcinoma: which patients benefit from surgical resection? *Ann Surg Oncol* 2008;15:1161–1168.

108. Shaikh T, et al. Contemporary trends in the utilization of radiotherapy in patients with renal cell carcinoma. *Urology* 2015;86:1165–1173.

109. van der Werf-Messing B. Proceedings: carcinoma of the kidney. *Cancer* 1973;32:1056–1061.

110. van der Werf-Messing B, van der Heul RO, Ledeboer RC. Renal cell carcinoma trial. *Strahlentherapie Sonderb* 1981;76:169–715.

111. Juusela H, et al. Preoperative irradiation in the treatment of renal adenocarcinoma. *Scand J Urol Nephrol* 1977;11:277–281.

112. Fugitt RB, Wu GS Martinelli LC. An evaluation of postoperative radiotherapy in hypernephroma treatment—a clinical trial. *Cancer* 1973;32:1332–1340.

113. Kjaer M, Frederiksen PL Engelholm SA. Postoperative radiotherapy in stage ii and iii renal adenocarcinoma. A randomized trial by the Copenhagen Renal Cancer Study Group. *Int J Radiat Oncol Biol Phys* 1987;13:665–672.

114. Aref I, Bociek RG Salhani D. Is post-operative radiation for renal cell carcinoma justified? *Radiother Oncol* 1997;43:155–157.

115. Yossepowitch O, et al. Positive surgical margins at partial nephrectomy: predictors and oncological outcomes. *J Urol* 2008;179:2158–2163.

116. Eminaga O, et al. Does postoperative radiation therapy impact survival in non-metastatic sarcomatoid renal cell carcinoma? A seer-based study. *Int Urol Nephrol* 2015;47:1653–1663.

117. Tunio MA, Hashmi A Rafi M. Need for a new trial to evaluate postoperative radiotherapy in renal cell carcinoma: a meta-analysis of randomized controlled trials. *Ann Oncol* 2010;21:1839–1845.

118. Staehler M, et al. Single fraction radiosurgery for the treatment of renal tumors. *J Urol* 2015;193:771–775.

119. Rades D, Heisterkamp C Schild SE. Do patients receiving whole-brain radiotherapy for brain metastases from renal cell carcinoma benefit from escalation of the radiation dose? *Int J Radiat Oncol Biol Phys* 2010;78:398–403.

120. Shuto T, et al. Treatment strategy for metastatic brain tumors from renal cell carcinoma: Selection of gamma knife surgery or craniotomy for control of growth and peritumoral edema. *J Neurooncol* 2010;98:169–175.

121. Kim WH, et al. Early significant tumor volume reduction after radiosurgery in brain metastases from renal cell carcinoma results in long-term survival. *Int J Radiat Oncol Biol Phys* 2012;82:1749–1755.

122. Kano H, et al. Outcome predictors of gamma knife radiosurgery for renal cell carcinoma metastases. *Neurosurgery* 2011;69:1232–1239.

123. Cochran DC, et al. The effect of targeted agents on outcomes in patients with brain metastases from renal cell carcinoma treated with gamma knife surgery. *J Neurosurg* 2012;116:978–983.

124. Kothari G, et al. Outcomes of stereotactic radiotherapy for cranial and extracranial metastatic renal cell carcinoma: a systematic review. *Acta Oncol* 2015;54:148–157.

125. Fossa SD, Kjolseth I Lund G. Radiotherapy of metastases from renal cancer. *Eur Urol* 1982;8:340–342.

126. Halperin EC Harisiadis L. The role of radiation therapy in the management of metastatic renal cell carcinoma. *Cancer* 1983;51:614–617.

127. Lee J, et al. A phase ii trial of palliative radiotherapy for metastatic renal cell carcinoma. *Cancer* 2005;104:1894–1900.

128. Onufrey V Mohiuddin M. Radiation therapy in the treatment of metastatic renal cell carcinoma. *Int J Radiat Oncol Biol Phys* 1985;11:2007–2009.

129. Gay HA, et al. Complete response in a cutaneous facial metastatic nodule from renal cell carcinoma after hypofractionated radiotherapy. *Dermatol Online J* 2007;13:6.

130. Zelefsky MJ, et al. Tumor control outcomes after hypofractionated and single-dose stereotactic image-guided intensity-modulated radiotherapy for extracranial metastases from renal cell carcinoma. *Int J Radiat Oncol Biol Phys* 2012;82:1744–1748.

131. Wersall PJ, et al. Extracranial stereotactic radiotherapy for primary and metastatic renal cell carcinoma. *Radiother Oncol* 2005;77:88–95.

132. Nguyen Q-N, et al. Management of spinal metastases from renal cell carcinoma using stereotactic body radiotherapy. *Int J Radiat Oncol Biol Phys* 2010;76:1185–1192.

133. Thibault I, et al. Spine stereotactic body radiotherapy for renal cell cancer spinal metastases: analysis of outcomes and risk of vertebral compression fracture. *J Neurosurg Spine* 2014;21:711–718.

134. Balagamwala EH, et al. Single-fraction stereotactic body radiotherapy for spinal metastases from renal cell carcinoma. *J Neurosurg Spine* 2012;17:556–564.

135. Amini A, et al. Local control rates of metastatic renal cell carcinoma (RCC) to the bone using stereotactic body radiation therapy: is RCC truly radioresistant? *Pract Radiat Oncol* 2015;5:e589–e596.

136. Wersall PJ, et al. Regression of non-irradiated metastases after extracranial stereotactic radiotherapy in metastatic renal cell carcinoma. *Acta Oncol* 2006;45:493–497.

137. Paly JJ, et al. Outcomes in a multi-institutional cohort of patients treated with intraoperative radiation therapy for advanced or recurrent renal cell carcinoma. *Int J Radiat Oncol Biol Phys* 2014;88:618–623.

138. Flaig TW, Spiess PE, Agarwal N, et al. *Bladder cancer NCCN Clinical Practice Guidelines in Oncology, vol. 2017, ed. Version 2.2017*. National Comprehensive Cancer Network, 2017.

139. Audenet F, et al. The role of chemotherapy in the treatment of urothelial cell carcinoma of the upper urinary tract (UUT-UCC). *Urol Oncol* 2013;31:407–413.

140. Clayman RV, Lange PH Fraley EE. Cancer of the upper urinary tract. In: Javadpour N, ed. *Principles and management of urologic cancer*, 2nd ed. Baltimore, MD: Williams & Wilkins, 1983.

141. Blacher EJ, et al. Squamous cell carcinoma of renal pelvis. *Urology* 1985;25:124–126.

142. Cozad SC, et al. Adjuvant radiotherapy in high stage transitional cell carcinoma of the renal pelvis and ureter. *Int J Radiat Oncol Biol Phys* 1992;24:743–745.

143. Chen B, et al. Radiotherapy may improve overall survival of patients with t3/t4 transitional cell carcinoma of the renal pelvis or ureter and delay bladder tumour relapse. *BMC Cancer* 2011;11:297.

144. Catton CN, et al. Transitional cell carcinoma of the renal pelvis and ureter; outcome and patterns of relapse in patients treated with postoperative radiation. *Urol Oncol* 1996;2:171–176.

145. Sternberg CN, et al. Seven year update of an EORTC phase III trial of high-dose intensity M-VAC chemotherapy and G-CSF versus classic M-VAC in advanced urothelial tract tumours. *Eur J Cancer* 2006;42:50–54.

146. Dawson LA, et al. Radiation-associated kidney injury. *Int J Radiat Oncol Biol Phys* 2010;76:S108–S115.

147. Kavanagh BD, et al. Radiation dose-volume effects in the stomach and small bowel. *Int J Radiat Oncol Biol Phys* 2010;76:S101–S107.

148. Pan CC, et al. Radiation-associated liver injury. *Int J Radiat Oncol Biol Phys* 2010;76:S94–S100.

149. Shrimali RK, Correa PD O'Rourke N. Low-dose palliative splenic irradiation in haematolymphoid malignancy. *J Med Imaging Radiat Oncol* 2008;52:297–302.

150. Brandner ED, et al. Abdominal organ motion measured using 4D CT. *Int J Radiat Oncol Biol Phys* 2006;65:554–560.

151. Schwartz LH, et al. Kidney mobility during respiration. *Radiother Oncol* 1994;32:84–86.

152. van Sornsen de Koste JR, et al. Renal mobility during uncoached quiet respiration: an analysis of 4dct scans. *Int J Radiat Oncol Biol Phys* 2006;64:799–803.

153. Reiff JE, et al. Changes in the size and location of kidneys from the supine to standing positions and the implications for block placement during total body irradiation. *Int J Radiat Oncol Biol Phys* 1999;45:447–449.

154. Stein M, et al. The value of postoperative irradiation in renal cancer. *Radiother Oncol* 1992;24:41–44.

155. Gay HA, et al. Isodose-based methodology for minimizing the morbidity and mortality of thoracic hypofractionated radiotherapy. *Radiother Oncol* 2009;91:369–378.

156. Lam JS, et al. Postoperative surveillance protocol for patients with localized and locally advanced renal cell carcinoma based on a validated prognostic nomogram and risk group stratification system. *J Urol* 2005;174:466–472; discussion 472; quiz 801.

157. Siva S, et al. Impact of stereotactic radiotherapy on kidney function in primary renal cell carcinoma: Establishing a dose-response relationship. *Radiother Oncol* 2016;118:540–546.

158. Yamamoto T, et al. Renal atrophy after stereotactic body radiotherapy for renal cell carcinoma. *Radiat Oncol* 2016;11:72.

159. Shuch B, et al. Defining early-onset kidney cancer: implications for germline and somatic mutation testing and clinical management. *J Clin Oncol* 2014;32:431–437.

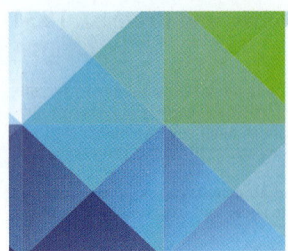

CHAPTER 68

Bladder Cancer

Carlos A. Perez

INTRODUCTION

This is an update of a chapter published by James et al.[1] in Principles and Practice of Radiation Oncology 6th edition.

Every aspect of the perceptions and management of bladder cancer requires change; departing from the use of the term "superficial" bladder cancer is the first step,[2] because the term is both inaccurate and implies an inappropriate lack of importance. In particular, given the very high costs to health care systems from long-term surveillance and treatment of the disease,[3] it is particularly surprising that there has not been more emphasis on the disease from health policy makers and pharmaceutical companies.

In addition, a rethinking of the view that cystectomy is the gold standard for invasive bladder cancer is long overdue. Comparisons of large surgical[4] and radiation therapy[5] series document similar long-term survival rates, and population-based studies do not appear to show any survival differences linked to the mode of treatment.[6] Furthermore, most large surgical series have median ages in the mid-60s,[4,7] well below the (rising) disease population median, suggesting the results may not be applicable to many or even most patients with invasive bladder cancer. Use of bladder preservation varies worldwide from around 10% in the United States[8] to 25% in Scandinavia[9] to around 50% in the United Kingdom.[10] Moreover, there is good evidence that older or less fit patients in low-volume centers are less likely to be referred for surgery, despite the likelihood of them being fit for radiation therapy.[8,9]

In contrast, recent large randomized radiation therapy series from the United Kingdom suggest that definitive radiation therapy with chemosensitization, either with low-dose chemotherapy[11] or with hypoxia-targeting agents,[12] is effective and well tolerated by elderly patients (median age in both studies was 72 to 73 years). Long-term functional outcomes with radiation therapy are excellent,[11–13] making it particularly suitable for less fit patients who may struggle with major surgery or a urinary diversion.

This chapter outlines the evidence base for the current therapeutic approaches to bladder cancer and in particular will examine the proposition that bladder preservation for muscle-invasive disease is an approach that merits continuous emphasis and re-evaluation.

ANATOMY OF THE BLADDER

The bladder is a hollow, muscular organ situated in the pelvis when empty but able to extend up into the abdomen when full, particularly in situations where bladder emptying is impeded. At birth, the pelvis is relatively small in comparison to the abdomen, and thus, the bladder has a larger abdominal component at birth and becomes more "pelvic" as growth and maturity proceed. By puberty, the bladder has migrated to the confines of the deepened true pelvis.

The bladder is described as having an apex, a superior surface, two inferolateral surfaces, a base or posterior surface, a trigone, and a neck. The apex reaches a short distance cephalad above the pubic bone and ends as a fibrous cord, the remnant of the fetal urachus, which connects the bladder to the allantois. The urachus lies anterior to the peritoneal cavity and is important as tumors can arise in the urachal remnant.

The superior surface is covered by the peritoneum, again an important anatomical feature as it means that there is bowel lying superiorly to the bladder, which is potentially a critical site to consider when planning radiotherapy, particularly in men. In women, it is associated with the uterus and ileum. The base of the bladder is posterior and is separated from the rectum by the vas deferens, seminal vesicles, and ureters in the male and by the uterus and vagina in the female. The seminal vesicles form a V-shaped structure at the base of the bladder, with the vas deferens entering the middle of the "V." The ureters enter into the bladder slightly superior and lateral to the seminal vesicles, with the vas deferens coursing above and in a caudal direction to the ureters. Again, these relations are critical as enlarging tumors either at the base or in the prostate can involve the ureters with consequent hydronephrosis. Inferiorly and laterally to the bladder lie the various pelvic bones and muscles: pubis, the levator ani, and obturator internus muscles. Within the pelvis, the lateral parts of the bladder are surrounded by loose connective tissue. Anteriorly, the bladder is separated from the pubic bone by the retropubic space. The inferior part of the bladder is described as the neck and is in continuity with the urethra and, very importantly, the prostate gland in males. The neck of the bladder is anchored in the pelvis, and the superior portions distend and expand upward as the bladder fills.

The mucosal lining of the bladder comprises a transitional epithelium that extends from the renal pelvis to the urethra. The most common tumors arising in the urinary system are transition cell (or urothelial) carcinomas (TCC or UC). These tumors can arise from anywhere within the urothelium, so diagnosis, treatment, and surveillance protocols must take account of this important biologic feature. As a distensible organ, the macroscopic appearance of the urothelium varies with distension from smooth and flat to folded when empty. A ridge called the interureteral fold lies between the ureteric orifices.

EPIDEMIOLOGY

Bladder cancer, with over 385,000 new cases reported worldwide in 2008[14] is a major cause of cancer morbidity and mortality. Median age at diagnosis is above 70 years, and as the tumor is often smoking related, many patients have significant comorbidity, posing risks for radical surgical approaches. Survival rates are poor, with around 45% of muscle-invasive cancer patients surviving 5 years irrespective of treatment modality.[4,5,7] Demographically, the industrializing nations will contribute to a significant rise in the global incidence of bladder UC,[15] with particularly large numbers likely in China given the rapid improvement in standards of living and the high prevalence of smoking. However, despite the decreasing incidence in developed nations, there remain specific challenges, mainly because of the aging population and increased life expectancy. Within two large cohorts separated by 15 years (1991 to 1992 and 2005 to 2010), researchers have recently demonstrated an increase in the median age at presentation of 4 years, with an increase from 13% to 24% in the proportion of patients over 80 years old.[16] Overall, around 75% to 80% of patients with bladder cancer are male, mostly reflecting historic trends in cigarette smoking.

There are well-known associations of squamous cell bladder carcinomas with bilharzia caused by *Schistosoma haematobium* infection in Africa, particularly in Egypt.[17] Aromatic amines, polycyclic aromatic and chlorinated hydrocarbons, arsenic-laced drinking water, aristolochic acid, cyclophosphamide exposure, and a range of industrial chemicals have been implicated in urothelial carcinogenesis. Importantly, as with most carcinogens, there are variations in individual susceptibility, and the basis of some of these polymorphisms regulating varied detoxification mechanisms has been identified.[18] With increasing awareness of these industrial associations, regulation of these processes means that these cases are becoming increasingly rare in the developed world. Their principal importance now is that those with industrially linked tumors may be entitled to compensation payments. In Egypt, there have been successful public health approaches to the control of *S. haematobium* infections, leading to a substantial decline in incidence and mortality from squamous carcinomas of the bladder.[19]

Within the developed world, the overwhelming majority of bladder tumors are now TCCs, and the main known causative factor is tobacco (particularly cigarette) smoking,[20–25] explaining approximately half of the cases in men and one-third of the cases in women in Europe (discussed in detail below). The relation between smoking and other prognostic factors is interesting, as it could give insight into biologic mechanisms of disease and, perhaps more importantly, have clinical implications by increasing our ability to identify patients at risk of more malignant disease.

NATURAL HISTORY

Non–Muscle-Invasive Bladder Cancer

Most cases (70% to 80%) present with non–muscle-invasive bladder cancer (NMIBC, stage Ta, T1, and carcinoma *in situ* [Tis]), which is rarely lethal, but shows a high recurrence rate of 50% to 70% after treatment by transurethral resection of the bladder tumor (TURBT).[26] In about 10% to 20% of patients with NMIBC, the disease progresses to muscle invasion (≥T2 lesions), which can lead to metastasis and death.[26] However, the majority of patients with NMIBC will die of other causes, given the typically advanced age at presentation and the strong association with cigarette smoking,[20–25] although it is worth noting that up to 21% of patients with Ta tumors and 49% of patients with T1 tumors will die from bladder cancer.[27] For patients with NMIBC, it has been observed that tumor grade and stage, and also tumor number, size, presence of carcinoma *in situ* (CIS), recurrence rate, and age at diagnosis are risk factors of progression.[28–30] The risk of both recurrence and progression necessitates lifelong follow-up for patients with bladder tumors. However, there are factors that predict a higher risk of progression (to invasion) as opposed to recurrence in lower-risk tumors, and the European Organisation for Research and Treatment of Cancer (EORTC) "bladder cancer calculator" quantifies the risk depending on the tumor characteristics imputed.[30]

Invasive Disease

Muscle-invasive bladder cancer has a poor prognosis because of a very high rate of occult metastatic disease at the time of diagnosis. Evidence for this comes from the high rate of death from metastasis after apparently successful surgery. Furthermore, reported 5-year survival rates with radiotherapy or surgery are remarkably similar at around 45% to 50%,[4,5] despite a higher rate of pelvic recurrence after radiation therapy versus surgery, suggesting that prognosis is driven by the presence, or otherwise, of metastases at the time of diagnosis, driven by tumor-related factors such as stage and grade.[6]

Metastatic Disease

A minority of patients (probably <10%) present with metastatic disease, carrying a poor prognosis; most patients with metastatic disease have had prior treatment for apparently localized disease. Overall survival from diagnosis of metastasis is difficult to ascertain as many patients receive only palliative treatment. A minority of patients are fit for systemic chemotherapy, and there are good data on outcomes with chemotherapy. In essence, extensive randomized studies, mostly carried out in the 1980s and 1990s, have demonstrated the superiority of cisplatinum-based combinations over those containing other drugs or cisplatinum alone.[31] Of the platinum-based combinations, methotrexate/vinblastine/doxorubicin (Adriamycin)/cisplatinum (MVAC)[32] and gemcitabine/cisplatinum (GC)[33] have proven to be superior to other combinations and broadly similar in efficacy to each other[34,35] (as reviewed by Hussain and James).[36] Median survival is 12 to 18 months, depending on the extent of disease and fitness of the patient. Intriguingly, however, a small minority of patients do appear to survive long term after chemotherapy for metastatic disease, but this percentage has sadly proved very hard to increase from that originally observed in the MVAC trials.

ETIOLOGY

The link between occupational exposure and an increased risk of urothelial cancer of the bladder was established more than a century ago when Rehn[37] reported on three cases of bladder cancer in a German chemical dye works in 1895.[38] During the following 40 years, similar reports appeared from around the world.[39] In 1938, Hueper et al.[39] demonstrated that when naphthylamine, an industrial arylamine used in the synthetic dye industry, was fed to dogs, it caused bladder carcinomas identical to the human disease. The link between industrial arylamines and bladder cancer was thus established and later confirmed by Case et al.[40] in 1954. These authors also identified an excess of bladder cancer in the tire industry, attributable to the use of 2-naphthylamine in the manufacture of rubber.[38,40] Around this time the "o-aminophenol hypothesis" of arylamine-induced human bladder cancer was proposed, suggesting that conjugation of aromatic amines by the liver and excretion in the urine with subsequent urinary reactions would liberate the carcinogen o-aminophenol.[41] Other workers later added to this hypothesis: arylamines are hydroxylated in the liver and conjugated with glucuronic acid, followed by excretion into urine and reliberalization of the active carcinogenic metabolite into the bladder lumen by urinary glucuronidases.[38,42,43] Slow acetylation by *N*-acetyltransferase, an enzyme involved in the metabolism of arylamines, has been shown to be a contributory risk factor for bladder carcinogenesis.[20,44,45]

Because of the widespread use of arylamines in textile dyes, hair dyes, and paint pigments, a number of high-risk occupations have been identified, including chemical, dye, textile, and rubber workers and painters and hairstylists.[21,46–48] In addition, the presence of various arylamines in tobacco smoke means that a significant proportion of bladder cancer cases can be attributed to cigarette smoking.[20–23] In fact, abandonment of the manufacture of many of these arylamines in the latter half of the 20th century means that smoking is currently the single most important cause of urothelial cancer.[24,49–51] Tobacco (particularly cigarette) smoking now explains approximately half of bladder cancer cases in men and one-third of cases in women in Europe. It has been demonstrated that an increased smoking frequency and duration and a lower age at initiation are associated with an increased risk of bladder cancer, whereas cessation seems to reduce the risk.[49] The relation between smoking and other prognostic factors is

Section III

interesting, as it could give insight into biologic mechanisms of disease and, perhaps more importantly, have clinical implications by increasing the ability to identify patients at risk of more malignant disease. Cigarette smoking also appears to be a risk factor for disease recurrence following a diagnosis of bladder UC,[49,52] although because of a lack of conclusive evidence, there is currently a low rate of physicians providing smoking cessation assistance.[49]

Studies also demonstrate a relation between *N*-acetyltransferase-2 slow acetylators and cigarette smoking, resulting in a further increase in the risk of bladder cancer, especially in those individuals with a high smoking intensity.[53–55] A similar relation has also been demonstrated with arylamine exposure.[56,57] A number of other susceptibility loci have also been identified, although such markers do not yet have sufficient discriminatory ability to be utilized for risk prediction in the general population or for prediction or prognostication in patients diagnosed with bladder cancer.[54,58,59]

CHRONIC INFLAMMATION AND BLADDER CANCER

Squamous metaplasia is considered a precursor of squamous cell carcinoma of the bladder and is a relatively common occurrence, especially on the trigone of the female bladder where a prevalence of up to 50% is reported.[60,61] Experimental evidence suggests that this does not occur by direct transformation of the superficial apical umbrella cells of the urothelium or by their dedifferentiation and redifferentiation; it is postulated that basal cells (probable stem cells) are selectively activated.[60] The normal urothelium is slowly proliferating, but urothelium undergoing squamous metaplasia becomes hyperplastic, and it may be that the hyperplasia component of urothelial squamous metaplasia is a major contributor to an enhanced risk of cancer formation.[60,61]

Squamous cell carcinoma and adenocarcinoma of the bladder often occur in the presence of chronic inflammation. In Africa and the Middle East, where these tumors are much more prevalent, the chronic inflammation occurs as a result of infestation with the parasite *S. haematobium* (bilharziasis), with a bladder carcinoma incidence of 2 to 4 per 100,000 in *S. haematobium* endemic areas.[62–64] This infestation can lead to malignancy through local tissue damage, mechanical irritation, bilharzial toxins, secondary bacterial infection, and the production of nitrosamines.[62,65] With liver involvement and subsequent liver dysfunction, tryptophan metabolism may be disturbed, resulting in excretion of carcinogenic metabolites.[62] In *S. haematobium*–infected individuals, the prevalence of squamous metaplasia rises significantly during the first 10 to 15 years of life, with a plateau at roughly constant levels thereafter (30% to 40% in males and 40% to 50% in females) when the active infection may have subsided.[61] It is suggested that proliferative changes in the bladder urothelium may become independent of ongoing infection after long periods of chronic *S. haematobium*–induced inflammation.[65,66] Severe metaplasia of the bladder may represent a precancerous transformation in some individuals, but in others, it may only represent a marker for the prolonged inflammation that is associated with a high cancer risk.[65] This sort of proliferative growth combined with the increased excretion or local formation of mutagens in the *S. haematobium*–inflamed bladder may significantly contribute to the onset of cancer formation, possibly involving mutations of the *p53* and *CDKN2* tumor suppressor genes.[65]

In Europe and North America, the stimulus of chronic bladder inflammation is usually chronic bacterial infection, bladder calculi, or long-term indwelling catheters.[67–70] A number of metaplastic conditions (squamous metaplasia, von Brunn nests, cystitis cystica, and cystitis glandularis)

may occur prior to frank malignant change, although the premalignant nature of some of these lesions is still unclear.[67–76]

Field Cancerization and Clonality

A fundamental characteristic of neoplasia is monoclonality, in which one transformed cell gives rise to daughter cells that all exhibit the same genetic changes that provided the initial growth advantages to the originally transformed parent cell.[77] Further genetic changes accumulate in subsequent daughter cells and provide additional growth advantages.[77] However, TCC behaves as a multifocal disease, often with multiple primary tumors and frequent recurrences that can occur anywhere in the urinary tract from the renal pelvis to the urethra. These observations gave rise to the idea of a "field defect" or "field cancerization," suggesting that the whole urothelium is exposed to the same urinary carcinogens, leading to the transformation of many independent separate urothelial cells and resulting in multiple tumors developing independently in multiple sites. Such tumors are thus genetically unrelated. An alternative explanation is that the multifocality of TCC arises as a result of a single carcinogenic insult to a single cell or group of cells. The progeny or clones of these cells spread throughout the bladder, either through intraepithelial migration or through cell shedding and reimplantation, leading to multiple synchronous and metachronous tumors.[77] These tumors are thus topographically distinct but are genetically related. This is the hypothesis of clonality.

Utilizing the relatively rudimentary technique of X-inactivation,[77–79] the early studies in this field appeared to show that the urothelium is derived from a small number of cells (200 to 300), which subsequently develop into larger patches; each patch is clonally related and possesses different predispositions to tumorigenesis.[80] Such stem cell–derived clonal units actively replenish the urothelium during aging.[81] Multiple synchronous and metachronous TCCs in the same patient appear to be clonally related when studied by X-inactivation.[77,79,82–85] However, these studies only provide a 50% probability that one particular TCC is related to the primary TCC, although that probability improves when multiple TCCs are analyzed. Clonal patch size also needs to be taken into consideration, and because of the large patch size of the urothelium (120 mm^2), X-inactivation studies are heavily biased toward demonstrating monoclonality.[78] Ideally, these studies should have taken into account the relation of the tumors to patch boundaries.[78] In addition, DNA methylation patterns change as a natural consequence of aging.[86] Therefore, although X-inactivation studies provided an early insight into the relative importance of the processes of clonality and field cancerization, they cannot be considered as entirely accurate and reliable. Similarly, using immunohistochemistry to study specific *p53* and *pRb* mutations cannot be considered to be wholly reliable for demonstrating monoclonality.

The accuracy of these investigations has been improved by utilizing newer and more sensitive techniques such as comparative genomic hybridization, fluorescence *in situ* hybridization, and loss of heterozygosity studies. These experiments revealed both monoclonality and oligoclonality in synchronous and metachronous TCCs. More recently, research has suggested that a genetic expression profile is established early in bladder tumor development and that this profile is stable and maintained in recurring tumors.[87–89] Majewski et al.[82] matched the clonal allelic losses in distinct chromosomal regions to specific phases of bladder neoplasia: these genetic changes mapped to six regions or "forerunner genes" involved in the early phases of bladder cancer development, representing critical hits driving bladder carcinogenesis. It is suggested that the clonal expansion, over vast expanses of the bladder mucosa, of urothelial cell populations containing losses of forerunner genes may represent the earliest molecular change in bladder carcinogenesis. A further wave of genetic "hits" within subregions of these clonally expanded cells leads to the first microscopically recognizable features of dysplasia, and a third and final wave is associated with the fully transformed phenotype of severe dysplasia or CIS.[88,90] The genetic changes map to six chromosomal regions that are suggested to represent the critical hits driving the development of bladder cancer.[88,90] In addition, Knowles et al.[85] have demonstrated that deletions of chromosome 9 occur in over half of bladder tumors of all grades and stages (9p, 51%; 9q, 57%). Loss of heterozygosity also occurs on 17p (32%), 11p (32%), 8p (23%), 4p (22%), and 13q (15%), and loss of heterozygosity of 5p, 8p, and 21q is significantly associated with worse grade and stage.[85] Genomic copy number alterations are also frequent in bladder TCC, with the most frequent changes involving complete or partial loss of 4q (83%) and gain of 20q (78%).[91] Other frequent losses are of 18q (65%), 8p (65%), 2q (61%), 6q (61%), 3p (56%), 13q (56%), 4p (52%), 6p (52%), 10p (52%), 10q (52%), and 5p (43%).[92]

Taken together, the studies described above show that multifocal TCCs are frequently monoclonal, whereas others show oligoclonality. The evidence for both theories is compelling (as reviewed by Duggan et al.[87]), with evidence supporting both the clonality and field cancerization theories. In reality, these theories are equally valid, with both processes seemingly often occurring simultaneously in the same patient.[83,84] In addition, many of these studies have demonstrated that deletions on chromosome 9p occur most frequently and early in transitional cell carcinogenesis with 17p13 losses (*p53* gene mutations) occurring in more advanced TCCs, shedding some light on the molecular pathology of bladder TCC.

Pathways to Muscle-Invasive and Non–Muscle-Invasive Bladder Cancer

A number of different approaches can be taken to describe the molecular alterations involved in bladder tumorigenesis (TCC). Some authors[93,94] have previously described such pathways in detail based on the six original "hallmarks of cancer" described by Hanahan and Weinberg[90] in 2000. In 2011, Hanahan and Weinberg[92] updated their original landmark review, describing genome instability and inflammation as underlying these hallmark changes and proposed "reprogramming of energy metabolism" and "evading immune destruction" as two emerging hallmarks with potential for generality. In addition, they reported that tumors exhibit another dimension of complexity by containing a repertoire of recruited, ostensibly normal cells that contribute to the acquisition of hallmark traits by creating the "tumor microenvironment." The particular timing and sequence of hallmark events can vary widely between tumors of the same type and within the same tumor, but ultimately, these hallmark capabilities of cancer will be reached.[95] In their 2011 update, Hanahan and Weinberg[92] also introduce the concept of "cancer stem cells," a concept that has existed for quite some time for hematopoietic malignancies.[96,97] Cancer stem cells are a subset of tumor cells that have the ability to self-renew and to generate all of the heterogeneous cells that comprise a tumor (properties that are analogous to a stem cell, the original cell of an organ, and responsible for organogenesis and organ maintenance).[96,98–101] It is proposed that these cells are responsible for tumorigenesis, tumor differentiation, tumor maintenance, tumor spread, and tumor relapse.[96,98–101] In the setting of bladder cancer, cancer stem cells appear to play a role in a subset of tumors, but their true significance has yet to be clarified.[99]

A number of other authors have also reviewed this field in detail,[102–107] and there is general consensus on a divergent pathway for the development of Ta/T1 disease and Tcis/T2+

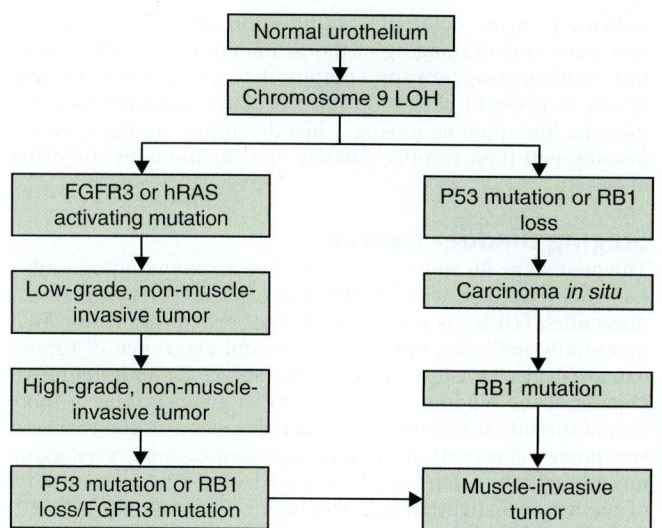

FIGURE 68.1. Pathways to development of bladder cancer. (Data from Pollard C, Smith SC, Theodorescu D. Molecular genesis of non-muscle-invasive urothelial carcinoma [NMIUC]. *Expert Rev Mol Med* 2010;12:e10.)

disease, as illustrated in Figure 68.1[108–114] (Leeds, UK); in their 2010 review, Goebell and Knowles[102] propose a third hypothetical pathway for the development of high-grade papillary tumors. Significant contributions to work in this field have been made by Knowles et al.[103]

A detailed examination of these pathways and related biomarkers is beyond the scope of this chapter. In addition, this is a rapidly changing field, and new developments appear frequently with the advent of high-throughput experimental platforms, including "deep sequencing,"[115] proteomics,[116,117] and metabolomics,[118] so readers are directed to the reviews cited above or to the latest work in this field.

SYMPTOMS AND SIGNS

The typical presenting symptoms of bladder cancer include painless, visible hematuria, infection, and storage symptoms. As the first of these is typically transient and the latter two are also attributable to prostate problems, patients often go undiagnosed for considerable periods.[27] Given the intermittent nature of the hematuria associated with bladder cancer, patients presenting with a convincing episode of hematuria require urgent assessment. Similar considerations apply to male patients with a urinary tract infection. Female patients present a more difficult problem because of the higher incidence of urinary infection and the lower risk of bladder cancer. Hematuria is also more likely to be misinterpreted in women of child-bearing age.

INVESTIGATION OF PATIENTS WITH BLADDER CANCER

This section is divided into the investigation of patients with suspected bladder cancer and the subsequent staging of those with an established diagnosis.

Suspected Bladder Cancer

In developed countries, most patients will be referred for evaluation because of hematuria or suspected bladder cancer. A minority may present via other routes (e.g., gynecologic clinics) or with metastatic symptoms (<10%). Hematuria clinics will generally include a clinical assessment, full blood count and biochemical profile, prostate-specific antigen (if indicated), urine cytologic examination, flexible cystoscopy, and some sort of imaging of the urothelium (e.g., ultrasound, intravenous urogram, or computed tomography [CT] urogram), which will vary with local practice and facilities.[119,120] Patients identified as having a bladder tumor on flexible cystoscopy will then require further investigations to stage the disease.

Staging Bladder Cancer

The next stage for most patients will be an examination under anesthetic coupled with TURBT. The presence or absence of a mass after TURBT is also an important prognostic factor as it potentially indicates either unsuccessful clearance of tumor, extravesical extension, or both. This serves as both definitive staging of the bladder lesion as well as a substantial proportion of the initial treatment. Pathologic review of the resected specimen will ascertain whether muscle invasion is present or not and whether there is CIS; these are the key determinants of further investigation and treatment. Patients with NMIBC, including CIS, do not usually require detailed further imaging, and treatment and surveillance are primarily by intravesical means. The main exception to this is patients with either extensive CIS or grade 3 lesions for whom additional cross-sectional imaging may be warranted. Patients with muscle-invasive bladder cancer (MIBC) will require detailed cross-sectional staging with CT or magnetic resonance imaging (MRI) of the chest, abdomen, and pelvis. If there are any features suggestive of bone metastasis (e.g., raised alkaline phosphatase, bone pain), an isotope bone scan will be indicated in addition.

A major confounding factor with imaging in bladder cancer is the effect of TURBT on the interpretation of the extent of the primary bladder tumor. Recent TURBT will cause perivesical changes that may be interpreted as extravesical spread. For similar reasons, enlarged pelvic nodes may be related to reactive rather than metastatic effects. On the other hand, changes such as infiltration of adjacent organs or hydronephrosis are likely to be reliable indicators of tumor stage and poor prognosis.

STAGING SYSTEM

The 2010 version of the UICC International Union Against Cancer's TNM system is the current, internationally used staging system,[120] and it is based on the size and extent of the primary tumor (T-stage), presence or absence of nodal (N), and metastatic (M) spread (Table 68.1). The TNM stage must be used in conjunction with the pathologic assessment of tumor removed at TURBT to decide on optimal therapy. Disappointingly, despite a substantial volume of research, no biomarkers have yet established themselves in clinical practice as either prognostic or predictive markers as has happened, for example, with estrogen receptor or *HER2* status in breast cancer. It is hoped that the wider availability of high-throughput systems such as proteomics, in-depth sequencing, and others to be developed will allow the development of such markers in the future.

The American Joint Committee on Cancer Staging Manual 8th edition published in 2017 basically uses the same TNM definitions, except for minor terminology variations.[121]

PATHOLOGY

In excess of 90% of bladder cancers are transitional cell carcinomas. Of the remainder, around 5% are squamous, although it should be noted that squamous differentiation is often present in poorly differentiated TCCs, so the extent to which these are genuinely distinct is open to question. As already noted, infestation with *S. haematobium* can lead to squamous cell carcinoma,

TABLE 68.1	TNM CLASSIFICATION OF TUMORS (2009)		
Tx	Primary tumor cannot be assessed		
T0	No evidence of primary tumor		
Ta	No invasive papillary carcinoma		
Tis	Carcinoma *in situ*: "flat tumor"		
T1	Tumor invades subepithelial connective tissue		
T2	Tumor invades muscle		
	T2a superficial muscle (inner half)		
	T2b deep muscle (outer half)		
T3	Tumor invades perivesical tissue:		
	T3a microscopically		
	T3b macroscopically (extravesical mass)		
T4	Tumor invades any of the following: prostate stroma, seminal vesicles, uterus, vagina, pelvic wall, abdominal wall		
	T4a tumor invades prostate, stroma, seminal vesicles, uterus, or vagina		
	T4b tumor invades pelvis or abdominal wall		
N0 regional lymph nodes	Defined as nodes of the true pelvis below the bifurcation of the common iliac arteries. Laterality does not affect the N classification		
Nx	Nodes cannot be assessed		
N0	No lymph node metastasis		
N1	Metastasis in a single lymph node in the true pelvis (hypogastric, obturator, external iliac, or presacral)		
N2	Metastasis in multiple lymph nodes in the true pelvis (hypogastric, obturator, external iliac, or presacral)		
N3	Metastasis in a common iliac lymph node(s)		
M—distant metastasis			
Mx	Cannot be assessed		
M0	No distant metastasis		
M1	Distant metastasis present		
Stage grouping			
Stage 0a	Ta	N0	M0
Stage 0is	Tis	N0	M0
Stage I	T1	N0	M0
Stage II	T2a,b	N0	M0
Stage III	T3a,b	N0	M0
	T4a	N0	M0
Stage IV	T4b	N0	M0
	Any T	N1, 2, 3	M0
	Any T	Any N	M1

From Sobin LH, Gospodarowicz M, Wittekind C. *TNM classification of malignant tumours.* 7th ed. Hoboken, NJ: Wiley-Blackwell, 2009. Copyright © 2010 Blackwell Publishing Ltd. Reprinted by permission of John Wiley & Sons, Inc.

but this is rapidly decreasing due to eradication programs. Small cell carcinoma is rare but important as it is generally very chemosensitive and treatment tends to follow schedules adapted from treating small cell lung cancer. Other tumor types include melanoma, carcinosarcoma, and adenocarcinoma (particularly in the urachal remnant). Typically, bladder TCCs will be graded using the standard TNM system of Gx (cannot be assessed) and then G1 through to G3 (well through to poorly differentiated).[120] CIS will frequently be found in addition to a tumor mass and critically affects treatment choices.

TREATMENT OF BLADDER CANCER

Non–Muscle-Invasive Bladder Cancer

Around 80% of patients with bladder cancer present with non–muscle-invasive disease. These are classified as Tis, Ta, and T1 by the TNM classification system. The gold standard for diagnosis is the resection of the lesion with adequate sampling of the detrusor muscle deep to the lesion (TURBT). This will give tissue for accurate staging of the bladder lesion as well as definitive treatment for the lesion. Recurrences after TURBT are found in up to 70% of patients undergoing surveillance, and more importantly, up to 15% of patients on surveillance will progress to muscle-invasive bladder cancer. At the time of diagnosis, the upper urinary tract also needs assessment. This can be done with intravenous urography, CT urography, or ultrasound. The incidence of upper tract tumors at the time of presentation with hematuria is only 1.8%, calling into question the use of contrast imaging for the group as a whole.[122] Ultrasound is now being used more frequently, with contrast imaging modalities being used for the higher-risk disease.

Prognostication and management strategy are based on accurate initial staging and grading of the disease. There can be variation in the interpretation of pathologic specimens, so review of pathology is recommended (European Association of Urology [EAU] guidelines).[123] If there is uncertainty over the pathology, a further early re-resection is indicated. The risk of residual tumor can be as high as 53% in T1 tumors.[124] If the disease is defined as NMIBC, it can be characterized as low, intermediate, or high risk, and this will dictate how the disease is managed (see below). The EORTC bladder cancer calculator provides a valuable online tool for doing this and determining follow-up frequency.[125]

Following resection of the tumor, there is good evidence that a single dose of mitomycin C administrated into the bladder for 1 hour within 24 hours of surgery will reduce the relative risk of recurrence by 24.2% but will not impact disease progression and disease survival.[125] Recurrences after TURBT are found in up to 70% of patients undergoing surveillance, and up to 15% of patients on surveillance will progress to muscle-invasive bladder cancer. Emerging endoscopic techniques employing photodynamic therapy aimed at improving diagnostic yield and thereby ultimately reducing the rates of recurrence and progression have demonstrated promising results.[126]

Low-risk tumors are single tumors that are <3 cm in diameter and are graded as G1 disease and staged as Ta with no evidence of CIS. These tumors have a 15% probability of recurrence and a 0.2% risk of progression at 1 year.[30] These patients should undergo a flexible cystoscopy 3 months after the initial resection, and if this is negative, a flexible cystoscopy should be undertaken 9 months later and then annually thereafter.

Intermediate- and high-risk tumors are defined using a scoring system based on a number of clinical and pathologic factors:

a. Number of tumors
b. Tumor size
c. Prior recurrence rate
d. T category
e. Presence of concurrent CIS
f. Tumor grade[127]

The high-risk tumors should be followed up with 3 monthly flexible cystoscopy for 2 years and 6 monthly for a further 5 years and then annually thereafter. Intermediate-risk tumors should be followed up using a surveillance regimen somewhere between that used for low- and high-risk diseases, which is adapted according to personal and subjective factors. The intermediate-risk tumors have up to a 38% probability of recurrence and a 5% risk of progression at 1 year. The high-risk tumors have a 61% probability of recurrence and a 17% risk of progression at 1 year.[30]

The use of flexible cystoscopy with urine cytology is the standard of bladder surveillance, with ongoing research into improving the sensitivity and specificity of flexible cystoscopy. There are a wide number of urinary biomarkers available such as NMP22, UroVysion (Abbott Laboratories, Abbott Park, Illinois), and ImmunoCyt (Scimedx, Denville, New Jersey). These agents suffer from high false-positive rates and variable sensitivity and are costly (as reviewed by Vrooman and Witjes[123]).

The presence of CIS in the bladder carries a 54% risk of disease progression without treatment.[128] Patients with high-risk tumors or CIS should be offered intravesical immunotherapy using bacille Calmette-Guérin (BCG) (EAU and American

Urology Association guidelines).[124,129] There are a variety of treatment schedules in the literature, but the authors recommend an intravesical treatment once a week for 6 weeks followed by a subsequent 3 weeks as an induction treatment. If there is no cystoscopic evidence of recurrence, the patient should then be offered ongoing maintenance BCG with 6-week courses of BCG every 3 to 6 months with regular cystoscopic surveillance. In a recent meta-analysis of trials with BCG maintenance, a 32% reduction in the risk of recurrence was seen for BCG compared with mitomycin C ($P < .0001$), whereas there was a 28% increase in the risk of recurrence ($P = .006$) for patients treated with BCG in the trials without BCG maintenance.[127] BCG is a very effective treatment, but not all patients with NMIBC should be treated with BCG because of the risk of toxicity. In a phase III study for NMIBC tumors using maintenance BCG therapy, 20.3% patients stopped BCG because of side effects, mostly local side effects; 68% who stopped because of side effects did so during the first 6 months. The choice of treatment depends on the patients' risk of recurrence and progression based on EORTC subgroups. The use of BCG does not alter the natural course of tumors in the low risk of recurrence subgroup and is therefore considered to be overtreatment. In patients with tumors at high risk of progression, for whom cystectomy is not carried out, BCG, including at least 1-year maintenance, is indicated. In patients at intermediate or high risk of recurrence and intermediate risk of progression, BCG with 1-year maintenance is more effective than chemotherapy for prevention of recurrence; however, it has more side effects than chemotherapy. For this reason, both BCG with maintenance and intravesical chemotherapy remain options. The final choice should reflect the individual patient's risk of recurrence and progression and the efficacy and side effects of each treatment modality (EAU guidelines). In treatment refractory disease, the patient should be offered radical treatment for the bladder.

Muscle-Invasive, Nonmetastatic Disease

For a review of recent guidelines and recommendations for broad therapeutic options in the multidisciplinary integrated management of invasive non–metastatic muscle-invasive bladder cancer by the American Urological Association (AUA), American Society of Clinical Oncology (ASCO), the American Society for Radiation Oncology (ASTRO) Society of Urologic oncology, and the European Association of Urology, the reader is referred to the original publications in the Journal of Clinical Oncology and the Journal of Oncology Practice.[126,130]

Relative Roles of Cystectomy and Bladder Preservation

Radiation therapy has been used as the primary treatment for muscle-invasive bladder cancer for many years, but utilization rates vary around the world from around 10% in the United States[8] to 25% in Scandinavia[128] to in excess of 50% in the United Kingdom.[10] There are no prospective randomized trials comparing surgery with radiation therapy, so the data on comparative efficacy can only be inferred indirectly. US authors in particular tend to refer to surgery as the gold standard of care, with bladder preservation with radiation therapy (with or without chemotherapy) being viewed as experimental. However, this opinion seems to be based on custom and practice and not on any hard comparative data. It is thus worth examining in some detail the data that exist on this topic. There is a solitary attempt using modern techniques to compare surgery with bladder preservation combining chemotherapy and radiotherapy. The UK SPARE trial (randomized trial of Selective Bladder Preservation against Radical Excision [cystectomy] in muscle-invasive T2/T3 transitional cell carcinoma of the bladder) was a feasibility study that has now closed due to poor accrual. These phase II and

Section III

III trials attempted to investigate the potential of using the response to neoadjuvant chemotherapy as a predictive tool for selecting patients for radiation therapy compared with the surgical standard. In the authors' experience, one of the problems with the trials was that the study used response to neoadjuvant chemotherapy to decide on suitability for bladder preservation. However, once this was explained to the patients in the information sheet, there were patients who had a good response but were reluctant to undergo surgery, particularly if the bladder was free of tumor at the interim cystoscopy.

Large population-based studies suggest that the main determinants of survival after diagnosis of bladder cancer are stage, grade, age, and to some extent social class. For example, Hayter et al.[6] studied patterns of care and outcomes in over 20,000 patients with bladder cancer in Ontario. They found significant variations in the use of cystectomy and radiation therapy between different districts but no evidence that these variations led to any differences in long-term outcomes. They concluded that bladder-sparing approaches were equivalent to surgery for invasive bladder cancer.

Another way to compare outcomes between surgery and radiation therapy is to look at large published series. In the United Kingdom, where both of these approaches are routinely employed, it is possible to compare the outcomes in Cancer Registry data. A recent paper from Munro et al.[10] examined outcomes in 458 patients with invasive bladder cancer treated in Yorkshire between 1993 and 1996. The ratio of cystectomy to radiation therapy was 1 to 3, reflecting UK practice at the time. Overall 10-year survival was similar between those who underwent radiation therapy (22%) and radical cystectomy (24%). Prognostic factors for inferior outcome at 10 years were female versus male, poor performance status, hydronephrosis, and increasing T-stage; treatment modality was not a factor in the prognosis.

One of the most widely quoted surgical series comes from the University of Southern California and reports the results of 1,054 patients undergoing cystectomy with overall 5- and 10-year survival rates of 60% and 43%, respectively. This series is discussed in detail below. However, this series included patients undergoing surgery for noninvasive tumors and excluded from the denominator 112 patients referred but deemed incurable at operation. If we look at the 5-year survival of those with invasive tumors, the rate drops to around 47% from the quoted 60%. A contemporary series of radiation therapy cases from Rödel et al.[5] reports 5- and 10-year survivals of 51% and 31% but included patients deemed inoperable.

Furthermore, if we analyze the outcomes in the surgical control arm in the U.S. Intergroup Neoadjuvant MVAC trial, the median survival was 38 months and the 5-year survival was 42%. Other relatively contemporary series quote similar 5-year survivals: for example, Dalbagni et al.[131] cite 45% overall and 65% disease-specific survival rates in a series of 300 patients. Furthermore, the only significant prognostic factors in this series were age, T-stage, and use or nonuse of neoadjuvant chemotherapy (see the Role of Systemic Therapy section). Data also exist from single-institution series with widespread use of both modalities. Kotwal et al.[132] report results on 169 patients treated between March 1996 and December 2000 in Leeds, United Kingdom. There were no differences in overall, cause-specific, and distant recurrence-free survival at 5 years between the two groups, despite the radiotherapy group being older (median age, 75.3 vs. 68.2 years). There were 31 local bladder recurrences in the radiation therapy group (24 of which were solitary and hence potentially suitable for salvage surgery), but no significant difference in distant recurrence-free survival. In another more recent (2002 to 2006) cohort, the median age of radiation therapy patients but not the cystectomy patients had increased to 78.4 from 75.3 years, respectively, whereas the age of those undergoing surgery remained similar at 67.9 and 68.2 years for surgery,

consistent with the aging trend in new bladder cancer cases. These authors concluded that although the patients undergoing radical cystectomy were significantly younger than the radiation therapy patients, treatment modality did not influence survival. They went on to state that radical radiotherapy is a viable treatment option for these patients, with equivalent long-term survival to surgery and the advantage of organ preservation.

Giacalone et al.[133] conducted an analysis of 465 patients with cT2e-T4a bladder cancer treated at a single institution with maximal transurethral resection of bladder tumor (TURBT) followed by concurrent cisplatin-based chemotherapy and RT. A subset of patients also received neoadjuvant chemotherapy. Repeat cystoscopy with biopsies was performed after 40 Gy. Patients with a complete response (CR) received consolidation chemoradiation to 64 to 65 Gy, and those with less than a CR or invasive recurrence were recommended to undergo salvage RC.

Median follow-up was 4.8 years for all patients and 7.5 years for surviving patients. Seventy-six percent of patients had a CR to induction chemoradiation, 84% after a visibly complete TURBT achieved a CR versus 59% with an incomplete TURBT ($P < .001$). When evaluated in 4-year intervals, the CR rate has improved from 64% in years 1986 to 1990 to 96% in years 2010 to 2012. One hundred twenty-five patients (27%) underwent salvage RC, 55 for less than CR and 70 for superficial or invasive recurrences. For those patients who achieved a CR, the 10-year actuarial rates for noninvasive, invasive, pelvic, and distant failures were 32%, 16%, 14%, and 29%, respectively. Five-, 10-, 15-, and 20-year DSS rates were 66%, 59%, 56%, and 50% (T2 Z 75%, 66%, 61%, and 58%; T3eT4a Z 50%, 45%, 45%, 36%), respectively.

Median OS was 6.4 years. Five-, 10-, 15-, and 20-year OS rates were 57%, 39%, 25%, and 18% (T2 Z 66%, 46%, 29%, 23%; T3eT4a Z 41%, 26%, 17%, 10%), respectively.

Neoadjuvant chemotherapy did not improve DSS or OS.

The authors noted this series represented one of the largest cohorts of MIBC treated with CMT and the data supported the high rates of CR and bladder preservation in patients receiving CMT and demonstrated long-term DSS similar to modern cystectomy series.

Using the National Cancer Database (NCDB), patients with AJCC clinical T2-T3, N0, and M0 urothelial carcinoma (MIBC) diagnosed between 2004 and 2013, Zhong et al.[134] carried out an analysis of patients treated with definitive intent with either radical cystectomy (with or without chemotherapy) or concurrent chemotherapy and radiation (bladder preservation) (BPCRT). Only patients documented to undergo a transurethral tumor resection followed by a definitive course of radiation with chemotherapy were included in this BPCRT cohort.

Among 8,454 MIBC patients, 7,276 (86%) underwent radical cystectomy with or without chemotherapy, and 1,178 (14%) underwent BPCRT. Patients undergoing BPCRT were significantly older (median age 77 vs. 68 years, $P < .001$) and had higher comorbidity scores (P Z 0.002). The median follow-up time was 4.5 years. The unadjusted 5-year OS rates were 45.0% and 31.8% for surgery and BPCRT cohorts, respectively ($P < .001$). Using matched propensity score analysis, there were 1,002 patients remaining in each cohort, and there was no significant difference in 5-year OS between the two groups (39.7% surgery vs. 32.4% BPCRT, P Z 0.10). BPCRT demonstrated similar survival outcomes compared to those treated with radical cystectomy with or without chemotherapy. In the absence of prospective randomized studies, these results may help guide decision-making for MIBC patients considering nonsurgical management options.

Vashista et al.[135] searched seven databases (PubMed, Scopus, EMBASE, Proquest, CINAHL, and ClinicalTrials. gov) for randomized, controlled trials and prospective and retrospective studies directly comparing RC with CMT from database inception to March 2016. They conducted a meta-analyses evaluating OS, DSS, and PFS with hazard ratios (HRs). Nineteen studies evaluating 12,380 subjects were selected. For the 8 studies encompassing 9,554 subjects eligible for meta-analyses, we found no difference in OS at 5 years (HR 0.96, favoring CMT) or 10 years (HR 1.02, favoring cystectomy). No difference was observed in DSS at 5 years (HR 0.83, favoring radiation) or 10 years (HR 1.17, favoring cystectomy), or PFS at 10 years (HR 0.85, favoring CMT). The cystectomy arms had higher rates of early major complications, whereas rates of minor complications were similar between the two treatments. In summary, this meta-analysis showed no differences in OS, DSS, or PFS between RC and CMT. Further randomized, controlled trials are necessary to identify the optimal treatment for specific patients.

The Surveillance, Epidemiology, and End Results (SEER) program was used by Wilhite et al.[136] to identify patients diagnosed from 1992 to 2013 with localized, muscle-invasive bladder (stages II to III) urothelial carcinoma, squamous cell carcinoma, or adenocarcinoma histology. Cystectomy was defined as partial or radical. Those who did not receive either cystectomy or RT were excluded. Treatment utilization patterns over time were assessed using Cochran-Armitage tests. Among 16,175 patients eligible for analysis, 11,917 (74%) and 4258 (26%) received cystectomy and RT, respectively. Patients who received RT were older (median age 79 vs. 68, $P < .01$), Over time, there was a statistically significant increase in the proportion of patients receiving RT relative to cystectomy (24% in 1992 to 2003 vs. 28% in 2004 to 2013, $P < .01$), despite median patient age throughout the study period remaining unchanged (71 for both 1992 to 2003 and 2004 to 2013). For RT, compared with patients diagnosed from 1992 to 2009, those diagnosed from 2010 to 2013 showed improved CSS (71% vs. 67% at 1 year, P Z 0.01; 51% vs. 40% at 3 years, $P < .01$) and OS (64% vs. 60% at 1 year, $P < .01$; 38% vs. 29% at 3 years, $P < .01$). In these SEER data, utilization of RT for localized, muscle-invasive bladder cancer increased relative to cystectomy from 1992 to 2013, despite the median age of treated patients over that period remaining unchanged. There was significant improvement in CSS and OS for patients receiving RT who were diagnosed from 2010 to 2013 compared with earlier years, support continued use of bladder preservation strategies utilizing RT.

Solanki et al.[137] conducted an electronic survey of US radiation oncologists regarding the management of patients with cT2-3N0M0 transitional cell muscle-invasive bladder cancer; 277 physicians completed the survey. Most respondents (58%) stated that they only treated 1 to 3 patients with bladder cancer in the prior year. Seventy-four percent of respondents primarily treated patients deemed unfit for cystectomy, whereas only 28% saw patients prior to cystectomy for consultation to discuss bladder preservation therapy. The majority of radiation oncologists (91%) used conventional fractionation instead of hypofractionation (7.6%), but more variability existed for radiation therapy targets. Sixty percent used a small-pelvis field, 29% used a whole-pelvis field, and 12% treated the bladder only. There was increased use of hypofractionation (29%) and bladder-only radiation therapy (34%) in patients who were not candidates for cystectomy or chemotherapy ($P < .001$). Cisplatin-based concurrent chemotherapy was most commonly preferred (89%). In noncisplatin candidates, most respondents preferred 5-fluorouracil plus mitomycin C (32%) or carboplatin (32%). IMRT use and midtreatment cystoscopic reevaluation were variable, whereas hyperfractionation use was low. Although there are areas of consistency, variability exists in many technical and practical aspects of treatment delivery. Further research and education are needed to determine the optimal radiation therapy target, dose/fractionation, and concurrent chemotherapy regimen.

Mitin et al.[138] performed a pooled analysis of 119 patients with muscle-invasive bladder cancer enrolled on NRG Oncology Radiation Therapy Oncology Group trials 9906 and 0233, who were classified as having a complete (T0) or near-complete (Ta or Tis) response after induction chemo-RT and completed consolidation with a total RT dose of at least 60 Gy.

One hundred one patients (85%) achieved T0, and 18 (15%) achieved Ta or Tis after induction chemo-RT and proceeded to consolidation. After a median follow-up of 5.9 years, 36 of 101 T0 patients (36%) versus 5 of 18 Ta or Tis patients (28%) experienced bladder recurrence (P Z .52). Thirteen patients among complete responders eventually required late salvage cystectomy for tumor recurrence, compared with 1 patient among near-complete responders. Disease-specific, bladder-intact, and overall survivals were not significantly different between T0 and Ta/Tis cases. Therefore, it is reasonable to recommend that patients with Ta or Tis after induction chemo-RT continue with bladder-sparing therapy with consolidation chemo-RT to full dose (60 to 64 Gy). Neoadjuvant chemotherapy randomized trials had been previously reported by the International Collaboration of Trialists.[139]

Walker et al.[140] reported on a Canadian survey of 64 urologists, 29 radiation oncologists (RO), and 26 medical oncologists (MO) on treatment of muscle-invasive bladder cancer. Participants reported comparable survival at 5 years with cystectomy (51%) and RT with concurrent chemotherapy (50%). Despite this, participants reported low RT referral/treatment rates: Urologists referred a median of 2/10 patients to RO; ROs treated a median of 5/10 patients referred; and MOs referred a median of 2/8 patients not referred to RO by urology.

A proportion of patients undergoing radiation therapy will relapse within the bladder and go on to salvage cystectomy. An important consideration, therefore, is whether cystectomy after radiation therapy can be carried out safely and whether the delay compromises survival. Again, there are no randomized data on this topic. However, UK surgeons in particular have good practical experience on this topic and have commented that neither prior chemotherapy nor radiation therapy compromises surgical salvage and that long-term results appear similar to primary cystectomy series.

Particularly intriguing in this regard is a comparison of survival rates following primary surgery or salvage surgery following failed radiation therapy from the Christie Hospital in Manchester, United Kingdom. The group examined the outcomes in 552 patients who underwent radical cystectomy between 1970 and 2005. Of these, 313 patients underwent primary radical cystectomy and 239 underwent salvage radical cystectomy following radiation failure. The median age was 62.5 years (range, 32.2 to 87.2) for the primary surgical group compared with 65.5 years for the salvage group. Overall 5-year survivals reported were 45.5% for the primary group and 42% for the salvage group, with cause-specific survivals of 51% and 50%, respectively. These differences persisted after stratification for stage, and the authors concluded that a policy of primary radiation therapy with surgical salvage did not compromise the long-term survival chances of patients.[139]

Clearly, there are surgical series with much higher survival rates than this in the literature. However, there are two factors accounting for this. One is case selection, the other is that these series are, to a degree, personal, so to publish results that appear inferior to other major centers is potentially a threat to a center's (or surgeon's) reputation and will tend to have a "ratchet" effect on published results. These data also suggest that the predominant prognosis driver in bladder cancer is the presence or absence of distant micrometastasis at diagnosis of invasive disease. The (relatively modest) effect of neoadjuvant chemotherapy tends to bear this out, particularly as the biggest effect in the Medical Research Council (MRC)/EORTC trial was on metastasis-free survival rather than pelvic tumor control rates.[139]

Section III

There is little in the way of randomized data on the efficacy of radiation therapy in either non–muscle-invasive disease or CIS. The only randomized trial on this topic comes from the United Kingdom and compared radiation therapy with surveillance for patients with a new diagnosis of pT1G3 NXM0 transitional cell carcinoma with unifocal disease and no CIS. Patients with multifocal disease or CIS were randomized between intravesical therapy and radiation therapy. There was no evidence of benefit from radiation therapy in terms of progression-free interval (hazard ratio [HR] 1.07; 95% confidence interval [CI], 0.65 to 1.74; $P = .785$), progression-free survival (HR 1.35; 95% CI, 0.92 to 1.98; $P = .133$), or overall survival (HR 1.32; 95% CI, 0.86 to 2.04; $P = .193$).[141] There is thus no indication for radiation therapy in these groups of patients.

In truth, surgery and radiation therapy do not compete but are complementary approaches of treatment of invasive bladder cancer. There are particular groups who appear to do poorly with primary radiation therapy, for example, those with poorly functioning bladders or extensive CIS in addition to their invasive disease. In the former case, radiation therapy is unlikely to improve bladder function; in the latter, the lack of effect of radiation therapy on CIS means that the patient remains at risk of further bladder intervention and ultimately cystectomy.[139] Similar considerations apply to patients with pT1G3 disease.[141] North American authors will also cite features such as hydronephrosis as a contraindication to radiation therapy.[142] However, hydronephrosis is also a poor prognostic factor for surgery and does not help in selecting patients one way or another.[6] On the other hand, there are many patients who may benefit from radical therapy but are poor surgical candidates, such as older patients, the obese, diabetics, poor anesthetic-risk patients, or those who may struggle with whatever form of neobladder is fashioned. Although large surgical series will include patients over age 80, these will typically comprise only a few percentage of the total, whereas, with a median age at diagnosis of bladder cancer in the middle to late 70s, there are probably many more who do not make it to surgery.

Surgery

Management of Invasive Bladder Cancer

Although the majority of patients present with NMIBC, 20% to 40% will either present with or ultimately develop muscle-invasive disease. Invasive bladder cancer is potentially lethal; if untreated, over 85% of patients will die of the disease within 2 years of diagnosis.[141] Furthermore, a certain percentage of patients with high-grade bladder tumors without involvement of the lamina propria will recur or progress or fail intravesical management, and they may be best treated with an earlier cystectomy when survival outcomes are optimal.[142] In these groups of patients, the 5-year survival rates after cystectomy exceed 80%.[143]

The rationale for an aggressive treatment approach employing radical cystectomy for high-grade, invasive bladder cancer is based on several important observations. First, the good long-term survival rates, coupled with the lowest local recurrences, are seen following a definitive surgical approach removing the primary bladder tumor and regional lymph nodes.[4,144,145] Although there are no randomized trials comparing radical cystectomy with bladder-preserving approaches, surgery remains the preferred treatment option for many clinicians for advanced, localized invasive bladder cancer.[144,145] Second, the morbidity and mortality of radical cystectomy has substantially improved over the past several decades.[144,146] Third, advocates say that radical cystectomy provides accurate pathologic staging of the primary bladder tumor (p stage) and regional lymph nodes, thus, selectively determining the need for adjuvant therapy based on precise

pathologic evaluation. However, it should be noted that the evidence base for adjuvant (as opposed to neoadjuvant) therapy is rather weak (see on the Role of Systemic Therapy section). For the abovementioned reasons, radical cystectomy has become a standard form of therapy for high-grade, invasive bladder cancer. Nonetheless, many articles on cystectomy emphasize the need for careful patient selection to achieve optimal results. Although this is undoubtedly true, it begs the question of what should be done with patients who do not meet these stringent selection standards but still need to be treated. This issue is rarely, if ever, addressed in cystectomy series publications.

The evolution and improvements in lower urinary tract reconstruction, particularly orthotopic diversion, have been major components in enhancing the quality of life of patients requiring cystectomy. Currently, most men and women can safely undergo orthotopic lower urinary tract reconstruction to the native, intact urethra following cystectomy,[147] although availability varies worldwide. Orthotopic reconstruction aims to mimic the native bladder in location and function, provides a continent means to store urine, and allows volitional voiding per urethra, although patients need to do this by coordinating opening the sphincter with a Valsalva maneuver, which does require training. The orthotopic neobladder eliminates the need for a cutaneous stoma, urostomy appliance, and the need for intermittent catheterization in most cases. These efforts have improved the quality of life of patients who require removal of their bladders and have also stimulated patients and physicians to consider radical cystectomy at an earlier more curable stage for high-grade, invasive bladder cancer.[148,149] A dedicated effort has been made to improve the surgical technique of radical cystectomy and to provide an acceptable form of urinary diversion, without compromise of a sound cancer operation.

Timing of cystectomy after the TURBT is important, and it has been demonstrated that a delay of more than 3 months undermines patient survival. This evidence forms the basis to negotiating resource needs with health care providers[150]. Certain technical issues regarding radical cystectomy and an appropriate lymph node dissection are critical to minimize local recurrence and positive surgical margins and to maximize cancer-specific survival.[151] Attention to surgical detail is important in optimizing the successful functional outcomes of orthotopic diversion by preserving the urinary sphincter mechanism and therefore continence. Finally, the observed associations between hospital volume and operative mortality are largely mediated by surgeon volume. Patients can often improve their chances of survival substantially, even at high-volume hospitals, by selecting surgeons who perform the operations frequently, as those centers that have adopted this strategy have demonstrated declining mortality in the past decade.[152,153]

Radical cystectomy by definition implies the *en bloc* removal of the pelvic–iliac lymph nodes along with the pelvic organs anterior to the rectum: the bladder, urachus, prostate, seminal vesicles, and visceral peritoneum in men and the bladder, urachus, ovaries, fallopian tubes, uterus, cervix, vaginal cuff, and the anterior pelvic peritoneum in women. An appropriate lymphadenectomy is an important component of radical cystectomy and is related to the clinical outcomes of patients with high-grade, invasive bladder cancer. Evidence suggests that a more extended lymphadenectomy is beneficial in both lymph node–positive and lymph node–negative patients with bladder cancer,[154-156] although this could be a surrogate for either case selection or surgical skill. Although the exact limits of the lymphadenectomy for patients with bladder cancer undergoing cystectomy are currently debated, the boundaries include initiation at the level of the inferior mesenteric artery (superior limits of dissection), extending laterally over the inferior vena cava or aorta to the genitofemoral nerve (lateral limits of dissection), and distally to the lymph node of Cloquet medially (on Cooper ligament) and the circumflex iliac vein laterally. This dissection includes bilaterally all obturator, hypogastric, presciatic, and presacral lymph nodes.[157,158] Removal of more than 15 lymph nodes has been postulated to be both sufficient for the evaluation of the lymph node status as well as beneficial for overall survival in retrospective studies.[158,159] However, potential interindividual differences in the number of pelvic and retroperitoneal lymph nodes and difficulties in processing of the removed tissue by pathologists are issues. Furthermore, the reality is that even in today's practice, the number of lymph nodes retrieved are low (<10) in a majority of patients (75%) and the chances are even lower if the patients are older, Hispanic (in the United States), and managed at low-volume, nonurban centers.[158] The true curative value of lymph node dissection and the optimal extent of dissection are both still unknown.

Technical variations from the standard cystectomy have been performed to improve patients' quality of life, including prostate-sparing cystectomy in order to preserve continence and potency. However, it carries a higher risk of missing unsuspected adenocarcinoma of the prostate. Coexistent prostate cancer and prostatic urothelial cancer are reported in 23% to 54% cases, of which 29% were clinically significant, leading to local recurrence and even metastasis.[160,161]

Radical cystectomy is an appropriate standard treatment for patients with high-grade, invasive bladder cancer. The clinical outcomes are presented in Table 68.2. These results should provide a benchmark for outcomes to which other therapies can be compared.

Both laparoscopic and robot-assisted cystectomy have been shown to be feasible and safe, but with a relatively shorter follow-up.[162-164] Despite an increased materials cost for a robotic-assisted cystectomy, it has been demonstrated to be cost-effective in a subgroup of patients undergoing ileal conduit when the impact of complications are considered in a single-institution series.[164,165]

Morbidity and Mortality of Radical Cystectomy and Lymphadenectomy

The early clinical results and outcomes with regard to the morbidity and mortality of radical cystectomy were disappointing. Lack of universal acceptance of this procedure was attributed to the considerable complication rate and the need for improvements in urinary diversion. Prior to 1970, perioperative complication rates of radical cystectomy were approximately 35%, with a mortality rate of nearly 20%. However, with contemporary medical, surgical, and anesthetic techniques, along with better patient selection, the mortality and morbidity from radical cystectomy have dramatically decreased (Table 68.2). Importantly, in high-volume centers, the administration of preoperative therapy (radiation or chemotherapy) and the form of urinary diversion performed (continent or incontinent) did not obviously increase the mortality rate of patients undergoing radical cystectomy.[142] The issue of the need to select patients for surgery complicates the comparison of bladder-sparing techniques, because frequently those not suitable for surgery will be the ones who appear in the radiotherapy-based series.

The early complication rate following radical cystectomy should not be underestimated in this elderly group of patients. The median age of patients undergoing cystectomy in a University of Southern California series was 66 years.[4] Of the 1,054 patients treated, 28% developed an early complication within the first 3 months of surgery. Early complications included all events related to the cystectomy, perioperative care, and urinary diversion. The administration of preoperative therapy (radiation or chemotherapy) and the form of urinary diversion did not significantly increase the early complication rate in these cystectomy patients. Most early complications following radical cystectomy are unrelated to the urinary diversion (85% diversion unrelated) and can be managed conservatively without the need for reoperation in approximately 90% of cases.[166] The most common early diversion-unrelated complication is dehydration, whereas the most common early diversion-related complication following radical cystectomy is prolonged urinary leakage. Overall, the most surgical complications after cystectomy are associated with urinary diversion in relation to the intestinal segments.[144,167]

Neoadjuvant chemotherapy is discussed in a later section, but it does not seem to increase the perioperative morbidity or mortality.[7,168] Preoperative radiation therapy is discussed below.

Radical cystectomy may appropriately be performed in carefully selected elderly patients[169]; however, this emphasis in the surgical literature on "careful selection" highlights as much the deficiencies as the efficacy of cystectomy as it emphasizes that the published results are not applicable to the entire population. It is emphasized that physiologic age may be more important than chronologic age when determining appropriate candidacy for radical cystectomy. Proper patient selection, strict attention to perioperative details, along with a dedicated and meticulous team-oriented surgical approach are critical components to minimize the morbidity and mortality of surgery and to ensure the best clinical outcomes in all patients following radical cystectomy.[166,170,171] A recommended approach from the authors' center previously pioneered by the Danish is adoption of an enhanced recovery pathway protocol (Fig. 68.2).[172]

Pathologic Stage and Subgroups

The pathologic stage of the primary bladder tumor and the presence of regional lymph node metastases are the most important survival determinants in patients undergoing cystectomy for bladder cancer.[4,145,147] These pathologic determinants may also be categorized into pathologic subgroups that provide risk stratification and direct the need for adjuvant therapy in the appropriately selected individual. Pathologic subgroups are defined as organ-confined, lymph node–negative tumors (P0, Pa, Pis, P1, P2a, P2b), nonorgan confined (extravesical) lymph node–negative tumors (P3, P4), and lymph node–positive disease (N+), representing 56%, 20%, and 24% of patients, respectively.[147] The 5- and 10-year recurrence-free survival rates for the entire group of 1,054 patients

TABLE 68.2 CYSTECTOMY OUTCOMES IN SELECTED SINGLE-INSTITUTION SERIES

Author (Reference)	Period (Year)	Number of Patients (Male/Female)	Median Age (Year)	Median Follow-Up (Year)	Histology	30-Day Mortality (%)	Pathologic Subgroup (%)		
							Organ Confined	Extravesical	Lymph Node Positive
Stein et al./USC[4]	1971–1997	1,054 (843/211)	66	10.2	TCC (94% high grade)	3	56	20	24
Madersbacher et al./Bern[144]	1985–2000	507 (400/107)	66	3.75	TCC (95% high grade)	7	43	33	24
Hautmann et al./Ulm[146]	1986–2003	788 (652/136)	64	2.9 y	TCC (82% high grade)	5	63	19	18

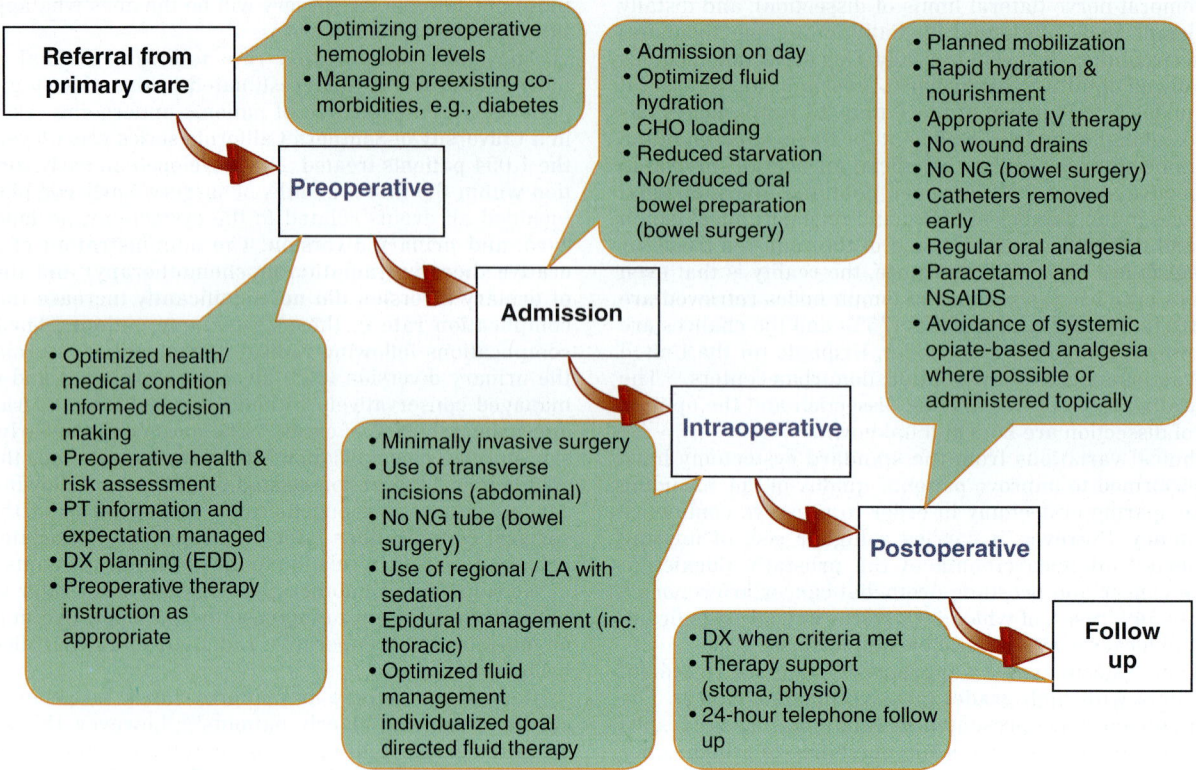

FIGURE 68.2. Schematic representation of the enhanced recovery program in patients undergoing a radical cystectomy.

in the University of Southern California series were 68% and 66%, respectively (Table 68.2). Most deaths occurred within the first 3 years following radical cystectomy and were attributed to cancer recurrence. However, with longer follow-up (>3 years), most deaths in this elderly group of patients were primarily related to comorbid diseases unrelated to bladder cancer. This underscores the effective and durable outcomes of radical cystectomy.

Molecular Biomarkers

It has been reported that patients who expressed high levels of meiotic recombination homolog (MRE11) on transurethral resection of the bladder tumor biopsy had a better response to radical RT (*P Z* .005). Also, studying other protein expression within the biopsy material, it was found that p16 was associated with poor prognosis after either RT or cystectomy. Tat-interactive protein (TIP60) was associated with disease-specific survival after cystectomy (*P Z* .001).

Further, telomeres protect the ends of chromosomes from degradation and fusion but are shortened during the DNA replication process. Shortening of telomeres is associated with chromosomal instability and may be related to an increased risk of bladder cancer, especially as bladder cancer is associated with lifestyle and occupational risk factors. In a study that analyzed the telomere length in leukocytes of 463 bladder cancer patients with both MIBC and non-MIBC (NMIBC), the main finding was that shortened telomere length was independently associated with overall and bladder cancer–specific survival. This association was maintained whether the bladder cancer was of high or low grade and whether or not it was muscle invasive.[173]

Bladder cancer therapy is rapidly evolving. There is accumulating evidence for the activity of programmed death 1 (PD-1) and programmed death ligand 1 (PD-L1) inhibitors, immunotherapeutic agents that reduce T-cell anergy. Gene expression profiles of bladder tumors suggest that there are several prognostic gene signatures present, which may predict

benefit from systemic chemotherapy[12] and may also predict response to immunotherapy[9]. Furthermore, the fundamental biology represented by gene expression may provide a context for mutationally driven tumors. One example is the enhanced peroxisome proliferator–activated receptor-γ expression observed in the luminal subtype, which is also enriched for fibroblast growth factor receptor 3 (FGFR3) mutations. Several datasets also support the activity of specific targeted agents in a mutation-dependent context. There is mounting substantial evidence for PD-1– and PD-L1–directed therapies, and a vigorous debate surrounds the use of PD-L1 immunohistochemical assessment to identify appropriate patients for therapy. Data from the phase II assessment of atezolizumab suggest the potential use of mutational load as a predictor of response. These preliminary findings support the recent recommendation by the NCCN Bladder Cancer Guidelines panel, which recommends molecular profiling of advanced bladder cancer.[174]

Organ-Confined, Lymph Node–Negative Tumors

In the University of Southern California series, 56% of patients demonstrated pathologically organ-confined, lymph node–negative tumor.[4] The outcomes in this pathologic subgroup were excellent (Table 68.3), with a 5- and 10-year recurrence-free survival of 85% and 82%, respectively. No significant survival differences were observed when comparing superficially noninvasive (Pis, Pa), lamina propria invasive (P1), and muscle-invasive (P2a, P2b) tumors as long as the tumor was confined to the bladder without evidence of lymph node involvement. Similar outcomes for patients with pathologic non–muscle-invasive bladder tumors following cystectomy have been previously reported.[4,146,175] Collectively, these data support the treatment of patients with surgery when a tumor is confined to the bladder, without evidence of extravesical extension or lymph node metastasis. Treatment delays in patients with invasive bladder cancer should be avoided. Evidence suggests that prolonged delays may lead to more advanced pathologic stage and decreased survival in patients

TABLE 68.3 SELECTED DATA FROM THE UNIVERSITY OF SOUTHERN CALIFORNIA BLADDER CANCER STUDY OF RADICAL CYSTECTOMY

Pathologic Stage[a]	Number of Patients	Probability Overall Survival (%)	
		5 Years	10 Years
T2a N0	94	77	57
T2b N0	98	64	44
T3 N0	135	49	29
T4a N0	79	44	23
Extravesical N0	214	47	27
All node negative pooled	808	69	49
All node positive pooled	246	31	23

[a]From reference 269.
Reprinted from Freiha F, Reese J, Torti FM. A randomized trial of radical cystectomy versus radical cystectomy plus cisplatin, vinblastine and methotrexate chemotherapy for muscle invasive bladder cancer. *J Urol* 1996;155(2):495–499. Copyright © 1996 American Urological Association, Inc. With permission.

with muscle-invasive bladder cancer.[150] Furthermore, caution should be taken in delaying definitive therapy in patients with high-risk, non–muscle-invasive bladder tumors or those with non–muscle-invasive tumors that have not appropriately responded to conservative forms of therapy.[1]

Extravesical, Lymph Node–Negative Tumors

Non–organ-confined (extravesical), lymph node–negative tumors were found in 20% of University of Southern California series patients undergoing cystectomy (Table 68.3). No obvious survival differences between extravesical P3 and P4 (node-negative) tumors were observed. The 5- and 10-year recurrence-free survival rates for this pathologic subgroup were 58% and 55%, respectively. Similar outcomes were reported by Madersbacher et al.[144] and Dhar et al.,[159] who demonstrated a 56% 5-year recurrence-free survival for the same pathologic subgroup. Patients with locally advanced tumors have higher recurrence rates and decreased survival compared with those with organ-confined, lymph node–negative tumors.[176] The 1997 AJCC TNM staging system used for these studies stratified extravesical tumor involvement (previously defined as pT3b) into microscopic (pT3a) and gross (pT3b) extravesical tumor extension. No significant difference was observed in the recurrence-free and overall survival in patients when evaluating for pT3a and pT3b extravesical extension.[176] The incidence of lymph node involvement was similar (~45%); however, the presence of lymph node involvement was associated with a higher risk of recurrence and worse survival compared with node-negative patients.

Lymph Node–Positive Disease

Perhaps one-fourth of patients in large cystectomy series will have positive lymph nodes (Tables 68.2 and 68.4). Although patients with lymph node tumor involvement are a high-risk group of patients, nearly one-third of these patients were alive at 5 years in the series by Stein et al..[4] It is possible that

the surgical approach employing an extended lymph node dissection provides some survival advantage in selected individuals with node-positive disease.[159] The role of adjuvant therapy in these patients is difficult to assess due to the absence of adequately powered trial data (see on the Role of Systemic Therapy section). In an analysis of lymph node–positive patients carried out by the University of Southern California group, the administration of adjuvant chemotherapy was a significant and independent predictor for recurrence and overall survival in this group[183]; however, case-mix effects will be prominent in this type of retrospective analysis as patients need to survive long enough and be fit enough to even start chemotherapy to figure in the analysis. Inevitably, this will bias results in favor of adjuvant chemotherapy by excluding those who died early or who never became fit enough postoperatively to receive chemotherapy. The authors own experience with attempting to recruit to adjuvant chemotherapy trials suggests that only the most fit patients are able to recover quickly enough postoperatively to undergo systemic chemotherapy, so these data are highly likely to be biased by underlying patient fitness. A further interesting feature of the BC2001 trial,[175] discussed in detail below, was that although no attempt was made to include pelvic nodes in the treatment field, the rate of nodal relapse was low at around 6% with radiotherapy alone, falling to 4% with chemoradiation. One possible interpretation of these data is that successful treatment of the primary, with either surgery or radiotherapy, may affect the subsequent behavior of low-volume nodal disease.

The prognosis in patients with lymph node–positive disease can be stratified by the number of lymph nodes involved (tumor burden), the stage of the primary tumor, and the presence of lymph node capsule perforation.[4] Patients with fewer than five positive lymph nodes among those with lymph node–positive organ-confined bladder tumors had a significantly improved recurrence-free survival rate.[4,156,157]

The number of lymph nodes involved with tumor and the extent of the lymph node dissection are both important variables for patients undergoing cystectomy for bladder cancer. Stein et al.[156] examined 246 patients with lymph node tumor involvement following radical cystectomy to evaluate other prognostic factors in this high-risk group. They used lymph node density to account for the extent of the lymph node dissection (number of lymph nodes removed) and the tumor burden (number of positive lymph nodes) following cystectomy for patients with lymph node–positive disease. Lymph node density as defined in this study was a significant and independent prognostic variable in patients with lymph node metastases. Future staging systems and the application of adjuvant therapy in clinical trials may consider applying these concepts to better stratify this high-risk group of patients.

Recurrence Following Radical Cystectomy

Recurrence following radical cystectomy for bladder cancer correlates well with the pathologic stage and subgroup.[4,144] With long-term follow-up (median, >10 years), recurrences in

TABLE 68.4 INCIDENCE OF LYMPH NODE METASTASIS FOLLOWING RADICAL CYSTECTOMY, CORRELATION TO PRIMARY TUMOR

Study (Reference)	Period (Year)	Number of Patients	Lymph Node Metastasis (%)	Bladder Tumor Stage[a] (%)				
				P0, Pis, Pa, P1	P2a	P2b	P3	P4
Poulsen et al.[177]	1990–1997	191	50[26]	2[4]	4[18]	7[25]	33[51]	4[43]
Vieweg et al.[176]	1980–1990	686	193[28]	10[10]	12[9]	22[23]	97[42]	52[41]
Leissner et al.[154]	1999–2002	290	81[28]	1[3]	5[13]	12[22]	53[43]	10[50]
Stein et al.[4]	1971–1997	1,054	246[24]	19[5]	21[18]	35[27]	113[44]	58[42]
Vazina et al.[178]	1992–2002	176	43[24]	1[179]	10[16]	–	20[180]	12[50]
Abdel-Latif et al.[181]	1997–1999	418	110[26]	3[179]	4[7]	29[25]	59[48]	15[182]
Madersbacher et al.[144]	1985–2000	507	124[24]	2[3]	26[17]	–	64[34]	32[41]
Hautmann et al.[146]	1986–2003	788	142[18]	2[2]	31[10]	–	73[41]	36[43]
Total		4,110	989[24]					

[a]From reference 262.
From American Joint Committee on Cancer. Urinary bladder. In: *AJCC cancer staging manual*. 5th ed. Philadelphia: Lippincott-Raven, 1997:241–243. With permission.

Section III

the University of Southern California series were classified as local (pelvic), distant, and urethral. Local recurrences were defined as those occurring within the soft tissue field of exenteration. Distant recurrences were defined as those occurring outside the pelvis, whereas urethral tumors were classified as a new primary tumor occurring in the retained urethra. Overall, 30% of all patients in the University of Southern California series experienced tumor recurrence.[4] The median time to any recurrence was 12 months, with 86% of all patients developing their recurrences within the first 3 years of cystectomy. Of the 311 patients who developed a recurrence, the median time to distant recurrence was 12 months, whereas the median time to local recurrence was 18 months. Late tumor recurrences, defined as 5 years or more after surgery, do occur and underscore the need for lifelong follow-up.

Pelvic (Locoregional) Recurrence

Pelvic recurrence rates of 6% to 9% are reported in large series,[144,146,175] with higher rates in tumors with extravesical spread or node-positive disease at cystectomy.[4]

In patients with muscle-invasive bladder cancer, locoregional failure (LRF) has been reported to occur in up to 20% of patients following radical cystectomy.

Reddy et al.[184] examined records in an institutional radical cystectomy database of 334 patients with pathologic T3-4 N0-1 bladder cancer after radical cystectomy and bilateral pelvic lymph node dissection. Of these, 46% received perioperative chemotherapy. The median follow-up was 11 months. On univariate analysis, margin status, pT stage, and pN stage were all associated with LRF ($P < .05$); however, on multivariate analysis, only pT and pN stages were significantly associated with LRF ($P < .05$). Three strata of risk were defined, including low-risk patients with pT3N0 disease, intermediate-risk patients with pT3N1 or pT4N0 disease, and high-risk patients with pT4N1 disease, who had a 2-year incidence of LRF of 12%, 33%, and 72%, respectively. The most common sites of pelvic relapse included the external and internal iliac lymph nodes (LNs) and obturator LN regions. Notably, 34% of patients with LRF had locoregional-only disease at the time of recurrence.

Metastatic (Distant) Recurrence

Recurrences following radical cystectomy are most commonly found at distant sites. This is consistent with the benefits observed in the neoadjuvant chemotherapy trials, where the maximum effect would be expected on low-volume, occult metastases rather than large-volume primary disease (discussed below). Distant recurrence rates of 20% to 35% are reported in large series (Table 68.5). However, overall death rates from bladder cancer are higher than this, so there would appear to be either underreporting of deaths in these series or the cases selected were not representative of wider experience.

Urethral Recurrence

Urethral tumor recurrence in patients with a history of bladder cancer following radical cystectomy represents a second manifestation of the multicentric defect of the primary transitional cell mucosa that led to the original bladder tumor. The term urethral recurrence is therefore somewhat misleading, suggesting a failure of definitive treatment of the bladder cancer. Most urethral tumors probably represent simply another occurrence of the transitional cell carcinoma in the remaining urothelium. Because radical cystectomy with orthotopic diversion has increasingly been performed, the fate of the retained urethra has become an increasingly important oncologic issue.

The advent of orthotopic lower urinary tract reconstruction has provided a more natural voiding pattern in patients following radical cystectomy. Approximately 85% of all patients undergoing cystectomy for TCC of the bladder at the University of Southern California research center receive an orthotopic neobladder substitute. From an oncologic perspective, only those with a positive surgical margin at the proximal urethra (distal to the apex of the prostate in men and just distal to the bladder neck in women) on intraoperative frozen section are absolutely excluded from orthotopic reconstruction. This enthusiasm to preserve the native urethra following radical cystectomy and allow for orthotopic reconstruction has rightfully increased concerns for a urethral recurrence in these patients.

Prior to the orthotopic era in women, urethral tumor recurrence was not an important oncologic issue because the entire urethra was removed at the time of cystectomy. With a better understanding of female pelvic anatomy and the innervation of the urinary sphincter and continence mechanism in women,[185] along with the identification of various pathologic risk factors for urethral tumor involvement in these patients, orthotopic diversion has now become a commonly performed form of urinary diversion in women following cystectomy.[183] Tumor involving the bladder neck is the most important risk factor for urethral tumor involvement in women.[186,187] Although bladder neck involvement is a significant risk factor for urethral tumors, not all women with tumor involving the bladder neck will have urethral tumors. Approximately 50% of female patients with tumor at the bladder neck will have an uninvolved urethra free of tumor. In this situation, the patient may potentially be considered an appropriate candidate for orthotopic diversion. Furthermore, intraoperative frozen-section analysis of the distal surgical margin is an accurate and reliable means to pathologically evaluate the proximal urethra.[187]

A growing population of male patients reconstructed to the urethra following cystectomy exists today. With longer follow-up, could this expose them to a greater risk for a urethral recurrence? The historical incidence of urethral recurrence in the retained urethra following cystectomy for bladder cancer ranges from 6% to 10%.[1] Specific clinical and pathologic risk factors that have been identified to provided risk assessment for urethral recurrence include multifocal tumors, CIS, tumor involvement of the prostate (particularly invasion of the prostatic stroma), and the form of urinary diversion (orthotopic or cutaneous) performed.[188–192]

Stein et al.[188] evaluated urethral recurrence in a large group of male patients undergoing radical cystectomy and urinary diversion for TCC of the bladder. In this study, the clinical and pathologic results of 768 consecutive male patients undergoing radical cystectomy with a median follow-up of 13 years were analyzed. Of these 768 patients, 397 men (51%) underwent an orthotopic diversion (median follow-up 10 years) and 371 men (49%) underwent a cutaneous diversion (median

TABLE 68.5 RECURRENCE-FREE SURVIVAL AND THE INCIDENCE OF RECURRENCE IN SELECTED STUDIES OF RADICAL CYSTECTOMY

Study (Reference)	Number of Patients	Median Follow-Up (Month)	Recurrence-Free Survival (%)		Recurrence (%)	
			5 Year	10 Year	Local	Distant
Stein et al./USC[4]	1,054	122	68	66	7.3	22.2
Madersbacher et al./Bern[144]	507	45	62	50	7.9	35.3
Hautmann et al./Ulm[146]	788	53	65	59	9.3	17.8
Yafi et al./Canada[175]	2,287	29	48	–	6.0	27.0

follow-up 19 years). Overall, 45 patients (7%) developed a urethral recurrence. The median time to a urethral recurrence was 2 years (range, 0.2 to 13.6 years). Of these 45 patients, 16 men (5%) had an orthotopic and 29 (9%) had a cutaneous form of urinary diversion. In this cohort of male patients, multiple risk factors were analyzed with regard to urethral recurrence. In a multivariate analysis, two important variables were identified that significantly increased the risk of a urethral tumor recurrence following cystectomy, including any prostate involvement and the form of urinary diversion. The estimated 5-year probability of a urethral recurrence was 5% without prostate involvement, which increased to 12% and 18% with superficial (prostatic urethra and ducts) and invasive (stroma) prostate involvement, respectively. Patients undergoing an orthotopic diversion demonstrated a statistically significantly lower risk of urethral recurrence compared with those undergoing a cutaneous form of urinary diversion.

The follow-up and management of the urethra in male patients treated for high-grade invasive bladder cancer is of importance. The indications and timing of a prophylactic urethrectomy in those undergoing cystectomy and a cutaneous diversion is debatable. It may include urethrectomy at the time of cystectomy based on preoperative clinical parameters or based on the intraoperative frozen-section analysis of the urethral margin or a delayed urethrectomy based on final pathologic evaluation of the cystectomy specimen. These issues are best detailed with the patient preoperatively ensuring proper informed consent.

Management of the Retained Urethra Following Cystectomy

Intraoperative frozen-section analysis of the proximal urethra by an experienced pathologist is a reliable and accurate means to determine indications for orthotopic diversion in all patients. It is good practice to proceed with an orthotopic neobladder in men and women whose intraoperative frozen section of the proximal urethra is free of tumor. This approach does not appear to increase the risk of a urethral recurrence in these patients.[1,193] Male patients with known prostatic tumor involvement should not necessarily be excluded from an orthotopic substitute if the intraoperative biopsy is normal. Similarly, female patients with bladder neck involvement should not necessarily be excluded from an orthotopic neobladder if the intraoperative biopsy is also normal. All patients should be carefully counseled regarding the need for follow-up, the long-term risks of a urethral recurrence, and the possible need for urethrectomy following cystectomy.

Salvage Cystectomy

Salvage cystectomy after prior radiation therapy was discussed above in the section comparing surgical with bladder-sparing approaches.

Summary of Surgical Therapy

Surgery is an important mode of therapy for invasive bladder cancer and undoubtedly can provide durable disease control for many patients with the disease. In addition, an integrated approach with other treatment modalities such as neoadjuvant chemotherapy and radiation therapy is essential if the best results are to be achieved in the entire patient population, especially those who are borderline fit for major surgery. Radical cystectomy probably provides the best local pelvic control of the disease and provides accurate evaluation of the primary bladder tumor along with the regional lymph nodes yielding important prognostic information. This, coupled with the evolution and successful application of orthotopic lower urinary tract reconstruction in both men and women, has provided patients a more physiologic and acceptable means to store and eliminate urine. However, most deaths from bladder

cancer still occur due to distant metastases, presumably present at the time of original surgery, so further improvements in outcome will depend on the development of both better systemic therapies and also predictive (as opposed to prognostic) markers that will allow better selection of therapies.

Radiation Therapy
External Beam Radiation Therapy

Whatever the merits or otherwise of radiation therapy as a treatment for bladder cancer, its use in the United States has declined since the 1980s, and the treatment is now used mainly in certain centers such as Boston in carefully selected patients rather than as a mainstream alternative to surgery. As discussed above, patterns vary worldwide with the US pattern of care predominating. Potential indications for radiation therapy are summarized in Table 68.6. Patients with radiologic node-positive or metastatic disease should be managed predominantly with either chemotherapy or palliative approaches such as local radiotherapy to bulk disease (see below). Patients with radiologic node-negative, muscle-invasive disease may be considered for radical radiotherapy. In North America, radiation therapy is administered as part of a package of care comprising maximal TURBT, chemotherapy, and radiation therapy, the so-called trimodality therapy (Fig. 68.3).[194,195]

The schedules used are complex but can be summarized as initial maximal TURBT followed by initial radiation therapy combined with synchronous chemotherapy, usually with cisplatinum followed by interim check cystoscopy. Patients experiencing a good response to treatment continue to consolidate chemoradiotherapy and then adjuvant polychemotherapy, usually with a cisplatinum base. Patients remain on long-term cystoscopic surveillance. Noninvasive recurrence can be managed by further TURBT and intravesical therapy. Those with isolated muscle-invasive recurrence or failure to respond (but with no systemic relapse) can undergo salvage cystectomy with or without further chemotherapy.

The optimal radiation therapy schedule has yet to be established. In North America, split schedules often used are 39 or 40 Gy in 1.8- or 2-Gy fractions with an interval cystoscopy; patients with responding disease proceed to a total dose of 64 to 68 Gy. Generally, these schedules achieve long-term survival comparable to surgical series. A significant risk of cystectomy remains, however, with 22% undergoing immediate cystectomy, 13% delayed cystectomy for local recurrence, and 65% retaining a functioning bladder.[195]

In some countries, particularly the United Kingdom and Australia, an alternative schema is used (Fig. 68.4). As in the trimodality approach, patients will undergo maximal TURBT for diagnostic and staging purposes. They can then be treated either with primary surgery (as elsewhere) or alternatively with either neoadjuvant chemotherapy or primary radiation therapy. The role of cystectomy was discussed above, and the evidence and use of neoadjuvant therapy is discussed in the section Role of Systemic Therapy. In the United Kingdom, the radiation therapy itself is given as a single definitive course,

TABLE 68.6 INDICATIONS FOR RADIATION THERAPY IN BLADDER CANCER

Stage	Recommendation
CIS, Ta, T1	No role for radiation therapy
T2-T4aN0M0	Potential role for radiation therapy, combined with synchronous chemotherapy if patient sufficiently fit (bladder preservation)
T any N1-3M0 or T any N any M1	No role for radical radiation therapy as sole treatment for stage IV disease. It may be worth considering, as part of "radical" palliation in combination with systemic chemotherapy. No randomized data on the use of radiation therapy in this setting beyond studies of fractionation

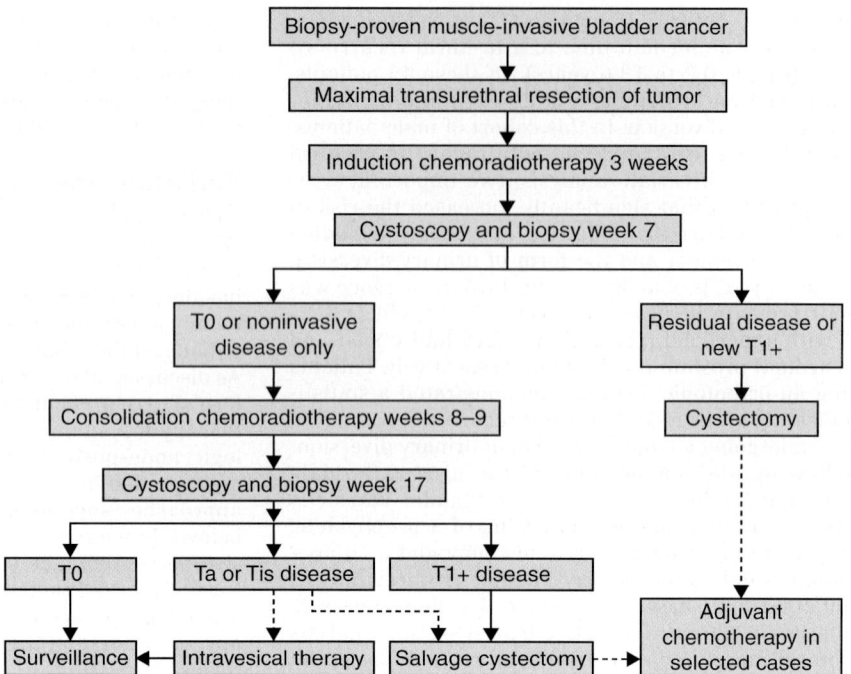

FIGURE 68.3. Trimodality therapy.

usually to the whole bladder, only with no attempt to treat the nodes (as discussed below). Typical dose schedules would be 64 Gy in 32 fractions or hypofractionated schedules such as 55 Gy in 20 fractions. Following radiation therapy, patients undergo cystoscopic surveillance as in the US model, with salvage cystectomy for isolated local failure.

There are key differences between these two approaches. The first and most obvious is that in most disease sites, definitive radiation therapy is not given as a split course but as a single continuously fractionated treatment as in the United Kingdom. To understand how this approach has arisen, it has to be understood that trimodality therapy is offered as an alternative to cystectomy in countries where the prevailing opinion is that surgery is the treatment of choice. Patients undergoing this treatment are offered what is termed selective bladder preservation, with the multiple checkpoints allowing early exit to surgery aimed at providing reassurance to surgeons in particular that the opportunity for cure is not being lost. The median ages (mid-60s) reported in studies using this approach reflect this patient selection and are similar to large surgical series.[4,134] The UK approach is completely different in this respect as there is a long tradition of using radical radiation therapy after TURBT, and the much older patient groups compared with surgical series reflect a different decision-making process in which younger, more fit patients are more likely to get surgery and older or less fit patients radiation therapy.[10,12,135,136,196] Interestingly, the long-term bladder preservation rates in older series seem similar to the rates for salvage cystectomy postradiotherapy occurring in approximately one-fourth of patients managed with radiation therapy alone at 10 years median follow-up,[197] with around two-thirds of

surviving patients retaining their bladders. The authors' own more recent chemoradiotherapy series suggests a higher rate of bladder preservation with the use of synchronous chemotherapy combined with full-dose radical radiation therapy.[11]

In summary, there are limited data exploring the effect of radiation therapy (RT) dose on outcomes in muscle-invasive bladder cancer (MIBC). As noted, most radiation oncologists use 60 to 70 Gy; many studies have used 64 to 66 Gy, but the optimal RT dose is not definitely known. Korpics et al.[198] conducted a retrospective cohort study of 843 patients with cT2-4 N0-3 M0 transitional cell MIBC treated with RT using the National Cancer Database. Patients were divided into dose groups: <50, 50 to 59, 60 to 66, and >66 Gy. A subgroup analysis was performed for patients treated with 60 to 66 Gy by dividing them into 3 groups (60 to 62, 63 to 64, and 65 to 66 Gy).

Median follow-up was 16.3 months; 267 patients (32%) received <50 Gy, 169 (20%) received 50 to 59 Gy, 376 (45%) patients received 60 to 66 Gy, and 31 (4%) patients received >66 Gy. Patients receiving concurrent chemoradiotherapy were more likely to receive an RT dose of 60 Gy ($P < .001$), and patients with higher T-stage were more likely to receive a lower RT dose (P Z 0.003).

Two-year OS rates, when divided by RT dose, were 26%, 31%, 56%, and 55%, respectively, for <50, 50 to 59, 60 to 66, and >66 Gy. Univariate analysis demonstrating increasing RT dose ($P < 0.001$) was associated with improved OS. On multivariate analysis (MVA), when compared to a dose of 60 to 66 Gy, <50 Gy (hazard ratio [HR] 2.36, $P < .001$), and 50 to 59 Gy (HR 1.72, $P < .001$) were associated with worse OS. Escalation of dose to higher than 66 Gy was not associated with OS

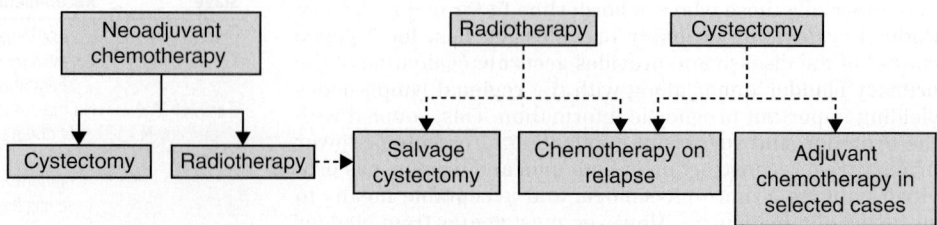

FIGURE 68.4. Integration of neoadjuvant chemotherapy, radiotherapy, and surgery in the United Kingdom.

(HR 1.01, P Z .977). In the subgroup of patients treated with 60 to 66 Gy, MVA revealed that compared to 65 to 66 Gy, there was worse OS with a dose of 60 to 62 Gy (HR 1.66, P Z .020), but no difference in OS with a dose of 63 to 64 Gy (HR 1.12, P Z .549).

The authors concluded that RT doses of <60 Gy are associated with worse OS in patients undergoing bladder RT and thus should be avoided in definitive treatment. Additionally, there is no survival advantage to increasing dose beyond 66 Gy. They felt that 63 to 66 Gy is the optimal RT dose when treating patients with bladder-preserving radiation therapy.

With regard to target volumes the usual practice is to treat the pelvis, including the iliac lymph nodes to the aortic bifurcation (L4-5 in most patients to doses, as noted above in the range of 50 Gy, with a volumes reduction encompassing the whole bladder to 60 Gy and an additional volume reduction targeted to residual gross tumor to complete 66 to 68 Gy.

Huddart et al.,[197] in a multicenter study, evaluated whether reducing radiation dose to uninvolved bladder while maintaining dose to the tumor would reduce side effects without impairing local control in the treatment of muscle-invasive bladder cancer. In this phase III multicenter trial, 219 patients were randomized to standard whole-bladder radiation therapy (sRT) or reduced high-dose volume radiation therapy (RHDVRT) that aimed to deliver full radiation dose to the tumor and 80% of maximum dose to the uninvolved bladder. Participants were also randomly assigned to receive radiation therapy alone or radiation therapy plus chemotherapy in a partial 2 x 2 factorial design (with a noninferiority margin of 10% at 2 years).

Overall incidence of late toxicity was less than predicted, with a cumulative 2-year Radiation Therapy Oncology Group grade 3/4 toxicity rate of 13% and no statistically significant differences between groups. The difference in 2-year locoregional recurrence-free rate (RHDVRT vs. sRT) was 6.4% under an intention to treat analysis and 2.6% in the "per protocol."

The authors concluded that RHDVRT did not result in a statistically significant reduction in late side effects compared with sRT, and noninferiority of locoregional control could not be concluded formally. However, overall low rates of clinically significant toxicity combined with low rates of invasive bladder cancer relapse confirmed that (chemo)radiation therapy is a valid option for the treatment of muscle-invasive bladder cancer.

Inter- and intrafraction anatomy changes in patients undergoing radiation therapy (RT) for bladder cancer (BC) are common and have been studied with implanted fiducial markers, 2D orthogonal films, and computed tomography (CT).

Fischer-Valuck et al.[199] assessed the soft tissue imaging capabilities of an integrated magnetic resonance image-guided RT (MR-IGRT) system to analyze daily positioning in a preliminary study of 14 patients with BC treated on a MR-IGRT system (ViewRay Corp, Sunnyvale, CA, USA). Patient setup was performed via volumetric MR imaging with a resolution of 0.15 × 0.15 cm. Alignment was performed according to skin marks and shifts assessed by comparing the treatment volume from the planning CT to the daily MR image. Two hundred forty pretreatment MR images were analyzed, and 3 shifts were recorded for each image.

The daily volumetric MR imaging allowed for accurate alignment and daily monitoring of bladder volume and normal tissue anatomy. Recorded shifts of the treated volume were 0.9 x 0.5 cm in the right/left direction, 0.7 x 0.3 cm in the anterior/posterior direction, and 0.7 x 0.4 cm in the craniocaudal direction. In 66 (28%) of cases, the vector shift was initially greater than the PTV margin. For 2 patients, pretreatment MR imaging showed the tumor reduced in size and dose to the bowel would have exceeded constraints, and treatment adaptation was performed to reduce normal tissue toxicity.

Using CTCAE criteria, no grade 3 or higher toxicities have been reported.

Adaptive radiation therapy is sparingly used in selected centers. Foroudi et al.[179] described a multicenter feasibility study at 12 departments of online adaptive radiotherapy, using a choice of three "plan of the day" for patients with muscle-invasive bladder cancer. Departments were activated if they were part of the pilot study or after a site-credentialing visit and real-time review of the first two cases from each department. Fifty-four patients (mean age 78 years, 43 males and 7 females) were recruited, with 50 proceeding to radiation therapy. The tumor stages included T1,[1] T2,[35] T3,[10] and T4.[4] One patient died of an unrelated cause during radiation therapy. The three adaptive plans were created before the 10th fraction in all cases. In 8 (16%) of the patients, a conventional plan using a "standard" CTV to PTV margin of 1.5 cm was used for one or more fractions where the pretreatment bladder CTV was larger than any of the three adaptive plans. The bladder CTV extended beyond the PTV on posttreatment imaging in 9 (18%) of the 49 patients. However, without further bladder filling control or imaging, a CTV to PTV margin of 7 mm is insufficient.

Treatment Results

It is difficult to compare results of older series to more contemporary ones for a number of reasons. First, staging systems have changed over the years, as have imaging techniques. Patients who may have been staged as organ confined in the early or pre-CT era may now be more accurately staged as more advanced with contemporary imaging. In contrast, surgical series will report accurate pathologic stage. It is well documented that more accurate staging will bring about a paradoxical improvement in reported results by stage because of upstaging of apparently early disease cases, the so-called Will Rogers phenomenon.[199] Treatment techniques in the past were obviously less refined, with little or no ability for conformal beam shaping, and hence, toxicity would have been higher. Nonetheless, it is clear from large series that tumor control could be attained in significant numbers of patients. For example, a study from Western General Hospital, Edinburgh, conducted between 1971 and 1982, reported treatment results from 963 patients. The reported stage mix was T1, 20%; T2, 32%; T3, 40%; and T4, 8%, with the administered dose of 55 Gy in 20 fractions—a widely used UK schedule. The overall 5- and 10-year survival rates were 30% and 18%, respectively.[179] This study reports tumor control at cystoscopy in 46% of patients, and this seems to be a pretty typical response rate with radiation therapy alone.

Similar control rates were reported in the radiation therapy–alone arm of the National Cancer Institute of Canada (NCIC) trial comparing radiation therapy with chemoradiotherapy with cisplatinum[198] and also in the radiation therapy–only arms at 2 years of the UK trials BCON[12] and BC2001[200] at 2 years. The latter two trials give an accurate reflection of the results of modern radiation therapy. They ran contemporaneously between 2000 and 2009 and between them recruited more than 800 patients from around 70 UK sites, including all major UK radiation therapy centers. Both trials had similar designs, including near identical entry criteria (essentially T2-4aN0M0, with a small number of T1G3 patients entered the BCON trial), the same control arms (definitive radiation therapy to bladder only to either 55 Gy in 20 fractions or 64 Gy in 32 fractions), and the same outcome measures (locoregional disease-free and overall survival). Both trials assessed both acute and late toxicities (Figs. 68.5 and 68.6). In addition, the BC2001 trial included an optional second randomization comparing whole-bladder radiation therapy with a reduced dose to uninvolved bladder of 80% of the isocenter dose. The BC2001 permitted

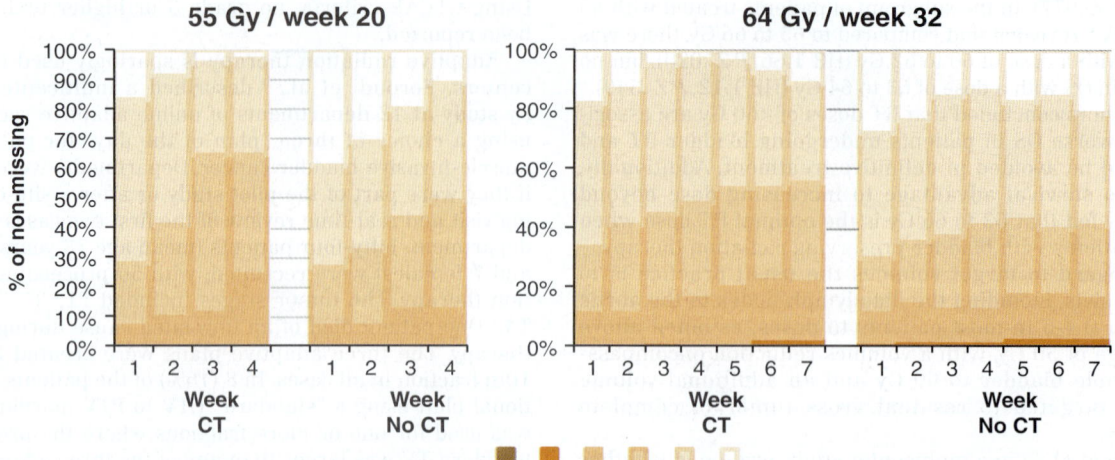

FIGURE 68.5. Acute toxicity of radiotherapy with and without synchronous chemotherapy. Graphs show worst grade of on-treatment toxicity by radiotherapy dose and week. *Darkest bars* indicate National Cancer Institute common terminology class grade 4; *white* indicates grade 0. Proportions with a grade 3 or 4 at any time on treatment: 64/178 (36.0%) chemotherapy (CT) versus 50/182 (27.5%). No CT-stratified chi-square test (*P* = .07).

neoadjuvant chemotherapy, which was a stratification factor. Around one-third of the chemoradiotherapy patients also received neoadjuvant chemotherapy.

The trials give a comprehensive insight into UK radiation therapy practice and great detail on outcomes. Median age in both trials was 73 to 74 years, with age range up to 90 years. Overall, around 40% of patients received 55 Gy in 20 fractions and 60% 64 Gy in 32 fractions. In both trials, over 95% of patients received at least 90% of the target dose in both arms, with no reduction associated with the two radiosensitizing treatments. Although the protocol recommended complete debulking at TURBT, this was only achieved in one-third to one-half of the cases, probably reflecting technical factors at surgery rather than deliberate intent.

The overall 5-year survival rate was 50% for radiation therapy plus carbogen and nicotinamide compared with 39% for radiation therapy alone (48% and 35%, respectively, if T1 tumors are excluded), with the greatest effect seen in T2 tumors. For BC2001, the estimated 5-year survival with radiation therapy alone was very similar at 34% (95% CI, 25% to 43%).

Toxicity

The toxicity of definitive radiation therapy varies with the dose and schedule used. Within BC2001 and BCON, there were two schedules: 55 Gy in 20 fractions and 64 Gy in 32 fractions. Acute toxicity is shown in Figure 68.5 for both schedules, with and without chemotherapy with 5-fluorouacil/mitomycin C.

The majority of patients experienced only grade 1 or 2 toxicity with very low rates of grade 4 events. Synchronous chemotherapy increased toxicity but was predominantly grade 1 or 2, with a nonstatistically significant effect on grade 3 or 4 events (27.5 vs. 36%; *P* = .07; boundary for significance set at 0.01 to reflect multiplicity of testing). The reduced-volume randomization failed to demonstrate a reduction in overall toxicity. However, when the volume of bowel irradiated was calculated, this did show a significant reduction; in an exploratory analysis, volume of bowel irradiated did correlate with the risk of grade 3 or 4 toxicity. There was no increase in acute toxicity observed in BC2001 if patients had received prior neoadjuvant chemotherapy.[200]

Treatment completion rates in both trials were very high, with an excess of 95% of patients receiving the prescribed

FIGURE 68.6. Late toxicity in the BC2001 trial. *Darkest bars* indicate Radiation Therapy Oncology Group (RTOG) grade 4; *white* indicates grade 0. Proportion of patients with grade 3 or 4 RTOG toxicity at any month during follow-up (6 months onward), up to 3 months before a recurrence: RT, 12.9% sRT versus 17.9% RHDV; odds ratio (95% confidence interval) 1.34 (0.55, 3.24); *P* = .52; CT, 8.3% CT versus 15.7% no CT; odds ratio 0.48 (0.21, 1.10); *P* = .07. Patients with no available assessment were excluded from analysis. CT, chemotherapy with radiotherapy; RT, radiotherapy; sRT, standard volume radiotherapy; RHDV, reduced high-dose volume radiotherapy.

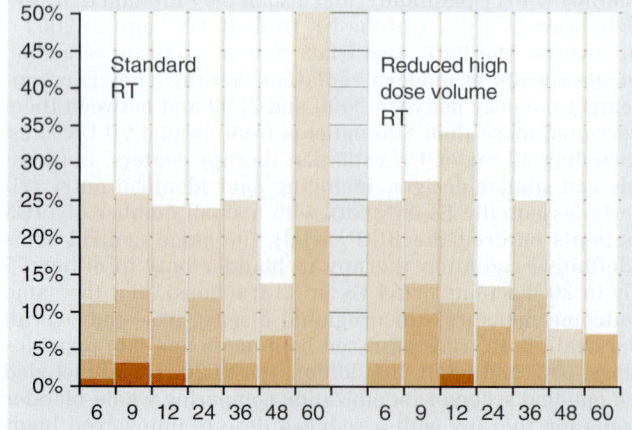
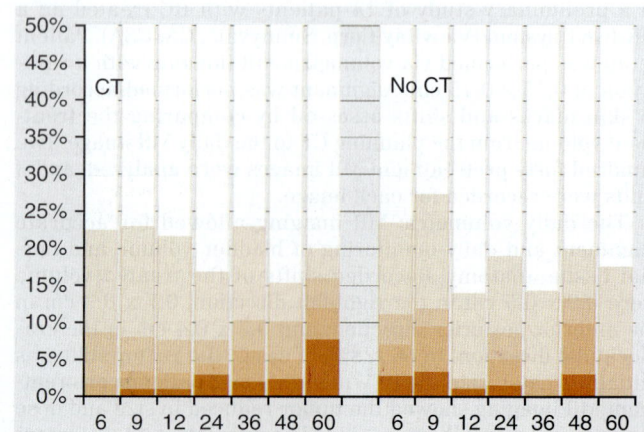

Month

dose. The majority of patients failing to complete did so for tumor-related reasons rather than toxicity. Late toxicity was of great interest in both trials and was analyzed somewhat differently. In BCON, the cumulative rates of grade 3 or 4 events were reported, which gives the worst-case scenario but does not reflect the overall toxicity at any given time point post treatment. BC2001 reports the toxicity rates at prespecified times.

There are a number of points of note here. First, late toxicity was the same with both randomizations in BC2001 (i.e., reduced-volume radiation therapy did not impact late toxicity). More significantly, the addition of synchronous chemotherapy also had no effect on reported late side effects. In addition, at any given point, 75% to 80% of patients report no late toxicity at all. This is supported by bladder capacity measurements in BC2001, which show a mean change in bladder volume at 1 and 2 years of <5 mL. Of those reported side effects, fewer than 5% report grade 4 events and fewer than 10% overall grade 3. Very similar findings pertain to the BCON trial.[12] In 2009, Efstathiou et al.[201] reported late toxicity results in 285 patients who had participated in four Radiation Therapy Oncology Group trimodality therapy trials. Overall 5.7% reported persistent late genitourinary and 1.9% gastrointestinal toxicity of grade 3 or above, consistent with the BCON and BC2001 results. The good toxicity and functional results associated with radiotherapy are borne out by surveys of quality of life and symptoms in cystectomy and radiotherapy patients carried out by Henningsohn et al. and others.[13,179,186,187,194,195,197–199,202–204] Furthermore, radiotherapy and cystectomy patients report different patterns of symptoms, with sexual dysfunction being more prominent in surgical patients and bowel symptoms more prominent in radiotherapy patients. The preservation of sexual function by radiotherapy is particularly striking given that the patients were an average of around 10 years older.

Lin et al.[205] analyzed 125,879 patients with stage II to IV, M0 bladder cancer diagnosed between 2004 and 2014 without a second primary malignancy identified from the National Cancer Database. Patients who received no treatment, cystectomy only, chemotherapy only, radiation only, radiation and cystectomy, or trimodality therapy were excluded from the analysis. There were 9,834 patients treated with cystectomy/chemo, and 4399 patients treated with chemo-RT (60 Gy to the bladder). Age ($P < .001$), sex ($P < .001$), race ($P < .001$), Charlson/Deyo Comorbidity Score (CDCS; $P < 0.001$), insurance status ($P < .001$), type of facility ($P < .001$), income ($P Z .05$), and stage ($P Z .005$) were significantly correlated with overall survival on univariate analyses. Prior to a matched pair analysis, patients treated with cystectomy/chemo were younger (mean: cystectomy/chemo 63.6 vs. chemo-RT 73.7, $P < .001$), had better performance status (CDCS 0: cystectomy/chemo 74.2% vs. chemo-RT 68.5%, $P < .001$), were privately insured (cystectomy/chemo 42.8% vs. chemo-RT 19.9%, $P < .001$), and were more likely female (cystectomy/chemo 32.7% vs. chemo-RT 28.4%, $P < .001$). Before a matched pair analysis, overall survival (OS) was significantly better for patients treated with cystectomy/chemo (3 years 50.9% and 5 years 41.4%) compared to chemo-RT (3 years 40.6% and 5 years 28.4%) ($P < .001$). A matched pair analysis matching age, sex, race, CDCS, insurance status, income, and stage produced 722 pairs ($N = 1,444$). After the matched pair analysis, OS was no longer significantly different between cystectomy/chemotherapy (3 years 47.3% and 5 years 37.8%) and chemo-RT (3 years 45.7% and 5 years 32%).

Effect of Synchronous Chemotherapy

There are a large number of phase I or II trials from North America,[20,194,195,198,202,203,206–209] mainland Europe,[5,210–212] and the United Kingdom that have examined various chemotherapy agents in combination with radiation therapy.[1] There are,

however, only a few trials reported in which radiotherapy alone is compared with radiotherapy with synchronous chemotherapy. The only randomized study using the trimodality therapy approach was carried out by the NCIC and reported in 1996.[192] This study compared radiation therapy to 40 Gy in 20 fractions with the same schedule combined with cisplatinum 100 mg/m^2 twice weekly ×3. Patients then underwent interim cystoscopy and either consolidation radiotherapy to 20 Gy in 10 fractions or cystectomy depending on response and fitness for surgery. Synchronous cisplatinum had no effect on the rate of distant metastasis, consistent with a lack of effect in neoadjuvant trials. The study, however, was relatively small and could only have detected very large effects. Concurrent cisplatinum had a highly significant effect on pelvic recurrence, with 25 of 48 control patients having a pelvic recurrence, compared with 15 of 51 cisplatinum-treated patients ($P = .036$; HR 0.50; 90% CI, 0.29 to 0.86). It should be noted that a similar platinum schedule given prior to radiation therapy had no effect whatsoever on recurrences, either local or distant.[1]

There are two randomized trials of radiosensitization using UK schedules: the BC2001 and BCON studies, as already discussed. These two large phase III randomized control trials reported results in 2009 to 2010. These trials used radiosensitization with either concurrent chemotherapy (BC2001) or carbogen and nicotinamide (BCON). BC2001 has shown a significant improvement in locoregional disease-free survival with concurrent 5 fluorouracil and mitomycin C of 34% (HR 0.66; 95% CI, 0.46 to 0.95) driven by a reduction of 47% in invasive locoregional recurrences (HR 0.53; $P = .007$), which is very similar to that observed in the NCIC trial with cisplatinum using the trimodality approach.[192] Figure 68.7 shows the Kaplan-Meier curves for invasive locoregional disease-free survival. Survival data show a trend toward an improvement in overall survival (HR 0.81; $P = .16$), although the data are immature. The BCON trial[12] with synchronous carbogen and nicotinamide narrowly failed to meet its primary endpoint of an improvement in local relapse-free survival (HR 0.87; 63% vs. 74%; $P = .1$) but did report an improvement in overall survival at 3 years (46% vs. 59%; HR 0.86; 95% CI, 0.745 to 0.996; $P = .04$).

Taken together, the trial data with chemoradiotherapy suggest good tolerability even in relatively elderly patients with excellent late toxicity profiles in the majority of patients whether treated with the North American trimodality approach or the UK single-treatment block.[1] The similar hazard ratios observed with cisplatinum and 5-fluorouacil/mitomycin C suggest that a range of chemotherapy approaches can probably be used with the selection based on toxicity. It is noteworthy that comparisons of platinum and 5-fluorouacil–based chemoradiotherapy combinations have been carried out in anal cancer, with the two approaches being similarly effective. The high rates of locoregional control seen make radical chemoradiotherapy a viable treatment option for many patients presenting with muscle-invasive bladder cancer.

Pattern of Failure

As already discussed above, a significant proportion of patients will experience locoregional failure and undergo salvage surgery. The BC2001 study gives a good indication of patterns of failure using the single-block approach to radical radiotherapy. A summary of relapse patterns in the chemoradiotherapy arm of the trial is shown in Figure 68.8.

There are a number of features of note here. First, the majority of locoregional failures are in the bladder, and there are more noninvasive than invasive recurrences. This underlines the need for regular surveillance postradiation therapy and the requirement for good integration of radiation therapy and surgical services if patients are to be managed by bladder

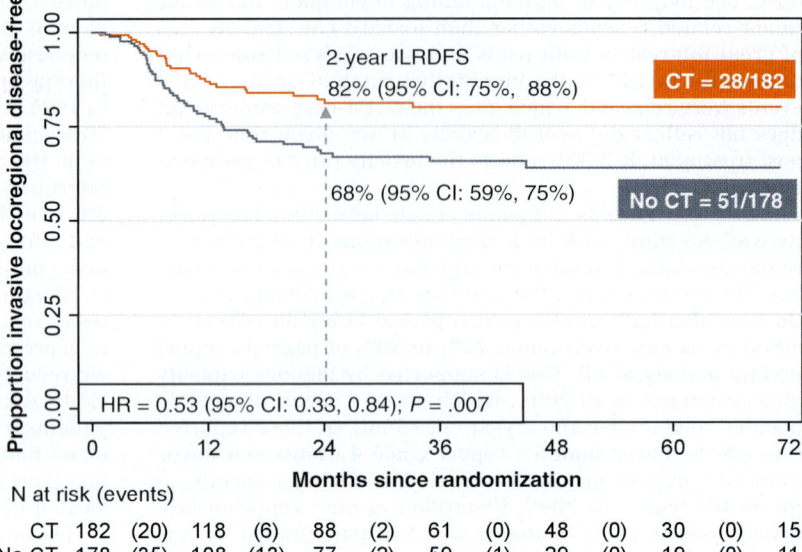

FIGURE 68.7. Invasive locoregional disease-free survival with or without chemotherapy.

N at risk (events)											
CT	182	(20)	118	(6)	88	(2)	61	(0)	48	(0)	30	(0)	15
No CT	178	(35)	108	(13)	77	(2)	59	(1)	29	(0)	19	(0)	11

conservation. In the authors' experience, the majority of non-invasive recurrences can be successfully managed conservatively without the need for cystectomy. For those with invasive recurrence, cystectomy remains an option if the patients are sufficiently fit. The low rate of nodal relapse in BC2001 is also of interest, as no attempt was made to include pelvic nodes in the field, although lower pelvic nodes would have been included in the treated volume. For improvement in the metastatic relapse rate, better systemic therapies must be found. However, the rate of second cancer is also notable and probably relates to the age of the patients and the historic high rate of tobacco consumption in the bladder cancer population.

Altered Fractionation Schedules

There are old data examining hyperfractionation in comparison to conventional treatment to 64 Gy in 32 fractions, both given as a split course. The data suggest an improvement with the hyperfractionated regimen; however, given the suboptimal nature of the control arm, it is hard to draw firm conclusions[1]. A study from the Royal Marsden Hospital compared 64 Gy in 32 fractions to 60.8 Gy in 32 fractions over 26 days in 228 patients.[213] Hypofractionated schedules are widely used in the United Kingdom and elsewhere for radical treatment and for palliation (as discussed below).

In Canada, Turgeon et al.[214] carried out a retrospective review of 24 patients 70 years or older treated with maximally

feasible TURBT followed by concomitant chemoradiation using hypofractionated IMRT, treated between January 2008 and August 2012.

The patients had histologically proven muscle-invasive transitional cell carcinoma of the bladder stage T2-T3N0M0 and were planned for a course of hypofractionated IMRT (50 Gy in 20 fractions). IMRT was delivered to the bladder volume only in 7 patients (29%). The remaining 17 patients received 50 Gy/20 fxs to the bladder and 40 Gy/20 fxs to the pelvic lymph nodes. All patients received concomitant chemotherapy either with gemcitabine 100 mg/m^2 weekly (21 patients) or cisplatin 40 mg/m^2 weekly.

Twenty-four patients with a median age of 79 years were eligible for our study. Nine patients refused cystectomy, and the remaining 15 were not considered medically fit for cystectomy. TURBT was not possible or judged incomplete by the urologist in five patients. Median follow-up was 16 months (range, 6 to 55 months). A cystoscopically and/or biopsy-proven complete response in the bladder was confirmed in 83% of the patients. Of the remaining patients, one of them underwent salvage cystectomy, and no disease was found in the bladder on histopathologic assessment. Seven patients recurred, four locoregionally and three with distant metastasis. Cancer-specific and the overall survival rates at 2 years were 74% and 63%, respectively. Grade 2 acute genitourinary (GU) and/or gastrointestinal (GI) toxicities occurred in 42%

FIGURE 68.8. Patterns of failure after chemoradiotherapy in BC2001.

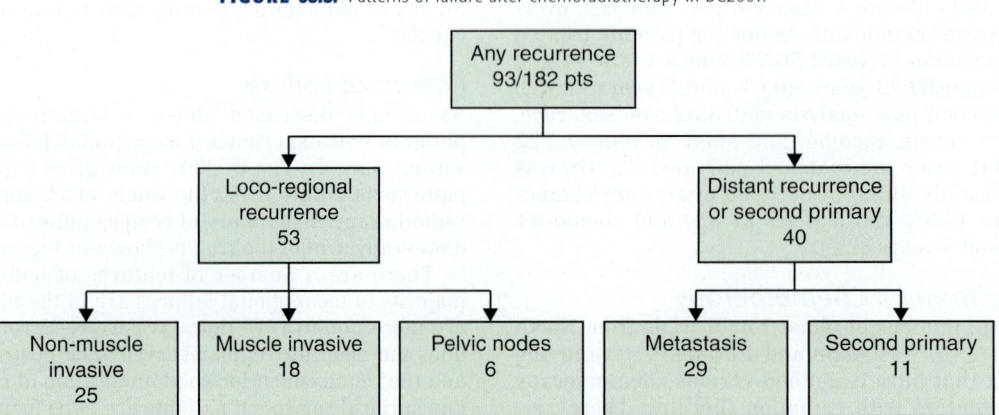

of the patients. A single patient had febrile neutropenia with combined grade 3 GU and GI acute toxicities. Grade 3 hematologic toxicity was seen in 13% of the patients. There was no grade 4 to 5 toxicity.

Hafeez et al.[215] reported on 55 patients with T2-T4aNx-2M0-1 bladder cancer not suitable for cystectomy or daily radiation therapy treatment. A plan of radiation therapy was used, treating the whole (empty) bladder to 36 Gy in 6 weekly fractions. Acute toxicity was assessed weekly during radiation therapy, at 6 and 12 weeks, and late toxicity was assessed at 6 and 12 months. Cystoscopy was used to assess local tumor control at 3 months.

Median age of the patients was 86 years. Eighty-seven percent of patients completed their prescribed course of radiation therapy. Genitourinary and gastrointestinal grade 3 acute toxicity was seen in 18% (10/55) and 4% (2/55) of patients, respectively. No grade 4 genitourinary or gastrointestinal toxicity was seen. Grade 3 late toxicity (any) at 6 and 12 months was seen in 6.5% (2/31) and 4.3% (1/23) of patients, respectively. Local tumor control after radiation therapy was 92% of assessed patients (60% total population). Cumulative incidence of local tumor progression at 1 year and 2 years for all patients was 7% and 17%, respectively. Overall survival at 1 year was 63%.

There are no modern trials comparing these schedules to 64 Gy in 32 fractions.

Harland et al[215a] conducted a multicenter randomized trial in the United Kingdom to determine the efficacy of radical radiation therapy in reducing the incidence of progression of pT1G3 transitional cell carcinoma of the bladder to muscle invasive disease and disease mortality.

Patients with a diagnosis of pT1G3 NXM0 transitional cell carcinoma with unifocal disease and no carcinoma in situ (group 1), or with multifocal disease and/or carcinoma in situ (group 2) were eligible for the trial. Patients in group 1 were randomized between observation and radiation therapy to the bladder, and in group 2 between intravesical therapy and radiation therapy.

A total of 210 patients from 37 centers in the United Kingdom were in the study (77 patients in group 1 and 133 patients in group 2); 6 patients were excluded because they were found to have pT2 disease by the reference pathologist. No evidence of an advantage with radiation therapy was found in terms of progression-free interval progression-free survival (hazard ratio 1.35) or overall survival (hazard ratio 1.32)There is no evidence that radiation therapy was better than conservative treatment.

Palliative Radiation Therapy

A prospective randomized trial was conducted in 500 patients to compare the outcome in two treatment groups. Group 1 received 35 Gy in 10 fractions and group 2 received 21 Gy in 3 fractions. Five hundred patients were recruited, but data on symptomatic improvement at 3 months were only available on 272 patients. Of these, 68% achieved symptomatic improvement (71% for 35 Gy, 64% for 21 Gy), with no evidence of a difference in efficacy or toxicity between the two arms. On the basis of these results, 21 Gy in 3 fractions is widely used in the United Kingdom as a palliative schedule. The data are congruent with other data on hypofractionation for palliation[1] as well as the growing trend for hypofractionation in other pelvic sites, in particular the prostate.

Preoperative Irradiation

Preoperative radiation therapy has been investigated in the past, but interest in the technique has waned, largely because none of the trials carried out showed any evidence of worthwhile benefit. In addition, the observed chemosensitivity of bladder cancer lead to a wave of neoadjuvant chemotherapy trials carried out in the 1980s and 1990s, effectively ending

interest in the technique. Given the subsequent improvements in both radiotherapy and surgical technique, it may be appropriate to revisit the possibility of combining surgery with radiotherapy, particularly given the apparent plateau in progress with systemic therapy since the licensing of gemcitabine more than 10 years ago. Most of the studies in the literature are old, retrospective, nonrandomized comparisons, and little can be concluded from them.

There are few randomized trials in the literature, and those that are available are also old, for the reasons outlined above. A study from the Royal Marsden Hospital randomized patients to preoperative radiation therapy to 40 Gy in 4 weeks followed by cystectomy, against definitive radiation therapy to 60 Gy in 6 weeks. The 5-year survival in patients receiving the combined therapy was 38% versus 29% for those treated with radiation therapy alone, the difference not reaching statistical significance. This trial of course did not compare radiotherapy plus surgery versus surgery alone and thus does not address the primary question in this section. However, it is noteworthy that no tumor was found in 31% of the cystectomy specimens, a similar complete response rate to that observed in the intergroup neoadjuvant MVAC study.[7] Similar response rates have been reported in other series.[1]

A second randomized study was carried out by the Memorial Sloan-Kettering Cancer Center in New York comparing radiation therapy to 40 Gy in 4 weeks followed by cystectomy 4 weeks later with a shorter 20 Gy in a 5-day course with immediate cystectomy modeled on the Swedish preoperative rectal cancer trials. Again, this study is not informative on the primary issue of the utility of adding irradiation to surgery but does demonstrate the feasibility and safety of such an approach. A retrospective review from the MD Anderson Cancer Center assessed the use of preoperative irradiation (50 Gy in 5 weeks) in patients with T3b bladder tumors. The 5-year local tumor control was 91% in the preoperative group (n = 92) compared with 72% for those treated with radical cystectomy alone (n = 43; P = .003).[1]

Parsons and Million[216] reviewed the results of retrospective studies and six prospective randomized trials on the use of preoperative irradiation. They concluded that the use of the technique may improve outcomes by up to 15% to 20% at 5 years. In particular, they noted that many preoperative radiotherapy series report pathologic complete response rates of around one-third, similar to that seen with neoadjuvant chemotherapy. There are no modern trials of preoperative radiation therapy, and the topic seems to be ripe for revisiting with modern techniques, particularly given the low long-term toxicity associated with chemoradiotherapy schedules, as summarized above.

Postoperative Radiation Therapy

As with many areas of bladder cancer practice, there are little in the way of randomized data on the use of adjuvant radiation therapy following surgery. When used, it is mostly based on the grounds of positive surgical margins or tumor spillage at surgery, where a high local recurrence rate can be anticipated.

Using the National Cancer Database (NCDB), Venigalla et al.[209] identified 46,380 patients diagnosed with nonmetastatic urothelial cell or squamous cell bladder cancer from 2004 to 2014 treated with radical cystectomy. Only 488 (1.1%) received adjuvant RT. In the overall cohort, administration of adjuvant RT was significantly associated with squamous cell carcinoma histology (P < .001), higher pathologic T-stage (P = .01), and positive surgical margins (P < .001). Other variables significantly associated with receipt of adjuvant RT included treatment at nonacademic facilities, receipt of chemotherapy, and earlier year of diagnosis. There were 2,766 patients in the positive surgical margin subgroup of which only 120 (4.3%) patients received adjuvant RT. Thus, in this pattern of care study, <5% of patients with positive surgical margins following radical cystectomy received adjuvant radiation therapy from 2004 to 2014 in the United States. A few studies combining pre- and postoperative irradiation have been published.[217]

With regard to radiation therapy technique in this cohort of patients, Baumann et al.[218] published a set of guidelines for postcystectomy irradiation, with emphasis on contouring of target volumes, which is challenging. The group proposed that patients at elevated risk for locoregional failure with negative margins should be treated to the pelvic nodes alone (internal/external iliac, distal common iliac, obturator, and presacral), whereas patients with positive margins should be treated to the pelvic nodes and cystectomy bed. Proposed OARs included the rectum, bowel space, bone marrow, and urinary diversion. Consensus language describing the CTVs and OARs was developed and externally validated.

With the use of neoadjuvant chemotherapy worldwide being at low levels, chemo-naive patients at high risk of recurrence can be offered adjuvant chemotherapy, although the evidence base for this approach is also somewhat lacking. What few data there are on radiation therapy suggests that limited doses are well tolerated. Given the more solid evidence base for neoadjuvant chemotherapy and the failure of adjuvant chemotherapy trials to accrue, the use of postoperative radiation therapy would also seem to be a topic well-worth revisiting with modern treatment techniques. An approach combining neoadjuvant chemotherapy, surgery, and adjuvant radiation therapy for patients at high risk of local recurrence would combine all three of the major bladder cancer treatment modalities in a novel fashion.

Electron Beam

Electron beams are only of interest in the context of intraoperative radiation therapy. The role of this modality for carcinoma of the bladder needs to be assessed in a prospective trial and cannot at present be recommended outside of a suitable study.

Neutron Beam

There are a small number of studies examining the use of neutrons beams for bladder cancer therapy. A single randomized trial failed to show a survival advantage but did show increased morbidity. There are currently no reasons to recommend neutron therapy for bladder cancer.[1]

Protons

There is scanty published information on the use of protons in the treatment of patients with muscle-invasive bladder cancer. The purpose of the present study is to retrospectively analyze the clinical outcomes of bladder preservation therapy using proton boost for muscle-invasive bladder cancer. Between August 1990 and February 2014, Kanuma et al.[180] treated 72 patients with stage T2-3N0M0 bladder cancer with concurrent chemoradiation therapy (CRT) as a bladder preservation therapy. Transurethral resection of the bladder tumor was performed, and pathologic examination for tumor invasion performed before CRT. Three cycles of intra-arterial chemotherapy consisting of MTX 30 mg/m² and CDDP 50 mg/m² were administered every 3 weeks during small-pelvis irradiation by x-ray (41.4 Gy/23 fractions). Upon completion of CRT, patients were evaluated by transurethral biopsy to confirm disappearance of cancer cells, and patients without residual tumor received boost irradiation (36.3 Gy equivalent/11 fractions) using proton beams. Median follow-up time was 36 months (range, 2 to 237 months).

Recurrences developed in 18 patients (25.0%); initial recurrence sites were bladder alone in 9, both bladder and distant organs in 2, lymph nodes in 4, distant organs alone in 2, and renal pelvis in 1. Recurrences at the bladder were observed in 11 cases (15.3%): seven tumors were noninvasive, and bladder function was preserved in 5 of them. Until the last follow-up,

9 patients died of disease recurrences, but 6 patients died of intercurrent diseases without any signs of recurrence. The 5-year rates of overall survival, local tumor control, and bladder preservation were 71.4%, 83.4%, and 86.3%, respectively. Treatment-related late toxicities grade 3 to 4 were observed in 3 patients: urinary hemorrhage, urethral stricture, and ureter stricture in each. There were no grade 3 gastrointestinal toxicities. Statistical analyses revealed that multiple tumors ($P Z$ .04), T3 ($P Z$ .014), and existence of hydronephrosis before treatment ($P Z$ .021) were prognostic factors for overall survival, and multiple tumors ($P < .001$) and tumor size ($P Z$ .02) had an impact on the local control rates.

Radiation Therapy Planning and Treatment Techniques

Patient Position and Immobilization

- The patient should be planned and treated in the same position; supine with arms on their chest. Knee and ankle immobilization should be used to ensure patient positioning is reproducible.
- The rectum should be empty of flatus and feces. The use of daily microenemas may be considered.
- Patients should be asked to empty the bladder 10 to 15 minutes prior to scanning.
- While breathing normally, the patient should have a CT scan performed with 3- to 5-mm slices. Patients are scanned from bottom of ischial tuberosities to 3 cm above the dome of the bladder or bottom of L5 (whichever is higher). A flattop CT scanner should be used.
- Neither intravenous nor oral contrast is thought to be of benefit in this instance.
- Reference tattoos should be made at the base of the abdomen and over each hip. The location of the tattoos should be marked on the planning scan by the use of radio-opaque markers to allow cross-referencing of planning scan and setup instructions.

Target Volumes or Field Localization

- The gross tumor volume can be difficult to define and should integrate information from the staging CT or MRI as well as the TURBT. MRI–CT fusion may be helpful, where available.
- The use of fiducial markers or contrast medium at the time of TURBT has been explored and may help identify tumor for image-guided adaptive radiation therapy.
- There are few data on the optimal radiation therapy volume. A standard approach is to define the planning target volume as the whole bladder, identified by its noninvolved outer bladder wall with a 1.5-cm margin plus extravesical extent of tumor with a 2-cm margin.
- All planning and treatment should be carried out with the bladder empty to minimize the risk of geographic miss and to keep the treated volumes as small as possible. Patients with significant residual volumes post voiding should be considered for planning and treatment with a catheter *in situ*, although this is likely to increase urinary toxicity.
- There are no data to support the routine irradiation of radiologically negative lymph nodes. The nodal relapse rate in the BC2001 trial, with planning target volume and clinical target volume defined as above, was only 3% in the chemoradiotherapy arm and 6% with radiation therapy only.

Brachytherapy

There is considerable historic literature on the use of brachytherapy, particularly from the Netherlands. Reported results seem to be very good, for example, van der Werf-Messing et al.[219] report the outcomes in 328 patients treated with 3 × 3.5 Gy external irradiation followed by a radium implant. Overall 5- and 10-year survival rates were 56% for T2 tumors and 39% and 13%, respectively, for T3 disease. Similar results have been obtained in more recent series with iridium-192 implants and manual afterloading.[220–222] There are also descriptions in the literature of the use of high dose rate afterloading, although one paper suggests that this may be less effective and more toxic than low dose rate treatment.[177] The striking feature of most of these series is the very low patient numbers and long time spans reported, suggesting that these techniques are only rarely used, even in centers with relevant expertise.

Recently, van der Steen-Banasik[223] reported on 57 patients with a T2 solitary bladder tumor treated with transurethral bladder resection followed by external beam irradiation to the bladder and regional iliac lymph nodes (40 Gy in 20 fractions, 5 fractions per week), and within 1 week interstitial HDR brachytherapy (BT), in selected cases combined with partial cystectomy and lymph node dissection. The BT catheters were placed via a transabdominal approach with robotic assistance from a Da Vinci robot. The fraction schedule for HDR was 10 fractions of 2.5 Gy, 3 fractions per day, which was calculated to be equivalent to a reference low dose rate schedule of 30 Gy in 60 hours.

Average postoperative hospitalization was 6 days, with minimal blood loss and no wound healing problems. Two patients had severe acute toxicity: 1 pulmonary embolism grade 4 and 1 cardiac death. Late toxicity was mild (2 urogenital grade 3 toxicity). The median follow-up was 2 years; the 2-year overall, disease-free, and disease-specific survival and local tumor control rates were 59%, 71%, 87%, and 82%, respectively.

As previously stated, the standard treatment for muscle-invasive bladder cancer (MIBC) is a radical cystectomy with pelvic lymph node dissection with or without neoadjuvant chemotherapy. In selected cases, a bladder-sparing approach is possible, with a limited surgical excision combined with external beam radiation therapy and brachytherapy. To perform brachytherapy, flexible catheters are implanted in the target volume of the bladder wall, which is done either by an open retropubic approach or by endoscopic surgical approach.

The largest experience for brachytherapy is with low dose rate and pulsed dose rate, although some short-term experience with high dose rate is also reported.

The main advantage for this technique is the conservation of bladder function, with comparable local tumor control as cystectomy series in selected cases.[221,222]

The GEC-ESTRO/ACROP (Groupe Européen de Curiethérapie-European Society for Radiotherapy and Oncology/Advisory Committee on Radiation Oncology Practice) published recommendations to perform bladder implants and brachytherapy as a treatment option for MIBC and techniques were described.[224]

Treatment of Patients with Uncommon Bladder Tumors

Squamous cell carcinoma is uncommon in the developed world, and many reported cases may in addition reflect sampling of squamous elements within a transitional cell carcinoma. As these tumors are often excluded from systemic therapy trials, there are few data on outcomes with treatment as most papers are retrospective collections of unconnected observations.[225,226] It appears that local failure may be more prevalent than distant relapse, but even that observation is based on very few cases. Urachal adenocarcinomas are extremely rare. Surgical resection with a partial cystectomy and *en bloc* resection of the urachal ligament with umbilicus are the treatment choices in the setting of localized disease. There is currently no definitive role for neoadjuvant or adjuvant chemotherapy in this tumor. Unfortunately, there are many patients who present with metastatic disease, which currently is not likely to be curable. There is no standard chemotherapy regimen for these patients.

Although squamous cell carcinoma (SCC) is represented in many of the studies on bladder preservation, some physicians may be reluctant to offer this approach to MIBC patients with this rare histology because of its perceived poor response to therapy and adverse outcomes in comparison to more common histologies of MIBC. Stokes et al.[227] queried the National Cancer Database (NCDB) for patients with T2-T4 or TX, N0M0 SCC of the urinary bladder diagnosed from 2004 to 2012 receiving both chemotherapy and high-dose radiation therapy (>55 Gy) without up-front cystectomy. Patients with urothelial cell carcinoma (UCC) were queried separately to serve as a comparison group.

Fifty-four SCC and 2,054 UCC patients were identified. SCC patients were more likely to be younger, female, or nonwhite and were more likely to have more advanced disease at presentation. Age >70, comorbidity score >0, and stage _T3 were associated with worse OS, whereas gender, race, insurance status, household income, facility type, chemotherapy (single vs. multiagent), and histology showed no association with OS. OS estimates were not significantly worse for SCC compared to UCC (5-year OS 25.4% vs. 33.3%; adjusted hazard ratio 1.34, P Z 0.12). Their conclusion was that OS did not significantly differ between SCC and UCC patients undergoing organ preservation for MIBC, whereas other prognostic factors were relevant in both groups.

Li et al.[228] evaluated the Surveillance, Epidemiology, and End Results (SEER) database (1998 to 2007) for patients with muscle-invasive (stage II to IV) SCC of the urinary bladder who underwent complete cystectomy. A total of 331 patients were included in the analysis; Majority were received cystectomy alone (n Z 297), whereas 10% (n Z 34) received postoperative RT. Factors associated with postoperative RT were younger age (pZ 0.03) and more advanced stage at diagnosis (P < 0.001). The addition of RT was not associated with an OS benefit (P Z 0.55). Median survival was 21 months for patients treated with cystectomy alone and 18 months for postoperative RT. Cox regression analysis confirmed the lack of improvement in OS among patients who received postoperative RT (P Z 0.47).

The lack of a survival benefit associated with postoperative RT suggests that RT for muscle-invasive SCC of the urinary bladder might be used with caution.

Carcinosarcoma is even more rare and appears to have a poor prognosis.[1] Similar considerations apply to small cell carcinoma (SCCB), although the consensus seems to be that metastasis is more likely and initial response to chemotherapy is usually good. These patients generally get treated along the same lines as small cell lung carcinoma, but the benefit of prophylactic cranial irradiation is unclear.[1,229–232]

Pasquier et al.[233] reported on a retrospective study at 15 Rare Cancer Network medical centers that contributed 107 cases of pure or mixed small cell carcinoma of the bladder, local, locoregional, and metastatic stages and age >18 years. Mean follow-up time was 4.4 years with 66% of these patients having pure SCCB. Seventy-two percent and 12% of the patients presented with T2-4N0M0 and T2-4N1-3M0 stages, respectively, and 16% presented with synchronous metastases. The most frequent curative treatments were radical surgery and chemotherapy, sequential chemotherapy and radiation therapy, and radical surgery alone. The median (interquartile range, IQR) OS and DFS times were 12.9 months (IQR, 7 to 32 months) and 9 months (IQR, 5 to 23 months), respectively. The metastatic, T2-4N0M0, and T2-4N1-3M0 groups differed significantly (P Z .001) in terms of median OS and DFS. In a multivariate analysis, impaired creatinine clearance (OS and DFS), clinical stage (OS and DFS), Karnofsky Performance Status <80 (OS), and pure SCC histology (OS) were independent and significant adverse prognostic factors. In the patients with nonmetastatic disease, the type of treatment (i.e., radical surgery with or without adjuvant chemotherapy vs. conservative treatment) did not significantly influence OS or DFS, suggesting that conservative treatment is appropriate in these patients.

ROLE OF SYSTEMIC THERAPY

Up to 50% of patients will develop metastatic disease. Bladder cancer is a chemosensitive disease, with responses reported to a range of agents. Systemic combination chemotherapy can be effective and result in tumor responses and symptom control. Overall response rates may be as high as 70%, with a median survival of approximately 12 to 14 months.[1,35] These agents were initially evaluated in the metastatic setting and subsequently in the neoadjuvant and adjuvant settings. However, despite over 30 years of research in the field, there remain many unanswered questions, including the role of adjuvant therapy and optimal second-line chemotherapy.

Neoadjuvant Chemotherapy

There are two principal rationales for neoadjuvant chemotherapy: first, to improve survival in patients with micrometastatic disease and, second, to preserve the bladder by shrinking the primary tumor to facilitate radiation therapy as an alternative definitive therapy to surgery.[1] The potential disadvantage of neoadjuvant chemotherapy, and a frequent reason cited for its nonuse, is the delay in definitive treatment (cystectomy or chemoradiotherapy), because this may lead to disease progression in a proportion of nonresponding patients who may conceivably become inoperable or unsuitable for radical organ preservation treatment. However, it is equally plausible that by undergoing neoadjuvant chemotherapy, these patients can be identified as those with biologically aggressive disease and therefore spared the morbidity of futile radical therapy. It should also be noted that a significant proportion, possibly up to two-thirds, of bladder cancer patients are elderly with multiple comorbidities and poor renal function and, therefore, unsuitable for neoadjuvant chemotherapy.[234] In the authors' experience, a patient who is considered fit for a radical cystectomy is likely to be fit for chemotherapy as well.

Chudhury et al.[234a] reported on 50 patients with transitional cell carcinoma, stage T2-3, N0, M0 after transurethral resection and magnetic resonance imaging treated with Gemcitabine IV (100 mg/m2 on days 1, 8, 15, and 22 of a 28-day RT schedule that delivered 52.5 Gy in 20 fractions). All patients completed RT; 46 tolerated all four cycles of gemcitabine. Two patients stopped after two cycles, and two stopped after three cycles, because of bowel toxicity. Forty-seven patients had a post-treatment cystoscopy; 44 (88%) achieved a complete endoscopic response. At a median follow-up of 36 months (range, 15 to 62 months), 36 patients were alive, and 32 of these had a functional and intact bladder. Fourteen patients died; seven died as a result of metastatic MIBC, five died as a result of intercurrent disease, and two died as a result of treatment-associated deaths. Four patients underwent cystectomy; three because of recurrent disease and one because of toxicity. One patient required a bowel resection for late toxicity. Using Kaplan-Meier analyses the 3-year cancer-specific survival was 82%, and overall survival was 75%.

There are two particularly key studies in the area of neoadjuvant chemotherapy. The South Western Oncology Group (SWOG) neoadjuvant study comparing surgery alone with 3 cycles of MVAC followed by surgery reported an estimated median survival of 6.2 versus 3.8 years in favor of patients having neoadjuvant chemotherapy ($P = .027$).[7,235] Updated results from the UK MRC/EORTC neoadjuvant chemotherapy trial, which used 3 cycles of cisplatinum, methotrexate, and vinblastine (CMV) prior to surgery or radiation therapy, show a statistically significant 16% reduction in the risk of death (HR 0.84; 95% CI, 0.72 to 0.99; $P = .037$), corresponding to an increase in 10-year survival from 30% to 36% after neoadjuvant chemotherapy.[236] In total, 976 patients with high-grade T2 to T4a urothelial bladder cancer accrued over 5.5 years from 106 institutions were randomly assigned to 3 cycles of neoadjuvant CMV chemotherapy ($n = 491$) or no chemotherapy ($n = 485$), followed by the institution's choice of definitive

therapy with either radical cystectomy or radiation therapy. Of patients in the chemotherapy and no chemotherapy groups, 42% and 43%, respectively, received radiation therapy alone as definitive therapy. Pathologic complete response with neoadjuvant chemotherapy was 33%. Overall survival at 3 years in the two groups was 55.5% versus 50%, respectively. The recent update, after 8 years of follow-up, showed an increase in 3-year survival from 50% to 56%, an increase in 10-year survival from 30% to 36%, and an increase in median survival time of 7 months (from 37 to 44 months) in CMV-treated patients compared with those treated with local therapy only. The SWOG study showed that of the 82% patients who underwent cystectomy, 38% had no evidence of disease pathologically. Patients who achieved pT0 status had a better prognosis than those who did not, although this difference may be accounted for by better disease biology rather than treatment effect. By definition, the SWOG study did not address organ preservation, because the mandated treatment plan was for surgery following neoadjuvant chemotherapy.

Meta-analyses show a 5% overall survival benefit at 5 years with cisplatin-containing regimens.[31] Thus, there have been two large randomized neoadjuvant studies in muscle-invasive bladder cancer, both showing significant survival advantage. Although many disciplines in cancer care would consider these data sufficient to change the standard of care, this does not seem to have taken place for the management of invasive bladder cancer.[235] The lack of widespread adoption of neoadjuvant chemotherapy may relate to the selected patients in clinical trials, not reflecting typical muscle-invasive bladder cancer patients who may be older or have impaired renal functions, which may limit the applicability of some chemotherapy regimens. GC,[33] standard,[7] or accelerated MVAC are widely used with definitive radical treatment (either surgery or radiotherapy/synchronous chemoradiotherapy) 4 to 6 weeks later. It is worth noting that these trials have been restricted to patients with well-preserved renal function (typically glomerular filtration rate >60 mL/min), thus excluding a significant proportion of bladder cancer patients who are elderly or have ureteric obstruction and therefore deemed unsuitable for neoadjuvant chemotherapy. This regimen requires in-patient or prolonged hydration and therefore has a significant impact on patient quality of life and health service resources. Level 1 evidence supports the use of cisplatin-based chemotherapy regimens in the neoadjuvant setting and for frontline therapy of patients with metastatic disease. In the second-line setting and beyond, there are no U.S. Food and Drug Administration–approved treatment options. The National Comprehensive Cancer Network (NCCN) guidelines list a variety of cytotoxic regimens, such as pemetrexed, paclitaxel, and docetaxel, all of which are supported by phase II trials[6]. These trials showed minimal benefit, with progression-free survival and overall survival generally ranging from 3 to 6 months and 6 to 9 months, respectively.[7]

Clinical trials investigating chemotherapy regimens that may broaden the spectrum of patients receiving cisplatin-based treatment have been conducted in palliative settings, for example, a split-dose regimen of cisplatin in combination with gemcitabine on days 1 and 8 of a 21-day schedule allowed safe treatment of patients with calculated glomerular filtration rate as low as 40 mL/min in the day case setting.[237] This regimen could be tested within a randomized clinical trial in the neoadjuvant setting and may go far in increasing the uptake of neoadjuvant chemotherapy. It is the responsibility of urology and oncology colleagues to work together to provide state-of-art care for our patients with muscle-invasive bladder cancer, which should include neoadjuvant chemotherapy prior to surgery or organ preservation therapy in fit patients.

Adjuvant Chemotherapy

Adjuvant chemotherapy has the potential advantage of enabling better patient selection based on the findings at surgical and pathologic staging. The major disadvantages,

TABLE 68.7 RANDOMIZED TRIALS OF ADJUVANT CHEMOTHERAPY

Author (Reference)	N	Standard Arm	Adjuvant Arm	Results
Skinner et al.[238]	91	Cystectomy	Cystectomy + CAP	Benefit, but few patients received planned therapy
Stockle et al.[239]	49	Cystectomy	Cystectomy + MVAC	Benefit, but limited trial size, premature closure, and no therapy upon relapse
Studer et al.[240]	77	Cystectomy	Cystectomy + cisplatinum	No benefit
Freiha et al.[241]	55	Cystectomy	Cystectomy + CMV	Benefit limited to relapse-free survival
Bono et al.[242]	83	Cystectomy	Cystectomy + CM	No benefit

CAP, cyclophosphamide/Adriamycin (doxorubicin)/cisplatin; CM, cisplatinum/methotrexate; CMV, cisplatinum/methotrexate/vinblastine; MVAC, methotrexate/vinblastine/doxorubicin (Adriamycin)/cisplatinum.

although, are the delay in systemic therapy and the inability to assess the response to chemotherapy in the absence of measurable disease. Randomized adjuvant chemotherapy studies (Table 68.7) have been conducted with the methodologic flaws of inadequate sample size, early closure, and suboptimal choice of chemotherapy, preventing a clear interpretation of the results. A systematic review and meta-analysis of updated individual patient data from all available randomized controlled trials in the adjuvant setting have been performed.[243] Updated data were collected, validated, and reanalyzed for 491 patients from 6 randomized controlled trials, representing 90% of all patients randomized in cisplatin-based combination chemotherapy trials and 66% of patients from all eligible trials. In view of this, the power of this meta-analysis was limited. The overall hazard ratio for survival of 0.75 (95% CI, 0.60 to 0.96; $P = .019$) suggests a 25% relative reduction in the risk of death favoring adjuvant chemotherapy. However, the impact of trials that stopped early of patients not receiving allocated treatments or not receiving salvage chemotherapy is less clear.[243] An Italian multicenter randomized phase III trial enrolled 194 patients (one-third of its target) with muscle-invasive TCC and assigned them to 4 cycles of GC or observation after cystectomy. The trial was stopped early because of poor accrual. After a median follow-up of 32.5 months, relapses were similar in both groups (43% vs. 45%) with no difference in disease-free survival. The 3-year overall survival was 67% for the chemotherapy arm and 48% for the observation arm and the 3-year disease-free survival was 47% and 35%, respectively, suggesting no statistically significant improvement in either survival rate with adjuvant GC in these patients.[1] A large phase III trial by EORTC (protocol 30994) evaluating observation versus adjuvant chemotherapy with one of the three chemotherapy regimens (GC, MVAC, or high-dose MVAC) in high-risk bladder cancer (pT3-4 and/or node-positive disease) was also prematurely closed due to poor accrual after enrollment of 278 of a planned 1,344 patients. This appropriately designed and sized study thus failed to conclusively address the issue of adjuvant chemotherapy following cystectomy. A possible reason for the failure of this trial was the tight window postsurgery for commencing chemotherapy. In the authors' experience, relatively few patients were able to enter the trial sufficiently soon because of slow postoperative recovery. This suggests that adjuvant chemotherapy may be less suitable than neoadjuvant chemotherapy in this patient population. The adjuvant chemotherapy question still requires international collaboration with an appropriately sized pragmatic study for a conclusive answer. In various disease sites, neoadjuvant chemotherapy followed by adjuvant chemotherapy is an acceptable norm with level I evidence. With an anticipated rise in uptake of neoadjuvant chemotherapy, patients with bladder cancer should not be precluded from this strategy where neoadjuvant chemotherapy is followed by radical treatment followed by a trial of adjuvant chemotherapy versus no chemotherapy in an appropriately sized phase III trial that meets its recruitment target, thus providing a definite answer for or against this strategy. Previous failures in meeting recruitment targets can be overcome by using better-tolerated regimens in common

use now and by extending the recruitment window from 12 to 16 weeks to allow full recovery post surgery and to allow more dose-intense adjuvant chemotherapy treatment.[1]

Chemotherapy Regimens in Metastatic Disease

Currently, systemic combination chemotherapy is the only treatment that may prolong survival in patients with metastatic disease. The chemosensitivity of bladder cancer is demonstrated by objective response rates of 12% to 73% and complete response rates of 0% to 35%. Although antitumor activity has been demonstrated with several single agents, the median survival associated with single-agent therapy is short (4 to 6 months).[1] Prior to the development of gemcitabine, a range of trials were done with doublet regimens, which typically showed median survival times of approximately 8 months.[244] The development of the four drug combination for MVAC chemotherapy extended this to over 12 months and became the established standard of care. The triplet combination CMV is also widely used but has not been compared with MVAC directly.[1]

The addition of paclitaxel to gemcitabine was evaluated in a phase III clinical trial by EORTC (protocol 30987), which enrolled 627 patients with advanced urothelial carcinoma. The regimens were well tolerated. Results showed that the GCP arm resulted in a higher rate of overall response rate (57% vs. 46%), CR (15% vs. 10%), and survival (15.7 vs. 12.8 months) compared with GC arm, but these differences were not statistically significant.[244]

Combination of docetaxel and cisplatin (DC) has been compared with MVAC in a multicenter phase III clinical trial by the Hellenic Cooperative Oncology Group.[245] Patients (n = 220) were randomly assigned to MVAC every 4 weeks versus docetaxel plus cisplatin every 3 weeks. Treatment with MVAC resulted in significantly superior response rate (54.2% vs. 37.4%), median time to progression (9.4 vs. 6.1 months), and median survival (14.2 vs. 9.3 months), suggesting that MVAC was superior to DC. Toxicity of MVAC was considerably lower than that previously reported for MVAC administered without granulocyte colony–stimulating factor. Currently, GC, MVAC, and high-dose MVAC with granulocyte colony–stimulating factor support are the acceptable standard of care as first-line chemotherapy in advanced or metastatic bladder cancer setting.

Second-Line Chemotherapy Treatment

The role of salvage chemotherapy after relapse following first-line chemotherapy remains an important subject of recent clinical trials. The enrollment in such trials is challenging in view of patients' poor performance status and deranged renal functions. Although various phase I or II studies have been reported, to date, there is only one completed phase III trial comparing vinflunine with best supportive care (BSC) alone. Patients (n = 370) were randomly assigned in a 2-to-1 ratio to receive vinflunine plus BSC (n = 253) or BSC alone (n = 117). Both arms were well balanced. Grade ≥3 toxicities for the vinflunine arm were neutropenia (50%), febrile neutropenia (6%), anemia (19%), fatigue (19%), and constipation (16%). A median survival advantage of 2.3 months (6.9 months for vinflunine plus BSC vs. 4.6 months for BSC) was achieved but was not statistically significant ($P = .287$). Cox multivariate analysis adjusting for prognostic factors showed a statistically significant effect of vinflunine on overall survival ($P = .036$), reducing the death risk by 23%. Objective response rate (8.6% vs. 0%), disease control (41.4% vs. 24.8%), and progression-free survival (3.0 vs. 1.5 months) were all statistically significant, favoring vinflunine. Because vinflunine was well tolerated, it is a reasonable second-line therapy option for patients with bladder cancer who have relapsed following cisplatin-based therapy.[246] Future second-line chemotherapy studies should incorporate vinflunine as the standard of care arm when testing any experimental treatment in a randomized trial.

Cost of Chemotherapy

In a retrospective study[247] using the SEER-Medicare dataset, first-line (1 L) and second-line (2 L) chemotherapy treatment patterns, health care visits, costs of health care in 2016 US dollars, and survival patterns were calculated from the index therapy date. Of 1215 patients diagnosed with advanced bladder cancer, 411 (33.8%) received 1 L chemotherapy and 189 (15.6%) subsequently received 2 L chemotherapy. During the 1 L and 2 L treatment courses, totals of 28.5 and 22.7 visits per patient were recorded, respectively. The total costs of cancer care during the 1 L and 2 L treatment courses were $36,790 and $26,730, respectively, of which more than $10,000 in costs were paid directly by the patient. Systemic therapy for bladder cancer is costly and should be weighed against the clinical outcomes likely to be achieved. Neither 1 L nor 2 L patients in this study experienced a median survival beyond 1 year following treatment initiation.

REFERENCES

1. James N, Bryan RT, Viney R, et al. Bladder cancer. In: Halperin EC, Wazer DE, Perez CA, et al. *Chapter 64 in principles and practice of radiation oncology*. 6th ed. Philadelphia: Wolters Kluwer Lippincott Williams & Wilkins, 2013:1259–1279.
2. Bryan RT, Wallace DM. Have we abandoned the "superficial" in bladder cancer? *Eur Urol* 2009;56(6):1091.
3. Riley GF, Potosky AL, Lubitz JD, et al. Medicare payments from diagnosis to death for elderly cancer patients by stage at diagnosis. *Med Care* 1995;33(8):828–841.
4. Stein JP, Lieskovsky G, Cote R, et al. Radical cystectomy in the treatment of invasive bladder cancer: long-term results in 1,054 patients. *J Clin Oncol* 2001;19(3):666–675.
5. Rödel C, Grabenbauer GG, Kuhn R, et al. Combined-modality treatment and selective organ preservation in invasive bladder cancer: long-term results [see comment]. *J Clin Oncol* 2002;20(14):3061–3071.
6. Hayter CR, Paszat LF, Groome PA, et al. The management and outcome of bladder carcinoma in Ontario, 1982–1994. *Cancer* 2000;89(1):142–151.
7. Grossman HB, Natale RB, Tangen CM, et al. Neoadjuvant chemotherapy plus cystectomy compared with cystectomy alone for locally advanced bladder cancer [see comment] [erratum appears in *N Engl J Med* 2003;349(19):1880]. *N Engl J Med* 2003;349(9):859–866.
8. Konety BR, Joslyn SA. Factors influencing aggressive therapy for bladder cancer: an analysis of data from the SEER program. *J Urol* 2003;170(5):1765–1771.
9. Sriplakich S, Jahnson S, Karlsson MG. Epidermal growth factor receptor expression: predictive value for the outcome after cystectomy for bladder cancer? *BJU Int* 1999;83(4):498–503.
10. Munro NP, Sundaram SK, Weston PM, et al. A 10-year retrospective review of a nonrandomized cohort of 458 patients undergoing radical radiotherapy or cystectomy in Yorkshire, UK. *Int J Radiat Oncol Biol Phys* 2010;77(1):119–124.
11. James ND, Hussain SA, Hall E, et al. Radiotherapy with or without chemotherapy in muscle-invasive bladder cancer. *N Engl J Med* 2012;366(16):1477–1488.
12. Hoskin PJ, Rojas AM, Bentzen SM, et al. Radiotherapy with concurrent carbogen and nicotinamide in bladder carcinoma. *J Clin Oncol* 2010;28(33):4912–4918.
13. Henningsohn L, Wijkstrom H, Dickman PW, et al. Distressful symptoms after radical radiotherapy for urinary bladder cancer. *Radiother Oncol* 2002;62(2):215–225.
14. International Agency for Research on Cancer. *GLOBOCAN 2008: Cancer incidence, mortality, and prevalence worldwide*. Available at: http://globocan.iarc.fr/.
15. Ploeg M, Aben KK, Kiemeney LA. The present and future burden of urinary bladder cancer in the world. *World J Urol* 2009;27(3):289–293.
16. Bryan RT, Zeegers MP, Bird D, et al. 20-years of bladder cancer research in the West Midlands: a comparison of two large cohorts. *J Urol* 2010;183:e196.
17. Zlotta AR, Cohen SM, Dinney C, et al. BCAN think tank session 1: overview of risks for and causes of bladder cancer. *Urol Oncol* 2010;28(3):329–333.
18. Volanis D, Kadiyska T, Galanis A, et al. Environmental factors and genetic susceptibility promote urinary bladder cancer. *Toxicol Lett* 2010;193(2):131–137.
19. Salem S, Mitchell RE, El-Alim El-Dorey A, et al. Successful control of schistosomiasis and the changing epidemiology of bladder cancer in Egypt. *BJU Int* 2011;107(2):206–211.
20. Hein DW. N-acetyltransferase 2 genetic polymorphism: effects of carcinogen and haplotype on urinary bladder cancer risk. *Oncogene* 2006;25(11):1649–1658.
21. Miller AB. The etiology of bladder cancer from the epidemiological viewpoint. *Cancer Res* 1977;37(8 Pt 2):2939–2942.
22. Hoffman D, Masuda Y, Wynder EL. Alpha-naphthylamine and beta-naphthylamine in cigarette smoke. *Nature* 1969;221(5177):255–256.
23. Lopez-Abente G, Gonzalez CA, Errezola M, et al. Tobacco smoke inhalation pattern, tobacco type, and bladder cancer in Spain. *Am J Epidemiol* 1991;134(8):830–839.
24. Claude J, Kunze E, Frentzel-Beyme R, et al. Life-style and occupational risk factors in cancer of the lower urinary tract. *Am J Epidemiol* 1986;124(4):578–589.
25. Kaufman DS, Shipley WU, Feldman AS. Bladder cancer. *Lancet* 2009;374(9685):239–249.
26. Wallace DM, Bryan RT, Dunn JA, et al. Delay and survival in bladder cancer. *BJU Int* 2002;89(9):868–878.
27. Kiemeney LA, Witjes JA, Verbeek AL, et al. The clinical epidemiology of superficial bladder cancer. Dutch South-East Cooperative Urological Group. *Br J Cancer* 1993;67(4):806–812.
28. Millan-Rodriguez F, Chechile-Toniolo G, Salvador-Bayarri J, et al. Multivariate analysis of the prognostic factors of primary superficial bladder cancer. *J Urol* 2000;163(1):73–78.
29. Sylvester RJ, van der Meijden AP, Oosterlinck W, et al. Predicting recurrence and progression in individual patients with stage Ta T1 bladder cancer using EORTC risk tables: a combined analysis of 2596 patients from seven EORTC trials. *Eur Urol* 2006;49(3):466–475.
30. Advanced Bladder Cancer (ABC) Meta-analysis Collaboration. Neoadjuvant chemotherapy in invasive bladder cancer: update of a systematic review and meta-analysis of individual patient data advanced bladder cancer (ABC) meta-analysis collaboration. *Eur Urol* 2005;48(2):202–205.
31. Sternberg CN, Yagoda A, Scher HI, et al. Preliminary results of M-VAC (methotrexate, vinblastine, doxorubicin and cisplatin) for transitional cell carcinoma of the urothelium. *J Urol* 1985;133(3):403–407.
32. Moore MJ, Winquist EW, Murray N, et al. Gemcitabine plus cisplatin, an active regimen in advanced urothelial cancer: a phase II trial of the National Cancer Institute of Canada Clinical Trials Group. *J Clin Oncol* 1999;17(9):2876–2881.
33. von der Maase H, Hansen SW, Roberts JT, et al. Gemcitabine and cisplatin versus methotrexate, vinblastine, doxorubicin, and cisplatin in advanced or metastatic bladder cancer: results of a large, randomized, multinational, multicenter, phase III study. *J Clin Oncol* 2000;18(17):3068–3077.
34. von der Maase H, Sengelov L, Roberts JT, et al. Long-term survival results of a randomized trial comparing gemcitabine plus cisplatin, with methotrexate, vinblastine, doxorubicin, plus cisplatin in patients with bladder cancer. *J Clin Oncol* 2005;23(21):4602–4608.
35. Hussain SA, James ND. The systemic treatment of advanced and metastatic bladder cancer. *Lancet Oncol* 2003;4(8):489–497.
36. Rehn L. Blasengeschwultse bei Fuchsein-arbeitern. *Arch Clin Chir* 1895;50:588–600.
37. Lower GMJ. Concepts in causality: chemically-induced human urinary bladder cancer. *Cancer* 1982;49:1056–1066.
38. Hueper WC, Wiley FH, Wolfe HD. Experimental production of bladder tumours in dogs by administration of beta-naphthylamine. *Indust Hyg Toxicol* 1938;20:46–84.
39. Case RAM, Hosker ME, McDonald DB, et al. Tumors of the urinary bladder in workmen engaged in the manufacture and use of certain dyestuff intermediates in the British chemical industry. Role of aniline, benzidine, alpha-naphthylamine, and beta-naphthylamine. *Br J Indust Med* 1954;11:75–104.
40. Clayson D. Working hypothesis for the mode of carcinogenesis of aromatic amines. *Br J Cancer* 1953;7:460–471.
41. King CM, Phillips B. Enzyme-catalyzed reactions of the carcinogen H-hydroxy-2-fluorenylacetamide with nucleic acid. *Science* 1968;159:1351–1353.
42. Radomski JL, Brill E. Bladder cancer induction by aromatic amines: role of N-hydroxy metabolites. *Science* 1970;167:992–993.
43. Risch A, Wallace DM, Bathers S, et al. Slow N-acetylation genotype is a susceptibility factor in occupational and smoking related bladder cancer. *Hum Mol Genet* 1995;4(2):231–236.
44. Probert JL, Persad RA, Greenwood RP, et al. Epidemiology of transitional cell carcinoma of the bladder: profile of an urban population in the south-west of England. *Br J Urol* 1998;82(5):660–666.
45. Morrison AS, Ahlbom A, Verhoek WG, et al. Occupation and bladder cancer in Boston, USA, Manchester, UK, and Nagoya, Japan. *J Epidemiol Commun Health* 1985;39(4):294–300.
46. Sorahan T, Hamilton L, Jackson JR. A further cohort study of workers employed at a factory manufacturing chemicals for the rubber industry, with special reference to the chemicals 2-mercaptobenzothiazole (MBT), aniline, phenyl-beta-naphthylamine and o-toluidine. *Occup Environ Med* 2000;57(2):106–115.
47. Guha N, Steenland NK, Merletti F, et al. Bladder cancer risk in painters: a meta-analysis. *Occup Environ Med* 2010;67(8):568–573.
48. Strope SA, Montie JE. The causal role of cigarette smoking in bladder cancer initiation and progression, and the role of urologists in smoking cessation. *J Urol* 2008;180(1):31–37.
49. Baris D, Karagas MR, Verrill C, et al. A case-control study of smoking and bladder cancer risk: emergent patterns over time. *J Natl Cancer Inst* 2009;101(22):1553–1561.
50. Freedman ND, Silverman DT, Hollenbeck AR, et al. Association between smoking and risk of bladder cancer among men and women. *JAMA* 2011;306(7):737–745.
51. Lammers RJ, Witjes WP, Hendricksen K, et al. Smoking status is a risk factor for recurrence after transurethral resection of non-muscle-invasive bladder cancer. *Eur Urol* 2011;60(4):713–720.
52. Moore LE, Baris DR, Figueroa JD, et al. GSTM1 null and NAT2 slow acetylation genotypes, smoking intensity and bladder cancer risk: results from the New England bladder cancer study and NAT2 meta-analysis. *Carcinogenesis* 2011;32(2):182–189.

53. Rothman N, Garcia-Closas M, Chatterjee N, et al. A multi-stage genome-wide association study of bladder cancer identifies multiple susceptibility loci. *Nat Genet* 2010;42(11):978–984.

54. Sanderson S, Salanti G, Higgins J. Joint effects of the *N*-acetyltransferase 1 and 2 (NAT1 and NAT2) genes and smoking on bladder carcinogenesis: a literature-based systematic HuGE review and evidence synthesis. *Am J Epidemiol* 2007;166(7):741–751.

55. Koutros S, Silverman DT, Baris D, et al. Hair dye use and risk of bladder cancer in the New England bladder cancer study. *Int J Cancer* 2011;129(12):2894–2904.

56. Yuan JM, Chan KK, Coetzee GA, et al. Genetic determinants in the metabolism of bladder carcinogens in relation to risk of bladder cancer. *Carcinogenesis* 2008;29(7):1386–1393.

57. Garcia-Closas M, Ye Y, Rothman N, et al. A genome-wide association study of bladder cancer identifies a new susceptibility locus within SLC14A1, a urea transporter gene on chromosome 18q12.3. *Hum Mol Genet* 2011;20(21):4282–4289.

58. Grotenhuis AJ, Vermeulen SH, Kiemeney LA. Germline genetic markers for urinary bladder cancer risk, prognosis and treatment response. *Future Oncol* 2010;6(9):1433–1460.

59. Liang FX, Bosland MC, Huang H, et al. Cellular basis of urothelial squamous metaplasia: roles of lineage heterogeneity and cell replacement. *J Cell Biol* 2005;171(5):835–844.

60. Hodder SL, Mahmoud AA, Sorenson K, et al. Predisposition to urinary tract epithelial metaplasia in *Schistosoma haematobium* infection. *Am J Trop Med Hyg* 2000;63(3–4):133–138.

61. Tawfik HN. Carcinoma of the urinary bladder associated with schistosomiasis in Egypt: the possible causal relationship. *Princess Takamatsu Symp* 1987;18:197–209.

62. Elem B, Patil PS. Pattern of urological malignancy in Zambia. A hospital-based histopathological study. *Br J Urol* 1991;67(1):37–39.

63. el-Mawla NG, el-Bolkainy MN, Khaled HM. Bladder cancer in Africa: update. *Semin Oncol* 2001;28(2):174–178.

64. Tricker AR, Mostafa MH, Spiegelhalder B, et al. Urinary excretion of nitrate, nitrite and *N*-nitroso compounds in Schistosomiasis and bilharzia bladder cancer patients. *Carcinogenesis* 1989;10(3):547–552.

65. Sheweita SA, Abu El-Maati MR, El-Shahat FG, et al. Changes in the expression of cytochrome P450 2E1 and the activity of carcinogen-metabolizing enzymes in *Schistosoma haematobium*-infected human bladder tissues. *Toxicology* 2001;162(1):43–52.

66. Davis CP, Cohen MS, Gruber MB, et al. Urothelial hyperplasia and neoplasia: a response to chronic urinary tract infections in rats. *J Urol* 1984;132(5):1025–1031.

67. Bullock PS, Thoni DE, Murphy WM. The significance of colonic mucosa (intestinal metaplasia) involving the urinary tract. *Cancer* 1987;59(12):2086–2090.

68. Delnay KM, Stonehill WH, Goldman H, et al. Bladder histological changes associated with chronic indwelling urinary catheter. *J Urol* 1999;161(4):1106–1108.

69. Wiener DP, Koss LG, Sablay B, et al. The prevalence and significance of Brunn's nests, cystitis cystica and squamous metaplasia in normal bladders. *J Urol* 1979;122(3):317–321.

70. Young RH, Bostwick DG. Florid cystitis glandularis of intestinal type with mucin extravasation: a mimic of adenocarcinoma. *Am J Surg Pathol* 1996;20(12):1462–1468.

71. Jacobs LB, Brooks JD, Epstein JI. Differentiation of colonic metaplasia from adenocarcinoma of urinary bladder. *Hum Pathol* 1997;28(10):1152–1157.

72. Sidransky D, Frost P, Von Eschenbach A, et al. Clonal origin bladder cancer. *N Engl J Med* 1992;326(11):737–740.

73. Novelli M, Cossu A, Oukrif D, et al. X-inactivation patch size in human female tissue confounds the assessment of tumor clonality. *Proc Natl Acad Sci U S A* 2003;100(6):3311–3314.

74. Chern HD, Becich MJ, Persad RA, et al. Clonal analysis of human recurrent superficial bladder cancer by immunohistochemistry of P53 and retinoblastoma proteins. *J Urol* 1996;156(5):1846–1849.

75. Gaisa NT, Graham TA, McDonald SA, et al. The human urothelium consists of multiple clonal units, each maintained by a stem cell. *J Pathol* 2011;225(2):163–171.

76. Simon R, Eltze E, Schafer KL, et al. Cytogenetic analysis of multifocal bladder cancer supports a monoclonal origin and intraepithelial spread of tumor cells. *Cancer Res* 2001;61(1):355–362.

77. Hartmann A, Rosner U, Schlake G, et al. Clonality and genetic divergence in multifocal low-grade superficial urothelial carcinoma as determined by chromosome 9 and p53 deletion analysis. *Lab Invest* 2000;80(5):709–718.

78. Hafner C, Knuechel R, Zanardo L, et al. Evidence for oligoclonality and tumor spread by intraluminal seeding in multifocal urothelial carcinomas of the upper and lower urinary tract. *Oncogene* 2001;20(35):4910–4915.

79. Steidl C, Simon R, Burger H, et al. Patterns of chromosomal aberrations in urinary bladder tumours and adjacent urothelium. *J Pathol* 2002;198(1):115–120.

80. Jones PA, Baylin SB. The fundamental role of epigenetic events in cancer. *Nat Rev Genet* 2002;3(6):415–428.

81. Lindgren D, Gudjonsson S, Jee KJ, et al. Recurrent and multiple bladder tumors show conserved expression profiles. *BMC Cancer* 2008;8:183.

82. Majewski T, Lee S, Jeong J, et al. Understanding the development of human bladder cancer by using a whole-organ genomic mapping strategy. *Lab Invest* 2008;88(7):694–721.

83. Bryan RT, Zeegers MP, James ND, et al. Biomarkers in bladder cancer. *BJU Int* 2009;105(5):608–613.

84. Crawford JM. The origins of bladder cancer. *Lab Invest* 2008;88(7):686–693.

85. Knowles MA, Elder PA, Williamson M, et al. Allelotype of human bladder cancer. *Cancer Res* 1994;54(2):531–538.

86. Hurst CD, Fiegler H, Carr P, et al. High-resolution analysis of genomic copy number alterations in bladder cancer by microarray-based comparative genomic hybridization. *Oncogene* 2004;23(12):2250–2263.

87. Duggan BJ, Gray SB, McKnight JJ, et al. Oligoclonality in bladder cancer: the implication for molecular therapies. *J Urol* 2004;171(1):419–425.

88. Bryan RT, Hussain SA, James ND, et al. Molecular pathways in bladder cancer: part 1. *BJU Int* 2005;95(4):485–490.

89. Bryan RT, Hussain SA, James ND, et al. Molecular pathways in bladder cancer: part 2. *BJU Int* 2005;95(4):491–496.

90. Hanahan D, Weinberg RA. The hallmarks of cancer. *Cell* 2000;100(1):57–70.

91. Reya T, Morrison SJ, Clarke MF, et al. Stem cells, cancer, and cancer stem cells. *Nature* 2001;414(6859):105–111.

92. Hanahan D, Weinberg RA. Hallmarks of cancer: the next generation. *Cell* 2011;144(5):646–674.

93. Brandt WD, Matsui W, Rosenberg JE, et al. Urothelial carcinoma: stem cells on the edge. *Cancer Metastasis Rev* 2009;28(3–4):291–304.

94. Bryan RT. Bladder cancer and cancer stem cells: basic science and implications for therapy. *Sci World J* 2011;11:1187–1194.

95. Gupta PB, Chaffer CL, Weinberg RA. Cancer stem cells: mirage or reality? *Nat Med* 2009;15(9):1010–1012.

96. Birkhahn M, Mitra AP, Cote RJ. Molecular markers for bladder cancer: the road to a multimarker approach. *Expert Rev Anticancer Ther* 2007;7(12):1717–1727.

97. Castillo-Martin M, Domingo-Domenech J, Karni-Schmidt O, et al. Molecular pathways of urothelial development and bladder tumorigenesis. *Urol Oncol* 2010;28(4):401–408.

98. Cheng L, Zhang S, MacLennan GT, et al. Bladder cancer: translating molecular genetic insights into clinical practice. *Hum Pathol* 2011;42(4):455–481.

99. Knowles MA. Molecular pathogenesis of bladder cancer. *Int J Clin Oncol* 2008;13(4):287–297.

100. Shariat SF, Karam JA, Lerner SP. Molecular markers in bladder cancer. *Curr Opin Urol* 2008;18(1):1–8.

101. Youssef RF, Mitra AP, Bartsch G Jr, et al. Molecular targets and targeted therapies in bladder cancer management. *World J Urol* 2009;27(1):9–20.

102. Goebell PJ, Knowles MA. Bladder cancer or bladder cancers? Genetically distinct malignant conditions of the urothelium. *Urol Oncol* 2010;28(4):409–428.

103. Knowles MA. Molecular genetics of bladder cancer. *Br J Urol* 1995;75(Suppl 1):57–66.

104. Knowles MA. Molecular genetics of bladder cancer: pathways of development and progression. *Cancer Surv* 1998;31:49–76.

105. Knowles MA. The genetics of transitional cell carcinoma: progress and potential clinical application. *BJU Int* 1999;84(4):412–427.

106. Knowles MA. What we could do now: molecular pathology of bladder cancer. *Mol Pathol* 2001;54(4):215–221.

107. Knowles MA. Molecular subtypes of bladder cancer: Jekyll and Hyde or chalk and cheese? *Carcinogenesis* 2006;27(3):361–373.

108. Knowles MA. Bladder cancer subtypes defined by genomic alterations. *Scand J Urol Nephrol Suppl* 2008;218:116–130.

109. Han Y, Chen J, Zhao X, et al. MicroRNA expression signatures of bladder cancer revealed by deep sequencing. *PLoS One* 2011;6(3):e18286.

110. Bryan RT, Wei W, Shimwell NJ, et al. Assessment of high-throughput high-resolution MALDI-TOF-MS of urinary peptides for the detection of muscle-invasive bladder cancer. *Proteomics Clin Appl* 2011;5(9–10):493–503.

111. Schiffer E, Vlahou A, Petrolekas A, et al. Prediction of muscle-invasive bladder cancer using urinary proteomics. *Clin Cancer Res* 2009;15(15):4935–4943.

112. Hawkins RD, Hon GC, Ren B. Next-generation genomics: an integrative approach. *Nat Rev Genet* 2010;11(7):476–486.

113. Edwards TJ, Dickinson AJ, Natale S, et al. A prospective analysis of the diagnostic yield resulting from the attendance of 4020 patients at a protocol-driven haematuria clinic. *BJU Int* 2006;97(2):301–305.

114. Khadra MH, Pickard RS, Charlton M, et al. A prospective analysis of 1,930 patients with hematuria to evaluate current diagnostic practice. *J Urol* 2000;163(2):524–527.

115. Sobin LH, Gospodarowicz MK, Wittekind C, eds. *UICC International Union Against Cancern TNM classification of malignant tumours*. 7th ed. Hoboken, NJ: Wiley-Blackwell, 2010.

116. Mostofi FK, Sobin LH, Torloni H. *Histological typing of urinary bladder tumours*. Geneva: World Health Organization, 1973.

117. 122. Goessl C, Knispel HH, Miller K, et al. Is routine excretory urography necessary at first diagnosis of bladder cancer? *J Urol* 1997;157(2):480–481.

118. European Association of Urology. Guidelines. 2011. Available at: http://www.uroweb.org/guidelines/online-guidelines/.

119. Miladi M, Peyromaure M, Zerbib M, et al. The value of a second transurethral resection in evaluating patients with bladder tumours. *Eur Urol* 2003;43(3):241–245.

120. European Organisation for Research and Treatment of Cancer. *Bladder cancer calculator*. Available at: http://www.eortc.be/tools/bladdercalculator/.

121. Amin MB, Edge SB, Brookland RK, eds. *AJCC American Joint Committee on Cancer staging manual*. 8th ed. Springer Nature, 2017:757.

122. Mowatt G, N'Dow J, Vale L, et al. Photodynamic diagnosis of bladder cancer compared with white light cystoscopy: systematic review and meta-analysis. *Int J Technol Assess Health Care* 2011;27(1):3–10.

123. Vrooman OP, Witjes JA. Urinary markers in bladder cancer. *Eur Urol* 2008;53(5):909–916.

124. American Urology Association. *Guidelines on management of bladder cancer*. Available at: http://www.auanet.org/content/guidelines-and-quality-care/clinical-guidelines.cfm?CFID=7269186&CFTOKEN=35fc09c207743 0ac-60CBB5BC-5056-9935-CB9E31CB2BE6EDED&jsessionid=8430be70f51e5 fd1550d764f6f755119572e.

125. van der Meijden AP, Sylvester RJ, Oosterlinck W, et al. Maintenance bacillus Calmette-Guerin for Ta T1 bladder tumors is not associated with increased toxicity: results from a European Organisation for Research and Treatment of Cancer Genito-Urinary Group phase III trial. *Eur Urol* 2003;44(4):429–434.

126. Milowsky MI, Rumble RB, Lee CT, et al. Guideline on muscle-invasive and metastatic bladder cancer (European Association of Urology Guideline): American Society of Clinical Oncology Clinical Practice Guideline Endorsement Summary. *J Oncol Pract* 2016;12:588–590.

Section
III

127. Malmstrom PU, Sylvester RJ, Crawford DE, et al. An individual patient data meta-analysis of the long-term outcome of randomised studies comparing intravesical mitomycin C versus bacillus Calmette-Guerin for non-muscle-invasive bladder cancer. *Eur Urol* 2009;56(2):247–256.

128. Jahnson S, Damm O, Hellsten S, et al. A population-based study of patterns of care for muscle-invasive bladder cancer in Sweden. *Scand J Urol Nephrol* 2009;43(4):271–276.

129. Huddart RA, Hall E, Lewis R, et al. Life and death of spare (selective bladder preservation against radical excision): reflections on why the spare trial closed. *BJU Int* 2010;106(6):753–755.

130. Chang SS, Bochner BH, Chou R, et al. Treatment of nonmetastatic muscle-invasive bladder cancer: American Urological Association/American Society of Clinical Oncology/American Society for Radiation Oncology/Society of Urologic Oncology Clinical Practice Guideline Summary. *J Oncol Pract* 2017;13:621–625.

131. Dalbagni G, Genega E, Hashibe M, et al. Cystectomy for bladder cancer: a contemporary series. *J Urol* 2001;165(4):1111–1116.

132. Kotwal S, Choudhury A, Johnston C, et al. Similar treatment outcomes for radical cystectomy and radical radiotherapy in invasive bladder cancer treated at a United Kingdom specialist treatment center. *Int J Radiat Oncol Biol Phys* 2008;70(2):456–463.

133. Giacalone NJ, Clayman RH, Efstathiou A, et al. Long-term outcomes after bladder-preserving combined modality therapy for patients with muscle-invasive bladder cancer. *Int J Radiat Oncol Biol Phys* 2015;93(3):S22–S23, Abstr 49.

134. Zhong J, Switchenko J, Jegadeesh N, et al. Comparison of outcomes in patients with muscle-invasive bladder cancer treated with radical cystectomy versus bladder-preserving chemoradiation. *Int J Radiat Oncol Biol Phys* 2016;96(2S):S93–S94.

135. Vashista V, Hanzhang W, Mazzone A, et al. Radical cystectomy compared to combined modality treatment for muscle-invasive bladder cancer: a systematic review and meta-analysis. *Int J Radiat Oncol Biol Phys* 2017;97:1002–1020.

136. Wilhite TJ, Routman D, Arnett ALH, et al. Increased utilization of external beam radiation therapy relative to cystectomy for localized, muscle-invasive bladder cancer: a SEER analysis. *Int J Radiat Oncol Biol Phys* 2017;99(2):E274–E275.

137. Solanki AA, Martin B, Korpics M, et al. Bladder-preserving therapy patterns of care: a survey of US radiation oncologists. *Int J Radiat Oncol Biol Phys* 2017;99:383–387.

138. Mitin T, George A, Zietman AL, et al. Long-term outcomes among patients who achieve complete or near-complete responses after the induction phase of bladder-preserving combined-modality therapy for muscle-invasive bladder cancer: a pooled analysis of NRG Oncology/RTOG 9906 and 0233. *Int J Radiat Oncol Biol Phys* 2016;94:67–74.

139. Neoadjuvant cisplatin, methotrexate, and vinblastine chemotherapy for muscle-invasive bladder cancer: a randomised controlled trial. International Collaboration of Trialists. *Lancet* 1999;354:533–540.

140. Walker M, French SD, Doiron RC, et al. Bladder-sparing radiotherapy for muscle-invasive bladder cancer: a survey of providers to determine barriers and enablers. *Radiother Oncol* 2017;125:351–356.

141. Prout GR, Marshall VF. The prognosis with untreated bladder tumors. *Cancer* 1956;9(3):551–558.

142. Michaelson MD, Shipley WU, Heney NM, et al. Selective bladder preservation for muscle-invasive transitional cell carcinoma of the urinary bladder. *Br J Cancer* 2004;90(3):578–581.

143. Shariat SF, Karakiewicz PI, Palapattu GS, et al. Outcomes of radical cystectomy for transitional cell carcinoma of the bladder: a contemporary series from the Bladder Cancer Research Consortium. *J Urol* 2006;176(6 Pt 1):2414–2422.

144. Madersbacher S, Hochreiter W, Burkhard F, et al. Radical cystectomy for bladder cancer today—a homogeneous series without neoadjuvant therapy. *J Clin Oncol* 2003;21(4):690–696.

145. Shelley MD, Barber J, Wilt T, et al. Surgery versus radiotherapy for muscle invasive bladder cancer. *Cochrane Database Syst Rev* 2002;1:CD002079.

146. Hautmann RE, de Petriconi RC, Volkmer BG. 25 years of experience with 1,000 neobladders: long-term complications. *J Urol* 2011;185(6):2207–2212.

147. Hautmann RE. Words of wisdom. Re: how close are we to knowing whether orthotopic bladder replacement surgery is the new gold standard? Evidence from a systematic review update. *Eur Urol* 2011;59(2):303–304.

148. Nagele U, Anastasiadis AG, Stenzl A, et al. Radical cystectomy with orthotopic neobladder for invasive bladder cancer: a critical analysis of long-term oncological, functional, and quality of life results. *World J Urol* 2012;30(6):725–732.

149. Herr H, Lee C, Chang S, et al. Standardization of radical cystectomy and pelvic lymph node dissection for bladder cancer: a collaborative group report. *J Urol* 2004;171(5):1823–1828.

150. Lee CT, Madii R, Daignault S, et al. Cystectomy delay more than 3 months from initial bladder cancer diagnosis results in decreased disease specific and overall survival. *J Urol* 2006;175(4):1262–1267.

151. Hadjizacharia P, Stein JP, Cai J, et al. The impact of positive soft tissue surgical margins following radical cystectomy for high-grade, invasive bladder cancer. *World J Urol* 2009;27(1):33–38.

152. Birkmeyer JD, Stukel TA, Siewers AE, et al. Surgeon volume and operative mortality in the United States. *N Engl J Med* 2003;349(22):2117–2127.

153. Finks JF, Osborne NH, Birkmeyer JD. Trends in hospital volume and operative mortality for high-risk surgery. *N Engl J Med* 2011;364(22):2128–2137.

154. Leissner J, Ghoneim MA, bol-Enein H, et al. Extended radical lymphadenectomy in patients with urothelial bladder cancer: results of a prospective multicenter study. *J Urol* 2004;171(1):139–144.

155. Stein JP. The role of lymphadenectomy in patients undergoing radical cystectomy for bladder cancer. *Curr Oncol Rep* 2007;9(3):213–221.

156. Stein JP, Cai J, Groshen S, et al. Risk factors for patients with pelvic lymph node metastases following radical cystectomy with en bloc pelvic lymphadenectomy: concept of lymph node density. *J Urol* 2003;170(1):35–41.

157. Stein JP, Quek ML, Skinner DG. Lymphadenectomy for invasive bladder cancer: I. Historical perspective and contemporary rationale. *BJU Int* 2006;97(2):227–231.

158. Stein JP, Quek ML, Skinner DG. Lymphadenectomy for invasive bladder cancer. II. Technical aspects and prognostic factors. *BJU Int* 2006;97(2):232–237.

159. Burkhard FC, Roth B, Zehnder P, et al. Lymphadenectomy for bladder cancer: indications and controversies. *Urol Clin North Am* 2011;38(4):397–405.

160. Studer UE, Collette L. Morbidity from pelvic lymphadenectomy in men undergoing radical prostatectomy. *Eur Urol* 2006;50(5):887–889.

161. Abdelhady M, Abusamra A, Pautler SE, et al. Clinically significant prostate cancer found incidentally in radical cystoprostatectomy specimens. *BJU Int* 2007;99(2):326–329.

162. Fleischmann A, Thalmann GN, Markwalder R, et al. Extracapsular extension of pelvic lymph node metastases from urothelial carcinoma of the bladder is an independent prognostic factor. *J Clin Oncol* 2005;23(10):2358–2365.

163. Pettus JA, Al-Ahmadie H, Barocas DA, et al. Risk assessment of prostatic pathology in patients undergoing radical cystoprostatectomy. *Eur Urol* 2008;53(2):370–375.

164. Nix J, Smith A, Kurpad R, et al. Prospective randomized controlled trial of robotic versus open radical cystectomy for bladder cancer: perioperative and pathologic results. *Eur Urol* 2011;57(2):196–201.

165. Smith A, Kurpad R, Lal A, et al. Cost analysis of robotic versus open radical cystectomy for bladder cancer. *J Urol* 2011;183(2):505–509.

166. Hollenbeck BK, Miller DC, Taub D, et al. Aggressive treatment for bladder cancer is associated with improved overall survival among patients 80 years old or older. *Urology* 2004;64(2):292–297.

167. Stein JP, Dunn MD, Quek ML, et al. The orthotopic T pouch ileal neobladder: experience with 209 patients. *J Urol* 2004;172(2):584–587.

168. Farnham SB, Cookson MS. Surgical complications of urinary diversion. *World J Urol* 2004;22(3):157–167.

169. Sherif A, Holmberg L, Rintala E, et al. Neoadjuvant cisplatinum based combination chemotherapy in patients with invasive bladder cancer: a combined analysis of two Nordic studies. *Eur Urol* 2004;45(3):297–303.

170. Koupparis AJ, Dunn J, Gillatt D, et al. Improvement of an enhanced recovery protocol for radical cystectomy. *BJMSU* 2011;3(6):237–240.

171. Melnyk M, Casey RG, Black P, et al. Enhanced recovery after surgery (ERAS) protocols: time to change practice? *Can Urol Assoc J* 2011;5(5):342–348.

172. Pruthi RS, Nielsen M, Smith A, et al. Fast track program in patients undergoing radical cystectomy: results in 362 consecutive patients. *J Am Coll Surg* 2011;210(1):93–99.

173. Choudury A. Molecular biomarkers in muscle-invasive bladder cancer. *Int J Radiat Oncol Biol Phys* 2015;92:705–706.

174. Pal SK, Agarwal N, Boorjian SA, et al. National comprehensive cancer network recommendations on molecular profiling of advanced bladder cancer. *J Clin Oncol* 2016;34:3346–3348.

175. Yafi FA, Aprikian AG, Chin JL, et al. Contemporary outcomes of 2287 patients with bladder cancer who were treated with radical cystectomy: a Canadian multicentre experience. *BJU Int* 2011;108(4):539–545.

176. Vieweg J, Gschwend JE, Herr HW, et al. Pelvic lymph node dissection can be curative in patients with node positive bladder cancer. *J Urol* 1999;161(2):449–454.

177. Poulsen AL, Horn T, Steven K. Radical cystectomy: extending the limits of pelvic lymph node dissection improves survival for patients with bladder cancer confined to the bladder wall. *J Urol* 1998;160(6 Pt 1):2015–2019.

178. Vazina A, Dugi D, Shariat SF, et al. Stage specific lymph node metastasis mapping in radical cystectomy specimens. *J Urol* 2004;171(5):1830–1834.

179. Foroudi F, Pham D, Rolfo A, et al. The outcome of a multi-centre feasibility study of online adaptive radiotherapy for muscle-invasive bladder cancer TROG 10.01 BOLART. *Radiother Oncol* 2014;111:316–320.

180. Kanuma R, Ishikawa H, Takaoka EI, et al. Bladder preservation therapy using proton boost concurrently combined with intra-arterial chemotherapy for invasive bladder. *Int J Radiat Oncol Biol Phys* 2015;93(3):E210, Abstr 2528.

181. Abdel-Latif M, Abol-Enein H, El-Baz M, et al. Nodal involvement in bladder cancer cases treated with radical cystectomy: incidence and prognosis. *J Urol* 2004;172(1):85–89.

182. Cooppan RM, Bhoola KD, Mayet FG. Schistosomiasis and bladder carcinoma in Natal. *S Afr Med J* 1984;66(22):841–843.

183. Stein JP, Ginsberg DA, Skinner DG. Indications and technique of the orthotopic neobladder in women. *Urol Clin North Am* 2002;29(3):725–734.

184. Reddy AV, Pariser JJ, Pearce SM, et al. Patterns of failure after radical cystectomy for pT3-4 bladder cancer: implications for adjuvant radiation therapy. *Int J Radiat Oncol Biol Phys* 2016;94:1031–1039.

185. Colleselli K, Stenzl A, Eder R, et al. The female urethral sphincter: a morphological and topographical study. *J Urol* 1998;160(1):49–54.

186. Henningsohn L, Wijkstrom H, Pedersen J, et al. Time after surgery, symptoms and well-being in survivors of urinary bladder cancer. *BJU Int* 2003;91(4):325–330.

187. Henningsohn L, Wijkstrom H, Dickman PW, et al. Distressful symptoms after radical cystectomy with urinary diversion for urinary bladder cancer: a Swedish population-based study. *Eur Urol* 2001;40(2):151–162.

188. Stein JP, Clark P, Miranda G, et al. Urethral tumor recurrence following cystectomy and urinary diversion: clinical and pathological characteristics in 768 male patients. *J Urol* 2005;173(4):1163–1168.

189. Hagan MP, Winter KA, Kaufman DS, et al. RTOG 97–06: initial report of a phase I-II trial of selective bladder conservation using TURBT, twice-daily accelerated irradiation sensitized with cisplatin, and adjuvant MCV combination chemotherapy. *Int J Radiat Oncol Biol Phys* 2003;57(3):665–672.

190. Mak RH, Zietman AL, Heney NM, et al. Bladder preservation: optimizing radiotherapy and integrated treatment strategies. *BJU Int* 2008;102(9 Pt B):1345–1353.

191. Kaufman DS, Winter KA, Shipley WU, et al. The initial results in muscle-invading bladder cancer of RTOG 95–06: phase I/II trial of transurethral surgery plus radiation therapy with concurrent cisplatin and 5-fluorouracil followed by selective bladder preservation or cystectomy depending on the initial response. *Oncologist* 2000;5(6):471–476.

192. Coppin CM, Gospodarowicz MK, James K, et al. Improved local control of invasive bladder cancer by concurrent cisplatin and preoperative or definitive

radiation. The National Cancer Institute of Canada Clinical Trials group. *J Clin Oncol* 1996;14(11):2901–2907.

193. Duncan W, Quilty PM. The results of a series of 963 patients with transitional cell carcinoma of the urinary bladder primarily treated by radical megavoltage X-ray therapy. *Radiother Oncol* 1986;7(4):299–310.

194. Shipley WU. Cisplatin and external beam radiation in patients with invasive bladder cancer. *Int J Radiat Oncol Biol Phys* 1989;16(6):1649–1650.

195. Prout GR Jr, Shipley WU, Kaufman DS, et al. Preliminary results in invasive bladder cancer with transurethral resection, neoadjuvant chemotherapy and combined pelvic irradiation plus cisplatin chemotherapy. *J Urol* 1990;144(5):1128–1134.

196. Stein JP, Cote RJ, Freeman JA, et al. Indications for lower urinary tract reconstruction in women after cystectomy for bladder cancer: a pathological review of female cystectomy specimens. *J Urol* 1995;154(4):1329–1333.

197. Huddart RA, Hall E, Hussain SA, et al. Randomized noninferiority trial of reduced high-dose volume versus standard volume radiation therapy for muscle-invasive bladder cancer: results of the BC2001 trial (CRUK/01/004). *Int J Radiat Oncol Biol Phys* 2013;87:261–268.

198. Korpics M, Blosk AM, Harkenrider MM, et al. The impact of radiation therapy dose on survival in patients with muscle-invasive bladder cancer: a population-based analysis. *Int J Radiat Oncol Biol Phys* 2016;96(2S):S183, Abstr 1045.

199. Fischer-Valuck BW, Green S, Mutic S, et al. Vector analysis of bladder cancer patient setup utilizing a magnetic resonance image guided radiation therapy (MR-IGRT) system. *Int J Radiat Oncol Biol Phys* 2016;96(2S):E261.

200. James N, Hussain SA, Hall E, et al. Results of a 2×2 phase III randomized trial of synchronous chemo-radiotherapy compared to radiotherapy alone and standard versus reduced high dose volume radiotherapy in muscle invasive bladder cancer. *J Clin Oncol* 2010;28(15S):(abstr 4517).

201. Efstathiou JA, Bae K, Shipley WU, et al. Late pelvic toxicity after bladder-sparing therapy in patients with invasive bladder cancer: RTOG 89-03, 95-06, 97-06, 99-06. *J Clin Oncol* 2009;27(25):4055–4061.

202. Shipley WU, Winter KA, Kaufman DS, et al. Phase III trial of neoadjuvant chemotherapy in patients with invasive bladder cancer treated with selective bladder preservation by combined radiation therapy and chemotherapy: initial results of Radiation Therapy Oncology Group 89–03. *J Clin Oncol* 1998;16(11):3576–3583.

203. Shipley WU, Kaufman DS, Heney NM, et al. An update of combined modality therapy for patients with muscle invading bladder cancer using selective bladder preservation or cystectomy. *J Urol* 1999;162(2):445–450.

204. Zietman AL, Shipley WU, Kaufman DS. Organ-conserving approaches to muscle-invasive bladder cancer: future alternatives to radical cystectomy. *Ann Med* 2000;32(1):34–42.

205. Lin HYD, Ye H, Krauss DJ. Muscle invasive bladder cancer survival after radical cystectomy or definitive chemoradiation: a National Cancer Database Matched Pair Analysis. *Int J Radiat Oncol Biol Phys* 2017;99(2):E252, Abstr 2602.

206. Miller LS. Bladder cancer: superiority of preoperative irradiation and cystectomy in clinical stages B2 and C. *Cancer* 1977;39(2 Suppl):973–980.

207. Whitmore WF Jr, Batata MA, Hilaris BS, et al. A comparative study of two preoperative radiation regimens with cystectomy for bladder cancer. *Cancer* 1977;40(3):1077–1086.

208. Cole CJ, Pollack A, Zagars GK, et al. Local control of muscle-invasive bladder cancer: preoperative radiotherapy and cystectomy versus cystectomy alone. *Int J Radiat Oncol Biol Phys* 1995;32(2):331–340.

209. Venigalla S, Chowdhry AK, Guttman DM. Adjuvant radiation therapy for positive surgical margins following radical cystectomy for bladder cancer: a National Patterns of Care Assessment. *Int J Radiat Oncol Biol Phys* 2017;99(2):E270, Abstr 2645.

210. Dunst J, Rödel C, Zietman A, et al. Bladder preservation in muscle-invasive bladder cancer by conservative surgery and radiochemotherapy. *Semin Surg Oncol* 2001;20(1):24–32.

211. Rödel C, Grabenbauer GG, Kuhn R, et al. Organ preservation in patients with invasive bladder cancer: initial results of an intensified protocol of transurethral surgery and radiation therapy plus concurrent cisplatin and 5-fluorouracil. *Int J Radiat Oncol Biol Phys* 2002;52(5):1303–1309.

212. Hussain SA, Moffitt DD, Glaholm J, et al. A phase II study of synchronous chemoradiotherapy for locally advanced bladder cancer. *Br J Cancer* 2001;85:16.

213. Horwich A, Dearnaley D, Huddart R, et al. A randomised trial of accelerated radiotherapy for localised invasive bladder cancer. *Radiother Oncol* 2005;75(1):34–43.

214. Turgeon GA, Souhami I, Cury FL, et al. Hypofractionation IMRT in combined modality treatment for bladder preservation in elderly patients with invasive bladder cancer. *Int J Radiat Oncol Biol Phys* 2013;87(2S):S399, Abstr 2511.

215. Hafeez S, Warren-Oseni K, McNair HA, et al. Prospective study delivering simultaneous integrated high-dose tumor boost (£70 Gy) with image guided adaptive radiation therapy for radical treatment of localized. *Int J Radiat Oncol Biol Phys* 2016;94:1022–1030.

215a. Harland SJ, Kynaston H, Grigor K, et al. A randomized trial of radical radiotherapy for the management of pT1G3 NXM0 transitional cell carcinoma of the bladder. *J Urol* 2007;178(3 Pt 1):807–813.

216. Parsons JT, Million RR. Planned preoperative irradiation in the management of clinical stage B2-C (T3) bladder carcinoma. *Int J Radiat Oncol Biol Phys* 1988;14(4):797–810.

217. Mohiuddin M, Kramer S, Newall J, et al. Combined pre- and postoperative adjuvant radiotherapy for bladder cancer: results of RTOG/Jefferson study. *Cancer* 1981;47(12):2840–2843.

218. Baumann BC, Bosch WR, Bahl A, et al. Development and validation of consensus contouring guidelines for adjuvant radiation therapy for bladder cancer after radical cystectomy. *Int J Radiat Oncol Biol Phys* 2016;96:79–85.

219. van der Werf-Messing BH, Menon RS, Hop WC. Carcinoma of the urinary bladder category T2, T3, NX, MO treated by interstitial radium implant. *Prog Clin Biol Res* 1988;260:511–524.

220. Van Poppel H, Lievens Y, Van Limbergen E, et al. Brachytherapy with iridium-192 for bladder cancer. *Eur Urol* 2000;37(5):605–608.

221. de Crevoisier R, Ammor A, Court B, et al. Bladder-conserving surgery and interstitial brachytherapy for lymph node negative transitional cell carcinoma of the urinary bladder: results of a 28-year single institution experience. *Radiother Oncol* 2004;72(2):147–157.

222. Pos FJ, Horenblas S, Lebesque J, et al. Low-dose-rate brachytherapy is superior to high-dose-rate brachytherapy for bladder cancer. *Int J Radiat Oncol Biol Phys* 2004;59(3):696–705.

223. van der Steen-Banasik E, Osterveld B, Wijburg C et al. The Curie Da Vinci connection: 5-years' experience with laparoscopic (robot-assisted) implantation for high-dose-rate brachytherapy of solitary T2 bladder tumors. *Int J Radiat Oncol Biol Phys* 2016;95:1439–1442.

224. Pieters BR, van der Steen-Banasik E, Smits GA et al. GEC-ESTRO/ACROP recommendations for performing bladder-sparing treatment with brachytherapy for muscle-invasive bladder carcinoma. *Radiother Oncol* 2017;122:340–346.

225. Kassouf W, Spiess PE, Siefker-Radtke A, et al. Outcome and patterns of recurrence of nonbilharzial pure squamous cell carcinoma of the bladder: a contemporary review of the University of Texas MD Anderson Cancer Center experience. *Cancer* 2007;110(4):764–769.

226. Kastritis E, Dimopoulos MA, Antoniou N, et al. The outcome of patients with advanced pure squamous or mixed squamous and transitional urothelial carcinomas following platinum-based chemotherapy. *Anticancer Res* 2006;26(5B):3865–3869.

227. Stokes A, Kessler ER, Wilson S, et al. Organ preservation for muscle-invasive squamous cell carcinoma of the urinary bladder in the United States. *Int J Radiat Oncol Biol Phys* 2017;99(2):S266, Abstr 2635.

228. Li B, Stessin A, Nori D, et al. The role of postcystectomy radiation in treatment of squamous cell carcinoma of the bladder: a SEER analysis. *Int J Radiat Oncol Biol Phys* 2014;90:S462, Abstr 2634.

229. Mukesh M, Cook N, Hollingdale AE, et al. Small cell carcinoma of the urinary bladder: a 15-year retrospective review of treatment and survival in the Anglian Cancer Network. *BJU Int* 2009;103(6):747–752.

230. Kaya AO, Coskun U, Yildiz R, et al. Primary pure small cell carcinoma of the urinary bladder that responded to carboplatin plus etoposide: a case report and review of the literature. *J BUON* 2009;14(4):703–706.

231. Ismaili N, Arifi S, Flechon A, et al. Small cell cancer of the bladder: pathology, diagnosis, treatment and prognosis. *Bull Cancer* 2009;96(6):E30–E44.

232. Bex A, de Vries R, Pos F, et al. Long-term survival after sequential chemoradiation for limited disease small cell carcinoma of the bladder. *World J Urol* 2009;27(1):101–106.

233. Pasquier D, Barney B, Sundar S, et al. Small cell carcinoma of the urinary bladder: a retrospective, multicenter rare cancer network study of 107 patients. *Int J Radiat Oncol Biol Phys* 2015;92:904–910.

234. Griffiths G, Hall R, Sylvester R, et al. International phase III trial assessing neoadjuvant cisplatin, methotrexate, and vinblastine chemotherapy for muscle-invasive bladder cancer: long-term results of the BA06 30894 trial. *J Clin Oncol* 2011;29(16):2171–2177.

234a. Choudhury A, Swindell R, Logue JP, et al. Phase II study of conformal hypofractionated radiotherapy with concurrent gemcitabine in muscle-invasive bladder cancer. *J Clin Oncol* 2011;29(6):733–738.

235. Bochner BH. Chemotherapy: standardizing the care of invasive bladder cancer. *Nat Rev Clin Oncol* 2011;8(8):454–455.

236. Sternberg CN, de Mulder PH, Schornagel JH, et al. Randomized phase III trial of high-dose-intensity methotrexate, vinblastine, doxorubicin, and cisplatin (MVAC) chemotherapy and recombinant human granulocyte colony-stimulating factor versus classic MVAC in advanced urothelial tract tumors: European Organization for Research and Treatment of Cancer Protocol no. 30924. *J Clin Oncol* 2001;19(10):2638–2646.

237. Hussain SA, Geh I, Riley P, et al. A phase I/II study of gemcitabine and cisplatin in metastatic or relapsed TCC of the bladder in an out-patient setting. *Proc Am Soc Clin Oncol* 2002;21:(abstr 2493).

238. Skinner DG, Daniels JR, Russell CA, et al. The role of adjuvant chemotherapy following cystectomy for invasive bladder cancer: a prospective comparative trial. *J Urol* 1991;145(3):459–464.

239. Stockle M, Meyenburg W, Wellek S, et al. Advanced bladder cancer (stages pT3b, pT4a, pN1 and pN2): improved survival after radical cystectomy and 3 adjuvant cycles of chemotherapy. Results of a controlled prospective study. *J Urol* 1992;148(2 Pt 1):302–306.

240. Studer UE, Bacchi M, Biedermann C, et al. Adjuvant cisplatin chemotherapy following cystectomy for bladder cancer: results of a prospective randomized trial. *J Urol* 1994;152(1):81–84.

241. Freiha F, Reese J, Torti FM. A randomized trial of radical cystectomy versus radical cystectomy plus cisplatin, vinblastine and methotrexate chemotherapy for muscle invasive bladder cancer. *J Urol* 1996;155(2):495–499.

242. Bono AV, Benvenuti C, Reali L, et al. Adjuvant chemotherapy in advanced bladder cancer. Italian Uro-Oncologic Cooperative Group. *Prog Clin Biol Res* 1989;303:533–540.

243. Advanced Bladder Cancer (ABC) Meta-analysis Collaboration. Adjuvant chemotherapy in invasive bladder cancer: a systematic review and meta-analysis of individual patient data Advanced Bladder Cancer (ABC) Meta-analysis Collaboration. *Eur Urol* 2005;48(2):189–199.

244. Bellmunt J, von der Maase H, Mead GM. Randomized phase III study comparing paclitaxel/cisplatin/gemcitabine (PCG) and gemcitabine/cisplatin (GC) in patients with locally advanced (LA) or metastatic (M) urothelial cancer without prior systemic therapy. American Society of Clinical Oncology Annual Meeting. Chicago; 2007. *J Clin Oncol* 2007;25(18S):(abstr LBA5030).

245. Bamias A, Aravantinos G, Deliveliotis C, et al. Docetaxel and cisplatin with granulocyte colony-stimulating factor (G-CSF) versus MVAC with G-CSF in advanced urothelial carcinoma: a multicenter, randomized, phase III study from the Hellenic Cooperative Oncology Group. *J Clin Oncol* 2004;22(2):220–228.

246. Bellmunt J, Theodore C, Demkov T, et al. Phase III trial of vinflunine plus best supportive care compared with best supportive care alone after a platinum-containing regimen in patients with advanced transitional cell carcinoma of the urothelial tract. *J Clin Oncol* 2009;27(27):4454–4461.

247. Kamat AM, Cao X, Jinghau H, et al. Costs of care for patients receiving chemotherapy for advanced bladder cancer. *J Clin Pathways* 2017;3:63–70.

CHAPTER 69

Low-Risk Prostate Cancer*

Carlos A. Perez, Jeff M. Michalski, and Michael J. Zelefsky

ANATOMY

Gross Anatomy and External Architecture

The prostate gland is an ovoid-shaped structure composed of fibrous, glandular, and muscular elements. It is located in the pelvis, adjacent to the rectum, bladder, dorsal and periprostatic venous complexes, pelvic sidewall musculature, the pelvic plexus, and cavernous nerves. Because of its shape, the prostate and the rectum curve away from each other as two convex surfaces. The prostate surrounds segments of the urethra before it passes through the genitourinary diaphragm (GUD; Fig. 69.1). Two of the five segments of the male urethra are the preprostatic urethra adjacent to the preprostatic sphincter and the prostatic urethra, which is placed from the verumontanum to the GUD. The paired seminal vesicles are situated posterosuperiorly to the prostate gland and secrete seminal fluid into the bilateral ductus deferens as they become the ejaculatory ducts. These ducts transverse the prostate to join the urethra at the verumontanum (Fig. 69.1, right). At this point, the urethra changes its angulation by bending 30 to 40 degrees anteriorly.

*This is an update of a chapter published by Zelefsky et al.[1] in the 6th edition of *Principles and Practice of Radiation Oncology*.

The prostate is contained within a thin, fibrous adherent capsule that is structurally continuous with the stroma of the gland. The apex of the gland rests above the GUD. The GUD surrounds the membranous sphincter and may vary in length and thickness. The puboprostatic ligaments extend anteriorly from the surface of the gland to the pubic symphysis. The prostate is separated from the rectum posteriorly by Denonvilliers fascia (rectovesical septum), which attaches above to the peritoneum and below to the GUD. It is this portion of the prostatic fascia that restricts posterior extension of prostatic carcinoma into the rectum. The lateral margins of the prostate are usually delineated against the levator ani muscles, forming the lateral prostatic sulci.

The anterior aspect of the prostate and the lateral pelvic floor are covered with the periprostatic fascia (Fig. 69.2). The endopelvic fascia lateral to the prostate gland contains neurovascular structures, including the venous plexus of Santorini, which is the primary drainage for the penis. This venous network, also referred to as the *dorsal vein complex*, covers the anterolateral surfaces of the prostate. The primary arterial blood supply to the prostate is via branches of the internal pudendal, inferior vesical, and middle hemorrhoidal arteries. The internal pudendal arteries also provide the blood flow to the penis. The nerves originate from the pelvic plexus, containing both sympathetic and parasympathetic fibers, and

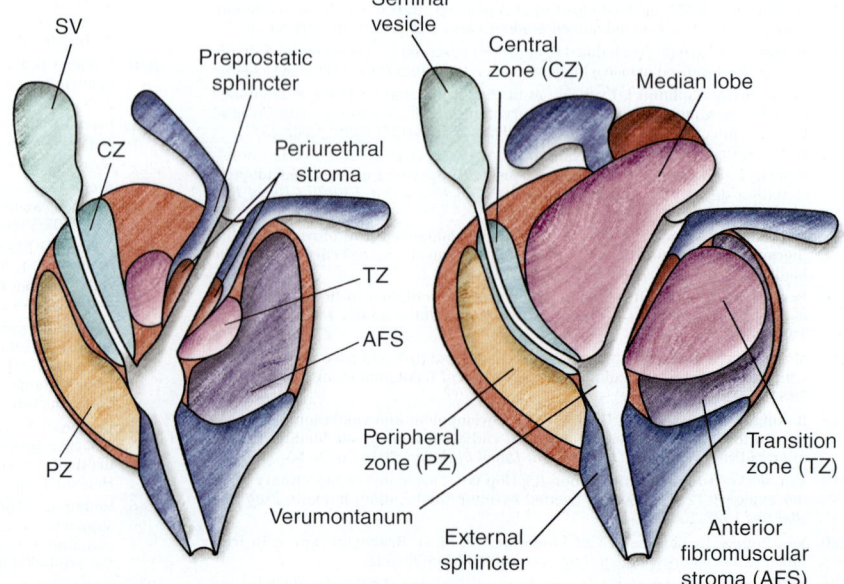

FIGURE 69.1. Zonal anatomy of the prostate. On the left, a young man with minimal transition zone (TZ) hypertrophy. Note that the preprostatic sphincter and periejaculatory duct zone (central zone of McLean) are clearly defined. On the right, an older man with TZ hypertrophy, which effaces the preprostatic sphincter and compresses the periejaculatory duct zone. AFS, anterior fibromuscular stroma; CZ, central zone; PZ, peripheral zone; SV, seminal vesicle. (Reprinted from McLaughlin PW, Troyer S, Berri S, et al. Functional anatomy of the prostate: implications for treatment planning. *Int J Radiat Oncol Biol Phys* 2005;63[2]:479–491. Copyright © 2005 Elsevier. With permission.)

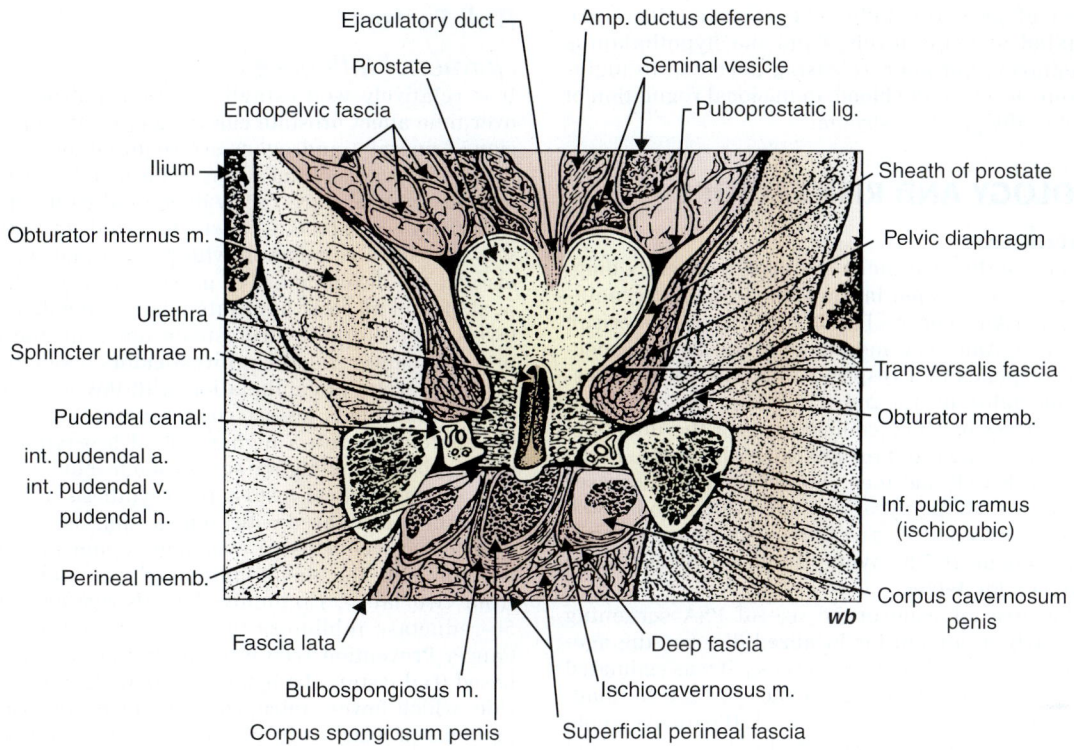

FIGURE 69.2. Frontal section of male pelvis at right angles to perineal membrane. (From Oelrich TM. The urethral sphincter muscle in the male. *Am J Anat* 1980;158[2]:229–246. Copyright © 1980 Wiley-Liss, Inc. Reprinted by permission of John Wiley & Sons, Inc.)

are distributed to the prostate, seminal vesicles, and the corpora cavernosa of the penis and urethra.

The prostatic apex is definable on diagnostic imaging and is very important anatomically for radiation therapy treatment planning. Although the apex and the GUD, which surrounds the membranous sphincter, are easily visualized on coronal magnetic resonance imaging (MRI), it is important to recognize that the level of the GUD from the apex to the penile bulb may vary because the absence of an apical capsule contributes to the difficulty in discrimination of the gland from the GUD during computed tomography (CT)-based treatment planning. Delineation of the neurovascular bundle is also limited on CT imaging.

Prostatic Zonal Anatomy

Zonal anatomy has essentially replaced lobar anatomy of the prostate. There are four zones of the prostate (Fig. 69.1): the peripheral zone (PZ), transition zone (TZ), central zone, and anterior fibromuscular stroma zone. The central zone that surrounds the ejaculatory ducts has marked histologic differences from the PZ. It is the PZ, extending across the entire posterior surface of the gland, that is palpated on rectal examination and is the location of most prostate cancers. The TZ is the location of benign prostatic hypertrophy. The anterior fibromuscular zone consists of an anterior band of fibromuscular tissue contiguous with bladder muscle and external sphincter. In young men, the PZ is the prominent zone, whereas the TZ becomes the dominant zone with age. It is important to note that there is no "median lobe" zone in this nomenclature, although such a "lobe" may be present in some prostate cancer patients and may have important implications for treatment planning and treatment selection. Histologically, the median lobe arises from the TZ or periurethral stroma, with varying proportions of fibrous, glandular, and muscle tissue.

Prostate Physiology

Histologically, the prostate consists of compound tubuloalveolar glands lined by two layers of cells. The glands are embedded in connective tissue comprising collagen and abundant smooth muscle that constitutes the prostatic stroma. This fibromuscular stroma functions both to control micturition by acting as a sphincter of the urethra and to express acidic prostatic secretions into the urethra by contracting during ejaculation.

The major function of the prostate is the production of seminal fluid that protects and nourishes the sperm after ejaculation. The prostate contributes approximately 30% to the seminal fluid, and the seminal vesicles, testicles, and bulbourethral glands provide the remaining 70%. Enzymes, including acid phosphatase and prostate-specific antigen (PSA), are secreted into the seminal fluid. PSA is a serine protease that is involved in the liquefaction of the seminal coagulum. Because PSA is produced primarily by benign and malignant prostatic epithelial cells and normally found at low concentrations in the serum, it is useful for prostate cancer screening and posttreatment monitoring of disease status.

The synthetic activity and growth of the prostate gland is regulated by androgens. The primary circulating androgen is testosterone. In the prostatic stroma, testosterone is converted to its active and more potent form, α-dihydrotestosterone, by 5-α-reductase. Secretory epithelial cells and stromal cells have intracellular androgen receptors. Dihydrotestosterone forms a complex with the dihydrotestosterone-binding domain of the androgen receptor, altering the structure of the DNA-binding domain such that it can reversibly bind DNA sequences known as *androgen response elements* in promoter or enhancer regions of androgen-regulated genes. The response includes stimulation of cell division, inhibition of apoptosis (programmed cell death), or cellular differentiation. In secretory epithelial cells, testosterone stimulation may result in the production and secretion of prostatic fluid. These mechanisms are tightly regulated at many levels, from the hypothalamus secreting luteinizing hormone–releasing hormone to maintain testosterone levels in the blood, to the local regulation of 5-α-reductase in the prostate stroma.

EPIDEMIOLOGY AND RISK FACTORS

Clinical Incidence

Adenocarcinoma of the prostate is the most frequently diagnosed visceral cancer of men in the United States, accounting for 33% of nonskin cancers. The lifetime risk for American White and African American men is 18% and 21%, respectively. This corresponds to a respective lifetime risk of prostate-specific mortality of 3% and 5%.[1,2] After large annual increases from 1988 to 1992, coinciding with the introduction of the PSA screening test, prostate cancer incidence in the United States leveled off and then showed modest decreases of approximately 1.9% per year between 2000 and 2008. Incidence rates between 1975 and 2015 were approximately 114 per 100,000 men, 107 for White, 186.8 for Black, 97 for Hispanic, and 54.8 for Asian[2]

Perhaps because of widespread use of PSA screening and effective early treatment for localized disease, the age-adjusted death rates have begun to decrease. It was estimated that 241,740 new cases of prostate cancer would be diagnosed in 2012, but only approximately 28,170 patients would die of the disease. This compares with 164,690 new cases and 29,430 estimated deaths in 2018.[2] Despite this encouraging incidence trend, carcinoma of the prostate remains the second greatest cause of male cancer mortality behind cancer of the lung and bronchus.[2]

Of the known or suspected risk factors for prostate cancer, the most important is age (Table 69.1).[3] The median age at diagnosis is 68 years, and the disease incidence escalates sharply with increasing age. The incidence among men aged 50 to 59 years is 1 in 58, increasing to 1 in 21 among men aged 60 to 69 years, and 1 in 12 among those aged 70 years and older.[2] According to autopsy data, 70% of men older than 80 years of age and 40% of men older than 50 years of age have pathologic evidence of cancer in the prostate.[4]

Although the risk for development of histologic evidence of cancer in the prostate is fairly constant across countries and races, there is considerable variability in the incidence of clinically evident disease and mortality among different populations worldwide and in the United States.[5]

The highest rates of prostate cancer are in Scandinavia, where it is the leading cause of male cancer death. The lowest recorded rates are in Asia. In the United States, incidence and mortality are higher among African Americans. The mortality rates of prostate cancer in Japan dramatically increased from 1960 to 2000 in all age groups before showing modest but sustained decreases from 2000 onward.[6]

TABLE 69.1 KNOWN OR SUSPECTED RISK FACTORS FOR PROSTATE CANCER

Factor	Effect on Prostate Cancer Risk
Age	Increase
African American race	Increase
Geography	Scandinavia, high; Asia, low
Family history	Increase
Dietary fat	Increase
Agent Orange	May increase
Vasectomy	No effect
Benign prostatic conditions	No effect
Sexually transmitted diseases	No effect
Tobacco	Inconclusive data
Androgens	Inconclusive data

Risk Factors

Hormonal Influences

It is relatively well established that androgenic influences over time affect prostate carcinogenesis and disease progression.[7] Generally, androgens are required for the development of prostate cancer, and it has been noted that men deficient in 2,5α-reductase are rarely diagnosed with benign prostatic hypertrophy or prostate cancer. In a study of 1,008 men, there was a positive correlation with plasma androstenedione levels and the development of prostate cancer.[8] However, Gann et al.[9] found no clear association between individual hormone levels, including dihydrotestosterone, and the incidence of prostatic cancer. Yet, these investigators noted that high levels of testosterone in combination with low levels of the serum protein that binds testosterone, sex hormone–binding globulin, correlated with a higher risk of prostate cancer. Meikle et al.[10] observed a higher sex hormone–binding globulin level and a higher rate of testosterone synthesis in men with prostate cancer compared with control subjects.

The most conclusive evidence supporting the hormonal influence in the development of prostate cancer comes from two large, randomized trials evaluating the use of 5α-reductase inhibitors in chemoprevention. The Prostate Cancer Prevention Trial was the first large-scale, population-based trial testing the hypothesis that treatment with finasteride, which lowers intraprostatic dihydrotestosterone levels, prevents prostate cancer.[11] In this trial, a total of 18,882 men ≥55 years old and with normal digital rectal examination (DRE) and PSA level ≤3.0 ng/mL were randomized to 7 years of finasteride (5 mg/d) or placebo. This study found that the prevalence of prostate cancer was reduced by 25% in men taking finasteride compared to placebo, with the prevalence of Gleason sum 7 to 10 tumors higher in the former group. The Reduction by Dutasteride of Prostate Cancer Events (REDUCE) trial randomized 8,231 men at high risk for prostate cancer (aged 50 to 60 years with a PSA of 2.5 to 10.0 or age ≥ 60 years with a PSA of 2.5 to 10.0 and a negative prostate biopsy within 6 months of enrollment) to dutasteride (0.5 mg daily) or placebo.[12] At 4 years, a relative risk reduction in the diagnosis or a subsequent prostate cancer of 22.8% was noted in men taking dutasteride, with a trend toward increased Gleason 8 to 10 tumors. For both trials, it remains controversial whether this increased risk of high Gleason tumors is real or artifactual. However, the U.S. Food and Drug Administration has declined to add chemoprevention of prostate cancer as an indication for finasteride and dutasteride.[13]

Dietary Influences

The development of prostate cancer may be attributed to both familial and environmental factors. Epidemiologic studies strongly suggest that a diet deficient in certain micronutrients is an important environmental risk factor. This has been supported through migration studies that indicate higher rates of prostate cancer in Asian men living in the United States compared with their counterparts in Japan or China.[14,15] It has been postulated that nutritional factors play a role in stimulating the progression of microscopic disease. Salient features of the "Western diet" that differ from the traditional Asian diet are high fat intake and low soy consumption. A Western diet has been associated with increased production of both androgens and estrogens and a vegetarian diet with lower levels.[16] Diets high in fat content may increase the relative risk of prostate cancer by a factor of 1.6 to 1.9.[17,18] In addition, several studies showed that men with diets high in fiber and presumably lower in fat have a decreased risk of prostate cancer.[19,20]

One prospective study found that the type of fat intake was directly related to risk of prostate cancer.[21] Red meat represented the food group with the strongest positive association with advanced cancer, with a relative risk of 2.64. Fat from dairy products (with the exception of butter) or fish was unrelated to risk. When analyzed by fatty acid type, only α-linolenic acid (an omega-3 fatty acid found in red meats and butter), and not linoleic acid (omega-6 fatty acid found in fish oil), was implicated, with an increase in risk for prostate cancer of more than threefold. Conversely, a subsequent Canadian case-controlled study suggested that saturated fat consumption, not α-linolenic acid consumption, may play a role in prostate cancer progression.[22] Finally, a Swedish study of 406 men with prostate cancer and 1,208 without it (control subjects) demonstrated that body mass index and total amount of food consumed were independent risk factors.[23]

Plant-based foods and their products, such as soy, tomatoes, cruciferous vegetables, and certain nutrients, are favorably associated with prostate cancer. It is believed that these dietary factors contribute to antioxidant effects against DNA and cell damage.

Several vitamins and trace nutrients, including selenium, vitamin E, and vitamin C, have garnered attention as potential protective agents. Early experimental and epidemiologic data supported the anticarcinogenic effects of selenium through apoptotic, angiogenic, or antioxidative pathways.[24] The Nutrition Prevention Trial identified a 50% reduction in prostate cancer risk in men blindly and randomly assigned selenium supplements compared with placebo.[25] Promising data for vitamin E as a protective agent were reported in the Finnish Alpha-Tocopherol, Beta-Carotene Cancer (ATBC) Prevention Study, which evaluated supplementation with vitamin E and beta-carotene in male smokers for chemoprevention of lung cancer.[26] Secondary analysis suggested a 32% reduction in prostate cancer risk among men randomized to receive vitamin E. However, a large, prospective, randomized trial failed to confirm these findings for selenium or vitamin E. The Selenium and Vitamin E Cancer Prevention (SELECT) Trial randomized 35,533 men to four arms: selenium (200 µg/d), vitamin E (400 IU/d rac-α-tocopheryl acetate), both selenium and vitamin E, or placebo only.[27] With a minimum follow-up of 7 years, the study identified no reduction in risk of prostate cancer with either vitamin E or selenium supplementation but identified an increased hazard ratio (1.17) for development of prostate cancer among men randomized to vitamin E alone. Vitamin E was contemporaneously evaluated in the randomized Physicians' Health Study II, which failed to demonstrate a reduction in prostate cancer incidence by supplementation with vitamin E or C.[28]

The beneficial effects of soy are attributed to isoflavones, one of several plant pigments found in soybeans. Isoflavones are a type of phytoestrogen compounds that have weak estrogenic, antiestrogenic, and antioxidant effects that may all be protective against progression of prostate cancer in humans. These isoflavones, most significantly genistein and daidzein, have been shown to inhibit the growth of prostate cancer cell lines in nude mice.[29] In particular, genistein has been shown to be a potent inhibitor of several steroid-metabolizing enzymes, such as aromatase, 5α-reductase, and 17β-hydroxysteroid dehydrogenase, as well as enzymes that are crucial to cellular proliferation, such as tyrosine kinase and topoisomerases I and II. Genistein is also an inhibitor of angiogenesis. It is estimated that Japanese men consume approximately 20 mg of isoflavones per day, whereas for Western men, the daily consumption is <1 mg/d. This is reflected in a mean plasma concentration of genistein of 180 ng/mL in Japanese men, compared with a level of <10 ng/mL for Western men.[30]

Another protective nutrient is lycopene present in tomatoes, processed tomato products, and other fruits, which is one of the most potent antioxidants among dietary carotenoids. Although the antioxidant properties of lycopene are believed to be primarily responsible for its beneficial effects, other mechanisms may also be involved. In a review of 72 epidemiologic studies that investigated a link between cancer risk

and consumption of tomato products, 57 linked tomato intake with a reduced risk; in 35 of those studies, the association was considered statistically significant.[31] Two large, prospective studies reported a decrease in prostate cancer risk with higher tomato product consumption.[32,33] Tomatoes were one of only four specific food items associated with significantly reduced prostate cancer risk in a prospective study of 14,000 Seventh-Day Adventist men.[33] A prospective study examined the relationship between the plasma concentration of several antioxidants and the risk for prostate cancer, using plasma samples obtained in the Physicians' Health Study. Higher serum and tissue lycopene levels were found to be inversely related to the incidence of prostate cancer development.[34] In a recent meta-analysis of 21 studies, high intake of tomatoes was associated with a 10% to 20% risk reduction in prostate cancer, with lower risk because of cooked versus raw tomatoes.[35] A summary of various epidemiologic studies indicating associations of various dietary factors to prostate cancer development and morality is shown in Table 69.2.

Familial Associations

A large cohort study of the Utah Mormon population demonstrated a positive family history of prostate cancer in 6.6% of families of probands with prostate cancer and only 2.2% of families of probands without prostate cancer.[36] A subsequent study using data from the Utah State Cancer Registry reported a familial relative risk of prostate cancer of 2.2.[37] Multiple studies have confirmed these findings, including a large case–control study from Johns Hopkins.[38] Extensive cancer pedigrees were obtained from 691 prostate cancer cases and 640 spouse control subjects showing a twofold increased risk in men with a family history of prostate cancer in a single first-degree relative. There was a fivefold risk if there were two affected relatives, and the relative risk rose to 11 for three first-degree relatives with prostate cancer.

In a Canadian study, the frequency of prostate cancer detected in men who had a first-degree relative with a history of prostate cancer was 2.6 times greater than for men without such a history.[39] Aprikian et al.,[40] in a study of 2,968 patients, noted that prostate cancer was detected in 40% (1,300 patients) of men with a family history of prostate cancer, compared with 29% of 769 men without a family history ($P < .0001$). In a review of the epidemiology of prostate cancer, Giovannucci[32] reported that approximately 9% of cases may

TABLE 69.2 NUTRITIONAL RISK FACTORS FOR PROSTATE CANCER INCIDENCE, RECURRENCE, AND MORTALITY

Food or Nutrient	Direction of Association with Prostate Cancer Risk	Direction of Association with Prostate Cancer Recurrence or Mortality	Overall Quality of Evidence
Selenium	Inverse		Strong
Tomato and lycopenes	Inverse	Inverse[a]	Good
Other carotenoids	Inverse	Inverse[a]	Good[a]
Vitamin E	Inverse (seen in smokers)	Inverse[a]	Good
Vitamin D	Inverse		Good
Calcium and dairy	Null to positive		Good
Red meat	Positive		Good
Fish/omega-3	Inverse	Inverse[a]	
Soy/isoflavones	Null to inverse	Null for PSA recurrence	Fair[a]
Tea/polyphenols	Null to inverse		Fair[a]
Zinc	Positive		Fair[a]
Heterocyclic amines	Positive		Fair[a]

[a]Limited data available.

Modified with permission from Chan JM, Gann PH, Giovannucci, EL. Role of diet in prostate cancer development and progression. *J Clin Oncol* 2005;23(32):8152–8160. Copyright © 2005 American Society of Clinical Oncology. All rights reserved.

TABLE 69.3 PARTIAL LIST OF PROSTATE CANCER SUSCEPTIBILITY GENES AND CANDIDATE GENES

Gene	Location	Alterations	Proposed Phenotypic Consequences
RNASEL/HPC1	1q24-25	Base substitutionsFour-base deletion leading to premature truncation	Encodes endoribonuclease Early age at diagnosis
ELAC2/HPC2	17p11	Base insertion leading to premature terminationBase substitutions	Unknown
MSR1	8p22-23	Base substitutions	Encodes subunit of class A macrophage-scavenger receptor
AR	Xq11-12	Polymorphic polyglutamine (CAG) and polyglycine (GGC) repeats	Encodes androgen receptor, and androgen dependent transcription factor
CYP17	10q24.3	Base substitutions in transcriptional promoter (T → C transition leading to a new Sp1 recognition site)	Encodes cytochrome P-450c17α, and enzymes that catalyzes key reactions in sex-steroid biosynthesis
SRD5A2	2p23	Base substitutions	Encodes the predominant 5-α-reductase in the prostate, converts testosterone to dihydrotestosterone
AMACR	5p13.2	Missense mutations	Unknown
BRCA2	13q12-13	Various	Possible link to higher Gleason score and stage at diagnosis
CHEK2	22q12.1	Frameshift/missense mutations	Unknown
HOXB13	17q21	Missense mutations in highly conserved functional domain	Early age at diagnosis
KFL6	10p15	DNA polymorphism	Leads to alternative splicing in encoded tumor suppressor gene
MMR genes (MLH1, MSH2, HSH6, PMS2)	Various	Various	Various
NBS1	8q21	Loss of heterozygosity in carriers	Role in DNA repair
HPCX	Xq27-28	Unknown	Unknown
CAPB	1p36	Unknown	Early age at diagnosis; association with CNS malignancies

Adapted from Nelson WG, De Marzo AM, Isaacs WB. Prostate cancer. *N Engl J Med* 2003;349:366–381; Langeberg WJ, Isaacs WB, Stanford JL. Genetic etiology of hereditary prostate cancer. *Front Biosci* 2007;12:4101–4110; Genetics of Prostate Cancer. www.cancer.gov. Accessed December 21, 2012.

be attributed directly to a family history, although this may be as high as 43% among men younger than 55 years of age.

Despite the familial clustering of prostate cancer observed in these epidemiologic studies, causation cannot be inferred, given the shared environmental factors among family members. Segregation analyses of cancer in multiple family members have been used to examine the role of genetic factors and inheritance patterns in prostate cancer. Segregation analysis is a statistical method used to determine the best-fitting model of inheritance for a particular disease in a study population. The largest segregation analysis of prostate cancer families suggested that the familial pattern was best explained by Mendelian inheritance of a rare, autosomal dominant gene in a subset of men with early-onset prostate cancer.[41] The allele is highly penetrant, accounting for cancer by age 85 years in 88% of carriers compared with only 5% of noncarriers. Although this gene appears to be responsible for many of the early-onset cases, only 9% of all prostate cancer cases are in patients with this genetic predisposition, a percentage similar to that seen in both hereditary breast and colon cancers. Twin studies have also been used in the analysis of prostate cancer inheritance and have shown four to five times higher concordance rates for monozygotic twins.[42]

Genetic and Molecular Influences

Progress in cytogenetic studies using polymerase chain reaction (PCR)-based polymorphism analysis has facilitated the identification of regions of the genome associated with various types of cancer. There is ongoing investigation into the role of chromosomal deletions, oncogenes, and tumor suppressor genes in the initiation and progression of prostate cancer. Emerging data from analysis of DNA from high-risk families suggest that specific high-risk alleles exist for prostate cancer, as they do for other tumors. A major susceptibility locus for prostate cancer on the long arm of chromosome 1 (1q24-25) was identified through a genome-wide scan.[43] The gene, *HPC1* (hereditary prostate cancer 1), has been linked

to families with multiple members affected with an early average age at diagnosis.[44] However, this association has not been identified in all studies. Subsequent studies have sought to identify additional susceptibility loci and germ-line mutations implicated in familial prostate cancer. A recent study by Ewing et al.[45] identified a recurrent mutation in HOXB13, a homeobox transcription factor gene involved in prostate development on the long arm of chromosome 17 (17q21-22) implicated in early-onset, familial prostate cancer. A number of other candidate susceptibility genes have been studied,[46] several of which are summarized in Table 69.3.

Research delving into the molecular physiology of the prostate gland has also uncovered specific DNA sequences that may be related to the occurrence and progression of prostate cancer. It is well known that prostate cancer cells, like their normal counterparts, are usually sensitive to androgens, and their growth depends on androgen-stimulated cell division. The androgen receptor gene contains a polymorphic CAG repeat sequence that encodes the portion of the receptor involved in DNA transcription. The length of the CAG repeat sequence was found to be inversely proportional to the activity of the androgen receptor; therefore, shorter CAG repeat sequences may be related to prostate cancer growth.[47] Giovannucci et al.,[48] in an analysis of the activity of the androgen receptor in men with prostate cancer, found that a shorter CAG repeat sequence in the androgen receptor gene predicts higher grade and more advanced stage of prostate cancer at diagnosis, as well as metastasis and mortality from the disease. Other studies found that the prevalence of short CAG repeats is higher among African Americans than Whites[49] and that these sequences are longest among Chinese men.[7]

In addition to these genetic alterations identified in prostate cancer, epigenetic changes such as abnormal DNA methylation have also been observed and may play a role in up-regulation or loss of expression of genes.[50] Millar et al.[51] observed that abnormal methylation of specific sites throughout the genome of prostate cancer cells leads to loss of glutathione *S*-transferase P1 (GSTP1) gene expression. The GSTP1 gene product is an enzyme that provides protection to mammalian cells against electrophilic metabolites of carcinogens and reactive oxygen species. Loss of GSTP1 may lead to a transition between proliferative inflammatory atrophy and prostatic intraepithelial neoplasia or prostate cancer.[52]

Other Risk Factors

Chronic or recurrent inflammation may have a role in the development of prostate cancer, as has been recognized in many other human cancers. In one large population-based study, prostate cancer risk was increased in men with a history of gonorrhea or syphilis (odds ratio [OR] 1.6; 95% confidence interval [CI] = 1.2 to 2.1).[53] A criticism of such epidemiologic studies is the bias that men with symptomatic prostatitis compared with men without it are more likely to seek out care with urologists, have an increased serum PSA test, and have prostate biopsies.[52]

Several commonly used medications have gained attention as potential chemopreventive agents, with particular interest in 5-hydroxy-3-methylglutaryl-coenzyme. Data for the effects of statin (a reductase inhibitor) use on subsequent risk of prostate cancer are conflicting, with some observational cohort studies and retrospective analyses suggesting a reduced risk of advanced prostate cancer,[54] reduced risk of death from prostate cancer,[55] and lower rates of relapse following radiotherapy[56] or radical prostatectomy (RP).[57] However, several large meta-analyses failed to identify a relationship between statin use and prostate cancer risk,[58,59] and no prospective, randomized studies have confirmed these observations.

Other risk factors for prostate cancer have been implicated but not corroborated. Several reports suggested an association between vasectomy and prostate cancer. In a prospective study of 10,055 vasectomized men and 37,800 nonvasectomized men, Giovannucci et al.[60] found an increased risk of 1.85 in the vasectomized men. In a retrospective study of 14,607 vasectomized or nonvasectomized men, the increased risk was 1.56.[61] In contrast, a population-based case–control study of 923 new cases of prostate cancer among men aged 40 to 74 years from the New Zealand Cancer Registry showed no association between prostate cancer and vasectomy.[62] Although there appears to be no definite etiologic relationship, it is possible that men undergoing vasectomy are more conscious of health care and more likely to be screened for prostate cancer.[63] Circumcision has not been correlated with development of prostate cancer.[64]

Armenian et al.,[65] in a study of 296 patients with benign prostatic hyperplasia diagnosed either histologically or clinically and 299 age-matched control subjects observed from 7 to 27 years, found the incidence of prostatic cancer to be 3.7 times higher in the hyperplasia group than in the control group. This association was not observed by others.[66]

Some studies correlated smoking with increased risk of prostate cancer,[67] whereas another study did not find a significant correlation.[68] In one analysis of 359 patients,[69] a greater tumor-specific mortality rate among smokers than nonsmokers with stage A and D tumors was observed. No occupational factors have been confirmed as risks, but some evidence suggests that occupational exposure to cadmium and some aspects of farming may increase risks moderately, although these factors would account for only a small proportion of the total cases. Japanese men exposed to atomic bomb explosions in Hiroshima and Nagasaki have not had a significantly higher incidence of prostatic cancer.[70]

NATURAL HISTORY

Local Growth Patterns

The studies of prostate morphology conducted by McNeal[71] showed that almost all prostatic carcinomas (>70%) develop in the PZ of the prostate, whereas benign prostatic hyperplasia (>90%) arises from the transition zone (TZ). In addition, examination of prostatectomy specimens revealed that small tumors tend to occur in the anteromedial gland, adjacent to the fibromuscular stroma, whereas larger, more advanced T-stage tumors are often located in the posterior gland near the prostatic capsule.[72,73]

Multifocality is characteristic of prostate cancer. On DRE, there may be one nodule or many, located unilaterally or bilaterally. Histologic and molecular studies of prostatectomy specimens of patients with prostate cancer have revealed that most contain a dominant or index tumor and one or more spatially separate, often heterogeneous, tumors.[74–77] Jewett[78]

reported that multiple foci of disease were found throughout the prostate in 77% of prostatectomy specimens. Wise et al.[79] noted that only 17% of 486 patients treated by radical retropubic prostatectomy had one carcinoma detected by 3-mm step-section histologic examination. Of the 83% with multifocal disease, secondary cancers were mostly small; 58% were <0.5 cm³ in volume. Qian et al.,[80] using fluorescence *in situ* hybridization to detect chromosomal abnormalities, found that an increasing incidence of chromosomal anomalies among specimens was positively correlated with progression from high-grade prostatic intraepithelial neoplasia to prostatic carcinoma. When lymph node involvement was present, there was usually evidence of one or more foci of the primary tumor sharing chromosomal anomalies with associated lymph node metastases, suggesting that just a single focus of carcinoma may give rise to metastases. This heterogeneity and multicentricity may account for the discrepancy between needle biopsy Gleason score and the grade determined from the dominant tumor in the prostatectomy specimen.

Tumors arising from the TZ tend to demonstrate a lower frequency of extracapsular extension and may harbor large volumes of disease with relatively high PSA levels but remain confined to the prostate. Despite a high PSA value (≥10 ng/mL), these tumors should be considered to have a favorable prognosis and be managed accordingly. Noguchi et al.[81] described the histologic characteristics of 148 cases of TZ prostate cancer from RP specimens. Seventy percent were clinical stage T1c, with a preoperative serum PSA of 10 ng/mL or greater in almost two-thirds of cases. Only 63% had a positive initial prostatic biopsy. On pathologic review, 80% had organ-confined disease, and more than one-third of cases had a cancer volume >6 mL. When compared with 79 PZ cancers matched by volume, there were no differences in percentage Gleason grade 4/5, serum PSA, or prostate weight, although differences in clinical stage T1c to T2c and organ-confined cancer were highly significant. The actuarial 5-year PSA relapse–free survival rate was 71.5% among men with TZ cancer, compared with 49.2% for those with PZ cancer.

PZ cancers tend to spread along the capsular surface of the gland and may extend through the capsule of the gland, invade seminal vesicles and periprostatic tissues, and involve the bladder neck or the rectum. Clinical stage closely correlated with risk of extracapsular extension and disease progression.[82–84] The incidence of microscopic tumor extension beyond the capsule of the gland (at the time of RP) in patients with clinically organ-confined disease ranges from 8% to 57%.[85,86] Oesterling et al.,[87] in an analysis of patients with stage T1c disease treated with RP, noted that 53% had pathologically organ-confined tumors, 35% had extracapsular extension, and 9% had seminal vesicle invasion. Of the last group, 66% had positive surgical margins, an incidence comparable with that for clinical stage T2 tumors. In a similar group of patients with T1c tumors, Epstein et al.[88] found that 34% had established extracapsular extension, 6% had seminal vesicle invasion, and 17% had positive surgical margins.

Pretreatment serum PSA is also predictive of extraprostatic extension and seminal vesicle invasion. The rate of organ-confined prostate cancer ranges from 53% to 67% for men with a PSA level between 4 and 10 ng/mL and from 31% to 56% for men with a PSA level between 10 and 20 ng/mL.[89–91] D'Amico et al.,[92] in a pathologic evaluation of 347 RP specimens, reported that none of 38 patients with PSA of ≤4 ng/mL had seminal vesicle involvement, in contrast to 6% of 144 patients with PSA of 4 to 10 ng/mL, 11% of 101 with PSA of 10 to 20 ng/mL, 36% of 45 with PSA of 20 to 40 ng/mL, and 42% of 19 with PSA of >40 ng/mL. The incidence of positive surgical margins for these PSA subgroups was 11%, 20%, 33%, 56%, and 63%, respectively. The incidence of seminal vesicle involvement also is associated with the level of PSA, the Gleason score, and the clinical stage.[93,94] Seminal vesicle involvement has been observed in from 10% of patients with A2 tumors to 30% of the patients with B2 lesions.[95,96]

Roach[97] proposed formulas based on analysis of RP specimens to estimate the probability of extracapsular extension (ECE+) and seminal vesicle involvement (SV+):

Regional Lymph Node Involvement

Tumor size and degree of differentiation affect the tendency of prostatic carcinoma to metastasize to regional lymphatics.[98,99] With an increasing number of patients being diagnosed in earlier stages (as a result of screening PSA), there has been a decreased incidence of lymph node metastases in patients with clinical stage T1c and T2 tumors.[100] In the low-risk prostate cancer patients, the risk of lymph node involvement is generally considered <10%.

Several groups[89,101–106] have developed models based on clinical or pathologic data that predict the risk of lymph node metastases. This information is important to decide whether a prostate cancer patient should be subjected to a staging lymphadenectomy (including laparoscopic technique) or considered for irradiation of the pelvic lymph nodes. Partin et al.[107] analyzed data from 703 patients and generated a nomogram for predicting nodal metastases based on three factors: clinical stage, preoperative PSA, and tumor biopsy grade. This model was validated in a larger multicenter study of 7,014 men and accurately predicted nodal metastases in 78% of patients.[108] The negative predictive value was 99%. Bluestein et al.[103] tested a model based on multivariate logistic regression analysis on 1,632 patients who underwent pelvic lymphadenectomy at the Mayo Clinic for staging of prostate cancer. Using this method, they determined that 29% of the patients with clinical stage T1a to T2c disease would have been spared pelvic lymphadenectomy with only a 3% rate of missed nodal metastases. Bishoff et al.[102] reported similar results demonstrating that 20% to 63% of patients with prostate cancer could be spared pelvic lymphadenectomy when accepting a 2% to 10% risk for missed nodal metastasis. These results suggest that many patients can be spared pelvic lymphadenectomy solely by analyzing preoperative PSA, Gleason grade, and clinical stage, without incurring an unacceptable risk for failing to identify regional metastasis.[109]

Stock et al.,[94] in a study of 99 patients who underwent laparoscopic lymph node dissection, correlated incidence of positive nodes with PSA, Gleason score, stage, and involvement of seminal vesicles. None of the patients with a Gleason score of 4 or lower, even those with PSA of >20 ng/mL, had positive pelvic lymph nodes, and 8% in the group with Gleason scores of 5 or 6 and PSA levels of 4 to 10 ng/mL had positive nodes. However, the incidence of positive lymph nodes increased significantly (to 24%) in patients with PSA of >20 ng/mL. These results are similar to those reported in patients treated with RP.[103,107]

In an analysis of 2,144 patients treated at two institutions, Rees et al.[110] noted that only 30 (2.2%) of 1,390 patients with a negative DRE and either PSA of 5 ng/mL or less, Gleason score of 5 or less, or a combination of PSA of <25 ng/mL and Gleason score of ≤7 had pelvic lymph node metastases.

Roach[97] suggested a formula based on pathologic findings in prostatectomy specimens to estimate the incidence of metastatic pelvic lymph nodes (nodes+).

Prognosis is closely related to the presence of regional lymph node metastases; patients with positive pelvic lymph nodes have a significantly greater probability (>85% at 10 years) for development of distant metastasis than those with negative nodes (<20%).[111] However, a single nodal metastasis is not an unfavorable prognostic sign. In a study by Cheng et al.,[112] 322 patients with positive lymph nodes after RP and bilateral pelvic lymphadenectomy were followed for a median of 6 years. Patients with prostate carcinoma who had multiple regional lymph node metastases had increased risk of death from disease, whereas patients with a single positive lymph

node appeared to have a more favorable prognosis after RP and immediate adjuvant hormonal therapy. Prout et al.,[113] in 92 patients with various stages of prostatic carcinoma, noted solitary lymph node metastasis in 11 (34%) of 32 patients with positive nodes. Bilateral pelvic lymph node involvement was present in 14 (58%) of 24 patients who had more than one metastatic lymph node. Only 2 (18%) of 11 patients with a single metastasis showed tumor progression, compared with 15 (76%) of 21 with multiple lymph node involvement. Golimbu et al.[114] noted a 10-year survival rate of 50% in patients with a single positive lymph node, compared with 20% for those with multiple lymph node involvement.

The prognostic significance of multiple involved lymph nodes should be considered with the extent of lymphadenectomy. Several studies have evaluated the anatomic extent of pelvic lymph node dissection on outcome.[115,116] At Johns Hopkins University Hospital, two surgeons performed 4,000 RP with or without an extended lymph node dissection. The extended dissection removed more lymph nodes (mean 12 vs. 9; $P < .0001$) and detected more lymph node–positive prostate cancer (3.2% vs. 1.1%; $P < .0001$) than more limited procedure. If disease was found involving <15% of the extracted lymph nodes, extended lymph node dissection resulted in a more favorable 5-year PSA progression-free survival (PFS). Thus, in certain subgroups, an extended dissection may be beneficial. In another study, the number and percentage of involved lymph nodes correlated with recurrence-free and overall survival.[116] These results need additional validation in prospectively controlled studies.

CLINICAL PRESENTATION AND DIAGNOSTIC WORKUP

Screening Methods and Markers

Although DRE is still an essential element in screening and assigning clinical stage, only 25% to 50% of men with an abnormal DRE have prostate cancer on biopsy. Moreover, because carcinoma of the prostate can be asymptomatic until attaining a significant size, if a patient presents with a palpable tumor, there is a significant risk that there already may be locally advanced or metastatic disease. With the advent of PSA screening, the diagnosis of prostate cancer may precede palpable disease on DRE and the symptoms of urinary obstruction or metastatic disease by many years. DRE is associated with 70% sensitivity and 50% specificity.[117] In fact, 70% of cancers detected by PSA screening are confined to the prostate, and 40% of cancers detected by PSA are not palpable.[86]

PSA, initially identified and purified from prostatic tissue by Wang et al.[118] in 1979, is a protein with a molecular weight of 33,000. PSA is detected not only in prostatic tissue (normal tissue, benign hyperplasia, and malignant tumors) and in seminal fluid but also in the sera of patients with prostatic cancer. It is localized in the cytoplasm of ductal epithelial cells and in secretory materials in ductal lamina.[119] PSA has been detected with immunohistochemical techniques in pancreas and salivary glands and in women; therefore, it is not absolutely specific for prostatic epithelium.[120]

Widespread use of PSA screening has come into question following publication of two landmark screening trials. The European Randomized Study of Screening for Prostate Cancer (ERSPC) randomized 162,387 men aged 50 to 74 years to PSA screening an average of once every 4 years or to no such screening.[121] At a median follow-up of 9 years, PSA screening showed a modest reduction in death from prostate cancer that would require screening of 1,410 men and treatment of 48 men to prevent one death from prostate cancer. The reduction in death from prostate cancer was apparent only in men aged 55 to 69 years. The contemporaneous U.S.-based Prostate, Lung, Colorectal, and Ovarian (PLCO) Cancer screening trial randomized 76,693 men aged 55 to 74 years to annual PSA testing for 6 years and annual DRE for 4 years versus no such screening.[122] At a median follow-up of 7 years, no difference in mortality was noted between the arms. As of August 2008, the U.S. Preventive Services Task Force recommended against PSA screening in men aged 75 years or older and concluded that current evidence is inadequate to make a PSA screening recommendation for men younger than the age of 75 years.[123] The American Urological Association continues to recommend annual DRE and PSA screening tests for men older than 40 years of age if their life expectancy is >10 years.[124]

Radioimmunoassays for prostatic acid phosphatase (PAP) have a sensitivity of approximately 10% and a specificity of about 90% for malignant tumors[117] and to a large extent have been superseded by PSA testing. Stamey et al.[125] reported PSA and PAP measurements by radioimmunoassay in 2,200 serum samples from 699 patients, 378 of whom were known to have prostatic carcinoma. PSA was elevated in 122 of 127 patients with newly diagnosed prostatic carcinoma, whereas PAP was elevated in only 57 patients with cancer and correlated less closely with tumor volume than did PSA. PSA was increased in 86% and PAP in 14% of the patients with benign prostatic hyperplasia.

After RP for cancer, PSA routinely declines to undetectable levels, with an associated half-life of 2.2 days. PAP, if initially elevated, normalizes within 24 hours after surgery. Several authors concluded that PSA is more sensitive than PAP and DRE in the detection of prostatic carcinoma and that PSA would be more useful in monitoring response and recurrence after therapy.[125-127] A caveat is that both PSA and PAP may be elevated in benign prostatic hyperplasia. Hudson et al.[126] reported that only 3% of 168 men with benign prostatic hyperplasia had PSA levels of >10 ng/mL, compared with 44% of 231 patients with prostatic carcinoma.

Several investigators[128-130] reported no significant impact of DRE on the plasma levels of PSA or PAP in patients with various prostatic abnormalities in whom blood samples were collected before, immediately after, and 30 minutes after rectal examination of the prostate. Others[131-133] detected a significant increase in PSA after DRE. Ornstein et al.[133] noted an increase in both total and free PSA in 31% and 48% of men, respectively, at 1 hour after DRE. Matzkin et al.[134] found no significant change in PSA levels after inserting a urethral catheter and maintaining it for several days. Yet, significant PSA elevation has been demonstrated after prostatic massage, transrectal ultrasonography (TRUS), prostate biopsy, and transurethral resection of the prostate (TURP).[130,131,135,136] The kinetics of serum PSA elevation after DRE and needle biopsy were investigated in a Dutch study with few participants.[137] Blood samples were taken at 1 and 30 minutes and 1, 3, 6, and 12 hours and then every 24 hours until 5 days had elapsed. The peak levels were between 30 and 60 minutes after DRE and returned to baseline 24 to 72 hours after the examination. There was a threefold increase in PSA after needle biopsy, and only two of seven patients had returned to their baseline PSA at 5 days. Studies reporting the effect of ejaculation on PSA also have contradictory results. Some authors found no effect at all,[138,139] whereas others demonstrated that ejaculation increased PSA levels in 87% of 64 men evaluated with serial determinations (at 1, 6, 24, and 48 hours).[140] A return to baseline was observed in 92% of subjects by 24 hours and in 97% by 48 hours.

Nadler et al.[141] quantified causes of elevated PSA in 148 men with PSA of >4 ng/mL (a finding suspect for cancer) and multiple negative biopsies. They were compared with 64 men who had a suspect DRE, multiple negative biopsies, and PSA of ≤4 ng/mL. Acute or chronic inflammation of the prostate was more prevalent in the high PSA group (63% vs. 27%; $P = .0001$). Patients with elevated PSA had significantly larger prostate volumes (median, 68 cm³) than those without PSA elevation (median, 32.5 cm³). Simultaneous regression analysis

TABLE 69.4 LIKELIHOOD OF DETECTING PROSTATE CANCER ON TRANSRECTAL BIOPSY FOR 2,054 MEN AGED 40 TO 80 YEARS AS A FUNCTION OF SERUM PSA LEVEL, INDEPENDENT OF DRE RESULT

	Likelihood at Given Age[a]			
PSA (ng/mL)	<50 Year	51–60 Years	61–70 Years	>71 Year
<2.5	10	14	17	23
2.6–4.0	11	15	19	24
4.1–6.0	12	16	21	26
6.1–10.0	14	18	23	29
10.1–20.0	17	23	31	37
>20.0	40	49	60	69

[a]Recorded at the time of PSA collection.
DRE, digital rectal examination; PSA, prostate-specific antigen. Ninety-five percent confidence intervals are within 2% to 12% for all probabilities.
Reprinted from Potter SR, Horniger W, Tinzl M, et al. Age, prostate-specific antigen, and digital rectal examination as determinants of the probability of having prostate cancer. *Urology* 2001;57(6):1100–1104. Copyright © 2001 Elsevier. With permission.

demonstrated that prostatic size accounted for 23%, inflammation for 7%, prostatic calculi for 3%, and nonisoechoic ultrasonographic lesions for 1% of the PSA serum variances.

The positive predictive value for PSA of >4 ng/mL ranges from 31% to 54%. A greater yield is observed when elevated PSA is coupled with positive ultrasonographic and rectal examinations (Tables 69.4 and 69.5).[142] The estimated rate of cancer detection by PSA screening ranges from 1.8% to 3.3%. The percentage of clinically localized tumors detected by PSA ranges from 81% to 97%. The percentage of pathologically localized tumors ranges from 36% to 91% and is significantly higher when serial PSA screening is done.

An important issue is the clinical significance of small tumors detected by PSA testing. Epstein et al.[88,143] identified a subset of patients with potentially biologically insignificant tumors among men with clinical stage T1c disease who underwent RP. On multivariate analysis, the best model predicting insignificant tumor was PSA density of <0.1 ng/mL per gram and no adverse pathologic findings on needle biopsy, or PSA density of 0.1 to 0.15 ng/mL per gram, with a low- to intermediate-grade cancer <3 mm found in only one needle biopsy core specimen. The positive predictive value of the model was 95%, with a negative predictive value of 66%.[88] Dugan et al.[144] offered a definition of clinically insignificant cancer as a tumor that gives rise to no more than 20 cm³ of cancerous tissue in the prostate by the time of expected death and a Gleason score of <4 in 40-year-old patients, 5 in 50- to 59-year-old patients, 6 in 60- to 69-year-old patients, and 7 in 70- to 79-year-old patients. Using these definitions, a review

TABLE 69.5 LIKELIHOOD OF DETECTING PROSTATE CANCER ON TRANSRECTAL BIOPSY FOR 2,054 MEN AGED 40 TO 80 YEARS AS A FUNCTION OF PATIENT AGE, SERUM PSA LEVEL, AND DRE FINDINGS

	Likelihood at Given Age[a]							
	<50 Year		51–60 Years		61–70 Years		71–80 Years	
PSA (ng/mL)	DRE–	DRE+	DRE–	DRE+	DRE–	DRE+	DRE–	DRE+
<2.5	9	37	12	39	15	42	20	44
2.6–4.0	9	41	12	42	16	44	20	47
4.1–6.0	10	41	14	44	17	47	22	48
6.1–10.0	11	–	15	48	19	50	25	42
10.1–20.0	13	55	19	54	25	58	31	60
>20.0	22	82	45	74	43	81	59	84

[a]Recorded at the time of PSA collection.
DRE, digital rectal examination; PSA, prostate-specific antigen. Ninety-five percent confidence intervals are within 2% to 12% for all probabilities.
Reprinted from Potter SR, Horniger W, Tinzl M, et al. Age, prostate-specific antigen, and digital rectal examination as determinants of the probability of having prostate cancer. *Urology* 2001;57(6):1100–1104. Copyright © 2001 Elsevier. With permission.

Section III

of 337 prostatectomy specimens showed that, for cancer volume doubling times of 2, 3, 4, and 6 years, clinically insignificant cancer was identified in 1 (0.3%), 13 (3.9%), 25 (7.4%), and 49 (14.5%) of specimens, respectively. Humphrey et al.[145] determined that in 11% to 30% of PSA-detected prostate cancers, the tumor volumes were <0.5 mL. Therefore, by these definitions, most men treated with RP or radiation therapy have clinically significant cancer.

The incidence of clinically unimportant cancers has been reported to be between 4% and 16%.[88,100,146,147] Researchers at the Fred Hutchinson Cancer Research Center developed a computer model to estimate the rates of prostate cancer overdiagnosis because of PSA testing. Using the National Cancer Institute's Surveillance, Epidemiology, and End Results (SEER) registry data as a comparison for their computer-generated incidence rates, they calculated overdiagnosis rates of 15% in whites and 37% in blacks. These men were predicted to have prostate cancer that would be detected only at autopsy.[148] Conversely, an epidemiologic study randomizing men from Göteborg, Sweden, to PSA screening or a control group demonstrated that screening did not lead to overdiagnosis of prostate cancer; rather, most cancers detected at PSA-guided screening would eventually develop into clinical, frequently fatal, disease.[149]

Although PSA screening–detected cancers may be smaller, they may harbor aggressive disease. Investigators from the Netherlands studied 121 RP specimens from screened patients and found that screening-detected specimens were more likely to be pathologically organ-confined tumors and to have Gleason scores of <8.[150] However, 60% of screening-detected tumors contained areas with high-grade cancer (Gleason pattern 4 or 5), and 50% had a Gleason score of 7, suggesting that most of these tumors are clinically important. Updated results from a study of expectant management of patients with nonpalpable prostate cancer believed to have small-volume disease showed a 6.5-year median survival free of intervention and a 33% intervention rate at a median of 2.2 years, with a median follow-up among the entire cohort of 2.7 years.[151] Increased PSA density and decreased percentage free PSA correlated with progression of disease. Ninety-two percent of patients had curable disease at the time of their diagnosis of progression. These investigators concluded that observation with close follow-up may be a reasonable alternative for older men with a high likelihood of harboring small-volume prostate cancer.

Refinements of the PSA screening test have been introduced to increase the sensitivity and specificity of the test. It was anticipated that such approaches would be able to more readily find curable cancers in younger men and to avoid unnecessary biopsies of benign hypertrophic disease in older men. Unfortunately, none of these modifications listed in the following sections has proven reliable enough alone on which to base a treatment decision for the individual patient.

Prostate-Specific Antigen Density

PSA density relies on the fact that cancers produce less PSA per cell than nonmalignant prostatic tissues. It is calculated by dividing the serum PSA concentration by the volume of the prostate gland measured by TRUS. A higher PSA density is associated with malignancy.

Prostate-Specific Antigen Velocity

Another method is to obtain serial PSA measurements and calculate the rate of rise in PSA, or PSA velocity. A rate of rise of >0.75 ng/mL per year has been associated with a higher frequency of cancer. Two large retrospective analyses suggested that a >2.0 ng/mL increase in PSA in the year prior to diagnosis is correlated with greater prostate cancer–specific mortality following radiotherapy[152] and RP[153] for localized prostate cancer, respectively.

Free Prostate-Specific Antigen

Serum tests for the molecular forms of PSA (free vs. complexed vs. total) have been developed to discriminate between elevated PSA levels from benign prostatic hyperplasia versus cancer. This is based on the concept that PSA exists in serum in a complexed form bound to either α_1-antichymotrypsin or α_2-macroglobulin, two extracellular protease inhibitors. Bound to α_1-antichymotrypsin or α_2-macroglobulin, the enzyme is inactive but still detectable using conventional immunoassays. In a study of free PSA, complexed PSA, and total PSA (free + complexed), the complexed-to-total ratio was higher and free PSA lower in patients with prostate cancer relative to those with benign prostatic hyperplasia.[154] Catalona et al.[155] reported on 113 patients with PSA levels between 4.1 and 10 ng/mL (63 with histologically confirmed benign prostatic hyperplasia, 30 with prostate cancer and enlarged gland, and 20 with cancer and a normal-sized gland). The median percentage of free PSA was 9.2% for men with cancer and a normal-sized gland, 15.9% for those with cancer and an enlarged gland, and 18.8% for those with benign prostatic hyperplasia ($P < .001$). Men with prostate cancer and either a normal or an enlarged gland had a significantly lower percentage of free PSA than men with benign prostatic hyperplasia only. At Washington University, a ratio of free to total PSA of ≤0.2 was most likely associated with prostate cancer and with higher percentages with benign prostatic hypertrophy. A ratio of ≤0.15 was associated with a higher Gleason score and poorer prognosis.[156]

Oesterling et al.[157] analyzed free, complexed, and total PSA in 422 healthy men aged 40 to 79 years. The respective recommended age-specific reference ranges (95th percentile) for the three forms were 0.5, 1, and 1 ng/mL for men aged 40 to 49 years; 0.7, 1.5, and 3 ng/mL for men aged 50 to 59 years; 1, 2, and 4 ng/mL for men aged 60 to 69 years; and 1.2, 3, and 5.5 ng/mL for men aged 70 to 79 years. Similar observations were made by investigators at Johns Hopkins.[158]

Reverse Transcriptase–Polymerase Chain Reaction Assay

Recent developments include using molecular biologic methods, particularly reverse transcriptase–PCR (RT-PCR), to measure markers by detecting low levels of messenger RNA (mRNA) for PSA and prostate-specific membrane antigen (PSMA) expressed by circulating metastatic prostate cancer cells.[159-163] The assay is highly specific because the only cells expressing PSA in the peripheral blood are circulating prostate cancer cells. However, there is a wide range of sensitivities of detection of PSA-expressing cells in the peripheral blood reported in the literature.[164]

Katz et al.,[165] in 94 patients on whom RT-PCR assay for PSA mRNA was performed, reported an enhanced reaction in 26 (72%) of 36 patients who had extraprostatic tumor at the time of surgery. The test was negative in 51 (88%) of 58 patients with organ-confined disease. Six months after surgery, an increased PSA level was noted in 19% and 2% of the two groups, respectively. This bioassay may have significant staging value in patients who are candidates for RP. Cama et al.[159] noted that, in contrast to the RT-PCR assay for PSA, the assay for PSMA did not correlate with pathologic stage of prostate cancer.

Oefelein et al.,[166] using RT-PCR for PSA, identified positive cells in 20 (91%) of 22 operative field samples, and 4 (25%) of 16 had evidence of intraoperative hematogenous dissemination ($P = .046$). Their results suggest that tumor cell spillage and, less frequently, hematogenous dissemination may be associated with operative manipulation of the prostate during RP and may potentially represent the mechanism of failure after this treatment.

Israeli et al.,[167] using the PCR assay, also reported circulating prostate tumor cells in 2 (6.7%) of 30 men. However, prostate-specific membrane primer assay demonstrated tumor cells in 19 (63%) of 30 patients. All 16 negative control subjects had negative PSA and PSMA PCR results. Using PSA mRNA as a marker for prostatic epithelial cells, Seiden et al.[168] noted that 5 of 65 patients with clinically localized carcinoma of the prostate had PSA mRNA–detectable cells by transcription and PCR. On the other hand, 10 of 20 patients with hormone-refractory and progressive prostate cancer also demonstrated the same increased frequency of PSA mRNA–detectable cells.

Overall, most studies report a 0% PSA rate by RT-PCR in negative control cases, whereas the positive rate in the metastatic group ranges between 31% and 88%.[163] However, 25% of men with localized prostate cancer who underwent RP and had specimen-confined disease had a positive PCR PSA assay.[165] These men would be denied surgery if it was concluded that circulating prostate cancer cells are synonymous with incurable disease. A new approach is to use a combination of primers to improve the overall staging accuracy of RT-PCR. Preliminary work from the Cleveland Clinic suggests that combining RT-PCR for PSA and PSMA may improve the staging accuracy.[169] Until the significance of a positive PCR assay is determined with long-term follow-up, RT-PCR remains experimental and should not change treatment recommendations.

Staging Workup

Patients with localized prostatic carcinoma are frequently asymptomatic; the diagnosis is often made with a screening PSA test. In the pre-PSA era, asymptomatic patients were diagnosed on the basis of palpating a firm prostate nodule on DRE. Patients with locally advanced tumors have presented with bladder outlet obstructive symptoms such as urinary hesitancy, decreased force of the urinary stream, and postvoid dribbling as the tumor impinges on the membranous urethra. Chronic obstruction and bladder distension can lead to decreased compliance of the detrusor muscle that is manifested by symptoms of urinary frequency, urgency, and nocturia. Very early-stage disease (T1a or T1b) may occasionally be diagnosed at TURP for symptoms of bladder outlet obstruction caused by benign prostatic hyperplasia. With local invasion into the urethra or ejaculatory ducts, patients may experience hematuria or hematospermia. As the disease penetrates the capsule of the prostate, there may be invasion into the neurovascular bundles that course along the lateral aspects of the prostate, leading to erectile dysfunction. Disseminated disease frequently manifests as bone pain from distant osseous metastases.

A complete clinical history and a general physical examination including DRE are mandatory. The DRE is best performed with a well-lubricated glove; the patient may be standing and bent over at the waist with his elbows resting comfortably on a firm surface or in the lateral decubitus position on the examining table. The examiner should note the size of the prostate gland, its overall consistency, the presence of any firm areas, and, currently, rarely, extraprostatic tumor extension. A typical neoplastic nodule of prostatic carcinoma is extremely firm, often not elevated above the surface of the gland, but surrounded by compressible prostatic tissue. The examiner should determine whether the lateral sulci are involved by tumor and also the degree of spread superiorly. In most patients, the seminal vesicles cannot be palpated as discrete structures, and the finding of a firm area extending above the prostate suggests that the seminal vesicles are involved by malignancy. Only approximately 50% of prostatic nodules found on DRE are confirmed to be malignant on biopsy.[78]

An abnormal DRE result, a consistently elevated PSA, or a combination of the two warrants a biopsy to establish a pathologic diagnosis. A TRUS-guided needle biopsy is the most common method for obtaining representative samples of the prostatic tissue. Ten to eighteen cores are taken, including cores from the base, mid, and apex bilaterally and additional cores from the midline and lateral PZ. If clinically indicated by obstructive symptoms, a separate biopsy of the TZ is taken. The pathology report frequently includes the length of each core and the length of each core that contains tumor.

Once the tissue diagnosis of prostate cancer is ascertained, the patient should undergo a staging workup including laboratory data such as a baseline PSA, complete blood count, and testosterone level. The standard tests required in the evaluation of patients with prostatic carcinoma are listed in Table 69.6. Although a chest radiograph is recommended, a study of 236 patients undergoing RP showed abnormal findings in only 28 (11.9%), mostly related to cardiac or pulmonary problems or arterial hypertension; one primary lung cancer was found.[170] According to the American College of Radiology appropriateness criteria, a chest radiograph should be performed as part of the initial staging only with suspected metastatic disease.[171]

Imaging Studies

Some diagnostic imaging studies have become an essential aspect of pretreatment evaluation and treatment selection. New techniques have allowed for more precise assessments of tumor location, volume, and extent, as well as biologic activity. As a result, clinical staging can be used more accurately as a prognostic factor for defining treatment options.

Transrectal Ultrasonography

The normal adult prostate imaged by TRUS appears as a symmetric, triangular, relatively homogeneous structure with an echogenic capsule. TRUS is used routinely for guidance during the transrectal biopsy and during prostate brachytherapy. However, only prostate cancers located in the PZ can be reliably detected by ultrasonography. Attempts to characterize adenocarcinoma by pattern on TRUS have indicated that prostate cancers can have variable echogenicities. Rifkin et al.,[172] in 443 men undergoing TRUS of the prostate, found 130 pathologically proven cancers and 313 cases of benign prostatic disease. Cancers were hyperechoic in 69% of the cases and had poorly defined margins, whereas benign lesions were hyperechoic in only 46% of the cases.

Chodak et al.,[173] in a prospective, randomized study of TRUS in 216 men, reported a sensitivity of 86% but a specificity of only 41%; tumors <1 cm were the most difficult to detect. For staging purposes, Rifkin et al.[172] found a sensitivity of only 60% using TRUS to distinguish between T2 and T3 lesions.

TABLE 69.6 DIAGNOSTIC WORKUP FOR CARCINOMA OF THE PROSTATE

Routine
  Clinical history and clinical examination
  Rectal examination
Laboratory
  Complete blood cell count, blood chemistry
  Serum prostate-specific antigen (total, free, percentage free)
  Plasma acid phosphatases (prostatic/total)
Radiographic imaging
  Magnetic resonance imaging with endorectal coil
  Radioisotope bone scan (prostate-specific antigen, >20)
  Computed tomography of the pelvis
  Chest radiograph (high risk for metastatic disease)
  Transrectal ultrasonography (for biopsy guidance)
Needle biopsy of the prostate (transrectal, transperineal)
Staging lymph node dissection (high risk for lymph node metastases)

From Edge SB, Byrd DR, Compton CC, et al., eds. *AJCC cancer staging handbook.* 7th ed. New York: Springer, 2010. Copyright © 2010 American Joint Committee on Cancer. Reproduced with permission of Springer International Publishing in the format Book via Copyright Clearance Center.

Computed Tomography

The primary role of CT in prostate cancer is for size determination of the prostate gland, radiation therapy treatment planning, and assessment of pelvic nodal metastases. Roach et al.[174] compared prostate volumes defined by MRI and CT and found a 32% increase in prostate volume when defined by noncontrast CT scan. Using image fusion, they identified four areas, including the posterior aspect, the posteroinferior apical aspect of the gland, the prostatic apex, and the neurovascular bundles, which tended to be areas of discrepancy between the two imaging modalities. Kagawa et al.,[175] using CT-MRI fusion software for planning three-dimensional conformal radiation therapy (3DCRT), demonstrated that MRI was clearly superior to CT in defining the prostate apex, neurovascular bundles, and anterior rectal wall. The discrepancy in prostate location between the two imaging studies was also greatest at the apex and base of the gland.

CT lacks the soft tissue resolution needed to detect intraprostatic disease, capsular extension, or seminal vesicle involvement. Moreover, for most patients with newly diagnosed prostate cancer, the incidence of positive lymph nodes is <5%; thus, there is little role for CT as a routine staging procedure.[176,177] CT identification of pelvic adenopathy depends on lymph node enlargement, and the correlation between nodal size and metastatic involvement is poor.[176,178,179]

Albertsen et al.[180] performed a population-based analysis to determine the positive yield of imaging studies performed on men with newly diagnosed prostate cancer. The positive yield of a CT scan was <12% for men with PSA of 4 to 20 ng/mL. More than 10% of men with PSA of >20 ng/mL and Gleason score of 6 or greater were likely to have CT scans positive for extracapsular or metastatic disease. For combinations of high Gleason scores and PSA of >50 ng/mL, the positive yield on CT scan was as high as 62%. Flanigan et al.[176] retrospectively studied 173 men who underwent preoperative CT scanning and found that none of the patients with a PSA of <25 ng/mL had an abnormality by CT scan. Of 33 patients with PSA levels of >25 ng/mL, 9 had nodal metastases, but only 3 (9%) of these 33 patients were correctly diagnosed by CT scanning. These authors concluded that routine preoperative CT scanning could not be justified in patients with a PSA of <25 ng/mL. Although the histologic incidence of positive pelvic lymph nodes is substantial when PSA levels exceed 25 ng/mL, the sensitivity of CT for detecting positive nodes is only approximately 30% to 35% even at these levels.[177]

Bone Scan

A close correlation exists between pretreatment PSA level and incidence of abnormal bone scan results.[181,182] Given the low risk of osseous metastasis in patients with early-stage prostate cancer, the yield of a bone scan is low unless the PSA is >20 ng/mL or the patient complains of bone pain. In a retrospective analysis of 589 patients with untreated carcinoma of the prostate and PSA levels of ≤20 ng/mL, Rees et al.[177] reported that only 3 (1%) of 274 patients evaluated by bone scan and 3 (1%) of 262 patients evaluated by CT scan had evidence of metastatic disease. Only 1 of 108 patients with a PSA of ≤10 ng/mL had metastatic disease, and no patient with a Gleason score of ≤5 had an abnormal bone scan or CT scan result or positive lymph nodes.

Huncharek and Muscat,[183] in an analysis of 265 patients with localized carcinoma of the prostate, noted that no patients with PSA of <4 ng/mL had a positive bone scan. In patients with PSA of 4.1 to 10 ng/mL and PSA of 10.1 to 20 ng/mL, 2.2% and 3.6%, respectively, had positive bone scans. In patients with PSA of >20 ng/mL, 6.7% had a positive bone scan.

Albertsen et al.[180] analyzed prospective data from the Prostate Cancer Outcomes Study from 1995 and found that physicians ordered bone scans for approximately two-thirds

and CT for one-third of all new patients. Less than 5% of the imaging studies yielded positive results. Only 1% of bone scans were positive for metastatic disease for men with PSA of <10 ng/mL and Gleason score of ≤6. Only men with PSA of >50 ng/mL and Gleason scores of 8 to 10 had positive yields on bone scan of >10%. The guidelines established by the American College of Radiology appropriateness criteria for pretreatment staging of clinically localized prostate cancer recommend that a radionuclide bone scan be considered only for patients with PSA of ≥20 ng/mL, T3-T4 disease, or Gleason score of ≥8 or for patients with skeletal symptoms.[171]

Falchook et al.[184] evaluated about 57,000 patients in the SEER–Medicare database diagnosed with prostate cancer from 2004 to 2007. They reported use of bone scans from the date of diagnosis to the earlier of treatment or 6 months. In patients who underwent bone scans, they noted use of bone-specific x-ray, CT, and MRI scans and bone biopsy within 3 months after bone scan. In all, 31% and 48% of patients with apparent low- and intermediate-risk prostate cancer underwent a bone scan; of these patients, 21% underwent subsequent x-rays, 7% CT, and 3% MRI scans. Bone biopsies were uncommonly performed. Overall, <1% of low- and intermediate-risk patients were found to have metastatic disease. The annual estimated Medicare cost for bone scans and downstream procedures was $11,300,000 for low- and intermediate-risk patients. For patients with apparent high-risk disease, only 62% received a bone scan, of whom 14% were found to have metastasis.

Thus, in this study, there was overuse of bone scans in patients with low- and intermediate-risk prostate cancers, which is unlikely to yield clinically actionable information and results in a potential Medicare waste. However, there was underuse of bone scans in high-risk patients for whom metastasis is more likely.

From a clinical standpoint, a baseline bone scan may be helpful before treatment with radiation therapy, especially in elderly patients or those with a history of arthritis, to document degenerative changes that may later be interpreted as metastatic osseous disease. Bone scintigraphy in routine follow-up has no value because PSA is more sensitive in detecting recurrence, and treatment of asymptomatic bone metastases (except in cases of impending pathologic fracture) cannot be justified. Periodic PSA assessment is adequate for follow-up of these patients, and bone scan should be limited to patients with rising PSA levels when clinically warranted.[184]

Magnetic Resonance Imaging

With the maturation of MRI technology, there have been significant improvements in MR technique and performance for imaging the prostate. Some of the recent advances include the use of multiparametric MRI (MP-MRI) that improve spatial resolution, analytic image correction software to eliminate artifacts, fast spin-echo imaging to reduce image acquisition time and provide higher signal-to-noise ratio, and magnetic resonance spectroscopy imaging (MRSI) to detect metabolic activity in the prostate.[185] Moreover, increasing reader experience has greatly improved the accuracy of MRI staging for prostate cancer. Strict MRI criteria for the diagnosis of extracapsular extension have been elucidated. Nevertheless, there is still interobserver variability, depending on the experience of the radiologist. One study demonstrated that the specificity for diagnosis of extracapsular extension was 93% for senior readers and 94% for junior readers, whereas sensitivity was only 50% for senior readers and 14% for junior readers.[186]

The appearance of the prostate and the information that can be gleaned for staging purposes depend on the MR technique used. On axial T1-weighted images, the prostate gland appears homogeneous and the zonal anatomy is not well appreciated.[187] However, there is a larger field of view, allowing for detection of locoregional adenopathy and suspected

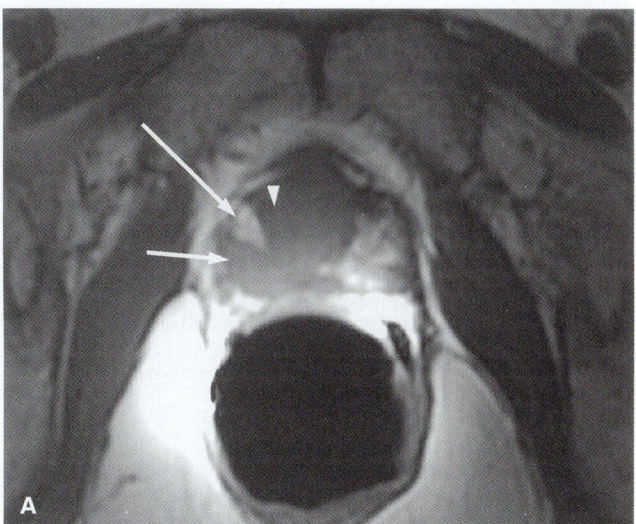
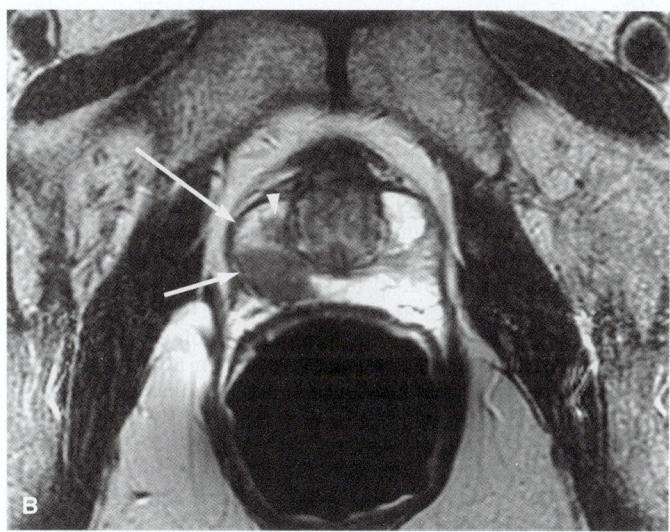

FIGURE 69.3. A: Normal T1-weighted axial magnetic resonance image. Age-related benign prostatic hyperplasia in the transition zone is evident (*long arrow*). The neurovascular bundles lie adjacent to the peripheral zone (*short arrow*). **B:** The T2-weighted axial image of the same level of the gland demonstrates areas of low signal intensity adjacent to the post-biopsy hemorrhage that are suspect for tumor (*short arrow* and *arrowhead*). This is an example of the hemorrhagic exclusion sign. (Courtesy of Steven Eberhardt, MD.)

bony lesions (Fig. 69.3A). Postbiopsy hemorrhage is evident on T1-weighted images as high T1 signal intensity (Fig. 69.3B), which may be in the prostate, seminal vesicles, or both. This is an important observation because hemorrhage may mimic tumor on T2-weighted images and because hemorrhage greatly limits the accuracy in the assessment of extracapsular extension.[188]

The zonal anatomy of the prostate is clearly depicted on axial and coronal T2-weighted images. The vas deferens and seminal vesicles are also discernible on T2-weighted axial and coronal images, whereas the neurovascular bundles can be seen best on axial images (Fig. 69.4).[187] The penile bulb is better imaged on T2-weighted coronal sections and is seen

much more accurately than with CT. The PZ is normally of high signal intensity, whereas tumor appears as low signal intensity. There are many other causes of low T2 signal intensity, including hemorrhage, prostatitis, hormone treatment, and radiation therapy. An area of low signal intensity can be attributed to hemorrhage if it causes high T1 signal intensity in the corresponding region. Low T2 signal intensity due to treatment (radiation or hormonal therapy) may be suspected when the signal change is diffuse and associated with a small, featureless prostate gland. Signs of extracapsular extension are a focal, irregular capsular bulge, asymmetry or invasion of the neurovascular bundles, and obliteration of the recto-prostatic angle.[186]

Magnetic Resonance Spectroscopy Imaging

Spectroscopy is based on the principle that the electron cloud surrounding different chemical compounds shields the resonant atoms of interest to varying degrees, depending on the specific atomic structure of the compound.[189] Because MRSI uses the same clinical MRI scanner, gradients, and radiofrequency coils as MRI, it can be added to an MRI examination, and the metabolic data can be overlaid directly on the corresponding anatomic images.[185] This modality is particularly useful in the prostate because there are metabolic compounds that localize to regions of the prostate and can be used to distinguish between normal prostate cells and malignant cells. Human prostatic glandular cells produce large amounts of citrate during cellular metabolism that are secreted into the prostatic fluid, yielding concentrations 240 to 1,300 times greater than blood plasma concentrations. High levels of citrate are found in the glandular regions of the prostate such as the PZ and lower levels in the transition and central zones. Choline is another metabolite found at intermediate levels in the normal prostate and seminal vesicles. On MRSI, regions of prostate cancer can be identified by differences in these two metabolite levels. A significant reduction in prostate citrate and a significant increase in prostate choline levels relative to the normal PZ have been observed.[185] The elevated levels of choline in prostate cancer may be attributed to the increased rate of cell proliferation, an increase in cell density in regions of cancer, and a change in the composition of the cell membrane leading to higher concentrations of choline-containing phospholipids.[185] The result of MRSI is a metabolic map of the

FIGURE 69.4. Normal T1-weighted axial magnetic resonance image. Age-related benign prostatic hyperplasia in the transition zone is evident (*long arrow*). The neurovascular bundles lie adjacent to the peripheral zone (*short arrow*). (Courtesy of Steven Eberhardt, MD.)

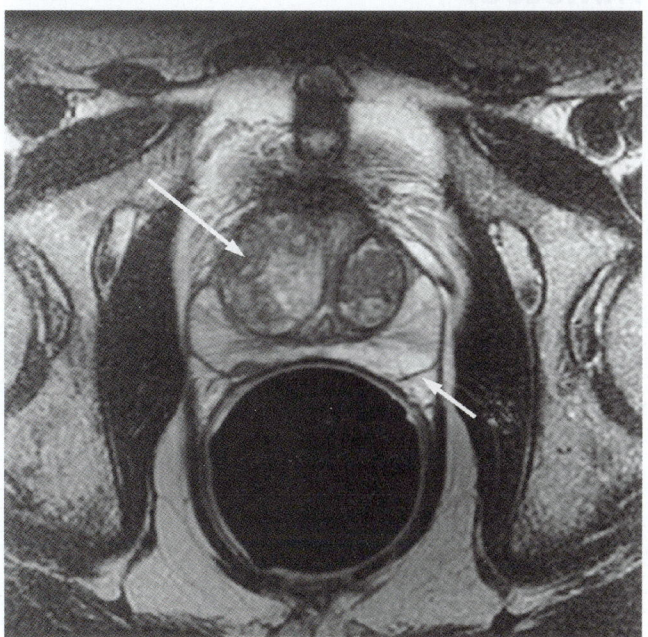

prostate corresponding to normal and abnormal metabolic activity that can be used to pinpoint the location of prostatic tumors. This is exceptionally useful for accurate localization of prostate tumors and, in particular, when distinguishing between tumor and postbiopsy hemorrhage, which obscures MRI interpretations of prostate cancer. Moreover, there is great potential for the use of this technique for follow-up after treatment and in the development of more focused therapy.

The contribution of metabolic information gleaned from MRSI to MR anatomic imaging has improved the diagnostic accuracy of MRI both in localizing and staging prostate cancer.[189] Investigators at the University of California, San Francisco,[190] assessed the accuracy of combined MRSI and MRI for tumor detection and localization in 62 patients by comparing preoperative imaging results with histopathologic step-section examination after prostatectomy. MRI tended to have a higher sensitivity and MRSI a higher specificity for detecting definite sites of cancer. The addition of MRSI significantly improved specificity over MRI alone. Compared with step-section pathology results, the specificity for tumor location with combined MRI and MRSI reached 91%. Combined MRI/MRSI allowed localization of cancer to a sextant of the prostate with a sensitivity of up to 95% compared with MRI alone when either MRI or MRSI was positive. Moreover, a study from the University of California, San Francisco,[191] found MRI and MRSI are comparable with biopsy in accurately localizing intraprostatic cancer and are more accurate than biopsy in the prostate apex.

In addition to improving prostate cancer localization, MRSI is complementary to MRI in staging and risk-stratifying patients with prostate cancer. Combined MRI/MRSI enhances the assessment of both extracapsular extension and seminal vesical invasion.[186] Furthermore, the addition of MRSI to MRI improves the accuracy of less experienced MRI readers and reduces interobserver variability in the diagnosis of extracapsular extension.[189] Emerging data suggest that metabolic information from MRSI may also be predictive of tumor aggressiveness. Preliminary MRI/MRSI studies have shown that citrate levels are lower in poorly differentiated prostate cancers, and choline levels may be elevated in more aggressive tumors with greater membrane phospholipid synthesis.[192]

RISK STRATIFICATION SYSTEMS AND STAGING CLASSIFICATION

Based on tumor stage, pretreatment PSA, and biopsy Gleason score, PZ prostate cancer is generally grouped according to one of several risk stratification models. These systems are useful to stratify disease-free survival, compare treatment results, and provide a means to appropriately recommend treatment options.[93] The most commonly used system is the prognostic risk grouping from the National Comprehensive Cancer Network (www.nccn.org), which defines low risk as PSA of ≤10 ng/mL, T1c-T2, and Gleason score of ≤6; intermediate risk as PSA of 10 to 20 or Gleason score of 7; and high risk as PSA of >20 ng/mL, Gleason score of 8 to 10, or any T3 disease.

Traditionally, clinical and pathologic staging systems were used alone to categorize outcome, but now they are primarily used as components in risk stratification systems. Nevertheless, it is critical to be familiar with the different updated staging systems in order to appropriately manage men with newly diagnosed prostate cancer. In 2010, the American Joint Committee on Cancer (AJCC) and International Union Against Cancer (UICC) updated the 2003 TNM classification system.[3] The TNM staging system is based on separate designations for the primary tumor, regional nodes, and distant metastases. All information that is available before first definitive treatment may be used for clinical staging, including imaging

TABLE 69.7 AMERICAN JOINT COMMITTEE ON CANCER 2010 TNM STAGING SYSTEM FOR PROSTATE CANCER

Primary Tumor (T)

TX	Primary tumor cannot be assessed
T0	No evidence of primary tumor
T1	Clinically inapparent tumor neither palpable
T1a	Tumor incidental histologic finding in 5% or less of tissue resected
T1b	Tumor incidental histologic finding in more than 5% of tissue resected
T1c	Tumor identified by needle biopsy found in one or both sides but not palpable
T2	Tumor is palpable and confined within the prostate
T2a	Tumor involves one-half of one side or less
T2b	Tumor involves more than one-half of one side but not both sides
T2c	Tumor involves both sides
T3	Extraprostatic tumor that is not fixed or does not invade adjacent structures
T3a	Extraprostatic extension (unilateral or bilateral)
T3b	Tumor invades seminal vesicle(s)
T4	Tumor is fixed or invades adjacent structures other than seminal vesicles, such as the external sphincter, rectum, bladder, levator muscles, and/or pelvic wall

Regional Lymph Nodes (N)

NX	Regional lymph nodes were not assessed
N0	No positive regional nodes
N1	Metastasis in regional nodes

Distant Metastasis (M)

M0	No distant metastasis
M1	Distant metastasis
M1a	Nonregional lymph node(s)
M1b	Metastasis in bone(s)
M1c	Metastasis in other site(s) or without bone disease

From Amin MB, Edge SB, Greene FL, et al., eds. *AJCC cancer staging manual*. 8th ed. New York: Springer, 2017. Reproduced with permission of Springer International Publishing in the format Book via Copyright Clearance Center.

studies. The 2010 staging system maintains many of the features of the 2003 systems but reclassifies microscopic invasion of the bladder neck (previously T4) as T3a and includes new Anatomic Stage/Prognostic Groups that incorporate both Gleason score and preoperative PSA. The 2017 AJCC/UICC staging system and the new anatomic stage/prognostic groups are outlined in Tables 69.7 and 69.9. The updated AJCC 2017 staging system has issued a new classification for histologic grading, as illustrated in Table 69.8.

PATHOLOGY

Adenocarcinoma, arising from peripheral acinar glands, is the most common tumor in the prostate. It is graded as well, moderately, or poorly differentiated according to cellular characteristics such as nuclear content, number of nuclei, pleomorphism, gland formation, and invasion of the stroma.[93]

Gleason[193,194] and Gleason and Mellinger[195] initially proposed a prognostic classification system based on the clinical stage and the degree of differentiation of primary and secondary morphologic patterns of the tumor, each graded from 1 to 5. Subsequently, only pathologic features were

TABLE 69.8 DEFINITION OF HISTOLOGIC GRADE

Grade Group	Gleason Score	Gleason Pattern
1	≤6	≤3 + 3
2	7	3 + 4
3	7	4 + 3
4	8	4 + 4
5	9 or 10	4 + 5, 5 + 4 or 5 + 5

Note: Recently, the Gleason system has been compressed into so-called Grade Groups.
From Amin MB, Edge SB, Greene FL, et al., eds. *AJCC cancer staging manual*. 8th ed. New York: Springer, 2017. Reproduced with permission of Springer International Publishing in the format Book via Copyright Clearance Center.

TABLE 69.9 AMERICAN JOINT COMMITTEE ON CANCER 2017 ANATOMIC STAGE PROGNOSTIC GROUPS

When T Is	And N Is	And M Is	And PSA Is	And Grade Group Is	Stage Group Is
cT1a-c cT2a	N0	M0	<10	I	I
pT2	N0	M0	<10	I	I
cT1a-c cT2a	N0	M0	≤10, <20	I	IIA
cT2b-c	N0	M0	<20	I	IIA
T1-2	N0	M0	<20	2	IIB
T1-2	N0	M0	<20	3	IIC
T1-2	N0	M0	<20	4	IIC
T1-2	N0	M0	>20	1-4	IIIA
T3-4	N0	M0	Any	1-4	IIIB
Any T	N0	M0	Any	5	IIIC
Any T	N1	M0	Any	Any	IVA
Any T	N0	M1	Any	≥8	IVB

Note: When either PSA or Grade Group is not available, grouping should be determined by T category and/or either PSA or Grade Group available.
From Amin MB, Edge SB, Greene FL, et al., eds. *AJCC cancer staging manual.* 8th ed. New York: Springer, 2017. Reproduced with permission of Springer International Publishing in the format Book via Copyright Clearance Center.

scored, resulting in the Gleason score that sums grades to yield nine discrete scores (range, 2 to 10). The Gleason score is one of the strongest predictors of biologic behavior in prostate cancer, including invasiveness and metastatic potential; however, it is limited by its subjectivity. There is significant interobserver and intraobserver variability reported using the Gleason grading system.[196] In addition, the treatment with hormonal therapy agents can affect the pathologist's ability to accurately identify a Gleason score.[197]

Moreover, grading errors may reflect sampling error because the needle biopsy samples a small fraction of the prostate gland, and the grade of cancer obtained on needle biopsy may not always be representative of the actual histologic subtype or degree of differentiation of the tumor. Most studies demonstrate a tendency of pathologists to undergrade biopsy specimens. Johnstone et al.[198] noted that, compared with subsequent RP specimens, the incidence of correct grading of prostatic carcinoma from needle biopsies was 71%, with 23% undergrading and 6% overgrading. In a study from Memorial Sloan Kettering Cancer Center (MSKCC), Gleason scores from 18-gauge needle biopsies were compared with radical retropubic prostatectomy specimens in 226 consecutive patients. The biopsy score was identical to the specimen score in 31% of cases, whereas 26% were discrepant by ≥2 Gleason scores. Overall, 54% of biopsies were undergraded and 15% were overgraded.[199] The University of Minnesota researchers found similar results from 466 patients.[200] The biopsy grade was the same as that of the prostatectomy specimen in 54% of the patients, with upgrading of the most common discordance in 75% of the well-differentiated tumors. When the biopsy grade was compared with the surgical pathologic stage, 49% of low-grade lesions and 82% of high-grade lesions in the biopsy had capsular penetration or locally advanced disease. A large, retrospective analysis[201] of the correlation between Gleason scores from biopsy and prostatectomy specimens and prediction of disease-free survival was carried out among 1,031 patients. Overall accuracy was 58.3%. When categorized by Gleason scores of <7, 7, and >7, patients with tumors of Gleason score <7 on prostatectomy specimens had a significant survival advantage over those with Gleason scores of <7 by biopsy, whereas disease-free survival was superior for patients with Gleason scores of >7 by biopsy than those with Gleason scores of >7 on prostatectomy specimens. The overall disease-free survival was similar among all patients with Gleason scores of 7. These data should be kept in mind when results of RP and irradiation are compared.

Predicting tumor extent and location using biopsy results was investigated by Humphrey et al.[145] in a correlative study of multiple parameters with pathologic features in 50 RP specimens. They noted that it was very difficult to predict tumor extent in the gland quadrants based on extent of tumor in the needle biopsy. There were 53 negative quadrant biopsies with carcinoma present in that quadrant in the RP specimen. Gregori et al.[202] evaluated the accuracy of sextant biopsies in predicting tumor location among 289 patients with clinically localized prostate cancer who underwent radical perineal prostatectomy. These investigators found that 33% of patients with a unilateral positive biopsy had cancer confined to one side of the gland, whereas 66% showed bilateral disease in the prostatectomy specimen.

The primary grade in the Gleason score provides additional prognostic information, particularly in Gleason score 7 prostate cancer. D'Amico et al.[203] studied pretreatment clinical and pathologic variables to predict time to postoperative PSA failure for patients with a PSA of <10 ng/mL and T1c or T2a disease. They noted that 5-year PSA failure-free survival rates were not statistically different for patients with a biopsy Gleason score of 2 to 6 versus 3 + 4 but were significantly different for patients with a biopsy Gleason score of 2 to 6 versus 4 + 3 or 2 to 6 versus 8 to 10. Five-year biochemical control rates were 79%, 81%, 62%, and 18% for patients with biopsy Gleason scores of 2 to 6 (no grade 4 or 5), 3 + 4, 4 + 3, and 8 to 10, respectively. Makarov et al.[204] at Johns Hopkins evaluated 537 patients with Gleason score 7 tumors on biopsy to determine whether Gleason score 3 + 4 = 7 and 4 + 3 = 7 cancers behave differently regardless of the number of positive cores. Five variables (3 + 4 versus 4 + 3, number of positive cores, PSA, age, and DRE) were analyzed with respect to pathologic findings after RP. Postoperative Gleason score and pathologic stage significantly correlated with preoperative PSA and preoperative Gleason scores of 4 + 3 versus 3 + 4 on biopsy.

Stamey[205] and Stamey et al.[206,207] emphasized that, with regard to natural history of prostate cancer and prognosis, it is not just the Gleason score that is important, but also how much of the tumor is present. In a study of histologic prognostic variables for PSA relapse among 372 men with prostate cancer followed for 3 years after retropubic prostatectomy, the most important variables predicting biochemical disease-free status for PZ cancers were percentage Gleason grade 4/5, cancer volume, serum PSA, and prostate weight.[207] Percentage Gleason grade 4/5, cancer location in the PZ, cancer volume, and lymph node involvement had prognostic value in large-volume prostate cancer. These investigators also noted that TZ cancers have a better prognosis than PZ tumors because they are separated from the neurovascular bundles and the ejaculatory ducts by the compressed surgical capsule caused by expanding benign hyperplastic nodules.[72] From the Stanford experience,[208] cancer location in the PZ and percentage Gleason grade 4/5 were the most powerful predictors of biochemical failure in men whose cancer was ≥6 cm³ and contained in the prostatic capsule. Preoperative serum PSA was not helpful in distinguishing biochemical failure rates in large-volume cancers regardless of whether they were organ confined.

D'Amico et al.[209,210] showed that the percentage of positive prostate biopsies added clinically significant information regarding time to PSA failure among 960 men with PSA-detected or clinically palpable prostate cancer treated with RP. Investigators at the University of Michigan,[211] in an analysis of preoperative factors, including clinical stage, PSA, biopsy Gleason score, greatest percentage of a biopsy core involved by cancer, number of biopsy cores containing cancer, and perineural invasion, found that only PSA, Gleason score, and greatest percentage of a biopsy core involved by cancer were highly predictive of PSA relapse-free survival on multivariate analysis. This additional prognostic information may identify patients who are candidates for adjuvant therapy after RP. In addition, with the use of radiation therapy, histologic features from prostatectomy specimens are not available to incorporate into prognostic models, and pretreatment risk stratification is important owing to the increasing use of nonsurgical treatment options.

Prostate core biopsy histologic features have been investigated for predicting extraprostatic extension and lymph node involvement. Researchers at the Mayo Clinic[212] compared biopsy specimen Gleason scores, percentage positive cores, and percentage surface area involved in all cores with pathologic stage determined from RP specimens. Multivariate analysis using these pathologic variables, in addition to patient age, clinical disease stage, and PSA, showed that the percentage of positive cores, initial serum PSA, and Gleason score of cancer in the needle biopsy were the only parameters that jointly predicted pathologic stage (T2 vs. T3 disease). Narayan et al.[105] used the combination of preoperative PSA plus biopsy Gleason score in 932 patients who had undergone pelvic lymphadenectomy to predict risk of positive pelvic lymph nodes. Patients with biopsy Gleason scores of ≤6 and preoperative PSA concentrations of ≤10 ng/mL had a <1% false-negative rate for pelvic lymph node metastases, suggesting that a staging pelvic lymphadenectomy is unnecessary.

Finally, the tumor histologic characteristics change with time and progression of disease. Cheng et al.[213] reported a trend toward histologic dedifferentiation when prostate carcinoma metastasized to regional lymph nodes. Among 242 patients treated with RP and pelvic lymphadenectomy at the Mayo Clinic, Gleason score in the lymph node metastases was higher than in the primary tumor in 45% of patients, lower in 12% of patients, and matched exactly in 43% of patients. The 5-year PFS rate was significantly different between patients with histologic dedifferentiation and those without dedifferentiation.

Other Histologic Subtypes

Periurethral duct carcinoma is a separate clinicopathologic entity, usually consisting of a transitional cell type of carcinoma, although a mixture of glandular and transitional cells is also observed.[214-216] Large anaplastic tumor cells cluster in the periurethral ducts and spread into the stroma. Frequent mitoses are seen.[217] This tumor does not invade the perineural spaces as commonly as does adenocarcinoma of the prostate.

Reese et al.[218] reviewed 49 patients with *transitional cell carcinoma* of the prostate; 29 patients had stromal invasion and 20 had transitional cell carcinoma in the prostatic ducts only. Lymph node metastases were found in 14 (54%) of 26 patients with stromal invasion, compared with 4 (24%) of 17 with duct/acinar involvement. The 5-year survival rates were 80% for stromal node–negative, 45% for ductal node–negative, 55% for ductal node–positive, and 30% for stromal node–positive patients.

Ductal adenocarcinoma arises rarely from the major ducts. These tumors are usually papillary and on microscopic sections are composed of tall columnar cells with eosinophilic cytoplasm that may resemble endometrial carcinoma.[51,219-221] Originally, this lesion was believed to originate in the prostatic utricle, a mullerian remnant[222]; however, most ductal adenocarcinomas are not derived from mullerian remnants and behave as acinar adenocarcinomas.[76]

Most reports point to aggressive behavior, with invasion of the prostatic stroma and the bladder neck and metastases to the lymph nodes, bone, and lung. In most series, the majority of patients die of the tumors within 4 years.[223,224] This tumor is moderately hormonally responsive and is sensitive to radiation therapy.[223] The treatment of choice is RP.[223,225] Kopelson et al.[215] reported a good prognosis in early stages; however, in stage C the 5-year survival rate was only 34.5%. They noted a 76% local tumor-control rate and a 58% 5-year survival

rate in patients treated with irradiation, in contrast to 14% local tumor control and 24% 5-year survival rates in patients not receiving this treatment. Brinker et al.[226] also observed a shortened average time to progression relative to a previous study group of men with acinar carcinoma among 58 patients treated with RP at Johns Hopkins.

Neuroendocrine tumors are a rare variant of a malignant tumor composed of small or carcinoid-like cells. Neuroendocrine cell substances found in these tumors include serotonin, neuron-specific enolase, chromogranin, calcitonin, and others. PAP and PSA are valuable to determine the prostatic origin of the tumor. Of 22 patients with stage T2 lesions, 4 died of the disease, and 3 of them had positive neuroendocrine cell findings.[227] Of 20 patients with stage T3, 5 died of the disease, and all 5 had positive neuroendocrine cell features

Mucinous carcinoma, not arising in major ducts or in the urethra, with positive histochemical stains for PAP, has been reported.[228]

Sarcomatoid carcinoma is a rare tumor and is difficult to distinguish from a true sarcoma. There is coexistence of prostatic adenocarcinoma with sarcomatoid components that have spindle cells with large pleomorphic hyperchromatic nuclei. The pattern is that of a high-grade sarcoma in most patients, similar to the malignant fibrous histiocytoma of soft tissues. Mitotic figures range from 6 to 36 per 10 high-power fields. In 12 patients reported by Shannon et al.,[229] tumor presentation was stage A or B in 4, C or D in 5, and unknown in 3 patients. Metastases data were available for 10 patients; the most common metastatic sites were the bone (7 patients), lymph nodes (2 patients), lung (2 patients), liver (1 patient), and skin (1 patient). Immunostaining or electron microscopy demonstrated epithelial differentiation in the sarcomatoid areas in 6 of 11 patients on whom these studies were performed. All 9 patients for whom follow-up data were available died of disease within 3 to 48 months after diagnosis. In 3 patients, sarcomatoid elements were part of the tumor at initial diagnosis; in the other 9, the sarcomatoid component was confirmed in subsequent evaluations after initial diagnosis (2 to 89 months). Four patients were treated with radiation therapy without beneficial result. These tumors are considered a very aggressive variant of prostatic adenocarcinoma.

Endometrioid tumors occasionally arise from the verumontanum. Endometrial glands and cells with numerous mitotic figures may be seen. These tumors may have an exophytic configuration in the prostatic urethra or infiltrate the adjacent tissues.

Adenoid cystic carcinoma is a rare tumor in the prostate (representing <0.1% of all tumors of this gland). The histologic appearance is similar to that of its salivary gland counterpart.

Other epithelial tumors, such as carcinoid or small cell carcinoma, have been reported in the prostate.[230,231] The experience with these lesions is very limited and, in most patients behavior, is highly aggressive and fatal.[232] A review of the literature showed that in 130 patients reported with small cell carcinoma of the prostate, the 2-year survival rate was 3.6%, the 3-year rate was 1.8%, and the 5-year rate was <1%.[233] A subsequent SEER database analysis of 241 cases of small cell carcinoma of the prostate identified 1- and 5-year overall survival of 47.9% and 14.3%, respectively.[234] Squamous cell carcinoma originating primarily in the prostate is rare.[235] Metastatic malignant tumors from other locations to the prostate are occasionally reported.[235,236]

Sarcomas (leiomyosarcoma, rhabdomyosarcoma, or fibrosarcoma) constitute approximately 0.1% of all primary neoplasms of the prostate.[217] Leiomyosarcoma is more common in middle-aged or older men, whereas rhabdomyosarcoma is found more frequently in younger patients. Several cases of malignant schwannoma have been described.[237] These tumors tend to invade lymphatics and blood vessels, causing widespread regional lymphatic and distant metastases.

Carcinosarcoma of the prostate constitutes 0.1% of prostatic neoplasms. A mixture of adenocarcinoma invading the stroma and sarcomatous elements is seen histologically; smooth or striated muscle, fibroblasts, or other mesenchymal malignant cells may be identified.

Primary lymphoma of the prostate is rare, with <100 cases having been reported. It accounted for only 0.1% of newly diagnosed lymphomas and only 0.09% of all prostatic neoplasias at MD Anderson Cancer Center.[238]

GENERAL MANAGEMENT IN THE UNITED STATES

The optimal management of clinically localized prostate cancer remains controversial and is often a source of confusion, frustration, and anxiety for many patients who are compelled to make a decision regarding a treatment intervention for their disease. The practitioner must be aware that the natural history of this tumor is variable and influenced by multiple prognostic factors. All of the various forms of therapy for prostate cancer can affect quality of life and sexual function in varying degrees. In the process of counseling and discussing therapeutic options, it is important for the radiation oncologist to present all available data regarding the natural history of this disease, prognostic significance of the diagnosis, potential therapeutic benefit of the various modalities, and immediate as well as late treatment-related sequelae. Life expectancy and quality of life considerations should be carefully discussed with the patient and spouse or significant other.

Based on the available data, when comparing patients with similar prognostic features, there are no significant differences in the biochemical and disease-free survival outcomes for patients with early-stage prostate cancer treated with active surveillance (AS), RP, high-dose external beam or stereotactic radiation therapy (EBRT or SBRT), or interstitial brachytherapy.[239-243] In the absence of randomized trials demonstrating superiority of one treatment over another, there are wide geographic variations in the preferred therapeutic intervention for early-stage prostate cancer practiced by urologists and radiation oncologists.

Observations from the Cancer of the Prostate Strategic Urologic Research Endeavor (CaPSURE) database—a registry of 11,000 men accrued from 36 community-based urologic practices across the United States—shed further light on practice patterns. Cooperberg et al.[244] reported that, in this cohort of patients, 50% elected to be treated with RP, 12% were treated with EBRT, 13% received brachytherapy, 4% received cryotherapy, and 14% were treated with primary ADT. In these patients, it was noted that among those with higher prognostic risk features, there was an increased use of primary ADT. Younger patients and especially those with low-risk disease were more often selected for prostatectomy. In addition to age playing a role in treatment selection, the presence of medical comorbidities, the socioeconomic status of the patient, and the personal practice trends of individual clinic treatment sites (irrespective of the patient's stage of disease) played important roles in treatment selection as well. There was an increasing trend observed for patients presenting at diagnosis with more favorable-risk disease in 2001 to 2002 (47%) compared with 1989 to 1990 (31%). A lower percentage of high-risk patients (defined as PSA of >20 ng/mL, Gleason 8 to 10 disease, or T3-T4 disease) was noted on initial presentation (15% compared with 41%) for 2000 to 2001 and 1989 to 1990, respectively.

A recent report[245] based on the SEER–Medicare linked database included 85,088 men with the diagnosis of prostate cancer at age 65 years and older. In this cohort of patients, 42% were treated with radiation therapy (RT), 21% were treated with RP, 17% were treated with primary ADT, and 20%

were followed expectantly. The authors also noted a strong association between the type of specialist seen (urologist vs. radiation oncologist vs. medical oncologist) and the primary therapy the patient had received. For patients who were 65 to 69 years old and evaluated by a urologist, 70% underwent a prostatectomy, whereas among patients who were 70 to 74 years old, surgery was selected in 45% of patients. In addition, among men who were seen by both a urologist and a radiation oncologist, RT radiation therapy was the most commonly used treatment modality (83% of this cohort). These data are consistent with prior studies showing that specialists more often made treatment recommendations favoring their particular specialty.

Within the practice of radiation oncology, there have been new trends in management and treatment delivery. Higher radiation doses and the use of adjunctive ADT with RT for various prognostic risk groups are more common than in the past. There has been a significant increase in the use of intensity-modulated radiation therapy (IMRT) for the treatment of localized prostate cancer and increasing use of image-guided radiation therapy (IGRT) with fiducial makers inserted into the prostate prior to therapy for daily target localization (cone-beam imaging), as well as the use of TomoTherapy prior to the administration of the daily fraction. In some institutions, there is increasing use of stereotactic external beam radiation therapy with regimens employing dose per fraction of 6.5 to 8 Gy for five treatments.

Zelefsky et al[246] reported the results of the Quality of Research Radiation Oncology (QRRO) group, which surveyed 414 patients with clinically localized prostate cancer treated with EBRT or brachytherapy that were selected from 45 institutions in the United States. Indicators used as specific measurable clinical performance measures to represent surrogates for quality of radiotherapy delivery included established measures, such as the use of prescription doses of ≥75 Gy for intermediate- and high-risk EBRT patients and androgen deprivation therapy (ADT) in conjunction with EBRT for patients with high-risk disease. Among favorable-risk patients, 72% were treated to ≥75 Gy. For high-risk EBRT patients, 60 (87%) were treated with ADT in conjunction with EBRT and 13% (n = 9) with radiotherapy alone. Among low- and intermediate-risk patients, 10% and 42%, respectively, were treated with ADT plus EBRT. For patients treated with EBRT, weekly electronic portal imaging was obtained as verification films without daily target localization in 35%, and the remaining 64% were treated with daily localization of the target, such as fiducial markers, cone-beam imaging, TomoTherapy, or intrafraction localization with a ferromagnetic marker device.

Active Surveillance

For selected patients with low-risk prostate cancer, expectant management (active surveillance) is an increasingly acceptable approach to avoid overtreatment and the potential morbidity associated with any therapy. Candidates for expectant management include those patients with low PSA values with relatively slow doubling times who have low-volume disease (5% core involvement) and Gleason score 6 disease based on biopsy findings. The long-term results of a phase III, randomized trial from the Scandinavian Prostate Cancer Group demonstrated a reduction in the cause-specific mortality with local therapy compared to an expectant management approach.[247] In this study, 695 men were included with early-stage T1 or T2 prostate cancer. The median follow-up was 12.8 years, the primary endpoint was death attributed to prostate cancer, and the secondary endpoint was overall survival. In the watchful-waiting group, 58% died, compared with 48% in the RP group (*P* = .007). The cumulative incidence of death directly related to prostate cancer was 14.6% in the surgery group versus 20.7% for the expectant management cohort.

The survival benefit was noted among low-risk patients, and this benefit was limited to patients who were younger than 65 years of age.

As noted by Choudhury in an editorial,[248] a United Kingdom landmark Prostate Testing for Cancer and Treatment (ProtecT) study was published in September 2016 in the NEJM.[249] The trial used a cohort of over 82,000 male patients who had undergone PSA screening, of whom 2,664 received a diagnosis of prostate cancer and oF whom 1,643 agreed to be randomized to either active surveillance, RP, or radical external beam radiation therapy (EBRT). From this cohort, 545 men were randomized to active surveillance, 545 to EBRT, and 553 to surgery. Analysis was on an intention-to-treat basis. The median age was 62 years (range, 50 to 69 years), the median PSA level was 4.6 mg/L (range, 3 to 19.9 mg/L), 77% of patients had a Gleason score of 6, and 76% of patients had T1c disease.

The active surveillance protocol was based on PSA levels alone with no routine imaging or repeat biopsies. A >50% increase in PSA level triggered review. EBRT was delivered as 74 Gy in 37 fractions using 3DCRT with ADT for 3 to 6 months. Failure was defined according to nadir plus 2 mg/L.

The primary outcome was prostate cancer mortality at 10 years. Secondary outcomes were all-cause mortality, rate of metastatic disease, clinical progression, primary treatment failure, and treatment complications.

The trial showed no difference in prostate cancer mortality ($P = .48$) or all-cause mortality ($P = .87$) among all three groups. However, disease progression as defined by metastatic disease, clinical T3 or T4 disease, or initiation of lifelong ADT was higher in the active surveillance group ($P < .001$).

As pointed out by Choudhury[248] although many investigators might say that this trial confirmed what is known, it did raise a number of interesting points. First, given that these patients form a younger age group than those men often seen in the clinic, not only are the death rates from prostate cancer very low at 10 years, with only 17 deaths overall (~1%), but all-cause mortality is also very low across all three groups (~10%).

Second, over half of the men assigned to active surveillance have undergone active treatment by 10 years, but 44% of men had undergone no treatment at all (Fig. 69.5) and had thus been spared any overtreatment. This is despite the fact that active surveillance protocols have evolved since the conception of this trial with the regular use of MP-MRI and repeat, often targeted biopsies.

A companion article describing patient-reported outcomes is of particular interest as a comparison of toxicity across the three groups.[250] Sexual and urinary outcomes are significantly worse with surgery, whereas the rate of bowel side effects is higher with EBRT. However, the long-term side effects after surgery are far from inconsequential, with approximately 1 in 5 men using urinary incontinence pads and a similar number unable to maintain an erection at 6 years. This does beg the question: If men are to be treated for their low-risk prostate cancer, is EBRT the treatment of choice? Surgeons will say that there has been an evolution in prostatectomy with robotic laparoscopic surgery and nerve-sparing techniques; however, there is little evidence that in the multicenter setting, late effects are significantly different in the modern era.[251] Conversely, there is significant evidence that with the advent of image-guided IMRT and brachytherapy, radiation therapy toxicity has decreased further since the conception of ProtecT.

The results of the Conventional or Hypofractionated High-Dose IMRT for Prostate cancer (CHHiP) trial have confirmed that hypofractionated radiation therapy is as effective as conventional radiation therapy, leading to a change of practice in the United Kingdom,[252] with EBRT being delivered in 4 weeks with minimal side effects and favorable long-term quality of life compared with prostatectomy; advocates of surgery for low-risk prostate cancer should be wary.

Taken alongside the results of other large treatment comparison studies, the Scandinavian Prostate Cancer Group Trial Number 4 (SPCG-4) and Prostate Cancer Intervention Versus Observation (PIVOT)[253] trials, the differences between the results and the advancement of prostate cancer care make drawing firm conclusions a challenge. However, all three studies suggest that active surveillance and active treatment both have roles in the management of low-risk prostate cancer. This trial, funded by the National Institute for Health Research, part of the National Health Service, has provided important data to inform decisions about the role of a prostate cancer screening program within the United Kingdom. Even now, there is still controversy as to whether routine screening using PSA levels should be introduced to improve outcomes from prostate cancer. Parallels are drawn with the NHS breast cancer and cervical cancer screening programs. Results from the Cluster Randomised Trial of PSA Testing for Prostate Cancer (CAP) study (ISRCTN9218725), which directly addresses screening, and the Prostate MRI Imaging Study (PROMIS) (ISRCTN16082556), which is due to report on diagnostic strategies, will be put together to recommend a suitable national strategy to manage the burden of prostate cancer in the United Kingdom. Current national guidance published by the UK National Institute for Health and Care Excellence in 2014 recommends active surveillance or radical treatment for

PROSTATE CANCER: 10 YEAR OUTCOME RANDOMIZED TRIAL (PROTECT)

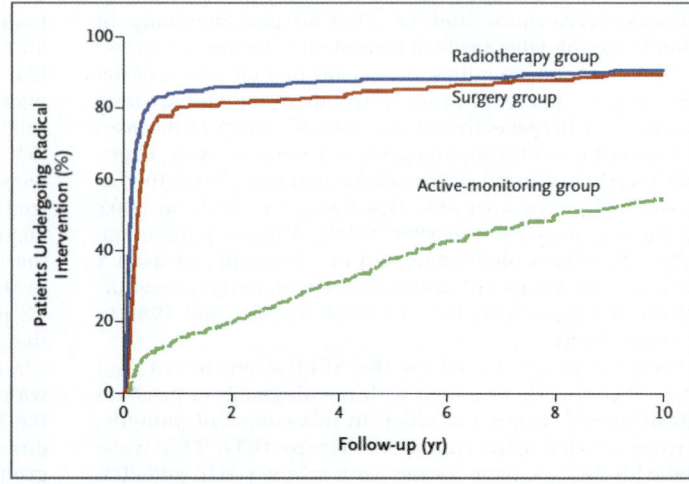

FIGURE 69.5. Cumulative probability of men undergoing definitive treatment intervention during the follow-up period, according to treatment group. (From Hamdy FC, Donovan JL, Lane JA, et al. 10-Year Outcomes after Monitoring, Surgery, or Radiotherapy for Localized Prostate Cancer. *N Engl J Med* 2016;375[15]:1415–1424. Copyright © 2016 Massachusetts Medical Society. Reprinted with permission from Massachusetts Medical Society.)

men with localized low- or intermediate-risk prostate cancer, involving a MP-MRI scan with PSA tests every 3 to 4 months for the first year and a repeat biopsy, followed by PSA tests every 3 to 6 months for the next 2 years and then every 6 months, with further imaging and biopsies if indicated. Definitive treatment is recommended for men with localized prostate cancer at high risk of tumor progression. RP, EBRT with hormone therapy in selected patients, and brachytherapy are all acceptable options. High-intensity ultrasound or cryotherapy was not recommended unless the patient is part of a clinical trial

Keeping men well informed of their options and considering individual preferences are key tenets of these guidelines. It is clear that patient information and careful selection are key. There are a number of studies seeking to address the role of genomic markers of both radiation therapy responses to tumor and normal tissues. Recent suggestions that molecular subgroups outside of the traditional prognostic factors can stratify patients more accurately need to be explored further. No definitive data on genetic or molecular markers in primary prostate cancer are available.[249]

The Prostate Cancer Intervention versus Observation Trial (PIVOT)[253] enrolled 761 US patients diagnosed by PSA screening. At 12-year follow-up, prostatectomy did not significantly reduce all-cause or prostate cancer–specific mortality compared with observation for localized prostate cancer in selected patients (T1-T2NxM0 with PSA <50 ng/mL, life expectancy of at least 10 years, negative bone scan for metastatic disease, and age no >75 years). Unlike the Scandinavian Prostate Cancer Group Study, the PIVOT study stratified overall survival and prostate cancer–specific survival by patient race; nearly one-third of study patients (233 of 761) were African American. The generalizability of PIVOT trial[253] conclusions to the contemporary US population has been questioned by a recent National Cancer Database analysis of PIVOT-eligible patients, which found that US men were younger, healthier, and more likely to have RP for higher-risk disease than men in the PIVOT trial.

Unfortunately, subsequent SEER-based work has indicated that the encouragement of deferring definitive intervention (RP or definitive radiation therapy) in favor of active surveillance may be deleterious for African American patients with low-risk prostate cancer. One study involving more than 51,000 men with low-risk prostate cancer (T1-T2a, Gleason score =6, and PSA = 10 ng/mL) found African American race to be an independently predictive risk factor for prostate cancer–specific mortality (43,792 Caucasian vs. 7,523 African American patients). Another analysis found that definitive intervention for screening detected, low-risk prostate cancer (T1c, Gleason score = 6, and PSA = 10 ng/mL) was more likely to occur in men who were Caucasian, married, and/or with high socioeconomic status.

As noted by McClelland et al.,[254] the absence of race-based results from two of these RCTs and questions about generalizability of PIVOT results to the general population (even more so to African American men), combined with findings from SEER, which examined more than 7,500 African Americans with low-risk prostate cancer, indicate that the results of active surveillance versus definitive intervention for clinically localized prostate cancer may not be as robust for African Americans as the RCTs indicate.

This situation sheds light on the dangers of interpreting RCT results independent of patient race or sociodemographic factors such as insurance status, when these factors have clearly influenced access to optimal care for cancers of the prostate and other organ systems. Recent work utilizing genomic sequencing samples from within The Cancer Genome Atlas has found Caucasians overrepresented in comparison with the US population, with samples from racial minorities being comparatively insufficient to detect moderately common mutational frequencies. The relatively low enrollment of racial minorities in cancer sequencing studies hinders the ability to detect race-specific targetable mutations, which could prove particularly pertinent for African Americans with prostate cancer.

The authors concluded that the findings from a low-risk prostate cancer population more than 30 times larger than the ProtecT study and 75 times larger than the Scandinavian Prostate Cancer Group and PIVOT studies should at minimum raise questions toward endorsing a blanket recommendation of delaying intervention for the sake of active surveillance for African Americans or other underrepresented ethnic groups (Hispanics, Native Americans) with low-risk prostate cancer.

Musunuru et al.[255] reported on 522 patients with low-risk prostate cancer (T1-T2a, Gleason score = 6, and PSA = 10 ng/mL) between 2006 and 2008 who were recruited to AS, low-dose rate brachytherapy (LDR BT), SABR, or standard EBRT. Out of the 522 patients, 178 opted for AS program, 76 for standard EBRT (76 Gy/38 fractions), and 83 for SABR (35 Gy/5 fractions) as part of a phase 2 trial, and 185 patients had LDR BT (I-125 implant-median dose of 145 Gy). Median follow-up was 51 months for the entire cohort; 10.1%, 16.85%, 6.02%, and 21.05% of the patients in AS, LDR, SABR, and EBRT groups had clinical T2 disease; median pretreatment PSAs for the four groups were 4.65, 5.66, 5.90, and 6.57 ng/mL ($P < .0001$). In the AS cohort, 38 patients (21.3%) underwent active treatment. Median time to treatment was 18.25 months (8 to 72 months). Among the 522 patients, 17 had biochemical failure. The 6-year bDFS was 96.1%. There was no difference in bDFS when stratified by clinical stage or pretreatment PSA. The results for 6-year bDFS were 97.7%, 93.2%, 97.4%, and 96.8% for the AS, LDR, SABR, and EBRT groups ($P = .28$). Hematochezia was observed in 2.24%, 3.13%, 7.14%, and 9.88% of the AS, LDR, SABR, and EBRT groups, respectively. Higher incidence of hematuria was noticed in the LDR BT cohort (11.98%), when compared to the other groups. Thus, AS, LDR, EBRT, and SABR were effective management options for low-risk prostate cancer patients.

The National Comprehensive Cancer Network (NCCN) recommends active surveillance (AS) for men with low-risk prostate cancer and life expectancy 10 years. Lester-Coll et al.[256] investigated trends and predictors of AS in a large national cohort of men with low-risk prostate cancer (nonmetastatic cT1eT2a, Gleason 6, and PSA < 10), in the National Cancer Database (NCDB) from 2010 to 2012. Management strategy and facility type (academic vs. nonacademic) were compared using univariable logistic regression. Additional covariates tested against management strategy included T-stage (T1c vs. T2a), age (<age 65 vs. 65 or older) Charlson/Deyo comorbidity score, location, insurance, rurality, race, education, and income.

Eighty-one thousand six hundred ninety men were identified, among whom 34,612 (42%) were evaluated at an academic center and 47,078 (58%) at a nonacademic center. Median age was 63.

Initial management was AS in 8,228 (10%), definitive treatment (DT) in 70,064 men (86%), and no treatment (NT) in 3,398 (4%). Patients evaluated at academic centers were significantly more likely than those at nonacademic centers to receive AS than DT or NT (15% vs. 7% AS, 81% vs. 89% DT, 4% vs. 4% NT, $P < .001$). After adjusting for age, T stage, insurance, and location, evaluation at an academic versus nonacademic facility was independently associated with increased odds of AS utilization (adjusted OR 1.91; 95% CI = 1.83 to 1.99, $P < .001$).

Treatment Techniques

Radical Prostatectomy

RP, initially described by Young[257] in 1905 and popularized by Jewett,[78] is a therapeutic option in selected patients, when the tumor is confined to the prostate. In the past, according to most urologists, it had a limited role in the management of gross extracapsular disease or seminal vesicle involvement or in the presence of lymph node metastases; however, more recently, there has been an increased use of surgery for locally advanced disease. Two approaches for the classic RP are used: retropubic and perineal. The procedure consists in complete removal of the prostate and its surrounding capsule together with the seminal vesicles, the ampulla, and the vas deferens. The prostate is removed completely by excision of the urethra at the prostatomembranous junction, leaving no residual prostatic tissue at the apex. The retropubic approach is preferred by many urologic surgeons as this procedure also facilitates access for performing a bilateral pelvic lymph node dissection.

In the last 5 to 10 years, there has been an increasing interest and practice of laparoscopic and robotic RP approaches in both the United States and Europe. Advantages cited for the use of the laparoscopic procedure versus the open approach include improved visualization of the anatomy optical magnification, less blood loss, less postoperative pain, and more rapid resumption of normal activities. Preliminary functional and oncologic outcomes with this approach compare favorably to those achieved with open RP approaches. The da Vinci robotic surgical system (Intuitive Surgical, Sunnyvale, CA) uses three multijoint robotic arms, with one arm controlling the binocular endoscope and the other arms controlling small-wristed instruments. This system is controlled by the surgeon, who can be in a remote location from the patient, seated at an operative console. The stereoscopic view of the operative field provides the surgeon three-dimensional visualization with a 10-fold magnification. In a comparison of open versus laparoscopic and robot-assisted RP (RARP) approaches, there were no significant differences in perioperative complication rates and tumor-control outcomes among the various surgical approaches. Among 239 patients evaluated with a median follow-up of 50 months, the 5-year biochemical control outcomes were 88% for open prostatectomy and 88% and 90% for laparoscopic and robotic-assisted prostatectomy, respectively. The incidence of positive margins also was similar among the different approaches. Long-term results of 184 patients treated with robot-assisted laparoscopic prostatectomy were reported by Suardi et al.[258] With a median follow-up of 67 months, the 7-year biochemical control rates for pathologic T2 and T3a and pathologic T3b disease were 85%, 84%, and 43% disease, respectively.

Radiation Therapy Techniques

Conformal and Intensity-Modulated Radiation Therapy Techniques

In the late 1980s, three-dimensional (also known as conformal) treatment techniques became increasingly available. CT-based images referenced to a reproducible patient position are used to localize the prostate and normal organs and to generate high-resolution 3D reconstructions of the patient anatomy. Treatment field directions are selected using beam's–eye view techniques, and the fields are shaped to conform to the patient's CT-defined target volume, thereby minimizing the volume of normal tissue irradiated. Conformal radiation therapy simulation, treatment planning, and delivery incorporate various additional maneuvers to reduce treatment uncertainties and enhance set-up reproducibility required during a protracted course of therapy.

IMRT is a refinement of 3D conformal techniques that uses treatment fields with highly irregular radiation intensity patterns to deliver exquisitely conformal radiation dose distributions.[259]

IMRT delivery is significantly more complex than 3D conformal delivery, requiring a computer-controlled beam-shaping multileaf collimator (MLC).

Simulation, Treatment Planning, Target, and Normal-Tissue Contouring

The techniques for simulation and treatment planning have been described in details in earlier chapters. Anatomical details and target volumes are defined in CT scan sections of 1 to 3 mm thickness. Although in the past prostate cancer patients were treated in the prone position at Memorial Sloan Kettering Cancer Center based on comparative studies[260] that demonstrated improved geometry of the normal anatomy juxtaposed to the prostate target, currently patients are routinely treated in the supine position. These changes were made based on the observation of less prostate motion observed in the supine compared to the prone position.[261] All patients undergo fiducial marker placement via transrectal ultrasound guidance 1 week prior to simulation. For immobilization, a thermoplastic mold is fabricated for simulation, CT scanning, and treatment to ensure that the patient is in the same treatment position during all procedures. The thermoplastic sheet is heated in warm water and molded to the patient's shape from the knees to midabdomen. Small sections of the mold are cut away to provide ports for marking and tattooing. The patient is scanned through an approximately 20- to 30-cm region around the prostate with a slice spacing and thickness of 3 mm. Before start of the CT planning study, several transverse images through the prostate and bladder are obtained to ensure that the rectal lumen is clearly visible, the bladder and rectum are not excessively filled, and the patient is properly positioned within the scan circle. With the use of the CT dataset, a "virtual simulation" is performed, using digitally reconstructed radiographs to localize the treatment area rather than conventional simulation films. The treatment isocenter is placed according to anatomic landmarks near the center of the prostate gland: midline, at the caudad aspect, and approximately 5 cm posterior to the symphysis pubis. The triangulation points for the isocenter are then tattooed, along with an additional alignment tattoo, along the sagittal line, approximately 10 cm superior to the isocenter. To ensure reproducible leg position, tattoos are placed on the back of the legs at the midshaft level, and the distance between the tattoos is recorded for future reference.

The clinical target volume (CTV) is defined as the prostate and seminal vesicles. The planning target volume (PTV) is defined as the CTV with a margin to account for physical uncertainties including set-up reproducibility and interfractional and intrafractional organ motion.

A 0.5- to 1-cm margin is added to the CTV to form the PTV in all directions except posteriorly at the interface with the rectum, where the margin is reduced to 0.5 cm. Clinically, these margins were found to provide adequate target coverage based on a serial CT scan study evaluating organ motion during a course of 3DCRT.[260] When using image-guided approaches with daily target localization, margins are reduced to 5 to 6 mm circumferentially around the CTV. Normal tissues identified on each CT slice include the inner and outer walls of the rectum and bladder, the femoral heads, and the outer skin surface. Portions of the small bowel or sigmoid colon within 1 cm of the PTV are also contoured and taken into consideration, if necessary, during planning. In addition, the central 1-cm diameter portion of the prostate encompassing the prostatic urethra is defined for dosimetric consideration and evaluation during high-dose IMRT planning.

Accurate anatomic delineation of the prostate and, in particular, the prostatic apex has been a topic of some controversy. Some have advocated urethrography at the time of simulation as a method to accurately localize the apex.[261] Mah et al.[262] performed sagittal MR scans immediately before and after urethrogram in 13 patients. No significant systematic motion of the prostate itself or the apex was observed, leading the authors to conclude that urethrography during simulation does not introduce localization error.

The contribution of MRI to improved accuracy and reproducibility of target localization in prostate cancer has also been well studied.[263] Roach et al.[174] evaluated 10 patients with both MR and CT images of the prostate and noted that the prostate volume was 32% larger when defined by noncontrast CT than when determined by MRI. Areas of disagreement tended to occur in the posterior and posteroinferior–apical portions of the prostate, the apex (because of disagreement between urethrography and MRI), and the regions corresponding to the neurovascular bundle. Rasch et al.[264] also observed differences in CT- and MR-defined volumes. On average, the prostate and seminal vesicle volume defined on CT was 40% larger than that defined on MR. The CT-defined prostate was 8 mm larger at the base of the seminal vesicles and 6 mm larger at the prostatic apex. This difference was found to be significantly larger than interobserver variation.

Contouring Techniques

There have been several reports documenting the variability of prostate-contouring techniques among practitioners.[1] McLaughlin et al.[265] provided an excellent demonstration of common contouring errors such as overestimation of the prostatic apex and underestimation of the prostatic base. The apex and the base in particular represent regions of the target volume that can be challenging to identify on CT images and better defined with MRI imaging. Two methods recommended include the inspection of lateral view projections of the contours to detect regions of the irregularities of the target geometry and improved recognition of the GUD elements. These elements are shown in the MRI representation of the GUD in Figure 69.6 and in the CT representation in Figure 69.7.

The beam weights are adjusted to obtain a uniform dose within the PTV and to place the hot spots away from the rectum. The plan was normalized so that the prescription isodose (95% to 100%) covers the PTV with a hot spot of 6% to 9% within the PTV. Although a small volume of the rectal wall close to the PTV is expected to receive the prescription dose or slightly higher, the rectal wall volume receiving 75.6 Gy or more should not exceed 20%. Other normal-tissue dose limits for these 3DCRT plans included limiting the maximum dose to the femurs to ≤48 Gy (90%), the maximum dose to large bowel to ≤60 Gy, and the maximum dose to small bowel to ≤50 Gy.

Most institutions performing IMRT planning set up templates that specify both the clinical goals of the dose distribution and initial target and normal tissue constraints for optimization. The MSKCC template for prostate IMRT planning to 81 Gy is shown in Table 69.10. Dose and dose–volume constraints for the PTV, PTV overlap with the rectum, and rectal and bladder walls are listed. It should be noted that constraint templates vary significantly among treatment planning systems; therefore, these constraints should be used only after a thorough evaluation on the user's system.

A variety of beam arrangements have been proposed for prostate IMRT treatment, including multifield axial or noncoplanar arrangements, in addition to intensity-modulated arc therapy.[266–268] Primarily because of concern about increased risk of secondary cancers from higher neutron doses associated with IMRT treatment at high energies,[269,270] 6-MV IMRT techniques are preferred for the treatment of prostate cancer. As shown by Pirzkall et al.,[271] however, a larger number of treatment fields may be necessary to achieve a dose distribution similar to that observed with 15-MV x-rays.

The MSKCC clinical goals used to evaluate the IMRT dose distributions and dose–volume histograms for prostate patients are outlined in Table 69.10. These dosimetric guidelines defining acceptable target coverage, dose uniformity, and normal-tissue doses have grown out of our 3DCRT and IMRT planning

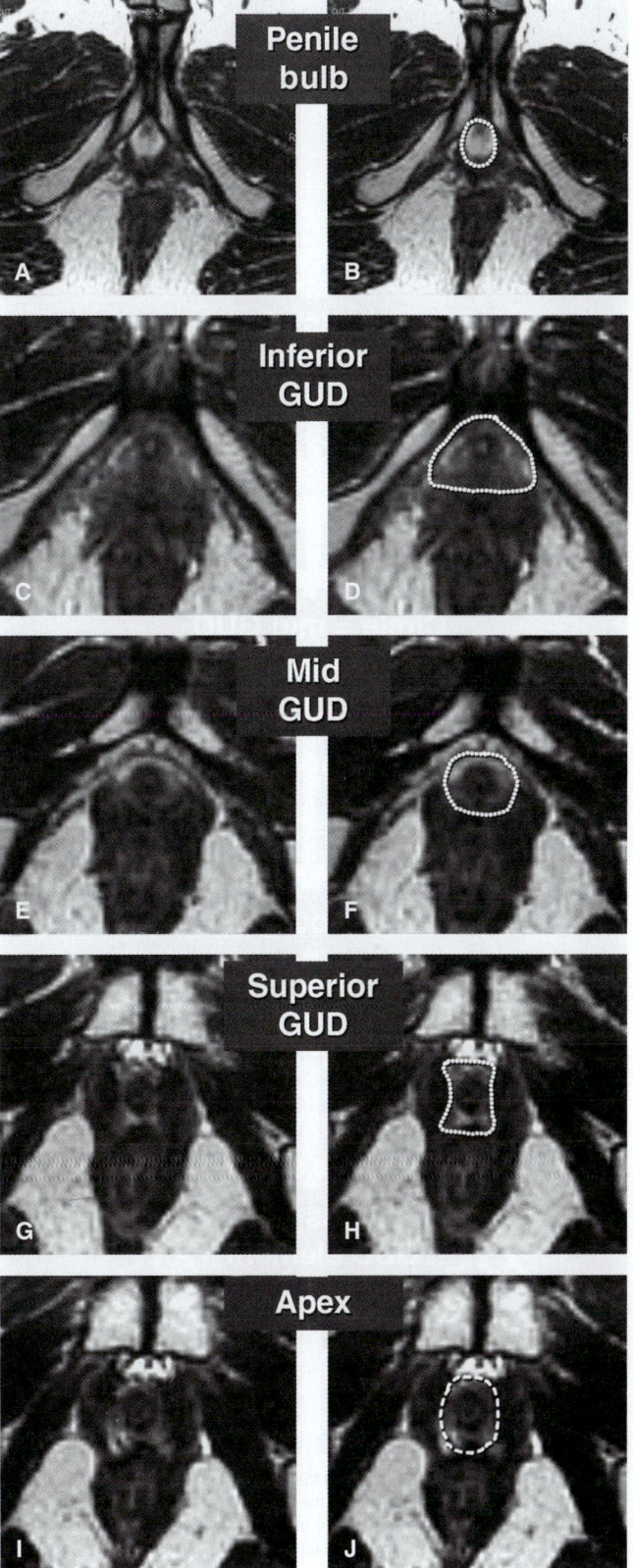

FIGURE 69.6. A–J: Representation of the genitourinary diaphragm on axial magnetic resonance imaging slices, demonstrating the anatomic configuration that can be used as a guide for contouring of the clinical prostate target volume. (Reprinted from McLaughlin PW, Evans C, Feng M, et al. Radiographic and anatomic basis for prostate contouring errors and methods to improve prostate contouring accuracy. *Int J Radiat Oncol Biol Phys* 2010;76[2]:369–378. Copyright © 2010 Elsevier. With permission.)

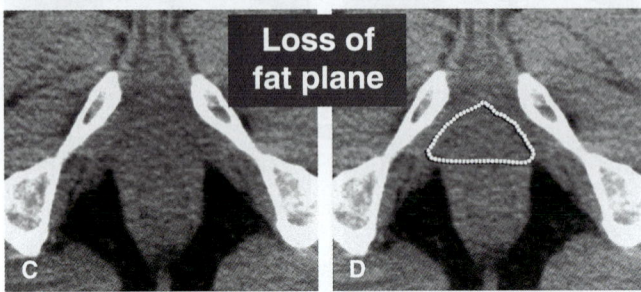

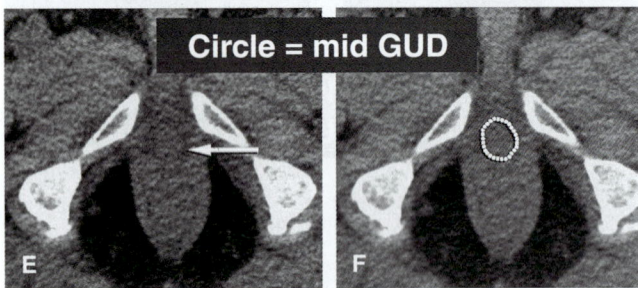

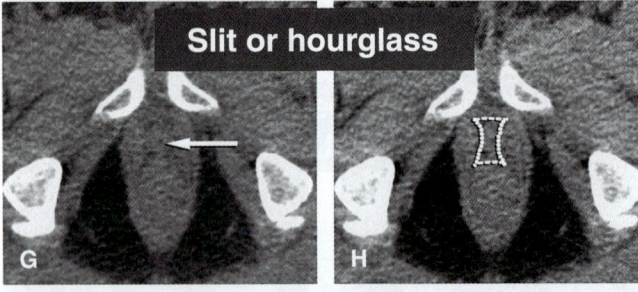

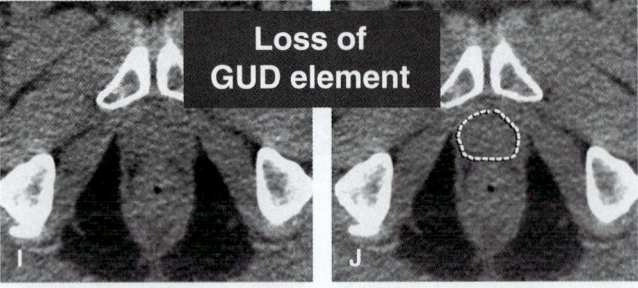

FIGURE 69.7. A–J: Representation of the genitourinary diaphragm on axial computed tomography slices, demonstrating the anatomic configuration that can be used as a guide for contouring of the clinical prostate target volume. (Reprinted from McLaughlin PW, Evans C, Feng M, et al. Radiographic and anatomic basis for prostate contouring errors and methods to improve prostate contouring accuracy. *Int J Radiat Oncol Biol Phys* 2010;76[2]:369–378. Copyright © 2010 Elsevier. With permission.)

experience during the last 20 years and include several refinements resulting from retrospective outcome and toxicity analyses from our institution. Most notably, studies by Skwarchuk et al.[272] and Jackson et al.[273] retrospectively evaluating the rectal wall dose–volume histograms for patients treated to 70.2 and 75.6 Gy using 3DCRT techniques found that, on average, patients with late rectal bleeding had significantly higher

TABLE 69.10 OPTIMIZATION CONSTRAINT TEMPLATE AND PLANNING GOALS FOR MEMORIAL SLOAN KETTERING CANCER CENTER 81-GY AND INTENSITY-MODULATED RADIATION THERAPY PROSTATE TREATMENT

Structure	Optimization Constraints[a]			Treatment Plan Goals[b]	
	Maximum Dose (Gy)/ Penalty	Minimum Dose (Gy)/ Penalty	Volume (%)	Dose (Gy)	Volume (%)
Planning target volume (excluding rectal overlap)	82.6/50	79.4/50	–	111% max	V₉₅ >90
Planning target volume and rectum					
Overlap region	77.8/20	75.3/10	–	–	–
Rectal wall	77/20	–	–	75.6	30
Rectal wall	32.4/20	–	30	47	53
Bladder wall	79.4/35	–	–	–	–
Bladder wall	32.4/20	–	30	40	60

[a]Optimization constraints = initial target and normal-tissue constraints entered into the IMRT optimization planning system.
[b]Treatment plan goals = dosimetric criteria used for evaluation and acceptance of an IMRT dose distribution.

rectal dose–volume histograms than patients who did not bleed. Both high- and intermediate-dose levels were found to be independently correlated with rectal bleeding. As a result of these studies, two rectal wall dose–volume histogram limits were implemented and are routinely enforced at MSKCC when treating prostate cancer: No more than 30% of the rectal wall may receive more than 75.6 Gy, and no more than 53% of the rectal wall can receive more than 47 Gy.

Typical dose distributions and dose–volume histograms for an 86.4-Gy IMRT plan are shown in Figure 69.8. The physician should carefully review the treatment plan and dose–volume histograms of the target and normal-tissue structures to select the optimal treatment plan for the patient. Target coverage should be carefully assessed, as well as the dose inhomogeneity and location of hot spots. In addition, careful attention should be given to determining whether the treatment plan adequately meets acceptable dose constraints for the rectum, bladder, and bowel.

Standard Prescription Doses for 3DCRT and IMRT

In general, 78 Gy with conventional fractionation is frequently used, although at MSKCC, 81 to 86 Gy has been delivered to favorable-risk patients using IMRT. Daily fractions of 1.8 to 2 Gy, five fractions per week, are routinely used. However, others have reported encouraging results with a hypofractionated scheme delivering 70 Gy with fractions of 2.5 Gy.[274,275] The dose is prescribed to an isodose line that encompasses as much of the PTV as possible while still respecting the target and normal-tissue goals listed in Table 69.10. Typically, at least 90% to 95% of the PTV receives the prescription dose.

Treatment Delivery and Organ Motion Control

Movement of the prostate during treatment or between treatment fractions has long been a concern for prostate radiation therapy. Many studies investigating interfractional and intrafractional motion of the prostate and seminal vesicles have been reported.[276–279] Most groups have measured prostate motion relative to bony landmarks through repeated imaging of implanted radiopaque markers or serial CT studies. Although the reported magnitude of motion has varied, relatively little motion in the lateral direction and potentially significant movement in the anterior–posterior and superior–inferior directions has been consistently reported. Many studies have also observed a correlation between prostate and seminal vesicle motion and rectal or bladder filling.

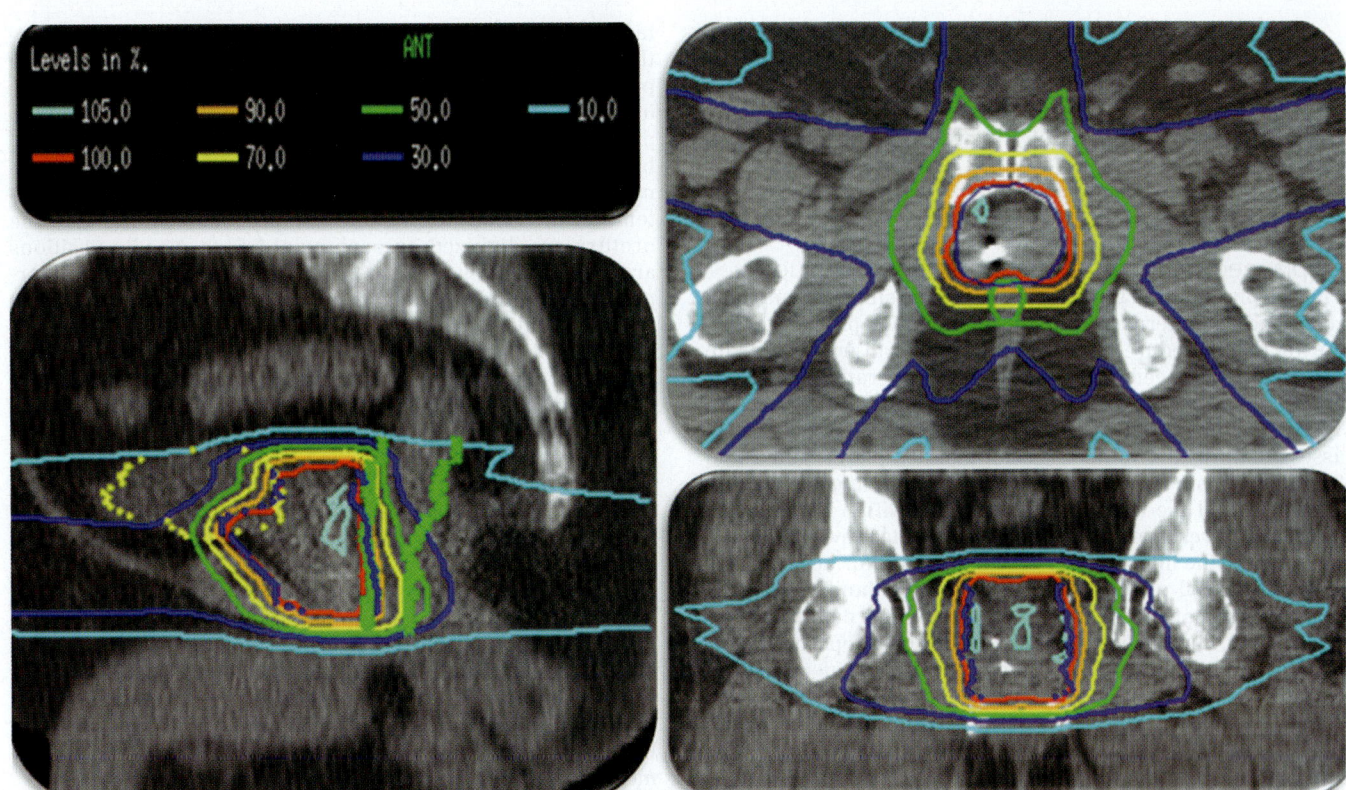

FIGURE 69.8. Dose distribution and dose–volume histogram display for a typical five-field intensity-modulated radiotherapy treatment plan whose prescription to the prostate target is 86.4 Gy. (Courtesy of Daniel Spratt MD.)

Interfractional prostate motion was studied in approximately 50 patients by Crook et al.[278] Gold seeds implanted in the prostate were visualized on kilovolt radiographs taken at the simulation and approximately midway through treatment. Minimal prostate motion was observed in the lateral directions (0.1 to 0.5 cm), but inferior displacements of 0.5 and 1.0 cm or more were observed in 43% and 11% of their patients. Average displacement in the posterior direction was 0.72, 0.62, and 0.46 cm for seeds placed at the seminal vesicles, posterior aspect of the prostate, or apex of the gland, respectively; 60% of patients showed >0.5-cm posterior displacement of the prostate base, and 30% showed >1 cm.

Zelefsky et al.[278a] obtained four serial CT studies for 50 patients (planning scan and three additional scans during the course of therapy). Prostate displacements in the anteroposterior and superior–inferior directions were most frequently observed. The mean prostate motion in the anterroposterior, superoinferior, and left–right directions was 1.2, 0.5, and 0.6 mm, respectively. Anterior–posterior movements were correlated with changes in rectal volume. Patients with large rectal volumes (>60 cm³) and large bladder volumes (>40 cm³) on the planning scan experienced a higher likelihood of having >3-mm systematic displacement of the prostate and seminal vesicles, leading the authors to conclude that these patients may require more generous PTV margins to ensure adequate CTV coverage. However, among patients without larger bladder and rectal volumes, a 1-cm margin around the CTV with a 6-mm margin at the prostate–rectal interface enclosed the posterior, anterior, superoinferior, and left–right aspects of the CTV within the prescription dose level with a probability of 90%, 100%, 99%, and 100%, respectively, indicating that the MSKCC margins provided adequate CTV coverage for most patients.

Intrafractional prostate motion was studied in 20 patients by Huang et al.[279] using pretreatment and posttreatment B-mode rectal ultrasound evaluations. Although the intrafractional motion was relatively insignificant in all directions, the predominant directions of motion were in the anterior and superior directions. Standard deviations of 0.4, 1.3, and 1.0 mm were observed in the lateral, anterior, and superior directions, respectively. Several methods have been developed to reduce uncertainty because of interfractional organ motion and thereby improve treatment delivery using computer-assisted transabdominal ultrasonography, radiopaque marker tracking, or CT/cone-beam image guidance. Recent technologic advances have opened up the possibility of acquiring pretreatment or posttreatment megavoltage or kilovoltage CT images directly on the linear accelerator (LINAC) with the patient in the treatment position, such as TomoTherapy. Langen et al.[280] compared three methods of registering megavoltage CT images from a TomoTherapy unit with the kilovoltage planning CT images and found that manual registration performed using implanted fiducial markers exhibited the least interobserver variability and agreed best with automatic registration computed from the center of mass of the three implanted fiducial markers. LINAC-based kilovoltage image guidance systems are routinely used now for image-guided therapy approaches. They possess capabilities for kilovoltage two-dimensional projection imaging (radiographs), fluoroscopy, and 3D cone-beam CT and are ideally suited for monitoring of interfractional and intrafractional motion.

Using intensity-modulated radiation therapy (IMRT, VMAT), 10-year biochemical control has been in the range of 85% to 88%, with acceptable morbidity. These recent technologic advances have allowed dose escalation, with improvement in the results of treatment. A study from MD Anderson Cancer Center showed that patients with favorable (low risk) prostate cancer treated with 78 Gy had a 10-year biochemical control of 88% compared to 63% in patients treated with 70 Gy. Grade 3 toxicity was 7% versus 1% respectively. A French multicenter trial compared 8,000 to 7,000 cGy in patients with various risk prognostic groupings. The 5-year BCFFR was 76.5% versus 67.9%, respectively. There was a trend toward more toxicity in the 8,000 cGy group (grade 3 rectal toxicity 6.5% and 1.5%, respectively).

In a study comparing 8-year outcomes of RP or EBRT, Kupelian et al. (Cleveland Clinic) reported on 1,054 patients who were treated with surgery and 628 with EBRT. With a median follow-up of 51 months, the PSA relapse-free survival was 72% and 70%, respectively.

Brachytherapy for Early-Stage Disease: Treatment Techniques

Preplanned Transperineal Implantation Techniques

The preplanning technique essentially attempts to map the seed-loading patterns prior to the implantation procedure, and during the procedure, the brachytherapist will try to simulate the preplanned needle positions with the operative conditions and settings. The technique can be summarized as follows: TRUS imaging is obtained before the planned procedure to assess the prostate volume. A computerized plan is generated from the transverse ultrasound images, producing isodose distributions and the ideal location of seeds within the gland to deliver the prescription dose to the prostate. Several days to weeks later, the implantation procedure is performed. Needles are then placed under ultrasonographic guidance through a perineal template according to the coordinates determined by the preplan. Radioactive seeds are individually deposited in the needle with the aid of an applicator or with preloaded seeds on a semirigid strand containing the preplanned number of seeds. In the latter case, this is accomplished by stabilizing the needle obturator that holds the seed column in a fixed position while the needle is withdrawn slowly, depositing a row or series of seeds within the gland. One of the inherent advantages of a stranded-seed approach is the reduction of seed migration and embolization to the lung compared with the use of free seeds. Among patients implanted with loose seeds, usually <2% of the implanted seeds are likely to migrate. There is no evidence of any adverse effect caused by seed embolization.[281]

Careful evaluation of the preplan with attention to dose–volume histogram analyses of both the target and normal tissues is essential to ensure that the dose to the urethra and rectum is within tolerance ranges and the prescription dose is being delivered to the prostate target. In a multi-institutional analysis, there remains a great deal of variability within preplans as to acceptable target volume, seed strength, dose homogeneity, treatment margins, and extracapsular seed placement, although prostate brachytherapy prescription doses are uniform.[282]

Intraoperative Planning Techniques for Prostate Brachytherapy

With the current availability of sophisticated treatment planning programs that can rapidly generate highly conformal dose distributions in the operating room, intraoperative planning for prostate brachytherapy is an attractive method. Intraoperative planning takes advantage of the opportunity of using real-time measurements of the prostate during the procedure, whereas preplanning is often performed several weeks before implantation, frequently under different conditions than the actual operative procedure. Subtle changes in the position of the ultrasound probe, as well as the distortion of the prostate associated with needle placement and subsequent edema, may result in profound changes in the shape of the gland compared with the preplanned prostatic contour. Consequently, intraoperative adjustments of seed and needle placements are frequently required using a preplanned technique, and the postplan CT-based dosimetry does not always correspond to the idealized preplan.

At MSKCC, intraoperative conformal optimization and planning for ultrasound-based transperineal implantation have been routinely used for well more than 10 years.[283] This technique involves a sophisticated optimization system that incorporates acceptable dose ranges allowed within the target, as well as dose constraints for the rectal wall and urethra. An ultrasound probe is positioned in the rectum, and the prostate and normal anatomies are identified. Needles are inserted through the perineal template at the periphery of the prostate. The prostate is subsequently scanned from apex to base, and these 0.5-cm images are transferred to the treatment planning system using a PC-based video capture system. On the computer monitor, the prostate contours and the urethra are digitized on each axial image. Needle positions are identified on each image, and their coordinates are incorporated into a genetic algorithm optimization program. After the optimization program identifies the optimal seed-loading pattern and the dose calculations are completed, isodose displays are superimposed on each transverse ultrasound image and carefully evaluated. Dose–volume histograms for the target volume, rectum, and urethra are also carefully assessed. For the intraoperative plan, the V_{100} for the prostate is set at 95% or higher, and the maximum urethral and rectal dose thresholds are set at <130% and 1 cm^3 <100% of the prescription doses, respectively. The entire planning process from the contouring of images to the generation of the seed-loading pattern requires approximately 10 minutes. Seeds are then loaded with a standard applicator. A cone-beam CT scan from a mobile unit is routinely used to obtain postimplantation dosimetric analysis while the patient is under anesthesia before the conclusion of the procedure to ensure optimal coverage of the target volume with the prescription dose. Figure 69.9 shows a postimplantation CT image used for dosimetric evaluation.

Dose, Isotope, and Activity Considerations for Prostate Brachytherapy

At present, the commonly used dose for LDR interstitial implantation when using ^{125}I is 144 Gy, prescribed to the isodose surface that completely encompasses the prostate as contoured from imaging studies. For ^{103}Pd, 125 Gy is the recommended prescription dose when the isotope is used as monotherapy.[284] There are clear physical differences between these two isotopes. The half-life of ^{125}I is 60 days, with mean photon energy of 27 keV and an initial dose rate of 7 cGy/h.

FIGURE 69.9. Postimplantation computed tomography scan after permanent transperineal ultrasound-guided seed implantation with urethral sparing.

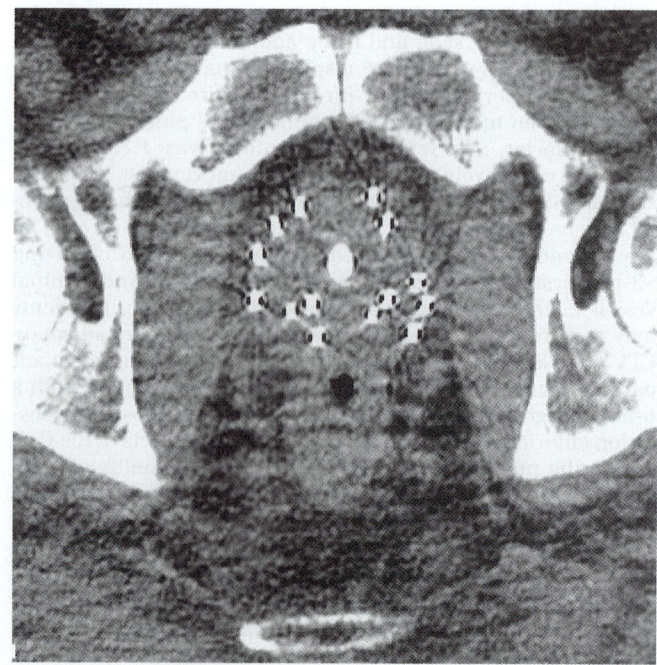

In contrast, the half-life of [103]Pd is 17 days, with mean photon energy of 21 keV and an initial dose rate of 19 cGy/h. Dosimetric analyses of treatment plans performed with either isotope have not revealed significant differences between them.[283] Most retrospective reports[286,287] failed to demonstrate any benefit in terms of local tumor control or long-term complications for either isotope. A randomized trial has been conducted comparing ^{125}I with [103]Pd for the treatment of early-stage prostate cancer. No differences in tumor-control outcomes have been noted between the two arms of the study. Preliminary findings from this study noted that patients treated with [103]Pd had more intense radiation prostatitis in the first month after implantation but recovered from their radiation-related symptoms sooner than ^{125}I patients, consistent with palladium's shorter half-life.[288] In a retrospective analysis, Kollmeier et al.[289] reported the outcome of patients treated with ^{125}I or [103]Pd in conjunction with supplemental EBRT. There were no differences in toxicity or PSA relapse–free survival outcomes between patients who received the [103]Pd or ^{125}I boost.

Postimplantation Dosimetric Evaluation

Postimplantation dosimetric evaluation after prostate brachytherapy is recommended as the standard assessment of the quality of permanent interstitial implantation used for the treatment of prostate cancer.[290] The adequacy of the target coverage with the intended prescription doses is evaluated with surrogate parameters such as volume of the prostate treated to 100% of the prescription dose (V_{100}) and the dose delivered to 90% of the prostate target (D_{90}). These parameters have been shown by several investigators to be associated with biochemical relapse and posttreatment biopsy outcomes.[291–294] Equally important, other parameters of implant quality measure the dose exposure to the urethra and rectum. These measurements have been correlated with postimplantation urinary and rectal-related toxicities.[295–298] Commercial software is routinely available to determine the coverage of the prostate and dose to critical normal-tissue structures. Isodose curves and dose–volume histograms produce a detailed analysis of the radiation dose distribution relative to the prostate and surrounding normal tissues. Postimplantation evaluation is performed on the day of the procedure or 30 days after the procedure. Although the latter time point takes advantage of assessments when prostate edema is less significant after the implant, with potential decreased underestimate of the prostate coverage with the prescription dose, assessments made on the day of the procedure provide more rapid feedback regarding the adequacy of the dose delivered to the prostate.

A summary of published dosimetric outcomes after LDR BT based on postimplantation CT-based dosimetric outcomes is shown in Table 69.11.

Postimplantation evaluation is a critical quality assurance procedure for prostate brachytherapy and provides important feedback to the brachytherapist concerning the quality of the implant, dose delivered to the prostate, and what corrections need to be made to optimize target coverage to reduce normal-tissue dosing. Stock et al.[299] reported that, among patients with low-risk disease who had an optimal dose based on retrospective postimplantation dosimetry evaluation from the day-30 CT scan ($D_{90} > 140$ Gy; $n = 49$), the PSA relapse–free survival at 8 years was 94%, compared to 75% for those who received lower-dose levels ($P = .02$). Investigators from Memorial Sloan Kettering Cancer Center recently demonstrated that higher D_{90} values based on the postimplantation dosimetric analysis from the CT taken on day 0 (the day of the procedure) also were associated with improved long-term biochemical control outcomes.[300] In that report, the 7-year PSA relapse–free survival was 99% compared to 89% for patients with $D_{90} > 140$ and <140 Gy, respectively ($P = .005$).

Safdieh et al.[301] noted that several studies have suggested that brachytherapy utilization has markedly decreased, coinciding with the recent increased utilization of IMRT, as well as an increase in urologist-owned centers. They investigated brachytherapy or EBRT utilization in patients with prostate cancer at a large, hospital-based registry (2004 to 2012) and were abstracted from the National Cancer Database (NCDB). To be included, men had to be clinically staged as T1c-T2aNx-0Mx-0, Gleason 6, PSA = 10.0 ng/mL.

There were 89,413 men included in this study, of which 37,054 (41.6%) received only EBRT and 52,089 received prostate brachytherapy. Of those who received brachytherapy, 47,710 (91.6%) received monotherapy and the remaining received brachytherapy as a boost to EBRT. The use of brachytherapy declined over time from 62.9% in 2004 to 51.3% in 2012 ($P < .001$).

This decline was noted in both academic facilities (from 60.8% in 2004 to 47.0% in 2012, $P < .001$) as well as non-academic facilities (from 63.7% in 2004 to 53.0% in 2012, $P < .001$). The use of IMRT increased during this same time period from 18.4% in 2004 to 38.2% in 2012 ($P < .001$). On multivariate analysis, treatment at an academic center (OR 0.89; 95% CI = 0.87 to 0.92, $P < .001$), increasing age, and years of diagnosis from 2006 to 2012 were significantly associated with reduced brachytherapy usage.

High dose rate (HDR) brachytherapy (iridium-192 sources) has been used in some institutions to treat patients with localized prostate cancer, including monotherapy. For techniques' description and dose schedules, the reader is referred to Chapters 27 and 28.

Results of Standard Treatment Interventions for Clinically Localized Prostate Cancer

Outcome with Radical Prostatectomy

Bianco et al.[302] reported the long-term outcomes of 1,963 patients who underwent RP, all performed by one surgeon. The positive margin rate was 12%. The overall 5- and 10-year biochemical tumor-control outcomes were 82% and 77%, respectively. Among patients with pretreatment PSA levels of 4 to 10, 10 to 20, and >20 ng/mL, the 10-year PSA relapse–free survival outcomes were 83%, 64%, and 47%, respectively. The overall cause-specific survival was 99% and 95%. At 24 months after surgery, 60% were potent, continent, and free of disease. Roehl et al.[302a] recently reported the outcome of 3,478 men who underwent RP for clinically localized prostate cancer at Washington University. In that report, the mean follow-up was 65 months.

TABLE 69.11 POSTIMPLANT COMPUTED TOMOGRAPHY–BASED DOSIMETRIC PARAMETERS WITH PERMANENT PROSTATE BRACHYTHERAPY: TARGET COVERAGE AND NORMAL-TISSUE DOSES

Institution	V_{100} (%)	D_{90} (Gy)	V_{150} (%)	Rectal Dose	Urethral Dose
BC Cancer Agency	Loose, 90	153	52.5	V_{100}, 1.29 cm³	NS
	Stranded, 91	152	60	V_{100}, 1.5 cm²	
Mt. Sinai Medical Center (New York)	94	175	56	D_{30}, 46 Gy	D_{30}, 209
				D_{10}, 117 Gy	D_{10}, 220
Wheeling Medical Center (West Virginia)	95	110	55	Mean, 78%	Mean, 120%
		167	68	Maximum, 115%	Maximum, 141%
Memorial Sloan Kettering Cancer Center	96	173	67	Mean, 32%	Mean, 103%
				Maximum, 72%	Maximum, 129%

NS, Not stated.

The overall biochemical recurrence (BCR) rate at 10 years was 32%, with a median time to failure of 28 months. The 10-year PSA relapse-free survival rates for patients with preoperative PSA levels of <2.6, 2.6 to 4, 4.1 to 10, and >10 ng/mL were 91%, 78%, 74%, and 49%, respectively. Multivariate analysis revealed that predictors for PSA relapse-free survival outcomes included the preoperative PSA level, clinical tumor stage, Gleason sum, pathologic stage, and treatment era. The 10-year cancer-specific and overall survival rates were 97% and 83%, respectively. The cancer-specific survival outcome was influenced by the pathologic stage (P < .004), Gleason sum (P = .004), and treatment era (P = .04).

Han et al.[304] reported the long-term outcome of RP from the Johns Hopkins Hospital. In that report, 2,091 men underwent RP. In this series, 79% of patients had PSA levels of <10 ng/mL, and 62% of the patients had Gleason scores of ≤6. The mean follow-up was 6.3 years. The overall 10- and 15-year PSA relapse-free survival outcomes were 85% and 79%, respectively. The 10-year PSA control rates for patients with preoperative PSA values of 0 to 4, 4 to 10, 10.1 to 20, and >20 ng/mL were 91%, 79%, 57%, and 48%, respectively.

Outcome with Conventional External Beam Radiation Therapy for Low-Risk Disease

Kuban et al.[305] reported the results of a large multi-institutional analysis comprising 4,839 patients with T1-T2 prostate cancer treated with EBRT between 1986 and 1995; no patient received neoadjuvant hormone therapy . The median follow-up was 6.3 years. Most of the patients included (70%) were treated with conventional EBRT, and 30% were treated with 3DCRT planning techniques. Prescription doses ranged from 60 to 78 Gy. For the cohort of patients treated to dose levels of <70 Gy, the median dose was 67 Gy; among those patients who received 70 Gy or more, the median dose in this cohort was 72 Gy. PSA failure as defined according to ASTRO definition was three consecutive rising PSA values above the nadir value. The overall 8-year PSA control rates for patients with pretreatment PSA values of 0 to 4, 4 to 9.9, 10 to 20, and >20 to 30 ng/mL were 80%, 60%, 46%, and 34%, respectively. The overall 8-year PSA control rates for patients with posttreatment nadir PSA values of 0 to 0.49, 0.5 to 0.99, 1 to 1.99, and ≥2.0 ng/mL were 93%, 88%, 86%, and 72%, respectively. Higher prescription dose levels of ≥72 Gy were associated with a significant decrease in PSA relapse rates, and these differences were most noted among patients with intermediate- and higher-risk disease. Although there was no apparent dose response for low-risk patients, the number of patients who received higher doses in this study was small.

Dose Escalation for Low-Risk Prostate Cancer

Phase III randomized trials and several single-institution trials have confirmed the advantage of high-dose CRT for patients with localized prostate cancer. These trials have shown long-term biochemical control advantages especially among patients with intermediate- and high-risk disease. More recently, however, updates of some these studies have indicated a benefit for the application of higher radiation dose levels even for patients with favorable-risk disease. The phase III trial from MD Anderson Hospital accrued 301 patients with T1-T3 prostate cancer, of whom 150 were treated to 70 Gy (conventional EBRT) and 151 were treated to 78 Gy (conventional EBRT followed by a 3D boost). The PSA relapse-free survival rates for the 78- and 70-Gy arms were 70% and 64%, respectively (P = .03). In a recent update of this trial,[306] a significant improvement in 8-year biochemical control was noted among low-risk patients who received 78 Gy compared to 70 Gy (88% vs. 63%; P = .042; Fig. 69.10).

Zietman et al.[307] reported the result of a randomized trial of 393 patients with T1-T2 prostate cancer with pretreatment PSA levels of <15 ng/mL. Patients were randomized to receive conventional EBRT to a dose level of 70.2 or 79.2 Gy. In both treatment arms, radiotherapy was delivered using a combination of photon and proton beams. The median follow-up in this study was 5.5 years. The 5-year PSA relapse-free survival rates for the low- and high-dose arms were 61% and 80%, respectively, which represented a 49% risk reduction in biochemical failure. What was most noteworthy in this trial was that a clear advantage for higher dose was observed among the subset of patients with low-risk disease, which represented the majority of patients accrued to the trial (PSA of <10 ng/mL, stage ≤ T2a, or Gleason score of <6). In this subgroup of patients, a significant advantage for higher doses was observed, with an associated 51% risk reduction in biochemical relapse (80% vs. 60% for higher vs. lower doses; P < .001).

The experience from MSKCC was reported by Zelefsky et al.[308] in 2,551 patients with T1-T3 prostate cancer treated with follow-up that extended beyond 20 years. The radiation dose was systematically increased from 64.8 to 86.4 Gy by increments of 5.4 Gy in consecutive groups of patients. This study also demonstrated an advantage for dose escalation in low-

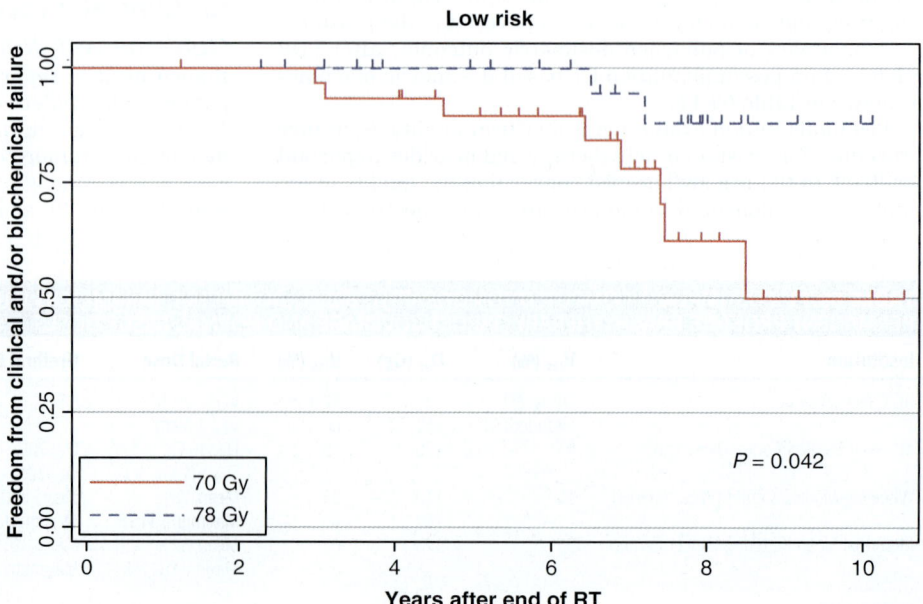

FIGURE 69.10. Freedom from biochemical failure for the subset of low-risk patients treated in the MD Anderson randomized trial with 78 versus 70 Gy. (Reprinted from Kuban DA, Tucker SL, Dong L, et al. Long-term results of the M. D. Anderson randomized dose-escalation trial for prostate cancer. *Int J Radiat Oncol Biol Phys* 2008;70[1]:67–74. Copyright © 2008 Elsevier. With permission.)

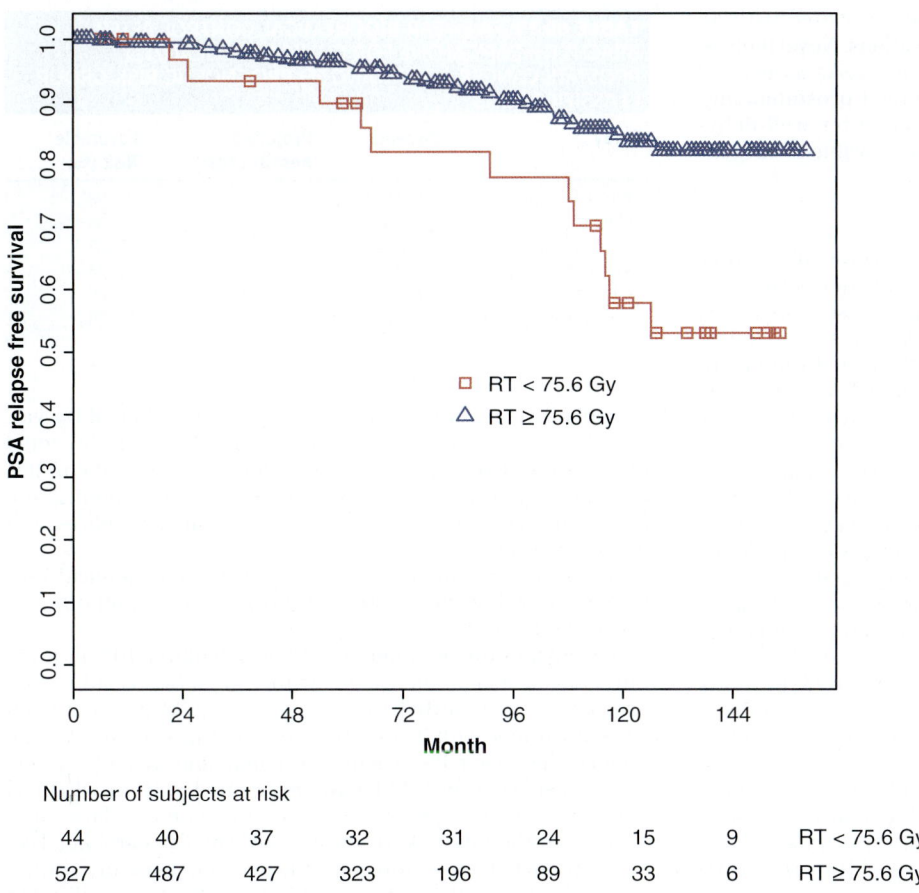

FIGURE 69.11 Memorial Sloan Kettering Cancer Center experience for prostate-specific antigen relapse-free survival outcomes for low-risk patients treated with 75.6 Gy and higher versus lower doses. (Reprinted from Zelefsky MJ, Chan H, Hunt M, et al. Long-term outcome of high dose intensity modulated radiation therapy for patients with clinically localized prostate cancer. *J Urol* 2006;176[4]:1415–1419. Copyright © 2006 American Urological Association. With permission.)

Number of subjects at risk

| 44 | 40 | 37 | 32 | 31 | 24 | 15 | 9 | RT < 75.6 Gy |
| 527 | 487 | 427 | 323 | 196 | 89 | 33 | 6 | RT ≥ 75.6 Gy |

risk patients. The 10-year PSA relapse-free survival among patients with low-risk disease who received dose levels of 75.6 Gy and higher was 84%, compared to 70% for patients who received lower-dose levels (P = .04; Fig. 69.11). In this report, there were no apparent differences in long-term outcomes among patients who received 81 versus 75.5 Gy for low-risk disease. Others did not demonstrate dose escalation advantages for low-risk disease,[309,310] but the follow-up was relatively limited in these studies. The 10-year biochemical outcomes from MSKCC patients for IMRT-treated patients have been reported.[311] The 10-year actuarial PSA relapse-free survival rates for favorable-, intermediate-, and unfavorable-risk group patients were 81%, 78%, and 62%, respectively. The 10-year actuarial distant metastases–free survival outcomes for favorable-, intermediate-, and unfavorable-risk group were 0%, 6%, and 10%, respectively. The 10-year actuarial risk of a prostate cancer–related death for favorable-, intermediate-, and unfavorable-risk group was 0%, 3%, and 14%.

Michalski et al.[312] reported the outcome of RTOG 94-06, which evaluated dose escalation using 3D conformal radiotherapy for patients with localized prostate cancer. Patients were accrued on five sequential dose levels: 68.4, 73.8, 79.2, 74, and 78 Gy. For patients with low-risk disease (n = 403), the 5-year PSA relapse-free survival outcomes for these respective dose levels were 68%, 73%, 67%, 84%, and 80%.

Comparison of EBRT Outcomes with Surgery for Early-Stage Prostate Cancer

Kupelian et al.[311] compared the 8-year outcomes of surgery and EBRT from the Cleveland Clinic. In this report, 1,054 patients were treated with surgery and 628 were treated with EBRT. Treatments (surgery or radiotherapy) were given between 1990 and 1998, and the median follow-up was 51 months. There were significant differences in the patient groups

because, in general, those treated with surgery were younger and had lower clinical stages, pretreatment PSA levels, and Gleason scores. The 8-year PSA relapse-free survival outcome for patients who underwent RP and EBRT was 72% and 70%, respectively (P = .01). Multivariate analysis demonstrated that the clinical stage, pretreatment PSA, biopsy Gleason score, use of neoadjuvant therapy, and year of treatment were all independent predictors of disease relapse, whereas the treatment modality (RT vs. surgery) did not influence likelihood of failure. These authors also noted a benefit for higher radiation doses in the favorable-risk subset of patients. Among favorable-risk patients who received 72 Gy or more, the 8-year PSA relapse-free survival outcome was similar (P = .08) to that of patients treated with RP and significantly better, in turn, than that of patients treated with RT to dose levels of <72 Gy (P < .001). Similarly, Zelefsky et al.[242] found similar distant metastases–free survival outcomes between high-dose IMRT and surgery for low-risk patients.

In the absence of randomized trials comparing surgery to RT, it is difficult to definitively make claims of the superiority of one treatment over another. It has been stated frequently that, whereas the results of radiation and radical surgery are comparable up to 10 years, there is a rapid decrement in the probabilities of both disease-free and overall survival after that time point among irradiated patients. However, such conclusions are likely erroneous owing to selection bias factors favoring a younger cohort with more favorable prognostic features who are more often chosen for surgery compared with radiation therapy. In addition, because of the lack of information in most radiation therapy series of the pathologic status of the lymph nodes, patients with microscopic nodal disease will likely be included in radiation therapy reports yet routinely excluded from surgical series. An additional argument posed for surgery is that if such an approach fails, salvage radiotherapy remains a viable option, whereas for those who fail radiotherapy, salvage surgery can be associated with an increased of risk of postoperative complications. Nevertheless, patients need to be informed that there are risks associated with salvage radiation therapy after a failed prostatectomy, and the likelihood of a successful outcome after well-delivered primary radiotherapy is high and comparable to surgery outcomes.

Outcome with Brachytherapy

Similar to the predictors of biochemical outcome after EBRT for prostate cancer, PSA relapse-free survival after permanent seed implantation depends on several prognostic variables, including the pretreatment PSA, biopsy Gleason score, clinical stage, and the implant dose delivered to the target volume. In general, among patients with pretreatment PSA of ≤10 ng/mL, permanent seed implantation alone is associated with excellent biochemical outcome and appears comparable with other local interventions. Fifteen-year outcomes were reported by Sylvester et al.[313] from 215 patients treated between 1988 and 1992. The PSA relapse-free survival outcomes were 86%, 80%, and 62% for favorable-, intermediate-, and high-risk patients, respectively. Similarly, Taira et al.[314] reported on 1,656 patients. For low-risk patients, the 7-year biochemical tumor control, cause-specific survival, and overall survival outcomes were noted to be 98.6%, 99%, and 77.5%, respectively.

Eleven institutions combined data on 2,693 patients treated with permanent interstitial brachytherapy monotherapy for T1-T2 prostate cancer.[294] Of these patients, 1,831 (68%) were treated with ^{125}I (median dose, 144 Gy) and 862 (32%) were treated with ^{103}Pd (median dose, 108 Gy). The median follow-up was 63 months. The 8-year PSA relapse-free survival outcomes for favorable-, intermediate-, and unfavorable-risk patients were 82%, 70%, and 48%, respectively ($P < .001$) according to the ASTRO consensus definition. Among patients in whom the dose to 90% of the prostate (D_{90}) was >130 Gy, the 8-year PSA relapse-free survival outcome was 90% compared with 73% for those with D_{90} dose levels of ≤130 Gy ($P < .001$). The PSA nadir value at 3 years after implantation was associated with the long-term biochemical outcome. The 8-year PSA relapse-free survival outcomes were 92%, 86%, 79%, and 67%, respectively, for patients who achieved PSA nadir values of 0 to 0.49, 0.5 to 0.99, 1.0 to 1.99, and >2.0 ng/mL ($P < .001$). Among patients who were free of biochemical relapse at 8 years, the median nadir level was 0.1 ng/mL, and 90% of these patients achieved a nadir PSA level of <0.6 ng/mL.

Stone et al.[315] reported on 2,111 patients who underwent brachytherapy followed for a median of 6 years. In this group, 56% of the patients were treated with ^{125}I, 10% were treated with ^{103}Pd, and 34% were treated with combined external beam radiotherapy and ^{103}Pd implant. Among low-risk patients, the PSA relapse-free survival outcome at 12 years was 88%. Significant predictors of long-term biochemical tumor control included the use of ADT ($P = .03$), pretreatment PSA level ($P = .026$), and a higher biologically effective dose ($P = .003$). Among patients who had a posttreatment biopsy 2 years after treatment, higher biologically effective dose levels were associated with improved local tumor-control outcomes.

In an update of the outcomes of real-time intraoperative planning at MSKCC reported by Zelefsky et al.,[300] 1,466 patients with prostate cancer were treated with permanent interstitial implantation using a transrectal ultrasound-guided approach. Real-time intraoperative treatment planning, which incorporated inverse planning optimization, was used. The 5-year PSA relapse-free survival outcomes for favorable- and intermediate-risk patients were 98% and 95%, respectively. In these patients, no dosimetric parameter was identified that influenced the biochemical outcome. For this cohort of patients, the use of androgen deprivation did not affect the long-term PSA relapse-free survival outcomes. Among patients treated with ^{125}I, improved biochemical

TABLE 69.12 FIVE-YEAR BIOCHEMICAL CONTROL AFTER BRACHYTHERAPY ALONE FOR CLINICALLY LOCALIZED PROSTATE CANCER ACCORDING TO PROGNOSTIC RISK GROUP CLASSIFICATIONS			
Study	Patients	Projected Results (Year)	Favorable Risk (%)
Taira et al.[314]	1,656	7	98
Sylvester et al.[313]	215	15	86
Multi-institutional[294]	2,693	8	82
Stone et al.[315]	2,111	12	88
Potters et al.[292]	1,449	12	89
Zelefsky et al.[300]	1,466	7	98

control outcomes were observed for patients who had D_{90} values of >140 Gy compared to lower doses. It should be noted that this improved biochemical control outcome based on this dosimetric parameter was observed for postimplantation, CT-based assessments made on the day of the procedure (and not 30 days later).

Table 69.12 summarizes the published biochemical outcomes after low dose rate interstitial seed implantation according to prognostic risk groups.

Brachytherapy with iodine-125 or palladium-103, in prostate cancer, has yielded comparable or better results than prostatectomy or EBRT. In a report of 2,693 patients from 11 institutions with T1-T2 tumors, for those with low-risk tumors, the 8 year PSA relapse-free outcome was 82%. Stone et al.[315] reported on 2,111 patients treated with brachytherapy. With a median follow-up of 6 years, the PSA relapse-free survival in the low-risk group was 88% at 12 years. Zelefsky et al. reported on 1,466 patients treated with interstitial brachytherapy with a 5-year PSA relapse-free survival in the group with favorable tumors of 98%. Equal results have been reported with HDR brachytherapy, usually combined with external beam irradiation.[300]

ACUTE AND LATE TREATMENT-RELATED SEQUELAE OF STANDARD TREATMENT INTERVENTIONS

Sequelae of Radical Prostatectomy

Complication rates after prostatectomy vary in the literature and recently have been shown to depend on the experience of the surgeon. Begg et al.[316] used the Medicare claim records from 11,522 patients who underwent prostatectomy between 1992 and 1996. Postoperative morbidity was found to be significantly reduced in hospitals that were considered to have high volume compared with lower-volume ones (27% vs. 32%; $P = .03$) and among surgeons with a high-volume practice compared to those with lower volumes (26% vs. 32%; $P < .001$).

Immediate intraoperative/postoperative complications include pelvic pain and transient incontinence. Although intraoperative blood loss can range from 300 to 4,000 mL, meticulous surgical technique should reduce blood loss. The operative mortality rate has been reported to be 1% to 2%, but in experienced hands, the incidence is a fraction of 1%. The incidence of postoperative stress incontinence ranges from 5% to 57%.

Catalona et al.[317] reported on the complication rates in 1,870 patients who underwent RP. They reported a 2% incidence of a thromboembolic event and a 4% incidence of an anastomotic stricture. Recovery of urinary continence depended on the age of the patient. Among patients in their 50s, 60s, and 70s, the likelihood of persistent urinary incontinence was 3%, 8%, and 13%, respectively. The incidence of impotence after bilateral and unilateral nerve-sparing surgery procedures was 53% and 32%, respectively. Bilateral nerve-sparing procedure was associated with improved potency preservation among patients who were younger than 70 years of age (71% vs. 48%; $P < .001$), whereas these differences were not significant in the older age group.

Bianco et al.[302] reported continence and potency outcomes in 1,472 patients who underwent surgery since 1991 and were operated on by a single surgeon. Among 1,288 patients who were continent prior to surgery, the actuarial likelihood of maintained continence was 91% at 12 months and 95% at 24 months. Of 785 patients with potency information available, the median time to erectile function recovery was 12 months, and the 2-year likelihood of potency preservation was 70%.

A large review from the Nationwide Inpatient Sample extracted from this dataset 11,889 patients who underwent RARP and compared the perioperative complication rates to 7,389 patients who underwent an open RP.[318] This analysis found that, among patients undergoing a RARP, significantly lower likelihoods for blood transfusions and intraoperative and postoperative complications were observed compared to the open prostatectomy procedure. In addition, a shorter duration of hospital stay was noted for the patients who underwent a RARP. However, one of the limitations of this retrospective study was the fact that these findings were not adjusted by the clinical stage of the patients and the surgeon's experience or volume, which play important roles in the frequency of surgical-related complications.

Sequelae of Conventional External Beam Radiation Therapy

EBRT delivered with conventional techniques is fairly well tolerated, although grade 2 or higher acute rectal morbidity (discomfort, tenesmus, diarrhea) or urinary symptoms (frequency, nocturia, urgency, dysuria) requiring medication occur in approximately 60% of patients. Symptoms usually appear during the 3rd week of treatment and resolve within days to weeks after treatment is completed. The incidence of late complications that develop ≥6 months after completion of treatment is significantly lower, whereas serious complications that require corrective surgical intervention are rare. In general, the incidence of chronic urinary sequelae (i.e., cystitis, hematuria, urethral stricture, or bladder contracture) using conformal treatment delivery techniques is <5%, and the incidence of grade 3 and 4 urinary-related complications requiring major surgical interventions or hospitalization is <1%. The incidence of chronic intestinal or rectal sequelae (chronic diarrhea, proctitis, or rectal bleeding) that requires medical management ranges from 3% to 10%, and <1% of grade 3 to 4 complications are observed after more targeted treatment delivery techniques such as IMRT and image-guided radiotherapy. Fecal urgency and incontinence are documented side effects after treatment and have been reported to occur in <2% of patients, occur less than once per week, and are often associated with incontinence for flatulence.[319] Most complications attributed to radiation therapy are observed within the first 3 to 4 years after treatment, and the likelihood of complications developing after 5 years is low. The risk of complications is increased when radiation doses exceed 72 Gy. Several factors have been associated with increased bowel or rectal toxicity after EBRT,[272,319–325] and these include the volume of the rectum exposed to higher doses of radiation, increasing age of the patient, concomitant use of ADT, and the presence of diabetes and inflammatory bowel disease. Even patients with a prior history of inflammatory bowel disease currently in remission may have significant increases of rectal toxicity, and alternative treatments should be considered for these patients. Among patients who undergo radiotherapy and experience acute rectal side effects, a higher incidence of late rectal toxicity has been observed.[323,325]

Michalski et al.[326] published a report on the toxicity outcomes of various risk groups enrolled in RTOG 9406, a phase I dose escalation study. The dose levels evaluated in this report included patients treated to the initial two dose levels of the study, 68.4 and 73.8 Gy. The median follow-up times in these subgroups ranged from 2.2 to 3.4 years. The acute grade 2 bowel/rectal toxicity rates ranged from 16% to 25%. The crude incidence of late bowel/rectal toxicities ranged from 2% to 8%. With a median follow-up of 2.5 years, the crude late grade 2 and 3 gastrointestinal (GI) toxicities for those patients treated to 78 Gy (2-Gy fractions) were 22% and 2%, respectively.

Storey et al.[327] reported late rectal toxicity among patients treated on the phase III trial form the MD Anderson Hospital. The 5-year actuarial risks of late grade 2 rectal toxicity for the 70- and 78-Gy dose level arms were 14% and 21%, respectively. In that report, the dose–volume histogram analyses of the patients treated to 78 Gy were analyzed to ascertain whether there were any predictive patterns for late rectal toxicity. These investigators reported a significant correlation for the percentage of the rectum treated to 70 Gy or higher and the likelihood of late rectal toxicity. Patients with >25% of the rectal wall treated to 70 Gy or higher had a 37% risk of grade 2 rectal toxicity, compared with 13% among patients who had <25% of the rectal wall exposed to these doses ($P = .05$). In an update of that experience, Kuban et al.[306] noted that the volume of rectum exposed to higher radiation doses was associated with the risk of rectal toxicity after external beam radiotherapy. The incidence of grade 2 rectal toxicity was 46% when >26% of the rectal volume was exposed to >70 Gy of the prescription dose. In contrast, among patients who had lower volume of rectum exposed to these dose levels, the incidence of grade 2 toxicity was significantly lower (14%).

Zelefsky et al.[328] reported the long-term tolerance of high-dose CRT at MSKCC. The 10-year actuarial rate of grade 2 or higher rectal toxicity was 9%. The use of IMRT significantly lowered the risk of grade 2 and higher toxicities from 13% to 5% ($P < .001$). This decline in rectal toxicity was observed despite the application of higher-dose levels of 81 Gy with IMRT compared to generally lower doses used with 3DCRT of 75.6 Gy (Fig. 69.12). In addition, patients who experienced acute GI side effects during treatment were six times more likely to experience late GI toxicities than were patients who did not experience such acute side effects (42% vs. 9%; $P < .001$). The 10-year incidence of grade 2 or higher late urinary toxicities was 15%, and the predictors for late toxicity included higher radiation doses and the presence of acute urinary symptoms during the course of EBRT. The 10-year toxicity outcomes of 81-Gy IMRT were recently updated by investigators from

FIGURE 69.12. Actuarial likelihood of late grade 2 or greater rectal toxicities or late grade 2 or greater rectal toxicities. (Reprinted from Zelefsky MJ, Chan H, Hunt M, et al. Long-term outcome of high dose intensity modulated radiation therapy for patients with clinically localized prostate cancer. *J Urol* 2006;176[4]:1415–1419. Copyright © 2006 American Urological Association. With permission.)

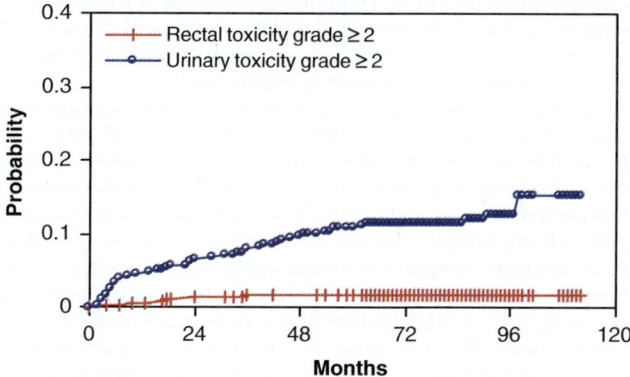

MSKCC.[329] The incidence of grade 2 and 3 GI toxicities was 2% and 1%, respectively. The 10-year actuarial incidence of grade 2 and higher urinary-related toxicities was 17%.

Peeters et al.[330] described the incidence of acute and late complications in a multicenter randomized trial comparing 68- to 78-Gy 3DCRT. The median follow-up was 31 months. The 3-year incidence of grade 2 and higher GI and genitourinary (GU) toxicities for the 68-Gy dose arm was 23% and 28.5%, respectively. The 3-year incidence of grade 2 and higher GI and GU toxicities for the 78-Gy dose arm was 26.5% and 30%, respectively. The differences were not significant. However, the authors did note a significant increase in grade 3 rectal toxicity requiring laser cauterization for the higher-dose arm. For patients treated to 78 Gy, the incidence of grade 3 rectal bleeding at 3 years was 10%, compared to 2% for those treated to 68 Gy. The following variables were found to be predictive of late GI toxicity: a history of abdominal surgery ($P < .001$) and the presence of pretreatment GI symptoms ($P = .001$). The following variables were predictive of late GU toxicity: pretreatment urinary symptoms ($P < .001$), the use of neoadjuvant ADT ($P < .001$), and prior transurethral resection of the prostate ($P = .006$).

Urethral strictures have been observed in 1.5% of 1,100 patients treated with 3DCRT. Grade 3 hematuria requiring fulguration was observed in <0.5% of the patients. Among patients who previously underwent a TURP, a 4% incidence of stricture development after 3DCRT was observed.[331] Other late urinary toxicities were not observed among patients with a prior history of a TURP. Lee et al.[332] observed a 2% incontinence rate among patients with a prior history of TURP who were treated with EBRT, compared with a 0.2% rate in patients without a prior TURP. At present, it does not appear that the use of IMRT has significantly reduced long-term urinary symptoms compared to conventional 3DCRT.

Potency Preservation with External Beam Radiation Therapy

The rates of erectile dysfunction after EBRT ranged from 6% to 84%.[333] The wide range of outcomes is a reflection of the varying assessment tools used and disparity in patient population, with heterogeneity of comorbidities, ages, and baseline functional status. Most studies show a progressive decline in erectile function with longer follow-ups, consistent with what is observed in an aging population with coexisting comorbidities such as hypertension, atherosclerotic heart disease, and diabetes. Investigators from the University of Chicago reported potency rates after EBRT.[334] With a median follow-up of 34 months, actuarial potency rates at 1, 20, 40, and 60 months were 96%, 75%, 59%, and 53%, respectively. In one report[335] comparing erectile function between patients who received 68 versus 78 Gy, no differences were observed between the different dose levels. Overall, in the studied cohort, the incidence of erectile dysfunction at 1 and 2 years after therapy was 27% and 36%, respectively. Aside from erectile dysfunction, other aspects of sexual dysfunction after radiotherapy include decreased volume of ejaculate, absence of ejaculate, decreased intensity of orgasm, and decreased libido. A summary of reported potency rates after treatment is shown in Table 69.13.

Significant limitations exist with the aforementioned reported potency preservation rates because the data are derived from retrospective analyses and information was often obtained without the use of validated questionnaires. Prospective studies suggest that when patients are assessed with validated tools, erectile dysfunction—defined as inability to achieve adequate erection sufficient for sexual intercourse—reaches 60% to 70%. What also complicates the interpretation of published incidence rates is the multifactorial nature of erectile dysfunction. The factors that impact erectile function include age, presence of medical comorbidities such

as cardiac disease and diabetes, antihypertensive medications, baseline erectile function, and the use of neoadjuvant and concurrent hormonal therapy. Pinkawa et al.[336] observed that the presence of spontaneous erection in evening or morning before treatment was a strong predictor for maintained erectile function after radiation therapy.

Radiation-mediated impotence is likely multifactorial. However, it has been observed that 63% of patients evaluated for impotence after radiation therapy were diagnosed as having arteriogenic dysfunction, whereas 31% had cavernosal dysfunction. Only 3% were believed to have neurogenic impotence.[336] Sildenafil administration results in significant improvement in erectile function.[337,338] In one report, sildenafil improved erectile function in 74% of patients who underwent 3DCRT (median dose, 75.6 Gy), whereas 22% of patients had no response.[338]

Low Dose Rate Brachytherapy: Acute and Late Toxicity

Urinary Toxicity

Acute urinary retention (AUR) is a known risk that can occur immediately after prostate brachytherapy, and the incidence varies in the literature. Roeloffzen et al.[339] recently reported the incidence and predictors of AUR in a cohort of 714 patients who were treated with ^{125}I brachytherapy. In 8% of patients, retention developed at a median of 30 days from the implantation procedure. In that report, multivariate analysis revealed that patients with prostate volume >35 cm^3 experienced a higher incidence of AUR compared to patients with smaller volumes (10.4% vs. 5.4%). In addition, those with higher International Prostate Symptom Scores (IPSS) had a higher likelihood of developing urinary retention, consistent with other reports. Other reports for AUR after low dose rate brachytherapy range from 5% to 15%.[340–342] There does not seem to be any relationship between dosimetric outcomes, such as urethral dose and V$_{150}$, and the incidence of AUR after brachytherapy because this condition seems to be more related to acute trauma and intraprostatic inflammation and edema. Consistent with this notion is the fact that some reports demonstrated that greater number of needles placed or seeds deposited is associated with higher rates of AUR.[340–342] In general, almost all patients after prostate brachytherapy develop acute urinary symptoms such as urinary frequency, urgency, and occasional urge incontinence. Depending on the isotope used, these symptoms often peak at 1 to 3 months after the procedure and subsequently gradually decline over the ensuing 3 to 6 months. Most patients significantly benefit with the use of an α-blocker, which ameliorates such symptoms in 60% to 70% of patients.

TABLE 69.13 INCIDENCE OF ERECTILE DYSFUNCTION AFTER RADIATION THERAPY FOR PROSTATE CANCER

Study	Treatment	Number of Patients	Follow-Up (Month)	Erectile Dysfunction Incidence (%)
Mameghan et al.	EBRT	42	55	45 at 2 y
Roach et al.	EBRT	60	21	38
Crook et al.	EBRT	158	33	35
Mantz et al.	EBRT	68	18	25 at 2 y
Zelefsky et al.	EBRT	544	42	39
Pilepich et al.	EBRT	230	54	72
Blasko et al.	BRT	469	38	≤70 y of age: 15 70 y of age: 50
Stock et al.	BRT	65	18	21
Zelefsky et al.	BRT	221	48	29
Merrick et al.	BRT	209	40	61 at 6 y

BRT, brachytherapy; EBRT, external beam radiation therapy.
Modified from Incrocci L, Slob AK, Levendag PC. Sexual (dys)function after radiotherapy for prostate cancer: a review. *Int J Radiat Oncol Biol Phys* 2002;52(3):681–693. Copyright © 2002 Elsevier. With permission.

Keyes et al.[343] reported on the acute and long-term urinary outcomes in 712 patients who were treated with ^{125}I permanent interstitial implantation who were followed for a median of 5 years. At 6 and 12 months after the procedure, approximately 37% and 23% experienced grade 2 acute urinary toxicities, and 4% and 2% experienced acute grade 3 urinary toxicities. Most urinary symptoms resolved within 12 months after the procedure, and significant residual toxicity was unusual. Multivariate analysis demonstrated that the use of ADT before implantation, higher baseline IPSS, and use of higher number of needles was associated with increased rates of grade 2 acute toxicity. The 5-year likelihood of developing late grade 2 and 3 urinary toxicities was 24% and 6%, respectively. Fewer than 1% of patients experienced a grade 4 urinary toxicity. In this report, predictors for increased risk of grade 2 or higher late urinary toxicity included the following variables: higher baseline IPSS, maximal postimplantation IPSS, presence of acute toxicity, and higher prostate V_{150}. The demonstration in this report that the V_{150} was an independent predictor of late urinary toxicity after brachytherapy highlights the importance of maintaining tight urethral dose constraints during the planning for brachytherapy. Urinary incontinence requiring pads was reported in <1% of treated patients. In a more recent report from MSKCC,[243] the 7-year incidence of grade 2 and 3 urinary toxicities after ^{125}I brachytherapy for low-risk patients was 15% and 2.2, respectively.

Rectal Tolerance

Zelefsky et al.[243] reported 5.1% and 1.1.% grade 2 and 3 late rectal toxicity, respectively, after prostate brachytherapy among 448 low-risk patients treated with ^{125}I implantation. Phan et al.[344] reported a 4% incidence of grade 2 rectal toxicity after permanent interstitial implantation and <1% incidence of grade 3 toxicity. In general, the incidence of grade 2 rectal toxicity after prostate brachytherapy ranges from 4% to 12%. Grade 3 or 4 rectal toxicity is unusual (<2%). Grade 2 symptoms manifest as rectal bleeding or increased mucous discharge. The onset of symptoms often peaks at 8 to 12 months and is self-limited in nature. Several reports noted that rectal bleeding is associated with the rectal dose and its volume exposed to a particular dose. Snyder et al.[297] noted that the rectal volume in cubic centimeters exposed to the prescription dose of 160 Gy correlated with the incidence of grade 2 proctitis. For patients with 0.8 cm³ or less of rectal volume exposed to the prescription dose, no patient developed proctitis; from 0.8 to 1.8 cm³, approximately 8% of patients developed rectal bleeding. However, among patients with >1.8 cm³ of the rectal volume exposed to 160 Gy, 25% of patients developed rectal toxicity. The American Brachytherapy Society recommends that rectal dose constraints should be maintained to restrict the dose to 1 cm of the rectum to the prescription dose or less to reduce the risk of rectal toxicity after brachytherapy.[345]

Erectile Function

Erectile dysfunction after brachytherapy has been reported to occur in from 20% to 80% of patients. The age of the patients, baseline function, and the presence of medical comorbidities play an important role in the likelihood of maintaining durable erectile function after therapy, as described earlier after EBRT. Stone et al.[346] noted a 62% potency preservation based on a patient questionnaire among patients who underwent brachytherapy and were potent prior to treatment. The median follow-up in that cohort was 7 years. Investigators from the Princess Margaret Hospital in Toronto reported a 93% of patients with good erectile function whose baseline function was considered potential prior to therapy.[347] In that cohort, 45% of patients who were potent after therapy required a phosphodiesterase inhibitor to maintain adequate posttreatment function.

The impact of short-course ADT in conjunction with brachytherapy on long-term erectile function is unclear. Some reports suggested that ADT produces only temporary deterioration in sexual function and with testosterone recovery the function returns.[348] Data from MSKCC suggest that the use of short-course ADT for the purpose of volume reduction among patients treated with brachytherapy was not associated with a higher incidence of ED compared to patients treated with brachytherapy alone.[243]

Taira et al.[349] evaluated posttreatment erectile function after brachytherapy in 226 men with adequate preimplantation erectile function. Adequate baseline function in this report was defined as an International Index of Erectile Function (IIEF-6) of >13 without pharmacologic support. The 7-year incidence of maintained erectile function was 56%. Posttreatment function depended on baseline pretreatment sexual function. Among patients with baseline IIEF scores of ≥24 and 18 to 23, the incidence of long-term erectile function preservation was 75% and 52%, respectively. Although not significant in a multivariate analysis, these investigators noted that higher doses delivered to 25% of the penile bulb created an added detrimental effect on long-term erectile function, especially among those baseline potent patients with lower IIEF scores or those who were of older age at the time of treatment. Excellent responses were observed with sildenafil citrate in the treatment of posttreatment impotence after brachytherapy, with response rates up to 85%.[350,351]

POSTIRRADIATION PROSTATE-SPECIFIC ANTIGEN

A transient increase of PSA during radiation therapy, even as soon as the first fraction, has been reported in some patients.[352,353] Because there is no prognostic significance to the PSA response during a course of radiation therapy, obtaining PSA levels during treatment is not necessary or recommended. PSA fluctuations are common in the follow-up period and have been termed *PSA bounce*. In one report,[354] 35% of patients after combined permanent interstitial implantation and EBRT experienced a transient rise in their PSA value after treatment. The median time from treatment to this bounce effect was 18 months, and 92% of the fluctuating levels were observed during the first 26 months after radiation therapy. These investigators reported fluctuations ranging from 0.11 to 15.8 ng/mL. Similar results have been reported by Cavanagh et al.[355] for patients treated with implantation alone or when combined with EBRT. Hanlon et al.[356] observed a PSA bounce effect in approximately one-third of patients treated with EBRT alone. In that series, the 5-year biochemical control rate for patients who experienced a PSA fluctuation was inferior to that in those patients who did not have a PSA bounce in their follow-up period (69% vs. 52%; $P = .02$). On the other hand, investigators from the MD Anderson Hospital[357] noted that, of 964 patients treated with EBRT, only 12% experienced a PSA bounce, and the 5-year PSA outcome was superior for those patients who experienced this PSA fluctuation compared with those who did not (82% vs. 58%; $P = .0001$).

Ciezki et al.[358] defined PSA bounce as an increased PSA level of at least 0.2 ng/mL greater than the nadir PSA with a subsequent PSA value declining back to the nadir level or lower. One hundred sixty-two patients were treated with a permanent ^{125}I implantation and followed for a minimum of 5 years. With this as the definition of a PSA bounce, almost half of the patients (46%) experienced this phenomenon. The authors observed that the patients who experienced this fluctuation were more likely to be younger and less likely to develop a biochemical relapse. The authors also noted that PSA bounces generally occurred much sooner after treatment than did a true PSA relapse. The median time to the first rise in PSA from the nadir was 15 months, compared with 30 months for an ASTRO-defined biochemical relapse or 22 months for a nadir +2-defined relapse. Other reports define PSA bounce in various ways, and for this reason, the literature needs to be interpreted with caution.[359]

Although a low absolute PSA level or nadir value after radiation therapy has prognostic significance for improved disease-free survival, it is difficult to assign a specific PSA cut-point or nadir level as a definition of biochemical relapse. Currently, the nadir + 2 definition (a rise by ≥2 ng/mL above the nadir PSA) is considered the standard definition for biochemical failure after EBRT with or without hormonal therapy. A consensus panel[360] also recommended that the date of failure be determined "at call" (not backdated). Several studies examined the significance of posttreatment PSA doubling time (PSADT). Following prostatectomy, in a single-institution experience, Pound et al.[361] noted that, for patients treated with RP, PSADT of <10 months predicted the development of metastatic disease. Zelefsky et al.[362] reported on the impact of PSADT in a cohort of patients who developed biochemical relapse after EBRT. The PSADT for favorable-, intermediate-, and unfavorable-risk patients who developed a biochemical failure was 20.0, 13.2, and 8.2 months, respectively ($P < .001$). The 3-year incidence of DM for patients with PSADT of 0 to 3, 3 to 6, 6 to 12, and >12 months was 49%, 41%, 20%, and 7%, respectively ($P < .001$). Patients with PSADT of 0 to 3 and 3 to 6 months demonstrated a 7.0 and 6.6 increased hazard of developing distant metastases or death, respectively, compared with patients with a doubling time of >12 months. Freedland et al.[363] noted that PSADT of <9 months correlated with prostate cancer–specific mortality but did not evaluate postprostatectomy PSADT as a surrogate for cause-specific survival. Using larger, multi-institutional databases, Albertsen et al.[180] and D'Amico et al.[364] noted that short PSADT correlated with an adverse effect on survival in patients treated with either prostatectomy or radiation therapy for prostate cancer.

Emerging data strongly correlate a rising PSA level with positive postirradiation prostate biopsies. Crook et al.[365] reported on 226 patients treated with conventional EBRT who underwent serial biopsies after treatment. At 13 months after radiation therapy, the incidence of a positive biopsy was 51%, but it decreased to 30% for biopsies obtained at 30 months. Posttreatment biopsies require an experienced pathologist to interpret because of the significant radiation effect that takes place in the prostate, which can easily be mistaken at times for residual disease. Immunohistochemical staining for high molecular weight keratin can often distinguish radiation atypia in benign glands from residual tumor.

Other Innovative Treatment Modalities

Recent developments in staging, predictive genomic testing, MP-MRI, and treatment techniques succinctly discussed on subsequent sections of this chapter, are influencing the management of patients with localized prostate cancer, including those in the low-risk group that opt for definitive treatment at diagnosis or who initially, in an active surveillance program, eventually require intervention because of tumor progression.

Genomic Testing and Molecular Biomarkers

The Genomic Prostate Score (GPS), based on the OncotypeDX Prostate Cancer assay, ranges from 0 to 100, with increasing scores indicating more biologically aggressive disease. Previous studies have validated it as a predictor of adverse pathology and BCR after RP. Van Den Eeden and colleagues[366] retrospectively assessed how the GPS predicted distant metastases and prostate cancer–specific death in 259 men with localized prostate cancer treated with RP between 1995 and 2010. During a median follow-up of 9.8 years, 64 prostate cancer–specific deaths, 79 metastatic events, and 117 BCRs occurred, according to an European Urology online report (Oct 6, 2017). Each 20-point increase in GPS was associated with a 2.34-fold increased risk of distant metastases, a 2.69-fold increased risk of prostate cancer–specific death, and a 2.11-fold increased risk of BCR, after adjustment for other variables. Among the four biologic pathways represented

in the GPS, down-regulation of androgen signaling and up-regulation of stromal response gene groups were most strongly associated with each outcome, although all four gene groups contributed to the prediction. The score predicted all three outcomes within clinically relevant subsets of patients by NCCN risk groups, age, race, and central biopsy Gleason score. One of the authors noted that "it was unclear which subset of patients might benefit most from this test, because men with low-risk prostate cancer have very high 10-year survival, and those with high-risk cancer are usually recommended for treatment. Furthermore, our study was limited to patients who had undergone RP, and it is unknown how the test may perform for those treated with radiation therapy or who undergo active surveillance." The authors commented that "several other genomic assays exist and have been validated to predict the risk of death from prostate cancer. In addition, other refined risk prediction tools include advanced imaging, such as multi-parametric MRI, that allows for more accurate clinical staging. Comparative studies are currently lacking, and may be increasingly important as we seek to understand how best to evaluate patients with newly diagnosed prostate cancer."

Prolaris is a panel of RNA cell cycle progression (CCP) genes measuring cancer proliferation. The primary endpoint of this test is the 10-year risk of prostate cancer death with conservative management. Cuzick et al.[367] examined the biopsy specimens from 761 men diagnosed with prostate cancer who were managed conservatively. After adjusting with PSA and Gleason score, CCP score was a significant predictor of prostate cancer death [hazard ratio (HR 1.65).

The Prolaris test measured on biopsy has also been shown to predict outcomes after radical treatment. Freedland et al.[368] reported on 141 men diagnosed with prostate cancer who received external beam radiation. CCP score was a significant predictor of BCR (HR 2.11, $P = .034$) after adjusting for PSA, Gleason score, positive cores, and use of hormonal therapy. There was also a statistically significant relationship with prostate cancer death on univariate analysis, but the number of events was small. Similarly, Bishoff et al.[369] showed that biopsy CCP scores were a significant predictor of BCR after RP (HR 1.47) in a multi-institutional cohort. It was also a significant predictor of metastatic disease on univariate analysis. Another recent study by Oderda et al.[370] in 52 Italian men treated by RP showed that mean Prolaris scores were −1.2, −0.444, and 0.208 in low-, intermediate-, and high-risk patients. Prolaris was a significant predictor of high-risk disease (odds ratio [OR], 5.73). Prolaris was also significantly associated with BCR on univariate but not multivariate analysis, although there were only 15 events.

Clinical utility studies have been performed using surveys, such as shown by Shore et al.[371] who surveyed 15 urologists about the influence of Prolaris results in 294 different cases, and they reported that approximately one-third of the results would potentially lead to changes in practice. Another study by Crawford et al.[372] reported changes from interventional to noninterventional management, and vice versa due to Prolaris results. Less is known about the long-term impact of changing initial management decisions on the basis of genomic test results or how these tests fit in a context with widespread MP-MRI use.

The Ontario (Canada) Technology Assessment[373] conducted a systematic review of the clinical and economic evidence of the CCP test in low- and intermediate-risk, localized prostate cancer in a medical and health economic databases search from 2010 to June or July 2016. For the review of clinical effectiveness, 3,021 citations were screened, and two before–after studies met their inclusion criteria. In one study, the results of the CCP test appeared to change the treatment plan (from initial to final plan) in 64.9% of cases overall (GRADE rating of the quality of evidence: very low). In the other study, the CCP test changed the treatment received in nearly half of cases overall, compared with the initial plan (GRADE: very low). No evidence was available on clinical outcomes of patients whose treatment was informed by CCP results. For the review of cost-effectiveness, 100 citations were identified and screened and no studies met the inclusion criteria. Patients viewed the test as potentially helpful but, because of the complexity of treatment decision-making, were unsure the test would ultimately change their treatment choices. The study found no evidence to demonstrate the impact of the Prolaris CCP test on patient-important clinical outcomes. The limited evidence available showed that the test appeared to provide information that, when considered in addition to clinical risk stratification, may change the treatment plan or actual treatment for some low- and intermediate-risk prostate cancer patients, but there are insufficient data to assess the cost-effectiveness of the CCP test.

The *OncotypeDx* prostate biopsy test calculates a GPS based on genes from four different pathways involved in prostate cancer: stromal response, androgen signaling, proliferation, and cellular organization. The primary endpoint of this test is to predict the risk of adverse disease at RP. Unlike Prolaris and Decipher (in postprostatectomy patients), OncotypeDx was designed for use with biopsy tissue and does not have a commercially available test for postprostatectomy risk stratification.

Klein et al.[374] defined the 17-gene panel for use in the OncotypeDx GPS and tested it in the biopsies of 395 men with low- to intermediate-risk prostate cancer. A 20-unit increase in GPS was associated with a significantly increased risk of high-grade and/or high-stage disease (OR 2.1; 95% CI = 1.4 to 3.2), after adjusting for the CAPRA score. Adding in a GPS measurement improved the discrimination of adverse disease compared with that of the CAPRA risk classification alone (area under the curve (AUC) 0.67 vs. 0.63). Cullen et al.[375] subsequently validated the OncotypeDx biopsy test in independent populations of men from military hospitals. On multivariable analysis adjusting for National Comprehensive Cancer Network (NCCN) risk group, a 20-unit increase in OncotypeDX GPS associated with 3.3× increased risk of adverse disease at RP and 2.7× increased risk of BCR. Badani et al.[376] reported that the GPS was discordant to the NCCN risk category in 39% of patients and that 18% of recommendations between active surveillance and treatment changed as a result of OncotypeDx. Clinicians also reported that the results increased their confidence in decisions.

Ehro et al.[377] using a transcriptome-wide assay developed a biomarker signature for patients assessed as low risk at diagnosis who are upgraded or upstaged following RP. Gene expression data of 56 RP samples from the Memorial Sloan Kettering Oncogenome Project (GSE21034) that met the low-risk criteria (i.e., biopsy Gleason score (GS) ≤ 6, clinical stage T1 or T2A, and preoperative PSA (preop PSA) ≤ 10 ng/mL) were used. Of these tumors, 31 underwent upgrading or upstaging (defined by pathologic GS ≥ 7 or a pathologic tumor stage > T3A). In the training set ($n = 29$), a median fold difference filter (MFD > 1.4) was applied to select features. The top 16 t-test ranked features were modeled with a K-nearest neighbor (KNN) classifier ($k = 3$), which predicted upgrading/upstaging events. The KNN was applied to the test set ($n = 27$) and achieved an area under the receiver operating characteristic curve (AUC) of 0.93, significantly better discrimination than preop PSA (AUC = 0.52) or tumor stage (AUC = 0.63). Compared to the null model's accuracy of 56%, the KNN correctly predicted 81% ($P < .005$) of the upgrading/upstaging events. In multivariable analysis with preop PSA, tumor stage, and age at diagnosis, the KNN remained the only significant ($P < .05$) factor with an odds ratio of 2.7. Validation studies of this signature in prospectively designed cohorts of active surveillance candidates have been underway to determine if the molecular signature can improve treatment and management decisions for low-risk PCa patients.

Multiparametric Magnetic Resonance Imaging (MP-MRI)

MP-MRI can visualize prostate tumor characteristics (extraprostatic extension (ECE), tumor volume, etc.) that can be predictive of final pathologic findings such as lymph node (LN) involvement, pathologic ECE (pECEs), and BCR, all pivotal factors in the decision-making process regarding treatment. Tumor contact length (TCL) is defined as the length of cancer in contact with the prostatic capsule. Kongnuyun et al.[378] evaluated the ability of 3T MP-MRI–determined TCL in predicting pECE, BCR, and LN in patients undergoing RP. All 1,260 patients who underwent a 3T MP-MRI at the NCI from 2007 to 2015 were retrospectively classed into no ECE, suspicious ECE (sECE), and frank ECE (fECE) based on MP-MRI findings. sECE was defined as tumor with capsular bulge on MRI, whereas fECE was clear capsular obliteration and tumor extension beyond the prostatic capsule. Demographic data were obtained on patients with fECE and sECE on MP-MRI with the presence of pECE, LN, and BCR status following RP from a single surgeon (PP) experience. The authors focused on 146 patients who had sECE (68) or fECE (78) on MP-MRI. Median PSA was 11.7 ng/mL. Logistic regression analysis showed that MP-MRI–determined TCL was predictive of ECE ($P = .01$), LN status ($P = .0001$) on final pathology, and BCR ($P = .05$) during follow-up. Patients with pECE had a longer median MP-MRI TCL (2.8 cm) compared to those without pECE (2.4 cm), $P = .04$. When analyzed individually, fECE correlated with pECE ($P = .05$), whereas s ECE did not correlate with pECE ($P = .11$). Although not statistically significant, the median MP-MRI TCL for sECE with pECE was still longer than in sECE with no pECE in the subgroup analysis.

Stereotactic Body Radiation Therapy

There has been increasing interest in the use of stereotactic body radiation therapy (SBRT) for the treatment of low- and intermediate-risk prostate cancer. SBRT has been used primarily in patients with low- (favorable) and intermediate-risk tumors. The main advantage is that the treatment, based on image-guided approaches with narrow margins, is delivered in 5 fractions (750 to 800 cGy per fraction), with lower doses to adjacent organs at risk, more convenient for the patient. Biochemical control has been comparable to standard IMRT and treatment morbidity has been low.

Freeman and King[379] reported the outcomes of 41 patients who were treated with SBRT to doses of 35 to 36.25 Gy in five fractions and followed for a median of 5 years. The 5-year PSA relapse–free survival outcome was 93%. The incidence of grade 2 late rectal and urinary toxicity was 2.5% and 7%, respectively. The incidence of grade 3 rectal and urinary toxicity was 0% and 2.5%, respectively. Katz et al.[380] reported on 304 patients with a limited follow-up of 2.5 years who were treated with 35 to 36.25 Gy. Among 206 patients with a minimum follow-up of 12 months, the incidence of grade 2 urinary and rectal toxicity was 5.8% and 2.9%, respectively. One late grade 3 urinary toxicity has been observed. No information was available regarding biochemical tumor control because of the limited follow-up observations in this report.

Boike et al.[381] recently reported the preliminary outcomes of a phase I dose escalation study for low- and intermediate-risk prostate cancer using SBRT. Cohorts of 15 patients were prospectively dose escalated from 45 to 50 Gy in 9-, 9.5-, and 10-Gy fractions. In these patients, a rectal balloon was routinely used to separate the posterior and lateral walls of the rectum and reduce the volume of rectal tissue exposed to the high doses of therapy. Patients were treated every other day to further reduce toxicity, as has been demonstrated in the Stanford experience with SBRT. The overall grade 2 and 3 rectal toxicities observed were 18% and 2%, respectively. The overall grade 2 and 3 urinary toxicities observed were 31%

and 4%, respectively. In the 50-Gy dose cohort, two patients developed grade 3 cystitis, which developed approximately 1 year after therapy, and one patient developed a grade 4 rectal injury. At MSKCC, a phase I dose escalation study has been underway in which patients with low- and intermediate-risk prostate cancer are being treated with SBRT using image-guided IMRT with margins of 5 mm around the prostate except at the prostate–rectal interface, where a 3-mm margin is used. Intrafraction tracking with a ferromagnetic marker is used for all patients, and the beam is interrupted upon organ motion exceeding 2 mm from the start position. The initial dose arm included 20 patients treated to 32.5 Gy in five fractions and subsequently to 35 Gy in five fractions. Patients are being treated to 37.5 Gy in five fractions with a final dose arm of 45 Gy in five fractions. Toxicity outcome is the primary endpoint, with a secondary endpoint of tumor control based on posttreatment biopsies performed at 2 years.

Katz and Kang[382] reported on 515 patients with organ-confined prostate cancer (471 T1c and 44 T2a, all N0M0) who received robotic radiosurgery SBRT. Mean PSA was 6.48 ng/mL; 343 were low-risk, 134 intermediate-risk and 38 high-risk. ADT was administered to 70 patients. One hundred fifty-eight patients received 3,500 cGy delivered in 5 daily fractions. The remaining patients, from all risk groups, received a total dose of 3,625 cGy in 5 daily fractions. At a median follow-up of 54 months (range, 9 to 79 months), 40 patients died of other unrelated causes and 33 were lost to follow-up. The median PSA at 60 months was 0.11 ng/mL. Biochemical failures occurred for 8 low-risk patients (none locally), 9 intermediate-risk patients (one locally), and 9 high-risk patients (2 proven local failures). The actuarial 6-year freedom from biochemical failure was 97.4%, 92%, and 70.4%, for the low-, intermediate-, and high-risk groups ($P < .001$). Late RTOG toxicity was mild with 4% grade 2 rectal, 7.8% grade 2 urinary, and 1.4% grade 3 urinary (all with 36.25 Gy). Late grade 2 urinary toxicity for 35 Gy was 5.1% versus 9.9% for 36.25 Gy. Sexual QOL declined by 23% at 6 to 12 months where it remains. Seventy-four percent and at 8 years 62% of the patients potent at baseline remain potent.

Meier et al.[383] described results in 309 patients with biopsy-proven adenocarcinoma of the prostate 172 low-risk (CS T1-T2a, Gleason 6, PSA < 10 ng/mL) and 137 intermediate-risk (CS T1c-T2b with either Gleason score 7 and PSA < 10 ng/mL or Gleason 6 and PSA between 10 and 20 ng/mL) treated with a nonisocentric robotic SBRT using real-time tracking of implanted fiducials, at 21 community, regional, and academic hospitals. The prostate dose was 40 Gy in 5 fractions of 8 Gy and seminal vesicles received 36.25 Gy. Normal tissues were rigidly constrained (rectal V_{36Gy} <1 cc; bladder V_{37Gy} <5 to 10 cc). No patient had concomitant or adjuvant androgen ablation therapy. Median follow-up was 61 months. Five grade 3+ toxicities (1.6%) were reported, far below the 10% rate deemed excessive. There were no grade 4 or 5 toxicities. All reported grade 3 GU toxicities occurred between 11 and 51 months after treatment. Five patients (1.6%) developed urinary retention, which required a temporary catheter placement. Seven patients were diagnosed with bladder cancers between 21 and 50 months after treatment. For the entire population, actuarial 5-year overall survival was 95.6%. Actuarial 5-year nadir +2 RFS was 97.1% for all patients and was 97.3% and 97.1% for the low- and intermediate-risk groups, respectively. Actuarial 5-year ASTRO RFS was 92.3% and 91.3% for these respective risk groups.

Dess et al.[384] evaluated sexual potency preservation in 830 men treated with SBRT in a prospective trial at a single institution. Prospective Health-Related Quality of Life (HRQOL) data were collected via the EPIC-26, including five major domains of urinary irritative, urinary incontinence, bowel, sexual, and hormonal.

The median age was 69 years old, 25% were low risk, 57% were intermediate risk, and 18% were high risk. Twenty

percent received ADT and 16% received supplemental standard fractionation radiation in addition to SBRT for higher-risk features. With a best possible score of 100, the mean baseline urinary irritative, urinary incontinence, bowel, sexual, and hormonal scores were 91, 87, 95, 53, and 92, respectively. Depending on the time point post-SBRT, between 10% and 15% of patients had 1× MID multidomain decline, and 1% to 5% of patients had 2× MID multidomain declines. On multivariable analysis, early toxicity in urinary incontinence, bowel, and hormonal domains predicted 3- and 12-month multidomain declines, with no consistent predictors at 2-, 3-, and 5-year time points.

Johnson et al.[385] evaluated bowel, urinary, and sexual patient-reported quality of life following treatment for prostate cancer with either moderately hypofractionated radiation therapy (<5 Gy/fraction) or SBRT (5 to 10 Gy/fraction). Three hundred and seventy-eight men who underwent moderate hypofractionation were compared to 534 men treated with SBRT.

After 1 year, patients receiving moderate hypofractionation were more likely to experience worsening in bowel symptoms (39.5%) when compared to SBRT (32.5%; $P = .06$), with a more substantive difference at 2 years (37.4% vs. 25.3%, respectively, $P = .002$).

Similarly, patients receiving moderate fractionation had worsening urinary symptom score compared to patients who underwent SBRT at 1 and 2 years (34.7% vs. 23.1%, $P < .001$; and 32.8% vs. 14.0%, $P < .001$, respectively). Patients receiving moderate hypofractionation had more frequent worsening in sexual symptom score, although the difference was nonsignificant at either 1 or 2 years (32.7% vs. 29.1%, $P = .30$; and 38.5% vs. 33%, $P = .18$, respectively). After adjusting for age, and cancer characteristics, patients receiving moderate hypofractionation were more likely to experience worse urinary symptoms scores than patients receiving SBRT at 2 years (OR 0.24; 95% CI = 0.07 to 0.79); there was no difference in likelihood of worsening bowel or sexual symptoms scores between groups at 1 or 2 years in the adjusted analysis.

Greco et al.[386] evaluated 86 hormone-naïve patients with low- and intermediate-risk PCa and an IPSS score <15 who were recruited to a phase I/II study of extreme hypofractionated IGRT to assess feasibility of urethral and rectal sparing. Minimum follow-up was 12 months. CT/MR fusion was used to delineate the CTV and organs-at-risk. Beacon transponders were placed inside the urethra via a preloaded Foley catheter at the time of simulation. Mean CTV was 49 cc (range 31 to 95) and CTV to PTV margin was 2 mm in all directions. The prescription dose was 9 Gy in five fractions delivered over 5 consecutive days. With a 2-mm expansion around the catheter, dose optimization was implemented to fulfill D_{1cc} < 36 Gy. Patients were treated with 10 MV FFF VMAT and an endorectal balloon (air filling of 150 cc) was used to mitigate prostate motion. Accurate patient setup was assisted by beacon transponders and confirmed by CBCT before treatment. Online tracking was used to monitor intrafractional motion, with a tolerance threshold of 2 mm in all directions. Quality of life was assessed using the Expanded Prostate Cancer Index Composite (EPIC-26) at baseline, 1 week, 1 month, every 3 months for the first year, and every 6 months thereafter. Patient compliance to treatment was excellent with all treatments completed in five consecutive sessions. Beacon transponders-detected target motion was compatible with the prescribed 2-mm CTV-PTV expansion. Median follow-up was 20 months (range, 12 to 31). Mean PSA at baseline was 9.2 ng/mL, reduced to 1.5, and 0.4 ng/mL at 12 and 24 months, respectively. There was 2.4% acute G2 urinary toxicity and no instances of acute G2 bowel toxicity.

Blacksburg et al.[387] reported on 773 patients with prostate cancer treated with robotic SBRT (35 Gy in 5 daily fractions) without the use of ADT. Mean age was 67 years; 43.2%, 47.7%, and 9.1% of patients had low-, intermediate-, and high-risk disease by NCCN risk stratification. The Gleason score was 6 in 50.5%, 7 in 42.0%, and 8 to 10 in 7.5%. The median pretreatment PSA was 5.73 ng/mL (range 1.2 to 68.18): At 30 months, the median PSA was 0.36, 0.41, and 0.40 ng/mL in low-, intermediate-, and high-risk patients. Despite a convergence in absolute PSA values at this time point, the shape of posttreatment PSA curves prior differs considerably based on Gleason score and initial PSA. At 12 months, 42.2%, 50.0%, and 70.8% of patients with low-, intermediate-, and high-risk disease have a PSA that has declined by at least 80% ($P < .0001$). 44.3%, 50.3%, and 66.7% of patients with Gleason scores 6, 7, and 8 to 10 experience this decline at the same time point ($P = .007$). 44.5% of patients with an initial PSA <10 ng/mL experience this decline as compared to 70.9% of those with an initial PSA >10 ng/mL ($P < .0001$).

Proton/Heavy Ion Particle Therapy

Proton or heavy ion therapy in localized prostate cancer is controversial. The main advantage of these modalities is that, because of their physical characteristics, the dose to the target in depth is optimized, with less radiation dose delivered to the normal structures in front and behind the target (bladder and rectum) and potential for dose escalation. Lee et al.[388] conducted a comparison of treatment plans in 27 prostate cancer patients treated at their proton center. Each patient had a photon IMRT backup plan independently designed. For comparison, opposed lateral proton beams were used to account for proton beam range uncertainties. All plans were designed to give 75.6 Gy or Cobalt Gray Equivalent (CGE) in 42 fractions to the entire CTV. Of these 27 pairs of clinically accepted plans, the mean doses to the prostate were 78.5 Gy for IMRT and 77.9 CGE for protons. On dose–volume histograms (DVH), the rectal wall dose was essentially identical for both plans between 45 to 73 Gy, but the proton plans were lower at doses lower than 45 Gy. The integral body dose was almost identical for doses higher than 50 Gy, but proton plans spared body dose below 30 Gy, which may be significant when considering the large absolute volume of tissue irradiated. The bladder wall DVHs were similar over 35 Gy (curves not shown for space). The proton plans gave a slightly higher dose between 40 and 75 Gy (maximum difference was at 60 Gy: 13.7% for IMRT and 16.2% for proton), but bladder wall dose <35 Gy was lower for proton plans. The proton treatment plans were almost identical to IMRT plans for target coverage and for normal tissues in higher-dose regions (i.e., >45 Gy); however, tissue sparing at lower doses was seen in all proton plans.

In a report by Choi et al.[389] comparing intensity-modulated proton therapy (IMPT) with scanning beam protons (PSPT) for the treatment of prostate cancer, the authors noted that IMPT significantly decreased the dose given to the rectum and the anterior rectal wall without sacrificing target coverage. This improvement was seen at all dose levels analyzed. The study showed that IMPT with scanning beam proton therapy offers an improved method of treating patients who need treatment to their prostate and seminal vesicles (i.e., patients with intermediate- and high-risk prostate cancers) over conventional passively scattered proton beam radiation therapy.

Biochemical and tumor control with protons or heavy ions is comparable to the results of dose escalation with IMRT/VMAT. The main benefit is in a lower rectal or urinary toxicity with protons, which has been reported as 1% to 2%.

In the absence of randomized trials comparing efficacy and toxicity to high-dose photon therapy, there is no cogent evidence supporting its superiority over other forms of EBRT. Investigators from Loma Linda reported the initial tumor-control outcomes and toxicity in 1,277 patients treated with early-stage disease with 74 CGE.[390] The authors noted excellent PSA relapse–free survival outcomes and low risks of late toxicity, although these findings appeared to be comparable to outcomes currently achieved with high-dose IMRT photon therapy. It should be noted that the Proton Radiation Oncology Group 95-09 randomized trial, which randomized patients to receive 79.2 CGE of proton therapy compared to 70.2 CGE, was testing the advantage of dose escalation. This study did not attempt to compare proton to photon therapy. Such a randomized trial is essential to elucidate the role of protons in the management of localized prostate cancer.

In a study of men treated with proton beam therapy (PBT) +/– ADT for localized prostate cancer enrolled on a prospective registry trial, patients received 75.6 Gy (RBE) in conventional fractionation; 344 men received proton scattered therapy(PSPT) and 79 IMPT. Both PSPT and IMPT confer favorable rates of grade 2 GI or GU toxicity with preservation of clinically meaningful sexual, urinary, and hormonal QOL at 48 months.

Takagi et al.[391] reported on 1,375 patients treated in Japan with protons for prostate cancer. The median follow-up period was 70 months (range, 4 to 145 months). For all patients, the 10-year overall survival (OS) and bRFS were 89.2% and 77.0%, respectively. The 10-year bRFS rates were 94.5%, 82.6%, 63.3%, and 45.5% for the low-, intermediate-, high-, and very high-risk groups, respectively. The cumulative grade 2 or greater late GI and GU toxicity rates were 4.1% and 5.4%, respectively.

Mendenhall et al.[392] reported on 211 prostate cancer patients treated with proton therapy (PT), 89 low-risk patients received 78 CGE in 39 fractions to the prostate, 82 intermediate-risk patients received 78 to 82 CGE on a dose escalation trial to the prostate and proximal seminal vesicles, and 40 high-risk patients received 78 CGE in 39 fractions with weekly concomitant docetaxel and 6 months of ADT. Twenty (22%) of the low-risk patients were "very low" risk according to recent National Comprehensive Cancer Network (NCCN) guidelines, and 28 (34%) of the intermediate-risk patients were unfavorable with PSA > 15, clinical stage T2C, or Gleason score 4 + 3. The median time of follow-up is 5.2 years (range, 0.1 to 6.0). Sixty-five patients required pre-PT urologic symptom management. Clinical and biochemical-free survival rates at 5 years for low-, intermediate-, and high-risk patients are 99%, 99%, and 76%, respectively, whereas overall survival rates are 93%, 88%, and 90%. Using Common Terminology Criteria for Adverse Events version 3.0 toxicity criteria, grade 3 GI toxicity has occurred in 1.4% of all patients and grade 3 GU toxicity in 5.3%. Patient-reported outcomes, including International Prostate Symptom Score (IPSS) and Expanded Prostate Index Composite 26 bowel, urinary continence, and urinary irritability, and sexual summary scores, have been excellent. Median pretreatment and 5-year posttreatment IPSS scores are 8 and 7. Median pretreatment and posttreatment 5-year scores are 95.8 and 93.8 for bowel summary, 100.0 and 100.0 for urinary continence, 93.8 and 93.8 for urinary irritability, and 61.0 and 40.2 for sexual summary.

Choi et al.[393] published a study of the combination of two prospective single-institution cohorts of prostate cancer patients treated with proton therapy. Outcomes were presented according to NCCN risk group. From 2006 to 2015, 1,869 prostate cancer patients were treated using proton therapy in these two cohorts, out of which 1,628 (87%) had sufficient follow-up for inclusion in the present analysis (low-risk [LR] 516, 31.7%, intermediate-risk [IR] 978, 60%, high-risk [HR] 134, 8.2%). Proton therapy delivered a median dose of 76 (range 75.6 to 78) Cobalt Gray Equivalent (CGE) in 2 CGE fractions according to risk group. Pelvic lymph nodes were not treated. Hormonal therapy was mostly used for IR (56.7%) and HR (96.3%) patients. The median follow-up was 4.1 years for the entire cohort and 4.4, 4.1 and 3.1 years for LR, IR, and HR patients, respectively. Two-/five-year overall survival rates were 100%/98.0% for LR, 99.2%/95.9% for IR and 99.2%/87.0% for HR ($P = .004$ for the differences between groups). Forty-four patients had died, of which twenty (45%) died because of prostate cancer (5-year prostate cancer–specific survival of 98% with no difference between groups, $P = .1$).

Five-year bPFS rates were 95.7%, 92.3%, and 80.7% for LR, IR, and HR, respectively (*P* = .0001) Five-year cPFS rates were 95.9%, 92.7%, and 78.0% for LR, IR, and HR, respectively (*P* = .0001).

Acute grade 2+ GU and GI toxicity occurred in 39.4% (*n* = 641) and 5.2% (*n* = 85) of the entire cohort, with only two grade 3 GU and no grade 3 GI toxicity. Five-year cumulative incidence of late grade 2+ GU and GI toxicity, defined as occurring 90 days or more after treatment, was 15.9% and /10.6%, respectively.

Late grade 3 and 4 GU toxicity occurred in 0.6% (*n* = 9) and 0.1% (*n* = 1) of patients, respectively, and late grade 3 and 4 GI toxicity occurred in 0.6% (*n* = 10) and 0.1% (*n* = 1) of patients, respectively.

Vargas et al.[394] reported on 82 patients with low-risk prostate cancer randomized to 38 Gy RBE in 5 treatments (*n* = 49) versus 79.2 Gy RBE in 44 treatments (*n* = 33). Randomization patient allocation scheme was 2:1 favoring the 38-Gy RBE arm. Proton therapy was administered using fiducial markers and daily image guidance. MRI registration for target delineation was mandatory for all cases. Adverse events (AE), Expanded Prostate Index Composite (EPIC) domains, and AUA were evaluated at various times. Median follow-up for both groups was 18 months, with 33 patients reaching follow-up of 2 years or more. Patient characteristics for both groups were similar, with most patients being T1c (84%) and all having a Gleason score of 6 and a PSA level of <10 (median, 5.6). Baseline median AUA was 5 for the 38-Gy RBE arm (range, 0 to 15) and for the 79.2-Gy RBE arm (range, 0 to 14). There was no difference between the 2 groups with regard to Expanded Prostate Index Composite (EPIC) urinary, bowel, or sexual function scores at 3, 6, 9, 12, 18, or 24 months.

The only significant difference was the International Prostate Symptom Score at 12 months, 8 for the 38-Gy RBE arm versus 5 for the 79.2-Gy RBE arm (*P* = .039), but there was no difference in the AUA scores at the other time points. No grade 3 or higher AEs were seen in either arm.

Ho et al.[395] at the same institution described quality of life in 255 men 60 years old and younger (143 low-risk, 106 intermediate-risk, and 6 high-risk patients) treated with definitive proton therapy for prostate cancer without ADT. Follow-up included serum PSA levels performed every 3 to 6 months with annual examinations by physicians.

Median follow-up was 5 years and 58% of men had 5-year Expanded Prostate Index Composite (EPIC) follow-up. The 5-year biochemical-free survival and overall survival rates were 98.6% and 99.2%, respectively. All three patients with biochemical progression (one high-risk and two intermediate-risk) were alive at 5 years without clinical progression, and none of the deaths were prostate cancer related.

Within the EPIC subscales, the urinary irritative/obstructive mean score initially declined from a baseline of 90 to 88 at 2 years that maintained for subsequent years. For the urinary incontinence mean score, a similar decline was noted from a baseline of 96 to 93 at 2 years that remained stable for subsequent years; additionally, only 1.4% of men required a pad at 2 years, which is unchanged at 5 years after treatment. The bowel habits mean score initially declined from a baseline of 96 to 88 at 1 year, which subsequently improved to 93 by the 5-year follow-up. The sexual mean score declined from a baseline of 84 to 69 after 2 years, which then stabilized for the subsequent years. Further, the potency rate declined rapidly from 90% to 71% over the first 2 years and then leveled off at 66% in the following 3 years. On multivariate analysis, only EPIC sexual summary score was a significant factor associated with potency (*P* = .0002). Five-year potency rates were 88%, 61%, and 40% for baseline sexual summary scores of 100, 99 to 68, and <68 (representing 75th, 50th, and 25th percentile, respectively).

Coen et al.[396] reported a case-matched analysis comparing high-dose EBRT for prostate cancer delivered on Proton Radiation Oncology Group (PROG) 95-09, a randomized trial,

with permanent prostate brachytherapy over the same era (1996 to 1999); 196 patients were accrued to the high-dose arm (79.2-Gray equivalent [GyE] using photons and protons) of PROG 95-09 at the Massachusetts General Hospital and Loma Linda University Medical Center. Entry criteria specified T1-T2 and PSA ≤ = 15 ng/mL. When Gleason score >7 was excluded, 177 men were left for case matching. At Massachusetts General Hospital, 203 similar patients were treated by a single brachytherapist from 1997 to 2002. Minimum follow-up was 3 years. Case matching, based on T-stage, Gleason score, PSA, and age resulted in 141 matches (282 patients). Median follow-up was 8.6 and 7.4 years for EBRT and brachytherapy, respectively.

Using the Phoenix definition, the 8-year BF rates were 7.7% and 16.1% for EBRT and brachytherapy, respectively (*P* = .42). A stratified analysis was performed by risk group. In the EBRT group, 113 and 28 patients were low- or intermediate-risk, respectively. In the brachytherapy group, 118 and 23 were in low- or intermediate-risk groups. When stratified by risk group, the BF rates were similar by either technique.

Habl et al.[397] reported a trial in Heidelberg, Germany, of 92 patients with localized prostate cancer randomized to receive either proton therapy (arm A) or carbon ion therapy (arm B) and were treated with a total dose of 66 Gy (relative biologic effectiveness [RBE]) administered in 20 fractions (single dose of 3.3 Gy [RBE]). Patients were stratified by the use of antihormone therapy. Primary endpoint was the combined assessment of safety and feasibility. Secondary endpoints were specific toxicities, PSA progression–free survival (PFS), overall survival (OS), and quality of life (QoL).

Ninety-one patients completed therapy and have had a median follow-up of 22.3 months. Among acute GU toxicities, grade 1 cystitis rates were 34.1% (39.1% in A; 28.9% in B) and 17.6% grade 2 (21.7% in A; 13.3% in B). Seven patients (8%) required urinary catheterization during treatment because of urinary retention, five of whom were in arm A. Regarding acute GI toxicities, two patients treated with protons developed grade 3 rectal fistulas. Grade 1 radiation proctitis occurred in 12.1% (13.0% in A; 11.1% in B) and grade 2 in 5.5% (8.7% in A; 2.2% in B). No statistically significant differences in toxicity profiles between arms were found. Reduced QoL was evident mainly in fatigue, pain, and urinary symptoms during therapy and 6 weeks thereafter. In conclusion, hypofractionated irradiation using either carbon ions or protons results in comparable acute toxicities and QoL parameters.

Because of the occurrence of gel in the rectal wall and the consecutive occurrence of two rectal fistulas, the authors stopped using the insertion of spacer gel.

Takagi et al.[398] reported on 1,375 consecutive patients treated at their institution between April 2003 and October 2012 with definitive proton therapy; 99% of the patients received 74.0 GyE in 37 fractions, 56% received neoadjuvant hormonal therapy, and 4% received adjuvant hormonal therapy. Patients were stratified by prognostic risk groups based on National Comprehensive Cancer Network (NCCN) criteria. The numbers of patients (%) were 249 (18.1%), 602 (43.8%), 499 (32.7%), and 75 (5.5%) in the low-, intermediate-, high-, and very high-risk groups, respectively. Biochemical failure was defined using the Phoenix consensus definition of the nadir PSA concentration plus 2 ng/mL.

The median follow-up period for the entire cohort was 70 months (range, 4 to 145 months). For all patients, the 5-/10-year OS and bRFS were 96.0%/82.3% and 89.2%/77.0%, respectively. The 5-/10-year bRFS rates were 98.7%/94.5%, 90.8%/82.6%, 85.6%/63.3%, and 65.6%/45.5% for the low-, intermediate-, high-, and very high-risk groups, respectively. The cumulative grade 2 or greater late GI and GU toxicity rates were 4.1% and 5.4%, respectively. In the univariate analysis, anticoagulant drugs (*P* = .04) and diabetes mellitus (*P* = .05) were predictive factors for grade 2 late GI and GU toxicities.

Iwata et al.[399] published a retrospective analysis of prostate cancer patients treated with proton therapy at seven centers in

Japan between January 2008 and December 2011. The inclusion criteria for this analysis were (a) histologically confirmed prostate cancer, (b) no lymph node or distant metastasis, (c) Japanese men, (d) no prior radiation therapy, (e) no castration-resistant prostate cancer, (f) minimum follow-up of 6 months for surviving patients, and (g) written informed consent.

A total of 2,091 patients were evaluated, 215 in the low-risk, 520 in the intermediate-risk, and 556 in the high-risk groups. The median follow-up period of surviving patients was 69 months (range: 7 to 107). In total, 98.8% of patients were treated using conventional fractionation (1.8 to 2.0 GyE) schedule (70 to 82 GyE/35 to 41 Fr), and 1.2% of patients were treated by hypofractionation schedule (63 to 66 GyE/21 to 22 Fr); 58.5% and 21.5% of patients received neoadjuvant and adjuvant ADT, respectively. The 5-year rates of bRFS and OS in the low-risk, intermediate-risk, and high risk patients were 97.0%, 91.1%, and 83.1% for bRFS and 98.4%, 96.8%, and 95.2% for OS, respectively. The incidence of grade 2 late GI and GU toxicities was 3.6% and 2.6%, retrospectively, but grade 3 toxicities were observed in only 6 and 4 patients, respectively.

Amini et al.[400] queried the National Cancer Database (NCDB) for men with localized (N0, M0) prostate cancer diagnosed between 2004 and 2013, treated with EBRT, with available data on EBRT modality (photon vs. protons-PBT). In total, 143,702 patients were evaluated with relatively few men receiving PBT (5,709 [4.0%]). Patients treated with PBT were generally younger, NCCN low-risk compared to intermediate- or high-risk, and white versus black race (0.66), with less comorbidity, lived in higher-income counties, and were more likely to travel >100 miles to the treatment. Annual PBT utilization during the study time period significantly increased in both total number and percentage of EBRT over time. PBT utilization increased most in men classified as NCCN low-risk (4% to 10.2%). The southern US region showed the largest PBT utilization increase over time (0% to 44% of all PBT).

With regard to use of protons in the treatment of patients with prostate cancer, Mehta et al.[401] reported on an analysis of patients treated by the Proton Collaborative Group in the United States. As of December 2014, the registry had been enrolling patients since July 2009 at an average of 66 per month. Patients with prostate cancer accounted for 91% of enrolled patients at the end of year 1; this dropped to 67%, 64%, 58%, 53%, and 48% by years 2 to 6, reflecting the increased use of protons for other conditions than prostate cancer (head and neck, lung, and pediatric patients). Mishra et al.[402] published a review of active PBT clinical trials from ClinicalTrials.gov and the World Health Organization International Clinical Trials Platform Registry.

A total of 122 active PBT clinical trials were identified, with target enrollment of >42,000 patients worldwide. Ninety-six trials (79%), with a median planned sample size of 68, were classified as interventional studies. Observational studies accounted for 21% of trials but 71% (n = 29,852) of planned patient enrollment. The most common PBT clinical trials focus on GI tract tumors (21%, n = 26), tumors of the central nervous system (15%, n = 18), and prostate cancer (12%, n = 15). Five active studies (lung, esophagus, head and neck, prostate, breast) will randomize patients between protons and photons, and three will randomize patients between protons and carbon ion therapy.

Focal Ultrasound Therapy

Focal ultrasound therapy is an emerging approach to the treatment of localized prostate cancer. Ghai et al.[403] reported the 6-month follow-up of a phase 1 trial of four patients treated with focal transrectal MRI-guided focused ultrasound in North America. The patients had PSA level of 10 ng/mL or less, tumor stage cT2a or less, and a Gleason score of 6 (3 + 3). Under MRI guidance and real-time monitoring with MR thermography, focused high-frequency ultrasound energy was delivered to ablate the target tissue. MRI and repeat transrectal ultrasound-guided biopsy were performed 6 months after treatment. All four patients had normal MRI findings in the treated regions (100%); biopsy showed that three patients (75%) were clear of disease in the treated regions, representing complete ablation of five target lesions (83%). It was concluded that MRI-guided focused ultrasound is a feasible method of noninvasively ablating low-risk prostate cancers with low morbidity.

Bolton et al.[404] created a centralized database—accessible only by nonurologist researchers—within a cancer epidemiology center, and a single researcher prospectively entered baseline, treatment, and clinical/biochemical follow-up data from all patients treated with HIFU in the state of Victoria over the study period. The study accrued 108 patients, of whom 103 had been staged as having clinically localized disease. Ninety-three patients (86.1%) had low- or intermediate-risk prostate cancer. Forty-four patients (40.5%) had persistent mild urinary incontinence at 3 months after treatment, and three of these ultimately underwent further surgical procedures to correct incontinence. Twenty-seven patients (25%) additionally experienced occasions of urinary retention in the first 3 months after treatment because of passage of tissue. Twenty-nine patients achieved a PSA level of <0.2 ng/mL at 3 months after HIFU. Fifty-six patients underwent post-HIFU prostate biopsy, and this was positive for residual cancer in 51 cases. Forty-five of the patients who had a positive post-HIFU biopsy underwent secondary treatment for prostate cancer. Oncologic control and complication outcomes in this cohort were inferior to those previously reported for HIFU in single-user series. Given the population-based multiuser nature of our series, the authors believed their observations are more likely to reflect the community outcomes that might be expected from widespread adoption of HIFU than generalizing from single-operator series. Ultrasound focal therapy for primary localized prostate cancer should remain investigational pending further study, according to a 2018 European Association of Urology (EAU) position paper (Eur Urol 2018, http://bit.ly/2E8q605).

REFERENCES

1. Zelefsky MJ, Daly ME, Valicenti RK. Chapter 65. Low-Risk Prostate Cancer. In: Halperin EC, Wazer DE, Perez CA, et al., eds. *Principles and Practice of Radiation Oncology*. 6th ed. Philadelphia, PA: Wolters Kluwer/Lippincott Williams & Wilkins, 2013:1280.
2. Siegel RL, Miller KD, Jemal A. Cancer statistics, 2018. *CA Cancer J Clin* 2018;68:7–30.
3. Centers for Disease Control and Prevention. Cancer among men. Available at: http://www.cdc.gov. Accessed February 2, 2012.
4. American Joint Committee on Cancer. Prostate cancer. In: Edge S, Byrd D, Compton C, et al., eds. *AJCC cancer staging manual*. 8th ed. New York: Springer, 2017:715–726.
5. Ross R, Coetzee G, Reichardt J, et al. Does the racial-ethnic variation in prostate cancer risk have a hormonal basis? *Cancer* 1995;75:1778–1782.
6. Matsuda T, Matsuda A. Time trends in prostate cancer mortality between 1950 and 2008 in Japan, the USA and Europe based on the WHO mortality database. *Jpn J Clin Oncol* 2011;41:1389.
7. Hsing AW, Gao YT, Wu G, et al. Polymorphic CAG and GGN repeat lengths in the androgen receptor gene and prostate cancer risk: a population-based case-control study in China. *Cancer Res* 2000;60:5111–5116.
8. Barrett-Connor E, Garland C, McPhillips JB, et al. A prospective, population-based study of androstenedione, estrogens, and prostatic cancer. *Cancer Res* 1990;50:169–173.
9. Gann PH, Hennekens CH, Ma J, et al. Prospective study of sex hormone levels and risk of prostate cancer. *J Natl Cancer Inst* 1996;88:1118–1126.
10. Meikle AW, Smith JA, Stringham JD. Production, clearance, and metabolism of testosterone in men with prostatic cancer. *Prostate* 1987;10:25–31.
11. Thompson IM, Goodman PJ, Tangen CM, et al. The influence of finasteride on the development of prostate cancer. *N Engl J Med* 2003;349:215–224.
12. Andriole GL, Bostwick DG, Brawley OW, et al. Effect of dutasteride on the risk of prostate cancer. *N Engl J Med* 2010;362:1192–1202.
13. U.S. Food and Drug Administration. Drug approvals and databases. Available at: http://www.fda.gov/Drugs/InformationOnDrugs/default.htm. Accessed February 2, 2012.
14. Muir CS, Nectoux J, Staszewski J. The epidemiology of prostatic cancer. Geographical distribution and time-trends. *Acta Oncol* 1991;30:133–140.
15. Shimizu H, Ross RK, Bernstein L, et al. Cancers of the prostate and breast among Japanese and white immigrants in Los Angeles County. *Br J Cancer* 1991;63:963–966.

16. Hill P, Wynder EL, Garbaczewski L, et al. Diet and urinary steroids in black and white North American men and black South African men. *Cancer Res* 1979;39:5101–5105.

17. Kaul L, Heshmat MY, Kovi J, et al. The role of diet in prostate cancer. *Nutr Cancer* 1987;9:123–128.

18. Severson RK, Grove JS, Nomura AM, et al. Body mass and prostatic cancer: a prospective study. *BMJ* 1988;297:713–715.

19. Mettlin C, Selenskas S, Natarajan N, et al. Beta-carotene and animal fats and their relationship to prostate cancer risk. A case-control study. *Cancer* 1989;64:605–612.

20. Slattery ML, Schumacher MC, West DW, et al. Food-consumption trends between adolescent and adult years and subsequent risk of prostate cancer. *Am J Clin Nutr* 1990;52:752–757.

21. Giovannucci E, Rimm EB, Colditz GA, et al. A prospective study of dietary fat and risk of prostate cancer. *J Natl Cancer Inst* 1993;85:1571–1579.

22. Bairati I, Meyer F, Fradet Y, et al. Dietary fat and advanced prostate cancer. *J Urol* 1998;159:1271–1275.

23. Gronberg H, Damber L, Damber JE. Total food consumption and body mass index in relation to prostate cancer risk: a case-control study in Sweden with prospectively collected exposure data. *J Urol* 1996;155:969–974.

24. Chan JM, Gann PH, Giovannucci EL. Role of diet in prostate cancer development and progression. *J Clin Oncol* 2005;23:8152–8160.

25. Duffield-Lillico AJ, Dalkin BL, Reid ME, et al. Selenium supplementation, baseline plasma selenium status and incidence of prostate cancer: an analysis of the complete treatment period of the Nutritional Prevention of Cancer Trial. *BJU Int* 2003;91:608–612.

26. Heinonen OP, Albanes D, Virtamo J, et al. Prostate cancer and supplementation with alpha-tocopherol and beta-carotene: incidence and mortality in a controlled trial. *J Natl Cancer Inst* 1998;90:440–446.

27. Klein EA, Thompson IM Jr, Tangen CM, et al. Vitamin E and the risk of prostate cancer: the Selenium and Vitamin E Cancer Prevention Trial (SELECT). *JAMA* 2011;306:1549–1556.

28. Gaziano JM, Glynn RJ, Christen WG, et al. Vitamins E and C in the prevention of prostate and total cancer in men: the Physicians' Health Study II randomized controlled trial. *JAMA* 2009;301:52–62.

29. Fair WR, Fleshner NE, Heston W. Cancer of the prostate: a nutritional disease? *Urology* 1997;50:840–848.

30. Griffiths K, Morton MS, Denis L. Certain aspects of molecular endocrinology that relate to the influence of dietary factors on the pathogenesis of prostate cancer. *Eur Urol* 1999;35:443–455.

31. Giovannucci E. Tomatoes, tomato-based products, lycopene, and cancer: review of the epidemiologic literature. *J Natl Cancer Inst* 1999;91:317–331.

32. Giovannucci E. Epidemiologic characteristics of prostate cancer. *Cancer* 1995;75:1766–1777.

33. Mills PK, Beeson WL, Phillips RL, et al. Cohort study of diet, lifestyle, and prostate cancer in Adventist men. *Cancer* 1989;64:598–604.

34. Gann PH, Ma J, Giovannucci E, et al. Lower prostate cancer risk in men with elevated plasma lycopene levels: results of a prospective analysis. *Cancer Res* 1999;59:1225–1230.

35. Etminan M, Takkouche B, Caamano-Isorna F. The role of tomato products and lycopene in the prevention of prostate cancer: a meta-analysis of observational studies. *Cancer Epidemiol Biomarkers Prev* 2004;13:340–345.

36. Woolf CM. An investigation of the familial aspects of carcinoma of the prostate. *Cancer* 1960;13:739–744.

37. Cannon L, Bishop D, Skolnick M, et al. Genetic epidemiology of prostate cancer in the Utah Mormon genealogy. *Cancer Surv* 1982;1:47–69.

38. Steinberg GD, Carter BS, Beaty TH, et al. Family history and the risk of prostate cancer. *Prostate* 1990;17:337–347.

39. Narod SA, Dupont A, Cusan L, et al. The impact of family history on early detection of prostate cancer. *Nat Med* 1995;1:99–101.

40. Aprikian AG, Bazinet M, Plante M, et al. Family history and the risk of prostatic carcinoma in a high risk group of urological patients. *J Urol* 1995;154:404–406.

41. Carter BS, Beaty TH, Steinberg GD, et al. Mendelian inheritance of familial prostate cancer. *Proc Natl Acad Sci U S A* 1992;89:3367–3371.

42. Gronberg H, Damber L, Damber JE. Studies of genetic factors in prostate cancer in a twin population. *J Urol* 1994;152:1484–1487.

43. Smith JR, Freije D, Carpten JD, et al. Major susceptibility locus for prostate cancer on chromosome 1 suggested by a genome-wide search. *Science* 1996;274:1371–1374.

44. Gronberg H, Isaacs SD, Smith JR, et al. Characteristics of prostate cancer in families potentially linked to the hereditary prostate cancer 1 (HPC1) locus. *JAMA* 1997;278:1251–1255.

45. Ewing CM, Ray AM, Lange EM, et al. Germline mutations in HOXB13 and prostate-cancer risk. *N Engl J Med* 2012;366:141–149.

46. Nelson WG, De Marzo AM, Isaacs WB. Prostate cancer. *N Engl J Med* 2003;349:366–381.

47. Chamberlain NL, Driver ED, Miesfeld RL. The length and location of CAG trinucleotide repeats in the androgen receptor N-terminal domain affect transactivation function. *Nucleic Acids Res* 1994;22:3181–3186.

48. Giovannucci E, Stampfer MJ, Krithivas K, et al. The CAG repeat within the androgen receptor gene and its relationship to prostate cancer. *Proc Natl Acad Sci U S A* 1997;94:3320–3323.

49. Irvine RA, Yu MC, Ross RK, et al. The CAG and GGC microsatellites of the androgen receptor gene are in linkage disequilibrium in men with prostate cancer. *Cancer Res* 1995;55:1937–1940.

50. Schmutte C, Jones PA. Involvement of DNA methylation in human carcinogenesis. *Biol Chem* 1998;379:377–388.

51. Millar DS, Ow KK, Paul CL, et al. Detailed methylation analysis of the glutathione S-transferase pi (GSTP1) gene in prostate cancer. *Oncogene* 1999;18:1313–1324.

52. Nelson WG, De Marzo AM, DeWeese TL, et al. The role of inflammation in the pathogenesis of prostate cancer. *J Urol* 2004;172:S6–S11.

53. Hayes RB, Pottern LM, Strickler H, et al. Sexual behaviour, STDs and risks for prostate cancer. *Br J Cancer* 2000;82:718–725.

54. Platz EA, Leitzmann MF, Visvanathan K, et al. Statin drugs and risk of advanced prostate cancer. *J Natl Cancer Inst* 2006;98:1819–1825.

55. Marcella SW, David A, Ohman-Strickland PA, et al. Statin use and fatal prostate cancer: A matched case-control study. *Cancer* 2012;118:4046–4052.

56. Gutt R, Tonlaar N, Kunnavakkam R, et al. Statin use and risk of prostate cancer recurrence in men treated with radiation therapy. *J Clin Oncol* 2010;28:2653–2659.

57. Hamilton RJ, Banez LL, Aronson WJ, et al. Statin medication use and the risk of biochemical recurrence after radical prostatectomy: results from the Shared Equal Access Regional Cancer Hospital (SEARCH) Database. *Cancer* 2010;116:3389–3398.

58. Dale KM, Coleman CI, Henyan NN, et al. Statins and cancer risk: a meta-analysis. *JAMA* 2006;295:74–80.

59. Browning DR, Martin RM. Statins and risk of cancer: a systematic review and metaanalysis. *Int J Cancer* 2007;120:833–843.

60. Giovannucci E, Ascherio A, Rimm EB, et al. A prospective cohort study of vasectomy and prostate cancer in US men. *JAMA* 1993;269:873–877.

61. Giovannucci E, Tosteson TD, Speizer FE, et al. A retrospective cohort study of vasectomy and prostate cancer in US men. *JAMA* 1993;269:878–882.

62. Cox B, Sneyd MJ, Paul C, et al. Vasectomy and risk of prostate cancer. *JAMA* 2002;287:3110–3115.

63. Howards SS, Peterson HB. Vasectomy and prostate cancer. Chance, bias, or a causal relationship? *JAMA* 1993;269:913–914.

64. Rotkin ID. Studies in the epidemiology of prostatic cancer: expanded sampling. *Cancer Treat Rep* 1977;61:173–180.

65. Armenian HK, Lilienfeld AM, Diamond EL, et al. Relation between benign prostatic hyperplasia and cancer of the prostate. A prospective and retrospective study. *Lancet* 1974;2:115–117.

66. Greenwald P, Kirmss V, Polan AK, et al. Cancer of the prostate among men with benign prostatic hyperplasia. *J Natl Cancer Inst* 1974;53:335–340.

67. Hsing AW, McLaughlin JK, Schuman LM, et al. Diet, tobacco use, and fatal prostate cancer: results from the Lutheran Brotherhood Cohort Study. *Cancer Res* 1990;50:6836–6840.

68. Fincham SM, Hill GB, Hanson J, et al. Epidemiology of prostatic cancer: a case-control study. *Prostate* 1990;17:189–206.

69. Daniell HW. A worse prognosis for smokers with prostate cancer. *J Urol* 1995;154:153–157.

70. Bean MA, Yatani R, Liu PI, et al. Prostatic carcinoma at autopsy in Hiroshima and Nagaski Japanese. *Cancer* 1973;32:498–506.

71. McNeal JE. Origin and development of carcinoma in the prostate. *Cancer* 1969;23:24–34.

72. McNeal JE. Cancer volume and site of origin of adenocarcinoma in the prostate: relationship to local and distant spread. *Hum Pathol* 1992;23:258–266.

73. McNeal JE, Price HM, Redwine EA, et al. Stage A versus stage B adenocarcinoma of the prostate: morphological comparison and biological significance. *J Urol* 1988;139:61–65.

74. Bostwick DG, Shan A, Qian J, et al. Independent origin of multiple foci of prostatic intraepithelial neoplasia: comparison with matched foci of prostate carcinoma. *Cancer* 1998;83:1995–2002.

75. Byar DP, Mostofi FK. Carcinoma of the prostate: prognostic evaluation of certain pathologic features in 208 radical prostatectomies. Examined by the step-section technique. *Cancer* 1972;30:5–13.

76. Greene LF, Farrow GM, Ravits JM, et al. Prostatic adenocarcinoma of ductal origin. *J Urol* 1979;121:303–305.

77. Qian J, Wollan P, Bostwick DG. The extent and multicentricity of high-grade prostatic intraepithelial neoplasia in clinically localized prostatic adenocarcinoma. *Hum Pathol* 1997;28:143–148.

78. Jewett HJ. The present status of radical prostatectomy for stages A and B prostatic cancer. *Urol Clin North Am* 1975;2:105–124.

79. Wise AM, Stamey TA, McNeal JE, et al. Morphologic and clinical significance of multifocal prostate cancers in radical prostatectomy specimens. *Urology* 2002;60:264–269.

80. Qian J, Bostwick DG, Takahashi S, et al. Chromosomal anomalies in prostatic intraepithelial neoplasia and carcinoma detected by fluorescence in situ hybridization. *Cancer Res* 1995;55:5408–5414.

81. Noguchi M, Stamey TA, Neal JE, et al. An analysis of 148 consecutive transition zone cancers: clinical and histological characteristics. *J Urol* 2000;163:1751–1755.

82. D'Amico AV, Whittington R, Malkowicz SB, et al. A multivariable analysis of clinical factors predicting for pathological features associated with local failure after radical prostatectomy for prostate cancer. *Int J Radiat Oncol Biol Phys* 1994;30:293–302.

83. Epstein JI, Pizov G, Walsh PC. Correlation of pathologic findings with progression after radical retropubic prostatectomy. *Cancer* 1993;71:3582–3593.

84. Rosen MA, Goldstone L, Lapin S, et al. Frequency and location of extracapsular extension and positive surgical margins in radical prostatectomy specimens. *J Urol* 1992;148:331–337.

85. Villers AA, McNeal JE, Freiha FS, et al. Development of prostatic carcinoma. Morphometric and pathologic features of early stages. *Acta Oncol* 1991;30:145–151.

86. Catalona WJ, Richie JP, Ahmann FR, et al. Comparison of digital rectal examination and serum prostate specific antigen in the early detection of prostate cancer: results of a multicenter clinical trial of 6,630 men. *J Urol* 1994;151:1283–1290.

87. Oesterling JE, Suman VJ, Zincke H, et al. PSA-detected (clinical stage T1c or B0) prostate cancer. Pathologically significant tumors. *Urol Clin North Am* 1993;20:687–693.

88. Epstein JI, Walsh PC, Carmichael M, et al. Pathologic and clinical findings to predict tumor extent of nonpalpable (stage T1 c) prostate cancer. *JAMA* 1994;271:368–374.

89. Narayan P, Gajendran V, Taylor SP, et al. The role of transrectal ultrasound-guided biopsy-based staging, preoperative serum prostate-specific antigen, and biopsy Gleason score in prediction of final pathologic diagnosis in prostate cancer. *Urology* 1995;46:205–212.

90. Partin AW, Kattan MW, Subong EN, et al. Combination of prostate-specific antigen, clinical stage, and Gleason score to predict pathological stage of localized prostate cancer. A multi-institutional update. *JAMA* 1997;277:1445–1451.

91. Perrotti M, Pantuck A, Rabbani F, et al. Review of staging modalities in clinically localized prostate cancer. *Urology* 1999;54:208–214.

92. D'Amico AV, Whittington R, Malkowicz SB, et al. A multivariate analysis of clinical and pathological factors that predict for prostate specific antigen failure after radical prostatectomy for prostate cancer. *J Urol* 1995;154:131–138.

93. D'Amico AV, Whittington R, Malkowicz SB, et al. Biochemical outcome after radical prostatectomy, external beam radiation therapy, or interstitial radiation therapy for clinically localized prostate cancer. *JAMA* 1998;280:969–974.

94. Stock RG, Stone NN, Ianuzzi C, et al. Seminal vesicle biopsy and laparoscopic pelvic lymph node dissection: implications for patient selection in the radiotherapeutic management of prostate cancer. *Int J Radiat Oncol Biol Phys* 1995;33:815–821.

95. Catalona WJ, Bigg SW. Nerve-sparing radical prostatectomy: evaluation of results after 250 patients. *J Urol* 1990;143:538–543.

96. Walsh PC. Radical retropubic prostatectomy with reduced morbidity: an anatomic approach. *NCI Monogr* 1988:133–137.

97. Roach M III Re: The use of prostate specific antigen, clinical stage and Gleason score to predict pathological stage in men with localized prostate cancer. *J Urol* 1993;150:1923–1924.

98. Fowler JE Jr, Whitmore WF Jr. The incidence and extent of pelvic lymph node metastases in apparently localized prostatic cancer. *Cancer* 1981;47:2941–2945.

99. Pisansky TM, Zincke H, Suman VJ, et al. Correlation of pretherapy prostate cancer characteristics with histologic findings from pelvic lymphadenectomy specimens. *Int J Radiat Oncol Biol Phys* 1996;34:33–39.

100. Ohori M, Wheeler TM, Dunn JK, et al. The pathological features and prognosis of prostate cancer detectable with current diagnostic tests. *J Urol* 1994;152:1714–1720.

101. Alagiri M, Colton MD, Seidmon EJ, et al. The staging pelvic lymphadenectomy: implications as an adjunctive procedure for clinically localized prostate cancer. *Br J Urol* 1997;80:243–246.

102. Bishoff JT, Reyes A, Thompson IM, et al. Pelvic lymphadenectomy can be omitted in selected patients with carcinoma of the prostate: development of a system of patient selection. *Urology* 1995;45:270–274.

103. Bluestein DL, Bostwick DG, Bergstralh EJ, et al. Eliminating the need for bilateral pelvic lymphadenectomy in select patients with prostate cancer. *J Urol* 1994;151:1315–1320.

104. Hoenig DM, Chi S, Porter C, et al. Risk of nodal metastases at laparoscopic pelvic lymphadenectomy using PSA, Gleason score, and clinical stage in men with localized prostate cancer. *J Endourol* 1997;11:263–265.

105. Narayan P, Fournier G, Gajendran V, et al. Utility of preoperative serum prostate-specific antigen concentration and biopsy Gleason score in predicting risk of pelvic lymph node metastases in prostate cancer. *Urology* 1994;44: 519–524.

106. Spevack L, Killion LT, West JC Jr, et al. Predicting the patient at low risk for lymph node metastasis with localized prostate cancer: an analysis of four statistical models. *Int J Radiat Oncol Biol Phys* 1996;34:543–547.

107. Partin AW, Yoo J, Carter HB, et al. The use of prostate specific antigen, clinical stage and Gleason score to predict pathological stage in men with localized prostate cancer. *J Urol* 1993;150:110–114.

108. Cagiannos I, Karakiewicz P, Eastham JA, et al. A preoperative nomogram identifying decreased risk of positive pelvic lymph nodes in patients with prostate cancer. *J Urol* 2003;170:1798–1803.

109. Link RE, Morton RA. Indications for pelvic lymphadenectomy in prostate cancer. *Urol Clin North Am* 2001;28:491–498.

110. Rees M, Campbell S, Klein E, et al. Validation of a model for predicting metastatic disease in the pelvic lymph nodes of patients with clinically localized prostate cancer (abstract). *J Urol* 1996;155:487.

111. Gervasi LA, Mata J, Easley JD, et al. Prognostic significance of lymph nodal metastases in prostate cancer. *J Urol* 1989;142:332–336.

112. Cheng L, Zincke H, Blute ML, et al. Risk of prostate carcinoma death in patients with lymph node metastasis. *Cancer* 2001;91:66–73.

113. Prout GR Jr, Heaney JA, Griffin PP, et al. Nodal involvement as a prognostic indicator in patients with prostatic carcinoma. *J Urol* 1980;124:226–231.

114. Golimbu M, Provet J, Al-Askari S, et al. Radical prostatectomy for stage D1 prostate cancer. Prognostic variables and results of treatment. *Urology* 1987;30:427–435.

115. Allaf ME, Palapattu GS, Trock BJ, et al. Anatomical extent of lymph node dissection: impact on men with clinically localized prostate cancer. *J Urol* 2004;172:1840–1844.

116. Daneshmand S, Quek ML, Stein JP, et al. Prognosis of patients with lymph node positive prostate cancer following radical prostatectomy: long-term results. *J Urol* 2004;172:2252–2255.

117. Catalona W. *Prostate cancer*. Orlando, FL: Grune & Stratton, 1984.

118. Wang MC, Valenzuela LA, Murphy GP, et al. Purification of a human prostate specific antigen. *Invest Urol* 1979;17:159–163.

119. Papsidero LD, Kuriyama M, Wang MC, et al. Prostate antigen: a marker for human prostate epithelial cells. *J Natl Cancer Inst* 1981;66:37–42.

120. Elgamal AA, Ectors NL, Sunardhi-Widyaputra S, et al. Detection of prostate specific antigen in pancreas and salivary glands: a potential impact on prostate cancer overestimation. *J Urol* 1996;156:464–468.

121. Schroder FH, Hugosson J, Roobol MJ, et al. Screening and prostate-cancer mortality in a randomized European study. *N Engl J Med* 2009;360:1320–1328.

122. Andriole GL, Crawford ED, Grubb RL III, et al. Mortality results from a randomized prostate-cancer screening trial. *N Engl J Med* 2009;360:1310–1319.

123. Lin K, Croswell JM, Koenig H, et al. *Prostate-specific antigen-based screening for prostate cancer: An evidence update for the U.S. Preventive Services Task Force*. Rockville, MD: Agency for Healthcare Research and Quality (US), 2011. Available at: http://www.ncbi.nlm.nih.gov/books/NBK82303/

124. Greene KL, Albertsen PC, Babaian RJ, et al. Prostate specific antigen best practice statement: 2009 update. *J Urol* 2009;182:2232–2241.

125. Stamey TA, Yang N, Hay AR, et al. Prostate-specific antigen as a serum marker for adenocarcinoma of the prostate. *N Engl J Med* 1987;317:909–916.

126. Hudson MA, Bahnson RR, Catalona WJ. Clinical use of prostate specific antigen in patients with prostate cancer. *J Urol* 1989;142:1011–1017.

127. Seamonds B, Yang N, Anderson K, et al. Evaluation of prostate-specific antigen and prostatic acid phosphatase as prostate cancer markers. *Urology* 1986;28:472–479.

128. McAleer JK, Gerson LW, McMahon D, et al. Effect of digital rectal examination (and ejaculation) on serum prostate-specific antigen after twenty-four hours. A randomized, prospective study. *Urology* 1993;41:111–112.

129. Serel TA, Cetin M, Delibas N, et al. Effect of transrectal ultrasonography of the prostate on serum prostate-specific antigen levels and free/total prostate-specific antigen ratio. *Urol Int* 2000;64:24–26.

130. Yuan JJ, Coplen DE, Petros JA, et al. Effects of rectal examination, prostatic massage, ultrasonography and needle biopsy on serum prostate specific antigen levels. *J Urol* 1992;147:810–814.

131. Collins GN, Martin PJ, Wynn-Davies A, et al. The effect of digital rectal examination, flexible cystoscopy and prostatic biopsy on free and total prostate specific antigen, and the free-to-total prostate specific antigen ratio in clinical practice. *J Urol* 1997;157:1744–1747.

132. Lechevallier E, Eghazarian C, Ortega JC, et al. Effect of digital rectal examination on serum complexed and free prostate-specific antigen and percentage of free prostate-specific antigen. *Urology* 1999;54:857–861.

133. Ornstein DK, Rao GS, Smith DS, et al. Effect of digital rectal examination and needle biopsy on serum total and percentage of free prostate specific antigen levels. *J Urol* 1997;157:195–198.

134. Matzkin H, Laufer M, Chen J, et al. Effect of elective prolonged urethral catheterization on serum prostate-specific antigen concentration. *Urology* 1996;48:63–66.

135. Klomp ML, Hendrikx AJ, Keyzer JJ. The effect of transrectal ultrasonography (TRUS) including digital rectal examination (DRE) of the prostate on the level of prostate specific antigen (PSA). *Br J Urol* 1994;73:71–74.

136. Oesterling JE, Rice DC, Glenski WJ, et al. Effect of cystoscopy, prostate biopsy, and transurethral resection of prostate on serum prostate-specific antigen concentration. *Urology* 1993;42:276–282.

137. Bossens MM, Van Straalen JP, De Reijke TM, et al. Kinetics of prostate-specific antigen after manipulation of the prostate. *Eur J Cancer* 1995;31A:682–685.

138. Heidenreich A, Vorreuther R, Neubauer S, et al. The influence of ejaculation on serum levels of prostate specific antigen. *J Urol* 1997;157:209–211.

139. Stenner J, Holthaus K, Mackenzie SH, et al. The effect of ejaculation on prostate-specific antigen in a prostate cancer-screening population. *Urology* 1998;51:455–459.

140. Tchetgen MB, Song JT, Strawderman M, et al. Ejaculation increases the serum prostate-specific antigen concentration. *Urology* 1996;47:511–516.

141. Nadler RB, Humphrey PA, Smith DS, et al. Effect of inflammation and benign prostatic hyperplasia on elevated serum prostate specific antigen levels. *J Urol* 1995;154:407–413.

142. De D, Brawer M. Screening for prostate cancer. In: Vogelzang N, Scardino P, Shipley W, et al., eds. *Comprehensive textbook of genitourinary oncology*. Philadelphia, PA: Lippincott Williams & Wilkins, 2000:654–672.

143. Epstein JI, Walsh PC, Brendler CB. Radical prostatectomy for impalpable prostate cancer: the Johns Hopkins experience with tumors found on transurethral resection (stages T1A and T1B) and on needle biopsy (stage T1C). *J Urol* 1994;152:1721–1729.

144. Dugan JA, Bostwick DG, Myers RP, et al. The definition and preoperative prediction of clinically insignificant prostate cancer. *JAMA* 1996;275:288–294.

145. Humphrey PA, Keetch DW, Smith DS, et al. Prospective characterization of pathological features of prostatic carcinomas detected via serum prostate specific antigen based screening. *J Urol* 1996;155:816–820.

146. Greene DR, Egawa S, Neerhut G, et al. The distribution of residual cancer in radical prostatectomy specimens in stage A prostate cancer. *J Urol* 1991;145:324–328.

147. Terris MK, McNeal JE, Stamey TA. Detection of clinically significant prostate cancer by transrectal ultrasound-guided systematic biopsies. *J Urol* 1992;148:829–832.

148. Etzioni R, Penson DF, Legler JM, et al. Overdiagnosis due to prostate-specific antigen screening: lessons from U.S. prostate cancer incidence trends. *J Natl Cancer Inst* 2002;94:981–990.

149. Hugosson J, Aus G, Becker C, et al. Would prostate cancer detected by screening with prostate-specific antigen develop into clinical cancer if left undiagnosed? A comparison of two population-based studies in Sweden. *BJU Int* 2000;85:1078–1084.

150. Hoedemaeker RF, Rietbergen JB, Kranse R, et al. Histopathological prostate cancer characteristics at radical prostatectomy after population based screening. *J Urol* 2000;164:411–415.

151. Tosoian JJ, Trock BJ, Landis P, et al. Active surveillance program for prostate cancer: an update of the Johns Hopkins experience. *J Clin Oncol* 2011;29:2185–2190.

152. D'Amico AV, Renshaw AA, Sussman B, et al. Pretreatment PSA velocity and risk of death from prostate cancer following external beam radiation therapy. *JAMA* 2005;294:440–447.

153. D'Amico AV, Chen MH, Roehl KA, et al. Preoperative PSA velocity and the risk of death from prostate cancer after radical prostatectomy. *N Engl J Med* 2004;351:125–135.

154. Marley GM, Miller MC, Kattan MW, et al. Free and complexed prostate-specific antigen serum ratios to predict probability of primary prostate cancer and benign prostatic hyperplasia. *Urology* 1996;48:16–22.

155. Catalona WJ, Smith DS, Wolfert RL, et al. Evaluation of percentage of free serum prostate-specific antigen to improve specificity of prostate cancer screening. *JAMA* 1995;274:1214–1220.

156. Arcangeli CG, Humphrey PA, Smith DS, et al. Percentage of free serum prostate-specific antigen as a predictor of pathologic features of prostate cancer in a screening population. *Urology* 1998;51:558–564; discussion 564–555.

157. Oesterling JE, Jacobsen SJ, Klee GG, et al. Free, complexed and total serum prostate specific antigen: the establishment of appropriate reference ranges for their concentrations and ratios. *J Urol* 1995;154:1090–1095.

158. Catalona WJ, Partin AW, Slawin KM, et al. Use of the percentage of free prostate-specific antigen to enhance differentiation of prostate cancer from benign prostatic disease: a prospective multicenter clinical trial. *JAMA* 1998;279:1542–1547.

159. Cama C, Olsson CA, Raffo AJ, et al. Molecular staging of prostate cancer. II. A comparison of the application of an enhanced reverse transcriptase polymerase chain reaction assay for prostate specific antigen versus prostate specific membrane antigen. *J Urol* 1995;153:1373–1378.

160. Chang SS, Gaudin PB, Reuter VE, et al. Prostate-specific membrane antigen: much more than a prostate cancer marker. *Mol Urol* 1999;3:313–320.

161. Ghossein RA, Osman I, Bhattacharya S, et al. Detection of prostatic specific membrane antigen messenger RNA using immunobead reverse transcriptase polymerase chain reaction. *Diagn Mol Pathol* 1999;8:59–65.

162. Kantoff PW, Halabi S, Farmer DA, et al. Prognostic significance of reverse transcriptase polymerase chain reaction for prostate-specific antigen in men with hormone-refractory prostate cancer. *J Clin Oncol* 2001;19:3025–3028.

163. Moreno JG, Gomella LG. Circulating prostate cancer cells detected by reverse transcription-polymerase chain reaction (RT-PCR): what do they mean? *Cancer Control* 1998;5:507–512.

164. Gomella LG, Raj GV, Moreno JG. Reverse transcriptase polymerase chain reaction for prostate specific antigen in the management of prostate cancer. *J Urol* 1997;158:326–337.

165. Katz AE, de Vries GM, Begg MD, et al. Enhanced reverse transcriptase-polymerase chain reaction for prostate specific antigen as an indicator of true pathologic stage in patients with prostate cancer. *Cancer* 1995;75:1642–1648.

166. Oefelein MG, Kaul K, Herz B, et al. Molecular detection of prostate epithelial cells from the surgical field and peripheral circulation during radical prostatectomy. *J Urol* 1996;155:238–242.

167. Israeli RS, Miller WH Jr, Su SL, et al. Sensitive detection of prostatic hematogenous tumor cell dissemination using prostate specific antigen and prostate specific membrane-derived primers in the polymerase chain reaction. *J Urol* 1995;153:573–577.

168. Seiden MV, Kantoff PW, Krithivas K, et al. Detection of circulating tumor cells in men with localized prostate cancer. *J Clin Oncol* 1994;12:2634–2639.

169. Grasso YZ, Gupta MK, Levin HS, et al. Combined nested RT-PCR assay for prostate-specific antigen and prostate-specific membrane antigen in prostate cancer patients: correlation with pathological stage. *Cancer Res* 1998;58:1456–1459.

170. Ranparia DJ, Hart L, Assimos DG. Utility of chest radiography and cystoscopy in the evaluation of patients with localized prostate cancer. *Urology* 1996;48:72–74.

171. Israel G, Francis I, Roach M, et al. *Pretreatment staging prostate cancer. American College of Radiology Appropriateness Criteria, ACR Web Site Edition*, 2009. Available at: http://www.acr.org/ac. Accessed February 2, 2012.

172. Rifkin MD, Zerhouni EA, Gatsonis CA, et al. Comparison of magnetic resonance imaging and ultrasonography in staging early prostate cancer. Results of a multi-institutional cooperative trial. *N Engl J Med* 1990;323:621–626.

173. Chodak GW, Wald V, Parmer E, et al. Comparison of digital examination and transrectal ultrasonography for the diagnosis of prostatic cancer. *J Urol* 1986;135:951–954.

174. Roach M 3rd, Faillace-Akazawa P, Malfatti C, et al. Prostate volumes defined by magnetic resonance imaging and computerized tomographic scans for three-dimensional conformal radiotherapy. *Int J Radiat Oncol Biol Phys* 1996;35:1011–1018.

175. Kagawa K, Lee WR, Schultheiss TE, et al. Initial clinical assessment of CT-MRI image fusion software in localization of the prostate for 3D conformal radiation therapy. *Int J Radiat Oncol Biol Phys* 1997;38:319–325.

176. Flanigan RC, McKay TC, Olson M, et al. Limited efficacy of preoperative computed tomographic scanning for the evaluation of lymph node metastasis in patients before radical prostatectomy. *Urology* 1996;48:428–432.

177. Rees M, McHugh T, Door R, et al. Assessment of the utility of bone scan, CT scan, and lymph node dissection in staging of patients with newly diagnosed prostate cancer (abstract). *J Urol* 1995;153:495.

178. Tiguert R, Gheiler EL, Tefilli MV, et al. Lymph node size does not correlate with the presence of prostate cancer metastasis. *Urology* 1999;53:367–371.

179. Wolf JS Jr, Cher M, Dall'era M, et al. The use and accuracy of cross-sectional imaging and fine needle aspiration cytology for detection of pelvic lymph node metastases before radical prostatectomy. *J Urol* 1995;153:993–999.

180. Albertsen PC, Hanley JA, Harlan LC, et al. The positive yield of imaging studies in the evaluation of men with newly diagnosed prostate cancer: a population based analysis. *J Urol* 2000;163:1138–1143.

181. Chybowski FM, Keller JJ, Bergstralh EJ, et al. Predicting radionuclide bone scan findings in patients with newly diagnosed, untreated prostate cancer: prostate specific antigen is superior to all other clinical parameters. *J Urol* 1991;145:313–318.

182. Lee N, Fawaaz R, Olsson CA, et al. Which patients with newly diagnosed prostate cancer need a radionuclide bone scan? An analysis based on 631 patients. *Int J Radiat Oncol Biol Phys* 2000;48:1443–1446

183. Huncharek M, Muscat J. Serum prostate-specific antigen as a predictor of radiographic staging studies in newly diagnosed prostate cancer. *Cancer Invest* 1995;13:31–35.

184. Falchook AD, Salloum RG, Hendrix LH, et al. Use of bone scan during initial prostate cancer workup, downstream procedures, and associated medicare costs. *Int J Radiat Oncol Biol Phys* 2014;89:243–248.

185. Kurhanewicz J, Vigneron DB, Males RG, et al. The prostate: MR imaging and spectroscopy. Present and future. *Radiol Clin North Am* 2000;38:115–138, viii–ix.

186. Yu KK, Hricak H, Alagappan R, et al. Detection of extracapsular extension of prostate carcinoma with endorectal and phased-array coil MR imaging: multivariate feature analysis. *Radiology* 1997;202:697–702.

187. Wefer A, Hricak H. Imaging and staging of prostate cancer. In: Kantoff P, D'Amico A, eds. *Prostate cancer: principles and practice*. Philadelphia, PA: Lippincott Williams & Wilkins, 2002:269–286.

188. White S, Hricak H, Forstner R, et al. Prostate cancer: effect of postbiopsy hemorrhage on interpretation of MR images. *Radiology* 1995;195:385–390.

189. Yu KK, Scheidler J, Hricak H, et al. Prostate cancer: prediction of extracapsular extension with endorectal MR imaging and three-dimensional proton MR spectroscopic imaging. *Radiology* 1999;213:481–488.

190. Wefer AE, Hricak H, Vigneron DB, et al. Sextant localization of prostate cancer: comparison of sextant biopsy, magnetic resonance imaging and magnetic resonance spectroscopic imaging with step section histology. *J Urol* 2000;164:400–404.

191. Scheidler J, Hricak H, Vigneron DB, et al. Prostate cancer: localization with three-dimensional proton MR spectroscopic imaging—clinicopathologic study. *Radiology* 1999;213:473–480.

192. Kurhanewicz J, Vigneron DB, Nelson SJ. Three-dimensional magnetic resonance spectroscopic imaging of brain and prostate cancer. *Neoplasia* 2000;2:166–189.

193. Gleason DF. Histologic grade, clinical stage, and patient age in prostate cancer. *NCI Monogr* 1988:15–18.

194. Gleason D., Veterans Administration Cooperative Urological Research Group. Histologic grading and clinical staging of prostatic carcinoma. In: Tannenbaum M, ed. *Urologic pathology: the prostate*. Philadelphia, PA: Lea & Febiger, 1977:171–198.

195. Gleason DF, Mellinger GT. Prediction of prognosis for prostatic adenocarcinoma by combined histological grading and clinical staging. *J Urol* 1974;111:58–64.

196. Cintra ML, Billis A. Histologic grading of prostatic adenocarcinoma: intraobserver reproducibility of the Mostofi, Gleason and Bocking grading systems. *Int Urol Nephrol* 1991;23:449–454.

197. Andriole G, Bostwick D, Civantos F, et al. The effects of 5alpha-reductase inhibitors on the natural history, detection and grading of prostate cancer: current state of knowledge. *J Urol* 2005;174:2098–2104.

198. Johnstone PA, Riffenburgh R, Saunders EL, et al. Grading inaccuracies in diagnostic biopsies revealing prostatic adenocarcinoma: implications for definitive radiation therapy. *Int J Radiat Oncol Biol Phys* 1995;32:479–482.

199. Cookson MS, Fleshner NE, Soloway SM, et al. Correlation between Gleason score of needle biopsy and radical prostatectomy specimen: accuracy and clinical implications. *J Urol* 1997;157:559–562.

200. Fernandes ET, Sundaram CP, Long R, et al. Biopsy Gleason score: how does it correlate with the final pathological diagnosis in prostate cancer? *Br J Urol* 1997;79:615–617.

201. Narain V, Bianco FJ Jr, Grignon DJ, et al. How accurately does prostate biopsy Gleason score predict pathologic findings and disease free survival? *Prostate* 2001;49:185–190.

202. Gregori A, Vieweg J, Dahm P, et al. Comparison of ultrasound-guided biopsies and prostatectomy specimens: predictive accuracy of Gleason score and tumor site. *Urol Int* 2001;66:66–71.

203. D'Amico AV, Renshaw AA, Schultz D, et al. The impact of the biopsy Gleason score on PSA outcome for prostate cancer patients with PSA < or = 10 ng/ml and T1c,2a: implications for patient selection for prostate-only therapy. *Int J Radiat Oncol Biol Phys* 1999;45:847–851.

204. Makarov DV, Sanderson H, Partin AW, et al. Gleason score 7 prostate cancer on needle biopsy: is the prognostic difference in Gleason scores 4 + 3 and 3 + 4 independent of the number of involved cores? *J Urol* 2002;167:2440–2442.

205. Stamey TA. Some concerns about prostate cancer location, Gleason grade, and postradiation doubling times. *Int J Radiat Oncol Biol Phys* 1995;33:967–968; discussion 972.

206. Stamey TA, McNeal JE, Yemoto CM, et al. Biological determinants of cancer progression in men with prostate cancer. *JAMA* 1999;281:1395–1400.

207. Stamey TA, Yemoto CM, McNeal JE, et al. Prostate cancer is highly predictable: a prognostic equation based on all morphological variables in radical prostatectomy specimens. *J Urol* 2000;163:1155–1160.

208. Noguchi M, Stamey TA, McNeal JE, et al. Preoperative serum prostate specific antigen does not reflect biochemical failure rates after radical prostatectomy in men with large volume cancers. *J Urol* 2000;164:1596–1600.

209. D'Amico AV, Whittington R, Malkowicz SB, et al. Clinical utility of percent-positive prostate biopsies in predicting biochemical outcome after radical prostatectomy or external-beam radiation therapy for patients with clinically localized prostate cancer. *Mol Urol* 2000;4:171–175; discussion 177.

210. D'Amico AV, Whittington R, Malkowicz SB, et al. Clinical utility of the percentage of positive prostate biopsies in defining biochemical outcome after radical prostatectomy for patients with clinically localized prostate cancer. *J Clin Oncol* 2000;18:1164–1172.

211. Nelson CP, Rubin MA, Strawderman M, et al. Preoperative parameters for predicting early prostate cancer recurrence after radical prostatectomy. *Urology* 2002;59:740–745; discussion 745–746.

212. Sebo TJ, Bock BJ, Cheville JC, et al. The percent of cores positive for cancer in prostate needle biopsy specimens is strongly predictive of tumor stage and volume at radical prostatectomy. *J Urol* 2000;163:174–178.

213. Cheng L, Slezak J, Bergstralh EJ, et al. Dedifferentiation in the metastatic progression of prostate carcinoma. *Cancer* 1999;86:657–663.

214. Bates HR, Jr. Transitional cell carcinoma of the prostate. *J Urol* 1969;101:206–207.

215. Kopelson G, Harisiadis L, Romas NA, et al. Periurethral prostatic duct carcinoma: clinical features and treatment results. *Cancer* 1978;42:2894–2902.

216. Matzkin H, Soloway MS, Hardeman S. Transitional cell carcinoma of the prostate. *J Urol* 1991;146:1207–1212.

217. Tannenbaum M. Histology of the prostate gland. In: Tannenbaum M, ed. *Urologic pathology: the prostate.* Philadelphia, PA: Lea & Febiger, 1977:312–315.

218. Reese JH, Freiha FS, Gelb AB, et al. Transitional cell carcinoma of the prostate in patients undergoing radical cystoprostatectomy. *J Urol* 1992;147:92–95.

219. Carney JA, Kelalis PP. Endometrial carcinoma of the prostatic utricle. *Am J Clin Pathol* 1973;60:565–569.

220. Tannenbaum M. Endometrial tumors and/or associated carcinomas of prostate. *Urology* 1975;6:372–375.

221. Zaloudek C, Williams JW, Kempson RL. "Endometrial" adenocarcinoma of the prostate: a distinctive tumor of probable prostatic duct origin. *Cancer* 1976;37:2255–2262.

222. Melicow MM, Tannenbaum M. Endometrial carcinoma of uterus masculinus (prostatic utricle). Report of 6 cases. *J Urol* 1971;106:892–902.

223. Colpaert C, Gentens P, Van Marck E. Ductal ("endometrioid") adenocarcinoma of the prostate. *Acta Urol Belg* 1998;66:29–32.

224. Kullu S, Ersev A, Simsek F, et al. Adenocarcinoma of the prostate with endometrioid features. *Int Urol Nephrol* 1991;23:577–580.

225. Wolfe JH, Lloyd-Davies RW. The management of transitional cell carcinoma in the prostate. *Br J Urol* 1981;53:253–257.

226. Brinker DA, Potter SR, Epstein JI. Ductal adenocarcinoma of the prostate diagnosed on needle biopsy: correlation with clinical and radical prostatectomy findings and progression. *Am J Surg Pathol* 1999;23:1471–1479.

227. Cohen RJ, Glezerson G, Haffejee Z. Neuro-endocrine cells—a new prognostic parameter in prostate cancer. *Br J Urol* 1991;68:258–262.

228. Epstein JI, Lieberman PH. Mucinous adenocarcinoma of the prostate gland. *Am J Surg Pathol* 1985;9:299–308.

229. Shannon RL, Ro JY, Grignon DJ, et al. Sarcomatoid carcinoma of the prostate. A clinicopathologic study of 12 patients. *Cancer* 1992;69:2676–2682.

230. Azumi N, Shibuya H, Ishikura M. Primary prostatic carcinoid tumor with intracytoplasmic prostatic acid phosphatase and prostate-specific antigen. *Am J Surg Pathol* 1984;8:545–550.

231. Ghali VS, Garcia RL. Prostatic adenocarcinoma with carcinoidal features producing adrenocorticotropic syndrome. Immunohistochemical study and review of the literature. *Cancer* 1984;54:1043–1048.

232. Small E, Prins G. Physiology and endocrinology of the prostate. In: Vogelzang N, Scardino P, Shipley W, et al., eds. *Comprehensive textbook of genitourinary oncology.* Baltimore, MD: Williams & Wilkins, 1996:600–620.

233. Abbas F, Civantos F, Benedetto P, et al. Small cell carcinoma of the bladder and prostate. *Urology* 1995;46:617–630.

234. Deorah S, Rao MB, Raman R, et al. Survival of patients with small cell carcinoma of the prostate during 1973–2003: a population-based study. *BJU Int* 2012;109(6):824–830.

235. Gray GF Jr, Marshall VF. Squamous carcinoma of the prostate. *J Urol* 1975;113:736–738.

236. Johnson DE, Chalbaud R, Ayala AG. Secondary tumors of the prostate. *J Urol* 1974;112:507–508.

237. Schuppler J. Malignant neurolemmoma of prostate gland. *J Urol* 1971;106:903–905.

238. Sarris A, Dimopoulos M, Pugh W, et al. Primary lymphoma of the prostate: good outcome with doxorubicin-based combination chemotherapy. *J Urol* 1995;153:1852–1854.

239. D'Amico AV, Whittington R, Kaplan I, et al. Equivalent biochemical failure-free survival after external beam radiation therapy or radical prostatectomy in patients with a pretreatment prostate specific antigen of >4–20 ng/ml. *Int J Radiat Oncol Biol Phys* 1997;37:1053–1058.

240. Kupelian P, Katcher J, Levin H, et al. External beam radiotherapy versus radical prostatectomy for clinical stage T1–2 prostate cancer: therapeutic implications of stratification by pretreatment PSA levels and biopsy Gleason scores. *Cancer J Sci Am* 1997;3:78–87.

241. Zelefsky MJ, Wallner KE, Ling CC, et al. Comparison of the 5-year outcome and morbidity of three-dimensional conformal radiotherapy versus transperineal permanent iodine-125 implantation for early-stage prostatic cancer. *J Clin Oncol* 1999;17:517–522.

242. Zelefsky MJ, Eastham JA, Cronin AM, et al. Metastasis after radical prostatectomy or external beam radiotherapy for patients with clinically localized prostate cancer: a comparison of clinical cohorts adjusted for case mix. *J Clin Oncol* 2010;28:1508–1513.

243. Zelefsky MJ, Yamada Y, Pei X, et al. Comparison of tumor control and toxicity outcomes of high-dose intensity-modulated radiotherapy and brachytherapy for patients with favorable risk prostate cancer. *Urology* 2011;77:986–990.

244. Cooperberg MR, Vickers AJ, Broering JM, et al. Comparative risk-adjusted mortality outcomes after primary surgery, radiotherapy, or androgen-deprivation therapy for localized prostate cancer. *Cancer* 2010;116:5226–5234.

245. Fowler FJ Jr, McNaughton Collins M, Albertsen PC, et al. Comparison of recommendations by urologists and radiation oncologists for treatment of clinically localized prostate cancer. *JAMA* 2000;283:3217–3222.

246. Zelefsky M, Lee W, Zietman A, et al. Evaluation of adherence to quality measures for prostate cancer radiotherapy in the United States from the Quality Research in Radiation Oncology (QRRO) survey. *Pract Radiat Oncol* 2013;3(1):2–8.

247. Bill-Axelson A, Holmberg L, Garmo H, et al. Radical prostatectomy versus watchful waiting in early prostate cancer. *N Engl J Med* 2014;370:932–942.

248. Choudhury A. Protecting low-risk prostate cancer. *Int J Radiat Oncol Biol Phys* 2017;99:515–517.

249. Hamdy FC, Donovan JL, Lane JA, et al. 10-Year outcomes after monitoring, surgery, or radiotherapy for localized prostate cancer. *N Engl J Med* 2016;375:1415–1424.

250. Donovan JL, Hamdy FC, Lane JA, et al. Patient-reported outcomes after monitoring, surgery, or radiotherapy for prostate cancer. *N Engl J Med* 2016;375:1425–1437.

251. Jackson MA, Bellas N, Siegrist T, et al. Experienced open vs early robotic-assisted laparoscopic radical prostatectomy: A 10-year prospective and retrospective comparison. *Urology* 2016;91:111–118.

252. Dearnaley D, Syndikus I, Mossop H, et al. Conventional versus hypofractionated high-dose intensity-modulated radiotherapy for prostate cancer: 5-Year outcomes of the randomised, non-inferiority, phase 3 CHHiP trial. *Lancet Oncol* 2016;17:1047–1060.

253. Wilt TJ, Brawer MK, Jones KM, et al. Radical prostatectomy versus observation for localized prostate cancer (PIVOT). *N Engl J Med* 2012;367:203–213.

254. McClelland S, Jaboin JJ, Mitin T Is advocacy for active surveillance over definitive intervention in low-risk prostate cancer applicable to African American patients? *Int J Radiat Oncol Biol Phys* 2017;99:1076–1077.

255. Musunuru HB, Sethukavalan P, Cheung P, et al. Comparison of active surveillance, low-dose-rate brachytherapy, stereotactic ablative body radiation therapy, and standard external beam in low-risk prostate cancer. *Int J Radiat Oncol Biol Phys* 2014;90(1S):S447.

256. Lester-Coll NH, Park HSM, Rutter CE, et al. Evaluation at academic centers increases the likelihood of active surveillance in low-risk prostate cancer. *Int J Radiat Oncol Biol Phys* 2015;93(3):S118.

257. Young H. The early diagnosis and radical cure of carcinoma of the prostate: Being a study of 40 cases and presentation of a radical operation which was carried out in four cases. *Bull Johns Hopkins Hosp* 1905;16:315–319.

258. Suardi N, Ficarra V, Willemsen P, et al. Long-term biochemical recurrence rates after robot-assisted radical prostatectomy: analysis of a single-center series of patients with a minimum follow-up of 5 years. *Urology* 2011;79:133–138.

259. Webb S. The physical basis of IMRT and inverse planning. *Br J Radiol* 2003;76:678–689.

260. Zelefsky MJ, Happersett L, Leibel SA, et al. The effect of treatment positioning on normal tissue dose in patients with prostate cancer treated with three-dimensional conformal radiotherapy. *Int J Radiat Oncol Biol Phys* 1997;37:13–19.

261. Bayley AJ, Catton CN, Haycocks T, et al. A randomized trial of supine vs. prone positioning in patients undergoing escalated dose conformal radiotherapy for prostate cancer. *Radiother Oncol* 2004;70:37–44.

262. Mah D, Freedman G, Movsas B, et al. To move or not to move: measurements of prostate motion by urethrography using MRI. *Int J Radiat Oncol Biol Phys* 2001;50:947–951.

263. Villeirs GM, Van Vaerenbergh K, Vakaet L, et al. Interobserver delineation variation using CT versus combined CT + MRI in intensity-modulated radiotherapy for prostate cancer. *Strahlenther Onkol* 2005;181:424–430.

264. Rasch C, Barillot I, Remeijer P, et al. Definition of the prostate in CT and MRI: a multi-observer study. *Int J Radiat Oncol Biol Phys* 1999;43:57–66.

265. McLaughlin PW, Evans C, Feng M, et al. Radiographic and anatomic basis for prostate contouring errors and methods to improve prostate contouring accuracy. *Int J Radiat Oncol Biol Phys* 2010;76:369–378.

266. Burman C, Chui CS, Kutcher G, et al. Planning, delivery, and quality assurance of intensity-modulated radiotherapy using dynamic multileaf collimator: a strategy for large-scale implementation for the treatment of carcinoma of the prostate. *Int J Radiat Oncol Biol Phys* 1997;39:863–873.

267. Price RA, Hanks GE, McNeeley SW, et al. Advantages of using noncoplanar vs. axial beam arrangements when treating prostate cancer with intensity-modulated radiation therapy and the step-and-shoot delivery method. *Int J Radiat Oncol Biol Phys* 2002;53:236–243.

268. Yu CX, Li XA, Ma L, et al. Clinical implementation of intensity-modulated arc therapy. *Int J Radiat Oncol Biol Phys* 2002;53:453–463.

269. Kry SF, Salehpour M, Followill DS, et al. Out-of-field photon and neutron dose equivalents from step-and-shoot intensity-modulated radiation therapy. *Int J Radiat Oncol Biol Phys* 2005;62:1204–1216.

270. Kry SF, Salehpour M, Followill DS, et al. The calculated risk of fatal secondary malignancies from intensity-modulated radiation therapy. *Int J Radiat Oncol Biol Phys* 2005;62:1195–1203.

271. Pirzkall A, Carol MP, Pickett B, et al. The effect of beam energy and number of fields on photon-based IMRT for deep-seated targets. *Int J Radiat Oncol Biol Phys* 2002;53:434–442.

272. Skwarchuk MW, Jackson A, Zelefsky MJ, et al. Late rectal toxicity after conformal radiotherapy of prostate cancer (I): multivariate analysis and dose-response. *Int J Radiat Oncol Biol Phys* 2000;47:103–113.

273. Jackson A, Skwarchuk MW, Zelefsky MJ, et al. Late rectal bleeding after conformal radiotherapy of prostate cancer. II. Volume effects and dose-volume histograms. *Int J Radiat Oncol Biol Phys* 2001;49:685–698.

274. Kupelian PA, Thakkar VV, Khuntia D, et al. Hypofractionated intensity-modulated radiotherapy (70 gy at 2.5 Gy per fraction) for localized prostate cancer: long-term outcomes. *Int J Radiat Oncol Biol Phys* 2005;63:1463–1468.

275. Pollack A, Hanlon AL, Horwitz EM, et al. Dosimetry and preliminary acute toxicity in the first 100 men treated for prostate cancer on a randomized hypofractionation dose escalation trial. *Int J Radiat Oncol Biol Phys* 2006;64:518–526.

276. Aubry JF, Beaulieu L, Girouard LM, et al. Measurements of intrafraction motion and interfraction and intrafraction rotation of prostate by three-dimensional analysis of daily portal imaging with radiopaque markers. *Int J Radiat Oncol Biol Phys* 2004;60:30–39.

277. Chung PW, Haycocks T, Brown T, et al. On-line aSi portal imaging of implanted fiducial markers for the reduction of interfraction error during conformal radiotherapy of prostate carcinoma. *Int J Radiat Oncol Biol Phys* 2004;60:329–334.

278. Crook JM, Raymond Y, Salhani D, et al. Prostate motion during standard radiotherapy as assessed by fiducial markers. *Radiother Oncol* 1995;37:35–42.

278a. Zelefsky MJ, Crean D, Mageras GS et al. Quantification and predictors of prostate position variability in 50 patients evaluated with multiple CT scans during conformal radiotherapy. *Radiother Oncol* 1999;50:225–234.

279. Huang E, Dong L, Chandra A, et al. Intrafraction prostate motion during IMRT for prostate cancer. *Int J Radiat Oncol Biol Phys* 2002;53:261–268.

280. Langen KM, Zhang Y, Andrews RD, et al. Initial experience with megavoltage (MV) CT guidance for daily prostate alignments. *Int J Radiat Oncol Biol Phys* 2005;62:1517–1524.
281. Older RA, Synder B, Krupski TL, et al. Radioactive implant migration in patients treated for localized prostate cancer with interstitial brachytherapy. *J Urol* 2001;165:1590–1592.
282. Merrick GS, Butler WM, Wallner KE, et al. Variability of prostate brachytherapy pre-implant dosimetry: a multi-institutional analysis. *Brachytherapy* 2005;4:241–251.
283. Zelefsky MJ, Yamada Y, Cohen G, et al. Postimplantation dosimetric analysis of permanent transperineal prostate implantation: improved dose distributions with an intraoperative computer-optimized conformal planning technique. *Int J Radiat Oncol Biol Phys* 2000;48:601–608.
284. Beyer D, Nath R, Butler W, et al. American Brachytherapy Society recommendations for clinical implementation of NIST-1999 standards for (103) palladium brachytherapy. The clinical research committee of the American Brachytherapy Society. *Int J Radiat Oncol Biol Phys* 2000;47:273–275.
285. Dicker AP, Lin CC, Leeper DB, et al. Isotope selection for permanent prostate implants? An evaluation of 103 Pd versus 125I based on radiobiological effectiveness and dosimetry. *Semin Urol Oncol* 2000;18:152–159.
286. Cha CM, Potters L, Ashley R, et al. Isotope selection for patients undergoing prostate brachytherapy. *Int J Radiat Oncol Biol Phys* 1999;45:391–395.
287. Merrick GS, Butler WM, Dorsey AT, et al. Potential role of various dosimetric quality indicators in prostate brachytherapy. *Int J Radiat Oncol Biol Phys* 1999;44:717–724.
288. Herstein A, Wallner K, Merrick G, et al. I-125 versus Pd-103 for low-risk prostate cancer: long-term morbidity outcomes from a prospective randomized multicenter controlled trial. *Cancer J* 2005;11:385–389.
289. Kollmeier MA, Pei X, Algur E, et al. A comparison of the impact of isotope ((125) I vs. (103)Pd) on toxicity and biochemical outcome after interstitial brachytherapy and external beam radiation therapy for clinically localized prostate cancer. *Brachytherapy* 2012;11:271–276.
290. Nag S, Bice W, DeWyngaert K, et al. The American Brachytherapy Society recommendations for permanent prostate brachytherapy postimplant dosimetric analysis. *Int J Radiat Oncol Biol Phys* 2000;46:221–230.
291. Ash D, Al-Qaisieh B, Bottomley D, et al. The correlation between D90 and outcome for I-125 seed implant monotherapy for localised prostate cancer. *Radiother Oncol* 2006;79:185–189.
292. Potters L, Morgenstern C, Calugaru E, et al. 12-year outcomes following permanent prostate brachytherapy in patients with clinically localized prostate cancer. *J Urol* 2005;173:1562–1566.
293. Stone NN, Stock RG, Unger P. Intermediate term biochemical-free progression and local control following 125iodine brachytherapy for prostate cancer. *J Urol* 2005;173:803–807.
294. Zelefsky M, Kuban D, Levy L, et al. Long-term multi-institutional analysis of stage T1-T2 prostate cancer treated with permanent brachytherapy (Abstract 56). *Int J Radiat Oncol Biol Phys* 2007;67:327–333.
295. Han BH, Wallner KE. Dosimetric and radiographic correlates to prostate brachytherapy-related rectal complications. *Int J Cancer* 2001;96:372–378.
296. Merrick GS, Butler WM, Wallner KE, et al. The impact of radiation dose to the urethra on brachytherapy-related dysuria. *Brachytherapy* 2005;4:45–50.
297. Snyder KM, Stock RG, Hong SM, et al. Defining the risk of developing grade 2 proctitis following 125I prostate brachytherapy using a rectal dose-volume histogram analysis. *Int J Radiat Oncol Biol Phys* 2001;50:335–341.
298. Zelefsky MJ, Yamada Y, Marion C, et al. Improved conformality and decreased toxicity with intraoperative computer-optimized transperineal ultrasound-guided prostate brachytherapy. *Int J Radiat Oncol Biol Phys* 2003;55:956–963.
299. Stock RG, Stone NN, Dahlal M, et al. What is the optimal dose for 125I prostate implants? A dose-response analysis of biochemical control, posttreatment prostate biopsies, and long-term urinary symptoms. *Brachytherapy* 2002;1:83–89.
300. Zelefsky MJ, Chou JF, Pei X, et al. Predicting biochemical tumor control after brachytherapy for clinically localized prostate cancer: the Memorial Sloan-Kettering Cancer Center experience. *Brachytherapy* 2012;11:245–249.
301. Safdieh J, Schwartz D, Osborn V et al Utilization of prostate brachytherapy for low-risk prostate cancer: is the decline overstated? *Int J Radiat Oncol Biol Phys* 2016;96(2):E242–E243, Abstr 2591.
302. Bianco FJ Jr, Scardino PT, Eastham JA. Radical prostatectomy: long-term cancer control and recovery of sexual and urinary function ("trifecta"). *Urology* 2005;66:83–94.
302a. Roehl KA, Han M, Ramos CG, et al. Cancer progression and survival rates following anatomica radical retropubic prostatectomy in 3,478 consecutive patients: long-term results. *J Urol* 2004;172:910–914.
303. Isbarn H, Wanner M, Salomon G, et al. Long-term data on the survival of patients with prostate cancer treated with radical prostatectomy in the prostate-specific antigen era. *BJU Int* 2010;106:37–43.
304. Han M, Partin AW, Zahurak M, et al. Biochemical (prostate specific antigen) recurrence probability following radical prostatectomy for clinically localized prostate cancer. *J Urol* 2003;169:517–523.
305. Kuban DA, Thames HD, Levy LB, et al. Long-term multi-institutional analysis of stage T1-T2 prostate cancer treated with radiotherapy in the PSA era. *Int J Radiat Oncol Biol Phys* 2003;57:915–928.
306. Kuban DA, Tucker SL, Dong L, et al. Long-term results of the M. D. Anderson randomized dose-escalation trial for prostate cancer. *Int J Radiat Oncol Biol Phys* 2008;70:67–74.
307. Zietman AL, DeSilvio ML, Slater JD, et al. Comparison of conventional-dose vs high-dose conformal radiation therapy in clinically localized adenocarcinoma of the prostate: a randomized controlled trial. *JAMA* 2005;294:1233–1239.
308. Zelefsky MJ, Pei X, Chou JF, et al. Dose escalation for prostate cancer radiotherapy: predictors of long-term biochemical tumor control and distant metastases-free survival outcomes. *Eur Urol* 2011;60:1133–1139.
309. Pollack A, Hanlon AL, Horwitz EM, et al. Prostate cancer radiotherapy dose response: an update of the Fox Chase experience. *J Urol* 2004;171:1132–1136.
310. Symon Z, Griffith KA, McLaughlin PW, et al. Dose escalation for localized prostate cancer: substantial benefit observed with 3D conformal therapy. *Int J Radiat Oncol Biol Phys* 2003;57:384–390.
311. Kupelian PA, Potters L, Khuntia D, et al. Radical prostatectomy, external beam radiotherapy <72 Gy, external beam radiotherapy > or = 72 Gy, permanent seed implantation, or combined seeds/external beam radiotherapy for stage T1-T2 prostate cancer. *Int J Radiat Oncol Biol Phys* 2004;58:25–33.
312. Michalski J, Winter K, Roach M, et al. Clinical outcome of patients treated with 3D conformal radiation therapy 3D-CRT for prostate cancer on RTOG 9406. *Int J Radiat Oncol Biol Phys* 2012;83:e363–e370.
313. Sylvester JE, Grimm PD, Wong J, et al. Fifteen-year biochemical relapse-free survival, cause-specific survival, and overall survival following I(125) prostate brachytherapy in clinically localized prostate cancer: Seattle experience. *Int J Radiat Oncol Biol Phys* 2011;81:376–381.
314. Taira AV, Merrick GS, Butler WM, et al. Long-term outcome for clinically localized prostate cancer treated with permanent interstitial brachytherapy. *Int J Radiat Oncol Biol Phys* 2011;79:1336–1342.
315. Stone NN, Stone MM, Rosenstein BS, et al. Influence of pretreatment and treatment factors on intermediate to long-term outcome after prostate brachytherapy. *J Urol* 2011;185:495–500.
316. Begg CB, Riedel ER, Bach PB, et al. Variations in morbidity after radical prostatectomy. *N Engl J Med* 2002;346:1138–1144.
317. Catalona WJ, Carvalhal GF, Mager DE, et al. Potency, continence and complication rates in 1,870 consecutive radical retropubic prostatectomies. *J Urol* 1999;162:433–438.
318. Trinh Q-D, Sammona J, Sun M, et al. Perioperative outcomes of robot-assisted radical prostatectomy compared with open radical prostatectomy: results from the Nationwide Inpatient Sample. *Eur Urol* 2012;61:679–685.
319. Geinitz H, Thamm R, Keller M, et al. Longitudinal study of intestinal symptoms and fecal continence in patients with conformal radiotherapy for prostate cancer. *Int J Radiat Oncol Biol Phys* 2011;79:1373–1380.
320. Herold DM, Hanlon AL, Hanks GE. Diabetes mellitus: a predictor for late radiation morbidity. *Int J Radiat Oncol Biol Phys* 1999;43:475–479.
321. Vavassori V, Fiorino C, Rancati T, et al. Predictors for rectal and intestinal acute toxicities during prostate cancer high-dose 3D-CRT: results of a prospective multicenter study. *Int J Radiat Oncol Biol Phys* 2007;67:1401–1410.
322. Huang EH, Pollack A, Levy L, et al. Late rectal toxicity: dose-volume effects of conformal radiotherapy for prostate cancer. *Int J Radiat Oncol Biol Phys* 2002;54:1314–1321.
323. Fiorino C, Sanguineti G, Cozzarini C, et al. Rectal dose-volume constraints in high-dose radiotherapy of localized prostate cancer. *Int J Radiat Oncol Biol Phys* 2003;57:953–962.
324. Heemsbergen WD, Peeters ST, Koper PC, et al. Acute and late gastrointestinal toxicity after radiotherapy in prostate cancer patients: consequential late damage. *Int J Radiat Oncol Biol Phys* 2006;66:3–10.
325. Zelefsky MJ, Chan H, Hunt M, et al. Long-term outcome of high dose intensity modulated radiation therapy for patients with clinically localized prostate cancer. *J Urol* 2006;176:1415–1419.
326. Michalski JM, Winter K, Purdy JA, et al. Toxicity after three-dimensional radiotherapy for prostate cancer on RTOG 9406 dose level V. *Int J Radiat Oncol Biol Phys* 2005;62:706–713.
327. Storey MR, Pollack A, Zagars G, et al. Complications from radiotherapy dose escalation in prostate cancer: preliminary results of a randomized trial. *Int J Radiat Oncol Biol Phys* 2000;48:635–642.
328. Zelefsky MJ, Levin EJ, Hunt M, et al. Incidence of late rectal and urinary toxicities after three-dimensional conformal radiotherapy and intensity-modulated radiotherapy for localized prostate cancer. *Int J Radiat Oncol Biol Phys* 2008;70:1124–1129.
329. Alicikus ZA, Yamada Y, Zhang Z, et al. Ten-year outcomes of high-dose, intensity-modulated radiotherapy for localized prostate cancer. *Cancer* 2011;117:1429–1437.
330. Peeters ST, Heemsbergen WD, van Putten WL, et al. Acute and late complications after radiotherapy for prostate cancer: results of a multicenter randomized trial comparing 68 Gy to 78 Gy. *Int J Radiat Oncol Biol Phys* 2005;61:1019–1034.
331. Sandhu AS, Zelefsky MJ, Lee HJ, et al. Long-term urinary toxicity after 3-dimensional conformal radiotherapy for prostate cancer in patients with prior history of transurethral resection. *Int J Radiat Oncol Biol Phys* 2000;48:643–647.
332. Lee WR, Schultheiss TE, Hanlon AL, et al. Urinary incontinence following external-beam radiotherapy for clinically localized prostate cancer. *Urology* 1996;48:95–99.
333. Incrocci L, Slob AK, Levendag PC. Sexual (dys)function after radiotherapy for prostate cancer: a review. *Int J Radiat Oncol Biol Phys* 2002;52:681–693.
334. Mantz CA, Nautiyal J, Awan A, et al. Potency preservation following conformal radiotherapy for localized prostate cancer: impact of neoadjuvant androgen blockade, treatment technique, and patient-related factors. *Cancer J Sci Am* 1999;5:230–236.
335. van der Wielen GJ, van Putten WL, Incrocci L. Sexual function after three-dimensional conformal radiotherapy for prostate cancer: results from a dose-escalation trial. *Int J Radiat Oncol Biol Phys* 2007;68:479–484.
336. Pinkawa M, Gagel B, Piroth MD, et al. Erectile dysfunction after external beam radiotherapy for prostate cancer. *Eur Urol* 2009;55:227–234.
337. Zelefsky MJ, Eid JF. Elucidating the etiology of erectile dysfunction after definitive therapy for prostatic cancer. *Int J Radiat Oncol Biol Phys* 1998;40:129–133.
338. Valicenti RK, Choi E, Chen C, et al. Sildenafil citrate effectively reverses sexual dysfunction induced by three-dimensional conformal radiation therapy. *Urology* 2001;57:769–773.
339. Roeloffzen EM, Battermann JJ, van Deursen MJ, et al. Influence of dose on risk of acute urinary retention after iodine-125 prostate brachytherapy. *Int J Radiat Oncol Biol Phys* 2011;80:1072–1079.
340. Ohashi T, Yorozu A, Toya K, et al. Predictive factors of acute urinary retention requiring catheterization following 125I prostate brachytherapy. *Jpn J Clin Oncol* 2006;36:285–289.

341. Keyes M, Schellenberg D, Moravan V, et al. Decline in urinary retention incidence in 805 patients after prostate brachytherapy: the effect of learning curve? *Int J Radiat Oncol Biol Phys* 2006;64:825–834.

342. Neill M, Studer G, Le L, et al. The nature and extent of urinary morbidity in relation to prostate brachytherapy urethral dosimetry. *Brachytherapy* 2007;6:173–179.

343. Keyes M, Miller S, Moravan V, et al. Predictive factors for acute and late urinary toxicity after permanent prostate brachytherapy: long-term outcome in 712 consecutive patients. *Int J Radiat Oncol Biol Phys* 2009;73:1023–1032.

344. Phan J, Swanson DA, Levy LB, et al. Late rectal complications after prostate brachytherapy for localized prostate cancer: incidence and management. *Cancer* 2009;115:1827–1839.

345. Davis BJ, Horwitz EM, Lee WR, et al. American Brachytherapy Society consensus guidelines for transrectal ultrasound-guided permanent prostate brachytherapy. *Brachytherapy* 2012;11:6–19.

346. Stone NN, Stock RG. Long-term urinary, sexual, and rectal morbidity in patients treated with iodine–125 prostate brachytherapy followed up for a minimum of 5 years. *Urology* 2007;69:338–342.

347. Gomez-Iturriaga Pina A, Crook J, Borg J, et al. Median 5 year follow-up of 125iodine brachytherapy as monotherapy in men aged < or = 55 years with favorable prostate cancer. *Urology* 2010;75:1412–1416.

348. Mabjeesh N, Chen J, Beri A, et al. Sexual function after permanent 125I-brachytherapy for prostate cancer. *Int J Impot Res* 2005;17:96–101.

349. Taira AV, Merrick GS, Galbreath RW, et al. Erectile function durability following permanent prostate brachytherapy. *Int J Radiat Oncol Biol Phys* 2009;75:639–648.

350. Merrick GS, Butler WM, Wallner KE, et al. Erectile function after prostate brachytherapy. *Int J Radiat Oncol Biol Phys* 2005;62:437–447.

351. Raina R, Agarwal A, Goyal KK, et al. Long-term potency after iodine–125 radiotherapy for prostate cancer and role of sildenafil citrate. *Urology* 2003;62:1103–1108.

352. Vijayakumar S, Quadri SF, Karrison TG, et al. Localized prostate cancer: use of serial prostate-specific antigen measurements during radiation therapy. *Radiology* 1992;184:271–274.

353. Zagars GK, Sherman NE, Babaian RJ. Prostate-specific antigen and external beam radiation therapy in prostate cancer. *Cancer* 1991;67:412–420.

354. Critz FA, Williams WH, Benton JB, et al. Prostate specific antigen bounce after radioactive seed implantation followed by external beam radiation for prostate cancer. *J Urol* 2000;163:1085–1089.

355. Cavanagh W, Blasko JC, Grimm PD, et al. Transient elevation of serum prostate-specific antigen following (125)I/(103)Pd brachytherapy for localized prostate cancer. *Semin Urol Oncol* 2000;18:160–165.

356. Hanlon AL, Pinover WH, Horwitz EM, et al. Patterns and fate of PSA bouncing following 3D-CRT. *Int J Radiat Oncol Biol Phys* 2001;50:845–849.

357. Rosser CJ, Kuban DA, Levy LB, et al. Prostate specific antigen bounce phenomenon after external beam radiation for clinically localized prostate cancer. *J Urol* 2002;168:2001–2005.

358. Ciezki JP, Reddy CA, Garcia J, et al. PSA kinetics after prostate brachytherapy: PSA bounce phenomenon and its implications for PSA doubling time. *Int J Radiat Oncol Biol Phys* 2006;64:512–517.

359. Zelefsky MJ. PSA bounce versus biochemical failure following prostate brachytherapy. *Nat Clin Pract Urol* 2006;3:578–579.

360. Roach M 3rd, Hanks G, Thames H Jr, et al. Defining biochemical failure following radiotherapy with or without hormonal therapy in men with clinically localized prostate cancer: recommendations of the RTOG-ASTRO Phoenix Consensus Conference. *Int J Radiat Oncol Biol Phys* 2006;65:965–974.

361. Pound CR, Partin AW, Eisenberger MA, et al. Natural history of progression after PSA elevation following radical prostatectomy. *JAMA* 1999;281:1591–1597.

362. Zelefsky MJ, Ben-Porat L, Scher HI, et al. Outcome predictors for the increasing PSA state after definitive external-beam radiotherapy for prostate cancer. *J Clin Oncol* 2005;23:826–831.

363. Freedland SJ, Humphreys EB, Mangold LA, et al. Risk of prostate cancer-specific mortality following biochemical recurrence after radical prostatectomy. *JAMA* 2005;294:433–439.

364. D'Amico AV, Cote K, Loffredo M, et al. Determinants of prostate cancer-specific survival after radiation therapy for patients with clinically localized prostate cancer. *J Clin Oncol* 2002;20:4567–4573.

365. Crook JM, Perry GA, Robertson S, et al. Routine prostate biopsies following radiotherapy for prostate cancer: results for 226 patients. *Urology* 1995;45:624–631.

366. Van Den Eeden SK, Lu R, Zhang N et al A Biopsy-based 17-gene genomic prostate score as a predictor of metastases and prostate cancer death in surgically treated men with clinically localized disease. *Eur Urol* 2018;73:129–138.

367. Cuzick J, Stone S, Fisher G, et al Validation of an RNA cell cycle progression score for predicting death from prostate cancer in a conservatively managed needle biopsy cohort. *Br J Cancer* 2015;113:382–389.

368. Freedland SJ, Gerber L, Reid J, et al. Prognostic utility of cell cycle progression score in men with prostate cancer after primary external beam radiation therapy. *Int J Radiat Oncol Biol Phys* 2013;86(5):848–853.

369. Bishoff JT, Freedland SJ, Gerber L, et al. Prognostic utility of the CCP score generated from biopsy in men treated with prostatectomy. *J Urol* 2014;192 (2):409.

370. Oderda M, Cozzi G, Barale M, et al. CCP-score improves the current risk assessment in newly diagnosed prostate cancer patients. *Eur Urol* 2016;15 (Suppl 3):e732.

371. Shore N, Boczko J, Kella N, et al. Impact of CCP test on personalizing treatment decisions: results from a prospective registry of newly diagnosed prostate cancer patients. *J Clin Oncol* 2015;33(15 Suppl 1).

372. Crawford ED, Shore N, Scardino PT, et al. Performance of CCP assay in an updated series of biopsy samples obtained from commercial testing. *J Clin Oncol* 2015;33(7 Suppl 1).

373. Health Quality Ontario. Prolaris cell cycle progression test for localized prostate cancer: a health technology assessment. *Ont Health Technol Assess Ser* 2017;17:1–75.

374. Klein, E.A., Cooperberg, M.R., Magi-Galluzzi, C. et al. A 17-gene assay to predict prostate cancer aggressiveness in the context of Gleason grade heterogeneity, tumor multifocality, and biopsy undersampling. *Eur Urol* 2014;66:550–560.

375. Cullen, J, Rosner, IL, Brand, TC, et al. A biopsy-based 17-gene Genomic Prostate Score predicts recurrence after radical prostatectomy and adverse surgical pathology in a racially diverse population of men with clinically low- and intermediate-risk prostate cancer. *Eur Urol* 2015;68:123–131.

376. Badani, K, Thompson, DJ, Buerki, C, et al. Impact of a genomic classifier of metastatic risk on postoperative treatment recommendations for prostate cancer patients: a report from the DECIDE study group. *Oncotarget* 2013;4:600–609.

377. Ehro N, Vergara IA, Buerki C, et al. Discovery of a biomarker signature that predicts upgrading or upstaging in patients with low-risk prostate cancer. *J Clin Oncol* 2012;30(37):(Abstract).

378. Kongnuyun M, George AK, Iyer A, et al Tumor contact length: A novel multiparametric MRI predictor of prostate cancer outcomes. *J Clin Oncol* 2016;34(2):61(Abstract).

379. Freeman DE, King CR. Stereotactic body radiotherapy for low-risk prostate cancer: five-year outcomes. *Radiat Oncol* 2011;6:3–9.

380. Katz A Stereotactic body radiation therapy offers a safe, non-invasive treatment for prostate cancer patients over 70 years old. *Int J Radiat Oncol Biol Phys* 2012;84(3): S361.

381. Boike TP, Cho L, Lotan Y, et al. A phase I dose escalation study of stereotactic body radiation therapy (SBRT) for low- and intermediate-risk prostate cancer. *Int J Radiat Oncol Biol Phys* 2009;75 (3): S80

382. Katz A, Kang J Stereotactic body radiation therapy for low-intermediate-, and high-risk prostate cancer: disease control and quality of life at 6 years. *Int J Radiat Oncol Biol Phys* 2013;87:S24–S25.

383. Meier R, Beckman G, Henning N, et al Five-year outcomes from a multicenter trial of stereotactic body radiation therapy for low- and intermediate-risk prostate cancer. *Int J Radiat Oncol Biol Phys* 2016;96(2S):S33, Abstr 74.

384. Dess RT, Jackson WC, Suy S, et al. Predictors of multidomain decline in health-related quality of life after stereotactic body radiation therapy (SBRT) for prostate cancer. *Int J Radiat Oncol Biol Phys* 2016;96(2S):S33, Abstr 75.

385. Johnson SB, Soulos PR, Shafman TD, et al. Patient-reported quality of life after stereotactic body radiation therapy versus moderate hypofractionation for clinically localized prostate cancer. *Int J Radiat Oncol Biol Phys* 2016;96(2):E242, Abstr 2590.

386. Greco C, Pares O, Pimentel N, et al. Phase 1/2 study of urethral and rectal sparing following extreme hypofractionated (5x9 Gy) stereotactic body radiation therapy in prostate cancer. *Int J Radiat Oncol Biol Phys* 2016;96(2):S33, Abstr 76.

387. Blacksburg SR, Witten MR, Katz AE, et al. Prostate-specific antigen kinetics after robotic radiosurgery based stereotactic body radiation therapy (SBRT): the effect of pretreatment clinical parameters. *Int J Radiat Oncol Biol Phys* 2016;96(2):S246, Abstr 2600.

388. Lee AK, Chi S, Nogueras Gonzalez G, et al. Long-term outcomes, toxicity, and quality of life after proton therapy for prostate cancer. *Int J Radiat Oncol Biol Phys* 2015;93(3):E207–E208, Poster Abstr 2521.

389. Choi S, Amin M, Palmer M, et al. Comparison of intensity modulated proton therapy (IMPT) to passively scattered proton therapy (PSPT) in the treatment of prostate cancer. *Int J Radiat Oncol Biol Phys* 2011;81(2):S154.

390. Slater JD, Rossi CJ Jr, Yonemoto LT, et al. Proton therapy for prostate cancer: the initial Loma Linda University experience. *Int J Radiat Oncol Biol Phys* 2004;59:348–352.

391. Takagi M. Mima M, Terashima K, et al. Long-term outcomes in patients treated with proton therapy for localized prostate cancer. *Int J Radiat Oncol Biol Phys* 2015;93:E186–E187, Abstr 2473.

392. Mendenhall NP, Hoppe BS, Nichols RC, et al Five-year outcomes from 3 prospective trials of image-guided proton therapy for prostate cancer. *Int J Radiat Oncol Biol Phys* 2014;88:596–602.

393. Choi S, Blanchard P, Ye R, et al Outcomes following proton therapy for the treatment of prostate cancer: efficacy and toxicity results from 2 prospective single institution cohorts. *Int J Radiat Oncol Biol Phys* 2017;99(2S):E221, Abstr 2531.

394. Vargas C, Hartsell WF, Dunn M, et al. Hypofractionated versus standard fractionated proton beam therapy for low-risk prostate cancer: interim results of a randomized trial, PCG GU 002. *Int J Radiat Oncol Biol Phys* 2015;93(3):S198, Abstr 1100.

395. Ho CK, Hoppe BS, Bryant CM, et al. Patient-reported quality of life and disease-specific outcomes five years following proton therapy for prostate cancer in men 60 years old and younger. *Int J Radiat Oncol Biol Phys* 2015;93(3):E488, Abstr 3219.

396. Coen JJ, Paly JJ, Niemierko A, et al. Long-term quality of life—outcome after proton beam monotherapy for localized prostate cancer. *Int J Radiat Oncol Biol Phys* 2012;82(2):e201–e209.

397. Habl G, Uhl M, Katayama S, et al Acute toxicity and quality of life in patients with prostate cancer treated with protons or carbon ions in a prospective randomized phase II study. The IPI trial. *Int J Radiat oncol Biol Phys* 2016;95:435–443.

398. Takagi M, Demizu Y, Terashima K, et al Long-term outcomes in patients treated with proton therapy for localized prostate cancer. *Cancer Med* 2017;6:2234–2243.

399. Iwata H, Ishikawa H, Takagi M, et al Long-term outcomes of proton therapy for prostate cancer in Japan: retrospective analysis of a multi-institutional survey. *Int J Radiat Oncol Biol Phys* 2017;99:E241–E242.

400. Amini A, Kavanagh BD, Raben D, et al. Proton beam therapy utilization and disparity in the united states for treatment of localized prostate cancer: a study of the National Cancer Data Base. *Int J Radiat Oncol Biol Phys* 2016;96(2):E244–E245.

401. Mehta MP, Dunn M, Hoppe BS, et al. Fact or fiction: proton beam therapy is primarily for patients with prostate cancer. *Int J Radiat oncol Biol Phys* 2015;93(3S):E353, Abstr 2879.

402. Mishra MV, Aggarwal S, Bentzen SM, et al Establishing evidence-based indications for proton therapy: an overview of current clinical trials. *Int J Radiat Oncol Biol Phys* 2017;97:228–235.

403. Ghai S. Real-time MRI-guided focused ultrasound for local therapy of locally confined low risk prostate cancer: Feasibility and preliminary results. *Am J Roentgenol* 2015;205:W177–W184.

404. Bolton D. A whole population multicenter series of high intensity ultrasound for management of localized prostate cancer. Outcomes and implications. *J Endourol* 2015;29:844–849.

Section III

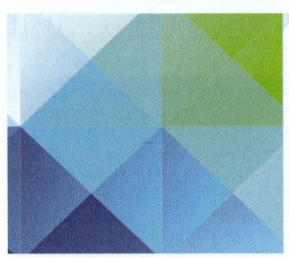

CHAPTER 70

Management of Intermediate- and High-Risk Prostate Cancer: What Do We Know?

Mack Roach III and Hans T. Chung

"It's not what you don't know that gets you into troubles, it's what you know for sure that ain't so"
Attributed to Mark Twain

INTRODUCTION

The management of clinically localized prostate cancer has changed considerably over the past 10 years. Fewer men are being treated for low-risk disease (e.g., prostate-specific antigen [PSA] < 10 ng/mL, Gleason score [GS] < 7, and T-stage < T2b), and more frequently, such men are being managed by active surveillance (AS).[1] Consequently, a higher percentage of men diagnosed with prostate cancer are now being treated with what is categorized as "intermediate-" to "high"-risk disease.[2] Concurrent with these developments, there has been a resurgence in enthusiasm among urologist for recommending radical prostatectomy (RP) as the treatment of choice for men with high-risk and locally advanced disease.[3,4] This trend appears to be in part fueled by plethora of post hoc retrospective studies.[5-7] This practice is not supported however by other recent studies that attempt to account for the "quality of care delivered" (defined as treatment delivered in compliance with National Comprehensive Cancer Network [NCCN] Guidelines) nor is it supported by the findings from contemporary phase III randomized trials.[2,8-13] This chapter was written in an attempt to bring clarity to the controversies surrounding the management of patients currently considered to have "intermediate-" and "high"-risk disease. We focus on the radiation-based therapeutic options and the evidence behind our recommendations. Since the last edition, a number of advances have been made in the technical delivery of radiation for prostate cancer, and some have now been established as "standard of care." Details on the management of low-risk prostate cancer can be found in Chapter 69.

CLINICAL PRESENTATION

Patients with intermediate- or high-risk prostate cancer may present with locoregional symptoms, but this is not common (although it appears to be increasingly common since PSA screening has become less popular). Lower urinary tract symptoms (LUTs) when seen may include nocturia, urinary frequency, urgency, decreased flow, incomplete voiding, intermittent flow, or hesitancy and occasionally erectile dysfunction (ED). Rarely, patients with bulky primary disease may present with urinary tract obstruction or difficulty in passing stool or even bloody stool. With increasing PSA and Gleason score, the risk of metastases increases. Metastatic spread is generally sequential, proceeding from the prostate to the periprostatic pelvic lymph nodes, but some appear to spread directly to the common iliac nodes and then to bone. Rarely, patients may present with renal failure, lymphedema of the lower extremities, and bone pain.

DEFINITIONS OF INTERMEDIATE- AND HIGH-RISK DISEASE

National Comprehensive Cancer Network–Defined Groups

Three prognostic factors have generally been used to define intermediate- and high-risk patients: (a) clinical T-stage (generally based on palpation [although imaging when compelling is included]), (b) the pretreatment PSA, and (c) the biopsy Gleason score (GS). To simplify treatment recommendations and prognostication, several risk classification schemes have been proposed by grouping patients who are thought to have similar biochemical and/or clinical outcomes.[14-17] The most widely recognized definitions for intermediate- to high-risk prostate cancers are that put forth by the NCCN.[2] This system represents a modification of the system proposed by D'Amico et al. However, the NCCN has modified subgroups to account for some of the heterogeneity in risk, by specifying that patients with multiple adverse factors "may be shifted into the next highest risk group."[18] Given the widespread acceptance of this system, for practical purposes, the readers should assume we are referring to this classification system throughout this chapter. Low risk is defined as meeting all the criteria: T1c to T2a, PSA <10 ng/mL, and Gleason score ≤6. Intermediate risk is defined as T2b to T2c, PSA 10 to 20 ng/mL, or GS = 7. High-risk (HR) prostate cancer is any of the following: ≥T3a, PSA >20 ng/mL, or GS 8 to 10.

Limitations of Risk Group Classifications and Other Risk Factors to Be Considered

Perhaps the greatest misunderstanding in using the risk groups based on PSA, GS, and stage is the implied assumption that each of these factors is roughly equally important. For example, a patient can be considered intermediate risk if either the clinical stage is T2b, PSA = 10 to 20, or the GS = 7. However, clinical T-stage is relatively subjective with a high degree or interobserver variability. Pretreatment PSA appears to be a strong predictor of biochemical (PSA) recurrence but a relatively weak predictor of cause-specific survival (CSS) and GS is the most powerful predictor of CSS, followed in importance by T-stage.[19] This has major implications for post hoc comparisons of the results of treatment wherein the distribution of these factors cannot be adequately controlled for.

Another major limitation of the risk groups most commonly used is their dependence on biochemical recurrence or PSA relapse after radiation therapy. In 1996, the American Society for Therapeutic Radiology and Oncology (ASTRO) developed a consensus definition of PSA relapse based on datasets of patients treated with external beam radiation therapy (EBRT) alone (i.e., no hormones).[20] After considerable scrutiny, it was determined that the first ASTRO definition was sensitive to follow-up bias, censoring artifact from backdating, and correlated poorly with clinical progression.[21] To address these issues, the RTOG-ASTRO cosponsored a conference in 2005 in Phoenix, Arizona, to develop a new definition, henceforth known as the Phoenix definition.[21] PSA relapse is defined as a rise of 2 ng/mL or more above the absolute PSA nadir. This definition was considered applicable only to patients treated with EBRT with or without short-term androgen deprivation therapy (ADT). The date of failure is taken at the time of meeting the definition and not backdated. Any salvage therapy initiated prior to meeting the criteria should also be declared as failure. With the Phoenix definition, sensitivity and specificity are 64% and 78%, respectively. This definition to date continues to be considered the standard definition for biochemical failure but should not be used to determine cure rates (e.g., compared to RP) nor should PSA that are consistently rising be ignored in men who could potentially benefit from salvage therapies.[21-23]

In addition to the T-stage, GS, and PSA, a number of other factors are known to impact outcomes. More than 10 years ago, a number of studies showed that the number and/or percentage of biopsy cores positive for prostate cancer (PPC) impacted the outcomes of patients treated definitively by RP or EBRT.[24,25] For example, status post RP, those patients with <34% PPC had similar outcomes as low-risk patients (5-year PSA control 85% vs. 91%, respectively), whereas patients with more than 50% PPC had similar outcomes as high-risk patients (5-year PSA control 30% vs. 43%, respectively). The prognostic significance of PPC has also been reported to extend to prostate cancer–specific mortality (PCSM) in intermediate-risk patients such that when stratified by ≤50% and >50% PPC, 7-year prostate cancer–specific survival was 100% versus 57% (*P* = .004), respectively.

The readers should be aware that there are a number of other limitations associated with attempting to use the risk groups described above to manage patients using the evidence from phase III randomized trials. Most importantly, essentially none of the mature trials on which our level I evidence is based were designed using the grouping systems described above. In fact, these trials generally included a heterogeneous mixture of relatively low- to very high-risk patients. To get around this problem, some investigators have attempted to leverage this mix of patients to create prognostics groupings directly from the patients included in the trials. For example, the Radiation Therapy Oncology Group (RTOG) conducted a meta-analysis based on multiple phase III trials.[14,26] In addition to the large sample size (>1,500 patients), long-term follow-up (out to 15 years), and study endpoints (PCSM and overall survival [OS]), it also incorporated central pathologic review.[14,26] Lessons learned from this meta-analysis (which were subsequently validated by the findings of multiple phase III trials) include the following: (a) the observation that low-risk patients (however defined) do not benefit from the addition of ADT; (b) patients with intermediate-risk disease benefitted from short-term ADT (e.g., 4 months), with no need for longer-term ADT; and (c) patients with high-risk

(HR) disease benefitted most from long-term ADT. The RTOG also subsequently demonstrated that older age (>70) patients were associated with a reduced risk of PCSM and metastases, even after adjusting for the expected increased risk of non–prostate cancer–specific mortality in this subgroup.[27]

There have been a number of very recent (and not so recent) attempts to incorporate biomarkers as prognostic and/or predictors of response to radiation therapy +/– ADT–based treatments.[28-32] Unfortunately, to date, none have been validated so as to provide actionable-based guidance. The critical need for validation is highlighted by the contradictory results noted following early impressive results associated with Bcl-2 and bax expression.[33,34] There is little doubt that one day not only will predictors of therapeutic outcomes be identified but radiation-induced complications as well.[28,35-39] In addition to cautionary notes surrounding the use of predictive markers for patients with intermediate- and high-risk disease, there are a few major cautionary notes related to patients treated on high-profile prospective randomized trials that are summarized in the next section below.

Cautionary Notes on Selected Phase III Randomized Prostate Cancer Trials

Much of the confusion concerning the optimum management of men with intermediate- to high-risk prostate cancer comes from the misinterpretation of high-profile phase III trials. There are several features that these trials have in common: (a) They tend to be underpowered for making evidenced-based conclusions concerning the management of high-risk disease; (b) the problems arising from the underpowered nature of these trials are exacerbated by patient heterogeneity; and (c) the findings appear to justify assertions (i.e., biases) that the investigators are seeking to prove. The underlying principle for these studies is that "if one wants to prove something does not work, make the study too small." Three examples of such high-profile trials suffering from these flaws are shown in Table 70.1.

#1 Beware of Randomized Trials that Are Too Small and Heterogeneous Patient Selection!

The conclusions of the PIVOT (Prostate Intervention Versus Observation Trial) suggest treatment is of limited value with the authors stating, "... After nearly 20 years of follow-up, among men with localized prostate cancer, surgery was not associated with significantly lower all-cause or prostate-cancer mortality than observation ...."[40] Although this trial does not explicitly address the issue of treatment of intermediate- and high-risk disease, it is relevant because the data actually strongly suggest a benefit, thus contradicting the conclusions

TABLE 70.1 SUMMARY OF CAUTIONARY NOTES ON RANDOMIZED TRIALS INCLUDING INTERMEDIATE-/HIGH-RISK PROSTATE CANCER			
First Au. (Ref.) (yr Published) Study	**No. Pts**	**Author's Conclusions**	**Why the Study Is Underpowered**
Wilt[40] 2017, PIVOT	731 (457)[a]		Underpowered based on their own plan to recruit 2,000 men but only recruited roughly 1/3 of this number
Nabid[41,42]	630	18 mo of ADT as effective as 36 mo	Criteria for high risk less evidence based (PSA >20 ng/mL) OS at 5 y 92% vs. 87% (*P* = .052) favoring 36 mo over 18 mo Because of the underpowered nature of the trial, known factors such as GS and T-stage were not significant either
Pommier[43] 2016, GETUG-01	446 (203)[b]	Pelvic node radiation did not improve outcomes	RTOG-9408 required 2,000 pts to show that 4 mo of ADT improved survival
James[44] STAMPEDE	1,917 (369)[c]	"Among men with locally advanced ... ADT plus abiraterone ... was associated with significantly higher rates of overall and failure-free survival than ADT alone ..."	No overall survival advantage for nonmetastatic patients, and no trend for benefits for men >70 y of age (median age for men treated on phase III trials involving RT). Thus, it remains unclear of the role of abiraterone in the setting of typical high-risk prostate cancer

[a]Intermediate and high risk (D'Amico).
[b]Number >15% risk of lymph node involvement.
[c]Node positive, non-metastatic.

in their abstract. Although it was grossly underpowered, the hazard ratios ranged from 0.54 to 0.69, and the differences reached borderline statistical sensitivity (0.08) for survival from death of any cause favoring treatment of patients with intermediate- and high-risk disease. Our assertion that this trial was underpowered is supported by the authors initial study design and comparisons to adequately powered phase III trials. In 1994, Wilt and Brawer described the launching of PIVOT and committed to recruiting 2,000 men. Given the low event rate expected with low-risk patients (42% of total cohort) and inclusion of men >65 years (68% of cohort recruited), even a trial of 2,000 men would be hard pressed to demonstrate a survival benefit. It is well known that active surveillance (AS) is the preferred approach for men with low-risk disease because the risk of death from prostate cancer is very low particularly in men older than 65 years of age. In addition, it is well known that the benefits of RP are most obvious in men <65 years of age. These investigators only recruited 1/3 of the planned accrual goal and still nearly had a positive trial. Thus, with the trends of the benefit favoring treatment for the most relevant subgroups, I consider this a positive trial supporting treatment and the authors' conclusions statistically invalid.

Another major underpowered trial reported by Nabid et al. argues for a shorter duration of long-term ADT suggesting that 18 months of ADT is as effective as 36 months in 630 men managed with EBRT.[41,42] Based on these data, some physicians have concluded that it has established a new standard of care for high-risk patients. However, the earlier trial that established that 36 months was superior to 6 months (Bolla et al.) recruited 50% more patients (*n* = 970). Should not a study lengthening ADT by 12 months require at least as many patients, particularly if they were lower risk (e.g., fewer T3 patients), to redefine the standard of care? Criteria for high risk in this study were less evidence based (PSA >20 ng/mL). Evidence that this study was underpowered is supported by the observation that known prognostic factors such as GS and T-stage were also not significant predictors of outcome. The desire to shorten the duration of ADT is admirable, and many patients would love to be spared the unnecessary use of ADT, but for most, a loss of life may be deemed an excessive price.

A third trial suffering from being underpowered and an unfortunate study design is GETUG-01 (Groupe d'Etude des Tumeurs Uro-Génitales). This French multicenter phase III reported by Pommier et al. concluded that there was no value to the use of prophylactic lymph nodal irradiation.[43] The fact is, not only was this trial grossly underpowered with only 203 men with a risk of lymph node involvement >15% (e.g., RTOG-9413 enrolled 1,200+ patients: RTOG-0924 targets 2,580), but *none* of the patients actually received "whole-pelvic" EBRT (see the discussion below) but instead were treated using a "mini-pelvic" technique.[45]

At the other end of the spectrum are studies suggesting a role for more aggressive drug therapy.[46] For example, although STAMPEDE (Systemic Therapy in Advancing or Metastatic Prostate Cancer: Evaluation of Drug Efficacy) was a rather large randomized trial (*n* = 1,917), its analysis is complicated by its very heterogeneous design. STAMPEDE included patients with metastatic and nonmetastatic disease (the latter including node + patients with high-risk localized prostate cancer), making it difficult to parse out who benefited the most. Per protocol, EBRT was mandated for patients with node-negative, nonmetastatic disease and "encouraged" for those with positive nodes. The primary outcome measure was overall survival, with failure-free survival (treatment failure was defined as radiologic, clinical, or PSA progression or death from prostate cancer), defined as an "intermediate primary outcome." The authors concluded that "Among men with locally advanced ... prostate cancer, ADT plus abiraterone ...

was associated with significantly higher rates of overall and failure-free survival than ADT alone ...." However, in fact, there is no overall survival advantage for "nonmetastatic" patients, and no trend for benefits for men >70 years of age (the median age for men treated on previous phase III RTOG trials involving RT and ADT). Thus, although encouraging it remains unclear of the role of abiraterone in the setting of typical high-risk prostate cancer managed with ADT and EBRT.

#2 Beware of Large Post Hoc Population-Based and Biased Retrospective Studies!

In addition to the problem of underpowered randomized trials, there are a large number of problematic post hoc studies comparing the outcomes following RP versus EBRT. Key characteristics of these have been the sizes of the databases used and efforts to use statistical methods to convince the readers that all meaningful biases have been accounted for so as to imply that the findings are likely to be accurate.

If a 700-patient, prospective randomized trial (PIVOT) can be published in the *New England Journal of Medicine* (twice) to show RP does not prolong survival compared to observation, why analyze 118,000 nonrandomized men with missing information and make clinically relevant conclusions? These studies tend to ignore or inadequately adjust for fundamental differences in patient selection (e.g., patient selection, existing baseline morbidity, a lack of modern radiation-based treatment techniques, and the use of ADT) and tend to be based on very large sample sizes (e.g., >50,000 to 100,000 or more), with no relevance to clinical medicine. These large sample sizes use hazard ratios (HR) that result in statistically significance but relatively small clinical differences. The potential for erroneous conclusions to be reached is quite high, given the absence in detailed patient level information (e.g., percent positive cores, bulkiness of disease). The practical reality is that the largest trials comparing survival outcomes after definitive treatment in men with localized disease conducted to date have included approximately 700 to 3,000 patients (e.g., PIVOT, PROTECT, RTOG-9408, RTOG-0924, CHHIP), so great caution must be taken in attempting to use post hoc analysis of cohorts of 7,500 to 118,000.[5,6,47] Small errors in the rate in attribution of cause of death and selection bias can easily explain biased conclusions.[10]

#3 Beware of Confusion Concerning the Evidence for the Importance of Radiation Dose and Volume!

We (radiation oncologist) have been a bit illogical, concerning our interpretation of the data from trials involving the three major "tweakable" interventions, namely, (a) radiation dose, (b) radiation volume, and (c) the use of ADT. Despite a plethora of trials involving dose-escalated radiation, all failing to prove that higher doses improve overall survival, high doses have become standard of care (see JNCI and NCCN guidelines). These studies have generally demonstrated improved biochemical control based on PSA but at increased cost and in some cases with increased toxicity. In contrast, the improvement in PSA associated with whole-pelvic radiation therapy (WPRT) demonstrated by the only adequately powered phase III trial, using an adequately sized pelvic field, has not convinced roughly 1/2 radiation oncologists to adopt this as standard for high-risk patients (personal communication, based on an informal audience survey). Even less logical is the willingness of radiation oncologists to look for reasons to shorten the duration or completely abandon ADT based on post hoc retrospective data, despite their lack of reliability. For example, numerous post hoc studies fail to show the value of ADT and tout the advantages of surgery compared to radiation but have not been borne out by randomized trials. Omitting ADT because "maybe, it would not be needed if higher doses of radiation were used" is potentially dangerous and should require a randomized trial to justify.

Novel Imaging Techniques: Implications of Nodal Imaging for Radiation Therapy

Until very recently, imaging contributed relatively little to the management of patients with clinically localized prostate cancer, such that the patient eligibility for RTOG trials has generally been based on palpation T-stage.[26] This philosophy is largely based on the fact that neither CT nor magnetic resonance imaging (MRI) has been shown to be sensitive or specific enough to be routinely used to rule out lymph node involvement.[48] In the absence of definitive evidence of the presence and location of lymph node involvement, a class solution is used to design radiation fields when WPRT is intended.[49,50] However, there are at least three major imaging approaches that may compliment the use of class solutions including (a) positron emission tomography (PET) imaging, (b) the use of lymphotropic nanoparticles, and (c) sentinel lymph node imaging.

PET imaging agents have recently grown in popularity with studies showing superior results compared to conventional imaging such as CT scans.[51] It also appears that prostate specific membrane antigen (PSMA)-based PET imaging may be as good or better than other available agents.[52] Higher detection rates have been observed with (68)Ga-PSMA PET/CT compared to choline PET/CT. Although PET (68)Ga PSMA-11 appears to have a higher detection rate than (11)C-choline for nodes and bones lesions, this comparison is complicated by the fact that there was a lack of concordance when applying both tracers.[53] However, there appear to be size limitations associated with this approach that hampers the sensitivity of PET imaging.[54] In one study, using a lymph nodal region-based analysis, the sensitivity of 68Ga-PSMA PET/CT was 56%, the specificity was 98%, and the positive predictive value (PPV) was 90%. Of note, the mean size of the false-negative nodes was 2.7 mm; thus, smaller nodes are likely to be missed.

Sentinel lymph node dissections are standard in a variety of cancer sites (e.g., breast cancer), but its application in prostate cancer has been very limited. Intraoperative gamma probe and dynamic lymphoscintigraphy appear to be a very sensitive approach for defining disease intraoperatively. For example, Wawroschek et al. reported that about a third of sentinel lymph nodes were in areas outside of a limited node dissection, such as the presacral, hypogastric, and pararectal regions.[55] Holl et al. also demonstrated that sentinel lymph node dissections guided by using radiolabeled nanocolloid were reliable in detecting positive nodes in over 2,000 patients.[56] Using a 2-day protocol, involving injection of a radioisotope injected into the prostate, combined with intraoperative scanning, they concluded that the detection rate was 97.6% and false-negative rate only 6%. Krengli et al. reported on the application of sentinel lymph node imaging (single-photon emission computed tomography [SPECT]) to pelvic radiation therapy for prostate cancer and reported that at least 25% of patients had nodes outside the standard nodal pelvic clinical target volume (CTV).[57] More recently, Chen et al. reported on a feasibility study performed at University of California San Francisco (UCSF) using sentinel lymph node image-guided intensity-modulated radiation therapy (IMRT) for prostate cancer and compared it to RTOG-based IMRT plans.[58] Patients were injected with ^{99m}Tc-sulfur colloid into six prostate locations and then imaged with SPECT to generate a lymphatic drainage map. Although all patients had sentinel nodes identified in the internal or external iliac nodal basins, 50% had sentinel nodes in the para-aortics. We concluded that RTOG consensus guidelines on pelvic lymph coverage would have included all relevant lymph nodes in only 30% of cases.

Guided by this sentinel nodal study we reported in comparative radiation therapy plans, there would have been no significant increase in the doses received by organs at risk.

Perhaps the most sensitive (but least available) diagnostic imaging test involves the use of lymphotropic superparamagnetic nanoparticles, which, combined with MRI, has been reported to be a very sensitive and specific test for detecting lymph node involvement.[59,60] It not only appears to be more specific than the "Roach equation" in assessing nodal involvement, but it can identify the location of disease. These nanoparticles are transported by lymphatic vessels, and filtered by lymph nodes. Lymph nodes that have been infiltrated by metastases will have distorted lymphatic flow and accumulate the nanoparticles. Of particular note, documented by histologic confirmation, 71% would not have met the MRI size criteria for malignancy. This imaging approach was associated with sensitivity in excess of 90% versus 35% with MRI alone ($P < .001$). When only nodes that were between 5 and 10 mm in diameter on the short axis were considered, the sensitivity increased from 28.5% to 96.4% ($P < .001$). Shih et al. proposed margins around major vessels as an alternative based on their studies because of the lack of availability of this imaging agent.[61] Dinniwell et al. proposed a pelvic nodal model based on nanoparticles and recommended CTV margins to the distal para-aortic (12 mm), common iliac (10 mm), external iliac (9 mm), and internal iliac (10 mm), drawn in continuity with a 12-mm expansion anterior to the sacrum and 22-mm expansion medial to the pelvic sidewall.[62] Unfortunately, despite great promise, this agent is currently only available in the Netherlands.[63]

MANAGEMENT OF PELVIC LYMPH NODAL DISEASE: THE RATIONALE AND EVIDENCE

The Rationale

Despite the improvements in the detection rate of lymph node involvement (LNI) provided by PET imaging agents, the ability of current imaging techniques to detect involved nodes is hampered by their sole reliance on size criteria.[54] The true incidence of clinically occult disease is generally much higher when sophisticated assays, imaging agents that have increased affinity to lymph nodes, and more extensive node dissections are performed. For example, Shariat et al. studied reverse-transcriptase polymerase chain reaction (RT-PCR) assay for human glandular kallikrein 2 (hK2) mRNA expression in *histopathologically* normal pelvic nodes in patients with pT3N0 prostate cancer.[64] Of the 199 evaluable men, 20% and 40% had positive and equivocal results, respectively. In multivariate analysis, a positive RT-PCR/hK2 result was associated with PSA progression, development of distant metastases, and PCSM.

When an extended pelvic lymph node dissection (including the nodes surrounding obturator vessels and internal iliac veins) is performed rather than the traditional limited dissection (or sampling), wherein the posterior extent is carried to the obturator nerve, more diseases are found. For example, Bader et al. conducted a prospective study of the anatomic extent of pelvic nodal involvement in a cohort of 365 men who underwent an extended lymph node dissection and radical prostatectomy.[65] The median number of nodes retrieved was 21. They used hematoxylin and eosin (H&E) stains to evaluate the extracted nodes, 24% of patients had node-positive disease, of which 49% of them had a PSA >20 ng/mL. The internal iliac nodes, which are not usually dissected in a limited dissection, were involved in 58% of men with node-positive disease. Of note, 19% of node-positive men had involved nodes that were exclusively found in the internal iliac region, suggesting that the lymphatic drainage of prostate cancer is variable. The rate of problematic lymphocele was 2%.

Another important consideration, when reviewing surgical studies, is whether H&E staining was performed or more sensitive analyses were included, such as immunohistochemistry (IHC) or RT-PCR. Heidenreich et al. reported on the incidence of lymph node involvement between standard and extended pelvic lymphadenectomies in 203 patients.[66] IHC staining was performed if the H&E findings were negative. There were more dissected nodes in the extended dissection group (28 vs. 11; P < .01), at the expense of longer operative time (179 vs. 125 minutes; P < .03). There were more than twice the number of patients with positive nodes (26% and 12%; P < .03) in the extended dissection group, with 42% of all metastases lying outside the planes of a limited dissection. In patients deemed as high risk (Gleason score 7 to 10 and PSA ≥10.6 ng/mL) for lymph node metastasis, 60.9% of patients had histologically positive nodes. There was no difference in pelvic lymphocele or postoperative complications between the two groups. Data reported by Briganti et al. also attempted to address the question concerning the optimal number of lymph nodes to be removed during a nodal dissection.[67] In a cohort of 858 men who were treated predominantly with an extended lymph node dissection and who had a median PSA of 5.8 ng/mL and 62% with GS ≤ 6 and approximately 25% GS = 7, based on a receiver operator curve (ROC) analysis, they concluded that the removal of 28 nodes yielded a 90% ability to detect LNI. They also concluded that assessment of 10 or fewer nodes was associated with a very high false-negative rate. This data highlight the shortcomings of studies postulating much lower rates of LNI involvement than suggested by the so-called Roach equation.[68–71]

Relevant to the rationale of recognizing the true incidence of LNI are circumstantial data to suggest that there may be a benefit of removing more involved lymph nodes even if they are occult. For example, retrospective study from Johns Hopkins, the pathologic findings and biochemical outcomes were compared between two high-volume surgeons, each of whom exclusively performed either limited (n = 1,865) or extended (n = 2,135) node dissections during radical prostatectomy.[72] As expected, the extended dissection group had more lymph nodes retrieved than the limited group (11.6 vs. 8.9 nodes; P < .0001). Yet the proportion of patients with involved nodes was also significantly higher in the extended dissection group (3.3% vs. 1.2%; P < .0001). When only patients with Gleason score 7 or 8 to 10 were considered, the difference was even more striking (8.2% vs. 2.4% and 23.2% vs. 8.9%, respectively). The relative risks of detecting a patient with involved nodes were remarkably similar, varying between 2.5 and 3 when adjusted by Gleason score, organ-confined status, seminal vesicle invasion (SVI), and surgical margin status. There was a trend in favor of the extended dissection group for 5-year biochemical recurrence-free survival (34.4% vs. 16.5%; P = .07). Among patients with <15% positive lymph nodes, the difference was more remarkable (42.9% vs. 10%; P = .01), suggesting a therapeutic benefit of an extended dissection in low-volume disease. Clinically significant lymphoceles occurred in only 0.3% in the extended dissection group. However, more recent studies have questioned the therapeutic value of more extensive dissection.[73]

On the basis of these studies, the NCCN guidelines recommend an extended lymph node dissection for all patients who have a predicted probability of lymph node metastases of >2% for both diagnostic and potentially therapeutic reasons.[2] Although there have been numerous nomograms to predict nodal involvement, most are derived from surgical data where only limited node dissections were performed.[74,75] Nomograms also have been developed using surgical data from patients who had an extended lymph node dissection to predict pelvic nodal involvement.[76] Despite these advances from a practical standpoint, because of its simplicity, it appears that the so-called Roach equation is still held relevant and has been validated with a cohort of over 3,000 patients treated with RP and

extended lymph node dissections.[71,77] Overall, the accuracy of this equation was found to be 80% in this cohort; however, Abdollah et al.[71] found that applying the recommended cutoff of ≥15% (to decide on whether to treat the pelvic nodes) might lead to missing about a third of patients with lymph node involvement, and thus, they recommended that the threshold be lowered to 6%.

Whole-Pelvic Radiation Therapy

Collectively, these studies argue that an extended node dissection may or may not yield a therapeutic benefit in the subgroup of patients with minimal nodal disease.[73] In the application of radiation with curative intent, this issue may have great relevance to prophylactic WPRT. Unfortunately, only one relevant large phase III trial has been completed to date, and although most retrospective studies have been supportive, some post hoc population-based studies have yielded conflicting results.[78–80] Much of this confusion concerning this issue stems from a misunderstanding of the data available from RTOG-9413.[81] Table 70.2 summarizes a body of selected literature addressing WPRT in patients with intermediate- to high-risk disease managed in the definitive and the postoperative setting.

RTOG-9413 was a landmark trial that featured a two-by-two factorial randomization scheme to either prostate-only radiation therapy (PORT) or WPRT followed by a prostate boost and either 4 months of neoadjuvant and concurrent hormones or 4 months of adjuvant ADT (AHT) at the completion of EBRT.[78] Patients with an estimated nodal risk of >15% or T2c to T4 with a Gleason score of ≥6 were eligible for the study. The 4-year progression-free survival was 54.2% and 47% in the combined WPRT arms and PORT arms (P = .02), respectively. When the four arms were analyzed separately, the neoadjuvant hormone and WPRT arm (59.6%) had a significantly better 4-year progression-free survival than the other three arms (44.3% to 49.8%; P = .008). Although there was no difference in acute (3% vs. 4%; P = .39) and late (2% vs. 2%; P = .85) grade 3 to 5 genitourinary (GU) morbidities, a trend toward increased acute (2% vs. 1%; P = .06) and late (1.7% vs. 0.6%; P = .09) grade 3 to 5 gastrointestinal (GI) morbidities was seen in the combined WPRT and prostate-only arms, respectively.

Although RTOG-9413 affirmed the role of WPRT and neoadjuvant hormonal therapy (NHT) in HR prostate cancer, there has been some lingering reluctance among some radiation oncologists, with many instead opting for "mini-pelvic" fields or omitting the pelvic field entirely.[101] To reinforce this notion of the volume dependence on control of microscopic nodal disease, we conducted a secondary post hoc secondary subset analysis of patients treated on RTOG-9413.[45] Because of the disparity in the time point at which the neoadjuvant and adjuvant ADT arms became susceptible to relapse (i.e., end of both radiation therapy and ADT), only patients (n = 649) who received NHT were included in this analysis. After stratifying by volume irradiated, the 7-year progression-free survival was 40%, 31%, and 27% in the groups that received whole-pelvic, mini-pelvic, and prostate-only radiation therapy, respectively (P = .02; Fig. 70.1). There was no difference in acute grade ≥3 genitourinary or gastrointestinal toxicities among the three volumes. No difference was seen in the incidence of late grade ≥3 genitourinary toxicities between the whole-pelvic, mini-pelvic, and prostate-only radiation therapy groups at 48 months (3.0%, 2.4%, and 0%, respectively; P = .24). There was a small but significant increase in the incidence of late grade ≥3 gastrointestinal toxicities with larger fields at 48 months (4.3%, 1.2%, and 0%, respectively; P = .006). Of note, 3D conformal radiation therapy (3DCRT), let alone IMRT, was not routinely performed in this study. It

TABLE 70.2 SELECTED STUDIES ASSESSING THE VALUE OF WPRT IN THE DEFINITIVE AND POSTOPERATIVE SETTINGS[a]

Authors (Chronologic)	Source	Study Design	Key Findings
Seaward[82,83]	UCSF	Retrospective single institutional analysis of patients undergoing prostate only or WPRT with and without hormonal therapy	WPRT (superior border L5-S1) associated with improved PSA control rate. Greatest benefit seen for those with risk between 15% and 30%
Pan[84]	U of Mich.	Compared men undergoing EBRT treated divided into three categories based on the estimated risk (Partin table) of LN involvement: 0–5%, >5–15%, and >15%	Benefit for WPRT in men with risk of lymph node involvement of 5–15% with an improved 2-year PSA control rate, 90.1% vs. 80.6% ($P = .02$)
Roach[78,85]	RTOG	Randomized trial ($n \sim 1,200$) compared sequence of ADT and WPRT vs. PO. Primary endpoint: PFS (PSA, clinical failure, death)	WPRT associated with improvement in PFS when preceded by combined hormonal blockade (CAB) but not when administered before CAB
Jacob[86]	Fox Chase	Retrospective study of patients with risk + LN >15% treated with "whole-" vs. "partial"-pelvic EBRT vs. PO fields ($n = 420$). Concluded no benefit to WPRT or ADT	None received WPRT (defined as defined by RTOG-9413). "Whole"-pelvic field use would have been included in PO arm of RTOG-9413
Pommier[43,87]	France	444 pts with T1b-T3N0M0 randomized to prostate +/− WPRT 46 Gy with superior border at S1-S2. Only 55% had LN risk <15%	None of the patients received WPRT (defined as top L5-S1); most low risk for lymph node involvement
Spiotto[88]	Stanford	Retrospective analysis of postop patients undergoing prostate only or WPRT with and without hormonal therapy	Use of WPRT associated with better PSA control with greatest benefit seen in patients with adverse features
Da Pozzo[89]	Italy	Retrospectively compared pts with + nodes with 129 treated with WPRT + ADT vs. 121 with ADT alone	Use of WPRT was a major predictor of PSA control ($P = .002$) and CSS ($P = .009$)
Aizer[90]	Yale	Retrospective review of 277 consecutive patients with estimated risk of lymph node involvement ≥15%	WPRT associated improved 4 y biochemical control rate (69.4% vs. 86.3%)
Milecki[91]	Poland	Retrospective analysis of HR prostate ca. with and without WPRT	Improved CSS with WPRT
Bittner[92]	USA	Compares PSA control CSS and OS among HR pts treated with brachytherapy and a mini-pelvic (MP) radiation therapy or WPRT	Trend toward improved PSA control, CSS, and OS with WPRT, most apparent among the ADT naive, who had improved OS
Mantini[93]	Italy	WPRT vs. PO in pts with HR prostate cancer treated with RT and long-term (>1 yr) ADT	Patients with >30% risk of + nodes had an improvement with WPRT ($P = .03$)
Moghanaki[94]	Virginia	WPRT vs. PBRT in the postoperative setting (pts excluded if they had + nodes or ADT)	In pts with PSA >/= 0.4 ng/mL, WPRT associated with a 53% reduction in PSA failure ($P = .031$)
Tward[95]	Utah	Evaluated EBRT on CSS and OS in cT1-T4, cN1, M0 prostate ca. using SEER data	Better 10-year CSS but not OS with EBRT with TNT 8 to prevent one death at 10 y
Amini[80]	Colorado	Compared WPRT vs. PORT for HR pts, using the NCDB in treated from 2004 to 2006, with propensity matching was performed	Authors concluded WPRT had no OS benefit vs. PORT. We conclude pts with WPRT had: higher T-stage, GS, PSA, ># adverse factors, and criteria for WPRT unknown
Braunstein[96]	Harvard	WPRT vs. PORT +/− ADT using a multi-institution cohort of 3,709 pts assessed all-cause mortality (ACM)	Authors concluded that WPRT and ADT were associated with a decrease in ACM, but the combination yielded no greater benefit, suggesting a shared mechanism treatment of micrometastatic nodal disease
Song[97]	Korea	Compared postop WPRT vs. PBRT in the salvage setting and propensity score matched	WPRT group had better PSA control vs. PBRT group (63.1% vs. 43.4%, $P = .034$)
Mason[98]	UK, Canada, USA	Reported prespecified final analysis of a randomized trial ADT vs. ADT + EBRT ($n = 1,205$)	Pts planned for WPRT showed a trend toward improved OS vs. PORT (HR = 0.70; $P = .12$) and DSS (HR = 0.53; $P = .098$)
James[99,100]	UK	Exploratory analysis using data from the STAMPEDE trial to assess the impact of RT on failure-free survival by nodal status	Failure-free survival outcomes favored planned use of RT for HR pts with N0M0 *and* N+M0 disease
	USA, multi-institutional	Explored WPRT +/− ADT vs. PORT PSA control using a data from 10 academic institutions	MVA showed both WPRT and ADT improved PSA control

[a]Studies in *blue* tend to argue against WPRT, whereas those in *black* tend to support it.
ADT, androgen depression therapy; CSS, cause-specific survival; EBRT, external beam radiation; HR, high risk; NCDB, National Cancer Database; OS, overall survival; PBRT, prostate bed radiation therapy; PFS, progression-free survival; PO, prostate only; pts, patients; SEER, surveillance, epidemiology and end results; TNT, the number needed to treat.

is conceivable that with either modality, late toxicities may be further decreased (Fig. 70.2).

The only other modern randomized trial is GETUG-01 (Groupe d'Etude des Tumeurs Uro-Génitales), which is a French multicenter phase III trial and was recently updated.[43] It randomized 444 patients with T1b-T3N0M0 prostate cancer to "WPRT" or PORT. Four to 8 months of neoadjuvant and concurrent hormones was not part of the protocol treatment for all patients. Patients were stratified based on estimated node involvement, and only those deemed to be high risk, defined as ≥T3, Gleason score ≥7, or PSA ≥3 times normal, for nodal involvement received hormones. The total prostate dose in the study was 66 to 70 Gy. With a median follow-up of 11 years, no significant difference was seen in progression-free survival between the WPRT and PORT arms. Although the results of GETUG-01 seem to contradict that of RTOG-9413, there are significant differences in the methodology of the two studies that warrant mention. First, more than half of the patients (~54%) had an estimated nodal risk of <15% ("Roach formula"), meaning that these patients had more favorable disease than those in RTOG-9413 and therefore would likely

not benefit from WPRT. Thus, this study was vastly underpowered, as is made a bit clearer, by considering this example. Suppose you designed a trial wherein the minimum eligibility was a risk of lymph node involvement >15%, such that the average risk for this cohort was 1/3rd. If you enrolled 1,200 patients, then 400 would really be the basis for the study outcome because only this number could potentially benefit. If the local recurrence rate was 50% (e.g., as might be expected after 66 Gy), then only 200 patients would be left to assess the merits of WPRT. This means that really only 100 patients would remain on the WPRT arm that could potentially benefit. If competing causes of death eliminated 50% of the patients, the remaining assessable patients would then be down to 50 per arm. Thus, even starting off with 1,200 patients, it would be challenging to assess the potential impact of WPRT. Clearly, GETUG-01, which only started out with 200 patients with a risk >15%, was not adequately powered to either disprove or prove the value of WPRT. Equally important, the protocol-defined pelvic fields were much smaller than those used in RTOG-9413. Specifically, the superior border was taken at the level of S1-S2 interspace, rather than L5-S1 interspace, which meant that a

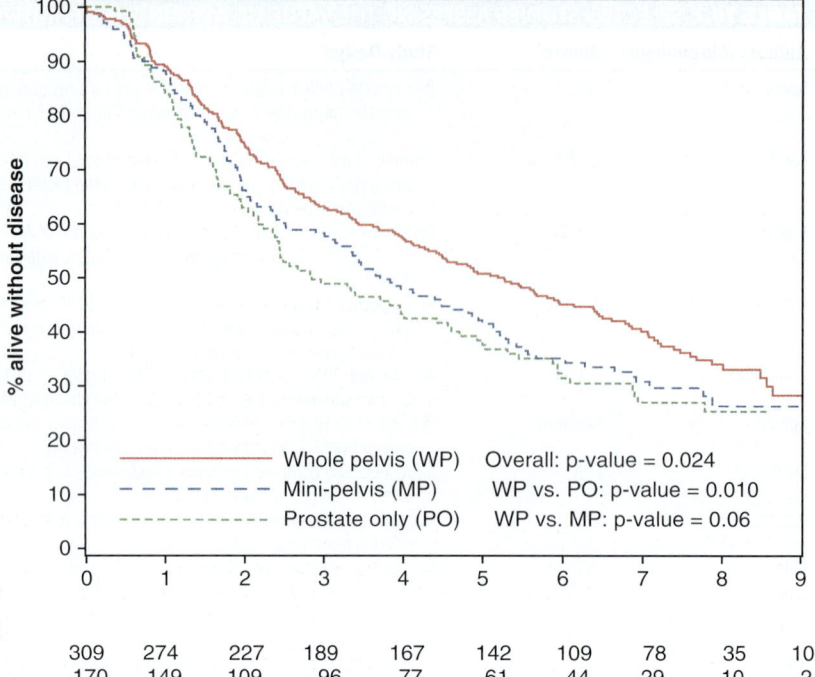

FIGURE 70.1. Progression-free survival of subgroup analysis of the Radiation Therapy Oncology Group (RTOG-9413) comparing whole-pelvic, mini-pelvic, and prostate-only radiotherapy. (Reprinted from Roach M III, DeSilvio M, Valicenti R, et al. Whole pelvic, "mini-pelvic" or prostate-only external beam radiotherapy after neoadjuvant and concurrent hormonal therapy in patients treated in the Radiation Therapy Oncology Group 9413 Trial. *Int J Radiat Oncol Biol Phys* 2006;66[3]:647–653. Copyright © 2006 Elsevier. With permission.)

At risk:

	0	1	2	3	4	5	6	7	8	9
WP	309	274	227	189	167	142	109	78	35	10
MP	170	149	109	96	77	61	44	29	10	2
PO	131	109	81	61	54	47	34	22	10	0

FIGURE 70.2. Isodose lines and dose–volume histogram from a representative patient treated with single-fraction 15 Gy high dose rate prostate brachytherapy with ultrasound-based planning. Twelve catheters were implanted. On dose–volume histogram, the prostate (*red line*), urethra (*blue line*), and rectum (*brown line*) are represented. (Courtesy of Gerard Morton, MD, Sunnybrook Odette Cancer Centre, University of Toronto, Toronto, Canada.)

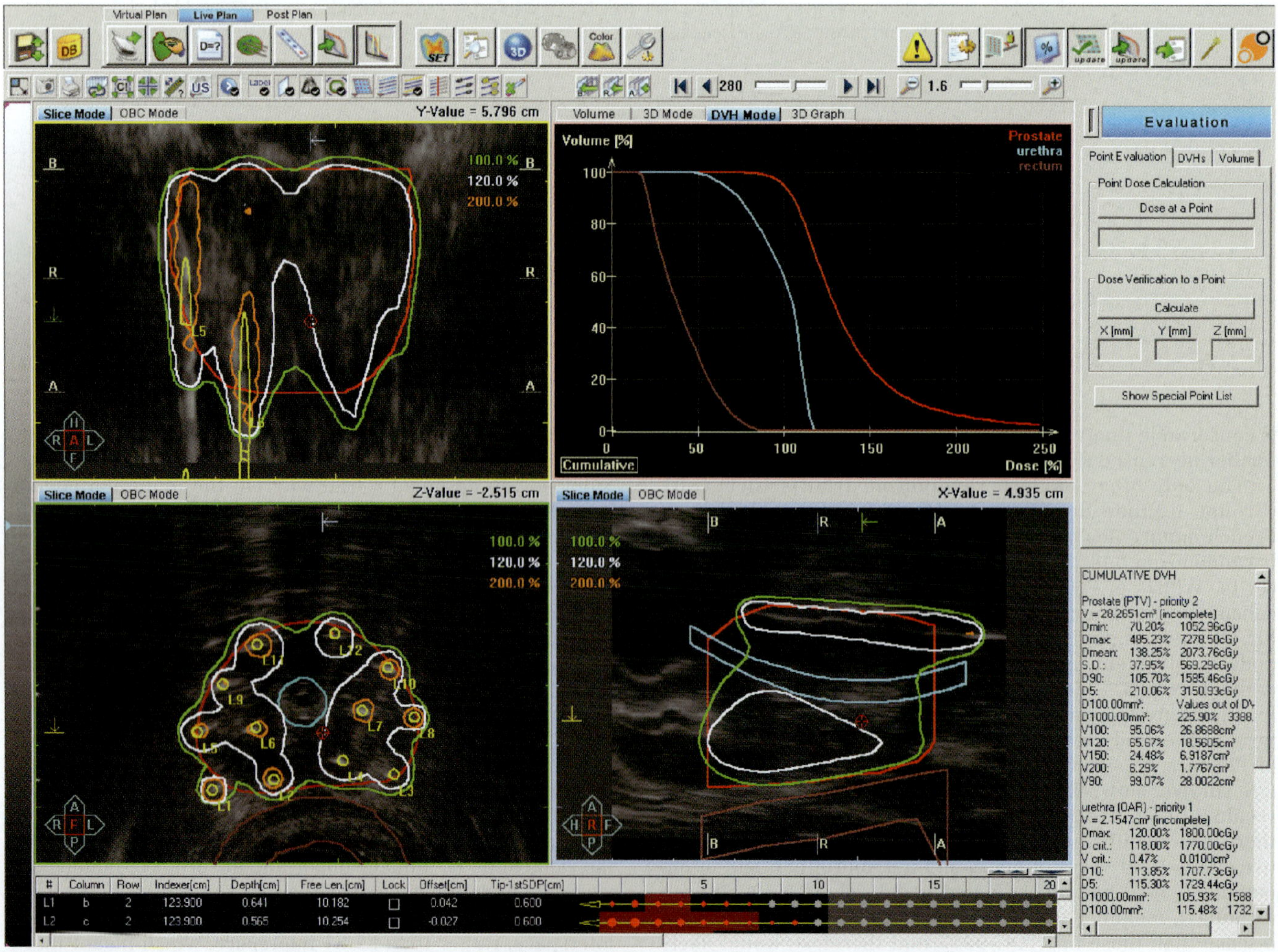

significant portion of the presacral and common iliac nodes were not treated. Thus, *none* of the patients included in this trial received WPRT in accordance with RTOG-9413, and *all* of the patients assigned to the "pelvic nodal" radiation arm would have been included in the PORT arm of RTOG-9413.

One of the most common questions regarding RTOG-9413 is whether the beneficial finding of NHT and WPRT still holds true in the dose escalation era where doses of more than 80 Gy to the prostate is given. For example, retrospective data from Fox Chase Cancer Center were used to investigate the effects of dose escalation, WPRT, and short-term hormones in the subgroup of patients who would otherwise be eligible for RTOG-9413 based on the inclusion criteria.[86] Multivariate results suggest that radiation dose (70 to 72.9 vs. 73 to 76.9 vs. ≥77 Gy), PSA, clinical T-stage, and Gleason score were significant predictors of biochemical failure, whereas short-term hormones and radiation field size were not. Despite being provocative, there are some shortcomings of this study, as pointed out by the authors, which merit closer attention. Although the inclusion criteria were identical to RTOG-9413, 42.4% and 31.4% of patients had a PSA <10 and 10 to 20 ng/mL (median PSA 10.95 ng/mL), respectively, whereas the median PSA in RTOG-9413 was 22.6 ng/mL. In addition, only 67 patients received neoadjuvant hormones. Radiation fields were prostate only, partial pelvis, and whole pelvis in 11.4%, 17.6%, and 71%, respectively. In the latter group, the whole-pelvic field extended superiorly to the inferior sacroiliac joints, which would not be considered adequate pelvic irradiation according to RTOG-9413, where a minimum unblocked field size of 16-by-16 cm was used. Because only 16% patients received NHT and none received WPRT (per RTOG-9413), there is a great potential for selection bias (patients treated with NHT may have had worse disease than those not receiving NHT). Thus, these data do not make a compelling argument against WPRT and NHT acquired from a large phase III trial.

When we designed NRG/RTOG-0924, we first identified a subset of patients from our original report of RTOG-9413 who appeared to have benefited the most from WPRT.[78,79] We also incorporated the percentage of positive biopsy cores into the eligibility criteria. Patients eligible for this study should have an estimated nodal risk of at least 15% and have either the following:

- Gleason score 7 to 10 and T1c-T2b and PSA < 50 ng/mL
- Gleason score 6 and (T2c-T4 or >50% biopsies) and PSA < 50 ng/mL
- Gleason score 6 and T1c-T2b and PSA >20 ng/mL

For NRG/RTOG-0924, we made the WPRT slightly larger and the PORT fields slightly smaller, and the phase I dose was 45 Gy in both arms and can be delivered with 3DCRT or IMRT. The phase II prostate boost can be achieved by IMRT (34.2 Gy; total dose 79.2 Gy), low dose rate (LDR) brachytherapy (110 Gy for iodine-125 [125I] and 100 Gy for palladium-103 [103Pd]), or high dose rate (HDR) brachytherapy (15 Gy in one fraction with iridium-192 [192Ir]). Patients will be stratified into 4 to 6 or 32 months of androgen suppression therapy.

The bottom-line concerning WPRT as summarized in Table 70.3 is as follows:

1. Most retrospective studies involving EBRT support the value of WPRT. Thus, there is no strong evidence to withhold WPRT based on retrospective data.
2. Every major RTOG and EORTC trial including high-risk patients with ADT included WPRT. Thus, there is no evidence that the results of these trials would be the same if WPRT was withheld.
3. The only large contemporary phase III randomized trial completed to date (RTOG-9413) continues with support an improved PSA control when NHT is added to WPRT compared to PORT. A larger confirmatory study with a survival endpoint is pending with >2,000 patients already enrolled.

RADIATION THERAPY TECHNIQUES: REGIONAL AND LOCAL

Boost Techniques: Options and Considerations

Over the past 20 years, the therapeutic options for definitive radiation in men with clinically localized disease have evolved immensely. At UCSF, favorable intermediate-risk patients are usually managed with monotherapy, a permanent prostate implant (PPI), a HDR implant, stereotactic body radiation therapy [SBRT] directed only at the prostate +/– the proximal SVs

TABLE 70.3 RADIATION THERAPY "PREFERRED" OPTIONS AND RELATIVE CONTRAINDICATIONS FOR PROSTATE CANCER AT UCSF (2017)

Type of Radiation Therapy	Year[a]	Primary Indications	Relative Contraindications
IGRT (intensity-modulated image-guided external beam radiation)[b]	Pre 1996	1. Combination therapy pre-/postboost treatment 2. Postop adjuvant treatment 3. Postop salvage treatment 4. Large TURP defects 5. Other options not covered by insurance 6. Patient preference	1. Previous full-dose radiation 2. Patient preference (e.g., logistically problematic) 3. Focal recurrence (favor focal treatments) 4. Technical issues (e.g., too large for CT scan but BT suitable) 5. Inflammatory bowel disease or connective tissue disorder 6. Noncompliant for many visits
PPI (permanent prostate implant) BT (brachytherapy)	1996	1. Monotherapy for low or favorable int. risk pts 2. Boost in clinically T1-T2 with IMRT 3. Focal salvage postrecurrence after IMRT 4. Focal salvage postrecurrence after PPI 5. Patient preference	1. Not a candidate for anesthesia 2. Discontinuation of anti-coagulation is unadvisable 3. Excessive pubic arch interference (PAI) 4. Excessively large TURP defect 5. Severe baseline urinary symptoms (e.g., urinary retention)
HDR (high dose rate) BT	1999	1. Monotherapy for low or favorable int. risk pts 2. Boost in clinically T1-T3 with IMRT 3. Focal salvage postrecurrence after IMRT 4. Pubic arch interference prohibiting PPI 5. Median lobe too large for SBRT 6. Insurance prohibits SBRT 7. Patient preference	1. Not a candidate for anesthesia 2. Discontinuation of anticoagulation is unadvisable 3. Excessive pubic arch interference 4. Excessively large TURP defect 5. Severe baseline urinary symptoms (e.g., urinary retention)
SBRT (stereo tactic body radiation therapy)	2005	1. Monotherapy for low- or favorable-risk pts 2. Boost for clinically T1-T4 with IMRT 3. Focal salvage in selected pts postrecurrences after IMRT when not a candidate for BT salvage 4. Patients presenting with obstruction because of locally advanced disease (e.g., "reverse" boost) 5. Patient preference (e.g., convenience)	1. Very large median lobe 2. Unable to lie still and flat for 45 min (e.g., tremor) 3. Poor localization because of metal artifacts (e.g., hip replacement, presence of PPI seeds) 4. Poor seed positioning ("too close") 5. Not covered by insurance 6. Protocol requires other treatments

[a]Approximate year program started at UCSF.
[b]Delivered with either conventional fractionation or hypofractionation.
"Primary": this term reflects the clinical nuances that go into the decisions concerning the use of various radiation options considered while practicing the "Art" of radiation therapy. There may be exceptions to what physicians decide to recommend to specific patients, but these "Primary" options as listed in this table reflect our typical considerations and our practice habits. It is recognized that for purposes of continuity of care and presumed clinical equivalence, patients who could be managed appropriately by more than one boost modality are more likely to be managed via the modality favor by the "clinical lead" radiation oncologist as listed above.

without ADT, or image-guided EBRT (IGRT). For patients with more unfavorable intermediate-risk disease, IGRT directed at periprostatic tissues (+/– the pelvic lymph nodes) is combined with an IGRT, a PPI, an HDR, or an SBRT boost +/– short-term ADT (e.g., 4 months), whereas for high-risk (HR) patients, long-term ADT (e.g., 2 to 3 years) with WPRT is usually recommended. Off study, the authors recommend prophylactic WPRT using IMRT to patients with an estimated nodal involvement of >15% and unfavorable intermediate- and high-risk prostate cancer. The authors recommend either adherence to the RTOG GU Radiation Oncology consensus statement on pelvic nodal volumes or use of a higher superior border.[49,102,103] If positive pelvic nodes are suggested by imaging (e.g., CT or PET), prophylactic para-aortic nodal treatment is usually added to WPRT.

The prostate boost is delivered with either an IMRT, a PPI, or an HDR brachytherapy, or an SBRT boost. Brachytherapy or SBRT are generally preferred by the authors because of their ability to deliver a higher biologic dose to the prostate. Brachytherapy can be performed either before or performed 1 to 3 weeks following pelvic radiation therapy. For T3 disease, the authors use an SBRT, HDR, or IMRT boost, which allows better coverage of extranodal disease than PPI boost. Table 70.3 summarizes some of the consideration when selecting the type of boost preferred for a given patient. Figures 70.3 and 70.4 provide a summary of some of the data supporting SBRT +/– ADT.[104] Based on the results of patients treated on RTOG-0232 comparing PPI to PPI + EBRT, the former is preferred in favorable intermediate-risk patients.[105]

FIGURE 70.3. Biochemical disease-free survival (bDFS) (Phoenix) of high-risk (HR) patients treated with stereotactic body radiation therapy (SBRT) boost, high dose rate (HDR) boost, external beam radiation therapy plus long-term androgen deprivation therapy (EBRT + LTADT), dose-escalated external beam radiation therapy (DE-EBRT), and low dose rate brachytherapy (LDR-BT) arm of the ASCENDE-RT trial. Data from the ASCENDE-RT trial were estimated from the Kaplan-Meier curve of bDFS for HR patients. Data for RTOG-9202 (EBRT + LTADT) were estimated from biochemical rate reported. *RTOG-9202 used the ASTRO definition for biochemical failure. **DE-EBRT arm of the ASCENDE-RT trial received 8 mo of neoadjuvant androgen deprivation therapy. (Modified from Gonzalez-Motta A, Roach M. Stereotactic body radiotherapy (SBRT) for high-risk prostate cancer: where are we now? *Pract Radiat Oncol* 2018;8[3]:185–202. Copyright © 2017 American Society for Radiation Oncology. With permission.[104])

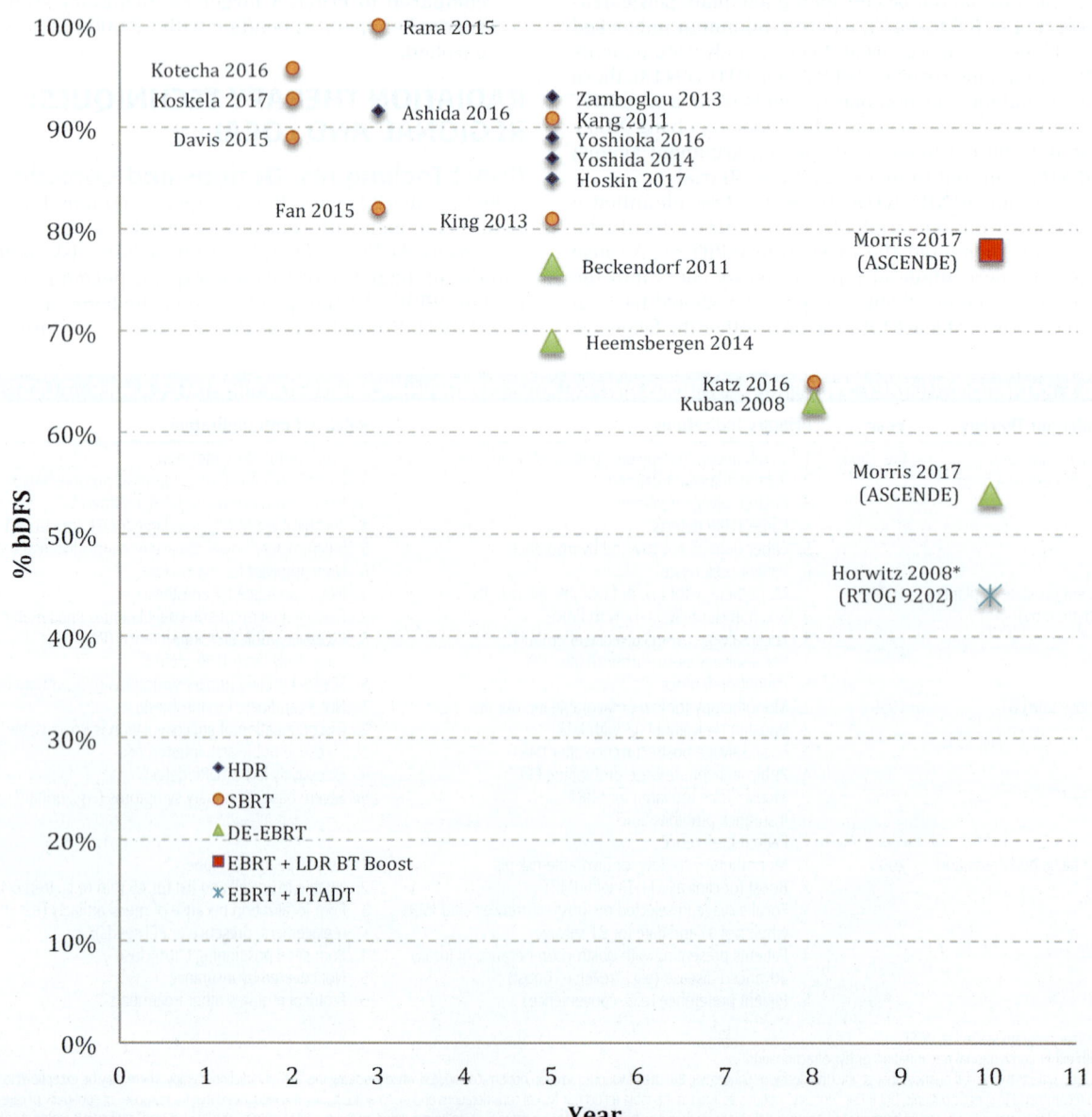

bDFS of High Risk patients treated with SBRT monotherapy, HDR monotherapy, DE-EBRT, EBRT + LDR BT Boost, EBRT+LTADT

Acute and late toxicity in SBRT, HDR, DE-EBRT and EBRT + LDR-BT Boost

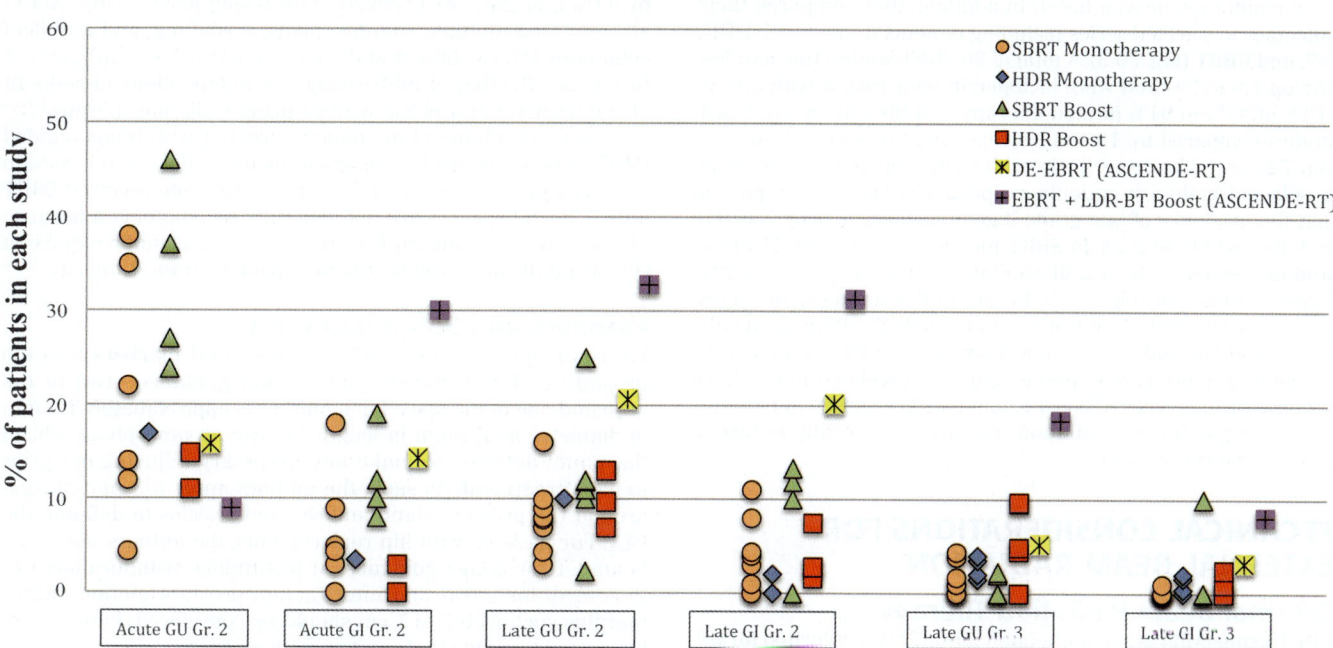

FIGURE 70.4. Acute and late toxicity reported in stereotactic body radiation therapy (SBRT), high dose rate (HDR) monotherapy, dose-escalated external beam radiation therapy (DE-EBRT), and low dose rate brachytherapy (LDR-BT) studies. Not all SBRT and HDR studies reported toxicity data. Three scales were used in the studies: the common terminology criteria for adverse events (CTCAE), the Radiation Therapy Oncology Group (RTOG) scale, and the LENT/SOMA (late effects normal tissue task force/subjective, objective, management, and analytic) scale. However, they were plotted together in the figure. (Modified from Gonzalez-Motta A, Roach M. Stereotactic body radiotherapy (SBRT) for high-risk prostate cancer: where are we now? *Pract Radiat Oncol* 2018;8[3]:185–202. Copyright © 2017 American Society for Radiation Oncology. With permission.[104])

Brachytherapy and Stereotactic Body Radiation Therapy Boost

Brachytherapy Boost

Notwithstanding the downsides that brachytherapy is an invasive procedure that requires anesthesia, additional resources, and expertise, the advantages of incorporating prostate brachytherapy as a means of boosting the dose to the prostate gland are compelling. First, the achievable biologically effective dose (BED) to the prostate far exceeds what can be achieved by IMRT, which appears to translate into a higher rate of local control and possibly cure. In addition to the recently reported ASCENDE-RT trial involving PPI boost there are a number of other comparative studies supportive of HDR brachytherapy boost as well.[106] For example, Hoskin et al. reported the results of their phase III trial comparing EBRT alone (55 Gy in 20 fractions) with combined EBRT (35.75 Gy in 13 fractions) followed by HDR prostate brachytherapy (17 Gy in 2 fractions over 24 hours) among 218 patients with clinically localized prostate cancer.[107] Biochemical control was significantly higher in patients treated with EBRT + HDR (P = .04). In multivariate analysis, risk category and ADT were significant covariates for risk of relapse. Of note perhaps because of the study size, there were no differences in OS. Fortunately, the incidence of severe late urinary and bowel morbidity was similar. In addition to apparently rendering improved PSA results, with a brachytherapy boost, the overall treatment time is usually less than the usual 8 weeks of conventionally fractionated x-ray therapy (XRT) and therefore more convenient for patients.

As compared to LDR brachytherapy, HDR brachytherapy yields the following advantages: greater flexibility in source positioning, adaption of dose to target and healthy organs, target volume–dose optimization, high-quality planning and dose distribution, lower risk of radiation exposition to health care personnel or public, and reduced cost. The potential

disadvantage of HDR is that it is often fractionated and takes more time and therefore may require more workload and careful coordination from the health care personnel. The indications of combined EBRT and brachytherapy boost are those with intermediate- or high-risk prostate cancer, particularly in patients who are relatively young and have high-volume disease. Relative contraindications to the use of a brachytherapy boost includes those with a large prostate (>60 cc), prior transurethral resection of the prostate with a large residual urethral defect, anticoagulation use, and significant urinary symptoms (i.e., International Prostate Symptom Score (IPSS) >20).

As noted previously, HDR brachytherapy may be performed before, during, or after the EBRT. The optimal HDR dose fractionation is currently unknown, and there is significant variability across centers. Nonetheless, there is a shift toward fewer implants, fewer fractions, and higher dose per fraction because of the radiobiologic advantage of high dose per fraction in prostate cancer. Reflecting this lack of consensus, RTOG-0815 and RTOG-0924 stipulate different HDR prescription doses. In RTOG-0815, the HDR brachytherapy boost may be performed during EBRT or within 1 week prior to its initiation or following its completion. The prescription is 21 Gy delivered in 2 equal fractions of 10.5 Gy, separated by at least 6 hours and given within 24 hours. In RTOG-0924, the implant may be done during EBRT or within 2 weeks prior to its initiation or following its completion. The prescription is 15 Gy in a single fraction. In both protocols, the dose constraints to the bladder is V75 <1 cc, rectum is V75 <1 cc, and urethra is V125 <1 cc and V150 is 0%.

SBRT Boost

More recently, there has been an increased interest in the use of SBRT as an alternative to the use of brachytherapy.[104] Gonzalez-Motta and Roach recently reviewed outcomes reported for patients with high-risk disease treated with SBRT as monotherapy or as a boost following EBRT.[104] Their systematic literature review was conducted to review the current evidence of biochemical disease-free survival (bDFS) and toxicity associated with the use of SBRT in high-risk prostate cancer either as monotherapy or as a boost. In addition, they compared their outcomes to selected series including patients treated with HDR, PPI, and EBRT (Fig. 70.3). A total of 20 SBRT studies (median follow-up 1.6 to 7 years) were included in their review with 5-year bDFS of 81% to 91% in monotherapy and 90% to 98% in boost studies compared to, 19 studies reporting bDFS of 85% to 93% and 72% to 93%, respectively, with HDR monotherapy or boost in selected high-risk patients, respectively. They also reported that the incidence of late grade 3 genitourinary toxicity was 0% to 4.4% and 0% to 2.3% in SBRT monotherapy and SBRT boost studies, respectively, not dissimilar to those seen with other forms of radiation (Fig. 70.4). Based on this analysis, outcomes appear to be similar with SBRT as with HDR, although ideally this should be validated in clinical trials. Table 70.3 summarizes the generally preferred options and the associated indications for how various types of boost techniques are chosen in patients undergoing definitive radiation therapy for clinically localized prostate cancer at UCSF.

TECHNICAL CONSIDERATIONS FOR EXTERNAL BEAM RADIATION

External Beam Radiation Therapy

EBRT using IMRT is recommended for optimal conformal target coverage and avoidance of rectum and bladder. At a minimum, the prostate, seminal vesicles, and periprostatic tissue should be irradiated. Inclusion of the first echelon lymph nodes (i.e., mini-pelvis) or the entire pelvic nodal contents (i.e., whole pelvis) may be considered, based on the estimated risk of involvement. The recommended EBRT dose is 45 to 50.4 Gy in 1.8 to 2.0 Gy per fraction. Generally speaking, the role of hypofractionated regimens has been less well defined in patients with unfavorable to higher-risk disease.[108–110] LDR brachytherapy boost may be performed either prior to starting the EBRT or 2 to 4 weeks after completing EBRT. The technique is identical to that of LDR brachytherapy as monotherapy (see Chapter 65). The American Brachytherapy Society recommends ([125])I and ([103])Pd doses of 100 to 110 Gy and 80 to 90 Gy, respectively.[111]

Prostate Motion and the Use of IGRT (Image-Guided IMRT)

The use of fiducial gold seed markers and daily electronic portal imaging (EPI) with online correction and/or the use of cone-beam computed tomography (CBCT) or endorectal balloons may be considered.[112,113] Well-placed marker migration was found to be minimal, with 79% within 1 mm and 96% within 1.5 mm. The latter results have been corroborated by Kupelian et al., who demonstrated that the average absolute variation in intermarker distance was 1.01 ± 1.03 mm.[114–116] Only 1% of the markers exhibited frequent movement, and it was found to be due to prostate deformation secondary to rectal filling. CBCT for online correction is gaining popularity as it allows for soft tissue matching and does not require an invasive procedure to implant fiducial markers. Moseley et al. compared kilovoltage CBCT with fiducial markers and EPI and found no significant difference as a means for image guidance.[113] Langen et al. described broadly two different types of intrafraction motions.[117,118] One is by a slow, small drift, usually posteriorly and inferiorly, that is thought to be associated with pelvic muscle relaxation or the gradual movement of rectal contents away from the prostate. Second is a sudden and transient motion, usually anteriorly and superiorly, that can be significant in extent and is thought to be due to peristalsis. In the cohort of 17 patients (550 fractions), the average proportion of the total treatment time that the prostate was displaced by >3 and >5 mm was 13.6% and 3.3%, respectively. However, when analyzed by patient-to-patient basis, the prostate was displaced by 36.2%

and 10.9%, respectively. An analysis of patients treated at UCSF, Chen et al. demonstrated that an isocenter shift of 5 or 10 mm in the superior direction could reduce nodal target coverage by 11% and 26%, respectively, with whole-pelvic IMRT. Xia et al. compared multiple adaptive plans, isoshifting, and multileaf collimator (MLC) shifting and concluded that MLC shifting was the most effective in addressing the independent movement of the prostate and pelvic nodes during radiation therapy.[119–121] In a study by Chung et al., patients treated with image-guided IMRT to pelvic nodes had significantly lower dose to the rectum and bladder and fewer toxicities than those who received IMRT only.[122] Rectal spacers are not generally recommended because of the potential concern for areas of extracapsular extension (ECE) and the observed marginal impact on grade 1 toxicity.[123,124]

Volumes and Setup Variation

We routinely place three fiducial gold seed markers into the prostate under transrectal ultrasound guidance—two in the base and one in the apex. Each marker is approximately 1.1 mm in diameter and 3 mm in length. We use an amorphous silicon flat panel detector to make any necessary adjustments prior to each treatment. As such, the authors apply a 3-mm margin around the prostate gland and seminal vesicles in defining the PTV. For patients with hip replacements, the authors use cone-beam CT for image guidance. At institutions without daily EPI to control for intra- and interfraction prostate motion, larger margins such as 0.5 to 1 cm should be considered. Patients are instructed to empty their rectum with an enema prior to simulation. Patients are told to maintain a full bladder during simulation and treatment. A retrograde urethrogram is no longer performed at UCSF to assist in identifying the apex of the gland, except in patients undergoing SBRT for whom an MRI is not possible or contraindicated. Three-millimeter slice thickness is used for the CT simulation. The critical organs that are contoured include the penile bulb, small bowel, rectum, bladder, and femoral heads. The entire rectum is contoured from the anus to the rectosigmoid junction. Rectal spacers are not recommended for patients with intermediate-risk and/or high-risk disease.

Intensity-Modulated Radiation Therapy Treatment Planning

For patients opting for definitive IMRT to the pelvis and prostate, the authors use a two- or three-phase plan. The first phase delivers 25 to 30 fractions of 1.8 Gy (total 45 to 60 Gy [the latter PET positive sites], superior border L4–L5 with node negative by imaging). Concurrently 2 Gy per fraction (total 54 to 56 Gy) to the seminal vesicles and prostate PTV. PET + nodes are boosted to 60 Gy and para-aortic nodes added if pelvic nodes are positive. The second phase is a cone-down boost to the prostate PTV alone with 12 fractions of 2.0 Gy per fraction. Therefore, the minimum total dose to the prostate (prescribed to the PTV) is 78 Gy. In postoperative patients opting for pelvic radiation therapy, the authors prescribe 25 fractions of 1.8 Gy to the nodes (total dose 45 Gy) and 2 Gy per fraction to the tumor bed PTV (total dose 50 Gy) and then 9 fractions of 2.0 Gy per fraction to the prostate bed (total minimal PTV dose 68 Gy).

Toxicity of Pelvic Intensity-Modulated Radiation Therapy

Since the previous edition, IMRT has been adopted as standard of care for pelvic nodal irradiation. For historical purposes, with conventional technique, pelvic irradiation is usually treated with a four-field box. The target volume usually includes the prostate, seminal vesicles, obturator, and proximal internal and external iliac nodal regions. Occasionally, common iliac, para-aortic, and even perirectal nodes are included in the initial target. The traditional field borders of the anteroposterior portals previously were as follows: superior at the L5-S1 interspace, inferior at 2 cm distal to the membranous urethra (defined by the apex of the urethrogram peak), and 1.5 to 2 cm lateral of the pelvic brim. More recently based on work involving sentinel lymph nodal imaging, we now recommend extending the superior border to L3-L4 or L4-L5 instead of L5-S1. Corner blocks are usually placed at all four corners to limit dose to the small bowel and femoral heads. In the lateral portals, the superior and inferior borders are placed at the same point as the anteroposterior portals; the anterior border is placed at the anterior most aspect of the pubic symphysis, and the posterior border is placed at the S2-S3 interspace. With CT planning, the prostate, seminal vesicles, rectum, small bowel, bladder, pelvic vessels, and penile bulb may be contoured to facilitate shielding of the rectum and small bowel.

Compared to conventional technique, IMRT allows unprecedented sparing of nearby critical structures like the rectum, small bowel, bladder, and femoral heads. In a study from UCSF, Wang-Chesebro et al. compared the nodal target coverage by conventional field borders with IMRT (Fig. 70.5).[125] The nodes that were contoured included the obturator, internal or external iliac, common iliac, and presacral regions. In the conventional four-field plan, only 70.3% of the nodal target volume received the prescription dose of 45 Gy, whereas 96.2% was covered in the IMRT plan (*P* = .002). Even worse, conventional field placement led to 20.2% of the nodal target volume to receive <80% of the prescription dose. The rectal and bladder volume receiving 95% of the prescribed dose was significantly reduced with IMRT, with an absolute reduction of 23% and 80%, respectively.

Whereas conventional technique involved simply placing field borders based on bony anatomy, IMRT requires the delineation of a nodal target volume based on vasculature. Investigators have used lymphotropic nanoparticle-enhanced MRI and ultra-small superparamagnetic iron oxide lymph node contrast agent, ferumoxtran-10, to develop nodal CTV models.[48] These MRI studies have formed the foundation for the RTOG Genitourinary Radiation Oncology Consensus on pelvic nodal CTV delineation, as shown in Figure 70.6.[49,103] However, the RTOG guidelines did not use sentinel lymph node imaging, which in a study by Chen et al. demonstrated that the RTOG pelvic nodal CTV included all identified sentinel lymph nodes in only 30% of patients.[58] In the same consensus, Lawton et al. recommended dose constraints to the rectum (V50 Gy ≤50%, V70 Gy ≤20%), bladder (V55 Gy ≤50%, V70 Gy ≤30%), femoral heads (V50 Gy <5%), and small bowel (maximum dose <52 Gy). Based on an extensive literature search, Chan et al. proposed guidelines on rectal dose constraints for patients receiving pelvic radiation therapy.[126]

ANDROGEN DEPRIVATION THERAPY AND RT: EVIDENCE AND INDICATIONS

EBRT Versus EBRT + ADT and ADT Versus ADT + EBRT

The optimal dose of radiation required to obtain a high level of local control while maintaining an acceptably low level of complications is not known. Several phase III randomized trials have compared conventional-dose with high-dose (76 to 82 Gy) EBRT, and although essentially all have demonstrated an improvement in PSA control, no survival advantage attributable to radiation dose were observed.[8,127,128] As expected, grade 3 GI toxicities appear to be worse with dose escalation. Of note, the Medical Research Council (MRC) RT01, Dutch CKVO96–10, and the Spanish trial permitted ADT.[127–129] The MRC and Spanish trials mandated ADT on both arms, yet dose escalation still appeared to be beneficial. This suggests that dose escalation alone cannot replace hormonal therapy as a strategy to improve cure and that both may be necessary in patients with intermediate- and high-risk disease. Recently, the RTOG (now NRG [NSAB, RTOG, and GoG]) completed accrual to RTOG-0815, a phase III multicenter trial evaluating the addition of 6 months of androgen blockade with dose-escalated radiation therapy, achieved by either 3DCRT or IMRT (79.2 Gy), combined low dose rate (110 Gy with ^{125}I or 100 Gy with ^{103}Pd) brachytherapy boost with 3DCRT or IMRT (45 Gy to the prostate and seminal vesicles), or combined HDR (2 fractions of 10.5 Gy per fractions); hopefully, this trial will finally fully address the question of the need for ADT when dose-escalated radiation is used. At UCSF, we have long favored brachytherapy boost (BT) for suitable patients treated with curative intent, based on the lower PSA nadir, degree of metabolic atrophy noted, and PSA control rates compared to any form of dose-escalated EBRT (including proton beam radiation therapy).[130–132] This philosophy seems to have been vindicated by the recent findings from the ASCENDE-RT trial, which confirmed a substantially higher PSA control rate with a LDR brachytherapy boost after ADT and EBRT compared to ADT and dose-escalated EBRT alone (see the discussion of brachytherapy below).[106]

Multiple phase III randomized controlled trials and several meta-analyses have been published in the peer reviewed literature that compared radiation therapy alone with radiation therapy and ADT.[8] At UCSF, the authors' practices regarding integrating pelvic radiation therapy and hormonal

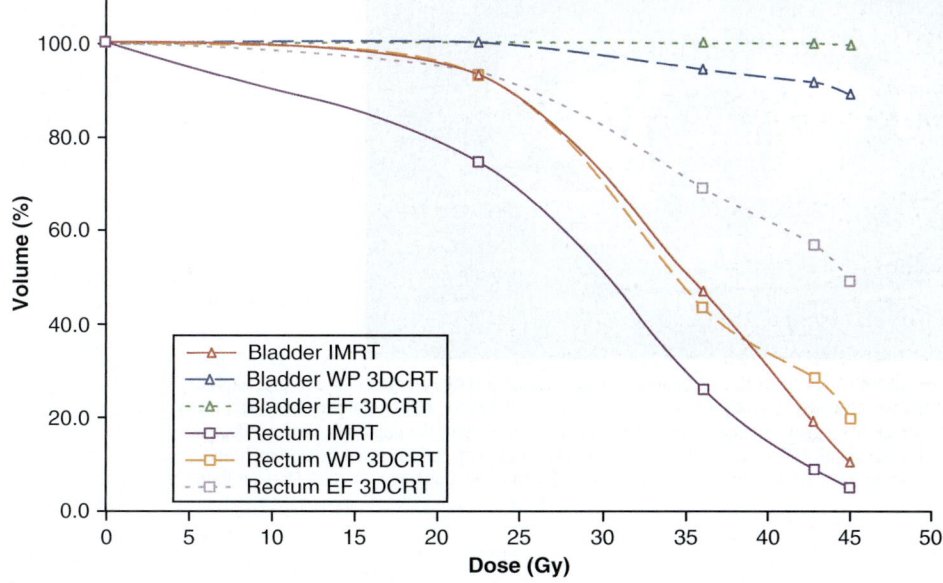

FIGURE 70.5. Comparison of dose–volume histograms for the rectum and bladder for whole-pelvic only phase using intensity-modulated radiotherapy (IMRT), whole-pelvic (WP) three-dimensional conformal radiotherapy (3DCRT), and extended-field (EF) 3DCRT plans. For both the bladder and rectum, IMRT significantly reduced V45, V42.75, V36, and V22.5 (*P* < .01 for all comparisons) compared to both WP and EF 3DCRT plans. (Reprinted from Wang-Chesebro A, Xia P, Coleman J, et al. Intensity-modulated radiotherapy improves lymph node coverage and dose to critical structures compared with three-dimensional conformal radiation therapy in clinically localized prostate cancer. *Int J Radiat Oncol Biol Phys* 2006;66[3]:654–662. Copyright © 2006 Elsevier. With permission.)

Section III

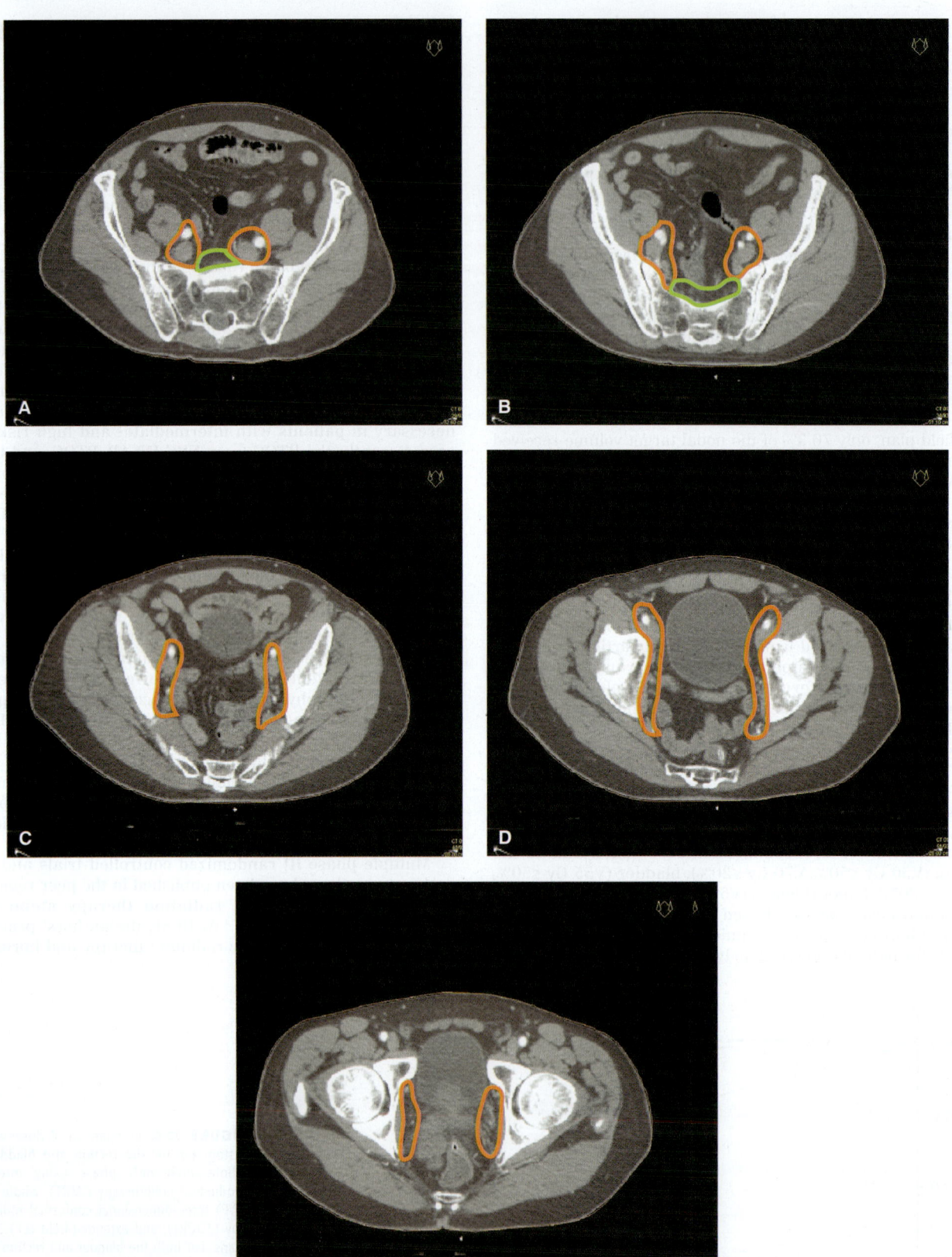

FIGURE 70.6. Representative pelvic lymph node clinical target volume contours of **(A)** common iliac and presacral at L5-S1; **(B)** external, internal, and presacral at S1-S3; **(C)** external and internal iliac below S3; **(D)** end of external iliac at top of femoral heads (bony landmark for the inguinal ligament); and **(E)** obturator at the top of the pubic symphysis. (Adapted from Lawton CA, Michalski J, El-Naga I, et al. RTOG GU radiation oncology specialists reach consensus on pelvic lymph node volumes for high-risk prostate cancer. *Int J Radiat Oncol Biol Phys* 2009;74[2]:383–387. Copyright © 2009 Elsevier. With permission.)

TABLE 70.4 GENERAL RECOMMENDATIONS FOR RADIATION THERAPY AND ADT

	Low Risk	Favorable Intermediate Risk	Unfavorable Intermediate Risk	High Risk
Active surveillance	Preferred	In highly selected patients	Only appropriate in those with a short life expectancy	Only appropriate in those with a very short life expectancy
Radiation therapy	PORT	PORT + ADT (4 mo)	WPRT + NHT (4 mo or longer in selected patients)	WPRT
ADT	Not indicated	Neoadjuvant and concurrent with EBRT (4 mo)	Neoadjuvant (2 mo)	Neoadjuvant (2 mo)
		Adjuvant (4 mo)	Concurrent +/− adjuvant	Concurrent + adjuvant (24–36 mo)
Other				+/− Second-generation ADT in selected patients*a*

*a*Age < 70, node +?
ADT, androgen deprivation therapy; PORT, prostate-only radiation therapy; WPRT, whole-pelvic radiation therapy.

therapy are summarized in Table 70.4. Whether the benefit of ADT remains in the current era of dose escalation is currently unclear and is the basis of the recently completed RTOG-0815. Previously, RTOG-9408 was designed to evaluate whether similar duration and timing of ADT (2 months neoadjuvant [NHT] and 2 months concurrent) could improve outcomes in patients with more favorable disease.[133] Among the 1,979 eligible patients, 54% had intermediate-risk disease and 11% had high-risk disease. All patients had prostate-only radiation therapy to 68.4 Gy, except for those with a PSA <10 ng/mL, Gleason score of 2 to 6, or negative lymph node dissection. The latter group received pelvic radiation therapy to 46.8 Gy and a total prostate dose of 66.6 Gy. With a median follow-up of 9.1 years, 10-year overall survival (57% vs. 62%; $P = .03$), PCSM (8% vs. 4%; $P = .001$), PSA failure (41% vs. 26%; $P < .001$), and distant metastases (8% vs. 6%; $P = .04$) were significantly in favor of the ADT arm. In *post hoc* analyses, the benefit in overall survival and PCSM appeared to be primarily among intermediate-risk patients. Two-year positive prostate biopsy rates (39% vs. 20%; $P < .001$) were significantly improved with ADT. The authors give 2 months of NHT using a luteinizing hormone–releasing hormone (LHRH) agonist and an antiandrogen.

In addition to NHT, 2 to 3 years of adjuvant ADT (e.g., LHRH agonist) is recommended for high-risk disease, but on occasion, lifelong androgen deprivation is used in patients with very high-risk disease (Table 70.4). Early trials demonstrated that for men with locally advanced disease, initial management with hormonal therapy resulted in a survival advantage when compared to deferred ADT.[8,134] Subsequently, numerous trials showed that the addition of ADT to EBRT improved survival for men with intermediate- and high-risk disease.[8] There is also clear level I evidence that EBRT + ADT renders a better survival than ADT alone for men with locally advanced disease.[135–137]

SEQUENCING, OPTIMAL TIMING, AND DURATION OF ADT AND RADIATION THERAPY

Sequence-Dependent Interactions Between ADT and EBRT

NHT by definition implies delivery of the hormone prior to definitive radiation, whereas adjuvant ADT (AHT) implies the initiation of hormonal therapy after the completion of radiation. Few studies have assessed the optimal sequence or precise duration of ADT. RTOG-9413 randomized 1,323 men to either receive 4 months of NHT (commenced 2 months prior to starting EBRT) compared to 4 months of AHT.[78] The authors noted sequence-dependent beneficial interactions, such that when NHT is used, PSA control favored the use of WPRT over PORT. However, NHT + WPRT was also associated with higher rates of late grade 3 GI toxicity at 10 years occurring in 5.1%, compared to 1.6 and 0.6% in both AHT groups and pts treated with NHT + PORT, respectively ($P = .0009$). Of note, when

PORT is used, AHT appears to be at least as effective as NHT. The mechanism by which these sequence-dependent interactions occurs is unknown.

Optimal Duration of Short-Term ADT

To date, there are at least eight randomized trials (two Canadian, one Irish, one Australian, two conducted in the United States [RTOG-9202, 9910], and two conducted by the EORTC) evaluating the optimal duration of ADT with a survival endpoint and an additional three randomized trials (two Canadian and one EORTC) with a PSA control endpoint.[8] The Canadian Urologic Oncology Group (CUOG) study randomized 378 patients to either 3 or 8 months of NHT plus EBRT, whereas the Irish Clinical Oncology Research Group designed a randomized study comparing 4 and 8 months of NHT with EBRT.[138,139] TROG compared 0 versus 3 versus 6 months ADT with EBRT, whereas RTOG-9910 compared 8 versus 28 weeks of NHT (total 4 vs. 9 months).[140,141] Taken together, these studies suggest that for patients with intermediate-risk disease, there is no reason to extend short-term ADT beyond 4 months when combined with EBRT.[8,26]

Optimal Duration of Long-Term ADT

A meta-analysis of RTOG trials suggested that long-term ADT was superior to short-term ADT for patients with high-risk disease.[26] This assertion has been subsequently confirmed by EORTC-22961 that compared 6 months with 36 months of adjuvant ADT in 1,113 patients with locally advanced prostate cancer and demonstrated the superiority of the latter.[142] RTOG-9202, another phase III trial, also demonstrated that the addition of 24 months of adjuvant ADT could improve outcome in high-risk patients, compared to short term (4 months).[143] Aside from overall survival, all other endpoints were significantly in favor of the long-term ADT arm: PCSM (83.9% vs. 88.7%; $P < .0001$), disease-free survival (13.2% vs. 22.5%; $P < .0001$), and biochemical control (31.9% vs. 48.1%; $P < .0001$). In subgroup analysis, again, patients with a Gleason score of 8 to 10 had a significant improvement in overall survival with long-term AST but not with a Gleason score of 2 to 7. The authors speculate that the absence in overall survival difference may be due to insufficient follow-up among patients with a Gleason score of 2 to 7. These data, as previously noted, are completely consistent with the meta-analysis of five consecutive RTOG randomized controlled prostate cancer trials (including RTOG-8531 and RTOG-8610), where 2,742 men were stratified into four previously identified risk groups based on Gleason score, clinical T-stage, and pelvic nodal involvement.[26]

Toxicities Associated with Androgen Deprivation Therapy

Having established that ADT improves survival when combined with radiation therapy, enthusiasm has been somewhat tempered by the increasing recognition of the potentially serious complications of ADT.[144] Some of these complications have been exaggerated.[145] What is clear is that the risk of fractures, fatigue, weight gain, osteoporosis, depression, decreased cognitive function, erectile dysfunction, loss of libido, gynecomastia, anemia, decreased high-density lipoprotein, insulin resistance, and hot flashes are increased with ADT. For example, in a study of 50,613 men with prostate cancer compiled from a linked database of Surveillance, Epidemiology, and End Results (SEER) and Medicare, the addition of ADT significantly increased the risk of any fracture from 12.6% to 19.4%; fractures requiring hospitalization similarly increased from 2.37% to 5.19%.[146]

More controversial is the issue of the impact of ADT on cardiovascular disease.[147-151] Some studies have raised the question of whether ADT, by way of increasing body fat and cholesterol levels, increases the risk of cardiovascular disease.[145] In an observational study of a population-based cohort of 73,196 patients with clinically localized prostate cancer, ADT was associated with an increased risk of incident diabetes (HR 1.44; $P < .001$), cardiovascular disease (HR 1.16; $P < .001$), myocardial infarction (HR 1.11; $P = .03$), and sudden cardiac death (HR 1.16; $P = .004$). However, data from randomized controlled trials of radiation therapy with or without ADT have not shown any increased cardiovascular disease, although these studies were not powered adequately.[152] The bottom-line is that if ADT increases the risk of cardiovascular disease, the risk is quite low and the subset of patients who are at risk are those with severe underlying cardiovascular disease.[148]

In addition to cardiovascular risk, another area to which much attention has been paid is the risk of the potential impact of ADT on the brain. For example, Nead et al. published a series of methodologically flawed studies that essentially ignore the tendency for men with declining mental status to be at greater risk for receiving ADT.[153,154] The best data suggest that the risk of damage to both the central nervous system and cardiovascular systems is low, such that with rare exceptions the benefits justify the risk.[152,155]

POSTOPERATIVE (AFTER A RADICAL PROSTATECTOMY) RADIATION THERAPY

Local Versus Distant Recurrence

A substantial number of men undergoing a radical prostatectomy will experience a recurrence with the only curative treatment afterward being postoperative radiation.[156] Positive surgical margins (PSM) and ECE are associated with increased risk of PSA and local recurrences. Rates of PSM have been reported to be 5% to 53%, with variations because of surgeon experience, surgical technique, preoperative PSA, clinical stage, and ECE.[157,158] In a multicenter study of 5,831 men treated with radical prostatectomy from eight international institutions, the 5-year biochemical control rates were 83.8% and 53.1% for men with negative and PSM, respectively ($P = .0001$).[159] In an analysis of patterns of treatment failure in the study by the South West Oncology Group, SWOG-8794, a randomized trial evaluating adjuvant radiation therapy (ART) in patients with adverse pathologic features (pT3a-b or PSM), the predominant site of failure was local rather than metastatic.[160] Overall, local failure was observed in 22% and 8% of patients in the observation and ART arms, respectively. In contrast, distant metastasis was observed in 16% and 7% of patients, respectively.

Many investigators have reported on the merits of Gleason score, time to PSA relapse, postradiation PSA nadir, and PSA doubling time (PSA-DT) after PSA failure as a predictor of distant metastases versus local recurrence and PCSM. Pound et al.[161] reported that time to PSA recurrence ≤2 years after surgery, Gleason score of 8 to 10, and PSA-DT ≤10 months predicted for metastatic disease. Lee et al.[162] reported similar findings, with a PSA-DT of <12 months and an interval of <12 months from end of radiation therapy to PSA rise as significant independent predictors of distant failure. In a multi-institutional analysis of 4,839 patients treated with

radiation therapy alone, PSA nadir and time to PSA nadir were significant independent predictors of biochemical and distant failure-free survival.[163] Eight-year biochemical control was 75%, 52%, 41%, and 18% and distant failure-free survival was 97%, 96%, 91%, and 73% with a PSA nadir of 0 to 0.49, 0.5 to 0.99, 1 to 1.99, and ≥2 ng/mL, respectively ($P < .0001$). A nomogram incorporating PSA-DT has been created to predict risk of distant metastases.[164]

Prostate Cancer–Specific Mortality

Sandler et al.[165] observed that a PSA-DT of <12 months had significantly greater PCSM than when it was >12 months. A study from Johns Hopkins found similar results with PSA-DT, Gleason score (≤7 vs. 8 to 10), and disease-free interval (≤3 vs. >3 years) independently associated with PCSM.[166] Compiled from two multi-institutional databases with a cumulative cohort of 8,669 men treated with surgery or radiation therapy, CaPSURE and CPDR, Zhou et al.[167] showed that a PSA-DT of <3 months ($P < .0001$) and Gleason score of 8 to 10 ($P < .0001$) were significantly associated with PCSM. Zelefsky et al.[168] reported that the postradiation therapy 2-year PSA nadir of ≤1.5 ng/mL was associated with a reduced risk of developing distant metastases and PCSM.

Adjuvant Radiation Therapy

The argument for ART is that patients with PSM or ECE after radical prostatectomy are at an increased risk of local recurrence. Yet it is also known that having either ECE or PSM does not necessarily mean that local recurrence is inevitable. Epstein et al.[159] reported on 617 men with clinically confined disease treated with radical prostatectomy and found that despite ECE, the 10-year progression-free survival was 58.4% to 67.7% depending on the extent. By the same token, 10-year progression-free survival was 54.9% in men with PSM. Progression was independently predicted by Gleason score, PSM, and ECE.

How common are PSM and ECE seen? In a large series from Memorial Sloan-Kettering Cancer Center and Baylor College of Medicine, the outcomes of 4,629 men with T1 to T3 prostate cancer were analyzed.[157] Overall, PSM were seen in 20% of cases (range 0% to 48%). ECE was observed in 30.1% of cases. When only surgeons who had contributed more than 10 cases were considered, the rate of PSM ranged from 10% to 48%. Independent predictors of PSM were PSA, Gleason score, ECE, the surgeon, and surgical volume.

Three large phase III trials, evaluating the merits of adjuvant versus expectant management in postoperative patients with PSM or pT3 disease, were reported.[169-171] EORTC-22911 consisted of 1,005 men with pT2-3N0 and at least one of the following risk factors: ECE, PSM, or SVI.[169] In the ART arm, radiation was commenced at a median of 90 days postoperative. ART consisted of 50 Gy in 25 fractions to a large volume that encompassed the surgical limits and subclinical disease, followed by 10 Gy boost given over 5 fractions to a reduced margin around the prostatic bed. The protocol salvage radiation therapy (SRT) dose fractionation was 70 Gy in 35 fractions. Toxicity was surprisingly mild. Radiation therapy was interrupted due to toxicities in only 3.1%, with diarrhea responsible in 8 of the 14 patients. In the ART arm, grade 3 diarrhea (5.3%) and urinary frequency (3.3%) were relatively low; the only grade 4 toxicity was urinary frequency (0.4%). There was no added risk of urinary incontinence with ART. Five-year biochemical progression-free survival was significantly improved from 52.6% to 74.0% ($P < .0001$) with ART, representing a 52% reduction in PSA relapse. The treatment benefit was significant for all postoperative prognostic factors, including negative surgical margins or absence of SVI and ECE. Long-term results, with a median follow-up of 10.6 years, were recently published and continued to support the use of ART.[172] The ART arm continued to have significantly improved biochemical progression-free survival (60.6% vs. 41.1%; HR 0.49, $P < .0001$). Similarly, 10-year cumulative rate of locoregional relapse was lower in the ART arm (7.3% vs. 16.6%; HR 0.45, $P < .001$). No difference in metastases-free or overall survival was observed, though it was not powered to detect a difference. However, the 10-year cumulative incidence of severe (grade 3) late toxicities (5.3% vs. 2.5%, $P = .052$) and late grade 2 or higher genitourinary toxicities (21.3% vs. 13.5%; $P = .003$) were higher in the ART arm. There was no significant difference in cumulative incidence of distant metastases ($P = .94$), prostate cancer mortality ($P = .34$), or overall survival ($P = .20$). In the wait-and-see arm, 275 patients had clinical or biochemical progression, of which 231 (84%) went on to receive active treatment and 155 (56%) received SRT at a median PSA of 1.7 ng/mL.

SWOG-8794 randomly assigned 425 node-negative patients initially treated with radical prostatectomy but found to have either PSM or pT3 (ECE and/or SVI) disease to ART or observation.[170] Central pathology review was performed in 73% of patients, and there was a 95% concordance with the community pathologist. Ninety percent of patients had ECE or PSM. Two-thirds of patients had a postoperative PSA <0.2 ng/mL. ART consisted of 60 to 64 Gy. Median PSA relapse-free survival was significantly longer with ART (10.3 vs. 3.1 years; HR 0.43; $P < .001$). Updated results have been published with a median follow-up of 12.6 years.[173] The 10-year distant metastasis-free survival (71% vs. 61%; HR 0.71; $P = .016$) and overall survival (74% vs. 66%; HR 0.72; $P = .023$) were significantly improved with ART. The median distant metastasis-free survival was prolonged from 12.9 to 14.7 years with ART, and overall survival from 13.3 to 15.2 years. On subgroup analyses, there was no interaction between the adverse pathologic features and treatment effect, and therefore, the benefit in distant metastasis-free survival was seen in all subsets. Among patients in the ART arm, those with an undetectable postoperative PSA had a significantly better 10-year distant metastasis-free survival (73% vs. 65%; $P = .03$) than those with a PSA >0.2 ng/mL. In the observation arm, only one-third of patients eventually received SRT, of which the median preradiation therapy PSA was 1.0 ng/mL. Hormonal therapy was initiated later (median 12.4 vs. 9.9 years) and less frequently (39% vs. 50%) in the ART arm. Complications observed in the ART arm included proctitis (3.3% vs. 0%), urethral stricture (17.8% vs. 9.5%), and total urinary incontinence (6.5% vs. 2.8%).

From the German Cancer Society, ARO-96–02/AUO-09/95 accrued 388 patients from 22 centers with pT3 or PSM to either ART (60 Gy in 2 Gy fractions) or observation.[171] In contrast to SWOG-8794 and EORTC-22911, only patients who achieved an undetectable postop PSA were included, 3DCRT planning was mandated, and central pathology review was required. In the initial report with a median follow-up of 54 months, using intention-to-treat analysis of only patients who achieved an undetectable postoperative PSA, ART significantly improved progression-free survival ($P < .0001$). When analyzed according to the received treatment, 5-year progression-free survival was 72% versus 54% in favor of ART ($P = .0015$; HR 0.53). ART was very well tolerated, with only 3% reporting acute grade 3 bladder toxicity and none with grade 3 rectal toxicity (12% had grade 2 rectal toxicity). Of note, the compliance in the ART arm was surprisingly poor—19% did not proceed with radiation therapy. Updated results with 10-year follow-up have since been published.[174] The 10-year progression-free survival was significantly better in the ART arm (56% vs. 35%; HR 0.51, $P < .0001$). However, despite longer follow-up, no difference in the development of distant metastases ($P = .53$) or overall survival ($P = .59$) was seen. The cumulative incidence of late grade 3 toxicities was 5.3% with ART and 2.5% with observation ($P = .052$). There was only one event of late grade 3 toxicity, which involved the bladder, and no late grade 4 GI or GU toxicities were observed.

A significant limitation of these three clinical trials was that they were conducted prior to the current era of ultrasensitive

PSA assays, which can detect PSA levels as low as 0.01 ng/mL. For instance, the ARO trial defined undetectable PSA as those <0.1 ng/mL, of which 59% had a PSA of >0.03 to 0.1 ng/mL. In the EORTC-22911 and SWOG-8794 studies, 11% and 34% of patients, respectively, had a postoperative PSA >0.2 ng/mL. In effect, a significant proportion of patients enrolled in these trials had "measurable disease" and thus received SRT.[175] Although there was an initial surge in enthusiasm in embracing ART, it has given way to increasing skepticism. In an observational study of postop patients identified by the National Cancer Data Base, which tracks outcomes on 71% of newly diagnosed cancer cases in the United State, 130,681 patients with at least one high-risk pathologic factor and diagnosed between 2004 and 2011 were analyzed.[176] The overall rate of ART was surprisingly low (9.9%) and did not change during the study period despite three randomized controlled trials demonstrating improved outcomes with ART. Similarly, SEER data of 35,361 postop patients diagnosed between 2004 and 2011 revealed that ART utilization remained low, 15.8% after March 2009 versus 13.5% before.[177]

Given the prevalence of ultrasensitive PSA assays, it is unclear whether a strategy of active surveillance with PSA tests and the early initiation of radiation therapy only when PSA has shown an upward trend can yield equivalent or better results. The advantage of such an approach is that perhaps the 50% of patients who do not relapse after surgery will be spared from radiation therapy. The disadvantage is that biochemical control and distant metastasis-free survival (SWOG-8794) may be compromised by waiting too long to intervene with definitive treatment, which could serve as a nidus for metastatic spread. In an editorial, King[175] showed that for every 0.1 ng/mL increment in postoperative PSA, there is an estimated 4% reduction in biochemical control. Nonetheless, the EORTC-22911, SWOG-8794, and ARO-96–02 provide consistent level I evidence that ART is better than expectant management in terms of biochemical control, at an acceptable toxicity. It remains to be seen whether with longer follow-up this translates into an improvement in survival. Accordingly, in 2013, the ASTRO/AUA published guidelines based on a systematic review on adjuvant and SRT.[178] The panel recommended that for those with adverse pathologic features (SVI, EPE, and PSM) should be counseled and that there is level I evidence that ART reduces the risk of biochemical recurrence, local recurrence, and clinical cancer progression.

Currently accruing are three key randomized phase III trials, RADICALS, RAVES, and GETUG-17, which are investigating ART versus early SRT. RADICALS, an MRC-led phase III trial, randomizes postoperative patients to immediate postoperative radiation therapy or early SRT.[179] RADICALS also has a hormone duration randomization substudy in which patients are randomized to radiation therapy alone or 6 months or 2 years of adjuvant hormones. Accrual was recently completed for RADICALS. RAVES is another phase III multicenter study being run in Australia and New Zealand that is randomizing patients to ART versus early SRT that is administered within 4 months following the first PSA ≥0.2 ng/mL.[180] GETUG-17 is a French study that is randomizing patients to ART and ADT versus early SRT with ADT.[181]

Salvage Radiation Therapy

As discussed earlier, the findings from EORTC-22911, SWOG-8794, and ARO-96–02/AUO-09/95 strongly advocate for the use of ART.[169-171] Accordingly, the ASTRO and AUA jointly recommended that SRT be offered to patients with biochemical recurrence, defined as a rising postop PSA ≥0.2 ng/mL with a second confirmatory level ≥ 0.2 ng/mL, or local recurrence after radical prostatectomy in the absence of distant metastases.[156] Yet none of these trials address the concept of early SRT given when the PSA is still low. The attraction of this strategy is that only half of the patients with adverse pathologic features will relapse and thus sparing them from unnecessary radiation. Furthermore, the observed benefit from ART as compared to SRT may have been augmented by some patients in the adjuvant arms who would have been cured with surgery alone.

An update of the often cited Stephenson predictive nomogram to estimate biochemical recurrence following SRT was recently published.[182,183] This was based on multi-institutional data of 2,460 patients. Unlike the initial nomogram, patients with pre-SRT PSA <0.2 ng/mL were included in the updated nomogram. The median pre-SRT PSA was 0.5 ng/mL, with 18% of patients <0.2 ng/mL. Higher pre-SRT PSA was associated with worse outcomes. The 5-year freedom from biochemical failure was 71%, 63%, 54%, 43%, and 37% for those with a pre-SRT PSA of 0.01 to 0.2, 0.21 to 0.50, 0.51 to 1.0, 1.01 to 2.0, and >2.0 ng/mL, respectively ($P < .001$). Similarly, the 10-year cumulative incidence of distant metastasis was 9%, 15%, 19%, 20%, and 37%, respectively ($P < .001$). Independent predictors of biochemical recurrence included higher pre-SRT PSA, higher Gleason score, presence of extraprostatic extension, SVI, negative surgical margins, lack of ADT, and SRT dose <66 Gy.

In the largest single-institution cohort of 1,106 patients treated with SRT, the 5- and 10-year cumulative incidence of biochemical recurrence was 50% and 64%, respectively.[184] On multivariate analysis, increasing tumor stage, Gleason score, pre-SRT PSA levels, SRT dose <68 Gy, and use of ADT were independent predictors of biochemical recurrence. Furthermore, patients with pre-SRT PSA >0.5 ng/mL had significantly higher 5-year rates of biochemical recurrence (56% vs. 42%, $P < .001$), distant metastases (14% vs. 7%, $P < .001$), and cause-specific mortality (4% vs. 1%, $P < .001$) as compared to those with pre-SRT PSA ≤0.5 ng/mL. Each doubling of pre-SRT PSA was associated with a 32% increase in the relative risk of distant metastases.

Using a multi-institutional cohort of 472 patients, Briganti et al. developed a nomogram to predict biochemical recurrence following early SRT, defined as PSA ≤0.5 ng/mL (median 0.24 ng/mL), for biochemical recurrence after previous radical prostatectomy.[185] All patients had an undetectable PSA after radical prostatectomy, but subsequently failed biochemically. With a median follow-up of 48 months, the 5-year biochemical recurrence-free survival after early SRT was 73.4%. On multivariate analysis, predictors of biochemical recurrence after early SRT included higher pathologic tumor stage, PSM, higher pathologic Gleason score, and higher pre-SRT PSA.

More recently, genomic classifiers are being developed to try to identify postop patients with adverse pathologic features who would benefit from ART. In a study by Dalela et al., they evaluated a risk stratification tool that included the Decipher multigene expression array score (GenomeDx Biosciences, Vancouver, British Columbia, Canada) with routine clinicopathologic features.[186] Their cohort included 512 postop patients with at least one pathologic adverse feature (≥ pT3a disease, PSM, or pathologic lymph node involvement) and received either ART or initial observation (with 42% subsequently receiving SRT). In multivariate analysis, in addition to Gleason score, pathologic pT3b-4 disease, and lymph node involvement, a high Decipher score was an independent predictor of higher risk of clinical recurrence. Based on these factors, a novel nomogram was created to identify those at higher risk of clinical recurrence and thus would benefit from ART, with a predictive accuracy of 85%. In another study of Decipher, Freedland et al. investigated whether it could predict for the subsequent development of metastatic disease in 170 postop patients treated with SRT for recurrence.[187] On multivariate analysis, the Decipher score was significantly predictive of metastases (HR 1.56, $P = .003$). By identifying patients at high risk of developing metastases, treatment intensification with hormonal therapy and/or systemic therapy can be explored. Likewise, patients with low risk of developing clinical recurrence or metastases could be observed.

While encouraging, external validation in larger prospective cohorts is needed.

As it stands, we have only retrospective data, though very large patient cohorts, that suggest that early SRT is more effective than later SRT, and this is likely due to reduced tumor burden.[182] Whether *early* SRT is as good as ART is unknown. As discussed earlier, RADICALS, RAVES, and GETUG-17 are three studies that will provide further insight into ART and early SRT.[179,180,188]

Androgen Suppression Therapy and Postoperative Radiation Therapy

Extrapolating from the benefits of shown in multiple phase III trials in the definitive setting, it is not surprising that ADT would be investigated in the postoperative setting. Recently, the results of RTOG-9601, a placebo-controlled phase III study to evaluate the addition of 2-years of antiandrogen therapy with SRT, were published.[189] Eligible patients included those with pathologic stage T2 with a PSM or T3 without nodal involvement. Patients were also required to have a detectable PSA of 0.2 to 4.0 ng/mL were eligible. Bicalutamide 150 mg daily for 24 months was used in the antiandrogen arm. The median follow-up among surviving patients was 13 years. The addition of antiandrogen significantly improved 12-year overall survival (76.3% vs. 71.3%; HR 0.77, $P = .04$), incidence of death from prostate cancer (5.8% vs. 13.4%, $P < .001$), cumulative incidence of metastatic prostate cancer (14.5% vs. 23.0%, $P = .005$), and biochemical recurrence (44.0% vs. 67.9%, $P < .001$). Post hoc subgroup analyses suggested that those with a PSA >1.5 ng/mL or a Gleason score of 7 had the greatest overall survival benefit. There was no difference in radiation-related acute or late toxicities. As expected, gynecomastia was more common in the antiandrogen arm and occurred in 69.7% of patients. Of note, antiandrogens alone are rarely used currently, replaced by gonadotropin-releasing hormone agonist and antagonist, and are no longer approved by the U.S. Food and Drug Administration.

GETUG-AFU16 was a phase III trial that randomized 743 postoperative patients undergoing SRT for biochemical recurrence to with or without 6 months of goserelin.[181] All patients had to have an undetectable postop PSA before biochemical recurrence. The PSA at time of randomization was <0.5 ng/mL in 80% of patients, with the upper limit of acceptance being 2 ng/mL. After a median follow-up of 63 months, the 5-year progression-free survival was significantly better in the hormone arm (80% vs. 62%, $P < .0001$). Independent predictors of disease progression were pre-SRT PSA >0.5 ng/mL, seminal vesicle involvement, negative surgical margins, and pre-SRT PSA doubling time <6 months. There was no significant difference in acute or late genitourinary and gastrointestinal adverse events between the two arms.

In postop patients with *very high-risk* clinicopathologic features, investigators are evaluating the addition of docetaxel to radiation therapy and ADT based on docetaxel improving survival in men with metastatic prostate cancer.[190] RTOG-0621 is a phase II study of 74 patients who had either a postop PSA nadir >0.2 ng/mL and a Gleason score ≥ 7 or a PSA nadir ≤0.2 ng/mL, Gleason score ≥8, and ≥pT3. Patients received 6 months of ADT, radiation therapy, and six cycles of docetaxel postradiation therapy. The 3-year freedom from progression was 73%. Although grade 3 to 4 hematologic toxicities were common, only 4.1% of patients developed febrile neutropenia. Currently accruing, the follow-up phase II/III trial is NRG-GU002, which is randomizing patients with a Gleason score ≥7 and postop PSA nadir ≥0.2 ng/mL to ART and ADT with or without adjuvant docetaxel.

In summary, the evidence to date suggests that the inclusion of hormonal therapy to postoperative radiation therapy may be beneficial, although the optimal type of hormones, duration, and timing remains unknown. The results of two important phase III studies, RTOG-0534 and RADICALS, will provide more clarity on the role and duration of ADT and postoperative radiation therapy. RTOG-0534 is a three-arm trial evaluating the role of short-term hormones (4 to 6 months) and pelvic radiation therapy in the salvage setting. RADICALS is a two-part study, with the hormone component randomizing patients to no hormones (i.e., radiation therapy alone), 6 months or 2 years of gonadotrophin-releasing hormone analogue.

Postoperative Radiation Therapy Dose

Currently, ART doses of 60 to 64 Gy and SRT doses of 66 to 70 Gy appear to be the most commonly used. The ASTRO/AUA guidelines recommend at least 64 to 65 Gy in the postop setting, with no distinction between adjuvant and salvage doses.[156] In a retrospective study by Cozzarini et al., 334 patients with adverse pathologic features and an undetectable postoperative PSA who received ART were analyzed for a dose response.[191] From 1993 to 2003, the radiation therapy dose gradually increased from 55.8 to 72 Gy. When stratified by dose (<70.2 Gy [median 66.6 Gy] vs. ≥ 70.2 Gy [median 70.2 Gy]), the high-dose group had significantly better 5-year biochemical relapse-free survival (83% vs. 71%; P = .001) and disease-free survival (94% vs. 88%; P = .005). In a systematic review, 71 studies (10,034 patients) of patients treated with SRT were identified.[192] The median radiation dose prescribed was 65.8 (range 60 to 76 Gy). A sigmoidal dose–response relationship was identified between SRT dose and relapse-free survival, with a TCD_{50} of 65.8 Gy and a 2.0% improvement with each additional Gy within a dose range of 60 to 70 Gy. Based on the sigmoidal dose–response curve, the relapse-free survival was 58.4% and 38.5% for 70 and 60 Gy, respectively. The initial results of the only randomized controlled dose escalation trial for SRT were recently published.[193] Patients with biochemical recurrence with a pre-radiation therapy PSA ≤ 2.0 ng/mL following radical prostatectomy were randomized to 64 or 70 Gy. There was no significant difference in acute grade 2 and 3 genitourinary or gastrointestinal toxicities between the two arms. No acute grade 4 to 5 toxicities were observed. However, on QOL questionnaires, a small but clinically relevant worsening in urinary symptoms was observed in the 70 Gy arm. Clinical outcomes are eagerly awaited. Open to accrual, NRG-GU003 is a randomized phase III trial of hypofractionated versus conventionally fractionated radiation therapy in postprostatectomy patients.

Postoperative Radiation Therapy Volume

Several consensus guidelines on delineation of the CTV in postop patients have been published, including RTOG and EORTC.[194-197] According to the RTOG contouring consensus guidelines, the limits of the prostatic fossa CTV are superior at the level of the caudal vas deferens remnant and inferior to >8 to 12 mm caudal to the vesicourethral anastomosis.[194] Above the pubic symphysis, the anterior border should include 1 to 2 cm of the posterior bladder wall, posterior border is the mesorectal fascia, and lateral border is the bounded by the sacrorectogenitopubic fascia. Below the superior border of the pubic symphysis, the anterior border is at the posterior aspect of the pubis, posterior border to the rectum, and lateral border extending to the levator ani.

Another area of research is the utility of elective nodal irradiation (ENI) in the postop setting, especially for those with higher-risk disease.[88,94,97,198] In a large multi-institutional retrospective study of 1,861 patients, ENI with SRT was associated with a significantly better 5-year freedom from biochemical failure of 62% versus 49% (P < .001).[100] The use of ADT with SRT was also associated with improved 5-year freedom from biochemical failure (55% vs. 50%, P = .012). Closed to accrual, RTOG-0534 is evaluating ENI and ADT in a three-arm study whereby patients would be randomized to prostate bed radiation therapy, prostate bed radiation therapy with 6 months of LHRH agonist, or ENI with 6 months of LHRH agonist.

University of California, San Francisco, Recommendations of Postoperative Radiation Therapy

We endorse the ASTRO/AUA guidelines whereby patients with adverse pathologic features should be jointly counseled by their urologist and radiation oncologist on the pros and cons of ART.[156] In those with an undetectable postop PSA of <0.02 ng/mL, we recommend observation with a PSA every 3 months. We would offer early SRT in those with two postop PSA readings above 0.2 ng/mL. The authors recommend adherence to the RTOG consensus guidelines on the definitions of CTV in the postoperative setting.[194] For adjuvant patients, the authors prescribe 68 Gy, whereas for salvage patients, the authors use 70.2 Gy, both of which are in 1.8-Gy fractions. WPRT, as defined by the RTOG contouring guidelines, to a dose of 45 Gy, is considered depending on the extent of pelvic lymph node dissection, presence of SVI, and the estimated nodal involvement. For both the prostate bed and ENI, we recommend IMRT technique with image guidance. There are now two phase III trials that support the addition of ADT with postop radiation therapy.[181,189] We recommend that those at higher risk of developing metastatic disease, including a detectable postop PSA, pre-SRT PSA >0.5 ng/mL, SVI, PSA doubling time <6 months, or node-positive disease, be considered for 4 to 6 months of LHRH. In addition, we favor image-guided radiation (IGRT) in the postoperative setting guided by the place of gold marker seeds at the anastomosis.[199]

CONCLUSIONS AND RECOMMENDATIONS

In conclusion, because of patient convenience, cost, and PSA control, we favor PPI, HDR, or SBRT monotherapy for patients with favorable intermediate-risk disease. For unfavorable risk disease, we favor short-term ADT (4 months) combined with IMRT and a boost with either PPI, HDR, or SBRT, with WPRT in selected patients. For high-risk patients, we favor long-term ADT (e.g., ≥28 months) combined with WPRT and an HDR, an SBRT, or a PPI boost. Image-guided techniques without rectal spacer are preferred at UCSF. In selected patients (age <70 years with node positive), additional systemic agents (e.g., abiraterone) are strongly considered. It remains to be determined if and when biomarkers or molecular assays or advances in imaging will help us refine what we mean by the categories that range from favorable intermediate- to very high-risk disease.[2] In the postoperative setting, we favor adjuvant or early salvage IMRT guided by ultrasensitive PSA monitoring combined with ADT.

REFERENCES

1. Ramey SJ, Agrawal S, Abramowitz MC, et al. Multi-institutional Evaluation of Elective Nodal Irradiation and/or Androgen Deprivation Therapy with Postprostatectomy Salvage Radiotherapy for Prostate Cancer. *Eur Urol* 2017.
2. Gonzalez-Motta A, Roach M, III. Stereotactic body radiation therapy (SBRT) for high-risk prostate cancer: where are we now? *Pract Radiat Oncol* 2018;8:185–202.
3. Tendulkar RD, Agrawal S, Gao T, et al. Contemporary Update of a Multi-Institutional Predictive Nomogram for Salvage Radiotherapy After Radical Prostatectomy. *J Clin Oncol* 2016;34:3648–3654.
4. Hager B, et al. Increasing use of radical prostatectomy for locally advanced prostate cancer in the USA and Germany: a comparative population-based study. *Prostate Cancer Prostatic Dis* 2017;20(1):61–66.
5. Wallis CJ, et al. Surgery versus radiotherapy for clinically-localized prostate cancer: a systematic review and meta-analysis. *Eur Urol* 2015;70(1):21–30.
6. Sooriakumaran P, et al. Comparative effectiveness of radical prostatectomy and radiotherapy in prostate cancer: observational study of mortality outcomes. *BMJ* 2014;348:g1502.
7. Feldman AS, et al. Morbidity and mortality of locally advanced prostate cancer: a population based analysis comparing radical prostatectomy versus external beam radiation. *J Urol* 2017;198(5):1061–1068.
8. Roach M 3rd, Thomas K. Overview of randomized controlled treatment trials for clinically localized prostate cancer: implications for active surveillance and the United States preventative task force report on screening? *J Natl Cancer Inst Monogr* 2012;2012(45):221–229.
9. Lazar AA, Lizarraga TL, Roach M 3rd. Re: Christopher JD Wallis, Refik Saskin, Richard Choo, et al. Surgery versus radiotherapy for clinically-localized prostate cancer: a systematic review and meta-analysis. *Eur Urol* 2016;70:21–30: Radical prostatectomy versus radiation for clinically localized prostate cancer: two systematic reviews and a randomized controlled trial. *Eur Urol* 2016;70(1):e13–e14.

Section III

10. Roach M 3rd, Ceron Lizarraga TL, Lazar AA. Radical prostatectomy versus radiation and androgen deprivation therapy for clinically localized prostate cancer: how good is the evidence? *Int J Radiat Oncol Biol Phys* 2015;93(5):1064–1070.

11. Lennernas B, et al. Radical prostatectomy versus high-dose irradiation in localized/locally advanced prostate cancer: a Swedish multicenter randomized trial with patient-reported outcomes. *Acta Oncol* 2015;54(6):875–881.

12. Hamdy FC, et al. 10-Year outcomes after monitoring, surgery, or radiotherapy for localized prostate cancer. *N Engl J Med* 2016;375:1415–1424.

13. Donovan JL, et al. Patient-reported outcomes after monitoring, surgery, or radiotherapy for prostate cancer. *N Engl J Med* 2016;375:1425–1437.

14. Roach M, et al. Four prognostic groups predict long-term survival from prostate cancer following radiotherapy alone on Radiation Therapy Oncology Group clinical trials. *Int J Radiat Oncol Biol Phys* 2000;47(3):609–615.

15. Kattan MW, et al. Pretreatment nomogram for predicting freedom from recurrence after permanent prostate brachytherapy in prostate cancer. *Urology* 2001;58(3):393–399.

16. Kattan MW, et al. Pretreatment nomogram that predicts 5-year probability of metastasis following three-dimensional conformal radiation therapy for localized prostate cancer. *J Clin Oncol* 2003;21:4568–4571.

17. Cooperberg MR, et al. The University of California, San Francisco Cancer of the Prostate Risk Assessment score: a straightforward and reliable preoperative predictor of disease recurrence after radical prostatectomy. *J Urol* 2005;173(6):1938–1942.

18. D'Amico AV, et al. Biochemical outcome after radical prostatectomy, external beam radiation therapy, or interstitial radiation therapy for clinically localized prostate cancer. *JAMA* 1998;280(11):969–974.

19. Roach M 3rd, et al. Defining high risk prostate cancer with risk groups and nomograms: implications for designing clinical trials. *J Urol* 2006;176(6 Pt 2):S16–S20.

20. ASTRO. Consensus statement: guidelines for PSA following radiation therapy. *Int J Radiat Oncol Biol Phys* 1997;37:1035–1041.

21. Roach M 3rd, et al. Defining biochemical failure following radiotherapy with or without hormonal therapy in men with clinically localized prostate cancer: recommendations of the RTOG-ASTRO Phoenix Consensus Conference. *Int J Radiat Oncol Biol Phys* 2006;65(4):965–974.

22. Aaronson DS, et al. Salvage permanent perineal radioactive-seed implantation for treating recurrence of localized prostate adenocarcinoma after external beam radiotherapy. *BJU Int* 2009;104(5):600–604.

23. Chen CP, et al. Salvage HDR brachytherapy for recurrent prostate cancer after previous definitive radiation therapy: 5-year outcomes. *Int J Radiat Oncol Biol Phys* 2013;86(2):324–329.

24. D'Amico AV, et al. Clinical utility of the percentage of positive prostate biopsies in defining biochemical outcome after radical prostatectomy for patients with clinically localized prostate cancer. *J Clin Oncol* 2000;18:1164–1172.

25. Kestin LL, et al. Percentage of positive biopsy cores as predictor of clinical outcome in prostate cancer treated with radiotherapy. *J Urol* 2002;168:1994–1999.

26. Roach M 3rd, et al. Predicting long-term survival, and the need for hormonal therapy: a meta-analysis of RTOG prostate cancer trials. *Int J Radiat Oncol Biol Phys* 2000;47(3):617–627.

27. Hamstra DA, et al. Older age predicts decreased metastasis and prostate cancer-specific death for men treated with radiation therapy: meta-analysis of Radiation Therapy Oncology Group trials. *Int J Radiat Oncol Biol Phys* 2011;81(5):1293–1301.

28. Zhao SG, et al. Associations of luminal and basal subtyping of prostate cancer with prognosis and response to androgen deprivation therapy. *JAMA Oncol* 2017;3(12):1663–1672.

29. Roach M 3rd, Waldman F, Pollack A. Predictive models in external beam radiotherapy for clinically localized prostate cancer. *Cancer* 2009;115(13 Suppl):3112–3120.

30. Zapatero A, et al. Predictive value of PAK6 and PSMB4 expression in patients with localized prostate cancer treated with dose-escalation radiation therapy and androgen deprivation therapy. *Urol Oncol* 2014;32(8):1327–1332.

31. Bouchaert P, et al. DNA-PKcs expression predicts response to radiotherapy in prostate cancer. *Int J Radiat Oncol Biol Phys* 2012;84(5):1179–1185.

32. Chan LW, et al. Urinary VEGF and MMP levels as predictive markers of 1-year progression-free survival in cancer patients treated with radiation therapy: a longitudinal study of protein kinetics throughout tumor progression and therapy. *J Clin Oncol* 2004;22(3):499–506.

33. Khor LY, et al. Bcl-2 and bax expression and prostate cancer outcome in men treated with radiotherapy in Radiation Therapy Oncology Group protocol 86–10. *Int J Radiat Oncol Biol Phys* 2006;66(1):25–30.

34. Mackey TJ, et al. Bcl-2/bax ratio as a predictive marker for therapeutic response to radiotherapy in patients with prostate cancer. *Urology* 1998;52(6):1085–1090.

35. Ahmed M, et al. Common genetic variation associated with increased susceptibility to prostate cancer does not increase risk of radiotherapy toxicity. *Br J Cancer* 2016;114(10):1165–1174.

36. Andreassen CN, et al. Individual patient data meta-analysis shows a significant association between the ATM rs1801516 SNP and toxicity after radiotherapy in 5456 breast and prostate cancer patients. *Radiother Oncol* 2016;121(3):431–439.

37. Kerns SL, et al. Meta-analysis of genome wide association studies identifies genetic markers of late toxicity following radiotherapy for prostate cancer. *EBioMedicine* 2016;10:150–163.

38. Oh JH, et al. Computational methods using genome-wide association studies to predict radiotherapy complications and to identify correlative molecular processes. *Sci Rep* 2017;7:43381.

39. Azria D, et al. Data-based radiation oncology: design of clinical trials in the toxicity biomarkers era. *Front Oncol* 2017;7:83.

40. Wilt TJ, et al. Follow-up of prostatectomy versus observation for early prostate cancer. *N Engl J Med* 2017;377(2):132–142.

41. Nabid A, Carrier N, Martin A-G, et al. High-risk prostate cancer treated with pelvic radiotherapy and 36 versus 18 months of androgen blockade: results of a phase III randomized study. In: Genitourinary Cancers Symposium Proceedings. 2013. Orlando, FL.

42. Nabid A, et al. Duration of androgen deprivation therapy in high risk prostate cancer: final results of a randomized phase III trial. *J Clin Oncol* 2017;35(15 Suppl):5008.

43. Pommier P, et al. Is there a role for pelvic irradiation in localized prostate adenocarcinoma? Update of the long-term survival results of the GETUG-01 randomized study. *Int J Radiat Oncol Biol Phys* 2016;96(4):759–769.

44. James ND, Spears MR, Sydes MR. Abiraterone in metastatic prostate cancer. *N Engl J Med* 2017;377(17):1696–1697.

45. Roach M 3rd, et al. Whole-pelvis, "mini-pelvis," or prostate-only external beam radiotherapy after neoadjuvant and concurrent hormonal therapy in patients treated in the Radiation Therapy Oncology Group 9413 trial. *Int J Radiat Oncol Biol Phys* 2006;66(3):647–653.

46. James ND, et al. Abiraterone for prostate cancer not previously treated with hormone therapy. *N Engl J Med* 2017;377:338–351.

47. Cooperberg MR, et al. Comparative risk-adjusted mortality outcomes after primary surgery, radiotherapy, or androgen-deprivation therapy for localized prostate cancer. *Cancer* 2010;116(22):5226–5234.

48. Roach M 3rd, et al. Diagnostic and therapeutic imaging for cancer: therapeutic considerations and future directions. *J Surg Oncol* 2011;103(6):587–601.

49. Lawton CA, et al. Variation in the definition of clinical target volumes for pelvic nodal conformal radiation therapy for prostate cancer. *Int J Radiat Oncol Biol Phys* 2009;74(2):377–382.

50. Harris VA, et al. Consensus guidelines and contouring atlas for pelvic node delineation in prostate and pelvic node intensity modulated radiation therapy. *Int J Radiat Oncol Biol Phys* 2015;92(4):874–883.

51. Maurer T, et al. Diagnostic efficacy of (68)Gallium-PSMA positron emission tomography compared to conventional imaging for lymph node staging of 130 consecutive patients with intermediate to high risk prostate cancer. *J Urol* 2016;195(5):1436–1443.

52. Afshar-Oromieh A, et al. Comparison of PET imaging with a (68)Ga-labelled PSMA ligand and (18)F-choline-based PET/CT for the diagnosis of recurrent prostate cancer. *Eur J Nucl Med Mol Imaging* 2014;41(1):11–20.

53. Schwenck J, et al. Comparison of (68)Ga-labelled PSMA-11 and (11)C-choline in the detection of prostate cancer metastases by PET/CT. *Eur J Nucl Med Mol Imaging* 2017;44(1):92–101.

54. van Leeuwen PJ, et al. Prospective evaluation of 68Gallium-prostate-specific membrane antigen positron emission tomography/computed tomography for preoperative lymph node staging in prostate cancer. *BJU Int* 2017;119(2):209–215.

55. Wawroschek F, et al. Radioisotope guided pelvic lymph node dissection for prostate cancer. *J Urol* 2001;166(5):1715–1719.

56. Holl G, et al. Validation of sentinel lymph node dissection in prostate cancer: experience in more than 2,000 patients. *Eur J Nucl Med Mol Imaging* 2009;36(9):1377–1382.

57. Krengli M, et al. Potential advantage of studying the lymphatic drainage by sentinel node technique and SPECT-CT image fusion for pelvic irradiation of prostate cancer. *Int J Radiat Oncol Biol Phys* 2006;66(4):1100–1104.

58. Chen CP, et al. Sentinel lymph node imaging guided IMRT for prostate cancer: individualized pelvic radiation therapy versus RTOG guidelines. *Adv Radiat Oncol* 2016;1(1):51–58.

59. Harisinghani MG, et al. Noninvasive detection of clinically occult lymph-node metastases in prostate cancer. *N Engl J Med* 2003;348:2491–2499.

60. Deserno WM, et al. Comparison of nodal risk formula and MR lymphography for predicting lymph node involvement in prostate cancer. *Int J Radiat Oncol Biol Phys* 2011;81(1):8–15.

61. Shih HA, et al. Mapping of nodal disease in locally advanced prostate cancer: rethinking the clinical target volume for pelvic nodal irradiation based on vascular rather than bony anatomy. *Int J Radiat Oncol Biol Phys* 2005;63:1262–1269.

62. Dinniwell R, et al. Pelvic lymph node topography for radiotherapy treatment planning from ferumoxtran-10 contrast-enhanced magnetic resonance imaging. *Int J Radiat Oncol Biol Phys* 2009;74(3):844–851.

63. Fortuin AS, et al. Ultra-small superparamagnetic iron oxides for metastatic lymph node detection: back on the block. *Wiley Interdiscip Rev Nanomed Nanobiotechnol* 2018;10(1).

64. Shariat SF, et al. Detection of clinically significant, occult prostate cancer metastases in lymph nodes using a splice variant-specific RT-PCR assay for human glandular kallikrein. *J Clin Oncol* 2003;21:1223–1231.

65. Bader P, et al. Is a limited lymph node dissection an adequate staging procedure for prostate cancer? *J Urol* 2002;168:514–518; discussion 518.

66. Heidenreich A, Varga Z, Von Knobloch R. Extended pelvic lymphadenectomy in patients undergoing radical prostatectomy: high incidence of lymph node metastasis. *J Urol* 2002;167:1681–1686.

67. Briganti A, et al. Critical assessment of ideal nodal yield at pelvic lymphadenectomy to accurately diagnose prostate cancer nodal metastasis in patients undergoing radical retropubic prostatectomy. *Urology* 2007;69(1):147–151.

68. Nguyen PL, et al. Predicting the risk of pelvic node involvement among men with prostate cancer in the contemporary era. *Int J Radiat Oncol Biol Phys* 2009;74(1):104–109.

69. Yu JB, Makarov DV, Gross C. A new formula for prostate cancer lymph node risk. *Int J Radiat Oncol Biol Phys* 2011;80(1):69–75.

70. Roach M 3rd. Re: The use of prostate specific antigen, clinical stage and Gleason score to predict pathological stage in men with localized prostate cancer. *J Urol* 1993;150(6):1923–1924.

71. Abdollah F, et al. Indications for pelvic nodal treatment in prostate cancer should change. Validation of the Roach formula in a large extended nodal dissection series. *Int J Radiat Oncol Biol Phys* 2012;83(2):624–629.

72. Allaf ME, et al. Anatomical extent of lymph node dissection: impact on men with clinically localized prostate cancer. *J Urol* 2004;172:1840–1844.

73. Colicchia M, et al. Therapeutic value of standard versus extended pelvic lymph node dissection during radical prostatectomy for high-risk prostate cancer. *Curr Urol Rep* 2017;18(7):51.

74. Weckermann D, et al. Incidence of positive pelvic lymph nodes in patients with prostate cancer, a prostate-specific antigen (PSA) level of < or = 10 ng/mL and biopsy Gleason score of < or = 6, and their influence on PSA progression-free survival after radical prostatectomy. *BJU Int* 2006;97:1173–1178.

75. Briganti A, et al. Validation of a nomogram predicting the probability of lymph node invasion based on the extent of pelvic lymphadenectomy in patients with clinically localized prostate cancer. *BJU Int* 2006;98(4):788–793.
76. Bandini M, et al. First North American validation and head-to-head comparison of four preoperative nomograms for prediction of lymph node invasion before radical prostatectomy. *BJU Int* 2017;121(4):592–599.
77. Roach M 3rd, et al. Predicting the risk of lymph node involvement using the pre-treatment prostate specific antigen and Gleason score in men with clinically localized prostate cancer. *Int J Radiat Oncol Biol Phys* 1994;28(1):33–37.
78. Roach M 3rd, et al. Phase III trial comparing whole-pelvic versus prostate-only radiotherapy and neoadjuvant versus adjuvant combined androgen suppression: Radiation Therapy Oncology Group 9413. *J Clin Oncol* 2003;21:1904–1911.
79. Morikawa LK, Roach M 3rd. Pelvic nodal radiotherapy in patients with unfavorable intermediate and high-risk prostate cancer: evidence, rationale, and future directions. *Int J Radiat Oncol Biol Phys* 2011;80(1):6–16.
80. Amini A, et al. Survival outcomes of whole-pelvic versus prostate-only radiation therapy for high-risk prostate cancer patients with use of the National Cancer Data Base. *Int J Radiat Oncol Biol Phys* 2015;93(5):1052–1063.
81. Lawton CA, et al. Long-term treatment sequelae after external beam irradiation with or without hormonal manipulation for adenocarcinoma of the prostate: analysis of Radiation Therapy Oncology Group studies 85-31, 86-10, and 92-02. *Int J Radiat Oncol Biol Phys* 2008;70(2):437–441.
82. Seaward SA, et al. Improved freedom from PSA failure with whole pelvic irradiation for high-risk prostate cancer. *Int J Radiat Oncol Biol Phys* 1998;42(5):1055–1062.
83. Seaward SA, et al. Identification of a high-risk clinically localized prostate cancer subgroup receiving maximum benefit from whole-pelvic irradiation. *Cancer J Sci Am* 1998;4:370–377.
84. Pan CC, et al. Influence of 3D-CRT pelvic irradiation on outcome in prostate cancer treated with external beam radiotherapy. *Int J Radiat Oncol Biol Phys* 2002;53:1139–1145.
85. Roach III M, Yan Y, Lawton CA, et al. Radiation Therapy Oncology Group (RTOG) 9413: A randomized trial comparing whole pelvic radiotherapy (WPRT) to prostate only (PORT) & neoadjuvant hormonal therapy (NHT) to adjuvant hormonal therapy (AHT). In: *Proceedings of the American Society for Radiation Oncology* 2013. Atlanta, GA: Elsevier.
86. Jacob R, et al. Role of prostate dose escalation in patients with greater than 15% risk of pelvic lymph node involvement. *Int J Radiat Oncol Biol Phys* 2005;61:695–701.
87. Pommier P, et al. Is there a role for pelvic irradiation in localized prostate adenocarcinoma? Preliminary results of GETUG-01. *J Clin Oncol* 2007;25(34):5366–5373.
88. Spiotto MT, Hancock SL, King CR. Radiotherapy after prostatectomy: improved biochemical relapse-free survival with whole pelvic compared with prostate bed only for high-risk patients. *Int J Radiat Oncol Biol Phys* 2007;69(1):54–61.
89. Da Pozzo LF, et al. Long-term follow-up of patients with prostate cancer and nodal metastases treated by pelvic lymphadenectomy and radical prostatectomy: the positive impact of adjuvant radiotherapy. *Eur Urol* 2009;55(5):1003–1011.
90. Aizer AA, et al. Whole pelvic radiotherapy versus prostate only radiotherapy in the management of locally advanced or aggressive prostate adenocarcinoma. *Int J Radiat Oncol Biol Phys* 2009;75(5):1344–1349.
91. Milecki P, et al. Benefit of whole pelvic radiotherapy combined with neoadjuvant androgen deprivation for the high-risk prostate cancer. *J Biomed Biotechnol* 2009;2009:625394.
92. Bittner N, et al. Whole-pelvis radiotherapy in combination with interstitial brachytherapy: does coverage of the pelvic lymph nodes improve treatment outcome in high-risk prostate cancer? *Int J Radiat Oncol Biol Phys* 2010;76(4):1078–1084.
93. Mantini G, et al. Effect of whole pelvic radiotherapy for patients with locally advanced prostate cancer treated with radiotherapy and long-term androgen deprivation therapy. *Int J Radiat Oncol Biol Phys* 2011;81(5):e721–e726.
94. Moghanaki D, et al. Elective irradiation of pelvic lymph nodes during postprostatectomy salvage radiotherapy. *Cancer* 2013;119(1):52–60.
95. Tward JD, Kokeny KE, Shrieve DC. Radiation therapy for clinically node-positive prostate adenocarcinoma is correlated with improved overall and prostate cancer-specific survival. *Pract Radiat Oncol* 2013;3(3):234–240.
96. Braunstein LZ, et al. Whole pelvis versus prostate-only radiotherapy with or without short-course androgen deprivation therapy and mortality risk. *Clin Genitourin Cancer* 2015;13(6):555–561.
97. Song C, et al. Elective pelvic versus prostate bed-only salvage radiotherapy following radical prostatectomy: a propensity score-matched analysis. *Strahlenther Onkol* 2015;191(10):801–809.
98. Mason MD, et al. Final report of the intergroup randomized study of combined androgen-deprivation therapy plus radiotherapy versus androgen-deprivation therapy alone in locally advanced prostate cancer. *J Clin Oncol* 2015;33(19):2143–2150.
99. James ND, et al. Failure-free survival and radiotherapy in patients with newly diagnosed nonmetastatic prostate cancer: data from patients in the control arm of the STAMPEDE trial. *JAMA Oncol* 2016;2(3):348–357.
100. Ramey SJ, et al. Multi-institutional evaluation of elective nodal irradiation and/or androgen deprivation therapy with postprostatectomy salvage radiotherapy for prostate cancer. *Eur Urol* 2017.
101. Nguyen PL, D'Amico AV. Targeting pelvic lymph nodes in men with intermediate- and high-risk prostate cancer despite two negative randomized trials. *J Clin Oncol* 2008;26(12):2055–2056; author reply 2056–7.
102. Lepinoy A, et al. Pattern of occult nodal relapse diagnosed with (18)F-fluorocholine PET/CT in prostate cancer patients with biochemical failure after prostate-only radiotherapy. *Radiother Oncol* 2014;111(1):120–125.
103. Lawton CA, et al. RTOG GU Radiation oncology specialists reach consensus on pelvic lymph node volumes for high-risk prostate cancer. *Int J Radiat Oncol Biol Phys* 2009;74(2):383–387.
104. Gonzalez-Motta A, Roach M. Stereotactic body radiotherapy (SBRT) for high-risk prostate cancer: where are we now? *Pract Radiat Oncol* 2017. In press.
105. Prestidge BR, Winter K, Sanda MG, et al. Initial report of NRG Oncology/RTOG 0232: A phase III study comparing combined external beam radiation and transperineal interstitial permanent brachytherapy with brachytherapy alone for selected patients with intermediate risk prostatic carcinoma. In: *Int J Radiat Biol* 2016. Boston, MA: Elsevier.
106. Morris WJ, et al. Androgen suppression combined with elective nodal and dose escalated radiation therapy (the ASCENDE-RT Trial): an analysis of survival endpoints for a randomized trial comparing a low-dose-rate brachytherapy boost to a dose-escalated external beam boost for high- and intermediate-risk prostate cancer. *Int J Radiat Oncol Biol Phys* 2017;98(2):275–285.
107. Hoskin PJ, et al. Randomised trial of external beam radiotherapy alone or combined with high-dose-rate brachytherapy boost for localised prostate cancer. *Radiother Oncol*, 2012;103(2):217–222.
108. Lee WR, et al. Randomized phase III noninferiority study comparing two radiotherapy fractionation schedules in patients with low-risk prostate cancer. *J Clin Oncol* 2016;34(20):2325–2332.
109. Lee WR. Hypofractionation for prostate cancer: tested and proven. *Lancet Oncol* 2016;17(8):1020–1022.
110. Dearnaley D, et al. Conventional versus hypofractionated high-dose intensity-modulated radiotherapy for prostate cancer: 5-year outcomes of the randomised, non-inferiority, phase 3 CHHiP trial. *Lancet Oncol* 2016;17(8):1047–1060.
111. Nag S, et al. The American Brachytherapy Society recommendations for permanent prostate brachytherapy postimplant dosimetric analysis. *Int J Radiat Oncol Biol Phys* 2000;46(1):221–230.
112. Schallenkamp JM, et al. Prostate position relative to pelvic bony anatomy based on intraprostatic gold markers and electronic portal imaging. *Int J Radiat Oncol Biol Phys* 2005;63(3):800–811.
113. Moseley DJ, et al. Comparison of localization performance with implanted fiducial markers and cone-beam computed tomography for on-line image-guided radiotherapy of the prostate. *Int J Radiat Oncol Biol Phys* 2007;67(3):942–953.
114. Kupelian P, et al. Multi-institutional clinical experience with the Calypso System in localization and continuous, real-time monitoring of the prostate gland during external radiotherapy. *Int J Radiat Oncol Biol Phys* 2007;67(4):1088–1098.
115. Kupelian PA, et al. Daily variations in the position of the prostate bed in patients with prostate cancer receiving postoperative external beam radiation therapy. *Int J Radiat Oncol Biol Phys* 2006;66(2):593–596.
116. Kupelian PA, et al. Image-guided radiotherapy for localized prostate cancer: treating a moving target. *Semin Radiat Oncol* 2008;18(1):58–66.
117. Langen KM, Jones DT. Organ motion and its management. *Int J Radiat Oncol Biol Phys* 2001;50:265–278.
118. Langen KM, et al. Observations on real-time prostate gland motion using electromagnetic tracking. *Int J Radiat Oncol Biol Phys* 2008;71(4):1084–1090.
119. Xia P, et al. Comparison of three strategies in management of independent movement of the prostate and pelvic lymph nodes. *Med Phys* 2010;37(9):5006–5013.
120. Qi P, et al. Offline multiple adaptive planning strategy for concurrent irradiation of the prostate and pelvic lymph nodes. *Med Phys* 2014;41(2):021704.
121. Ludlum E, et al. An algorithm for shifting MLC shapes to adjust for daily prostate movement during concurrent treatment with pelvic lymph nodes. *Med Phys* 2007;34(12):4750–4756.
122. Chung HT, et al. Does image-guided radiotherapy improve toxicity profile in whole pelvic-treated high-risk prostate cancer? Comparison between IG-IMRT and IMRT. *Int J Radiat Oncol Biol Phys* 2009;73(1):53–60.
123. Mariados N, et al. Hydrogel spacer prospective multicenter randomized controlled pivotal trial: dosimetric and clinical effects of perirectal spacer application in men undergoing prostate image guided intensity modulated radiation therapy. *Int J Radiat Oncol Biol Phys* 2015;92(5):971–977.
124. Hamstra DA, et al. Continued benefit to rectal separation for prostate radiation therapy: final results of a phase III trial. *Int J Radiat Oncol Biol Phys* 2017;97(5):976–985.
125. Wang-Chesebro A, et al. Intensity-modulated radiotherapy improves lymph node coverage and dose to critical structures compared with three-dimensional conformal radiation therapy in clinically localized prostate cancer. *Int J Radiat Oncol Biol Phys* 2006;66(3):654–662.
126. Chan LW, et al. Proposed rectal dose constraints for patients undergoing definitive whole pelvic radiotherapy for clinically localized prostate cancer. *Int J Radiat Oncol Biol Phys* 2008;72(1):69–77.
127. Zapatero A, et al. High-dose radiotherapy with short-term or long-term androgen deprivation in localised prostate cancer (DART01/05 GICOR): a randomised, controlled, phase 3 trial. *Lancet Oncol* 2015;16(3):320–327.
128. Dearnaley DP, et al. Escalated-dose versus standard-dose conformal radiotherapy in prostate cancer: first results from the MRC RT01 randomised controlled trial. *Lancet Oncol* 2007;8(6):475–487.
129. Peeters ST, et al. Dose–response in radiotherapy for localized prostate cancer: results of the Dutch multicenter randomized phase III trial comparing 68 Gy of radiotherapy with 78 Gy. *J Clin Oncol* 2006;24:1990–1996.
130. Pickett B, Kurhanewicz J, Pouliot J, et al. Efficacy of high dose external beam radiotherapy (EBRT) compared to permanent prostate implant (PPI) in treating low risk prostate cancer based on endorectal magnetic resonance spectroscopy imaging (MRSI) and PSA. In: *Int J Rad Bio Phys* 2004. Atlanta, GA: Elsevier.
131. Pickett B, et al. Time to metabolic atrophy after permanent prostate seed implantation based on magnetic resonance spectroscopic imaging. *Int J Radiat Oncol Biol Phys* 2004;59:665–673.
132. Jabbari S, et al. Equivalent biochemical control and improved prostate-specific antigen nadir after permanent prostate seed implant brachytherapy versus high-dose three-dimensional conformal radiotherapy and high-dose conformal proton beam radiotherapy boost. *Int J Radiat Oncol Biol Phys* 2010;76(1):36–42.
133. Jones CU, et al. Radiotherapy and short-term androgen deprivation for localized prostate cancer. *N Engl J Med* 2011;365(2):107–118.
134. Immediate versus deferred treatment for advanced prostatic cancer: initial results of the Medical Research Council Trial. The Medical Research Council Prostate Cancer Working Party Investigators Group. *Br J Urol* 1997;79(2):235–246.
135. Fossa SD, et al. Ten- and 15-yr prostate cancer-specific mortality in patients with nonmetastatic locally advanced or aggressive intermediate prostate cancer, randomized to lifelong endocrine treatment alone or combined with radiotherapy: final results of the Scandinavian prostate cancer group-7. *Eur Urol*, 2016;70(4):684–691.

136. Warde P, et al. Combined androgen deprivation therapy and radiation therapy for locally advanced prostate cancer: a randomised, phase 3 trial. *Lancet,* 2011;378(9809):2104–2111.

137. Brundage M, et al. Impact of radiotherapy when added to androgen-deprivation therapy for locally advanced prostate cancer: long-term quality-of-life outcomes from the NCIC CTG PR3/MRC PR07 randomized trial. *J Clin Oncol* 2015;33(19):2151–2157.

138. Crook J, et al. Final report of multicenter Canadian Phase III randomized trial of 3 versus 8 months of neoadjuvant androgen deprivation therapy before conventional-dose radiotherapy for clinically localized prostate cancer. *Int J Radiat Oncol Biol Phys* 2009;73(2):327–333.

139. Armstrong JG, et al. A randomized trial (Irish clinical oncology research group 97-01) comparing short versus protracted neoadjuvant hormonal therapy before radiotherapy for localized prostate cancer. *Int J Radiat Oncol Biol Phys* 2011;81(1):35–45.

140. Denham JW, et al. Short-term neoadjuvant androgen deprivation and radiotherapy for locally advanced prostate cancer: 10-year data from the TROG 96.01 randomised trial. *Lancet Oncol* 2011;12(5):451–459.

141. Pisansky TM, et al. Duration of androgen suppression before radiotherapy for localized prostate cancer: Radiation Therapy Oncology Group randomized clinical trial 9910. *J Clin Oncol* 2015;33(4):332–339.

142. Bolla M, et al. Duration of androgen suppression in the treatment of prostate cancer. *N Engl J Med* 2009;360(24):2516–2527.

143. Hanks GE, et al. Phase III trial of long-term adjuvant androgen deprivation after neoadjuvant hormonal cytoreduction and radiotherapy in locally advanced carcinoma of the prostate: the Radiation Therapy Oncology Group Protocol 92-02. *J Clin Oncol* 2003;21:3972–3978.

144. Keating NL, O'Malley AJ, Smith MR. Diabetes and cardiovascular disease during androgen deprivation therapy for prostate cancer. *J Clin Oncol* 2006;24(27):4448–4456.

145. Roach M 3rd. Regarding the influence of adjuvant suppression therapy for prostate cancer on the frequency and timing of fatal myocardial infarction: how real is the risk? *J Clin Oncol* 2007;25(33):5325–5326; author reply 5326.

146. Shahinian VB, et al. Risk of fracture after androgen deprivation for prostate cancer. *N Engl J Med* 2005;352:154–164.

147. Gandaglia G, et al. The impact of androgen-deprivation therapy (ADT) on the risk of cardiovascular (CV) events in patients with non-metastatic prostate cancer: a population-based study. *BJU Int* 2014;114(6b):E82–E89.

148. Nanda A, et al. Cardiovascular comorbidity and mortality in men with prostate cancer treated with brachytherapy-based radiation with or without hormonal therapy. *Int J Radiat Oncol Biol Phys* 2013;85(5):e209–e215.

149. Muraleedharan V, et al. Testosterone deficiency is associated with increased risk of mortality and testosterone replacement improves survival in men with type 2 diabetes. *Eur J Endocrinol* 2013;169(6):725–733.

150. Lester-Coll NH, et al. Death from high-risk prostate cancer versus cardiovascular mortality with hormonal therapy: a decision analysis. *Cancer* 2013;119(10):1808–1815.

151. Zapatero A, et al. Androgen deprivation and radiotherapy in patients with prostate cancer and cardiovascular risk factors: clinical controversies. *Clin Transl Oncol* 2015;17(3):223–229.

152. Nguyen PL, et al. Association of androgen deprivation therapy with cardiovascular death in patients with prostate cancer: a meta-analysis of randomized trials. *JAMA* 2011;306(21):2359–2366.

153. Nead KT, et al. Androgen deprivation therapy and future Alzheimer's disease risk. *J Clin Oncol* 2016;34(6):566–571.

154. Nead KT, et al. Association between androgen deprivation therapy and risk of dementia. *JAMA Oncol* 2017;3(1):49–55.

155. Baik SH, Kury FSP, McDonald CJ. Risk of Alzheimer's disease among senior Medicare beneficiaries treated with androgen deprivation therapy for prostate cancer. *J Clin Oncol* 2017;35(30):3401–3409.

156. Valicenti RK, et al. Adjuvant and salvage radiation therapy after prostatectomy: American Society for Radiation Oncology/American Urological Association guidelines. *Int J Radiat Oncol Biol Phys* 2013;86(5):822–828.

157. Eastham JA, et al. Variations among individual surgeons in the rate of positive surgical margins in radical prostatectomy specimens. *J Urol* 2003;170(6 Pt 1):2292–2295.

158. Wieder JA, Soloway MS. Incidence, etiology, location, prevention and treatment of positive surgical margins after radical prostatectomy for prostate cancer. *J Urol* 1998;160(2):299–315.

159. Epstein JI, et al. Prediction of progression following radical prostatectomy. A multivariate analysis of 721 men with long-term follow-up. *Am J Surg Pathol* 1996;20(3):286–292.

160. Swanson GP, et al. Predominant treatment failure in postprostatectomy patients is local: analysis of patterns of treatment failure in SWOG 8794. *J Clin Oncol* 2007;25(16):2225–2229.

161. Pound CR, et al. Natural history of progression after PSA elevation following radical prostatectomy. *JAMA* 1999;281:1591–1597.

162. Lee F, et al. Long-term follow-up of stages T2–T3 prostate cancer pretreated with androgen ablation therapy prior to radical prostatectomy. *Anticancer Res* 1997;17(3A):1507–1510.

163. Ray ME, et al. PSA nadir predicts biochemical and distant failures after external beam radiotherapy for prostate cancer: a multi-institutional analysis. *Int J Radiat Oncol Biol Phys* 2006;64(4):1140–1150.

164. Slovin SF, et al. Time to detectable metastatic disease in patients with rising prostate-specific antigen values following surgery or radiation therapy. *Clin Cancer Res* 2005;11(24 Pt 1):8669–8673.

165. Sandler HM, et al. Overall survival after prostate-specific-antigen-detected recurrence following conformal radiation therapy. *Int J Radiat Oncol Biol Phys* 2000;48(3):629–633.

166. Freedland SJ, et al. Risk of prostate cancer-specific mortality following biochemical recurrence after radical prostatectomy. *JAMA* 2005;294:433–439.

167. Zhou P, et al. Predictors of prostate cancer-specific mortality after radical prostatectomy or radiation therapy. *J Clin Oncol* 2005;23(28):6992–6998.

168. Zelefsky MJ, et al. Postradiotherapy 2-year prostate-specific antigen nadir as a predictor of long-term prostate cancer mortality. *Int J Radiat Oncol Biol Phys* 2009;75(5):1350–1356.

169. Bolla M, et al. Postoperative radiotherapy after radical prostatectomy: a randomised controlled trial (EORTC trial 22911). *Lancet* 2005;366:572–578.

170. Thompson IM Jr, et al. Adjuvant radiotherapy for pathologically advanced prostate cancer: a randomized clinical trial. *JAMA* 2006;296(19):2329–2335.

171. Wiegel T, et al. Phase III postoperative adjuvant radiotherapy after radical prostatectomy compared with radical prostatectomy alone in pT3 prostate cancer with postoperative undetectable prostate-specific antigen: ARO 96-02/AUO AP 09/95. *J Clin Oncol* 2009;27(18):2924–2930.

172. Bolla M, et al. Postoperative radiotherapy after radical prostatectomy for high-risk prostate cancer: long-term results of a randomised controlled trial (EORTC trial 22911). *Lancet* 2012;380(9858):2018–2027.

173. Thompson IM, et al. Adjuvant radiotherapy for pathological T3N0M0 prostate cancer significantly reduces risk of metastases and improves survival: long-term followup of a randomized clinical trial. *J Urol* 2009;181(3):956–962.

174. Wiegel T, et al. Adjuvant radiotherapy versus wait-and-see after radical prostatectomy: 10-year follow-up of the ARO 96-02/AUO AP 09/95 trial. *Eur Urol* 2014;66(2):243–250.

175. King CR. Adjuvant radiotherapy after prostatectomy: does waiting for a detectable prostate-specific antigen level make sense? *Int J Radiat Oncol Biol Phys* 2011;80(1):1–3.

176. Kalbasi A, et al. Low rates of adjuvant radiation in patients with nonmetastatic prostate cancer with high-risk pathologic features. *Cancer* 2014;120(19):3089–3096.

177. Mahal BA, et al. National trends in the recommendation of radiotherapy after prostatectomy for prostate cancer before and after the reporting of a survival benefit in March 2009. *Clin Genitourin Cancer* 2015;13(3):e167–e172.

178. Thompson IM, et al. Adjuvant and salvage radiotherapy after prostatectomy: AUA/ASTRO guideline. *J Urol* 2013;190(2):441–449.

179. Parker C, et al. Radiotherapy and androgen deprivation in combination after local surgery (RADICALS): a new Medical Research Council/National Cancer Institute of Canada phase III trial of adjuvant treatment after radical prostatectomy. *BJU Int* 2007;99(6):1376–1379.

180. Pearse M, et al. A phase III trial to investigate the timing of radiotherapy for prostate cancer with high-risk features: background and rationale of the radiotherapy—adjuvant versus early salvage (RAVES) trial. *BJU Int* 2014;113(Suppl 2):7–12.

181. Carrie C, et al. Salvage radiotherapy with or without short-term hormone therapy for rising prostate-specific antigen concentration after radical prostatectomy (GETUG-AFU 16): a randomised, multicentre, open-label phase 3 trial. *Lancet Oncol* 2016;17(6):747–756.

182. Stephenson AJ, et al. Predicting the outcome of salvage radiation therapy for recurrent prostate cancer after radical prostatectomy. *J Clin Oncol* 2007;25(15):2035–2041.

183. Tendulkar RD, et al. Contemporary update of a multi-institutional predictive nomogram for salvage radiotherapy after radical prostatectomy. *J Clin Oncol* 2016.

184. Stish BJ, et al. Improved metastasis-free and survival outcomes with early salvage radiotherapy in men with detectable prostate-specific antigen after prostatectomy for prostate cancer. *J Clin Oncol* 2016;34(32):3864–3871.

185. Briganti A, et al. Prediction of outcome following early salvage radiotherapy among patients with biochemical recurrence after radical prostatectomy. *Eur Urol* 2014;66(3):479–486.

186. Dalela D, et al. Genomic classifier augments the role of pathological features in identifying optimal candidates for adjuvant radiation therapy in patients with prostate cancer: development and internal validation of a multivariable prognostic model. *J Clin Oncol* 2017;35(18):1982–1990.

187. Freedland SJ, et al. Utilization of a genomic classifier for prediction of metastasis following salvage radiation therapy after radical prostatectomy. *Eur Urol* 2016;70(4):588–596.

188. Richaud P, et al. [Postoperative radiotherapy of prostate cancer]. *Cancer Radiother* 2010;14(6–7):500–503.

189. Shipley WU, et al. Radiation with or without antiandrogen therapy in recurrent prostate cancer. *N Engl J Med* 2017;376(5):417–428.

190. Hurwitz MD, et al. Adjuvant radiation therapy, androgen deprivation, and docetaxel for high-risk prostate cancer postprostatectomy: results of NRG oncology/RTOG study 0621. *Cancer* 2017;123(13):2489–2496.

191. Cozzarini C, et al. Need for high radiation dose (> or = 70 Gy) in early postoperative irradiation after radical prostatectomy: a single-institution analysis of 334 high-risk, node-negative patients. *Int J Radiat Oncol Biol Phys* 2009;75(4):966–974.

192. King CR. The dose–response of salvage radiotherapy following radical prostatectomy: a systematic review and meta-analysis. *Radiother Oncol* 2016;121(2):199–203.

193. Ghadjar P, et al. Acute toxicity and quality of life after dose-intensified salvage radiation therapy for biochemically recurrent prostate cancer after prostatectomy: first results of the randomized trial SAKK 09/10. *J Clin Oncol* 2015;33(35):4158–4166.

194. Michalski JM, et al. Development of RTOG consensus guidelines for the definition of the clinical target volume for postoperative conformal radiation therapy for prostate cancer. *Int J Radiat Oncol Biol Phys* 2010;76(2):361–368.

195. Sidhom MA, et al. Post-prostatectomy radiation therapy: consensus guidelines of the Australian and New Zealand Radiation Oncology Genito-Urinary Group. *Radiother Oncol* 2008;88(1):10–19.

196. Wiltshire KL, et al. Anatomic boundaries of the clinical target volume (prostate bed) after radical prostatectomy. *Int J Radiat Oncol Biol Phys* 2007;69(4):1090–1099.

197. Poortmans P, et al. Guidelines for target volume definition in post-operative radiotherapy for prostate cancer, on behalf of the EORTC Radiation Oncology Group. *Radiother Oncol* 2007;84(2):121–127.

198. Kim BS, et al. Effect of pelvic lymph node irradiation in salvage therapy for patients with prostate cancer with a biochemical relapse following radical prostatectomy. *Clin Prostate Cancer* 2004;3(2):93–97.

199. Schiffner DC, et al. Daily electronic portal imaging of implanted gold seed fiducials in patients undergoing radiotherapy after radical prostatectomy. *Int J Radiat Oncol Biol Phys* 2007;67(2):610–619.

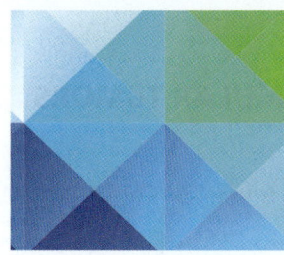

CHAPTER 71

Testicular Cancer

Lucas C. Mendez and Gerard C. Morton

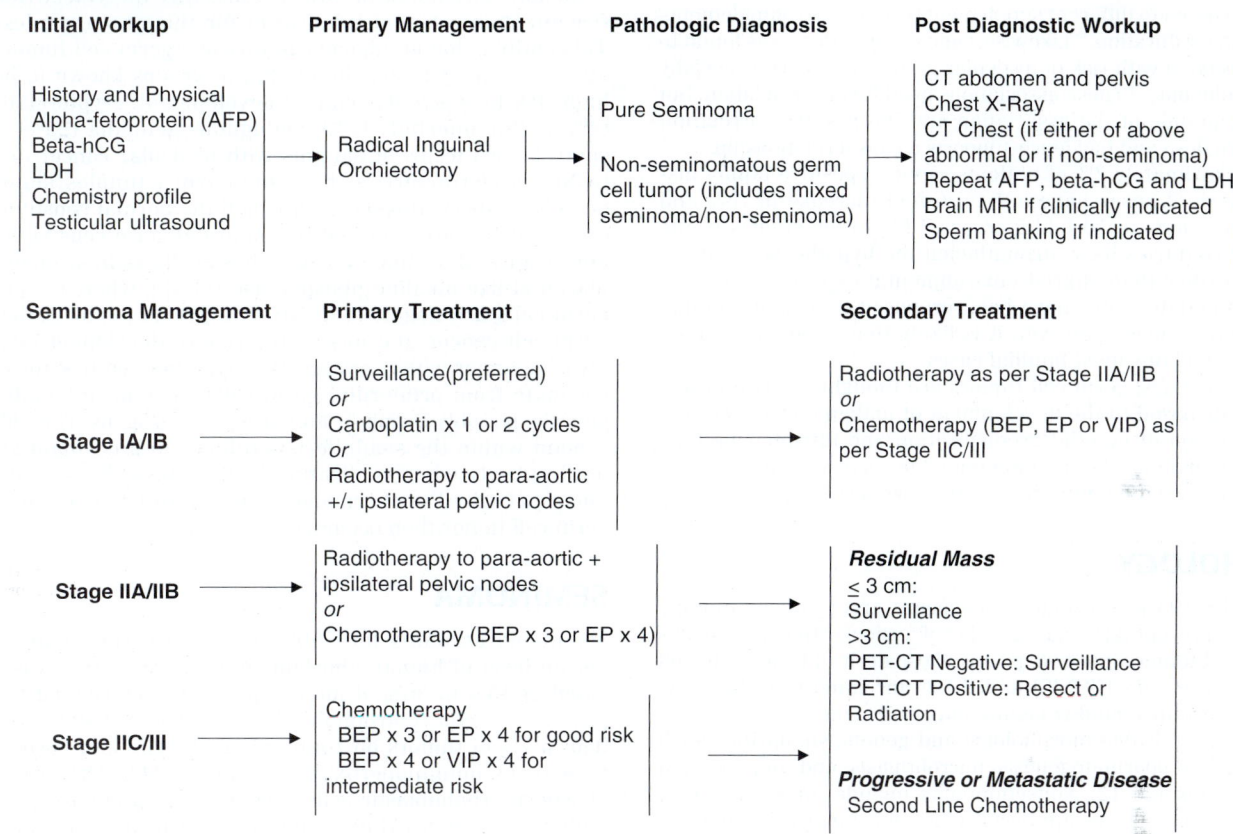

Initial Workup

History and Physical
Alpha-fetoprotein (AFP)
Beta-hCG
LDH
Chemistry profile
Testicular ultrasound

Primary Management

Radical Inguinal
Orchiectomy

Pathologic Diagnosis

Pure Seminoma

Non-seminomatous germ
cell tumor (includes mixed
seminoma/non-seminoma)

Post Diagnostic Workup

CT abdomen and pelvis
Chest X-Ray
CT Chest (if either of above
abnormal or if non-seminoma)
Repeat AFP, beta-hCG and LDH
Brain MRI if clinically indicated
Sperm banking if indicated

Seminoma Management

Primary Treatment

Secondary Treatment

Stage IA/IB

Surveillance(preferred)
or
Carboplatin x 1 or 2 cycles
or
Radiotherapy to para-aortic
+/- ipsilateral pelvic nodes

Radiotherapy as per Stage IIA/IIB
or
Chemotherapy (BEP, EP or VIP) as
per Stage IIC/III

Stage IIA/IIB

Radiotherapy to para-aortic +
ipsilateral pelvic nodes
or
Chemotherapy (BEP x 3 or EP x 4)

Residual Mass
≤ 3 cm:
Surveillance
>3 cm:
PET-CT Negative: Surveillance
PET-CT Positive: Resect or
Radiation

Stage IIC/III

Chemotherapy
BEP x 3 or EP x 4 for good risk
BEP x 4 or VIP x 4 for
intermediate risk

Progressive or Metastatic Disease
Second Line Chemotherapy

ALGORITHM 71.1

EPIDEMIOLOGY

Testicular cancer is the most common malignancy among young men in North America and most Western European Countries, although accounts for only 1% of all male tumors.[1] More than 95% of testicular cancers are germ cell tumors, with almost equal division between seminomas and nonseminomas. Seminomas are most commonly diagnosed between the ages of 30 and 34 years, whereas nonseminomas are usually diagnosed 5 to 10 years earlier. Other histologies such as sex cord–stromal tumors and lymphomas are less frequent, although the latter is the most common testicular malignancy in men older than 60 years.[2] It is estimated that just under 9,000 new cases of testicular cancer are diagnosed annually in the United States, with approximately 400 deaths.[1]

There is marked variation in incidence worldwide. The highest incidence occurs in Northern and Western European countries (up to 9 per 100,000) and the lowest in Asian and African populations (<1 per 100,000).[3,4] In North America, incidence rates are highest among Caucasians and lowest among African Americans, with an overall increase in age-adjusted incidence rate in the United States of 72% between 1975 and 2004.[5,6] A similar increased incidence has been reported in Europe and Australasia.[7-9] Over the past 30 years, the global incidence of testicular cancer has doubled with the highest annual increase seen in developed countries.[10] Despite the increased incidence of both seminoma and nonseminoma, there has been a significant reduction of mortality and improvement in survival. The most dramatic reduction in mortality occurred in the 1970s with the introduction of cisplatin-based chemotherapy.[11,12] The 10-year survival for seminoma increased from 81% in 1970 to 1979 to 95% in 2000 to 2002; that for nonseminoma increased from 54% to 92%.[13]

A history of undescended testicle has long been recognized as a risk factor for the development of testicular cancer. There is also an increased risk of malignancy in the normally descended contralateral testicle. The relative risk is estimated to be 6 in the undescended testicle and 2 in the contralateral testicle.[14] The mechanism of the increased risk is unclear. It is hypothesized that a common etiologic agent predisposes both to testicular maldescent and subsequent malignancy (uterine theory). Nevertheless, it is also possible that the maldescended testicle is subject to a hostile and malignancy-inducing environment (position theory). If that were the case, orchiopexy during the prepubertal phase would be expected to reduce the risk of testicular cancer. However, the relative risk of developing testicular cancer remains higher than in the general population even after early orchiopexy.

The temporal and geographic variation in incidence rates strongly suggests environmental etiologic factors. Male infertility is associated with an increased risk of testicular cancer, and infertile men with abnormal semen analyses have a 20-fold greater risk of testicular cancer than the general population.[15] The increasing incidence has paralleled decline in semen quality over the past several decades.[16,17] This has led to the hypothesis that poor semen quality, testicular cancer, cryptorchidism, and hypospadias represent a testicular dysgenesis syndrome as a result of disruption of gonadal development during embryonal development.[18] Various exogenous hormonal disruptors (e.g., exogenous estrogens) have been proposed, although with no conclusive evidence implicating one particular agent.

A few modifiable environmental exposures have been identified as possible risk factors for testicular cancer. Men who have used muscle-building supplements were found to have an increased incidence of testicular cancer. The association was greatest in men who started supplement use at a younger age were exposed to different supplement types or used supplements for a longer duration.[19] Likewise, cannabis exposure was found to be associated with risk of testicular germ cell tumors, especially nonseminomas.[20] These associations need further validation, but the magnitude of the association and the positive correlation between dose and incidence supports a causal relationship.

Approximately 2% of patients report a positive family history. Sons of cases have a 4- to 6-fold increase in risk and brothers an 8- to 10-fold increase.[21] Migration studies in the Nordic countries have strengthened the hypothesis of shared genes rather than shared environmental exposure, and several candidate genes have been proposed to explain familial testicular cancer; however, it is likely that no single genetic change explains most familial cases.

In summary, germ cell tumors are thought to arise in testes predisposed to the development of malignancy owing to a combination of familial predisposition and intrauterine hormonal imbalance, later compounded by environmental factors and manifested by impaired spermatogenesis.

PATHOLOGY

More than 95% of testicular neoplasms are germ cell tumors. The most recent WHO classification of testicular tumors[22] divides germ cell tumors into two groups: those derived from germ cell neoplasia in situ (GCNIS) and those unrelated to GCNIS. The former group includes seminomas and nonseminomas that share recognizable morphologic and genetic similarities such as impaired spermatogenesis, microlithiasis, and amplification of chromosome 12. Nonseminomas include embryonal carcinoma, yolk sac (postpubertal type), teratoma (postpubertal type), choriocarcinoma, and mixed germ cell tumors. The group not derived from GCNIS is heterogeneous and includes spermatocytic tumor, prepubertal teratoma, and yolk sac tumors. Sex cord–stromal tumors make up the remaining 3% to 4% of testicular neoplasms, and most are benign (Table 71.1).

TABLE 71.1 CLASSIFICATION OF TUMORS OF THE TESTIS
Germ Cell Tumors Derived from Germ Cell Neoplasia *In Situ*
Germ cell neoplasia *in situ*
Seminoma
Seminoma with syncytiotrophoblast cells
Nonseminomatous germ cell tumors
Embryonal carcinoma
Yolk sac tumor, postpubertal type
Teratoma, postpubertal type
Teratoma with somatic-type malignancy
Trophoblastic tumors
Mixed germ cell tumors
Regressed germ cell tumor
Germ Cell Tumors Unrelated to Germ Cell Neoplasia *In Situ*
Spermatocytic tumor
Yolk sac tumor, prepubertal type
Teratoma, prepubertal type
Mixed teratoma and yolk sac tumor, prepubertal type
Sex Cord–Stromal Tumors
Leydig cell tumor
Sertoli cell tumor
Granulosa cell tumor
Tumors in the fibroma–thecoma group
Mixed sex cord–stromal tumor
Unclassified sex cord–stromal group
Gonadoblastoma

CLASSIFICATION OF TESTICULAR TUMORS

Germ Cell Tumors

Tumors Derived from Germ Cell Neoplasia In Situ

Germ Cell Neoplasia In Situ

GCNIS, previously called intratubular germ cell neoplasia or testicular carcinoma in situ, is currently the World Health Organization recommended term for this precursor lesion. This entity is found adjacent to invasive germ cell tumors in >95% of cases and also in all clinical groups known to be at high risk for testicular cancer development: cryptorchidism (2% to 4%), infertility (1%), ambiguous genitalia (25%), and contralateral testes of patients with testicular cancer (5%).[23] GCNIS is characterized by seminiferous tubules showing decreased spermatogenesis in which the normal constituents of the tubules are replaced by abnormal germ cells with the appearance of seminoma cells. These cells stain strongly for placental-like alkaline phosphatase (PLAP), whereas normal germ cells are negative. GCNIS is a precursor to testicular germ cell cancer and has a 50% risk of developing into an invasive tumor within 5 years. It is hypothesized that the cells originate from primordial germ cells early during embryogenesis, possibly owing to an excess of estrogens. They likely remain within the seminiferous tubules in a dormant stage until puberty when replication begins, possibly as a consequence of raised sex hormone levels. Transition to an invasive germ cell tumor then occurs.

SEMINOMA

Seminoma accounts for >50% of all germ cell neoplasms. Serum level of human chorionic gonadotropin (HCG) is elevated in 15% to 30% of men at presentation, related to the presence of syncytiotrophoblastic cells. These may be identified in 7% of tumors on routine hematoxylin and eosin sections or by immunoperoxidase stains in 24%. The presence of syncytiotrophoblastic cells does not alter prognosis. Serum alpha-fetoprotein (AFP) is not elevated in pure seminoma. Grossly, seminoma is a soft tan-colored diffuse multinodular mass. Focal necrosis is sometimes present. A prominent lymphocytic infiltrate is commonly seen within the fibrous stroma. More than 90% of seminomas will stain positive for PLAP.

NONSEMINOMATOUS GERM CELL TUMORS

Nonseminomatous germ cell tumors (NSGCTs) usually contain a mixture of germ cell types (embryonal, yolk sac, teratoma, and choriocarcinoma), although tumors comprised of just one component may also be found. Commonly, NSGCTs are heterogeneous and present with considerable amount of necrosis and hemorrhage on gross examination.

Embryonal carcinoma is the most common component in mixed tumors, and AFP- and HCG-positive cells are present in 33% and 20%, respectively. Postpubertal yolk sac tumors rarely occur in a pure form and have a complex histology. High levels of AFP are usually present. Postpubertal teratoma has marked morphologic differences from the prepubertal type with a predominantly solid appearance, disordered tissue arrangement, and frequent mitotic figures.[24] This tumor is not associated with elevated AFP or HCG and presents with distant metastasis in approximately 20% of the cases. Trophoblastic tumors have choriocarcinoma as the main component. This is the least common type of pure NSGCT and is present in about 4% of mixed tumors. It is particularly aggressive, almost always metastatic at diagnosis, often to brain, and is associated with high levels of HCG. Seminomatous components are also common in mixed tumors, and serum markers (AFP and HCG) are elevated depending on the relative germ cell elements present.

Tumors Unrelated to Germ Cell Neoplasia
In Situ

This heterogeneous group of tumors lacks association with GCNIS and abnormalities on chromosome 12. These include spermatocytic tumor, prepubertal-type yolk sac tumor, and prepubertal-type teratoma.

Spermatocytic Tumor

Previously known as spermatocytic seminoma, the spermatocytic tumor accounts for 2% of testicular tumors. It tends to occur in an older age group at a mean age of 54 years. The new nomenclature better differentiates this from seminoma, which reflects its different origin and natural history. Spermatocytic tumor is confined to the testes, is not associated with elevated HCG levels,[25] and is almost always cured by orchiectomy alone. Bilaterality occurs in 10%, and metastasis is rare. The cell of origin of the spermatocytic tumor is probably the postpubertal mature spermatogonia that acquires abnormal proliferative capacity. Spermatocytic tumor does not contain glycogen, stains negative for PLAP and is not associated with GCNIS. It has a unique amplification on chromosome 9 and is not associated with other germ cell tumors.[26,27]

Yolk Sac Tumor and Teratoma, Prepubertal Type

Prepubertal-type yolk sac tumor is the commonest type of germ cell testicular cancer in infants and children and is associated with high levels of AFP. This malignancy arises from a distinct pathway to the postpubertal-type yolk sac tumors although has no significant morphologic difference. The prepubertal teratoma is composed of somatic elements from ectoderm, mesoderm, and endoderm. These tumors lack cytologic atypia and arise from a germ cell line that has not undergone malignant transformation. Both prepubertal yolk sac tumor and teratoma are less aggressive and have a better prognosis than the postpubertal versions.

ANATOMY AND NATURAL HISTORY

In the developing embryo, the testes originate from the genital ridge located near the second lumbar vertebra. Accompanied by their blood supply and lymphatics, they descend into the scrotum via the inguinal canal. As a result, the primary lymphatic drainage from the testis is to the retroperitoneal lymph nodes. The lymphatic vessels first drain into the collecting trunks at the hilum of the testicle. These lymphatic trunks accompany the testicular artery, vein, and spermatic cord through the internal inguinal ring and then continue proximally to the retroperitoneal lymph nodes. The retroperitoneal lymph nodes are situated anterior to the T11 to L4 vertebral bodies, concentrated at the L1-3 level. On the left, the lymphatics drain primarily into the preaortic and paraaortic lymph nodes around the left renal hilum and from there to the interaortocaval nodes (Fig. 71.1A). On the right, the first nodes involved are usually in the precaval or interaortocaval region, followed by the preaortic lymph nodes (Fig. 71.1B). Contralateral spread is mainly seen with right-sided tumors and rarely with left-sided tumors. Exclusive metastasis in the contralateral nodes (without ipsilateral involvement) is rare.

From the retroperitoneal nodes, the lymph drains into the cisterna chyli, thoracic duct, posterior mediastinum, and left supraclavicular fossa. The thoracic duct drains into the left subclavian vein in the left supraclavicular region. In 5% to 10% of patients, drainage into the right supraclavicular area can occur.

Aberrant lymphatic drainage may occur in the event of previous scrotal or inguinal surgery. Hernia repair alters the drainage of the testicle. The testicular lymphatic vessels anastomose with the regional lymph vessels, resulting in drainage into the ipsilateral inguinal and iliac lymph nodes. In addition, the testicular trunks may abandon the spermatic vessels at the internal inguinal ring and pass posteriorly and superiorly into the external iliac lymph nodes. The scrotum drains directly into the inguinal and external iliac lymph nodes.

FIGURE 71.1. A: The left testis drains primarily by lymphatics along the left testicular vein (*LTV*) to lymph nodes inferior to the left renal vessels (*LRV*). Left paraaortic (*PaA*), preaortic (*PreA*), and interaortocaval (*IAC*) nodes are most commonly involved. Less commonly, nodal involvement may be found inferior to bifurcation of the aorta (*Ao*) or inferior vena cava (*IVC*), or superior to the renal vessels. **B:** Primary lymphatic drainage from the right testis (*arrow*) is along the right testicular vein (*RTV*) to precaval (*PreCa*) and then to interaortocaval and preaortic nodes. Less commonly, preaortic, right common iliac, or right external iliac (*RFI*) nodes are involved.

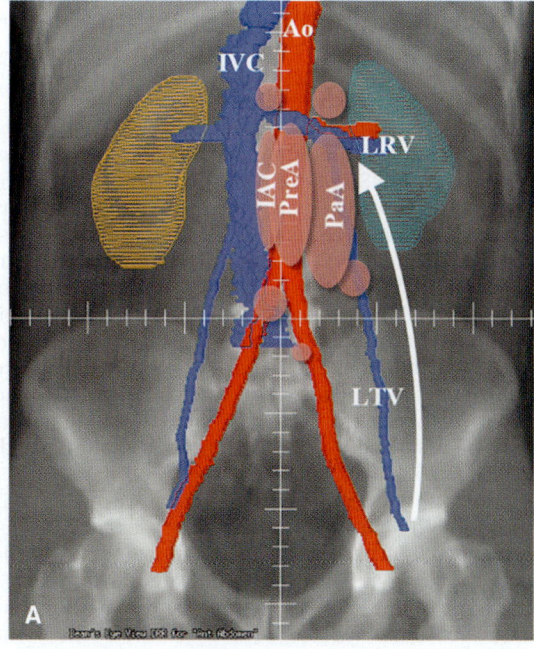
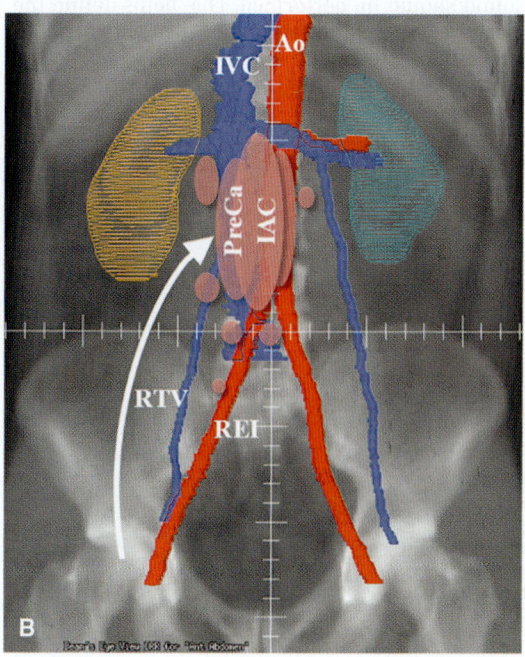

Therefore, direct invasion of the tunica vaginalis or scrotum could result in spread to pelvic and inguinal nodes.

Seminoma has an orderly and predictable pattern of spread. Locoregional lymphatics are the first site of metastatic disease. From the retroperitoneal lymph nodes, seminoma spreads proximally to involve the next echelon—the mediastinal lymph nodes—and then the supraclavicular lymph nodes. Very occasionally, metastases from retroperitoneal lymph nodes can drain directly via the thoracic duct to the supraclavicular fossa, resulting in supraclavicular metastases in the absence of mediastinal disease. Hematogenous metastases are rare in pure seminoma, being much more common with NSGCT. Lung is the most common site of distant disease, although bone, liver, and brain may also be involved.

CLINICAL PRESENTATION AND DIAGNOSTIC WORKUP

A testicular tumor usually presents as a painless swelling in the scrotum, however, pain, heaviness, and tenderness at presentation are not uncommon. Disease in the lymph nodes of the retroperitoneum may produce back pain or abdominal swelling. Widely disseminated parenchymal disease in lungs, liver, bone, or brain is rare but, if present, may produce systemic symptoms. Gynecomastia is a rare presentation of embryonal carcinoma that may be seen in association with the very uncommon sex cord–stromal tumors. Gynecomastia and hyperthyroidism may rarely result from high levels of HCG produced by the tumor. Occasionally, patients present with metastatic germ cell malignancies diagnosed by biopsy or elevated levels of serum tumor markers without evidence of a palpable mass in the testis. Occult primary disease in the testis is often detected by testicular ultrasound. If there is no evidence of a primary tumor in the testis, a diagnosis of an extratesticular germ cell tumor—usually mediastinal, retroperitoneal, or pineal—may be made.

DIAGNOSTIC WORKUP (TABLE 71.2)

A complete history should be taken, including information about previous inguinal or scrotal surgery, cryptorchidism, retractile testes, and orchidopexy. The physical examination should pay special attention to possible sites of lymph node metastases. The presence or absence of gynecomastia is an important observation. If testicular tumor is suspected, testicular ultrasound should be performed. This helps define the origin of the scrotal mass as the vast majority of extratesticular lesions are benign.[28] Testicular tumor usually appears as a solid mass within the testis, often with associated testicular

TABLE 71.2 DIAGNOSTIC WORKUP FOR TUMORS OF THE TESTIS
General
History (document cryptorchidism and previous inguinal or scrotal surgery)
Physical examination
Laboratory Studies
Complete blood count
Biochemistry profile (including lactate dehydrogenase)
Serum assays
α-Fetoprotein (AFP)
β-Human chorionic gonadotropin (β-HCG)
Surgery
Radical inguinal orchiectomy
Diagnostic Radiology
Chest x-ray films, posterior/anterior and lateral views
Computed tomography (CT) scan of the abdomen and pelvis
CT scan of the chest for nonseminomas and stage II seminomas
Bilateral testicular ultrasound
Special Study
Semen analysis

microlithiasis. The contralateral testis should be examined clinically and by ultrasound. Inguinal biopsy of the contralateral testis may sometimes be considered during surgery if atrophy, cryptorchidism, or suspicious abnormalities on ultrasound are found. Radical orchiectomy through an inguinal incision is diagnostic and removes the primary tumor.

Laboratory Studies

A routine complete blood count and chemistry screen, including renal function tests, should be performed. Pulmonary or renal function tests should be performed for patients who may receive bleomycin or combination chemotherapy. NSGCTs of the testes are uniquely associated with reliable serum tumor markers: the β-subunit of human chorionic gonadotropin (β-HCG) and AFP. One or both of these serum markers are elevated in 80% to 85% of patients with disseminated nonseminomatous disease. These markers are important prognostic factors and contribute to cancer staging.

The metabolic half-life of AFP is approximately 5 days and for β-HCG is approximately 18 to 24 hours. Although β-HCG may be modestly elevated in 15% to 30% of patients with pure seminomas, usually any elevation of AFP connotes nonseminomatous disease. In the setting of elevated AFP with pure seminoma seen in the pathology specimen, an undetected nonseminomatous focus may be assumed, and the clinical management should follow accordingly. Serum tumor markers may be elevated in other circumstances or conditions, such as laboratory error, cross-reactivity with luteinizing hormone, marijuana use, hepatitis, or development of antibodies to the glycoproteins. Serum lactate dehydrogenase (LDH), although nonspecific, is elevated in 80% of patients with advanced testicular cancer and has prognostic value.

If a testicular cancer is suspected, serum tumor markers should be assayed before and after orchiectomy, and interpretation of the levels of markers should take into account their metabolic half-lives. Serum tumor markers can document persistent or recurrent cancer after surgery or chemotherapy and may predict the responsiveness of nonseminomas to treatment. The level of β-HCG should decrease by $\geq$90% every 21 days with each successful treatment cycle of chemotherapy. A slow decline in β-HCG after treatment may imply suboptimal response to chemotherapy, permitting early implementation of salvage therapy before the development of overt resistance to chemotherapy. The decline of AFP is less predictable.

Semen analysis and banking of sperm should be considered for patients in whom treatment is likely to compromise fertility. With newer technologies, it is possible to retrieve and bank sperm even with poorer-quality sperm.

Radiographic Studies

Investigations should routinely include chest x-ray films for all patients and computed tomography (CT) of the thorax for any patient with NSGCTs of the testis. CT scans of the abdomen and pelvis should be performed to evaluate the retroperitoneal nodal areas and assess the liver. A thoracic CT scan should also be performed in seminoma patients with an abnormal abdominal CT scan or chest x-ray. Magnetic resonance imaging (MRI) of the brain and bone scan are indicated if symptoms are present. Brain MRI is also indicated for choriocarcinoma.

CT of abdomen and pelvis relies on nodal size to assess the retroperitoneal nodes, with a sensitivity of 40% and a specificity of 95% using a 1-cm threshold.[29] A higher accuracy level can be achieved if a 7- to 8-mm threshold is used[30]; however, there is considerable overlap between the size of normal and abnormal lymph nodes using either size limit. CT therefore has limited ability to exclude the presence of disease, although enlarged lymph nodes in the appropriate clinical context (location, laterality, disease parameters) are very likely to be truly positive. Likewise, lymph nodes with certain morphologic features, such as central necrosis and rounded shape, are considered more suspicious.[31] MRI appears equivalent to CT in determining the size and location of retroperitoneal adenopathy and generally is performed in patients in whom iodinated contrast is contraindicated. Fluorodeoxyglucose–positron emission tomography (FDG-PET) scan has a slightly higher sensitivity (66%) than CT with a comparable specificity (98%). It has little role in initial disease staging but may have a role where CT is questionable.[29] It is unable to detect lesions <5 mm in size or teratomas of any size owing to their very low metabolic activity. It also has an important role in evaluating residual retroperitoneal disease following chemotherapy.

In ultrasound imaging, a solid intratesticular mass associated with internal vasculature suggests tumor. Testicular Doppler ultrasonography has a high accuracy in detecting malignancy, with both sensitivity and specificity over 90%.[32] Ultrasonography is not reliable in predicting tumor histology, but in general, seminomas are commonly hypoechoic and homogeneous, whereas calcifications and heterogeneity in echotexture are more often seen in NSGCTs. Baseline ultrasonography of the remaining testis should also be performed. If the contralateral testis is atrophic and the patient is <30 years of age, then there is a 30% risk of GCNIS. Biopsy of the contralateral testis is suggested by some authorities in this setting.

STAGING AND PROGNOSTIC FACTORS

Patients are staged according to the American Joint Committee on Cancer (AJCC) criteria as indicated in Table 71.3, which incorporates features of the primary tumor (T), node (N), metastasis (M), and level of serum tumor markers (S).[33]

TABLE 71.3 AMERICAN JOINT COMMITTEE ON CANCER 2010 STAGING FOR TESTICULAR CANCER

Primary Tumor (T) (Pathologic Classification)

pTx	Primary tumor cannot be assessed
pT0	No evidence of primary tumor (scar, etc.)
pTis	Intratubular, noninvasive
pT1	Tumor limited to testis and epididymis, no vascular/lymphatic invasion
pT2	Tumor limited to testis and epididymis, with vascular/lymphatic invasion or involvement of the tunica vaginalis
pT3	Tumor invades spermatic cord
pT4	Tumor invades scrotum

Lymph Node (N)

N0	No regional node metastasis
N1	Metastasis in single or multiple nodes ≤2 cm in greatest dimension
N2	Metastasis in single or multiple nodes 2–5 cm greatest dimension
N3	Metastasis in lymph nodes >5 cm in maximum diameter

Distant Metastasis (M)

M0	No distant metastasis
M1a	Nonregional lymph node or pulmonary metastasis
M1b	Nonpulmonary visceral metastasis

Serum Tumor Markers (S)

Sx	Serum tumor markers not performed
S0	Serum tumor markers within normal limits
S1	LDH <1.5 × N and HCG <5,000 and AFP <1,000
S2	LDH 1.5–10 × N or HCG 5,000–50,000 or AFP 1,000–10,000
S3	LDH >10 × N or HCG >50,000 or AFP >10,000

Staging Groupings

IA	T1, N0, M0, S0
IB	T2-4, N0, M0, S0
IS	Any T, N0, M0, S1-3
IIA	Any T, N1, M0, S0/1
IIB	Any T, N2, M0, S0/1
IIC	Any T, N3, M0, S0/1
IIIA	Any T, Any N, M1a, S0/1
IIIB	Any T, Any N, M1a, S2
IIIC	Any T, Any N, M1b or S3

AFP, alpha-fetoprotein; HCG, human chorionic gonadotropin; LDH, lactate dehydrogenase; N, node. From Edge SB, Byrd DR, Compton CC, et al., eds. *AJCC cancer staging manual.* 7th ed. New York: Springer, 2010. Copyright © 2010 American Joint Committee on Cancer. Reproduced with permission of Springer in the format Book via Copyright Clearance Center.

TABLE 71.4 INTERNATIONAL GERM CELL CANCER COLLABORATIVE GROUP CONSENSUS CLASSIFICATION OF METASTATIC GERM CELL CANCER[a]

Nonseminoma	Seminoma
Good prognosis group with all of the following:	
Testis/retroperitoneal primary	Any primary site
No nonpulmonary visceral metastases	No nonpulmonary visceral metastases
AFP < 1,000 ng/mL	Normal AFP
HCG < 5,000 IU/L	Any HCG
LDH < 1.5 × normal	Any LDH
Intermediate prognosis group with all of the following:	
Testis/retroperitoneal primary	Any primary site
No nonpulmonary visceral metastases	Nonpulmonary visceral metastases
Intermediate markers:	
AFP > 1,000 and <10,000 ng/mL *or*	Normal AFP
HCG > 5,000 and <50,000 IU/L *or*	Any HCG
LDH > 1.5× and <10× normal	Any LDH
Poor prognosis group with any of the following:	
Mediastinal primary *or*	
Nonpulmonary visceral metastases *or*	
AFP > 10,000 ng/mL *or*	
HCG > 50,000 IU/L *or*	
LDH > 10× normal	

[a]Survival at 5 years is approximately 91%, 80%, and 50% for good, intermediate, and poor prognostic groups, respectively.
AFP, alpha-fetoprotein; HCG, human chorionic gonadotropin; LDH, lactate dehydrogenase. From International Germ Cell Consensus Classification: a prognostic factor-based staging system for metastatic germ cell cancers. International Germ Cell Cancer Collaborative Group. *J Clin Oncol* 1997;15(2):594–603. Reprinted with permission. Copyright © 1997 American Society of Clinical Oncology. All rights reserved.

Approximately 80% of seminoma patients and 50% to 60% of nonseminoma patients have stage I disease at presentation. For stage I seminoma, tumor size (>4 cm) and rete testis invasion are the most commonly reported predictors of recurrence. For nonseminomas, T stage, extensive embryonal component, and lymphovascular invasion are prognostic. Increased age is an adverse prognostic factor for patients diagnosed with all stages of testicular cancer.[34]

The International Germ Cell Cancer Collaborative Group (IGCCCG) developed a widely accepted classification system for patients with metastatic germ cell malignancies,[35] which has been incorporated into the TNM system (Table 71.4). The prognostic classification is based on data collected on approximately 6,000 patients with metastatic germ cell tumor from 10 countries during the platinum era. The classification was internally and prospectively validated on a subsequent cohort of patients. The factors most strongly associated with a poor prognosis were mediastinal primary, nonpulmonary visceral metastases, or grossly elevated tumor markers (AFP >10,000 ng/mL, HCG >50,000 IU/L, or LDH >10 times normal). Patients with NSGCT were divided into three prognostic groups (good, intermediate, and poor prognosis) and seminomas into either good or intermediate prognostic groups (Table 71.3). The good prognosis group comprised >50% of all patients with metastatic NSGCTs and 90% of seminomas and was associated with a 5-year survival >90%. The intermediate prognosis group comprised 25% to 30% of patients and had a 5-year survival of 80%. The poor prognosis group comprised 15% to 20% of patients with NSGCT and had a 5-year survival of approximately 50%.

GENERAL MANAGEMENT

The initial management of a suspected malignant germ cell tumor of the testis consists of obtaining serum AFP and β-HCG measurements and then performing a radical (inguinal) orchiectomy with division of the spermatic cord at the internal inguinal ring. In this procedure, the involved testis is removed en bloc with the spermatic cord, enclosed by the tunica layers through an inguinal incision, minimizing the chance of tumor spillage. Historically, it had been thought that scrotal violation (transscrotal orchiectomy, open testicular biopsy, or fine needle aspiration) compromised prognosis. Scrotal violation is associated with a slight increase in local recurrence rate compared with inguinal orchiectomy (2.9% vs. 0.4%, respectively) but is not associated with any difference in distant recurrence rates or overall survival.[36] Orchiectomy is both diagnostic and therapeutic. Further management depends on pathologic diagnosis and the stage and extent of disease. Radiation treatment plays a significant role in the management of seminomas. Nonseminomatous tumors are generally managed by cisplatin-based combination chemotherapy and/or surgical resection.[37] A detailed discussion of the management of nonseminomatous tumors is beyond the scope of this chapter.

SEMINOMA

Stage I

Most patients with stage I seminoma are cured by orchiectomy alone, and approximately 20% will relapse if no adjuvant therapy is offered. Either adjuvant radiation therapy or adjuvant chemotherapy with single-agent carboplatin is associated with a disease-free survival >95% and disease-specific survival approaching 100%.[38] Surveillance, with treatment at time of relapse, is associated with a similar survival outcome and allows 80% of patients to avoid morbidity of treatment.[39]

Surveillance

Surveillance has become the management strategy of choice for most men with stage I seminoma. A survey of Canadian radiation oncologists in 2006 revealed that 56% felt surveillance was the preferred management.[40] Kollmansberger et al. document the increasing use of surveillance for managing patients with stage I seminoma in a population-based cohort from British Columbia, Canada, and Oregon.[41] Between 1999 and 2008, the proportion of patients receiving adjuvant radiation therapy decreased from 50% to 9%, and the proportion being managed by surveillance increased from 47% to 87%. A similar trend was seen in the United States by Matulewicz et al. through analysis of the National Cancer Data Base.[42] The authors reported that the use of surveillance for stage I seminoma increased from 24.7% in 1998 to 2000 to 61.2% in 2010 to 2012.

The reported series (Table 71.5) include >2,400 patients, and all report similar rates, timing, and patterns of recurrence.[41,43–51] When managed by surveillance, up to 20% of patients will relapse at a median time of around 14 months. Over 90% of relapses occur in the first 3 years. Given the small event rate in the individual reports, Warde et al.[52] performed a pooled analysis from four series (PMH, Royal Marsden Hospital [RMH], Royal London Hospital, and the Danish Testicular Cancer Study Group). Individual patient data on 638 stage I seminoma patients managed by surveillance were

obtained. With a median follow-up time of 7 years, the 5- and 10-year relapse-free rates were 82.3% and 78.7%, respectively. Most relapses (69%) occurred within the first 2 years of surgery, whereas 7% relapsed beyond 6 years. The 5-year cause-specific survival was 99.3%. A more recent pooled analysis[53] of databases from Sweden and Norway, the Princess Margaret Cancer Centre, British Columbia and Oregon, Bart's Cancer Institute, and the University of Oxford reported similar findings. With a median follow-up time of 52 months, relapse occurred in 13% of 1,344 stage 1 seminoma patients at a median of 14 months. No patient died from seminoma, although one patient died from complications of treatment.

Almost all patients (99%) who relapse after surveillance are classified by IGCCCG in the good risk category, and the predominant site of relapse is in the retroperitoneum (76% to 94%). Approximately 5% to 15% of patients relapse in the mediastinum or lungs, with inguinal relapse described in 3% to 11%, usually only after previous scrotal interference. Some variability is reported in management at the time of relapse. Traditionally, most (74% to 82% of patients in the older series) were initially managed by radiation therapy, with a second relapse occurring in about 10% (6% to 16%). Second relapse almost always occurred at distant sites with a 90% to 95% rate of successfully salvage with chemotherapy. More recent series describe a greater use of chemotherapy as initial salvage treatment. In the population-based study from the Swedish Norwegian Testicular Cancer Study Group (SWENOTECA), cisplatin-based combination chemotherapy as salvage treatment was given to 89% of relapsing patients,[51] with further relapse in only 1 of 58 patients. Kollmansberger et al.[41] report the use of salvage chemotherapy in 68% of relapsing patients in the British Columbia and Oregon Testis Cancer Program database. No further relapse occurred in the 32 patients managed by chemotherapy, whereas relapse occurred in 3 of 15 patients who received salvage radiotherapy. Although salvage chemotherapy is effective, it is associated with greater toxicity than salvage radiotherapy.

In the pooled analysis,[52] tumor size, rete testis invasion, and lymphovascular invasion were predictive of relapse on univariate analysis. On multivariate analysis, tumor size (hazard ratio [HR] 2.0) and rete testis invasion (HR 1.7) remained significant. The relapse-free rate decreased from 87.8% for tumors <4 cm without rete testis invasion to 68.5% for tumors >4 cm with rete testis invasion. Tyldesley et al.[54] also noted the importance of size >4 cm and rete testis invasion, reporting a 5-year relapse-free rate of 86%, 71%, and 50% in patients with no risk factor, one risk factor, or both risk factors, respectively. Choo et al.[47] reported a reduction in 10-year relapse-free rate from 86% to 52% with rete testis invasion. These risk factors were recently validated by the SWENOTECAVII study.[55] In this prospective and population-based protocol, a significant difference in relapse was seen between patients with no risk factor (4%) and patients with these 1 to 2 factors (15.5%) managed by surveillance.

TABLE 71.5 PATTERNS OF RECURRENCE FOR STAGE I SEMINOMA MANAGED BY SURVEILLANCE

Author (Reference)	Number	Median Follow-Up (Months)	Relapse-Free Survival (%)	Proportion Relapsing in Retroperitoneum (%)	Disease-Specific Survival (%)	Median Time to Relapse (Months)
Kollmannsberger et al.[41]	313	34	81	–	100	14
von der Maase et al.[43]	261	48	80	94	99	14
Chung et al.[44]	203	110	82	91	99.5	17
Francis et al.[45]	120	55	82	94	100	4
Daugaard et al.[46]	394	60	83	87	100	13
Choo et al.[47]	88	145	80	76	100	14
Cummins et al.[48]	164	160	87	82	98.7	16
Aparico et al.[49]	143	52	84	84	100	11
Kamba et al.[50]	186	45	79	79	100	21
Tandstad et al.[51]	512	60	86	94	99.8	17

Based on pattern and timing of relapse, a reasonable surveillance policy involves assessments every 4 to 6 months in the first 2 years, six monthly assessments in years 3 to 5, and annual assessments until year 10. Assessment should include physical examination and abdominopelvic CT. Serum markers may be included for the first 2 years if initially elevated.

Although chest x-ray was routinely used in most surveillance series, no relapse was detected on chest x-ray alone. Therefore, some authors suggest omitting routine chest imaging from the follow-up schedule.[56] The use of low dose CT,[57] less intensive imaging protocol,[58] and MRI are being investigated to further reduce long-term radiation exposure.

Surveillance is a more costly approach to management than adjuvant nodal irradiation owing largely to the increased number of radiologic investigations,[59] although leading to less overall treatment burden to patients than upfront treatment.[60] Surveillance should be conducted only with a compliant patient and with an understanding that because of the risk of late relapse, the patient should be monitored for at least 10 years. Although there is no randomized trial comparing surveillance and adjuvant treatment, the survival rate of 99.5% from the large surveillance series indicates that this therapeutic option produces a result equivalent to that achieved with immediate adjuvant treatment and is a safe and effective alternative management, provided that guidelines are followed. Moreover, a recent analysis with a median follow-up time over 14 years has shown that patients with stage I seminoma managed by surveillance have comparable survival to that of the general population.[61]

Adjuvant Radiation Therapy

In the past, the standard postoperative management of patients with stage I seminoma has been adjuvant radiation therapy to the paraaortic and ipsilateral pelvic lymph nodes (the "dog-leg" or "hockey stick" radiation field). This is a highly effective treatment, with a reported relapse rate between 1% and 5% and a disease-specific survival of 100% in many mature series[51,62-72] (Table 71.6) without the need for ongoing abdominal imaging.[73] With the realization that most of the relapses on surveillance occur in the paraaortic region, many have adopted smaller radiation target volumes to reduce treatment toxicity. Series that treat just the paraaortics report a higher rate of failure in the pelvic nodes; however, the disease-free survival is minimally compromised. A multicenter single-arm trial of paraaortic radiotherapy was reported by the German Testicular Cancer Study Group, which included 721 patients with stage I seminoma.[68] Disease-free survival at 8 years was 95%. Of 26 recurrences, 21 were within infradiaphragmatic lymph nodes beyond the treatment volume (mostly ipsilateral pelvic), with no in-field recurrences. The Medical Research Council (MRC) performed a randomized controlled trial comparing classic dog-leg irradiation to paraaortic irradiation in stage I seminoma.[72] Those with previous ipsilateral inguinal or scrotal surgery were excluded. Radiation therapy was better tolerated in the paraaortic alone arm with a reduction in the severity and frequency of acute gastrointestinal and hematologic toxicity. At a median follow-up of 4.5 years, there was no difference in the 3-year relapse-free survival or overall survival. For those in the paraaortic radiation therapy arm, the pelvis was the most frequent site of recurrence, whereas the pelvis was a rare site of recurrence in those in the paraaortic and ipsilateral pelvic radiotherapy arm. A retrospective review showed that the median size of pelvic nodal recurrence was 7.3 cm (range, 2.8 to 13 cm) if CT scans were not included in the follow-up schedule of patients treated with paraaortic radiation therapy.[74]

Given that nearly all recurrences following paraaortic radiation therapy are in the lower common iliac or upper external iliac nodes, a common approach is to use a modified dog leg wherein the inferior border is placed at the midpelvic level. This encompasses the nodal areas at risk while further reducing volume of normal tissue irradiated.[75]

Adjuvant Chemotherapy

Adjuvant chemotherapy using single-agent carboplatin was proposed as a less toxic approach than radiotherapy for stage I seminoma. For men with advanced seminoma, carboplatin has long been known to have significant efficacy with relatively low toxicity.[76] It was logical to investigate the use of one or two cycles of carboplatin as adjuvant treatment following orchiectomy.[77-79] With a median follow-up of 75 months, Steiner et al.[80] reported a 5-year relapse-free survival of 98.1% in a population of 276 men with stage I seminoma treated with two cycles of carboplatin. Aparicio et al.[49] described a risk-adaptive strategy wherein patients with stage I seminoma deemed at low risk of recurrence were managed with surveillance, and those considered at higher risk based on large tumor size or rete testis invasion received two cycles of carboplatin. With a median follow-up of 34 months, the 5-year disease-free survival following carboplatin was 96.2%. In light of the higher (9.3%) relapse rate reported with one course of carboplatin in patients with 1 to 2 risk factors from the SWENOTECA VII study, two cycles of carboplatin seem more appropriate for higher-risk patients.[55]

Recurrence following adjuvant carboplatin tends to be in the retroperitoneum and can be salvaged with cisplatin-based chemotherapy in approximately 85% of the cases[81] resulting in an overall disease-specific survival approaching 100%. Between 2001 and 2006, the use of single-course carboplatin following orchiectomy for stage I seminoma increased

TABLE 71.6 RATE OF RELAPSE AND LOCATION FOR STAGE I SEMINOMA MANAGED BY ADJUVANT RADIOTHERAPY

Author (Reference)	Number	Median Follow-Up (Years)	Radiation Dose (Gy)	Fields	Number Relapsing	Paraaortic	Pelvic/Inguinal	Distant	Cause-Specific Survival (%)
Tandstad et al.[51]	481	6.1	25.2	DL	4 (0.8%)	2	0	2	100
Fossa et al.[62]	365	9.1	36–40	DL	13 (4%)	1	7	6	99
Bauman et al.[63]	169	7.5	30	DL	5 (3%)	1	0	4	100
Logue et al.[64]	431	5.2	20	PA	15 (3%)	1	9	5	99
Santoni et al.[65]	487	10	30	DL, PA	21 (4%)	4	8	9	—
Niazi et al.[66]	71	6.25	25	PA	1 (1%)	0	1	0	100%
Melchior et al.[67]	87	7.7	36	DL	3 (3%)	0	0	3	100%
Classen et al.[68]	721	5.1	26	PA	26 (4%)	6	21	5	99.6
Bruns et al.[69]	80	7.1	20	Mini PA	4 (5%)	1	3	0	100
Jones et al.[70]	313	5.1	30	PA (88%)	10 (3%)	2	6	2	100
	312		20	PA (89%)	11 (3%)	1	3	7	99.7
Oliver et al.[71]	904	6.5	20–30	PA (86%)	33 (4%)	3	11	19	99.9
Fossa et al.[72]	236	4.5	30	DL	9 (4%)	0	0	9	100
	242			PA	9 (4%)	1	2	4	99.3

DL, dog leg; PA, paraaortic.

from 0% to 70% in Sweden and Norway.[51] Over the same time period, the use of adjuvant radiotherapy decreased from 40% to 5%. The relapse risk with chemotherapy was higher than that following radiotherapy (3.9% vs. 0.8%); however, overall survival was the same. In the British Columbia/Oregon database,[41] 73 patients received either one or two cycles of carboplatin, with only one relapse, yielding a relapse-free survival probability of 98% and a cause-specific survival of 100%.

The MRC performed a randomized comparison of single-agent carboplatin and nodal irradiation in stage I seminoma.[71] Almost 1,500 patients from 14 European countries were randomized to receive either adjuvant radiation therapy or one injection of carboplatin. Radiation was limited to paraaortic fields in 87%, and the remainder also had inclusion of the ipsilateral pelvic nodes. Information on tumor size and rete testis invasion was not detailed. With a median follow-up time of 6.5 years, the 5-year relapse-free survival rates were similar at 96.0% and 94.7% in the radiation therapy and carboplatin arms, respectively. In the adjuvant radiation therapy arm, the most common site of recurrence was either distant (57%) or in the pelvic nodes (31%). In the carboplatin arm, most of the relapses (74%) were in paraaortic nodes. Only one death from testicular cancer occurred in the radiation therapy group, with no cancer-related deaths in the chemotherapy group. An 80% reduction in the rate of contralateral testicular cancer was seen in the carboplatin arm (2 vs. 15 cases). Long-term toxicity (e.g., risk of leukemia) is unknown; however, the regimen is well tolerated acutely with only mild myelotoxicity. Powles et al.[82] found no increased risk of death from circulatory disease or risk of second malignancy in a cohort of 199 patients who received adjuvant carboplatin and were followed for a median of 9 years.

Mead et al.[38] analyzed mature results of three randomized noninferiority MRC clinical trials for stage I seminoma, which included nearly 2,500 patients. They concluded that either radiation therapy or carboplatin was a reasonable adjuvant therapy. It is clear that the survival of patients with stage I seminoma approaches 100%, no matter what treatment strategy is employed. The goal of management is to limit treatment morbidity without compromising chance of cure. For the compliant patient, surveillance is probably the option of choice. For patients not suitable for surveillance, adjuvant radiation therapy or adjuvant chemotherapy significantly reduces the risk of relapse. There are, however, limited data on the long-term efficacy or toxicity of adjuvant carboplatin. Furthermore, ongoing surveillance of the retroperitoneal nodes will still be required.

Stage II

For patients with stage II seminoma, the recommended treatment depends on the bulk of retroperitoneal nodal disease. Radiation therapy, 25 to 35 Gy, is the treatment of choice for patients with stage IIA or IIB seminoma. Irradiation of the paraaortic and ipsilateral pelvic nodes is a highly effective treatment strategy with a recurrence rate <10% (Table 71.7) and a disease-specific survival rate of 97% to 100%.[63,83-91] The most common site of relapse following infradiaphragmatic radiation therapy is in the supraclavicular fossa or mediastinum. In the past, some authors[85] recommended prophylactic supraclavicular irradiation. However, the proportion of patients destined to relapse exclusively in the supraclavicular fossa is <5%, and results with infradiaphragmatic irradiation alone with chemotherapy as salvage are excellent.[92]

No clinical trial has prospectively compared radiation therapy with cisplatin-based chemotherapy in stage II disease. Recently, a study using the U.S. National Cancer Database[93] compared these treatment strategies in stage II patients and suggested a lower overall survival for multiagent chemotherapy in stage IIA disease, with no differences found in stage IIB patients. Better local control and less toxicity associated

TABLE 71.7 RELAPSE RATE FOLLOWING INFRADIAPHRAGMATIC +/− MEDIASTINAL RADIOTHERAPY BY NODAL STAGE FOR STAGE II SEMINOMA

Author (Reference)	Stage IIA (≤2 cm)		Stage IIB (2–5 cm)		Stage IIC (>5 cm)	
	N	Relapses	N	Relapses	N	Relapses
Bauman et al.[63]	29	2	10	1	4	2
Chung et al.[83]	49	4	30	4	16	10
Classen et al.[84]	66	2	21	2	–	–
Zagars et al.[85]	6	0	38	5	25	3
Patterson et al.[86]	46	6	34	9	–	–
Whipple et al.[87]	31	2	14	3	–	–
Vallis et al.[88]	26	1	22	2	5	2
Dosmann and Zagars[89]	55	7	13	4	–	–
Mason and Kearsley[90]	–	–	25	1	24	6
Evensen et al.[91]	6	0	18	1	49	11
Total	**314**	**24 (8%)**	**225**	**32 (14%)**	**123**	**34 (28%)**

with radiation therapy are possible explanations. Other series have reported conflicting results and indicated equivalence between both treatment strategies in patients with stage IIA disease.[94,95] Although it is clear that most patients with stage IIA/B seminoma can be cured with cisplatin-based chemotherapy, greater levels of toxicity are expected with this treatment than that associated with radiotherapy alone.[96] Radiation therapy is therefore considered the preferred treatment for nonbulky stage II seminomas.

Disease control rates for stage IIA/B seminoma with single-agent carboplatin appear inferior to that with radiation therapy. A phase II study by the German Testicular Cancer Study Group[78] delivered three or four cycles of carboplatin to patients with stage IIA or stage IIB seminoma, respectively. The overall failure rate was 18%, with all relapses occurring in the retroperitoneum. A few authors have retrospectively assessed the benefit of a combined approach using neoadjuvant carboplatin followed by radiation therapy in patients with stage IIA/B seminomas.[86,97] Although these results are not definitive, this strategy appears to reduce the rate of relapses and may be a promising approach, especially for bulkier disease.

Factors other than stage may be considered in selection of treatment strategy after orchiectomy in stage II seminoma. A greater number of retroperitoneal nodal metastases may suggest an overall greater bulk of disease, indicating a higher likelihood for distant metastasis. Furthermore, Domont et al.[98] have reported that nodal diameter ≥ 3 cm on CT is associated with higher risk of distant failure following local therapy and suggested that these patients would be better managed with systemic treatment. The risk of distant metastasis is likely proportional to the extent of disease seen in the retroperitoneal nodes, and this should be taken into account when deciding which strategy to follow.

Patients with stage IIC retroperitoneal disease (nodes > 5 cm) are usually managed with systemic chemotherapy. Radiation therapy remains a treatment option; however, the relapse rate of >30% is considered by many to be excessive. Chung et al.[83] reported recurrence in 10 of 16 patients with stage IIC disease managed with radiation therapy compared to only one relapse in a similar group of 23 patients managed by chemotherapy. The choice of modality is also influenced by the size and location of the retroperitoneal nodal mass. If the mass is centrally located and does not overlie most of one kidney or significantly overlap the liver, primary radiation therapy remains an option. If the location of the mass is such that the irradiation volume covers most of one kidney or significant volumes of the liver, then the potential morbidity of radiation therapy can be avoided by the use of primary cisplatin-containing combination chemotherapy (usually etoposide/cisplatin [EP] or bleomycin/etoposide/cisplatin [BEP]). For nodal disease >10 cm in diameter, the relapse rate is >40% with radiotherapy and such patients should be managed with systemic chemotherapy.

For the rare patient with stage III disease (i.e., supradiaphragmatic nodal disease or dissemination to parenchymal organs), or those with relapse following radiation therapy, the current standard therapy is three courses of BEP or four courses of EP chemotherapy. These patients are classified into either a good prognosis or intermediate prognosis group by the International Germ Cell Cancer Collaborative Group Consensus Classification, depending on the absence or presence of nonpulmonary visceral metastases, respectively. The 5-year survival is around 91% for good prognosis patients and 80% for intermediate prognosis patients. Despite initial favorable reports, single-agent carboplatin is not as effective as cisplatin-based combination treatment. In a pooled analysis of two randomized trials of 361 patients with metastatic seminoma, Bokemeyer et al.[99] reported an inferior progression-free (72% vs. 92%) and overall (89% vs. 94%) survival with carboplatin.

Residual Mass

For patients with stage II or III disease treated with primary chemotherapy, residual masses are present at 1 month in up to 80% of patients. Most of these then gradually regress over a period of several months. Flechon et al.[100] reported that 50% of residual masses disappeared on follow-up, and viable cancer cells were found only in masses >3 cm in size. Management strategies involve the use of consolidative radiotherapy, surgical resection, or observation. In an effort to define the role of postchemotherapy radiation therapy, the MRC Testicular Tumour Working Party conducted a retrospective review of patients with advanced seminoma managed by chemotherapy from 10 European centers.[101] Of 302 patients identified, 174 (58%) had residual masses on completion of chemotherapy, with a subsequent 3-year progression-free survival of 85%. Approximately half of these patients underwent postchemotherapy radiation therapy, with selection based predominantly on institutional preference. Radiation therapy did not significantly influence risk of progression, contributing an absolute increase in progression-free survival of only 2.3%. Instead, the most important prognostic factors for progression were the presence of prechemotherapy visceral metastases or raised LDH, or persistent visceral metastases postchemotherapy. At St. Bartholomew's Hospital, 43 of 107 patients (40%) with advanced seminoma had a residual mass postchemotherapy.[102] Positive histology was found in 3 of 19 patients (15%) who underwent surgical exploration, whereas relapse at the site of the mass occurred in 3 other patients observed. Residual disease was only found in masses >3 cm in size. Of the 107 patients, 98 patients (92%) remained alive and free from recurrence. The largest report of surgical resection following chemotherapy comes from the Memorial Sloan-Kettering Cancer Center.[103] A total of 55 patients with advanced seminoma underwent resection or biopsy of residual mass within 4 weeks of chemotherapy. Of 27 patients with a mass >3 cm, 8 patients (30%) had residual tumor. No viable tumor was found in any of the 28 patients with a residual mass <3 cm in maximal diameter.

From the reports discussed, it is clear that observation alone is adequate for a residual mass <3 cm in size. Two patterns of response to chemotherapy are evident on CT: the residual mass may be well defined with discrete borders or the mass may have indistinct borders merging into surrounding structures and resembling a fibrous plaque. The former are more amenable to surgical resection. Furthermore, if the tumor is well defined on CT and measures >3 cm in greatest dimension, positive histology can be found in 50%. It is reasonable to resect these masses. If the mass is poorly defined, even if >3 cm, the chance of finding positive histology is <10%. Resecting such a mass is hazardous, with risk of great vessel, ureteric, and small bowel injury. These should be observed.

FDG-PET scans have been shown to reliably predict the presence of viable disease in retroperitoneal masses postchemotherapy in seminomas. This diagnostic examination has a high accuracy in identifying persistent disease, which is greater than CT.[104] De Santis et al.[105] evaluated the efficacy of FDG-PET by analyzing 51 patients with 56 postchemotherapy lesions. The FDG-PET correctly identified 54 lesions with two false-negative results, both in nodes <3 cm. For the whole cohort, this test sensitivity was 80%, but FDG-PET accuracy for residual masses >3 cm was 100%. Based on this result, authors estimated that 45% to 73% of patients with >3 cm residual mass would be overtreated with surgery if FDG-PET information is not taken into account, as a negative scan may be reliably used as a tool for avoiding surgical resection. FDG-PET should be performed 6 weeks after day 21 of the last chemotherapy cycle, as earlier imaging has a higher risk of false-positive results.

Bilateral Testicular Cancer

Testicular cancer is bilateral in up to 5% of cases, with one-third being synchronous and two-thirds being metachronous.[106] Although bilateral orchiectomy is an effective management strategy in synchronous disease, the option of testis-sparing surgery and postoperative radiation therapy has emerged as an alternative.[107] Partial orchiectomy may be considered for selected patients with bilateral disease or a solitary testicle. Ideally, tumors should be <2 cm in size and have negative surgical margins for invasive disease. Postoperative radiotherapy to a dose of 18 to 20 Gy is usually administered to the residual testicle to eradicate GCNIS, which is found in >80% of cases.[108,109] Observation alone has also been reported.[110] In either case, some degree of hormonal dysfunction is common, and many patients may still require lifelong testosterone replacement. Patients with testicular cancer are at a higher risk of developing contralateral malignant disease. In consequence, some authors advocate performing a biopsy of the contralateral testis during the radical orchiectomy procedure for early diagnosis of GCNIS or invasive disease. However, routine biopsy of the contralateral testicle has not been shown to significantly reduce the incidence of metachronous germ cell malignancy.[111] In the setting of GCNIS identified by the biopsy, a course of radiation therapy may be considered to the contralateral testis for treatment of the *in situ* component of the neoplasia, as patients with GCNIS almost invariably progress to invasive cancer. In this setting, a low dose of radiation is able to preserve some function of the Leydig cells and avoid progression of disease.

RADIATION THERAPY TECHNIQUE

Target Volume and Field Borders

For stage I disease, the clinical target volume (CTV) encompasses the interaortocaval, preaortic, and paraaortic nodes (Fig. 71.1). The left renal hilar nodes are included for left-sided tumors. The ipsilateral external iliac and common iliac nodes may also be included, particularly if there is concern about aberrant drainage. Inclusion of the inguinal scar, inguinal lymph nodes, or hemiscrotum is not routinely warranted. For stage II disease, a gross tumor volume is identified from diagnostic imaging, and the CTV also usually includes the ipsilateral pelvic nodes.

The planning target volume (PTV) includes the CTV plus a margin to account for positional and setup uncertainties. To cover the known location of the retroperitoneal and iliac

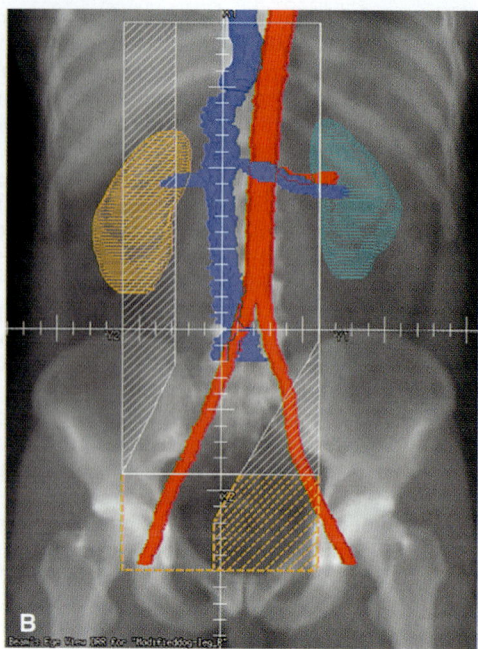

FIGURE 71.2. For stage I seminoma, a modified "dog-leg" field is used to encompass nodal regions at risk. The superior border is placed at the upper border of T10 or T11 and the inferior border at the superior aspect of the acetabulum. Traditionally, the inferior border was placed at the superior obturator foramen (indicated in *orange*) to include all external iliac nodes. These nodes are rarely involved, and using a higher border as indicated will reduce toxicity. If paraaortic fields are to be used, the inferior border is placed at the bottom of L5. The left renal hilum is included for left-sided tumors **(A)** but not for tumors on the right **(B)**.

lymph nodes with an appropriate margin, standard anatomic field borders have been used. This is commonly referred to as the dog-leg or hockey stick field. Classically, the superior border is placed between the T9 and T10 vertebral bodies, with the inferior border at the top of the obturator foramen. A modified approach is now commonly used wherein the superior border is placed between T10 and T11, and the inferior border is placed at the superior aspect of the acetabulum (Fig. 71.2). The field is approximately 9 cm wide in the paraaortic region and usually covers the transverse processes. On the left, the lateral border is extended to include the left renal hilum, and customized shielding is positioned to reduce the amount of kidney irradiated. Field width here is typically 11 to 12 cm. At the mid-L4 level, the field is extended laterally to cover the ipsilateral external iliac nodes. Multileaf collimators are used to define the field shape. If retroperitoneal nodes alone are to be treated, the superior and lateral borders are as described previously, and the inferior border is placed at the L5/S1 disc space. Some report using a lower superior border, T10-11, and a higher inferior border, the bottom of L4.[69]

Once these borders are placed, the planning CT can be used to ensure adequate coverage of the target volume. Distance from the PTV to the field border is 8 to 15 mm depending on field size, energy, separation, and shielding. It should be noted that there is often a distance of several centimeters between the cranial and caudal field edges and the 95% isodose, which is related to the large field size and variability in separation.

In stage II disease, the PTV includes the same CTV as for stage I disease with an appropriate margin. Care must be taken to include the gross nodal disease in the CTV (Fig. 71.3). If the lymphadenopathy is >4 cm in size, a boost to gross disease is commonly used. This may be delivered either concurrently or sequentially. The advantage of a sequential approach is that it allows for reduction in disease volume and less irradiation of normal tissues. This is particularly appropriate where the initial disease is large and overlies the kidney.

A study has analyzed the location of metastatic lymph nodes relative to vascular structures in stage II or stage I patients presenting with nodal relapse after surveillance. Authors found, after analyzing 90 patients, that almost all detected nodes were contained within a 2.5-cm posterior and

lateral margin and a 2.1-cm anterior margin from the arterial vasculature. No positive nodes were identified above the L1 level.[75] Although requiring further validation, this suggests that the classic field borders based on bony anatomy treats a larger volume than required and modification, for example, by lowering the superior border, may be considered in the future.

Simulation and Treatment Planning

A volumetric planning CT scan is acquired with the patient supine and arms at the sides. Testicular shielding (often in the form of a clamshell device) is used. Utilization of a CT-based

FIGURE 71.3. Stage IIA and stage IIB seminomas may be treated with a traditional or modified dog leg to a dose of 25 Gy in 20 fractions, with a boost of 10 Gy in 5 fractions to nodes >3 cm in diameter.

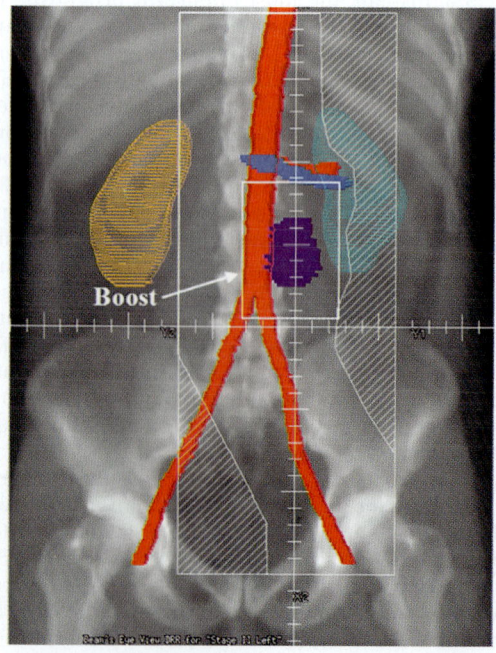

planning technique enables visualization of the location of the lymph node regions, adjacent tissues, and critical normal structures including the kidneys and liver. In addition, the beam's eye view (BEV) allows evaluation of the coverage of the PTV, and shielding can be appropriately placed. Treatment is delivered with a linear accelerator using anterior and posterior parallel-opposed fields. Depending on the separation, 6- to 18-MV photons are utilized. More elegant treatment techniques using intensity-modulated radiotherapy (IMRT) to cover the target volume with greater sparing of organs at risk are described.[112] Although IMRT enables reduction of dose to organs at risk (stomach, bowel, bone marrow), it may increase low radiation doses to surrounding normal tissues, and it is not clear how this is reflected in reduction of early or late side effects of treatment, including risk of second malignancy.

Dose and Fractionation
Stage I Seminoma
Radiation doses between 20 and 40 Gy at 1.25 to 2 Gy per fraction have been reported. A dose of 25 Gy in 20 fractions has been the most commonly used dose/fractionation at North American institutions,[113] with close to 100% control of retroperitoneal disease. The United Kingdom's MRC (MRC TE18) completed a randomized controlled trial of 30 Gy in 15 fractions over 3 weeks or 20 Gy in 10 fractions over 2 weeks.[70] Relapse-free survival was similar in both groups. Acutely, there was significantly more moderate or severe lethargy and inability to carry out normal work in the group that received 30 Gy. However, by 12 weeks, there were no differences between the two groups.

Stage II Seminoma
In general, patients with stage II seminoma should have the ipsilateral pelvic nodes treated. The optimal radiation dose is yet to be determined, and several regimens are used. One regimen of 25 Gy in 20 fractions is frequently used with a boost (10 Gy in 5 to 8 fractions) to the residual mass for lymphadenopathy >2 to 3 cm.[83] Alternatively, 30 Gy in 15 fractions for stage IIA and 36 Gy in 18 fractions for stage IIB seminoma have been shown to provide excellent local control.[84]

Testicular Shielding
During a fractionated course of radiotherapy to the retroperitoneal and ipsilateral iliac lymph nodes, the dose to the remaining testis ranges between 0.3 and 1.5 Gy. Dose received strongly depends on distance from the testicle to field edge. Several effective shielding devices have been described to reduce dose received by the testicle to <1% of the midplane dose.[114-116] Most departments use simple forms of gonadal shielding, such as the clamshell device, which consists of a cup that is 1 cm thick. This shields the testicle from low-energy scattered photons and effectively reduces the testicular dose by a factor of 4.

RESULTS OF THERAPY
Seminoma
The outcome of treatment depends on the stage and extent of disease at presentation. Age >40 years at diagnosis is also an adverse prognostic factor.[34] For stage I disease, routine irradiation of the paraaortic and ipsilateral pelvic nodes results in 10-year relapse-free survival rates of 96% to 98%. Approximately 1% to 4% of patients relapse after infradiaphragmatic irradiation, usually within the first 3 years. The sites of relapse are usually evenly distributed between the

mediastinum and distant sites. Occasional relapses occur as nonseminomatous germ cell malignancies, even after careful review of the initial tumor has shown a pure seminoma. Deaths from stage I seminoma are extremely rare. Most relapsing patients are salvaged with subsequent treatment, usually chemotherapy. Cause-specific survival rates in the large series are 99% to 100%.

The outcome for patients with stage II disease treated with infradiaphragmatic irradiation is shown in Table 71.7. Disease-free survival is approximately 92% and 86% for patients with stage IIA and IIB disease, respectively. Relapse most commonly occurs in the mediastinum, supraclavicular nodes, and lungs. Cisplatin-based chemotherapy is able to salvage in excess of 80% of the relapses, leading to a 5-year cause-specific survival of 96% to 100%. The relapse rate for patients with stage IIC disease managed by primary radiotherapy is >30%, and these patients are best managed with initial chemotherapy. Because of the ability to salvage patients who relapse following radiotherapy with cisplatin-based combination chemotherapy, the survival results following primary radiotherapy or chemotherapy as initial therapy even in patients with bulkier nodal disease are comparable. The potential toxicities of each approach must be evaluated for each patient, along with other factors influencing the choice of therapy.

Cisplatin-based chemotherapy (BEP × 3 fractions or EP × 4 fractions) is the standard treatment for patients with stage III seminoma, as well as for those with retroperitoneal masses >5 cm. Mencel et al.[117] reported that 93% of 142 patients with advanced seminoma achieved a favorable response to platinum-based chemotherapy, with an overall progression-free survival of 86%.

SEQUELAE OF TREATMENT
Radiation Therapy
The long-term sequelae of standard infradiaphragmatic irradiation for stages I and IIA disease are related to the dose of radiation used. There appears to be no curative advantage for doses >25 Gy; however, there is an increase in toxicity. In the MRC randomized trial comparing 30 Gy in 15 fractions delivered to either dog-leg or paraaortic fields, 33 of 478 patients (7%) were diagnosed with a peptic ulcer during follow-up. The occurrence rate was similar in both treatment arms. Very few patients report diarrhea as a long-term consequence, and most patients report a satisfactory quality of life, with a maintained body image and few side effects.[70]

Approximately 50% of patients with testicular seminoma have some degree of impairment in spermatogenesis at the time of presentation. Exposure of the remaining testis to therapeutic irradiation may further impair fertility, and the degree of impairment is dose dependent. Available data suggest that hormonal function and spermatogenesis may be compromised at dose levels as low as 0.5 Gy and those cumulative doses >2 Gy probably lead to permanent injury.[118] Hahn et al.[119] reported the induction of aspermia in 10 of 14 patients who received >65 cGy to the remaining testis. Aspermia was not detected at doses <50 cGy. Recovery of sperm in the semen occurred in most within 30 to 80 weeks of radiation therapy. A detailed assessment of fertility and sexual function was performed in the Southwest Oncology Group Study 8711 in a series of men following orchidectomy and radiation therapy for seminoma.[120] Fourteen of 26 patients (54%) were subfertile at baseline, with a sperm count <20,000/mL. The average prescribed dose was 26 Gy in 1.6-Gy fractions, delivering a median dose of 79 cGy to the remaining testis. With a testicular dose below the median, the sperm count tended to drop to a nadir value around

6 months, with recovery of fertility by 12 months. With higher testicular dose, recovery of sperm count was further delayed. Jacobsen et al.[121] reported a 50% reduction in sperm count at 1 year in 21 men following dog-leg radiation therapy (median testis dose, 32 cGy). No change in sperm count was noted in 24 men treated with paraaortic fields (median testis dose 9 cGy). Dog-leg radiation therapy also results in an elevation of serum follicle-stimulating hormone (FSH) levels, with no change in serum testosterone. FSH levels are highest within 6 months of radiation therapy and return to normal within 3 years. With current radiation techniques, most men will have return to baseline sperm concentrations and hormone levels with minimal impact on fertility.

Patients are at the increased risk of developing a second primary malignancy following treatment for testicular cancer.[122-124] Travis et al.[125] investigated the occurrence of second malignancies among >40,000 men who had undergone treatment for a testicular cancer between 1943 and 2001 from 14 population-based cancer registries in North America and Europe. The risk of developing a second solid tumor among 10-year survivors was almost twice that of the general population, with a relative risk (RR) of 1.9. The risk remained elevated for 35 years, with the highest risk for cancers of the stomach (RR 4.0), pancreas (RR 3.6), and bladder (RR 2.7). There was also an increased risk of developing cancers of the lung, esophagus, colon, and pleura. An increased risk was found for both seminomas and nonseminomas and in patients treated with radiation therapy alone (RR 2.0), chemotherapy alone (RR 1.8), and both modalities (RR 2.9). A case–control study of leukemia risk in a cohort of 18,567 patients treated for testicular cancer between 1970 and 1993 has also been reported.[126] Radiation therapy (mean dose 12.6 Gy to bone marrow) without chemotherapy was associated with a threefold elevated risk of leukemia. Risk increased with increasing dose of radiation to bone marrow largely associated with the use of mediastinal irradiation. The cumulative dose of cisplatin was also predictive of excess leukemia risk, being 3.2 with the commonly administered dose. In absolute terms, it is estimated that 25 Gy to the retroperitoneum would result in 9 excess cases of leukemia in 10,000 patients followed for 15 years. Commonly used doses of cisplatin might result in 16 excess cases. Although treatment factors are strongly implicated in the development of second primary malignancies following treatment, an excess risk of second cancers is seen even among testicular cancer patients who have just been observed. An increased rate of spontaneous chromosomal translocations is seen in lymphocytes of patients with early-stage seminoma compared to healthy controls.[127] Following adjuvant radiation therapy, the translocation rate increases before returning to preradiotherapy levels at around 30 months.[128] It is hypothesized that this genomic instability may be a predisposing factor toward malignancy development.

Long-term survivors following radiation therapy for seminoma are also at increased risk of death related to cardiac disease, even without mediastinal irradiation,[129] with a cardiac standardized mortality ratio of 1.85 in patients followed out beyond 15 years. One suggested explanation for the increased risk of cardiovascular deaths relates to the higher prevalence of diabetes in patients previously treated with radiation therapy to the paraaortic site.[130]

Chemotherapy

Cisplatin-based chemotherapy is associated with alopecia and the potential for substantial nausea and vomiting. Modern antiemetics have improved gastrointestinal reactions. Serious short-term problems are myelosuppression, bleomycin-induced pulmonary fibrosis, and rarely cisplatin nephrotoxicity. Myelosuppression and pulmonary fibrosis are fatal in 0.5% to 4% of treated patients. A recently recognized effect of chemotherapy used in the treatment of germ cell tumors is the risk of secondary malignancy. As discussed previously, the cumulative dose of cisplatin strongly correlates with the risk of subsequent malignancy.[126] Etoposide exposure increases the risk of leukemia. Morphologically, these leukemias are usually monocytic or myelomonocytic. Characteristic chromosomal translocations are frequently but not invariably present. The onset of leukemia is ordinarily closer to chemotherapy exposure than is the typical leukemia induced by alkylating agents.

Other late toxicities reported include high-tone hearing loss, neurotoxicity, Raynaud phenomenon, ischemic heart disease, hypertension, renal dysfunction, and pulmonary toxicity. In an observational study of 1,800 men treated with cisplatin-based chemotherapy for testicular cancer, Brydoy et al.[131] noted long-term Raynaud-like phenomena in 39%, paraesthesia in 29%, hearing impairment in 22%, and troubling tinnitus in 22%. Long-term fertility seems little impaired following chemotherapy.[132] BEP causes immediate azoospermia; however, with time, more than half of patients may recover normal or near-normal spermatogenesis.[133] The paternity rate following two to four cycles of BEP is 70% to 85%.[134,135] Symptomatic hormone dysfunction only occurs with high cumulative doses of cisplatin,[136] although subclinical endocrine abnormalities are more common.[137]

REFERENCES

1. Siegel RL, Miller KD, Jemal A. Cancer Statistics, 2017. CA Cancer J Clin 2017;67(1):7–30.
2. Vitolo U, Ferreri AJ, Zucca E. Primary testicular lymphoma. Crit Rev Oncol Hematol 2008;65(2):183–189.
3. Chia VM, Quraishi SM, Devesa SS, et al. International trends in the incidence of testicular cancer, 1973–2002. Cancer Epidemiol Biomarkers Prev 2010;19(5):1151–1159.
4. Rosen A, Jayram G, Drazer M, et al. Global trends in testicular cancer incidence and mortality. Eur Urol 2011;60(2):374–379.
5. Holmes L, Escalante C, Garrison O, et al. Testicular cancer incidence trends in the USA (1975–2004): plateau or shifting racial paradigm. Public Health 2008;122(9):862–872.
6. Bray F, Ferlay J, Devesa SS, et al. Interpreting the international trends in testicular seminoma and nonseminoma incidence. Nat Clin Pract Urol 2006;3(10):532–543.
7. Baade P, Carrière P, Fritschi L. Trends in testicular germ cell cancer incidence in Australia. Cancer Causes Control 2008;19(10):1043–1049.
8. Manecksha RP, Fitzpatrick JM. Epidemiology of testicular cancer. BJU Int 2009;104(9 Pt B):1329–1333.
9. Sarfati D, Shaw C, Blakely T, et al. Ethnic and socioeconomic trends in testicular cancer incidence in New Zealand. Int J Cancer 2011;128(7):1683–1691.
10. Shanmugalingam T, Soultati A, Chowdhury S, et al. Global incidence and outcome of testicular cancer. Clin Epidemiol 2013;5:417–427.
11. Bosetti C, Bertuccio P, Chatenoud L, et al. Trends in mortality from urologic cancers in Europe, 1970–2008. Eur Urol 2011;60(1):1–15.
12. Bertuccio P, Malvezzi M, Chatenoud L, et al. Testicular cancer mortality in the Americas, 1980–2003. Cancer 2007;109(4):776–779.
13. Verhoeven RH, Coebergh JW, Kiemeney LA, et al. Testicular cancer: trends in mortality are well explained by changes in treatment and survival in the southern Netherlands since 1970. Eur J Cancer 2007;43(17):2553–2558.
14. Akre O, Pettersson A, Richiardi L. Risk of contralateral testicular cancer among men with unilaterally undescended testis: a meta analysis. Int J Cancer 2009;124(3):687–689.
15. Raman JD, Nobert CF, Goldstein M. Increased incidence of testicular cancer in men presenting with infertility and abnormal semen analysis. J Urol 2005;174(5):1819–22; discussion 1822.
16. Jørgensen N, Asklund C, Carlsen E, et al. Coordinated European investigations of semen quality: results from studies of Scandinavian young men is a matter of concern. Int J Androl 2006;29(1):54–61; discussion 105.
17. Jørgensen N, Vierula M, Jacobsen R, et al. Recent adverse trends in semen quality and testis cancer incidence among Finnish men. Int J Androl 2011;34(4 Pt 2):e37–e48.
18. Skakkebaek NE, Rajpert-De Meyts E, Main KM. Testicular dysgenesis syndrome: an increasingly common developmental disorder with environmental aspects. Hum Reprod 2001;16(5):972–978.
19. Li N, Hauser R, Holford T, et al. Muscle-building supplement use and increased risk of testicular germ cell cancer in men from Connecticut and Massachusetts. Br J Cancer 2015;112(7):1247–1250.

20. Gurney J, Shaw C, Stanley J, et al. Cannabis exposure and risk of testicular cancer: a systematic review and meta-analysis. *BMC Cancer* 2015;15:897.

21. Greene MH, Kratz CP, Mai PL, et al. Familial testicular germ cell tumors in adults: 2010 summary of genetic risk factors and clinical phenotype. *Endocr Relat Cancer* 2010;17(2):R109–R121.

22. Moch H, Cubilla AL, Humphrey PA, et al. The 2016 WHO Classification of Tumours of the Urinary System and Male Genital Organs-Part A: Renal, Penile, and Testicular Tumours. *Eur Urol* 2016;70(1):93–105.

23. Dieckmann KP, Skakkebaek NE. Carcinoma in situ of the testis: review of biological and clinical features. *Int J Cancer* 1999;83(6):815–822.

24. Cheng L, Lyu B, Roth LM. Perspectives on testicular germ cell neoplasms. *Hum Pathol* 2017;59:10–25.

25. Bomeisl PE, MacLennan GT. Spermatocytic seminoma. *J Urol* 2007;177(2):734.

26. Aggarwal N, Parwani AV. Spermatocytic seminoma. *Arch Pathol Lab Med* 2009;133(12):1985–1988.

27. Looijenga LH. Spermatocytic seminoma: toward further understanding of pathogenesis. *J Pathol* 2011;224(4):431–433.

28. Kim W, Rosen MA, Langer JE, et al. US MR imaging correlation in pathologic conditions of the scrotum. *Radiographics* 2007;27(5):1239–1253.

29. de Wit M, Brenner W, Hartmann M, et al. [18F]-FDG-PET in clinical stage I/II non-seminomatous germ cell tumours: results of the German multicentre trial. *Ann Oncol* 2008;19(9):1619–1623.

30. Hudolin T, Kastelan Z, Knezevic N, et al. Correlation between retroperitoneal lymph node size and presence of metastases in nonseminomatous germ cell tumors. *Int J Surg Pathol* 2012;20(1):15–18.

31. McMahon CJ, Rofsky NM, Pedrosa I. Lymphatic metastases from pelvic tumors: anatomic classification, characterization, and staging. *Radiology* 2010;254(1):31–46.

32. Schwerk WB, Schwerk WN, Rodeck G. Testicular tumors: prospective analysis of real-time US patterns and abdominal staging. *Radiology* 1987;164(2):369–374.

33. American Joint Committee on Cancer. *AJCC cancer staging manual.* 7th ed. New York, NY: Springer, 2010.

34. Fosså SD, Cvancarova M, Chen L, et al. Adverse prognostic factors for testicular cancer-specific survival: a population-based study of 27,948 patients. *J Clin Oncol* 2011;29(8):963–970.

35. International Germ Cell Consensus Classification: a prognostic factor-based staging system for metastatic germ cell cancers. International Germ Cell Cancer Collaborative Group. *J Clin Oncol* 1997;15(2):594–603.

36. Capelouto CC, Clark PE, Ransil BJ, et al. A review of scrotal violation in testicular cancer: is adjuvant local therapy necessary. *J Urol* 1995;153(3 Pt 2):981–985.

37. Albers P, Albrecht W, Algaba F, et al. Guidelines on Testicular Cancer: 2015 Update. *Eur Urol.* 2015;68(6):1054–1068.

38. Mead GM, Fossa SD, Oliver RT, et al. Randomized trials in 2466 patients with stage I seminoma: patterns of relapse and follow-up. *J Natl Cancer Inst* 2011;103(3):241–249.

39. Chung P, Mayhew LA, Warde P, et al.; Genitourinary CDSGOCCOPIE-bC. Management of stage I seminomatous testicular cancer: a systematic review. *Clin Oncol (R Coll Radiol)* 2010;22(1):6–16.

40. Alomary I, Samant R, Genest P, et al. The preferred treatment for stage I seminoma: a survey of Canadian radiation oncologists. *Clin Oncol (R Coll Radiol)* 2006;18(9):696–9; discussion 693.

41. Kollmannsberger C, Tyldesley S, Moore C, et al. Evolution in management of testicular seminoma: population-based outcomes with selective utilization of active therapies. *Ann Oncol* 2011;22(4):808–814.

42. Matulewicz RS, Oberlin DT, Sheinfeld J, et al. The Evolving Management of Patients with Clinical Stage I Seminoma. *Urology* 2016;98:113–119.

43. von der Maase H, Specht L, Jacobsen GK, et al. Surveillance following orchidectomy for stage I seminoma of the testis. *Eur J Cancer* 1993;29A(14):1931–1934.

44. Chung P, Parker C, Panzarella T, et al. Surveillance in stage I testicular seminoma—risk of late relapse. *Can J Urol* 2002;9(5):1637–1640.

45. Francis R, Bower M, Brunström G, et al. Surveillance for stage I testicular germ cell tumours: results and cost benefit analysis of management options. *Eur J Cancer* 2000;36(15):1925–1932.

46. Daugaard G, Petersen PM, Rørth M. Surveillance in stage I testicular cancer. *APMIS* 2003;111(1):76–83; discussion 83.

47. Choo R, Thomas G, Woo T, et al. Long-term outcome of postorchiectomy surveillance for Stage I testicular seminoma. *Int J Radiat Oncol Biol Phys* 2005;61(3):736–740.

48. Cummins S, Yau T, Huddart R, et al. Surveillance in stage I seminoma patients: a long-term assessment. *Eur Urol* 2010;57(4):673–678.

49. Aparicio J, Germà JR, García del Muro X, et al. Risk-adapted management for patients with clinical stage I seminoma: the Second Spanish Germ Cell Cancer Cooperative Group study. *J Clin Oncol* 2005;23(34):8717–8723.

50. Kamba T, Kamoto T, Okubo K, et al. Outcome of different post-orchiectomy management for stage I seminoma: Japanese multi-institutional study including 425 patients. *Int J Urol* 2010;17(12):980–987.

51. Tandstad T, Smaaland R, Solberg A, et al. Management of seminomatous testicular cancer: a binational prospective population-based study from the Swedish Norwegian testicular cancer study group. *J Clin Oncol* 2011;29(6):719–725.

52. Warde P, Specht L, Horwich A, et al. Prognostic factors for relapse in stage I seminoma managed by surveillance: a pooled analysis. *J Clin Oncol* 2002;20(22):4448–4452.

53. Kollmannsberger C, Tandstad T, Bedard PL, et al. Patterns of relapse in patients with clinical stage I testicular cancer managed with active surveillance. *J Clin Oncol* 2015;33(1):51–57.

54. Tyldesley S, Voduc D, McKenzie M, et al. Surveillance of stage I testicular seminoma: British Columbia Cancer Agency Experience 1992 to 2002. *Urology* 2006;67(3):594–598.

55. Tandstad T, Ståhl O, Dahl O, et al. Treatment of stage I seminoma, with one course of adjuvant carboplatin or surveillance, risk-adapted recommendations implementing patient autonomy: a report from the Swedish and Norwegian Testicular Cancer Group (SWENOTECA). *Ann Oncol* 2016;27(7):1299–1304.

56. Tolan S, Vesprini D, Jewett MA, et al. No role for routine chest radiography in stage I seminoma surveillance. *Eur Urol* 2010;57(3):474–479.

57. O'Malley ME, Chung P, Haider M, et al. Comparison of low dose with standard dose abdominal/pelvic multidetector CT in patients with stage 1 testicular cancer under surveillance. *Eur Radiol* 2010;20(7):1624–1630.

58. Cafferty FH, Gabe R, Huddart RA, et al. UK management practices in stage I seminoma and the Medical Research Council Trial of Imaging and Schedule in Seminoma Testis managed with surveillance. *Clin Oncol (R Coll Radiol)* 2012;24(1):25–29.

59. Cox JA, Gajjar SR, Lanni TB, et al. Cost analysis of adjuvant management strategies in early stage (stage I) testicular seminoma. *Res Rep Urol* 2015;7:1–7.

60. Leung E, Warde P, Jewett M, et al. Treatment burden in stage I seminoma: a comparison of surveillance and adjuvant radiation therapy. *BJU Int* 2013;112(8):1088–1095.

61. Kier MG, Hansen MK, Lauritsen J, et al. Second Malignant Neoplasms and Cause of Death in Patients With Germ Cell Cancer: A Danish Nationwide Cohort Study. *JAMA Oncol* 2016;2(12):1624–1627.

62. Fosså SD, Aass N, Kaalhus O. Radiotherapy for testicular seminoma stage I: treatment results and long-term post-irradiation morbidity in 365 patients. *Int J Radiat Oncol Biol Phys* 1989;16(2):383–388.

63. Bauman GS, Venkatesan VM, Ago CT, et al. Postoperative radiotherapy for Stage I/II seminoma: results for 212 patients. *Int J Radiat Oncol Biol Phys* 1998;42(2):313–317.

64. Logue JP, Harris MA, Livsey JE, et al. Short course para-aortic radiation for stage I seminoma of the testis. *Int J Radiat Oncol Biol Phys* 2003;57(5):1304–1309.

65. Santoni R, Barbera F, Bertoni F, et al. Stage I seminoma of the testis: a bi-institutional retrospective analysis of patients treated with radiation therapy only. *BJU Int* 2003;92(1):47–52; discussion 52.

66. Niazi TM, Souhami L, Sultanem K, et al. Long-term results of para-aortic irradiation for patients with stage I seminoma of the testis. *Int J Radiat Oncol Biol Phys* 2005;61(3):741–744.

67. Melchior D, Hammer P, Fimmers R, et al. Long term results and morbidity of paraaortic compared with paraaortic and iliac adjuvant radiation in clinical stage I seminoma. *Anticancer Res* 2001;21(4B):2989–2993.

68. Classen J, Schmidberger H, Meisner C, et al. Para-aortic irradiation for stage I testicular seminoma: results of a prospective study in 675 patients. A trial of the German testicular cancer study group (GTCSG). *Br J Cancer* 2004;90(12):2305–2311.

69. Bruns F, Bremer M, Meyer A, et al. Adjuvant radiotherapy in stage I seminoma: is there a role for further reduction of treatment volume. *Acta Oncol* 2005;44(2):142–148.

70. Jones WG, Fossa SD, Mead GM, et al. Randomized trial of 30 versus 20 Gy in the adjuvant treatment of stage I Testicular Seminoma: a report on Medical Research Council Trial TE18, European Organisation for the Research and Treatment of Cancer Trial 30942 (ISRCTN18525328). *J Clin Oncol* 2005;23(6):1200–1208.

71. Oliver RT, Mead GM, Rustin GJ, et al. Randomized trial of carboplatin versus radiotherapy for stage I seminoma: mature results on relapse and contralateral testis cancer rates in MRC TE19/EORTC 30982 study (ISRCTN27163214). *J Clin Oncol* 2011;29(8):957–962.

72. Fosså SD, Horwich A, Russell JM, et al. Optimal planning target volume for stage I testicular seminoma: a Medical Research Council randomized trial. Medical Research Council Testicular Tumor Working Group. *J Clin Oncol* 1999;17(4):1146.

73. Souchon R, Hartmann M, Krege S, et al. Interdisciplinary evidence-based recommendations for the follow-up of early stage seminomatous germ cell cancer patients. *Strahlenther Onkol* 2011;187(3):158–166.

74. Livsey JE, Taylor B, Mobarek N, et al. Patterns of relapse following radiotherapy for stage I seminoma of the testis: implications for follow-up. *Clin Oncol (R Coll Radiol)* 2001;13(4):296–300.

75. Paly JJ, Efstathiou JA, Hedgire SS, et al. Mapping patterns of nodal metastases in seminoma: rethinking radiotherapy fields. *Radiother Oncol* 2013;106(1):64–68.

76. Horwich A, Dearnaley DP, Duchesne GM, et al. Simple nontoxic treatment of advanced metastatic seminoma with carboplatin. *J Clin Oncol* 1989;7(8):1150–1156.

77. Dieckmann KP, Krain J, Küster J, et al. Adjuvant carboplatin treatment for seminoma clinical stage I. *J Cancer Res Clin Oncol* 1996;122(1):63–66.

78. Krege S, Boergermann C, Baschek R, et al. Single agent carboplatin for CS IIA/B testicular seminoma. A phase II study of the German Testicular Cancer Study Group (GTCSG). *Ann Oncol* 2006;17(2):276–280.

79. Reiter WJ, Brodowicz T, Alavi S, et al. Twelve-year experience with two courses of adjuvant single-agent carboplatin therapy for clinical stage I seminoma. *J Clin Oncol* 2001;19(1):101–104.

80. Steiner H, Scheiber K, Berger AP, et al. Retrospective multicentre study of carboplatin monotherapy for clinical stage I seminoma. *BJU Int* 2011;107(7):1074–1079.

81. Fischer S, Tandstad T, Wheater M, et al. Outcome of Men With Relapse After Adjuvant Carboplatin for Clinical Stage I Seminoma. *J Clin Oncol* 2017;35(2):194–200.

82. Powles T, Robinson D, Shamash J, et al. The long-term risks of adjuvant carboplatin treatment for stage I seminoma of the testis. *Ann Oncol* 2008;19(3):443–447.

83. Chung PW, Gospodarowicz MK, Panzarella T, et al. Stage II testicular seminoma: patterns of recurrence and outcome of treatment. *Eur Urol* 2004;45(6):754–59; discussion 759.

84. Classen J, Schmidberger H, Meisner C, et al. Radiotherapy for stages IIA/B testicular seminoma: final report of a prospective multicenter clinical trial. *J Clin Oncol* 2003;21(6):1101–1106.

85. Zagars GK, Pollack A. Radiotherapy for stage II testicular seminoma. *Int J Radiat Oncol Biol Phys* 2001;51(3):643–649.

86. Patterson H, Norman AR, Mitra SS, et al. Combination carboplatin and radiotherapy in the management of stage II testicular seminoma: comparison with radiotherapy treatment alone. *Radiother Oncol* 2001;59(1):5–11.

87. Whipple GL, Sagerman RH, van Rooy EM. Long-term evaluation of postorchiectomy radiotherapy for stage II seminoma. *Am J Clin Oncol* 1997;20(2):196–201.

88. Vallis KA, Howard GC, Duncan W, et al. Radiotherapy for stages I and II testicular seminoma: results and morbidity in 238 patients. *Br J Radiol* 1995;68(808):400–405.

89. Dosmann MA, Zagars GK. Post-orchiectomy radiotherapy for stages I and II testicular seminoma. *Int J Radiat Oncol Biol Phys* 1993;26(3):381–390.

90. Mason BR, Kearsley JH. Radiotherapy for stage 2 testicular seminoma: the prognostic influence of tumor bulk. *J Clin Oncol* 1988;6(12):1856–1862.

91. Evensen JF, Fossa SD, Kjellevold K, et al. Testicular seminoma: analysis of treatment and failure for stage II disease. *Radiother Oncol* 1985;4(1):55–61.

92. Chung PW, Warde PR, Panzarella T, et al. Appropriate radiation volume for stage IIA/B testicular seminoma. *Int J Radiat Oncol Biol Phys* 2003;56(3):746–748.

93. Glaser SM, Vargo JA, Balasubramani GK, et al. Stage II Testicular Seminoma: Patterns of Care and Survival by Treatment Strategy *Clin Oncol (R Coll Radiol)* 2016;28(8):513–521.

94. Garcia-del-Muro X, Maroto P, Gumà J, et al. Chemotherapy as an alternative to radiotherapy in the treatment of stage IIA and IIB testicular seminoma: a Spanish Germ Cell Cancer Group Study. *J Clin Oncol* 2008;26(33):5416–5421.

95. Giannatempo P, Greco T, Mariani L, et al. Radiotherapy or chemotherapy for clinical stage IIA and IIB seminoma: a systematic review and meta-analysis of patient outcomes. *Ann Oncol* 2015;26(4):657–668.

96. Giannis M, Aristotelis B, Vassiliki K, et al. Cisplatin-based chemotherapy for advanced seminoma: report of 52 cases treated in two institutions. *J Cancer Res Clin Oncol* 2009;135(11):1495–1500.

97. Horwich A, Dearnaley DP, Sohaib A, et al. Neoadjuvant carboplatin before radiotherapy in stage IIA and IIB seminoma. *Ann Oncol* 2013;24(8):2104–2107.

98. Domont J, Massard C, Patrikidou A, et al. A risk-adapted strategy of radiotherapy or cisplatin-based chemotherapy in stage II seminoma. *Urol Oncol* 2013;31(5):697–705.

99. Bokemeyer C, Kollmannsberger C, Stenning S, et al. Metastatic seminoma treated with either single agent carboplatin or cisplatin-based combination chemotherapy: a pooled analysis of two randomised trials. *Br J Cancer* 2004;91(4):683–687.

100. Flechon A, Bompas E, Biron P, et al. Management of post-chemotherapy residual masses in advanced seminoma. *J Urol* 2002;168(5):1975–1979.

101. Duchesne GM, Stenning SP, Aass N, et al. Radiotherapy after chemotherapy for metastatic seminoma—a diminishing role. MRC Testicular Tumour Working Party. *Eur J Cancer* 1997;33(6):829–835.

102. Ravi R, Ong J, Oliver RT, et al. The management of residual masses after chemotherapy in metastatic seminoma. *BJU Int* 1999;83(6):649–653.

103. Herr HW, Sheinfeld J, Puc HS, et al. Surgery for a post-chemotherapy residual mass in seminoma. *J Urol* 1997;157(3):860–862.

104. Becherer A, De Santis M, Karanikas G, et al. FDG PET is superior to CT in the prediction of viable tumour in post-chemotherapy seminoma residuals. *Eur J Radiol* 2005;54(2):284–288.

105. De Santis M, Becherer A, Bokemeyer C, et al. 2-18fluoro-deoxy-D-glucose positron emission tomography is a reliable predictor for viable tumor in post-chemotherapy seminoma: an update of the prospective multicentric SEMPET trial. *J Clin Oncol* 2004;22(6):1034–1039.

106. Klatte T, de Martino M, Arensmeier K, et al. Management and outcome of bilateral testicular germ cell tumors: a 25-year single center experience. *Int J Urol* 2008;15(9):821–826.

107. Bazzi WM, Raheem OA, Stroup SP, et al. Partial orchiectomy and testis intratubular germ cell neoplasia: world literature review. *Urol Ann* 2011;3 115–118.

108. Huyghe E, Soulie M, Escourrou G, et al. Conservative management of small testicular tumors relative to carcinoma in situ prevalence. *J Urol* 2005;173(3):820–823.

109. Heidenreich A, Weissbach L, Höltl W, et al. Organ sparing surgery for malignant germ cell tumor of the testis. *J Urol* 2001;166(6):2161–2165.

110. Lawrentschuk N, Zuniga A, Grabowksi AC, et al. Partial orchiectomy for presumed malignancy in patients with a solitary testis due to a prior germ cell tumor: a large North American experience. *J Urol* 2011;185(2):508–513.

111. Kier MG, Lauritsen J, Almstrup K, et al. Screening for carcinoma in situ in the contralateral testicle in patients with testicular cancer: a population-based study. *Ann Oncol* 2015;26(4):737–742.

112. Zilli T, Boudreau C, Doucet R, et al. Bone marrow-sparing intensity-modulated radiation therapy for Stage I seminoma. *Acta Oncol* 2011;50(4):555–562.

113. Choo R, Sandler H, Warde P, et al. Survey of radiation oncologists: practice patterns of the management of stage I seminoma of testis in Canada and a selected group in the United States. *Can J Urol* 2002;9(2):1479–1485.

114. Fraass BA, Kinsella TJ, Harrington FS, et al. Peripheral dose to the testes: the design and clinical use of a practical and effective gonadal shield. *Int J Radiat Oncol Biol Phys* 1985;11(3):609–615.

115. Bieri S, Rouzaud M, Miralbell R. Seminoma of the testis: is scrotal shielding necessary when radiotherapy is limited to the para-aortic nodes? *Radiother Oncol* 1999;50(3):349–353.

116. Ravichandran R, Binukumar JP, Kannadhasan S, et al. Testicular shield for para-aortic radiotherapy and estimation of gonad doses. *J Med Phys* 2008;33(4):158–161.

117. Mencel PJ, Motzer RJ, Mazumdar M, et al. Advanced seminoma: treatment results, survival, and prognostic factors in 142 patients. *J Clin Oncol* 1994;12(1):120–126.

118. Hansen PV, Trykker H, Svennekjaer IL, et al. Long-term recovery of spermatogenesis after radiotherapy in patients with testicular cancer. *Radiother Oncol* 1990;18(2):117–125.

119. Hahn EW, Feingold SM, Simpson L, et al. Recovery from aspermia induced by low-dose radiation in seminoma patients. *Cancer* 1982;50(2):337–340.

120. Gordon W, Siegmund K, Stanisic TH, et al. A study of reproductive function in patients with seminoma treated with radiotherapy and orchidectomy: (SWOG-8711). Southwest Oncology Group. *Int J Radiat Oncol Biol Phys* 1997;38(1):83–94.

121. Jacobsen KD, Olsen DR, Fosså K, et al. External beam abdominal radiotherapy in patients with seminoma stage I: field type, testicular dose, and spermatogenesis. *Int J Radiat Oncol Biol Phys* 1997;38(1):95–102.

122. Fatigante L, Ducci F, Campoccia S, et al. Long-term results in patients affected by testicular seminoma treated with radiotherapy: risk of second malignancies. *Tumori* 2005;91(2):144–150.

123. Robinson D, Moller H, Horwich A. Mortality and incidence of second cancers following treatment for testicular cancer. *Br J Cancer* 2007;96(3):529–533.

124. Hauptmann M, Fossa SD, Stovall M, et al. Increased stomach cancer risk following radiotherapy for testicular cancer. *Br J Cancer* 2015;112(1):44–51.

125. Travis LB, Fosså SD, Schonfeld SJ, et al. Second cancers among 40,576 testicular cancer patients: focus on long-term survivors. *J Natl Cancer Inst* 2005;97(18):1354–1365.

126. Travis LB, Andersson M, Gospodarowicz M, et al. Treatment-associated leukemia following testicular cancer. *J Natl Cancer Inst* 2000;92(14):1165–1171.

127. Schmidberger H, Virsik-Koepp P, Rave-Fränk M, et al. Reciprocal translocations in patients with testicular seminoma before and after radiotherapy. *Int J Radiat Oncol Biol Phys* 2001;50(4):857–864.

128. Müller I, Geinitz H, Braselmann H, et al. Time-course of radiation-induced chromosomal aberrations in tumor patients after radiotherapy. *Int J Radiat Oncol Biol Phys* 2005;63(4):1214–1220.

129. Zagars GK, Ballo MT, Lee AK, et al. Mortality after cure of testicular seminoma. *J Clin Oncol* 2004;22(4):640–647.

130. Haugnes HS, Wethal T, Aass N, et al. Cardiovascular risk factors and morbidity in long-term survivors of testicular cancer: a 20-year follow-up study. *J Clin Oncol* 2010;28(30):4649–4657.

131. Brydøy M, Oldenburg J, Klepp O, et al. Observational study of prevalence of long-term Raynaud-like phenomena and neurological side effects in testicular cancer survivors. *J Natl Cancer Inst* 2009;101(24):1682–1695.

132. Kim C, McGlynn KA, McCorkle R, et al. Fertility among testicular cancer survivors: a case-control study in the U.S. *J Cancer Surviv* 2010;4(3):266–273.

133. Stephenson WT, Poirier SM, Rubin L, et al. Evaluation of reproductive capacity in germ cell tumor patients following treatment with cisplatin, etoposide, and bleomycin. *J Clin Oncol* 1995;13(9):2278–2280.

134. Fosså SD, Oldenburg J, Dahl AA. Short- and long-term morbidity after treatment for testicular cancer. *BJU Int* 2009;104(9 Pt B):1418–1422.

135. Brydøy M, Fosså SD, Klepp O, et al. Paternity and testicular function among testicular cancer survivors treated with two to four cycles of cisplatin-based chemotherapy. *Eur Urol* 2010;58(1):134–140.

136. Gerl A, Mühlbayer D, Hansmann G, et al. The impact of chemotherapy on Leydig cell function in long term survivors of germ cell tumors. *Cancer* 2001;91(7):1297–1303.

137. Huddart RA, Norman A, Moynihan C, et al. Fertility, gonadal and sexual function in survivors of testicular cancer. *Br J Cancer* 2005;93(2):200–207.

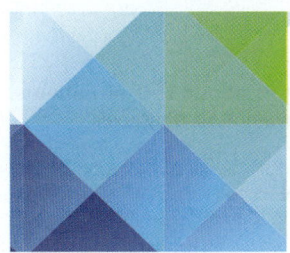

C H A P T E R   7 2

Cancer of the Penis and Male Urethra

Hiram A. Gay and David B. Mansur

ANATOMY

The basic structural components of the penis include two corpora cavernosa and the corpus spongiosum. These are encased in a dense fascia (Buck fascia), which is separated from the skin by a layer of loose connective tissue. Distally, the corpus spongiosum expands into the glans penis, which is covered by a skin fold known as the prepuce. The skin extends over and is firmly attached to the glans.

The male urethra is composed of a mucous membrane and the submucosa. It extends from the bladder neck to the external urethral meatus. The posterior urethra is subdivided into the membranous urethra, the portion passing through the urogenital diaphragm, and the prostatic urethra, which passes through the prostate. The anterior urethra passes through the corpus spongiosum and is subdivided into fossa navicularis (a widening within the glans); the penile urethra, which passes through the pendulous part of the penis; and the bulbous urethra, the dilated proximal portion of the anterior urethra. The prostatic urethra is covered by transitional epithelium only. The distal portion of the anterior urethra is covered by stratified squamous epithelium, which changes proximally to pseudostratified columnar epithelium. The columnar epithelium gradually changes into transitional epithelium in the membranous urethra.

The lymphatic channels of the prepuce and the skin of the shaft drain into the superficial inguinal nodes located above the fascia lata. The rich anastomotic network of the lymphatics within the penis and at the base of the penis means that for practical purposes, lymphatic drainage may be considered bilateral. There is some disagreement as to whether the glans and the deep penile structures drain into the superficial or deep inguinal lymph nodes (those under the fascia lata). The so-called sentinel nodes located above and medial to the junction of the epigastric and saphenous veins have been identified as the primary drainage sites in carcinoma of the penis.[1] Selective biopsy of this group of nodes is of obvious importance in assessment of tumor extent, because, if they are not involved by tumor, a complete nodal dissection may not be necessary. The reliability of this procedure has not been supported by some.[2,3] Catalona[4] found that biopsy of the sentinel nodes showed false-negative results in 10% of Cabanas's[5] cases who died of carcinoma.

The lymphatics of the fossa navicularis and the penile urethra follow the lymphatics of the penis to the superficial and deep inguinal lymph nodes. The lymphatics of the bulbomembranous and prostatic urethra may follow three routes. Some pass under the pubic symphysis to the external iliac nodes, some go to the obturator and internal iliac nodes, and others end in the presacral lymph nodes. The pelvic (iliac) lymph nodes are rarely involved in the absence of inguinal lymph node involvement.[6]

EPIDEMIOLOGY AND RISK FACTORS

Penile Cancer

In the United States, in 2017, the estimated number of new cases of penis and other genital cancers was 2,120, with 360 deaths. This accounts for <1% of cancer in males in the United States.[7] In the European Union, the annual number of males that develop penile cancer is estimated at 3,100, which is equivalent to an age-standardized rate (ASR) of 12 per million males. The 5-year relative survival rate is 69%. Squamous cell carcinoma is the predominant morphologic entity.[8]

A systematic review and meta-analysis showed that men circumcised in childhood/adolescence are at substantially reduced risk of invasive penile cancer, and this effect could be mediated partly through an effect on phimosis. In contrast, there was some evidence that circumcision in adulthood was associated with an increased risk of invasive penile cancer.[9] A trade-off analysis of routine newborn circumcision was performed on the Comprehensive Hospital Abstract Reporting System for Washington State. Routine newborn circumcisions performed over 9 years (1987 to 1996) were retrospectively examined. Of 354,297 male infants born during the study period, 37% were circumcised during their newborn stay. Overall, 0.2% of circumcised children and 0.01% of uncircumcised children had complications potentially associated with circumcision. The authors estimated that almost two complications can be expected for every case of penile cancer prevented.[10]

A study of 1,010 penile invasive cancers diagnosed between 1983 and 2011 from 25 countries showed that between one-quarter and one-third of penile cancers are related to human papillomavirus (HPV). HPV16 was the most frequent HPV type detected in HPV-positive cancers.[11] A Brazilian study of 110 asymptomatic men and 30 patients who underwent circumcision because of phimosis showed that HPV was present in 46% of patients with phimosis, of whom 50% were high-risk phenotypes. They detected a significantly high rate of HPV genital infection in patients presenting with phimosis compared with asymptomatic men. The prevalence of high-risk HPV genotypes in patients with phimosis was also statistically significant.[12]

The quadrivalent vaccine against HPV serotypes 6, 11, 16, and 18 has been approved for females aged 9 to 26 years to prevent cervical cancer. Based on the demonstrated ability to significantly decrease the incidence of penile lesions (primarily HPV-6– and HPV-11–associated genital warts) in young men, the U.S. Food and Drug Administration also approved the use of the vaccine in males aged 9 to 26 years. Because the incidence of penile cancer in the United States is much lower than that of genital warts, the reduction in penile cancer incidence is expected to be low. Perhaps the greatest benefit of vaccination of young men in the United States would be the reduced HPV infection rate in the overall population and subsequent reduced transmission to females at risk for cervical cancer.[13] Other potential strategies for the prevention of penile cancer could include smoking cessation and hygienic measures.[14]

Urethral Cancer

Carcinoma of the male urethra is also rare. Each year, around 650 individuals in the European Union develop cancer of the urethra. The ASR for cancer of the urethra is 1.1 (males 1.6; females 0.6) per million inhabitants, respectively. The 5-year relative survival rate for cancer of the urethra is 54%. Transitional cell carcinoma (TCC) is the predominant morphologic entity of cancer of the urethra.[8]

There are no recognized racial or geographic predisposing factors. Although the etiology remains unknown, there seems to be some correlation between the incidence of carcinoma of the urethra and chronic irritation (infection, venereal diseases, strictures). Some evidence suggests that some cases of female urethral carcinoma may originate from Skene glands.[15] Significant past medical history of male urethra cancer patients includes venereal disease (24% to 37%), urethral stricture (35% to 54%), urethral trauma (7%), and urethral polyps (2%).[16,17] The part of the urethra covered by the transitional epithelium (prostatic and membranous urethra) may be susceptible to the same carcinogenic factors that affect the bladder and the upper urinary tract. Average age at presentation of these tumors is 58 to 60 years, although 10% occur in men younger than 40 years.[5,17]

NATURAL HISTORY

Penile Cancer

Most carcinomas of the penis start within the preputial area, arising in the glans, coronal sulcus, or the prepuce itself. Lesions arising in the skin of the shaft are rare. In most patients, carcinoma of the penis is characterized by slow locoregional progression. The penis is handled and observed daily, yet there is often significant debate as to when patient recognition and medical diagnosis should have occurred. The patient experiences fear and embarrassment, which probably contributes to delayed diagnosis. Therefore, expeditious diagnosis of all penile lesions should be the rule. Extensive primary lesions may involve the corpora cavernosa or even the abdominal wall. The inguinal lymph nodes are the most common site of metastatic spread. Pathologic evidence of nodal metastases is reported in about 35% of all patients and in approximately 50% of those with palpable lymph nodes.[5,18–20]

Distant metastases are uncommon (about 10%), even in patients with advanced locoregional disease, and usually occur in patients with inguinal lymph node involvement. These patients often die of septic complications, erosion of large vessels in the groin, or a combination of the two.

Tumors can also metastasize to the penis. Most common primary sites are the genitourinary tract (mostly bladder urothelial carcinoma and prostatic adenocarcinoma) and the lower gastrointestinal tract (rectal and sigmoid colon adenocarcinomas). Secondary tumors tend to be localized in the penile shaft and to invade the vascular spaces of erectile tissues, with corpora cavernosa involvement in most of the cases. For patients with penile metastasis, cancer-related death rate is high and the prognosis is dismal.[21]

Urethral Cancer

The natural history of carcinoma of the anterior urethra in the male is similar to that of carcinoma of the penis. Approximately 40% of tumors originate in the anterior urethra.[16] Many tumors are low grade and progress slowly at primary and regional sites rather than spread to distal areas. Tumors of the penile urethra spread to the inguinal lymph nodes first, whereas those of the bulbomembranous and prostatic urethra metastasize first to the pelvic lymph nodes. Approximately one-third of men will present with either clinically or pathologically involved lymph nodes.[16]

Urethral cancers tend to spread by direct extension to adjacent structures. Invasion into the vascular space of the corpus spongiosum in the periurethral tissues is common. Malignancies beginning in the bulbomembranous urethra often invade the deep structures of the perineum, including the urogenital diaphragm, prostate, and adjacent skin. In the majority of prostatic urethral tumors, the bulk of the prostate gland is invaded at the time of diagnosis. Hematogenous spread is uncommon except in advanced regional disease. Kaplan

et al.[17] reported distant metastases in about 15% of patients, and most had corpora cavernosa invasion at diagnosis.

CLINICAL PRESENTATION

Penile Cancer

Carcinoma of the penis may present as either an infiltrative–ulcerative or an exophytic papillary lesion. Figure 72.1 demonstrates the localization of penile tumors in 259 patients from 14 cancer institutes in France. The glans and the prepuce were the predominant sites of the primary lesion, whereas tumors of the shaft were rare.[22] Assessment of the primary lesion may be obscured by the presence of phimosis. Secondary infection and associated foul smell are quite common. Urethral obstruction is an unusual symptom of carcinoma of the penis. The most common presenting symptom is a mass, which occurs in over two-thirds of patients. Ulceration is also common, occurring in approximately half of patients.[20,23] In a collective series of 552 patients with penile carcinoma, the presenting symptoms were mass lesions (78%), pain or itching (12%), bleeding (7%), groin mass (7%), and urinary symptoms (4%).[24–26] Inguinal lymph nodes are palpable on presentation in 30% to 45% of patients[5,18,19,25,27,28]; however, only half contain tumor.[19,20] Enlargement of the lymph nodes is often related to inflammatory (infectious) processes. Administration of antibiotics over several weeks results in regression of inguinal lymph nodes in a substantial proportion of cases, and many have advocated this practice before the status of the regional lymph nodes is definitively assessed. Conversely, between 20% and 40% of patients with clinically negative inguinal lymph nodes have occult metastases.[3,29–32]

Urethral Cancer

Patients with urethral carcinoma most commonly present with obstructive symptoms (43%). Other presenting signs and symptoms include mass (28%), bleeding (20%), abscess (20%), and irritative symptoms (20%).[16] These symptoms are often attributed to urethritis or urethral stricture, which may precede the development of urethral carcinoma and may also result in delay in diagnosis. The majority of urethral carcinomas occur in the bulbomembranous (posterior) region (61%), and tumors

FIGURE 72.1. Localization of the primary tumor in 259 patients; each circle represents one anatomic compartment. Intersections indicate involvement of two or three compartments. Unknown: two. (Reprinted from Rozan R, Albuisson E, Giraud B, et al. Interstitial brachytherapy for penile carcinoma: a multicentric survey [259 patients]. *Radiother Oncol* 1995;36[2]:83–93. Copyright © 1995 Elsevier Ireland Ltd. With permission.)

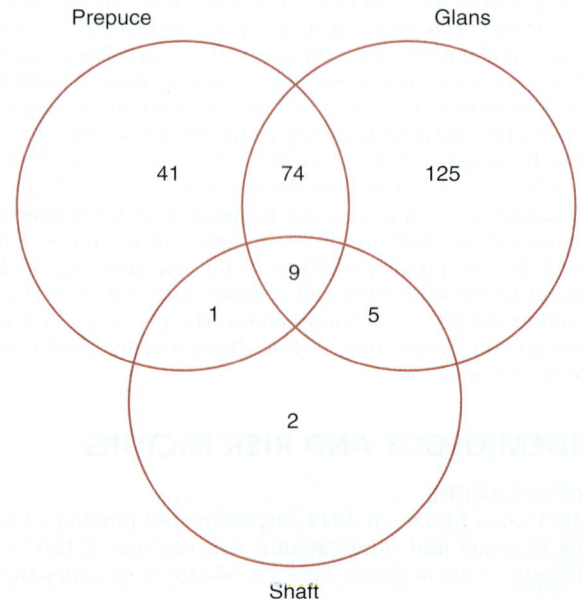

in this location have a worse prognosis compared with those arising in the anterior urethra.[16]

DIAGNOSTIC WORKUP

In penile and urethral cancers, imaging plays a crucial role in enhancing the precision of clinical staging and facilitating optimal surgical planning. High-resolution magnetic resonance imaging (MRI) now represents the gold standard for evaluating the primary tumor and its local extension. Lymphotropic nanoparticle–enhanced MRI and dynamic sentinel lymph node biopsy (DSNB) combined with FNA seem to be superior for imaging regional lymph nodes. Positron emission tomography/computed tomography (PET/CT) has shown great promise for the detection of distant metastases.[33]

Penile Cancer

See Table 72.1 for the diagnostic workup of penile cancer based on the Penile Cancer National Comprehensive Cancer Network (NCCN) Guidelines.

On MRI, penile tumors are best evaluated on T2-weighted images because of the superior contrast resolution between the hypointense fascial layers and the adjacent hyperintense corporal bodies. Squamous cell carcinomas typically appear as hypointense lesions when compared to the adjacent corpora. On MRI, nonsquamous variants of penile cancer can appear different from squamous carcinomas. Although penile cancers enhance with gadolinium, the normal corporal bodies enhance even more, which makes contrast enhancement less useful.[33]

The presence of central nodal necrosis and/or an irregular nodal border of the regional lymph nodes on preoperative CT images are accurate and reproducible (sensitivity of 95% [21 of 22] and a specificity of 82% [31 of 38]) criteria to identify high-risk pathologic node-positive penile cancer.[34]

Sentinel lymph node biopsy with a radiotracer (Tc-99m nanocolloid) is a reliable method with low morbidity that is associated with a low-radiation burden for clinical staff. The false-negative rate and morbidity were <5%.[35]

Limited prospective data regarding the use of PET with CT are available, but preliminary results show encouraging sensitivity (88%) and specificity (98%) in evaluating inguinal lymph nodes[36] and a diagnostic accuracy of 96% in evaluating pelvic lymph nodes in patients with known inguinal metastases.[37]

Urethral Cancer

See Table 72.2 for the diagnostic workup of urethral cancer based on the Bladder Cancer NCCN guidelines.[38]

A cystourethroscopy is essential for urethral primaries. Inguinal lymph nodes should be thoroughly evaluated. CT is useful in the identification of enlarged pelvic and periaortic lymph nodes in patients with involved inguinal lymph nodes.[33]

TABLE 72.1 DIAGNOSTIC WORKUP FOR PENILE CANCER
General
History and physical examination
• Risk factors: balanitis, chronic inflammation, penile trauma, tobacco use, lichen sclerosus, poor hygiene, sexually transmitted disease
• Primary characteristics: diameter, location, number of lesions, morphology (papillary, nodular, ulcerous, or flat), relationship to other structures (submucosal, corpus spongiosum and/or corpora cavernosa, urethra)
• Lymph node characteristics: diameter, unilateral or bilateral, number, relationship to other structures, mobility or fixation, skin involvement
Punch, excisional, or incisional biopsy
Palpable lymph nodes: abdominal and pelvic MRI or CT with contrast unless contraindicated and chest imaging (CT or x-ray). Percutaneous lymph node biopsy, ultrasound or CT guided.

CT, computed tomography; MRI, magnetic resonance imaging.

TABLE 72.2 DIAGNOSTIC WORKUP FOR URETHRAL CANCER
General
History and physical examination
Cystourethroscopy, examination under anesthesia, transurethral resection, or transvaginal biopsy
Radiographic Studies
MRI of pelvis with and without contrast
Palpable lymph nodes: chest, abdominal, and pelvic CT with contrast. Lymph node biopsy.

CT, computed tomography; MRI, magnetic resonance imaging.

On MRI, urethral tumors tend to show a decreased signal intensity relative to that of the surrounding normal corporal tissue on T1- and T2-weighted images. Malignant lesions usually enhance with gadolinium.[33]

STAGING

Penile Cancer

The American Joint Committee on Cancer (AJCC) staging systems for carcinoma of the penis and urethra are shown in Tables 72.3 and 72.4, respectively.[39]

PATHOLOGIC CLASSIFICATION

Penile Cancer

The World Health Organization (WHO) classifies malignant epithelial tumors of the penis as squamous cell carcinoma (basaloid, warty [condylomatous], verrucous, papillary NOS, sarcomatous, mixed, and adenosquamous carcinoma), Merkel cell carcinoma, small cell carcinoma of neuroendocrine type, sebaceous carcinoma, clear cell carcinoma, and basal cell carcinoma.[40] Basaloid carcinoma has a poor prognosis and frequently early inguinal nodal metastases. Warty carcinoma has a good prognosis with rare metastases. Verrucous carcinoma has a good prognosis with no metastases. Papillary carcinoma has a good prognosis with rare metastases. Sarcomatous carcinoma has a very poor prognosis with early vascular metastases. Mixed carcinoma has a heterogeneous prognosis. Adenosquamous carcinoma occurs in the central and perimeatal glans, is high grade with a high metastatic potential but low mortality.[41]

Most malignant penile tumors are well differentiated squamous cell carcinomas.[42] Although an apparent adverse prognostic effect of anaplasia has been reported in some series,[18] others found no significant correlation between histologic grade and survival.[25,43]

Bowen disease is squamous cell carcinoma *in situ* that may involve the shaft of the penis as well as the hairy skin of the inguinal and suprapubic area. Clinically, the lesion is a solitary, dull-red plaque with areas of crusting and oozing. Approximately 25% to 50% of patients with this disease have a concomitant visceral malignancy.[6]

Erythroplasia of Queyrat is an epidermoid carcinoma *in situ* that involves the mucosal or mucocutaneous areas of the prepuce or glans.[42] It appears as a reddened, elevated, or ulcerated lesion. Graham and Helwig[44] reported that 10 of 100 patients presenting with erythroplasia of Queyrat had invasive squamous cell carcinoma at diagnosis. Mikhail[45] reported on 5 of 15 patients with the same presentation. Erythroplasia of Queyrat is not as frequently associated with internal malignancies as Bowen disease.[40]

Basal cell carcinoma is infrequently reported, accounting for 1% to 2% of all cases of penile cancers.[41,42]

Extramammary Paget disease is a rare intraepithelial apocrine carcinoma. The most common sites are the scrotum, inguinal folds, and perineal region.[45] The lesion has a propensity to metastasize, necessitating frequent assessment

Section III

TABLE 72.3 2017 PENIS CANCER TNM STAGING AJCC UICC

Penis

T category	T Criteria
TX	Primary tumor cannot be assessed
T0	No evidence of primary tumor
Tis	Carcinoma in situ (penile intraepithelial neoplasia [PeIN])
Ta	Noninvasive localized squamous cell carcinoma
T1	Glans: Tumor invades the lamina propria
	Foreskin: Tumor invades dermis, lamina propria, or dartos fascia
	Shaft: Tumor invades connective tissue between epidermis and corpora regardless of location
	All sites with or without lymphovascular invasion or perineural invasion and is or is not high grade
T1a	Tumor is without lymphovascular invasion or perineural invasion and is not high grade (i.e., grade 3 or sarcomatoid)
T1b	Tumor exhibits lymphovascular invasion and/or perineural invasion or is high grade (i.e., grade 3 or sarcomatoid)
T2	Tumor invades into corpus spongiosum (either glans or ventral shaft) with or without urethral invasion
T3	Tumor invades into corpora cavernosum (including tunica albuginea) with or without urethral invasion.
T4	Tumor invades other adjacent structures (i.e., scrotum, prostate, pubic bone)

Regional Lymph Nodes (N)[a]

Clinical N (cN)

cN Category	cN Criteria
cNX	Regional lymph nodes cannot be assessed
cN0	No palpable or visibly enlarged inguinal lymph nodes
cN1	Palpable mobile unilateral inguinal lymph node
cN2	Palpable mobile ≥2 unilateral inguinal nodes or bilateral inguinal lymph nodes
cN3	Palpable fixed inguinal nodal mass or pelvic lymphadenopathy unilateral or bilateral

Clinical N (pN)

pN Category	pN Criteria
pNX	Lymph node metastases cannot be established
pN0	No lymph node metastasis
pN1	≤2 unilateral inguinal metastases; no ENE
pN2	≥3 unilateral inguinal metastases or bilateral inguinal metastases
pN3	ENE of lymph node metastases or pelvic lymph node metastases

M Category	M criteria
M0	No distant metastasis
M1	Distant metastasis present

AJCC Prognostic Stage Groups

0is	Tis	N0	M0
0a	Ta	N0	M0
I	T1a	N0	M0
IIA	T1b or T2	N0	M0
IIB	T3	N0	M0
IIIA	T1–T3	N1	M0
IIIB	T1–T3	N2	M0
IV	T4	Any N	M0
	Any T	N3	M0
	Any T	Any N	M1

Histologic grade (G)

GX	Grade cannot be assessed
G1	Well differentiated
G2	Moderately differentiated
G3	Poorly differentiated/high grade

[a]The regional lymph nodes are as follows: superficial and deep inguinal lymph nodes, pelvic nodes (NOS), and pelvic nodes (specified): external iliac, internal iliac (also called hypogastric), and obturator. From AJCC. Penis. In: Amin MB, Edge SB, Greene FL, et al., eds. *AJCC cancer staging manual.* 8th ed. New York: Springer, 2017:701–714. Reproduced with permission of Springer International Publishing in the format Book via Copyright Clearance Center.

TABLE 72.4 2017 URETHRA CANCER TNM STAGING AJCC UICC

Male Penile Urethra and Female Urethra

T category	T Criteria
TX	Primary tumor cannot be assessed
T0	No evidence of primary tumor
Ta	Noninvasive papillary carcinoma
Tis	Carcinoma in situ
T1	Tumor invades subepithelial connective tissue
T2	Tumor invades any of the following: corpus spongiosum, periurethral muscle
T3	Tumor invades any of the following: corpus cavernosum, anterior vagina
T4	Tumor invades other adjacent organs (e.g., invasion of the bladder wall)

Prostatic Urethra

T category	T Criteria
Tis	Carcinoma in situ involving the prostatic urethra or periurethral or prostatic ducts without stromal invasion
T1	Tumor invades urethral subepithelial connective tissue immediately underlying the urothelium
T2	Tumor invades the prostatic stroma surrounding ducts either by direct extension from the urothelial surface or by invasion from prostatic ducts
T3	Tumor invades the periprostatic fat
T4	Tumor invades other adjacent organs (e.g., extraprostatic invasion of the bladder wall, rectal wall)

N Category	N Criteria
NX	Regional lymph nodes cannot be assessed
N0	No regional lymph node metastasis
N1	Single regional node metastasis in the inguinal region or true pelvis (perivesical, obturator, internal [hypogastric] and external iliac), or presacral lymph node
N2	Multiple regional lymph node metastasis in the inguinal region or true pelvis (perivesical, obturator, internal [hypogastric] and external iliac) or presacral lymph node

M Category	M criteria
M0	No distant metastasis
M1	Distant metastasis

AJCC Prognostic Stage Groups

0is	Tis	N0	M0
0a	Ta	N0	M0
I	T1	N0	M0
II	T2	N0	M0
III	T1 or T2	N1	M0
	T3	N0 or N1	M0
IV	T4	N0 or N1	M0
	Any T	N2	M0
	Any T	Any N	M1

Histologic grade (G) Urothelial Carcinoma

LG	Low grade
HG	High grade

Squamous Cell Carcinoma and Adenocarcinoma

GX	Grade cannot be assessed
G1	Well differentiated
G2	Moderately differentiated
G3	Poorly differentiated

[a]The regional lymph nodes are as follows: superficial and deep inguinal lymph nodes, pelvic nodes (NOS), and pelvic nodes (specified): external iliac, internal iliac (also called hypogastric), and obturator. From AJCC. Urethra. In: Amin MB, Edge SB, Greene FL, et al., eds. *AJCC cancer staging manual.* 8th ed. New York: Springer, 2017:767–776. Reproduced with permission of Springer International Publishing in the format Book via Copyright Clearance Center.

of regional nodes. Radiation therapy has been recommended as palliative treatment.[45]

Soft tissue tumors are uncommon. Approximately half of the tumors are benign and may include angiomatous, neurogenous, myogenous, fibrous, and lymphoreticular tumors.[46,47] Most soft tissue tumors occur on the shaft and are malignant.

Primary lymphoma of the penis was reported in one patient with Peyronie disease, without other evidence of lymphomatous involvement. Five cases of secondary involvement of the penis by lymphoma were reported in the literature.[48]

Cancers metastatic to the penis are rare and usually represent late, advanced carcinomatosis. The most common neoplasms metastasizing to the penis are from the genitourinary organs, followed by the gastrointestinal and respiratory systems (Table 72.5). The predominant cell type is carcinoma, occurring in 202 of 219 cases.[49] Sarcomas and tumors of unknown histologic type are rare. A palpable mass, swelling,

TABLE 72.5 PRIMARY MALIGNANCIES ASSOCIATED WITH SECONDARY CANCERS OF THE PENIS IN 219 PATIENTS

Site of Primary Malignancy	Number of Patients
Genitourinary Tract	
Bladder	65
Prostate	65
Kidney	23
Testis	10
Ureter	1
Gastrointestinal Tract	
Rectum/sigmoid	34
Colon	1
Anus	1
Liver	1
Pancreas	1
Respiratory Tract	
Lungs	8
Nasopharynx	1
Other	
Lymphosarcoma/reticulum cell sarcoma	4
Bone	2
Burkitt lymphoma	1
Skin (malignant melanoma)	1

From Powell BL, Craig JB, Muss HB. Secondary malignancies of the penis and epididymis: a case report and review of the literature. *J Clin Oncol* 1985;3(1):110–116. Reprinted with permission. Copyright © 1985 American Society of Clinical Oncology. All rights reserved.

nodule, or skin change frequently occurs. Priapism as an initial presenting feature or subsequent development occurs in 40% of patients.[49]

Urethral Cancer

The histologic subtypes in the Memorial Sloan Kettering Cancer Center series of urethral cancers included squamous cell carcinoma (52%), TCC (33%), epidermoid carcinoma (11%), adenocarcinoma (2%), and anaplastic carcinoma (2%).[16] Primary malignant melanoma arising from the urethra has been reported.[50,51] The frequency of histologic type varies with site. Over 90% of carcinomas of the prostatic urethra are of transitional cell type. Adenocarcinomas occur only in the bulbomembranous urethra.

PROGNOSTIC FACTORS

Penile Cancer

The principal prognostic factors in carcinoma of the penis are extent of the primary lesion and status of the lymph nodes.[23,52] The incidence of nodal involvement is related to the size, location, and grade of the primary lesion. Invasion of deep-seated structures (corpora cavernosa) carries a high risk of deep inguinal node involvement.

A study of 212 penile cancer cases in the Netherlands showed a statistically significant difference in the 5-year disease-specific survival between the high-risk HPV-negative group (82%) and the high-risk HPV-positive group (96%).[53] In addition, p16 positivity, a surrogate for HPV infection, confers an improved prognosis and has excellent interobserver reproducibility.[54]

Tumor-free regional nodes imply an excellent (80% to 90%) long-term survival or cure.[19,28,52] Patients with involvement of the inguinal nodes fare considerably worse, and only 40% to 50% survive long term.[19,28,52,55] Pelvic lymph node involvement implies a still worse prognosis; <20% of these patients survive.[5,19,25] Gerbaulet and Lambin[56] reported the results of 109 patients with carcinoma of penis at Institut Gustave Roussy. The actuarial survival rates of patients with negative nodes were 82% at 5 years and 59% at 10 years. For patients with positive nodes, the survival rates were 36% and 18%, respectively. The number of positive lymph nodes has also been

reported to have prognostic significance. Brkovic et al.[57] reported a 5-year survival rate of 71% in patients with solitary inguinal lymph node metastasis compared with 33% in patients with multiple positive inguinal nodes.

Tumor differentiation was shown to be an important prognostic factor by Fraley et al.[58] None of 9 patients with carcinoma *in situ*, 1 of 20 with well differentiated, 5 of 13 with moderately differentiated, and 3 of 4 with poorly differentiated lesions died of their tumors. Other investigators have confirmed the prognostic significance of tumor grade.[23,52,59,60]

Carcinoma of the penis has been reported to have greater propensity to metastasize and poorer prognosis in patients younger than 50 years of age[58] and patients older than 65 years of age.[59] Soria et al.[23] reported younger age at presentation adversely affected disease-free survival, but not overall survival. Conversely, Marcial et al.[61] observed no difference in survival in relation to age.

An epithelial–mesenchymal transition (EMT) phenotype at the invasion front of squamous cell carcinoma of the penis confers a worse prognosis. EMT is a process that allows polarized epithelial cells to undergo biochemical, molecular, and morphologic changes that affect the acquisition of a mesenchymal cell phenotype with increased migration, tissue invasion, and resistance to apoptosis. A retrospective study of 149 penile cancers showed that the 10-year overall survival and cancer-specific survival (CSS) rates in patients with presence or absence of complete EMT status were 38.0% and 55.6% and 48.0% and 91.9%, respectively.[62] Activation of mTOR signaling may contribute to penile squamous cell carcinoma progression and aggressive behavior.[63] CD44 levels and patterns of expression can be considered as markers for penile squamous cell carcinoma aggressiveness and may serve as predictive markers for lymph node metastases.[64]

Predictors of cancer-specific mortality after disease recurrence in patients with squamous cell carcinoma of the penis include shorter time to disease recurrence, lymph node metastasis at the time of initial treatment, and regional recurrence.[65]

Urethral Cancer

A SEER database study of 2,065 men from 1988 to 2006 showed that advanced age, higher grade, higher T stage, systemic metastases, other histology versus TCC, and no surgery versus radical resection were predictors of death and death from disease. Adenocarcinoma was associated with a lower likelihood of death and death from disease as compared with TCC. Nodal metastasis was a predictor of death. Surgery had a better outcome than radiation for stage T2 to T4 nonmetastatic disease.[66]

Another SEER database study of 722 women from 1983 to 2008 showed that advanced age, T stage, node-positive disease, nonsquamous histologic features, and black race were associated with reduced CSS. Surgical resection was associated with a longer CSS. Black women presented with more advanced tumors and had a shorter CSS than white women.[67]

Overall prognosis in males with carcinoma of the urethra varies considerably with location of the primary lesion.[16,68–73] Distal lesions generally have a prognosis similar to that of carcinoma of the penis. Lesions of the bulbomembranous urethra are usually quite extensive and are associated with a dismal prognosis. Dalbagni et al.[16] reported a 5-year overall survival of 69% in patients with anterior tumors compared with 26% in patients with posterior tumors. Other prognostic factors included lymph node status and histology (superficial vs. invasive). A study of an international cohort of 154 patients with primary urethral cancer showed that clinical nodal stage is a critical parameter for outcomes.[74] Tumors of the prostatic urethra show prognostic features similar to those in bladder carcinoma. Superficial lesions have a good prognosis and may be managed with transurethral resection.[71] Deeply invasive tumors have a greater tendency to develop inguinal or pelvic lymph node and distant metastases.

GENERAL MANAGEMENT

Penile Cancer

General Treatment Approach

According to the NCCN Guidelines for Penile Cancer, clinical Tis, Ta, and T1 penile cancer lesions may be amenable to organ-sparing approaches like topical therapy (5-FU or imiquimod), laser therapy, glansectomy, wide local excision, and Mohs micrographic surgery. For T1 G1 to G2 tumors, interstitial brachytherapy (preferred) or external beam radiation therapy (EBRT) can be considered (category 2B). Circumcision should always precede RT to prevent radiation-related complications. For T1 G3 to G4 or T2 tumors smaller than 4 cm with negative nodes, interstitial brachytherapy and EBRT ± inguinal lymph node RT are options after circumcision. Tumors 4 cm or larger or node-positive disease that is unresectable, circumcision followed by chemoradiotherapy, and carefully selected patients may be amenable to brachytherapy. Postsurgical RT to the primary tumor site may be considered for positive margins.[75]

If the patient is unable or unwilling to undergo surgical management, prophylactic EBRT to the lymph nodes should be considered. Patients with pN2 to N3 disease, a pelvic lymph node dissection (PLND) with or without adjuvant chemotherapy or chemoradiotherapy should be considered. Definitive chemoradiotherapy is also an option. Postoperative RT or chemoRT may be considered after PLND, particularly in the setting of a positive surgical margin, viable cancer in multiple inguinal or pelvic lymph nodes, and/or extranodal extension on pathology.[75]

The International Penile Advanced Cancer Trial (InPACT; NCT02305654) sponsored by the Institute of Cancer Research (United Kingdom) will consist of two randomizations. The first randomization relates to the inguinal management has three arms: therapeutic inguinal node dissection (arm A), neoadjuvant chemotherapy followed by therapeutic inguinal node dissection (arm B), and neoadjuvant chemoradiotherapy followed by therapeutic inguinal node dissection (arm C). Patients who have a pathologic high risk defined as ≥3 nodes or extranodal spread undergo a second randomization: arm A and arm B are randomized between adjuvant chemoradiotherapy and prophylactic PLND followed by adjuvant chemoradiotherapy, and arm C is randomized between surveillance and prophylactic PLND. Neoadjuvant chemotherapy consists of up to four cycles of paclitaxel, ifosfamide, and cisplatin (TIP), and concurrent chemoradiotherapy uses cisplatin.[76]

Conservative Therapies

Treatment for carcinoma *in situ* and very small penile carcinomas includes topical imiquimod and 5-fluorouracil (5-FU).[77] For larger lesions, conservative laser surgery[78] or Mohs micrographic surgery is used.[79]

Surgery

Treatment of patients with carcinoma of the penis is generally performed in two phases: initial management of the primary tumor and later treatment of the regional lymphatics. According to the NCCN Guidelines, organ-sparing surgical interventions at the primary site may range from laser therapy, wide local excision, glansectomy, and Mohs micrographic surgery. Partial or total penectomy should be considered for high-grade primary penile tumors or tumors invading the corpora cavernosum.[75]

In very advanced proximal tumors, more aggressive resections such as total emasculation (penectomy, scrotectomy, orchiectomy) or cystoprostatectomy may be indicated. Although surgical resection is a highly effective and an expedient treatment modality in most cases, it may not be acceptable to sexually active patients. Radical surgery, especially total penectomy, may be psychologically devastating to the patient. The ideal surgical procedure removes the disease with adequate margins while preserving sexual and urinary function, although this is not always possible because of the extent of disease. The high local recurrence rates described in some reports with limited surgery[80,81] illustrate the need for careful patient selection in choosing a surgical approach.

Lesions confined to the prepuce may be treated with wide circumcision. Microsurgical techniques have shown local excision to be an acceptable and desirable option with small superficial lesions. A local control rate of 92% was achieved in 29 patients with a 5-year survival rate of 81% for stage I and 57% for stage II lesions.[82] It is possible for some patients to remain sexually active after partial penectomy. Jensen[83] reported 45% of patients with 4 to 6 cm and 25% of patients with 2 to 4 cm of penile stump could perform sexual intercourse. D'Ancona et al.[84] evaluated the quality of life in 14 patients treated with partial penectomy. Sexual function was reported to be normal or only slightly decreased in 64% of patients. Complete loss of sexual function was reported in 14% of patients.

Surgical Treatment of Inguinal Lymph Nodes

According to the NCCN Guidelines, standard or modified inguinal lymph node dissection (ILND) or DSNB is indicated in patients with high-risk features for nodal metastases: lymphovascular invasion, ≥pT1G3 or ≥T2, or >50% poorly differentiated. If DSNB is positive, then ILND is recommended. PLND should be considered at the time or following ILND in patients with ≥2 positive inguinal nodes on the ipsilateral ILND site or extranodal extension on pathology. A bilateral PLND should be considered at the time or following ILND in patients with ≥4 positive inguinal nodes total.[75]

The clinical evaluation of inguinal lymph nodes in men with cancer of the penis is unreliable. Several series have shown the sensitivity of clinical staging of the nodes to be 40% to 60% and false-negative rates to be 10% to 20%.[3,4] McDougal et al.[85] reported the correlation between clinical findings and pathologic positivity of inguinal nodes in patients with penile carcinoma. For tumors with no invasion or superficial invasion, moderately or well differentiated, only 12% of clinically enlarged inguinal nodes were pathologically positive. However, 78% to 88% of invasive or poorly differentiated tumors metastasized to inguinal nodes regardless of clinical findings. In a prospective study involving 37 patients with clinically negative groins, Solsona et al.[32] have demonstrated the predictive value of histologic grade and T stage in predicting the likelihood of occult-positive lymph nodes. Three groups were identified: low, intermediate, and high risk with an incidence of occult-positive nodes of 0%, 33%, and 83%, respectively (Table 72.6).

Radiation Therapy

The primary advantage of radiation therapy is organ preservation. According to the NCCN Guidelines for Penile Cancer, T1 to T2 tumors <4 cm can be managed with circumcision followed by brachytherapy alone (category 2B), EBRT (category 2B), or EBRT with concurrent chemotherapy (category 3) to

TABLE 72.6 T STAGE AND GRADE PREDICT THE RISK OF OCCULT-POSITIVE LYMPH NODES

Risk Group		Occult-Positive Lymph Nodes (%)
Low	Tis, T1 grade 1	0/13 (0)
Intermediate	T1 grade 2–3 T2 grade 1	4/12 (33.3)
High	T2 grade 2 T2–T3 grade 3	10/12 (83.3)

Reprinted from Solsona E, Iborra I, Rubio J, et al. Prospective validation of the association of local tumor stage and grade as a predictive factor for occult lymph node micrometastasis in patients with penile carcinoma and clinically negative inguinal lymph nodes. *J Urol* 2001;165(5):1506–1509. Copyright © 2001 American Urological Association, Inc. With permission.

a total dose of 65 to 70 Gy with conventional fractionation. Prophylactic EBRT to the inguinal lymph nodes may be considered for nonsurgical candidates or those who decline surgery.[75]

T1 to T2 tumors ≥4 cm can be managed with circumcision followed by EBRT with concurrent chemotherapy (category 3) to 45 to 50.4 Gy to a portion of or the whole penile shaft depending on the extent of the lesion plus pelvic lymph nodes, followed by a boost to the primary lesion to 60 to 70 Gy with conventional fractionation. Brachytherapy alone may be considered in select cases.[75]

T3 to T4 or N-positive tumors (surgically unresectable) can be managed with circumcision followed by 45 to 50.4 Gy to the whole penile shaft, pelvic lymph nodes, and bilateral inguinal lymph nodes followed by a boost to the primary lesion to 60 to 70 Gy with conventional fractionation.[75]

If the margins are positive following penectomy, postsurgical EBRT to 60 to 70 Gy to the primary tumor site and surgical scar is recommended. Bilateral inguinal lymph nodes and pelvic lymph nodes may be treated if no or inadequate lymph node dissection. Brachytherapy may be considered in select cases.[75]

Palliative courses of 20 Gy in 5 fractions or 30 Gy in 10 fractions are acceptable for painful metastases. A short course is unlikely effectively palliate advanced locoregional disease. If the patient's general condition permits, a more prolonged fractionation, especially with the addition of chemotherapy, such as low-dose weekly cisplatin, may produce longer-lasting benefit.[86]

Chemotherapy

The use of systemic chemotherapy as either an adjuvant or concomitantly with radiation therapy has not been fully investigated in patients with penile cancer. Modern multiagent chemotherapy regimens have overall response rates ranging from 15% to 55% in patients with advanced disease (Table 72.7). Additional clinical trials are needed to adequately define the role of chemotherapy in the management of cancer of the penis.

Preoperative paclitaxel/ifosfamide/cisplatin (TIP) can yield clinically significant responses among patients with regionally advanced penile cancer. About 50% of such patients with an objective response to chemotherapy who undergo consolidative lymphadenectomy will remain alive at 5 years.[93] Cetuximab has antitumor activity in metastatic penile cancer and may enhance the effect of cisplatin-based chemotherapy.[94]

According to the NCCN Guidelines, the preferred chemotherapy regimens are TIP and 5-FU + cisplatin (not recommended neoadjuvantly). For chemoradiotherapy, cisplatin ± 5-FU is preferred with mitomycin C + 5-FU or capecitabine (palliation) as alternatives.[75]

Urethral Cancer

The primary mode of therapy for carcinoma of the male urethra is surgical excision. According to the NCCN Guidelines, patients with clinical Tis, Ta, or T1 tumors should be managed with a transurethral resection followed by intraurethral chemotherapy or BCG in selected cases.[38]

Clinical T2 tumors of the male pendulous urethra can be managed with a distal urethrectomy or partial penectomy. Positive margins are managed with further surgery, radiotherapy, or chemoradiotherapy (preferred). Clinical T2 tumors of the male bulbar urethra are managed with urethrectomy with or without cystoprostatectomy. Subsequently, pathologic T3 to T4 or N1 to N2 tumors can be considered for adjuvant chemoradiotherapy or chemotherapy. Clinical T2 tumors of the female urethra can be treated with chemoradiotherapy or urethrectomy plus cystectomy.[38]

Clinical T3 and T4 tumors that are cN0 can receive neoadjuvant chemotherapy and consolidation with surgery or radiotherapy, chemoradiotherapy, or radiotherapy. Clinical T3 and T4 tumors that are cN1 or cN2 can be treated with radiotherapy preferably with chemotherapy (especially for squamous cell carcinoma), chemotherapy, or chemoradiotherapy followed by consideration of consolidative surgery.

Because of the rarity of this disease, comparison of the cure rates with radiation therapy or surgery is difficult. The principal advantage of radiotherapy is organ preservation. Noninvasive carcinoma of the proximal urethra can be treated with transurethral resection. In lesions of the distal urethra, results with either penectomy or radiation therapy are similar to those for carcinoma of the penis, and the 5-year survival rates are comparable (50% to 60%).[95] Involved regional lymph nodes are treated with lymphadenectomy.

Most patients, however, present with advanced invasive lesions, which are difficult to manage with either radical surgery or radiation therapy. The major problem is the high rate of local recurrence. In an attempt to improve the locoregional control rate, extended resections encompassing the inferior pubic rami, prostate, bladder, and perineum have been performed after preoperative radiation therapy.

Chemotherapy

Gheiler et al.[50] reported their experience with multimodality treatment of 21 patients (10 women, 11 men) with urethral carcinoma. Treatment consisted of cisplatin- and 5-FU-based chemotherapy for squamous cell carcinoma and concomitant external beam irradiations. Patients with TCC were treated with concomitant methotrexate, vinblastine, Adriamycin (doxorubicin), and cisplatin. Some patients underwent surgical resection following chemoradiation. With a median follow-up of 42 months, the overall disease-free survival rate was 62%. Of significance is the pathologic complete response rate of 87.5% in eight women undergoing resection following chemoradiation. Another retrospective study of 29 males with urethral cancer treated with 2 cycles of 5-fluorouracil and mitomycin C with concurrent EBRT to the genitalia, perineum, and inguinal and external iliac lymph nodes showed that 79% had a complete response to treatment, whereas the rest did not respond and died of their disease. Of the complete responders, 42% had

Author (Reference)	Agents	n	PR (%)	CR (%)	Median Survival (mo)	Fatal Toxicity (%)
Corral et al. (87)	Bleomycin Cisplatin Methotrexate	29	41	14	11.5	3.4
Di Lorenzo et al. (88)	Cisplatin 5-FU	78	32	0	8	0
Di Lorenzo et al. (89)	Paclitaxel	25	20	0	5.25	0
Hass et al. (90)	Bleomycin Cisplatin Methotrexate	40	20	12.5	7	12.5
Kattan et al. (91)	Varied (platinum based)	13	8	8	7.6	—
Pagliaro et al. (92)	Paclitaxel Ifosfamide Cisplatin	30	40	10	17.1	0

TABLE 72.7 MULTIAGENT CHEMOTHERAPY IN ADVANCED PENILE CARCINOMA

CR, complete response; PR, partial response.

disease recurrence at a median of 12.5 months. The 5-year overall, disease-specific, and disease-free survival rates were 52%, 68%, and 43%, respectively.[96]

A series of 124 patients with primary urethral cancer treated between 1993 and 2012 from 10 referral centers showed that those who received neoadjuvant chemotherapy or neoadjuvant chemoradiotherapy with adjuvant chemotherapy for cT3 and/or cN+ tumors appeared to demonstrate improved survival compared with those who underwent upfront surgery with or without adjuvant chemotherapy. Proximal tumor location correlated with an inferior 3-year relapse-free survival and overall survival.[97]

RADIATION THERAPY TECHNIQUES

Penile Cancer

If indicated, circumcision must be performed before radiation therapy is initiated. The purpose of this procedure is to minimize radiation therapy–associated morbidity: swelling, irritation of the skin, moist desquamation, and secondary infection.

Although external beam therapy has become prevalent in the treatment of the primary lesion in carcinoma of the penis, plastic molds or interstitial implants are still used.

External Beam Radiation Therapy

External beam therapy requires specially designed accessories (including bolus) necessary to achieve homogeneous dose distribution to the entire penis. Frequently, a plastic box with a central circular opening that can be fitted over the penis is used. The space between the skin and the box must be filled with tissue-equivalent material (Fig. 72.2). This box can then be treated with parallel-opposed megavoltage beams. An alternative to the box technique is the use of a water-filled container to envelop the penis while the patient is in a prone position.[98]

Another more complex device consists of a Perspex tube attached to a baseplate resting on the skin.[99] This is placed as close as possible to the base of the penis, and a flexible tube is connected to a vacuum pump. The suction effect keeps the penis in a fixed position during treatment. Appropriate bolus is placed outside the tube. The patient can also be treated in the prone position, with the penis hanging through a small hole placed in the Perspex's cylinder.

Regional lymphatics may be treated with external beam radiotherapy. Both groins should be irradiated. The fields should include inguinal *and* pelvic (external iliac and

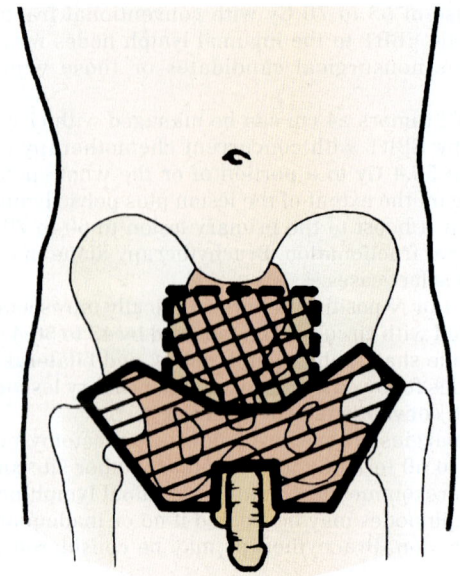

FIGURE 72.3. Portals encompassing inguinal and pelvic lymph nodes.

hypogastric) lymph nodes (Fig. 72.3). The posterior pelvis may be partially spared by anterior loading of the beams. Depending on the extent of the nodal disease and the proximity of the detectable tumor to the skin surface or the presence of skin invasion, application of a bolus to the inguinal area should be considered. Techniques such as intensity-modulated radiation therapy (IMRT) may allow for the treatment of the inguinal lymph nodes and/or pelvic lymph nodes while sparing the bladder, small and large bowel, and rectum. Primary lesions should be boosted with 2-cm margins. Treatment doses are discussed in the previous "Radiation Therapy" section.

Brachytherapy

For detailed coverage of this topic, we refer the reader to the American Brachytherapy Society-Groupe Européen de Curiethérapie-European Society of Therapeutic Radiation Oncology (ABS-GEC-ESTRO) consensus statement for penile brachytherapy. Tumors that are of clinical stage T1b or T2 and <4 cm in maximum diameter are most suitable for primary brachytherapy. Lesions confined to the glans are ideal, but those with minor extension across the coronal sulcus are also

FIGURE 72.2. A: View from above of plastic box with central cylinder for external irradiation of the penis. Patient is treated in the prone position. The penis is placed in the central cylinder, and water is used to fill the surrounding volume in the box. Depth dose is calculated at the central point of box. **B:** Lateral view.

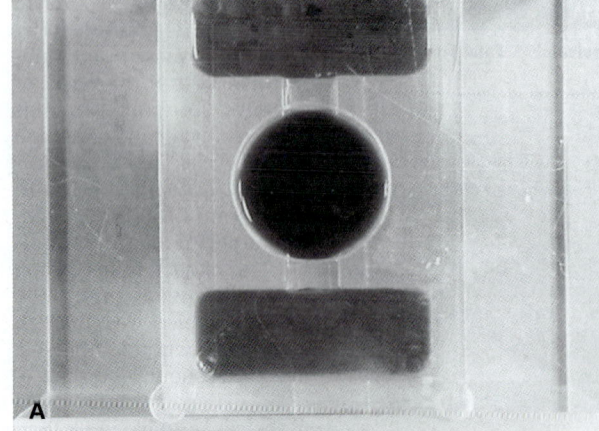

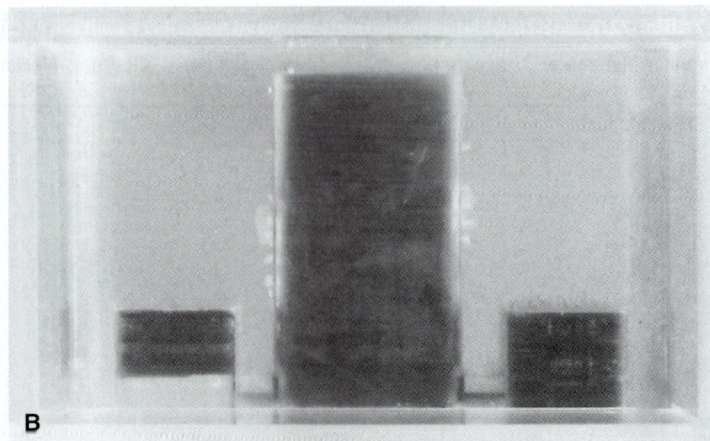

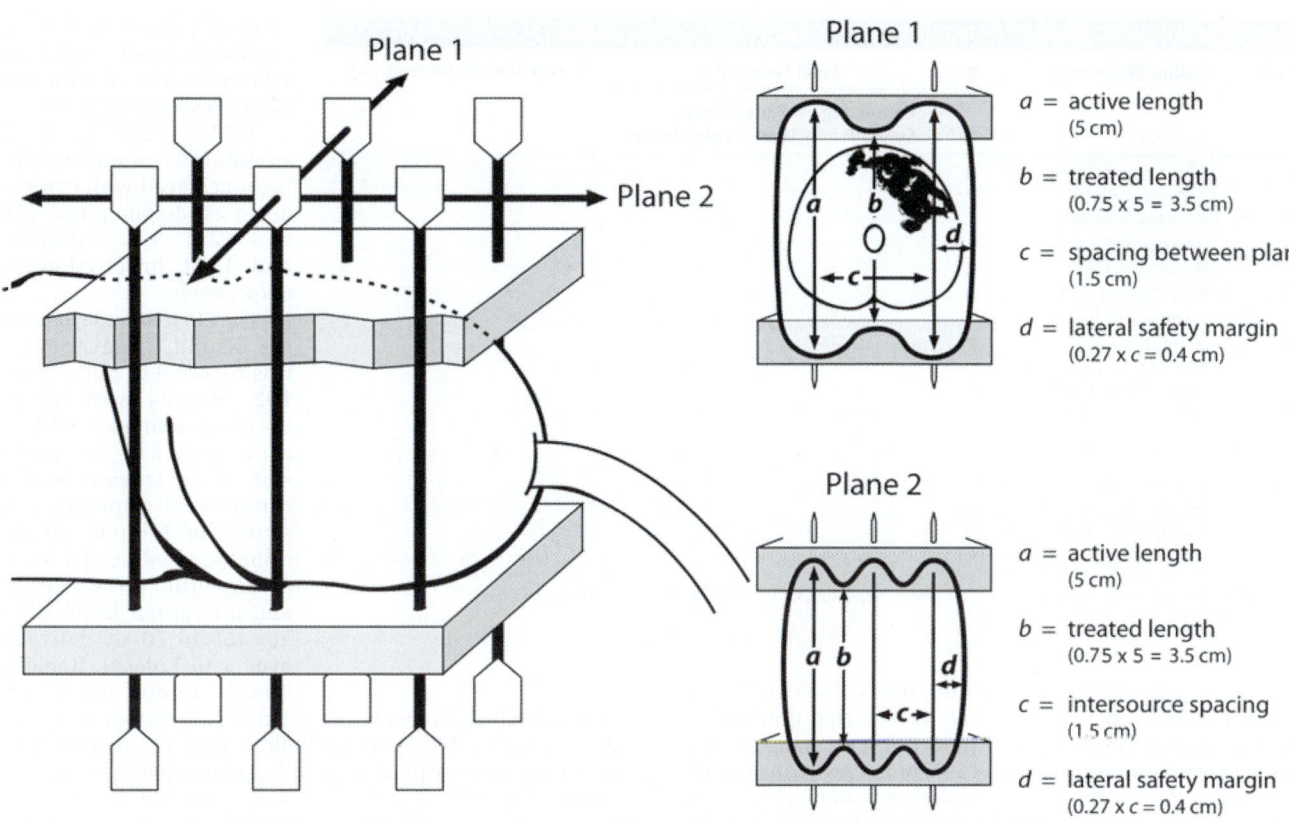

FIGURE 72.4. Schematic of a 2-plane, 6-needle implant showing the prescription isodose coverage according to the Paris System rules. (Reprinted from Crook JM, Haie-Meder C, Demanes DJ, et al. American Brachytherapy Society-Groupe Européen de Curiethérapie-European Society of Therapeutic Radiation Oncology (ABS-GEC-ESTRO) consensus statement for penile brachytherapy. *Brachytherapy* 2013;12[3]:191–198. Copyright © 2013 American Brachytherapy Society. With permission.)

suitable provided the extension can be covered with no more than one additional plane of needles.[100]

The low-dose rate (LDR) prescribed dose is generally 60 Gy at 0.5 to 0.6 Gy/h with the treatment completed in about 5 days. For pulsed dose rate (PDR) treatments, pulses equivalent to the hourly dose rate of an LDR implant are delivered every hour.

According to the Paris System, prescription for LDR and PDR is to 85% of the dose rate minima between the planes (Fig. 72.4).[100]

ABS-GEC-ESTRO experts concluded that high-dose rate (HDR) fractionation volume implants of 3.2 Gy twice daily for a total of 38.4 Gy in 6 days is well tolerated (Figs. 72.5 and 72.6). The interval between fractions should be at least 6 hours.

FIGURE 72.5. Interstitial implant showing the templates and needles in place. A layer of tissue-equivalent bolus material is seen on the left side of the photograph (patient's right) with an overlying plane of needles, to ensure that full dose is delivered to the skin surface. (Reprinted from Crook J. The role of radiotherapy in the management of penile cancer. *Curr Probl Cancer.* 2015;39[3]:158–165. Copyright © 2015 Elsevier. With permission.)

FIGURE 72.6. 3D printing can be used to make a custom mold fitted with catheters for delivery of the high-dose rate (HDR) source. This device would be applied twice per day for 5 days and is used to treat superficial cancers where no more than 5-mm depth of treatment is required. 3D, 3-dimensional. (Photo courtesy of Dr. Gerard Morton, Department of Radiation Oncology, Odette Cancer Center, University of Toronto. Reprinted from Crook J. The role of radiotherapy in the management of penile cancer. *Curr Probl Cancer* 2015;39[3]:158–165. Copyright © 2015 Elsevier. With permission.)

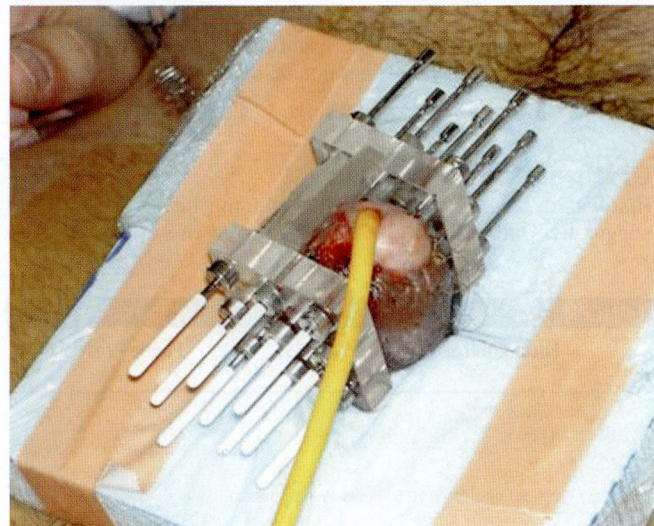

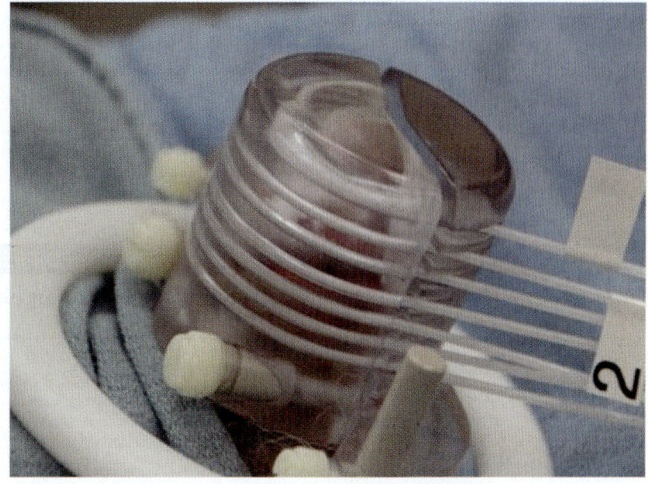

TABLE 72.8 SURGICAL RESULTS IN PATIENTS WITH CARCINOMA OF THE PENIS

T Stage	Author (Reference)	n	Local Failure (%)		5-Year Overall Survival (%)
			Conserving Surgery[a]	Partial/Total Penile Amputation	
T1	Brkovic et al. (57)	22	56	0	77
	Feldman et al. (101)	28	21	–	–
	Horenblas et al. (81)	–	10	–	–
	Lindegaard et al. (59)	41	–	–	72
T2	Brkovic et al. (57)	23	100	18	70
	Horenblas et al. (81)	–	32	–	–
	Lindegaard et al. (59)	26	–	–	55
T3/T4	Brkovic et al. (57)	6	–	–	0
	Horenblas (81)	–	100	–	–
	Lindegaard et al. (54)	6	–	–	10
T1–T3	Philippou et al. (102)	179	T1: 6.8 T2: 10.3 T3: 13.0	–	–
T1–T4	Lindegaard et al. (59)	63	35	5	–
	Derakhshani et al. (20)	42	–	–	78
	Zouhair et al. (103)[b]	16	–	25	–
	Lopes et al. (55)	145	–	–	54

[a]Includes wide excision, Mohs micrographic surgery, laser ablation, radical circumcision, partial glansectomy, and local excision.
[b]All patients treated with postoperative radiation therapy.

Penile necrosis has been observed after doses of 3.5 to 3.75 Gy × 12 Gy in 6 days, but this risk may be reduced if attention is paid to dose homogeneity and the V125 (percentage of the planning target volume receiving 125% of the prescribed dose) is <40% and the V150 is <20%. To decrease the incidence of urethral strictures, the urethra V115 should be <10% and the V90 <95% of the volume. Confluent areas of the skin receiving >125% of the prescription will reduce the risk of skin necrosis. CT-based planning is mandatory for HDR 192Ir penile brachytherapy, with three-dimensional delineation of the gross tumor volume, clinical target volume, skin, and urethra.[100]

Urethral Cancer

Radiation therapy for carcinoma of the anterior (distal) urethra is quite similar to that for carcinoma of the penis; lesions of the bulbomembranous urethra can be treated with a set of parallel-opposed fields covering the groins and the pelvis, followed by perineal and inguinal boost. Lesions of the prostatic urethra can be treated with techniques and doses similar to those used for carcinoma of the prostate.

RESULTS

Penile Cancer

At many institutions, patients with carcinoma of the penis are treated surgically. A summary of selected modern surgical series is presented in Table 72.8. Ornellas et al.[31] reported the results of 350 patients treated with surgery alone. Five-year disease-free survival was 62% for patients treated with immediate lymphadenectomy versus 8% for those treated with delayed lymphadenectomy. For all node-negative patients, 5-year disease-free survival was 87% compared with 29% for node-positive patients. Boon et al.[104] reported tumor control in

13 of 16 patients (81%) with carcinoma in situ or T1 and T2 tumors treated with wide local excision and lasers.

Tables 72.9 to 72.11 summarize tumor control rates achieved with external beam irradiation alone, LDR and PDR brachytherapy, and HDR brachytherapy, respectively.

The 20-year experience of the Institut Gustave Roussy was reported by Soria et al.[23] 102 patients with tumors <4 cm in diameter with <1 cm corpora cavernosa invasion were treated with a conservative approach consisting of limited surgery (biopsy, local excision, or therapeutic circumcision) and interstitial brachytherapy (65 to 70 Gy delivered over 5 to 7 days). Regional lymph nodes were not treated electively but were dissected in patients with clinically enlarged nodes. With a median follow-up of 111 months, local tumor recurrence rate was 25%. A regional nodal recurrence developed in 21% of patients. Disease-free survival at 5 and 10 years was 56% and 42%, respectively. Overall survival at 5 and 10 years was 63% and 50%, respectively.

Irradiation of the involved regional lymph nodes in patients with carcinoma of the penis results in permanent control and cure in a substantial proportion of patients. In the classic series of Staubitz et al.,[43] 13 patients with proven involvement of regional lymph nodes received radiation therapy to these nodes. Five of 13 (38%) survived 5 years. Mazeron et al.[111] described tumor control in 8 of 9 patients with stage T1, 21 of 27 with T2, and 10 of 14 with T3 tumors treated with ^{192}Ir, using the Paris dosimetry system, to deliver doses of 60 to 70 Gy to the 85% minimal tumor isodose. The tumor-free 5-year actuarial survival rate was 63%. The penis was preserved in 75% of patients with a follow-up of 8 years. Thirty-seven patients received no prophylactic treatment to the inguinal nodes, and only two (one with a T2 and another with a T3 lesion) later developed inguinal lymph node metastases treated by inguinal node dissection and postoperative irradiation. One patient was alive with no evidence of disease at 10 years. Five patients with metastases to the lymph nodes at the time of diagnosis were treated with therapeutic nodal dissection and postoperative irradiation. Four patients had uncontrolled lymph node metastases, and all 5 died with distant disease.

Urethral Cancer

Historically, men with urethral carcinoma have been treated surgically. Dalbagni et al.[16] have reported the outcome of 46

TABLE 72.9 RESULTS OF EXTERNAL BEAM RADIOTHERAPY FOR PENILE CANCER

References	n	Follow-Up (mo) Med (range)	Dose (Gy)	Local Control	5-Year CSS	Penile Preservation
Sarin et al.[105]	59	62 (2–269)	60/30	55%	66%	50%
Zouhair et al.[103]	23	12 (5–139)	45–74 Gy in 25–37 fxs.	41%	–	36%

CSS, cause-specific survival (© 2015 Juanita Crook; licensee X[s]).
Reprinted from Crook J. The role of radiotherapy in the management of penile cancer. *Curr Probl Cancer* 2015;39(3):158–165. Copyright © 2015 Elsevier. With permission.

TABLE 72.10 RESULTS OF LDR AND PDR BRACHYTHERAPY FOR PENILE CANCER

References	Number of Patients	Dose (Gy)	Mean Follow-Up in Mo (range)	% 5-Year Local Control (y)	% 5-Year + Cancer-Specific Survival (y)[a]	Complications	% Penile Preservation (y)
Chaudhary et al. 106	23	50	21 (4–117)	70 (8)		0% necrosis and 9% stenosis	70 (8)
de Crevoisier et al. 107	144	65	68 (6–348)	80 (10)	92 (10)	26% necrosis and 29% stenosis	72 (10)
Crook et al. 108	67	60	48 (6–194)	87 (5) 72 (10)	83.6 (10)	12% necrosis and 9% stenosis	67 (10)
Delannes et al. 109	51	50–65	65 (12–144)	86 crude	85	23% necrosis and 45% stenosis	75
Kiltie et al. 110	31	63.5	61.5	81	85.4	8% necrosis and 44% stenosis	75
Mazeron et al. 111	50	60–70	36–96+	78 crude		6% necrosis and 19% stenosis	74
Rozan et al. 22	184	63	139	86	88	21% necrosis and 45% stenosis	78
Soria et al. 23	102	61–70	111	77	72	Not stated	72 (6)

[a]Corrected for intercurrent death (© 2013 Crook et al.; licensee X[100]).

Reprinted from Crook JM, Haie-Meder C, Demanes DJ, et al. American Brachytherapy Society-Groupe Européen de Curiethérapie-European Society of Therapeutic Radiation Oncology (ABS-GEC-ESTRO) consensus statement for penile brachytherapy. *Brachytherapy* 2013;12(3):191–198. Copyright © 2013 American Brachytherapy Society. With permission.

patients with carcinoma of the anterior and bulbar urethra treated at the Memorial Sloan Kettering Cancer Center. The majority of patients were treated with definitive surgery. With a median follow-up of 125 months, the local control rate was 51%. The 5-year overall survival was 42%. Improved survival was seen in patients with anterior lesions (69%) compared with those with posterior lesions (26%).

Bracken et al.[114] described results in 11 patients with tumors at or anterior to the penoscrotal junction, 8 of which were epidermoid carcinoma, 2 TCC, and 1 melanoma. Three of four patients treated with total penectomy and perineal urethrostomy had tumor control. Partial penectomy controlled the local tumor in two patients. The patient with melanoma had a local recurrence after operation. Two patients were treated with radiation therapy and a third with a combination of preoperative irradiation (45 Gy) and total penectomy. In all of these patients, tumor recurred locally. In four patients with inguinal lymph node metastases, the regional disease was controlled by bilateral lymphadenectomy. All six patients in whom local and regional tumor was controlled remain alive and disease free at 1 to 20 years. In 16 patients, the urethral tumors arose posterior to the penoscrotal junction: 13 lesions were squamous cell carcinoma, 2 transitional cell, and 1 adenocarcinoma. Penectomy was performed in five patients, all of whom had tumor control and no evidence of recurrence 5 to 29 months after therapy. Two patients treated with local excision died of disease 14 and 18 months after surgery. Irradiation was used in three patients unsuccessfully, and all died of cancer 13 to 31 months after therapy.

Kaplan et al.[17] reported on 29 patients treated at Northwestern University and reviewed the literature. In their analysis, lesions of the distal urethra carried the best prognosis and those in the bulbomembranous urethra the worst. Five-year survival rates were 22% (16 of 71 patients) with tumors in the distal urethra, 10% (10 of 99 patients) with bulbomembranous urethra lesions, and 25% (4 of 16 patients) with prostatic urethra tumors. Radiation therapy was infrequently used for these patients. Table 72.12 demonstrates equivalent local tumor control with either definitive radiation therapy or *en bloc* resection.

The combination of radiation therapy and chemotherapy using 5-FU and mitomycin C has been reported for urethral carcinoma for organ preservation in locally advanced tumors. Reports by Baskin and Turzan,[117] Johnson et al.,[118] Licht et al.,[119] and Shah et al.[120] support the efficacy of this combination for squamous cell carcinoma of the male and female urethra. Cleveland Clinic[119] reported results of patients with locally advanced squamous cell carcinoma of the urethra treated with concomitant chemoirradiation including 5-FU (1 g/m² intravenous infusion on days 1 to 4 and days 29 to 32) and mitomycin C (50 mg/m² bolus intravenous injection on day 1). External beam irradiation (30 Gy in 15 fractions) to the pelvis and inguinal lymph nodes began on day 1. An additional 20-Gy tumor boost was given. Complete response was obtained in three patients, who remained disease free after 43 months of follow-up. A patient with a T2N2M0 lesion treated with 30 Gy died of myocardial infarction several months after radiation therapy. Chemotherapy was well tolerated and required no dose reduction or delay in treatment. One grade 3 acute toxicity (skin reaction) occurred that did not compromise the therapeutic plan. One patient developed urethral stricture that was managed successfully with urethral dilatation.

As previously described in this chapter, the largest chemoradiation experience for urethral carcinoma is the Wayne

TABLE 72.11 RESULTS OF HDR BRACHYTHERAPY FOR PENILE CANCER

References	n	Follow-Up (mo) Med (range)	Dose (Gy)	Local Control	CSS (y)	Penile Preservation
Petera et al.[112]	10	20	51 Gy, 3 Gy twice daily	100%	100% (5 y)	100%
Sharma et al.[113]	14	22 (6–40)	42–45 Gy, 3 Gy twice daily	86%	83% (3 y)	93%

CSS, cause-specific survival (© 2015 Juanita Crook; licensee X[86]).

Reprinted from Crook J. The role of radiotherapy in the management of penile cancer. *Curr Probl Cancer* 2015;39(3):158–165. Copyright © 2015 Elsevier. With permission.

TABLE 72.12 LOCAL TUMOR CONTROL OF MALE URETHRAL CARCINOMA WITH RADIATION THERAPY OR *EN BLOC* RESECTION

Author (Reference)	Number of Patients	Number Controlled
Radiation Therapy		
Hopkins et al. (115)	1	1
Kaplan et al. (17)	11	9
Raghavaiah (95)	2	2
En Bloc Resection		
Anderson and McAninch (116)	2	1
Klein et al. (70)	7	5
Kaplan et al. (17)	28	25

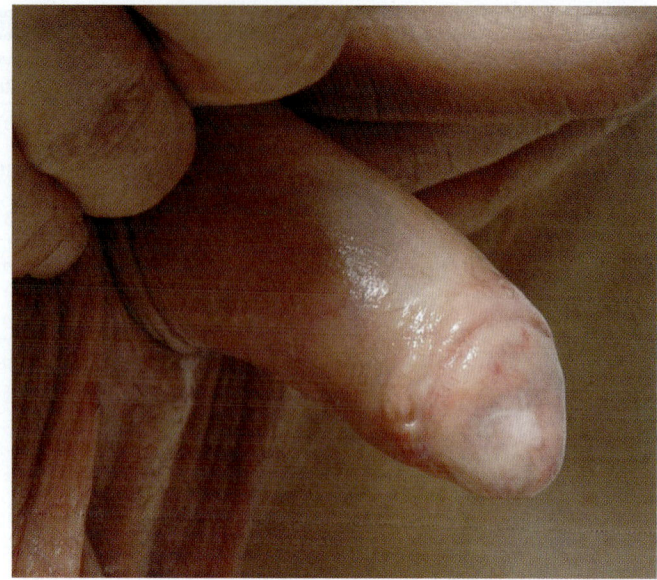

FIGURE 72.7. Telangiectasia and area of hypopigmentation 6 years after pulsed dose rate brachytherapy. (Reprinted from Crook JM, Haie-Meder C, Demanes DJ, et al. American Brachytherapy Society-Groupe Européen de Curiethérapie-European Society of Therapeutic Radiation Oncology (ABS-GEC-ESTRO) consensus statement for penile brachytherapy. *Brachytherapy* 2013;12[3]:191–198. Copyright © 2013 American Brachytherapy Society. With permission.)

State experience.[50] Concomitant 5-FU and cisplatin were used for squamous cell carcinoma, whereas concomitant methotrexate, vinblastine, doxorubicin, and cisplatin (MVAC) were used for TCC. A pathologic complete response was reported in 87.5% of women undergoing resection following chemoradiation. With a median follow-up of 42 months, the overall disease-free survival rate was 62%.

SEQUELAE OF TREATMENT

Irradiation of the penis produces a brisk erythema, dry or moist desquamation, and swelling of the subcutaneous tissue of the shaft in virtually all patients. Although quite uncomfortable, these are reversible reactions that subside with conservative treatment within a few weeks. Telangiectasia is a common late consequence of radiation therapy and is usually asymptomatic (Figs. 72.7 and 72.8).

In the reported LDR and PDR brachytherapy series, stenosis occurs in 9% to 45% of patients and necrosis in 0% to 26% of patients (see Table 72.10).[22,23,106–111] This incidence compares favorably with the incidence of urethral stricture following penectomy.[20] Most strictures following radiation therapy are at the meatus.

Lymphedema of the legs has been reported following inguinal and pelvic radiation therapy, but the role of irradiation in the development of this complication remains controversial. Many patients with this symptom have active disease in the lymphatics that may be responsible for lymphatic blockage.

Routine use of a meatal dilator in the healing phase and for a few months beyond can decrease the rate of meatal stenosis. Soft tissue ulceration is more frequent in larger and more deeply invasive cancers but will usually heal with conservative measures such as attention to hygiene, topical antibiotics, or steroid creams.[86] More severe cases may respond to a course of hyperbaric oxygen.[121]

FIGURE 72.8. A: Squamous cell carcinoma of the balanopreputial region with extension into the glands (stage I). Patient was treated with 120-kVp x-rays, 0.3-mm Cu half-value layer, receiving 60-Gy skin dose in 5 weeks. **B:** Same patient 4 years later with no evidence of disease. Telangiectasia is present.

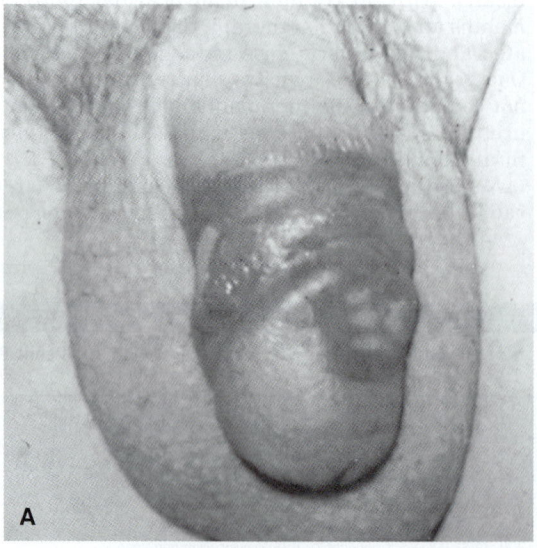

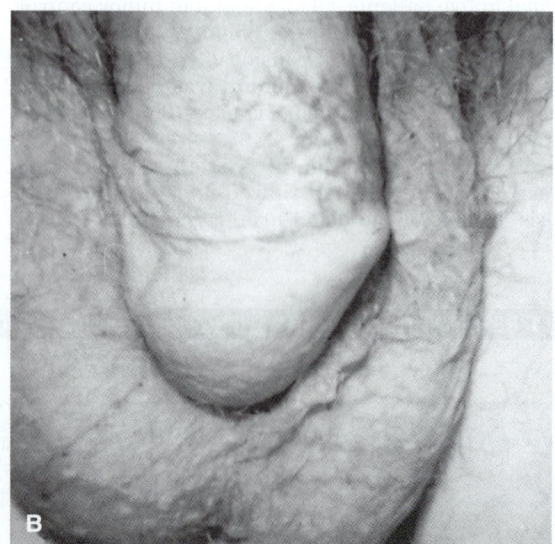

Of all male genitourinary cancers, penile cancer poses the greatest threat to sexual function and carries the most devastating psychological impact of penectomy. Despite recent advances in treatment, sexual function is not likely to be adequately preserved in some patients. These patients and their partners need information about the physical impairments after surgical intervention and should be taught adjustment skills prior to undertaking treatment. Referral to a trained sexual consultant or therapist for help is indicated.

REFERENCES

1. Senthil Kumar MP, Ananthakrishnan N, Prema V. Predicting regional lymph node metastasis in carcinoma of the penis: a comparison between fine-needle aspiration cytology, sentinel lymph node biopsy and medial inguinal lymph node biopsy. *Br J Urol* 1998;81(3):453–457.
2. Perinetti E, Crane DB, Catalona WJ. Unreliability of sentinel lymph node biopsy for staging penile carcinoma. *J Urol* 1980;124(5):734–735.
3. Persky L. Commentary: problems and management of squamous cell carcinoma of the penis. In: Whitehead E, Leiter E, eds. *Current operative urology.* Philadelphia: Harper & Row, 1984:1180–1183.
4. Catalona WJ. Modified inguinal lymphadenectomy for carcinoma of the penis with preservation of saphenous veins: technique and preliminary results. *J Urol* 1988;140(2):306–310.
5. Cabanas RM. An approach for the treatment of penile carcinoma. *Cancer* 1977;39(2):456–466.
6. Crawford E, Dawkins C. Cancer of the penis. In: Skinner D, Lieskovsky G, eds. *Diagnosis and management of genitourinary cancer.* Philadelphia: W. B. Saunders Co., 1988:549–563.
7. Siegel RL, Miller KD, Jemal A. Cancer statistics, 2017. *CA Cancer J Clin* 2017;67(1):7–30.
8. Visser O, et al. Incidence and survival of rare urogenital cancers in Europe. *Eur J Cancer* 2012;48(4):456–464.
9. Larke NL, et al. Male circumcision and penile cancer: a systematic review and meta-analysis. *Cancer Causes Control* 2011;22(8):1097–1110.
10. Christakis DA, et al. A trade-off analysis of routine newborn circumcision. *Pediatrics* 2000;105(1 Pt 3):246–249.
11. Alemany L, et al. Role of human papillomavirus in penile carcinomas worldwide. *Eur Urol* 2016;69(5):953–961.
12. Afonso LA, et al. High risk human papillomavirus infection of the foreskin in asymptomatic men and patients with phimosis. *J Urol* 2016;195(6):1784–1789.
13. Barroso LF II, Wilkin T. Human papillomavirus vaccination in males: the state of the science. *Curr Infect Dis Rep* 2011;13(2):175–181.
14. Minhas S, et al. Penile cancer—prevention and premalignant conditions. *Urology* 2010;76(2 Suppl 1):S24–S35.
15. Reis LO, et al. Female urethral carcinoma: evidences to origin from Skene's glands. *Urol Oncol* 2011;29(2):218–223.
16. Dalbagni G, et al. Male urethral carcinoma: analysis of treatment outcome. *Urology* 1999;53(6):1126–1132.
17. Kaplan GW, Bulkey GJ, Grayhack JT. Carcinoma of the male urethra. *J Urol* 1967;98(3):365–371.
18. Ekström T, Edsmyr F. Cancer of the penis; a clinical study of 229 cases. *Acta Chir Scand* 1958;115(1–2):25–45.
19. de Kernion JB, et al. Proceedings: carcinoma of the penis. *Cancer* 1973;32(5):1256–1262.
20. Derakhshani P, et al. Results and 10-year follow-up in patients with squamous cell carcinoma of the penis. *Urol Int* 1999;62(4):238–244.
21. Chaux A, et al. Metastatic tumors to the penis: a report of 17 cases and review of the literature. *Int J Surg Pathol* 2011;19(5):597–606.
22. Rozan R, et al. Interstitial brachytherapy for penile carcinoma: a multicentric survey (259 patients). *Radiother Oncol* 1995;36(2):83–93.
23. Soria JC, et al. Squamous cell carcinoma of the penis: multivariate analysis of prognostic factors and natural history in monocentric study with a conservative policy. *Ann Oncol* 1997;8(11):1089–1098.
24. Haddad FS. Re: cavernosography in diagnosis of metastatic tumors of the penis: 5 new cases and a review of the literature. *J Urol* 1989;141(4):959–960.
25. Hardner GJ, et al. Carcinoma of the penis: analysis of therapy in 100 consecutive cases. *J Urol* 1972;108(3):428–430.
26. Narayana AS, et al. Carcinoma of the penis: analysis of 219 cases. *Cancer* 1982;49(10):2185–2191.
27. Gursel EO, et al. Penile cancer. *Urology* 1973;1(6):569–578.
28. Skinner DG, Leadbetter WF, Kelley SB. The surgical management of squamous cell carcinoma of the penis. *J Urol* 1972;107(2):273–277.
29. Derrick FC Jr, et al. Epidermoid carcinoma of the penis: computer analysis of 87 cases. *J Urol* 1973;110(3):303–305.
30. Grabstald H, Kelley CD. Radiation therapy of penile cancer: six to ten-year follow-up. *Urology* 1980;15(6):575–576.
31. Ornellas AA, et al. Surgical treatment of invasive squamous cell carcinoma of the penis: retrospective analysis of 350 cases. *J Urol* 1994;151(5):1244–1249.
32. Solsona E, et al. Prospective validation of the association of local tumor stage and grade as a predictive factor for occult lymph node micrometastasis in patients with penile carcinoma and clinically negative inguinal lymph nodes. *J Urol* 2001;165(5):1506–1509.
33. Stewart SB, Leder RA, Inman BA. Imaging tumors of the penis and urethra. *Urol Clin North Am* 2010;37(3):353–367.
34. Graafland NM, et al. Identification of high risk pathological node positive penile carcinoma: value of preoperative computerized tomography imaging. *J Urol* 2011;185(3):881–887.
35. Lützen U, et al. 10-Year experience regarding the reliability and morbidity of radio guided lymph node biopsy in penile cancer patients and the associated radiation exposure of medical staff in this procedure. *BMC Urol* 2016;16(1):47.
36. Schlenker B, et al. Detection of inguinal lymph node involvement in penile squamous cell carcinoma by 18F-fluorodeoxyglucose PET/CT: a prospective single-center study. *Urol Oncol* 2012;30(1):55–59.
37. Graafland NM, et al. Scanning with 18F-FDG-PET/CT for detection of pelvic nodal involvement in inguinal node-positive penile carcinoma. *Eur Urol* 2009;56(2):339–345.
38. Bladder Cancer. *NCCN Clinical Practice Guidelines in Oncology 2017 [cited 2017 4/20/2017]; Version 2.2017.* Available at: https://www.nccn.org/professionals/physician_gls/pdf/bladder.pdf
39. American Joint Committee on Cancer. In: *AJCC cancer staging handbook.* Chicago, IL: AJCC, 2010.
40. Cancer, I.A.f.R.o. *WHO classification of tumours of the urinary system and male genital organs.* 4th ed. IARC WHO Classification of Tumours, 2016.
41. Hakenberg OW, et al. EAU guidelines on penile cancer: 2014 update. *Eur Urol* 2015;67(1):142–150.
42. Barnes RD, et al. Carcinoma of the penis—the Groote Schuur Hospital experience. *J R Coll Surg Edinb* 1989;34(1):44–46.
43. Staubitz WJ, Lent MH, Oberkircher OJ. Carcinoma of the penis. *Cancer* 1955;8(2):371–378.
44. Graham JH, Helwig EB. Erythroplasia of Queyrat. A clinicopathologic and histochemical study. *Cancer* 1973;32(6):1396–1414.
45. Mikhail GR. Cancers, precancers, and pseudocancers on the male genitalia. A review of clinical appearances, histopathology, and management. *J Dermatol Surg Oncol* 1980;6(12):1027–1035.
46. Dehner LP, Smith BH. Soft tissue tumors of the penis. A clinicopathologic study of 46 cases. *Cancer* 1970;25(6):1431–1447.
47. Macaluso JN Jr, Sullivan JW, Tomberlin S. Glomus tumor of glans penis. *Urology* 1985;25(4):409–410.
48. Yu GS, Nseyo UO, Carson JW. Primary penile lymphoma in a patient with Peyronie's disease. *J Urol* 1989;142(4):1076–1077.
49. Powell BL, Craig JB, Muss HB. Secondary malignancies of the penis and epididymis: a case report and review of the literature. *J Clin Oncol* 1985;3(1):110–116.
50. Gheiler EL, et al. Management of primary urethral cancer. *Urology* 1998;52(3):487–493.
51. Oliva E, et al. Primary malignant melanoma of the urethra: a clinicopathologic analysis of 15 cases. *Am J Surg Pathol* 2000;24(6):785–796.
52. Villavicencio H, et al. Grade, local stage and growth pattern as prognostic factors in carcinoma of the penis. *Eur Urol* 1997;32(4):442–447.
53. Djajadiningrat RS, et al. Human papillomavirus prevalence in invasive penile cancer and association with clinical outcome. *J Urol* 2015;193(2):526–531.
54. Gunia S, et al. p16(INK4a) is a marker of good prognosis for primary invasive penile squamous cell carcinoma: a multi-institutional study. *J Urol* 2012;187(3):899–907.
55. Lopes A, et al. Prognostic factors in carcinoma of the penis: multivariate analysis of 145 patients treated with amputation and lymphadenectomy. *J Urol* 1996;156(5):1637–1642.
56. Gerbaulet A, Lambin P. Radiation therapy of cancer of the penis. Indications, advantages, and pitfalls. *Urol Clin North Am* 1992;19(2):325–332.
57. Brkovic D, et al. Surgical treatment of invasive penile cancer—the Heidelberg experience from 1968 to 1994. *Eur Urol* 1997;31(3):339–342.
58. Fraley EE, et al. Cancer of the penis. Prognosis and treatment plans. *Cancer* 1985;55(7):1618–1624.
59. Lindegaard JC, et al. A retrospective analysis of 82 cases of cancer of the penis. *Br J Urol* 1996;77(6):883–890.
60. Salaverria JC, et al. Conservative treatment of carcinoma of the penis. *Br J Urol* 1979;51(1):32–37.
61. Marcial VA, et al. Carcinoma of the penis. *Radiology* 1962;79:209–220.
62. da Cunha IW, et al. Epithelial-mesenchymal transition (EMT) phenotype at invasion front of squamous cell carcinoma of the penis influences oncological outcomes. *Urol Oncol* 2016;34(10):433.e19–433.e26.
63. Ferrandiz-Pulido C, et al. mTOR signaling pathway in penile squamous cell carcinoma: pmTOR and peIF4E over expression correlate with aggressive tumor behavior. *J Urol* 2013;190(6):2288–2295.
64. Minardi D, et al. Prognostic value of CD44 expression in penile squamous cell carcinoma: a pilot study. *Cell Oncol* 2012;35(5):377–384.
65. Rieken M, et al. Predictors of cancer-specific mortality after disease recurrence in patients with squamous cell carcinoma of the penis. *Eur Urol* 2014;66(5):811–814.
66. Rabbani F. Prognostic factors in male urethral cancer. *Cancer* 2011;117(11):2426–2434.
67. Champ CE, et al. Prognostic factors and outcomes after definitive treatment of female urethral cancer: a population-based analysis. *Urology* 2012;80(2):374–381.

Section III

68. Grabstald H. Controversies concerning lymph node dissection for cancer of the penis. *Urol Clin North Am* 1980;7(3):793–799.

69. Kearsley JH, Roberts SJ, Kynaston B. Curative radiotherapy for stage IV carcinoma of the penis. *Med J Aust* 1986;145(9):474–475.

70. Klein FA, et al. Inferior pubic rami resection with en bloc radical excision for invasive proximal urethral carcinoma. *Cancer* 1983;51(7):1238–1242.

71. Konnak JW. Conservative management of low grade neoplasms of the male urethra: a preliminary report. *J Urol* 1980;123(2):175–177.

72. Mandler JI, Pool TL. Primary carcinoma of the male urethra. *J Urol* 1966;96(1):67–72.

73. Mullin EM, Anderson EE, Paulson DF. Carcinoma of the male urethra. *J Urol* 1974;112(5):610–613.

74. Gakis G, et al. Prognostic factors and outcomes in primary urethral cancer: results from the international collaboration on primary urethral carcinoma. *World J Urol* 2016;34(1):97–103.

75. Penile Cancer. *NCCN Clinical Practice Guidelines in Oncology 2017 [cited 2017 5/3/2017]; Version 2.2017.* Available at: https://www.nccn.org/professionals/physician_gls/pdf/penile.pdf

76. Crook J. Radiotherapy approaches for locally advanced penile cancer: neoadjuvant and adjuvant. *Curr Opin Urol* 2017;27(1):62–67.

77. Shapiro D, et al. Contemporary management of localized penile cancer. *Expert Rev Anticancer Ther* 2011;11(1):29–36.

78. Solsona E, et al. New developments in the treatment of localized penile cancer. *Urology* 2010;76(2 Suppl 1):S36–S42.

79. Salvioni R, et al. Penile cancer. *Urol Oncol* 2009;27(6):677–685.

80. Hanash KA, et al. Carcinoma of the penis: a clinicopathologic study. *J Urol* 1970;104(2):291–297.

81. Horenblas S, et al. Squamous cell carcinoma of the penis. II. Treatment of the primary tumor. *J Urol* 1992;147(6):1533–1538.

82. Mohs FE, et al. Microscopically controlled surgery in the treatment of carcinoma of the penis. *J Urol* 1985;133(6):961–966.

83. Jensen MO. Cancer of the penis in Denmark 1942 to 1962 (511 cases). *Dan Med Bull* 1977;24(2):66–72.

84. D'Ancona CA, et al. Quality of life after partial penectomy for penile carcinoma. *Urology* 1997;50(4):593–596.

85. McDougal WS, et al. Treatment of carcinoma of the penis: the case for primary lymphadenectomy. *J Urol* 1986;136(1):38–41.

86. Crook J. The role of radiotherapy in the management of penile cancer. *Curr Probl Cancer* 2015;39(3):158–165.

87. Corral DA, et al. Combination chemotherapy for metastatic or locally advanced genitourinary squamous cell carcinoma: a phase II study of methotrexate, cisplatin and bleomycin. *J Urol* 1998;160(5):1770–1774.

88. Di Lorenzo G, et al. Cisplatin and 5-fluorouracil in inoperable, stage IV squamous cell carcinoma of the penis. *BJU Int* 2012;110(11 Pt B):E661–E666.

89. Di Lorenzo G, et al. Paclitaxel in pretreated metastatic penile cancer: final results of a phase 2 study. *Eur Urol* 2011;60(6):1280–1284.

90. Haas GP, et al. Cisplatin, methotrexate and bleomycin for the treatment of carcinoma of the penis: a Southwest Oncology Group study. *J Urol* 1999;161(6):1823–1825.

91. Kattan J, et al. Penile cancer chemotherapy: twelve years' experience at Institut Gustave-Roussy. *Urology* 1993;42(5):559–562.

92. Pagliaro LC, et al. Neoadjuvant paclitaxel, ifosfamide, and cisplatin chemotherapy for metastatic penile cancer: a phase II study. *J Clin Oncol* 2010;28(24):3851–3857.

93. Dickstein RJ, et al. Prognostic factors influencing survival from regionally advanced squamous cell carcinoma of the penis after preoperative chemotherapy. *BJU Int* 2016;117(1):118–125.

94. Carthon BC, et al. Epidermal growth factor receptor-targeted therapy in locally advanced or metastatic squamous cell carcinoma of the penis. *BJU Int* 2014;113(6):871–877.

95. Raghavaiah NV. Radiotherapy in the treatment of carcinoma of the male urethra. *Cancer* 1978;41(4):1313–1316.

96. Kent M, et al. Combined chemoradiation as primary treatment for invasive male urethral cancer. *J Urol* 2015;193(2):532–537.

97. Gakis G, et al. Impact of perioperative chemotherapy on survival in patients with advanced primary urethral cancer: results of the international collaboration on primary urethral carcinoma. *Ann Oncol* 2015;26(8):1754–1759.

98. Sagerman RH, et al. External-beam irradiation of carcinoma of the penis. *Radiology* 1984;152(1):183–185.

99. Franzen L, et al. A technical device for irradiation in carcinoma of the penis. *Acta Oncol* 1987;26(1):77–78.

100. Crook JM, et al. American Brachytherapy Society-Groupe Européen de Curiethérapie-European Society of Therapeutic Radiation Oncology (ABS-GEC-ESTRO) consensus statement for penile brachytherapy. *Brachytherapy* 2013;12(3):191–198.

101. Feldman AS, McDougal WS. Long-term outcome of excisional organ sparing surgery for carcinoma of the penis. *J Urol* 2011;186(4):1303–1307.

102. Philippou P, et al. Conservative surgery for squamous cell carcinoma of the penis: resection margins and long-term oncological control. *J Urol* 2012;188(3):803–808.

103. Zouhair A, et al. Radiation therapy alone or combined surgery and radiation therapy in squamous-cell carcinoma of the penis? *Eur J Cancer* 2001;37(2):198–203.

104. Boon TA. Sapphire probe laser surgery for localized carcinoma of the penis. *Eur J Surg Oncol* 1988;14(3):193–195.

105. Sarin R, et al. Treatment results and prognostic factors in 101 men treated for squamous carcinoma of the penis. *Int J Radiat Oncol Biol Phys* 1997;38(4):713–722.

106. Chaudhary AJ, et al. Interstitial brachytherapy in carcinoma of the penis. *Strahlenther Onkol* 1999;175(1):17–20.

107. de Crevoisier R, et al. Long-term results of brachytherapy for carcinoma of the penis confined to the glans (N- or NX). *Int J Radiat Oncol Biol Phys* 2009;74(4):1150–1156.

108. Crook J, Ma C, Grimard L. Radiation therapy in the management of the primary penile tumor: an update. *World J Urol* 2009;27(2):189–196.

109. Delannes M, et al. Iridium-192 interstitial therapy for squamous cell carcinoma of the penis. *Int J Radiat Oncol Biol Phys* 1992;24(3):479–483.

110. Kiltie AE, et al. Iridium-192 implantation for node-negative carcinoma of the penis: the Cookridge Hospital experience. *Clin Oncol (R Coll Radiol)* 2000;12(1):25–31.

111. Mazeron JJ, et al. Interstitial radiation therapy for carcinoma of the penis using iridium 192 wires: the Henri Mondor experience (1970–1979). *Int J Radiat Oncol Biol Phys* 1984;10(10):1891–1895.

112. Petera J, et al. High-dose rate brachytherapy in the treatment of penile carcinoma—first experience. *Brachytherapy* 2011;10(2):136–140.

113. Sharma DN, et al. High-dose-rate interstitial brachytherapy for T1-T2-stage penile carcinoma: short-term results. *Brachytherapy* 2014;13(5):481–487.

114. Bracken RB, Henry R, Ordonez N. Primary carcinoma of the male urethra. *South Med J* 1980;73(8):1003–1005.

115. Hopkins SC, Nag SK, Soloway MS. Primary carcinoma of male urethra. *Urology* 1984;23(2):128–133.

116. Anderson KA, McAninch JW. Primary squamous cell carcinoma of anterior male urethra. *Urology* 1984;23(2):134–140.

117. Baskin LS, Turzan C. Carcinoma of male urethra: management of locally advanced disease with combined chemotherapy, radiotherapy, and penile-preserving surgery. *Urology* 1992;39(1):21–25.

118. Johnson DW, et al. Low dose combined chemotherapy/radiotherapy in the management of locally advanced urethral squamous cell carcinoma. *J Urol* 1989;141(3):615–616.

119. Licht MR, et al. Combination radiation and chemotherapy for the treatment of squamous cell carcinoma of the male and female urethra. *J Urol* 1995;153(6):1918–1920.

120. Shah AB, et al. Squamous cell cancer of female urethra. Successful treatment with chemoradiotherapy. *Urology* 1985;25(3):284–286.

121. Gomez-Iturriaga A, et al. The efficacy of hyperbaric oxygen therapy in the treatment of medically refractory soft tissue necrosis after penile brachytherapy. *Brachytherapy* 2011;10(6):491–497.

PART I
Gynecologic

CHAPTER 73
Uterine Cervix

Akila N. Viswanathan

ANATOMY

The uterus is a hollow, thick-walled, pear-shaped, muscular organ located in the pelvis above the vagina, behind the bladder, and in front of the rectum (Fig. 73.1). On average, it is approximately 7 to 8 cm long, 5 to 7 cm wide, and 2 to 3 cm thick.

The uterus is divided into the uterine corpus superiorly and the uterine cervix inferiorly, with the most superior part of the corpus also known as the fundus and the middle portion of the corpus known as the body. The fundus is located superior to the line joining the entrance of the fallopian tubes. The body

FIGURE 73.1. Anatomy of the pelvis. (Anatomical Chart Company, Lexington, SC.)

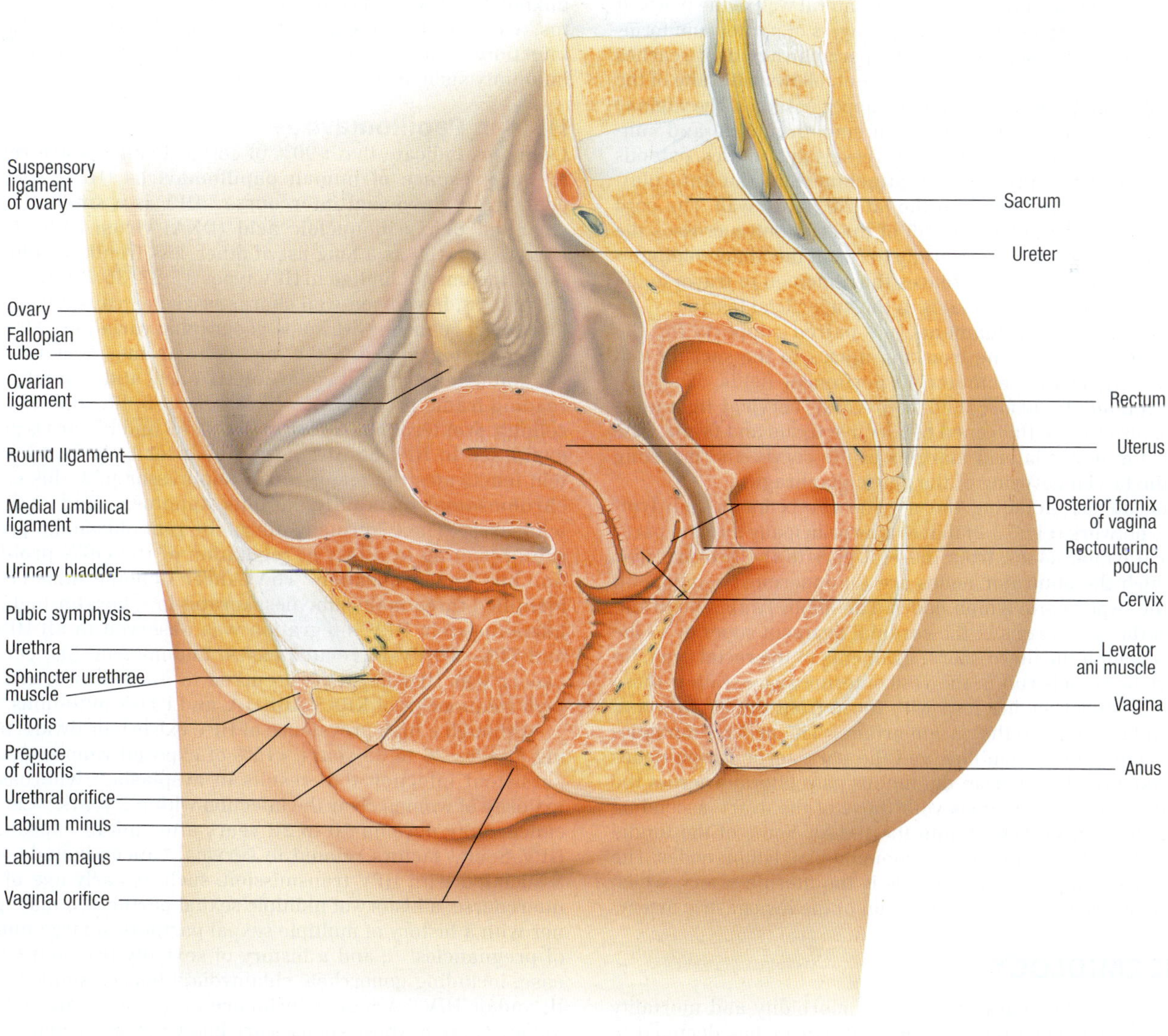

of the uterus is enclosed between layers of the broad ligament and is freely mobile. The regions of the body where the fallopian tubes enter are called the cornua. The most inferior, slightly constricted, portion of the uterus is called the isthmus or lower uterine segment (LUS). The cervix rests inferior to the LUS.

The uterus is usually bent anteriorly (anteflexed) between the cervix and the uterine body. The entire uterine cervix structure is normally bent anteriorly (anteverted) in the pelvis. The uterus may be posteriorly retroverted, especially in older women who have a small uterus. The wall of the uterus has three layers: the outer serosal layer; the middle myometrium, which is approximately 12 to 15 mm of muscle through which the main blood vessels and nerves flow; and the inner coat called the endometrium.

The cervix measures approximately 3 by 3 cm and is predominantly a fibrous organ. The cervix is divided into an upper or supravaginal portion, above the ring containing the endocervical canal, and the vaginal portion, projecting in the vaginal vault. Central in the rounded vaginal region is the external os, bounded by the anterior and posterior lips of the cervix, extending inward to the internal os, the endocervical canal, and endometrial canal.

The uterus is partially covered by peritoneum in its fundal and posterior portions; its anterior and lateral surfaces are related to the bladder and the broad ligaments, respectively. It is attached to the surrounding structures in the pelvis by two pairs of ligaments—the broad and the round ligaments. The broad ligament is a double layer of peritoneum extending from the lateral margin of the uterus to the lateral wall of the pelvis. It contains the fallopian tubes. The two layers of peritoneum forming the broad ligament enclose the parametrium as it reaches the uterus. Inferiorly, the broad ligament follows the plane of the pelvic floor and ends medially in the upper portion of the vagina.[1]

The round ligament, a band of smooth muscle and connective tissue that contains small vessels and nerves, extends forward horizontally from its attachment in the anterolateral portion of the uterus to the lateral pelvic wall. The cord ascending from the lateral wall of the true pelvis crosses the pelvic brim and extends laterally to reach the abdominoinguinal ring, through which it leaves the abdomen to traverse the inguinal canal and terminates in the superficial fascia.

The uterosacral ligaments are paired supports for the lower uterus, extending from the uterus to the sacrum and running along the rectouterine peritoneal fields.[1] The cardinal ligaments, also called transverse cervical ligaments (Mackenrodt), are thickened connective tissue and fascia arising at the upper lateral margins of the cervix and inserting into the fascial covering of the pelvic diaphragm.

The uterus including the uterine cervix has a rich lymphatic network (Fig. 73.2) that drains principally into the paracervical lymph nodes; from there, it goes to the external iliac (of which the obturator nodes are the innermost component) and the hypogastric lymph nodes. The major lymphatic drainage of the cervix runs in the cardinal ligament superior to the ureter, and in the utero-sacral ligaments to the rectal area. No lymphatic vessels run in the vesicouterine space, rather those from the upper vagina fuse with those from the bladder and extend laterally into the parametrium.[1a] The pelvic lymphatics drain into the common iliac and the para-aortic lymph nodes (PALNs). Lymphatics from the fundus pass laterally across the broad ligament continuous with those of the ovary, ascending along the ovarian vessels into the PALNs. Some of the fundal lymphatics also drain into the common iliac lymph nodes. The main artery supplying the uterus is the uterine artery, which originates from the anterior division of the hypogastric artery.

EPIDEMIOLOGY

Over the last 80 years, the relative morbidity and mortality of locally advanced invasive cervical cancer has declined in the United States and Europe because of effective screening and treatment of preinvasive lesions.[2] In the United States, 50% of women who develop cervical cancer have never been screened, and another 10% have not been screened within the previous 5 years. However, in the last decade, incidence rates of invasive carcinoma have remained relatively constant due to population growth and aging. The American Cancer Society estimates in 2018 that approximately 13,240 new cases of invasive carcinoma of the cervix arise in the United States and about 4,170 deaths will occur per year, in addition to >60,000 cases of carcinoma in situ.[3]

Worldwide, cervical cancer remains the most common gynecologic cancer and the fourth most common malignancy in women, with over 526,000 women globally developing this tumor as reported in 2015 and 239,000 dying of the disease every year.[4] Adjusting for population growth and aging, the global incidence rate for cervical cancer declined by 1.2% from 2005–2015.[4a] The majority of cases are in Africa, because of the paucity of screening measures and the prevalence of immunodeficiency because of human immunodeficiency virus (HIV). Unfortunately, it often affects young women, resulting in loss of the ability to bear future children. An economic analysis from India demonstrates the economic benefit to treating women with cervical cancer with MR-based advances.[5]

Cervical cancer is more common in areas where women have less access to screening, including parts of Asia, Africa, and Central and South America. Whether regional differences in predisposition to developing cervical cancer exist is debated because it is impossible to adequately correct for unknown and known confounders, such as socioeconomic status, access to health care, parity, smoking, presence of other infections, immune status, and other factors affecting host immunity such as nutritional status.[6]

Human Papillomavirus

Estimates indicate that >90% of cervical cancers are related to the presence of human papillomavirus (HPV) and are contracted via sexual intercourse.[7] HPV is a small, double-stranded deoxyribonucleic acid (DNA) virus; HPV-16 and HPV-18, as well as a long list of other, less frequent subtypes, including but not limited to HPV types 31, 33, 35, 39, 45, 51, 52, 56, and 58, have been well characterized as causative agents for cervical cancer, with some geographic variation.[8] The HPV genome integrates into the host cell chromosomes in cervical epithelial cells and codes for six early and two late open reading frame proteins, of which three (E5, E6, and E7) alter cellular proliferation. Two viral genes, E6 and E7, are typically expressed in HPV-positive cervical cancer cells. The E6 protein inactivates the major tumor suppressor p53; this causes chromosomal instability, inhibits apoptosis, and activates telomerase. The E7 protein affects the retinoblastoma protein (Rb), resulting in a loss of regulation of the cell's proliferation and immortalization.[9] The Cancer Genome Atlas (TCGA) identified three main subtypes: keratin-low, keratin-high, and adenoma-rich. HPV integration was observed in all HPV-18 and 76% of HPV-16 related cases. Endometrial-like cervical cancer was HPV-negative, occurred in 5% of cases, and had high frequencies of KRAS, ARID1A, and PTEN mutations.[9a]

Although a high prevalence of HPV exists worldwide, peaking at ages 25 to 35 years, <15% of exposed women develop persistent infection that results in dysplasia,[10] whereas the majority of women clear the infection within 2 years.[11] Cervical cancer may develop 10 to 20 years after initial exposure to HPV. Social factors related to cervical cancer include those associated with HPV transmission, such as early age of first intercourse; a history of multiple sexual partners; a male partner with a history of multiple sexual partners; a large number of pregnancies[12,13]; and a history of sexually transmitted disease, including gonorrhea, chlamydia,[14] herpes simplex virus II, and/or HIV.[15] A higher incidence of cervical cancer exists among women whose spouses are known or suspected to have had higher exposure to HPV[16] or whose partners have a history

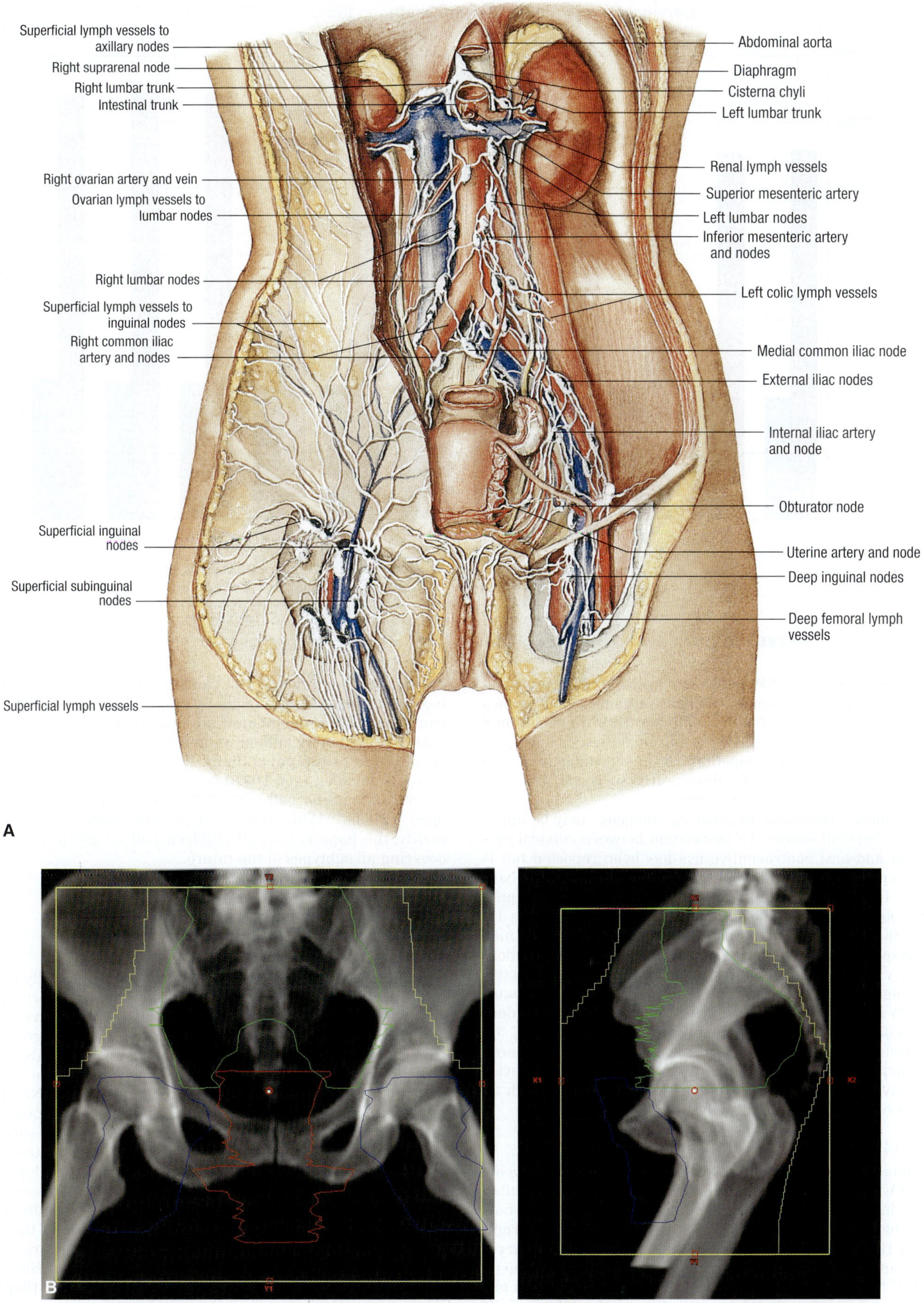

Superficial lymph vessels to axillary nodes

Right suprarenal node

Right lumbar trunk

Intestinal trunk

Right ovarian artery and vein

Ovarian lymph vessels to lumbar nodes

Right lumbar nodes

Superficial lymph vessels to inguinal nodes

Right common iliac artery and nodes

Superficial inguinal nodes

Superficial subinguinal nodes

Superficial lymph vessels

Abdominal aorta

Diaphragm

Cisterna chyli

Left lumbar trunk

Renal lymph vessels

Superior mesenteric artery

Left lumbar nodes

Inferior mesenteric artery and nodes

Left colic lymph vessels

Medial common iliac node

External iliac nodes

Internal iliac artery and node

Obturator node

Uterine artery and node

Deep inguinal nodes

Deep femoral lymph vessels

A

B

FIGURE 73.2. A: Lymph vessels and lymph nodes of the cervix and the body of the uterus. (Anatomical Chart Company, Lexington, SC.) **B:** Three-dimensional reconstruction of location of pelvic and common iliac lymph nodes outlined on CT scans in patients with carcinoma involving the distal vagina, requiring inguinal node coverage. Treatment portal is shown.

(Continued)

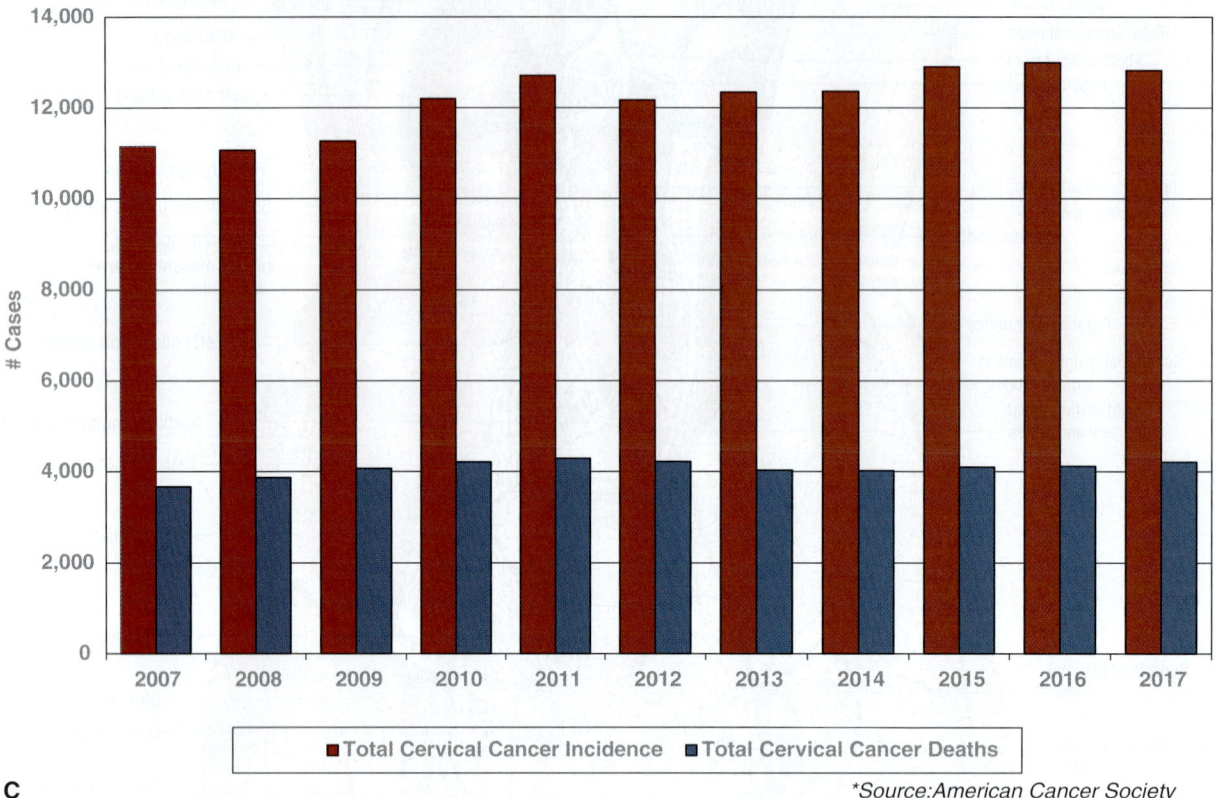

Cervical Cancer Incidence and Deaths in the USA, 2007-2017*

*Source:American Cancer Society

C

FIGURE 73.2. (*Continued*) **C:** The incidence of cervical cancer increased slightly in the United States from 2007 to 2017.

of penile carcinoma.[17,18] Whether circumcision may be protective to women is controversial[19] because circumcision may be a surrogate for unknown factors related to HPV transmission.[20] The integration pattern of HPV as episomal (best), single-copy or multiple-copy tandem repetition, or undetectable (worst) is a strong prognostic factor for disease-free survival (DFS) after radiation therapy in cervical cancer.[21]

Chemical,[22] hormonal, or other carcinogens[23] may be implicated in cervical cancer. An association between cervical carcinoma and oral contraceptive use has been reported but is considered controversial.[24] Prenatal exposure to diethylstilbestrol (DES) is linked to the development of clear cell adenocarcinoma, although the overall incidence is small (0.14 to 1.4 per 1,000 DES-exposed women).[25–27] Cigarette smoking may increase the risk of cervical cancer.[28] However, passive smoking may not be an independent factor in the absence of active smoking.[29] A review of >50 studies considers smoking a cofactor for HPV infection and carcinogenesis,[30] although one study does not confirm this.[16] Current smoking (relative risk [RR] = 1.55) and younger age at HPV exposure (RR = 1.75) are considered risk factors among HIV-positive women.[31] Intrauterine device use may decrease cervical cancer risk, potentially through an increase in cellular immunity triggered by the device.[32]

HPV Vaccination

The quadrivalent human papillomavirus recombinant vaccine for HPV types 6, 11, 16, and 18, first approved in the United States in 2006 for girls and women ages 9 to 26 years, is now available for boys ages 9 to 26 years, with the goal of eradicating HPV-related gynecologic, penile, anal, and oropharyngeal cancers. A second vaccine with strong immunogenicity to HPV types 16 and 18, approved for girls 9 to 25 years old, is more frequently administered in Europe. In 2015, results of a 9 valent HPV vaccine were reported, showing significant activity against HPV types 31, 33, 45, 52, and 58 in addition to 6, 11, 16, and 18.[33] Although its development is a major

advance in the prevention of cancer, vaccine implementation has been hindered worldwide by cost and access. To date, 64 countries have implemented national HPV vaccination programs. A total of 59 million women have received at least one dose, (1·7% of the population). In more developed regions, 33·6% of females aged 10–20 years received the full course of vaccine, compared with only 2·7% (of females in less developed regions.[33a] With an increase in understanding and availability, the hope is that all children will be given a vaccine covering all subtypes in the future.

NATURAL HISTORY AND PATTERNS OF SPREAD

Squamous cell carcinoma of the uterine cervix usually originates at the squamous columnar junction (transformation zone) of the endocervical canal and portion of the cervix.

Cellular transformation follows a stepwise progression from normal to higher levels of dysplasia. Of patients diagnosed with cervical intraepithelial neoplasia (CIN) type 1, 60% have regression of the lesion, and of those with CIN2, 40% regress. Higher levels of dysplasia are more likely to progress to cancer, particularly in the presence of cofactors such as smoking or impaired immunity. Although progression typically takes 10 to 20 years,[34] in some instances, a rapid development of carcinoma may be associated with aggressive disease.

The development of a malignant phenotype results from cells that break through the basement membrane of the epithelium and invade the cervical stroma. Invasion may result in spread to pelvic lymph nodes or other, more distant sites.[35] If the cells are detected at this stage by a Papanicolaou (Pap) or thin preparation test, appropriate minimally invasive therapy may suffice. However, if the lesion progresses, it may present as a superficial ulceration or exophytic tumor in the ectocervix or with extensive infiltration of the endocervix. If untreated, the tumor may spread to the adjacent vaginal fornices, paracervical or parametrial tissues,[36] or adjacent organs, including the bladder, the rectum, or both. Landoni et al.[37] studied 230 patients with clinical stage IB and IIA tumors treated with radical hysterectomy with pelvic lymphadenectomy and noted that the tumor spread endocervically equally in all directions. Tumor extension into the vesicocervical ligament (anterior parametrium) was noted in 23% of cases, into the uterosacral ligaments (posterior parametrium) and the rectovaginal septum in approximately 15%, and into the parametria in 28% to 34% of cases. Paracervical extension was related to the depth of stromal invasion, tumor size, lymphatic invasion, and presence of lymph node metastasis.

Approximately 10% to 30% of patients with carcinoma of the uterine cervix have extension into the LUS and the endometrial cavity.[38] Decreased survival rates and a greater incidence of distant metastases were reported by Perez et al.[38] and Chao et al.[39] in patients with stromal endometrial invasion (EI) or replacement of normal endometrium by cervical carcinoma. Regional lymphatic or hematogenous spread may occur and increases with stage, although dissemination does not always follow an orderly sequence, and occasionally, a small primary tumor may be seen infiltrating the pelvic lymph nodes, invading the bladder or rectum, or metastasizing distantly.

Both adjacent parametrial and pelvic lymph nodes may be involved. Girardi et al.[40] analyzed 359 radical hysterectomy specimens and found positive parametrial nodes in 280 patients (78%); the incidence of positive nodes was 11.4% in stage IB and 21.5% in stage IIB disease. With negative parametrial nodes, only 26% of patients had positive iliac lymph nodes, whereas 81% of patients with positive parametrial lymph nodes also had pelvic node metastases. These data underscore the need to irradiate the parametrial tissues or carry out a complete bilateral pelvic lymphadenectomy with a radical hysterectomy in patients with invasive cervical carcinoma.

Spread of carcinoma of the cervix may progress to the obturator lymph nodes, considered a medial group of the external iliac chain, to other external iliac nodes, and to the hypogastric lymph nodes. From these, there may be tumor metastasis to the common iliac or PALNs.[41] The incidence of metastasis to pelvic or PALNs for various stages of the disease is listed in Tables 73.1 and 73.2. In one study, pelvic lymph nodes were dissected in 225 patients with cervical carcinoma treated with radical hysterectomy; positive pelvic nodes were identified in 13 of 91 women (14.2%) with stage IB and IIA, 16 of 81 (19.8%) with stage IIB, and 11 of 40 (28%) with stage IIIB diseases.[56] The most commonly involved groups were the parametrial, obturator, external iliac, and common iliac nodes (Fig. 73.3). PALNs were involved in 3 of 91 patients (3.3%) with stage IB or IIA tumors 4 cm or less and in 5 of 38 patients (13.1%) with stage IIB or III disease.

Spread through the venous plexus and the paracervical veins resulting in hematogenous dissemination, though infrequent, is relatively common with more advanced stages. In an analysis of 322 patients in whom distant metastases developed, the most frequently observed metastatic sites were the

TABLE 73.1 INCIDENCE OF PELVIC NODE METASTASES IN CARCINOMA OF THE UTERINE CERVIX

Authors (Reference)	Stage I (%)	Stage II (%)	Stage III (%)
No Irradiation			
Alvarez et al.[42]	12	–	–
Delgado et al.[43]	16	–	–
Piver and Chung[44]	27	–	–
Fine et al.[45]	–	23	37
Wharton et al.[46]	38	35	33
Huang et al.[47]	24	37	–
Canton-Romero et al.[48]	11	–	–
Sentinel Node			
Gortzak-Uzan et al.[49]	17	–	–
Positron Emission Tomography/Computed Tomography			
Leblanc et al.[50]	34	16	
Postirradiation Lymphadenectomy			
Perez et al.[51]	7	–	–

Modified from Perez CA, DiSaia PJ, Knapp RC, et al. Gynecologic tumors. In: DeVita VT Jr, Hellman S, Rosenberg SA, eds. *Cancer: principles and practice of oncology*. 2nd ed. Philadelphia, PA: JB Lippincott, 1985:1013–1041. With permission.

lung (21%), PALNs (11%), abdominal cavity (8%), and supraclavicular lymph nodes (7%).[57] Bone metastases occurred in 16% of patients, most commonly to the lumbar and thoracic spine (Table 73.3). Spinal epidural compression from metastatic tumor, often involving lumbar segments, can occur rarely,[58] and metastases to the brain and the heart have been reported, although it is unusual to have spread to the brain without evidence of pulmonary metastases already present,[59] even for small cell carcinoma of the cervix.[60]

PAP SMEAR SCREENING

The American College of Obstetrics and Gynecology guidelines published in 2009[61] state that Pap smear screening should begin at age 21 years regardless of sexual activity status and continue every 2 years until age 30 years; then, if there are three normal consecutive Pap smears and no history of CIN2, CIN3, DES exposure, or HIV infection and the woman is not otherwise immunocompromised, screening should be every 3 years. The US Preventive Services Task Force and American College of Obstetricians and Gynecologists (ACOG) updated recommendations in 2012.[62] Instead of every 2 years, the recommendation is now to repeat the exam every 3 years until age 30. HPV testing is not recommended for women younger than age 30. After age 30, women have the option of having Pap smears every 3 years, of having Pap with HPV testing every 5 years. At age 65, women can stop having Pap smears as long as their routine screening was within the past 10 years, with normal results. Women who have had a hysterectomy for benign reasons and have no history of high-grade squamous intraepithelial lesion may discontinue testing. Women who have been treated for CIN2 or CIN3 need annual screening for at least 20 years. Those who have had a hysterectomy and a history of CIN2/CIN3 should continue to undergo screening with annual pelvic exams.

When obtaining the Pap smear, special attention should be directed to not using a lubricating agent (warm water on the speculum will suffice), to obtaining good "scrapings" from the cervix and vaginal posterior fornix (without blood), and to using a small brush to obtain an endocervical sample. The patient should be instructed not to cleanse with a douche

TABLE 73.2 METASTASES TO PARA-AORTIC LYMPH NODES IN CARCINOMA OF THE UTERINE CERVIX

Author (Reference)	Stage IB (%)	Stage IIA (%)	Stage IIB (%)	Stage IIIA (%)	Stage IIIB (%)	Stage IV (%)
Lagasse et al.[52]	8/143 (8)	4/22 (18)	19/58 (33)	0/3 (0)	19/61 (31)	1/4 (25)
Nelson et al.[53]	–	–	5/31 (16)	–	13/28 (46)	–
Piver et al.[54]	–	–	6/46 (13)	–	18/49 (37)	4/7 (57)
Wharton et al.[46]	0/21 (0)	0/10 (0)	10/47 (21)	–	14/42 (33)	–
Huang et al.[47]	7/89 (8)	–	12/48 (25)	–	–	–
Rutledge et al.[55]	9/177 (6)	–	–	–	–	–
Leblanc et al.[50]	2/43 (2)	1/9 (11)	5/46 (10)	–	3/13 (23)	3/10 (30)

Percentages are in parentheses.
Modified from Hoskins WJ, Perez CA, Young RC. Gynecologic tumors. In: DeVita VT Jr, Hellman S, Rosenberg SA, eds. *Cancer: principles and practice of oncology*. 3rd ed. Philadelphia, PA: JB Lippincott, 1989:1013–1041. With permission.

Section III

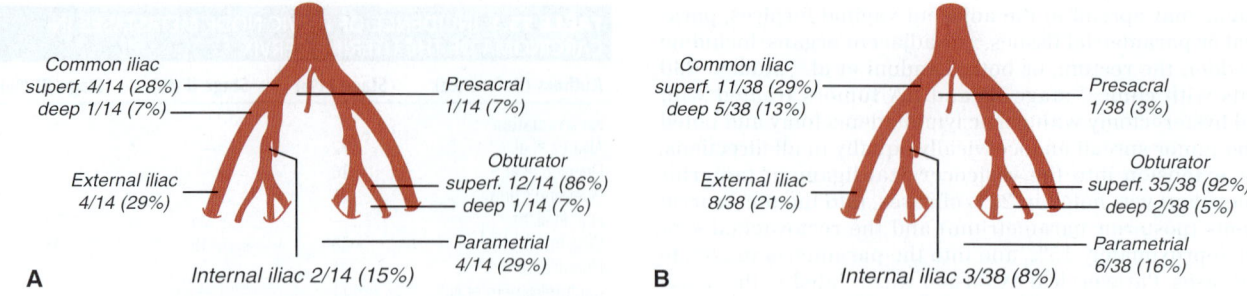

FIGURE 73.3. Distribution of pelvic node metastases in 14 patients with stage IB to IIA cervical cancers, tumor size <4 cm **(A)**, and 38 patients with locally advanced cervical cancer treated with neoadjuvant chemotherapy **(B)**. (Reprinted from Benedetti-Panici P, Maneschi F, Scambia G, et al. Lymphatic spread of cervical cancer: an anatomical and pathological study based on 225 radical hysterectomies with systematic pelvic and aortic lymphadenectomy. *Gynecol Oncol* 1996;62[1]:19–24. Copyright © 1996 Academic Press. With permission.)

before the examination, and if indicated, specimens should be obtained to check for trichomonas. If the cytologic smear shows atypia or mild dysplasia (class II), it should be repeated no sooner than 2 weeks after the initial test to allow representative cellular exfoliation to occur. Guidelines for reporting results of cervical and vaginal cytology were promulgated in 1988. The Bethesda system eliminated the classes of Pap cytology. The correlation between the cytologic diagnosis and subsequent histologic examination is >90%.[63] This system was modified in 1991 and in 2001.[64]

CLINICAL PRESENTATION

Cervical cancer in the United States is most frequently identified during routine gynecologic examination. Intraepithelial or early invasive carcinoma of the cervix may be detected by cytologic smears before symptoms appear; Pap smear, colposcopy and biopsies, and HPV testing have high specificity and sensitivity. Visible lesions present with an exophytic mass or a barrel-shaped cervix because of an endocervical lesion. Patients may present complaining of metrorrhagia (intermenstrual bleeding), menorrhagia (heavier menstrual flow), or postcoital bleeding. If chronic bleeding occurs, the patient may complain of fatigue or other symptoms related to anemia.

In cases with more advanced disease, bowel obstruction, renal failure, foul-smelling serosanguineous or yellowish vaginal discharge, pelvic pain, flank and/or leg pain, rectal bleeding, obstipation, dysuria, hematuria, or persistent edema of lower extremities because of lymphatic/venous blockade by pelvic sidewall disease may occur. Pain in the pelvis or hypogastrium may be caused by tumor necrosis or associated pelvic inflammatory disease. In patients with pain in the lumbosacral area, the possibility of PALN involvement

with extension into the lumbosacral roots or hydronephrosis should be considered.

DIAGNOSTIC WORKUP

When a patient presents with an abnormal smear or if abnormal squamous cells of undetermined significance (ASCUS) are detected but HPV status is negative, follow-up in 1 year is recommended. If the second smear reveals ASCUS, regardless of HPV status, colposcopy is recommended. When both ASCUS and HPV are present or adenocarcinoma *in situ* or a squamous intraepithelial lesion is identified, directed biopsies at the time of colposcopy should be carried out. Endocervical curettage may be performed except in pregnant women. If the biopsy results are negative, the procedure should be repeated in 6 months, and if they are positive, a conization should be performed.

Patients presenting with low-grade squamous intraepithelial lesions (LSIL) on cytology are further triaged based on age and HPV status. Women age 30 and older with LSIL and positive HPV are evaluated with colposcopy; those with LSIL and negative HPV testing are recommended to follow up in 1 year with repeat cervical and HPV cotesting rather than colposcopy. Women younger than age 30 with LSIL are managed based on cytology alone. Guidelines for management of abnormal cervical cytology in women age 21 to 24 have been revised recently, based on the higher prevalence of HPV infection and low risk of cervical cancer in this population. For younger women, ASCUS or LSIL on cervical cytology is managed with repeat cytology at 12 months.[65]

Results from a large-scale cervical cancer screening trial, conducted over a span of 15 years from Mumbai, India, were reported. Over 75,000 women were screened every 2 years using visual inspection and acetic acid vinegar. There was a significant 31% reduction in cervical cancer mortality in the screening group, compared with the control group. The 7% reduction in all-cause mortality in the screening group did not reach significance. These results suggest acetic acid screening can be utilized in places that lack standard Pap smear screening and treatment resources.[66]

Patients who present with a clinically visible lesion should be jointly evaluated by the radiation and gynecologic oncologists. After obtaining a careful clinical history and performing a general physical examination, with attention to the inguinal and supraclavicular (nodal) areas, abdomen, and liver, a careful pelvic examination should be carried out with as little discomfort to the patient as possible without compromising the thoroughness of the evaluation.[67] Pelvic examination should include inspection of the external genitalia, vagina, and uterine cervix, a rectal examination, and bimanual palpation of the pelvis. Pelvic examination under anesthesia (EUA) is a universally accepted component in the evaluation and clinical

TABLE 73.3 CARCINOMA OF THE UTERINE CERVIX (MALLINCKRODT INSTITUTE OF RADIOLOGY 1959–1986): ANATOMIC SITE OF FIRST METASTASIS

Site	Number of Patients with Distant Metastases (*n* = 322)
Lung	69 (21%)
Para-aortic nodes	37 (11%)
Abdominal cavity	26 (8%)
Supraclavicular nodes	21 (7%)
Spine	21 (7%)
Gastrointestinal tract	14 (4%)
Liver	13 (4%)
Inguinal nodes	10 (3%)
Miscellaneous	111 (35%)

Reprinted from Fagundes H, Perez CA, Grigsby PW, et al. Distant metastases after irradiation alone in carcinoma of the uterine cervix. *Int J Radiat Oncol Biol Phys* 1992;24(2):197–204. Copyright © 1992 Elsevier. With permission.

staging of patients in order to provide a pain-free examination that allows a clearer estimation of parametrial or sidewall tumor extension. In countries in which magnetic resonance imaging (MRI) is available, this may be used to assist with assessing tumor extension beyond the lower cervix, and in many institutions, it has replaced the EUA. Cystoscopy or rectosigmoidoscopy should be performed in all patients with symptoms consistent with presence of a fistula of the urinary or lower gastrointestinal tract, patients with clinical stage IIB, III, or IVA disease who cannot undergo an MRI, or patients with an MRI suspicious for bladder or bowel invasion. The diagnostic procedures for carcinoma of the cervix are presented in Table 73.4.

Conization/Loop Excision

Conization involves a conical removal of a large portion of the ectocervix and endocervix. Cold knife cone biopsy specimens should always be obtained with a scalpel or other appropriate instrument. At least 50% of the endocervical canal should be removed without compromising the internal sphincter. Curettage of the remaining endocervical canal should be carried out.

Conization must be performed in the following situations: no gross lesion of the cervix is noted and an endocervical tumor is suspected; the entire lesion cannot be seen with the colposcope; diagnosis of microinvasive carcinoma is made on biopsy; discrepancies are found between the cytologic and the histologic appearances of the lesion; or the patient is not reliable for all necessary follow-up. With careful selection of patients who have a negative positron emission tomography (PET) scan and an MRI with a central lesion <2 cm in width, knife conization with lymphadenectomy may be considered for fertility preservation. Laser conization and loop diathermy excision are frequently done in an office setting as an alternative to conization; loop excision is less expensive and more reliable than laser conization.

Biopsy

Multiple punch biopsies of a grossly visible lesion should be adequate to confirm the diagnosis of invasive carcinoma. Specimens should be obtained from any suspect area and from all four quadrants of the cervix and from any suspect areas in the vagina. It is important to obtain tissue from the periphery of the lesion with some adjoining normal tissue;

biopsy specimens from central ulcerated or necrotic areas may not be adequate for diagnosis. Dilation and curettage is not required if the biopsy confirms a diagnosis of invasive disease.

Laboratory Studies

For invasive carcinoma, patients should have the following laboratory studies: complete peripheral blood evaluation, including hemogram, white blood cell count, and differential and platelet count; blood chemistry profile, with particular attention to blood urea nitrogen and creatinine; liver function values; and urinalysis.

Imaging Studies

In countries where three-dimensional (3D) imaging is not routinely available, FIGO recommended evaluation for patients with cervical cancer includes a chest radiograph to assess for lung metastases and an intravenous pyelogram (IVP) to determine whether hydronephrosis is present. The IVP in many countries has been replaced by computed tomography (CT) scan of the pelvis and abdomen with intravenous (IV) contrast material or by PET–CT scan. In places where CT is not available, patients with stage IIB, III, and IVA diseases who have symptoms in the colon and rectum may benefit from a barium enema. A skeletal survey may be performed to determine whether bone metastases are present. Historically, pedal lymphangiography was used to assess lymph node involvement in the pelvic or para-aortic nodes with mixed results.[68,69] The number of physicians trained to perform lymphangiography has declined in the United States, and instead, PET scan is preferred.

Since the 1990s, the use of CT scanning has rapidly increased worldwide. A CT provides diagnostic information about the presence of metastases, enlarged lymph nodes, and the primary tumor. On a CT scan, the cervical tumor may be seen as an enlarged, irregular, hypoechoic cervix or as a mass with ill-defined margins. Parametrial regions appear dense when involved, and uterosacral involvement may be seen. Lymph nodes appear enlarged, with most >1 cm on axial dimension considered pathologic. The overall accuracy of CT scanning in staging cervical cancer ranges from 63% to 88%.[68,70] In the detection of lymph node abnormalities, the overall accuracy of conventional CT scanning is 77% to 85%, with sensitivity of 44% and specificity of 93%.[71]

In order to correlate radiographic and surgical findings, Camilien et al.[72] reported on 61 patients with carcinoma of the cervix who had both preoperative CT scans and exploratory laparotomy; results showed that 75% of the enlarged pelvic lymph nodes on CT contained metastases, and 97% of patients with negative nodes on CT scan had pathologically negative findings (specificity of 97%). However, histologically positive pelvic nodes were often missed on CT scan (sensitivity of 25%). The CT scan is more valuable in evaluation of the PALNs (specificity of 100% and sensitivity of 67%).

Several studies evaluated the role of CT or PET–CT with regard to para-aortic nodal detection (Table 73.5). The ACRIN6671/GOG0233 trial enrolled 109 patients with PET and pathology available; sensitivity of PET was 0.5 and for diagnostic CT was 0.42 ($P = .052$).[75] Heller et al.[76] conducted a prospective evaluation of 320 patients with stage IIB to IVA carcinomas of the cervix entered into a Gynecologic Oncology Group (GOG) protocol in which preoperative CT scan, lymphangiography, and ultrasonography of the aortic area were performed. Para-aortic node dissection was done in patients with negative staging studies. Lymphangiography, CT scan, and ultrasonography had false-negative frequencies for pelvic lymph node evaluation of 14.2%, 25%, and 30%, respectively. The sensitivity was 79% for lymphangiography, 34% for CT scan, and 19% for ultrasonography, and the specificity ratings were 73%, 96%, and 99%, respectively.

TABLE 73.4 DIAGNOSTIC WORKUP FOR CARCINOMA OF THE UTERINE CERVIX

General
History
Physical examination, including bimanual pelvic and rectal examinations

Diagnostic Procedures
Cytologic smears (Papanicolaou) if not bleeding
Colposcopy
Conization (subclinical tumor)
Punch biopsies (edge of gross tumor, four quadrants)
Dilation and curettage
Cystoscopy, rectosigmoidoscopy (stages IIB, III, and IVA)

Radiographic Studies
Standard
Chest radiography
Intravenous pyelography
Barium enema
Computed tomography
Magnetic resonance imaging
Positron emission tomography scan

Laboratory Studies
Complete blood count
Blood chemistry
Urinalysis

TABLE 73.5 COMPUTED TOMOGRAPHY AND POSITRON EMISSION TOMOGRAPHY IN THE EVALUATION OF PARA-AORTIC NODES

Author (Reference)	Number of Cases	FIGO Stage	Sensitivity (%)	Specificity (%)	Accuracy (%)
Kilcheski et al.[73]	36	I–IV	–	80	–
Camilien et al.[72]	51	IB–IIA	67	100	100
Camilien et al.[72]	10	IIB–IV	67	100	90
PET–CT					
Leblanc et al.[50]	125	IB2–IIA	33.3	94.2	–
Yildirim et al.[74]	16	IIB–IVA	50	83.3	–

FIGO, International Federation of Gynecology and Obstetrics.
Modified from Camilien L, Gordon D, Fruchter RG, et al. Predictive value of computerized tomography in the presurgical evaluation of primary carcinoma of the cervix. *Gynecol Oncol* 1988;30(2):209–215. Copyright © 1988 Elsevier. With permission.

Ultrasonography, therefore, is not reliable in preoperative detection of lymph node metastases, but it has limited value in evaluating extrauterine tumor involvement. Ultrasound (US) has a primary role in assisting with intracavitary brachytherapy applicator insertion and may detect uterine perforation, allowing for proper positioning, which is critical for adequate dosing and affects survival.[77,78] PET has a higher sensitivity than CT and higher specificity than MR in detecting bone metastases.[79]

Magnetic Resonance Imaging

MRI is frequently used for the initial assessment of the cervical tumor and of extracervical tumor extension,[80] often in lieu of an EUA. MRI is contraindicated in patients with pacemakers/ICDs, cochlear implants, metallic prostheses, metallic fragments from prior accidents, or large vascular clips. On T2-weighted images, a cervical cancer may be seen as a mass of intermediate to high signal intensity, usually of greater intensity than the fibrocervical stroma. On T1-weighted images, tumors are usually isointense with the normal cervix and may not be seen[81] but can increase in intensity with the administration of IV contrast. Abnormal, irregular cervical margins, prominent parametrial strands, exocentric parametrial enlargement, and loss of parametrial fat planes on T1-weighted images or high signal in the parametria or cardinal/uterosacral ligaments on T2-weighted images are indicative of more extensive tumors.[70,80,82] Parametrial tumor may be identified as brighter regions on T2-weighted images when compared to the low signal intensity of the cervix and uterine ligaments.

Pretreatment tumor staging and volume were assessed by EUA, transrectal ultrasonography (TRUS), and MRI in 60 patients with invasive carcinoma of the cervix.[83] TRUS and MRI assigned the same tumor stage in only 30% of patients, and EUA and MRI agreed on tumor stage in an additional 27%. In cases of disagreement, the MRI staging correlated better with outcome than TRUS or EUA. Sixty-two percent of patients with enlarged lymph nodes on pretreatment MRI either died or had tumor recurrence or metastases. MRI was superior to both TRUS and EUA in assessing the full extent of bulky tumors and lymph node enlargement.

Postema et al.[84] compared MRI with pelvic examination (including under general anesthesia in selected patients) and surgicopathologic findings in 103 patients with invasive cervical carcinoma. MRI was better at identifying extracervical tumor spread, but it had more false-positive results. The pelvic examination led to correct treatment decisions in 89% of patients. In a study by Hansen et al.,[85] clinical assessment (done according to International Federation of Gynecology and Obstetrics [FIGO] recommendations) was superior to low-field MRI with contrast enhancement in staging cervical cancer in 95 women who had both within 2 weeks after clinical diagnosis; the clinical staging correctly classified 57 patients (accuracy, 92%) compared with 52 for MRI (accuracy, 84%).

A prospective study by the American College of Radiology Imaging Network compared clinical examination, CT, and MRI.[71] MRI was significantly better than clinical examination or CT for detecting uterine body involvement or measuring tumor size,[86] but no method was accurate at evaluating the cervical stroma. MRI was significantly better[87] at detecting the tumor and parametrial involvement. MRI also somewhat increased detection of involved lymph nodes.[71]

The tumor is less likely to be as visible on MRI for adenocarcinoma cases, compared to squamous cell cancer. Haider et al.[88] evaluated 56 patients with adenocarcinoma involving the cervix using MRI and noted that 42 (75%) had a visible mass. Kodaira et al.[89] reviewed records of 84 patients with stage II cancer evaluated by MRI. The 5-year DFS rate of patients with maximal tumor size (D_{max}) of ≥50 mm was significantly lower than that for patients with $D_{max} < 50$ mm (46% vs. 88%; $P < .0001$).

Ebner et al.[90] reviewed MRI findings in 12 women with recurrent pelvic tumors and 10 with a fibrotic mass (confirmed by laparotomy or biopsy in 21 patients). They were able to differentiate between the two processes accurately in most instances. However, it is highly desirable to confirm abnormal or suspect lymph node radiographic findings with CT-guided fine-needle aspiration biopsies.

Corn et al.[91] evaluated endorectal coil MRI in 18 patients with stage IB to IIIB cervical carcinoma; in 7 patients, tumors were a higher stage by endorectal coil MRI because of proximal vaginal involvement or the combination of proximal vaginal involvement and parametrial extension. Compared with those who had a dark or intermediate signal, patients with bright signal characteristics tended to present with earlier stages, were less likely to have anemia, and were more likely to have complete response to external beam radiation.

Radiation-induced changes detected over the course of radiation may predict local recurrence and survival. Mayr et al.[92] studied 34 patients with cervical cancer of various FIGO stages who underwent 1.5-T MRI before and after radiation therapy. Tumor volumetry (3D measurements) based on T2-weighted images quantified the tumor regression rate. Sequential tumor volumetry using MR imaging may be a very effective measure of the responsiveness of cervical cancer to irradiation. MRI dynamic contrast enhancement (DCE) during the first 2 weeks of radiation therapy may provide early prediction of tumor regression rate. In seven patients, tumor regression rates ranged from 2% to 15.2% per day and correlated positively with changes in both peak and mean tumor enhancement ($P < .01$). Hatano et al.[93] evaluated MRI in 42 patients with advanced cervical cancer treated with external beam irradiation and high–dose rate (HDR) brachytherapy. In biopsies performed immediately after radiation therapy (RT), no residual cancer was found in 36 patients (86%). The simultaneous MRI study demonstrated no high signal intensity on T2-weighted images in 28 patients (75%). A high signal intensity area was observed in 14 patients, and this disappeared 3 months after RT in 8 patients with a negative biopsy. The sensitivity, specificity, and accuracy of MRI tumor response studies at 3 months after radiation therapy were 100%. MRI studies performed after 30 Gy of external beam irradiation and 3 months after all radiation therapy predicted local tumor control. Similar studies were published by Gong et al.[94] and van de Bunt et al.[95] Furthermore, MRI is useful in providing accurate target volume definition in brachytherapy treatment planning (Fig. 73.4).[96]

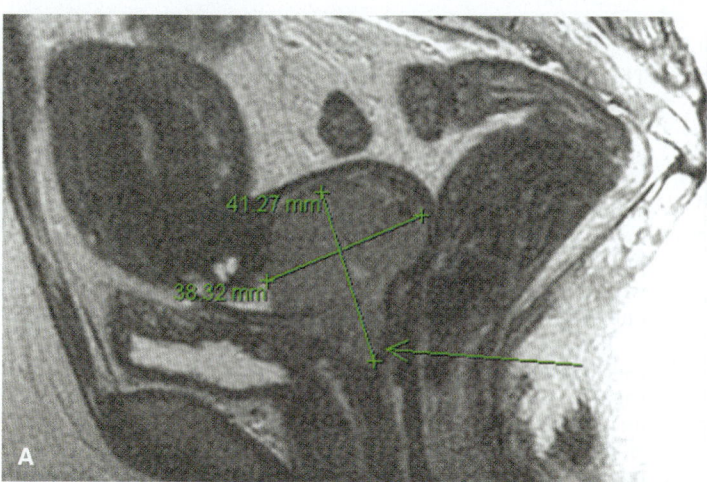
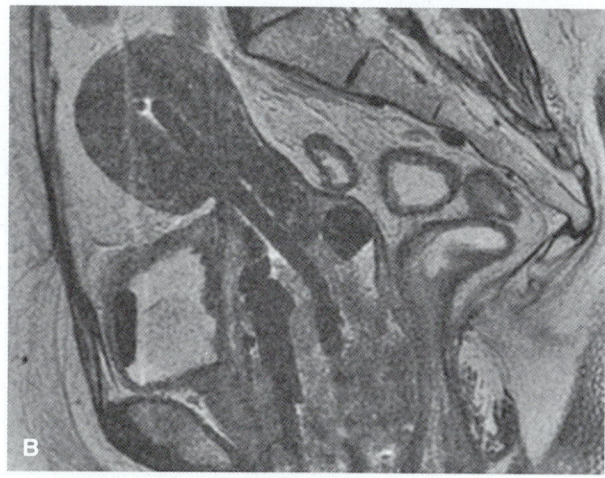

FIGURE 73.4. **A:** Magnetic resonance imaging (MRI) at diagnosis showing an enlarged cervical tumor. **B:** MRI with tandem and ring brachytherapy applicator in place showing dramatic shrinkage of the tumor after concurrent chemotherapy with external beam radiation.

Positron Emission Tomography

PET scanning is increasingly used in the evaluation of patients with malignant neoplasia, including invasive cervical cancer, using 2-[18F]-fluoro-2-deoxy-D-glucose (FDG). Rose et al.[97] observed uptake in 91% of the primary tumors in 32 patients with locally advanced carcinoma of the cervix. Squamous cell carcinoma is more often FDG avid than is adenocarcinoma. Compared with surgical staging, PET scanning had a sensitivity of 75% and a specificity of 92% in detecting para-aortic metastasis.[98] PET–CT provides highly accurate localization of focal radiotracer uptake, which significantly improves the diagnostic accuracy compared with PET or CT alone. Diagnostic PET images may be fused with simulation CT images to ensure accurate radiation dose coverage of the target and any PET-avid lymph nodes (Fig. 73.5). Care must be taken in interpretation because physiologic FDG excretion into the urinary bladder may result in false-positive assessment of the primary tumor, and ureters may be contoured as lymph nodes; therefore, tracing the ureters and complete bladder voiding prior to imaging are recommended.

Grigsby et al.[98] compared CT and FDG-PET scanning for lymph node staging in 101 patients with carcinoma of the cervix. CT demonstrated abnormally enlarged pelvic lymph nodes in 20 patients and PALNs in 7, whereas PET demonstrated abnormal FDG uptake in pelvic lymph nodes in 67, in PALNs in 21, and in supraclavicular lymph nodes in 8. The 2-year progression-free survival (PFS) rate, based solely on para-aortic lymph node status, was 64% in CT-negative and PET-negative patients, 18% in CT-negative and PET-positive patients, and 14% in CT-positive and PET-positive patients (P < .0001). The most significant prognostic factor for PFS was the presence of positive PALNs on PET imaging (P = .025). Among 76 patients with no abnormal FDG uptake, the 2-year survival rate was 86%, with persistent abnormal uptake in 40%; there were no survivors among patients who developed new sites of abnormal uptake.[99] In a follow-up study of 152 patients, the authors reported a 5-year cause-specific survival (CSS) rate of 80% in 114 patients without abnormalities on posttherapy FDG-PET versus 32% in 20 patients with persistent uptake and no survivors among 18 patients with new

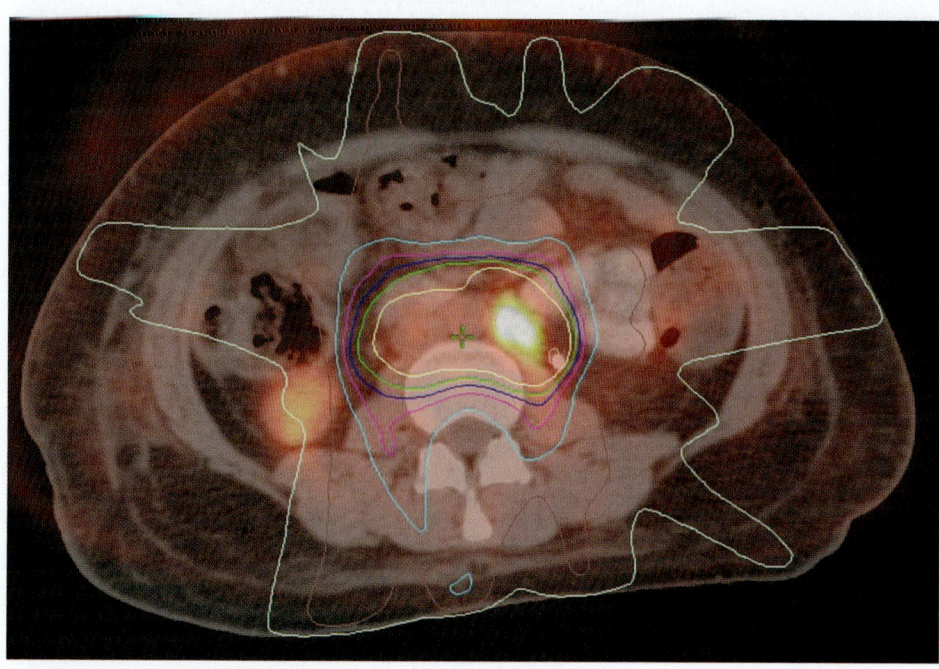

FIGURE 73.5. A fusion of a diagnostic positron emission tomography (PET) scan with simulation CT delineates the hypermetabolic lymph nodes, allowing for radiation dose escalation. In this case, the entire para-aortic chain received 45 Gy, followed by a sequential boost to the PET-avid node with a 7-mm margin to approximately 65 Gy. Caution is necessary to protect small bowel and kidneys when escalating dose to an enlarget para-aortic node.

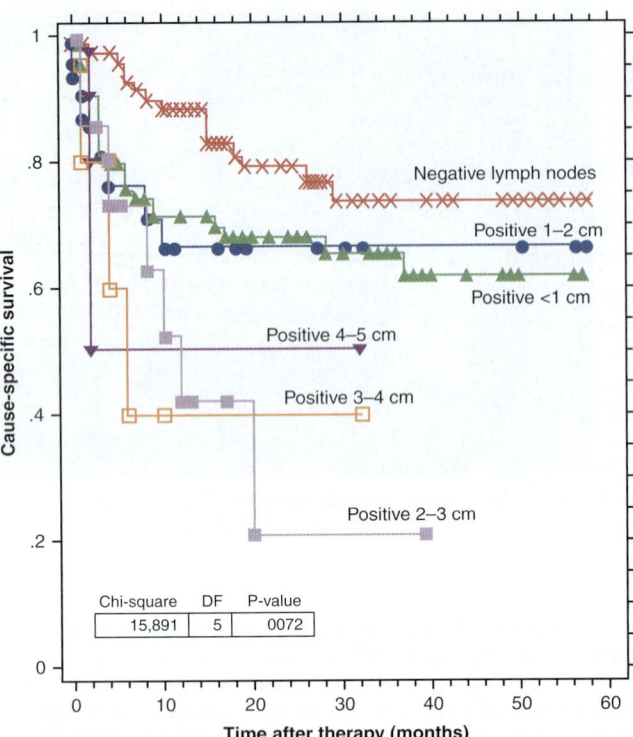

FIGURE 73.6. Cause-specific survival in patients with carcinoma of the cervix correlated with pelvic lymph node status on posttreatment 2-[924F]fluoro-2-deoxy-D-glucose/positron emission tomography. (Reprinted from Grigsby PW, Singh AK, Siegel BA, et al., Lymph node control in cervical cancer. *Int J Radiat Oncol Biol Phys* 2004;59[3]:706–712. Copyright © 2004 Elsevier. With permission.)

sites of abnormal uptake.[100] In another study, Grigsby et al.[101] noted in 208 patients a close correlation between radiation doses, number and size of positive lymph nodes, and outcome (treatment failures and survival; Fig. 73.6). Hope et al.[102] performed FDG-PET scans in 58 patients with cervical carcinoma who had an endometrial biopsy or dilation and curettage; 36 (64%) had pathologic EI. Pelvic lymph node metastasis was more commonly detected in this group than in patients without EI (70% vs. 23%; *P* < .001), as were para-aortic and supraclavicular nodal metastasis (30% vs. 0%; *P* = .006). Furthermore, 2-year survival rates were 78% versus 58%, and overall survival rates were 92% versus 65%, respectively (*P* = .047). Lin et al.,[103] using FDG-PET in 32 patients with cervical carcinoma, observed a reduction in physiologic tumor volume of 50% occurring within 20 days from the initiation of radiation therapy.

Kidd et al.[104–108] demonstrated that maximum standardized uptake value (SUV max) is an independent predictor of death from cervical cancer and is associated with persistent disease. Similarly, the SUV of the pelvic node predicts pelvic disease recurrence. Survival rates are worse with supraclavicular nodal PET positivity; PALN metastases portend a survival rate between those of pelvic node and supraclavicular positivity. The detection of supraclavicular metastases on FDG-PET at diagnosis and its relationship to clinical outcome for 186 cervical cancer patients was reported by Tran et al.[109] Fourteen patients (8%) had abnormal FDG uptake in left supraclavicular lymph nodes without palpable disease, confirmed on biopsy; six were treated with palliative intent, and seven received definitive irradiation and concurrent chemotherapy. The median overall survival was 7.5 months; all patients developed distant metastases. After external beam radiation is finished, an FDG-PET scan provides important information about posttreatment uptake and is prognostic with regard to outcome.[110–113]

STAGING

The FIGO staging system is based on clinical evaluation (inspection, palpation, colposcopy); roentgenographic examination of the chest, kidneys, and skeleton; and endocervical curettage and biopsies. Lymphangiograms, arteriograms, imaging findings, and laparoscopy or laparotomy findings should not be used for clinical staging. The 2009 FIGO staging system for cervical cancer has one modification from the previous version: Stage IIA has been divided into stage IIA1, with tumors invading into the upper vagina but ≤4 cm in size, and stage IIA2, with tumors >4 cm in size.[114]

Patients with hydronephrosis or a nonfunctioning kidney ascribed to extension of the tumor are classified as stage IIIB regardless of the pelvic findings. Other prognostic factors, such as endometrial extension of cervical carcinoma, stromal invasion, lymphatic/vascular permeation, and involvement of the lateral parametrium (as opposed to the medial parametrium) in stage IIB, are not included in the staging system. Suspected invasion of the bladder or rectum should be confirmed by biopsy. Bullous edema of the bladder and swelling of the mucosa of the rectum are not accepted as definitive criteria for staging. For a lesion to be classified as stage IIIB based on tumor extension without hydronephrosis, the tumor should extend to the lateral pelvic wall, although fixation is not required.

A parallel tumor-node-metastasis (TNM) staging system is published by the American Joint Committee on Cancer[115]; however, this system requires nodal staging, which is not feasible in many settings, and radiologic nodal information is not available to most patients with cervical cancer worldwide. The FIGO system remains the standard staging system, given the lack of 3D imaging to determine nodal status in countries with the highest incidence of cervical cancer. All histologic types should be included. When there is a disagreement regarding the staging, the earlier stage should be recorded (Table 73.6 and Fig. 73.7).

TABLE 73.6 FIGO STAGING OF CARCINOMA OF THE UTERINE CERVIX

Primary Tumor (T)	
I	Cervical carcinoma confined to the uterus (extension to the corpus should be disregarded)
IA	Preclinical invasive carcinoma, diagnosed by microscopy only
IA1	Minimal microscopic stromal invasion
IA2	Tumor with an invasive component ≤5 mm in depth taken from the base of the epithelium and ≤7 mm in horizontal spread
IB	Clinical lesions confined to the cervix or preclinical lesions greater than IA
IB1	Clinical lesions ≤4 cm in size
IB2	Clinical lesions ≤4 cm in size
II	Cervical carcinoma invades beyond the uterus but not to the pelvic wall or to the lower one-third of the vagina
IIA	Tumor in the upper two-thirds of the vagina without parametrial invasion
IIA1	Tumor in the upper two-thirds of the vagina without parametrial invasion, ≤4 cm in greatest dimension
IIA2	Tumor in the upper two-thirds of the vagina without parametrial invasion, >4 cm in greatest dimension
IIB	Tumor with parametrial invasion
III	Cervical carcinoma extends to the pelvic wall and/or involves lower one-third of the vagina and/or causes hydronephrosis or nonfunctioning kidney
IIIA	Tumor involves lower one-third of the vagina, with no extension to the pelvic wall
IIIB	Tumor extends to the pelvic wall and/or causes hydronephrosis or nonfunctioning kidney
IVA*a*	Tumor invades mucosa of the bladder or rectum and/or extends beyond the true pelvis
IVB	Distant metastasis

*a*Presence of bullous edema is not sufficient evidence to classify a tumor as T4.
FIGO, International Federation of Gynecology and Obstetrics.

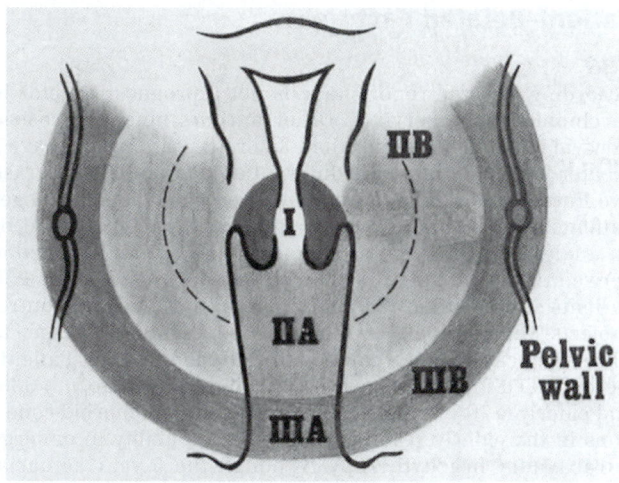

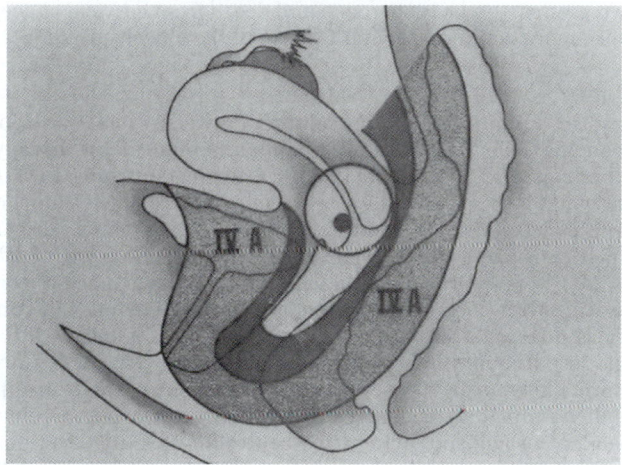

FIGURE 73.7. Diagrammatic representation of various anatomic stages of carcinoma of the uterine cervix, according to the FIGO classification. Stage IIA has been divided into stage IIA1, with tumors invading into the upper vagina but ≤4 cm in size, and stage IIA2, with tumors >4 cm in size.

PATHOLOGIC CLASSIFICATION

More than 90% of tumors are squamous cell carcinoma. Approximately 7% to 10% are classified as adenocarcinoma, and 1% to 2% are the clear cell mesonephric type. Squamous cell (or epidermoid) carcinoma is composed of cores and nests of epithelial cells arranged randomly; cells show central keratinization with pearls and sometimes necrosis. Nonkeratinizing tumors may be seen. Electron microscopy may show desmosomes and tonofilaments. Squamous cell carcinomas are divided into three types: large-cell keratinizing, nonkeratinizing, and small cell carcinomas. They are subdivided according to the degree of differentiation into well, moderately, or poorly differentiated.

Verrucous carcinoma is a variant of a very well-differentiated squamous cell carcinoma that characteristically has a tendency to recur locally but not to metastasize.[116] Mitotic activity is very low. It may be difficult to discriminate verrucous carcinoma from a giant condyloma with cytologic atypia or from a well-differentiated invasive squamous carcinoma. Microscopically, verrucous carcinoma is exophytic, with an undulating, hyperkeratotic surface; the deep margin is composed of large, bulbous masses that invade along a wide front in a "pushing" fashion.

Adenocarcinoma arises from the cylindrical mucosa of the endocervix or the mucus-secreting endocervical glands. Mucinous is the most common subtype of adenocarcinoma. This endocervical adenocarcinoma may form mucosal glands lined by high columnar cells and produce tubular folds oriented in many directions. In another subtype, cells resemble those of the intestines; the epithelium tends to be pseudostratified and may contain goblet cells. The third variant is the signet-ring cell adenocarcinoma, which is rare and usually mixed with the endocervical or intestinal patterns.

Endometrioid carcinoma is the most common cell type of endocervical adenocarcinoma; the cells resemble those of the endometrium, and the presence of intracytoplasmic mucin in some cells may be seen in a substantial proportion of tumors. The World Health Organization recommends that endometrioid or endocervical types of adenocarcinoma be graded according to their architecture, based on the degree of gland formation.[117]

Sometimes, it is difficult to differentiate a primary endocervical adenocarcinoma from an endometrial tumor. In the future, genomic analyses may provide information to guide classification. Drescher et al.[118] described a higher incidence of involvement of the uterine corpus and the regional lymph nodes in 21 patients with adenocarcinoma compared with a similar number of patients with squamous cell carcinoma. Chao et al.[119] and Contag et al.[120] described the use of microarray analysis for gene profiling (cDNA/RNA) to understand the molecular features of these tumors, which could aid in their classification. HPV has been identified in some subtypes of adenocarcinoma of the cervix.[121]

Adenoma malignum is a rare form of cervical cancer that is difficult to diagnose and often highly malignant and refractory to treatment.[122] Adenoma malignum is associated with Peutz-Jeghers syndrome and has an ominous natural history, with few reported cures.[123] Adenosquamous carcinoma is also relatively rare (2% to 5%) and consists of intermingled epithelial cell cores with squamous features and glandular structures. The squamous component is frequently nonkeratinizing. If the squamous component is benign metaplasia, the tumor is called adenoacanthoma.

Glassy-cell carcinoma (1% to 2%) is considered a poorly differentiated adenosquamous tumor; it is rare and highly malignant. Survival is poor after surgery or irradiation. Ulbright and Gersell,[124] in five cases of glassy-cell carcinoma evaluated by light and electron microscopy, described both glandular and squamous differentiation. Littman et al.[125] reported only 4 of 13 patients, the majority with stage II disease, surviving 5 years (6 had extrapelvic failures). Piura et al.[126] reported on five patients with cervical glassy-cell carcinoma, three with stage IB1 disease. All three patients were alive without disease 4, 12, and 18 months after diagnosis.

Adenoid cystic carcinoma is a rare variant of adenocarcinoma of the cervix (<1%), with an appearance similar to its counterparts in the salivary gland or the bronchial tree.[127] The tumor is composed of nests and nodules of small carcinoma cells with a few characteristic cribriform patterns. Immunohistochemical findings for type IV collagen and laminin reveal intercellular cylinders composed of basement membrane material in the solid area without a cribriform pattern. They are locally aggressive and prone to metastasize.[128]

Clear cell carcinoma (mesonephric), not related to DES exposure, comprises approximately 2% primary cervical adenocarcinomas and is believed to arise in mesonephric remnants.[26] These tumors are submucosal, composed of clear and "hobnail" cells, and may grow in a tubular, glandular, papillary, or solid pattern. They appear at any age, with one-third occurring in women younger than 30 years of age. The clear cell is characterized by a voluminous cytoplasm filled with glycogen and the hobnail cell by single-cell apical projections into the neoplastic lumina. These tumors tend to be deeply positioned, with the bulk of the lesion on the stroma forming tubular structures, diffusely infiltrating the cervical stroma.

Cervical malignant mixed Müllerian tumors, compared with their counterparts in the corpus, are more commonly confined at presentation and may have a better prognosis.

Clement et al.[129] described the clinicopathologic features with mixed Müllerian tumors of the cervix in nine patients. Gross examination revealed polypoid or pedunculated masses that invaded the cervical wall in 50% of the hysterectomy specimens. On microscopic examination, five tumors contained basaloid carcinoma or squamous cell carcinoma and four contained adenocarcinoma. In seven tumors, the sarcomatous component was homologous, usually resembling fibrosarcoma or endometrial stromal sarcoma, and two tumors contained heterologous sarcomatous elements.

Small cell carcinoma of the cervix, according to some authors, arises from endocervical argyrophilic cells or their precursors, multipotential neuroendocrine cells; however, some small cell tumors do not contain morphologic evidence of neuroendocrine origin. Nuclear molding, absence of nucleoli, cell necrosis, and high mitotic activity are common. One-third to one-half stain positively for neuroendocrine markers such as chromogranin, serotonin, synaptophysin, or somatostatin.[60] In the majority of patients, the cervical stroma is extensively infiltrated by single small, round cells.[130] Lymphatic and vascular invasion are significantly more common in small cell carcinomas (noted in 58% of patients with stage IB disease; 40% of these patients had lymph node metastases at the time of radical surgery).[131] HPV-18 has been detected in the majority of these tumors.[132]

Van Nagell et al.,[133] in an analysis of 25 patients, noted a 5-year survival rate of 54% for all stages of small cell carcinoma, compared with 68% for matched large-cell nonkeratinizing squamous cell and 74% for keratinizing squamous cell carcinomas. Viswanathan et al.[60] studied 21 patients. All were confirmed after central pathology review to stain positively for chromogranin, synaptophysin, or CD56. The median time to first relapse from the initiation of treatment was 8.4 months. No patient had brain metastases as the sole site of first recurrence. However, two patients developed brain metastases concurrently with lung metastases. The overall survival rate was 29% at 5 years; none of the patients who had disease more extensive than stage IB1 or clinical evidence of lymph node metastases survived their disease. Similar 5 year overall survival of 29% was reported in 487 patients in the SEER registry.[133a]

Basaloid carcinoma or adenoid basal carcinoma, an extremely uncommon tumor, is characterized by nests or cords of small basaloid cells, prominent peripheral palisading of cells in the tumor nests, no significant stromal reaction or capillary space invasion, and an infiltrating growth pattern. Some authors have suggested a slow growth pattern with limited local invasiveness and low probability of lymph node metastases.[134] Prognosis is excellent.[135]

Primary sarcomas of the cervix have been occasionally described (e.g., leiomyosarcoma, rhabdomyosarcoma, stromal sarcoma, carcinosarcoma).[136] Malignant lymphomas, primary or secondary in the cervix, have been sporadically reported. They should be treated like other lymphomas.[137] Melanoma of the cervix is similarly extremely rare and difficult to cure despite attempts at radical surgery. Metastasis of distant tumors to the uterine cervix is rare (about 4% of all tumors) and should be considered in the differential diagnosis. Metastases to the cervix from the breast, ovary, and kidney have been reported.[138–140]

PROGNOSTIC AND PREDICTIVE FACTORS

The NRG/GOG combined data from randomized trials of chemoradiotherapy and created nomograms predicting progression-free survival, overall survival, and pelvic recurrence in locally advanced cervical cancer. Multivariable analysis of 2,042 patients identified histology, race/ethnicity, performance status, tumor size, stage, grade, pelvic node status, and treatment with cisplatin-based chemotherapy concurrently as significant measures for outcomes.[141]

Patient-Related Factors

Age

According to some reports, age is not a prognostic factor in carcinoma of the cervix.[142] Other authors noted decreased survival in women younger than 35 or 40 years,[143] who have a greater frequency of poorly differentiated tumors. In contrast, two European studies showed improved outcome for younger patients.[144] This apparent contradiction may be explained by an analysis by Rutledge et al.,[145] who showed an interaction between age and stage in the relative hazard plots for 250 patients younger than 35 years of age and matched control subjects. Mitchell et al.[146] evaluated 398 patients with stage I to III cervical carcinoma treated with radiation therapy. Patients were divided into non-elderly (35 to 69 years of age; n = 338) and elderly (≥70 years of age; n = 60) groups. Comorbid conditions in the elderly resulted in diminished ability to undergo intracavitary brachytherapy. Although the 5-year actuarial disease-free survival and CSS rates were comparable in the two groups, tumor recurrence and death from cervical cancer were more common beyond 5 years in the elderly group.

Race/Socioeconomic Status

Several authors noted a correlation between racial or socioeconomic characteristics of patients and outcome of therapy. Mundt et al.[147] examined factors affecting outcome in 316 African American and 94 white patients undergoing RT for cervical cancer. With a median follow-up of 72.4 months, African Americans had a trend toward poorer 8-year CSS rates (47.9% vs. 60.6%; P = .10) compared with white patients. Factors correlating with poor outcome, including lower hemoglobin (Hb) levels during RT (P = .001), lower median income (P = .001), and less frequent intracavitary brachytherapy (P = .09), were more likely to be present in the African American group. Multivariate analysis demonstrated that race was not an independent prognostic factor after controlling for differences in patient, tumor, and treatment factors. In a report on 452 white and 124 African American women with stage II or III cancer of the cervix treated with RT alone, Grigsby et al.[148] observed 5-year CSS rates of 66% and 61% (P = .56) for those with stage II and of 38% and 47% (P = 0.34) for those with stage III disease, respectively. Overall survival rates for stage II for the two racial groups were different (60% and 51%, respectively; P = .02) and may be related to non–cancer-related comorbidity factors.

Brooks et al.[149] evaluated 1,009 patients with invasive carcinoma of the cervix: 606 white, 354 African American, and 5% "other" races. African Americans were more likely to have Medicaid or to be uninsured (44% vs. 23%; P = .001) and were more likely to be admitted for an emergency or for a cancer-related complication (P = .036), to have comorbid illness (P = .001), to be admitted for a transfusion (P = .01), or to be treated with radiation rather than surgery (P = .001). Racial differences existed in patterns of admission, type of therapy, and severity of illness.

Moreover, in an analysis of the 1994 Patterns of Care study of 471 cases of squamous cell carcinoma treated in the United States and a randomly selected 215 additional cases from 17 institutions that admitted >40% minority patients, women who lived in low-income neighborhoods, who had only Medicaid coverage, or who were treated at large academic or minority-rich institutions tended to have a poorer initial performance status, higher-stage or bulky central tumor, and a lower pretreatment hemoglobin level.[150]

General Medical Factors

Anemia and Tumor Hypoxia

Although stage, tumor volume, histologic type of the lesion, and vascular or lymphatic invasion are known to affect the prognosis of patients with cervical carcinoma, whether hemoglobin levels contribute to patient prognosis is controversial. Many radiation oncologists routinely administer red blood cell transfusions (RBCTs) to correct anemia before treatment with radiation therapy. This may have a generally favorable effect on the patient's sense of well-being and energy level and an impact on tumor radiosensitivity. Typically, patients receive transfusion to maintain hemoglobin levels >12 to 12.5 g/dL.

Hirst[151] emphasized that in animal tumor models, the opportunity to affect radiosensitivity by blood transfusion is transient. Blood transfusion is in general beneficial to the anemic patient with cancer, but it must be given as soon as possible before the first radiation dose to maximize its effects. Accounting for both the normal pulmonary and peripheral circulation and parallel flow through tumor tissue, Kavanagh et al.[152] calculated that decreasing hemoglobin–oxygen affinity should render a quantitatively greater decrease in radiobiologically hypoxic regions than what has been measured after the use of transfusions alone.[153]

Investigators have reported worse outcomes for patients whose tumors have either a median partial pressure of oxygen (Po_2) level, measured using polarographic needle electrodes for direct tumor tissue oxygen measurements, of <10 mm Hg[154] or a high percentage of Po_2 measurements <5 mm Hg.[155,156] Comparisons of intratumoral oxygen measurements before and after external beam radiation therapy have usually indicated a trend toward improved oxygenation after radiation therapy,[157,158] but the significance of posttreatment measurements is unclear.[159] Hypoxic tumors are more likely to recur locoregionally than well-oxygenated tumors regardless of whether surgery or radiation therapy is the primary local treatment.[154]

Haensgen et al.[160] analyzed 70 patients with stage IIB to IVA cervical cancer treated with external beam radiotherapy (EBRT) and brachytherapy. *In vivo* oxygenation was measured with an Eppendorf probe, and patient hemoglobin levels were recorded. Patients with a hemoglobin level of <11 g/dL had a 3-year survival rate of 27%, compared with 62% for those with a hemoglobin level of ≥11 g/dL (P = .006). Combining hypoxia and tp53 allowed stratification of subgroups with differing 3-year survival rates: 79% for tp53 (n = 10) and 47% for tp53 without hypoxia (n = 44).

A randomized trial reported by Bush[161] on 132 patients with stage IIB to III cervical cancer required the control arm to receive transfusions only if the hemoglobin level dropped to <10 g/dL, whereas the experimental arm had to maintain the hemoglobin level ≥12.5 g/dL. The results suggested an improved outcome for patients in the experimental arm who received transfusion; however, there was not a statistically significant difference in outcome between treatment arms when compared using an intent-to-treat analysis.[162] Second, the randomization was not stratified according to the potentially confounding influence of tumor size. Finally, the thresholds for transfusion were based on anemia during therapy, not the initial hemoglobin. Thomas[163] reviewed the Canadian experience and found that in 605 eligible patients with cervical cancer, 25% received blood transfusions, most frequently when Hb was <100 g/L. On multivariate analysis, baseline Hb was not a significant prognostic factor, but average weekly nadir during radiation therapy was significant, those with values >120 g/L having lower incidences of local relapse and distant metastasis and a better 5-year survival rate.

Dunst et al.[164] showed that pretreatment anemia had a significant impact on 3-year relapse rates (6% in 20 patients with Hb of >13 g/dL, 15% in 47 with Hb between 11 and 13 g/dL, and 67% in 20 with Hb of <11 g/dL). The 3-year survival rate was 38% in patients with poorly oxygenated tumors, compared to 68% in patients with higher Po_2 (P = .02). Munstedt et al.,[165] in a study of 183 patients who received adjuvant RT after radical surgery, noted that those with Hb of <11 g/dL had

lower recurrence-free and overall survival rates, primarily in a subgroup of women who had inadequate surgery.

In a retrospective review of >600 patients treated at seven different cancer centers in Canada, Grogan et al.[166] observed that the patients who maintained an average weekly hemoglobin level of >12 g/dL with or without transfusions had a significantly higher 5-year survival rate than patients with lower average weekly hemoglobin levels, regardless of the hemoglobin at presentation.

Kapp et al.[167] reported on 204 patients who received RBCT during RT when Hb level was <11 g/dL. Patients whose Hb was corrected (18.5%) had outcomes similar to those of nontransfused patients. However, nonresponders to RBCT had decreased tumor control and survival rates. Vaupel et al.,[168] in a review of published data, concluded that maximum oxygenation of tumors is expected with Hb in the range of 12 to 14 g/dL for women and that higher Hb levels may not be better.

A large retrospective review of 2,454 patients with cervical cancer showed on univariate analysis that low hemoglobin levels were significantly associated with central recurrence, distant metastases, and disease-specific survival. On multivariate analysis, a hemoglobin level of <10 g/dL during RT was found to be significant for lower DSS (HR 1.28) and freedom from distant metastases (HR 1.33), but not freedom from central recurrence. In a subset analysis of patients receiving chemoradiation, transfusion did not provide a benefit.[169]

Recombinant human erythropoietin is not routinely recommended as an alternative means of sustaining or raising hemoglobin levels during radiation therapy. Thrombotic complications[170] and the lack of any survival benefit[171] mitigate the utility of this as a therapeutic intervention.

Other Medical Factors

Jenkin and Stryker[172] observed a higher incidence of pelvic recurrences and complications in patients with arterial hypertension (diastolic pressure of >110 mm Hg). Kapp and Lawrence[173] reported on 398 patients. Patients with temperatures of >101°F had a higher incidence of distant metastases and a lower survival rate. In patients with cervical cancer screened for HIV and treated with RT, Campbell et al.[174] observed a 4.2% positive HIV rate. These patients had more-advanced tumors. The duration of remission was shorter than in the HIV-negative group. RT had no effect on the HIV titers. Women who are HIV positive or have acquired immunodeficiency syndrome associated with *in situ* or invasive carcinoma of the cervix are at a higher risk for tumor recurrence after treatment and death as a consequence of the malignant process.[175,176]

Evidence continues to mount that increasing levels of plasma micronutrients are associated with a decreasing risk of cervical cancer. Increasing serum lycopene and α- and γ-tocopherol levels and higher intake of dark green and deep yellow vegetables and fruit were significantly inversely associated with cancer.[177-179] Women should be counseled to eat a well-balanced diet, particularly those at high risk for developing cervical cancer.

The neutrophil-to-lymphocyte ratio has been shown to be prognostic, with an NLR > 2.95 associated with a worse OS (HR 1.65, P < .001) and EFS (HR 1.57, P < .001).[180]

Tumor Factors

HPV Subtype

HPV-16 and HPV-18 are the most frequent HPV subtypes worldwide. Studies have reported a higher risk of lymph node and other distant metastases with HPV-18 compared to HPV-16.[181,182] Wang et al.[183] studied 1,010 patients with cervical cancer after radiotherapy between 1993 and 2000. The HPV genotypes were determined by a gene chip that can detect 38 types of HPV. A total of 25 genotypes of HPV were detected in

992 specimens, of which 8 types that predominated were HPV types 16, 58, 18, 33, 52, 39, 31, and 45. Two high-risk HPV species were identified: α-7 (HPV types 18, 39, 45) and α-9 (HPV types 16, 31, 33, 52, 58). Risk groups determined included the high-risk group, which consisted of patients without HPV infection or those infected with the α-7 species only. The medium-risk group included patients coinfected with the α-7 and α-9 species.

Tumor Volume

There is a close correlation between depth of stromal invasion, tumor size, and incidence of parametrial and pelvic node metastases and survival in patients with cervical cancer.[42,43] In a study of women treated with radical hysterectomy, the 5-year DFS rate was 90% in 181 patients with stage IB1 ($\leq$4 cm) and 72.8% in 48 patients with stage IB2 disease ($P = .02$).[184]

Toita et al.,[185] in a review of 70 patients with stage IIB and IIIB carcinoma of the uterine cervix treated with RT alone, reported no significant correlation of 5-year DFS with size of the cervical tumor <60 mm (70% to 85%); however, in patients with tumor $\geq$60 mm, the 5-year DFS was 28.6%. Piver and Chung[44] showed a greater incidence of lymphatic and distant metastasis and lower survival rates in patients with bulky and barrel-shaped stage IB and IIA tumors treated by radical hysterectomy. In addition, a higher incidence of pelvic recurrences and distant metastases and a decreased survival rate were reported by Fletcher,[186] Eifel et al.,[187] and Perez et al.[188] in patients with larger tumors treated with irradiation. In stages IB and IIA, higher radiation doses improved local tumor control.[189,190]

Furthermore, Leveque et al.,[191] in patients with stage I to II adenocarcinoma of the cervix treated with RT alone or combined with radical surgery, noted that FIGO stage and pelvic node involvement were the most important parameters influencing overall survival. Silver et al.,[192] in 93 patients with stage I adenocarcinoma of the cervix, described patient age and tumor grade as significant prognostic variables for survival ($P < .01$ and .01, respectively); tumor size was significant ($P < .01$) for survival and PFS.

In contrast, Grigsby et al.,[193] in patients with stage IB and IIA carcinoma of the cervix treated with preoperative irradiation and radical or conservative hysterectomy, observed no correlation of tumor volume with outcome. The 5-year pelvic failure rates for stage IB were 16% for tumors <3 cm and 9% for larger tumors ($P = .90$) and for stage IIA were 22% for tumors <3 or >3 cm ($P = .75$).

Several retrospective studies demonstrated decreased survival and a greater incidence of distant metastases in patients with endometrial extension of a primary cervical carcinoma (endometrial stromal invasion or replacement of the endometrium by tumor only).[38] Grimard et al.[194] on the other hand, confirmed these findings only in patients with stage IB tumors but not in more advanced stages. Similar findings were noted by Noguchi et al.[195] Patients without uterine body invasion had a 5-year survival rate of 92.4%, compared with 53.8% in patients with invasion.

Perez et al.[190] in an update of a previous report[188] reviewed 1,499 patients (stages IA to IVA) treated with definitive irradiation (combination of external beam irradiation plus two intracavitary insertions to deliver doses of 70 to 90 Gy to point A). There was a close correlation between tumor size and extent and pelvic tumor control, incidence of distant metastasis, and DFS in all stages.

Impact of Histology on Outcomes

Several series have questioned whether adenocarcinoma has a worse prognosis than squamous cell carcinoma. A Surveillance, Epidemiology, and End Results (SEER) analysis of women with stage IB to IVB cervical cancer treated between 1988 and 2005 stratified 24,562 women by squamous cell carcinoma (77%), adenocarcinoma, or adenosquamous histology. Patients with adenocarcinoma were younger and presented with early-stage disease ($P < .0001$). For both early and advanced stage diseases, women with adenocarcinoma had an increased likelihood of dying from disease compared to those with squamous neoplasms (HR 1.39 and HR 1.21, respectively).[196]

In a retrospective analysis of 1,671 patients accrued on prior prospective GOG trials with locally advanced cervical carcinoma treated with either radiation alone or chemoradiation, a total of 70 adenocarcinoma patients treated with radiation alone had a borderline poorer survival difference ($P = .0499$) compared to 647 patients with squamous cell carcinoma. In patients treated with concurrent chemoradiation, 112 adenocarcinoma patients had no difference in overall survival ($P = .47$) compared to 842 patients with squamous cell carcinoma. The authors conclude that in the era of chemoradiation, no difference in outcome exists between squamous cell and adenocarcinoma in this large retrospective analysis.[197]

Margin Status After Radical Hysterectomy

In addition to the known high-risk factors of positive margins, positive parametrial spread, and/or positive lymph nodes and the intermediate-risk factors of depth of stromal invasion, lymphovascular invasion, and tumor size, small series have indicated the significance of close margin status.[198,199] Viswanathan et al.[200] studied 284 patients after radical hysterectomy (RH) and central pathology review. The crude rates for any recurrence were 11%, 20%, and 38% for patients with negative ($\geq$1 cm), close (>0 and <1 cm), and positive margins, respectively. Postoperative RT decreased the rate of local recurrence (LR) from 10% to 0% for negative, 17% to 0% for close, and 50% to 25% for positive margins. The significant predictors of decreased relapse-free survival on univariate analysis were the depth of tumor invasion (hazard ratio [HR] = 2.14/cm increase, $P = .007$), positive margins (HR = 3.92, $P = .02$), tumor size (HR = 1.3/cm increase, $P = .02$), lymphovascular invasion (HR = 2.19, $P = .03$), and margin status (HR = 0.002/increasing millimeter from cancer for those with close margins, $P = .03$).

Histologic Grade

Most reports have shown no significant correlation of survival or tumor behavior with the degree of differentiation of squamous cell carcinoma or adenocarcinoma of the cervix.[201–203] Alfsen et al.[201] analyzed 417 adenocarcinomas and 88 other nonsquamous cell carcinomas of the cervix; on multivariate analysis, small cell histology, corpus infiltration, vascular invasion, and positive lymph nodes were significant prognostic variables. Although Reagan and Fu[204] demonstrated prognostic value of histologic differentiation in patients treated with irradiation, Crissman et al.[205] failed to observe a correlation between histologic parameters and patient survival. In the era of chemoradiation, Monk et al.[206] showed no significant impact of histology or grade on survival in postoperative cervical cancer patients with other high-risk features.

Lymph Node Ratio

In a review of 95 patients with stage I to II cervical cancer treated with a radical hysterectomy and pelvic and/or paraaortic lymphadenectomy, the ratio of involved lymph nodes was associated on multivariate analysis with worse survival. A ratio of positive to negative of >7.6% had an HR of 3.96 ($P = .01$).[197]

Treatment Duration

In patients treated with radiation therapy, overall treatment time (OTT) should be as short as possible, and any planned or unplanned interruptions or delays should be avoided. Timely integration of external beam and intracavitary irradiation in

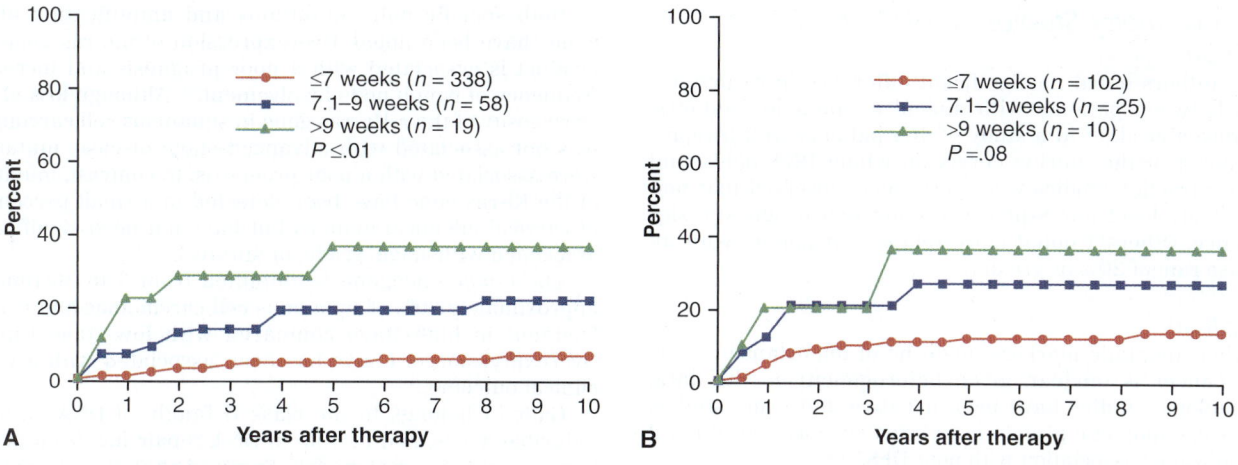

FIGURE 73.8. Pelvic failure rate correlated with length of treatment in stage IB **(A)** and IIA **(B)** carcinomas of the uterine cervix. (Reprinted from Perez CA, Grigsby PW, Castro-Vita H, et al. Carcinoma of the uterine cervix: I. Impact of prolongation of treatment time and timing of brachytherapy on outcome of radiation therapy. *Int J Radiat Oncol Biol Phys* 1995;32[5]: 1275–1288. Copyright © 1995 Elsevier. With permission.)

patients with carcinoma of the uterine cervix is an important factor in improving pelvic tumor control (Fig. 73.8).[207] Several studies described lower pelvic tumor control and survival rates in invasive carcinoma of the uterine cervix when the overall time in a course of irradiation is prolonged.[142,208–210] Chatani et al.,[211] In 216 patients with stage IIB to III cervical carcinoma treated with a combination of external beam and HDR brachytherapy, noted that OTT was the most highly significant factor for local tumor control in multivariate analysis (P = .0005). For relapse-free survival, stage classification (P = .0001), OTT (P = .0035), and hemoglobin level (P = .0174) were the three most important prognostic factors; there was no relationship between treatment time and late complications.

Whether treatment duration has an impact in the era of chemoradiation has been assessed. Shaverdian et al. analyzed 480 cervical cancer patients treated either with RT alone or with chemoradiation (CRT). In patients treated with RT, a treatment duration of 62 days or greater was not associated with a decreased DFS (HR 1.42, P = .086) nor was CRT.[212] In a retrospective review of 488 patients all treated with CT or MR image-based brachytherapy in the retroEmbrace study, D_{90} dose, clinical target volume (CTV) volume, and longer OTT were associated with local control.[213]

Fyles et al.[208] reported approximately 1% loss of tumor control per day of prolongation of treatment time beyond 30 days in 830 patients with cervical carcinoma treated with irradiation alone. Lanciano et al.,[210] in an analysis of 837 patients with squamous cell carcinoma of the cervix from the Patterns of Care Study who were treated with irradiation and received doses of 66 Gy or greater, described a 4-year actuarial in-field recurrence increase from 6% to 20% when total treatment time increased from 6 weeks or fewer to 10 weeks (P = .0001); this translated into significantly decreased survival. Girinsky et al.,[209] in 386 patients with stage IIB or III carcinoma of the cervix, also observed that the 10-year local recurrence–free survival rate decreased when OTT exceeded 52 days. A 1.1% loss of pelvic tumor control per day was also observed in their regression analysis.

Perez et al.,[214] in 1,330 patients treated with definitive irradiation, noted a major impact of prolongation of treatment time on pelvic tumor control in stages IB, IIA, and IIB. In stage III, although the rate of pelvic failure was higher with prolongation of treatment time, the difference was not statistically significant. There was also a strong correlation between OTT and survival. Regression analysis confirmed previous reports that prolongation of OTT resulted in an increased failure rate of 0.59% per day in stage IB and IIA and 0.86% per day in

stage IIB disease. Performance of all intracavitary insertions within 4.5 weeks from initiation of irradiation yielded lower pelvic failure rates (8.8% vs. 18% in stage IIB tumors; $P \le .01$).

Biomarkers

Several studies assessed various biologic markers to determine whether they are prognostic; however, the majority suffered from not having multivariate analyses to determine whether these may be valid independent factors. Noordhuis et al.,[215] in a systematic review of 42 studies with 82 cell biologic markers, reported that on univariate analysis, 34 biologic markers showed a relation with survival, 27 of which were independently associated with survival.

Angiogenesis and Hypoxia

Angiogenesis—the formation of new blood vessels—relies on the presence of proangiogenic growth factors, such as vascular endothelial growth factor (VEGF). As new blood vessels form, they deliver nutrients and oxygen to the cancerous cells. As tumors expand, the newly formed blood vessels may no longer reach the central portions of the tumor, and a hypoxic core develops. Hypoxia-inducible factor (HIF-1α) and HIF-2α regulate the response to hypoxic stress; HIF-1α but not HIF-2α has been associated with poor DFS.[216–219] The HIF-2α/CD68 ratio was correlated with poor DFS.[219] One study found that VEGF decreased overall survival.[220,221] Loncaster et al.,[220] in a retrospective study of 100 patients, found that VEGF expression in tumor biopsies in advanced carcinoma of the cervix was associated with a poor prognosis. Level of thymidine phosphorylase,[221] which increases hypoxic conditions, similarly was associated with poor outcomes. Nitric oxide synthase[222] and carbonic anhydrase (CA) may be prognostic for a poor outcome. In particular, CA9 is related to poor DFS.[223,224] CA12, in contrast, was related to metastasis-free survival.[225]

Microvessel count is higher in patients with cervical neoplasia than in control patients and higher in patients who experience posttreatment recurrences. Obermair et al.,[226] in 166 patients with stage IB cervical cancer, observed a 5-year survival rate of 89.7% in 102 patients whose tumors had a microvessel density of 20 per field or less and 63% in 64 patients whose tumors had a microvessel density of >20 per field (log rank P < .0001). In a multivariate Cox model, microvessel density, lymph node involvement, tumor size, and the application of radiation therapy were independent prognostic factors for survival. Similar findings were reported by Cooper et al.[227]

Section III

Flow Cytometry Studies on DNA and Growth Fraction

Some authors noted no significant difference in recurrence rates between patients with diploid or aneuploid tumors. Kristensen et al.,[228] in a study of 465 patients with invasive carcinoma of the uterine cervix on whom DNA index and S-phase fraction studies were performed, observed that neither ploidy level nor S-phase fraction had prognostic significance. Others[229] noted more relapses in tumors with an S-phase rate of 20% or greater.

Apoptosis

Whether apoptotic markers might be of importance in cervical cancer is unclear, given heterogeneity in the data. Morphologic studies have been negative, but some studies evaluating apoptotic protein expression such as that of Bcl-2 and p63 show association with poor DFS.[230,231]

Ohno et al.[232] studied 20 patients before and after administration of 9 Gy and found an increase in apoptotic cell index and Bax protein. Wootipoom et al.,[230] in 174 patients with cervical cancer, noted Bax, Bcl-2, and p53 expression in 68.4%, 25.9%, and 77.6% of the cases, respectively. Bax expression was associated with better survival, whereas Bcl-2 expression was associated with poor survival. Jain et al.[233] also found that neither Bcl-2 nor p53 expression was an independent predictor of outcome in locally advanced cervical cancer.

The p53 gene controls entry into the S-phase of the cell cycle. Mukherjee et al.[234] analyzed radioresistant cervical cancer cases and found that 15% had positivity for Bcl-2 and p21 proteins and 34% showed mutant p53 protein. None of the radiosensitive tumors were positive for these proteins. Seventy-five percent of the radiosensitive tumors were positive for the Bax antibody, whereas 81% of the radioresistant tumors were negative for Bax ($P < .01$). Kainz et al.,[235] in a study of 109 surgically treated patients, and Ebara et al.,[236] in 46 patients with stage IIIB squamous cell carcinoma of the cervix treated with RT alone, noted no significant difference in outcome when correlated with p53 protein expression.

Cell Cycle and Cellular Oncogenes

Cerciello et al.,[237] in 40 patients with stage IIA to IIIB cervix cancer treated with RT without chemotherapy, obtained biopsies before and after five fractions of RT. They observed significant changes in the cell cycle of cervical cancer, indicating intact G2/M checkpoint function, leading to the expectation that targeting compounds interfering with G2/M transition may enhance the effect of irradiation on cervix cancer.

In patients with carcinoma of the uterine cervix treated with irradiation, Tsang et al.,[238] observed that the most significant factors for DFS were large tumor size ($P = .01$), low hemoglobin ($P = .01$), labeling index (LI) flow cytometry (DFS, 67% for LI < 7%; 33% for LI ≥ 7%; $P = .03$), and potential doubling time (T_{pot}; 66% for $T_{pot} > 5$ days, 35% for $T_{pot} \leq 5$ days; $P = .04$). For small tumors (<6 cm in diameter), either a high LI (>7%) or a high apoptotic index (>1%) was associated with poorer DFS. West et al.[239] evaluated the intrinsic radiosensitivity of 145 tumor biopsies from patients with cervical carcinoma (in vitro survival fraction at 2 Gy using a clonogenic assay). Diploid tumors tended to be more radioresistant than aneuploid tumors ($P = .07$).

The p27/Kip1 gene inhibits a variety of cyclin-dependent kinase complexes and regulates cell growth. Oka et al.[240] studied 202 biopsy specimens obtained from 77 patients with squamous cell carcinoma of the cervix before and during RT for expression of p27 and p53 proteins. A high p27 LI before radiation therapy was associated significantly with good disease-free and metastasis-free survival rates. A high p53 LI before irradiation was associated with poor overall survival.

Both specific point mutations and amplification of *ras* genes have been noted. Overexpression of the ras gene p21 product is associated with a poor prognosis and increased frequency of lymph node involvement.[241] Although loss of heterozygosity of the c-Ha-ras gene in squamous cell carcinomas was not associated with advanced-stage disease, mutations were associated with a poor prognosis. In contrast, mutations of the Ki-ras gene have been detected in a small percentage of cervical adenocarcinomas but have not been significantly associated with stage, grade, or survival.[242,243]

The c-*myc* oncogene is amplified from 3 to 30 times in approximately 20% of squamous cell carcinomas and is more frequent in high-stage compared with low-stage tumors. Overexpression of c-myc has been associated with a worse clinical outcome.[244,245]

Gadd45 belongs to the class II family of DNA damage–inducible genes, and its role in DNA repair has been proven in many experimental models. Santucci et al.,[246] in 14 patients with cervical cancer, found a correlation between the lack of gadd45 induction and a clinical response to irradiation (both local tumor control and DFS) when a dose ranging from 18 to 25 Gy was delivered to the pelvis.

CD34 is an antigen present in hemopoietic progenitor cells and is a sensitive marker for endothelial cells. In 62 patients with cervical cancer evaluated by Vieira et al.,[247] CD34 reactivity and higher microvessel density were associated with squamous cell carcinoma. CD109 is a cell surface protein that was found to be expressed in cervical cancer more than in endometrial adenocarcinoma.[248]

Cytokeratin Markers and the Epidermal Growth Factor Receptor Pathway

Altered expression of c-ercB-2 (HER2) protein was shown to have prognostic significance in adenocarcinoma but not in squamous cell carcinoma of the cervix.[249] HER1, as well as coexpression of epidermal growth factor receptor and HER2, has been associated with poor DFS.[250] PTEN mutations have also been associated with poor prognosis.[251]

In 80 patients with carcinoma of the cervix, expression of cytokeratin 10 and 13 and involucrin was found in 24%, 64%, and 53%, respectively.[252] There was no difference in the expression of cytokeratin or involucrin between patients with positive or negative lymph nodes, although in the lymph node–positive group, survival was higher in patients lacking cytokeratin 13 expression ($P = .02$).

Squamous Cell Carcinoma Antigen and Carcinoembryonic Antigen

Tsai et al.,[253] in 117 patients with adenocarcinoma of the cervix, 28 of whom had preoperative carcinoembryonic antigen (CEA) levels of >5 ng/mL, noted a correlation with larger tumor size, deeper cervical invasion, and lymphovascular invasion ($P < .001$). A Spanish study of 96 patients with invasive carcinoma of the cervix and 7 with intraepithelial neoplasia showed elevated CEA levels in 33%, CA 19.9 in 32%, and CA 125 in 21.5% of patients.[254] Specificity for each tumor marker was 98%. Increased CEA and CA 19.9 levels were found with more advanced stages of the disease and in patients with adenocarcinoma compared with squamous cell carcinoma. At follow-up, all cases of progressive tumor or recurrence were detected by elevation of one of the three antigens. Specificity during follow-up was 92% for CEA and CA 125 and 92.6% for CA 19.9.

In a study of 272 patients with invasive carcinoma of the cervix with 1,053 samples, Bolli et al.[255] noted an elevation of squamous cell carcinoma antigen (SCC-Ag) before treatment in 53% of 103 patients, increasing with advancing tumor stage at diagnosis. In 70 patients with recurrent tumor, 81% had elevated SCC-Ag. Ngan et al.[256] also identified elevation of serum SCC-Ag in 62% of 308 women with carcinoma of the cervix. Posttreatment SCC-Ag levels were raised in 69 patients (22.4%), and this was associated with a <5% 5-year survival rate, in contrast to 87% in women with normal SCC-Ag levels.

Hong et al.,[257] in 401 patients with stage I to IV squamous cell carcinoma of the cervix treated with RT, noted that the preirradiation SCC-Ag level strongly correlated with disease stage. A persistently elevated SCC-Ag level 3 months after RT was a stronger predictor for treatment failure than residual induration by pelvic examination, and it was associated with a higher incidence of distant metastasis.

Similarly, Micke et al.,[258] in 141 patients with cervical cancer treated with RT, noted that the pretherapy serum level of SCC-Ag was elevated in 72% (>2 ng/mL). Patients with an SCC-Ag of <7.2 U/mL had better tumor response than those with higher levels. After RT, 98% of patients in complete remission and 87% of those in partial remission had a serum level below the cutoff. In recurrent tumors, 82% of patients had a significant increase in serum levels before clinical manifestation of relapse (≤ 0.001). Hong et al.,[259] in 1,031 patients with squamous cell cervical cancer treated with RT with or without chemotherapy, noted that independent risk factors for local relapse were advanced stage and age <45 years; 5-year local relapse–free survival was higher (90%) if squamous cell carcinoma antigen was <2. This antigen may be a useful marker in the prognosis of patients with carcinoma of the uterine cervix. Huang et al.[260,261] noted that SCC-Ag and CEA were predictive of para-aortic node failure. Markovina et al. note that SCC-Ag is a significant independent predictor of positive post-therapy FDG-PET/CT, recurrence and death.[261a]

Epstein-Barr Virus, Transforming Growth Factor, β-Integrin, and Other Markers

Activity of Epstein-Barr virus antigen–specific killer T cells and shedding of Epstein-Barr virus were evaluated in 55 patients with carcinoma of the cervix.[262] Activity was decreased in patients with cervical carcinoma compared with control patients; it became increasingly lower as the clinical stage of the disease advanced, and activity after treatment was clearly related to patient survival. These data may indicate an imbalance in local immunity against viral infection and impairment of T-cell immunity in patients with advanced cervical carcinoma.

In 79 patients undergoing radiation therapy for carcinoma of the cervix, pretreatment transforming growth factor-β_1 (TGF-β_1) levels were a significant prognostic factor for survival and local tumor control. There were weak significant correlations of TGF-β_1 levels with disease stage and the levels of circulating tumor markers (CA 125).[263] Hazelbag et al.[264] also assessed TGF-β_1 and plasminogen activator inhibitor (PAI-1) expression in 108 specimens of cervical carcinoma and noted that TGF was not associated with worse prognosis, whereas PAI-1 was.

Gruber et al.,[265] in biopsies of 82 patients with cervical cancer, found that β_3-integrin was expressed in 50 (61%) and correlated it with higher incidence of locoregional recurrences and decreased survival.

Cyclooxygenase-2

Gaffney et al.,[266] in 24 patients with carcinoma of the cervix treated with RT, observed that 5-year overall survival rates for tumors with low versus high COX-2 values were 75% and 35%, respectively ($P = .021$). COX-2 staining intensity was found to correlate positively with tumor size ($P = .022$).

Kim et al.[267] screened 84 patients with stage IIB squamous cell and 21 with adenocarcinoma cervical cancer and found COX-2 expression more frequently in the adenocarcinoma group (57% vs. 24%; $P = .007$). The 5-year survival rate was 83% for COX-2–negative and 57% for COX-2–positive patients, regardless of histologic subtype ($P = .001$). Pyo et al.[268] also showed that expression of COX-2 and coexpression of COX-2

and thymidine phosphorylase were correlated with high locoregional recurrence and lower survival. Moreover, Kang et al.,[269] in 84 patients with cervix adenocarcinoma, observed a higher incidence of lymph node metastasis and decreased survival with elevated expression of COX-2.

Hormonal Receptors

Suzuki et al.[270] investigated the expression of estrogen receptors and progesterone receptors (PgRs) in biopsy specimens from cervical tumors before RT in 44 patients with cervical adenocarcinoma and 22 with adenosquamous cell carcinomas. Staining for estrogen receptors or PgR was positive in 12 patients (19%). The estrogen receptor status did not correlate with the local tumor control, disease-free survival, or CSS. The DFS rate of PgR-positive patients was significantly higher than that of PgR-negative patients ($P = .044$), but PgR status was not statistically significant in relation to 5-year CSS or local tumor control.

Cancer Genome Atlas

Using RNA sequencing and whole exome DNA sequencing, several mutations have been reported in cervical cancer.[271] Notable APOBEC mutagenesis patterns and novel significantly mutated genes in SHKBP1, ERBB3, CASP8, HLA-A, and TGFBR2 were identified. Amplifications in PD-L1 and PD-L2 and BCAR4 were also noted. Categories of cervical cancer were defined as endometrial like (predominantly HPV-negative), keratin-low squamous, keratin-high squamous, and adenocarcinoma-rich subgroups.[272]

TECHNIQUES USED FOR TREATMENT

Preinvasive Disease

Patients with CIN may be candidates for observation or treatment. CIN1-2 has a spontaneous regression rate in 1 to 3 years of >50%,[273] and therefore, observation may be an appropriate course. For patients with persistent dysplasia, cryotherapy has a very low complication rate and is highly successful but may be less effective than laser ablation for high-grade dysplasia.[274] Patients with no visible lesion undergo frequent serial exams. Cold knife conization (CKC) may be used for diagnostic and therapeutic intent, with side effects of bleeding, cellulitis, cervical stenosis, or loss of cervical competence. Loop electrosurgical excision procedure (LEEP) has become popular, although bleeding and stenosis may occur; pregnancy outcomes may be better with LEEP than with CKC.[275–277]

Invasive Disease

Surgical Techniques

Simple Conization

In patients with minimal invasion, no parametrial involvement, and small tumor size, simple conization with lymphadenectomy has been reported. Although only 36 patients were studied, after a median follow-up of 66 months, only 1 pelvic nodal relapse was observed.[278]

Radical Trachelectomy

Described in the 1960s,[279] trachelectomy entails removal of the cervix entirely. Radical trachelectomy also removes the parametrial tissue. As a means of fertility preservation in early-stage cervical cancer patients,[280] trachelectomy should be combined with preoperative PET imaging to confirm no nodal involvement and with MRI to confirm no endocervical canal extension of tumor into the uterus.[281] A laparoscopic lymphadenectomy should accompany the trachelectomy to confirm no nodal involvement. A non-absorbable cerclage is placed around the uterine isthmus. Radical abdominal trachelectomy also may result in successful fertility preservation.[282] Selection criteria for a trachelectomy include those patients requesting fertility-sparing surgery; age <40 years; stage IA1, IA2, or IB1 with no nodal involvement detected on MRI or PET scan; squamous cell or adenocarcinoma with a lesion <2 cm; no lymphovascular invasion on initial biopsy; and no upper endocervical involvement. The main site for recurrence is the central pelvis (average 5% risk), at the cervicouterine junction, or in the adjacent parametrial tissue. In a retrospective review of 29 patients with stage IB1 disease with tumor size 2 cm or greater treated with radical trachelectomy, patients with high-risk features were taken to immediate hysterectomy, and 21% required chemoradiation. A total of nine patients (31%) were able to undergo a fertility-sparing procedure, with one recurrence at a median follow-up of 44 months.[283] If high- or intermediate-risk features are present (i.e., presence of positive lymph nodes or positive margins) after a trachelectomy, radiation should be performed without requiring a completion hysterectomy. Leaving the uterus intact results in less small-bowel dose; radiation or chemoradiation followed by image-based brachytherapy with an attenuated dose based on amount of residual disease in the uterus is feasible in order to minimize bladder and rectal dose.[283a]

Types of Hysterectomy

Several types of hysterectomy are used in the management of carcinoma of the uterine cervix (Table 73.7).[284]

Total (extrafascial) abdominal hysterectomy (class I) consists of removal of the cervix and adjacent tissues, as well as a small cuff of the upper vagina in a plane outside the pubocervical fascia. There is minimal disturbance of the ureters and the trigone of the bladder. This may be the surgical treatment of choice for stage IA1 cervical cancer.

The use of a radical hysterectomy for cervical cancer was first described by Wertheim in 1912.[285] In a modified radical extended hysterectomy (class II), the cervix and upper vagina are removed, including paracervical tissues, and the ureters are dissected in the paracervical tunnel to their point of entry into the bladder. Because the ureters are unsheathed and retracted laterally, parametrial and paracervical tissue can be safely removed medial to the ureter. This operation is performed with a lymphadenectomy. This is the most common surgical approach selected for stage IA2 cervical cancer.

Radical abdominal hysterectomy (class III) with bilateral pelvic lymphadenectomy consists of a wider resection of the parametrial tissues to the pelvic wall, with dissection of the ureters and mobilization of the bladder, as well as of the rectum to allow for more extensive removal of tissues. This approach was described by Meigs in 1944.[286] In addition, a vaginal cuff of at least 2 to 3 cm is always included in the procedure, as well as the uterosacral ligaments.[284] A bilateral pelvic lymphadenectomy is usually carried out. This operation is often referred to as the Wertheim or Meigs procedure. The extended radical hysterectomy (class IV) includes complete dissection of the ureter from the vesicouterine ligament, sacrifice of the superior vesicle artery, and removal of the upper three-fourths of the vagina. Because of the high rate of fistula and significant morbidity, it is rarely used.[284] In 2007, after a consensus conference in Japan, a new classification system was released based only on the lateral extent of the resection.[287] Four levels of hysterectomy are described (A to D) and four levels of lymphadenectomy (1 to 4). The levels of lymph node dissection include the internal and external iliac (level 1), common iliac and presacral (level 2), aortic intramesenteric (level 3), and aortic infrarenal (level 4). The levels of primary tumor resection include the following:

Type A: Extrafascial hysterectomy, with minimum resection of the paracervix medial to the ureter and minimal vaginal resection <1 cm, without removal of the paracolpos.

Type B: Modified radical hysterectomy with partial resection of the vesicouterine and uterosacral ligaments, unroofing of the ureter, transection of the parametrial tissue at the ureter, and removal of at least 1 cm of the vagina. This type is divided into B1, without removal of paracervical lymph nodes, and B2, with removal of lateral paracervical nodes.

Type C: Classic radical hysterectomy, variant in which the entire uterosacral and vesicouterine ligaments are removed, 1.5 to 2 cm of the vagina with paracolpos is excised, and neuronal preservation is critical.

Type D: Includes the complete radical hysterectomy and resects tissues to the pelvis sidewall, including the hypogastric (internal iliac) vessels, and exposes the sciatic nerve (type D1). Type D2 also removes the fascial and lateral muscles, called the laterally extended endopelvic resection.

Pelvic Exenteration

Pelvic exenteration has been used for en masse removal of the pelvic viscera for recurrent carcinoma of the cervix. Modern radiation therapy with concurrent chemotherapy results in high complete response rates and has made residual extensive disease a rare indication for exenteration. Patients with adjacent organ invasion are given a course of radical concurrent chemoradiation, followed by interstitial brachytherapy, with exenteration reserved for salvage.[288-290]

This operation, which is not done as a palliative procedure, consists of a radical hysterectomy, pelvic lymph node dissection, and removal of the bladder (anterior exenteration), removal of the rectosigmoid colon (posterior exenteration), or both (total exenteration). The ileum or sigmoid has been the usual means of achieving urinary diversion. Because some patients have a pelvic recurrence after radiation therapy, the bowel is used for the urinary conduit. Proof that there is no fixation to the pelvic wall and no extension of disease beyond the pelvis is mandatory. Metastases outside the pelvis, including those in PALNs or any viscera, are absolute contraindications to the procedure. Bilateral ureteral obstruction secondary to

TABLE 73.7 TYPES OF ABDOMINAL HYSTERECTOMY

	Intrafascial	Extrafascial Type I	Modified Radical Type II	Radical Type III–IV[a]
Cervical fascia	Partially removed	Completely removed	———	———
Vaginal cuff removal	None	Small rim removed	Proximal 1–2 cm removed	Upper one-third to one-half removed
Bladder	Partially mobilized		———	Mobilized
Rectum	Not mobilized	Rectovaginal septum partially mobilized	———	Mobilized
Ureters	Not mobilized	———	Unroofed in the ureteral tunnel	Completely dissected to the bladder entry
Cardinal ligaments	Resected medial to the ureters	———	Resected at level of the ureter	Resected at pelvic the sidewall
Uterosacral ligaments	Resected at level of the cervix	———	Partially resected	Resected at postpelvic insertion
Uterus	Removed	———	———	———
Cervix	Partially removed	Completely removed	———	———

[a]Type IV, extended radical hysterectomy (partial removal of the bladder and/or ureter), in addition to type III.

TABLE 73.8 CARCINOMA OF THE UTERINE CERVIX: SURVIVAL AFTER STAGING LAPAROTOMY

Stage	Explored		Not Explored	
	Number of Patients	Percentage Surviving	Number of Patients	Percentage Surviving
IIB	31	64.5	14	92.8
IIIA–IIIB	28	57.1	10	60.0

Reprinted from Nelson JH, Macasaet MA, Lu T, et al. The incidence and significance of paraaortic lymph node metastases in late invasive carcinoma of the cervix. *Am J Obstet Gynecol* 1974;118(6):749–756. Copyright © 1974 Elsevier. With permission.

tumor is also a relative contraindication.[291] Patients with sacroiliac or hip pain or leg edema rarely benefit from this procedure and should be excluded on a clinical basis.

Pretreatment Surgical Nodal Assessment

Exploratory laparotomy and nodal staging to evaluate the presence of metastases to the pelvic or para-aortic nodes may provide diagnostic information but has not had a demonstrated impact on survival (Table 73.8). In a prospective evaluation of 290 patients with carcinoma of the cervix[52] para-aortic node metastases were found in 19 of 58 patients (32.8%) with clinical stage IIB and 19 of 61 (31.1%) with stage IIIB disease. A number of studies compared the significance of para-aortic nodal metastases with other clinical and surgical findings with regard to PFS and overall survival.[292] In 626 patients treated on GOG randomized studies, the RR associated with positive para-aortic nodes was 11.0 for time to recurrence and 6.2 for survival time. In addition to the significant increase in risk of regional relapses, patients with para-aortic nodal metastasis are more likely to have extrapelvic failure.[293]

Cosin et al.[294] reviewed 266 patients with locally advanced cervical carcinoma who underwent extraperitoneal pelvic and para-aortic lymphadenectomy before RT. Patients were divided into four groups: group A had negative lymph nodes; B, resected, microscopic lymph node metastases; C, macroscopically positive lymph nodes that were resectable at the time of surgery; and D, unresectable lymph nodes. Lymph node metastases were detected in 50% of patients. All patients received pelvic EBRT (pre–intensity-modulated radiation therapy [IMRT] era) and brachytherapy; patients with lymph node metastases received extended-field irradiation. Five- and 10-year DFS rates were similar for all patients in groups B and C. All patients in group D recurred. There was a 10.5% incidence of severe radiation-related morbidity and a 1.1% incidence of treatment-related deaths.

The potential benefit of surgical nodal debulking followed by irradiation has been studied.[295] Potish et al.[296] noted that more than half of the patients with advanced cervical cancer with grossly positive pelvic nodes that were debulked survived, compared with none with unresectable lymph nodes, findings closely paralleling those of Inoue and Morita[297]; however, these studies predated the ability to implement dose escalation with IMRT to the involved nodes. Nonetheless, surgical debulking of nodes decreases the dose of radiation required to these regions. The use of high-energy photon beams and limitation

of the tumor dose to extended volumes in the para-aortic region for those with completely resected but positive nodes to 45 to 50 Gy decrease the probability of complications. IMRT also enhances the sparing of adjacent abdominal normal tissues.[298,299] However, if node dissection is not feasible or would result in a treatment delay, patients may successfully be managed with IMRT with dose escalation to approximately 60 to 65 Gy to the grossly enlarged lymph nodes.[101,300–302]

Complication risk may be high (Table 73.9), particularly when patients are treated with postresection RT. One study showed an 11.5% incidence of major primarily small-bowel complications with transperitoneal compared with 3.9% in the extraperitoneal lymphadenectomy group (P = .03).[303] Transperitoneal lymphadenectomy should be avoided.[45,304]

Because of a high rate of complications, preirradiation laparotomy was discontinued at the MD Anderson Cancer Center. The status of the lymph nodes is investigated with lymphangiography and verified when possible with percutaneous transabdominal needle biopsy. Wharton et al.[46] reported on 120 patients who had preirradiation celiotomy; 16 had fatal complications, and 32 had major intestinal complications. Most patients with positive lymph nodes died with distant metastasis. More recently, PET–CT followed by biopsy may be a useful approach. In one series of 60 patients without evidence of PALN involvement on preoperative CT or MRI, patients underwent a preoperative PET–CT followed by surgery. Twenty-six patients had a negative PET–CT, of whom 3 (12%) had positive nodes pathologically. Of the 27 with positive pelvic but negative para-aortic nodes on PET–CT, 6 (22%) had pathologically positive para-aortic nodes, indicating a sensitivity of 36% and a specificity of 96%. In another study, 125 patients had a PET–CT followed by para-aortic lymphadenectomy.[50] Seventeen percent had positive para-aortic metastases, 66% of whom had a negative PET–CT. The sensitivity and specificity of PET–CT were 33% and 94%, respectively. Morbidity of the surgery was 7%, and there was no delay in initiating chemoradiotherapy. A Cochrane overview of pretreatment surgical para-aortic lymph node assessment in stage IB2 to IVA cervical cancer identified one randomized trial of 61 women that favored CT or MRI over surgical staging.[305,306] Alternatively, para-aortic node sampling may be performed through a laparoscopic approach; the procedure is well tolerated, recovery is prompt, and yield is adequate.[307,308]

Aside from para-aortic nodes, supraclavicular metastases may rarely be involved. Perez-Mesa and Spratt[309] found no supraclavicular node metastasis in 73 consecutive patients with various stages of cervical carcinoma. Manetta et al.[310] also did not detect scalene node metastasis in 24 patients with recurrent carcinoma of the cervix evaluated for exploration and possible pelvic exenteration. There is no indication for removal of the supraclavicular nodes.

Sentinel Lymph Node Biopsy

Sentinel lymph node (SLN) studies show mixed results, with a 20% false-negative rate and a 50% incidence of other pelvic metastases.[311] However, the method allows for aborting surgery and pursuing RT instead. Sentinel node biopsy in patients with cervical cancer is used in several institutions; a seven-center prospective study analyzed 139 patients and detected 454 SLNs. Intraoperative examination did not detect micrometastasis or isolated tumor cells. Other techniques, such as molecular assays, may improve SLN assessment in the future.[312,313] The SENTICOL study[314] injected 145 stage IA1 to

TABLE 73.9 COMPLICATION RATE FOR PRETHERAPY SURGICAL STAGING

	Transperitoneal (122/189; 64.6%)		Retroperitoneal (67/189; 35.4%)	
	Prior Laparotomy (n = 52), Group 1	No Prior Laparotomy (n = 70), Group 2	Prior Laparotomy (n = 27), Group 3	No Prior Laparotomy (n = 40), Group 4
Complications per group	32 (61.5%)	25 (37.9%)	8 (29.6%)	1 (2.5%)
Percentage of total complications (n = 66)	48.5	37.9	12.1	1.5

Reprinted from Fine BA, Hempling RE, Piver MS, et al. Severe radiation morbidity in carcinoma of the cervix: impact of pretherapy surgical staging and previous surgery. *Int J Radiat Oncol Biol Phys* 1995;31(4):717–723. Copyright © 1995 Elsevier. With permission.

IB1 cervical cancer patients with combined technetium-99 and patent blue. The sensitivity (92%) and lack of false-negative results were favorable, but SLN biopsy was reliable only when SLNs were detected bilaterally.

Ovarian Transposition

In premenopausal women, surgery and radiation may directly impact gonadal function. For women with early-stage cervical cancer who undergo a radical hysterectomy, ovarian function may be preserved. In patients who require postoperative radiation, transposition of ovarian tissue outside of the radiation field may help to preserve ovarian function, although even low doses to the ovaries may cause acute ovarian failure (Fig. 73.9). In women who require radical radiation to the uterus and ovarian tissue, counseling before treatment begins with a fertility expert in reproductive endocrinology may be of benefit if an intervention such as egg retrieval is desired. Care must be taken to ensure that any potential intervention does not delay the initiation of curative treatment. In addition, women with early-stage cervical cancer have an approximately 1% risk of ovarian metastasis with squamous cell carcinoma and 5% risk with adenocarcinoma. Therefore, women should be counseled on the potential risks of recurrence with ovarian preservation.[315]

In a survey of 124 patients who had undergone radical hysterectomy and lymphadenectomy with ovarian transposition, 68 responders were premenopausal at the time of surgery. Six of 30 women (20%) with ovarian preservation experienced early hormonal failure (5 had one ovary, and 1 patient had both preserved).[316] Combined modality therapy affects ovarian function more than operation alone.[317] Anderson et al.[318] noted that only 4 of 24 patients (17%) with ovarian transposition who received postoperative pelvic irradiation had continued ovarian function. Feeney et al.[319] reported on 132 patients on whom lateral ovarian transposition was performed at the time of radical hysterectomy; 28 patients received postoperative pelvic irradiation. Fourteen of 28 patients (50%) who received pelvic irradiation had evidence of ovarian failure, in contrast to 3 of 104 patients (2.9%) on whom ovarian transposition was performed, without postoperative irradiation. Buekers et al.[320] also evaluated ovarian function in 102 patients with cervical cancer, 83 of whom underwent radical hysterectomy and 19 of whom had a staging laparotomy, all with ovarian preservation (80 included ovarian transposition); 26 patients received postoperative radiation therapy. After ovarian transposition without RT, 98% of patients retained ovarian function for a mean of 126 months, with menopause at a mean age of 45.8 years. When ovarian transposition and RT were added, 41% retained ovarian function for a mean of 43 months and experienced menopause at a mean age of 36.6 years.

Morice et al.[321] reported on 107 patients treated for cervical cancer with radical hysterectomy and lymphadenectomy, 104 of whom (98%) had ovarian transposition to the paracolic gutters performed. Preservation of ovarian function was achieved in 100% for patients treated exclusively by surgery, 90% for those treated by postoperative vaginal brachytherapy, and 60% for patients treated by postoperative EBRT and vaginal brachytherapy.

Ovarian transposition or oophoropexy has been performed using laparoscopy, achieving continued hormonal function in 68% (8 of 11) and 50% (3 of 6) of the patients.[322] Mean follow-up was 8.5 years, and mean radiation absorbed dose to the displaced ovaries was 26 Gy. Stockle et al.[323] performed laparoscopic lateral ovarian transposition during staging lymphadenectomy in 11 patients with carcinoma of the cervix treated with brachytherapy (11 cases), EBRT (9 cases), and chemotherapy (2 cases). Ovarian preservation was achieved in 30% of the cases. Age was the most predictive factor for ovarian function preservation. Pahisa et al.[324] performed laparoscopic ovarian transposition on 29 FIGO stage IB1 cervical cancer patients. After a mean follow-up of 44 months, ovarian function was preserved in 93% of the nonirradiated and 64% of the irradiated patients.

Radiation Therapy Techniques

Since the early 1900s, radiation has been used in the curative management of cervical cancer, with a combination of external beam and brachytherapy resulting in the highest survival rates. Over the ensuing 100 years, treatment planning techniques have evolved, as has the equipment used for treatment. Several methods have been developed to aid with conformality and normal-tissue sparing. External irradiation is used to treat the whole pelvis. Structures treated include the uterus and cervix or, in the postoperative cases, the tumor bed, the vagina, the parametrial tissue, and the pelvic lymph nodes, including the internal, external, and common iliac nodes. In selected cases, the PALNs may be treated. In patients with locally advanced disease, in addition to external beam radiation, treatment of central disease (cervix, vagina, and medial

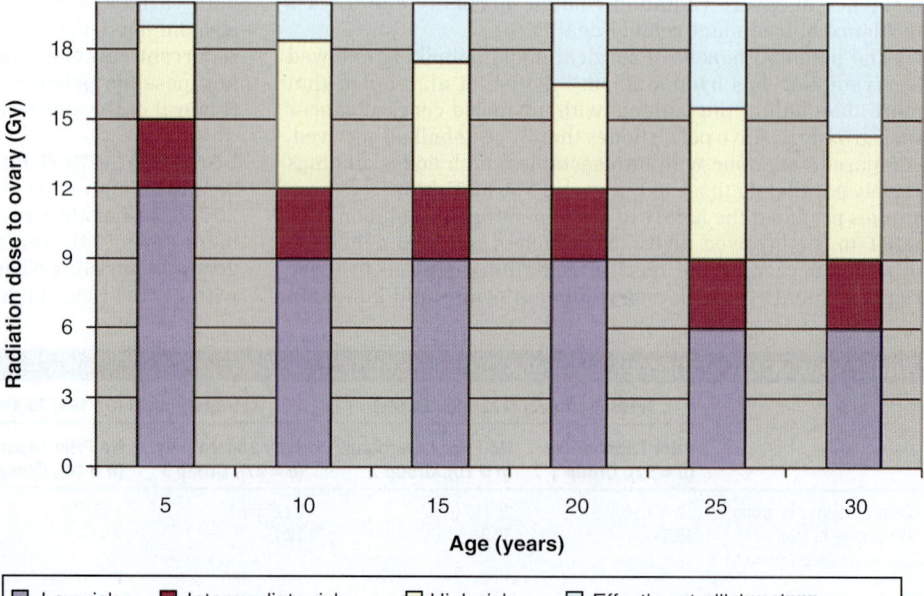

FIGURE 73.9. Risk of developing acute ovarian failure, defined as ovarian failure within 5 years, stratified by age and radiation dose to the ovary. (Reprinted from Wo JY, Viswanathan AN. Impact of radiotherapy on fertility, pregnancy, and neonatal outcomes in female cancer patients. *Int J Radiat Oncol Biol Phys* 2009;73[5]:1304–1312. Copyright © 2009 Elsevier. With permission.)

parametria) relies heavily on dose given with intracavitary sources through brachytherapy. The techniques described apply, with some individualization, to most patients with locally advanced cervical carcinoma.

External Beam Irradiation

External beam treatments may be routinely administered to cervical cancer patients with stages IB2 to IVA in a curative fashion. Patients with stages IA to IB1 may be considered for external beam treatment if they are deemed inoperable or prefer to avoid surgery. Patients with stage IVB disease may receive palliative radiation to the pelvis for selected indications such as to stop vaginal bleeding, relieve pain, or alleviate urethral obstruction from extrinsic compression. External beam radiation covers the primary cervical tumor; treats any adjacent parametrial or uterosacral, uterine, or vaginal extension; and, most important, addresses microscopic disease present in pelvic lymph nodes. In treatment of invasive carcinoma of the uterine cervix, it is important to deliver adequate doses of irradiation not only to the primary tumor but also to the pelvic lymph nodes to maximize tumor control.

The initiation of external beam radiation typically precedes brachytherapy. Although brachytherapy may be interdigitated with external beam treatment, based on the desire to minimize the duration of treatment, the brachytherapy dose to the normal tissues may be better optimized after maximal tumor shrinkage; therefore, many institutions prefer to wait until the completion of 45-Gy treatment before initiating brachytherapy, particularly for patients with large tumors.

Patient Positioning

Patients may be positioned in either the supine position for stability or the prone position on a belly board. The prone position aids in shifting the small bowel out of the pelvis.

In patients who have had a hysterectomy, the small bowel may drop into the pelvic area. For those patients treated for cervical cancer with an intact cervix, the small bowel often lies superior to the uterus and above the pelvic brim, creating less need to shift the bowel out of the pelvis. For patients receiving IMRT, because of stability of the pelvis, the supine position is typically preferred with immobilization devices surrounding the pelvis to ensure minimal motion during treatment. IV contrast may be helpful to localize the pelvic vessels for contouring but is not routinely used in most centers. Oral contrast delineates the small bowel. Rectal contrast and placement of a Foley catheter for bladder contrast are not considered necessary in the majority of cases that use CT simulation because the outer wall of these normal-tissue structures can be contoured without contrast on CT.

Plain X-Ray Simulation

If CT is not available, simple plain film simulation may be performed. The standard plain radiographic simulation to the pelvis with x-rays, typically using opposed anterior–posterior/posterior–anterior (AP-PA) fields, results in comprehensive coverage of all pelvic regions. Because of the lack of visible soft tissue detail, contrast may be placed using barium in the rectum, a vaginal tube in the vagina, and/or a wire marker over surgical scars. The superior border is set at the L4-L5 interspace in order to cover the common iliac lymph nodes and the lateral borders 1.5 to 2 cm from the pelvic brim, and the inferior border covers at least the obturator foramen (Fig. 73.10). More commonly in patients with large tumors, the inferior border extends to the ischial tuberosities. When there is vaginal involvement, the entire length of this organ should be treated down to the introitus. It is very important to identify the distal extension of the tumor at the time of simulation by placing a radiopaque clip or bead on

FIGURE 73.10. A: Anteroposterior simulation film of the pelvis illustrating portals used for external irradiation. The 15 by 15 cm portals at source-to-skin distance are used for stage IB (*broken line*), and 18 by 15 cm portals are used for more advanced disease (*solid line*). This allows better coverage of the common iliac lymph nodes. The distal margin is usually placed at the bottom of the obturator foramina. **B:** Diagram of pelvic portals used in external irradiation of carcinoma of uterine cervix. Standard portal for stage IB tumors is outlined (*solid line indicated as A*). When the common iliac nodes are to be covered, the upper margin is extended to the L4-L5 space (*indicated in section B*). If there is vaginal tumor extension, the lower margin of the field is drawn at the introitus (*indicated in section C*).

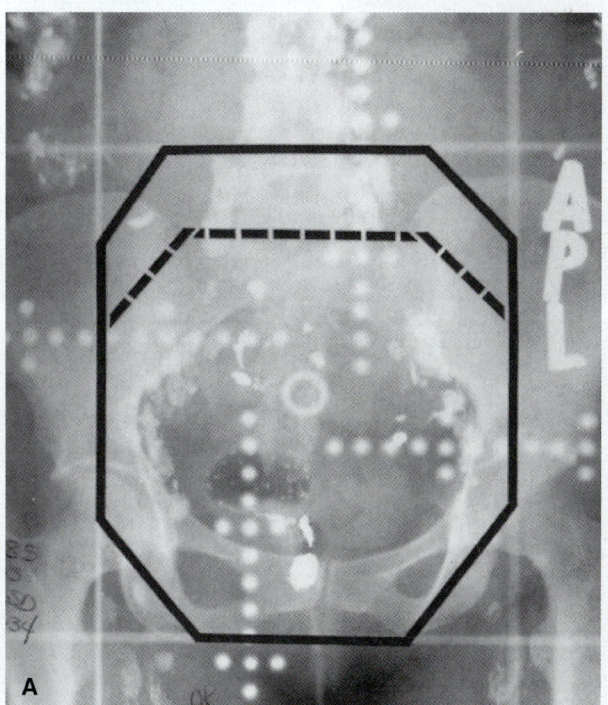

A

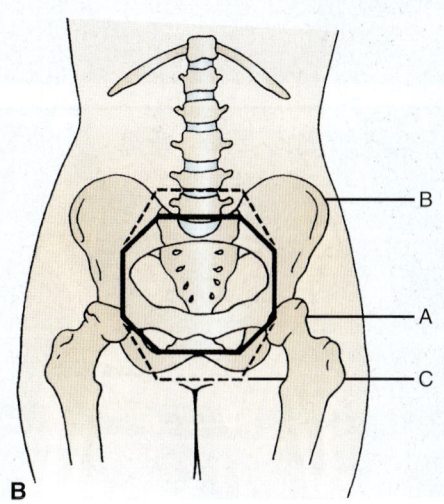

B

the vaginal wall or inserting a small fiducial marker in the vagina. When the tumor involves the distal half of the vagina, the portals should be modified to cover the inguinal lymph nodes because of the increased probability of metastases (see Fig. 73.2).

For the lateral field borders, in both postoperative and intact cervix settings, the posterior border must be set in such a way that the entire sacrum is covered because the uterosacral ligaments are at high risk for harboring microscopic extension. The uterosacral ligaments insert onto the sacrum, and therefore, the posterior block should ensure coverage of the entire sacrum. The anterior border on the lateral field should be set at a vertical line anterior to the pubic symphysis, because the external iliac lymph nodes must be covered.

For patients with para-aortic nodal involvement, simple plain film simulation followed by AP-PA treatments to the para-aortic nodal chain may overdose the kidneys, spinal cord, and small bowel. Dose escalation to para-aortic nodes to approximately >45 Gy is not feasible with AP-PA fields, given potential bowel complications. The use of four fields, including AP-PA and two lateral fields, is implemented as an alternative to AP-PA alone as a way to reduce some of the dose to the anterior small bowel. Patients receive oral barium approximately 30 minutes before the simulation to ensure blockage of as much small bowel as feasible superiorly. The superior border covers the renal hilum, often at the T12-L1 interspace, and the inferior borders cover the obturator foramen, unless there is distal vaginal or inguinal node involvement. For the para-aortic portion of the field, the anterior border rests 2 cm in front of the vertebral body or enlarged nodes as contoured, and posteriorly, the border bisects the midvertebral body. The pelvic portion mimics that described

for the four-field pelvic setup. The use of lateral fields allows a decrease in dose to the small bowel, but care must be taken to include all structures of interest.[325–327]

Three-Dimensional Conformal Treatment Planning

CT simulation allows direct assessment of the pelvic vessels and by adjacent location the para-aortic and pelvic nodes. Oral contrast is beneficial to identify the small bowel. Cerrobend customized blocks or multileaf collimator blocking is used on each field to block the radiation to selected areas, including the skin, muscle, soft tissue, anterior small bowel, and portions of the anus and lower rectum (Fig. 73.11).

The superior border is set based on the CT-visualized bifurcation of the common iliac nodes into the external and internal iliac nodes, which may lie as high as the L3-L4 interspace. If patients have positive pelvic nodes based on PET imaging, the superior border may be shifted to either the superior border of the common iliac nodes or the superior aspect of the renal hilum to treat the para-aortic nodes. In postoperative cases in which the patient has had an extensive surgical staging, the superior border may be reduced to the L5-S1 interspace. Similar to plain x-ray simulation, in patients with vaginal involvement, the inferior border is extended to cover 2 cm below the lowest extent of disease, which may lie in the vulvar tissue, and in such cases, the inguinal lymph nodes are treated, resulting in a wider AP field.

On the lateral fields, the anterior border covers the front of the pubic symphysis. Bonin et al.,[328] in a review of 22 patients on whom detailed anatomic mapping of the anatomy of the pelvic lymph nodes was carried out by lymphangiography,

FIGURE 73.11. Anterior–posterior and lateral digitally reconstructed radiograph simulation film of the pelvis, illustrating portals used for external irradiation with the patient in the prone position on a belly board to minimize small-bowel dose. Pelvic lymph nodes are indicated in their approximate position. The uterus, cervix, and vagina are contoured to ensure adequate coverage.

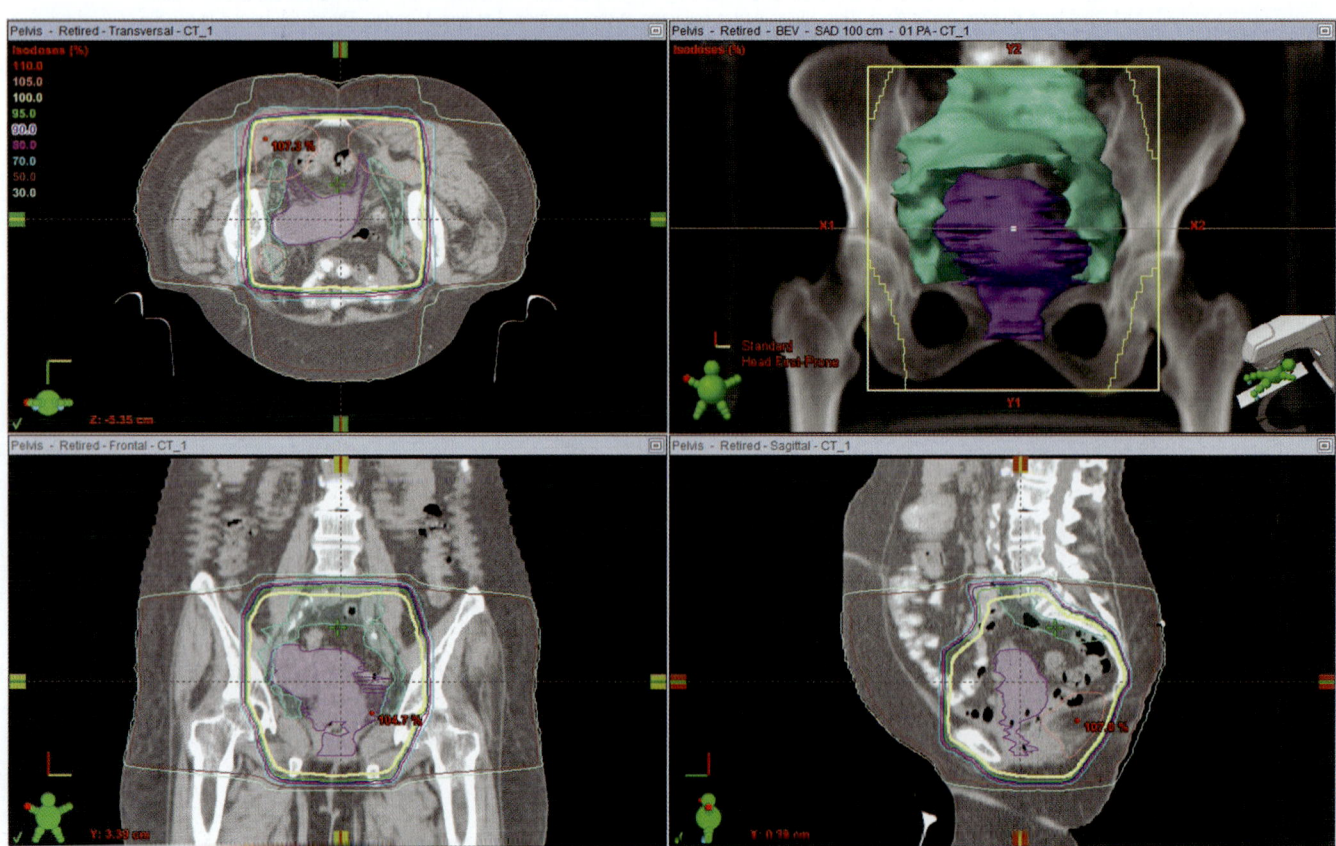

concluded that if the criteria for adequacy of standard pelvic fields as defined in prior clinical trials were applied (anteroposterior: 1.5-cm margin on the pelvic rim; lateral field anterior edge is a vertical line anterior to the pubic symphysis and posterior border), 10 patients (45%) would have had inadequate nodal coverage in the irradiation fields. The incompletely irradiated lymph nodes were in the lowest lateral external iliac group. However, CT simulation with contouring may prevent omission of these nodes.

For the lateral borders in postoperative and intact cervix cases, posterior coverage of the entire sacral hollow is imperative. Zunino et al.[329] reviewed the appropriateness of radiation therapy box technique for cancer of the cervix in 35 sagittal MRIs and 10 lymphangiograms. If the posterior border were to be placed at the S2-S3 interspace, for 50% of the patients with FIGO IB and in 67% with stage IIA disease, the posterior border of the lateral field would not adequately encompass the planning target volume (PTV). In stage IIB, the posterior border was inadequate in eight patients (42%). In patients with stage IIB and IVA disease, the PTV was not encompassed. Furthermore, Knocke et al.[330] used standard simulator planning guided by bony landmarks for pelvic irradiation in 20 patients with primary cervical carcinoma, stages I to III, using a four-field box technique. After defining the PTV with a 3D planning system, they compared the field configuration of the simulator planning with a second one based on the defined PTV. They evaluated the ability of the PTV to encompass the treatment volume (International Commission on Radiation Units and Measurements [ICRU]). Planning by simulation resulted in 1 geographic miss, and in 10 more cases, the coverage of the PTV by the treatment volume was inadequate.

Finlay et al.[331] contoured pelvic blood vessels on CT scans as surrogates for lymph nodes in 43 patients and found this to be more accurate than bony landmarks for field delineation. In total, 95% of patients planned with conventional fields had inadequate coverage of some portion of lymph node coverage, whereas 56% additional normal tissue was treated that did not require radiation. Therefore, most centers implement 3D simulation when feasible. Taylor et al.[332] used MRI to outline the pelvic lymph nodes in 20 patients and noted that with margins of 10 mm, nodal coverage was 94% and with 15 mm, 99%; with a modified 7-mm margin, they ensured 99% nodal coverage with less volume of small bowel at risk.

In the postoperative setting, van den Berg et al.,[333] using 47 lymphangiograms and 15 CT scans, asked radiation oncologists (n = 17) to define the CTV and PTV and to delineate on simulation films the RT treatment portals to be used after a radical hysterectomy with lymph node dissection for stage IB or IIA cervical carcinoma with positive iliac lymph nodes. Large variations were observed in the portals used and in treatment techniques. From the digitized films, it appeared that in 50% of the cases, the defined PTV was not covered adequately. Furthermore, 71% of the treatment plans would not cover the lateral borders of the reference PTV sufficiently. Thus, there is a need for careful adherence to standardized guidelines.

Treatment techniques may have an effect on outcome. Yamazaki et al.[334] compared 34 patients with cervical cancer treated with irregularly shaped four-field whole-pelvis radiation therapy using CT simulation and 40 patients receiving whole-pelvis EBRT with parallel-opposed fields in a nonrandomized study of postoperative radiation therapy consisting of 50 Gy in 25 fractions in 6 weeks. With a mean follow-up of 60 months, the actuarial 5-year pelvic tumor control was 94% with the two-field technique and 100% for the irregularly shaped four-field technique. The incidence of grade 2 or 3 bowel complications in the irregularly shaped technique group (2.9%, 1 of 34) was significantly lower than that in the two-field technique group (17.5%, 7 of 40; $P < .05$).

Burnett et al.[335] described a prosthetic silicone plastic device that is filled with saline and Renografin for x-ray visualization (capacity between 750 and 1,500 mL) to conform to the pelvis and exclude the small bowel from the irradiated volume. The device remains in place throughout the radiation therapy course and is removed through a small incision after draining the contents of the prosthesis. Seven devices had been placed to date of the report. In the postoperative period, there was one pulmonary embolism. All seven patients completed planned radiation therapy. The devices have been removed with no adhesions to the prosthesis.

Intensity-Modulated Radiation

IMRT was developed using the techniques required for inverse planning. That is, one starts with the necessary dose around the target and then works backward to develop the requisite beam intensities. IMRT spatially modulates the intensity of the beam using the motion of multileaf collimators. Because of the increasing use of intensity-modulated or image-guided radiation therapy (IMRT/IGRT) including volumetric arc therapy (VMAT) in the treatment of patients with gynecologic malignancies, there is growing emphasis on imaging the pelvic anatomic structures, including lymph nodes, for treatment planning.[336] IMRT may reduce the amount of small bowel and bone marrow that receives the full dose of radiation.

The use of IMRT has been standardized in the postoperative setting and is more frequently used for intact cervix cases though caution must be exercised to cover the full uterosacral ligaments and to provide a large enough anterior margin to account for shifts in uterine anatomy. What constitutes adequate margins in the intact cervix setting continues to be a matter of concern, given significant organ motion during treatment. Uncertainties in the definition of target volumes arise using 3D techniques. Bladder filling and rectal filling changes require accurate definition of margins for the PTV.[337] Beadle et al.[338] found that mean maximum changes in the center of the cervix were 2.1, 1.6, and 0.82 cm in the superior–inferior, anterior–posterior, and right–left lateral dimensions, respectively. Mean maximum changes in the perimeter of the cervix were 2.3 and 1.3 cm in the superior and inferior, 1.7 and 1.8 cm in the anterior and posterior, and 0.76 and 0.94 cm in the right and left lateral directions, respectively. Haripotepornkul et al.[339] found in 10 women with locally advanced cervical cancer that within and between radiation treatments, cervical motion averages approximately 3 mm but may be up to 18 mm in any given direction. The mean intrafractional movements in cervical seed positions in the lateral, vertical, and AP directions were 1.6 mm (standard deviation [SD] ± 2.0), 2.6 mm (SD ± 2.4), and 2.9 mm (SD ± 2.7), respectively, with a range from 0 to 15 mm for each direction. The mean interfractional movements in the lateral, vertical, and AP directions were 1.9 mm (SD ± 1.9), 4.1 mm (SD ± 3.2), and 4.2 mm (SD ± 3.5), respectively, with a range from 0 to 18 mm for each direction. Tyagi et al.[340] show that a uniform CTV planning treatment volume margin of 15 mm would not encompass the cervical CTV in 32% of fractions. with IMRT, there is a need for continual replanning (at least every other week), given rapid tumor regression and internal-organ motion.[341-343] The dosimetric effect of organ motion during intact IMRT for cervical cancer was studied in 10 patients. With 10- to 15-mm PTV margins, significant CTV underdosing was identified during treatment, primarily because of changes in bladder volume. Larger margins of up to 2–3 cm in the AP direction and bladder volumes at 150 to 300 cc are recommended.[344]

After a CT and/or MRI scan for simulation, the images are brought into a treatment planning workstation. Contouring the gross tumor volume (GTV) on MRI may include the uterus, cervix, and/or vagina. Lim et al.[345] had 19 experts in gynecologic radiation oncology contour a case of locally advanced cervical cancer on axial MRI of the pelvis. Substantial Simultaneous Truth and Performance Level Estimation (STAPLE) agreement sensitivity and specificity values were seen for GTV delineation (0.84 and 0.96, respectively) with a kappa statistic of 0.68 ($P < .0001$). Agreement for delineation of cervix, uterus, vagina, and parametria was moderate. The greatest variability in physician contouring was in the parametrial tissue.[345]

The CTV for the pelvic lymph nodes was based on the Radiation Therapy Oncology Group (RTOG) atlas for the female postoperative pelvis.[346] An example of dose distribution achieved with supine IMRT pelvic irradiation is illustrated in Figure 73.12. Fiducial markers may be placed in the apex of the vagina for identification on CT scan and show up to 3.5 cm of vaginal cuff motion during treatment.[347] Therefore, for postoperative patients, the vagina is contoured using a full-bladder CT scan fused to an empty-bladder CT scan to account for vaginal mobility because of differences in bladder filling.[348] This vaginal target volume has been referred to as an integrated target volume (ITV). The expansion of the CTV and/or ITV to the PTV is necessary, although given the movement of the uterus, the exact amount of margin is a matter of debate. Generous margins of approximately 2 to 3 cm are considered, particularly in the regions of the uterus and cervix or in the postoperative case around the ITV vagina. In order to cover the uterosacral ligaments, the rectum cannot be spared. Rectal filling with gas may change the position of the anterior rectal wall over 5 cm during treatment. Dose constraints required for an optimal IMRT plan have not been standardized. In the RTOG postoperative clinical trial 0921 using IMRT,[349] a PTV of 7 mm around the nodal contours is recommended, and the dose is prescribed to cover 97% of the vaginal PTV and nodal PTV. A volume of 0.03 cc within any PTV should not receive >110% of the prescribed dose. No more than 0.03 cc of any PTV will receive <93% of its prescribed dose. Any contiguous volume of 0.03 cc or larger of the tissue outside the vaginal/nodal PTVs must not receive >110% of the dose prescribed to the vaginal/nodal PTV; for normal tissues, the small/large bowel (30% of the entire bowel volume must not receive >40 Gy), rectum/sigmoid (60% of the rectosigmoid volume must receive ≤40 Gy), bladder (35% of the bladder volume must receive ≤45 Gy), and femoral head (15% of the femoral head volume must receive <35 Gy) constraints are being tested in RTOG 0921. Careful attention must be paid to all normal-tissue organ motion because the bladder and rectum may have 3- to 5-cm shifts because of filling changes in a short time frame.

For patients that have had a diagnostic PET or MRI before the simulation, these images may be registered to create a fused dataset for contouring, particularly when a nodal boost is required. This allows the physician to visualize areas of PET enhancement or tumor volume, as seen on the MRI, onto the simulation films. Grigsby et al.[350] use a PET-defined target volume contoured with a metabolically active tumor specified at the 40% threshold. Normal-tissue structures, including the rectum, sigmoid, bladder, and small bowel, are routinely contoured for patients treated with IMRT who will be undergoing a nodal boost in order to limit the dose received primarily to the small bowel. Based on an overview of published data, the absolute volume of small bowel receiving ≥15 Gy should be held to <120 cc when possible to minimize severe acute toxicity if delineating the contours of bowel loops themselves. Alternatively, if the entire volume of peritoneal space in which the small bowel can move is delineated, the volume receiving >45 Gy should be <195 cc when possible.[351] For the rectum, dose–volume constraints selected as a conservative starting point that have not yet been validated for 3D treatment planning include $V_{50} < 50\%$, $V_{60} < 35\%$, $V_{65} < 25\%$, $V_{70} < 20\%$, and $V_{75} < 15\%$.[352] No dose constraint for external beam planning for the bladder could be identified, although the limits for prostate cancer may be adopted for gynecologic IMRT, including a dose constraint of no more than 15% of the volume to receive a dose >80 Gy, no more than 25% of the volume to receive a dose >75 Gy, no more than 35% of the volume to receive a dose >70 Gy, or no more than 50% of the volume to receive a dose >65 Gy.[353]

Imaging may guide more accurate definition of lymph nodes.[332] Portelance et al.[299] carried out IMRT as well as conventional planning with two- and four-field techniques in 10 patients. Prescription was 45 Gy in 25 fractions to the uterus and the pelvic and PALNs. All IMRT plans were normalized to obtain a full coverage of the cervix with the 95% isodose curve (Fig. 73.13A). The volumes of the small bowel receiving the prescribed dose (45 Gy) with IMRT para-aortic–only technique were, with four fields, 11%; with seven fields, 15%; and with nine fields, 13.5% (Fig. 73.13B). These dose distributions were all significantly better than with two-field or four-field conventional techniques ($P < .05$). Ahmed et al.[354] arrived at similar conclusions in five patients with para-aortic node metastasis, and they demonstrated the feasibility of escalating the dose to 60 Gy while sparing the kidneys, spinal cord, small bowel, and bone marrow. Heron et al.,[355] in a study of 10 patients, showed that with IMRT there was a reduction of 52% in the small-bowel volume receiving >30 Gy and a decrease of 66% for the rectum and 36% for the bladder compared with 3D radiation therapy. D'Souza et al.,[356] in 10 patients, also noted a reduction of small-bowel volume (33%) with IMRT compared with four-field pelvic RT; however, small volumes of bowel received 55 to 60 Gy with the IMRT plans. Positioning the patient prone on a belly board was shown to reduce the volume of small-bowel irradiated. However, patients on a belly board may have large daily anatomic shifts that make prone IMRT unreproducible.[357]

Brixey et al.[358] and Lujan et al.[359] also used IMRT planning to spare the bone marrow of patients with gynecologic tumors. Brixey et al.,[358] in 36 patients, noted no significant difference in hematologic toxicity with IMRT or conventional RT alone; however, in patients receiving chemotherapy, less grade 2 white blood cell toxicity was observed with IMRT (31.2% vs. 60%, respectively). PET-detected bone marrow was spared using an atlas.[360] In a single-arm phase II study of 83 patients, with median follow-up of 26.0 months, the incidence of grade ≥3 neutropenia and clinically significant GI toxicity was 19.3% (95% confidence interval [CI], 12.2% to 29.0%) and 12.0% (95% CI, 6.7% to 20.8%), respectively. Compared with patients treated without IG-IMRT ($n = 48$), those treated with IG-IMRT ($n = 35$) had a significantly lower incidence of grade ≥3 neutropenia (8.6% vs. 27.1%; 2-sided χ^2 $P = .035$) and nonsignificantly lower incidence of grade ≥3 leukopenia (25.7% vs. 41.7%; $P = .13$) and any grade ≥3 hematologic toxicity (31.4% vs. 43.8%; $P = .25$).[361]

FIGURE 73.12. Intensity-modulated radiation therapy treatment plan for external irradiation of pelvic lymph nodes while sparing organs at risk. Note margins required to cover uterosacral ligaments posteriorly while accounting for organ motion with daily cone beam imaging.

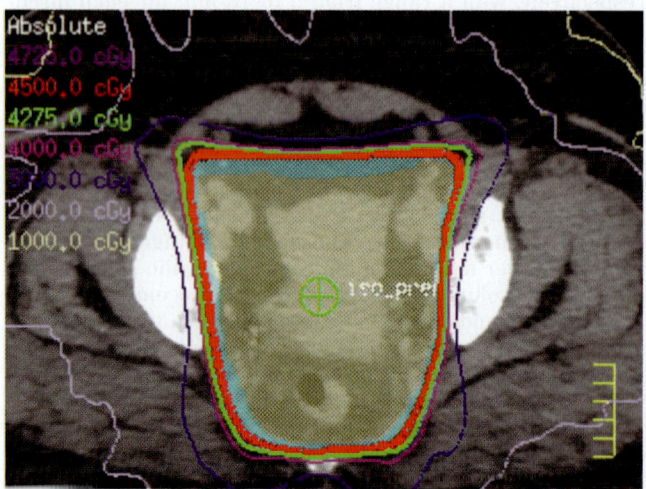

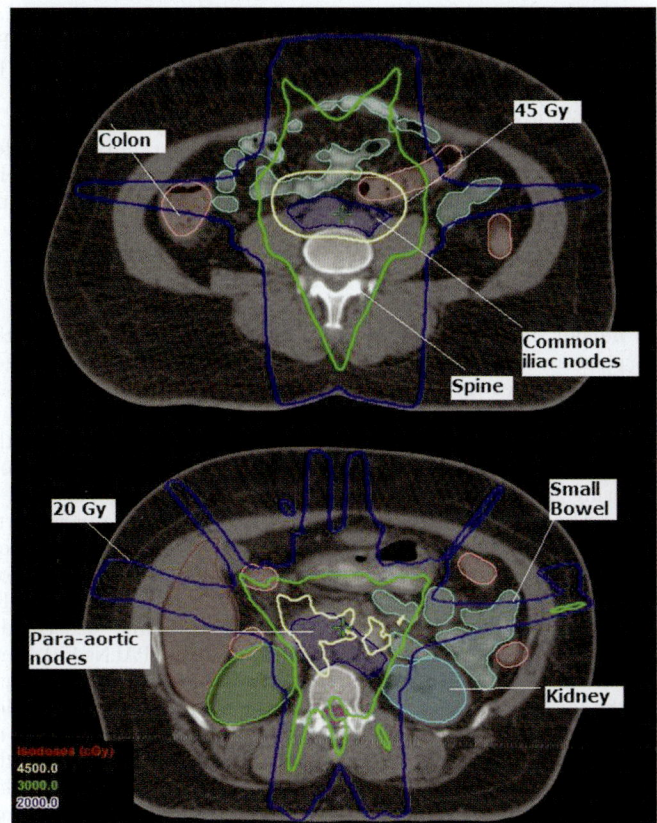

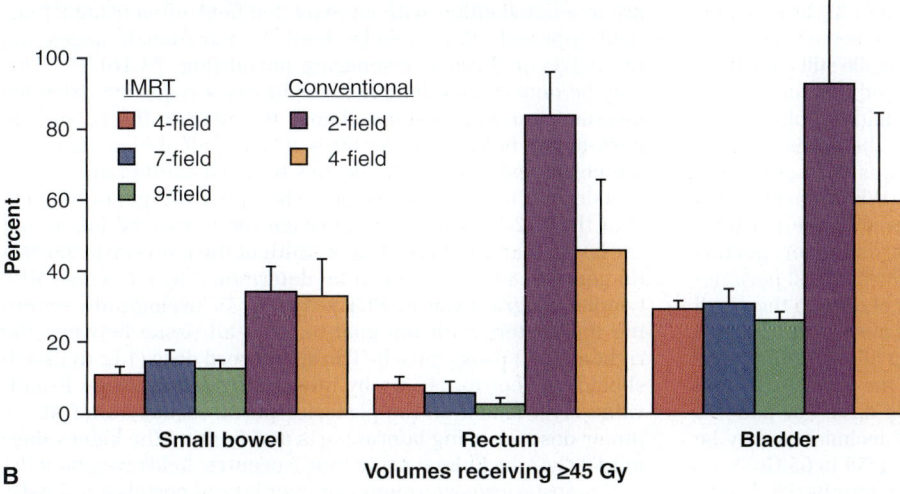

FIGURE 73.13. A: Axial views of IMRT dose distribution. **B:** The functional volume of the small bowel, rectum, and bladder receiving ≥45 Gy with IMRT or conventional techniques when 100% of the target volume (uterus) receives ≥95% of the prescription dose (45 Gy). (Reprinted from Portelance L, Chao KSC, Grigsby PW, et al. Intensity-modulated radiation therapy [(IMRT)] reduces small bowel and bladder doses in patients with cervical cancer receiving pelvic and para-aortic irradiation. *Int J Radiat Oncol Biol Phys* 2001;51[1]:261–266. Copyright © 2001 Elsevier. With permission.)

Hasselle et al.[362] report on 111 patients treated with multiple different approaches, including 22 treated with postoperative IMRT, 8 with IMRT followed by intracavitary brachytherapy and adjuvant hysterectomy, and 81 with IMRT followed by planned intracavitary brachytherapy. Median follow-up time was 27 months. Acute and late grade 3 toxicity or higher was 2% (95% CI, 0% to 7%) and 7% (95% CI, 2% to 13%), respectively. Guerrero et al.[363] proposed using an IMRT simultaneous integrated boost (SIB) as an alternative to conventional whole-pelvis irradiation and used the linear quadratic equation to calculate equivalent uniform dose in multiple plans. However, a report by Kavanagh et al.[364] found that accelerated fractionation caused an unacceptably high rate of complications. A combination of an SIB to approximately 50 Gy followed by a sequential boost to 60 to 65 Gy has been shown to be feasible to both pelvic and para-aortic

nodes. Caution in the pelvis when also administering brachytherapy is required to ensure bowel dose is limited, and in the para-aortic region, rapid shrinkage of the tumor may result in movement of bowel into the boost field, and replanning immediately prior to beginning the sequential portion of the boost is recommended.[365,366]

Postoperative IMRT with cisplatin was reported in 34 patients with stage IA2 to IIA cervical cancer; 5 year disease-free and overall survival was 91%. One patient (2.9%) had a grade 3 side effect (proctitis).[367]

Although IMRT has dosimetric advantages over conventional RT, IMRT exposes a greater amount of normal tissues to lower irradiation levels, which has the potential to increase the incidence of radiation-induced second cancers,[368] a phenomenon already described with conventional RT techniques.[369]

Image-Guided Radiation Therapy

Although not always available, daily cone-beam CT imaging for in-room image-guided RT (IGRT) permits visualization of bladder and rectum.[370] Particularly in cases with a large, mobile uterus, such as is seen in young women, if an extended field is used and there is concern that the uterus may be out of the field, this may be instituted helpful to confirm full coverage of the CTV daily. When IMRT is used for locally advanced cervical cancer, the priority should be to treat with wide margins, so that the field mimics that of a 3D conformal (four-field) plan in order to ensure no increase in the risk of local recurrence.[340] IGRT daily may demonstrate organ motion, but criteria for replanning have not been defined.

Stereotactic body radiotherapy (SBRT) uses highly conformal treatments with large fraction sizes and in selected cases has been considered for a nodal boost of an isolated para-aortic node, although care must be taken to treat the entire para-aortic chain to 45 Gy with IMRT or 4 Field (4F) prior to considering an SBRT boost in order to ensure eradication of adjacent micrometastatic disease.[371] SBRT should not be used instead of brachytherapy, given the significant increase in normal-tissue doses with SBRT compared to brachytherapy.[372]

Midline Shielding in AP-PA Portals and Use of a Parametrial Boost

Depending on the institution and brachytherapy dose administered, midline shielding with rectangular or specially designed blocks has been traditionally used for a portion of the external beam dose delivered with the AP-PA ports.[326] Midline blocks may be individualized, based on the point A isodose line or a rectangular block of approximately 4-cm width. In one series, overall survival and incidence of chronic complications were not related to the type of shielding.[373] However, in the era of 3D brachytherapy planning, the use of a midline block has been questioned because it may result in tumor underdosing while still contributing significant dose to the bladder, sigmoid, and rectum.[374]

Several institutions reported placing a midline block after a full course of external beam treatment to the pelvis in order to boost the parametria or nodes for patients with persistent disease after approximately 45 to 50 Gy. When parametrial tumor persists, 50 to 60 Gy may be delivered to the parametria, with reduced anteroposterior/posteroanterior portals (8 by 12 cm for unilateral and 12 by 12 cm for bilateral parametrial coverage). However, careful estimation of dose to the small bowel, sigmoid, and rectum is needed. In the modern era, the use of highly conformal boosts with 3D planning allows an increase in normal-tissue sparing. Contours on CT of the parametrial and nodal region allow more precise tailoring of dose. For patients with enlarged nodes, when available, IMRT techniques may be best at providing conformal dose escalation to 54 to 65 Gy.

Similarly, with 3D brachytherapy and computerized optimization as available with high HDR or pulsed dose rate (PDR) brachytherapy, the physician may cover the adjacent parametria using large enough fraction sizes that an additional external beam boost is not needed. When one prescribes HDR brachytherapy, the per fraction nodal dose is approximately 25% of prescription. In one study, the per fraction dose to the pelvic lymph nodes by HDR brachytherapy, when the high-risk clinical target volume (HR-CTV) received 5.5 Gy per fraction, was 1.4 Gy per fraction. Therefore, HDR brachytherapy may obviate the need for a parametrial boost, given the high per fraction dose to the parametria and pelvic sidewall.[374]

In a comparison of three different approaches, Fenkell et al.[375] reported on parametrial boost with midline shielding in six patients with locally advanced cervical cancer (IIB to IIIB) treated with definitive chemoradiotherapy and MRI-guided brachytherapy. A three-phase plan was modeled: 45-Gy (1.8 Gy per fraction) four-field box, 9-Gy (1.8 Gy per fraction) midline-shielded anteroposterior/posteroanterior fields (MBB), and intracavitary MRI-guided brachytherapy boost of 28 Gy (7 Gy per fraction). Midline shields 3, 4, and 5 cm wide were simulated for each patient. Brachytherapy and MBB plans were volumetrically summed. After a 4-cm MBB, HR-CTV D_{90} remained <85 Gy in all cases (mean, 74 Gy; range, 64 to 82 Gy). Bladder, rectum, or sigmoid D_{2cc} increased by >50% of the boost dose in four of six patients. The authors concluded that a midline block may not be beneficial in patients receiving 3D image-planned brachytherapy with adequate optimization of dose to the tumor and away from the normal tissues.

Para-aortic Lymph Node Irradiation

If para-aortic node metastases are enlarged or suspected to harbor disease, patients are treated with 45 to 50 Gy to the para-aortic area plus a sequential 5- to 10-Gy boost to enlarged lymph nodes through reduced lateral or rotational portals.[302] If feasible, 3D planning with IMRT treatment is preferred to spare normal tissues, superiorly covering above the level of the renal hilum or the highest extent of disease and inferiorly covering 2 cm below the lowest extent of disease (Fig. 73.14).

The use of IMRT has allowed dose escalation to para-aortic nodes, particularly unresectable nodes. Clinical reports show excellent control of disease with dose escalation, with one report demonstrating an 85% 2-year nodal control rate after IMRT with a median dose of 63 Gy.[376] Esthappan et al.[298] described a technique using CT and FDG-PET to treat the PALNs (50.4 and 59.4 Gy) with IMRT (Fig. 73.15). Acceptable dose distribution of the target volumes and sparing of the stomach, liver, and colon were achieved. Sparing of the spinal cord was dependent on the number and arrangements of the beams, as it was for the small bowel, sparing of which was limited because of overlap with the target volume. Adjusting the number of beams and prescription parameters minimally improved kidney sparing.

When only conventional techniques are available, the PALNs are irradiated either with an extended field, often using a four-field approach, that includes both the para-aortic nodes and the pelvis or through a separate portal (Fig. 73.16).[326,377] This may be done as one long field, or in cases requiring extended distance, one may instead choose to separate the pelvic and para-aortic fields. This requires a "gap calculation" between the pelvic and para-aortic portals to avoid overlap and excessive dose to the small intestines. The upper margin of the field is at the T12-L1 interspace to reach the infrarenal hilum and the lower margin at L5-S1. The width of the para-aortic portals (in general, 8 to 10 cm) can be determined by CT scans, MRI, lymphangiography, FDG-PET scans, or IV pyelography outlining the ureters with the goal to treat all tissue between the right and left psoas muscle. The spinal cord dose (T12 to L2-L3) should be kept to <45 Gy by interposing a 2-cm-wide 5–half-value-layer shield on the posterior portal (usually after 40-Gy tumor dose) or using lateral ports and limiting the kidney dose to <18 Gy. A technique using four isocentric fields weighted 2:1 anteroposterior/posteroanterior over lateral portals and 1.8-Gy fractions was described by Russell et al.[378] to deliver high-dose therapy (56 to 61 Gy). Kodaira et al.[379] evaluated a four-field para-aortic irradiation technique with 10-MV photons (mean, 50.4 Gy) in 97 patients with cervical cancer. The 5-year CSS rate was 32.2%. Grade 1 or 2 stomach and duodenum sequelae developed in 26.8%, grade 2 sequelae of small bowel in 3.1%, and grade 2 sequelae of bone in 3.1%. Rates of toxicity with IMRT are lower though dose escalation with a simultaneous integrated boost to large nodes next to the duodenum must be done with caution given the risk of duodenal perforation.[302]

Beam Energies

For IMRT, 6-MV energy is used to provide the most homogeneous dose. However, in conventional irradiation, because of the thickness of the pelvis, high-energy photon beams (10 MV or higher) are especially suited for this treatment. They decrease the dose of radiation delivered to the peripheral normal tissues (particularly bladder and rectum) and provide a more homogeneous dose distribution in the central pelvis.

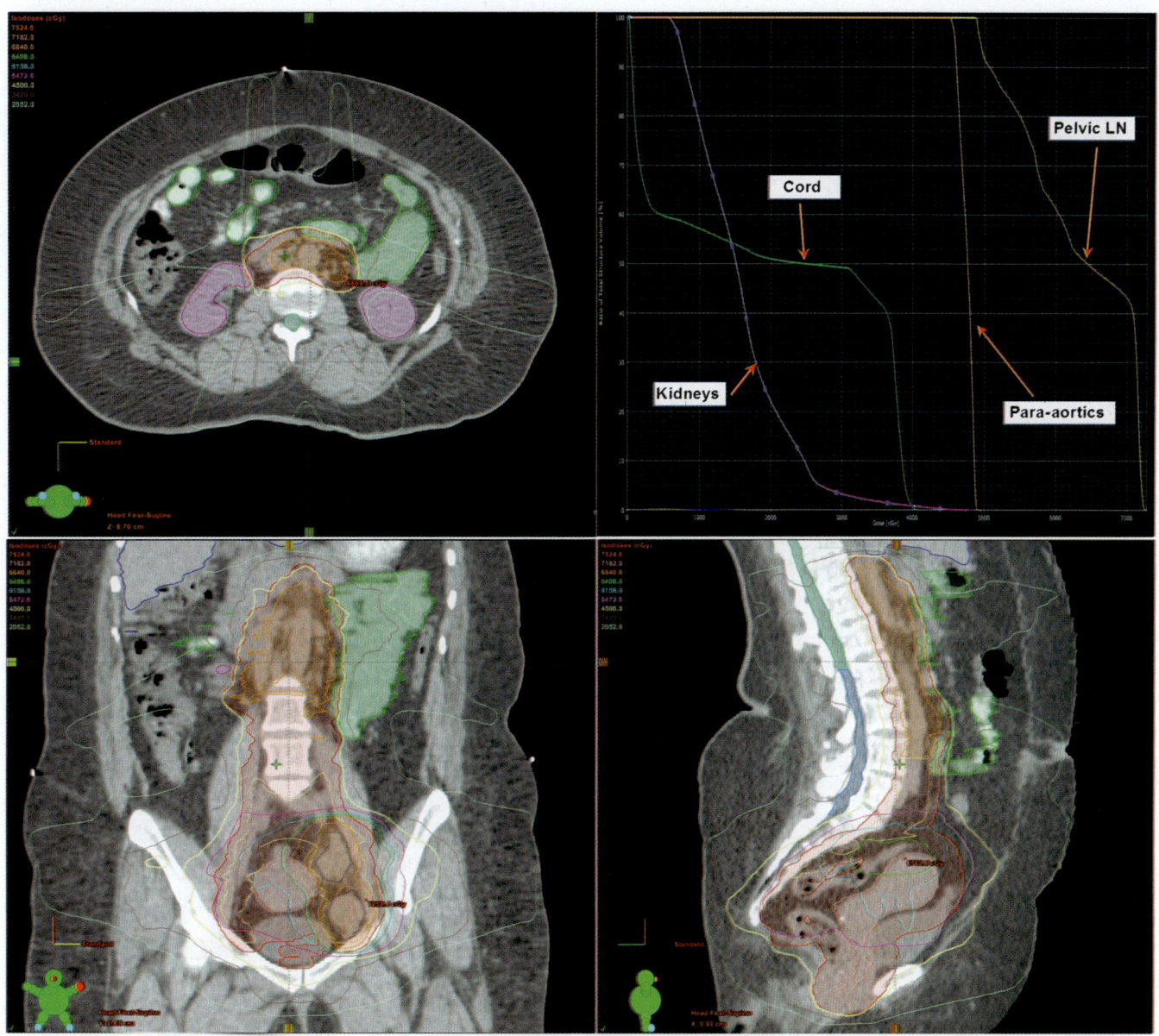

FIGURE 73.14. Extended-field IMRT for external irradiation of uterine cervix and pelvic and para-aortic lymph nodes. Dose–volume histogram values for the spinal cord, kidneys, para-aortic nodes, and pelvic node boost are shown for a patient who had an unresectable 4-cm pelvic lymph node.

With lower-energy photons ([65]Co or 4- to 6-MV x-rays), higher maximum doses must be given, and more complicated field arrangements should be used to achieve the same midplane tumor dose (three-field or four-field pelvic box or rotational techniques) while minimizing the dose to the bladder and rectum and to avoid subcutaneous fibrosis (Fig. 73.17).[380] Biggs and Russell[381] noted that the presence of a metallic prosthesis when using lateral fields or a box pelvic irradiation technique may result in a dose decrease of approximately 2% for 25-MV x-rays and average increases of 2% for 10-MV x-rays and 5% for [65]Co. Allt[382] and Johns,[383] in an update of a randomized study, reported better pelvic tumor control and survival and fewer complications in 65 patients with stage IIB and III cervical carcinomas treated with 23-MV photons compared with 61 treated with external irradiation with [65]Co in addition to brachytherapy in both groups. In contrast, Holcomb et al.[380] compared outcome of 195 patients with stage IIB and IVA cervical carcinomas treated with [65]Co radiation therapy (group 1) and 53 treated with linear accelerators (group 2). There was no significant difference in overall survival, although there was a trend toward increasing pelvic recurrence in the [65]Co

group (50.8%) compared with group 2 (35.8%; P = .08). Mixed beam external radiation with neutrons and photons resulted in unacceptably high toxicity rates and is not recommended.[384] Similarly, carbon ion therapy was reported but resulted in major intestinal complications.[385]

Hyperfractionated or Accelerated Hyperfractionated Radiation Therapy

MacLeod et al.[386] reported on a phase II trial of 61 patients with locally advanced cervical cancer treated with accelerated hyperfractionated radiation therapy (1.25 Gy administered twice daily at least 6 hours apart to a total pelvic dose of 57.5 Gy). A boost dose was administered with either low–dose rate (LDR) brachytherapy or EBRT to a smaller volume. Thirty patients had acute toxicity that required regular medication. One patient died of acute treatment-related toxicity. The overall 5-year survival was 27%, relapse-free survival was 36%, and actuarial local tumor control was 66%. There were eight severe late complications observed in seven patients, who required surgical intervention (actuarial rate of 27%). Five patients also required total hip replacement.

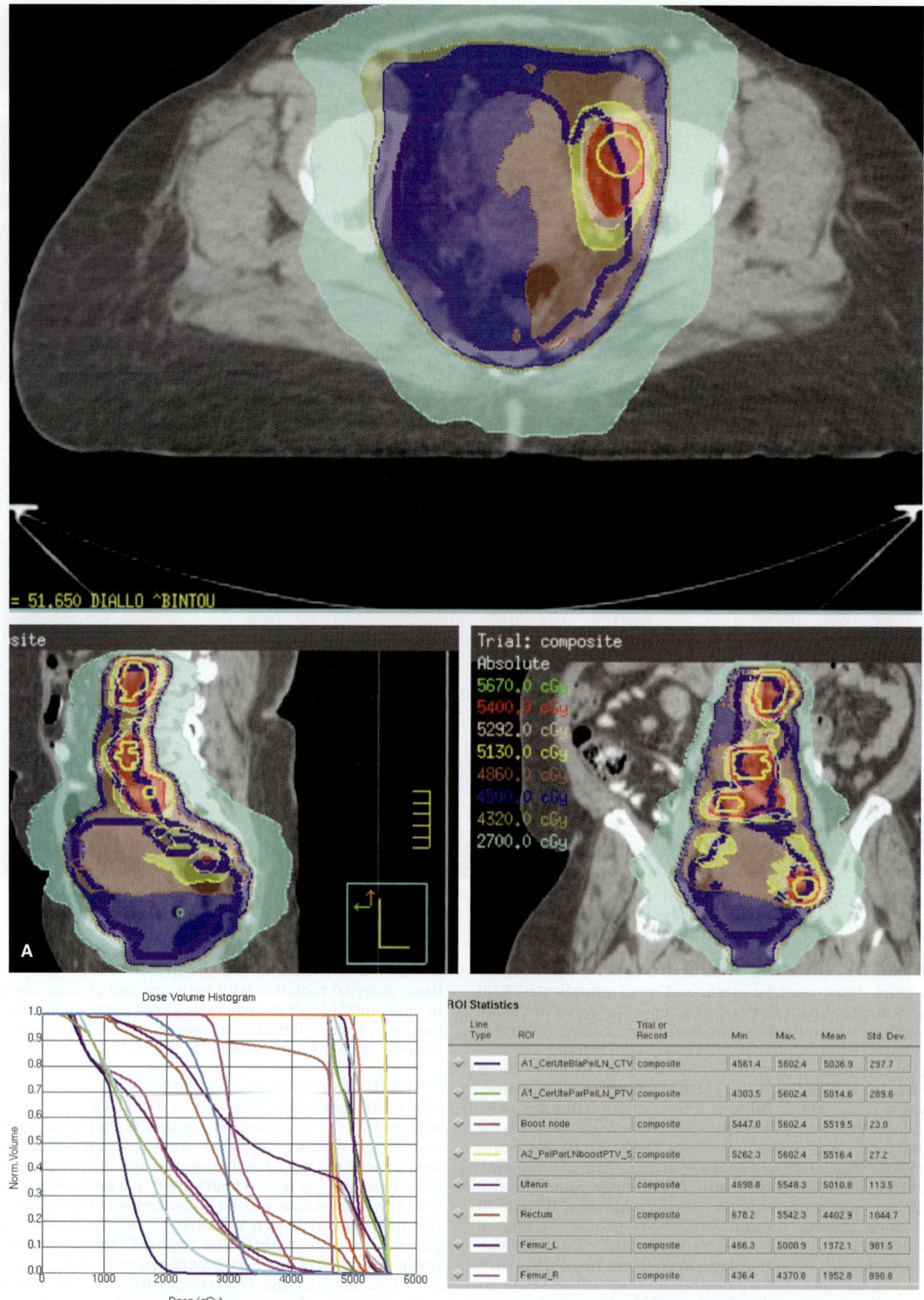

FIGURE 73.15. **A:** Example of treatment plan with IMRT for irradiation of para-aortic lymph nodes. **B:** Dose–volume histogram illustrating sparing of kidney and small intestine and dose escalation with nodal boost. (Reprinted from Mutic S, Malyapa RS, Grigsby PW, et al. PET-guided IMRT for cervical carcinoma with positive para-aortic lymph nodes—a dose-escalation treatment planning study. *Int J Radiat Oncol Biol Phys* 2003;55[1]:28–35. Copyright © 2003 Elsevier. With permission.)

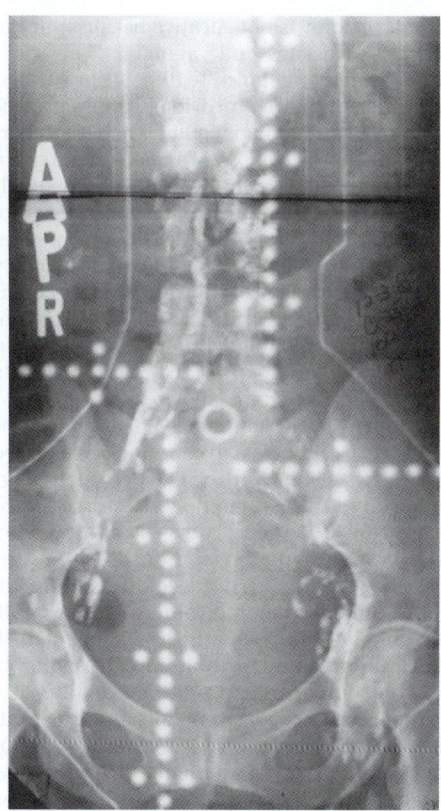

FIGURE 73.16. Extended field simulated with conventional plain films for external irradiation of pelvic and para-aortic lymph nodes.

Another study reported on 30 patients with stage II or III cervical cancer randomized to receive either hyperfractionation (15 patients) or conventional fractionation (15 patients).[387] At 5 years, two patients in the hyperfractionation group and eight patients in the conventional treatment group had recurrent tumor (*P* = .04). Delayed bowel complications (grade 2 and 3) occurred in nine women in the hyperfractionation group and two patients in the conventional group (*P* = 0.0006).

RTOG 88-05 conducted a phase II trial of hyperfractionation (1.2 Gy to the whole pelvis twice daily at 4- to 6-hour intervals, 5 days/week) with brachytherapy in 81 patients with locally advanced carcinoma of the cervix. Total dose to the whole pelvis was 24 to 48 Gy, followed by one or two LDR intracavitary

applications to deliver 85 Gy at point A and 65 Gy to the lateral pelvic nodes. Grigsby et al.[388] updated the results and noted that external irradiation was completed in 71 cases (88%). The 5-year cumulative rate of grade 3 and 4 late effects for patients with stage IB2 or IIB tumors was 7% and at 8 years was 10%, and with stage III or IVA disease, it was 12% at 5 years. The absolute survival was 48% at 8 years, and DFS was 33%. Comparison with historical control patients treated on other RTOG studies showed equivalent rates of pelvic tumor control, survival, and grade 3 and 4 toxicities at 3, 5, and 8 years, respectively.

Calkins et al.[389] assessed the toxicities of multiple daily fractionated (twice-daily, 1.2-Gy fractions) whole-pelvis radiation plus concurrent chemotherapy for locally advanced carcinoma of the cervix. In the first study (GOG 8801), for 38 patients, hydroxyurea was given orally (80 mg/kg to a maximum of 6 g) at least 2 hours before irradiation, twice every week. In the second study (GOG 8901), for 30 patients, cisplatin and fluorouracil (5-FU) were used concomitantly with RT. Acute toxicity was primarily enteric and appeared to be dose related. The maximum tolerated dose of whole-pelvis radiation that could be delivered in a hyperfractionated setting with concomitant chemotherapy was 57.6 Gy in 48 fractions, followed by brachytherapy.

Thomas et al.[390] conducted a four-arm study in which 234 women with bulky stage IB to IVA cervical cancer were randomized to receive either standard RT (EBRT and brachytherapy to deliver 90 Gy to point A) with or without a 4-day infusion of 5-FU (1 g/m²) on days 1 to 5 and 22 to 25 or partially hyperfractionated RT with or without the same chemotherapy regimen. The partially hyperfractionated regimen delivered two fractions, 6 hours apart, on the first 4 days of treatment, coinciding with the infusion of 5-FU. The addition of 5-FU did not improve pelvic tumor control (37% to 75% at 5 years) or overall survival. However, this study closed without reaching target patient accrual. A concomitant boost technique was reported by Kavanagh et al.[364] but had an unacceptably high rate (8 of 20 patients) of late complications.

GENERAL MANAGEMENT

Carcinoma *In Situ*

Patients with persistent high-grade carcinoma *in situ* are usually treated with a total abdominal hysterectomy with or without a small portion of the upper vagina removed. The decision to remove the ovaries depends on the age of the patient and status of the ovaries. Occasionally, when the patient wishes to have more children, carcinoma *in situ* may be treated

FIGURE 73.17. Example of isodose curves of 4F box irradiation of the pelvis with high-energy photons and CT-based high–dose rate brachytherapy optimized to cover the tumor and minimize dose to the bladder and rectum. **A:** Axial. **B:** Coronal view.

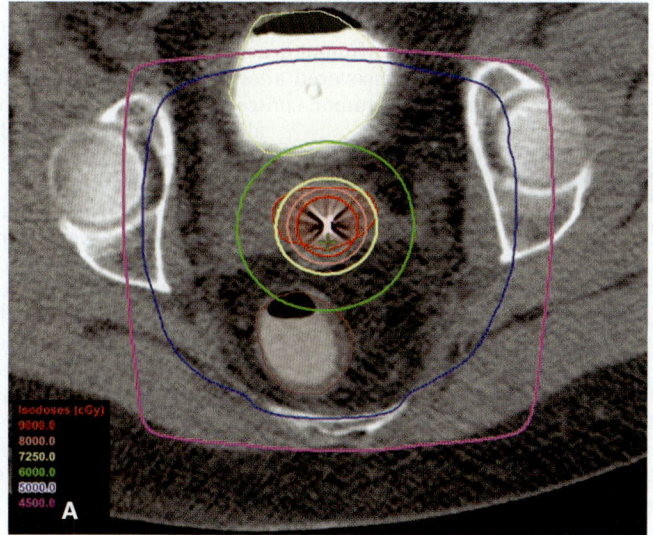

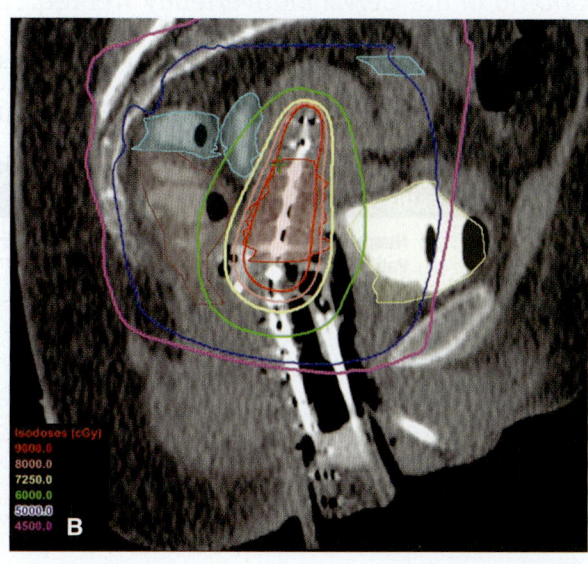

conservatively with a therapeutic conization,[391] laser therapy, or cryotherapy.[392] This approach should be judiciously selected when the extent of tumor allows it and the patient is reliable for continued follow-up.[393] Conization microscopic margins are critical in decision-making regarding a conservative approach or proceeding with a hysterectomy. A therapeutic hysterectomy can be performed 6 weeks after the conization.

Irradiation may be useful for the treatment of carcinoma *in situ*, particularly in patients with strong medical contraindications to surgery or when there is extension of the lesion to the vaginal wall or multifocal carcinoma *in situ* in both the cervix and the vagina.[326,394] In a group of 26 patients with carcinoma *in situ* treated at Washington University with intracavitary brachytherapy alone (~5,000 milligram-hours [mgh], 45 Gy to point A with LDR) with tandem and ovoids, no recurrences were recorded[395] Ogino et al.[396] used HDR brachytherapy in 14 patients with grade 3 cervical and 6 with grade 3 vaginal intraepithelial neoplasia (3 with microinvasion) and 6 with recurrent CIN after hysterectomy. Seventeen patients were treated with HDR brachytherapy alone and three in combination with EBRT without surgery. The mean dose of HDR brachytherapy was 26.1 Gy (range, 20 to 30 Gy) prescribed at point A for intact uterus, at 1 cm superior to the vaginal apex, or 1 cm beyond the vaginal mucosa for lesions of the vaginal stump. At mean follow-up of 90 months, 14 patients were alive and 6 had died from intercurrent disease; none had recurrent disease. Rectal bleeding occurred in three patients and subsided spontaneously. Moderate and severe vaginal reactions were noted in two patients in whom the treatment included the entire vagina.

Invasive Disease

Based on available resources globally and the stage of disease, a debate continues among those who advocate radical surgery,[326,397,398] those who favor radiation, and those who favor chemoRT for the treatment of carcinoma of the uterine cervix. Patients should be treated with close collaboration between the gynecologic oncologist and the radiation oncologist, and an integrated team approach should be vigorously pursued. In countries with access to RT facilities and financial resources to supply chemotherapy, the use of concurrent chemoRT represents the accepted standard for patients with stage IB2 to IVA cervical cancer. For earlier-stage patients, the use of either surgery or chemoRT is recommended. The most recent survey of patterns of radiotherapy practice again documented a rise in the use of cisplatin-based concurrent chemoRT in patients with advanced stages, from 63% in 1999 to 74% in 2007.[177,399,400] Moreover, Barbera et al.[401] also reported a significant increase in the use of chemoRT in Canada after the *U.S. National Cancer Institute Bulletin* on the subject.[402]

Carcinoma of the Cervix Inadvertently Treated with a Simple Hysterectomy

Occasionally, a simple or total abdominal hysterectomy is performed and invasive carcinoma of the cervix is incidentally found in the surgical specimen. In general, extrafascial abdominal hysterectomy is not curative because the paravaginal or paracervical soft tissues and vaginal cuff are not removed. Furthermore, it may be technically difficult to perform an adequate radical operation after previous simple hysterectomy. If only microinvasive carcinoma is found when a total or extrafascial hysterectomy with a wide cuff is performed, no additional therapy is necessary for lesions with deeper stromal invasion; at most, one or two vaginal intracavitary insertions to deliver a 65-Gy LDR mucosal dose (or 7 Gy × six fractions prescribed at the vaginal surface or 5 Gy at 0.5 cm × six fractions with HDR brachytherapy) to the vault are sufficient. If a less comprehensive resection was carried out, it is critical that these patients receive radiation therapy immediately with or without concurrent chemotherapy, depending on the risk factors present pathologically when their postoperative status allows it because the prognosis is worse if postoperative irradiation is not administered.

In patients with fully invasive tumor, therapy consists of approximately 40 to 45 Gy to the whole pelvis with cylinder brachytherapy to the vaginal vault for an approximately 60-Gy mucosal dose. If there is gross tumor present in the vaginal vault or parametrium, the dose to the whole pelvis should be 45 Gy with concurrent weekly cisplatin chemotherapy, followed by an additional parametrial dose of 10 to 20 Gy. An intracavitary insertion should be performed. If there is gross residual tumor, an interstitial implant should be carried out to selectively increase the dose to this volume.

Several studies have reported results of postoperative external beam irradiation after conservative surgery (Table 73.10). Andras et al.[403] reported on 148 patients, 90 of whom were available for 10-year evaluation, who were divided into five groups, depending on tumor extent when therapy was instituted. The majority of patients were treated with 50-Gy total-pelvis irradiation (with 10-Gy parametrial boost through reduced fields), at times combined with vaginal vault intracavitary irradiation. Eight major complications were noted in 148 patients.

Ampil et al.[405] described results in 44 patients receiving postoperative irradiation after hysterectomy for stage IB and IIA carcinoma of the uterine cervix (15 patients treated with radical hysterectomy). Their 5-year results were 80% local tumor control and 63% overall survival. In three patients treated with intracavitary vaginal cuff irradiation only, two had tumor control.

Green and Morse[406] reported 9 of 30 patients (30%) surviving 5 years after definitive radiation therapy for treatment of invasive cervical carcinoma after simple hysterectomy. The same authors noted that 14 of 32 patients retreated with another surgical procedure, usually a Wertheim hysterectomy, died within 5 years. They pointed out that the 5-year cure rate was 30% in patients treated within 1 year after the hysterectomy but was only 16% in those treated after 1 year. Thus, the time at which the patient is treated and the volume of tumor are important prognostic factors.

Crane and Schneider[407] described results in 18 patients treated with RT (with or without brachytherapy) for invasive carcinoma of the cervix discovered after simple hysterectomy. The 10-year actuarial local tumor control was 88%, and the overall survival rate was 93%. Huerta Bahena et al.,[408] in 59 patients with carcinoma of the cervix incidentally found in simple hysterectomy specimens (27 with gross residual tumor) who were treated with postoperative RT, reported a 3-year survival of 59%; factors affecting prognosis included gross residual tumor, time between hysterectomy and irradiation >6 months, RT doses <50 Gy, and histologic tumor type.

TABLE 73.10 RESULTS OF POSTOPERATIVE EXTERNAL BEAM IRRADIATION AFTER CONSERVATIVE HYSTERECTOMY IN EARLY-STAGE CARCINOMA OF THE CERVIX[a]

Author (Reference)	Number of Patients	Local Control (%)	Survival Percentage	Survival Months	Severe Complications (%)[b]
Andras et al.[403]	80[c]	89	89	60	4
Ampil et al.[58]	27[c]	89	70	60	4
Saibishkumar et al.[384]	105	72	55	60	12
Sharma et al.[404]	83	70	62	60	6

[a]Patients with postsurgery gross residual or recurrent disease before irradiation were excluded from the total number of cited cases.
[b]Remedial surgery was performed because of bowel or bladder damage in some patients in some series.
[c]All or some of the patients had additional vaginal cuff irradiation.
Modified from Ampil F, Datta R, Datta S. Elective postoperative external radiotherapy after hysterectomy in early-stage carcinoma of the cervix: is additional vaginal cuff irradiation necessary? *Cancer* 1987;60(3):280–288. Copyright © 1987 American Cancer Society. Reprinted by permission of John Wiley & Sons, Inc.

Münstedt et al.[409] reported on 119 patients who received postoperative RT after radical hysterectomy and 80 who received it after simple hysterectomy. There was a trend toward better survival in the radical hysterectomy group, but the authors concluded that postoperative RT is a good treatment in patients with invasive cervical cancer who undergo a simple hysterectomy. In another report of 105 patients with invasive cervical carcinoma found in inadequate surgery specimens treated with postoperative RT, 5-year pelvic tumor control was 72% and the survival rate was 55%. Late rectal toxicity was 19%, bladder toxicity was 4.8%, and small-bowel toxicity was 14.3%.[410]

In a series of 147 patients treated at Asan Medical Center in Korea, 48 patients with stage IA1 lesions did not receive further treatment. Another 99 patients had stage IA2 to IIA lesions incidentally identified. Of these, 26 received no further therapy, 44 had either radiation or chemoradiation, and 29 had a radical parametrectomy. For patients with stage IA1 disease who were observed, 0% relapsed, whereas 35% of patients with stage IA2 to IIA disease who were observed suffered from a recurrence.[411] Either radical parametrectomy or radiation is required for patients with stage IA2 or higher cancer after a simple hysterectomy. However, these treatments increase the risk of side effects[412] including for those patients receiving robotic parametrectomy.[413]

Stage IA

The definition of microinvasive (stage IA) carcinoma of the cervix includes invasive carcinoma diagnosed only by microscopy. Conization is mandatory for a more accurate diagnosis. According to Kolstad,[414] lesions <1 mm in depth can be treated with conization, provided all margins are tumor-free and continued careful follow-up is instituted. Raspagliesi et al.[415] used margins of 8 to 10 mm as guidelines for clearance in conization. Smaller margins and lymphovascular invasion in addition to depth of invasion were prognostic factors for recurrence.

Tumor volume in the stroma may be a more reliable criterion than depth of invasion to arrive at a definition of stage IA. Vascular space involvement does not impact stage. Depth of invasion and tumor confluence have been identified as prognostic factors that should be taken into consideration in the planning of therapy.[416]

Early invasive carcinoma of the cervix (stage IA2) is usually treated with a total abdominal or modified radical hysterectomy or in some cases with simple conization[278] or radical trachelectomy.[417] Inoperable patients may be treated with intracavitary radioactive sources alone with 6,500 to 8,000 mgh, 60 to 75 Gy to point A, in two LDR insertions, respectively, or with the equivalent dose using HDR brachytherapy, approximately 10 fractions of 5 Gy per fraction. In 47 patients with microinvasive carcinoma treated at Washington University—20 with intracavitary therapy only and 27 patients with combined external irradiation and intracavitary brachytherapy—only 1 patient had a pelvic recurrence and distant metastases 10 years later; the 5-year DFS rate was 96%.[397]

When the depth of penetration of the stroma by tumor is <3 mm, the incidence of lymph node metastasis is 1% or less, and a lymph node dissection or pelvic external irradiation is not warranted.[326,397] With more extensive lesions, a Wertheim radical hysterectomy with pelvic lymphadenectomy is the preferred treatment. Tumor control with all treatment methods is >95%, with patients eventually dying of intercurrent disease. Gadducci et al.[418] treated 30 patients with conization and 82 with total and 54 with radical hysterectomy; the recurrence rates were 10%, 4.9%, and 9.3%, respectively. None of 67 patients subjected to lymphadenectomy had positive pelvic nodes. In 98 patients with adenocarcinoma of the cervix, none of 48 with depth of invasion (DOI) of ≤5 mm had involved parametria or positive nodes, in contrast to 6 of 36 (16%) with DOI of >5 mm.[419]

Vaginal trachelectomy (removal of the cervix) and laparoscopic lymphadenectomy have been used to treat young patients with microinvasive carcinoma to preserve fertility.

The overall incidence of central recurrence is approximately 5%.[395] Webb et al.[420] analyzed lymph node status and survival rates of women with microinvasive cervical adenocarcinoma (FIGO stages IA1 and IA2) from the SEER database between 1988 and 1997. Among reported cases, 131 had stage IA1 and 170 had stage IA2 disease. Simple hysterectomy was done in 54 women with IA1 and in 64 women with IA2 disease and radical hysterectomy in 50 and 83 women, respectively. Only 1 of 140 women who had lymphadenectomy had a single positive lymph node. There were 4 tumor-related deaths (1 with IA1 and 3 with IA2 disease). The survival rate was 98.7%.

Stages IB to IIA

The choice of definitive irradiation or radical surgery for stage IB and IIA carcinoma of the cervix remains controversial, and the preference for one procedure over another depends primarily on the impact on the patient's fertility and on the institution, the gynecologic oncologist or radiation oncologist involved, the general condition of the patient, and characteristics of the lesion. An operation has been preferred by some in young women to preserve the ovaries, attempting to prevent premature menopause. However, in some reports,[318] ovarian function preservation has been observed in only 50% to 60% of surgically treated patients not receiving irradiation. Postmenopausal patients may have a survival benefit with chemoradiation and avoid the operative risks. When therapeutic results in invasive carcinoma of the cervix are evaluated, a direct comparison of surgically treated or irradiated patients is fraught with many uncertainties, including patient selection, reporting of surgical cases using staging determined by laparotomy findings, and different treatment techniques.[421] In particular, in the modern era when concurrent chemoradiation is known to be superior to radiation alone, a direct comparison of chemoradiation versus surgery in early-stage cervical cancer is needed.

Surgery provides an opportunity for a thorough pelvic and abdominal evaluation. However, surgical staging has not been shown to improve overall patient survival.[46,53] Kupets et al.[422] assessed the value of debulking large nodes and concluded that the incremental overall benefit by stage was small. Delgado et al.[43] described a GOG study in which 1,125 patients were registered before surgery; 80 were ineligible after strict pathology review, and an additional 129 patients were explored, but the hysterectomy was abandoned because of intraoperative complications in 49 patients or extent of disease beyond the uterus in 80 patients. In the era of MRI, surgeons may rely on imaging findings to screen for operability. The impact of patient selection in results of surgical series was illustrated by Whitney and Stehman[423] who evaluated the frequency with which intended radical hysterectomy for cervical cancer is abandoned and the outcomes for those selected patients. In 1,127 patients with stage IB carcinoma of the cervix entered on GOG Protocol 49, 98 women (8.7%) were found at surgery to have extrauterine disease, and the proposed radical operation was abandoned. Subgroups of patients with extrapelvic disease[34] and pelvic extension[419] including grossly positive pelvic nodes,[42] other pelvic implants,[424] and gross serosal extension[130] were identified. Sixty-three (93%) patients subsequently underwent pelvic radiation therapy and brachytherapy. Para-aortic fields were added for eight patients who were found to have positive para-aortic nodes. The DFS was shorter for patients whose radical procedure was abandoned than for those patients who underwent radical hysterectomy.

The important contribution of external beam irradiation to improve pelvic tumor control in larger lesions has been documented. Hamberger et al.,[425] in 151 patients with stage IA or IB lesions <1 cm in diameter treated with intracavitary therapy alone to high doses (8,640, 9,340, and 13,680 mgh), noted no failures in 41 patients with stage IA disease and only 4 of 93 patients (4%) with stage IB, small-volume disease. However,

3 of 17 patients (18%) with more extensive stage IB lesions, treated with intracavitary therapy only, had regional failures. Only 3 of 151 patients (0.2%) had grade 3 complications.

Volterrani and Lombardi[426] reported 5-year survival of 82.6% in 23 patients with occult stage IB carcinoma of the cervix treated with intracavitary[251] Ra only (7,500 mgh), in contrast to only 64.8% with larger stage IB tumors and 50% with stage II. Unfortunately, the authors did not report the exact location of the failures. It is obvious that intracavitary therapy alone is grossly inadequate to irradiate larger primary tumors, including stage IB1.

With EBRT and brachytherapy without chemotherapy, the usual 5-year survival rate for stage IB is 86% to 92% and for stage IIA is approximately 75%.[410] Late toxicity was observed in 1% to 2% of patients. Concurrent chemotherapy significantly improves survival, including in stage IB to IIA disease. In RTOG 90-01, for the subset of 272 stage IB to IIA patients, the 8-year overall survival was 55% with RT alone versus 78% with concurrent chemoradiation (P < .001).[427]

Randomized Studies: Surgery Versus Radiation

Few randomized trials have compared the results of radical hysterectomy with definitive RT, and none have compared surgery to chemoradiation. Outcome between radiation alone versus surgery is comparable. Newton[428] and Roddick and Greenlaw[429] reported, in prospectively randomized studies, equivalent survival and pelvic recurrence rates in patients with stage IB and IIA carcinoma of the uterine cervix treated with a radical hysterectomy or irradiation alone. Landoni et al.[37] published results of a prospective, randomized trial of radiation therapy versus surgery; 469 women with stage IB and IIA cervical carcinoma were referred for treatment and 343 were randomized (172 to surgery and 171 to radiation therapy). Postoperative irradiation was delivered after surgery for women with surgical stage pT2b or greater, <3 mm of cervical stromal invasion and cut-through margins, or positive pelvic nodes. Scheduled treatment was delivered to 169 and 158 women, respectively; 62 of 114 women with cervical diameters of <4 cm and 46 of 55 women with >4 cm received radiation therapy. After a median follow-up of 87 months (range, 57 to 120 months), 5-year overall survival and DFS rates were nearly identical in the surgery and radiation therapy groups (83% and 74%, respectively); recurrent disease developed in 86 women: 42 (25%) in the surgery group and 44 (26%) in the radiation therapy group (Fig. 73.18). Forty-eight patients (28%) in the surgery group had severe morbidity, compared with 19 (12%) in the radiation therapy group (P = .0004; Table 73.11). The combination of surgery and radiation therapy had the worst morbidity, especially urologic complications.

Of note, no randomized study has compared chemoRT to radical hysterectomy, although chemoRT has a significant survival advantage over RT alone for patients with stage IB to IIA cervical cancer.[430] In a meta-analysis looking at the value

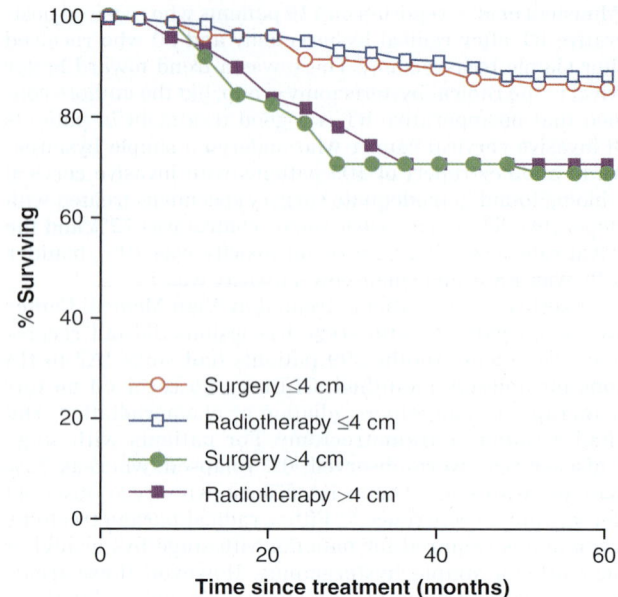

FIGURE 73.18. Overall actuarial survival of patients with carcinoma of the cervix randomized to treatment with radical surgery or radiation therapy according to treatment group and cervical diameter. (Reprinted from Landoni F, Maneo A, Colombo A, et al. Randomised study of radical surgery versus radiotherapy for stage IB-IIA cervical cancer. *Lancet* 1997;350[9077]:535–540. Copyright © 1997 Elsevier. With permission.)

of adjuvant cisplatin-based chemotherapy after radical hysterectomy, radiation therapy, or both for patients with stage IA2, IB1, or IIA cervical cancer, three randomized clinical trials were evaluated.[430] Two of the three trials showed a significant benefit compared to adjuvant chemotherapy concurrent with radiation, with a reduced risk of death (HR = 0.56, 95% CI = 0.36 to 0.87). No benefit was seen when chemotherapy was given prior to radiotherapy.

Neoadjuvant chemotherapy plus surgery does not improve survival over surgery alone.[431] In a meta-analysis of six trials, although there was an improvement in PFS with neoadjuvant chemotherapy (HR = 0.76, 95% CI = 0.62 to 0.94, P = .01), this did not translate into an overall survival benefit. Another meta-analysis reviewed 18 trials with locally advanced cervical cancer patients treated with neoadjuvant chemotherapy before radiation or surgery or both and excluded concurrent chemoradiation trials; it showed significant heterogeneity and no conclusive results.[432]

Nonrandomized Studies Comparing Surgery to Radiation

Keilbinska et al.,[433] in a long-term study of 792 women treated with irradiation and 789 women treated with hysterectomy and/or irradiation for stage I cervical carcinoma, found no

TABLE 73.11 RANDOMIZED TRIAL OF RADICAL SURGERY OR IRRADIATION IN STAGE I TO II CERVICAL CANCERS: RELAPSES AND MORBIDITY

| | Surgery | | | | | | Radiation Therapy Alone | |
| | Surgery Only | | Surgery Plus Radiation Therapy | | | | | |
	≤4 cm	>4 cm	≤4 cm	>4 cm	Total ≤4 cm	>4 cm	≤4 cm	>4 cm
Number of patients[a]	53 (52)	9 (9)	62 (62)	46	115 (114)	55 (55)	114 (105)	54 (53)
Relapses	7 (13%)	2 (22%)	15 (26%)	17 (37%)	23 (20%)	19 (34%)	21 (18%)	23 (42%)
Pelvic	4	2	7	9	11	11	12	16
Distant morbidity	3	—	9	8	12	8	9	7
Grade 2–3[b]	16 (31%)	3 (33%)	18 (29%)	11 (24%)	34 (30%)	14 (25%)	13 (12%)	6 (11%)
Short term	10 (16%)	—	22 (20%)	—	32 (19%)	—	11 (7%)	—
Long term	15 (24%)	—	31 (29%)	—	46 (27%)	—	25 (16%)	—

[a]Parentheses show number of patients who actually received this treatment instead of intention to treat.
[b]Percentage calculated for number of patients who actually received treatment.
Reprinted from Landoni F, Maneo A, Colombo A, et al. Randomised study of radical surgery versus radiotherapy for stage IB-IIA cervical cancer. *Lancet* 1997;350(9077):535–540. Copyright © 1997 Elsevier. With permission.

difference in survival, general health, incidence of recurrent carcinoma, or appearance of second primary malignancies. Piver et al.[434] treated 103 women with stage IB cervical carcinoma with either radical hysterectomy and pelvic lymphadenectomy (if tumor was <3 cm in greatest diameter) or irradiation (tumor of >3 cm or medically inoperable). The 5-year DFS rate was 92.3% for the surgical group and 91.1% for the radiation therapy group. Equivalent overall 5-year survival rates were noted. Einhorn et al.,[435] in a nonrandomized study, observed a 100% 5-year survival rate in 49 patients with stage IB disease receiving combined therapy in comparison with 81% in 64 patients treated with irradiation alone. No difference was observed in 25 patients with stage IIA tumor treated with combined therapy and 40 patients treated with irradiation alone (5-year survival rate, 75%).

Perez et al.[51] reported on a prospectively randomized study of 118 patients with stage IB or IIA carcinoma of the uterine cervix in which patients were treated with RT alone or irradiation and surgery (20 Gy to the whole pelvis, one intracavitary insertion for 5,000 to 6,000 mgh, followed by a radical hysterectomy with pelvic lymphadenectomy 2 to 6 weeks later). In stage IB, the 5-year tumor-free survival was 80% and 82% (P = .23), respectively, and in stage IIA, it was 56% and 79%, respectively (P = .13). The incidence of grade 2 or 3 complications for radiation alone was 13.8% and with preoperative irradiation and surgery was 11%. Subsequently, Perez et al.[436] described results in 415 patients with stage IB or limited stage IIB treated with preoperative or postoperative irradiation and surgery. The 10-year CSS rate for patients with stage IB nonbulky tumors treated with irradiation alone or irradiation combined with surgery was 84% with either modality. With bulky tumors (>5 cm), the 10-year rates were 61% and 68%, respectively (P = .5). For patients with stage IIA nonbulky tumors, the 10-year CSS rates were 66% and 71%, respectively, and with bulky tumors, 69% and 44%, respectively (P = .05). In patients with stage IIB nonbulky tumors treated with irradiation alone or combined with surgery, the 10-year CSS rates were 72% and 65%, respectively. In stage IB and IIA disease after a hysterectomy and lymphadenectomy (even combined with irradiation), patients with metastatic lymph nodes have survival rates that are approximately 50% of those of patients with negative nodes.[437]

Randomized Trials of Postoperative Radiation Therapy or Chemoradiation After Radical Hysterectomy

Patients who have undergone radical hysterectomy with no preoperative radiation therapy are considered for postoperative chemoradiation therapy if they have high-risk prognostic factors, which include positive pelvic lymph nodes, as are patients with negative nodes who have microscopic positive margins of resection or parametrial involvement.[438]

Patients with any two of deep stromal invasion, vascular/lymphatic permeation, and large tumor size are candidates for postoperative radiation.[439] These patients have an intermediate risk of failure.[43] Whether to add concurrent chemotherapy to postoperative radiation in the intermediate-risk group is being tested in an accruing randomized trial; many institutions routinely implement chemoRT for intermediate-risk patients. Song et al.[440] reported a 20-year experience in stage IB to IIA cervical cancer patients with intermediate-risk factors (two or more of deep stromal invasion, lymphovascular invasion, and large tumor size) who received postoperative RT or chemoradiation. Chemoradiation significantly decreased pelvic recurrence and distant metastases; there was no difference in acute or chronic grade 3 and 4 gastrointestinal side effects.

One randomized study showed improved recurrence-free survival with postoperative pelvic irradiation (46 to 50.4 Gy in 23 to 28 fractions) after radical surgery in the presence of positive pelvic nodes or node-negative high-risk factors in women with stage IB cervical cancer treated by radical hysterectomy and pelvic lymphadenectomy. There were 277 eligible patients with at least two of the following risk factors: greater than one-third stromal invasion, capillary lymphatic space involvement, and large clinical tumor diameter; 137 patients were randomized to pelvic radiation therapy and 140 to no further treatment. The results were updated by Rotman et al.[441]; 24 (17%) patients in the irradiation group and 43 (30.7%) in the no-further-treatment group had cancer recurrences. In the radiation therapy group, 27 patients died of cancer, and in the no-further-treatment group 40 died from cancer. There was a statistically significant reduction in risk of recurrence in the irradiation group, with recurrence-free rates at 2 years of 88% versus 79% for the irradiation and no-further-treatment groups, respectively. Overall survival difference did not reach statistical difference (P = .074; Fig. 73.19). Severe or life-threatening (GOG grade 3 or 4) adverse effects occurred in 9 patients (6.6%) in the radiation therapy group and 3 (2.1%) in the observation group. A meta-analysis of trials including stage IB1 to IIA cervical cancer found that women who received postoperative radiation had a significantly lower risk of disease progression at 5 years (RR = 0.6, 95% CI = 0.4 to 0.9). The risk of serious adverse events was not significantly higher if women received radiotherapy rather than no further treatment, possibly because the rate of adverse events was low.[442]

FIGURE 73.19. Recurrence-free survival **(A)** and overall survival **(B)** of patients with stage IB carcinoma of the cervix, correlated with treatment method. (Reprinted from Rotman M, Sedlis A, Piedmonte MR. A phase III randomized trial of postoperative pelvic irradiation in patients with stage IB cervical carcinoma with poor prognostic features: follow up of a Gynecologic Oncology Group study. *Int J Radiat Oncol Biol Phys* 2006;65[1]:169–176. Copyright © 2006 Elsevier. With permission.)

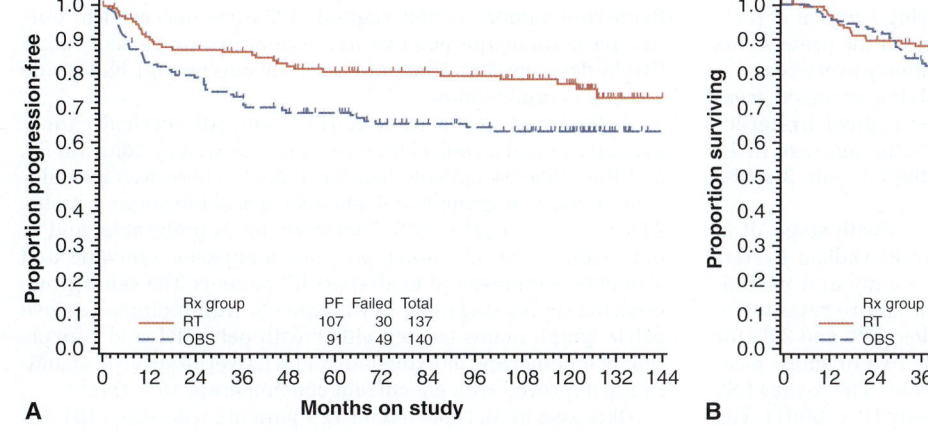

Rx group	PF	Failed	Total
RT	107	30	137
OBS	91	49	140

A Months on study

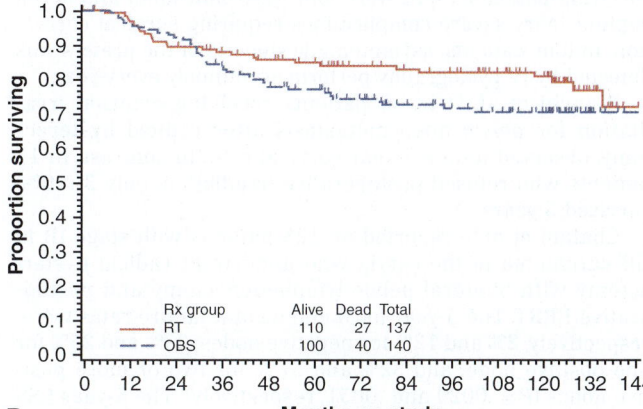

Rx group	Alive	Dead	Total
RT	110	27	137
OBS	100	40	140

B Months on study

Sundfør et al.[443] conducted a randomized study in which 122 patients with stage IIA and 20 patients with stage IIB cervix cancer were treated with intracavitary radium followed by either radical pelvic surgery including lymphadenectomy (group A, 72 patients) or EBRT (40 Gy) to the pelvis (group B, 70 patients). Postoperative RT (40 to 50 Gy) was given to patients in group A found to have node metastasis at operation. Fourteen patients in group A and 23 in group B died of recurrent cancer. The 10-year survival was 84% and 69%, respectively.

Nonrandomized Trials of Postoperative Radiation Therapy or Chemoradiation After Radical Hysterectomy

Snijders-Keilholz et al.[444] described results in 233 women who underwent radical hysterectomy for stage I or IIA cervical carcinoma; 156 were treated with surgery alone, and 77 received adjuvant radiation therapy for tumor-related high-risk prognostic factors. The most important prognostic factor for survival and DFS was pelvic lymph node positivity; additional factors were depth of invasion and positive surgical margins. Twelve patients recurred after surgery alone, all in the pelvis (100%). Of the 23 recurrences after surgery and adjuvant radiation therapy, 13 were in the pelvis (56%; $P = .003$). Ten patients with poor prognostic factors and negative nodes received adjuvant radiation therapy, and none of these patients recurred. The incidence of severe gastrointestinal radiation-related side effects was 2%. The incidence of lymphedema of the leg was 11%, which was similar to that in the surgery-alone group.

Garipagaoglu et al.[445] investigated prognostic factors in 100 patients with stage IB or IIA cervical carcinoma treated with radical hysterectomy and postoperative irradiation. The 5-year overall survival, DFS, and pelvic tumor control rates were 83.6%, 82.8%, and 91.8%, respectively. Pelvic lymph node metastasis ($P = .008$), interval between surgery and irradiation ($P = .001$), overall radiation therapy time ($P = .007$), and tumor size ($P = .028$) were significant factors for pelvic tumor control, as well as for overall survival.

Lahousen et al.[446] reported on a GOG prospectively randomized, multicenter trial in which patients with stage IB or IIB cervical cancer treated with radical hysterectomy who had pelvic lymph node metastases or vascular invasion randomly received adjuvant chemotherapy (400 mg/m^2 carboplatin and 30 mg bleomycin), external pelvic radiation therapy, or no further treatment. After a median follow-up of 4.1 years (range, 2 to 7 years), there were no statistically significant differences ($P = .9539$) in DFS rates among the three treatment arms, suggesting that adjuvant chemotherapy or radiation does not improve survival or recurrence rates in high-risk patients with cervical cancer after radical hysterectomy.

González González et al.[447] reported that in 89 patients with stage IB or IIA cervical cancer with positive lymph nodes receiving postoperative irradiation, the 5- and 10-year survival rates were 60% and 51%, respectively. By comparison, 43 patients with negative lymph nodes had a survival rate of 85%. In the surviving patients, there were four gastrointestinal and seven genitourinary severe complications requiring surgical correction. In four patients, asymptomatic stenosis of the ureters was detected by IV pyelography performed routinely every year.

Bianchi et al.,[448] in 60 patients receiving external irradiation for pelvic node metastasis after radical hysterectomy, observed a 65% 5-year survival rate. In contrast, in 15 patients who refused postoperative irradiation, only 3 (20%) survived 5 years.

Chatani et al.[449] reported on 128 patients with stage IB to IIB carcinoma of the cervix who underwent radical hysterectomy with bilateral pelvic lymphadenectomy and postoperative EBRT. The 5-year local and distant failure rates were, respectively, 2% and 12% for negative nodes, 23% and 25% for one positive node, and 32% and 57%, for two or more positive nodes ($P = .0029$ and .0051, respectively). The 5-year CSS rates were 90%, 59%, and 42%, respectively ($P = .0001$). The most common complication was lymphedema of the lower extremity, experienced by half of the patients (42% at 5 years and 49% at 10 years).

Uno et al.[450] evaluated results of postradical hysterectomy irradiation in 98 patients with stage IB to IIB cervical cancer; all of the patients had at least one pathologic risk factor for pelvic recurrence. The 5-year overall survival was 82%. There were pelvic recurrences in 5 cases and distant metastases in 15 cases. The 5-year overall survival rates for patients with or without pelvic lymph node metastasis were 76% and 89%, respectively ($P = .018$).

Kinney et al.[451] compared results of therapy in 82 patients with stage IB or IIA carcinoma of the cervix found to have pelvic lymph node metastases at Wertheim hysterectomy and bilateral lymphadenectomy without additional adjuvant therapy with 103 similar patients who received 50 Gy to the pelvis after surgery. The 5-year survival rate was 72% for the surgery-only patients and 64% for the group receiving adjuvant irradiation. The incidences of pelvic recurrence were 67% and 27%, respectively. The lack of impact on overall survival in the irradiated patients is most likely related to a higher incidence of distant metastases, which may be a reflection of shorter survival time and more high-risk patients. In 117 patients treated with radical hysterectomy and pelvic lymphadenectomy, histologically proven nodal metastatic disease was detected in 51 patients (44%; squamous cell in 35 and nonsquamous in 16). Nodal involvement was bilateral in 24 patients (47%).[452] PALN dissection was performed in 14 patients, and 5 had tumor involvement. Postoperative pelvic irradiation was administered to 29 of 51 patients (51.2 Gy, two fractions). Extended fields to the para-aortic area were used in six patients. The 5-year survival rates were 33% for the group receiving irradiation and 50% for the nonirradiated group. Only one patient treated with postoperative irradiation had a pelvic failure, in contrast to seven patients not irradiated.

Inoue and Morita[297] described results in 72 patients treated with extended-field irradiation after radical surgery for nodal metastases with stage IB (37 patients), IIA (6 patients), and IIB (29 patients) cervical cancers. The median dose to PALNs was 43.5 Gy and to the pelvis was 45 Gy. The 5-year DFS rates were 72% in 61 patients with squamous cell carcinoma and 27% in 11 patients with nonsquamous cell carcinoma. The 10-year DFS rates were 88% for 22 patients with one positive node, 67% for 15 patients with two or three positive nodes, 64% for 16 patients with four to 17 positive nodes, and 20% for 10 patients with unresectable lymph nodes. Nineteen severe complications occurred in 17 patients; 5 were attributed to surgery, 5 to irradiation, and 9 to both modalities. Four patients (5%) died of severe complications. Another six patients (8%) underwent major abdominal surgery for rectovaginal and ureterovaginal fistulas.

Mitsuhashi et al.[453] described an analysis of 108 patients with carcinoma of the cervix treated with postoperative EBRT to the pelvis followed by intravaginal cone boost with electron beam to the vaginal cuff. The 5-year CSS rates were 89% for 89 patients undergoing elective radiation therapy and 56% for 19 patients undergoing salvage irradiation ($P < .001$). Recurrent tumors at the vaginal cuff were observed in only two patients in the elective irradiation group. Vesicovaginal fistula developed in four patients; only one patient had grade 2 rectal complications.

A Japanese group treated 189 stage IIB cervical cancer patients; 95 had a radical hysterectomy followed by adjuvant RT, and the other 94 patients had RT alone.[454] There was a significant increase in grade 3 to 4 late toxicities in the surgery group, 24% versus 10%, $P = .048$. Therefore, RT is preferable, and in the modern era, chemoRT provides a superior outcome and should be administered to all stage IIB patients. The same group reported on 55 stage IA2 to IIB patients with multiple positive pelvic lymph nodes treated either with pelvic RT and concurrent chemotherapy or extended-field RT. Overall survival significantly improved with concurrent chemotherapy ($P = .03$).[455]

Okazawa et al. reported on 129 patients with stage IB1-IIB cervical cancer and showed significant improvement in PFS and OS with chemoradiation compared to RT. Patients with deep stromal invasion also had an improved PFS compared to observation.[456] A meta-analysis of 397 women with early-stage cervical cancer showed that postoperative RT reduced disease progression (RR 0.58, 95% CI 0.37 to 0.91).[457]

Lee et al.[458] retrospectively compared 201 stage IB1 to IIB cervical cancer patients who had a radical hysterectomy with pelvic lymph node dissection followed by adjuvant concurrent weekly cisplatin to triweekly combination chemotherapy. With a median follow-up of 52 months, the weekly cisplatin group had the same therapeutic effect with less toxicity. The 5-year disease-free and overall survival were 82% and 81%, respectively, for patients treated with weekly cisplatin chemotherapy versus 74% and 79% for those treated with triweekly combination chemotherapy (P = NS). Leukopenia, neutropenia, thrombocytopenia, anemia, and hepatopathy were significantly more common in the triweekly combination chemotherapy group.

Postoperative External Beam Radiation Dose

When metastatic pelvic lymph nodes are present, treatment has consisted of 45 Gy to the whole pelvis delivered with a four-field technique with concurrent weekly cisplatin. If gross residual disease is present, dose escalation to 54 to 65 Gy, depending on small-bowel dose limits (e.g., $D_{5cc} < 55$ Gy), may be considered with a sequential IMRT nodal boost.[101] Patients with positive common iliac or para-aortic node metastases should receive 45 Gy to the entire para-aortic region with the superior border covering the renal hilum, with consideration of a boost to the tumor bed. If gross residual nodal disease is left, a nodal boost up to 65 Gy with IMRT is particularly suited to treat these patients.[301,302]

In patients for whom postoperative irradiation is indicated for deep stromal invasion in the cervix or close or positive surgical margins, an alternative is to deliver 45-Gy pelvic external irradiation in combination with an intracavitary insertion (LDR, PDR, or HDR) and LDR equivalent dose of 65 Gy to the vaginal mucosa, using colpostats or a cylinder.[459] At some institutions, external irradiation alone (50 Gy to the midplane of the pelvis) with a four-field box technique has been used. Hong et al.[199] recommended, for node-negative patients with high-risk factors, to irradiate only the low pelvis (median dose, 50 Gy), which resulted in a reduction of grade 3 small-bowel morbidity (3 of 149 = 2%) in comparison with patients treated to the whole pelvis (6 of 79 = 8%). Five-year disease-specific survival was 84% and 86%, respectively.

Postoperative Intracavitary High–Dose Rate Brachytherapy

Depending on the extent of surgical resection of the vagina, the vaginal cuff may be at risk for recurrence. There is no clear agreement on the indications for vaginal brachytherapy after radical hysterectomy, although adjuvant vaginal brachytherapy for cervical cancer is most commonly used as a boost after EBRT, particularly in patients with positive margins.[460] Based on the American Brachytherapy Society guidelines, vaginal cuff boost should be considered in patients with a less-than-radical hysterectomy, close or positive margins, large or deeply invasive tumors, parametrial or vaginal involvement, or extensive lymphovascular invasion.[459] Consideration of postoperative vaginal intracavitary brachytherapy after external beam therapy is recommended for patients with carcinoma at the vaginal margin of resection.[326] If parametrial margins were close or positive, defined by either surgical clips or in the region of the surgical tumor bed, an external beam dose of at least 54 Gy for close margins and higher for positive margins is recommended.

In patients receiving postoperative irradiation, extreme care should be exercised in designing treatment techniques, including intracavitary insertions; because of the surgical extirpation of the uterus, the bladder and rectosigmoid may be closer to the radioactive sources than in the patient with an intact uterus. Furthermore, vascular supply may be affected by the surgical procedure, and adhesions can prevent mobilization of the small-bowel loops that may be fixed in the pelvis. HDR brachytherapy after surgery is particularly suited for patients with cervical cancer because it prevents the prolonged immobilization required for LDR brachytherapy. In some patients at higher risk for parametrial tumor or lymph node metastases, HDR brachytherapy is combined with external beam pelvic irradiation.

Hart et al.[461] described results in 83 patients who received postoperative RT for early-stage cervical cancer with positive surgical margins, positive pelvic or PALNs, lymphovascular space invasion, or deep stromal invasion or for disease discovered incidentally at simple hysterectomy. Twenty-eight patients were treated with LDR brachytherapy with or without EBRT and 55 with EBRT to the pelvis and HDR intracavitary. Of these 83 patients, 66 were evaluable (20 LDR and 46 HDR patients). Mean follow-up time was 101 months for the LDR group and 42 for the HDR group. The 5-year DFS rates were 89% and 72%, and local tumor control rates were 90% (18 of 20) and 89% (41 of 46), respectively. Three of 20 patients (15%) receiving LDR and 4 of 46 (9%) receiving HDR experienced grade 2 or 3 late treatment-related complications. No patient in either group had grade 4 or 5 complications.

Busch et al.[462] studied the outcome of 68 patients with cervical carcinoma; 48 were treated with radical hysterectomy and, because of risk factors, with postoperative RT (group 1), and 20 patients (group 2) were pretreated with standard hysterectomy and then admitted to the hospital for postoperative radiation therapy of the whole pelvis. Postoperative pelvic RT consisted of 39.6 Gy (box technique) and 6-Gy external beam therapy to the pelvic lymph nodes, sparing the midline, plus two HDR applications (7.5 Gy each). Survival, locoregional tumor control, and metastatic disease rates were nearly identical in both groups. Patients with positive lymph nodes had a worse prognosis (75% 3-year survival rate).

Atkovar et al.[463] described results in 126 patients treated with postoperative irradiation (median of 50 Gy in 5 weeks); 37 received vaginal cuff HDR brachytherapy (three fractions of 8 to 10 Gy at 5 mm, weekly). Overall survival and DFS and locoregional tumor control rates were 71%, 69.9%, and 78.1%, respectively. Grade 2 and 3 complications developed in 5.5% of patients. Survival was the same in 67 patients treated with total abdominal hysterectomy and bilateral salpingo-oophorectomy and in 59 patients treated with radical hysterectomy and pelvic lymphadenectomy.

Stages IB2 to IVA: Chemoradiation

Patients with stage IB2 to IVA tumors are treated with irradiation including external beam and brachytherapy combined with concurrent chemotherapy. Numerous reports have been published on the concomitant use of irradiation and cytotoxic agents (hydroxyurea, cisplatin, and 5-FU, in some trials combined with mitomycin C) administered to obtain a radiosensitizing effect.[464–466] Cisplatin is one of the most active cytotoxic agents in squamous cell carcinoma of the uterine cervix.[467] When cisplatin and irradiation are used concomitantly, substantial enhancement of cell killing is observed. Coughlin and Richmond[465] and Douple[468] suggested two mechanisms for radiation enhancement by cisplatin: (a) in hypoxic or oxygenated cells, free radicals with altered binding of cisplatin to DNA are formed at the time of irradiation, and (b) interaction inhibits repair of sublethal damage.

It is important, however, that patients complete the full course of 45 Gy with, ideally, five to six weekly doses of cisplatin or two doses of cisplatin and 5-FU every 3 weeks. In a study of 41 patients who had weekly biopsies while receiving RT and chemotherapy for cervix cancer, increased tumor cell proliferation and accelerated repopulation was observed within 2 weeks from the initiation of therapy. Patients with a sustained yield and high S-phase fraction for 2 or more weeks were at increased risk for tumor progression.[469]

Green et al.,[470] in a search of medical databases for randomized trials of cervical cancer that compared RT with or without concurrent chemotherapy, identified 19 trials comprising 4,580 randomized patients, and they were the subjects of the meta-analysis. Concomitant chemotherapy and radiation improved tumor control and overall survival (RR = 0.71; P < .0001) and PFS (RR = 0.61; P < .0001). The benefit was maximal in early-stage (I and II) disease. The absolute survival benefit was 12%. Patients receiving chemoirradiation had a higher incidence of grade 3 or 4 hematologic and gastrointestinal toxicities.

Patients with stage IVA disease (bladder and/or rectal invasion) can be treated either with higher doses of external radiation to the whole pelvis with concurrent chemotherapy followed by intracavitary or interstitial insertions (total dose to point A with LDR brachytherapy about 90 Gy) and additional parametrial irradiation or with pelvic exenteration.[471] Niibe et al.,[472] in an analysis of 179 patients with stage IIIB adenocarcinoma, suggested that an optimal dose for large tumors was a total biologic effective dose of >100 Gy.

A prospective single-arm trial, RTOG 0116, treated patients with positive para-aortic or high common iliac lymph nodes with extended-field radiation combined with cisplatin chemotherapy followed by brachytherapy.[473] IMRT was not allowed. The trial showed that this regimen is feasible, but the late grade 3 and 4 toxicity rate was 40%. There was no reduction in acute toxicity with the addition of amifostine.[474] The use of extended-field IMRT has been shown to reduce the risk of gastrointestinal toxicity in two retrospective series reports[302,475] and may be of benefit to patients with positive common or PALNs requiring extended-field radiation with concurrent chemotherapy.

In countries or circumstances where a wait time exists and patients cannot immediately start on concurrent chemoradiation, induction chemotherapy may be considered. An alternative to cisplatin in this situation may be concurrent nedaplatin, which did not cause any nephrotoxicity in an analysis of 104 patients.[476]

Randomized Trials of Chemoradiation

Results from several cooperative oncology groups demonstrated that cisplatin-based chemotherapy, when given concurrently with RT, prolongs survival in women with locally advanced cervical cancers (Table 73.12), as well as in women with stage I to IIA disease who have metastatic disease in the pelvic lymph nodes, positive parametrial disease, or positive surgical margins at the time of primary surgery.[480]

The GOG conducted randomized Protocol 85, in which patients with carcinoma of the cervix, a clinical stage of IIB to

IVA, and negative para-aortic nodes were treated with external pelvic irradiation (51 Gy) combined with 30 Gy to point A with LDR brachytherapy.[478] One hundred twenty-seven patients received 5-FU (IV infusion, 1 g/m² for 4 days) and cisplatin (50 mg/m² IV) on days 1, 29, and 30 to 33, and 191 patients received hydroxyurea (80 mg/kg orally twice weekly). With a median follow-up for survivors of 8.7 years, the 5-year survival rate in the cisplatin/5-FU arm was 60%, compared with 47% for women in the hydroxyurea arm.

After completion of GOG 85, the group opened GOG 120[479,481] for the same patient population, which was a three-arm randomized trial comparing irradiation plus hydroxyurea versus irradiation plus weekly cisplatin versus irradiation plus hydroxyurea, cisplatin, and 5-FU. In 526 evaluable patients with a median follow-up for survivors of 106 months, the 5- and 10-year survival rates for women in both the weekly cisplatin and irradiation arm and the irradiation, 5-FU, and cisplatin arm were 60% and 53%, respectively, compared with 40% and 34% in the hydroxyurea and irradiation arm (P ≤ .01). Overall survival was also significantly better in the two patient groups receiving cisplatin. Hematologic toxicity was greater in the group treated with the three drugs compared with cisplatin or hydroxyurea alone.

The RTOG conducted a randomized study of 389 patients with stage IB to IIA of >5 cm, proven positive pelvic lymph nodes, or stage IIB to IVA carcinoma of the cervix in which patients were treated with either pelvic and para-aortic irradiation (best arm of RTOG Protocol 79-20) or pelvic irradiation and three cycles of concomitant chemotherapy with cisplatin (75 mg/m²) and 4-day infusion of 5-FU (1,000 mg/m² per day).[482] Results were updated by Eifel et al.[427] with a median follow-up of 6.6 years for 228 survivors, the 8-year overall survival rate for women on the irradiation and cisplatin/5-FU arm was 67% versus 41% in the irradiation-only arm (P < .0001). DFS rates were 66% and 36%, respectively. There were no significant differences in late complications in the treatment groups.

Southwest Oncology Group 8797 was a study for women with FIGO stage IA2, IB, or IIA carcinoma of the cervix with metastatic disease in the pelvic lymph nodes, positive parametrial involvement, or positive surgical margins at the time of primary radical hysterectomy with total pelvic lymphadenectomy. Patients had confirmed negative PALNs; if the PALNs were not sampled, the patients had confirmed negative common iliac lymph nodes. One hundred twenty-seven patients were randomized to treatment with pelvic EBRT with 5-FU infusion and cisplatin, and 116 were treated with irradiation alone. The 3-year survival for women on the adjuvant

TABLE 73.12 DETAILS OF THE TREATMENT PROTOCOLS OF THE FIVE RANDOMIZED TRIALS THAT FORMED THE BASIS OF THE NATIONAL CANCER INSTITUTE ANNOUNCEMENT

Author (Reference)	Number of Patients	Tumor Stage	Surgical Staging	Control Arm	Investigational Arm
Keys et al.[477] (GOG 123)	369	Bulky IB (≥4 cm)	Completion hysterectomy	XRT	XRT + cisplatin (40 mg/m² IV weekly × 6 wk)
Whitney et al.[478] (GOG 85)	368	IIB, III, IVA	Yes	XRT + hydroxyurea (80 mg/kg PO 2×/wk)	XRT + cisplatin (50 mg/m² IV days 1, 28) + 5-FU infusion (1 g/m² per day, days 2–5, 30–33)
Rose et al.[479] (GOG 120)	526	IIB, III, IVA	Yes	XRT + hydroxyurea (3 g/m² PO 2×/wk)	XRT + cisplatin (40 mg/m² weekly × 6 wk) versus XRT + cisplatin (50 mg/m² IV days 1, 29) + 5-FU infusion (1 g/m² per day, days 1–4, 29–33) + hydroxyurea PO (2 g/m² 2×/wk × 6 wk)
Eifel et al.[427] (RTOG 90-01)	389	IIB, III, IVA, IB, IIA + tumor ≥5 cm or positive pelvic nodes	Yes	XRT (pelvic + para-aortic)	XRT + cisplatin (75 mg/m² IV day 1) + 5-FU infusion (1 g/m² per day, days 1–5 × 3 q3 wk)
Peters et al.[438] (GOG 109)	243	IA2, IB, IIA (pathologic stage) + positive pelvic nodes and/or positive margins and/or microscopic involvement of parametria	Yes	XRT	XRT + cisplatin (70 mg/m² IV) + 5-FU infusion (1 g/m² days 1–5 × 4 q3 wk)

5-FU, 5-fluorouracil; PO, orally; XRT, pelvic external radiation therapy.
Modified from Viswanathan AN. Advances in the use of radiation for gynecologic cancers. *Hematol Oncol Clin North Am* 2012;26(1):157–168. Copyright © 2012 Elsevier. With permission.

cisplatin/5-FU and RT arm was 87%, compared with 77% for women on the pelvic irradiation arm.[438] The difference was statistically significant. An updated analysis with 5.2-year median follow-up reported 5-year overall survival of 80% versus 66%, favoring postoperative chemoradiation in high-risk patients.[206]

In GOG 123, 369 women were enrolled. One hundred eighty-three women with bulky (≥4 cm) stage IB carcinoma of the cervix with negative pelvic and para-aortic nodes radiographically or surgically determined were randomized to be treated with pelvic EBRT and brachytherapy, followed by extrafascial hysterectomy, and 186 received EBRT and brachytherapy with weekly cisplatin (40 mg/m²; total dose not to exceed 70 mg/week) followed by extrafascial hysterectomy.[477] In an updated analysis with median follow-up of 101 months[483] the 6-year PFS rate for women treated with irradiation and cisplatin was 71%, compared with 60% for those treated with RT alone, after adjusting for age and tumor size (P < .004). The unadjusted 6-year overall survival rates were 78% and 64%, respectively (P < .015).

The results of randomized trials using concurrent chemoradiation are summarized in Table 73.13.[486] Curtin et al.[487] completed a small phase III trial in which 89 patients with high-risk stage IB or IIA undergoing radical hysterectomy and pelvic node dissection were randomized to be treated with postoperative cisplatin/bleomycin alone (44 patients) or combined with pelvic RT (45 patients). There were 9 and 10 recurrences, respectively, and survival was equivalent.

On the other hand, Pearcey et al.[484] reported on a Canadian randomized study in which 127 patients with stage IB to IIA of >5 cm or IIB carcinoma of the cervix were randomized to be treated with cisplatin (40 mg/m² weekly) and RT, and 126 patients were treated with RT alone (50.4 Gy to the pelvis combined with brachytherapy). With a median follow-up of 65 months, the 5-year survival rates were 59% and 56%, respectively (P = .43). There was a somewhat greater incidence of significant late morbidity in the RT-alone group (12% vs. 6%; P = .08). Possible explanations for the discrepancy in results between the five US trials[402] and the Canadian study were analyzed by Lehman and Thomas.[480] Some theories include that a higher percentage of early-stage patients were accrued, who therefore had less of a difference in survival, given that the baseline survival rate for both arms was quite high; and that treatment time was short for both arms,

again minimizing the difference in improving survival in the chemotherapy arm. This was the smallest of the randomized chemoradiation trials, and although the HR was reduced, given the factors equalizing the two arms, a larger number of patients would have possibly shown a significant difference.

A 2005 update of a meta-analysis of concomitant chemotherapy and radiation therapy found 24 trials and concluded that chemoradiation improves overall survival and PFS, whether or not cisplatin was used, with absolute benefits of 10% and 13%, respectively.[488] Similarly, a 2008 meta-analysis of the 13 trials that compared chemoradiotherapy to radiation found that there was a 6% improvement in 5-year survival with concurrent chemoradiation (HR 0.81, P < .001). The effect was attributed to a reduction in both local and distant recurrence. Chemoradiation increased acute hematologic and gastrointestinal toxicity, but no confirmation was made about a difference in late toxicity.[489]

In the United States, weekly cisplatin has become the preferred approach, with less toxicity than an every 3-week regimen and increased likelihood of completing the treatment on schedule. The number of completed cycles of weekly treatment was shown by Nugent et al.[490] to be predictive of survival. One hundred eighteen patients with locally advanced cervical cancer (stages IB2 to IVA) were treated with combination weekly cisplatin (40 mg/m²) and radiation between 2003 and 2007. Thirty percent of patients completed fewer than six cycles of chemotherapy. In multivariate analyses, the number of chemotherapy cycles was independently predictive of progression-free survival (PFS) and overall survival (OS). Patients who received fewer than six cycles of cisplatin had a worse PFS (HR = 2.65; 95% CI = 1.35 to 5.17; P = .0045) and OS (HR = 4.47; 95% CI = 1.83 to 10.9; P = .001). Advanced stage, longer time to RT completion, and absence of brachytherapy were also associated with decreased OS and PFS (P < .05). Similar results were found when analysis was conducted using a breakpoint of at least but not less than five chemotherapy cycles. The authors concluded that aggressive supportive care to minimize missed chemotherapy treatments may improve survival after chemoradiation. A retrospective review[491] questioned whether cervical cancer patients should receive cisplatin 20 mg/m² × 5 days every 21 days concomitant with RT or weekly 40 mg/m² weekly concomitant with RT, given that an advantage with regard to both acute toxicity and PFS was seen in the 5-day regimen.

TABLE 73.13 RANDOMIZED STUDIES OF CONCURRENT CHEMOIRRADIATION IN CERVICAL CARCINOMA

Author (Reference)	Drugs	Number of Patients	Median Follow-Up Time (Year)	Survival		
				Chemoradiation Therapy (%)	Radiation Therapy (%)	P
Chemoirradiation Versus Radiation Alone						
Eifel et al.[399] (RTOG 9001)[a]	CF	389	6.6	67	41	<.0001
Keys et al.[477]; Stehman et al.[483] (GOG 123)	C	369	8.4	78	64	<.015
Peters et al.[438] (SWOG 8797)	CF	243	5.2	80	66	NR
Pearcey et al.[484] (NCIC)	C	253	6.9	62	58	.53
Comparative Trials of Chemoirradiation Regimens						
Whitney et al.[478] (GOG 85)	CF vs. H	368	8.7	55 CF	43 H	.018
Rose et al.[479] (GOG 120)	C vs. H	526	8.8	5 yr, 60; 10 yr, 53	5 y, 40; 10 yr, 34	.002
	CHF vs. H			5 yr, 61; 10 yr, 53	5 yr, 40; 10 yr, 34	.002
Comparative Trials of Chemotherapy Regimens						
Lanciano et al.[485] (GOG 165)[b]	F vs. C	316	3.4	64	55	NR

[a]Eight-year results.
[b]Trial terminated early because of higher risk of treatment failure and higher mortality with 5-fluorouracil (HR = 1.37, 95% CI = 0.96–1.97).
C, cisplatin; F, 5-fluorouracil; GOG, Gynecologic Oncology Group; H, hydroxyurea; RTOG, Radiation Therapy Oncology Group; SWOG, Southwest Oncology Group.
Modified from Viswanathan AN. Advances in the use of radiation for gynecologic cancers. *Hematol Oncol Clin North Am* 2012;26(1):157–168. Copyright © 2012 Elsevier. With permission.

High-risk patients may benefit from adjuvant chemo-therapy after chemoRT. A randomized trial of 515 cases of stage IIB to IVA cervical carcinomas treated with concurrent gemcitabine plus cisplatin followed by adjuvant gemcitabine and cisplatin compared to standard concurrent cisplatin with radiation showed a significant 3-year PFS benefit of 74% versus 65% ($P = .03$), as well as one in overall survival (HR = 0.68, 95% CI = 0.49 to 0.65).[492] Grade 3 and 4 toxicities were higher in the extended-chemotherapy arm, including two deaths. A trial comparing "outback" Carboplatin/Taxol chemotherapy completed accrual.

Alternatives to Concurrent Cisplatin-Based Chemoradiation

In GOG Protocol 165, patients with stage IIB to IVA cervical cancers received either radiation therapy and concurrent weekly cisplatin (40 mg/m²) or radiation therapy and a protracted venous infusion (PVI) of 5-FU. Lanciano et al.[485] reported that the study was prematurely closed after an interim analysis showed a failure rate 35% higher and would not result in improved DFS with PVI 5-FU/RT compared with weekly cisplatin.

Lorvidhaya et al.[493] reported on 673 patients with predominant stage IIB and IIIB disease randomized to receive either irradiation alone or combined with chemotherapy administered in an adjuvant, concurrent, or adjuvant and concurrent schedule. Concomitant chemotherapy consisted of mitomycin C (10 mg/m²) given on days 1 and 30 and oral 5-FU (300 mg/m² per day) given on days 1 to 14 and 42 to 56. Adjuvant chemotherapy consisted of three cycles of oral 5-FU (200 mg/day) given for 4 weeks, with a 2-week rest every 6 weeks. With a median follow-up of 25 months, there was a statistically significant improvement in DFS for all patients who received chemotherapy/RT, regardless of the timing of administration of the chemotherapy. However, the authors did not state the radiation dose delivered with brachytherapy, the total dose prescribed to point A, or the OTT. In the absence of this information, the adequacy of the radiation therapy cannot be evaluated, and we cannot assume that the results of this study apply to all patients treated with irradiation.

In a randomized trial comparing monthly fluorouracil and cisplatin versus weekly cisplatin concurrent with pelvic radiation, Kim et al.[494] enrolled 158 stage IIB and IVA patients. With a median follow-up of 39 months, the acute grade 3 and 4 hematologic toxicities were significantly worse in the fluorouracil/cisplatin arm, 43% versus 26% ($P = .04$). The trial was not powered to detect a survival difference, and no difference in the overall survival or PFS was noted.

Tseng et al.[495] published results of a study in which patients with advanced carcinoma of the cervix were randomly assigned to either RT alone or concurrent chemotherapy (cisplatin, vincristine, and bleomycin every 3 weeks for a total of four courses) and RT. After a median follow-up of 46.8 months, the DFS and actuarial survival rates were 51.7% and 61.7% in the concurrent group and 53.2% and 64.5% in the RT group, respectively ($P = .27$). Treatment-related toxicity was higher with the combination therapy compared with irradiation alone (36.7% vs. 17.7%; $P = .02$).

Several small phase II studies have been performed showing no advantage to weekly paclitaxel over weekly cisplatin[496] and too high toxicity with concomitant cisplatin–paclitaxel.[497] Concurrent weekly carboplatin alone has been shown in many studies to be feasible[498] including in the elderly; it is also an alternative in patients that have an elevated creatinine. Docetaxel and carboplatin concurrent with radiation was also found to be a feasible regimen.[499]

The GOG carried out a trial of irradiation with either concomitant hydroxyurea (HOU) or a placebo in patients with stage IIIB or IVA cervix cancer.[500] The study was criticized because patients were not surgically staged, half of the 190

patients were not evaluable, and radiation doses were low.[326] Piver et al.[501] published an update of a study of 130 patients (13 with PALN metastasis), 75 of whom were surgically staged. Of 66 patients who underwent surgical staging, 33 received hydroxyurea and 33 a placebo in combination with irradiation. Of the patients who did not have surgical staging, 27 received hydroxyurea and 37 received placebo. The 2-year survival was higher in the HOU group. Symonds et al.,[502] in a review of seven randomized trials, found no evidence to support the use of hydroxyurea with RT in cervix cancer.

In larger randomized trial by the GOG reported by Stehman et al.,[503] 296 surgically staged patients with stage IIB to IVA disease and negative para-aortic nodes were randomized to irradiation plus either hydroxyurea (139 patients) or misonidazole (157 patients). Survival was not statistically different between the regimens, with 33.8% deaths in the hydroxyurea group and 38.9% deaths in the misonidazole group ($P = .25$). Failure limited to the pelvis occurred in 18% of patients in the hydroxyurea group and 23.6% in the misonidazole group. Of note, in a randomized RTOG trial of patients with stage III disease, Leibel et al.[504] and Overgaard et al.[505] reported lower survival in patients receiving misonidazole than in the patients treated with irradiation alone.

Grigsby et al.[506] published results of an RTOG study in which 120 patients with carcinoma of the cervix were randomized to receive irradiation alone or combined with misonidazole. The 5-year PFS was 22% and 29%, respectively. These findings are similar to those reported by Overgaard et al.[505] who, in a randomized study of 331 patients with carcinoma of the cervix treated with either misonidazole or a placebo and irradiation, found no significant difference in local tumor control (50% vs. 54%), DFS (47% vs. 46%), or crude survival (39% vs. 45%). Immunotherapy studies are ongoing.

Nonrandomized Studies of Chemotherapy and Irradiation

Numerous preliminary reports have been published on results of neoadjuvant/concomitant use of cisplatin and 5-FU, with or without mitomycin C, combined with irradiation to treat patients with locally advanced or recurrent carcinoma of the cervix.[507]

Trials with Cisplatin, 5-Fluorouracil, or Both

Perez and Grigsby[508] reported on 58 patients with locally advanced carcinoma of the cervix treated with concurrent 5-FU/cisplatin and irradiation and compared the results with 257 patients with similar stages treated with irradiation alone during the same period. Pelvic tumor control and disease-free survival and CSS were comparable. The incidence of rectal and bladder fistula was 7% in the chemoirradiation group and 4% with irradiation alone ($P = .61$).

Park et al.[466] described results in 113 patients with high-risk invasive cervical carcinoma treated with cisplatin and 5-FU. For adenocarcinoma, doxorubicin (45 mg/m² IV) was added. The patients subsequently received radiation therapy (not described in the publication). For patients with stage I or II tumors >4 cm, the 5-year survival rate was 78.3% with chemoirradiation and was 48% for 77 patients treated with RT alone ($P < .01$). For stages III and IV, the rates were 69.1% and 57.4%, respectively. Toxicity with combined chemoirradiation was not significantly enhanced compared with irradiation alone.

Sardi et al.[509] reported results of three courses of cisplatin, vincristine, and bleomycin (days 1 to 3) at 10-day intervals combined with RT in 205 unselected patients with stage IB cervix cancer (tumors >2 cm) who were divided at random into two groups treated with surgery and RT or neoadjuvant chemotherapy, surgery, and irradiation. After 67 months, no difference in survival was seen in patients with tumors 2 to 4 cm in both groups (77% for control patients vs. 82% with neoadjuvant chemotherapy), but statistically significant differences were seen in bulky tumors (>4 cm): 61% versus 80% in favor of neoadjuvant chemotherapy.

Souhami et al.[510] treated 50 patients with bulky, locally advanced carcinoma of the cervix with a combination of weekly cisplatin (30 mg/m²) concurrent with RT. At 44 months, the actuarial survival rate was 65%, the total pelvic failure rate was 26%, and the distant metastasis rate was 24%. The incidence of late gastrointestinal toxicity was high, with 10 rectal ulcers (4 colostomies required for severe bleeding), 2 rectovaginal fistulas, and 2 small-bowel obstructions.

Park et al.[511] treated patients with stage I and II carcinomas of the cervix >4 cm with RT alone or concurrent or sequential chemoradiation with cisplatin and 5-FU. The 30-month survival rates were 100% with concurrent chemoirradiation, 89.5% with sequential treatment, and 79.5% with irradiation alone (*P* < .05).

Lee et al.[512] treated 40 women with cervix cancer using 50-Gy EBRT and brachytherapy; in 25 cases, three concurrent cycles of cisplatin/5-FU were given, and in 15 cases, six cycles of consolidation chemotherapy were given. There was no difference in 2-year survival between the two groups (98% to 100%). Grade 2 or greater hematologic toxicity was more frequent in the consolidation patients.

Grigsby et al.,[513] in a prospective study of 65 patients with cervical cancer and node negative on FDG-PET treated with RT alone (15 patients) or combined with concurrent weekly cisplatin (50 patients), noted a 5-year CSS of 78% and 74%, respectively. Severe complications included 1 rectovaginal fistula and 1 rectal stricture in the concurrent chemotherapy/RT group and 1 chemotherapy-related death.

Trials with Carboplatin

Katanyoo et al.[498] reported 148 patients with stage IIB to IVA cervical cancers treated with concurrent weekly carboplatin (100 mg/m² or area under the curve 2) for a median of six cycles and radiation. Among the 142 responders, 36 experienced recurrences: pelvic recurrences in 7 (4.7%), distant failure in 25 (16.9%), and both pelvic and distant in 4 (2.7%). The 2- and 5-year PFS rates were 75.1% and 63.0%, respectively, with the corresponding 2- and 5-year overall survival rates of 81.9% and 63.5%. No grade 3 or 4 hematologic and nonhematologic toxicities were observed during treatment in any patients. Late grade 3 to 4 gastrointestinal or genitourinary toxicities were 10.1% and 0.7%, respectively.

Cetina et al.[514] looked at the use of weekly carboplatin in 59 elderly, diabetic, and/or hypertensive stage IB2 to IIIB cervical cancer patients. All patients completed radiation and 80% received five of six planned cycles, with 83% reaching a complete response. With a median follow-up of 20 months, 33% relapsed, and the 3-year overall survival rate was 63%. Although the regimen is safe and tolerable, it may have reduced efficacy compared to weekly cisplatin.

Trials with Mitomycin C or Tirapazamine

Mitomycin C acts as an alkylating agent and inhibits DNA and RNA synthesis. Activation of mitomycin C is increased in hypoxic conditions, and thus, it acts as a hypoxic radiosensitizer. Interstitial pneumonitis and pulmonary fibrosis are usually related to the dose of drug. Use of IV dexamethasone before administration of the drug may prevent pulmonary toxicity.

Christie et al.[464] described results in three groups of patients with stage IIB and III carcinomas of the cervix treated with pelvic irradiation and an intracavitary insertion combined with chemotherapy. Group A (64 patients) received 5-FU infusion during the first and last weeks of irradiation combined with mitomycin C (10 mg/m² IV). Group B (29 patients) received 5-FU without mitomycin C, and group C (84 patients) received irradiation alone. With median follow-up of 7.2 years, the 5-year survival rates were 56%, 32%, and 36%,

and the local tumor control was 73%, 53%, and 50%, respectively. Toxicity was greater in group A (36% grades 3 and 4) compared with the 5-FU and irradiation group (14%) and the irradiation-alone group (20%).

Roberts et al.[515] reported on a trial in which 160 patients with locally advanced cervical cancer were randomized to receive RT alone (82 patients) or RT with concomitant mitomycin C (78 patients). The 4-year actuarial survival was 72% and 56%, respectively (*P* = .13), and the local recurrence–free survival rate was 78% and 63%, respectively (*P* = .11). There were no treatment-related deaths. No excess in nonhematologic toxicity has been observed with combined mitomycin C and irradiation.

Tirapazamine, a radiation sensitizer with selective cytotoxic effect on hypoxic cells, was combined with cisplatin in 56 patients with recurrent or metastatic cancer. After six cycles given every 21 days, 4 complete and 13 partial responses were noted. Overall 6-month survival was 56%. Better response was seen in patients who had not received radiosensitizing chemotherapy previously.[516]

Besides the usual hematologic and pelvic toxicity described in many of these studies with chemoradiation, Wun et al.,[517] in a retrospective analysis of 75 patients with gynecologic cancer who received erythropoietin and chemotherapy/RT, noted that 17 had upper- or lower-extremity thrombosis, in contrast to 2 of 72 who did not receive erythropoietin. Of note, Anders et al.,[518] in a review of the literature, reported that 6 of 128 patients (4.7%) treated with chemotherapy/RT without erythropoietin developed grade 4 or 5 thrombosis toxicity.

Trial with Bevacizumab Concurrent with RT

RTOG 0417 treated patients with once-weekly cisplatin (40 mg/m²) chemotherapy and standard pelvic radiotherapy and brachytherapy. Bevacizumab was administered at 10 mg/kg intravenously every 2 weeks for three cycles. A total of 49 patients were evaluable. The median follow-up was 12.4 months (range, 4.6 to 31.4 months). There were no treatment-related serious adverse events. There were 15 (31%) protocol-specified, treatment-related adverse events within 90 days of treatment start; the most common were hematologic (12 of 15; 80%). Eighteen (37%) occurred during treatment or follow-up at any time.[519] An update with 3.8 years follow-up (range 0.8 to 6 years) showed a 3-year OS 81.3%, DFS 68.7%, and LRF 23.2%, with 26.5% grade 3 adverse events (mainly hematologic) and 10.2% grade 4 events.[520]

Trial with Epidermal Growth Factor Receptor Inhibition Concurrent with RT

Nogueira-Rodrigues et al.[521] reported a phase I study administering escalating doses of erlotinib (50/100/150 mg) combined with cisplatin (40 mg/m², weekly, five cycles) and radiotherapy (external beam, 4,500 cGy in 25 fractions, followed by four fractions/600 cGy weekly of brachytherapy) in squamous cell cervical carcinoma patients, stages IIB to IIIB. Fifteen patients were enrolled, 3 at dose level (DL) 50 mg, 4 at DL 100 mg, and 8 at DL 150 mg. Three patients did not complete the planned schedule. One patient at DL 100 mg withdrew informed consent because of grade 2 rash; at DL 150 mg, 1 patient presented with Raynaud syndrome and had cisplatin interrupted, and another patient presented with grade 4 hepatotoxicity. The latter was interpreted as dose-limiting toxicity, and a new cohort of 150 mg was started. No further grade 4 toxicity occurred. Grade 3 toxicity occurred in six cases: diarrhea in three patients, rash in two patients, and leukopenia in one patient. Treatment did not lead to limiting infield toxicity.

Intra-arterial Chemotherapy

Intra-arterial infusion of chemotherapeutic agents in cervical carcinoma was used for some years based on the distinct arterial supply to the tumor-bearing area. Unfortunately, the responses have been uncommon and short, and the toxicity and complication rates have been significant.[522]

Onishi et al.[523] evaluated intra-arterial cisplatin through catheters inserted into both internal iliac arteries in cervix carcinoma. Patients were randomized into a concurrent intra-arterial infusion of cisplatin with RT (18 patients) or RT alone (15 patients). Five-year overall survival rates were 44.4% and 50%, respectively. In the group receiving intra-arterial infusion, grade 3 or 4 late bowel complications were seen in 44% and grade 3 or 4 myelosuppression in 33%, significantly more than in the RT group.

Neoadjuvant Chemotherapy

Thomas[524] summarized the rationale and potential limitations of neoadjuvant chemotherapy in carcinoma of the cervix. Although response rates to the chemotherapy are between 30% and 85%, none of the studies showed an advantage for pelvic tumor control or survival.[525-532] Colombo et al.,[533] in a review of the literature, concluded that the role of neoadjuvant chemotherapy followed by radiation and by concomitant chemotherapy or by surgery is controversial because no significant advantages in survival or local control have been shown, and receiving upfront chemotherapy may compromise immune status and the patient's ability to receive definitive treatment with radiation or surgery.

Souhami et al.[534] randomized 107 patients with stage IIIB carcinoma of the cervix to treatment with irradiation alone or combined with bleomycin, vincristine, mitomycin, and cisplatin. The overall 5-year survival rate for the neoadjuvant-treated patients was 23%, in contrast to 39% for those treated with irradiation alone (P = .02). Locoregional and distant failure rates were similar in both groups.

Kumar et al.[535] reported a randomized trial in which 94 patients with carcinoma of the cervix were treated with chemotherapy (two cycles of bleomycin, ifosfamide–mesna, and cisplatin) followed by RT, and 90 patients were treated with irradiation alone. In the chemotherapy/RT group, 32-month survival was 63% for stage IIB and 50% for stage III, and in the RT group, the rate was 59% for stage IIB and 27% for stage IIIB tumors (differences not statistically significant). There was no difference in radiation-induced toxicity between the two groups.

In a Swedish study,[531] 47 patients with carcinoma of the cervix were randomized to be treated with irradiation alone (64.8 Gy, 1.8-Gy fractions) and 47 with a combination of three cycles of cisplatin and 5 days of 5-FU administered every third week, followed by the same pelvic irradiation. The 5-year DFS rates were 70% with chemoirradiation and 57% with irradiation alone (P = .07). The incidences of pelvic recurrence were 60% and 47%, respectively, and for distant metastasis, they were 19% and 35%, respectively. Two patients in the chemoirradiation and 1 in the irradiation-alone group died as a consequence of therapy.

Response to Chemotherapy Alone for Patients with Metastatic or Recurrent Disease

Cisplatin has been combined with other cytotoxic agents. Long et al.[536] conducted a randomized study comparing methotrexate, vinblastine, doxorubicin, and cisplatin (MVAC), cisplatin/topotecan, or cisplatin alone in patients with advanced cervical cancer. The MVAC arm was closed after 4 deaths in 63 patients. In 294 patients assigned to the other arms, response rate was 27% for cisplatin/topotecan and 13% for cisplatin alone, with median survival of 9.4 and 6.5 months, respectively.

Paclitaxel, a natural product found initially in the bark of the western yew tree, produces depolymerization and irreversible bundling of tubulin in the cell. It has been shown to have a radiosensitizing effect and may also be considered for patients with metastatic disease. Rose et al.[537] reported on a phase II study of 44 patients in which the starting dose was paclitaxel (135 mg/m², maximum 170 mg/m²) infused over 24 hours, followed by cisplatin (75 mg/m²) every 21 days. Forty patients (90.9%) had received prior radiation therapy. A median of six courses of chemotherapy was given. Of the 41 assessable patients, 5 (12.2%) had a complete response and 14 (34.1%) had a partial response. Vinorelbine is a semisynthetic derivative of vinblastine. In a phase II trial in patients with prior irradiation, a 28% response rate was observed.[538] Other trials used the drug as neoadjuvant chemotherapy; in 42 patients, 2 complete and 17 partial responses (45%) were observed.[539,540]

Irinotecan and topotecan are camptothecin derivatives whose cytotoxic mechanism is believed to target topoisomerase I.[541] An international phase II trial reported a similar 21% response rate in patients predominantly with prior irradiation (1 complete and 8 partial responses among 42 patients).[542]

Gemcitabine, a nucleoside analogue, showed a 4.5% partial response and 36% stable disease in 22 patients.[543] In combination with cisplatin, it was evaluated in 32 women with previously treated cervix cancer (initial dose 800 mg/m² on days 1 and 8, then every 28 days); there were 7 (22%) partial responses and 12 stable disease responses.[544]

A phase II trial of docetaxel and gemcitabine showed an overall response rate of 21%. With a median survival of 7 months, 39% were alive at 1 year. Docetaxel combined with carboplatin has been shown to have a 25% response rate.[499]

A four-arm comparison of cisplatin/paclitaxel versus cisplatin/vinorelbine, cisplatin/gemcitabine, or cisplatin/topotecan found that the standard arm of cisplatin/paclitaxel remained the best option for patients with stage IVB, recurrent or persistent cervical carcinoma.[545]

In a phase II GOG study of cetuximab 400 mg/m² initial dose followed by 250 mg/m² weekly until disease progression or prohibitive toxicity, 38 patients (15%) had no progression for at least 6 months. The median OS was 7 months. When cetuximab was combined with cisplatin, no additional benefit beyond cisplatin was identified.[546]

Ifosfamide, paclitaxel, and carboplatin as a triple regimen showed a 33% objective complete or partial response, with an overall median survival of 10 months.[547] Antiangiogenic tyrosine kinase inhibitors pazopanib and lapatinib were tested in 230 patients with stage IVB persistent/recurrent cervical carcinoma. An improvement in progression-free and overall survival was seen with pazopanib.[548] A trial of PD-1 positive cervical cancer treated with immunotherapy is ongoing.

Studies with Radiation Alone

For patients unable to tolerate concurrent chemotherapy or in countries where chemotherapy is not readily available, radiation alone may be used as an alternative to chemoradiation. Mendenhall et al.[549] analyzed 1,211 patients treated with radiation alone with a minimum follow-up of 3 years. In patients with stage IB and IIA disease, there was no significant correlation between doses to these points and pelvic tumor control. In stage IIB, doses of <6,000 cGy to point A correlated with a high pelvic failure rate (8 of 12, 66.7%) in contrast to doses of 6,000 to 9,000 cGy (61 of 261, 23.4%) or higher than 9,000 cGy (10 of 74, 13.5%) (P = 0.01). In stage III, the pelvic failure rate with doses below 6,000 cGy to point A was 72% (18 of 25) compared to 39% (71 of 180) for 6,000 to 9,000 cGy or 35% (27 of 77) with doses above 9,000 cGy (P ≤ .01).

Thoms et al.[550] reported on 363 patients with bulky endocervical carcinoma treated with curative intent (246 with irradiation alone and 117 with irradiation and surgery); 10-year survival was 45% and 64%, respectively. In a subset of 48 patients with similar tumors treated with irradiation alone and 45 treated with irradiation and surgery, the 10-year survival rates were comparable, and the pelvic tumor control rates were 90% and 87%, respectively.

Eifel et al.[189] evaluated 1,526 patients, of whom 371 had tumors 6 cm or greater. There were biases in treatment selection, but a statistically significantly higher 10-year survival rate was noted in patients treated with irradiation and surgery (64% vs. 45%). Tumor diameter was highly significant as a prognostic factor, and the authors concluded that only patients with lesions >8 cm in diameter benefited from adjuvant hysterectomy. In the same study, 98 patients with stage IB and IIB bulky endocervical carcinomas (≥6 cm in diameter) were treated with RT alone. Twenty-four patients received <6,000 mgh of intracavitary treatment, and 73 received higher doses. Despite having somewhat more favorably treated tumors, patients who received <6,000 mgh had a higher rate of pelvic recurrence at 5 years (33%) than those who received higher doses (16%; P = .03). Actuarial 5-year survival rates were 44% and 60% for low- and high-dose groups, respectively (P = .14).

Kim et al.[551] assessed the prognostic factors for pelvic tumor control in 40 patients with FIGO stage IB or IIA carcinoma and 25 patients with stage IIB carcinoma classified as barrel shaped (i.e., at least 5 cm in diameter) treated with curative intent. Seventy-two percent were treated with RT alone and 28% with RT and extrafascial hysterectomy. The extent of tumor regression after external beam radiation therapy correlated with the likelihood of local tumor control (P = .02). For patients treated with radiation therapy alone, increased brachytherapy dose was associated with better local tumor control. The 10-year overall and CSS rates were 53% and 68%, respectively, and did not differ significantly between treatment groups.

Paley et al.[552] reported on 57 patients with barrel-shaped (mean diameter, 5 to 9 cm) cervical carcinoma treated with preoperative EBRT and BT (mean dose to point A, 79.6 Gy) followed by extrafascial hysterectomy 6 to 8 weeks later. Residual disease was present in 35 (61%) of the hysterectomy specimens; tumor sterilization correlated significantly with the mean dose to point A (P = .016). Ninety-five percent of the patients with negative specimens remained clinically free of disease at their last follow-up versus 31% of those with residual disease (P < .001).

The GOG and RTOG conducted a randomized phase III clinical trial in which 282 patients with carcinoma of the cervix measuring 4 cm or greater (exophytic or barrel shaped) were treated with either external beam and intracavitary irradiation or a slightly lower dose of intracavitary irradiation and the same pelvic EBRT followed by an extrafascial hysterectomy.[553] The survival rates were 61.4% for irradiation alone and 64.4% for the combined irradiation and surgery group. The incidence of recurrences was 43.3% in the irradiation group compared to 34.5% with combined therapy (P = .081). The incidence of local recurrences was 25.8% and 14.4%, respectively. The incidence of grade 3 and 4 sequelae of therapy was 10.5% and 9.8%, respectively. Thus, the addition of hysterectomy to standard irradiation did not significantly affect survival, although there was a small reduction in the local recurrence rate. When combined therapy is used, the dose of irradiation delivered to the lymph nodes, the time of the operation, and the pathologic examination of the specimens are critical in determining the presence of postirradiation residual tumor.

Perez et al.[38] noted that in patients with primary carcinoma of the uterine cervix who had endometrial stromal invasion or tumor only in the curettings, the addition of a hysterectomy did not improve the survival rate because most of the patients failed at distant sites.

For stage IIB tumors treated with irradiation alone, the 5-year survival rate is 60% to 65%. The pelvic failure rate ranges from 18% to 39%. In an analysis of the Patterns of Care Study in 157 patients who had stage IIB disease, Coia et al.[554] reported a better 4-year survival rate (67% and 54%)

and infield tumor control rate (78% and 68%) in patients with unilateral versus bilateral parametrial involvement, respectively. Similarly, in a review of 1,178 patients with stage IIB disease, the 5-year survival rates were 70% with medial parametrial and 58% with lateral parametrial involvement (P = .004).[555] Kim et al.,[556] in patients with stage IIB disease, found a correlation of point A dose and incidence of pelvic failures.

In stage IIIB carcinoma, the 5-year survival rates range from 25% to 48%, and pelvic failure rates range from 38% to 50%.[186,557] Hanks et al.,[558] reporting on the Patterns of Care Study, noted a 28% probability of 5-year survival in patients with stage III carcinoma of the cervix treated in a large number of facilities in the United States versus 60% survival in selected large centers (extended survey). Later, Komaki et al.[559] reported a significant increase in local pelvic tumor control (69%) in patients with stage III carcinoma of the cervix treated in 1983, compared with 37% and 49% in earlier periods (P = .03). The 5-year survival rate increased from 25% to 47% (P = .02). The improvement in pelvic tumor control may be associated with higher external beam doses but more likely is related to the substantial increase in the percentage of patients receiving brachytherapy (96%) and more careful dosimetry and dose calculations for intracavitary therapy. They noted a decrease in major complications from 15% in the 1973 and 13% in the 1978. Patterns of Care Surveys to 7% in 1983. Montana et al.[560] reported that calculation of doses to the bladder and rectum were performed in 80% and 76% of patients, respectively, in the 1983 survey, which may also have resulted in decreased toxicity.

Arthur et al.,[561] in 89 patients with stage IIIB carcinoma of the cervix treated with external irradiation and brachytherapy, observed a locoregional tumor control rate of 22.5% and a DFS rate of 15% in 16 patients treated with 78 Gy or lower doses to point A, in comparison with 53% and 47%, respectively, in 24 patients receiving higher doses.

Horiot et al.[562] reported the results of a French cooperative study of 1,383 patients with invasive carcinoma of the uterus treated with irradiation alone following the MD Anderson Hospital treatment guidelines. Survival and locoregional tumor control were similar in both groups, except in stage III, in which the pelvic and central failure rates were lower in the French patients, may be because of different tumor volumes or socioeconomic factors. Major urinary complications were noted in 2% of the patients. Grade 3 bowel complications occurred in 3% of the patients with stage I and IIA diseases and in 7% of patients with stage IIB and III diseases. Barillot et al.[563] updated the results in 642 patients; the analysis was divided into three periods: 1970 to 1978 (use of standard prescriptions), 1979 to 1984 (implementation of individual adjustments), and 1985 to 1994 (systematic individual adjustments). There was a significant reduction of the external radiation dose (>40 Gy in 47% of patients before 1979 vs. 36% after 1984), use of parametrial boost (55% vs. 39%), use of vaginal cylinder (28% vs. 11.5%), and combined intracavitary and external irradiation volume (842 vs. 503 cm³ on average). The 5-year actuarial toxicity rates were as follows: grade 2, 23.5%; grade 3, 10%; and grade 4, 3%. The three main predictive factors for rectal and bladder sequelae were increased external radiation dose, higher dose rate at reference points, and whole-vagina brachytherapy.

Marcial et al.[564] described results of a randomized trial in 301 patients with stage IIB, III, and IVA carcinomas of the uterine cervix treated with split-course irradiation (10 fractions of 2.5 Gy, five weekly doses up to 25 Gy, followed by a rest period of 2 weeks, and an additional 25 Gy delivered in the same manner) or continuous irradiation (30 fractions of 1.7 Gy daily, five times per week, total dose 51 Gy) combined with LDR brachytherapy for 30 Gy to point A. There was no significant difference in tumor control, acute or late complications, or survival in the two groups.

In patients with stage IVA disease, the 5-year survival rates range from 18% to 34%, and pelvic failures from 60% to 80% after definitive irradiation.[288] Million et al.[289] reported 18 of 53 patients (34%) with bladder involvement surviving without disease after definitive irradiation, results comparable with those obtained with exenteration. Kramer et al.[288] reported on 48 patients with stage IVA carcinoma of the cervix treated with definitive RT. Patients with minimal parametrial involvement had a 5-year survival rate of 46%, compared with only 5% for those with extensive parametrial tumor. The major complication rate was 22%, consisting mostly of vesicovaginal fistula in five patients.

Crozier et al.[565] described equivalent 5-year survival rates after salvage pelvic exenteration (37% in 35 patients with adenocarcinoma and 39% in 70 patients with squamous cell carcinoma). In the adenocarcinoma group, 14 of 22 patients and, in the squamous cell carcinoma group, 14 of 30 patients had distant metastases after pelvic exenteration.

Combination of Irradiation and Surgery

Preoperative Chemoirradiation

Bulky endocervical tumors and the so-called barrel-shaped cervix have a higher incidence of central recurrence, pelvic and PALN metastases, and distant dissemination.[566] When using plain x-ray point-based planning for brachytherapy, because of the inability of intracavitary sources to encompass the entire tumor in a high-dose volume, larger doses of external radiation to the whole pelvis, extrafascial hysterectomy, or both have been advocated to improve therapeutic results.[4] Alternatively, the use of 3D planning for the brachytherapy component significantly improves survival,[567] and the ability to dose escalate because of a more precise dose delivery improves local control.[568] In rare cases with large residual after 45 Gy external beam, an Extrafascial hysterectomy may be considered 6 to 12 weeks after completion of preoperative irradiation (45 Gy to the whole pelvis and one intracavitary LDR insertion for 5,500 mgh, delivering approximately 50 Gy to point A, with a total dose to point A of 70 Gy, or the equivalent dose in HDR, approximately three fractions of 6 Gy per fraction). Higher doses of irradiation alone yield equivalent pelvic tumor control and survival rates.[189]

Keys et al.[477] reported on 183 women with bulky (≥4 cm) stage IB carcinoma of the cervix with negative pelvic and para-aortic nodes radiographically treated with pelvic EBRT and brachytherapy, followed by extrafascial hysterectomy, or EBRT and brachytherapy (to 70 Gy) with weekly cisplatin followed by extrafascial hysterectomy. A significant survival advantage was seen with the combination of concurrent chemoradiation. However, in comparison to other trials, the survival was not significantly improved with the addition of a hysterectomy. The use of PET scanning to determine residual disease allows selection of patients who may be appropriate candidates for a hysterectomy after completion of external beam treatment.[111] Therefore, patients should receive definitive doses of chemoradiation, with hysterectomy reserved for salvage in patients with either gross residual disease or PET-positive disease that is biopsy proven at 3 months after completion of radiation. A subsequent reanalysis including GOG 123 and GOG 71 analyzed 464 patients allocated to pelvic radiation (75 Gy, $n = 291$) plus hysterectomy or to pelvic radiation (75 Gy) and cisplatin (40 mg/m^2, $n = 176$) plus hysterectomy. A benefit to chemoradiation was seen for patients who had a poor response.[569]

Morice et al.[570] reported a randomized trial of 61 patients treated with adjuvant hysterectomy versus none after EBRT with concurrent weekly cisplatin and vaginal brachytherapy (15 Gy to intermediate-risk CTV) for stage IB2 or II cervical cancer. Hysterectomy increased the number of deaths, with an 11% nonsignificant survival advantage in the no-hysterectomy arm (86% vs. 97%). As a result of this trial, routine adjuvant hysterectomy is no longer practiced for patients who have no residual disease at 6 weeks after chemoradiation.

Motton et al.[571] retrospectively reviewed 171 patients treated with chemoradiation followed by simple extrafascial hysterectomy or extended hysterectomy. There was no difference in survival or complication rate based on type of surgery. Lèguevaque et al.[572] reported on 111 patients treated with or without adjuvant hysterectomy after chemoradiation; there was no advantage to overall survival, but there was a significant difference in recurrence rates.

Touboul et al.[573] reported on toxicities for 150 patients with stage IB2 to IVA cervical cancers treated at Institut Gustave Roussy (IGR) with extrafascial versus modified radical hysterectomy after chemoradiation. After a median follow-up of 3.6 years, 15% had grade 2 or greater side effects, including lymphedema, ureteral fistula, bowel fistula, and iliac and vessel rupture. There were two postoperative deaths. Modified radical versus extrafascial hysterectomy had a higher odds ratio (OR) for complications of 2.4 ($P = .04$), as did the presence of residual disease.

Elective Para-Aortic Lymph Node Irradiation

Rotman et al.[441] updated results of an RTOG randomized study of 337 patients with stage IIB carcinoma of the uterine cervix with no clinical or radiographic evidence of para-aortic lymphadenopathy who, in addition to standard pelvic irradiation, were randomized to electively receive or not 45 Gy to the para-aortic region (1.6- to 1.8-Gy fractions). The 10-year survival rate was 55% for patients receiving elective para-aortic irradiation and 44% for those treated to the pelvis only ($P = .02$). The locoregional tumor control rate was similar (69% in the para-aortic node–irradiated group and 65% for the pelvis-irradiated group). The 10-year grade 4 or 5 (major) complication rate was 8% in the group receiving para-aortic irradiation, compared with 4% in patients treated with pelvic irradiation alone ($P = .06$).

A similar randomized study was reported by Haie et al.[574] and the European Organization for Research and Treatment of Cancer (EORTC) on 441 patients with cervical carcinoma, including stage III, who had no evidence of PALN involvement. In the study group, the para-aortic area either received or did not receive 45 Gy with external beam irradiation. No statistically significant difference was found between the two treatment arms with regard to local tumor control, distant metastases, or survival. However, the incidence of para-aortic and distant metastases without pelvic failure was significantly higher in patients receiving pelvic irradiation alone. The incidence of small-bowel injury was 0.9% in the pelvic irradiation group and 2.3% in the pelvic plus para-aortic irradiation group. A severe complication rate of 9% was observed in patients receiving para-aortic irradiation, compared with 4.8% in those treated to the pelvis only.

Sood et al.[575] treated 54 patients with cervix cancer using extended fields (45 Gy) and HDR brachytherapy; 44 received concurrent cisplatin (20 mg/m^2 per day for 5 days during weeks 1 and 4 and once after the second HDR insertion). During a median follow-up of 28 months, six patients had died. The 3-year local tumor control was 100% and 85%, respectively. Late toxicity was 10% and 6%, respectively.

Huang et al.[260] assessed 758 patients and found that 38 (5%) and 42 (6%) had isolated and nonisolated PALN recurrences after a median follow-up of 50 months (range, 2 to 159 months), respectively. The 3- and 5-year overall survival rate after PALN recurrence was 35% and 28%, respectively, with those with isolated recurrences faring better than those with a nonisolated recurrence ($P < .001$). An SCC-Ag level of >40 ng/mL

($P < .001$), advanced parametrial involvement (score 4 to 6; $P = .002$), and the presence of pelvic lymphadenopathy ($P = .007$) were independent factors associated with PALN relapse on multivariate analysis. This group subsequently identified pretreatment CEA of ≥ 10 ng/mL as an additional risk factor of PALN relapse after definitive concurrent chemoradiation therapy (CCRT) for SCC of the uterine cervix in patients with pretreatment SCC-Ag levels of <10 ng/mL.[261] The role of prophylactic para-aortic radiation, particularly in patients with large tumor size, parametrial involvement, or involved pelvic lymph nodes, must be carefully weighed against the potential toxicities of para-aortic radiation.

METASTASES TO PARA-AORTIC LYMPH NODES

PALN metastases are frequently combined with distant dissemination but are clinically apparent in only 10% to 20% of patients who have recurrences.

Varia et al.[576] reported on GOG Protocol 125, in which 87 patients with biopsy-confirmed PALNs from cervical cancer were treated with extended-field irradiation (45 Gy in 1.5-Gy fractions) and higher doses to the pelvis (~80 Gy to point A) in combination with 5-FU and cisplatin. The 3-year PFS rate was 33%, and the overall survival rate was 39%. Grade 3 and 4 hematologic toxicities were noted in 13 patients (15%) and chronic proctitis in 3 (3.5%), and 4 patients (4.6%) required surgery for rectal complications.

Nelson et al.[53] reported on 104 patients with stage II and III cervical carcinomas who had exploratory laparotomy and PALN biopsies; 12.5% of patients had stage IIA disease, 14.9% had stage IIB disease, and 38.4% had stage III disease and had PALN metastases. They were treated with 60 Gy to the para-aortic region. Within 4 years, 50% of these patients had distant metastases, and only 1 out of 13 was alive. There was no significant increase in complications in the patients receiving para-aortic irradiation (39% and 32%). The authors concluded that the main goal of exploratory laparotomy and PALN biopsy is to define the extent of disease.

Lovecchio et al.[577] noted a 50% 5-year survival rate in 36 patients with stage IB and IIA cervical carcinomas who had histologically confirmed PALN metastases treated with RT (including 45 Gy to the PALNs). Fourteen of 31 evaluable patients had pelvic recurrences (12 combined with distant metastases). Unfortunately, the authors did not specify how many patients had para-aortic recurrences, although they reported four abdominal failures.

Stryker and Mortel[578] determined survival after extended-field treatment of PALN metastasis plus brachytherapy or pelvic boost in 35 patients; 5-year survival was 41.7% for 12 patients with microscopic PALN metastasis and 26.1% for 23 patients with grossly enlarged lymph nodes. Three patients (8.6%) had grade 4 morbidity.

Grigsby et al.[579] reviewed 43 patients with cervical cancer and biopsy-proven positive PALN treated with external irradiation to the pelvis and para-aortic regions (45 to 50 Gy) combined with brachytherapy. The 5-year overall survival rate was 32%, and the CSS rate was 49%. Tumor recurrence occurred in 20 patients (3 in the pelvis, 9 in pelvis and distant metastasis, and 8 in distant metastasis only). Severe grade 3 complications occurred in 2 patients (1 had an enterovaginal fistula and the other had radiation myelitis).

Hacker et al.,[580] in 437 patients with invasive cervical carcinoma, 222 of whom were treated with radical hysterectomy and lymphadenectomy, identified 34 in whom resection of bulky pelvic or PALNs was carried out without a complete lymphadenectomy. Thirty-three patients received pelvic external irradiation, and 28 combined pelvic and para-aortic extended-field irradiation (50.4 Gy in 1.8-Gy fractions using a four-field technique). Four cycles of cisplatin were administered to 23 patients. The 5-year survival was 80% in patients with pelvic and common iliac nodes and 48% in those with positive PALNs. Serious long-term morbidity occurred in 6 patients (18%). Radiation enteritis was observed in 5 patients, leading to small-bowel obstruction necessitating resection.

Grigsby et al.[581] evaluated twice-daily external irradiation to the pelvis and para-aortic nodes (1.2 Gy at 4- to 6-hour intervals, 5 days/week) combined with brachytherapy and concurrent chemotherapy in 29 patients with carcinoma of the cervix and positive PALNs. EBRT doses were 24 to 48 Gy to the whole pelvis, 12 to 36 Gy parametrial boost, and 48 Gy to the para-aortics, with additional boost to a total dose of 54 to 58 Gy to known metastatic para-aortic sites. One or two LDR brachytherapy applications were performed to deliver a total dose of 85 Gy to point A. Cisplatin (75 mg/m², days 1 and 22) and 5-FU (1,000 mg/m² per 24 hours for 4 days, days 1 and 22) were given for two or three cycles. Hyperfractionated external radiation therapy was completed in 86% (25 of 29). Radiation therapy toxicity was grade 2 in 34%, grade 3 in 21%, and grade 4 in 28%. An unacceptably high rate (31%, 9 of 29) of grade 4 nonhematologic toxicity was recorded. With a median follow-up of 18.9 months, at 2 years, the overall survival rate was 47%, and the probability of locoregional failure was 49%.

Malfetano et al.[582] treated 67 patients with carcinoma of the cervix (44 with stage IIB and 23 with stage III disease) with cisplatin (1 mg/kg up to 60 mg weekly) and extended-field radiation therapy, including the para-aortic nodes, and brachytherapy; 75% were alive without evidence of disease with a mean follow-up of 47.5 months.

Chou et al.[583] treated 19 patients with isolated PALN metastasis from cervix cancer, 14 of them with chemoradiation, 4 with chemotherapy, and 1 with irradiation alone. Seven of the 14 patients receiving chemoradiation survived.

Goodman et al.[584] compiled survival statistics on patients with PALN metastasis and found an average 5-year survival rate of approximately 40%.

Toxicity to the small bowel and duodenum is important to consider when treating para-aortic nodes. In a retrospective study of 14 cervical cancer and 39 endometrial cancer patients treated to the para-aortic nodes with extended-field (EF) IMRT, 6.5% developed acute and 6.5% developed late $\geq$ grade 3 GI toxicity. Planning constraints were set as small bowel (contrast-enhanced loops) at ideal 5 cc < 55 Gy and maximum at 30 cc < 55Gy. No patients experience duodenal toxicity.[302] In 105 patients with enlarged para-aortic nodes (PAN), 36% had cervical cancer; the 3-year rate of duodenal toxicity was 11.7%, with fatal events in two patients because of perforation. The recommended $V_{55} < 15$ cc resulted in 7% toxicity, whereas $V_{55} > 15$ cc resulted in 48% toxicity.[589] A retrospective analysis of 103 patients with cervical cancer and PAN metastases, demonstrated factors associated with improved DSS included concurrent chemoradiation ($P = .001$), baseline PET imaging ($P = .01$), and treatment of PANs with IMRT ($P = .02$). The crude rate of grade 3 or higher late treatment-related adverse effects was 17%.[590] Simultaneous integrate boost to 50-54 Gy followed by a sequential boost to 60-65 Gy has been demonstrated, with adherence to small bowel dose constraints.[590a,590b]

CARCINOMA OF THE CERVICAL STUMP

A supracervical hysterectomy, which removes the uterus and leaves the cervix behind, may be performed for benign conditions of the uterus. The use of subtotal hysterectomy has declined, given the persistent risk of cervical cancer arising in the remnant tissue and the difficulty of managing cancer of the cervical stump.

Section III

It is important to divide carcinoma of the cervical stump into true, when the first symptom occurs 3 or more years after subtotal hysterectomy, or coincidental, when the symptoms are noticed before the third postoperative year. This separation is important because the prognosis for true carcinoma of the stump is significantly better than for coincidental lesions, in which carcinoma was probably present when the hysterectomy was performed.[326]

The natural history and patterns of spread of carcinoma of the cervical stump are similar to those of the cervix in the intact uterus. The diagnostic workup, clinical staging, and basic principles of therapy are the same. Treatment also follows similar paradigms. When surgery is indicated for early stage I tumors, it may be more difficult because of the previous surgical procedures and the presence of adhesions in the pelvis. With radiation therapy, external beam treatments are identical, although small bowel may be adherent to the superior portion of the cervix because of scar tissue, and using the prone position, as well as having the patient maintain a full bladder for treatment, may aid in attempting to move the small bowel out of the radiated field. Whole-pelvic radiation is recommended, with the superior border set at the level of the bifurcation of the common iliac nodes as determined by a CT simulation, or at the L4-L5 interspace for those planned with plain film radiographs. A dose of 45 Gy in 1.8-Gy fractions over 5 weeks is the most commonly recommended dose, with concurrent weekly cisplatin at 40 mg/m^2 given for five doses. For brachytherapy, if >2 cm of the endocervical canal remain, it is best to insert a short tandem surrounded by ovoids, a ring, or, if indicated because of vaginal extension or lateral extension, interstitial catheters. For LDR insertions, as many sources as technically feasible should be inserted in the remaining cervical canal. For HDR brachytherapy, the tandem should extend from the cervical os superiorly to the full extent of the canal. When there is no opportunity to insert any sources in the cervical canal, an interstitial implant to bring the tumor dose to approximately 80 to 90 Gy for brachytherapy after completing a standard dose of 45 Gy to the whole pelvis is recommended while monitoring the radiation dose to the organs at risk (OAR). The use of external beam radiation alone is not recommended due to the significant mobility of the cervix because of bladder motion, the low dose tolerance of the surrounding small bowel, and the high dose of radiation necessary for cure in patients with bulky disease. Total dose (external and LDR intracavitary brachytherapy) to the upper vaginal mucosa should not exceed 150 Gy, and tolerance doses to small volumes (D$_{2cc}$) of the bladder (90 to 100 Gy) or rectum and sigmoid (70 to 75 Gy) should be carefully monitored.

The 5-year survival rate for carcinoma of the cervical stump treated with irradiation is similar to that reported for patients with carcinoma of the intact uterus.[591,592] The anatomic sites of failure and the incidence of recurrences are similar to those of patients in whom the uterus is intact. Distant metastases also follow the same distribution. In 253 patients with carcinoma of the cervical stump treated at MD Anderson Cancer Center, median survival was 203, 140, and 32 months for stages I, II, and III, respectively.[593] Kovalic et al.[591] reported on 70 patients with carcinoma of the surgical stump treated with irradiation; 16 also underwent a surgical procedure. The 10-year DFS was 79% for stage IB, 66% for stage IIB, and 39% for stage IIIB disease. The pelvic failure rates were 10%, 9%, and 50%, respectively. Major gastrointestinal complications were noted in 9% of patients and urinary complications in 3.8%. The results are comparable with those seen in patients treated for invasive carcinoma of the cervix with an intact uterus.

Hannoun-Levi et al.[594] published results in 77 patients treated for carcinoma of the cervical stump. Treatment consisted of a combination of EBRT and brachytherapy, and in a few cases, patients underwent surgery or interstitial brachytherapy. Three-year pelvic tumor control was achieved in 59 of 77 patients (76.6%); tumor control probabilities were 77%, 73.7%, and 56% in patients with stage I, II, and III tumors, respectively. Late complications were grade 2 in 5 patients (6.5%); grade 3 in 1 patient (1.3%), and grade 4 in 2 patients (2.6%).

Hellstrom et al.[595] published a retrospective study of 145 patients treated for carcinoma of the cervical stump, representing 2.2% of all cervical cancers. Three control cases to each case were matched from the cohort of cases with cervical carcinoma with intact uterus. The dose of irradiation from the intracavitary application given to the stump cancers was lower than for comparable cases with intact uterus. Long-term prognosis for squamous cell carcinoma of the uterine stump was comparable to that of the ordinary cervical carcinomas. Stump adenocarcinomas had a worse prognosis compared with adenocarcinoma of the intact uterus (P < .07) and with squamous cell carcinoma stump (P = .05). The complication rate was higher for stump cancer cases compared with that for cervical cancers with an intact uterus.

Because of the close proximity of the bladder, rectum, and small intestine to the intracavitary sources and to the often higher doses of external beam irradiation given to the whole pelvis, complications are somewhat more frequent than in carcinoma of the cervix with an intact uterus. Care in brachytherapy treatment planning, including the use of 3D-based treatment planning to minimize dose to the normal tissues, should be considered.

SMALL CELL CARCINOMA OF THE CERVIX

Small cell carcinoma of the cervix, like its counterparts in the lung and other anatomic locations, has a high proliferation rate and marked propensity for regional lymph node and distant metastases. Miller et al.[596] demonstrated that all small cell carcinomas of the cervix are aneuploid, compared with only 30% of large-cell nonkeratinizing squamous carcinomas. The incidence of lymphatic vascular space invasion is 80% to 90%, and that of lymph node metastases has been reported to be 40% to 67%.[597] These patients must be evaluated in conjunction with a medical oncologist; the workup should include bone marrow aspiration biopsy of the iliac crest and other tests to rule out metastatic spread. Furthermore, the basic therapy should include a combination of cytotoxic agents with pelvic EBRT and intracavitary brachytherapy to doses similar to those used in squamous cell carcinoma, although some patients have been treated with radical surgery. If bleeding is present, prompt institution of radiation therapy with concurrent chemotherapy is necessary. Patients have extremely poor outcomes, with the only reported survivors having had triple-modality therapy of small tumors treated by radical hysterectomy, concurrent chemoRT, and adjuvant chemotherapy. Prophylactic cranial irradiation is not indicated because cervix cancer will most commonly spread first to lung and then to brain.

Patients with small cell carcinoma of the cervix are treated with the same irradiation techniques as outlined for other histologic varieties of cervical carcinoma in combination with multiagent chemotherapy, including external beam radiation to 45 Gy, followed by nodal boost if PET-positive nodes are identified, followed by brachytherapy. The most frequently prescribed drugs are cisplatin and etoposide (VP-16) every 3 weeks.[598] Hoskins et al.[599] used a multimodality regimen of four cycles of cisplatin and etoposide with concurrent locoregional RT in 11 women with small cell carcinoma of the cervix. The 3-year overall and failure-free survival rates were 28%. Four patients were alive in first remission; the remaining seven died (two from toxicity, five from cancer). Toxicity of therapy was significant, with 70% experiencing severe neutropenia; 40% were admitted to the hospital for emesis control.

Twelve patients with small cell carcinoma of the cervix were treated with radical hysterectomy (five received postoperative RT for lymph node metastases and two for close margins). With a mean follow-up of 73 months, the DFS rate was 36.4%, compared with 71.6% for patients with non–small cell carcinoma.[597] Four of five patients who received postoperative irradiation died with pelvic recurrence, and three also had disseminated metastases. However, only those with small lesions or those who received adjuvant irradiation were cured.

Delaloge et al.[600] reported only 2 of 10 patients with neuroendocrine small cell carcinoma of the cervix surviving at 13 and 53 months after treatment, which included surgery, irradiation, and cisplatin/etoposide combination chemotherapy.

Boruta et al.[601] reviewed results in 11 of their and 23 other patients with early-stage[601] neuroendocrine cervical carcinoma identified by a Medline search. Lymphovascular space invasion was present in 21 of 27 patients (78%) (7 unknown), and 15 of 29 (52%) had lymph node metastases. Fifteen patients were treated with cisplatin/etoposide (PE), 7 with vincristine/doxorubicin/cyclophosphamide (VAC), 2 with alternating cycles of VAC and PE, and 10 with other chemotherapy regimens. Twenty women were treated with radiation therapy. The presence of lymph node metastases was a poor prognostic factor (*P* < .001). PE and VAC chemotherapy were associated with increased survival (*P* < .01).

ADENOCARCINOMA OF THE CERVIX

Squamous cell carcinoma accounts for 80% of cervical cancers, adenocarcinoma for 15%, and adenosquamous carcinoma for 3% to 5%. SEER data from 1972 to 2002 suggest that the incidence of cervical adenocarcinoma is rising, but based on SEER data, cause-specific mortality is not significantly different than that for SCC.[602] Adenocarcinoma has been linked to HPV-18, which has a higher rate of nodal and distant metastases than HPV-16.[183] Despite a slower regression after irradiation, reflecting cellular kinetics and slow growth, no difference in tumor control or survival has been observed in adenocarcinomas compared with squamous cell carcinomas[603,604] although prognosis is related to clinical stage, volume of disease, and dose of irradiation.[605] Because of the predilection for endocervical involvement in adenocarcinoma, a combination of irradiation and conservative hysterectomy has been advocated by some authors[606] although results are comparable with those obtained with irradiation alone.[603] Given a lower toxicity profile with chemoRT, this is preferable to a planned course of RT alone followed by hysterectomy upfront. Patients who have residual disease after chemoRT may be candidates for adjuvant hysterectomy.

Grigsby et al.[603] found no difference in 5-year DFS in patients with adenocarcinoma of the cervix (AC) compared with SCC treated with RT alone or combined with surgery. In contrast, Eifel et al.[607] reported that overall 5-year survival rates for patients with SCC and AC were 81% and 72%, respectively (*P* < .01). Patients with AC had a maximum cervical diameter of <4 cm more often than did those with SCC (53% vs. 47%). For 903 patients with tumors of ≥4 cm, 73% of those with SCC survived ≥5 years, compared with only 59% of those with AC (*P* < .01). Although there was no significant difference in the rate of pelvic disease recurrence for patients with AC or SCC tumors of ≥4 cm (17% vs. 13%; *P* = .16), the rate of distant metastases was greater for patients with AC (37% vs. 21%; *P* < .01). For patients with tumors of ≥4 cm, prognosis was strongly correlated with tumor size (*P* < .01) and lymphangiogram findings (*P* < .01) but not with age (*P* = .58) or tumor morphology (exophytic vs. endocervical; *P* = .33); a trend

toward better survival in 165 patients who underwent adjuvant hysterectomy (78% vs. 71%) was not significant (*P* = .09). Multivariate analysis confirmed a highly significant independent association between histology and survival; patients with tumors ≥4 cm in diameter that were AC had an estimated risk of death 1.9 times that of patients with SCC (*P* < .01).

Nakano et al.[608] studied 58 patients with adenocarcinoma of the cervix treated with LDR or HDR brachytherapy and external pelvic irradiation. The 10-year survival rates for stages I, II, III, and IV were 85.7%, 60%, 27.6%, and 9.1%, respectively. The local tumor control rate with HDR treatment was 45.5%, significantly lower than with LDR (85.7%) or mixed–dose rate treatments (72.7%). Kilgore et al.,[604] in a study of 162 patients with adenocarcinoma compared with matched patients with squamous cell carcinoma, found that clinical stage and lesion size were the most important prognostic factors. In patients with stage I tumors, no significant difference in survival was found when they were treated with radical surgery, irradiation alone, or irradiation combined with hysterectomy. In contrast, Kjorstad et al.[609] reported a worse 5-year survival rate in 102 patients with adenocarcinoma (51%) compared with that of 1,900 patients with squamous cell or other differentiated carcinomas (68%).

A Cochrane database review[610] found only one randomized trial, the Landoni study, in which a small subgroup analysis that was not powered to detect a difference showed an apparent improvement with surgery, although the majority of patients required adjuvant RT, rather than chemoradiation, which increases the rates of toxicity. Adenocarcinoma predicts worse OS on multivariate analysis (HR = 2.68, 95% CI = 1.9 to 3.8). Primary chemoradiation is considered the standard regimen for patients with locally advanced cervical adenocarcinoma.

Huang et al.[611] reported on 318 stage IB to IIB postoperative cervical cancer patients, 202 (63.5%) with SCC and 116 (36.5%) with AC/atypical squamous cells (ASC), treated by radical hysterectomy and adjuvant RT/concurrent chemoRT (CCRT). The 5-year relapse-free survival rates for SCC and AC/ASC patients were 83.4% and 66.5%, respectively (*P* < .001). Distant metastasis was the major failure pattern in both groups. After multivariate analysis, prognostic factors for local recurrence included younger age, parametrial invasion, AC/ASC histology, and positive resection margin; for distant recurrence, they included parametrial invasion, lymph node metastasis, and AC/ASC histology. Compared with SCC patients, those with AC/ASC had higher local relapse rates for the intermediate-risk group but a higher distant metastasis rate for the high-risk group. Postoperative CCRT tended to improve survival for intermediate-risk but not for high-risk AC/ASC patients.

A SEER analysis showed that patients with adenocarcinoma had an increased risk of dying compared to squamous cell carcinoma patients.[196] A review of GOG prospective trial patients showed that there was no difference between adenocarcinoma and squamous cell carcinoma if patients received chemoradiation.[197]

TREATMENT OF ELDERLY PATIENTS

Oguchi et al.[612] reported on 23 patients 90 years of age or older treated for cervix carcinoma. Definitive radiation therapy was completed in 13 of the patients, and local tumor control at 6 months was attained in 9 patients. Palliative RT was completed in 7 of 11, and palliation was observed in 9 patients (81%). Seven patients were alive for 15 to 67 months. Fourteen patients died because of intercurrent disease or senility associated with active cancer and 2 because of senility without evidence of cancer. The 2-year overall and relapse-free survival rates were 30% and 21%, respectively.

CARCINOMA OF THE CERVIX AND PREGNANCY

The concurrent presence of carcinoma *in situ* or invasive carcinoma of the uterine cervix and pregnancy, although rare, poses a therapeutic dilemma to gynecologic and radiation oncologists. Reported incidence is approximately 1 to 10 per 10,000 pregnancies.[613] In the United States, the incidence has decreased. Norstrom et al.,[614] in Sweden, found that cervical cancer was diagnosed in 33 women in association with pregnancy (incidence, 11.1 cases per 100,000 deliveries and 7.5 per 100,000 pregnancies). Abnormal bleeding was the symptom that led to diagnosis in 54.5% of the women; 45.5% were asymptomatic but had an abnormal cervicovaginal cytologic test result (39.4%) or abnormal vaginal examination (6.1%) in association with pregnancy. During the follow-up, 1 of 12 women with cervix cancer in the first trimester, 4 of 12 in the third trimester, and 2 of 9 postpartum died of the disease. Primary surgery was used more frequently than radiation therapy.

For carcinoma *in situ*, if the pregnancy is allowed to reach full term, confirmation of the diagnosis by colposcopy and conservative management with monthly Pap smears constitutes the best approach. Conization has frequently been performed. Punch biopsies can be obtained, but the diagnostic accuracy is less reliable. As many as 50% of the patients have residual carcinoma *in situ* after delivery.

In patients with invasive carcinoma, the lesion is usually clinically apparent. Multiple punch biopsies are adequate to confirm the diagnosis. Management is individualized based on tumor size and stage, patient age, and desires of the patient (or couple) regarding the pregnancy. The majority of patients with cervical cancer diagnosed during pregnancy (~75%) have stage I tumors.[613,615,616]

Women with tumors diagnosed early in pregnancy are often recommended to abort the fetus. Because there is a greater need to institute therapy as soon as possible, the accepted method of treatment in patients in the first 6 months of pregnancy is to carry out definitive surgery or radiation therapy, as indicated by the stage of the disease, with resultant loss of the fetus. An abortifacient may be administered before initiating radiation to ensure fetal demise and delivery of the placenta prior to initiation of treatment. The whole pelvis is irradiated (40 to 45 Gy in 4 to 5 weeks). However, in one series of 45 patients, 27% did not abort spontaneously and surgical evacuation was required[617]; misoprostol may be administered as an alternative to surgical evacuation after failed spontaneous abortion.[618] After this dose of radiation, careful evacuation of the uterus and LDR (or equivalent-dose HDR) brachytherapy may be performed under general anesthesia. If a radical hysterectomy is performed and positive pelvic lymph nodes are found, the usual postoperative irradiation, including external beam with or without intracavitary insertion, should be carried out.

If the woman refuses abortion, serial MRI scans at 2- to 3-month intervals to ensure no growth or spread to lymph nodes is recommended. Neoadjuvant chemotherapy may be considered in selected patients.[619] Sorosky et al. reported on eight pregnant women with stage I carcinoma of the cervix who had declined immediate therapy and followed until the late third trimester; a cesarean section–radical hysterectomy was performed, with delay in therapy ranging from 3 to 40 weeks during the pregnancies. There was no clinical progression of the disease with follow-up of 33 months.

When patients are diagnosed in midpregnancy (second trimester), consideration to keeping the pregnancy and treating with chemotherapy is given. A French series reported five cases between 2002 and 2009.[620] Three patients received neoadjuvant chemotherapy; one patient died of cancer. A Chinese report described treatment of two patients with neoadjuvant paclitaxel and cisplatin as feasible.[621]

Occasionally in late pregnancy (final trimester), if tumors are small and an MRI confirms no lymph node involvement, definitive therapy is postponed until after imminent delivery. In a review of the literature, intentional treatment delay was associated with a recurrence rate of 4%.[392] Greer et al.[325] noted that in 600 infants without congenital abnormalities, when stage IB cervical carcinoma was diagnosed during pregnancy and fetal survival was chosen, the neonatal mortality rate decreased from 30% when the fetus was delivered at 26 to 27 weeks to 2.7% when the fetus was allowed to mature to 34 to 35 weeks. In the third trimester of pregnancy, some gynecologic oncologists prefer a postpartum cesarean section, combined with a radical hysterectomy and lymphadenectomy followed by radiation for high-risk features when present. However, some authors report that vaginal delivery has no detrimental effect on the prognosis.[622]

Patients who require high doses of pelvic irradiation should be counseled regarding the permanent loss of reproductive capability, not only because of ovarian ablation (which happens with doses of 8 Gy or higher) but also as a consequence of radiation effects in the uterus.[623,624]

Survival is the same regardless of the trimester of the pregnancy in which definitive treatment is instituted. Creasman et al.[622] reported on 48 patients treated by irradiation, 45 by irradiation followed by surgery, and 5 with radical hysterectomy alone. The survival was comparable with that of nonpregnant patients for similar stages. The survival rate for patients with stage I disease was comparable whether vaginal delivery was allowed or a cesarean section was performed (~85% in stage I and 50% to 64% in stage II). In addition, the percentage of infants surviving (>80%) was the same in both groups.

Sood et al.[624] performed a retrospective analysis of 26 women with cervical carcinoma diagnosed during pregnancy and treated primarily with radiation therapy (mean dose, 46.7 Gy) and LDR intracavitary radiation (mean dose, 56.5 Gy to point A). These cases were matched with 26 nonpregnant control patients based on age, histology, stage, treatment, and year of treatment. There were no statistically significant differences in recurrence rates or survival between the pregnant group and the control patients. Short-term toxicity was comparable in pregnant and nonpregnant patients. Long-term complication rates were 12% in pregnant patients and 27% in control patients, but this difference was not statistically significant. Most complications were likely related to radiation techniques (particularly the predominance of ^{60}Co).

Sood et al.[625] compared the prognosis of 56 women who had cervical cancer diagnosed during pregnancy and 27 who were diagnosed within 6 months after delivery. Control patients (cervical cancer diagnosed at least 5 years since last delivery) were matched one to one with cases based on age, histology, stage, treatment, and time of treatment. Among the postpartum women, 11 were treated with radical hysterectomies and 14 with radiation therapy, and 2 with stage IA1 disease were treated with vaginal hysterectomies. One of seven patients who had cesarean sections had a local and distant recurrence. In contrast, 10 of 17 (59%) patients who delivered vaginally had recurrences ($P = .04$). In multivariate analysis, vaginal delivery was the most significant predictor of recurrence, followed by high tumor stage. Survival for patients diagnosed in the postpartum period was significantly worse than for control patients and for those diagnosed during pregnancy. The authors concluded that pregnant women with cervical cancer should be delivered by cesarean section.

Jones et al.[626] published a survey by the American College of Surgeons that evaluated management of invasive cervical carcinoma in 161 pregnant patients; 86 were treated with surgery alone, 30 with radiation therapy alone, and 45 with a combination of the 2 modalities. Approximately one-third of patients were diagnosed in each trimester. The 5-year survival was 94.6% for patients diagnosed in the first trimester, 76.9% for the second, and 68.9% for the third. The prognosis of patients with invasive carcinoma of the cervix associated with pregnancy was similar to that of nonpregnant patients. There was no significant difference in 5-year survival between the patients delivered by cesarean section and by normal vaginal delivery.

Senekjian et al.[627] reported no difference in survival or patterns of failure in 24 women who were pregnant at the time of diagnosis of clear cell adenocarcinoma of the cervix and vagina compared with 408 who had never been pregnant. The 5- and 10-year actuarial survival rates were 86% and 68% for the pregnant patients and 87% and 79% for the patients who had not been pregnant, respectively.

The practice popularized 30 years ago of administering a "restraining dose of radium" and deferring definitive radiation therapy until delivery is carried out should be strongly rejected. Strauss[628] reported 2 of 11 infants being born with microcephaly in addition to other complications such as alopecia, facial deformity, eye damage, and chromosomal abnormalities after this procedure.

BRACHYTHERAPY

After the discovery of radium in 1898 by the Curies, publications followed describing use of the first glass radium capsule in 1904 and a metal brachytherapy applicator for cervical cancer in 1905.[629] The incorporation of brachytherapy after external beam treatment arose from the recognition that tumor control probability correlated with radiation dose and cancer volume.[630] Evidence confirms that brachytherapy as used for dose escalation after external beam treatment for cervical cancer significantly improves survival.[558,631-634] Therefore, brachytherapy is a standard part of the treatment of locally advanced (stages IB2 to IVA) cervical cancer after external beam radiation; brachytherapy alone may be used as primary treatment for selected cases with early-stage (stages IA to IB1) cervical cancer.[635] The increasing complexity of brachytherapy administration, including the use of complex imaging, mandates implementation of careful quality assurance measures and a culture of open communication to ensure safe practices in the clinic.[635]

Dose Rate

The ICRU in its Report 38[636] defines brachytherapy dose rate as follows: LDR, 0.4 to 2 Gy/hour; medium dose rate (MDR) or PDR, 2 to 12 Gy/hour; and HDR, >12 Gy/hour. For LDR, the most commonly used isotope is ^{144}Cs, and for PDR and HDR, it is ^{206}Ir. The use of HDR has significantly increased in the United States, from 13% in the 1996–1999 Quality Research in Radiation Oncology (formerly known as the Patterns of Care) survey to 62% in the 2007–2009 survey.[400,637] In other US, European, and Japanese surveys of gynecologic brachytherapy practitioners, approximately 85% state that they use HDR brachytherapy,[638-640] whereas in Canada, the reported use is 68% HDR, 10% PDR, and 23% LDR.[641] The dose delivered per fraction for HDR and proportion of dose delivered with external beam versus brachytherapy vary substantially in different centers around the world.[639]

Most institutions in the United States have either LDR or HDR brachytherapy available. Larger centers may have LDR, PDR, and/or HDR. Overall, outcomes are similar regardless of dose rate, with the caveat that for HDR, 3D imaging should be incorporated to ensure coverage of the tumor, particularly for large-volume disease.[642] Several studies demonstrate worse

survival for stage IIIB cervical cancer treated with HDR because of initiating the treatment early in the course of external beam therapy[643] when the tumor mass was >4 cm and therefore a prescription to point A did not cover the tumor volume or by not using 3D planning to cover large residual disease.[644]

Biology of High–Dose Rate Brachytherapy for Cervical Carcinoma: Equivalent Dose in 2 Gy and Biologically Effective Dose

To achieve tumor control using HDR equivalent to that with LDR brachytherapy, attention to the dose/fractionation schedule and to normal tissue doses is mandatory.[645-647] The linear-quadratic (LQ) model provides calculation estimates of biologically equivalent dose taking into account dose rate, dose per fraction, and OTT.[648,649] For comparison of LDR to HDR, the LQ model doses are normalized to an equivalent dose in 2 Gy (EQD2).[650,651] The α/β ratio is a critical component of the LQ model.[651] For cervix cancer, an α/β ratio of 10 Gy is used for tumor and an α/β of 3 Gy is used for normal tissues,[652] which may have inherent inaccuracies in generalizability[653] although an α/β ratio of 3 Gy for the rectum has been correlated with late rectal complications.[654-656]

Spreadsheets to assist with HDR EQD2 dose conversions are available from the American Brachytherapy Society (www.americanbrachytherapy.org/guidelines). The values derived are not actual doses but biologically effective ones that take into consideration dose rate and effect of fraction size.[657]

Although use of a detailed EQD2 conversion is preferred, an approximation of these values was proposed by Orton et al.[647] with an LDR-to-HDR reduction factor of 0.54 to 0.6 (Table 73.14) and by Patel et al.[644] with a similar correction factor of 0.58. These conversion factors are valid when three to five HDR fractions are used, but with a higher number of fractions (six to eight), the conversion factor is closer to 0.75. Therefore, use of the EQD2 worksheet is recommended for consistency.

The importance of adopting biologically based equivalent doses when switching from LDR to HDR brachytherapy is exemplified in a report by Newman[658] on 115 patients treated with external irradiation (40 to 50 Gy) and manual afterloading cesium sources delivering 60 Gy to point A with a dose rate of 0.75 Gy/hour, or a Selectron device with 40-mCi sources, which delivered from 0.75 to 1 Gy/hour to point A. Because of the increased dose rate, the total intracavitary dose was reduced by 20%. Grade 3 genitourinary and gastrointestinal complications were observed in 3 of 87 patients (3.4%) treated with LDR, in contrast to 30 of 132 patients (22.7%) treated with the Selectron HDR sources. No significant differences in local tumor control and survival were found.

TABLE 73.14 MEAN VALUES OF THE NUMBER OF FRACTIONS, DOSE/FRACTION TO POINT A (FOR HIGH DOSE RATE) AND TREATMENT TIME, DOSE RATE FOR LOW DOSE RATE (WITH STANDARD ERRORS), AND THE RATIO OF TOTAL DOSES

Stage	HDR		LDR		Ratio of Total Doses (HDR/LDR)
	Fractions	Dose Per Fraction (Gy)	Treatment Time (Hour)	Dose Rate (Gy/Hour)	
I	5.3 ± 0.40	7.6 ± 0.40	75.4 ± 7.3	0.87 ± 0.14	0.60 ± 0.13
II	4.7 ± 0.30	7.4 ± 0.30	80.2 ± 7.0	0.80 ± 0.11	0.54 ± 0.10
III	4.6 ± 0.40	7.4 ± 0.40	77.3 ± 8.9	0.87 ± 0.14	0.50 ± 0.11
IV	4.7 ± 0.70	7.5 ± 0.60	79.6 ± 18.5	0.89 ± 0.27	0.50 ± 0.21
All	4.82 ± 0.21	7.45 ± 0.20	78.1 ± 4.4	0.85 ± 0.07	0.54 ± 0.06

HDR, high dose rate; LDR, low dose rate.
Reprinted from Orton CG, Seyedsadr M, Somany A. Comparison of high and low-dose rate remote afterloading for cervix cancer and the importance of fractionation. *Int J Radiat Oncol Biol Phys* 1991;21(6):1425–1434. Copyright © 1991 Elsevier. With permission.

Figure 73.20 illustrates the late normal-tissue effect, which is proportional to log cell kill, and the relationship to the number of HDR treatment fractions.[659] Each solid curve is calculated assuming the same log cell kill. Late damage rises sharply as the number of HDR fractions is decreased. When these curves are above the dashed lines that represent the maximum late effect of 70 Gy of LDR brachytherapy given at 0.5 Gy/hour, the risk of late complications increases. Displacing the bladder and rectum away from the HDR sources for the short duration of therapy may offset the radiobiologic disadvantage of using a few brachytherapy fractions.[647]

Brachytherapy Process: Preparation and Timing

Standard procedures for pretreatment evaluation, imaging, anesthesia use, and treatment duration should follow accepted general principles in the guidelines published by the American Brachytherapy Society in 2012.[635,660,661] Planning the course of brachytherapy should begin at the time of initial presentation. An examination at diagnosis assessing disease extension and tumor size should be recorded. Periodic examinations during external beam treatment should be performed to monitor response. For patients receiving concurrent chemoradiation, rapid shrinkage should be expected because treatment may regress the tumor to 70% to 80% of the pretherapeutic volume. Therefore, a clinical gynecologic examination at the time of brachytherapy is also important.[662,663] Inserting radiopaque marker seeds ("fiducials") at the time of diagnosis that mark the inferior, lateral, and superior extension of a vaginal tumor may aid in identifying regions requiring dose escalation with brachytherapy even after complete regression during external beam treatment.

Treatment schedules integrating external beam irradiation and brachytherapy were initially designed with regard to the disease stage and volume.[664] For LDR, insertion of the applicator may be done after all external beam finishes, with the caveat that one or two insertions may be required, approximately 1 week apart. All treatments, including external beam treatment and brachytherapy, should finish 8 weeks from the initiation of radiation.[207]

The optimal time–dose–fractionation scheme and the technique for remote control afterloading intracavitary brachytherapy for cervical cancer have yet to be established through systematic clinical trials. For HDR or PDR brachytherapy, the applicator insertion and treatment may commence after external beam treatment finishes, to ensure optimal geometry with normal tissues far from the applicator. Alternatively, the physician may choose to insert the applicator for treatment as early as during the second week of external radiation if the tumor is small enough, to minimize total treatment time. However, brachytherapy and external beam treatments are not given on the same day.

Applicator Selection

The tandem and ovoid applicator provides radiation dose covering the cervix, uterus, inner parametria, and approximately 1 to 2 cm of the upper vagina. The tandem and ring applicator has a slightly narrower dose distribution, but with HDR, the dose distribution may be optimized and mimics that obtained with the tandem and ovoid applicator. For patients with a very narrow vagina because of stricturing, a tandem and cylinder applicator may be the only option available. However, this applicator provides insufficient dosing to the parametrial tissue and should be used with caution. For patients with large tumors with residual bulky disease after external beam radiation or those with vaginal extension, fistulae, or pelvic sidewall invasion, a combination of tandem/ring or ovoid with interstitial applicator or tandem/interstitial applicator alone may be inserted.

Applicator Insertion

General guidelines from the American Brachytherapy Society should be followed.[635] The patient receives appropriate anesthesia for pain management. In the lithotomy position, the perineum is sterilely prepped and draped. The Foley catheter is inserted into the bladder. The catheter is clamped and the

FIGURE 73.20. Relationship between number of high–dose rate (HDR) fractions and late normal tissue effects. *Solid lines* show the increase in normal-tissue late effects as the number of HDR fractions used to treat cervical cancer decreases. *Dotted lines* indicate the maximum level of late damage calculated for conventional low–dose rate brachytherapy of 70 Gy at 0.5 Gy/hour for 140 hours and an arbitrary level 5% above this. The intersection of the *solid lines* with the *dotted lines* indicates the number of HDR fractions needed to give equal late normal-tissue effects. In this model, the dose to late-responding tissues should be kept at 83% of the tumor dose when treating with four to six HDR fractions. (Modified from Fowler JF. The radiobiology of brachytherapy. In: Martinez AA, Orton CG, Mould RF, eds. *Brachytherapy HDR and LDR*. Leersum, Netherlands: Nucletron International BV, 1990:121–137; with permission.)

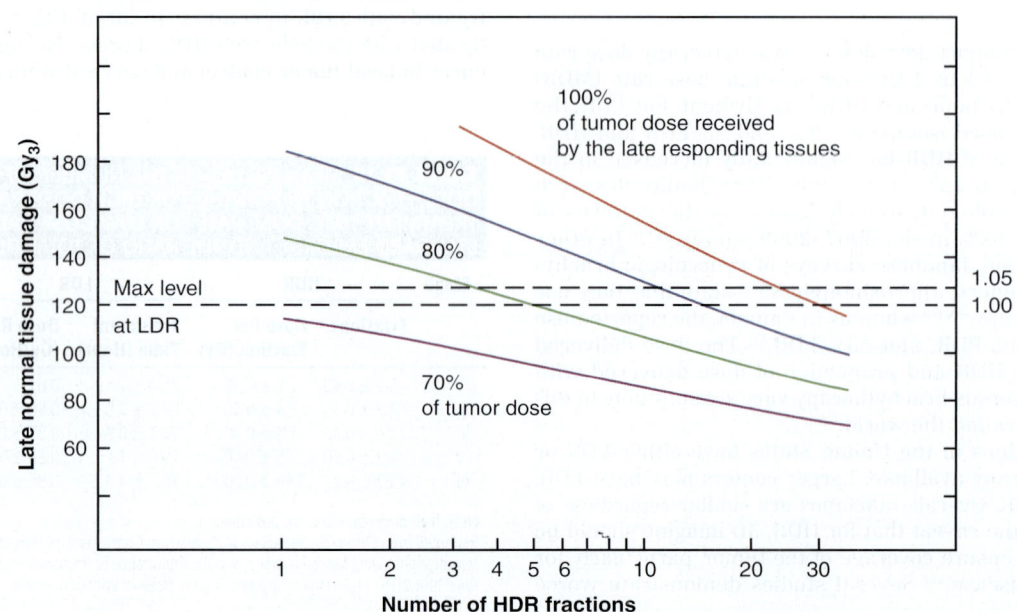

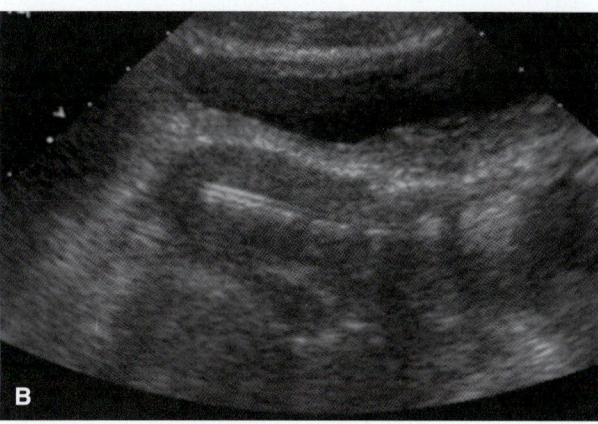

FIGURE 73.21. Ultrasound used during intrauterine tandem insertion can ensure proper placement into the intrauterine canal and shorten overall procedure time. **A:** Ultrasound depicts that the tandem is placed in the posterior myometrium. **B:** Ultrasound directs the tandem into the intrauterine canal.

bladder filled with 150 to 200 cc of saline if US is used. US with a transabdominal probe can significantly speed up the insertion process and assist with accurate placement because the uterine canal is often clearly visible after instilling fluid in the bladder (Fig. 73.21). Transabdominal US can measure uterine width and height in patients who do not have large fibroids or tumor volumes that greatly distort uterine configuration.[665] US does not define the target volume as clearly as MRI but may be used to assist with 3D-based planning when CT or MRI is unavailable.[666] Transrectal US may assist with interstitial brachytherapy when other imaging modalities are not available. For interstitial insertions, CT or MRI may be used during the insertion process iteratively using real-time guidance to ensure proper tumor coverage and no inadvertent insertions into the rectum or bladder.[667] After tandem and ovoid or tandem and ring applicator placement, vaginal packing covered with lubricant gel is placed in the vagina to separate the bladder and rectum, which also helps to maintain applicator position.

Applicator Position

An experienced brachytherapist has greater familiarity with applicator insertion and evaluation.[399] Applicator position is a critical determinant of dose specification[637,668] and pelvic control.[78,669] As Fletcher[566] emphasized, conditions for an adequate intracavitary insertion include the following:

1. The geometry of the insertion must prevent underdosing around the cervix.
2. Sufficient dose must be delivered to the paracervical areas.
3. Vaginal mucosal, bladder, and rectal tolerance doses must be respected.

For LDR Fletcher-Suit applicators, Potish et al.[670] used linear least-squares regression to show that although there was a moderately good correlation between the milligram-hours and dose to point A, it was markedly affected by the position of the colpostats and the tandem. A review of plain films of 808 LDR intracavitary applications in 396 cervical cancer patients treated at MD Anderson[671] quantified acceptable implant geometry. The median distance from the tandem to the sacrum was 4 cm, or one-third the distance from the pubis to the sacrum. The distance between the vaginal ovoids and cervical marker seeds was 7 mm, and the median distance between the tandem and the posterior edge of the ovoids was 50% of the ovoid length. In 92% of insertions, vaginal packing was posterior to or within 5 mm of a line that passed through the posterior edge of the ovoids, parallel to the tandem. The median doses to point A and rectal, bladder, and vaginal surface reference points were 87, 68, 70, and 125 Gy, respectively. Analysis of

the LDR and HDR brachytherapy positions for 103 patients enrolled on RTOG trials 0116 and 0128 found that patients with unacceptable symmetry of ovoids to the tandem had a significantly higher risk of LR than patients in the acceptable group (HR = 2.67; 95% CI = 1.11 to 6.45; P = .03).[78] Patients with displacement of ovoids in relation to the cervical os had a significantly increased risk of LR (HR = 2.50; 95% CI = 1.05 to 5.93; P = .04) and a lower DFS rate (HR = 2.28; 95% CI = 1.18 to 4.41; P = .01). Inappropriate placement of packing resulted in a lower DFS rate (HR = 2.06; 95% CI = 1.08Y3.92; P = .03).

Imaging After Insertion

For LDR brachytherapy, active sources may be inserted after the films have been reviewed and the position of the applicators judged to be satisfactory.[78,671] Placing a small amount of contrast into the bladder and rectum before CT or plain film may clarify the location of these structures.

When a CT scan is obtained after applicator insertion, it also verifies proper placement (no perforation) and analyzes cervix and normal-tissue location in relationship to brachytherapy dose distribution.[638] CT provides a reasonable estimate of the location of the uterus and cervix. The CT contours of the cervix overestimate the tumor contours compared to an MRI, although the additional width contoured on a CT may not be of detriment to the patient because cervical cancer tends to spread laterally along the parametrial tissues.[672] CT depicts changes in the OAR related to tumor shrinkage, organ motion, and the location of the brachytherapy applicator in relation to the uterus. However, separating the OAR, such as the sigmoid or the small bowel from portions of the uterus or cervix, may be difficult on CT, given the lack of contrast. OAR dosimetry based on CT is similar to that based on MRI when optimized similarly.[673] CT may not provide sufficient detail of the tumor if selected dose escalation is required, such as in cases with large residual tumors. In the vast majority of cases, however, it should suffice.[674–676] The uterus and cervix cannot be distinguished as separate structures on a CT, whereas they can on an MRI. Therefore, CT-based contouring guidelines recommend delineating the entire cervix and uterus.[672]

In a multicenter study, MR imaging was significantly better than CT for tumor visualization and detection of parametrial involvement.[87] Other advantages of MR include multiplanar capability and excellent soft tissue contrast resolution. The strength of a magnet in an MR scanner is expressed by a unit of measurement referred to as a tesla (T). Higher field strength produces a better overall signal-to-noise ratio and more accurate imaging.

Regardless of whether a plain film radiograph, CT, or MR is obtained after insertion to aid treatment planning, in order to properly visualize the apparatus, radiopaque markers should be inserted to identify source position to aid with dosimetric planning. Identifying the applicator using either a radiopaque marker inserted into it or for interstitial cases undergoing MR, a special 3-T MR sequence may be used to create artifact that allows the tip of the needle to appear as a balloon on the sagittal image and as a cross on the axial images.[677]

Dose Specification

Point A

Several methods for specifying dose in brachytherapy evolved over the 20th century.

Because of the limited availability of 3D imaging worldwide and a 100-year history of plain film radiography, the majority of institutions internationally use point-based dosimetry based on the ICRU 38 nomenclature[636] defining point A rather than prescribing dose to a tumor volume.[638] Other institutions use a system of milligram-hours, whereas others consider the volume of the region of interest. Based on the general principles guidelines for cervical cancer brachytherapy published by the American Brachytherapy Society and the ICRU report, the point A definition was updated in 2012.[635] To determine point A, connect a line through the center of each ovoid or the lateral most dwell position in the ring; extend this line superiorly along the radius of the ovoids (or ring), and then move an additional 2 cm superior along the tandem. From this point, extend out 2 cm on each side laterally on a line perpendicular to the tandem (Fig. 73.22). For tandem and cylinders, begin at the flange or cervical marking seed and move 2 cm superiorly along the tandem and then 2 cm laterally.

Three-dimensional image-based brachytherapy treatment planning precisely defines the tumor and aids with the precision of radiation dose delivery, which may reduce the dose to the normal tissues and reduce toxicity.[678] In the era of increasing use of HDR brachytherapy, proper applicator placement and precise estimation of the location of the normal tissue is critical. When 3D imaging is available, point-based radiographic dosimetry has limited utility for the dose adaptation required for HDR brachytherapy because point A may overestimate or underestimate the tumor dose based on 3D imaging.[679,679] Kim et al.[680] found that dose to point A was significantly lower than the D_{90} for HR-CTV calculated using 3D image-based optimization. With imaging, one may visualize the tumor volume and conform dose to the volume,

which may result in the dose to point A being lower than the prescription 100% isodose line (covering a smaller tumor volume) or a higher-than-prescription dose to point A because of a large tumor volume extending beyond the boundaries of point A. The tumor coverage relies on tumor volume at the time of brachytherapy, with larger tumors requiring greater optimization to be adequately covered by the prescribed isodose line.[679,681,682] The dose to point A should be reported to ensure consistency in terminology between centers.[683]

Accurate delineation of the tumor and OAR is critical for precise treatment planning (Fig. 73.23). Because of the rapid falloff of dose, imprecise contouring can dramatically change dosing to normal-tissue structures. Formal contouring education programs reduce the variability of interobserver contours.[684]

Computed Tomography Imaging for Brachytherapy Contouring

A CT scan can define a CTV with the lateral borders of the cervix and any parametrial extension defined based on suspicious regions seen on the scan. CT-contouring guidelines should be followed.[672] Uterosacral ligaments may be visualized on CT, and if detected, they should be included in the CTV contours. No GTV may be identified on CT. The superior border of the cervix is not defined, but instead, the entire tandem length is planned and the top dwell is optimized off the sigmoid to reduce bowel dose.

Magnetic Resonance Imaging for Brachytherapy Contouring

For MR-based contouring, the Groupe Europeen Curietherapy-European Society for Therapeutic Radiation Oncology (GEC-ESTRO) guidelines[662,663] delineate volumes for MR. The recommended volumes include the GTV, including all T2-bright areas of enhancement; the HR-CTV, which is the entire cervix, any regions of high to intermediate signal intensity in the parametria, uterus, or vagina, and any residual disease detected on clinical examination at the time of brachytherapy; and the intermediate-risk clinical target volume (IR-CTV), which subtracts out the OARs but includes the tumor extension at the time of diagnosis, adding 1 cm to the HR-CTV volume. The IR-CTV defines regions with potential microscopic seeding of tumor cells (Fig. 73.24).[652] Lang et al.,[650] in a multicenter study, confirmed the feasibility of these recommendations, with total doses to point A from both BT and EBRT ranging from 85 to 91 Gy and to CTV from 69 to 73 cGy. Doses to OAR were comparable to those obtained with standard dosimetric methods, although they were more accurately determined with dose–volume histograms (DVHs).

The American Brachytherapy Society conducted a survey on the use of image-based brachytherapy in 2007[638] and updated this in 2014. Of 219 respondents in 2014, 13% obtain an MR after the first fraction of brachytherapy, and 7% with subsequent fractions, whereas 6% use MR for every fraction. The majority (52%) specify dose to a contoured volume rather than to point A.[685]

A panel of gynecologic radiation oncologists generated a 95% consensus volume contouring atlas to delineate the CTV in locally advanced cervical cancer. Patients with parametrial extension benefitted most from MR at the time of brachytherapy, particularly those with an apparent complete response.[686] The atlas is available online at https://www.nrgoncology.org/Scientific-Program/Center-for-Innovation-in-Radiation-Oncology/GYN-Cervical-Brachytherapy.

Dose–Volume Histogram Reporting

With MR-planned brachytherapy, the most common dose–volume parameters reported for target structures of the entire cervix and any residual disease at the time of brachytherapy,

FIGURE 73.22. Definition of point A shown on a tandem and ovoid applicator based on the American Brachytherapy Society 2012 Guidelines for Cervical Cancer.

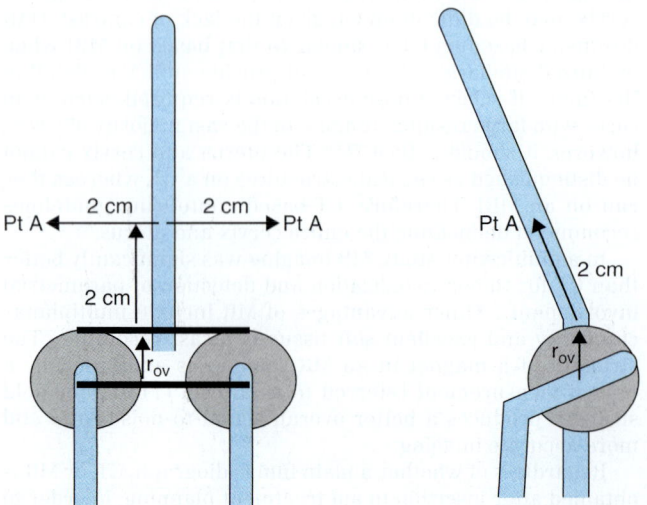

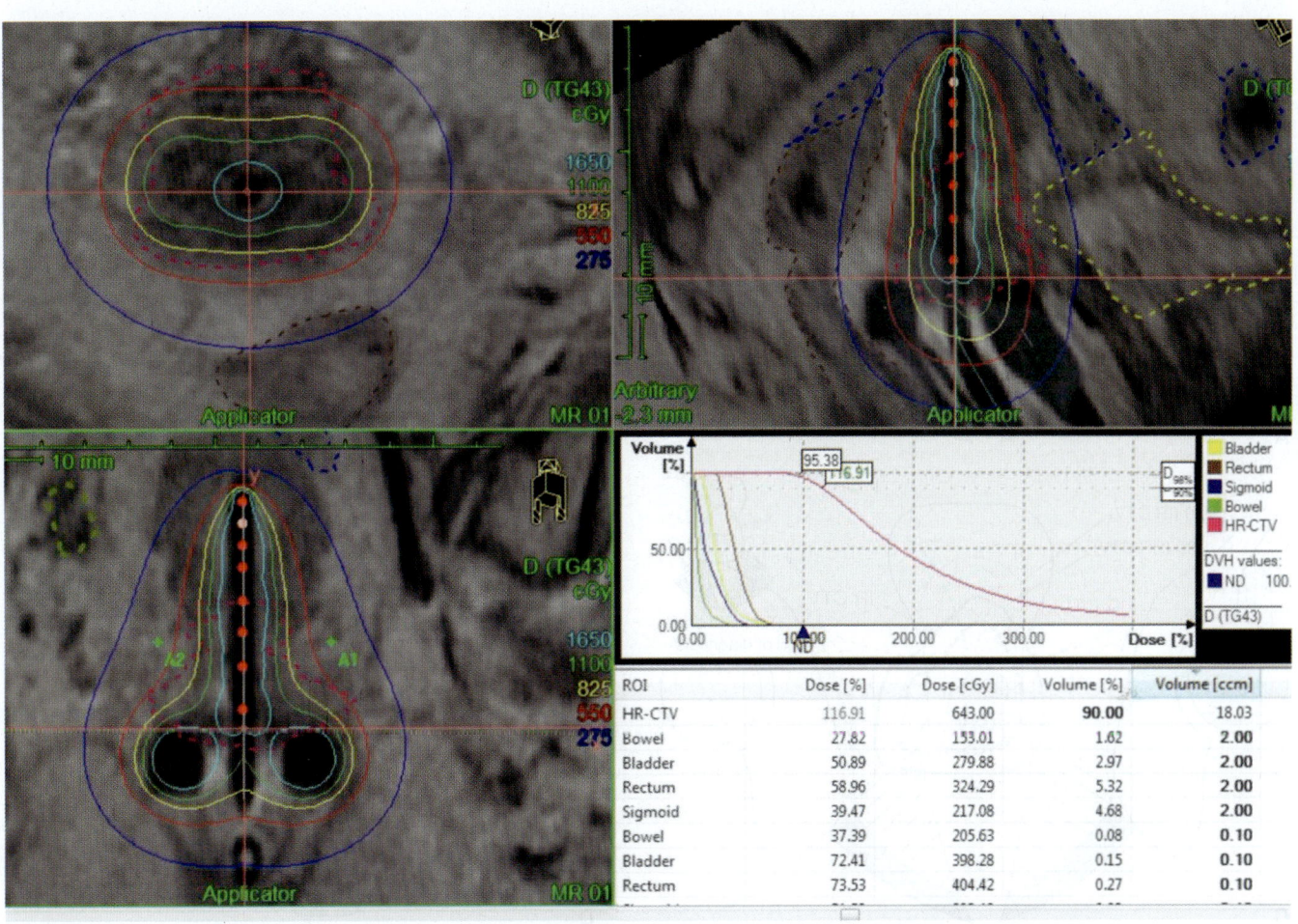

ROI	Dose [%]	Dose [cGy]	Volume [%]	Volume [ccm]
HR-CTV	116.91	643.00	**90.00**	18.03
Bowel	27.82	153.01	1.62	2.00
Bladder	50.89	279.88	2.97	2.00
Rectum	58.96	324.29	5.32	2.00
Sigmoid	39.47	217.08	4.68	2.00
Bowel	37.39	205.63	0.08	0.10
Bladder	72.41	398.28	0.15	0.10
Rectum	73.53	404.42	0.27	0.10

FIGURE 73.23. Tandem and ring implant showing the use of three-dimensional (magnetic resonance or computed tomography) imaging to adequately cover the high-risk clinical target volume (HR-CTV) while minimizing dose to the organs at risk (OAR)—the rectum, sigmoid, and bladder. Dose–volume histograms record the D_{2cc} limits to the OAR. The dose at point A is recorded but varies between patients based on optimization of the HR-CTV and OAR.

the HR-CTV, are D_{90}, defined as the dose received by at least 90% of the target volume, D_{100}, and V_{100}, based on the GEC-ESTRO recommendations.[687,688] The cumulative D_{90} equals the sum of D_{90} values from the individual fractions plus the dose from a homogeneous 3D conformal external beam treatment. D_{100}, the minimum target dose, may be more sensitive to inaccuracies in contouring and dose calculation. V_{100} assesses dose coverage of the whole target volume and is 100% when the entire target is covered by the prescribed dose. V_{150} and V_{200} are often reported in interstitial brachytherapy. One may report these for CT, although the dimensions of the target will differ significantly from the absolute dimensions on MR, and the CT contour of the HR-CTV will include the cervix, residual areas in the parametria or uterosacral ligaments, and part of the uterus because the superior border of the cervix is not visible.[672] CT contours are more accurate if an MRI can be performed immediately before or with the first fraction of brachytherapy.[689] In both CT and MRI, prescribed dose is based on the physician's directive of the dose intended for the target volume, that is, the volume covered by the 100% isodose line, and point A should be recorded. Several institutions have validated the use of these guidelines with HDR, LDR, or PDR brachytherapy.[682,689–693]

With 3D imaging, one may define the surrounding normal tissue structures as the OAR, including the rectum, sigmoid, and bladder. With 2D imaging, the ICRU 38 report requires only reporting point estimates for the rectum and bladder because the sigmoid cannot easily be visualized.[636] However, the ICRU bladder point may underestimate maximum doses to

the OAR, in particular for the bladder[694,695]; it is less likely that rectal doses will be incorrectly estimated. Numerous publications correlate the ICRU point dose and the probability of late complications for bladder and rectum.[696,697] Nevertheless, DVH metrics may provide a more reliable predictor of long-term complications.[698] In a review of 50 patients treated with LDR or HDR brachytherapy who then had a CT for treatment planning, the closest point of the sigmoid was related to sigmoid dose but varied in proximity to the tandem up to 40% between fractions, with a median distance of 1.7 cm. No sigmoid toxicity was noted after a median follow-up of 31 months.

Kapp et al.[699] analyzed 720 [206]Ir HDR applications in 331 patients with gynecologic tumors to evaluate the dose to normal tissues. CT-based dosimetry showed that the maximum doses to bladder and rectum were generally higher than those obtained from orthogonal films, with an average ratio of 1.44 for the bladder neck, 2.42 for the bladder base, and 1.37 for the rectum. The ratio of bladder–base dose to bladder–neck dose was 1.5 for intracervical and 1.46 for intravaginal applications. If conventional methods are used for dosimetry, the authors recommended that doses to the bladder base should be routinely calculated because single-point measurements at the bladder neck seriously underestimate the dose to the bladder. In addition, the rectal dose should be determined at several points over the length of the implant because of the wide range of anatomic variations.

Eich et al.,[700] in 11 applications of HDR brachytherapy for cervical carcinoma, calculated doses to ICRU points on

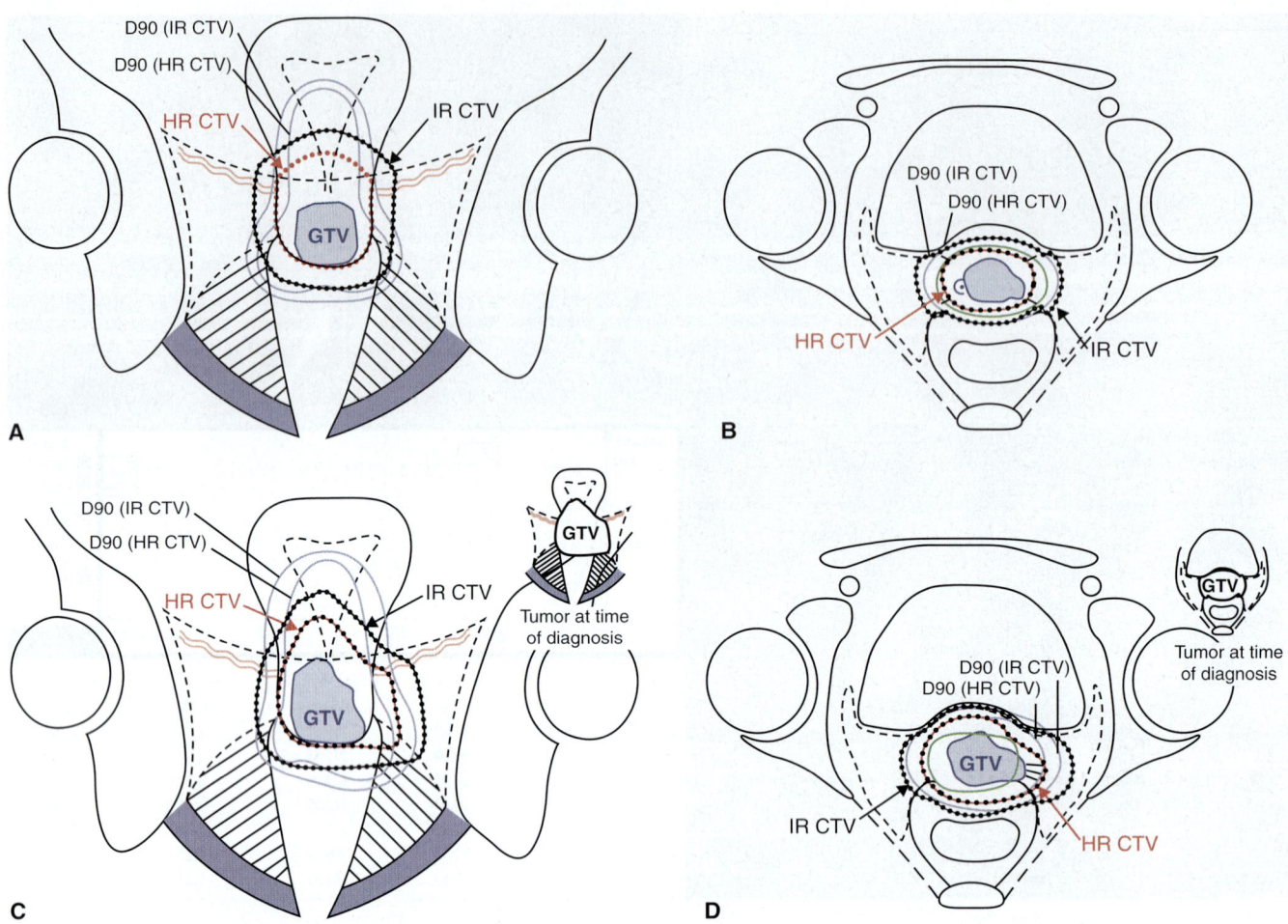

FIGURE 73.24. Diagrammatic representation of gross tumor volume (GTV) and clinical target volume (CTV) for three-dimensional treatment planning in carcinoma of the uterine cervix. Coronal (**A** and **C**) and transverse (**B** and **D**) sections for limited (**A** and **B**) and advanced (**C** and **D**) disease (*gray zones in left parametrium*). (Reprinted from Potter R, Haie-Meder C, Limbergen EV, et al. Recommendations from gynaecological (GYN) GEC ESTRO working group (II): Concepts and terms in 3D image-based treatment planning in cervix brachytherapy-3D dose volume parameters and aspects of 3D image-based anatomy, radiation physics, radiobiology. *Radiother Oncol* 2006;78[1]:67–77. Copyright © 2005 Elsevier Ireland Ltd. With permission.)

orthogonal radiographs, and the doses at rectum reference points were compared with *in vivo* measurements. The *in vivo* measurements were 1.5 Gy below the doses determined for the ICRU rectum reference point (4.05 ± 0.68 vs. 6.11 ± 1.63 Gy). The advantage of *in vivo* dosimetry is the possibility to determine rectal dose during radiation. The advantages of computer-aided planning at ICRU reference points are that calculations are available before radiation and they can be taken into account for treatment planning.

Pelloski et al.[701] compared CT-based volumetric calculations and ICRU reference point radiation doses in 60 patients with cervix cancer treated with LDR brachytherapy. Of 118 insertions performed, 93 were evaluated, and the minimal doses delivered to the 2 or 3 cm of bladder or rectum (DBV2 and DRV2, respectively) were determined on a DVH. They concluded that the ICRU dose was a reasonable surrogate for the DRV2 but not for the DBV2. Furthermore, these calculations may not be applicable to other treatment guidelines or intracavitary applicators.

Patil et al.[702] found significant correlations between ICRU point doses to the bladder and rectum and volumetric doses, particularly the D_{2cc}. However, there was significant variability, and they concluded that 3D imaging is essential to properly assess doses to the OAR.

Both CT- and MR-based OAR dosimetry report similar cumulative DVH parameters, including D_{2cc} and $D_{0.1cc}$. The D_{2cc} is the minimum dose received by the most exposed 2-cm³ volume of the analyzed organ. For CT-based brachytherapy,

contrast placed in the OAR may cause some artifact, resulting in some variation in contouring the wall of the organ. MR-based brachytherapy relies less on contrast because the organ wall may be more clearly visualized. Wachter-Gerstner et al.[703] analyzed the correlation between DVHs for the bladder and rectum and found that D_{2cc} served as a good estimate for doses to the organ wall, whereas D_{5cc} was less reliable as it changes more based on filling status. Rectal wall thickness did not significantly affect D_{2cc}.[704]

Based on CT dosimetry, Koom et al.[705] showed that more severe rectal side effects (endoscopy score >2) occurred in patients with a higher D_{2cc}. Seventy-one patients with FIGO stage IB to IIIB uterine cervical cancers had CT-based HDR intracavitary brachytherapy. The mean values of the DVH parameters and ICRU rectal point ($\alpha/\beta = 3$) were significantly greater in patients with a score of >2 than in those with a score of <2 at 12 months after brachytherapy (ICRU, 71 Gy vs. 66 Gy [*P* = .02]; $D_{0.1cc}$, 93 vs. 85 Gy [*P* = .04]; D_{1cc}, 80 vs. 73 Gy [*P* = .02]; D_{2cc}, 75 vs. 69 Gy [*P* = .02]). The probability of a score of >2 was significantly correlated with the DVH parameters and ICRU rectal point (ICRU, *P* = .03; $D_{0.1cc}$, *P* = .05; D_{1cc}, *P* = .02; D_{2cc}, *P* = .02).

For MR-based dosimetry, Georg et al.[698] tested the predictive value of dose–volume parameters for late effects of the rectum, sigmoid colon, and bladder using the D_{2cc}, D_{1cc}, and $D_{0.1cc}$ of these three OARs for 141 cervical cancer patients treated with tandem and ring HDR brachytherapy after EBRT. The mean D_{2cc} values for bladder, rectum, and sigmoid were 95 ± 22, 65 ±

12, and 62 ± 12 Gy, respectively. This study confirmed that D_{2cc} was a predictor of late toxicity for the rectum and bladder. A rectoscopy study[706] was done in 35 patients in which EQD2 (α/β = 3 Gy) of the $D_{0.1cc}$, D_{1cc}, and D_{2cc} of the rectum was recorded. After a mean follow-up time of 18 months, telangiectasia was found in 26 patients (74%), and 5 had ulceration that corresponded to the $D_{0.1cc}$ of the anterior rectal wall. The D_{2cc} was higher in patients with rectoscopy score of >3 compared to <3 (72 ± 6 vs. 62 ± 7 Gy; P < .001) and in symptomatic versus asymptomatic patients (72 ± 6 vs. 63 ± 8 Gy; P < .001).

Mazeron et al. described late rectal morbidity in 960 patients treated with MR-based brachytherapy in the EMBRACE study. With a median follow-up of 2 years, rectal events peaked at 2 years post treatment. The total crude rate of events was 28%, including 18% proctitis, 16% bleeding, 1% stenosis, and 1% fistula. Rectal dose morbidity was 6% 60 Gy, 8% 65 Gy, 10% 70 Gy, and 13% 75 Gy. The authors conclude that a D_{2cc} < 65 Gy results in a <10% risk of rectal toxicity.[707]

For interstitial brachytherapy, in which a much longer portion of the anterior rectal wall is treated as part of the target volume, D_{2cc} > 62 Gy predicted for late toxicity.[708] The development of mucosal and clinical changes in the rectum seems to follow a clear dose effect and volume effect. For patients receiving interstitial brachytherapy who require treatment to the entire vaginal length, the dose to the rectum should be reduced as much as possible without compromising target coverage.

The dose given to the vagina is also associated with vaginal toxicity,[709] with a threshold of 108 Gy analyzed in one study.[710]

3D Treatment Planning for Pulsed and High Dose Rate Brachytherapy

Treatment planning for PDR and HDR brachytherapy can be accomplished by a variety of techniques. Treatment planning for LDR is covered in a separate chapter. For cervical cancer, customized optimization of source loading for each HDR insertion is recommended (Fig. 73.25), given significant changes in tumor and OAR dosimetry between fractions.[664,711]

FIGURE 73.25. A: Coronal view of a CT-planned tandem and ring applicator with standard HDR loading (to point A). **B:** Tandem and ring treatment plan optimized to maximize tumor coverage and minimize the dose to the organs at risk (OAR) including the rectum (*brown*), sigmoid (*blue*), and bladder (*yellow*). **C:** Sagittal CT of the standard plan at point A. **D:** Sagittal CT image of the optimized plan showing the reduction in OAR dose. **E:** Cervical stump cancer showing an MR-planned tandem and interstitial brachytherapy implant without HDR optimization. **F:** Optimized tandem and interstitial plan cover the posterior border of the cervical stump while minimizing dose to the bladder and rectum.

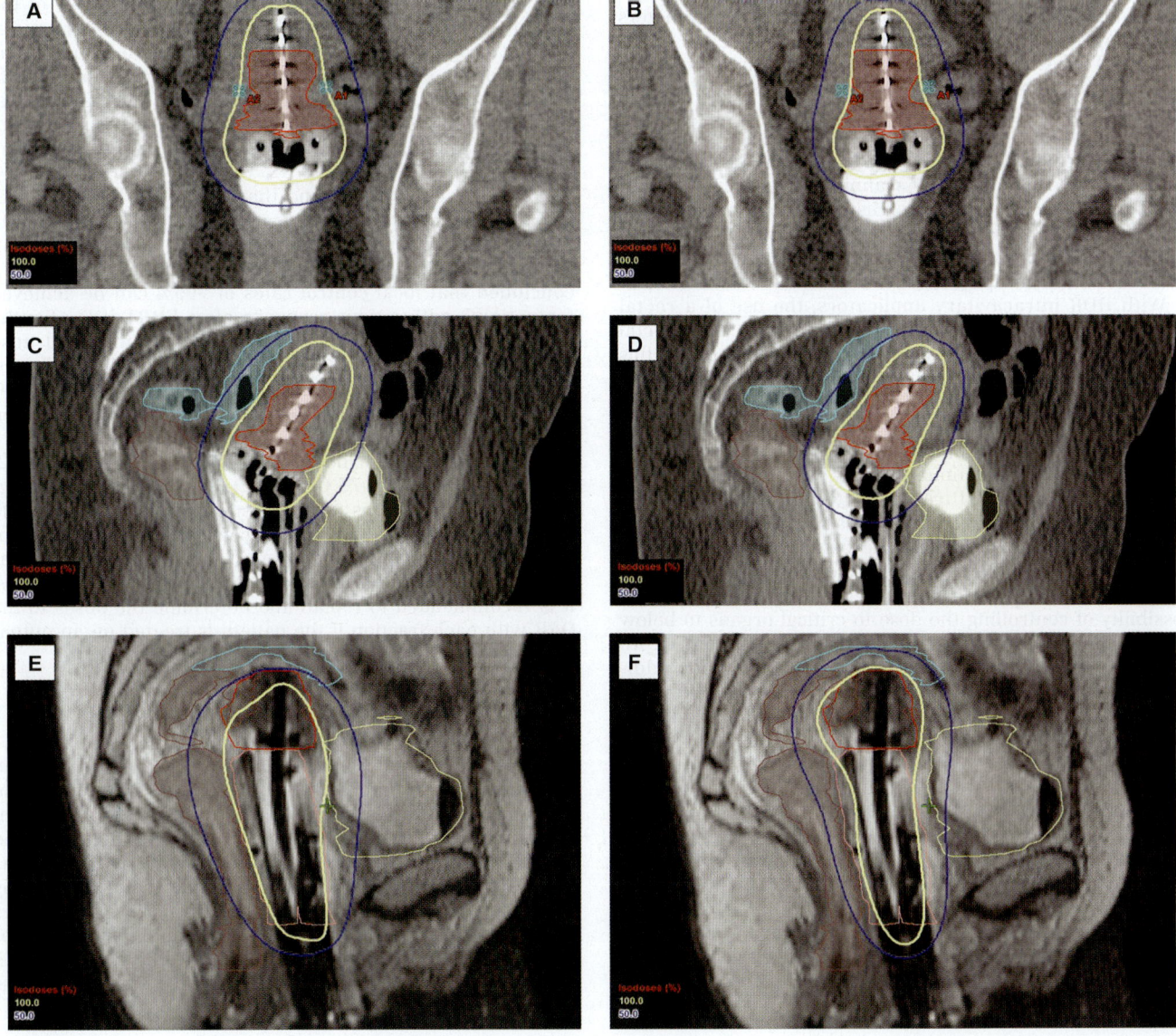

Section III

Himmelmann et al.[712] described individualized computer treatment optimization of source position and the dwell time for each position. Customized planning does increase the time needed for planning and requires experience on the part of the physics and dosimetry staff.[713]

CT-Based Treatment Planning

Fellner et al.[714] compared treatment planning for cervical carcinoma based on CT sections and 3D dose computations or, when these techniques were not available, dose evaluation based on orthogonal radiographs. The CT-based planning provides information on target and organ volumes and DVHs. The radiography-based planning provides dimensions and doses only at selected points. For the study, 28 patients with 35 applications receiving HDR treatment with ^{206}Ir were investigated. For a dose prescription of 7 Gy at point A, 83% (44 cm^3) of the CTV received at least 7 Gy.

Gebara et al.[715] estimated the external, internal, and common iliac dose rates using 3D CT-based dose calculations in tandem and ovoid brachytherapy in 30 patients with carcinoma of the uterine cervix treated with LDR brachytherapy using a CT-compatible Fletcher-Suit-Delclos device. Thirty-six implants were performed, and the authors concluded that the point B dose is similar to the maximum common iliac nodal dose. With HDR brachytherapy, the dose to the pelvic lymph nodes is approximately 25% of the per fraction dose.[374]

Dewitt et al.,[716] in 15 patients with cervical cancer, defined target and OAR for planning of HDR brachytherapy and established guidelines for volume and dose constraint parameters using image-guided inverse treatment planning.

Careful assessment of the quality of brachytherapy and dose distributions is critical. Suyama et al.[717] analyzed the minimal radiation dose to the peripheral area of the cervix in relation to local tumor failure using CT images taken at the time of intracavitary brachytherapy in 80 patients with carcinoma of the cervix. After CT scanning, isodose curves were superimposed on the CT images. Histograms of both the minimum percentage peripheral dose and the dose to the cervical area showed significant correlation in the local tumor control and local failure groups ($P < .001$).

With HDR intracavitary applicators, the use of a rectal retractor has been shown to substantially reduce the rectal dose.[647] Lee et al.,[718] in a study of 15 patients, found that this reduction was significant only in the subgroup who received >70% of the prescription dose ($P < .05$).

Wanderas et al.[719] reviewed data from 19 patients (72 fractions) retrospectively. Standard library plans were compared to individually optimized plans using a Fletcher HDR applicator. For standard treatment planning, the tolerance dose limits were exceeded in the bladder, rectum, and sigmoid in 26%, 4%, and 15% of the plans, respectively. This was observed most often for the smallest target volumes. The individualized planning of the delivered treatment gave the possibility of controlling the dose to critical organs to below certain limits. The dose was still prescribed to point A. An increase in target dose coverage was achieved when additional individual optimization was performed while keeping the dose to the OARs below predefined limits. Relatively low average target coverage was seen, however, especially for the largest volumes.

MR-Based Treatment Planning

Basic principles of MR imaging during brachytherapy have been described.[720] Several institutions have reported the dosimetric advantages of MR-based brachytherapy, with reduction in OAR doses with optimization.[682,691,721–723] Tanderup et al.[721] showed that point A dose was a poor surrogate of HR-CTV dose, and MR-based planning improved target coverage and reduced OAR dose. Starting with a standard plan is important

for consistency because relative uniformity of the dose distribution should be maintained.[724]

A comparison of MR to US was reported by Van Dyk et al.[666] for 71 patients, showing comparability between the two modalities in terms of target volume and rectal point dose. Mahantshetty et al.[725] similarly confirmed the feasibility of US for institutions that do not have easy access to MR or CT. One study hypothesizes that US may be more similar to MR than CT.[726]

Recommended Doses

Stage IA (microinvasive) tumors are treated with intracavitary therapy only. LDR dose is approximately 60 Gy in one insertion or 75 to 80 Gy in two insertions to point A, or with HDR an equivalent dose, with one or two fractions per week. This may be given in approximately 5 Gy per fraction for 10 fractions or other regimens based on normal-tissue exposure.

For stage IB to IVA cervical cancers in the United States, the most common EBRT dose treats the elective pelvic nodes to 45 to 50 Gy given in 1.8 Gy per fraction.[635] Some institutions instead use lower doses of whole-pelvis external irradiation (20 to 40 Gy) in addition to parametrial doses to complete 50 to 60 Gy to the involved parametrial tissues or nodal regions for more advanced stages. Brachytherapy follows, with a goal EQD2 dose of 80 to 90 Gy to point A or to the HR-CTV. For LDR, intracavitary treatment for approximately 4,000 to 5,000 mgh (36 to 50 Gy to point A at 60 cGy/hour) is given, depending on the tumor volume and stage and age of the patient. Fyles et al.[159] identified FIGO stage as the most significant prognostic factor in 965 patients with invasive carcinoma of the cervix, followed by dose of irradiation to point A and overall time of radiation therapy. The 10-year survival rate was 62% in 743 patients receiving doses to point A of 85 Gy or higher, in contrast to 53% for 222 patients receiving lower doses.

For HDR, one study found that a dose to the HR-CTV of >87 Gy resulted in a local recurrence rate of 4% compared to 20% for D$_{90}$ < 87 Gy when the tumor was >5 cm and using an HDR tandem/ring or tandem/ring/interstitial approach. They concluded that local control rates of >95% can be achieved for patients with a poor response after EBRT if D$_{90}$ for the HR-CTV is 87 Gy or higher.[727] The IR-CTV intended dose should be approximately 60 Gy EQD2. In the United States, the most common regimen uses five fractions (5 to 6 Gy per fraction), with two fractions per week, 24 to 48 hours between fractions.

DVH constraints for both PDR and HDR are 90 Gy (EQD2) for bladder and 70 to 75 Gy (EQD2) for both rectum and sigmoid as minimal doses to the most exposed D$_{2cc}$ of the OAR. There are no generally accepted constraints for the 0.1-cm^3 level. Given the rapid regression of the tumor and the dramatic change in the location and size of the normal tissues, it is recommended to replan and determine the doses to the OAR with each fraction if the patient is treated on an outpatient basis.[711]

Dose Fractionation in High Dose Rate Brachytherapy

The relationship between dose and fractionation for HDR and LDR intracavitary irradiation of stage I and II carcinoma of the cervix was examined by Arai et al.[681] The dose rate at point A was 2 to 3 Gy/minute (120 to 180 Gy/hour) for HDR and 0.6 to 0.9 Gy/hour for LDR irradiation. Concurrent EBRT was given to the whole pelvis (23 to 30 Gy), followed by 25 to 30 Gy with central shielding, along with brachytherapy. The authors concluded that the optimal dose fractionation schedules for HDR brachytherapy were 28 ± 3 Gy in 4 to 5 fractions, 34 ± 4 Gy in 8 to 10 fractions, or 40 ± 5 Gy in 12 to 14 fractions at point A. Petereit and Pearcey,[656] based on their preliminary results and published reports in the literature, recommend doses of 45 to 50.5 Gy in a 1.8-Gy per fraction external beam followed by HDR with either 5.5 or 6 Gy per fraction in the era before the standardization of chemoradiation. Since the implementation of concurrent chemoradiation, several institutions in the United States have standardized the use of 5.5 Gy for five fractions, given some concerns about rectal toxicity with 6 Gy per fraction.[728]

Chatani et al.[729] described a study in which 165 patients with carcinoma of the cervix were randomized to an HDR brachytherapy point A dose of 6 Gy (group A) or 7.5 Gy (group B) per fraction, both combined with external irradiation. The 5-year local failure rate was 16% in both groups, and distant failure rates were 23% and 29%, respectively ($P = .2955$). Moderate to severe complications requiring treatment were comparable (six patients, 7%) in the two groups.

Hama et al.[730] compared the effectiveness and safety of once- versus twice-weekly HDR brachytherapy for cervical cancer in 124 patients treated with EBRT (50 Gy); 74 patients (group A) were treated with one HDR brachytherapy insertion weekly (three fractions of 7 Gy each to point A), and 50 patients (group B) were treated twice weekly (six fractions of 4.5 Gy each to point A). Overall survival rates were 65.2% and 65.3%, respectively ($P = .96$). Local recurrence–free survival rates were 69% for group A and 90% for group B ($P < .001$). The rate of grade 2 (moderate) and grade 3 (severe) complications was significantly lower for group B (6%) versus 32% in group A ($P < .001$).

Mayer et al.[731] compared HDR BT in two schedules used to treat 210 patients with cervix cancer—one sequential (SRT), consisting of four fractions of 8 Gy followed by EBRT, and the other continuous (CRT), consisting of five fractions of 6 Gy one session per week integrated with EBRT (four fractions per week). Total dose to point A was 68 to 70 Gy. PFS was 71% with CRT versus 56% with SRT ($P > 0.05$). Late bladder and rectal morbidity were 13% in the CRT group and 25% in the SRT group ($P = .037$), related to the higher dose per fraction (8 Gy).

Nam and Ahn[732] compared, in a randomized study of 46 patients, two schedules of HDR BT (10 fractions of 3 Gy or five fractions of 5 Gy) followed by a small BT boost to residual tumor in combination with EBRT (30.6 Gy to whole pelvis and 14.4 Gy to parametria with midline block). Three-year pelvic tumor control was 90% in both groups, and disease-specific survival was 90.5% and 84.9% ($P = .64$), respectively. Late grade 2 and greater bladder or rectal morbidity was 23.8% and 9.1%, respectively ($P = .24$).

Liu et al.[733] based on the LQ model, developed isoeffect tables to convert traditional LDR doses and number of fractions to point A to HDR brachytherapy; depending on dose rate, different dose values can be calculated for various fractionation schedules. They predicted that, using therapeutic gain ratio, similar results would be obtained with either brachytherapy modality with two to four fractions of LDR and four to seven fractions of HDR.

The optimal time–dose–fractionation scheme for HDR brachytherapy for cervical cancer has yet to be established. In an international survey from the Gynecologic Cancer Intergroup, 28 different fractionation regimens were used by international cooperative group members (Table 73.15); the most common was 6 Gy for five fractions after 45 Gy.[639] The American Brachytherapy Society published recommendations for HDR brachytherapy for carcinoma of the cervix.[660] Each institution should follow a consistent treatment policy, including complete documentation of treatment parameters and correlation with clinical outcome (pelvic tumor control, survival, and complications). The goals are to treat point A to at least a total LDR equivalent

TABLE 73.15 HIGH DOSE RATE BRACHYTHERAPY DOSE AND FRACTIONATION REGIMENS WORLDWIDE

Percentage Respondents (Number)	Dose/Fraction	Number of Fractions	EQD2
Standard Fractionation for Stage IB to IIA Cervical Cancers			
18% (12)	6	5	40
15% (9)	6	4	32
12% (7)	7	3	29.75
8% (5)	5	6	37.5
8% (5)	7	4	39.7
5% (3)	5	5	31.25
5% (3)	5.5	5	35.52
Standard Fractionation for Stage IIB to IVA Cervical Cancers			
23% (14)	6	5	40
10% (7)	7	4	40
10% (7)	7	3	30
8% (5)	6	4	32
7% (4)	5.5	5	35.5
5% (3)	5	6	37.5
5% (3)	7	6	59.5
5% (3)	6	3	24
5% (3)	8	3	36

Gynecologic Cancer Intergroup physicians worldwide who use high–dose rate (HDR) brachytherapy for cervical cancer were queried regarding the specific fractionation regimen that they routinely implement for stage IB to IIA and stage IIB to IVA cervical cancer patients. Results are shown for regimens reported by three or more respondents. The most common external beam dose was 45 Gy in 1.8 Gy per fraction, followed by five fractions of 5 to 6 Gy per fraction. The EQD2 formula was used to convert the HDR dose and number of fractionations and does not include the external beam dose contribution.

Modified from Viswanathan AN, Creutzberg CL, Craighead P, et al. International brachytherapy practice patterns: a survey of the Gynecologic Cancer Intergroup (GCIG). *Int J Radiat Oncol Biol Phys* 2012;82(1):250–255. Copyright © 2012 Elsevier. With permission.

of 80 to 85 Gy for early-stage disease and 85 to 90 Gy for advanced-stage disease. The pelvic sidewall dose recommendations are 50 to 55 Gy for early lesions and 55 to 65 Gy for advanced ones. As with LDR BT, every attempt should be made to keep the bladder and rectal doses to <100 Gy and 75 Gy LDR-equivalent doses, respectively. Interstitial brachytherapy should be considered when the tumor cannot be optimally encompassed by intracavitary brachytherapy. Some suggested dose and fractionation schemes for combining the external beam radiation therapy with HDR brachytherapy for each stage of disease have been presented by the American Brachytherapy Society, although they have not been thoroughly tested. The responsibility for the medical decisions ultimately rests with the treating radiation oncologist. Petereit and Pearcey,[656] in a review of 24 HDR dose fractionation schedules published in the last three decades, found no dose relationship for either tumor control or late morbidity. Viswanathan et al.,[639] for the Gynecologic Cancer Intergroup, found significant international variation in the HDR dose/fractionation regimens reported, but aside from Japan, where the ratio of HDR brachytherapy dose to external beam is higher, there was consistency in converted EQD2 doses administered.

Clinical Outcomes of Brachytherapy

Randomized Studies Comparing HDR to LDR Using Plain X-Ray Dosimetry

Four randomized trials (Table 73.16) and a meta-analysis summarizing the results of these have been published comparing HDR and LDR brachytherapy for carcinoma of the cervix.[737,738] Teshima et al.[734] reported on a prospective, randomized study of 430 patients with carcinoma of the uterine cervix treated with either LDR (171 patients) or HDR (259 patients) brachytherapy combined with external irradiation. Cause-specific and overall survival rates were comparable for each clinical stage

Section III

TABLE 73.16 RANDOMIZED TRIAL RESULTS OF TOXICITY AND OVERALL AND DISEASE-FREE SURVIVAL COMPARING HDR AND LDR

Author (Reference)	Stage	Overall Survival (%)[a]		Disease-Free Survival (%)[a]		Toxicity (%)[b]	
		HDR	LDR	HDR	LDR	HDR	LDR
Patel et al.[644]	Stage I, <3 cm	100	100	85	81	0.4	2.4
	Stage II, <3 cm	82	82	71	66		
	Stage I, >3 cm	87	88	75	70		
	Stage II, >3 cm	74	78	63	60		
	Stage III	71	76	43	50		
Teshima et al.[734]	Stage I	66	89[c]	85	93	7	3
	Stage II	61	73	73	78		
	Stage III	47	45	53	47		
Hareyama et al.[735]	Stage II	89	100	69	87	7.5	16.2
	Stage III	69	70	51	60		
Lertsanguansinchai et al.[736d]	Stage IIB	65	74	65	76	5	4
	Stage IIIB	71	63	74	59		

[a]Five-year results unless otherwise stated.
[b]Grade 3 to 5 rectal and bladder toxicities combined.
[c]Statistically significant difference.
[d]Three-year results.
HDR, high dose rate; LDR, low dose rate.
From Stewart AJ, Viswanathan AN. Current controversies in high-dose-rate versus low-dose-rate brachytherapy for cervical cancer. *Cancer* 2006;107(5):908–915. Copyright © 2006 American Cancer Society. Reprinted by permission of John Wiley & Sons, Inc.

For bladder, rectosigmoid, and small-bowel complications, the RR was 1.33 (95% CI = 0.53 to 3.34), 1.00 (95% CI = 0.52 to 1.91), and 3.37 (95% CI = 1.06 to 10.72), respectively, indicating no significant differences except for increased small-bowel complications with HDR (P = .04). Of note, none of the randomized studies used 3D imaging to optimize away from normal tissues.

The use of 3D imaging to guide brachytherapy treatment planning has allowed optimization of HDR and PDR brachytherapy, thereby reducing the high per fraction doses to the normal tissues that might potentially cause significant side effects. A retrospective comparison of LDR and HDR with pretreatment MRI used for tumor volume determination showed a significant reduction in complications with HDR when image-based planning was implemented.[739] Similarly, the use of 3D imaging optimizes tumor coverage, which is critical with fractionated HDR therapy.

with either modality, except for stage I overall survival. The conversion factor of total intracavitary dose from LDR to HDR was 0.5 to 0.53. With HDR, four fractions usually were delivered, and with LDR, two fractions. The incidence of pelvic failures was comparable in both groups. The incidence of grade 2 and 3 morbidity was somewhat higher in the HDR group (~10%) than in the LDR group (4%; P = .002).

Patel et al.[644] published a randomized trial of 482 patients with invasive squamous cell carcinoma of the cervix. The overall local tumor control rate with LDR brachytherapy was 79.7%, compared with 75.8% with HDR. The 5-year survival rates were 73% with LDR and 78% with HDR in stage I, 62% and 64%, respectively, in stage II, and 50% and 43% in stage III. The only statistically significant difference was the incidence of overall rectal complications, which was 19.9% for LDR, compared with 6.4% for HDR. However, the incidences of more severe grade 3 and 4 complications were not significantly different (2.5% and 0.4%, respectively). Bladder morbidity was similar in both groups.

Hareyama et al.[735] conducted a randomized study in 132 patients with stage II or IIIB cervical carcinoma treated with LDR or HDR BT and identical pelvic EBRT. The conversion factor from LDR to HDR was 0.588. The 5-year DSS with HDR for stages II and IIIB was 69% and 51%, respectively, and with LDR it was 87% and 60%, respectively. Pelvic tumor control for stage II and III was 89% and 73% with HDR and 100% and 70% with LDR, respectively, and grade 3 or greater morbidity was 10% and 13%, respectively (differences were not statistically significant).

Lertsanguansinchai et al.[736] randomized 237 patients with cervical cancer to be treated with LDR (109 patients) or HDR (112 patients) brachytherapy and EBRT. Median follow-up was 40 and 37 months, respectively. Three-year pelvic tumor control was 89% and 86.4%, respectively, and relapse-free survival was 69% in both groups. Grade 3 or 4 morbidity was noted in 2.8% of LDR and 7.1% of HDR patients (P = .23).

A meta-analysis[738] including these four trials reported a pooled RR for HDR versus LDR of 0.95 (95% CI = 0.79 to 1.15), 0.93 (95% CI = 0.84 to 1.04), and 0.79 (95% CI = 0.52 to 1.20) for 3-, 5-, and 10-year overall survival rates and 0.95 (95% CI = 0.84 to 1.07) and 1.02 (CI = 0.88 to 1.19) for 5- and 10-year DSS rates. For local control rates, the RR was 0.95 (95% CI = 0.86 to 1.05) and 0.95 (95% CI = 0.87 to 1.05) at 3 and 5 years, respectively.

tion in complications with HDR when image-based planning was implemented.[739] Similarly, the use of 3D imaging optimizes tumor coverage, which is critical with fractionated HDR therapy.

Prospective Data Using Point A Dosimetry

Haie-Meder et al.,[740] in 204 patients with cervical cancer randomized to receive one of two preoperative LDR brachytherapy procedures (0.4 or 0.8 Gy/hour), noted similar local tumor control (93%) and overall survival (85%) rates at 2 years with either dose rate. Grade 3 late complications were observed in 7% of patients treated with 0.4 Gy/hour and in 13% of patients treated with 0.8 Gy/hour. There was 1 small-bowel obstruction in the 0.4-Gy/hour group (1%), in contrast with 5 (5%) in the 0.8-Gy/hour group. Vesicovaginal fistulas were observed in 2% and 4%, respectively.

A prospective study in Japan of stage I and II cervical cancer with tumors <4 cm (by T2 MRI) and no lymphadenopathy treated 60 patients with whole-pelvis EBRT 20 Gy/10 fractions with midline block followed by 30 Gy/15 fractions and HDR 24 Gy/4 fractions (at point A).[741] The cumulative BED was 62 Gy (α/β = 10) at point A, lower than that reported by any other institution worldwide. Median tumor diameter was 28 mm (range, 6 to 39 mm). Median OTT was 43 days. Median follow-up was 49 months (range, 7 to 72 months). Seven patients developed recurrences: three patients had pelvic recurrences (two central, one nodal), and four patients had distant metastases. The 2-year disease-free and overall survival rates were 90% (95% CI = 82% to 98%) and 95% (95% CI = 89% to 100%), respectively. The 2-year late complication rates (according to RTOG/EORTC grade ≥ 1) were 18% (95% CI = 8% to 28%) for large intestine/rectum, 4% (95% CI = 0% to 8%) for small intestine, and 0% for bladder. No cases grade ≥3 were observed for genitourinary/gastrointestinal late complications.

The prospective French STIC trial[742] reported patients treated with x-ray simulation compared to 3D-based planning. A total of 705 patients with stage IB to IIIB cervical cancers were enrolled. Toxicity and survival were significantly improved with 3D-based treatment planning. Plain film–based 2-year local control was 74% for patients treated with chemoradiation and LDR or PDR brachytherapy. Detailed results are shown in Table 73.17.

TABLE 73.17 CLINICAL OUTCOMES WITH THREE-DIMENSIONAL PLANNED BRACHYTHERAPY

Institution (Years Reported)	Number of Patients	Mode of Treatment	Stage	Imaging During BT	Median Follow-Up (Year)	Local Control (%)	Disease-Specific Survival (%)	Overall Survival (%)	Late Grade 3–4 Toxicity (%) (Number)
French STIC (2005–2007)[742,a]	705	—	IB–IIIB	—	2	—	—	—	—
	76	Preop LDR or PDR	—	X-ray	—	92[b]	87[b]	95[b]	14.6[b]
	89	Preop PDR	—	CT	—	100[b]	90[b]	96[b]	8.9[b]
	142	Preop ChRT/LDR or PDR	—	X-ray	—	85[b]	73[b]	85[b]	12.5[b]
	163	Preop ChRT/PDR	—	CT	—	93[b]	77[b]	86[b]	8.8[b]
	118	ChRT/LDR or PDR	—	X-ray	—	74[b]	55[b]	65[b]	22.7[b]
	117	ChRT/PDR	—	CT	—	78.5[b]	60[b]	74[b]	2.6[b]
Vienna (1993–1997)[743]	189	EB/HDR	IA–IVB	CT	2.8	78[c]	68[c]	58[c]	(3 GU), (4 GI), (31 V)[c]
Vienna (1998–2003)[744]	145	EB ± Ch[d]-HDR	IA–IVA	MR	4.3	85[c]	68[c]	58[c]	(3 GU), (4 GI), (5 V)[c]
Vienna (2001–2008)[690]	156	EB ± Ch[e]-HDR	IA–IVA	MR	3.5	95[c]	74[c]	68[c]	(3 GU), (5 GI), (2 V)[c]
UPMC (2007–2010)[689]	44	ChRT/HDR	IB–IIIB	CT + MR	0.6	88[b]	85[b]	86[b]	0
Addenbrooke (2005–2007)[745]	28	ChRT/HDR	IB1–IIIB	CT	1.9	96[c]	81[c]	—	14 (3 GI)[c]
IGR (2000–2004)[746]	39	Preop LDR	IB1–IIB	MR	4.4	9[f]	86[f]	94[f]	0
IGR (2000–2004)[692]	84	ChRT/LDR	IB2–IVB	MR	4.4	89[f]	52[f]	57[f]	(3 GU; 1 GI)[f]
IGR (2004–2006)[688]	45	ChRT/PDR	IB–IVA	MR	2.2	100[b]	73[b]	78[b]	(1 Fi)[+]
BW/DFCC (2004–2011)[747]	115	ChRT/HDR	IB–IIIB	CT	1.8	93[b]	83[b]	78[b]	—

[a]Prospective trial.
[b]Two years.
[c]Three years.
[d]Ch administered to 55%.
[e]Ch administered to 73%.
[f]Four years.
BW/DFCC, Brigham and Women's/Dana-Farber Cancer Center; Ch, concurrent cisplatin chemotherapy; ChRT, concurrent cisplatin with external beam radiotherapy; CT, computed tomography; EB, external beam; Fi, fistula; GI, gastrointestinal; GU, genitourinary; HDR, high–dose rate brachytherapy; IGR, Institut Gustave Roussy; LDR, low–dose rate brachytherapy; MR, magnetic resonance imaging; PDR, pulsed dose rate brachytherapy; Preop, preoperative therapy; STIC, Soutien aux Thérapeutiques Innovantes et Couteuses; UPMC, University of Pittsburgh Medical Center; V, vaginal.

Retrospective Data Using Point A Dosimetry for Low Dose Rate Brachytherapy

Fowler[748] analyzed results in 270 patients with carcinoma of the cervix treated with either 75 cGy/hour from manually loaded cesium or 150 cGy/hour by remote afterloading. There was an increase in grade 3 late complications from 4% to 22%, in spite of a reduction of 20% in dose, implying a rather large difference in biologic effect between the two systems. The effect of the increased dose rate was also described by Leborgne et al.[749] LQ modeling was used to calculate biologically effective doses in the clinical protocols used. When the LDR was doubled, it was called MDR. The maximum ratios calculated for the biologic effective doses of 16 Gy at MDR to 20 Gy at LDR were 1.06 to 1.15, assuming $\alpha/\beta = 4$ to 2 Gy, the latter being an unlikely extreme for rectal or urinary complications. The theoretically ideal dose reduction factors, calculated using the $t_{1/2}$ values derived from the clinical data, are in the range of 24% to 29% instead of 20%.

Rodrigus et al.[750] analyzed late complications in 143 patients with cervical cancer treated with two different brachytherapy schedules and external radiation. Seventy-seven patients had two intracavitary applications with a dose rate of 0.54 Gy/hour and 66 patients with that of 1.07 Gy/hour. Because of the expected increase in complications with the higher dose rate, the latter dose per application was reduced from 25 to 20 Gy. Late intestinal and urinary complications were scored in 49 of 77 and 46 of 68 patients, respectively. Actuarial estimates at 5 years showed 42% and 54.1% late intestinal complications and 16.9% and 24.1% late urinary complications, respectively. Thus, despite the dose reduction, there was a clear dose rate effect on late morbidity. These studies emphasize the importance of the dose rate of brachytherapy in carcinoma of the cervix.

Rotmensch et al.[751] compared the outcome in 140 patients with early-stage cervical cancer undergoing whole-pelvis radiation therapy with one versus two LDR intracavitary brachytherapy applications. The two groups had similar 5-year local tumor control (P = .83), disease-free (P = .23), and cause-specific (P = .29) survival. Late complications were similar in the two groups. These results support the use of a single LDR application in patients with early-stage disease undergoing definitive radiation therapy after 45-Gy external beam pelvic irradiation.

In a retrospective analysis, Perez et al.[190] noted that in patients with cervical cancer treated with radiation therapy alone for stage IB tumors <2 cm in diameter, the pelvic failure rate <10% with LDR doses of 70 to 80 Gy to point A, whereas for larger lesions, even doses of 85 to 90 Gy resulted in 25% to 37% pelvic failure rates. In stage IIB with LDR doses of 70 Gy to point A, the pelvic failure rate was approximately 50%, compared with 20% in nonbulky and 30% in bulky tumors with doses >80 Gy. In stage III unilateral lesions, the pelvic failure rate was approximately 50% with 70 Gy or less to point A versus 35% with higher doses, and in bilateral or bulky tumors, it was 60% with doses <70 Gy and 50% with higher doses.

A study from France reported on preoperative LDR followed by radical surgery with lymph node dissection for 257 patients with stage IB1, IIA, and IIB cervical cancers of <4 cm.[752] Residual tumor was identified in 44% of patients, whereas 4.3% of patients had parametrial invasion and 17.9% of patients had lymph node involvement. Late complications of grade 2 occurred in 7.4% and of grade 3 in 2.7% of patients. Five-year actuarial overall survival and DFS were 83% (CI = 78.3 to 87.5) and 80.9% (CI = 76.3 to 85.7), respectively. In multivariate analysis, lymph node involvement, parametrial involvement, and smoking factors significantly affected overall survival and DFS rates.

Retrospective Results Using Point A with Pulsed Dose Rate Brachytherapy

Rogers et al.[753] treated 52 patients with cervical carcinoma, 31 of whom had staging laparotomy before radiation therapy. Brachytherapy was interstitial in 18 patients and intracavitary in 28. The median EBRT pelvis dose was 45 Gy in 25 fractions. Median total doses were 75.8 Gy to the implant volume with interstitial and 84.1 Gy to the A points with intracavitary at a median dose rate of 0.55 Gy per pulse per hour. Six patients had laparotomy-documented para-aortic node involvement and received EBRT to this site (45 Gy in 25 fractions). Thirty patients received concomitant weekly cisplatin chemotherapy (40 mg/m²). With a median follow-up of 25 months, the actuarial 4-year DFS rates were 66% for the entire group (100% for stage IB, 69% for stage II, 68% for stage III/IVA, and 43% in patients treated for recurrences after surgery). Grade 4 complications occurred in 2 patients (4.3%). One patient (2.2%) had a grade 3 complication (frequent hematuria), and 5 (10.9%) had grade 2 complications.

Kaneyasu et al.[754] treated 419 patients with squamous cell carcinoma of the cervix from 1969 to 1999 with LDR or MDR. LDR required overnight admission, whereas MDR was given over approximately 5 hours on an outpatient basis. The 5-year overall survival rates for stages I, II, III, and IVA in the LDR group were, respectively, 78%, 72%, 55%, and 34% versus 100%, 68%, 52%, and 42% in the MDR group (not statistically different). The actuarial rates of late complications of grade 2 or greater at 5 years for the rectum, bladder, and small intestine in the LDR group were 11.1%, 5.8%, and 2.0%, respectively, whereas for the MDR group, they were 11.7%, 4.2%, and 2.6%, respectively (not significantly different).

El-Baradie et al.[755] published a prospective study in which 45 patients with carcinoma of the uterine cervix were randomly allocated to either HDR or MDR. The external beam radiation dose was the same in the two groups. The point A dose rate correction factor from LDR to HDR was 0.53, and that from LDR to MDR 0.6. The 3-year survival and locoregional tumor control rates for both modalities were equivalent (respectively 62% and 67% for HDR and 68% and 74% for MDR). The rectal and bladder complication rates were the same in both groups (29% at 3 years). Tanaka et al.[756] also compared HDR and MDR brachytherapy in 150 and 56 patients, respectively. The survival was equivalent in the two groups; grade 2 or greater late toxicity tended to be higher in the HDR group (14% vs. 6%, respectively).

Bachtiary et al.[757] reported on 109 patients treated with LDR BT and 57 who received PDR BT. The 3-year overall survival and DFS rates were 70% and 57% for the LDR group and 82% and 70% for the PDR group, respectively (P = .25

and .19). The 3-year probability rate for late grade 3 or worse toxicity was 7.4% for LDR BT patients and 7.6% for PDR BT patients (P = .69) and was 6.9% and 7.6%, respectively, for concurrent chemotherapy versus none (P = .69).

Rath et al.[758] reported on 48 patients treated with PDR brachytherapy (ICRT) and pelvic irradiation. A single session delivered a dose of 27 Gy to point A by PDR (hourly pulse, 70 cGy). Ten patients had disease recurrence (five each in stage IIB and stage IIIB). Eight patients had pelvic failure, one had bone metastases, and one had supraclavicular node metastases. Overall, the grade III to IV late toxicity rate at 50 months was 6%. For the median follow-up period of 15 months, the actuarial recurrence-free survival in stages I to II was 82% and in stages III to IV was 78%.

Retrospective Results with Point A Using High Dose Rate Brachytherapy

Many nonrandomized studies compared the results of HDR with those of historic or concurrent control patients receiving LDR at the same institution.[645,664,712,759-761] HDR in patients with stage IIIB disease or large tumors must be used cautiously because the brachytherapy prescription dose should cover the tumor volume and avoid the normal tissues as much as possible (Table 73.18). Although it is generally recommended not to give concurrent chemotherapy on the day of HDR brachytherapy[635] several studies indicate that HDR does not increase toxicity in patients treated with chemoradiation (Table 73.19). Most studies used point A as a reference point, although the definition of point A may have differed from center to center.

A retrospective population-based cohort study of all uterine cervix cancer cases in Saskatchewan diagnosed between 1985 and 2001 had 107 LDR and 37 HDR cases with similar stage distribution. The 5-year CSS rate was 56% for HDR and 67% for LDR (P = .72). Acute toxicities were diarrhea (60%) and abdominal cramps (12.5%), and chronic toxicities were vaginal stenosis (5.5%) and small-bowel obstruction (4%).[778]

Petereit et al.[643] reported on 191 patients receiving LDR brachytherapy and 173 receiving HDR brachytherapy with equivalent external beam radiation therapy techniques. Pelvic tumor control and survival rates were comparable with the two techniques, except in stage III; in this subgroup, outcome was better with LDR brachytherapy, but this may have been related to a lower HDR equivalent dose administered. In an analysis of 198 patients treated with LDR brachytherapy, the 3-year survival rate was 66% versus 77% for 40 patients treated with HDR brachytherapy.[768] Pelvic tumor control rates were 80% and 77%, respectively. The incidences of complications requiring hospitalization or surgery were 10% (20 of 198) and 2.5% (1 of 40), respectively.

Kapp et al.,[779] in a study of 181 patients with FIGO stage IB to IV carcinomas of the cervix, documented that prognostic factors for patients treated with HDR

TABLE 73.18 STAGE III OVERALL SURVIVAL, PELVIC CONTROL, AND TOXICITY IN RETROSPECTIVE SERIES

	Low Dose Rate			High Dose Rate			
	Number	Overall Survival[a] (%)	Pelvic Control (%)	Toxicity[b] (%)	Number	Overall Survival (%)	Pelvic Control (%)	Toxicity[b] (%)
Akine et al.[424c,d]	212	38	61	–	37	54	64	–
Arai et al.[683c,d]	143	46.5	–	–	508	52.2	–	–
Falkenberg et al.[762c,e,f]	23	45	72	4.8	6	33	83	3.5
Ferrigno et al.[763d]	69	**46**[g]	58	**4.7**[g]	56	**36**[g]	50	**0.8**[g]
Hsu et al.[764d]	73	50.2	–	–	30	51.1 (7) 42.9 (4)	–	–
Kim et al.[765d]	8	35.7	–	–	16	43.8	–	–
Kucera et al.[766e]	212	**37.3**[g]	–	–	78	**53.8**[g]	–	9.0
Okkan et al.[767c,d]	21	47.3	53	–	98	31.6	45	–
Orton et al.[647d]	1464	42.6	–	–	2721	47.2	–	–
Petereit et al.[643c,e]	50	**58**[g]	**75**[g]	–	50	**33**[g]	**44**[g]	–
Sarkaria et al.[768e]	57	46	63	7.0	12	58	50	2.5
Lorvidhaya et al.[769c,d]	–	–	–	–	675	47.8	68.8	8.3
Sakata et al.[770d]	–	–	–	–	48	–	63	–
Souhami et al.[771c]	–	–	–	–	77	42	–	–
Wong et al.[772c,d]	–	–	–	–	51	25	63.2	–

[a]Combined grade 3 to 5 rectal and bladder late complications, reported for all stages.
[b]Stage IIIB results.
[c]Five-year results.
[d]Three-year results.
[e]Cause-specific survival reported.
[f]Statistically significant differences in bold.
[g]Six- and four-fraction results.

From Stewart AJ, Viswanathan AN. Current controversies in high-dose-rate versus low-dose-rate brachytherapy for cervical cancer. *Cancer* 2006;107(5):908–915. Copyright © 2006 American Cancer Society. Reprinted by permission of John Wiley & Sons, Inc.

TABLE 73.19 FRACTIONATION AND TOXICITY OF HIGH–DOSE RATE AND CONCURRENT CHEMOTHERAPY

	High Dose Rate		Toxicity (%)[a]		Follow-Up (Month)
	Dose (Gy)	Number of Fractions	No Chemotherapy	Chemotherapy	
Tseng et al.[495b]	4.3	6	6.5 (GI)3.2 (GU)	10 (GI)3.3 (GU)	47
Pearcey et al.[484b,c]	8	3	9 (GI)7 (GU)	5 (GI)10 (GU)	82
Sood et al.[773d]	9	2	5 (GI)	5 (GI)	36
Saibishkumar et al.[774d]	9	2	(GI)1.0 (GU)	1.8 (GI)0 (GU)	39
Sood et al.[775d]	9	2	10	6	28
Ozsaran et al.[776e]	8.5–9	1–2	0	0	20
Souhami et al.[510e]	10	3		28 (GI)6 (GU)	27
Strauss et al.[777e]	7	5		3.7 (GI)3.7 (GU)	19

[a]Grade 3 to 5 late complications.
[b]Prospective, randomized trial.
[c]Includes high, medium, and low dose rate.
[d]Retrospective comparison of patients treated with and without chemotherapy.
[e]Retrospective review, all patients received chemotherapy.
GI, gastrointestinal; GU, genitourinary.
From Stewart AJ, Viswanathan AN. Current controversies in high-dose-rate versus low-dose-rate brachytherapy for cervical cancer. *Cancer* 2006;107(5):908–915. Copyright © 2006 American Cancer Society. Reprinted by permission of John Wiley & Sons, Inc.

are similar to those in previous series with LDR brachytherapy. In multivariate analysis, tumor size was the most powerful factor for pelvic tumor control and incidence of distant metastasis.

Ferrigno et al.[763] carried out a retrospective study of 190 patients treated with LDR and 118 with HDR brachytherapy in combination with pelvic EBRT for cervical cancer. For stage I or II patients, there was no difference in outcome; however, in the stage III group, local tumor control was 58% with LDR and 50% with HDR ($P = .19$), and DFS was 49% versus 37% ($P = .03$). At 5 years, rectal sequelae were 16% versus 8% ($P = .03$), bladder sequelae were 6% and 3% ($P = .13$), and small-bowel sequelae were 4.6% and 8.9% ($P = .17$).

Falkenberg et al.[762] reviewed 160 patients, 103 treated with LDR and 57 treated with HDR from 1990 to 2000. Locoregional control was 78% for LDR and 76% for HDR ($P = .96$); overall survival was 60% for LDR versus 55% for HDR ($P = .48$) at 3 years. Late complications were reported in 2 HDR patients (3.5%) and 5 LDR patients (4.8%).

Orton et al.[647] noted that dose per fraction of HDR brachytherapy significantly influenced toxicity. Morbidity rates were significantly lower for point A doses/fractions of 7 Gy or less for both severe (1.28% vs. 3.44%; $P < .0001$) and moderate plus severe injuries (7.58% vs. 19.51%; $P < .001$). The effect of dose/fractionation on cure rates was equivocal.

Kuske et al.[780] described a method to improve target coverage and locoregional tumor control with HDR tandem and ovoid applications by which HDR endocavitary and interstitial brachytherapy are applied in the same session for tumors with a lateral expansion of 25 mm or more from the axis of the cervical canal. Seventy-six combined applications were given to 41 patients. With a follow-up average of 23 months, in stage IIB tumors, 3-year DFS was 75%. No severe early or persistent late complications were observed. Combined applicators with the tandem and ring with interstitial[781] and tandem and ovoid with interstitial[693,782] are now available for HDR brachytherapy.

Forrest et al.[728] presented the results of 122 patients treated with EBRT followed by 6 Gy per fraction for five fractions of HDR. They reported a 2-year DFS rate of 70% and grade 3/4 toxicity rate of 14% (13 patients). The median time to recurrence was 8 months (range, 2 to 22 months) and to toxicity was 10 months (range, 4 to 27 months). They concluded that the high toxicity of this regimen should prompt consideration of dose reduction in BT dose or use of 3D imaging to shape the dose. Several institutions in the United States now report 5.5 Gy × five fractions instead of 6 Gy per fraction for patients treated with chemoradiation.[638,639]

Anker et al.[783] treated 65 patients with HDR with 6 Gy × fractions, and 45 patients had the top dwells retracted as the tumor regressed. With a median follow-up of 24.5 months, the 3-year overall, disease-free distant metastases–free survival, and local control rates were 67%, 76%, 79%, and 97%, respectively. Acute and actuarial 3-year late grade 3 toxicity or greater occurred in 24.6% and 17% of patients, respectively.

Le Pechoux et al.[784] treated 130 patients with cervical cancer with HDR brachytherapy (for stage I, 30 Gy in 6 weekly sessions) in combination with EBRT (50-Gy mean dose with midline shielding). Patients with more advanced disease received four sessions of biweekly brachytherapy for a total dose of 18 to 24 Gy and external irradiation (20 to 30 Gy to the whole pelvis, 50 to 66 Gy to parametria with midline shielding). The 5-year survival rates were 82% for patients with stage IIB and 47% with stage IIIB disease. There were 4 rectovaginal or vesicovaginal fistulas and 1 case of proctitis requiring colostomy. Survival, local tumor control, and morbidity were equivalent in 76 patients treated with 6 Gy once a week and in 54 patients receiving twice-weekly brachytherapy of 5 Gy per session.

Hsu et al.[764] dosed 92 patients with cancer of the cervix with HDR brachytherapy, six fractions of 7 Gy per fraction (42 Gy) at point A (HDR-6); 57 received four fractions of 8 Gy per fraction (32 Gy) at point A (HDR-4). A twice-daily program was used for all patients receiving HDR in two split courses. A historic control group of 259 patients was treated with LDR brachytherapy (40 Gy in two split courses). All patients received whole-pelvis external irradiation of 36 to 45 Gy (mostly 40 Gy) before brachytherapy. Five-year local tumor control rates were equivalent in the three groups (82%, 85.5% for HDR, and 89.5% for LDR). Five-year survival rates were also comparable (67.7%, 77.9%, and 74.1%, respectively). However, late complications were lower in the HDR-4 group, which received treatment more biologically equivalent to the LDR regimen, than in patients in the HDR-6 group (11% vs. 25.6%).

Selke et al.[785] published results in 187 patients with primary carcinoma of the cervix treated with whole-pelvis irradiation (46 Gy) and HDR brachytherapy with a dose rate to point A of 1.6 Gy/minute, decreasing to approximately 0.8 Gy/minute at the end of the 5-year study. Three HDR fractions (8 to 10 Gy to point A per fraction) were concurrently administered with the last 2 to 3 weeks of external irradiation. The 5-year actuarial survival rates were 72% for stage IB, 65% for IIA, 66% for IIB, 66% for IIIA, and 45% for stage IIIB. With a median follow-up of 54 months, 23 patients had 25 complications; 13 (7.6%) were grade 3 or 4. Rectal complications were significantly higher in patients who received a total rectal dose of >54 Gy ($P = .045$).

Choi et al.[786] treated 136 patients with carcinoma of the cervix with external beam whole-pelvis irradiation (46 Gy in 23 fractions) and three weekly applications of HDR brachytherapy of 7 or 8 Gy per fraction to point A. The actuarial 5-year survival was 85% in stage IB, 64% in stage IIA, 70% in stage IIB, and 53% in stage IIIB. Grade 3 or higher complications occurred in 3% to 7% of the patients.

The most significant determinants of severe rectal complications were the addition of a lower vaginal tandem ($P < .01$), uterine tandem length >5 cm, a total biologically effective dose to the rectum of >120 Gy, and stage III disease.

Kagei et al.[787] reported on 217 patients with carcinoma of the cervix (71 patients with stage II and 146 with stage III disease) who received whole-pelvis EBRT (40 Gy in 20 fractions or 39.6 Gy in 22 fractions) and an additional 10 Gy in five fractions to the parametria followed by HDR brachytherapy. Cause-specific 5-year survival rates were 77% for stage II and 50% for stage III. Pelvic failure rates were 13% and 36%, respectively. The rates of severe (grade 4) late complications were 2% for the rectum, 1% for the small intestine or sigmoid colon, and 1% for the bladder.

Takeshi et al.[788] treated 265 patients with stage III cervical carcinoma with external beam radiation therapy (50.3 Gy) and intracavitary HDR brachytherapy (19.8 Gy). The 5-year overall survival, relapse-free survival, and locoregional event–free rates were 50.7%, 57.1%, and 71.2%, respectively. The 5-year incidence of major complications was 2.6% for bladder and 8.3% for rectum. The radiation dose in the subgroup with rectal complications was significantly greater than that in the subgroup without complications.

Wang et al.[789] reported treatment results in 173 patients with cervical carcinoma treated with HDR brachytherapy and whole-pelvis irradiation (40 to 44 Gy in 20 to 22 fractions) followed by pelvic wall boost (6 to 14 Gy in three to seven fractions with central shielding). HDR brachytherapy delivered 7.2 Gy to point A in each of three applications 1 to 2 weeks apart. Five-year pelvic tumor control rates were 94%, 87%, and 72% for stages IIA, IIB to IIIA, and IIIB to IVA, respectively. Five-year actuarial survival rates were 79%, 59%, and 41%, respectively. Sixty-six patients (38%) had rectal complications, and 19 (11%) had bladder complications. The 5-year actuarial rectal complication rates were 15%, 4%, and 3% for grades 2, 3, and 4, respectively.

Lorvidhaya et al.[769] reported the results in 1,992 patients with carcinoma of the cervix treated by external irradiation and HDR brachytherapy. There were 211 patients with stage IB, 225 with stage IIA, 902 with stage IIB, 14 with stage IIIA, 675 with stage IIIB, 16 with stage IVA, and 16 (0.8%) patients with stage IVB. With a median follow-up of 96 months, the actuarial 5-year DFS rates were 70%, 59.4%, 46.1%, 32.3%, 7.8%, and 23,1%, respectively. The late complication rates (RTOG) for bowel and bladder combined were 7% for grade 3 and 1.9% for grade 4 complications.

Leborgne et al.[790] described a 4-year pelvic control rate of 93% and a DFS rate of 88% for 59 patients with stage IB to IIA disease. All were treated with 18 Gy to the whole pelvis and 22 Gy to the parametria combined with six HDR fractions (14 Gy/hour to point A) of 7 Gy to point A, two in each treatment day, with 6-hour interfraction intervals. The corresponding parameters for 29 patients with stage IIB disease were 79%, 75%, and 75%. The actuarial 4-year late grade 2 and 3 complication rate was 4.7%.

In 1,148 patients with squamous cell cervical cancer treated with external RT and HDR brachytherapy with 22 years median of follow-up, the 10-year pelvic tumor control was 93% for stage IB, 82% for stage II, and 75% for stage III.[791] CSS was 89%, 74%, and 59%, respectively. Major sequelae were 4.4% in the rectosigmoid, 0.9% in the bladder, and 3.3% in the small intestine. Nakano et al.[792] subsequently presented a study of 210 patients with stage IIIB cervical cancer from eight Asian countries treated from 1996 to 1998 with radiation and brachytherapy. Though follow-up was difficult to obtain, the reported 5-year major complication rates were 6% in the HDR group and 10% in the LDR group. The 5-year overall survival rates were 51.1% in the HDR group and 57.5% in the LDR group.

Novetsky et al.[793] presented data on 77 patients treated with external beam with concomitant cisplatin followed by two HDR brachytherapy fractions of 9 Gy each. Median follow-up was 3.5 years. The local control rate was 88% for stages IB2/II and 68% for stages III/IV. Grade 3/4 gastrointestinal acute symptoms occurred in 47%. Grade 3/4 late toxicities occurred in 5 (6%) patients. Patel et al.[794] describe 104 cervical cancer patients treated with external beam and HDR, either 9 Gy for two fractions or 6.8 Gy for three fractions, each fraction 1 week apart. Median follow-up was 31 months. The 3-year actuarial local control was 81.35% with 9 Gy versus 65.18% with 6.8 Gy ($P = .04$). The 3-year actuarial risk of developing any grade 3 or worse late toxicity was 7.47% with 9 Gy and 3.57% with 6 Gy ($P = 0.3$).

Prospective Trial with CT or MR Compared to X-Ray

The clinical outcome results from institutions using CT- or MR-based treatment planning for cervical cancer brachytherapy are listed in Table 73.17. The French STIC trial[793] collected data from 20 centers prospectively and stratified to 2D versus 3D (mainly with CT) brachytherapy. A total of 705 patients were treated with one of three arms: (a) brachytherapy followed by surgery (stage IB1, 165 patients); (b) EBRT plus chemotherapy, BT, then surgery (305 patients); or (c) EBRT plus chemotherapy and then BT (235 patients). For the 235 patients treated with concurrent chemoradiation and then brachytherapy, 2-year overall survival was 74% for 3D versus 65% for 2D ($P = .27$); DFS was 60% versus 55% ($P = .09$); local regional relapse–free survival was 70% versus 61% ($P = .001$), and local-only relapse–free survival was 79% versus 74% ($P = .003$). Toxicity was reduced overall from 23% with 2D to 2.6% with 3D ($P = .002$); urinary from 9% in 2D to 1% with 3D ($P = .02$), gastrointestinal from 9% to 0% ($P = 0.17$), and gynecologic from 15% to 1% ($P = .01$).

Retrospective Comparison of CT to MR-Planned Brachytherapy

Three studies compared CT to MRI contouring for HDR tandem and ring brachytherapy. Wachter-Gerstner et al.[795] compared MR-based plans in 15 patients to those derived with either CT or orthogonal films. CT and MR enabled higher dose to the target volume with similar OAR dosing. Viswanathan et al.[672] compared CT contours to MR contours based on a standard set of guidelines; the CT contours were larger in width, but no other significant differences in DVHs were identified. A report by Eskander et al.[673] of 10 patients treated with an MR for the first fraction only, showed that CT volumes had a greater length on the coronal plane, whereas MR images had a greater height on the sagittal plane. No differences were found in DVH parameters after optimization.[673] Similar to the Eskander et al.[673] study, using an MR for the first fraction and CT for subsequent fractions, Beriwal et al.[689] treated 44 patients with 5- to 6-Gy per fraction HDR after EBRT. Ninety-three percent had a complete response by PET at 3 months. Of those with a CR, 2 had a local recurrence at 6 and 8 months. With a median follow-up of 8 months (range, 2.5 to 38 months), 2-year local control, disease-specific, and overall survival rates were 88%, 85%, and 86%, respectively.

One study compared CT to MR interstitial based brachytherapy for cervical cancer and showed 2-year LC rates for MR-based and CT-based treatments as 96% and 87%, respectively (log-rank $P = .65$). At 2 years, OS was significantly better in the MR-guided cohort (84% vs. 56%, $P = .036$). On multivariate analysis, squamous histology was associated with longer OS (HR 0.23, 95% CI 0.07 to 0.72) in a model with MR BT (HR 0.35, 95% CI 0.08 to 1.18). There was no difference in toxicities between CT and MR BT.[796]

Retrospective Results with CT-Planned Brachytherapy

Potter et al.[743] reported results in 189 patients treated with HDR brachytherapy and EBRT (48.6 to 50 Gy). Small tumors were treated with five to six fractions of 7 Gy at point A (25 Gy in the brachytherapy volume), which is isoeffective to 76 to 86 Gy at point A. Large tumors received three to four fractions of 7 Gy after 50 Gy of EBRT, which is isoeffective to 82 to 92 Gy at point A. Three-dimensional treatment planning for brachytherapy was based on conventional x-rays and in 181 of 189 patients on CT scan. The mean brachytherapy dose was 16.2 Gy at the ICRU rectum reference point and 14.4 Gy at the ICRU bladder point. Taking into account the dose for EBRT, the mean isoeffective dose at the ICRU rectum reference point was 69.9 Gy. After a mean follow-up of 34 months, the actuarial pelvic control rate was 78% and the late complication rate for grades 3 and 4 was 2.9% for bladder, 4% for bowel, 6.1% for rectum, and 30.6% for the vagina (shortening and obliteration).

CT-based clinical outcomes were reported by the Addenbrooke's Hospital. Twenty-eight patients had HDR, 8 Gy × 3, CT-planned brachytherapy.[745] The 3-year actuarial cancer-specific survival rate in this group was 81%, with a pelvic control rate of 96%. Five of the 28 patients died of para-aortic or other distant disease, 1 of them being the only one with local recurrence presenting as a malignant vesicovaginal fistula. In 24 patients, $D_{90} \geq 74$ Gy was achieved. The only patient with local recurrence had $D_{90} = 63.8$ Gy, which was a 20% improvement over historical non–image-guided controls.

At Brigham and Women's Hospital, 115 stage IB to IVA cervical cancer patients had CT-planned brachytherapy and were treated with 595 fractions of 5.5- to 6-Gy per fraction HDR brachytherapy.[747] The 2-year local relapse rate was 6.9%. The 2-year disease-specific survival was 83%, and overall survival rate was 78%.

Cho et al. reported on 128 patients treated with CT-based brachytherapy. The 2-year LC rate was 96%, PFS was 88%, and OS was 88%. No patients had LR only. Point A was 85% of prescription for tumors <4 cm and decreased approximately 3% over 5 fractions compared to 90% of prescription for tumors >4 cm that decreased approximately 4%.[747]

Retrospective Results with MR-Planned LDR Brachytherapy

An initial report of MRI during intracavitary gynecologic brachytherapy was published in 1992 from the University of Michigan by Schoeppel et al.[797] Three patients had CT and MRI with their first of two intracavitary implants. A CT- and MR-compatible Fletcher applicator was used. CT could not distinguish the tumor with as much clarity as MR. Tardivon et al.[798] at IGR treated 10 patients with MR evaluation of the tumor during intracavitary brachytherapy for cervical and vaginal cancer and found that in 7 cases MR findings were concordant with clinical examination. MR was useful to determine the tumor/applicator relationship and distinguish the adjacent OAR.

A review was published of 39 patients treated at IGR with MRI-guided LDR brachytherapy in the preoperative setting.[746] A total dose of 60 Gy to the IR-CTV was followed 6 weeks later by extrafascial hysterectomy and bilateral salpingo-oophorectomy with pelvic node dissection. Adjuvant chemoradiation was delivered to patients with pelvic lymph node involvement. After a median follow-up of 4.4 years (range, 2.6 to 6.6 years), there were no central recurrences; 1 local recurrence occurred in the lateral pelvis (2.6%). The 4-year actuarial overall and DFS rates were 94% and 86%, respectively. The 2- and 4-year actuarial local relapse–free survival rates were 94% and 91%, respectively. Haie-Meder et al.[692] subsequently published a series of 84 patients treated with LDR MR-planned brachytherapy after chemoradiation. With a

median follow-up of 53 months (range, 31 to 79 months), the 4-year overall survival and DFS rates were 57 (95% CI = 43 to 69) and 52% (95% CI = 40 to 64), respectively. Thirty-nine late complications occurred in 28 patients (33.3%): 13 bladder, 7 rectal, 5 small bowel, 4 urethral, 3 colic, 2 vaginal, 1 pelvic fibrosis, and 4 others. Four grade 3 delayed complications were observed, and no grade 4 complication occurred.

Retrospective Results with MR-Planned PDR or HDR Brachytherapy

With a 0.2-T MRI at the Medical University of Vienna, 145 patients with stage IB to IVA cervical cancer were treated with four fractions of 7-Gy HDR from 1998 to 2003.[744] Complete remission was achieved in 138 patients (95%), with 7 patients having locally persistent or progressive disease in the central ($n = 5$) or noncentral ($n = 2$) pelvis. With a median follow-up of 40 months, the 4-year local control rate was 83%, compared to 63% for historical controls. A subsequent analysis of 156 patients treated from 2001 to 2008 with MR-based brachytherapy was reviewed.[690] Local control was 98% for tumors 2 to 5 cm and 92% for tumors >5 cm. Overall survival, however, was 72% for tumors 2 to 5 cm and 65% for tumors >5 cm, indicating that despite the increase in local control with MR-based brachytherapy, death from distant metastases remains a problem in patients with large-volume cancer.

Investigators at the IGR reported on 45 patients treated between 2004 and 2006 with a tandem and mold technique using PDR brachytherapy and MR-based contouring.[688] Until recently at IGR, surgery was often performed after brachytherapy if disease was suspected on clinical examination. A dose of ≥15 Gy (after EBRT) was prescribed to the IR-CTV. The dose to the HR-CTV was approximately 250% of the dose to the IR-CTV (i.e., 80 Gy to the HR-CTV). With a median follow-up of 26 months, the 2-year overall and DFS rates were 78% and 73%, respectively. At Tata Memorial Hospital in India, 24 patients with squamous cell carcinoma were treated with MRI-based HDR. With a median follow-up of 12 months,[799] two patients had local failures.[653] Other European centers[682,691,693] and one Canadian center[800] reported feasibility data for MR-based cervical cancer brachytherapy, showing a reduction in the normal-tissue toxicity rate. When implementing 0.5- to 1.5-T MR-based tandem/ring or tandem/ovoid brachytherapy with MRI, specific guidelines for MR use should be followed.[720]

Toxicities

Table 73.17 lists general toxicities in series using CT- or MR-planned brachytherapy. In the Medical University of Vienna series reporting patients treated from 2001 to 2008, 73% received concurrent cisplatin chemotherapy.[690] A total of 11 grade 3 and 4 late events were recorded in 143 patients. With a median follow-up of 3.5 years, the actuarial grade 3 and 4 late morbidity at 3 and 5 years was, respectively, as follows: gastrointestinal, 4% and 4%; urinary, 2% and 3%; and vaginal, 1% and 3%. Two patients developed massive rectal bleeding requiring transfusions. Three patients required stoma (grade 4) for rectal wall ulceration, resulting in a fistula, a rectal perforation, and a rectovaginal fistula. Three patients developed grade 3 urinary frequency or urgency. Three patients experienced grade 3 or 4 coaptation of the vagina.

At IGR, of the 45 patients studied,[688] 23 and 2 developed acute grade 1 or 2 and grade 3 complications, respectively; 21 patients presented with delayed grade 1 or 2 complications. One other patient presented with a grade 3 vesicovaginal fistula. No grade 4 or greater complications, whether acute or delayed, were observed. In the IGR experience with LDR brachytherapy from 2000 to 2004, 39 late complications were reported; 13 bladder, 7 rectal, 5 small bowel, 4 urethral, 3 colic, 2 vaginal, 1 pelvic fibrosis, and 4 others. Grade 3 complications were 1 rectal, 2 bladder, and 1 urethral. Tan et al.[745]

reported on 28 patients treated with CT-guided brachytherapy for stage IB to IIIB cervix cancer. Their overall actuarial 3-year grade 3 and 4 morbidity rate was 14%. Two patients had grade 3 abdominal pain and 1 had a colovaginal fistula. Overall, the data indicate that a potential reduction in morbidity appears to be a benefit of image-guided brachytherapy. Advocating for contouring bowel as a separate organ at risk during image-based brachytherapy, a report of 32 patients showed that when bowel was present around the brachytherapy applicator, contouring the bowel reduced the D_{2cc} optimized dose.

Template-Based Interstitial Brachytherapy

Interstitial implants with [240]Ra, [144]Cs needles, or [206]Ir afterloading plastic catheters to limited tumor volumes are helpful in specific clinical situations. Indications include large residual bulky cervical tumors after external beam treatment, residual tumor with sidewall invasion, vaginal extension, presence of a fistula and/or adjacent organ invasion, or a prior supracervical hysterectomy (Fig. 73.26). Syed-Neblett[801] and Martinez et al.[802] perineal applicators are the most commonly selected. Methods for insertion have been described.[635] A tandem should be inserted when a uterus is present.[803] If the os is not visible, US guidance to determine the proper placement of the tandem is advised.[804] A ring applicator modified to allow simultaneous insertion of interstitial needles[687] and ovoid application with interstitial needles have been described.[693]

Traditionally, plain x-ray films are used for brachytherapy treatment planning. Determination of normal tissue doses and optimization is not feasible, and the risk of complications is high. In these cases, consideration of laparoscopic approaches is recommended.[635] Syed et al.[801] reported on 185 locally advanced cervical cancer patients treated with LDR interstitial brachytherapy from 1977 to 1997. Patients received external beam treatment to 50.4 Gy, followed by interstitial brachytherapy to 40 to 50 Gy. Local control was 82%; 5-year DFS rates were 65%, 67%, 49%, and 17% for patients with stage IB, II, III, and IV disease, respectively. Eighteen (10%) of the 185 patients developed RTOG grade 3 or 4 late complications.

Clinical outcomes using traditional techniques have been reported by several institutions. Thirty patients with stage IIB and 37 patients with stage III carcinoma received interstitial irradiation in the parametrium to supplement the dose delivered by external beam treatment and intracavitary brachytherapy. Despite the fact that the patients treated with interstitial implant were in a high-risk group, local tumor control was comparable to that of patients treated with standard techniques.[190] Pierquin et al.[805] described locoregional

recurrences in 6% of 53 patients with T1, 11% in 47 patients with T2, and 42% of 19 patients with T3 primary tumors of the uterine cervix treated with a combination of external beam irradiation and the Creteil method for interstitial implantation of [206]Ir sources in a plastic cervical–vaginal moulage and a uterine tandem. Prempree[806] reported a 96% local tumor control rate and 61% 5-year DFS rate in 23 patients with stage IIIB carcinoma of the cervix treated with a combination of external irradiation and intracavitary and interstitial implants to the parametrium. Overall, major complications were noted in 8% of the patients. Martinez et al.,[802] using the Martinez Universal Perineal Interstitial applicator, treated 37 patients with advanced or recurrent carcinoma of the cervix and 26 with vaginal–urethral tumors. Doses of approximately 35 Gy were given, in addition to external irradiation (36 Gy to the whole pelvis and 14 Gy to the pelvic sidewall). They reported 6 local failures in the patients with cervical lesions and 5 in the group with vaginal–urethral tumors. The overall complication rate was 5.1%. Nag et al.[807] reported on 31 patients with carcinoma of the cervix treated with external beam radiation therapy and fluoroscopically guided interstitial brachytherapy. With a median follow-up of 36 months, 16 patients (51%) with cervical had no local recurrence. The 5-year actuarial survival rate was 34%. Only 1 patient experienced grade 3 complications (2.5%).

Fallon et al. reported on 315 patients treated from 1992 to 2009 with interstitial brachytherapy. The 10-year local control was 87% and late grade GU and GI toxicities were 4.8% G3 and 5.4% G4.[808]

Recio et al.[809] used laparoscopy at the time of interstitial brachytherapy in six patients with FIGO stage IIB to IVA cervical carcinomas after completion of whole-pelvis radiation; a total of 98 needles were inserted to deliver a median interstitial brachytherapy dose of 20 Gy. Eleven perforations in the pelvic peritoneum or bladder were identified during surgery in five of the six patients, leading to immediate repositioning of needles. No acute or short-term morbidity related to the procedure was noted.

Sharma et al.[810] presented results on 42 patients treated from 2005 to 2007 in a prospective study of two weekly sessions of 10 Gy, 1 week after finishing external beam radiation. Median follow-up was 23 months. Delayed toxicity was 9%. The 3-year overall survival for all stages was 47%, and the 3-year recurrence-free survival for stages IIB, IIIB, and IVA was 67%, 34%, and 20%, respectively. Sharma et al.[811] also reported on the use of transrectal US to assist with insertion of the interstitial needles.

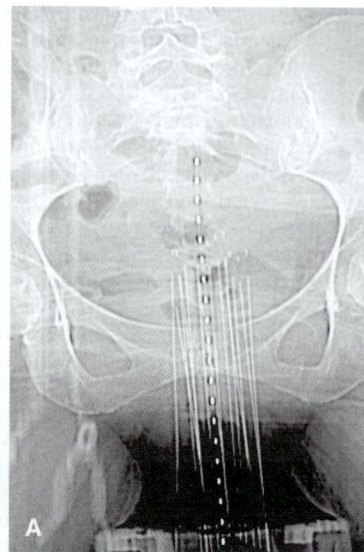
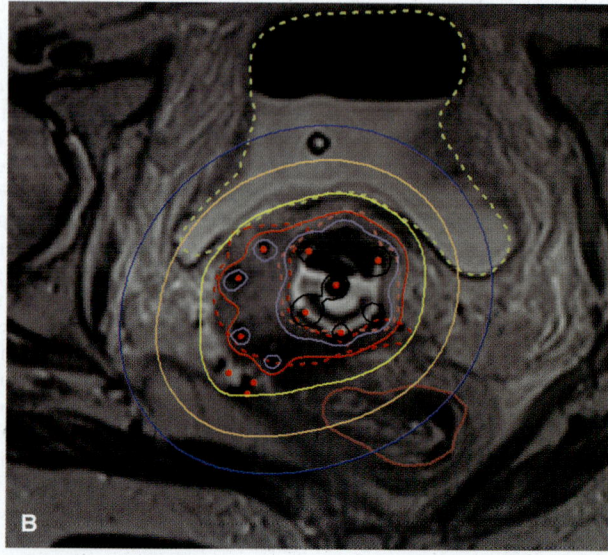

FIGURE 73.26. A: Picture of anterior scout CT showing a template-based interstitial brachytherapy application. **B:** Magnetic resonance imaging during interstitial needle insertion in a patient with stage IIIB cervical cancer ensures proper placement of the catheters adjacent to the tandem. The 100% isodose line is in *yellow*.

With image-based planning including either a CT[674,675] or an MRI,[667] the physician evaluates the placement of the needles and may choose either to not treat specific catheters or to lower the dose given through catheters close to normal-tissue structures. An approximate 11% rate of bowel insertion and a long-term fistula rate of 4% to 10% have been reported in studies using CT for planning after insertion.[674,675] When a physician has the facility to insert the applicator in a CT or MR suite while the patient is under anesthesia, an iterative process of image-guided needle insertion ensures proper placement of the catheters and prevents an inadvertent insertion into a surrounding normal-tissue structure, such as the rectum, sigmoid, or bladder.[667]

Dose optimization with either PDR or HDR may improve the normal-tissue doses for interstitial therapy for some patients. The University of Pittsburgh reported on 11 cervical cancer patients treated with CT-guided HDR interstitial brachytherapy (5 fractions of 3.5 Gy per fraction).[812] From 1998 to 2004, interstitial brachytherapy was chosen for cases with distorted anatomy or extensive vaginal disease. The 5-year actuarial local control rate was 63%. No patient had acute grade 3 or 4 toxicity. Grade 3 or 4 late toxicity occurred in 1 patient, with a 5-year actuarial rate of 7%. Three patients had late grade 2 rectal toxicity, and 1 patient had grade 2 small-bowel toxicity.

Dimopoulos et al.[781] reported on the use of tandem/ring with short interstitial needles and MR-planned HDR brachytherapy for 22 cervical cancer patients followed for a median of 20 months, no grade 3 or 4 toxicities were noted, and 1 patient had a local recurrence. Nomden et al.[782] described the use of tandem/ovoid application with short interstitial needles for the second insertion with MR-planned PDR brachytherapy for 20 cervical cancer patients. They compared the first insertion with just a tandem and ovoid applicator to the second insertion, which included the addition of interstitial needles. There was an average increase in dose of 4.4 Gy (SD 2.3), with better coverage of the HR-CTV with the second insertion.

A prospective cohort of MR-guided interstitial brachytherapy showed a local control rate of 96%. In a comparison of CT- to MR-based brachytherapy, no difference in toxicities were noted, whereas MR had superior outcomes.[796] A systematic review of 672 patients described a local control rate of 79% with image-based planning.[813]

Mikami et al.[814] analyzed needle applicator displacement in 10 patients treated with 30 Gy HDR in five fractions and found on daily CT scans an average of 1 to 2 mm of caudal displacement. Shifts of >3 mm were replanned. Shukla et al.[815] presented data on 20 patients with cervical cancer treated with interstitial brachytherapy who underwent every-other-fraction CT imaging. The mean needle displacement was 2.5 (range, 0 to 7.4), 17.4 (range, 0 to 27.9), 1.7 (range, 0 to 6.7), 2.1 (range, 0 to 9.5), 1.7 (range, 0 to 9.3), and 0.6 mm (range, 0 to 7.8 mm) in cranial, caudal, anterior, posterior, right, and left directions, respectively. The mean displacement in the caudal direction was higher between days 1 and 2 than that between days 2 and 3 (13.4 vs. 3.8 mm; $P = .01$). Damato et al.,[816] in a study of 10 patients treated with interstitial brachytherapy, found on average that <1-cm displacements and deformations of the implant occurred over the course of treatment. The most significant dosimetric consequences were due to changes in organ filling rather than catheter shifts. Proper quality assurance methodologies should be in place to detect shifts that can potentially result in inadvertent insertion into normal tissue.

Brachytherapy in the Elderly

Magné et al.[817] reported on 113 patients with median age of 76 years (range, 70.7 to 94.4 years) treated by conventional LDR BT as a part of their treatment. For rectal complications, grade 1/2, 3/4, and 5 (fatal) crude incidences were 19.4% (22 of 113), 1.8% (2 of 113) and 0.9% (1 of 113), respectively. Acute

toxicity death occurred in 1 patient with major diarrhea associated with a hemodynamic shock. For small-bowel complications, grade 1/2 and 3/4 crude incidences were 3.5% (4 of 113) and 0.9% (1 of 113), respectively. For urinary tract complications, grade 1/2 and 3/4 crude incidences were 11.5% (13/113) and 2.7% (3/113), respectively. With a median follow-up of 3.1 years, 10 patients developed distant metastases, and 10 others had local relapses. The 3-year specific overall survival rate was 88.6% (95% CI = 77 to 92), and the corresponding DFS rate was 81% (95% CI = 72 to 88). Age did not influence the effectiveness of BT in elderly patients, and BT should be considered whenever possible, even in elderly patients presenting with a cervix cancer.

Image-Guided Brachytherapy Versus External Beam Boost

Studies of external beam treatment as an alternative boost instead of brachytherapy demonstrate significantly inferior survival rates compared to those that use brachytherapy. In a SEER analysis, 63% of 7,359 women received brachytherapy in combination with EBRT, and 37% received EBRT alone. The brachytherapy utilization rate decreased from 83% in 1988 to 58% in 2009 ($P < .001$). In a propensity score-matched cohort, brachytherapy treatment was associated with higher 4-year CSS (64.3% vs. 51.5%, $P < .001$) and overall survival (OS; 58.2% vs. 46.2%, $P < .001$). Brachytherapy treatment was independently associated with better CSS (HR, 0.64; 95% CI, 0.57 to 0.71) and OS (HR 0.66; 95% CI, 0.60 to 0.74).[818,819] In the study of the NCDB, only 44% of patients received standard of care therapy; black patients were less likely to receive no boost or brachytherapy.[820] The use of US enables tandem placement in most cases, even when the os cannot be identified, and should be attempted for difficult cases. Barraclough et al.[821] reported on 44 patients with cervical cancer who did not receive brachytherapy and were treated with EBRT to 54 to 70 Gy via a 3D conformal boost. After a median follow-up of 2.3 years, 48% relapsed, with 16 of 21 developing a central recurrence. The 5-year overall survival rate was 49%, which is much lower than for brachytherapy-treated patients.

The dosimetry of brachytherapy cannot be adequately mimicked by external beam techniques. A treatment planning report compared inversely planned EBRT with photons (IMRT/SBRT) and protons (IMPT) to 3D MRI-guided brachytherapy.[822] EBRT was planned to deliver the highest possible doses to the PTV while respecting D_{2cc} limits from brachytherapy, assuming the same fractionation. Volumes receiving 60 Gy (in equivalent dose in 2-Gy fractions) were approximately twice as large for IMRT compared with brachytherapy, and the high central tumor dose was lower than that seen with brachytherapy. Both IMRT and protons were inferior to 3D image-based brachytherapy.

With IMRT, there is a need for replanning because of rapid tumor regression[341–343] and an increase in integral dose, with normal tissues throughout the pelvis receiving more radiation than with brachytherapy. Given the large movement and the increased dose to the normal tissues resulting in an increase in normal-tissue toxicity, highly conformal (IMRT, IGRT, SBRT) methods for boosting the cervix are not routinely recommended. Every effort should be made to use image guidance to insert a tandem into the uterus in order to provide adequate brachytherapy doses for all cervical cancer cases receiving radiation.

External Beam Irradiation Alone

Occasionally, brachytherapy procedures cannot be performed because of medical reasons or unusual anatomic configuration of the pelvis or the tumor (i.e., extensive lesion, inability to identify the cervical canal). These patients may be treated with higher doses of external beam irradiation alone, although survival is significantly worse than when brachytherapy is implemented, and normal-tissue toxicity is higher due to the excessive dose to the rectum and bowel. Therefore, every attempt to treat with brachytherapy should be made because brachytherapy moves with the patient and provides high regions of dose in the central regions of the tumor. With IMRT, a significantly higher normal-tissue dose is administered, and the desired high central regions of radiation cannot safely be administered.

Coia et al.,[554] in an analysis of 565 patients with various stages of cervical carcinoma treated in the Patterns of Care Study, reported better survival (67%) and pelvic tumor control (78%) for patients treated with external irradiation and brachytherapy than for patients who had no intracavitary brachytherapy applications (36% 4-year survival rate and 47% infield failure rate). Patients treated with two intracavitary applications had a higher 4-year survival rate (73%) and infield tumor control rate (83%) than those receiving only one application (60% 4-year survival rate and 71% infield tumor control rate).

Hanks et al.[558] and Montana et al.[557] reported a higher incidence of central pelvic recurrences in patients with stage III cervical carcinoma treated with external beam therapy alone than in patients receiving brachytherapy in addition to external beam irradiation (Table 73.20). The incidence of major complications was similar in both groups of patients.

Akine et al.[824] treated 104 patients with carcinoma of the uterine cervix with external irradiation alone (anteroposterior–posteroanterior or four-field box techniques) because of inability to perform intracavitary brachytherapy. Average doses delivered were 50 Gy to the whole pelvis, followed by additional doses with reduced portals to deliver a total of 60.8 Gy in 6 weeks, 72.3 Gy in 7.5 weeks, or 80.5 Gy in 8 weeks, with a daily dose of 1.9 or 2 Gy. The local tumor control rate was 27% for stage II, 19% for stage III, and 15% for stage IVA disease. The 5-year survival rates were 36%, 17%, and 5%, respectively. Four patients had major complications (usually proctitis) that required surgical treatment, and one patient died of rectal bleeding. Eight of 23 patients treated with conformal therapy had control of the tumor and survived 5 years without major complications. Saibishkumar et al.[825] treated 146 patients with cervix cancer with EBRT alone (60 to 66 Gy) because of unsuitability for brachytherapy; 5-year pelvic tumor control was 21.9% and DFS was 11.6%.

Cost-Effectiveness of LDR Versus HDR Brachytherapy

Wright et al.[826] developed a questionnaire to elicit patient preference for two brachytherapy methods (one LDR or three HDR fractions and two HDR or five HDR fractions, assuming both methods to be isoeffective). The questionnaire was completed by 90 female staff members at their center, 18 previously treated patients, and 20 newly diagnosed patients.

When both methods were assumed to be isoeffective, only 34% of the 38 patients preferred three HDR fractions to one LDR fraction. However, when HDR was assumed to be 2% more curative or 6% less toxic, 50% said they would prefer the HDR therapy. Both preference and strength of preference for LDR were significantly associated with a greater traveling distance for treatments. More studies on resource utilization[827] are needed.

Alternative Isotopes

Californium has been proposed as an alternative to iridium as the radioactive isotope. Maruyama and Muir[828] reported on 41 patients with stage IB cervix cancer treated with 40 to 50 Gy to the whole pelvis followed by a 5- to 15-Gy boost to the lateral pelvic wall and a single ^{268}Cf-neutron brachytherapy insertion in approximately 8 hours. Nearly total tumor clearance was achieved in >90% of the patients; tumor regression was more rapid in the ^{268}Cf group than in similar patients treated with ^{144}Cs and the same external beam irradiation dose.

FOLLOW-UP

After treatment, patients should be regularly followed by both the radiation and the gynecologic oncologist. Careful history taking and a complete physical and pelvic/rectal examination usually are performed every month for the first 3 months after completion of irradiation, every 3 months for the remainder of the first year, every 4 months the second year, every 6 months during the third through the fifth year, and yearly thereafter. The use of Pap smears for cervical and vaginal cytology as a follow-up study is controversial because of postirradiation cellular morphology that renders it difficult to distinguish postirradiation changes from residual or recurrent malignant cells.[829,830] DNA analysis of postirradiation cytologic smears demonstrating atypia or dysplasia may provide ancillary information.[831]

Rintala et al.[832] evaluated the reliability of cytologic analysis and atypia after radiation therapy in 89 patients treated for cervical carcinoma. A total of 697 Pap smears were taken; during the follow-up, 44 patients had recurrent disease, which was local in 17 (39%) cases. The rate of false-positive samples was only 3%. Radiation-induced atypia was detected in 28% of the Pap smears taken during the first 4 months after radiation therapy, and its incidence decreased thereafter. In 1,000 patients treated with either surgery or radiation therapy at the MD Anderson Cancer Center for stage IB cervical cancer posttreatment, Pap smears did not detect a single asymptomatic recurrence among 133 patients with recurrent disease.[833]

The presence of apparently viable tumor cells in the cytologic smear 3 months after irradiation should be evaluated with cervical biopsies, dilation and curettage, and careful EUA, as indicated.

Complete blood counts and chemistry profile tests are obtained as clinically indicated. Chest radiography is commonly obtained on a yearly basis, usually for the first 5 years posttreatment, although its value to detect curable lung metastasis is not proven. If radiographs are consistently negative, obtaining them every other year thereafter may be sufficient.

Other imaging studies, such as CT, MRI, PET scanning, or bone scans, are obtained when clinically warranted. When persistent or recurrent tumor is suspected, biopsies should be obtained for histologic confirmation. If a biopsy is positive, immediate treatment should be instituted, as is discussed later.

Usually, hematometra after radiation therapy for cervical carcinoma is related to recurrent disease but occasionally may be related to estrogen replacement therapy, endometrial activity, or fibrosis and obliteration of the endocervix.[834]

TABLE 73.20 CARCINOMA OF THE UTERINE CERVIX: INCIDENCE OF CENTRAL/PELVIC RECURRENCES CORRELATED WITH METHOD OF THERAPY

Author (Reference)	Stage	Incidence of Pelvic Failures		P
		External Beam Only	External Beam and Intracavitary	
Hanks et al.[558]	III	33/38 (86%)	55/109 (50%)	.0002
Montana et al.[557]	III	14/35 (40%)	12/37 (32%)	.6725
Coia et al.[554]	I, II, III	(53%)	(22%)	<.0100
Longsdon and Eifel[823a]	IIIB	641 (45%)	266 (24%)	<.0001

[a]Five-year disease-free survival.
Modified from Stehman FR, Perez CA, Kurman RJ, et al. Uterine cervix. In: Hoskins WJ, Perez CA, Young RC, eds. *Principles and practice of gynecologic oncology*. 3rd ed. Philadelphia, PA: Lippincott Williams & Wilkins, 2000:841–918. With permission.

TREATMENT OF RECURRENT CARCINOMA OF THE CERVIX

After Previous Surgery

Radiation may salvage approximately 50% of patients with localized pelvic recurrences after surgery alone. A combination of whole-pelvis external irradiation (45 to 50 Gy) with concurrent chemotherapy followed by interstitial brachytherapy is recommended. If the tumor lies outside of an accessible region for brachytherapy, dose escalation with conformal or IMRT techniques may be attempted, depending on the location of the tumor and the need to protect the bowel, with at least 65 to 70 Gy necessary for adequate control. In the setting of recurrent disease, the total mucosal dose from the external and brachytherapy can approach 140 Gy to the upper vagina and 95 Gy to the distal vagina without a high risk.[835] With interstitial brachytherapy, doses of 20 to 35 Gy are administered with single, double-plane, or volume implants, for a total tumor dose of approximately 80 Gy, depending on the extent of the tumor.

Larson et al.[836] observed 27 recurrences (11%) in 249 patients treated with radical hysterectomy and pelvic lymphadenectomy for stage IB carcinoma of the cervix; 17 (63%) had tumor recurrence in the pelvis or vulva; the other 10 patients had recurrences outside the pelvis. Eight of 15 patients (53%) treated with irradiation for an isolated recurrence in the pelvis or vulvar region were tumor-free between 10 and 126 months after treatment of the recurrence (median, 48 months).

Ijaz et al.[837] reported on 50 patients treated with RT for an isolated pelvic recurrence of cervical carcinoma after radical hysterectomy; 7 patients were treated with palliative intent using hypofractionated RT. The remaining 43 patients were treated with curative intent, 33 with RT only and 10 with cisplatin-based chemoirradiation. The overall 5-year survival rate was 33% for all 50 patients, 39% for the 43 patients treated with curative intent, and 25% for patients with isolated sidewall recurrences treated with curative intent. Three patients experienced late treatment complications.

Hille et al.[838] described results in 17 patients with recurrent cervix cancer (9 had a complete microscopically incomplete resection) treated with EBRT and brachytherapy to 50 to 65 Gy. The 5-year pelvic tumor control was 48%, and relapse-free survival was 24%.

After Definitive Irradiation

Reirradiation of previously irradiated patients must be undertaken with extreme caution. It is very important to analyze the techniques used in the initial treatment (beam energy, volume, doses delivered with external or intracavitary irradiation). In addition, the period of time between the two treatments must be taken into consideration because it is postulated that some repair of the initial damage may take place in the interval. In general, external irradiation for recurrent tumor is given to limited volumes (40 to 45 Gy, 1.8-Gy tumor dose per fraction, preferentially using lateral portals). Occasionally, intracavitary or interstitial irradiation can be used to treat relatively circumscribed recurrences.

Sommers et al.[839] described the results of retreatment in 376 patients with recurrent carcinoma of the uterine cervix. Ninety-one patients received irradiation, mostly external (86.8%), occasionally combined with brachytherapy (7.7%) to control bleeding of central recurrences; brachytherapy alone was administered in 5.5% of patients. The usual dose for recurrent pelvic masses was 40 to 45 Gy, and for PALN metastases, it was 45 to 50 Gy in 5 weeks. Other metastatic sites were treated with 35 to 40 Gy in 3 to 4 weeks. Pelvic exenteration was attempted in 23 patients, only 10 of whom were deemed to be operable (43.5%), but it was completed in only 7. The probability of 5-year survival after treatment for recurrence was 30% with combined surgery and external irradiation, 12% with surgery alone, and 4% with external irradiation alone. The 5-year survival rate for 10 patients who underwent pelvic exenteration was 16%. Only 1% of the untreated patients survived 5 years. Six of 140 patients (4.3%) experienced grade 2 or 3 complications.

Selected patients with limited pelvic recurrences not fixed to the pelvic wall and without evidence of extrapelvic metastases can be potentially salvaged by radical hysterectomy or pelvic exenteration. Coleman et al.[840] described results in 50 patients who underwent radical hysterectomy for persistent (18 patients) or recurrent (32 patients) cervical cancer after primary radiation therapy. Lymph node metastases were identified in 5 of 39 patients (13%) in whom the lymph nodes were evaluated. The 5- and 10-year survival rates were 72% and 60%, respectively.

In 65 patients on whom pelvic exenteration was carried out at Memorial Sloan-Kettering Cancer Center, the 5-year survival rate was 23%.[841] The operative mortality rate was 9.2%. The authors pointed out that the significant mortality and morbidity associated with this procedure preclude its use as palliative therapy.

Urinary diversion, either by nephrostomy or ileal bladder, may be of palliative value in patients with either recurrent carcinoma in the pelvis or complications. It must be kept in mind that diversion may prolong life but runs the risk of denying a terminally ill patient with cancer the oblivion and insensibility of uremia.

Kastritis et al.[842] treated 200 patients with stage IV or recurrent cervix cancer with cisplatin-based chemotherapy; response rate was 43.5% in 142 patients with squamous cell and 53.5% in 58 patients with nonsquamous tumors (P = .79). Median survival was 11.57 and 19 months, respectively. Tinker et al.[843] treated 25 women for recurrent cervical cancer with carboplatin–paclitaxel and noted a 20% cure rate and 20% progression rate, with median survival of 21 months. Brewer et al.,[544] in 32 women, all of whom had previous chemotherapy and 29 of whom had previous RT, used cisplatin and gemcitabine, with a progression rate of 22% and median time to progression of 3.5 months.

GOG 240 was a four-arm randomized trial of 452 women with recurrent or metastatic cervical cancer randomized to cisplatin and paclitaxel, or topotecan and paclitaxel, either alone or in combination with 15 mg/kg of bevacizumab. There was a significant improvement of median survival with the addition of bevacizumab, from 13.3 to 17 months (P = .0035), but with higher toxicities (grade 3 to 4 bleeding 5%, thromboembolism 9%, and GI fistula 3%).[844]

Para-aortic Lymph Node Recurrences

Isolated recurrences in the para-aortic nodes after pelvic irradiation have been described in about 3% of patients, and some may be salvaged with aggressive therapy. The advent of IMRT makes treatment easier, with less morbidity.

Kim et al.[585] treated 12 patients with isolated PALN metastasis with hyperfractionated RT (60 Gy in 1.2-Gy fractions twice a day) and concurrent cisplatin–paclitaxel. Fields extended from the superior plate of T12 to the lower plate of L5. Three-year survival was 19%. Grade 3 or 4 hematologic toxicity developed in two patients. Singh et al.[586] detected 14 isolated PALN metastases in 816 patients previously treated with RT; these women were subsequently treated with RT to the PALNs combined with concurrent chemotherapy. Seven patients survived 5 years.

In a review of 1,955 patients treated with RT for cervix cancer, Jhingran et al.[845] identified 120 patients with recurrent tumor above the pelvic fields. Initially, 10 had common iliac and 5 had para-aortic node involvement. In 104 patients, recurrences were immediately adjacent to the upper borders of the RT fields. In 15 patients treated with curative intent for the PALN recurrence, 5-year survival was 25%.

Section III

Intraoperative Irradiation

Intraoperative radiation therapy (IORT) has been used for treatment of locally advanced and recurrent carcinoma of the cervix, with 3-year survival rates of 8% to 21% as reported by Mahé et al.[846] and Garton et al.,[847] and a 5-year survival rate of 33% in 14 patients described by Kinney et al.[452] Patient selection may have had an impact on the different results. Abe and Shibamoto[848] noted that central recurrences, particularly in nonirradiated patients, and resection of the gross recurrent tumor in irradiated patients improve the benefit from IORT. Significant toxicity included peripheral nerve injury and ureteral stenosis (with doses >15 to 20 Gy).

IORT was used in 70 patients with pelvic recurrences in a European cooperative study.[846] Complete tumor resection was carried out in 30 patients, partial in 37, and unspecified in 3. Sixty-five patients had electron beam therapy (12 to 25 MeV), with mean doses of 18 Gy (10 to 25 Gy) after gross complete resection and 19 Gy (10 to 30 Gy) after partial resection. The 3-year overall survival rate was 8%. Grade 2 or 3 toxicity was observed in 19/70 patients (27%), with 10 complications being related to IORT.

Martinez Monge et al.[849] reported a study of IORT in 26 patients with recurrent gynecologic tumors, some relapsing after full-dose radiation therapy (group 1) or after surgery (group 2). Cervical carcinoma was the initial tumor site of involvement in 18 patients. Treatment consisted of maximal surgical resection and IORT (10 to 25 Gy) to high-risk areas. Patients not previously irradiated also received external beam irradiation (with or without chemotherapy) before or after surgery. There was 1 IORT-related incidence of motor neuropathy. The local tumor control rates were 33% and 77%; the 4-year actuarial survival for group 1 was 7%, and the 6-year actuarial survival rate for group 2 was 33%.

In another study, 42 patients with stage IIA to IVA cervical cancers initially received 50.4 Gy of pelvic external beam radiation with concurrent cisplatin and 5-fluorouracil.[850] Patients then underwent radical surgery 6 to 8 weeks later with IORT. The 5-year DFS and OS were 46% and 49%, respectively, which are inferior to reported results with standard concurrent chemoradiation followed by brachytherapy without surgery or IORT. Therefore, this regimen remains of questionable value in potentially curable patients.

URGENT BLEEDING AND PALLIATIVE IRRADIATION

Frequently, the radiation oncologist is faced with the challenge of treating a patient with stage IVB or recurrent carcinoma requiring palliation of pelvic pain or bleeding. Tumors respond rapidly to radiation, and bleeding usually resolves within a few days of treatment. If vaginal bleeding is the main concern, several possibilities may be effective. In a descriptive review of eight papers that presented palliative treatment data,[851] five papers were found to report using 10 Gy per fraction, with the best resolution of bleeding and/or pain when each 10-Gy fraction was given at 3- to 4-week intervals for a total of three fractions. Alternatively, common palliative regimens used in other sites of the body, such as 4 Gy for five or six fractions or 3 Gy for 10 fractions, or a Quad shot regimen may be implemented. Patients who present with a new diagnosis may be treated with 3 to 4 Gy for two or three fractions, followed by standard 1.8 Gy to approximately 39.6 Gy and then brachytherapy. Alternatively, patients may receive 1 to 2 days of 1.8 Gy twice a day, switching to once-a-day treatment with 1.8 Gy per fraction after bleeding has stopped on day 2 or 3, completing treatment after 45 Gy and then commencing routine brachytherapy.

A single LDR intracavitary insertion with tandem and colpostats for approximately 6,000 mgh (55 Gy to point A) may be used for palliation. If irradiation was delivered previously, lower intracavitary doses should be prescribed (4,000 to 5,000 mgh). Grigsby et al.[852] used two fractions of HDR brachytherapy with a ring applicator (once weekly) with control of bleeding in 14 of 15 patients.

Several high-dose fractionation schedules with external beam radiation have been used. Spanos et al.[853] reported on a phase II study of daily multifractionated split-course irradiation in 142 patients with recurrent or metastatic disease in the pelvis. Irradiation consisted of 3.7 Gy per fraction given twice daily for 2 consecutive days, repeated at 3- to 6-week intervals for a total of three courses, aiming at a total tumor dose of 44.4 Gy. Occasionally, this regimen was combined with an LDR intracavitary insertion (4,500 mgh), blocking the midline for the last 14.4-Gy external dose. Twenty-seven patients survived >1 year. There were only two recorded cases of grade 3 toxicity (lower gastrointestinal tract). This study was expanded to a phase III protocol randomizing 136 patients between a short (2 weeks) or a longer (4 weeks) rest period between the split courses of irradiation.[854] There was a trend toward increased acute toxicity in patients with shorter rest periods (5 of 58 vs. 0 of 68; $P = .07$). Late toxicity was not significantly different in the two groups. Pelvic tumor response was comparable in both groups (34% vs. 26%). Spanos et al.[853] reported a 6% complication rate in 290 patients treated in RTOG Protocol 85-02. No patient receiving <30 Gy experienced late toxicity. There was no significant difference in the incidence of complications for patients with a 2- or 4-week rest ($P = .47$).

IRRADIATION AND HYPERTHERMIA

Because of technical limitations in the delivery of adequate heat to large parts of the body such as the pelvis, the use of hyperthermia in the treatment of carcinoma of the uterine cervix has been rare. Hornback et al.[855] described a nonrandomized study in which the combination of microwave hyperthermia (433 MHz) and irradiation resulted in improved pelvic tumor control (72%) in a group of 79 patients with stage IIIB carcinoma compared with previously irradiated historic control patients (53%). However, 5-year survival rates were comparable in both groups (22% to 30%).

Sharma et al.[856] reported a 70% DFS rate at 18 months in 20 patients with stage IIB or III carcinoma of the uterine cervix treated with a combination of irradiation and hyperthermia (13.5 MHz, 42°C to 43°C, 30 minutes before irradiation) in comparison with a 50% DFS rate in 22 patients treated with irradiation alone. The grade 3 complication rate (8%) was similar in both groups.

Dinges et al.[857] treated 18 patients with advanced carcinoma of the cervix with RT plus hyperthermia (in the first and fourth weeks, two regional hyperthermia treatments were applied). The acute toxicity was low and similar to that with RT alone. The local tumor control was 48% at 2 years.

Harima et al.[858] evaluated radiation therapy or thermoirradiation (three sessions of hyperthermia) for stage IIIB cervical carcinoma; two groups of 20 patients each were randomly divided. A complete response was achieved in 50% (10 of 20) in the RT group versus 80% (16 of 20) in the thermoirradiation group ($P = .048$). The 3-year overall survival and DFS rates for the patients who were treated with thermoirradiation (58.2% and 63.6%) were better than with RT (48.1% and 45%), but differences were not statistically significant. The 3-year local relapse–free survival rate of the patients who were treated with thermoirradiation (79.7%) was significantly better than that of the patients treated with irradiation alone (48.5%; $P = .048$). Thermoirradiation was well tolerated and did not add to either acute or long-term toxicity over radiation alone.

Vasanthan et al.[859] reported on 110 patients with locally advanced cervix cancer randomized to treatment with RT alone or combined with hyperthermia (minimum five sessions, 60 minutes each, once weekly). Overall 3-year pelvic tumor control was 68.5% and survival was 73.2%, with no difference in either group, although survival was lower in the patients with stage IIB treated with hyperthermia. Acute toxicity was 18% (10 of 55) in the hyperthermia patients and 4% (2 of 55) with RT alone. Late toxicity was not different in the two arms.

A Cochrane database review identified six randomized, controlled trials published between 1987 and 2009 comparing RT versus combined hyperthermia and RT. The results show 74% of patients had stage IIIB cervical cancer. A significantly higher complete response rate (RR = 0.56, 95% CI = 0.39 to 0.79) and lower local recurrence rate (HR = 0.48, 95% CI = 0.37 to 0.63) and improved overall survival (HR = 0.67, 95% CI = 0.45 to 0.99) with no difference in acute or late grade 3 to 4 toxicity were seen for patients treated with combined therapy.[860] Catheter-based US devices provide a method to deliver heat with HDR brachytherapy, but clinical results are not yet available.[861]

SIDE EFFECTS: SURGERY AND RADIATION

Descriptions of sequelae vary among institutions because toxicity-grading scales are not uniform and the scoring system for complications is not clearly stated in all reports. Surgical side effects alone depend on the extent of surgery and the amount of disease. Radical hysterectomy alone may cause long-term side effects such as urinary retention requiring chronic suprapubic catheter placement, sciatic nerve injury, postoperative seroma or hematoma formation, pelvic pain, or, when lymphadenectomy is performed, lifelong edema. Oophorectomy also may induce menopause; hysterectomy removes the ability to carry a pregnancy, and removal of a portion of the vagina may significantly change sexual function if vaginal shortening is severe.

With improved anesthesia, surgical techniques, and antibiotic therapy, the mortality rate for radical hysterectomy with pelvic lymphadenectomy has decreased to 1% or less. The most frequent sequela after radical hysterectomy is urinary dysfunction as a result of partial denervation of the detrusor muscle. Patients may have various degrees of loss of bladder sensation, inability to initiate voiding, residual urine retention, and incontinence.

In 375 patients treated with a modified radical hysterectomy for various gynecologic disorders, Magrina et al.[862] observed some form of postoperative (within 42 days of surgery) complications in 89 patients (24%). Patients who had a pelvic lymphadenectomy experienced a greater incidence of lower extremity lymphedema than those who did not undergo this procedure. Preoperative or postoperative pelvic irradiation was a significant predisposing factor for urinary tract infection, lymphedema, and bowel obstruction in these patients compared with those who did not receive pelvic irradiation.

Some loss of defecatory urge associated with chronic rectal dysfunction was observed by Barnes et al.[863] after radical hysterectomy. Manometric studies suggest a disruption of the spinal arcs controlling defecation.

Other complications include ureterovaginal fistula (the incidence of which has decreased to <3%), hemorrhage, infection, bowel obstruction, stricture and fibrosis of the intestine or rectosigmoid colon, and bladder and rectovaginal fistulas. Postsurgical complications are usually more amenable to correction than are late complications after irradiation.

When postoperative radiation therapy is given to selected patients, further complications of the additional therapy are expected. The main areas of side effects because of radiation are bowel, bladder, skin, and sexual function.[864] Because of intestinal adhesions to denuded surfaces in the pelvis, enteric complications, such as obstruction, fistula, or dysfunction, were observed in 24% of patients reported by Fiorica et al.[865] Other investigators, however, have reported no increase in the incidence of severe complications in patients treated with postoperative irradiation.[419,866]

Lower body mass index (BMI) is correlated with an increase in toxicity. A total of 404 patients with stage IB1 cervical cancer with positive lymph nodes or stage IB2 or higher were treated from 1998 to 2008. A BMI of <18.5 was associated with a decreased overall survival (HR = 2.37, P < .01). Grade 3 and 4 complications appeared to trend higher; overall, 17% versus 14%; specifically, for fistula, 11% versus 9% (P = .05), for bowel obstruction, 33% versus 4% (P < .01), and for lymphedema, 5.6% versus 1.2% (P = .02).[867]

Montz et al.[868] evaluated bowel obstruction in 98 patients undergoing radical hysterectomy for a nonadnexal gynecologic malignancy. The incidence of small-bowel obstruction was significantly higher (P < .05) in patients who received concomitant radiation therapy (20%). None of these patients had recurrent disease at the time of small-bowel obstruction. Findings at surgery consisted of minimal incisional adhesions but extensive matted small-bowel loops adherent to the pelvic operative sites.

When irradiation is combined with surgery, the complication rate tends to be somewhat higher, particularly because of injury to the ureter or the bladder (ureteral stricture or ureterovaginal or vesicovaginal fistula).[869] The dose of irradiation, technique, and type of surgical procedure performed are important in determining the morbidity of combined therapy. Jacobs et al.,[870] in 102 patients with invasive cervical carcinoma treated with low-dose preoperative irradiation and radical hysterectomy with lymphadenectomy or high-dose preoperative irradiation and conservative extrafascial hysterectomy, noted a major complication rate of 5%. After combined treatment, some degree of lymphedema may be observed (30% to 40%).

A significant number of complications are associated with pretherapy staging laparotomy, particularly if irradiation (>55 Gy) is given to metastatic PALNs. The incidence of complications is between 5% and 20%, depending on the extent of the PALN dissection, use of transperitoneal or retroperitoneal approach for the operation, and dose of irradiation given.[46]

Late Sequelae: Overall

The incidence of major late sequelae of radiation therapy for stage I and IIA carcinomas of the cervix ranges from 3% to 5% and for stages IIB and III between 10% and 15%. The most frequent major sequelae for the various stages are listed in Tables 73.21 and 73.22. Injury to the gastrointestinal tract usually appears within the first 2 years after radiation therapy, whereas complications of the urinary tract are seen more frequently 3 to 5 years after treatment.[609,871] Pedersen et al.,[872] in a review of morbidity of radiation therapy in 442 patients with cervical cancer stages IIB, III, and IVA, recommended that actuarial estimates rather than frequency of sequelae be reported to avoid underestimation of risks of late morbidity after radiation therapy in long-term survivors. In fact, Eifel et al.,[869] in 1,784 patients with stage IB carcinoma of the cervix, noted that the greatest risk of sequelae is in the first 3 years after therapy. The risk of rectal complications declined after the first 2 years of follow-up to 0.6%/year, whereas the risk of major urinary tract complications for survivors continued at 0.3%/year, with a 20-year actuarial risk of major complications of 14.4%.

Montana et al.[557], Perez et al.,[873] and Pourquier et al.[874] noted a greater incidence of complications with higher doses of irradiation. Perez et al.[871] and Pourquier et al.[874] reported that with doses <75 to 80 Gy delivered to limited volumes, grade 2 and 3 complications in the urinary tract and

TABLE 73.21 CARCINOMA OF THE UTERINE CERVIX: GRADE 2 SEQUELAE (WASHINGTON UNIVERSITY, 1959–1989)

	Stage				
	IB	IIA	IIB	III	IVA
Total number of patients treated	415	137	391	326	23
Number of complications	51 (12%)	14 (10%)	65 (17%)	38 (12%)	3 (13%)
Rectum–Bowel	–	–	–	–	–
Rectal stricture	–	1	2	1	1
Proctitis	8	1	13	6	–
Rectal ulcer	1	–	–	2	1
Diverticulitis	–	–	1	–	–
Small-bowel obstruction	2	–	3	4	–
Malabsorption	3	–	1	1	–
Urinary	–	–	–	–	–
Chronic cystitis	–	2	12	4	–
Bladder ulcer	3	1	2	1	–
Incontinence	1	–	1	–	–
Urethral stricture	2	–	1	–	–
Extensive cystocele	–	–	–	3	–
Other					
Vaginal stenosis	21	4	7	6	1
Vault necrosis	8	2	2	5	–
Postoperative pelvic abscess	1	–	1	2	–
Lymphocyst	–	–	2	2	–
Pulmonary embolus	–	–	1	–	–
Subcutaneous fibrosis	1	–	–	–	–
Leg edema	–	–	7	3	–
Hemorrhage	–	–	1	–	–
Thrombosis of pelvic blood vessels	–	1	–	–	–
Arteriosclerosis	1	–	8	2	–
Thrombophlebitis	–	–	1	–	–
Pelvic fibrosis	–	1	–	–	–
Acute pelvic cellulitis	–	1	–	–	–
Neuritis	–	–	–	1	–

TABLE 73.22 CARCINOMA OF THE UTERINE CERVIX: GRADE 3 SEQUELAE (WASHINGTON UNIVERSITY, 1959–1989)

	Stage				
	IB	IIA	IIB	III	IVA
Total number of patients treated	415	137	391	326	23
Number of complications	26 (6%)	23 (17%)	57 (15%)	45 (14%)	2 (9%)
Rectum–Rectosigmoid					
Rectovaginal fistula	4	2	8	12	1
Rectouterine fistula	1	–	–	–	–
Colovaginal fistula	–	–	1	–	–
Rectal stricture	3	4	4	2	–
Proctitis	2	2	6	2	–
Rectal ulcer	–	–	1	–	–
Sigmoid perforation	1	–	3	1	–
Small Bowel					
Small-bowel obstruction	3	5	12	8	–
Small-bowel perforation	–	–	2	1	–
Enterocolic fistula	1	–	–	–	–
Enterocutaneous fistula	–	1	–	1	–
Enterovaginal fistula	–	–	1	–	–
Enteritis/cachexia	–	–	–	1	–
Urinary					
Vesicovaginal fistula	3	2	6	9	2
Ureterovaginal fistula	–	–	–	1	–
Cystitis	2	–	–	–	–
Bladder ulcer	–	–	–	1	–
Ureteral stricture	5	5	9	4	–
Other					
Postoperative pelvic abscess	–	–	1	1	–
Pulmonary embolus	–	–	1	–	–
Hemorrhage	–	–	1	2	–
Pelvic infection	1	–	–	–	–
Neuritis	–	1	1	–	–

rectosigmoid were approximately 5%. However, the incidence increased to >10% with higher doses of irradiation to these organs (Fig. 73.27). Doses >60 Gy were also correlated with a greater incidence of small-bowel injury (Fig. 73.28). The same analysis showed that patients who experienced sequelae of therapy had slightly better survival rates than patients without any complications. This was related to improved tumor control with higher doses of irradiation.[871]

Perez et al.[873] quantitated the effect of total doses of irradiation, dose rate, and ratio of doses to bladder or rectum and point A on sequelae in 1,456 patients treated for cervical cancer with external beam irradiation plus two LDR intracavitary insertions to deliver 70 to 90 Gy to point A. Median follow-up was 11 years. In stage IB, the frequency of grade 2 morbidity was 9%, and in grade 3, it was 5%; in stages IIA, IIB, III, and IVA, the frequency of grade 2 morbidity was 10% to 12% and that of grade 3 was 10%. The most frequent grade 2 urinary/rectal sequelae were cystitis and proctitis (0.7% to 3%). The most common grade 3 sequelae were vesicovaginal fistula (0.6% to 2% in patients with stage I to III tumors), rectovaginal fistula (0.8% to 3%), and intestinal obstruction (0.8% to 4%). In the bladder, doses <80 Gy correlated with a <3% incidence of morbidity, which was 5% with higher doses (P = .31). In the rectosigmoid, the incidence of significant morbidity was <4% with doses <75 Gy and increased to 9% with higher doses. For the small intestine, the incidence of morbidity was <1% with 50 Gy or less, 2% with 50 to 60 Gy, and 5% with higher doses to the lateral pelvic wall (P = .04). Multivariate analysis showed that dose to the rectal point was the only factor influencing rectosigmoid sequelae and dose to the bladder point affected bladder morbidity.

In a review of the Patterns of Care Study, Lanciano et al.[875] observed a 5-year actuarial rate of 14% for major late complications in 1,558 patients treated with irradiation for invasive carcinoma of the cervix. Women <40 years of age or with a history of prior surgery or laparotomy for staging had a greater incidence of significant morbidity (15% to 18% vs. 8% to 9%). In addition, EBRT dose per fraction of >2 Gy, paracentral doses of 85 Gy or greater, and lateral parametrial doses >60 Gy were independently associated with a higher complication rate.

Lee et al.,[876] using 3-Gy fractions with EBRT, calculated the rectal point dose in the anterior wall at the level of the cervical os and noted that total higher BED (142.7 Gy) was associated with more frequent rectal sequelae compared with BED of <131 Gy.

Mitchell et al.[146] evaluated 398 patients with stage I to III cervical carcinomas treated with radiation therapy. Patients were divided into nonelderly (35 to 69 years of age; n = 338) and elderly (≥70 years of age; n = 60) groups. The frequency and severity of acute and chronic sequelae were equivalent in both groups.

Gastrointestinal Toxicity

When late radiation proctitis occurs, initial treatment is the same as for acute proctitis. If the symptoms and rectal bleeding persist, laser treatment of rectal telangiectasis or ulcers is frequently beneficial. Roche et al.[877] treated six patients with hemorrhagic radiation-induced proctitis using outpatient intrarectal application of formaldehyde 4%. In four cases, the bleeding ceased after the first formaldehyde application; two patients continued to bleed, but another application 3 weeks later definitively controlled the hemorrhage. There were no complications, such as burns or late stenosis

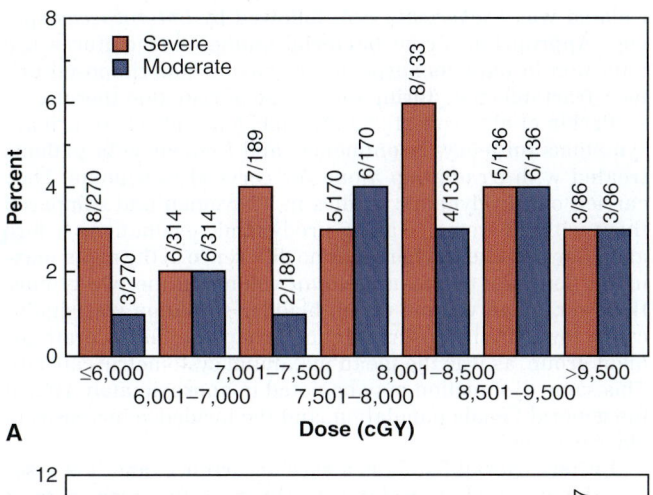

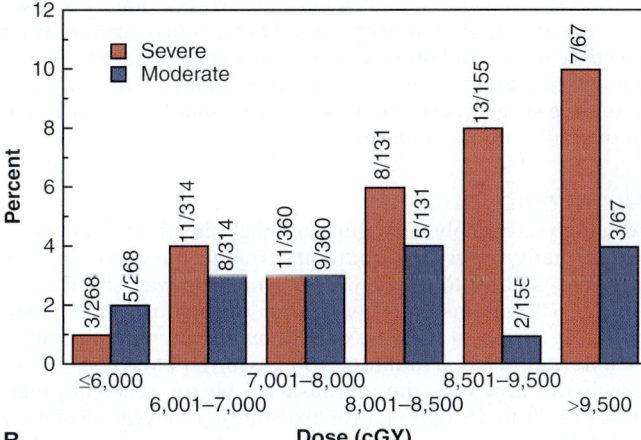

FIGURE 73.27. Incidence of moderate or severe genitourinary **(A)** or rectosigmoid **(B)** complications in patients with carcinoma of the uterine cervix (all stages) treated with irradiation alone (external and brachytherapy). A greater frequency of complications is noted with maximum doses of >75 to 80 Gy to the bladder or rectum.

of the deep layers of the rectum, and this technique was well tolerated. Rubinstein et al.[878] and Seow-Choen et al.[866] also reported treatment of radiation proctitis with a similar technique. Patients are sedated, a local anesthetic block is administered, and a sponge moistened with 4% formalin is applied for 4 minutes to each bleeding area of the rectum. Care is taken to protect the perianal skin from any caustic effects of the formalin.

FIGURE 73.28. Incidence of moderate or severe complications in small intestine correlated with doses of irradiation.

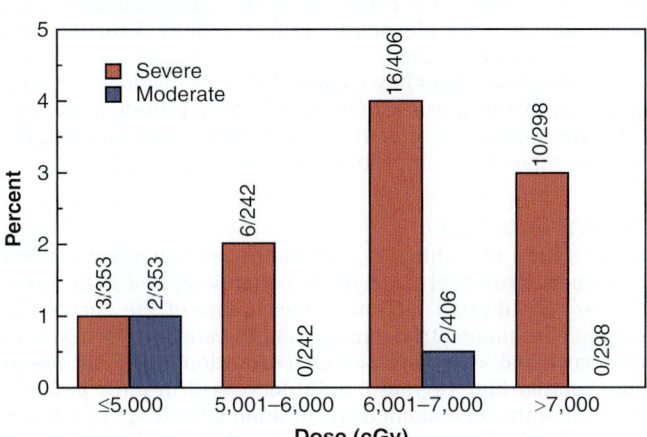

Occasionally, a colostomy is necessary if conservation management fails. The importance of performing colonoscopy in patients with rectal bleeding to exclude other lesions in the colon, including polyps or cancer, is emphasized. If routine screening colonoscopy is not urgent, unless there is a medical reason, the colonoscopy may be postponed until 1 year after pelvic radiation to ensure no issues with poor wound healing, bleeding, or ulceration secondary to biopsy performed at the time of colonoscopy.

Anal incontinence is occasionally observed. This sequela must be assessed in light of a report by Nelson et al.,[879] who in a survey of 6,959 nonirradiated patients, identified 153 (2.2%) who reported anal incontinence, without specific etiology. Thirty percent of incontinent subjects were >65 years of age, and 63% were women. Of those with anal incontinence, 36% were incontinent to solid feces, 54% to liquid feces, and 60% to gas.

Kim et al.[880] investigated the effects of radiation on anorectal function using manometry in 24 patients with carcinoma of the uterine cervix who had late radiation proctitis. These data were compared with those from 24 age-matched nonirradiated female volunteers. Regardless of the severity of proctitis symptoms, 75% of irradiated patients exhibited abnormal manometric parameters for sensory or motor functions. Radiation damage to nerves and to the external sphincter muscle was considered to be an important cause of motor dysfunction.

Quilty[881] noted a greater incidence of pelvic complications in patients treated with higher doses to the whole pelvis (40 to 50 Gy). The author commented that the intracavitary radium dose was not correlated with severe complications. Similar observations were made by Stryker et al.[882] who recorded a 9% incidence of fistulas and a 14% incidence of grade 2 and 3 complications in 132 patients after delivery of 50 Gy or higher to the whole pelvis (1.8-Gy daily dose) combined with intracavitary insertion. They recommended that the whole-pelvis dose should not exceed 40 to 45 Gy when doses of approximately 40 Gy are delivered to point A with LDR intracavitary insertions.

Kuske et al.[780] reported results of therapy in 99 patients with carcinoma of the cervix on whom minicolpostats were used and noted a 15% incidence of grade 2 and 3 complications, which was higher than the 8% incidence noted in a similar group of patients treated with regular colpostats during the same period (P = .08).

Perez et al.[871] reported that the incidence and type of complications with interstitial therapy were approximately the same as in patients treated with intracavitary technique only. In contrast, Kasibhatla et al.[883] noted 6% small-bowel obstruction in 36 women with gynecologic cancer treated with EBRT and interstitial brachytherapy, which was aggravated by previous abdominopelvic surgery. The 3-year risk of rectovaginal fistula was 18%, and it was significantly higher in patients who received total doses of >76 Gy (100% vs. 7%; P = .009).

Irradiation of the PALNs has been reported to cause increased morbidity, particularly if it is done after transperitoneal staging para-aortic lymphadenectomy. In a randomized study reported by Rotman et al.,[884] a somewhat higher incidence of grade 2 and 3 complications was reported in 170 patients (10 complications) given 45 Gy to the para-aortic area in addition to standard pelvic irradiation, compared with 5 complications in 167 patients treated by pelvic irradiation only. The incidence of fatal (grade 5) complications was 4 and 1, respectively. In a similar randomized study by Haie et al.[574] for the EORTC, the incidence of grade 3 small-bowel injury was 2.3% in the para-aortic irradiation group and 0.9% in the pelvic irradiation–only group. The overall incidences of severe complications were 9% and 4.8%, respectively.

Willett et al.[885] reported on 28 patients with inflammatory bowel disease (10 with Crohn disease, 18 with ulcerative colitis) who underwent external beam abdominal or pelvic irradiation. Patients were treated either by specialized techniques (16 patients) to minimize small- and large-bowel irradiation or by conventional approaches (12 patients). The overall incidence of severe toxicity was 46% (13 of 28 patients), and 6 patients (21%) experienced severe acute toxicity necessitating cessation of radiation therapy. Late toxicity requiring hospitalization or surgical intervention was observed in 8 of 28 patients (29%). For patients treated with conventional approaches, the 5-year actuarial rate of late toxicity was 73% versus 23% for patients treated by specialized techniques (P = .02). In patients with inflammatory bowel disease, abdominal or pelvic irradiation must be used judiciously.

In contrast, Song et al.,[440] in a review of 24 patients with a history of inflammatory bowel disease who received RT (median dose of 45 Gy in 1.8- to 3-Gy fractions) to fields encompassing some portion of the gastrointestinal tract, noted that 5 patients (21%) experienced acute intestinal toxicity of grade 3 or greater and 2 (8%) had grade 3 or greater late intestinal toxicity. Fifteen patients also received concurrent chemotherapy. The authors believed that the gastrointestinal toxicity in these patients was more modest than generally perceived. Tiersten and Saltz[886] noted that five patients with inflammatory bowel disease and gastrointestinal malignancy completed planned radiation therapy (30 to 54 Gy), usually with concurrent 5-FU, without difficulty.

Salama et al.[475] reported preliminary observations on acute toxicity with extended-field IMRT in 13 patients with gynecologic cancer. With median follow-up of 11 months, 2 patients treated with chemoradiation experienced grade 3 or higher morbidity, and 1 (with a history of previous surgeries) developed small-bowel obstruction.

Levenback et al.[887] identified 116 of 1,784 patients (6.5%) with stage IB carcinoma of the cervix treated with irradiation in whom hemorrhagic cystitis developed, 23% grade 2 (repeated minor bleeding) and 18% grade 3 (hospitalization required for medical management). The median interval to onset of hematuria was 35.5 months. The risk of severe hematuria requiring surgical intervention was 1.4% at 10 years and 2.3% at 20 years. Minor episodes of hematuria are managed by antibiotic therapy. Cystoscopic, laser, or cautery treatment of bleeding points is indicated. Clot evacuation and continuous bladder irrigation are important elements in the acute management of patients with heavy bleeding. Occasionally, a urinary diversion is required for intractable severe hematuria.

Genitourinary Toxicity

Ureteral stricture at 20 years was observed in 2.5% of 1,784 patients with stage IB carcinoma of the cervix treated with irradiation (274 followed for up to 20 years or longer).[888] The most common presenting symptoms were flank pain and urinary tract infection. In 5 patients, ureteral stricture was complicated by a vesicovaginal fistula. Seven of 43 patients who had no evidence of cancer and had hydroureter or hydronephrosis died of radiation complications. Treatment of ureteral stenosis may consist of stenting or resection of the fibrotic segment and reimplantation of the ureter with either ureteroneocystostomy or ureteroileocystostomy. In approximately half of the patients, diversion of urinary stream and ileal conduits are necessary. Occasionally, a nephrectomy is performed for removal of a nonfunctional kidney. Buglione et al.[889] reported a 10% incidence of late urinary morbidity and 1% ureteral fibrosis, grade III or IV, in 191 patients. They postulated the role of TGF-β_1 in the activation of fibroblasts and remodeling of extracellular matrix, which may be important in the induction of these sequelae.

Patients with gynecologic malignancies, including those receiving radiation therapy, are prone to development of urinary tract infections. Prasad et al.[890] collected 216 urine samples from 36 patients receiving pelvic irradiation, 12 of whom had urinary tract infection. The most common organism

isolated was *Escherichia coli*, followed by *Enterococcus* species. Appropriate urine bacterial studies and cultures are indicated in patients suspected of having superimposed urinary tract infection during the course of radiation therapy.

Parkin et al.[891] reported a 26% incidence of severe urinary symptoms (urgency, incontinence, and frequency) in patients treated with irradiation alone for cervical carcinoma. They carried out urodynamic studies in 42 women and compared them with 28 women having urodynamic evaluations before and after treatment. There was no difference in the mean maximum flow rate or mean *residual* volume in the two groups. However, mean volume of full bladder sensation was significantly lower in the postirradiation group than in the pretreatment group, as was the mean maximum cystometric capacity. This same dysfunction may be noted in approximately 10% of the general female population, and the incidence increases in older women.[326]

Ureteroarterial fistula is a rare occurrence, and it is associated with a high mortality rate. When profuse urinary tract bleeding occurs in patients previously diagnosed with a gynecologic malignancy and treated with radiation therapy and extensive surgery, ureteroarterial fistula should be considered in the differential diagnoses.[892]

Neurologic Toxicity

Although extremely rare, lumbosacral plexopathy has been occasionally reported in patients treated for pelvic tumors with doses of 60 to 67.5 Gy. This syndrome was observed in 4 of 2,410 patients with cervical or endometrial carcinoma receiving 45 Gy to the PALNs (without spinal cord shielding) or external pelvic irradiation (60 Gy to the parametria) and brachytherapy, with the lumbosacral plexus receiving total doses of 70 to 79 Gy.[893] Lower extremity paralysis secondary to lumbosacral plexopathy was reported in one patient after standard radiation therapy for cervical cancer.[894]

Patients previously reported as having radiation myelopathy to the lumbar spine may have suffered a lumbar and sacral nerve plexopathy instead of or in addition to the spinal cord injury. The differential diagnosis of plexopathy with recurrent tumors is sometimes difficult. In a comparison of 20 patients with lumbosacral plexopathy after irradiation and 30 patients with plexus damage from pelvic malignancy, Thomas et al.[895] noted that indolent leg weakness occurred early in radiation-induced plexopathy (pain occurred initially in 10% of patients, although ultimately it was present in 50%), whereas pain was most frequently associated with tumor plexopathy. Muscular weakness, numbness, and paresthesia are common in both groups. Electromyography showed abnormal myokymic discharges in 57% of patients, whereas this finding was very unusual in tumor-induced plexopathy. CT is extremely helpful in the detection of pelvic masses or bone destruction caused by tumor. The authors also reported extensive retroperitoneal fibrosis of the lumbosacral plexus in two patients and femoral nerve fibrosis with plexopathy in one patient. Although cystometrograms have demonstrated bladder atonicity in some cases, several authors have failed to observe bladder or rectal sphincter disturbances. Unfortunately, as in radiation myelopathy, the neurologic deficit is irreversible, and no effective therapy other than supportive care has been found.

Sexual Function

Other types of clinically significant sequelae have been described. Bruner et al.,[896] in 90 patients treated with intracavitary irradiation for either carcinoma of the cervix (42 patients) or endometrial carcinoma (48 patients), 78 of whom also received external pelvic irradiation (44.5-Gy mean dose), noted that vaginal length decreased in most patients (at 24 months, in endometrial carcinoma from 8.8 to 7.8 cm, and in cervical carcinoma from 7.6 to 6.2 cm). Pretreatment sexual activity was reported by 31% of women in comparison with 43% after treatment. However, 22% of women reported a decrease in sexual frequency and 37% a decrease in sexual satisfaction. This was correlated with increased dyspareunia, which was noted in 31% of women treated for carcinoma of the cervix and 44% of those treated for endometrial carcinoma. Grigsby et al.[897] described complex problems with sexual adjustment in women with gynecologic tumors treated with radiation therapy, with decreased frequency of sexual intercourse, desire, orgasm, and enjoyment of intercourse in 16% to 47% of patients.

Lammerink et al. published a systemic review of 20 studies on sexual functioning of cervical cancer survivors. Survivors had a higher rate of dyspareunia compared to controls, with pain during intercourse reported more frequently and for a longer duration of time in patients treated with radiotherapy.[898]

Regular vaginal dilation is widely recommended to maintain vaginal health and sexual functioning; however, the compliance rate with this recommendation is not consistent. In a study to test the effectiveness of an "information–motivation–behavior skills" model, the intervention improved the use of vaginal dilation after radiotherapy and decreased fear about sex after treatment.[899] There was no evidence that the experimental intervention improved global sexual health. Jensen et al.[900] described persistent sexual dysfunction throughout 2 years after RT in 118 women; 85% had low or no sexual interest, 35% had lack of vaginal lubrication, and 55% had mild to severe dyspareunia. However, 63% of the sexually active patients before RT remained active, although with decreased frequency.

Radiation causes ovarian failure with a cessation of menses over a 6-month to 1-year period after treatment. Radiation also causes uterine fibrosis in a dose-dependent fashion. The dose required for radical cervical cancer treatment causes sufficient uterine fibrosis that even if a woman were to become pregnant through embryo donation, the pregnancy terminates as a stillbirth because of insufficient uterine distensibility.[623,775]

Bone Toxicity

Grigsby et al.,[901] in 1,313 patients with gynecologic tumors treated with radiation therapy, identified 207 who received pelvic irradiation to the inguinal areas, including the hips. Femoral neck fractures developed in 10 patients (4.8%); 4 were bilateral. The cumulative actuarial incidence of fracture was 11% at 5 years and 15% at 10 years. Most of the fractures occurred in patients receiving 45 to 63 Gy, and although radiation dose could not be correlated with the occurrence of fracture, no fractures were noted in patients receiving <42 Gy. Cigarette smoking and osteoporosis were significant prognostic factors for increased risk of fracture.

A retrospective cohort study using SEER cancer registry data linked to Medicare claims data analyzed 6,428 women of age 65 years and older diagnosed with pelvic malignancies from 1986 through 1999, and compared results for women who did ($n = 2,855$) with those who did not ($n = 3,573$) undergo radiation therapy. Results demonstrated that women who underwent radiation therapy were more likely to have a pelvic fracture than women who did not undergo radiation therapy. The cumulative 5-year fracture rate was 8.2% versus 5.9% in women with cervical cancer; the difference was statistically significant, and most fractures (90%) were hip fractures.[902] Concurrent chemoradiation may result in a higher risk than for patients treated with RT alone because the highest fracture rates were seen in patients with anal carcinoma treated with concurrent chemoradiation.

Blomlie et al.[903] reported radiation-induced insufficiency fractures of the pelvis on MRI (characterized by edema on T1-weighted images) in 16 of 18 women (9 premenopausal and 9 postmenopausal) with advanced cervical carcinoma. During the study, the fractures associated with edema

subsided without treatment in 41 of 52 (79%) lesions in 15 of 16 (94%) patients. Moreno et al.[904] described eight patients with pelvic cancer who developed insufficiency fractures after pelvic irradiation, with an average onset of 13.7 months after treatment. The bone and CT scan showed abnormalities in the sacroiliac joint in all cases and in the pubis in three cases. In five patients, the initial diagnosis was incorrectly labeled as bone metastases. In patients over 50 years old, a sacrum D50% reduced from 40Gy to 35 Gy EQD2 reduced fracture risk from 45% to 22%.[905]

Huh et al.[906] reported on 463 patients treated for cervical cancer with RT alone, 1.7% of whom developed insufficiency fractures between 7 and 19 months (median, 12 months) after treatment. All had resolution of symptoms within <1 year with conservative therapy, including nonsteroidal anti-inflammatory medication and rest.

The most common complaint is persistent low back pain. Insufficiency fractures may be falsely diagnosed as metastases on PET–CT. The most common form of treatment is conservative management, followed by sacroplasty with polymethylmethacrylate. Bye et al.[907] assessed health-related quality of life (HRQOL) at 3 to 4 years after pelvic radiation therapy for carcinoma of the endometrium and cervix in 94 survivors, 79 (84%) of whom answered a survey. The treated women scored lower than the general population on role functioning (81.5 vs. 90.6; $P < .01$) and higher on diarrhea (23.8 vs. 9.5; $P < .01$). Compared with pretreatment conditions, an increase in cases with pain in the lower back, hips, and thighs was seen and was associated with deterioration in HRQOL.

Toxicities Related to Brachytherapy

Descriptions of sequelae vary among institutions because toxicity-grading scales are not uniform and the scoring system for complications is not clearly stated in all reports. It is helpful to institute preventive measures when initiating radiation; for example, Dusenbery et al.[908] reported 21 (6.4%) life-threatening complications in 327 of 462 patient implants. Lanciano et al.,[909] in 95 tandem and ovoid insertions for cervical cancer in 91 patients and for endometrial cancer in 4, observed 2 uterine perforations and a vaginal laceration in 2 patients. Twenty-four percent of implants in 16 patients were associated with temperatures >100.5°F. Five implants (5%) were removed because of presumed sepsis, pulmonary disease, arterial hypotension, change in mental status, and myocardial infarction.

Jhingran and Eifel,[910] in 4,043 patients with carcinoma of the cervix who had undergone 7,662 intracavitary procedures, observed 11 (0.3%) documented or suspected thromboembolisms, resulting in 4 deaths; the incidence of postimplant thromboembolism did not decrease significantly with the routine use of minidose heparin prophylaxis. Other life-threatening perioperative complications included myocardial infarction (1 death in 5 patients), cerebrovascular accident (2 patients), congestive heart failure (3 patients), and halothane liver toxicity (2 deaths). Intraoperative complications included uterine perforation (2.8%) and vaginal laceration (0.3%), which occurred more frequently in patients 60 years of age or older ($P < .01$).

Wollschlaeger et al.[911] reported morbidity during hospitalization in 128 patients with cervical carcinoma undergoing 110 LDR intracavitary brachytherapy insertions. Forty-two implants (24.7%) were associated with acute problems; the most common were fever/infection (14.1%) or gastrointestinal problems (5.9%).

Acute gastrointestinal side effects of pelvic irradiation include diarrhea, abdominal cramping, rectal discomfort, and occasionally rectal bleeding, which may be caused by transient enteroproctitis. Patients with hemorrhoids may experience discomfort earlier than other patients. Diarrhea and abdominal cramping can be controlled with the oral administration of diphenoxylate hydrochloride, with loperamide, atropine sulfate, or opium preparations or emollients such as kaolin and pectin. Proctitis and rectal discomfort can be alleviated by small enemas with hydrocortisone and anti-inflammatory suppositories containing bismuth, benzyl benzoate, zinc oxide, or Peruvian balsam. Some suppositories contain cortisone. Small enemas with cod liver oil are also effective. A low-residue diet with no grease or spices and increased fiber in the stool (psyllium, polycarbophil) usually helps to decrease gastrointestinal symptoms.

Genitourinary symptoms secondary to cystourethritis are dysuria, frequency, and nocturia. The urine is usually clear, although there may be microscopic or even gross hematuria. Methenamine mandelate and antispasmodics such as phenazopyridine hydrochloride or a smooth muscle antispasmodic such as flavoxate hydrochloride, hyoscyamine sulfate, oxybutynin chloride, or tolterodine tartrate can relieve symptoms. Fluid intake should be at least 2,000 to 2,500 mL daily. Urinary tract infections may occur; diagnosis should be established with appropriate urine culture studies, including sensitivity to sulfonamides and antibiotics. Therapy should be promptly instituted.

Erythema and dry or moist desquamation may develop in the perineum or intergluteal fold. Proper skin hygiene and topical application of petroleum jelly, petrolatum, or lanolin should relieve these symptoms. U.S.P. zinc oxide ointment and intensive skin care may be needed for severe cases.

Management of acute radiation vaginitis includes douching every day or at least three times weekly with a 1:5 mixture of hydrogen peroxide and water. Douching should be continued on a weekly basis until the mucositis has resolved or for 2 or 3 months as necessary. Superficial ulceration of the vagina responds to topical (intravaginal) estrogen creams, which stimulate epithelial regeneration within 3 months after irradiation. Use of vaginal dilators several times daily, started during the course of treatment, prevents vaginal stenosis. Psychoeducational intervention and motivation improve the compliance in use of dilators.[912] More severe necrosis may require debridement on a weekly basis until healing takes place. Judicious use of biopsies is recommended to rule out persistent or recurrent cancer.

Petereit et al.[913] reported 16 acute events (9.5%) in 169 patients treated with HDR brachytherapy (128 with cervical cancer also receiving external irradiation and 41 medically inoperable endometrial carcinomas). The overall 30-day morbidity rate for the patients with cervical cancer was 5.5%, and the 30-day mortality rate was 1.6% (2 patients; 1 died of pulmonary edema 12 days after first HDR insertion and the other had enteritis and died in a nursing home).

The complication rates for HDR and LDR techniques are usually equivalent.[645,647] Petereit et al.[643] observed a 12% 3-year actuarial overall toxicity (2.6% genitourinary and 5.6% rectum) with LDR, compared to 15% overall (3% genitourinary and 4.6% rectum) with HDR brachytherapy. However, in the series by Cikaric,[759] the rectal complication rate was significantly higher in the LDR group. Bladder complication rates reported, in general, are lower than rectal complication rates; again, except for the series by Cikaric[759] showing a higher complication rate with the LDR technique, there were no significant differences with the two techniques.

Ogino et al.,[914] in 253 patients with invasive carcinoma of the cervix treated with HDR brachytherapy, noted that grade 4 rectal complications were not observed in patients with a time–dose factor of <130 or biologic equivalent dose of <147, assuming an α/β ratio of 3 Gy for late reactions.

Spontaneous intraperitoneal rupture of the urinary bladder, an extremely rare event, was reported by Fujikawa et al.[915] after radiation therapy for cervical cancer in 6 of 148 patients treated with HDR intracavitary brachytherapy combined with EBRT. All 6 patients underwent laparotomy and repair of the perforation; however, rerupture of the bladder occurred in 3 of these patients.

Clark et al.[916] reported on 43 patients treated with pelvic EBRT (46 Gy) and three HDR intracavitary treatments given weekly combined with concomitant chemotherapy (cisplatin, 30 mg/m² weekly) for advanced carcinoma of the cervix. At 40 months after treatment, 9 of 13 patients who received a dose to the rectal reference point greater than the prescribed point A dose had a 46% actuarial rate of serious (grade 3 and 4) rectal complications, compared with 14% in the remainder. A strong dose response was observed, with a threshold for complications at a brachytherapy dose of 8 Gy per fraction.

Hyperbaric Oxygen

In 13 patients with hemorrhagic cystitis treated with hyperbaric oxygen, all but 1 experienced durable cessation of hematuria.[917] Lee et al.[918] also noted that, in 16 of 20 patients (80%) with hemorrhagic radiation cystitis, significant improvement was observed after treatment with hyperbaric oxygen at 2.5 atm (44 sessions).

Several reports evaluated the efficacy of hyperbaric oxygen combined with irradiation in the treatment of a variety of human tumors, including carcinoma of the uterine cervix. Watson et al.,[919] in a randomized clinical trial of 320 patients (stages III to IVA), reported a 5-year survival rate of 33% in the oxygen-treated group in contrast to 27% in the control group treated in normal air (P = .08). The local recurrence rate was 33% in the 161 patients treated with oxygen and 53% in 159 patients treated in normal air (P < .001). Morbidity in the patients treated with oxygen was greater (20 severe and 13 moderate complications) than in those treated in normal air (6 severe and 8 moderate complications, respectively). The difference was particularly striking in the bowel (13 and 2 severe complications, respectively).

Dische et al.[920] reviewed the data in a randomized study of patients with advanced carcinoma of the cervix treated with radiation therapy and hyperbaric oxygen or air and noted that the patients treated with oxygen had improved survival at Mount Vernon and Glasgow but not at Cape Town. Data from the three centers were merged, and analysis showed that local tumor control was significantly worse in patients treated in normal air who had a prior blood transfusion, but in the oxygen group, this effect was reversed. The same interaction was noted in the survival results (P = .042).

A trial reported by Fletcher[186] in which 233 patients with stage IIB, III, and IV carcinomas of the cervix were randomized to be treated with irradiation in normal air or with hyperbaric oxygen demonstrated no significant benefit in survival or tumor control (20 of 109 patients treated with oxygen failed in the pelvis, in contrast to 29 of 124 treated in normal air). Furthermore, morbidity was greater (26 complications) in patients treated with hyperbaric oxygen compared with the control group (15 complications).

Dische et al.[920] published results of a four-arm randomized trial of hyperbaric oxygen and radiation therapy of stage IIB and III carcinomas of the cervix in which 335 patients were randomized to treatment in 10 or 28 fractions in hyperbaric oxygen or in normal air. Data from 327 cases were analyzed. There was no advantage in tumor control with the use of hyperbaric oxygen. There was an increase in late radiation morbidity when treatment was given in hyperbaric oxygen rather than in normal air, and when using 10 fractions, a total dose of 45 Gy rather than 40 Gy was administered.

No definite conclusions can be drawn concerning the use of hyperbaric oxygen in carcinoma of the cervix. It is possible that hyperbaric oxygen administered with fewer high-dose fractions may be more efficacious than when combined with conventional dose and fractionation schemes. The trials reported have not shown an increased incidence of distant metastasis, which has been observed in a clinical study and in some animal experiments.[921]

Hormonal Replacement After Treatment of Cervical Cancer

After pelvic irradiation or bilateral salpingo-oophorectomy, usually carried out with a radical hysterectomy in patients treated for carcinoma of the uterine cervix, symptoms of menopause may occur. They can be treated with replacement hormones, although some gynecologists have expressed reservations. During the past 25 years, hormonal replacement therapy has been shown to reduce the risk of cardiovascular diseases, osteoporotic fractures, and colon carcinoma. On the other hand, there is a significant increase of the risk in breast cancer with prolonged use of estrogen plus progesterone for >5 years. Consideration may be given to progesterone alone, which does not increase the risk of endometrial cancer but has potential thromboembolic risks.[922]

Burger et al.[923] concluded that squamous cell cancers of the cervix, vulva, and vagina are unlikely to be influenced by hormonal replacement therapy. In a study of women 50 years of age or younger with ovarian cancer, estrogen replacement therapy did not have a negative influence on DFS. Long-term hormonal replacement therapy in women treated for a gynecologic cancer must be based on the medical history of and discussion of risk with the individual patient (and her family when warranted). Usually, 0.625 to 1.25 mg of coagulated estrogen daily is sufficient.[924]

Second Malignancy

The risk for induction of secondary primary cancers by pelvic irradiation is low, and many potential confounders either are unknown or may not be fully accounted for, given the available information.[925] Using the population-based cancer registries of Denmark, Finland, Norway, Sweden, and the United States, Chaturvedi et al.[926] found a significantly increased cancer risk in both SCC and AC survivors, with standardized incidence ratio of 1.31 (95% CI = 1.29 to 1.34) and 1.29 (95% CI = 1.22 to 1.38), respectively. The risk of smoking-related lung cancer was higher in the SCC than in the AC population, whereas second malignancies of the colon, soft tissue, melanoma, and non-Hodgkin lymphoma were higher in the AC population. Similarly, 1-year survivors of cervical cancer had an increased risk of HPV-related cancers, including pharynx, genital, and anal cancers. Higher HRs for second cancer of the rectum, anus, bladder, and genital sites was seen for younger patients, with a 40-year cumulative risk of any second cancer of 22% for women diagnosed with cervical cancer before age 50 years versus 16% for those diagnosed at age >50 years.[927] In contrast, Lee et al.[928] observed no significant increase in the incidence of second malignancies in patients irradiated for carcinoma of the cervix in comparison with the Connecticut Tumor Registry prevailing rates.

Boice et al.,[369] in a review of 68,730 women with carcinoma of the cervix treated with radiation therapy, observed a second malignant tumor in 3,324, compared with 3,063 expected (4.8% increase; $P < .001$). The excess was concentrated in the lung, other genital organs, the bladder, and the rectum. In addition, in 10,817 women with invasive cervical cancer not treated with irradiation, 479 secondary malignant tumors were observed versus 435 expected (4.4%; $P = .02$). Thus, the incidence of secondary tumors in women treated for carcinoma of the cervix with or without irradiation is only slightly greater than in the general population. Pelvic organs receiving a high dose of irradiation appear to have a somewhat greater incidence of a second primary.

Storm,[929] in a comprehensive analysis of the Danish Cancer Registry data of 24,970 women with invasive cervical cancer and 19,470 with carcinoma *in situ* of the cervix treated between 1943 and 1982, noted a small overall excess of secondary primary cancers in the lung, stomach, pancreas, rectum, and bladder and connective tissue sarcomas, although there was a decreased incidence of breast cancer in the irradiated patients compared with nonirradiated patients (attributable to ovarian ablation by radiation therapy). In the patients irradiated for invasive carcinoma, there was an excess of 64 cases per 10,000 women per year of tumors in organs close to or at an intermediate distance from the cervix, reaching a maximum after 30 years or longer of follow-up. A high risk for development of acute nonlymphatic leukemia was observed in irradiated patients with carcinoma *in situ* but not in those with invasive lesions. This could be explained by the lower doses of irradiation delivered to the bone marrow in the *in situ* tumors treated with brachytherapy alone, with greater induction of mutations and less cell killing, which may be responsible for the leukemogenic effect. Decreased risk was noted for tumors of the brain, myeloma of the skin, and tumors of the colon other than rectal.

In a study of 117,830 women diagnosed with cervical carcinoma *in situ* and 17,556 with invasive cervical carcinoma in Sweden, treatment not specified and *in situ* lesions traditionally treated with surgery alone, there was an increased incidence (RR = 2.3 to 3) of second primary tumors in the anus, rectum, urinary bladder, pancreas, esophagus, and lung compared with the standardized incidence rate for all women.[930] The data showed consistent increases in suggested targets for HPV at tobacco-related sites. A contributing role for a depressed immune response was considered.

Werner-Wasik et al.,[931] in an analysis of 125 women with stage I and II carcinomas of the cervix treated with radiation therapy, observed 11 secondary primary tumors in 10 patients (4 breast, 2 lung, and 1 each of myeloma, non-Hodgkin lymphoma, bladder, thyroid, and vulva). All secondary primary tumors were located outside the irradiation fields. The increased RR of breast cancer in these patients was 2.64, higher than reported by Boice et al.[369]

In an analysis of 199,268 individuals by Wright et al.,[932] the risk of secondary leukemia increased 72% in patients who received pelvic radiotherapy, with a peak at 5 to 10 years after treatment; there was no increased risk of multiple myeloma. Mark et al.[933] identified 13 of 114 patients diagnosed with uterine sarcoma who had a prior history of pelvic irradiation (doses of 40 to 80 Gy). Criteria for radiation-induced sarcomas included a prior history of pelvic irradiation, a latent period of several years, development of sarcoma within previously irradiated field, and histologic confirmation of malignancy. Histologic types of tumor were mixed Müllerian in 6, leiomyosarcoma in 4 patients, endometrial stroma sarcoma in 1, fibrosarcoma in 1, and angiosarcoma in 1. Sarcoma developed in the uterus in 12 patients and at the vaginal cuff in 1 patient. Ten patients were treated with surgery and 2 with radiation therapy. The 5-year DFS rate after salvage therapy was 17%.

In a theoretical analysis of IMRT risk in postoperative cases relative to 3D conformal radiotherapy, the estimated increase in second cancer risk was 6% for 6-MV IMRT and 26% for 18 MV IMRT, with large increases in organs away from the primary beam and skin because with IMRT a much larger volume of skin was exposed.[934]

Seidman et al.[935] reviewed 15 cases of second malignancies after pelvic radiation; 5 were HPV-related vaginal primary tumors. The average latency period for development was approximately 20 years.

Kleinerman et al. reviewed 53,547 5-year survivors of cervical cancer from 5 population-based cancer registries. Over 90% were treated with radiation; there was a significant, linear dose–response relationship for the risk of stomach cancer (OR 4.2 for dose of 5Gy or higher).[936]

SELECTED REFERENCES

A full list of references for this chapter is available online.

REFERENCES

1. Anson BJ, McVay CB. *Surgical anatomy. 5th ed.* Philadelphia: W. B. Saunders, 1971, 800–835.

1a. Kraima AC, Derks M, Smit NN, et al. Lymphatic drainage pathways from the cervix uteri: implications for radical hysterectomy? *Gynecol Oncol* 2014;132(1):107–113.

2. WHO. *Age-standardized incidence rates of cervical cancer.* 2009.

3. *Cancer facts and figures.* Atlanta, GA: American Cancer Society, 2017.

4. World Health Organization. Globocan 2012: Estimated cancer incidence, mortality and prevalence worldwide in 2012. http://globocan.iarc.fr/Pages/fact_sheets_cancer.aspx. Accessed July 8, 2017.

4a. Global Burden of Disease Cancer Collaboration, Fitzmaurice C, Allen C, Barber RM, et al. Global, regional, and national cancer incidence, mortality, years of life lost, years lived with disability, and disability-adjusted life-years for 32 Cancer Groups, 1990 to 2015: a systematic analysis for the global burden of disease study. *JAMA Oncol* 2017;3(4):524–548. doi:10.1001/jamaoncol.2016.5688.

5. Chakraborty S, Mahantshetty U, Chopra S, et al. Income generated by women treated with magnetic resonance imaging-based brachytherapy: a simulation study evaluating the macroeconomic benefits of implementing a high-end technology in a public sector healthcare setting. *Brachytherapy* 2017;16(5):981–987. doi:10.1016/j.brachy.2017.05.003.

6. Hochman A, Ratzkowski E, Schreiber H. Incidence of carcinoma of the cervix in Jewish women in Israel. *Br J Cancer* 1955;9(3):358–364.

7. Bosch FX, Lorincz A, Munoz N, et al. The causal relation between human papillomavirus and cervical cancer. *J Clin Pathol* 2002;55:244–265.

8. World Health Organization. Human papillomavirus and related cancers, 2010. Available at: http://apps.who.int/hpvcentre/statistics/dynamic/ico/country_pdf/XWX.pdf?CFID=5541015. Accessed March 1, 2012

9. zur Hausen H. Papillomaviruses causing cancer: evasion from host-cell control in early events in carcinogenesis. *J Natl Cancer Inst* 2000;92(9):690–698.

9a. Cancer Genome Atlas Research Network. Integrated genomic and molecular characterization of cervical cancer. *Nature* 2017;543(7645):378–384. doi:10.1038/nature21386.

10. Franco EL, Villa LL, Sobrinho JP, et al. Epidemiology of acquisition and clearance of cervical human papillomavirus infection in women from a high-risk area for cervical cancer. *J Infect Dis* 1999;180(5):1415–1423.

11. Ho GY, Bierman R, Beardsley L, et al. Natural history of cervicovaginal papillomavirus infection in young women. *N Engl J Med* 1998;338(7):423–428.

12. Christopherson WM, Parker JE. Relation of cervical cancer to early marriage and childbearing. *N Engl J Med* 1965;273:235–239.

13. Keighley E. Carcinoma of the cervix among prostitutes in a women's prison. *Br J Vener Dis* 1968;44:254–255.

14. Vriend HJ, Boot HJ, van der Sande MA; Medical Microbiological Laboratories, Municipal Health Services. Type-specific human papillomavirus infections among young heterosexual male and female STI clinic attendees. *Sex Transm Dis* 2012;39(1):72–78.

15. Nahmias AJ, Naib ZM, Josey WE. Epidemiological studies relating genital herpetic infection to cervical carcinoma. *Cancer Res* 1974;34:1111–1117.

16. Agarwal SS, Sehgal A, Sardana S, et al. Role of male behavior in cervical carcinogenesis among women with one lifetime sexual partner. *Cancer* 1993;72:1666–1669.

17. Iversen T, Tretli S, Johansen A, et al. Squamous cell carcinoma of the penis and of the cervix, vulva and vagina in spouses: is there any relationship? an epidemiological study from Norway, 1960–92. *Br J Cancer* 1997;76:658–660.

18. Boon ME, Susanti I, Tasche MJ, et al. Human papillomavirus (HPV)-associated male and female genital carcinomas in a Hindu population. the male as vector and victim. *Cancer* 1989;64:559–565.

19. Terris M, Wilson F, Nelson JH Jr. Relation of circumcision to cancer of the cervix. *Am J Obstet Gynecol* 1973;117(8):1056–1066.

20. Lynch HT, Watson P, Lynch JF. Hereditary ovarian cancer: heterogeneity in age at onset. *Cancer* 1993;71(Suppl):573–581.

21. Joo J, Shin HJ, Park B, et al. Integration pattern of human papillomavirus is a strong prognostic factor for disease-free survival after radiation therapy in cervical cancer patients. *Int J Radiat Oncol Biol Phys* 2017;98(3):654–661.

22. Joneja MG, Coulson DB. Histopathology and cytogenetics of tumors induced by the application of 7,12-dimethybenz(a)anthracene (DMBA) in mouse cervix. *Eur J Cancer* 1973;9:367–374.

23. Drill VA. Oral contraceptives: relations to mammary cancer, benign breast lesions, and cervical cancer. *Annu Rev Pharmacol* 1975;15:367–385.

24. Green J, Berrington de Gonzalez A, Smith JS, et al. Human papillomavirus infection and use of oral contraceptives. *Br J Cancer* 2003;88:1713–1720.

25. Kaminski PF, Maier RC. Clear cell adenocarcinoma of the cervix unrelated to diethylstilbestrol exposure. *Obstet Gynecol* 1983;62:720–727.

26. Herbst AL, Cole PL. Epidemiologic and clinical aspects of clear cell adenocarcinoma in young women. In: *Gynecology.* Chicago, IL: American College of Obstetrics Gynecology, 1978:2–7.

27. Becker TM, Wheeler CM, McGough NS, et al. Sexually transmitted diseases and other risk factors for cervical dysplasia among southwestern Hispanic and non-Hispanic white women. *JAMA* 1994;271:1181–1188.

28. Gram IT, Austin H, Stalsberg H. Cigarette smoking and the incidence of cervical intraepithelial neoplasia, grade III, and cancer of the cervix uteri. *Am J Epidemiol* 1992;135(4):341–346.

29. Louie KS, Castellsague X, de Sanjose S, et al. Smoking and passive smoking in cervical cancer risk: pooled analysis of couples from the IARC multicentric case-control studies. *Cancer Epidemiol Biomarkers Prev* 2011;20(7):1379–1390.

30. Szarewski A. Smoking and cervical neoplasia: a review of the evidence. *J Epidemiol Biostat* 1998;3:229–256.

31. Palefsky JM, Minkoff H, Kalish LA, et al. Cervicovaginal human papillomavirus infection in human immunodeficiency virus-1 (HIV)-positive and high-risk HIV-negative women. *J Natl Cancer Inst* 1999;91:226–236.

32. Castellsague X, Diaz M, Vaccarella S, et al. Intrauterine device use, cervical infection with human papillomavirus, and risk of cervical cancer: a pooled analysis of 26 epidemiological studies. *Lancet Oncol* 2011;12(11):1023–1031.

33. Joura EA, Giuliano AR, Iversen OE, et al. A 9-valent HPV vaccine against infection and intraepithelial neoplasia in women. *N Engl J Med* 2015;372(8):711–723.

33a. Bruni L, Diaz M, Barrionuevo-Rosas L, et al. Global estimates of human papillomavirus vaccination coverage by region and income level: a pooled analysis. *Lancet Glob Health* 2016;4:e453–e463.

34. Barron BA, Richart RM. Statistical model of the natural history of cervical carcinoma. II. Estimates of the transition time from dysplasia to carcinoma in situ. *J Natl Cancer Inst* 1970;45:1025–1030.

35. Bohm JW, Krupp PJ, Lee FY, et al. Lymph node metastasis in microinvasive epidermoid cancer of the cervix. *Obstet Gynecol* 1976;48:65–67.

36. Inoue T, Okumura M. Prognostic significance of parametrial extension in patients with cervical carcinoma stages IB, IIA, and IIB. A study of 628 cases treated by radical hysterectomy and lymphadenectomy with or without postoperative irradiation. *Cancer* 1984;54:1714–1719.

37. Landoni F, Maneo A, Colombo A, et al. Randomised study of radical surgery versus radiotherapy for stage Ib-IIa cervical cancer. *Lancet* 1997;350:535–540.

38. Perez CA, Camel HM, Askin F, et al. Endometrial extension of carcinoma of the uterine cervix: a prognostic factor that may modify staging. *Cancer* 1981;48(1):170–180.

39. Chao KSC, Grigsby PW, Mutch D, et al. Prognostic factors for distant metastasis in carcinoma of the cervix with endometrial extension. *J Brachyther Int* 2000;16:181–186.

40. Girardi F, Lichtenegger W, Tamussino K, et al. The importance of parametrial lymph nodes in the treatment of cervical cancer. *Gynecol Oncol* 1989;34:206–211.

41. Henriksen E. The lymphatic spread of carcinoma of the cervix and of the body of the uterus; a study of 420 necropsies. *Obstet Gynecol* 1949;58:924–942.

42. Alvarez RD, Soong SJ, Kinney WK, et al. Identification of prognostic factors and risk groups in patients found to have nodal metastasis at the time of radical hysterectomy for early-stage squamous carcinoma of the cervix. *Gynecol Oncol* 1989;35:130–135.

43. Delgado G, Bundy BN, Fowler WC, et al. A prospective surgical pathological study of stage I squamous carcinoma of the cervix: a gynecologic oncology group study. *Gynecol Oncol* 1989;35:314–320.

44. Piver MS, Chung WS. Prognostic significance of cervical lesion size and pelvic node metastases in cervical carcinoma. *Obstet Gynecol* 1975;46:507–510.

45. Fine BA, Hempling RE, Piver MS, et al. Severe radiation morbidity in carcinoma of the cervix: impact of pretherapy surgical staging and previous surgery. *Int J Radiat Oncol Biol Phys* 1995;31:717–723.

46. Wharton JT, Jones HWI, Day TG, et al. Preirradiation celiotomy and extended field irradiation for invasive carcinoma of the cervix. *Obstet Gynecol* 1977;49:333–338.

47. Huang H, Liu J, Li Y, et al. Metastasis to deep obturator and para-aortic lymph nodes in 649 patients with cervical carcinoma. *Eur J Surg Oncol* 2011;37:978–983.

48. Canton-Romero J, Anaya-Prado R, Rodriguez-Garcia H, et al. Laparoscopic radical hysterectomy with the use of a modified uterine manipulator for the management of stage IB1 cervix cancer. *J Obstet Gynaecol* 2010;30:49–52.

49. Gortzak-Uzan L, Jimenez W, Nofech-Mozes S, et al. Sentinel lymph node biopsy vs. pelvic lymphadenectomy in early stage cervical cancer: is it time to change the gold standard? *Gynecol Oncol* 2010;116:28–32.

50. Leblanc E, Gauthier H, Querleu D, et al. Accuracy of 18-fluoro-2-deoxy-D-glucose positron emission tomography in the pretherapeutic detection of occult para-aortic node involvement in patients with a locally advanced cervical carcinoma. *Ann Surg Oncol* 2011;18(8):2302–2309.

51. Perez CA, Camel HM, Kao MS, et al. Randomized study of preoperative radiation and surgery or irradiation alone in the treatment of stage IB and IIA carcinoma of the uterine cervix: final report. *Gynecol Oncol* 1987;27:129–140.

52. Lagasse LD, Creasman WT, Shingleton HM, et al. Results and complications of operative staging in cervical cancer: experience of the Gynecologic Oncology Group. *Gynecol Oncol* 1980;9:90–98.

53. Nelson JH Jr, Boyce J, Macasaet M, et al. Incidence, significance, and follow-up of para-aortic lymph node metastases in late invasive carcinoma of the cervix. *Obstet Gynecol* 1977;128:336–340.

54. Piver MS, Barlow JJ, Krishnamsetty R. Five-year survival (with no evidence of disease) in patients with biopsy-confirmed aortic node metastasis from cervical carcinoma. *Obstet Gynecol* 1981;139:575–578.

55. Rutledge TL, Kamelle SA, Tillmanns TD, et al. A comparison of stages IB1 and IB2 cervical cancers treated with radical hysterectomy. is size the real difference? *Gynecol Oncol* 2004;95:70–76.

56. Benedetti-Panici P, Maneschi F, Scambia G, et al. Lymphatic spread of cervical cancer: an anatomical and pathological study based on 225 radical hysterectomies with systematic pelvic and aortic lymphadenectomy. *Gynecol Oncol* 1996;62:19–24.

57. Fagundes H, Perez CA, Grigsby PW, et al. Distant metastases after irradiation alone in carcinoma of the uterine cervix. *Int J Radiat Oncol Biol Phys* 1992;24:197–204.

58. Ampil FL, Apple S, Bell MC. Spinal epidural compression complicating cancer of the cervix: review of seven cases. *Eur J Gynaecol Oncol* 1998;19:105–107.

59. Mahmoud-Ahmed A, Suh JH, Barnett GH, et al. Tumor distribution and survival in six patients with brain metastases from cervical carcinoma. *Gynecol Oncol* 2001;81:196–200.

60. Viswanathan AN, Deavers MT, Jhingran A, et al. Small cell neuroendocrine carcinoma of the cervix: outcome and patterns of recurrence. *Gynecol Oncol.* 2004;93(1):27–33.

61. American College of Obstetricians and Gynecologists. *Guidelines for women's health care: a resource manual*, Washington, DC: Author, 2009.

62. Committee on Practice Bulletins-Gynecology. ACOG Practice Bulletin Number 131: screening for cervical cancer. *Obstet Gynecol* 2012;120(5):1222–1238.

63. Kern W, Zivolich MR. The accuracy and consistency of the cytologic classification of squamous lesions of the uterine cervix. *Acta Cytol* 1977;21(4):519–523.

64. Solomon D, Davey D, Kurman R, et al. The 2001 Bethesda system: terminology for reporting results of cervical cytology. *JAMA* 2002;287:2114–2119.

65. Massad LS, Einstein MH, Huh WK, et al. 2012 Updated consensus guidelines for the management of abnormal cervical cancer screening tests and cancer precursors. *J Low Genit Tract Dis* 2013;17(5 Suppl 1):S1–S27.

66. Shastri SS, Mittra I, Mishra GA, et al. Effect of VIA screening by primary health workers: randomized controlled study in Mumbai, India. *J Natl Cancer Inst* 2014;106(3):dju009.

67. Novak ER, Jones GS, Jones HW. *Novak's textbook of gynecology.* Williams and Wilkins,1970.

68. Kim SH, Choi BI, Han JK, et al. Preoperative staging of uterine cervical carcinoma: comparison of CT and MRI in 99 patients. *J Comput Assist Tomogr* 1993;17(4):633–640.

69. Lagasse LD, Ballon SC, Berman MS, et al. Pretreatment lymphangiography and operative evaluation in carcinoma of the cervix. *Obstet Gynecol* 1979;134:219–224.

70. Kim SH, Han MC. Invasion of the urinary bladder by uterine cervical carcinoma: evaluation with MR imaging. *AJR Am J Roentgenol* 1997;168:393–397.

71. Mitchell DG, Snyder B, Coakley F, et al. Early invasive cervical cancer: MRI and CT predictors of lymphatic metastases in the ACRIN 6651/GOG 183 intergroup study. *Gynecol Oncol* 2009;112(1):95–103.

72. Camilien L, Gordon D, Fruchter RG, et al. Predictive value of computerized tomography in the presurgical evaluation of primary carcinoma of the cervix. *Gynecol Oncol* 1988;30:209–215.

73 Kilcheski TS, Arger PH, Mulhern CB, et al. Role of computed tomography in the presurgical evaluation of carcinoma of the cervix. *J Comput Assist Tomogr* 1981;5:378–383.

74. Yildirim Y, Sehirali S, Avci ME, et al. Integrated PET/CT for the evaluation of para-aortic nodal metastasis in locally advanced cervical cancer patients with negative conventional CT findings. *Gynecol Oncol* 2008;108:154–159.

75. Atri M, Zhang Z, Dehdashti F, et al. Utility of PET-CT to evaluate retroperitoneal lymph node metastasis in advanced cervical cancer: results of ACRIN6671/GOG0233 trial. *Gynecol Oncol* 2016;142(3):413–419.

76. Heller PB, Malfetano JH, Bundy BN, et al. Clinical-pathologic study of stage IIB, III, and IVA carcinoma of the cervix: extended diagnostic evaluation for para-aortic node metastasis—a gynecologic oncology group study. *Gynecol Oncol* 1990;38:425–430.

77. Wong F, Bhimji S. The usefulness of ultrasonography in intracavitary radiotherapy using selectron applicators. *Int J Radiat Oncol Biol Phys* 1990;19:477–482.

78. Viswanathan AN, Moughan J, Small W, et al. The quality of cervical cancer brachytherapy implantation and the impact on local recurrence and disease-free survival in Radiation Therapy Oncology Group prospective trials 0116 and 0128. *Int J Gynecol Cancer* 2012;22:123–131.

79. Liu FY, Yen TC, Chen MY, et al. Detection of hematogenous bone metastasis in cervical cancer: 18F-fluorodeoxyglucose-positron emission tomography versus computed tomography and magnetic resonance imaging. *Cancer* 2009;115(23):5470–5480.

80. Hricak H, Powell CB, Yu KK, et al. Invasive cervical carcinoma: role of MR imaging in pretreatment work-up—cost minimization and diagnostic efficacy analysis. *Radiology* 1996;198:403–409.

81. Ascher SM, Cooper C, Scoutt L, et al. Diagnostic imaging techniques in gynecologic oncology. In: Hoskins WJ, Perez CA, Young RC, eds. *Principles and practice of gynecologic oncology.* 4th ed. Philadelphia: Lippincott Williams & Wilkins, 2005:223–266.

82. Sironi S, Belloni C, Taccagni GL, et al. Carcinoma of the cervix: value of MR imaging in detecting parametrial involvement. *AJR Am J Roentgenol* 1991;156:753–756.

83. Hawnaur JM, Johnson RJ, Carrington BM, et al. Predictive value of clinical examination, transrectal ultrasound and magnetic resonance imaging prior to radiotherapy in carcinoma of the cervix. *Br J Radiol* 1998;71:819–827.

84. Postema S, Pattynama PM, van den Berg-Huysmans A, et al. Effect of MRI on therapeutic decisions in invasive cervical carcinoma. Direct comparison with the pelvic examination as a preoperative test. *Gynecol Oncol* 2000;79:485–489.

85. Hansen MA, Pedersen PH, Andreasson B, et al. Staging uterine cervical carcinoma with low-field MR imaging. *Acta Radiol* 2000;41:647–652.

86. Mitchell DG, Snyder B, Coakley F, et al. Early invasive cervical cancer: tumor delineation by magnetic resonance imaging, computed tomography, and clinical examination, verified by pathologic results, in the ACRIN 6651/GOG 183 intergroup study. *J Clin Oncol* 2006;24(36):5687–5694.

87. Hricak H, Gatsonis C, Coakley FV, et al. Early invasive cervical cancer: CT and MR imaging in preoperative evaluation—ACRIN/GOG comparative study of diagnostic performance and interobserver variability. *Radiology* 2007;245(2):491–498.

88. Haider MA, Patlas M, Jhaveri K, et al. Adenocarcinoma involving the uterine cervix: magnetic resonance imaging findings in tumours of endometrial, compared with cervical, origin. *Can Assoc Radiol J* 2006;57:43–48.

89. Kodaira T, Fuwa N, Kamata M, et al. Clinical assessment by MRI for patients with stage II cervical carcinoma treated by radiation alone in multicenter analysis: are all patients with stage II disease suitable candidates for chemoradiotherapy? *Int J Radiat Oncol Biol Phys* 2002;52:627–636.

90. Ebner F, Kressel HY, Mintz MC, et al. Tumor recurrence versus fibrosis in the female pelvis: differentiation with MR imaging at 1.5 T. *Radiology* 1988;166:333–340.

91. Corn BW, Schnall MD, Milestone B, et al. Signal characteristics of tumors shown by high-resolution endorectal coil magnetic resonance imaging may predict outcome among patients with cervical carcinoma treated with irradiation. A preliminary study. *Cancer* 1996;78:2535–2542.

92. Mayr NA, Yuh WT, Magnotta VA, et al. Tumor perfusion studies using fast magnetic resonance imaging technique in advanced cervical cancer: a new noninvasive predictive assay. *Int J Radiat Oncol Biol Phys* 1996;36:623–633.

93. Hatano K, Sekiya Y, Araki H, et al. Evaluation of the therapeutic effect of radiotherapy on cervical cancer using magnetic resonance imaging. *Int J Radiat Oncol Biol Phys* 1999;45:639–644.

94. Gong QY, Brunt JN, Romaniuk CS, et al. Contrast enhanced dynamic MRI of cervical carcinoma during radiotherapy: early prediction of tumour regression rate. *Br J Radiol* 1999;72:1177–1184.

95. van de Bunt L, van der Heide UA, Ketelaars M, et al. Conventional, conformal, and intensity-modulated radiation therapy treatment planning of external beam radiotherapy for cervical cancer: the impact of tumor regression. *Int J Radiat Oncol Biol Phys* 2006;64:189–196.

96. Dimopoulos JC, Schard G, Berger D, et al. Systematic evaluation of MRI findings in different stages of treatment of cervical cancer: potential of MRI on delineation of target, pathoanatomic structures, and organs at risk. *Int J Radiat Oncol Biol Phys* 2006;64:1380–1388.

97. Rose PG, Adler LP, Rodriguez M, et al. Positron emission tomography for evaluating para-aortic nodal metastasis in locally advanced cervical cancer before surgical staging: a surgicopathologic study. *J Clin Oncol* 1999;17:41–45.

98. Grigsby PW, Siegel BA, Dehdashti F. Lymph node staging by positron emission tomography in patients with carcinoma of the cervix. *J Clin Oncol* 2001;19:3745–3749.

99. Grigsby PW, Siegel BA, Dehdashti F, et al. Posttherapy surveillance monitoring of cervical cancer by FDG-PET. *Int J Radiat Oncol Biol Phys* 2003;55:907–913.

100. Grigsby PW, Siegel BA, Dehdashti F, et al. Posttherapy [18F] fluorodeoxyglucose positron emission tomography in carcinoma of the cervix: response and outcome. *J Clin Oncol* 2004;22:2167–2171.

101. Grigsby PW, Singh AK, Siegel BA, et al. Lymph node control in cervical cancer. *Int J Radiat Oncol Biol Phys* 2004;59:706–712.

102. Hope AJ, Saha P, Grigsby PW. FDG-PET in carcinoma of the uterine cervix with endometrial extension. *Cancer* 2006;106:196–200.

103. Lin LL, Yang Z, Mutic S, et al. FDG-PET imaging for the assessment of physiologic volume response during radiotherapy in cervix cancer. *Int J Radiat Oncol Biol Phys* 2006;65:177–181.

104. Kidd EA, Grigsby PW. Intratumoral metabolic heterogeneity of cervical cancer. *Clin Cancer Res* 2008;14:5236–5241.

105. Kidd EA, Siegel BA, Dehdashti F, et al. The standardized uptake value for F-18 fluorodeoxyglucose is a sensitive predictive biomarker for cervical cancer treatment response and survival. *Cancer* 2007;110:1738–1744.

106. Kidd EA, Siegel BA, Dehdashti F, et al. Pelvic lymph node F-18 fluorodeoxyglucose uptake as a prognostic biomarker in newly diagnosed patients with locally advanced cervical cancer. *Cancer* 2010;116:1469–1475.

107. Kidd EA, Siegel BA, Dehdashti F, et al. Lymph node staging by positron emission tomography in cervical cancer: relationship to prognosis. *J Clin Oncol* 2010;28:2108–2113.

108. Kidd EA, Spencer CR, Huettner PC, et al. Cervical cancer histology and tumor differentiation affect 18F-fluorodeoxyglucose uptake. *Cancer* 2009;115:3548–3554.

109. Tran BN, Grigsby PW, Dehdashti F, et al. Occult supraclavicular lymph node metastasis identified by FDG-PET in patients with carcinoma of the uterine cervix. *Gynecol Oncol* 2003;90:572–576.

110. Schwarz JK, Grigsby PW, Dehdashti F, et al. The role of 18F-FDG PET in assessing therapy response in cancer of the cervix and ovaries. *J Nucl Med* 2009;50(Suppl 1):64S–73S.

111. Schwarz JK, Lin LL, Siegel BA, et al. 18-F-fluorodeoxyglucose-positron emission tomography evaluation of early metabolic response during radiation therapy for cervical cancer. *Int J Radiat Oncol Biol Phys* 2008;72:1502–1507.

112. Schwarz JK, Siegel BA, Dehdashti F, et al. Association of posttherapy positron emission tomography with tumor response and survival in cervical carcinoma. *JAMA* 2007;298:2289–2295.

113. Schwarz JK, Siegel BA, Dehdashti F, et al. Metabolic response on posttherapy FDG-PET predicts patterns of failure after radiotherapy for cervical cancer. *Int J Radiat Oncol Biol Phys* 2012;83(1):185–190.

114. Horn LC, Fischer U, Raptis G, et al. Tumor size is of prognostic value in surgically treated FIGO stage II cervical cancer. *Gynecol Oncol* 2007;107(2):310–315.

115. American Joint Committee on Cancer. *AJCC cancer staging handbook.* 7th ed. New York: Springer, 2010.

116. Kraus FT, Perezmesa C. Verrucous carcinoma. Clinical and pathologic study of 105 cases involving oral cavity, larynx and genitalia. *Cancer* 1966;19:26–38.

117. Look KY, Brunetto VL, Clarke-Pearson D, et al. An analysis of cell type in patients with surgically staged stage IB carcinoma of the cervix: a Gynecologic Oncology Group study. *Gynecol Oncol* 1996;63:304–311.

118. Drescher CW, Hopkins MP, Roberts JA. Comparison of the pattern of metastatic spread of squamous cell cancer and adenocarcinoma of the uterine cervix. *Gynecol Oncol* 1989;33:340–343.

Section III

119. Chao A, Wang TH, Lee YS, et al. Molecular characterization of adenocarcinoma and squamous carcinoma of the uterine cervix using microarray analysis of gene expression. *Int J Cancer* 2006;119:91–98.

120. Contag SA, Gostout BS, Clayton AC, et al. Comparison of gene expression in squamous cell carcinoma and adenocarcinoma of the uterine cervix. *Gynecol Oncol* 2004;95:610–617.

121. An HJ, Kim KR, Kim IS, et al. Prevalence of human papillomavirus DNA in various histological subtypes of cervical adenocarcinoma: a population-based study. *Mod Pathol* 2005;18:528–534.

122. Silverberg SG, Hurt WG. Minimal deviation adenocarcinoma ("adenoma malignum") of the cervix: a reappraisal. *Obstet Gynecol* 1975;121:971–975.

123. Srivatsa PJ, Keeney GL, Podratz KC. Disseminated cervical adenoma malignum and bilateral ovarian sex cord tumors with annular tubules associated with Peutz-Jeghers syndrome. *Gynecol Oncol* 1994;53(2):256–264.

124. Ulbright TM, Gersell DJ. Glassy cell carcinoma of the uterine cervix. A light and electron microscopic study of five cases. *Cancer* 1983;51:2255–2263.

125. Littman P, Clement PB, Henriksen B, et al. Glassy cell carcinoma of the cervix. *Cancer* 1976;37:2238–2246.

126. Piura B, Rabinovich A, Meirovitz M, et al. Glassy cell carcinoma of the uterine cervix. *J Surg Oncol* 1999;72:206–210.

127. Gordon HW, McMahon NJ, Agliozzo CM, et al. Adenoid cystic (cylindromatous) carcinoma of the uterine cervix: report of two cases. *Am J Clin Pathol* 1972;58:51–57.

128. Nishida M, Nasu K, Takai N, et al. Adenoid cystic carcinoma of the uterine cervix. *Int J Clin Oncol* 2005;10:198–200.

129. Clement PB, Zubovits JT, Young RH, et al. Malignant Müllerian mixed tumors of the uterine cervix: a report of nine cases of a neoplasm with morphology often different from its counterpart in the corpus. *Int J Gynecol Pathol* 1998;17:211–222.

130. Abeler VM, Holm R, Nesland JM, et al. Small cell carcinoma of the cervix. A clinicopathologic study of 26 patients. *Cancer* 1994;73:672–677.

131. Gersell DJ, Mazoujian G, Mutch DG, et al. Small-cell undifferentiated carcinoma of the cervix. A clinicopathologic, ultrastructural, and immunocytochemical study of 15 cases. *Am J Surg Pathol* 1988;12:684–698.

132. Ishida GM, Kato N, Hayasaka T, et al. Small cell neuroendocrine carcinomas of the uterine cervix: a histological, immunohistochemical, and molecular genetic study. *Int J Gynecol Pathol* 2004;23:366–372.

133. Van Nagell JR Jr, Powell DE, Gallion HH, et al. Small cell carcinoma of the uterine cervix. *Cancer* 1988;62:1586–1593.

133a. Zhou J, Wu SG, Sun JY, et al. Clinicopathological features of small cell carcinoma of the uterine cervix in the surveillance, epidemiology, and end results database. *Oncotarget* 2017;8(25):40425–40433. doi:10.18632/oncotarget.16390.

134. Daroca PJ Jr, Dhurandhar HN. Basaloid carcinoma of uterine cervix. *Am J Surg Pathol* 1980;4:235–239.

135. Layton-Henry J, Scurry J, Planner R, et al. Cervical adenoid basal carcinoma: five cases and literature review. *Int J Gynecol Cancer* 1996;6:193–199.

136. Toyoshima M, Okamura C, Niikura H, et al. Epithelioid leiomyosarcoma of the uterine cervix: a case report and review of the literature. *Gynecol Oncol* 2005;97:957–960.

137. el Omari-Alaoui H, Kebdani T, Benjaafar N, et al. [Non-Hodgkin's lymphoma of the uterus: apropos of 4 cases and review of the literature]. *Cancer Radiother* 2002;6:39–45.

138. Bozaci EA, Atabekoglu C, Sertcelik A, et al. Metachronous metastases from renal cell carcinoma to uterine cervix and vagina: case report and review of literature. *Gynecol Oncol* 2005;99:232–235.

139. Pauer HU, Viereck V, Burfeind P, et al. Uterine cervical metastasis of breast cancer: a rare complication that may be overlooked. *Onkologie* 2003;26:58–60.

140. Shimada M, Kigawa J, Nishimura R, et al. Ovarian metastasis in carcinoma of the uterine cervix. *Gynecol Oncol* 2006;101:234–237.

141. Rose PG, Java J, Whitney CW, et al. Nomograms predicting progression-free survival, overall survival, and pelvic recurrence in locally advanced cervical cancer developed from an analysis of identifiable prognostic factors in patients from NRG Oncology/Gynecologic Oncology Group Randomized Trials of chemoradiotherapy. *J Clin Oncol* 2015;33(19):2136–2142.

142. Delaloye JF, Pampallona S, Coucke PA, et al. Younger age as a bad prognostic factor in patients with carcinoma of the cervix. *Eur J Obstet Gynecol Reprod Biol* 1996;64:201–205.

143. Dattoli MJ, Gretz HF, Beller U, et al. Analysis of multiple prognostic factors in patients with stage IB cervical cancer: age as a major determinant. *Int J Radiat Oncol Biol Phys* 1989;17:41–47.

144. Meanwell CA, Kelly KA, Wilson S, et al. Young age as a prognostic factor in cervical cancer: analysis of population based data from 10,022 cases. *Br Med J (Clin Res Ed)* 1988;296:386–391.

145. Rutledge FN, Mitchell MF, Munsell M, et al. Youth as a prognostic factor in carcinoma of the cervix: a matched analysis. *Gynecol Oncol* 1992;44:123–130.

146. Mitchell PA, Waggoner S, Rotmensch J, et al. Cervical cancer in the elderly treated with radiation therapy. *Gynecol Oncol* 1998;71:291–298.

147. Mundt AJ, Connell PP, Campbell T, et al. Race and clinical outcome in patients with carcinoma of the uterine cervix treated with radiation therapy. *Gynecol Oncol* 1998;71:151–158.

148. Grigsby PW, Hall-Daniels L, Baker S, et al. Comparison of clinical outcome in black and white women treated with radiotherapy for cervical carcinoma. *Gynecol Oncol* 2000;79:357–361.

149. Brooks SE, Chen TT, Ghosh A, et al. Cervical cancer outcomes analysis: impact of age, race, and comorbid illness on hospitalizations for invasive carcinoma of the cervix. *Gynecol Oncol* 2000;79:107–115.

150. Katz A, Eifel PJ, Moughan J, et al. Socioeconomic characteristics of patients with squamous cell carcinoma of the uterine cervix treated with radiotherapy in the 1992 to 1994 patterns of care study. *Int J Radiat Oncol Biol Phys* 2000;47:443–450.

151. Hirst DG. Anemia: a problem or an opportunity in radiotherapy? *Int J Radiat Oncol Biol Phys* 1986;12:2009–2017.

152. Kavanagh BD, Secomb TW, Hsu R, et al. A theoretical model for the effects of reduced hemoglobin-oxygen affinity on tumor oxygenation. *Int J Radiat Oncol Biol Phys* 2002;53:172–179.

153. Sundfør K, Lyng H, Kongsgard UL, et al. Polarographic measurement of pO2 in cervix carcinoma. *Gynecol Oncol* 1997;64:230–236.

154. Hockel M, Schlenger K, Mitze M, et al. Hypoxia and radiation response in human tumors. *Semin Radiat Oncol* 1996;6:3–9.

155. Knocke TH, Weitmann HD, Feldmann HJ, et al. Intratumoral pO2-measurements as predictive assay in the treatment of carcinoma of the uterine cervix. *Radiother Oncol* 1999;53:99–104.

156. Rofstad EK, Sundfor K, Lyng H, et al. Hypoxia-induced treatment failure in advanced squamous cell carcinoma of the uterine cervix is primarily due to hypoxia-induced radiation resistance rather than hypoxia-induced metastasis. *Br J Cancer* 2000;83:354–359.

157. Cooper RA, West CM, Logue JP, et al. Changes in oxygenation during radiotherapy in carcinoma of the cervix. *Int J Radiat Oncol Biol Phys* 1999;45:119–126.

158. Dunst J, Hansgen G, Lautenschlager C, et al. Oxygenation of cervical cancers during radiotherapy and radiotherapy + cis-retinoic acid/interferon. *Int J Radiat Oncol Biol Phys* 1999;43:367–373.

159. Fyles AW, Pintilie M, Kirkbride P, et al. Prognostic factors in patients with cervix cancer treated by radiation therapy: results of a multiple regression analysis. *Radiother Oncol* 1995;35:107–117.

160. Haensgen G, Krause U, Becker A, et al. Tumor hypoxia, p53, and prognosis in cervical cancers. *Int J Radiat Oncol Biol Phys* 2001;50:865–872.

161. Bush RS. The significance of anemia in clinical radiation therapy. *Int J Radiat Oncol Biol Phys* 1986;12:2047–2050.

162. Fyles AW, Milosevic M, Pintilie M, et al. Anemia, hypoxia and transfusion in patients with cervix cancer: a review. *Radiother Oncol* 2000;57:13–19.

163. Thomas G. In: The effect of hemoglobin level on radiotherapy outcomes: The Canadian experience. *Seminars in oncology*. Elsevier, 2001:60–65.

164. Dunst J, Kuhnt T, Strauss HG, et al. Anemia in cervical cancers: impact on survival, patterns of relapse, and association with hypoxia and angiogenesis. *Int J Radiat Oncol Biol Phys* 2003;56:778–787.

165. Munstedt K, Johnson P, Bohlmann MK, et al. Adjuvant radiotherapy in carcinomas of the uterine cervix: the prognostic value of hemoglobin levels. *Int J Gynecol Cancer* 2005;15:285–291.

166. Grogan M, Thomas GM, Melamed I, et al. The importance of hemoglobin levels during radiotherapy for carcinoma of the cervix. *Cancer* 1999;86:1528–1536.

167. Kapp KS, Poschauko J, Geyer E, et al. Evaluation of the effect of routine packed red blood cell transfusion in anemic cervix cancer patients treated with radical radiotherapy. *Int J Radiat Oncol Biol Phys* 2002;54:58–66.

168. Vaupel P, Mayer A, Hockel M. Impact of hemoglobin levels on tumor oxygenation: the higher, the better? *Strahlenther Onkol* 2006;182:63–71.

169. Bishop AJ, Allen PK, Klopp AH, et al. Relationship between low hemoglobin levels and outcomes after treatment with radiation or chemoradiation in patients with cervical cancer: has the impact of anemia been overstated? *Int J Radiat Oncol Biol Phys* 2015;91(1):196–205.

170. Thomas G, Ali S, Hoebers FJ, et al. Phase III trial to evaluate the efficacy of maintaining hemoglobin levels above 12.0 g/dL with erythropoietin vs above 10.0 g/dL without erythropoietin in anemic patients receiving concurrent radiation and cisplatin for cervical cancer. *Gynecol Oncol* 2008;108(2):317–325.

171. Blohmer J, Paepke S, Sehouli J, et al. Randomized phase III trial of sequential adjuvant chemoradiotherapy with or without erythropoietin alfa in patients with high-risk cervical cancer: results of the NOGGO-AGO intergroup study. *J Clin Oncol* 2011;29(28):3791–3797.

172. Jenkin R, Stryker J. The influence of the blood pressure on survival in cancer of the cervix. *Br J Radiol* 1968;41(492):913–920.

173. Kapp DS, Lawrence R. Temperature elevation during brachytherapy for carcinoma of the uterine cervix: adverse effect on survival and enhancement of distant metastasis. *Int J Radiat Oncol Biol Phys* 1984;10:2281–2292.

174. Campbell OB, Arowojolu AO, Adu FD, et al. Human immunodeficiency virus antibody in patients with cancer of the uterine cervix undergoing radiotherapy: clinical stages, histological grade and outcome of radiotherapy. *J Obstet Gynaecol* 1999;19:403–405.

175. Klevens RM, Fleming PL, Mays MA, et al. Characteristics of women with AIDS and invasive cervical cancer. *Obstet Gynecol* 1996;88:269–273.

176. Wright TC Jr, Ellerbrock TV, Chiasson MA, et al. Cervical intraepithelial neoplasia in women infected with human immunodeficiency virus: prevalence, risk factors, and validity of Papanicolaou smears. New York Cervical Disease Study. *Obstet Gynecol* 1994;84:591–597.

177. Tomita LY, Costa MC, Andreoli MAA, et al. Diet and serum micronutrients in relation to cervical neoplasia and cancer among low-income Brazilian women. *Int J Cancer* 2010;126(3):703–714.

178. Cho H, Kim MK, Lee JK, et al. Relationship of serum antioxidant micronutrients and sociodemographic factors to cervical neoplasia: a case-control study. *Clin Chem Lab Med* 2009;47(8):1005–1012.

179. Goodman MT, Kiviat N, McDuffie K, et al. The association of plasma micronutrients with the risk of cervical dysplasia in hawaii. *Cancer Epidemiol Biomarkers Prev* 1998;7(6):537–544.

180. Ethier JL, Desautels DN, Templeton AJ, et al. Is the neutrophil-to-lymphocyte ratio prognostic of survival outcomes in gynecologic cancers? A systematic review and meta-analysis. *Gynecol Oncol* 2017;145(3):584–594.

181. Lai C, Chang C, Huang H, et al. Role of human papillomavirus genotype in prognosis of early-stage cervical cancer undergoing primary surgery. *J Clin Oncol* 2007;25(24):3628–3634.

182. Lai C, Huang H, Hsueh S, et al. Human papillomavirus genotype in cervical cancer: a population-based study. *Int J Cancer* 2007;120(9):1999–2006.

183. Wang CC, Lai CH, Huang HJ, et al. Clinical effect of human papillomavirus genotypes in patients with cervical cancer undergoing primary radiotherapy. *Int J Radiat Oncol Biol Phys* 2010;78:1111–1120.

184. Finan MA, DeCesare S, Fiorica JV, et al. Radical hysterectomy for stage IB1 vs IB2 carcinoma of the cervix: does the new staging system predict morbidity and survival? *Gynecol Oncol* 1996;62:139–147.

185. Toita T, Nakano M, Higashi M, et al. Prognostic value of cervical size and pelvic lymph node status assessed by computed tomography for patients with uterine cervical cancer treated by radical radiation therapy. *Int J Radiat Oncol Biol Phys* 1995;33:843–849.

186. Fletcher GH. Cancer of the uterine cervix. Janeway lecture, 1970. *Am J Roentgenol* 1971;111(2):224–242.

187. Eifel PJ, Morris M, Wharton JT, et al. The influence of tumor size and morphology on the outcome of patients with FIGO stage IB squamous cell carcinoma of the uterine cervix. *Int J Radiat Oncol Biol Phys* 1994;29:9–16.

188. Perez CA, Grigsby PW, Nene SM, et al. Effect of tumor size on the prognosis of carcinoma of the uterine cervix treated with irradiation alone. *Cancer* 1992;69:2796–2806.

189. Eifel PJ, Thoms WW Jr, Smith TL, et al. The relationship between brachytherapy dose and outcome in patients with bulky endocervical tumors treated with radiation alone. *Int J Radiat Oncol Biol Phys* 1994;28:113–118.

190. Perez CA, Grigsby PW, Chao KS, et al. Tumor size, irradiation dose, and long-term outcome of carcinoma of uterine cervix. *Int J Radiat Oncol Biol Phys* 1998;41:307–317.

191. Leveque J, Laurent JF, Burtin F, et al. Prognostic factors of the uterine cervix adenocarcinoma. *Eur J Obstet Gynecol Reprod Biol* 1998;80:209–214.

192. Silver DF, Hempling RE, Piver MS, et al. Stage I adenocarcinoma of the cervix: does lesion size affect treatment options and prognosis? *Am J Clin Oncol* 1998;21:431–435.

193. Grigsby PW, Perez CA, Chao KS, et al. Lack of effect of tumor size on the prognosis of carcinoma of the uterine cervix stage IB and IIA treated with preoperative irradiation and surgery. *Int J Radiat Oncol Biol Phys* 1999;45: 645–651.

194. Grimard L, Genest P, Girard A, et al. Prognostic significance of endometrial extension in carcinoma of the cervix. *Gynecol Oncol* 1986;31:301–309.

195. Noguchi H, Shiozawa I, Kitahara T, et al. Uterine body invasion of carcinoma of the uterine cervix as seen from surgical specimens. *Gynecol Oncol* 1988;30:173–182.

196. Galic V, Herzog TJ, Lewin SN, et al. Prognostic significance of adenocarcinoma histology in women with cervical cancer. *Gynecol Oncol* 2012;125(2): 287–291.

197. Rose PG, Java JJ, Whitney CW, et al. Locally advanced adenocarcinoma and adenosquamous carcinomas of the cervix compared to squamous cell carcinomas of the cervix in Gynecologic Oncology Group trials of cisplatin-based chemoradiation. *Gynecol Oncol* 2014;135(2):208–212.

198. Estape RE, Angioli R, Madrigal M, et al. Close vaginal margins as a prognostic factor after radical hysterectomy. *Gynecol Oncol* 1998;68:229–232.

199. Hong JH, Tsai CS, Lai CH, et al. Postoperative low-pelvic irradiation for stage I-IIA cervical cancer patients with risk factors other than pelvic lymph node metastasis. *Int J Radiat Oncol Biol Phys* 2002;53:1284–1290.

200. Viswanathan AN, Lee H, Hanson E, et al. Influence of margin status and radiation on recurrence after radical hysterectomy in stage IB cervical cancer. *Int J Radiat Oncol Biol Phys* 2006;65:1501–1507.

201. Alfsen GC, Kristensen GB, Skovlund E, et al. Histologic subtype has minor importance for overall survival in patients with adenocarcinoma of the uterine cervix: a population-based study of prognostic factors in 505 patients with non-squamous cell carcinomas of the cervix. *Cancer* 2001;92:2471–2483.

202. Chen F, Trapido EJ, Davis K. Differences in stage at presentation of breast and gynecologic cancers among whites, blacks, and Hispanics. *Cancer* 1994;73:2838–2842.

203. Waldenstrom AC, Horvath G. Survival of patients with adenocarcinoma of the uterine cervix in western Sweden. *Int J Gynecol Cancer* 1999;9: 18–23.

204. Reagan JW, Fu YS. Histologic types and prognosis of cancers of the uterine cervix. *Int J Radiat Oncol Biol Phys* 1979;5:1015–1020.

205. Crissman JD, Budhraja M, Aron BS, et al. Histopathologic prognostic factors in stage II and III squamous cell carcinoma of the uterine cervix. an evaluation of 91 patients treated primarily with radiation therapy. *Int J Gynecol Pathol* 1987;6:97–103.

206. Monk BJ, Wang J, Im S, et al. Rethinking the use of radiation and chemotherapy after radical hysterectomy: a clinical-pathologic analysis of a Gynecologic Oncology Group/Southwest Oncology Group/Radiation Therapy Oncology Group trial. *Gynecol Oncol* 2005;96:721–728.

207. Petereit DG, Sarkaria JN, Chappell R, et al. The adverse effect of treatment prolongation in cervical carcinoma. *Int J Radiat Oncol Biol Phys* 1995;32:1301–1307.

208. Fyles A, Keane TJ, Barton M, et al. The effect of treatment duration in the local control of cervix cancer. *Radiother Oncol* 1992;25:273–279.

209. Girinsky T, Rey A, Roche B, et al. Overall treatment time in advanced cervical carcinomas: a critical parameter in treatment outcome. *Int J Radiat Oncol Biol Phys* 1993;27:1051–1056.

210. Lanciano RM, Pajak TF, Martz K, et al. The influence of treatment time on outcome for squamous cell cancer of the uterine cervix treated with radiation: a patterns-of-care study. *Int J Radiat Oncol Biol Phys* 1993;25: 391–397.

211. Chatani M, Matayoshi Y, Masaki N, et al. High-dose rate intracavitary irradiation for carcinoma of the uterine cervix. The adverse effect of treatment prolongation. *Strahlenther Onkol* 1997;173:379–384.

212. Shaverdian N, Gondi V, Sklenar KL, et al. Effects of treatment duration during concomitant chemoradiation therapy for cervical cancer. *Int J Radiat Oncol Biol Phys* 2013;86(3):562–568.

213. Tanderup K, Fokdal LU, Sturdza A, et al. Effect of tumor dose, volume and overall treatment time on local control after radiochemotherapy including MRI guided brachytherapy of locally advanced cervical cancer. *Radiother Oncol* 2016;120(3):441–446.

214. Perez CA, Grigsby PW, Castro-Vita H, et al. Carcinoma of the uterine cervix. II. Lack of impact of prolongation of overall treatment time on morbidity of radiation therapy. *Int J Radiat Oncol Biol Phys* 1996;34:3–11.

215. Noordhuis MG, Eijsink JJ, Roossink F, et al. Prognostic cell biological markers in cervical cancer patients primarily treated with (chemo) radiation: a systematic review. *Int J Radiat Oncol Biol Phys* 2011;79(2):325–334.

216. Bachtiary B, Schindl M, Potter R, et al. Overexpression of hypoxia-inducible factor 1alpha indicates diminished response to radiotherapy and unfavorable prognosis in patients receiving radical radiotherapy for cervical cancer. *Clin Cancer Res* 2003;9:2234–2240.

217. Burri P, Djonov V, Aebersold DM, et al. Significant correlation of hypoxia-inducible factor-1α with treatment outcome in cervical cancer treated with radical radiotherapy. *Int J Radiat Oncol Biol Phys* 2003;56(2):494–501.

218. Hutchison GJ, Valentine HR, Loncaster JA, et al. Hypoxia-inducible factor 1alpha expression as an intrinsic marker of hypoxia: correlation with tumor oxygen, pimonidazole measurements, and outcome in locally advanced carcinoma of the cervix. *Clin Cancer Res* 2004;10(24):8405–8412.

219. Kawanaka T, Kubo A, Ikushima H, et al. Prognostic significance of HIF-2α expression on tumor infiltrating macrophages in patients with uterine cervical cancer undergoing radiotherapy. *J Med Invest* 2008;55(1-2):78–86.

220. Loncaster JA, Cooper RA, Logue JP, et al. Vascular endothelial growth factor (VEGF) expression is a prognostic factor for radiotherapy outcome in advanced carcinoma of the cervix. *Br J Cancer* 2000;83:620–625.

221. Kabuubi P, Loncaster JA, Davidson SE, et al. No relationship between thymidine phosphorylase (TP, PD-ECGF) expression and hypoxia in carcinoma of the cervix. *Br J Cancer* 2006;94(1):115–120.

222. Chen HH, Su W, Chou C, et al. Increased expression of nitric oxide synthase and cyclooxygenase-2 is associated with poor survival in cervical cancer treated with radiotherapy. *Int J Radiat Oncol Biol Phys* 2005;63(4):1093–1100.

223. Lee S, Shin H, Han I, et al. Tumor carbonic anhydrase 9 expression is associated with the presence of lymph node metastases in uterine cervical cancer. *Cancer Sci* 2007;98(3):329–333.

224. Loncaster JA, Harris AL, Davidson SE, et al. Carbonic anhydrase (CA IX) expression, a potential new intrinsic marker of hypoxia: correlations with tumor oxygen measurements and prognosis in locally advanced carcinoma of the cervix. *Cancer Res* 2001;61(17):6394–6399.

225. Kim J, Shin H, Kim T, et al. Tumor-associated carbonic anhydrases are linked to metastases in primary cervical cancer. *J Cancer Res Clin Oncol* 2006;132(5):302–308.

226. Obermair A, Wanner C, Bilgi S, et al. Tumor angiogenesis in stage IB cervical cancer: correlation of microvessel density with survival. *Obstet Gynecol* 1998;178:314–319.

227. Cooper RA, Wilks DP, Logue JP, et al. High tumor angiogenesis is associated with poorer survival in carcinoma of the cervix treated with radiotherapy. *Clin Cancer Res* 1998;4:2795–2800.

228. Kristensen GB, Kaern J, Abeler VM, et al. No prognostic impact of flow-cytometric measured DNA ploidy and S-phase fraction in cancer of the uterine cervix: a prospective study of 465 patients. *Gynecol Oncol* 1995;57:79–85.

229. Strang P, Eklund G, Stendahl U, et al. S-phase rate as a predictor of early recurrences in carcinoma of the uterine cervix. *Anticancer Res* 1987;7: 807–810.

230. Wootipoom V, Lekhyananda N, Phungrassami T, et al. Prognostic significance of bax, bcl-2, and p53 expressions in cervical squamous cell carcinoma treated by radiotherapy. *Gynecol Oncol* 2004;94:636–642.

231. Cho NH, Kim YB, Park TK, et al. P63 and EGFR as prognostic predictors in stage IIB radiation-treated cervical squamous cell carcinoma. *Gynecol Oncol* 2003;91(2):346–353.

232. Ohno T, Nakano T, Niibe Y, et al. Bax protein expression correlates with radiation-induced apoptosis in radiation therapy for cervical carcinoma. *Cancer* 1998;83:103–110.

233. Jain D, Srinivasan R, Patel FD, et al. Evaluation of p53 and bcl-2 expression as prognostic markers in invasive cervical carcinoma stage IIb/III patients treated by radiotherapy. *Gynecol Oncol* 2003;88:22–28.

234. Mukherjee G, Freeman A, Moore R, et al. Biologic factors and response to radiotherapy in carcinoma of the cervix. *Int J Gynecol Cancer* 2001;11:187–193.

235. Kainz C, Kohlberger P, Gitsch G, et al. Mutant p53 in patients with invasive cervical cancer stages IB to IIB. *Gynecol Oncol* 1995;57:212–214.

236. Ebara T, Mitsuhashi N, Saito Y, et al. Prognostic significance of immunohistochemically detected p53 protein expression in stage IIIB squamous cell carcinoma of the uterine cervix treated with radiation therapy alone. *Gynecol Oncol* 1996;63:216–218.

237. Cerciello F, Hofstetter B, Fatah SA, et al. G2/M cell cycle checkpoint is functional in cervical cancer patients after initiation of external beam radiotherapy. *Int J Radiat Oncol Biol Phys* 2005;62:1390–1398.

238. Tsang RW, Wong CS, Fyles AW, et al. Tumour proliferation and apoptosis in human uterine cervix carcinoma II: correlations with clinical outcome. *Radiother Oncol* 1999;50:93–101.

239. West CM, Davidson SE, Burt PA, et al. The intrinsic radiosensitivity of cervical carcinoma: correlations with clinical data. *Int J Radiat Oncol Biol Phys* 1995;31:841–846.

240. Oka K, Suzuki Y, Nakano T. Expression of p27 and p53 in cervical squamous cell carcinoma patients treated with radiotherapy alone: radiotherapeutic effect and prognosis. *Cancer* 2000;88:2766–2773.

241. Hayashi Y, Hachisuga T, Iwasaka T, et al. Expression of ras oncogene product and EGF receptor in cervical squamous cell carcinomas and its relationship to lymph node involvement. *Gynecol Oncol* 1991;40:147–151.

242. Koulos JP, Wright TC, Mitchell MF, et al. Relationships between c-Ki-ras mutations, HPV types, and prognostic indicators in invasive endocervical adenocarcinomas. *Gynecol Oncol* 1993;48:364–369.

243. Lee JH, Lee SK, Yang MH, et al. Expression and mutation of H-ras in uterine cervical cancer. *Gynecol Oncol* 1996;62:49–54.

244. Iwasaka T, Yokoyama M, Oh-uchida M, et al. Detection of human papillomavirus genome and analysis of expression of c-myc and Ha-ras oncogenes in invasive cervical carcinomas. *Gynecol Oncol* 1992;46:298–303.

245. Riou G, Barrois M, Le MG, et al. C-myc proto-oncogene expression and prognosis in early carcinoma of the uterine cervix. *Lancet* 1987;1:761–763.

246. Santucci MA, Barbieri E, Frezza G, et al. Radiation-induced gadd45 expression correlates with clinical response to radiotherapy of cervical carcinoma. *Int J Radiat Oncol Biol Phys* 2000;46:411–416.

247. Vieira SC, Silva BB, Pinto GA, et al. CD34 as a marker for evaluating angiogenesis in cervical cancer. *Pathol Res Pract* 2005;201:313–318.

248. Zhang JM, Hashimoto M, Kawai K, et al. CD109 expression in squamous cell carcinoma of the uterine cervix. *Pathol Int* 2005;55:165–169.

249. Mandai M, Konishi I, Koshiyama M, et al. Altered expression of nm23-H1 and c-erbB-2 proteins have prognostic significance in adenocarcinoma but not in squamous cell carcinoma of the uterine cervix. *Cancer* 1995;75:2523–2529.

250. Perez-Regadera J, Sanchez-Munoz A, De-la-Cruz J, et al. Negative prognostic impact of the coexpression of epidermal growth factor receptor and c-erbB-2 in locally advanced cervical cancer. *Oncology* 2009;76(2):133–141.

251. Harima Y, Sawada S, Nagata K, et al. Mutation of the PTEN gene in advanced cervical cancer correlated with tumor progression and poor outcome after radiotherapy. *Int J Oncol* 2001;18(3):493–497.

252. van Bommel PF, Kenemans P, Helmerhorst TJ, et al. Expression of cytokeratin 10, 13, and involucrin as prognostic factors in low stage squamous cell carcinoma of the uterine cervix. *Cancer* 1994;74:2314–2320.

253. Tsai CC, Lin H, Huang EY, et al. The role of the preoperative serum carcinoembryonic antigen level in early-stage adenocarcinoma of the uterine cervix. *Gynecol Oncol* 2004;94:363–367.

254. Borras G, Molina R, Xercavins J, et al. Tumor antigens CA 19.9, CA 125, and CEA in carcinoma of the uterine cervix. *Gynecol Oncol* 1995;57:205–211.

255. Bolli JA, Doering DL, Bosscher JR, et al. Squamous cell carcinoma antigen: clinical utility in squamous cell carcinoma of the uterine cervix. *Gynecol Oncol* 1994;55:169–173.

256. Ngan HY, Cheng GTS, Cheng D, al e. Post-treatment serial serum squamous cell carcinoma antigen (SCC) in the monitoring of squamous cell carcinoma of the cervix. *Int J Gynecol Cancer* 1996;6:115–119.

257. Hong JH, Tsai CS, Chang JT, et al. The prognostic significance of pre- and post-treatment SCC levels in patients with squamous cell carcinoma of the cervix treated by radiotherapy. *Int J Radiat Oncol Biol Phys* 1998;41:823–830.

258. Micke O, Bruns F, Schafer U, et al. The impact of squamous cell carcinoma (SCC) antigen in patients with advanced cancer of uterine cervix treated with (chemo-)radiotherapy. *Anticancer Res* 2005;25:1663–1666.

259. Hong JH, Tsai CS, Lai CH, et al. Risk stratification of patients with advanced squamous cell carcinoma of cervix treated by radiotherapy alone. *Int J Radiat Oncol Biol Phys* 2005;63:492–499.

260. Huang EY, Wang CJ, Chen HC, et al. Multivariate analysis of para-aortic lymph node recurrence after definitive radiotherapy for stage IB-IVA squamous cell carcinoma of uterine cervix. *Int J Radiat Oncol Biol Phys* 2008;72(3):834–842.

261. Huang EY, Huang YJ, Chanchien CC, et al. Pretreatment carcinoembryonic antigen level is a risk factor for para-aortic lymph node recurrence in addition to squamous cell carcinoma antigen following definitive concurrent chemoradiotherapy for squamous cell carcinoma of the uterine cervix. *Radiat Oncol* 2012;7:13, doi:10.1186/1748-717X-7-13.

261a. Markovina S, Wang S, Henke LE, et al. Serum squamous cell carcinoma antigen as an early indicator of response during therapy of cervical cancer. *Br J Cancer* 2018;118(1):72–78. doi:10.1038/bjc.2017.390.

262. Kitano Y, Fujisaki S, Nakamura N, et al. Immunological disorder against the Epstein-Barr virus infection and prognosis in patients with cervical carcinoma. *Gynecol Oncol* 1995;57:150–157.

263. Dickson J, Davidson SE, Hunter RD, et al. Pretreatment plasma TGF beta 1 levels are prognostic for survival but not morbidity following radiation therapy of carcinoma of the cervix. *Int J Radiat Oncol Biol Phys* 2000;48:991–995.

264. Hazelbag S, Kenter GG, Gorter A, et al. Prognostic relevance of TGF-beta1 and PAI-1 in cervical cancer. *Int J Cancer* 2004;112:1020–1028.

265. Gruber G, Hess J, Stiefel C, et al. Correlation between the tumoral expression of beta3-integrin and outcome in cervical cancer patients who had undergone radiotherapy. *Br J Cancer* 2005;92:41–46.

266. Gaffney DK, Holden J, Davis M, et al. Elevated cyclooxygenase-2 expression correlates with diminished survival in carcinoma of the cervix treated with radiotherapy. *Int J Radiat Oncol Biol Phys* 2001;49:1213–1217.

267. Kim YB, Kim GE, Pyo HR, et al. Differential cyclooxygenase-2 expression in squamous cell carcinoma and adenocarcinoma of the uterine cervix. *Int J Radiat Oncol Biol Phys* 2004;60:822–829.

268. Pyo H, Kim YB, Cho NH, et al. Coexpression of cyclooxygenase-2 and thymidine phosphorylase as a prognostic indicator in patients with FIGO stage IIB squamous cell carcinoma of uterine cervix treated with radiotherapy and concurrent chemotherapy. *Int J Radiat Oncol Biol Phys* 2005;62:725–732.

269. Kang S, Kim MH, Park IA, et al. Elevation of cyclooxygenase-2 is related to lymph node metastasis in adenocarcinoma of uterine cervix. *Cancer Lett* 2006;237:305–311.

270. Suzuki Y, Nakano T, Arai T, et al. Progesterone receptor is a favorable prognostic factor of radiation therapy for adenocarcinoma of the uterine cervix. *Int J Radiat Oncol Biol Phys* 2000;47:1229–1234.

271. Ojesina AI, Lichtenstein L, Freeman SS, et al. Landscape of genomic alterations in cervical carcinomas. *Nature* 2014;506(7488):371–375.

272. Cancer Genome Atlas Research Network; Albert Einstein College of Medicine; Analytical Biological Services, et al. Integrated genomic and molecular characterization of cervical cancer. *Nature* 2017;543(7645):378–384.

273. Nasiell K, Roger V, Nasiell M. Behavior of mild cervical dysplasia during long-term follow-up. *Obstet Gynecol* 1986;67(5):665–669.

274. Ferenczy A. Management of patients with high grade squamous intraepithelial lesions. *Cancer* 1995;76(10 Suppl):1928–1933.

275. Michelin MA, Merino LM, Franco CA, et al. Pregnancy outcome after treatment of cervical intraepithelial neoplasia by the loop electrosurgical excision procedure and cold knife conization. *Clin Exp Obstet Gynecol* 2009;36(1):17–19.

276. Kyrgiou M, Koliopoulos G, Martin-Hirsch P, et al. Obstetric outcomes after conservative treatment for intraepithelial or early invasive cervical lesions: systematic review and meta-analysis. *Lancet* 2006;367(9509):489–498.

277. Arbyn M, Kyrgiou M, Simoens C, et al. Perinatal mortality and other severe adverse pregnancy outcomes associated with treatment of cervical intraepithelial neoplasia: meta-analysis. *BMJ* 2008;337:a1284.

278. Maneo A, Sideri M, Scambia G, et al. Simple conization and lymphadenectomy for the conservative treatment of stage IB1 cervical cancer. An Italian experience. *Gynecol Oncol* 2011;123(3):557–560.

279. Riva HL, Hefner JD, Marchetti AA, et al. Prophylactic trachelectomy of cervical stump: two hundred and twelve cases. *South Med J* 1961;54:1082–1084.

280. Dargent D, Mathevet P. Schauta's vaginal hysterectomy combined with laparoscopic lymphadenectomy. *Baillieres Clin Obstet Gynaecol* 1995;9(4):691–705.

281. Peppercorn PD, Jeyarajah AR, Woolas R, et al. Role of MR imaging in the selection of patients with early cervical carcinoma for fertility-preserving surgery: initial experience. *Radiology* 1999;212(2):395–399.

282. Smith JR, Boyle DC, Corless DJ, et al. Abdominal radical trachelectomy: a new surgical technique for the conservative management of cervical carcinoma. *Br J Obstet Gynaecol* 1997;104(10):1196–1200.

283. Wethington SL, Sonoda Y, Park KJ, et al. Expanding the indications for radical trachelectomy: a report on 29 patients with stage IB1 tumors measuring 2 to 4 centimeters. *Int J Gynecol Cancer* 2013;23(6):1092–1098.

283a. Hazell SZ, Stone RL, Lin JY, et al. Adjuvant therapy after radical trachelectomy for stage I cervical cancer. *Gynecol Oncol Rep* 2018;25:15–18.

284. Piver MS, Rutledge F, Smith JP. Five classes of extended hysterectomy for women with cervical cancer. *Obstet Gynecol* 1974;44:265–272.

285. Wertheim E. The extended abdominal operation for carcinoma uteri (based on 500 operative cases). *Am J Obstet Gynecol* 1912:169–173.

286. Meigs J. Carcinoma of the cervix: the Wertheim operation. *Gynecol Obstet* 1944:195–199.

287. Querleu D, Morrow CP. Classification of radical hysterectomy. *Lancet Oncol* 2008;9(3):297–303.

288. Kramer C, Peschel RE, Goldberg N, et al. Radiation treatment of FIGO stage IVA carcinoma of the cervix. *Gynecol Oncol* 1989;32:323–326.

289. Million RR, Rutledge F, Fletcher GH. Stage IV carcinoma of the cervix with bladder invasion. *Obstet Gynecol* 1972;113:239–246.

290. Upadhyay SK, Symonds RP, Haelterman M, et al. The treatment of stage IV carcinoma of cervix by radical dose radiotherapy. *Radiother Oncol* 1988;11:15–19.

291. Van Dyke AH, Van Nagell JR Jr. The prognostic significance of ureteral obstruction in patients with recurrent carcinoma of the cervix uteri. *Surg Gynecol Obstet* 1975;141:371–373.

292. Stehman FB, Bundy BN, DiSaia PJ, et al. Carcinoma of the cervix treated with radiation therapy. I. A multi-variate analysis of prognostic variables in the gynecologic oncology group. *Cancer* 1991;67:2776–2785.

293. Berman ML, Keys H, Creasman W, et al. Survival and patterns of recurrence in cervical cancer metastatic to periaortic lymph nodes (a gynecologic oncology group study). *Gynecol Oncol* 1984;19:8–16.

294. Cosin JA, Fowler JM, Chen MD, et al. Pretreatment surgical staging of patients with cervical carcinoma: the case for lymph node debulking. *Cancer* 1998;82:2241–2248.

295. Potish RA. Surgical staging, extended field radiation, and enteric morbidity in the treatment of cervix cancer. *Int J Radiat Oncol Biol Phys* 1995;31:1009–1010.

296. Potish RA, Downey GO, Adcock LL, et al. The role of surgical debulking in cancer of the uterine cervix. *Int J Radiat Oncol Biol Phys* 1989;17:979–984.

297. Inoue T, Morita K. Long-term observation of patients treated by postoperative extended-field irradiation for nodal metastases from cervical carcinoma stages IB, IIA, and IIB. *Gynecol Oncol* 1995;58:4–10.

298. Esthappan J, Mutic S, Malyapa RS, et al. Treatment planning guidelines regarding the use of CT/PET-guided IMRT for cervical carcinoma with positive para-aortic lymph nodes. *Int J Radiat Oncol Biol Phys* 2004;58:1289–1297.

299. Portelance L, Chao KS, Grigsby PW, et al. Intensity-modulated radiation therapy (IMRT) reduces small bowel, rectum, and bladder doses in patients with cervical cancer receiving pelvic and para-aortic irradiation. *Int J Radiat Oncol Biol Phys* 2001;51:261–266.

300. Mutic S, Malyapa RS, Grigsby PW, et al. PET-guided IMRT for cervical carcinoma with positive para-aortic lymph nodes-a dose-escalation treatment planning study. *Int J Radiat Oncol Biol Phys* 2003;55:28–35.

301. Esthappan J, Chaudhari S, Santanam L, et al. Prospective clinical trial of positron emission tomography/computed tomography image-guided intensity-modulated radiation therapy for cervical carcinoma with positive para-aortic lymph nodes. *Int J Radiat Oncol Biol Phys* 2008;72:1134–1139.

302. Poorvu PD, Sadow CA, Townamchai K, et al. Duodenal and other gastrointestinal toxicity in cervical and endometrial cancer treated with extended-field

intensity modulated radiation therapy to paraaortic lymph nodes. *Int J Radiat Oncol Biol Phys* 2013;85(5):1262–1268.

303. Weiser EB, Bundy BN, Hoskins WJ, et al. Extraperitoneal versus transperitoneal selective paraaortic lymphadenectomy in the pretreatment surgical staging of advanced cervical carcinoma (a gynecologic oncology group study). *Gynecol Oncol* 1989;33:283–289.

304. Berman ML, Lagasse LD, Watring WG, et al. The operative evaluation of patients with cervical carcinoma by an extraperitoneal approach. *Obstet Gynecol* 1977;50(6):658–664.

305. Brockbank E, Kokka F, Bryant A, et al. Pre-treatment surgical para-aortic lymph node assessment in locally advanced cervical cancer. *Cochrane Database Syst Rev* 2011;(4):CD008217. doi(4):CD008217.

306. Lai CH, Huang KG, Hong JH, et al. Randomized trial of surgical staging (extraperitoneal or laparoscopic) versus clinical staging in locally advanced cervical cancer. *Gynecol Oncol* 2003;89(1):160–167.

307. Fowler JM, Carter JR, Carlson JW, et al. Lymph node yield from laparoscopic lymphadenectomy in cervical cancer: a comparative study. *Gynecol Oncol* 1993;51:187–192.

308. Ramirez PT, Jhingran A, Macapinlac HA, et al. Laparoscopic extraperitoneal para-aortic lymphadenectomy in locally advanced cervical cancer: a prospective correlation of surgical findings with positron emission tomography/computed tomography findings. *Cancer* 2011;117:1928–1934.

309. Perez-Mesa C, Spratt JS. Scalene node biopsy in the pretreatment staging of carcinoma of the cervix uteri. *Obstet Gynecol* 1976;125:93–95.

310. Manetta A, Podczaski ES, Larson JE, et al. Scalene lymph node biopsy in the preoperative evaluation of patients with recurrent cervical cancer. *Gynecol Oncol* 1989;33:332–334.

311. Chereau E, Feron JG, Ballester M, et al. Contribution of pelvic and para-aortic lymphadenectomy with sentinel node biopsy in patients with IB2-IIB cervical cancer. *Br J Cancer* 2012;106(1):39–44.

312. Di Stefano AB, Acquaviva G, Garozzo G, et al. Lymph node mapping and sentinel node detection in patients with cervical carcinoma: a 2-year experience. *Gynecol Oncol* 2005;99:671–679.

313. Bats AS, Buenerd A, Querleu D, et al. Diagnostic value of intraoperative examination of sentinel lymph node in early cervical cancer: a prospective, multicenter study. *Gynecol Oncol* 2011;123(2):230–235.

314. Lecuru F, Mathevet P, Querleu D, et al. Bilateral negative sentinel nodes accurately predict absence of lymph node metastasis in early cervical cancer: results of the SENTICOL study. *J Clin Oncol* 2011;29(13):1686–1691.

315. Yamamoto R, Okamoto K, Yukiharu T, et al. A study of risk factors for ovarian metastases in stage Ib-IIIb cervical carcinoma and analysis of ovarian function after a transposition. *Gynecol Oncol* 2001;82(2):312–316.

316. Parker M, Bosscher J, Barnhill D, et al. Ovarian management during radical hysterectomy in the premenopausal patient. *Obstet Gynecol* 1993;82:187–190.

317. Flay LD, Matthews JH. The effects of radiotherapy and surgery on the sexual function of women treated for cervical cancer. *Int J Radiat Oncol Biol Phys* 1995;31:399–404.

318. Anderson B, LaPolla J, Turner D, et al. Ovarian transposition in cervical cancer. *Gynecol Oncol* 1993;49:206–214.

319. Feeney DD, Moore DH, Look KY, et al. The fate of the ovaries after radical hysterectomy and ovarian transposition. *Gynecol Oncol* 1995;56:3–7.

320. Buekers TE, Anderson B, Sorosky JI, et al. Ovarian function after surgical treatment for cervical cancer. *Gynecol Oncol* 2001;80:85–88.

321. Morice P, Juncker L, Rey A, et al. Ovarian transposition for patients with cervical carcinoma treated by radiosurgical combination. *Fertil Steril* 2000;74:743–748.

322. Le Bouedec G, Rabishong B, Canis M, et al. Ovarian transposition by laparoscopy in young women before curietherapy for cervical cancer. *J Gynecol Obstet Biol Reprod* 2000;29:564–570.

323. Stockle E, Verdier G, Thomas L, et al. Functional outcome of laparoscopically transposed ovaries in the multidisciplinary treatment of cervical cancers. analysis of risk factors. *J Gynecol Obstet Biol Reprod* 1996;25:244–252.

324. Pahisa J, Martinez-Roman S, Martinez-Zamora MA, et al. Laparoscopic ovarian transposition in patients with early cervical cancer. *Int J Gynecol Cancer* 2008;18(3):584–589.

325. Greer BE, Koh WJ, Figge DC, et al. Gynecologic radiotherapy fields defined by intraoperative measurements. *Gynecol Oncol* 1990;38:421–424.

326. Perez CA, Kavanagh BD. Uterine cervix. In: Perez CA, Brady LW, Halperin EC, Schmidt-Ulrich RK, eds. *Principles and practice of radiation oncology*. Philadelphia: Lippincott Williams & Wilkins, 2004:1800–1915.

327. Russell AH, Walter JP, Anderson MW, et al. Sagittal magnetic resonance imaging in the design of lateral radiation treatment portals for patients with locally advanced squamous cancer of the cervix. *Int J Radiat Oncol Biol Phys* 1992;23:449–455.

328. Bonin SR, Lanciano RM, Corn BW, et al. Bony landmarks are not an adequate substitute for lymphangiography in defining pelvic lymph node location for the treatment of cervical cancer with radiotherapy. *Int J Radiat Oncol Biol Phys* 1996;34:167–172.

329. Zunino S, Rosato O, Lucino S, et al. Anatomic study of the pelvis in carcinoma of the uterine cervix as related to the box technique. *Int J Radiat Oncol Biol Phys* 1999;44:53–59.

330. Knocke TH, Pokrajac B, Fellner C, et al. A comparison of CT-supported 3D planning with simulator planning in the pelvic irradiation of primary cervical carcinoma. *Strahlenther Onkol* 1999;175:68–73.

331. Finlay MH, Ackerman I, Tirona RG, et al. Use of CT simulation for treatment of cervical cancer to assess the adequacy of lymph node coverage of conventional pelvic fields based on bony landmarks. *Int J Radiat Oncol Biol Phys* 2006;64:205–209.

332. Taylor A, Rockall AG, Reznek RH, et al. Mapping pelvic lymph nodes: guidelines for delineation in intensity-modulated radiotherapy. *Int J Radiat Oncol Biol Phys* 2005;63(5):1604–1612.

333. van den Berg HA, Olofsen-van Acht MJ, van Santvoort JP, et al. Definition and validation of a reference target volume in early stage node-positive cervical carcinoma, based on lymphangiograms and CT-scans. *Radiother Oncol* 2000;54:163–170.

334. Yamazaki A, Shirato H, Nishioka T, et al. Reduction of late complications after irregularly shaped four-field whole pelvic radiotherapy using computed tomographic simulation compared with parallel-opposed whole pelvic radiotherapy. *Jpn J Clin Oncol* 2000;30:180–184.

335. Burnett AF, Coe FL, Klement V, et al. The use of a pelvic displacement prosthesis to exclude the small intestine from the radiation field following radical hysterectomy. *Gynecol Oncol* 2000;79:438–443.

336. Bouchard M, Nadeau S, Germain I, et al. Anatomy-based MLC field optimization for the treatment of gynecologic malignancies. *Int J Radiat Oncol Biol Phys* 2005;63:S344–S345.

337. Han Y, Shin EH, Huh SJ, et al. Interfractional dose variation during intensity-modulated radiation therapy for cervical cancer assessed by weekly CT evaluation. *Int J Radiat Oncol Biol Phys* 2006;65:617–623.

338. Beadle BM, Jhingran A, Salehpour M, et al. Cervix regression and motion during the course of external beam chemoradiation for cervical cancer. *Int J Radiat Oncol Biol Phys* 2009;73:235–241.

339. Haripotepornkul NH, Nath SK, Scanderbeg D, et al. Evaluation of intra- and inter-fraction movement of the cervix during intensity modulated radiation therapy. *Radiother Oncol* 2011;98:347–351.

340. Tyagi N, Lewis JH, Yashar CM, et al. Daily online cone beam computed tomography to assess interfractional motion in patients with intact cervical cancer. *Int J Radiat Oncol Biol Phys* 2011;80:273–280.

341. Lim K, Chan P, Dinniwell R, et al. Cervical cancer regression measured using weekly magnetic resonance imaging during fractionated radiotherapy: radiobiologic modeling and correlation with tumor hypoxia. *Int J Radiat Oncol Biol Phys* 2008;70:126–133.

342. Lee CM, Shrieve DC, Gaffney DK. Rapid involution and mobility of carcinoma of the cervix. *Int J Radiat Oncol Biol Phys* 2004;58:625–630.

343. van de Bunt L, Jürgenliemk-Schulz IM, de Kort GA, et al. Motion and deformation of the target volumes during IMRT for cervical cancer: what margins do we need? *Radiother Oncol* 2008;88(2):233–240.

344. Eminowicz G, Rompokos V, Stacey C, et al. Understanding the impact of pelvic organ motion on dose delivered to target volumes during IMRT for cervical cancer. *Radiother Oncol* 2017;122(1):116–121.

345. Lim K, Small W Jr, Portelance L, et al. Consensus guidelines for delineation of clinical target volume for intensity-modulated pelvic radiotherapy for the definitive treatment of cervix cancer. *Int J Radiat Oncol Biol Phys* 2011;79: 348–355.

346. Small W Jr, Mell LK, Anderson P, et al. Consensus guidelines for delineation of clinical target volume for intensity-modulated pelvic radiotherapy in postoperative treatment of endometrial and cervical cancer. *Int J Radiat Oncol Biol Phys* 2008;71:428–434.

347. Ma DJ, Michaletz-Lorenz M, Goddu SM, et al. Magnitude of interfractional vaginal cuff movement: implications for external irradiation. *Int J Radiat Oncol Biol Phys* 2012;82(4):1439–1444.

348. Jhingran A, Salehpour M, Sam M, et al. Vaginal motion and bladder and rectal volumes during pelvic intensity-modulated radiation therapy after hysterectomy. *Int J Radiat Oncol Biol Phys* 2012;82(1):256–262.

349. Viswanathan A, Moughan J, Miller B, et al. A phase 2 study of postoperative intensity modulated radiation therapy (IMRT) with concurrent cisplatin and bevacizumab (Bev) followed by carboplatin and paclitaxel for patients with endometrial cancer: one-year results from RTOG 0921. *Int J Radiat Oncol Biol Phys* 2013;87(2):S4–S5.

350. Miller TR, Grigsby PW. Measurement of tumor volume by PET to evaluate prognosis in patients with advanced cervical cancer treated by radiation therapy. *Int J Radiat Oncol Biol Phys* 2002;53:353–359.

351. Kavanagh BD, Pan CC, Dawson LA, et al. Radiation dose–volume effects in the stomach and small bowel. *Int J Radiat Oncol Biol Phys* 2010;76(3):S101–S107.

352. Michalski JM, Gay H, Jackson A, et al. Radiation dose–volume effects in radiation-induced rectal injury. *Int J Radiat Oncol Biol Phys* 2010;76(3): S123–S129.

353. Viswanathan AN, Yorke ED, Marks LB, et al. Radiation dose-volume effects of the urinary bladder. *Int J Radiat Oncol Biol Phys* 2010;76:S116–S122.

354. Ahmed RS, Kim RY, Duan J, et al. IMRT dose escalation for positive para-aortic lymph nodes in patients with locally advanced cervical cancer while reducing dose to bone marrow and other organs at risk. *Int J Radiat Oncol Biol Phys* 2004;60:505–512.

355. Heron DE, Gersten K, Selvaraj RN, et al. Conventional 3D conformal versus intensity-modulated radiotherapy for the adjuvant treatment of gynecologic malignancies: a comparative dosimetric study of dose-volume histograms. *Gynecol Oncol* 2003;91:39–45.

356. D'Souza WD, Ahamad AA, Iyer RB, et al. Feasibility of dose escalation using intensity-modulated radiotherapy in posthysterectomy cervical carcinoma. *Int J Radiat Oncol Biol Phys* 2005;61:1062–1070.

357. Adli M, Mayr NA, Kaiser HS, et al. Does prone positioning reduce small bowel dose in pelvic radiation with intensity-modulated radiotherapy for gynecologic cancer? *Int J Radiat Oncol Biol Phys* 2003;57:230–238.

358. Brixey CJ, Roeske JC, Lujan AE, et al. Impact of intensity-modulated radiotherapy on acute hematologic toxicity in women with gynecologic malignancies. *Int J Radiat Oncol Biol Phys* 2002;54:1388–1396.

359. Lujan AE, Mundt AJ, Yamada SD, et al. Intensity-modulated radiotherapy as a means of reducing dose to bone marrow in gynecologic patients receiving whole pelvic radiotherapy. *Int J Radiat Oncol Biol Phys* 2003;57:516–521.

360. Li N, Noticewala SS, Williamson CW, et al. Feasibility of atlas-based active bone marrow sparing intensity modulated radiation therapy for cervical cancer. *Radiother Oncol* 2017;123(2):325–330.

361. Mell LK, Sirak I, Wei L, et al. Bone marrow-sparing intensity modulated radiation therapy with concurrent cisplatin for stage IB-IVA cervical cancer: an International Multicenter Phase II Clinical Trial (INTERTECC-2). *Int J Radiat Oncol Biol Phys* 2017;97(3):536–545.

362. Hasselle MD, Rose BS, Kochanski JD, et al. Clinical outcomes of intensity-modulated pelvic radiation therapy for carcinoma of the cervix. *Int J Radiat Oncol Biol Phys* 2011;80:1436–1445.

363. Guerrero M, Li XA, Ma L, et al. Simultaneous integrated intensity-modulated radiotherapy boost for locally advanced gynecological cancer: radiobiological and dosimetric considerations. *Int J Radiat Oncol Biol Phys* 2005;62(3):933–939.

364. Kavanagh BD, Gieschen HL, Schmidt-Ullrich R, et al. A pilot study of concomitant boost accelerated superfractionated radiotherapy for stage III cancer of the uterine cervix. *Int J Radiat Oncol Biol Phys* 1997;38:561–568.

365. Boyle J, Craciunescu O, Steffey B, et al. Methods, safety, and early clinical outcomes of dose escalation using simultaneous integrated and sequential boosts in patients with locally advanced gynecologic malignancies. *Gynecol Oncol* 2014;135(2):239–243.

366. Vargo JA, Kim H, Choi S, et al. Extended field intensity modulated radiation therapy with concomitant boost for lymph node-positive cervical cancer: analysis of regional control and recurrence patterns in the positron emission tomography/computed tomography era. *Int J Radiat Oncol Biol Phys* 2014;90(5):1091–1098.

367. Folkert MR, Shih KK, Abu-Rustum NR, et al. Postoperative pelvic intensity-modulated radiotherapy and concurrent chemotherapy in intermediate- and high-risk cervical cancer. *Gynecol Oncol* 2013;128(2):288–293.

368. Hall EJ. Intensity-modulated radiation therapy, protons, and the risk of second cancers. *Int J Radiat Oncol Biol Phys* 2006;65:1–7.

369. Boice JD Jr, Day NE, Andersen A, et al. Second cancers following radiation treatment for cervical cancer. An international collaboration among cancer registries. *J Natl Cancer Inst* 1985;74:955–975.

370. Kamrava M, Mell LK, Yashar CM. In-room image-guided radiation therapy for cervical cancers. *Gynecol Cancer* 2011;2(3):357.

371. Higginson DS, Morris DE, Jones EL, et al. Stereotactic body radiotherapy (SBRT): technological innovation and application in gynecologic oncology. *Gynecol Oncol* 2011;120(3):404–412.

372. Viswanathan AN. Image-guided brachytherapy in cervical cancer. *Gynecol Cancer* 2011;2(3):371.

373. Wolfson AH, Abdel-Wahab M, Markoe AM, et al. A quantitative assessment of standard vs. customized midline shield construction for invasive cervical carcinoma. *Int J Radiat Oncol Biol Phys* 1997;37:237–242.

374. Lee LJ, Sadow CA, Russell A, et al. Correlation of point B and lymph node dose in 3D-planned high-dose-rate cervical cancer brachytherapy. *Int J Radiat Oncol Biol Phys* 2009;75:803–809.

375. Fenkell L, Assenholt M, Nielsen SK, et al. Parametrial boost using midline shielding results in an unpredictable dose to tumor and organs at risk in combined external beam radiotherapy and brachytherapy for locally advanced cervical cancer. *Int J Radiat Oncol Biol Phys* 2011;79:1572–1579.

376. Townamchai K, Lee L, Poorvu P, et al. Clinical outcomes with dose escalation using intensity modulated radiation therapy for node-positive endometrial and cervical cancer. *Int J Radiat Oncol Biol Phys* 2012;84(3):S454.

377. Podczaski E, Stryker JA, Kaminski P, et al. Extended-field radiation therapy for carcinoma of the cervix. *Cancer* 1990;66:251–258.

378. Russell AH, Jones DC, Russell KJ, et al. High dose para-aortic lymph node irradiation for gynecologic cancer: technique, toxicity, and results. *Int J Radiat Oncol Biol Phys* 1987;13:267–271.

379. Kodaira T, Karasawa K, Shimizu T, et al. Clinical efficacy of applying four-field portals to paraaortic irradiation in the treatment of cervical carcinoma. *Radiat Oncol Investig* 1999;7:170–177.

380. Holcomb K, Gabbur N, Tucker T, et al. 60Cobalt vs. linear accelerator in the treatment of locally advanced cervix carcinoma: a comparison of survival and recurrence patterns. *Eur J Gynaecol Oncol* 2001;22:16–19.

381. Biggs PJ, Russell MD. Effect of a femoral head prosthesis on megavoltage beam radiotherapy. *Int J Radiat Oncol Biol Phys* 1988;14:581–586.

382. Allt WE. Supervoltage radiation treatment in advanced cancer of the uterine cervix. A preliminary report. *Can Med Assoc J* 1969;100:792–797.

383. Johns HE. Optimization of energy and equipment. In: Kramer S, Suntharalingam N, Zinniger GF, eds. *High energy photons and electrons: clinical application in cancer management.* New York: John Wiley & Sons, Inc.; 1976:333–345.

384. Maor MH, Gillespie BW, Peters LJ, et al. Neutron therapy in cervical cancer: results of a phase III RTOG study. *Int J Radiat Oncol Biol Phys* 1988;14:885–891.

385. Kato S, Ohno T, Tsujii H, et al. Dose escalation study of carbon ion radiotherapy for locally advanced carcinoma of the uterine cervix. *Int J Radiat Oncol Biol Phys* 2006;65:388–397.

386. MacLeod C, Bernshaw D, Leung S, et al. Accelerated hyperfractionated radiotherapy for locally advanced cervix cancer. *Int J Radiat Oncol Biol Phys.* 1999;44(3):519–524.

387. Viswanathan FR, Varghese C, Peedicayil A, et al. Hyperfractionation in carcinoma of the cervix: tumor control and late bowel complications. *Int J Radiat Oncol Biol Phys* 1999;45(3):653–656.

388. Grigsby PW, Heydon K, Mutch DG, et al. Long term follow up of radiation therapy oncology group 92–10; cervical cancer with positive para-aortic lymph nodes. *Int J Radiat Oncol Biol Phys* 2001;51:982–987.

389. Calkins AR, Harrison CR, Fowler WC, et al. Hyperfractionated radiation therapy plus chemotherapy in locally advanced cervical cancer: results of two phase I dose-escalation gynecologic oncology group trials. *Gynecol Oncol* 1999;75:349–355.

390. Thomas G, Dembo A, Ackerman I, et al. A randomized trial of standard versus partially hyperfractionated radiation with or without concurrent 5-fluouracil in locally advanced cervical cancer. *Gynecol Oncol* 1998;69:137–145.

391. Bjerre B, Eliasson G, Linell F, et al. Conization as only treatment of carcinoma in situ of the uterine cervix. *Obstet Gynecol* 1976;125:143–152.

392. Randall ME, Michael H, Ver Morken J, et al. Uterine cervix. In: Hoskins WJ, Perez CA, Young RC, eds. *Principles and practice of gynecologic oncology.* 4th ed. Philadelphia: Lippincott Williams & Wilkins, 2005:743–822.

393. Christopherson WM, Gray LA, Parker JE. Microinvasive carcinoma of the uterine cervix: a long-term followup study of eighty cases. *Cancer* 1976;38:629–632.

394. Delregato JA, Cox JD. Transvaginal roentgen therapy in the conservative management of carcinoma in situ of the uterine cervix. *Radiology* 1965;84:1090–1095.

395. Grigsby PW, Perez CA. Radiotherapy alone for medically inoperable carcinoma of the cervix: stage IA and carcinoma in situ. *Int J Radiat Oncol Biol Phys* 1991;21:375–378.

396. Ogino I, Kitamura T, Okajima H, et al. High-dose-rate intracavitary brachytherapy in the management of cervical and vaginal intraepithelial neoplasia. *Int J Radiat Oncol Biol Phys* 1998;40:881–887.

397. Brunschwig A. The surgical treatment of cancer of the cervix: stage I and II. *Am J Roentgenol Radium Ther Nucl Med* 1968;102:147–151.

398. Liu W, Meigs JV. Radical hysterectomy and pelvic lymphadenectomy; a review of 473 cases including 244 for primary invasive carcinoma of the cervix. *Obstet Gynecol* 1955;69:1–32.

399. Eifel PJ, Moughan J, Erickson B, et al. Patterns of radiotherapy practice for patients with carcinoma of the uterine cervix: a patterns of care study. *Int J Radiat Oncol Biol Phys* 2004;60:1144–1153.

400. Eifel P, Khalid N, Erickson B, et al. Patterns of radiotherapy practice for patients treated for intact cervical cancer in 2005–2007: a QRRO study. *Int J Radiat Oncol Biol Phys* 2010;78(3):S119–S120.

401. Barbera L, Paszat L, Thomas G, et al. The rapid uptake of concurrent chemotherapy for cervix cancer patients treated with curative radiation. *Int J Radiat Oncol Biol Phys* 2006;64:1389–1394.

402. National Cancer Institute. *Concurrent chemoradiotherapy for cervical cancer. Clinical announcement.* Washington, DC: National Cancer Institute, 1999.

403. Andras EJ, Fletcher G, Rutledge F. Radiotherapy of carcinoma of the cervix following simple hysterectomy. *Obstet Gynecol* 1973;115:647–655.

404. Sharma DN, Rath GK, Kumar S, et al. Postoperative radiotherapy following inadvertent simple hysterectomy versus radical hysterectomy for cervical carcinoma. *Asian Pac J Cancer Prev* 2011;12:1537–1541.

405. Ampil F, Datta R, Datta S. Elective postoperative external radiotherapy after hysterectomy in early-stage carcinoma of the cervix. Is additional vaginal cuff irradiation necessary? *Cancer* 1987;60:280–288.

406. Green TH Jr, Morse WJ Jr. Management of invasive cervical cancer following inadvertent simple hysterectomy. *Obstet Gynecol* 1969;33:763–769.

407. Crane CH, Schneider BF. Occult carcinoma discovered after simple hysterectomy treated with postoperative radiotherapy. *Int J Radiat Oncol Biol Phys* 1999;43:1049–1053.

408. Huerta Bahena J, Labastida Almendaro S, Cortez Arroyo H, et al. [Postoperative radiotherapy in patients with invasive uterine cervix cancer treated previously with simple hysterectomy. Results from the Hospital de Oncologia, Centro Médico Nacional SXXI.]. *Ginecol Obstet Mex* 2003;71:304–311.

409. Münstedt K, Johnson P, von Georgi R, et al. Consequences of inadvertent, suboptimal primary surgery in carcinoma of the uterine cervix. *Gynecol Oncol* 2004;94(2):515–520.

410. Saibishkumar EP, Patel FD, Ghoshal S, et al. Results of salvage radiotherapy after inadequate surgery in invasive cervical carcinoma patients: a retrospective analysis. *Int J Radiat Oncol Biol Phys* 2005;63:828–833.

411. Park JY, Kim DY, Kim JH, et al. Management of occult invasive cervical cancer found after simple hysterectomy. *Ann Oncol* 2010;21(5):994–1000.

412. Smith KB, Amdur RJ, Yeung AR, et al. Postoperative radiotherapy for cervix cancer incidentally discovered after a simple hysterectomy for either benign conditions or noninvasive pathology. *Am J Clin Oncol* 2010;33(3):229–232.

413. Ramirez PT, Schmeler KM, Wolf JK, et al. Robotic radical parametrectomy and pelvic lymphadenectomy in patients with invasive cervical cancer. *Gynecol Oncol* 2008;111(1):18–21.

414. Kolstad P. Follow-up study of 232 patients with stage Ia1 and 411 patients with stage Ia2 squamous cell carcinoma of the cervix (microinvasive carcinoma). *Gynecol Oncol* 1989;33:265–272.

415. Raspagliesi F, Ditto A, Quattrone P, et al. Prognostic factors in microinvasive cervical squamous cell cancer: long-term results. *Int J Gynecol Cancer* 2005;15:88–93.

416. Benson WL, Norris HJ. A critical review of the frequency of lymph node metastasis and death from microinvasive carcinoma of the cervix. *Obstet Gynecol* 1977;49:632–638.

417. Abu-Rustum NR, Sonoda Y. Fertility-sparing surgery in early-stage cervical cancer: indications and applications. *J Natl Compr Canc Netw* 2010;8(12):1435–1438.

418. Gadducci A, Sartori E, Maggino T, et al. The clinical outcome of patients with stage Ia1 and Ia2 squamous cell carcinoma of the uterine cervix: a cooperation task force (CTF) study. *Eur J Gynaecol Oncol* 2003;24:513–516.

419. Balega J, Michael H, Hurteau J, et al. The risk of nodal metastasis in early adenocarcinoma of the uterine cervix. *Int J Gynecol Cancer* 2004;14:104–109.

420. Webb JC, Key CR, Qualls CR, et al. Population-based study of microinvasive adenocarcinoma of the uterine cervix. *Obstet Gynecol* 2001;97:701–706.

421. Zola P, Volpe T, Castelli G, et al. Is the published literature a reliable guide for deciding between alternative treatments for patients with early cervical cancer? *Int J Radiat Oncol Biol Phys* 1989;16:785–797.

422. Kupets R, Thomas GM, Covens A. Is there a role for pelvic lymph node debulking in advanced cervical cancer? *Gynecol Oncol* 2002;87:163–170.

423. Whitney CW, Stehman FB. The abandoned radical hysterectomy: a gynecologic oncology group study. *Gynecol Oncol* 2000;79:350–356.

424. Akine Y, Arimoto H, Ogino T, et al. High-dose-rate intracavitary irradiation in the treatment of carcinoma of the uterine cervix: early experience with 84 patients. *Int J Radiat Oncol Biol Phys* 1988;14:893–898.

425. Hamberger AD, Fletcher GH, Wharton JT. Results of treatment of early stage I carcinoma of the uterine cervix with intracavitary radium alone. *Cancer* 1978;41:980–985.

426. Volterrani F, Lombardi F. Long term results of radium therapy in cervical cancer. *Int J Radiat Oncol Biol Phys* 1980;6:565–570.

427. Eifel PJ, Winter K, Morris M, et al. Pelvic irradiation with concurrent chemotherapy versus pelvic and para-aortic irradiation for high risk cervical cancer: an update of radiation therapy oncology group trial (RTOG) 90-01. *J Clin Oncol* 2004;22:872–880.

428. Newton M. Radical hysterectomy or radiotherapy for stage I cervical cancer. A prospective comparison with 5 and 10 years follow-up. *Obstet Gynecol* 1975;123:535–542.

429. Roddick JW Jr, Greenelaw RH. Treatment of cervical cancer. A randomized study of operation and radiation. *Obstet Gynecol* 1971;109:754–764.

430. Rosa DD, Medeiros LR, Edelweiss MI, et al. Adjuvant platinum-based chemotherapy for early stage cervical cancer. *Cochrane Database Syst Rev* 2012;(6):CD005342. doi(6):CD005342.

431. Rydzewska L, Tierney J, Vale CL, et al. Neoadjuvant chemotherapy plus surgery versus surgery for cervical cancer. *Cochrane Database Syst Rev* 2012;12:CD007406.

432. Neoadjuvant Chemotherapy for Locally Advanced Cervical Cancer Meta-analysis Collaboration. Neoadjuvant chemotherapy for locally advanced cervical cancer: a systematic review and meta-analysis of individual patient data from 21 randomised trials. *Eur J Cancer* 2003;39(17):2470–2486.

433. Keilbinska S, Ludwika, Tarlowska, Fraczek O. Studies of mortality and health status in women cured of cancer of the cervix uteri comparison of long-term results of radiotherapy and combined surgery and radiotherapy. *Cancer* 1973;32:245–252.

434. Piver MS, Marchetti DL, Patton T, et al. Radical hysterectomy and pelvic lymphadenectomy versus radiation therapy for small (less than or equal to 3 cm) stage IB cervical carcinoma. *Am J Clin Oncol* 1988;11:21–24.

435. Einhorn N, Patek E, Sjöberg B. Outcome of different treatment modalities in cervix carcinoma stage IB and IIA. *Cancer* 1985;55:949–955.

436. Perez CA, Grigsby PW, Camel HM, et al. Irradiation alone or combined with surgery in stage IB, IIA, and IIB carcinoma of uterine cervix: update of a nonrandomized comparison. *Int J Radiat Oncol Biol Phys* 1995;31:703–716.

437. Jobson VW, Girtanner RE, Averette HE. Therapy and survival of early invasive carcinoma of the cervix uteri with metastases to the pelvic nodes. *Surg Gynecol Obstet* 1980;151:27–29.

438. Peters WA, Liu PY, Barrett RJ, et al. Concurrent chemotherapy and pelvic radiation therapy compared with pelvic radiation therapy alone as adjuvant therapy after radical surgery in high-risk early-stage cancer of the cervix. *J Clin Oncol.* 2000;18:1606–1613.

439. Sedlis A, Bundy BN, Rotman MZ, et al. A randomized trial of pelvic radiation therapy versus no further therapy in selected patients with stage IB carcinoma of the cervix after radical hysterectomy and pelvic lymphadenectomy: a gynecologic oncology group study. *Gynecol Oncol* 1999;73:177–183.

440. Song S, Song C, Kim HJ, et al. 20 year experience of postoperative radiotherapy in IB-IIA cervical cancer patients with intermediate risk factors: impact of treatment period and concurrent chemotherapy. *Gynecol Oncol* 2012;124(1):63–67.

441. Rotman M, Sedlis A, Piedmonte MR, et al. A phase III randomized trial of postoperative pelvic irradiation in stage IB cervical carcinoma with poor prognostic features: follow-up of a gynecologic oncology group study. *Int J Radiat Oncol Biol Phys* 2006;65:169–176.

442. Rogers L, Siu S, Luesley D, et al. Adjuvant radiotherapy and chemoradiation after surgery for cervical cancer. *Cochrane Database Syst Rev* 2009;4;CD007583.

443. Sundfør K, Trope CG, Kjorstad KE. Radical radiotherapy versus brachytherapy plus surgery in carcinoma of the cervix 2A and 2B—long-term results from a randomized study 1968–1980. *Acta Oncol* 1996;35(Suppl 8):99–107.

444. Snijders-Keilholz A, Hellebrekers BW, Zwinderman AH, et al. Adjuvant radiotherapy following radical hysterectomy for patients with early-stage cervical carcinoma (1984–1996). *Radiother Oncol* 1999;51:161–167.

445. Garipagaoglu M, Tulunay G, Kose MF, et al. Prognostic factors in stage IB-IIA cervical carcinomas treated with postoperative radiotherapy. *Eur J Gynaecol Oncol* 1999;20:131–135.

446. Lahousen M, Haas J, Pickel H, et al. Chemotherapy versus radiotherapy versus observation for high-risk cervical carcinoma after radical hysterectomy: a randomized, prospective, multicenter trial. *Gynecol Oncol* 1999;73:196–201.

447. González González D, Ketting BW, van Bunningen B, et al. Carcinoma of the uterine cervix stage IB and IIA: results of postoperative irradiation in patients with microscopic infiltration in the parametrium and/or lymph node metastasis. *Int J Radiat Oncol Biol Phys* 1989;16:389–395.

448. Bianchi UA, Sartori E, Pecorelli S, et al. Treatment of primary invasive cervical cancer. Considerations on 997 consecutive cases. *Eur J Gynaecol Oncol* 1988;9:47–53.

449. Chatani M, Nose T, Masaki N, et al. Adjuvant radiotherapy after radical hysterectomy of the cervical cancer. Prognostic factors and complications. *Strahlenther Onkol* 1998;174:504–509.

450. Uno T, Ito H, Itami J, et al. Postoperative radiation therapy for stage IB-IIB carcinoma of the cervix with poor prognostic factors. *Anticancer Res* 2000;20:2235–2239.

451. Kinney WK, Alvarez RD, Reid GC, et al. Value of adjuvant whole-pelvis irradiation after Wertheim hysterectomy for early-stage squamous carcinoma of the cervix with pelvic nodal metastasis: a matched-control study. *Gynecol Oncol* 1989;34:258–262.

452. Kinney WK, Hodge DO, Egorshin EV, et al. Surgical treatment of patients with stages IB and IIA carcinoma of the cervix and palpably positive pelvic lymph nodes. *Gynecol Oncol* 1995;57:145–149.

453. Mitsuhashi N, Takahashi M, Yamakawa M, et al. Results of postoperative radiation therapy for patients with carcinoma of the uterine cervix: evaluation of intravaginal cone boost with an electron beam. *Gynecol Oncol* 1995;57:321–326.

454. Mabuchi S, Okazawa M, Isohashi F, et al. Radical hysterectomy with adjuvant radiotherapy versus definitive radiotherapy alone for FIGO stage IIB cervical cancer. *Gynecol Oncol* 2011;123(2):241–247.

455. Mabuchi S, Okazawa M, Isohashi F, et al. Postoperative whole pelvic radiotherapy plus concurrent chemotherapy versus extended-field irradiation for early-stage cervical cancer patients with multiple pelvic lymph node metastases. *Gynecol Oncol* 2011;120(1):94–100.

456. Okazawa M, Mabuchi S, Isohashi F, et al. Impact of the addition of concurrent chemotherapy to pelvic radiotherapy in surgically treated stage IB1-IIB cervical cancer patients with intermediate-risk or high-risk factors: a 13-year experience. *Int J Gynecol Cancer* 2013;23(3):567–575.

457. Rogers L, Siu SS, Luesley D, et al. Radiotherapy and chemoradiation after surgery for early cervical cancer. *Cochrane Database Syst Rev* 2012;(5):CD007583. doi(5):CD007583.

458. Lee HN, Lee KH, Lee DW, et al. Weekly cisplatin therapy compared with tri-weekly combination chemotherapy as concurrent adjuvant chemoradiation therapy after radical hysterectomy for cervical cancer. *Int J Gynecol Cancer* 2011;21(1):128–136.

459. Small W Jr, Beriwal S, Demanes DJ, et al. American brachytherapy society consensus guidelines for adjuvant vaginal cuff brachytherapy after hysterectomy. *Brachytherapy* 2012;11(1):58–67.

460. Mitra D, Klopp AH, Viswanathan AN. Pros and cons of vaginal brachytherapy after external beam radiation therapy in endometrial cancer. *Gynecol Oncol* 2016;140(1):167–175.

461. Hart K, Han I, Deppe G, et al, Postoperative radiation for cervical cancer with pathologic risk factors. *Int J Radiat Oncol Biol Phys* 1997;37:833–838.

462. Busch M, Rath W, Schaffer M, et al. Results of postoperative radiotherapy of cervix carcinoma after radical versus non radical hysterectomy. *Radiol Med* 1997;93:110–114.

463. Atkovar G, Uzel O, Ozsahin M, et al. Postoperative radiotherapy in carcinoma of the cervix: treatment results and prognostic factors. *Radiother Oncol* 1995;35:198–205.

464. Christie DR, Bull CA, Gebski V, et al. Concurrent 5-fluorouracil, mitomycin C and irradiation in locally advanced cervix cancer. *Radiother Oncol* 1995;37:181–189.

465. Coughlin CT, Richmond RC. Biologic and clinical developments of cisplatin combined with radiation: concepts, utility, projections for new trials, and the emergence of carboplatin. *Semin Oncol* 1989;16:31–43.

466. Park TK, Choi DH, Kim SN, et al. Role of induction chemotherapy in invasive cervical cancer. *Gynecol Oncol* 1991;41:107–112.

467. Rotman MZ. Chemoirradiation: a new initiative in cancer treatment. 1991 RSNA annual oration in radiation oncology. *Radiology* 1992;184:319–327.

468. Douple EB. Platinum-radiation interactions. *NCI Monogr* 1988;6:315–319.

469. Durand RE, Aquino-Parsons C. Predicting response to treatment in human cancers of the uterine cervix: sequential biopsies during external beam radiotherapy. *Int J Radiat Oncol Biol Phys* 2004;58:555–560.

470. Green JA, Kirwan JM, Tierney JF, et al. Survival and recurrence after concomitant chemotherapy and radiotherapy for cancer of the uterine cervix: a systematic review and meta-analysis. *Lancet* 2001;358:781–786.

471. Deckers PJ, Ketcham AS, Sugerbaker EV, et al. Pelvic exenteration for primary carcinoma of the uterine cervix. *Obstet Gynecol* 1971;37:647–659.

472. Niibe Y, Hayakawa K, Kanai T, et al. Optimal dose for stage IIIB adenocarcinoma of the uterine cervix on the basis of biological effective dose. *Eur J Gynaecol Oncol* 2006;27:47–49.

473. Small W Jr, Winter K, Levenback C, et al. Extended-field irradiation and intracavitary brachytherapy combined with cisplatin chemotherapy for cervical cancer with positive para-aortic or high common iliac lymph nodes: results of ARM 1 of RTOG 0116. *Int J Radiat Oncol Biol Phys* 2007;68:1081–1087.

474. Small W Jr, Winter K, Levenback C, et al. Extended-field irradiation and intracavitary brachytherapy combined with cisplatin and amifostine for cervical cancer with positive para-aortic or high common iliac lymph nodes: results of arm II of radiation therapy oncology group (RTOG) 0116. *Int J Gynecol Cancer.* 2011;21:1266–1275.

475. Salama JK, Mundt AJ, Roeske J, et al. Preliminary outcome and toxicity report of extended-field, intensity-modulated radiation therapy for gynecologic malignancies. *Int J Radiat Oncol Biol Phys* 2006;65(4):1170–1176.

476. Yin M, Zhang H, Li H, et al. The toxicity and long-term efficacy of nedaplatin and paclitaxel treatment as neoadjuvant chemotherapy for locally advanced cervical cancer. *J Surg Oncol* 2012;105(2):206–211.

477. Keys HM, Bundy BN, Stehman FB, et al. Cisplatin, radiation, and adjuvant hysterectomy compared with radiation and adjuvant hysterectomy for bulky stage IB cervical carcinoma. *N Engl J Med* 1999;340:1154–1161.

478. Whitney CW, Sause W, Bundy BN, et al. Randomized comparison of fluorouracil plus cisplatin versus hydroxyurea as an adjunct to radiation therapy in stage IIB-IVA carcinoma of the cervix with negative para-aortic lymph nodes: a gynecologic oncology group and southwest oncology group study. *J Clin Oncol* 1999;17:1339–1348.

Section
III

479. Rose PG, Bundy BN, Watkins EB, et al. Concurrent cisplatin-based radiotherapy and chemotherapy for locally advanced cervical cancer. *N Engl J Med* 1999;340:1144–1153.

480. Lehman M, Thomas G. Is concurrent chemotherapy and radiotherapy the new standard of care for locally advanced cervical cancer? *Int J Gynecol Cancer* 2001;11:87–99.

481. Rose PG, Ali S, Watkins E, et al. Long-term follow-up of a randomized trial comparing concurrent single agent cisplatin, cisplatin-based combination chemotherapy, or hydroxyurea during pelvic irradiation for locally advanced cervical cancer: a gynecologic oncology group study. *J Clin Oncol* 2007;25(19):2804–2810.

482. Morris M, Eifel PJ, Lu J, et al. Pelvic radiation with concurrent chemotherapy compared with pelvic and para-aortic radiation for high-risk cervical cancer. *N Engl J Med* 1999;340:1137–1143.

483. Stehman FB, Ali S, Keys HM, et al. Radiation therapy with or without weekly cisplatin for bulky stage 1B cervical carcinoma: follow-up of a gynecologic oncology group trial. *Obstet Gynecol* 2007;197(5):503. e1, 503. e6.

484. Pearcey R, Brundage M, Drouin P, et al. Phase III trial comparing radical radiotherapy with and without cisplatin chemotherapy in patients with advanced squamous cell cancer of the cervix. *J Clin Oncol* 2002;20:966–972.

485. Lanciano R, Calkins A, Bundy BN, et al. Randomized comparison of weekly cisplatin or protracted venous infusion of fluorouracil in combination with pelvic radiation in advanced cervix cancer: a gynecologic oncology group study. *J Clin Oncol* 2005;23:8289–8295.

486. Rose PG, Eifel PJ. Combined radiation therapy and chemotherapy for carcinoma of the cervix. *Cancer J* 2001;7:86–94.

487. Curtin JP, Hoskins WJ, Venkatraman ES, et al. Adjuvant chemotherapy versus chemotherapy plus pelvic irradiation for high-risk cervical cancer patients after radical hysterectomy and pelvic lymphadenectomy (RH-PLND): a randomized phase III trial. *Gynecol Oncol* 1996;61:3–10.

488. Green JA, Kirwan JJ, Tierney J, et al. Concomitant chemotherapy and radiation therapy for cancer of the uterine cervix. *Cochrane Database Syst Rev* 2005;20:CD002225.

489. Chemoradiotherapy for Cervical Cancer Meta-Analysis Collaboration. Reducing uncertainties about the effects of chemoradiotherapy for cervical cancer: a systematic review and meta-analysis of individual patient data from 18 randomized trials. *J Clin Oncol* 2008;26(35):5802–5812.

490. Nugent EK, Case AS, Hoff JT, et al. Chemoradiation in locally advanced cervical carcinoma: an analysis of cisplatin dosing and other clinical prognostic factors. *Gynecol Oncol* 2010;116(3):438–441.

491. Einstein MH, Novetsky AP, Garg M, et al. Survival and toxicity differences between 5-day and weekly cisplatin in patients with locally advanced cervical cancer. *Cancer* 2007;109(1):48–53.

492. Duenas-Gonzalez A, Zarba JJ, Patel F, et al. Phase III, open-label, randomized study comparing concurrent gemcitabine plus cisplatin and radiation followed by adjuvant gemcitabine and cisplatin versus concurrent cisplatin and radiation in patients with stage IIB to IVA carcinoma of the cervix. *J Clin Oncol* 2011;29:1678–1685.

493. Lorvidhaya V, Tonusin A, Sukthomya W, et al. Induction chemotherapy and irradiation in advanced carcinoma of the cervix. *Gan To Kagaku Ryoho* 1995;22(Suppl 3):244–251.

494. Kim YS, Shin SS, Nam JH, et al. Prospective randomized comparison of monthly fluorouracil and cisplatin versus weekly cisplatin concurrent with pelvic radiotherapy and high-dose rate brachytherapy for locally advanced cervical cancer. *Gynecol Oncol* 2008;108(1):195–200.

495. Tseng CJ, Chang CT, Lai CH, et al. A randomized trial of concurrent chemoradiotherapy versus radiotherapy in advanced carcinoma of the uterine cervix. *Gynecol Oncol* 1997;66:52–58.

496. Geara FB, Shamseddine A, Khalil A, et al. A phase II randomized trial comparing radiotherapy with concurrent weekly cisplatin or weekly paclitaxel in patients with advanced cervical cancer. *Radiat Oncol* 2010;5(1):84.

497. Martinez-Monge R, Gaztanaga M, Aramendia JM, et al. A phase II trial of less than 7 weeks of concomitant cisplatin-paclitaxel chemoradiation in locally advanced cervical cancer. *Int J Gynecol Cancer* 2010;20:133–140.

498. Katanyoo K, Tangjitgamol S, Chongthanakorn M, et al. Treatment outcomes of concurrent weekly carboplatin with radiation therapy in locally advanced cervical cancer patients. *Gynecol Oncol* 2011;123(3):571–576.

499. Takekida S, Fujiwara K, Nagao S, et al. Phase II study of combination chemotherapy with docetaxel and carboplatin for locally advanced or recurrent cervical cancer. *Int J Gynecol Cancer* 2010;20(9):1563–1568.

500. Hreshchyshyn MM, Aron BS, Boronow RC, et al. Hydroxyurea or placebo combined with radiation to treat stages IIIB and IV cervical cancer confined to the pelvis. *Int J Radiat Oncol Biol Phys* 1979;5:317–322.

501. Piver MS, Barlow JJ, Vongtama V, et al. Hydroxyurea as a radiation sensitizer in women with carcinoma of the uterine cervix. *Obstet Gynecol* 1977;129:379–383.

502. Symonds RP, Collingwood M, Kirwan J, et al. Concomitant hydroxyurea plus radiotherapy versus radiotherapy for carcinoma of the uterine cervix: a systematic review. *Cancer Treat Rev* 2004;30:405–414.

503. Stehman FB, Bundy BN, Thomas G, et al. Hydroxyurea versus misonidazole with radiation in cervical carcinoma: long-term follow-up of a gynecologic oncology group trial. *J Clin Oncol* 1993;11:1523–1528.

504. Leibel S, Bauer M, Wasserman T, et al. Radiotherapy with or without misonidazole for patients with stage IIIB or stage IVA squamous cell carcinoma of the uterine cervix: preliminary report of a radiation therapy oncology group randomized trial. *Int J Radiat Oncol Biol Phys* 1987;13:541–549.

505. Overgaard J, Bentzen SM, Kolstad P, et al. Misonidazole combined with radiotherapy in the treatment of carcinoma of the uterine cervix. *Int J Radiat Oncol Biol Phys* 1989;16:1069–1072.

506. Grigsby PW, Winter K, Wasserman TH, et al. Irradiation with or without misonidazole for patients with stages IIIB and IVA carcinoma of the cervix: final results of RTOG 80-05. Radiation therapy oncology group. *Int J Radiat Oncol Biol Phys* 1999;44:513–517.

507. Bonomi P, Blessing J, Ball H, et al. A phase II evaluation of cisplatin and 5-fluorouracil in patients with advanced squamous cell carcinoma of the cervix: a gynecologic oncology group study. *Gynecol Oncol* 1989;37:354–358.

508. Perez CA, Grigsby PW. Adjuvant chemotherapy and irradiation in locally advanced squamous cell carcinoma of the uterine cervix. *PPGO Updates* 1993;1:1–20.

509. Sardi JE, Giaroli A, Sananes C, et al. Long-term follow-up of the first randomized trial using neoadjuvant chemotherapy in stage Ib squamous carcinoma of the cervix: the final results. *Gynecol Oncol* 1997;67:61–69.

510. Souhami L, Seymour R, Roman TN, et al. Weekly cisplatin plus external beam radiotherapy and high dose rate brachytherapy in patients with locally advanced carcinoma of the cervix. *Int J Radiat Oncol Biol Phys* 1993;27:871–878.

511. Park TK, Lee SK, Kim SN, et al. Combined chemotherapy and radiation for bulky stages I–II cervical cancer: comparison of concurrent and sequential regimens. *Gynecol Oncol* 1993;50:196–201.

512. Lee JW, Kim BG, Lee SJ, et al. Preliminary results of consolidation chemotherapy following concurrent chemoradiation after radical surgery in high-risk early-stage carcinoma of the uterine cervix. *Clin Oncol (R Coll Radiol)* 2005;17:412–417.

513. Grigsby PW, Mutch DG, Rader J, et al. Lack of benefit of concurrent chemotherapy in patients with cervical cancer and negative lymph nodes by FDG-PET. *Int J Radiat Oncol Biol Phys* 2005;61:444–449.

514. Cetina L, Garcia-Arias A, Uribe Mde J, et al. Concurrent chemoradiation with carboplatin for elderly, diabetic and hypertensive patients with locally advanced cervical cancer. *Eur J Gynaecol Oncol* 2008;29(6):608–612.

515. Roberts KB, Urdaneta N, Vera R, et al. Interim results of a randomized trial of mitomycin C as an adjunct to radical radiotherapy in the treatment of locally advanced squamous-cell carcinoma of the cervix. *Int J Cancer* 2000;90:206–223.

516. Smith HO, Jiang CS, Weiss GR, et al. Tirapazamine plus cisplatin in advanced or recurrent carcinoma of the uterine cervix: a southwest oncology group study. *Int J Gynecol Cancer* 2006;16:298–305.

517. Wun T, Law L, Harvey D, et al. Increased incidence of symptomatic venous thrombosis in patients with cervical carcinoma treated with concurrent chemotherapy, radiation, and erythropoietin. *Cancer* 2003;98:1514–1520.

518. Anders JC, Grigsby PW, Singh AK. Cisplatin chemotherapy (without erythropoietin) and risk of life-threatening thromboembolic events in carcinoma of the uterine cervix: the tip of the iceberg? A review of the literature *Radiat Oncol* 2006;1:14.

519. Schefter TE, Winter K, Kwon JS, et al. A phase II study of bevacizumab in combination with definitive radiotherapy and cisplatin chemotherapy in untreated patients with locally advanced cervical carcinoma: preliminary results of RTOG 0417. *Int J Radiat Oncol Biol Phys* 2012;83(4):1179–1184.

520. Schefter T, Winter K, Kwon JS, et al. RTOG 0417: efficacy of bevacizumab in combination with definitive radiation therapy and cisplatin chemotherapy in untreated patients with locally advanced cervical carcinoma. *Int J Radiat Oncol Biol Phys* 2014;88(1):101–105.

521. Nogueira-Rodrigues A, do Carmo CC, Viegas C, et al. Phase I trial of erlotinib combined with cisplatin and radiotherapy for patients with locally advanced cervical squamous cell cancer. *Clin Cancer Res* 2008;14(19):6324–6329.

522. Morris M, Eifel PJ, Burke TW, et al. Treatment of locally advanced cervical cancer with concurrent radiation and intra-arterial chemotherapy. *Gynecol Oncol* 1995;57:72–78.

523. Onishi H, Yamaguchi M, Kuriyama K, et al. Effect of concurrent intra-arterial infusion of platinum drugs for patients with stage III or IV uterine cervical cancer treated with radical radiation therapy. *Cancer J Sci Am* 2000;6:40–45.

524. Thomas GM. *Is neoadjuvant chemotherapy a useful strategy for the treatment of stage 1B cervix cancer?*. *Gynecol Oncol* 1993;49(2):153–155.

525. Benedetti-Panici P, Greggi S, Colombo A, et al. Neoadjuvant chemotherapy and radical surgery versus exclusive radiotherapy in locally advanced squamous cell cervical cancer: results from the Italian multicenter randomized study. *J Clin Oncol* 2002;20:179–188.

526. Chang TC, Lai CH, Hong JH, et al. Randomized trial of neoadjuvant cisplatin, vincristine, bleomycin, and radical hysterectomy versus radiation therapy for bulky stage IB and IIA cervical cancer. *J Clin Oncol* 2000;18:1740–1747.

527. Chauvergne J, Lhomme C, Rohart J, et al. Neoadjuvant chemotherapy of stage IIb or III cancers of the uterine cervix. long-term results of a multicenter randomized trial of 151 patients. *Bull Cancer* 1993;80:1069–1079.

528. Herod J, Burton A, Buxton J, et al. A randomised, prospective, phase III clinical trial of primary bleomycin, ifosfamide and cisplatin (BIP) chemotherapy followed by radiotherapy versus radiotherapy alone in inoperable cancer of the cervix. *Ann Oncol* 2000;11:1175–1181.

529. Kumar L, Grover R, Pokharel YH, et al. Neoadjuvant chemotherapy in locally advanced cervical cancer: two randomised studies. *Aust N Z J Med* 1998;28:387–390.

530. Leborgne F, Leborgne JH, Doldan R, et al. Induction chemotherapy and radiotherapy of advanced cancer of the cervix: a pilot study and phase III randomized trial. *Int J Radiat Oncol Biol Phys* 1997;37:343–350.

531. Sundfør K, Trope CG, Hogberg T, et al. Radiotherapy and neoadjuvant chemotherapy for cervical carcinoma. A randomized multicenter study of sequential cisplatin and 5-fluorouracil and radiotherapy in advanced cervical carcinoma stage 3B and 4A. *Cancer* 1996;77:2371–2378.

532. Symonds RP, Habeshaw T, Reed NS, et al. The Scottish and Manchester randomised trial of neo-adjuvant chemotherapy for advanced cervical cancer. *Eur J Cancer* 2000;36(8):994–1001.

533. Colombo A, Landoni F, Maneo A, et al. Neoadjuvant chemotherapy to radiation and concurrent chemoradiation for locally advanced squamous cell carcinoma of the cervix: a review of the recent literature. *Tumori* 1998;84:229–237.

534. Souhami L, Gil RA, Allan SE, et al. A randomized trial of chemotherapy followed by pelvic radiation therapy in stage IIIB carcinoma of the cervix. *J Clin Oncol* 1991;9:970–977.

535. Kumar L, Kaushal R, Nandy M, et al. Chemotherapy followed by radiotherapy versus radiotherapy alone in locally advanced cervical cancer: a randomized study. *Gynecol Oncol* 1994;54:307–315.

536. Long HJ III, Bundy BN, Grendys EC, et al. Randomized phase III trial of cisplatin with or without topotecan in carcinoma of the uterine cervix: a gynecologic oncology group study. *J Clin Oncol* 2005;23:4626–4633.

537. Rose PG, Blessing JA, Gershenson DM, et al. Paclitaxel and cisplatin as first-line therapy in recurrent or advanced squamous cell carcinoma of the cervix: a gynecologic oncology group study. *J Clin Oncol* 1999;17:2676–2680.

538. Gebbia V, Caruso M, Testa A, et al. Vinorelbine and cisplatin for the treatment of recurrent and/or metastatic carcinoma of the uterine cervix. *Oncology* 2002;63(1):31–37.

539. Lacava JA, Leone BA, Machiavelli M, et al. Vinorelbine as neoadjuvant chemotherapy in advanced cervical carcinoma. *J Clin Oncol* 1997;15:604–609.

540. Morris M, Brader KR, Levenback C, et al. Phase II study of vinorelbine in advanced and recurrent squamous cell carcinoma of the cervix. *J Clin Oncol* 1998;16:1094–1098.

541. Umesaki N, Fujii T, Nishimura R, et al. Phase II study of irinotecan combined with mitomycin-C for advanced or recurrent squamous cell carcinoma of the uterine cervix: the JGOG study. *Gynecol Oncol* 2004;95:127–132.

542. Verschraegen CF, Levy T, Kudelka AP, et al. Phase II study of irinotecan in prior chemotherapy-treated squamous cell carcinoma of the cervix. *J Clin Oncol* 1997;15:625–631.

543. Schilder RJ, Blessing J, Cohn DE. Evaluation of gemcitabine in previously treated patients with non-squamous cell carcinoma of the cervix: a phase II study of the Gynecologic Oncology Group. *Gynecol Oncol* 2005;96:103–107.

544. Brewer CA, Blessing JA, Nagourney RA, et al. Cisplatin plus gemcitabine in previously treated squamous cell carcinoma of the cervix: a phase II study of the gynecologic oncology group. *Gynecol Oncol* 2006;100:385–388.

545. Monk BJ, Sill MW, McMeekin DS, et al. Phase III trial of four cisplatin-containing doublet combinations in stage IVB, recurrent, or persistent cervical carcinoma: a gynecologic oncology group study. *J Clin Oncol* 2009;27(28):4649–4655.

546. Farley J, Sill MW, Birrer M, et al. Phase II study of cisplatin plus cetuximab in advanced, recurrent, and previously treated cancers of the cervix and evaluation of epidermal growth factor receptor immunohistochemical expression: a gynecologic oncology group study. *Gynecol Oncol* 2011;121(2):303–308.

547. Downs LS Jr, Chura JC, Argenta PA, Judson PL, et al. Ifosfamide, paclitaxel, and carboplatin, a novel triplet regimen for advanced, recurrent, or persistent carcinoma of the cervix: a phase II trial. *Gynecol Oncol* 2011;120(2):265–269.

548. Monk BJ, Mas Lopez L, Zarba JJ, et al. Phase II, open-label study of pazopanib or lapatinib monotherapy compared with pazopanib plus lapatinib combination therapy in patients with advanced and recurrent cervical cancer. *J Clin Oncol* 2010;28(22):3562–3569.

549. Mendenhall WM, McCarty PJ, Morgan LS, et al. Stage IB or IIA-B carcinoma of the intact uterine cervix greater than or equal to 6 cm in diameter: is adjuvant extrafascial hysterectomy beneficial? *Int J Radiat Oncol Biol Phys* 1991;21:899–904.

550. Thoms WW Jr, Eifel PJ, Smith TL, et al. Bulky endocervical carcinoma: a 23-year experience. *Int J Radiat Oncol Biol Phys* 1992;23:491–499.

551. Kim HK, Silver B, Berkowitz R, et al. Bulky, barrel-shaped cervical carcinoma (stages IB, IIA, IIB): the prognostic factors for pelvic control and treatment outcome. *Am J Clin Oncol* 1999;22:232–236.

552. Paley PJ, Goff BA, Minudri R, et al. The prognostic significance of radiation dose and residual tumor in the treatment of barrel-shaped endophytic cervical carcinoma. *Gynecol Oncol* 2000;76:373–379.

553. Keys H, Bundy B, Stehman FB, et al. Adjuvant hysterectomy after radiation therapy reduces detection of local recurrence in "bulky" stage IB cervical cancer without improving survival: results of a prospective randomized GOG trial. *Cancer J Sci Am* 1997;3:117.

554. Coia L, Won M, Lanciano R, et al. The patterns of care outcome study for cancer of the uterine cervix. results of the second national practice survey. *Cancer* 1990;66:2451–2456.

555. Russell AH, Koh WJ, Markette K, et al. Radical reirradiation for recurrent or second primary carcinoma of the female reproductive tract. *Gynecol Oncol* 1987;27:226–232.

556. Kim RY, Trotti A, Wu CJ, et al. Radiation alone in the treatment of cancer of the uterine cervix: analysis of pelvic failure and dose response relationship. *Int J Radiat Oncol Biol Phys* 1989;17:973–978.

557. Montana GS, Fowler WC, Varia MA, et al. Carcinoma of the cervix, stage III. Results of radiation therapy. *Cancer* 1986;57:148–154.

558. Hanks GE, Herring DF, Kramer S. Patterns of care outcome studies. results of the national practice in cancer of the cervix. *Cancer* 1983;51:959–967.

559. Komaki R, Brickner TJ, Hanlon AL, et al. Long-term results of treatment of cervical carcinoma in the united states in 1973, 1978, and 1983: patterns of care study (PCS). *Int J Radiat Oncol Biol Phys* 1995;31:973–982.

560. Montana GS, Hanlon AL, Brickner TJ, et al. Carcinoma of the cervix: patterns of care studies: review of 1978, 1983, and 1988–1989 surveys. *Int J Radiat Oncol Biol Phys* 1995;32:1481–1486.

561. Arthur D, Kaufam N, Schmidt-Ullrich R, et al. Heuristically derived tumor burden score as a prognostic factor for stage IIIB carcinoma of the cervix. *Int J Radiat Oncol Biol Phys* 1995;34:743–751.

562. Horiot JC, Pigneux J, Pourquier H, et al. Radiotherapy alone in carcinoma of the intact uterine cervix according to G. H. Fletcher guidelines: a French cooperative study of 1383 cases. *Int J Radiat Oncol Biol Phys* 1988;14:605–611.

563. Barillot I, Horiot JC, Maingon P, et al. Impact on treatment outcome and late effects of customized treatment planning in cervix carcinomas: baseline results to compare new strategies. *Int J Radiat Oncol Biol Phys* 2000;48:189–200.

564. Marcial VA, Amato DA, Marks RD, et al. Split-course versus continuous pelvis irradiation in carcinoma of the uterine cervix: a prospective randomized clinical trial of the radiation therapy oncology group. *Int J Radiat Oncol Biol Phys* 1983;9:431–436.

565. Crozier M, Morris M, Levenback C, et al. Pelvic exenteration for adenocarcinoma of the uterine cervix. *Gynecol Oncol* 1995;58:74–78.

566. Fletcher G. *Textbook of radiotherapy*. 3rd ed. Philadelphia: Lea & Febiger, 1980:180–218, 103–179.

567. Charra-Brunaud C, Harter V, Delannes M, et al. Impact of 3D image-based PDR brachytherapy on outcome of patients treated for cervix carcinoma in France: results of the French STIC prospective study. *Radiother Oncol* 2012;103:305–313.

568. Dimopoulos JC, Potter R, Lang S, et al. Dose-effect relationship for local control of cervical cancer by magnetic resonance image-guided brachytherapy. *Radiother Oncol* 2009;93:311–315.

569. Kunos C, Ali S, Abdul-Karim FW, et al. Posttherapy residual disease associates with long-term survival after chemoradiation for bulky stage 1B cervical carcinoma: a gynecologic oncology group study. *Am J Obstet Gynecol* 2010;203(4):351.e1–351.e8.

570. Morice P, Rouanet P, Rey A, et al. Results of the GYNECO 02 study, an FNCLCC phase III trial comparing hysterectomy with no hysterectomy in patients with a (clinical and radiological) complete response after chemoradiation therapy for stage IB2 or II cervical cancer. *Oncologist* 2012;17(1):64–71.

571. Motton S, Houvenaeghel G, Delannes M, et al. Results of surgery after concurrent chemoradiotherapy in advanced cervical cancer: comparison of extended hysterectomy and extrafascial hysterectomy. *Int J Gynecol Cancer* 2010;20(2):268–275.

572. Lèguevaque P, Motton S, Delannes M, et al. Completion surgery or not after concurrent chemoradiotherapy for locally advanced cervical cancer? *Eur J Obstet Gynecol Reprod Biol* 2011;155(2):188–192.

573. Touboul C, Uzan C, Mauguen A, et al. Prognostic factors and morbidities after completion surgery in patients undergoing initial chemoradiation therapy for locally advanced cervical cancer. *Oncologist* 2010;15:405–415.

574. Haie C, Pejovic MH, Gerbaulet A, et al. Is prophylactic para-aortic irradiation worthwhile in the treatment of advanced cervical carcinoma? Results of a controlled clinical trial of the EORTC radiotherapy group. *Radiother Oncol* 1988;11:101–112.

575. Sood BM, Gorla GR, Garg M, et al. Extended-field radiotherapy and high-dose-rate brachytherapy in carcinoma of the uterine cervix: clinical experience with and without concomitant chemotherapy. *Cancer* 2003;97:1781–1788.

576. Varia MA, Bundy BN, Deppe G, et al. Cervical carcinoma metastatic to para-aortic nodes: extended field radiation therapy with concomitant 5-fluorouracil and cisplatin chemotherapy: a gynecologic oncology group study. *Int J Radiat Oncol Biol Phys* 1998;42:1015–1023.

577. Lovecchio JL, Averette HE, Donato D, et al. 5-year survival of patients with periaortic nodal metastases in clinical stage IB and IIA cervical carcinoma. *Gynecol Oncol* 1989;34:43–45.

578. Stryker JA, Mortel R. Survival following extended field irradiation in carcinoma of cervix metastatic to para-aortic lymph nodes. *Gynecol Oncol* 2000;79:399–405.

579. Grigsby PW, Perez CA, Chao KS, et al. Radiation therapy for carcinoma of the cervix with biopsy-proven positive para-aortic lymph nodes. *Int J Radiat Oncol Biol Phys* 2001;49:733–738.

580. Hacker NF, Wain GV, Nicklin JL. Resection of bulky positive lymph nodes in patients with cervical carcinoma. *Int J Gynecol Cancer* 1995;5:250–256.

581. Grigsby PW, Lu JD, Mutch DG, et al. Twice-daily fractionation of external irradiation with brachytherapy and chemotherapy in carcinoma of the cervix with positive para-aortic lymph nodes: phase II study of the radiation therapy oncology group 92–10. *Int J Radiat Oncol Biol Phys* 1998;41:817–822.

582. Malfetano JH, Keys H, Cunningham MJ, et al. Extended field radiation and cisplatin for stage IIB and IIIB cervical carcinoma. *Gynecol Oncol* 1997;67:203–207.

583. Chou HH, Wang CC, Lai CH, et al. Isolated paraaortic lymph node recurrence after definitive irradiation for cervical carcinoma. *Int J Radiat Oncol Biol Phys* 2001;51:442–448.

584. Goodman HM, Niloff JM, Nelson JR, et al. Cervical malignancies. In: Knapp RC, Berkowitz RS, eds. *Gynecologic oncology*. New York: MacMillan, 1986: 225–273.

585. Kim JS, Kim SY, Kim KH, et al. Hyperfractionated radiotherapy with concurrent chemotherapy for para-aortic lymph node recurrence in carcinoma of the cervix. *Int J Radiat Oncol Biol Phys* 2003;55:1247–1253.

586. Singh AK, Grigsby PW, Rader JS, et al. Cervix carcinoma, concurrent chemoradiotherapy, and salvage of isolated paraaortic lymph node recurrence. *Int J Radiat Oncol Biol Phys* 2005;61:450–455.

587. Kim YS, Kim JH, Ahn SD, et al. High-dose extended-field irradiation and high-dose-rate brachytherapy with concurrent chemotherapy for cervical cancer with positive para-aortic lymph nodes. *Int J Radiat Oncol Biol Phys* 2009;74:1522–1528.

588. Rajasooriyar C, Van Dyk S, Bernshaw D, et al. Patterns of failure and treatment-related toxicity in advanced cervical cancer patients treated using extended field radiotherapy with curative intent. *Int J Radiat Oncol Biol Phys* 2011;80:422–428.

589. Verma J, Sulman EP, Jhingran A, et al. Dosimetric predictors of duodenal toxicity after intensity modulated radiation therapy for treatment of the para-aortic nodes in gynecologic cancer. *Int J Radiat Oncol Biol Phys* 2014;88(2):357–362.

590. Osborne EM, Klopp AH, Jhingran A, et al. Impact of treatment year on survival and adverse effects in patients with cervical cancer and paraortic lymph node metastases treated with definitive extended-field radiation therapy. *Pract Radiat Oncol* 2017;7(3):e165–e173.

590a. Boyle J, Craciunescu O, Steffey B, et al. Methods, safety, and early clinical outcomes of dose escalation using simultaneous integrated and sequential boosts

Section III

in patients with locally advanced gynecologic malignancies. *Gynecol Oncol* 2014;135(2):239–243. doi:10.1016/j.ygyno.2014.08.037.

590b. Vargo JA, Kim H, Choi S, et al. Extended field intensity modulated radiation therapy with concomitant boost for lymph node-positive cervical cancer: analysis of regional control and recurrence patterns in the positron emission tomography/computed tomography era. *Int J Radiat Oncol Biol Phys* 2014;90(5):1091–1098. doi:10.1016/j.ijrobp.2014.08.013.

591. Kovalic JJ, Grigsby PW, Perez CA, et al. Cervical stump carcinoma. *Int J Radiat Oncol Biol Phys* 1991;20:933–938.

592. Wolff JP, Lacour J, Chassagne D, et al. Cancer of the cervical stump. study of 173 patients. *Obstet Gynecol* 1972;39:10–16.

593. Miller BE, Copeland LJ, Hamberger AD, et al. Carcinoma of the cervical stump. *Gynecol Oncol* 1984;18:100–108.

594. Hannoun-Levi J, Peiffert D, Hoffstetter S, et al. Carcinoma of the cervical stump: retrospective analysis of 77 cases. *Radiother Oncol* 1997;43:147–153.

595. Hellstrom AC, Sigurjonson T, Pettersson F. Carcinoma of the cervical stump. The radiumhemmet series 1959–1987. Treatment and prognosis. *Acta Obstet Gynecol Scand* 2001;80:152–157.

596. Miller B, Dockter M, el Torky M, et al. Small cell carcinoma of the cervix: a clinical and flow-cytometric study. *Gynecol Oncol* 1991;42:27–33.

597. Sevin BU, Method MW, Nadji M, et al. Efficacy of radical hysterectomy as treatment for patients with small cell carcinoma of the cervix. *Cancer* 1996;77:1489–1493.

598. Morris M, Gershenson DM, Eifel P, et al. Treatment of small cell carcinoma of the cervix with cisplatin, doxorubicin, and etoposide. *Gynecol Oncol* 1992;47:62–65.

599. Hoskins PJ, Wong F, Swenerton KD, et al. Small cell carcinoma of the cervix treated with concurrent radiotherapy, cisplatin, and etoposide. *Gynecol Oncol* 1995;56:218–225.

600. Delaloge S, Pautier P, Kerbrat P, et al. Neuroendocrine small cell carcinoma of the uterine cervix: what disease? What treatment? report of ten cases and a review of the literature. *Clin Oncol (R Coll Radiol)* 2000;12:357–362.

601. Boruta DM II, Schorge JO, Duska LA, et al. Multimodality therapy in early-stage neuroendocrine carcinoma of the uterine cervix. *Gynecol Oncol* 2001;81: 82–87.

602. Vinh-Hung V, Bourgain C, Vlastos G, et al. Prognostic value of histopathology and trends in cervical cancer: a SEER population study. *BMC Cancer* 2007;7:164.

603. Grigsby PW, Perez CA, Kuske RR, et al. Adenocarcinoma of the uterine cervix: lack of evidence for a poor prognosis. *Radiother Oncol* 1988;12:289–296.

604. Kilgore LC, Soong SJ, Gore H, et al. Analysis of prognostic features in adenocarcinoma of the cervix. *Gynecol Oncol* 1988;31:137–153.

605. Eifel PJ, Morris M, Oswald MJ, et al. Adenocarcinoma of the uterine cervix: prognosis and patterns of failure of 367 cases treated at the M. D. Anderson Cancer Center between 1965 and 1985. *Cancer* 1990;65:2507–2514.

606. Rutledge FN, Galakatos AE, Wharton JT, et al. Adenocarcinoma of the uterine cervix. *Obstet Gynecol* 1975;122:236–245.

607. Eifel PJ, Burke TW, Morris M, et al. Adenocarcinoma as an independent risk factor for disease recurrence in patients with stage IB cervical carcinoma. *Gynecol Oncol* 1995;59:38–44.

608. Nakano T, Arai T, Morita S, et al. Radiation therapy alone for adenocarcinoma of the uterine cervix. *Int J Radiat Oncol Biol Phys* 1995;32:1331–1336.

609. Kjorstad KE, Martimbeau PW, Iversen T. Stage IB carcinoma of the cervix, the Norwegian radium hospital: results and complications. III. Urinary and gastrointestinal complications. *Gynecol Oncol* 1983;15:42–47.

610. Baalbergen A, Veenstra Y, Stalpers LL, et al. Primary surgery versus primary radiation therapy with or without chemotherapy for early adenocarcinoma of the uterine cervix. *Cochrane Database Syst Rev* 2010;(1):CD006248.

611. Huang Y, Wang C, Tsai C, et al. Clinical behaviors and outcomes for adenocarcinoma or adenosquamous carcinoma of cervix treated by radical hysterectomy and adjuvant radiotherapy or chemoradiotherapy. *Int J Radiat Oncol Biol Phys* 2012;84(2):420–427.

612. Oguchi M, Ikeda H, Watanabe T, et al. Experiences of 23 patients > or = 90 years of age treated with radiation therapy. *Int J Radiat Oncol Biol Phys* 1998;41:407–413.

613. Duggan B, Muderspach LI, Roman L, et al. Cervical cancer in pregnancy: reporting on planned delay in therapy *Obstet Gynecol* 1993;82:598–602.

614. Norstrom A, Jansson I, Andersson H. Carcinoma of the uterine cervix in pregnancy. A study of the incidence and treatment in the western region of Sweden 1973 to 1992. *Acta Obstet Gynecol Scand* 1997;76:583–589.

615. Hopkins MP, Morley GW. The prognosis and management of cervical cancer associated with pregnancy. *Obstet Gynecol* 1992;80:9–13.

616. Monk BJ, Montz FJ. Invasive cervical cancer complicating intrauterine pregnancy: treatment with radical hysterectomy. *Obstet Gynecol* 1992;80:199–203.

617. Sood AK, Sorosky JI, Krogman S, et al. Surgical management of cervical cancer complicating pregnancy: a case-control study. *Gynecol Oncol* 1996;63:294–298.

618. Ostrom K, Ben-Arie A, Edwards C, et al. Uterine evacuation with misoprostol during radiotherapy for cervical cancer in pregnancy. *Int J Gynecol Cancer.* 2003;13(3):340–343.

619. Tewari K, Cappuccini F, Gambino A, et al. Neoadjuvant chemotherapy in the treatment of locally advanced cervical carcinoma in pregnancy. *Cancer* 1998;82(8):1529–1534.

620. Carillon MA, Emmanuelli V, Castelain B, et al. Management of pregnant women with advanced cervical cancer: about five cases observed in Lille from 2002 till 2009. Evaluation of practices referring to the new French recommendations of 2008. *J Gynecol Obstet Biol Reprod (Paris)* 2011;40(6):514–521.

621. Li J, Wang LJ, Zhang BZ, et al. Neoadjuvant chemotherapy with paclitaxel plus platinum for invasive cervical cancer in pregnancy: two case report and literature review. *Arch Gynecol Obstet* 2011;284(3):779–783.

622. Creasman WT, Rutledge FN, Fletcher GH. Carcinoma of the cervix associated with pregnancy. *Obstet Gynecol* 1970;36:495–501.

623. Wo JY, Viswanathan AN. Impact of radiotherapy on fertility, pregnancy, and neonatal outcomes in female cancer patients. *Int J Radiat Oncol Biol Phys* 2009;73(5):1304–1312.

624. Sood AK, Sorosky JI, Mayr N, et al. Radiotherapeutic management of cervical carcinoma that complicates pregnancy. *Cancer* 1997;80:1073–1078.

625. Sood AK, Sorosky JI, Mayr N, et al. Cervical cancer diagnosed shortly after pregnancy: prognostic variables and delivery routes. *Obstet Gynecol* 2000;95:832–838.

626. Jones WB, Shingleton HM, Russell A, et al. Cervical carcinoma and pregnancy. A national patterns of care study of the American College of Surgeons. *Cancer* 1996;77:1479–1488.

627. Senekjian EK, Hubby M, Bell DA, et al. Clear cell adenocarcinoma (CCA) of the vagina and cervix in association with pregnancy. *Gynecol Oncol* 1986;24:207–219.

628. Strauss A. Irradiation of carcinoma of the cervix uteri in pregnancy. *Am J Roentgenol Radium Ther Nucl Med* 1940;43:552–566.

629. Mould RF. Invited review: the early years of radiotherapy with emphasis on X-ray and radium apparatus. *Br J Radiol* 1995;68(810):567–582.

630. Fletcher GH, Shukovsky LJ. The interplay of radiocurability and tolerance in the irradiation of human cancers. *J Radiol Electrol Med Nucl* 1975;56(5): 383–400.

631. Montana GS, Fowler WC, Varia MA, et al. Analysis of results of radiation therapy for stage II carcinoma of the cervix. *Cancer* 1985;55(5):956–962.

632. Lanciano RM, Martz K, Coia LR, et al. Tumor and treatment factors improving outcome in stage III-B cervix cancer. *Int J Radiat Oncol Biol Phys* 1991;20:95–100.

633. Lanciano RM, Won M, Coia L, et al. Pretreatment and treatment factors associated with improved outcome in squamous cell carcinoma of the uterine cervix: a final report of the 1973 and 1978 patterns of care studies. *Int J Radiat Oncol Biol Phys* 1991;20:667–676.

634. Montana GS, Martz KL, Hanks GE. Patterns and sites of failure in cervix cancer treated in the U.S.A. in 1978. *Int J Radiat Oncol Biol Phys* 1991;20:87–93.

635. Viswanathan AN, Thomadsen B; American Brachytherapy Society Cervical Cancer Recommendations Committee. American brachytherapy society consensus guidelines for locally advanced carcinoma of the cervix. part I: general principles. *Brachytherapy* 2012;11(1):33–46.

636. International Commission on Radiation Units, and Measurements. *Dose and volume specifications for reporting intracavitary therapy in gynecology.* Bethesda, MD: International Commission on Radiation Units and Measurements, 1985.

637. Erickson B, Eifel P, Moughan J, et al. Patterns of brachytherapy practice for patients with carcinoma of the cervix (1996–1999): a patterns of care study. *Int J Radiat Oncol Biol Phys* 2005;63:1083–1092.

638. Viswanathan AN, Erickson BA. Three-dimensional imaging in gynecologic brachytherapy: a survey of the American Brachytherapy Society. *Int J Radiat Oncol Biol Phys* 2010;76:104–109.

639. Viswanathan AN, Creutzberg CL, Craighead P, et al. International brachytherapy practice patterns: a survey of the gynecologic cancer intergroup (GCIG). *Int J Radiat Oncol Biol Phys* 2012;82:250–255.

640. Tomita N, Toita T, Kodaira T, et al. Patterns of radiotherapy practice for patients with cervical cancer in Japan, 2003–2005: changing trends in the pattern of care process. *Int J Radiat Oncol Biol Phys* 2012;83(5):1506–1513.

641. Pavamani S, D'Souza DP, Portelance L, et al. Image-guided brachytherapy for cervical cancer: a Canadian brachytherapy group survey. *Brachytherapy* 2011;10:345–351.

642. Stewart AJ, Viswanathan AN. Current controversies in high-dose-rate versus low-dose-rate brachytherapy for cervical cancer. *Cancer* 2006;107: 908–915.

643. Petereit DG, Sarkaria JN, Potter DM, et al. High-dose-rate versus low-dose-rate brachytherapy in the treatment of cervical cancer: analysis of tumor recurrence—the university of Wisconsin experience. *Int J Radiat Oncol Biol Phys* 1999;45:1267–1274.

644. Patel FD, Sharma SC, Negi PS, et al. Low dose rate vs. high dose rate brachytherapy in the treatment of carcinoma of the uterine cervix: a clinical trial. *Int J Radiat Oncol Biol Phys* 1994;28:335–341.

645. Fu KK, Phillips TL. High-dose-rate versus low-dose-rate intracavitary brachytherapy for carcinoma of the cervix. *Int J Radiat Oncol Biol Phys* 1990;19(3):791–796.

646. Hall EJ, Brenner DJ. The dose-rate effect revisited: radiobiological considerations of importance in radiotherapy. *Int J Radiat Oncol Biol Phys* 1991;21:1403–1414.

647. Orton CG, Seyedsadr M, Somnay A. Comparison of high and low dose rate remote afterloading for cervix cancer and the importance of fractionation. *Int J Radiat Oncol Biol Phys* 1991;21:1425–1434.

648. Dale RG. The application of the linear-quadratic dose-effect equation to fractionated and protracted radiotherapy. *Br J Radiol* 1985;58:515–528.

649. Joiner M. The linear quadratic approach to fractionation. *Basic Clin Radiobiol* 1993:55–64.

650. Lang S, Nulens A, Briot E, et al. Intercomparison of treatment concepts for MR image assisted brachytherapy of cervical carcinoma based on GYN GEC-ESTRO recommendations. *Radiother Oncol* 2006;78:185–193.

651. Bentzen SM, Joiner MC. The linear-quadratic approach in clinical practice. *Basic Clin Radiobiol* 2009;4:120–134.

652. Potter R, Haie-Meder C, Van Limbergen E, et al. Recommendations from gynaecological (GYN) GEC ESTRO working group (II): concepts and terms in 3D image-based treatment planning in cervix cancer brachytherapy-3D dose volume parameters and aspects of 3D image-based anatomy, radiation physics, radiobiology. *Radiother Oncol* 2006;78:67–77.

653. Sturdza A, Pötter R. Outcomes related to the disease and the use of 3D-based external beam radiation and image-guided brachytherapy. In: Viswanathan AN, Kirisits C, Erickson B, Potter R, eds. *Gynecologic radiation therapy: novel approaches to image-guidance and management*. Berlin, Germany: Springer, 2011:263–282.
654. Noda SE, Ohno T, Kato S, et al. Late rectal complications evaluated by computed tomography-based dose calculations in patients with cervical carcinoma undergoing high-dose-rate brachytherapy. *Int J Radiat Oncol Biol Phys* 2007;69:118–124.
655. Clark BG, Souhami L, Roman TN, et al. The prediction of late rectal complications in patients treated with high dose-rate brachytherapy for carcinoma of the cervix. *Int J Radiat Oncol Biol Phys* 1997;38:989.
656. Petereit DG, Pearcey R. Literature analysis of high dose rate brachytherapy fractionation schedules in the treatment of cervical cancer: is there an optimal fractionation schedule? *Int J Radiat Oncol Biol Phys* 1999;43:359–366.
657. Lang S, Kirisits C, Dimopoulos J, et al. Treatment planning for MRI assisted brachytherapy of gynecologic malignancies based on total dose constraints. *Int J Radiat Oncol Biol Phys* 2007;69(2):619–627.
658. Newman G. Increased morbidity following the introduction of remote afterloading, with increased dose rate, for cancer of the cervix. *Radiother Oncol* 1996;39:97–103.
659. Fowler JF, Martinez AA, Orton CG, et al. The radiobiology of radiotherapy. In: Martinez AA, Orton CG, Mould RF, eds. *Brachytherapy HDR and LDR*. Columbia: Nucletron, 1990:121–137.
660. Viswanathan AN, Beriwal S, De Los Santos JF, et al. American brachytherapy society consensus guidelines for locally advanced carcinoma of the cervix. Part II: high-dose-rate brachytherapy. *Brachytherapy* 2012;11(1): 47–52.
661. Lee LJ, Das IJ, Higgins SA, et al. American brachytherapy society consensus guidelines for locally advanced carcinoma of the cervix. Part III: low-dose-rate and pulsed-dose-rate brachytherapy. *Brachytherapy* 2012;11(1):53–57.
662. Haie-Meder C, Potter R, Van Limbergen E, et al. Recommendations from gynaecological (GYN) GEC-ESTRO working group (I): concepts and terms in 3D image based 3D treatment planning in cervix cancer brachytherapy with emphasis on MRI assessment of GTV and CTV. *Radiother Oncol* 2005;74:235–245.
663. Potter R, Dimopoulos J, Kirisits C, et al. Recommendations for image-based intracavitary brachytherapy of cervix cancer: the GYN GEC ESTRO working group point of view: in regard to Nag et al. (Int J Radiat Oncol Biol Phys 2004;60:1160–1172). *Int J Radiat Oncol Biol Phys* 2005;62:293–295; author reply 295–6.
664. Arai T, Morita S, Iinuma T, et al. Radiation treatment of cervix cancer using the high dose rate remote afterloading intracavitary irradiation: an analysis of the correlation between optimal dose range and fractionation. *Jpn J Cancer Clin* 1979;25:605–612.
665. Watkins JM, Kearney PL, Opfermann KJ, et al. Ultrasound-guided tandem placement for low-dose-rate brachytherapy in advanced cervical cancer minimizes risk of intraoperative uterine perforation. *Ultrasound Obstet Gynecol* 2011;37(2):241–244.
666. Van Dyk S, Narayan K, Fisher R, et al. Conformal brachytherapy planning for cervical cancer using transabdominal ultrasound. *Int J Radiat Oncol Biol Phys* 2009;75:64–70.
667. Viswanathan AN, Cormack R, Holloway CL, et al. Magnetic resonance-guided interstitial therapy for vaginal recurrence of endometrial cancer. *Int J Radiat Oncol Biol Phys* 2006;66:91–99.
668. Potish RA. The effect of applicator geometry on dose specification in cervical cancer. *Int J Radiat Oncol Biol Phys* 1990;18(6):1513–1520.
669. Corn BW, Hanlon AL, Pajak TF, et al. Technically accurate intracavitary insertions improve pelvic control and survival among patients with locally advanced carcinoma of the uterine cervix. *Gynecol Oncol* 1994;53:294–300.
670. Potish RA, Deibel FC Jr, Khan FM. The relationship between milligram-hours and dose to point A in carcinoma of the cervix. *Radiology* 1982;145: 479–483.
671. Katz A, Eifel PJ. Quantification of intracavitary brachytherapy parameters and correlation with outcome in patients with carcinoma of the cervix. *Int J Radiat Oncol Biol Phys* 2000;48:1417–1425.
672. Viswanathan AN, Dimopoulos J, Kirisits C, et al. Computed tomography versus magnetic resonance imaging-based contouring in cervical cancer brachytherapy: results of a prospective trial and preliminary guidelines for standardized contours. *Int J Radiat Oncol Biol Phys* 2007;68:491–498.
673. Eskander RN, Scanderbeg D, Saenz CC, et al. Comparison of computed tomography and magnetic resonance imaging in cervical cancer brachytherapy target and normal tissue contouring. *Int J Gynecol Cancer* 2010;20: 47–53.
674. Eisbruch A, Johnston CM, Martel MK, et al. Customized gynecologic interstitial implants: CT-based planning, dose evaluation, and optimization aided by laparotomy. *Int J Radiat Oncol Biol Phys* 1998;40:1087–1093.
675. Erickson B, Albano K, Gillin M. CT-guided interstitial implantation of gynecologic malignancies. *Int J Radiat Oncol Biol Phys* 1996;36:699–709.
676. Holloway CL, Racine ML, Cormack RA, et al. Sigmoid dose using 3D imaging in cervical-cancer brachytherapy. *Radiother Oncol* 2009;93:307–310.
677. Kapur T, Egger J, Damato A, et al. 3-T MR-guided brachytherapy for gynecologic malignancies. *Magn Reson Imaging* 2012;30:1279–1290.
678. Petric P, Pötter R, Van Limbergen E, et al. Adaptive contouring of the target volume and organs at risk. In: Viswanathan AN, Kirisits C, Erickson B, Potter R, eds. *Gynecologic radiation therapy: novel approaches to image-guidance and management*. Berlin, Germany: Springer, 2011:99–118.
679. Kim RY, Pareek P. Radiography-based treatment planning compared with computed tomography (CT)-based treatment planning for intracavitary brachytherapy in cancer of the cervix: analysis of dose-volume histograms. *Brachytherapy* 2003;2:200–206.
680. Kim H, Beriwal S, Houser C, et al. Dosimetric analysis of 3D image-guided HDR brachytherapy planning for the treatment of cervical cancer: is point A-based dose prescription still valid in image-guided brachytherapy? *Med Dosim* 2011;36(2):166–170.
681. Arai T, Morita S, Iinuma T, et al. Radiation treatment of cervix cancer using the high dose rate remote afterloading intracavitary irradiation: an analysis of the correlation between optimal dose range and fractionation. *Jpn J Cancer Clin* 1979;25:605–612.
682. Lindegaard JC, Tanderup K, Nielsen SK, et al. MRI-guided 3D optimization significantly improves DVH parameters of pulsed-dose-rate brachytherapy in locally advanced cervical cancer. *Int J Radiat Oncol Biol Phys* 2008;71:756–764.
683. Arai T, Nakano T, Morita S, et al. High-dose-rate remote afterloading intracavitary radiation therapy for cancer of the uterine cervix. A 20-year experience. *Cancer.* 1992;69:175–180.
684. Petric P, Dimopoulos J, Kirisits C, et al. Inter- and intraobserver variation in HR-CTV contouring: intercomparison of transverse and paratransverse image orientation in 3D-MRI assisted cervix cancer brachytherapy. *Radiother Oncol.* 2008;89(2):164–171.
685. Grover S, Harkenrider MM, Cho LP, et al. Image guided cervical brachytherapy: 2014 survey of the American Brachytherapy Society. *Int J Radiat Oncol Biol Phys* 2016;94(3):598–604.
686. Viswanathan AN, Erickson B, Gaffney DK, et al. Comparison and consensus guidelines for delineation of clinical target volume for CT- and MR-based brachytherapy in locally advanced cervical cancer. *Int J Radiat Oncol Biol Phys* 2014;90(2):320–328.
687. Kirisits C, Lang S, Dimopoulos J, et al. The Vienna applicator for combined intracavitary and interstitial brachytherapy of cervical cancer: design, application, treatment planning, and dosimetric results. *Int J Radiat Oncol Biol Phys* 2006;65:624–630.
688. Chargari C, Magne N, Dumas I, et al. Physics contributions and clinical outcome with 3D-MRI-based pulsed-dose-rate intracavitary brachytherapy in cervical cancer patients. *Int J Radiat Oncol Biol Phys* 2009;74:133–139.
689. Beriwal S, Kannan N, Kim H, et al. Three-dimensional high dose rate intracavitary image-guided brachytherapy for the treatment of cervical cancer using a hybrid magnetic resonance imaging/computed tomography approach: feasibility and early results. *Clin Oncol (R Coll Radiol)* 2011;23(10): 685–690.
690. Potter R, Georg P, Dimopoulos JC, et al. Clinical outcome of protocol based image (MRI) guided adaptive brachytherapy combined with 3D conformal radiotherapy with or without chemotherapy in patients with locally advanced cervical cancer. *Radiother Oncol* 2011;100:116–123.
691. De Brabandere M, Mousa AG, Nulens A, et al. Potential of dose optimisation in MRI-based PDR brachytherapy of cervix carcinoma. *Radiother Oncol* 2008;88:217–226.
692. Haie-Meder C, Chargari C, Rey A, et al. MRI-based low dose-rate brachytherapy experience in locally advanced cervical cancer patients initially treated by concomitant chemoradiotherapy. *Radiother Oncol* 2010;96:161–165.
693. Jurgenliemk-Schulz IM, Tersteeg RJ, Roesink JM, et al. MRI-guided treatment-planning optimisation in intracavitary or combined intracavitary/interstitial PDR brachytherapy using tandem ovoid applicators in locally advanced cervical cancer. *Radiother Oncol* 2009;93(2):322–330.
694. Ling CC, Schell MC, Working KR, et al. CT-assisted assessment of bladder and rectum dose in gynecological implants. *Int J Radiat Oncol Biol Physics* 1987;13:1577–1582.
695. Schoeppel SL, LaVigne ML, Martel MK, et al. Three-dimensional treatment planning of intracavitary gynecologic implants: analysis of ten cases and implications for dose specification. *Int J Radiat Oncol Biol Phys* 1994;28:277–283.
696. Kim HJ, Kim S, Ha SW, et al. Are doses to ICRU reference points valuable for predicting late rectal and bladder morbidity after definitive radiotherapy in uterine cervix cancer? *Tumori* 2008;94(3):327–332.
697. Chen SW, Liang JA, Yeh LS, et al. Comparative study of reference points by dosimetric analyses for late complications after uniform external radiotherapy and high-dose-rate brachytherapy for cervical cancer. *Int J Radiat Oncol Biol Phys* 2004;60:663–671.
698. Georg P, Lang S, Dimopoulos JC, et al. Dose-volume histogram parameters and late side effects in magnetic resonance image-guided adaptive cervical cancer brachytherapy. *Int J Radiat Oncol Biol Phys* 2011;79:356–362.
699. Kapp KS, Stuecklschweiger GF, Kapp DS, et al. Dosimetry of intracavitary placements for uterine and cervical carcinoma: results of orthogonal film, TLD, and CT-assisted techniques. *Radiother Oncol* 1992;24:137–146.
700. Eich HT, Haverkamp U, Micke O, et al. Dosimetric analysis at ICRU reference points in HDR-brachytherapy of cervical carcinoma. *Rontgenpraxis* 2000;53:62–66.
701. Pelloski CE, Palmer M, Chronowski GM, et al. Comparison between CT-based volumetric calculations and ICRU reference-point estimates of radiation doses delivered to bladder and rectum during intracavitary radiotherapy for cervical cancer. *Int J Radiat Oncol Biol Phys* 2005;62:131–137.
702. Patil VM, Patel FD, Chakraborty S, et al. Can point doses predict volumetric dose to rectum and bladder: a CT-based planning study in high dose rate intracavitary brachytherapy of cervical carcinoma? *Br J Radiol* 2011;84(1001):441–448.
703. Wachter-Gerstner N, Wachter S, Reinstadler E, et al. Bladder and rectum dose defined from MRI based treatment planning for cervix cancer brachytherapy: comparison of dose-volume histograms for organ contours and organ wall, comparison with ICRU rectum and bladder reference point. *Radiother Oncol* 2003;68:269–276.
704. Olszewska AM, Saarnak AE, de Boer RW, et al. Comparison of dose-volume histograms and dose-wall histograms of the rectum of patients treated with intracavitary brachytherapy. *Radiother Oncol* 2001;61:83–85.
705. Koom WS, Sohn DK, Kim JY, et al. Computed tomography-based high-dose-rate intracavitary brachytherapy for uterine cervical cancer: preliminary demonstration of correlation between dose-volume parameters and rectal mucosal changes observed by flexible sigmoidoscopy. *Int J Radiat Oncol Biol Phys* 2007;68(5):1446–1454

706. Georg P, Kirisits C, Goldner G, et al. Correlation of dose-volume parameters, endoscopic and clinical rectal side effects in cervix cancer patients treated with definitive radiotherapy including MRI-based brachytherapy. *Radiother Oncol* 2009;91:173–180.

707. Mazeron R, Fokdal LU, Kirchheiner K, et al. Dose-volume effect relationships for late rectal morbidity in patients treated with chemoradiation and MRI-guided adaptive brachytherapy for locally advanced cervical cancer: results from the prospective multicenter EMBRACE study. *Radiother Oncol* 2016;120(3):412–419.

708. Lee LJ, Viswanathan AN. Predictors of toxicity following image-guided high dose rate interstitial brachytherapy for gynecologic cancer. *Int J Radiat Oncol Biol Phys* 2012;84(5):1192–1197.

709. Kirchheiner K, Nout RA, Tanderup K, et al. Manifestation pattern of early-late vaginal morbidity after definitive radiation (chemo)therapy and image-guided adaptive brachytherapy for locally advanced cervical cancer: an analysis from the EMBRACE study. *Int J Radiat Oncol Biol Phys* 2014;89(1):88–95.

710. Susko M, Craciunescu O, Meltsner S, et al. Vaginal dose is associated with toxicity in image guided tandem ring or ovoid-based brachytherapy. *Int J Radiat Oncol Biol Phys* 2016;94(5):1099–1105.

711. Kirisits C, Lang S, Dimopoulos J, et al. Uncertainties when using only one MRI-based treatment plan for subsequent high-dose-rate tandem and ring applications in brachytherapy of cervix cancer. *Radiother Oncol* 2006;81:269–275.

712. Himmelmann A, Holmberg E, Jansson I, et al. The effect of postoperative external radiotherapy on cervical carcinoma stage IB and IIA. *Gynecol Oncol* 1985;22:73–84.

713. Thomadsen BR, Shahabi S, Stitt JA, et al. High dose rate intracavitary brachytherapy for carcinoma of the cervix: the Madison System: II procedural and physical considerations. *Int J Radiat Oncol Biol Phys* 1992;24:349–357.

714. Fellner C, Potter R, Knocke TH, et al. Comparison of radiography- and computed tomography-based treatment planning in cervix cancer in brachytherapy with specific attention to some quality assurance aspects. *Radiother Oncol* 2001;58:53–62.

715. Gebara WJ, Weeks KJ, Jones EL, et al. Carcinoma of the uterine cervix: a 3D—CT analysis of dose to the internal, external and common iliac nodes in tandem and ovoid applications. *Radiother Oncol* 2000;56:43–48.

716. Dewitt KD, Hsu IC, Speight J, et al. 3D inverse treatment planning for the tandem and ovoid applicator in cervical cancer. *Int J Radiat Oncol Biol Phys* 2005;63:1270–1274.

717. Suyama S, Nakaguchi T, Kawakami K, et al. Computed tomography analysis of causes of local failure in radiotherapy for cervical carcinoma. *Cancer* 1998;83:1956–1965.

718. Lee KC, Kim TH, Choi JH, et al. Use of the rectal retractor to reduce the rectal dose in high dose rate intracavitary brachytherapy for a carcinoma of the uterine cervix. *Yonsei Med J* 2004;45:113–122.

719. Wanderas AD, Sundset M, Langdal I, et al. Adaptive brachytherapy of cervical cancer, comparison of conventional point A and CT based individual treatment planning. *Acta Oncol* 2012;51(3):345–354.

720. Dimopoulos JC, Petrow P, Tanderup K, et al. Recommendations from gynaecological (GYN) GEC-ESTRO working group (IV): basic principles and parameters for MR imaging within the frame of image based adaptive cervix cancer brachytherapy. *Radiother Oncol.* 2012;103(1):113–122.

721. Tanderup K, Nielsen SK, Nyvang GB, et al. From point A to the sculpted pear: MR image guidance significantly improves tumour dose and sparing of organs at risk in brachytherapy of cervical cancer. *Radiother Oncol* 2010;94:173–180.

722. Mahantshetty U, Swamidas J, Khanna N, et al. Magnetic resonance image-based dose volume parameters and clinical outcome with high dose rate brachytherapy in cervical cancers—a validation of GYN GEC-ESTRO brachytherapy recommendations. *Clin Oncol (R Coll Radiol)* 2011;23:376–377.

723. Mahantshetty U, Swamidas J, Khanna N, et al. Reporting and validation of gynaecological Groupe Euopeen de Curietherapie European Society for Therapeutic Radiology and Oncology (ESTRO) brachytherapy recommendations for MR image-based dose volume parameters and clinical outcome with high dose-rate brachytherapy in cervical cancers: a single-institution initial experience. *Int J Gynecol Cancer* 2011;21:1110–1116.

724. Jurgenliemk-Schulz I, Lang S, Tanderup K, et al. Variation of treatment planning parameters (D90 HR-CTV, D 2cc for OAR) for cervical cancer tandem ring brachytherapy in a multicentre setting: comparison of standard planning and 3D image guided optimisation based on a joint protocol for dose-volume constraints. *Radiother Oncol* 2010;94:339–345.

725. Mahantshetty U, Khanna N, Swamidas J, et al. Trans-abdominal ultrasound (US) and magnetic resonance imaging (MRI) correlation for conformal intracavitary brachytherapy in carcinoma of the uterine cervix. *Radiother Oncol* 2012;102:130–134.

726. Schmid MP, Nesvacil N, Potter R, et al. Transrectal ultrasound for image-guided adaptive brachytherapy in cervix cancer—an alternative to MRI for target definition? *Radiother Oncol* 2016;120(3):467–472.

727. Dimopoulos JC, Lang S, Kirisits C, et al. Dose-volume histogram parameters and local tumor control in magnetic resonance image-guided cervical cancer brachytherapy. *Int J Radiat Oncol Biol Phys* 2009;75:56–63.

728. Forrest JL, Ackerman I, Barbera L, et al. Patient outcome study of concurrent chemoradiation, external beam radiotherapy, and high-dose rate brachytherapy in locally advanced carcinoma of the cervix. *Int J Gynecol Cancer* 2010;20:1074–1078.

729. Chatani M, Matayoshi Y, Masaki N, et al. A prospective randomized study concerning the point A dose in high-dose rate intracavitary therapy for carcinoma of the uterine cervix. the final results. *Strahlenther Onkol* 1994;170:636–642.

730. Hama Y, Uematsu M, Nagata I, et al. Carcinoma of the uterine cervix: twice- versus once-weekly high-dose-rate brachytherapy. *Radiology* 2001;219:207–212.

731. Mayer A, Nemeskeri C, Petnehazi C, et al. Primary radiotherapy of stage IIA/B-IIIB cervical carcinoma. A comparison of continuous versus sequential regimens. *Strahlenther Onkol* 2004;180:209–215.

732. Nam TK, Ahn SJ. A prospective randomized study on two dose fractionation regimens of high-dose-rate brachytherapy for carcinoma of the uterine cervix: comparison of efficacies and toxicities between two regimens. *J Korean Med Sci* 2004;19:87–94.

733. Liu WS, Yen SH, Chang CH, et al. Determination of the appropriate fraction number and size of the HDR brachytherapy for cervical cancer. *Gynecol Oncol* 1996;60:295–300.

734. Teshima T, Inoue T, Ikeda H, et al, High-dose rate and low-dose rate intracavitary therapy for carcinoma of the uterine cervix final results of Osaka University Hospital. *Cancer* 1993;72:2409–2414.

735. Hareyama M, Sakata K, Oouchi A, et al. High-dose-rate versus low-dose-rate intracavitary therapy for carcinoma of the uterine cervix: a randomized trial. *Cancer* 2002;94:117–124.

736. Lertsanguansinchai P, Lertbutsayanukul C, Shotelersuk K, et al. Phase III randomized trial comparing LDR and HDR brachytherapy in treatment of cervical carcinoma. *Int J Radiat Oncol Biol Phys* 2004;59:1424–1431.

737. Gupta BD, Ayyagara S, Sharma SC, et al. Carcinoma of the cervix: optimal time-dose-fractionation of HDR brachytherapy and comparison with conventional dose-rate brachytherapy. In: Mould RF, ed. *Brachytherapy from radium to optimization.* Leersum, The Netherlands: Nucletron International BV, 1989:307–308.

738. Wang X, Liu R, Ma B, et al. High dose rate versus low dose rate intracavity brachytherapy for locally advanced uterine cervix cancer. *Cochrane Database Syst Rev* 2010;(7):CD007563.

739. Narayan K, van Dyk S, Bernshaw D, et al. Comparative study of LDR (Manchester system) and HDR image-guided conformal brachytherapy of cervical cancer: patterns of failure, late complications, and survival. *Int J Radiat Oncol Biol Phys* 2009;74:1529–1535.

740. Haie-Meder C, Kramar A, Lambin P, et al. Analysis of complications in a prospective randomized trial comparing two brachytherapy low dose rates in cervical carcinoma. *Int J Radiat Oncol Biol Phys* 1994;29:953–960.

741. Toita T, Kato S, Niibe Y, et al. Prospective multi-institutional study of definitive radiotherapy with high-dose-rate intracavitary brachytherapy in patients with nonbulky (<4-cm) stage I and II uterine cervical cancer (JAROG0401/JROSG04-2). *Int J Radiat Oncol Biol Phys* 2012;82:e49–e56.

742. Charra-Brunaud C, Harter V, Delannes M, et al. Impact of 3D image-based PDR brachytherapy on outcome of patients treated for cervix carcinoma in France: results of the national STIC prospective study. *Radiother Oncol* 2012.

743. Potter R, Knocke TH, Fellner C, et al. Definitive radiotherapy based on HDR brachytherapy with iridium 192 in uterine cervix carcinoma: report on the Vienna University Hospital findings (1993–1997) compared to the preceding period in the context of ICRU 38 recommendations. *Cancer Radiother* 2000;4:159–172.

744. Potter R, Dimopoulos J, Georg P, et al. Clinical impact of MRI assisted dose volume adaptation and dose escalation in brachytherapy of locally advanced cervix cancer. *Radiother Oncol* 2007;83:148–155.

745. Tan LT, Coles CE, Hart C, et al. Clinical impact of computed tomography-based image-guided brachytherapy for cervix cancer using the tandem-ring applicator—the Addenbrooke's experience. *Clin Oncol (R Coll Radiol)* 2009;21:175–182.

746. Haie-Meder C, Chargari C, Rey A, et al. DVH parameters and outcome for patients with early-stage cervical cancer treated with preoperative MRI-based low dose rate brachytherapy followed by surgery. *Radiother Oncol* 2009;93:316–321.

747. Cho LP, Manuel M, Catalano P, et al. Outcomes with volume-based dose specification in CT-planned high-dose-rate brachytherapy for stage I–II cervical carcinoma: a 10-year institutional experience. *Gynecol Oncol* 2016;143(3):545–551.

748. Fowler JF. Dose reduction factors when increasing dose rate in LDR or MDR brachytherapy of carcinoma of the cervix. *Radiother Oncol* 1997;45:49–54.

749. Leborgne F, Fowler JF, Leborgne JH, et al. Fractionation in medium dose rate brachytherapy of cancer of the cervix. *Int J Radiat Oncol Biol Phys* 1996;35:907–914.

750. Rodrigus P, De Winter K, Venselaar JL, et al. Evaluation of late morbidity in patients with carcinoma of the uterine cervix following a dose rate change. *Radiother Oncol* 1997;42:137–141.

751. Rotmensch J, Connell PP, Yamada D, et al. One versus two intracavitary brachytherapy applications in early-stage cervical cancer patients undergoing definitive radiation therapy. *Gynecol Oncol* 2000;78:32–38.

752. Ngo C, Alran S, Plancher C, et al. Outcome in early cervical cancer following pre-operative low dose rate brachytherapy: a ten-year follow up of 257 patients treated at a single institution. *Gynecol Oncol* 2011;123:248–252.

753. Rogers CL, Freel JH, Speiser BL. Pulsed low dose rate brachytherapy for uterine cervix carcinoma. *Int J Radiat Oncol Biol Phys* 1999;43:95–100.

754. Kaneyasu Y, Kita M, Okawa T, et al. Treatment outcome of medium-dose-rate intracavitary brachytherapy for carcinoma of the uterine cervix: comparison with low-dose-rate intracavitary brachytherapy. *Int J Radiat Oncol Biol Phys* 2012;84(1):137–145.

755. El-Baradie M, Inoue T, Murayama S, et al. HDR and MDR intracavitary treatment for carcinoma of the uterine cervix. A prospective randomized study. *Strahlenther Onkol* 1997;173:155–162.

756. Tanaka E, Suzuki O, Oh RJ, et al. Intracavitary brachytherapy for carcinoma of the uterine cervix—comparison of HDR (ir-192) and MDR (cs-137). *Radiat Med* 2006;24:50–57.

757. Bachtiary B, Dewitt A, Pintilie M, et al. Comparison of late toxicity between continuous low-dose-rate and pulsed-dose-rate brachytherapy in cervical cancer patients. *Int J Radiat Oncol Biol Phys* 2005;63:1077–1082.

758. Rath GK, Sharma DN, Julka PK, et al. Pulsed-dose-rate intracavitary brachytherapy for cervical carcinoma: the AIIMS experience. *Am J Clin Oncol* 2010;33:238–241.

759. Cikaric S. Radiation therapy of cervical carcinoma using either HDR or LDR afterloading: comparison of 5-year results and complications. *Strahlenther Onkol (Suppl)* 1988;82:119–122.
760. Glaser FH. Comparison of HDR afterloading with 192Ir versus conventional radium therapy in cervix cancer: 5-year results and complications. *Strahlenther Onkol (Suppl)* 1988;82:106–113.
761. Joslin CAF. High-activity source afterloading in gynecologic cancer and its future prospects. *Endocuriether Hypertherm Oncol* 1989;5:69–81.
762. Falkenberg E, Kim RY, Meleth S, et al. Low-dose-rate vs. high-dose-rate intracavitary brachytherapy for carcinoma of the cervix: the University of Alabama at Birmingham (UAB) experience. *Brachytherapy* 2006;5:49–55.
763. Ferrigno R, Nishimoto IN, Novaes PE, et al. Comparison of low and high dose rate brachytherapy in the treatment of uterine cervix cancer. Retrospective analysis of two sequential series. *Int J Radiat Oncol Biol Phys* 2005;62:1108–1116.
764. Hsu WL, Wu CJ, Jen YM, et al. Twice-per-day fractionated high versus continuous low dose rate intracavitary therapy in the radical treatment of cervical cancer: a nonrandomized comparison of treatment results. *Int J Radiat Oncol Biol Phys* 1995;32:1425–1431.
765. Kim WC, Kim GE, Suh CO, et al. High versus low dose rate intracavitary irradiation for adenocarcinoma of the uterine cervix. *Jpn J Clin Oncol* 2001;31:432–437.
766. Kucera H, Potter R, Knocke TH, et al. High dose versus low dose rate brachytherapy in definitive radiotherapy of cervical cancer. *Wien Klin Wochenschr* 2001;113:58–62.
767. Okkan S, Atkovar G, Sahinler I, et al. Results and complications of high dose rate and low dose rate brachytherapy in carcinoma of the cervix: Cerrahpasa experience. *Radiother Oncol* 2003;67:97–105.
768. Sarkaria JN, Petereit DG, Stitt JA, et al. A comparison of the efficacy and complication rates of low dose-rate versus high dose-rate brachytherapy in the treatment of uterine cervical carcinoma. *Int J Radiat Oncol Biol Phys* 1994;30:75–82; discussion 247.
769. Lorvidhaya V, Tonusin A, Changwiwit W, et al. High dose rate afterloading brachytherapy in carcinoma of the cervix: an experience of 1992 patients. *Int J Radiat Oncol Biol Phys* 2000;46:1185–1191.
770. Sakata KI, Nagakura H, Oouchi A, et al. High dose rate intracavitary brachytherapy: results of analyses of late rectal complications. *Int J Radiat Oncol Biol Phys* 2002;54:1369–1376.
771. Souhami L, Corns R, Duclos M, et al. Long-term results of high-dose rate brachytherapy in cervix cancer using a small number of fractions. *Gynecol Oncol* 2005;97:508–513.
772. Wong FC, Tung SY, Leung TW, et al. Treatment results of high-dose-rate remote afterloading brachytherapy for cervical cancer and retrospective comparison of two regimens. *Int J Radiat Oncol Biol Phys* 2003;55:1254–1264.
773. Sood BM, Gorla G, Gupta S, et al. Two fractions of high-dose-rate brachytherapy in the management of cervix cancer: clinical experience with and without chemotherapy. *Int J Radiat Oncol Biol Phys* 2002;53:702–706.
774. Saibishkumar EP, Patel FD, Sharma SC. Results of a phase II trial of concurrent chemoradiation in the treatment of locally advanced carcinoma of uterine cervix: an experience from India. *Bull Cancer* 2005;92:E7–E12.
775. Viswanathan AN. Childhood cancer survivors: stillbirth and neonatal death. *Lancet* 2010;376:570–572.
776. Ozsaran Z, Yalman D, Yurut V, et al. Radiochemotherapy for patients with locally advanced cervical cancer: early results. *Eur J Gynaecol Oncol* 2003;24:191–194.
777. Strauss HG, Kuhnt T, Laban C, et al. Chemoradiation in cervical cancer with cisplatin and high dose rate brachytherapy combined with external beam radiotherapy results of a phase II study. *Strahlenther Onkol* 2002;178:378–385.
778. Mahmud A, Brydon B, Tonita J, et al. A population-based study of cervix cancer: incidence, management and outcome in the Canadian Province of Saskatchewan. *Clin Oncol (R Coll Radiol)* 2011;23:691–695.
779. Kapp KS, Stuecklschweiger GF, Kapp DS, et al. Prognostic factors in patients with carcinoma of the uterine cervix treated with external beam irradiation and IR-192 high-dose-rate brachytherapy. *Int J Radiat Oncol Biol Phys* 1998;42:531–540.
780. Kuske RR, Perez CA, Jacobs AJ, et al. Mini-colpostats in the treatment of carcinoma of the uterine cervix. *Int J Radiat Oncol Biol Phys* 1988;14:899–906.
781. Dimopoulos JC, Kirisits C, Petric P, et al. The Vienna applicator for combined intracavitary and interstitial brachytherapy of cervical cancer: clinical feasibility and preliminary results. *Int J Radiat Oncol Biol Phys* 2006;66:83–90.
782. Nomden CN, de Leeuw AA, Moerland MA, et al. Clinical use of the Utrecht applicator for combined intracavitary/interstitial brachytherapy treatment in locally advanced cervical cancer. *Int J Radiat Oncol Biol Phys* 2012;82(4):1424–1430.
783. Anker CJ, Cachoeira CV, Boucher KM, et al. Does the entire uterus need to be treated in cancer of the cervix? Role of adaptive brachytherapy. *Int J Radiat Oncol Biol Phys* 2010;76:704–712.
784. Le Pechoux C, Akine Y, Sumi M, et al. High dose rate brachytherapy for carcinoma of the uterine cervix: comparison of two different fractionation regimens. *Int J Radiat Oncol Biol Phys* 1995;31:735–741.
785. Selke P, Roman TN, Souhami L, et al. Treatment results of high dose rate brachytherapy in patients with carcinoma of the cervix. *Int J Radiat Oncol Biol Phys* 1993;27:803–809.
786. Choi P, Teo P, Foo W, et al. High-dose rate remote afterloading irradiation of carcinoma of the cervix in Hong Kong: unexpectedly high complication rate. *Clin Oncol* 1992;4:186–191.
787. Kagei K, Shirato H, Nishioka T, et al. High-dose-rate intracavitary irradiation using linear source arrangement for stage II and III squamous cell carcinoma of the uterine cervix. *Radiother Oncol* 1998;47:207–213.
788. Takeshi K, Katsuyuki K, Yoshiaki T, et al. Definitive radiotherapy combined with high-dose-rate brachytherapy for stage III carcinoma of the uterine cervix: retrospective analysis of prognostic factors concerning patient characteristics and treatment parameters. *Int J Radiat Oncol Biol Phys* 1998;41:319–327.
789. Wang CJ, Leung SW, Chen HC, et al. High-dose-rate intracavitary brachytherapy (HDR-IC) in treatment of cervical carcinoma: 5-year results and implication of increased low-grade rectal complication on initiation of an HDR-IC fractionation scheme. *Int J Radiat Oncol Biol Phys* 1997;38:391–398.
790. Leborgne F, Leborgne JH, Zubizarreta E, et al. High dose rate brachytherapy at 14Gy per hour to point A: preliminary results of a prospectively designed schedule for cancer of the cervix based on the linear-quadratic model. *Int J Gynecol Cancer* 2001;11:445–453.
791. Nakano T, Kato S, Ohno T, et al. Long-term results of high-dose rate intracavitary brachytherapy for squamous cell carcinoma of the uterine cervix. *Cancer* 2005;103:92–101.
792. Nakano T, Kato S, Cao J, et al. A regional cooperative clinical study of radiotherapy for cervical cancer in east and south-east Asian countries. *Radiother Oncol* 2007;84:314–319.
793. Novetsky AP, Einstein MH, Goldberg GL, et al. Efficacy and toxicity of concomitant cisplatin with external beam pelvic radiotherapy and two high-dose-rate brachytherapy insertions for the treatment of locally advanced cervical cancer. *Gynecol Oncol* 2007;105:635–640.
794. Patel FD, Kumar P, Karunanidhi G, et al. Optimization of high-dose-rate intracavitary brachytherapy schedule in the treatment of carcinoma of the cervix. *Brachytherapy* 2011;10:147–153.
795. Wachter-Gerstner N, Wachter S, Reinstadler E, et al. The impact of sectional imaging on dose escalation in endocavitary HDR-brachytherapy of cervical cancer: results of a prospective comparative trial. *Radiother Oncol* 2003;68:51–59.
796. Kamran SC, Manuel MM, Cho LP, et al. Comparison of outcomes for MR-guided versus CT-guided high-dose-rate interstitial brachytherapy in women with locally advanced carcinoma of the cervix. *Gynecol Oncol* 2017;145(2): 284–290.
797. Schoeppel SL, Ellis JH, LaVigne ML, et al. Magnetic resonance imaging during intracavitary gynecologic brachytherapy. *Int J Radiat Oncol Biol Phys* 1992;23:169–174.
798. Tardivon AA, Kinkel K, Lartigau E, et al. MR imaging during intracavitary brachytherapy of vaginal and cervical cancer: preliminary results. *Radiographics* 1996;16:1363–1370.
799. Cozzi L, Dinshaw KA, Shrivastava SK, et al. A treatment planning study comparing volumetric arc modulation with RapidArc and fixed field IMRT for cervix uteri radiotherapy. *Radiother Oncol* 2008;89:180–191.
800. Zwahlen D, Jezioranski J, Chan P, et al. Magnetic resonance imaging-guided intracavitary brachytherapy for cancer of the cervix. *Int J Radiat Oncol Biol Phys* 2009;74:1157–1164.
801. Syed AM, Feder BH. Technique of after-loading interstitial implants. *Radiol Clin* 1977;46:458–475.
802. Martinez A, Edmundson GK, Cox RS, et al. Combination of external beam irradiation and multiple-site perineal applicator (MUPIT) for treatment of locally advanced or recurrent prostatic, anorectal, and gynecologic malignancies. *Int J Radiat Oncol Biol Phys* 1985;11:391–398.
803. Viswanathan AN, Cormack R, Rawal B, et al. Increasing brachytherapy dose predicts survival for interstitial and tandem-based radiation for stage IIIB cervical cancer. *Int J Gynecol Cancer* 2009;19:1402–1406.
804. Small W Jr, Strauss JB, Hwang CS, et al. Should uterine tandem applicators ever be placed without ultrasound guidance? No: a brief report and review of the literature. *Int J Gynecol Cancer* 2011;21:941–944.
805. Pierquin B, Marinello G, Mege JP, et al. Intracavitary irradiation of carcinomas of the uterus and cervix: the Creteil method. *Int J Radiat Oncol Biol Phys* 1988;15:1465–1473.
806. Prempree T. Parametrial implant in stage III B cancer of the cervix. III. A five-year study. *Cancer* 1983;52:748–750.
807. Nag S, Martinez-Monge R, Selman AE, et al. Interstitial brachytherapy in the management of primary carcinoma of the cervix and vagina. *Gynecol Oncol* 1998;70:27–32.
808. Fallon J, Park SJ, Yang L, et al. Long term results from a prospective database on high dose rate (HDR) interstitial brachytherapy for primary cervical carcinoma. *Gynecol Oncol.* 2016.
809. Recio FO, Piver MS, Hempling RE, et al. Laparoscopic-assisted application of interstitial brachytherapy for locally advanced cervical carcinoma: results of a pilot study. *Int J Radiat Oncol Biol Phys* 1998;40:411–414.
810. Sharma DN, Rath GK, Thulkar S, et al. High-dose rate interstitial brachytherapy using two weekly sessions of 10 Gy each for patients with locally advanced cervical carcinoma. *Brachytherapy* 2011;10:242–248.
811. Sharma DN, Rath GK, Thulkar S, et al. Use of transrectal ultrasound for high dose rate interstitial brachytherapy for patients of carcinoma of uterine cervix. *J Gynecol Oncol* 2010;21:12–17.
812. Beriwal S, Bhatnagar A, Heron DE, et al. High-dose-rate interstitial brachytherapy for gynecologic malignancies. *Brachytherapy* 2006;5:218–222.
813. Mendez LC, Weiss Y, D'Souza D, et al. Three-dimensional-guided perineal-based interstitial brachytherapy in cervical cancer: a systematic review of technique, local control and toxicities. *Radiother Oncol* 2017;123(2):312–318.
814. Mikami M, Yoshida K, Takenaka T, et al. Daily computed tomography measurement of needle applicator displacement during high-dose-rate interstitial brachytherapy for previously untreated uterine cervical cancer. *Brachytherapy* 2011;10:318–324.
815. Shukla P, Chopra S, Engineer R, et al. Quality assurance of multifractionated pelvic interstitial brachytherapy for postoperative recurrences of cervical cancers: a prospective study. *Int J Radiat Oncol Biol Phys* 2012;82:e617–e622.
816. Damato A, Cormack R, Viswanathan AN. Characterization of implant displacement and deformation in gynecologic interstitial brachytherapy. *Brachytheraphy* 2014;13(1):100–109.
817. Magné N, Mancy NC, Chajon E, et al. Patterns of care and outcome in elderly cervical cancer patients: a special focus on brachytherapy. *Radiother Oncol* 2009;91:197–201.

818. Han K, Milosevic M, Fyles A, et al. Trends in the utilization of brachytherapy in cervical cancer in the united states. *Int J Radiat Oncol Biol Phys* 2013;87(1):111–119.

819. Han K, Viswanathan AN. Brachytherapy in gynecologic cancers: why is it underused? *Curr Oncol Rep* 2016;18(4):26.

820. Robin TP, Amini A, Schefter TE, et al. Disparities in standard of care treatment and associated survival decrement in patients with locally advanced cervical cancer. *Gynecol Oncol* 2016;143(2):319–325.

821. Barraclough LH, Swindell R, Livsey JE, et al. External beam boost for cancer of the cervix uteri when intracavitary therapy cannot be performed. *Int J Radiat Oncol Biol Phys* 2008;71:772–778.

822. Georg D, Kirisits C, Hillbrand M, et al. Image-guided radiotherapy for cervix cancer: high-tech external beam therapy versus high-tech brachytherapy. *Int J Radiat Oncol Biol Phys* 2008;71:1272–1278.

823. Logsdon MD, Eifel PJ. FIGO IIIB squamous cell carcinoma of the cervix: an analysis of prognostic factors emphasizing the balance between external beam and intracavitary radiation therapy. *Int J Radiat Oncol Biol Phys* 1999;43:763–775.

824. Akine Y, Hashida I, Kajiura Y, et al. Carcinoma of the uterine cervix treated with external irradiation alone. *Int J Radiat Oncol Biol Phys* 1986;12:1611–1616.

825. Saibishkumar EP, Patel FD, Sharma SC, et al. Results of external-beam radiotherapy alone in invasive cancer of the uterine cervix: a retrospective analysis. *Clin Oncol (R Coll Radiol)* 2006;18:46–51.

826. Wright J, Jones G, Whelan T, et al. Patient preference for high or low dose rate brachytherapy in carcinoma of the cervix. *Radiother Oncol* 1994;33:187–194.

827. Bastin K, Buchler D, Stitt J, et al. Resource utilization. high dose rate versus low dose rate brachytherapy for gynecologic cancer. *Am J Clin Oncol* 1993;16:256–263.

828. Maruyama Y, Muir W. Human cervical cancer clearance after 252Cf neutron brachytherapy versus conventional photon brachytherapy. *Am J Clin Oncol* 1984;7:347–352.

829. Marcial VA, Blanco MS, De Leon E. Persistent tumor cells in the vaginal smear during the first year after radiation therapy of carcinoma of the uterine cervix. prognostic significance. *Am J Roentgenol Radium Ther Nucl Med* 1968;102:170–175.

830. Soisson AP, Geszler G, Soper JT, et al. A comparison of symptomatology, physical examination, and vaginal cytology in the detection of recurrent cervical carcinoma after radical hysterectomy. *Obstet Gynecol* 1990;76:106–109.

831. Davey DD, Zaleski S, Sattich M, et al. Prognostic significance of DNA cytometry of postirradiation cervicovaginal smears. *Cancer* 1998;84:11–16.

832. Rintala MA, Rantanen VT, Salmi TA, et al. PAP smear after radiation therapy for cervical carcinoma. *Anticancer Res* 1997;17:3747–3750.

833. Bodurka-Bevers D, Morris M, Eifel PJ, et al. Posttherapy surveillance of women with cervical cancer: an outcomes analysis. *Gynecol Oncol* 2000;78:187–193.

834. Vernooij CB, Kruitwagen RF, Rodrigus P, et al. Hematometra after radiotherapy for cervical carcinoma. *Gynecol Oncol* 1997;67:325–327.

835. Hintz BL, Kagan AR, Chan P, et al. Radiation tolerance of the vaginal mucosa. *Int J Radiat Oncol Biol Phys* 1980;6:711–716.

836. Larson DM, Copeland LJ, Stringer CA, et al. Recurrent cervical carcinoma after radical hysterectomy. *Gynecol Oncol* 1988;30:381–387.

837. Ijaz T, Eifel PJ, Burke T, et al. Radiation therapy of pelvic recurrence after radical hysterectomy for cervical carcinoma. *Gynecol Oncol* 1998;70:241–246.

838. Hille A, Weiss E, Hess CF. Therapeutic outcome and prognostic factors in the radiotherapy of recurrences of cervical carcinoma following surgery. *Strahlenther Onkol* 2003;179:742–747.

839. Sommers GM, Grigsby PW, Perez CA, et al. Outcome of recurrent cervical carcinoma following definitive irradiation. *Gynecol Oncol* 1989;35:150–155.

840. Coleman RL, Keeney ED, Freedman RA, et al. Radical hysterectomy after radiotherapy for recurrent carcinoma of the uterine cervix. *Gynecol Oncol* 1994;55:29–35.

841. Lawhead RA Jr, Clark DG, Smith DH, et al. Pelvic exenteration for recurrent or persistent gynecologic malignancies: a 10-year review of the Memorial Sloan-Kettering Cancer Center experience (1972–1981). *Gynecol Oncol* 1989;33:279–282.

842. Kastritis E, Bamias A, Efstathiou E, et al. The outcome of advanced or recurrent non-squamous carcinoma of the uterine cervix after platinum-based combination chemotherapy. *Gynecol Oncol* 2005;99:376–382.

843. Tinker AV, Bhagat K, Swenerton KD, et al. Carboplatin and paclitaxel for advanced and recurrent cervical carcinoma: the British Columbia Cancer Agency experience. *Gynecol Oncol* 2005;98:54–58.

844. Penson RT, Huang HQ, Wenzel LB, et al. Bevacizumab for advanced cervical cancer: patient-reported outcomes of a randomised, phase 3 trial (NRG oncology-gynecologic oncology group protocol 240). *Lancet Oncol* 2015;16(3):301–311.

845. Jhingran A, Yom SS, Zang X, et al. Recurrence above the radiotherapy field after definitive treatment of cervix cancer. *Int J Radiat Oncol Biol Phys* 2005;63:S217–S218.

846. Mahé MA, Gerard JP, Dubois JB, et al. Intraoperative radiation therapy in recurrent carcinoma of the uterine cervix: report of the French intraoperative group on 70 patients. *Int J Radiat Oncol Biol Phys* 1996;34:21–26.

847. Garton GR, Gunderson LL, Webb MJ, et al. Intraoperative radiation therapy in gynecologic cancer: the Mayo Clinic experience. *Gynecol Oncol* 1993;48:328–332.

848. Abe M, Shibamoto Y. The usefulness of intraoperative radiation therapy in the treatment of pelvic recurrence of cervical cancer. *Int J Radiat Oncol Biol Phys* 1996;34:513–514.

849. Martinez Monge R, Jurado M, Azinovic I, et al. Intraoperative radiotherapy in recurrent gynecological cancer. *Radiother Oncol* 1993:127–133.

850. Giorda G, Boz G, Gadducci A, et al. Multimodality approach in extra cervical locally advanced cervical cancer: chemoradiation, surgery and intra-operative radiation therapy. A phase II trial. *Eur J Surg Oncol* 2011;37:442–447.

851. van Lonkhuijzen L, Thomas G. Palliative radiotherapy for cervical carcinoma, a systematic review. *Radiother Oncol* 2011;98:287–291.

852. Grigsby PW, Portelance L, Williamson JF. High dose ratio (HDR) cervical ring applicator to control bleeding from cervical carcinoma. *Int J Gynecol Cancer* 2002;12(1):18–21.

853. Spanos WJ Jr, Clery M, Perez CA, et al. Late effect of multiple daily fraction palliation schedule for advanced pelvic malignancies (RTOG 8502). *Int J Radiat Oncol Biol Phys* 1994;29(5):961–967.

854. Spanos WJ, Perez CA, Marcus S, et al. Effect of rest interval on tumor and normal tissue response—a report of phase III study of accelerated split course palliative radiation for advanced pelvic malignancies (RTOG-8502). *Int J Radiat Oncol Biol Phys* 1993;25:399–403.

855. Hornback NB, Shupe RE, Shidnia H, et al. Advanced stage IIIB cancer of the cervix treatment by hyperthermia and radiation. *Gynecol Oncol* 1986;23:160–167.

856. Sharma S. A prospective randomized study of local hyperthermia as a supplement and radiosensitizer in the treatment of carcinoma of the cervix with radiotherapy. *Endocuriether Hyperthermia Oncol* 1989;5:151–159.

857. Dinges S, Harder C, Wurm R, et al. Combined treatment of inoperable carcinomas of the uterine cervix with radiotherapy and regional hyperthermia. Results of a phase II trial. *Strahlenther Onkol* 1998;174:517–521.

858. Harima Y, Nagata K, Harima K, et al. A randomized clinical trial of radiation therapy versus thermoradiotherapy in stage IIIB cervical carcinoma. *Int J Hyperthermia* 2001;17:97–105.

859. Vasanthan A, Mitsumori M, Park JH, et al. Regional hyperthermia combined with radiotherapy for uterine cervical cancers: a multi-institutional prospective randomized trial of the international atomic energy agency. *Int J Radiat Oncol Biol Phys* 2005;61:145–153.

860. Lutgens L, van der Zee J, Pijls-Johannesma M, et al. Combined use of hyperthermia and radiation therapy for treating locally advanced cervix carcinoma. *Cochrane Database Syst Rev* 2010;(1):CD006377.

861. Wootton JH, Prakash P, Hsu IC, et al. Implant strategies for endocervical and interstitial ultrasound hyperthermia adjunct to HDR brachytherapy for the treatment of cervical cancer. *Phys Med Biol* 2011;56:3967–3984.

862. Magrina JF, Goodrich MA, Weaver AL, et al. Modified radical hysterectomy: morbidity and mortality. *Gynecol Oncol* 1995;59:277–282.

863. Barnes W, Waggoner S, Delgado G, et al. Manometric characterization of rectal dysfunction following radical hysterectomy. *Gynecol Oncol* 1991;42:116–119.

864. Viswanathan AN, Lee LJ, Eswara JR, et al. Complications of pelvic radiation in patients treated for gynecologic malignancies. *Cancer* 2014;120(24):3870–3883.

865. Fiorica JV, Roberts WS, Greenberg H, et al. Morbidity and survival patterns in patients after radical hysterectomy and postoperative adjuvant pelvic radiotherapy. *Gynecol Oncol* 1990;36:343–347.

866. Seow-Choen F, Goh HS, Eu KW, et al. A simple and effective treatment for hemorrhagic radiation proctitis using formalin. *Dis Colon Rectum* 1993;36:135–138.

867. Kizer NT, Thaker PH, Gao F, et al. The effects of body mass index on complications and survival outcomes in patients with cervical carcinoma undergoing curative chemoradiation therapy. *Cancer* 2011;117:948–956.

868. Montz FJ, Holschneider CH, Solh S, et al. Small bowel obstruction following radical hysterectomy: risk factors, incidence, and operative findings. *Gynecol Oncol* 1994;53:114–120.

869. Eifel PJ, Levenback C, Wharton JT, et al. Time course and incidence of late complications in patients treated with radiation therapy for FIGO stage IB carcinoma of the uterine cervix. *Int J Radiat Oncol Biol Phys* 1995;32:1289–1300.

870. Jacobs AJ, Perez CA, Camel HM, et al. Complications in patients receiving both irradiation and radical hysterectomy for carcinoma of the uterine cervix. *Gynecol Oncol* 1985;22:273–280.

871. Perez CA, Breaux S, Bedwinek JM, et al. Radiation therapy alone in the treatment of carcinoma of the uterine cervix. II. Analysis of complications. *Cancer* 1984;54:235–246.

872. Pedersen D, Bentzen SM, Overgaard J. Early and late radiotherapeutic morbidity in 442 consecutive patients with locally advanced carcinoma of the uterine cervix. *Int J Radiat Oncol Biol Phys* 1994;29:941–952.

873. Perez CA, Grigsby PW, Lockett MA, et al. Radiation therapy morbidity in carcinoma of the uterine cervix: dosimetric and clinical correlation. *Int J Radiat Oncol Biol Phys* 1999;44:855–866.

874. Pourquier H, Dubois JB, Delard R. Cancer of the uterine cervix: dosimetric guidelines for prevention of late rectal and rectosigmoid complications as a result of radiotherapeutic treatment. *Int J Radiat Oncol Biol Phys* 1982;8:1887–1895.

875. Lanciano RM, Martz K, Montana GS, et al. Influence of age, prior abdominal surgery, fraction size, and dose on complications after radiation therapy for squamous cell cancer of the uterine cervix. A patterns of care study. *Cancer* 1992;69:2124–2130.

876. Lee SW, Suh CO, Chung EJ, et al. Dose optimization of fractionated external radiation and high dose rate intracavitary brachytherapy for FIGO stage IB uterine cervical carcinoma. *Int J Radiat Oncol Biol Phys* 2002;52:1338–1344.

877. Roche B, Chautems R, Marti MC. Application of formaldehyde for treatment of hemorrhagic radiation-induced proctitis. *World J Surg* 1996;20:1092, 1094; discussion 1094–5.

878. Rubinstein E, Ibsen T, Rasmussen RB, et al. Formalin treatment of radiation-induced hemorrhagic proctitis. *Am J Gastroenterol* 1986;81:44–45.

879. Nelson R, Norton N, Cautley E, et al. Community-based prevalence of anal incontinence. *JAMA* 1995;274:559–561.

880. Kim GE, Lim JJ, Park W, et al. Sensory and motor dysfunction assessed by anorectal manometry in uterine cervical carcinoma patients with radiation-induced late rectal complication. *Int J Radiat Oncol Biol Phys* 1998;41:835–841.

881. Quilty PM. A report of late rectosigmoid morbidity in patients with advanced cancer of the cervix, treated by a six week pelvic brick technique. *Clin Radiol* 1988;39:297–300.

882. Stryker JA, Bartholomew M, Velkley DE, et al. Bladder and rectal complications following radiotherapy for cervix cancer. *Gynecol Oncol* 1988;29:1–11.

883. Kasibhatla M, Clough RW, Montana GS, et al. Predictors of severe gastrointestinal toxicity after external beam radiotherapy and interstitial brachytherapy for advanced or recurrent gynecologic malignancies. *Int J Radiat Oncol Biol Phys* 2006;65:398–403.

884. Rotman M, Pajak TF, Choi K, et al. Prophylactic extended-field irradiation of para-aortic lymph nodes in stages IIB and bulky IB and IIA cervical carcinomas. ten-year treatment results of RTOG 79-20. *JAMA* 1995;274:387–393.

885. Willett CG, Ooi CJ, Zietman AL, et al. Acute and late toxicity of patients with inflammatory bowel disease undergoing irradiation for abdominal and pelvic neoplasms. *Int J Radiat Oncol Biol Phys* 2000;46:995–998.

886. Tiersten A, Saltz LB. Influence of inflammatory bowel disease on the ability of patients to tolerate systemic fluorouracil-based chemotherapy. *J Clin Oncol* 1996;14:2043–2046.

887. Levenback C, Eifel PJ, Burke TW, et al. Hemorrhagic cystitis following radiotherapy for stage Ib cancer of the cervix. *Gynecol Oncol* 1994;55:206–210.

888. McIntyre JF, Eifel PJ, Levenback C, et al. Ureteral stricture as a late complication of radiotherapy for stage IB carcinoma of the uterine cervix. *Cancer* 1995;75:836–843.

889. Buglione M, Toninelli M, Pietta N, et al. Post-radiation pelvic disease and ureteral stenosis: physiopathology and evolution in the patient treated for cervical carcinoma. review of the literature and experience of the radium institute]. *Arch Ital Urol Androl* 2002;74:6–11.

890. Prasad KN, Pradhan S, Datta NR. Urinary tract infection in patients of gynecological malignancies undergoing external pelvic radiotherapy. *Gynecol Oncol* 1995;57:380–382.

891. Parkin DE, Davis JA, Symonds RP. Urodynamic findings following radiotherapy for cervical carcinoma. *Br J Urol* 1988;61:213–217.

892. DePasquale SE, Mylonas I, Falkenberry SS. Fatal recurrent ureteroarterial fistulas after exenteration for cervical cancer. *Gynecol Oncol* 2001;82:192–196.

893. Georgiou A, Grigsby PW, Perez CA. Radiation induced lumbosacral plexopathy in gynecologic tumors: clinical findings and dosimetric analysis. *Int J Radiat Oncol Biol Phys* 1993;26:479–482.

894. Abu-Rustum N, Rajbhandari D, Glusman S, et al. Acute lower extremity paralysis following radiation therapy for cervical cancer. *Gynecol Oncol* 1999;75:152–154.

895. Thomas JE, Cascino TL, Earle JD. Differential diagnosis between radiation and tumor plexopathy of the pelvis. *Neurology* 1985;35:1–7.

896. Bruner DW, Lanciano R, Keegan M, et al. Vaginal stenosis and sexual function following intracavitary radiation for the treatment of cervical and endometrial carcinoma. *Int J Radiat Oncol Biol Phys* 1993;27:825–830.

897. Grigsby PW, Russell A, Bruner D, et al. Late injury of cancer therapy on the female reproductive tract. *Int J Radiat Oncol Biol Phys* 1995;31:1281–1299.

898. Lammerink EA, de Bock GH, Pras E, et al. Sexual functioning of cervical cancer survivors: a review with a female perspective. *Maturitas* 2012;72(4):296–304.

899. Robinson JW, Faris PD, Scott CB. Psychoeducational group increases vaginal dilation for younger women and reduces sexual fears for women of all ages with gynecological carcinoma treated with radiotherapy. *Int J Radiat Oncol Biol Phys* 1999;44:497–506.

900. Jensen PT, Groenvold M, Klee MC, et al. Longitudinal study of sexual function and vaginal changes after radiotherapy for cervical cancer. *Int J Radiat Oncol Biol Phys* 2003;56:937–949.

901. Grigsby PW, Roberts HL, Perez CA. Femoral neck fracture following groin irradiation. *Int J Radiat Oncol Biol Phys* 1995;32:63–67.

902. Baxter NN, Habermann EB, Tepper JE, et al. Risk of pelvic fractures in older women following pelvic irradiation. *JAMA* 2005;294:2587–2593.

903. Blomlie V, Rofstad EK, Talle K, et al. Incidence of radiation-induced insufficiency fractures of the female pelvis: evaluation with MR imaging. *AJR Am J Roentgenol* 1996;167:1205–1210.

904. Moreno A, Clemente J, Crespo C, et al. Pelvic insufficiency fractures in patients with pelvic irradiation. *Int J Radiat Oncol Biol Phys* 1999;44:61–66.

905. Ramlov A, Pedersen EM, Rohl L, et al. Risk factors for pelvic insufficiency fractures in locally advanced cervical cancer following intensity modulated radiation therapy. *Int J Radiat Oncol Biol Phys.* 2017;97(5):1032–1039.

906. Huh SJ, Kim B, Kang MK, et al. Pelvic insufficiency fracture after pelvic irradiation in uterine cervix cancer. *Gynecol Oncol* 2002;86:264–268.

907. Bye A, Trope C, Loge JH, et al. Health-related quality of life and occurrence of intestinal side effects after pelvic radiotherapy—evaluation of long-term effects of diagnosis and treatment. *Acta Oncol* 2000;39:173–180.

908. Dusenbery KE, Carson LF, Potish RA. Perioperative morbidity and mortality of gynecologic brachytherapy. *Cancer* 1991;67:2786–2790.

909. Lanciano R, Corn B, Martin E, et al. Perioperative morbidity of intracavitary gynecologic brachytherapy. *Int J Radiat Oncol Biol Phys* 1994;29:969–974.

910. Jhingran A, Eifel PJ. Perioperative and postoperative complications of intracavitary radiation for FIGO stage I–III carcinoma of the cervix. *Int J Radiat Oncol Biol Phys* 2000;46:1177–1183.

911. Wollschlaeger K, Connell PP, Waggoner S, et al. Acute problems during low-dose-rate intracavitary brachytherapy for cervical carcinoma. *Gynecol Oncol* 2000;76:67–72.

912. Jeffries SA, Robinson JW, Craighead PS, et al. An effective group psychoeducational intervention for improving compliance with vaginal dilation: a randomized controlled trial. *Int J Radiat Oncol Biol Phys* 2006;65:404–411.

913. Petereit DG, Sarkaria JN, Chappell RJ. Perioperative morbidity and mortality of high-dose-rate gynecologic brachytherapy. *Int J Radiat Oncol Biol Phys* 1998;42:1025–1031.

914. Ogino I, Kitamura T, Okamoto N, et al. Late rectal complication following high dose rate intracavitary brachytherapy in cancer of the cervix. *Int J Radiat Oncol Biol Phys* 1995;31:725–734.

915. Fujikawa K, Yamamichi F, Nonomura M, et al. Spontaneous rupture of the urinary bladder is not a rare complication of radiotherapy for cervical cancer: report of six cases. *Gynecol Oncol* 1999;73:439–442.

916. Clark BG, Souhami L, Roman TN, et al. Rectal complications in patients with carcinoma of the cervix treated with concomitant cisplatin and external beam irradiation with high-dose-rate brachytherapy: a dosimetric analysis. *Int J Radiat Oncol Biol Phys* 1994;28:1243–1250.

917. Weiss JP, Mattei DM, Neville EC, et al. Primary treatment of radiation-induced hemorrhagic cystitis with hyperbaric oxygen: 10-year experience. *J Urol* 1994;151:1514–1517.

918. Lee HC, Liu CS, Chiao C, et al. Hyperbaric oxygen therapy in hemorrhagic radiation cystitis: a report of 20 cases. *Undersea Hyperb Med* 1994;21:321–327.

919. Watson ER, Halnan KE, Dische S, et al. Hyperbaric oxygen and radiotherapy: a medical research council trial in carcinoma of the cervix. *Br J Radiol* 1978;51:879–887.

920. Dische S, Saunders MI, Sealy R, et al. Carcinoma of the cervix and the use of hyperbaric oxygen with radiotherapy: a report of a randomised controlled trial. *Radiother Oncol* 1999;53:93–98.

921. Johnson RJ, Walton RJ. Sequential study on the effect of the addition of hyperbaric oxygen on the 5 year survival rates of carcinoma of the cervix treated with conventional fractional irradiations. *Am J Roentgenol Radium Ther Nucl Med* 1974;120:111–117.

922. Taylor HS, Manson JE. Update in hormone therapy use in menopause. *J Clin Endocrinol Metab* 2011;96:255–264.

923. Burger CW, van Leeuwen FE, Scheele F, et al. Hormone replacement therapy in women treated for gynaecological malignancy. *Maturitas* 1999;32:69–76.

924. Sadan O, Frohlich EP, Driscoll JA, et al. Is it safe to prescribe hormonal contraception and replacement therapy to patients with premalignant and malignant uterine cervices? *Gynecol Oncol* 1989;34:159–163.

925. Tominaga K, Koyama Y, Sasagawa M, et al. A follow-up study of patients with cervical cancer after resection, with special emphasis on the incidence of second primary cancers. *Gynecol Oncol* 1995;56:71–74.

926. Chaturvedi AK, Kleinerman RA, Hildesheim A, et al. Second cancers after squamous cell carcinoma and adenocarcinoma of the cervix. *J Clin Oncol* 2009;27:967–973.

927. Chaturvedi AK, Engels EA, Gilbert ES, et al. Second cancers among 104,760 survivors of cervical cancer: evaluation of long-term risk. *J Natl Cancer Inst* 2007;99:1634–1643.

928. Lee JY, Perez CA, Ettinger N, et al. The risk of second primaries subsequent to irradiation for cervix cancer. *Int J Radiat Oncol Biol Phys* 1982;8:207–211.

929. Storm HH. Second primary cancer after treatment for cervical cancer. late effects after radiotherapy. *Cancer* 1988;61:679–688.

930. Hemminki K, Dong C, Vaittinen P. Second primary cancer after in situ and invasive cervical cancer. *Epidemiology* 2000;11:457–461.

931. Werner-Wasik M, Schmid CH, Bornstein LE, et al. Increased risk of second malignant neoplasms outside radiation fields in patients with cervical carcinoma. *Cancer* 1995;75:2281–2285.

932. Wright JD, St Clair CM, Deutsch I, et al. Pelvic radiotherapy and the risk of secondary leukemia and multiple myeloma. *Cancer* 2010;116:2486–2492.

933. Mark RJ, Poen J, Tran LM, et al. Postirradiation sarcoma of the gynecologic tract. A report of 13 cases and a discussion of the risk of radiation-induced gynecologic malignancies. *Am J Clin Oncol* 1996;19:59–64.

934. Zwahlen DR, Ruben JD, Jones P, et al. Effect of intensity-modulated pelvic radiotherapy on second cancer risk in the postoperative treatment of endometrial and cervical cancer. *Int J Radiat Oncol Biol Phys* 2009;74:539–545.

935. Seidman JD, Kumar D, Cosin JA, et al. Carcinomas of the female genital tract occurring after pelvic irradiation: a report of 15 cases. *Int J Gynecol Pathol* 2006;25:293–297.

936. Kleinerman RA, Smith SA, Holowaty E, et al. Radiation dose and subsequent risk for stomach cancer in long-term survivors of cervical cancer. *Int J Radiat Oncol Biol Phys* 2013;86(5):922–929.

Section
III

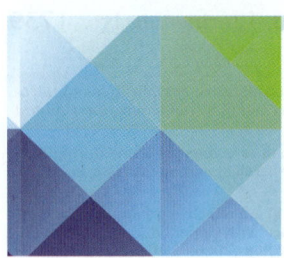

CHAPTER 74

Endometrial Cancer

Kaled M. Alektiar

ANATOMY

The uterus is a hollow, muscular organ located in the true pelvis between the bladder and the rectum. The average adult uterus is about 8 cm long, 5 cm wide, and 2.5 cm thick. It is divided into the fundus, body (corpus), and cervix. The junction between the body and cervix is called the isthmus. The fundus is pierced at each cornu by the fallopian tubes. The uterine surface is partially covered by peritoneum. The uterine cavity is lined by endometrium, made up of columnar cells forming many tubular glands. The thickness of the endometrium varies during the menstrual cycle, but by the end of menstruation, it should be 2 to 3 mm in thickness. The wall of the uterus is composed of myometrium, consisting of smooth muscle fibers. The major supports of the uterus are the broad, round, uterosacral and cardinal ligaments. The major blood supply to the uterus is the uterine artery, which enters the uterus at the isthmus after it crosses over the ureter. The lymphatic drainage for the body of the uterus is mainly to the obturator and internal and external iliac lymph nodes. The lymphatics from the fundus accompany the ovarian artery and drain into the para-aortic lymph nodes.

EPIDEMIOLOGY AND RISK FACTORS

Endometrial cancer is the most common gynecologic cancer and the fourth most frequently diagnosed cancer in women in the United States. According to 2018 cancer statistics, the estimated number of newly diagnosed cases is 63,230, with a probability of 1 in every 35 women (2.8%) developing it during her lifetime.[1] Although it is a cancer that affects predominantly postmenopausal women, 14% are diagnosed in premenopausal women, with 5% being younger than 40 years.[2] The expected number of deaths from endometrial cancer in 2018 is 11,350, making it the sixth leading cause of death from cancer in women. Recent estimates on the death rate from endometrial cancer seemed to indicate that the rate is on the rise, by about 2% per year.[1]

The incidence of endometrial cancer is higher in more developed areas of the world (5.5%) compared to less developed countries (4.2%), indicating a possible influence of environmental factors on the incidence of this disease.[3] The exact etiology of endometrial cancer remains unknown, but several risk factors have been associated with it, chiefly unopposed estrogen. It is well established that endometrial cancer risk is increased among women who have high circulating levels of bioavailable estrogens and low levels of progesterone, so that the mitogenic effect of estrogens is insufficiently counterbalanced by the opposing effect of progesterone.[4] The source of unopposed estrogen could be endogenous or exogenous. Regarding endogenous estrogen,[5] in a nested case–control study of 93,676 postmenopausal women, parent estrogens (estrone and estradiol) were positively related to endometrial cancer risk, with the highest risk observed for unconjugated estradiol (OR 5th vs. 1st quintile = 6.19; 95% confidence interval [CI], 2.95 to 13.03, Ptrend = 0.0001). The association with unconjugated estradiol was stronger for type I than type II tumors (Phet = 0.01). Lifetime cumulative number of menstrual cycles, that is, menstruation span, is associated with

increased risk of developing endometrial cancer. This is due to the fact that endometrial cell proliferation increases during the follicular phase, which is the longest in the menstrual cycle. Thus, *early age at menarche* (estimated relative risk [RR], 1.5 to 2) and *late age at menopause* (RR, 2 to 3), examples of increased menstruation span, are risk factors for endometrial cancer.[6] *Nulliparity* (RR, 3) is also associated with increased risk of endometrial cancer[6] due in part to anovulatory menstrual cycles. *Obesity* is a significant risk factor for endometrial cancer, with estimation that 38.4% of endometrial cancer worldwide could be attributed to high body mass index (BMI).[7] The increase in endometrial cancer risk is mainly through changes in endogenous hormone metabolism. After menopause, when ovarian production of both estrogen and progesterone ceases, the major source of estrogen is via peripheral conversion, mostly within adipose tissue, of androgens that continue being produced by the adrenal glands and ovaries. Thus, with obesity, there is an increase in the amount of bioavailable estrogens in the circulation and the endometrial tissue.[4] Obesity may also influence endometrial cancer risk via chronic hyperinsulinemia, which appears to be a key factor for the development of ovarian hyperandrogenism, associated with anovulation and progesterone deficiency, especially for premenopausal women.[8] *Non–insulin-dependent diabetes mellitus* and *hypertension* (RR, 1 to 3) also increases the risk of endometrial cancer. This is often believed to be secondary to obesity, but there are data showing that these risk factors could be independent of obesity.[9] With regard to exogenous estrogen, it is well established that the use of *estrogen-only hormone replacement therapy* and *sequential oral contraceptives* greatly increases endometrial cancer risk, whereas combined preparations, that is, those that contain a progestogen as well as estrogen throughout the treatment period, have a protective effect (RR, 0.3 to 0.5).[10,11] The use of *tamoxifen* in patients with breast cancer has been associated with increased risk of endometrial cancer. The mechanism of action of tamoxifen is in competition with that of endogenous estrogen for estrogen receptors. In premenopausal women, tamoxifen has an antiestrogenic effect, but in postmenopausal women, it has a weak estrogenic effect because of the up-regulation of estrogen receptors. In a meta-analysis on adjuvant tamoxifen and endometrial cancer, for patients who were <55 years of age, there was little absolute risk compared to patients of 55 to 69 years of age, for whom the 15-year incidence was 3.8% in the tamoxifen group versus 1.1% in the control group (absolute increase 2.6% [standard error 0.6], 95% CI = 1.4 to 3.8), highlighting the influence of age and the length of its use on the risk of endometrial cancer from tamoxifen use.[12,13] Initial data seemed to indicate that the majority of endometrial cancers associated with tamoxifen use were of early stage with favorable features.[14] More recent data, however, show a change in the profile of these endometrial cancers, with a rise in the rate of serous, clear cell, carcinosarcoma, and sarcoma types.[15] Inherited genetic predisposition, especially in the setting of hereditary nonpolyposis colorectal cancer (HNPCC), probably accounts for <5% of all endometrial cancer cases. Mutations in one of the four mismatch repair (MMR) genes *hMLH1, hMSH2, hMSH6,* or *hPMS2* have been identified in patients with Lynch syndrome.

Although HNPCC is thought of primarily in terms of risk of developing colorectal cancer, it is important to note that lifetime cumulative risk of endometrial cancer for women with HNPCC is 40% to 60%, which equals or exceeds their risk of colorectal cancer.[16] There seems to be a high rate of lower uterine segment involvement (LUSI) in patients with HNPCC-associated endometrial cancer.[17]

CLINICAL PRESENTATION AND NATURAL HISTORY

The most common presentation for endometrial cancer is postmenopausal vaginal bleeding, which is reported by 80% to 90% of patients. The incidence of endometrial cancer in women presenting with postmenopausal bleeding is only 10% to 15%. This incidence, however, could range from 1% up to 25%, depending on patient age and the presence of other risk factors. In a report of a total of 3,548 women presenting with postmenopausal vaginal bleeding, 201 (6%) had a diagnosis of endometrial carcinoma. Use of a multiple logistic regression model showed that recurrent episodes of bleeding (odds ratio [OR], 3.64), a history of diabetes (OR, 1.48), older age (1.06), and high body mass index (OR, 1.07) increased the risk of endometrial malignancy when corrected for other characteristics.[18] Other patterns of presentations include vaginal discharge, abnormal Papanicolaou smear, or thickened endometrium on routine transvaginal ultrasound. For patients with advanced disease, they may present with urinary or rectal bleeding, constipation, pain, lower extremity lymphedema, abdominal distension due to ascites, and cough and/or hemoptysis.

The International Federation of Gynecology and Obstetrics (FIGO) annual report[19] showed that the 5-year survival rate for 8,110 patients with endometrial cancer treated between 1999 and 2001 was 80%. Such excellent outcome is a reflection of the fact that the majority of patients are diagnosed with early-stage disease. The tumor was limited to the corpus uteri in 71% of cases, involved the cervix in 12%, and extended beyond the uterus, but short of distant spread in 13%. For patients with disease limited to the endometrium or with <50% myometrial invasion, the 5-year survival rate was 91%. However, the rate dropped to 66% when disease extended to adnexa/serosa/positive peritoneal cytology, to 57% with regional lymph node involvement, to 25.5% with bladder or rectal involvement, and to 20% with distant spread. For clinically staged patients, the 5-year survival rate ranged from 67% for early-stage disease down to 15% for advanced disease. Mass screening for endometrial cancer in women at average risk or

increased risk due to a history of unopposed estrogen therapy, tamoxifen therapy, late menopause, nulliparity, infertility or failure to ovulate, obesity, diabetes, or hypertension is not recommended. American Cancer Society (ACS) recommends that women at average and increased risk should be informed about risks and symptoms (in particular, unexpected bleeding and spotting) of endometrial cancer at the onset of menopause and should be strongly encouraged to immediately report these symptoms to their physician. However, screening has been recommended by the ACS for women who carry, or are related to carriers of, the HNPCC mutation, starting at age 35 years, including annual transvaginal ultrasound and endometrial biopsy.[20] Prophylactic hysterectomy and bilateral salpingo-oophorectomy (BSO) once childbearing is completed have been shown to effectively reduce the risk of endometrial cancer in patients with HNPCC and should be strongly considered.[21]

DIAGNOSTIC WORKUP

Endometrial tissue sampling remains the gold standard by which the diagnosis of endometrial cancer is established. This is achieved via biopsy or dilation and curettage (D&C). *Endometrial biopsy,* which can be easily performed in the office with a Pipelle or similar device, is the preferred approach. Its sensitivity in detecting endometrial cancer in postmenopausal women is 99.6% compared to 91% in premenopausal women. Its specificity is >98% for both groups.[22] If the patient is undergoing hysterectomy, routine D&C is not necessary after an office Pipelle sampling has documented malignancy. However, if symptoms persist, the office sampling is inadequate, or the patient is being considered for conservative fertility-sparing approaches, a D&C should be performed. In addition, D&C provides more reliable assessments of final pathologic findings in hysterectomy specimens, mainly with regard to tumor grade.[23] Given that the incidence of endometrial cancer in women with postmenopausal bleeding is only 10% to 15%, it is unclear how feasible it is to perform endometrial sampling on every patient. *Transvaginal ultrasonography* (TVU) may be considered as a useful tool to assess patient's vaginal bleeding. Normal endometrium looks thin and homogeneously hyperechoic, but it is thickened and heterogeneous, with hyperplasia, polyps, and cancer[24] as shown in Figure 74.1. The consensus statement from the Society of Radiologists in Ultrasound defines an endometrial thickness of 5 mm or greater as being abnormal.[25] If the thickness of the endometrium is <5 mm, the risk of endometrial cancer is minimal; the false-negative rate is about 4%. If the TVU is

FIGURE 74.1. Sagittal view of the uterus on transvaginal ultrasound. **A:** Normal thin endometrium (*arrow*). **B:** Thickened endometrium (*arrow*).

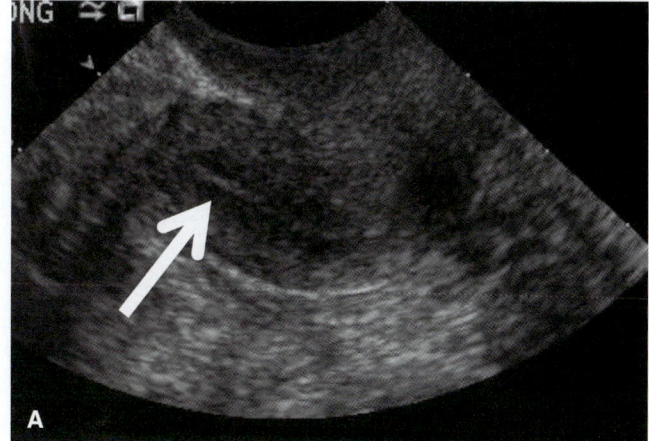
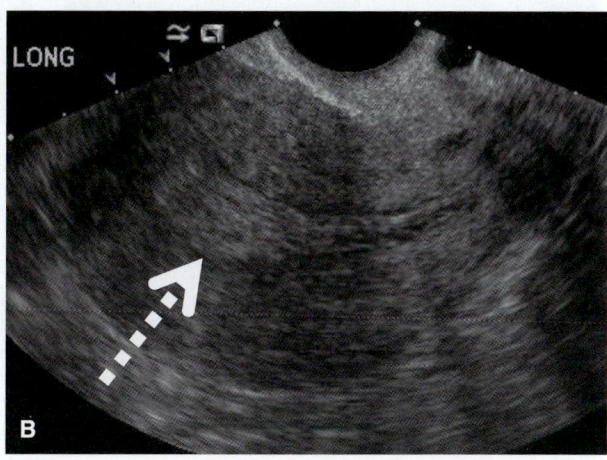

abnormal but the biopsy is negative/nondiagnostic or the uterine cavity is inaccessible, then *saline infusion sonography* or *hysteroscopy*[26,27] should be considered to help exclude intracavitary lesions, especially polyps that might contain cancer. In addition, these methods are also helpful in premenopausal women, for whom the accuracy of TVU is limited because the endometrial thickness fluctuates, depending on the level of female hormones. The potential downside to saline infusion or hysteroscopy is that there have been reports that the insufflation of the distending medium into the canal has been associated with an increase in positive peritoneal cytology, although the prognostic implications are unclear of such positive cytology "induced" by sampling.[28] Several imaging studies are available to define the extent of disease preoperatively.[29] Good-quality pelvic *computed tomography* (CT) scans obtained with oral and intravenous contrast can demonstrate the extent of the endometrial tumor. The endometrial carcinoma is a hypodense mass relative to the normal myometrium and may be seen as a diffuse, circumscribed vegetative or polypoidal mass within the uterine cavity. CT is helpful in assessing regional and distant metastasis. *Magnetic resonance imaging* (MRI) is considered the most accurate imaging study to assess tumor extension in endometrial cancer, especially myometrial invasion.[30,31] Dynamic contrast-enhanced (DCE) and diffusion-weighted (DW) MRI are equivalent in detecting deep myometrial invasion.[32] A clear junctional zone or preservation of a sharp delineation between the tumor and the myometrium implies disease limited to the endometrium. Disease characterized by disruption of the junctional zone, increased–signal-intensity tumor in the inner half of the myometrium with preservation of the outer myometrium, or both correlates with superficial myometrial invasion. If there is extension of the high–signal-intensity tumor into the outer myometrium with preservation of a peripheral rim of normal, intact myometrium, then that is considered deep myometrial invasion (Fig. 74.2). MRI also helps to delineate tumor extension into the cervix. The normal cervical stroma is hypointense on T2-weighted images and is replaced by intermediate–signal-intensity tumor in cases of invasion.[33] The reported sensitivity of MRI in detecting lymph node metastasis is on average 43.5% and the specificity is 95.9%.[31] *Positron emission tomography (PET)/CT* is also being used in endometrial cancer.[34]

There seems to be little benefit in assessing the primary tumor extension. With regard to regional lymph node metastasis, the reported sensitivity is 72% and the specificity is 94%. The main advantage of PET-CT over other imaging modalities is its accuracy in detecting distant metastasis.[33] The FIGO staging for endometrial cancer is a surgical staging, and thus, preoperative imaging studies (except chest x-rays) are not part of the staging. *Cancer antigen 125* (CA-125) serum levels could be elevated in patients with endometrial cancer. Kim et al.[35] in a review of 413 patients found that 23.9% of patients had >35 U/mL serum CA-125 levels. Hsieh et al.[36] found that preoperative levels of >40 U/mL correlated significantly with regional lymph node metastasis and suggested that such levels could be used as an indication for full-pelvic and para-aortic lymphadenectomy at the time of surgical staging in the absence of metastatic disease.

Pathologic Classification

Endometrial Hyperplasia

The diagnostic criterion for hyperplasia is an increase in the number and size of proliferating glands. The International Society of Gynecologic Pathologists standardized the subclassification of endometrial hyperplasia. In simple hyperplasia, there is only glandular proliferation and enlargement with increased stromal cellularity. This rarely progresses to carcinoma (<1%). Complex hyperplasia is characterized by back-to-back proliferation of glands with intraluminal papillae, epithelial pseudostratification, and few mitotic figures. If there is no cytologic atypia, the risk of malignant degeneration is again quite low, on the order of 3%. Any proliferation demonstrating cytologic abnormalities (in cellular or nuclear morphology) is classified as atypical hyperplasia. Atypical hyperplasia has a much higher risk of progression to an invasive carcinoma—8% for simple atypical hyperplasia, increasing to 29% for complex hyperplasia associated with atypia.[37] The Gynecologic Oncology Group (GOG) conducted a prospective trial in which all patients with atypical hyperplasia of the uterus underwent an immediate hysterectomy. The rate of underlying concurrent carcinoma in the uterus was 42.6% in these patients.[38] The standard recommended treatment for atypical hyperplasia of the uterus is hysterectomy if

FIGURE 74.2. Sagittal magnetic resonance imaging view of the uterus. **A:** Normal uterus. **B:** Deep myometrial invasion (*arrows*).

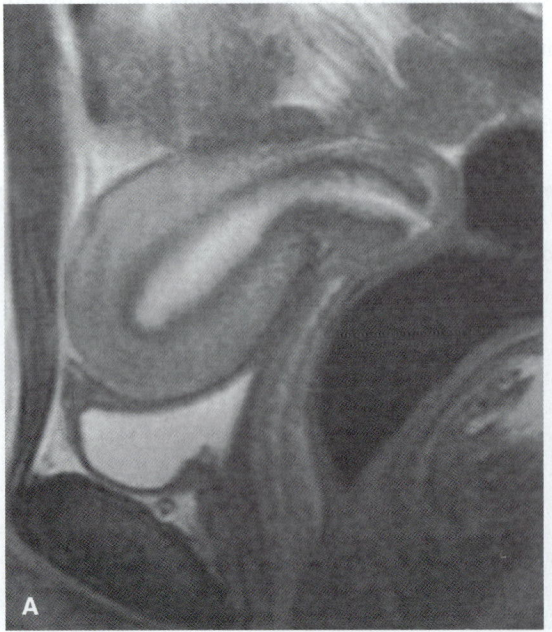

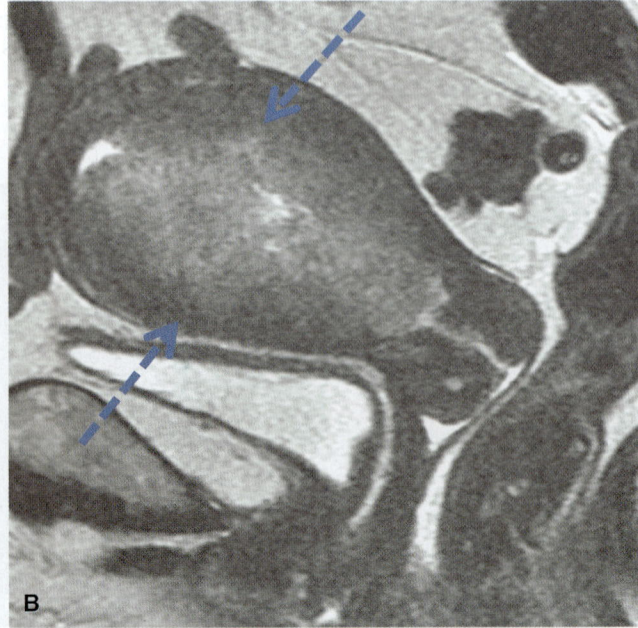

TABLE 74.1 PATHOLOGIC CLASSIFICATON OF ENDOMETRIAL CANCERS

Endometrioid adenocarcinoma
  Not otherwise specified
  Villoglandular
  Secretory adenocarcinoma
  Ciliated carcinoma
  Adenocarcinoma with squamous differentiation
Uterine papillary serous
Clear cell carcinoma
Mucinous carcinoma
Squamous cell carcinoma
Transitional cell carcinoma
Mixed cell type
Undifferentiated carcinoma
Metastatic carcinoma to the endometrium

childbearing is complete and the patient has no other contraindications to surgery. In patients who desire future fertility or have an absolute contraindication to surgery, progestational therapies may be used with caution.[39]

Carcinoma of the Endometrium
Endometrioid Carcinoma
Endometrioid adenocarcinoma is the most common endometrial carcinoma, constituting 75% to 80% of all cases (Table 74.1). The classic histologic appearance is that of marked glandular proliferation with back-to-back proliferation of

glands and little intervening stroma (Fig. 74.3A). The name endometrioid is derived from resemblance to proliferative-phase endometrium. Architectural grading is determined by the amount of solid mass of tumor cells compared to well-defined glands. Grade 1 is an endometrioid cancer in which <5% of the tumor growth is in solid sheets. Grade 2 is an adenocarcinoma in which 6% to 50% of the tumor is composed of solid sheets of cells. Grade 3 occurs when >50% of the tumor is made up of solid sheets. Nuclear grading is determined by the nuclear shape, size, chromatin distribution, and size of the nucleoli. The grading is primarily driven by the architectural grading, but if there is marked nuclear atypia in an otherwise grade 2 architectural grading, it should be increased to grade 3. Within endometrioid adenocarcinoma, the subtypes are endometrioid carcinoma not otherwise specified (NOS), endometrioid carcinoma with squamous differentiation, villoglandular endometrioid carcinoma, secretory carcinoma, and a ciliated cell variant.[40] Most of the endometrioid adenocarcinomas are designated NOS. Foci of squamous differentiation are often found with endometrioid adenocarcinoma. The squamous component could be benign, with the designation of adenoacanthoma, or malignant, in which case it is called adenosquamous carcinoma. Such designations have not been very useful, however, because the degree of differentiation of the squamous component parallels that of the glandular architectural grading. Therefore, most gynecologic pathologists use the term *adenocarcinoma with squamous differentiation*. Other subtypes of endometrioid adenocarcinoma include the relatively common *villoglandular carcinoma*,

FIGURE 74.3. Different histologic types of endometrial cancer. **A:** Endometrioid. **B:** Papillary serous. **C:** Clear cell. **D:** Carcinosarcoma (heterologous; chondrosarcoma).

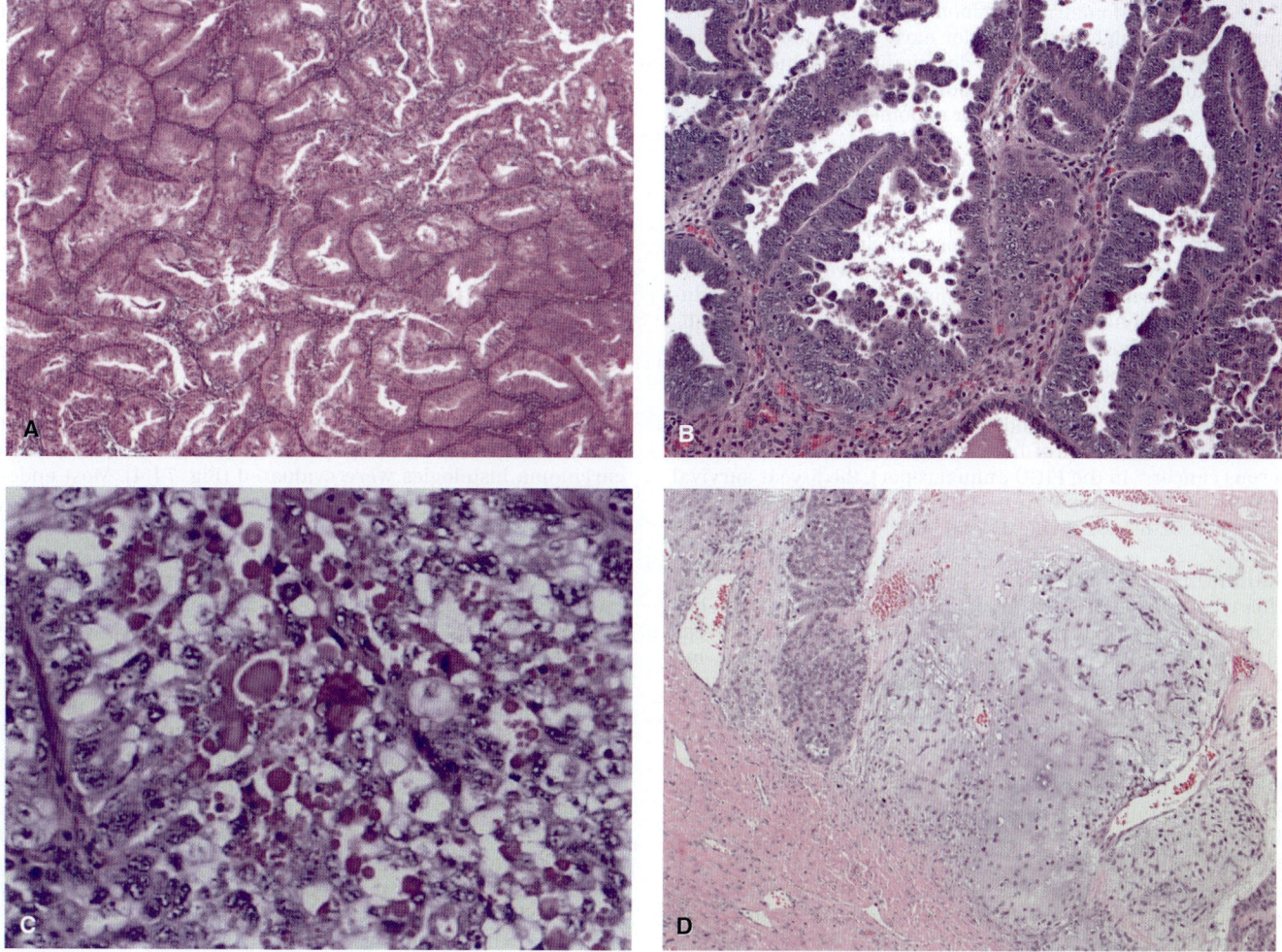

which grows in a papillary fashion. The prognosis of this sub-type is similar to that of low-grade endometrioid cancer, and it must not be confused with serous carcinoma because of its papillary features. *Secretory carcinoma,* which represents <2% of all endometrial carcinomas, is characterized by a very well-differentiated glandular pattern with much intracellular glycogen, thus resembling early secretory endometrium. Although the cells have clear cytoplasm, their histologic and cytologic features are different from those of clear cell carcinoma. *Ciliated carcinoma* is a very rare subtype, characterized by the presence of ciliated cells comprising >75% of the tumor specimen. It is usually associated with a history of prior estrogen use, and the prognosis is quite good, because most are well differentiated.

Mucinous Carcinoma

This designation requires >50% of the tumor cells to be mucinous. These cells are carcinoembryonic antigen positive and are laden with mucin, which stains positively with mucicarmine and periodic acid–Schiff stains but is diastase resistant. Because of the resemblance to endocervical adenocarcinoma, it is essential to exclude it by endocervical curettage. Mucinous carcinomas are usually well differentiated and have the same prognosis as ordinary endometrioid carcinomas.

Serous Carcinoma

Serous carcinomas, also known as papillary serous cancers, resemble ovary cancer in terms of histology and to some extent in terms of behavior. The mere presence of papillary structure is not diagnostic because other histologic types may have papilla as well. However, the presence of marked cellular atypia in addition to papilla distinguishes serous carcinoma from others (Fig. 74.3B). Psammoma bodies are found in up to 33% of cases. The incidence of serous endometrial cancer is about 11.4% that of endometrial carcinomas.[41] This is an aggressive subtype, with a high propensity for early lymphatic and intraperitoneal dissemination, often despite little myometrial penetration. In the FIGO annual report, the 5-year survival rate was 52.6% compared to 83.2% for endometrioid carcinoma.[19]

Clear Cell Carcinoma

Clear cell carcinoma of the endometrium resembles renal carcinoma, but its origin from mullerian structures is now well established. Unlike vaginal and cervical clear cell carcinoma, it is not related to intrauterine diethylstilbestrol exposure. The microscopic structure may vary from solid patterns to glandular differentiation (Fig. 74.3C). In the latter pattern, small cells resembling "hobnail" cells line spaces and glands. These are cells that extruded their cytoplasm, leaving bare nuclei that protrude into the glandular lumens. The rate of clear cell carcinoma is about 3.5% of endometrial carcinomas.[41] The prognosis of this cancer is in between that of endometrioid and serous cancer.[42] In the FIGO annual report, the 5-year survival rate was 62.5% compared to 83.2% for endometrioid carcinoma and 52.6% for serous carcinoma.[19]

Squamous Carcinoma

This type of cancer is extremely rare, and the diagnosis has to be made after the exclusion of cervical origin. The 5-year survival rate based on the FOGO report is 68.9% overall, but the prognosis is poor for patients with extrauterine disease or distant spread.[19]

Undifferentiated Carcinoma

The World Health Organization classification describes endometrial undifferentiated carcinomas as "malignant poorly differentiated endometrial carcinomas, lacking any evidence of differentiation" without any further characterization.[43] Undifferentiated carcinomas can also be associated with an endometrioid carcinoma component, and such tumors have been referred to as "dedifferentiated carcinomas," which is

being recognized with increased frequency. Some of these tumors may belong to the spectrum of gynecologic neoplasms seen in the setting of microsatellite instability and possibly Lynch syndrome.[44]

Mixed Histology

Mixed cell–type endometrial cancer composed of two or more pure types was observed in 4.5% of patients in GOG 210 study.[41] By convention, in order to be designated as mixed, the other cell-type component has to comprise at least 10% of the tumor. Except for mixed endometrioid and serous or clear cell carcinoma, the clinical significance of mixed cell type is questionable.

Simultaneous Tumors

Occasionally identical tumor type, mainly endometrioid histology, can be discovered in the ovary and endometrium. Usually, the site of the largest tumor is assigned the primary origin, but at times, true primary endometrial and ovarian malignancies may coexist.[45] If the endometrial tumor is <5 cm in diameter, well differentiated, with no vascular invasion, limited to less than the middle one-third of the myometrium, and the ovarian lesions are bilateral, it is more likely that there are two concomitant primary tumors. Genetic profiling may represent a powerful tool in clinical practice for distinguishing between metastatic and dual primaries in patients with simultaneous ovarian/endometrial cancer and for predicting disease outcome.[46]

Molecular Biology

Several investigators pointed out that there are two distinct types of endometrial cancer.[47,48] In type I endometrial cancer, there is strong correlation with prior estrogen stimulation. The cancers in this category are often indolent in nature, with minimal myometrial invasion and low-grade histology. They affect premenopausal and perimenopausal women. Type II endometrial cancer often affects postmenopausal women with no prior history of estrogen stimulation. The histology of the tumors is often high grade, such as serous or clear cell cancers with deep invasion, and at a more advanced stage at the time of presentation.[2] What is intriguing is the fact that at the molecular level, the existence of two distinct types of endometrial cancer seems to be validated.[49] The most frequently altered molecular pathway in type I endometrial carcinomas is the PI3 K/PTEN/AKT pathway, which is dysregulated by oncogenic mutations, PTEN loss of function, and/or overexpression of upstream tyrosine kinase growth factor receptors, leading to uncontrolled cell proliferation and survival. On the other hand, the main pathway alterations in type II endometrial cancers involve the tumor suppressors p53. However, the findings from the Cancer Genome Atlas (TCGA) have revolutionized our understanding of endometrial cancer.[50] In that study, the genomic landscape of endometrioid and serous carcinoma histologies were evaluated (Fig. 74.4). Most endometrioid tumors had frequent mutations in PTEN, CTNNB1, PIK3CA, ARID1A, and KRAS, novel mutations in the SWI/SNF chromatin remodeling complex gene ARID5B, and few copy number alterations or TP53 mutations. Uterine serous tumors and about 25% of high-grade endometrioid tumors (serous-like) had frequent TP53 mutations and extensive copy number alterations, but few deoxyribonucleic acid (DNA) methylation changes, and low estrogen receptor/progesterone receptor levels. A subset of endometrioid tumors (about 10%) that was identified had a markedly increased mutation frequency and newly identified hotspot mutations in the exonuclease domain of *POLE*. Based on these results, endometrial cancers can be classified into four categories: POLE ultramutated, microsatellite instability hypermutated, copy number low, and copy number high. The somatic copy number alterations (SCNAs) analysis showed that most endometrioid tumors have few SCNAs, whereas most serous and serous-like tumors (endometrioid) exhibit extensive SCNAs.

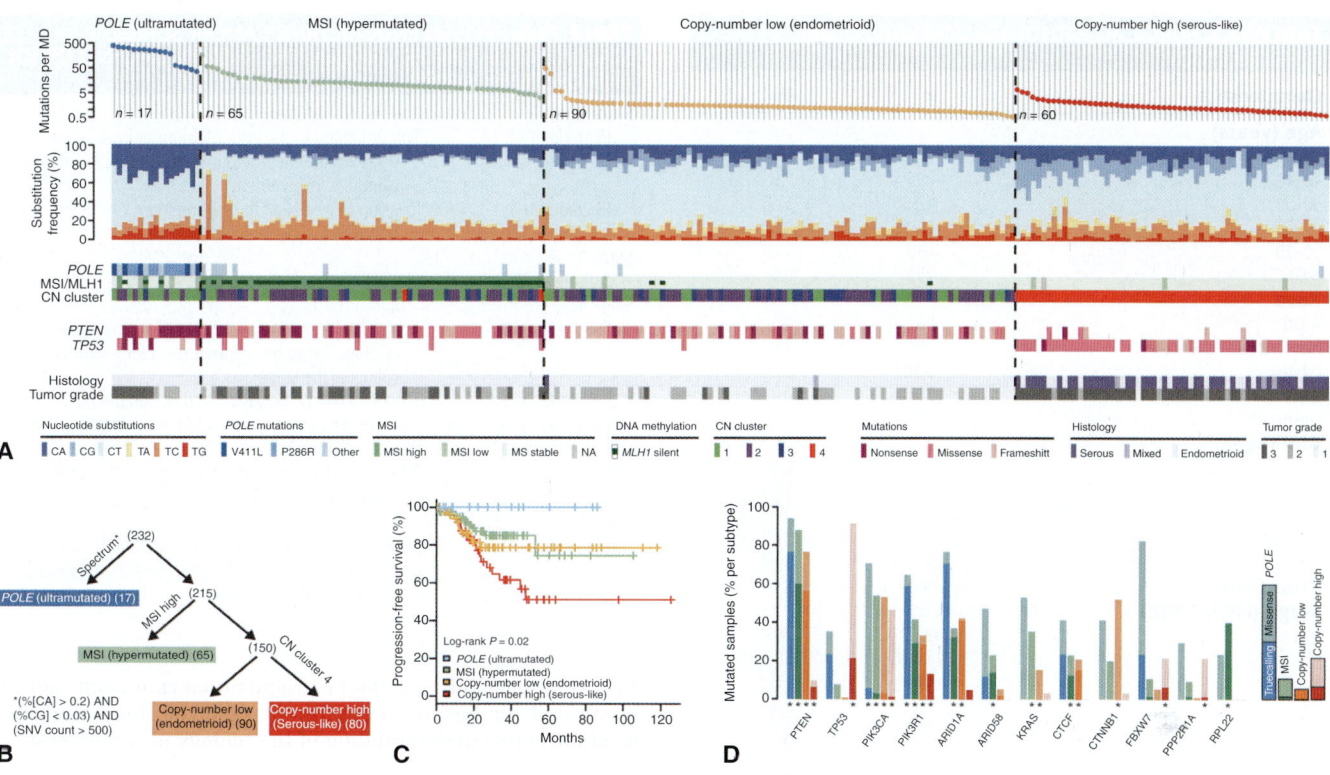

FIGURE 74.4. Genomic landscape of endometrial cancer.

Genomic analysis of clear cell carcinoma of the uterus demonstrated that, akin to endometrioid carcinomas, there are four gnomically distinct groups: POLE, MMR-deficient tumors, copy number low, and copy number high.[51]

STAGING

Before 1988, the staging system for endometrial cancer was clinical. Stage I was tumor limited to the uterus, with IA designation if the length was ≤8 cm and IB if it was >8 cm. Stage II was for when cervix was involved, stage III when disease extension beyond uterus/cervix was limited to the true pelvis, and stage IV when it extended beyond the true pelvis or involved bladder or rectum (IVA) or distant spread (IVB). This system is applicable to the few patients who cannot have surgery and are treated with definitive radiation. Using the FOGO 1988 staging system, Creasman et al. reported a GOG 210 study on 5,855 patients with endometrial cancer who underwent hysterectomy/BSO and peritoneal cytology.[41] During the initial phase of the study of 3,715 patients, enrollment was unrestricted, but in the later phase, enrollment was restricted to patients (n = 2,151) with adverse features, such as non-endometrioid histologies, non-Caucasian race, and preoperative imaging suggestive of deep myometrial invasion, and such histologies were as follows: endometrioid (grade 1 was 37.8%, grade 2 was 26.3%, and grade 3 was 9.7%), serous 11.4%, clear cell 3.5%, and mixed 4.5%. The rate of positive peritoneal cytology was 8.9% and that of adnexal involvement was 8.6%. The breakdown by stage (FIGO 1988) was as follows: IA 24.8%, IB 38.4%, IC 11.2%, IIA 2.3%, IIB 4.4%, IIIA 4.6%, IIIB 0.2%, IIIC 9.8%, and IV 4.4% (Table 74.2).

In 2009, the FIGO staging system was modified.[52] Patients who formerly were staged as IB, that is, <50% myometrial invasion, are now considered IA. Patients with >50% myometrial invasion are designated as stage IB. Endocervical glandular involvement no longer affects staging; only patients with cervical stromal invasion are considered stage II. Having positive peritoneal cytology no longer affects stag-

ing. Parametrial extension is now considered IIIB. Patients with stage IIIC are now subdivided into IIIC1 if pelvic nodes are involved and IIIC2 if para-aortic nodes are involved (Table 74.3). The discriminating power of the new FIGO staging system is being debated. Page et al.[53] evaluated 10,839 cases from 1998 to 2006 using the Surveillance, Epidemiology, and End Results (SEER) Program. The analysis demonstrated the usefulness of two divisions rather than three for stage I in the new FIGO staging system. In contrast, a study from Memorial Sloan Kettering Cancer Center (MSKCC) of 1,307 patients with FIGO 1988 stage I disease showed that the revised system for stage I did not improve its predictive ability over the 1988 system.[54]

Prognostic Factors

Several clinicopathologic factors have been identified in patients with endometrial carcinoma to help predict the prognosis and individualize the treatment plan. At MSKCC, a nomogram was developed for predicting overall survival of women with endometrial cancer (n = 1,735) after primary therapy.[55] Use of five prognostic factors—age, grade, histologic type, number of lymph nodes removed, and FIGO 1988 surgical stage—predicted OS with high concordance probability. Postoperative Radiation Therapy in Endometrial Cancer (PORTEC) group also developed nomogram for predicting recurrence in FIGO stage I disease.[56]

Age

The influence of older age on worse outcome has been well established. The adverse impact of older age is often explained by pointing out that older patients tend to present with aggressive histology and more advanced disease and are generally treated less aggressively. What is intriguing, however, is that the strongest correlation between older age and poor outcome is seen in patients with otherwise favorable characteristics. Furthermore, the adverse impact of advanced age on outcome persists even when elderly patients are treated as aggressively as their younger counterparts.[57,58]

TABLE 74.2 SURGICAL–PATHOLOGIC FINDINGS FROM GOG 120 STUDY

Characteristics	n	%
Age (years)		
<40	92	2.5
40–49	293	7.9
50–59	1,165	31.4
60–69	1,212	32.6
70–79	698	18.8
>80	255	6.9
Race		
Asian	50	1.3
Black/African American	294	7.9
White	3,307	89.0
Other	25	0.7
Unknown	39	1.0
BMI (kg/m²)		
<18.5	20	0.5
18.5–24.9	609	16.4
25.0–29.9	833	22.4
30.0–34.9	786	21.2
>35	1,449	39.0
Prior Cancers	305	8.2
Stage (FIGO 1988)		
IA	922	24.8
IB	1,426	38.4
IC	416	11.2
IIA	85	2.3
IIB	162	4.4
IIIA	169	4.6
IIIB	9	0.2
IIIC	364	9.8
IV	162	4.4
Histology, Grade		
Endometrioid, grade 1	1,403	37.8
Endometrioid, grade 2	978	26.3
Endometrioid, grade 3	360	9.7
Serous	423	11.4
Clear cell	129	3.5
Carcinosarcoma	153	4.1
Mixed	168	4.5
Other	101	2.7
Myometrial Invasion		
Endometrium only	899	24.2
Inner half	1,823	49.1
Outer half	863	23.2
Serosa	114	3.1
Positive Peritoneal Cytology	330	8.9
Adnexa Involvement	318	8.6
Pelvic Node Metastasis	363	9.8
Aortic Node Metastasis	188	5.1
Other Extrauterine Metastasis	396	10.7
Lymphovascular Involvement	842	22.7

TABLE 74.3 REVISED ENDOMETRIAL CANCER SURGICAL STAGING SYSTEM: INTERNATIONAL FEDERATION OF GYNECOLOGY AND OBSTETRICS 2009

Stage I	
IA grades 1–3	Tumor limited to the endometrium or invasion to <50% of the myometrium (includes endocervical glandular involvement)
IB grades 1–3	Invasion to ≥50% of the myometrium (includes endocervical glandular involvement)
Stage II	
II grades 1–3	Cervical stromal invasion
Stage III	
IIIA grades 1–3	Tumor invades uterine serosa or adnexa (positive cytology has to be reported separately without changing the stage)
IIIB grades 1–3	Tumor involving the vagina and/or parametria
IIIC grades 1–3	Pelvic or para-aortic lymph nodal involvement
IIIC1 grades 1–3	Pelvic nodal involvement only
IIIC2 grades 1–3	Para-aortic nodal involvement with or without pelvic nodal involvement
Stage IV	
IVA grades 1–3	Invasion of bladder, bowel mucosa, or both
IVB	Distant metastases, including intra-abdominal spread or inguinal lymph nodes

11.2%, respectively. The higher recurrence rate could not be accounted for based on treatment received, indicating the need for better understanding of the biology of this disease.[59]

Histologic Subtype

According to the FIGO annual report, the 5-year survival rate was 83.2% for endometrioid adenocarcinoma, compared to 52.6% for serous cancer and 62.5% for clear cell cancer in 8,033 surgically staged patients. Patients with endometrioid histology have surgical stage III to IV disease only in 13.8% of patients, compared to 41.7% with serous and 33% with clear cell carcinoma, which could explain the worse outcome. However, the influence of histology was seen even in patients with surgical stage I disease ($n = 5,285$), for whom 5-year survival dropped from 90% for endometrioid histology to 79.9% with serous and 85.1% with clear cell carcinoma.[19]

Grade

Tumor grade is one of the most sensitive indicators of prognosis. Grade directly affects the depth of myometrial penetration and the frequency of lymph node involvement. In GOG 210 report by Cresman et al.,[41] the rate of deep myometrial invasion was 15% for grade 1, 25% for grade 2, and 38% for grade 3. The rate of positive pelvic and para-aortic node based on depth of invasion and histology is shown in Table 74.4. In the FIGO annual report,[19] grade 3 was an independent predictor of poor survival on multivariate analysis within each stage—stages I (HR, 2.45), II (HR, 2.14), III (HR, 2.44), and IV (HR, 2.55). The recognition that about 25% of grade 3 endometrioid histology has copy number high mutations, that is, serous-like, further highlight the impact of genomic stratification on prognosis.[50]

Race

The incidence of endometrial cancer is lower in African American than white women, yet the rate of high-risk features in this group is higher. In a GOG study, 24.3% of African Americans presented with stage III as opposed to 17.6% for white and the histology was serous in 24.4% as opposed to

TABLE 74.4 RATE OF PELVIC AND PARAORTIC METASTASIS BASED ON HISTOLOGY AND DEPTH OF INVASION

Depth of Invasion	EG1 Pel/PA%	EG2 Pel/PA%	EG3 Pel/PA%	Serous Pel/PA%	Clear Cell Pel/PA%
Endometrium only	0.8/0	1.6/1.1	1.7/0	7.9/4.2	1.3/0
Inner half	2.0/1.3	3.9/1.7	3.9/0.8	18.3/11.3	15.5/6.4
Outer half	15.4/6.9	16.8/8.4	29.1/14.5	44.3/32.4	40.5/28.4
Serosa	42.9/28.6	50/33.3	67.6/43.2	66.7/61.5	70/60

E, endometrioid; G, grade; PA, para-aortic; Pel, pelvic.

Myometrial Invasion

Regardless of grade, only 1.7% of tumors limited to the endometrium had lymph nodal involvement, as compared with 29% pelvic and 14.5% para-aortic involvement with deep penetration.[41] Before the 1988 FIGO staging system, the depth of invasion had been reported as none or inner, middle, or outer one-third of the myometrium. The 1988 FIGO staging system subdivided myometrial invasion into none or inner or outer half. Under that staging system, for patients with <50% myometrial invasion, it seems that invasion to less than versus greater than one-third is not a significant predictor of outcome.[60] In the current 2009 FIGO staging system, depth of invasion in stage I is divided into two categories: A (no or <50% myometrial invasion) and B (>50% invasion).

Lymphovascular Invasion

In GOG 210 study,[41] the rate of lymphovascular invasion (LVI) was 22.7%. The presence of LVI increased the rate of positive pelvic node from 4.1% to 37.5%, and para-aortic node from 2.3% to 23.8%. LVI is also associated with higher rate of relapse in the vagina[61] and a poorer outcome especially if it was substantial.[62] The presence of LVI needs to be viewed in the context of other risk factors so that its mere presence does not trigger excessive therapy.[63]

Lower Uterine Segment Involvement

The presence of LUSI is associated with worse outcome. In a study of 481 surgically staged endometrioid endometrial cancers (FIGO stage I to II), LUSI was present in 223 cases (46.4%) and was associated with both decreased disease-free survival (P = .02) and overall survival (P = .01) in univariate analysis.[64] There seems to be a high rate of LUSI in patients with HNPCC-associated endometrial cancer.[65]

Cervical Involvement

In the 1988 FIGO staging system, cervical involvement was divided into IIA when limited to endocervical glandular involvement and IIB when it involves the cervical stroma. According to the FIGO report, the 5-year survival for stage IIA was very good (89.9% for grade 1 and 83.7% for grade 2). In contrast, the corresponding figures for stage IIB were 81.2% and 76.9%, respectively.[19] This led to a change in the 2009 FIGO staging system, in which only cervical stromal invasion is considered stage II. Although the prognosis of the old stage IIA grades 1 and 2 approximated stage I rather than stage IIB, it is important to note that in the same FIGO annual report, patients with stage IIA grade 3 did not fare as well; their 5-year survival was 68.3%, which was worse than that for IC grade 3 (74.9%) and similar to that for IIB grade 3 (64.9%).

Peritoneal Cytology

In the 2009 FIGO staging, having positive peritoneal cytology is no longer considered stage IIIA. The reason for the change is due to lack of clear correlation between positive cytology and outcome for early-stage endometrial cancer. However, the true prognostic significance of positive peritoneal cytology on outcome cannot be devoid of the influence of surgical techniques or other prognostic factors. There is some suggestion of a higher rate of positive cytology for patients undergoing laparoscopic hysterectomy, because of manipulation of the uterine cavity. In a randomized trial[66] trying to address this issue, the rate of positive cytology was 7.2% when manipulator was used compared to 1.8% when it was not, but that difference was not statistically significant (P = .147). In GOG 210 study, positive peritoneal cytology was found in 11.3% of patients undergoing surgical staging. This was associated with 31.8% pelvic lymph node involvement and 22.7% para-aortic node involvement.[41] Histology also impacts the rate of positive

cytology: 7.7% for endometrioid histology compared to 20.2% for nonendometrioid histologies.[42] In patients with early-stage disease (low-grade endometrioid histology, minimal invasion), the influence of positive peritoneal cytology on outcome is not evident.[67] In contrast, for patients with stage III disease, having positive cytology affects prognosis significantly and needs to be taken into account.[68]

Adnexal/Serosal Involvement

In GOG 210 study,[41] the rate of positive adnexal involvement was 8.6%. The rate of positive pelvic node with such involvement is 41%, and for para-aortic is 31.4%. Jobsen et al.[69] reported on 46 patients with isolated adnexal involvement and 21 with isolated serosal involvement. There was no statistically significant difference in outcome between adnexal and serosal involvement. The 5-year disease-free survival was 76.4% versus 59.6% (P = ns), and the disease-specific survival (DSS) was 76.3% and 75.4%, respectively.

Pelvic and Para-aortic Lymph Node Involvement

The pattern of lymphatic spread in endometrial cancer is different than that in cervical cancer. In endometrial cancer, a simultaneous spread to both pelvic and para-aortic nodes could occur, whereas in cervical cancer, the spread to para-aortic nodes is almost always secondary to pelvic lymph node involvement. Overall, about 12.6% of patients with stage I and occult stage II endometrial cancer have pelvic nodal involvement. This increases to 27.7%, 41%, and 45.7% with deep myometrial invasion, adnexal involvement, and extrauterine spread, respectively.[41] Lymph node involvement is a major predictor of outcome; the 5-year disease-free survival rates drop to 65% to 70% in patients with pelvic lymph node involvement as their only risk factor.[70] In GOG 210 study, the rate of para-aortic nodal metastases is about 7.2%.[41] The biggest risk factor for para-aortic node involvement is the presence of pelvic nodal metastases. The 5-year disease-free survival rates drop to about 30% in this subpopulation.[70]

Molecular Prognostic Factors

In the TCGA report on endometrial cancer,[50] there was a correlation between prognosis and genomic group (Fig. 74.4). In the PORTEC trials, patients with *POLE* mutations had excellent prognosis, with very low risk of recurrence, which could be attributed to its high mutational burden.[71] On the other end of the spectrum, patients with copy number high had the worst prognosis in the TCGA report.[50] The recognition that about 25% of grade 3 endometrioid adenocarcinoma (serous-like) do belong to the copy number high group (mainly serous) further highlight the prognostic importance of genomic classifications of endometrial cancer.[72] Patients with CTNNB1 (β catenin) mutations do significantly worse even in patients with early-stage endometrioid histology.[73] Analysis of GOG 210 showed that in endometrioid adenocarcinoma of the uterus, the presence of MMR defects was associated with higher rate of LVI and higher-grade cancers. But interestingly, MMR defects were not associated with significantly worse prognosis.[74]

SURGICAL MANAGEMENT

Surgery is the main treatment for endometrial cancer. It consists of simple hysterectomy, BSO, and inspection of the pelvic and abdominal cavities, with biopsy of any suspicious extrauterine lesions, accompanied by peritoneal washings. The FIGO staging system did not say that obtaining peritoneal washings is no longer required but only that the finding does not alter the stage. Surgical assessment of lymph nodes ranges from palpation, biopsy of suspicious nodes, to pelvic and para-aortic lymphadenectomy.

Section
III

Hysterectomy

There are several approaches to simple hysterectomy, also known as extrafascial hysterectomy, but in the main, it consists of removal of the entire uterine corpus and cervix without contiguous parametrial tissue. The pubocervical fascia is entered, and the ureters are not unroofed. *Total abdominal hysterectomy/BSO* (TAH/BSO) is the most prevalent and time-tested form of simple hysterectomy in endometrial cancer. It is an abdominal approach, usually via a vertical midline incision that allows thorough exploration of intra-abdominal and pelvic cavities. The main drawback of TAH/BSO is that it is a laparotomy-based approach, in a group of patients with pre-existing comorbidities such as obesity, hypertension, and diabetes. Therefore, it is not surprising that minimally invasive surgery, whether laparoscopically or robotically, has gained a great deal of acceptance in the surgical management of endometrial cancer. In *laparoscopic vaginal hysterectomy/BSO* (LAVH/BSO), the uterus is removed vaginally rather than abdominally. The benefit of using the laparoscope is to enable the surgeon to have a thorough intra-abdominal exploration and to perform BSO, which is difficult to accomplish with just a vaginal hysterectomy. The GOG completed a trial in which patients with clinical stage I to occult IIA uterine cancer were randomly assigned to laparoscopy ($n = 1,696$) or open laparotomy ($n = 920$), including hysterectomy, salpingo-oophorectomy, pelvic cytology, and pelvic and para-aortic lymphadenectomy. The main study endpoints were 6-week morbidity and mortality, hospital length of stay, conversion from laparoscopy to laparotomy, recurrence-free survival, site of recurrence, and patient-reported quality of life outcomes.[75] Laparoscopy had fewer moderate to severe postoperative adverse events than laparotomy (14% vs. 21%, respectively; $P < .0001$). Hospitalization of >2 days was significantly lower in laparoscopy than in laparotomy patients (52% vs. 94%, respectively; $P < .0001$). The conversion rate to laparotomy was 25.8%. With a median follow-up time of 59 months for 2,181 patients still alive, there were 309 recurrences (laparoscopy 210, laparotomy 99) and 350 deaths (laparoscopy 229, laparotomy 121). The estimated 5-year recurrence rate was 11.61% in the laparotomy arm and 13.68% for laparoscopy. The estimated 5-year overall survival rate was 89.8% for laparoscopy and 89.8% for laparotomy. The study demonstrated that surgical treatment of endometrial cancer can be performed laparoscopically with relatively small differences in recurrence rates (estimated difference at 3 years, 1.14%). These results, combined with improved quality of life and decreased complications associated with laparoscopy, are reassuring to patients and allow surgeons to reasonably suggest this method as a means to surgically treat and stage patients with presumed early-stage uterine cancers.[76] In recent years, *robotic-assisted hysterectomy/BSO* has emerged as an alternative minimally invasive surgery in endometrial cancer. It affords many advantages, including three-dimensional visualization, increased freedom of instrument movement, and enhanced ergonomics and surgeon comfort. The question of difference in cost is under debate debatable.[77] *Radical hysterectomy* is not routinely performed in endometrial cancer because of low incidence of parametrial involvement. There is no evidence to show that the cure rates are any better with such radical operations. The possible exception to this might be in patients with gross cervical involvement.[78]

Surgical Assessment of Lymph Nodes

The question of which patients need routine surgical lymph nodal staging and, if so, to what extent is a matter of great debate. The uncertainty about lymphadenectomy relates to whether the benefit from it is prognostic rather than therapeutic. Those who advocate for *no lymphadenectomy* and limit nodal assessment to inspection and removal of any enlarged/suspicious pelvic or para-aortic nodes cite the lack of documented survival advantages to lymphadenectomy. Furthermore, patients who have adverse pathologic features that increase the risk of microscopic lymph node metastasis are generally offered adjuvant pelvic radiation. Advocates for *full-pelvic and para-aortic lymph node sampling* on the other end of the spectrum reason that surgical staging is the most accurate method to assess the extent of disease and that the sensitivity and specificity of palpation of lymph nodes are only 72% and 81%, respectively.[79] Lymphadenectomy in endometrial cancer includes removal of the fat pads surrounding the major vessels in the abdomen and pelvis without skeletonizing them. According to the GOG surgical guidelines, pelvic lymph nodes are to be removed from the distal one-half of the common iliac artery down to the circumflex iliac vein, and nodal tissue is to be removed anterior to the obturator nerve and surrounding the iliac arteries and vein. The para-aortic nodes include those overlying the vena cava, between the vena cava and aorta, and to the left of the aorta. The cephalad boundary of the para-aortic specimen is generally, but not limited to, the inferior mesenteric artery, and the distal boundary is the midpoint of the common iliac artery. For the sampling to be adequate, five lymphatic stations from each side need to be removed—para-aortic, common iliac, internal iliac, external iliac, and obturator—or a total of 10 nodes.[41]

Two trials addressed the role of lymphadenectomy. The first was an Italian study[80] in which 514 eligible patients with preoperative FIGO stage I endometrial carcinoma were randomly assigned to undergo pelvic lymphadenectomy ($n = 264$) or no lymphadenectomy ($n = 250$). The median number of lymph nodes removed was 30 in the pelvic lymphadenectomy arm. Both early and late postoperative complications occurred more frequently in patients who had received pelvic systematic lymphadenectomy (81 patients in the lymphadenectomy arm and 34 patients in the no-lymphadenectomy arm; $P = .001$). Lymphadenectomy improved surgical staging, as statistically significantly more patients with lymph node metastases were found in the lymphadenectomy arm than in the no-lymphadenectomy arm (13.3% vs. 3.2%; $P < .001$). At a median follow-up of 49 months, the 5-year disease-free and overall survival rates in an intention-to-treat analysis were similar between arms (81.0% and 85.9% in the lymphadenectomy arm and 81.7% and 90.0% in the no-lymphadenectomy arm, respectively). In the second trial (Medical Research Council [MRC]/A Study in the Treatment of Endometrial Cancer [ASTEC]), patients with endometrial cancer believed preoperatively to be confined to the uterine corpus were first randomized to standard surgery consisting of hysterectomy/BSO, pelvic washing, and palpation of para-aortic nodes ($n = 704$) or to lymphadenectomy ($n = 704$). In the lymphadenectomy group, patients underwent standard surgery plus systematic dissection of iliac and obturator nodes.[81] If the nodes could not be dissected, sampling of suspect nodes was recommended. Whether to dissect the para-aortic nodes was left to the discretion of the surgeon. After a median follow-up of 37 months, 191 women (88 standard surgery group, 103 lymphadenectomy group) had died, with an absolute difference in 5-year overall survival of 1% (95% CI = 4 to 6) and an absolute difference in 5-year recurrence-free survival of 6%. The conclusion from both trials was that pelvic lymphadenectomy significantly improved surgical staging, that is, it is a good prognosticator, but it did not improve disease-free or overall survival. *Optional lymphadenectomy* is another approach, in which preoperative tumor grading with intraoperative assessment of depth of myometrial invasion, as well as histologic subtype, is frequently used to decide whether lymph node dissection is necessary at the time of hysterectomy. With such a policy, patients with grade 3 disease or serous or clear cell histology and those with deep myometrial invasion on frozen section will undergo lymphadenectomy. Opponents of this

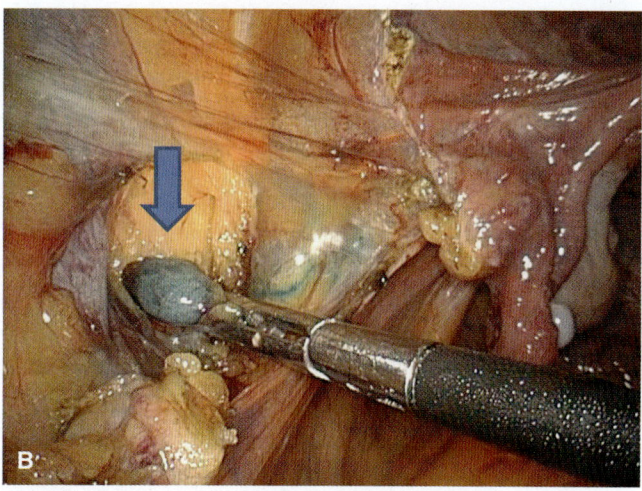

FIGURE 74.5. Comparison of nodal dissection **(A)** to sentinel node biopsy **(B)**. Solid *arrow* points to the blue dye in the sentinel node.

selective lymphadenectomy approach point out that depth of invasion on frozen section correlated with final pathology in only 67% of cases.[82] With regard to grade, preoperative FIGO grade 1 diagnosis correlates with final grade diagnosis in only 85% of cases of endometrial cancer.[23]

As a trade-off between lymphadenectomy and no surgical assessment at all in patients with endometrial cancer, there has growing interest in adopting a *sentinel lymph node (SLN) mapping* approach similar to that in breast cancer (Fig. 74.5). In a report from MSKCC, 266 patients with endometrial cancer underwent SLN mapping. At least one sentinel node was identified in 84% of cases. Location of SLN was in the pelvis in 94% of cases, in the pelvis and para-aortic in 5%, and in the para-aortic in 1%. Positive nodes were diagnosed in 12% of patients.[83] In a recent report of a prospective study[84] of 385 patients, 86% had successful mapping of at least one SLN. Positive node rate was 12%, with nodal metastases being identified in the SLNs in 97% of these 36 patients, yielding a sensitivity to detect node-positive disease of 97.2% (95% CI 85·0 to 100) and a negative predictive value of 99.6% (97.9 to 100). It is important to note that if a patient did not have bilateral mapping, a side-specific lymphadenectomy needs to be performed on the site that failed to map, because one reason for failed mapping might be due to the presence of nodal metastasis. In addition, any suspicious node on inspection needs to be removed even if it did not map. With such encouraging results, SLN mapping is gaining more acceptance in the staging of endometrioid adenocarcinoma for sure. This approach is gaining acceptance not only in the gynecologic oncology community[85,86] but also in other histologies. In a prospective study of 123 patients with grade 3 endometrioid histology, serous, clear cell, and carcinosarcoma, all underwent sentinel node mapping followed by lymphadenectomy. Overall, sentinel node detection rate was 89%, with an overall sensitivity of 95% and false-negative rate of 5% (1/20). The rate of positive node was 23% with only 1 patient having negative sentinel nodes but positive nonsentinel node.[87]

ROLE OF RADIATION

Radiation therapy plays a significant role in the management of endometrial cancer. It is often used as an adjuvant treatment after surgery (which will be discussed here) or as definitive treatment for patients who are medically inoperable or with local recurrence (which will be discussed later). In the past, most patients were treated with preoperative intracavitary brachytherapy with or without external beam

radiotherapy, followed by hysterectomy. This approach is not without its merit, especially in patients with gross cervical involvement. However, most patients nowadays undergo surgery first; then, depending on the prognostic features obtained from the pathology review, the need for radiotherapy is determined. In recent years, there has been a plethora of data from prospective, randomized trials addressing several aspects of the management of endometrial cancer. However, unlike in cervical cancer, for which the data from the majority of the randomized trials pointed in the same direction, that is, chemoradiation is better than radiotherapy (RT) alone, the data in endometrial cancer are less conclusive. Therefore, it is important for radiation oncologists to be familiar with the methodology of these studies so that objections to the use of any form of adjuvant RT can be addressed with facts.

Role of RT in Stages I and II

Treatment options for patients with early-stage endometrial cancer after hysterectomy include observation, intravaginal RT, or pelvic RT. At MSKCC, intravaginal RT is the preferred approach for most patients because it provides the best therapeutic ratio. As the discussion will demonstrate, observation may have the best morbidity profile, but it does not provide the best therapeutic ratio because of the increased risk of local recurrence. Pelvic RT, on the other hand, although very effective in reducing recurrence, has a higher morbidity profile than intravaginal RT. The results of prospective, randomized trials will be discussed first, and then, treatment recommendations based on risk factors will follow.

Results of RT Randomized Trials

There are six randomized trials regarding the role of adjuvant RT in early-stage endometrial cancer, mainly pertaining to endometrioid histology and conducted in the "modern" era.

Observation Versus Pelvic RT

Three randomized trials compared pelvic RT to observation in early-stage endometrial cancer. The first trial was the PORTEC trial, which randomized 715 patients after TAH and BSO to observation or pelvic RT.[88] Patients included were those with stage (FIGO 1988) IB grades 2 and 3 and those with IC grades 1 and 2. Those with IB grade 1 and those with IC grade 3 were excluded because it was felt that adjuvant RT was not indicated for the former and most physicians would not omit it for the latter. No lymph node sampling was done, and the dose of pelvic RT was 46 Gy at 2 Gy per fraction. At 5 years, there was a statistically significant difference in the rates of vaginal/pelvic recurrence in favor of adjuvant pelvic RT (14% vs. 4%; $P < .001$). Overall survival, however, was not different between the two groups (81% RT vs. 85% surgery; $P = .31$), and the complications with pelvic RT were significantly higher (25% vs. 6%; $P < .0001$). In addition, many of the patients who relapsed locally after surgery alone were successfully salvaged with subsequent definitive RT. The second randomized trial was GOG 99. There were 190 patients with stage (FIGO 1988) IB to IIB (grades 1 to 3), who all underwent TAH/BSO, pelvic washing, and pelvic/para-aortic lymph node sampling and then were randomized to observation versus pelvic RT to a dose of 50.4 Gy at 1.8 Gy per fraction.[89] At 2 years, there was a statistically significant difference in the rates of relapse in favor of the adjuvant pelvic RT arm (3% vs. 12%; $P = .007$). The 2-year estimated incidence of isolated vaginal/pelvic recurrence was 1.6% in the RT group and 7.4% in the surgery-alone group. There was, however, no significant difference in 4-year overall survival (92% RT vs. 86% with surgery alone; $P = .557$), but there were more complications with pelvic RT. The third trial consisted of two trials with separate randomizations consolidated into one intergroup trial. One trial was conducted by the MRC and the other by the National Cancer Institute of Canada (NCIC). Furthermore, the MRC ASTEC trial in itself consisted of two trials with separate randomizations designed to answer a surgical as well as a radiation question.[90] The surgical question was discussed earlier and regarded the need for lymphadenectomy in clinical localized endometrial cancer. The radiation question was whether pelvic RT is needed. Intermediate- or high-risk early-stage patients were then randomized to observation or pelvic RT. Intermediate risk included stage (FIGO 1988) IA grade 3, IB grade 3, IC grades 1 and 2, and IIA grades 1 and 2. High risk included IC grade 3, IIA grade 3, and IA to IIA serous and clear cell tumors. Patients who had positive pelvic nodes (stage IIIC) were allowed but not those with cervical stromal invasion (IIB). The pelvic RT was given to a total dose of 40 to 46 Gy in 20 to 25 fractions over 4 to 5 weeks. Intravaginal RT was permitted regardless of the pelvic RT randomization as long as it was the stated policy for the treating center to do so. The recommended dose was 4 Gy in two fractions prescribed to a depth of 0.5 cm treating the upper one-third of the vagina when using high dose rate (HDR) and 15 Gy when using low dose rate. The NCIC had a similar design but with a few exceptions. Patients with stage IIA serous or clear cell carcinoma were excluded, as were those with positive nodes. The dose of pelvic RT was 45 Gy in 25 fractions, and intravaginal brachytherapy was permitted in accordance with local practice.

Of the 905 patients (789 MRC and 116 NCIC) in the trial, 453 were randomized to observation and 452 to pelvic RT. The two arms were balanced except for more high-risk patients (113; 25%) in the observation arm than in the pelvic RT arm (89; 20%). There were 137 (32%) patients in the observation arm in whom nodes were removed, and 5 (4%) had positive nodes. In the pelvic RT arm, 159 (38%) had nodes removed, and 6 (4%) were positive. In the observation arm, 228 (51%) patients received intravaginal RT, 7 (2%) received pelvic and intravaginal RT, 3 (1%) received pelvic RT, and 3 (1%) were unknown. Only 212 (47%) received no form of adjuvant RT. Conversely, in the pelvic RT arm, 24 (5%) did not receive any adjuvant RT, 10 (2%) received intravaginal RT, and 2 (0.4%) were unknown. Combined intravaginal and pelvic RT was given to 232 (52%) patients, and only 184 (41%) received pelvic RT alone. The primary endpoint of this study was overall survival. With a median follow-up of 58 months, the 5-year overall survival was 84% in both arms ($P = .77$). The 5-year cumulative incidence for isolated vaginal or pelvic recurrence was 6.1% in the observation group and 3.2% in the pelvic RT group. This difference was statistically significant ($P = .2$)

with a HR of 0.46 (95% CI = 0.24 to 0.89). The rate of any acute toxicity was 27% in the observation arm compared to 57% for pelvic RT. Similarly, late toxicity was more prevalent in the pelvic RT compared to observation (61% vs. 45%, respectively).

The triad of lack of overall survival advantage, increased toxicity, and high salvage rate of local recurrence for patients who are observed has led some to conclude that all forms of adjuvant RT, not simply pelvic RT, should be abandoned. The morbidity of pelvic RT and the validity of omitting adjuvant RT in favor of RT for salvage policy will be discussed later in the chapter. With regard to overall survival, it is considered the gold standard for primary endpoint in many randomized trials in oncology, but for early-stage endometrial cancer, it is perhaps unattainable with adjuvant RT for two reasons. First, many of the patients have other, competing causes of death such as hypertension, diabetes, and obesity. In the PORTEC trial, the 8-year actuarial rates of intercurrent death were 19.7% in the RT arm and 15.6% in the surgery-alone arm.[91] Endometrial cancer–related deaths in comparison were only 9.6% and 7.5%, respectively. Similarly, in the GOG 99 trial,[89] approximately half of the deaths were due to causes other than endometrial cancer or treatment (surgery alone, 19 of 36; RT, 15 of 30). This led the authors of GOG 99 to write, "With this number of intercurrent deaths in both arms, even if RT reduces the risk of endometrial cancer-related deaths, the size of this trial is not adequate to reliably detect an overall survival difference." That is why overall survival was not the primary endpoint in GOG99 but rather the disease-free interval, which was significantly different in favor of adjuvant pelvic RT over surgery alone.[89] Therefore, it is not unreasonable to conclude that neither PORTEC nor GOG 99 was large enough to conclusively show whether adjuvant pelvic RT affected overall survival. The second difficult hurdle for adjuvant RT to overcome when discussing overall survival has to do with its localized nature. In the MRC/NCIC trial, the rate of first vaginal/pelvic recurrence was reduced from 11.4% ($n = 37$ of 453) in the observation arm to 2.8% ($n = 13$ of 452) with pelvic RT. Adjuvant pelvic RT, however, did not affect distant spread; the rate of first distant spread was 8.1% ($n = 37$ of 453) in the observation compared to 9% ($n = 41$ of 452) in the pelvic RT arm.[90] One would expect adjuvant RT to make a difference in overall survival only when systemic therapy has an effect on the rate of distant spread. This is exactly the story learned from postoperative chest wall irradiation in breast cancer. Because pelvic RT significantly improved local control, albeit with increased toxicity, why not replace it with intravaginal RT rather than advocating observation for all early-stage endometrial cancer?

Observation Versus Intravaginal RT

In a trial reported by Sorbe et al.,[92] 645 patients with stage (FIGO 1988) IA to IB grades 1 and 2 endometrioid adenocarcinoma were randomized after surgery to observation ($n = 326$) or intravaginal RT ($n = 319$). Surgery consisted of TAH/BSO (laparoscopic surgery was allowed), pelvic washing, and removal of enlarged nodes. The dose and type of intravaginal RT varied among the six centers participating in this trial, but 347 of 645 patients were treated with HDR to 18 Gy in six fractions. The proximal upper two-thirds of the vagina was treated with the dose prescribed to 0.5 cm from the surface of the cylinder. The rate of vaginal recurrence was 3.1% in the observation arm compared to 1.2% for the intravaginal RT arm ($P = .114$). The rate of pelvic recurrence was 0.9% in the observation arm and 0.3% in the treatment arm ($P = .326$). No significance difference was seen between the two arms in terms of overall survival. There was significantly more grade 1 vaginal toxicity with intravaginal RT (8.8% vs. 1.5%; $P = .00004$). There was no significant difference in gastrointestinal (GI) or genitourinary toxicity.

Pelvic RT Versus Intravaginal RT

In the PORTEC-2 trial, 427 patients were randomized to pelvic RT (n = 214) or intravaginal RT (n = 213). Patients enrolled were those with stage (FIGO 1988) IB grade 3 and >60 years old, IC grades 1 and 2 and >60 years old, and IIA grades 1 and 2 of all ages but with <50% myometrial invasion. During surgery, patients underwent TAH/BSO, pelvic washing, and removal of suspicious pelvic or para-aortic lymph nodes. Routine lymphadenectomy was not performed. The dose of pelvic RT was 46 Gy given in 23 fractions. Intravaginal RT was delivered using a cylinder to treat the upper half of the vagina. The dose was prescribed to 0.5 cm from the surface of the cylinder. Three types of brachytherapy were used: HDR to 21 Gy in three fractions, low dose rate to 30 Gy at 0.5 to 0.7 Gy/h, and medium dose rate to 28 Gy at 1 Gy/h. With a median follow-up of 36 months, the 3-year vaginal recurrence rates were 0.9% in the intravaginal RT arm and 1.9% in the pelvic RT arm (P = .97). The pelvic recurrence was significantly different; the 3-year rate was 3.5% in the intravaginal RT arm compared to 0.6% in the pelvic RT arm (P = .03). The corresponding rates of isolated pelvic recurrence, however, were not significant: 0.6% versus 1.2%, respectively (P = .54). There was no significant difference in disease-free or overall survival between the two arms. The rate of grades 1 and 2 acute GI toxicity was 53% versus 12% in favor of intravaginal RT (P < .001). This trial showed that intravaginal RT alone is sufficient to control vaginal recurrence even in patients with intermediate- to high-risk features.[93]

In the Swedish trial reported by Sorbe et al.,[94] patients with stage (FIGO 1988) I endometrioid adenocarcinoma with at least one of the risk factors grade 3, ≥50% myometrial invasion, or DNA aneuploidy were randomized to adjuvant intravaginal RT (IVRT; n = 263) or pelvic and IVRT (n = 264). Lymphadenectomy was required. There was no difference in vaginal recurrence, which was 2.7% (7 of 263) in the IVRT-alone arm compared to 1.9% (5 of 264) in the combined arm (P = .555). Pelvic recurrence rate, however, was different: 5.3% in the IVRT arm compared to 0.4% in the pelvic plus IVRT arm (P = .0006). There was no significant difference in overall survival between the two arms (90% vs. 89%, respectively). The toxicity was significantly higher in the combined arm compared to IVRT alone.

Radiation Treatment Recommendations for Early-Stage Disease Based on Risk Factors

Based on the results of these trials in early-stage endometrial cancer, it is clear that pelvic RT is an excessive treatment for most of those patients. Therefore, the treatment recommendations should be individualized based on risk factors. When deciding on whether to recommend observation, intravaginal RT, or pelvic RT, the risk of vaginal recurrence and pelvic recurrence should be assessed separately. With respect to vaginal recurrence, the data from randomized trials indicate that adjuvant intravaginal RT alone is sufficient to control potential microscopic disease in the vagina. The PORTEC-2 trial showed that intravaginal RT is as good as pelvic RT in controlling vaginal recurrence (0.9% vs. 1.9%, respectively; P = .97) despite the fact that patients included in this trial were at high risk for vaginal recurrence based on age ≥60 years old, deep myometrial invasion, or endocervical gland involvement.[93] The data from the Swedish randomized trial further confirmed that when it comes to vaginal control, IVRT alone is sufficient.[94] The vaginal recurrence was 2.9% in the IVRT arm compared to 1.9% (P = .555) in the pelvic plus intravaginal RT arm. How best to reduce pelvic recurrence is more controversial. For patients at low risk of having pelvic lymph node involvement, that is, endometrioid grade 1 or 2 with no or minimal myometrial invasion, neither lymphadenectomy nor pelvic RT is likely to be of significant benefit because of

low rate of pelvic node involvement.[41] Those who are at higher risk of having lymph node involvement may need to have their lymph nodes surgically assessed to ensure that they are pathologically negative or receive pelvic RT to control potential microscopic disease. However, the two PORTEC trials, as well as the Swedish trial, showed that the risk of pelvic recurrence was only 2% to 6% even in the absence of lymphadenectomy.[88,93,94] This low rate of pelvic recurrence, coupled with the lack of survival advantage to lymphadenectomy and pelvic RT, raises the question of whether either approach is needed for the majority of patients with early-stage endometrial cancer. In the eyes of many, having LVI is almost indicative of nodal involvement. Cohn et al.[95] correlated LVI and the risk of positive pelvic nodes in 366 surgically staged patients. The rate of LVI was 25%, and the rate of positive pelvic nodes was 13%. Patients with LVI were significantly more likely to have nodal metastasis (35 of 92 vs. 11 of 274; P < .001). However, the influence of LVI on pelvic nodal metastasis was the strongest in patients with deep myometrial invasion and high grade. Data from MSKCC on 126 patients with endometrioid FIGO (1988) stages IB to IIB and LVI also showed that the mere presence of LVI should not be a trigger for giving pelvic RT, especially when patients had lymphadenectomy. Patients were divided into two groups: those from the old era, when treatment was often pelvic RT, and those from the modern era, when patients were more often treated with lymphadenectomy and intravaginal RT.[63] The rate of pelvic relapse for patients with LVI was 7% in the old era compared to 3% (P = .3) in the modern era.

No Myometrial Invasion, Grades 1 and 2

The risk of vaginal recurrence is almost negligible. Straughn et al.[96] reported no vaginal recurrence in 103 such patients treated with surgery alone. Pelvic lymph nodal positivity was ≤3%. The 5-year progression-free survival (PFS) rate in this group was on the order of 95% to 98%. It is unlikely that postoperative pelvic or intravaginal RT would add anything to the final outcome, and therefore, radiation is not routinely recommended to this group of patients.

No Myometrial Invasion, Grade 3

In GOG study 210, there were only 69 patients out of 5,866 (1.1%) with disease limited to endometrium and had grade endometrioid histology, making it difficult to draw any meaningful conclusion.[41] Straughn et al.[96] reported on eight patients with stage IA grade 3 disease treated with surgery alone, with two of patients developing isolated vaginal recurrence. The risk of lymph node metastasis in this group of patients is about (1.7%) in GOG 210 study.[41] At MSKCC, these patients are offered either intravaginal RT alone or observation.

Less than 50% Myometrial Invasion, Grades 1 and 2

This group of patients constitutes the most common stage subgroup of all endometrial cancers. Straughn et al.[96] reported a 3% (9 of 296) risk of vaginal recurrence when surgery alone was done. In the surgery-alone arm of the PORTEC-1 trial,[88] the 5-year vaginal recurrence rate for patients with <50% myometrial invasion grade 2 was 5%. In a randomized trial reported by Sorbe et al.,[92] the vaginal recurrence rate was 3.1% for those in the observation arm compared to 1.2% for those in the intravaginal RT arm (P = .114). The trial was designed to detect a difference of 1% versus 5% in the vaginal recurrence rate in the two groups. The data were not reported separately based on whether myometrial invasion was present or not, making it difficult to determine the true impact of intravaginal RT on the rate of vaginal recurrence in patients with myometrial invasion. Data from MSKCC on 233 patients with <50% myometrial invasion grade 1 or 2 showed a vaginal recurrence rate of only 1% using intravaginal RT alone.[97,98] In addition, Sorbe et al.[99] reported on 110 patients with IB grade 1 or 2 who were part of a prospective, randomized trial evaluating two different intravaginal RT doses; the rate of vaginal recurrence was 0.9%. The risk of pelvic recurrence was only 1.8%, even though lymphadenectomy was not required. This low rate of pelvic recurrence is similar to those reported by Straughn et al.[96] of 0.3% (1 of 296) and by Horowitz et al.[100] of 0% (0 of 62) in the setting of lymphadenectomy. This indicates that pelvic RT is of limited use, and therefore, it seems reasonable to suggest that either observation or intravaginal RT is a reasonable option for patients with grade 1 or 2 and <50% myometrial invasion.

However, when deciding on whether adjuvant RT is needed, it is important to address two issues. First, older patients tend to have higher rates of relapse. In the study by Straughn et al.,[96] 8 of the 10 vaginal/pelvic recurrences were in patients ≥60 years old. In the randomized trial by Sorbe et al.[92] comparing adjuvant intravaginal RT to observation, patients with vaginal recurrences were significantly (P = .018) older (mean age, 68.6 years) than patients without vaginal recurrences (mean, 62.6 years). Second, patients with LVI have a higher chance of vaginal recurrence, as demonstrated by Mariani et al.[61] who reported on 508 patients with endometrial cancer limited to the corpus treated with surgery alone. The presence of LVI significantly increased the vaginal relapse rate from 3% to 7% (P = .02). The rate of vaginal relapse would have been even higher if patients without myometrial invasion (152 of 508) had been excluded because LVI is exceedingly rare in patients without myometrial invasion. At MSKCC, patients who are ≥60 years old or have LVI are recommended to have intravaginal RT.

Greater Than 50% Myometrial Invasion, Grade 3

Some advocate observation for patients with <50% myometrial invasion grade 3, yet the 5-year vaginal recurrence rate in PORTEC-1 was 14% for such patients treated with surgery alone compared to none for those treated with pelvic RT.[88] Perhaps a better choice for those patients is intravaginal RT. The incidence of positive pelvic lymph nodes at time of surgery in this subset of patients is about 3.9%. In the PORTEC-1 trial, none of the 37 patients with grade 3 disease and <50% myometrial invasion who were treated with TAH/BSO alone relapsed in the pelvis.[88] At MSKCC, intravaginal RT is recommended for this subset of patients irrespective of whether lymphadenectomy was performed.

Fifty Percent or Greater Myometrial Invasion, Grades 1 and 2

The risk of vaginal recurrence with surgery alone in this group of patients is not minimal. In the PORTEC-1 trial,[88] the 5-year vaginal recurrence for patients with ≥50% myometrial invasion treated with surgery alone was 10% for those with grade 1 and 13% for grade 2. The corresponding 5-year vaginal recurrence rates for patients treated with pelvic RT were 1% and 2%, respectively. With regard to pelvic control, the 5-year pelvic recurrence for patients with ≥50% myometrial invasion treated with surgery alone was 2% for grade 1 and 6% for grade 2. The data from the PORTEC-2 trial[93] and the Swedish trial[94] in which patients with ≥50% myometrial invasion grade 1 or 2 were included indicate that the omission of pelvic RT increased the risk of pelvic recurrence. In PORTEC-2 trial,[93] the 3-year rate was 3.5% in the intravaginal RT arm compared to 0.6% in the pelvic RT arm (P = .03). In the Swedish trial,[94] the pelvic recurrence rate was 5.3% in the IVRT arm compared to 0.4% in the pelvic plus intravaginal RT arm (P = .0006). At MSKCC, most of these patients undergo SLN mapping, and if the nodes are pathologically negative, they undergo intravaginal RT alone.

Fifty Percent or Greater Myometrial Invasion and Grade 3

In GOG 210, the risk of finding positive lymph nodes in this group of patients was 29.1.[41] Such patients were not enrolled in the PORTEC trials because it was felt that omitting pelvic RT when lymphadenectomy was not performed could not be justified. In the registry study reported by Creutzberg et al.,[101] 99 patients with ≥50% myometrial invasion grade 3 were treated with postoperative pelvic RT. The 5-year rate of vaginal recurrence was 5%, that of pelvic recurrence was 8%, and that of distant relapse was 31%. Very few investigators would recommend surgery alone for these patients. In fact, an argument could be made that pelvic RT might be needed even after a negative lymphadenectomy, especially for older patients and those with LVI. In GOG 99 trial, factors associated with an increased recurrence rate (25% at 5 years) were identified using proportional hazards regression modeling of historical data from GOG 33.[89] These factors were (a) increasing age, (b) moderate to poorly differentiated tumor grade, (c) presence of LVI, and (d) outer one-third myometrial invasion. From the results of that analysis, a subgroup of patients with high intermediate risk (HIR) was defined as follows: (a) at least 70 years of age with only one of the other risk factors, (b) at least 50 years of age with any two of the other risk factors, or (c) any age with all three of the other risk factors. Those on the RT arm demonstrated a somewhat lower overall death rate when compared to those on the observation arm (relative hazard [RH] = 0.73, 90% CI = 0.43 to 1.26) in the HIR subgroup. AT MSKCC, patients with deep myometrial invasion grade 3 who are HIR per GOG 99 are offered postoperative pelvic RT. If they are not HIR, which is not that common in this subset of patients, they could be considered for intravaginal RT, but only in the setting of adequate surgical lymph node assessment.

Cervical Involvement

Gross cervical involvement increases the risk of parametrial extension as well as spread to pelvic lymph nodes in a fashion similar to primary cervical cancer. Such patients could undergo radical hysterectomy and pelvic lymph node dissection or preoperative radiation including pelvic radiation and intracavitary brachytherapy followed by simple hysterectomy. The FOGO 2009 staging system only recognizes cervical stromal invasion, and not endocervical gland involvement, as being stage II. But it is important to note that patients with endocervical gland involvement were included in POTEC 2 trial comparing pelvic RT to intravaginal RT.

There are also emerging data on the role of intravaginal RT alone in highly selected patients with cervical stromal invasion. Elsheaikh et al. reported on 27 patients treated with intravaginal RT. There were no vaginal recurrence and only 1 pelvic recurrence.[102,103] At MSKCC, patients with endocervical glandular involvement are often treated with IVRT. For patients with cervical stromal invasion grade 1 and 2 and the depth of cervical stromal invasion <50%, intravaginal RT could be offered if they underwent adequate surgical lymph node assessment. For those with grade 3 or deep cervical stromal invasion, pelvic RT is recommended irrespective of lymphadenectomy. Table 74.5 shows overall treatment recommendations for early-stage endometrioid adenocarcinoma at MSKCC.

ROLE OF SYSTEMIC THERAPY

Hormonal therapy has been used in the treatment of recurrent/advanced endometrial cancer for many years. Agents used include megestrol acetate (Megace), medroxyprogesterone acetate (Provera), and, to a lesser extent, tamoxifen.[104–106] The response rate ranges from 9% to 33%, with an overall survival

TABLE 74.5 TREATMENT RECOMMENDATIONS AT MEMORIAL SLOAN KETTERING CANCER CENTER FOR STAGE I AND II PATIENTS WITH ENDOMETRIOID ADENOCARCINOMA

Extent/Grade	1	2	3
No MI invasion	Observation	Observation	IVRT or observation[a]
<50% MI	IVRT or observation[a]	IVRT or observation[a]	IVRT
≥50% MI	IVRT	IVRT	IVRT or IMRT[b]
Endocervical gland	IVRT	IVRT	IVRT or IMRT[b]
CSI <50%	IVRT	IVRT	IVRT or IMRT[b]
CSI >50%	IMRT	IMRT	IMRT

[a]Observation is offered to patients <60 years old and without lymph node invasion.
[b]IMRT if high to intermediate risk.
CSI, cervical stromal invasion; IMRT, intensity-modulated radiotherapy; IVRT, intravaginal radiotherapy; MI, myometrial invasion.

of 6 to 14 months. In GOG 107, doxorubicin was compared to doxorubicin and cisplatin.[107] The response rate was 42% versus 25% ($P = .004$), and the progression-free interval was 5.7 versus 3.8 months ($P = .014$) in favor of combination chemotherapy. However, this did not translate into overall survival advantage (9 vs. 9.2 months). In GOG 177 trial,[108] doxorubicin/cisplatin was compared to doxorubicin/cisplatin/paclitaxel. The three-drug regimen was superior in terms of response rate (57% vs. 34%, $P < .01$), progression-free interval (8.3 vs. 5.3 months, $P < .01$), and survival (15.3 vs. 12.3 months, $P = .037$).

With the widespread use of chemotherapy in the recurrent/advanced setting, its use in the adjuvant setting has also started to increase and to challenge the role of adjuvant RT. There are several randomized trials addressing the role of adjuvant chemotherapy in advanced endometrial cancer.

Chemotherapy Versus RT Trials

There are three randomized trials comparing adjuvant chemotherapy to radiation. The Japanese Gynecology Oncology Group (JGOG) trial randomized 385 patients with stage (FIGO 1988) IC to III (25% with stage III) endometrial cancer to pelvic radiation (193 patients) or to chemotherapy (192 patients).[109] The surgery was hysterectomy with optional lymphadenectomy. The dose of pelvic RT was 45 to 50 Gy using open anteroposterior/posteroanterior (AP/PA) fields. Chemotherapy consisted of cyclophosphamide (333 mg/m²), cisplatin (50 mg/m²), and doxorubicin (40 mg/m²) every 4 weeks for three cycles or more. There was no significant difference in progression-free ($P = .726$) or overall survival rate ($P = .462$) between the two groups. A trial from Italy had a similar design, in which 340 patients with stage (FIGO 1988) IC grade 3, stage II grade 3, and stage III (two-thirds of patients) were randomized to radiation or to chemotherapy.[110] With a median follow-up of 95.5 months, the 5-year disease-free survival rate was 63% in both arms ($P = .44$) and the 5-year overall survival rate was 69% in the radiation arm and 66% in the chemotherapy arm ($P = .77$). Again, there was no significant difference in outcome despite using five cycles of Cytoxan, cisplatin, and doxorubicin. In GOG 122, 396 patients with stage (FIGO 1988) III to IV disease were randomized to whole-abdomen radiation ($n = 202$) versus doxorubicin/cisplatin ($n = 194$) for eight cycles. Progression-free survival was the primary endpoint of this study. With a median follow-up of 74 months, there was significant improvement in both progression-free (50% vs. 38%; $P = .007$) and overall survival rate (55% vs. 42%; $P = .004$), respectively, in favor of chemotherapy.[111] However, before concluding that chemotherapy alone is the answer, a closer examination of the data is warranted. The overall absolute rate of relapse was 54% in the radiation arm compared to 50% in the chemotherapy arm, a small difference, if any, and yet the corresponding 5-year PFS rates were 38% and 50% ($P = .007$), respectively. The reason for the discrepancy is that in this study, there was stage imbalance, in which there were

more stage IIIA patients in the RT arm (28.2%) than in the chemotherapy arm (18%). Conversely, there were more patients with stage IIIC disease in the chemotherapy arm (51.5%) than in the RT arm (44.6%). Therefore, the 5-year disease-free survival rate for the chemotherapy arm was increased from 42% to 50%, which became significantly different than the RT arm (50% vs. 38%, $P = .007$) rather than 42% versus 38%, which is not likely to be significant. The 5-year overall survival rate in the chemotherapy arm was 55% compared to 42% for the RT arm ($P = .004$). What are we to make of the significant difference in overall survival? There were 15 deaths unrelated to endometrial cancer or protocol treatment in the radiation arm compared to only six in the chemotherapy arm, raising a question about whether the two arms of the study were truly balanced, especially because no stratification was performed in that trial.[111] The results of GOG 122 have led to the adoption of adjuvant chemotherapy as the preferred treatment for stage III endometrial cancer. It is important to note, however, that GOG 122, JGOG, and the Italian study all showed no significant difference in the patterns of relapse between RT and chemotherapy. If one were to use the unadjusted PFS from GOG 122, then all three randomized trials failed to show that adjuvant chemotherapy is superior to adjuvant RT.

Chemoradiation Versus RT Trials

There are four randomized trials comparing adjuvant chemoradiation to radiation (Table 74.6). In the first trial from Finland,[112] 156 patients with stage (FIGO 1988) IA or IB grade 3 ($n = 28$) or stage IC to IIIA grade 1 to 3 ($n = 128$) were postoperatively randomized to receive radiotherapy (56 Gy) only ($n = 72$) or radiotherapy combined with three cycles of cisplatin (50 mg/m²), epirubicin (60 mg/m²), and cyclophosphamide (500 mg/m²) chemotherapy ($n = 84$). The disease-specific overall 5-year survival was 84.7% in the RT arm versus 82.1% in the chemoradiation arm ($P = .148$). The second trial reported by Hogberg et al.[113] is two trials (Mario Negri Gynecologic Oncology Group [MaNGO] and Nordic Society of Gynecological Oncology [NSGO]/European Organisation for Research and Treatment of Cancer [EORTC]) combined in one report. In the MaNGO trial, there were 157 patients (two-thirds were stage III); 76 were randomized to postoperative pelvic RT (45 Gy) and 80 to chemotherapy followed by pelvic RT. The chemotherapy consisted of three cycles of doxorubicin (60 mg/m²) and cisplatin (50 mg/m²). The 5-year PFS was 61% in the RT group compared to 74% for the chemoradiation group, but that difference was not significant ($P = .1$). The 5-year overall survival (OS) was also not significant (73% vs. 78%, respectively; $P = .41$). In the NSGO/EORTC trial, 383 patients were randomized to RT ($n = 191$) versus RT and chemotherapy ($n = 187$). The type of chemotherapy varied, and only a handful of patients were stage III. The 5-year PFS was better for the chemoradiation arm (79% vs. 72% for RT; $P = .04$), but OS was not significantly better (83% vs. 76%, respectively; $P = .1$).

The third trial is GOG 249 trial, where 601 patients with stage I to II high- to intermediate-risk endometrioid adenocarcinoma and all stage I to II serous or clear cell carcinoma were

TABLE 74.6 EFFECT OF CHEMORADIATION COMPARED TO RADIATION ON OUTCOME IN HIGH-RISK ENDOMETRIAL CANCER

	Finland	NSGO	MaNGO	GOG 249	PORTEC-3
PFS	↔	↑	↔	↔	↔ stage I–II ↑ stage III
OS	↔	↔	↔	↔	↔

Gynecologic Oncology Group (GOG) 249 compared chemotherapy plus intravaginal RT to pelvic RT, whereas the Finland trial, Nordic Society of Gynecological Oncology (NSGO), Mario Negri Gynecologic Oncology Group (MaNGO), and PORTEC-3 compared chemotherapy plus pelvic RT to pelvic RT.
OS, overall survival; PFS, progression-free survival.
↔, chemoradiation equivalent to pelvic RT; ↑, chemoradiation better than pelvic RT.

Section III

randomized to either pelvic RT (45 Gy) or intravaginal RT plus 3 cycles of carboplatin/paclitaxel. With median follow-up of 53 months, the 3-year recurrence-free survival was 82% in both arms. The overall survival rate was 91% in the pelvic RT arm compared to 88% for the chemotherapy and intravaginal RT arm. There was no significant difference in rate of vaginal relapse or distant metastasis. There was a higher rate of pelvic recurrence in the chemotherapy arm compared to pelvic RT (25 vs. 6 patients). Toxicity was also higher in the chemotherapy arm.[114] The fourth trial is PORTEC-3, which included stage III patients as well as high-risk early-stage disease. There were 660 patients who were randomized to either pelvic RT (46.8 Gy) or pelvic RT with concurrent cisplatin (50 mg/m^2) on weeks 1 and 4 followed by 4 cycles of carboplatin/paclitaxel.[115] With a median follow-up time of 60.2 months, the 5-year OS was 81.8% for chemoradiation arm versus 76.7% for RT arm; HR 0.79 (95% CI = 0.57 to 1.12, P = .183). The corresponding 5-year failure-free survival rates were 75.5% versus 68.9%, respectively, with an HR of 0.77 (0.58 to 1.03, P = .078).

Chemoradiation Versus Chemotherapy Trial

In GOG 258 trial, 736 patients with stage III and IVA endometrial cancer or stage I to II (but with positive cytology) were randomized to 6 cycles of carboplatin/paclitaxel versus postoperative external beam RT with concurrent cisplatin (50 mg/m^2) on weeks 1 and 4 followed by 4 cycles of carboplatin/paclitaxel.[116] With a median follow-up of 47 months, the 5-year recurrence-free survival was about 58% in both arms. The 5-year overall survival was 73% in the chemotherapy-alone arm compared to 70% for the chemoradiation arm. When comparing the chemoradiation arm to chemotherapy-alone arm, there were some differences in the rates of relapse: vaginal recurrence (3% vs. 7%), pelvic/para-aortic (10% vs. 19%), and distant (27% vs. 21%), respectively.

Systemic Therapy Recommendations Based on Risk Factors

When considering the use of adjuvant chemotherapy in endometrial cancer based on risk factors, one need to pay attention to whether we are dealing with an isolated as opposed to multiple risk factors. This is particularly important when dealing with FIGO 2009 stage III disease.

Early-Stage High-Risk Endometrioid Adenocarcinoma

In GOG 249 randomized trial[114] limited to high-risk stage I to II disease, 71% of patients had endometrioid histology. In PORTEC-3, patients with stage I (grade 3 with deep myometrial invasion and/or LVI) as well as stage II were included (55%); endometrioid histology was seen in 71% of patients.[115] In both trials, the addition of chemotherapy did not impact outcome of particularly distant metastasis, which was equivalent in GOG 249 and only slightly less in PORTEC-3 (23.1% for chemoradiation vs. 29.7% for pelvic RT; P = .077). Therefore, routine use of adjuvant chemotherapy in addition to radiation could not be recommended for all high-risk early-stage endometrioid adenocarcinoma.

Early-Stage Serous and Clear Cell Cancer

Serous cancer and to a lesser extent clear cell cancer tend to spread in a fashion similar to ovarian cancer, with a high propensity for upper abdominal relapse. Therefore, it is important to perform comprehensive surgical staging because of the high rate of surgical upstaging. For serous endometrial cancer, the preferred approach is intravaginal RT plus carboplatin/paclitaxel.[98,117,118] In a report from MSKCC on 41 patients with stage I to II (all had negative peritoneal cytology) treated as such, with a median follow-up time of 58 months, the 5-year disease-free and overall survival rates were 85% and 90%, respectively.[118] The 5-year actuarial recurrence rates were 9%

in the pelvis, 5% in the para-aortic nodes, and 10% at distant sites. None of the patients developed vaginal recurrence. In a subsequent report, the presence of deep myometrial invasion and/or cervical stromal invasion was associated with higher rate of pelvic recurrence.[98] This issue raises the question of whether pelvic RT alone or in combination with chemotherapy should be considered for such a subset of early-stage serous cancers. More mature data from PORTEC-3 and GOG 249 may shed more light on the role of pelvic RT in this histology. At MSKCC, most patients with early-stage serous endometrial cancer disease who are surgically staged are treated with intravaginal RT interdigitated with 6 cycles of concurrent carboplatin/paclitaxel. Treatment recommendations for clear cell carcinoma often mirror those for serous, but it is debatable if that is always warranted. When outcome of early-stage serous was compared to that with clear cell, the 5-year relapse-free and overall survival were identical despite the fact that only 38% of patients received adjuvant chemotherapy in the clear cell group compared to 67% with serous, P = .02.[119] At MSKCC, patient with early-stage clear cell carcinoma are treated with intravaginal RT and concurrent carboplatin/paclitaxel being reserved for those with deep invasion or cervical involvement.

Stage IIIA

The results of postoperative external beam RT in patients with isolated adnexal or serosal involvement are generally good. However, the rate of distant relapse is still 26% to 33%, indicating the need for adjuvant systemic therapy.[69] Furthermore, patients with more than one site of involvement, that is, multiple risk factors, do worse. Jobson et al.[120] reported on 141 patients with IIIA endometrioid adenocarcinoma (patients with isolated positive peritoneal cytology were excluded) treated with postoperative RT. The risk of abdominal relapse was 12.4% (11 of 89) for patients with one site of involvement compared to 36.5% (19 of 52) for more than one site (P < .001). Distant metastasis rate was 23.9% (21 of 89) compared to 34.6% (18 of 52), respectively. The 5-year DSS was 70.4% for one involved site compared to 43.3% for more than one (P = .001). On multivariate analysis, grade 3 (HR, 2.5; P = .045) and more than one site involvement (HR, 2.2; P = .012) were independent predictors of poor DSS. In the ongoing debate on whether chemotherapy alone is better than chemoradiation in patients with stage III, it is in this group of patients with multiple sites of involvement especially with positive peritoneal cytology and/or aggressive histologies[68,121] in which chemotherapy plus intravaginal RT might be a better choice than combining with pelvic RT.

Stage IIIC

The outcome of patients with isolated lymph node involvement (especially pelvic nodes), treated with postoperative pelvic RT is relatively good.[70] At MSKCC, we recommend external beam radiation with concurrent cisplatin followed by carboplatin/paclitaxel to try to reduce the risk of recurrence even further. Milgrom et al.[122] reported on 40 patients with stage III (82% were IIIC) treated with such an approach. With a median follow-up time of 49 months, the 5-year freedom from relapse was 79% and overall survival 85%. The rate of vaginal recurrence was 3%, pelvic recurrence 3%, para-aortic 11%, peritoneal 5%, and other distant 11%.

Because stage IIIC is the most common subset in stage III disease (73% of patients in GOG 258), a discussion here about how to reconcile the data from GOG 258 and those from PORTEC-3 (stage III subset 45%) is in order. In PORTEC-3, the 5-year failure-free survival was 58% for RT alone compared to 69% for chemoradiation (P = .032) in stage III patients. The corresponding rates for OS were 70% and 79% respectively.[115] In GOG 258, the 5-year relapse-free survival was about 58% in both arms and overall survival was 70% in the chemoradiation arm and 73% in the chemotherapy-alone arm.[116] The question then becomes: Why was the rate of overall survival and relapse-free survival of the radiation-alone arm in PORTEC-3 for patients with stage III similar to both arms of in GOG 258? The answer might be found in the different inclusion criteria: GOG 258 allowed for patients with <2 cm gross residual disease (17 patients with 11/17 developing recurrence), whereas POTEC 3 excluded patients with gross residual disease.

As mentioned above in stage IIIA, the presence of *multiple risk factors* in stage IIIC has been shown to be a predictor of poor outcome.[123] In a recent SEER review, Garg et al.[124] showed that for patients with stage IIIC disease (*n* = 2,559), the 5-year DSS was 67%, which dropped to 43% when extranodal involvement (i.e., positive washing, adnexa/serosal, and vaginal/parametrial involvement) was present (*P* < .001). At MSKCC, such patients are treated with full systemic chemotherapy plus intravaginal RT rather than external beam and concurrent chemotherapy.

RADIATION THERAPY TECHNIQUES

Intravaginal Radiation

The purpose of this treatment modality is to deliver the highest dose of radiation to the vaginal mucosa while limiting the dose to the surrounding normal structures such as the bladder, rectum, and small intestines. HDR brachytherapy using ^{192}Ir sources is the preferred method of delivering intravaginal RT. The type of applicator used is generally a cylinder. The treatment is given on an outpatient basis without the need for anesthesia and without the radiation exposure to medical personnel. At MSKCC, patients start their treatment 4 to 6 weeks postoperatively, depending on the vaginal cuff healing. It takes longer for the vaginal cuff to heal [125] after LAVH/BSO and robotic hysterectomy than after TAH/BSO. The treatment is given in three fractions of 7 Gy to a total dose of 21 Gy. The interval between each fraction is 1 to 2 weeks. When intravaginal RT is given with chemotherapy, it is given concurrently but not during the week when the patient is receiving their chemotherapy. The dose is prescribed to a 0.5-cm depth from the mucosal surface (Fig. 74.6). The treatment is usually delivered using a 3-cm-diameter cylinder to treat a 4- to 7-cm length of the vagina, depending on depth of invasion and tumor grade. For patients with grade 3, serous or clear cell carcinoma, the length of vagina treated is generally 7 cm (assuming an average length of vagina after simple hysterectomy of about 10 cm). This is done to account for potential submucosal extension that may lead to relapse in the distal periurethral region with these aggressive histologies. For patients with grade 1 or 2 endometrioid adenocarcinoma, the treated vaginal length increases from 4 cm if myometrial invasion is <50%, to 5 cm for >50% myometrial invasion, and to 6 cm for cervical involvement. Occasionally, the dose per fraction is lowered to 6 Gy instead of 7 Gy if the diameter of the cylinder is <3 cm. This is usually done to avoid a very high dose of radiation to the vaginal mucosa. The dose per fraction is also lowered to 4 to 5 Gy when pelvic radiation is added.

External Beam Radiation

Conventional RT

At the time of simulation for *pelvic* RT, the small bowel is opacified using oral contrast, a vaginal marker is used to define the vaginal cuff, and the rectum is opacified with barium or CT-compatible contrasts. Patients are usually placed in the prone position to displace the small intestines from the radiation field. The target volume consists of the pelvic lymph nodes, including obturator, external, internal, and lower common iliac groups and the proximal two-thirds of the vagina. The presacral nodes are not included unless patients have gross cervical involvement. High-energy linear accelerators (15 MV) are preferred because of their sparing of the skin and subcutaneous tissue. The ideal beam arrangement with conventional radiation is the four-field pelvic-box technique to reduce the dose to the small intestines and to some extent the bladder and rectum. For AP/PA fields, the superior border is L5-S1, the inferior border is the bottom of the obturator foramina, and the lateral border is 2 cm beyond the widest point of the inlet of the true bony pelvis. For lateral fields, the anterior border is in front of the pubis symphysis and the posterior border at least at S2-S3. The superior and inferior borders are the same for the AP/PA fields. All fields are treated daily to a dose of 1.8 Gy. A total dose of 50.4 Gy is generally given when pelvic radiation is used alone, or 45 Gy when combined with intravaginal RT.

When para-aortic nodes are involved, *extended field* RT is used, and CT simulation is crucial for accurate delineation of the kidneys, small bowel, and liver in addition to nodal target. The latter should include, in addition to the pelvic nodes, the pericaval, interaortocaval, and para-aortic areas, defined by contrast-enhanced blood vessels. The preferred approach is the four-field box technique rather than AP/PA in order

FIGURE 74.6. Dose distribution with intravaginal radiation therapy (prescription dose 7 Gy in *solid yellow*). **A:** Sagittal view. **B:** Axial view.

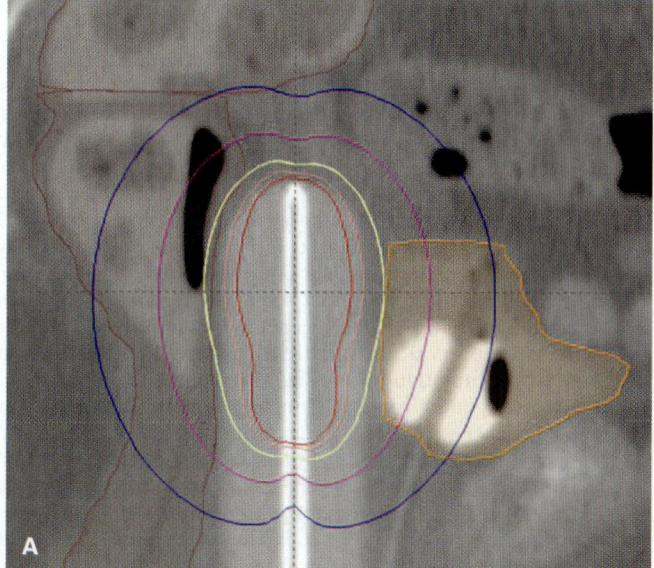

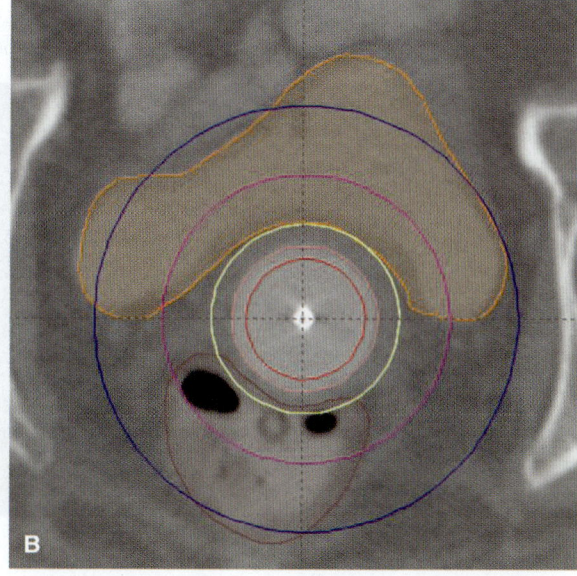

to lower the dose to the small intestines. However, attention should be paid to the dose that the kidneys might receive with the four-field arrangement. The lower border is the same as in pelvic radiation, but the upper border is extended usually to the T12-L1 interspace. The typical dose is 45.0 Gy at 1.8 Gy or 1.5 Gy if patients develop acute GI toxicity.

Intensity-Modulated RT

At MSKCC, postoperative intensity-modulated RT (IMRT) is used for most patients with endometrial cancer who need pelvic or extended field radiation (Fig. 74.7). At the time of simulation, patients are placed in the prone (pelvic) or supine (extended) position and immobilized using Aquaplast. Oral and rectal contrasts are used to better visualize the small and large intestines. In addition, contrast is inserted in the vaginal cuff to better visualize the upper vagina. Because pelvic lymph nodes are poorly visualized by CT when normal, they should be defined by encompassing the contrast-enhanced blood vessels. Taylor et al.[126] found that a modified 7-mm margin around contrast-enhanced vessels offers a good surrogate target for pelvic lymph nodes. Small et al.[127] reported on consensus guidelines for delineation of clinical target volume (CTV) for intensity-modulated pelvic radiotherapy in postoperative treatment of endometrial and cervical cancer. A modified 7-mm margin (excluding bowel and muscles) is recommended around the iliac vessels to create nodal CTV. To create nodal planning target volume (PTV), an additional expansion of 7 mm all around nodal CTV is generally recommended. At MSKCC, vaginal PTV is created by outlining the contrast-enhanced vaginal cuff and adding a 3-cm margin axially and 2 cm superior and inferior to account for the impact of bladder and rectal filling, as well as of vaginal motion.[128] An alternative approach would be to simulate patient with bladder full and bladder empty and create an ITV. The Radiation Oncology Cooperative Group (RTOGO) established dose constrains for using postoperative IMRT in endometrial cancer.[129] For bladder, <35% receives ≥45 Gy; rectum, <60% receives ≥45 Gy; small bowel, <30% receives ≥40 Gy; femoral heads, <15% receives ≥30 Gy; and any ≤1% or ≤1 mL receives >110% prescribed dose normal tissue.

Data on outcome with postoperative IMRT in endometrial cancer are encouraging. He et al. reported on 129 patients (77% stage I to II). With median follow-up of 57 months, the 5-year DFS in the subset of patients with stage I to II (n = 98) was 85.7% for those with low intermediate risk and 71.6 for high intermediate risk. The corresponding rates for overall survival were 91.7% and 76.2%, respectively.[130] Shih et al. reported on 46 patients with high-risk endometrial cancer patients treated with postoperative IMRT. With a median follow-up of

52 months, the 5-year disease-free and overall survival rate in stage III (n = 36) were 84% and 95%, respectively.[131]

COMPLICATIONS OF TREATMENT

Surgery

In PORTEC-1 trial,[88] the rate of complications in the surgery-alone arm was very low (6%). Surgical toxicity data are generally collected within 30 days of surgery, that is, before patients were enrolled in the trial. Therefore, it is important to assess surgical toxicity from trials addressing a surgical question. In the GOG LAP2 trial comparing laparotomy to laproscopy,[75] the rate of intraoperative complications was 8% versus 10%, respectively (P = .106). More importantly, the rate of postoperative (within 6 weeks of surgery) grade 2 or greater complications was 21% for laparotomy versus 14% for laparoscopy (P < .001). In the Italian randomized trial comparing hysterectomy to hysterectomy and lymphadenectomy, both early and late postoperative complications occurred significantly more frequently in the lymphadenectomy patients (81 of 264; 30.6%) than for hysterectomy alone (34 of 250, 13.6%; P = .001). Most of the difference in morbidity was due to lymphoceles and lymphedema, which occurred in 35 patients in the lymphadenectomy arm and 4 patients in the no-lymphadenectomy arm.[79]

Radiation

Intravaginal RT

The main advantage of intravaginal brachytherapy is its ability to deliver a relatively high dose of radiation to the vagina while limiting the dose to the surrounding normal structures, such as the bowels and bladder. In PORTEC-2 trial, the long-term health-related quality of life (HRQL) analysis showed at 7 years, clinically relevant fecal leakage was reported by 10.6% in the pelvic RT group versus 1.8% for IVRT (P = .03), diarrhea by 8.4% versus 0.9% (P = .04), limitations due to bowel symptoms by 10.5% versus 1.8% (P = .001), and bowel urgency by 23.3% versus 6.6% (P < .001). Urinary urgency was reported by 39.3% of pelvic RT patients, 25.5% for IVRT, P = .05. No difference in sexual activity was seen between treatment arms.[132] However, such a low rate of severe complications cannot be taken for granted because special attention needs to be paid to the depth of prescription, the dose per fraction, the length of vagina treated, and the diameter of the cylinder used. Sorbe and Smeds[133] reported a 15% late complication rate and a very high incidence of vaginal stenosis after postoperative high dose rate intravaginal irradiation. This was attributed to the high dose per fraction of 6 to 9 Gy; moreover, this dose was prescribed at a depth of 10 mm from the surface of the cylinder, resulting in very high vaginal mucosal, bladder, and rectal doses. Adherence to vaginal dilator use[134] after IVRT as well as routine use of vaginal lubricants and moisturizers may further reduce the rate of vaginal stenosis.

In a cohort of 104 patients with early-stage endometrial cancer treated with surgery and IVRT, Female Sexual Function Index (FSFI) questionnaires were used to quantify levels of sexual functioning.[107] Sexual dysfunction defined as an FSFI score of <26 was reported by 81% of respondents. Multivariate analysis isolated factors associated with lower FSFI scores, including having laparotomy as opposed to minimally invasive surgery (effect size, −7.1 points; P < .001), lack of vaginal lubricant use (effect size, −4.4 points; P = .040), and short time interval (<6 months) from hysterectomy to questionnaire completion (effect size, −4.6 points; P = .059).

In a subsequent report[135] from MSKCC, 205 early-stage endometrial cancer survivors (>1 year from surgery) completed questionnaires containing the EuroQol (EQ5D) and the FSFI. A total of 136 (66.3%) underwent surgery alone, and 69 (33.7%) received additional IVRT. A majority of patients (80%) met criteria for sexual dysfunction by FSFI <26.5. The two groups were well balanced with respect to demographics, comorbidities, and baseline

FIGURE 74.7. Pelvic intensity-modulated radiation therapy dose distribution. Outlined iliac vessels are shown in *pink* and nodal planning target volume in *yellow*.

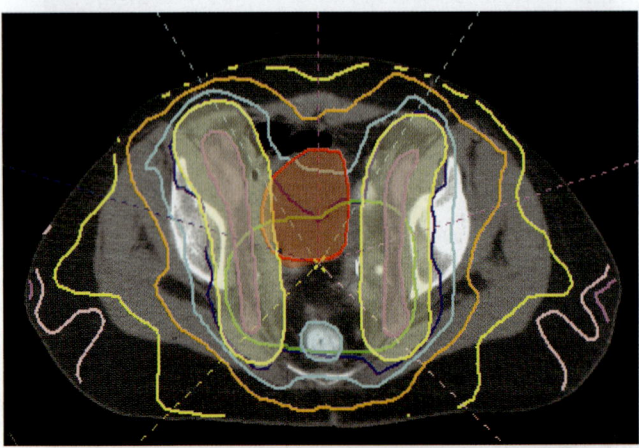

50.4 40.0 30.0 20.0 10.0 5.0 Gy

sexual activity. Controlling for age and surgery type (open vs. minimally invasive), IVRT was not associated with poorer health state or sexual function. Receipt of laparotomy was associated with both poorer health state and sexual function (P = .0156 and P = .0247, respectively). These studies highlight the fact endometrial cancer patients whether treated with surgery alone or with additional IVRT, when compared to the index population (healthy women ages 18 to 74), all scores were low.

Pelvic Radiation

In the PORTEC-1 randomized trial,[136] the overall (grades 1 to 4) rate of late complications was 26% in the RT group compared to 4% in the observation group (P < .0001). Most of the late complications in the RT group, however, were grades 1 and 2 (22%), and only 3% were grades 3 and 4. It is also important to note that many patients in this trial were treated with AP/PA fields, for which the overall rate of complications was 30%, compared to 21% for those treated with the four-field box (P = .06). In GOG 99 when lymphadenectomy was performed, chronic lymphedema was seen in 2.5% of the patients randomized to surgery alone compared to 5% with postoperative pelvic RT.[89] There is an increased awareness of sacral insufficiency fractures (SIFs) as a potential complication of pelvic RT in gynecologic cancers. In a report from MSKCC, 222 patients were treated with postoperative pelvic RT.[137] In the subset of endometrial cancer (n = 144), the 5-year rate of SIF was 5.7%. Risk of secondary malignancies is often cited as one of the main reasons to avoid pelvic RT in endometrial cancer patients; however, when PORTEC-1 and PORTEC-2 trials were combined, there was no clear evidence of increased risk.[138]

The use of IMRT seems to be associated with less risk of obstruction (BO). In a report from MSKCC on 224 patients (152 with endometrial cancer) treated with postoperative radiation,[139] the 5-year rate of BO in the IMRT group was 0.9% compared to 9.3% for 3-D RT (P = .006). Patients with BMI ≥30kg/m^2 were less likely to develop BO (2.6% vs. 8.3; P = .03). On multivariate analysis, only IMRT retained its significance as an independent predictor of less BO (P = .022).

In PORTEC-3 trial, the addition of chemotherapy to radiation showed increased physician and patient-reported toxicities. However, by 24 months, results equalized, with the exception of persistence of patient-reported sensory neurologic symptoms in 25% of patients in the chemoradiation arm.[140]

Definitive Radiation for Inoperable Disease

In medically inoperable patients with endometrial cancer, radiation is an effective alternative to surgery. These patients are usually treated in a fashion similar to those with cervical cancer by using intracavitary applicators with or without pelvic radiation. In a systematic review of twenty-five reports of patients treated with RT as single treatment, the 5-year DSS was 78.5%. External beam radiation therapy (EBRT) combined with brachytherapy (BT) was used in 1,278 patients (47.4%), BT alone in 1383 patients (51.3%), and EBRT alone in 33 patients (1.2%). The average rate of grade 3 or worse late toxicity was 3.7% for EBRT + BT, 2.8% for BT alone, and 1.2% for EBRT alone.[141] The American Brachytherapy Society established general guideline recommendations regarding HDR alone or in combination with external beam RT in terms of prescription point (2 cm from the central axis at the midpoint along the intrauterine sources), number of fractions, dose per fraction, combination with EBRT, and optimization. Patients with stage IIIB disease (vaginal involvement), an uncommon presentation, are usually not surgical candidates and are also treated with definitive radiation, including a combination of external beam and intracavitary/interstitial radiotherapy tailored to the extent of their disease.[142]

For patients with clinical stage I grade 1 or 2 and no evidence of myometrial invasion or lymph node metastasis on MRI, intracavitary brachytherapy alone is sufficient. Gephardt et al. reported on 45 patients with grade 1 to 2, clinical stage I endometrial adenocarcinoma, <50% myometrial invasion, and tumor ≤2 cm treated with 5 to 6 fractions HDR intracavitary brachytherapy to a median total dose of 37.5Gy. Median follow-up among living patients was 18.6 months. The 2-year local control, cancer-specific survival, and overall survival rates were 90%, 86%, and 97%, respectively. No grade 3+ acute or late toxicity was observed.[143] In another report, 43 consecutive patients with endometrial cancer FIGO stages I to III were treated definitively with HDR brachytherapy with or without EBRT.[144] Mean follow-up was 29.7 months. Median BMI was 50.2 kg/m^2. The 2-year overall survival was 65.2%. The 2-year cumulative incidence of pelvic and distant failures was 8.3% and 13.5%, respectively. Grade 3 disease was associated with a higher risk of all failures (hazard ratio [HR], 4.67; P = .044). The incidence of acute grade 3 GI/GU toxicities was 4.6%.

Radiation Therapy for Local Recurrence

Radiation therapy can be curative in a select group of patients with small vaginal recurrences who have not received prior radiation. Creutzberg et al. reported on survival after relapse based on the PORTEC-1 randomized trial.[91] In patients who were initially randomized to surgery alone (n = 46 of 360), the 5-year survival after vaginal relapse was 65%. However, before adopting salvage radiation as a treatment policy for all early-stage endometrial cancer, a few aspects of this trial need to be addressed. First, the 5-year survival rate from the PORTEC trial is much higher than what is reported in the literature.[145-148] Most likely, the vaginal recurrences in this trial were detected very early, unlike the situation for patients in the community. The extent and size of local recurrence in endometrial cancer are very significant predictors of outcome.[148] Second, this high rate of salvage pertains only to isolated vaginal recurrence. The rate of survival at 3 years for pelvic recurrence in the PORTEC-1 trial[91] was 0%. Third, although the trial does not mention any data on complications, it is not unrealistic to expect a higher complication rate than what is normally seen with adjuvant radiation. With salvage radiation, external beam RT and brachytherapy are often combined, and the doses of radiation required are much higher than those used with adjuvant radiation. The study from MD Anderson Cancer Center by Jhingran et al.[145] clearly highlights these issues. They reported on 91 patients who were treated with definitive radiation for isolated vaginal recurrence. The 5-year local control and overall survival rates were 75% and 43%, respectively. The median dose of radiation was 75 Gy, which often included external radiation and brachytherapy. The rate of grade 4 complications (requiring surgery) was 9%. Thus, when talking with a patient about adjuvant radiation versus radiation reserved for salvage, these issues need to be addressed and compared to the excellent local control and low morbidity obtained with adjuvant intravaginal brachytherapy. In a recent report from the University of Pittsburgh,[149] 41 patients were treated with HDR brachytherapy using image-based planning with contouring/optimization with each fraction to a median dose of 23.75 Gy in 5 fractions. Brachytherapy was combined with pelvic IMRT in 90% of patients to a dose of 45 Gy. At a median follow-up of 18 months, the 3-year local control, distant control, recurrence-free survival, and overall survival were 95%, 61%, 68%, and 67%. The 3-year rate of grade 3 or higher late toxicity was 8%. This indicates that even with more modern techniques, the morbidity of salvage RT cannot be ignored.

With the increased use of IMRT, salvage rate of nodal recurrence in endometrial cancer is better. In a report by Ho et al., 38 patients with endometrial cancer who had no prior external beam radiation were treated definitively using IMRT for regionally confined pelvic or para-aortic nodal recurrences. Chemotherapy was given to 33 out of 38. The total dose of IMRT was 64.7Gy (range 59 to 73 Gy). The 2-year survival was 71%. Three patients (8%) experienced grade 3 to 4 late GI toxicity.[150]

UTERINE CARCINOSARCOMA

Uterine carcinosarcoma (UCS) is no longer considered a uterine sarcoma. In GOG 210, UCS represented about 4.1 of endometrial cancinomas.[41] Molecular evaluation of UCS revealed that frequent mutations were found in TP53, PTEN, PIK3CA, PPP2R1A, FBXW7, and KRAS, similar to endometrioid and serous uterine carcinomas. The range of epithelial-to-mesenchymal transition EMT scores in UCS was the largest among all tumor types studied via TCGA. UCSs shared proteomic features with gynecologic carcinomas and sarcomas with intermediate EMT features.[151]

The etiology of UCS is not well established but seems to share some similarity with endometrial adenocarcinoma. History of prior pelvic radiation has been reported in some patients with carcinosarcoma.[152] These neoplasms are often bulky, necrotic, and deeply invasive. The epithelial component is generally serous carcinoma. Homologous tumors have stroma that contains cell types normally seen in the uterus, in contrast to heterologous tumors, which may contain striated muscle cells (rhabdomyosarcoma), cartilage (chondrosarcoma), and bone (osteogenic sarcoma) (Figure 74.3D).

The main treatment is surgery, and these patients should undergo comprehensive surgical staging similar to that with serous cancer. Pelvic nodal metastasis is seen in 21.1%, and in para-aortic node in 15.2% of patients.[41] For carcinosarcomas, the 2009 staging system for carcinomas of the endometrium is used, recognizing the similarity in patterns of spread.

With regard to the role of *adjuvant radiation*, the EORTC performed a prospective, randomized trial addressing the role of postoperative pelvic RT in stages I to II uterine sarcomas. There were a total of 224 patients in the trial who underwent TAH/BSO, and 166 who had peritoneal washings. Lymphadenectomy was optional. There were 91 carcinosarcomas included in that study; the rate of pelvic recurrence only was 4% in the pelvic RT arm compared to 24% for the surgery-alone arm. The corresponding rates for any local recurrence were 24% and 47%, respectively, for this subset of patients.[153]

Adjuvant chemotherapy has been evaluated mainly in carcinosarcoma. Sutton et al.[154] reported on 65 patients with completely resected stage I or II carcinosarcoma of the uterus treated with adjuvant ifosfamide and cisplatin. None of the patients received adjuvant RT. Overall 5-year survival was 62%. Initial site of relapse was vaginal apex in 6 of 65 and pelvis in 4 of 64, suggesting that a combined chemoradiation approach might be ideal. GOG-150 is a phase III randomized study of whole abdominal RT versus three cycles of cisplatin, ifosfamide, and mesna (CIM). Eligible patients ($n = 206$) included those with stages I to IV UCS, no >1-cm postsurgical residuum, and/or no extra-abdominal spread. Stage distribution was as follows: I, 64 (31%); II, 26 (13%); III, 92 (45%); and IV, 24 (12%). The estimated crude probability of recurring within 5 years was 58% for chemotherapy and 52% for RT. Adjusting for stage and age, the recurrence rate was 21% lower for chemotherapy patients than for RT patients (RH, 0.789; 95% CI = 0.530 to 1.176; $P = .245$, two-tailed test). The estimated death rate was 29% lower in the chemotherapy group (RH, 0.712; 95% CI = 0.484 to 1.048; $P = .085$, two-tailed test). The conclusion was that there was not a statistically significant advantage in recurrence rate or survival for adjuvant chemotherapy over RT in patients with UCS. However, the observed differences favor the use of combination chemotherapy in future trials. The rate of vaginal recurrence was 4 of 105 (3.8%) in the WAI compared to 10 of 101 (9.9%). The corresponding abdominal relapse rates were 27.6% (29 of 105) and 18.8% (19 of 101). There was no difference in pelvic recurrence between the two arms. The rates of lung metastasis (14 of 105 vs. 14 of 101, respectively) or other distant sites (13 of 101 vs. 10 of 101, respectively) were similar. Analysis of the patterns of relapse from this trial also indicates the need for chemoradiation in patients with stage I to III carcinosarcoma.[155]

The use of intravaginal RT and chemotherapy is appealing in stage I to II carcinosarcoma. Desai et al. reported on 60 patients with stage I to II UCS and compared them to 112 stage I to II serous endometrial cancers.[156] Adjuvant therapy was to 90% of patients. With a median follow-up of 48 months, outcomes were better for serous versus UCS: 5-year actuarial rates of recurrence (17% vs. 45%; $P < .001$), disease-specific mortality (11% vs. 30%; $P = .016$), and all-cause mortality (12% vs. 34%; $P = .007$). However, in a subgroup analysis of 111 patients (77 serous, 34 UCS) who receive IVRT and chemotherapy, UCS no longer was associated significantly with increased recurrence (29% vs. 15%, $P = .18$), disease-specific mortality (22% vs. 10%, $P = .39$), or all-cause mortality (22% vs. 10%, $P = .45$). This indicates that when early-stage UCS were treated aggressively, their outcome were not significantly different than serous endometrial cancer.

At MSKCC, patients with surgical stage I or II carcinosarcoma are treated with intravaginal RT and chemotherapy. Most stage III patients are treated in a similar fashion with few exceptions when extrauterine disease is limited to nodal disease. Then, consideration is given to concurrent pelvic RT/cisplatin followed by carboplatin/paclitaxel.

UTERINE SARCOMA

Uterine sarcomas are uncommon, representing about 3% to 7% of all uterine cancers.[157] The most common histology is leiomyosarcoma, followed by endometrial stromal sarcoma (resemble proliferative-phase endometrial stroma), undifferentiated uterine sarcoma, and adenosarcoma (benign epithelial component and low-grade sarcoma). Age-related incidences vary among the histologic types. The mean age at diagnosis for endometrial stromal sarcoma is 41 years, for leiomyosarcoma 53.5 years, and for adenosarcoma 57.4 years. Little is known about the risk factors for uterine sarcomas. Most uterine sarcomas present with vaginal bleeding, but leiomyosarcomas are more commonly discovered incidentally after simple hysterectomy for presumed uterine leiomyomata.

Pathology and Staging

Endometrial stromal sarcomas are generally divided into endometrial stromal sarcomas, which are low grade by definition, and undifferentiated endometrial sarcoma, which are high grade. Tumor cells in endometrial stromal sarcoma resemble those found in the stroma of proliferative endometrial lining. In contrast, tumor cells in undifferentiated endometrial stromal sarcoma do not resemble endometrial stroma. *Leiomyosarcomas* of the uterus have a fleshy appearance, often with areas of necrosis. They display nuclear atypia, high mitotic rates, and areas of coagulative tumor necrosis. *Adenosarcomas* have two components—a benign epithelial tumor and a malignant mesenchymal component (generally low-grade sarcoma that resembles endometrial stroma). Sarcomatous overgrowth, defined as the presence of pure sarcoma, usually of high grade and without a glandular component, occupying at least 25% of the tumor, has been reported in 33% of uterine adenosarcomas.[157] The 2009 FIGO staging recognizes the uniqueness of each uterine sarcoma. For leiomyosarcomas and endometrial stromal sarcomas, the staging system recognizes the importance of tumor size on outcome. For adenosarcomas, the new staging system recognizes the importance of depth of myometrial invasion.

Management

The main treatment for uterine sarcoma is *surgery* in a similar fashion to endometrial adenocarcinoma. The extent of surgical staging varies, depending on the risk of lymph node involvement. Nodal metastases are seen in <5% of leiomyosarcoma unless there is obvious extrauterine disease.[158] For stromal sarcomas, dos Santos et al.[159] reported a 19% (7 of 36) rate of nodal metastasis. The rate of occult metastasis was only 10%. The corresponding rates from the literature review were 10.1% and 8.1%, respectively. Thus, patients with endometrial stromal sarcomas and adenosarcomas might benefit from lymph node sampling. On the other hand, for patients with leiomyosarcomas, the rate of nodal involvement is too low to justify routine lymphadenectomy.

With regard to the role of *adjuvant radiation*, the EORTC performed a prospective, randomized trial addressing the role of postoperative pelvic RT in stage I to II uterine sarcomas.[153] There were a total of 224 patients in the trial who underwent TAH/BSO, and 166 who had peritoneal washings. Lymphadenectomy was optional. There were 103 leiomyosarcomas (LMSs) and 28 endometrial stromal sarcomas. The 5-year cumulative incidence of locoregional recurrence was 18.8% in the pelvic RT arm compared to 35.9% in the surgery-alone arm. That difference was statistically significant ($P = .0013$). The 5-year cumulative incidence of distant relapse was 45.3% for the pelvic RT and 33.6% for surgery alone, but the difference was not statistically significant ($P = .2569$). There was no significant difference in progression-free ($P = .3254$) or overall survival ($P = .923$) between the two arms. For LMS patients, the rate of pelvic recurrence only was 2% in the pelvic RT compared to 14% in patients treated with surgery alone, and for any local recurrence, it was 20% versus 24%. It is important to note that the primary endpoint of this trial was pelvic control, which it met ($P = .0013$). The study was not powered to detect a significant difference in PFS or OS. Sampath et al.[160] performed a retrospective review of uterine sarcoma patients using the National Oncology Database. The impact of adjuvant radiation was assessed in patients who presented with nonmetastatic disease and underwent definitive surgery ($n = 2,206$). For endometrial stromal sarcoma, the rate was 97% with RT (109) versus 93% for surgery alone ($n = 252$; $P < .05$). For LMS, it was 98% for RT ($n = 131$) compared to 84% with surgery alone ($n = 398$; $P < .01$).

For patients with leiomyosarcomas, the main treatment is surgery, and the role of adjuvant treatment, whether RT or chemotherapy, is not well defined. The high rate of distant relapse in these patients overshadows any local control benefit attained with adjuvant RT. These patients should be encouraged to participate in trials assessing the role of chemotherapy and/or targeted therapy. For patients with low-grade endometrial stromal sarcomas, observation is feasible, because most are hormonally sensitive and generally behave in an indolent manner, with long disease-free intervals. For those with undifferentiated endometrial sarcomas, adjuvant pelvic RT is reasonable. For patients with adenosarcomas, especially with sarcomatous overgrowth, adjuvant pelvic RT is also reasonable.

REFERENCES

1. Siegel RL, Miller KD, Jemal A. Cancer statistics, 2018. *CA Cancer J Clin* 2018;68(1):7–30.
2. Morice P, Leary A, Creutzberg C, et al. Endometrial cancer. *Lancet* 2016;387(10023):1094–1108.
3. Amant F, Mirza MR, Koskas M, et al. Cancer of the corpus uteri. *Int J Gynaecol Obstet* 2015;131(Suppl 2):S96–S104.
4. Allen NE, Key TJ, Dossus L, et al. Endogenous sex hormones and endometrial cancer risk in women in the European Prospective Investigation into Cancer and Nutrition (EPIC). *Endocr Relat Cancer* 2008;15(2):485–497.
5. Brinton LA, Trabert B, Anderson GL, et al. Serum estrogens and estrogen metabolites and endometrial cancer risk among postmenopausal women. *Cancer Epidemiol Biomarkers Prev* 2016;25(7):1081–1089.
6. Zucchetto A, Serraino D, Polesel J, et al. Hormone-related factors and gynecological conditions in relation to endometrial cancer risk. *Eur J Cancer Prev* 2009;18(4):316–321.
7. Pearson-Stuttard J, Zhou B, Kontis V, et al. Worldwide burden of cancer attributable to diabetes and high body-mass index: a comparative risk assessment. *Lancet Diabetes Endocrinol* 2018;6:95–104. pii: S2213-8587(17)30366-2.
8. Dossus L, Allen N, Kaaks R, et al. Reproductive risk factors and endometrial cancer: the European Prospective Investigation into Cancer and Nutrition. *Int J Cancer* 2010;127:442–451.
9. Esposito K, Chiodini P, Capuano A, et al. Metabolic syndrome and endometrial cancer: a meta-analysis. *Endocrine* 2014;45(1):28–36.
10. Sjögren LL, Mørch LS, Løkkegaard E. Hormone replacement therapy and the risk of endometrial cancer: a systematic review. *Maturitas* 2016;91:25–35.
11. Simin J, Tamimi R, Lagergren J, et al. Menopausal hormone therapy and cancer risk: an overestimated risk? *Eur J Cancer* 2017;84:60–68.
12. Davies C, Godwin J, Gray R, et al; Early Breast Cancer Trialists' Collaborative Group (EBCTCG). Relevance of breast cancer hormone receptors and other factors to the efficacy of adjuvant tamoxifen: patient-level meta-analysis of randomised trials. *Lancet* 2011;378(9793):771–784.
13. Davies C, Pan H, Godwin J, et al. Long-term effects of continuing adjuvant tamoxifen to 10 years versus stopping at 5 years after diagnosis of oestrogen receptor-positive breast cancer: ATLAS, a randomised trial. Adjuvant Tamoxifen: Longer Against Shorter (ATLAS) Collaborative Group [published erratum appears in Lancet 2013;381:804]. *Lancet* 2013;381:805–816.
14. Fisher B, Costantino J, Wickerham DL, et al. Tamoxifen for the prevention of breast cancer: current status of the National Surgical Adjuvant Breast and Bowel Project P-1 study. *J Natl Cancer Inst* 2005;97:1652–1662.
15. Bland AE, Calingaert B, Secord AA, et al. Relationship between tamoxifen use and high risk endometrial cancer histologic types. *Gynecol Oncol* 2009;112(1):150–154.
16. Meyer LA, Broaddus RR, Lu KH. Endometrial cancer and Lynch syndrome: clinical and pathologic considerations. *Cancer Control* 2009;16(1):14–22.
17. Westin SN, Lacour RA, Urbauer DL, et al. Carcinoma of the lower uterine segment: a newly described association with Lynch syndrome. *J Clin Oncol* 2008;26(36):5965–5971.
18. Burbos N, Musonda P, Duncan TJ, et al. Estimating the risk of endometrial cancer in symptomatic postmenopausal women: a novel clinical prediction model based on patients' characteristics. *Int J Gynecol Cancer* 2011;21(3):500–506.
19. Creasman WT, Odicino F, Maisonneuve P, et al. Carcinoma of the corpus uteri. FIGO 26th Annual Report on the Results of Treatment in Gynecological Cancer. *Int J Gynaecol Obstet* 2006;95(Suppl 1):S105–S143.
20. Smith RA, Andrews KS, Brooks D, et al. Cancer screening in the United States, 2017: a review of current American Cancer Society guidelines and current issues in cancer screening. *CA Cancer J Clin* 2017;67(2):100–121.
21. Schmeler KM, Lynch HT, Chen L, et al. Prophylactic surgery to reduce the risk of gynecologic cancers in the Lynch syndrome. *N Engl J Med* 2006;354:261.
22. Dijkhuizen FP, Mol BW, Brolmann HA, et al. The accuracy of endometrial sampling in the diagnosis of patients with endometrial carcinoma and hyperplasia: a meta-analysis. *Cancer* 2000;89:1765–1772.
23. Leitao MM Jr, Kehoe S, Barakat RR, et al. Comparison of D&C and office endometrial biopsy accuracy in patients with FIGO grade 1 endometrial adenocarcinoma. *Gynecol Oncol* 2009;113:105.
24. Bell DJ, Pannu HK. Radiological assessment of gynecologic malignancies. *Obstet Gynecol Clin North Am* 2011;38(1):45–68.
25. Goldstein RB, Bree RL, Benson CB, et al. Evaluation of the women with postmenopausal bleeding: society of radiologists in ultrasound-sponsored consensus conference statement. *J Ultrasound Med* 2001;20:1025–1036.
26. de Kroon CD, Jansen FW. Saline infusion sonography in women with abnormal uterine bleeding: an update of recent findings. *Curr Opin Obstet Gynecol* 2006;18(6):653–657.
27. Visser NCM, Reijnen C, Massuger LFAG, et al. Accuracy of endometrial sampling in endometrial carcinoma: a systematic review and meta-analysis. *Obstet Gynecol* 2017;130(4):803–813.
28. Bradley WH, Boente MP, Brooker D, et al. Hysteroscopy and cytology in endometrial cancer. *Obstet Gynecol* 2004;104:1030–1033.
29. Haldorsen IS, Salvesen HB. What is the best preoperative imaging for endometrial cancer? *Curr Oncol Rep* 2016;18(4):25.
30. Wu LM, Xu JR, Gu HY, et al. Predictive value of T2-weighted imaging and contrast-enhanced MR imaging in assessing myometrial invasion in endometrial cancer: a pooled analysis of prospective studies. *Eur Radiol* 2013;23(2):435–449.
31. Luomaranta A, Leminen A, Loukovaara M. Magnetic resonance imaging in the assessment of high-risk features of endometrial carcinoma: a meta-analysis. *Int J Gynecol Cancer* 2015;25(5):837–842.
32. Andreano A, Rechichi G, Rebora P, et al. MR diffusion imaging for preoperative staging of myometrial invasion in patients with endometrial cancer: a systematic review and meta-analysis. *Eur Radiol* 2014;24(6):1327–1338.
33. Gee MS, Atri M, Bandos AI, et al. Identification of distant metastatic disease in uterine cervical and endometrial cancers with FDG PET/CT: analysis from the ACRIN 6671/GOG 0233 multicenter trial. *Radiology* 2018;287:176–187.
34. Bollineni VR, Ytre-Hauge S, Bollineni-Balabay O, et al. High diagnostic value of 18F-FDG PET/CT in endometrial cancer: systematic review and meta-analysis of the literature. *J Nucl Med* 2016;57(6):879–885.
35. Kim HS, Park CY, Lee JM, et al. Evaluation of serum CA-125 levels for preoperative counselling in endometrioid endometrial cancer: a multi-centre study. *Gynecol Oncol* 2010;118:283–288.
36. Hsieh CH, ChangChien CC, Lin H, et al. Can a preoperative CA 125 level be a criterion for full pelvic lymphadenectomy in surgical staging of endometrial cancer? *Gynecol Oncol* 2002;86:28–33.
37. Kurman RJ, Kaminski PF, Norris HJ. The behavior of endometrial hyperplasia. A long-term study of "untreated" hyperplasia in 170 patients. *Cancer* 1985;56:403.
38. Trimble CL, Kauderer J, Zaino R, et al. Concurrent endometrial carcinoma in women with a biopsy diagnosis of atypical endometrial hyperplasia: a Gynecologic Oncology Group Study. *Cancer* 2006;106:812.
39. Leitao MM Jr, Chi DS. Fertility-sparing options for patients with gynecologic malignancies. *Oncologist* 2005;10:613.
40. Silverberg SG, Kurman RJ, Nogales F, et al. Epithelial tumors and related lesions. In: Tavassoli FA, Devilee P, eds. *Tumors of the breast and female genital organs: World Health organization classification of tumours*. Lyon, France: IARC Press, 2003:227.
41. Creasman WT, Ali S, Mutch DG, et al. Surgical-pathological findings in type 1 and 2 endometrial cancer: an NRG Oncology/Gynecologic Oncology Group study on GOG-210 protocol. *Gynecol Oncol* 2017;145(3):519–525.
42. Fader AN, Java J, Tenney M, et al. Impact of histology and surgical approach on survival among women with early-stage, high-grade uterine cancer: an NRG Oncology/Gynecologic Oncology Group ancillary analysis. *Gynecol Oncol* 2016;143(3):460–465.

43. Kurman RJ, Carcangiu ML, Herrington CS, et al. *WHO classification of tumours of female reproductive organs.* Lyon, France: IARC, 2014.

44. Tafe LJ, Garg K, Chew I, et al. Endometrial and ovarian carcinomas with undifferentiated components: clinically aggressive and frequently underrecognized neoplasms. *Mod Pathol* 2010;23(6):781–789.

45. Williams MG, Bandera EV, Demissie K, et al. Synchronous primary ovarian and endometrial cancers: a population-based assessment of survival. *Obstet Gynecol* 2009;113(4):783–789.

46. Schultheis AM, Ng CK, De Filippo MR, et al. Massively parallel sequencing-based clonality analysis of synchronous endometrioid endometrial and ovarian carcinomas. *J Natl Cancer Inst* 2016;108(6):djv427.

47. Bokhman JV. Two pathogenetic types of endometrial carcinoma. *Gynecol Oncol* 1983;15:10.

48. Deligdisch L, Holinka CF. Endometrial carcinoma: two diseases? *Cancer Detect Prev* 1987;10:237.

49. Dedes KJ, Wetterskog D, Ashworth A, et al. Emerging therapeutic targets in endometrial cancer. *Nat Rev Clin Oncol* 2011;8(5):261–271.

50. Cancer Genome Atlas Research Network, Kandoth C, Schultz N, Cherniack AD, et al. Integrated genomic characterization of endometrial carcinoma. *Nature* 2013;497(7447):67–73.

51. DeLair DF, Burke KA, Selenica P, et al. The genetic landscape of endometrial clear cell carcinomas. *J Pathol* 2017;243(2):230–241.

52. International Federation of Gynecology and Obstetrics. Revised FIGO staging for carcinoma of the vulva, cervix, and endometrium. *Int J Gynecol Obstet* 2009;105:103.

53. Page BR, Pappas L, Cooke EW, et al. Does the FIGO 2009 endometrial cancer staging system more accurately correlate with clinical outcome in different histologies? Revised staging, endometrial cancer, histology. *Int J Gynecol Cancer* 2012;22(4):593–598.

54. Abu-Rustum NR, Zhou Q, Iasonos A, et al. The revised 2009 FIGO staging system for endometrial cancer: should the 1988 FIGO stages IA and IB be altered? *Int J Gynecol Cancer* 2011;21(3):511–516.

55. Abu-Rustum NR, Zhou Q, Gomez JD, et al. A nomogram for predicting overall survival of women with endometrial cancer following primary therapy: toward improving individualized cancer care. *Gynecol Oncol* 2010;116(3):399–403.

56. Creutzberg CL, van Stiphout RG, Nout RA, et al. Nomograms for prediction of outcome with or without adjuvant radiation therapy for patients with endometrial cancer: a pooled analysis of PORTEC-1 and PORTEC-2 trials. *Int J Radiat Oncol Biol Phys* 2015;91(3):530–539.

57. Alektiar KM, Venkatraman E, Abu-Rustum N, et al. Is endometrial carcinoma intrinsically more aggressive in elderly patients? *Cancer* 2003;98(11):2368–2377.

58. Bishop EA, Java JJ, Moore KN, et al. Pathologic and treatment outcomes among a geriatric population of endometrial cancer patients: an NRG Oncology/Gynecologic Oncology Group Ancillary Data Analysis of LAP2. *Int J Gynecol Cancer* 2017;27(4):730–737.

59. Felix AS, Brasky TM, Cohn DE, et al. Endometrial carcinoma recurrence according to race and ethnicity: an NRG Oncology/Gynecologic Oncology Group 210 Study. *Int J Cancer* 2018;142(6):1102–1115.

60. Alektiar KM, McKee A, Lin O, et al. The significance of the amount of myometrial invasion in patients with stage IB endometrial carcinoma. *Cancer* 2002;95:316–321.

61. Mariani A, Dowdy SC, Keeney GL, et al. Predictors of vaginal relapse in stage I endometrial cancer. *Gynecol Oncol* 2005;97:820–827.

62. Bosse T, Peters EE, Creutzberg CL, et al. Substantial lymph-vascular space invasion (LVSI) is a significant risk factor for recurrence in endometrial cancer--A pooled analysis of PORTEC 1 and 2 trials. *Eur J Cancer* 2015;51(13):1742–1750.

63. Croog VJ, Abu-Rustum NR, Barakat RR, et al. Adjuvant radiation for early stage endometrial cancer with lymphovascular invasion. *Gynecol Oncol* 2008;111(1):49–54.

64. Kizer NT, Gao F, Guntupalli S, et al. Lower uterine segment involvement is associated with poor outcomes in early-stage endometrioid endometrial carcinoma. *Ann Surg Oncol* 2011;18(5):1419–1424.

65. Rossi L, Le Frere-Belda MA, Laurent-Puig P, et al. Clinicopathologic characteristics of endometrial cancer in Lynch syndrome: a French Multicenter Study. *Int J Gynecol Cancer* 2017;27(5):953–960.

66. Lee M, Kim YT, Kim SW, et al. Effects of uterine manipulation on surgical outcomes in laparoscopic management of endometrial cancer: a prospective randomized clinical trial. *Int J Gynecol Cancer* 2013;23(2):372–379.

67. Scott SA, van der Zanden C, Cai E, et al. Prognostic significance of peritoneal cytology in low-intermediate risk endometrial cancer. *Gynecol Oncol* 2017;145(2):262–268.

68. Milgrom SA, Kollmeier MA, Abu-Rustum NR, et al. Positive peritoneal cytology is highly predictive of prognosis and relapse patterns in stage III (FIGO 2009) endometrial cancer. *Gynecol Oncol* 2013;130(1):49–53.

69. Jobsen JJ, Naudin Ten Cate L, Lybeert ML, et al. Outcome of endometrial cancer stage IIIA with adnexa or serosal involvement only. *Obstet Gynecol Int* 2011;2011:962518.

70. Morrow CP, Bundy BN, Kurman RJ, et al. Relationship between surgical-pathological risk factors and outcome in clinical stage I and II carcinoma of the endometrium: a Gynecologic Oncology Group study. *Gynecol Oncol* 1991;40:55–65.

71. Stelloo E, Nout RA, Osse EM, et al. Improved risk assessment by integrating molecular and clinicopathological factors in early-stage endometrial cancer-combined analysis of the PORTEC cohorts. *Clin Cancer Res* 2016;22(16):4215–4224.

72. Cosgrove CM, Tritchler DL, Cohn DE, et al. An NRG Oncology/GOG study of molecular classification for risk prediction in endometrioid endometrial cancer. *Gynecol Oncol* 2018;148(1):174–180.

73. Kurnit KC, Kim GN, Fellman BM, et al. CTNNB1 (beta-catenin) mutation identifies low grade, early stage endometrial cancer patients at increased risk of recurrence. *Mod Pathol* 2017;30(7):1032–1041.

74. McMeekin DS, Tritchler DL, Cohn DE, et al. Clinicopathologic significance of mismatch repair defects in endometrial cancer: an NRG Oncology/Gynecologic Oncology Group Study. *J Clin Oncol* 2016;34(25):3062–3068.

75. Walker JL, Piedmonte MR, Spirtos NM, et al. Laparoscopy compared with laparotomy for comprehensive surgical staging of uterine cancer: gynecologic Oncology Group Study LAP2. *J Clin Oncol* 2009;27(32):5331–5336.

76. Walker JL, Piedmonte MR, Spirtos NM, et al. Recurrence and survival after random assignment to laparoscopy versus laparotomy for comprehensive surgical staging uterine cancer: gynecology Oncology Group LAP2 study. *J Clin Oncol* 2012;30(7):695–700.

77. Wright JD, Burke WM, Wilde ET, et al. Comparative effectiveness of robotic versus laparoscopic hysterectomy for endometrial cancer. *J Clin Oncol* 2012;30(8):783–791.

78. Mariani A, Webb MJ, Keeney GL, et al. Role of wide/radical hysterectomy and pelvic lymph node dissection in endometrial cancer with cervical involvement. *Gynecol Oncol* 2001;83:72.

79. Arango HA, Hoffman MS, Roberts WS, et al. Accuracy of lymph node palpation to determine need for lymphadenectomy in gynecologic malignancies. *Obstet Gynecol* 2000;95(4):553–556.

80. Benedetti Panici P, Basile S, Maneschi F, et al. Systematic pelvic lymphadenectomy versus no lymphadenectomy in early-stage endometrial carcinoma: randomized clinical trial. *J Natl Cancer Inst* 2008;100(23):1707–1716.

81. ASTEC Study Group. Efficacy of systematic pelvic lymphadenectomy in endometrial cancer (MRC ASTEC trial): a randomised study. *Lancet* 2009;373(9658):125–136.

82. Case AS, Rocconi RP, Straughn JM Jr, et al. A prospective blinded evaluation of the accuracy of frozen section for the surgical management of endometrial cancer. *Obstet Gynecol* 2006;108(6):1375–1379.

83. Khoury-Collado F, Murray MP, Hensley ML, et al. Sentinel lymph node mapping for endometrial cancer improves the detection of metastatic disease to regional lymph nodes. *Gynecol Oncol* 2011;122(2):251–254.

84. Rossi EC, Kowalski LD, Scalici J, et al. A comparison of sentinel lymph node biopsy to lymphadenectomy for endometrial cancer staging (FIRES trial): a multicentre, prospective, cohort study. *Lancet Oncol* 2017;18(3):384–392.

85. Ballester M, Dubernard G, Lécuru F, et al. Detection rate and diagnostic accuracy of sentinel-node biopsy in early stage endometrial cancer: a prospective multicentre study (SENTI-ENDO). *Lancet Oncol* 2011;12(5):469–476.

86. Holloway RW, Abu-Rustum NR, Backes FJ, et al. Sentinel lymph node mapping and staging in endometrial cancer: a Society of Gynecologic Oncology literature review with consensus recommendations. *Gynecol Oncol* 2017;146(2):405–415.

87. Soliman PT, Westin SN, Dioun S, et al. A prospective validation study of sentinel lymph node mapping for high-risk endometrial cancer. *Gynecol Oncol* 2017;146(2):234–239.

88. Creutzberg CL, van Putten WL, Koper PC, et al. Surgery and postoperative radiotherapy versus surgery alone for patients with stage-1 endometrial carcinoma: multicentre randomised trial. PORTEC Study Group. Post Operative Radiation Therapy in Endometrial Carcinoma. *Lancet* 2000;355:1404–1411.

89. Keys HM, Roberts JA, Brunetto VL, et al. A phase III trial of surgery with or without adjunctive external pelvic radiation therapy in intermediate risk endometrial adenocarcinoma: a Gynecologic Oncology Group study. *Gynecol Oncol* 2004;92(3):744–751.

90. Blake P, Swart AM, Otron J, et al. Adjuvant external beam radiotherapy in the treatment of endometrial cancer (MRC ASTEC and NCIC CTG EN.5 randomised trials): pooled trial results, systematic review, and meta-analysis. *Lancet* 2009;373(9658):137–146.

91. Creutzberg CL, van Putten WL, Koper PC, et al. Survival after relapse in patients with endometrial cancer: results from a randomized trial. *Gynecol Oncol* 2003;89:201–209.

92. Sorbe B, Nordström B, Mäenpää J, et al. Intravaginal brachytherapy in FIGO stage I low-risk endometrial cancer: a controlled randomized study. *Int J Gynecol Cancer* 2009;19(5):873–878.

93. Nout RA, Smit VT, Putter H, et al; PORTEC Study Group. Vaginal brachytherapy versus pelvic external beam radiotherapy for patients with endometrial cancer of high-intermediate risk (PORTEC-2): an open-label, non-inferiority, randomised trial. *Lancet* 2010;375(9717):816–823.

94. Sorbe B, Horvath G, Andersson H, et al. External pelvic and vaginal irradiation versus vaginal irradiation alone as postoperative therapy in medium-risk endometrial carcinoma—a prospective randomized study. *Int J Radiat Oncol Biol Phys* 2012;82(3):1249–1255.

95. Cohn DE, Horowitz NS, Mutch DG, et al. Should the presence of lymphovascular space involvement be used to assign patients to adjuvant therapy following hysterectomy for unstaged endometrial cancer? *Gynecol Oncol* 2002;87:243–246.

96. Straughn JM Jr, Huh WK, Kelly FJ, et al. Conservative management of stage I endometrial carcinoma after surgical staging. *Gynecol Oncol* 2002;84(2):194–200.

97. Alektiar KM, McKee A, Venkatraman E, et al. Intravaginal high-dose-rate brachytherapy for Stage IB (FIGO Grade 1, 2) endometrial cancer. *Int J Radiat Oncol Biol Phys* 2002;53(3):707–713.

98. Desai NB, Kiess AP, Kollmeier MA, et al. Patterns of relapse in stage I-II uterine papillary serous carcinoma treated with adjuvant intravaginal radiation (IVRT) with or without chemotherapy. *Gynecol Oncol* 2013;131(3):604–608.

99. Sorbe B, Straumits A, Karlsson L. Intravaginal high-dose-rate brachytherapy for stage I endometrial cancer: a randomized study of two dose-per-fraction levels. *Int J Radiat Oncol Biol Phys* 2005;62(5):1385–1389.

100. Horowitz NS, Peters WA III, Smith MR, et al. Adjuvant high dose rate vaginal brachytherapy as treatment of stage I and II endometrial carcinoma. *Obstet Gynecol* 2002;99:235–240.

101. Creutzberg CL, van Putten WL, Warlam-Rodenhuis CC, et al. Outcome of high-risk stage IC, grade 3, compared with stage I endometrial carcinoma patients: the Postoperative Radiation Therapy in Endometrial Carcinoma Trial. *J Clin Oncol* 2004;22:1234–1241.

102. Elshaikh MA, Al-Wahab Z, Mahdi H, et al. Recurrence patterns and survival endpoints in women with stage II uterine endometrioid carcinoma: a multi-institution study. *Gynecol Oncol* 2015;136(2):235–239.

103. Thigpen JT, Brady MF, Alvarez RD, et al. Oral medroxyprogesterone acetate in the treatment of advanced or recurrent endometrial carcinoma: a dose–response study by the Gynecologic Oncology Group. *J Clin Oncol* 1999;17:1736–1744.
104. Thigpen T, Brady MF, Homesley HD, et al. Tamoxifen in the treatment of advanced or recurrent endometrial carcinoma: a Gynecologic Oncology Group study. *J Clin Oncol* 2001;19:364–367.
105. Whitney CW, Brunetto VL, Zaino RJ, et al. Phase II study of medroxyprogesterone acetate plus tamoxifen in advanced endometrial carcinoma: a Gynecologic Oncology Group study. *Gynecol Oncol* 2004;92:4–9.
106. Thigpen JT, Brady MF, Homesley HD, et al. Phase III trial of doxorubicin with or without cisplatin in advanced endometrial carcinoma: a gynecologic oncology group study. *J Clin Oncol* 2004;22:3902–3908.
107. Damast S, Alektiar KM, Goldfarb S, et al. Sexual functioning among endometrial cancer patients treated with adjuvant high-dose-rate intra-vaginal radiation therapy. *Int J Radiat Oncol Biol Phys* 2012;84(2):e187–e193.
108. Fleming GF, Brunetto VL, Cella D, et al. Phase III trial of doxorubicin plus cisplatin with or without paclitaxel plus filgrastim in advanced endometrial carcinoma: a Gynecologic Oncology Group Study. *J Clin Oncol* 2004;22:2159–2166.
109. Susumu N, Sagae S, Udagawa Y, et al. Randomized phase III trial of pelvic radiotherapy versus cisplatin-based combined chemotherapy in patients with intermediate- and high-risk endometrial cancer: a Japanese Gynecologic Oncology Group study. *Gynecol Oncol* 2008;108(1):226–233.
110. Maggi R, Lissoni A, Spina F, et al. Adjuvant chemotherapy vs radiotherapy in high-risk endometrial carcinoma: results of a randomised trial. *Br J Cancer* 2006;95(3):266–271.
111. Randall ME, Filiaci VL, Muss H, et al. Randomized phase III trial of whole-abdominal irradiation versus doxorubicin and cisplatin chemotherapy in advanced endometrial carcinoma: a Gynecologic Oncology Group Study. *J Clin Oncol* 2006;24(1):36–44.
112. Kuoppala T, Mäenpää J, Tomas E, et al. Surgically staged high-risk endometrial cancer: randomized study of adjuvant radiotherapy alone versus sequential chemo-radiotherapy. *Gynecol Oncol* 2008;110(2):190–195.
113. Hogberg T, Signorelli M, de Oliveira CF, et al. Sequential adjuvant chemotherapy and radiotherapy in endometrial cancer—results from two randomised studies. *Eur J Cancer* 2010;46(13):2422–2431.
114. Randall M, Filiaci V, McMeekin D, et al. A Phase 3 Trial of Pelvic Radiation Therapy Versus Vaginal Cuff Brachytherapy Followed by Paclitaxel/Carboplatin Chemotherapy in Patients with High-Risk, Early-Stage Endometrial Cancer: A Gynecology Oncology Group Study. *Int J Radiat Oncol Biol Phys* 2017;99:1313.
115. de Boer SM, Powell ME, Mileshkin L, et al: Adjuvant chemoradiotherapy versus radiotherapy alone for women with high-risk endometrial cancer (PORTEC-3): final results of an international, open-label, multicentre, randomised, phase 3 trial. *Lancet Oncol* 2018;19:295–309.
116. Matei D, Filiaci VL, Randall M, et al. A randomized phase III trial of cisplatin and tumor volume directed irradiation followed by carboplatin and paclitaxel vs. carboplatin and paclitaxel for optimally debulked, advanced endometrial carcinoma. *J Clin Oncol* 2017;35:5505–5505.
117. Alektiar KM, Makker V, Abu-Rustum NR, et al. Concurrent carboplatin/paclitaxel and intravaginal radiation in surgical stage I-II serous endometrial cancer. *Gynecol Oncol* 2009;112(1):142–145.
118. Kiess AP, Damast S, Makker V, et al. Five-year outcomes of adjuvant carboplatin/paclitaxel chemotherapy and intravaginal radiation for stage I-II papillary serous endometrial cancer. *Gynecol Oncol* 2012;127(2):321–325.
119. Yang J. Abstract. ASTRO 2015.
120. Jobsen JJ, ten Cate LN, Lybeert ML, et al. The number of metastatic sites for stage IIIA endometrial carcinoma, endometrioid cell type, is a strong negative prognostic factor. *Gynecol Oncol* 2010;117(1):32–36.
121. Milgrom SA, Kollmeier MA, Abu-Rustum NR, et al. Quantifying the risk of recurrence and death in stage III (FIGO 2009) endometrial cancer. *Gynecol Oncol* 2014;134(2):297–301.
122. Milgrom SA, Kollmeier MA, Abu-Rustum NR, et al. Postoperative external beam radiation therapy and concurrent cisplatin followed by carboplatin/paclitaxel for stage III (FIGO 2009) endometrial cancer. *Gynecol Oncol* 2013;130(3):436–440.
123. Mariani A, Webb MJ, Keeney GL, et al. Stage IIIC endometrioid corpus cancer includes distinct subgroups. *Gynecol Oncol* 2002;87:112–117.
124. Garg G, Morris RT, Solomon L, et al. Evaluating the significance of location of lymph node metastasis and extranodal disease in women with stage IIIC endometrial cancer. *Gynecol Oncol* 2011;123(2):208–213.
125. Stahl JM, Park HS, Silasi DA, et al. Influence of robotic-assisted laparoscopic hysterectomy on vaginal cuff healing and brachytherapy initiation in endometrial carcinoma patients. *Pract Radiat Oncol* 2016;6(4):226–232.
126. Taylor A, Rockall AG, Reznek RH, et al. Mapping pelvic lymph nodes: guidelines for delineation in intensity-modulated radiotherapy. *Int J Radiat Oncol Biol Phys* 2005;63:1604–1612.
127. Small W Jr, Mell LK, Anderson P, et al. Consensus guidelines for delineation of clinical target volume for intensity-modulated pelvic radiotherapy in postoperative treatment of endometrial and cervical cancer. *Int J Radiat Oncol Biol Phys* 2008;71(2):428–434.
128. Ahamad A, D'Souza W, Salehpour M, et al. Intensity-modulated radiation therapy after hysterectomy: comparison with conventional treatment and sensitivity of the normal-tissue-sparing effect to margin size. *Int J Radiat Oncol Biol Phys* 2005;62:1117–1124.
129. Jhingran A, Winter K, Portelance L, et al. A phase II study of intensity modulated radiation therapy to the pelvis for postoperative patients with endometrial carcinoma: radiation therapy oncology group trial 0418. *Int J Radiat Oncol Biol Phys* 2012;84(1):e23–e28.
130. He S, Gill BS, Heron DE, et al. Long-term outcomes using adjuvant pelvic intensity modulated radiation therapy (IMRT) for endometrial carcinoma. *Pract Radiat Oncol* 2017;7(1):19–25.
131. Shih KK, Milgrom SA, Abu-Rustum NR, et al. Postoperative pelvic intensity-modulated radiotherapy in high risk endometrial cancer. *Gynecol Oncol* 2013;128(3):535–539.
132. de Boer SM, Nout RA, Jürgenliemk-Schulz IM, et al. Long-term impact of endometrial cancer diagnosis and treatment on health-related quality of life and cancer survivorship: results from the randomized PORTEC-2 trial. *Int J Radiat Oncol Biol Phys* 2015;93(4):797–809.
133. Sorbe BG, Smeds AC. Postoperative vaginal irradiation with high dose rate afterloading technique in endometrial carcinoma stage I. *Int J Radiat Oncol Biol Phys* 1990;18:305–314.
134. Law E, Kelvin JF, Thom B, et al. Prospective study of vaginal dilator use adherence and efficacy following radiotherapy. *Radiother Oncol* 2015;116(1):149–155.
135. Damast S, Alektiar K, Eaton A, et al. Comparative patient-centered outcomes (health state and adverse sexual symptoms) between adjuvant brachytherapy versus no adjuvant brachytherapy in early stage endometrial cancer. *Ann Surg Oncol* 2014;21(8):2740–2754.
136. Creutzberg CL, van Putten WL, Koper PC, et al; The Postoperative Radiation Therapy in Endometrial Carcinoma. The morbidity of treatment for patients with stage I endometrial cancer: results from a randomized trial. *Int J Radiat Oncol Biol Phys* 2001;51(5):1246–1255.
137. Shih KK, Folkert MR, Kollmeier MA, et al. Pelvic insufficiency fractures in patients with cervical and endometrial cancer treated with postoperative pelvic radiation. *Gynecol Oncol* 2013;128(3):540–543.
138. Wiltink LM, Nout RA, Fiocco M, et al. No increased risk of second cancer after radiotherapy in patients treated for rectal or endometrial cancer in the randomized TME, PORTEC-1, and PORTEC-2 trials. *J Clin Oncol* 2015;33(15):1640–1646.
139. Shih KK, Hajj C, Kollmeier M, et al. Impact of postoperative intensity-modulated radiation therapy (IMRT) on the rate of bowel obstruction in gynecologic malignancy. *Gynecol Oncol* 2016;143(1):18–21.
140. de Boer SM, Powell ME, Mileshkin L, et al; PORTEC study group. Toxicity and quality of life after adjuvant chemoradiotherapy versus radiotherapy alone for women with high-risk endometrial cancer (PORTEC-3): an open-label, multicentre, randomised, phase 3 trial. *Lancet Oncol* 2016;17(8):1114–1126.
141. van der Steen-Banasik E, Christiaens M, Shash E, et al; European Organisation for Research and Treatment of Cancer, Gynaecological Cancer Group (EORTC-GCG). Systemic review: radiation therapy alone in medical non-operable endometrial carcinoma. *Eur J Cancer* 2016;65:172–181.
142. Schwarz JK, Beriwal S, Esthappan J, et al. Consensus statement for brachytherapy for the treatment of medically inoperable endometrial cancer. *Brachytherapy* 2015;14(5):587–599.
143. Gebhardt B, Gill B, Glaser S, et al. Image-guided tandem and cylinder brachytherapy as monotherapy for definitive treatment of inoperable endometrial carcinoma. *Gynecol Oncol* 2017;147(2):302–308.
144. Acharya S, Esthappan J, Badiyan S, et al. Medically inoperable endometrial cancer in patients with a high body mass index (BMI): patterns of failure after 3-D image-based high dose rate (HDR) brachytherapy. *Radiother Oncol* 2016;118(1):167–172.
145. Jhingran A, Burke TW, Eifel PJ. Definitive radiotherapy for patients with isolated vaginal recurrence of endometrial carcinoma after hysterectomy. *Int J Radiat Oncol Biol Phys* 2003;56:1366–1372.
146. Lin LL, Grigsby PW, Powell MA, et al. Definitive radiotherapy in the management of isolated vaginal recurrences of endometrial cancer. *Int J Radiat Oncol Biol Phys* 2005;63:500–504.
147. Wylie J, Irwin C, Pintilie M, et al. Results of radical radiotherapy for recurrent endometrial cancer. *Gynecol Oncol* 2000;77:66–72.
148. Jereczek-Fossa B, Badzio A, Jassem J. Recurrent endometrial cancer after surgery alone: results of salvage radiotherapy. *Int J Radiat Oncol Biol Phys* 2000;48(2):405–413.
149. Vargo JA, Kim H, Houser CJ, et al. Definitive salvage for vaginal recurrence of endometrial cancer: the impact of modern intensity-modulated-radiotherapy with image-based HDR brachytherapy and the interplay of the PORTEC 1 risk stratification. *Radiother Oncol* 2014;113(1):126–131.
150. Ho JC, Allen PK, Jhingran A, et al. Management of nodal recurrences of endometrial cancer with IMRT. Management of nodal recurrences of endometrial cancer with IMRT. *Gynecol Oncol* 2015;139(1):40–46.
151. Cherniack AD, Shen H, Walter V, et al. Integrated molecular characterization of uterine carcinosarcoma. *Cancer Cell* 2017;31(3):411–423.
152. Pothuri B, Ramondetta L, Eifel P, et al. Radiation-associated endometrial cancers are prognostically unfavorable tumors: a clinicopathologic comparison with 527 sporadic endometrial cancers. *Gynecol Oncol* 2006;103(3):948–951.
153. Reed NS, Mangioni C, Malmström H, et al; European Organisation for Research and Treatment of Cancer Gynaecological Cancer Group. Phase III randomised study to evaluate the role of adjuvant pelvic radiotherapy in the treatment of uterine sarcomas stages I and II: an European Organisation for Research and Treatment of Cancer Gynaecological Cancer Group Study (protocol 55874). *Eur J Cancer* 2008;44(6):808–818.
154. Sutton G, Kauderer J, Carson LF, et al; Gynecologic Oncology Group. Adjuvant ifosfamide and cisplatin in patients with completely resected stage I or II carcinosarcomas (mixed mesodermal tumors) of the uterus: a Gynecologic Oncology Group study. *Gynecol Oncol* 2005;96(3):630–634.
155. Wolfson AH, Brady MF, Rocereto T, et al. A gynecologic oncology group randomized phase III trial of whole abdominal irradiation (WAI) versus cisplatin-ifosfamide and mesna (CIM) as post-surgical therapy in stage I-IV carcinosarcoma (CS) of the uterus. *Gynecol Oncol* 2007;107(2):177–185.
156. Desai NB, Kollmeier MA, Makker V, et al. Comparison of outcomes in early stage uterine carcinosarcoma and uterine serous carcinoma. *Gynecol Oncol* 2014;135(1):49–53.
157. Benson C, Miah AB. Uterine sarcoma—current perspectives. *Int J Womens Health* 2017;9:597–606.
158. Leitao MM, Sonoda Y, Brennan MF, et al. Incidence of lymph node and ovarian metastases in leiomyosarcoma of the uterus. *Gynecol Oncol* 2003;91:209–212.
159. Dos Santos LA, Garg K, Diaz JP, et al. Incidence of lymph node and adnexal metastasis in endometrial stromal sarcoma. *Gynecol Oncol* 2011;121(2):319–322.
160. Sampath S, Schultheiss TE, Ryu JK, et al. The role of adjuvant radiation in uterine sarcomas. *Int J Radiat Oncol Biol Phys* 2010;76(3):728–734.

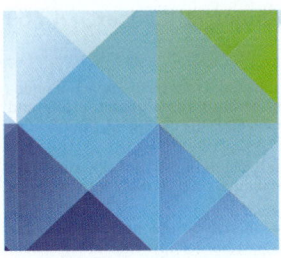

CHAPTER 75

Ovarian and Fallopian Tube Cancer

Larissa Lee, Ross Stuart Berkowitz, and Ursula A. Matulonis

INTRODUCTION

Ovarian neoplasms encompass a wide array of benign and malignant tumors with diverse histologic cell types, clinical features, and survival outcomes. Primary malignant tumors of the ovary include the epithelial ovarian cancers, germ cell tumors, and sex cord tumors. Low malignant potential (LMP) tumors of the ovary are noninvasive epithelial tumors often confined to the ovary, although extraovarian tumor implants may be detected. Metastases to the ovary occur from other primary malignancies including uterine, gastrointestinal (Krukenberg tumors), and breast cancers. Primary lymphoma, sarcoma, and melanoma of the ovary are rare. Relative to its incidence, epithelial ovarian cancers have substantially high mortality because effective screening tools are lacking; only 25% are detected as stage I at diagnosis, and current therapies for advanced cancer, although improving, have approached a therapeutic plateau. Surgery is the mainstay for diagnosis, staging, and the initial treatment for ovarian cancer. Platinum-based chemotherapy is indicated for patients with high-risk or advanced disease. Novel agents, such as antiangiogenics and poly (ADP-ribose) polymerase (PARP) inhibitors, are under active investigation in the adjuvant and/

or recurrent setting. The use of whole-abdomen irradiation (WAI) or intraperitoneal (IP) radioisotopes is primarily historical, and radiation therapy now has a limited role in the management of ovarian cancer. Nonetheless, palliative radiotherapy may be of significant benefit for symptomatic disease relapse or select patients with localized recurrence.

ANATOMY

In premenopausal women, the ovaries are almond-shaped, gray–pink solid organs that measure approximately 4 × 2.5 × 1 cm, with an average weight of 4 to 5 g. After menopause, the ovaries atrophy and become nonfunctional and smaller in size. When normally positioned, the ovary is attached by the mesovarium to the broad ligament that covers the uterus and fallopian tubes. The infundibular pelvic, or suspensory, ligament extends from the surface of the ovary to the lateral pelvic wall, forming the superior and lateral aspect of the broad ligament (Fig. 75.1). The blood supply of the ovary is derived from the ovarian arteries, which arise from the aorta immediately below the level of the renal arteries and course through the retroperitoneum and infundibular pelvic ligaments. The

FIGURE 75.1. Anatomy of the ovary and female reproductive tract. (Asset provided by the Anatomical Chart Company.)

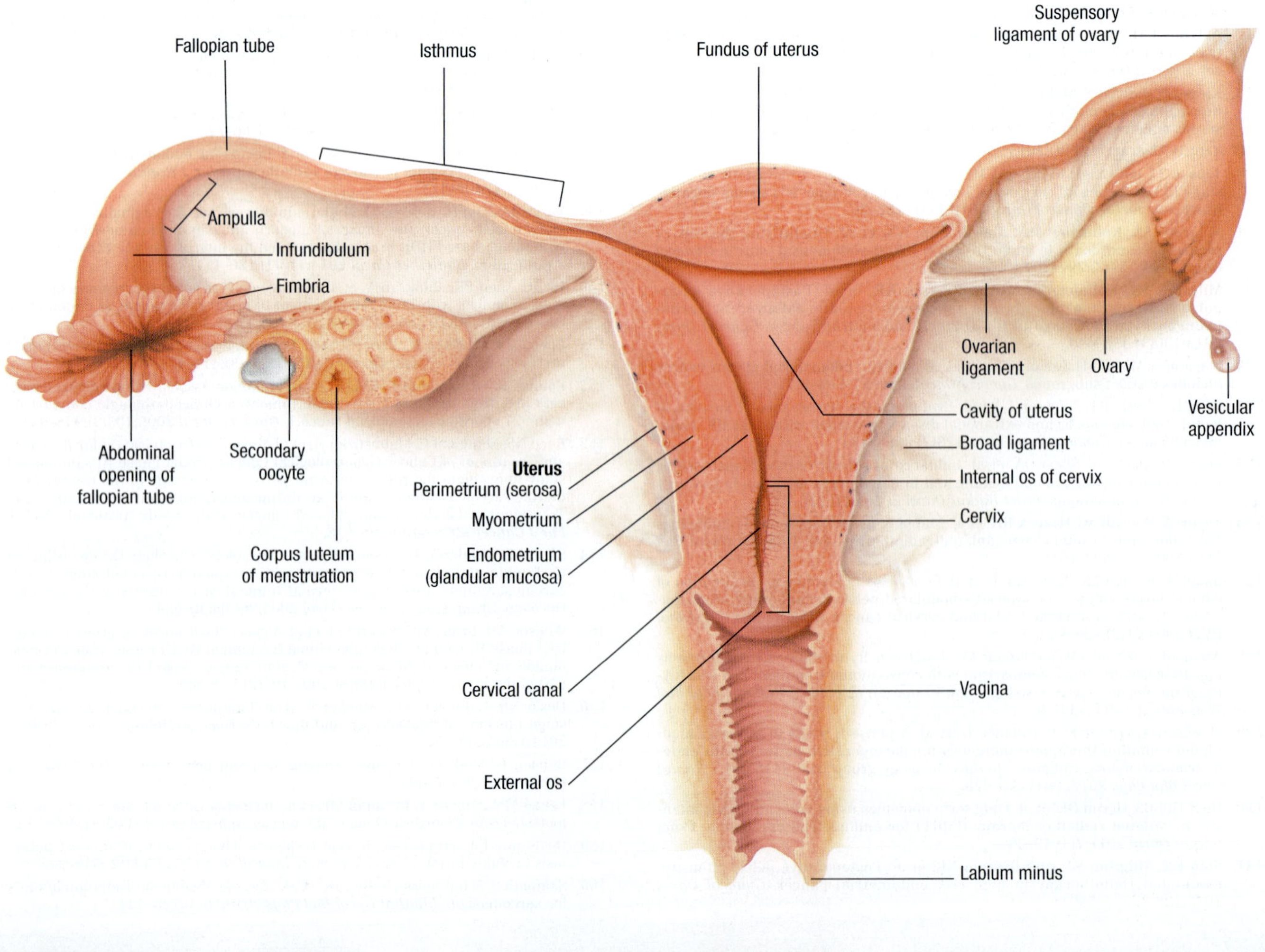

venous return of the ovary empties to the renal vein on the left and directly to the vena cava on the right. The primary lymphatic drainage of the ovary parallels the course of the ovarian veins, with secondary lymphatic flow passing through the inguinal canal and to the iliac nodal system.[1] Histologically, the outer cortex of the ovary is covered by a layer of pseudo-columnar or cuboidal epithelium, termed the germinal epithelium of Waldeyer or ovarian surface epithelium (OSE). The inner medulla consists of a superficial tunica albuginea and dense stromal tissue filled with blood vessels and spindled, "muscle-like" connective tissue. Within the medulla, maturing follicles are present throughout the various layers.

The fallopian tubes are positioned horizontally within the superior part of the broad ligament and extend from the superior–posterior portion of the uterine fundus to the ovaries. The fallopian tubes are hollow, muscular viscera that are in direct communication with the peritoneal cavity. The ovarian artery anastomoses with the uterine artery to supply the fallopian tube, and venous drainage is through the pampiniform plexus to the ovarian vein and uterine plexus. The mucosa of the fallopian tube contains a rich network of intercommunicating lymphatic sinusoids that anastomose with adjacent organs and drain into the ovarian lymphatics and para-aortic and iliac lymph nodes.[2] The fallopian tubes consist of four separate histologic layers: the mucosa, submucosa, muscularis (external longitudinal and inner circular layers), and outer serosal layer, which is continuous with the visceral peritoneum of the uterus. The mucosa is intricately folded, with the number of folds increasing from the interstitial portion to the ampulla. The epithelium is composed mainly of ciliated cells and secretory cells. Cyclic changes are evident in the tubal epithelium, similar to those of the endometrium, in response to estrogen and progesterone.

EPIDEMIOLOGY

Ovarian cancer is the second most common gynecologic malignancy in the United States after endometrial cancer. Approximately 22,440 women in the United States received a diagnosis of epithelial ovarian cancer in 2017, and 14,080 died of the disease[3,4] (Fig. 75.2). Ovarian cancer represents the fifth leading cause of cancer-related death in US women, following lung, breast, colorectal, and pancreatic cancers. The lifetime risk of ovarian cancer is approximately 1 in 77 women with

a median age at diagnosis of 63 years; >80% of women are diagnosed after the age of 40 years.[5] The incidence of ovarian cancer rises with increasing age and peaks in the eighth decade of life. Differences in race and ethnicity are apparent in the age-adjusted annual incidence per 100,000 women, which in 2010 to 2014 was highest for White women (12.2), followed by Hispanic (10.6), American Indian/Alaska Native (9.5), Black (9.4), and Asian/Pacific Islanders (9.5).[5] The incidence of ovarian cancer also varies significantly by geography, with the highest rates in North America and northern Europe, which are three to seven times higher than that observed in Japan.[6] Survival rates for ovarian cancer have been increasing in the United States since 1975, when the 5-year survival rate reported by the Surveillance, Epidemiology, and End Results (SEER) program was 34%, which has increased to 47% in 2009.[5]

Primary cancer of the fallopian tube was once considered a rare disease, accounting for 0.2% to 0.5% of female gynecologic malignancies. However, the true incidence has likely been underestimated considering a large proportion of extra-uterine high-grade serous carcinomas may actually originate in the fimbriated end of the fallopian tube.[7,8] Precursor lesions, known as serous tubal intraepithelial carcinomas (STICs), have been detected in the fallopian tubes of prophylactic salpingo-oophorectomy specimens from high-risk patients. The model of the fallopian tube as the primary site of origin for extrauterine high-grade serous carcinoma is supported by epidemiologic, morphologic, and genetic data, as discussed later.

PATHOGENESIS

The female reproductive tract originates from the müllerian ducts, which are paired embryologic structures of mesodermal origin that give rise to the fallopian tubes, uterus, cervix, and upper vagina. Ovarian tissue is composed of embryonic yolk sac cells that give rise to the ova or germ cells, stromal cells that produce the steroid hormones, and mesothelium that provides the epithelial covering for the follicle cysts. These cell types give rise to germ cell tumors, sex cord–stromal tumors, and the epithelial tumors of the ovary, respectively. The traditional view of ovarian cancer pathogenesis is that all tumor subtypes arise from the OSE. In the "incessant ovulation hypothesis," ovarian cancer develops from an aberrant repair process as a result of repeated rupture of

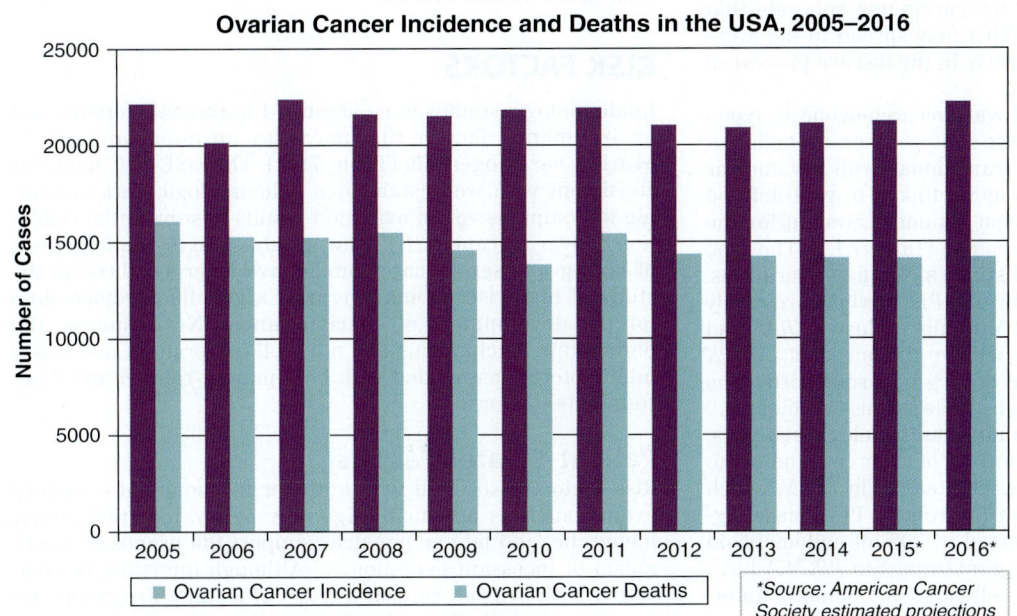

FIGURE 75.2. Ovarian cancer incidence and deaths in the United States from 2005 to 2016. (Courtesy of the American Cancer Society.)

Section III

the surface epithelium during each ovulatory cycle, thought to produce inflammation and scarring that serves as a nidus for carcinogenesis.[9–11] A second proposed mechanism is related to hormonal and reproductive factors such as persistent exposure to gonadotropins and elevated estradiol levels that stimulate malignant transformation.[12,13] Strong evidence exists that many borderline tumors and low-grade carcinomas of the ovary arise from cortical inclusion cysts (CICs) within the ovarian parenchyma. These benign cysts are composed of müllerian epithelium that closely resembles the fallopian tube. CICs are thought to result from invaginations of the OSE into the ovarian stroma through repeated ovulation and aging, acquiring a müllerian phenotype through metaplasia.[8] An alternate explanation is that remnants of müllerian-derived epithelia from the fallopian tube may adhere to the ovarian surface and become incorporated into CICs in a process known as endosalpingiosis. Nonetheless, as a result of hormone exposure, damage repair processes, and inflammation within the ovary, neoplastic transformation gives rise to a variety of müllerian cell type differentiations, including serous carcinomas that resemble the fallopian tube, mucinous tumors as seen in the endocervix, endometrioid tumors from the endometrium, and glycogen-rich clear cell cancers similar to secretory-phase endometrial glands.

High-grade serous ovarian carcinomas are infrequently associated with benign or borderline precursor lesions within the ovary, a contradiction of the OSE–CIC model. Furthermore, high-grade serous carcinomas of the ovary share distinct morphologic and genetic characteristics with high-grade serous carcinomas of other extrauterine sites, including serous fallopian tube carcinoma and primary peritoneal serous carcinoma. In this context, a second model of ovarian carcinogenesis has emerged with the recognition of the distal fallopian tube as the primary site of origin for many high-grade serous carcinomas. With rigorous pathologic processing, occult fallopian tube cancer has been detected in the fimbria of prophylactic salpingo-oophorectomy specimens from high-risk patients.[14,15] Furthermore, STICs have been found in a large proportion of high-grade serous carcinomas initially designated as primary ovarian cancers.[16] An adenoma–carcinoma sequence has since been described that involves a dysplastic tubal precursor lesion with loss of p53 detectable by immunohistochemical staining ("p53 signature") with progression to a STIC characterized by increased proliferation, followed by the development of frank invasive serous carcinoma.[7,17] The concept of the fallopian tube as the primary site of high-grade serous carcinoma suggests that previously undetected serous STICs may spread to the adjacent ovary or peritoneal cavity early in the disease process of serous carcinogenesis.

In the two-pathway model of ovarian carcinogenesis, type I tumors include all major histologic subtypes (serous, endometrioid, mucinous, clear cell, and transitional) with low nuclear and architectural grade that may be linked to well-defined benign precursor lesions, and type II tumors account for the bulk of high-grade serous carcinomas (Table 75.1). The type I tumors are associated with distinct molecular alterations, such as mutations in *KRAS*, *BRAF*, and *PTEN*, which are rarely found in type II serous tumors.[18] Mutually exclusive *KRAS* and *BRAF* mutations, both of which activate the oncogenic *MAPK* signaling pathway, are observed in 65% of serous borderline tumors but are rarely seen in high-grade serous carcinomas.[19] *KRAS* mutations also occur in müllerian histologic subtypes, including 60% of mucinous, 5% to 16% of clear cell, and 4% to 5% of endometrioid carcinomas.[18] Mutations in *PTEN*, which lead to constitutive activation of the related PI3 kinase signaling pathway, have been detected in 20% of endometrioid carcinomas,[20] whereas activating mutations in *PIK3CA* have been identified in 30% of clear cell cancers.[21] Somatic mutations in *ARID1A*, a novel tumor suppressor gene, have been

TABLE 75.1 TWO-PATHWAY MODEL OF EPITHELIAL OVARIAN CARCINOGENESIS

Type 1	Type 2
All müllerian subtypes (serous, endometrioid, mucinous, clear cell, transitional)	High-grade serous carcinoma
Usually low grade	High grade
Linked to benign or borderline precursor lesions	Associated with serous tubal intraepithelial carcinomas (STICs)
KRAS or *BRAF* mutation (MAPK pathway)	Inactivation of *BRCA* pathway
PTEN or *PIK3CA* mutation (PI3K pathway)	
ARID1A mutation, loss of BAF250a expression	
Wild-type p53 status	High frequency of p53 mutation
Chromosomally stable	Widespread DNA copy number change
Frequently platinum insensitive	Usually platinum sensitive

Adapted by permission from Nature: Bowtell DD. The genesis and evolution of high-grade serous ovarian cancer. *Nat Rev Cancer* 2010;10(11):803–808. Copyright © 2010 Springer Nature.

identified in 46% of ovarian clear cell cancers and 30% of endometrioid cancers. *ARID1A* mutation and corresponding loss of BAF250a expression, a key component in chromatin remodeling, were also seen in preneoplastic lesions and may represent an early event in the transformation of endometriosis.[22] In contrast, type II tumors exhibit a high frequency of p53 mutation and widespread DNA copy number change. Inactivation of the BRCA pathway, a critical component of DNA repair by homologous recombination, is also a hallmark of high-grade serous carcinomas.[23] Disruption of the BRCA pathway by germline or somatic mutation, epigenetic silencing, or microRNA regulation has been observed in >50% of serous cancers,[24] and functional assays show defective formation of homologous recombination repair foci following DNA damage.[25]

Angiogenesis plays an important role in normal ovarian function, as heavy vascularization occurs at the beginning of each ovulatory cycle with predictable variation in the serum levels of vascular endothelial growth factor (VEGF). Epithelial ovarian cancers frequently overexpress VEGF, fibroblast growth factor, platelet-derived growth factor (PDGF), and angiopoietin.[26] In preclinical models, expression of VEGF provides a survival advantage to transformed cells of the ovary. Other studies have found an association between preoperative serum VEGF level and clinical outcome.[27] Targeting the tumor microenvironment in ovarian cancer is an attractive treatment strategy given the inherent genomic instability of high-grade serous cancers.

RISK FACTORS

Epidemiologic studies have identified hormonal, genetic, and environmental factors that may play an important role in ovarian carcinogenesis (Table 75.2). The OSE–CIC model is consistent with well-established epidemiologic data indicating that suppression of ovulation results in substantial reduction of ovarian cancer risk. New insights into the pathogenesis of high-grade serous carcinomas have emerged through the study of high-risk populations with a genetic predisposition for the development of ovarian cancer. Nevertheless, the pathogenic mechanisms are not well understood and likely multifactorial, associated with both patient-related and environmental factors.

Patient-Related Factors

Risk factors associated with a higher frequency of ovulatory events, such as advancing age, low parity, infertility, early menarche, and late menopause, support the proposed mechanism of incessant ovulation.[28–31] Although infertility is associated with ovarian cancer, the use of fertility drugs has not been conclusively linked.[32–34] Suppression of ovulatory events

TABLE 75.2 FACTORS INFLUENCING THE RISK OF OVARIAN CANCER

Factor	Estimated Risk (%)	Estimated Relative Risk
Baseline lifetime risk	1.4	1
Race		
White	12.2 per 100,000	–
Hispanic or American Indian	10.6 per 100,000	–
African American	9.4 per 100,000	–
Risk factors		
Family history	9.4	5–7
BRCA1 mutation	35–46	18–29
BRCA2 mutation	13–23	16–19
Lynch II/HPNCC	3–14	6–7
Infertility	–	2–5
Obesity	–	1.1–4
Nulliparity	–	2–3
Late menopause	–	1.5–2
Early menarche	–	1–1.5
Unopposed estrogen use	–	1.2–2
Protective factors		
Multiparity	–	0.4–0.6
Oral contraceptive use	–	0.7
Hysterectomy or tubal ligation	–	0.6–0.7

HPNCC, hereditary nonpolyposis colorectal cancer.
Adapted from Holschneider CH, Berek JS. Ovarian cancer: epidemiology, biology, and prognostic factors. *Semin Surg Oncol* 2000;19(1):3–10. Copyright © 2000 Wiley-Liss, Inc. Reprinted by permission of John Wiley & Sons, Inc.

from pregnancy, breast feeding, and oral contraceptive use may explain the observed protective benefit.[30,31,35] With oral contraceptive use for 4, 8, or 12 years, the risk of ovarian cancer is reduced by 40%, 53%, and 60%, respectively.[36] In a collaborative meta-analysis of 45 epidemiologic studies from 21 countries, the use of oral contraceptives was significantly associated with a decreased risk of ovarian cancer in ever users (hazard ratio [HR] 0.73, $P < .0001$), with larger reductions observed for longer duration of use.[37] The authors conclude that 200,000 ovarian cancers and 100,000 deaths have been prevented since the introduction of oral contraceptives 50 years ago.

Other patient-related risk factors such as polycystic ovarian disease and endometriosis may act through hormonal mechanisms attributable to elevated gonadotropins or by chronic inflammation. In a meta-analysis of eight case–control studies, women with polycystic ovarian disease had a 2.5-fold increase in ovarian cancer risk.[38] Endometriosis has been shown to be an independent risk factor for ovarian cancer with an estimated rate of malignant transformation of 2.5%.[39] Ovarian cancers that arise from endometriosis are most often low-grade tumors with endometrioid or clear cell histology and are associated with a better prognosis.[40] Altered hormonal levels such as elevated androgens may also increase risk, whereas progestins have been shown to be protective.[41] Large prospective cohort studies have demonstrated an increase in ovarian cancer risk and mortality with the use of exogenous estrogen and hormone replacement therapy.[42–44] Surgical procedures, including hysterectomy and tubal ligation, are independently associated with a 34% reduction each in ovarian cancer risk, although the protective mechanism is unknown.[29,45–47] Chronic inflammatory conditions such as pelvic inflammatory disease and tuberculous salpingitis were once believed to be causative factors in the development of fallopian tube malignancies, although this theory remains unproven.

Genetic Factors

Heredity tumors account for 10% to 15% of all ovarian cancers, and family history is the strongest risk factor after increasing age.[48,49] The risk of developing ovarian cancer in the general population is approximately 1.4%, whereas the lifetime risk for a woman with one first-degree family member with ovarian cancer is 5% and climbs to 7% with two first-degree relatives. If a hereditary syndrome is present, the lifetime risk is on the order of 25% to 50% with an age of diagnosis approximately 10 years younger than women with sporadic disease.[50]

Three distinct familial ovarian cancer syndromes have been identified by pedigree analysis with autosomal dominant patterns of inheritance.[51,52] *BRCA1* and *BRCA2* mutations are the most common genetic alterations, with up to 90% of all hereditary cases associated with a deleterious mutation of the *BRCA1* gene, located on chromosome 17q21, or the *BRCA2* gene, located on chromosome 13q22. The lifetime risk of ovarian cancer is approximately 40% in *BRCA1* mutation carriers and 18% in *BRCA2* mutation carriers.[53] BRCA-associated ovarian cancers are most frequently invasive serous adenocarcinomas and less likely borderline or mucinous tumors.[54] Mutation carriers are also more likely to present with advanced-stage disease and have poorly differentiated tumors.[55] Nonetheless, *BRCA1* or *BRCA2* mutation carriers have a more favorable clinical course with a significantly longer recurrence-free and overall survival compared to noncarriers. The improved outcome appears related to a higher sensitivity to platinum chemotherapy across first and subsequent lines of treatment.[56–60]

The importance of the fallopian tube in the pathogenesis of extrauterine serous carcinoma was initially recognized in *BRCA1* and *BRCA2* mutation carriers. In a prospective study of 483 *BRCA1* mutation carriers, the incidence of fallopian tube cancer was reported as 120 times that of the general population.[61] High-grade serous primary peritoneal carcinomas are also frequently observed in mutation carriers.[62] Further attention was focused on the fallopian tube as the primary site of origin following reports of epithelial dysplasia and occult serous carcinomas in prophylactic salpingo-oophorectomy specimens from mutation carriers.[63–66] In contrast to the standard pathologic sampling of the ampullary region of the fallopian tube in ovarian cancer cases, more extensive complete sectioning of the tube revealed an abundance of lesions in the fimbria of the distal tube.[14–16] The detection of early serous carcinomas, or STICs, lent further support to the emerging concept of the fallopian tube as the primary site for extrauterine serous carcinoma. In this context, the National Comprehensive Cancer Network (NCCN) guidelines recommend that any woman with a diagnosis of ovarian, fallopian tube, or primary peritoneal carcinoma be referred to a cancer genetics professional for consideration of BRCA mutation testing.[67] BRCA screening in a population of women with non-mucinous ovarian cancer detected germline mutations in 14% of women, including 22% with high-grade serous cancer, reinforcing the importance of offering testing to all patients.[68]

Hereditary nonpolyposis colorectal syndrome, or Lynch type II cancer syndrome, is responsible for the remaining 10% of hereditary ovarian cancers.[69] In this syndrome, germline mutations of DNA mismatch repair genes lead to an increased risk of colorectal, stomach, endometrial, and ovarian cancer owing to underlying microsatellite instability. A total of seven mismatch repair genes have been identified with mutations in *MLH1* and *MSH2* accounting for 90% of the observed mutations in Lynch syndrome families.[70,71] Mutations in *MSH6* and *PMS2* have been reported in the remaining 10% of families, whereas alterations in the remaining three identified genes are uncommonly observed. Inactivating mutations in specific genes may modify the underlying cancer predisposition. Women with *MSH6* mutations are twice as likely to develop endometrial cancer compared to carriers of *MSH2* or *MLH1* gene mutations, which are the most common alterations underlying colorectal cancer risk.[72] Women with *MSH2* gene mutations have been shown to have a risk of epithelial ovarian cancer twice that of *MLH1* carriers. In contrast to *BRCA1* and *BRCA2* mutation carriers, women with Lynch syndrome may present with a variety of non-serous epithelial tumor types, including endometrioid and clear cell histologies. Ovarian cancer associated with Lynch syndrome is more often diagnosed at an earlier stage with well- to moderately differentiated tumor grade. The lifetime risk of ovarian cancer in women with Lynch syndrome is estimated at 3% to 14% and is most commonly diagnosed in the fifth decade of life.[73] In women with a family or personal history suggestive of Lynch syndrome, tumor testing may be performed by microsatellite instability analysis or immunohistochemical staining for mismatch repair genes. Direct sequencing of the mismatch repair genes is used for detection of germline mutations. Other less common germline mutations have been identified by genomic sequencing and involve the following genes: *PALB2, BARD1, BRIP1, RAD51C, RAD51D, MSH2, MLH1, PMS2,* and *MSH6.*[74]

Other genetic disorders linked with nonepithelial ovarian cancers include Peutz-Jeghers syndrome, which is associated with an increased risk of sex cord–stromal tumors, and gonadal dysgenesis, associated with dysgerminomas and gonadoblastomas.

Environmental Factors

Environmental or physical causes of ovarian cancer have been investigated through numerous case–control studies. Women in developing countries have a lower incidence of ovarian cancer than those living in industrialized nations,[75] although, to date, no specific chemical carcinogens have been identified. Chronic exposure to asbestos-related products, including talc products, has long been implicated in the development of ovarian cancer.[76] The Nurses' Health Study reported a modestly elevated risk of invasive serous cancers with talc use (relative risk [RR] 1.4), although no association was detected with overall ovarian cancer risk.[77] The development of mucinous ovarian cancer has been found to be associated with cigarette smoking (RR 2 to 2.2) but not other epithelial subtypes.[78,79]

Dietary and metabolic factors have also been explored in large population-based studies as possible contributors to ovarian cancer risk. To date, there have been no consistent associations of coffee or alcohol consumption with increased risk. Large epidemiologic studies also showed no relationship between consumption of animal fat and the development of ovarian cancer.[80,81] In a Swedish population–based cohort study of the effect of body mass index on cancer risk in >35,000 women, a 36% higher risk of cancer was observed in obese women (body mass index ≥ 30) relative to women with body mass index in the normal range (18.5 to 25); cancer sites most strongly related to obesity were endometrium, ovary (risk for top quartile 2.09; 95% confidence interval [CI], 1.13 to 4.13), and colon.[82] Obesity has also been associated with increased ovarian cancer mortality in a large prospective study of adults in the United States.[83] There is no clear relationship between exercise and ovarian cancer risk.

SCREENING

In the absence of a reliable screening test, most women with ovarian cancer are diagnosed with advanced-stage disease. In contrast to women with localized disease (stage I/II) who have estimated 5-year survival rates of 70% to 90%, overall survival for women with advanced disease (stage III/IV) is poor, ranging from 20% to 45% (Table 75.3). The low sensitivity and specificity of the available screening modalities and the low prevalence of the disease in the general population have hindered the development of a robust screening test. Recent screening approaches have been associated with a low positive predictive value and unacceptable false-positive rates without impacting disease mortality in the general population or high-risk groups.

TABLE 75.3 EPITHELIAL OVARIAN CANCER STAGE DISTRIBUTION AND SURVIVAL BY STAGE

FIGO Stage	Patients (*n* = 4,825) (%)	5-Year Overall Survival (%)
IA	13	90
IB	1	86
IC	14	83
IIA	2	71
IIB	2	66
IIC	5	71
IIIA	3	47
IIIB	6	42
IIIC	42	33
IV	13	19

FIGO, International Federation of Gynecology and Obstetrics.
Adapted from Heintz APM, Odicino F, Maisonneuve P, et al. Carcinoma of the ovary. FIGO 26th Annual Report on the Results of Treatment in Gynecological Cancer. *Int J Gynaecol Obstet* 2006;95(Suppl 1):S161–S192. Copyright © 2006 International Federation of Gynecology and Obstetrics. Reprinted by permission of John Wiley & Sons, Inc.

Several screening strategies have been investigated, including pelvic exam, the serum tumor marker CA-125, and transvaginal ultrasound (TVUS), either alone or in combination.[84] CA-125 values >35 U/mL are observed in 80% of patients with epithelial ovarian cancer, including 90% of women with advanced-stage disease, but only in 50% of early-stage patients.[85] CA-125 is nonspecific for ovarian cancer, as it can be elevated in benign gynecologic and non-gynecologic conditions, including endometriosis, uterine leiomyoma, cirrhosis, pelvic inflammatory disease, the presence of pleural or peritoneal fluid, as well as endometrial carcinoma and non-gynecologic cancers of the breast, lung, and pancreas. Screening with CA-125 alone has been found to lack specificity in an average-risk population of postmenopausal women. Ultrasound alone is able to detect early-stage disease in an average-risk population,[86–88] although the significant false-positive rate remains a concern. In a United Kingdom multimodality screening study, diagnostic surgeries were performed nine times more frequently to detect one cancer in the group screened by TVUS alone compared to multimodality screening (CA-125 and TVUS).[89]

Several large screening trials currently in progress in the United States, United Kingdom, and Japan have been designed to assess reduction in mortality with early detection of ovarian cancer. The Prostate, Lung, Colorectal, and Ovarian Cancer (PLCO) screening trial in the United States randomized 78,216 women aged 55 to 74 to annual screening with CA-125 and TVUS versus usual medical care. Following baseline screening, 570 surgical procedures, including 325 laparotomies, were performed; 29 tumors were detected, 9 of which were of LMP.[90] The positive predictive value for the detection of invasive ovarian cancer was 3.7% for an abnormal CA-125, 1.0% for an abnormal TVUS, and 23.5% for both. Publication of the mortality data with 12-year follow-up showed no difference in the stage of cancer detected by screening (90% stage III or IV) and no reduction in cause-specific or overall mortality for women who underwent screening.[91] Furthermore, diagnostic evaluation for women with false-positive screening resulted in a serious complication rate of 15%.

A second trial, the United Kingdom Collaborative Trial of Ovarian Cancer Screening (UKCTOCS), has accrued >200,000 postmenopausal women to evaluate multimodality screening with TVUS and serum CA-125. In the prevalence screen, the sensitivity, specificity, and positive predictive values of multimodality screening for invasive epithelial ovarian and tubal cancers were 89.5%, 99.8%, and 35.1%, respectively.[89] The initial results of baseline screening were more promising than the US study, with 43% of invasive cancers detected as stage I or II, which may reflect differences in study design and the diagnostic algorithm. However, after a median follow-up of 11 years, a significant mortality reduction with multimodality screening was not observed.[92] The multicenter, randomized Japanese study utilizes a similar screening strategy with TVUS and CA-125 and has accrued >80,000 women. Unlike the US and UK trials, there was a nonsignificant trend for the detection of more stage I cancers in the screened population (63% vs. 38%), although mortality rates have not yet been reported.[93]

The present data do not support routine screening for ovarian cancer in the general population. All of the North American expert groups, including the U.S. Preventive Services Task Force, the American College of Obstetricians and Gynecologists (ACOG), the Society of Gynecologic Oncologists (SGO), and the Canadian Task Force on the Periodic Health Examination, recommend against routine screening in asymptomatic women. The incidence of ovarian cancer is relatively low in the general population; thus, the concerns for false-positive screening and the associated risks of exploratory surgery are significant.[94] However, women at high risk for ovarian cancer with *BRCA1* or *BRCA2* mutations or hereditary nonpolyposis colorectal syndrome could potentially benefit from chemoprevention; screening with pelvic examinations, TVUS, and CA-125 on a biannual or annual basis; or prophylactic surgery.[95] Although the efficacy of screening has been disappointing in the high-risk population,[96] some physicians will follow women with high risk factors, such as *BRCA* mutation or family history, with pelvic exam, CA-125, and TVUS. The U.S. National Institutes of Health Consensus Development Panel recommends that prophylactic salpingo-oophorectomy be considered in women with ovarian cancer syndromes at age 35 years or after childbearing is complete, as the risk reduction with salpingo-oophorectomy is 80%.[98,99] Removal of the ovaries also reduces the risk of breast cancer in BRCA mutation carriers.[100]

HISTOLOGIC CLASSIFICATION

The World Health Organization and International Federation of Gynecology and Obstetrics (FIGO) have adopted a unified classification of the common epithelial, germ cell, sex cord, and stromal tumors[101,102] (Table 75.4). Most ovarian malignancies (60% to 65%) are epithelial, with germ cell tumors (20%), sex cord–stromal tumors (5%), and metastases to the ovary (5% to 10%) accounting for the remainder.[103] Serous tumors are most common, comprising 50% to 60% of epithelial tumors. Other subtypes include mucinous carcinoma in 10%; endometrioid carcinoma, 8%; clear cell carcinoma, 3% to 5%; transitional, 3% to 5%; and undifferentiated carcinoma, 1%. Bilateral presentation occurs frequently in epithelial tumors, most commonly in serous tumors followed by endometrioid (15%) and mucinous tumors (5% to 10%).

High-grade serous carcinomas are often widely disseminated at diagnosis and account for most deaths from ovarian, tubal, and peritoneal cancers. In contrast, 5-year survival for low-grade serous carcinoma is 85%. Most serous tumors present as large ovarian masses and grossly appear nodular with multiple papillary projections and cysts filled with clear serous fluid. A two-tiered grading system separates high-grade serous carcinomas from low-grade tumors,[104,105] which have a similar prolonged natural history to noninvasive borderline tumors, or tumors of LMP.[106] As discussed previously, there is increasing evidence that high-grade serous carcinomas originate in the fimbria of the fallopian tube and may spread rapidly to the adjacent ovary and peritoneal sites. Low-grade tumors appear to follow a stepwise progression from borderline tumor to invasive carcinoma and involve molecular pathways distinct from their high-grade counterparts.[107–109] Although treatment is similar for all serous tumors, low-grade tumors have been shown to be less responsive to chemotherapy.[106,110,111]

TABLE 75.4 WORLD HEALTH ORGANIZATION CLASSIFICATION OF OVARIAN TUMORS

Serous low-grade carcinoma
Serous high-grade carcinoma
Mucinous carcinoma
Endometrioid carcinoma
Clear cell carcinoma
Malignant Brenner tumor
Seromucinous carcinoma
Undifferentiated carcinoma
Germ cell tumors
  Dysgerminoma
  Yolk sac tumor
  Embryonal carcinoma
  Non-gestational choriocarcinoma
  Mature teratoma
  Immature teratoma
  Mixed germ cell tumor
Germ cell and sex cord–stromal tumors
  Mixed germ cell–sex cord–stromal tumor, unclassified
  Gonadoblastoma
Sex cord–stromal tumors
  Pure sex cord tumors
    Adult granulosa cell tumor
    Juvenile granulosa cell tumor
    Sertoli cell tumor
    Sex cord tumor with annular tubules
  Pure stromal tumors
    Fibroma
    Cellular fibroma
    Thecoma
    Luteinized thecoma associated with sclerosing peritonitis
    Fibrosarcoma
    Sclerosing stromal tumor
    Signet-ring stromal tumor
    Microcystic stromal tumor
    Leydig cell tumor
    Steroid cell tumor
Mixed sex cord–stromal tumors
  Sertoli-Leydig cell tumors
  Sex cord–stromal tumors, NOS
Monodermal teratoma and somatic-type tumors arising from a dermoid cyst
  Struma ovarii
  Carcinoid
  Neuroectodermal-type tumors
  Sebaceous tumors
  Carcinomas
Mixed epithelial and mesenchymal tumors
  Carcinosarcoma
  Adenosarcoma

LMP or borderline tumors have nuclear abnormalities and mitotic activity intermediate between benign and malignant tumors of similar cell type but lack stromal invasion (Fig. 75.3). Borderline tumors are a subcategory of ovarian malignancies that account for 10% to 20% of all epithelial neoplasms.[112,113] The prognosis, surgical approach, and postoperative treatment recommendations are vastly different as compared with those of their invasive counterparts. The majority of LMPs (75%) present with stage I disease, which directly contrasts with the 75% advanced stages in the invasive epithelial tumors. The 5- and 10-year survival rates for women with LMP tumors are >95%. Significant heterogeneity exists in the biologic behavior of borderline tumors. Women with nonlocalized LMP tumors of the ovary have decreased survival compared to those with localized LMP tumors but is similar to that of women with localized, well-differentiated epithelial ovarian carcinoma.[114] Other pathologic features that affect prognosis include the cell type, tumor stage, implant type (invasive vs. noninvasive), the presence of micropapillary architecture, and microinvasion. Extensive sampling of all pathologic specimens is required to firmly establish the diagnosis.

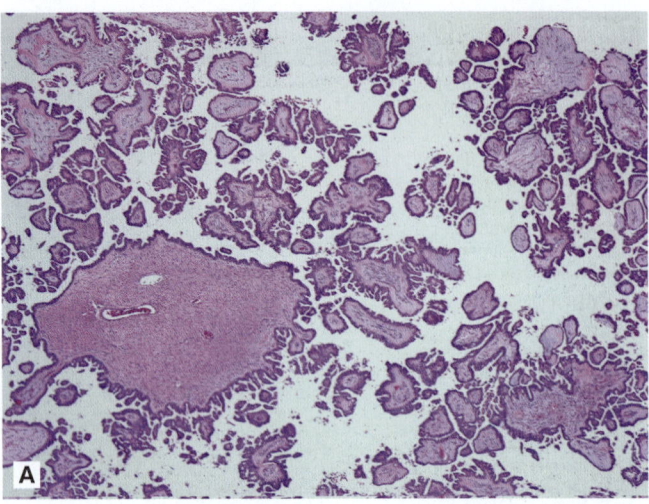
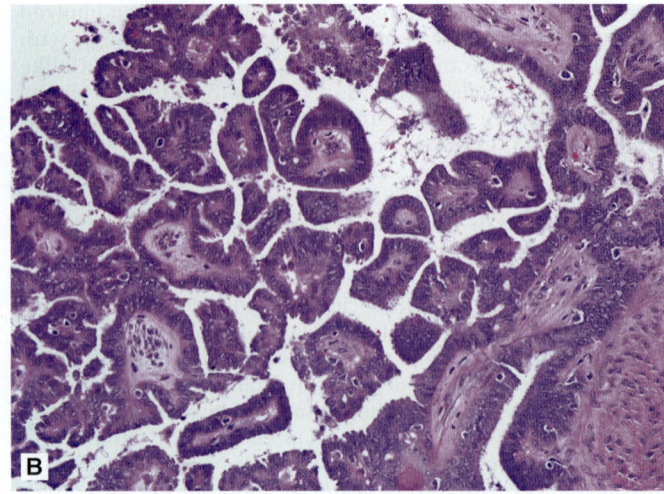

FIGURE 75.3. Serous tumor of low malignant potential of the ovary at low power **(A)** and high power **(B)**. At low power, note the progressively branching papillary fronds with fibrovascular support and detached papillary clusters; at high power, note the serous epithelium with nuclear hyperchromasia and cytologic atypia. By definition, there is no destructive stromal invasion.

Most endometrioid and clear cell carcinomas arise in foci of endometriosis and follow an adenoma to borderline tumor to carcinoma sequence. Endometrioid carcinoma of the ovary resembles its endometrial counterpart (Fig. 75.4), and synchronous primary cancers are detected in 10% of women with ovarian cancer and 5% of women with endometrial cancer.[115] Bilateral ovarian involvement, small multinodular ovaries, and surface and hilar spread suggest metastatic involvement from an endometrial primary, particularly if the endometrial tumor is high grade, deeply invasive, and associated with lymphovascular invasion. A large, cystic, unilateral tumor of low grade arising in a focus of endometriosis likely represents a primary ovarian tumor. Endometrioid tumors appear to have a better prognosis than serous cancers regardless of tumor stage.[116] Multiple synchronous primary tumors may represent a field defect related to endometriosis, which is associated with improved survival.[117]

Mucinous tumors follow a similar progression from cystadenoma to borderline tumor prior to invasion. All subtypes are more likely to be diagnosed when confined to the ovary. Mucinous cancers may grow to a very large size, often measuring up to 20 cm in diameter and filled with large pockets of thick, necrotic, mucinous debris.[118,119] Ovarian mucinous tumors closely resemble mucin-secreting tumors originating from other sites—most commonly the gastrointestinal tract. The pathologic distinction between primary and metastatic mucinous carcinoma may be challenging, despite the use of immunohistochemical analysis. Further clinical evaluation is often required to exclude a clinically occult non-ovarian primary source. Secondary involvement of the ovary may also occur in association with pseudomyxoma peritonei arising from a low-grade tumor often of appendiceal origin.[120]

Clear cell carcinoma is characterized by clear and hobnail cells with a similar histologic appearance to clear cell carcinoma of the kidney, endometrium, and vagina. Ovarian clear cell carcinoma is often seen in association with venous thromboembolism and hypercalcemia. Although more likely to be stage I than serous carcinoma, clear cell histology is associated with a lower response rate to platinum-based chemotherapy, higher recurrence rate, and worse survival.[121] The transitional cell tumors, including Brenner tumors, are benign in most cases (98%) and carry a favorable prognosis.

FIGURE 75.4. Endometrioid adenocarcinoma of the ovary. **A:** At low power, note the tumor composed of back-to-back endometrioid glands. **B:** At high power, note the squamous metaplasia, commonly seen in this epithelial variant. Assignment of tumor grade is based on similar criteria as for carcinomas arising in the endometrium. This tumor would qualify as well differentiated or grade 1.

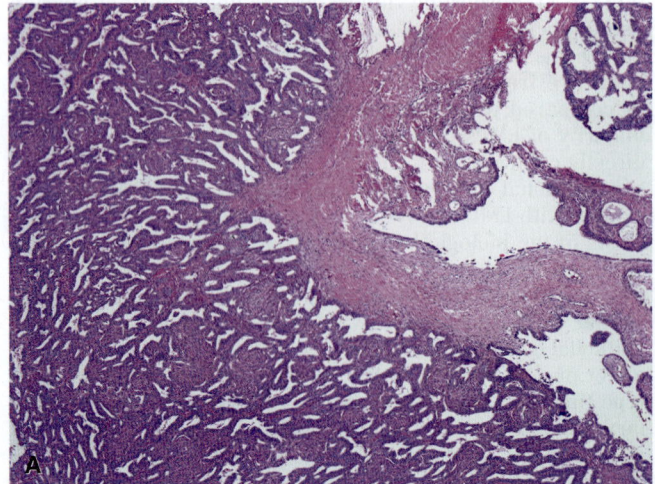
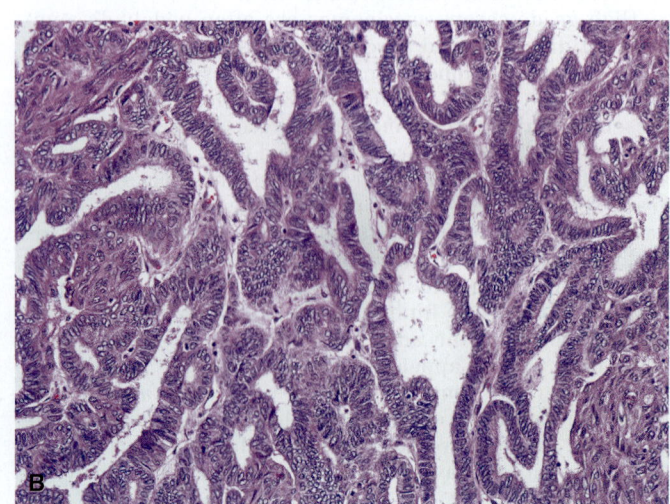

Ovarian germ cell tumors comprise <5% of ovarian malignancies and are classified by the World Health Organization (Table 75.4). Dysgerminomas are the most common of the germ cell tumors and occur bilaterally in 10% to 20% of cases. The other germ cell tumor types are typically unilateral. Endodermal sinus tumors, also known as yolk sac tumors, are characterized by Schiller-Duval bodies. Embryonal carcinomas are rare and tend to occur in younger populations; they may be seen with nongestational choriocarcinomas as part of mixed germ cell tumors (10% of all germ cell tumors). Immature teratomas are characterized by immature elements from the germ layers. The grade, treatment recommendations, and outcome are directed by the amount of immature neural elements.

Sex cord–stromal tumors are also classified by the World Health Organization (Table 75.4), with granulosa cell tumors being the most common (70%). Histologically, the granulosa cell tumors are composed of granulosa cells that have a pale, grooved, "coffee bean" nucleus or a rosette of cells surrounding eosinophilic material, a Call-Exner body. Thecomas (hormonally active) and fibromas (hormonally inactive) are both clinically benign tumors and are most common in middle-age women.

The most common histopathology of primary fallopian tube malignancies is papillary serous adenocarcinoma. Other less common müllerian subtypes include endometrioid, clear cell, and malignant mixed müllerian tumors.[122,123] Rare reports of squamous cell carcinoma, immature teratoma, glassy cell tumor, and sarcoma have also been described. Benign tumors are found even less frequently than malignant neoplasms. Metastatic involvement of the fallopian tube is reported in up to 12% of women with uterine cancer and 4% with cervical cancer.[124,125]

PATTERNS OF SPREAD

The primary mode of spread for epithelial ovarian and fallopian tube cancers is transperitoneal, as malignant cells exfoliate into the peritoneal cavity. Intraperitoneal spread is favored by intestinal peristalsis and negative hydrostatic pressure below the diaphragm. The exfoliated tumor cells follow the intra-abdominal fluid stream passing along the paracolic gutters toward the diaphragm, predominately on the right side, before implantation on any peritoneal surface.[126,127] Metastatic deposits are frequently seen in the posterior cul-de-sac, paracolic gutters, diaphragmatic surfaces, liver capsule, intestinal surfaces, and omentum. Metastases may also be found in the uterus or contralateral ovary from peritoneal spread or flow through the fallopian tubes. Dense tumor "caking" can cause infiltration into the abdominal organs creating a mass effect on the omentum, ureter, bowel, liver, pancreas, spleen, or adrenals, resulting in advanced disease stage at presentation with associated ascites.

Lymphatic drainage constitutes the second most common pattern of spread. The lymphatic capillaries of the ovary converge on the hilus and follow the ovarian blood vessels in the infundibular ligament to drain to the para-aortic nodes at the level of the renal hilum. Lymphatics also drain along the broad ligament to the hypogastric and external iliac nodes in the pelvis. Less frequently, spread can occur to the inguinal nodes via the round ligament.[128] Approximately 10% to 15% of women with disease that appears confined to the ovary have para-aortic lymph node involvement,[129] which becomes increasingly common in advanced-stage disease. Because of the rich lymphatic supply of the fallopian tubes, lymph node involvement is common even in the absence of tubal musculature involvement.[130] Pelvic and para-aortic lymph node involvement has been reported in 10% to 30% of women with fallopian tube cancer at diagnosis.[131]

Transdiaphragmatic spread occurs to the pleural cavity and is the most common finding in stage IV disease. Hematogenous spread is infrequent at the time of presentation, with only 2% to 3% of patients with parenchymal liver or lung disease. Brain metastasis is also rare. However, >50% of recurrences occur both within and outside the peritoneal cavity at the time of treatment failure.

CLINICAL PRESENTATION

As ovarian cancer has insidious growth and is asymptomatic in early-stage disease, most women do not present until symptoms arise from advanced disease progression. Vague gastrointestinal complaints of dyspepsia, nausea, early satiety, bloating, constipation, or obstipation are common presenting symptoms, as are genitourinary symptoms including frequency, urgency, or incontinence. Other ill-defined symptoms include fatigue, back pain, pain with intercourse, and menstrual irregularities. These nonspecific symptoms can be present for several months but may not trigger diagnostic evaluation until after the symptoms fail to clear with other medical therapy.[132] Detection of early-stage disease may occur by palpation of an asymptomatic adnexal mass on routine examination, although most adnexal masses require moderate size for palpation. In premenopausal women, most of these masses are benign, as ovarian cancer represents <5% of adnexal neoplasms. An adnexal mass in a postmenopausal woman has a higher likelihood of malignancy, and surgical exploration is often indicated. Physical examination findings such as a fixed pelvic mass, palpable upper abdominal mass, and ascites are highly suggestive of an ovarian malignancy. According to a consensus statement on the symptoms of ovarian cancer published by the Gynecologic Cancer Foundation, SGO, and American Cancer Society, new and persistent symptoms of bloating, pelvic or abdominal pain, difficulty eating, early satiety, or urinary urgency or frequency should prompt women to seek medical evaluation.

A portion of women with fallopian tube carcinoma may present with early clinical signs and symptoms. Two triads have been described as pathognomonic for fallopian tube malignancy: (a) pelvic pain, pelvic mass, and leukorrhea and (b) vaginal bleeding, vaginal discharge, and lower abdominal pain. However, the percentage of patients presenting with either triad of symptoms has been reported as low as 11%.[133] Another classic sign—hydrops tubae profluens—is a sudden emptying of accumulated fluid in the distended fallopian tube that causes profuse, watery, serosanguineous vaginal discharge. The discharge is often accompanied by a decrease in pelvic mass size on physical examination. In a meta-analysis of 122 patients with primary fallopian tube cancer, hydrops tubae profluens was a presenting sign in only 9%.[124] In other series,[127,130] it has been specifically reported that neither a triad nor hydrops tubae profluens was present in any of the patients reviewed. When clinically apparent, the fallopian tube may be dilated and mimic more benign pathologic processes such as hydrosalpinx, pyosalpinx, or hematosalpinx.[134] In more advanced disease with tubal wall invasion, extension of a necrotic mass to involve the ovary may give the initial impression of a tuboovarian abscess.

Germ cell and stromal cell malignancies present at an earlier stage than epithelial ovarian or fallopian tube cancers, often related to abdominal discomfort or symptoms of excessive estrogen or androgen production. Granulosa cell tumors may lead to precocious puberty in young girls, and Sertoli-Leydig cell tumors may cause virilization.

DIAGNOSTIC WORKUP

Evaluation of a pelvic mass will be influenced by the patient's age, clinical presentation, and imaging features. An ovarian mass is more likely to be a malignant neoplasm in the pediatric, perimenopausal, and postmenopausal age groups and benign during the reproductive years. Ultrasound is often the first, noninvasive step for the evaluation of a pelvic mass. Sonographic characteristics suggestive of malignancy include irregular borders, a solid component that is not hyperechoic and often nodular or papillary, Doppler demonstration of flow in the solid component, dense multiple irregular septa (>2 to 3 mm), and the presence of ascites, peritoneal masses, enlarged nodes, or matted bowel. Computed tomography (CT) or magnetic resonance imaging (MRI) of the abdomen and pelvis (performed with contrast) may be useful preoperatively to assess disease extent for surgical planning.[135–137] FDG-PET-CT may also be used to characterize indeterminate lesions and has increased sensitivity for the detection of occult metastatic disease when compared with CT alone or MRI, although further study is warranted.[97,138,139] Although limited as a screening tool,[140] an elevated CA-125 level may suggest more advanced or greater bulk of disease and high-grade serous histology but in general is a weak predictor of surgical resection.[141,142] Human chorionic gonadotropin (β-hCG), α-fetoprotein (AFP), total inhibin, and lactate dehydrogenase levels may aid in the diagnosis of and treatment for nonepithelial germ cell ovarian tumors, particularly in women younger than age 35 years with a pelvic mass.[143,144]

Other conditions may mimic ovarian cancer in their presentation, including colon, gastric, and appendiceal carcinomas as well as metastatic breast cancer and primary lymphoma.[145] Although ideally the primary site of disease is determined in the preoperative setting, the diagnosis often cannot be made accurately until the time of surgery, and frozen section pathologic evaluation may guide surgical approach. Among gynecologic malignancies, primary endometrial and cervical cancer may also present with an adnexal mass, and synchronous tumors of the ovary and endometrium have been reported in up to 10% of women, often in the setting of Lynch syndrome or an estrogen-secreting tumor.[115,146] Primary malignancies of the fallopian tube have been difficult to diagnose prior to surgical exploration, as the clinical presentation may be similar to that of salpingitis, ovarian abscess, pelvic inflammatory disease, or even ectopic pregnancy. Occult tubal primaries may be detected only by careful pathologic processing of the fimbriated tubal end.[147]

Referral to a gynecologic oncologist should be considered for any woman with a suspicious pelvic mass, family history of ovarian or fallopian tube cancer, or elevated CA 125.[148] Initial evaluation should include a thorough history and full physical and pelvic examination, laboratory studies (complete blood count, chemistries), and imaging (abdominal and pelvic CT/MRI, directed ultrasound, chest x-ray, or CT). The NCCN guidelines do not recommend the use of biomarkers such as CA-125 or HE4 for determining the status of an undiagnosed pelvic mass.[140] However, a baseline CA-125 drawn prior to surgery may be useful in follow-up to evaluate treatment response and monitor for recurrence. Further evaluation with mammography, upper gastrointestinal endoscopy, or colonoscopy may be indicated in some scenarios to exclude an extraovarian primary cancer.[149] If possible, fine needle aspirate (FNA) for diagnostic purposes should be avoided in patients with presumed early-stage disease to prevent cyst rupture and tumor spillage, although it is often necessary in patients with bulky, nonoperable disease. Comorbid conditions may prompt additional evaluations, including cardiac risk assessment, pulmonary function testing, and nutritional evaluation.

SURGICAL STAGING

Surgical advances in staging and the therapeutic benefit of a maximal safe tumor resection have improved the progression-free and overall survival of women with ovarian cancer over the past two decades. Surgical staging for ovarian cancer is based on the FIGO staging system as shown in Table 75.5,[150]

TABLE 75.5 FIGO STAGING FOR OVARIAN, FALLOPIAN TUBAL, AND PERITONEAL CARCINOMA

Stage I Tumor limited to the ovaries or fallopian tube(s)

IA Tumor limited to 1 ovary; ascites and peritoneal washings negative for malignant cells. No tumor on the external surface of ovary or fallopian tube; ovarian capsule intact

IB Tumor limited to both ovaries or fallopian tubes; ascites and peritoneal washings negative for malignant cells. No tumor on the external surfaces of ovaries or fallopian tubes; ovarian capsules intact

IC Tumor stage IA or IB, and including any of the following:
   IC1: Surgical spill of ovarian or fallopian tube contents
   IC2: Ovarian capsule ruptured before surgery, or tumor on surface of the ovaries or fallopian tube(s)
   IC3: Ascites or peritoneal washings positive for malignant cells

Stage II Tumor involving 1 or both ovaries with pelvic extension or primary peritoneal cancer

IIA Extension and/or implants on the uterus and/or fallopian tubes and/or ovaries

IIB Extension to other intraperitoneal pelvic tissues (below pelvic brim)

Stage III Tumor involving 1 or both ovaries or fallopian tubes, or primary peritoneal cancer, with pathologically confirmed peritoneal implants outside the pelvis and/or positive retroperitoneal lymph nodes

IIIA Tumor grossly limited to the true pelvis, but with pathologically confirmed retroperitoneal lymph nodes or microscopic seeding of extrapelvic peritoneal surfaces (above the pelvic brim)
   IIIA1: Positive retroperitoneal lymph nodes only
   IIIA2: Microscopic seeding of extrapelvic peritoneal sites, with or without retroperitoneal nodal involvement

IIIB Macroscopic peritoneal metastases involving extrapelvic peritoneal surfaces up to 2 cm in greatest dimension, with or without retroperitoneal nodal involvement

IIIC Macroscopic peritoneal metastases involving extrapelvic surfaces more than 2 cm in greatest dimension, with or without retroperitoneal nodal involvement. Tumor may extend to the capsule of the liver or spleen without parenchymal involvement.

Stage IV Presence of distant metastasis outside the peritoneal cavity.
   IVA: Pleural effusion with positive cytology
   IVB: Parenchymal metastasis (including the liver and spleen) and metastases to extra-abdominal organs, including the inguinal lymph nodes and nodal basins outside the abdomen and pelvis

FIGO, International Federation of Gynecology and Obstetrics.
Reprinted from Prat J; FIGO Committee on Gynecologic Oncology. Staging classification for cancer of the ovary, fallopian tube, and peritoneum. *Int J Gynaecol Obstet* 2014;124(1):1–5. Copyright © 2013 International Federation of Gynecology and Obstetrics. With permission.

which was updated in 2014 and approved by the American Joint Committee on Cancer. In 2018, the FIGO/AJCC staging guidelines will combine staging for ovarian and fallopian tube carcinoma.

Comprehensive surgical staging is the mainstay of diagnosis and initial treatment for ovarian, fallopian tube, and peritoneal cancers.[140] Based on improved outcomes, surgical staging and cytoreduction should be performed by a gynecologic oncologist.[151,152] In apparent early-stage cancers, surgical evaluation is required for accurate pathologic staging to guide adjuvant treatment recommendations. In patients with advanced disease, surgery represents the initial treatment by providing optimal cytoreduction. Comprehensive surgical staging begins with an exploratory laparotomy via a vertical midline incision followed by collection of peritoneal washings or any ascitic fluid for cytology. Select patients with early-stage disease may be candidates for minimally invasive procedures if performed by an experienced gynecologic oncologist.[153–155] The surgeon performs a thorough inspection of all visceral and peritoneal surfaces within the abdomen and pelvis, with particular attention to the intestinal serosal surfaces, mesentery, paracolic gutters, hemidiaphragms, gallbladder, and liver. Any peritoneal surface or adhesion that is suspicious for metastasis should be excised of biopsied. In the absence of suspicious areas, random peritoneal biopsies should be taken from the pelvis, paracolic gutters, and/or undersurfaces of the hemidiaphragms.[140] Total hysterectomy, bilateral salpingo-oophorectomy, and omentectomy should be performed with intact removal of the adnexal mass when possible. NCCN guidelines state that pelvic and para-aortic nodal dissection should be performed in patients with pelvic-confined disease or extrapelvic implants measuring 2 cm or less (presumed stage IIIB disease), although recent level 1 data suggest that there is not a therapeutic benefit for lymphadenectomy in clinically node-negative patients with advanced disease.[156] Every effort should be made to achieve maximal cytoreduction of all gross disease in the pelvis, abdomen, and retroperitoneum.[157] In patients with advanced disease, bowel resection and/or appendectomy, diaphragm stripping, splenectomy, partial cystectomy and/or ureteroneocystostomy, partial hepatectomy, partial gastrectomy, cholecystectomy, and/or distal pancreatectomy may be considered. In the operative report, the surgeon should describe the following: (1) the extent of initial disease prior to cytoreduction; (2) the amount of residual disease following cytoreduction; and (3) whether a complete or incomplete resection was performed (including a description of the size and number of residual lesions).[140,158] In select cases, preservation of the contralateral unaffected ovary and the uterus can be achieved in young women wishing to retain fertility who have stage I (stage 1A or 1C, but not 1B) and/or low-risk tumors (early-stage, low-grade invasive tumors, LMP/borderline lesions, or malignant stromal or germ cell tumors).[140,159,160] In the setting of unilateral salpingo-oophorectomy, comprehensive surgical staging should be performed to exclude occult disease. Exceptions to upfront surgical management include patients with significant medical comorbidities who are poor operative candidates and patients with a complex ovarian cyst where extraovarian disease has not been excluded. Neoadjuvant chemotherapy followed by interval cytoreduction may be considered in patients with bulky stage III or IV disease. Before initiation of neoadjuvant chemotherapy, the pathologic diagnosis should be confirmed by biopsy, FNA, or paracentesis. The NCCN guidelines recommend that patients who are evaluated for neoadjuvant chemotherapy be seen by a fellowship-trained gynecologic oncologist before being deemed a nonsurgical candidate.[140]

PROGNOSTIC FACTORS

Tumor stage, grade, histology, and optimal cytoreduction by a trained gynecologic oncologist are the most important determinants of survival for ovarian and fallopian tube cancer. Patients with FIGO stage 1A disease who have negative staging laparotomy have 5-year survival rates of 80% to 90%. If extrapelvic disease is detected at the time of surgical staging, the patient is upstaged to stage III disease with corresponding 5-year survival rates of 30% to 50%. Primary or interval cytoreductive surgery should be performed by a gynecologic oncologist based on published evidence of a 6- to 9-month median survival benefit.[151,152,161]

The volume of residual disease after primary surgery is also an important determinant of outcome.[162–167] The extent of cytoreduction may be defined as complete, no gross visible disease; optimal, residual disease that is 1 cm or less in maximal tumor diameter (GOG definition); or suboptimal, residual tumor nodules greater than 1 cm. Patients who have optimal cytoreduction of tumor have a 22-month improvement in median survival compared to those with suboptimal resection. In a meta-analysis of 18 studies, which included over 13,000 women with stage IIB or higher ovarian, tubal, or peritoneal carcinoma, each 10% increase in the proportion of patients undergoing complete cytoreduction showed a 2.3-month increase in median survival when compared to a 1.8-month increase for those with optimal cytoreduction.[167] Complete cytoreduction has also been associated with improved response to chemotherapy and less platinum resistance.[166,168] Preoperative CA-125 measurement is not independently prognostic, as it likely reflects disease burden. In

contrast, the half-life and nadir of CA-125 during induction chemotherapy are associated with improved outcome in ovarian and fallopian tube cancers.[123,169–173]

Although a strong correlation exists between histologic grade and stage, grade has independent prognostic significance, particularly in early-stage disease. Survival rates for stage I disease with grade 1, 2, or 3 tumors are 96%, 78%, and 62%, respectively.[174] The impact of histologic subtype on survival is less robust owing to other more important clinical variables, including stage, grade, and volume of disease. Patients with mucinous and endometrioid subtypes have improved survival rates compared to serous adenocarcinoma, predominately related to the earlier stage at presentation. Clear cell carcinomas appear to be more aggressive than other epithelial malignancies. The 5-year survival rate for stage I clear cell carcinoma is 60% and for other stages is <15%.[121] Younger patients also have a more favorable prognosis, as they are more likely to have tumors of lower grade and less aggressive histology, as well as better baseline performance status.[175]

MANAGEMENT OF EPITHELIAL TUMORS

Treatment for ovarian and fallopian tube cancer depends largely on the stage and grade of disease at presentation. Table 75.6 presents a general schematic for treatment recommendations for women with epithelial ovarian, fallopian tube, and primary peritoneal cancer.

Early-Stage Disease

Surgical Therapy
Comprehensive surgical staging should be performed in all women with apparent early-stage disease to confirm that the cancer is confined to the adnexa. Fertility-sparing surgery with unilateral salpingo-oophorectomy may be considered in a small subset of women with stage IA disease if the contralateral ovary is normal in appearance.[176] In addition to abdominal exploration and full surgical staging, endometrial biopsy should be considered to sample the endometrium.

Postoperative Management
Early studies by the Gynecologic Oncology Group (GOG) and others have identified a small subgroup of patients with well-to moderately differentiated (grade 1 or 2) stage IA and IB tumors who have a low risk of relapse and may not require adjuvant therapy.[177,178] The NCCN guidelines state that women with early-stage (FIGO IA or IB) grade 1 endometrioid carcinoma of the ovary may be treated with surgical resection and observation with expected 5-year survival rates on the

TABLE 75.6 SCHEMATIC OF THE PRIMARY TREATMENT FOR EPITHELIAL OVARIAN CANCER	
Low risk, early stage	
Stage IA/B, grade 1	Observation
Stage IA/B, grade 2	Observation or IV taxane/carboplatin for 3–6 cycles
High risk, early stage	
Stage IC, all grades	IV taxane/carboplatin for 3–6 cycles
Stage IA/B, grade 3	IV taxane/carboplatin for 3–6 cycles
Stage II	IV taxane/carboplatin for 6 cycles
	IP chemotherapy in optimally cytoreduced patients
Advanced stage	
Optimal cytoreduced stage III	IP chemotherapy
	IV taxane/carboplatin for 6 cycles
	Clinical trial
Suboptimal cytoreduced stage III/IV	IV taxane/carboplatin for 6 cycles
	Clinical trial
	Interval cytoreduction if indicated by tumor response and resectability

IP, intraperitoneal; IV, intravenous.

Section III

order of 90%.[140,179] If observation is considered for women with early-stage grade 2 disease, full surgical staging should be performed.

Adjuvant Chemotherapy

Women with early-stage disease and a less favorable prognosis include patients with grade 3 tumors, clear cell histology, or disease extension beyond the ovarian capsule, positive peritoneal cytology, or pelvic extension or implants (stage IC or II). Various adjuvant treatment approaches have been investigated to improve clinical outcomes, although the optimal management remains controversial. Few randomized trials have been conducted in this population, and they have been limited by small sample size and lack of power to demonstrate a survival advantage.

Nonetheless, two large multi-institutional trials conducted in Europe randomized women with early-stage ovarian cancer to platinum-based chemotherapy or observation following surgery (Table 75.7). The International Collaborative Ovarian Neoplasm 1 (ICON1) trial enrolled 477 women with FIGO IA-C ovarian cancer inclusive of all tumor grades and histologic subtypes.[180] Adjuvant chemotherapy consisted of six cycles of a platinum-based regimen per institutional preference. With a median follow-up of 9.2 years, 10-year recurrence-free survival was 67% for the chemotherapy arm and 57% for observation (HR 0.7, $P = .02$).[181] Overall survival also favored the chemotherapy group (72% vs. 64%, $P = .06$). When stratified by histology and grade, the largest benefit for adjuvant chemotherapy was seen in patients with high-risk disease, defined as FIGO stage IA grade 3, stages IB or IC grades 2 and 3, or any clear cell histology. HRs for recurrence and death for the high-risk subset were 0.52 and 0.48, respectively (both $P < .01$). The second trial, Adjuvant Chemotherapy in Ovarian Neoplasm (ACTION), assigned 448 women with early-stage ovarian cancer to four to six cycles of platinum-based adjuvant chemotherapy or observation following surgery. Women with FIGO IA grade 2 and 3 diseases, all stages IC-IIA, or any clear cell histology were eligible for the trial. Recurrence-free survival, but not overall survival, was significantly improved in the chemotherapy group (70% vs. 62% at 10 years).[182,183] The greatest benefit was seen in the subset of women with non-optimal surgical staging. In a combined analysis of the ICON1 and ACTION trials, adjuvant chemotherapy was associated with significantly improved overall survival at 5 years (82% vs. 74%) compared to observation.[184]

The GOG conducted a randomized trial to determine the optimal duration of adjuvant chemotherapy in women with high-risk, surgical stage I disease by comparing three versus six cycles of carboplatin and Taxol chemotherapy.[185] Rates of recurrence (25% vs. 20%) and overall survival (81% vs. 83%) were similar at 5 years for three and six cycles of

chemotherapy, although six cycles were associated with significantly more toxicity, including neuropathy, granulocytopenia, and anemia. However, subset analysis revealed a significantly lower risk of recurrence for women with serous tumors.[186] At 5 years, recurrence-free survival for women with serous tumors was 83% for six cycles of chemotherapy versus 60% for three cycles (HR 0.33, $P = .04$). Overall survival was also improved at 5 years (86% vs. 73%), although not statistically significant.

Adjuvant Whole-Abdomen Irradiation

WAI was an accepted standard modality in the adjuvant postoperative treatment for completely resected ovarian cancer; however, its use declined significantly after 1975. The practical advantage of WAI was the ability to treat all of the peritoneal surfaces within the abdomen and pelvis, although the delivered dose was limited by the relatively low tolerance of the liver and kidneys. Interest in WAI was established following the publication from Princess Margaret Hospital of a randomized comparison of 147 patients with FIGO IB, II, or III debulked ovarian cancer who received WAI with a pelvic boost or pelvic radiotherapy followed by chlorambucil.[187] WAI significantly improved 10-year survival rates over limited pelvic radiotherapy and chemotherapy (64% vs. 40%, respectively). The greatest magnitude of the survival benefit was observed in patients with <2 cm of residual disease (10-year survival 78% vs. 51%, respectively). No significant benefit was observed in patients with extensive residual tumor.

Subsequent randomized studies did not find a benefit for WAI compared to combined adjuvant treatment modalities. A multi-institutional trial by the National Cancer Institute of Canada (NCIC) randomized 257 high-risk stage I or optimally debulked stage II or III patients to receive melphalan, WAI, or IP phosphorus 32 (^{32}P).[188] All patients had previously received 22.5 Gy to the pelvis prior to study entry. The WAI arm delivered 22.5 Gy to the abdomen in 2.25-Gy fractions. Actuarial 10-year survival rates failed to demonstrate a statistically significant difference among all groups.[189] A second study from the Danish Ovarian Cancer Group (DACOVA) reported similar outcomes for women who received adjuvant WAI versus pelvic radiotherapy with cyclophosphamide or melphalan (4-year survival, 63% vs. 55%, respectively).[190]

WAI has also been shown to be comparable to single agent or combination chemotherapy in the adjuvant setting. A prospective study from the MD Anderson Cancer Center randomized 149 women with stage I through III ovarian cancer and <2 cm of residual disease to WAI or melphalan.[191] WAI was delivered by a moving strip technique with a pelvic boost. Overall survival at 5 years was 71% for WAI and 72% for the melphalan arm. Severe late gastrointestinal toxicity requiring surgical intervention was reported in 14% of patients who

TABLE 75.7	RANDOMIZED STUDIES OF ADJUVANT CHEMOTHERAPY IN EARLY-STAGE OVARIAN CANCER						
Trial	Stage	Study Design	Number of Patients	5-Year DFS%	5-Year OS%	Notes
Observation vs. Chemotherapy						
GOG (1990)	IA, IB grades 1–2	Observation	44	91	94	No survival difference; optimal staging
		Melphalan	48	98	98	
ICON1 (2003, 2007)	I/II	Observation	236	62	70	Largest benefit for high-risk group; no surgical staging
		Platinum-based	241	73[a]	79[a]	
ACTION (2003, 2010)	IA, IB grades 2–3 IC–IIA all grades Clear cell	Observation	224	68	78	Optimal staging in 1/3
		Platinum-based	224	76[a]	85	
Duration of Chemotherapy						
GOG (2006, 2010)	IA, IB grade 3 IC–II all grades Clear cell	3 cycles CT	232	75	81	No survival difference; greatest benefit for serous tumors
		6 cycles CT	225	80	83	

ACTION, Adjuvant Chemotherapy in Ovarian Neoplasm; CT, carboplatin and paclitaxel; DFS, disease-free survival; GOG, Gynecologic Oncology Group; ICON1, International Collaborative Ovarian Neoplasm 1; OS, overall survival.
[a]Statistically significant.

received WAI, attributed to the moving strip technique that delivered excessive pelvic dose. A second prospective trial from the Northwest Oncologic Cooperative Group of Italy randomized 70 women with early-stage high-risk disease to adjuvant WAI or six cycles of cisplatin plus cyclophosphamide. Despite protocol violations in the assigned treatment groups, there was no difference in relapse-free or overall survival when analyzed by treatment received.[192] From these studies, WAI appears equivalent to chemotherapy when delivered in patients with optimally debulked disease but is no longer used. Further escalation of WAI to 27.5 Gy does not appear to provide additional survival benefit.[193]

The role of consolidative radiotherapy in patients with stage I or II disease and clear cell, endometrioid or mucinous histology has recently been raised by population-based studies. In a multicenter retrospective study of 241 patients with stage I and II ovarian clear cell carcinoma, consolidative radiation was associated with a 20% benefit in disease-free survival at 5 years for patients with stage IC or II disease.[194] Following surgical staging, patients were treated with either three cycles of carboplatin and paclitaxel followed by WAI (45 Gy to pelvis and 22.5 Gy to whole abdomen) or six cycles of chemotherapy alone. The survival benefit was most pronounced among patients with negative or unknown peritoneal cytology. Similar results were also seen for patients with stage I or II ovarian cancer of endometrioid, clear cell, and mucinous subtypes in a larger analysis of this population-based study, which reported a 40% reduction in disease-specific mortality and 43% reduction in overall mortality with the addition of consolidative radiotherapy. A survival benefit with the addition of consolidative radiotherapy was not observed in patients with stage II disease or serous tumors.[195] However, at this time, there is no level 1 evidence to support the role of adjuvant or consolidative radiation for patients with early-stage disease and non-serous histology.

Adjuvant Intraperitoneal Phosphorus 32

IP instillation of ^{32}P was extensively studied as an alternative to external beam radiotherapy but is no longer in clinical use. In high-risk, early-stage ovarian cancer patients, randomized trials of adjuvant IP ^{32}P versus chemotherapy from the GOG and Norwegian Radium Hospital found no significant differences in disease-free or overall survival in a population with high-risk early-stage disease.[178,196,197] Given a higher incidence of bowel toxicity and limitations of delivery, ^{32}P has largely been replaced by platinum and taxane combination chemotherapy as the adjuvant treatment for early-stage and advanced disease.

Advanced-Stage Disease

Surgical Considerations

Optimal or complete cytoreduction is one of the most important prognostic factors for survival in patients with advanced-stage ovarian cancer. Cytoreductive surgery in advanced-stage disease may improve the patient's disease-related symptoms such as abdominal pain and early satiety and allow for the ability to maintain nutritional status. Optimal cytoreduction may also enhance chemotherapy delivery and response by removal of large hypoxic tumor masses. Bowel resection may be required to remove metastatic implants involving the bowel mesentery or serosa. Extensive upper abdominal surgery, including splenectomy, partial hepatectomy, partial gastrectomy, partial cystectomy and/or ureteroneocystostomy, cholecystectomy, distal pancreatectomy, and/or diaphragmatic resection, also results in prolonged palliation and improved survival.[157,198,199] Select patients may be potential candidates for intraperitoneal chemotherapy, as discussed below, and consideration should be given to placement of an IP catheter at the time of surgery. Laparoscopy may be utilized to identify

which patients with advanced ovarian cancer have the greatest likelihood of attaining complete cytoreduction with primary surgery.[200,201] However, based upon the evaluation of 2,655 patients in GOG182, patients with larger tumor burden still have worse survival despite aggressive surgery attaining no residual disease.[202]

Second-look laparotomy (SLL) was introduced to assess the extent of residual disease following cytoreductive surgery and adjuvant chemotherapy. Up to 20% to 50% of patients may have residual disease after adjuvant therapy that was not detected on physical examination or by CA-125 levels or imaging. Although SLL demonstrated the prognostic importance of a pathologic remission, it was not found to have a therapeutic benefit in a GOG trial of 800 patients.[203] Therefore, second-look evaluations for the purposes of determining therapy, and not for interval cytoreduction, should be reserved for women enrolled in clinical trials.

Several studies have evaluated the importance of interval cytoreduction following an initial attempt at surgical debulking. In a randomized trial by the European Organisation for Research and Treatment of Cancer (EORTC), 319 women with suboptimally debulked disease (>1 cm residual) were assigned to six cycles of cisplatin/cyclophosphamide chemotherapy or interval cytoreduction after three cycles of chemotherapy, followed by additional three cycles.[204] Progression-free and overall survival were significantly improved with interval cytoreduction (median overall survival 26 vs. 20 months, $P = .04$) without increased surgical morbidity. However, a subsequent GOG trial of 550 women failed to reproduce these results.[205] Following a suboptimal resection in the GOG trial, patients were randomized to three cycles of cisplatin and paclitaxel followed by interval debulking or chemotherapy alone for a maximum of six cycles in both arms. The absence of a survival benefit may be attributable to differences in the chemotherapy used or more aggressive initial surgical management by gynecologic oncologists in the GOG trial. The NCCN guidelines state that patients should be evaluated for potential interval cytoreduction before the fourth cycle of neoadjuvant chemotherapy.[140]

The role of neoadjuvant chemotherapy has been explored in a randomized EORTC/NCIC trial of 670 women with stage IIIC and IV ovarian, fallopian tube, or primary peritoneal cancer randomized to initial surgical debulking followed by six cycles of cisplatin-based chemotherapy or interval debulking after three cycles, followed by three additional cycles.[206] The cohort had extensive bulky disease, with >60% of patients with metastases >10 cm. Although progression-free and overall survival were similar between the two groups, interval surgery achieved optimal cytoreduction more often (81% vs. 42%) and with fewer surgical complications. A major criticism of the trial is that the median survival was significantly lower than that of recently reported US trials (approximately 30 months compared to overall survival averages of 50 months),[207,208] which may be related to selection of higher-risk patients. In a retrospective analysis of the EORTC/NCIC trial, patients with stage IVB disease and bulky tumors had better 5-year survival rates with neoadjuvant therapy, whereas those with stage IIIC and less bulky tumors had a greater survival benefit with upfront surgery.[209] NCCN guidelines state that neoadjuvant chemotherapy may be considered for patients with bulky stage III to IV disease who are not surgical candidates following assessment by a gynecologic oncologist.[140] However, more data will be necessary prior to recommending neoadjuvant chemotherapy in patients with potentially resectable ovarian cancer, as upfront debulking surgery remains the treatment of choice in the United States. In a single US institutional series of 586 patients with advanced ovarian cancer, upfront debulking surgery was associated with an improved median overall survival of 72 months compared to 43 months for those selected for treatment with neoadjuvant chemotherapy.[210]

Section III

Chemotherapy for Advanced-Stage Disease

Platinum agents are the most active class of compounds in the adjuvant treatment for ovarian cancer. Before 1980, alkylating-based regimens such as cyclophosphamide and doxorubicin were used with clinical response rates of 15% to 20%. GOG 47 demonstrated an improvement in clinical complete response rates (51% vs. 26%) and progression-free survival (13 vs. 8 months) with the addition of cisplatin to cyclophosphamide and doxorubicin. Cisplatin has since been used extensively in both single-agent and multidrug studies. A meta-analysis of 49 trials from the Advanced Ovarian Cancer Trialists' Group found that platinum combination chemotherapy improved survival rates over the same nonplatinum regimen (HR 0.88, 95% CI 0.79 to 0.98) and nonplatinum monotherapy (HR 0.93, 95% CI 0.83 to 1.05).[211] The women in the nonplatinum groups routinely received platinum chemotherapy at the time of relapse, likely obscuring the magnitude of the benefit. This meta-analysis also incorporated data from 11 trials that directly compared carboplatin and cisplatin, either as single agents or in combination with other drugs, which suggested no difference in efficacy between the two agents. Carboplatin clearly has fewer treatment-related side effects, including less nephrotoxicity, neurotoxicity, and emetogenic potential, and is considered standard of care. However, carboplatin does have more associated myelosuppression, primarily thrombocytopenia, which is cumulative and may be dose limiting.

In addition to platinum compounds, taxanes have become a cornerstone of the treatment schemas for women with epithelial ovarian cancer. GOG 111 was a randomized study comparing cisplatin and paclitaxel with cisplatin and cyclophosphamide in women with suboptimally debulked, large-volume ovarian cancer. The paclitaxel-containing arm demonstrated improved clinical response rates (73% vs. 60%), progression-free survival (18 vs. 13 months), and overall survival (38 vs. 24 months).[212] A second GOG study of 614 women with advanced disease and suboptimal resection compared single-agent cisplatin to 24-hour infusion of paclitaxel and to the combination of paclitaxel and cisplatin.[213] Cisplatin alone or in combination with paclitaxel resulted in improved clinical response rates and progression-free survival, although overall survival was similar in the three arms. Combination chemotherapy also had lower cumulative toxicity. As several trials have demonstrated the comparable efficacy of cisplatin and carboplatin, combination of carboplatin and paclitaxel has become the preferred first-line chemotherapy regimen. Although the standard dosing of intravenous carboplatin and paclitaxel is every 21 days, a phase III trial from Japan demonstrated significant gains in progression-free and overall survival with a dose-dense regimen of weekly paclitaxel in combination with carboplatin given every 3 weeks[214,215] (Table 75.8). Grade 3 or 4 anemia was more common in the dose-dense arm, although other toxicities were similar. In the GOG-262 trial, weekly paclitaxel was associated with an increase in progression-free survival that was 3.9 months longer than that observed with paclitaxel administered every 3 weeks among patients who did not receive bevacizumab.[216] Carboplatin and docetaxel are also an acceptable first-line alternative and may be considered for patients at high risk for neuropathy.[217] In elderly patients or those with poor performance status, weekly paclitaxel and carboplatin may be considered.[218] Phase III trials have failed to show a benefit for the addition of a third cytotoxic agent to the carboplatin and paclitaxel regimen. GOG 182-ICON5 was a five-arm randomized trial of 4,312 women that compared the addition of gemcitabine, liposomal doxorubicin, or topotecan to carboplatin and paclitaxel. There were no improvements in progression-free or overall survival with any experimental regimen.[219] The recommended intravenous regimens accepted by a consensus of the NCCN panel include (1) paclitaxel and carboplatin given every 3 weeks for six cycles, (2) dose-dense weekly paclitaxel plus carboplatin every 3 weeks for six cycles, (3) weekly paclitaxel and carboplatin for 18 weeks, and (4) docetaxel and carboplatin every 3 weeks for six cycles.[140]

The role of novel biologics in the first-line treatment for ovarian, fallopian tube, and primary peritoneal cancers is under active investigation. Antiangiogenics have demonstrated activity in the recurrent treatment setting, and the addition of bevacizumab to conventional first-line chemotherapy has been tested in two randomized trials. Bevacizumab is a humanized monoclonal antibody directed against the VEGF receptor that may inhibit tumor angiogenesis and improve chemotherapy delivery. GOG 218 reported that the addition of concurrent and maintenance bevacizumab for 15 months significantly improved progression-free survival compared to six cycles of carboplatin and paclitaxel alone (14.1 vs. 10.3 months).[220] The benefit was not seen in the group who received concurrent bevacizumab without maintenance therapy. Rates of hypertension, gastrointestinal perforation, and fistula formation were higher with the use of bevacizumab. With a median follow-up of 17.4 months, overall survival was similar between the treatment arms, as was quality of life. In a subsequent analysis, women with ascites who received bevacizumab maintenance regimen had significantly improved progression-free and overall survival.[221] The ICON7 trial also reported a progression-free but not overall survival benefit with concurrent bevacizumab and carboplatin/paclitaxel chemotherapy when compared to chemotherapy alone although the absolute benefit was modest (2.4 months).[222] The greatest benefit was observed in patients at high risk for progression, defined as FIGO stage IV or >1 cm of residual disease and FIGO stage III (median progression-free survival of 16 vs. 10.5 months). In an updated analysis, the addition of bevacizumab

---

TABLE 75.8 RANDOMIZED STUDIES OF ADJUVANT CHEMOTHERAPY IN ADVANCED-STAGE OVARIAN CANCER

Trial	Stage	Study Design	Number of Patients	Median PFS (Months)	Median OS (Months)	Notes
GOG 172 (2006)	III	IP/IV cisplatin/paclitaxel	415	23.6	65.6	Greater toxicity in IP/IV arm
	≤1 cm residual	IV cisplatin/paclitaxel		18.3[a]	49.7[a]	
Japanese GOG (2009, update 2013)	II–IV	Dose-dense CT	631	28.2	100.5	More anemia with dose-dense schedule
		CT (every 21 d)		17.5[a]	62.2[a]	
GOG 218 (2010)	III–IV	CT	1,873	10.3	39.3	Higher rates of hypertension, GI perforation, and fistula
		+ c. bevacizumab		11.2	38.7	
		+ c/m. bevacizumab		14.1[a]	39.7	
ICON7 (2010)	High risk I–II	CT	1,528	17.4	–	Greatest benefit in high-risk subset
	III–IV	+ c/m. bevacizumab		19.8[a]		

c., concurrent; CT, carboplatin and paclitaxel; GI, gastrointestinal; ICON7, International Collaborative Ovarian Neoplasm 7; IP, intraperitoneal; IV, intravenous; m., maintenance; OS, overall survival; PFS, progression-free survival.
[a]Statistically significant.

did not increase overall survival in the whole study population, although patients with a poor prognosis had a significantly longer survival time with bevacizumab (39.3 months) compared to those who received chemotherapy alone (34.5 months).[223] Concerns about cost and lack of an overall survival and/or quality of life benefit have tempered the widespread adoption of bevacizumab to the first-line chemotherapy backbone. The NCCN Ovarian Cancer Panel has included the addition of bevacizumab to upfront therapy with carboplatin/paclitaxel and maintenance therapy with a Category 2B recommendation.[140]

Several VEGFR tyrosine kinase inhibitors (TKIs) have been evaluated in the concurrent and/or maintenance setting in the upfront treatment of ovarian cancer. A phase III trial of the oral antiangiogenic nintedanib (BIBF 1120) in combination with carboplatin and paclitaxel reported a significant benefit in progression-free survival (17.2 vs. 16.6 months), although a higher rate of serious adverse gastrointestinal events were observed when compared to chemotherapy alone.[224] Pazopanib, a potent multitargeted TKI against VEGF receptor, PDGF receptor, and c-Kit, was evaluated as maintenance therapy following surgical debulking and first-line chemotherapy in a randomized phase III trial of 940 patients (AGOOVAR 16 trial).[225] The addition of maintenance pazopanib resulted in a median progression-free survival benefit of 5.6 months at the expense of increased toxicity, and no overall survival difference was observed.

Intraperitoneal Chemotherapy

Because of the unique peritoneal dissemination of epithelial ovarian and fallopian tube cancer, there has been a significant interest in evaluating IP administration of chemotherapy, which allows for a severalfold increase in drug concentration compared to systemic delivery. However, penetration into tumor tissue may be limited such that therapy is best suited for patients with minimal residual disease after surgical cytoreduction. The National Cancer Institute published a consensus statement in 2006 stating that IP chemotherapy should be offered to every woman with optimally debulked advanced-stage ovarian cancer based on the findings of GOG 172 (Table 75.8), which showed a progression-free and overall survival benefit to IP chemotherapy when compared with intravenous therapy alone (23.6 vs. 18.3 months and 65.6 vs. 49.7 months, respectively).[207] In women with stage III disease, survival was significantly increased by 16 months after IP therapy using cisplatin/paclitaxel when compared to standard intravenous therapy (65.6 vs. 49.7 months). Only 42% of patients completed all six cycles of IP chemotherapy owing to treatment-related toxicity and catheter-related complications, which included gastrointestinal events, abdominal pain, metabolic abnormalities, neuropathy, catheter infection, and blockage. Despite the higher incidence of toxicity, additional support for IP chemotherapy is derived from a meta-analysis of eight trials comparing IP to intravenous administration of platinum-based chemotherapy. IP delivery resulted in a 22% decrease in the risk of death, which translated into a 12-month median survival benefit.[226] NCCN guidelines recommend that all patients with stage III cancer with optimal cytoreduction (<1 cm residual disease) received intravenous/IP chemotherapy. Women with stage II disease may also receive IP chemotherapy, although randomized evidence has not yet been published.[140] Despite the clinical advisory, IP chemotherapy has not been consistently adopted for treatment in women with optimally cytoreduced ovarian cancer given the technical demands and increased toxicity. Patients with poor performance status, medical comorbidities, stage IV disease, or advanced age may not tolerate the IP regimen. The feasibility and effectiveness of IP carboplatin have been evaluated in the phase III GOG 252 study comparing a modified GOG 172 intravenous/IP cisplatin/paclitaxel regimen with a lowered cisplatin dose to IP carboplatin/weekly paclitaxel as well as intravenous carboplatin/weekly paclitaxel (dose-dense regimen). All three arms receive concurrent and maintenance bevacizumab for 1 year. Preliminary results have not shown a significant difference in progression-free survival for the IP chemotherapy compared to intravenous alone, which was 33.8 months for patients with complete cytoreduction and stage III disease, when compared to 60.4 months in GOG 172.[227]

CONSOLIDATIVE THERAPY FOR EPITHELIAL OVARIAN CANCER

Consolidative radiotherapy was introduced in hopes of eradicating subclinical residual disease in women who remain at high risk for relapse following surgical cytoreduction and adjuvant chemotherapy. Despite a negative SLL, 30% to 50% of women with confirmed clinical remission ultimately relapse, most commonly in the pelvis or upper abdomen. Consolidative WAI as well as IP radiocolloid have been evaluated in several studies, although randomized data are currently lacking. Radiotherapy is not currently used as consolidative treatment for ovarian or fallopian tube carcinomas, although it may have a role in the salvage or palliative treatment of select cases.

Consolidative Whole-Abdomen Irradiation

The efficacy of WAI has been demonstrated in early-stage patients with minimal residual disease (<2 cm) after cytoreductive surgery. A few early, prospective randomized trials have evaluated the role of consolidative WAI compared to extended chemotherapy in patients with advanced-stage disease (stage III/IV) after initial surgical cytoreduction, adjuvant chemotherapy, and SLL. In all of these trials, disease-free and overall survival rates were not found to be significantly different between WAI and chemotherapy.[228–230] A possible limitation of these trials was that women with macroscopic residual disease after SLL were eligible for enrollment.

Two trials have evaluated consolidative WAI in patients with complete clinical or pathologic remission following cytoreductive surgery and adjuvant chemotherapy. A randomized study from Austria demonstrated improved disease-free and overall survival for consolidative WAI, with the greatest benefit seen in stage III patients.[231] The Swedish-Norwegian Ovarian Cancer Study Group recently reported their long-term results from a randomized trial of stage III patients.[232] Following primary cytoreductive surgery and four cycles of cisplatin-based chemotherapy, women with complete remission at second-look surgery were randomized to WAI, six additional cycles of chemotherapy, or observation (if pathologic remission confirmed). In the subgroup with pathologic remission, WAI improved progression-free survival compared to chemotherapy or no further therapy (56%, 36%, and 35%, respectively). Overall survival was not statistically different, although statistical power was limited because only 172 (23%) of 742 enrolled patients were randomized to consolidative treatment.

WAI does not appear to compromise the ability for patients to receive and tolerate salvage chemotherapy following relapse, as recently reported in a phase II study from Princess Margaret Hospital.[233] However, the long-term complication rate using conventional radiotherapy techniques is significant. In a multicenter retrospective study from France with a median follow-up of 14 years, late symptomatic enteritis occurred in 20% of patients, of which 8% required surgical intervention for bowel obstruction, and death related to bowel complications occurred in 4%.[234] At this time, WAI is not included in the NCCN guidelines as a treatment recommendation for initial or consolidative treatment in ovarian cancer.[140]

Consolidative Intraperitoneal Phosphorus 32

Randomized data evaluating IP ^{32}P as consolidative treatment following SLL are limited. The Norwegian Radium Hospital randomized 50 patients with stage IA high grade and IB through III disease and negative SLL to ^{32}P versus observation and found no significant difference between the arms.[196] The GOG also conducted a prospective randomized trial of 202 stage III patients with complete clinical remission and microscopically negative disease at SLL.[235] Compared with patients who received no further therapy, those who received [32]P (15 mCi) within 10 days of SLL did not have improved 5-year disease-free survival (36% vs. 42%, respectively) or overall survival (63% vs. 67%, respectively).

Recurrent Ovarian Cancer

Women in clinical remission following initial adjuvant treatment for ovarian cancer may be followed with a combination of physical examination, serial CA-125 levels, and/or abdominal and pelvic CT. Detection of early relapse by a rising CA-125 is fairly specific, although the lead time between biochemical and clinical progression may be up to 6 months. Patients should also be educated about the signs and symptoms of recurrence, such as pelvic pain, bloating, early satiety, obstruction, weight loss, and fatigue.[140] Second-line chemotherapy is not curative; thus, the timing of salvage therapy is controversial. The EORTC conducted a randomized trial of early versus delayed treatment for relapsed ovarian cancer that showed no difference in overall survival between the arms and a decrement in quality of life.[236] These findings have not been widely adopted in the United States owing to criticisms regarding the study design, including lack of stratification by known prognostic factors and nonstandard second-line therapies. The NCCN panel encourages physicians to discuss the pros and cons of CA-125 monitoring with their patients and the implications regarding early treatment and quality of life.

Chemotherapy

The selection of second-line chemotherapy for recurrent ovarian cancer is based on the interval to disease relapse and determination of platinum sensitivity or resistance. The intent of recurrence therapy is to decrease tumor burden, control symptoms, improve progression-free survival, and/or increase length or quality of life. Patients who experience an early recurrence within 6 months of the completion of initial chemotherapy, have stable disease, or progress during initial induction chemotherapy are considered platinum-resistant with low likelihood of cure. Women who suffer an early recurrence do have treatment options, including second-line chemotherapy agents (topotecan, weekly paclitaxel, pegylated liposomal doxorubicin, gemcitabine, oral etoposide, docetaxel), hormonal therapies, targeted therapeutics, and the opportunity to participate in clinical trials. For women with a late recurrence, retreatment with a platinum-based combination is a reasonable option, and the longer the disease-free interval, the higher the response rate to the agents. Preferred platinum-based combinations include carboplatin/paclitaxel, carboplatin/liposomal doxorubicin, carboplatin/weekly paclitaxel, carboplatin/docetaxel, carboplatin/gemcitabine, or cisplatin/gemcitabine.[140] With the exception of those women who have a prolonged disease-free interval, the opportunity for a meaningful second remission is low, and one needs to carefully balance quality of life, chemotherapy-related toxicity, cost, and the patient's goals of care. Several randomized phase III studies are testing the role of antiangiogenics in the recurrent setting with combination chemotherapy. The AURELIA trial evaluated bevacizumab in combination with liposomal doxorubicin, weekly paclitaxel, or topotecan compared to chemotherapy alone in patients with platinum-resistant ovarian

cancer. The addition of bevacizumab resulted in a statistically significant progression-free survival benefit (6.7 vs. 3.4 months) and nonsignificant overall survival benefit (16.6 vs. 13.3 months) when compared to chemotherapy alone.[237] As the gastrointestinal perforation rate in the bevacizumab arm was 2.2%, these combination regimens are contraindicated in patients at increased risk. In the OCEANS trial, the addition of bevacizumab to carboplatin/gemcitabine chemotherapy resulted in improved response rates (79% vs. 57%) and progression-free survival (median 12.4 vs. 8.4 months) in women with platinum-sensitive recurrent disease.[238] In the final survival analysis, there was not a significant increase in overall survival with the addition of bevacizumab when compared to chemotherapy alone (33.6 vs. 32.9 months).[239] A third large multi-institutional trial of 674 women evaluated the role of secondary surgical cytoreduction and bevacizumab in women with recurrent platinum-sensitive ovarian cancer and found that the addition of bevacizumab followed by maintenance therapy until progression improved median overall survival by sensitivity analysis.[240] Phase II studies of bevacizumab have demonstrated single-agent activity in patients with platinum-resistant recurrent ovarian cancer with response rates of 15% to 20%.[241,242] However, one of these studies reported a gastrointestinal perforation rate of 11% in a heavily pretreated population. Based on the phase III trials discussed above, the NCCN panel recommends combination regimens with bevacizumab for patients with platinum-resistant recurrent ovarian cancer, although there is less consensus for those with platinum-sensitive disease.

Emerging data are confirming the activity of PARP inhibitors in select patients with recurrent ovarian cancer. This new class of targeted therapy inhibits key enzymes involved in DNA repair and has been shown to be particularly active in treating cancers in BRCA mutation carriers. In the setting of BRCA deficiency, PARP inhibition results in accumulation of double-strand DNA breaks that are lethal to tumor cells through a mechanism known as synthetic lethality. A substantial number of patients with ovarian cancer have been found to have BRCA-deficient tumors related to germline or somatic mutation, epigenetic silencing, or alteration in microRNA levels. Olaparib has shown single-agent response rates ranging from 28% to 41% depending on dose and BRCA mutation status. In a phase II of 298 patients with germline BRCA1/2 mutation and advanced cancer, olaparib resulted in an overall response rate of 31% for those with platinum-resistant ovarian cancer.[243] In the platinum-sensitive setting, olaparib maintenance therapy resulted in progression-free survival benefit of 8.4 months compared to 4.8 months with placebo for women with relapsed ovarian cancer, although an overall survival benefit was not observed.[244] Single-agent olaparib is now recommended as recurrence therapy for patients with advanced ovarian cancer who have a germline BRCA mutation and received three or more lines of chemotherapy.[140] Olaparib maintenance therapy was recently granted FDA approval based on the results of the SOLO-2 trial, which showed a significant improvement in progression-free survival in patients with germline BRCA-mutated, platinum-sensitive recurrent ovarian cancer when compared to placebo.[245] Two other PARP inhibitors have also been recently granted FDA approval. In the NOVA trial, patients with recurrent epithelial, fallopian tube, or primary peritoneal cancer were stratified by germline BRCA mutation status and randomized to either niraparib or placebo following complete or partial response to platinum-based chemotherapy. Maintenance niraparib resulted in a significant improvement in progression-free survival, with the greatest benefit among patients with germline BRCA mutations.[246] Rucaparib was granted accelerated approval for patients with germline or somatic BRCA mutation who have been treated with two or more chemotherapy regimens. BRCA mutation status was determined by a next-generation sequencing diagnostic test. The overall response rate in a single-arm open-label clinical trial was 54% and ranged from 66% for patients with platinum-sensitive disease to 25% for those platinum-resistant.[247]

In summary, there are three PARP inhibitors that are FDA-approved for recurrent ovarian cancer that clinicians may select from: (1) olaparib for patients with recurrent germline BRCA-mutated ovarian cancer who have received three or more prior lines of chemotherapy or as maintenance therapy following response to platinum therapy for those with platinum-sensitive recurrence, (2) rucaparib for patients with BRCA-mutated ovarian cancer (either deleterious tumor or germline mutation) who have received at least two prior lines of chemotherapy, and (3) niraparib for platinum-sensitive recurrent ovarian cancer patients as maintenance therapy following response to platinum-based chemotherapy, regardless of BRCA or tumor homologous recombination status. Further studies of PARP inhibitor agents as single agents and in combination therapy are under way in patients with platinum-sensitive and platinum-resistant disease.

A number of TKIs have been tested in the recurrent setting as single agents with demonstrated response rates of 3% to 29%.[27,248] These agents include cediranib (targets VEGF receptor and c-Kit), sunitinib (targets VEGF receptor, c-Kit, PDGF receptor, RET, and FLT-3), sorafenib (targets VEGF receptor, c-Kit, RAF, and PDGF receptor-b), ENMD2076 (targets VEGF receptor and aurora A), pazopanib (targets VEGF receptor, PDGF receptor, and c-Kit), trebananib (inhibits binding of angiopoietins 1 and 2 to the Tie2 receptor), and cabozantinib (targets VEGF receptor and c-MET). In the phase III ICON 6 trial, patients with platinum-sensitive recurrent ovarian cancer were randomized to platinum-based chemotherapy with or without cediranib as concurrent and/or maintenance therapy. The addition of maintenance cediranib showed a significant progression-free survival benefit, although at the expense of increased toxicity.[249] Trebananib has also been tested in the phase 3 setting with weekly single-agent paclitaxel and, similar to other agents in its class, resulted in prolonged progression-free survival, but with higher rates of serious adverse events, treatment discontinuation, and chronic edema.[250] Combinatorial therapy with PARP and VEGF inhibition has also been explored with promising results in a phase II study,[251] and large phase III evaluations are underway.

Palliative Surgery

Secondary cytoreductive surgery with the intent of prolonging survival may benefit a select subset of patients with a long disease-free interval, good performance status, and single or few sites of recurrence.[252,253] A recently reported phase III trial randomized 407 women with platinum-sensitive disease at the time of first relapse to cytoreduction followed by second-line chemotherapy versus chemotherapy alone. Eligible patients had an excellent performance status, volume of ascites of 500 cc or less, and complete cytoreduction at diagnosis. The median progression-free survival was 21 versus 13.9 months in favor of surgery. The primary endpoint of overall survival will be reported in subsequent analysis.[254] Palliative surgery may also be considered in women who present with symptomatic tumor masses or intestinal obstruction. However, the risk of perioperative mortality and reobstruction is significant, and the patient's medical condition, performance status, and anticipated life expectancy should be carefully considered before operative intervention. For patients who are not surgical candidates, percutaneous decompression and intravenous hydration with consideration of palliative chemotherapy and/or hospice referral may be appropriate.

Palliative Radiation Treatment

Radiation therapy may be an effective palliative treatment modality in settings where localized recurrences are causing significant symptoms that are unresponsive to systemic therapy. Symptoms such as bleeding, pain, or obstruction in the pelvis, groin, abdomen, or chest may be palliated with an abbreviated course of radiation treatment. Clinical response rates have been reported in the range of 70% to 100%, with complete clinical response rates of 30% to 70% and a median duration of 5 to 11 months.[255–259] Palliative radiotherapy is effective even in patients heavily pretreated with systemic or IP chemotherapy. Pain relief and cessation of bleeding are achieved in >80% of patients and symptoms from bowel or ureteral obstruction in 60% to 75%.[260] A recent report found that response rates to palliative radiation did not vary among patients with platinum-resistant versus platinum-sensitive disease either at the time of diagnosis or time of radiation treatment. However, patients with clear cell ovarian cancer had lower clinical response rates when compared to those with serous or endometrioid cell types, although these patients may still experience symptomatic relief with radiation.[261] When delivered locally to symptomatic sites, radiation therapy appears to be of significant and durable benefit and should be considered for palliative purposes in select patients with symptomatic relapses, particularly in those who are refractory to chemotherapy.

The role of salvage radiotherapy in select patients with isolated pelvic recurrences has been suggested by several reports. In a series by Firat and Erickson,[262] 28 patients with recurrent or persistent disease involving the vagina and/or rectum received palliative radiotherapy delivered by external beam radiotherapy, brachytherapy, or a combination of both. Bleeding was controlled in all cases, and 79% achieved a complete symptomatic response. Of the 21 patients with no evidence of liver or extra-abdominal disease, 2-year survival was 57% compared to 0% for the 7 patients with liver and extra-abdominal metastases at the time of radiotherapy. In the group of 14 patients with pelvic-confined disease, 5 patients had recurrences in the upper abdomen and 4 patients were long-term survivors >5 years after radiotherapy administration. A second study by Albuquerque et al.[263] evaluated the outcomes of 20 women treated with salvage radiotherapy for isolated extraperitoneal recurrence. Most recurrences were in the pelvis, although 3 patients had regional nodal recurrences and 1 patient had an abdominal wall recurrence. The median delivered dose to a tumor-directed volume was 50.4 Gy, and a brachytherapy boost was delivered in select cases. Local recurrence–free survival at 2 years was 89% for patients with optimal debulking prior to radiotherapy compared to 42% for patients with suboptimal debulking or gross residual disease. The corresponding disease-free survival rates at 3 years were 72% and 22%, and overall survival rates at 5 years were 50% and 19%, respectively. In a large single institutional series of 102 patients with epithelial ovarian cancer who received salvage involved–field radiotherapy, 5-year rates of progression-free and overall survival were 40% and 24%, respectively, with an infield control rate of 71%. Of note, the time interval to relapse and subsequent chemotherapy was prolonged following radiation treatment compared to the time interval to relapse before radiation. Furthermore, 25 patients did not experience relapse for a median of 61 months, and patients with clear cell histology had the highest rates of progression-free and overall survival after salvage radiation therapy.[264] Given the exceptional local control rates, minimal toxicity, and long-term survival, select patients with isolated extraperitoneal recurrences may be appropriate candidates for salvage involved–field radiation treatment.

Ovarian cancer metastatic to the brain is a rare occurrence reported in <1% of patients in autopsy cases and in 2%

of clinical series.[265,266] More recent series have suggested an increased incidence as chemotherapy regimens have become more effective.[266] Nonetheless, long-term prognosis is poor, as brain metastases are often a late manifestation of advanced disease, with a median survival time <12 months. In a series of 24 patients with metastatic brain disease treated with whole-brain radiotherapy, stereotactic radiosurgery (SRS), or a combination of whole-brain radiotherapy and SRS, median survival was 8.5 months. Patients with solitary metastatic lesions had significantly improved survival compared to those with multiple metastases, 17 versus 6 months, respectively.[267] Platinum sensitivity was also recently identified as an important prognostic factor in women with metastatic brain involvement from ovarian cancer. In an analysis of 4,277 women treated at six German hospitals, 74 patients (1.7%) had clinical documentation of brain metastases, of which 61 patients received radiotherapy alone or in combination with surgical resection and chemotherapy.[268] On multivariate analysis, platinum sensitivity (HR 0.23) and good performance status (HR 0.45) were associated with improved survival, whereas multiple lesions (HR 4.4) and low tumor grade (HR 3.1) were associated with adverse outcome. Although the extent of extracranial disease was not associated with outcome in this study, it is unclear whether the prognostic importance of platinum sensitivity was related to control of intracranial or systemic disease. In a retrospective analysis from the MITO (Multicenter Italian Trials in Ovarian cancer) group that included 174 women with epithelial ovarian cancer, most of which had platinum-sensitive disease, the presence of extracranial disease (HR 1.8), older age (1.7), monotherapy (HR 2.6), and multiple brain metastasis (HR 1.9) were associated with worse overall survival following a diagnosis of brain metastases.[269]

SPECIALIZED RADIATION THERAPY TECHNIQUES

Whole-Abdominal Radiation Therapy

The clinical target volume for WAI includes the entire peritoneum from the diaphragm to the pelvic floor, encompassing both the visceral and parietal surfaces as well as the pelvic and para-aortic nodes. Conventionally, large anterior and posterior fields have been used. The simulation technique requires attention to the excursion of the diaphragm at the superior margin during respiration to ensure appropriate coverage. The field should encompass the pouch of Douglas inferiorly as well as the lateral extent of the peritoneal margins, which may be located outside the pelvic brim in obese patients. Fluoroscopy may be used to assess the range of quiet respiratory motion. Alternatively, image fusion of CT scans obtained at inspiration and expiration or throughout the respiratory cycle (four-dimensional [4D] CT) may be used to design the treatment fields. Extended source to skin distance may be required in some patients to ensure adequate coverage. Organs at risk that are dose limiting include the kidneys, liver, small and large bowel, and bone marrow. Kidney doses are limited to 15 Gy with customized blocking, and whole-liver tolerance is 30 Gy. The standard whole-abdomen dose is 30 Gy delivered in 1.2- to 1.5-Gy fractions. An additional boost may be delivered to the pelvis and para-aortic lymph nodes to 45 to 50 Gy, depending on the clinical requirements. Patients will need to be monitored for acute gastrointestinal and hematologic toxicity as well as nutritional support.

The use of intensity-modulated radiation therapy (IMRT) to deliver WAI has been proposed as a means to reduce the radiation dose to the bone marrow and kidneys to decrease the incidence of myelotoxicity and renal damage. Dosimetric analysis has demonstrated improved planning target volume (PTV) coverage and significant dose reductions to bones with equivalent kidney sparing using dynamic multileaf collimator IMRT

when compared with conventional fields.[270] The PTV receiving 95% of the prescribed dose improved from 72% to 84%, and the volume of pelvic bones receiving >21 Gy was reduced by a relative 60% from 86% to 35%. Dose inhomogeneity, however, increased slightly, with small regions of underdosing near the kidneys. Similar improvements in PTV dose coverage were reported in a study using IMRT arc therapy.[271] It remains to be seen whether the dosimetric advantages gained from WAI–IMRT will translate to a significant and clinically relevant benefit. Furthermore, technical considerations must be considered with great care given the complex anatomy and delineation of the peritoneal cavity boundaries. Patient breathing motion and setup uncertainties will also need to be addressed. Early-phase clinical trials assessing the feasibility and toxicity of WAI–IMRT as consolidation following optimal cytoreduction and platinum-based chemotherapy are ongoing.[272]

Intraoperative Radiation for Ovarian Cancer

Several studies have suggested that intraoperative radiation therapy (IORT) as part of salvage surgery for locally recurrent gynecologic cancers, including ovarian cancer, may improve local–regional control and overall survival.[273–277] The largest IORT retrospective study to date that reported results of 22 ovarian cancer patients treated with IORT (median dose, 12 Gy; range, 9 to 14 Gy) suggests that the addition of IORT to cytoreductive surgery may potentially improve local–regional control and achieve palliation in highly selected patients with locally recurrent ovarian cancer.[273] Various sites were treated, most commonly the pelvic sidewall. Most patients received additional treatment after IORT, including WAI, pelvic and/or inguinal radiation, and chemotherapy. Local–regional control was achieved in 68% of patients, with a median time to recurrence of 14 months and 5-year disease-free survival of 18% and overall survival of 22%. Overall treatment-related grade 3 toxicities occurred in 41%. Bowel obstruction occurred in seven patients, all of whom received postoperative WAI and two of whom also had a component of local–regional relapse. No long-term neurologic sequelae were reported.

SEQUELAE OF TREATMENT

Acute Toxicity

Acute toxicity from WAI is common but rarely severe. The use of large radiation fields that encompass multiple abdominal organs, including the liver, kidneys, gastrointestinal tract, bladder, spleen, lungs, and pancreas, contributes to the development of predictable side effects. Gastrointestinal side effects are the most common acute and subacute toxicities encountered with WAI given the large volume of bowel within the treatment field. Up to 75% of patients treated with WAI experience mild to moderate diarrhea; severe diarrhea requiring hospitalization and intravenous hydration is seen in 10% of patients. Limiting bowel exposure through the use of shielding or appropriately timed field reductions can minimize or prevent this toxicity. Approximately 60% to 70% may also experience nausea, particularly early during treatment, although emesis occurs infrequently. Premedication with antiemetic therapy 30 to 60 minutes prior to treatment may help to mitigate this side effect. Routine intravenous hydration to prevent dehydration is also recommended. Appetite loss accompanied by weight loss is a frequent concern. It is thus essential to closely monitor and ensure proper nutrition to avoid malnourishment and dehydration that may result in hospitalization and treatment interruption.

Clinically significant liver damage is extremely rare with appropriate shielding.[278] Approximately 50% of patients will develop transiently elevated alkaline phosphatase levels; however, symptomatic hepatitis occurs in <1%.[279] Hematologic toxicity including leukopenia and thrombocytopenia occurs in

10% to 20% of patients, although significant drops in blood counts causing treatment interruption are rare. Splenic damage may occur even at low radiation doses because of the exquisite radiosensitivity of the spleen, resulting in transient reduction in platelet counts.

Urethritis and bladder spasm from pelvic irradiation may occur and should be treated symptomatically. Adequate and careful shielding of the kidneys to limit the delivered dose to <15 Gy is critical to minimize renal damage and failure. Stricture of the ureters or urethra is rare, occurring in <1% of cases and is usually not seen until 3 to 6 months postradiation. Because treatment to the entire peritoneal cavity with adequate margins requires extension of fields above the diaphragm, inclusion of the lung bases bilaterally is required. Chest radiographs may show fibrosis or bibasilar pneumonitis in 5% to 20% of patients but is generally self-limited and rarely symptomatic.

Late Toxicity

Late toxicities following WAI were more common with the moving strip technique than with the open-field technique, primarily because of the higher doses and hot spots that were generated. High radiation doses can exceed normal organ tolerances, leading to permanent organ damage and failure. Chronic gastrointestinal damage (i.e., bloating, intermittent diarrhea) occurs in <5% of treated patients. The overall incidence of bowel obstruction has been reported to be 5% to 10% at 5 years in cases in which IP ^{32}P or WAI is used independently. Approximately 50% of these patients who develop bowel obstructions will require surgical intervention (incidence, 3% to 5%); however, recent data suggest that this incidence may be higher and closer to 10% in long-term survivors at 10 years.[234] Bowel obstructions occur more frequently with doses >45 Gy and in patients with gapped or abutted split fields. In addition, adhesions in the peritoneal cavity and the combination of additional pelvic radiation to ^{32}P or WAI may double the risk of significant bowel complications up to 20% to 25%.[188,196] As with most anatomic sites, escalating doses of radiation come with an increase in rate and degree of toxicity. Major bowel complications from 10 pooled series of 1,098 patients reported an incidence of 1.4% with abdominal dose of 22.5 Gy compared with 14% with 30 Gy.[279]

MANAGEMENT OF GERM CELL TUMORS

In general, the presentation and management of nonepithelial tumors are similar to those of their epithelial counterparts, as patients usually experience vaginal bleeding, abdominal bloating, or pain and typically require surgical intervention and chemotherapy. On presentation, routine workup is identical to that for other ovarian cancers as outlined previously. Pretreatment AFP and β-hCG levels are of particular importance in diagnosis and treatment. An elevated β-hCG with a normal AFP is strongly suggestive of dysgerminoma. Lactate dehydrogenase and CA-125 levels should also be drawn, as the germ cell tumors may have several tumor markers that can be followed (Table 75.9). Variations in surgical manage-

ment and adjuvant chemotherapy and radiation do exist among the nonepithelial tumors, and treatments should consider the patient's desire to maintain fertility while offering the greatest chance for cure.

Most ovarian neoplasms diagnosed in children and adolescents are germ cell tumors, with approximately two-thirds of these tumors being malignant at the time of diagnosis. Germ cell tumors comprise 20% of all ovarian neoplasms and 2% to 5% of all ovarian malignancies. The most common germ cell tumor is the mature cystic teratoma (also the most common ovarian neoplasm); however, fortunately, only the minority contain a malignancy or immature elements.

Dysgerminoma

Dysgerminoma is the most common of the malignant germ cell tumors and also has the highest bilaterality rate (20%), with 10% of the ovaries being grossly involved and 10% being microscopically involved. As shown in Table 75.9, dysgerminomas may secrete lactate dehydrogenase and have elevated β-hCG levels. Most women with dysgerminomas receive a diagnosis of early-stage disease, and 80% present before the age of 30 years. In many instances, young women affected by this disease wish to maintain fertility after therapy. The high rate of contralateral disease confers a greater risk with conservative surgical therapy. Comprehensive staging is recommended as initial surgery for patients who do not desire fertility preservation, although may be omitted in children or adolescents.[110]

Postoperative therapy for patients with dysgerminoma can be separated into those women with stage I disease and those with disease of a more advanced stage. Women with stage I dysgerminoma may be monitored closely without compromising cure. Approximately 15% to 25% of these women will experience a recurrence, although successful salvage treatment with chemotherapy results in survival rates close to 100%. For women with more advanced-stage disease, chemotherapy with three to four cycles of BEP (bleomycin, etoposide, and cisplatin) is recommended.[280] In a report from MD Anderson Cancer Center, >95% of the patients with ovarian dysgerminoma were free from relapse at a median of 7 years follow-up.[281] Of the 16 women treated with fertility-sparing surgery, 10 patients maintained menstrual function during chemotherapy and 13 patients returned to their prechemotherapy baseline. Five pregnancies were reported, and two of the women had difficulty conceiving.

Dysgerminomas are unique in that they are exquisitely radiosensitive tumors. Radiotherapy may be considered for patients who are not candidates for platinum-based chemotherapy. The appropriate radiation dose for dysgerminoma is 25 Gy in 12 to 14 fractions with a boost of 10 Gy for gross residual disease. However, radiotherapy will affect ovarian function and fertility, which must be taken into consideration when recommending adjuvant radiation therapy in a young patient.

Other Germ Cell Tumors

Nondysgerminomas are almost always unilateral. For apparent early-stage disease, unilateral salpingo-oophorectomy appears to be as effective as more extensive surgery. Patients with stage I grade 1 immature teratomas usually require no further therapy after unilateral salpingo-oophorectomy. All others, including stage I grade 2 and 3 immature teratoma, should be treated with three or four cycles of BEP chemotherapy.[140] Because of the low number of diagnosed cases, large-scale studies comparing adjuvant therapy are uncommon.

Extrapolation of data regarding the efficacy of chemotherapeutic regimens in treatment for nonseminomatous testicular germ cell tumors has had a great impact on treatment in patients with nondysgerminoma ovarian germ cell

TABLE 75.9 SERUM MARKERS FOR OVARIAN GERM CELL TUMORS			
Tumor Type	AFP	hCG	LDH
Dysgerminoma	−	+/−	+
Choriocarcinoma	−	+	−
Endodermal sinus tumor	+	−	−
Immature teratoma	+/−	−	−
Mixed germ cell tumor	+/−	+/−	+/−
Embryonal carcinoma	+/−	+	−
Polyembryoma	+/−	+	−

AFP, α-fetoprotein; hCG, human chorionic gonadotropin; LDH, lactate dehydrogenase.

tumors. Patients with less well-differentiated tumors and all those with endodermal sinus tumor, embryonal carcinoma, choriocarcinoma, or mixed germ cell tumors should receive adjuvant postoperative chemotherapy. Various regimens have been used, including VAC (vincristine, dactinomycin, and cyclophosphamide), PVC (cisplatin, vincristine, and cyclophosphamide), and CVB (cyclophosphamide, vincristine, and bleomycin). The BEP regimen was prospectively evaluated by the GOG in patients with completely resected, surgically staged I, II, and III disease and resulted in a 96% disease-free survival rate.[282] NCCN guidelines recommend three to four courses of BEP as the standard treatment for well-staged patients with resected ovarian germ cell tumors. Six cycles of chemotherapy may be considered for patients with gross residual or stage IV disease.

Management of Sex Cord–Stromal Tumors

Sex cord–stromal tumors derive from the intraovarian matrix of mesenchymal and connective tissue elements that supports the germ cells. The most common sex cord–stromal tumors are the granulosa cell tumors, derived from the sex cord cells along with Sertoli cell tumors. The mesenchymal derivatives include fibromas, thecal cell tumors, and Leydig cell tumors. These tumors are responsible for <5% of all ovarian malignancies but account for 90% of all functioning ovarian neoplasms. One-third of the tumors will produce estrogen, progesterone, testosterone, or other androgens. This hormonal expression may lead to presenting signs and symptoms such as precocious puberty, postmenopausal bleeding, hirsutism, or virilization. Sex cord–stromal tumors can develop in women of any age (with the granulosa cell tumors having a bimodal age distribution) with a peak incidence in postmenopausal women around 50 years of age. These tumors typically behave in a benign fashion with LMP. Surgery remains the mainstay of treatment; however, occasionally, postoperative therapy is required, although these tumors are considered relatively insensitive.

Adult granulosa cell tumors account for 95% of all granulosa cell tumors. Most women are diagnosed after 30 years of age, with a median age of 52 years. Abdominal pain, distension, and vaginal bleeding are the most common signs and symptoms. Because of the relative state of estrogen excess produced by these tumors, 25% of women will also have concomitant endometrial pathology, such as hyperplasia or adenocarcinoma.[283] These tumors tend to be large with an average diameter of 12 cm. If a granulosa cell tumor is suspected preoperatively, inhibin A and B levels may be elevated and useful in narrowing the differential diagnosis. Ninety percent of patients present with stage I disease, and the tumors are typically unilateral in 90% of cases. Stage is the most important prognostic factor for granulosa cell tumors; other factors include tumor rupture, stage IC disease, poorly differentiated tumor, and tumor size >10 to 15 cm. The 10-year survival for women with stage I disease is approximately 90%, with 15% to 25% of stage I patients ultimately suffering a disease recurrence. The 10-year survival for women with advanced-stage disease is 26% to 49%.

Juvenile granulosa cell tumors are rare, although they account for 90% of the granulosa cell tumors that occur in prepubertal girls and women <30 years of age.[284] Similar to the adult form, the juvenile tumors may also secrete estrogen; therefore, the prepubertal girls may present with isosexual precocious puberty. This may be the most dramatic presentation; however, the most common presentation is that of an abdominal mass. As with the adult variant, the juvenile variant is rarely bilateral, with bilaterality occurring in only 5% of cases. More than 90% of cases will be stage I at the time of diagnosis, and other prognostic factors apply as with the adult variant. The 5-year survival rate is 95%, and the prognosis remains poor with advanced-stage or recurrent disease.

Most granulosa cell tumors are unilateral and can be treated with fertility-preserving therapy consisting of unilateral salpingo-oophorectomy and appropriate surgical staging. Given the rarity of pelvic and para-aortic nodal involvement, lymphadenectomy may be omitted for patients with stage IA or IC disease.[140] Endometrial sampling should be performed in all women retaining their uterus, as these tumors may be associated with concomitant hyperplasia or adenocarcinoma. In women not wishing to preserve fertility or those who are postmenopausal, complete hysterectomy with bilateral salpingo-oophorectomy is the procedure of choice. Surgery alone is typically curative. However, risk factors for relapse that should be considered in adjuvant treatment for stage I disease include tumor rupture, stage IC disease, poorly differentiated tumor, and tumor size >10 to 15 cm. Adjuvant treatment options for high-risk stage I and advanced-stage disease include observation or consideration of platinum-based chemotherapy.[140] Radiation therapy may also be considered for patients with stage II to IV tumors and localized disease. Inhibin levels, if initially elevated, may be a useful tumor marker for surveillance of patients under observation.[285]

FUTURE DIRECTIONS

Ovarian cancer represents a spectrum of distinct disease processes, ranging from noninvasive borderline tumors to disseminated high-grade serous carcinomas. The cell of origin may be extraovarian in a large proportion of cases, as many high-grade serous carcinomas appear to originate in the distal fallopian tube. Clear cell, endometrioid, and mucinous cancers may arise from metaplastic transformation of the OSE, although an extraovarian origin has been proposed. Recent insights from molecular and genomic studies also support the concept of distinct biologic subtypes of ovarian cancer. Gene expression profiling has revealed greater similarity between ovarian clear cell carcinoma and renal clear cell carcinoma than other ovarian subtypes.[286] High-grade serous carcinoma shares genomic and transcriptional features with the basal subtype of breast cancer, characterized by a BRCA-deficient phenotype.[23] Driver mutations that activate the PI3 kinase signaling pathway and mutations in the tumor suppressor *ARID1A* have been identified in endometrioid and clear cell ovarian cancers, which share a strong epidemiologic link with endometriosis.

The recognition of distinct ovarian cancer subtypes has implications for prevention, early detection, clinical trial design, and the identification of new therapeutic targets, particularly for advanced-stage and recurrent disease. Results from the large screening trials of postmenopausal women in the United States, United Kingdom, and Japan using CA-125 and TVUS do not at present support routine screening for ovarian and fallopian tube cancer in the general population. Future screening strategies may focus on women at greatest genetic risk by high-throughput sequencing and mutation testing. Genome-wide association studies have recently identified new ovarian cancer risk loci.[287,288] Novel screening strategies will also be needed to detect precursor lesions within the fallopian tube, particularly for high-grade serous carcinomas. It is not yet known whether prophylactic salpingectomy without removal of the ovaries is an acceptable prevention strategy for premenopausal women with familial ovarian cancer syndromes. Clinical trials will soon incorporate targeted therapies with blood and imaging biomarkers to assess pathway inhibition and accurately measure disease response. Trial endpoints should also include robust quality-of-life tools to assess the effect of palliative chemotherapy on symptom control as well as evaluation of its toxicity. Although no longer used in the initial management of ovarian cancer, the role of radiation therapy in palliation remains of significant importance for symptomatic recurrence, particularly for women with chemotherapy–refractory disease.

REFERENCES

1. Janovski NA, Paramanandhan TL. Ovarian tumors. Tumors and tumor-like conditions of the ovaries, fallopian tubes and ligaments of the uterus. *Major Probl Obstet Gynecol* 1973;4:1–245.
2. Kol S, Gal D, Friedman M, et al. Preoperative diagnosis of fallopian tube carcinoma by transvaginal sonography and CA-125. *Gynecol Oncol* 1990;37(1):129–131.
3. Siegel R, Miller K, Jemal A. Cancer statistics, 2017. *CA Cancer J Clin* 2017;67(1):7–30.
4. American Cancer Society. *Cancer facts and figures 2017.* Available at: https://www.cancer.org/content/dam/cancer-org/research/cancer-facts-and-statistics/annual-cancer-facts-and-figures/2017/cancer-facts-and-figures-2017.pdf
5. Howlader N, Noone AM, Krapcho M, et al. *SEER cancer statistics review, 1975–2014.* Bethesda, MD: National Cancer Institute. Available at: http://seer.cancer.gov/csr/1975_2014/.
6. Daly M, Obrams GI. Epidemiology and risk assessment for ovarian cancer. *Semin Oncol* 1998;25(3):255–264.
7. Levanon K, Crum C, Drapkin R. New insights into the pathogenesis of serous ovarian cancer and its clinical impact. *J Clin Oncol* 2008;26(32):5284–5293.
8. Karst AM, Drapkin R. Ovarian cancer pathogenesis: a model in evolution. *J Oncol* 2010;2010:932371.
9. Fathalla MF. Incessant ovulation—a factor in ovarian neoplasia? *Lancet* 1971;2(7716):163.
10. Casagrande JT, Louie EW, Pike MC, et al. "Incessant ovulation" and ovarian cancer. *Lancet* 1979;2(8135):170–173.
11. Fleming JS, Beaugie CR, Haviv I, et al. Incessant ovulation, inflammation and epithelial ovarian carcinogenesis: revisiting old hypotheses. *Mol Cell Endocrinol* 2006;247(1–2):4–21.
12. Choi JH, Wong AS, Huang HF, et al. Gonadotropins and ovarian cancer. *Endocr Rev* 2007;28(4):440–461.
13. Cramer DW, Welch WR. Determinants of ovarian cancer risk. II. Inferences regarding pathogenesis. *J Natl Cancer Inst* 1983;71(4):717–721.
14. Medeiros F, Muto MG, Lee Y, et al. The tubal fimbria is a preferred site for early adenocarcinoma in women with familial ovarian cancer syndrome. *Am J Surg Pathol* 2006;30(2):230–236.
15. Callahan MJ, Crum CP, Medeiros F, et al. Primary fallopian tube malignancies in BRCA-positive women undergoing surgery for ovarian cancer risk reduction. *J Clin Oncol* 2007;25(25):3985–3990.
16. Kindelberger DW, Lee Y, Miron A, et al. Intraepithelial carcinoma of the fimbria and pelvic serous carcinoma: evidence for a causal relationship. *Am J Surg Pathol* 2007;31(2):161–169.
17. Lee Y, Miron A, Drapkin R, et al. A candidate precursor to serous carcinoma that originates in the distal fallopian tube. *J Pathol* 2007;211(1):26–35.
18. Shih Ie M, Kurman RJ. Ovarian tumorigenesis: a proposed model based on morphological and molecular genetic analysis. *Am J Pathol* 2004;164(5):1511–1518.
19. Singer G, Oldt R III, Cohen Y, et al. Mutations in BRAF and KRAS characterize the development of low-grade ovarian serous carcinoma. *J Natl Cancer Inst* 2003;95(6):484–486.
20. Obata K, Morland SJ, Watson RH, et al. Frequent PTEN/MMAC mutations in endometrioid but not serous or mucinous epithelial ovarian tumors. *Cancer Res* 1998;58(10):2095–2097.
21. Kuo KT, Mao TL, Jones S, et al. Frequent activating mutations of PIK3CA in ovarian clear cell carcinoma. *Am J Pathol* 2009;174(5):1597–1601.
22. Wiegand KC, Shah SP, Al-Agha OM, et al. ARID1A mutations in endometriosis-associated ovarian carcinomas. *N Engl J Med* 2011;363(16):1532–1543.
23. Bowtell DD. The genesis and evolution of high-grade serous ovarian cancer. *Nat Rev Cancer* 2010;10(11):803–808.
24. Integrated genomic analyses of ovarian carcinoma. *Nature* 2011;474(7353):609–615.
25. Mukhopadhyay A, Elattar A, Cerbinskaite A, et al. Development of a functional assay for homologous recombination status in primary cultures of epithelial ovarian tumor and correlation with sensitivity to poly(ADP-ribose) polymerase inhibitors. *Clin Cancer Res* 2010;16(8):2344–2351.
26. Martin L, Schilder R. Novel approaches in advancing the treatment of epithelial ovarian cancer: the role of angiogenesis inhibition. *J Clin Oncol* 2007;25(20):2894–2901.
27. Liu J, Matulonis UA. Anti-angiogenic agents in ovarian cancer: dawn of a new era? *Curr Oncol Rep* 2011;13(6):450–458.
28. Negri E, Franceschi S, Tzonou A, et al. Pooled analysis of 3 European case–control studies: I. Reproductive factors and risk of epithelial ovarian cancer. *Int J Cancer* 1991;49(1):50–56.
29. Whittemore AS, Harris R, Itnyre J. Characteristics relating to ovarian cancer risk: collaborative analysis of 12 US case–control studies. IV. The pathogenesis of epithelial ovarian cancer. Collaborative Ovarian Cancer Group. *Am J Epidemiol* 1992;136(10):1212–1220.
30. Titus-Ernstoff L, Perez K, Cramer DW, et al. Menstrual and reproductive factors in relation to ovarian cancer risk. *Br J Cancer* 2001;84(5):714–721.
31. Ness RB, Grisso JA, Cottreau C, et al. Factors related to inflammation of the ovarian epithelium and risk of ovarian cancer. *Epidemiology* 2000;11(2):111–117.
32. Mahdavi A, Pejovic T, Nezhat F. Induction of ovulation and ovarian cancer: a critical review of the literature. *Fertil Steril* 2006;85(4):819–826.
33. Brinton LA, Lamb EJ, Moghissi KS, et al. Ovarian cancer risk after the use of ovulation-stimulating drugs. *Obstet Gynecol* 2004;103(6):1194–1203.
34. Kashyap S, Moher D, Fung MF, et al. Assisted reproductive technology and the incidence of ovarian cancer: a meta-analysis. *Obstet Gynecol* 2004;103(4):785–794.
35. Hinkula M, Pukkala E, Kyyronen P, et al. Incidence of ovarian cancer of grand multiparous women—a population-based study in Finland. *Gynecol Oncol* 2006;103(1):207–211.
36. Schlesselman JJ. Net effect of oral contraceptive use on the risk of cancer in women in the United States. *Obstet Gynecol* 1995;85(5 Pt 1):793–801.
37. Beral V, Doll R, Hermon C, et al. Ovarian cancer and oral contraceptives: collaborative reanalysis of data from 45 epidemiological studies including 23,257 women with ovarian cancer and 87,303 controls. *Lancet* 2008;371(9609):303–314.
38. Chittenden BG, Fullerton G, Maheshwari A, et al. Polycystic ovary syndrome and the risk of gynaecological cancer: a systematic review. *Reprod Biomed Online* 2009;19(3):398–405.
39. Van Gorp T, Amant F, Neven P, et al. Endometriosis and the development of malignant tumours of the pelvis. A review of literature. *Best Pract Res Clin Obstet Gynaecol* 2004;18(2):349–371.
40. Orezzoli JP, Russell AH, Oliva E, et al. Prognostic implication of endometriosis in clear cell carcinoma of the ovary. *Gynecol Oncol* 2008;110(3):336–344.
41. Risch HA. Hormonal etiology of epithelial ovarian cancer, with a hypothesis concerning the role of androgens and progesterone. *J Natl Cancer Inst* 1998;90(23):1774–1786.
42. Lacey JV Jr, Mink PJ, Lubin JH, et al. Menopausal hormone replacement therapy and risk of ovarian cancer. *JAMA* 2002;288(3):334–341.
43. Rodriguez C, Patel AV, Calle EE, et al. Estrogen replacement therapy and ovarian cancer mortality in a large prospective study of US women. *JAMA* 2001;285(11):1460–1465.
44. Beral V, Bull D, Green J, et al. Ovarian cancer and hormone replacement therapy in the Million Women Study. *Lancet* 2007;369(9574):1703–1710.
45. Narod SA, Sun P, Ghadirian P, et al. Tubal ligation and risk of ovarian cancer in carriers of BRCA1 or BRCA2 mutations: a case–control study. *Lancet* 2001;357(9267):1467–1470.
46. Cibula D, Widschwendter M, Majek O, et al. Tubal ligation and the risk of ovarian cancer: review and meta-analysis. *Hum Reprod Update* 2011;17(1):55–67.
47. Hankinson SE, Hunter DJ, Colditz GA, et al. Tubal ligation, hysterectomy, and risk of ovarian cancer. A prospective study. *JAMA* 1993;270(23):2813–2818.
48. Bergfeldt K, Rydh B, Granath F, et al. Risk of ovarian cancer in breast-cancer patients with a family history of breast or ovarian cancer: a population based cohort study. *Lancet* 2002;360(9337):891–894.
49. Pal T, Permuth-Wey J, Betts JA, et al. BRCA1 and BRCA2 mutations account for a large proportion of ovarian carcinoma cases. *Cancer* 2005;104(12):2807–2816.
50. Kerlikowske K, Brown JS, Grady DG. Should women with familial ovarian cancer undergo prophylactic oophorectomy? *Obstet Gynecol* 1992;80(4):700–707.
51. Lynch HT, Bewtra C, Lynch JF. Familial ovarian carcinoma. Clinical nuances. *Am J Med* 1986;81(6):1073–1076.
52. Lynch HT, Fitzsimmons ML, Conway TA, et al. Hereditary carcinoma of the ovary and associated cancers: a study of two families. *Gynecol Oncol* 1990;36(1):48–55.
53. Chen S, Parmigiani G. Meta-analysis of BRCA1 and BRCA2 penetrance. *J Clin Oncol* 2007;25(11):1329–1333.
54. Lakhani SR, Manek S, Penault-Llorca F, et al. Pathology of ovarian cancers in BRCA1 and BRCA2 carriers. *Clin Cancer Res* 2004;10(7):2473–2481.
55. Bolton K, Chenevix-Trench G, Goh C, et al. Association between BRCA1 and BRCA2 mutations and survival in women with invasive epithelial ovarian cancer. *JAMA* 2012;307(4):382–389.
56. Rubin SC, Benjamin I, Behbakht K, et al. Clinical and pathological features of ovarian cancer in women with germ-line mutations of BRCA1. *N Engl J Med* 1996;335(19):1413–1416.
57. Tan DS, Rothermundt C, Thomas K, et al. "BRCAness" syndrome in ovarian cancer: a case–control study describing the clinical features and outcome of patients with epithelial ovarian cancer associated with BRCA1 and BRCA2 mutations. *J Clin Oncol* 2008;26(34):5530–5536.
58. Chetrit A, Hirsh-Yechezkel G, Ben-David Y, et al. Effect of BRCA1/2 mutations on long-term survival of patients with invasive ovarian cancer: the national Israeli study of ovarian cancer. *J Clin Oncol* 2008;26(1):20–25.
59. Cass I, Baldwin RL, Varkey T, et al. Improved survival in women with BRCA-associated ovarian carcinoma. *Cancer* 2003;97(9):2187–2195.
60. Boyd J, Sonoda Y, Federici MG, et al. Clinicopathologic features of BRCA-linked and sporadic ovarian cancer. *JAMA* 2000;283(17):2260–2265.
61. Brose MS, Rebbeck TR, Calzone KA, et al. Cancer risk estimates for BRCA1 mutation carriers identified in a risk evaluation program. *J Natl Cancer Inst* 2002;94(18):1365–1372.
62. Piek JM, Torrenga B, Hermsen B, et al. Histopathological characteristics of BRCA1- and BRCA2-associated intraperitoneal cancer: a clinic-based study. *Fam Cancer* 2003;2(2):73–78.
63. Finch A, Shaw P, Rosen B, et al. Clinical and pathologic findings of prophylactic salpingo-oophorectomies in 159 BRCA1 and BRCA2 carriers. *Gynecol Oncol* 2006;100(1):58–64.
64. Piek JM, van Diest PJ, Zweemer RP, et al. Dysplastic changes in prophylactically removed fallopian tubes of women predisposed to developing ovarian cancer. *J Pathol* 2001;195(4):451–456.
65. Carcangiu ML, Radice P, Manoukian S, et al. Atypical epithelial proliferation in fallopian tubes in prophylactic salpingo-oophorectomy specimens from BRCA1 and BRCA2 germline mutation carriers. *Int J Gynecol Pathol* 2004;23(1):35–40.
66. Leeper K, Garcia R, Swisher E, et al. Pathologic findings in prophylactic oophorectomy specimens in high-risk women. *Gynecol Oncol* 2002;87(1):52–56.
67. National Comprehensive Cancer Network. *Genetic/familial high-risk assessment: breast and ovarian. NCCN Clinical Practice Guidelines in Oncology (NCCN Guidelines) 2012.* Available at: http://www.nccn.org

Section III

68. Alsop K, Fereday S, Meldrum C, et al. BRCA mutation frequency and patterns of treatment response in BRCA mutation-positive women with ovarian cancer: a report from the Australian Ovarian Cancer Study Group. *J Clin Oncol* 2012;30(21):2654–2663.

69. Lynch HT, Smyrk T. Hereditary nonpolyposis colorectal cancer (Lynch syndrome). An updated review. *Cancer* 1996;78(6):1149–1167.

70. Pal T, Permuth-Wey J, Sellers TA. A review of the clinical relevance of mismatch-repair deficiency in ovarian cancer. *Cancer* 2008;113(4):733–742.

71. Shulman LP. Hereditary breast and ovarian cancer (HBOC): clinical features and counseling for BRCA1 and BRCA2, Lynch syndrome, Cowden syndrome, and Li-Fraumeni syndrome. *Obstet Gynecol Clin North Am* 2010;37(1):109–133.

72. Wijnen J, de Leeuw W, Vasen H, et al. Familial endometrial cancer in female carriers of MSH6 germline mutations. *Nat Genet* 1999;23(2):142–144.

73. Barrow E, Robinson L, Alduaij W, et al. Cumulative lifetime incidence of extracolonic cancers in Lynch syndrome: a report of 121 families with proven mutations. *Clin Genet* 2009;75(2):141–149.

74. Norquist BM, Harrell MI, Brady MF, et al. Inherited mutations in women with ovarian carcinoma. *JAMA Oncol* 2016;2(4):482–490.

75. Jemal A, Bray F, Center MM, et al. Global cancer statistics. *CA Cancer J Clin* 2011;61(2):69–90.

76. Keal EE. Asbestosis and abdominal neoplasms. *Lancet* 1960;2(7162):1211–1216.

77. Gertig DM, Hunter DJ, Cramer DW, et al. Prospective study of talc use and ovarian cancer. *J Natl Cancer Inst* 2000;92(3):249–252.

78. Jordan SJ, Whiteman DC, Purdie DM, et al. Does smoking increase risk of ovarian cancer? A systematic review. *Gynecol Oncol* 2006;103(3):1122–1129.

79. Tworoger SS, Gertig DM, Gates MA, et al. Caffeine, alcohol, smoking, and the risk of incident epithelial ovarian cancer. *Cancer* 2008;112(5):1169–1177.

80. Chang ET, Lee VS, Canchola AJ, et al. Diet and risk of ovarian cancer in the California Teachers Study cohort. *Am J Epidemiol* 2007;165(7):802–813.

81. Schulz M, Nothlings U, Allen N, et al. No association of consumption of animal foods with risk of ovarian cancer. *Cancer Epidemiol Biomarkers Prev* 2007;16(4):852–855.

82. Lukanova A, Bjor O, Kaaks R, et al. Body mass index and cancer: results from the Northern Sweden Health and Disease Cohort. *Int J Cancer* 2006;118(2):458–466.

83. Calle EE, Rodriguez C, Walker-Thurmond K, et al. Overweight, obesity, and mortality from cancer in a prospectively studied cohort of U.S. adults. *N Engl J Med* 2003;348(17):1625–1638.

84. Chu CS, Rubin SC. Screening for ovarian cancer in the general population. *Best Pract Res Clin Obstet Gynaecol* 2006;20(2):307–320.

85. Bast RC Jr, Klug TL, St John E, et al. A radioimmunoassay using a monoclonal antibody to monitor the course of epithelial ovarian cancer. *N Engl J Med* 1983;309(15):883–887.

86. Tailor A, Bourne TH, Campbell S, et al. Results from an ultrasound-based familial ovarian cancer screening clinic: a 10-year observational study. *Ultrasound Obstet Gynecol* 2003;21(4):378–385.

87. Van Nagell JR Jr, DePriest PD, Reedy MB, et al. The efficacy of transvaginal sonographic screening in asymptomatic women at risk for ovarian cancer. *Gynecol Oncol* 2000;77(3):350–356.

88. Van Nagell JR Jr, DePriest PD, Ueland FR, et al. Ovarian cancer screening with annual transvaginal sonography: findings of 25,000 women screened. *Cancer* 2007;109(9):1887–1896.

89. Menon U, Gentry-Maharaj A, Hallett R, et al. Sensitivity and specificity of multimodal and ultrasound screening for ovarian cancer, and stage distribution of detected cancers: results of the prevalence screen of the UK Collaborative Trial of Ovarian Cancer Screening (UKCTOCS). *Lancet Oncol* 2009;10(4):327–340.

90. Buys SS, Partridge E, Greene MH, et al. Ovarian cancer screening in the Prostate, Lung, Colorectal and Ovarian (PLCO) cancer screening trial: findings from the initial screen of a randomized trial. *Am J Obstet Gynecol* 2005;193(5):1630–1639.

91. Buys SS, Partridge E, Black A, et al. Effect of screening on ovarian cancer mortality: the Prostate, Lung, Colorectal and Ovarian (PLCO) Cancer Screening Randomized Controlled Trial. *JAMA* 2011;305(22):2295–2303.

92. Jacobs IJ, Menon U, Ryan A, et al. Ovarian cancer screening and mortality in the UK Collaborative Trial of Ovarian Cancer Screening (UKCTOCS): a randomised controlled trial. *Lancet* 2016;387(10022):945–956.

93. Kobayashi H, Yamada Y, Sado T, et al. A randomized study of screening for ovarian cancer: a multicenter study in Japan. *Int J Gynecol Cancer* 2008;18(3):414–420.

94. Moyer VA; on behalf of the U.S. Preventive Services Task Force. Screening for ovarian cancer: U.S. preventive services task force reaffirmation recommendation statement. *Ann Intern Med* 2012;157(12):900–904.

95. Burke W, Daly M, Garber J, et al. Recommendations for follow-up care of individuals with an inherited predisposition to cancer. II. BRCA1 and BRCA2. Cancer Genetics Studies Consortium. *JAMA* 1997;277(12):997–1003.

96. Bourne TH, Campbell S, Reynolds K, et al. The potential role of serum CA 125 in an ultrasound-based screening program for familial ovarian cancer. *Gynecol Oncol* 1994;52(3):379–385.

97. Risum S, Høgdall C, Loft A, et al. The diagnostic value of PET/CT for primary ovarian cancer—a prospective study. *Gynecol Oncol* 2007;105(1):145–149.

98. National Institutes of Health Consensus Development Conference Statement. Ovarian cancer: screening, treatment, and follow-up. *Gynecol Oncol* 1994;55(3 Pt 2):S4–S14.

99. Finch A, Beiner M, Lubinski J, et al. Salpingo-oophorectomy and the risk of ovarian, fallopian tube, and peritoneal cancers in women with a BRCA1 or BRCA2 mutation. *JAMA* 2006;296(2):185–192.

100. Kramer JL, Velazquez IA, Chen BE, et al. Prophylactic oophorectomy reduces breast cancer penetrance during prospective, long-term follow-up of BRCA1 mutation carriers. *J Clin Oncol* 2005;23(34):8629–8635.

101. Kurman RJ, Carcangiu ML, Herrington CS, et al. *World Health Organization Classification of Tumours of the Female Reproductive Organs.* Lyon: IARC, 2014.

102. Meinhold-Heerlein I, Fotopoulou C, Harter P, et al. Statement by the Kommission Ovar of the AGO: the new FIGO and WHO classifications of ovarian, fallopian tube and primary peritoneal cancer. *Geburtshilfe Frauenheilkd* 2015;75:1021–1027.

103. Seidman JD, Horkayne-Szakaly I, Haiba M, et al. The histologic type and stage distribution of ovarian carcinomas of surface epithelial origin. *Int J Gynecol Pathol* 2004;23(1):41–44.

104. Malpica A, Deavers MT, Lu K, et al. Grading ovarian serous carcinoma using a two-tier system. *Am J Surg Pathol* 2004;28(4):496–504.

105. Silverberg SG. Histopathologic grading of ovarian carcinoma: a review and proposal. *Int J Gynecol Pathol* 2000;19(1):7–15.

106. Gershenson DM, Sun CC, Lu KH, et al. Clinical behavior of stage II-IV low-grade serous carcinoma of the ovary. *Obstet Gynecol* 2006;108(2):361–368.

107. Bonome T, Lee JY, Park DC, et al. Expression profiling of serous low malignant potential, low-grade, and high-grade tumors of the ovary. *Cancer Res* 2005;65(22):10602–10612.

108. Meinhold-Heerlein I, Bauerschlag D, Hilpert F, et al. Molecular and prognostic distinction between serous ovarian carcinomas of varying grade and malignant potential. *Oncogene* 2005;24(6):1053–1065.

109. Singer G, Stohr R, Cope L, et al. Patterns of p53 mutations separate ovarian serous borderline tumors and low- and high-grade carcinomas and provide support for a new model of ovarian carcinogenesis: a mutational analysis with immunohistochemical correlation. *Am J Surg Pathol* 2005;29(2):218–224.

110. Gershenson DM, Sun CC, Bodurka D, et al. Recurrent low-grade serous ovarian carcinoma is relatively chemoresistant. *Gynecol Oncol* 2009;114(1):48–52.

111. Schmeler KM, Sun CC, Bodurka DC, et al. Neoadjuvant chemotherapy for low-grade serous carcinoma of the ovary or peritoneum. *Gynecol Oncol* 2008;108(3):510–514.

112. Pecorelli S, Odicino F, Maisonneuve P, et al. FIGO annual report of the results of treatment in gynaecological cancer. Carcinoma of the ovary. *J Epidemiol Biostat* 1998;3(75):75–102.

113. Skirnisdottir I, Garmo H, Wilander E, et al. Borderline ovarian tumors in Sweden 1960–2005: trends in incidence and age at diagnosis compared to ovarian cancer. *Int J Cancer* 2008;123(8):1897–1901.

114. Sherman ME, Mink PJ, Curtis R, et al. Survival among women with borderline ovarian tumors and ovarian carcinoma: a population-based analysis. *Cancer* 2004;100(5):1045–1052.

115. Soliman PT, Slomovitz BM, Broaddus RR, et al. Synchronous primary cancers of the endometrium and ovary: a single institution review of 84 cases. *Gynecol Oncol* 2004;94(2):456–462.

116. Storey DJ, Rush R, Stewart M, et al. Endometrioid epithelial ovarian cancer: 20 years of prospectively collected data from a single center. *Cancer* 2008;112(10):2211–2220.

117. Zaino R, Whitney C, Brady MF, et al. Simultaneously detected endometrial and ovarian carcinomas—a prospective clinicopathologic study of 74 cases: a Gynecologic Oncology Group study. *Gynecol Oncol* 2001;83(2):355–362.

118. Seidman JD, Ronnett BM, Kurman RJ. Pathology of borderline (low malignant potential) ovarian tumours. *Best Pract Res Clin Obstet Gynaecol* 2002;16(4):499–512.

119. Yemelyanova AV, Vang R, Judson K, et al. Distinction of primary and metastatic mucinous tumors involving the ovary: analysis of size and laterality data by primary site with reevaluation of an algorithm for tumor classification. *Am J Surg Pathol* 2008;32(1):128–138.

120. Hart WR. Mucinous tumors of the ovary: a review. *Int J Gynecol Pathol* 2005;24(1):4–25.

121. Sugiyama T, Kamura T, Kigawa J, et al. Clinical characteristics of clear cell carcinoma of the ovary: a distinct histologic type with poor prognosis and resistance to platinum-based chemotherapy. *Cancer* 2000;88(11):2584–2589.

122. Alvarado-Cabrero I, Young RH, Vamvakas EC, et al. Carcinoma of the fallopian tube: a clinicopathological study of 105 cases with observations on staging and prognostic factors. *Gynecol Oncol* 1999;72(3):367–379.

123. Baekelandt M, Jorunn Nesbakken A, Kristensen GB, et al. Carcinoma of the fallopian tube. *Cancer* 2000;89(10):2076–2084.

124. Nordin AJ. Primary carcinoma of the fallopian tube: a 20-year literature review. *Obstet Gynecol Surv* 1994;49(5):349–361.

125. Anbrokh GB, Anbrokh YM. Morphology of metastatic cancer of the fallopian tube in uterine cervix carcinoma. *Neoplasma* 1975;22(1):73–79.

126. Pickel H, Lahousen M, Stettner H, et al. The spread of ovarian cancer. *Baillieres Clin Obstet Gynaecol* 1989;3(1):3–12.

127. Roberts JA, Lifshitz S. Primary adenocarcinoma of the fallopian tube. *Gynecol Oncol* 1982;13(3):301–308.

128. Piver MS, Nitz U, Bender HG. Malignancies of the ovaries. In: Vahrson H, ed. *Radiation oncology of gynecological cancers.* Berlin, Germany: Springer, 1997:297–396.

129. Piver MS, Barlow JJ, Lele SB. Incidence of subclinical metastasis in stage I and II ovarian carcinoma. *Obstet Gynecol* 1978;52(1):100–104.

130. Sedlis A. Carcinoma of the fallopian tube. *Surg Clin North Am* 1978;58(1):121–129.

131. Maxson WZ, Stehman FB, Ulbright TM, et al. Primary carcinoma of the fallopian tube: evidence for activity of cisplatin combination therapy. *Gynecol Oncol* 1987;26(3):305–313.

132. Yawn BP, Barrette BA, Wollan PC. Ovarian cancer: the neglected diagnosis. *Mayo Clin Proc* 2004;79(10):1277–1282.

133. Hanton EM, Malkasian GD Jr, Dahlin DC, et al. Primary carcinoma of the fallopian tube. *Am J Obstet Gynecol* 1966;94(6):832–839.

134. Anbrokh YM. Macroscopic characteristics of cancer of the fallopian tube. *Neoplasma* 1970;17(5):557–564.

135. Dodge JE, Covens AL, Lacchetti C, et al. Management of a suspicious adnexal mass: a clinical practice guideline. *Curr Oncol* 2012;19(4):e244–e257.

136. Harris RD, Javitt MC, Glanc P, et al. ACR Appropriateness Criteria® clinically suspected adnexal mass. *Ultrasound Q* 2013;29(1):79–86.

137. American College of Obstetricians and Gynecologists. ACOG Practice Bulletin. Management of adnexal masses. *Obstet Gynecol* 2007;110(1):201–214.

138. Castellucci P, Perrone AM, Picchio M, et al. Diagnostic accuracy of 18F-FDG PET/CT in characterizing ovarian lesions and staging ovarian cancer: correlation with transvaginal ultrasonography, computed tomography, and histology. *Nucl Med Commun* 2007;28(8):589–595.

139. Yamamoto Y, Oguri H, Yamada R, et al. Preoperative evaluation of pelvic masses with combined 18F-fluorodeoxyglucose position emission tomographic and computed tomography. *Int J Gynaecol Obstet* 2008;102:124–127.

140. National Comprehensive Cancer Network. *Ovarian cancer including fallopian tube cancer and primary peritoneal cancer. NCCN Clinical Practice Guidelines in Oncology (NCCN Guidelines) 2017*. Available at: http://www.nccn.org.

141. Memarzadeh S, Lee SB, Berek JS, et al. CA125 levels are a weak predictor of optimal cytoreductive surgery in patients with advanced epithelial ovarian cancer. *Int J Gynecol Cancer* 2003;13(2):120–124.

142. Cooper BC, Sood AK, Davis CS, et al. Preoperative CA 125 levels: an independent prognostic factor for epithelial ovarian cancer. *Obstet Gynecol* 2002;100(1):59–64.

143. Gregory JJ, Jr, Finlay JL. Alpha-fetoprotein and beta-human chorionic gonadotropin: their clinical significance as tumor markers. *Drugs* 1999;57:463–467.

144. Kawai M, Furuhashi Y, Kano T, et al. Alpha-fetoprotein in malignant germ cells tumors of the ovary. *Gynecol Oncol* 1990;39:160–166.

145. Young RH. From Krukenberg to today: the ever present problems posed by metastatic tumors in the ovary. Part II. *Adv Anat Pathol* 2007;14(3):149–177.

146. Zaino R, Whitney C, Brady MF, et al. Simultaneously detected endometrial and ovarian carcinomas—a prospective clinicopathologic study of 74 cases: a gynecologic oncology group study. *Gynecol Oncol* 2001;83(2):355.

147. Gilks B, Movahedi-Lankarani S, Baker PM, et al. *Protocol for the examination of specimens from patients with carcinoma of the ovary or fallopian tube: based on the AJCC/UICC TNM*. 7th ed. Northfield, Illinois: College of American Pathologists; 2016.

148. American College of Obstetricians and Gynecologists. ACOG Committee Opinion: number 280, December 2002. The role of the generalist obstetrician-gynecologist in the early detection of ovarian cancer. *Gynecol Oncol* 2002;87(3):237–239.

149. Ledermann JA, Luvero D, Shafer A, et al. Gynecologic Cancer InterGroup (GCIG) consensus review for mucinous ovarian carcinoma. *Int J Gynecol Cancer* 2014;24(9 Suppl 3):S14–S19.

150. Prat J, FIGO guidelines: staging classification for cancer of the ovary, fallopian tube, and peritoneum. *Int J Gynaecol Obstet* 2014;124:1–5.

151. Earle CC, Schrag D, Neville BA, et al. Effect of surgeon specialty on processes of care and outcomes for ovarian cancer patients. *J Natl Cancer Inst* 2006;98(3):172–180.

152. Du Bois A, Quinn M, Thigpen T, et al. 2004 consensus statements on the management of ovarian cancer: final document of the 3rd International Gynecologic Cancer Intergroup Ovarian Cancer Consensus Conference (GCIG OCCC 2004). *Ann Oncol* 2005;16(Suppl 8):viii7–viii12.

153. Schorge JO, Eisenhauer EE, Chi DS. Current surgical management of ovarian cancer. *Hematol Oncol Clin North Am* 2012;26(1):93–109.

154. Park JY, Kim DY, Suh DS, et al. Comparison of laparoscopy and laparotomy in surgical staging of early-stage ovarian and fallopian tubal cancer. *Ann Surg Oncol* 2008;15(7):2012–2019.

155. Covens AL, Dodge JE, Lacchetti C, et al. Surgical management of a suspicious adnexal mass: a systematic review. *Gynecol Oncol* 2012;126(1):149–156.

156. Harter P, Sehouli J, Lorusso D, et al. LION: lymphadenectomy in ovarian neoplasms—a prospective randomized AGO study group led gynecologic cancer intergroup trial. *J Clin Oncol* 2017:35.

157. Chi DS, Eisenhauser EL, Zivanovic O, et al. Improved progression-free and overall survival in advanced ovarian cancer as a result of a change in surgical paradigm. *Gynecol Oncol* 2009;114:26–31.

158. Cliby WA, Powell MA, Al-Hammadi N, et al. Ovarian cancer in the United States: contemporary patterns of care associated with improved survival. *Gynecol Oncol* 2015;136(1):11–17.

159. Wright JD, Shah M, Mathew L, et al. Fertility preservation in young women with epithelial ovarian cancer. *Cancer* 2009;115(18):4118–4126.

160. Satoh T, Hatae M, Watanabe Y, et al. Outcomes of fertility-sparing surgery for stage I epithelial ovarian cancer: a proposal for patient selection. *J Clin Oncol* 2010;28(10):1727–1732.

161. Giede KC, Kieser K, Dodge J, et al. Who should operate on patients with ovarian cancer? An evidence-based review. *Gynecol Oncol* 2005;99(2):447–461.

162. Hoskins WJ, McGuire WP, Brady MF, et al. The effect of diameter of largest residual disease on survival after primary cytoreductive surgery in patients with suboptimal residual epithelial ovarian carcinoma. *Am J Obstet Gynecol* 1994;170(4):974–979; discussion 9–80.

163. Eisenkop SM, Friedman RL, Wang HJ. Complete cytoreductive surgery is feasible and maximizes survival in patients with advanced epithelial ovarian cancer: a prospective study. *Gynecol Oncol* 1998;69(2):103–108.

164. Winter WE III, Maxwell GL, Tian C, et al. Prognostic factors for stage III epithelial ovarian cancer: a Gynecologic Oncology Group study. *J Clin Oncol* 2007;25(24):3621–3627.

165. Hoskins WJ, Bundy BN, Thigpen JT, et al. The influence of cytoreductive surgery on recurrence-free interval and survival in small-volume stage III epithelial ovarian cancer: a Gynecologic Oncology Group study. *Gynecol Oncol* 1992;47(2):159–166.

166. Elattar A, Bryant A, Winter-Roach BA, et al. Optimal primary surgical treatment for advanced epithelial ovarian cancer. *Cochrane Database Syst Rev* 2011;(8):CD007565. doi: 10.1002/14651858.CD007565.pub2.

167. Chang SJ, Hodeib M, Chang J, et al. Survival impact of complete cytoreduction to no gross residual disease for advanced-stage ovarian cancer: a meta-analysis. *Gynecol Oncol* 2013;130(3):493–498.

168. Eisenhauer EL, Abu-Rustum NR, Sonoda Y, et al. The effect of maximal surgical cytoreduction on sensitivity to platinum-taxane chemotherapy and subsequent survival in patients with advanced ovarian cancer. *Gynecol Oncol* 2008;108(2):276–281.

169. Fayers PM, Rustin G, Wood R, et al. The prognostic value of serum CA 125 in patients with advanced ovarian carcinoma: an analysis of 573 patients by the Medical Research Council Working Party on Gynaecological Cancer. *Int J Gynecol Cancer* 1993;3(5):285–292.

170. Riedinger JM, Wafflart J, Ricolleau G, et al. CA 125 half-life and CA 125 nadir during induction chemotherapy are independent predictors of epithelial ovarian cancer outcome: results of a French multicentric study. *Ann Oncol* 2006;17(8):1234–1238.

171. Hefler LA, Rosen AC, Graf AH, et al. The clinical value of serum concentrations of cancer antigen 125 in patients with primary fallopian tube carcinoma: a multicenter study. *Cancer* 2000;89(7):1555–1560.

172. Zorn KK, Tian C, McGuire WP, et al. The prognostic value of pretreatment CA 125 in patients with advanced ovarian carcinoma: a Gynecologic Oncology Group study. *Cancer* 2009;115(5):1028–1035.

173. Makar AP, Kristensen GB, Kaern J, et al. Prognostic value of pre- and postoperative serum CA 125 levels in ovarian cancer: new aspects and multivariate analysis. *Obstet Gynecol* 1992;79(6):1002–1010.

174. Carey MS, Dembo AJ, Simm JE, et al. Testing the validity of a prognostic classification in patients with surgically optimal ovarian carcinoma: a 15-year review. *Int J Gynecol Cancer* 1993;3(1):24–35.

175. Klar M, Hasenburg A, Hasanov M, et al. Prognostic factors in young ovarian cancer patients: An analysis of four prospective phase III intergroup trials of the AGO Study Group, GINECO and NSGO. *Eur J Cancer* 2016;66:114.

176. Maltaris T, Boehm D, Dittrich R, et al. Reproduction beyond cancer: a message of hope for young women. *Gynecol Oncol* 2006;103(3):1109–1121.

177. Vergote I, De Brabanter J, Fyles A, et al. Prognostic importance of degree of differentiation and cyst rupture in stage I invasive epithelial ovarian carcinoma. *Lancet* 2001;357(9251):176–182.

178. Young RC, Walton LA, Ellenberg SS, et al. Adjuvant therapy in stage I and stage II epithelial ovarian cancer. Results of two prospective randomized trials. *N Engl J Med* 1990;322(15):1021–1027.

179. Winter-Roach BA, Kitchener HC, Dickinson HO. Adjuvant (post-surgery) chemotherapy for early stage epithelial ovarian cancer. *Cochrane Database Syst Rev* 2009;(3):CD004706.

180. Colombo N, Guthrie D, Chiari S, et al. International Collaborative Ovarian Neoplasm trial 1: a randomized trial of adjuvant chemotherapy in women with early-stage ovarian cancer. *J Natl Cancer Inst* 2003;95(2):125–132.

181. Swart A. Long-term follow-up of women enrolled in a randomized trial of adjuvant chemotherapy for early stage ovarian cancer (ICON1). *J Clin Oncol* 2007;25(Suppl 18):5509.

182. Trimbos B, Timmers P, Pecorelli S, et al. Surgical staging and treatment of early ovarian cancer: long-term analysis from a randomized trial. *J Natl Cancer Inst* 2010;102(13):982–987.

183. Trimbos JB, Vergote I, Bolis G, et al. Impact of adjuvant chemotherapy and surgical staging in early-stage ovarian carcinoma: European Organisation for Research and Treatment of Cancer-Adjuvant ChemoTherapy in Ovarian Neoplasm trial. *J Natl Cancer Inst* 2003;95(2):113–125.

184. Trimbos JB, Parmar M, Vergote I, et al. International Collaborative Ovarian Neoplasm trial 1 and Adjuvant ChemoTherapy in Ovarian Neoplasm trial: two parallel randomized phase III trials of adjuvant chemotherapy in patients with early-stage ovarian carcinoma. *J Natl Cancer Inst* 2003;95(2):105–112.

185. Bell J, Brady MF, Young RC, et al. Randomized phase III trial of three versus six cycles of adjuvant carboplatin and paclitaxel in early stage epithelial ovarian carcinoma: a Gynecologic Oncology Group study. *Gynecol Oncol* 2006;102(3):432–439.

186. Chan JK, Tian C, Fleming GF, et al. The potential benefit of 6 vs. 3 cycles of chemotherapy in subsets of women with early-stage high-risk epithelial ovarian cancer: an exploratory analysis of a Gynecologic Oncology Group study. *Gynecol Oncol* 2010;116(3):301–306.

187. Dembo AJ, Bush RS, Beale FA, et al. Ovarian carcinoma: improved survival following abdominopelvic irradiation in patients with a completed pelvic operation. *Am J Obstet Gynecol* 1979;134(7):793–800.

188. Klaassen D, Shelley W, Starreveld A, et al. Early stage ovarian cancer: a randomized clinical trial comparing whole abdominal radiotherapy, melphalan, and intraperitoneal chromic phosphate: a National Cancer Institute of Canada Clinical Trials Group report. *J Clin Oncol* 1988;6(8):1254–1263.

189. Dent SF, Klaassen D, Pater JL, et al. Second primary malignancies following the treatment of early stage ovarian cancer: update of a study by the National Cancer Institute of Canada—Clinical Trials Group (NCIC-CTG). *Ann Oncol* 2000;11(1):65–68.

190. Sell A, Bertelsen K, Andersen JE, et al. Randomized study of whole-abdomen irradiation versus pelvic irradiation plus cyclophosphamide in treatment of early ovarian cancer. *Gynecol Oncol* 1990;37(3):367–373.

191. Smith JP, Rutledge FN, Delclos L. Postoperative treatment of early cancer of the ovary: a random trial between postoperative irradiation and chemotherapy. *Natl Cancer Inst Monogr* 1975;42:149–153.

192. Chiara S, Conte P, Franzone P, et al. High-risk early-stage ovarian cancer. Randomized clinical trial comparing cisplatin plus cyclophosphamide versus whole abdominal radiotherapy. *Am J Clin Oncol* 1994;17(1):72–76.
193. Fyles AW, Thomas GM, Pintilie M, et al. A randomized study of two doses of abdominopelvic radiation therapy for patients with optimally debulked stage I, II, and III ovarian cancer. *Int J Radiat Oncol Biol Phys* 1998;41(3): 543–549.
194. Hoskins PJ, Le N, Gilks B, et al. Low-stage ovarian clear cell carcinoma: population-based outcomes in British Columbia, Canada, with evidence for a survival benefit as a result of irradiation. *J Clin Oncol* 2012;30(14):1656–1662.
195. Swenerton KD, Santos JL, Gilks CB, et al. Histotype predicts the curative potential of radiotherapy: the example of ovarian cancers. *Ann Oncol* 2011;22(2):341–347.
196. Vergote IB, Winderen M, De Vos LN, et al. Intraperitoneal radioactive phosphorus therapy in ovarian carcinoma. Analysis of 313 patients treated primarily or at second-look laparotomy. *Cancer* 1993;71(7):2250–2260.
197. Young RC, Brady MF, Nieberg RK, et al. Adjuvant treatment for early ovarian cancer: a randomized phase III trial of intraperitoneal 32P or intravenous cyclophosphamide and cisplatin—a Gynecologic Oncology Group study. *J Clin Oncol* 2003;21(23):4350–4355.
198. Eisenhauer EL, Abu-Rustum NR, Sonoda Y, et al. The addition of extensive upper abdominal surgery to achieve optimal cytoreduction improves survival in patients with stages IIIC-IV epithelial ovarian cancer. *Gynecol Oncol* 2006;103(3):1083–1090.
199. Wimberger P, Lehmann N, Kimmig R, et al. Prognostic factors for complete debulking in advanced ovarian cancer and its impact on survival. An exploratory analysis of a prospectively randomized phase III study of the Arbeitsgemeinschaft Gynaekologische Onkologie Ovarian Cancer Study Group (AGO-OVAR). *Gynecol Oncol* 2007;106(1):69–74.
200. Rutten MJ, van Mears HS, van de Vrie R, et al. Laparoscopy to predict the result of primary cytoreductive surgery in patients with advanced ovarian cancer: a randomized controlled trial. *J Clin Oncol* 2017;35(6):613–621.
201. Gomez-Higaldo NR, Martinez-Cannon BA, Nick AM, et al. Predictors of optimal cytoreduction in patients with newly diagnosed advanced-stage epithelial ovarian cancer: time to incorporate laparoscopic assessment into standard of care. *Gynecol Oncol* 2015;137(3):553–558.
202. Horowitz NS, Miller A, Rungruang B, et al. Does aggressive surgery improve outcomes? Interaction between preoperative disease burden and complex surgery in patients with advanced-stage ovarian cancer: an analysis of GOG 182. *J Clin Oncol* 2015;33(8):937–943.
203. Greer BE, Bundy BN, Ozols RF, et al. Implications of second-look laparotomy in the context of optimally resected stage III ovarian cancer: a non-randomized comparison using an explanatory analysis: a Gynecologic Oncology Group study. *Gynecol Oncol* 2005;99(1):71–79.
204. Van der Burg ME, van Lent M, Buyse M, et al. The effect of debulking surgery after induction chemotherapy on the prognosis in advanced epithelial ovarian cancer. Gynecological Cancer Cooperative Group of the European Organization for Research and Treatment of Cancer. *N Engl J Med* 1995;332(10): 629–634.
205. Rose PG, Nerenstone S, Brady MF, et al. Secondary surgical cytoreduction for advanced ovarian carcinoma. *N Engl J Med* 2004;351(24):2489–2497.
206. Vergote I, Trope CG, Amant F, et al. Neoadjuvant chemotherapy or primary surgery in stage IIIC or IV ovarian cancer. *N Engl J Med* 2010;363(10):943–953.
207. Armstrong DK, Bundy B, Wenzel L, et al. Intraperitoneal cisplatin and paclitaxel in ovarian cancer. *N Engl J Med* 2006;354(1):34–43.
208. Chi DS, Musa F, Dao F, et al. An analysis of patients with bulky advanced stage ovarian, tubal, and peritoneal carcinoma treated with primary debulking surgery (PDS) during an identical time period as the randomized EORTC-NCIC trial of PDS vs neoadjuvant chemotherapy (NACT). *Gynecol Oncol* 2012;124(1):10–14.
209. van Meurs HS, Tajik P, Hof MH, et al. Which patients benefit most from primary surgery or neoadjuvant chemotherapy in stage IIIC or IV ovarian cancer? An exploratory analysis of the European Organisation for Research and Treatment of Cancer 55971 randomised trial. *Eur J Cancer* 2013;49(15):3191–3201.
210. Mueller JJ, Zhou QC, Iasonos A, et al. Neoadjuvant chemotherapy and primary debulking surgery utilization for advanced-stage ovarian cancer at a comprehensive cancer center. *Gynecol Oncol* 2016;140(3):436–442.
211. Chemotherapy for advanced ovarian cancer. Advanced Ovarian Cancer Trialists Group. *Cochrane Database Syst Rev* 2000;(2):CD001418.
212. McGuire WP, Hoskins WJ, Brady MF, et al. Cyclophosphamide and cisplatin compared with paclitaxel and cisplatin in patients with stage III and stage IV ovarian cancer. *N Engl J Med* 1996;334(1):1–6.
213. Muggia FM, Braly PS, Brady MF, et al. Phase III randomized study of cisplatin versus paclitaxel versus cisplatin and paclitaxel in patients with suboptimal stage III or IV ovarian cancer: a Gynecologic Oncology Group study. *J Clin Oncol* 2000;18(1):106–115.
214. Katsumata N, Yasuda M, Takahashi F, et al. Dose-dense paclitaxel once a week in combination with carboplatin every 3 weeks for advanced ovarian cancer: a phase 3, open-label, randomised controlled trial. *Lancet* 2009;374(9698):1331–1338.
215. Katsumata N, Yasuda M, Isonishi S, et al. Long-term results of dose-dense paclitaxel and carboplatin versus conventional paclitaxel and carboplatin for treatment of advanced epithelial ovarian, fallopian tube, or primary peritoneal cancer (JGOG 3016): a randomised, controlled, open-label trial. *Lancet Oncol* 2013;14(10):1020–1026.
216. Chan JK, Brady MF, Penson RT, et al. Weekly vs. every-3-week paclitaxel and carboplatin for ovarian cancer. *N Engl J Med* 2016;374:738–748.
217. Vasey PA, Jayson GC, Gordon A, et al. Phase III randomized trial of docetaxel-carboplatin versus paclitaxel-carboplatin as first-line chemotherapy for ovarian carcinoma. *J Natl Cancer Inst* 2004;96(22):1682–1691.
218. Pignata S, Scambia G, Katsaros D, et al. Carboplatin plus paclitaxel once a week versus every 3 weeks in patients with advanced ovarian cancer (MITO-7): a randomised, multicentre, open-label, phase 3 trial. *Lancet Oncol* 2014;15(4):396–405.
219. Bookman MA, Brady MF, McGuire WP, et al. Evaluation of new platinum-based treatment regimens in advanced-stage ovarian cancer: a phase III trial of the Gynecologic Cancer Intergroup. *J Clin Oncol* 2009;27(9):1419–1425.
220. Burger R, Brady M, Bookman M, et al. Incorporation of bevacizumab in the primary treatment of ovarian cancer. *N Engl J Med* 2011;365(26):2473–2483.
221. Ferriss JS, Java JJ, Bookman MA, et al. Ascites predicts treatment benefit of bevacizumab in front-line therapy of advanced epithelial ovarian, fallopian tube and peritoneal cancers: an NRG Oncology/GOG study. *Gynecol Oncol* 2015;139(1):17–22.
222. Perren T, Swart AM, Pfisterer J, et al. A phase 3 trial of bevacizumab in ovarian cancer. *N Engl J Med* 2011;365(26):2484–2496.
223. Oza AM, Cook AD, Pfisterer J, et al. Standard chemotherapy with or without bevacizumab for women with newly diagnosed ovarian cancer (ICON7): overall survival results of a phase 3 randomised trial. *Lancet Oncol* 2015;16(8):928–936.
224. Du Bois A, Kirstensen G, Ray-Coquard I, et al. Standard first-line chemotherapy with or without nintedanib for advanced ovarian cancer (AGO-OVAR 12): a randomised, double-blind, placebo-controlled phase 3 trial. *Lancet Oncol* 2016;17(1):78–89.
225. du Bois A, Floquet A, Kim JW, et al. Incorporation of pazopanib in maintenance therapy of ovarian cancer. *J Clin Oncol* 2014;32(30):3374–82.
226. Jaaback K, Johnson N. Intraperitoneal chemotherapy for the initial management of primary epithelial ovarian cancer. *Cochrane Database Syst Rev* 2006;(1):CD005340.
227. Walker JL, Brady MF, DiSilvestro PA, et al. A phase III trial of bevacizumab with IV versus IP chemotherapy in ovarian, fallopian tube, and peritoneal carcinoma NCI-supplied agent(s): A GOG/NRG trial (GOG 252). *2016 Society of Gynecologic Oncology Annual Meeting. Late-breaking abstract 6. Presented March 21, 2016.*
228. Bruzzone M, Repetto L, Chiara S, et al. Chemotherapy versus radiotherapy in the management of ovarian cancer patients with pathological complete response or minimal residual disease at second look. *Gynecol Oncol* 1990;38(3):392–395.
229. Lambert HE, Rustin GJ, Gregory WM, et al. A randomized trial comparing single-agent carboplatin with carboplatin followed by radiotherapy for advanced ovarian cancer: a North Thames Ovary Group study. *J Clin Oncol* 1993;11(3):440–448.
230. Lawton F, Luesley D, Blackledge G, et al. A randomized trial comparing whole abdominal radiotherapy with chemotherapy following cisplatinum cytoreduction in epithelial ovarian cancer. West Midlands Ovarian Cancer Group Trial II. *Clin Oncol (R Coll Radiol)* 1990;2(1):4–9.
231. Pickel H, Lahousen M, Petru E, et al. Consolidation radiotherapy after carboplatin-based chemotherapy in radically operated advanced ovarian cancer. *Gynecol Oncol* 1999;72(2):215–219.
232. Sorbe B. Consolidation treatment of advanced (FIGO stage III) ovarian carcinoma in complete surgical remission after induction chemotherapy: a randomized, controlled, clinical trial comparing whole abdominal radiotherapy, chemotherapy, and no further treatment. *Int J Gynecol Cancer* 2003;13(3):278–286.
233. Dinniwell R, Lock M, Pintilie M, et al. Consolidative abdominopelvic radiotherapy after surgery and carboplatin/paclitaxel chemotherapy for epithelial ovarian cancer. *Int J Radiat Oncol Biol Phys* 2005;62(1):104–110.
234. Petit T, Velten M, d'Hombres A, et al. Long-term survival of 106 stage III ovarian cancer patients with minimal residual disease after second-look laparotomy and consolidation radiotherapy. *Gynecol Oncol* 2007;104(1):104–108.
235. Varia MA, Stehman FB, Bundy BN, et al. Intraperitoneal radioactive phosphorus (32P) versus observation after negative second-look laparotomy for stage III ovarian carcinoma: a randomized trial of the Gynecologic Oncology Group. *J Clin Oncol* 2003;21(15):2849–2855.
236. Rustin GJ, van der Burg ME, Griffin CL, et al. Early versus delayed treatment of relapsed ovarian cancer (MRC OV05/EORTC 55955): a randomised trial. *Lancet* 2010;376(9747):1155–1163.
237. Pujade-Lauraine E, Hilpert F, Weber B, et al. Bevacizumab combined with chemotherapy for platinum-resistant recurrent ovarian cancer: The AURELIA open-label randomized phase III trial. *J Clin Oncol* 2014;32(13): 1302–1308.
238. Aghajanian C, Blank SV, Goff BA, et al. OCEANS: a randomized, double-blind, placebo-controlled phase III trial of chemotherapy with or without bevacizumab in patients with platinum-sensitive recurrent epithelial ovarian, primary peritoneal, or fallopian tube cancer. *J Clin Oncol* 2012;30(17): 2039–2045.
239. Aghajanian C, Goff B, Nycum LR, et al. Final overall survival and safety analysis of OCEANS, a phase 3 trial of chemotherapy with or without bevacizumab in patients with platinum-sensitive recurrent ovarian cancer. *Gynecol Oncol* 2015;139(1):10–16.
240. Coleman RL, Brady MF, Herzog TJ, et al. Bevacizumab and paclitaxel-carboplatin chemotherapy and secondary cytoreduction in recurrent, platinum-sensitive ovarian cancer (NRG Oncology/Gynecologic Oncology Group study GOG-0213): a multicentre, open-label, randomised, phase 3 trial. *Lancet Oncol* 2017;18(6):779–791.
241. Burger RA, Sill MW, Monk BJ, et al. Phase II trial of bevacizumab in persistent or recurrent epithelial ovarian cancer or primary peritoneal cancer: a Gynecologic Oncology Group Study. *J Clin Oncol* 2007;25(33):5165–5171.
242. Cannistra SA, Matulonis UA, Penson RT, et al. Phase II study of bevacizumab in patients with platinum-resistant ovarian cancer or peritoneal serous cancer. *J Clin Oncol* 2007;25(33):5180–5186.

243. Kaufman B, Shapira-Frommer R, Schmutzler RK, et al. Olaparib monotherapy in patients with advanced cancer and a germline BRCA1/2 mutation. *J Clin Oncol* 2015;33(3):244–250.

244. Ledermann J, Harter P, Gourley C,, et al. Olaparib maintenance therapy in platinum-sensitive relapsed ovarian cancer. *N Engl J Med* 2012;366(15): 1382–1392.

245. Pujade-Lauraine E, Ledermann JA, Penson RT, et al. Treatment with olaparib monotherapy in the maintenance setting significantly improves progression-free survival in patients with platinum-sensitive relapsed ovarian cancer: Results from the phase III SOLO2 study. *Presented at the Society of Gynecologic Oncology Annual Meeting on Women's Cancer (SGO), March 12–15. National Harbor, MD.*

246. Mirza MR, Monk BJ, Herrstedt J, et al. Niraparib maintenance therapy in platinum-sensitive, recurrent ovarian cancer. *N Engl J Med* 2016;375(22):2154–2164.

247. Balasubramaniam S, Beaver JA, Horton S, et al. FDA approval summary: rucaparib for the treatment of patients with deleterious BRCA mutation-associated advanced ovarian cancer. *Clin Cancer Res* 2017;23(23):7165–7170.

248. Horowitz N, Matulonis UA. New biologic agents for the treatment of gynecologic cancers. *Hematol Oncol Clin North Am* 2012;26(1):133–156.

249. Ledermann JA, Embleton AC, Raja F, et al. Cediranib in patients with relapsed platinum-sensitive ovarian cancer (ICON6): a randomised, double-blind, placebo-controlled phase 3 trial. *Lancet* 2016;387:1066–1074.

250. Monk BJ, Poveda A, Vergote I, et al. Anti-angiopoietin therapy with trebananib for recurrent ovarian cancer (TRINOVA-1): a randomised, multicentre, double-blind, placebo-controlled phase 3 trial. *Lancet Oncol* 2014;15: 799–808.

251. Liu JF, Barry WT, Birrer M, et al. Combination cediranib and olaparib versus olaparib alone for women with recurrent platinum-sensitive ovarian cancer: a randomised phase 2 study. *Lancet Oncol* 2014;15(11):1207–1214.

252. Hauspy J, Covens A. Cytoreductive surgery for recurrent ovarian cancer. *Curr Opin Obstet Gynecol* 2007;19(1):15–21.

253. Bristow RE, Puri I, Chi DS. Cytoreductive surgery for recurrent ovarian cancer: a meta-analysis. *Gynecol Oncol* 2009;112(1):265–274.

254. DuBois A, Vergote I, Ferron G, et al. Randomized controlled phase III study evaluating the impact of secondary cytoreductive surgery in recurrent ovarian cancer: AGO DESKTOP III/ENGOT ov20. *J Clin Oncol* 2017;35(Suppl):abstr 5501.

255. Gelblum D, Mychalczak B, Almadrones L, et al. Palliative benefit of external-beam radiation in the management of platinum refractory epithelial ovarian carcinoma. *Gynecol Oncol* 1998;69(1):36–41.

256. May LF, Belinson JL, Roland TA. Palliative benefit of radiation therapy in advanced ovarian cancer. *Gynecol Oncol* 1990;37(3):408–411.

257. Tinger A, Waldron T, Peluso N, et al. Effective palliative radiation therapy in advanced and recurrent ovarian carcinoma. *Int J Radiat Oncol Biol Phys* 2001;51(5):1256–1263.

258. Corn BW, Lanciano RM, Boente M, et al. Recurrent ovarian cancer: effective radiotherapeutic palliation after chemotherapy failure. *Cancer* 1994;74(11):2979–2983.

259. E C, Quon M, Gallant V, et al. Effective palliative radiotherapy for symptomatic recurrent or residual ovarian cancer. *Gynecol Oncol* 2006;102:204–209.

260. De Meerleer G, Vandecasteele K, Ost P, et al. Whole abdominopelvic radiotherapy using intensity-modulated arc therapy in the palliative treatment of chemotherapy-resistant ovarian cancer with bulky peritoneal disease: a single-institution experience. *Int J Radiat Oncol Biol Phys* 2011;79(3):775–781.

261. Jiang G, Balboni T, Taylor A, et al. Palliative radiation therapy for recurrent ovarian cancer: efficacy and predictors of clinical response. *Int J Gynec Cancer* 2018;28(1):43–50.

262. Firat S, Erickson B. Selective irradiation for the treatment of recurrent ovarian carcinoma involving the vagina or rectum. *Gynecol Oncol* 2001;80(2):213–220.

263. Albuquerque KV, Singla R, Potkul RK, et al. Impact of tumor volume-directed involved field radiation therapy integrated in the management of recurrent ovarian cancer. *Gynecol Oncol* 2005;96(3):701–704.

264. Brown AP, Jhingran A, Klopp AH, et al. Involved-field radiation therapy for locoregionally recurrent ovarian cancer. *Gynecol Oncol* 2013;130(2):300–305.

265. Mayer RJ, Berkowitz RS, Griffiths CT. Central nervous system involvement by ovarian carcinoma: a complication of prolonged survival with metastatic disease. *Cancer* 1978;41(2):776–783.

266. Cormio G, Maneo A, Parma G, et al. Central nervous system metastases in patients with ovarian carcinoma. A report of 23 cases and a literature review. *Ann Oncol* 1995;6(6):571–574.

267. Ratner ES, Toy E, O'Malley DM, et al. Brain metastases in epithelial ovarian and primary peritoneal carcinoma. *Int J Gynecol Cancer* 2009;19(5):856–859.

268. Sehouli J, Pietzner K, Harter P, et al. Prognostic role of platinum sensitivity in patients with brain metastases from ovarian cancer: results of a German multicenter study. *Ann Oncol* 2011;21(11):2201–2205.

269. Marchetti C, Ferrandina G, Cormio G, et al. Brain metastases in patients with EOC: clinico-pathological and prognostic factors. A multicentric retrospective analysis from the MITO group (MITO 19). *Gynecol Oncol* 2016;143(3):532–538.

270. Hong L, Alektiar K, Chui C, et al. IMRT of large fields: whole-abdomen irradiation. *Int J Radiat Oncol Biol Phys* 2002;54(1):278–289.

271. Duthoy W, De Gersem W, Vergote K, et al. Whole abdominopelvic radiotherapy (WAPRT) using intensity-modulated arc therapy (IMAT): first clinical experience. *Int J Radiat Oncol Biol Phys* 2003;57(4):1019–1032.

272. Rochet N, Kieser M, Sterzing F, et al. Phase II study evaluating consolidation whole abdominal intensity-modulated radiotherapy (IMRT) in patients with advanced ovarian cancer stage FIGO III—the OVAR-IMRT-02 Study. *BMC Cancer* 2011;11:41.

273. Yap OW, Kapp DS, Teng NN, et al. Intraoperative radiation therapy in recurrent ovarian cancer. *Int J Radiat Oncol Biol Phys* 2005;63(4):1114–1121.

274. Del Carmen MG, McIntyre JF, Fuller AF, et al. Intraoperative radiation therapy in the treatment of pelvic gynecologic malignancies: a review of fifteen cases. *Gynecol Oncol* 2000;79(3):457–462.

275. Garton GR, Gunderson LL, Webb MJ, et al. Intraoperative radiation therapy in gynecologic cancer: update of the experience at a single institution. *Int J Radiat Oncol Biol Phys* 1997;37(4):839–843.

276. Haddock MG, Petersen IA, Webb MJ, et al. IORT for locally advanced gynecological malignancies. *Front Radiat Ther Oncol* 1997;31:256–259.

277. Konski AA, Neisler J, Phibbs G, et al. A pilot study investigating intraoperative electron beam irradiation in the treatment of ovarian malignancies. *Gynecol Oncol* 1990;38(1):121–124.

278. Lund B, Hansen M, Lundvall F, et al. Intestinal obstruction in patients with advanced carcinoma of the ovaries treated with combination chemotherapy. *Surg Gynecol Obstet* 1989;169(3):213–218.

279. Thomas GM, Dembo AJ. Integrating radiation therapy into the management of ovarian cancer. *Cancer* 1993;71(4 Suppl):1710–1718.

280. Williams SD, Blessing JA, Hatch KD, et al. Chemotherapy of advanced dysgerminoma: trials of the Gynecologic Oncology Group. *J Clin Oncol* 1991;9(11):1950–1955.

281. Brewer M, Gershenson DM, Herzog CE, et al. Outcome and reproductive function after chemotherapy for ovarian dysgerminoma. *J Clin Oncol* 1999;17(9):2670–2675.

282. Williams S, Blessing JA, Liao SY, et al. Adjuvant therapy of ovarian germ cell tumors with cisplatin, etoposide, and bleomycin: a trial of the Gynecologic Oncology Group. *J Clin Oncol* 1994;12(4):701–706.

283. Miller BE, Barron BA, Wan JY, et al. Prognostic factors in adult granulosa cell tumor of the ovary. *Cancer* 1997;79(10):1951–1955.

284. Young RH, Dickersin GR, Scully RE. Juvenile granulosa cell tumor of the ovary. A clinicopathological analysis of 125 cases. *Am J Surg Pathol* 1984;8(8):575–596.

285. Boggess JF, Soules MR, Goff BA, et al. Serum inhibin and disease status in women with ovarian granulosa cell tumors. *Gynecol Oncol* 1997;64(1):64–69.

286. Zorn KK, Bonome T, Gangi L, et al. Gene expression profiles of serous, endometrioid, and clear cell subtypes of ovarian and endometrial cancer. *Clin Cancer Res* 2005;11(18):6422–6430.

287. Bolton KL, Tyrer J, Song H, et al. Common variants at 19p13 are associated with susceptibility to ovarian cancer. *Nat Genet* 2010;42(10):880–884.

288. Song H, Ramus SJ, Tyrer J, et al. A genome-wide association study identifies a new ovarian cancer susceptibility locus on 9p22.2. *Nat Genet* 2009;41(9):996–1000.

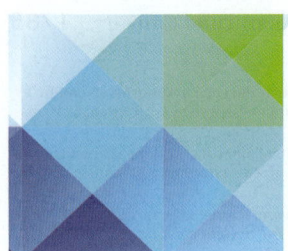

CHAPTER 76

Vaginal Cancer

Josephine Kang, Stephanie L. Wethington, and Akila N. Viswanathan

TREATMENT SCHEMATIC

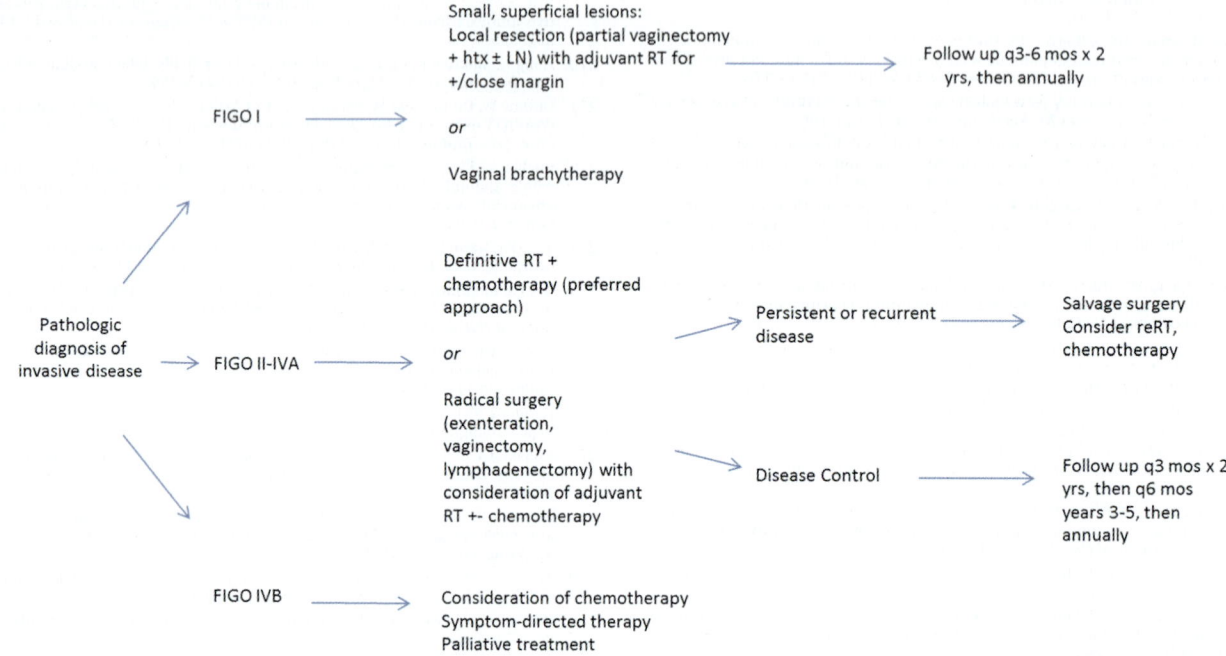

ANATOMY

The vagina is a fibromuscular tube that extends from the cervix down to the vestibule, or cleft, between the labia minora. The average length of the vagina is 3 to 4 inches or 7.5 cm. It lies dorsal to the urethra and bladder base and ventral to the rectum. Invaginations between the vaginal mucosa and cervix form the anterior, posterior, and lateral fornices. Embryologically, the vagina is believed to be of dual origin, with the upper third derived from the uterine canal, whereas the lower two-thirds are derived from the urogenital sinus.[1]

Proximally, the vagina joins the uterine cervix at an angle, and, as a result, the posterior vaginal wall is longer than the anterior wall (Fig. 76.1). The proximal posterior vaginal wall is separated from the rectum by the rectovaginal septum or fascia. The overlying peritoneal reflection forms the posterior cul de sac, also known as the pouch of Douglas. Invaginations between the vaginal mucosa and cervix form the anterior, posterior, and lateral fornices. Laterally, the vagina is adjacent to the pelvic fascia and levator ani muscles. Inferiorly, the vagina extends through the urogenital diaphragm to lie dorsal to the urethra and ventral to the rectum. The fibromuscular perineal body separates the vagina from the anal canal. At the introitus, the vagina has a perforated fold of thin connective tissue and mucous membrane known as the hymen.

The vaginal wall is comprised of the mucosa, muscularis, and adventitia. The innermost lining of the vagina is formed by a nonkeratinizing, stratified squamous epithelium overlying a basement membrane. This epithelial mucosa lacks glandular structures and instead receives lubrication from mucous secretions originating in the cervix. Underneath the mucosa is the connective tissue composed of elastin and a thick muscularis layer composed of two layers of smooth muscle. The inner layer is arranged circularly, whereas the outer layer is arranged longitudinally. This muscular layer is covered by the third layer, a thin adventitia that merges with neighboring organs.

The vagina has a complex, extensive network of lymphatic drainage, with vessels that course through the submucosal and muscularis layer (Fig. 76.2). The proximal portion drains primarily via cervical lymphatics. The proximal anterior vagina drains along cervical channels to the internal iliac and parametrial nodes and the proximal posterior vagina drains into the inferior gluteal, presacral, and anorectal nodes. The distal aspect of the vagina drains into the superficial inguinal nodes, and ultimately to the pelvic nodes, following drainage patterns of the vulva. Lesions in the midvagina have been shown to drain either way.[2] Lesions infiltrating the rectovaginal septum may spread to the pararectal and presacral nodes because there are multiple interconnections between the lymphatic channels, and pattern of drainage cannot be reliably predicted based on location of the primary tumor.

The vagina is supplied by the vaginal artery, which arises from the cervical branch of the uterine artery and runs lateral to the vagina until it anastomoses distally with the inferior vesical and middle rectal arteries. The venous plexus runs parallel to the arteries, draining into the internal iliac vein. The vaginal vault is innervated by the lumbar plexus and pudendal nerve, with branches from sacral roots 2 to 4.[3]

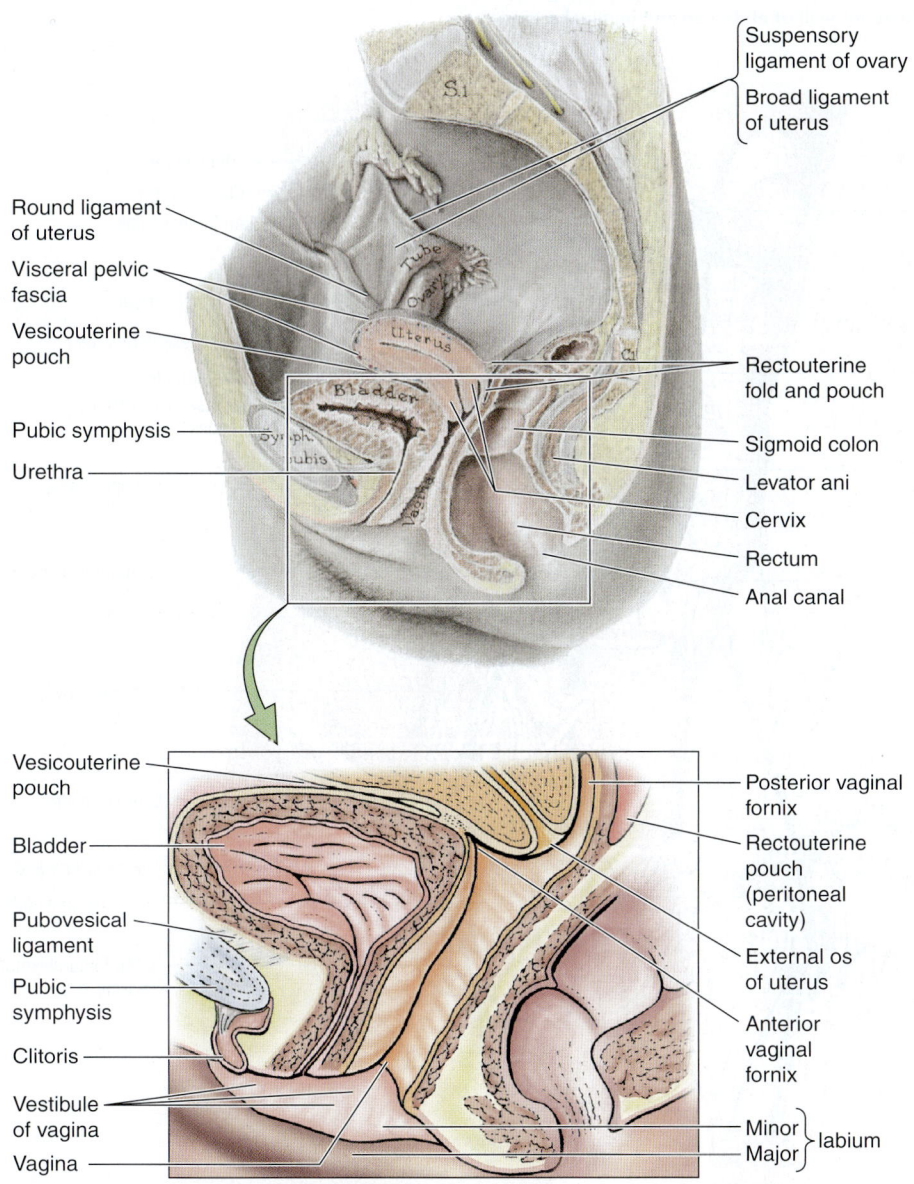

FIGURE 76.1. Anatomy of female pelvis.

EPIDEMIOLOGY, PRESENTATION AND MANAGEMENT

Primary vaginal cancer is a rare malignancy, constituting 1% to 2% of all gynecologic malignancies. There are approximately 4,600 new cases and 950 deaths from primary vaginal cancer in the United States every year.[4]

The majority of malignant lesions in the vagina are attributable to direct spread or metastases from other gynecologic malignancies. According to the staging system set by the International Federation of Obstetrics and Gynecology (FIGO), any tumor involving both the vagina and cervix should be classified as a cervical carcinoma. Similarly, any tumor involving both the vagina and vulva is to be classified as a vulvar carcinoma.[5] A malignant vaginal lesion in a patient with prior history of invasive cervical carcinoma within the past 5 years also excludes diagnosis as a primary vaginal cancer.[6] As a result, only a minority of vaginal carcinoma cases meet the criteria of being a primary vaginal cancer.

The peak incidence of primary vaginal cancer is in the sixth and seventh decade of life. According to data from the Surveillance, Epidemiology, and End Results (SEER) program,[7] 2,149 women in the United States were diagnosed with primary vaginal cancer from 1990 to 2004. The mean age at diagnosis was 65 +/– 14 years and incidence rates increased with age. There has been an overall decrease in the incidence of primary vaginal tumors, possibly secondary to earlier detection and to implementation of strict exclusion criteria in the FIGO staging system.

According to the SEER study by Shah et al.,[7] most women diagnosed with primary vaginal cancer are non-Hispanic whites (66%), followed by African Americans (14%), Hispanic whites (12%), Asian/Pacific Islanders (7%), and others (1%). Incidence rates were highest for African American women (1.24/100,000 person-years) and lowest for Asian/Pacific Islanders (0.64/100,000 person-years).

A review of five series, encompassing a total of 1,375 cases of vaginal cancer, reported a FIGO stage distribution as follows: 26% stage I, 37% stage II, 24% stage III, and 13% stage IV.[8] Consistent with this, the National Cancer Database (NCDB) review by Creasman et al.,[9] for the period of 1985 to 1994, revealed 3,244 cases of invasive primary vaginal carcinoma, with 24% of patients presenting with American Joint Committee on Cancer (AJCC) stage I disease, 20% AJCC stage II, 24% AJCC stages III-IV, and 32% unknown. Most tumors were moderately (28%) or poorly (28%) differentiated at presentation.

Posterior wall of abdomen and inguinal region

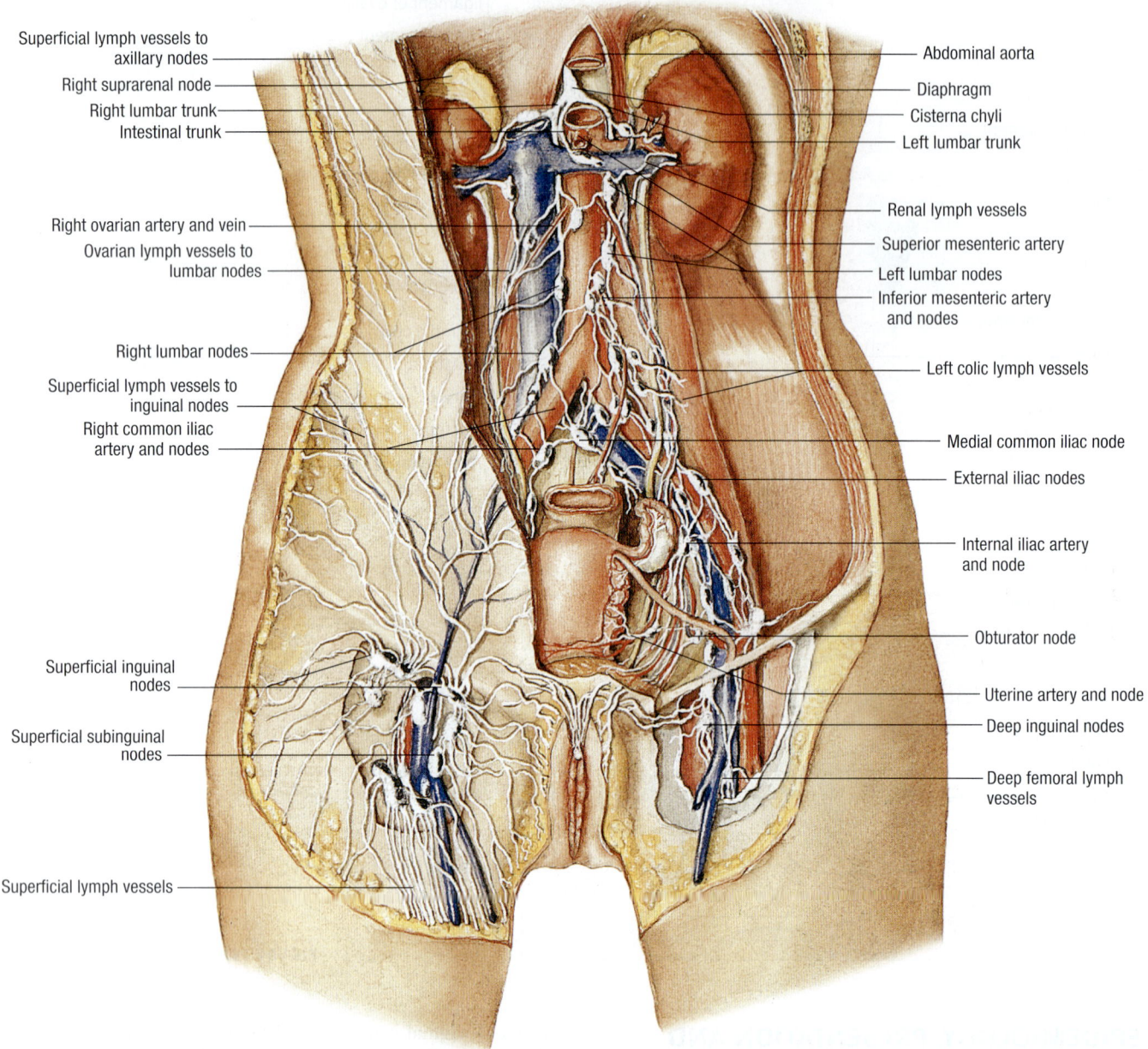

Superficial lymph vessels to axillary nodes

Right suprarenal node

Right lumbar trunk

Intestinal trunk

Right ovarian artery and vein

Ovarian lymph vessels to lumbar nodes

Right lumbar nodes

Superficial lymph vessels to inguinal nodes

Right common iliac artery and nodes

Superficial inguinal nodes

Superficial subinguinal nodes

Superficial lymph vessels

Abdominal aorta

Diaphragm

Cisterna chyli

Left lumbar trunk

Renal lymph vessels

Superior mesenteric artery

Left lumbar nodes

Inferior mesenteric artery and nodes

Left colic lymph vessels

Medial common iliac node

External iliac nodes

Internal iliac artery and node

Obturator node

Uterine artery and node

Deep inguinal nodes

Deep femoral lymph vessels

FIGURE 76.2. Lymphatic drainage of the vagina.

Because of the low incidence, treatment recommendations are based on results from relatively small retrospective series comprised of heterogeneous patient populations and treatments, and it remains unlikely that randomized clinical trials will be feasible.

Vaginal Intraepithelial Neoplasia

It is hypothesized that vaginal intraepithelial neoplasia (VAIN) is a precursor lesion to squamous cell carcinoma of the vagina.[10] There has been a steady increase in the diagnosis of VAIN over the past several decades, perhaps because of a combination of increased cytologic screening, awareness, and incidence of human papillomavirus (HPV). VAIN is defined as atypical of squamous cells without evidence of stromal invasion and was first reported by Hummer and colleagues in 1933.[10]

VAIN is further classified into low grade (VAIN 1) and high grade (VAIN 2 to 3). VAIN 1 is characterized by cytomorphologic changes limited to the upper one-third of the epithelium. Such changes include nuclear enlargement, nuclear hyperchromasia, cytoplasmic halos, and occasional binucleation. VAIN 2 to 3 is characterized by cytomorphologic changes in the basal keratinocytes, including nuclear pleomorphism, nuclear hyperchromasia and crowding, and mitotic figures (including atypical forms). VAIN 2 and 3 are distinguished by depth of cytologic change. Cytologic changes confined to the lower two-thirds of the epithelium are designated VAIN 2, whereas changes involving the full thickness of the epithelium are VAIN 3. Carcinoma *in situ* encompasses the full epithelial thickness and is included under VAIN 3.

The overall incidence of VAIN is estimated to be 0.2 to 0.3 cases per 100,000, with peak incidence found in women who are 40 and 60 years of age.[10] The incidence of VAIN 3, or *in situ* vaginal cancer, is estimated to be 0.1 per 100,000 women with peak incidence between ages 70 and 79, according to data from the US Centers for Disease Control and

Prevention's National Program of Cancer Registries and the National Cancer Institute's SEER Program.[11]

VAIN is typically asymptomatic.[12] As a result, many cases are detected after cytologic evaluation as part of surveillance in patients with a history of CIN or invasive cervical carcinoma.

Although the likelihood of VAIN progressing to invasive disease is difficult to predict for individual cases, multiple clinical series have demonstrated a significant overall increase in risk of invasive vaginal cancer after a diagnosis of VAIN. Several retrospective studies have demonstrated a range of 2% to 20% of patients with VAIN progressing to invasive vaginal cancer.[12,13] The rate of occult invasive disease in patients with VAIN 3 has been reported to be as high as 28%.[14] The risk of malignant transformation in VAIN 1 and 2 is less clearly elucidated.

Risk Factors

HPV is implicated in development of VAIN, though the relationship between HPV and development of intraepithelial neoplasia has been best demonstrated for cervical lesions. HPV 16 and 18 are the most prevalent subtypes associated with VAIN. It is estimated that HPV 16/18 is identified in 40% of VAIN 1 and 60% of high-grade VAIN 2/3 cases.[15] With widespread implementation of HPV vaccination, it is anticipated that the incidence of VAIN will start to decline. It is predicted that HPV vaccination will ultimately prevent up to 70% of VAIN cases.[16]

The diagnosis of VAIN is often associated with prior or concurrent neoplasia elsewhere in the lower genital tract. Multiple series suggest approximately 50% to 90% of patients with VAIN have concurrent or prior history of intraepithelial neoplasia or carcinoma of the cervix or vulva.[13,17,18]

Treatment Options for VAIN

In general, women with low-grade VAIN can be offered close surveillance, as lesions often regress spontaneously. In a study by Aho et al.,[13] 78% of patients with VAIN 1 or VAIN 2 had spontaneous regression of disease without treatment. Over time, however, VAIN 1 can recur; in one series, up to 54% of patients with VAIN 1 who were observed ultimately developed recurrent, persistent or progressive disease,[10] at a median time of 17 months. High-grade VAIN has a higher likelihood of occult invasive disease and progression to invasive disease [14,19] and is typically treated aggressively. There is currently no consensus on optimal treatment modality for patients with high-grade VAIN. Treatment approaches include local excision, partial or total vaginectomy, laser vaporization, electrocoagulation, topical 5% fluorouracil administration, topical 5% imiquimod, and radiation.[18-26] Reported success rates for different approaches range from 48% to 100% for laser vaporization,[27,28] 52% to 100% for colpectomy,[14,19,29] 75% to 100% for topical 5-FU,[20,30-34] 57% to 86% for topical 5% imiquimod,[26] and 83% to 100% for radiation[22,35-38] (Table 76.1). Given the breadth of available therapies, an individualized approach to patient management is advised, with consideration given to the patient's overall health, desire to preserve sexual function, candidacy for surgery, disease multifocality, and prior treatment failures.

Surgical and Ablative Therapies

Surgical excision for VAIN is an option in select cases, particularly for vaginal vault lesions or lesions close to the introitus. Approaches include wide local excision, partial vaginectomy and, in rare cases, total vaginectomy for highly extensive disease, which provides the advantage of obtaining a complete pathologic diagnosis. Most resections can be performed through a transvaginal approach. Smaller lesions can be excised or ablated using a cold-knife approach, electrosurgical loop excision, laser, or via ultrasonic surgical aspiration.[55-57]

Location of VAIN in the vaginal vault or posthysterectomy suture recesses may require partial vaginectomy for complete resection, as redundancy of the vaginal mucosa makes it difficult to rule out occult disease with biopsy alone. Multifocal or extensive lesions may require a more extensive approach, such as total vaginectomy with or without skin grafting.[19]

Overall, series looking specifically at upper vaginectomy report control rates of 68% to 88%.[14,19,29,58]

Potential complications depend on the extent and method of surgical resection and range from vaginal shortening and stenosis to standard postoperative morbidity associated with abdominal procedures such as injury to bowel or bladder. Complication rates of upper vaginectomy have been variably reported; in the series by Indermaur, there was a 9% complication rate. It should be noted that patients with a history of radiation treatment are at higher risk of postoperative complications, with a higher rate of fistula formation reported in one study.[17]

Topical Treatments

Topical treatments include topical 5-fluorouracil (5-FU) and 5% imiquimod cream, with response rates of 41% to 88% for 5-FU and 50% to 86% for imiquimod.[22,30-32,34,53,54,59] Imiquimod increases levels of interferon alpha, interleukin 12, and tumor necrosis factor[53] thought to result in immunomodulation of the vaginal mucosa. Long-term efficacy is unknown as well as response rates in immunocompromised patients.

Topical therapies have been utilized in patients with early-stage lesions, multifocal disease, or multiple comorbidities rendering them nonideal surgical candidates. Topical creams are favored in management of young, HPV-positive women presenting with multifocal lesions. Topical applications have also been utilized prior to surgery, to reduce lesion size and improve stripping of neoplastic epithelial cells from underlying stroma.[18] Side effects of topical treatments include local irritation, burning, and ulceration.[31,32]

Radiation Therapy

In general, radiation is reserved for patients who relapse after more conservative treatments, and/or have VAIN 3, particularly if there is an *in situ* disease component. Numerous small series over the past 20 to 30 years have reported control rates ranging from 80% to 100%.[12,22-24,35-37,60] Drawbacks to radiation include potential undertreatment of occult invasive disease, the risk of secondary malignancy, and long-term morbidity, although there are no prospective data available regarding the impact of treatment on sexual function and quality of life. High–dose rate (HDR), medium–dose rate (MDR), and low–dose rate (LDR) techniques have been reported with acceptable results, although it is difficult to compare regimens because of small patient numbers, generally short follow-up times and overall nonuniformity among series.

Overall, excellent local control and low toxicity have been reported for LDR brachytherapy. LDR treatment is delivered with an intracavitary vaginal cylinder using cesium-137. Typically, a dose of 60 Gy is prescribed to the vaginal mucosa, but a wide range of doses, depending on depth of dose prescription, as well as a variety of techniques, have been reported.[22,35,36,41] Chyle et al.[40] prescribed 70 to 80 Gy to the vaginal surface and reported a 17% recurrence rate at 10 years in their series of 37 patients. Perez et al.[41] treated patients to the vaginal surface with a dose of 60 to 70 Gy and reported 1 recurrence out of 20 patients. The recurrence occurred in the distal vagina and was noted to be a marginal recurrence. Blanchard et al.[35] published a series on 28 patients with VAIN 3 treated at Institut Gustave Roussy from 1985 to 2008. Patients were treated with LDR brachytherapy, using a vaginal mold technique, to dose of 60 Gy prescribed 5 mm below the vaginal surface; 18 patients received treatment to

TABLE 76.1 VAGINAL INTRAEPITHELIAL NEOPLASIA OUTCOMES BY TREATMENT MODALITY

Series	Follow-Up	No. of Pts	% Recurrence	Comments
Radiation				
Prempree[39]		7	0%	ICB 70–80 Gy
Chyle[40]		37	17%	ICB or orthovoltage radiation
MacLeod[38]	46 mo (mean)	14	14%	HDR-ICB, 34–45 Gy to vaginal surface, 4–10 fx
Ogino[37]	13–153 mo	6	0%	HDR-ICB, mean dose 23.3 Gy
Perez[41]		20	6%	ICB 60–70 Gy
Graham[24]	77 mo	22	14%	MDR-ICB, 48 Gy to point Z
Blanchard[35]	79 mo	28	7%	LDR, 60 Gy to 5 mm below mucosa
Song[42]	48 mo	34	6%	HDR-ICB, 40 Gy in 8 fx
Zolciak-Siwinska[43]	39 mo	20	10%	HDR-ICB, 6–7.5 Gy × 3–5 fx
Surgery				
Benedet[44]	>5 y	136	25%	WLE, PV, TV
Lenehan[12]	5–112 mo	19	16%	PV, TV
Ireland[45]	3 mo to 11 y	25	4%	PV, TV
Hoffman[14]	6–73 mo	32	17%	PV; 28% invasive cancer
Fanning[46]	1.8 y	15	0%	PV; 6.6% invasive cancer
Cheng[17]	1–124 mo	35	34%	WLE
Dodge[47]	>7 mo	13	0%	PV
Indermaur[19]	2–9 mo	105	12%	PV, 12% invasive cancer
Terzakis[48]	24 mo	23	25%	
Gunderson[10]	1–194 mo	44	27%	PV, LE
Laser Therapy				
Jobson[49]	6–27 mo	24	17%	
Audet-LaPoint[50]	7–85 mo	32	28%	3.8% invasive cancer at excision
Hoffman[27]				3 of 11 w/invasive cancer at recurrence
Diakomanolis[29]	2.2 y (mean)	26	42%	
Campagnutta[51]	35–82 mo	25	32%	
Dodge[47]	13–90 mo	39	23%	
Jobson[49]	>7 mo	42	38%	
Perrotta[52]	12–78 mo	21	14%	
Gunderson[10]	1–194 mo	34	47%	
Topical 5-FU				
Woodruff[31]	3–7 y	9	11%	1%–2% 5-FU q mo
Petrilli[20]	2–60 mo	15	20%	BID × 5 d
Kirwan[34]	4–42 mo	14	7%	q wk × 10 wk
Krebs[30]	12–84 mo	37	19%	q wk × 10 wk
Audet-Lapointe[50]	9–42 mo	12	17%	q d × 5 d
Dodge[47]	>7 mo	22	59%	
Topical imiquimod				
Diakomonolis[53]		3	See note	3× weekly × 8 wk
				3 pts with high-grade disease, therapy revealed regression to VAIN1 (n = 2) or cure (n = 1)
Buck[54]		56	14%	0.25 g qwk × 3 wk

HDR, high-dose rate; ICB, intracavitary brachytherapy; LDR, low-dose rate; MDR, medium-dose rate; PV, partial vaginectomy; TV, total vaginectomy; WLE, wide local excision.

the upper half of the vagina, 6 were treated to the upper two-thirds, and 4 were treated to the whole vaginal length. With a median follow-up time of 41 months, the authors report only 1 in-field recurrence, with a 10-year local control rate of 93%. Treatment with LDR brachytherapy is overall well tolerated; in the Perez series, there was only 1 grade 3 urinary complication among 40 patients with VAIN 3 or stage 1 vaginal cancer treated with LDR.[41]

There are limited data on use of MDR brachytherapy treatment for VAIN. Graham et al.[24] reviewed their experience using MDR intracavitary brachytherapy for VAIN 3 at the Beatson Oncology Centre in Glasgow, UK. Using a MDR Selectron, 48 Gy was prescribed 0.5 cm lateral to the ovoid surface (point Z) over two insertions, spaced 1 week apart. Ovoids were chosen over vaginal cylinder placement in order to adequately cover epithelium sutured into the superolateral vagina at hysterectomy. With a median follow-up duration of 77 months, recurrent/residual VAIN 3 was documented in 3 patients, and 2 of these patients subsequently clinently developed invasive or microinvasive vaginal carcinoma. One other patient developed late progression 14 years after treatment.

Several series have reported promising results for HDR brachytherapy, with disease-free survival rates of 90% or greater. Ogino et al.[37] reported their experience treating 6 patients with VAIN 3 at Kanagawa Cancer Center from 1983 to 1993, with a mean dose of 23.3 Gy (range, 15 to 30 Gy); most treatments were delivered in 5 fractions using two ovoids, with dose calculated to a point 1 cm superior to the vaginal apex. Lesions distal to the vaginal vault had doses calculated 1 cm beyond the plane of the vaginal cylinder in order to deliver adequate dose to the entire vagina. Median follow-up was 90.5 months, with no evidence of disease recurrence in the treated patients. MacLeod et al.[38] reviewed their experience treating 14 patients with VAIN 3 from 1985 to 1995. Total dose was 34 to 45 Gy to the vaginal surface, in 8.5-Gy fractions delivered twice a week, or 4.5-Gy fractions delivered four times a week. One patient developed invasive cancer, and 1 patient had persistent VAIN 3. There were no major acute toxicities, and 2 patients developed late grade 3 vaginal atrophy and stenosis. According to one study that evaluated toxicity after use of HDR brachytherapy for VAIN in 20 patients, with utilization of the CTCAE scale, a biologically equivalent dose of 70 Gy or greater results in significantly greater toxicity. The most commonly seen toxicities were decreased libido, vaginal discharge, dryness, mucositis, stenosis, and vaginitis.[43]

Malignant Tumors of the Vagina: Squamous Cell Carcinoma

Clinical Presentation

Symptoms

Up to 20% of women are asymptomatic at the time of diagnosis,[61] with lesions detected via cytologic screening or by speculum examination. Squamous cell carcinoma accounts for 65% to 85% of vaginal cancer cases,[7] and the greatest proportion of women present with stage I disease (36%). Up to 65% of patients with vaginal cancer present with irregular vaginal bleeding as their primary symptom.[61,62] Vaginal discharge is the second most common symptom, occurring in 10% to 15% of patients. Less frequent symptoms, associated with locally advanced disease, include the presence of a mass; pain; urinary symptoms including frequency, dysuria, or hematuria;

or gastrointestinal complaints such as tenesmus, constipation, or melena. Because of the proximity of anterior wall lesions to the urethra and bladder, urinary symptoms can be seen more commonly in vaginal cancer than in cervical cancer.

Location

Vaginal cancer most frequently involves the superior one-third of the vaginal canal, with series reporting 50% to 83% of cases occurring in this region.[58,63–66] There is approximately equal involvement of the middle and inferior thirds,[58] although some studies suggest that involvement of the lower third is more common than involvement of the middle third.[61,63] The lateral walls are less frequently involved. Tumors may exhibit an exophytic or ulcerative, infiltrating growth pattern.

A high proportion of patients have a history of prior hysterectomy. Involvement of the cervix (if present) or vulva at the time of diagnosis excludes classification as a primary vaginal cancer. Lesions can extend radially, either into the lumen to form exophytic masses or through the vaginal wall to invade surrounding musculature and organs. Anterior wall lesions can infiltrate the vesicovaginal septum and/or urethra. Posterior wall lesions can infiltrate the rectovaginal septum and involve the rectal mucosa. Advanced disease can extend laterally toward the parametrium and paracolpal tissues or into the urogenital diaphragm, levator ani muscles, or pelvic fascia and eventually to the pelvic side wall.

Advanced or recurrent disease can present with distant metastases. The most frequent site of hematogenous metastasis is the lung, with less commonly noted sites being liver and bone.[40] In a series by Perez et al.,[67] the incidence of distant metastasis was 16% for stage I, 31% for stage II, 46% for stage IIB, 62% for stage III, and 50% for stage IV. Some histologies may have a higher likelihood of distant metastases than others. Chyle et al.[40] noted a higher incidence of distant metastases in patients with adenocarcinoma (48%) than in those with SCC (10%), with correspondingly lower 10-year survival rates (20% vs. 50%).

Histopathology

Grossly, SCC of the vagina can present as nodular, ulcerated, indurated, exophytic, or endophytic lesions. Histologically, tumors are graded as well, moderate or poorly differentiated and have been described as keratinizing, nonkeratinizing, basaloid, warty, or verrucous. The majority of these lesions are nonkeratinizing and moderately differentiated.[68] It is not possible to histologically distinguish a primary vaginal SCC from recurrent cervical or vulvar carcinoma.

Verrucous carcinoma is a distinct histologic variant of vaginal SCC[69] that typically presents as a well-circumscribed, soft, cauliflower-like mass that is microscopically well differentiated, with a papillary growth pattern and acanthotic epithelium. There is surface maturation with parakeratosis or hyperkeratosis without koilocytosis. This variant of SCC exhibits less aggressive behavior and rarely metastasizes.[69] It is also resistant to radiation and often transforms to a more aggressive histology if treated with radiation. Therefore, it should be considered as a distinct entity separate from other vaginal SCC.

Sarcomatoid squamous cell carcinoma is a rare subset of vaginal SCC, comprising 2% of all cases. It is characterized by spindle-shaped neoplastic cells that can initially be mistaken for sarcoma. However, positive stains for cytokeratin help distinguish sarcomatoid SCC as a poorly differentiated variant of vaginal SCC.[70]

Patterns of Lymphatic Drainage

The vagina has a complex pattern of lymphatic drainage, with multiple interconnections. The upper vagina drains to the obturator and hypogastric nodes, similar to the cervix.

The lower vagina drains to the inguinal, femoral, and external iliac nodes, and posteriorly situated lesions can drain to the inferior gluteal, presacral, or perirectal nodes. Lymphatic channels in the mucosa run parallel to networks of channels in the submucosa and muscular layer, ultimately converging to form trunks at the vaginal wall periphery, which subsequently drain to major pelvic nodal groups.

Because of considerable crossover drainage, the location of the primary tumor is not a reliable indicator of drainage site. Frumovitz et al. utilized lymphoscintigraphy to determine patterns of lymphatic drainage in 14 women diagnosed with primary vaginal cancers[71] and found a substantial degree of anomalous drainage, resulting in a change in radiation treatment for 33% of patients. For example, among 4 women with lesions located in the upper third of the vagina, which is predicted to drain along the cervical lymphatic chains to the pelvis, 2 (50%) were found to have a sentinel node in the inguinal region. Among 5 women with lesions located at the vaginal introitus, a location predicted to drain along the vulvar lymphatic chains to the inguinal triangle, 3 (60%) were found to have a sentinel node in the pelvis.

The risk of nodal involvement increases significantly with stage. At diagnosis, up to 20% of patients have clinically positive inguinal nodes, with reported ranges of 5.3% to 20%.[41,67] Sparse data on nodal metastases are derived from series in which exploratory laparotomies and lymphadenectomies were performed.[72] However, the true incidence of positive lymph nodes is difficult to determine because most patients receive treatment with radiation therapy and do not undergo surgical lymphadenectomy. The incidence of lymph node involvement has been reported to be 0% to 14% in stage I and 21% to 32% in stage II disease.[72–74] The incidence of nodal involvement in stages III and IV has been reported to be as high as 78% and 83%, respectively.[63]

The risk of nodal failure increases significantly if there is local recurrence. Chyle et al.[40] reported 10-year inguinal and pelvic failure rates of 16% and 28%, respectively, in patients with local recurrence, in contrast to 2% and 4%, respectively, in patients without local recurrence.

Staging

The AJCC[75] and FIGO[5] systems are used to stage vaginal cancer (Tables 76.2 and 76.3). Primary vaginal melanomas and lymphomas are staged according to the AJCC staging systems for melanomas and lymphomas, respectively.[75]

For patients with a prior gynecologic malignancy, a 5-year period free of disease is generally considered adequate to allow for distinction between recurrent disease and a new primary vaginal cancer. FIGO no longer recognizes carcinoma *in situ* as stage 0.

TABLE 76.2 INTERNATIONAL FEDERATION OF GYNECOLOGY AND OBSTETRICS STAGING SYSTEM FOR CARCINOMA OF THE VAGINA

Stage	Description
Stage I	Carcinoma is limited to vaginal wall.
Stage II	Carcinoma has involved the subvaginal tissue but has not extended to the pelvic wall.
Stage III	Carcinoma has extended to the pelvic wall.[a]
Stage IV	Carcinoma has extended beyond the true pelvic or has involved the mucosa of the bladder or rectum; bullous edema as such does not permit a case to be allotted to stage IV.
Stage IVA	Tumor invades the bladder and/or rectal mucosa and/or direct extension beyond the true pelvis.

[a]Pelvic wall is defined as muscle, fascia, neurovascular structures, or skeletal portions of the bony pelvis. From FIGO Committee on Gynecologic Oncology. Current FIGO staging for cancer of the vagina, fallopian tube, ovary, and gestational trophoblastic neoplasia. *Int J Gynaecol Obstet* 2009;105(1):3–4. Copyright © 2009 International Federation of Gynecology and Obstetrics. Reprinted by permission of John Wiley & Sons, Inc..

TABLE 76.3 AMERICAN JOINT COMMISSION ON CANCER STAGING OF VAGINAL CANCER 7TH EDITION

Primary Tumor (T)

Tx	Primary tumor cannot be assessed.
T0	No evidence of primary tumor
Tis/0	Carcinoma *in situ*
T1/I	Tumor confined to the vagina
T2/II	Tumor invades paravaginal tissues but not to the pelvic wall.
T3/III	Tumor extends to the pelvic wall*.
T4/IVA	Tumor invades the mucosa of the bladder or rectum and/or extends beyond the pelvis (bullous edema is not sufficient to classify a tumor as T4).

Regional Lymph Nodes (N)

Nx	Regional lymph nodes cannot be assessed.
N0	No regional lymph nodes
N1/IVB	Pelvic or inguinal lymph node metastasis

Distant Metastasis (M)

Mx	Distant metastasis cannot be assessed.
M0	No distant metastasis
M1/IVB	Distant metastasis

Stage Groupings

Stage 0	Tis N0 M0
Stage I	T1 N0 M0
Stage II	T2 N0 M0
Stage III	T1–3 N1 M0, T3 N0 M0
Stage IVA	T4, any N, M0
Stage IVB	Any T, any N, M1

*Pelvic wall is defined as muscle, fascia, neurovascular structures, or skeletal portions of the bony pelvis.
From Edge SB, Byrd DR, Compton CC, et al., eds. *AJCC cancer staging manual.* 7th ed. New York: Springer, 2010. Copyright © 2010 American Joint Committee on Cancer. Reproduced with permission of Springer in the format Book via Copyright Clearance Center.

Stage I disease is defined as limited to the vaginal wall, and stage II disease involves subvaginal tissue without extension to the pelvic wall. Discriminating between stages I and II can be subjective; thin tumors <0.5 cm are generally classified as stage I, with thicker infiltrating tumors or those with paravaginal nodularity classified as stage II. Perez et al. proposed a modification to the FIGO system in 1973, distinguishing tumors with paravaginal submucosal extension only (stage IIA) from tumors with parametrial infiltration (stage IIB).[41] The study reported a 20% 5-year survival difference (55% vs. 35%) between stages IIA and IIB. This modification has not been adopted into FIGO staging. However, some investigators consider the distinction to be prognostically relevant.[39,67] Stage III disease extends to the pelvic sidewall or involves lymph nodes, whereas stage IV disease reflects spread to the bladder, bowel, or distant sites.

Diagnostic Workup

The diagnostic workup should start with a thorough history and physical examination. During speculum examination, the speculum blades can obscure the anterior and posterior walls, so it is essential to rotate the speculum for visualization of all four walls from the introitus to the apex. Bimanual examination, with careful digital palpation, should be performed, assessing for parametrial and pelvic side wall involvement and invasion of tumor to the rectal mucosa. Complete assessment of tumor extent and assessment of vaginal walls are facilitated by examination under anesthesia.

Inguinal nodes should be palpated for disease involvement, particularly if the primary lesion is situated in the lower portion of the vagina, as 5% to 20% of patients have been reported to have involved inguinal nodes at presentation.[41,67] Suspicious nodes warrant a biopsy. Laboratory tests include a complete blood count with differential and assessment of renal and hepatic function.

A definitive diagnosis is achieved with biopsy of suspected lesions, which can present as an exophytic mass, plaque, or ulcer. If a lesion is not visible in the setting of

abnormal cytology, colposcopy with acetic acid, followed by Lugol iodine stain, is conducted. Biopsies of white epithelium or atypical vascularity should be obtained after application of acetic acid. Iodine will identify Schiller-positive regions, which are nonstaining and should correspond with areas identified following application of acetic acid. Adequate biopsies should include the cervix, if present, to rule out a cervical primary. Patients can present with multiple regions of abnormality.

FIGO staging of vaginal cancer is clinical and allows chest x-ray, intravenous pyelography (IVP), barium enema, cystoscopy, and proctosigmoidoscopy. FIGO encourages the utilization of more advanced imaging modalities, such as computed tomographic (CT) imaging, magnetic resonance imaging (MRI), and positron emission tomography (PET), as guidance for treatment, though imaging findings cannot be used to reassign stage.[76] Cystoscopy or proctosigmoidoscopy may be necessary in patients with symptoms suggestive of bladder or rectal infiltration. CT of the pelvis is obtained in place of IVP to assess the renal parenchyma and also to obtain information on the extent of local disease and lymph node status. MRI can provide salient treatment planning information by characterizing extent of invasion and differentiating malignant tumor, which is isointense to muscle on T1, and hyperintense on T2, from normal structures and/or fibrosis.[77] Advantages of MRI over other imaging modalities include superior soft tissue contrast resolution, allowing accurate assessment of tumor volume and extent of local invasion and accurate assessment of pelvic nodal involvement. In general, MRI is regarded as superior to CT for staging of gynecologic malignancies and should be obtained when available.

Positron emission tomography (PET) has shown efficacy in detecting the extent of primary tumor and abnormal lymph nodes in vaginal cancer with higher sensitivity than CT (Fig. 76.3), as is the case with cervical carcinoma.[78,79] Primary vaginal carcinoma and metastatic lesions demonstrate avid uptake of 2-[fluorine 18] fluoro-2-deoxy-D-glucose (FDG). In one study, 23 patients with primary vaginal carcinoma received both PET and CT during staging. CT identified the primary tumor in only 43% of patients, whereas PET identified the tumor in 100%. PET identified suspicious uptake in groin and pelvic nodes in 8 of 23 patients, compared to 4/23 with CT. Treatment planning was modified in 14% of patients because of findings from PET, and the authors concluded that PET detects primary tumor and abnormal lymph nodes more often than CT.[78] Another series compared detection of suspicious lymph nodes using PET/CT versus MRI and CT; PET/CT outperformed both MRI and CT, resulting in a change in management in 36% of cases.[79] It is important that the patient have an empty bladder prior to imaging, as physiologic FDG activity in a filled bladder can potentially interfere with accurate estimation of vaginal involvement. In practice, most patients undergo planning for radiation treatment with multiple imaging modalities.

Risk Factors

Risk factors for primary vaginal SCC are similar to VAIN and cervical neoplasia. Commonly cited factors include HPV infection and/or history of cervical or vulvar intraepithelial neoplasia, immunosuppression, multiple sexual partners, smoking, and early age at first intercourse.

It is believed that majority of cases of vaginal cancer can be attributed to HPV infection. According to a meta-analyses comprised of 14 studies, the overall HPV prevalence was 70% for vaginal carcinomas, with the most common subtypes as follows: HPV 16 (53.7%), HPV 18 (7.6%), and HPV 31 (5.6%). Multiple subtypes of HPV were identified in 3.4% of vaginal carcinoma cases.[80] In a population-based case control study of 156 women with VAIN or invasive cancer, HPV DNA was detectable in 80% of patients with *in situ* disease and 60% of

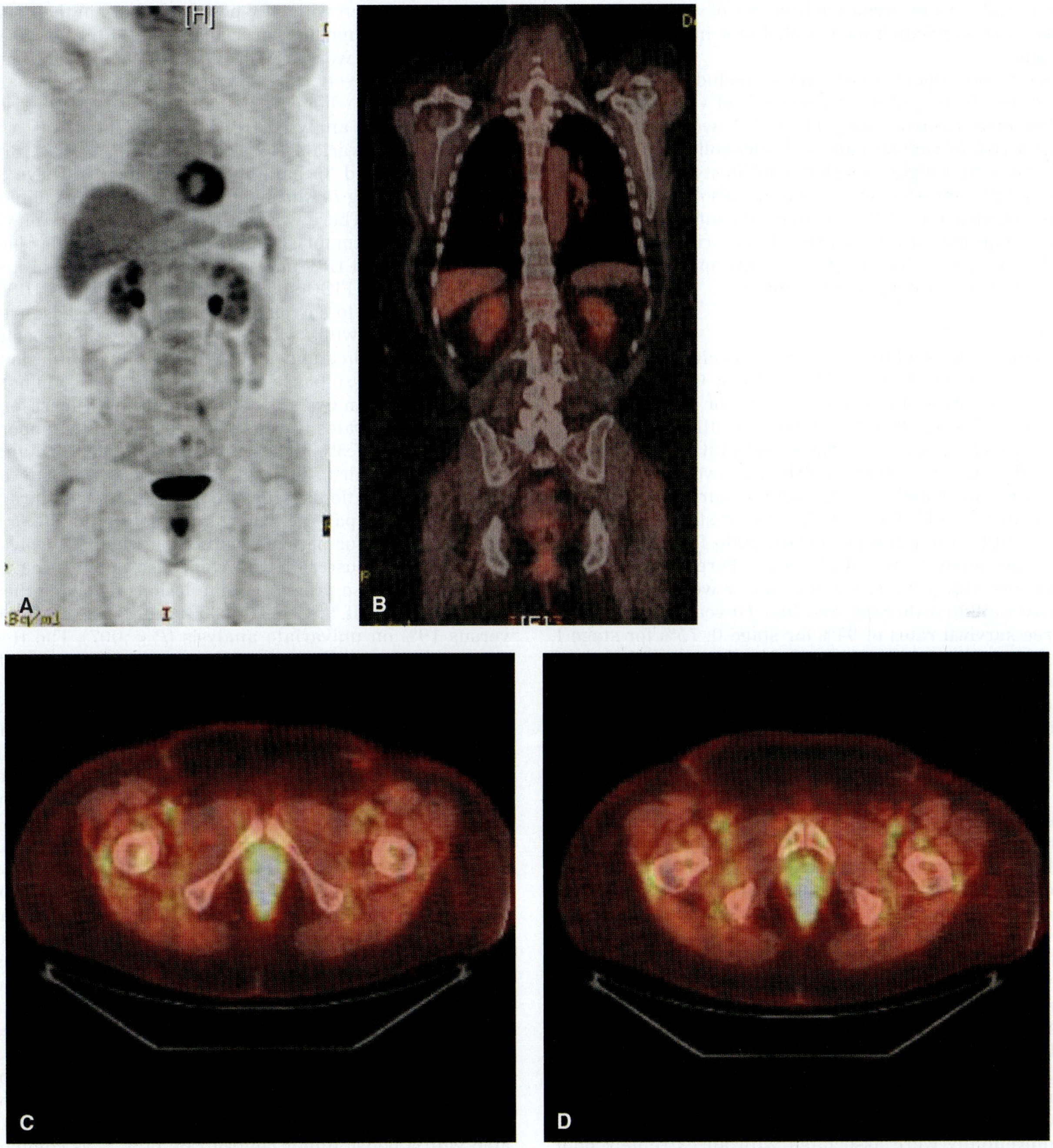

FIGURE 76.3. CT/PET fusion images of vaginal carcinoma. Coronal **(A, B)** and axial **(C, D)** images of a localized invasive vaginal carcinoma, extending into the central and lower 1/3 portion of the vagina above the introitus.

those with invasive disease, and 30% of patients reported a history of treatment for invasive malignancy, most commonly cervix, or *in situ* anogenital neoplasia.[81]

Patients with a history of cervical cancer have a significantly higher risk of developing *in situ* as well as invasive carcinoma of the vagina. Studies suggest that 10% to 50% of patients with a history of VAIN or invasive carcinoma of the vagina have undergone treatment for *in situ* or invasive cervical carcinoma,[12,40,61,67,82–86] with the interval from treatment of cervical disease to development of vaginal carcinoma averaging approximately 14 years.[61,72] Early hysterectomy appears to be a risk factor in some studies, if performed for malignant or premalignant disease.[81,87]

The role of ionizing radiation to the pelvis in the development of vaginal carcinoma is unclear, with conflicting reports. According to one study which analyzed 1,200 patients treated over a 20-year period for carcinoma of the cervix, prior RT was not shown to result in increased secondary pelvic neoplasms.[88] A second study by Boice et al.,[89] however, reported a 14-fold increased risk of vaginal cancer in women with a history of pelvic irradiation before the age of 45, with a significant dose–response relationship.

Another risk factor is chronic irritation of the vaginal mucosa, resulting in chronic inflammation, hyperkeratosis, thickening, and acanthosis,[90] with subsequent metaplastic and dysplastic changes; however, this is not proven. Although older studies showed that more vaginal cancers arise from the posterior vaginal wall, other studies report approximately equal distribution of invasive carcinomas on the anterior and posterior walls,[58,61,63,64,91] arguing against the theory that pooling of irritating substances in the posterior fornix contributes to development of vaginal cancers, particularly on the posterior wall. Chronic irritation from use of vaginal pessaries has also been implicated as a contributor in vaginal cancer development.[92]

Other, lesser reported risk factors include low socioeconomic status, history of genital warts, and vaginal trauma.[93] A larger case–control study of 36,856 women found an increased risk of vaginal cancer in alcoholic women, likely associated with a higher incidence of lifestyle factors, such as promiscuity and smoking, which are also associated with a higher incidence of HPV infection. HIV-infected and other immunocompromised women are at higher risk of developing vaginal carcinoma, which tends to behave more aggressively than in the immunocompetent patients.[90]

Prognostic Factors

Stage at time of presentation is the most significant prognostic factor.[7,41,84,94] According to an NCDB study by Creasman et al.,[9] 5-year survival rates are as follows: 96% for stage 0, 73% for stage I, 58% for stage II, and 36% for stage III/IV disease.

The series by Shah et al.,[7] based on SEER data for women diagnosed between 1990 and 2004, also reveals the correlation between stage and outcome, with 5-year disease-specific survival rates of 84% for stage I, 75% for stage II, and 57% for stage III/IV; the adjusted hazard ratio for mortality, on multivariate analysis, was 4.67. In the Perez et al. series,[67] 165 patients with primary vaginal cancer were treated with definitive radiation therapy, and had 10-year actuarial disease-free survival rates of 94% for stage 0, 75% for stage I, 55% for stage IIA, 43% for stage IIB, 32% for stage III, and 0% for stage IV.[95]

Size of the initial lesion is a prognostic factor that has shown significance in several series. The SEER database study,[7] which included 2,149 women with primary vaginal cancer, noted a significantly lower 5-year survival rate in women with tumors 4 cm or larger than in women with tumors smaller than 4 cm (65% vs. 84%); however, size information was missing for 52% of women. After multivariate analysis, the women with the larger tumors had an adjusted hazard ratio of 1.71 for mortality. Chyle et al.[40] in their review of 301 patients treated at M.D. Anderson Cancer Center (MDACC) from 1953 to 1991 found that women with lesions larger than 5 cm in maximum diameter had a significantly higher 10-year local recurrence rate than those with smaller lesions (40% vs. 20%). The series by Hellman et al.,[94] with 314 patients treated at the Karolinska University Hospital from 1956 to 1996, found only three factors to independently predict for poor survival on multivariate analysis: advanced age, tumor size greater than or equal to 4 cm, and advanced stage. Tumors comprising two-thirds or more of the vagina and tumors growing circumferentially were associated with an extremely poor prognosis. The series by Tran et al.,[96] which reviewed records of 78 patients with SCC treated at Stanford University Medical Center from 1959 to 2005, also found size to be a prognostic factor for disease-free survival on multivariate analysis, along with stage, prior hysterectomy, and pretreatment hemoglobin level. Smaller series by Tjalma et al.[97] and Kirkbride et al.[84] also describe adverse outcomes with larger tumor size. Other series have failed to show significance, but likely are hindered by small numbers, difficulties in accurate assessment of size, and treatment heterogeneity.

Extent of vaginal canal involvement has also been examined and found to be significant, perhaps because it is a surrogate for tumor size. In a series by Stock et al.,[64] which examined 100 cases of primary vaginal carcinoma treated at Magee-Women's Hospital from 1962 to 1992, patients with involvement of one-third of the vaginal canal or less had a significantly higher 5-year disease-free survival rate (61%) than patients with more extensive involvement (25%).

Several studies suggest HPV status is an indicator of favorable prognosis. Fuste et al. found a trend toward longer survival in women with HPV-positive tumors in their series of 32 patients, with median survival times of 113.9 months versus 19.7 months for women with HPV-positive and HPV-negative tumors, respectively (P = .15).[98] Alonso et al.[99] evaluated 57 total patients, of whom 70.2% had evidence of high-risk HPV. On multivariate analysis, HPV-positive status was a favorable prognostic variable for OS (HR 0.35, P = .038). Brunner et al.[100] evaluated 35 patients with primary invasive SCC of the vagina. Using *in situ* hybridization, HPV was detected in 51.4% of cases. There was no significant influence on clinical stage, grade or tumor size, nor did prognosis differ between HPV-positive and HPV-negative tumors. However, in a subset of patients with FIGO stage III or higher disease, HPV positivity was found to correlate with improved disease-free and overall survival, with P values of .004 and .023, respectively.

There is conflicting evidence on the impact of lesion location on prognosis; it has been noted in some[40,65,101] but not all[66,67] reports. In an analysis of 110 patients by Kucera et al.,[102] 5-year survival rates were 60% for lesions of the upper third of the vagina, 37.5% for lesions of the middle third and 37% for the lower third. Chyle et al.[40] noted a 17% rate of pelvic relapse in patients with tumors in the upper third of the vagina, 36% for patients with tumors in the middle or lower third, and 42% for patients with whole-vaginal involvement. Lesions in the posterior wall were also noted to be associated with a worse prognosis than lesions involving the anterior vaginal wall,[40] with 10-year recurrence rates of 32% versus 19% on univariate analysis (P < .007). The Hellman series,[94] however, found no difference in prognosis between the anterior and posterior tumors. Similarly, histologic grade has been found to be an independent significant predictor of survival in several series[65,84,101] but not others.[94] Hellman et al. evaluated the impact of tumor grade and other histopathologic variables (mitotic activity, koilocytosis, growth in vessels, lymphocytic reactions) and found no correlation with survival.

Several series suggest there is a correlation between older age and decreased survival.[10,94,101] For example, age was also noted to be a significant prognostic factor in the Urbanski et al. series,[101] with 5-year survival rates of 83% for patients younger than 60 compared to 25% for those 60 years of age or older (P < .0001). Age >60 years was negatively associated with survival in the series by Gunderson et al., which examined a total of 110 patients (HR 2.16; P = .0339). Other series have failed to demonstrate the statistical significance of age.[41,103]

For patients treated with radiation, treatment time may be a significant factor impacting tumor control.[104,105] Lee et al.[105] found overall treatment time of 9 weeks or less to be associated with a pelvic tumor control rate of 97% as compared to 57% for treatment time > 9 weeks (P < .01). Pingley et al. also noted a correlation between treatment time and outcome; patients receiving brachytherapy within 4 weeks of external beam radiation therapy (EBRT) had a 5-year disease-free survival rate of 60%, compared to a 30% rate in patients who had an interval >4 weeks.[104]

Other possible prognostic factors include hemoglobin levels, prior hysterectomy, and smoking status. Tran et al. reviewed records of 78 patients with primary SCC of the vagina treated at Stanford University Hospital, and found a hemoglobin level <12.5 g/dL prior to definitive treatment to be prognostic for worse pelvic control and disease-specific survival[73]; 5-year disease-specific survival rates were 55% for women with Hg levels <12.5 g/dL and 76% for those with levels greater than or equal to 12.5 g/dL. This remained significant after multivariate analysis, along with prior hysterectomy, stage, and tumor size. The study by Tran et al.[96] is the first to identify prior hysterectomy as a favorable prognostic factor on multivariate analysis. This may reflect more rigorous surveillance in posthysterectomy patients, resulting in tumors discovered at an earlier stage, or may be a reflection of less overall vaginal tissue as a substrate for tumorigenesis. Two subsequent studies have identified hysterectomy as a significant prognostic factor but only in univariate analysis.[40,94]

Treatment: Surgery

For most patients with invasive vaginal cancer, surgery has a limited role and radiation is the treatment of choice. Because of the rarity of these lesions, and required individualization of treatment, it is recommended that patients are referred to a tertiary center with experienced practitioners. In general, surgery is considered beneficial only in carefully selected patients. Typically, amenable lesions are small, superficially invasive and well-demarcated, and localized to the upper vagina. For patients who have previously undergone hysterectomy, a radical upper vaginectomy and pelvic lymphadenectomy can be considered. If the uterus is present, a radical hysterectomy (which include upper vaginectomy and radical parametrectomy) with lymph node assessment could be considered, particularly for patients with a lesion in the posterior proximal vagina.[6] Regardless of surgical procedure, wide negative margins are necessary.

Older surgical series often required pelvic exenteration in 40% to 50% of cases to obtain negative margins.[63,72] Invasive anterior wall lesions may require anterior exenteration, which removes the vagina, urethra, and bladder. Posterior exenteration requires resection of the vagina and rectum. Deeply invasive, circumferential lesions may require a total exenteration in order to achieve clear margins. If positive margins, adjuvant radiation should be offered. Lesions that extend to the inferior vagina require a total vaginectomy with radical hysterectomy, pelvic lymphadenectomy, and possibly vulvovaginectomy and inguinofemoral lymphadenectomy.[61,63,64,83] It is not uncommon for relatively small lesions to invade the rectum or urethra early in the disease course, given the close proximity of the vagina to these structures. Given the potentially devastating functional results associated with radical surgery, definitive radiation is the treatment of choice for most patients with invasive vaginal cancer and has largely replaced surgery as the primary therapeutic modality.

Exenterative surgical procedures can be a considered for previously irradiated patients with a pelvic confined tumor who cannot receive further radiation.

Patients with advanced disease are typically not candidates for curative intent surgery because of difficulty achieving negative margins, morbidity of resection, and metastatic disease.

Reported 5-year overall survival rates for stage I vaginal cancer treated with surgery range from 75% to 100% (Table 76.4).[9,64,72,83,97,107] The distinction between stage I and II

disease is made clinically, based on physical examination, and can be subject to variability. The NCDB review for cancers of the vagina noted superior survival rates in patients treated with surgery,[9] though this likely reflects selection of healthier patients with good performance status for radical surgery. A more recent analysis utilizing the SEER database[7] found women with stage I disease treated with surgery only to have a lower risk of mortality than those treated with radiation only, combined modalities or no treatment; however, this difference did not reach statistical significance. For stage II vaginal cancer patients, there was a similar trend toward increased mortality in women who did not have surgery alone as their primary treatment modality, but values once again did not reach statistical significance in their multivariate adjusted model.

Ling et al., in a small series consisting of 4 patients with stage I disease, report their experience using laparoscopic radical hysterectomy with vaginectomy and reconstruction of the vagina.[108] With follow-up times ranging from 40 to 54 months, they report all patients to be free of disease, with satisfactory sexual function. The authors suggest that laparoscopic surgery can be an option for select patients with early-stage disease, with good outcomes.

Other series also report excellent results with primary surgical therapy, though authors acknowledge bias resulting from selection of healthier patients with less extensive disease for primary surgery over radiation. In a review of 100 cases by Stock et al.,[64] with 85 SCC cases, surgical treatment was noted to be a significantly favorable prognostic factor for disease-free survival (63%), compared to treatment with radiation alone (26%). This benefit appears to skew from the advanced stage patients and potentially therefore with a selection bias. For stage I patients, disease-free survival rates were 56% and 80% for patients treated with surgery versus radiation, respectively. For stage II patients, survival rates were 68% and 31% after surgery and radiation, respectively, though this likely reflects selection bias, with patients with more extensive involvement offered radiation. Overall 5-year survival was 47%. Stock et al. concluded that surgery consisting of radical hysterectomy, pelvic lymphadenectomy, and upper vaginectomy could be reasonable for stage I lesions and select stage II lesions, with radiation being the preferred primary modality for patients with stage IIB disease. It should be noted, however, that 23 of 33 stage II patients (70%) treated with surgery required a total vaginectomy or exenterative procedure, which carries significant morbidity and functional impairment.

Smaller series also support use of surgery in select patients with early-stage disease. Tjalma et al.[97] reported on 55 cases of primary vaginal SCC. Of 27 patients with stage I disease, 26 received surgery, with 4 subsequently receiving some form of adjuvant radiation. With a median follow-up time of 45 months, 5-year survival was reported to be 91%. Otton et al.,[107] in their retrospective review of 70 patients with stage I to II vaginal carcinoma, treated at Queensland Centre for Gynaecological Cancer between 1982 and 1998, report that patients treated with surgery alone, or a combination of surgery and radiation, had significantly longer survival times than patients treated

TABLE 76.4 OUTCOMES AFTER PRIMARY SURGERY IN EARLY-STAGE VAGINAL CANCER

Series	Stage	No. of Pts	Outcomes	Comments
Jain (2010–2015)[106]	I	10	1 y DFS 89%	6 pts received adjuvant treatment for + margins/nodes
	II	1	1 y OS 100%	2 RV; 5 TV; 4 PV
Tjalma (1974–1999)[97]	I	26	5 y OS 91%	4 pts received adjuvant RT
				5 LE, 19 HTX, 2 EXT
Creasman (1985–1994)[9]	I	76	5 y OS 90%	
	II	34	5 y OS 70%	
Otton (1982–1998)[107]	I	8	5 y OS 100%	6 PV; 2 HTX + removal of vaginal cuff
Stock (1962–1992)[64]	I	17	5 y DFS 56%	6 LE, 7 PV, 4 RV
	II	33	5 y DFS 68%	6 EXT, 17 RV, 8 PV, 2 LE
Davis (1960–1987)[72]	I/II	52	5 y OS 85%	21 EXT
Rubin (1957–1980)[63]	I/II	9	5 y OS 75%	
Ball (1947–1978)[83]	I	19	5 y OS 84%	4 EXT
	II	8	5 y OS 63%	1 EXT

DFS, disease-free survival; EXT, exenteration; HTX, hysterectomy; LE, local excision; OS, overall survival; pts, patients; PV, partial vaginectomy; RV, radical vaginectomy; TV, total vaginectomy.

with radiation alone. The authors suggest that surgery may be effective in a select subset of patients with small, localized tumors that permit clear surgical margins. Peters et al.[66] reviewed records of 86 patients with vaginal carcinoma, including 68 SCC cases, treated at the University of Michigan Medical Center. Twelve selected patients had surgery as primary therapy, with a 75% survival rate. Similarly, Rubin et al.[63] reported on 8 patients with stage I or II disease who received surgery as primary treatment; 5-year survival was 75%, and the overall local control rate for the stage I patients was 80%, suggesting that highly selected patients can achieve excellent outcomes with surgery. Davis et al.[72] reported on 89 patients with vaginal carcinoma, treated primarily at the Mayo Clinic from 1960 to 1987. A total of 52 patients were treated with surgery as primary therapy, with 5-year survival of 85%, compared to 65% for patients who received radiation alone. In the stage II patients, the 5-year survival rates were 49%, 50%, and 69% for surgery, radiation, and combined treatment with surgery and radiation, respectively. However, treatment modalities cannot be effectively compared using retrospective series, given selection biases.

A case report documented the use of neoadjuvant chemotherapy consisting of bleomycin and cisplatin, followed by radical surgery, for 1 patient with stage II SCC of the vagina. The patient was free of disease, with satisfactory sexual function, at 30 months.[109] However, larger series of patients treated with this approach, with longer follow-up, are necessary to further evaluate the feasibility of this treatment.

Another approach that has been proposed involves neoadjuvant chemotherapy followed by radical surgery.[109,110] Benedetti et al. reported results on 11 patients with stage II SCC of the vagina,[110] treated with using three cycles of neoadjuvant paclitaxel and cisplatin followed by surgical resection. Ninety-one percent of patients obtained a partial or complete response to neoadjuvant chemotherapy; 27% achieved a complete response. All patients had disease-free resection margins after surgery, and only 1 patient had positive lymph nodes. At a median follow-up time of 75 months, 10 of 11 patients (91%) were alive, and of those, 8 (73%) were free of disease. Postoperative complications were mild.

Advanced vaginal cancers are generally treated with definitive radiation in combination with chemotherapy. The use of combined modality treatment is imputed from the cervical cancer literature. Several series report their experience using surgery for advanced stage III or IV patients, with most cases requiring radical excision, typically pelvic exenteration.[61,63,64,83] Control rates, at best, are around 50%, even with highly selected patients.

Treatment: Radiation

For most patients, radiation is the treatment of choice given the desire for organ preservation and the significant morbidity that may be incurred by exenterative surgery. It is important to individualize radiation therapy techniques based on size, depth, and location of the lesion. The outcomes of retrospective series on use of radiation for vaginal cancer are summarized in Table 76.5 and in detail below.

Stage I

For very small, superficial tumors, brachytherapy alone can be considered, but appropriate patient selection is critical. Reported local control rates range from 62% to 100%.[62,65,67,85,91,101,111,121] Perez et al.[41] reported pelvic tumor control of 88% in patients with stage I disease who received

TABLE 76.5 OUTCOMES BY STAGE FOR VAGINAL CANCER TREATED WITH PRIMARY RADIATION, +/− CHEMOTHERAPY

Series	Outcome	Stage I	Stage II	Stage III	Stage IV	Treatment	Notes
Kanayama (1993–2012)[111]	3 y OS	81%	86%	83% (St III = IV combined)		EBRT + BT ($n = 9$), EBRT ($n = 8$), BT ($n = 7$); 12% CRT	
Chang (1976–2011)[112]	5 y OS	75%	69%	68%	69%	EBRT + BT ($n = 112$), EBRT ($n = 22$), BT ($n = 4$)	CRT 41%
Miyamoto (1972–2009)[113]	3 y OS	56% (Combined I–IV)				RT ± S	CRT 31%
Damast (1998–2008)[114]	5 y OS	67% (St I–II combined)				EBRT + MRI-based BT; 40% CRT	
Beriwal (2000–2006)[115]	2 y crude LC		100%	100%	100%	EBRT + HDR BT	
Lian (1986–2006)[116]	5 y DSS	90%	87%	32%	26%	EBRT + BT ($n = 28$), EBRT ($n = 17$), BT ($n = 4$), S + RT ($n = 6$)	
Tran (1959–2005)[96]	5 y PC	83%	76%	62%	26%	EBRT + BT ($n = 43$), EBRT ($n = 22$), BT ($n = 10$)	
	5 y DSS	92%	68%	44%	30%		
Shah (1990–2004)[7]	5 y DSS	84%	75%	57%		RT and/or S	
de Crevoisier (1970–2001)[117]	5 y PC	79%		62%		EBRT and/or BT	
Frank (1970–2000)[62]	5 y PC	86%	84%	71%		EBRT + BT ($n = 119$), EBRT ($n = 63$)	
Mock (1986–1999)[60]	5 y DSS	92%	57%	59%	0%	EBRT + BT ($n = 55$), EBRT ($n = 5$), BT ($n = 26$)	
Hellman (1956–1996)[94]	5 y DSS	75%	36%	36%	20%, 0%[a]	RT and/or S	
Creasman (1985–1994)[9]	5 y OS	73%	58%	36%		RT and/or S	
Stryker (1976–1994)[118]	5 y DSS	78%	63%	33%	50%	EBRT + BT ($n = 25$), EBRT ($n = 7$), BT ($n = 2$)	
Stock (1962–1992)[64]	5 y LC	72%	62%	0%	21%	RT and/or S	
	5 y DFS	67%	53%	0%	15%		
Fine (1963–1991)[119]	5 y OS	42%	68%	58%	0%	EBRT and/or BT	
Perez (1953–1991)[67]	PC	85%	66%, 56%[b]	65%	27%	EBRT and/or BT	
	10 y DFS	80%	55%, 35%[b]	38%	0%		
Chyle (1953–1991)[40]	10 y PC	84%	75%	60%	40%	EBRT + BT ($n = 121$), EBRT ($n = 95$), BT ($n = 26$)	
	10 y OS	55%	51%	37%	40%	Transvaginal cone ($n = 2$)	
Lee (1964–1990)[120]	5 y PC	87%	88%, 68%[b]	80%	67%	EBRT and/or BT	
	5 y CSS	94%	80%, 39%[b]	79%	62%		
Kirkbride (1974–1989)[84]	5 y DSS	72%	70%	53%	42%	RT and/or S	
Dixit (1985–1989)[103]	2 y DSS	100%	70%	19%	0%	EBRT and/or BT	
Urbanski (1965–1988)[101]	5 y DFS	73%	54%	23%	0%	EBRT + BT ($n = 77$), EBRT ($n = 15$), BT ($n = 11$)	
Kucera (1975–1984)[102]	5 y OS	81%	44%	35%	32%, 0%[a]	EBRT and/or BT	
Rubin (1958–1980)[63]	5 y OS	75%	48%	54%	15%	RT and/or S	

BT, brachytherapy of any form; CRT, chemoradiation; CSS, cause-specific survival; DFS, disease-free survival; DSS, disease-specific survival; EBRT, external beam radiation therapy; HDR, high-dose rate; LC, local control; OS, overall survival; PC, pelvic control; RT, radiotherapy (any form); S, surgery.
[a]Outcomes for stages IVA, IVB, respectively.
[b]Outcomes for stages IIA, IIB, respectively.

brachytherapy alone, using a dose of 60 to 70 Gy, prescribed 5 mm beyond the plane of the implant or vaginal mucosa, with a vaginal surface dose of 80 to 120 Gy. Notably, tumor control in stage I vaginal carcinoma was similar to brachytherapy alone, versus brachytherapy plus EBRT. This observation is consistent with reports from some groups,[41,102,122] but not others.[62,111] Other series suggest high locoregional failure rates with brachytherapy alone. Kanayama et al. report 3 out of 8 (38%) patients with stage I vaginal cancer, treated with brachytherapy alone, developed lymph node recurrence. Frank et al.[62] reported on 21 patients with stage I disease who were treated with local radiation only, without regional node coverage. Nine received brachytherapy alone, 11 received EBRT with or without brachytherapy, and 1 received local EBRT using a transvaginal orthovoltage cone. Three of 9 patients treated with brachytherapy alone developed recurrent disease in the pelvis, resulting in a 10-year pelvic disease control rate of 67%. Patients who received EBRT with or without brachytherapy did not have pelvic recurrences. A pelvic relapse rate of 18% at 10 years was noted by Frank et al.,[62] with all pelvic failures occurring in patients treated with brachytherapy alone. Overall, results suggest caution should be taken when brachytherapy alone is used without prophylactic lymph node irradiation, given fairly high rates of lymph node recurrence. Appropriate patient selection is critical when utilizing brachytherapy alone as primary treatment, particularly since the distinction between stage I and II is based on clinical exam and can vary between providers.

With LDR, treatment can be delivered in two applications, with the first designed to treat the entire vaginal wall and a second application to cover the tumor volume. When HDR brachytherapy is the primary treatment, the entire length of the vagina is typically treated to a mucosal dose of 60 to 65 Gy, with an additional mucosal dose of 20 to 30 Gy delivered to the area of tumor involvement.[123] Treatment can be delivered with a shielded vaginal cylinder or with a multichannel HDR cylinder to treat the tumor with a 2-cm margin and block uninvolved mucosal surfaces.[124] HDR can also be used to treat superficial lesions.

Use of a multichannel HDR cylinder is an alternative technique with favorable local control and low toxicity. The standard multichannel HDR cylinder is comprised of a central channel with 6 to 12 peripheral channels, allowing preferential dosing to the target while decreasing dose to normal structures. Vargo et al.[125] reported their outcomes for 41 patients with vaginal cancer treated with this technique to median EQD2 (equivalent dose in 2 Gy fractions) of 77.1 Gy. Definitive treatment consisted of EBRT followed by brachytherapy. The majority (71%) of patients had FIGO 1 disease. At 2 years, there was 93% local control, and 4% overall late grade 3 or higher toxicity, demonstrating comparable results to historical treatments. A tumor thickness cutoff of 5 mm for the apex and posterior vagina, and 7 mm for other locations was utilized.

Guidelines from the American Brachytherapy Society recommend a cumulative D90 (dose to 90% of volume) EQD2 of 70 to 85 Gy prescribed to the vaginal tumor.[126] Various regimens can be utilized to achieve this dose, with commonly utilized schedules of 45 Gy in 25 fractions EBRT followed by HDR brachytherapy in 5 fractions of 4.5 to 5.5 Gy (EQD2 = 71.4 to 79.8 Gy) or 9 to 10 fractions of 3 Gy (EQD2 = 73.5 to 76.8 Gy).

Poorly differentiated or extensively infiltrating stage I lesions should be treated with a combination of EBRT and brachytherapy. Given possible underestimation of submucosal disease and/or nodal disease, resulting in a potentially high likelihood of recurrence with brachytherapy alone, some groups recommend incorporating EBRT into treatment of all stage I patients, except for those with very small, superficial

lesions.[62,111] Damast et al. reported outcomes for early-stage vaginal cancer treated with a combination of EBRT and MRI-based intracavitary brachytherapy between 1998 and 2008.[114] With mean EBRT dose of 45, followed by intracavitary HDR brachytherapy, 5-year overall survival, disease-specific survival, and local failure-free survival were 67%, 80%, and 90%, respectively. Notably, 60% of patients had a complete response after EBRT; of this group, there were no recurrences. Concurrent cisplatin was used as a radiosensitizer in 40% of patients.

Actuarial 5-year survival rates for stage I disease range from 60% to 85%.[7,62,67,96] Disease-specific survival rates for stage I disease, treated with definitive radiation, range from 75% to 95%.[40,41,86] The 10-year pelvic relapse rate, comprised of local, pelvic nodal, and inguinal nodal failures, was noted to be 16% by Frank et al. for stage I patients.[62] Most failures are locoregional. Distant metastases are uncommon and occur in about 5% of patients.[41,72,121]

Stage II

Stage II vaginal carcinoma involves the subvaginal tissue but does not extend to the pelvic side wall. The primary treatment for stage II disease is radiation, most commonly as a combination of EBRT followed by vaginal brachytherapy; chemotherapy is typically considered. Outcomes with brachytherapy alone have been poor; thus, this approach is not recommended. With brachytherapy alone, Perez et al.[41] noted a 36% pelvic tumor control rate in stage II patients, compared to 67% in patients treated with a combination of EBRT and brachytherapy. The benefit of combining EBRT and brachytherapy, as opposed to using either alone, has been shown in other series as well.[40,64]

During EBRT, the pelvis generally receives 45 to 50.4 Gy in 1.8 Gy fractions, with consideration of a parametrial boost if there is extensive primary infiltration or high suspicion of nodal disease. Inguinal lymph nodes are included in a modified whole pelvic field for lesions involving the distal one-third of the vaginal canal.

Subsequent brachytherapy should be carefully delivered to ensure adequate coverage of tumor volume. An interstitial technique, ideally with three-dimensional (3D) imaging for treatment planning, is required for tumors >5 mm in depth.[85] Extensive tumors, or deeply infiltrating tumors with nondistinct margins, may be poor candidates for brachytherapy. In such cases, boosting tumors with conformal techniques or intensity-modulated radiation therapy (IMRT) can be considered and may yield better outcomes than suboptimal brachytherapy.[62] The tumor volume should receive a minimum of 75 to 80 Gy using combined EBRT and brachytherapy. Fleming et al.[127] and Puthawala et al.[128] both report improved outcomes with higher doses of 80 to 100 Gy.

The 5-year survival rate for patients with stage II disease treated with RT alone ranges from 35% to 70% for stage IIA and 35% to 60% for stage IIB.[29,129,130] Pelvic relapse at 10 years has been reported to be 25% by Frank et al., consistent with recent series reporting 5-year pelvic control rates ranging from 76% to 84%.[62,96] The likelihood of distant metastasis is higher for stage IIB lesions compared to stage IIA,[67,122] with overall reported rates ranging from 22% to 46%.[67,72]

Stages III and IVA

Locally advanced vaginal cancer is treated with a combined modality approach of radiation and chemotherapy, extrapolating from favorable outcomes with use of CRT in cervical cancer patients.[131,132] Radiation is delivered as pelvic EBRT, followed by additional parametrial boost when warranted. If adequate tumor coverage can be achieved without undue toxicity, interstitial brachytherapy is employed to deliver a minimum tumor dose of 75 to 80 Gy. If brachytherapy is not feasible because of extensive tumor infiltration of the rectovaginal septum or bladder, a shrinking field technique or IMRT have been used to deliver additional dose to the primary lesion.[133,134] The overall cure rate for patients with stage III disease ranges from 30% to 50%. Stage IVA carries a worse prognosis. In highly selected patients with small volume stage IV disease, pelvic exenteration can yield good long-term control; however, in practice, EBRT remains the primary treatment.[7,9,41,62-64,101]

Five-year actuarial survival rates for women with stage III disease range from 25% to 58%,[7,9] with local failure rates of 30% to 75%.[62,67,96] Outcomes for stage IV disease are worse, with survival rates of 0% to 40%.[40,64,119] Despite treatment with EBRT and brachytherapy, only 20% to 30% of patients with stage III to IV disease achieve local control. Pelvic recurrences occur more often than distant recurrences.[62]

Role of Combined Chemotherapy and Radiation

Chemotherapy has been incorporated with radiation for treatment of vaginal cancer, extrapolating from studies in cervical cancer showing improved progression-free and overall survival when cisplatin is added to RT.[41,131,132,135,136] Given rarity of vaginal cancer, there are no randomized trials comparing radiation alone to radiation plus chemotherapy.

Retrospective series are limited by small numbers or inclusion of other cancers, such as cervical and vulvar carcinomas. Nonetheless, the majority of retrospective studies suggest that a combined modality approach is feasible and may yield improved outcomes. These studies are summarized as follows (Table 76.6).

An NCDB study identified 13,689 women with primary vaginal cancer treated between 1998 and 2011 and explored the impact of concurrent chemoradiation on survival.[141] Median survival with chemotherapy and radiation was significantly longer, compared to radiation alone (56.2 months vs. 41.2 months, $P < .0005$). It was noted that only 48.6% of all patients received chemotherapy, but there was a consistent trend toward increased use of concurrent chemoradiation from 20% to 59.1% between 1998 and 2011.

Ghia et al.[142] published a retrospective patterns of care analysis using the SEER database, analyzing data from women with primary vaginal cancer treated with EBRT and/or brachytherapy between 1991 and 2005. Of the 326 women in the study cohort, 80.4% had SCC. It was noted that CRT was used in 7.5% of patients treated before 1999 compared to 36.1% of those treated afterward ($P < .001$). Cisplatin was the most frequently utilized agent, accounting for 59% of CRT treatments. Chemotherapy was significantly less likely to be used in conjunction with radiation for

women older than 80 years of age; otherwise, there was no difference for race, stage, grade, histologic diagnosis, comorbidities, or brachytherapy use. On multivariate analysis, CRT was not found to correlate with improved cause-specific or overall survival.

In a retrospective analysis of 71 patients with primary vaginal cancer treated at Dana-Farber Cancer Institute/Brigham and Women's Hospital from 1972 to 2009, 51 patients were treated with radiation alone and 20 were treated with CRT and RT.[136] Of patients treated with chemosensitization during radiation, 85% of patients received weekly cisplatin chemotherapy, whereas the remainder received either carboplatin or 5-FU. Three-year actuarial overall survival and disease-free survival was 56% for the RT alone group, compared to 79% for the CRT group ($P = .01$). Three-year disease-free survival was 43% for the RT alone group, compared to 73% for the CRT group ($P = .01$). At a median follow up of 3 years, tumor relapse was seen in 15% of patients treated with CRT compared to 45% of patients treated with radiation alone ($P = .03$). On multivariate analysis, the addition of chemotherapy was a significant predictor of DFS (HR 0.31).

Evans et al.[143] reported the use of radiation with 5-fluorouracil (5-FU) and mitomycin C (MMC) in 7 patients with vaginal cancer. Four out of 7 patients were free of disease with follow-up times ranging from 19 to 39 months. Roberts et al.[144] reported results for 7 patients with vaginal cancer treated with concurrent 5-FU, cisplatin, and radiation. Three patients received interstitial brachytherapy after EBRT, and 2 patients received intracavitary brachytherapy after EBRT. Eighty-five percent of patients achieved a complete response initially. Ultimately, 61% recurred, with a median time to recurrence of 6 months. There were 3 local recurrences and 1 distant metastasis and the 5-year overall survival rate was 22%. Kirkbride et al.[84] reported on the use of concurrent 5-FU, with or without MMC, in 26 of 153 patients with vaginal carcinoma treated at Princess Margaret Hospital. Seventy-seven percent of the patients had stage III/IV disease. Radiation was EBRT followed by interstitial or intracavitary brachytherapy to a total dose of 62 to 74 Gy. The 5-year survival rate was 50%. Dalrymple et al.[137] reported results using 5-FU–based chemotherapy in combination with radiation for treatment of primary SCC of the vagina. Thirteen of 14 patients (93%) had stage I or II disease. The median dose of radiation was 63 Gy, achieved using EBRT alone or EBRT with intracavitary brachytherapy. The 5-year survival rate was 86% for all patients, and 9 patients were free of disease with a median follow-up time of 100 months, suggesting that good local control can be achieved despite the use of lower radiation doses. There was a 31% rate of severe bowel complications reported, with 2 deaths as a result of bowel obstruction.

A retrospective series from MDACC by Frank et al.[62] included 9 patients with stage II to IVA SCC of the vagina treated with radiation therapy and concurrent cisplatin-based CRT. With a mean follow-up time of 129 months, improved local control with the use of chemotherapy was noted; with 44% of patients treated with concurrent CRT remaining free of disease. Samant et al. published a review of 12 vaginal cancer patients, Stage II to IVA, treated with concurrent weekly cisplatin at a dose of 40 mg/m² for 5 weeks.[139]

TABLE 76.6 OUTCOMES AFTER COMBINED CHEMORADIATION IN VAGINAL CANCER

Series	Stage	Outcomes	Notes
Miyamoto (1972–2009)[136]	St I, n = 18; St II, n = 19; St III, n = 8, St IVA, n = 6	3 y OS 79%	RT + cis, 5FU or carboplatin
Dalrymple (1986–1996)[137]	St I, n = 1; St II, n = 10; St III, n = 1	NED n = 9 (FU 74–168 mo); DOD n = 1 (12 mo); DID n = 4 (46–109 mo)	RT + 5-FU, cis/5FU or MMC
Gunderson (1990–2004)[138]	St I, n = 31; St II, n = 30; St III/IV, n = 69	4 y OS 64% (stage I), 40% (stage II) 12% (stage III/IV)	CRT, n = 87; S + CRT, n = 43
Samant (1999–2004)[139]	St II, n = 6; St III, n = 4; St IVA, n = 2	5 y OS 66%	RT + cis
Nashiro (2002–2005)[140]	St II, n = 2; St III, n = 1; St IVA, n = 3	DOD n = 1 (25 mo); NED n = 4 (FU 19–54 mo); AWD n = 1 (FU 19 mo)	RT + cis or cis/5FU

AC, adenocarcinoma; AWD, alive with disease; B, brachytherapy; cis, cisplatin; CRT, chemoradiation; DID, died of intercurrent disease; DOD, died of disease; EBRT, external beam radiation therapy; FU, fluorouracil; 5-FU, 5-fluorouracil; LR PFS, locoregional progression-free survival; MMC, mitomycin; NED, no evidence of disease; OS, overall survival; SCC, squamous cell carcinoma.

Patients received concurrent EBRT to a median dose of 45 Gy, with LDR interstitial or an HDR intracavitary brachytherapy boost of median dose 30 Gy. Six patients had stage II disease, 4 had stage III disease, and 2 had stage IVA. Ten of 12 patients (83%) had SCC; the other 2 had adenocarcinoma. Overall, treatment was well tolerated, with 92% of patients completing therapy as prescribed. Two of 10 patients who received interstitial brachytherapy required surgery for fistula repair. The 5-year overall survival, progression-free survival, and locoregional progression-free survival rates were 66%, 75%, and 92%, respectively, supporting use of concurrent weekly cisplatin therapy. A small series of 6 patients treated with CRT at the University of the Ryukyus was reported by Nashiro et al. All patients received EBRT to 50 Gy, followed by either a boost with shrinking fields (n = 4) or intracavitary brachytherapy (n = 2). Radiation was delivered with two to three cycles of cisplatin. Two patients had stage II, 1 had stage III, and 3 had stage IVA disease. All 6 achieved a complete response, and 4 of 6 patients remained free of disease at follow-up times of 18 to 55 months.

Outcomes

In general, the rate of locoregional recurrence ranges from 10% to 20% for stage I and 30% to 40% for stage II. Patients with advanced disease often have persistent disease despite treatment. In a series by Dixit et al.,[103] 68% of failures in stage III patients were due to persistent disease. Most treatment failures occur within 5 years, with a median time to recurrence of 6 to 12 months,[62,145] and local recurrence is the most common pattern of treatment failure in the majority of published series. Extravaginal recurrences in the pelvic lymph nodes are less common. The reported rates of distant metastasis vary, ranging from 7% to 33% and usually occur later in the course of disease, with approximately half of all distant metastases presenting at the time of local recurrence.[67,85,103,146]

According to SEER-based data, outcomes for vaginal cancer may be improving. A recent study by Shah et al.[7] analyzed records from the SEER database of 2,149 women diagnosed with primary vaginal cancer between 1990 and 2004. The risk of mortality is noted to have decreased over time, with a 17% decrease in the risk of death for women diagnosed after 2,000 relative to those diagnosed between 1990 and 1994. The authors reported 5-year disease-specific survival rates of 84% for stage I, 75% for stage II, and 57% for stage III to IV. An older study by Creasman et al.[9] focused on 4,885 women diagnosed with vaginal cancer between 1985 and 1994 and reported 5-year survival rates of 96% for stage 0, 73% for stage I, 58% for stage II, and 36% for stages III–IV, with 85% of invasive cases being SCC.

Melanoma

Vaginal melanomas comprise approximately 4% of all primary vaginal cancers,[9] with just over 100 new cases of vaginal melanoma reported each year in the United States. Melanomas arising from the vaginal mucosa are thought to originate from mucosal melanocytes in regions of melanosis or from atypical melanocytic hyperplasia.

The incidence of vaginal melanoma has remained stable and is reported to be approximately 0.26 per million.[147] The majority of reported cases are in Caucasian women; one study of 37 women with primary melanoma of the vagina reported 84% of patients to be Caucasian, and only 3% African American.[148] According to a report by Hu et al.[149] analyzing SEER data from 1992 to 2005 on 125 cases of vaginal melanoma with known race/ethnicity, there is no significant difference in incidence rate of vaginal melanoma between Caucasian and African American women, with a white/black ratio of 1.02 after age adjustment. In the report by Creasman et al.,[9] most patients were of advanced age at presentation, with only 23% of patients diagnosed before the age of 60; 28%

were diagnosed between the ages of 60 and 69, 28% were diagnosed between the ages of 70 and 79, and 22% were diagnosed at age 80 or older.

Grossly, melanoma of the vagina tends to be pigmented and may present as a dark mass, plaque, or ulceration; multifocal presentation is also common. In a case series of 37 women with primary vaginal melanoma reported by Frumovitz et al.,[148] median tumor size at presentation was 3 cm (range, 0.4 to 5 cm), with median depth of invasion of 7 mm (range, 1 to 21 mm). Twenty-one percent of patients presented with multifocal disease. Twenty-four patients (65%) presented with lesions in the distal third of the vagina or introitus. The most common appearance is polypoid nodular.[150] The most common location at presentation is the anterior vaginal wall and lower one-third of the vagina.[148]

Microscopically, tumors may be composed of epithelioid, spindle, or nevus-like cells, with variable morphology, and stain frequently positive for S-100 protein, HMB-45, and melan A. When S-100 is negative or only focally positive, tyrosinase and MART-1 are useful markers. Poorly differentiated tumors may be difficult to distinguish from carcinomas or sarcomas. Tumor thickness correlates with prognosis and is measured by the methods of Breslow.[151]

Vaginal melanoma is a high malignant disease with a propensity for early hematogenous spread. The most common presenting symptoms reported have been slight vaginal bleeding and vaginal discharge which is usually blood-tinged, foul smelling, or purulent.[152] Reid et al. reviewed 115 patients with primary melanoma of the vagina, found depth of invasion and lesion size >3 cm to be negative prognostic factors.[153] Stage was not found to be prognostic for outcome, but only 42 of the 115 patients had this information available. Compared to women with SCC, patients with vaginal melanoma have a significant 1.5-fold increased risk of mortality.[7]

Treatment Options

Primary vaginal melanoma is uncommon and treatment outcomes for only a small number of patients have been reported.[148,152,154–157] As a result, it is difficult to make definitive treatment recommendations. Treatments used in published series include wide local excision, radical surgery, radiation and chemotherapy, or a combination of modalities.

Some authors advocate incorporation of radical surgical resection into the treatment paradigm, when feasible.[158,159] The rationale for favoring surgery over radiation is based upon the observation that melanoma tends to be radioresistant. Geisler et al.[158] recommend primary pelvic exenteration for vaginal melanomas with >3 mm invasion, reporting a 5-year survival rate of 50% if pelvic nodes are free of disease. Morrow and DiSaia,[160] in their review of gynecologic melanoma, recommend radical surgery based on a review of the literature revealing 3 out of 19 long-term survivors after exenteration with wide local excision. Chung et al.[154] reviewed 19 cases of primary vaginal melanoma treated between 1934 and 1976. All patients who received wide local excision developed recurrence. Five-year survival was only 21%. Miner et al.[161] reported on 35 patients treated at Memorial Sloan-Kettering Cancer Center from 1977 to 2001. Sixty-nine percent underwent surgery, which was either *en bloc* removal of the involved pelvic organs, wide excision, or total vaginectomy, with elective pelvic lymph node dissection in 74% of cases. Thirty-one percent of patients received definitive radiation. Primary surgical therapy was significantly associated with a longer overall survival time (25 months vs. 13 months). Recurrence-free survival was not found to correlate with surgical extent. A study by Huang et al. found 5-year overall survival to be 32% but as high as 47% in patients who underwent surgical treatment.[162]

The goal of surgical excision should be complete resection with a negative margin. Drawing on the general melanoma guidelines this would be between 0.5 and 2 cm depending on the Breslow thickness of the primary tumor. Given the close proximity of the bladder and rectum, a wide local excision can rarely achieve this. Because of the risk of metastatic disease and the aggressive nature of the tumor, however, several series comparing radical surgery and local excision find equivalent outcomes.[152,155,163,164]

The role of surgical lymphadenectomy, lymph node sampling or sentinel lymph node mapping is not established in vaginal cancer given the vast variability in lymphatic drainage and substantial morbidity in the form of lymphedema that could result from sampling of both the inguinal and pelvic nodal basins. Lymphadenectomy could be considered in patients with nodal disease with the goal of locoregional control.

The use of wide local excision followed by postoperative EBRT and brachytherapy has been proposed. Bonner et al.[165] reported on nine cases of vaginal melanoma. Three patients were treated with wide local excision and 6 underwent radical surgery. All 9 patients developed locoregional recurrence. As a result, the authors suggest adding pelvic radiation therapy to improve local control. A more recent review by Frumovitz et al.[148] reported that radiation after wide local excision can reduce local recurrences. However, most patients develop distant metastases, most commonly in the lungs and liver. New advanced in immunotherapy hold promise for changing the outcomes of patients and evolving the management of patients with melanoma. There is no general recommendation for the treatment of primary vaginal melanoma. When radiation is administered, vaginal melanoma is treated similarly to vaginal carcinoma, with volumes and doses ranging from 50 Gy for subclinical disease to 75 Gy for gross tumor.

Retrospective data suggest that radiation may improve local control for vaginal melanoma.[152,166] Among the few long-term survivors reported in the literature are a handful of patients who were treated with radiation. Harwood and Cummings[167] described a complete response in 4 patients with vaginal melanoma treated with radiation, although two subsequently relapsed. Rogo et al.,[168] in their series of 22 cases of vulvovaginal melanoma, reported comparable results for surgery and radiation, with 8 patients (36%) alive 5 years after treatment. Petru et al.,[166] in their series documenting 14 patients treated for primary malignant melanoma of the vagina, noted that 3 of 9 patients treated with radiation, either as primary treatment ($n = 2$) or in the postoperative setting ($n = 1$), survived longer than 5 years. Median overall survival for all patients was 10 months, with a 5-year disease-free survival rate of 14% and an overall survival rate of 21%.

Frumovitz et al., in their review of 37 women with stage I melanoma of the vagina treated at MDACC between 1980 and 2009, report very poor prognosis even in this group of patients with localized disease, with a 5-year overall survival rate of 20%. In that study, 10% of patients received nonsurgical treatment with radiation, chemotherapy, or both. Patients treated surgically had significantly longer survival times compared to those treated nonsurgically. Radiation delivered after wide local excision reduced local recurrence and demonstrated a trend toward longer survival times, from 16.1 to 29.4 months.[169] A study by Xia et al. evaluated 44 women, diagnosed and treated for vaginal melanoma between 2002 and 2011.[157] There was no difference in overall survival between local excision and radical surgery. However, the authors note increased progression-free survival with the addition of adjuvant chemotherapy and radiation (8.6 months vs. 16.0 months, $P = .038$). Given the high rates of distant metastases, chemotherapy has been used, either alone or in conjunction with radiation.[148,170] Other reports have described the use of immunotherapy after surgery.[162]

Recommendations for the use of adjuvant chemotherapy for vaginal melanoma derive from the general melanoma literature where multiple agents have been the focus of investigation. One of the first drugs used was interferon alpha, which

was been found to bring an improvement in recurrence-free survival with no overall survival benefit. More recently in a phase II study, patients treated with surgery followed by adjuvant temozolomide in combination with cisplatin were noted to have a 48.7-month overall survival, superior to IFN-α (40.4 months) or observation (21.2 months) ($P < .01$). Further studies are ongoing.[171]

Effectiveness of targeted molecular therapies and immunotherapy in cutaneous melanoma has significantly expanded the options for patients with advanced melanoma. Approved therapies for advanced, unresectable melanomas include ipilimumab (antibody against cytotoxic T-lymphocyte–associated protein 4 [CTLA-4]), nivolumab (inhibitor of programmed cell death 1 [PD-1] protein), pembrolizumab (PD-1 inhibitor), vemurafenib (B-raf proto-oncogene serine/threonine kinase [BRAF] inhibitor), dabrafenib (BRAF inhibitor) and trametinib (mitogen-activated protein kinase kinase [MEK] inhibitor). However, it is difficult to extrapolate the effectiveness of these therapies for cutaneous melanoma to vaginal melanoma, and there are no specific trials that have validated efficacy of these regimens in vaginal melanoma. Testing of tumors for BRAF, NRAS, and c-KIT can be used to guide therapy. There appears to be high levels of PD-1 and PDL-1 expression in both vaginal and vulvar melanomas, suggesting utilization of immunotherapy may have efficacy for this disease.[129]

Regardless of primary treatment, outcomes have been disappointing. Overall prognosis is poor, with historic 5-year survival rates ranging from 5% to 30% regardless of treatment modality or extent of surgical resection.[153,154,156] There is a high rate of distant metastases, ranging from 66% to 100%.[154,172]

Sarcoma

Sarcomas represent 3% of all primary vaginal cancers.[9] In a report based on data from the NCDB between 1985 and 1994,[9] there were 135 cases of primary vaginal sarcoma of heterogeneous histologies and varying age. Twenty-two percent of patients were under 14 years of age, with a median age at presentation of approximately 50 years. Consistent with this, a recent analysis of the Surveillance, Epidemiology, and End Results (SEER) database identified 221 patients with primary vaginal sarcoma, diagnosed between 1988 and 2010, with mean age of 54.9.[173] Compared to other vaginal cancers, sarcomas tended to be larger, with decreased likelihood of lymph node involvement, and more likely to be treated with primary surgery without radiation. It was estimated that, after adjusting for other variables, vaginal sarcomas had a 69% greater risk of cancer-related mortality when compared to squamous cell carcinoma.

Vaginal sarcoma most frequently presents as an asymptomatic vaginal mass.[174] In one series, this was the most frequent symptom, found in 35% of patients, followed by vaginal, rectal or bladder pain (26%), bleeding, or serosanguinous discharge from the vagina or rectum (18%), leucorrhea (9%), dyspareunia (7%), or difficulty in micturition (7%).

Leiomyosarcoma is the most common histology in adults, representing up to 65% of all vaginal sarcoma cases; however, overall numbers are very small, with <150 published reports in the literature.[174] Vaginal leiomyosarcomas originate from the smooth muscle of the vaginal wall but may also develop from smooth muscle cells in tissues adjacent to the vagina. Leiomyosarcomas have a predilection for the posterior vaginal wall, with published reports suggesting approximately 43% to 45% in the posterior vagina, 17% to 21% anteriorly, and 34% to 39% laterally.[174,175]

Grossly, patients present with a palpable submucosal nodule, although advanced tumors may demonstrate palpable necrosis or exophytic polypoid tissue.[176] Criteria to distinguish between benign leiomyoma and leiomyosarcoma include the mitotic index, cytologic atypia, and coagulative tumor necrosis.[176a] Because of considerable variation in smooth muscle tumors from area to area, adequate sampling is recommended to achieve an accurate diagnosis. Microscopically, leiomyosarcomas demonstrate interlacing bundles of spindle-shaped cells, with blunt-ended nuclei and fibrillar cytoplasm.[152,177] Leiomyosarcomas are also aggressive; they undergo early hematogenous dissemination, recur locally[9,174] and demonstrate pulmonary metastases.[178]

Other less common histologies include endometrial stromal sarcoma and angiosarcoma.[179,180] Fewer than ten cases of angiosarcoma of the vagina have been reported in the literature.[181,182] A history of pelvic radiation is a risk factor for pelvic sarcomas, particularly angiosarcoma.[180] In the pediatric population, embryonal rhabdomyosarcoma/sarcoma botryoides is the most common histology,[183] with 90% of cases occurring in children younger than 5 years of age.[184]

Prognostic Factors

Review of the literature indicates that vaginal sarcomas undergo early hematogenous dissemination as well as frequent local recurrence. Pulmonary metastases are common.[174,175] Adverse prognostic factors for vaginal sarcoma include high histologic grade, stage, size >3 cm, infiltrative borders, and cytologic atypia.[178]

Treatment Options

Despite surgery and the use of adjuvant RT in select cases, sarcoma patients sustain poor outcomes because of a high incidence of local recurrence and distant metastasis. Locoregional control is especially important for vaginal leiomyosarcoma. The addition of systemic treatment, typically with doxorubicin, is standard for leiomyosarcoma.[185] Postoperative radiation therapy has been used to manage soft tissue sarcomas in other sites, to reduce locoregional recurrence rates.[186] Results from adjuvant radiation for high-grade sarcoma in other regions of the body have been extrapolated to vaginal cancer. In patients with involved margins, high doses above 62.5 Gy are generally required to achieve local control.[187]

A series by Peters et al.[188] reported on 17 cases, comprised of 10 patients with leiomyosarcoma, 4 with MMT, and 3 with other types of sarcomas. There were only 3 patients alive and free of disease with follow-up times of 84 to 161 months. All 3 patients had undergone pelvic exenteration. Patients who received other forms of primary therapy all died of recurrence, with the pelvis as the first site of recurrence in all cases. In 50% of cases, the pelvis was the only site of failure, stressing the importance of local treatment. Overall survival of 8 and 10 years following wide local excision has been reported.[175]

Outcomes

In the SEER analysis, 5-year survival was 89% for stage I and under 50% for stage II vaginal sarcomas of all types.[173] Other series describe similarly poor outcomes. Five-year survival was 36% for patients with leiomyosarcoma in the Peters et al. series.[188]

Malignant Mixed Müllerian Tumors

Mixed müllerian tumors (MMT), also called carcinosarcomas, are highly aggressive, biphasic neoplasms composed of an epithelial component as well as a sarcomatous component. The epithelial component in vaginal MMT is most often SCC.[179] The sarcomatous component can be composed of fibroblasts and smooth muscle or includes cartilage, striated muscle, bone, and other heterologous tissues. The metaplastic carcinoma theory suggests that there is a common cell of origin for MMT, with carcinoma giving rise to the sarcomatous component via metaplasia.[189] The most common differential diagnosis is sarcomatoid carcinoma. The spindle and carcinomatous components are positive for cytokeratin in sarcomatous carcinoma, whereas MMT demonstrates a sarcomatous component that is positive for vimentin, with the carcinomatous component positive for cytokeratin.[179] The first case of vaginal MMT was described in 1975 by Davis et al.[190]; since then, only 11 cases have been reported in the literature, with age ranging from 57 to 74 years.[179,191-194] At least one case report of MMT of the vagina detected high-risk HPV in both the carcinomatous and sarcomatous component, suggesting that some vaginal MMTs may be related to HPV.[191]

The survival rate for patients with MMT was even lower, at 17%. There are only a few case reports and small series detailing treatment of primary vaginal MMT. Neesham et al.[193] published a case report of a 74-year-old patient treated with wide local excision and radiation for a 5.5-cm stage I MMT. She developed distant metastases within 6 months of local therapy. Analysis of patterns of failure suggests that local therapy does not have a significant impact on survival because of early distant spread. For that reason, chemotherapy is typically administered after surgery for MMT in other sites and should be considered for primary vaginal lesions, along with adjuvant radiation as warranted. Platinum-based chemotherapy has been used for MMT occurring elsewhere in the pelvis. It has not yet been determined whether platinum agents are best administered alone or in combination with other agents. Combination regimens include a paclitaxel with either ifosfamide or a platinum agent.[195-197]

Clear Cell Adenocarcinoma

Epidemiology

Clear cell adenocarcinoma of the vagina was first reported in 1971 by Herbst and Scully,[198] who documented six cases of primary vaginal clear cell carcinoma in patients 15 to 22 years of age: five of the six had been exposed to the synthetic estrogen DES *in utero* during the first trimester. This was the first report suggesting that *in utero* exposure to DES, prescribed during the mid-1940s to 1960s for high-risk pregnancies, could result in an increased risk of clear cell adenocarcinoma. DES-related clear cell adenocarcinoma presents at a young age, with studies documenting median age at presentation to be within the second or third decade of life.[198]

Studies suggest that there is a bimodal distribution for clear cell adenocarcinoma of the vagina, with the first peak containing young women with a mean age of 26, most of whom were exposed to DES *in utero*, and a second peak containing women with a mean age of 71 years, not exposed to DES.[198] The majority of patients present with stage I to II disease.[198,199] DES-related clear cell adenocarcinoma is rarely seen today, as DES is no longer administered to pregnant women.

Risk Factors

In 45% to 95% of cases, clear cell adenocarcinoma of the vagina is associated with vaginal adenosis, defined as the abnormal presence of glandular epithelium in the vagina.[200,201] Vaginal adenosis has three patterns: endocervical, tuboendometrial, and embryonic.[169,201,202] Grossly, vaginal adenosis appears as red, velvety, grapelike clusters in the vagina. Glandular columnar epithelium of müllerian type either appears beneath the squamous epithelium or replaces it, undergoing progressive squamous metaplasia.[203] Vaginal adenosis is believed to be a precursor lesion to clear cell adenocarcinoma of the vagina. It is a common histologic abnormality in women who have been exposed to DES *in utero*, presenting in up to 95% of such women.[200,201]

The risk of developing clear cell adenocarcinoma in DES-exposed women is estimated to be 1 in 1,000,[199] suggesting that there are multiple factors contributing to pathogenesis.

However, it is not strictly confined to this population; there are rare, sporadic cases of primary adenocarcinoma of the vagina that is not associated with DES exposure.[204]

Histopathology

Clear cell adenocarcinoma of the vagina is most often located in the upper third of the anterior vagina and can vary greatly in size. Grossly, they exhibit exophytic growth and are superficially invasive.[205] Microscopically, they are composed of vacuolated, glycogen-rich cells, hence the term clear cell carcinoma. The most common histologic pattern is tubulocystic, although solid, papillary, and mixed cell patterns have also been described.[74,206] Cells are cuboidal or columnar in shape, with large, atypical protruding nuclei, rimmed by a small amount of vacuolated cytoplasm.

Clinical Presentation

Patients with clear cell adenocarcinoma most often present with abnormal vaginal bleeding,[198] which is found in 50% to 75% of cases. Cytology is not reliable, revealing abnormality in only 33% of cases; therefore, careful assessment of the entire vaginal vault to assess for submucosal irregularity is recommended, in addition to four-quadrant cytologic assessment.[207] The cervix should be carefully inspected, as clear cell adenocarcinoma can arise from this region as well. Abnormal discharge, urinary symptoms, and lower gastrointestinal complaints can also be noted, particularly in advanced cases. The differential diagnosis of vaginal adenocarcinoma is often challenging, because it must be distinguished from metastases from distant sites.

Prognostic Factors

Prognostic variables associated with worse survival include advanced stage, nontubulocystic pattern of histology, size >3 cm, and depth of invasion >3 mm.[205] A study of 21 women with clear cell carcinoma of the vagina and cervix reported overexpression of wild-type p53 to be associated with a more favorable prognosis.[208] Primary adenocarcinoma of the vagina not associated with DES exposure is extremely rare, with poor outcomes. In a review of 26 such cases by Frank et al., 5-year overall survival was 34%, worse than in patients with SCC.[209] A recent series described 5 cases of clear cell adenocarcinoma in patients without prior DES exposure, treated between 1990 and 2013.[210] Patients were all older than 40 years of age. There was high incidence of distant spread, especially to the lungs. Overall survival at 5 years was 55%.

Treatment Options

The optimal management of clear cell adenocarcinoma is unclear. There are several published series on DES-related clear cell adenocarcinomas[74,130,205,211,212] using conventional treatments similar to those used for squamous cell carcinoma of the vagina for stage I and II disease, including surgery with radical hysterectomy, vaginectomy, and lymphadenectomy with construction of a neovagina or definitive radiation with consideration of radiosensitizing concurrent chemotherapy.[113,213] In these series, there has been an emphasis on preservation of ovarian and vaginal function, because of the earlier age at diagnosis in DES-exposed patients. According to data from the United States Registry for Research on Hormonal Transplacental Carcinogenesis, approximately one-half of all vaginal clear cell adenocarcinoma cases were treated with radical surgery alone as primary therapy.[214]

Wharton et al. report the use of intracavitary or transvaginal irradiation for early-stage disease, with excellent tumor control and preservation of ovarian function.[215] Herbst et al.[216] reported on 142 cases of stage I clear cell adenocarcinoma.

For the 117 patients treated with radical surgery, there was an 8% risk of recurrence and 87% overall survival. For patients treated with radiation, there was a 36% risk of recurrence. The authors acknowledge that it is difficult to compare surgery to radiation, as radiation was most likely used in patients with larger lesions less amenable to resection.

A series by Senekjian et al.[212] reported on 219 cases of stage I clear cell vaginal adenocarcinoma. Forty-three patients received local therapy alone, consisting of vaginectomy, local excision, or local irradiation with or without excision, and the rest had conventional radical surgery. At 10 years, the actuarial survival rates were equivalent (88% vs. 90%) for patients who received local therapy only and those treated conventionally, respectively. However, the actuarial recurrence rate was significantly higher (40% vs. 13%) with local excision alone. Patients who received local irradiation, with or without local excision, had decreased local recurrence compared to those treated with excision alone ($P < .03$).

A subsequent series by Senekjian et al. reviewed 76 cases of stage II clear cell adenocarcinoma.[74] The 10-year overall survival rate was 65%. The 5-year survival rates were 80% for patients treated with surgery, 87% for patients treated with radiation, and 85% for patients treated with both. The authors advocate treatment with combination EBRT and brachytherapy for stage II disease, with surgery reserved for smaller, more easily resectable lesions in the upper vagina. The use of pelvic exenteration for primary and recurrent lesions has been reported by Senekjian et al.[130] Survival outcomes were comparable to those of patients treated with other modalities. Thus, to minimize morbidity and preserve quality of life, exenterative approaches are advocated only for patients with disease recurrence after radiation. The 5-year survival rate after pelvic relapse is reported to be 40% by Herbst et al.[211]

Most recurrences occur within 3 years of therapy, although recurrences occurring 10 to 20 years after treatment have been reported.[217] Most recurrences are local or locoregional, with approximately one-third detected at distant sites, most commonly in the lungs or extrapelvic lymph nodes, although there have been rare cases of CNS metastases manifesting years after treatment.[218] The 10-year actuarial survival rate for clear cell adenocarcinoma of the vagina is 79%. For stage I and II disease, survival rates are 90% and 80%, respectively.

Other Adenocarcinomas

The majority of adenocarcinomas that present in the vagina are attributed to metastatic spread from other sites. Vaginal metastases from adenocarcinoma of the breast, kidneys, or other gynecologic primary sites have been described.[219-221] Primary non–clear cell adenocarcinoma of the vagina is extremely rare and occurs predominantly in postmenopausal women. Histologic variants include endometrioid, mucinous, mesonephric, and papillary serous adenocarcinoma. Vaginal endometrioid adenocarcinoma is the most common non–clear cell subtype and presents most often in women with a history of endometriosis. Only a handful of case reports or series have been published in detail about endometrioid adenocarcinoma of the vagina.[222-226] In one series of 18 cases of primary vaginal endometrioid adenocarcinoma,[222] 10 cases arose from the apex. Fourteen out of 18 cases had vaginal endometriosis, important in indicating a primary vaginal tumor rather than secondary spread from the endothelium. Median age at presentation was 57, with a range from 45 to 81 years. There have been case reports of mucinous adenocarcinoma of the vagina,[227-229] with at least one arising from a focus of endocervicosis.[230]

On gross exam, endometrioid adenocarcinomas can be polypoid, papillary, rough, granular, fungating, exophytic, or flat, and most arise from the superior aspect of the vagina.

Microscopically, tumors display a predominant component of typical endometrioid carcinoma, with tubular glands lined by columnar cells with moderate amounts of eosinophilic cytoplasm and large elongated nuclei. Only a handful of cases of mucinous adenocarcinoma have been described,[220,227–229] including rare cases arising in neovaginas[231] or arising from endocervicosis.[230] Mesonephric adenocarcinoma arises from mesonephric duct remnants situated in the lateral vaginal wall.[232,233] Primary papillary serous adenocarcinoma of the vagina has rarely been reported.[234]

Lymphoma

Lymphomas of the female genital tract are rare, accounting for only 1% of all primary extranodal lymphomas.[235] Lymphomas of the vagina are exceedingly uncommon, with fewer than 30 cases reported in the literature thus far.[236–249] In one review from the Armed Forces Institute of Pathology, only 4 of 9,500 cases of lymphoma were determined to originate from the vagina.[250] Diffuse large B-cell lymphoma is the most common histology, though there have also been reports of lymphoplasmacytic, Burkitt, and mucosa-associated lymphoid tissue (MALT) lymphomas.[241]

On exam, tumor is typically palpable, with infiltrative thickening and/or ulceration of the vaginal wall.[248] Immunohistochemical analyses are valuable techniques for confirming diagnosis, with tumors typically expressing CD20.[242,249] The most common symptom at presentation is vaginal bleeding. Leukemic infiltrates may be difficult to distinguish from lymphoma; therefore chloroacetate esterase or myeloperoxidase staining may be useful. Though there is no established treatment protocol for primary lymphoma of the vagina, it seems reasonable to extrapolate from results for extranodal lymphomas elsewhere in the body and to use similar chemotherapeutic and response-based radiation regimens. For patients wishing to retain fertility, chemotherapy alone may be an option in select cases.

If diagnosed at an early stage, the prognosis for vaginal lymphoma is excellent, with 5-year survival rates ranging up to 90%. Of 10 cases reported in the literature between 1994 and 2007, all patients except 1 were cured of disease after treatment with chemotherapy or a combination of radiation and chemotherapy.[240,242,246,247,251–254] Follow-up periods for these 10 case reports ranged from 6 to 120 months and 1 patient died from other causes. Eight patients had Ann Arbor stage IEA disease, 1 had IIEA, and 1 did not have stage reported. The most common chemotherapy regimen was cyclophosphamide, doxorubicin, vincristine, and prednisone (CHOP). Complete remission was also achieved using methotrexate, doxorubicin, cyclophosphamide, vincristine, prednisone, and bleomycin (MACOP-B) in 1 patient. Half of the patients did not receive radiation because of an excellent response with chemotherapy alone.

Small Cell Carcinoma of the Vagina and Other Rare Histologies

Primary small cell carcinoma of the vagina is an exceedingly rare entity, with fewer than 25 cases reported in the literature.[255] Mean age at diagnosis is 59 years, with poor outcome because of early widespread dissemination. Eighty-five percent of patients die within 1 year of diagnosis.[256,257] Neuroendocrine differentiation is often manifested by secretory granules, argyrophilia, and expression of neuroendocrine markers,[258,259] staining positive for cytokeratin, neuron-specific enolase, chromogranin A, and serotonin. Thyroid transcription factor 1 can also be positive, and should not be used to differentiate primary from metastatic disease.[260] Microscopically, it is indistinguishable from that of the lung. These tumors can occur in pure form or be associated with squamous or glandular elements.[256,258] Ectopic Cushing's

syndrome has been documented to occur in primary small cell carcinoma of the vagina.[259] Treatment typically follows general principles for small cell carcinomas of the cervix, with aggressive therapy, including combination cisplatin-based chemotherapy, radiation therapy, brachytherapy, and surgery if feasible indicated.

Vaginal paraganglioma is a rare neuroendocrine tumor, with <10 cases reported in the literature in younger women, with median age at presentation of 31 years.[261–263] It is thought to be an indolent tumor, managed surgically. The tumor can manifest with catecholamine secretion, similar to paragangliomas elsewhere in the body.[261]

Adenosquamous carcinoma of the vagina is also uncommon. Microscopically, tumor cells are composed of glandular and squamous elements. One case report described adenosquamous carcinoma associated with small cell carcinoma of the endometrium in a 64-year-old female.[264] Treatment similarly follows general approaches for squamous cell carcinoma of the vagina, including consideration of combination chemoradiation for patients with gross disease.

RADIOTHERAPY TECHNIQUES

Definitive treatment of primary vaginal cancer with radiation typically involves a combination of EBRT and brachytherapy. The use of 3D-based imaging to guide brachytherapy treatment planning is evolving, and recent results for vaginal cancer show excellent outcomes.[265,266] Because of advances in conformal radiation therapy, tumor dose can be escalated, whereas the dose to surrounding normal structures, such as small bowel, rectum, bladder, urethra, and the femoral heads, can be minimized. Brachytherapy can be delivered via intracavitary or interstitial approaches, using LDR or HDR techniques.

External Beam Radiotherapy

In general, when radiation is delivered as primary therapy, EBRT is prescribed prior to or, in rare select cases, without brachytherapy for a subset of patients with stage I and all patients with stages II to IVA disease. The treatment technique, dose prescription, and selection of the appropriate energy level must be individualized for each patient.

At time of simulation, it may be helpful to identify the distal tumor margin with a radio-opaque marker. Unless contraindicated, the use of oral and intravenous contrast can be helpful, allowing delineation of vascular structures and facilitating the contouring of the bladder, small bowel, and rectum. CT simulation allows contouring of vessels as a surrogate for lymph node localization, allowing more precise and individualized field delineation relative to pelvic bony anatomy.[267] When available, fusion of diagnostic pelvic MRI or PET-CT to the treatment planning CT can assist in defining the tumor (Fig. 76.3). If inguinal nodes are to be treated, a "frog leg" position to expose the groin region can be considered.

Three-Dimensional Conformal Treatment

The use of 3-D imaging for treatment planning has increased dramatically over the past two decades and is currently used at almost all centers for simulation and treatment planning. This allows treatment fields to be tailored to a patient's specific anatomy.

The target volume for EBRT is influenced by diagnostic imaging results and stage of disease. Treatment fields are designed to ensure coverage of the vagina and common iliac, external iliac, hypogastric, and obturator lymph nodes. A standard field has the L5-S1 interspace as the superior border, which ensures coverage of retroperitoneal nodes that lie caudal to the common iliac bifurcation.[268] However, because many initial failures occur predominantly in the vagina, paracolpos, and parametria, some authors suggest setting the superior border 1 to 2 cm superior to the inferior margin of the sacroiliac joints in patients with negative imaging of regional nodes, in order to minimize treatment toxicity.[269] If there are positive pelvic lymph nodes, the superior border should be raised to the L4-L5 interspace or higher in order to cover the common iliac nodes. The inferior border lies at the introitus to ensure coverage of the entire vagina or 4 cm distal to the most caudal aspect of the vaginal tumor. Lateral borders are 1.5 to 2.0 cm lateral to the pelvic brim. Lateral fields, when utilized, should extend anteriorly to the pubic symphysis and posteriorly to the junction of the S2-S3 interspace. The border should be extended accordingly to include the inguinal nodes, if warranted. The dose to the inguinal nodes should be calculated during treatment planning, to ensure appropriate coverage. When designing treatment fields, the interconnectivity of vaginal lymph node drainage should be kept in mind. Unexpected nodal drainage is possible and should be considered. In a study of 14 women with vaginal cancer who received pretreatment lymphatic mapping with sentinel lymph node identification, 2 out of 4 women with a lesion in the upper one-third of the vagina were found to have a sentinel lymph node in the inguinal region.[71]

Several techniques can be considered when treating the inguinal region, to minimize dose to the femoral heads. An electron boost can be used to raise the inguinal dose to appropriate levels. Alternately, unequally weighted beams (2:1, AP:PA) or a combination of low- and high-energy photons (4 to 6 MV AP; 15 to 18 MV PA) can be used. Another method uses a wide AP and a narrow PA field, with a daily photon boost to the inguinal nodes delivered with asymmetric collimator jaws.[270]

The gross tumor volume (GTV) is defined as the extent of gross disease found on clinical examination, as well as palpable lymph nodes and suspicious lymph nodes and regions seen on CT, MRI, and/or PET. The GTV is expanded by 1 to 2 cm to form the clinical target volume (CTV), which also includes the entire length of the vagina, paravaginal tissue up to the pelvic sidewall, and bilateral pelvic lymph nodes. Visualization of vessels allows approximation of lymph node locations. The pelvic nodal CTV can be defined as a 1- to 2-cm margin around blood vessels and should include the common iliac, external iliac, internal iliac, obturator, perirectal, and presacral lymph node regions. For distal vaginal involvement, inguinal lymph nodes are commonly included, with the inferior border set at the lowest aspect of the ischial tuberosity or lesser trochanter. The CTV is expanded by 1 cm to form the planning target volume (PTV). The small bowel, bladder, and rectum are contoured and doses to normal structures calculated.

Standard dose to the pelvis is 45 to 50.4 Gy in 1.8-Gy fractions, followed in select cases by a parametrial boost ranging from 50 to 65 Gy. Elective nodal irradiation of the inguinal nodes may be delivered to 45 to 50 Gy. Gross nodal disease should receive 60 to 65 Gy, if feasible, using conformal therapy. For clinically palpable inguinal nodes, this can be achieved with reduced portals, using low-energy photons or electrons.

The location of the tumor, size, and extent of disease and treatment response are factors to be taken into consideration when individualizing treatment for each patient. After EBRT to the pelvis, tumors of the vaginal apex >0.5 cm in depth should be considered for interstitial brachytherapy or external beam boost; tumors <0.5 cm should be treated with intracavitary brachytherapy. Depending on location, tumors of the midvagina can be treated with external beam boost or considered for freehand interstitial brachytherapy, particularly if they are located anteriorly or laterally. Tumors of the distal vagina are also amenable to treatment with interstitial brachytherapy, especially if the tumor is relatively confined.

In general, brachytherapy is delivered upon completion of EBRT and allows dose escalation to the vaginal tumor to 70 to 80 Gy.

Intensity-Modulated Radiation Therapy

Intensity-modulated radiation therapy (IMRT) may allow dose escalation to gross disease in areas such as inguinal or pelvic lymph nodes, diffusely infiltrative disease, or sidewall tumors inaccessible to brachytherapy. Shrinking field techniques, or IMRT, can be used for dose escalation if brachytherapy is not feasible.[271,272] In such circumstances, a total dose of 70 to 75 Gy minimum should be delivered to gross disease. Higher doses are difficult to achieve without substantially increasing the risk of toxicity to adjacent normal tissues such as urethra, bladder, and rectum. Typical IMRT input parameters based on those used for postoperative endometrial cancer for the Radiation Therapy Oncology Group (RTOG) trial 0921 include ≤30% of small bowel to receive ≤40 Gy, with a dose to 2 cm³ of the small bowel (D2cc) maximum of 55 Gy; ≤35% of bladder to receive ≤40 Gy with a D2cc maximum of 90 Gy; ≤60% of the rectum and sigmoid to receive ≤40 Gy with a D2cc maximum of 70 to 75 Gy; and the femoral heads 15% to receive ≤35 Gy. The IMRT plans are optimized to minimize the volume of PTV that receives more than 110% of the prescribed dose.[273]

When utilizing IMRT technique, it is important to take into account the possibility of significant shifts in tumor position because of constant normal tissue changes and rapid tumor regression. As a result, we recommend contouring an integrated vaginal volume (IVV), which reflects the CTV volume, paying close attention to rectal and bladder filling, and contouring the position of the vagina with both bladder full and bladder empty (Fig. 76.4).[274] A PTV margin of 1 to 1.5 cm is recommended given the degree of motion and uncertainties in target definition.

Brachytherapy

The utilization of brachytherapy should be considered for all patients with vaginal cancer who are undergoing radiation, unless they are unable to tolerate the procedure. According to a SEER database analysis spanning the years 1974 to 2011, the use of brachytherapy as a boost or definitive treatment provided a disease-specific and overall survival benefit across all FIGO stages of primary vaginal cancer.[275] An NCDB study spanning 2004 to 2011 found the use of brachytherapy as a boost in vaginal cancer has been declining, however, from 87.7% in 2004 to 68.4% in 2011 (*P* < .001), with increase in use of IMRT boost from 4.5% to 23.5%.[276] Treatment at a high-volume facility predicted for greater likelihood of brachytherapy as a boost.

Intracavitary brachytherapy as monotherapy can be considered for patients with VAIN and highly selected patients with minimally invasive stage I disease. In most cases, brachytherapy is offered after EBRT to boost the cumulative dose to a minimum of 70 to 80 Gy. Tumor response to EBRT is used to assess suitability for intracavitary or interstitial brachytherapy. In general, patients with superficial disease that is 5 mm in thickness or less can receive intracavitary treatment, whereas thicker lesions require interstitial brachytherapy in order to achieve adequate dose coverage. Image-based interstitial brachytherapy technique should be utilized to optimize target dose delivery and minimize dose to organs at risk; this has been shown to maximize disease control compared to non–image-based techniques.[277]

Intracavitary Brachytherapy: Low Dose Rate

Intracavitary brachytherapy can be delivered with low dose rate or high dose rate technique. Low dose rate intracavitary brachytherapy (LDR-ICB) is most commonly performed using a vaginal cylinder loaded with cesium-137 radioactive

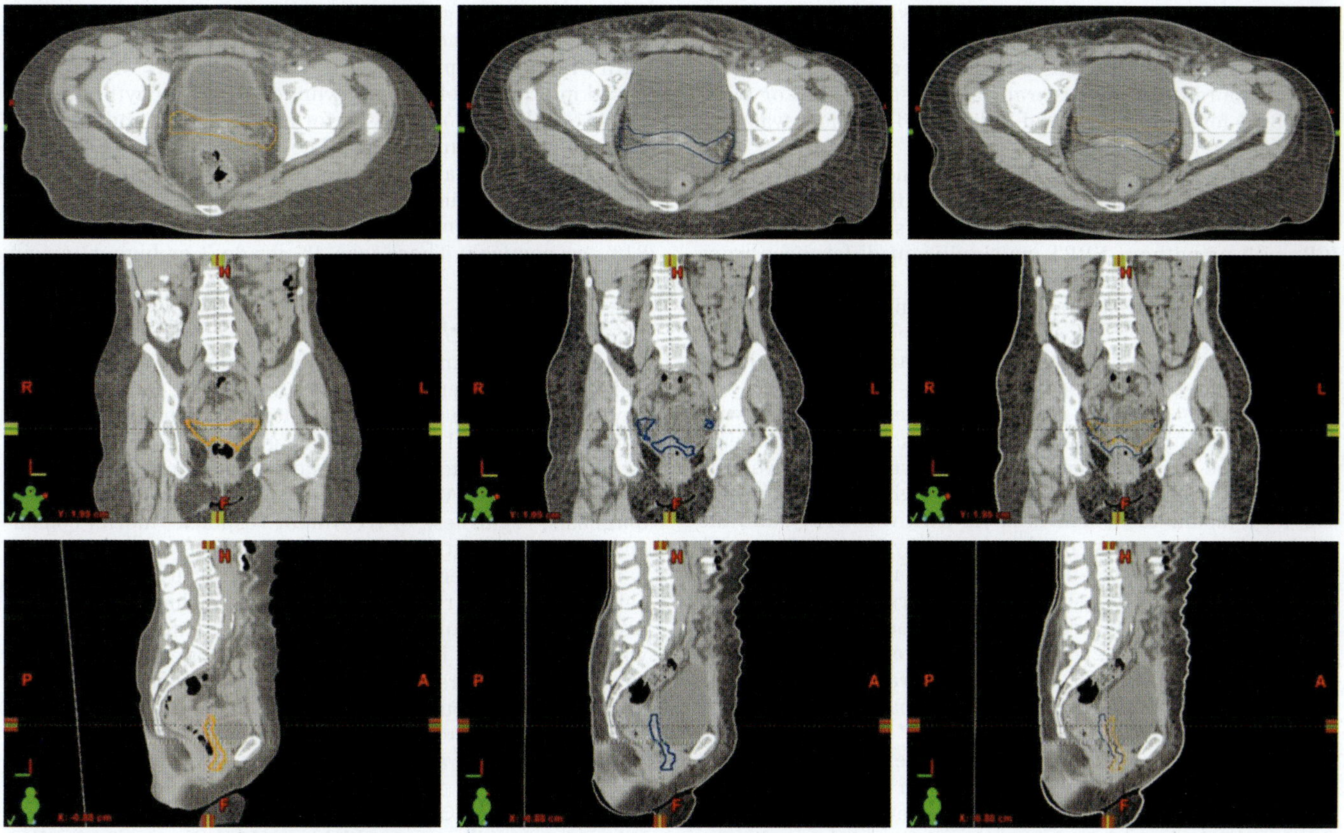

FIGURE 76.4. Displacement of the vagina with bladder filling. Axial, coronal, and sagittal images are shown for the same patient. The *left panel* shows a relatively empty bladder, with vaginal cuff contoured in *yellow*. *Middle panel* shows a full bladder, with vaginal cuff contoured in *blue*. *Right panel* shows a full bladder with the two vaginal contours superimposed, demonstrating the posterior deviation of the vaginal cuff that occurs with bladder filling.

sources. Use of LDR remote control afterloading can be utilized to minimize radiation exposure to hospital personnel.

A variety of vaginal applicators are available, such as Burnett, Bloedorn, Delclos[278] or MIRALVA.[279,280] Some cylinders have lead shielding to protect regions of the vagina, bladder, and rectum. Most applicators come in different diameters, and the largest diameter cylinder that can be comfortably accommodated by the patient should be used to improve the ratio of mucosa to tumor dose.

Typically, two to three cesium sources are placed along the central tandem of the cylinder, and labia are sutured closed to secure the implant during the treatment. To minimize skin toxicity, it is important to avoid placing a source over the vulva. With appropriate selection of dose specification points, a uniform dose distribution can be achieved over the entire length of the vagina. In cases where disease is localized to the upper vagina or vaginal fornices, an intrauterine tandem can be used to anchor the vaginal cylinder or be used with vaginal colpostats. Vaginal colpostats alone can be used to treat the upper vagina. Some institutions report good results using custom vaginal molds.[281]

A retrospective series by Pingley et al.[104] reported their experience treating 134 women with primary vaginal cancer ranging from stage I to IV; intracavitary brachytherapy was delivered using LDR technique. Only the 75 patients who completed treatment were analyzed. Most patients received EBRT to 50 Gy, and 59 of 75 patients received subsequent brachytherapy (30 with LDR-ICB, 29 interstitial). The 5-year disease-free survival rate in patients treated with LDR-ICB was 53% and was 30% for patients who did not receive brachytherapy. Patients who received brachytherapy within

4 weeks of EBRT had a disease-free survival rate of 60%, compared to 30% in those who did not, suggesting that a shorter interval between EBRT and brachytherapy is preferable.

Intracavitary Brachytherapy: High Dose Rate

High dose rate intracavitary brachytherapy (HDR-ICB) is typically performed using iridium-192, with applicators that are similar to those described for LDR. HDR-ICB delivers treatment over a span of several minutes and has the potential advantages of limiting exposure to caregivers, as well as the ability to optimize dose distribution through varying dwell times.[282,283] The largest cylinder that a patient can comfortably tolerate should be selected.

Compared to LDR radiation, there is theoretically less potential sublethal damage repair and thus an increased likelihood of normal tissue toxicity. However, this has not been demonstrated in vaginal cancer, nor in cervical cancer, where multiple prospective and retrospective studies have failed to note any significant difference in local control, survival, or toxicity outcomes between HDR and LDR brachytherapy.[284]

Several single-institution studies with small numbers of patients have reported their outcomes for HDR brachytherapy and are summarized below.

The largest series of HDR brachytherapy for vaginal cancer is from Vienna by Mock et al.[60] and reported on 86 patients. Patients with stage 0 to stage II disease received treatment with intracavitary HDR brachytherapy alone (*n* = 26). Prescribed dose per fraction ranged from 5 to 8 Gy, with a mean dose of 7 Gy, and the number of insertions ranged from

2 to 6, with a median of 5. In that series, the 5-year recurrence-free survival rates were 100%, 77%, and 50% for stages 0, I, and II, respectively. The authors noted similar local failure rates for HDR brachytherapy administered with or without EBRT, for both stage I and II disease. Treatment was well tolerated.

Kucera et al.[285] described their experience with 80 patients who received treatment with HDR-ICB, with or without EBRT. Compared to a historical group of patients treated with LDR-ICB, with or without EBRT, no significant differences were noted for local and distant recurrences or rate of complications. Three-year actuarial overall and disease-specific survival rates were 51% and 61%, respectively. Three-year disease-specific survival rates for stage I and stage II patients were 83% and 66%, respectively.

Stock et al.[91] reported results for 49 patients treated with primary carcinoma of the vagina. Of this group, 15 patients were treated with EBRT and HDR brachytherapy for vaginal carcinoma, with dose per treatment ranging from 3 to 8 Gy. The total median dose delivered via HDR was 21 Gy, and the total median tumor dose overall was 63 Gy. No significant difference in outcome was noted between patients treated with LDR versus HDR. Five-year actuarial survival was reported to be 50% in the HDR brachytherapy group. In comparison, the 5-year survival rate for patients who received EBRT alone (n-11) was 9% ($P < .001$), with a higher rate of stage IV disease in the EBRT-alone group (36%) compared to the brachytherapy group (5%).

Nanavati et al.[286] published their experience treating 13 patients with primary vaginal cancer with EBRT to 45 Gy followed by HDR-ICB of 20 to 28 Gy, delivered in 3 to 4 fractions, and calculated 0.5 cm from the surface of the applicator. All 13 patients achieved a complete response; with a median follow-up time of 2.6 years, the local control rate was 92%. No grade 3 or 4 acute or chronic intestinal or bladder toxicity was noted during this short follow-up period, but 46% of patients developed moderate to severe vaginal stenosis. All patients had stage I or stage II disease, and the authors concluded that EBRT plus HDR-ICB is an acceptable treatment with a high response rate, good local control and survival, and minimal toxicity.

Damast et al.[114] reported outcomes for 10 patients with small-volume, stage I to II primary vaginal cancer, treated with pelvic EBRT (mean dose 45 Gy), followed by MRI-based HDR- or LDR-ICB. For HDR, the total dose ranged from 18 to 21 Gy in 3 to 5 fractions, prescribed to 5 to 10 mm depth. In general, the entire vagina was treated to minimum EQD2 dose of 60 Gy, with additional boost to higher risk areas to at least 75 Gy. If warranted, partially shielded cylinders were utilized to reduce dose to uninvolved vaginal tissue. Concurrent cisplatin was considered for stage II patients; 40% received CRT. At median follow up of 60 months, the authors document 5-year local failure-free survival of 90% and disease-specific survival of 80%. One patient with approximately 5-mm-thick residual tumor after EBRT developed local recurrence; no patients with a complete response after EBRT developed local recurrence following ICB.

Beriwal et al.[115] described their experience using intracavitary HDR brachytherapy in 5 patients with either primary or recurrent vaginal cancer treated between 2000 and 2006. The median dose for intracavitary brachytherapy was 20 Gy in 3 to 5 fractions, prescribed 0.5 cm from the surface of the applicator. One patient received intracavitary brachytherapy only, because of prior radiation therapy with EBRT and HDR brachytherapy. Interpretation is limited because of short follow-up, and the results are combined with interstitial brachytherapy patients but suggest that EBRT followed by HDR brachytherapy is efficacious and safe.

The use of image-based HDR-ICB was reported by Vargo et al.,[125] in a series of 41 patients with vaginal cancer treated with chemotherapy and definitive radiation with image-based multichannel vaginal cylinder HDR brachytherapy. CT (41%) or MRI (59%) was used for each fraction, and high-risk clinical target volume drawn. The median dose to 90% of the high-risk clinical target volume was 77.1 Gy (equivalent dose of 2 Gy per fraction), and outcomes were favorable, with 2-year local, regional, and distant control of 93%, 100%, and 81%, respectively. There was 4% grade 3 or higher toxicity at 2 years.

Interstitial Brachytherapy

According to the American Brachytherapy Society Consensus Guidelines for interstitial brachytherapy for vaginal cancer, any lesions >5 mm in thickness after EBRT should be considered for interstitial BT, and image guidance is recommended to minimize dose to normal organs and optimize dose to the target volume.[126] Any paravaginal extension at the time of diagnosis, regardless of treatment response, merits consideration of interstitial brachytherapy, as a vaginal cylinder is unable to deliver sufficient coverage to this region. Other candidates for interstitial brachytherapy include patients with lesions thicker than 5 mm, distal vaginal extension, or those with a vagina that is unable to accommodate standard intracavitary applicators. When possible, image-based interstitial brachytherapy should be utilized, as outcomes are superior to non–image-based techniques.[277] Further details of the procedure and planning are below.

Preoperative Assessment

When determining tumor thickness, MRI is superior to other imaging modalities. T1- with gadolinium and T2-weighted MRI should be obtained if possible after EBRT to assess residual disease.[124] Contrast, such as ultrasound gel placed to distend the vagina, may also aid in visualization of the tumor. Clinical examination provides an imprecise estimate of tumor thickness. An exam under anesthesia can be performed after EBRT; placement of gold fiducial markers can be considered to mark the proximal and distal end of residual disease. Use of a radio-opaque marker in the vagina placed at the time of diagnosis and after external beam will facilitate assessment of the lesion on CT imaging.

The patient should be assessed for general, epidural or spinal anesthesia. When feasible, a combination of general anesthesia during the insertion followed by an epidural patient-controlled anesthesia approach that continues during the entire inpatient hospitalization maximizes pain relief. Epidural anesthesia allows the patient to control the degree of pelvic anesthesia while avoiding the systemic effects, somnolence, and potential mental status changes that may occur with a peripheral patient-controlled anesthesia device. Patients with a history of laminectomy, significant degenerative disease, or labile blood pressure are suboptimal candidates for epidural anesthesia.

Patients on anticoagulation with medications such as warfarin should switch to low molecular weight (LMR) heparin approximately 1 week prior to the procedure, and LMR heparin may be discontinued 24 hours prior to insertion time and be withheld during the duration of the implant, though subcutaneous heparin for thrombosis prophylaxis may be initiated after the procedure is completed. Patients may have a gentle bowel preparation orally or an enema before the procedure.

Applicator Selection

Template systems are available to secure the position of the needles in the target volumes and include the Syed-Neblett template, the modified Syed-Neblett, and the MUPIT (Martinez Universal Perineal Interstitial Template).[287]

These systems consist of a perineal template, a vaginal cylindrical obturator, and hollow guides for loading radionuclide sources. The perineal template requires suturing to perineal skin. The vaginal obturator allows for placement of a tandem, making it possible to combine interstitial with intracavitary treatment if desired. Lower vaginal tumors may be suitable for freehand technique, if the mass can be readily visualized and palpated.

Procedure

The insertion procedure is performed with the patient in a dorsal lithotomy position. A sterile setup is used at the time of insertion. A Foley catheter is placed for bladder drainage.

A digital and speculum examination allows assessment of vaginal width, tumor size and location, amount and thickness of residual parametrial or paravaginal disease, and presence of any fistulas. For patients with an intact uterus, a central tandem may be inserted to anchor the applicator. A vaginal central plastic cylindrical is placed over the tandem and secured. The template, which contains multiple openings through which needles can be inserted, is placed onto the perineum. The tumor volume is implanted by inserting the needles through the holes of the template, with the goal of covering the GTV with a 1- to 2-cm margin, utilizing 3-D imaging afterward to confirm proper needle location and uniform dose distribution around the tumor volume. Generally speaking, needles should extend approximately 5 to 10 mm past the disease, with 10 mm between each needle.[124] The physician should be mindful that slight needle displacement can occur when legs are lowered back to the supine position.

When possible, utilizing image guidance to perform implants is ideal in order to improve target localization and guide needle placement. Available modalities include laparoscopic guidance, ultrasound, CT, and MRI. Results with these various techniques are summarized below.

Several investigators have used laparoscopic guidance or laparotomy[288-290] to improve the accuracy and safety of interstitial implant placement. With open laparotomy, the bladder and urethra can be visualized during needle placement. The bladder and rectum can be protected either by using slings or tissue expanders or by lysis of adhesions. Disaia and Creasman[291] described the creation of an "omental carpet," where a section of omentum is placed along the descending colon into the pelvis in order to separate the bladder and rectum from the implant and prevent small bowel adhesions. If laparotomy is performed in a two-application course of treatment, it is typically done for the first application only. As expected, there is higher associated morbidity with the use of laparotomy compared to other techniques, as a result of increased operative time, longer postoperative recovery, risk of bleeding, and ileus.

Laparascopic visualization is an alternative to open laparotomy that has also been reported. Though laparoscopy is less invasive, both laparoscopic approaches and open laparotomy are limited by an inability to visualize extraperitoneal structures, such as parts of the bladder, uterus, and cervix, as well as the vagina and paravaginal tissues. However, these techniques can be considered when CT or MRI are not available during brachytherapy, to avoid needle insertion through the small bowel and sigmoid.

Stock et al. reported results using real-time transrectal ultrasound as visualization.[288] The ultrasound probe was brought into close proximity to the vagina, parametria, and cervix, and the longitudinal mode of the ultrasound probe was useful in determining the optimum depth of needle insertion. Transverse imaging was utilized during the procedure to ensure coverage of the target area and

avoid entry into bladder, rectum, or small bowel. Using this technique, invasive laparotomy or laparoscopy was able to be avoided.

In general, temporary implants are preferred over permanent implants because of their relative safety/simplicity, cost-effectiveness, easy applicability, readily controlled distribution of sources, and easier modification of dose distribution. HDR interstitial brachytherapy has the advantage of limiting exposure to caregivers and visitors and offers the ability to optimize dose distribution using 3-D image-based treatment planning.[265,283] Use of permanent radioactive implants using gold-198 or iodine-125 have also been reported for smaller volume disease,[292] and can be considered for select patients; reports suggest long-lasting control can be achieved with appropriate selection of patients..

Image-Guided Brachytherapy

The use of 3-D imaging during HDR brachytherapy has increased with the rise of CT and MR availability and has been a favored approach when available because of lower morbidity and invasiveness compared to historic approaches.[293] Only a few institutions have access to real-time image guidance during brachytherapy[294]; most scan patients after insertion is complete, with subsequent readjustment as needed. It is not feasible at many institutions to obtain an MRI at the time of brachytherapy. A diagnostic MRI obtained after EBRT prior to brachytherapy can be used instead to assist with treatment planning. MRI provides superior tumor delineation, whereas CT images can cause overestimation of tumor extension.[295]

The integration of 3D imaging during the brachytherapy procedure allows determination of depth and location of insertion and enables repositioning if perforation into the bladder or rectum is detected. Treatment planning based on 3D imaging allows high dose to be delivered to the tumor volume, while sparing critical adjacent organs. The use of 3D image-based HDR brachytherapy has been shown to improve local control and decrease treatment-related toxicities.[277,296] There are fewer published reports on 3D HDR brachytherapy for primary vaginal cancer, but results suggest similar outcomes.[266,277]

Dosimetry

Given close proximity of the rectum and bladder, it is important to minimize treatment toxicity by avoiding overdose of critical normal structures. However, underdosing the target volume is also a serious risk; thus, it is critical to optimize target localization and needle placement.[297]

Vaginal cancer with gross residual disease at the time of brachytherapy is prescribed a cumulative EQD2 dose of 70 to 90 Gy, with 60 Gy prescribed to the entire vaginal surface. Special care should be taken to minimize the dose to the bowel, which often lies in close proximity to gross disease. Image-based planning software, when available, allows the dose to conform to the target areas while avoiding organs at risk. As a result, optimal dose distribution can be achieved. Image-guided technique should be utilized when possible to reduce toxicity and improve local control.

Proposed dose schedules for HDR interstitial brachytherapy, depending on dose of initial EBRT, have been released by the American Brachytherapy Society[126] (Table 76.7). The number of fractions range from 3 to 10 with goal of delivering total EQD2 of over 70 Gy to the CTV. Given the difficulty of insertion, physicians may insert the applicator once and treat patients over a several day inpatient hospitalization. Twice-a-day regimens range from 9 to 10 fractions of 200 to 300 cGy per fraction, BID, or 3 to 6 fractions, ranging from 450 to 650 cGy,

TABLE 76.7 DOSE SCHEDULES FOR HDR INTERSTITIAL BRACHYTHERAPY IN COMBINATION WITH EBRT, AS PROPOSED BY THE AMERICAN BRACHYTHERAPY SOCIETY CONSENSUS GUIDELINES FOR INTERSTITIAL BRACHYTHERAPY FOR VAGINAL CANCER

EBRT		HDR		EQD2
Total Dose	**# Fx**	**Dose per Fx**	**# Fx**	**CTV**
36 Gy[a]	18	5.0 Gy	6	72.9
		5.5 Gy	6	87
39.6 Gy[a]	22	5.0 Gy	6	76.4
		5.5 Gy	6	81.5
45 Gy	25	3.0 Gy	9	73.6
		3.0 Gy	10	76.8
		4.5 Gy	5	71.5
		5.0 Gy	5	75.5
		5.5 Gy	5	79.8
		7.0 Gy	3	74.1
50.4 Gy	28	4.0 Gy	5	72.9
		4.5 Gy	5	76.8
		5.0 Gy	5	80.9
		7.0 Gy	3	79.4

[a]Assumes midline block after 36–39.6 Gy, with total pelvic dose to 50.4 Gy.
EBRT, external beam radiation therapy; EQD2, equivalent dose in 2 Gy fractions; Fx, fractions; HDR, high-dose rate.
Modified from Beriwal S, Demanes DJ, Erickson B, et al. American Brachytherapy Society consensus guidelines for interstitial brachytherapy for vaginal cancer. *Brachytherapy* 2012;11(1):68–75. Copyright © 2012 American Brachytherapy Society. With permission.

BID, with at least 6 hours between fractions. It is also feasible to perform two separate insertions with two hospitalizations required.

For CT- or MRI-based 3D treatment planning, the D90, D100, V100, V150, and V200 are parameters used to describe tumor volumes and the doses to those volumes. D90 and D100 are defined as the minimum dose delivered to 90% and 100% of the volume, respectively. V100, V150, and V200 are defined as the volumes receiving 100%, 150%, and 200% of the prescribed physical dose, respectively.[298] Figure 76.5 depicts a representative isodose distribution.

When MRI-guided adaptive brachytherapy is utilized, the high-risk CTV (HRCTV) is defined as clinically palpable disease, plus any residual disease seen on MRI, and the entire circumference of the adjacent vagina at the level of the residual tumor. The intermediate-risk CTV (IRCTV) includes the region of initial tumor extension and the remaining vagina, in order to encompass potential submucosal tumor spread. The low-risk CTV (LRCTV) is the remaining vagina.

The bladder, rectum, sigmoid, urethra, and small bowel are contoured as volumes at risk, and the D2cc and D0.1cc calculated.[299] The recommended maximum equivalent dose in 2-Gy fractions (EQD2) D2cc to the rectum and sigmoid is 70 to 75 Gy and should be <70 Gy when feasible.[126] Maximum EQD2 D2cc for the bladder should be 90 Gy. There are no DVH parameters specific to the female urethra, but in general, the D2cc should be comparable to parameters for the bladder and rectum. The small bowel dose can be limited with use of a full bladder; some institutions limit the EQD2 maximum point dose to 60 to 65 Gy.[124] A study from Brigham and Women's Hospital reported the incidence of grade 3 or higher complication rates in 51 women undergoing HDR 3D-planned interstitial brachytherapy.[120] Median D2cc for the bladder, rectum, and sigmoid were 64.6, 61.0, and 51.9 Gy, respectively. The actuarial rates of grade 3 to 4 complications at 2 years were 20% gastrointestinal, 9% vaginal, 6% skin, 3% musculoskeletal, and 2% lymphatic. The D2cc for the rectum was significantly higher in patients with grade 2 or more gastrointestinal toxicity. On univariate analysis, D2cc and D0.1cc for the rectum and sigmoid, tumor size, and tumor volume at the time of brachytherapy were

associated with gastrointestinal complications. This analysis validated the recommended D0.1 cc and D2cc for the rectum and sigmoid.

Precautions for Interstitial Patients

Appropriate measures should be taken to reduce likelihood of needle displacement during hospitalization. Patients should be instructed to remain in bed, with head of the bed raised no more than 15 degrees. To ensure there has been no needle displacement between fractions, the needle length protruding the template can be measured and validated prior to every treatment.

Skin care is also critical. Given risk of decubitus ulcer, it is advisable to utilize an air mattress, when available. To minimize skin abrasion, gauze or Duoderm can be placed between the template and perineal skin.

To prevent development of a deep vein thrombosis, patients should receive subcutaneous heparin and pneumoboots.

Patients should be seen in follow-up 2 to 4 weeks after implant removal for a skin check, then at 3-month intervals up to a year, and then every 6 months. Dilute hydrogen peroxide douching is advised for patients with tissue necrosis development. Antibiotics with anaerobic coverage are recommended if a malodorous discharge accompanies the necrosis. Hyperbaric oxygen should be considered for those that have been proven on biopsy not to have recurrent disease.

Outcomes with Interstitial Technique

There are only a handful of series describing outcomes for vaginal cancer treated with interstitial brachytherapy. They are summarized below.

The use of MRI-guided adaptive brachytherapy in locally advanced vaginal cancer was reported by Dimopoulos et al.[300] with excellent outcomes, supporting the use of the following parameters for image-guided adaptive brachytherapy: for HRCTV, D90 of ≥85 Gy; for IRCTV, D90 approximately 60 Gy; and for LRCTV, D90 of approximately 50 Gy. Thirteen patients with stage II to IV disease were treated. Mean D2cc doses to the bladder, urethra, rectum, and sigmoid colon were 80, 76, 70, and 60 Gy, respectively. Toxicity was acceptable, with two fistulas reported and one case of periurethral necrosis. The 3-year local control and overall survival rates were 92% and 85%, respectively, with a mean D90 to the HRCTV of 86 (±13) Gy. Consistent with these promising outcomes, image-guided interstitial brachytherapy results were reported by Manuel et al.,[277] with 2-year local control, disease-free interval, and overall survival of 93%, 86%, and 82%, respectively, in their cohort of 72 patients. Patients were treated with image-guided (n = 50) or non–image-guided (n = 25) technique treated during the time period of 1973 to 2014.[266] With the use of image-guided technique, there was a trend toward improved disease-free survival (2-year DFS 77% vs. 42%, respectively; P = .072), improved overall survival (84% vs. 47%; P = .26), and decreased gastrointestinal and genitourinary toxicity, supporting incorporation of CT and/or MRI as image guidance when available.

Kushner et al.[301] reported outcomes of HDR brachytherapy in 19 patients with primary vaginal cancer. Two-dimensional (2D) treatment planning was performed, with interstitial brachytherapy delivered to 8 patients at a median dose of 23 Gy in 4 fractions. The 2-year overall survival rate for patients for all patients was 66.1%. Three patients (15.8%) had serious late effects, including ureteral stenosis, vaginal necrosis, and small-bowel obstruction; 2 of these patients were treated with interstitial brachytherapy.

A series by Tewari et al.[302] reviewed long-term results using interstitial brachytherapy, with or without EBRT, in

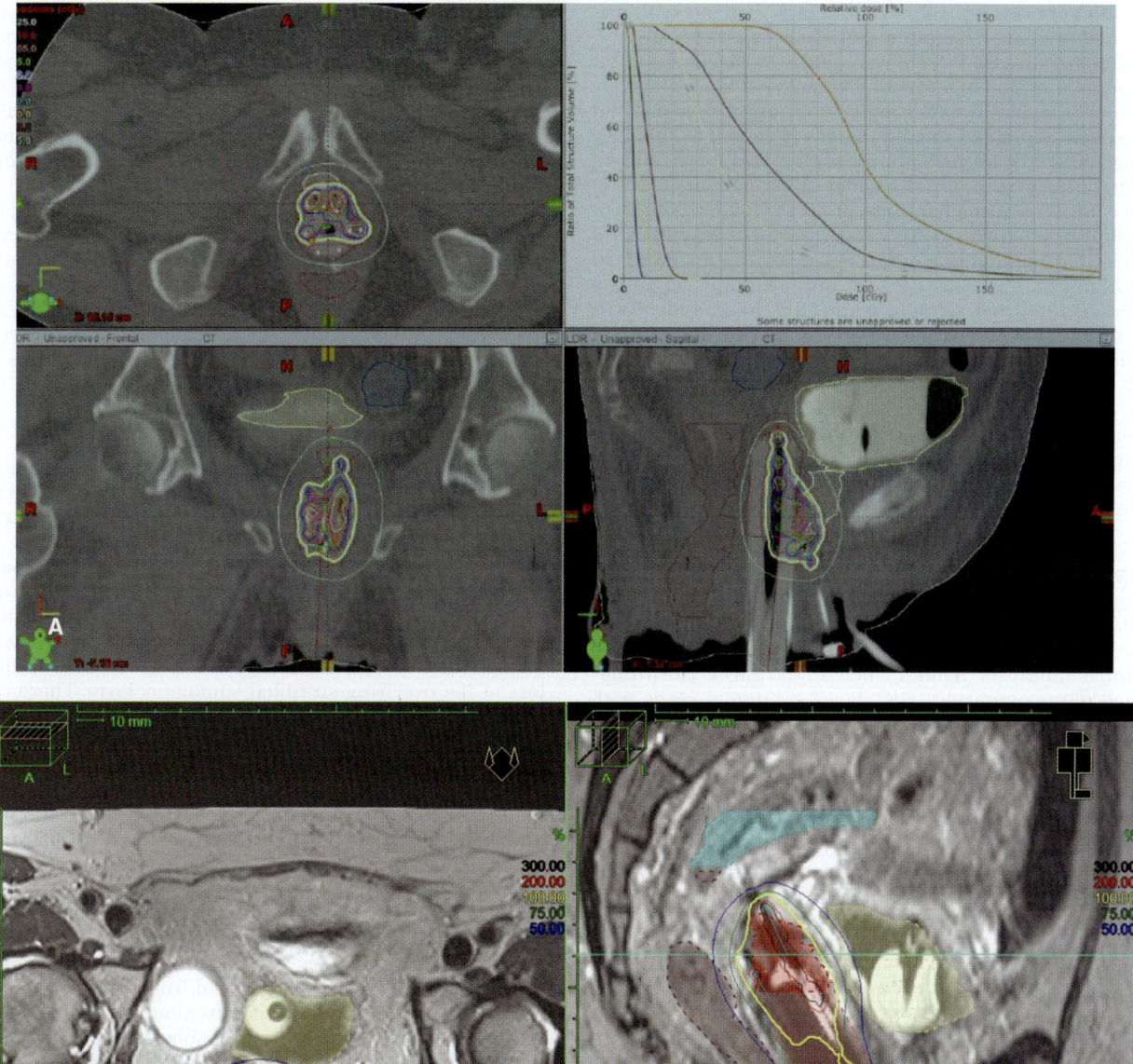

FIGURE 76.5. Interstitial implantation of a vaginal tumor. **A:** Axial, coronal, and sagittal isodose distributions are depicted with dose–volume histogram. **B:** Isodose distributions for a vaginal tumor on axial and sagittal MRI.

71 patients with primary vaginal cancer. A Syed-Neblett template was used with an interstitial iridium-192 afterloading technique. Patients received a minimum of 20 Gy via implant, with a total tumor dose of approximately 80 Gy. With a median follow-up time of 66 months, 5-year disease-free survival rates were reported to be 100%, 60%, 61%, 30%, and 0% for stages I, IIA, IIB, III, and IV patients, respectively. Significant complications were noted in 13% of patients and included

necrosis, fistula, and small-bowel obstruction. Overall, 75% of patients achieved local control.

Beriwal et al. describe results using 3-D image–based HDR interstitial brachytherapy[265] at the University of Pittsburgh Cancer Institute. A total of 30 patients with primary vaginal cancer (*n* = 17) or recurrent gynecologic cancer to the vagina (*n* = 13) were treated using the Syed-Neblett template, with CT scan done after placement of needles for confirmation and treatment planning. Of the subset of 17 patients with primary vaginal cancer, the numbers of patients with stage I, II, III, and IVA disease were 2, 9, 5, and 1, respectively. Fifty-three percent of patients received concurrent chemotherapy with weekly cisplatin at 40 mg/m^2 and apical lesions had laparoscopic guidance during needle placement. The CTV and organs at risk were contoured on CT scan for treatment planning after placement of needles. Most patients (93.3%) received EBRT to a median dose of 45 Gy, followed by HDR interstitial brachytherapy at 3.75 to 5 Gy per fraction in 5 fractions to a median dose of 21.3 Gy. Overall median D90 to the high-risk CTV was 74.3 Gy, and median D2cc to the bladder, rectum, and sigmoid were 58.5, 57.2, and 50 Gy, respectively, showing excellent sparing of critical organs. At a median follow-up time of 16.7 months, the 2-year locoregional control and overall survival rates were 78.8% and 70.2%, respectively, suggesting good local control. Overall, the treatment was fairly well tolerated. There were no grade 3 or higher gastrointestinal complications. One patient developed late grade 3 vaginal ulceration and another had grade 4 vaginal necrosis.

Brachytherapy Versus External Beam Boost

In select circumstances when patients are not appropriate candidates for brachytherapy, IMRT can be considered as an alternative for boost to residual gross disease. A retrospective dosimetric analysis from Princess Margaret Hospital[303] reported data comparing IMRT boost treatment plans with conventional and 4-field radiation boost plans for 12 patients with cervical ($n = 8$), endometrial ($n = 2$), or vaginal ($n = 2$) cancer. IMRT conferred a significant improvement in dose conformity, with overall improvement in rectal and bladder dose-volume distributions, relative to conformal radiation, though inferior to brachytherapy. However, when comparing an ideal photon or proton external beam boost to brachytherapy, brachytherapy provided the best coverage and normal tissue sparing.[304]

Barraclough et al.[305] used an EBRT boost in 21 patients with cervical cancer who could not undergo intracavitary brachytherapy. A 3-D conformal boost was used to deliver a total dose of 54 to 70 Gy. With a median follow-up time of 2.3 years, 48% of patients had recurrent disease, with central recurrence in 16 of 21 patients, significantly higher than 3% to 4% local recurrence rates reported with MR-planned brachytherapy. These results are dramatically inferior to those reported with brachytherapy, suggesting that external beam boosts should only be considered as an alternative when brachytherapy is not feasible.

Stereotactic body radiotherapy (SBRT) is a relatively newer treatment modality with very little data to support its use. A review by Higginson et al.[306] reported on 2 vaginal cancer patients treated with a SBRT boost instead of brachytherapy. Fiducials were placed into the paravaginal, parametrial, or cervical tissues during outpatient clinical examination. The 2 patients with vaginal cancer received 40 to 45 Gy EBRT followed by 25 Gy in 5 fractions of SBRT; 1 patient had a local recurrence at 5 months, and another developed distant disease 17 months posttreatment. Toxicity included one acute grade 2 cystitis and one late grade 3 rectal bleeding.

Treatment Toxicity and Management

Acute Toxicity

The bladder and rectum are located in close proximity to the vagina and it is common for patients to develop acute bowel and urinary toxicity during treatment.[307] Increased urinary frequency, urgency, and dysuria can be managed with phenazopyridine, a urinary tract analgesic, as well

as oral anticholinergic and antispasmodic medications. Antidiarrheal medications such as loperamide, or in more severe cases, tincture of opium, should be prescribed for symptom management early in the development of symptoms. Irritation of the anal mucosa can cause exacerbation of hemorrhoids and occasional hemorrhagic spotting and discomfort with defecation; topical hemorrhoidal ointments or suppositories can be used.

Acute irritation of the vaginal mucosa can be managed symptomatically through hygiene, recognition and treatment of infection, and pain control. Sitz baths and topical ointments may be useful for radiation dermatitis, and both topical and oral analgesics can be prescribed for mucositis and general discomfort during radiation and immediately thereafter. As *Candida* can exacerbate vaginitis, there should be a low threshold for starting antifungal medications.

Late Toxicity

Late toxicity after radiation can manifest as rectovaginal or vesicovaginal fistulas, strictures in the rectum or vagina, premature menopause from radiation exposure to the ovaries, or cystitis, proctitis, or necrosis of the soft tissue or bone.

Clinically, vaginal stenosis and shortening can manifest several months after radiation, although presentation as late as 15 years posttreatment has been documented.[308] Pathologic changes in the vaginal mucosa after radiation treatment include marked mucosal atrophy with epithelial thinning and loss of the overlying stratified squamous layer. There can be hyalinization and collagenization of submucosal connective tissues, with fibrosis of the muscular layer and vasculature. Such changes result in compromised oxygenation of injured tissues, promoting ulceration and fistula formation. It is common to find cytologic abnormalities within the first 6 months after radiation, and it is important to distinguish postradiation atypia from new or recurrent malignancy during posttreatment follow-up.[309]

Regular use of a vaginal dilator to decrease stenosis and shortening should be recommended shortly after completion of radiation treatment, as it is difficult to reverse stenosis and shortening once fibrosis has ensued. Topical estrogen, applied three times a week for 6 to 9 months after radiation, was shown in a randomized controlled trial published in 1975 to reduce the incidence of stenosis, dyspareunia, and cytologic changes in vaginal epithelium.[310] However, because of a small potential for systemic absorption with untoward effects on endometrial proliferation, the use of topical estrogens is not favored for patients.

Radiation necrosis can be conservatively managed with local debridement, peroxide douches, antimicrobials, and estrogen. There is some evidence that hyperbaric oxygen can facilitate healing, with a >50% reduction in vaginal ulceration noted in one series.[311] Fistulas present more of a treatment challenge. Despite the use of interventions such as urinary or fecal diversions, additional surgical correction is often required for effective management, particularly in the case of rectovaginal fistulas.[312]

PATTERNS OF FAILURE

Most treatment failures occur within 5 years, with a median time to recurrence of 6 to 12 months,[62,145] and local recurrence is the most common pattern of treatment failure in the majority of published series. Extravaginal recurrences in the pelvic lymph nodes are less common.

Overall outcomes, by stage, are shown in Table 76.5. In general, the rate of locoregional recurrence ranges from 10% to 20% for stage I and 30% to 40% for stage II. Patients with advanced disease often have persistent disease despite treatment, up to 68% according to one series.[103] The reported rates of distant metastasis vary, ranging from 7% to 33% and usually occur later in the course of disease, with approximately half of all distant metastases presenting at the time of local recurrence.[67,85,103,146]

GENERAL MANAGEMENT, TREATMENT OPTIONS, AND OUTCOME—SPECIAL SCENARIOS

The Posthysterectomy Patient

Approximately 60% of patients with primary vaginal cancer have had a prior hysterectomy. This likely reflects patients with a history of cervical neoplasia and carcinoma requiring surgical management.[313,314] Finding methods to improve target positioning during EBRT becomes especially important as treatment delivery becomes increasingly more conformal.

After hysterectomy, the small bowel tends to fall lower into the pelvis, increasing the likelihood of it being irradiated during treatment. There is also daily variation in vaginal vault position. A study by Jhingran et al.[274] evaluated the variations in vaginal vault position and bladder and rectal volumes in posthysterectomy patients undergoing IMRT and found significant variations in the position of the vaginal vault depending on bladder and rectal filling. Patients were instructed to have a full bladder prior to radiation treatment; however, the study showed a median difference of 247 cc despite this. It is likely that bladder movement impacts vaginal position. For patients with fiducial markers placed in the vagina, the median movement during treatment was 0.59 cm in the right-left direction, 1.46 cm in the anterior–posterior direction, and 1.2 cm in the superior–inferior direction. Thus, it is important to be mindful of target movement when delineating the treatment volume.

To minimize uncertainly, the treating physician can fuse planning CT scans taken with full and empty bladder in order to estimate the potential range of target volume positions during treatment. Another approach, though less practical, is to fill the bladder with a fixed volume of saline using a Foley catheter immediately prior to treatment or to utilize fiducial markers for daily localization.

History of Prior Pelvic Radiation

Up to 10% to 50% of patients with VAIN or invasive carcinoma of the vagina have a previous diagnosis of cervical carcinoma,[12,40,61,67,82–86] with average time interval of 14 years between diagnosis of cervical disease to development of vaginal carcinoma.[61,72] As a result, a proportion of patients with vaginal cancer have history of prior pelvic radiation. Reirradiation can be considered in this setting, but there is an increased risk of toxicity, particularly radionecrosis and fistula formation. Xiang-E et al.[315] published a series on 73 patients with a history of radiation treatment for cervical carcinoma who received a second diagnosis of vaginal malignancy 5 to 30 years later. All patients received EBRT and brachytherapy for treatment of their initial cancer. Reirradiation for the vaginal malignancy was planned according to site and volume of the vaginal tumor and location and dose of the prior radiation. Patients received brachytherapy, using either radium delivered to the tumor base (30 to 40 Gy in 3 to 5 fractions) or HDR with cobalt-60 to the tumor base (20 to 35 Gy in 3 to 5 fractions), followed by a dose to 0.5 cm below the vaginal mucosa at 20 to 30 Gy in 4 to 6 fractions delivered using a vaginal mold. For involvement of the vulva or groin, patients additionally received EBRT to a dose of 30 to 40 Gy. Most patients received radiation alone; 11 also received chemotherapy, most typically cisplatin based. The 5-year survival rate was 40.3% and 3 patients survived more than 15 years. There were significant side effects with reirradiation: 18 of

73 patients developed radionecrosis. Other side effects included 1 (1.4%) vesicovaginal fistula and 8 (11%) rectovaginal fistulas, hematuria (12.3%), and moderate to severe rectal sequelae (13.6%).

Beriwal et al. reported on the use of HDR interstitial and intracavitary brachytherapy for 5 patients with recurrent vaginal cancer with history of prior pelvic radiation.[115] Significant grade 3 or higher toxicities were noted in patients who received total EQD2 dose above 140 Gy. Median time from prior radiation to recurrence was 4 years (range, 6 months to 18 years). The recurrence was within 2 cm of the prior field in 2 patients and within the previous field for 4 patients. All patients received EBRT to a median dose of 45 Gy, followed by brachytherapy. For the 4 patients with prior overlapping fields, the cumulative EQD2 to the vaginal mucosa ranged from 120.7 to 154.54 Gy. Of these patients, one developed a rectovaginal fistula 2 years after treatment, and another developed chronic vaginal ulceration with vaginal shortening to 2 cm; the EQD2 values were 142.98 and 154 Gy, respectively.

Carcinoma of the Neovagina

The neovagina is a surgically constructed vaginal canal, typically described in patients with congenitally deformed or absent genitalia or patients desiring reconstruction of a functional vaginal after surgery for gynecologic malignancy. Various methods have been utilized for neovaginal construction, including split skin grafts, myocutaneous flaps, and formation of an artificial canal between the rectum and vagina.[316] Given its overall rarity, there are very few reports of in situ or invasive carcinoma arising in the neovagina.

A review of published literature reveals six published reports of carcinoma in situ.[317–322] The period of development of carcinoma in situ ranged from 6 months to 20 years after constructive surgery. Invasive carcinoma of the neovagina tends to be poorly differentiated, and majority of reported cases have been SCC. All reported patients have presented with large tumor masses and evidence of rapid progression, with poor overall outcomes.[231,323,324]

Treatment options include radiation, with or without an attempt at radical resection, and, in select cases, lymph node dissection. Of 16 reported cases from a review by Steiner et al.,[316] 9 received primary radiation alone, 1 received radiation followed by exenteration and intraoperative radiation, and 4 underwent exenteration. Recurrence status was not documented for all patients. Three were found to have rapid disease recurrence within several months. Two patients were free of disease at 10 and 18 months, respectively. One patient had a recurrence-free interval of 3 years but died a year later from disease.

Though there is no optimal treatment, resection followed by consideration of adjuvant radiation is preferable to definitive radiation alone, as surgery can offer full pathologic diagnosis. The extent of disease, patient characteristics, and treatment goals should be used to guide the choice of treatment.

Salvage Therapy for Recurrent or Persistent Disease

For patients with recurrent or persistent disease, it is important to determine whether there is a reasonable chance of cure with salvage treatment or whether the primary goal is palliation. Thus, multiple factors, including histology, sites and extent of recurrence, disease-free interval, patient age, comorbidities, and overall performance status, must be considered.

Early-stage lesions that recur after radiation therapy can be surgically salvaged. A retrospective review of pelvic exenteration for recurrent gynecologic malignancies at University of California Los Angeles Medical Center from 1956 to 2001 reported survival rates for patients with recurrent cervical and vaginal cancer to be 73% at 1 year and 54% at 5 years.[325]

Patients with tumor persistence or recurrence after limited surgical procedures can be considered for more extensive surgery. If not, systemic chemotherapy and/or radiation can be administered.

Recurrent disease in advanced stage patients is more challenging to treat. Most patients have received prior EBRT and thus have options limited to radical surgery or, in patients with localized disease, reirradiation. For patients with small pelvic recurrences, reirradiation with intracavitary or interstitial brachytherapy has been reported, with control rates between 50% and 75% and grade 3 or higher complication rates between 7% and 15%.[115,315,326-329] Beriwal et al. evaluated HDR brachytherapy for primary and recurrent vaginal malignancy. In the subset of patients with a previous malignancy, crude local control rates were 100% for patients without prior radiation and 67% for patients with a history of radiation.

Palliative Therapy

Local treatment can provide symptomatic benefit for patients with advanced disease, who have no curative options. Advanced disease can result in vaginal bleeding, pelvic pain, lymphedema, and visceral obstruction. Vaginal bleeding is a common symptom, which can become brisk if tumor erodes into a larger vessel. Large fractions of radiation delivered initially during the treatment course may be useful in achieving hemostasis for such cases. Other options include embolization, infusion of vasopressin, and balloon catheterization for severe hemodynamic losses.

FOLLOW-UP

Recommendations for posttreatment surveillance are based on Society of Gynecologic Oncologist (SGO) guidelines for gynecologic malignancies.[330] Patients with early-stage lesions, treated with surgery alone, can be followed every 6 months for 2 years, then annually thereafter. Patients with more advanced lesions are at higher risk of recurrence and are recommended follow up every 3 months for the first 2 years, then 6 months for the next 3 years, and annually thereafter.

There is insufficient evidence to support the use of regular cervical or vaginal cytology to detect cancer recurrence. However, the SGO recommends annual cytology as surveillance to detect lower genital tract dysplasia. The routine use of CT or PET as surveillance is not recommended.

SUMMARY

Vaginal cancer is a rare disease, accounting for 1% to 2% of all gynecologic malignancies. Treatment options depend on stage. For early-stage disease, definitive surgery and radiation are efficacious; more advanced disease is generally managed with a combination of chemotherapy and radiation.

REFERENCES

1. Cunha GR. The dual origin of vaginal epithelium. *Am J Anat* 1975;143(3): 387–392.
2. Benson RC. Cancer of the female genital tract. *CA Cancer J Clin* 1968;18(1):2–13.
3. Sedlis A, Robboy SJ. Diseases of the vagina. In: Kurman RJ, ed. *Blaustein's pathology of the female genital tract.* New York: Springer-Verlag, 1987: 98–140.
4. Siegel RL, Miller KD, Jemal A. Cancer statistics, 2016. *CA Cancer J Clin* 2016;66(1):7–30.
5. FIGO Committee on Gynecologic Oncology. Current FIGO staging for cancer of the vagina, fallopian tube, ovary, and gestational trophoblastic neoplasia. *Int J Gynaecol Obstet* 2009;105(1):3–4.
6. Hacker NF, Eifel PJ, van der Velden J. Cancer of the vagina. *Int J Gynaecol Obstet* 2012;119(Suppl 2):S97–S99.
7. Shah CA, et al. Factors affecting risk of mortality in women with vaginal cancer. *Obstet Gynecol* 2009;113(5):1038–1045.
8. Berek JS, Hacker NH. *Berek & Hacker's gynecologic oncology.* 5th ed. Philadelphia: Lippincott Williams & Wilkins, 2009.
9. Creasman WT, Phillips JL, Menck HR. The National Cancer Data Base report on cancer of the vagina. *Cancer* 1998;83(5):1033–1040.
10. Gunderson CC, et al. A contemporary analysis of epidemiology and management of vaginal intraepithelial neoplasia. *Am J Obstet Gynecol* 2013;208(5): 410 e1–410 e6.
11. Watson M, Saraiya M, Wu X. Update of HPV-associated female genital cancers in the United States, 1999–2004. *J Womens Health* 2009;18(11):1731–1738.
12. Lenehan PM, Meffe F, Lickrish GM. Vaginal intraepithelial neoplasia: biologic aspects and management. *Obstet Gynecol* 1986;68(3):333–337.
13. Aho M, et al. Natural history of vaginal intraepithelial neoplasia. *Cancer* 1991;68(1):195–197.
14. Hoffman MS, et al. Upper vaginectomy for in situ and occult, superficially invasive carcinoma of the vagina. *Am J Obstet Gynecol* 1992;166(1 Pt 1):30–33.
15. Smith JS, et al. Human papillomavirus type-distribution in vulvar and vaginal cancers and their associated precursors. *Obstet Gynecol* 2009;113(4):917–924.
16. Dillner J, et al. Four year efficacy of prophylactic human papillomavirus quadrivalent vaccine against low grade cervical, vulvar, and vaginal intraepithelial neoplasia and anogenital warts: randomised controlled trial. *Br Med J* 2010;341:c3493.
17. Cheng D, et al. Wide local excision (WLE) for vaginal intraepithelial neoplasia (VAIN). *Acta Obstet Gynecol Scand* 1999;78(7):648–652.
18. Sillman FH, et al. Vaginal intraepithelial neoplasia: risk factors for persistence, recurrence, and invasion and its management. *Am J Obstet Gynecol* 1997;176(1 Pt 1):93–99.
19. Indermaur MD, et al. Upper vaginectomy for the treatment of vaginal intraepithelial neoplasia. *Am J Obstet Gynecol* 2005;193(2):577–580; discussion 580–581.
20. Petrilli ES, et al. Vaginal intraepithelial neoplasia: biologic aspects and treatment with topical 5-fluorouracil and the carbon dioxide laser. *Am J Obstet Gynecol* 1980;138(3):321–328.
21. Boonlikit S, Noinual N. Vaginal intraepithelial neoplasia: a retrospective analysis of clinical features and colpohistology. *J Obstet Gynaecol Res* 2010;36(1):94–100.
22. Murta EF, et al. Vaginal intraepithelial neoplasia: clinical-therapeutic analysis of 33 cases. *Arch Gynecol Obstet* 2005;272(4):261–264.
23. Rome RM, England PG. Management of vaginal intraepithelial neoplasia: a series of 132 cases with long-term follow-up. *Int J Gynecol Cancer* 2000;10(5):382–390.
24. Graham K, et al. 20-Year retrospective review of medium dose rate intracavitary brachytherapy in VAIN3. *Gynecol Oncol* 2007;106(1):105–111.
25. Diakomanolis E, et al. Vaginal intraepithelial neoplasia: report of 102 cases. *Eur J Gynaecol Oncol* 2002;23(5):457–459.
26. de Witte CJ, et al. Imiquimod in cervical, vaginal and vulvar intraepithelial neoplasia: a review. *Gynecol Oncol* 2015;139(2):377–384.
27. Hoffman MS, et al. Laser vaporization of grade 3 vaginal intraepithelial neoplasia. *Am J Obstet Gynecol* 1991;165(5 Pt 1):1342–1344.
28. Townsend DE, et al. Treatment of vaginal carcinoma in situ with the carbon dioxide laser. *Am J Obstet Gynecol* 1982;143(5):565–568.
29. Diakomanolis E, et al. Treatment of vaginal intraepithelial neoplasia with laser ablation and upper vaginectomy. *Gynecol Obstet Invest* 2002;54(1):17–20.
30. Krebs HB. Treatment of vaginal intraepithelial neoplasia with laser and topical 5-fluorouracil. *Obstet Gynecol* 1989;73(4):657–660.
31. Woodruff JD, Parmley TH, Julian CG. Topical 5-fluorouracil in the treatment of vaginal carcinoma-in-situ. *Gynecol Oncol* 1975;3(2):124–132.
32. Caglar H, Hertzog RW, Hreshchyshyn MM. Topical 5-fluorouracil treatment of vaginal intraepithelial neoplasia. *Obstet Gynecol* 1981;58(5):580–583.
33. Daly JW, Ellis GF. Treatment of vaginal dysplasia and carcinoma in situ with topical 5-fluorouracil. *Obstet Gynecol* 1980;55(3):350–352.
34. Kirwan P, Naftalin NJ. Topical 5-fluorouracil in the treatment of vaginal intraepithelial neoplasia. *Br J Obstet Gynaecol* 1985;92(3):287–291.
35. Blanchard P, et al. Low-dose-rate definitive brachytherapy for high-grade vaginal intraepithelial neoplasia. *Oncologist* 2011;16(2):182–188.
36. Woodman CB, Mould JJ, Jordan JA. Radiotherapy in the management of vaginal intraepithelial neoplasia after hysterectomy. *Br J Obstet Gynaecol* 1988;95(10):976–979.
37. Ogino I, et al. High-dose-rate intracavitary brachytherapy in the management of cervical and vaginal intraepithelial neoplasia. *Int J Radiat Oncol Biol Phys* 1998;40(4):881–887.
38. MacLeod C, et al. High-dose-rate brachytherapy in the management of high-grade intraepithelial neoplasia of the vagina. *Gynecol Oncol* 1997;65(1):74–77.
39. Prempree T, et al. Radiation management of primary carcinoma of the vagina. *Cancer* 1977;40(1):109–118.
40. Chyle V, et al. Definitive radiotherapy for carcinoma of the vagina: outcome and prognostic factors. *Int J Radiat Oncol Biol Phys* 1996;35(5):891–905.
41. Perez CA, et al. Factors affecting long-term outcome of irradiation in carcinoma of the vagina. *Int J Radiat Oncol Biol Phys* 1999;44(1):37–45.
42. Song JH, et al. High-dose-rate brachytherapy for the treatment of vaginal intraepithelial neoplasia. *Cancer Res Treat* 2014;46(1):74–80.
43. Zolciak-Siwinska A, et al. Brachytherapy for vaginal intraepithelial neoplasia. *Eur J Obstet Gynecol Reprod Biol* 2015;194:73–77.
44. Benedet JL, Sanders BH. Carcinoma in situ of the vagina. *Am J Obstet Gynecol* 1984;148(5):695–700.
45. Ireland D, Monaghan JM. The management of the patient with abnormal vaginal cytology following hysterectomy. *Br J Obstet Gynaecol* 1988;95(10):973–975.
46. Fanning J, Manahan KJ, McLean SA. Loop electrosurgical excision procedure for partial upper vaginectomy. *Am J Obstet Gynecol* 1999;181(6):1382–1385.

47. Dodge JA, et al. Clinical features and risk of recurrence among patients with vaginal intraepithelial neoplasia. *Gynecol Oncol* 2001;83(2):363–369.

48. Terzakis E, et al. Loop electrosurgical excision procedure in Greek patients with vaginal intraepithelial neoplasia and history of cervical cancer. *Eur J Gynaecol Oncol* 2011;32(5):530–533.

49. Jobson VW, Homesley HD. Treatment of vaginal intraepithelial neoplasia with the carbon dioxide laser. *Obstet Gynecol* 1983;62(1):90–93.

50. Audet-Lapointe P, et al. Vaginal intraepithelial neoplasia. *Gynecol Oncol* 1990;36(2):232–239.

51. Campagnutta E, et al. Treatment of vaginal intraepithelial neoplasia (VAIN) with the carbon dioxide laser. *Clin Exp Obstet Gynecol* 1999;26(2):127–130.

52. Perrotta M, et al. Use of CO_2 laser vaporization for the treatment of high-grade vaginal intraepithelial neoplasia. *J Low Genit Tract Dis* 2013;17(1):23–27.

53. Diakomanolis E, Haidopoulos D, Stefanidis K. Treatment of high-grade vaginal intraepithelial neoplasia with imiquimod cream. *N Engl J Med* 2002; 347(5):374.

54. Buck HW, Guth KJ. Treatment of vaginal intraepithelial neoplasia (primarily low grade) with imiquimod 5% cream. *J Low Genit Tract Dis* 2003;7(4):290–293.

55. Patsner B. Treatment of vaginal dysplasia with loop excision: report of five cases. *Am J Obstet Gynecol* 1993;169(1):179–180.

56. von Gruenigen VE, et al. Surgical treatments for vulvar and vaginal dysplasia: a randomized controlled trial. *Obstet Gynecol* 2007;109(4):942–947.

57. Robinson JB, et al. Cavitational ultrasonic surgical aspiration for the treatment of vaginal intraepithelial neoplasia. *Gynecol Oncol* 2000;78(2):235–241.

58. Benedet JL, et al. Primary invasive carcinoma of the vagina. *Obstet Gynecol* 1983;62(6):715–719.

59. Iavazzo C, et al. Imiquimod for treatment of vulvar and vaginal intraepithelial neoplasia. *Int J Gynaecol Obstet* 2008;101(1):3–10.

60. Mock U, et al. High-dose-rate (HDR) brachytherapy with or without external beam radiotherapy in the treatment of primary vaginal carcinoma: long-term results and side effects. *Int J Radiat Oncol Biol Phys* 2003;56(4):950–957.

61. Gallup DG, et al. Invasive squamous cell carcinoma of the vagina: a 14-year study. *Obstet Gynecol* 1987;69(5):782–785.

62. Frank SJ, et al. Definitive radiation therapy for squamous cell carcinoma of the vagina. *Int J Radiat Oncol Biol Phys* 2005;62(1):138–147.

63. Rubin SC, Young J, Mikuta JJ. Squamous carcinoma of the vagina: treatment, complications, and long-term follow-up. *Gynecol Oncol* 1985;20(3): 346–353.

64. Stock RG, Chen AS, Seski J. A 30-year experience in the management of primary carcinoma of the vagina: analysis of prognostic factors and treatment modalities. *Gynecol Oncol* 1995;56(1):45–52.

65. Kucera H, Vavra N. Radiation management of primary carcinoma of the vagina: clinical and histopathological variables associated with survival. *Gynecol Oncol* 1991;40(1):12–16.

66. Peters WA III, Kumar NB, Morley GW. Carcinoma of the vagina. Factors influencing treatment outcome. *Cancer* 1985;55(4):892–897.

67. Perez CA, et al. Definitive irradiation in carcinoma of the vagina: long-term evaluation of results. *Int J Radiat Oncol Biol Phys* 1988;15(6):1283–1290.

68. Perez CA, et al. Radiation therapy in carcinoma of the vagina. *Obstet Gynecol* 1974;44(6):862–872.

69. Vayrynen M, et al. Verrucous squamous cell carcinoma of the female genital tract. Report of three cases and survey of the literature. *Int J Gynaecol Obstet* 1981;19(5):351–356.

70. Raptis S, Haber G, Ferenczy A. Vaginal squamous cell carcinoma with sarcomatoid spindle cell features. *Gynecol Oncol* 1993;49(1):100–106.

71. Frumovitz M, et al. Lymphatic mapping and sentinel lymph node detection in women with vaginal cancer. *Gynecol Oncol* 2008;108(3):478–481.

72. Davis KP, et al. Invasive vaginal carcinoma: analysis of early-stage disease. *Gynecol Oncol* 1991;42(2):131–136.

73. Al-Kurdi M, Monaghan JM. Thirty-two years experience in management of primary tumours of the vagina. *Br J Obstet Gynaecol* 1981;88(11):1145–1150.

74. Senekjian EK, et al. An evaluation of stage II vaginal clear cell adenocarcinoma according to substages. *Gynecol Oncol* 1988;31(1):56–64.

75. Edge SB, et al, eds. *AJCC cancer staging manual.* 6th ed. Berlin, Germany: Springer, 2010.

76. Lee LJ, et al. ACR appropriateness criteria management of vaginal cancer. *Oncology (Williston Park)* 2013;27(11):1166–1173.

77. Taylor MB, et al. Magnetic resonance imaging of primary vaginal carcinoma. *Clin Radiol* 2007;62(6):549–555.

78. Lamoreaux WT, et al. FDG-PET evaluation of vaginal carcinoma. *Int J Radiat Oncol Biol Phys* 2005;62(3):733–737.

79. Robertson NL, et al. The impact of FDG-PET/CT in the management of patients with vulvar and vaginal cancer. *Gynecol Oncol* 2016;140(3):420–424.

80. De Vuyst H, et al. Prevalence and type distribution of human papillomavirus in carcinoma and intraepithelial neoplasia of the vulva, vagina and anus: a meta-analysis. *Int J Cancer* 2009;124(7):1626–1636.

81. Daling JR, et al. A population-based study of squamous cell vaginal cancer: HPV and cofactors. *Gynecol Oncol* 2002;84(2):263–270.

82. Andersen ES. Primary carcinoma of the vagina: a study of 29 cases. *Gynecol Oncol* 1989;33(3):317–320.

83. Ball HG, Berman ML. Management of primary vaginal carcinoma. *Gynecol Oncol* 1982;14(2):154–163.

84. Kirkbride P, et al. Carcinoma of the vagina—experience at the Princess Margaret Hospital (1974–1989). *Gynecol Oncol* 1995;56(3):435–443.

85. Leung S, Sexton M. Radical radiation therapy for carcinoma of the vagina—impact of treatment modalities on outcome: Peter MacCallum Cancer Institute experience 1970–1990. *Int J Radiat Oncol Biol Phys* 1993;25(3):413–418.

86. Spirtos NM, et al. Radiation therapy for primary squamous cell carcinoma of the vagina: Stanford University experience. *Gynecol Oncol* 1989;35(1):20–26.

87. Herman JM, Homesley HD, Dignan MB. Is hysterectomy a risk factor for vaginal cancer? *JAMA* 1986;256(5):601–603.

88. Lee JY, et al. The risk of second primaries subsequent to irradiation for cervix cancer. *Int J Radiat Oncol Biol Phys* 1982;8(2):207–211.

89. Boice JD Jr, et al. Radiation dose and second cancer risk in patients treated for cancer of the cervix. *Radiat Res* 1988;116(1):3–55.

90. Merino MJ. Vaginal cancer: the role of infectious and environmental factors. *Am J Obstet Gynecol* 1991;165(4 Pt 2):1255–1262.

91. Stock RG, et al. The importance of brachytherapy technique in the management of primary carcinoma of the vagina. *Int J Radiat Oncol Biol Phys* 1992;24(4):747–753.

92. Jain A, Majoko F, Freites O. How innocent is the vaginal pessary? Two cases of vaginal cancer associated with pessary use. *J Obstet Gynaecol* 2006;26(8): 829–830.

93. Schiffman M, Kjaer SK. Chapter 2. Natural history of anogenital human papillomavirus infection and neoplasia. *J Natl Cancer Inst Monogr* 2003;(31): 14–19.

94. Hellman K, et al. Clinical and histopathologic factors related to prognosis in primary squamous cell carcinoma of the vagina. *Int J Gynecol Cancer* 2006;16(3):1201–1211.

95. Herbst AL, Green TH Jr, Ulfelder H. Primary carcinoma of the vagina. An analysis of 68 cases. *Am J Obstet Gynecol* 1970;106(2):210–218.

96. Tran PT, et al. Prognostic factors for outcomes and complications for primary squamous cell carcinoma of the vagina treated with radiation. *Gynecol Oncol* 2007;105(3):641–649.

97. Tjalma WA, et al. The role of surgery in invasive squamous carcinoma of the vagina. *Gynecol Oncol* 2001;81(3):360–365.

98. Fuste V, et al. Primary squamous cell carcinoma of the vagina: human papillomavirus detection, p16 (INK4A) overexpression and clinicopathological correlations. *Histopathology* 2010;57(6):907–916.

99. Alonso I, et al. Human papillomavirus as a favorable prognostic biomarker in squamous cell carcinomas of the vagina. *Gynecol Oncol* 2012;125(1): 194–199.

100. Brunner AH, et al. The prognostic role of human papillomavirus in patients with vaginal cancer. *Int J Gynecol Cancer* 2011;21(5):923–929.

101. Urbanski K, et al. Primary invasive vaginal carcinoma treated with radiotherapy: analysis of prognostic factors. *Gynecol Oncol* 1996;60(1):16–21.

102. Kucera H, et al. Radiotherapy of primary carcinoma of the vagina: management and results of different therapy schemes. *Gynecol Oncol* 1985;21(1):87–93.

103. Dixit S, Singhal S, Baboo HA. Squamous cell carcinoma of the vagina: a review of 70 cases. *Gynecol Oncol* 1993;48(1):80–87.

104. Pingley S, et al. Primary carcinoma of the vagina: Tata Memorial Hospital experience. *Int J Radiat Oncol Biol Phys* 2000;46(1):101–108.

105. Lee WR, et al. Radiotherapy alone for carcinoma of the vagina: the importance of overall treatment time. *Int J Radiat Oncol Biol Phys* 1994;29(5):983–988.

106. Jain V, et al. Role of radical surgery in early stages of vaginal cancer—our experience. *Int J Gynecol Cancer* 2016;26(6):1176–1181.

107. Otton GR, et al. Early-stage vaginal carcinoma—an analysis of 70 patients. *Int J Gynecol Cancer* 2004;14(2):304–310.

108. Ling B, et al. Laparoscopic radical hysterectomy with vaginectomy and reconstruction of vagina in patients with stage I of primary vaginal carcinoma. *Gynecol Oncol* 2008;109(1):92–96.

109. Lv L, et al. Neoadjuvant chemotherapy followed by radical surgery and reconstruction of the vagina in a patient with stage II primary vaginal squamous carcinoma. *J Obstet Gynaecol Res* 2010;36(6):1245–1248.

110. Benedetti Panici P, et al. Neoadjuvant chemotherapy followed by radical surgery in patients affected by vaginal carcinoma. *Gynecol Oncol* 2008;111(2):307–311.

111. Kanayama N, et al. Definitive radiotherapy for primary vaginal cancer: correlation between treatment patterns and recurrence rate. *J Radiat Res* 2015;56(2):346–353.

112. Chang JH, et al. Definitive treatment of primary vaginal cancer with radiotherapy: multi-institutional retrospective study of the Korean Radiation Oncology Group (KROG 12-09). *J Gynecol Oncol* 2016;27(2):e17.

113. Miyamoto DT, Tanaka CK, Viswanathan AN. Concurrent chemoradiation improves survival in patients with vaginal cancer. In 52nd American Society for Therapeutic Radiology and Oncology Annual Meeting. San Diego, CA, 2010.

114. Damast S, et al. Treatment of early stage vaginal cancer with EBRT and MRI-based intracavitary brachytherapy: a retrospective case review. *Gynecol Oncol Rep* 2016;17:89–92.

115. Beriwal S, et al. High-dose rate brachytherapy (HDRB) for primary or recurrent cancer in the vagina. *Radiat Oncol* 2008;3:7.

116. Lian J, et al. Twenty-year review of radiotherapy for vaginal cancer: an institutional experience. *Gynecol Oncol* 2008;111(2):298–306.

117. de Crevoisier R, et al. Exclusive radiotherapy for primary squamous cell carcinoma of the vagina. *Radiother Oncol* 2007;85(3):362–370.

118. Stryker JA. Radiotherapy for vaginal carcinoma: a 23-year review. *Br J Radiol* 2000;73(875):1200–1205.

119. Fine BA, et al. The curative potential of radiation therapy in the treatment of primary vaginal carcinoma. *Am J Clin Oncol* 1996;19(1):39–44.

120. Lee LJ, Viswanathan AN. Predictors of toxicity after image-guided high-dose-rate interstitial brachytherapy for gynecologic cancer. *Int J Radiat Oncol Biol Phys* 2012;84(5):1192–1197.

121. Dancuart F, et al. Primary squamous cell carcinoma of the vagina treated by radiotherapy: a failures analysis—the M.D. Anderson Hospital experience 1955–1982. *Int J Radiat Oncol Biol Phys* 1988;14(4):745–749.

Section III

122. Prempree T, Amornmarn R. Radiation treatment of primary carcinoma of the vagina. Patterns of failures after definitive therapy. *Acta Radiol Oncol* 1985;24(1):51–56.

123. Perez CA, Korba A, Sharma S. Dosimetric considerations in irradiation of carcinoma of the vagina. *Int J Radiat Oncol Biol Phys* 1977;2(7–8):639–649.

124. Glaser SM, Beriwal S. Brachytherapy for malignancies of the vagina in the 3D era. *J Contemp Brachyther* 2015;7(4):312–318.

125. Vargo JA, et al. Image-based multichannel vaginal cylinder brachytherapy for vaginal cancer. *Brachytherapy* 2015;14(1):9–15.

126. Beriwal S, et al. American Brachytherapy Society consensus guidelines for interstitial brachytherapy for vaginal cancer. *Brachytherapy* 2012;11(1):68–75.

127. Fleming P, et al. Description of an afterloading 192Ir interstitial-intracavitary technique in the treatment of carcinoma of the vagina. *Obstet Gynecol* 1980;55(4):525–530.

128. Puthawala A, et al. Integrated external and interstitial radiation therapy for primary carcinoma of the vagina. *Obstet Gynecol* 1983;62(3):367–372.

129. Hou JY, et al. Vulvar and vaginal melanoma: A unique subclass of mucosal melanoma based on a comprehensive molecular analysis of 51 cases compared with 2253 cases of nongynecologic melanoma. *Cancer* 2017;123(8):1333–1344.

130. Senekjian EK, Frey K, Herbst AL. Pelvic exenteration in clear cell adenocarcinoma of the vagina and cervix. *Gynecol Oncol* 1989;34(3):413–416.

131. Morris M, et al. Pelvic radiation with concurrent chemotherapy compared with pelvic and para-aortic radiation for high-risk cervical cancer. *N Engl J Med* 1999;340(15):1137–1143.

132. Rose PG, et al. Concurrent cisplatin-based radiotherapy and chemotherapy for locally advanced cervical cancer. *N Engl J Med* 1999;340(15):1144–1153.

133. Mundt AJ, et al. Intensity-modulated whole pelvic radiotherapy in women with gynecologic malignancies. *Int J Radiat Oncol Biol Phys* 2002;52(5):1330–1337.

134. Mundt AJ, Mell LK, Roeske JC. Preliminary analysis of chronic gastrointestinal toxicity in gynecology patients treated with intensity-modulated whole pelvic radiation therapy. *Int J Radiat Oncol Biol Phys* 2003;56(5):1354–1360.

135. Keys HM, et al. Cisplatin, radiation, and adjuvant hysterectomy compared with radiation and adjuvant hysterectomy for bulky stage IB cervical carcinoma. *N Engl J Med* 1999;340(15):1154–1161.

136. Miyamoto DT, Viswanathan AN. Concurrent chemoradiation for vaginal cancer. *PLoS One* 2013;8(6):e65048.

137. Dalrymple JL, et al. Chemoradiation for primary invasive squamous carcinoma of the vagina. *Int J Gynecol Cancer* 2004;14(1):110–117.

138. Gunderson CC, et al. Vaginal cancer: the experience from 2 large academic centers during a 15-year period. *J Low Genit Tract Dis* 2013;17(4):409–413.

139. Samant R, et al. Primary vaginal cancer treated with concurrent chemoradiation using Cis-platinum. *Int J Radiat Oncol Biol Phys* 2007;69(3):746–750.

140. Nashiro T, et al. Concurrent chemoradiation for locally advanced squamous cell carcinoma of the vagina: case series and literature review. *Int J Clin Oncol* 2008;13(4):335–339.

141. Rajagopalan MS, et al. Adoption and impact of concurrent chemoradiation therapy for vaginal cancer: a National Cancer Data Base (NCDB) study. *Gynecol Oncol* 2014;135(3):495–502.

142. Ghia AJ, et al. Primary vaginal cancer and chemoradiotherapy: a patterns-of-care analysis. *Int J Gynecol Cancer* 2011;21(2):378–384.

143. Evans LS, et al. Concomitant 5-fluorouracil, mitomycin-C, and radiotherapy for advanced gynecologic malignancies. *Int J Radiat Oncol Biol Phys* 1988;15(4):901–906.

144. Roberts WS, et al. Further experience with radiation therapy and concomitant intravenous chemotherapy in advanced carcinoma of the lower female genital tract. *Gynecol Oncol* 1991;43(3):233–236.

145. Tabata T, et al. Treatment failure in vaginal cancer. *Gynecol Oncol* 2002;84(2):309–314.

146. Houghton CR, Iversen T. Squamous cell carcinoma of the vagina: a clinical study of the location of the tumor. *Gynecol Oncol* 1982;13(3):365–372.

147. Weinstock MA. Malignant melanoma of the vulva and vagina in the United States: patterns of incidence and population-based estimates of survival. *Am J Obstet Gynecol* 1994;171(5):1225–1230.

148. Frumovitz M, et al. Primary malignant melanoma of the vagina. *Obstet Gynecol* 2010;116(6):1358–1365.

149. Hu DN, Yu GP, McCormick SA. Population-based incidence of vulvar and vaginal melanoma in various races and ethnic groups with comparisons to other site-specific melanomas. *Melanoma Res* 2010;20(2):153–158.

150. Gupta JC, et al. Primary melanoma of the vagina. *J Obstet Gynaecol Br Commonw* 1964;71:801–803.

151. Breslow A. Tumor thickness, level of invasion and node dissection in stage I cutaneous melanoma. *Ann Surg* 1975;182(5):572–575.

152. Irvin WP Jr, et al. Malignant melanoma of the vagina and locoregional control: radical surgery revisited. *Gynecol Oncol* 1998;71(3):476–480.

153. Reid GC, et al. Primary melanoma of the vagina: a clinicopathologic analysis. *Obstet Gynecol* 1989;74(2):190–199.

154. Chung AF, et al. Malignant melanoma of the vagina—report of 19 cases. *Obstet Gynecol* 1980;55(6):720–727.

155. Buchanan DJ, Schlaerth J, Kurosaki T. Primary vaginal melanoma: thirteen-year disease-free survival after wide local excision and review of recent literature. *Am J Obstet Gynecol* 1998;178(6):1177–1184.

156. Van Nostrand KM, et al. Primary vaginal melanoma: improved survival with radical pelvic surgery. *Gynecol Oncol* 1994;55(2):234–237.

157. Xia L, et al. Primary malignant melanoma of the vagina: a retrospective clinicopathologic study of 44 cases. *Int J Gynecol Cancer* 2014;24(1):149–155.

158. Geisler JP, et al. Pelvic exenteration for malignant melanomas of the vagina or urethra with over 3 mm of invasion. *Gynecol Oncol* 1995;59(3):338–341.

159. Stellato G, et al. Primary malignant melanoma of the vagina: case report. *Eur J Gynaecol Oncol* 1998;19(2):186–188.

160. Morrow CP, DiSaia PJ. Malignant melanoma of the female genitalia: a clinical analysis. *Obstet Gynecol Surv* 1976;31(4):233–271.

161. Miner TJ, et al. Primary vaginal melanoma: a critical analysis of therapy. *Ann Surg Oncol* 2004;11(1):34–39.

162. Huang Q, et al. Clinical outcome of 31 patients with primary malignant melanoma of the vagina. *J Gynecol Oncol* 2013;24(4):330–335.

163. DeMatos P, Tyler D, Seigler HF. Mucosal melanoma of the female genitalia: a clinicopathologic study of forty-three cases at Duke University Medical Center. *Surgery* 1998;124(1):38–48.

164. Cobellis L, et al. Malignant melanoma of the vagina. A report of 15 cases. *Eur J Gynaecol Oncol* 2000;21(3):295–297.

165. Bonner JA, et al. The management of vaginal melanoma. *Cancer* 1988;62(9):2066–2072.

166. Petru E, et al. Primary malignant melanoma of the vagina: long-term remission following radiation therapy. *Gynecol Oncol* 1998;70(1):23–26.

167. Harwood AR, Cummings BJ. Radiotherapy for mucosal melanomas. *Int J Radiat Oncol Biol Phys* 1982;8(7):1121–1126.

168. Rogo KO, et al. Conservative surgery for vulvovaginal melanoma. *Eur J Gynaecol Oncol* 1991;12(2):113–119.

169. Robboy SJ, et al. Atypical vaginal adenosis and cervical ectropion. Association with clear cell adenocarcinoma in diethylstilbestrol-exposed offspring. *Cancer* 1984;54(5):869–875.

170. Brand E, et al. Vulvovaginal melanoma: report of seven cases and literature review. *Gynecol Oncol* 1989;33(1):54–60.

171. Lian B, et al. Phase II randomized trial comparing high-dose IFN-alpha2b with temozolomide plus cisplatin as systemic adjuvant therapy for resected mucosal melanoma. *Clin Cancer Res* 2013;19(16):4488–4498.

172. Norris HJ, Taylor HB. Melanomas of the vagina. *Am J Clin Pathol* 1966;46(4):420–426.

173. Ghezelayagh T, Rauh-Hain JA, Growdon WB. Comparing mortality of vaginal sarcoma, squamous cell carcinoma, and adenocarcinoma in the surveillance, epidemiology, and end results database. *Obstet Gynecol* 2015;125(6):1353–1361.

174. Ahram J, Lemus R, Schiavello HJ. Leiomyosarcoma of the vagina: case report and literature review. *Int J Gynecol Cancer* 2006;16(2):884–891.

175. Ciaravino G, et al. Primary leiomyosarcoma of the vagina. A case report and literature review. *Int J Gynecol Cancer* 2000;10(4):340–347.

176. Suh MJ, Park DC. Leiomyosarcoma of the vagina: a case report and review from the literature. *J Gynecol Oncol* 2008;19(4):261–264.

176a. Bell SW, Kempson RL, Hendrickson MR. Problematic uterine smooth muscle neoplasms: a clinicopathologic study of 213 cases. *Am J Surg Pathol* 1994;18:535–558.

177. Tavassoli FA, Norris HJ. Smooth muscle tumors of the vagina. *Obstet Gynecol* 1979;53(6):689–693.

178. Curtin JP, et al. Soft-tissue sarcoma of the vagina and vulva: a clinicopathologic study. *Obstet Gynecol* 1995;86(2):269–272.

179. Ahuja A, et al. Primary mixed mullerian tumor of the vagina—a case report with review of the literature. *Pathol Res Pract* 2011;207(4):253–255.

180. Prempree T, et al. Angiosarcoma of the vagina: a clinicopathologic report. A reappraisal of the radiation treatment of angiosarcomas of the female genital tract. *Cancer* 1983;51(4):618–622.

181. McAdam JA, Stewart F, Reid R. Vaginal epithelioid angiosarcoma. *J Clin Pathol* 1998;51(12):928–930.

182. Tohya T, et al. Angiosarcoma of the vagina. A light and electron microscopy study. *Acta Obstet Gynecol Scand* 1991;70(2):169–172.

183. Hays DM, et al. Sarcomas of the vagina and uterus: the Intergroup Rhabdomyosarcoma Study. *J Pediatr Surg* 1985;20(6):718–724.

184. Magne N, et al. Vulval and vaginal rhabdomyosarcoma in children: update and reappraisal of Institut Gustave Roussy brachytherapy experience. *Int J Radiat Oncol Biol Phys* 2008;72(3):878–883.

185. Nielsen OS, et al. High-dose epirubicin is not an alternative to standard-dose doxorubicin in the treatment of advanced soft tissue sarcomas. A study of the EORTC soft tissue and bone sarcoma group. *Br J Cancer* 1998;78(12):1634–1639.

186. Suit HD, et al. Treatment of the patient with stage M0 soft tissue sarcoma. *J Clin Oncol* 1988;6(5):854–862.

187. Fein DA, et al. Management of extremity soft tissue sarcomas with limb-sparing surgery and postoperative irradiation: do total dose, overall treatment time, and the surgery-radiotherapy interval impact on local control? *Int J Radiat Oncol Biol Phys* 1995;32(4):969–976.

188. Peters WA III, et al. Primary sarcoma of the adult vagina: a clinicopathologic study. *Obstet Gynecol* 1985;65(5):699–704.

189. Kounelis S, et al. Carcinosarcomas (malignant mixed mullerian tumors) of the female genital tract: comparative molecular analysis of epithelial and mesenchymal components. *Hum Pathol* 1998;29(1):82–87.

190. Davis PC, Franklin EW III. Cancer of the vagina. *South Med J* 1975;68(10):1239–1242.

191. Sebenik M, et al. Malignant mixed mullerian tumor of the vagina: case report with review of the literature, immunohistochemical study, and evaluation for human papilloma virus. *Hum Pathol* 2007;38(8):1282–1288.

192. Sotiropoulou M, et al. Primary malignant mixed mullerian tumor of the vagina immunohistochemically confirmed. *Arch Gynecol Obstet* 2005;271(3):264–266.

193. Neesham D, Kerdemelidis P, Scurry J. Primary malignant mixed Mullerian tumor of the vagina. *Gynecol Oncol* 1998;70(2):303–307.

194. Shibata R, et al. Primary carcinosarcoma of the vagina. *Pathol Int* 2003;53(2):106–110.

195. Leiser AL, et al. Carcinosarcoma of the ovary treated with platinum and taxane: the memorial Sloan-Kettering Cancer Center experience. *Gynecol Oncol* 2007;105(3):657–661.

196. Mok JE, et al. Malignant mixed mullerian tumors of the ovary: experience with cytoreductive surgery and platinum-based combination chemotherapy. *Int J Gynecol Cancer* 2006;16(1):101–105.

197. Rutledge TL, et al. Carcinosarcoma of the ovary—a case series. *Gynecol Oncol* 2006;100(1):128–132.

198. Herbst AL, Ulfelder H, Poskanzer DC. Adenocarcinoma of the vagina. Association of maternal stilbestrol therapy with tumor appearance in young women. *N Engl J Med* 1971;284(15):878–881.

199. Melnick S, et al. Rates and risks of diethylstilbestrol-related clear-cell adenocarcinoma of the vagina and cervix. An update. *N Engl J Med* 1987;316(9):514–516.

200. Robboy SJ, Scully RE, Herbst AL. Pathology of vaginal and cervical abnormalities associated with prenatal exposure to diethylstilbestrol (des). *J Reprod Med* 1975;15(1):13–18.

201. Robboy SJ, et al. Topographic relation of cervical ectropion and vaginal adenosis to clear cell adenocarcinoma. *Obstet Gynecol* 1982;60(5):546–551.

202. Verloop J, Rookus MA, van Leeuwen FE. Prevalence of gynecologic cancer in women exposed to diethylstilbestrol in utero. *N Engl J Med* 2000;342(24):1838–1839.

203. Robboy SJ, et al. Dysplasia and cytologic findings in 4,589 young women enrolled in diethylstilbestrol-adenosis (DESAD) project. *Am J Obstet Gynecol* 1981;140(5):579–586.

204. Robboy SJ, et al. Vaginal adenosis in women born prior to the diethylstilbestrol era. *Hum Pathol* 1986;17(5):488–492.

205. Herbst AL, et al. Clear-cell adenocarcinoma of the vagina and cervix in girls: analysis of 170 registry cases. *Am J Obstet Gynecol* 1974;119(5):713–724.

206. Jones WB, et al. Clear-cell adenocarcinoma of the lower genital tract: Memorial Hospital 1974–1984. *Obstet Gynecol* 1987;70(4):573–577.

207. Hanselaar AG, et al. Clear cell adenocarcinoma of the vagina and cervix. A report of the Central Netherlands Registry with emphasis on early detection and prognosis. *Cancer* 1991;67(7):1971–1978.

208. Waggoner SE, et al. p53 protein expression and gene analysis in clear cell adenocarcinoma of the vagina and cervix. *Gynecol Oncol* 1996;60(3):339–344.

209. Frank SJ, et al. Primary adenocarcinoma of the vagina not associated with diethylstilbestrol (DES) exposure. *Gynecol Oncol* 2007;105(2):470–474.

210. Nomura H, et al. Clinical characteristics of non-squamous cell carcinoma of the vagina. *Int J Gynecol Cancer* 2015;25(2):320–324.

211. Herbst AL, et al. An analysis of 346 cases of clear cell adenocarcinoma of the vagina and cervix with emphasis on recurrence and survival. *Gynecol Oncol* 1979;7(2):111–122.

212. Senekjian EK, et al. Local therapy in stage I clear cell adenocarcinoma of the vagina. *Cancer* 1987;60(6):1319–1324.

213. Guiou M, et al. Primary clear cell adenocarcinoma of the rectovaginal septum treated with concurrent chemoradiation therapy: a case report. *Int J Gynecol Cancer* 2008;18(5):1118–1121.

214. Waggoner SE, et al. Influence of in utero diethylstilbestrol exposure on the prognosis and biologic behavior of vaginal clear-cell adenocarcinoma. *Gynecol Oncol* 1994;55(2):238–244.

215. Wharton JT, et al. Vaginal intraepithelial neoplasia and vaginal cancer. *Obstet Gynecol Clin North Am* 1996;23(2):325–345.

216. Herbst AL, et al. Epidemiologic aspects and factors related to survival in 384 Registry cases of clear cell adenocarcinoma of the vagina and cervix. *Am J Obstet Gynecol* 1979;135(7):876–886.

217. Fishman DA, et al. Late recurrences of vaginal clear cell adenocarcinoma. *Gynecol Oncol* 1996;62(1):128–132.

218. Lin LM, et al. Diethylstilbestrol (DES)-induced clear cell adenocarcinoma of the vagina metastasizing to the brain. *Gynecol Oncol* 2007;105(1):273–276.

219. Tarraza HM Jr, et al. Vaginal metastases from renal cell carcinoma: report of four cases and review of the literature. *Eur J Gynaecol Oncol* 1998;19(1):14–18.

220. Saitoh M, et al. Primary mucinous adenocarcinoma of the vagina: possibility of differentiating from metastatic adenocarcinomas. *Pathol Int* 2005;55(6):372–375.

221. Nag S, et al. Perineal template interstitial brachytherapy salvage for recurrent endometrial adenocarcinoma metastatic to the vagina. *Gynecol Oncol* 1997;66(1):16–19.

222. Staats PN, Clement PB, Young RH. Primary endometrioid adenocarcinoma of the vagina: a clinicopathologic study of 18 cases. *Am J Surg Pathol* 2007;31(10):1490–1501.

223. Nomoto K, et al. Endometrioid adenocarcinoma of the vagina with a microglandular pattern arising from endometriosis after hysterectomy. *Pathol Int* 2010;60(9):636–641.

224. Adjetey V, Ganesan R, Downey GP. Primary vaginal endometrioid carcinoma following unopposed estrogen administration. *J Obstet Gynaecol* 2003;23(3):316–317.

225. Eckert R, Eckert R. Adenocarcinoma arising in endometriosis. *Am Fam Physician* 2000;62(4):734, 736.

226. Tewari DS, et al. Primary invasive vaginal cancer in the setting of the Mayer-Rokitansky-Kuster-Hauser syndrome. *Gynecol Oncol* 2002;85(2):384–387.

227. Ebrahim S, et al. Primary mucinous adenocarcinoma of the vagina. *Gynecol Oncol* 2001;80(1):89–92.

228. Nasu K, et al. Primary mucinous adenocarcinoma of the vagina. *Eur J Gynaecol Oncol* 2010;31(6):679–681.

229. Werner D, et al. Primary adenocarcinoma of the vagina with mucinous-enteric differentiation: a report of two cases with associated vaginal adenosis without history of diethylstilbestrol exposure. *J Low Genit Tract Dis* 2004;8(1):38–42.

230. McCluggage WG, Price JH, Dobbs SP. Primary adenocarcinoma of the vagina arising in endocervicosis. *Int J Gynecol Pathol* 2001;20(4):399–402.

231. Hiroi H, et al. Mucinous adenocarcinoma arising in a neovagina using the sigmoid colon thirty years after operation: a case report. *J Surg Oncol* 2001;77(1):61–64.

232. Droegemueller W, Makowski EL, Taylor ES. Vaginal mesonephric adenocarcinoma in two prepubertal children. *Am J Dis Child* 1970;119(2):168–170.

233. Shaaban MM. Primary adenocarcinoma of the vagina of mesonephric pattern. Report of a case and review of literatur. *Aust N Zeal J Obstet Gynaecol* 1970;10(1):55–58.

234. Riva C, et al. Primary serous papillary adenocarcinoma of the vagina: a case report. *Int J Gynecol Pathol* 1997;16(3):286–290.

235. Ferry JA, Young RH. Malignant lymphoma, pseudolymphoma, and hematopoietic disorders of the female genital tract. *Pathol Annu* 1991;26(Pt 1):227–263.

236. Mahendran SM. Primary non-Hodgkin's lymphoma of the vagina masquerading as a uterine fibroid in pregnancy. *J Obstet Gynaecol* 2008;28(4):456–458.

237. Hussein IY, et al. Primary non-Hodgkin's lymphoma of the vagina. *J Obstet Gynaecol* 2007;27(7):752.

238. Cohn DE, et al. Non-Hodgkin's lymphoma mimicking gynecological malignancies of the vagina and cervix: a report of four cases. *Int J Gynecol Cancer* 2007;17(1):274–279.

239. Zafar M, et al. Primary non-Hodgkin's lymphoma of vagina associated with pregnancy. *J Coll Physicians Surg Pak* 2006;16(6):424–425.

240. Garavaglia E, et al. Primary stage I-IIE non-Hodgkin's lymphoma of uterine cervix and upper vagina: evidence for a conservative approach in a study on three patients. *Gynecol Oncol* 2005;97(1):214–218.

241. Yoshinaga K, et al. A case of primary mucosa-associated lymphoid tissue lymphoma of the vagina. *Hum Pathol* 2004;35(9):1164–1166.

242. Engin H, et al. Successful treatment of primary non-Hodgkin's lymphoma of the vagina with chemotherapy. *Arch Gynecol Obstet* 2004;269(3):208–210.

243. Raspagliesi F, et al. Primary non-Hodgkin's lymphoma of the vagina. *Haematologica* 2000;85(6):666–667.

244. Vang R, et al. Non-Hodgkin's lymphoma involving the vagina: a clinicopathologic analysis of 14 patients. *Am J Surg Pathol* 2000;24(5):719–725.

245. Guarini A, et al. Primary non Hodgkin's lymphoma of the vagina. *Leuk Lymphoma* 1999;35(5–6):619–622.

246. Skinnider BF, et al. Primary non-Hodgkin's lymphoma and malakoplakia of the vagina: a case report. *Hum Pathol* 1999;30(7):871–874.

247. Hoffkes HG, et al. Primary non-Hodgkin's lymphoma of the vagina. Case report and review of the literature. *Ann Hematol* 1995;70(5):273–276.

248. Lonardi F, et al. Primary lymphoma of the vagina. A case report. *Haematologica* 1994;79(2):182–183.

249. Harris NL, Scully RE. Malignant lymphoma and granulocytic sarcoma of the uterus and vagina. A clinicopathologic analysis of 27 cases. *Cancer* 1984;53(11):2530–2545.

250. Chorlton I, et al. Primary malignant reticuloendothelial disease involving the vagina, cervix, and corpus uteri. *Obstet Gynecol* 1974;44(5):735–748.

251. McNicholas MM, Fennelly JJ, MacErlaine DP. Imaging of primary vaginal lymphoma. *Clin Radiol* 1994;49(2):130–132.

252. Domingo S, et al. Epstein-Barr virus positivity in primary vaginal lymphoma. *Gynecol Oncol* 2004;95(3):719–721.

253. Pham DC, Guthrie TH, Ndubisi B. HIV-associated primary cervical non-Hodgkin's lymphoma and two other cases of primary pelvic non-Hodgkin's lymphoma. *Gynecol Oncol* 2003;90(1):204–206.

254. Signorelli M, et al. Conservative management in primary genital lymphomas: the role of chemotherapy. *Gynecol Oncol* 2007;104(2):416–421.

255. Gardner GJ, Reidy-Lagunes D, Gehrig PA. Neuroendocrine tumors of the gynecologic tract: a Society of Gynecologic Oncology (SGO) clinical document. *Gynecol Oncol* 2011;122(1):190–198.

256. Kaminski JM, et al. Primary small cell carcinoma of the vagina. *Gynecol Oncol* 2003;88(3):451–455.

257. Elsaleh H, et al. Small cell carcinoma of the vagina. *Australas Radiol* 2000;44(3):336–337.

258. Ulich TR, et al. Endocrine and tumor differentiation markers in poorly differentiated small-cell carcinoids of the cervix and vagina. *Arch Pathol Lab Med* 1986;110(11):1054–1057.

259. Crowder S, Tuller E. Small cell carcinoma of the female genital tract. *Semin Oncol* 2007;34(1):57–63.

260. Bing Z, et al. Primary small cell neuroendocrine carcinoma of the vagina: a clinicopathologic study. *Arch Pathol Lab Med* 2004;128(8):857–862.

261. Cai T, et al. Paraganglioma of the vagina: a case report and review of the literature. *Onco Targets Ther* 2014;7:965–968.

262. Hassan A, et al. Paraganglioma of the vagina: report of a case, including immunohistochemical and ultrastructural findings. *Int J Gynecol Pathol* 2003;22(4):404–406.

263. Shen JG, et al. Vaginal paraganglioma presenting as a gynecologic mass: case report. *Eur J Gynaecol Oncol* 2008;29(2):184–185.

264. Tohya T, et al. Small cell carcinoma of the endometrium associated with adenosquamous carcinoma: a light and electron microscopic study. *Gynecol Oncol* 1986;25(3):363–371.

265. Beriwal S, et al. 3D image-based HDR interstitial brachytherapy for vaginal cancer. *Brachytherapy* 2012;11(3):176–180.

266. Manuel M, et al. Are clinical outcomes improved with image guided interstitial brachytherapy for vaginal cancer? *Int J Radiat Oncol Biol Phys* 2015;93(3):E285–E286.

267. Finlay MH, et al. Use of CT simulation for treatment of cervical cancer to assess the adequacy of lymph node coverage of conventional pelvic fields based on bony landmarks. *Int J Radiat Oncol Biol Phys* 2006;64(1):205–209.

268. McAlpine J, et al. Radiation fields in gynecologic oncology: correlation of soft tissue (surgical) to radiologic landmarks. *Gynecol Oncol* 2004;92(1):25–30.

269. Yeh AM, et al. Patterns of failure in squamous cell carcinoma of the vagina treated with definitive radiotherapy alone: what is the appropriate treatment volume? *Int J Cancer* 2001;96(Suppl):109–116.

270. Dittmer PH, Randall ME. A technique for inguinal node boost using photon fields defined by asymmetric collimator jaws. *Radiother Oncol* 2001;59(1):61–64.

271. Roeske JC, et al. Intensity-modulated whole pelvic radiation therapy in patients with gynecologic malignancies. *Int J Radiat Oncol Biol Phys* 2000; 48(5):1613–1621.

272. Mundt AJ, Roeske JC, Lujan AE. Intensity-modulated radiation therapy in gynecologic malignancies. *Med Dosim* 2002;27(2):131–136.

273. Viswanathan AN, et al., eds. *Gynecologic radiation therapy: novel approaches to image-guidance and management.* 1st ed. Heidelberg, Germany: Springer-Verlag, 2011.

274. Jhingran A, et al. Vaginal motion and bladder and rectal volumes during pelvic intensity-modulated radiation therapy after hysterectomy. *Int J Radiat Oncol Biol Phys* 2012;82(1):256–262.

275. Orton A, et al. Brachytherapy improves survival in primary vaginal cancer. *Gynecol Oncol* 2016;141(3):501–506.

276. Rajagopalan MS, et al. Patterns of care and brachytherapy boost utilization for vaginal cancer in the United States. *Pract Radiat Oncol* 2015;5(1): 56–61.

277. Manuel MM, et al. Outcomes with image-based interstitial brachytherapy for vaginal cancer. *Radiother Oncol* 2016;120(3):486–492.

278. Delclos L, et al. Minicolpostats, dome cylinders, other additions and improvements of the Fletcher-suit afterloadable system: indications and limitations of their use. *Int J Radiat Oncol Biol Phys* 1980;6(9):1195–1206.

279. Perez CA, Slessinger E, Grigsby PW. Design of an afterloading vaginal applicator (MIRALVA). *Int J Radiat Oncol Biol Phys* 1990;18(6):1503–1508.

280. Slessinger ED, et al. Dosimetry and dose specification for a new gynecological brachytherapy applicator. *Int J Radiat Oncol Biol Phys* 1992;22(5): 1117–1124.

281. Bertoni F, Bertoni G, Bignardi M. Vaginal molds for intracavitary curietherapy: a new method of preparation. *Int J Radiat Oncol Biol Phys* 1983;9(10):1579–1582.

282. Nag S, et al. The American Brachytherapy Society recommendations for high-dose-rate brachytherapy for carcinoma of the cervix. *Int J Radiat Oncol Biol Phys* 2000;48(1):201–211.

283. Orton CG. High-dose-rate brachytherapy may be radiobiologically superior to low-dose rate due to slow repair of late-responding normal tissue cells. *Int J Radiat Oncol Biol Phys* 2001;49(1):183–189.

284. Stewart AJ, Viswanathan AC. Current controversies in high-dose-rate versus low-dose-rate brachytherapy for cervical cancer. *Cancer* 2006;107: 908–915.

285. Kucera H, et al. Radiotherapy alone for invasive vaginal cancer: outcome with intracavitary high dose rate brachytherapy versus conventional low dose rate brachytherapy. *Acta Obstet Gynecol Scand* 2001;80(4):355–360.

286. Nanavati PJ, et al. High-dose-rate brachytherapy in primary stage I and II vaginal cancer. *Gynecol Oncol* 1993;51(1):67–71.

287. Martinez A, Cox RS, Edmundson GK. A multiple-site perineal applicator (MUPIT) for treatment of prostatic, anorectal, and gynecologic malignancies. *Int J Radiat Oncol Biol Phys* 1984;10(2):297–305.

288. Stock RG, et al. A new technique for performing Syed-Neblett template interstitial implants for gynecologic malignancies using transrectal-ultrasound guidance. *Int J Radiat Oncol Biol Phys* 1997;37(4):819–825.

289. Orr JW Jr, et al. Surgically (laparotomy/laparoscopy) guided placement of high dose rate interstitial irradiation catheters (LG-HDRT): technique and outcome. *Gynecol Oncol* 2006;100(1):145–148.

290. Paley PJ, et al. A new technique for performing Syed template interstitial implants for anterior vaginal tumors using an open retropubic approach. *Gynecol Oncol* 1999;73(1):121–125.

291. Disaia PJ, Creasman WT. *Clinical gynecologic oncology.* 4th ed. St. Louis, MO: Mosby, 1993.

292. Randall ME, et al. Interstitial reirradiation for recurrent gynecologic malignancies: results and analysis of prognostic factors. *Gynecol Oncol* 1993;48(1): 23–31.

293. Viswanathan AN, Erickson BA. Three-dimensional imaging in gynecologic brachytherapy: a survey of the American Brachytherapy Society. *Int J Radiat Oncol Biol Phys* 2010;76(1):104–109.

294. Viswanathan AN, et al. Magnetic resonance-guided interstitial therapy for vaginal recurrence of endometrial cancer. *Int J Radiat Oncol Biol Phys* 2006;66(1):91–99.

295. Viswanathan AN, et al. Computed tomography versus magnetic resonance imaging-based contouring in cervical cancer brachytherapy: results of a prospective trial and preliminary guidelines for standardized contours. *Int J Radiat Oncol Biol Phys* 2007;68(2):491–498.

296. Holloway CL, et al. Sigmoid dose using 3D imaging in cervical-cancer brachytherapy. *Radiother Oncol* 2009;93(2):307–310.

297. Subak LL, et al. Cervical carcinoma: computed tomography and magnetic resonance imaging for preoperative staging. *Obstet Gynecol* 1995;86(1):43–50.

298. Potter R, et al. Recommendations from gynaecological (GYN) GEC ESTRO working group (II): concepts and terms in 3D image-based treatment planning in cervix cancer brachytherapy-3D dose volume parameters and aspects of 3D image-based anatomy, radiation physics, radiobiology. *Radiother Oncol* 2006;78(1):67–77.

299. Kirisits C, et al. Dose and volume parameters for MRI-based treatment planning in intracavitary brachytherapy for cervical cancer. *Int J Radiat Oncol Biol Phys* 2005;62(3):901–911.

300. Dimopoulos JC, et al. Treatment of locally advanced vaginal cancer with radiochemotherapy and magnetic resonance image-guided adaptive brachytherapy: dose-volume parameters and first clinical results. *Int J Radiat Oncol Biol Phys* 2012;82(5):1880–1888.

301. Kushner DM, et al. High dose rate (192)Ir afterloading brachytherapy for cancer of the vagina. *Br J Radiol* 2003;76(910):719–725.

302. Tewari K, et al. Interstitial brachytherapy for vaginal recurrences of endometrial carcinoma. *Gynecol Oncol* 1999;74(3):416–422.

303. Chan P, et al. Dosimetric comparison of intensity-modulated, conformal, and four-field pelvic radiotherapy boost plans for gynecologic cancer: a retrospective planning study. *Radiat Oncol* 2006;1:13.

304. Georg D, et al. Image-guided radiotherapy for cervix cancer: high-tech external beam therapy versus high-tech brachytherapy. *Int J Radiat Oncol Biol Phys* 2008;71(4):1272–1278.

305. Barraclough LH, et al. External beam boost for cancer of the cervix uteri when intracavitary therapy cannot be performed. *Int J Radiat Oncol Biol Phys* 2008;71(3):772–778.

306. Higginson DS, et al. Stereotactic body radiotherapy (SBRT): technological innovation and application in gynecologic oncology. *Gynecol Oncol* 2011;120(3):404–412.

307. Shrieve DC, Loeffler JS, eds. *Human radiation injury.* 1st ed. Philadelphia: Lippincott Williams & Wilkins, 2011.

308. Eifel PJ, et al. Time course and incidence of late complications in patients treated with radiation therapy for FIGO stage IB carcinoma of the uterine cervix. *Int J Radiat Oncol Biol Phys* 1995;32(5):1289–1300.

309. Gupta S, Gupta YN, Sanyal B. Radiation changes in vaginal and cervical cytology in carcinoma of the cervix uteri. *J Surg Oncol* 1982;19(2):71–73.

310. Pitkin RM, Buchsbaum HJ, Lenz H. Estrogen and the irradiated vagina. *Obstet Gynecol* 1975;46(2):243–245.

311. Fink D, et al. Hyperbaric oxygen therapy for delayed radiation injuries in gynecological cancers. *Int J Gynecol Cancer* 2006;16(2):638–642.

312. Piekarski JH, et al. Does fecal diversion offer any chance for spontaneous closure of the radiation-induced rectovaginal fistula? *Int J Gynecol Cancer* 2008;18(1):66–70.

313. Manetta A, et al. Primary invasive carcinoma of the vagina. *Obstet Gynecol* 1988;72(1):77–81.

314. Mawson AR. The place of hysterectomy in the management of benign uterine disease. *HMO Pract* 1996;10(2):69–74.

315. Xiang EW, et al. Treatment of late recurrent vaginal malignancy after initial radiotherapy for carcinoma of the cervix: an analysis of 73 cases. *Gynecol Oncol* 1998;69(2):125–129.

316. Steiner E, et al. Carcinoma of the neovagina: case report and review of the literature. *Gynecol Oncol* 2002;84(1):171–175.

317. Lathrop JC, Ree HJ, McDuff HC Jr. Intraepithelial neoplasia of the neovagina. *Obstet Gynecol* 1985;65(3, Suppl):91S–94S.

318. Gallup DG, Castle CA, Stock RJ. Recurrent carcinoma in situ of the vagina following split-thickness skin graft vaginoplasty. *Gynecol Oncol* 1987;26(1):98–102.

319. Imrie JE, et al. Intraepithelial neoplasia arising in an artificial vagina. Case report. *Br J Obstet Gynaecol* 1986;93(8):886–888.

320. Wheelock JB, Schneider V, Goplerud DR. Malignancy arising in the transplanted vagina. *South Med J* 1986;79(12):1585–1587.

321. Lowe MP, Ault KA, Sood AK. Recurrent carcinoma in situ of a neovagina. *Gynecol Oncol* 2001;80(3):403–404.

322. Guven S, et al. Recurrence of high-grade squamous intraepithelial neoplasia in neovagina: case report and review of the literature. *Int J Gynecol Cancer* 2005;15(6):1179–1182.

323. Rotmensch J, et al. Carcinoma arising in the neovagina: case report and review of the literature. *Obstet Gynecol* 1983;61(4):534–536.

324. Munkarah A, et al. Mucinous adenocarcinoma arising in a neovagina. *Gynecol Oncol* 1994;52(2):272–275.

325. Berek JS, et al. Pelvic exenteration for recurrent gynecologic malignancy: survival and morbidity analysis of the 45-year experience at UCLA. *Gynecol Oncol* 2005;99(1):153–159.

326. Russell AH, et al. Radical reirradiation for recurrent or second primary carcinoma of the female reproductive tract. *Gynecol Oncol* 1987;27(2):226–232.

327. Randall ME, Barrett RJ. Interstitial irradiation in the management of recurrent carcinoma of the cervix after previous radiation therapy. *N C Med J* 1988;49(6):306–308.

328. Gupta AK, et al. Iridium-192 transperineal interstitial brachytherapy for locally advanced or recurrent gynecological malignancies. *Int J Radiat Oncol Biol Phys* 1999;43(5):1055–1060.

329. Charra C, et al. Outcome of treatment of upper third vaginal recurrences of cervical and endometrial carcinomas with interstitial brachytherapy. *Int J Radiat Oncol Biol Phys* 1998;40(2):421–426.

330. Salani R, et al. Posttreatment surveillance and diagnosis of recurrence in women with gynecologic malignancies: Society of Gynecologic Oncologists recommendations. *Am J Obstet Gynecol* 2011;204(6):466–478.

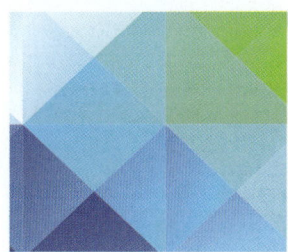

CHAPTER 77

Female Urethra

Tony Y. Eng

INTRODUCTION

Primary urethral carcinoma is a rare tumor, accounting for <1% of all malignancies. Although previous data suggested that urethral cancer was more common in women than men, a recent Surveillance, Epidemiology, and End Results (SEER) study reports that primary urethral cancer is more common in men.[1] The ratio of female to male predominance is approximately 1:3. Because of its rarity and lack of prospective data, optimal management of female urethral cancer is based on retrospective data and depends on the clinical stage, tumor location, extent of nodal involvement, patient's health status, and treatment preference.

ANATOMY

The female urethra is approximately 3 to 4 cm long and 0.6 cm in resting diameter. It is embedded in the anterior vaginal wall behind the pubis symphysis, extending inferiorly and anteriorly from the urinary bladder through the urogenital diaphragm to the vestibule, where it forms the urethral meatus. Because of the proximity of the pubis symphysis, a small curve is formed with an anterior concavity. The lower distal half of the urethra is considered the anterior urethra, and the upper proximal half is considered the posterior urethra. Figure 77.1 illustrates the urethra and adjacent organs in the female pelvis.

The wall of the urethra consists of three layers. The muscular layer is continuous with that of the bladder. At the vesicular end of the urethra, this muscular wall forms the internal sphincter. The voluntary urethral sphincter is at the plane of the urogenital diaphragm. A thin layer of erectile tissue consisting of a plexus of veins and muscle fibers forms the middle layer of the wall. The inner layer is the mucous membrane, which is continuous with the bladder proximally and with the vulva distally. This membrane consists of transitional epithelium near the bladder but distally changes to

FIGURE 77.1. MR T1-weighted sagittal image of the female pelvis.

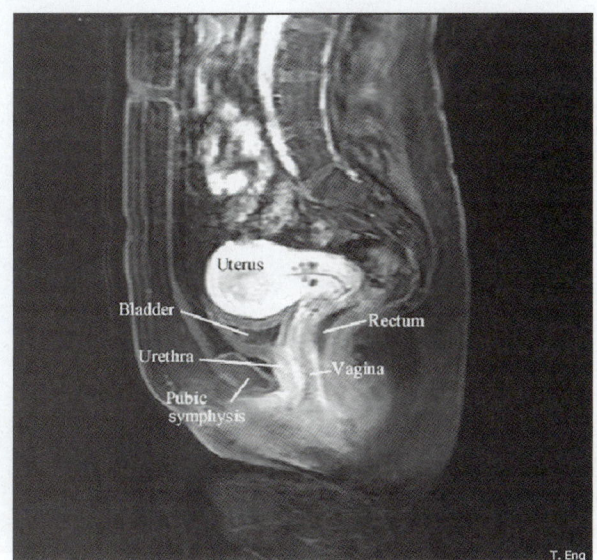

nonkeratinizing stratified squamous epithelium and pseudostratified columnar epithelium. The distal urethra also contains small mucous recesses and periurethral or Skene glands, most of which are in the region of the meatus.

The lymphatic drainage of the distal urethra and urethral meatus parallels that of the vulva to the superficial and deep inguinal and external iliac lymph nodes. The primary drainage of the posterior or entire urethra is mainly to the obturator and internal and external iliac nodes.

EPIDEMIOLOGY AND ETIOLOGY

The SEER database for 1973 to 2002 identified a total of 1,615 cases of primary urethral carcinoma, of which 540 were women.[1] The overall annual incidence was 1.5 per million for women (4.3 per million for men). Although previous observation suggests that this cancer is more common in white women than in black women,[2,3] the SEER data show the incidence to be higher for African Americans and increase steadily with age. As carcinoma of the urethra is rare in women, only a few cases are seen annually at major cancer centers.[4-6] Carcinoma of the female urethra makes up 0.02% of all cancers in women and accounts for approximately 0.1% of all gynecologic cancers.[7,8] The average patient age at the time of diagnosis is 60 years, with most patients between 50 and 80 years of age.[1,2,9-11]

Although chronic infection and local irritation have been proposed, the etiology of female urethral cancer remains obscure. Unlike other transitional cell carcinoma of the urinary tract, there is no reported correlation between cigarette smoking and urethral carcinoma. Wiener and Walther[12] analyzed archival surgical specimens of women with urethral carcinoma. Human papillomavirus (HPV) was detected in 10 of 17 patients with invasive disease. HPV type 16 was found in eight patients. Eight women with squamous cell carcinoma and two with transitional cell carcinoma had HPV. Female urethral cancer may also be associated with urethral diverticula.[13-15] Figure 77.2 illustrates a carcinoma arising within a urethral diverticulum. Patients with transitional cell carcinoma of the bladder, especially the bladder neck, may have a higher risk of developing urethral cancer either synchronously or metachronously.[16,17]

NATURAL HISTORY

Most urethral cancers are clinically aggressive and historically carry a poor prognosis. During the later stages, cancers of the middle or posterior urethra tend to extend upward into the urinary bladder, downward to invade the remainder of the urethra, and posteriorly into the vaginal mucosa. Lesions involving the anterior urethra account for approximately 30% of all cases.[9,18]

Regional lymph node involvement is uncommon in early tumors (stage 0) of the urethral meatus. Advanced tumors (stages II and III) of the urethra have been associated with a 35% to 50% incidence of inguinal or pelvic lymph node involvement.[6,10,19-21] Bilateral nodal involvement occurs in approximately one-third of patients with positive nodes. Grabstald[9] confirmed nodal involvement in 24 of 25 patients with clinically palpable nodes. In his series of patients with

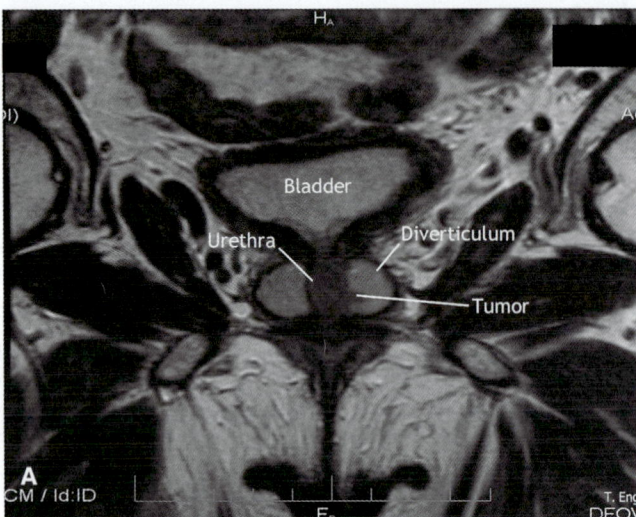
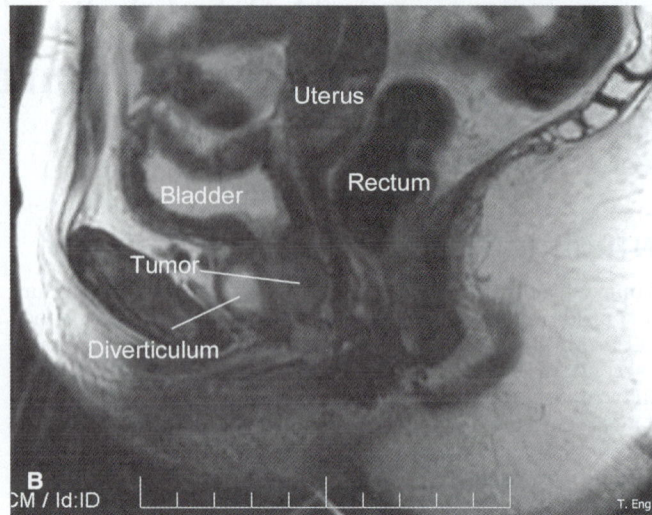

FIGURE 77.2. Coronal **(A)** and sagittal **(B)** T2-weighted MR images demonstrate a large diverticulum surrounding the urethra with a tumor mass arising within the confines of the diverticulum posteriorly that results in an impression at the vagina.

advanced disease, 26 underwent pelvic lymph node sampling and 13 (50%) had nodal involvement.

Distant metastases are found in approximately 10% of patients at presentation, and approximately 30% to 50% ultimately die of distant disease. The most common sites of metastasis are lung, liver, bone, and brain.[9,22]

CLINICAL PRESENTATION

A majority of patients with urethral cancer present with some degree of irritative or obstructive urethral symptoms.[23] Bleeding (hematuria) or spotting is the prevailing presenting sign in 50% to 60% of patients.[2,24,25] Approximately 30% to 50% of patients experience pain or irritative symptoms, difficulty urinating, and frequent micturition. Urinary retention and overflow incontinence may occur in advanced cases. Less frequently cited signs and symptoms are a mass in the introitus (10% to 20% of patients), dyspareunia, perineal pain, and inguinal lymphadenopathy.[20,22] Urethrovaginal and vesicovaginal fistulas may develop in advanced, neglected cases.

Small tumors involving the urethral meatus are often mistakenly diagnosed as urethral caruncle; a benign, inflammatory lesion; or a prolapse of the mucosa through the urethral orifice. As the lesion progresses, it enlarges and eventually ulcerates.[22] Tumors may arise in a urethral diverticulum.[15,26,27] Larger lesions of the distal urethra are readily identified on inspection (Fig. 77.3). Tumors occupying the proximal urethra may produce a fusiform enlargement that can be palpated during pelvic examination.

DIAGNOSTIC WORKUP

An outline for the diagnostic workup for carcinoma of the female urethra is presented in Table 77.1. A routine history and general physical examination should be performed for all patients. A detailed pelvic examination under anesthesia is necessary to fully evaluate the clinical extent of the disease. This examination can be performed at the time of urethroscopy and cystoscopy. Urine cytologic analyses have a high false-negative rate.[28] The definitive diagnosis is made by punch or incisional biopsy.

Routine radiographic evaluation should include chest radiographs, an intravenous urogram, and a computed tomography (CT) scan of the abdomen and pelvis[29,30] (Fig. 77.4).

Barium enema can be cost-effective for patients with symptoms of advanced disease. Magnetic resonance imaging (MRI) of the pelvis helps delineate the tumor extent, especially when an endourethral coil is used (Fig. 77.2). It provides a discrete view of the muscular layers of the urethra.[31,32] Additional complementary studies include interactive virtual urethrography and ultrasonography that can help detect a urethral diverticulum without contrast agent filling.[33] Multidetector CT voiding urethrography yields real-time urethral images during micturition.

Currently, there are no studies addressing the role of PET-FDG (positron emission tomography with fluorodeoxyglucose) scan in urethral cancer. Perhaps, some genitourinary tumors do not accumulate sufficient FDG, which may not be a useful tracer for the detection of primary genitourinary tumors because of its physiologic excretion in the urine.[34] However, PET scans may potentially be useful for identifying nodal and distant sites of disease, especially in patients with equivocal findings on conventional imaging.[35–37]

FIGURE 77.3. A meatal carcinoma of the urethra in a 68-year-old white woman presenting with hematuria.

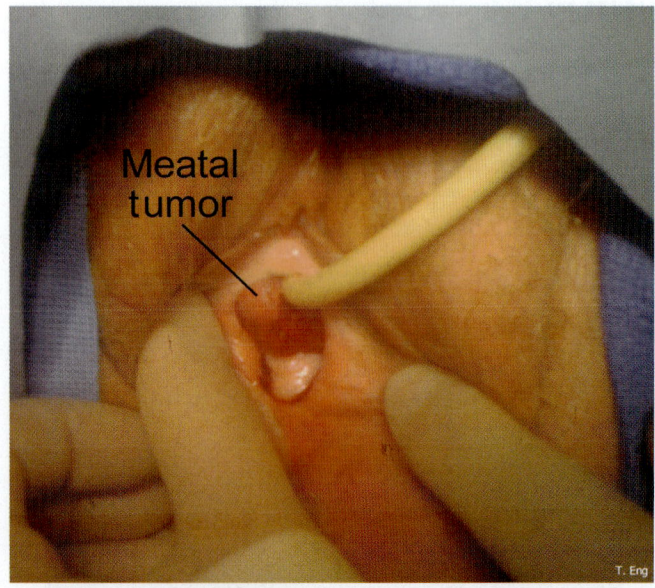

TABLE 77.1 DIAGNOSTIC WORKUP FOR CARCINOMA OF THE FEMALE URETHRA

General
History
Physical examination, including detailed pelvic examination under anesthesia
Special procedures
  Punch biopsy
  Urethroscopy
  Cystoscopy
  Rectosigmoidoscopy (advanced stages or if symptomatic)
Radiographic evaluation
  Standard
  Chest radiographs
  Intravenous urography
  CT scan (abdomen and pelvis)
  Magnetic resonance imaging
  Complementary
  Bone scan (if symptomatic or elevated alkaline phosphatase)
  Barium enema (if symptomatic or advanced stages)
  Ultrasound
  Urethrography
Laboratory evaluation
  Complete blood count
  Chemistry profile
  Urinalysis

TABLE 77.2 PROPOSED CLINICAL STAGING SYSTEM FOR CARCINOMA OF THE FEMALE URETHRA

Tumor Stage	Characteristics
I	Disease limited to distal one-half of urethra
II	Disease involving entire urethra, with extension to periurethral tissues, but not involving vulva or bladder neck
III	
A	Disease involving urethra and vulva
B	Disease invading vaginal mucosa
C	Disease involving urethra and bladder neck
IV	
A	Disease invading parametrium or paracolpium
B	Metastasis
B1	Inguinal lymph nodes
B2	Pelvic lymph nodes
B3	Para-aortic nodes
B4	Distant metastasis

From Prempree T, Amornmarn R, Patanaphan V. Radiation therapy in primary carcinoma of the female urethra: II. An update on results. *Cancer* 1984;54(4):729–733. Copyright © 1984 American Cancer Society. Reprinted by permission of John Wiley & Sons, Inc..

STAGING SYSTEMS

Clinical staging is based on findings on physical examination, chest x-ray, and CT scan of the abdomen and pelvis. Many attempts have been made to formulate a staging system for carcinoma of the urethra. Urethral tumors can be classified in two groups: those involving the distal half of the urethra and those located in the proximal or entire urethra. Most authors have found that this classification correctly depicts the feasibility of treatment and the prognosis. A staging system based on location has been proposed by Prempree et al.[38] (Table 77.2). The current TNM staging system of the American Joint Committee on Cancer[39] is shown in Table 77.3.

PATHOLOGIC CLASSIFICATION

As the urethra is lined by transitional cells proximally and stratified squamous cells distally, transitional cell carcinoma occurs typically in the proximal urethra, whereas squamous cell carcinoma occurs frequently in the distal urethra. The SEER data report the most common histologic type is transitional cell carcinoma followed by squamous cell and adenocarcinoma.[1] However, most published series suggest

that squamous cell carcinoma is the most common histologic type in cancer of the female urethra, representing more than 50% of all cases whereas transitional cell carcinoma and adenocarcinoma represent approximately 15% to 20% and 10% to 15%, respectively.[14,40,41] The remainder of the histologic types include adenoid cystic carcinoma, melanoma, clear cell adenocarcinoma, anaplastic tumors, Kaposi sarcoma, lymphomas, and metastatic lesions.[5,35,42–45]

PROGNOSTIC FACTORS

Conventional prognostic factors such as grade and histology have not been consistently predictive for recurrence or survival for female urethral cancer. In the literature, some of the most important factors in determining prognosis and survival are stage, depth of invasion, tumor size, and anatomic location.[2,14,20,28,46,47] The 1983 to 2008 SEER database shows that advance age, T stage, node positivity, nonsquamous histology, and black race were associated with reduced cause-specific survival.[48] Dalbagni et al.[2] showed that primary stage was one of the major independent predictors of survival in 72 female

TABLE 77.3 TNM CLASSIFICATION OF CARCINOMA OF THE URETHRA (MALE OR FEMALE)

Primary Tumor (T)

TX	Primary tumor cannot be assessed
T0	No evidence of primary tumor
Ta	Noninvasive papillary carcinoma
Tis	Carcinoma *in situ*
T1	Tumor invades subepithelial connective tissue
T2	Tumor invades any of the following: corpus spongiosum, periurethral muscle
T3	Tumor invades any of the following: corpus cavernosum, anterior vagina
T4	Tumor invades other adjacent organs (e.g., invasion of the bladder wall)

Regional Lymph Nodes (N)

NX	Regional lymph nodes cannot be assessed
N0	No regional lymph node metastasis
N1	Single lymph node metastasis in the inguinal region or true pelvis [perivesical, obturator, internal (hypogastric) and external iliac], or presacral lymph node
N2	Multiple regional lymph node metastasis in the inguinal region or true pelvis [perivesical, obturator, internal (hypogastric) and external iliac], or presacral lymph node

Distant Metastasis (M)

M0	No distant metastasis
M1	Distant metastasis

From Amin MB, Edge SB, Greene FL, et al., eds. *AJCC cancer staging manual.* 8th ed. New York: Springer, 2017. Reproduced with permission of Springer International Publishing in the format Book via Copyright Clearance Center.

FIGURE 77.4. Transaxial CT image of a patient with urethral cancer illustrating the periurethral and anterior vaginal wall expansion and deviation of the urethra (*arrow*).

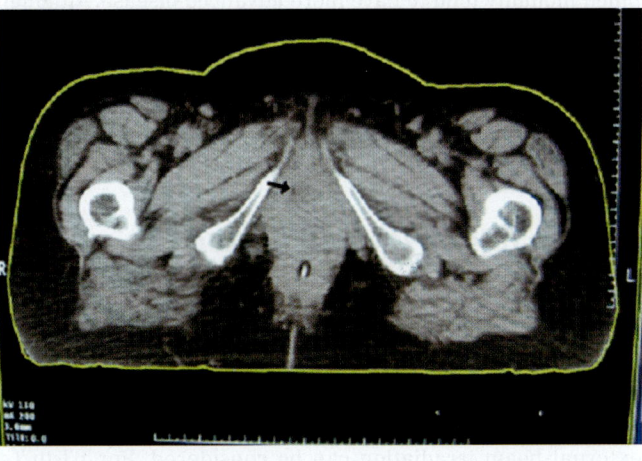

patients with a 5-year survival of 83% for low-stage tumors and 33% for high-stage tumors.

Lesions located in the meatus or distal urethra tend to be superficial, with a better prognosis; lesions in the posterior urethra are often deeply invasive and tend to have a worse prognosis.[8] Most investigators found that patients with advanced-stage disease do poorly, often irrespective of their treatment.[2,23,47,49]

Grigsby and associates[24,50] demonstrated a worsening prognosis with increased tumor size. The 5-year progression-free survival was 81% for patients with lesions <2 cm, compared with 37% for those with lesions 2 to 4 cm and 7% for patients with lesions >4 cm (P = .0001). For lesions confined to the proximal urethra, local control was observed in all four patients. However, patients with tumors involving the distal urethra had a 5-year progression–survival rate of 69%, and there was a 12% survival rate for those with involvement of the entire free urethra (P = .0001). Patients with meatal tumors, if diagnosed early and treated appropriately, can achieve an 80% to 90% survival rate (Figs. 77.5 and 77.6).[24] Bladder neck involvement, parametrial extension, and inguinal lymph node involvement have been identified as poor prognostic factors.

Several investigators found that the use of brachytherapy improves local control. Milosevic et al.[51] reported that patients who were treated with external beam therapy only were 4.2 times more likely to recur locally independent of other prognostic factors, compared with those who received brachytherapy as a component of management. Similarly, in a study of six patients with locally advanced urethral carcinoma, Dalbagni et al.[52] noted that high-dose intraoperative brachytherapy followed by external beam radiation appeared to improve local control.

The histology of the primary lesion appears to be less important as a prognostic factor in determining response to therapy and survival. Patients with adenocarcinoma have been reported to have a good prognosis, but most studies have shown no difference in survival among patients with adenocarcinoma, squamous cell carcinoma, and transitional cell carcinoma.[9,13,38,46] Grigsby[24] found a worse prognosis in patients with adenocarcinoma. Primary melanoma of the urethra, although rare, has a very poor prognosis.[53–55]

GENERAL MANAGEMENT

Although various therapeutic approaches have been advocated for the management of carcinoma of the female urethra, there are no established therapeutic guidelines. The variety of treatments reflects the dimensions and locations

FIGURE 77.5. Progression-free survival correlated with tumor size. (From Grigsby PW, Herr HW. Urethral tumors. In: Vogelzang J, Scardino PT, Shipley WU, et al., eds. *Comprehensive textbook of genitourinary oncology.* Baltimore, MD: Williams & Wilkins, 1996:1117–1123. With permission.)

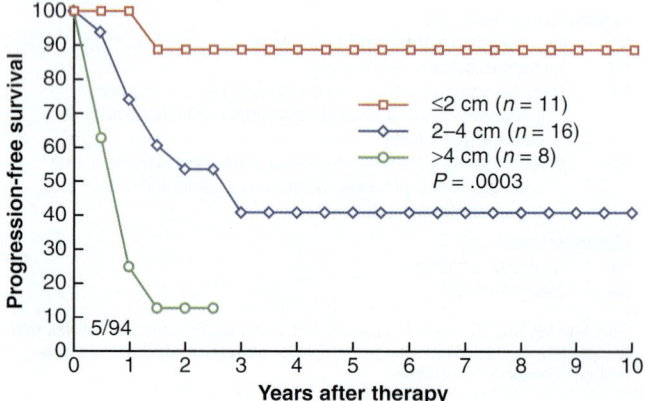

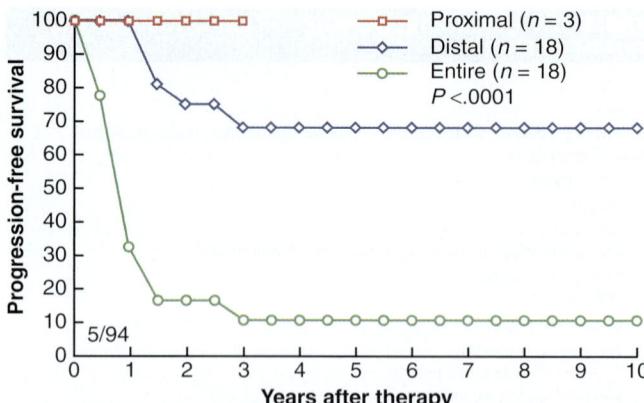

FIGURE 77.6. Progression-free survival correlated with tumor location. (From Grigsby PW, Herr HW. Urethral tumors. In: Vogelzang J, Scardino PT, Shipley WU, et al., eds. *Comprehensive textbook of genitourinary oncology.* Baltimore, MD: Williams & Wilkins, 1996:1117–1123. With permission.)

of disease and the approaches of the treating physicians.[3] In general, surgical resection is a primary mode of treatment.[56] Radical urethral resection with urinary diversion and pelvic lymphadenectomy is commonly performed for lesions not involving the bladder neck. However, early-stage lesions of limited extent may be amenable to organ-sparing radiation therapy or conservative surgical management with or without adjuvant radiation therapy to minimize the morbidity associated with surgical intervention. Surgical approaches include neodymium:yttrium–aluminum–garnet (Nd:YAG) laser coagulation,[57] Mohs micrographic surgery, and partial or total urethrectomy.[41] Radiation therapy may include external-beam radiation, interstitial brachytherapy, or a combination of these treatments.[58] For patients who are medically nonsurgical candidates because of potential risks of anesthesia, outpatient high–dose rate (HDR) intracavitary and intraluminal brachytherapy may be an option.[52,59]

Multimodality Therapy

For patients with locally invasive urethral carcinoma, anterior exenteration may be required. Although most available data are insufficient, in patients with more advanced disease, some authors have advocated adjuvant radiation therapy and/or combined irradiation and chemotherapy including 5-fluorouracil, cisplatin, vinblastine, epirubicin, carboplatin, bleomycin, methotrexate, or mitomycin C after surgical extirpation.[56,60–63] A subgroup of patients with positive nodes may also benefit from preoperative cisplatin-based chemotherapy.[64]

Multimodality therapy appears to achieve similar or better overall results, even though those patients who receive combined modality tend to have more advanced disease. Although most studies included a small number of patients, those patients who received combined therapy seem to have better disease-free survival.[14,47,49] Combination therapy often consists of either chemotherapy with radiotherapy or radiotherapy with surgery. Combined chemotherapy and radiation therapy for locally advanced urethral cancer has shown a reasonable response in several reports.[47,49,60,62,65]

Anterior (Distal) Urethral Cancer

For stage 0 and I (Ta, Tis, or small T1) lesions, open excision, electroexcision, fulguration, and laser (Nd:YAG or CO₂) coagulation are possible for tumors at the meatus or with *in situ* involvement of the distal urethra (stage 0). For larger and more invasive lesions (stage T1 and T2), surgical resection of the distal third of the urethra is often adequate. Alternately, interstitial irradiation or a combination of interstitial and external-beam irradiation can be considered. For T3 to T4 or recurrent anterior urethral lesions previously treated by local excision or radiation therapy, anterior exenteration and urinary diversion may be curative. Adjuvant radiation therapy may be required, depending on surgical findings.

If a limited number of inguinal nodes are involved, ipsilateral node dissection or irradiation is indicated because cure is still achievable. If no inguinal adenopathy exists, node dissection is not recommended, but prophylactic groin irradiation is recommended for patients with invasive lesions.[5,46]

Posterior (Proximal) Urethral Cancer

Cancers of the posterior or entire urethra are usually associated with invasion of the bladder, a high incidence of inguinal and pelvic lymph node metastases, and a worse prognosis. For lesions <2 cm, radical resection, definitive radiation therapy, or combined treatment may provide adequate control.[50] However, for larger lesions or locally advanced disease, the best results have been achieved with preoperative irradiation, exenterative surgery, and urinary diversion. Pelvic lymphadenectomy is performed and inguinal node dissection may be indicated if the inguinal nodes are involved. In selected patients, it is possible to remove part of the pubis symphysis and the inferior pubic rami to maximize the surgical margin. A transpubic approach has been advocated by Golimbu et al.[66] Perineal closure and vaginal reconstruction can be accomplished with the use of myocutaneous flaps. Hedden et al.[67] have advocated the use of bladder-sparing surgery with or without irradiation.

Recurrent Urethral Cancer

In most cases, locally recurrent urethral cancer after surgery alone should be considered for combination radiation therapy and wider surgical resection. Locally recurrent urethral cancer after radiation therapy should be treated by surgical excision. For those who are not surgical candidates, local reirradiation (i.e., hyperfractionated intensity-modulated radiation therapy or brachytherapy) may be considered if radiation tolerance has not been exceeded. Patients with metastatic urethral cancer should be considered for investigational chemotherapy protocols. Palliative radiation therapy may provide good symptomatic relief.

RADIATION THERAPY TECHNIQUES

Small meatal and distal urethral lesions are curable with limited therapy. Interstitial implants have been the usual method for treating meatal carcinomas. Radioactive needles, forming a double-plane or a volume implant, have been used (Fig. 77.7). Both low–dose rate (LDR) and HDR afterloading implants using ^{192}Ir have replaced radium.[7,52,59] For early localized disease without involvement of adjacent organs, a volume implant composed of 8 to 12 needles arranged in an arc around the urethral orifice is used (Fig. 77.8). Radiographs may be used to verify needle placement (Fig. 77.9). Computer planning with CT-based simulation and 3-D treatment planning should be the standard of care to spare the adjacent normal organs. A dose of 60 to 70 Gy (LDR) should be given in 6 to 7 days (0.4 to 0.5 Gy/h to the target volume) when an implant alone is used.

Alternatively, in patients with small localized disease receiving radiation therapy alone, noninvasive intracavitary or intraluminal HDR brachytherapy without sedation or anesthesia after pelvic external beam radiation has been used.[47,59] Figure 77.10 illustrates an intraluminal HDR brachytherapy using a Foley catheter. The resultant conformal radiation dose covers the periurethral tissue well while sparing the surrounding normal structures. At the University of Texas Health Science Center in San Antonio, we deliver 500 to 600 cGy at twice a week, 3 days apart, to a total dose of 2,400 to 2,500 cGy with good response.

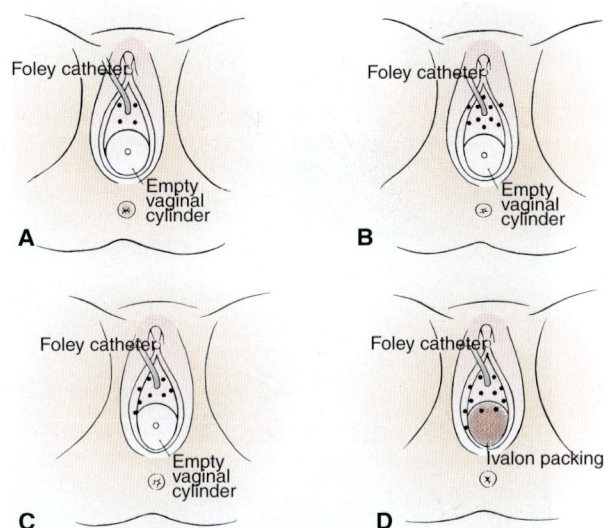

FIGURE 77.7. Diagrams of implants. **A:** Tumor limited to the urethra. **B:** Tumor extending to the periurethral tissues or originating in the periurethral glands. **C:** Tumor extending into the vagina or labia minora. **D:** Tumor involving the suburethral area. (Reprinted from Delclos L. Carcinoma of the female urethra. In: Johnson DE, Boileau MA, eds. *Genitourinary tumors: fundamental principles and surgical techniques.* New York: Grune & Stratton, 1982:275–286. Copyright © 1982 Elsevier. With permission.)

Large tumors or advanced disease extending into the labia, vagina, entire urethra, or base of the bladder should not be treated with an implant alone. For these patients, a combination of external-beam irradiation and implant is recommended.[51,59,68] The external-beam portal should flash the perineum to cover the entire urethra. The conventional portal should be wide enough to cover the inguinal nodes and should extend cephalad to the L5-S1 interspace to include the pelvic nodes (Fig. 77.11).[69] A bolus, appropriate for the photon energy used, should be added to the groin when inguinal nodes are positive. This technique minimizes the hazard of groin failure due to underdosing of gross tumor. Hahn et al.[70] have demonstrated the importance of treating the inguinal lymph nodes in all patients. The whole pelvis is treated to a dose of 45 to 50 Gy. A boost of 10 to 15 Gy is delivered to positive groin nodes through reduced anteroposterior fields.

After pelvic radiation therapy, the primary tumor can be treated with a vaginal cylinder to bring the dose to the entire urethra to approximately 60 Gy. An interstitial implant is administered to raise the total tumor dose to 70 to 80 Gy. For

FIGURE 77.8. A template used for a curved, double-plane implant that surrounds the urethra. The closed-end flexible catheters inserted in the periurethral or vaginal tissues are glued to the template, which is sutured to the skin. The catheters are afterloaded with [192]Ir.

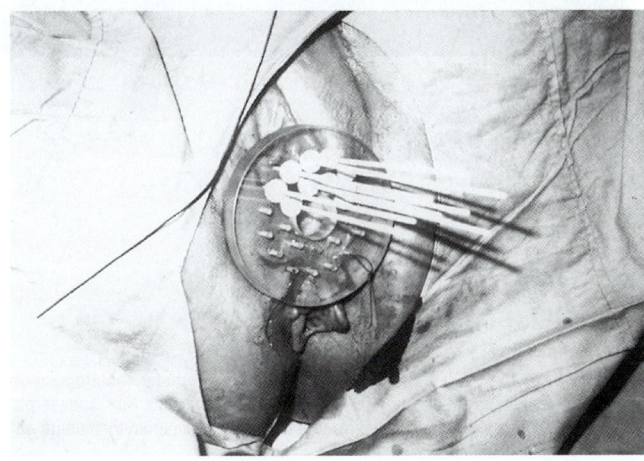

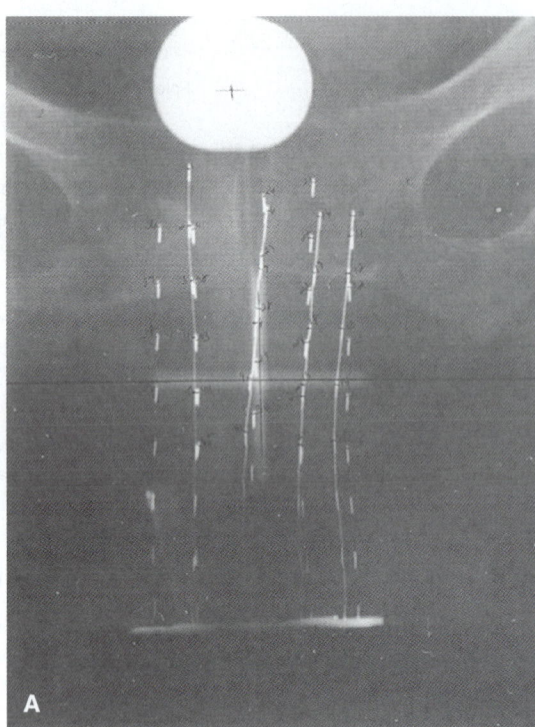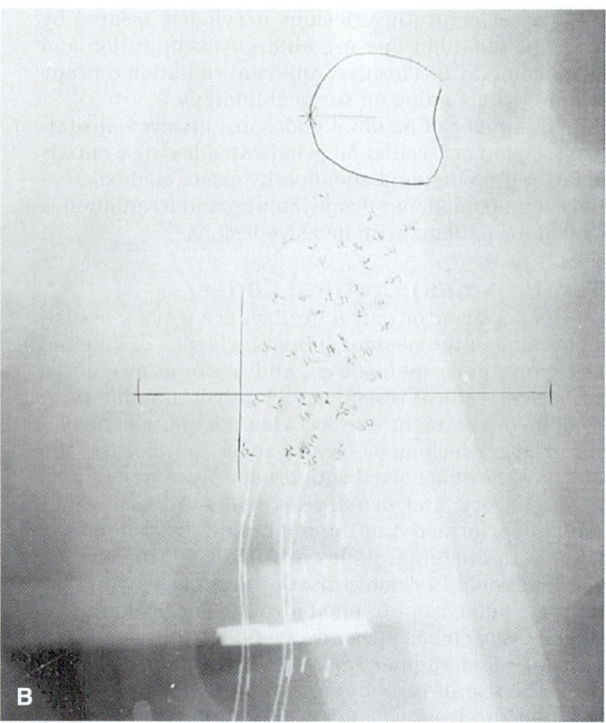

FIGURE 77.9. Anteroposterior **(A)** and lateral **(B)** simulation radiographs with dummy seeds in place. Contrast material is used to inflate the balloon of the urinary catheter, which is used to localize the bladder.

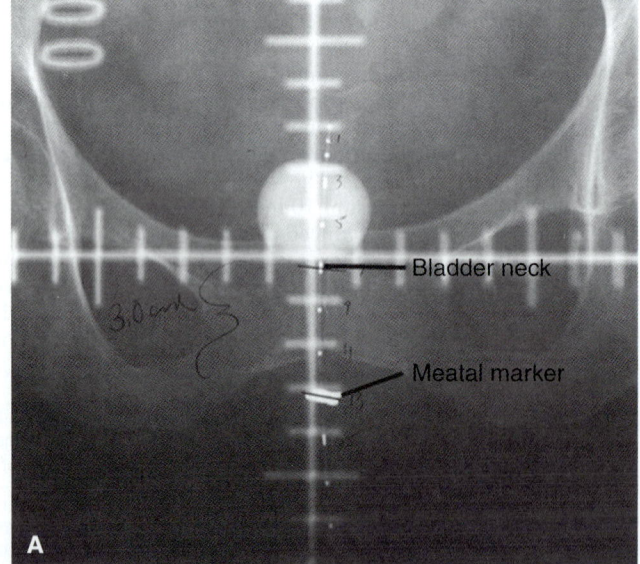

Bladder neck

Meatal marker

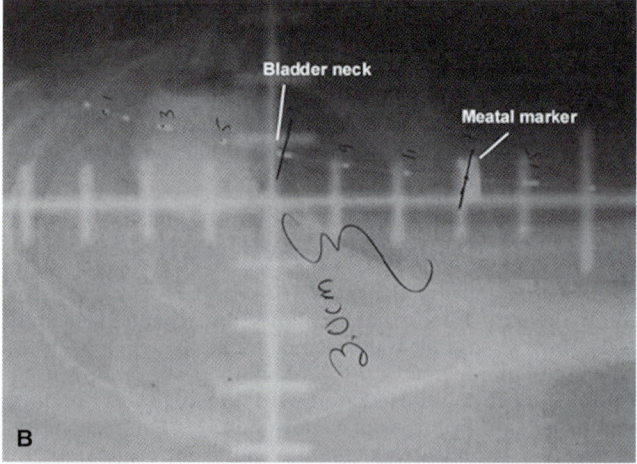

Bladder neck

Meatal marker

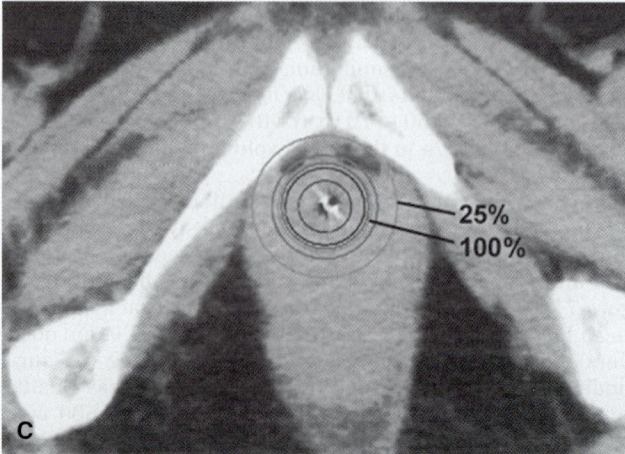

25%
100%

FIGURE 77.10. HDR brachytherapy with a Foley catheter. Anteroposterior **(A)** and lateral simulation films **(B)**, and transaxial CT image with isodose plan **(C)**. The resultant uniformed, steep isodose lines cover the periurethral tissue well.

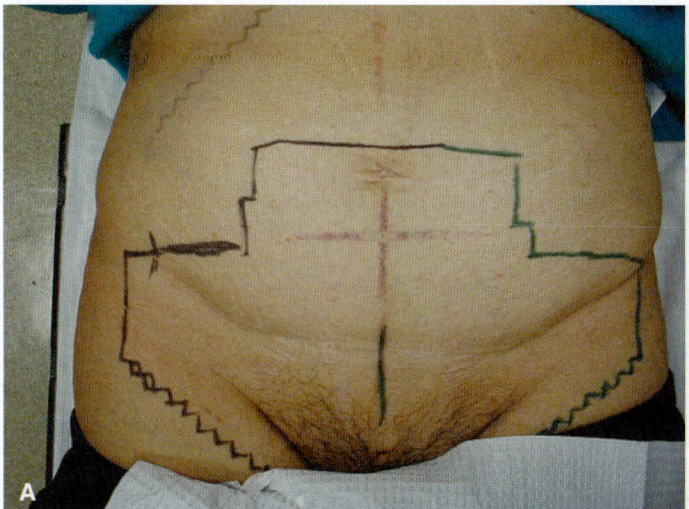
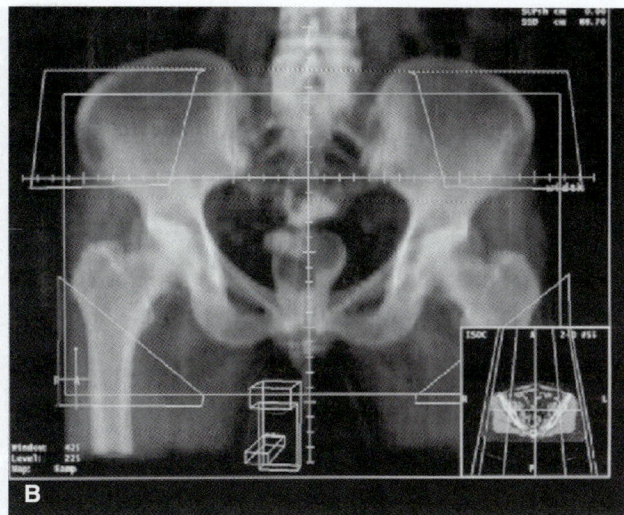
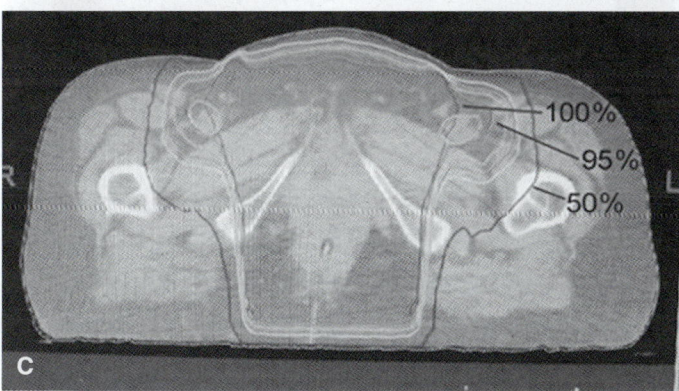

FIGURE 77.11. Whole pelvis and inguinal field. External skin marking **(A)** and anteroposterior simulation film **(B)** of a pelvic portal showing the lateral extension to cover the inguinal lymph nodes, and the isodose plan **(C)**.

patients undergoing postoperative therapy, the tumor bed is treated after pelvic radiation therapy with an additional 10 to 15 Gy using interstitial brachytherapy.[52] Intracavitary irradiation with the vaginal cylinder and an interstitial implant are almost never used simultaneously because of the resultant high dose rate at the vaginal mucosa interface of the intracavitary and interstitial implant fields. A vaginal cylinder with partial shielding posteriorly can be used in select patients. Gerbaulet et al.[71] have demonstrated the use of a catheter or a vaginal mold applicator for intraluminal/intracavitary brachytherapy and needles or guide gutters for interstitial brachytherapy.

At the University of Texas Health Science Center in San Antonio, we commonly deliver external beam therapy, 4,500 to 5,040 cGy, to the primary tumor and pelvic lymphatics using intensity-modulated radiation therapy technique (IMRT) with CT image guidance (Fig. 77.12). This is followed by interstitial HDR brachytherapy, 500 to 600 cGy twice a day, 6 hours apart. A vaginal cylinder is always employed to provide spatial protection of the posterior vagina and rectum. The HDR brachytherapy is repeated in one week to achieve a total dose of 2,000 to 2,400 cGy (Fig. 77.13). The major advantage of interstitial HDR brachytherapy is geometric or volume optimization by changing the dwell time and dwell position of the radioactive source along the afterloading catheter so that the target volume is well covered with good conformity while the doses to the vaginal mucosa and surround structures are kept below their tolerances. Modification of dose and fractionation may be made depending on the tumor size and response to external beam therapy. The HDR brachytherapy is performed as an outpatient treatment.

One of the limiting factors in the use of external-beam irradiation is the tolerance of the perineal and vulva skin (i.e.,

confluent moist desquamation). Extensive disease combined with advanced age can be a formidable obstacle to completing the irradiation course. Proper radiation therapy techniques and diligent personal hygiene and individualized skin care during and after treatment are necessary if patients are to complete the course of treatment.

RESULTS OF THERAPY

The SEER 1983 to 2008 database identified 722 women with urethral cancer.[48] The median overall survival was 42 months, and the 5- and 10- year overall survival was 43% and 32% respectively. The median cause-specific survival was 78 months, and the 5- and 10-year cause-specific survival was 53% and 46%, respectively. Table 77.4 summarizes the recent treatment results from various institutions. Depending on the various prognostic and treatment factors, the 5-year overall survival and cause-specific survival rates range from 32% to 59% and 40% to 61%, respectively. The recurrence rates range from 58% to 64%.

Surgery

There is a paucity of long-term outcome data. In general, female urethral cancers are clinically aggressive with high recurrence and poor survival rates.[2,9,14,21,49] DiMarco et al.[23] reviewed 53 female patients with primary urethral carcinoma undergoing partial urethrectomy or radical extirpation. The estimated 10-year cancer-specific survival was 60%. In a study of 72 patients treated at Memorial Sloan Kettering Cancer Center between 1925 and 1994, the 5-year disease-specific survival was 89% for low-stage tumors and 33% for high-stage tumors.[2] The overall survival was 78% and 22%, respectively, as shown in Table 77.4.

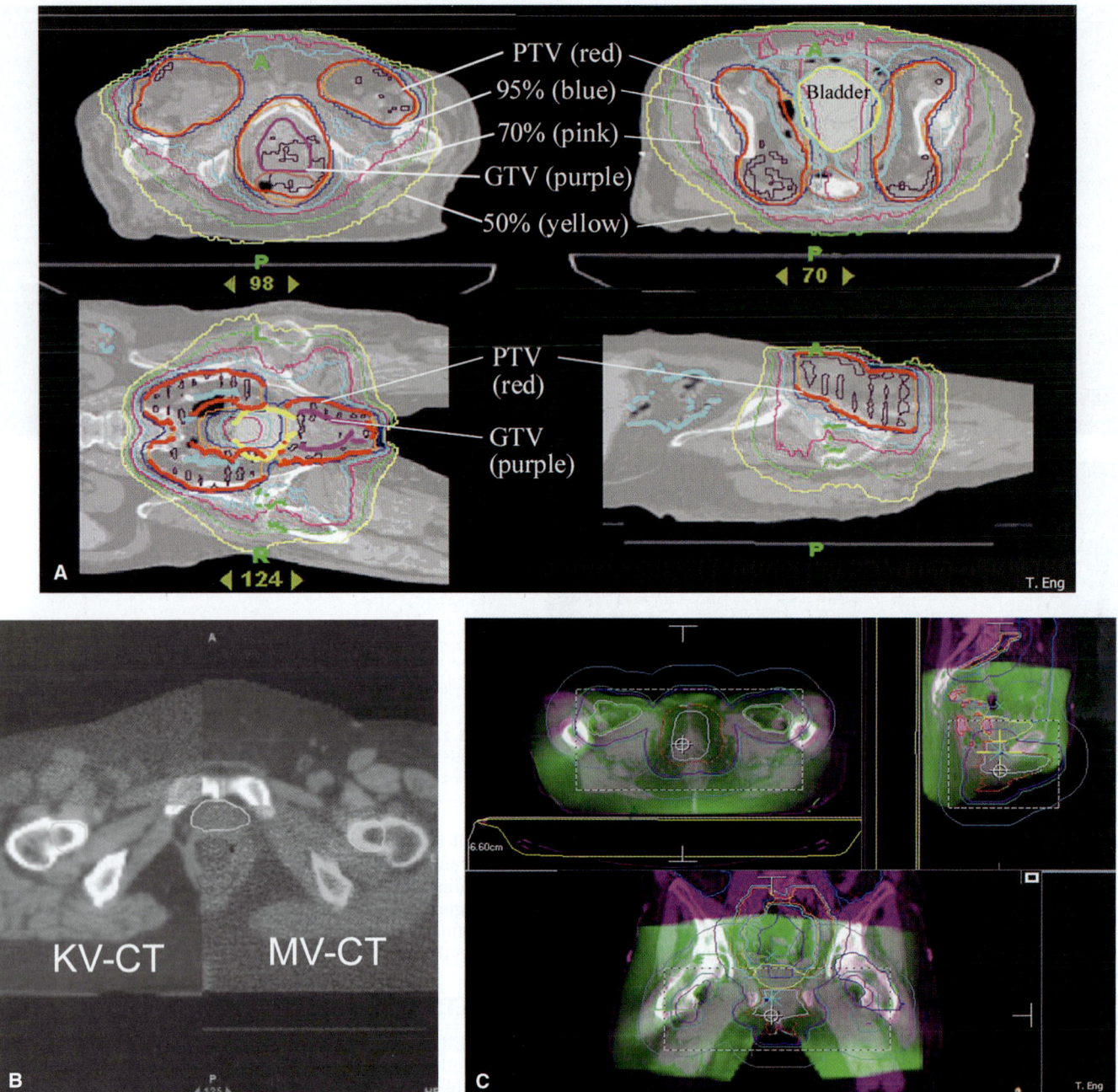

FIGURE 77.12. Pelvic IMRT plan. It shows a conformal dose distribution covering the lymphatics and primary target volume or the planning target volume (PTV) and gross tumor volume (GTV) **(A)**. Daily matching of MV-CT with the reference planning CT (KV-CT) **(B)** or CBCT **(C)** images is done prior to each treatment.

Five of seven patients with early meatal tumors were cured of disease in the series reported by Grabstald[9] after partial urethrectomy. In the remaining two patients, both local recurrences and distant metastases developed. Bracken et al.[46] reported local control in just one of four patients treated with local excision only for distal urethral lesions. Peterson et al.[22] reported on two patients in whom squamous cell carcinomas were excised successfully. In the same series, a patient with adenocarcinoma treated with local excision had a local recurrence and left inguinal adenopathy 4 years later.

Grabstald et al.[20] performed radical surgery on 15 patients with advanced disease; there were only 3 survivors at 5 years. Peterson et al.[22] performed radical surgery on seven patients, three of whom were still alive at 5 years. Primary radical cystectomy with anterior vaginectomy and total urethrectomy was performed on eight patients by Mayer et al.[74] Three of these patients were free of disease at 1, 4, and 11 years.

Radiation Therapy

Although DiMarco et al.[23] found that adjuvant radiation did not improve local control or survival in the study of 53 female patients with urethral carcinoma, treatment selection bias may have played a role as the higher-stage tumors tended to receive adjuvant radiation therapy. Eng et al.[47] reported only one of six patients with low-stage disease was referred for adjuvant radiation therapy, whereas four of five patients with advanced disease received radiation therapy. The one who did not receive radiation died 10 months after surgery. Case review of early-stage urethral cancer treated with external beam radiotherapy, brachytherapy, or a combination of both seems to have equivalent results as surgery alone.[52,58,65,69]

Control of tumors of the urethral meatus or the distal urethra with irradiation alone is often satisfactory. Early meatal tumors have cure rates of 70% to 90%.[38] Chu[19] reported a 5-year progression-free survival rate of 64% for 11 patients

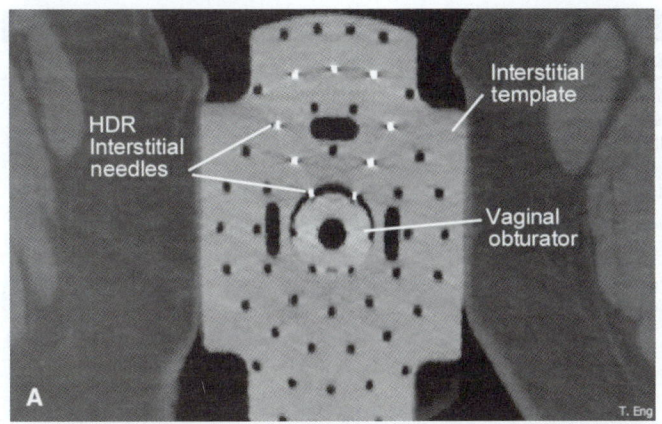

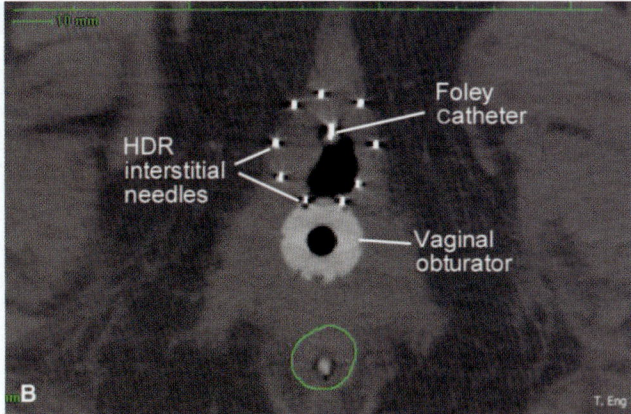

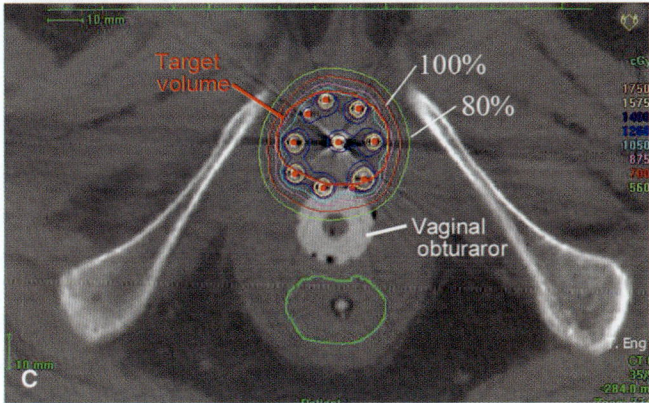

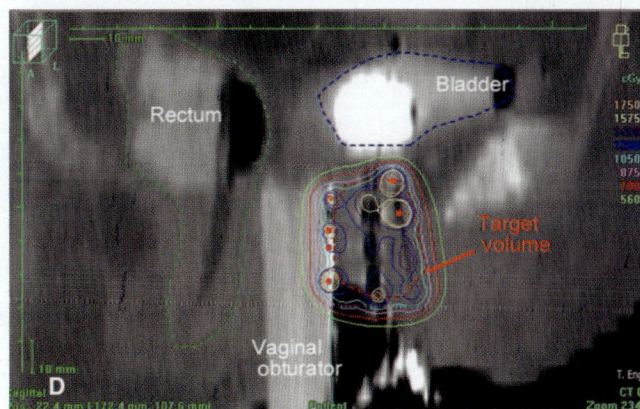

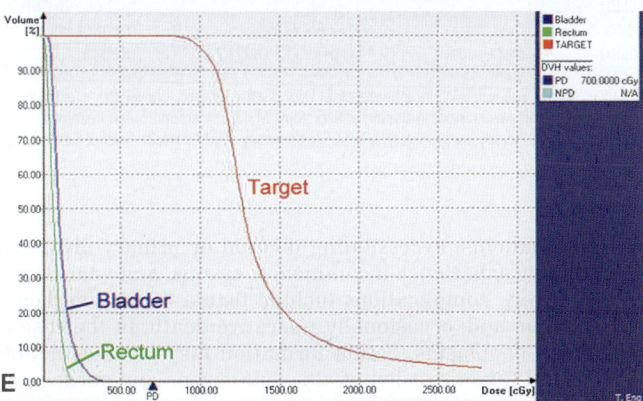

FIGURE 77.13. HDR interstitial brachytherapy. An interstitial template with a vaginal obturator is used to guide the needle placement **(A)**. The needles surround the urethra at approximately 1 cm distance **(B)**. With proper optimization, the resultant dose distribution conforms to the target volume while sparing all the surrounding organs **(C** and **D)**. Dose–volume histogram (DVH) shows a large dose separation of the target from the bladder and rectum **(E)**.

with tumor involvement of the anterior urethra treated with irradiation alone. Prempree et al.[38] treated three patients with stage I disease with interstitial irradiation alone (50 to 65 Gy) and achieved local control in all three. In the same series, two of four patients with stage II disease achieved local control and were alive 5 years after treatment. Weghaupt et al.[8] reported a 5-year survival rate of 71% for 42 patients with cancer of the anterior urethra. Their doses ranged from 55 to 70 Gy from intracavitary and external irradiation. Princess Margaret Hospital reported an 87% relapse-free survival rate in patients with stage I or II disease.[51] The majority of patients with small primary tumors received brachytherapy as a component of their treatment. Patients receiving brachytherapy and external-beam radiation therapy had a median total dose of 65 Gy.

Tumors of the proximal urethra or the entire urethra are more difficult to treat. The overall local control rate is 20% to 30%. Bracken et al.[46] treated 81 patients, and the 5-year survival rate was approximately 25% for patients with stage III and 20% for those with stage IV disease. Princess

Margaret Hospital reported stage III and IV tumors to have cause-specific survival rates of 26% and 16%, respectively.[40] Weghaupt et al.[8] reported a 5-year survival rate of 50% among 20 patients with tumor involvement of the posterior urethra who received irradiation alone or preoperative irradiation and surgery. Garden et al.[3] treated 86 patients with irradiation only after excision or biopsy of the primary lesion. Radiation doses ranged from 40 to 106 Gy (median, 65 Gy). The 5-year disease-specific survival rate was 49%, and the 5-year local control rate was 64%. Preoperative irradiation combined with radical surgery is an approach used by Klein et al.[21] They treated five women in this manner and achieved a 5-year survival rate of 40%. Dalbagni et al.[52] used anterior pelvic exenteration with intraoperative tumor bed interstitial brachytherapy using ^{192}Ir, followed several weeks later by pelvic external beam radiation therapy. A variety of chemosensitizing agents were used. The median brachytherapy dose was 15 Gy, and pelvic radiation therapy given was 45 Gy. Local control was achieved in four of six women with T2 and T4 disease.

TABLE 77.4 FEMALE URETHRA TREATMENT SUMMARY

Authors/Site/Year	Patients	Stage	Treatment	Radiation Dose (Gy)	Follow-Up (y)	Results	Prognostic Factors
Eng et al. UTHSCSA 2017[72]	18	Tis-3, N0-2, M0-1	5 part urethrectomy 3 surg ± RT ± chemo 5 RT ± brachy 5 RT/chemo ± brachy	30–68 primary 50 nodes 25 HDR brachy	7.1 (mean)	5-y OS 56% 5-y CSS 61%	Stage
Kang et al. Seoul National University 2015[73]	19	T1-4, N0-N+, M0-1	7 surg 7 surg ± RT ± chemo 3 RT ± chemo 2 biopsy only	No details	7.2 (median)	5-y RFS 34.8% 5-y CSS, 58.9% 5-y OS 58.9% Recurrence rate 57.9%	Stage, nodal status
Thyavihally et al. Tata Memorial 2005[28]	18	T1-4, N0-N+, M0	2 LE/RT 4 exent 4 exent/RT 4 RT 4 palliative RT/chemo	45–50 pelvis 20–25 boost	1.5–5.8	5-y OS 33% (45%, distal vs. 16%, proximal lesions; 50%, low vs. 0% high stage)	Stage, disease site
DiMarco et al. Mayo Clinic 2004[23]	53	pT1-3, N0-N+	26 part urethrectomy 27 exent (20 adj RT/3 brachy/3 chemo)	20–60 (50, median)	12.8 (mean)	10-y CSS 60% 10-y CS 42% LR 15 pts, DM 2 pts, LR + DM 10 pts	Path stage, nodal status, partial urethrectomy
Milosevic et al. PMH 2000[51]	34	T1-4, N0-N+, M0	5 brachy 14 RT 15 RT + brachy	35 brachy (median) 50 RT (median)		LR 62% 7 y AS 41% 7 y CSS 45%	Brachy, size
Dalbagni et al. MSKCC 1998[2]	72	Tx-4, Nx-N+	42 exent/part urethrectomy 25 RT/brachy 10 preop RT	No details	7.1 (median)	5-y OS 32% (78%, low vs. 22%, high stage) 5-y DSS 46% (89%, low vs. 33%, high stage)	Stage, nodal status, surgery type, disease site
Grigsby MIR 1998[24]	44	T1-4, N0-2	7 surg 25 RT 12 surg + RT	30–73.68 Adj RT (50.4 median) 12–70 RT (42.59 median) 20–95 brachy (42.72 median)	8.25 (mean)	5-y OS 42% 5-y DSS 40% (89%, 36%, 19% for <2, 2–4, >4 cm) LR 8 pts, LR + DM 15 pts, DM 4 pts	Size and histology
Garden et al. MDA 1993[3]	97	T1-4, N0-N+	86 LE + RT: (35 RT + brachy, 21 RT, 30 brachy) 11 preop RT	40–106 RT (65 median) 45–75 brachy (60 median)	8.75 (median)	5-y AS 41% 10-y AS 31% 15-y AS 22% LC 64% (RT only)	Local extension, fixation, involvement of entire urethra

adj, adjuvant; AS, actuarial survival; brachy, brachytherapy; chemo, chemotherapy; CS, crude survival; CSS, cancer-specific survival; DM, distant metastasis; DSS, disease-specific survival; exent, exenteration; HDR, high dose rate; LC, local control; LE, local excision; LR, local recurrence; MDA, MD Anderson Cancer Center; MIR, Mallinckrodt Institution of Radiology; MSKCC, Memorial Sloan Kettering Cancer Center; OS, overall survival; part, partial; preop, preoperative; pts, patients; PMH, Princess Margaret Hospital; RT, radiation therapy; surg, surgery; UTHSCSA, University of Texas Health Science Center at San Antonio; y, year.

Chemotherapy and Multimodality

Dayyani et al.[64] reported the response rate of 72% in 36 patients with locally advanced urethral cancer who had received definitive or preoperative platinum-based chemotherapy. The median overall survival was 25.6 months. Gheiler et al.[49] reported a disease-free survival rate of 60% in selected patients with advanced T3 or higher disease treated with a multimodality regimen consisting of neoadjuvant chemotherapy and radiation therapy. A phase 2 study has shown the combination of ifosfamide, paclitaxel, and cisplatin used in 45 patients with advanced transitional carcinoma of the urothelial tract is well tolerated and results in a median survival of 20 months.[75] Similar encouraging results have been reported in patients with advanced urethral cancer receiving concomitant fluorouracil, mitomycin C, and radiation therapy.[60,61,76]

SEQUELAE OF THERAPY

Complications as a result of surgery, irradiation, or combined-modality therapy vary greatly, from 0% to 42%, because of different tumor stages, the extent of surgery, and various irradiation doses.[10,19,24,67,77] In general, more aggressive treatment is expected to result in a higher complication rate. Garden et al.[3] reported that 27 of 55 patients (49%) achieving local control had complications, including urethral stenosis, fistula, necrosis, cystitis, and hemorrhage. Urethral strictures develop in some patients, necessitating dilation or urinary diversion. Others may experience incontinence, cystitis, and vaginal stenosis. Severe complications include fistula formation, bowel obstruction, and, occasionally, operative death. In the case of advanced neoplasms, fistula formation may be unavoidable because of tumor erosion of adjacent organs and subsequent tumor necrosis. Unlike the male counterpart, the physical loss of the female urethra is not uniformly associated with sexual impotence; nevertheless, the associated treatment side effects and negative self-image may affect sexual function and quality of life.

FUTURE DIRECTION

Early detection and intervention provide the best chance of organ preservation and cure. Although most clinical information comes from retrospective case series accumulated over a long span of time using various treatment modalities, multimodality shows encouraging results and should always be considered, especially in patients with locally advanced or metastatic disease. Clinical trials are clearly needed to obtain prospective data. Improved knowledge of tumor and normal tissue radiobiology along with continued technologic advances in external-beam radiation therapy and brachytherapy delivery will maximize organ preservation and minimize some of the treatment-related complications.

REFERENCES

1. Swartz MA, Porter MP, Lin DW, et al. Incidence of primary urethral carcinoma in the United States. *Urology* 2006;68(6):1164–1168.
2. Dalbagni G, Zhang ZF, Lacombe L, et al. Female urethral carcinoma: an analysis of treatment outcome and a plea for a standardized management strategy. *Br J Urol* 1998;82(6):835–841.
3. Garden AS, Zagars GK, Delclos L. Primary carcinoma of the female urethra. Results of radiation therapy. *Cancer* 1993;71(10):3102–3108.
4. Levine RL. Urethral cancer. *Cancer* 1980;45(7 Suppl):1965–1972.
5. Sailer SL, Shipley WU, Wang CC. Carcinoma of the female urethra: a review of results with radiation therapy. *J Urol* 1988;140(1):1–5.
6. Srinivas V, Khan SA. Female urethral cancer—an overview. *Int Urol Nephrol* 1987;19(4):423–427.
7. Johnson DE, O'Connell JR. Primary carcinoma of female urethra. *Urology* 1983;21(1):42–45.
8. Weghaupt K, Gerstner GJ, Kucera H. Radiation therapy for primary carcinoma of the female urethra: a survey over 25 years. *Gynecol Oncol* 1984;17(1):58–63.
9. Grabstald H. Proceedings: tumors of the urethra in men and women. *Cancer* 1973;32(5):1236–1255.
10. Pointon RC, Poole-Wilson DS. Primary carcinoma of the urethra. *Br J Urol* 1968;40(6):682–693.
11. Turner AG, Hendry WF. Primary carcinoma of the female urethra. *Br J Urol* 1980;52(6):549–554.
12. Wiener JS, Walther PJ. A high association of oncogenic human papillomaviruses with carcinomas of the female urethra: polymerase chain reaction-based analysis of multiple histological types. *J Urol* 1994;151(1):49–53.
13. Nakamura Y, Takahashi M, Suga A, et al. A case of adenocarcinoma arising within a urethral diverticulum diagnosed only by the surgical specimen. *Gynecol Obstet Invest* 1995;40(1):69–70.
14. Narayan P, Konety B. Surgical treatment of female urethral carcinoma. *Urol Clin North Am* 1992;19(2):373–382.
15. Rajan N, Tucci P, Mallouh C, et al. Carcinoma in female urethral diverticulum: case reports and review of management. *J Urol* 1993;150(6):1911–1914.
16. Chen ME, Pisters LL, Malpica A, et al. Risk of urethral, vaginal and cervical involvement in patients undergoing radical cystectomy for bladder cancer: results of a contemporary cystectomy series from M. D. Anderson Cancer Center. *J Urol* 1997;157(6):2120–2123.
17. De Paepe ME, Andre R, Mahadevia P. Urethral involvement in female patients with bladder cancer. A study of 22 cystectomy specimens. *Cancer* 1990;65(5):1237–1241.
18. Taggart CG, Castro JR, Rutledge FN. Carcinoma of the female urethra. *Am J Roentgenol Radium Ther Nucl Med* 1972;114(1):145–151.
19. Chu AM. Female urethral carcinoma. *Radiology* 1973;107(3):627–630.
20. Grabstald H, Hilaris B, Henschke U, et al. Cancer of the female urethra. *JAMA* 1966;197(11):835–842.
21. Klein FA, Whitmore WF, Herr HW, et al. Inferior pubic rami resection with en bloc radical excision for invasive proximal urethral carcinoma. *Cancer* 1983;51(7):1238–1242.
22. Peterson DT, Dockerty MB, Utz DC, et al. The peril of primary carcinoma of the urethra in women. *J Urol* 1973;110(1):72–75.
23. Dimarco DS, Dimarco CS, Zincke H, et al. Surgical treatment for local control of female urethral carcinoma. *Urol Oncol* 2004;22(5):404–409.
24. Grigsby PW. Carcinoma of the urethra in women. *Int J Radiat Oncol Biol Phys* 1998;41(3):535–541.
25. Moinuddin Ali M, Klein FA, Hazra TA. Primary female urethral carcinoma. A retrospective comparison of different treatment techniques. *Cancer* 1988;62(1):54–57.
26. Nakatsuka S, Taguchi I, Nagatomo T, et al. A case of clear cell adenocarcinoma arising from the urethral diverticulum: utility of urinary cytology and immunohistochemistry. *Cytojournal* 2012;9:11.
27. Hruby G, Choo R, Lehman M, et al. Female clear cell adenocarcinoma arising within a urethral diverticulum. *Can J Urol* 2000;7(6):1160–1163.
28. Thyavihally YB, Wuntkal R, Bakshi G, et al. Primary carcinoma of the female urethra: single center experience of 18 cases. *Jpn J Clin Oncol* 2005;35(2):84–87.
29. Hricak H, Secaf E, Buckley DW, et al. Female urethra: MR imaging. *Radiology* 1991;178(2):527–535.
30. Morikawa K, Togashi K, Minami S, et al. MR and CT appearance of urethral clear cell adenocarcinoma in a woman. *J Comput Assist Tomogr* 1995;19(6):1001–1003.
31. Fisher M, Hricak H, Reinhold C, et al. Female urethral carcinoma: MRI staging. *AJR Am J Roentgenol* 1985;144(3):603–604.
32. Quick HH, Serfaty JM, Pannu HK, et al. Endourethral MRI. *Magn Reson Med* 2001;45(1):138–146.
33. Chou CP, Levenson RB, Elsayes KM, et al. Imaging of female urethral diverticulum: an update. *Radiographics* 2008;28(7):1917–1930.
34. Fanti S, Nanni C, Ambrosini V, et al. PET in genitourinary tract cancers. *Q J Nucl Med Mol Imaging* 2007;51(3):260–271.
35. Nguyen BD. Clear cell adenocarcinoma of the urethra: 18 F-FDG PET/CT imaging. *Clin Nucl Med* 2015;40(3):241–243.
36. Larson SM, Schoder H. Advances in positron emission tomography applications for urologic cancers. *Curr Opin Urol* 2008;18(1):65–70.
37. Shvarts O, Han KR, Seltzer M, et al. Positron emission tomography in urologic oncology. *Cancer Control* 2002;9(4):335–342.
38. Prempree T, Amornmarn R, Patanaphan V. Radiation therapy in primary carcinoma of the female urethra. II. An update on results. *Cancer* 1984;54(4):729–733.
39. Amin MB, Edge SB, Greene FL, et al. *AJCC cancer staging manual.* 8th ed. Switzerland: Springer Nature, 2017.
40. Meis JM, Ayala AG, Johnson DE. Adenocarcinoma of the urethra in women. A clinicopathologic study. *Cancer* 1987;60(5):1038–1052.
41. Nash PA, Bihrle R, Gleason PE, et al. Mohs' micrographic surgery and distal urethrectomy with immediate urethral reconstruction for glanular carcinoma in situ with significant urethral extension. *Urology* 1996;47(1):108–110.
42. Ali SZ, Smilari TF, Gal D, et al. Primary adenoid cystic carcinoma of Skene's glands. *Gynecol Oncol* 1995;57(2):257–261.
43. Pandey PK, Vijay MK, Goel H, et al. Primary malignant melanoma of female urethra: a rare neoplasm. *J Cancer Res Ther* 2014;10(3):758–760.
44. Inuzuka S, Koga S, Imanishi D, et al. Primary malignant lymphoma of the female urethra. *Anticancer Res* 2003;23(3C):2925–2927.
45. Millan-Rodriguez F, Montlleo-Gonzalez M, Rosales-Bordes A, et al. Kaposi's sarcoma of the urethral meatus: management by urethral dilatation. *Br J Urol* 1995;75(4):558.
46. Bracken RB, Johnson DE, Miller LS, et al. Primary carcinoma of the female urethra. *J Urol* 1976;116(2):188–192.
47. Eng TY, Naguib M, Galang T, et al. Retrospective study of the treatment of urethral cancer. *Am J Clin Oncol* 2003;26(6):558–562.
48. Champ CE, Hegarty SE, Shen X, et al. Prognostic factors and outcomes after definitive treatment of female urethral cancer: a population-based analysis. *Urology* 2012;80(2):374–381.
49. Gheiler EL, Tefilli MV, Tiguert R, et al. Management of primary urethral cancer. *Urology* 1998;52(3):487–493.
50. Grigsby PW, Corn BW. Localized urethral tumors in women: indications for conservative versus exenterative therapies. *J Urol* 1992;147(6):1516–1520.
51. Milosevic MF, Warde PR, Banerjee D, et al. Urethral carcinoma in women: results of treatment with primary radiotherapy. *Radiother Oncol* 2000;56(1):29–35.
52. Dalbagni G, Donat SM, Eschwege P, et al. Results of high dose rate brachytherapy, anterior pelvic exenteration and external beam radiotherapy for carcinoma of the female urethra. *J Urol* 2001;166(5):1759–1761.
53. Aragona F, Maio G, Piazza R, et al. Primary malignant melanoma of the female urethra: a case report. *Int Urol Nephrol* 1995;27(1):107–111.
54. DiMarco DS, DiMarco CS, Zincke H, et al. Outcome of surgical treatment for primary malignant melanoma of the female urethra. *J Urol* 2004;171(2 Pt 1):765–767.
55. Barbagli G, Natali A, Urso C, et al. Primary malignant melanoma of the female urethra: a case report with immunohistochemical findings. *Urol Int* 1988;43(2):110–112.
56. Karnes RJ, Breau RH, Lightner DJ. Surgery for urethral cancer. *Urol Clin North Am* 2010;37(3):445–457.
57. Dann T, Schuller J, Schmeller NT, et al. Treatment of distal urethral cancer by laser coagulation. *Urologe A* 1989;28(5):296–299.
58. Micaily B, Dzeda MF, Miyamoto CT, et al. Brachytherapy for cancer of the female urethra. *Semin Surg Oncol* 1997;13(3):208–214.
59. Kuettel MR, Parda DS, Harter KW, et al. Treatment of female urethral carcinoma in medically inoperable patients using external beam irradiation and high dose rate intracavitary brachytherapy. *J Urol* 1997;157(5):1669–1671.
60. Hara I, Hikosaka S, Eto H, et al. Successful treatment for squamous cell carcinoma of the female urethra with combined radio- and chemotherapy. *Int J Urol* 2004;11(8):678–682.
61. Johnson DW, Kessler JF, Ferrigni RG, et al. Low dose combined chemotherapy/radiotherapy in the management of locally advanced urethral squamous cell carcinoma. *J Urol* 1989;141(3):615–616.
62. Licht MR, Klein EA, Bukowski R, et al. Combination radiation and chemotherapy for the treatment of squamous cell carcinoma of the male and female urethra. *J Urol* 1995;153(6):1918–1920.
63. Skarlos DV, Aravantinos G, Linardou E, et al. Chemotherapy with methotrexate, vinblastine, epirubicin and carboplatin (Carbo-MVE) in transitional cell urothelial cancer. A Hellenic Co-Operative Oncology Group study. *Eur Urol* 1997;31(4):420–427.
64. Dayyani F, Pettaway CA, Kamat AM, et al. Retrospective analysis of survival outcomes and the role of cisplatin-based chemotherapy in patients with urethral carcinomas referred to medical oncologists. *Urol Oncol* 2013;31(7):1171–1177.
65. Koontz BF, Lee WR. Carcinoma of the urethra: radiation oncology. *Urol Clin North Am* 2010;37(3):459–466.
66. Golimbu M, al-Askari S, Morales P. Transpubic approach for lower urinary tract surgery: a 15-year experience. *J Urol* 1990;143(1):72–76.
67. Hedden RJ, Husseinzadeh N, Bracken RB. Bladder sparing surgery for locally advanced female urethral cancer. *J Urol* 1993;150(4):1135–1137.
68. Libby B, Chao D, Schneider BF. Non-surgical treatment of primary female urethral cancer. *Rare Tumors* 2010;2(3):e55.
69. Foens CS, Hussey DH, Staples JJ, et al. A comparison of the roles of surgery and radiation therapy in the management of carcinoma of the female urethra. *Int J Radiat Oncol Biol Phys* 1991;21(4):961–968.
70. Hahn P, Krepart G, Malaker K. Carcinoma of female urethra. Manitoba experience: 1958–1987. *Urology* 1991;37(2):106–109.
71. Gerbaulet A, Haie-Meder C, Marsiglia H, et al. Brachytherapy in cancer of the urethra. *Ann Urol (Paris)* 1994;28(6–7):312–317.
72. Eng TY, Chen TW, Patel AJ, et al. Treatment and Outcomes of Primary Urethra Cancer. *Am J Clin Oncol* May 2017. [Epub ahead of print].
73. Kang M, Jeong CW, Kwak C, et al. Survival outcomes and predictive factors for female urethral cancer: long-term experience with Korean patients. *J Korean Med Sci* 2015;30(8):1143–1149.
74. Mayer R, Fowler JE Jr, Clayton M. Localized urethral cancer in women. *Cancer* 1987;60(7):1548–1551.
75. Bajorin DF, McCaffrey JA, Dodd PM, et al. Ifosfamide, paclitaxel, and cisplatin for patients with advanced transitional cell carcinoma of the urothelial tract: final report of a phase II trial evaluating two dosing schedules. *Cancer* 2000;88(7):1671–1678.
76. Shah AB, Kalra JK, Silber L, et al. Squamous cell cancer of female urethra. Successful treatment with chemoradiotherapy. *Urology* 1985;25(3):284–286.
77. Benson RC Jr, Tunca JC, Buchler DA, et al. Primary carcinoma of the female urethra. *Gynecol Oncol* 1982;14(3):313–318.

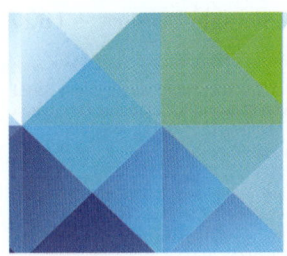

CHAPTER 78

Carcinoma of the Vulva

Junzo P. Chino, Brittany A. Davidson, and Gustavo S. Montana

ANATOMY

Vulva

The vulva is composed of the mons pubis, clitoris, labia majora and minora, vaginal vestibule, and their supporting subcutaneous tissues. The vulva blends with the urinary meatus anteriorly and with the perineum and anus posteriorly. The mons pubis consists of prominent tissue located anteriorly to the pubic symphysis. The labia majora are two elongated skin folds that course posteriorly from the mons pubis and blend into the perineal body. The skin of the labia majora is pigmented and contains hair follicles and sebaceous glands. The labia minora are a smaller pair of skin folds located between the labia majora. Anteriorly, the labia minora separates into two components that course above and below the clitoris, fusing with those of the opposite side to form the prepuce and frenulum, respectively. The skin of the labia minora contains numerous sebaceous glands but no hair follicles and has no underlying adipose tissue. The clitoris is 2 to 3 cm anterior to the urethral meatus and is supported externally by the fusion of the labia minora.

The vaginal introitus is demarcated laterally by the labia minora and posteriorly by the perineal body. Anteriorly, numerous small vestibular glands are located beneath the mucosa and open onto its surface adjacent to the urethral meatus. The Bartholin glands (or greater vestibular glands) are two small mucus-secreting glands situated within the subcutaneous tissue in the posterior aspect of the labia majora. The ducts of the Bartholin glands open onto the posterolateral portion of the introitus. The Skene glands (or paraurethral glands) open in the anterior aspect of the introitus but can be variable in location. The perineal body is a 3- to 4-cm band of skin that separates the vaginal introitus from the anus and forms the posterior margin of the vulva with the fusion of the labia minora, the fourchette.

Lymphatic Drainage

The inguinofemoral nodes are located within the triangle formed by the inguinal ligament superiorly, the border of the sartorius muscle laterally, and the border of the adductor longus muscle medially. There are superficial inguinal lymph nodes that lie along the saphenous vein and its branches between Camper fascia and the cribriform fascia overlying the femoral vessels. There are usually three to five deep nodes, the most superior of which, Cloquet node, is located under the inguinal ligament. Lymph drains from these nodes into the external and common iliac pelvic lymph nodes.

Lymphatic drainage is specific to the location of a vulvar lesion. Labial lesions drain into the superficial inguinal and femoral lymph nodes, and then penetrate the cribriform fascia and reach the deep femoral nodes. Lesions of the fourchette and perineum follow the lymphatics of the labia. Lymphatic drainage from the glans clitoris or perineal body enters either unilateral or bilateral superficial femoral nodes or the deep femoral and pelvic lymph nodes. Some lymphatics originating in the clitoris enter the pelvis directly, bypassing the femoral nodes to connect with the obturator and external iliac lymph nodes, though, in practice, the pelvic lymph nodes are rarely involved without synchronous involvement of the inguinal nodes (Fig. 78.1).

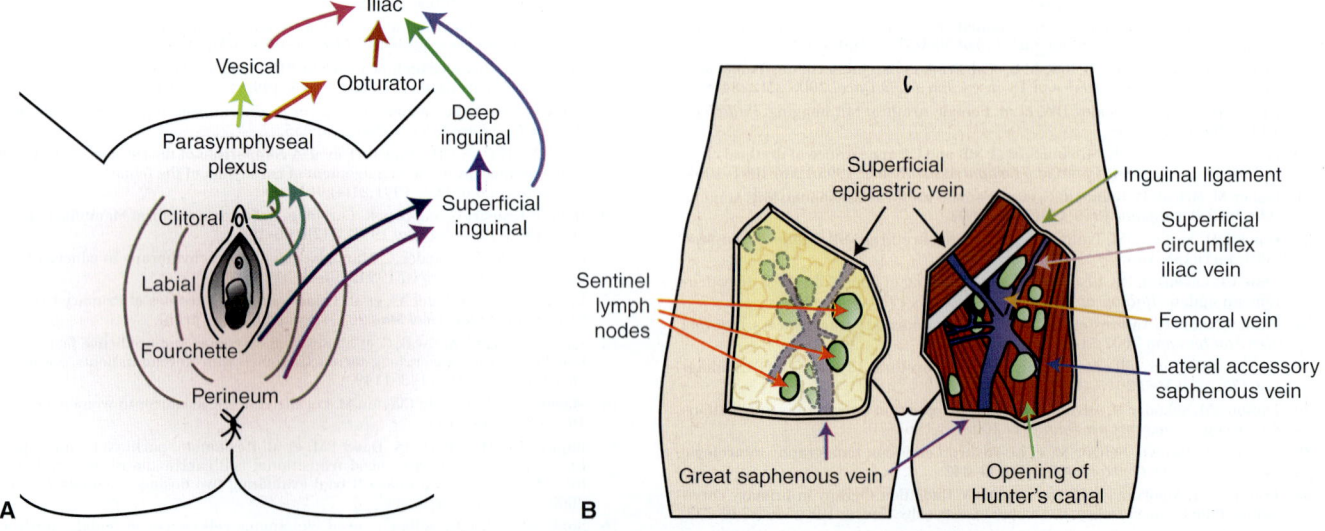

FIGURE 78.1. A: The lymphatic drainage of the vulva initially flows to the superficial inguinal nodes and then to the deep femoral and iliac group. Drainage from midline structures may flow directly beneath the symphysis to the pelvic nodes. (Modified from Plentl AA, Friedman EA, eds. *Lymphatic system of the female genitalia*. Philadelphia: WB Saunders, 1971. Copyright © 1971 Elsevier. With permission.) **B:** The superficial inguinal lymph nodes comprise 8 to 10 subcutaneous nodes located between the Camper fascia and the cribriform fascia. These nodes are immediately adjacent to the saphenous vein and its branches. (Modified from DiSaia PJ, Creasman WT, Rich WM. An alternative approach to early cancer of the vulva. *Am J Obstet Gynecol* 1979;133[7]:825–832. Copyright © 1979 Elsevier. With permission.)

EPIDEMIOLOGY

Vulvar cancer is a rare malignancy that represents <1% of all the cancers diagnosed in women and <5% of all gynecologic neoplasms. In the United States, it is estimated that there were 6,020 new cases in 2017, with 1,150 deaths due to the disease.[1] The incidence is 2.5 cases per 100,000 women; however, this incidence increases to 15.5 per 100,000 in women of age >75 years.[2] The incidence is slightly lower in black women (2.1 per 100,000) compared with whites (2.8 per 100,000).

There are two primary mechanisms believed to be involved in the carcinogenesis of this disease: human papillomavirus (HPV) and vulvar dystrophy, including lichen sclerosus (LS) and squamous hyperplasia. HPV DNA can be identified in between 30% and 40% of invasive vulvar cancers, with 16, 18, and 33 being the predominant subtypes.[3] This is in contrast to vulvar intraepithelial neoplasia (VIN), from which HPV can be isolated in 70% to 90% of lesions. Because HPV infection is related to numerous other cancers of the anogenital region (e.g., cervical cancer and anal canal cancer), the risk factors are similar: previous diagnosis of genital warts, multiple sexual partners, smoking history, previous abnormal Papanicolaou test, and immune suppression.[4] LS is often associated with the remaining HPV-negative cancers, although there is no histopathologic evidence of direct transformation.[5] Women with existing LS have a 5% to 7% risk of developing invasive disease, with risk increasing with older age and concurrent VIN (up to 19% risk of invasive cancer at 10 years).[6,7] The evidence for VIN as an obligate precursor to invasive vulvar disease, however, is less compelling than that established between cervical intraepithelial neoplasia and cervical cancer. Only one-third of vulvar cancers have an associated VIN-3 lesion, and only 5% to 7% of women with an existing VIN lesion will subsequently be diagnosed with invasive disease.[8]

VIN may in fact be divisible into two general types, depending on the lesion dependence (or independence) from HPV.[9] Usual-type VIN (uVIN) is often HPV driven and occurs in younger women with HPV risk factors. Differentiated-type VIN (dVIN) arises in the setting of LS and other chronic inflammatory processes and is associated with older age. These differing precursor lesions may then transform into two distinct classifications of squamous carcinoma: keratinizing squamous carcinomas (KSCs) arising from dVIN and basaloid squamous carcinomas (BSCs) arising from uVIN.[10] KSC is more common (80% of cases), and p53 mutations may play a role in pathogenesis in a subset of these neoplasms, whereas p16 is rarely positive indicating a lack of association with HPV.[11,12] BSC, in contrast, is less common (20% of cases), and staining for p53 is often negative, whereas p16 is often positive because of its association with HPV. Similar to findings related to HPV-related cancers in other sites, HPV-driven lesions (uVIN and BSC) portend a better prognosis.[13] Overexpression of p16 may also be associated with an improved prognosis, even when high-risk HPV DNA is not detected.[14]

PATHOLOGY

Squamous Carcinoma

Eighty to ninety percent of invasive disease of the vulva is squamous cell carcinoma (Fig. 78.2),[15] arising within squamous epithelium, within or adjacent to areas of epithelial abnormalities or of premalignant conditions such as LS, erythroplasia of Queyrat, and Bowen disease.[16] The depth of invasion, critical for appropriate staging and management, is defined as the distance from the epithelial stromal junction of the most superficial adjacent dermal papillae to the deepest point of invasion. Tumor thickness is measured from the overlying surface epithelium, or the bottom of the granular layer if the surface is keratinized, to the deepest point of invasion as specified by the International Society of Gynecological Pathologists.[17]

There are three recognizable types of growth pattern of squamous carcinoma: confluent, compact, and spray or finger-like growth. Confluent growth is defined as a tumor mass composed of interconnected tumor >1 mm in dimension. This type of growth is characteristic for being deeply invasive with associated stromal desmoplasia. Compact growth is associated with well-differentiated tumors, which maintain continuity with the overlying epithelium, infiltrating as a well-defined and circumscribed tumor mass, which rarely invades the vascular space. Histologically, the tumor cells resemble squamous cells of adjacent and overlaying epithelium. The spray or finger-like growth pattern is characterized by a trabecular appearance with small islands of poorly differentiated tumor cells found within the dermis or submucosa, deeper than the main tumor mass. This growth pattern

FIGURE 78.2. Squamous cell carcinoma of the vulva. **A:** Squamous cell carcinoma with ulceration, arising from the right labia minora. This elderly woman had no apparent predisposing disease. **B:** Photomicrograph of invasive keratinizing squamous cell carcinoma of the vulva. Note the keratin pearls. (Courtesy of Dr. Stanley Robboy, Duke University Medical Center, Durham, NC.)

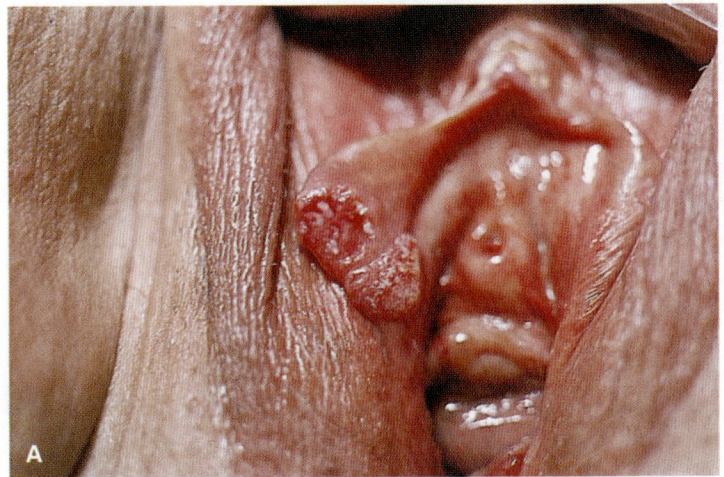

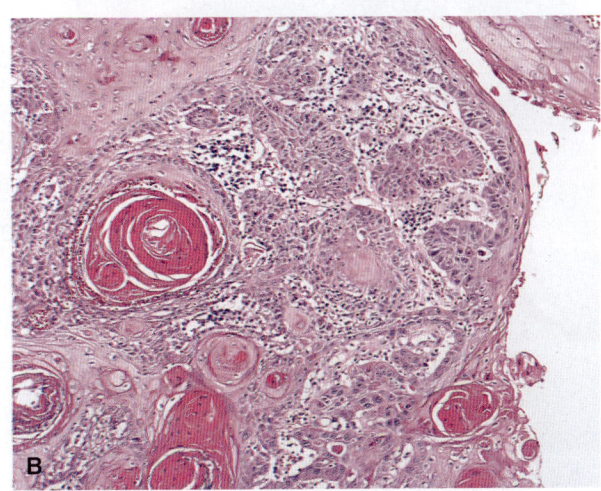

is often associated with desmoplastic stromal response and a lymphocytic inflammatory infiltrate. Vascular space involvement is seen more commonly with this growth pattern than with tumors with a compact pattern.[18]

UNCOMMON HISTOLOGIC TYPES AND MANAGEMENT

Melanoma

Malignant melanoma of the vulva accounts for approximately 10% of all primary tumors of the vulva, with a peak incidence in the sixth and seventh decades (Fig. 78.3).[19,20] Sometimes, the tumor arises in a preexisting pigmented lesion, and in these cases, the differential diagnosis includes benign vulvar melanosis and pigmented VIN. Vulvar melanomas can be subclassified into three specific categories: superficial spreading malignant melanoma, nodular melanoma, and acral lentiginous melanoma. As is the case for melanomas arising in other mucosal sites, the level of invasion, tumor thickness, and nodal evaluations dictate the therapy and determine the prognosis.[21] Compared to nongynecologic melanomas, BRAF and KIT mutations are more frequently detected in vulvar and vaginal melanomas, and PD-L1 and PD-1 may be more frequently expressed, having implications for targeted therapies and immunmodulation.[22]

The prognosis is poor, with a 5-year overall survival of approximately 35%, and is worse in patients who have one or more of the following features: deep invasion, ulceration, nodular growth pattern, epithelioid cell type, and high mitotic rate.[23–25] The prognosis is also worse in older patients. Primary surgical excision with nodal evaluation is preferred if possible, with adjuvant radiotherapy for nodal disease or close margins at the primary site. In a study of 32 patients treated at the Royal Marsden Hospital in London, there was no difference in the outcome between patients treated with wide local excision and those treated with more radical surgical procedures.[26] Radiation may be considered for patients with positive margins or positive lymph nodes or for palliation of symptoms. As with melanomas of other sites, the prognosis is guarded because of a propensity for distant metastasis.

Adenocarcinoma

Adenocarcinomas of the vulva arise predominantly in the Bartholin glands, although apocrine, eccrine, and Skene glands can also be the site of origin. In the rare instances when adenocarcinomas arise in the absence of glandular tissue, they may be of cloacogenic origin. Carcinoma of the Bartholin gland is seen more frequently in older women and is often solid and deeply infiltrative. The overlying epidermis or mucosa may remain intact, leading to misinterpretation as a benign process. Other histopathologic types are mucinous, papillary, mucoepidermoid, adenosquamous, and transitional. The transition from normal to malignant glandular tissue can be recognized in some cases. Adenocarcinomas often present with more locally advanced disease and metastases to the inguinofemoral lymph nodes.

The general approach to treatment, however, follows squamous cell carcinomas, with initial surgery with tailored adjuvant radiation therapy for resectable disease, and multimodality therapies for advanced stages. Survival after treatment is comparable to stage-matched squamous cell cancers.[27] The role of radiation for Bartholin gland carcinoma has been studied by Copeland et al. and Leuchter et al.[28,29] These two studies suggest that adjuvant radiation to the vulva and regional nodes after conservative surgery may decrease local recurrence, with 7% recurrence with radiation and 27% recurrence without it in the Copeland et al. study. Five-year survival of 67% was reported by Cardosi et al. in patients who were found to have close margins and were treated with primary surgery and adjuvant radiation.[30]

FIGURE 78.3. Melanoma of the vulva. **A:** A nodular, elevated, and darkly pigmented lesion arising from the right labia majora. **B:** Photomicrograph of invasive melanoma, with melanin apparent in portions of the tumor. (Courtesy of Dr. Stanley Robboy, Duke University Medical Center, Durham, NC.)

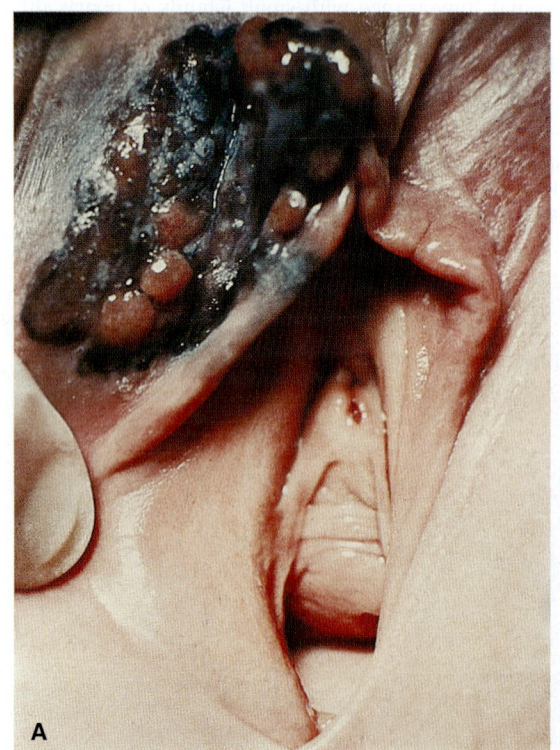

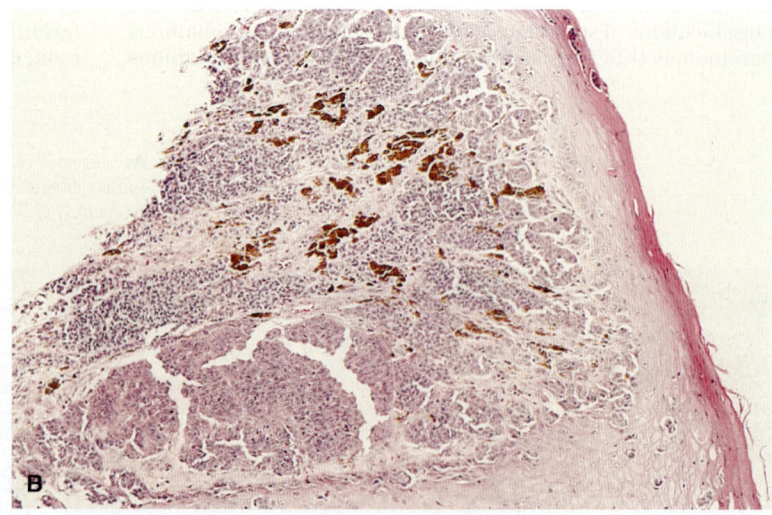

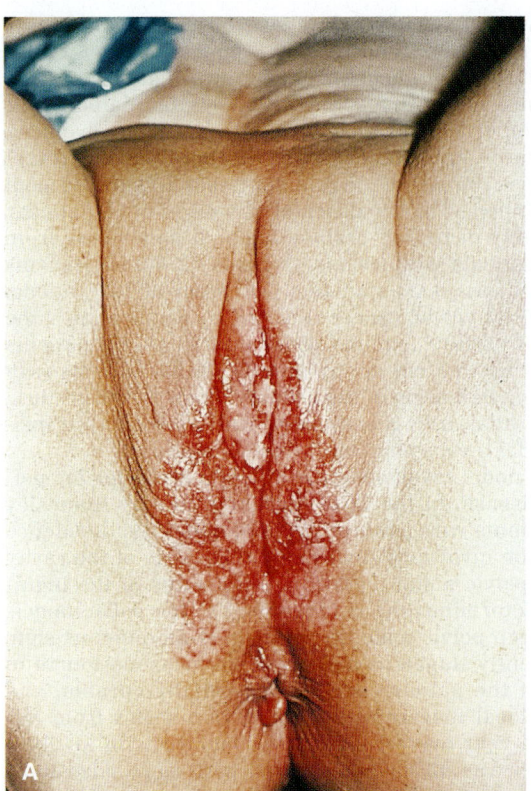

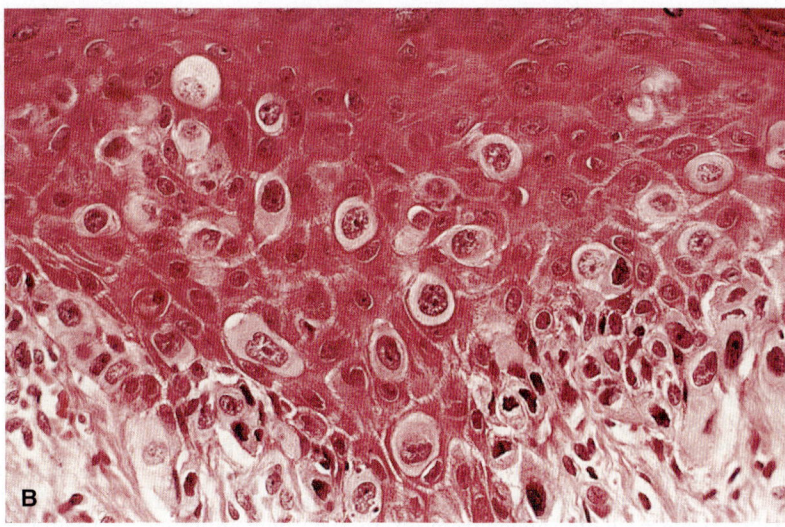

FIGURE 78.4. Paget disease of the vulva. **A:** Photo of extensive perineal disease, extending to the perianal skin. **B:** Photomicrograph of intraepithelial Paget cells, with copious pale cytoplasm, occurring singly or in small clusters and appearing slightly larger than neighboring squamous cells (Courtesy of Dr. Stanley Robboy, Duke University Medical Center, Durham, NC.)

Paget Disease of the Vulva

Paget disease of the vulva (intraepithelial adenocarcinoma) is seen most often in postmenopausal, older white women. The disease varies in appearance, but most often, it presents as an eczematoid, red can, or weeping lesion, and it can be mistakenly diagnosed as eczema or contact dermatitis (Fig. 78.4). The lesion may be flat, raised, or ulcerated and may appear whitish (leukoplakia), red (erythroplastic), or hyperpigmented. This condition has a typical histologic pattern and often stains positive for carcinoembryonic antigen. Vulvar Paget disease is associated with invasive carcinoma in 10% to 20% of the cases.[31,32] The invasive disease may be an underlying adenocarcinoma of the apocrine or Bartholin glands, or it may be an adenocarcinoma arising elsewhere in the anogenital region. Management is generally focused on maximal safe resection, though radiotherapy is an effective therapy for recurrent or unresectable disease.[33] Topical imiquimod also shows promise as an effective nonoperative therapy.[34]

Verrucous Carcinoma

Verrucous carcinomas of the vulva are uncommon, usually diagnosed in the fifth or sixth decade of life. They are locally invasive tumors that present as fungating, ulcerative masses. Histologically, these tumors are often well differentiated and have a low incidence of metastasis to lymph nodes. In instances when the lesion is in early stage, excellent results are obtained with radical wide excision.[35] Inguinofemoral dissections are not recommended routinely because of the rarity of nodal metastases.

The literature regarding vulvar verrucous carcinomas consists largely of case reports, with the exception of the series by Japaze et al.[36] This study was based on 24 patients, 17 of whom were treated with surgery only and 7 of whom were treated with surgery and radiation. In the surgery group, only 1 patient developed recurrence and died as a result of it. In the radiation group, 4 patients developed recurrence, and all died from the disease. Although it is difficult to draw conclusions from this small series, there are no convincing data to recommend the routine use of radiotherapy for this disease. In addition, there is no sufficient evidence to support the notion that radiation induces anaplastic transformation.[37]

Other Histologies

Other vulvar malignancies arising from epidermal cell types are rare. Merkel cell tumors (neuroendocrine carcinomas) are aggressive locally, have a high incidence of distant metastasis, and carry a poor prognosis. Basal cell carcinomas, on the other hand, seldom spread to lymph nodes and are appropriately treated with wide excision alone.[38] Transitional cell carcinomas may arise from the Bartholin glands or may also represent metastasis from the bladder and/or lower urinary tract.

Leiomyosarcomas are the most common subtypes of vulvar sarcoma followed by malignant fibrous histiocytomas, epithelioid sarcomas, and rhabdomyosarcomas. Rhabdomyosarcomas of the vulva require combination therapy, chemotherapy, and radiation, as per rhabdomyosarcoma protocols of other sites. Results of treatment with other sarcomas of the vulva are unpredictable, and wide resection and/or radical radiotherapy should be considered, given the relative inactivity of chemotherapy.

CLINICAL PRESENTATION

Vulvar pruritus is the most common presenting symptom, often associated with bleeding, pain, or discharge. If there is a visible lesion on physical examination, a biopsy is required to distinguish it from other vulvar lesions such as dystrophia, benign condylomata, and VIN. Unfortunately, many women have a long delay in diagnosis due to denial or minimization of symptoms and may present with a locally advanced tumor by the time of initial evaluation. These lesions may also present with symptoms related to the invasion of regional structures, including difficulty with urination or defecation. Metastatic disease is an uncommon presenting symptom because the primary lesion is usually much more problematic, although consequences of groin and distant disease may also be seen at presentation.

PATTERNS OF DISEASE AND SPREAD

Primary Site

Approximately 70% of vulvar malignancies arise in the labia majora and minora, 15% in the clitoris, 5% in the perineum and fourchette, 5% in the prepuce Bartholin glands and urethra, and 5% are too extensive at presentation to classify.[39]

Lymphatic Spread

High-grade tumors with "spray" growth pattern and lymphatic space invasion have a proclivity to spread to the regional lymphatic nodes. The superficial inguinofemoral lymph nodes are the first echelon, followed by the deep inguinofemoral nodes. For well-lateralized lesions, metastasis to the contralateral inguinal or pelvic lymph nodes is unusual in the absence of ipsilateral inguinofemoral node involvement. Lesions of the clitoris or urethra can spread directly to pelvic lymph nodes, although this is rare without inguinal node involvement.[40,41]

The frequency of inguinal lymph node metastasis in surgically staged patients ranges from 6% to 50%, depending on tumor invasion and extent of disease (Table 78.1).[42–46] Physical examination alone is inaccurate to assess lymph node involvement: Plentl and Friedman reported a 62% incidence of lymph node metastases in patients with clinically palpable adenopathy and 35% involvement in patients without clinically palpable adenopathy.[39] In the Gynecologic Oncology Group (GOG) protocol 36, Homesley reported that 24% of the patients with clinically negative inguinal nodes were found to have nodal metastasis on final pathology. When the lymph nodes were clinically suspicious, 76% of the patients had histologically positive nodes.

Multiple clinical and histologic features of the primary tumor are associated with nodal metastasis, including tumor thickness, histologic grade, capillary-like space involvement, depth of invasion, location of the tumor, and tumor size.[47,48] Rutledge et al.[48] also described the adverse effect on local control and survival of tumor size, clinical stage, positive inguinal or pelvic nodes, and positive margins at the primary site. When the tumor thickness is ≤1 mm, the probability of nodal metastasis is ≤3%, but with a tumor thickness ≥5 mm, the probability increases to 33.3%. Depth of invasion of 1, 2, and 3 mm corresponds to a 4.3%, 7.8%, and 17% incidence of nodal involvement, respectively. It should be noted that thickness of the epithelium in the vulva varies significantly from one area to another, in some areas being >0.8 mm thick, which can influence the relative value given to tumor thickness and depth of invasion. Measuring tumor thickness in superficially ulcerated tumors can be misleading and may lead to underestimating the depth of invasion. Perineural invasion correlates strongly with lymph node metastasis.[49]

In analysis of the GOG database on carcinoma of the vulva, several clinical and histologic tumor characteristics were identified as predictors of nodal involvement. In order of importance, these are clinical node status (palpable vs. nonpalpable), grade, capillary lymphatic space involvement, tumor thickness, and patient's age.[47,50,51] There is also a correlation between the size of the primary tumor and involvement of the lymph nodes. In Donaldson et al.'s series of 66 patients, the probability of having positive inguinal nodes rose from 18.9% for patients with lesions <3 cm to 72.4% for patients with primary tumors ≥3 cm.[43] In a GOG study of 267 patients with superficial vulvar cancer reported by Sedlis et al.[47], the frequency of positive inguinal nodes was 18.1% for patients with lesions up to 3 cm in size and 29.3% for patients with lesions ≥3 cm. Extension of the primary tumor to the urethra, vagina, and anal area is associated with an increased incidence of nodal involvement and worse prognosis.

Inguinal nodal involvement is a strong predictor for pelvic nodal disease. In the GOG study reported by Homesley et al. of patients with positive inguinal nodes, the incidence of pelvic node involvement was 28%.[52] Because of the rarity of isolated pelvic nodal metastasis, the status of the inguinal nodes determines the management of the pelvic nodes. Although deep pelvic node involvement is an ominous sign, and is currently staged as metastatic disease, one-fourth to one-third of the patients are still potentially curable, and aggressive local therapy is indicated. In a series from MD Anderson, 5-year overall survival for women with involved pelvic nodes was 43% when treated with aggressive local therapy.[53]

Distant Metastases

Hematogenous dissemination generally occurs late in the natural history of the disease, with the most common sites being the lungs, liver, and bones. The overall survival is limited in these cases to a median of approximately 6 months.[54]

PROGNOSTIC FACTORS

Lymph node metastasis is the most important prognostic factor in patients with vulvar cancer. The presence of inguinal node metastases is accompanied by a 50% reduction in long-term survival.[55] Lymph node extracapsular tumor extension has been noted in several series, and it is known to have a negative effect on prognosis. Origoni et al.[56] evaluated the significance of the size of the metastases in the lymph nodes, the number of positive lymph nodes, and the extracapsular extension (ECE) of the disease and found that the presence of any one of these factors worsened the prognosis. Extracapsular tumor extension as an independent adverse prognostic factor on survival was also described by van der Velden et al.[57]

Pelvic nodal metastasis has an even more profound negative effect on survival.[58] Although deep pelvic node involvement is an ominous sign, and is currently staged as metastatic disease, one-fourth to one-third of the patients are still potentially curable, and aggressive local therapy is indicated. In a series from MD Anderson, 5-year overall survival for women with involved pelvic nodes was 43% when treated with aggressive local therapy.[53]

In an analysis of formalin-fixed tissue specimens, Heaps et al.[59] demonstrated a sharp rise in the incidence of local recurrence for tumors with microscopic, surgical margins <8 mm. This corresponds to a margin of 1 cm in fresh, unfixed tissue. Although the frequency of local recurrences correlates with the adequacy of the margins of the surgical resection, when dealing with larger or thicker tumors or when they involve midline structures, adequate surgical margins may be difficult to obtain.

TABLE 78.1 INCIDENCE OF LYMPH NODE INVOLVEMENT CORRELATED WITH PRIMARY TUMOR SIZE AND EXTENT

Primary Tumor Size and Depth of Invasion	Number of Patients	Number of Patients with Positive Lymph Nodes (%)
Depth		
<1 mm	120	0 (0)
1.1–2 mm	121	8 (6.6)
2.1–3 mm	97	8 (8.2)
3.1–4 mm	50	11 (22)
4.1–5 mm	40	10 (25)
Size		
>5 mm	32	12 (37.5)
>2 cm	168	77 (45.8)
Any size of primary tumor extending beyond the vulva	70	38 (54.2)

Adapted from Perez CA, Grigsby PW, Chao C. Vulva. In: Perez CA, Brady LW, eds. *Principles and practice of radiation oncology.* 3rd ed. Philadelphia: Lippincott-Raven, 1997.

Kurzl and Masserer[60] analyzed 124 patients with various stages of vulvar carcinoma treated with simple vulvectomy alone and local/inguinal irradiation. They found that age, disassociated growth, lymphatic spread, thickness, and ulceration of the primary tumor were important prognostic factors. In a detailed analysis of a GOG clinicopathologic study of 558 women with vulvar cancer, two significant risk factors were identified that predispose for recurrence in the vulva: tumor size >4 cm and capillary lymphatic space involvement.[50] If either of these factors was present, the risk of local recurrence after radical vulvectomy was 21%, but if neither factor was present, the risk of local recurrence was only 9%. In this study, the depth of invasion did not predict for vulvar failure.

HPV-positive or p16-positive cancers may have a better prognosis, as described above in the epidemiology section.

INITIAL EVALUATION

A thorough examination of the genitourinary system is warranted in all women with vulvar cancer because the disease may be multifocal. Examination of the vagina, cervix, perianal skin, and anal canal is of particular importance in order to delineate the extent of disease and to identify synchronous lesions. Special attention as well is paid to the inguinofemoral basins for clinical detection of lymphatic spread.

Imaging studies may not be necessary in early lesions that may be approached with surgery as the first treatment modality. However, imaging in women with locally advanced disease or with clinically suspicious lymph nodes helps the clinician select the most appropriate treatment. Computed tomography (CT) scans can identify suspicious lymphadenopathy in the inguinofemoral chains, pelvis, or para-aortic regions.[61] Contrast-enhanced magnetic resonance imaging (MRI) is also helpful to delineate the primary lesion and contributes to the evaluation of inguinal lymph nodes, with a sensitivity of 80% and a specificity of 88%.[62] Clinically or radiographically detected inguinal nodes may be evaluated with ultrasound-guided fine needle aspiration, though a negative result does not rule out involvement.[63] Fluorodeoxyglucose (FDG) positron emission tomography (PET) has been used to evaluate the groin prior to surgical evaluation, with a sensitivity of 67% and a specificity of 95%.[64] FDG-PET at diagnosis may change the prior clinical impression in up to 50% of cases.[65] It should be noted that the sensitivities of all imaging modalities available are insufficient to omit surgical evaluation in women with a high risk of nodal involvement.

STAGING

The staging system first adopted in 1983 was based entirely on clinical findings. The system was modified in 1988 to give the clinical status of the nodes more importance. In 1997, the staging was revised again to create a separate category for minimally invasive lesions, stage IA, emphasizing the need for histologic assessment of the inguinal nodes in all patients presenting with primary tumors with >1 mm depth of invasion.

The most recent Federation of Gynecology and Obstetrics (FIGO) staging revision was performed in 2009 and contains significant changes from the 1988 framework (Table 78.2).[17,66] Stage IB now includes primary lesions >2 cm in size (previously stage II), and stage II includes lesions with involvement of adjacent perineal structures (previously stage III). Stage III is now divided into three substages, reflecting the importance of the number and size of inguinal nodes involved and the prognostic significance of ECE. Presence of pelvic nodal metastases remains stage IVB disease.

TABLE 78.2 VULVAR CANCER: 2009 AMERICAN JOINT COMMITTEE ON CANCER (AJCC) STAGING AND CORRESPONDING INTERNATIONAL FIGO STAGING

2009 AJCC			FIGO
Tis	Carcinoma *in situ*		–
T1a	Confined to the vulva/perineum, size ≤2 cm, stromal invasion ≤1 mm	N0	IA
T1b	Confined to the vulva/perineum, size >2 cm or stromal invasion >1 mm	N0	IB
T2	Adjacent spread to distal one-third urethra and/or vagina or anus	N0	II
T3	Extension to proximal two-thirds urethra and/or vagina, bladder/rectal mucosa, or fixation to pubic bones		IVA
N1a	1–2 lymph nodes involved, all <5 mm		IIIA
N1b	1 lymph node involved, ≥5 mm		IIIA
N2a	3 or more lymph nodes involved, all <5 mm		IIIB
N2b	2 or more lymph nodes involved, ≥5 mm		IIIB
N2c	Any lymph nodes involved with ECE		IIIC
N3	Fixed or ulcerated lymph nodes		IVA
M1	Distant metastasis (including pelvic lymph node metastasis).		IVB

According to the AJCC, femoral and inguinal nodes are considered regional spread, whereas iliac nodes are considered distant metastasis.

From Edge SB, Byrd DR, Compton CC, et al., eds. *AJCC cancer staging handbook*. 7th ed. New York: Springer, 2010. Copyright © 2010 American Joint Committee on Cancer. Reproduced with permission of Springer International Publishing in the format Book via Copyright Clearance Center.

MANAGEMENT OVERVIEW

Many factors make the treatment of carcinoma of the vulva challenging. Many women with this disease are older and have comorbidities. The tumor, by virtue of its location, can easily involve adjacent organs such as the bladder and the rectum, and the frequency of nodal involvement is high. Because of its relatively low incidence, most published reports consist of small and heterogeneous groups of patients. Management of carcinoma of the vulva is further complicated by the major psychosexual impact that the disease itself and its treatment can have on patients. For the aforementioned reasons, it has been difficult to study this disease and to develop general treatment guidelines.

The management of vulvar carcinoma has undergone very significant changes in the last few decades. En bloc resection of the primary tumor and a full inguinal node dissection used to be the standard of care, but this is no longer the case. Extensive surgery has been replaced by multimodality therapy, with the surgery being more tailored to the extent of the disease. This change is in large measure due to the recognition of the morbidity associated with radical surgery, the improved results achieved with multimodality therapy, and the recognition of the negative impact that radical surgery can have on sexual function and body image.[67–69] Although radical surgery retains a very important place in the management of vulvar cancer, it is no longer the initial and mainstay of treatment. The likelihood of controlling the primary tumor with surgery largely depends on the adequacy of the margins of resection, and it is not necessary to remove the entire vulva. A clear margin of ≥8 mm in all directions is sufficient to achieve a high rate of local control of the primary tumor.[59]

There have been refinements in the surgical technique that have made the procedures more tolerable. Examples of such improvements include primary closure of the perineal wound, the use of myocutaneous flaps to close the surgical defect in the inguinal area, and the use of separate incisions for the resection of the primary tumor and the inguinal nodes. These developments have resulted in a decrease in operative mortality and morbidity.

Section III

In recent decades, there have been also significant advances in all aspects of radiation therapy that apply to the treatment of carcinoma of the vulva. The technical resources available now make it possible to deliver effective doses of radiation to the vulvovaginal and inguinal regions with less acute and late morbidity. With high-photon energy units, well-collimated fields, multileaf collimators, electron beams of different energies, and intensity-modulated radiation therapy (IMRT), radiation is now delivered to the primary disease and lymph nodes with precise account of the differences in contour, tissue thickness, and extent of the disease. It is possible to tailor the treatment to the specified treatment volume while keeping the dose to the normal tissues within acceptable limits of tolerance. Brachytherapy may also be used as primary treatment in very selected cases or in combination with external beam to bring the dose higher to limited volumes.

Perhaps the most significant advance of recent decades in the management of cancer patients is the use of more than one treatment modality concurrently or sequentially. Chemotherapy, radiation, and surgery in sequence and/or in combination lessen the impact of any one modality and can lead to functional organ preservation with comparable or improved local tumor control and survival (Fig. 78.5).

SURGERY

Wide Local Excision, Radical Vulvectomy, and Exenteration

In the past, even patients with early-stage IB disease were considered to have diffuse disease, and a radical vulvectomy was considered the standard of care, yielding 90% survival rates but with considerable physical and emotional sequelae. Although there is a lack of prospective data comparing radical local excisions versus more extensive radical vulvectomies, several retrospective studies reveal no difference in recurrence or survival outcomes.[70] For T1 and smaller T2 lesions (<4 cm) with ≤ 1-mm invasion, a wide local excision is recommended without inguinofemoral node evaluation given the risk of nodal involvement in these cases is <1%.[71] For tumors with >1-mm invasion, a more radical excision with an inguinofemoral groin node evaluation is recommended. If these tumors are well lateralized (>2 cm from the midline), only an ipsilateral groin evaluation is necessary; however, for midline lesions, bilateral groin node evaluation is recommended.[72]

At surgical resection, the depth of the excision should be to the deep perineal fascia or periosteum of the pubis for more anterior lesions. Excision of 2-cm margins of grossly

FIGURE 78.5. Treatment algorithm.

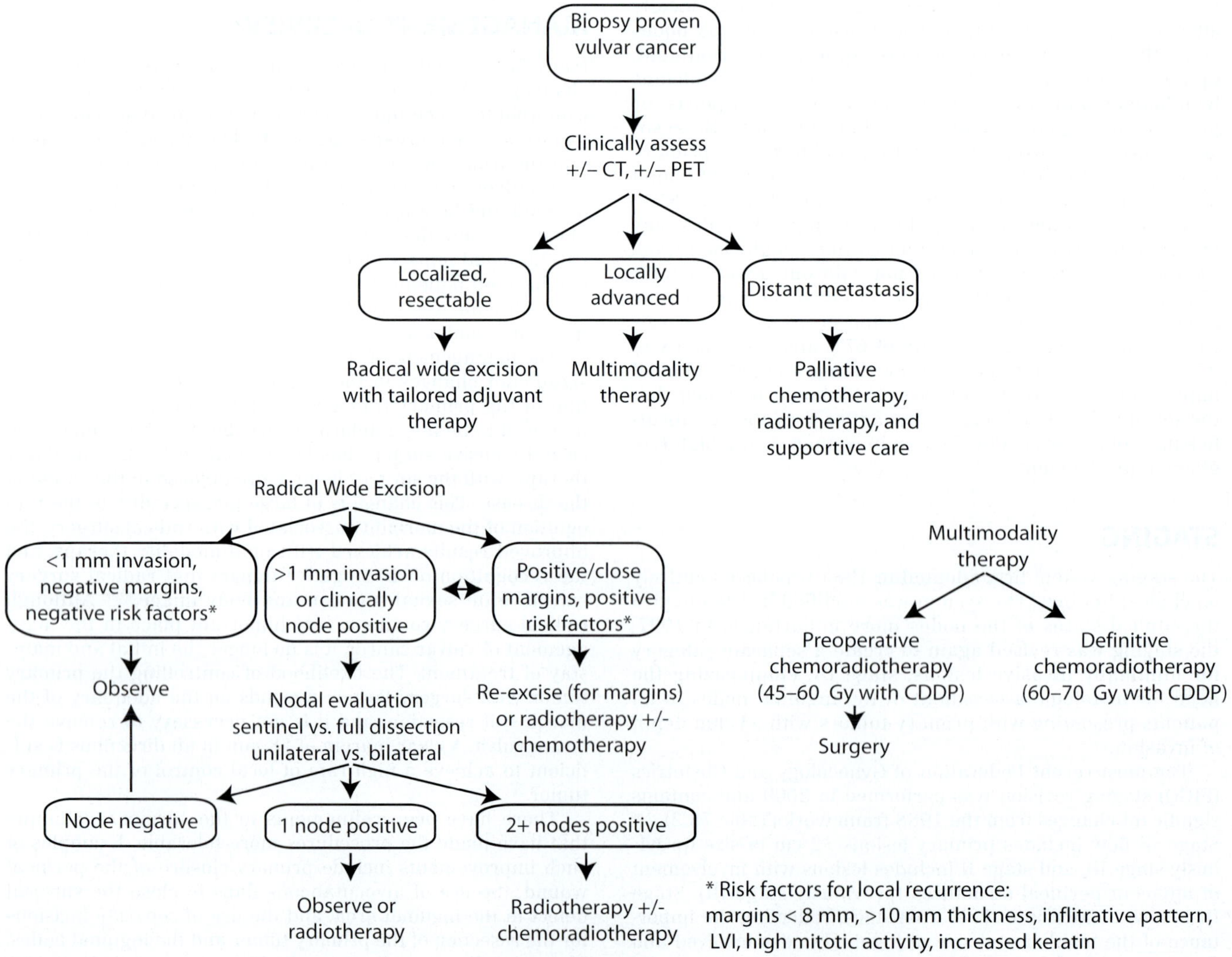

* Risk factors for local recurrence:
margins < 8 mm, >10 mm thickness, inflitrative pattern, LVI, high mitotic activity, increased keratin

normal-appearing tissue is recommended when possible, with a goal of obtaining at least 1-cm microscopic margins in fresh tissue, and ≥8 mm following tissue processing. If the tumor involves or abuts the clitoris, preservation of this structure may not be possible.

Radical vulvectomy is reserved for patients with large or multifocal lesions in whom preservation of normal vulvar tissue is not possible or would not serve a functional or reconstructive benefit. When the anus, vagina, or urethra is involved by malignancy, extended radical vulvectomy or pelvic exenteration is required to clear the disease surgically.[73,74] Surgery alone for patients with advanced disease yielded disappointing results, stimulating interest in multimodality treatment in the mid to late 1980s.[75,76]

Surgical Evaluation of Inguinofemoral Lymph Nodes

Attention to risk factors for nodal involvement is critical as inguinal recurrences are very difficult to treat and a full inguinofemoral node dissection can be quite morbid. The main complications of groin surgery are wound breakdown, infection, and lower extremity lymphedema. Although wound breakdown will often heal successfully by secondary intention, chronic lower extremity edema is very difficult to deal with and can lead to significant long-term disability. To reduce the frequency and the severity of these complications, an effort is made to identify patients in whom the extent of the node dissection can be decreased or eliminated altogether without compromising the likelihood of control of the disease.

As mentioned previously, patients with small (<2-cm diameter) superficial squamous cell carcinomas with a depth of invasion 1 mm or less and no lymph vascular invasion have a very low risk of nodal involvement, and the groin dissection may be omitted.[77] For lesions with >1-mm invasion, groin node assessment should be performed in the form of superficial inguinal lymphadenectomy or sentinel node procedure. Small (<4 cm), lateralized lesions (>2 cm from the midline) may be treated by unilateral groin evaluation, whereas for midline and clitoral lesions, both groins should be assessed. For patients undergoing primary surgery, palpable inguinal nodes should be removed if present.

The need to perform bilateral inguinal node dissection in patients with unilateral vulvar lesions, as well as the need to dissect the deep nodes whenever a superficial node dissection is carried out, has been re-examined in light of the additive morbidity of each procedure. When bilateral superficial and deep inguinal node dissections are performed, the potential for wound breakdown and lower extremity lymphedema increases. When a unilateral dissection is indicated and nodes are found to be negative, a contralateral node dissection is not required because of the low likelihood of contralateral metastasis.[78,79] The deep inguinal node dissection is usually omitted, based on the fact that if the superficial nodes are free of tumor, the deep nodes are rarely involved.[80] However, control of the disease in the lymph nodes is of utmost importance because many women who develop groin recurrences will die as a result of the recurrence.[81]

Women with fixed or ulcerated inguinal nodes are rarely curable with surgery alone. These patients should have a biopsy to document the nodal involvement and should be treated with combined radiation and chemotherapy, either primarily or in a preoperative fashion as discussed below.

Sentinel Lymph Node Dissection

Assessment of the groin nodes may be accomplished via full superficial inguinal dissection or alternatively via a sentinel lymph node procedure alone if performed by groups experienced with this technique. In the multicenter Groningen International Study on Sentinel Nodes in Vulvar Cancer (GROINSS-V), a sentinel node procedure using radioactive tracer and blue dye was performed in 623 groins and resulted in a 2.3% groin recurrence rate following a negative sentinel node.[82] This compares favorably to the 5% ipsilateral groin recurrence rate following negative full superficial inguinal dissection in a prospective GOG study of low-risk vulvar cancer.[81] Patients who underwent a sentinel but not a full node dissection had significantly lower groin wound breakdown (12% vs. 34%) compared to those who went on to a full inguinofemoral dissection following the sentinel procedure. Long-term follow-up of the GROINSS-V trial demonstrated 5- and 10-year recurrence rates of 24.6% and 36.4% for sentinel node–negative patients versus 33.2% and 46.4% in patients who had positive sentinel nodes with subsequent completion inguinofemoral node dissection.[83] Optimal lesions for sentinel node procedures are those with small (<4 cm), unifocal lesions with surgeons who have performed at least 10 prior sentinel procedures under supervision. If a sentinel node approach is undertaken, it is recommended that the sentinel nodes be evaluated prior to vulvar resection to avoid disruption of lymphatic channels emanating from the tumor. If no sentinel node is found, a full inguinofemoral lymphadenectomy is recommended.

The GOG 88 protocol tested whether radiation therapy alone could supplant nodal dissections after vulvectomy.[84] Women with clinically negative nodes after radical vulvectomy were randomized between 50 Gy to the bilateral inguinal regions or a lymph node dissection with selective radiation delivered to those with positive nodes. The radiation-alone arm had increased recurrences within the inguinal regions (at 2 years: 32% RT alone vs. 6% nodal dissection, $P = .033$), with an associated decrement in overall survival as well (59% RT alone vs. 90% nodal dissection, $P = .035$). Although the depth of the inguinal nodes to which the radiation dose was prescribed may account for the difference in local control and survival, surgical management of the lymph nodes remains the standard of care.[85]

Intraoperative diagnosis of inguinal node metastasis necessitates further diagnostic or therapeutic procedures. Because there is no established sentinel node metastasis size cutoff below which withholding further treatment of the groin can be considered safe, all women in whom a sentinel node is found to be positive a full ipsilateral groin dissection and/or radiotherapy to the groin should be considered.[86] The GROINSS-VII/GOG 270 study is ongoing and evaluates groin radiotherapy versus completion inguinofemoral lymphadenectomy in this population.[87] In an interim analysis of this study, excessive recurrences were found in sentinel nodes with macrometastases (>2 mm) or ECE (20%), compared to those without either factor (2%), causing these subjects to be excluded from radiation alone. Particular care should be taken therefore with these risk factors, and completion dissection should be considered.

In the case of a non–sentinel node metastasis that is diagnosed intraoperatively, the options are to dissect the deep nodes as well as the opposite groin or to cover both groins with adjuvant radiotherapy. Standard adjuvant treatment for inguinal node metastasis consists of both inguinal and pelvic radiotherapies.[52] In the situation where an ipsilateral inguinal node is found to be positive for metastatic disease, nodal assessment of the contralateral groin versus radiation should be considered.

Pelvic Lymph Nodes

Patients with clinically or pathologically positive groin nodes are at risk for having contralateral groin and pelvic nodal involvement. Thus, the status of the groin nodes is to be taken into consideration when determining the management of the pelvic nodes. The randomized GOG trial of pelvic node dissection versus pelvic node radiation showed that control of the disease in the pelvis could be achieved with either form of therapy.[52] Radiation to the pelvic nodes is generally preferred over surgery as women in need of treatment to the pelvis often also require radiation to the primary and/or inguinal nodes.

ADJUVANT RADIATION THERAPY

In the setting of early invasive disease treated with wide local excision, radiation to the tumor bed may be advised to prevent local recurrence. As noted previously, pathologic features associated with higher risk of local recurrence at the primary site include lymphatic–vascular invasion (LVI), depth of invasion >5 mm, margins <8 mm, and microscopically positive margins.[59] Faul et al.[88] reported a retrospective study of 62 patients with close (≤8 mm) or positive surgical margins that found that local recurrence was significantly reduced from 58% with observation to 16% with postoperative radiation. Although postoperative radiation reduces the incidence of local recurrence, some may be salvaged with surgery, resulting in equivalent survival and long-term control. However, in the absence of randomized trials, women with positive margins, margins <8 mm, deep invasion, and/or LVI should also be considered for adjuvant radiation.

The role of radiation in the management of inguinal and pelvic nodes was evaluated in the GOG 37 trial reported in 1986.[52] In this trial, women underwent bilateral inguinal lymphadenectomy, and those with positive groin nodes were randomized to either pelvic lymphadenectomy or radiation to the pelvis and bilateral groins. The radiation group had significantly lower groin recurrence rate, 5%, compared to 24% for the group that did not receive radiation. This translated into a 2-year significant survival benefit of 68% versus 54% (P = .03) in favor of the group that received postoperative radiation. Subgroup analysis of this study showed that the benefit was seen primarily in patients with more than one pathologically positive node. An update of this trial, suggested that if the ratio of involved nodes to submitted nodes was >20%, may be a better selection of this higher-risk cohort, which benefits most from radiation.[89] An analysis of the Surveillance, Epidemiology, and End Results databases in patients with one node positive revealed a significant survival difference in patients with <12 nodes submitted, supporting the hypothesis that the benefit of radiation may be greater in patients with an insufficient nodal dissection.[90] However, based on the entry criteria for the GOG 37 study, adjuvant radiation to the pelvis and both groins should be considered for all patients with nodal involvement.

All women with ECE of tumor in the nodes or with residual disease in the inguinal areas should receive postoperative radiation to the pelvis and inguinal areas, because of the increased risk recurrence at the primary and the lymph nodes.[57] When the surgical margins are clear and there is no pathologic indication to treat the vulva, a midline block can be used to avoid the reaction and the sequelae of the treatment to the vulvar area, though consideration should be paid to local risk factors. A series from Dusenbery et al. found the probability of vulvar recurrence to be 48% when midline blocks were used; however, the vulvar recurrence rates in GOG 37 and GOG 88 were only 4% to 9%.[52,84,91]

Adjuvant radiation therapy to the primary site may be delivered with either photons or en face electrons with bolus. When treating a large area of the vulva and groins, AP/PA photon fields may be used; however, increasing data suggest that use of IMRT may be equally effective with much less morbidity. Further details in regard to treatment planning may be found later in the chapter. The elective volume (grossly uninvolved nodal basins) can be treated to 45 to 50.4 Gy. When microscopic disease in the primary tumor area is suspected, a dose of 55 Gy is recommended. When there is ECE of tumor in the lymph nodes, the dose to the groins can be carried up to 60 Gy. If there is gross residual disease postsurgery, the dose to the area should be brought to a minimum of 65 to 70 Gy, a dose used for definitive therapy.

The GOG 37 study required treatment to both groins; however, in the dissection arm of GOG 88, only the ipsilateral groin and hemipelvis were treated suggesting that with well-lateralized lesions, ipsilateral-only treatment may be effective. In a small series of 20 women undergoing ipsilateral radiation alone (44 Gy in 2 Gy fractions), no contralateral recurrences were observed.[92] In fact, the *ipsilateral* recurrence rate was quite high (45% crude rate), suggesting that 44 Gy is an insufficient dose.

The use of adjuvant chemotherapy with radiation therapy, either sequentially or concurrent, has not be tested prospectively. A National Cancer Database (NCDB) study found that adjuvant chemotherapy has been used more frequently since 1999 (11% in 1998 to 41% in 2006) and that the use of chemotherapy is associated with improved overall survival (HR 0.62, 95% CI 0.48 to 0.79).[93] Unfortunately, no details are available in regard to the nature and timing of chemotherapy; however, concurrent cisplatin at 40 mg/m² weekly may be a reasonable extrapolation from the cervical cancer literature for women with higher risk of recurrence (≥2 nodes positive).

PREOPERATIVE RADIATION THERAPY WITH CONCURRENT CHEMOTHERAPY

As the treatment for vulvar cancer has evolved with the goals of decreasing the sequelae of radical surgery and to maximize functional outcome, multimodality therapies have become the standard of care, particularly for patients with advanced stages of disease.[94] After initial concurrent chemoradiation and healing of the reaction, the response to the therapy at the primary site and the lymph nodes is assessed. If there is complete clinical regression of the disease at the site of the primary, one option is to perform biopsies of the primary site, foregoing resection if there is a pathologic complete response.[95] In general, it is recommended to carry out an inguinal dissection as well, as residual disease may be found in lymph nodes.[94] It also should be noted that whereas recurrences at the primary site are potentially salvageable, nodal recurrences, particularly after any prior irradiation, are often fatal.

Preoperative chemoradiation was tested in the phase II GOG 101 trial for patients with advanced primary and/or nodal disease.[94,95] Radiation treatment consisted of 170 cGy twice daily on days 1 to 4 and 170 cGy once a day on day 5 and days 8 to 12, for a dose of 2,380 cGy. Cisplatin, 50 mg/m², was given on day 1, and 5-FU, 1,000 mg/m² by a 24-h infusion, daily on days 1 to 4. The combined cycle of chemotherapy and radiation was repeated after about a 2-week break, thus delivering a total radiation dose of 4,760 cGy. In the locally advanced cohort, the pCR rate was 34% and R0 resections were possible in 77% of subjects. 55% were alive and without disease at last follow-up. In the group of women with advanced nodal disease, the nodes became resectable in 83%, with a pCR rate of 40% in those who underwent surgery, with 43% of the patients being alive and disease free at last follow-up.

The follow-up phase II GOG 205 study enrolled women with T3 or T4 tumors, treated with a total dose of 5,760 cGy (180 cGy/fraction) and weekly cisplatin (40 mg/m²), with no planned treatment breaks.[96] Sixty-nine percent of women were able to complete the protocol per plan, 64% achieved a complete response, and 50% had a pCR on surgical biopsy. Overall survival at 2 years (estimated from curves provided in the manuscript) was 40% for those with no or partial clinical response, 62% for those with a complete clinical response, and

81% for those with a complete pathologic response. As this regimen compares favorably with the prior 101 protocol, it is currently the preferred approach for preoperative therapy.

The next GOG/NRG study (GOG 279) to examine vulvar cancer utilizes a dose of 45 to 50 Gy to the elective nodal volume and 64 Gy to the vulva and gross nodal disease, with a combination of weekly cisplatin and gemcitabine.[97] Dissection is performed upfront for patients with initially resectable nodal disease, and further surgery is reserved for any residual disease after 6 to 8 weeks post treatment.

DEFINITIVE RADIATION THERAPY

The standard of care for early lesions is surgical resection; however, selected patients with small central lesions may be considered for definitive radiation, particularly when the lesions are in close proximity to the urethra, clitoris, or anus. There are few published series of radiation alone used as definitive therapy for vulvar cancer.[98–100] The reported series include patients with recurrent disease postsurgery and patients who are not medically suitable for surgery or have declined it. In Ellis's series of 65 patients treated with brachytherapy and or external beam, the crude 5-year survival rate was 23%, with crude local control in 40%.[98] Slevin and Pointon[100] reported on the results of 58 patients treated also with brachytherapy and/or external beam, depending on the extent of the disease. The crude 5-year survival rate was 26% with a similar local tumor control rate of 40%. These series reflect the difficulty of achieving appropriate curative doses for gross disease with radiation alone.

Selected patients with a low risk of having nodal involvement (<1-mm invasion, or negative lymph node dissection, or sentinel node biopsy) may be treated to the vulvar area alone. The treatment may be delivered using electrons, low-energy photons, or IMRT. When the treatment is given with electrons only, a generous margin around the primary tumor should be used because the dose decreases toward the periphery of the field. Bolus material should be used also to avoid underdosing the surface of the tumor.

Brachytherapy has been used for inoperable vulvar cancer and as a boost to the primary tumor and/or to the lymph nodes. The efficacy of this treatment is difficult to evaluate because of the variability of the clinical situation in which this type of treatment may be employed. Vulvar necrosis

was reported in up to one-third of the patients.[98] A series from the Centre Alexis Vautrin Institute in France describes 34 patients, 21 with primary and 13 with recurrent disease, treated with brachytherapy only.[99] The median brachytherapy dose was 60 Gy, with a range of 53 to 88 Gy. In the group of 21 patients who underwent brachytherapy as primary treatment, 3 patients developed locoregional recurrence, for a 5-year local control rate of 80% and a disease-specific survival of 70%. In the group of 13 patients who were treated for recurrence, 8 developed local recurrence, with or without disease at other sites, for a local control rate of 19%. Of the entire group of 34 patients, 5 developed necrosis. This relatively low complication rate most likely reflects that extensive experience and high quality of the brachytherapy carried out in this institution. The authors of this study advocate brachytherapy for primary vulvar cancer if the patient refuses surgery or if surgery is contraindicated. Nonetheless, because of the significant risk of necrosis, the use of brachytherapy should be limited to very selected cases and performed by experienced practitioners.

DEFINITIVE CHEMORADIATION THERAPY

Definitive chemoradiation is used for patients with advanced tumors considered unresectable at presentation or for patients who are medically inoperable (Table 78.3). This may be used when the tumor does not become resectable in the midst of preoperative intent chemoradiation or as an upfront alternative to surgically based treatment. In these patients, chemotherapy should be continued throughout the entire course of radiation for the purpose of radiosensitization of the tumor in the treatment volume and possible eradication of subclinical disease outside of the radiation field. With appropriate field reductions, the radiation dose should be brought up to 60 to 70 Gy. The total dose to certain areas is dependent upon the location and extent or bulk of the disease, the response to the therapy, and the estimated tolerance of the area requiring the high radiation dose. Often, it is the tolerance of normal tissue that limits the dose to ≤65 Gy.

There is little in the way of comparative prospective trials for chemotherapy selection with concurrent treatment; however, a retrospective series from Dana-Farber/Brigham and Women's Cancer Center and Massachusetts General Hospital does shed some light.[101] In this series of 44 women, 24 of

TABLE 78.3	STUDIES OF CONCURRENT RADIATION AND COMBINATION CHEMOTHERAPY AS PRIMARY TREATMENT FOR ADVANCED VULVAR CANCER						
Authors	**Number of Patients**	**Chemotherapy**	**Radiation Therapy Dose (Gy)**	**Number of Posttreatment Surgeries**	**Median and Range of Follow-up (mo)**	**Clinical Complete Response (%)**	**Clinical Outcome (%)**
Moore et al.[96]	58	P	57.6	34	NS	64	NS
Mak et al.[101]	16	P	50	4	32	60	62 (2 y DFS)
Mak et al.[87]	28	F + P/M	55	6	32	58	56 (2 y DFS)
Tans et al.[102]	28[a]	F + M	60	NS	42	72[a]	71[a] (4 y PFS)
Beriwal et al.[103]	42	P ± F	46.4	33	29	51	66 (3 y LC)
Montana et al.[94]	46	F + P	47.6	38	78 (56–89)	NS	54 (crude NED)
Moore et al.[95]	71	F + P	47.6	64	45	48	63 (crude NED)
Landoni et al.[104]	58[a]	F + M	54	42	(4–48)	27[a]	49[a] (crude NED)
Lupi et al.[105]	24	F + M	54	22	34 (22–73)	42	55 (5 y OS)
Wahlen et al.[106]	19	F ± M	45–50	6	(3–67)	53	89 (5y DSS)
Sebag-Montefiore et al.[107]	37	F + M	45	14	NS	47	37 (2 y OS)
Koh et al.[108]	17	F ± P/M	54	10	(1–75)	53	49 (5 y DSS)
Russell et al.[109]	18	F + P	46.8–72	1	24 (2–52)	89	75 (crude NED)
Natesan et al.[110]	25	P ± F/M	64Gy	3 (salvage only)	26	NS	71 (3 y OS) 65 (3 y LC)

DFS, disease-free survival; DSS, disease-specific survival; F, 5-fluorouracil; M, mitomycin C; NS, not stated; NED, no evidence of disease; OS, overall survival; P, cisplatin; PFS, progression-free survival.
[a]Includes patients treated for recurrent disease.

whom were treated definitively without surgery, 16 received weekly platinum-based regimens, and 28 received a 5-FU–based regimen every 3 to 4 weeks. The 2-year overall survival (74% platinum, 70% 5-FU), disease-free survival (62% platinum, 56% 5-FU), and locoregional recurrence (31% platinum, 33% 5-FU) were no different. The grade 3 or higher skin toxicity was higher with weekly platinum (62% platinum, 32% 5-FU), but the nonskin toxicity was higher with 5-FU (13% platinum, 46% 5-FU). Given these data and the results of GOG 101 of weekly platinum in preoperative treatment (discussed above), weekly platinum at 40 mg/m² is a reasonable option for concurrent treatment.[96]

There are no prospective data comparing chemoradiotherapy alone and combined with surgery; however, an NCDB study has examined survival after both strategies have been reported.[111] In the overall cohort, women undergoing primary radiation had overall survival at 3 years of 42% compared to 57% with radiation plus surgery. However, when limiting the definitive cohort to those who received concurrent chemotherapy and radiation to doses ≥55 Gy, the survival improved to 57%, comparable to preoperative approaches. Although there are multiple possible confounders not captured in the NCDB, these data suggest that initial chemotherapy and radiation may be used initially with surgery reserved for salvage.

TREATMENT VOLUME AND TECHNIQUE

Simulation and Target Delineation

Appropriate identification of the targets of treatment is a challenging but critical process in vulvar cancer. CT- or MR-based 3-D planning is essential to establish the location, extent, and depth of the inguinal and pelvic nodal basins, as well as the primary. Specific components of each individual's treatment volume depend on the clinical scenario and are discussed above.

At the time of simulation, markers should be placed on the primary, the lymph nodes, and scars from previous surgery to document the extent of the disease. "Frog-leg" positioning may be used to reduce skin folds in the inguinal regions, though this may be less important if IMRT is used. Advanced immobilization devices such as a cradle can be considered, though, for some, the cradle itself may become uncomfortable during treatment because of the expected skin reaction.

Bubble wrap or bariatric slings may also be used to reduce skin folds, particularly in patients with a pronounced panniculus. Bolus is often critical over the vulva and groins, which may be applied at the time of simulation or applied "virtually" at the time of treatment planning—however, obtaining good contact against the skin at all points to eliminate significant air gap is challenging. Use of wet gauze, towels, or impregnated gauze may be necessary. Placement of bolus should be confirmed at the time of treatment, either through direct inspection of setup or the use of onboard imaging such as a cone beam, if available.

The primary vulvar lesion (pGTV) may be hard to identify on CT imaging alone, making the use of radiopaque markers critical. MRI and PET imaging if available may also aid in the identification of the primary lesion. When defining a primary PTV, ample margins (1.5 to 2 cm) should be placed to account for microscopic spread of disease and the potential variations in daily setup. Additional clinical tumor volume (CTV) coverage of the vagina should be added for lesions that involve the introitus. The uterus, if present, is not usually target.

The nodal targets include the inguinal basins, which should be defined based on anatomic compartment; symmetric margins around the vessels are inadequate, leading to undertreatment medially and overtreatment to deep structures.[112] This compartment is defined by:

Lateral: The medial border of the iliopsoas
Medial: The lateral border of adductor longus or medial end of pectineus
Posterior: The iliopsoas muscle laterally and anterior aspect of the pectineus muscle medially
Anterior: The anterior edge of sartorius muscle (Fig. 78.6).

The pelvic nodes are often also targets of treatment and include the obturator and external and internal iliac chains, defined in a manner similar to uterine or cervical disease. Common iliac nodes or para-aortic basins may be added if there are nodes positive in the more distal echelons. Presacral basins are usually not target, unless there is involvement of the anal canal or rectum.

Consensus contours are now available to guide treatment and may be very helpful particularly when more conformal techniques such as IMRT are used.[113]

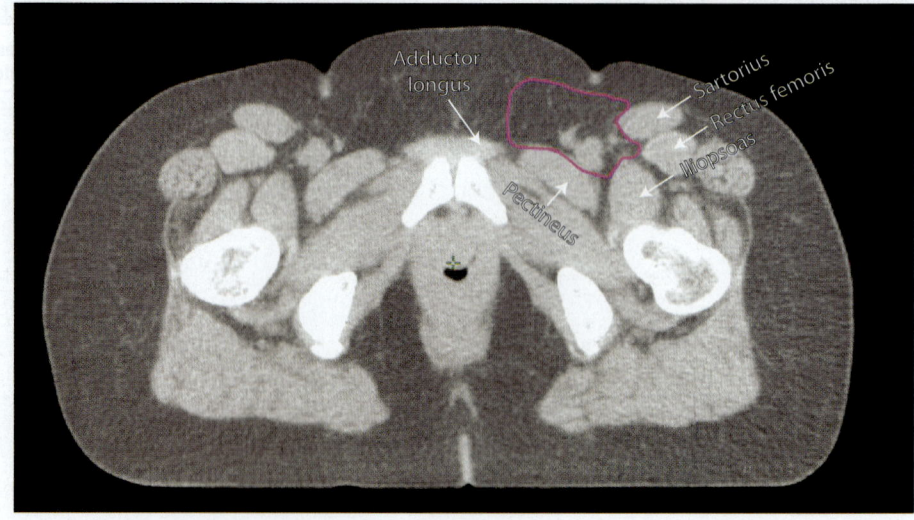

FIGURE 78.6. Example of a CTV for inguinal treatment (*purple contour*). The lateral border is the medial edge of the iliopsoas. The medial border is the lateral extent of the adductor longus or medial end of pectineus. The posterior border is bounded by the iliopsoas muscle laterally and anterior aspect of the pectineus muscle medially. The anterior border is carried over from the anterior edge of sartorius muscle. All benign nodes also should be included, and the inferior extent should extend 1 to 2 cm below the vulva and perineum.

2-D and 3-D Conformal Treatment

Medium- or high-energy photon beams with anteroposterior/posteroanterior (AP/PA) fields with the patient in the supine position are recommended for the 3-D delivery of external beam. The superior border of the pelvic field should extend to the middle of the sacroiliac joints to cover the external and internal iliac nodes. If a patient has internal or external iliac node involvement, the superior border should be extended to the L3/L4 interspace to cover the common iliac nodes. The inferior border should cover the entire vulva and the most superficial, inferior inguinal nodes. Laterally, the pelvic field extends 2 cm laterally to the widest point of the pelvic inlet. Although there are no data regarding scar recurrences, it is common practice to include the inguinal node dissection scars in the radiation field.

Depending on whether the inguinofemoral lymph nodes and/or pelvic lymph nodes are to be included in the radiation volume, different field configurations may be used. To reduce the dose to the femoral heads while delivering an adequate dose to the inguinal nodes, various techniques are available.

One approach is to use a wide AP field that includes the pelvic and inguinal areas, with a narrow PA field covering only the pelvis and sparing the femoral heads. The photon fields are weighted equally, and the inguinal dose is supplemented by separate anterior electron fields matched to the pelvic field (Fig. 78.7). Bolus material should be used to ensure adequate dose to the superficial portions of the groin.

An alternative method consists of using a wide AP field and narrow PA field, with a partial transmission block placed in the central portion of the AP field. The desired dose at a specified depth is delivered to the inguinal nodes through the AP field.[114] The degree of central anterior beam attenuation is calculated so that the midpoint of the pelvis receives equal doses from the AP and PA beams. This technique eliminates the dosimetric problems of photon/electron field matching, as well as the potential for daily setup variation, but the design of a precise partial transmission block is difficult.

Another method consists in using matched AP/PA fields to include the primary and the pelvic nodes and treating the groins through separate anterior electron fields. This approach has the advantage of relatively easy setup, but the main drawback is ensuring an adequate dose at the match line, particularly when the match line is over gross disease. An example of an AP radiation field encompassing the inguinal/femoral and pelvic lymph nodes is shown in Figure 78.8.

Moran et al.[115] described a modified segmental boost technique using multileaf collimators with a single-isocenter technique and a wide AP field to cover the vulva, pelvis, and groins and a narrow PA field to cover the vulva and pelvis. The supplemental anterior photon groin fields are angled such that the central axis is coplanar with the divergence from the PA field. The medial blocking of the groin fields is designed to match the divergence from the PA field. This technique provides a more homogeneous dose distribution and is easier to reproduce on a daily basis.

Intensity-Modulated Radiotherapy

Intensity-modulated radiotherapy (IMRT) is now often used to treat the pelvis and inguinal nodes.[103,116,117] Beriwal et al.[116] reported 15 patients treated with IMRT using a median of 7 fields. The CTV was defined as a 1- to 2-cm margin around bilateral external iliac, internal iliac, and inguinofemoral nodes, as well as a 1-cm margin around the entire vulvar region. Gross tumor was also expanded by 1 cm for the CTV. The planning treatment volume was defined as 1-cm margin beyond the CTV, and the prescription dose was 43 to 48 Gy for preoperative treatment and 50 Gy for postoperative treatment, delivered partly on a twice-daily schedule. This early experience yielded reasonable clinical response, with 13 of 15 patients having no evidence of disease at last follow-up. This technique also resulted in improved dose conformality and lower doses to normal structures, including the rectum, bladder, small bowel, and femoral heads. The most recent update of this series found a pCR rate of 48%, 3-year overall survival of 61%, and 3-year local recurrence–free survival of 66%.[103] These results are comparable to the GOG 101 results and cause less acute skin toxicity than 2D or 3D techniques.

It must be noted that careful quality assurance is required when using IMRT. In particular, care should be placed to ensure that the surface of the vulvar tumor receives adequate dose. This may be accomplished by creating a "virtual flash" during treatment planning, where the PTV is expanded out of the skin by 1 to 2 cm, with additional placement of virtual tissue equivalent to allow for dose buildup. This protects against underdosing the tumor surface if there is superior displacement of the patient during treatment. Placement of thermoluminescent dosimetry chips or similar in the inguinal and perineum areas is recommended to document the dose given to the skin and target areas (Fig. 78.9).

FIGURE 78.7. Treatment borders demonstrating the wide anterior field (*outer border*) and the narrow posterior field (*shaded region*).

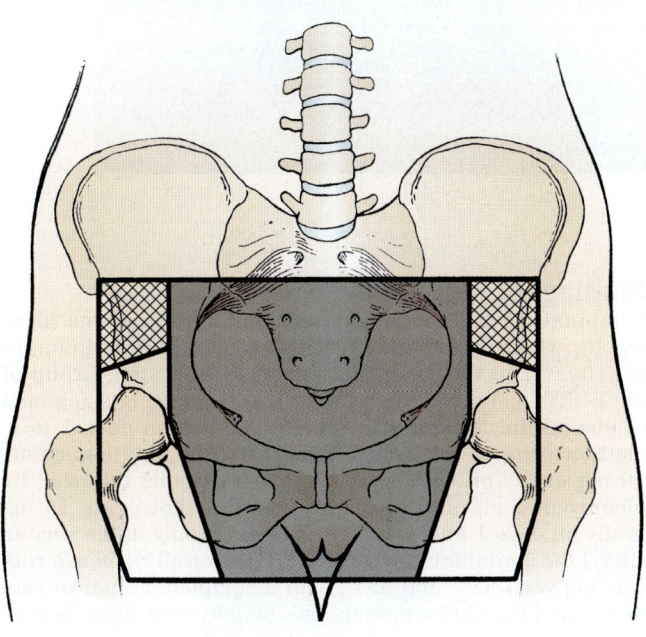

CHEMOTHERAPY

The use of chemotherapy alone is usually reserved for patients having advanced, inoperable, or recurrent disease. Limited data exist given the rarity of this tumor type and the diversity of treatment regimens used in small, single-institution studies.

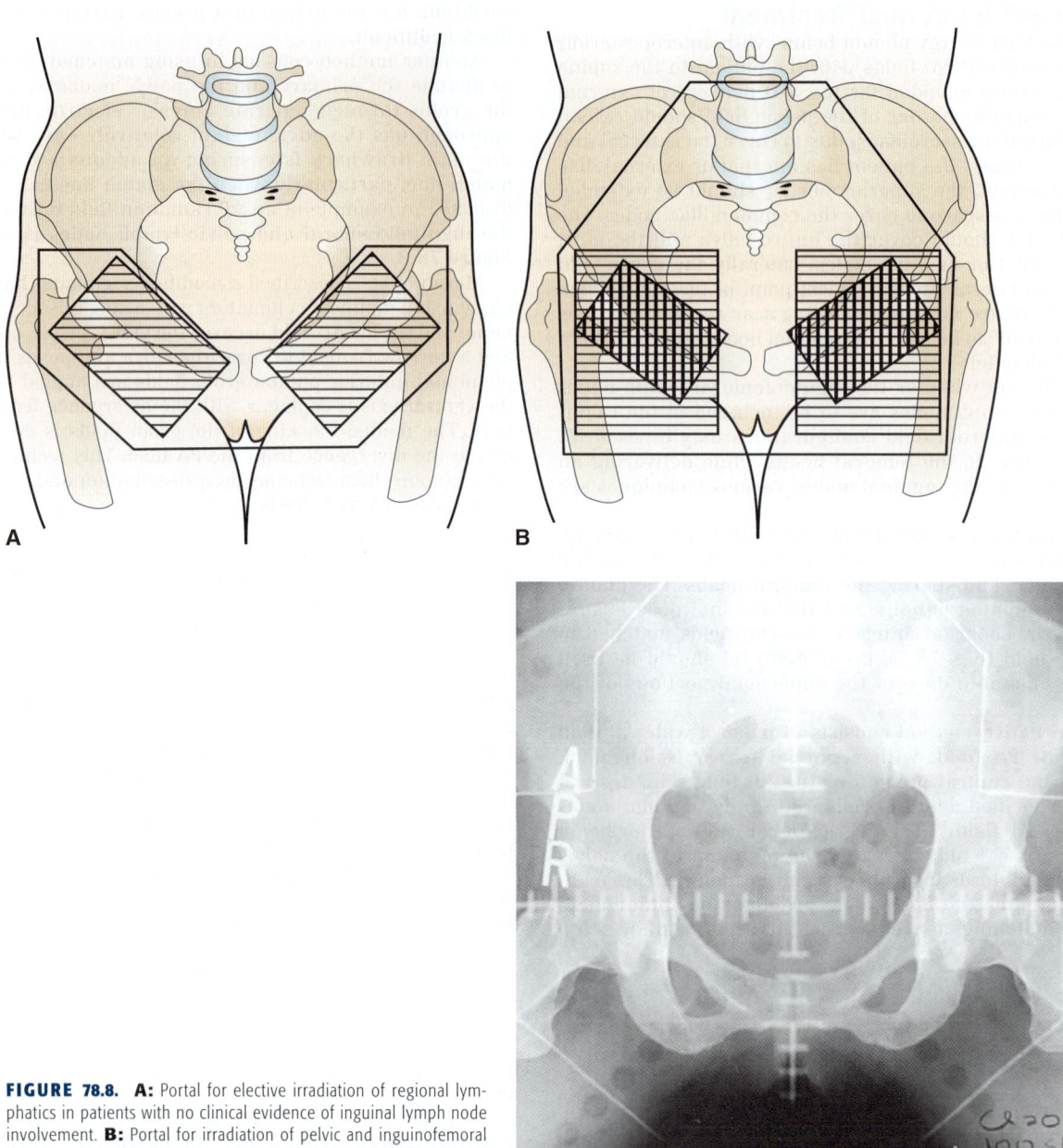

FIGURE 78.8.   **A:** Portal for elective irradiation of regional lymphatics in patients with no clinical evidence of inguinal lymph node involvement. **B:** Portal for irradiation of pelvic and inguinofemoral lymph nodes and vulvar area. A final boost to the positive inguinal lymph nodes may be given with a reduced field. **C:** Simulation film of portal covering pelvic and inguinofemoral lymph nodes and vulva.

Single-Agent Chemotherapy

There is limited experience with single-agent chemotherapy for the treatment of vulvar cancer (Table 78.4). The single agents cisplatin, piperazinedione, mitoxantrone, and etoposide have all been evaluated prospectively by the GOG with disappointing results.[123-125] Paclitaxel has moderate activity, with a 14% response rate described in a phase II trial of the European Organization for Radiation Therapy and Chemotherapy (EORTC).[54] Bleomycin has been tested in older studies as a single agent in both the neoadjuvant and recurrent settings with a high initial response rate.[126,127] Limited objective responses have also been reported in a small number of patients with doxorubicin.[128]

Multiagent Regimens

Combination chemotherapy regimens have included bleomycin, which is associated with considerable pulmonary toxicity.[129] The Gynecological Cancer Cooperative Group of the EORTC conducted two phase II studies using a regimen of bleomycin, 5 mg intramuscularly, given on days 1 to 5, methotrexate 15 mg orally on days 1 and 4, and lomustine, 40 mg orally on days 5 to 7 in the 1st week, followed by bleomycin 5 mg intramuscularly and methotrexate 15 mg orally on days 1 and 4 (modified to day 1 only in the second study) for 5 additional weeks.[119,120] The overall response rate was between 55% and 65%, with a complete response rate of 8% to 11%. Unfortunately, the toxicity was high. Severe mucositis was noted in up to 21% of patients, 13% had severe infections, and up to 7% developed severe pulmonary toxicity, with one death in each of the two studies possibly due to pulmonary toxicity. Other severe toxicities included nausea/vomiting and hematologic, renal, and mucocutaneous reactions. A group of prospective studies evaluated cisplatin, bleomycin, and methotrexate in the neoadjuvant setting and reported a 10% response rate of the primary tumor but a 67% response rate of nodal disease after two cycles of treatment.[121]

In other small series, combinations of cisplatin with a second agent such as vinorelbine or 5-fluorouracil showed significant activity.[118,130] In a recent small report of neoadjuvant chemotherapy with cisplatin and 5-fluorouracil, at least a partial response was observed in all 10 patients. Of interest, three patients were treated with cisplatin alone in the same series with no responses.[118]

Biologic Agents

The epidermal growth factor receptor (EGFR) is a tyrosine kinase overexpressed in many squamous cell carcinomas of the vulva.[131] Erlotinib, an EGFR inhibitor, was reported to have significant activity in a case report, leading to the development of a phase II trial of this agent for women with lesions amenable to surgery or chemoradiation (cohort 1) or metastatic measurable disease.[132] The overall clinical benefit rate was 67.5% with 27.5% experiencing partial responses and 40% with stable disease. Responses, however, were of short duration. Rare but significant grade 3-4 toxicities included diarrhea/electrolyte abnormalities, ischemic colitis, and renal failure.[133] In one other case report, the EGFR inhibitor cetuximab elicited a partial response when administered in combination with cisplatin.[134] Further studies may elucidate the role of EGRF-targeted agents and other biologics in the treatment of this disease.

In conclusion, paclitaxel and erlotinib are single agents showing activity against advanced vulvar cancer in phase II studies. Combination chemotherapy regimens, particularly those including cisplatin and 5-fluorouracil, yield improved response rates, but they are associated with significant toxicity. Bleomycin as single agent and in combination also appears to have activity but with risk of significant pulmonary toxicity. In the recurrent or metastatic setting, the choice of regimen requires consideration of single agents having modest activity but low toxicity versus combination regimens that carry both higher response and toxicity rates.

TREATMENT SEQUELAE

The adverse effects of treatment can be classified as acute or chronic and depend on the treatment modality or modalities used, as well as the intensity of the treatment. With early-stage disease and appropriately limited surgery to the primary site, the acute surgical complications are relatively minor and essentially consist of wound infection and hematomas. With more extensive surgery, the frequency and degree of the complications can be far more significant. With single "longhorn" or "butterfly" incisions for bilateral inguinal lymphadenectomies and for resection of the primary, wound infection, necrosis, and breakdown occurred in as many as 50% to 85% of the cases. Since the use of separate incisions was adopted, the incidence of groin wound infection, necrosis, and breakdown has decreased dramatically to a low as 15%.[44,135] Other potential complications of surgery include wound infections, seromas, hemorrhage, deep vein thrombosis, pulmonary embolism, osteitis pubis, and loss of sensory perception in the anterior aspect of the thigh secondary to femoral nerve injury.

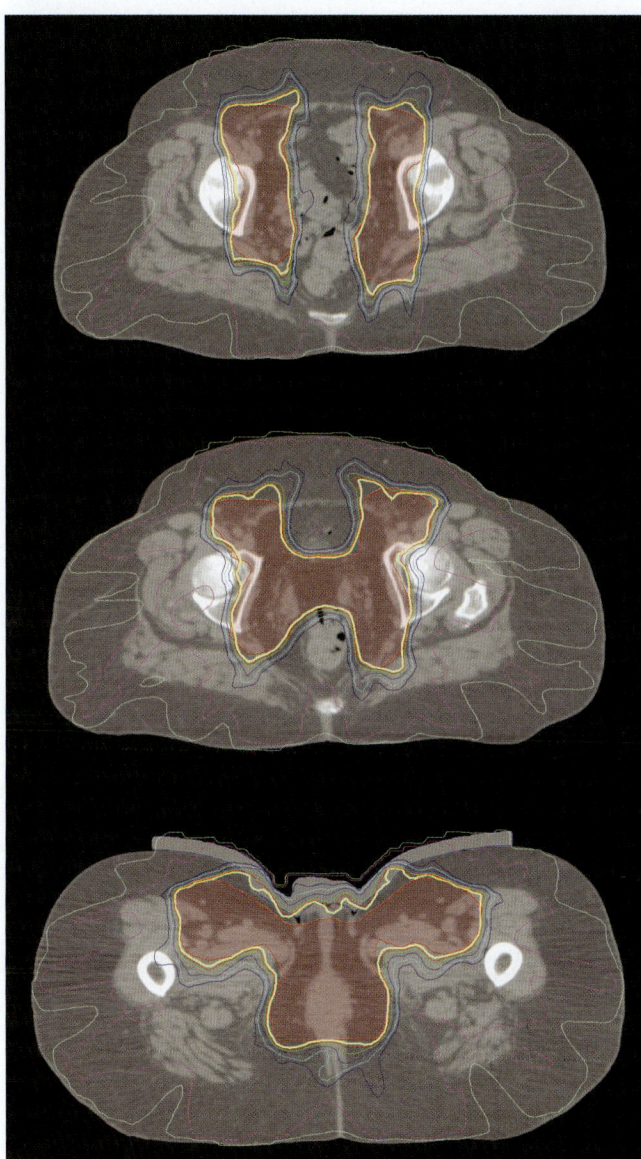

FIGURE 78.9. IMRT for vulvar cancer. This patient had a lesion of the posterior portion of the labia minora, involving the fourchette and the distal vagina. Three axial views are shown of the conformality of the 100% isodose line (*yellow*) and the planning treatment volume contour (*shaded red volume*). The central dose in the middle axial level is the superior margin for the vagina, added in this case because of the distal vaginal involvement.

TABLE 78.4 CHEMOTHERAPY FOR VULVAR CANCER

Authors	Number of Patients	Regimen	Partial Response (Number of Patients)	Complete Response (Number of Patients)
Geisler et al.[118]	9	FP	5	4
Geisler et al.[118]	3	P	0	0
Wagenaar et al.[119]	25	BMC	12	2
Durrant et al.[120]	31	BMC	15	3
Benedetti-Panici et al.[121]	21	PBM	Tumor, 2 Node, 3	Tumor, 0 Node, 11
Belinson et al.[122]	3	BOMP	0	0

BMC, bleomycin, methotrexate, CCNU; BOMP, bleomycin, vincristine, mitomycin C, cisplatin; FP, 5-fluorouracil, cisplatin; P, cisplatin; PBM, cisplatin, bleomycin, methotrexate.

The most significant chronic surgical complication is edema of the lower extremities. Lymphedema is related to the extent of the lymphadenectomy, and it is therefore more likely to occur with a deep inguinal node dissection. The incidence of lymphedema may be as high as 69%.[135,136] Lymphedema can be progressive and very difficult to manage. Early referral for physical therapy is indicated to prevent progression and stimulate regression of symptoms. Other chronic complications reported are chronic cellulitis of the inguinal areas, stenosis of the introitus, femoral hernias, and rectovaginal or rectoperineal fistulas.

The most significant acute morbidity of radiation, alone or in combination with chemotherapy, is the mucocutaneous reaction in the vulva, perineum, and inguinal folds that may develop early during the course of the treatment. The severity of the reaction depends upon the radiation fractionation schema used and the type of chemotherapy employed. The degree of reaction may be such that a treatment interruption is unavoidable. Topical agents, such as zinc oxide preparations, may be helpful; however, this preparation must be off the skin during radiation treatments because it can exacerbate the skin reaction. Sitz baths with sodium bicarbonate may also aid in the cleansing and soothing of the affected skin. Treatment of candidal infections with appropriate antifungal agents should be provided as required. Narcotic pain medications may also be required in the final weeks of treatment.

Acute hematologic toxicity is common and depends upon the type and intensity of the chemotherapy used. Decreased leukocytes may be managed well with colony-stimulating factors, and blood transfusions may be necessary for anemia. Chemotherapy dose adjustments or interruptions are sometimes required. Severe hematologic toxicity can lead to septicemia, with fatal consequences in some instances.[94,109]

The late complications of chemotherapy/radiation and surgery combined include telangiectasis and atrophy of the skin and mucosa of the vulva, dryness of the mucosa of the vagina and vulva, and narrowing of the vaginal introitus. Avascular necrosis of the femoral head is rare, even when AP/PA photon fields that include the inguinal nodes are used. In the GOG combined-modality study for patients with advanced disease, only one patient developed avascular necrosis of the femoral head.[94] In this study, there were two instances of injury to the femoral artery. In one patient, necrosis of the femoral artery occurred immediately following surgery and was fatal. The second patient required femoral artery angioplasty.

Besides the generally recognized complications seen with surgery, radiation, and/or chemotherapy, the treatment of carcinoma of the vulva has significant psychosexual consequences. In some instances, these consequences can be far greater than expected when considering the type and extent of the therapy given. The psychosexual impact of the treatment has been studied by some investigators, but it has not received the attention that it merits, possibly because of the difficulty in its nature and impact.[87] In a study by Andersen et al.[137] of 42 patients, most of whom were treated with conservative surgery, with wide local excision in 32 patients and simple vulvectomy in 10, there was a two- to threefold increase in the frequency of sexual dysfunction from the pretreatment level. In this study, 30% of the patients were sexually inactive at follow-up. Andersen and Hacker[138] also reported that vulvar surgery has a significant impact on sexual functioning and body image even when intercourse remains possible. As might be expected, after pelvic exenteration, patients also experience significant sexual dysfunction,

even when a neovagina is created. Ostomies necessitated by exenteration have a significant detrimental impact on quality of life.[139] The concern for the significant impact of radical surgery on patients with carcinoma of the vulva has been the principal reason for the development of multimodality therapy. Organ preservation, maintenance of function, and improved body image with reasonable control of the disease can be achieved in women with this disease, particularly when the disease is in an early stage.

REFERENCES

1. American Cancer Society. *Cancer facts & figures.* Atlanta, GA: American Cancer Society, 2017.
2. National Cancer Institute. *Fast Stats: an interactive tool for access to SEER statistics.* Bethesda: National Cancer Institute, 2017.
3. de Sanjose S, Alemany L, Ordi J, et al. Worldwide human papillomavirus genotype attribution in over 2000 cases of intraepithelial and invasive lesions of the vulva. *Eur J Cancer* 2013;49:3450–3461.
4. Brinton LA, Thistle JE, Liao LM, et al. Epidemiology of vulvar neoplasia in the NIH-AARP Study. *Gynecol Oncol* 2017;145(2):298–304.
5. Trietsch MD, Nooij LS, Gaarenstroom KN, et al. Genetic and epigenetic changes in vulvar squamous cell carcinoma and its precursor lesions: a review of the current literature. *Gynecol Oncol* 2015;136:143–157.
6. Bleeker MC, Visser PJ, Overbeek LI, et al. Lichen sclerosus: incidence and risk of vulvar squamous cell carcinoma. *Cancer Epidemiol Biomarkers Prev* 2016;25:1224–1230.
7. Halonen P, Jakobsson M, Heikinheimo O, et al. Lichen sclerosus and risk of cancer. *Int J Cancer* 2017;140:1998–2002.
8. van Seters M, van Beurden M, de Craen AJ. Is the assumed natural history of vulvar intraepithelial neoplasia III based on enough evidence? A systematic review of 3322 published patients. *Gynecol Oncol* 2005;97:645–651.
9. Hoang LN, Park KJ, Soslow RA, et al. Squamous precursor lesions of the vulva: current classification and diagnostic challenges. *Pathology* 2016;48:291–302.
10. Trimble CL, Hildesheim A, Brinton LA, et al. Heterogeneous etiology of squamous carcinoma of the vulva. *Obstet Gynecol* 1996;87:59–64.
11. Toki T, Kurman RJ, Park JS, et al. Probable nonpapillomavirus etiology of squamous cell carcinoma of the vulva in older women: a clinicopathologic study using in situ hybridization and polymerase chain reaction. *Int J Gynecol Pathol* 1991;10:107–125.
12. Santos M, Landolfi S, Olivella A, et al. p16 overexpression identifies HPV-positive vulvar squamous cell carcinomas. *Am J Surg Pathol* 2006;30:1347–1356.
13. McAlpine JN, Leung S, Cheng A, et al. HPV-independent vulvar squamous cell carcinoma has a worse prognosis than HPV-associated disease: a retrospective cohort study. *Histopathology* 2017;1(2):238–246.
14. Sznurkowski JJ, Zawrocki A, Biernat W. The overexpression of p16 is not a surrogate marker for high-risk human papilloma virus genotypes and predicts clinical outcomes for vulvar cancer. *BMC Cancer* 2016;16:465.
15. Hunter DJ. Carcinoma of the vulva: a review of 361 patients. *Gynecol Oncol* 1975;3:117–123.
16. Carlson JA, Ambros R, Malfetano J, et al. Vulvar lichen sclerosus and squamous cell carcinoma: a cohort, case control, and investigational study with historical perspective; implications for chronic inflammation and sclerosis in the development of neoplasia. *Hum Pathol* 1998;29:932–948.
17. Pecorelli S. Revised FIGO staging for carcinoma of the vulva, cervix, and endometrium. *Int J Gynaecol Obstet* 2009;105:103–104.
18. Wilkinson EJ, Rico MJ, Pierson KK. Microinvasive carcinoma of the vulva. *Int J Gynecol Pathol* 1982;1:29–39.
19. Creasman WT, Phillips JL, Menck HR. A survey of hospital management practices for vulvar melanoma. *J Am Coll Surg* 1999;188:670–675.
20. Stang A, Streller B, Eisinger B, et al. Population-based incidence rates of malignant melanoma of the vulva in Germany. *Gynecol Oncol* 2005;96:216–221.
21. Irvin WP Jr, Legallo RL, Stoler MH, et al. Vulvar melanoma: a retrospective analysis and literature review. *Gynecol Oncol* 2001;83:457–465.
22. Hou JY, Baptiste C, Hombalegowda RB, et al. Vulvar and vaginal melanoma: a unique subclass of mucosal melanoma based on a comprehensive molecular analysis of 51 cases compared with 2253 cases of nongynecologic melanoma. *Cancer* 2017;123:1333–1344.
23. Bradgate MG, Rollason TP, McConkey CC, et al. Malignant melanoma of the vulva: a clinicopathological study of 50 women. *Br J Obstet Gynaecol* 1990;97:124–133.
24. Raber G, Mempel V, Jackisch C, et al. Malignant melanoma of the vulva. Report of 89 patients. *Cancer* 1996;78:2353–2358.
25. Podratz KC, Gaffey TA, Symmonds RE, et al. Melanoma of the vulva: an update. *Gynecol Oncol* 1983;16:153–168.
26. Davidson T, Kissin M, Westbury G. Vulvo-vaginal melanoma—should radical surgery be abandoned? *Br J Obstet Gynaecol* 1987;94:473–476.
27. van der Linden M, Schuurman M, Bulten J, et al. Incidence and survival of glandular vulvar malignancies in the Netherlands. *Gynecol Oncol* 2017;144:553–557.

28. Copeland LJ, Sneige N, Gershenson DM, et al. Bartholin gland carcinoma. *Obstet Gynecol* 1986;67:794–801.

29. Leuchter RS, Hacker NF, Voet RL, et al. Primary carcinoma of the Bartholin gland: a report of 14 cases and review of the literature. *Obstet Gynecol* 1982;60:361–368.

30. Cardosi RJ, Speights A, Fiorica JV, et al. Bartholin's gland carcinoma: a 15-year experience. *Gynecol Oncol* 2001;82:247–251.

31. Pierie JP, Choudry U, Muzikansky A, et al. Prognosis and management of extra-mammary Paget's disease and the association with secondary malignancies. *J Am Coll Surg* 2003;196:45–50.

32. MacLean AB, Makwana M, Ellis PE, et al. The management of Paget's disease of the vulva. *J Obstet Gynaecol* 2004;24:124–128.

33. Tolia M, Tsoukalas N, Sofoudis C, et al. Primary extramammary invasive Paget's vulvar disease: what is the standard, what are the challenges and what is the future for radiotherapy? *BMC Cancer* 2016;16:563.

34. Cowan RA, Black DR, Hoang LN, et al. A pilot study of topical imiquimod therapy for the treatment of recurrent extramammary Paget's disease. *Gynecol Oncol* 2016;142:139–143.

35. Liu G, Li Q, Shang X, et al. Verrucous carcinoma of the vulva: a 20 year retrospective study and literature review. *J Low Genit Tract Dis* 2016;20:114–118.

36. Japaze H, Van Dinh T, Woodruff JD. Verrucous carcinoma of the vulva: study of 24 cases. *Obstet Gynecol* 1982;60:462–466.

37. Kraus FT, Perezmesa C. Verrucous carcinoma. Clinical and pathologic study of 105 cases involving oral cavity, larynx and genitalia. *Cancer* 1966;19:26–38.

38. de Giorgi V, Salvini C, Massi D, et al. Vulvar basal cell carcinoma: retrospective study and review of literature. *Gynecol Oncol* 2005;97:192–194.

39. Plentl A, Friedman E. *Lymphatic system of the female genitalia: the morphologic basis of oncologic diagnosis and therapy.* Philadelphia: WB Saunders, 1971.

40. Franklin EW III, Rutledge FD. Prognostic factors in epidermoid carcinoma of the vulva. *Obstet Gynecol* 1971;37:892–901.

41. Krupp PJ, Bohm JW. Lymph gland metastases in invasive squamous cell cancer of the vulva. *Am J Obstet Gynecol* 1978;130:943–952.

42. Boutselis JG. Radical vulvectomy for invasive squamous cell carcinoma of the vulva. *Obstet Gynecol* 1972;39:827–836.

43. Donaldson ES, Powell DE, Hanson MB, et al. Prognostic parameters in invasive vulvar cancer. *Gynecol Oncol* 1981;11:184–190.

44. Hacker NF, Leuchter RS, Berek JS, et al. Radical vulvectomy and bilateral inguinal lymphadenectomy through separate groin incisions. *Obstet Gynecol* 1981;58:574–579.

45. Parker RT, Duncan I, Rampone J, et al. Operative management of early invasive epidermoid carcinoma of the vulva. *Am J Obstet Gynecol* 1975;123:349–355.

46. Rutledge F, Smith JP, Franklin EW. Carcinoma of the vulva. *Am J Obstet Gynecol* 1970;106:1117–1130.

47. Sedlis A, Homesley H, Bundy BN, et al. Positive groin lymph nodes in superficial squamous cell vulvar cancer. A Gynecologic Oncology Group Study. *Am J Obstet Gynecol* 1987;156:1159–1164.

48. Berman ML, Soper JT, Creasman WT, et al. Conservative surgical management of superficially invasive stage I vulvar carcinoma. *Gynecol Oncol* 1989;35:352–357.

49. Rowley KC, Gallion HH, Donaldson ES, et al. Prognostic factors in early vulvar cancer. *Gynecol Oncol* 1988;31:43–49.

50. Homesley HD, Bundy BN, Sedlis A, et al. Assessment of current International Federation of Gynecology and Obstetrics staging of vulvar carcinoma relative to prognostic factors for survival (a Gynecologic Oncology Group study). *Am J Obstet Gynecol* 1991;164:997–1003; discussion: 1003–1004.

51. Homesley HD, Bundy BN, Sedlis A, et al. Prognostic factors for groin node metastasis in squamous cell carcinoma of the vulva (a Gynecologic Oncology Group study). *Gynecol Oncol* 1993;49:279–283.

52. Homesley HD, Bundy BN, Sedlis A, et al. Radiation therapy versus pelvic node resection for carcinoma of the vulva with positive groin nodes. *Obstet Gynecol* 1986;68:733–740.

53. Thaker NG, Klopp AH, Jhingran A, et al. Survival outcomes for patients with stage IVB vulvar cancer with grossly positive pelvic lymph nodes: time to reconsider the FIGO staging system? *Gynecol Oncol* 2015;136:269–273.

54. Witteveen PO, van der Velden J, Vergote I, et al. Phase II study on paclitaxel in patients with recurrent, metastatic or locally advanced vulvar cancer not amenable to surgery or radiotherapy: a study of the EORTC-GCG (European Organisation for Research and Treatment of Cancer—Gynaecological Cancer Group). *Ann Oncol* 2009;20:1511–1516.

55. Farias-Eisner R, Cirisano FD, Grouse D, et al. Conservative and individualized surgery for early squamous carcinoma of the vulva: the treatment of choice for stage I and II (T1-2 N0-1 M0) disease. *Gynecol Oncol* 1994;53:55–58.

56. Origoni M, Sideri M, Garsia S, et al. Prognostic value of pathological patterns of lymph node positivity in squamous cell carcinoma of the vulva stage III and IVA FIGO. *Gynecol Oncol* 1992;45:313–316.

57. van der Velden J, van Lindert AC, Lammes FB, et al. Extracapsular growth of lymph node metastases in squamous cell carcinoma of the vulva. The impact on recurrence and survival. *Cancer* 1995;75:2885–2890.

58. Curry SL, Wharton JT, Rutledge F. Positive lymph nodes in vulvar squamous carcinoma. *Gynecol Oncol* 1980;9:63–67.

59. Heaps JM, Fu YS, Montz FJ, et al. Surgical-pathologic variables predictive of local recurrence in squamous cell carcinoma of the vulva. *Gynecol Oncol* 1990;38:309–314.

60. Kurzl R, Messerer D. Prognostic factors in squamous cell carcinoma of the vulva: a multivariate analysis. *Gynecol Oncol* 1989;32:143–150.

61. Mann WJ, Baim R, Patsner B, et al. The value of CT scanning in the management of patients with gynecologic malignancies. *Arch Gynecol Obstet* 1989;246:15–25.

62. Kataoka MY, Sala E, Baldwin P, et al. The accuracy of magnetic resonance imaging in staging of vulvar cancer: a retrospective multi-centre study. *Gynecol Oncol* 2010;117:82–87.

63. Land R, Herod J, Moskovic E, et al. Routine computerized tomography scanning, groin ultrasound with or without fine needle aspiration cytology in the surgical management of primary squamous cell carcinoma of the vulva. *Int J Gynecol Cancer* 2006;16:312–317.

64. Cohn DE, Dehdashti F, Gibb RK, et al. Prospective evaluation of positron emission tomography for the detection of groin node metastases from vulvar cancer. *Gynecol Oncol* 2002;85:179–184.

65. Robertson NL, Hricak H, Sonoda Y, et al. The impact of FDG-PET/CT in the management of patients with vulvar and vaginal cancer. *Gynecol Oncol* 2016;140:420–424.

66. Hacker NF. Revised FIGO staging for carcinoma of the vulva. *Int J Gynaecol Obstet* 2009;105:105–106.

67. Grimm D, Eulenburg C, Brummer O, et al. Sexual activity and function after surgical treatment in patients with (pre)invasive vulvar lesions. *Support Care Cancer* 2016;24:419–428.

68. Grimm D, Hasenburg A, Eulenburg C, et al. Sexual activity and function in patients with gynecological malignancies after completed treatment. *Int J Gynecol Cancer* 2015;25:1134–1141.

69. Barlow EL, Hacker NF, Hussain R, et al. Sexuality and body image following treatment for early-stage vulvar cancer: a qualitative study. *J Adv Nurs* 2014;70:1856–1866.

70. Ansink A, van der Velden J. Surgical interventions for early squamous cell carcinoma of the vulva. *Cochrane Database Syst Rev* 2000:CD002036.

71. Hacker NF, Van der Velden J. Conservative management of early vulvar cancer. *Cancer* 1993;71:1673–1677.

72. Koh WJ, Greer BE, Abu-Rustum NR, et al. Vulvar cancer, version 1.2017, NCCN clinical practice guidelines in oncology. *J Natl Compr Canc Netw* 2017;15:92–120.

73. Cavanagh D, Shepherd JH. The place of pelvic exenteration in the primary management of advanced carcinoma of the vulva. *Gynecol Oncol* 1982;13:318–322.

74. Phillips B, Buchsbaum HJ, Lifshitz S. Pelvic exenteration for vulvovaginal carcinoma. *Am J Obstet Gynecol* 1981;141:1038–1044.

75. Boronow RC. Combined therapy as an alternative to exenteration for locally advanced vulvo-vaginal cancer: rationale and results. *Cancer* 1982;49:1085–1091.

76. Levin W, Goldberg G, Altaras M, et al. The use of concomitant chemotherapy and radiotherapy prior to surgery in advanced stage carcinoma of the vulva. *Gynecol Oncol* 1986;25:20–25.

77. Iversen T, Abeler V, Aalders J. Individualized treatment of stage I carcinoma of the vulva. *Obstet Gynecol* 1981;57:85–89.

78. DeSimone CP, Van Ness JS, Cooper AL, et al. The treatment of lateral T1 and T2 squamous cell carcinomas of the vulva confined to the labium majus or minus. *Gynecol Oncol* 2007;104:390–395.

79. Gonzalez Bosquet J, Magrina JF, Magtibay PM, et al. Patterns of inguinal groin metastases in squamous cell carcinoma of the vulva. *Gynecol Oncol* 2007;105:742–746.

80. DiSaia PJ, Creasman WT, Rich WM. An alternate approach to early cancer of the vulva. *Am J Obstet Gynecol* 1979;133:825–832.

81. Stehman FB, Bundy BN, Dvoretsky PM, et al. Early stage I carcinoma of the vulva treated with ipsilateral superficial inguinal lymphadenectomy and modified radical hemivulvectomy: a prospective study of the Gynecologic Oncology Group. *Obstet Gynecol* 1992;79:490–497.

82. Van der Zee AG, Oonk MH, De Hullu JA, et al. Sentinel node dissection is safe in the treatment of early-stage vulvar cancer. *J Clin Oncol* 2008;26:884–889.

83. Te Grootenhuis NC, van der Zee AG, van Doorn HC, et al. Sentinel nodes in vulvar cancer: long-term follow-up of the GROningen INternational Study on Sentinel nodes in Vulvar cancer (GROINSS-V) I. *Gynecol Oncol* 2016;140:8–14.

84. Stehman FB, Bundy BN, Thomas G, et al. Groin dissection versus groin radiation in carcinoma of the vulva: a Gynecologic Oncology Group study. *Int J Radiat Oncol Biol Phys* 1992;24:389–396.

85. Koh WJ, Chiu M, Stelzer KJ, et al. Femoral vessel depth and the implications for groin node radiation. *Int J Radiat Oncol Biol Phys* 1993;27:969–974.

86. Oonk MH, van Hemel BM, Hollema H, et al. Size of sentinel-node metastasis and chances of non-sentinel-node involvement and survival in early stage vulvar cancer: results from GROINSS-V, a multicentre observational study. *Lancet Oncol* 2010;11:646–652.

87. Van der Zee AG. GROningen INternational Study on Sentinel nodes in Vulvar Cancer, (GROINSS-V) II An Observational Study: GROINS-V II Protocol Amendment: Comprehensive Cancer Centre North Netherlands; 2012. Available at: http://www.dgog.nl/images/stories/studies/groinssvii/groinssviistudyproto-colversion07052011.pdf.

88. Faul CM, Mirmow D, Huang Q, et al. Adjuvant radiation for vulvar carcinoma: improved local control. *Int J Radiat Oncol Biol Phys* 1997;38:381–389.

89. Kunos C, Simpkins F, Gibbons H, et al. Radiation therapy compared with pelvic node resection for node-positive vulvar cancer: a randomized controlled trial. *Obstet Gynecol* 2009;114:537–546.

90. Parthasarathy A, Cheung MK, Osann K, et al. The benefit of adjuvant radiation therapy in single-node-positive squamous cell vulvar carcinoma. *Gynecol Oncol* 2006;103:1095–1099.

Section III

91. Dusenbery KE, Carlson JW, LaPorte RM, et al. Radical vulvectomy with post-operative irradiation for vulvar cancer: therapeutic implications of a central block. *Int J Radiat Oncol Biol Phys* 1994;29:989–998.

92. Jackson KS, Fankam EF, Das N, et al. Unilateral groin and pelvic irradiation for unilaterally node-positive women with vulval carcinoma. *Int J Gynecol Cancer* 2006;16:283–287.

93. Gill BS, Bernard ME, Lin JF, et al. Impact of adjuvant chemotherapy with radiation for node-positive vulvar cancer: a National Cancer Data Base (NCDB) analysis. *Gynecol Oncol* 2015;137:365–372.

94. Montana GS, Thomas GM, Moore DH, et al. Preoperative chemo-radiation for carcinoma of the vulva with N2/N3 nodes: a gynecologic oncology group study. *Int J Radiat Oncol Biol Phys* 2000;48:1007–1013.

95. Moore DH, Thomas GM, Montana GS, et al. Preoperative chemoradiation for advanced vulvar cancer: a phase II study of the Gynecologic Oncology Group. *Int J Radiat Oncol Biol Phys* 1998;42:79–85.

96. Moore DH, Ali S, Koh WJ, et al. A phase II trial of radiation therapy and weekly cisplatin chemotherapy for the treatment of locally-advanced squamous cell carcinoma of the vulva: a gynecologic oncology group study. *Gynecol Oncol* 2012;124:529–533.

97. The Gynecologic Oncology Group. Protocol GOG-279. A Phase II trial evaluating cisplatin and gemcitabine concurrent with intensity modulated radiation therapy (IMRT) in the treatment of locally advanced squamous cell carcinoma of the vulva: the Gynecologic Oncology Group; 2012.

98. Ellis F. Cancer of the vulva treated by radiation; an analysis of 127 cases. *Br J Radiol* 1949;22:513–520.

99. Pohar S, Hoffstetter S, Peiffert D, et al. Effectiveness of brachytherapy in treating carcinoma of the vulva. *Int J Radiat Oncol Biol Phys* 1995;32:1455–1460.

100. Slevin NJ, Pointon RC. Radical radiotherapy for carcinoma of the vulva. *Br J Radiol* 1989;62:145–147.

101. Mak RH, Halasz LM, Tanaka CK, et al. Outcomes after radiation therapy with concurrent weekly platinum-based chemotherapy or every-3-4-week 5-fluorouracil-containing regimens for squamous cell carcinoma of the vulva. *Gynecol Oncol* 2011;120:101–107.

102. Tans L, Ansink AC, van Rooij PH, et al. The role of chemo-radiotherapy in the management of locally advanced carcinoma of the vulva: single institutional experience and review of literature. *Am J Clin Oncol* 2011;34:22–26.

103. Beriwal S, Shukla G, Shinde A, et al. Preoperative intensity modulated radiation therapy and chemotherapy for locally advanced vulvar carcinoma: analysis of pattern of relapse. *Int J Radiat Oncol Biol Phys* 2013;85:1269–1274.

104. Landoni F, Maneo A, Zanetta G, et al. Concurrent preoperative chemotherapy with 5-fluorouracil and mitomycin C and radiotherapy (FUMIR) followed by limited surgery in locally advanced and recurrent vulvar carcinoma. *Gynecol Oncol* 1996;61:321–327.

105. Lupi G, Raspagliesi F, Zucali R, et al. Combined preoperative chemoradiotherapy followed by radical surgery in locally advanced vulvar carcinoma. A pilot study. *Cancer* 1996;77:1472–1478.

106. Wahlen SA, Slater JD, Wagner RJ, et al. Concurrent radiation therapy and chemotherapy in the treatment of primary squamous cell carcinoma of the vulva. *Cancer* 1995;75:2289–2294.

107. Sebag-Montefiore DJ, McLean C, Arnott SJ, et al. Treatment of advanced carcinoma of the vulva with chemoradiotherapy—can exenterative surgery be avoided? *Int J Gynecol Cancer* 1994;4:150–155.

108. Koh WJ, Wallace HJ III, Greer BE, et al. Combined radiotherapy and chemotherapy in the management of local-regionally advanced vulvar cancer. *Int J Radiat Oncol Biol Phys* 1993;26:809–816.

109. Russell AH, Mesic JB, Scudder SA, et al. Synchronous radiation and cytotoxic chemotherapy for locally advanced or recurrent squamous cancer of the vulva. *Gynecol Oncol* 1992;47:14–20.

110. Natesan D, Susko M, Havrilesky L, et al. Definitive Chemoradiotherapy for Vulvar Cancer. *Int J Gynecol Cancer* 2016;26:1699–1705.

111. Natesan D, Hong JC, Foote J, et al. Primary versus preoperative radiation for locally advanced vulvar cancer. *Int J Gynecol Cancer* 2017;27(4):794–804.

112. Kim CH, Olson AC, Kim H, et al. Contouring inguinal and femoral nodes; how much margin is needed around the vessels? *Pract Radiat Oncol* 2012;2:274–278.

113. Gaffney DK, King B, Viswanathan AN, et al. Consensus recommendations for radiation therapy contouring and treatment of vulvar carcinoma. *Int J Radiat Oncol Biol Phys* 2016;95:1191–1200.

114. Kalend AM, Park TL, Wu A, et al. Clinical use of a wing field with transmission block for the pelvis including the inguinal node. *Int J Radiat Oncol Biol Phys* 1990;19:153–158.

115. Moran M, Lund MW, Ahmad M, et al. Improved treatment of pelvis and inguinal nodes using modified segmental boost technique: dosimetric evaluation. *Int J Radiat Oncol Biol Phys* 2004;59:1523–1530.

116. Beriwal S, Heron DE, Kim H, et al. Intensity-modulated radiotherapy for the treatment of vulvar carcinoma: a comparative dosimetric study with early clinical outcome. *Int J Radiat Oncol Biol Phys* 2006;64:1395–1400.

117. Beriwal S, Coon D, Heron DE, et al. Preoperative intensity-modulated radiotherapy and chemotherapy for locally advanced vulvar carcinoma. *Gynecol Oncol* 2008;109:291–295.

118. Geisler JP, Manahan KJ, Buller RE. Neoadjuvant chemotherapy in vulvar cancer: avoiding primary exenteration. *Gynecol Oncol* 2006;100:53–57.

119. Wagenaar HC, Colombo N, Vergote I, et al. Bleomycin, methotrexate, and CCNU in locally advanced or recurrent, inoperable, squamous-cell carcinoma of the vulva: an EORTC Gynaecological Cancer Cooperative Group Study. European Organization for Research and Treatment of Cancer. *Gynecol Oncol* 2001;81:348–354.

120. Durrant KR, Mangioni C, Lacave AJ, et al. Bleomycin, methotrexate, and CCNU in advanced inoperable squamous cell carcinoma of the vulva: a phase II study of the EORTC Gynaecological Cancer Cooperative Group (GCCG). *Gynecol Oncol* 1990;37:359–362.

121. Benedetti-Panici P, Greggi S, Scambia G, et al. Cisplatin (P), bleomycin (B), and methotrexate (M) preoperative chemotherapy in locally advanced vulvar carcinoma. *Gynecol Oncol* 1993;50:49–53.

122. Belinson JL, Stewart JA, Richards AL, et al. Bleomycin, vincristine, mitomycin-C, and cisplatin in the management of gynecological squamous cell carcinomas. *Gynecol Oncol* 1985;20:387–393.

123. Thigpen JT, Blessing JA, Fowler WC Jr, et al. Phase II trials of cisplatin and piperazinedione as single agents in the treatment of advanced or recurrent non-squamous cell carcinoma of the cervix: a Gynecologic Oncology Group Study. *Cancer Treat Rep* 1986;70:1097–1100.

124. Muss HB, Bundy BN, Christopherson WA. Mitoxantrone in the treatment of advanced vulvar and vaginal carcinoma. A gynecologic oncology group study. *Am J Clin Oncol* 1989;12:142–144.

125. Slayton RE, Blessing JA, Beecham J, et al. Phase II trial of etoposide in the management of advanced or recurrent squamous cell carcinoma of the vulva and carcinoma of the vagina: a Gynecologic Oncology Group Study. *Cancer Treat Rep* 1987;71:869–870.

126. Domingues AP, Mota F, Durao M, et al. Neoadjuvant chemotherapy in advanced vulvar cancer. *Int J Gynecol Cancer* 2010;20:294–298.

127. Trope C, Johnsson JE, Larsson G, et al. Bleomycin alone or combined with mitomycin C in treatment of advanced or recurrent squamous cell carcinoma of the vulva. *Cancer Treat Rep* 1980;64:639–642.

128. Deppe G, Bruckner HW, Cohen CJ. Adriamycin treatment of advanced vulvar carcinoma. *Obstet Gynecol* 1977;50:13s–14s.

129. Chambers SK, Flynn SD, Del Prete SA, et al. Bleomycin, vincristine, mitomycin C, and cis-platinum in gynecologic squamous cell carcinomas: a high incidence of pulmonary toxicity. *Gynecol Oncol* 1989;32:303–309.

130. Cormio G, Loizzi V, Gissi F, et al. Cisplatin and vinorelbine chemotherapy in recurrent vulvar carcinoma. *Oncology* 2009;77:281–284.

131. Johnson GA, Mannel R, Khalifa M, et al. Epidermal growth factor receptor in vulvar malignancies and its relationship to metastasis and patient survival. *Gynecol Oncol* 1997;65:425–429.

132. Olawaiye A, Lee LM, Krasner C, et al. Treatment of squamous cell vulvar cancer with the anti-EGFR tyrosine kinase inhibitor Tarceva. *Gynecol Oncol* 2007;106:628–630.

133. Horowitz NS, Olawaiye AB, Borger DR, et al. Phase II trial of erlotinib in women with squamous cell carcinoma of the vulva. *Gynecol Oncol* 2012;127:141–146.

134. Richard SD, Krivak TC, Beriwal S, et al. Recurrent metastatic vulvar carcinoma treated with cisplatin plus cetuximab. *Int J Gynecol Cancer* 2008;18:1132–1135.

135. Podratz KC, Symmonds RE, Taylor WF, et al. Carcinoma of the vulva: analysis of treatment and survival. *Obstet Gynecol* 1983;61:63–74.

136. Gould N, Kamelle S, Tillmanns T, et al. Predictors of complications after inguinal lymphadenectomy. *Gynecol Oncol* 2001;82:329–332.

137. Andersen BL, Turnquist D, LaPolla J, et al. Sexual functioning after treatment of in situ vulvar cancer: preliminary report. *Obstet Gynecol* 1988;71:15–19.

138. Andersen BL, Hacker NF. Psychosexual adjustment after vulvar surgery. *Obstet Gynecol* 1983;62:457–462.

139. Dessole M, Petrillo M, Lucidi A, et al. Quality of life in women after pelvic exenteration for gynecological malignancies: a multicentric study. *Int J Gynecol Cancer* 2018;28:267–273.

CHAPTER 79

Retroperitoneum

Meng Xu-Welliver, Eric D. Miller, Joel L. Mayerson, Brian A. Van Tine,
and Jeffrey C. Buchsbaum

Primary tumors of the retroperitoneum are rare and account for 0.1% to 0.2% of all malignancies[1–3] with up to 80% of lesions being malignant.[4] A retroperitoneal lesion was first reported by Morgagni in 1761 following an autopsy[5] with additional work by Pack and Tabah demonstrating the variety of histologies that can originate from the retroperitoneum.[3] This chapter focuses on lesions that primarily arise from tissues in the retroperitoneum.

ANATOMY

The anatomy of the retroperitoneum has been described in detail by Burkill et al.[6] and reviewed by Osman et al.[7] and shown in Figure 79.1. In summary, the anterior border of the retroperitoneal compartment is the posterior parietal peritoneum and the posterior border is the transversalis fascia. Superiorly, it extends to the diaphragm and inferiorly to the superior aspect of the pelvic diaphragm formed by the levator ani and coccygeus muscles. The retroperitoneum can be divided into three compartments: the anterior pararenal, the perirenal, and the posterior pararenal spaces. The anterior pararenal compartment is bordered anteriorly by the posterior parietal peritoneum, posteriorly by the anterior renal fascia, and laterally by the lateroconal fascia and contains the ascending and descending colon, the pancreas, and second portion of the duodenum. The perirenal compartment is located between the anterior and posterior renal fascia and contains the kidneys and adrenal glands. It is shaped like an inverted cone and superiorly abuts the bare liver on the right and the subdiaphragmatic space on the left. The posterior pararenal compartment is located between the posterior renal fascia and the transversalis fascia and contains fat without any visceral organs. Below the level of the kidneys, the anterior and posterior pararenal compartments combine to form the infrarenal retroperitoneal space, which communicates with the pelvis inferiorly.[4] The aorta and inferior vena cava are contained within the great vessel space that is a primarily fat-containing region immediately anterior to the vertebral bodies and psoas muscles.[4]

EPIDEMIOLOGY

The population incidence of retroperitoneal tumors is based on two population studies and is estimated to be 3 per million persons.[1,2] The age range of patients varied between 3 and 83 years with half of the patients diagnosed between the ages of 60 and 80. There was no significant difference in frequency observed between males and females.[2]

The age at diagnosis of several large series of patients with primary retroperitoneal tumors is shown in Figure 79.2.[1–3,8,9] Two peak age periods are seen with the first peak occurring

during the first decade of life generally caused by neuroblastoma or germ cell tumors, and a second peak occurring during the sixth decade generally caused by mesenchymal lesions. These histologies are outlined in Figure 79.3. Lawenda and Johnstone performed a comprehensive review of the Surveillance Epidemiology and End Results (SEER) public use registry focusing on retroperitoneal tumors.[10] As seen in the

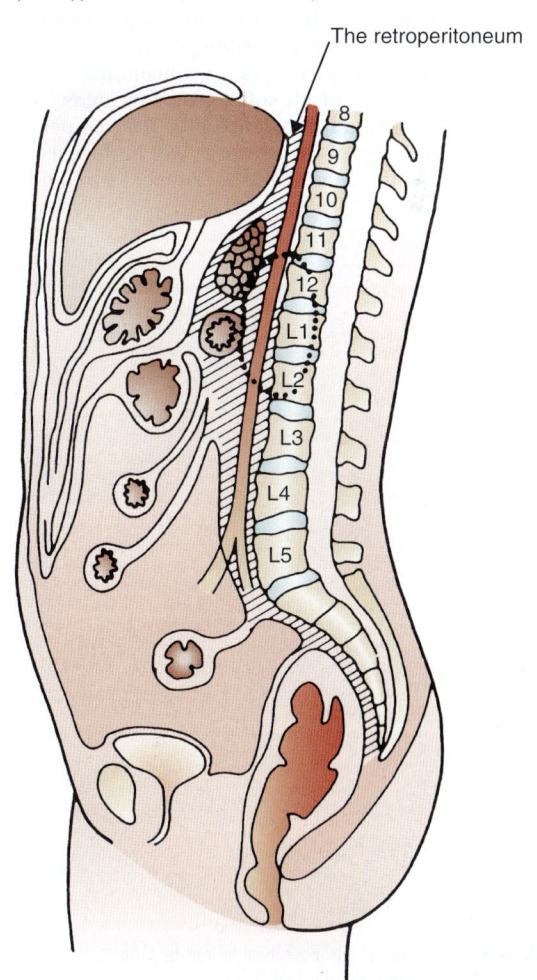

FIGURE 79.1. Sagittal view of trunk, showing the retroperitoneal space (*shaded area*). The kidney is outlined by *dots*. (From Wasserman TH, Tepper JE. Retroperitoneum. In: Perez CA, Brady LW, eds. *Principles and practice of radiation oncology*. 3rd ed. Philadelphia: Lippincott-Raven, 1997:1943–1956.)

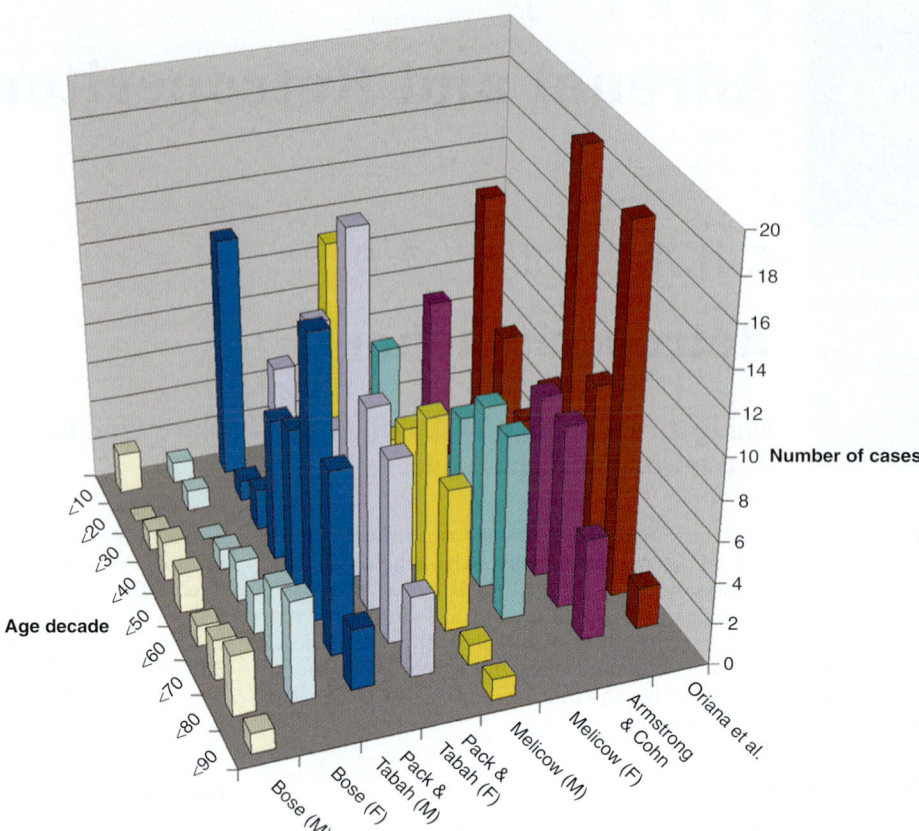

FIGURE 79.2. Age at diagnosis of malignant retroperitoneal tumors (pooled data from multiple series).

results of this review in Table 79.1, soft tissue sarcomas constitute a major portion of retroperitoneal tumors. However, in general, retroperitoneal sarcomas are uncommon representing approximately 15% of all soft tissue sarcomas[11] with an average estimated annual incidence of 2.7 cases per million persons.[12] The majority of this chapter will be focused on the diagnosis and management of retroperitoneal sarcomas.

NATURAL HISTORY

With such varied neoplasms occurring in the retroperitoneum, the natural history is primarily dependent on histology. As the retroperitoneum is a potential space, neoplasms in this region can become quite large, weigh over 50 kg, and cause displacement or compression of adjacent organs prior to diagnosis.

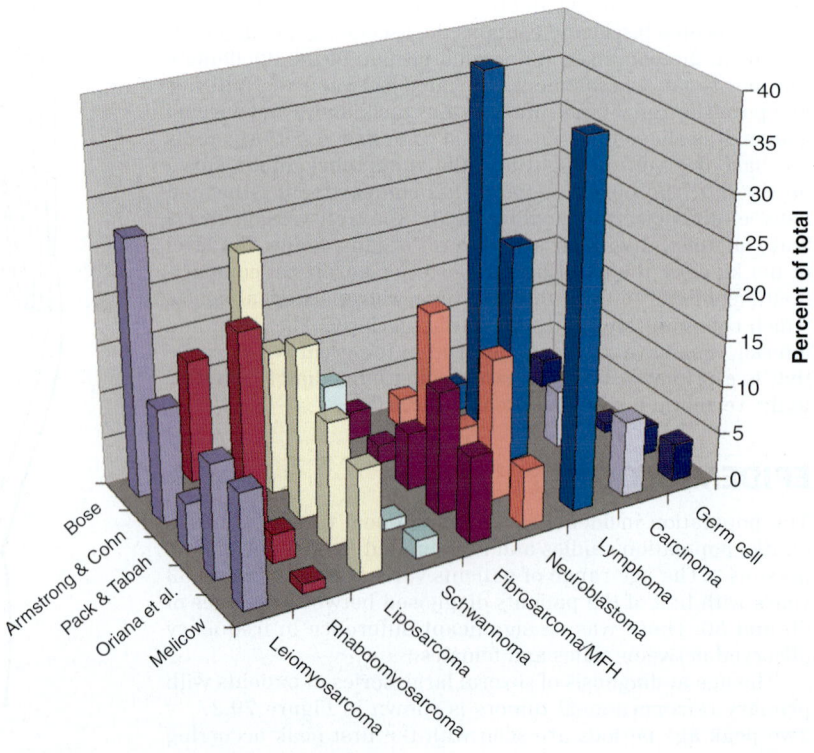

FIGURE 79.3. Percentage of retroperitoneal lesions by histology (pooled data from multiple published series).

TABLE 79.1 SURVEILLANCE, EPIDEMIOLOGY, AND END RESULTS DATA: RETROPERITONEAL MALIGNANCIES, 2002

Patient Data (*n* = 162)	Number	Percent
Patient sex		
Male	78	48
Female	84	52
Patient race		
White	128	79
Black	16	9.9
Other	17	10.5
Unknown	1	0.06
Histologic derivation		
Soft tissue sarcoma	126	77.8
Sympathetic nervous system	14	8.6
Epithelial	7	4.3
Germ cell	5	3
Renal	1	0.06
Other (unspecified)	9	5.6

CLINICAL PRESENTATION

Table 79.2 outlines pooled data regarding signs and symptoms at presentation of retroperitoneal tumors. In general, presentation involves a mass or abdominal pain in the majority of cases.

DIAGNOSTIC WORKUP

Retroperitoneal tumors include a diverse group of both benign and malignant neoplasms that may be primary or secondary in origin.[7] Imaging serves an important role in differentiating retroperitoneal masses with computed tomography (CT) and magnetic resonance imaging (MRI) serving as the primary imaging modalities. Although the differential diagnosis is broad, certain imaging characteristics such as fat content, necrotic changes, contrast enhancement, presence of calcifications and/or cysts, and appearance on T1- and T2-weighted images all provide clues to narrow the differential diagnosis.[4] For example, in retroperitoneal liposarcoma, the most common subtype,[13] tumors appear as a hypoattenuating lesion on CT because of the fat content and are indistinguishable from a benign lipoma.[4,7] On MRI, a well-differentiated liposarcoma demonstrates high signal intensity on T1, intermediate signal on T2, and loss of fat signal intensity on fat-suppressed images and may be contrast enhancing.[4,7] However, in a dedifferentiated liposarcoma, both fat and solid components are observed with occasional associated calcifications.[4] Leiomyosarcomas, the second most common subtype,[13] appear on CT as either homogeneously solid, but larger tumors may develop areas of necrosis and hemorrhage.[4] On MRI, these tumors demonstrate low T1 signal intensity and intermediate to high T2 signal intensity depending on the presence of necrosis with peripheral and heterogeneous contrast enhancement.[4,14] In general, retroperitoneal neoplasms can be divided into either solid or cystic tumors based on their imaging appearance.[7] Solid tumors fall into three main categories including mesodermal, neurogenic, or extragonadal germ cell origin, whereas cystic tumors include cystic changes in solid neoplasms as well as cystic lymphangioma, cystic teratoma, cystadenoma, cystadenocarcinoma, and cystic mesothelioma.[7]

As part of the primary workup, in addition to imaging the primary tumor with a CT of the abdomen/pelvis with intravenous (IV) contrast, a CT chest should also be obtained to evaluate for metastatic disease. MRI of the abdomen/pelvis with IV contrast can also be considered to further classify the lesion and evaluate extent of disease. Imaging with 18-fluorine–labeled 2-deoxy-2-fluoro-D-glucose (^{18}F-FDG-PET) is not routinely performed for retroperitoneal sarcomas but may be useful for evaluating the extent of distant metastasis during initial staging if the primary lesion is PET avid in the first place.[15]

A definitive diagnosis is obtained with a biopsy and should be performed unless preoperative treatment is not planned. Image-guided core needle biopsy is recommended with multiple cores obtained for histologic and molecular subtyping.[16] Both fine needle aspiration and laparotomy with open biopsy should be avoided. Ideally, biopsy of a solid, well-perfused portion of the tumor should be performed rather than an area of necrosis.[16]

RETROPERITONEAL SARCOMA GENERAL MANAGEMENT

Because of the rarity of retroperitoneal sarcoma, patients should be evaluated at high-volume centers with expertise in sarcoma by a multidisciplinary team including surgical oncology, radiation oncology, and medical oncology.[17] Based on guidelines presented by the National Comprehensive Cancer Network (NCCN, Version 2.2017), the first decision point is assessing if the patient is resectable or unresectable.[18] Surgical resection is the primary treatment for retroperitoneal sarcoma and is the only potentially curative option for localized and resectable disease. Criteria for unresectable tumors may include extensive major vessel involvement including the root of the mesentery, spinal cord involvement, peritoneal implants, and distant metastasis.[19] Achieving an R0 resection of a retroperitoneal sarcoma is often challenging due to the size and anatomic location of the tumor. Based on a review by Mendenhall et al.,[13] which includes data from 4 large institutional series, the rate of complete resection, which includes R0 and R1 resections, was 50% to 67%. Patients who have an R1 resection are at increased risk of local recurrence[20] with recent data from the National Cancer Database (NCDB) suggesting inferior survival as well.[21] Surgical resection often involves resection of adjacent organs to achieve complete extirpation of the tumor. Liberal visceral en bloc resections may increase morbidity but also have been associated with higher rates of local control and potentially an improvement in overall survival based on retrospective data although this practice has not yet been widely adopted.[22,23]

Although a number of retrospective studies have shown a local control benefit with adjuvant external beam radiotherapy (EBRT) following resection,[24–26] there are no randomized trials comparing surgery with and without adjuvant EBRT. Similarly, several nonrandomized prospective studies[27,28] have demonstrated acceptable local control and toxicity in patients with retroperitoneal sarcomas treated with preoperative radiation therapy although no prospective randomized trials have been performed. Currently, the European Organisation for Research and Treatment of Cancer (EORTC 62092-22092) is conducting a prospective, randomized phase III study in

TABLE 79.2 PRESENTING COMPLAINTS (%) OF PATIENTS WITH RETROPERITONEAL LESIONS (POOLED FROM LITERATURE SOURCES)

Sign/Symptom	Bose[2] (*n* = 30)	Pack and Tabah[3] (*n* = 120)	Oriana et al.[9] (*n* = 56)
Mass	83	31	42
Abdominal pain	60	51	42[a]
Back pain	20	7	
Weight loss	35	3	12
Anorexia	20	NS	9
Nausea/vomiting	20	20	8
Lower extremity edema	17	7	9

[a]Indicates all patients with pain as presenting sign.
NS, data not stated.

patients with retroperitoneal sarcoma comparing patients treated with surgery alone to patients treated with preoperative radiation therapy (either 3-D conformal or intensity-modulated radiation therapy [IMRT]) followed by surgery, known as the STRASS trial.[29] A prior similar study conducted by the American College of Surgeons Oncology Group (ACOSOG Z9031) closed prematurely due to poor accrual.[30] Preoperative radiation therapy has several advantages over postoperative treatment. In the preoperative setting, the tumor is more clearly defined and the target volume is smaller because the entire operative bed must be included in the postoperative setting, which may reduce normal tissue toxicity. The tumor typically displaces adjacent normal tissues including bowel, kidney, and liver out of the target volume. In the postoperative setting, these organs may fall into the resection cavity making it difficult to deliver therapeutic postoperative radiation therapy doses. Finally, there is a theoretical radiobiologic advantage in treating a tumor with an intact vascular supply as it renders the tumor more sensitive to radiation therapy.

For patients with a resectable intermediate- or high-grade retroperitoneal sarcomas, preoperative radiation therapy should be considered prior to resection. If available, intraoperative radiation therapy (IORT) can also be considered to deliver a boost to the resection site to help improve local control. Based on the NCCN guidelines, for patients with unresectable or borderline resectable tumors, downstaging can be attempted using preoperative radiation therapy, combination chemotherapy with doxorubicin/ifosfamide/mesna (AIM), or chemoradiation.[18] Repeat imaging with CT chest/abdomen/pelvis with or without MRI abdomen/pelvis should then be performed to evaluate the treatment response and to verify that the patient has not developed metastasis. If the tumor progresses or the patient develops metastatic disease, palliative care can be considered, which may involve any combination of chemotherapy, radiation therapy, surgery to help control symptoms,[31] or other supportive care.[18] In patients with unresectable tumors, particle therapy may provide durable local control.[32]

Following preoperative radiation therapy in the definitive setting, surgical resection is typically delayed 3 to 8 weeks with radiographic restaging performed to assess for metastases and treatment response. In the setting of a positive microscopic margin (R1 resection) following preoperative radiation therapy, a postoperative external beam radiation therapy boost can be considered but is discouraged.[18] In general, postoperative radiation therapy is discouraged in the NCCN guidelines with the recommendation for observation following surgical resection with consideration of preoperative EBRT in the event of a local recurrence.[18] However, postoperative EBRT should be considered in the situation where a local recurrence would cause significant morbidity because of a critical anatomic location. For patients who undergo a resection where gross residual disease is present (R2 resection), re-resection should be discussed, if possible.

Unlike extremity sarcomas where the majority of first recurrences are distant, retroperitoneal sarcomas tend to fail locally with a 5-year local control of approximately 50%.[13] In the setting of recurrent disease, patients who did not receive prior radiation therapy should be considered for preoperative radiation. Repeat resection should be offered, if possible, as patients who completed resection for recurrent disease had improved survival based on a large retrospective study from the Trans-Atlantic Retroperitoneal Sarcoma Working Group.[33] IORT can also be considered in an attempt to improve the chances of local control in the recurrent setting.[34–36]

Patients who present with or develop metastatic disease should be managed on a case-by-case basis. Any combination of chemotherapy, radiation therapy, surgery to palliate symptoms, and other supportive care is appropriate.[18]

Following definitive treatment, patients should undergo physical exam with imaging every 3 to 6 months for the first 2

to 3 years.[18] For the next 2 years, the patient should undergo physical exam and imaging every 6 months, and then annually after that. Imaging should include CT or MRI of the abdomen/pelvis with chest x-ray or CT of the chest also included.

A histology-based retroperitoneal sarcoma prognostic system identifies retroperitoneal sarcoma into three prognostic groups, and it can be used in both primary and recurrent retroperitoneal sarcoma. Distinct risk stratification is necessary for specific assessment of prognosis and decision regarding individualized adjuvant therapy.[37] Some authors recommend the formulation of a liposarcoma-specific postoperative nomogram based on histologic subtypes, which provides more accurate survival predictions for patients with primary retroperitoneal sarcoma.[38] Well-differentiated and dedifferentiated liposarcoma differ significantly in their biologic behavior and are treated by different surgical approaches at MD Anderson.[39] Researchers at the center recommend that the American Joint Committee on Cancer soft tissue sarcoma staging system needs to incorporate the primary site, histologic subtype, margin status, and recurrence to further shed light on prognosis.[40]

CHEMOTHERAPY

Adjuvant chemotherapy is controversial in the management of adult patients with macroscopically completely resected retroperitoneal soft tissue sarcomas. Retrospective analysis of both preoperative[41] or postoperative[19,42–44] chemotherapy has yet to demonstrate overall survival benefit. In a National Cancer Institute trial, patients with STSs were randomized to chemotherapy or observation following resection; some patients had postoperative irradiation.[45] Among patients who were assigned to chemotherapy, survival was favorably affected in those with extremity tumors. However, patients with head and neck and truncal lesions (including retroperitoneal sarcomas) did not benefit; the 5-year survival rate was approximately 40% in both arms. Similar findings were reported in a large meta-analysis of patients with STS.[46]

The use of neoadjuvant or adjuvant chemotherapy is not standard in the management of nonmetastatic adult retroperitoneal STSs. Neoadjuvant chemotherapy has been primarily studied in the setting of high-grade, extremity STSs. Pisters et al.[47] demonstrated feasibility of using preoperative concurrent doxorubicin and EBRT (18 to 50.4 Gy), followed by resection and IORT (15 Gy) in patients with RPS. An R0 or R1 resection was possible in 90% of the patients who went to surgery (83%). Newer studies have shown that doxorubicin-based adjuvant chemotherapy significantly improves local and distant recurrence in localized resectable soft tissue sarcoma.[48] Newer agents, such as olaratumab,[49] are currently being tested in the neoadjuvant setting to see if overall survival can be improved. Overall, treatment with chemotherapy is not recommended outside clinical protocols.

RADIATION THERAPY TECHNIQUES

External Beam Radiation Therapy

In patients where radiation therapy is recommended, preoperative radiation therapy is the preferred approach. Treatment guidelines based on the consensus of an international expert panel for preoperative radiation therapy of retroperitoneal sarcoma have been published by Baldini et al.[17] Suitable candidates for preoperative radiation therapy include patients with unifocal or localized tumors that are amenable to an R0 resection and where delivery of 50 to 50.4 Gy to the tumor while meeting the dose objectives for the adjacent normal structures is feasible. Patients with symptoms requiring urgent surgical intervention should not be considered for preoperative radiation therapy. Prior to any therapy, the surgical and radiation oncologist should work together to develop a consensus plan. In the setting of kidney or liver involvement where surgical resection may involve either a nephrectomy or partial hepatectomy, or where radiation therapy may result in impaired function of one kidney, preliminary studies need to be performed to ensure adequate function in the remaining kidney or liver. Further, in the setting of a nephrectomy or partial hepatectomy, care should be taken to minimize the radiation dose to the remaining kidney and/or liver. Kidney function can be evaluated using a renal perfusion study, whereas the liver can be evaluated using serum liver chemistries.

CT simulation should be performed with the patient in the supine position with arms up using an Alpha Cradle with/without a wing board or equivalent custom immobilization device to allow reproducible setup during treatment. Both oral and intravenous contrast should be considered for the simulation scan to better delineate the tumor and adjacent normal structures including bowel. A four-dimensional CT should be performed to evaluate tumor motion during the respiratory cycle with more motion anticipated in superiorly located tumors in the abdomen.[50] For patients with more than 1 cm of motion, motion management techniques should be considered such as active breathing control, respiratory gating, or end-expiration breath hold. To aid with target and organ at risk delineation, registration of the free-breathing planning CT with diagnostic studies should be performed. Useful diagnostic studies may include a diagnostic CT and/or T1-weighted postcontrast MRI. Data on the use of [18] F-FDG-PET in the staging of retroperitoneal sarcoma and for use in radiation therapy treatment planning are currently limited with more data likely to emerge in the coming years.

Target Delineation/Organs at Risk

Target volumes for retroperitoneal sarcomas are included in the international expert panel consensus guidelines from Baldini et al.[17] For upper abdominal tumors where a four-dimensional (4-D) computed tomography (CT) simulation is performed, the gross tumor volume (GTV) is delineated, and an internal gross tumor volume (iGTV) is made based on the motion of the GTV throughout the respiratory cycle. The internal target volume (ITV) is made using a 1.5-cm uniform expansion of the iGTV edited off of uninvolved bone, kidney, and liver. The ITV volume should expand 5 mm into the bowel and any air cavities and should be cropped away from uninvolved skin per institutional guidelines. If the tumor extends into the inguinal canal, the inferior expansion of the iGTV to make the ITV should be 3 cm. For an upper abdominal tumor where a 4-D CT simulation is not performed, the GTV should be expanded by 2 to 2.5 cm in the superior–inferior direction and 1.5 to 2 cm radially. The CTV should be edited off of the interfaces in the same manner as the ITV in the upper abdomen case where a 4-D scan is obtained. For tumors below the level of the iliac crest, the GTV can be expanded 1.5 cm uniformly and edited off of the interfaces as mentioned above to create the CTV. In all cases, the planning target volume (PTV), which accounts for setup error and patient movement, should be based off of imaging frequency and institutional guidelines. The standard preoperative dose is 50.4 Gy in 1.8 Gy fractions or 50 Gy in 25 fractions. The delivery of a boost dose to the areas considered to be at high risk for a positive margin has been reported.[51] However, this approach remains experimental and is the subject of a currently accruing phase I/II trial at Massachusetts General Hospital.[52] In the setting of a positive surgical margin following preoperative EBRT, a postoperative EBRT boost may be considered. In this situation, a boost of 16 to 18 Gy for microscopic disease and 20 to 26 Gy for gross residual disease should be considered being certain to observe the limits of adjacent normal tissues.[18]

In the postoperative setting, the treatment volumes are generally larger with a larger volume of normal tissue in the treatment field as the bowel and other organs initially displaced by the tumor fall into the resection cavity. Temporary tissue expanders have been used in a limited number of studies to displace bowel and other organs at risk out of the treatment volume.[34,53] Target delineation in the postoperative setting is challenging and no consensus guidelines exist. Ideally, preoperative imaging is available and can be registered with the CT simulation scan. Postoperative diagnostic studies should also be considered to evaluate for residual disease. In the event where an R1 or R2 resection is expected, clips placed in the areas at highest risk for positive margins/residual disease aid greatly in target delineation. In general, the preoperative GTV and any surgical clips should be included in the post-treatment volume. CTV expansion volumes should be limited to exclude fascial and peritoneal boundaries not violated by tumor. Again, the PTV is based on the method of immobilization and institutional guidelines. The larger treatment field is generally treated to a dose of 50.4 Gy in 1.8 Gy fractions or 50 Gy in 25 fractions with a limited boost field based on the presence of residual disease and proximity to organs at risk. Based on the NCCN guidelines, a 10 to 16 Gy boost is recommended in the setting of negative margins, 16 to 18 Gy for microscopically positive margins, and 20 to 26 Gy for gross residual disease.[18] The total dose is generally limited by the tolerance of adjacent normal tissues. Particle therapy such as protons may be advantageous in the postoperative setting by permitting delivery of a therapeutic radiation dose to the PTV while sparing abutting organs and tissues. This remains the subject of active investigation.

Adjacent organs at risk include liver, stomach, bowel including duodenum, small and large bowel, kidneys, spinal cord, testicles, ovaries, bladder, rectum, and femoral heads. To aid in normal organ contouring, consensus guidelines and an atlas are available from the Radiation Therapy Oncology Group.[54] Again, the consensus guidelines for preoperative radiation therapy for retroperitoneal sarcoma includes a summary of constraints for organs at risk primarily derived from Quantitative Analysis of Normal Tissue Effects in the Clinic (QUANTEC) data.[17,55] In brief, no more than 100% of the stomach should receive ≥45 Gy, the mean bilateral kidney dose is 15 to 18 Gy, and no more than 15% of the remaining kidney should receive >18 Gy if one kidney is removed. For the small/large bowel contoured as the peritoneal cavity, no more than 195 cm³ should receive >45 Gy. The mean residual liver dose should be limited to <26 Gy and the spinal cord dose should be <50 Gy.

Treatment Planning and Delivery

For radiation therapy planning using photons, intensity-modulated radiation therapy (IMRT) is preferred over 3-D conformal radiation because of increased conformality with decreased dose to adjacent organs at risk.[56] Swanson et al.[56] determined the optimal radiation therapy technique for the treatment of retroperitoneal sarcomas by comparing plans prepared using 3-D conformal proton radiation therapy, IMRT, and 3-D conformal photon radiation therapy. The IMRT and conformal proton plans were more conformal than the 3-D photon plans. Furthermore, the IMRT and proton plans provided a lower bowel and kidney dose than the 3-D photon plans.

Based on the results of Wong et al., which demonstrated volumetric changes and significant interfraction displacement during preoperative radiation therapy for retroperitoneal sarcoma, daily image-guided radiation therapy should be considered where soft tissue is clearly visible such as cone-beam CT.[17,50] Prophylactic antiemetics should be considered for the patient depending on the location of the tumor.

Additional Radiation Techniques

IORT refers to the delivery of either brachytherapy or external beam irradiation to a target area, whereas the area is exposed during surgery. IORT is typically used to deliver a focal boost to areas of concern such as close or positive margins. The advantages of IORT include the ability to directly visualize the area of concern and manually remove normal tissues from the field or shield them prior to treatment delivery. When electron beams are used (IOERT), typical doses range from 10 Gy for completely resected tumors with negative margins, 12.5 to 15 Gy for positive microscopic margins, and 15 to 20 Gy for gross residual disease.[57] Typical electron energies range from 9 to 15 MeV based on the desired depth of penetration.

IORT can also be delivered using high dose rate intraoperative irradiation (HDR-IORT) as previously described in detail by Harrison et al.[58,59] For HDR-IORT, following displacement of normal tissue from the field of interest, a Harrison-Anderson-Mick (HAM) applicator (an array of catheters spaced 1 cm apart in a silicone rubber pad) is secured in the target region and a dose of 10 to 20 Gy at a tissue depth of 5 to 10 mm is typically delivered.[57] Following delivery of IORT, the applicators are removed from the target region, and the surgeon continues with the case. The advantages and disadvantages of each IORT technique have been previously summarized.[57] HDR-IORT allows for delivery of more conformal treatments along curved surfaces secondary to the flexible nature of the HAM applicator, the ability to treat large fields without field matching, and the ability to deliver radiation therapy to areas that may not necessarily be accessible with IOERT. HDR-IORT is limited to treating target areas ≤0.5 cm thick. IOERT can treat both superficial and deeper targets by varying the electron energy employed for treatment. Treatment with IOERT is also generally shorter than HDR-IORT, thus decreasing the overall procedure time.

RESULTS OF THERAPY

Surgical resection remains the only curative treatment for patients with retroperitoneal sarcomas, although local control rates with resection alone remain poor. Because of both the size and proximity of retroperitoneal sarcomas to critical organs, margin negative resections are difficult to achieve. Locoregional failure is the predominant pattern of failure,[13,60] and failure to achieve local control is the major cause of death in patients with retroperitoneal sarcoma.[61] A large retrospective series from Memorial Sloan Kettering reported on 231 patients with primary retroperitoneal sarcoma that was resectable.[62] Of the 231 patients, 185 (80%) were able to undergo a gross total resection. Patients with a gross total resection were found to have a statistically significant increase in survival compared to those who underwent incomplete resection, 103 versus 18 months. No difference in survival was observed between patients with unresectable disease and patients who underwent incomplete resection. For patients with localized, completely excised retroperitoneal sarcoma, 5-year overall survival is 49% to 70% with selected studies summarized in Table 79.3.

TABLE 79.4 LOCAL RECURRENCE IN PATIENTS WITH OR WITHOUT POSTOPERATIVE RADIATION THERAPY (PORT) FOLLOWING A COMPLETE RESECTION

Study	Local Recurrence with PORT (%)	Local Recurrence without PORT (%)	P Value
Ferrario and Karakousis[63]	38 (at 41 mo)	53 (at 41 mo)	.16
Stoeckle et al.[24]	45 (5 y)	77 (5 y)	.0021
Catton et al.[60]	103 mo to LRF	30 mo to LRF	.02

LRF, locoregional failure.

Patients with positive microscopic margins are at increased risk of local recurrence[20] based on retrospective data with a recent study from the NCDB demonstrating a survival advantage in patients able to achieve an R0 resection versus R1 resection, 92 and 70 months, respectively.[21] As part of the analysis, preoperative radiation therapy was associated with an increased probability of R0 resection. A number of retrospective studies demonstrate an improvement in local control with postoperative radiation therapy with select studies summarized in Table 79.4. In the report by Stoeckle et al.,[24] patients with complete excision had a significant reduction in local recurrence risk when treated with received postoperative radiation therapy (median dose = 50 Gy) compared to those not treated with adjuvant radiation therapy (relative risk, 3.36; P = .0021). However, no improvement in overall survival on multivariate analysis was observed. Catton et al.[60] found that adjuvant radiation therapy for patients who had a complete resection increased the time to locoregional relapse, from 30 months (no radiation) to 103 months (P = .06). Again, radiation did not have an impact on survival.

Preoperative radiation therapy is preferred over postoperative radiation therapy because of improved target delineation, a smaller treatment volume, and the potential for displacement of normal tissues by the tumor. Preoperative radiation therapy has been evaluated in the prospective setting with small nonrandomized studies.[27,28] Pawlik et al.[28] reported the results of two prospective studies performed at MD Anderson. Patients with intermediate- or high-grade retroperitoneal sarcoma were treated with preoperative radiation therapy with a median dose of 45 Gy followed by surgical resection. Nearly 90% of the patients completed the planned radiation course with a complete resection achieved in 95% of patients. For the patients who had a complete resection, the 5-year local recurrence-free and overall survival rates were 60% and 61%, respectively. A separate NCDB study was performed comparing patients with retroperitoneal sarcoma treated with surgery alone versus pre- or postoperative radiation therapy. An improvement in overall survival was observed in the patients treated with either preoperative (HR 0.70; 95% CI 0.59 to 0.82; P < .0001) or postoperative (HR 0.78; 95% CI 0.70 to 0.85; P < .0001) radiation therapy compared to patients treated with surgery alone.[65] Hopefully, there will be a definitive answer regarding the role of preoperative radiation therapy in the

TABLE 79.3 COMPLETE RESECTION AND SURVIVAL IN PATIENTS WITH NONMETASTATIC (M0) RETROPERITONEAL SARCOMA (RPS)

Study	Complete Resection (%)	Local Recurrence (%)	Overall Survival (%)	LR with Incomplete Excision (%)	Overall Survival with Incomplete Excision (%)
Ferrario and Karakousis[63]	95	Primary RPS: 41	Primary RPS: 65 (5 y), 56 (10 y)		
		Recurrent: 61	Recurrent: 53 (5 y), 34 (10 y)		
Stoeckle et al.[24]	65	57 (5 y)	49 (5 y)		
Lewis et al.[62]	Primary RPS: 67		70 (5 y); median, 103 mo		Median, 18 mo
Catton et al.[60]	43	50 (5 y); 82 (10 y)	55 (5 y); 22 (10 y)	86 (5 y); 95 (10 y)	15 (5 y); 10 (10 y)
Gronchi et al.[64]	88	Primary RPS: 37 Recurrent: 72	54 (5 y); 27 (10 y)		

retroperitoneal sarcoma by completion of EORTC 62092, the STRASS trial.

IORT is used by some centers to deliver a boost to the resection cavity to improve local control. A prospective randomized trial was performed by the National Cancer Institute to evaluate the benefit of gross total resection with IORT followed by postoperative EBRT compared to gross total resection and postoperative EBRT alone.[66] IORT was delivered with electrons with an energy of 11 to 15 MeV delivered in a single dose of 20 Gy. For patients treated with IORT, the postoperative EBRT dose was 35 to 40 Gy delivered in 1.5 to 1.8 Gy fractions. For patients treated with postoperative EBRT alone, the dose was 50 to 55 Gy delivered in 1.5 to 1.8 Gy fractions. For patients treated in the IORT arm, significantly fewer locoregional recurrences were observed compared to the postoperative EBRT alone arm. No difference in survival was observed between the two arms. Additional nonrandomized studies summarized in Table 79.5 have demonstrated excellent local control with the use of IORT and EBRT with acceptable toxicity.

Patients with unresectable disease have a poor prognosis. Surgery may be considered to palliate symptoms. A retrospective study from Memorial Sloan Kettering was performed to evaluate patients with retroperitoneal sarcoma who underwent palliative procedures.[68] Patients most frequently underwent a procedure because of gastrointestinal (GI) symptoms (44% of patients). Overall, about 50% of patients were symptom-free at 100 days postprocedure, but only 23% of patients with GI obstructive symptoms were symptom-free at 100 days. The postoperative morbidity was 29%, and the postoperative mortality was 12%. Particle therapy can also be considered for patients with unresectable disease. Serizawa reported on a small series of patients with unresectable retroperitoneal sarcoma treated with carbon ion radiotherapy.[32] The patient cohort included both primary and recurrent disease with doses ranging from 52.8 to 73.6 GyE in 16 fractions. The local control rates at 2 and 5 years were 77% and 69%, respectively, with a 2- and 5-year overall survival of 75% and 50%, respectively. No grade ≥3 toxicities were observed.

Recurrence is common, and there are minimal data to guide management in the recurrent setting.[33] A large retrospective series from the Trans-Atlantic Retroperitoneal Sarcoma Working Group evaluated postrelapse outcomes in 408 patients.[33] For patients with a local recurrence only, the median time from initial resection to recurrence was 23 months. Repeat resection was performed in 48% of patients with chemotherapy and radiation therapy given to 31% and 18% of patients, respectively. Following local recurrence, the median overall survival was 33 months and the 5-year overall survival was 29% with repeat resection and longer time interval to recurrence found to be significant predictors for survival. Treatment with radiation therapy trended for significance. The 5-year overall survival for patients who underwent repeat resection was 43% versus 11% for those not able to undergo repeat resection. The 5-year overall survival for patients with distant metastasis and those with local recurrence and distant metastasis was 20% and 14%, respectively. For patients with distant metastasis only, resection of the distant metastasis was found to be a significant predictor of improved disease-specific survival. For patients with both a local recurrence and distant metastasis, patients who completed resection of the recurrent disease had longer survival than those who did not.

TREATMENT SEQUELAE

Acute symptoms from EBRT of the retroperitoneum include fatigue, radiation dermatitis, nausea, vomiting, and diarrhea. For large radiation fields where the adjacent spine is included, a significant portion of bone marrow may also be included and anemia, neutropenia, and thrombocytopenia may occur. At minimum, weekly monitoring of vital signs

TABLE 79.5 OUTCOMES WITH EXTERNAL BEAM RADIOTHERAPY (EBRT) + INTRAOPERATIVE RADIOTHERAPY (IORT) BOOST FOLLOWING RESECTION OF PRIMARY AND RECURRENT RETROPERITONEAL SARCOMA (RPS)

Study	Median EBRT Dose (Gy)	Median IORT Dose (Gy)	Local Recurrence (%)	Overall Survival (%)	Toxicity (%)
Petersen et al.[67]	Primary RPS: 48.6 (postop) Recurrent: 45 (postop)	Primary RPS: 12.5 Recurrent: 15	Primary RPS: 0 (CE), 8 (micro), 40 (gross); 5-y LC Recurrent: 0 (CE), 64 (micro), 33 (gross)	Primary RPS: 62 (CE), 54 (micro), 29 (gross); 5 y-OS Recurrent: 80 (CE), 44 (micro), 45 (gross)	Chronic enteritis (16); grade 3–4 GI complications (18); fistula formation (18); neuropathy (mild, 12; moderate/ severe, 21)
Sindelar et al.[66]	IORT arm: 35–40 (postop); EBRT alone arm: 50–55 (postop)	20	IORT arm: time to in-field local recurrence: >127 mo EBRT alone arm: 38 mo (P < .05)	IORT arm: 45 mo EBRT alone arm: 52 (P = .39)	IORT arm: chronic enteritis (13); neuropathy (mild, 13; 47% moderate/severe, 47) EBRT alone arm: chronic enteritis (50), fistula formation (25); neuropathy (mild, 6; moderate/severe, 0)
Gieschen et al.[36]	45–50.4 (preop)	10 (CE), 12.5–15 (micro), 15–20 (gross)	Complete excision: EBRT + IORT: 17 (5 y); EBRT alone: 39 (5 y)	Complete excision: EBRT + IORT: 74 (5 y); EBRT alone: 30 (5 y)	Neuropathy (19), hydronephrosis (19), vaginal fistula (6), ureteral fistula (6), small bowel obstruction (6)
Alektiar et al.[34]	45–50.4 (postop)	12–15 (HDR, Ir-192)	Complete excision: EBRT + IORT: 29 (5 y) primary RPS; 39 (5 y) recurrent; 44% (5 y) total IORT alone: NR (5 y) primary RPS; 67 (5 y) recurrent; 50% (5 y) total	Primary RPS: 75 (5 y) Recurrent: 30 (5 y)	Bowel obstruction (18), fistula (9), neuropathy (mild, 6; moderate/severe, 0), ureteral injury (3)
Petersen et al.[67]	Primary RPS: 48.6 (postop) Recurrent: 45 (postop)	Primary RPS: 12.5 Recurrent: 15	Primary RPS: 0 (CE), 8 (micro), 40 (gross); 5-y LC Recurrent: 0 (CE), 64 (micro), 33 (gross)	Primary RPS: 62 (CE), 54 (micro), 29 (gross); 5 y-OS Recurrent: 80 (CE), 44 (micro), 45 (gross)	Chronic enteritis (16); grade 3–4 GI complications (18); fistula formation (18); neuropathy (mild, 12; moderate/severe, 21)

CE, complete excision; GI, gastrointestinal; gross, gross residual disease; HDR, high dose rate; LC, local control; micro, microscopic residual disease; NR, not reported; OS, overall survival.

should be performed and monitoring of blood counts should be considered. Reported postoperative complications include bleeding, impaired wound healing or dehiscence, infection, myocardial infarction, and death.[27,67]

Late toxicities of surgery and radiation include small bowel enteritis, stricture, perforation, fistula, and obstruction. Development of nephritis is possible after radiation doses >30 Gy with resultant hypertension. Late complications are associated with the number of laparotomies to which the patient has been subjected and to the radiation dose and volume.[69] A lower incidence of enteritis has been reported with the use of EBRT and an IORT boost compared with EBRT alone, as the bowel is able to be moved from the field resulting in a lower radiation dose[66] (Table 79.5). Overlap of adjacent IORT fields can increase the risk of neuropathy and ureteral injury.[27,36,67] As discussed previously, preoperative radiation therapy is the preferred approach over postoperative radiation therapy because of a more favorable toxicity profile and ease of target delineation.[17] Proton therapy may also allow decreased dose to the bowel resulting in a decrease in acute and late toxicity.[70]

Callegaro et al.[71] performed a cross-sectional study to assess the long-term morbidity of patients treated for retroperitoneal sarcoma. Patients were evaluated for lower limb function using the Lower Extremity Functional Scale (LEFS) and pain was assessed using the Brief Pain Inventory–Short Form, both self-report questionnaires. Radiation therapy and chemotherapy were used in 28.8% and 51.4% of patients, respectively. Overall, sensory impairment of the limbs was reported in 76% of patients with a median LEFS score of 60 out of a maximum 80 (high function) indicating overall good motor function. Mean pain scores varied from 1.23 to 2.68 out of a maximum of 10 (bad pain) indicating mild pain overall. No difference in median creatinine levels on multivariate analysis was observed in patients requiring nephrectomy compared to those who did not.

LYMPHOMAS

Lymphomas frequently involve the retroperitoneum with the predominant histologic variant being non-Hodgkin lymphoma. Workup generally includes CT and/or MRI and 18F-FDG-PET. On CT, lymphomas appear as a homogeneous mass that generally spreads between normal structures occasionally causing displacement, but generally not resulting in compression.[4] On MRI, lymphomas are isointense on T1 and iso- to hyperintense on T2-weighted images with patchy contrast enhancement.[4] PET imaging is also generally used with FDG avidity dependent on histologic subtype.[72] A definitive diagnosis requires a tissue biopsy that can be difficult in the retroperitoneum. An image-guided needle biopsy is to be used over fine needle aspiration for diagnostic purposes if no other superficial lymph nodes are accessible and also because sarcoma is in the differential.[73] Flow cytometry and immunohistochemical stains are used to confirm the diagnosis of lymphoma. The diagnosis, staging, and management of retroperitoneal lymphoma are similar to that of other lymphoma sites and are discussed elsewhere in this text. As with all retroperitoneal tumors, radiation doses and treatment volumes may be limited by adjacent normal tissues.

OTHER LESIONS

Neuroblastoma is the most common solid extracranial tumor in children and the most common cancer in infants younger than 12 months, though this can occur rarely in adults.[74] In the United States, approximately 650 new cases are diagnosed per year[75] with a prevalence of 1 case per 7,000 live births and an incidence of 10.54 cases per 1 million per year in children younger than 15 years.[74] Ninety percent of cases are diagnosed in children <5 years of age with about 37% diagnosed as infants.[74] Neuroblastoma accounts for approximately 15% of all pediatric cancer fatalities. This tumor is extraordinarily

uncommon in adults with an estimated incidence of 0.2 per million population in those aged 30 to 39.[76] The paradigm for treatment of neuroblastoma includes combination therapy with chemotherapy, surgery, and radiotherapy in advanced-stage disease, which is most commonly found in adults.[77]

Wilms tumor (WT) or nephroblastoma is the most common intra-abdominal malignancy of childhood with an incidence of 7.1 cases per 1 million children younger than age 15 years with approximately 650 cases diagnosed in the United States each year.[74] It is the second most common extracranial solid neoplasm of childhood and the most common renal malignancy in children.[78] In contrast, it is an uncommon malignancy in patients ≥16 years of age with an estimated incidence of 0.2 per million population.[79,80] Adults frequently present with flank pain and painless hematuria,[81] whereas children are more likely to present with painless hematuria and/or a palpable abdominal mass.[74] The treatment and outcomes of patients with adult Wilms tumor (AWT) remain controversial with no standard therapy yet developed.[82] Kalapurakal et al.[83] reported the outcomes of 23 adults (>16 years of age) treated on Children Oncology Group (COG) protocols (National Wilms Tumor Study Group; NWTS 4 and 5) and found no difference between the adults and their pediatric counterparts. Similarly, the International Society of Pediatric Oncology (SIOP) published results from an SIOP retrospective review of 30 AWT patients >16 years of age with comparable results between adults and children.[81] Conversely, Izawa et al.[84] reported on 128 AWT patients from SIOP as well as individual institutional reports and concluded that the outcomes in adults were inferior to that of children. A SEER study by Ali et al.[85] concluded that the outcome in 152 AWT patients was worse than in children. Overall survival at 5 years was 69% in AWT versus 88% in children (P < .001). On multivariate analysis, adult status (≥16 years), SEER stage, treatment era (before 1990), and lack of surgical staging of lymph nodes were significant prognostic factors in this cohort. A consensus statement by an international group of childhood renal experts was published that recommends adoption of the pediatric paradigm for treatment of AWT patients including surgical resection, chemotherapy agents depending on stage and histologic subtype, and local therapy with irradiation depending on the stage of disease.[82] Furthermore, patients <30 years old are included on the current COG WT studies. The toxicities of treatment (severe acute neuropathy, grade 4 hematologic toxicity) in AWT patients may be somewhat higher than in the pediatric population but are thought to be reasonable in view of the high response rates.[81]

Retroperitoneal schwannomas are a rare tumor, accounting for approximately 4% of retroperitoneal tumors, but are the most common benign tumor found in this location.[86,87] They belong in the family of peripheral nerve sheath tumors, which in addition to schwannomas includes neurofibromas, solitary circumscribed neuromas, and perineuriomas.[88] Schwannomas may occur in any nerve trunk in the body with the exception of cranial nerves 1 and 2 (which are not covered by Schwann cells) and are most commonly found at peripheral nerve sites of the upper extremities and cranial nerves with only 0.3% to 3.2% of all schwannomas occurring in the retroperitoneum.[88] Benign schwannomas are associated neurofibromatosis 2 (NF2) in approximately 5% to 18% of NF2 patients, presenting most commonly between 20 and 50 years of age.[89] They are slow-growing nonaggressive tumors that displace rather than invade normal tissues and often form large, well-circumscribed masses.[87,88] They may display cystic degeneration, calcification, hemorrhage, and hyalinization on imaging studies. In several moderate to large series, there appears to be a slight female patient propensity and the tumors are often diagnosed incidentally during radiologic examinations for unrelated symptoms.[90,91] Bone changes may occur in tumors adjacent to the spine with invasion into nerve roots or the spinal canal, which may lead to neurologic symptoms including paresthesias, weakness, and pain. MRI examinations are the preferred method of imaging these soft tissue neoplasms although CT scanning may be necessary to better visualize potential bone abnormalities particularly in the spine. Because these tumors are frequently quite vascular, some investigators do not recommend the use of CT-guided biopsies because of the risk of hemorrhage.[92] Whenever feasible, complete surgical resection with negative margins is the treatment of choice although adjuvant radiation therapy may be necessary for incompletely excised sacral schwannomas.[93] NF1 patients have a particularly high risk of developing STS, particularly and malignant peripheral nerve sheath tumors (MPNST), often with an aggressive clinical presentation and poor outcome.[94]

Aggressive fibromatosis, also referred to as desmoid tumors, is a rare fibroblastic neoplasm that arises from deep musculoaponeurotic connective tissue and has an incidence of 2 to 4 cases per million population,[95] occurring either sporadically or associated with familial adenomatous polyposis (FAP).[96–99] Ten to 30% of patients with FAP eventually develop desmoid tumors with the majority occurring in either the extremities or abdomen/retroperitoneum.[100–102] They occur slightly more frequently in women than in men.[103] Although benign in nature, they are locally aggressive and may infiltrate critical structures. Complete surgical resection is the mainstay of treatment, but because the local recurrence rate and morbidity from resection can be high, some patients are now managed with observation and close clinical radiologic follow-up per NCCN guidelines. Local recurrence is common even in the setting of a wide local resection in up to 40% of patients depending on the series.[104–107] Postoperative radiotherapy and/or chemotherapy may be indicated when a complete surgical resection is not achieved or is not feasible or in multiple recurrent disease, though some institutions have been adopting a watch-and-wait approach to the treatment of desmoids as they are an indolent disease. The data are variable regarding the dose and treatment volumes for this disease; however, most reported series suggest that a dose of 50 to 60 Gy with margins of 5 to 7 cm is appropriate.[107,108] Doses >56 Gy may not be necessary to control gross disease.[108] A meta-analysis by Nuyttens et al., which included data from 22 studies, suggested that local control was improved with adjuvant radiation therapy compared to surgery alone; local control after surgery alone was 72% (R0) and 41% (R1 and R2) compared to 94% (R0) and 75% (R1 and R2) after surgery and adjuvant radiation.[107] In patients with unresectable disease, radiation therapy alone is effective in providing long-term local control in up to 80% of patients.[107,109] Systemic therapy may also play a role in unresectable, incompletely resected, or recurrent disease. Systemic therapy options include both cytotoxic and noncytotoxic agents including anthracyclines, hormonal therapy, nonsteroidal anti-inflammatory drugs, imatinib, and clinical trials with agents like sorafinib.[110]

Extragonadal germ cell tumors (EGCTs) account for approximately 1% to 5% of all germ cell tumors and occur in the retroperitoneum as the second most common extra

gonadal site in adults after the mediastinum.[111] Primary retroperitoneal germ cell tumors account for approximately 5% of all primary malignant retroperitoneal tumors in adults.[112] It is believed that these tumors arise from primordial germ cells, which are displaced during their migration along the urogenital ridge to the gonads.[111] When they occur in the retroperitoneum, they are considered to be metastases from an occult or "burned out" gonadal primary until proven otherwise. EGCTs are most typically found in children or young adults and mostly arise in midline locations. The majority of these tumors occur in young men, and the majority are nonseminomatous germ cell tumors (NSGCTs) rather than seminomatous germ cell tumors (SGCTs).[111] In young women, the histologic varieties are dysgerminomas and nondysgerminomas. NSGCTs include the following histologies: teratoma, embryonal carcinoma, endodermal sinus tumor (yolk sac tumor), choriocarcinoma, and mixed histologies. Any proportion of nonseminomatous component is enough to classify a tumor as an NSGCT. NSGCTs generally have a much more aggressive course than do SGCTs. Serum markers, although nonspecific, may help to categorize the histology and can be useful for following both response to therapy and the presence of recurrence. Beta human chorionic gonadotropin (β-HCG) is elevated in choriocarcinoma and embryonal carcinoma and in approximately 10% to 15% of SGCTs.[113] Serum α-fetoprotein is elevated in endodermal sinus tumors and embryonal carcinomas. These tumors often present as large masses in the retroperitoneum and frequently displace, compress, or encase abdominal vessels. There are no distinguishing features by imaging to differentiate germ cell tumors from other retroperitoneal masses; thus, image-guided biopsy is necessary. Gonadal primaries must be ruled out using high-resolution ultrasound.[114] A biopsy of the gonads appears to be unnecessary in the presence of a negative ultrasound. Common sites of metastases are liver, bone, brain, and lungs. The prognosis of retroperitoneal SGCTs and their mediastinal counterparts are similar; however, retroperitoneal NSGCTs actually have a better prognosis than those occurring in the mediastinum.[111]

The treatment for EGCTs has evolved over past 10 to 15 years from the use of primary radiotherapy for SGCTs to the more commonly recommended treatment of platinum-based chemotherapy regimens.[111] Treatment paradigms for early-stage SGCT and NSGCT are covered elsewhere in this book. The International Germ Cell Cancer Collaborative Group established a classification system for assessing prognosis in NSGCT and SGCT[115] (Table 79.6), which is used to guide treatment decisions. For patients with a retroperitoneal SGCT, the preferred treatment approach is systemic chemotherapy using a cisplatin-based regimen similar to a patient with advanced testicular SGCT. In an international retrospective review of EGCTs, patients with retroperitoneal SGCTs had an overall survival of approximately 90% with the majority of patients treated with chemotherapy alone.[111] Patients treated

TABLE 79.6 THE INTERNATIONAL GERM CELL CANCER COLLABORATIVE GROUP CLASSIFICATION SYSTEM FOR ASSESSING PROGNOSIS IN NSGCT AND SGCT[115]

Tumor	Good Prognosis	Intermediate Prognosis	Poor Prognosis
NSGCT	• Testis/retroperitoneal primary, no nonpulmonary visceral metastases, AFP <1,000 ng/mL, β-hCG <1,000 IU/L, and LDH <1.5 × upper limit of normal • 5-y PFS, 89% • 5-y survival rate, 92%	• Testis/retroperitoneal primary, no nonpulmonary visceral metastases, AFP >1,000 ng/mL and <10,000 ng/mL and/or β-hCG 5,000–50,000 IU/L and/or LDH >1.5 × normal to 10 × normal • 5-y PFS, 75% • 5-y survival rate, 92%	• Indicated by any of the following: mediastinal primary, nonpulmonary visceral metastases or AFP >10,000 ng/mL, β-hCG >50,000 IU/L, or LDH >10 × normal • 5-y PFS, 41% • 5-y survival rate, 48%
Seminoma	• Any primary site, no nonpulmonary visceral metastases, normal AFP, any β-hCG, any LDH • 5-y PFS, 92% • 5-y survival rate, 88%	• Any primary site, nonpulmonary visceral metastases, normal AFP, any β-hCG, any LDH • 5-y PFS, 67% • 5-y survival rate, 72%	• No patients classified as having poor prognosis

From International Germ Cell Consensus Classification: a prognostic factor-based staging system for metastatic germ cell cancers. International Germ Cell Cancer Collaborative Group. *J Clin Oncol* 1997;15(2):594–603. Reprinted with permission. Copyright © 1997 American Society of Clinical Oncology. All rights reserved.

with primary radiation therapy had an inferior progression-free survival compared to patients treated with either chemotherapy alone or chemotherapy plus radiation therapy.[111] For retroperitoneal NSGCTs, the preferred treatment is also cisplatin-based chemotherapy as in a testicular NSGCT with the number of cycles dependent on if the patient is in the good or intermediate/poor prognosis group (Table 79.6). Residual masses should then be resected. In the international retrospective review of EGCTs, patients with retroperitoneal NSGCTs were primarily treated with primary chemotherapy with 45% of patients undergoing a secondary surgery for residual disease.[111] The 5-year overall survival for patients with retroperitoneal NSGCTs was 62%.[111]

CONCLUSIONS

The retroperitoneum is a challenging space for clinicians with a wide variety of possible histologies and adjacent normal tissues limiting therapeutic options. Advances in imaging have improved the ability to characterize these lesions, although ultimately, a histologic diagnosis is necessary. In general, treatment is driven by histology. For the majority of neoplasms in the retroperitoneum, evaluation by a multidisciplinary team is necessary. Radiation therapy technology advances, including the use of intensity-modulated radiation therapy and particle therapy, have improved the ability to deliver a therapeutic radiation dose to the tumor in this challenging space while sparing abutting organs at risk. Although much progress has been made with advances in surgery, systemic therapy, and radiation therapy, patient outcomes remain poor, thus, additional advancements need to be made including more prospective multi-institutional studies.

REFERENCES

1. Armstrong JR, Cohn I, Jr. Primary malignant tumors of the retroperitoneum. *Nebr State Med J* 1965;50:520–524.
2. Bose B. Primary malignant retroperitoneal tumours: analysis of 30 cases. *Can J Surg* 1979;22:215–220.
3. Pack GT, Tabah EJ. Primary retroperitoneal tumors: a study of 120 cases. *Int Abstr Surg* 1954;99:313–341.
4. Rajiah P, et al. Imaging of uncommon retroperitoneal masses. *Radiographics* 2011;31:949–976, doi:10.1148/rg.314095132.
5. Pemberton J de J, Whitlock M. Large retroperitoneal lipoma. *Surg Clin North Am* 1934;14:601.
6. Burkill GJC, Healy JC. Anatomy of the Retroperitoneum. *Imaging* 2000;12:10–20.
7. Osman S et al. A comprehensive review of the retroperitoneal anatomy, neoplasms, and pattern of disease spread. *Curr Probl Diagn Radiol* 2013;42:191–208, doi:10.1067/j.cpradiol.2013.02.001.
8. Melicow MM. Primary tumors of the retroperitoneum; a clinicopathologic analysis of 162 cases; review of the literature and tables of classification. *J Int Coll Surg* 1953;19:401–449.
9. Oriana S, Bonardi P, Preda F. Primary retroperitoneal tumors. *Tumori* 1977;63:397–405.
10. Ries LAG, Eisner MP, Kosary CL. *SEER-cancer statistics review*, 1975–2002, http://seer.cancer.gov/csr/1975_2002/.
11. Lawrence W Jr, et al. Adult soft tissue sarcomas. A pattern of care survey of the American College of Surgeons. *Ann Surg* 1987;205:349–359.
12. Porter GA, Baxter NN, Pisters PW. Retroperitoneal sarcoma: a population-based analysis of epidemiology, surgery, and radiotherapy. *Cancer* 2006;106:1610–1616, doi:10.1002/cncr.21761.
13. Mendenhall WM, et al. Retroperitoneal soft tissue sarcoma. *Cancer* 2005;104:669–675, doi:10.1002/cncr.21264.
14. O'Sullivan PJ, Harris AC, Munk PL. Radiological imaging features of non-uterine leiomyosarcoma. *Br J Radiol* 2008;81:73–81, doi:10.1259/bjr/18595145.
15. Roberge D, Hickeson M, Charest M, et al. Initial McGill experience with fluorodeoxyglucose PET/CT staging of soft-tissue sarcoma. *Curr Oncol* 2010;17:18–22.
16. Trans-Atlantic, R. P. S. W. G. Management of primary retroperitoneal sarcoma (RPS) in the adult: a consensus approach from the Trans-Atlantic RPS Working Group. *Ann Surg Oncol* 2015;22:256–263, doi:10.1245/s10434-014-3965-2.
17. Baldini EH, et al. Treatment guidelines for preoperative radiation therapy for retroperitoneal sarcoma: preliminary consensus of an international expert panel. *Int J Radiat Oncol Biol Phys* 2015;92:602–612, doi:10.1016/j.ijrobp.2015.02.013.
18. Ohnstad HO, et al. MDM2 antagonist Nutlin-3a potentiates antitumour activity of cytotoxic drugs in sarcoma cell lines. *BMC Cancer* 2011;11:211:1–11, doi:10.1186/1471-2407-11-211.
19. Jaques DP, Coit DG, Hajdu SI, et al. Management of primary and recurrent soft-tissue sarcoma of the retroperitoneum. *Ann Surg* 1990;212:51–59.
20. Lehnert T, et al. Primary and locally recurrent retroperitoneal soft-tissue sarcoma: local control and survival. *Eur J Surg Oncol* 2009;35:986–993, doi:10.1016/j.ejso.2008.11.003.
21. Stahl JM, et al. The effect of microscopic margin status on survival in adult retroperitoneal soft tissue sarcomas. *Eur J Surg Oncol* 2017;43:168–174, doi:10.1016/j.ejso.2016.05.031.
22. Gronchi A, et al. Aggressive surgical policies in a retrospectively reviewed single-institution case series of retroperitoneal soft tissue sarcoma patients. *J Clin Oncol* 2009;27:24–30, doi:10.1200/JCO.2008.17.8871.
23. Gronchi A, et al. Frontline extended surgery is associated with improved survival in retroperitoneal low- to intermediate-grade soft tissue sarcomas. *Annals Oncol* 2012;23:1067–1073, doi:10.1093/annonc/mdr323.
24. Stoeckle E, et al. Prognostic factors in retroperitoneal sarcoma: a multivariate analysis of a series of 165 patients of the French Cancer Center Federation Sarcoma Group. *Cancer* 2001;92:359–368.
25. van Doorn RC, et al. Resectable retroperitoneal soft tissue sarcomas. The effect of extent of resection and postoperative radiation therapy on local tumor control. *Cancer* 1994;73:637–642.
26. Heslin MJ, et al. Prognostic factors associated with long-term survival for retroperitoneal sarcoma: implications for management. *J Clin Oncol* 1997;15:2832–2839, doi:10.1200/jco.1997.15.8.2832.
27. Jones JJ, et al. Initial results of a trial of preoperative external-beam radiation therapy and postoperative brachytherapy for retroperitoneal sarcoma. *Ann Surg Oncol* 2002;9:346–354.
28. Pawlik TM, et al. Long-term results of two prospective trials of preoperative external beam radiotherapy for localized intermediate- or high-grade retroperitoneal soft tissue sarcoma. *Ann Surg Oncol* 2006;13:508–517, doi:10.1245/ASO.2006.05.035.
29. EORTC, E. O. f. R. a. T. o. C. *A phase III randomized study of preoperative radiotherapy plus surgery versus surgery alone for patients with retroperitoneal sarcoma (RPS)*, https://www.clinicaltrials.gov/ct2/show/NCT01344018.
30. ACOSOG. *A phase III randomized study of preoperative radiation plus surgery versus surgery alone for patients with retroperitoneal sarcomas (RPS)*, https://www.clinicaltrials.gov/ct2/show/NCT00091351.
31. Shibata D, Lewis JJ, Leung DH, et al. Is there a role for incomplete resection in the management of retroperitoneal liposarcomas? *J Am Coll Surg* 2001;193:373–379.
32. Serizawa I et al. Carbon ion radiotherapy for unresectable retroperitoneal sarcomas. *Int J Radiat Oncol Biol Phys* 2009;75:1105–1110, doi:10.1016/j.ijrobp.2008.12.019.
33. MacNeill AJ, et al. Post-relapse outcomes after primary extended resection of retroperitoneal sarcoma: a report from the Trans-Atlantic RPS Working Group. *Cancer* 2017, doi:10.1002/cncr.30572.
34. Alektiar KM, Hu K, Anderson L, et al. High-dose-rate intraoperative radiation therapy (HDR-IORT) for retroperitoneal sarcomas. *Int J Radiat Oncol Biol Phys* 2000;47:157–163.
35. Dziewirski W, et al. Surgery combined with intraoperative brachytherapy in the treatment of retroperitoneal sarcomas. *Ann Surg Oncol* 2006;13:245–252, doi:10.1245/ASO.2006.03.026.
36. Gieschen HL et al. Long-term results of intraoperative electron beam radiotherapy for primary and recurrent retroperitoneal soft tissue sarcoma. *Int J Radiat Oncol Biol Phys* 2001;50:127–131.
37. Anaya DA, et al. Establishing prognosis in retroperitoneal sarcoma: a new histology-based paradigm. *Ann Surg Oncol* 2009;16:667–675, doi:10.1245/s10434-008-0250-2.
38. Dalal KM, Kattan MW, Antonescu CR, et al. Subtype specific prognostic nomogram for patients with primary liposarcoma of the retroperitoneum, extremity, or trunk. *Ann Surg* 2006;244:381–391, doi:10.1097/01.sla.0000234795.98607.00.
39. Lahat G, et al. Resectable well-differentiated versus dedifferentiated liposarcomas: two different diseases possibly requiring different treatment approaches. *Ann Surg Oncol* 2008;15:1585–1593, doi:10.1245/s10434-007-9805-x.
40. Lahat G, et al. New perspectives for staging and prognosis in soft tissue sarcoma. *Ann Surg Oncol* 2008;15:2739–2748, doi:10.1245/s10434-008-9970-6.
41. Storm FK, Eilber FR, Mirra J, et al Retroperitoneal sarcomas: a reappraisal of treatment. *J Surg Oncol* 1981;17:1–7.
42. Bevilacqua RG, Rogatko A, Hajdu SI, et al. Prognostic factors in primary retroperitoneal soft-tissue sarcomas. *Arch Surg* 1991;126:328–334.
43. Karakousis CP, Velez AF, Emrich LJ. Management of retroperitoneal sarcomas and patient survival. *Am J Surg* 1985;150:376–380.
44. Glenn J, et al. A randomized, prospective trial of adjuvant chemotherapy in adults with soft tissue sarcomas of the head and neck, breast, and trunk. *Cancer* 1985;55:1206–1214.
45. Rosenberg SA. Prospective randomized trials demonstrating the efficacy of adjuvant chemotherapy in adult patients with soft tissue sarcomas. *Cancer Treat Rep* 1984;68:1067–1078.
46. Sarcoma Meta-analysis Collaboration. Adjuvant chemotherapy for localised resectable soft-tissue sarcoma of adults: meta-analysis of individual data. *Lancet* 1997;350:1647–1654, doi:S0140673697081658 [pii].
47. Pisters PW, et al. Phase I trial of preoperative concurrent doxorubicin and radiation therapy, surgical resection, and intraoperative electron-beam radiation therapy for patients with localized resectable sarcoma. *J Clin Oncol* 2003;21:3092–3097, doi:10.1200/JCO.2003.01.143.
48. Adjuvant chemotherapy for localised resectable soft tissue sarcoma in adults. Sarcoma Meta-analysis Collaboration (SMAC). *Cochrane Database Syst Rev* 2000;(4):CD001419.
49. Tap DW, Jones RL, Chmielowski B, et al. A randomized phase Ib/II study evaluating the safety and efficacy of olaratumab (IMC-3G3), a human anti-platelet-derived growth factor α (PDGFRα) monoclonal antibody, with or without doxorubicin (Dox), in advanced soft tissue sarcoma (STS). *J Clin Oncol* 2015;33(suppl; abstr 10501).

50. Wong P, et al. Spatial and volumetric changes of retroperitoneal sarcomas during pre-operative radiotherapy. *Radiother Oncol* 2014;112:308–313, doi:10.1016/j.radonc.2014.08.004.

51. Tzeng CW, et al. Preoperative radiation therapy with selective dose escalation to the margin at risk for retroperitoneal sarcoma. *Cancer* 2006;107:371–379, doi:10.1002/cncr.22005.

52. Vassilev LT, et al. In vivo activation of the p53 pathway by small-molecule antagonists of MDM2. *Science* 2004;303:844–848, doi:10.1126/science.1092472.

53. Park H, et al. Tissue expander placement and adjuvant radiotherapy after surgical resection of retroperitoneal liposarcoma offers improved local control. *Medicine* 2016;95:e4435, doi:10.1097/MD.0000000000004435.

54. Jabbour SK, et al. Upper abdominal normal organ contouring guidelines and atlas: a Radiation Therapy Oncology Group consensus. *Pract Radiat Oncol* 2014;4:82–89, doi:10.1016/j.prro.2013.06.004.

55. Marks LB, et al. Use of normal tissue complication probability models in the clinic. *Int J Radiat Oncol Biol Phys* 2010;76:S10–S19, doi:10.1016/j.ijrobp.2009.07.1754.

56. Swanson EL, et al. Comparison of three-dimensional (3D) conformal proton radiotherapy (RT), 3D conformal photon RT, and intensity-modulated RT for retroperitoneal and intra-abdominal sarcomas. *Int J Radiat Oncol Biol Phys* 2012;83:1549–1557, doi:10.1016/j.ijrobp.2011.10.014.

57. Czito B, Donohue J, Willett CG, et al., eds. *Intraoperative irradiation.* Springer, 2011 (Ch. 17).

58. Harrison LB, Enker WE, Anderson LL. High-dose-rate intraoperative radiation therapy for colorectal cancer. *Oncology (Williston Park)* 1995;9:737–741; discussion 742–738 passim.

59. Harrison LB, Enker WE, Anderson LL. High-dose-rate intraoperative radiation therapy for colorectal cancer. *Oncology (Williston Park)* 1995;9:679–683.

60. Catton CN, et al. Outcome and prognosis in retroperitoneal soft tissue sarcoma. *Int J Radiat Oncol Biol Phys* 1994;29:1005–1010.

61. Hassan I, et al. Operative management of primary retroperitoneal sarcomas: a reappraisal of an institutional experience. *Ann Surg* 2004;239:244–250, doi:10.1097/01.sla.0000108670.31446.54.

62. Lewis JJ, Leung D, Woodruff JM, et al. Retroperitoneal soft-tissue sarcoma: analysis of 500 patients treated and followed at a single institution. *Ann Surg* 1998;228:355–365.

63. Ferrario T, Karakousis CP. Retroperitoneal sarcomas: grade and survival. *Arch Surg* 2003;138:248–251.

64. Gronchi A, et al. Retroperitoneal soft tissue sarcomas: patterns of recurrence in 167 patients treated at a single institution. *Cancer* 2004;100:2448–2455, doi:10.1002/cncr.20269.

65. Nussbaum DP, et al. Preoperative or postoperative radiotherapy versus surgery alone for retroperitoneal sarcoma: a case-control, propensity score-matched analysis of a nationwide clinical oncology database. *Lancet Oncol* 2016;17:966–975, doi:10.1016/S1470-2045(16)30050-X.

66. Sindelar WF, et al. Intraoperative radiotherapy in retroperitoneal sarcomas. Final results of a prospective, randomized, clinical trial. *Arch Surg* 1993;128:402–410.

67. Petersen IA, et al. Use of intraoperative electron beam radiotherapy in the management of retroperitoneal soft tissue sarcomas. *Int J Radiat Oncol Biol Phys* 2002;52:469–475.

68. Yeh JJ, Singer S, Brennan MF, et al. Effectiveness of palliative procedures for intra-abdominal sarcomas. *Ann Surg Oncol* 2005;12:1084–1089, doi:10.1245/ASO.2005.03.016.

69. Kepka L, DeLaney TF, Suit HD, et al. Results of radiation therapy for unresected soft-tissue sarcomas. *Int J Radiat Oncol Biol Phys* 2005;63:852–859, doi:10.1016/j.ijrobp.2005.03.004.

70. Hug EB, et al. Conformal proton radiation treatment for retroperitoneal neuroblastoma: introduction of a novel technique. *Med Pediatr Oncol* 2001;37:36–41, doi:10.1002/mpo.1160.

71. Callegaro D, et al. Long-term morbidity after multivisceral resection for retroperitoneal sarcoma. *Br J Surg* 2015;102:1079–1087, doi:10.1002/bjs.9829.

72. Weiler-Sagie M, et al. (18)F-FDG avidity in lymphoma readdressed: a study of 766 patients. *J Nucl Med* 2010;51:25–30, doi:10.2967/jnumed.109.067892.

73. Zangos S, et al. MR-guided biopsies of lesions in the retroperitoneal space: technique and results. *Eur Radiol* 2006;16:307–312, doi:10.1007/s00330-005-2870-2.

74. Neuroblastoma Treatment (PDQ®): Health Professional Version in *PDQ Cancer Information Summaries* 2002.

75. Gurney JG, et al. Infant cancer in the U.S.: histology-specific incidence and trends, 1973 to 1992. *J Pediatr Hematol Oncol* 1997;19:428–432.

76. Davis S, Rogers MA, Pendergrass TW. The incidence and epidemiologic characteristics of neuroblastoma in the United States. *Am J Epidemiol* 1987;126:1063–1074.

77. Godkhindi VM, Basade MM, Khan K, et al. Adult neuroblastoma-case report and literature review. *J Clin Diagn Res* 2016;10:ED01–ED02, doi:10.7860/JCDR/2016/20237.9080.

78. Breslow N, Olshan A, Beckwith JB, et al. Epidemiology of Wilms tumor. *Med Pediatr Oncol* 1993;21:172–181.

79. Merten DF, Yang SS, Bernstein J. Wilms' tumor in adolescence. *Cancer* 1976;37:1532–1538.

80. Mitry E, et al. Incidence of and survival from Wilms' tumour in adults in Europe: data from the EUROCARE study. *Eur J Cancer* 2006;42:2363–2368, doi:10.1016/j.ejca.2006.04.009.

81. Reinhard H, et al. Wilms' tumor in adults: results of the Society of Pediatric Oncology (SIOP) 93-01/Society for Pediatric Oncology and Hematology (GPOH) Study. *J Clin Oncol* 2004;22, 4500–4506, doi:10.1200/JCO.2004.12.099.

82. Segers H, et al. Management of adults with Wilms' tumor: recommendations based on international consensus. *Expert Rev Anticancer Ther* 2011;11:1105–1113, doi:10.1586/era.11.76.

83. Kalapurakal JA, et al. Treatment outcomes in adults with favorable histologic type Wilms tumor-an update from the National Wilms Tumor Study Group. *Int J Radiat Oncol Biol Phys* 2004;60:1379–1384, doi:10.1016/j.ijrobp.2004.05.057.

84. Izawa JI, et al. Prognostic variables in adult Wilms tumour. *Can J Surg* 2008;51:252–256.

85. Ali AN, Diaz R, Shu HK, et al. Surveillance, epidemiology and end results (SEER) program comparison of adult and pediatric Wilms' tumor. *Cancer* 2012;118:2541–2551, doi:10.1002/cncr.26554.

86. Nah YW, et al. Benign retroperitoneal schwannoma: surgical consideration. *Hepato-Gastroenterology* 2005;52:1681–1684.

87. Theodosopoulos T, et al. Special problems encountering surgical management of large retroperitoneal schwannomas. *World J Surg Oncol* 2008;6:107, doi:10.1186/1477-7819-6-107.

88. Strauss DC, Qureshi YA, Hayes AJ, et al. Management of benign retroperitoneal schwannomas: a single-center experience. *Am J Surg* 2011;202:194–198, doi:10.1016/j.amjsurg.2010.06.036.

89. Antiheimo J, Hu K, Anderson L, et al. Population based analysis of sporadic and type 2 neurofibromatosis-associated meningiomas and schwannomas. *Neurology* 2000;54:71–76.

90. Hughes MJ, Thomas JM, Fisher C, et al. Imaging features of retroperitoneal and pelvic schwannomas. *Clin Radiol* 2005;60:886–893, doi:10.1016/j.crad.2005.01.016.

91. Li Q, Gao C, Juzi JT, et al. Analysis of 82 cases of retroperitoneal schwannoma. *ANZ J Surg* 2007;77:237–240, doi:10.1111/j.1445-2197.2007.04025.x.

92. Daneshman S, Youssefzadeh D, Chamie K, et al. Benign retroperitoneal schwannoma: a case series and review of the literature. *Urology* 2003;62:993–997.

93. Carli M, et al. Pediatric malignant peripheral nerve sheath tumor: the Italian and German soft tissue sarcoma cooperative group. *J Clin Oncol* 2005;23:8422–8430, doi:10.1200/JCO.2005.01.4886.

94. Ferrari A, et al. Soft-tissue sarcomas in children and adolescents with neurofibromatosis type 1. *Cancer* 2007;109:1406–1412, doi:10.1002/cncr.22533.

95. Reitamo JJ, Hayry P, Nykyri E, et al. The desmoid tumor. I. Incidence, sex-, age- and anatomical distribution in the Finnish population. *Am J Clin Pathol* 1982;77:665–673.

96. Reitamo JJ, Scheinin TM, Hayry P. The desmoid syndrome. New aspects in the cause, pathogenesis and treatment of the desmoid tumor. *Am J Surg* 1986;151:230–237.

97. Nieuwenhuis MH, et al. A nation-wide study comparing sporadic and familial adenomatous polyposis-related desmoid-type fibromatoses. *Int J Cancer* 2011;129:256–261, doi:10.1002/ijc.25664.

98. Latchford AR, Sturt NJ, Neale K, et al. A 10-year review of surgery for desmoid disease associated with familial adenomatous polyposis. *Br J Surg* 2006;93:1258–1264, doi:10.1002/bjs.5425.

99. Ferenc T, et al. Aggressive fibromatosis (desmoid tumors): definition, occurrence, pathology, diagnostic problems, clinical behavior, genetic background. *Pol J Pathol* 2006;57:5–15.

100. de Camargo VP, et al. Clinical outcomes of systemic therapy for patients with deep fibromatosis (desmoid tumor). *Cancer* 2010;116:2258–2265, doi:10.1002/cncr.25089.

101. Meazza C, Alaggio R, Ferrari A. Aggressive fibromatosis in children: a changing approach. *Minerva Pediatr* 2011;63:305–318.

102. Meazza C, et al. Aggressive fibromatosis in children and adolescents: the Italian experience. *Cancer* 2010;116:233–240, doi:10.1002/cncr.24679.

103. Mankin HJ, Hornicek FJ, Springfield DS. Extra-abdominal desmoid tumors: a report of 234 cases. *J Surg Oncol* 2010;102:380–384, doi:10.1002/jso.21433.

104. Mullen JT, et al. Desmoid tumor: analysis of prognostic factors and outcomes in a surgical series. *Ann Surg Oncol* 2012;19:4028–4035, doi:10.1245/s10434-012-2638-2.

105. Huang K, Fu H, Shi YQ, et al. Prognostic factors for extra-abdominal and abdominal wall desmoids: a 20-year experience at a single institution. *J Surg Oncol* 2009;100:563–569, doi:10.1002/jso.21384.

106. Ballo MT, Zagars GK, Pollack A, et al. Desmoid tumor: prognostic factors and outcome after surgery, radiation therapy, or combined surgery and radiation therapy. *J Clin Oncol* 1999;17:158–167, doi:10.1200/JCO.1999.17.1.158.

107. Nuyttens JJ, Rust PF, Thomas CR Jr, et al. Surgery versus radiation therapy for patients with aggressive fibromatosis or desmoid tumors: a comparative review of 22 articles. *Cancer* 2000;88:1517–1523.

108. Ballo MT, Zagars GK, Pollack A. Radiation therapy in the management of desmoid tumors. *Int J Radiat Oncol Biol Phys* 1998;42:1007–1014.

109. Micke O, Seegenschmiedt MH. Radiation therapy for aggressive fibromatosis (desmoid tumors): results of a national patterns of care study. *Int J Radiat Oncol Biol Phys* 2005;61:882–891, doi:10.1016/j.ijrobp.2004.07.705.

110. Kasper B, et al. Management of sporadic desmoid-type fibromatosis: a European consensus approach based on patients' and professionals' expertise – a sarcoma patients EuroNet and European Organisation for Research and Treatment of Cancer/Soft Tissue and Bone Sarcoma Group initiative. *Eur J Cancer* 2015;51:127–136, doi:10.1016/j.ejca.2014.11.005.

111. Bokemeyer C, et al. Extragonadal germ cell tumors of the mediastinum and retroperitoneum: results from an international analysis. *J Clin Oncol* 2002;20:1864–1873.

112. Sangster GP, et al. The gamut of primary retroperitoneal masses: multimodality evaluation with pathologic correlation. *Abdom Imaging* 2016;41:1411–1430, doi:10.1007/s00261-016-0735-6.

113. Shinagare AB, Jagannathan JP, Ramaiya NH, et al. Adult extragonadal germ cell tumors. *Am J Roentgenol* 2010;195:W274–280, doi:10.2214/AJR.09.4103.

114. Bohle A, Studer UE, Sonntag RW, et al. Primary or secondary extragonadal germ cell tumors? *J Urol* 1986;135:939–943.

115. International Germ Cell Cancer Collaborative Group. International Germ Cell Consensus Classification: a prognostic factor-based staging system for metastatic germ cell cancers. *J Clin Oncol* 1997;15:594–603.

Section III

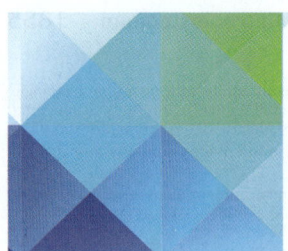

CHAPTER 80

Adrenal Cancer

Filip T. Troicki and John J. Coen

ANATOMY

The paired suprarenal (adrenal) glands are located between the superomedial aspects of the kidney and the diaphragmatic crura. They are surrounded by connective tissue containing perinephric fat. The glands are enclosed by renal fascia but separated from the kidneys by fibrous tissue. The triangular right gland relates to the diaphragm posteriorly and the inferior vena cava and liver anteriorly. The semilunar left adrenal gland is positioned in the middle of the left crux of the diaphragm. The omental bursa separates it from the stomach. It is also related to the spleen and pancreas.[1]

The endocrine function of the adrenal glands necessitates an abundant blood supply. The superior suprarenal arteries are derived from the inferior phrenic artery, the middle suprarenal arteries from the abdominal aorta near the origin of the superior mesenteric artery, and the inferior suprarenal arteries from the renal artery. A large central vein leaves the anterior surface of the gland at the hilum. The shorter right suprarenal vein drains into the inferior vena cava, and the longer left suprarenal vein drains into the left renal vein.[1]

The lymphatic drainage follows the arterial supply and is predominantly to lumbar lymph nodes. The superior lymphatic trunks end in aortocaval lymph nodes located near the origin of the celiac plexus. The inferior lymphatic trunks end in lateroaortic nodes above the renal pedicle. Some trunks may pass through the diaphragm, following the splanchnic nerves, ending in retroaortic nodes in the posterior mediastinum. On the right, some lymphatic trunks may penetrate the liver.[2]

The adrenal gland is composed of a central catecholamine-producing medulla enveloped by the steroid-secreting cortex. Although they are in intimate contact, they represent two functionally separate organs with different embryologic origins.

EPIDEMIOLOGY

Adrenal Cortical Tumors

Adrenocortical tumors are rare. Benign tumors are more common, occurring in 1% to 8% of the general population, and the incidence of carcinoma is approximately 1 per million population in the United States.[3,4] There are approximately 75 to 115 new cases per year.[5] Adrenal cortex carcinoma deaths account for 0.2% of all yearly cancer deaths. There is a bimodal age distribution with disease peaks before the age of 5 years and in the fourth to fifth decades of life.

Overall, adrenocortical carcinoma (ACC) is slightly more common in women than in men. Nonfunctional carcinomas occur in an older age population (>30 years old) and are more common in men (3:2 male-to-female ratio), although functional tumors are more common in women (7:3 female-to-male ratio) and younger patients. As they frequently present with symptoms related to hormone production, functional tumors are usually detected at an early stage.

Although most cases of ACC are sporadic, it has been described as a component of several hereditary cancer syndromes, including Li-Fraumeni syndrome (breast cancer, soft tissue and bone sarcoma, brain tumors, and ACC), Beckwith-Wiedemann syndrome (Wilms tumor, neuroblastoma, hepatoblastoma, and ACC), multiple endocrine neoplasia type I (MEN-I) (parathyroid, pituitary and pancreatic neuroendocrine tumors, and adrenal adenomas and carcinomas), and SBLA syndrome (sarcoma, breast, lung, ACC, and other tumors).[6–9] A role for p53 mutations in sporadic ACC is suspected.

Adrenal Medulla Tumors

Ganglioneuromas are rare, benign tumors of the adrenal medulla seen in children and young adults.[10,11] Neuroblastoma is the most common malignant tumor of the adrenal gland in children, accounting for 90% of all cases.[3,12]

Pheochromocytomas and functional ganglioneuromas (or extra-adrenal pheochromocytomas) are rare tumors that rise from chromaffin cells in the adrenal medulla and elsewhere. They secrete catecholamines and cause intermittent, episodic, or sustained hypertension. Pheochromocytomas have an estimated prevalence of 0.1% in hypertensive patients.[13] In autopsy series, there is a 0.01% to 0.1% prevalence of unsuspected pheochromocytomas. Extra-adrenal tumors are more commonly malignant.[14] Estimates of the incidence of malignancy in pheochromocytoma range from 5% to 46% in different series.[15,16] Approximately 400 new cases of malignant pheochromocytomas are expected each year in the United States.[17,18]

Pheochromocytomas may be associated with a variety of endocrine and nonendocrine inherited disorders. Bilateral pheochromocytomas are a component of multiple endocrine neoplasia type IIa (MEN-IIA) syndrome (pheochromocytoma, medullary thyroid carcinoma, and parathyroid hyperplasia) or MEN-IIB syndrome in which they are associated with marfanoid habitus, mucosal neuromas, and medullary thyroid carcinoma. Pheochromocytomas occur in 25% of patients with von Hippel-Lindau syndrome and <1% of patients with neurofibromatosis and von Recklinghausen disease.[19,20]

NATURAL HISTORY

Fifty-nine percent of adrenal cortex tumors are functional, the left-to-right ratio is approximately 1:1, and 2.4% are bilateral.[21] Diagnosis is frequently delayed because of the rarity of disease and the deep retroperitoneal location of the adrenal glands.[22]

Nonfunctioning ACCs are typically larger tumors, >6 cm, whereas functioning tumors tend to be discovered at an earlier stage (for TNM staging, see Table 80.1). Incidentally discovered adrenal masses <3 cm are rarely malignant. ACC is an aggressive malignancy that frequently violates the tumor capsule and invades surrounding tissues. It metastasizes to lungs, liver, brain, and regional lymph nodes. Many patients present with widespread metastasis; most of these patients die within 6 months of diagnosis. This situation is especially

TABLE 80.1 TNM STAGING FOR ACC

Tumor (T)
T1: Tumor ≤5 cm in size; invasion absent
T2: Tumor >5 cm in size; invasion absent
T3: Tumor outside adrenal in fat
T4: Tumor invading adjacent organs

Lymph Nodes (N)
N0: No positive lymph nodes
N1: Positive lymph nodes

Metastases (M)
M0: No distant metastases
M1: Distant metastases
Stage I–T1, N0, M0
Stage II–T2, N0, M0
Stage III–T1, N1, M0, T2, N1, M0, T3, N1, M0
Stage IV–T3, N1, M0, T4, N1, M0, any T, any N, M1

From Edge SB, Byrd DR, Compton CC, et al., eds. *AJCC cancer staging manual.* 7th ed. New York: Springer, 2010. Copyright © 2010 American Joint Committee on Cancer. Reproduced with permission of Springer in the format Book via Copyright Clearance Center.

TABLE 80.2 DIAGNOSTIC WORKUP FOR ADRENAL TUMORS

General
  History
  Physical examination
Radiology
  Chest CT
  Abdominal CT with thin cuts
  MRI
  Ultrasonography
  Angiographic studies
Nuclear medicine studies
  Fluorodeoxyglucose positron emission tomography
Laboratory studies
  Complete blood count, blood chemistry, urinalysis
  Serum and urine cortisol (adrenal cortical tumors)
  Serum and urine catecholamines (pheochromocytoma)

CT, computed tomography; MRI, magnetic resonance imaging.

common in the pediatric population. For all stages, the 5-year overall survival is only 20% to 25%.[22]

Malignant pheochromocytomas exhibit a similar pattern of spread but also metastasize to bone. They are equally common in men and women. The average age of presentation is 40 to 50 years old, but these carcinomas may also occur in children.

CLINICAL PRESENTATION

Functional adrenocortical tumors most frequently secrete cortisol and androgens, resulting in Cushing syndrome, virilization, and hypertension. Estrogen or aldosterone production is less common. Approximately 60% of ACCs are functional. In a child, virilization is the most common symptom of ACC, and Cushing syndrome is relatively uncommon. By contrast, adults usually present with either Cushing syndrome alone or mixed with virilization. Patients with nonfunctioning tumors present with nonspecific symptoms related to tumor burden, including abdominal fullness, early satiety, pain, weight loss, weakness, fever, or an abdominal mass. Nonfunctioning ACCs are more common in older patients and tend to progress more rapidly. An increasing number of adrenal tumors are incidentally discovered during abdominal imaging in the absence of any symptoms.

Pheochromocytomas arising in the setting of an inherited disorder occur in the adrenal medulla in 90% of cases, as compared with 75% of sporadic pheochromocytomas. When associated with MEN-II syndromes, 80% are bilateral. A tumor >5 cm more commonly has a malignant course than a smaller lesion. Serum catecholamines and urinary metanephrine and vanillylmandelic acid levels are elevated in 90% of pheochromocytomas. These patients present with a range of symptoms from mild labile hypertension to sudden cardiac death secondary to hypertensive crisis, myocardial infarction, or cerebrovascular accident. The classic triad of symptoms consists of episodic headaches, diaphoresis, and tachycardia.[8,23] About half of patients have paroxysmal hypertension, and others have sustained hypertension. Pheochromocytomas may also present with normal blood pressure in 5% to 15%. Other symptoms may include pallor, palpitations, panic attack symptoms, or generalized weakness. Orthostatic hypertension may occur in association with hypovolemia.

DIAGNOSTIC WORKUP AND STAGING

Patients with adrenal gland tumors should be evaluated for other primary tumors, because metastasis to the adrenal gland is common. In metastatic tumors that are not adrenal in origin, a biopsy is recommended. Prior to obtaining a biopsy, however, pheochromocytomas must be ruled out by measuring the fractionated plasma-free metanephrine, as well as the 24-hour urine fractionated metanephrines and catecholamines. Low suspicion for pheochromocytoma either clinically or biochemically should steer providers toward obtaining an adrenal biopsy. Furthermore, any patient with a suspected adrenal tumor should be screened for hormonal hypersecretion, including cortisol, aldosterone, and catecholamine secretion (Table 80.2). As hypercortisolism is the most frequent abnormality, serum cortisol, a 24-hour urinary cortisol, and an overnight dexamethasone suppression test should be obtained.

Morphologic evaluation of the adrenal glands with computed tomography (CT) of the abdomen should be performed as per adrenal protocol. CT of the abdomen with thin cuts through the adrenal gland is the imaging test of choice for the evaluation of adrenal tumors. Carcinomas can mimic adenomas but are characterized by larger size, irregular margins, and heterogeneous enhancement. They may also demonstrate tumor necrosis and cystic degeneration. Local invasion, tumor extension into the vena cava, as well as lymph node or other metastases are often seen in advanced ACC. Magnetic resonance imaging (MRI) is useful in the evaluation of adrenal tumors (Fig. 80.1). ACC

FIGURE 80.1. T2-weighted magnetic resonance image of a 35-year-old woman with a left adrenal carcinoma.

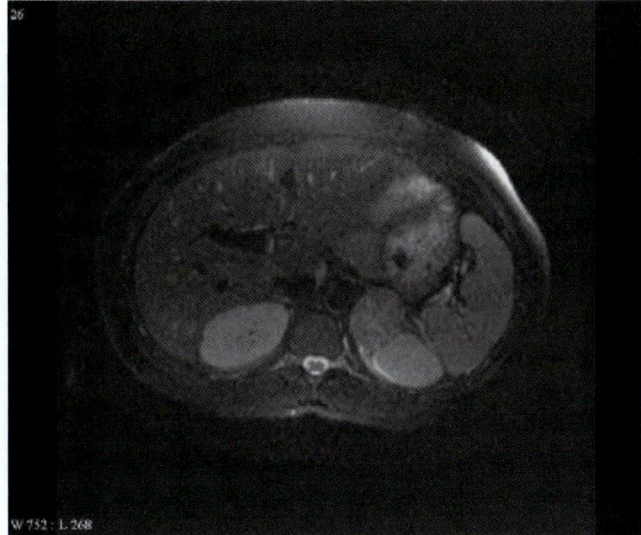

and pheochromocytomas are hyperintense on T2-weighted images, and venous invasion is better imaged on MRI. If there is still question of vascular invasion, an angiographic study can be performed preoperatively, either selective arteriography or vena cavography. Fluorodeoxyglucose positron emission tomography may be useful in differentiating benign from malignant lesions. It may also serve as an additional staging study for patients with known ACC. A chest CT should also be performed.

Evaluation of the patient's adrenal function is indicated if there is no suspicion of adrenal metastasis. Workup for hyperaldosteronism, Cushing syndrome, and pheochromocytoma should be performed when clinically indicated. The diagnosis of pheochromocytoma is confirmed by measurements of urinary and plasma fractionated metanephrines and catecholamines. Medication-induced elevation of metanephrine levels is common and should be evaluated prior to initiating further costly workup. Levels of metanephrine four times the normal limit are diagnostic of pheochromocytoma, and biochemical confirmation of disease is followed by imaging to locate the tumor. Other scans, including the OctreoScan (Mallinckrodt Inc., St. Louis, MO) and a bone scan, may be indicated if metastatic disease is suspected.

Levels of plasma aldosterone (high) and renin (low) activity should be assessed when suspecting primary aldosteronism (hyperaldosteronism). The ratio of aldosterone to renin above 30 is suggestive of hyperaldosteronism and should be confirmed with saline suppression or salt loading tests, and electrolytes should be measured. Although malignant hyperaldosteronism is rare, these patients require an open adrenalectomy to prevent tumor rupture. In benign cases of hyperaldosteronism, adrenal vein sampling for aldosterone is considered standard of care.

Patients with Cushing syndrome require an evaluation of serum levels of corticotropin, cortisol, as well as the sex steroid dehydroepiandrosterone sulfate (DHEA-S). If cortisol levels are elevated, a confirmatory test with dexamethasone suppression is recommended. It is important to remember that elevated corticotropin levels do not indicate adrenal origin, and further workup is necessary to look for primary causes of increased corticotropin. Benign adrenal tumors can be removed laparoscopically. Patients who present with Cushing syndrome in the presence of large (>4 cm), inhomogeneous, or invasive masses should be suspected to have malignant tumors, and imaging of the chest, abdomen, and pelvis is warranted to look for metastasis.

Pathologic Classification

Tumors <6 cm are more likely adenomas, although some smaller tumors may be malignant (Table 80.3). In order to establish stability of an adrenal mass, imaging should be repeated in 6 to 12 months for benign-appearing adenomas measuring <4 cm, and 3 to 6 months for larger lesions up to 6 cm. Hemorrhage and necrosis may be observed macroscopically in carcinomas. Numerous mitotic figures and cellular undifferentiation are common microscopic findings. Larger size, vascular invasion, or invasion of surrounding tissues and numerous mitotic figures are poor prognostic features.[24]

Pheochromocytomas have malignant features in <10% of cases. Macroscopically, they tend to be encapsulated with areas of cystic change, hemorrhage, and necrosis. The capsule is frequently invaded, but that does not constitute malignant change. Benign and malignant pheochromocytomas may appear identical histologically. The only absolute criterion for malignancy is metastasis.[9] Histologically, cell size, nuclear size, and arrangement of cells are variable. A

TABLE 80.3 CLASSIFICATION OF ADRENAL TUMORS
Adrenal cortex
Adenoma
Functioning
Nonfunctioning
Carcinoma
Adrenal medulla
Ganglioneuroma
Pheochromocytoma
Neuroblastoma
Mixed type (ganglioneuroblastoma)
Connective tissue tumors
Myelolipomas
Lipomas
Myomas
Angiomas
Fibromas
Fibrosarcoma

twisted cell cord pattern, basophilic or cytophilic staining with fine intracytoplasmic pigment granules, and periodic acid–Schiff staining of secretory droplets aid in the diagnosis.

GENERAL MANAGEMENT

Benign tumors are nonfunctioning and are most often found incidentally. After the benign nature of these tumors is confirmed, small tumors can be left untreated and can be followed up by repeat imaging 6 to 12 months after diagnosis to confirm their stability. Larger tumors (>4 cm) should be followed up with imaging in 3 to 6 months after diagnosis. A small benign mass that grows at the rate of >1 cm/year can be removed electively, but any significant growth of a larger mass should alert the clinician to a potentially malignant nature of the tumor and adrenalectomy is recommended in that case.

Nonfunctioning adrenal tumors that are >4 cm, are heterogeneous, or have irregular margins are suspicious for adrenal carcinomas. Surgery with removal of adjacent lymph nodes is the primary treatment for ACC. Complete resection, such as an open adrenalectomy, is the only treatment that offers long-term disease-free survival, but it is not always feasible.[25] For patients with a macroscopically complete resection, a margin-free resection is a strong predictor for survival. Efforts to avoid tumor spillage are warranted, and the tumor capsule should remain intact. Invasion or adherence of adjacent structures often necessitates *en bloc* resection of the kidney or spleen, partial hepatectomy, or pancreatectomy. The presence of tumor thrombus in the renal vein or vena cava does not preclude resection. A lymphadenectomy is often included. An extensive regional lymph node dissection has not been shown to have any impact on overall survival (OS) or disease specific survival (DSS).[26] For patients with localized disease who have high-risk features, such as positive margins, rupture of capsule, high grade, or large size, postoperative radiation should be considered. The role of tumor debulking in the presence of metastatic disease is not clear. Incomplete resection of the primary tumor or metastatic disease not amenable to surgery is associated with a poor prognosis. Still, tumor debulking may help control hormonal oversecretion or relieve local symptoms in certain cases. Even with a complete resection, local recurrence and metastatic disease are common. For isolated distant metastases and locally unresectable disease, cytoreductive resection with or without radiation is recommended.

The role of radiation in the management of ACC is not well defined. It has been proposed as adjuvant therapy in high-grade adrenal carcinoma as well as after complete resection or as management of microscopic residual disease. One series reports a 10-year crude survival rate of 33% for surgical resection followed by adjuvant radiation.[27] External radiation results in good response rates and effective palliation in patients with residual macroscopic disease or bone or nodal metastasis.[18,28]

Mitotane, a chemical congener of the insecticide DDT (dichlorodiphenyltrichloroethane), is an adrenolytic compound with specific activity on the adrenal cortex. It is the chemotherapeutic agent most commonly used in the management of ACC. In patients with measurable disease, overall response rates of 14% to 36% have been reported, but most studies have reported no significant survival benefit.[29] The largest retrospective study from Italy and Germany that included 177 patients with resected ACC (stages I to III) showed improvements in disease-free survival and overall survival.[30] Unfortunately, responses are usually partial and transient, with only an occasional complete remission.[21] The role of mitotane as adjuvant therapy after complete surgical resection is questionable. Despite limited supporting data, it is frequently employed in this setting, given the high rates of locoregional and distant recurrence. Serum levels of mitotane are monitored in order to optimize therapy because objective response in the metastatic setting was associated with higher serum levels (>14 mg/L). Unfortunately, increased toxicity is also associated with higher serum levels. Side effects are predominantly gastrointestinal, particularly nausea, but anorexia and diarrhea also occur. Although less common, central nervous system toxicity can include lethargy, somnolence, ataxia, dizziness, or confusion.

Single-agent chemotherapy has proven disappointing in the management of ACC. Doxorubicin and cisplatin have both been evaluated as single-agent therapy and in combination with mitotane. Neither drug was efficacious.[31] Multiagent chemotherapy has shown more promise. A multicenter phase II study by the Italian Group for the Study of Adrenal Cancer demonstrated 49% overall response rate using a regimen of etoposide, doxorubicin, and cisplatin in combination with mitotane. The regimen was well tolerated. The most common side effects were gastrointestinal. The time to progression in responding patients was 2 years.[6] Inclusion of mitotane in a multidrug regimen is rational as ACCs are prone to multidrug resistance mediated by the multidrug resistance-1/P glycoprotein drug pump, whose mechanism is inhibited by mitotane. This multidrug regimen is worthy of further study.

Surgical resection is the definitive management of pheochromocytoma, but it is a high-risk procedure. Cardiovascular and hemodynamic parameters must be monitored closely. Preoperative medical therapy is aimed at controlling hypertension and expanding intravascular volume. Preoperative pharmacologic preparation typically includes combined α- and β-adrenergic blockade.

In patients with undiagnosed pheochromocytomas who undergo surgery for other reasons, surgical mortality rates are high because of lethal hypertensive crisis and multiorgan failure.[32] In the largest series of 147 patients undergoing surgery for pheochromocytoma, perioperative mortality and morbidity rates were 2.4% and 24%, respectively.[33] Although it results in rapid symptomatic control, surgical removal of a pheochromocytoma does not always lead to a longtime cure. In a large series of 176 patients, pheochromocytoma recurred in 16% of patients. Half of these recurrences were malignant.[34] In patients

with bilateral pheochromocytomas, usually in the setting of an inherited syndrome, bilateral adrenalectomy is recommended. Hormone replacement is required in this setting. Although not curative, debulking surgery for control of symptoms is the primary therapy for malignant pheochromocytoma.

The radioisotope iodine-131 metaiodobenzylguanidine (^{131}I-MIBG) has been used as a therapeutic agent in malignant pheochromocytomas that demonstrate avid uptake of the agent. Investigators have reported partial responses, based on biochemical response as well as decreased tumor volume, ranging from 18% to 82%.[35-37] Symptomatic improvement was observed in responding patients with regard to both painful metastases and manifestations of increased catecholamine levels. Partial remissions are usually temporary, with some patients relapsing between doses of MIBG. In other patients, sustained partial remissions have been noted with durable palliation extending 2 to 3 years.[36,38] Prolonged survival has been associated with measurable responses and higher administered doses of MIBG (>500 mCi).[39] Toxicity includes bone marrow toxicity (particularly thrombocytopenia), nausea, and vomiting.

Combination chemotherapy with cyclophosphamide, vincristine, and dacarbazine has shown efficacy in a small study. In 14 treated patients, the clinical and biochemical response rates were 57% and 79%, respectively. Response was associated with objective improvement in performance status and blood pressure, and treatment was well tolerated.[40]

RADIATION THERAPY TECHNIQUES

The role of radiation in the management of ACC is controversial. Locoregional disease control remains a major problem in this disease, and some reports suggest that external radiation may reduce recurrence rates.

In the primary management of ACC, external radiation may play a role preoperatively for unresectable tumors, postoperatively for patients with residual disease or high risk of local failure, or as definitive therapy for patients who are medically unfit for surgery. Radiation is also effective in the palliative setting for bone and nodal metastases.

For patients with macroscopic or unresectable disease, doses of 50 to 60 Gy delivered during 5 to 6 weeks should be considered. Initial fields should encompass the gross tumor with adequate margins as well as the regional lymph nodes, which should include the contralateral para-aortic lymph nodes. Dose to regional nodes can be limited to 45 Gy when they are not macroscopically involved. Care should be taken to limit dose to the spinal cord, kidneys, liver, and small bowel. For macroscopic disease for which high dose is desired, conformal techniques and intensity-modulated radiation should be considered. For patients receiving postoperative treatment for high-risk or microscopic disease, doses of 45 to 54 Gy are appropriate. The role of stereotactic body radiotherapy (SBRT) for primary adrenal tumors has not been established, although it's gaining popularity for metastatic disease to the adrenal gland. A handful of case series have shown potential efficacy of SBRT for primary adrenal tumors that are unresectable because of comorbidities or patient preference. SBRT utilization for oligometastatic disease to the adrenal gland is increasing across institutions. The popularity of SBRT is mainly based on results of case series and retrospective reviews, which show good local control rates ranging from 60% to 70% at year 1 and between

40% and 50% at year 2.[41] No prospective randomized trials are available to compare the efficacy of SBRT against a surgical resection.

In the palliative setting, doses of 30 to 40 Gy given during the course of 2 to 3 weeks are reasonable. In patients with painful bone metastases, hypofractionated regimens should be considered for patients with poor performance status or otherwise limited life expectancy.

External beam radiation is limited to a palliative role in the management of pheochromocytomas.

FOLLOW-UP

Patients with pheochromocytomas should have frequent follow-up that includes a thorough history and physical examination with an evaluation of vital signs and plasma markers. This should be done every 6 months for the first 3 years starting around 3 months postsurgery and annually thereafter. Advanced or persistent disease may require more frequent follow-up and symptom management.

REFERENCES

1. Moore K, Agur A. *Essential clinical anatomy.* Baltimore, MD: Lippincott Williams & Wilkins, 2002:182–185.
2. Rouvière H. *Anatomie des lymphatiques de l'homme.* Paris: Masson, 1932.
3. Dunnick NR. Adrenal carcinoma. *Radiol Clin North Am* 1994;32:99–108.
4. McClennan BL. Oncologic imaging. Staging and follow-up of renal and adrenal carcinoma. *Cancer* 1991;67:1199–1208.
5. Shambaugh E, Ryan R. *Summary staging guide for the cancer surveillance, epidemiology and end results reporting (SEER) program.* Rockville, MD: US Dept of Health and Human Services, Public Health Service, 1977.
6. Berruti A, Terzolo M, Sperone P, et al. Etoposide, doxorubicin and cisplatin plus mitotane in the treatment of advanced adrenocortical carcinoma: a large prospective phase II trial. *Endocr Relat Cancer* 2005;12:657–666.
7. Bravo EL. Evolving concepts in the pathophysiology, diagnosis, and treatment of pheochromocytoma. *Endocr Rev* 1994;15:356–368.
8. Bravo EL. Pheochromocytoma: new concepts and future trends. *Kidney Int* 1991;40:544–556.
9. Cotran A, Kumar V, Robbins SL. *Robbins pathologic basis of disease.* 5th ed. Philadelphia: WB Saunders, 1994:1161–1164.
10. Hubbard MM, Husami TW, Abumrad NN. Nonfunctioning adrenal tumors. Dilemmas in management. *Am Surg* 1989;55:516–522.
11. De Maria M, Barbiera F, Bonadonna F, et al. Diseases of the adrenal medulla. *Rays* 1992;17:62–86.
12. Miller RW, Fraumeni JF Jr, Hill JA. Neuroblastoma: epidemiologic approach to its origin. *Am J Dis Child* 1968;115:253–261.
13. Beard CM, Sheps SG, Kurland LT, et al. Occurrence of pheochromocytoma in Rochester, Minnesota, 1950 through 1979. *Mayo Clin Proc* 1983;58:802–804.
14. Melicow MM. One hundred cases of pheochromocytoma (107 tumors) at the Columbia-Presbyterian Medical Center, 1926–1976: a clinicopathological analysis. *Cancer* 1987;40:1987–2004.
15. Beierwaltes WH, Sisson JC, Shapiro B. Malignant potential of pheochromocytoma. *Proc Am Acad Cancer Res* 1986;27:617.
16. Cryer PE. Pheochromocytoma. *Clin Endocrinol Metab* 1985;14:203–220.
17. Javadpour N, Woltering EA, Brennan MF. Adrenal neoplasms. *Curr Probl Surg* 1980;17:1–52.
18. Percarpio B, Knowlton AH. Radiation therapy of adrenal cortical carcinoma. *Acta Radiol Ther Phys Biol* 1976;15:288–292.
19. Loughlin KR, Gittes RF. Urological management of patients with von Hippel-Lindau's disease. *J Urol* 1986;136:789–791.
20. Nakagawara A, Ikeda K, Tsuneyoshi M, et al. Malignant pheochromocytoma with ganglioneuroblastoma elements in a patient with von Recklinghausen's disease. *Cancer* 1985;55:2794–2798.
21. Wooten MD, King DK. Adrenal cortical carcinoma. Epidemiology and treatment with mitotane and a review of the literature. *Cancer* 1993;72:3145–3155.
22. Haak HR, Hermans J, van de Velde CJ, et al. Optimal treatment of adrenocortical carcinoma with mitotane: results in a consecutive series of 96 patients. *Br J Cancer* 1994;69:947–951.
23. Stein PP, Black HR. A simplified diagnostic approach to pheochromocytoma. A review of the literature and report of one institution's experience. *Medicine* 1991;70:46–66.
24. King DR, Lack EE. Adrenal cortical carcinoma: a clinical and pathologic study of 49 cases. *Cancer* 1979;44:239–244.
25. Livhits M, Li N, Yeh MW, et al. Surgery is associated with improved survival for adrenocortical cancer, even in metastatic disease. *Surgery* 2014;156(6):1531–1541.
26. Saade N, Sadler C, Goldfarb M. Impact of regional lymph node dissection on disease specific survival in adrenal cortical carcinoma. *Horm Metab Res* 2015;47(11): 820–825.
27. Magee BJ, Gattamaneni HR, Pearson D. Adrenal cortical carcinoma: survival after radiotherapy. *Clin Radiol* 1987;38:587–588.
28. Markoe AM, Serber W, Micaily B, et al. Radiation therapy for adjunctive treatment of adrenal cortical carcinoma. *Am J Clin Oncol* 1991;14:170–174.
29. Pommier RF, Brennan MF. An eleven-year experience with adrenocortical carcinoma. *Surgery* 1992;112:963–971.
30. Terzolo M, Angeli A, Fassnacht M, et al. Adjuvant mitotane treatment for adrenocortical carcinoma. *N Engl J Med* 2007;356:2372–2380.
31. Ahlman H, Khorram-Manesh A, Jansson S, et al. Cytotoxic treatment of adrenocortical carcinoma. *World J Surg* 2001;25:927–933.
32. Lo CY, Lam KY, Wat MS, et al. Adrenal pheochromocytoma remains a frequently overlooked diagnosis. *Am J Surg* 2000;179:212–215.
33. Plouin PF, Duclos JM, Soppelsa F, et al. Factors associated with perioperative morbidity and mortality in patients with pheochromocytoma: analysis of 165 operations at a single center. *J Clin Endocr Metab* 2001;86:1480–1486.
34. Amar L, Servais A, Gimenez-Roqueplo AP, et al. Year of diagnosis, features at presentation, and risk of recurrence in patients with pheochromocytoma or secreting paraganglioma. *J Clin Endocr Metab* 2005;90:2110–2116.
35. Shapiro B, Gross MD, Shulkin B. Radioisotope diagnosis and therapy of malignant pheochromocytoma. *Trends Endocrinol Metab* 2001;12:469–475.
36. Shapiro B, Sisson JC, Wieland DM, et al. Radiopharmaceutical therapy of malignant pheochromocytoma with [131I]metaiodobenzylguanidine: results from ten years of experience. *J Nucl Biol Med* 1991;35:269–276.
37. Sidhu S, Sywak M, Robinson B, et al. Adrenocortical cancer: recent clinical and molecular advances. *Curr Opin Oncol* 2004;16:13–18.
38. Loh KC, Fitzgerald PA, Matthay KK, et al. The treatment of malignant pheochromocytoma with iodine-131 metaiodobenzylguanidine (131I-MIBG): a comprehensive review of 116 reported patients. *J Endocrinol Invest* 1997;20:648–658.
39. Safford SD, Coleman RE, Gockerman JP, et al. Iodine-131 metaiodobenzylguanidine is an effective treatment for malignant pheochromocytoma and paraganglioma. *Surgery* 2003;134:956–962.
40. Averbuch SD, Steakley CS, Young RC, et al. Malignant pheochromocytoma: effective treatment with a combination of cyclophosphamide, vincristine, and dacarbazine. *Ann Intern Med* 1988;109:267–273.
41. Guiou M, Mayr NA, Kim EY. Stereotactic body radiotherapy for adrenal metastases from lung cancer. *J Radiat Oncol* 2012;1(2):155.

CHAPTER 81

Hodgkin Lymphoma

Richard T. Hoppe and Bradford S. Hoppe

INTRODUCTION

The management of Hodgkin lymphoma (HL) continues to evolve. Since the last edition of this text, functional imaging has become standard for initial staging and end-of-treatment response evaluation as well as to assess early response to therapy and define adaptive approaches to therapy intensification and deintensification. Recent clinical trials in adaptive therapy have established a role for chemotherapy alone in early-stage disease following a favorable response on interim positron emission tomography (PET). New, more precise techniques for radiation therapy delivery have been devised and adopted, and guidelines for radiation field design have been endorsed by professional societies. New systemic agents have been approved by the U.S. Food and Drug Administration. Large prospective, randomized clinical trials have allowed us to refine treatments, and data regarding late effects continue to influence the development of management approaches.

ANATOMY

HL almost always begins in the lymph nodes. Over 80% of patients present with cervical lymph node involvement and over 50% have mediastinal disease. Disease can extend into extralymphatic sites, such as lung, pericardium, and soft tissue, but solitary extralymphatic involvement without nodal disease is rare.

EPIDEMIOLOGY AND RISK FACTORS

The reported incidence of HL is just below 3 per 100,000 with a slight male predominance (1.2:1). It accounts for 0.56% of all cancers diagnosed, but only 0.23% of all cancer deaths in the United States each year, a death rate that decreased by more than one-third between 1990 and 2006 (0.85 per 100,000 to 0.56 per 100,000).[1] Although HL is rare in children <10 years of age, it is the most common diagnosed malignancy among 15- to 19-year-olds.[2] The median age of patients at the time of diagnosis is 26 years. Its incidence shows a bimodal peak as a function of age.[3] The early peak, from ages 25 to 30 years, shows an incidence of approximately 5.5 per 100,000 per year. A second peak, from age 75 to 80 years, shows a similar incidence.

Geographic clusters of patients with HL have been reported, but these are likely coincidental.[4] Inherited risk has also been reported among first-degree relatives.[5,6] A relation between HL and previous infection with Epstein-Barr virus (EBV) has been proposed,[7] and Weiss et al.[8] identified components of the EBV genome in the cellular DNA of Reed-Sternberg (R-S) cells in lymph nodes involved by HL. The risk for development of HL is 2.55 times higher among individuals with a history of infectious mononucleosis than among noninfected control subjects.[9] Several series have demonstrated an association between EBV infection and mixed cellularity HL (MCHL), especially among children in developing countries.[10] However, the precise relationship between EBV infection and development of HL remains undefined. Recently, data have emerged suggesting that people with human immunodeficiency virus and AIDS are at a higher risk of developing HL.[11] Studies attempting to link occupational exposures or other etiologic factors with the development of HL have been inconclusive or contradictory.[4]

NATURAL HISTORY AND CLINICAL PRESENTATION

Patients with HL usually present with painless lymphadenopathy. Some note systemic symptoms such as unexplained fevers, drenching night sweats, weight loss, generalized pruritus, fatigue, and alcohol-induced pain in tissues involved by HL. Still other patients are diagnosed after detection of a mediastinal mass on a routine chest radiograph.

Sites of involvement are typically contiguous, although occasional skip areas occur.[12,13] The theory of contiguity of spread and the development of treatment programs with radiation that included treatment of uninvolved sites were important conceptual advances in the treatment of HL in the latter half of the 20th century.

HL can extend from the lymph nodes to adjacent organs, as when it spreads from enlarged mediastinal or bronchopulmonary (pulmonary hilar) nodes directly into the pulmonary parenchyma. It can also be hematogenous, as with nodular disease in the liver or multiple bony sites. Involved bones can undergo blastic changes, especially those in the vertebrae (creating the classic "ivory vertebra" on plain radiographs), pelvis, sternum, or ribs.

The likelihood of disseminated disease, including bone marrow and liver involvement, increases with increased splenic involvement.[14,15] HL rarely involves the Waldeyer lymphoid region or the gut-associated lymphoid tissues such as Peyer patches. It also rarely involves the upper aerodigestive tract, central nervous system, and skin.[12]

The rapidity of HL's growth and spread varies. Disease can evolve over several years, as demonstrated on serial radiographs or suspected by clinical history, and it is uncommon to document progression during evaluation and staging.

Three "B symptoms" are included as part of the staging system for HL (see later discussion). They are fever, drenching night sweats, and significant weight loss (10% of baseline weight). One-third of patients present with 1 of these symptoms. Fevers may present in the classic waxing-and-waning Pel-Ebstein pattern. Drenching night sweats may require a change of bedclothes. The B symptoms can occur even in patients with relatively limited disease (stage II), but they are uncommon in stage I disease.

Historically, children fare better with treatment than adults, so different treatment strategies have been developed for children (see Chapter 93).[16,17] More recently, results from adult treatment programs have been as successful as those in children. Older adults (>60 years) have a worse prognosis, often secondary to intercurrent illness or an inability to tolerate standard therapies, especially bleomycin, anthracyclines, and extended-field irradiation.[18,19] In fact, a recent report of older adults demonstrated a 5% treatment-related mortality rate following four cycles of ABVD (doxorubicin, bleomycin, vinblastine, dacarbazine).[19]

If HL is diagnosed during pregnancy, special treatment considerations are warranted; however, no evidence exists that pregnancy affects the natural course of the disease.[20–22] Many women become pregnant after successful treatment. Among patients infected with human immunodeficiency virus type 1, HL tends to behave differently, with a poorer prognosis.[23,24]

DIAGNOSTIC WORKUP

Diagnostic and staging procedures commonly used for HL are listed in Table 81.1. Patient age and intercurrent disease may influence the selection of staging studies.[25–27]

Hematologic evaluation may reveal anemia, leukocytosis, lymphopenia, or thrombocytosis, common paraneoplastic effects stimulated by cytokines. Anemia, lymphopenia, leukocytosis, and hypoalbuminemia are adverse prognostic factors, especially in patients with advanced disease (stages III to IV).[28] The serum alkaline phosphatase level can serve as a nonspecific marker of tumor activity or hepatic, bone marrow, or bone disease. The erythrocyte sedimentation rate (ESR) is a prognostic factor for patients with limited disease (stages I to II).[29] Other useful markers include lactate dehydrogenase and β_2-microglobulin levels.

Radiographic evaluation should include posterior–anterior (PA) and lateral chest radiographs. Mediastinal adenopathy can be measured by dividing the maximum width of the mediastinal mass by the maximum intrathoracic diameter (near the level of the diaphragm) on a standing PA chest radiograph, as shown in Figure 81.1. When this ratio exceeds 1:3, the disease is defined as bulky, which affects assignment to many

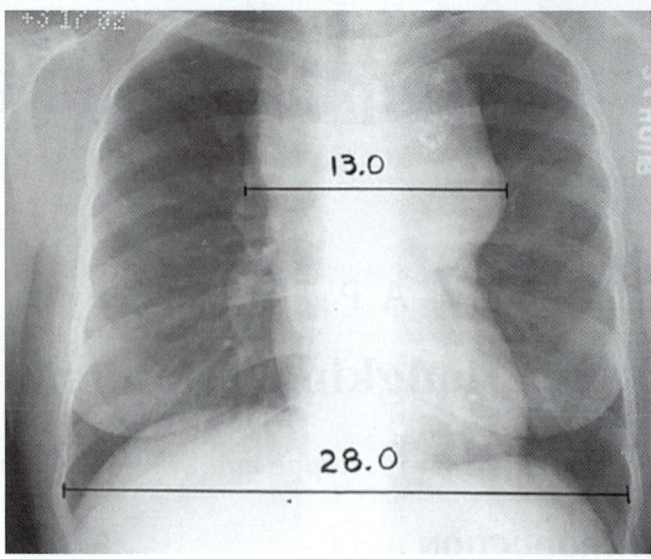

FIGURE 81.1. The mediastinal mass ratio (MMR). This ratio is defined as the maximum single horizontal mediastinal mass measurement divided by the maximum intrathoracic diameter, which is usually near the diaphragm. In this example, MMR = 13.0/28.0 = 0.46.

clinical trials. Other definitions of bulky mediastinal adenopathy include a mass >10 cm and a ratio of mediastinal mass to the chest diameter at T5-T6 exceeding 0.35 (employed in European Organization for the Treatment of Cancer [EORTC] clinical trials). Contrast-enhanced (diagnostic) computed tomography (CT) scans of the chest, abdomen, and pelvis may reveal adenopathy or organ involvement. If irradiation to the cervical nodes is being considered, a CT scan of the neck can help identify their precise location for treatment planning. Lymph nodes larger than 1.5 cm on CT scan are considered enlarged.[27] Although splenomegaly or hepatomegaly alone do not suggest involvement of HL (in the absence of confirmatory findings on a contrast-enhanced CT scan or 2-fluoro-2-deoxy-D-glucose (FDG)-PET scan), a spleen over 13-cm long is considered likely involved per the current staging system.[27]

PET using FDG with fused CT images (PET-CT scan) has become essential to staging HL. Omitting PET-CT as part of staging can negatively influence outcomes, especially as they pertain to designing radiation treatment fields.[30] Tissues affected by HL are intensely FDG-avid, and FDG-PET is more sensitive than CT for detecting disease.[31] FDG's uptake pattern in bone defines whether bone or bone marrow is involved, obviating the need for a bone marrow biopsy.[32,33] The overall incidence of bone marrow involvement in HL is only approximately 5%.

PET-CT is an essential study for response assessment, is particularly useful for evaluating residual masses detected by CT scanning, and can be a useful prognostic indicator when repeated after some chemotherapy has been administered (*vide infra* interim PET-CT).[26,27] The 5-point Deauville score is used to evaluate the degree of response to therapy, based on the comparison of active disease to levels in the liver and mediastinal blood pool (Table 81.2).

TABLE 81.1 DIAGNOSTIC AND STAGING PROCEDURES FOR HL

History
Systemic B symptoms: unexplained fever, drenching night sweats, weight loss
  >10% of body weight in the last 6 mo.
Other symptoms: alcohol intolerance, pruritus, respiratory problems, fatigue

Physical Examination
Palpable nodes (note number, size, location, shape, consistency, mobility)
Palpable viscera

Laboratory Studies
Complete blood count, differential, platelets
ESR
Serum albumin, lactate dehydrogenase, liver function studies
Blood urea nitrogen, creatinine
If indicated:
  Pregnancy test in women of child-bearing age
  Pulmonary function studies
  Cardiac ejection fraction
  HIV testing

Imaging
Chest radiograph: posterior–anterior and lateral
Contrast-enhanced CT scan of thorax, abdomen, and pelvis
Contrast-enhanced CT scan of the neck (if neck irradiation is indicated)
Integrated PET-CT scan (skull base to midthigh)

TABLE 81.2 DEAUVILLE FIVE-POINT SCALE FOR ASSESSING TREATMENT RESPONSE ON PET-CT

Score	PET-CT Scan Result
1	No uptake
2	Uptake ≤ mediastinum
3	Uptake > mediastinum but ≤ liver
4	Uptake moderately higher than liver
5	Uptake markedly higher than liver and/or new lesions
X	New areas of uptake unlikely to be related to lymphoma

PET-CT, positron emission tomography–computed tomography.

TABLE 81.3 THE ANN ARBOR STAGING CLASSIFICATION FOR HODGKIN DISEASE

Stage I	Involvement of a single lymph node region
Stage II	Involvement of two or more lymph node regions on the same side of the diaphragm (II) or localized involvement of an extralymphatic organ or site and one or more lymph node regions on the same side of the diaphragm (IIE)
Stage III	Involvement of lymph node regions on both sides of the diaphragm (III), which can be accompanied by involvement of the spleen (IIIS) or by localized involvement of an extralymphatic organ or site (IIIE) or by both (IIISE)
Stage IV	Diffuse or disseminated involvement of one or more extralymphatic organs or tissues, with or without associated lymph node involvement

Note: The absence or presence of fever, night sweats, and/or unexplained loss of 10% or more body weight in the 6 mo before diagnosis is denoted by the suffix letter A or B, respectively. The Cotswolds system used X to designate bulky disease, variably defined, but including a mediastinal mass width exceeding 1/3 of the thoracic ratio at the T5-T6 interspace and any disease >10 cm.[35] The Lugano system recommended deleting X and instead noting the size of the largest node.[27]

Although not widely used, magnetic resonance imaging (MRI) is an alternative to chest or abdominal–pelvic CT scanning for initial staging. Its main value is in the staging evaluation of pregnant women (without contrast) and children. Furthermore, it can be incorporated with FDG-PET to generate fused PET-MRI scans.[21,34]

STAGING

The Ann Arbor staging system for HL, used since 1971, was modified in the Cotswolds, England, in 1989[35] and in Lugano, Switzerland, in 2014[27] (see Table 81.3).[36] The lymphoid regions as defined in the Ann Arbor staging system are shown in Figure 81.2. Although somewhat arbitrary in their borders,

FIGURE 81.2. The lymph node regions as defined in the Ann Arbor staging system. Note that the ipsilateral supraclavicular, cervical, preauricular, and occipital nodes are defined as a single region. The mediastinum and pulmonary hila are defined as separate regions. The infraclavicular region corresponds to the subpectoral nodes. The GHSG and EORTC define the lymph node regions slightly differently. Both combine the hilar and mediastinal regions. The GHSG also combines subpectoral with cervical, whereas the EORTC combines subpectoral with axilla. (Reprinted from Hoppe RT. The non-Hodgkin lymphomas: pathology, staging, treatment. *Curr Probl Cancer* 1987;11[6]:364–434. Copyright © 1987 Elsevier. With permission.)

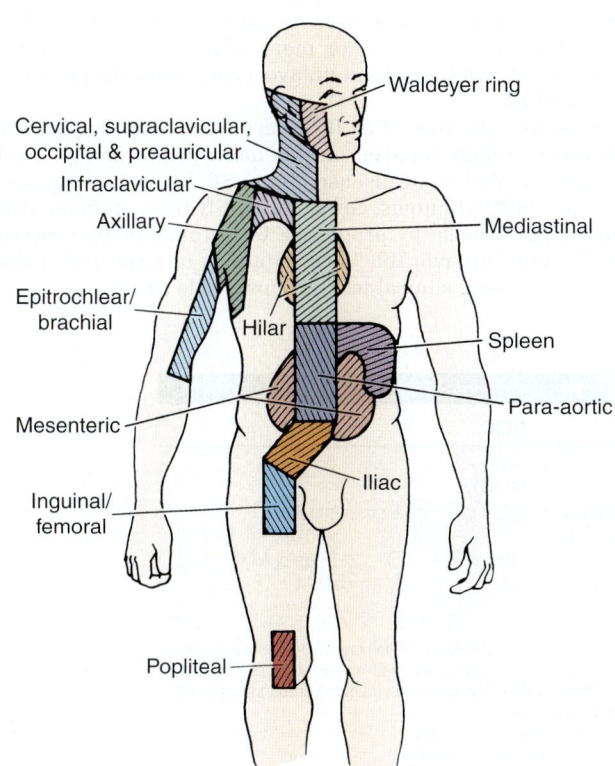

these definitions reliably describe the extent of disease and help define clinical risk groups for clinical trial assignment. Defining the "E" lesion has always been a challenge. The Cotswolds system attempts to clarify it as direct disease extension from any nodal site that can be encompassed by a radiation field; however, some scenarios are more complex.[37] The final stage reflects the distribution of disease as observed on physical examination and imaging studies, with or without B symptoms.

PATHOLOGIC CLASSIFICATION

The World Health Organization (WHO) defines two major categories of HL: classic HL and nodular lymphocyte–predominant HL (NLPHL).[38]

Classic HL is characterized by its signature neoplastic cell, the R-S cell. Morphologically, the R-S cell is binucleate with a prominent, centrally located nucleolus in each nucleus, a well-demarcated nuclear membrane, and eosinophilic cytoplasm with a perinuclear halo. R-S cells usually account for <1% of the cells in a lymph node involved by HL. The components of the microenvironment include lymphoid cells, eosinophils, plasma cells, and other normal inflammatory cells.[39]

R-S cells probably originate from B-lineage cells at various stages of development, including pre–B-cell and germinal center B-cell origin. Interactions of these cells with the cells of the microenvironment are complex.[40] In most instances, the R-S cells stain positively with the lymphocyte activation marker CD30, with PAX5 (dimly), and with variable expression of the antigranulocyte monoclonal antibody CD15. CD20, a marker of mature B cells, is expressed on some tumor cells with variable intensity in as many as 40% of cases. They stain negatively with CD45, ALK, and J chain.[41] Nearly all R-S cells express the PD-1 ligand.[41] The expression of CD30 and PDL-1 open opportunities for targeted therapy of classic HL.

Classic HL is divided into four histologic subtypes. *Nodular sclerosis HL* (NSHL) is the most common histologic subtype diagnosed in developed countries. Involved nodes often have a thickened capsule and are traversed by broad bands of birefringent collagen that surround nodules of cells consisting of lymphocytes, eosinophils, plasma cells, and tissue histiocytes intermixed with a variable proportion of atypical mononuclear cells, inflammatory cells, and R-S cells. The syncytial variant of NSHL refers to cases of prominent cellular aggregates of atypical cells and histiocytes. Patients with NSHL typically present in the clinic with mediastinal involvement, and one-third have B symptoms. It is more common among women, especially young ones. The natural history of NSHL is favorable.

Mixed cellularity Hodgkin lymphoma (MCHL) is characterized by lymph nodes that are diffusely effaced by lymphocytes, eosinophils, plasma cells, inflammatory cells, and relatively abundant atypical mononuclear and R-S cells. Patients with MCHL usually present with advanced disease and tend to be slightly older than those with NSHL. The natural history of MCHL is less favorable than that of NSHL.

Lymphocyte-rich Hodgkin lymphoma (LRHL)[42,43] typically has a nodular growth pattern but may be diffuse. In the past, many cases of LRHL were confused with lymphocyte-predominant HL (LPHL); however, the staining characteristics of the malignant cells in LRHL are consistent with those of classic HL. The clinical characteristics of patients affected by LRHL resemble those of NLPHL: early stage, absence of B symptoms, and excellent prognosis.

Lymphocyte-depleted Hodgkin lymphoma (LDHL) varies in its microscopic appearance but reveals a paucity of normal-appearing cells and an abundance of abnormal mononuclear cells, R-S cells, and R-S variants. Differentiating LDHL from anaplastic large cell lymphoma is challenging, especially because both are CD30 positive.[44] It is an exceedingly uncommon subtype of HL. It tends to occur in older patients and is more likely to be associated with advanced disease and

TABLE 81.4 MAJOR HISTOLOGIC SUBTYPES CORRELATED WITH CLINICAL CHARACTERISTICS OF 615 ADULT PATIENTS TREATED FOR HL AT STANFORD UNIVERSITY (1989 TO 2011)

	NLPHL	NSHL	MCHL
Number of patients (%)	40 (7)	468 (76)	49 (8)
Age (y)			
Range	15–85	15–83	17–81
Median	45	30	35
Male to female ratio	23:17	228:241	32:17
Stage			
I (%)	14 (36)	30 (6)	10 (21)
II (%)	14 (36)	272 (58)	14 (29)
III (%)	11 (28)	89 (19)	12 (25)
IV (%)	0	78 (17)	12 (25)
B symptoms (%)	4 (10)	147 (31)	16 (33)

MCHL, mixed cellularity Hodgkin lymphoma; NLPHL, nodular lymphocyte–predominant Hodgkin lymphoma; NSHL, nodular sclerosis Hodgkin lymphoma.

B symptoms. It has the worst prognosis of all histologic subtypes of HL.[45]

Nodular lymphocyte–predominant Hodgkin lymphoma (NLPHL) has recently been subdivided into six entities based on morphology and immunohistochemistry characteristics termed typical and variant histologies.[46,47] It is characterized by having many more normal-appearing lymphocytes than abnormal cells. Unlike the other subtypes of HL, the abnormal cells ("L and H cells" or "popcorn cells") are strongly reactive for CD20, CD45, CD79a, and PAX5 and negative for CD15 and CD30.[39,41] NLPHL is often diagnosed in young people who present with early-stage disease, usually in a solitary peripheral nodal site. Systemic symptoms are uncommon (<10%). The natural history is the most favorable of the histologic subtypes. Some patients demonstrate a pattern of late relapse but good survival, resembling that observed in the follicular (B-cell) lymphomas. For up to 14% of patients, NLPHL will transform into an aggressive B-cell lymphoma as part of its natural history.[48,49] Patients with a variant histology, versus those with typical NLPHL, are at greater risk for transformation[47] and are also more likely to present with advanced disease and experience disease relapse. A reactive process termed *progressive transformation of germinal centers* may be observed either before, with, or after the diagnosis of NLPHL.[50,51]

Table 81.4 summarizes the characteristics of patients treated at Stanford University (California) from 1989 to 2010 stratified by the major histologic subtypes and represents most large centers in the United States and Western Europe. Histologic subtype distribution and clinical behavior will differ for patients in South America, Asia, Africa, Eastern Europe, and even some parts of the United States, with a higher ratio of unfavorable histologic subtypes and more aggressive clinical behavior in economically developing regions.[52,53]

TABLE 81.5 INTERNATIONAL PROGNOSTIC SCORE FOR ADVANCED HL

Factor	Unfavorable Covariate
Serum albumin	<4 g/dL
Hemoglobin	<10.5 g/dL
Sex	Male
Age	≥45 y
Stage	IV (Ann Arbor)
Leukocyte count	≥15,000/mm^3
Lymphocyte count	<600/mm^3 or <8% of white count

PROGNOSTIC FACTORS AND THERAPEUTIC IMPLICATIONS

In HL, prognostic factors are important for defining therapy and predicting outcome. Histologic subtypes have little impact on therapy, except when identifying NLPHL for which different treatment algorithms apply.[25] Although large series report a slightly worse outcome for men than women,[1] gender influences treatment choice more because of potential reproductive complications than outcome (see "Sequelae of Treatment").

Although it is probably safe to argue that Ann Arbor stage is the greatest determinant of therapy, and that early data show that stage has a marked impact on prognosis, current management programs blur its influence. For many patients, disease bulk influences treatment selection, especially bulky mediastinal disease. In general, the risk of relapse after treatment with single-modality therapy is high and, therefore, combined modality therapy has been standard for patients with bulky disease.[25,54]

An important international study evaluated a series of prognostic factors among 5,141 patients with advanced-stage HL (Table 81.5).[28] Seven factors were identified, each of which had an independent yet similar relationship with prognosis. Unfavorable factors included male gender, age >45 years, Ann Arbor stage IV, hemoglobin level <10.5 g/dL, white cell count >15,000/mL, lymphocyte count <8% or absolute lymphocyte count <600, and albumin <4 g/dL. This International Prognostic Score is now used to assign patients to clinical trials. Patients with three or more adverse risk factors are often considered to be in an unfavorable prognostic group for advanced HL.

Patients with stage I or II disease often have only one or two adverse factors based on this index. Other factors, such as number of sites of disease, age, ESR, bulky disease, and presence of B symptoms, can help stratify these patients with early-stage disease by prognosis. Unfortunately, the criteria for defining "unfavorable" presentations of stage I to II disease vary among clinical trial groups (Table 81.6).

TABLE 81.6 DEFINITION OF "UNFAVORABLE" STAGE I TO II HL

	EORTC	GHSG^a	NCIC	NCCN
Age (y)	≥50	—	≥40	—
Histology	—	—	MC/LD	—
ESR/B symptoms	≥30 mm with any B sx. ≥50 mm without B sx.	≥30 mm with any B sx. ≥50 mm without B sx.	≥50 mm or any B sx.	Any B sx >50 mm
Mediastinal mass	MTR ≥ 0.35	MMR > 0.33	MMR > 0.33	10 cm or MMR > 0.33
Number of nodal regions	>3^b	>2^c	>3	>3
E lesion	—	Any	—	—

E, extralymphatic; EORTC, European Organization for Research and Treatment of Cancer; ESR, erythrocyte sedimentation rate; GHSG, German Hodgkin Study Group; LD, lymphocyte depleted; MC, mixed cellularity; MMR, maximum mediastinal width/maximum chest width on chest x-ray; MTR, maximum mediastinal width/chest width at T5-T6 on chest x-ray; NCCN, National Cancer Center Network; NCIC, National Cancer Institute, Canada; sx, symptoms. Patients with one or more of these factors were considered to have "unfavorable" stage I to II disease.
^{a}Patients with B symptoms and either E lesion or large mediastinal mass treated in advanced disease clinical trials.
^{b}Mediastinum and both hila considered as a single region; subpectoral and ipsilateral axilla considered a single region.
^{c}Mediastinum and both hila considered as a single region; subpectoral and ipsilateral cervical/supraclavicular considered a single region.

GENERAL MANAGEMENT

Radiation Therapy

Radiation therapy is the most effective therapeutic agent for treating HL and has been used in its management for over a century.[55] The optimal irradiation technique includes meticulous pretreatment evaluation of disease sites, precise simulation and immobilization, individually contoured treatment volumes according to the location of a patient's tumor configuration, radiation exposure to all adjacent organs at risk (ORAs) that is as low as reasonably achievable (ALARA), an adequate target dose, a multifield fractionated regimen, and image guidance during therapy. Outcomes are best maximized and risks minimized through scrupulous attention to every detail of therapy.[56]

Chemotherapy

The standard drug combinations in use worldwide for the primary treatment of HL are ABVD[57,58] and bleomycin, etoposide, doxorubicin, cyclophosphamide, vincristine, procarbazine, and prednisone (BEACOPP), which includes baseline, escalated, and 14-day schedules.[59] Another combination, specifically devised to minimize toxicity and that is used with radiation, is nitrogen mustard, bleomycin, doxorubicin, vinblastine, vincristine, etoposide, prednisone (Stanford V).[60]

Table 81.7 summarizes the doses and scheduling of these drug combinations.[61]

Targeted Therapy

New systemic agents have been approved by the Food and Drug Administration for the treatment of HL. These include brentuximab vedotin (BV) and the checkpoint inhibitors nivolumab[62] and pembrolizumab.[63] BV is an anti-CD30 monoclonal antibody linked to an antitubulin agent. BV has demonstrated efficacy in CD30+ lymphomas, including HL and anaplastic large-cell lymphoma. It is approved for patients whose disease recurs after stem cell transplantation and is being introduced in clinical trials to define its potential in other settings.[64] Because of overlapping pulmonary toxicity, however, bleomycin is removed from any drug combination that includes BV, so trials of primary therapy with an ABVD backbone typically incorporate BV-AVD.

Owing to the ETHERA trial, BV has been approved as a maintenance therapy following autologous hematopoietic cell transplant.[65] Pembrolizumab is approved for patients with disease that is chemoresistant or has relapsed after three or more lines of therapy, and nivolumab is approved for patients whose disease has relapsed or progressed after autologous hematopoietic cell transplant and posttransplant brentuximab.

Combined Modality Therapy

Combined modality therapy has become the most common form of general management for patients with HL. Modern treatment protocols can include irradiation of all initially involved sites, bulky sites only, slowly responding sites, or sites of incomplete response to chemotherapy. In general, irradiation of all initially involved sites is indicated when combined with abbreviated chemotherapy in early-stage HL. Treatment of just high-risk areas, such as bulky disease, slowly responding disease, or incompletely responding disease, is reserved for more advanced-stage disease treated with definitive chemotherapy (i.e., six cycles of ABVD, 12 weeks of Stanford V, or six cycles of escalated BEACOPP).

RADIATION THERAPY TECHNIQUES

The principal objective of radiation therapy in HL is to treat regions at high risk for containing disease to a dose associated with a high likelihood of tumor eradication, meanwhile keeping the dose to adjacent tissues and organs ALARA. Thoughtful evaluation of all imaging studies, especially diagnostic CT and integrated PET-CT scans; precise simulation with appropriate immobilization and consideration of organ motion; detailed treatment planning; and effective and conformal treatment delivery, including image guidance, treatment verification, and appropriate quality assurance measures are requisite to achieving the best outcomes.[56]

Simulation

Patient positioning for simulation must allow for patient comfort, daily reproducibility, displacement of ORAs (such as breasts) beyond the treatment field, impact of positioning on target delineation, and feasibility of treatment delivery. For patients with low neck and mediastinal involvement, a headrest with a face mask that extends the head can help pull the chin superiorly and beyond the radiation field. However, a headrest and face mask can also introduce uncertainties when fusing with the prechemotherapy PET-CT scan, which often is done with the head flexed on a pillow for comfort. Arm position, in general, is more comfortable at the patient's side or slightly akimbo and affects whether breast tissue falls inferior/laterally or beyond the field, especially when combined with an inclined board and immobilization bag. Conversely, patients with axillary, infraclavicular, or subpectoral involvement may have smaller target volumes with less uncertainty when their arm position resembles that in the prechemotherapy PET-CT scan because defining the target is challenging after chemotherapy. In these circumstances, the best position in which to treat the patient may be with arms above the head in an immobilization bag, which helps with reproducibility and with reducing the dose to the lungs. Occasionally, the prechemotherapy CT imaging is performed with arms up, whereas the PET-CT scan is performed with arms down, providing both options to optimize treatment.

With proton therapy, some immobilization devices can hinder the path of the particle beam and compromise beam selection, a concern that should be evaluated with physics and dosimetry before simulation.

Simulation should be done with intravenous contrast to help define the interface between normal soft tissues and residual disease. Furthermore, it can be helpful in identifying the cardiac substructures.

TABLE 81.7 COMMON DRUG COMBINATIONS USED IN THE TREATMENT OF HL

Drug Combination and Cycle Duration	Agents	Dose (mg/m²)	Route	Treatment Day(s)
ABVD, 28 d	Doxorubicin[a]	25	IV	1, 15
	Bleomycin	10	IV	1, 15
	Vinblastine	6	IV	1, 15
	Dacarbazine	375	IV	1, 15
Stanford V, 28 d	Doxorubicin[a]	25	IV	1, 15
	Vinblastine	6	IV	1, 15
	Nitrogen mustard	6	IV	1
	Vincristine[b]	1.4	IV	8, 22
	Bleomycin	5	IV	8, 22
	Etoposide	60	IV	15, 16
	Prednisone	40	PO	Every other day
BEACOPP, 21 d	Bleomycin	10	IV	8
	Etoposide	100 (200)[c]	IV	1–3
	Doxorubicin[a]	25 (35)[c]	IV	1
	Cyclophosphamide	650 (1250)[c]	IV	1
	Vincristine[b]	1.4	IV	8
	Procarbazine	100	PO	1–7
	Prednisone	40	PO	1–14
	G-CSF		SC	8–14

IV, intravenous; PO, oral; SC, subcutaneous.
[a]Adriamycin.
[b]Maximum, 2 mg.
[c]Higher dose is for escalated BEACOPP.

Section III

Motion Management

Patients with mediastinal involvement must undergo motion management strategies with the use of a 4-dimensional (4D) CT scan or deep-inspiration breath hold (DIBH) technique. For sites below the diaphragm, respiration management may be necessary. For example, when splenic irradiation is required, a 4D treatment planning scan can help define the phase in the respiratory cycle that allows for the most sparing of the heart, left lung, or left kidney. Retroperitoneal and pelvic nodes, in contrast, tend to not require motion management.

4D CT scans acquire imaging throughout the full 10 phases of the respiratory cycle, allowing us to assess the margin to add to the clinical target volume (CTV) that will account for normal respiratory motion. This internal treatment volume (ITV) margin can be an expansion of the CTV on the average scan of the 4D CT scan or independently drawn as the ITV, ensuring coverage of all 10 phases of the scan. In some cases, respiratory gating can be used to minimize the ITV margin.

Alternatively, DIBH is a technique that results in reduced doses to the lungs and heart for patients with mediastinal involvement.[66] DIBH can spare additional volume of the lungs when treating superior mediastinal disease. Additionally, DIBH pulls the heart medially and down, away from mediastinal disease located above the heart. Figure 81.3 demonstrates this effect. In most cases, DIBH is likely to reduce the lung and heart doses, but in cases with extensive lower mediastinal involvement including cardiophrenic nodes, the relative benefit of DIBH may diminish.[67]

Various techniques of DIBH have been described.[66,68,69] Important concepts to consider with DIBH include breath hold reproducibility, the patient's ability to maintain the breath hold or multiple breath holds during treatment, and the breath hold's impact on contouring.

Involved-Node and Involved-Site Radiotherapy

The classic field configurations for HL treatment with radiotherapy alone have included the mantle and inverted Y. However, clinical trials have shown the equivalence of "involved field" treatment (IFRT) with "extended-field" or "subtotal lymphoid" irradiation as part of combined modality therapy programs; thus, IFRT was adopted as the standard for combined modality therapy in clinical trials.[70–72] Field reductions and three-dimensional (3-D) target-volume definitions comprise the loosely described techniques for "intelligent-field radiation therapy" and "modified IFRT." The more clearly defined "involved-node radiotherapy" (INRT)[73] and "involved-site" irradiation (ISRT)[56] have become the standard of care in clinical practice and more recent clinical trials. INRT, as defined by Girinsky et al. for the EORTC-GELA Lymphoma Group, requires prechemotherapy diagnostic CT and PET-CT imaging with the patient in the treatment position, postchemotherapy contrast-enhanced CT simulation, and fusion of the prechemotherapy and postchemotherapy images.[73–75] The fields are designed to treat only the initially involved nodes with some modifications to avoid OARs. This gross tumor volume (GTV) then becomes the CTV, and a 1-cm expansion of the CTV defines the planning target volume (PTV).

When components of this planning process are missing—perhaps the pretreatment PET-CT scan was not done in the treatment position, there is poor registration between scans, or the CT simulation scan was done without intravenous contrast—it may be impossible to treat such strictly defined INRT fields. However, field reduction is still possible to what has been termed ISRT.[56]

ISRT volumes will vary depending on the clinical situation and treatment protocol. In general, because of the use of abbreviated chemotherapy (i.e., two to four cycles of ABVD or 8 weeks Stanford V), patients with favorable early-stage HL receive ISRT to all initial sites of disease after completing chemotherapy.

For patients treated with radiotherapy alone (i.e., NLPHL), the ISRT CTV should be increased to include sites of potential subclinical disease. In practice, this would mean an additional 2- to 5-cm margin within the lymphatic stations superior and inferior to the initially involved disease on PET-CT imaging, taking into account the OARs

Among patients with unfavorable early-stage HL, ISRT to all sites of disease should be used when abbreviated chemotherapy has been delivered; however, for those who receive more intensive chemotherapy, certain complete responding areas that could result in an unacceptable dose to an OAR if included could be omitted (i.e., cardiophrenic nodes or axillary lymph nodes in a young woman could be omitted if she has had a complete response [CR] by CT scan). Patients with stage III/IV disease are more likely to receive ISRT to sites of

FIGURE 81.3. ISRT treatment plans for a patient with extensive mediastinal HL during free breathing *(left)* and inspiration breath hold *(right)*. The mean radiotherapy lung dose with free breathing was 15.7 Gy; with inspiration breath hold, it was 11.2 Gy. (Reprinted from Specht L, Yahalom J, Illidge T, et al. Modern radiation therapy for Hodgkin lymphoma: field and dose guidelines from the international lymphoma radiation oncology group (ILROG). *Int J Radiat Oncol Biol Phys* 2014;89[4]: 854–862. Copyright © 2014 Elsevier. With permission.)

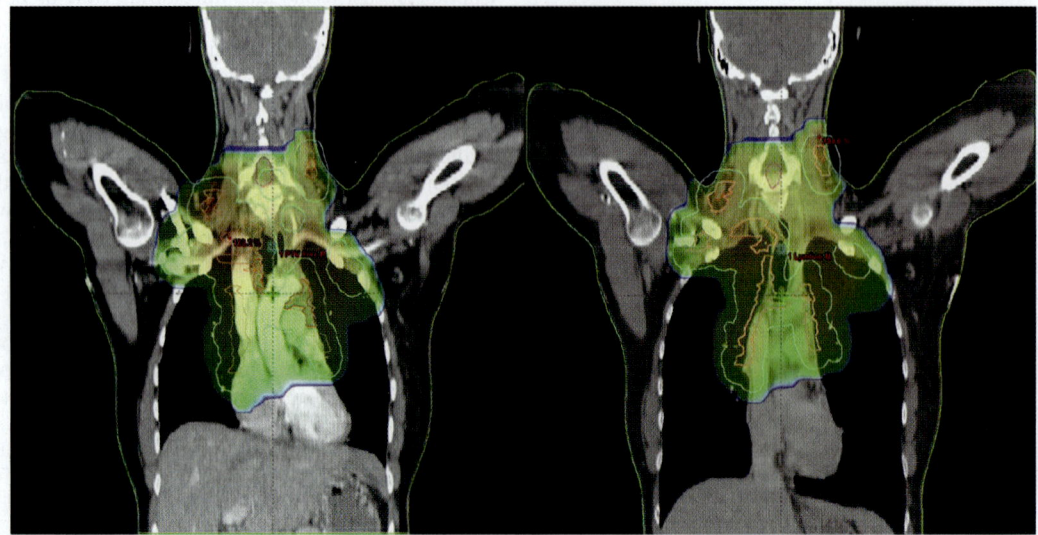

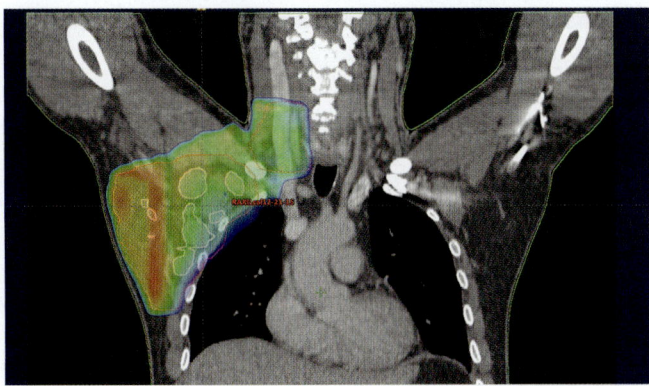

FIGURE 81.4. ISRT treatment plan for a 50-year-old man with stage IIA NLPHL involving the right axillary and subpectoral nodes. Note the extension of the field into the right supraclavicular fossa to treat possible subclinical disease in that location. Thick orange lines outline the PET-positive nodes (GTV); the thin orange line represents the PTV.

initially bulky disease or sites of slow or incomplete response to chemotherapy.

Design of ISRT Fields

The GTV (or prechemotherapy GTV) is based on localizing the initially positive lymph nodes (and extranodal sites) on the staging PET-CT scan fused to the treatment planning CT. When radiation therapy is the sole treatment modality, it is simple to identify the GTV, especially after PET-CT simulation. This may be the case for treating patients with primary radiotherapy for nodular LPHL (Figs. 81.4 and 81.5).[56]

For the more common situation of combined modality treatment, the CTV includes the entire initial disease volume but is modified (reduced) to exclude uninvolved normal organs (e.g., lungs, bones, muscles, great vessels) and to accommodate shrinking lymph node masses following chemotherapy, especially in the chest. The CTV can be expanded based on the quality of the initial imaging or owing to concerns of subclinical disease (Fig. 81.6). For initially large mediastinal masses, the postchemotherapy treatment fields should conform to

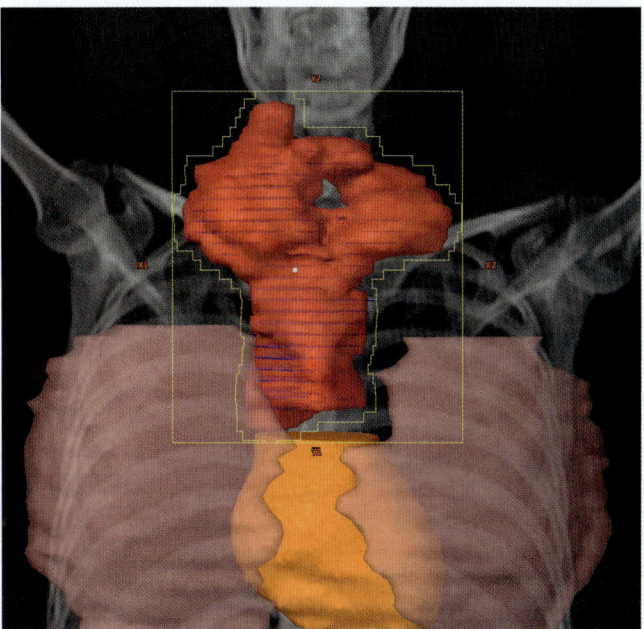

FIGURE 81.6. Involved-site 3-D radiotherapy AP/PA field design and treatment plan for a 28-year-old woman with stage II NSHL involving the right neck, bilateral supraclavicular, and superior mediastinum. *Faint blue horizontal lines*, GTV; *red*, PTV; *orange*, heart; *pink*, breasts.

the width of only the residual disease (absent any pulmonary parenchymal extension), and the superior and inferior field margins should encompass the initial extent of disease with the margin previously noted (Fig. 81.7).[56] Adjacent organ dose constraints may also mean reducing the CTV. The PTV is an expansion of the CTV based on day-to-day set-up uncertainties.

FIGURE 81.7. A 28-year-old man with massive mediastinal NSHL and right supraclavicular disease, following completion of chemotherapy, with a negative PET scan. *White*, pretreatment PET-positive disease; *black*, postchemotherapy residual abnormality on CT. Multileaf collimators define the ISRT field.

FIGURE 81.5. ISRT field for treating unilateral pelvic nodes, in this case for a 34-year-old man with stage IIA lymphocyte predominance HL. The initial PET-positive nodes (GTV) are shown in blue. The treatment field includes margins superiorly and inferiorly to include potential areas of microscopic spread, in this case approximately 5 cm cephalad and approximately 3 cm caudad.

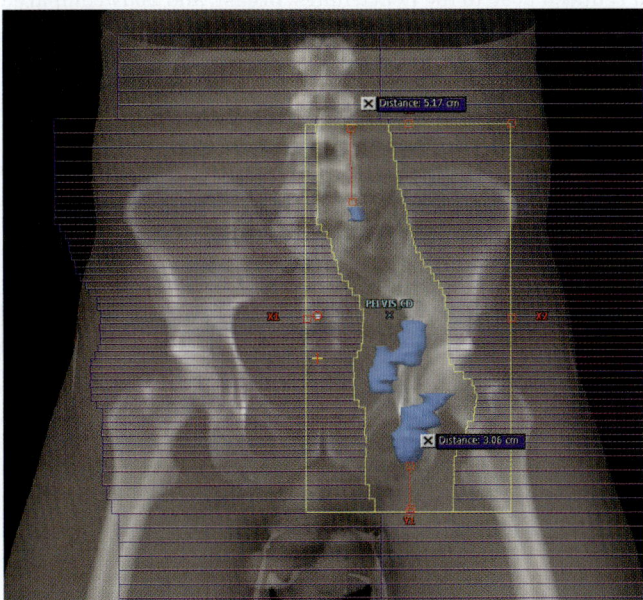

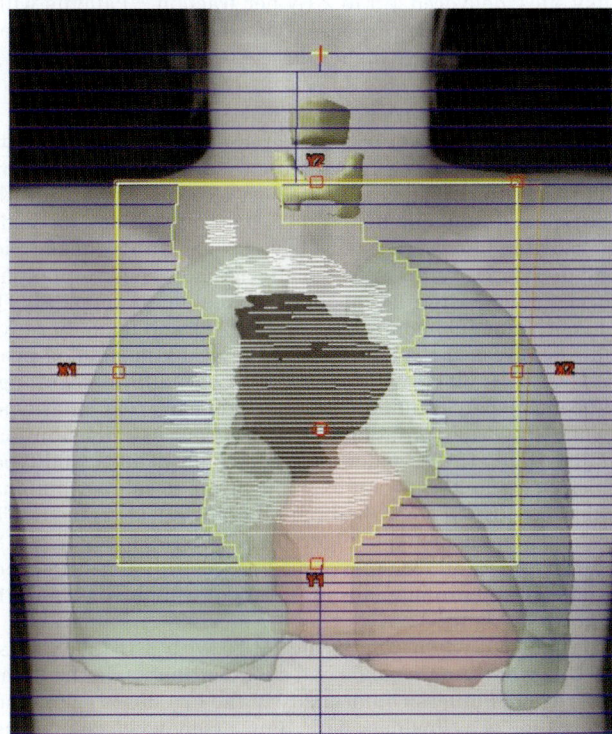

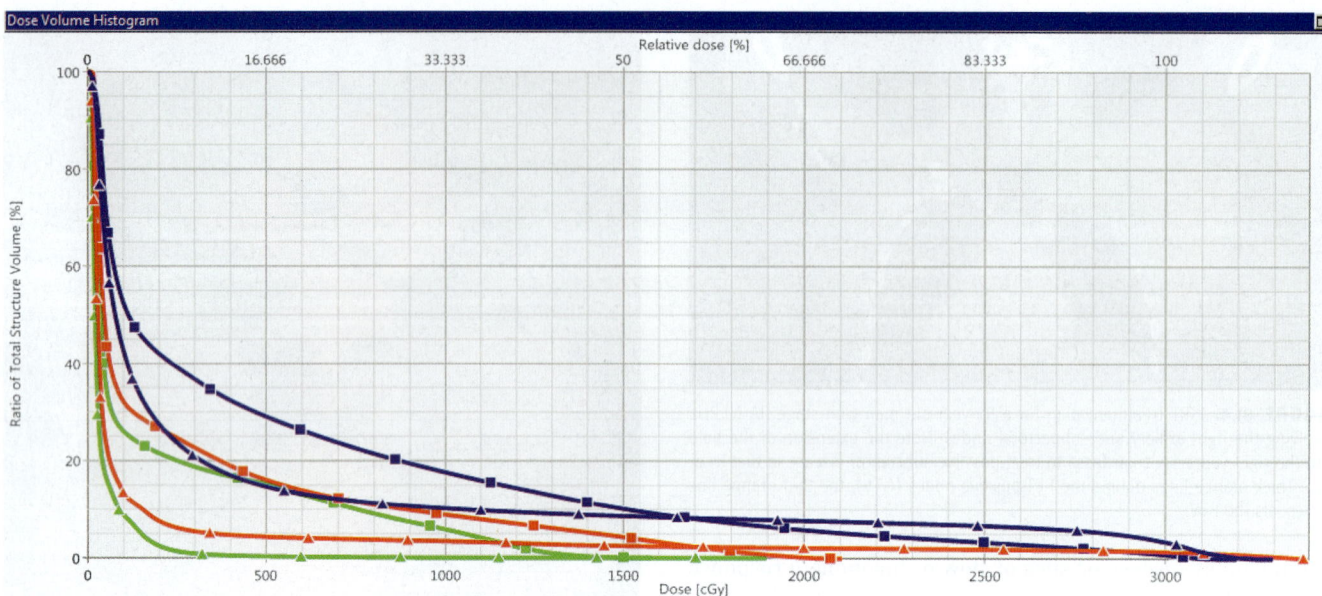

FIGURE 81.8. For the patient displayed in Figure 81.6, DVHs for a 3-D AP/PA treatment plan (*triangles*) and an intensity-modulated radiotherapy plan (*squares*). *Blue*, combined lungs; *red*, right breast; *green*, left breast. The 3-D plan was chosen for this patient because the mean dose and V_4 to the breasts were less than in the IMRT plan, whereas the V_{20} and V_{30} for the lungs were similar. (See also Table 81.8.)

Radiation Dose

In the uncommon scenario that radiation therapy alone is used for the treatment of HL (most commonly for NLPHL), the National Cancer Center Network (NCCN) Guidelines recommend a dose of 30 to 36 Gy to involved sites and 25 to 30 Gy to sites of potential subclinical involvement, delivered in 1.5- to 2-Gy fractions.[25] More commonly, however, radiation therapy is as a component of a combined modality approach, with chemotherapy expected to eradicate subclinical disease, and radiation playing a role in eradicating disease in involved sites. Doses vary considerably among trials, depending on the prognostic category of patients, disease bulk, and chemotherapy regimen. The dose ranges considered acceptable per the NCCN are 20 to 30 Gy for nonbulky and 30 to 36 Gy for bulky sites, delivered 1.5 to 2 Gy per fraction.[25] Patients with incomplete metabolic response (Deauville 4, 5) following chemotherapy can receive higher doses (36 to 45 Gy).

Radiation Delivery

Historically, irradiation was delivered after 2-D or 3-D treatment planning, typically with opposed anterior–posterior (AP)/PA treatment fields. Over the last 15 years, however, with more refined radiation fields and 3-D target delineation, modern radiation delivery systems have helped with reducing the radiation dose to the OARs. Such techniques require photon-based systems (intensity-modulated radiation therapy [IMRT], volumetric modulated arc therapy [VMAT], and tomo therapy) and proton-based systems (3-D and intensity-modulated proton therapy [IMPT]) with passive scatter, uniform scanning, and pencil beam scanning. The benefit of each treatment type depends on various factors, including disease distribution relative to the OARs, patient age and comorbidities, and type of prior chemotherapy. An example of the dose distributions achieved with 3-D conformal radiotherapy (CRT) versus IMRT for the patient depicted in Figure 81.6 is shown in Figure 81.8 and Table 81.8. An example of the dose distributions achieved with IMRT and proton plans for a patient with mediastinal HL is shown in Figure 81.9.

In general, when comparing IMRT with 3-D CRT plans, IMRT delivers a more conformal dose distribution in the high-dose region, but less conformality in the low-dose region and the creation of a "low-dose bath." Conversely, when comparing proton therapy techniques with 3-D CRT, protons deliver a more conformal dose distribution in both the high- and low-dose ranges.

Among patients with high cervical disease, IMRT or protons can be useful in reducing the radiation dose to the parotid glands and oral cavity. But the radiation dose to the thyroid warrants consideration because the low-dose bath of IMRT can increase its exposure to radiation compared with conventional 3-D CRT.

For most patients with involvement of the mediastinum and/or axilla, IMRT can improve dose–volume histogram (DVH) criteria for the heart, coronary arteries, esophagus, and lungs, compared with 3-D CRT. The dose-sparing effects for these normal tissues may be dramatic when using IMRT and will lead to adopting an IMRT plan (Fig. 81.9). The low-dose bath that puts larger volumes of normal tissue at risk for the development of secondary cancer[76,77] or pneumonitis[78] is often overshadowed by the significant sparing of the heart and coronary arteries with the IMRT plan. Proton therapy allows for a reduced dose to the heart, lungs, breast, and body compared with either IMRT or 3-D CRT techniques[77,79] without generating a low-dose bath (Fig. 81.10).

Infradiaphragmatic radiation may also benefit from the use of IMRT or proton therapy, especially when the spleen is irradiated, to help minimize the radiation dose to the heart, stomach, pancreas, and left kidney.[80,81]

IMRT and proton therapy are also useful in patients reirradiated for relapsed disease close to or within a previously treated area.[82]

TABLE 81.8 DOSE TO KEY ORAS FOR THE PATIENT SHOWN IN FIGURE 81.6 AND DVHS DISPLAYED IN FIGURE 81.8

Organ at Risk	IMRT Plan	3-D AP/PA Plan
Right breast V_4	19%	5%
Right breast mean dose	2.5 Gy	1.3 Gy
Left breast V_4	17%	0.5%
Left breast mean dose	1.9 Gy	0.04 Gy
Combined lung V_5	29%	15%
Combined lung mean dose	4.8 Gy	3.8 Gy

3-D, 3-dimensional; AP, anterior–posterior; IMRT, intensity-modulated radiation therapy; PA, posterior–anterior.

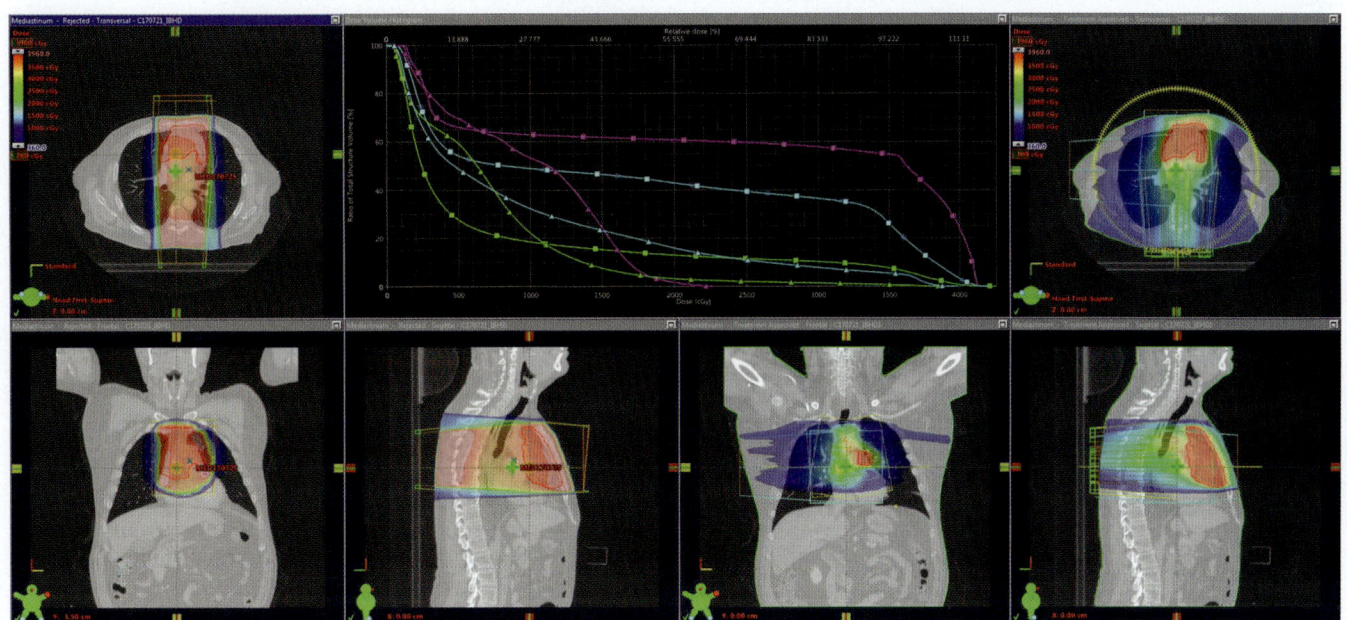

FIGURE 81.9. Comparison plans for 3-D conformal AP/PA fields and IMRT for a 45-year-old man with bulky mediastinal disease. In the DVH panel, *squares* show the 3-D plan and *triangles* indicate the IMRT plan. The *green lines* show a larger low dose–volume to the lungs for the IMRT plan, but there is a much lower dose to the heart (*light blue*) and LAD artery (*pink*). The IMRT plan was selected.

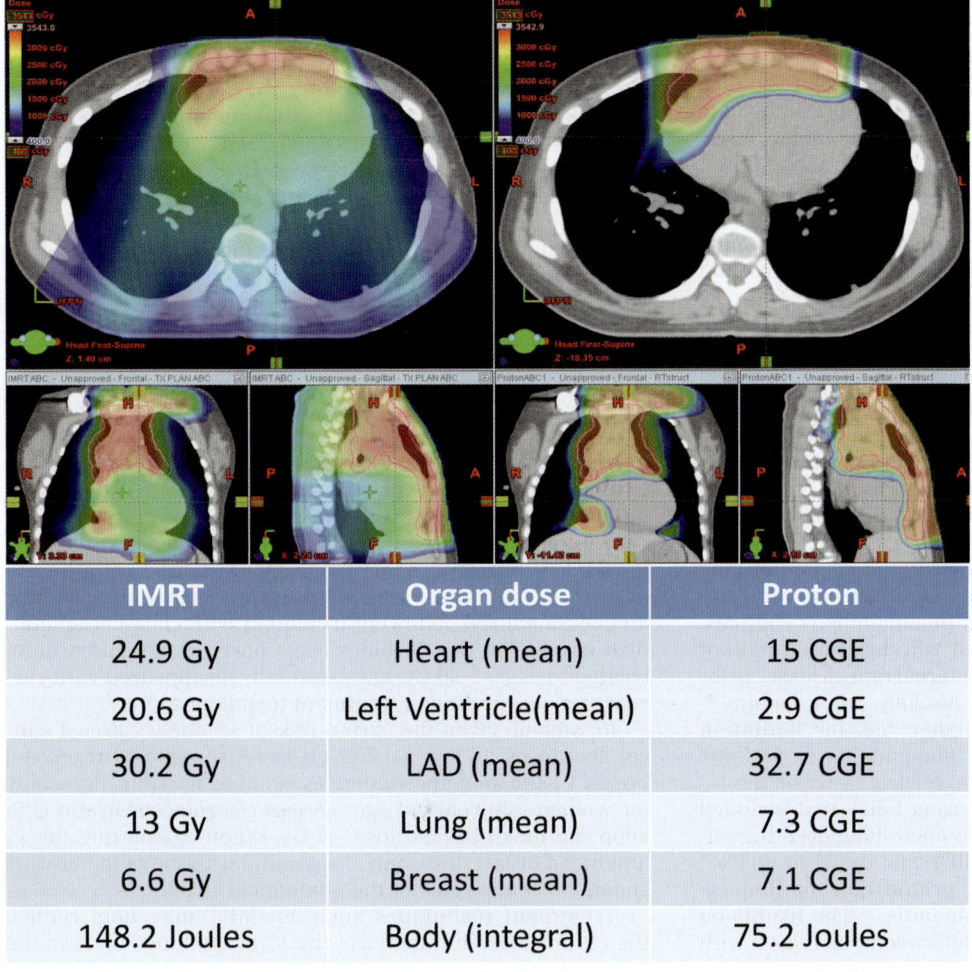

IMRT	Organ dose	Proton
24.9 Gy	Heart (mean)	15 CGE
20.6 Gy	Left Ventricle(mean)	2.9 CGE
30.2 Gy	LAD (mean)	32.7 CGE
13 Gy	Lung (mean)	7.3 CGE
6.6 Gy	Breast (mean)	7.1 CGE
148.2 Joules	Body (integral)	75.2 Joules

FIGURE 81.10. Color-wash dose distribution comparisons for two different plans for treating bulky mediastinal HL in a 30-year-old woman. **Left:** IMRT; **Right:** proton therapy. Both plans were done in breath hold.

Clinical results using these modern radiation technologies are beginning to emerge, but, thus far, they only demonstrate clinical effectiveness in regard to disease control and acceptable rates of acute toxicities. Investigators at three centers have reported their experiences using IMRT for HL (N = 40 to 60 patients), observing excellent relapse-free survival (~95%).[75,83,84] Similar results have been found by investigators at proton therapy institutes, some of whom conducted a small prospective clinical trial. In a combined analysis of academic and community proton centers where patients received consolidative proton therapy, the 3-year event-free survival rate was approximately 95% for patients with a CR before radiation.[85,86] The true benefit of these technologies won't be realized for at least two decades, when late toxicities become apparent. Until then, radiation oncologists should utilize all tools available to them to minimize the dose to the OARs and, therefore, minimize acute and late toxicities.

IMRT, VMAT, and Tomotherapy for Mediastinal Disease

Various techniques exist for delivering IMRT, VMAT, and tomotherapy.[83] Cella et al. reported comparison planning using forward-planned IMRT wherein the treatment fields were chosen to mimic an AP/PA field arrangement and then compared with a 7-field IMRT plan or tomotherapy. The forward-planned IMRT was better at reducing the radiation dose to the lungs and breast, but the 7-field IMRT plan and the tomotherapy plan were better at sparing the heart. Accordingly, the optimal treatment approach should be individually tailored to address potential toxicities.

Proton Therapy

Several techniques exist for delivering proton therapy, including passive scatter, uniform scanning, and pencil beam scanning with single-field optimization or multifield optimization. Several important factors should be considered when proton therapy is employed.[77] Guidelines are currently under development. When disease extends low and anterior to the heart, one should utilize anterior beams and avoid using posterior beams that traverse the heart unnecessarily. Similarly, for disease extending low and posterior to the heart, one should utilize posterior beams and avoid using anterior beams that traverse the heart unnecessarily.[87]

Organs at Risk

The dose range used for HL (20 to 36 Gy) is below the threshold tolerance for most organs; however, intrathoracic structures can be affected by these doses, and careful review of DVHs is warranted to minimize both acute and late effects. Table 81.9 provides a summary of published data on radiation doses to various OARs and their impact on the risk of acute and late toxicity.

The risk for pneumonitis is related to the volume of lung irradiated, total dose, and fraction size. The relationship between mean lung dose or V_x and pneumonitis is complex, can vary for different diseases, and will depend on patient age, smoking history, presence of intercurrent disease, prior chemotherapy, prior surgery, and possibly other factors.[102] Some investigators identified a higher risk for Radiation Therapy Oncology Group grade 2 pneumonitis in patients with HL when the mean lung dose exceeded 14 Gy or the V_{20} exceeded 35%.[103] In another study using IMRT that included RTOG grade 1 to 3 pneumonitis, the mean lung dose threshold was set at 13.5 Gy, the V_{20} to <30%, and the V_5 to <55%.[78] Conversely, a recent report using proton therapy demonstrated no significant risk of pneumonitis.[104] The likelihood of radiation-related pulmonary complications increases with the use of bleomycin,[105] although the impact of total bleomycin dose, which varies significantly with different drug combinations, has not been well defined. For example, the bleomycin dose after six cycles of ABVD is 120 u/m², whereas with 12 weeks of Stanford V, it is only 30 u/m². Bleomycin dose may influence lung DVH parameters following chemotherapy. Following Stanford V chemotherapy, an acceptable threshold to minimize the risk of radiation pneumonitis is a mean lung dose of 17 Gy. When used alongside high-dose therapies and autologous hematopoietic cell transplants, the risk of pneumonitis with radiotherapy increases and lower-dose constraints are warranted. New targeted agents, such as BV, nivolumab, and pembrolizumab, also may be associated with a higher risk of pneumonitis and should be used cautiously with mediastinal radiotherapy until further data are generated. BV should not be used in conjunction with bleomycin because of the high pneumonitis risk.[64]

With respect to carcinogenesis, because data indicate that lung cancer risk increases after doses as low as 5 Gy, it is reasonable to define and minimize the lung V_5 if multiple plans are reviewed, taking into account potential toxicity to other organs.[90] The lung cancer risk is also increased by the use of alkylating agent chemotherapy or procarbazine.[106,107]

The criteria for cardiac dose tolerance are less well defined. Tolerances are influenced by lifestyle; comorbidities such as diabetes mellitus, hyperlipidemia, and hypertension; family history; and prior treatment with cardiotoxic drugs like doxorubicin. In a large analysis of Dutch patients treated before 1996 (with lymphoma radiation fields and doses that are no longer employed), patients who received mediastinal irradiation had a 4- to 6-fold increased standardized incidence ratio of cardiovascular disease.[95] In a more detailed comparison of coronary heart disease and mean heart dose (MHD), the excess relative risk (ERR) was 7.4% per Gy of MHD.[96] The ERR was negligible with an MHD <5 Gy and was approximately 2 for an MHD of 12 Gy, a dose which should be achievable in most patients with contemporary treatment techniques. Although the MHD has been used as a surrogate for the likelihood of developing secondary cardiac effects, the dose to individual subunits of the heart is more likely to define the true cardiac risks. Therefore, effort should be made to contour all of the cardiac subunits using one of the standard cardiac atlases as a guide.[108] It is likely the dose to the left anterior descending (LAD) coronary artery and left ventricle is the most important; however, it is only recently that the dose to these structures has been contoured and measured, so limited retrospective data are available regarding acceptable threshold doses. The best approach is to keep the dose ALARA. With respect to valvular disease, the ERR is increased only minimally for valve doses up to approximately 20 Gy, but with a steep increase in risk thereafter.[97] Congestive heart failure risk is demonstrable when the left ventricular mean dose exceeds 15 Gy, or V_{30} is ≥50%, but the greatest increase in risk for congestive heart failure is associated with the use of anthracycline-based chemotherapy.[98] Acute pericarditis, an occasional risk following treatment with classical mantle-field irradiation that includes large parts of the pericardium treated to doses >30 Gy, has essentially disappeared with current standard radiation treatment techniques.

In women, given the excess risk of secondary breast cancer for doses as low as 4 Gy, it is reasonable to track the breast V_4 and keep the volume as small as possible, especially for women <30 years of age.[89] A less rigorous constraint is to keep the mean breast dose <4 Gy. When calculating the V_4 and mean breast dose, only the glandular tissue of the breasts should be contoured, not the anatomical structures.

Treatment techniques such as IMRT may help reduce the cardiac dose but increase the V_5 to the lungs or V_4 to the

TABLE 81.9 SUMMARY OF STUDIES DESCRIBING THE RISK OF SECONDARY CANCERS, CARDIOVASCULAR DISEASE, PULMONARY TOXICITY, AND ENDOCRINOPATHIES AMONG PATIENTS TREATED WITH RADIATION THERAPY FOR HL

	Outcome	Referent Group	Risk (95% Confidence Interval)
Second Cancers			
Castellino et al., 2011[88]	Fatal second malignant neoplasms	No RT	<30 Gy[a]: HR 1.9 (0.4–8.7)
			≥30 Gy[a]: HR 7.4 (1.8–30.3)
Travis et al., 2003[89]	Incidence of breast cancer	0–3.9 Gy[b]	4.0–6.9 Gy: RR 1.8 (0–4.5)
			7.0–23.1 Gy: RR 4.1 (1.4–12.3)
			23.2–27.9 Gy: RR 2.0 (0.7–5.9)
			28.0–37.1 Gy: RR 6.8 (2.3–22.3)
			37.2–40.4 Gy: RR 4.0 (1.3–13.4)
			40.5–61.3 Gy: RR 8.0 (2.6–26.4)
			[≥4 Gy: RR 3.2 (1.4–8.2)]
Travis et al., 2002[90] and Gilbert et al., 2003[91]	Incidence of lung cancer	<5 Gy[b]	>0–4.9: Gy RR 1.3 (0.3–4.9)
			5.0–14.9: Gy RR 4.1 (0.7–22)
			15.0–29.9: Gy RR 2.5 (0.1–16.1)
			30.0–39.9: Gy RR 8.6 (2.9–30)
			≥40 Gy: RR 7.2 (2.2–28)
			[≥5 Gy: RR 5.9 (2.7–13.5)]
Morton et al., 2014[92]	Incidence of esophageal cancer	<30 Gy[b]	≥30 Gy: RR 4.3 (1.5–15.3)
Morton et al., 2013[93]	Incidence of stomach cancer	0 Gy[b]	0.1–0.9 Gy: RR 1.3 (0.4–4.1)
			1.0–4.9 Gy: RR 1.0 (0.3–3.5)
			5.0–24.9 Gy: RR 0.5 (0.1–2.7)
			25.0–34.9 Gy: RR 4.6 (1.2–20.5)
			35.0–39.9 Gy: RR 8.2 (2.6–29.7)
			≥40 Gy: RR 4.2 (1.2–15.6)
			[≥25 Gy vs. <25 Gy: RR 5.8 (3.0–12.3)]
Dores et al., 2014[94]	Incidence of pancreatic cancer	<10 Gy[b]	≥10 Gy: RR 4.3 (1.7–15)
Cardiovascular			
van Nimwegen et al., 2015[95]	Incidence of any cardiac event	No RT	>0–29 Gy[a]: HR 2.3 (1.3–3.8)
			30–35 Gy[a]: HR 3.1 (2.3–4.2)
			≥36 Gy[a]: HR 3.8 (3.0–5.0)
van Nimwegen et al., 2016[96]	Incidence of MI/angina	No RT	>0–5 Gy[b]: RR 1.14 (0.62–2.10)
			5–14 Gy: RR 2.14 (1.28–3.58)
			15–19 Gy: RR 2.76 (2.10–3.59)
			20–24 Gy: RR 2.79 (2.23–3.49)
			25–34 Gy: RR 3.21 (2.52–4.09)
			35–45 Gy: RR 2.54 (0.96–6.69)
Cutter et al., 2015[97]	Incidence of valvular heart disease	No RT	≤30 Gy[b]: RR 1.4 (0.5–3.8)
			31–35 Gy: RR 3.1 (1.7–5.6)
			36–40 Gy: RR 5.4 (3.9–7.7)
			>40 Gy: RR 11.8 (4.9–28.5)
			P_{trend} < 0.001 (nonlinearity)
van Nimwegen et al., 2017[98]	Incidence of congestive heart failure	No RT	1–15 Gy[b]: RR 1.27 (0.86–1.89)
			16–20 Gy: RR 1.65 (0.98–2.77)
			21–25 Gy: RR 3.84 (1.97–7.47)
			≥26 Gy: RR 4.39 (2.00–9.65)
			P_{trend} < 0.001
Pulmonary Complications			
Ng et al., 2008[99]	Decline in %DLCO	N/A	MLD ≥ 13 Gy or V_{20} ≥ 33% = 60% persistently declined %DLCO
Endocrinopathies			
van Nimwegen et al., 2015[100]	Diabetes	General population	≥36 Gy para-aortic/spleen HR 2.3 (1.54–3.44)
			≥36 Gy para-aortic alone HR 1.82 (1.02–3.25)
Cella et al., 2013[101]	Hypothyroidism	N/A	Cumulative risk (median follow-up 32 mo):
			V_{30} ≤ 62.5% = 11.5%
			V_{30} > 62.5% = 70.8%

%DLCO, percentage-predicted carbon monoxide–diffusing capacity; AER, absolute excess risk; CCSS, Childhood Cancer Survivor Study; CI, confidence interval; CT, chemotherapy; ERR, excess relative risk; Gy, Gray; HR, hazard ratio; MI, myocardial infarction; RR, relative risk; RT, radiotherapy; SMR, standardized mortality ratio; TIA, transient ischemic attack; yo, years old.
[a]Prescribed dose.
[b]Estimated dose to where late outcome occurred.
[c]No evidence of departure from linearity.
Modified from Tseng YD, Cutter DJ, Plastaras JP, et al. Evidence-based review on the use of proton therapy in lymphoma from the Particle Therapy Cooperative Group (PTCOG) Lymphoma Subcommittee. *Int J Radiat Oncol Biol Phys* 2017;99(4):825–842. Copyright © 2017 Elsevier. With permission.

breasts, potentially resulting in a higher risk for secondary cancer in those organs (Figs. 81.6 and 81.7). This is not a problem when using proton therapy.[77]

In treating retroperitoneal nodes or the spleen, the organ at greatest risk is the left kidney. QUANTEC data recommend that the mean kidney dose (bilateral) should be <18 Gy, which should always be achievable in the context of treating HL.[109] In women who require pelvic nodal irradiation, the dose to the ovaries must be considered, as they are near the iliac nodes. Occasionally, an oophoropexy is necessary to provide sufficient ovarian protection. If an oophoropexy is performed, the surgeon should clip the superior and inferior poles of the ovary for precise localization on simulation scans. The menopausal effect of irradiation on the ovaries is dependent upon a woman's age. At age 20, the mean sterilizing dose is 15 Gy, but it drops to 12 Gy at age 30 and 8 Gy at age 40.[110] Alkylator agent chemotherapy, such as is in BEACOPP, will induce menopause in >50% of women, also correlating with age.[111] Among men, the possibility of inadvertent testicular irradiation is most likely to occur when the inguinal–femoral nodes are treated. This dose can be readily reduced 3- to 10-fold by use of a "clamshell" testicular shield.

Hypothyroidism is a common complication following cervical/supraclavicular node irradiation, as the thyroid cannot be spared completely because of involvement of those nodes. Data regarding dose–volume risks are limited. One analysis showed that the risk of developing hypothyroidism is only 11.5% if the V_{30} is ≤62.5 and 70.8% if the V_{30} is >62.5.[101]

A summary of the OAR dose constraints is displayed in Table 81.9.

RESULTS OF THERAPY

HL is responsive to both irradiation and chemotherapy, and a variety of regimens can achieve similar survival rates. However, significant differences in freedom from relapse rates and potential complications of therapy can occur. The results described in the following sections emphasize treatment programs that adhere to the NCCN Guidelines.[25] Clinical trial results that have helped define the current standards are shown in Tables 81.10 to 81.12.

Interim PET-CT

The utility of PET-CT imaging as a prognostic indicator after two cycles of chemotherapy was first demonstrated in patients with stage III to IV HL.[127] Patients with a positive interim PET study had a significantly higher risk for relapse than patients with a negative study, regardless of their initial international prognostic score. The impact on patients with stage I to II disease is less clear, and most patients with stage I to II disease will do well regardless of interim PET studies.[128,129] Nevertheless, interim PET is

employed in current clinical trials for all stages of HL and has also become standard in clinical practice and treatment guidelines.[25]

Favorable Prognosis Stage I to IIA Classic HL

Favorable presentation of stage I to II disease usually excludes patients with systemic (B) symptoms or large mediastinal adenopathy. Some clinical trial groups also exclude patients with an elevated ESR (≥50), extralymphatic extension (E lesion), multiple sites of disease (>2 or 3), older age (≥50 years), or unfavorable histology (mixed cellularity or lymphocyte depleted) and treat them according to algorithms for intermediate prognosis disease (Table 81.10).

In favorable prognostic groups, patients are treated with either chemotherapy alone or combined modality therapy. According to trials by the German Hodgkin Study Group (GHSG), patients with just one or two disease sites, an ESR < 50, and no extranodal disease can be treated with just two cycles of ABVD followed by 20 Gy ISRT.[114,130] For patients who do not fit these criteria, standard combined modality therapy programs can include four cycles of ABVD followed by 30 Gy ISRT[120] or, if the interim PET is negative (Deauville 1 or 2), three cycles of ABVD followed by 30 Gy ISRT.[116,131] Another option for these patients is 8 weeks of Stanford V followed by 30 Gy ISRT.[113]

After a positive interim PET following two cycles of ABVD, and absent progressive disease, additional treatment can include two additional cycles of ABVD (total four) plus 30 Gy ISRT[131] or treatment escalation to two cycles of escalated BEACOPP followed by 30 Gy ISRT.[116] Outcomes for any of these approaches are excellent (Table 81.10).

Owing to concerns for late radiation-related toxicity, clinical trials have evaluated the role of ABVD alone as treatment for patients with favorable disease presentations. The NCIC-CTG HD.6 trial was the first large trial to compare ABVD alone to combined modality therapy.[132] This trial has been criticized for including subtotal lymphoid radiation rather than IFRT or ISRT in the combined modality arm. However, the outcome of

TABLE 81.10 SELECTED CLINICAL TRIALS IN STAGE I TO II FAVORABLE HL

Clinical Trial (Reference)	Accrual	Median Age	Median F-U (mo)	Treatment	Interim PET	N	FFDP/FFP/ FFTF/PFS % (y)	OS % (y)	Comments
NCIC-CTG HD.6 Meyer et al., 2012[112]	1994–2002	35	136	4 ABVD	CR/CRu on CT	69	95 FFDP (5)	94 (12)	Excluded B symptoms, LMA. 70% of patients were ≥40 years, ESR ≥ 50, MC/LD histology, or >3 sites.
				6 ABVD	PR on CT	108	81 FFDP (5)		
Stanford G4 Advani et al., 2013[113]	1995–2001	30	127	8 wk Stanford V + 30 Gy IFRT	Not done	87	95.0 FFP (5)	98.0 (5)	Excluded LMA, B symptoms, abdominal disease. 48% of patients unfavorable by GHSG criteria; 38% of patients unfavorable by EORTC criteria
GHSG HD10 Engert et al., 2010[114]	1998–2003	36	90	2 ABVD + 20 Gy IFRT	Not done	299	91.2 FFTF (5) 91.6 PFS (5)	96.6 (5)	Excluded >2 sites, E lesion, ESR ≥50 or ESR ≥30 with B sx, LMA
UK RAPID Radford et al., 2015[115]	2003–2010	34	60	3 ABVD + 30 Gy IFRT	Negative[a] (D1–D2)	209	94.6 PFS (3) ITT 97.1 PFS (3) AT	97.1 (3)	Excluded B symptoms, LMA. 32% of patients unfavorable by GHSG criteria; 38% of patients unfavorable by EORTC criteria
				3 ABVD	Negative[a] (D1–D2)	211	90.8 PFS (3) ITT 90.8 PFS (3) AT	99 (3)	
				4 ABVD + 30 Gy IFRT	Positive[a] (D3–D5)	145	87.6 PFS (3)		
EORTC/LYSA/FIL H10F Andre et al., 2017[116]	2006–2011	31	60	3 ABVD + 30 Gy INRT	Negative[b] (D1–D2)	412	99.0 PFS (5)	100 (5)	Excluded >3 sites, age ≥ 50, ESR ≥ 50 or ESR ≥ 30 with B sx, MC/LD histology, LMA
		30		4 ABVD	Negative[b] (D1–D2)	238	87.1 PFS (5)	99.6 (5)	
		30	54	3 ABVD + 30 Gy INRT	Positive[b] (D3–D5)	54	77.4 PFS (5)	89.3 (5)	PFS and OS for PET+ include 43 H10F and 126 H10U.
		30		2 ABVD + 2 BEACOPP-esc + 30 Gy INRT	Positive[b] (D3–D5)	43	90.6 PFS (5)	96 (5)	

AT, as treated; CR, complete response; CRu, complete response undefined; D, Deauville 5-point scale; EFS, event-free survival; EORTC, European Organization for the Research and Treatment of Cancer; F-U, follow-up; FFDP, freedom from disease progression; FFP, freedom from progression; FFS, failure-free survival; FFTF, freedom from treatment failure; GHSG, German Hodgkin Study Group; IF, involved field; ITT, intent to treat; LMA, large mediastinal adenopathy; NCIC-CTG, National Cancer Institute of Canada Clinical Trials Group; NR, not reported; OS, overall survival; PFS, progression-free survival; PR, partial response; RT, radiation therapy; sx, symptoms; UK, United Kingdom.
Selection criteria vary widely. See text and original papers for details. For drug combination definitions, see Table 81.7.
[a]Interim PET after 3 ABVD.
[b]Interim PET after 2 ABVD.

TABLE 81.11 SELECTED CLINICAL TRIALS IN STAGE I TO II UNFAVORABLE HL

Clinical Trial (Reference)	Accrual	Median Age	Median F-U (mo)	Treatment	Interim PET	N	5-y EFS/FFTF FFS/PFS (%)	5-y OS (%)	Comments
EORTC H9U Ferme et al., 2017[117]	1998–2002	31	91	6 ABVD + 30 Gy IFRT	Not done	256	89.9 EFS	94	Included >3 sites, age ≥ 50, ESR ≥ 50 or ESR ≥ 30 with B sx, MC/LD histology, or LMA
		30	88	4 ABVD + 30 Gy IFRT		259	85.9 EFS	93	
		31	90	4 BEACOPP-base + 30 Gy IFRT		233	88.8 EFS	93	
GHSG HD11 Eich et al., 2010[118]	1998–2003	35	82	4 ABVD + 30Gy IFRT	Not done	356	85.3 FFTF	94.3	Included >2 sites, E lesion, ESR ≥ 50 or ESR ≥ 30 with B sx, or LMA. Excluded B symptoms + LMA or Bsx + E lesion (treated as advanced-stage disease)
		35		4 ABVD + 20Gy IFRT		347	81.1 FFTF	93.8	
		36		4 BEACOPP-base + 30 Gy IFRT		341	87.0 FFTF	94.6	
		36		4 BEACOPP-base + 20 Gy IFRT		351	86.8 FFTF	95.1	
ECOG E2496 Advani et al., 2015[119]	1999–2006	31	78	6–8 ABVD + 36 Gy RT	Not done	135	85 FFS	96	Included LMA only 52% of patients had B sx; 13% had E lesions.
		29		12 wk Stanford V + 36 Gy RT		129	79 FFS	92	
GHSG HD14 von Tresckow et al., 2012[120]	2003–2008	32	43	4 ABVD + 30 Gy IFRT	Not done	765	88 FFTF	97	Included >2 sites, E lesion, ESR ≥ 50 or ESR ≥ 30 with B sx, LMA. Excluded B symptoms + LMA or Bsx + E lesion (treated as advanced-stage disease)
				2 BEACOPP-esc + 2 ABVD + 30 Gy IFRT		763	95 FFTF	97	
EORTC H10U Andre et al., 2017[116]	2006–2011	32	61	4 ABVD + 30 Gy INRT	Negative (D1–D2)	512	92.1 PFS	96.7	Included >3 sites, age ≥ 50, ESR ≥ 50 or ESR ≥ 30 with B sx, MC/LD histology, LMA
		31		6 ABVD	Negative (D1–D2)	302	89.6 PFS	98.3	
		30	54	4 ABVD + 30 Gy INRT	Positive (D3–D5)	138	77.4 PFS	89.3	PFS and OS for PET+ include 43 H10F and 126 H10U
		30		2 ABVD + 2 BEACOPP-esc + 30 Gy INRT	Positive (D3–D5)	126	90.6 PFS	96	

CR, complete response; CRu, complete response undefined; D, Deauville 5-point scale; ECOG, Eastern Cooperative Oncology Group; EFS, event-free survival; EORTC, European Organization for the Research and Treatment of Cancer; F-U, follow-up; FFP, freedom from progression; FFS, failure-free survival; FFTF, freedom from treatment failure; GHSG, German Hodgkin Study Group; IF, involved field; IN, involved node; NR, not reported; OS, overall survival; PFS, progression-free survival; PR, partial response; RT, radiation therapy; sx, symptoms; UK, United Kingdom.
Selection criteria vary widely. See text and original papers for details. For drug combination definitions, see Table 81.7.

treatment with ABVD alone at 12 years yielded a 94% survival rate, 87% progression-free survival (PFS) rate, and 85% event-free survival rate. These findings set the stage for other trials of ABVD alone (three or four cycles total after a negative interim PET) versus combined modality therapy (Table 81.10).[116,131] The details related to the outcomes of these studies can influence their interpretation. Ultimately, the difference in PFS or event-free survival is approximately 6% to 12%, favoring management with combined modality therapy. The median follow-up of these trials has been too short to know whether differences in survival truly exist, owing to either the late effects of radiation or salvage therapy required for relapse. Nevertheless, the smaller radiation fields and lower doses now used compared to previous trials should result in a lower risk of radiation-related late effects. Selecting the right treatment for these patients depends on many variables,

TABLE 81.12 SELECTED CLINICAL TRIALS IN ADVANCED-STAGE HL

Clinical Trial (Reference)	Accrual	Median Age	Median F-U (mo)	Treatment	Interim PET	N	% Stage II	% RT	EFS/FFTF/ PFS % (y)	OS % (y)	Comments
EORTC 20884 Aleman et al., 2007[121]	1989–2000	32	79	6 MOPP-ABV	CR on EOT CT	161	0	0	84 EFS (5)	91 (5)	
		36		6 MOPP-ABV+ 24 Gy IFRT	CR on EOT CT	172	0	100	79 EFS (5)	85 (5)	
		30		8 MOPP-ABV+ 30 Gy IFRT	PR on EOT CT	250	0	100	79 EFS (5)	87 (5)	
ECOG E2496 Gordon et al., 2013[122]	1999–2006	33	77	6–8 ABVD±RT	Not done	395	35	41	74 FFS (5)	88 (5)	ABVD RT 36 Gy to large mediastinal disease only
				12 wk Stanford V+RT		399	36	75	71 FFS (5)	88 (5)	Stanford V RT 36 Gy to large mediastinal, nodes >2.5 cm, and involved spleen
EORTC 20012 Carde et al., 2016[123]	2002–2010	35	43	8 ABVD	Not done	275	0.4	0	63.7 EFS (4)	86.7 (4)	
				4 BEACOPP-esc+4 BEACOPP-base		274			69.3 EFS (4)	90.3 (4)	
GHSG HD15 Engert et al., 2012[124]	2003–2008	33	48	8 BEACOPP-esc	Not done	705	17	9	84.4 FFTF (5)	91.9 (5)	30 Gy RT to 2.5 cm residual disease that was PET+ @end of chemo. 4-yr PFS PET-92.6%; PFS PET+ 86.2%
		34		6 BEACOPP-esc		711	15	12	89.3 FFTF (5)	95.3 (5)	
		33		8 BEACOPP-14		710	15	11	85.4 FFTF (5)	94.5 (5)	
UK RATHL Johnson et al., 2016[125]	2008–2012	32	41	2 ABVD+4 ABVD	Negative (D1–D3)	470	41.5	2.6	85.7 PFS (3)	97.2 (3)	
		33		2 ABVD+4 AVD	Negative (D1–D3)	465	42.4	4.3	84.4 PFS (3)	97.6 (3)	
		32		2ABVD+BEACOPP*	Positive (D4–D5)	172	42.4		67.5 PFS (3)	87.8 (3)	*4BEACOPP-esc or 6BEACOPP-14
SWOG S0816 Press et al., 2016[126]	2010–2012	32	40	6 ABVD	Negative (D1–D3)	271	0	0	82 PFS (2)	NR	
		32	40	2 ABVD+6 BEACOPP-esc	Positive (D4–D5)	49			64 PFS (2)	NR	

base, baseline; D, Deauville 5-point scale; ECOG, Eastern Cooperative Oncology Group; EFS, event-free survival; EORTC, European Organization for the Research and Treatment of Cancer; EOT, end of chemotherapy; esc, escalated; F-U, follow-up; FFP, freedom from progression; FFS, failure-free survival; FFTF, freedom from treatment failure; GHSG, German Hodgkin Study Group; IF, involved field; NR, not reported; OS, overall survival; PFS, progression-free survival; PR, partial response; RT, radiation therapy; SWOG, Southwest Oncology Group; UK, United Kingdom.
Selection criteria vary widely. See text and original papers for details. For drug combination definitions, see Table 81.7.

and patient education and engagement are encouraged. For example, a young woman with mediastinal and axillary node involvement might choose the risk of relapse with ABVD alone over the risk of breast cancer from combined modality therapy. The opposite may be true for a patient with neck and superior mediastinal involvement, for which the heart and breasts would receive little radiation exposure.

Subdiaphragmatic involvement is seen in fewer than 10% of patients with stage I or II HL. For patients in whom disease is nonbulky and limited to pelvic lymph nodes with or without extension into the lower para-aortic nodes, the same general treatment principles apply as for supradiaphragmatic disease. In general, the outcome of treatment for these patients resembles that of patients with supradiaphragmatic disease.[133,134]

Patients with bulky abdominal presentations or those with involvement of the spleen are typically treated according to guidelines for "unfavorable" stage I or II disease or for stage III or IV disease.

Stage I to IIA Nodular Lymphocyte–Predominant HL

Contrary to the experience with classic HL, patients with limited presentation of NLPHL can achieve long-term disease-free survival after treatment with limited irradiation (IFRT) alone.[135-138] In contemporary terms, we use ISRT, but ISRT is defined somewhat differently than in the classic HL sense, which is treatment with combined modality therapy. The CTV expansion must account for possible microscopic spread beyond the lymph nodes clinically observed on PET-CT imaging (Fig. 81.5). For a patient who presents with unilateral level I or IIA disease, the CTV should be expanded to include ipsilateral levels IIB, III, and even IV. For a femoral node presentation, the CTV should include at least a 5-cm extension along the lymphatic chains superiorly and a 2-cm extension inferiorly.[139] The usual dose for NLPHL is 30 to 36 Gy. Doses below 30 Gy have been evaluated, but responses have not been as durable as with conventional doses.[140] Retrospective data from the GHSG show a 4-year PFS rate of 93.2% and an 8-year overall survival (OS) rate of 99% for patients with stage I NLPHL treated with IFRT.[137] There was no benefit from extending the radiation fields or adding chemotherapy. Single-institution results for treatment of stage I to II disease with radiation therapy alone include a 10- to 15-year PFS rate of 75% to 82% and 10-year OS rate of 83% to 100%.[135,136,141,142] In general, the results for PFS are a bit inferior for stage II versus stage I disease, but long-term survival rates are similar.

At some treatment centers, management resembling that for classic HL is preferred, utilizing combined modality therapy.[142] With combined modality therapy, the chemotherapy delivered can be ABVD (with or without rituximab), but evidence exists that alkylator-based chemotherapy may be superior for this histologic subtype.[143]

Based on these data, ESMO and NCCN guidelines reflect a preference for ISRT alone in stage I disease and, per NCCN, limited stage II disease.[25,54] For stage II disease, combined modality therapy is preferred, unless it is nonbulky and with no more than two contiguous sites involved.

Unfavorable Prognosis Stage I to II Classic HL

This category includes a diverse patient group. Unfavorable factors in different series nearly always include patients with B symptoms or bulky mediastinal disease (variably defined). Additional factors include more than two or three involved nodal regions, ESR above 50, age over 40 years, unfavorable histology (mixed cellularity or lymphocyte depleted), and extranodal disease (Table 81.11).

Based on consensus data, the most commonly used treatment for stage I or II HL with large mediastinal adenopathy is combined modality therapy with four to six cycles of ABVD plus 30 Gy ISRT. The expected FFP is 80% to 90%.[70,120,130] The EORTC H9U study showed no significant benefit to six cycles

compared with four cycles of ABVD[144] when given with RT. An essential concern with this treatment program is the potential for overlapping toxicities with doxorubicin, bleomycin, and irradiation (i.e., cardiac and pulmonary effects).

Although ABVD remains the standard chemotherapy for this clinical presentation, both Stanford V and BEACOPP regimens have been evaluated in clinical trials. The GHSG HD11 trial for patients with intermediate prognosis—which included patients with large mediastinal adenopathy, elevated ESR, extranodal disease, or more than two sites of involvement—randomized the chemotherapy to baseline BEACOPP versus ABVD and the IFRT dose to 20 versus 30 Gy.[118] Twenty percent of patients had bulky mediastinal disease. This trial demonstrated that 20 Gy was sufficient if BEACOPP chemotherapy was used but inadequate following ABVD. Nevertheless, owing to the greater toxicity of BEACOPP, ABVD × 4 plus 30 Gy IFRT became the standard arm of the next trial, the GHSG HD14.[120]

The Stanford V regimen has been used for patients with large mediastinal adenopathy. The 12-week chemotherapy program is followed by irradiation (30 to 36 Gy) to all sites >5 cm. In the setting of large mediastinal adenopathy, this program included irradiation of the mediastinum, bilateral hilar, and supraclavicular areas.[145] The Eastern Cooperative Oncology Group (ECOG) compared treatment with ABVD × 6 to 8 versus Stanford V × 12 weeks, in both cases followed by 36-Gy irradiation to the mediastinum and bilateral hilar and supraclavicular areas (the E2496 trial). Of the patients, 100% had bulky mediastinal involvement. There were no significant differences in 5-year OS (95% and 92%) or failure-free survival (FFS; 85% and 77%) for the two treatment arms.[119]

Clinical trials groups have investigated the use of chemotherapy alone in patients with stage I to II disease and unfavorable characteristics. The RAPID trial, cited above, excluded patients with large mediastinal adenopathy or B symptoms, but 32% of its patients were judged unfavorable by GHSG criteria and 38% by EORTC criteria.[131] Results were not reported separately for those different cohorts, however. The EORTC H10U trial evaluated the use of interim PET-CT to define a group of patients who might be treated effectively with ABVD chemotherapy alone.[116] In this trial, 40% of patients had bulky mediastinal disease (mediastinal–thoracic ratio ≥0.35 at the T5-T6 interspace). Patients with a negative interim PET were randomized to 4 additional ABVD or 2 ABVD + INRT. Among the patients randomized to treatment with ABVD alone, the 5-year PFS rate was 89.6% versus 92.1% with combined modality therapy. No subset analysis was performed to analyze the impact of specific unfavorable characteristics.

In the same trial, there was a benefit to escalated BEACOPP following an interim positive PET scan. All patients then received INRT. Patients whose treatment was escalated had a significantly improved 5-year PFS compared to those who continued ABVD + INRT (90.6% vs. 77.4%). The OS difference (96% vs. 89.3%) was not statistically significant ($p = .062$)

Approximately 15% to 20% of patients with stage I or II disease exhibit B symptoms. In general, these patients are managed analogous to those with stage III to IV disease. However, given the limited anatomic extent of disease with stage I to II, there is a strong argument for the inclusion of consolidative ISRT for these patients, as is recommended by the ESMO and NCCN.[25,54]

Stage III to IV Classic HL

Chemotherapy is the mainstay of treatment for patients with stage III to IV HL. The landmark study informing chemotherapy programs was the prospective, randomized clinical trial conducted by the Cancer and Leukemia Group B. Patients with stage III$_2$A, IIIB, or IV HL were randomly assigned to treatment with MOPP (six to eight cycles), MOPP/ABVD (12 months), or ABVD (six to eight cycles). Treatment results with MOPP/ABVD and ABVD were equivalent, and both were superior to MOPP alone. Among the 115 patients treated with ABVD chemotherapy, the CR rate was 82%, the 5-year FFS rate was 61%, and the OS rate was 73%.[58] More recently, the "gold standard" of ABVD has been challenged by the GHSG, which developed the BEACOPP regimen and has demonstrated in a series of trials that results using escalated BEACOPP (often including irradiation) are superior to those achieved with ABVD. The GHSG HD9 trial compared escalated BEACOPP, baseline BEACOPP, and COPP/ABVD.[146] Outcomes were best in the escalated BEACOPP arm, with a 5-year freedom from treatment failure (FFTF) rate of 87% and an OS rate of 91%. However, in an Italian multi-institutional study that compared an initial treatment strategy of ABVD (four to eight cycles) with BEACOPP (four escalated plus four baseline cycles), which took into account the possibility of autologous stem cell transplant as salvage therapy, there was no significant difference in 7-year freedom from second progression or OS (89% vs. 84%), and severe adverse events were more likely in the BEACOPP group.[147] In general, comparisons of escalated BEACOPP and ABVD chemotherapy show an advantage to escalated BEACOPP with respect to PFS, but no difference in OS (Table 81.12).

The value of treatment adaption based on interim PET results has been evaluated in advanced disease. Both the RATHL study[125] and the SWOG S0816[126] trial used escalated BEACOPP for PET-positive patients. Although escalated BEACOPP improved patient outcomes, neither trial had a comparison arm for continued treatment with ABVD. An important conclusion of the RATHL study was that patients with a negative interim PET scan could have bleomycin removed from cycles three to six of ABVD without compromising outcomes.

Because 70% of patients who receive chemotherapy alone relapse exclusively in sites of initial disease, combined modality therapy may be recommended for those with stage III to IV disease.[148] In addition to their low accrual, early trials evaluating the use of radiation in this setting were poorly designed and relied on chemotherapy programs that are no longer thought optimal. Nevertheless, trials of systemic therapy for advanced disease continue to include the selective use of consolidative irradiation.[146,147,149]

The EORTC–Groupe Pierre-et-Marie Curie H34 (20884) trial evaluated the role of radiation in advanced disease by treating patients with six to eight cycles of nitrogen mustard, vincristine, procarbazine, prednisone, Adriamycin, bleomycin, and vinblastine chemotherapy (MOPP-ABV).[150] Those who achieved a CR (57%) were randomized to no further therapy versus 25 Gy IFRT. No differences in FFTF or OS were identified. A detailed evaluation of causes of death revealed an unusually high rate of secondary myelodysplasia in the group randomized to combined modality therapy, but a similar risk was not observed in the nonrandomized patients, all of whom received irradiation to a higher dose! Most importantly, this trial demonstrated the important contribution radiation therapy made to the outcomes of the 43% of patients who did not exhibit a CR on CT. These patients received 30 Gy IFRT. The subsequent FFTF and OS rates for this group closely paralleled those for patients who had achieved a CR, suggesting value to adding IFRT when only a partial response has been achieved.[121]

Although the value of consolidative irradiation after CR to conventional chemotherapy (ABVD or BEACOPP) has not been proven, programs of attenuated chemotherapy in which radiation therapy is an essential component exist. The Stanford V program includes only 12 weeks of chemotherapy, with highly attenuated total doses for some drugs (see Table 81.7). Compared to six cycles of ABVD, it includes only 50% of the cumulative dose of doxorubicin (Adriamycin) and 25% of the cumulative dose of bleomycin. Radiation therapy (30 to 36 Gy) is routinely added to initially bulky (>5 cm) sites of disease as well as to macroscopic splenic involvement and commences 2 to 3 weeks after completing chemotherapy. The results of this approach have been excellent.[122,145,151] A similar study that did not employ the same guidelines for radiotherapy, however, showed much worse outcome, proving the importance of radiotherapy.[152] The ECOG E2496 trial compared management

with ABVD versus Stanford V for patients with advanced-stage or locally advanced disease. There was no difference in 5-year FFS (73% for ABVD, 71% for Stanford V) or OS (88% for ABVD, 87% for Stanford V).[122] The United Kingdom National Cancer Research Institute Lymphoma Group Study ISRCTN 64141244 also showed no difference between ABVD and Stanford V.[153]

The use of PET to identify patients with advanced disease who might benefit from RT was incorporated into the GHSG HD15 trial.[124] In this trial, patients with residual abnormalities on CT scan ≥2.5 cm underwent PET imaging. Only if the PET scan was positive did they receive local RT to that site. This strategy proved effective as the patients who were PET positive enjoyed a 5-year PFS rate of 86.2%. Although this outcome was statistically inferior to that in the PET-negative population (5-year PFS, 92.6%), these patients might otherwise be considered "chemotherapy resistant" and go on to autologous hematopoietic cell transplant. Clearly, that does not seem necessary in this setting.

A general conclusion regarding the role of combined modality therapy compared with chemotherapy alone for patients with stage III to IV disease is that patients who achieve a CR to a full course of conventional chemotherapy experience no proven benefit from adding radiotherapy. However, irradiation is often selectively added to such programs, especially for patients with bulky disease or sites of suspected residual disease. Furthermore, attenuated chemotherapy programs may confer a benefit by adding radiotherapy, and outcomes of patients who achieve only a partial response to chemotherapy may benefit from added radiotherapy. Ultimately, improvements in imaging and evaluations of early response to chemotherapy with FDG-PET or other diagnostic tests may help identify a subset of patients who would benefit reliably from consolidative radiotherapy (see section on "Current Clinical Trials").

Pediatric Patients

Most contemporary programs for managing pediatric HL rely on clinical staging. They employ chemotherapy alone or combined modality therapy with low-dose irradiation because higher doses are associated with an unacceptably high risk of growth impairment and late effects.[16] Radiotherapy doses in children should not exceed 15 to 30 Gy. Regardless of stage, children treated with these programs experience 5-year OS rates of approximately 90% and relapse-free survival rates exceeding 80%.[154-158] The management of children with HL is dealt with more comprehensively in Chapter 93.

Older Adult Patients

Treating HL in older patients (>60 years) is challenging because they often have less favorable histologies and a worse performance status.[159-161] They are also more likely to have intercurrent disease that compromises the aggressive management programs used for younger patients. Overall outcomes for patients ≥60 years old are comparably poor.[159] Chemotherapy programs must often be modified to minimize cardiac or pulmonary toxicity, and the hematologic reserve in elderly patients requires dose reductions or premature discontinuation.[162] Bleomycin should be avoided, and BEACOPP should not be used in patients over 60 years old.[163] Drug combinations better tolerated by older adults include ChlVPP,[164] procarbazine, Alkeran, and vinblastine,[165] and vinblastine, bleomycin, and methotrexate (used primarily for stages I to II).[166] Patients receiving radiotherapy may require slower fractionation programs and must be observed carefully for signs of weight loss or general decline in performance status. Extended fields are more difficult to tolerate than limited ones.[167]

Treatment for Relapse

Treatment for relapse must be individualized. Initial disease characteristics, initial treatment and response duration, relapse sites, and general patient status must be considered in developing an effective secondary treatment program. The conventional salvage therapy for most patients who were treated initially with chemotherapy alone or combined modality therapy is high-dose chemotherapy followed by autologous hematopoietic cell transplantation, which is effective in approximately 50% of patients.[168,169] Allotransplantation is not used often for relapsed HL but can be considered after an unsuccessful autotransplant or when disease is refractory to both conventional chemotherapy and biologic agents. Reduced-intensity conditioning regimens appear to be safer than myeloablative regimens.[170]

An increasing dilemma is the management of patients who present with stage I to II disease and are treated with abbreviated chemotherapy only, such as three cycles of ABVD. In these patients, relapse may be restricted to initial sites of disease.[171] In the RAPID trial, for example, only 7 of 22 patients whose disease relapsed after 3 cycles of ABVD went on to an autologous transplant. Five were treated with radiotherapy alone, four with chemotherapy alone, and six with combined modality therapy. Although more evidence is needed to define the best "salvage" regimens for these patients, it has become apparent that autologous transplant can be avoided in many situations.

The Role of Radiation Therapy in Hematopoietic Cell Transplantation

Radiation therapy can be incorporated into high-dose therapy/hematopoietic cell transplantation programs for relapsed or refractory HL. Fractionated TBI is sometimes used, but its value is debatable. Often, relapse is locoregional rather than systemic. Data suggest that radiotherapy doses resembling those used for total-body irradiation (12 to 15 Gy) are likely to eradicate disease in only approximately 20% of treated sites.[12] Thus, radiation should be limited to sites of failure or sites at high risk for disease, such as initially bulky ones.

Other considerations relevant to the issue of radiation therapy are its timing (pretransplant or posttransplant), field design, and dose. The advantages of using radiation therapy as cytoreductive treatment before high-dose therapy are that it can effectively reduce the tumor burden before high-dose treatment and the risk of interruption or delay of the locoregional radiation therapy is minimal. The primary disadvantages include potential delay of the high-dose therapy and the potential overlapping toxicities of the locoregional irradiation and high-dose therapy, including mucositis and pneumonitis.[172]

Many published series of high-dose therapy for HL have included locoregional irradiation in selected patients, usually after transplant.[173] The range of intervals from transplant to irradiation varies from 1 to 4 months. Often, the fields treated include sites of bulky disease (variably defined) at the time of relapse or sites that remain positive on PET imaging before the transplant. Some fields included all sites involved at the time of relapse.

In these studies, radiation doses ranged from 18 to 40 Gy. In general, lower doses were employed when initially nonbulky disease was included in the treatment or when there was a CR to high-dose therapy.

The use of locoregional irradiation in high-dose therapy programs can alter disease patterns and reduce the failure risk. At Stanford University, 49 patients with relapsed stage I to III disease underwent high-dose therapy and received IFRT as a component of their salvage treatment.[174] Investigators observed 3-year freedom from relapse, OS, and event-free survival rates of 100%, 85%, and 85%, respectively, compared with only 67%, 60%, and 54%, respectively, for patients who received high-dose chemotherapy alone. The difference in freedom from relapse was statistically significant ($p = .04$). The same was observed in a cohort of patients who received transplants at several centers.[175,176] The International Lymphoma Radiation Oncology Group has developed radiation treatment guidelines for patients undergoing hematopoietic cell transplantation.[176a]

FOLLOW-UP

All studies that initially yielded abnormal results (e.g., blood work and imaging) should be repeated upon completing therapy to document the patient's response to treatment. The Lugano response criteria mandate PET-CT imaging immediately following therapy for this purpose.[26,27] Earlier challenges with interpreting residual mediastinal abnormality after therapy have been obviated by the adoption of FDG-PET imaging as a posttreatment assessment tool, so concern can be limited to those patients with residual PET activity.[177]

The follow-up interval is typically every 3 to 6 months during the first 2 years and every 6 to 12 months thereafter.[25] The most important component of follow-up is an interim history and physical examination, which help to identify two-thirds of relapses.[178] Relapses can be detected by enlarged nodes or when the initial symptoms return, such as night sweats, pruritus, or alcohol intolerance. If ESR, serum albumin, and other serum marker studies were abnormal at presentation, they can be repeated, although they rarely suggest disease recurrence without clinical symptoms or physical findings.[179] Given the effectiveness of primary therapy for HL, the low rate of relapse, the risk for "false-positive" imaging studies, and the expense to the health care enterprise, the value of routine imaging has become debatable and guidelines remain nonspecific.[178,180,181] The NCCN Guidelines endorse up to 3 CT scans in the first 2 years after therapy.[182,183] Surveillance PET imaging is not indicated because of the high likelihood of false-positive findings, radiation exposure, and economic costs.[184-186]

In virtually every case, the first episode of relapse should be documented by biopsy. Inflammatory disease, progressive transformation of germinal centers, or the rebound growth of the thymus in young patients are other reactive processes that can be confused with recurrent HL. All of these processes can be FDG-avid on PET imaging.

Long-term follow-up helps detect late effects and ensures health maintenance. Serum thyroxine (T_4) and sensitive thyroid-stimulating hormone (TSH) levels should be obtained at least annually in patients who received radiation to the neck to detect subclinical hypothyroidism.

Cardiovascular risk factors should be managed aggressively, especially for patients exposed to thoracic radiation or Adriamycin chemotherapy. The NCCN Guidelines[25] recommend annual fasting blood sugar and biannual lipid panels and a stress echocardiogram, and carotid ultrasound should be done 10 years after treatment. Women exposed to thoracic radiation should initiate routine mammographic screenings 8 years after therapy or at age 40, whichever occurs first. Also, women treated before 30 years old should undergo both routine mammography and magnetic resonance mammography annually. Surveillance for other malignancies should conform to the American Cancer Society guidelines. Annual immunization against influenza is recommended.

SEQUELAE OF TREATMENT

Depending on the fields treated, the acute side effects of radiotherapy can include mild skin reactions, sore throat, an altered sense of taste, dysphagia, reflux symptoms, dry cough, nausea, occasional vomiting, diarrhea, and blood count suppression. Most of these sequelae can be managed symptomatically. Complications that arise in the early phase of the follow-up program can include mild radiation pneumonitis, radiation pericarditis, hypothyroidism, herpes zoster, Lhermitte sign, and xerostomia.

Radiation pneumonitis can develop within 6 to 12 weeks after completing mantle irradiation. After classic mantle therapy, <5% of patients experience symptomatic pneumonitis, manifested by cough, fever, pleuritic chest pain, and an infiltrate on chest radiography that usually conforms to the radiotherapy fields; this rate has been reported as higher following IMRT[78] and lower following proton therapy.[104] Symptomatic management is usually sufficient; however, some patients require treatment with corticosteroids, usually beginning with a daily dose of 40 to 60 mg of prednisone (or other corticosteroid equivalent). Corticosteroid therapy is a 4- to 6-week commitment at minimum, with slow, careful tapering to avoid exacerbation of symptoms.

Subclinical hypothyroidism develops in as many as half of patients who receive doses above 30 Gy to the neck.[187] It can be detected by elevated TSH levels even in the presence of a normal T_4 level. Thyroid replacement therapy with L-thyroxine is recommended, with an initial dose of up to 0.1 mg/d. The T_4 and TSH values are monitored regularly to adjust dose. Evidence suggests that thyroid replacement therapy in this setting reduces the risk of developing benign thyroid nodules.[188] It is likely that newer treatment techniques with lower doses and better shielding of the thyroid gland will result in decreased risk.

Herpes zoster can occur either during or within the first few years of HL treatment in 10% to 15% of patients.[189] The outbreak is usually limited to one or two contiguous dermatomes. Cutaneous dissemination is uncommon, and visceral involvement is extremely rare. If the cutaneous eruption is identified within 72 hours of onset, treatment with acyclovir (800 mg five times per day for 7 to 10 days or another antiviral equivalent) can be initiated. Acyclovir can limit the duration and intensity of the infection and decrease the likelihood of cutaneous or visceral dissemination. Currently, zoster vaccine immunization is not recommended for patients treated for lymphoma (www.cdc.gov/vaccines).

Lhermitte sign develops in approximately 10% to 15% of patients after radiation therapy to a significant length of the spinal cord via AP/PA fields. It is more likely to occur among patients who have been treated with vinca alkaloids (vincristine and vinblastine). It is marked by paresthesias that extends into the arms and legs on neck flexion and can be related to transient demyelinization of the spinal cord. Its onset is usually 1 to 2 months after completing mantle therapy and typically resolves spontaneously after 2 to 6 months. This sequela is not related to the more serious problem of transverse myelitis and is much less common among patients treated with IMRT or proton therapy, for whom the spinal cord doses are much lower.

Significant xerostomia can follow irradiation of the Waldeyer lymphoid region or the bilateral submandibular regions, which is rarely necessary, and permanent attention to dental care is required for these patients. Frequent dental prophylaxis and use of fluoride supplements are recommended.

An uncommon but potentially serious complication is overwhelming sepsis after splenectomy or splenic irradiation.[190,191] The most serious infections occur with gram-positive organisms, including *Streptococcus pneumoniae*, meningococci, and *Haemophilus* strains. Immunizing against these organisms minimizes risk. Patients can be immunized upon diagnosing the HL. Recommendations vary for the immunization of patients who have been previously treated but not immunized. Recent data suggest that patients can develop adequate antibody titers to *H. influenzae* type b-conjugate, 4-valent meningococcal polysaccharide vaccine, and 23-valent pneumococcal polysaccharide vaccine 2 after treatment.[192] Reimmunization is recommended for every 5 to 7 years. Fortunately, sepsis has become even more rare with the declining use of staging laparotomy and splenic irradiation.

An important concern of many patients with HL is the possible effect of treatment on reproductive potential. In men, pelvic irradiation can be followed by azoospermia if no special precautions are taken to shield the testes. With the appropriate testicular shielding, however, azoospermia is typically transient, and sperm counts will recover to fertile levels.[193] Chemotherapy programs such as MOPP, MOPP-like combinations that include alkylating agents and procarbazine, or BEACOPP will cause sterility in most men. However, the ABVD

and Stanford V regimens seem to preserve male fertility.[145,194] Among women, the risk for infertility is influenced by patient age. When undergoing radiotherapy, despite proper oophoropexy and well-planned pelvic treatment fields, the scattered dose may be sufficient to affect ovarian function and cause menopausal symptoms in women >30 years old.[195] In younger women, radiotherapy may not have an immediate effect on reproductivity but can eventually cause premature menopause. Similarly, chemotherapy with alkylating agents will not typically affect menstruation in women younger than 25 years old, but women above 30 years may see changes; also, premature menopause may occur.[111,196] In contrast to MOPP and BEACOPP, the ABVD and Stanford V combinations appear to preserve female fertility.[145,194]

An uncommon but significant treatment complication is the "dropped-head syndrome" secondary to cervical muscle atrophy that occurs in just some patients treated with high-dose irradiation (>36 Gy) to the neck.[197] This is a late risk, not usually apparent until >10 years after therapy. Management of this problem is challenging, with varying responses to physical therapy and use of a "soft collar." Surgical intervention has been attempted in some patients.[198] The use of contemporary therapies should obviate this risk.

Long-term follow-up is essential to identifying significant adverse late treatment complications in all patients.[199-202] The most important long-term concerns are secondary malignancies[107] and cardiovascular disease.[96]

Secondary malignancies include leukemia, lymphoma, and solid tumors. In a large series by Schaapveld et al., the standardized incidence ratio for developing a second malignancy after treatment for HL was 4.6, with 121.8 excess cancer cases per 10,000 patients per year.[107] Breast cancer was the greatest contributor to excess risk, followed by lung cancer, gastrointestinal tract cancers, and non-HLs. The highest (relative) risks were for thyroid cancer, soft tissue sarcoma, mesothelioma, and non-HL. Patients were also at an elevated risk of developing esophageal, gastric, pancreatic, and lung cancers as well as leukemia. These data were gathered in an earlier era of larger radiation fields, higher doses, and alkylating agent chemotherapy; therefore, risks are likely much lower now with the current management programs.[76,203-205] Secondary solid tumors, which have a latency of at least 7 to 10 years, are largely attributable to radiation therapy, although chemotherapy plays a part, especially with secondary lung cancers and gastrointestinal tract cancers.[93,106,107]

Myelodysplastic syndrome or acute myelogenous leukemia can develop after treatment that includes alkylating agents, procarbazine, or etoposide (e.g., MOPP or BEACOPP) after a latency of 3 to 7 years. During the era when alkylating agent chemotherapy was commonly used, the relative and absolute risks for this complication were 9.5 and 6.1, respectively.[107] Leukemia after treatment with irradiation alone is unusual.

Secondary lymphomas are usually of the diffuse large-cell B-cell type. The latent interval is typically over 5 years. The relative risk is 13.4, and the absolute excess risk is 16.0.[107] The development of secondary lymphomas does not seem to be related to any specific component of therapy but can be related to underlying immunosuppression.

A recent study of >1,000 women below age 51 years when treated for HL reported a 5.6-fold increased risk for developing invasive breast cancer compared with the general population of women (absolute excess risk, 57 cases per 10,000 persons per year).[204] The increased risk was primarily among women younger than 40 years at the time they were treated, and the risk was greater for women treated to a full mantle field compared with mediastinal irradiation only. The risk can also be related to radiation dose. Travis et al.[89] reported that doses exceeding 4 Gy were associated with an increased risk for developing a secondary cancer.

The lung cancer risk after irradiation exposure is also dose related, with an increased risk for lung cancer following doses as low as 5 Gy.[90] In addition, it has been clearly demonstrated that the lung cancer risk is extraordinarily high among irradiated patients who continue to smoke after treatment.[206] Because of this inordinately high risk for lung cancer, patients who continue to smoke after treatment should be urged to stop and encouraged to enter smoking cessation programs.

Potential cardiac complications following treatment for HL include pericarditis (which can occur during therapy), valvular dysfunction, conduction abnormalities, coronary artery disease, and ventricular dysfunction.[96] Radiation pericarditis is a potential risk if a large portion of the pericardium is treated, which is uncommon in the current management programs; it presents as an acute febrile syndrome associated with chest pain and friction rub, an asymptomatic pericardial effusion diagnosed by chest radiograph or echocardiogram, or constrictive pericarditis or tamponade. Mild manifestations can be managed with conservative medical treatment including analgesics and nonsteroidal anti-inflammatory agents; it usually clears within a few weeks. Although rare, tamponade or constrictive pericarditis is the most serious and can require surgical intervention.

Long-term cardiovascular sequelae result in increased morbidity and mortality.[96] Coronary heart disease for patients increases 2.5-fold for those who receive an MHD of 20 Gy. The use of Adriamycin did not increase this risk, although it did increase the risk for congestive heart failure nearly 3-fold.[98] Compared with the general population, the risk for cardiac morbidity requiring hospitalization is 2.77-fold for patients treated with both mediastinal irradiation and Adriamycin and 1.82-fold following mediastinal irradiation alone.[207] Screening studies have shown a significant risk of asymptomatic coronary artery disease, although optimal screening guidelines for patients after mediastinal irradiation have not been clearly defined.[208] Aggressive management of hypertension, diabetes, and serum lipid abnormalities is recommended for all patients.[25,209]

Another group of sequelae involves psychosocial problems, fatigue, marital difficulties, and employment issues.[210-212] Identifying these problems can promote the development of rehabilitation programs to anticipate and deal with these issues early in the course of treatment.

CURRENT CLINICAL TRIALS

Two clinical trials are evaluating reduced therapy for patients with negative PET scans after two cycles of ABVD. In the GHSG HD16 trial, patients without risk factors receive two cycles of ABVD chemotherapy followed by an interim PET. In the standard treatment arm, all patients receive 20 Gy IFRT, independent of the PET result. In the experimental arm, PET-positive patients are irradiated with 20 Gy IFRT and those with a negative FDG-PET receive no further treatment (two cycles of ABVD total). In the CALGB/Alliance 50604 trial, following a negative interim PET, all patients receive just two additional cycles of ABVD (no randomization).

Most current clinical trials emphasize the use of novel systemic therapies, including BV and the checkpoint inhibitors. The LCCC 1115 trial includes patients with stage I to II nonbulky disease. Following two cycles of ABVD and an interim PET, patients receive up to four additional cycles of ABVD, based on initial risk factors. This is followed by six doses of brentuximab and another PET scan. Only patients with a positive scan (Deauville ≥3) receive local irradiation. All other patients are observed.

The Memorial Sloan Kettering Cancer Center (New York, NY) 13-034 trial[213] includes patients with stage I to II disease and unfavorable characteristics. All patients receive two cycles of BV and AVD (no bleomycin, BV-AVD), followed by an interim PET and two more cycles of the same systemic therapy and another PET. Those who are PET-negative proceed to ISRT.

The GHSG proposed a phase II trial as a follow-up study to the HD16 trial for patients with early-stage favorable HL without risk factors. All patients will be treated with a checkpoint inhibitor (anti-PD1 antibody) combined with 20 Gy of ISRT. They will be randomized to either concurrent or sequential (anti-PD1 followed by ISRT) treatment. No patient will receive conventional chemotherapy. For patients with stage I to II disease with risk factors, the proposed randomized arms will be four cycles of nivolumab plus AVD followed by 30 Gy ISRT versus nivolumab monotherapy followed by two cycles of nivolumab–AVD, two cycles of AVD, and then consolidation with 30 Gy ISRT.

In patients with advanced disease, the ECHELON-1 industry-sponsored international study randomized patients to primary therapy with ABVD or BV-AVD. Recently reported, this trial showed an improved 2-year modified progression-free survival for BV-AVD, but no difference in survival.[214] Another, nonrandomized trial tests the effectiveness of nivolumab + AVD as induction therapy for patients with stage IIB or III to IV disease.

For patients with relapsed disease who are otherwise candidates for treatment with high-dose chemotherapy followed by autologous hematopoietic cell transplantation, combined BV and nivolumab is being evaluated as an alternative to high-dose chemotherapy for cytoreduction before transplant.

REFERENCES

1. Jemal A, Siegel R, Xu J, et al. Cancer statistics, 2010. *CA Cancer J Clin* 2010;60:277–300.
2. Ward E, DeSantis C, Robbins A, et al. Childhood and adolescent cancer statistics, 2014. *CA Cancer J Clin* 2014;64:83–103.
3. Mueller N, Grufferman S, Chang E. The epidemiology of Hodgkin lymphoma. In: Hoppe R, Armitage J, Diehl V, eds. *Hodgkin lymphoma*. Philadelphia, PA: Lippincott Williams & Wilkins, 2007:7–24
4. Grufferman S, Delzell E. Epidemiology of Hodgkin's disease. *Epidemiol Rev* 1984;6:76–106.
5. Kharazmi E, Fallah M, Pukkala E, et al. Risk of familial classical Hodgkin lymphoma by relationship, histology, age, and sex: a joint study from five Nordic countries. *Blood* 2015;126:1990–1995.
6. Mack TM, Cozen W, Shibata DK, et al. Concordance for Hodgkin's disease in identical twins suggesting genetic susceptibility to the young-adult form of the disease. *N Engl J Med* 1995;332:413–418.
7. Ambinder RF, Weiss LM. Association of Epstein-Barr virus with Hodgkin lymphoma. In: Hoppe R, Armitage J, Diehl V, eds. *Hodgkin lymphoma*. Philadelphia, PA: Lippincott Williams & Wilkins, 2007:25–42
8. Weiss LM, Movahed LA, Warnke RA, et al. Detection of Epstein-Barr viral genomes in Reed-Sternberg cells of Hodgkin's disease. *N Engl J Med* 1989;320:502–506.
9. Hjalgrim H, Askling J, Sorensen P, et al. Risk of Hodgkin's disease and other cancers after infectious mononucleosis. *J Natl Cancer Inst* 2000;92:1522–1528.
10. Glaser SL, Lin RJ, Stewart SL, et al. Epstein-Barr virus-associated Hodgkin's disease: epidemiologic characteristics in international data. *Int J Cancer* 1997;70:375–382.
11. Shiels MS, Pfeiffer RM, Gail MH, et al. Cancer burden in the HIV-infected population in the United States. *J Natl Cancer Inst* 2011;103:753–762.
12. Kaplan H. *Hodgkin disease*. Cambridge, UK: Harvard University Press, 1980.
13. Rosenberg SA, Kaplan HS. Evidence for an orderly progression in the spread of Hodgkin's disease. *Cancer Res* 1966;26:1225–1231.
14. Kaplan HS. On the natural history, treatment, and prognosis of Hodgkin's disease. *Harvey Lect* 1968;64:215–259.
15. Hoppe RT, Cox RS, Rosenberg SA, et al. Prognostic factors in pathologic stage III Hodgkin's disease. *Cancer Treat Rep* 1982;66:743–749.
16. Kelly KM, Hodgson D, Appel B, et al. Children's Oncology Group's 2013 blueprint for research: Hodgkin lymphoma. *Pediatr Blood Cancer* 2013;60:972–978.
17. Mauz-Korholz C, Metzger ML, Kelly KM, et al. Pediatric Hodgkin Lymphoma. *J Clin Oncol* 2015;33:2975–2985.
18. Boll B, Goergen H, Behringer K, et al. Bleomycin in older early-stage favorable Hodgkin lymphoma patients: analysis of the German Hodgkin Study Group (GHSG) HD10 and HD13 trials. *Blood* 2016;127:2189–2192.
19. Boll B, Gorgen H, Fuchs M, et al. ABVD in older patients with early-stage Hodgkin lymphoma treated within the German Hodgkin Study Group HD10 and HD11 trials. *J Clin Oncol* 2013;31:1522–1529.
20. Lambe M, Hsieh CC, Tsaih SW, et al. Childbearing and the risk of Hodgkin's disease. *Cancer Epidemiol Biomarkers Prev* 1998;7:831–834.
21. Portlock CS, Yahalom J. The management of Hodgkin lymphoma during pregnancy. In: Hoppe R, Armitage J, Diehl V, eds. *Hodgkin lymphoma*. Philadelphia, PA: Lippincott Williams & Wilkins, 2007:419–26
22. Mazonakis M, Varveris H, Fasoulaki M, et al. Radiotherapy of Hodgkin's disease in early pregnancy: embryo dose measurements. *Radiother Oncol* 2003;66:333–339.
23. Olszewski AJ, Castillo JJ. Outcomes of HIV-associated Hodgkin lymphoma in the era of antiretroviral therapy. *AIDS* 2016;30:787–796.
24. Tirelli U, Errante D, Dolcetti R, et al. Hodgkin's disease and human immunodeficiency virus infection: clinicopathologic and virologic features of 114 patients from the Italian Cooperative Group on AIDS and Tumors. *J Clin Oncol* 1995;13:1758–1767.
25. National Comprehensive Cancer Guidelines: Hodgkin lymphoma. 2017. Available at: https://www.nccn.org/professionals/physician_gls/pdf/hodgkins.pdf. Accessed April 13, 2017.

26. Barrington SF, Mikhaeel NG, Kostakoglu L, et al. Role of imaging in the staging and response assessment of lymphoma: consensus of the International Conference on Malignant Lymphomas Imaging Working Group. *J Clin Oncol* 2014;32:3048–3058.
27. Cheson BD, Fisher RI, Barrington SF, et al. Recommendations for initial evaluation, staging, and response assessment of Hodgkin and non-Hodgkin lymphoma: the Lugano classification. *J Clin Oncol* 2014;32:3059–3068.
28. Hasenclever D, Diehl V. A prognostic score for advanced Hodgkin's disease. International Prognostic Factors Project on Advanced Hodgkin's Disease. *N Engl J Med* 1998;339:1506–1514.
29. Henry-Amar M, Friedman S, Hayat M, et al. Erythrocyte sedimentation rate predicts early relapse and survival in early-stage Hodgkin disease. The EORTC Lymphoma Cooperative Group. *Ann Intern Med* 1991;114:361–365.
30. Figura N, Flampouri S, Mendenhall NP, et al. Importance of baseline PET/CT imaging on radiation field design and relapse rates in patients with Hodgkin lymphoma. *Adv Radiat Oncol* 2017;2:197–203.
31. Partridge S, Timothy A, O'Doherty MJ, et al. 2-Fluorine-18-fluoro-2-deoxy-D glucose positron emission tomography in the pretreatment staging of Hodgkin's disease: influence on patient management in a single institution. *Ann Oncol* 2000;11:1273–1279.
32. El-Galaly TC, d'Amore F, Mylam KJ, et al. Routine bone marrow biopsy has little or no therapeutic consequence for positron emission tomography/computed tomography-staged treatment-naive patients with Hodgkin lymphoma. *J Clin Oncol* 2012;30:4508–4514.
33. Purz S, Mauz-Korholz C, Korholz D, et al. [18F]Fluorodeoxyglucose positron emission tomography for detection of bone marrow involvement in children and adolescents with Hodgkin's lymphoma. *J Clin Oncol* 2011;29:3523–3528.
34. Afaq A, Fraioli F, Sidhu H, et al. Comparison of PET/MRI with PET/CT in the evaluation of disease status in lymphoma. *Clin Nucl Med* 2017;42:e1–e7.
35. Lister TA, Crowther D, Sutcliffe SB, et al. Report of a committee convened to discuss the evaluation and staging of patients with Hodgkin's disease: Cotswolds meeting. *J Clin Oncol* 1989;7:1630–1636.
36. Carbone PP, Kaplan HS, Musshoff K, et al. Report of the committee on Hodgkin's disease staging classification. *Cancer Res* 1971;31:1860–1861.
37. Connors JM, Klimo P. Is it an E lesion or stage IV? An unsettled issue in Hodgkin's disease staging. *J Clin Oncol* 1984;2:1421–1423.
38. Swerdlow SH, Campo E, Harris NL, et al. (eds.) *WHO classification of tumours of haematopoietic and lymphoid tissues*. 4th ed. Lyon, France: IARC, 2017.
39. Weiss LM, Warnke RA, Hansmann ML. Pathology of Hodgkin lymphoma. In: Hoppe R, Armitage J, Diehl V, eds. *Hodgkin lymphoma*. Philadelphia, PA: Lippincott Williams & Wilkins, 2007:43–72.
40. Kuppers R, Engert A, Hansmann ML. Hodgkin lymphoma. *J Clin Invest* 2012;122:3439–3447.
41. Roemer MG, Advani RH, Ligon AH, et al. PD-L1 and PD-L2 genetic alterations define classical Hodgkin lymphoma and predict outcome. *J Clin Oncol* 2016;34:2690–2697.
42. Shimabukuro-Vornhagen A, Haverkamp H, Engert A, et al. Lymphocyte-rich classical Hodgkin's lymphoma: clinical presentation and treatment outcome in 100 patients treated within German Hodgkin's Study Group trials. *J Clin Oncol* 2005;23:5739–5745.
43. Anagnostopoulos I. Lymphocyte-rich classical Hodgkin lymphoma. In: Swerdlow SH, Campo E, Harris NL, et al., eds. *WHO classification of tumours of haematopoietic and lymphoid tissues*. 4th ed. Lyon, France: IARC, 2008.
44. Benharroch D. Lymphocyte-depleted classical Hodgkin lymphoma. In: Swerdlow SH, Campo E, Harris NL, et al., eds. *WHO classification of tumours of haematopoietic and lymphoid Tissues*. 4th ed. Lyon, France: IARC, 2008.
45. Klimm B, Franklin J, Stein H, et al. Lymphocyte-depleted classical Hodgkin's lymphoma: a comprehensive analysis from the German Hodgkin study group. *J Clin Oncol* 2011;29:3914–3920.
46. Fan Z, Natkunam Y, Bair E, et al. Characterization of variant patterns of nodular lymphocyte predominant Hodgkin lymphoma with immunohistologic and clinical correlation. *Am J Surg Pathol* 2003;27:1346–1356.
47. Hartmann S, Eichenauer DA, Plutschow A, et al. The prognostic impact of variant histology in nodular lymphocyte-predominant Hodgkin lymphoma: a report from the German Hodgkin Study Group (GHSG). *Blood* 2013;122:4246–4252; quiz 92.
48. Al-Mansour M, Connors JM, Gascoyne RD, et al. Transformation to aggressive lymphoma in nodular lymphocyte-predominant Hodgkin's lymphoma. *J Clin Oncol* 2010;28:793–799.
49. Kenderian SS, Habermann TM, Macon WR, et al. Large B-cell transformation in nodular lymphocyte-predominant Hodgkin lymphoma: 40-year experience from a single institution. *Blood* 2016;127:1960–1966.
50. Hansmann ML, Fellbaum C, Hui PK, et al. Progressive transformation of germinal centers with and without association to Hodgkin's disease. *Am J Clin Pathol* 1990;93:219–226.
51. Poppema S. Nodular lymphocyte predominant Hodgkin lymphoma. In: Swerdlow SH, Campo E, Harris NL, et al., eds. *WHO classification of tumours of haematopoietic and lymphoid tissues*. 4th ed. Lyon, France: IARC, 2008.
52. Hu E, Hufford S, Lukes R, et al. Third-World Hodgkin's disease at Los Angeles County-University of Southern California Medical Center. *J Clin Oncol* 1988;6:1285–1292.
53. Jacobs P. Hodgkin lymphoma in developing countries: an African perspective with a note on Asia and Latin America. In: Hoppe R, Armitage J, Diehl V, eds. *Hodgkin Lymphoma*. Philadelphia, PA: Lippincott Williams & Wilkins, 2007:427–448.
54. Eichenauer DA, Engert A, Andre M, et al. Hodgkin's lymphoma: ESMO Clinical Practice Guidelines for diagnosis, treatment and follow-up. *Ann Oncol* 2014;25(Suppl 3):iii70–iii75.
55. Pusey WA. Cases of sarcoma and of Hodgkin's disease treated by exposures to X-rays: a preliminary report. *JAMA* 1902;38:166–169.
56. Specht L, Yahalom J, Illidge T, et al. Modern radiation therapy for Hodgkin lymphoma: field and dose guidelines from the international lymphoma radiation oncology group (ILROG). *Int J Radiat Oncol Biol Phys* 2014;89:854–862.
57. Bonadonna G. Chemotherapy strategies to improve the control of Hodgkin's disease: the Richard and Hinda Rosenthal Foundation Award Lecture. *Cancer Res* 1982;42:4309–4320.
58. Canellos GP, Anderson JR, Propert KJ, et al. Chemotherapy of advanced Hodgkin's disease with MOPP, ABVD, or MOPP alternating with ABVD. *N Engl J Med* 1992;327:1478–1484.
59. Diehl V, Fuchs M. Early, intermediate and advanced Hodgkin's lymphoma: modern treatment strategies. *Ann Oncol* 2007;18(Suppl 9):ix71–ix79.
60. Bartlett NL, Rosenberg SA, Hoppe RT, et al. Brief chemotherapy, Stanford V, and adjuvant radiotherapy for bulky or advanced-stage Hodgkin's disease: a preliminary report. *J Clin Oncol* 1995;13:1080–1088.
61. Hough R, Hancock BW. Principles of chemotherapy in Hodgkin lymphoma. In: Hoppe R, Armitage J, Diehl V, eds. *Hodgkin lymphoma*. Philadelphia, PA: Lippincott Williams & Wilkins, 2007:189–204.
62. Younes A, Santoro A, Shipp M, et al. Nivolumab for classical Hodgkin's lymphoma after failure of both autologous stem-cell transplantation and brentuximab vedotin: a multicentre, multicohort, single-arm phase 2 trial. *Lancet Oncol* 2016;17:1283–1294.
63. Armand P, Shipp MA, Ribrag V, et al. Programmed death-1 blockade with pembrolizumab in patients with classical Hodgkin lymphoma after brentuximab vedotin failure. *J Clin Oncol* 2016;34:3733–3739.
64. Younes A. CD30-targeted antibody therapy. *Curr Opin Oncol* 2011;23:587–593.
65. Moskowitz CH, Nademanee A, Masszi T, et al. Brentuximab vedotin as consolidation therapy after autologous stem-cell transplantation in patients with Hodgkin's lymphoma at risk of relapse or progression (AETHERA): a randomised, double-blind, placebo-controlled, phase 3 trial. *Lancet* 2015;385:1853–1862.
66. Paumier A, Ghalibafian M, Gilmore J, et al. Dosimetric benefits of intensity-modulated radiotherapy combined with the deep-inspiration breath-hold technique in patients with mediastinal Hodgkin's lymphoma. *Int J Radiat Oncol Biol Phys* 2012;82:1522–1527.
67. Hoppe BS, Mendenhall NP, Louis D, et al. Comparing breath hold and free breathing during intensity-modulated radiation therapy and proton therapy in patients with mediastinal Hodgkin lymphoma. *Int J Particle Ther* 2017;3(4):492–496.
68. Petersen PM, Aznar MC, Berthelsen AK, et al. Prospective phase II trial of image-guided radiotherapy in Hodgkin lymphoma: benefit of deep inspiration breath-hold. *Acta Oncol* 2015;54:60–66.
69. Charpentier AM, Conrad T, Sykes J, et al. Active breathing control for patients receiving mediastinal radiation therapy for lymphoma: Impact on normal tissue dose. *Pract Radiat Oncol* 2014;4:174–180.
70. Bonadonna G, Bonfante V, Viviani S, et al. ABVD plus subtotal nodal versus involved-field radiotherapy in early-stage Hodgkin's disease: long-term results. *J Clin Oncol* 2004;22:2835–2841.
71. Engert A, Schiller P, Josting A, et al. Involved-field radiotherapy is equally effective and less toxic compared with extended-field radiotherapy after four cycles of chemotherapy in patients with early-stage unfavorable Hodgkin's lymphoma: results of the HD8 trial of the German Hodgkin's Lymphoma Study Group. *J Clin Oncol* 2003;21:3601–3608.
72. Ferme C, Eghbali H, Meerwaldt JH, et al. Chemotherapy plus involved-field radiation in early-stage Hodgkin's disease. *N Engl J Med* 2007;357:1916–1927.
73. Girinsky T, van der Maazen R, Specht L, et al. Involved-node radiotherapy (INRT) in patients with early Hodgkin lymphoma: concepts and guidelines. *Radiother Oncol* 2006;79:270–277.
74. Girinsky T, Ghalibafian M, Bonniaud G, et al. Is FDG-PET scan in patients with early stage Hodgkin lymphoma of any value in the implementation of the involved-node radiotherapy concept and dose painting? *Radiother Oncol* 2007;85:178–186.
75. Paumier A, Ghalibafian M, Beaudre A, et al. Involved-node radiotherapy and modern radiation treatment techniques in patients with Hodgkin lymphoma. *Int J Radiat Oncol Biol Phys* 2011;80:199–205.
76. Weber DC, Johanson S, Peguret N, et al. Predicted risk of radiation-induced cancers after involved field and involved node radiotherapy with or without intensity modulation for early-stage Hodgkin lymphoma in female patients. *Int J Radiat Oncol Biol Phys* 2011;81:490–497.
77. Tseng YD, Cutter DJ, Plastara JP, et al. Evidence-based review on the use of proton therapy in lymphoma from the Particle Therapy Cooperative Group Lymphoma Subcommittee. *Int J Radiat Oncol Biol Phys* 2017;99(4):825–842.
78. Pinnix CC, Smith GL, Milgrom S, et al. Predictors of radiation pneumonitis in patients receiving intensity modulated radiation therapy for Hodgkin and non-Hodgkin lymphoma. *Int J Radiat Oncol Biol Phys* 2015;92:175–182.
79. Hoppe BS, Flampouri S, Zaiden R, et al. Involved-node proton therapy in combined modality therapy for Hodgkin lymphoma: results of a phase 2 study. *Int J Radiat Oncol Biol Phys* 2014;89:1053–1059.
80. Sachsman S, Hoppe BS, Mendenhall NP, et al. Proton therapy to the subdiaphragmatic region in the management of patients with Hodgkin lymphoma. *Leuk Lymphoma* 2015;56:2019–2024.
81. Holtzman AL, Hoppe BS, Li Z, et al. Advancing the therapeutic index in stage III/IV pediatric Hodgkin lymphoma with proton therapy. *Int J Particle Ther* 2014;1:343–356.
82. Plastaras JP, Berman AT, Freedman GM. Special cases for proton beam radiotherapy: re-irradiation, lymphoma, and breast cancer. *Semin Oncol* 2014;41:807–819.
83. Filippi AR, Ciammella P, Piva C, et al. Involved-site image-guided intensity modulated versus 3D conformal radiation therapy in early stage supradiaphragmatic Hodgkin lymphoma. *Int J Radiat Oncol Biol Phys* 2014;89:370–375.
84. Lu NN, Li YX, Wu RY, et al. Dosimetric and clinical outcomes of involved-field intensity-modulated radiotherapy after chemotherapy for early-stage Hodgkin's lymphoma with mediastinal involvement. *Int J Radiat Oncol Biol Phys* 2012;84:210–216.
85. Wray J, Flampouri S, Slayton W, et al. Proton therapy for pediatric Hodgkin lymphoma. *Pediatr Blood Cancer* 2016;63:1522–1526.
86. Hoppe BS, Hill-Kayser CE, Tseng YD, et al. Consolidative proton therapy after chemotherapy for patients with Hodgkin lymphoma. *Ann Oncol* 2017;28(9):2179–2184.
87. Hoppe BS, Flampouri S, Li Z, et al. Cardiac sparing with proton therapy in consolidative radiation therapy for Hodgkin lymphoma. *Leuk Lymphoma* 2010;51:1559–1562.
88. Castellino SM, Geiger AM, Mertens AC, et al. Morbidity and mortality in long-term survivors of Hodgkin lymphoma: a report from the Childhood Cancer Survivor Study. *Blood* 2011;117:1806–1816.

89. Travis LB, Hill DA, Dores GM, et al. Breast cancer following radiotherapy and chemotherapy among young women with Hodgkin disease. *JAMA* 2003;290:465–475.

90. Travis LB, Gospodarowicz M, Curtis RE, et al. Lung cancer following chemotherapy and radiotherapy for Hodgkin's disease. *J Natl Cancer Inst* 2002;94:182–192.

91. Gilbert ES, Stovall M, Gospodarowicz M, et al. Lung cancer after treatment for Hodgkin's disease: focus on radiation effects. *Radiat Res* 2003;159:161–173.

92. Morton LM, Gilbert ES, Stovall M, et al. Risk of esophageal cancer following radiotherapy for Hodgkin lymphoma. *Haematologica* 2014;99:e193–e196.

93. Morton LM, Dores GM, Curtis RE, et al. Stomach cancer risk after treatment for Hodgkin lymphoma. *J Clin Oncol* 2013;31:3369–3377.

94. Dores GM, Curtis RE, van Leeuwen FE, et al. Pancreatic cancer risk after treatment of Hodgkin lymphoma. *Ann Oncol* 2014;25:2073–2079.

95. van Nimwegen FA, Schaapveld M, Janus CP, et al. Cardiovascular disease after Hodgkin lymphoma treatment: 40-year disease risk. *JAMA Intern Med* 2015;175:1007–1017.

96. van Nimwegen FA, Schaapveld M, Cutter DJ, et al. Radiation dose-response relationship for risk of coronary heart disease in survivors of Hodgkin lymphoma. *J Clin Oncol* 2016;34:235–243.

97. Cutter DJ, Schaapveld M, Darby SC, et al. Risk of valvular heart disease after treatment for Hodgkin lymphoma. *J Natl Cancer Inst* 2015;107.

98. van Nimwegen FA, Ntentas G, Darby SC, et al. Risk of heart failure in survivors of Hodgkin lymphoma: effects of cardiac exposure to radiation and anthracyclines. *Blood* 2017;129:2257–2265.

99. Ng AK, Li S, Neuberg D, et al. A prospective study of pulmonary function in Hodgkin's lymphoma patients. *Ann Oncol* 2008;19:1754–1758.

100. van Nimwegen FA, Schaapveld M, Janus CP, et al. Risk of diabetes mellitus in long-term survivors of Hodgkin lymphoma. *J Clin Oncol* 2014;32:3257–3263.

101. Cella L, Conson M, Caterino M, et al. Thyroid V30 predicts radiation-induced hypothyroidism in patients treated with sequential chemo-radiotherapy for Hodgkin's lymphoma. *Int J Radiat Oncol Biol Phys* 2012;82:1802–1808.

102. Marks LB, Bentzen SM, Deasy JO, et al. Radiation dose-volume effects in the lung. *Int J Radiat Oncol Biol Phys* 2010;76:S70–S76.

103. Koh ES, Sun A, Tran TH, et al. Clinical dose-volume histogram analysis in predicting radiation pneumonitis in Hodgkin's lymphoma. *Int J Radiat Oncol Biol Phys* 2006;66:223–228.

104. Nanda R, Flampouri S, Mendenhall NP, et al. Pulmonary toxicity following proton therapy for thoracic lymphoma. *Int J Radiat Oncol Biol Phys* 2017;99(2):494–497.

105. Cosset JM, Henry-Amar M, Meerwaldt JH. Long-term toxicity of early stages of Hodgkin's disease therapy: the EORTC experience. EORTC Lymphoma Cooperative Group. *Ann Oncol* 1991;2(Suppl 2):77–82.

106. Swerdlow AJ, Higgins CD, Smith P, et al. Second cancer risk after chemotherapy for Hodgkin's lymphoma: a collaborative British cohort study. *J Clin Oncol* 2011;29:4096–4104.

107. Schaapveld M, Aleman BM, van Eggermond AM, et al. Second cancer risk up to 40 years after treatment for Hodgkin's lymphoma. *N Engl J Med* 2015;373:2499–2511.

108. Duane F, Aznar MC, Bartlett F, et al. A cardiac contouring atlas for radiotherapy. *Radiother Oncol* 2017;122:416–422.

109. Dawson LA, Kavanagh BD, Paulino AC, et al. Radiation-associated kidney injury. *Int J Radiat Oncol Biol Phys* 2010;76:S108–S115.

110. Wallace WH, Thomson AB, Saran F, et al. Predicting age of ovarian failure after radiation to a field that includes the ovaries. *Int J Radiat Oncol Biol Phys* 2005;62:738–744.

111. Behringer K, Mueller H, Goergen H, et al. Gonadal function and fertility in survivors after Hodgkin lymphoma treatment within the German Hodgkin Study Group HD13 to HD15 trials. *J Clin Oncol* 2013;31:231–239.

112. Meyer RM, Gospodarowicz MK, Connors JM, et al. ABVD alone versus radiation-based therapy in limited-stage Hodgkin's lymphoma. *N Engl J Med* 2012;366:399–408.

113. Advani RH, Hoppe RT, Baer D, et al. Efficacy of abbreviated Stanford V chemotherapy and involved-field radiotherapy in early-stage Hodgkin lymphoma: mature results of the G4 trial. *Ann Oncol* 2013;24:1044–1048.

114. Engert A, Plutschow A, Eich HT, et al. Reduced treatment intensity in patients with early-stage Hodgkin's lymphoma. *N Engl J Med* 2010;363:640–652.

115. Radford J, Illidge T, Barrington S. PET-directed therapy for Hodgkin's lymphoma. *N Engl J Med* 2015;373:392.

116. Andre MPE, Girinsky T, Federico M, et al. Early positron emission tomography response-adapted treatment in stage I and II Hodgkin lymphoma: final results of the randomized EORTC/LYSA/FIL H10 Trial. *J Clin Oncol* 2017;35:1786–1794.

117. Noordijk EM, Carde P, Dupouy N, et al. Combined-modality therapy for clinical stage I or II Hodgkin's lymphoma: long-term results of the European Organisation for Research and Treatment of Cancer H7 randomized controlled trials. *J Clin Oncol* 2006;24:3128–3135.

118. Eich HT, Diehl V, Gorgen H, et al. Intensified chemotherapy and dose-reduced involved-field radiotherapy in patients with early unfavorable Hodgkin's lymphoma: final analysis of the German Hodgkin Study Group HD11 trial. *J Clin Oncol* 2010;28:4199–4206.

119. Advani RH, Hong F, Fisher RI, et al. Randomized phase III trial comparing ABVD plus radiotherapy with the Stanford V regimen in patients with stages I or II locally extensive, bulky mediastinal Hodgkin lymphoma: a subset analysis of the North American Intergroup E2496 Trial. *J Clin Oncol* 2015;33:1936–1942.

120. von Tresckow B, Plutschow A, Fuchs M, et al. Dose-intensification in early unfavorable Hodgkin's lymphoma: final analysis of the German Hodgkin Study Group HD14 trial. *J Clin Oncol* 2012;30:907–913.

121. Aleman BM, Raemaekers JM, Tomisic R, et al. Involved-field radiotherapy for patients in partial remission after chemotherapy for advanced Hodgkin's lymphoma. *Int J Radiat Oncol Biol Phys* 2007;67:19–30.

122. Gordon LI, Hong F, Fisher RI, et al. Randomized phase III trial of ABVD versus Stanford V with or without radiation therapy in locally extensive and advanced-stage Hodgkin lymphoma: an intergroup study coordinated by the Eastern Cooperative Oncology Group (E2496). *J Clin Oncol* 2013;31:684–691.

123. Carde P, Karrasch M, Fortpied C, et al. Eight cycles of ABVD versus four cycles of BEACOPPescalated plus four cycles of BEACOPPbaseline in stage III to IV, International Prognostic Score >/= 3, high-risk Hodgkin lymphoma: first results of the Phase III EORTC 20012 Intergroup Trial. *J Clin Oncol* 2016;34:2028–2036.

124. Engert A, Haverkamp H, Kobe C, et al. Reduced-intensity chemotherapy and PET-guided radiotherapy in patients with advanced stage Hodgkin's lymphoma (HD15 trial): a randomised, open-label, phase 3 non-inferiority trial. *Lancet* 2012;379:1791–1799.

125. Johnson P, Federico M, Kirkwood A, et al. Adapted treatment guided by interim PET-CT scan in advanced Hodgkin's lymphoma. *N Engl J Med* 2016;374:2419–2429.

126. Press OW, Li H, Schoder H, et al. US Intergroup trial of response-adapted therapy for stage III to IV Hodgkin lymphoma using early interim fluorodeoxyglucose-positron emission tomography imaging: Southwest Oncology Group S0816. *J Clin Oncol* 2016;34:2020–2027.

127. Gallamini A, Hutchings M, Rigacci L, et al. Early interim 2-[18F]fluoro-2-deoxy-D-glucose positron emission tomography is prognostically superior to international prognostic score in advanced-stage Hodgkin's lymphoma: a report from a joint Italian-Danish study. *J Clin Oncol* 2007;25:3746–3752.

128. Simontacchi G, Filippi AR, Ciammella P, et al. Interim PET after two ABVD cycles in early-stage Hodgkin lymphoma: outcomes following the continuation of chemotherapy plus radiotherapy. *Int J Radiat Oncol Biol Phys* 2015;92:1077–1083.

129. Barnes JA, LaCasce AS, Zukotynski K, et al. End-of-treatment but not interim PET scan predicts outcome in nonbulky limited-stage Hodgkin's lymphoma. *Ann Oncol* 2011;22:910–915.

130. Sasse S, Brockelmann PJ, Goergen H, et al. Long-term follow-up of contemporary treatment in early-stage Hodgkin lymphoma: updated analyses of the German Hodgkin Study Group HD7, HD8, HD10, and HD11 Trials. *J Clin Oncol* 2017;35:1999–2007.

131. Radford J, Illidge T, Counsell N, et al. Results of a trial of PET-directed therapy for early-stage Hodgkin's lymphoma. *N Engl J Med* 2015;372:1598–1607.

132. Meyer RM, Gospodarowicz MK, Connors JM, et al. Randomized comparison of ABVD chemotherapy with a strategy that includes radiation therapy in patients with limited-stage Hodgkin's lymphoma: National Cancer Institute of Canada Clinical Trials Group and the Eastern Cooperative Oncology Group. *J Clin Oncol* 2005;23:4634–4642.

133. Darabi K, Sieber M, Chaitowitz M, et al. Infradiaphragmatic versus supradiaphragmatic Hodgkin lymphoma: a retrospective review of 1,114 patients. *Leuk Lymphoma* 2005;46:1715–1720.

134. Vassilakopoulos TP, Angelopoulou MK, Siakantaris MP, et al. Pure infradiaphragmatic Hodgkin's lymphoma. Clinical features, prognostic factor and comparison with supradiaphragmatic disease. *Haematologica* 2006;91:32–9.

135. Chen RC, Chin MS, Ng AK, et al. Early-stage, lymphocyte-predominant Hodgkin's lymphoma: patient outcomes from a large, single-institution series with long follow-up. *J Clin Oncol* 2010;28:136–141.

136. Wirth A, Yuen K, Barton M, et al. Long-term outcome after radiotherapy alone for lymphocyte-predominant Hodgkin lymphoma: a retrospective multicenter study of the Australasian Radiation Oncology Lymphoma Group. *Cancer* 2005;104:1221–1229.

137. Eichenauer DA, Plutschow A, Fuchs M, et al. Long-term course of patients with stage IA nodular lymphocyte-predominant Hodgkin lymphoma: a report from the German Hodgkin Study Group. *J Clin Oncol* 2015;33:2857–2862.

138. Advani RH, Hoppe RT. How I treat nodular lymphocyte predominant Hodgkin lymphoma. *Blood* 2013;122:4182–4188.

139. Hoppe BS, Hoppe RT. Expert radiation oncologist interpretations of involved-site radiation therapy guidelines in the management of Hodgkin lymphoma. *Int J Radiat Oncol Biol Phys* 2015;92:40–45.

140. Haas RL, Girinsky T, Aleman BM, et al. Low-dose involved-field radiotherapy as alternative treatment of nodular lymphocyte predominance Hodgkin's lymphoma. *Int J Radiat Oncol Biol Phys* 2009;74:1199–1202.

141. Wilder RB, Schlembach PJ, Jones D, et al. European Organization for Research and Treatment of Cancer and Groupe d'Etude des Lymphomes de l'Adulte very favorable and favorable, lymphocyte-predominant Hodgkin disease. *Cancer* 2002;94:1731–1738.

142. Savage KJ, Skinnider B, Al-Mansour M, et al. Treating limited-stage nodular lymphocyte predominant Hodgkin lymphoma similarly to classical Hodgkin lymphoma with ABVD may improve outcome. *Blood* 2011;118:4585–4590.

143. Canellos GP, Mauch P. What is the appropriate systemic chemotherapy for lymphocyte-predominant Hodgkin's lymphoma? *J Clin Oncol* 2010;28:e8.

144. Ferme C, Thomas J, Brice P, et al. ABVD or BEACOPPbaseline along with involved-field radiotherapy in early-stage Hodgkin Lymphoma with risk factors: Results of the European Organisation for Research and Treatment of Cancer (EORTC)-Groupe d'Etude des Lymphomes de l'Adulte (GELA) H9-U intergroup randomised trial. *Eur J Cancer* 2017;81:45–55.

145. Horning SJ, Hoppe RT, Breslin S, et al. Stanford V and radiotherapy for locally extensive and advanced Hodgkin's disease: mature results of a prospective clinical trial. *J Clin Oncol* 2002;20:630–637.

146. Diehl V, Franklin J, Pfreundschuh M, et al. Standard and increased-dose BEACOPP chemotherapy compared with COPP-ABVD for advanced Hodgkin's disease. *N Engl J Med* 2003;348:2386–2395.

147. Viviani S, Zinzani PL, Rambaldi A, et al. ABVD versus BEACOPP for Hodgkin's lymphoma when high-dose salvage is planned. *N Engl J Med* 2011;365:203–212.

148. Dhakal S, Biswas T, Liesveld JL, et al. Patterns and timing of initial relapse in patients subsequently undergoing transplantation for Hodgkin's lymphoma. *Int J Radiat Oncol Biol Phys* 2009;75:188–192.

149. Johnson PW, Sydes MR, Hancock BW, et al. Consolidation radiotherapy in patients with advanced Hodgkin's lymphoma: survival data from the UKLG LY09 randomized controlled trial (ISRCTN97144519). *J Clin Oncol* 2010;28:3352–3359.

150. Aleman BM, Raemaekers JM, Tirelli U, et al. Involved-field radiotherapy for advanced Hodgkin's lymphoma. *N Engl J Med* 2003;348:2396–2406.

151. Edwards-Bennett SM, Jacks LM, Moskowitz CH, et al. Stanford V program for locally extensive and advanced Hodgkin lymphoma: the Memorial Sloan-Kettering Cancer Center experience. *Ann Oncol* 2010;21:574–581.

152. Chisesi T, Bellei M, Luminari S, et al. Long-term follow-up analysis of HD9601 trial comparing ABVD versus Stanford V versus MOPP/EBV/CAD in patients with newly diagnosed advanced-stage Hodgkin's lymphoma: a study from the Intergruppo Italiano Linfomi. *J Clin Oncol* 2011;29:4227–4233.

153. Hoskin PJ, Lowry L, Horwich A, et al. Randomized comparison of the Stanford V regimen and ABVD in the treatment of advanced Hodgkin's lymphoma: United Kingdom National Cancer Research Institute Lymphoma Group Study ISRCTN 64141244. *J Clin Oncol* 2009;27:5390–5396.

154. Hudson MM, Krasin M, Link MP, et al. Risk-adapted, combined-modality therapy with VAMP/COP and response-based, involved-field radiation for unfavorable pediatric Hodgkin's disease. *J Clin Oncol* 2004;22:4541–4550.

155. Donaldson SS, Hudson MM, Lamborn KR, et al. VAMP and low-dose, involved-field radiation for children and adolescents with favorable, early-stage Hodgkin's disease: results of a prospective clinical trial. *J Clin Oncol* 2002;20:3081–3087.

156. Nachman JB, Sposto R, Herzog P, et al. Randomized comparison of low-dose involved-field radiotherapy and no radiotherapy for children with Hodgkin's disease who achieve a complete response to chemotherapy. *J Clin Oncol* 2002;20:3765–3771.

157. Ruhl U, Albrecht M, Dieckmann K, et al. Response-adapted radiotherapy in the treatment of pediatric Hodgkin's disease: an interim report at 5 years of the German GPOH-HD 95 trial. *Int J Radiat Oncol Biol Phys* 2001;51:1209–1218.

158. Mauz-Korholz C, Gorde-Grosjean S, Hasenclever D, et al. Resection alone in 58 children with limited stage, lymphocyte-predominant Hodgkin lymphoma-experience from the European network group on pediatric Hodgkin lymphoma. *Cancer* 2007;110:179–185.

159. Evens AM, Hong F, Gordon LI, et al. The efficacy and tolerability of Adriamycin, bleomycin, vinblastine, dacarbazine and Stanford V in older Hodgkin lymphoma patients: a comprehensive analysis from the North American intergroup trial E2496. *Br J Haematol* 2013;161:76–86.

160. Austin-Seymour MM, Hoppe RT, Cox RS, et al. Hodgkin's disease in patients over sixty years old. *Ann Intern Med* 1984;100:13–8.

161. Diaz-Pavon JR, Cabanillas F, Majlis A, et al. Outcome of Hodgkin's disease in elderly patients. *Hematol Oncol* 1995;13:19–27.

162. Engert A, Ballova V, Haverkamp H, et al. Hodgkin's lymphoma in elderly patients: a comprehensive retrospective analysis from the German Hodgkin's Study Group. *J Clin Oncol* 2005;23:5052–5060.

163. Wongso D, Fuchs M, Plutschow A, et al. Treatment-related mortality in patients with advanced-stage Hodgkin lymphoma: an analysis of the German Hodgkin Study Group. *J Clin Oncol* 2013;31:2819–2824.

164. Selby P, Patel P, Milan S, et al. ChlVPP combination chemotherapy for Hodgkin's disease: long-term results. *Br J Cancer* 1990;62:279–285.

165. Horning SJ, Ang PT, Hoppe RT, et al. The Stanford experience with combined procarbazine, Alkeran and vinblastine (PAVe) and radiotherapy for locally extensive and advanced stage Hodgkin's disease. *Ann Oncol* 1992;3:747–754.

166. Zinzani PL, Magagnoli M, Bendandi M, et al. Efficacy of the VBM regimen in the treatment of elderly patients with Hodgkin's disease. *Haematologica* 2000;85:729–732.

167. Klimm B, Eich HT, Haverkamp H, et al. Poorer outcome of elderly patients treated with extended-field radiotherapy compared with involved-field radiotherapy after chemotherapy for Hodgkin's lymphoma: an analysis from the German Hodgkin Study Group. *Ann Oncol* 2007;18:357–363.

168. von Tresckow B, Moskowitz CH. Treatment of relapsed and refractory Hodgkin lymphoma. *Semin Hematol* 2016;53:180–185.

169. Linch DC, Winfield D, Goldstone AH, et al. Dose intensification with autologous bone-marrow transplantation in relapsed and resistant Hodgkin's disease: results of a BNLI randomised trial. *Lancet* 1993;341:1051–1054.

170. Sureda A, Robinson S, Canals C, et al. Reduced-intensity conditioning compared with conventional allogeneic stem-cell transplantation in relapsed or refractory Hodgkin's lymphoma: an analysis from the Lymphoma Working Party of the European Group for Blood and Marrow Transplantation. *J Clin Oncol* 2008;26:455–462.

171. Shahidi M, Kamangari N, Ashley S, et al. Site of relapse after chemotherapy alone for stage I and II Hodgkin's disease. *Radiother Oncol* 2006;78:1–5.

172. Tsang RW, Gospodarowicz MK, Sutcliffe SB, et al. Thoracic radiation therapy before autologous bone marrow transplantation in relapsed or refractory Hodgkin's disease. PMH Lymphoma Group, and the Toronto Autologous BMT Group. *Eur J Cancer* 1999;35:73–8.

173. Ferme C, Mounier N, Divine M, et al. Intensive salvage therapy with high-dose chemotherapy for patients with advanced Hodgkin's disease in relapse or failure after initial chemotherapy: results of the Groupe d'Etudes des Lymphomes de l'Adulte H89 trial. *J Clin Oncol* 2002;20:467–475.

174. Poen JC, Hoppe RT, Horning SJ. High-dose therapy and autologous bone marrow transplantation for relapsed/refractory Hodgkin's disease: the impact of involved field radiotherapy on patterns of failure and survival. *Int J Radiat Oncol Biol Phys* 1996;36:3–12.

175. Lancet JE, Rapoport AP, Brasacchio R, et al. Autotransplantation for relapsed or refractory Hodgkin's disease: long-term follow-up and analysis of prognostic factors. *Bone Marrow Transplant* 1998;22:265–271.

176. Kahn S, Flowers C, Xu Z, et al. Does the addition of involved field radiotherapy to high-dose chemotherapy and stem cell transplantation improve outcomes for patients with relapsed/refractory Hodgkin lymphoma? *Int J Radiat Oncol Biol Phys* 2011;81:175–180.

177. Weihrauch MR, Re D, Scheidhauer K, et al. Thoracic positron emission tomography using 18F-fluorodeoxyglucose for the evaluation of residual mediastinal Hodgkin disease. *Blood* 2001;98:2930–2934.

178. Dryver ET, Jernstrom H, Tompkins K, et al. Follow-up of patients with Hodgkin's disease following curative treatment: the routine CT scan is of little value. *Br J Cancer* 2003;89:482–486.

179. Torrey MJ, Poen JC, Hoppe RT. Detection of relapse in early-stage Hodgkin's disease: role of routine follow-up studies. *J Clin Oncol* 1997;15:1123–1130.

180. Thompson CA, Charlson ME, Schenkein E, et al. Surveillance CT scans are a source of anxiety and fear of recurrence in long-term lymphoma survivors. *Ann Oncol* 2010;21:2262–2266.

181. Guadagnolo BA, Punglia RS, Kuntz KM, et al. Cost-effectiveness analysis of computerized tomography in the routine follow-up of patients after primary treatment for Hodgkin's disease. *J Clin Oncol* 2006;24:4116–4122.

182. Bestawros A, Foltz L, Srour N, et al. Patients' and physicians' roles in detecting recurrent Hodgkin lymphoma following complete remission. *Ann Oncol* 2013;24:1359–1363.

183. Pingali SR, Jewell SW, Havlat L, et al. Limited utility of routine surveillance imaging for classical Hodgkin lymphoma patients in first complete remission. *Cancer* 2014;120:2122–2129.

184. Dann EJ, Berkahn L, Mashiach T, et al. Hodgkin lymphoma patients in first remission: routine positron emission tomography/computerized tomography imaging is not superior to clinical follow-up for patients with no residual mass. *Br J Haematol* 2014;164:694–700.

185. Lee AI, Zuckerman DS, Van den Abbeele AD, et al. Surveillance imaging of Hodgkin lymphoma patients in first remission: a clinical and economic analysis. *Cancer* 2010;116:3835–3842.

186. El-Galaly TC, Mylam KJ, Brown P, et al. Positron emission tomography/computed tomography surveillance in patients with Hodgkin lymphoma in first remission has a low positive predictive value and high costs. *Haematologica* 2012;97:931–936.

187. Hancock SL, Cox RS, McDougall IR. Thyroid diseases after treatment of Hodgkin's disease. *N Engl J Med* 1991;325:599–605.

188. Fogelfeld L, Wiviott MB, Shore-Freedman E, et al. Recurrence of thyroid nodules after surgical removal in patients irradiated in childhood for benign conditions. *N Engl J Med* 1989;320:835–840.

189. Guinee VF, Guido JJ, Pfalzgraf KA, et al. The incidence of herpes zoster in patients with Hodgkin's disease. An analysis of prognostic factors. *Cancer* 1985;56:642–648.

190. Dailey MO, Coleman CN, Kaplan HS. Radiation-induced splenic atrophy in patients with Hodgkin's disease and non-Hodgkin's lymphomas. *N Engl J Med* 1980;302:215–217.

191. Donaldson SS, Moore MR, Rosenberg SA, et al. Characterization of postsplenectomy bacteremia among patients with and without lymphoma. *N Engl J Med* 1972;287:69–71.

192. Molrine DC, George S, Tarbell N, et al. Antibody responses to polysaccharide and polysaccharide-conjugate vaccines after treatment of Hodgkin disease. *Ann Intern Med* 1995;123:828–834.

193. Pedrick TJ, Hoppe RT. Recovery of spermatogenesis following pelvic irradiation for Hodgkin's disease. *Int J Radiat Oncol Biol Phys* 1986;12:117–121.

194. Viviani S, Santoro A, Ragni G, et al. Gonadal toxicity after combination chemotherapy for Hodgkin's disease. Comparative results of MOPP vs ABVD. *Eur J Cancer Clin Oncol* 1985;21:601–605.

195. Horning SJ, Hoppe RT, Hancock SL, et al. Vinblastine, bleomycin, and methotrexate: an effective adjuvant in favorable Hodgkin's disease. *J Clin Oncol* 1988;6:1822–1831.

196. Horning SJ, Hoppe RT, Kaplan HS, et al. Female reproductive potential after treatment for Hodgkin's disease. *N Engl J Med* 1981;304:1377–1382.

197. van Leeuwen-Segarceanu EM, Dorresteijn LD, Pillen S, et al. Progressive muscle atrophy and weakness after treatment by mantle field radiotherapy in Hodgkin lymphoma survivors. *Int J Radiat Oncol Biol Phys* 2012;82:612–618.

198. Gerling MC, Bohlman HH. Dropped head deformity due to cervical myopathy: surgical treatment outcomes and complications spanning twenty years. *Spine (Phila Pa 1976)* 2008;33:E739–E745.

199. Favier O, Heutte N, Stamatoullas-Bastard A, et al. Survival after Hodgkin lymphoma: causes of death and excess mortality in patients treated in 8 consecutive trials. *Cancer* 2009;115:1680–1691.

200. Chow LM, Nathan PC, Hodgson DC, et al. Survival and late effects in children with Hodgkin's lymphoma treated with MOPP/ABV and low-dose, extended-field irradiation. *J Clin Oncol* 2006;24:5735–5741.

201. Greenfield DM, Wright J, Brown JE, et al. High incidence of late effects found in Hodgkin's lymphoma survivors, following recall for breast cancer screening. *Br J Cancer* 2006;94:469–472.

202. Hoppe RT. Hodgkin's disease: complications of therapy and excess mortality. *Ann Oncol* 1997;8(Suppl 1):115–118.

203. Schneider U, Lomax A, Lombriser N. Comparative risk assessment of secondary cancer incidence after treatment of Hodgkin's disease with photon and proton radiation. *Radiat Res* 2000;154:382–388.

204. De Bruin ML, Sparidans J, van't Veer MB, et al. Breast cancer risk in female survivors of Hodgkin's lymphoma: lower risk after smaller radiation volumes. *J Clin Oncol* 2009;27:4239–4246.

205. Hodgson DC, Koh ES, Tran TH, et al. Individualized estimates of second cancer risks after contemporary radiation therapy for Hodgkin lymphoma. *Cancer* 2007;110:2576–2586.

206. Travis LB, Gilbert E. Lung cancer after Hodgkin lymphoma: the roles of chemotherapy, radiotherapy and tobacco use. *Radiat Res* 2005;163:695–696.

207. Myrehaug S, Pintilie M, Tsang R, et al. Cardiac morbidity following modern treatment for Hodgkin lymphoma: supra-additive cardiotoxicity of doxorubicin and radiation therapy. *Leuk Lymphoma* 2008;49:1486–1493.

208. Heidenreich PA, Schnittger I, Strauss HW, et al. Screening for coronary artery disease after mediastinal irradiation for Hodgkin's disease. *J Clin Oncol* 2007;25:43–49.

209. Chen AB, Punglia RS, Kuntz KM, et al. Cost effectiveness and screening interval of lipid screening in Hodgkin's lymphoma survivors. *J Clin Oncol* 2009;27:5383–5389.

210. Fobair P, Hoppe RT, Bloom J, et al. Psychosocial problems among survivors of Hodgkin's disease. *J Clin Oncol* 1986;4:805–814.

211. Hjermstad MJ, Fossa SD, Oldervoll L, et al. Fatigue in long-term Hodgkin's disease survivors: a follow-up study. *J Clin Oncol* 2005;23:6587–6595.

212. Ng AK, Li S, Recklitis C, et al. A comparison between long-term survivors of Hodgkin's disease and their siblings on fatigue level and factors predicting for increased fatigue. *Ann Oncol* 2005;16:1949–1955.

213. Kumar A, Casulo C, Yahalom J, et al. Brentuximab vedotin and AVD followed by involved-site radiotherapy in early stage, unfavorable risk Hodgkin lymphoma. *Blood* 2016;128:1458–1464.

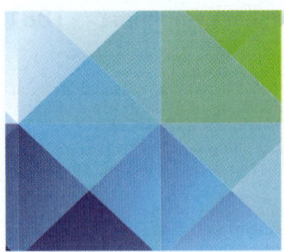

CHAPTER 82

Non-Hodgkin Lymphomas

Chris R. Kelsey, Jeremy M. Brownstein, Grace J. Kim, and Leonard R. Prosnitz

Non-Hodgkin lymphomas (NHLs) are a heterogeneous group of malignancies of the lymphoid system characterized by an abnormal clonal proliferation of B cells, T cells, or NK (natural killer) cells. Scientific knowledge regarding NHL has increased dramatically in the last several decades, resulting in significant advances in the spheres of molecular biology and immunobiology leading to new histopathologic classifications and therapies. Chemotherapy, immunotherapy, and radiation therapy (RT) all play important roles in the management of NHL.

There are currently approximately 70 distinct NHL entities within the 2016 WHO classification. A description of all the varieties of NHL is not practical and beyond the scope of this chapter. We focus on the most common entities including diffuse large B-cell lymphoma (DLBCL), follicular lymphoma (FL), marginal zone lymphoma (MZL), mantle cell lymphoma (MCL), primary central nervous system lymphoma (PCNSL), and peripheral T-cell lymphomas (PTCLs) including extranodal NK/T-cell lymphoma, nasal type. Other entities less frequently encountered by radiation oncologists are also briefly discussed.

EPIDEMIOLOGY

The US age-adjusted incidence rate for NHL was 19.5 per 100,000 between 2009 and 2013, according to the Surveillance, Epidemiology, and End Results (SEER) Program of the National Cancer Institute. In 2017, the projected number of new NHL cases in the United States is 72,240 comprising 4.3% of new cancer diagnoses; deaths from NHL are projected at 20,140. NHL is primarily a disease of older populations with a median age of 65 at diagnosis.[1] In 2012, worldwide estimated incidence was 386,000 new cases and 200,000 deaths.[2] International NHL incidence rates vary, with the highest incidence rates in North America, Europe, and Australia/New Zealand. The lowest rates have been reported in Asia, Central America, the Caribbean, and West Africa.[3]

Between 1975 and 2000, there was a striking increase in new cases of NHL with incidence rates nearly doubling. New cases peaked at 21.3/100,000 in 2010 and have since subtly decreased to 20/100,000 in 2014.[1] The US mortality rate rose from 5.6/100,000 to 8.2/100,000 between 1975 and 2000. Since a peak of 8.9/100,000 in 1997, the mortality rate has steadily declined with most recent SEER data reporting 5.7/100,000 deaths in 2014.[1]

The increased incidence of NHL in the late 20th century has been attributed to several factors including advances in molecular diagnostic techniques, aging of the population, immunosuppression from human immunodeficiency virus (HIV), infectious agents, and occupational/environmental exposures.[4] There are likely other contributing factors, which remain unknown at present.

ETIOLOGY

Several genetic diseases, environmental exposures, and infectious agents have been associated with the development of lymphoma. Additionally, a family history of hematologic malignancy appears to be an important risk factor for lymphoma. Specifically, a family history of leukemia is associated with development of PTCL, chronic lymphocytic leukemia/small lymphocytic lymphoma (CLL/SLL), and MCL. A family history of NHL is associated with an increased risk of all forms of NHL.

Immune Disorders

The frequency of NHL is greatly increased in immunocompromised patients. The two most common clinical circumstances are among HIV-infected patients and solid organ transplant recipients, both associated with prolonged immunosuppression.[5,6] Between 1996 and 2009, the cumulative incidence of NHL among those infected with HIV was 4.5%—the highest of any malignancy.[7] Among those who died from NHL between 2005 and 2012, 4.2% were infected with HIV. Burkitt lymphoma (BL), DLBCL, and PCNSL are the most frequent lymphomas among those infected with HIV and are considered AIDS-defining illnesses.[8] The introduction of highly active antiretroviral therapy (HAART) has resulted in the decline in NHL incidence and mortality among those infected with HIV. This trend is seen in most HIV-associated NHL subtypes apart from BL whose incidence has subtly increased since the advent of HAART. This may be explained by BL's unique pathogenesis, which is dependent on an intact immune system capable of producing germinal centers.[9]

Immunosuppression caused by organ transplantation and end-stage renal disease is also associated with increased risk of NHL. A large registry study in Sweden found that solid organ transplant recipients and dialysis patients had an incidence of NHL 7.9 and 5.1 times that of the general population, respectively.[10] Additionally, those with rare inherited immunodeficiency disorders such as X-linked lymphoproliferative syndrome, common variable immunodeficiency, Wiskott-Aldrich syndrome, and ataxia telangiectasia experience up to a 7% lifetime risk for development of NHL.[11]

NHL is more common among those with certain autoimmune diseases. Sjögren disease is strongly associated with increased incidence of MZL.[12] Sjögren disease is also associated with DLBCL, as are other B-cell–activating autoimmune diseases such as autoimmune hemolytic anemia, systemic lupus erythematosus, and rheumatoid arthritis.[13–15] Unsurprisingly, T-cell–activating autoimmune disorders such as celiac disease are associated with T-cell lymphomas, as are chronic skin diseases such as psoriasis, bullous pemphigoid, and atopic dermatitis.[14,16]

Infectious Agents

Epstein-Barr virus (EBV), a member of the herpes family, has been implicated in the pathogenesis of several lymphomas. The EBV viral genome can be found within tumor cells of nearly every endemic BL case, 40% of HIV-associated BL and 10% to 15% of sporadic BL.[17,18] Given that the distribution of BL in equatorial Africa closely overlaps that of holoendemic malaria, many have suspected that *Plasmodium falciparum* infection may also play a role in the development of BL.[19,20] The molecular basis for this link remained elusive until evidence recently emerged suggesting *P. falciparum* may work synergistically with EBV to increase the likelihood of malignant transformation within germinal centers.[21–23] EBV infection is also implicated in the development of DLBCL, PCNSL, plasmablastic lymphoma, primary effusion lymphoma, and NK/T-cell lymphoma, nasal type.[24]

The human T-cell lymphotropic virus type 1 (HTLV-1) is an RNA virus that is endemic in Japan, the Caribbean, intertropical Africa, South America, and Papua New Guinea.[25] Infection with HTLV-1 conveys a 5% lifetime risk of developing adult T-cell leukemia/lymphoma, though the risk is substantially lower for those infected after adolescence.[26] Human herpes virus 8 (HHV-8), the causative agent of Kaposi sarcoma, is associated with several rare lymphoproliferative diseases, including primary effusion lymphoma, which can occur in immunosuppressed individuals with or without HIV infection.[27]

Hepatitis C virus (HCV) is the leading cause of both chronic hepatitis and hepatocellular carcinoma worldwide.[28] A large analysis of seven case–control studies through the InterLymph Consortium indicates that HCV infection is associated with a two- to threefold increased incidence of DLBCL, lymphoplasmacytic lymphoma, and MZL.[29]

MZL is peculiar among the NHLs in its association with localized bacterial infections. Specifically, there is a strong causal link between infection with *Helicobacter pylori* (*H. pylori*) and the development of gastric MALT lymphoma (mucosa-associated lymphoma tissue). Infection with this organism is found in over 90% of patients with gastric MALT.[30] Moreover, successful eradication of *H. pylori* with antibiotic therapy in localized gastric MALT results in complete remission in 62% of patients.[31]

The role of other bacterial infections in nongastric MALT is controversial.[32] Several studies document a strong association between *Chlamydia psittaci* (*C. psittaci*) and ocular adnexal MALT. In a series of 40 patients from Northern Italy, *C. psittaci* DNA was found in 80% of cases, compared with 0% found in nonneoplastic orbital biopsies.[33] However, another series including 142 patients from Europe, Asia, and North America found *C. psittaci* in only 22% of cases. Although this differed significantly from the prevalence of *C. psittaci* in nonneoplastic biopsies and non-MALT lymphoma biopsies (10% and 9%, respectively), there was marked geographic heterogeneity, suggesting that the association may be variable and dependent on other factors such as the prevalence of infection within the region's population.[34] *Borrelia burgdorferi* and *Campylobacter jejuni* have been linked to cutaneous MZL and immunoproliferative small intestine disease/MZL of the small bowel, respectively. However, the data supporting these associations are based on anecdotal reports and small case series.[35] *There remains no clear role for the use of antibiotics in the treatment of nongastric MZL.*

Environmental and Occupational Exposures

Many occupations have been associated with a higher risk of developing NHL. A recent pooled analysis from the InterLymph Consortium demonstrated an increased incidence of NHL in farmworkers (OR 1.19; 95% CI [1.01 to 1.36]), women's hairdressers (OR 1.34; [1.02 to 1.75]), charworkers/cleaners (OR 1.17; [1.01 to 1.36]), spray painters (OR 2.07; [1.30 to 3.29]), electrical wiremen (OR 1.24; [1.00 to 1.54]), and carpenters (OR 1.42; [1.04 to 1.93]).[36] Several other studies have documented an increased incidence of NHL among teachers,[37–39] though this association was not borne out in the aforementioned InterLymph Consortium analyses.[16,36] Exposure to solvents such as benzene, toluene, xylene, and styrene are linked to development of FL.[40] Exposure to individual pesticides has been extensively studied with conflicting results.[41]

The connection between cigarette smoking and lymphoma is controversial. A large meta-analysis found a subtle association between cigarette smoking and development of NHL (OR 1.05; [1.00 to 1.09]).[42] A second large meta-analysis found an association only among female smokers (OR 1.40; [1.14 to 1.73]),[43] although several large studies detected no association.[16,44,45]

The data concerning UV radiation are conflicting as well with some studies suggesting a positive association between increased sun exposure with NHL,[46–48] whereas other studies suggest that sunlight may be protective.[49] Ionizing radiation exposure is associated with development of leukemia and many solid tumors. However, the link to the development of NHL is tenuous. Large analyses of atomic bomb survivors, radiologic technologist, and those who have received therapeutic radiation have not detected any association with NHL.[50–52] Conversely, a large Dutch study evaluating 3,905 survivors of Hodgkin lymphoma (HL) treated between 1965 and 2000 found a significantly increased risk of developing NHL among those who underwent mantle field/supradiaphragmatic RT compared to those who received no radiation treatment, though the absolute excess risk was small.[53]

PATHOLOGY

NHL comprises numerous disease entities, often difficult to diagnosis, with a correspondingly complex histopathologic classification that has changed relatively frequently over the years. The predecessor to the currently utilized World Health Organization (WHO) classification was the Working Formulation.[54] It subdivided NHL into low-grade, intermediate-grade, high-grade, and miscellaneous entities. Such groupings were convenient and appeared clinically useful, but represented an oversimplification and did not account for several distinct clinical–pathologic entities.

The WHO 2008 classification divided NHL into B-cell, T-cell, and NK cell neoplasms.[55] Substantive revisions were published in 2016 (Table 82.1).[56] These specific entities are distinguished on the basis of reproducibly identifiable morphologic, immunologic, and genetic characteristics. Combining pathologic findings with clinical presentation is required to distinguish some entities (e.g., CD30+ lymphoproliferative disorders). The specific diseases described may be either indolent or aggressive in behavior. Within a given disease, there may be a range of behaviors (e.g., anaplastic large-cell lymphoma [ALCL]). Similarly, the histologic grade and the biologic behavior may vary within a specific disease entity (e.g., FL). The WHO classification describes new disease categories not clearly recognized in the Working Formulation, notably MZL, MCL, PTCLs, ALCL, and primary mediastinal large B-cell lymphoma.

It must be emphasized that lymphoma pathology is complex with a long history of interobserver disagreement. The National Comprehensive Cancer Network (NCCN) guidelines describe as "essential" specialized hematopathology review of all slides and adequate immunophenotyping to establish the diagnosis.[57] Fine needle aspiration alone is rarely acceptable for the initial diagnosis of lymphoma because of lack of nodal architecture.[58] Specific pathologic features for each lymphoma subtype will be discussed under the relevant disease sections.

TABLE 82.1 2016 WHO CLASSIFICATION OF MATURE LYMPHOID NEOPLASMS[a]
Mature B-cell Neoplasms
Chronic lymphocytic leukemia/small lymphocytic lymphoma
Monoclonal B-cell lymphocytosis
B-cell prolymphocytic leukemia
Splenic marginal zone lymphoma
Hairy cell leukemia
Splenic B-cell lymphoma/leukemia, unclassifiable
Splenic diffuse red pulp small B-cell lymphoma
Hairy cell leukemia variant
Lymphoplasmacytic lymphoma
Waldenstrom macroglobulinemia
Monoclonal gammopathy of undetermined significance (MGUS), IgM
μ Heavy chain disease

(Continued)

Section III

TABLE 82.1 2016 WHO CLASSIFICATION OF MATURE LYMPHOID NEOPLASMS*ᵃ* (Continued)

γ Heavy chain disease
α Heavy chain disease
Monoclonal gammopathy of undetermined significance (MGUS), IgG/A
Plasma cell myeloma
Solitary plasmacytoma of bone
Extraosseous plasmacytoma
Monoclonal immunoglobulin deposition diseases
Extranodal marginal zone lymphoma of mucosa-associated lymphoid tissue (MALT lymphoma)
Nodal marginal zone lymphoma
    Pediatric nodal marginal zone lymphoma
Follicular lymphoma
    In situ follicular neoplasia
    Duodenal-type follicular lymphoma
Large B-cell lymphoma with IRF4 rearrangement
Primary cutaneous follicle center lymphoma
Mantle cell lymphoma
    In situ mantle cell neoplasia
Diffuse large B-cell lymphoma (DLBCL), NOS
    Germinal center B-cell type
    Activated B-cell type
T-cell/histiocyte-rich large B-cell lymphoma
Primary DLBCL of the central nervous system (CNS)
Primary cutaneous DLBCL, leg type
EBV+ DLBCL, NOS
EBV+ mucocutaneous ulcer
DLBCL associated with chronic inflammation
Lymphomatoid granulomatosis
Primary mediastinal (thymic) large B-cell lymphoma
Intravascular large B-cell lymphoma
ALK+ large B-cell lymphoma
Plasmablastic lymphoma
Primary effusion lymphoma
HHV8+ DLBCL, NOS
Burkitt lymphoma
Burkitt-like lymphoma with 11q aberration
High-grade B-cell lymphoma, with MYC and BCL2 and/or BCL6 rearrangements
High-grade B-cell lymphoma, NOS
B-cell lymphoma, unclassifiable, with features intermediate between DLBCL and classical Hodgkin lymphoma

Mature T and NK Neoplasms
T-cell prolymphocytic leukemia
T-cell large granular lymphocytic leukemia
Chronic lymphoproliferative disorder of NK cells
Aggressive NK-cell leukemia
Systemic EBV+ T-cell lymphoma of childhood
Hydroa vacciniformelike lymphoproliferative disorder
Adult T-cell lymphoma/leukemia
Extranodal NK/T-cell lymphoma, nasal type
Enteropathy-associated T-cell lymphoma
Monomorphic epitheliotropic intestinal T-cell lymphoma
Indolent T-cell lymphoproliferative disorder of the GI tract
Hepatosplenic T-cell lymphoma
Subcutaneous panniculitislike T-cell lymphoma
Mycosis fungoides
Sezary syndrome
Primary cutaneous CD30+ T-cell lymphoproliferative disorders
    Lymphomatoid papulosis
    Primary cutaneous anaplastic large-cell lymphoma
Primary cutaneous γδ T-cell lymphoma
Primary cutaneous CD8+ aggressive epidermotropic cytotoxic T-cell lymphoma
Primary cutaneous acral CD8+ T-cell lymphoma
Primary cutaneous CD4-positive small/medium T-cell lymphoproliferative disorder
Peripheral T-cell lymphoma, NOS
Angioimmunoblastic T-cell lymphoma
Follicular T-cell lymphoma
Nodal peripheral T-cell lymphoma with TFH phenotype
Anaplastic large-cell lymphoma, ALK+
Anaplastic large-cell lymphoma, ALK−
Breast implant–associated anaplastic large-cell lymphoma

ᵃExcludes Hodgkin lymphoma, posttransplant lymphoproliferative disorders, and histiocytic/dendritic cell neoplasms.
Republished with permission of American Society of Hematology from Swerdlow SH, Campo E, Pileri SA, et al. The 2016 revision of the World Health Organization classification of lymphoid neoplasms. Blood 2016;127(20):2375–2390; permission conveyed through Copyright Clearance Center, Inc.[36]

CLINICAL FEATURES AND EVALUATION

Clinical Presentation

NHL is predominantly a disease of older adults, in contrast to HL, with a median age at presentation of approximately 65 years.[1] There is a slight male preponderance (55% to 60% male). NHL may involve lymph nodes in almost any area of the body but may also present at extranodal sites, in contrast to HL in which extranodal presentation is rare.

The clinical features differ somewhat depending on the histology. For patients with primarily nodal disease, presentation is typically an asymptomatic lump in the neck or inguinal–femoral regions. Axillary involvement is somewhat less common. Patients with FL frequently give a history of waxing and waning of lymph nodes, sometimes over several years. Although patients with nodal presentations may initially appear to have localized disease, subsequent staging evaluation usually results in assignment to a more advanced stage, particularly in patients with FL. Most nodal presentations of NHL are asymptomatic. B symptoms including unexplained fevers, drenching night sweats, and >10% weight loss are much less frequently encountered than in HL, are not prognostic, and usually do not influence choice of treatment.

Patients with extranodal presentations are likely to have symptoms related to the organ in question (e.g., the stomach or head and neck sites). Extranodal involvement is common in DLBCL, occurring in approximately 50% of patients with early-stage disease[59] and approximately 70% of all patients.[60] With the exception of bone marrow involvement, extranodal disease is relatively rare with FL. Extranodal presentation is the rule for MZL. Considering patients with DLBCL, primary extranodal disease, stage for stage, is managed in the same fashion as primary nodal disease and has a virtually identical outcome. There are a few notable exceptions such as primary CNS lymphoma and testicular DLBCL; the latter has a special tendency to spread to the contralateral testis and CNS.[61]

Initial diagnosis of lymphoma is made on appropriate histologic tissue preferably by an experienced hematopathologist and is dependent on morphology, immunohistochemistry, flow cytometry, and, in some instances, appropriate molecular studies. As stated, a fine needle aspirate rarely provides sufficient tissue for diagnosis of a new lymphoma.[58] An incisional or excisional biopsy is ideal; sometimes, a core needle biopsy is sufficient.

Evaluation and Staging

It is important to define the extent of disease at presentation to allow for appropriate therapeutic decisions (Table 82.2). One begins with a careful history and physical examination, a truism but often neglected in the age of extensive and readily

TABLE 82.2 CLINICAL, LABORATORY, AND RADIOLOGIC EVALUATION OF PATIENTS WITH NHLᵃ

History and physical examination including performance status
Incisional/excisional biopsy with appropriate hematopathology review
Blood studies
    Complete blood count
    Comprehensive metabolic panel
    Lactate dehydrogenase
    Pregnancy test in women of child-bearing age
    Hepatitis serologies and HIV testing (as indicated)
Imaging evaluation
    Positron emission tomography/computed tomography with contrast (preferred)
    Computed tomography scan of the chest, abdomen, pelvis with contrast (head and neck as indicated)
Bone marrow aspirate and biopsy (as indicated)

HIV, human immunodeficiency virus.
ᵃAdditional tests may be necessary based on underlying histology and presentation.

available imaging. The history should record the presence or absence of B symptoms, performance status, growth history of any lymph node enlargement, and any specific symptoms suggestive of extranodal disease. All peripheral nodal areas including the epitrochlear nodes and Waldeyer ring should be examined clinically and enlarged nodes measured with readily available inexpensive calipers and the largest diameter of any enlarged nodes recorded.

Laboratory procedures include complete blood count, metabolic panel, LDH, $\beta2$ microglobulin, and hepatitis B and HIV antibodies in selected patients.

In the United States and much of the developed world, PET-CT is now the imaging procedure of choice for FDG-avid lymphomas, which comprise the great majority of NHLs. The CT aspect of the PET-CT examination should be performed with contrast in a similar fashion to a regular diagnostic CT scan. If PET-CT is not available, routine CT examination will suffice. A regular chest x-ray is no longer recommended because of the greater accuracy and sensitivity of CT.[62]

Routine bone marrow biopsy has been standard in lymphoma evaluation for many years, but the high sensitivity of PET-CT for bone marrow involvement in DLBCL is calling this practice into question for that entity.[62] If a PET-CT indicates marrow involvement in DLBCL, a confirmatory bone marrow biopsy is not recommended. There are considerably less data, however, for other histologies, particularly FL where bone marrow biopsy remains standard of practice and is particularly important in patients with ostensible stage I or II disease who are candidates for curative radiotherapy.

In the past, staging systems for lymphoma were primarily the Ann Arbor system and the Cotswolds modification, but they have been superseded by the Lugano classification (Table 82.3). For NHL, A and B subtypes have been dropped because of the infrequency of systemic symptomatology, the unclear influence on prognosis, and the usual lack of relevance for management decisions. Tumor bulk is no longer a part of the staging system because of the lack of consensus as to what constitutes bulky disease as well as the uncertain influence of bulk on prognosis in the current therapeutic era. The Lugano recommendation is simply to record the largest diameter of a given nodal site.[62]

Response Assessment

Response assessment should include clinical evaluation with repeat history and physical examination and appropriate imaging studies. If available, PET-CT is the most accurate imaging modality for response assessment as well as

TABLE 82.3 REVISED STAGING SYSTEM—THE LUGANO CLASSIFICATION

Stage	Involvement	Extranodal (E) Status[a]
Limited		
I	One node or a group of adjacent nodes	Single extranodal lesion without nodal involvement
II	Two or more nodal groups on the same side of the diaphragm	Stage I/II by nodal extent with limited contiguous extranodal involvement
II bulky	II as above with "bulky" disease[b]	N/A
Advanced		
III	Nodes on both sides of the diaphragm; nodes above the diaphragm with spleen involvement	N/A
IV	Additional noncontiguous extralymphatic involvement	N/A

[a]Tonsils, Waldeyer ring, and spleen are considered nodal tissue.
[b]Definition of bulky disease in DLBCL not validated but 6 to 10 cm generally accepted.
Adapted with permission from Cheson BD, Fisher RI, Barrington SF, et al. Recommendations for initial evaluation, staging, and response assessment of Hodgkin and non-Hodgkin lymphoma: the Lugano classification. *J Clin Oncol* 2014;32(27):3059–3068. Copyright © 2014 American Society of Clinical Oncology. All rights reserved.

TABLE 82.4 DEAUVILLE CRITERIA (PET-CT 5-POINT SCALE)

Score	Definition
Deauville 1	No uptake above background
Deauville 2	Uptake ≤ mediastinal blood pool
Deauville 3	Uptake > mediastinal blood pool but ≤ liver
Deauville 4	Uptake moderately increased compared to the liver
Deauville 5	Uptake markedly increased compared to the liver or new sites of disease

Adapted by permission from Springer: Barrington SF, Qian W, Somer EJ, et al. Concordance between four European centres of PET reporting criteria designed for use in multicentre trials in Hodgkin lymphoma. *Eur J Nucl Med Mol Imaging* 2010;37(10):1824–1833. Copyright © 2010 Springer-Verlag.

the initial evaluation. Use of PET-CT eliminates the need for the category CRu (complete response uncertain), a situation observed with static CT imaging in which tumor masses were observed to have decreased in size but had not completely disappeared, raising the question of whether viable tumor remained. End-of-treatment assessment is probably most accurate and most meaningful.

Responses may be divided into complete, partial, no response or stable disease, and progressive disease. Detailed descriptions of response criteria were described at the Lugano meeting.[62] A complete metabolic response is defined as absence of all palpable disease, and a PET score of 1, 2, or 3 utilizing the 5-point scale or Deauville criteria, with or without a residual mass on static CT imaging (Table 82.4). A partial metabolic response is defined as a score of 4 or 5 but with reduced uptake compared with original scans. Similarly, on CT imaging, a partial remission indicates >50% decrease in measurable disease. No response or stable disease suggests no change in lesion size on static imaging and no significant change in FDG uptake. Progressive disease is a worsening of these findings.

The term partial response can be somewhat misleading. A Deauville score of 4 or 5 at the completion of therapy strongly suggests treatment failure even if uptake has been reduced from baseline. It is often advisable, however, to confirm the presence of active disease histologically with biopsy in patients with a partial metabolic response if major therapeutic changes are contemplated (e.g., stem cell transplantation). The use of radiotherapy in the circumstance of partial metabolic response is discussed in the individual disease sections.

Imaging response assessment is also frequently carried out midway through the course of therapy, so-called interim PET imaging. Many studies of interim PET-CT have been carried out, particularly in DLBCL, suggesting that an interim positive PET-CT (Deauville 4 or 5) predicts for a worse outcome. Thus far, however, there is no conclusive evidence that changing treatment according to the interim PET findings improves outcome. This question is currently under active investigation.

For the less aggressive histologies such as FL, data regarding the role of interim PET are sparse but do not suggest any particular benefit. Considering the generally incurable nature of advanced FL, if the patient is doing clinically well at the completion of therapy, the value of extensive imaging can be questioned.

Follow-Up and Routine Surveillance

Follow-up procedures and routine surveillance studies have been infrequently addressed in the literature. NCCN guidelines suggest a history and physical and routine laboratory assessment every 3 to 6 months for 5 years and then annually as indicated.[57] Routine surveillance PET scanning is not recommended. CT imaging can be considered depending on underlying histology and clinical presentation but is of unclear benefit.

Detection of relapse is most relevant for DLBCL where curative therapy is available, most notably a stem cell transplant. The NCCN does point out, however, that even for DLBCL,

Section III

there is no evidence demonstrating improved survival outcome with early detection of relapse. Further, the great majority of relapses are associated with clinical symptoms or abnormal physical findings. It is rare to discover recurrent disease on a routine imaging study in a patient who is clinically well with a normal exam.

Curative potential also exists for recurrent MZL. Relapses often occur at sites prone to development of MZL such as the orbit, skin, or head and neck area, are often localized, and respond well to a second course of radiotherapy. Such patients may well be long-term survivors—whether they are truly cured is controversial.

For most other histologic varieties of NHL, particularly FL, the detection of recurrence is less relevant. Generalized FL is still regarded as incurable (in contrast to localized FL). Relapse after treatment of localized FL is almost always generalized. An ostensibly localized nodal recurrence on the opposite side of the diaphragm, for example, would be considered generalized disease. Of course, if the disease was generalized at onset, it remains so at relapse, even if the recurrence is ostensibly localized to a nodal area. Because generalized FL is often observed without treatment until specific criteria for initiating therapy are met, there is little rationale for aggressive attempts at early detection of relapse in an asymptomatic patient with a normal exam.

DIFFUSE LARGE B-CELL LYMPHOMA

DLBCL, the most common type of NHL (30% of all cases in North America and Western Europe),[64] comprises a heterogeneous group of neoplasms with multiple morphologic variants and subtypes described in the current WHO classification.[55] Distinct subtypes include PCNSL, primary cutaneous DLBCL, leg type, T-cell/histiocyte-rich large B-cell lymphoma, and EBV-positive DLBCL of the elderly. Further, numerous other NHL entities arise from large B cells including primary mediastinal (thymic) large B-cell lymphoma (PMBCL).

Pathology

DLBCL is a neoplasm of large, transformed B cells with a diffuse growth pattern that totally or partially effaces the nodal architecture. The proposed normal counterparts are peripheral B cells of either germinal center or postgerminal center (activated B cell) origin. Indeed, DNA microarray analyses using fresh frozen tissue show that unique molecular subgroups exist, which include a germinal center B-cell (GCB) subgroup and an activated B-cell (ABC) subgroup.[65,66] PMBCL also has a unique molecular signature that closely resembles classical HL.[67] Assays utilizing immunohistochemistry to identify molecular subgroups, using formalin-fixed, paraffin-embedded tissue, have also been developed.[68–73] No single algorithm using immunohistochemistry is perfect in regard to predicting gene expression profiling results, though each divides patients into groups with different survival outcomes. Treatment tailored to molecular subclassification of this disease is currently being evaluated in prospective studies and is not routinely practiced.

DLBCL express one or more pan B-cell markers (CD19, CD20, CD22, and CD79a) and often surface and/or cytoplasmic immunoglobulin.[74] *MYC*, *BCL2*, and/or *BCL6* gene rearrangements are present in a minority of patients with DLBCL. However, DLBCL with gene rearrangements of *MYC* (a potent oncogene) together with a translocation of *BCL2* (an antiapoptotic gene), or less frequently *BCL6*, is now referred to as a double-hit lymphoma. If all three genes are rearranged, it is referred to as a triple-hit lymphoma. Approximately 5% to 10% of patients with DLBCL have double-hit or triple-hit genetics, which carries a particularly poor prognosis, despite the fact that the molecular subgroup is typically the

GCB-like.[75,76] Similarly, other patients, typically with an ABC-like subtype, have overexpression by immunohistochemistry of MYC and BCL2 and/or BCL6, without the accompanying gene rearrangements. Such DLBCLs are referred to as double or triple expressors. Such patients also have a worse prognosis, though more favorable than double-hit lymphomas.[77]

Clinical Presentation

DLBCL is primarily a disease of older adults, with a median age of 64 years and a slight preponderance of men (55%). B symptoms are present in approximately one-third of patients but are not prognostic, and current guidelines do not recommend including an "A" or "B" staging designation, as is done for HL.[62] Just over half the patients (55%) have localized disease (stages I or II). As is opposed to localized FL, where nodal presentations are predominant, about half of patients with stage I to II DLBCL present with extranodal disease. Patients most often present with an enlarging peripheral nodal mass or with symptoms related to a primary extranodal site of involvement.

Prognostic Factors

The International Non-Hodgkin's Lymphoma Prognostic Factors project examined data on 2,031 patients, all with aggressive histology NHL.[60,78] Two indices were developed, the International Prognostic Index (IPI) and the age-adjusted IPI, because age was found to be a highly significant prognostic variable (>60 vs. ≤60 years). For the IPI, five prognostic variables were found to be significant: age, performance status, stage, number of extranodal sites, and LDH (Table 82.5). The relative risks of these factors were low, ranging from 1.47 for stage to 1.96 for age. Five-year survival was 73%, 51%, 43%, and 26% when 0 to 1, 2, 3, and 4 to 5 risk factors were present. When patients were divided by age, three factors remained independently significant: performance status, stage, and LDH.

The IPI was designed in the prerituximab era. In the last 10 to 15 years, multiple randomized studies have shown that rituximab significantly improves survival when combined with standard combination chemotherapy.[81–83] Using data from three prospective trials, the German High-Grade Non-Hodgkin's Lymphoma Study Group found the IPI to retain prognostic significance in the rituximab era.[84] Adding approximately 10% survival to each IPI subgroup approximates outcomes when rituximab is added to combination chemotherapy.

TABLE 82.5 PROGNOSTIC INDICES—DIFFUSE LARGE B-CELL LYMPHOMA AND FOLLICULAR LYMPHOMA

Prognostic Index	Risk Factors	Score (Number of Factors)	Outcome
Diffuse Large B-Cell Lymphoma			
IPI[60]	Age > 60 y	Low (0–1)	73% (5-year survival)
	Performance status ≥ 2	Low Intermediate (2)	51%
	Stage III-IV	High Intermediate (3)	43%
	Elevated LDH	High (4–5)	26%
	>1 extranodal site		
Follicular Lymphoma			
FLIPI[79]	Age ≥ 60 y	Low (0–1)	71% (10-year survival)
	>4 nodal sites	Intermediate (2)	51%
	Elevated LDH	High (≥3)	36%
	Stage III-IV		
	Hemoglobin <12 g/dL		
FLIPI-2[80]	Age > 60 y	Low (0)	80% (5-year PFS)
	B2M elevated	Intermediate (1–2)	51%
	Hemoglobin <12 g/dL	High (≥3)	19%
	BM involvement		
	Nodal diameter >6 cm		

β2M, beta-2 microglobulin; BM, bone marrow; FLIPI, Follicular Lymphoma International Prognostic Index; IPI, International Prognostic Index; LDH, lactate dehydrogenase; PFS, progression-free survival.

As mentioned previously, several pathologic factors carry prognostic implications. Distinct subgroups of DLBCL, based on different cells of origin, can be identified using either gene expression profiling[85] or immunohistochemistry.[68–73] The GCB subtype has a more favorable prognosis compared with the ABC subtype (defined using gene expression profiling) or non–GCB-like subtype (defined using immunohistochemistry).[65,86] Additional molecular signatures that appear to influence tumor behavior have also been proposed.[66] Also, double-expressor, and particularly double-hit, lymphomas carry a worse prognosis.[75,76]

Both interim and postchemotherapy PET-CT assessments also carry prognostic importance. Although PET-CT interpretation was not standardized in most of these studies, in current practice, the 5-point scale (Deauville criteria) should be utilized.[62] In numerous studies, residual PET-positive disease after the completion of chemotherapy alone in aggressive NHLs (mostly DLBCL) is associated with a high risk of disease progression.[87–90] For example, in the setting of advanced DLBCL with PET-positive disease after chemotherapy without rituximab, the risk of progression was 100% in a series by Mikhaeel et al. ($n = 9$)[88] and Spaepen et al. ($n = 26$).[87] Similarly, poor outcomes have been noted when a posttreatment PET-CT is still positive after R-CHOP (rituximab, cyclophosphamide, doxorubicin, vincristine, prednisone).[91] Outcomes appear to be much better when RT is administered in this clinical setting.[92,93]

Achievement of a negative PET-CT early in the course of therapy (after 2 to 3 cycles) is associated with improved progression-free survival (PFS), but not always overall survival (OS),[91] compared with a positive interim PET-CT.[89,91,94–97] For example, in a study by Safar et al., 3-year progression-free and OS were 84% and 88%, respectively, in patients achieving a negative PET-CT after 2 cycles of chemotherapy plus rituximab.[97] This compared with 47% and 62%, respectively, in patients who were still PET positive. Interim PET-CT response appears to have prognostic significance in both the low- and high-risk IPI groups[89,96] but may be less prognostic in the ABC subtype compared with the germinal center-like subtype.[98]. Although the negative predictive value of interim PET-CT is high, the positive predictive value is relatively low. When compared with interim response assessment, postchemotherapy PET-CT response appears to be more prognostic, particularly in terms of the positive predictive value.[91,95,99]

Clinical Management

Chemoimmunotherapy, with or without consolidation RT, is standard in all stages of DLBCL. Perhaps, the most promising innovation in the last several decades in the treatment of B-cell NHLs, including DLBCL, has been the development of effective immunotherapy. DLBCL expresses the B-cell antigen CD20, which led to the genetic engineering of the human chimeric anti-CD20 antibody rituximab. In contrast to prior murine-derived monoclonal antibodies, rituximab is quite well tolerated in humans. Rituximab was the first antibody of any type FDA approved (1997) for the treatment of any human malignancy. Multiple phase III trials have now demonstrated the value of adding rituximab to standard CHOP.

The GELA study compared CHOP alone with rituximab and CHOP in 399 patients over age 60.[81] PFS improved from 30% to 54% and 5-year OS from 45% to 58%. Similarly, a European cooperative trial compared R-CHOP and CHOP in 824 patients aged 18 to 60 with stages II to IV DLBCL.[82] Three-year PFS was 79% in the R-CHOP group compared with 59% in the CHOP group. Three-year OS was 93% and 84%, respectively. In this trial, unlike the GELA trial, RT was given to select patients with bulky disease and/or extranodal disease. These studies have led to the rapid adaptation of R-CHOP as standard initial therapy of DLBCL for all stages of disease. The effect of the addition of rituximab is so substantial as to

force a re-evaluation of prognostic factors as well as other adjuvant therapies (such as stem cell transplantation or RT) in the rituximab era.

The most widely used chemotherapy combination is CHOP. An older randomized study by the Southwest Oncology Group (SWOG) demonstrated that CHOP was just as effective, less costly, and with fewer side effects than more aggressive regimens that demonstrated promise in phase II studies.[100] A more recent randomized trial demonstrated that R-CHOP was just as effective as the more aggressive regimen DA-EPOCH-R (dose adjusted, etoposide, prednisolone, vincristine, cyclophosphamide, doxorubicin, rituximab).[101] Thus, R-CHOP remains the standard regimen for DLBCL.

Stage I to II DLBCL

In the prechemotherapy era, early-stage DLBCL was treated with RT alone.[102–108] The doses of RT varied widely from 30 to 60 Gy. Field sizes and arrangements also varied widely, but, in general, involved field RT was used. The complete response rate was high, usually >80% with 10-year PFS and OS ranging from 30% to 60%, depending on the mix of patients and prognostic variables. The pattern of failure in these series was primarily distal, either organ involvement or nodal sites remote from the primary site. Patients with both nodal and extranodal diseases were included in these series and appeared to have equivalent prognoses. Stage II patients did worse than stage I with a long-term PFS in the range of 25%, in contrast to patients with stage I disease where PFS was higher (50% to 60%).

In the late 1970s and early 1980s, efforts to improve upon these results by the addition of chemotherapy were begun. With combination chemotherapy plus RT, complete response rates of approximately 90% were reported with PFS and OS in the range of 70% to 85%.[109–112] The chemotherapy regimen as well as the number of cycles varied, as did the doses of RT. None of the trials used rituximab as part of the therapy (now standard) nor was functional imaging employed for assessment of response.

After improved outcomes were seen with the addition of chemotherapy, the question was raised whether RT was still necessary. Multiple randomized studies in early-stage DLBCL have been conducted comparing chemotherapy with a combined modality program (Table 82.6).[59,113,115–117,119] Interpretation of the trials can be challenging, given their individual peculiarities. Only one, unpublished to date, included rituximab or functional imaging. A brief summary of each of the trials follows.

The SWOG S8736 study compared brief CHOP chemotherapy (3 cycles) plus RT (40 to 55 Gy) to a more extended CHOP regimen (8 cycles) without RT.[113] Both PFS (77% vs. 64%) and OS (82% vs. 72%) at 5 years were improved in the combined modality arm with less toxicity. However, after median follow-up of almost 18 years, no significant differences were apparent, because of late systemic relapses in the arm with only 3 cycles of CHOP. Interestingly, a continual pattern of relapse was noted in both arms throughout the follow-up period.[114] Long-term data from the phase II SWOG S0014 trial evaluating 3 cycles of R-CHOP + RT also demonstrated a continuous risk of relapse over time.[114] Thus, brief chemotherapy may provide insufficient systemic treatment for most patients with DLBCL.

The Eastern Cooperative Oncology Group (ECOG) 1484 study evaluated whether consolidation RT (30 Gy) would reduce the risk of relapse in the setting of extended chemotherapy (8 cycles of CHOP in this case).[59] The primary outcome was PFS which was significantly improved with the addition of RT (73% with consolidation RT vs. 56% with observation at 6 years) ($P = .05$). No difference in OS was noted, though the study was not powered to evaluate this. This study suggests that consolidation RT provides benefit even after an extended course of chemotherapy.

TABLE 82.6 RANDOMIZED TRIALS OF CHEMOTHERAPY OR COMBINED MODALITY THERAPY FOR EARLY-STAGE DLBCL

Study	n	Disease Characteristics	Randomization	Progression-Free Survival[a]	Comments
SWOG[113,114]	401	I	CHOP × 8	64%	No difference with long f/u
		II (nonbulky)	CHOP × 3 + RT	77% (P = .03)	
ECOG[59]	172	I (high-risk)	CHOP × 8	56%	Only patients in CR by CT randomized
		II	CHOP × 8 + RT	73%[b] (P = .05)	
GELA 93-4[115]	576	I–II without risk factors	CHOP × 4	61%	Only patients ≥ 60 years old
			CHOP × 4 + RT	64% (P = .6)	
GELA 93-1[116]	647	I–II without risk factors	ACVBP × 3[c]	82%	Only patients ≤ 61 years old
			CHOP × 3 + RT	74% (P < .01)	
IELSG[117]	44	I–II gastric DLBCL	CHOP[d]	82%	Closed early because of poor accrual
			CHOP[d] + RT	100% (P = .04)	
LYSA/GOELAMS[118]	301	I–II nonbulky	R-CHOP × 4–6	87%	PET-CT imaging utilized
			R-CHOP × 4–6 + RT	88% (P = .13)	

ACVBP, doxorubicin, cyclophosphamide, vindesine, bleomycin, and prednisone; CHOP, cyclophosphamide, adriamycin, vincristine, prednisone; DLBCL, diffuse large B-cell lymphoma; ECOG, Eastern Cooperative Oncology Group; GELA, Groupe d'Étude des Lymphomes de l'Adulte; IELSG, International Extranodal Lymphoma Study Group; The Lymphoma Study Association/The French Acute Leukemia and Blood Diseases West–East Group; RT, radiation therapy; SWOG, Southwest Oncology Group.
[a]5 y unless otherwise noted.
[b]6 years.
[c]Plus consolidation chemotherapy with methotrexate, etoposide, ifosfamide, and cytarabine.
[d]CHOP or CHOP-like chemotherapy.

The Groupe d'Etudes des Lymphomes de l'Adulte (GELA) 93-4 enrolled older patients (>60 years) with early-stage disease without adverse risk factors.[115] Crude rates of local failure were less with RT (18% vs. 7%). However, neither PFS nor OS was improved with consolidation RT (40 Gy) after 4 cycles of chemotherapy. This study has been criticized by protocol violations (12% of patients did not receive RT) and delays in starting RT (median of 35 days after last cycle of chemotherapy). This study also suggests that older patients, especially those with favorable prognostic factors and/or medical comorbidities, may derive less benefit from consolidation RT.

GELA 93-1 demonstrated that an aggressive chemotherapy regimen (induction ACVBP [doxorubicin, cyclophosphamide, vindesine, bleomycin, prednisone] followed by consolidation methotrexate, etoposide, ifosfamide, and cytarabine) was superior to CHOP plus RT but at the expense of significantly increased toxicity.[116] Despite the apparent advantage of the aggressive chemotherapy program, it has not been generally adopted due to its toxicity profile.

Finally, the International Extranodal Lymphoma Study Group (IELSG) enrolled a small number of patients with gastric DLBCL to CHOP versus CHOP plus RT. PFS was improved with the combined approach.[117]

A randomized study from the LYSA/GOELAMS group compared 4 to 6 cycles of R-CHOP with and without RT (40 Gy) in stage I to II nonbulky DLBCL who achieved a complete response by PET-CT.[118] Event-free survival at 5 years was 87% with R-CHOP versus 91% with R-CHOP plus RT (P = .13). There were no local failures in the arm receiving RT, whereas approximately 50% of failures in the no-RT arm failed at original sites of disease involvement. Most patients in this study had low-risk disease by the IPI. To date, this study has only been presented in abstract form.

In summary, the results from the randomized studies are mixed. The majority of the randomized studies (excepting the LYSA/GOELAMS trial) did not employ rituximab or PET-CT imaging, which is a significant limitation. However, using data from the modern era, the advantage of combined modality therapy has been observed using large databases including SEER,[120] NCCN,[121] and NCDB (National Cancer Database),[122,123] in addition to a large single institutional experience.[124] Given the modest doses employed (~30 Gy), high rates of local control after RT (~95%),[59,92,115] and predominance of data showing a benefit for consolidation RT, we favor a combined modality approach.

Stage III to IV DLBCL

The mainstay of treatment of advanced DLBCL is clearly systemic chemoimmunotherapy, typically R-CHOP, with 5-year survival of approximately 60%.[81] Many strategies have been explored to improve upon CHOP and R-CHOP including more chemotherapy cycles,[125] dose dense chemotherapy,[126,127] more intensive chemotherapy regimens,[100,101] maintenance rituximab,[83] and high-dose chemotherapy (HDC) and autologous stem cell transplant (ASCT).[128] None have consistently improved survival compared with standard R-CHOP. A comparatively unexplored approach is the use of consolidation RT in combination with chemotherapy for advanced DLBCL. One rational for the use of consolidation RT is the tendency of patients with advanced lymphoma to relapse at sites of original involvement and, in particular, sites of original bulk.[129–131] In view of the efficacy of combined modality therapy in localized disease, exploration of its value in more advanced disease appears worthwhile.

Several institutional series have evaluated the role of consolidation RT in advanced DLBCL. In the prerituximab era, series from M.D. Anderson[129] and Milan[130] both demonstrated improved local control and PFS with the additional of RT. Although OS was improved in the Milan series, which only included patients with disease >6 cm, survival was not improved in the M.D. Anderson series. In the rituximab era, series from M.D. Anderson,[132] Duke,[133] and Emory[134] have demonstrated improvements in local control[133,134] and survival[132,134] with consolidation RT, even when patients are in complete response by PET-CT. The Duke series suggests such benefits can be accomplished with low doses of radiation that are well tolerated with a low risk of long-term complications (~20 Gy).

Results from prospective studies have demonstrated the benefit of consolidation RT in the presence of bulky disease. The RICOVER-60 trial was a four-arm randomized study comparing different chemotherapy regimens. Consolidation RT was delivered to sites of initial bulk (≥7.5 cm) or extranodal disease. At the conclusion of the trial, an additional cohort was accrued and treated with the most effective regimen from the randomized trial (R-CHOP-14 × 6 cycles) but without consolidation RT (referred to as the RICOVER-noRTh trial). When comparing the two arms receiving the same chemotherapy regimen, the addition of consolidation RT improved both PFS (75% vs. 61%, P < .001) and OS (90% vs. 65%, P = .001).[135] Similarly, the German UNFOLDER trial (NCT00278408) prematurely closed the R-CHOP arms not receiving consolidation RT because of excess relapses in those with bulky disease (≥7.5 cm). Results from this trial have not yet been published. Other circumstances that may warrant consideration of consolidation RT include limited skeletal disease,[136] partial response to chemotherapy,[92,93,137] and limited presentations (e.g., mediastinal and upper retroperitoneal disease).

Relapsed and Refractory DLBCL

There has been a great interest in the application of HDC with ASCT in the treatment of malignant lymphomas, primarily in the setting of relapsed or refractory disease. Alternatively, an allogeneic transplant may be carried out in individuals with a suitable matched donor. In this procedure, it is hoped that the infused donor stem cells will additionally mount an immunologic attack on the tumor. Allogeneic transplantation may be preceded by full-dose (myeloablative) chemotherapy designed to have not only an antitumor effect but also to condition the patient for the infusion of the donor cells, or it may be preceded by a nonmyeloablative or reduced intensity conditioning (RIC) program designed primarily to enable the recipient to accept the donor stem cells. In this latter situation, the major antitumor effect is postulated to derive from the infused donor stem cells. Nonmyeloablative allogeneic transplants are associated with a much lower treatment-related mortality (10% to 20%) compared with myeloablative allogeneic transplants (40% to 50%).[138,139] Total-body irradiation is often a component of the conditioning program with doses varying quite widely from 2 to 4 Gy in nonmyeloablative regimens to 12 to 13.5 Gy in ablative regimens. An expert committee of the American Society for Blood and Marrow Transplantation has recently issued guidelines surrounding autologous and allogeneic transplantation.[140]

In general, ASCT has been investigated in three types of situations: (1) patients who have been treated with conventional chemotherapy and then relapsed, (2) patients who fail conventional chemotherapy from the onset (so-called primary refractory disease), and (3) patients who have responded well to primary chemotherapy but are considered at high risk for relapse. The most widely accepted use is for the treatment of patients with DLBCL who have relapsed following initial CHOP or R-CHOP chemotherapy.

In a phase III trial from the Parma group, patients with DLBCL who had relapsed following initial CHOP chemotherapy and who were responsive to a salvage program (dexamethasone, cisplatin, cytarabine) were then randomly assigned to receive either four additional cycles of DHAP or a HDC program with ASCT.[141] Those receiving ASCT had a markedly improved PFS (46% vs. 12%) and OS (53% vs. 32%), compared with those getting conventional chemotherapy. Note that in both arms of this trial, RT to original bulky sites of disease (≥5 cm) was utilized, dose of 35 Gy in 20 fractions in the conventional chemotherapy arm and 26 Gy in 1.3 Gy fractions bid in the ASCT arm. All patients in the Parma trial were younger than 60 years of age. Those with a short remission after initial chemotherapy had a worse outcome.[142]

The Parma trial has led to the adaptation of ASCT as standard of care for patients <60 years of age with DLBCL relapsing after initial chemotherapy. Note that the Parma trial is the only phase III investigation of relapsed DLBCL patients ever done. It is also important to recognize that in this as well as almost all other transplant trials, patients who do not respond to the initial salvage program do poorly with subsequent HDC and are not considered good candidates. More recently, PET-CT imaging is the preferred method to define response; those with a persistently positive PET-CT after a salvage program (Deauville 4) do poorly with HDC.[143,144]

Patients with primary refractory disease (i.e., those who are chemotherapy induction failures) should be managed similar to relapsed disease and proceed with salvage chemotherapy, typically R-ICE (rituximab, ifosfamide, carboplatin, etoposide) or R-DHAP (rituximab, dexamethasone, cytarabine, cisplatin). If a good response is achieved to salvage chemotherapy, ideally a complete response by PET-CT, then outcomes with subsequent stem cell transplantation are relatively good.[145] Those with primary progressive disease generally have a poor prognosis, however.

The role of RT in patients undergoing stem cell transplant, either autologous or allogeneic, is undefined.[146] The rationale for RT lies in the observation that most treatment failures after transplant occur at sites of initial involvement. As mentioned above, consolidation RT was employed in the landmark Parma trial. It is also commonly used at a number of institutions, usually directed at bulk disease sites present before the start of salvage chemotherapy but with considerable interinstitutional variation and without a clear definition of what constitutes bulk disease. We recommend doses of 20 to 30 Gy for those patients who have not received prior RT, depending on clinical circumstances and also dependent on whether or not TBI is planned as part of the conditioning regimen.

Palliation

For patients with relapsed/refractory disease, RT is an effective modality to achieve palliation of symptomatic disease. Although doses of 24 to 30 Gy are most commonly utilized, low-dose RT (2 Gy × 2) may be reasonable in select circumstances. Response rates of 50% to 80% have been reported with 2 Gy × 2 with a median time to progression of about 1 year.[147,148] Larger and more durable responses are likely achieved with more traditional dosing schemes.

RT Dose and Field Design

The dose of RT in a combined modality treatment program depends principally on the stage of disease and response to chemotherapy. For patients with stage I to II disease, the standard dose is 30 Gy when a complete response (Deauville 1 to 3) has been achieved by PET-CT after chemoimmunotherapy, typically R-CHOP. A British National Lymphoma Investigation randomized study showed no difference in freedom from local progression, PFS, or OS between 30 Gy and 40 to 45 Gy.[149] Numerous other studies have shown high (~95%) rates of local control when approximately 30 Gy of RT is given after a complete response by CT or PET-CT to systemic therapy Gy.[59,92,93,112,132,150]

Even smaller doses may suffice with more effective systemic therapy, including rituximab-based regimens. A phase II study from Duke University recently completed accrual evaluating 20 Gy in the setting of a complete response by PET-CT after R-CHOP. The primary endpoint was local control. Preliminary results, with a median follow-up of 34 months, demonstrated no local failures with PFS at 3 and 5 years of 92% and 78%, respectively.[151]

For patients who have persistent PET-positive disease (Deauville 4), higher doses of consolidation RT may be required to achieve optimal local control (≥40 Gy)[92,93] (Fig. 82.1). In the unusual circumstance when RT alone is pursued for patients with localized disease, a dose of 40 Gy is recommended. There is little evidence for doses above 40 Gy.

In regard to field design, detailed guidelines from the International Lymphoma Radiation Oncology Group are available.[152,153] These guidelines recommend treatment using "involved-site" principles. Involved-site radiation therapy (ISRT) involves creating a clinical target volume that consists of the prechemotherapy extent of disease, adjusted to exclude uninvolved normal tissues after chemotherapy, and expanded to account for uncertainties in recreating the prechemotherapy extent of disease (anatomical changes, patient positioning differences between diagnostic PET-CT and planning CT scan,

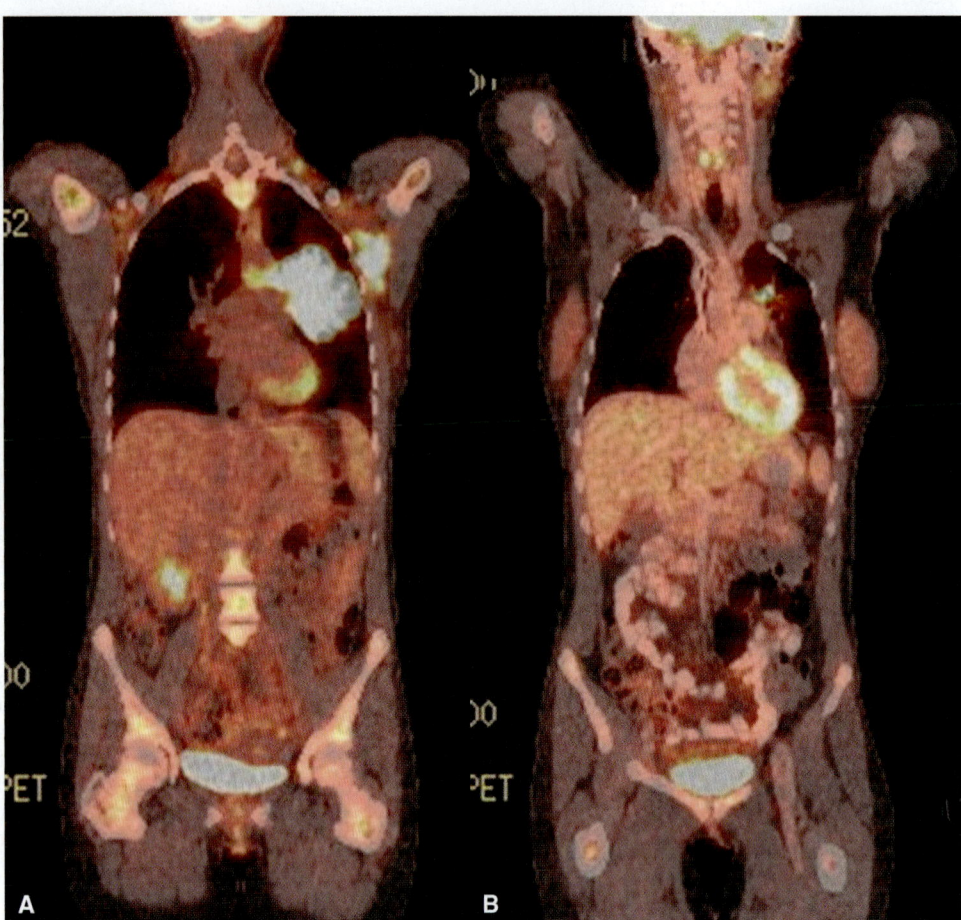

FIGURE 82.1. Fused coronal positron emission tomography/computed tomography (PET-CT) images of a patient with diffuse large B-cell lymphoma before **(A)** and after **(B)** chemoimmunotherapy. The postchemotherapy PET-CT was scored as a Deauville 4 (uptake above the liver) in the left hilum. Biopsy confirmed persistent disease.

imaging uncertainties, etc.). A planning target volume is then created to account for setup variation and potential organ motion. Such recommendations are supported by prior studies demonstrating that the dominant pattern of failure after combined modality therapy is usually disseminated disease, with a small percentage with local failure.[113] On the other hand, after chemotherapy alone, more local failure occurs.[113,154] Failure in nodal areas adjacent to the original disease is uncommon.

For patients with localized disease (stage I to II), all sites of original involvement should be treated. For patients with advanced disease (stage III to IV), treatment fields should be customized. In those with reasonably limited presentations, consolidation of all sites of original involvement is favored. When this is not practical, treatment of select sites may be more prudent. This may include original sites of bulk, limited skeletal involvement, or a site that failed to achieve a complete response to chemotherapy.

FOLLICULAR LYMPHOMA

FL is the second most common NHL in the United States and Western Europe, comprising approximately 20% of cases. It is the most common "indolent" lymphoma.

Pathology

FL is a tumor of follicle center B cells (centrocytes and centroblasts) with a follicular (nodular) pattern that morphologically is similar to normal germinal centers. The neoplastic follicles may be present in the entire tumor, or the lymphoma may contain a diffuse component as well. FL is graded based on morphology. There is a predominance of small cleaved cells (centrocytes), grade 1; a mixture of small cleaved and large cells, grade 2; or predominantly large cells (centroblasts), grade 3. In the WHO classification, the number of large cells per high-powered field is used to assign grades (0 to 5, 5 to 15, >15 for grades 1 to 3, respectively). Grade 3 is further subdivided into 3A and 3B with the latter characterized by an absence of centrocytes. Grade 1, 2, and 3A FLs are all closely related with similar biologic behavior and response to therapy. FL grade 3B, however, has a clinical course very similar to DLBCL and is usually managed as such.[155]

The tumor cells of FL are usually surface immunoglobulin positive and express pan B-cell–associated antigens (CD19, CD20), CD21, and CD10 (60% of the time), but lack CD5. Most cases are BCL-2 positive; nuclear BCL-6 is expressed by at least some of the neoplastic cells. The (14;18) translocation is characteristic for FL and together with the BCL-2 rearrangement is present in approximately 85% of cases. It is frequently absent, however, in FL grade 3B, further supporting the biologic distinctiveness of this category.

Recently, inactivating mutations of MLL-2 have been found in over 80% of FL patients, interfering with the ability of MLL-2 to activate gene transcription through H3K4 methylation.[156]

Clinical Presentation

FL primarily affects older adults (median age 65 years). There is a slight female preponderance. Most patients present with painless peripheral lymphadenopathy involving cervical, axillary, or inguinal–femoral regions. There may often be a history of spontaneous waxing and waning of lymph node size. Constitutional B symptoms of fever, sweats, or weight loss are uncommon. In contrast to DLBCL, approximately 80% of patients present with generalized disease, most often with stage IV disease. The bone marrow is the principle extranodal organ involved. The presence of minimal bone marrow involvement as determined by BCL-2/IgH rearrangement detected by polymerase chain reaction (PCR) is much more common, found probably in the majority of stage I to II patients. The significance of this finding is uncertain and is not presently used to change the staging of such patients.

In contrast to DLBCL, localized extranodal presentation of FL is uncommon, reported in only 6% of the ILSG series.[157] A unique but uncommon variant of FL is extranodal presentation in the intestinal tract, usually the duodenum, usually stage I.[158] The WHO has classified duodenal FL as a separate entity, but the biologic behavior is very similar to localized FL at other sites.

The principle indicated imaging study is the PET-CT scan. Although FL is typically less FDG-avid than DLBCL, increased uptake is still seen in about 90% to 95% of cases.[159] Bone marrow biopsy should be performed in all patients thought to have early-stage disease given the high incidence of involvement. PET-CT is less accurate in detecting bone marrow involvement than in DLBCL. For patients with advanced disease, a bone marrow can be pursued if the results will change clinical management.

Large-cell transformation to DLBCL occurs in approximately 30% of patients with FL at a rate of approximately 2% per year.[160] This should be suspected if LDH levels are rising, B symptoms develop, extranodal sites become involved, disproportionate growth occurs, or high SUVmax is observed (>10).[161] The prognosis after transformation is generally not good but better in the rituximab era, with a median survival of 50 months following transformation. The outlook is better with an increasing interval between FL diagnosis and the occurrence of transformation.

Prognostic Factors

Subsequent to the development of the widely used IPI for DLBCL, attempts were made to apply it to FL, but here, it was less useful because most patients fell into a favorable prognostic category. Additional efforts to address this problem led to the development of the FLIPI, the follicular lymphoma IPI[79] (Table 82.5). The initial database included 4,167 patients with FL diagnosed between the years 1985 and 1992 (the prerituximab era). Five adverse prognostic factors were identified on multivariate analysis, age (>60 vs. <60 years), stage (I/II vs. III/IV), hemoglobin level (<12 g/dL vs. ≥12 g/dL), number of nodal areas (>4 vs. ≤4), and finally serum LDH. Low-risk patients had 0 to 1 adverse factors, intermediate risk 2 factors, and poor risk 3 or more. Patients were divided approximately equally between the three groups with good separation in terms of OS (Table 82.5).

The FLIPI was subsequently modified to take into account the advent of rituximab leading to the FLIPI-2 categorization.[80] That index identified age, elevated $\beta 2$ microglobulin

(B2M), hemoglobin, bone marrow involvement, and lymph node diameter >6 cm as independent risk factors for PFS (OS data not as yet available) (Table 82.5).

Recently, a third prognostic index is under development utilizing genetic risk factors as well and known as the M7-FLIPI.[162] This model integrates the mutational status of seven genes known to be important in FL.

As with DLBCL, interim and posttreatment PET-CT response appears to have prognostic significance, particularly posttreatment PET response.[163,164] Limited studies on interim PET scanning have suggested no benefit from this.[164,165]

Clinical Management

The majority of patients with FL present with advanced stage disease. Advanced FL is still considered incurable despite advances in chemoimmunotherapy in the last several years with resulting prolongation of both PFS and OS. For the minority of patients who present with localized disease, a subset varyingly reported to range from 20% to 32%, local radiotherapy has curative potential.

Stage I to II FL

A large number of retrospective studies have shown a high rate of local disease control with approximately 50% of patients achieving long-term survival without relapse in early-stage FL. Selected series are shown in Table 82.7. The great majority of patients in these series have been staged and treated in an era prior to widespread use of modern imaging technology, particularly PET-CT scanning. With modern staging including PET-CT, its likely results would be even better. Unfortunately, there are no prospective phase III studies demonstrating the value of definitive radiotherapy, most likely because of the relative infrequency of localized FL at presentation and the necessity for a study with very long follow-up.

Several comments about the series listed in Table 82.7 are in order:

1. Most of the studies shown are older, which gives them the advantage of long follow-up but the disadvantage of lack of modern staging (PET-CT). Further, most of the series included some patients with other low-grade lymphoma histologies other than FL, although the great majority were FL.

2. The radiation doses used varied widely from 16 to 50 Gy, although most patients received in the neighborhood of 30 Gy. None of the series report detailed dose response data. In general, there appeared to be no dose response demonstrated, with >90% local control with doses in the 30 Gy range.

3. The field sizes also varied considerably with somewhat different definitions than are now used. In brief, involved

Study	Year	Number of Patients	Radiation Fields	Radiation Dose (Gy)	Failure-Free Survival % (10 Years)	Overall Survival % (10 Years)
Vaughan Hudson[107]	1996	208	NS	35	47	71–84[a]
MacManus[166]	1996	177	IF, EF, TNI	34–55	44	64
Stuschke[167]	1997	117	ER, TNI	36	59	86
Wilder[168]	2001	80	IF, EF	26–50	57	65
Petersen[169]	2004	460	IF	16–47	41	62
Guadagnolo[170]	2006	106	IF, EF	30–42	46	75
Pugh[171]	2010	2,222	NS	NS	NS	62–79[a]
Campbell[172]	2010	237	IN, EF	20–40	49	66–82[a]
Vargo[173]	2015	10,613	NS	NS	NS	68

TABLE 82.7 RADIOTHERAPY FOR STAGE I/II FOLLICULAR LYMPHOMA

EF, extended field; IF, involved field; IN, involved nodal; NS, not specified; TNI, total nodal irradiation.
[a]Overall survival and cause-specific survival.

field radiation, in which the nodal area in question was treated with a generous margin, appeared to be as effective as larger fields.

4. Ten-year PFS is remarkably close to 50% in all of the series. There was more variation in the OS, which generally ranged from about 60% to 80% depending on whether lymphoma-only deaths were counted or all deaths because of any cause. In general, the risk of a patient with stage I/II FL treated with radiation alone *dying of lymphoma* at 10 years was approximately 20%.

5. As can be inferred by the high local control rate of approximately 90%, the great majority of relapses were at distant sites from the original disease, not adjacent nodal areas. This has led directly to the practice of irradiating only the involved nodal site with a generous margin. Importantly, few relapses were observed after 10 years with a general flattening of the PFS curve.

The largest series in the literature is the report from Pugh et al.[171] The SEER database forms the basis of this study. 6558 patients were identified from 1973 to 2004 with localized FL. 2,222 (34%) of these patients were treated with initial radiotherapy. No details as to radiation fields or dose are available. Compared with patients from the SEER database who received no radiotherapy, cause-specific survival was improved in the radiation group at 10 years from 65% to 79%. Survival at 10 years was 60% in the radiated patients and 50% in those not receiving radiotherapy.

On the basis of these studies, radiotherapy remains the treatment of choice for early-stage FL. Most of the patients in these series had stage I disease or contiguous stage II disease. For noncontiguous stage II disease, the data are sparse. Many centers individualize the treatment of such patients rather than automatically treating with radiotherapy.

Small series of patients with localized disease have been observed without treatment with apparently favorable results.[174] Experience with this approach, however, is quite limited. NCCN guidelines recommend radiotherapy as the standard approach for localized disease with observation reserved for selected patients in whom there might be a concern for the ability to tolerate radiotherapy.[57]

Despite the above data and NCCN and ESMO guidelines[175] endorsing radiotherapy as the preferred initial management, the use of radiation in patients with early-stage FL continues to decline. In the Pugh study, only 24% of patients with localized disease received radiotherapy as initial treatment.[171] In the National LymphoCare study, 23% of patients with stage I FL received radiotherapy alone.[176] The remainder of the patients were treated in a variety of ways including rituximab plus chemotherapy (30%), rituximab alone (13%), and observation (29%). OS at 5 years was approximately 90% in all treatment groups.

Adjuvant systemic therapy after definitive RT in early-stage FL has been infrequently studied. In the prerituximab era, there were four randomized trials.[109,110,177,178] Three of the trials had only small numbers of patients as part of a larger trial including patients with DLBCL. In brief, no benefit was seen in FL for the use of systemic therapy along with radiation. A larger British National Lymphoma Investigation of adjuvant chlorambucil was similarly negative.[177]

In the rituximab era, two retrospective trials have looked at this question, both of which were relatively small.[179] They suggested benefit for adjuvant systemic therapy, but the numbers are small and the follow-up short. A recent multicenter prospective phase III trial randomized 150 patients with limited-stage FL to radiotherapy alone or with addition of systemic therapy (CVP).[180] Of the 75 patients randomized to the latter, only 31 received rituximab-containing chemotherapy with a benefit in PFS seen in the latter. No OS benefits were

seen. Thus, outside of a clinical trial, this approach cannot be recommended.

Stage III and IV FL

Advanced FL is still considered an incurable disease with survival curves that never become parallel to that of the corresponding normal population. The clinical course, however, is often prolonged with multiple effective therapeutic agents available. Because of the relatively indolent nature of advanced FL, a strategy of initial observation without therapy was introduced first at Stanford University.[181] It was later confirmed with randomized trials that this approach did not adversely affect long-term survival.[182] It should be cautioned that these trials were performed in the prerituximab era. Nonetheless, the strategy of "watchful waiting" has gained widespread acceptance. NCCN guidelines consider observation the "standard practice for patients with advanced stage low tumor burden FL."[57] Tumor burden has generally been assessed with the GELF criteria in which any one of the following signifies a high tumor burden: (1) three distinct nodal sites each $\geq$ 3 cm, (2) a single nodal site $\geq$ 7 cm, (3) symptomatic splenomegaly, (4) organ compression or compromise, (5) pleural effusions or ascites, (6) B symptoms, and (7) elevated LDH or beta-2 microglobulin.[183]

One nonrandomized study in the rituximab era, the FL2 registry study of the International Follicular Lymphoma Prognostic Factor Project, compared outcomes in 107 patients with a low tumor burden initially observed with 242 patients of similar tumor burden who were treated with a rituximab-containing regimen. Five-year OS and freedom from relapse were not statistically different in the two groups.[184]

One randomized trial has compared single-agent rituximab to the watch and wait policy. At 3 years, the proportion of patients without progression was 33% in the watch and wait group, approximately 70% in the rituximab-treated patients. OS did not differ, however.

Another algorithm divides patients with advanced stage disease into four categories: asymptomatic or symptomatic with a low tumor burden or high tumor burden, the tumor burden defined as above under the GELF criteria. For asymptomatic patients with a low tumor burden, the proposed therapeutic strategies are either observation or treatment with single-agent rituximab. For asymptomatic patients with a high tumor burden, proposed therapeutic choices are observation or chemotherapy along with rituximab. For symptomatic patients with low tumor burden, treatment choices include single-agent rituximab or in combination with chemotherapy. For high tumor burden symptomatic patients, the preferred strategy is rituximab-containing chemotherapy with maintenance rituximab. In this decision-making process, there is room for considerable individualization with consideration for the patient's age, comorbidities, predicted life expectancy, and general patient preference.[185]

The majority of patients for whom systemic therapy is desirable will receive rituximab in combination with chemotherapy. In the last two decades, the addition of rituximab to chemotherapy constitutes a major therapeutic advance. Its use has been associated with increased response rates, duration of response, and improvement in PFS at a minimum. One recent meta-analysis suggests a benefit in OS as well, although longer follow-up is needed.[186]

Multiple chemotherapy combinations have been studied in combination with rituximab. These include CHOP, CVP, and fludarabine. In brief, no one drug program when combined with rituximab has demonstrated superiority over another. Recently, however, the alkylating agent bendamustine has been introduced for therapy of FL in combination with rituximab. A phase III trial from the Study Group Indolent Lymphoma (SCIL) compared bendamustine–rituximab (BR) to R-CHOP and demonstrated increased efficacy and reduced toxicity with the BR combination.[187] This improved efficacy was manifested by prolongation of PFS and improved response rates, but, as is so often the case with FL, no differences in survival were found. A second study, a randomized phase III noninferiority trial (BRIGHT study), indicated the equivalence of BR to R-CHOP or R-CVP with, however, somewhat different toxicity profiles.[188] Because the BR combination appears to be generally significantly less toxic, this has led to the rapid adaptation in the United States of BR as first-line systemic therapy for advanced stage FL patients who require treatment.

Another novel strategy for first-line treatment has involved combining rituximab with the immunomodulatory agent lenalidomide. An overall response rate of 98% was reported by M.D. Anderson investigators with a 3-year PFS of 78% with acceptable toxicity.[189] This particular approach is now being compared in phase III trials to more standard chemotherapy with rituximab.

The use of maintenance rituximab after chemoimmunotherapy has gained widespread acceptance following a large phase III intergroup trial (PRIMA study).[190] In this trial, patients with previously untreated FL who had responded to chemoimmunotherapy were randomly assigned 2 years of maintenance with rituximab or placebo. With short follow-up, the 2-year PFS in the rituximab maintenance arm was 75% compared with 58% in the observation arm. There was a slight increase in adverse events in the maintenance arm. There was no difference in OS. Thus, the benefit of rituximab maintenance is unclear but is being increasingly employed.

Given the radiosensitivity of FL and the effectiveness of rituximab, therapy with a radiolabeled monoclonal anti-CD20 antibody is an attractive option. High response rates, PFS, and OS have been reported, both in localized and advanced stage FLs.[191,192] Toxicity has generally been minimal and limited to reversible myelosuppression, although late development of myelodysplastic syndrome (MDS) is a concern.[193]

Initially, there were two such products investigated and on the market, but in the United States, only one is still available, [90]y-ibritumomab tiuxetan. This drug is a combination of the beta-emitting isotope [90]y, linked to rituximab. Its use has been recently extensively reviewed.[193a] A recent international trial of [90]y-ibritumomab as first-line therapy for advanced disease revealed an overall response rate of 94% with a CR of 58%.[194] The 3-year PFS was 58% and OS 95%. Toxicity was minimal and limited to hematologic effects.

In addition to its use as initial therapy, radioimmunotherapy (RIT) has been studied as maintenance or consolidation treatment after initial chemotherapy. In a phase III multicenter European trial, a tripling of the median PFS was observed from 13 to 36 months.[195] However, when R-CHOP was directly compared to CHOP followed by RIT, no difference was found.[196]

Thus, the role of RIT remains uncertain. It is an attractive option for patients needing systemic treatment who might not tolerate conventional R-chemotherapy. It has not been explored as consolidation treatment after R-CHOP. Finally, RIT has never been studied as consolidation treatment after curative radiotherapy for localized disease.

Treatment of Relapsed, Refractory, or Transformed FL

Patients who relapse after initial therapy of localized FL almost always have generalized disease, even if the area of relapse is ostensibly localized. For example, patients who initially present with localized disease above the diaphragm and who sustain a relapse inferior to the diaphragm are considered to have generalized disease, even if there is no evidence of supradiaphragmatic disease at the time of the infradiaphragmatic relapse. These patients should be re-evaluated in a similar fashion to those who present with advanced disease, as has been already discussed. Similarly, patients who presented with advanced disease and relapse after initial therapy should be re-evaluated in a similar fashion as they were at the time of diagnosis. Are they symptomatic, what is the extent of the tumor burden, do they meet the GELF criteria for treatment, what is the goal of therapy, what are the patient preferences, and finally what is the patient's overall medical condition. Answers to these questions will guide the therapeutic choices.

At the time of relapse, biopsy of a new disease site is appropriate to rule out transformation to a more aggressive histology. Restaging is usually appropriate as well with the procedures mentioned above including routine blood studies, LDH, β2 microglobulin, and PET-CT scan. A bone marrow examination is less important in the presence of known generalized disease.

For patients relapsing with limited extent of disease, low-dose palliative radiotherapy, to 4 Gy total, should be strongly considered. Such low doses have been found to be remarkably effective (see below). Side effects are minimal—1% grade 3 to 4 toxicity. Unfortunately, low-dose palliative radiotherapy is often overlooked in the management of generalized disease.

For patients with generalized disease who do require systemic therapy, the choice of agents is greatly influenced by what prior therapy the patient has received. For example, if the initial systemic therapy was BR, it would be logic to proceed with R-CHOP or vice versa. If the patient has not received RIT, that may have a significant role to play. A new anti-CD20 antibody, obinutuzumab, may be employed.[197] A new class of drugs, phosphatidylinositol 3-kinase (P13K) inhibitors, has been developed. Idelalisib, a selective oral inhibitor of P13K, has been studied in relapsing disease with an overall response rate of 57%.[198]

Finally, stem cell transplantation has been extensively studied in FL, both autologous (ASCT) and allogeneic. In the only phase III trial to compare ASCT to conventional chemotherapy in relapsed FL, patients appeared to demonstrate a higher PFS and OS when treated with ASCT.[199] However, the procedure is not believed to be curative for relapsed disease, in contrast to the situation with DLBCL. Allogeneic transplantation may have curative potential, but its use has been hindered by the high treatment-related mortality of approximately 40% at 3 years for a full myeloablative transplant and a treatment-related mortality of up to 20% even for the reduced intensity conditioning transplant, as well as the logistical difficulties of finding a matched donor. In a recent NCCN database retrospective analysis, however, 3-year OS for allogeneic SCT versus autologous SCT was 87% versus 61%.[200] It should be noted that neither ASCT nor allogeneic SCT has any proven role in the initial treatment of generalized FL, such as consolidation therapy for patients in first remission.

Histologic transformation to DLBCL occurs in approximately 2% to 3% of patients per year and historically has been associated with a poor clinical outcome. The prognosis directly relates to the number of prior therapies the patient has received with a much poorer outlook in those with multiple prior therapies. Aggressive chemotherapy has most often been employed in this situation. In selected patients in a Canadian trial, treated after transformation by induction chemotherapy followed by HDC and ASCT, a 5-year survival of 65% has been reported.[201]

Radiation Dose and Field Size

As can be seen from Table 82.7, the dose of radiotherapy employed in older retrospective studies varied widely from approximately 20 to 44 Gy with local control being achieved in over 90% of patients irrespective of dose. Retrospective dose analyses reported from the Princess Margaret Hospital and the University of Florida suggested local control rates over 90% with doses in the range of 25 to 35 Gy at the Princess Margaret[202] and 30 Gy at the University of Florida.[203]

These discrepancies led to the performance of a large prospective trial by the British National Lymphoma Investigation comparing 24 Gy to 40 to 45 Gy.[149] This is one of the few prospective phase III trials of different radiotherapy doses in any disease. In brief, no differences were observed in any measured outcome, either local control, PFS, or OS between the two different doses employed. This study made no mention of bulk of disease. Such patients appeared to have been included. There is no information as to whether their outcome was any different from those with small-volume disease.

This study has led to the widespread adoption of 24 to 30 Gy as the appropriate dose for curative treatment of FL and other so-called indolent lymphomas. Most centers stay within this dose range irrespective of the bulk of disease but would probably give 30 Gy for bulk disease (variably defined) and only exceed this dose if the clinical response was not satisfactory. Doses around 24 Gy are typically employed when there is concern for normal tissue toxicity, such as when irradiating the eye. One could argue for only treating to 24 Gy in all cases of localized FL irrespective of site, but 30 Gy remains a popular option, given the long experience with this dose and its excellent safety profile.

Even lower doses (2 to 4 Gy) have been found to be quite effective in the palliation of advanced FL. Response rates of 80% to 90% have been reported with a median duration of response ranging from 22 to 45 months.[204–206] These data have led some to propose the use of very low doses of 2 to 4 Gy as appropriate for curative treatment of limited-stage FL, leading to a randomized trial involving 548 patients who were prospectively allocated to receive either 4 or 24 Gy.[205] In 40% of these patients, the treatment was curative in intent and 60% palliative. PFS at 2 years was superior in both the curative and palliative cases for the 24 Gy dose. Thus, 24 to 30 Gy remains the standard dose for curative therapy of localized FL with 2 to 4 Gy reserved for palliation of advanced disease.

The choice of an appropriate radiation field size for localized FL is more complex. Prospective randomized trials addressing this issue do not exist. The field sizes used in the studies in the table were highly variable with no suggestion of a different outcome related to field size. Almost none of the studies employed modern imaging techniques in either the initial diagnosis or subsequent therapy. CT-based three-dimensional treatment planning was carried out in almost none of these studies, yet alone IMRT. The only trial that looked at involved nodal radiotherapy or involved-site radiotherapy and compared it with larger fields was the Campbell trial from British Columbia.[172] This trial had a relatively large number of patients. No difference was observed in the treatment outcome depending on field size. Additional evidence for small fields derives from the patterns of failure in limited-stage FL patients treated with radiotherapy alone. Most recurrence is at distant sites, either nodal, extranodal, or both, very seldom at adjacent nodal areas or within the radiation field.

Extensive guidelines for both radiation field size and target definition and radiation doses have been developed by the International Lymphoma Radiation Oncology Group[153] (Fig. 82.2). Most patients with FL will not have received preradiation systemic therapy, but for those who may have, the target volume is the initial extent of disease prior to any therapeutic intervention. Modern imaging techniques should be used to define the extent of disease, preferably a PET-CT scan. The involved area should be treated with a generous margin, not well defined in the literature and highly dependent on the clinical situation. For example, the margin may be greater

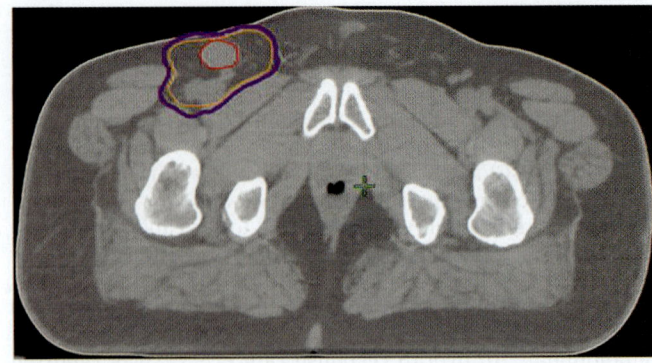

FIGURE 82.2. Stage I follicular lymphoma of a right inguinal lymph node treated with radiation therapy alone using involved-site principles. The gross tumor volume is contoured in *red*. The clinical target volume (*orange*) includes the immediate area at risk of harboring microscopic disease. The planning target volume (*purple*) includes a small margin to account for daily set-up error.

when the disease is not close to important normal organs or tissues. It may be prudent to increase the margin to account for respiratory motion if the latter is not compensated for in some other fashion, such as 4-D planning. For localized FL, the margins should probably be a little larger than customary for localized DLBCL in which the patient is receiving systemic therapy in almost all instances. Patients with localized FL may receive systemic therapy as well, but the lack of proven effectiveness for systemic therapy in this disease would suggest more generous margins to account for subclinical microscopic disease than might be the case for a more aggressive histology such as DLBCL.

Most patients with localized FL have peripheral nodal areas involved such as the neck or inguinal–femoral regions. Usually, relatively simple field arrangements such as AP-PA will suffice, but 3-D planning or IMRT should be considered depending on individual circumstances.

MARGINAL ZONE LYMPHOMAS

MZL accounts for approximately 10% of all cases of NHL. MZL entities include nodal MZL, splenic MZL, and extranodal MZL of mucosa-associated lymphoid tissue (MALT). MALT as a distinct clinical pathologic type of lymphoma was first described in 1983,[207] is the most frequent MZL entity encountered in clinical practice, and will be the focus of the following section. A brief synopsis of nodal and splenic MZL is also included.

Pathology

MALT lymphoma is characterized by a polymorphous infiltrate of marginal zone (centrocyte-like) B cells, small lymphocytes, monocytoid B cells, and plasma cells, as well as rare large basophilic blast cells (centroblast- or immunoblast-like).[208] In epithelial tissues, the marginal zone B cells typically infiltrate the epithelium forming lymphoepithelial lesions defined by invasion and partial obstruction of mucosal glands by tumor cells.[209] Although transformed large cells are typically present, they are in the minority. If present in large numbers, a diagnosis of DLBCL is warranted.

The tumor cells express pan B-cell–associated antigens including CD19, CD20, CD22, and CD79a, but there is no specific marker for MALT at present. However, lack of CD5 (positive in CLL/SLL and MCL), CD10 (positive in FL), and cyclin D1 (positive in MCL) expression helps distinguish MALT from other small B-cell lymphomas.[210]

Clinical Presentation

Two-thirds to three-fourths of patients have stage I or II disease, usually stage I. The most common locations for MALT lymphoma are the stomach, orbit, and skin.[211] Other less common anatomic sites include the parotid, breast, thyroid, and lung. Involvement of paired organs simultaneously, or less commonly two distinct extranodal sites, is occasionally encountered. With such scenarios, it is best to stage each site separately as opposed to making a stage IV designation. Such patients may be treated with local RT to both paired sites with long-term disease control.[212]

The most common site of MALT is the stomach. A unique feature of gastric MALT is the association with *H. pylori* infection, initially reported by Isaacson's group.[30,213] *H. pylori* can be identified in up to 92% of patients.[30] Lymphoid tissue is not normally present in the stomach, but in response to an antigenic stimulus brought about by *H. pylori*, normally, present T cells in the gastric mucosa attract a B-cell population, giving rise to lymphoid follicles and, after prolonged antigenic stimulation, lymphomas.[214]

Recently, an association with bacterial infection for MALT at sites other than the stomach has been described.[215] *Chlamydia psittaci* has been found in many cases of ocular adnexal lymphoma. Additionally, *B. burgdorferi* and *C. jejuni* have been associated with MZL arising in the skin and small intestine, respectively.[215,216] This association is somewhat controversial, however, and unlike gastric MALT, the standard initial treatment for these conditions remains local radiotherapy, as opposed to antibiotics, with very high rates of complete response and local control in excess of 90%, similar to what has been reported for gastric MALT.[217,218]

Patients with orbital MALT typically present with mass lesions in the bulbar or palpebral conjunctivae, described in the literature as "salmon pink" in color. Tumors of the retrobulbar region may present with swelling, proptosis, double vision, and/or other associated disturbances in function of the extraocular muscles. Bilaterality is not unusual, occurring in 10% to 15% of cases. Similar to salivary gland and skin tumors, this does not adversely affect prognosis.

Prognostic Factors

The primary prognostic factor is disease site. MALT arising in paired organs (e.g., orbit or salivary gland) appears to have a higher risk of relapse compared with that arising in a single organ (e.g., stomach or thyroid).[211,217,219] Relapse after RT for cutaneous MZL is also rather frequent.[220]

Treatment of gastric MALT with antibiotics is a special consideration. Predictive factors associated with a lower chance of achieving and maintaining a complete response after antibiotic therapy include deep gastric wall invasion,[221-223] nodal involvement,[223,224] and the translocation t(11;18).[225,226]

Clinical Management

First-line treatment for localized MALT lymphoma should be RT, with the exception of *H. pylori*–positive gastric MALT lymphoma. Complete response rates approach 100% with doses approximately 24 to 30 Gy.[219] Local failure is rare.[211] The overall prognosis of patients with localized MALT lymphoma treated with RT is generally excellent with >90% 5-year survival, although relapses occur in approximately 25% of patients.[211,219,227] Relapses rarely develop within nodal areas but rather sites prone to MALT development. Many such relapses are localized, often in the contralateral paired organ, and after appropriate treatment, often further RT alone, long-term survival is excellent.

For patients with gastric MALT lymphoma, antibiotic treatment is indicated in the presence of *H. pylori* infection. Eradication of *H. pylori* is near universal after antibiotics. A frequently recommended combination is omeprazole, metronidazole, and clarithromycin.[228] A complete response is achieved in approximately 80% of patients, though this may take up to 2 years or longer to achieve.[225] As long as the

lymphoma is regressing on serial endoscopy, a watch and wait policy is appropriate.

Of patients achieving a complete response to antibiotics, approximately 30% will relapse. Many such relapses are subclinical and only apparent on histologic examination of random biopsies performed during upper endoscopy. Continued observation and monitoring is preferred for these patients as many will subsequently revert to a histologic complete response.[31,225]

For patients who are *H. pylori* negative, do not respond to or relapse clinically after antibiotics, the treatment of choice is RT. Long-term progression-free and OS exceeds 90%.[219] Interestingly, the original B-cell clone is also detected frequently after RT for gastric MALT lymphoma but without an associated risk of relapse.[229]

Orbital MZL has been associated with the bacterium *C. psittaci*.[33] A trial of antibiotic therapy has been suggested for patients in whom this organism is identified,[230] but a meta-analysis has shown highly variable results of antibiotic therapy with an overall incidence of *C. psittaci* of 23%.[231] It has also been suggested that observation only is a reasonable strategy. In a Japanese series of 36 patients, 70% did not require treatment with a median follow-up of 7 years.[232] However, for stage I orbital MALT, RT remains the standard of care.

Radiation Dose and Field Design

Detailed radiation field and dose guidelines for extranodal lymphomas, including MALT, have recently been published.[152] For MALT lymphoma, particularly gastric MALT, local control rates of 95% to 100% are achieved with doses of approximately 30 Gy.[219,233] Similar results, although in smaller numbers, are available for MZL at sites other than the stomach.[217,234] A small number of patients with MALT were included in the randomized British National Lymphoma Investigation demonstrating similar clinical outcomes with 24 Gy compared to 40 to 45 Gy.[149] Thus, in general, a dose of 24 to 30 Gy is recommended for localized MALT lymphoma with lower doses (24 Gy) preferred for orbital and parotid presentations.

For stage IE gastric MALT lymphoma, the entire stomach should be included in the clinical target volume. Both 3-D and intensity-modulated RT can be utilized to minimize dose to the heart, liver, and kidneys. Clinicians must be mindful of several characteristics of the stomach that can make IMRT problematic. First, the shape and position of the stomach in the upper abdomen often change from day to day. The patient should fast for 3 to 4 hours before simulation and treatment. Daily cone-beam CTs with soft tissue matching can be helpful in some situations, but in others, the clinical target volume from the planning CT scan simply cannot be matched to the stomach as visualized on the cone-beam CT because of these variations. Second, the stomach typically moves significantly during the respiratory cycle necessitating some form of active respiratory management, especially if IMRT is utilized.

Often, simple AP/PA fields will exclude most of the liver and left kidney depending on the patient's anatomy. When this is unsatisfactory, one helpful 3-D approach is to use a single isocenter, half-beam block technique with the isocenter position at the top of the kidneys. AP/PA (or slightly obliqued) fields are utilized superiorly to treat the upper stomach (while avoiding almost all of the liver) with more obliqued fields (sometimes very close to laterals) utilized inferiorly to avoid the posteriorly positioned kidneys. When treating the entire stomach, 1.5-Gy daily fractions with prophylactic antiemetics are helpful to minimize nausea.

For conjunctival MALT, a single en face electron field provides appropriate coverage of the conjunctiva while minimizing dose to the lacrimal gland and posterior globe. It is usually appropriate to treat the entire conjunctiva. A lens shield is occasionally used to prevent cataracts but may increase marginal misses. We generally do not use one. Well-circumscribed orbital lesions elsewhere can be managed with either a 3-D or IMRT approach. Target volumes are somewhat controversial. Some authors suggest the entire orbit be treated to avoid marginal misses.[235,236] Depending on the size and location, partial orbit coverage may also be reasonable. With doses of approximately 24 Gy, cataract formation is the principle risk, occurring in 20% to 30% of patients,[236] which, however, can be easily corrected surgically. Some dryness may result from inclusion in the field of a portion of the lacrimal gland and meibomian glands.

As mentioned, orbital MZL may involve both eyes at presentation. Under these circumstances, RT alone remains the treatment of choice, with careful attention to treatment planning and prescribed dose to minimize eye complications. For MALT lymphomas of the thyroid and parotid, treatment of the entire gland is generally advisable, given the multifocality of the disease.

In the unusual circumstance of disseminated MALT lymphoma, treatment generally follows the guidelines for advanced FL. Chemotherapy is palliative and reserved for patients with generalized disease who are symptomatic. MALT lymphomas also respond well to rituximab.[237] Asymptomatic individuals with generalized disease should be considered for observation, similar to patients with generalized FL because the course is so often indolent. Patients with generalized disease with symptoms because of a localized tumor mass may be easily palliated with modest doses of RT (e.g., 2 Gy × 2) to the mass in question. That approach is often superior to systemic chemotherapy. There is no role for chemotherapy or rituximab in localized disease.

Splenic and Nodal Marginal Zone Lymphoma

Splenic MZL patients usually present with splenomegaly.[238-240] Almost all have stage IV disease, principally because of bone marrow or blood involvement. The disease is relatively indolent with three-quarters of patients alive at 5 years, but a more aggressive subset does exist. Observation is typically pursued for asymptomatic patients. When symptomatic, splenectomy, rituximab, or chemoimmunotherapy are all options. Nodal MZL generally presents like FL, with widespread nodal disease. For the rare patient with localized disease, definitive RT (24 to 30 Gy) is recommended.

MANTLE CELL LYMPHOMA

MCL was first distinguished in the 1980s by Weisenburger et al.,[241] who described a type of FL in which there were wide mantles of malignant cells around apparently benign germinal centers. It was thought to represent a variant of FL and was classified under the Working Formulation as a low-grade lymphoma. Its behavior, however, is more characteristic of aggressive disease. MCL represents about 7% of all NHL.[64]

Pathology

Additional features of this disease have been recognized since Weisenburger and colleagues' original description. It is a neoplasm of small- to medium-sized B cells with irregular nuclei that resemble the cleaved cells (centrocytes) of germinal centers. The morphologic pattern may be diffuse, nodular, a mantle zone, or some combination thereof.[242]

Tumor cells are typically CD5 positive, CD23 negative, CD20 positive, and CD10 negative. A characteristic cytogenetic abnormality is t(11;14) involving the *BCL-1* gene and resulting in the overexpression of cyclin D1. The product of the cyclin D1 gene can be detected in paraffin-embedded tissue sections with the immunoperoxidase technique and is useful in distinguishing MCL from other lymphoma variants.[243,244]

Immunophenotyping studies are useful in confirming malignancy (light-chain restriction) and in excluding other B-cell histologies such as chronic lymphocytic leukemia (CD5+) and FLs (CD10+).[210]

Clinical Presentation

MCL has a 74% male preponderance and a median age of 63 years.[157,245] Eighty percent of patients have stage III or IV disease at onset. IPI scores are high, with 23% of patients with a score of 4 or 5, 54% 2 or 3, and only 23% 0 or 1. In common with FL, the organ most likely to be involved is the bone marrow, which is positive in two-thirds of patients at the time of diagnosis. Gastrointestinal tract involvement is frequent as well.[246] CNS is occasionally encountered, particularly those with blastoid histology or elevated LDH.[247]

Prognostic Factors

Although originally classified among the low-grade/indolent lymphomas, the clinical course for MCL is unfavorable in the great majority of patients. The 5-year survival rate in the ILSG project was only 27%, with a PFS rate of 11%.[157] This PFS rate is, in fact, among the worst for virtually any type of lymphoma. The survival pattern of MCL resembles advanced FL in its response to therapy and PFS (i.e., no plateauing of the PFS curve and thus no indication of cure), but DLBCL in its OS (i.e., much shorter than FL).[248-251] A proportion of MCL patients have a more indolent course, but identifying these patients prospectively can be challenging.

A simple prognostic scoring has continued utility: the MIPI or MCL IPI.[252] This index uses four parameters: age, performance status, LDH, and leukocyte count. The MIPI score allows discrimination into three prognostic subgroups: median survival was not reached in the low-risk group with a 5-year OS of 60%, but was 51 and 29 months in the intermediate- and high-risk groups, respectively. Multiple reports have shown consistent reliability of the MIPI prognostic scoring that has had independent significance over pathologic, molecular-based, and clinical/therapeutic predictors.[253]

Clinical Management

Chemoimmunotherapy is the standard initial treatment for all stages of MCL. Rituximab is generally combined with chemotherapy regimens as it is CD20+.[254,255] There is no standard treatment regimen for MCL. The choice of chemotherapy regimen is often guided by age and performance status. Both aggressive (e.g., R-hyperCVAD [rituximab, cyclophosphamide, vincristine, doxorubicin, dexamethasone, cytarabine, and methotrexate]) and less aggressive (R-CHOP, BR [bendamustine and rituximab]),[187] regimens are available. HDC and ASCT are often pursued in patients who achieve a complete response to first-time therapy. For patients not eligible for transplant, maintenance rituximab should be considered.[256]

Patients with localized MCL (stage I or II) are seldom encountered. One small series from British Columbia has been reported.[257] Of 26 patients reviewed, 17 received RT with or without chemotherapy and 9 patients received chemotherapy or were observed. RT was associated with improved PFS (68% vs. 11%, *P* = .002). This finding was corroborated by a large NCDB database analysis.[258] Thus, for early-stage disease, we recommend a combined modality approach. RT is also very effective palliation for patients with advanced disease.[259] Modest doses (4 to 10 Gy) are typically sufficient in the palliative setting.

Radiation Dose and Field Design

For the minority of patients presenting with localized (stage I to II) disease, we recommend consolidation RT after chemoimmunotherapy. In the setting of a complete response by PET-CT, a dose of 30 Gy is appropriate. Treatment of the original site of disease with a margin, following involved-site principles, is recommended.

PRIMARY CNS LYMPHOMA

PCNSL comprises all primary intracerebral or intraocular lymphomas. The incidence of PCNSL has been increasing for several decades.[260] This increase is only partially attributable to HIV-associated cases, with a significant rise in immunocompetent patients.

Pathology

The majority of PCNSL are of B-cell lineage, typically DLBCL though T-cell histology,[261] lymphoblastic, and Burkitt lymphomas are occasionally encountered.[262] In immunocompromised patients, the lymphoma is virtually always associated with EBV[263] but is rare in immunocompetent patients.

Clinical Presentation

The median age at presentation is 55 years for immunocompetent patients and 31 years for patients with HIV-associated disease. Neurologic symptoms are usually of brief duration, 3 months or less. Specific neurologic deficits depend on tumor location. Generalized symptomatology such as altered mental status, seizures, and symptoms of increased intracranial pressure such as headache, nausea, and vomiting may occur. Immunocompetent patients are more likely to have localized neurologic deficits, in contrast to patients with HIV infection who more often have diffuse disease with generalized symptomatology.[264,265]

Radiologic imaging often suggests the diagnosis. PCNSL is usually isodense or hyperdense on nonenhanced CT scans, in contradistinction to other primary brain tumors or metastatic lesions. The preferred imaging modality for PCNSL is MRI, which can detect up to 10% of lesions missed by CT. Lesions appear isointense to hypointense on T1-weighted images, and approximately 50% are hyperintense on T2-weighted imaging. Homogeneous contrast enhancement is commonly seen in immunocompetent patients.[266] Despite the appearance of a focal mass on CT or MRI imaging, diffuse parenchymal infiltration is often present, underestimated by imaging. The majority of PCNSL occur in a periventricular distribution, involving the corpus callosum, thalamus, or basal ganglia. In patients with HIV infection, disease is often multifocal in the brain and may be difficult to distinguish from CNS infections.[264]

At diagnosis, although most patients with PCNSL have a solitary brain lesion, the presence of leptomeningeal and ocular involvement is seen in approximately 33% and 20% of cases, respectively. Evaluation of these areas is indicated, including lumbar puncture (if the intracranial pressure is not increased and it can be done safely) and full ophthalmologic evaluation. Staging to evaluate for extracranial disease is appropriate.[264,267]

Prognostic Factors

Almost all studies reveal age and performance status to be important independent prognostic factors. A prognostic model developed at Memorial Sloan-Kettering from 338 patients with PCNSL incorporates age and Karnofsky performance status dividing patients into three prognostic classes with distinct survivals. Class 1 includes patients < 50 years with a median survival of 8.5 years. Class 2 patients are ≥50 years with good performance status (KPS ≥ 70) with median survival of 3.2 years. Class 3 includes patients ≥ 50 years with poor performance status (KPS < 70) with median survival of 1 year.[268] The International Extranodal Lymphoma Study Group (IELSG) has

also reported elevated LDH, increased CSF protein, and tumor location within the deep regions of the brain as significant prognostic variables.[268–270]

Clinical Management

The role of surgery in the management of PCNSL is limited to establishing the diagnosis, preferably by stereotactic biopsy. PCNSL is usually not amenable to surgical resection because of deep location, involvement of critical structures, and its microscopically widespread infiltrative nature. Occasionally, surgical decompression and shunt placement are necessary for relief of increased intracranial pressure. CSF analysis, including immunoglobulin gene rearrangement studies, can identify clonal populations to confirm the diagnosis of PCNSL.[271] Corticosteroids, commonly used to alleviate symptoms including intracranial pressure, have a direct antitumor effect.[267] Tumor regression may lead to difficulties in establishing diagnosis. Accordingly, steroids should be withheld if possible until after biopsy if the diagnosis of lymphoma is suspected.

The management of PCNSL has evolved over recent years. Historically, the treatment was whole-brain radiation therapy (WBRT) alone to address the disease's multifocal nature. Results were poor, however, despite the known radiosensitivity of DLBCL outside the CNS. Two representative series from Radiation Therapy Oncology Group (RTOG) and Princess Margaret Hospital report median survivals of 12.2 and 17 months, respectively, with 5-year survival rates of 10% to 20%.[272,273] Although the tumor initially responds to RT, regrowth is inevitable and uncontrolled disease in the brain is the primary cause of death. Attempts at dose escalation beyond 50 Gy resulted in high toxicity rates without improvements in survival.[273]

Given the poor results achieved with RT alone and the chemo-responsiveness of lymphomas generally, evaluation of systemic chemotherapy for PCNSL was soon undertaken. Initial programs consisted of CHOP and variations on that combination. Despite the efficacy of this combination in NHL outside the CNS, the results in PCNSL have been disappointing.[274] Other studies have come to similar conclusions. This lack of efficacy may be due to the failure of many drugs to penetrate the blood–brain barrier (BBB).

Methotrexate (MTX), particularly in high doses, is known to penetrate the BBB. It was first used for treatment of PCNSL in 1980 with subsequent use becoming widespread.[264] There has been much variability in dosage, scheduling, and combinations with intrathecal methotrexate and other cytotoxics such as cytarabine, vincristine, thiotepa, temozolomide, and rituximab. The phase II RTOG 9310 study treated patients with combination chemotherapy, including high-dose MTX and WBRT. The 5-year OS was 32% with PFS of 25%, results better than historically obtained with RT alone.[275]

The primary concern with the combination of high-dose MTX and full-dose WBRT is neurotoxicity.[276,277] Neurologic complications can arise as early as 3 months post treatment with symptoms of attention deficit, ataxia, urinary incontinence, and memory impairment, which may ultimately lead to dementia.[278] Patients older than age 60 seem to be at highest risk. A multiinstitutional retrospective series reported a 30% actuarial rate of neurotoxicity overall, with patients >60 years having a 58% risk at 7 years.[279] Given higher neurologic toxicity rates in the elderly, many institutions treat this subset of patients with chemotherapy alone.[280,281]

An alternative approach is reduced-dose WBRT. The Memorial Sloan-Kettering group has reduced the dose to 23.4 Gy for patients achieving complete response to rituximab and MTX-based chemotherapy with promising results.[282] Median PFS and OS for all patients enrolled on the study were 3.3 and 6.6 years, respectively. For those patients who achieved a complete response and received reduced-dose WBRT, the 5-year OS was 80%. Significant post-WBRT neurotoxicity was not observed.

The largest phase III study in this disease was conducted in Germany and sought to evaluate the role of WBRT after high-dose MTX-based regimens. The dose of WBRT was 45 Gy. The study was hampered by poor protocol compliance and a complicated trial design. Although PFS was improved with WBRT, there was no difference in OS.[283]

Future areas of research include additional chemotherapeutic drugs in combination with high-dose MTX. Regimens including cytarabine and rituximab have been reported in the literature.[284,285] A recent randomized phase II trial with the International Extranodal Lymphoma Study Group-32 demonstrated that the MATRix regimen, methotrexate, cytarabine, thiotepa, and rituximab, had superior complete response rate versus methotrexate and cytarabine alone, 49% versus 23%.[284]

HDC with ASCT has also been evaluated. Soussain et al. reported 96% CR after HDC and ASCT. Two-year OS was 45% among the entire cohort and 69% among the 27 patients undergoing HDC and ASCT.[286] Additional studies have evaluated the use of HDC and ASCT, many in combination with WBRT, in newly diagnosed PCNSL.[287-292] A randomized trial for patients <60 years old comparing WBRT or HDC–ASCT as consolidation after high-dose MTX is ongoing.[278]

To conclude, the role of WBRT after high-dose MTX is controversial, particularly in patients achieving a complete response to chemotherapy and in those >60 years old. It seems clear that 45-Gy WBRT results in unacceptable toxicity in older patients and perhaps in younger ones as well. Given the overall unsatisfactory results with chemotherapy alone, the addition of low-dose RT (23.4 Gy) to chemotherapy for patients achieving a complete response remains a promising approach. Several trials are ongoing that may help delineate the role of WBRT in PCNSL–RTOG 1114, PRECIS, and IELSG 32.

Radiation Dose and Field Design

Radiation field design is a standard whole-brain field with a couple of adjustments. Because the CSF surrounds optic apparatus and is contiguous with the intracranial cavity, with the vitreous space frequently involved, the posterior globes should be encompassed in the RT field. In addition, the inferior border of the field should be at the C1/C2 vertebral body to cover the obex, where the fourth ventricle narrows to become the central canal of the spinal cord (Fig. 82.3). Prophylactic RT to the spine is not recommended.

FIGURE 82.3. Whole-brain radiation fields to treat primary CNS lymphoma. Note the isocenter is placed at the lens and the posterior globe is included in the field.

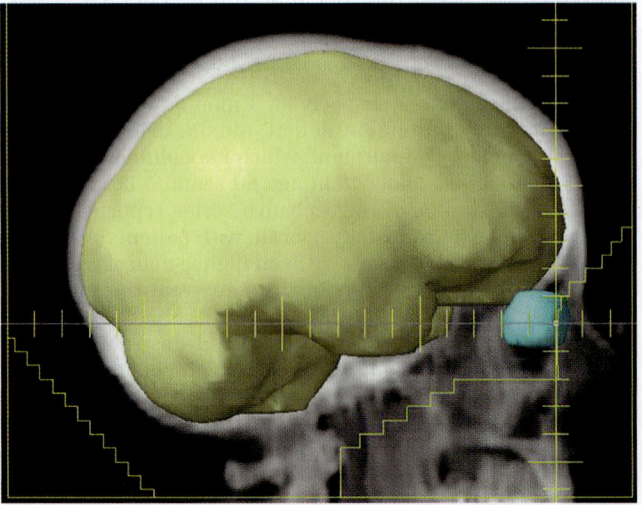

PERIPHERAL T-CELL LYMPHOMAS

The PTCLs are the group most confusing to clinicians. The term PTCL is often misinterpreted. It refers not to the anatomic distribution of the lymphomas but to their origin, from so-called peripheral or mature T cells outside the thymus, as opposed to thymic (precursor) T lymphocytes. The T-cell and NK lymphomas collectively make up approximately 10% of all NHL.[293] Their frequency is quite different, however, by geographic locale with a roughly 5% to 10% incidence of PTCL in North America compared with 15% to 20% in Asia.[294] They are a diverse group that includes nearly 30 distinct entities (Table 82.1).

Pathology

PTCL, not otherwise specified (NOS), typically contains a mixture of medium and/or large cells with many mitotic figures. The architectural pattern is diffuse. T-cell–associated antigens (CD2, CD3, CD4) are variably expressed, and oftentimes, the T-cell antigens CD5 and CD7 are lost. A CD4+/CD8– phenotype is typical in nodal cases.[55] B-cell–associated antigens are lacking. The T-cell receptor genes (*TCR*) are usually but not always rearranged. T-cell receptor beta-chain is typically expressed distinguishing PTCL from NK and $\gamma\delta$ T-cell lymphomas.

A special variant of PTCL is anaplastic large-cell lymphoma (ALCL).[295,296] In the ILSG project, this comprised 2% of all NHL.[64] The tumor is usually composed of large cells with round, pleomorphic, or horseshoe-shaped nuclei with single or multiple prominent nucleoli and abundant cytoplasm, giving the cells an epithelial or histiocyte-like appearance. The cells express CD30 (Ki-1) and usually express CD25 and either T-cell or null lineage–specific antigens.[296] CD30 was originally recognized on HL cells. In some cases, there may be confusion between ALCL and HL, but distinction between the two on the basis of immunophenotyping and morphology is usually possible. The WHO recognizes two distinct entities—ALK-positive ALCL and ALK-negative ALCL, with the former characterized by overexpression of anaplastic lymphoma kinase (ALK-1) protein, typically from a chromosomal translocation [t(2:5)].[297] Approximately 60% of cases overexpress the ALK protein; such cases have a better prognosis than ALK-negative cases (except primary cutaneous ALCL which is invariably ALK negative but has an excellent prognosis).

Extranodal NK/T-cell lymphomas are characterized by a diffuse lymphomatous infiltrate with an angiocentric pattern. Necrosis is common and attributed to vascular obstruction by lymphoma cells, though chemokines and cytokines may also be contributory. CD56, though not specific for NK cells, is generally expressed with extranodal NK/T-cell lymphoma. Cytotoxic molecules including granzyme B and perforin are also positive. Epstein-Barr virus analyses, preferably *in situ* hybridization, are mandatory and should be positive. No specific translocations have been observed for this disease.

Clinical Presentation

The most common T-cell lymphoma in North America is PTCL NOS, accounting for about one-third of cases (vs. ~20% in Asia).[298,299] This is a disease of older adults with a median age of 60 years with a slight male predominance. Both nodal and extranodal disease is common in a similar fashion to B-cell lymphoma. In contrast to DLBCL, however, the great majority of patients (70%) have stage III or IV disease at diagnosis, and overall the outlook is considerably worse. The International T-Cell Lymphoma Project reported 10-year survivals in the range of 20%.[300]

ALCL consists of both a systemic malignancy, typically presenting with widespread involvement of lymph nodes and extranodal sites, and a type limited to the skin (primary cutaneous ALCL).[296,301-305] The systemic type may in turn be separated into those patients who are ALK positive and those who do not overexpress this protein. The clinical features and prognosis differ widely among these two categories. Patients with ALK-positive ALCL are predominantly young men and, despite advanced stage disease, respond well to combination chemotherapy with 10-year survival rates of approximately 70%.[297,306] ALCL in children/young adults is usually ALK positive.[296] ALK-negative patients, in contrast, tend to be older with a more nearly equal male to female ratio, with a long-term OS of approximately 20%.

Cutaneous ALCL constitutes a special situation.[301] It is almost invariably ALK-negative but carries an excellent prognosis. It is often difficult to distinguish from benign lymphomatoid papulosis (LyP). The latter may spontaneously remit and tends to run a benign clinical course over many years. ALCL of the skin is quite responsive and highly curable with localized radiotherapy[307] (see Chapter 83). Chemotherapy generally has no role.

Extranodal NK/T-cell lymphoma is a T-cell lymphoma of special interest. This lymphoma has a variety of names in the older literature, including angiocentric lymphoma, midline malignant reticulosis, polymorphic reticulosis, and lethal midline granuloma. It is much more frequent in Asia (about 22% of T-cell lymphomas) than in the United States and associated with EBV.[308] In contrast to most lymphomas, tissue destruction of the nasal/facial area is common. The response to chemotherapy and radiotherapy is variable and slow, in contrast to the usual rapid response observed in most other lymphomas.[309] The disease appears to progress primarily locally with only a small predilection for regional or systemic failure.[310]

A provisional entity in the current WHO classification is breast implant–associated ALCL.[56] Initially described in 1997, it often presents as an accumulation of fluid between the implant and the fibrous capsule. Given the rarity of this presentation, the optimal management remains largely unknown though capsulectomy, and removal of the implant appears to be essential.[311] Outcomes for those with disease confined within the fibrous capsule are excellent with surgery alone.

Prognostic Factors

Two prognostic scores are commonly utilized for PTCL NOS including the IPI and the Prognostic Index for PTCL-U (PIT). The IPI, primarily utilized for DLBCL, has also been shown to be prognostic in PTCL.[298] The PIT identified four factors on multivariate analysis including three that are also contained in the IPI—age ≥ 60 years, elevated LDH, and ECOG performance ≥ 2. The novel factor was bone marrow involvement.[312] Five-year survival was 33% with 0 to 2 risk factors and 18% for 3 or 4 risk factors. Patients with stage I to II disease, although quite uncommon, also appear to have a more favorable prognosis.[313]

Several studies have shown that survival is significantly better with ALK-positive ALCL compared with ALK-negative ALCL.[297,306,314,315] The International Peripheral T-cell Lymphoma Project demonstrated that ALK-positive ALCL has the most favorable prognosis among all T and NK histologies, followed by ALK-negative ALCL.[299] The heterogeneity and complexity of ALCL well illustrate past difficulties of attempting to group lymphomas in categories of low, intermediate, and high grade, indolent or aggressive, and favorable or unfavorable, on the basis of histologic appearance alone, because all ALCL appears aggressive histologically. There remains some uncertainty whether ALK expression is independently prognostic or simply correlates with other favorable factors (e.g., young age). A recent report from the Groupe d'Etude

des Lymphomes de l'Adulte demonstrated elevated β2 microglobulin and older age as independent prognostic factors, but not ALK status.[314] ALK was also not independently prognostic in the study by Suzuki et al.[316] However, other reports have demonstrated independent prognostic significance of ALK.[297,306]

For extranodal NK/T-cell lymphomas, age ≥ 60 years, stage III to IV disease, distant lymph node involvement, and nonnasal type disease are unfavorable prognostic factors. A validated prognostic index stratifies patients into low-, intermediate-, and high-risk cohorts with 0, 1, or ≥ 2 risk factors.[317] In a study of 527 patients, 3-year OS was 81%, 62%, and 25%, respectively. Detectable EBV DNA in the circulating blood at diagnosis also appeared to be a negative prognostic factor.

Clinical Management

For PTCL NOS and ALCL, CHOP is probably the most commonly employed regimen in the United States. For younger patients, the addition of etoposide (CHOEP) can be considered.[318] Because this is a T-cell lymphoma, there is no role for rituximab. For the minority of patients who present with stage I to II PTCL[298,319] or ALCL,[320] consolidation RT after chemotherapy is recommended. Three-year PFS and OS were 50% and 33% in early-stage PTCL NOS with combined modality therapy versus 23% and 15% with chemotherapy alone, in one small series.[319]

The optimal treatment of localized NK/T-cell lymphoma, nasal type, is not established. Treatment approaches have consisted of RT alone, chemotherapy alone, and the two combined. With RT alone, approximately two-thirds of patients achieved CR,[310,321,322] but half of those relapsed. The prognosis appears somewhat worse for stage II than stage I.[322]

The contribution of chemotherapy to the management of NK/T-cell lymphoma is unclear. When treated initially with CHOP-like regimens, CR occurs in only a minority of patients,[309,322-324] in contrast to the results seen with most other lymphomas. Japanese and Korean investigators have reported the use of concurrent chemotherapy and radiation with encouraging results.[325,326] The Japanese series used concurrent dexamethasone, etoposide, carboplatin, and ifosfamide with a dose of 50 Gy. The CR rate was 77% and the 2-year survival 78% compared with historical controls of 45%.[325] The Korean series employed concurrent cisplatin and radiation (40 to 50 Gy), followed by 3 cycles of cisplatin, dexamethasone, ifosfamide, and etoposide. The CR rate was 83%, the 3-year survival 86%.[326] In both series, the number of patients was small (33 and 30 patients, respectively), but the results are quite promising and worthy of further study. Sequential chemoradiation regimens using pegaspargase (e.g., SMILE, GELOX) can also be considered. There are no data, particularly from the United States, to recommend one regimen over another at this point.

RT Dose and Field Design

Doses and field sizes of RT for PTCL NOS and ALCL should approximate those for DLBCL. For extranodal NK/T-cell lymphomas, nasal type, higher doses of RT are generally employed. With RT alone, the recommended tumor dose is 50 to 56 Gy. When RT is given with concurrent or sequential chemotherapy, doses of 45 to 56 Gy can be considered. In general, adhering to published protocols, in relation to both dose and field, is prudent, given the rarity of this disease. IMRT is often, but not always, required given the proximity of the tumor to critical structures such as the optic apparatus, parotid glands, and brain and brainstem (Fig. 82.4). More detailed recommendations have been published by the International Lymphoma Radiation Oncology Group.[152]

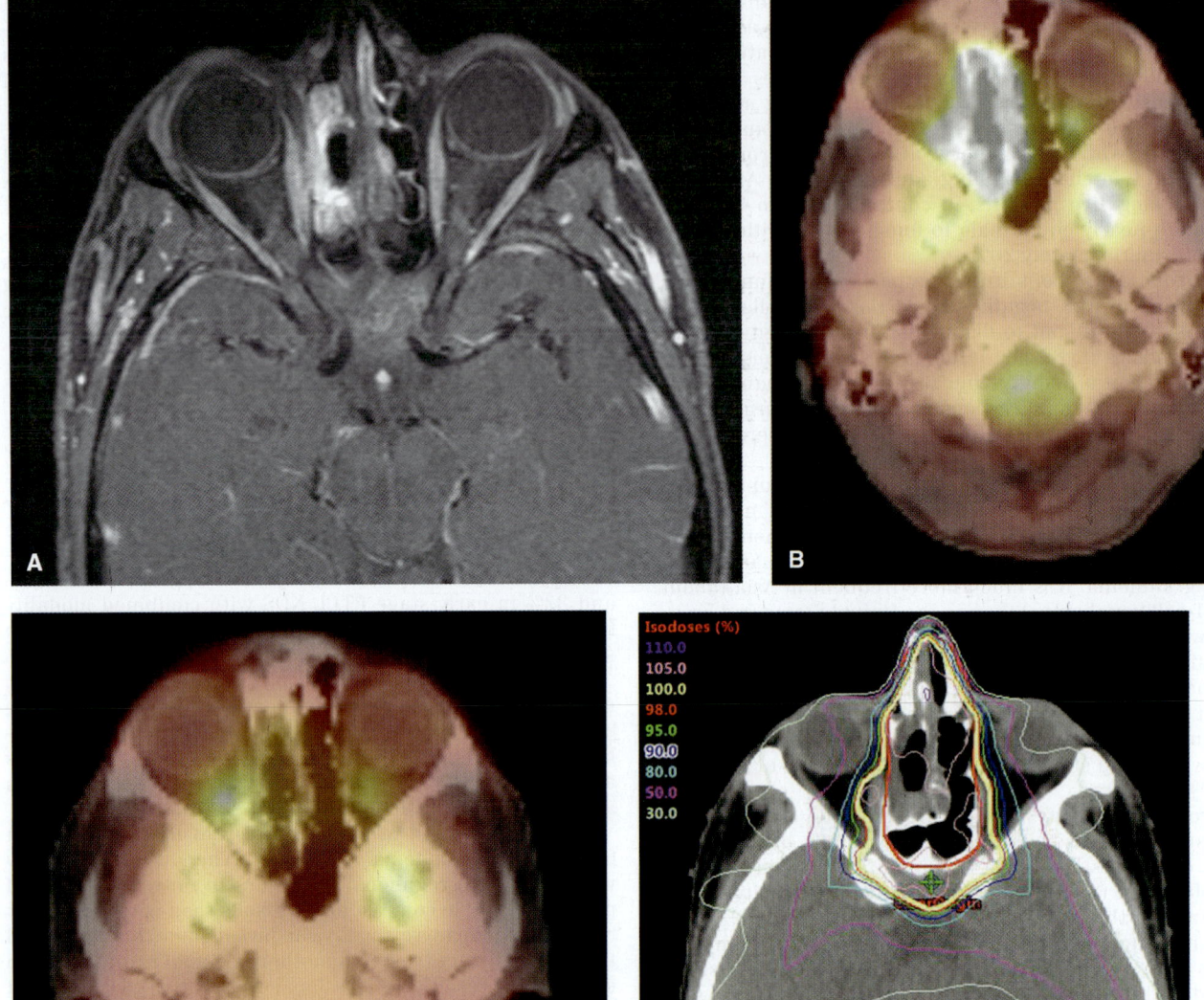

FIGURE 82.4. IE NK/T-cell lymphoma of the left nasal cavity and ethmoid sinuses on MRI **(A)** and PET-CT **(B)**. The patient achieved a complete response **(C)** by PET-CT (Deauville 2) after SMILE chemotherapy (dexamethasone, methotrexate, ifosfamide, pegaspargase, etoposide). He then received consolidation RT **(D)** to 50 Gy. The clinical target volume (*red contour*) included bilateral nasal cavities and ethmoid sinuses.

PRIMARY MEDIASTINAL (THYMIC) LARGE B-CELL LYMPHOMA

Primary mediastinal (thymic) large B-cell lymphoma (PMBCL) comprises about 2% of all NHL and is believed to arise from thymic medullary B cells. Although the histologic appearance can vary, compartmentalizing alveolar fibrosis is a common feature. PMBCL expresses pan B-cell antigens, including CD20, but are negative for surface immunoglobulin. CD30 is present in a majority of patients but stains weaker than classical

HL.[55] Microarray studies have revealed a unique molecular signature for PMBCL with a resemblance to nodular sclerosis HL.[327] The disease affects primarily young women (median age 37) and is generally confined to the anterior mediastinum, sometimes with supraclavicular or cervical adenopathy. When grouped according to the IPI, the prognosis is similar to that of DLBCL generally, perhaps a bit more favorable[327,328] with a plateau observed in the PFS curve after 18 to 24 months.[328]

PMBCL is typically managed with standard chemotherapy (R-CHOP) plus consolidation RT (30 Gy) or more intensive chemotherapy (DA-EPOCH-R) without RT.[329,330] Omission of RT with DA-EPOCH-R is primarily based on phase II[331] and retrospective data,[330] and more studies are needed. The failure of DA-EPOCH-R to improve outcomes compared with R-CHOP in DLBCL NOS should temper enthusiasm of this regimen in PMBCL until more data are available.[101] An ongoing randomized trial (IELSG-37, NCT01599559) is evaluating the role of RT when a complete metabolic response is achieved to R-CHOP-like regimens. As this disease presents in a similar fashion to nodular sclerosis HL, with a gene expression profile more closely aligned with HL then DLBCL, a combined modality approach is still reasonable with R-CHOP, perhaps utilizing a lower dose of consolidation RT (20 Gy) if a complete response is achieved by PET-CT.

T-CELL/HISTIOCYTE-RICH LARGE B-CELL LYMPHOMA

T-cell/histiocyte-rich B-cell lymphoma consists of large malignant B cells with a florid background of inflammatory T cells, with or without histiocytes. Clinically, it occurs in a younger population compared with DLBCL, generally with a male predominance.[332,333] This entity is also more likely to present with B symptoms and involve the spleen, liver, and bone marrow. Treatment recommendations are similar to DLBCL, not otherwise specified.

CHRONIC LYMPHOCYTIC LEUKEMIA/ SMALL LYMPHOCYTIC LYMPHOMA

CLL/SLL represents a spectrum of hematopoietic neoplasia involving an overproliferation of mature B cells, typically afflicting the elderly. A diagnosis of CLL requires the presence of $> 5.0 \times 10^9$/L monoclonal CLL cells in the peripheral blood with or without lymph node/splenic involvement, whereas a diagnosis of SLL includes CLL involvement of the lymph nodes and/or spleen in the absence of a lymphocytosis $>5.0 \times 10^9$/L.[334] Monoclonal B lymphocytosis is a third entity seen in healthy asymptomatic adults who have a monoclonal B-cell lymphocytosis $<5.0 \times 10^9$/L with no evidence of cytopenias, splenic, or nodal involvement. Histologically, CLL cells have a similar appearance to mature lymphocytes with scant cytoplasm, a dense nuclei, and no discernible nucleoli.[335] During the tissue preparation process, CLL cells are more prone to rupture than healthy lymphocytes forming "smudge cells" (Gumprecht phenomenon). There is some evidence to suggest that an increased percentage of these cells present on peripheral smear conveys a poor prognosis.[336]

CLL/SLL is most commonly diagnosed following an elevated WBC discovered during a routine office visit. In symptomatic patients, 80% present with lymphadenopathy and 60% with splenomegaly. Less common symptoms include weight loss, bleeding, infections, and anemia, which are usually indicative of advanced disease.[337]

Diagnosis of CLL is made by flow cytometry of peripheral blood, which should confirm a monoclonal B-cell population. A typical immunophenotype of CLL is CD5+, CD10-, CD20 dim, and CD23+. FISH analysis for t(11:14) is helpful to distinguish it from MCL, which is included in the differential diagnosis of CD5+ B-cell neoplasms.[338] If analysis of peripheral blood confirms CLL, a bone marrow biopsy is not required. A diagnosis of SLL can similarly be made with flow cytometry of a biopsied lymph node or with immunohistochemistry for the above cell surface makers. Workup for CLL/SLL should include history (with specific inquiry into the presence of B symptoms) and physical exam (with focus on node-bearing areas, liver and spleen). Imaging with a CT chest/abdomen/pelvis may be helpful to characterize the extent of disease, but PET-CT is

typically not recommended in CLL unless Richter transformation is suspected.[339]

The modified Rai staging system stratifies CLL patients into risk categories as follows: low-risk disease is confined to marrow and blood; intermediate risk includes presence of lymphadenopathy, splenomegaly, or hepatomegaly; and high risk includes thrombocytopenia or anemia. Approximately 30% present with low-risk disease and 10% present with high-risk disease.[337] The Binet system separates patients by the number of sites involved: Stage A includes two or fewer sites; stage B includes three or more sites; and stage C includes those with cytopenias.[335] Additionally, the Ann Arbor staging may be applied for lymph node–only disease.

In the 1990s, the mutational status of the variable region of the immunoglobulin heavy chain (IgH) was identified as a prognostic marker. Somatic mutation of the IgH naturally occurs as part of B-cell maturation in the germinal centers. In CLL, those with an unmutated IgH (i.e., >98% homology with the germ line) have a worse prognosis than mutated IgH independent of stage.[340] Elevated expression of cell surface proteins Zap70 (>20%), CD38 (>30%), and CD49d (>30%), as well as elevated serum levels of β2 microglobulin (>3.5 mg/L), and thymidine kinase (>10 U/L) have all been associated with a worse prognosis.[341] The advent of interphase FISH and next-generation genetic sequencing has led to a better understanding of the cytogenetic and mutational underpinnings of CLL and has improved prognostic stratification. An integrated mutational and cytogenetic analysis by Rossi et al. yielded four prognostic groups: very low risk (del13q14) with 10-year survival of 69.3%—similar to general population, low risk (normal genetics or trisomy 12) with 10-year survival of 57%; intermediate risk (NOTCH1 mut, SF3B1 mut, and/or del11q22-23) with 10-year survival 37%, and high risk (TP53 or BIRC3 abnormalities) with 10-year survival 29%.[342,343]

For asymptomatic CLL/SLL patients with low- or intermediate-risk disease, observation is usually advised until the development of symptoms, anemia or thrombocytopenia. In progressive or high-risk disease, first-line chemotherapy with fludarabine, cyclophosphamide, and rituximab is recommended for young and fit patients, whereas bendamustine and rituximab are recommended for those >65 or with significant comorbidities.[344,345] Response to chemotherapy is poor in patients with p53 mutations or del17p. Ibrutinib monotherapy may have activity in this population.[346]

Definitive RT is preferred in the treatment of localized SLL (stage I), which is seldom encountered. Radiation technique is similar to that of other indolent NHLs. The recommended total dose is 24 to 30 Gy, and treatment volumes should follow involved-site principles similar to FL. Like FL, RT can be used to palliate symptomatic lymphadenopathy in CLL/SLL. A small series of 14 patients with symptomatic SLL was treated with 2 Gy × 2 with involved field radiation, resulting in an overall response rate of 85% with a median time to local progression of 14 months.[204] The regimen can be safely repeated if symptoms recur.

POSTTRANSPLANT LYMPHOPROLIFERATIVE DISORDERS

The number and the success of solid organ and hematopoietic stem cell transplants have increased with corresponding improvements in OS. Unfortunately, with long-term immunosuppression, posttransplant lymphoproliferative disorders (PTLD) are being increasingly diagnosed. EBV is implicated in the majority of cases (50% to 80%), especially if PTLD occurs within 2 years of transplantation. All other non-EBV cases of PTLD are of unknown etiology.[347]

During the diagnostic workup, infection with lymphoplasmacytic infiltrations, graft rejection, graft-versus-host disease, and/or recurrence from a previous lymphoma should be ruled out. Pathology presents on a spectrum and is divided into four main categories: (1) early lesions, (2) polymorphic PTLD, (3) monomorphic PTLD, and (4) classic HL-like PTLD. The most common subtypes are posttransplant DLBCL, BL, and plasmablastic lymphoma.

The prognosis of PTLD is poor compared to immunocompetent counterparts with similar histologies. Five-year OS ranges from 40% to 60%. The IPI can be used in patients with PTLD to predict outcomes. Other various prognostic indices have been developed as well but ultimately are fraught with validation inconsistencies. Still, older age, advanced disease, poor KPS, elevated LDH, and CNS involvement are consistently associated with inferior outcomes.[348]

In solid organ PTLD, reduction of immunosuppression should be considered, which can lead to responses in about 10% of people within a matter of weeks. Caution should be taken to prevent graft rejection or graft-versus-host disease. If no response is achieved with immunosuppression reduction, rituximab can be considered for CD20+ PTLDs. Overall response rates are approximately 40%, and complete response rates can be almost 30% with little risk of treatment-related mortality.[349] Chemotherapy can also provide good responses but are associated with increased toxicity. A phase II study demonstrated that the combination of rituximab and CHOP is an effective combination with up to a 90% response rate and a 68% complete response rate.[350] Mortality from chemotherapy remains a significant risk in PTLD.[350,351]

Radiation is reserved for localized disease (consolidation after chemotherapy or as a definitive modality) or in palliative situations. Involved site radiation principles with appropriate doses depending on the underlying histology are recommended.

REFERENCES

1. Howlader N, Noone AM, Krapcho M, et al. SEER Cancer Statistics Review, 1975–2013, 2016; http://seer.cancer.gov/csr/1975_2013/. Accessed January 12, 2017.
2. Ferlay J SI, Ervik M, Dikshit R, et al. GLOBOCAN 2012 v1.0, Cancer Incidence and Mortality Worldwide: IARC CancerBase No. 11 [Internet], 2013; http://globocan.iarc.fr. Accessed January 12, 2017.
3. Torre LA, Bray F, Siegel RL, et al. Global cancer statistics, 2012. *CA Cancer J Clin* 2015;65(2):87–108.
4. Dave SS, Wright G, Tan B, et al. Prediction of survival in follicular lymphoma based on molecular features of tumor-infiltrating immune cells. *N Engl J Med* 2004;351(21):2159–2169.
5. Behler CM, Kaplan LD. Advances in the management of HIV-related non-Hodgkin lymphoma. *Curr Opin Oncol* 2006;18(5):437–443.
6. Gottschalk S, Rooney CM, Heslop HE. Post-transplant lymphoproliferative disorders. *Annu Rev Med* 2005;56:29–44.
7. Silverberg MJ, Lau B, Achenbach CJ, et al. Cumulative incidence of cancer among persons with HIV in North America: a cohort study. *Ann Intern Med* 2015;163(7):507–518.
8. Gibson TM, Morton LM, Shiels MS, et al. Risk of non-Hodgkin lymphoma subtypes in HIV-infected people during the HAART era: a population-based study. *Aids* 2014;28(15):2313–2318.
9. Howlader N, Shiels MS, Mariotto AB, et al. Contributions of HIV to Non-Hodgkin Lymphoma Mortality Trends in the United States. *Cancer Epidemiol Biomarkers Prev* 2016;25(9):1289–1296.
10. Hortlund M, Arroyo Muhr LS, Storm H, et al. Cancer risks after solid organ transplantation and after long-term dialysis. *Int J Cancer* 2017;140(5):1091–1101.
11. Tran H, Nourse J, Hall S, et al. Immunodeficiency-associated lymphomas. *Blood Rev* 2008;22(5):261–281.
12. Johnsen SJ, Brun JG, Goransson LG, et al. Risk of non-Hodgkin's lymphoma in primary Sjogren's syndrome: a population-based study. *Arthritis Care Res* 2013;65(5):816–821.
13. Yadlapati S, Efthimiou P. Autoimmune/inflammatory arthritis associated lymphomas: who is at risk? *Biomed Res Int* 2016;2016:8631061.
14. Engels EA, Parsons R, Besson C, et al. Comprehensive evaluation of medical conditions associated with risk of non-Hodgkin lymphoma using medicare claims ("MedWAS"). *Cancer Epidemiol Biomarkers Prev* 2016;25(7):1105–1113.
15. Anderson LA, Gadalla S, Morton LM, et al. Population-based study of autoimmune conditions and the risk of specific lymphoid malignancies. *Int J Cancer* 2009;125(2):398–405.
16. Morton LM, Slager SL, Cerhan JR, et al. Etiologic heterogeneity among non-Hodgkin lymphoma subtypes: the InterLymph Non-Hodgkin Lymphoma Subtypes Project. *J Natl Cancer Inst Monogr* 2014;2014(48):130–144.
17. Gromminger S, Mautner J, Bornkamm GW. Burkitt lymphoma: the role of Epstein-Barr virus revisited. *Br J Haematol* 2012;156(6):719–729.
18. Vockerodt M, Yap LF, Shannon-Lowe C, et al. The Epstein-Barr virus and the pathogenesis of lymphoma. *J Pathol* 2015;235(2):312–322.
19. Dalldorf G. Lymphomas of African children with different forms or environmental influences. *JAMA* 1962;181:1026–1028.
20. Burkitt DP. Epidemiology of Burkitt's lymphoma. *Proc R Soc Med* 1971;64(9):909–910.
21. Thorley-Lawson D, Deitsch KW, Duca KA, et al. The link between *Plasmodium falciparum* malaria and endemic Burkitt's lymphoma—new insight into a 50-year-old enigma. *PLoS Pathog* 2016;12(1):e1005331.
22. Robbiani DF, Deroubaix S, Feldhahn N, et al. Plasmodium infection promotes genomic instability and AID-dependent B cell lymphoma. *Cell* 2015;162(4):727–737.
23. Torgbor C, Awuah P, Deitsch K, et al. A multifactorial role for *P. falciparum* malaria in endemic Burkitt's lymphoma pathogenesis. *PLoS Pathog* 2014;10(5):e1004170.
24. Grywalska E, Rolinski J. Epstein-Barr virus–associated lymphomas. *Semin Oncol* 2015;42(2):291–303.
25. Proietti FA, Carneiro-Proietti AB, Catalan-Soares BC, et al. Global epidemiology of HTLV-I infection and associated diseases. *Oncogene* 2005;24(39):6058–6068.
26. Ishitsuka K, Tamura K. Human T-cell leukaemia virus type I and adult T-cell leukaemia-lymphoma. *Lancet Oncol* 2014;15(11):e517–e526.
27. Sunil M, Reid E, Lechowicz MJ. Update on HHV-8-associated malignancies. *Curr Infect Dis Rep* 2010;12(2):147–154.
28. Goossens N, Hoshida Y. Hepatitis C virus-induced hepatocellular carcinoma. *Clin Mol Hepatol* 2015;21(2):105–114.
29. de Sanjose S, Benavente Y, Vajdic CM, et al. Hepatitis C and non-Hodgkin lymphoma among 4784 cases and 6269 controls from the International Lymphoma Epidemiology Consortium. *Clin Gastroenterol Hepatol* 2008;6(4):451–458.
30. Wotherspoon AC, Ortiz-Hidalgo C, Falzon MR, et al. Helicobacter pylori-associated gastritis and primary B-cell gastric lymphoma. *Lancet* 1991;338(8776):1175–1176.
31. Fischbach W, Goebeler-Kolve ME, Dragosics B, et al. Long term outcome of patients with gastric marginal zone B cell lymphoma of mucosa associated lymphoid tissue (MALT) following exclusive Helicobacter pylori eradication therapy: experience from a large prospective series. *Gut* 2004;53(1):34–37.
32. Collina F, De Chiara A, De Renzo A, et al. Chlamydia psittaci in ocular adnexa MALT lymphoma: a possible role in lymphomagenesis and a different geographical distribution. *Infect Agent Cancer* 2012;7:8.
33. Ferreri AJ, Guidoboni M, Ponzoni M, et al. Evidence for an association between Chlamydia psittaci and ocular adnexal lymphomas. *J Natl Cancer Inst* 2004;96(8):586–594.
34. Chanudet E, Zhou Y, Bacon CM, et al. Chlamydia psittaci is variably associated with ocular adnexal MALT lymphoma in different geographical regions. *J Pathol* 2006;209(3):344–351.
35. Ferreri AJ, Govi S, Ponzoni M. Marginal zone lymphomas and infectious agents. *Semin Cancer Biol* 2013;23(6):431–440.
36. t'Mannetje A, De Roos AJ, Boffetta P, et al. Occupation and risk of non-Hodgkin lymphoma and its subtypes: a pooled analysis from the InterLymph Consortium. *Environ Health Perspect* 2016;124(4):396–405.
37. Chia SE, Wong KY, Tai BC. Occupation and risk of non-Hodgkin's lymphoma in Singapore. *Occup Med* 2012;62(1):29–33.
38. Boffetta P, de Vocht F. Occupation and the risk of non-Hodgkin lymphoma. *Cancer Epidemiol Biomarkers Prev* 2007;16(3):369–372.
39. Zheng T, Blair A, Zhang Y, et al. Occupation and risk of non-Hodgkin's lymphoma and chronic lymphocytic leukemia. *J Occup Environ Med* 2002;44(5):469–474.
40. Cocco P, t'Mannetje A, Fadda D, et al. Occupational exposure to solvents and risk of lymphoma subtypes: results from the Epilymph case-control study. *Occup Environ Med* 2010;67(5):341–347.
41. Bassig BA, Lan Q, Rothman N, et al. Current understanding of lifestyle and environmental factors and risk of non-hodgkin lymphoma: an epidemiological update. *J Cancer Epidemiol* 2012;2012:978930.
42. Sergentanis TN, Kanavidis P, Michelakos T, et al. Cigarette smoking and risk of lymphoma in adults: a comprehensive meta-analysis on Hodgkin and non-Hodgkin disease. *Eur J Cancer Prev* 2013;22(2):131–150.
43. Castillo JJ, Dalia S. Cigarette smoking is associated with a small increase in the incidence of non-Hodgkin lymphoma: a meta-analysis of 24 observational studies. *Leuk Lymphoma* 2012;53(10):1911–1919.
44. Schollkopf C, Smedby KE, Hjalgrim H, et al. Cigarette smoking and risk of non-Hodgkin's lymphoma—a population-based case-control study. *Cancer Epidemiol Biomarkers Prev* 2005;14(7):1791–1796.
45. Willett EV, Smith AG, Dovey GJ, et al. Tobacco and alcohol consumption and the risk of non-Hodgkin lymphoma. *Cancer Causes Control* 2004;15(8):771–780.
46. Adami J, Gridley G, Nyren O, et al. Sunlight and non-Hodgkin's lymphoma: a population-based cohort study in Sweden. *Int J Cancer* 1999;80(5):641–645.
47. Bertrand KA, Chang ET, Abel GA, et al. Sunlight exposure, vitamin D, and risk of non-Hodgkin lymphoma in the Nurses' Health Study. *Cancer Causes Control* 2011;22(12):1731–1741.
48. Zhang Y, Holford TR, Leaderer B, et al. Ultraviolet radiation exposure and risk of non-Hodgkin's lymphoma. *Am J Epidemiol* 2007;165(11):1255–1264.
49. Kricker A, Armstrong BK, Hughes AM, et al. Personal sun exposure and risk of non Hodgkin lymphoma: a pooled analysis from the Interlymph Consortium. *Int J Cancer* 2008;122(1):144–154.
50. Boice JD Jr, Morin MM, Glass AG, et al. Diagnostic x-ray procedures and risk of leukemia, lymphoma, and multiple myeloma. *JAMA* 1991;265(10):1290–1294.
51. Shimizu Y, Kato H, Schull WJ. Studies of the mortality of A-bomb survivors. 9. Mortality, 1950–1985: Part 2. Cancer mortality based on the recently revised doses (DS86). *Radiat Res* 1990;121(2):120–141.
52. Sigurdson AJ, Doody MM, Rao RS, et al. Cancer incidence in the US radiologic technologists health study, 1983–1998. *Cancer* 2003;97(12):3080–3089.

53. Schaapveld M, Aleman BM, van Eggermond AM, et al. Second cancer risk up to 40 years after treatment for Hodgkin's lymphoma. *N Engl J Med* 2015;373(26):2499–2511.

54. National Cancer Institute sponsored study of classifications of non-Hodgkin's lymphomas: summary and description of a working formulation for clinical usage. The Non-Hodgkin's Lymphoma Pathologic Classification Project. *Cancer* 1982;49(10):2112–2135.

55. Swerdlow SH, Campo E, Harris NL, et al., eds. *WHO classification of tumours of haematopoietic and lymphoid tissues*. 4th ed. Lyon, France: International Agency for Research on Cancer; 2008.

56. Swerdlow SH, Campo E, Pileri SA, et al. The 2016 revision of the World Health Organization classification of lymphoid neoplasms. *Blood* 2016;127(20):2375–2390.

57. Network NCC. B-Cell Lymphomas (Version 3.2017). 2017; https://www.nccn.org/professionals/physician_gls/f_guidelines.asp#b-cell. Accessed April 27, 2017.

58. Hehn ST, Grogan TM, Miller TP. Utility of fine-needle aspiration as a diagnostic technique in lymphoma. *J Clin Oncol* 2004;22(15):3046–3052.

59. Horning SJ, Weller E, Kim K, et al. Chemotherapy with or without radiotherapy in limited-stage diffuse aggressive non-Hodgkin's lymphoma: Eastern Cooperative Oncology Group study 1484. *J Clin Oncol* 2004;22(15):3032–3038.

60. A predictive model for aggressive non-Hodgkin's lymphoma. The International Non-Hodgkin's Lymphoma Prognostic Factors Project. *N Engl J Med* 1993;329(14):987–994.

61. Zucca E, Conconi A, Mughal TI, et al. Patterns of outcome and prognostic factors in primary large-cell lymphoma of the testis in a survey by the International Extranodal Lymphoma Study Group. *J Clin Oncol* 2003;21(1):20–27.

62. Cheson BD, Fisher RI, Barrington SF, et al. Recommendations for initial evaluation, staging, and response assessment of Hodgkin and non-Hodgkin lymphoma: the Lugano classification. *J Clin Oncol* 2014;32(27):3059–3068.

63. Barrington SF, Qian W, Somer EJ, et al. Concordance between four European centres of PET reporting criteria designed for use in multicentre trials in Hodgkin lymphoma. *Eur J Nucl Med Mol Imaging* 2010;37(10):1824–1833.

64. Armitage JO, Weisenburger DD. New approach to classifying non-Hodgkin's lymphomas: clinical features of the major histologic subtypes. Non-Hodgkin's Lymphoma Classification Project. *J Clin Oncol* 1998;16(8):2780–2795.

65. Alizadeh AA, Eisen MB, Davis RE, et al. Distinct types of diffuse large B-cell lymphoma identified by gene expression profiling. *Nature* 2000;403(6769):503–511.

66. Rosenwald A, Wright G, Chan WC, et al. The use of molecular profiling to predict survival after chemotherapy for diffuse large-B-cell lymphoma. *N Engl J Med* 2002;346(25):1937–1947.

67. Rosenwald A, Wright G, Leroy K, et al. Molecular diagnosis of primary mediastinal B cell lymphoma identifies a clinically favorable subgroup of diffuse large B cell lymphoma related to Hodgkin lymphoma. *J Exp Med* 2003;198(6):851–862.

68. Hans CP, Weisenburger DD, Greiner TC, et al. Confirmation of the molecular classification of diffuse large B-cell lymphoma by immunohistochemistry using a tissue microarray. *Blood* 2004;103(1):275–282.

69. Choi WW, Weisenburger DD, Greiner TC, et al. A new immunostain algorithm classifies diffuse large B-cell lymphoma into molecular subtypes with high accuracy. *Clin Cancer Res* 2009;15(17):5494–5502.

70. Muris JJ, Meijer CJ, Vos W, et al. Immunohistochemical profiling based on Bcl-2, CD10 and MUM1 expression improves risk stratification in patients with primary nodal diffuse large B cell lymphoma. *J Pathol* 2006;208(5):714–723.

71. Natkunam Y, Farinha P, Hsi ED, et al. LMO2 protein expression predicts survival in patients with diffuse large B-cell lymphoma treated with anthracycline-based chemotherapy with and without rituximab. *J Clin Oncol* 2008;26(3):447–454.

72. Nyman H, Jerkeman M, Karjalainen-Lindsberg ML, et al. Prognostic impact of activated B-cell focused classification in diffuse large B-cell lymphoma patients treated with R-CHOP. *Mod Pathol* 2009;22(8):1094–1101.

73. Meyer PN, Fu K, Greiner TC, et al. Immunohistochemical methods for predicting cell of origin and survival in patients with diffuse large B-cell lymphoma treated with rituximab. *J Clin Oncol* 2011;29(2):200–207.

74. Borowitz MJ, Bray R, Gascoyne R, et al. U.S.-Canadian Consensus recommendations on the immunophenotypic analysis of hematologic neoplasia by flow cytometry: data analysis and interpretation. *Cytometry* 1997;30(5):236–244.

75. Aukema SM, Siebert R, Schuuring E, et al. Double-hit B-cell lymphomas. *Blood* 2011;117(8):2319–2331.

76. Oki Y, Noorani M, Lin P, et al. Double hit lymphoma: the MD Anderson Cancer Center clinical experience. *Br J Haematol* 2014;166(6):891–901.

77. Green TM, Young KH, Visco C, et al. Immunohistochemical double-hit score is a strong predictor of outcome in patients with diffuse large B-cell lymphoma treated with rituximab plus cyclophosphamide, doxorubicin, vincristine, and prednisone. *J Clin Oncol* 2012;30(28):3460–3467.

78. Shipp MA. Prognostic factors in aggressive non-Hodgkin's lymphoma: who has "high-risk" disease? *Blood* 1994;83(5):1165–1173.

79. Solal-Celigny P, Roy P, Colombat P, et al. Follicular lymphoma international prognostic index. *Blood* 2004;104(5):1258–1265.

80. Federico M, Bellei M, Marcheselli L, et al. Follicular lymphoma international prognostic index 2: a new prognostic index for follicular lymphoma developed by the international follicular lymphoma prognostic factor project. *J Clin Oncol* 2009;27(27):4555–4562.

81. Feugier P, Van Hoof A, Sebban C, et al. Long-term results of the R-CHOP study in the treatment of elderly patients with diffuse large B-cell lymphoma: a study by the Groupe d'Etude des Lymphomes de l'Adulte. *J Clin Oncol* 2005;23(18):4117–4126.

82. Pfreundschuh M, Trumper L, Osterborg A, et al. CHOP-like chemotherapy plus rituximab versus CHOP-like chemotherapy alone in young patients with good-prognosis diffuse large-B-cell lymphoma: a randomised controlled trial by the MabThera International Trial (MInT) Group. *Lancet Oncol* 2006;7(5):379–391.

83. Habermann TM, Weller EA, Morrison VA, et al. Rituximab-CHOP versus CHOP alone or with maintenance rituximab in older patients with diffuse large B-cell lymphoma. *J Clin Oncol* 2006;24(19):3121–3127.

84. Ziepert M, Hasenclever D, Kuhnt E, et al. Standard International prognostic index remains a valid predictor of outcome for patients with aggressive CD20+ B-cell lymphoma in the rituximab era. *J Clin Oncol* 2010;28(14):2373–2380.

85. Alizadeh AA, Eisen MB, Davis RE, et al. Distinct types of diffuse large B-cell lymphoma identified by gene expression profiling. *Nature* 2000;403(6769):503–511.

86. Lenz G, Wright G, Dave SS, et al. Stromal gene signatures in large-B-cell lymphomas. *N Engl J Med* 2008;359(22):2313–2323.

87. Spaepen K, Stroobants S, Dupont P, et al. Prognostic value of positron emission tomography (PET) with fluorine-18 fluorodeoxyglucose ([18F]FDG) after first-line chemotherapy in non-Hodgkin's lymphoma: is [18F]FDG-PET a valid alternative to conventional diagnostic methods? *J Clin Oncol* 2001;19(2):414–419.

88. Mikhaeel NG, Timothy AR, O'Doherty MJ, et al. 18-FDG-PET as a prognostic indicator in the treatment of aggressive Non-Hodgkin's Lymphoma-comparison with CT. *Leuk Lymphoma* 2000;39(5–6):543–553.

89. Haioun C, Itti E, Rahmouni A, et al. [18F]fluoro-2-deoxy-D-glucose positron emission tomography (FDG-PET) in aggressive lymphoma: an early prognostic tool for predicting patient outcome. *Blood* 2005;106(4):1376–1381.

90. Juweid ME, Wiseman GA, Vose JM, et al. Response assessment of aggressive non-Hodgkin's lymphoma by integrated International Workshop Criteria and fluorine-18-fluorodeoxyglucose positron emission tomography. *J Clin Oncol* 2005;23(21):4652–4661.

91. Mamot C, Klingbiel D, Hitz F, et al. Final Results of a Prospective Evaluation of the Predictive Value of Interim Positron Emission Tomography in Patients With Diffuse Large B-Cell Lymphoma Treated With R-CHOP-14 (SAKK 38/07). *J Clin Oncol* 2015;33(23):2523–2529.

92. Dorth JA, Chino JP, Prosnitz LR, et al. The impact of radiation therapy in patients with diffuse large B-cell lymphoma with positive post-chemotherapy FDG-PET or gallium-67 scans. *Ann Oncol* 2011;22(2):405–410.

93. Halasz LM, Jacene HA, Catalano PJ, et al. Combined modality treatment for PET-positive non-Hodgkin lymphoma: favorable outcomes of combined modality treatment for patients with non-Hodgkin lymphoma and positive interim or postchemotherapy FDG-PET. *Int J Radiat Oncol Biol Phys* 2012;83(5):e647–e654.

94. Zinzani PL, Gandolfi L, Broccoli A, et al. Midtreatment 18F-fluorodeoxyglucose positron-emission tomography in aggressive non-Hodgkin lymphoma. *Cancer* 2011;117(5):1010–1018.

95. Cashen AF, Dehdashti F, Luo J, et al. 18F-FDG PET/CT for early response assessment in diffuse large B-cell lymphoma: poor predictive value of international harmonization project interpretation. *J Nucl Med* 2011;52(3):386–392.

96. Yang DH, Min JJ, Song HC, et al. Prognostic significance of interim (1)(8)F-FDG PET/CT after three or four cycles of R-CHOP chemotherapy in the treatment of diffuse large B-cell lymphoma. *Eur J Cancer* 2011;47(9):1312–1318.

97. Safar V, Dupuis J, Itti E, et al. Interim [18F]fluorodeoxyglucose positron emission tomography scan in diffuse large B-cell lymphoma treated with anthracycline-based chemotherapy plus rituximab. *J Clin Oncol* 2012;30(2):184–190.

98. Kim J, Lee JO, Paik JH, et al. Different predictive values of interim 18F-FDG PET/CT in germinal center like and non-germinal center like diffuse large B-cell lymphoma. *Ann Nucl Med* 2017;31(1):1–11.

99. Pregno P, Chiappella A, Bello M, et al. Interim 18-FDG-PET/CT failed to predict the outcome in diffuse large B-cell lymphoma patients treated at the diagnosis with rituximab-CHOP. *Blood* 2012;119(9):2066–2073.

100. Fisher RI, Gaynor ER, Dahlberg S, et al. Comparison of a standard regimen (CHOP) with three intensive chemotherapy regimens for advanced non-Hodgkin's lymphoma. *N Engl J Med* 1993;328(14):1002–1006.

101. Wilson W, Sin-Ho J, Pitcher BN, et al. Phase III randomized study of R-CHOP versus DA-EPOCH_R and molecular analysis of untreated diffuse large B-cell lymphoma: CALGB/Alliance 50303. *Blood* 2016;128:469.

102. Bush RS, Gospodarowicz M. The place of radiation therapy in the management of patients with localized non-Hodgkin's lymphoma. In: Rosenberg SA, Kaplan HS, eds. *Malignant lymphomas: etiology, immunology, pathology, treatment*. New York: Academic Press, 1982.

103. Chen MG, Prosnitz LR, Gonzalez-Serva A, et al. Results of radiotherapy in control of stage I and II non-Hodgkin's lymphoma. *Cancer* 1979;43(4):1245–1254.

104. Kamath SS, Marcus RB Jr, Lynch JW, et al. The impact of radiotherapy dose and other treatment-related and clinical factors on in-field control in stage I and II non-Hodgkin's lymphoma. *Int J Radiat Oncol Biol Phys* 1999;44(3):563–568.

105. Kaminski MS, Coleman CN, Colby TV, et al. Factors predicting survival in adults with stage I and II large-cell lymphoma treated with primary radiation therapy. *Ann Intern Med* 1986;104(6):747–756.

106. van der Maazen RW, Noordijk EM, Thomas J, et al. Combined modality treatment is the treatment of choice for stage I/IE intermediate and high grade non-Hodgkin's lymphomas. *Radiother Oncol* 1998;49(1):1–7.

107. Vaughan Hudson B, Vaughan Hudson G, MacLennan KA, et al. Clinical stage 1 non-Hodgkin's lymphoma: long-term follow-up of patients treated by the British National Lymphoma Investigation with radiotherapy alone as initial therapy. *Br J Cancer* 1994;69(6):1088–1093.

108. Wylie JP, Cowan RA, Deakin DP. The role of radiotherapy in the treatment of localised intermediate and high grade non-Hodgkin's lymphoma in elderly patients. *Radiother Oncol* 1998;49(1):9–14.

109. Monfardini S, Banfi A, Bonadonna G, et al. Improved five year survival after combined radiotherapy-chemotherapy for stage I-II non-Hodgkin's lymphoma. *Int J Radiat Oncol Biol Phys* 1980;6(2):125–134.

110. Nissen NI, Ersboll J, Hansen HS, et al. A randomized study of radiotherapy versus radiotherapy plus chemotherapy in stage I-II non-Hodgkin's lymphomas. *Cancer* 1983;52(1):1–7.

111. Prestidge BR, Horning SJ, Hoppe RT. Combined modality therapy for stage I-II large cell lymphoma. *Int J Radiat Oncol Biol Phys* 1988;15(3):633–639.

112. Shenkier TN, Voss N, Fairey R, et al. Brief chemotherapy and involved-region irradiation for limited-stage diffuse large-cell lymphoma: an 18-year experience from the British Columbia Cancer Agency. *J Clin Oncol* 2002;20(1):197–204.

113. Miller TP, Dahlberg S, Cassady JR, et al. Chemotherapy alone compared with chemotherapy plus radiotherapy for localized intermediate- and high-grade non-Hodgkin's lymphoma. *N Engl J Med* 1998;339(1):21–26.

114. Stephens DM, Li H, LeBlanc ML, et al. Continued risk of relapse independent of treatment modality in limited-stage diffuse large B-cell lymphoma: final and long-term analysis of Southwest Oncology Group Study S8736. *J Clin Oncol* 2016;34(25):2997–3004.

115. Bonnet C, Fillet G, Mounier N, et al. CHOP alone compared with CHOP plus radiotherapy for localized aggressive lymphoma in elderly patients: a study by the Groupe d'Etude des Lymphomes de l'Adulte. *J Clin Oncol* 2007;25(7):787–792.

116. Reyes F, Lepage E, Ganem G, et al. ACVBP versus CHOP plus radiotherapy for localized aggressive lymphoma. *N Engl J Med* 2005;352(12):1197–1205.

117. Martinelli G, Gigli F, Calabrese L, et al. Early stage gastric diffuse large B-cell lymphomas: results of a randomized trial comparing chemotherapy alone versus chemotherapy + involved field radiotherapy (IELSG 4) [corrected]. *Leuk Lymphoma* 2009;50(6):925–931.

118. Lamy T, Damaj G, Gyan E, et al. R-CHOP with or without radiotherapy in non-bulky limited-stage diffuse large B cell lymphoma (DLBCL): preliminary results of the prospective randomized phase III 02-03 trial from the LYSA/GOELAMS. *Blood* 2014;124 (Abstract 393).

119. Miller TP, LeBlanc M, Spier C. CHOP alone compared to CHOP plus radiotherapy for early stage aggressive non-Hodgkin's lymphomas: update of the Southwest Oncology Group (SWOG) randomized trial. *Blood* 2001;98:724s.

120. Ballonoff A, Rusthoven KE, Schwer A, et al. Outcomes and effect of radiotherapy in patients with stage I or II diffuse large B-cell lymphoma: a surveillance, epidemiology, and end results analysis. *Int J Radiat Oncol Biol Phys* 2008;72(5):1465–1471.

121. Dabaja BS, Vanderplas AM, Crosby-Thompson AL, et al. Radiation for diffuse large B-cell lymphoma in the rituximab era: analysis of the National Comprehensive Cancer Network lymphoma outcomes project. *Cancer* 2015;121(7):1032–1039.

122. Parikh RR, Yahalom J. Older patients with early-stage diffuse large B-cell lymphoma: the role of consolidation radiotherapy after chemoimmunotherapy. *Leuk Lymphoma* 2017;58(3):614–622.

123. Vargo JA, Gill BS, Balasubramani GK, et al. Treatment selection and survival outcomes in early-stage diffuse large B-cell lymphoma: do we still need consolidative radiotherapy? *J Clin Oncol* 2015;33(32):3710–3717.

124. Phan J, Mazloom A, Medeiros LJ, et al. Benefit of consolidative radiation therapy in patients with diffuse large B-cell lymphoma treated with R-CHOP chemotherapy. *J Clin Oncol* 2010;28(27):4170–4176.

125. Pfreundschuh M, Schubert J, Ziepert M, et al. Six versus eight cycles of bi-weekly CHOP-14 with or without rituximab in elderly patients with aggressive CD20+ B-cell lymphomas: a randomised controlled trial (RICOVER-60). *Lancet Oncol* 2008;9(2):105–116.

126. Cunningham D, Hawkes EA, Jack A, et al. Rituximab plus cyclophosphamide, doxorubicin, vincristine, and prednisolone in patients with newly diagnosed diffuse large B-cell non-Hodgkin lymphoma: a phase 3 comparison of dose intensification with 14-day versus 21-day cycles. *Lancet* 2013;381(9880):1817–1826.

127. Delarue R, Tilly H, Mounier N, et al. Dose-dense rituximab-CHOP compared with standard rituximab-CHOP in elderly patients with diffuse large B-cell lymphoma (the LNH03-6B study): a randomised phase 3 trial. *Lancet Oncol* 2013;14(6):525–533.

128. Stiff PJ, Unger JM, Cook JR, et al. Autologous transplantation as consolidation for aggressive non-Hodgkin's lymphoma. *N Engl J Med* 2013;369(18):1681–1690.

129. Schlembach PJ, Wilder RB, Tucker SL, et al. Impact of involved field radiotherapy after CHOP-based chemotherapy on stage III-IV, intermediate grade and large-cell immunoblastic lymphomas. *Int J Radiat Oncol Biol Phys* 2000;48(4):1107–1110.

130. Ferreri AJ, Dell'Oro S, Reni M, et al. Consolidation radiotherapy to bulky or semibulky lesions in the management of stage III-IV diffuse large B cell lymphomas. *Oncology* 2000;58(3):219–226.

131. Jegadeesh N, Rajpara R, Esiashvili N, et al. Predictors of local recurrence after rituximab-based chemotherapy alone in stage III and IV diffuse large B-cell lymphoma: guiding decisions for consolidative radiation. *Int J Radiat Oncol Biol Phys* 2015;92(1):107–112.

132. Phan J, Mazloom A, Medeiros J, et al. Benefit of consolidative radiation therapy in patients with diffuse large B-cell lymphoma treated with R-CHOP chemotherapy. *J Clin Oncol* 2010;28(27):4170–4176.

133. Dorth JA, Prosnitz LR, Broadwater G, et al. Impact of consolidation radiation therapy in stage III-IV diffuse large B-cell lymphoma with negative post-chemotherapy radiologic imaging. *Int J Radiat Oncol Biol Phys* 2012;84(3):762–767.

134. Shi Z, Das S, Okwan-Duodu D, et al. Patterns of failure in advanced stage diffuse large B-cell lymphoma patients after complete response to R-CHOP immunochemotherapy and the emerging role of consolidative radiation therapy. *Int J Radiat Oncol Biol Phys* 2013;86(3):569–577.

135. Held G, Murawski N, Ziepert M, et al. Role of radiotherapy to bulky disease in elderly patients with aggressive B-cell lymphoma. *J Clin Oncol* 2014;32(11):1112–1118.

136. Held G, Zeynalova S, Murawski N, et al. Impact of rituximab and radiotherapy on outcome of patients with aggressive B-cell lymphoma and skeletal involvement. *J Clin Oncol* 2013;31(32):4115–4122.

137. Sehn LH, Klasa R, Shenkier T, et al. Long-term experience with PET-guided consolidative radiation therapy (XRT) in patients with advanced stage diffuse large B-cell lymphoma (DLBCL) treated with R-CHOP. *Hematol Oncol* 2013;31:96–150.

138. Baron F, Maris MB, Sandmaier BM, et al. Graft-versus-tumor effects after allogeneic hematopoietic cell transplantation with nonmyeloablative conditioning. *J Clin Oncol* 2005;23(9):1993–2003.

139. Dean RM, Bishop MR. Allogeneic hematopoietic stem cell transplantation for lymphoma. *Clin Lymphoma* 2004;4(4):238–249.

140. Oliansky DM, Czuczman M, Fisher RI, et al. The role of cytotoxic therapy with hematopoietic stem cell transplantation in the treatment of diffuse large B cell lymphoma: update of the 2001 evidence-based review. *Biol Blood Marrow Transplant* 2011;17(1):20–47 e30.

141. Philip T, Guglielmi C, Hagenbeek A, et al. Autologous bone marrow transplantation as compared with salvage chemotherapy in relapses of chemotherapy-sensitive non-Hodgkin's lymphoma. *N Engl J Med* 1995;333(23):1540–1545.

142. Guglielmi C, Gomez F, Philip T, et al. Time to relapse has prognostic value in patients with aggressive lymphoma enrolled onto the Parma trial. *J Clin Oncol* 1998;16(10):3264–3269.

143. Dickinson M, Hoyt R, Roberts AW, et al. Improved survival for relapsed diffuse large B cell lymphoma is predicted by a negative pre-transplant FDG-PET scan following salvage chemotherapy. *Br J Haematol* 2010;150(1):39–45.

144. Sauter CS, Matasar MJ, Meikle J, et al. Prognostic value of FDG-PET prior to autologous stem cell transplantation for relapsed and refractory diffuse large B-cell lymphoma. *Blood* 2015;125(16):2579–2581.

145. Vardhana SA, Sauter CS, Matasar MJ, et al. Outcomes of primary refractory diffuse large B-cell lymphoma (DLBCL) treated with salvage chemotherapy and intention to transplant in the rituximab era. *Br J Haematol* 2016.

146. Kelsey CR, Beaven AW, Diehl LF, et al. Radiation therapy in the management of diffuse large B-cell lymphoma: still relevant? *Oncology (Williston Park)* 2010;24(13):1204–1212.

147. Haas RL, Poortmans P, de Jong D, et al. Effective palliation by low dose local radiotherapy for recurrent and/or chemotherapy refractory non-follicular lymphoma patients. *Eur J Cancer* 2005;41(12):1724–1730.

148. Murthy V, Thomas K, Foo K, et al. Efficacy of palliative low-dose involved-field radiation therapy in advanced lymphoma: a phase II study. *Clin Lymphoma Myeloma* 2008;8(4):241–245.

149. Lowry L, Smith P, Qian W, et al. Reduced dose radiotherapy for local control in non-Hodgkin lymphoma: A randomised phase III trial. *Radiother Oncol* 2011;100(1):86–92.

150. Krol AD, Berenschot HW, Doekharan D, et al. Cyclophosphamide, doxorubicin, vincristine and prednisone chemotherapy and radiotherapy for stage I intermediate or high grade non-Hodgkin's lymphomas: results of a strategy that adapts radiotherapy dose to the response after chemotherapy. *Radiother Oncol* 2001;58(3):251–255.

151. Kelsey C, Beaven AW, Diehl LF, et al. Phase 2 study of dose-reduced consolidation radiation therapy in patients with diffuse large B-cell lymphoma. *Proceedings of ASTRO*. 2017.

152. Yahalom J, Illidge T, Specht L, et al. Modern radiation therapy for extranodal lymphomas: field and dose guidelines from the International Lymphoma Radiation Oncology Group. *Int J Radiat Oncol Biol Phys* 2015;92(1):11–31.

153. Illidge T, Specht L, Yahalom J, et al. Modern radiation therapy for nodal non-Hodgkin lymphoma-target definition and dose guidelines from the International Lymphoma Radiation Oncology Group. *Int J Radiat Oncol Biol Phys* 2014;89(1):49–58.

154. Miller TP, Jones SE. Initial chemotherapy for clinically localized lymphomas of unfavorable histology. *Blood* 1983;62(2):413–418.

155. Wahlin BE, Yri OE, Kimby E, et al. Clinical significance of the WHO grades of follicular lymphoma in a population-based cohort of 505 patients with long follow-up times. *Br J Haematol* 2012;156(2):225–233.

156. Morin RD, Mendez-Lago M, Mungall AJ, et al. Frequent mutation of histone-modifying genes in non-Hodgkin lymphoma. *Nature* 2011;476(7360):298–303.

157. A clinical evaluation of the International Lymphoma Study Group classification of non-Hodgkin's lymphoma. The Non-Hodgkin's Lymphoma Classification Project. *Blood* 1997;89(11):3909–3918.

158. Schmatz AI, Streubel B, Kretschmer-Chott E, et al. Primary follicular lymphoma of the duodenum is a distinct mucosal/submucosal variant of follicular lymphoma: a retrospective study of 63 cases. *J Clin Oncol* 2011;29(11):1445–1451.

159. Barrington SF, Mikhaeel NG. PET scans for staging and restaging in diffuse large B-cell and follicular lymphomas. *Curr Hematol Malig Rep* 2016;11(3):185–195.

160. Link BK, Maurer MJ, Nowakowski GS, et al. Rates and outcomes of follicular lymphoma transformation in the immunochemotherapy era: a report from the University of Iowa/MayoClinic Specialized Program of Research Excellence Molecular Epidemiology Resource. *J Clin Oncol* 2013;31(26):3272–3278.

161. Noy A, Schoder H, Gonen M, et al. The majority of transformed lymphomas have high standardized uptake values (SUVs) on positron emission tomography (PET) scanning similar to diffuse large B-cell lymphoma (DLBCL). *Ann Oncol* 2009;20(3):508–512.

162. Pastore A, Jurinovic V, Kridel R, et al. Integration of gene mutations in risk prognostication for patients receiving first-line immunochemotherapy for follicular lymphoma: a retrospective analysis of a prospective clinical trial and validation in a population-based registry. *Lancet Oncol* 2015;16(9):1111–1122.

163. Dupuis J, Berriolo-Riedinger A, Julian A, et al. Impact of [(18)F]fluorodeoxyglucose positron emission tomography response evaluation in patients with high-tumor burden follicular lymphoma treated with immunochemotherapy: a prospective study from the Groupe d'Etudes des Lymphomes de l'Adulte and GOELAMS. *J Clin Oncol* 2012;30(35):4317–4322.

164. Adams HJ, Nievelstein RA, Kwee TC. Prognostic value of interim and end-of-treatment FDG-PET in follicular lymphoma: a systematic review. *Ann Hematol* 2016;95(1):11–18.

165. Adams HJ, Kwee TC. No convincing evidence to support postinduction FDG-PET in follicular lymphoma. *Ann Hematol* 2016;95(12):2085–2086.

166. Mac Manus MP, Hoppe RT. Is radiotherapy curative for stage I and II low-grade follicular lymphoma? Results of a long-term follow-up study of patients treated at Stanford University. *J Clin Oncol* 1996;14(4):1282–1290.

167. Stuschke M, Hoederath A, Sack H, et al. Extended field and total central lymphatic radiotherapy in the treatment of early stage lymph node centroblastic-centrocytic lymphomas: results of a prospective multicenter study. Study Group NHL-frühe Stadien. *Cancer* 1997;80(12):2273–2284.

168. Wilder RB, Jones D, Tucker SL, et al. Long-term results with radiotherapy for Stage I-II follicular lymphomas. *Int J Radiat Oncol Biol Phys* 2001;51(5):1219–1227.

292. Montemurro M, Kiefer T, Schuler F, et al. Primary central nervous system lymphoma treated with high-dose methotrexate, high-dose busulfan/thiotepa, autologous stem-cell transplantation and response-adapted whole-brain radiotherapy: results of the multicenter Ostdeutsche Studiengruppe Hamato-Onkologie OSHO-53 phase II study. *Ann Oncol* 2007;18(4):665–671.

293. Rudiger T, Weisenburger DD, Anderson JR, et al. Peripheral T-cell lymphoma (excluding anaplastic large-cell lymphoma): results from the Non-Hodgkin's Lymphoma Classification Project. *Ann Oncol* 2002;13(1):140–149.

294. Anderson JR, Armitage JO, Weisenburger DD. Epidemiology of the non-Hodgkin's lymphomas: distributions of the major subtypes differ by geographic locations. Non-Hodgkin's Lymphoma Classification Project. *Ann Oncol* 1998;9(7):717–720.

295. Kutok JL, Aster JC. Molecular biology of anaplastic lymphoma kinase-positive anaplastic large-cell lymphoma. *J Clin Oncol* 2002;20(17):3691–3702.

296. Stein H, Foss HD, Durkop H, et al. CD30(+) anaplastic large cell lymphoma: a review of its histopathologic, genetic, and clinical features. *Blood* 2000;96(12):3681–3695.

297. Falini B, Pileri S, Zinzani PL, et al. ALK+ lymphoma: clinico-pathological findings and outcome. *Blood* 1999;93(8):2697–2706.

298. Weisenburger DD, Savage KJ, Harris NL, et al. Peripheral T-cell lymphoma, not otherwise specified: a report of 340 cases from the International Peripheral T-cell Lymphoma Project. *Blood* 2011;117(12):3402–3408.

299. Vose J, Armitage J, Weisenburger D, et al. International peripheral T-cell and natural killer/T-cell lymphoma study: pathology findings and clinical outcomes. *J Clin Oncol* 2008;26(25):4124–4130.

300. Vose J, Armitage J, Weisenburger D. International peripheral T-cell and natural killer/T-cell lymphoma study: pathology findings and clinical outcomes. *J Clin Oncol* 2008;26(25):4124–4130.

301. Bekkenk MW, Geelen FA, van Voorst Vader PC, et al. Primary and secondary cutaneous CD30(+) lymphoproliferative disorders: a report from the Dutch Cutaneous Lymphoma Group on the long-term follow-up data of 219 patients and guidelines for diagnosis and treatment. *Blood* 2000;95(12):3653–3661.

302. Kadin ME, Carpenter C. Systemic and primary cutaneous anaplastic large cell lymphomas. *Semin Hematol* 2003;40(3):244–256.

303. Shulman LN, Frisard B, Antin JH, et al. Primary Ki-1 anaplastic large-cell lymphoma in adults: clinical characteristics and therapeutic outcome. *J Clin Oncol* 1993;11(5):937–942.

304. Weisenburger DD, Anderson JR, Diebold J, et al. Systemic anaplastic large-cell lymphoma: results from the non-Hodgkin's lymphoma classification project. *Am J Hematol* 2001;67(3):172–178.

305. Zinzani PL, Bendandi M, Martelli M, et al. Anaplastic large-cell lymphoma: clinical and prognostic evaluation of 90 adult patients. *J Clin Oncol* 1996;14(3):955–962.

306. Gascoyne RD, Aoun P, Wu D, et al. Prognostic significance of anaplastic lymphoma kinase (ALK) protein expression in adults with anaplastic large cell lymphoma. *Blood* 1999;93(11):3913–3921.

307. Kaufmann TP, Coleman M, Nisce LZ. Ki-1 skin lymphoproliferative disorders: management with radiation therapy. *Cancer Invest* 1997;15(2):91–97.

308. Niedobitek G, Meru N, Delecluse HJ. Epstein-Barr virus infection and human malignancies. *Int J Exp Pathol* 2001;82(3):149–170.

309. Cheung MM, Chan JK, Lau WH, et al. Early stage nasal NK/T-cell lymphoma: clinical outcome, prognostic factors, and the effect of treatment modality. *Int J Radiat Oncol Biol Phys* 2002;54(1):182–190.

310. Kim GE, Cho JH, Yang WI, et al. Angiocentric lymphoma of the head and neck: patterns of systemic failure after radiation treatment. *J Clin Oncol* 2000;18(1):54–63.

311. Clemens MW, Medeiros LJ, Butler CE, et al. Complete surgical excision is essential for the management of patients with breast implant-associated anaplastic large-cell lymphoma. *J Clin Oncol* 2016;34(2):160–168.

312. Gallamini A, Stelitano C, Calvi R, et al. Peripheral T-cell lymphoma unspecified (PTCL-U): a new prognostic model from a retrospective multicentric clinical study. *Blood* 2004;103(7):2474–2479.

313. Abramson JS, Feldman T, Kroll-Desrosiers AR, et al. Peripheral T-cell lymphomas in a large US multicenter cohort: prognostication in the modern era including impact of frontline therapy. *Ann Oncol* 2014;25(11):2211–2217.

314. Sibon D, Fournier M, Briere J, et al. Long-term outcome of adults with systemic anaplastic large-cell lymphoma treated within the Groupe d'Etude des Lymphomes de l'Adulte Trials. *J Clin Oncol* 2012;30(32):3939–3946.

315. Savage KJ, Harris NL, Vose JM, et al. ALK-anaplastic large-cell lymphoma is clinically and immunophenotypically different from both ALK+ ALCL and peripheral T-cell lymphoma, not otherwise specified: report from the International Peripheral T-Cell Lymphoma Project. *Blood* 2008;111(12):5496–5504.

316. Suzuki R, Kagami Y, Takeuchi K, et al. Prognostic significance of CD56 expression for ALK-positive and ALK-negative anaplastic large-cell lymphoma of T/null cell phenotype. *Blood* 2000;96(9):2993–3000.

317. Kim SJ, Yoon DH, Jaccard A, et al. A prognostic index for natural killer cell lymphoma after non-anthracycline-based treatment: a multicentre, retrospective analysis. *Lancet Oncol* 2016;17(3):389–400.

318. Schmitz N, Trumper L, Ziepert M, et al. Treatment and prognosis of mature T-cell and NK-cell lymphoma: an analysis of patients with T-cell lymphoma treated in studies of the German High-Grade Non-Hodgkin Lymphoma Study Group. *Blood* 2010;116(18):3418–3425.

319. Zhang XM, Li YX, Wang WH, et al. Survival advantage with the addition of radiation therapy to chemotherapy in early stage peripheral T-cell lymphoma, not otherwise specified. *Int J Radiat Oncol Biol Phys* 2013;85(4):1051–1056.

320. Zhang XM, Li YX, Wang WH, et al. Favorable outcome with doxorubicin-based chemotherapy and radiotherapy for adult patients with early stage primary systemic anaplastic large-cell lymphoma. *Eur J Haematol* 2013;90(3):195–201.

321. Kim WS, Song SY, Ahn YC, et al. CHOP followed by involved field radiation: is it optimal for localized nasal natural killer/T-cell lymphoma? *Ann Oncol* 2001;12(3):349–352.

322. Liang R, Todd D, Chan TK, et al. Treatment outcome and prognostic factors for primary nasal lymphoma. *J Clin Oncol* 1995;13(3):666–670.

323. Li YX, Yao B, Jin J, et al. Radiotherapy as primary treatment for stage IE and IIE nasal natural killer/T-cell lymphoma. *J Clin Oncol* 2006;24(1):181–189.

324. Ribrag V, Ell Hajj M, Janot F, et al. Early locoregional high-dose radiotherapy is associated with long-term disease control in localized primary angiocentric lymphoma of the nose and nasopharynx. *Leukemia* 2001;15(7):1123–1126.

325. Yamaguchi M, Tobinai K, Oguchi M, et al. Phase I/II study of concurrent chemoradiotherapy for localized nasal natural killer/T-cell lymphoma: Japan Clinical Oncology Group Study JCOG0211. *J Clin Oncol* 2009;27(33):5594–5600.

326. Kim SJ, Kim K, Kim BS, et al. Phase II trial of concurrent radiation and weekly cisplatin followed by VIPD chemotherapy in newly diagnosed, stage IE to IIE, nasal, extranodal NK/T-Cell Lymphoma: Consortium for Improving Survival of Lymphoma study. *J Clin Oncol* 2009;27(35):6027–6032.

327. Savage KJ, Monti S, Kutok JL, et al. The molecular signature of mediastinal large B-cell lymphoma differs from that of other diffuse large B-cell lymphomas and shares features with classical Hodgkin lymphoma. *Blood* 2003;102(12):3871–3879.

328. Savage KJ, Al-Rajhi N, Voss N, et al. Favorable outcome of primary mediastinal large B-cell lymphoma in a single institution: the British Columbia experience. *Ann Oncol* 2006;17(1):123–130.

329. Vitolo U, Seymour JF, Martelli M, et al. Extranodal diffuse large B-cell lymphoma (DLBCL) and primary mediastinal B-cell lymphoma: ESMO Clinical Practice Guidelines for diagnosis, treatment and follow-up. *Ann Oncol* 2016;27(Suppl 5):v91–v102.

330. Binkley MS, Hiniker SM, Wu S, et al. A single-institution retrospective analysis of outcomes for stage I-II primary mediastinal large B-cell lymphoma treated with immunochemotherapy with or without radiotherapy. *Leuk Lymphoma* 2016;57(3):604–608.

331. Dunleavy K, Pittaluga S, Maeda LS, et al. Dose-adjusted EPOCH-rituximab therapy in primary mediastinal B-cell lymphoma. *N Engl J Med* 2013;368(15):1408–1416.

332. Achten R, Verhoef G, Vanuytsel L, et al. T-cell/histiocyte-rich large B-cell lymphoma: a distinct clinicopathologic entity. *J Clin Oncol* 2002;20(5):1269–1277.

333. Bouabdallah R, Mounier N, Guettier C, et al. T-cell/histiocyte-rich large B-cell lymphomas and classical diffuse large B-cell lymphomas have similar outcome after chemotherapy: a matched-control analysis. *J Clin Oncol* 2003;21(7):1271–1277.

334. Campo E, Swerdlow SH, Harris NL, et al. The 2008 WHO classification of lymphoid neoplasms and beyond: evolving concepts and practical applications. *Blood* 2011;117(19):5019–5032.

335. Hallek M, Cheson BD, Catovsky D, et al. Guidelines for the diagnosis and treatment of chronic lymphocytic leukemia: a report from the International Workshop on Chronic Lymphocytic Leukemia updating the National Cancer Institute-Working Group 1996 guidelines. *Blood* 2008;111(12):5446–5456.

336. Nowakowski GS, Hoyer JD, Shanafelt TD, et al. Percentage of smudge cells on routine blood smear predicts survival in chronic lymphocytic leukemia. *J Clin Oncol* 2009;27(11):1844–1849.

337. Redaelli A, Laskin BL, Stephens JM, et al. The clinical and epidemiological burden of chronic lymphocytic leukaemia. *Eur J Cancer Care* 2004;13(3):279–287.

338. Craig FE, Foon KA. Flow cytometric immunophenotyping for hematologic neoplasms. *Blood* 2008;111(8):3941–3967.

339. Bruzzi JF, Macapinlac H, Tsimberidou AM, et al. Detection of Richter's transformation of chronic lymphocytic leukemia by PET/CT. *J Nucl Med* 2006;47(8):1267–1273.

340. Hamblin TJ, Davis Z, Gardiner A, et al. Unmutated Ig V(H) genes are associated with a more aggressive form of chronic lymphocytic leukemia. *Blood* 1999;94(6):1848–1854.

341. Rai KR, Jain P. Chronic lymphocytic leukemia (CLL)—then and now. *Am J Hematol* 2016;91(3):330–340.

342. Foa R, Del Giudice I, Guarini A, et al. Clinical implications of the molecular genetics of chronic lymphocytic leukemia. *Haematologica* 2013;98(5):675–685.

343. Rossi D, Rasi S, Spina V, et al. Integrated mutational and cytogenetic analysis identifies new prognostic subgroups in chronic lymphocytic leukemia. *Blood* 2013;121(8):1403–1412.

344. Eichhorst B, Fink AM, Bahlo J, et al. First-line chemoimmunotherapy with bendamustine and rituximab versus fludarabine, cyclophosphamide, and rituximab in patients with advanced chronic lymphocytic leukaemia (CLL10): an international, open-label, randomised, phase 3, non-inferiority trial. *Lancet Oncol* 2016;17(7):928–942.

345. Reynolds C, Di Bella N, Lyons RM, et al. A phase III trial of fludarabine, cyclophosphamide, and rituximab vs. pentostatin, cyclophosphamide, and rituximab in B-cell chronic lymphocytic leukemia. *Invest New Drugs* 2012;30(3):1232–1240.

346. Wiestner A, Farooqui M, Valdez J, et al. Single agent ibrutinib (PCI-32765) is highly effective in chronic lymphocytic leukaemia patients with 17p deletion. *Hematol Oncol* 2013;31:98.

347. Morscio J, Tousseyn T. Recent insights in the pathogenesis of post-transplantation lymphoproliferative disorders. *World J Transplant* 2016;6(3):505–516.

348. Dharnidharka VR, Webster AC, Martinez OM, et al. Post-transplant lymphoproliferative disorders. *Nat Rev Dis Primers* 2016;2:15088.

349. Choquet S, Leblond V, Herbrecht R, et al. Efficacy and safety of rituximab in B-cell post-transplantation lymphoproliferative disorders: results of a prospective multicenter phase 2 study. *Blood* 2006;107(8):3053–3057.

350. Trappe R, Oertel S, Leblond V, et al. Sequential treatment with rituximab followed by CHOP chemotherapy in adult B-cell post-transplant lymphoproliferative disorder (PTLD): the prospective international multicentre phase 2 PTLD-1 trial. *Lancet Oncol* 2012;13(2):196–206.

351. Choquet S, Trappe R, Leblond V, et al. CHOP-21 for the treatment of post-transplant lymphoproliferative disorders (PTLD) following solid organ transplantation. *Haematologica* 2007;92(2):273–274.

Section III

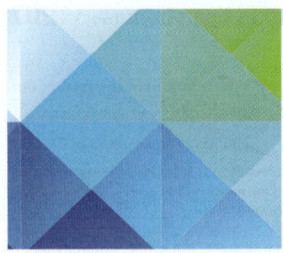

CHAPTER 83

Primary Cutaneous Lymphomas

James E. Hansen, Youn H. Kim, Richard T. Hoppe, and Lynn D. Wilson

INTRODUCTION

Primary cutaneous lymphoma is defined by an accumulation of malignant lymphoid cells in the skin without evidence of extracutaneous disease at the time of diagnosis. The distinction between a primary cutaneous lymphoma and a nodal lymphoma with secondary cutaneous involvement is important and markedly impacts evaluation, staging, prognosis, and therapeutic management. The term *primary cutaneous lymphoma* encompasses a heterogeneous group of extranodal non-Hodgkin lymphomas, and in 2005, the World Health Organization (WHO) and European Organisation for Research and Treatment of Cancer (EORTC) endorsed a consensus classification system that defines three categories of primary cutaneous lymphomas: cutaneous T-cell and NK-cell lymphomas, cutaneous B-cell lymphomas, and precursor hematologic neoplasms/immature hematologic malignancies (Table 83.1).[1] This chapter will review the primary cutaneous lymphomas in the context of this consensus system. A slightly modified classification system was released by the WHO in 2008.[2]

CUTANEOUS T-CELL AND NK-CELL LYMPHOMAS

Cutaneous T-cell lymphoma (CTCL) is the most common primary cutaneous lymphoma. In the United States, 71% of the 3,884 cases of primary cutaneous lymphoma diagnosed during 2001 to 2005 were CTCL.[3] Similarly, 78% of primary cutaneous lymphoma diagnoses recorded in the Dutch and Austrian Cutaneous Lymphoma Group registry over 1986 to 2002[1] and 85% of diagnoses in the Central Cutaneous Lymphoma Registry of the German Society of Dermatology over 1999 to 2004 were CTCL.[4]

CTCL subtypes include mycosis fungoides (MF); CD30+ lymphoproliferative disorders; extranodal NK-/T-cell lymphoma, nasal type; subcutaneous panniculitis-like T-cell lymphoma; adult T-cell leukemia/lymphoma; and primary cutaneous peripheral T-cell lymphomas. MF is the most common CTCL, responsible for 54% of CTCL diagnoses in the United States over 2001 to 2005.[3] CD30+ T-cell lymphoproliferative disorders and cutaneous peripheral T-cell lymphomas represent the majority of the remaining cases of CTCL. The remaining CTCL subtypes are extremely rare and represent <1% of primary cutaneous lymphomas.

Mycosis Fungoides

MF is the archetype cutaneous lymphoma. The first case of MF was reported in 1806 by the French dermatologist Jean-Louis-Marc Alibert in his atlas of dermatoses, *Descriptions des maladies de la peau* (Fig. 83.1). After Alibert released his depiction of MF, approximately 300 similar cases were reported over the next decade, and in modern times, approximately 1,500 new cases of MF were diagnosed during 2001 to 2005.[3] MF is a disease of skin-homing CD4+ T-helper cells[5] and is most commonly diagnosed in men (male:female ratio of 1.6 to 2.0:1) with a median age at diagnosis of 55 to 60.[1] Significant advances in MF therapy have been made over the past 200 years, but the precise etiology responsible for the development of MF remains elusive.

Cutaneous Disease

Pruritus, either diffuse or localized to areas of involved skin, is the most common symptom associated with MF. Ulcerated lesions may also cause patients significant pain. Cutaneous lesions in classic (or Alibert-Bazin) MF follow a predictable evolutionary course, and a consensus statement from the International Society for Cutaneous Lymphomas (ISCL), U.S. Cutaneous Lymphoma Consortium (USCLC), and EORTC defines the lesions found in distinct phases of MF.[6] In the *premycotic phase,* a small number of red, scaled, macular or patchlike lesions develop in sun-shielded areas of the skin such as the trunk, pelvis, and extremities. These early lesions are unstable and usually regress, followed by development of new lesions. Biopsies of premycotic lesions are rarely diagnostic because of a paucity of malignant lymphocytes in the lesion. With increased deposition of malignant T cells in the skin, the lesions become increasingly durable, and persistent cutaneous patches are characteristic of the *patch phase.* The ISCL/USCLC/EORTC consensus definition of an MF patch is "any size lesion without induration or significant elevation above the surrounding uninvolved skin: poikiloderma may be present."[6] As the lesions become more densely infiltrated by both malignant and reactive lymphocytes, they evolve into plaques with thickened and raised borders in the *plaque phase* of classic MF. Plaques are defined by the ISCL/USCLC/EORTC as "any size lesion that is elevated or indurated: crusting or poikiloderma may be present."[6] Plaques may evolve into cutaneous tumors, which the ISCL/USCLC/EORTC defines as "any solid or nodular lesion ≥1 cm in diameter with evidence of deep infiltration in the skin and/or vertical growth."[6] The presence of cutaneous tumors designates the tumor phase of MF. MF may also progress to or present with erythroderma, in which a diffuse erythema involves >80% of the skin surface area.[6] Representative images of patches, plaques, tumors, and erythroderma are shown in Figure 83.2.

Leukemic CTCL and the Sézary Syndrome

In rare CTCL cases, circulating malignant T cells are identified in the peripheral blood. This phenomenon, sometimes referred to as leukemic CTCL or the Sézary syndrome (SS), most commonly occurs in association with erythroderma but may occur in patients with minimal cutaneous disease.[1] The circulating malignant T cells (also called Sézary cells) are atypical T cells with hyperconvoluted nuclei seen at analysis of peripheral buffy coat smear. The circulating cells most commonly possess a CD4+/CD7− or CD4+/CD26− immunophenotype, and flow cytometry allows for quantification of the proportion of circulating malignant T cells. In addition, presence of a dominant circulating malignant clone may be demonstrated by evaluation of the T-cell receptor (TCR) by polymerase chain reaction (PCR) or Southern blotting. The degree of tumor burden in the peripheral blood is denoted as B0 (≤5% atypical or Sézary cells seen on examination of buffy coat smear), B1 (>5% of cells on buffy coat analysis are atypical, but further criteria meeting

TABLE 83.1 WHO/EORTC CLASSIFICATION[1]

Cutaneous T-Cell and NK-/T-Cell Lymphomas
Mycosis fungoides and variants (folliculotropic mycosis fungoides, pagetoid reticulosis, and granulomatous slack skin)
Sézary syndrome
CD30+ lymphoproliferative disorders (primary cutaneous anaplastic large-cell lymphoma and lymphomatoid papulosis)
Extranodal NK-/T-cell lymphoma, nasal type
Subcutaneous panniculitis-like T-cell lymphoma
Primary cutaneous peripheral T-cell lymphoma, unspecified
Primary cutaneous aggressive epidermotropic CD8+ T-cell lymphoma (provisional)
Primary cutaneous $\gamma\delta$ T-cell lymphoma (provisional)
Primary cutaneous CD4+ small-/medium-sized pleomorphic T-cell lymphoma (provisional)

Cutaneous B-Cell Lymphomas
Primary cutaneous marginal zone lymphoma
Primary cutaneous follicle center lymphoma
Primary cutaneous diffuse large B-cell lymphoma, leg type
Primary cutaneous diffuse large B-cell lymphoma, other

Precursor Hematologic Neoplasm
CD4+/CD56+ hematodermic neoplasm (blastic NK-cell lymphoma)

Republished with permission of American Society of Hematology from Willemze R, Jaffe ES, Burg G, et al. WHO-EORTC classification for cutaneous lymphomas. *Blood* 2005;105(10):3768–3785; permission conveyed through Copyright Clearance Center, Inc.

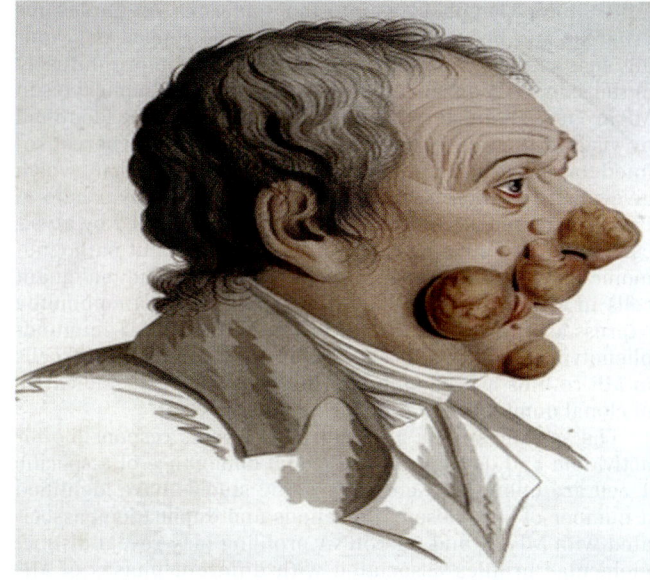

FIGURE 83.1. Pian fungoide, from Jean-Louis-Marc Alibert's atlas of dermatoses, *Descriptions des Maladies de la Peau.*

B2 disease are not met), or B2 (combination of presence of a dominant T-cell clone in the peripheral blood identified by PCR or Southern blot and ≥1,000 Sézary cells/mm,³ an increased amount of CD3+ or CD4+ T cells with CD4:CD8 ratios >10, or increased quantities of abnormal T cells defined as loss of CD7 in >40% of cells or CD26 in >30% of cells).⁶ If peripheral blood is evaluated for a circulating clone by PCR or Southern blot, B0 or B1 disease may be stratified into B0a or B1a (absence of circulating clone) or B0b or B1b (presence of circulating clone). The mechanism responsible for the development of leukemic disease in MF is unknown and in some cases may simply reflect disease progression. In other cases, erythroderma and circulating cell disease develop simultaneously, which has historically been referred to as SS. The distinction between SS and erythrodermic MF with leukemic involvement (or SS syndrome preceded by MF) has been a point of controversy, and it remains unclear whether the two diseases are distinct or merely variants of one another. At present, SS is specifically defined as the combination of erythroderma with B2 disease.⁶

Extracutaneous Disease

In advanced stages of disease, MF may progress to involve regional or distant lymph nodes or extracutaneous organ systems (most commonly the lungs, oral cavity, pharynx, or central nervous system), and these sites may cause patients significant pain or functional impairment.⁷ Of note, in advanced cases of MF, the extent of cutaneous or extracutaneous disease may vary significantly in patients of the same clinical stage. Clinical trials that report results by stage alone may therefore be difficult to interpret. The ISCL/USCLC/EORTC consensus statement on clinical endpoints and response criteria should facilitate improved communication of the degree of disease and response to treatment in future clinical trials.⁶

Molecular and Cellular Pathophysiology

Examination of early-phase MF lesions by hematoxylin and eosin staining commonly reveals epidermotropism, a profound

Patch   *Plaque*

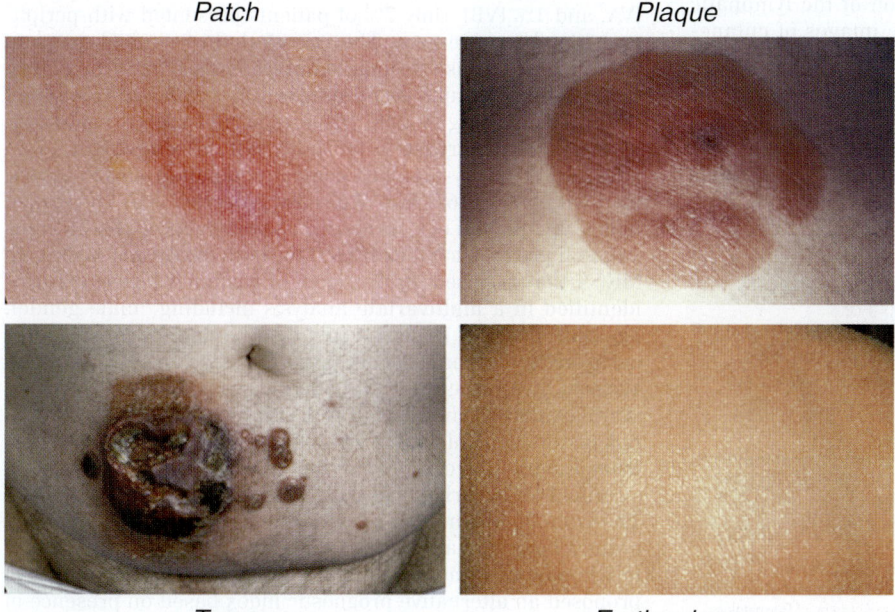

Tumor   *Erythroderma*

FIGURE 83.2. Representative images of cutaneous lesions in mycosis fungoides. (From Smith BD, Wilson LD. Management of mycosis fungoides. Part 1. Diagnosis, staging, and prognosis. *Oncology* 2003;17[9]:1281–1288. Reprinted by permission of Benjamin D. Smith.)

Section III

infiltration of lymphocytes into the epidermis. As the lesions progress and become thickened, epidermotropism is gradually lost as the lymphocytes begin to localize more diffusely in the skin. Only a fraction of the skin-homing lymphocytes in MF are malignant, and the malignant T cells may be identified by visualization of their small to medium-sized hyperconvoluted (or cerebriform) nuclei and surrounding lacunae, which give them the impression of being surrounded by a halo. A Pautrier microabscess (Langerhans cell surrounded by atypical T cells in the epidermis) is a less common but pathognomonic histologic finding associated with MF.[1,5] The malignant cells in MF are CD4+ T-helper cells, which most commonly express a CD3+, CD4+, CD45RO+, CLA+, and CCR4+ immunophenotype. Evaluation of the TCR profile of malignant T cells in MF reveals a predominant TCR rearrangement indicative of clonal dominance in a majority of cases.

The specific stimuli and molecular events responsible for activation and development of clonal dominance of a specific T cell are unknown. Genetic profiling studies have identified a number of chromosomal deletions and duplications associated with MF/SS, and microRNA profiling may reveal distinct molecular profiles associated with different phases of MF. More recently, whole exome/genome sequencing of leukemic CTCL cells revealed mutations of interest involving 17 genes associated with a range of cellular functions including TCR and NF-kB signaling pathways, chromatin remodeling, and DNA repair. In addition to any molecular aberrations intrinsic to the malignant T cells, the cutaneous microenvironment is also likely to play a key role in the development and maintenance of disease.[5,8–12]

Diagnosis and Evaluation

Evaluation of a patient with suspected or recently diagnosed MF should include a comprehensive history/physical examination, biopsy of cutaneous lesion(s) and suspicious lymph nodes, and appropriate laboratory and imaging studies. The ISCL has designed a diagnostic algorithm for early-stage MF (not applicable to MF variants) (Table 83.2),[13] and specific recommendations for patient evaluation have been released by the ISCL/EORTC.[14,15]

History and Physical Examination

The duration of symptoms, evolutionary course of cutaneous disease, and presence or absence of B symptoms should be determined. The percentage of body surface area involved by disease and presence or absence of cutaneous tumors should be documented, and a thorough evaluation of the lymphatic system should be performed. Appropriate images of cutaneous lesions should be recorded so that disease progression or response to therapy may be monitored.

Skin Biopsy

Biopsies should be taken from a minimum of two distinct sites of disease. Lesions of the greatest induration will be most likely to yield a diagnosis because of greater numbers of malignant cells. However, scaled lesions are more likely to show epidermotropism. Tissue should be evaluated with hematoxylin and eosin staining, immunostaining for surface marker expression profiles (including CD2, CD3, CD4, CD5, CD7, CD8, CD20, CD30, CD26, CD56, TIA1, granzyme B, βF1), and PCR for clonal TCR rearrangement. Slides should be reviewed by a dermatopathologist.

Excisional biopsies of enlarged or otherwise suspicious lymph nodes (fixed or matted lymph nodes, or lymph nodes ≥1.5 cm or ≥1 cm in the head and neck) should be evaluated as described previously. When multiple suspicious lymph nodes are encountered, the choice of lymph node to be excised should be based on size, fluorodeoxyglucose (FDG) avidity, and location, with priority given to the largest lymph node draining an affected area of skin or the lymph node with the highest standardized uptake value (SUV) on positron emission tomography (PET) scan. If all other factors are equal, priority should be given first to cervical nodes, followed by axillary and then inguinal nodes.[14,15]

Laboratory and Imaging Studies

Laboratory studies should include a complete blood count, chemistry panel, liver function tests, and lactate dehydrogenase (LDH). Examination of the peripheral blood for circulating disease by PCR and flow cytometry should also be considered, particularly for patients with erythroderma and nodal or extracutaneous disease. Bone marrow biopsy should be considered if peripheral blood or extracutaneous organs are found to harbor disease.[14,15] Computed tomography (CT) of the chest, abdomen, and pelvis is recommended in the evaluation of all patients with MF with the exception of patients with patch/plaque disease limited to 10% or less of the body surface area. In these cases, a chest x-ray or nodal ultrasound may suffice. PET scanning was shown to be more sensitive than CT in identifying involved lymph nodes, and the role of PET in MF continues to evolve.[16]

Staging and Prognosis

MF is presently staged using the modified TNMB system proposed by the ISCL/EORTC (Table 83.3).[14] Based on a review of 525 patients with MF (staged using the previous 1979 TNMB system), the majority of patients present with early-stage disease (30% IA, 25% IB, 11% IIA, 16% IIB, 3% IIIA, 8% IIIB, 6% IVA, and 1% IVB). Only 7% of patients presented with peripheral blood involvement. The correlation of clinical stage to overall and disease-specific survival is presented in Figure 83.3.[7] Similar results were obtained in a validation study of the current staging system.[17] Of note, stage IA MF is not associated with any increase in mortality risk in comparison to an age- and ethnicity-matched control population and is associated with only a 16% rate of disease progression at 20 years of follow-up.[7] Benton et al. proposed a cutaneous lymphoma international prognostic index (CLIPi) for both early- and late-stage MF/SS that is based on presence of certain adverse features identified in a multivariate analysis including "male gender, age >60, plaques, folliculotropic disease and stage N1/Nx for early stage, and male gender, age >60, stages B1/B2, N2/3 and visceral involvement for late stage disease."[18] The CLIPi then stratifies patients into low (0 to 1 risk factors), intermediate (2 risk factors), and high (3 to 5 risk factors) risk groups.[18] A report from Emory University indicates that the CLIPi successfully stratified their early-stage but not late-stage MF/SS patients.[19] The Cutaneous Lymphoma International Consortium conducted a multi-institutional and international study of potential prognostic factors in advanced-stage (IIB to IV) MF/SS and have proposed an alternative prognostic index based on presence of four risk factors (stage IV disease, age >60, elevated LDH, and

TABLE 83.2 DIAGNOSTIC CRITERIA FOR EARLY-STAGE MYCOSIS FUNGOIDES[a,13]

Clinical	Immunopathologic
Persistent and/or progressive patches and plaques plus: 1. Non-sun-exposed location 2. Size/shape variation 3. Poikiloderma *Scoring:* Two points if two or more criteria met. One point if only one criterion met.	1. CD2, 3, 5 <50% of T cells 2. CD7 <10% of T cells 3. Epidermal discordance from expression of CD2, 3, 5, or 7 on dermal T cells *Scoring:* One point if any criterion met.
Molecular/Biologic	**Histopathologic**
1. Clonal TCR gene rearrangement *Scoring:* One point if present.	1. Epidermotropism without spongiosis 2. Lymphoid atypia *Scoring:* One point for each.

[a]Not applicable to mycosis fungoides variants. Diagnosis made with 4 points or more.
Reprinted from Pimpinelli N, Olsen EA, Santucci M, et al. Defining early mycosis fungoides. *J Am Acad Dermatol* 2005;53(6):1053–1063. Copyright © 2005 American Academy of Dermatology, Inc. With permission.

TABLE 83.3 ISCL/EORTC REVISIONS TO MYCOSIS FUNGOIDES STAGING[14]

T Stage	N Stage
T1: Limited patches, papules, and/or plaques covering <10% of the skin surface. May further stratify into T1a (patch only) vs. T1b (plaque/patch)	N0: No clinically abnormal peripheral lymph nodes; biopsy not required
T2: Patches, papules, or plaques covering ≥10% of the skin surface. May further stratify into T2a (patch only) vs. T2b (plaque/patch).	N1: Clinically abnormal peripheral lymph nodes; histopathology Dutch grade 1 or NCI LN0–2 (N1a, clone negative; N1b, clone positive)
T3: One or more tumors (≥1-cm diameter)	N2: Clinically abnormal peripheral lymph nodes; histopathology Dutch grade 2 or NCI LN3
T4: Confluence of erythema covering >80% body surface area	N3: Clinically abnormal peripheral lymph nodes; histopathology Dutch grades 3 or 4 or NCI LN4; clone positive or negative
	NX: Clinically abnormal peripheral lymph nodes; no histologic confirmation

B Stage	M Stage
B0: Absence of significant blood involvement: <5% of peripheral blood lymphocytes are atypical (Sézary) cells	M0: No visceral organ involvement
B1: Low blood tumor burden: >5% of peripheral blood lymphocytes are atypical (Sézary) cells, but does not meet B2 criteria	M1: Visceral involvement (must have pathology confirmation and organ involved should be specified)
B2: High blood tumor burden: ≥1,000/mL Sézary cells with positive clone	

Staging Groups

IA: T1 N0 M0 B0–1	IIA: T1–2 N1–2 M0 B0
IIIA: T4 N0–2 M0 B0	IVA1: T1–4 N0–2 M0 B0–2
IB: T2 N0 M0 B0–1	IIB: T3 N0–2 M0 B0–1
IIIB: T4 N0–2 M0 B1	IVA2: T1–4 N3 M0 B0–2
	IVB: T1–4 N0–3 M1 B0–2

Republished with permission of American Society of Hematology from Olsen E, Vonderheid E, Pimpinelli N, et al. Revisions to the staging and classification of mycosis fungoides and Sezary syndrome: a proposal of the International Society for Cutaneous Lymphomas (ISCL) and the Cutaneous Lymphoma Task Force of the European Organization of Research and Treatment of Cancer (EORTC). *Blood* 2007;110(6):1713–1722; permission conveyed through Copyright Clearance Center, Inc.

large-cell transformation in the skin). Based on these factors, patients are stratified into low (0 to 1 risk factor; 67.8% 5-year survival), intermediate (2 risk factors; 43.5% 5-year survival), or high (3 to 4 risk factors; 27.6% 5-year survival) risk groups.[20] Overall, these studies underscore the complexities and difficulties inherent to developing accurate prognostic indices for such rare disease entities. A prospective international effort

FIGURE 83.3. Overall **(A)** and disease-specific **(B)** survival in mycosis fungoides by stage. (Reproduced with permission from Kim YH, Liu HL, Mraz-Gernhard S, et al. Long-term outcome of 525 patients with mycosis fungoides and Sezary syndrome: Clinical Prognostic Factors and Risk for Disease Progression. *Arch Dermatol* 2003;139[7]: 857–866. Copyright © 2003 American Medical Association. All rights reserved.)

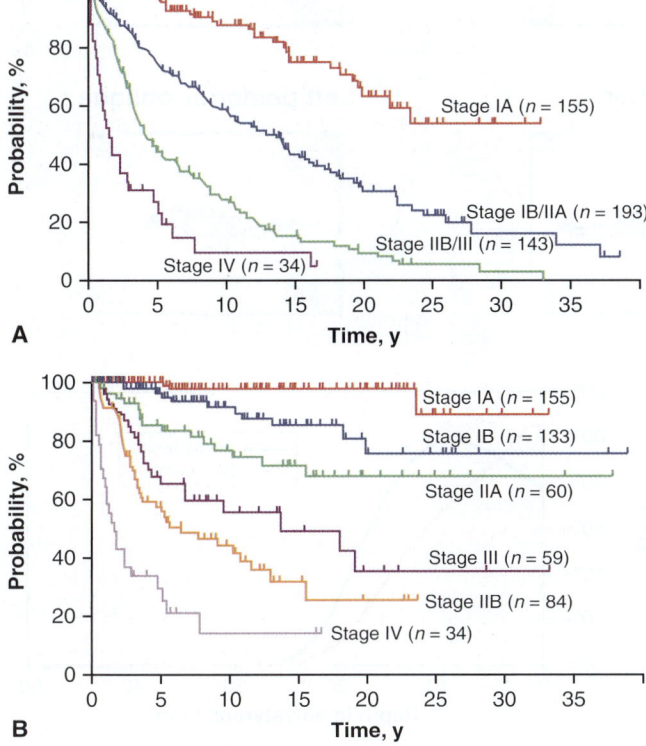

(PROCLIPI) has been initiated to define better the prognostic factors for patients with advanced disease (stage IIB or greater).

Skin-Directed Therapy

MF is not generally considered to be curable, although extended periods of disease-free survival after treatment have been reported. Efforts to treat MF are primarily focused on preventing progression and ameliorating symptoms. In early-stage disease, a number of skin-directed treatments are effective and should be considered as first-line therapy. Topical therapies include corticosteroids (complete response [CR] rates of 63% for T1 and 25% for T2 disease),[21] nitrogen mustard (CR rates of 76% to 80% for stage IA and 35% to 68% for stage IB),[22] carmustine (CR rates of 86% for T1 and 47% for T2 disease),[23] and bexarotene gel (CR rate of 21% in early-stage MF).[24] Phototherapy with narrow-band ultraviolet B (NB-UVB) (54% CR in stages IA or IB)[25] or psoralen + UVA (PUVA) (CR rate of 65%)[26] is also frequently used. However, the most effective skin-directed therapy for MF is ionizing radiation.

Ionizing radiation is well suited to the treatment of cutaneous lymphoma. Lymphocytes are highly radiosensitive, and radiation doses may be effectively limited to the epidermis and dermis by appropriate selection of photon or electron energies. Options for irradiation include local superficial irradiation or irradiation of the entirety of the skin via total skin electron beam therapy (TSEBT). The International Lymphoma Radiation Oncology Group recently reported their suggested guidelines for field and dose selection.[27]

Local Superficial Irradiation

A small portion (5%) of patients with stage IA MF present with "minimal" disease, defined as a solitary lesion or two to three MF lesions clustered sufficiently close to one another that they are amenable to treatment with a single or abutting radiation fields.[28] For these patients, treatment with local superficial irradiation may be considered. Treatment fields should be designed to encompass the entirety of the lesion (determined by visual inspection, palpation, and/or appropriate imaging) with a 1- to 2-cm margin, with use of a lead or Cerrobend cutout to conform field borders to the anatomy of the cutaneous lesion. Skin collimation can also be incorporated. Treatment is most commonly provided with electrons, with energies (usually 6 to 16 MeV) carefully selected to optimize dose penetration. Bolus is usually required with the lower-energy electrons (6 to 9 MeV) in order to

TABLE 83.4 EORTC TECHNICAL RECOMMENDATIONS FOR TSEBT[29]

The primary target in TSEBT is the epidermis, adnexal structures, and dermis.

The goal of treatment (either by primary or supplemental treatments) is to deliver a dose of 26–28 Gy to a depth of 4 mm below the skin surface, which usually translates to a truncal dose of 31–36 Gy.

Treatment should be provided in 30–36 fractions (1–1.2 Gy/fraction) over 6–10 wk. Fraction sizes should not exceed 2–2.5 Gy because of increased acute and late side effects.

The 80% isodose line should extend to 4 mm below the skin surface, the dose 20 mm deep to the skin must be <20% of the maximum dose at skin, and the dose at curved skin sites must not exceed 120% of the prescribed skin dose.

Patient positioning is critical, and patients must be positioned in a manner to maximize unfolding of the skin. A minimum of six treatment positions is recommended.

The optimal source-to-patient distance is 3–8 m, and dose should be homogenous to within 10% across the entire vertical and lateral dimensions of the beam at the patient's surface.

The globe of the eye must be limited to <15% of the maximum skin dose, and photon contamination at the bone marrow must be limited to <0.7 Gy.

Reprinted from Jones GW, Kacinski BM, Wilson LD, et al. Total skin electron radiation in the management of mycosis fungoides: Consensus of the European Organization for Research and Treatment of Cancer (EORTC) Cutaneous Lymphoma Project Group. *J Am Acad Dermatol* 2002;47(3):364–370. Copyright © 2002 American Academy of Dermatology, Inc. With permission.

maximize the dose at the skin surface. The EORTC recommends that the 80% isodose line is set at the deep border of the dermis,[29] which is commonly at a depth of approximately 4.5 mm.

Local superficial radiation is very effective in generating a CR for patients with "minimal" stage IA MF. In a review of 21 patients with "minimal" stage IA MF treated with local superficial radiation (superficial or orthovoltage x-rays or megavoltage electrons) to doses ranging from 20 to 40 Gy in four to five or 10 to 15 fractions, Wilson et al.[28] found a CR rate of 97%. Importantly, review of the recurrence rates associated

with different total doses of local superficial radiation revealed a 25% local recurrence rate (two of eight fields) with treatment to 20 Gy and an 8% local recurrence rate (two of 25 fields) with treatment to 20 to 40 Gy. Similarly, Cotter et al.[30] reported a local recurrence rate of 42% for fields treated to 10 Gy or less, but 0% for fields treated to >30 Gy. More recently, treatment to 8 Gy in one or two fractions has been shown to yield a CR rate of 92 to 94%.[31,32] Based on these studies, it is recommended that "minimal" stage IA (i.e., unilesional or up to three closely approximated sites) MF lesions are treated to a dose of 30 to 36 Gy, and treatment as low as 8 Gy in one or two fractions may be considered as a palliative treatment. Side effects of local superficial radiation are usually limited to mild dermatitis, local alopecia, and pigmentation changes.

Total Skin Electron Beam Therapy
Technique

TSEBT is technically challenging and should only be attempted in centers with special expertise in its provision, including skilled physics support. EORTC recommendations regarding the technical aspects of TSEBT are presented in Table 83.4. Modern TSEBT is usually accomplished with 6- to 9-MeV electrons generated by a medical linear accelerator directed at a patient standing behind a polycarbonate screen, 3.8 m from the linear accelerator head. The polycarbonate screen scatters the incident electron beam and contributes to an improved surface dose. Treatment is provided in "cycles," with one cycle composed of treatment of the patient in six different positions (Fig. 83.4A) over 2 days (three positions each day). Typically, a dose of 2 Gy is provided to the entirety of the skin during one cycle, and two cycles are usually administered per week. Treatment in six positions optimizes dose distribution at the skin surface (Fig. 83.4B). At Yale and Stanford, the anterior, right posterior oblique, and left posterior

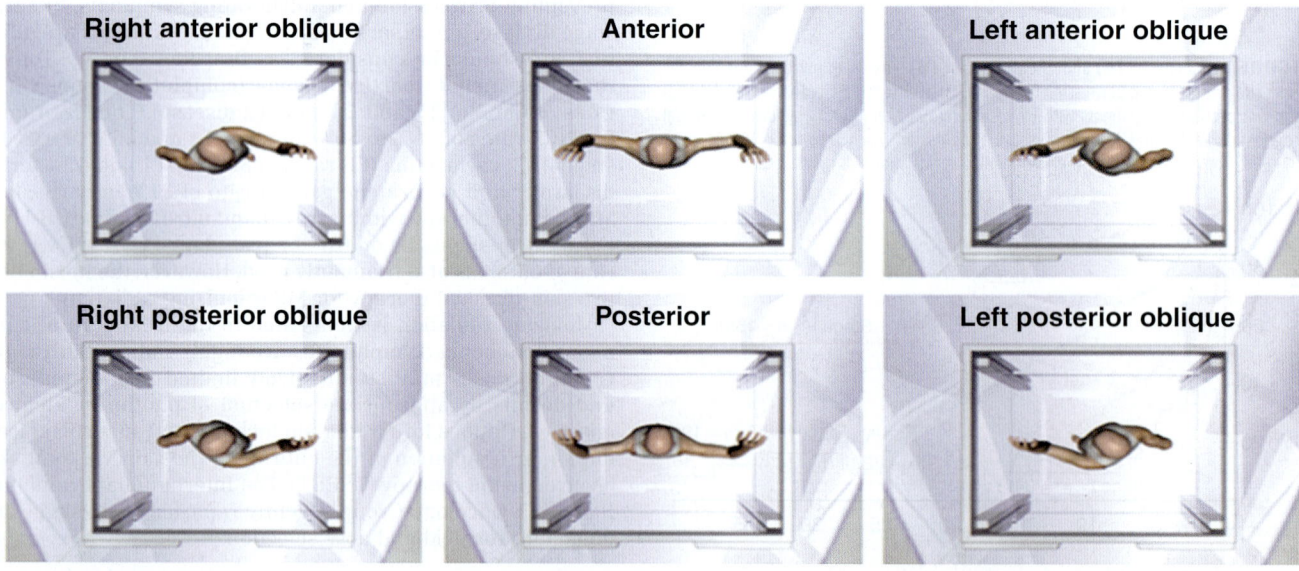

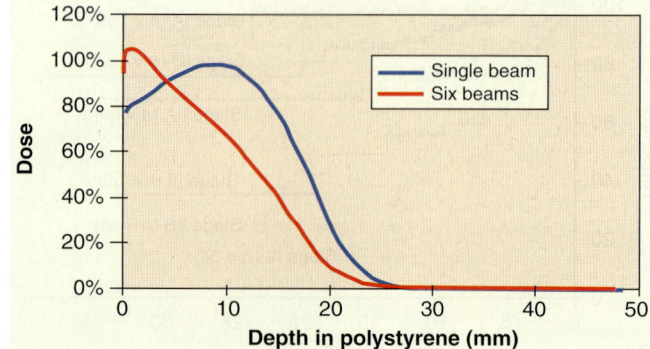

FIGURE 83.4.   A: The six total skin electron beam therapy (TSEBT) treatment positions as viewed from above. Images not to scale. **B:** Comparison of depth dose profiles associated with a single treatment position (*blue curve*) versus six treatment positions (*red curve*). (**A**, Courtesy of Christian Chang, www.christianchang.com, printed with permission from the artist. **B**, From Smith BD, Wilson LD. Management of mycosis fungoides: Part 2. Treatment. *Oncology* 2003;17[10]:1419–1428. Reprinted by permission of Benjamin D. Smith.)

oblique positions are treated on cycle day 1, and the posterior, right anterior oblique, and left anterior oblique positions on cycle day 2.[33,34] When the patient stands in a treatment position, a dual-field technique is used to deliver treatment to a superior and inferior field by angling the gantry 16 to 17.5 degrees above and below horizontal, respectively, the specific angle dependent upon individual machine characteristics (Fig. 83.5). Treatment to the six positions using the dual-field technique, which is in use at Yale and Stanford, delivers maximum dose to a depth of 1 mm, 80% dose to 6 to 7 mm, and 20% dose to 12.5 mm.[33,34]

Dose and Fractionation

Sublethal damage repair does not appear to be a major factor in determining the response of MF to ionizing radiation,[35] and modern TSEBT is provided with a relatively protracted course of two cycles per week for 9 weeks, which provides a total dose of 36 Gy to the skin surface. The total radiation dose appears to be directly associated with CR rates, with 18% CR with treatment to <10 Gy, 55% CR with treatment to 10 to 20 Gy, 66% CR with treatment to 20 to 25 Gy, 75% CR with treatment to 25 to 30 Gy, and 94% CR with treatment to 30 to 36 Gy.[36] However, lower doses yield impressive rates of overall response (defined as a >50% reduction in cutaneous disease), overall survival, progression-free survival, and relapse-free survival rates. Relapse rates are relatively high even in patients in which a CR is obtained, and the absolute benefit of a CR relative to the increased side effects at higher doses of TSEBT is unclear. The application of reduced-dose TSEBT (10 to 20 Gy) in combination with additional therapies may be a viable alternative to the current standard of 36 Gy.[37,38]

Two prospective trials of low-dose (10 to 12 Gy) TSEBT have been reported.[38,39] In the Stanford/MD Anderson trial, 33 patients with stage IB to IIIA disease were treated with 12 Gy TSEBT over 3 weeks. The CR rate was only 27%, but the overall response rate was 88%. The duration of clinical benefit (time to which another total skin therapy or systemic therapy was required for management) was 70.7 weeks.[38] This approach of management with TSEBT allows more frequent use of this very effective modality for the duration of a patient's illness, which is often many years. In addition, the toxicity is significantly less than with conventional dose treatment.

Supplemental Treatments

The six treatment positions in TSEBT maximize unfolding of the skin and exposure of the skin surface to the incident electron beam, but areas such as the soles of the feet, perineum, and scalp remain obscured and require supplemental doses to ensure that a minimum of 20 to 28 Gy is administered to a depth of approximately 4 mm. Supplemental treatment to these areas may be accomplished by the use of 120-kV superficial photons with half-value layer (HVL) 4.2-mm Al or low-energy (6 MeV) electrons with 1-cm bolus to treat the soles of the feet (1 Gy/fraction) and the perineum (1 Gy/fraction). In some setups, the scalp is treated by placing an angled electron reflector above the patient,[33] but supplemental boosting is an alternative approach that is incorporated in some centers. Additional areas that may need supplemental dose include thick cutaneous tumors and skin folds secondary to body habitus, and the need for supplemental dose to such areas is based on the judgment of the radiation oncologist.[33,34]

Side Effects

In a review of perceptions of MF therapy, patients overall considered TSEBT to be a more difficult treatment to endure

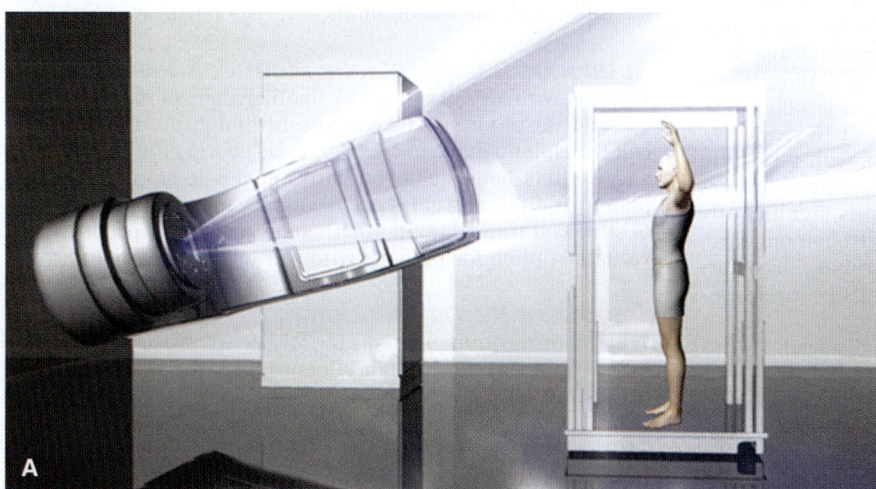

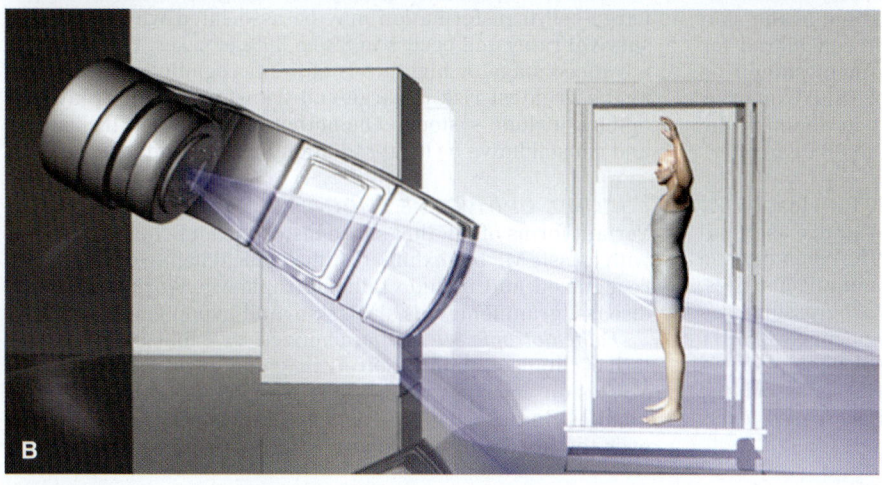

FIGURE 83.5. Dual-field technique for total skin electron beam therapy (TSEBT). **A:** Treatment of superior field. **B:** Treatment of inferior field. Images not to scale. (Courtesy of Christian Chang, www.christianchang.com, printed with permission from the artist.)

as compared to other treatments,[40] and it is important that patients are advised that symptoms such as pruritus and cutaneous erythema may be exacerbated during therapy. Additional acute side effects that commonly occur include xerosis, dry desquamation, extremity edema, blister/bullae formation over the lower extremities, alopecia (including hair of the scalp, eyebrows, eyelashes, and body), and nail changes (nails may ultimately be lost but usually regrow). Hypohydrosis secondary to damage to sweat glands may occur. Similarly, dryness and irritation of the nasal mucosa may result in nose bleeds. Gynecomastia is a rare occurrence. Late/chronic side effects are minimal and include cataract formation, chronic xerosis, persistent alopecia, dystrophic nails, telangiectasia, and secondary skin cancers including squamous and basal cell carcinomas and melanomas. Clinicians should be vigilant for the possibility of active cutaneous infection during the course of therapy.[29,41-45]

In an effort to minimize side effects, areas that are most susceptible to TSEBT such as the eyes, lips, hands, fingernails, feet, and testes are blocked during certain cycles of treatment. Shielding of the eye and lens may be accomplished by a combination of internal/external shields, selected based upon the proximity of clinical disease. Usually, if internal eyeshields are used, they are used for only a portion of the therapy (7 to 20 Gy). The lips, hands, and fingernails may be blocked by lead mitts or fingernail shields as clinical circumstances warrant. The feet may be blocked by footboards for a portion of the treatment. A testicular shield may be used during perineal boost treatments.[33]

Clinical Efficacy

TSEBT is very effective, particularly for early-stage disease. TSEBT yields a CR rate of >90% with a 15-year relapse-free survival of 40% in patients with T1 disease, although it is no longer recommended for such limited disease.[36] Of note, patients with recurrent disease after a course of TSEBT most commonly have disease restricted to <5% of the skin surface area, and these recurrences are therefore amenable to local salvage therapy with topical therapy or limited superficial radiation. When successful salvage of such limited recurrences is taken into account, relapse-free survival improves to 70% at 15 years.[46-48]

In T2 disease, TSEBT is similarly effective, with a CR rate of 76% to 90% and a 50% relapse-free survival rate at 5 years and 10% at 10 years. Relapse-free survival is significantly improved by addition of adjuvant PUVA or nitrogen mustard. Specifically, adjuvant PUVA improves 5-year relapse-free survival to 85%, and nitrogen mustard improves 10-year relapse-free survival to 40%.[29,48-50]

When cutaneous tumors are present (T3 disease), TSEBT is less effective but still yields an impressive CR rate of 44% to 54% of patients, much greater than any other single modality. Adjuvant treatment should be considered, and retrospective studies suggest that nitrogen mustard may increase the durability of response. Alternatively, a combination of nitrogen mustard and local superficial radiation may be considered for tumors localized to a small percentage of the skin surface.[48,50,51] Supplemental boosts should be considered for patients with tumors, and such boost treatment should be provided concomitantly with the initiation of TSEBT or prior to its initiation. The purpose of the boost is to diminish the thickness of the lesion so that electrons from TSEBT can effectively penetrate the entire lesion.

In erythrodermic MF (T4 disease), TSEBT yields a 70% to 100% response rate (for patients with T4N0 disease) and 5-year progression-free survival of 25% to 69%. When disease involves the peripheral circulation or extracutaneous sites, TSEBT is less effective and response and progression-free survival rates decrease to 74% and 36%, respectively. TSEBT appears to be synergistic with extracorporeal photopheresis (ECP), and the combination of TSEBT and ECP is associated with improved disease-specific survival and decreased levels of circulating malignant cells.[51-55]

Palliative Radiotherapy

Symptomatic nodal or visceral disease may be effectively palliated by a brief course of localized radiotherapy, usually to a total dose of 12 to 30 Gy. If this treatment is given in conjunction with a course of TSEBT, a similar dose may be used. In the subset of patients that develop extensive recurrence of cutaneous disease after a previous course of TSEBT, additional courses of TSEBT to lower total doses can be considered and have proven effective in studies at Yale and Stanford.[56,57]

Systemic Therapy

Skin-directed therapy should be attempted first for patients with early-stage disease, but in patients with advanced or refractory disease, systemic therapy may be considered. Options for systemic therapy include oral bexarotene (response rate up to 54% in refractory CTCL at a dose of 300 mg/m², and bexarotene may be used in combination with other therapies),[58,59] denileukin diftitox (a fusion protein consisting of interleukin-2 and a portion of the diphtheria toxin that yields an overall response rate of 30% in refractory CTCL),[60] histone deacetylase inhibitors (such as vorinostat and romidepsin, 30% response rate in refractory CTCL),[61,62] alemtuzumab (a monoclonal antibody targeted against the CD52 surface marker with a 38% overall response rate in relapsed or refractory CTCL and 86% response rate in SS),[63,64] interferon-α2a (IFN-α) (a biologic modifier with a response rate of 40% to 80% in CTCL as a single agent and with synergistic activity with other MF therapies),[65-71] ECP (associated with improvement in peripheral blood and skin involvement, especially in those with T4 disease),[72] brentuximab vedotin,[73] and cytotoxic chemotherapy (single-agent chemotherapy with agents such as purine or nucleoside analogs, liposomal doxorubicin, and antifolate agents, including methotrexate and pralatrexate, is preferred because no distinct advantages have been identified with the use of multiagent regimens).[74-80]

Autologous or Allogeneic Stem Cell Transplant

Patients with MF/SS refractory to other therapies may be considered for stem cell transplant. Although autologous stem cell transplants have not proven to be overly effective, greater success has been achieved with allogeneic stem cell transplants. Additional studies are necessary to fully define the role of stem cell transplant in MF. This approach may prove to be a valuable option for patients with refractory disease.[81-85]

Treatment Recommendations by Stage

Treatment recommendations for MF/SS are presented by stage in Table 83.5.[82] The National Comprehensive Cancer Network (NCCN) has also published treatment guidelines for MF/SS.[86]

Transformed Disease

In some cases, large-cell transformation of MF may occur, which is identified on biopsy by >25% large cells in the sample. Large-cell transformation may be associated with decreased survival rates and occurs in 8% to 39% of cases. Patients with advanced stage or high levels of β₂-microglobulin or LDH are at the greatest risk of large-cell transformation. Treatment options include systemic chemotherapy, stem cell transplant, and consolidative or local radiation for localized disease.[82]

Variants of Mycosis Fungoides

Variant forms of MF that share histologic and clinical features with classic MF but exhibit distinct clinical behavior have been recognized and include folliculotropic MF, Woringer-Kolopp disease, granulomatous slack skin, and hypopigmented MF.

Folliculotropic MF is characterized by a folliculotropic pattern of cutaneous infiltration of malignant T cells. Folliculotropic MF lesions present as patches, plaques, or tumors or may manifest in an acneiform pattern. Lesions primarily develop over the head and neck and are rarely found over the trunk.

TABLE 83.5 RECOMMENDATIONS FOR TREATMENT OF MF BY STAGE

Stage	First-Line Therapies	Options for Refractory or Relapsed Disease
"Minimal" IA	Local superficial irradiation	Consider standard-stage IA first-line therapies
IA, IB, IIA	Expectant observation (for stage IA)	Second course TSEBT
	Topical therapies (corticosteroids, nitrogen mustard, BCNU, bexarotene)	Oral bexarotene
		IFN-α
		Low-dose MTX
	Phototherapy (PUVA, NB-UVB)	Vorinostat
		Denileukin diftitox
	TSEBT (consider adjuvant PUVA or nitrogen mustard)	Clinical trials
		NOTE: Chemotherapy is not recommended
IIB	TSEBT (consider boosts to cutaneous tumors and adjuvant PUVA or nitrogen mustard)	Second course TSEBT
		Oral bexarotene
		Vorinostat
	IFN-α	Denileukin diftitox
	PUVA	Clinical trials
		Chemotherapy
IIIA, IIIB, leukemic CTCL or SS	TSEBT + ECP	Second course TSEBT
	ECP alone	Oral bexarotene
	IFN-α	Vorinostat
	PUVA + IFN-α	Denileukin diftitox
	MTX	Alemtuzumab
		Clinical trials
		Chemotherapy
		Allogeneic stem cell transplant
IVA(1–2), IVB	Chemotherapy	Allogeneic stem cell transplant
	TSEBT for palliation	
	Oral bexarotene	
	Denileukin diftitox	
	IFN-α	
	Vorinostat	
	Romidepsin	
	Low-dose MTX	
	Clinical trials	

BCNU, bis-chloroethylnitrosourea; CTCL, cutaneous T-cell lymphoma; ECP, extracorporeal photopheresis; IFN-α, interferon-alpha; MTX, methotrexate; NB-UVB, narrowband ultraviolet B; PUVA, psoralen plus ultraviolet A; SS, Sézary syndrome; TSEBT, total skin electron beam therapy.

Localized alopecia secondary to the folliculotropic pattern is common. Folliculotropic MF is associated with a 15-year survival of 41% for early-stage disease. Early-stage disease may be treated with PUVA combined with bexarotene or IFN-α. Local radiation therapy may be advantageous because it can effectively treat to deeper depths of involvement seen in this variant. Advanced-stage disease is minimally responsive to cytotoxic chemotherapy, and alternate options such as irradiation or allogeneic stem cell transplant should be considered.[1,87,88]

Woringer-Kolopp disease (pagetoid reticulosis) is characterized by a solitary erythematous and scaling cutaneous patch on an extremity. Biopsy results are similar to classic MF, and the malignant T cells commonly carry a CD3+/CD4+/CD8− or CD3+/CD4−/CD8+ immunophenotype. If CD8+ disease is identified, it is important to consider the alternative diagnosis of CD8+ aggressive peripheral CTCL, and the distinction between these diagnoses is made by the aggressiveness of disease. Specifically, as compared to CD8+ aggressive peripheral CTCL, Woringer-Kolopp disease is very slowly progressive and carries an excellent prognosis. Treatment options include skin-directed therapies such as corticosteroids, nitrogen mustard, resection, or local irradiation. Local radiation may be very successful in achieving long-term local control even in locally very advanced disease. In rare cases of diffuse or refractory disease, irradiation is also recommended.[1,89]

Granulomatous slack skin (GSS) is an extremely rare variant of MF, with <100 cases reported in the literature. It is characterized by cutaneous infiltration of a clonal population of malignant T cells coupled with a granulomatous infiltration. The granulomatous infiltrate ultimately causes destruction of local elastin fibers and impairs the structural integrity and elasticity of the skin, which results in loose or "slack" skin. This loosening of the skin is most commonly observed in the axilla, groin, neck, and breast. Although GSS is itself an indolent disease, it is associated with an increased incidence of secondary lymphomas, most commonly Hodgkin lymphoma or MF. Given the rarity of this disease, it is difficult to make definitive recommendations regarding therapy, but surgical resection or local superficial radiation may be effective.[1,90]

Hypopigmented MF presents at an earlier age (childhood or adolescence) than classic MF and is characterized by development of hypopigmented patches frequently over the trunk or extremities. In contrast to classic MF, the malignant T cells are often CD8+. Treatment and disease course are otherwise similar to classic MF.[91,92]

Non–Mycosis Fungoides Cutaneous T-Cell Lymphoma
Staging
In 2007, the ISCL and EORTC presented a new TNM staging system for non-MF/SS cutaneous lymphomas (Table 83.6).[93]

CD30+ Lymphoproliferative Disorders
A review of the SEER registry identified 268 cases of primary cutaneous CD30+ lymphoproliferative disorders recorded between 1974 and 2004 (58% male and 42% female patients). The median age of diagnosis was 61, and population-matched 3-year relative survival was 87%, with 5-year disease-specific survival 92%. Localization of disease in the head and neck appears to be a negative prognostic factor.[94] The primary cutaneous CD30+ lymphoproliferative disorders recognized by the WHO/EORTC are primary cutaneous anaplastic large-cell

TABLE 83.6 ISCL/EORTC TNM CLASSIFICATION OF CUTANEOUS LYMPHOMA OTHER THAN MF/SS[93]

T Stage	N Stage	M Stage
T1: Solitary skin involvement	N0: No clinical or pathologic lymph node involvement	M0: No evidence of extracutaneous non–lymph node disease
T1a: A solitary lesion <5 cm in diameter	N1: Involvement of 1 peripheral lymph node region that drains an area of current or prior skin involvement	M1: Extracutaneous non–lymph node disease present
T1b: A solitary lesion >5 cm in diameter		
T2: Regional skin involvement: multiple lesions limited to 1 body region or 2 contiguous body regions	N2: Involvement of 2 or more peripheral lymph node regions or involvement of any lymph node region that does not drain an area of current or prior skin involvement	
T2a: All-disease-encompassing in a <15-cm-diameter circular area		
T2b: All-disease-encompassing in a >15- and <30-cm-diameter circular area	N3: Involvement of central lymph nodes	
T2c: All-disease-encompassing in a >30-cm-diameter circular area		
T3: Generalized skin involvement		
T3a: Multiple lesions involving 2 noncontiguous body regions		
T3b: Multiple lesions involving ≥3 body regions		

Republished with permission of American Society of Hematology from Kim YH, Willemze R, Pimpinelli N, et al. TNM classification system for primary cutaneous lymphomas other than mycosis fungoides and Sezary syndrome: a proposal of the International Society for Cutaneous Lymphomas (ISCL) and the Cutaneous Lymphoma Task Force of the European Organization of Research and Treatment of Cancer (EORTC). *Blood* 2007;110(2):479–484; permission conveyed through Copyright Clearance Center, Inc.

Section III

lymphoma and lymphomatoid papulosis.[1] These cannot be differentiated histologically. It is essential to take a careful clinical history to document the distribution of lesions and their clinical course (e.g., history of spontaneous regression). The diagnosis is a clinicopathologic one. The EORTC, ISCL, and USCLC have provided consensus recommendations regarding the evaluation and treatment of primary cutaneous CD30+ lymphoproliferative disorders.[95]

Primary cutaneous anaplastic large-cell lymphoma (C-ALCL) is characterized by development of cutaneous plaques, nodules, or tumors that are usually solitary or clustered into a localized area. Multifocal disease is uncommon (occurring in only 20% of patients), and lymph nodes are involved in only 10% of cases. Extracutaneous disease is rarely found. C-ALCL is most commonly diagnosed in males, with a male:female ratio of 2–3:1. When disease is localized to the skin and regional lymph nodes, prognoses are excellent, with anticipated 5-year overall survival and 10-year disease-specific survival rates of 90%. Progression to extracutaneous disease is associated with overall survival, and extensive limb disease (defined as "initial presentation or progression to multiple skin tumors in 1 limb or contiguous body regions")[96] is associated with disease-specific survival. Biopsies of C-ALCL lesions reveal a diffuse infiltration of large anaplastic CD4+ T cells, and at least 75% of these anaplastic T cells express CD30. Similar to MF, clonal dominance is frequently detected by PCR evaluation for TCR rearrangement.[1]

Limited resection or local superficial irradiation is very effective in controlling localized cutaneous disease, and low-dose methotrexate may be considered when widespread cutaneous disease precludes simple resection or irradiation. Local superficial radiation to a dose of 34 to 44 Gy was associated with a 100% CR rate,[97] but more recent data suggest that lower doses such as 20 Gy may be adequate.[98] In rare cases in which extracutaneous disease is found, doxorubicin-based chemotherapy should be considered.

Of note, prior to initiating therapy, it is critically important to verify that C-ALCL has been correctly distinguished from the more common systemic ALCL. Molecular studies to evaluate the presence of the (2:5)(p23;q35) chromosomal translocation and expression of anaplastic lymphoma kinase (ALK) or epithelial membrane antigen (EMA) are useful in making this distinction, because the (2:5) translocation and expression of ALK and EMA are found in systemic ALCL but rarely found in C-ALCL.[1,99]

Lymphomatoid papulosis (LyP) carries an excellent prognosis, with a 5-year overall survival rate of 100%. However, 15% to 20% of patients with LyP will develop MF, C-ALCL, or a Hodgkin lymphoma. LyP is characterized by development of violaceous papular or papulonodular lesions over the trunk or extremities, which typically regress after 3 to 12 weeks, often leaving a residual scar. Biopsy of LyP cutaneous lesions reveals epidermotropic atypical CD3+/CD4+/CD8– lymphocytes, and clonal TCR rearrangement is identified in 60% to 70% of cases. Three distinct histologic subtypes are recognized: LyP A, B, and C. LyP A (characterized by large multinucleated CD30+ cells intermixed with an inflammatory infiltrate) and C (characterized by large CD30+ cells with minimal inflammatory infiltrate) represent 90% of cases. In contrast to types A and C, atypical lymphocytes in LyP B are CD3+/CD4+/CD30–, reminiscent of MF.[1]

Aggressive therapies such as chemotherapy or radiation should be avoided in LyP. In the rare patient with a large cutaneous burden of disease, skin-directed therapy with PUVA or a topical chemotherapy agent may be considered. In addition, low-dose oral methotrexate may be effective in suppressing the development of new lesions and should be considered if previous LyP lesions caused significant scarring.[1]

Extranodal NK-/T-Cell Lymphoma, Nasal Type
Extranodal NK-/T-cell lymphoma, nasal type most commonly arises in the nasal cavity and nasopharynx but in select cases

may present with cutaneous plaques or tumors over the extremities and trunk and is therefore included in the WHO/EORTC classification of cutaneous lymphomas. Biopsy of a cutaneous lesion reveals a dense lymphoid infiltrate, which may exhibit an epidermotropic component. The malignant cells are most commonly NK in origin with a CD3–/CD2+/CD56+ immunophenotype, but on occasion, the malignant cells are derived from cytotoxic T cells. Epstein-Barr virus (EBV) is directly associated with disease development, and cutaneous lesions are nearly always EBV+. Consistent with an EBV-mediated pathophysiology, the disease occurs more commonly in geographic distributions in which EBV is endemic (Central America, South America, South Asia). The TCR usually remains in germline configuration when the malignant cells are of NK-cell origin, but clonal TCR rearrangement may be observed in cases in which the malignant cells are derived from cytotoxic T cells. Optimal treatment regimens for cutaneous extranodal NK-/T-cell lymphoma, nasal type have not yet been determined. Treatment with extended field radiotherapy to a median dose of 50 Gy yields a CR rate of 95.4% in early-stage disease, but local or distant recurrences are common and adjuvant therapy with L-asparaginase and other regimens should be considered. Advanced-stage disease is treated primarily with chemotherapy.[1,100–102]

Subcutaneous Panniculitis-like T-Cell Lymphoma
Subcutaneous panniculitis-like T-cell lymphoma presents with subcutaneous nodules and/or plaques, which are commonly localized over the legs or trunk. Biopsy reveals a lymphoid infiltrate composed primarily of malignant cytotoxic CD8+ T cells. Prior to the establishment of the WHO/EORTC classification system, α/β and γ/δ T-cell forms of disease were each recognized as subcutaneous panniculitis-like T-cell lymphoma. However, γ/δ T-cell lymphoma is now recognized as a distinct, more aggressive disease and is categorized as a primary cutaneous peripheral T-cell lymphoma. The 5-year survival of the less aggressive α/β disease approaches 80%, and treatment involves combinations of corticosteroids and radiation, and potentially chemotherapy for refractory disease.[1] Notably, presence of the hemophagocytic syndrome predicts a worse prognosis.

Adult T-Cell Leukemia/Lymphoma
Infection with the human T-lymphotropic virus 1 (HTLV-1) may result in adult T-cell leukemia/lymphoma in approximately 1% to 5% individuals, and patients may develop associated cutaneous disease characterized by papules, plaques, and tumors. In smoldering disease, cutaneous lesions may be the only sign of pathology. Chemotherapy is the primary therapy for acute adult T-cell leukemia/lymphoma, while smoldering cases may be treated with skin-directed therapies.[1]

Primary Cutaneous Peripheral T-Cell Lymphoma
Additional CTCLs that do not fit into the previously discussed categories are grouped as "primary cutaneous peripheral T-cell lymphomas," and provisional subsets of this category described by the WHO/EORTC include primary cutaneous aggressive epidermotropic CD8+ cytotoxic T-cell lymphoma (characterized by cutaneous papules/plaques, nodules, and tumors with ulceration and a propensity for extracutaneous spread of disease; of note, it has recently been proposed that CD8+ should be removed from the naming of this disease entity in order to allow inclusion of diseases of similar behavior that is CD8- or has variability in TCR expression status),[103] cutaneous γ/δ T-cell lymphoma (most commonly characterized by subcutaneous plaques or tumors in the extremities), primary cutaneous CD4+ small/medium-sized pleomorphic T-cell lymphoma (usually presents as a single cutaneous plaque or tumor on the head and neck or upper trunk and has an indolent clinical behavior), and primary cutaneous peripheral T-cell lymphoma, unspecified (most commonly presents as solitary or generalized

nodules). The primary cutaneous peripheral T-cell lymphomas are primarily treated with chemotherapy or allogeneic stem cell transplantation, with the exception of primary cutaneous CD4+ small/medium-sized pleomorphic T-cell lymphoma, which may be treated with local resection or radiation.[1]

CUTANEOUS B-CELL LYMPHOMAS

Primary cutaneous B-cell lymphoma (PCBCL) was first recognized as a distinct clinical entity in 1981 and accounts for only 29% of the 3,884 cases of primary cutaneous lymphoma diagnosed in the United States during 2001 to 2005.[3] The WHO/EORTC classification system recognizes three primary categories of CBCL: primary cutaneous marginal zone B-cell lymphoma (PCMZL), primary cutaneous follicle center B-cell lymphoma (PCFCL), and primary cutaneous diffuse large B-cell lymphoma, leg type (PCLBCL-LT).[1] Of the CBCL cases diagnosed in the United States in 2001 to 2005, the most common subtype was primary cutaneous DLBCL (40%, of which only 23% were of leg type), followed closely by cutaneous follicle center lymphoma (30%) and cutaneous marginal zone B-cell lymphoma (25%).[3] However, it should be noted that the histopathologic criteria for PLCBCL changed upon adoption of the WHO/EORTC consensus system, and it is likely that most of the PLCBCL cases diagnosed during 2001 to 2005 would now be reclassified as PCFCL. In a recent review, 65% of CBCL cases classified as DLBCL using the older WHO criteria were found to be PCFCL under the current WHO/EORTC classification.[104]

Primary Cutaneous Marginal Zone B-Cell Lymphoma

PCMZL commonly presents with isolated or multifocal red or violaceous papules, plaques, and/or nodules on the trunk or extremities. The malignant cells are marginal zone B cells with a CD20+/CD79a+/CD5−/CD10− immunophenotype. Biopsies reveal an infiltrate composed of numerous lymphoid cells including marginal zone B cells, lymphoplasmacytoid cells, plasma cells, centroblast-like and immunoblast-like cells, reactive T cells, and reactive germinal centers. The prognosis for patients with PCMZL is excellent, and extracutaneous disease is rarely seen. Five-year overall survival rates of approximately 99% are expected, and cutaneous disease is very responsive to therapy. Cutaneous relapses are common but do not predict decreased survival.[1]

Primary Cutaneous Follicle Center Lymphoma

In contrast to PCMZL, PCFCL frequently presents with solitary or clustered plaques and tumors on the scalp, forehead, and trunk. Biopsy reveals a nodular or diffuse lymphoid infiltrate containing varying proportions of centrocytes, centroblasts, and reactive T cells growing in patterns ranging from follicular to diffuse. Similar to PCMZL, the malignant cells in PCFCL are of a CD20+/CD79a+ immunophenotype. Clonal rearrangement of immunoglobulin genes is usually observed. Importantly, the chromosomal translocation t(14:18) is infrequently seen in PCFCL, and therefore, detection of this translocation should prompt consideration of a nodal or systemic follicular lymphoma. Similar to PCMZL, cutaneous lesions respond well to treatment, but rates of cutaneous relapse are relatively high at 20% overall. Extracutaneous disease is detected in 5% to 10% of patients, and bone marrow biopsy is an important component of evaluation. The 5-year overall survival rate for PCFCL is estimated at 95%.[1]

Primary Cutaneous Diffuse Large B-Cell Lymphoma, Leg Type

PCLBCL, leg type, most commonly presents with violaceous cutaneous tumors over the lower extremities. Despite the nomenclature, anatomic restriction to the legs is not a requirement, and in rare cases, PCLBCL, leg type, may be found in other cutaneous sites than the leg. The disease is characterized by diffuse lymphoid infiltrates with a predominance of centroblasts and immunoblasts, with absence of any significant numbers of centrocytes being a key distinguishing feature from PCFCL. A CD20+, CD79a+, Bcl-6+/−, CD10−, Bcl-2+, MUM-1+, and FOXP1+ immunophenotype is usually observed. In contrast to PCMZL and PCFCL, both cutaneous relapses and development of extracutaneous disease are common, and the 5-year overall survival is decreased to 50%. A very small subset of PCLBCL (such as intravascular PCLBCL or anaplastic or plasmablastic PCLBCL) is categorized as "PCLBCL, other."[1]

Diagnosis and Evaluation

Evaluation of patients with suspected PCBCL should follow the basic protocol recommended by ISCL/USCLC/EORTC previously discussed.[13] In addition, a bone marrow biopsy is needed for PCBCL-LT and should be strongly considered in PCFCL (rate of bone marrow involvement may be as high as 11%). In other cases the need for bone marrow biopsy is left to the discretion of the treating physician. A further component to evaluation of PCBCL in European nations includes evaluation for *Borrelia burgdorferi* infection.[1,105] The *Borrelia* subspecies *Borrelia afzelii* that appears to be the causative organism is not found in the United States.[106]

Staging and Prognosis

PCBCLs should be staged in accordance with the ISCL/EORTC staging system for non-MF/SS cutaneous lymphomas (Table 83.6). A cutaneous B-cell lymphoma prognostic index (CBCL-PI) was developed by correlating outcome data from the Surveillance, Epidemiology, and End Results (SEER) database with PCBCL histology and anatomic location (Table 83.7).[107] Four prognostic groups (IA, IB, II, III) were defined by the CBCL-PI based on specific combinations of histology and anatomic location. However, as described earlier, the histologic criteria in use during the years on which the CBCL-PI is based (1973 to 2001) were changed with the 2005 release of the WHO/EORTC consensus classification system,[1] and the CBCL-PI should be used with caution when modern histopathologic classification criteria are used.

In 2011, the International Extranodal Lymphoma Study Group (IELSG) released the CLIPi for indolent CBCL. Independent prognostic factors associated with progression-free survival included serum LDH, morphology (nodule vs. other), and number of distinct cutaneous sites of disease (greater than two). One point is scored for each factor, and patients are grouped into low risk (score 0), intermediate risk (score 1), and high risk (score 2 or 3) with associated 5-year progression-free survival rates of 91%, 64%, and 48%, respectively.[108] The clinical utility of this prognostic system in determining risk-adapted therapy remains unclear.

Treatment

No prospective randomized clinical trial data are available to help guide treatment decisions, but the ISCL/EORTC recently performed an extensive survey of the literature pertaining to treatment of the PCBCLs and published consensus recommendations.[109] The NCCN has also published treatment guidelines for PCBCLs.[110]

PCMZL and PCFCL

PCMZL and PCFCL are not expected to be associated with decreased survival relative to control populations (although PCFCL arising in the leg may have a worsened prognosis under the WHO/EORTC classification), and therefore, side effects of proposed treatments should be carefully considered. Treatment options include local superficial irradiation, surgical excision, intralesional IFN-α, local and systemic rituximab, antibiotics (where *B. burgdorferi* is endemic), and chemotherapy.

Section III

TABLE 83.7 CUTANEOUS B-CELL LYMPHOMA PROGNOSTIC INDEX

CBCL-PI Group[107]	Histology	Site	% 5-Year OS	% Relative 5-Year OS
IA	Any indolent	Any	81	94
IB	Diffuse large B cell	Favorable	72	96
II	Diffuse large B cell	Unfavorable	48	60
	Immunoblastic diffuse large B cell	Favorable		
III	Immunoblastic diffuse large B cell	Unfavorable	27	34

CBCL-PI, cutaneous B-cell lymphoma prognostic index; OS, overall survival.

Local Superficial Irradiation. In the ISCL/EORTC literature review, 132 patients with PCMZL treated with local superficial irradiation were identified, and a 99% CR rate was observed. Doses ranged from 30 to 45 Gy, and field margins ranged from 1 to 5 cm. Although cutaneous relapse of disease occurred in 46% of patients, extracutaneous progression occurred in only 2% of patients. For PCFCL, 460 patients treated with radiation were reviewed, and the CR rate was 99% with a 30% relapse rate. Doses ranged from 20 to 54 Gy and margins were 0.5 to 5+ cm. Current guidelines suggest that for definitive therapy, a dose of 24 to 30 Gy is sufficient, with treatment margins of 1 to 1.5 cm.[27] Recently, local superficial irradiation to 4 Gy in two fractions was shown to yield a 72% CR rate for PCMZL and PCFCL and is recommended as a palliative dose.[25,109]

Surgery. *Excision* is associated with a 99% CR rate and 43% cutaneous relapse rate in PCMZL and a 98% CR rate and 40% cutaneous relapse rate in PCFCL.[109]

IFN-α. Intralesional IFN-α yields a 100% CR rate and 25% local relapse rate for PCMZL and a 100% CR rate and 29% local relapse rate for PCFCL.[109]

Rituximab. Systemic rituximab (monoclonal antibody targeted against CD20) has proven effective as a treatment for non-Hodgkin lymphomas and has been applied to the treatment of PCBCL. In a review of five patients with PCMZL treated with systemic rituximab, the overall response rate was 60%, and in 10 patients with PCFCL treated with systemic rituximab, a 100% overall response rate and 80% CR rate was observed. Intralesional rituximab may also be effective, with a reported CR rate of 89% in nine patients with PCMZL, but with a high relapse rate of 62%. Twelve patients with PCFCL treated with intralesional rituximab had a CR rate of 83% with 40% relapse.[111] This is a useful modality for patients who have extensive skin involvement.

Chemotherapy. Single-agent treatment with chlorambucil was evaluated in 14 patients with PCMZL, and a CR rate of 64% with 33% relapse rate was observed. Multiagent chemotherapy with cyclophosphamide, doxorubicin, vincristine, and prednisone (CHOP) was also evaluated in 33 patients with PCMZL, and an 85% CR rate with 57% relapse rate was observed. In 104 patients with PCFCL treated with CHOP or CHOP-like regimens, an 85% CR rate with 48% relapse rate was reported.[109]

ISCL/EORTC Recommendations. For patients who have only one or a few lesions clustered in one region, radiation (30 Gy or more) using a margin of 1 to 1.5 cm is highly effective. Patients presenting with a single small lesion may be treated with resection alone. Scattered lesions that cannot easily be encompassed in one or a few radiation fields may be carefully observed, with treatment reserved for only the most concerning or symptomatic sites. In the setting of diffuse disease, systemic rituximab should be considered. Of note, cutaneous relapses are common, and relapsed disease often responds to retreatment and does not predict for worsened overall survival rate.[109]

PCLBCL, Leg Type (PCBCL-LT)
PCLBCL-LT is a significantly more aggressive entity in comparison to PCMZL and PCFCL. The primary treatment options that are used in therapy for PCBCL-LT are radiation, rituximab, and multiagent chemotherapy.

Local Superficial Irradiation. The ISCL/EORTC literature review found 101 patients with PCLBCL-LT treated with radiation. In contrast to the more indolent lymphomas in which CR rates were close to 100%, the CR rate for PCLBCL-LT was lower at 88%. The rate of cutaneous relapse rate was high (58%), and even more concerning, 30% of patients were found to have extracutaneous progression of disease.

Rituximab. Systemic rituximab in PCLBCL-LT has been investigated (dose 375 mg/m² weekly for 4 to 8 weeks) and yielded a CR rate of 38%. Relapse rates are as yet unknown, and additional follow-up is necessary.[109]

Chemotherapy. Multiagent chemotherapy regimens have been tested in PCLBCL-LT, and in 32 patients treated with CHOP or CHOP-like regimens, an 81% CR rate has been observed. However, despite aggressive therapy, relapse rates remain high at 54%.[109]

ISCL/EORTC Recommendations. Based on the aggressive nature of PCLBCL-LT and its propensity to develop extracutaneous disease, recommended treatment in patients able to tolerate multiagent chemotherapy is R-CHOP, with the possible addition of local superficial radiation to distinct cutaneous lesions. In the subset of patients unable to tolerate a multiagent course of chemotherapy, systemic rituximab may be considered. Alternatively, an aggressive course of radiation to all cutaneous sites of disease may be considered, but relapse is expected.[109]

PRECURSOR HEMATOLOGIC NEOPLASMS

The third category of cutaneous lymphomas in the WHO/EORTC system is precursor hematologic neoplasms/immature hematologic malignancies. At present, this category primarily references CD4+/CD56+ hematodermic neoplasm (also referred to as blastic NK-cell lymphoma or blastic plasmacytoid dendritic cell neoplasm), which is characterized by development of red or violaceous cutaneous nodules. Biopsy reveals cutaneous infiltration of abnormal cells with an appearance reminiscent of lymphoblasts and myeloblasts. The origin of the tumor cells in CD4+/CD56+ hematodermic neoplasm is unclear. Immunohistochemistry indicates that the tumor cells lack CD3 and CD8 and express both CD4 and CD56. The expression of CD56 initially led investigators to believe these cells were of NK origin. However, the concomitant expression of CD4 and CD56 is unusual, and further exploration led to the identification of expression of CD123 and TCL1 in these tumor cells, which suggests a possible origin in plasmacytoid dendritic cells. Examination of TCR status in these cells indicates it remains in germline configuration, providing further support for the notion that these cells are not derived from a B- or T-cell lineage. CD4+/CD56+ hematodermic neoplasm is an aggressive malignancy, and it is common for patients to harbor nodal or systemic disease at diagnosis. Because of the propensity for systemic spread of disease, skin-directed therapies are usually unlikely to control disease and chemotherapy is often necessary. Although chemotherapy may induce remission of disease, the duration of remission is typically relatively brief and median survival is only 14 months.[1]

Summary

The primary cutaneous lymphomas are a diverse group of extranodal non-Hodgkin lymphomas, each with distinct biologic activity. A correct histopathologic diagnosis is critical to the determination of appropriate management. Although significant advances in therapy have been made since the recognition of MF in 1806, numerous questions remain unanswered regarding the pathophysiology and optimal treatment of the cutaneous lymphomas. Advances in genomic profiling of the cutaneous lymphomas may yield greater insight into the molecular bases of these diseases and help identify better and more individualized therapies. Recent efforts to develop improved prognostic indices and uniform criteria for classification of disease and response to treatment should facilitate ongoing international collaborations. Because of the rarity of these diseases, large multi-institutional collaborative efforts are critical to the advancement of our understanding of the primary cutaneous lymphomas.

REFERENCES

1. Willemze R, Jaffe ES, Burg G, et al. WHO-EORTC classification for cutaneous lymphomas. *Blood* 2005;105:3768–3785.
2. *WHO classification of tumours of haematopoeitic and lymphoid tissues*. 4th ed. Lyon, France: IARC, 2008.
3. Bradford PT, Devesa SS, Anderson WS, et al. Cutaneous lymphoma incidence patterns in the United States: a population-based study of 3884 cases. *Blood* 2009;113(21):5064–5073.
4. Assaf C, Gellrich S, Steinhoff M, et al. Cutaneous lymphomas in Germany: an analysis of the Central Cutaneous Lymphoma Registry of the German Society of Dermatology (DDG). *J Dtsch Dermatol Ges* 2007;5(8):662–668.
5. Girardi M, Heald PW, Wilson LD. The pathogenesis of mycosis fungoides. *N Engl J Med* 2004;350:1978–1988.
6. Olsen EA, Whittaker S, Kim YH, et al. Clinical end points and response criteria in mycosis fungoides and Sezary syndrome: a consensus statement of the International Society for Cutaneous Lymphomas, the United States Cutaneous Lymphoma Consortium, and the Cutaneous Lymphoma Task Force of the European Organisation for Research and Treatment of Cancer. *J Clin Oncol* 2011;29(18):2598–2607.
7. Kim YH, Liu HL, Mraz-Gernhard S, et al. Long-term outcome of 525 patients with mycosis fungoides and Sezary syndrome. *Arch Dermatol* 2003;139:857–866.
8. Salgado R, Servitje O, Gallardo F, et al. Oligonucleotide array-CGH identifies genomic subgroups and prognostic markers for tumor stage mycosis fungoides. *J Invest Dermatol* 2010;130(4):1126–1135.
9. Van Doorn R, van Kester MS, Dijkman R, et al. Oncogenomic analysis of mycosis fungoides reveals major differences with Sezary syndrome. *Blood* 2009;113(1):127–136.
10. Ballabio E, Mitchell T, van Kester MS, et al. MicroRNA expression in Sezary syndrome: identification, function, and diagnostic potential. *Blood* 2010;116(7):1105–1113.
11. van Kester MS, Ballabio E, Benner MF, et al. miRNA expression profiling of mycosis fungoides. *Mol Oncol* 2011;5(3):273–280.
12. Choi J, Goh G, Walradt T, et al. Genomic landscape of cutaneous T cell lymphoma. *Nat Genet* 2015;47(9):1011–1019.
13. Pimpinelli N, Olsen EA, Santucci M, et al. Defining early mycosis fungoides. *J Am Acad Dermatol* 2005;53(6):1053–1063.
14. Olsen E, Vonderheid E, Pimpinelli N, et al. Revisions to the staging and classification of mycosis fungoides and Sezary syndrome: a proposal of the International Society for Cutaneous Lymphomas (ISCL) and the Cutaneous Lymphoma Task Force of the European Organization of Research and Treatment of Cancer (EORTC). *Blood* 2007;110(6):1713–1722.
15. Trautinger F, Eder J, Assaf C, et al. European Organisation for Research and Treatment of Cancer consensus recommendations for the treatment of mycosis fungoides/Sezary syndrome—update 2017. *Eur J Cancer* 2017;77:57–74.
16. Tsai EY, Taur A, Espinosa L, et al. Staging accuracy in mycosis fungoides and Sezary syndrome using integrated positron emission tomography and computed tomography. *Arch Dermatol* 2006;142(5):577–584.
17. Agar NS, Wedgeworth E, Crichton S, et al. Survival outcomes and prognostic factors in mycosis fungoides/Sezary syndrome: validation of the revised International Society for Cutaneous Lymphomas/European Organisation for Research and Treatment of Cancer staging proposal. *J Clin Oncol* 2010;28:4730–4739.
18. Benton EC, Crichton S, Taplur R, et al. A cutaneous lymphoma international prognostic index (CLIPi) for mycosis fungoides and Sezary syndrome. *Eur J Cancer* 2013;49(19):2859–2868.
19. Danish HH, Liu S, Jhaveri J, et al. Validation of cutaneous lymphoma international prognostic index (CLIPI) for mycosis fungoides and Sezary syndrome. *Leuk Lymphoma* 2016;57(12):2813–2819.
20. Scarisbrick JJ, Prince HM, Vermeer MH, et al. Cutaneous lymphoma international consortium study of outcome in advanced stages of mycosis fungoides and Sezary syndrome: effect of specific prognostic markers on survival and development of a prognostic model. *J Clin Oncol* 2015;33(32):3766–3773.
21. Zackheim HS, Kashani-Sabet M, Amin S. Topical corticosteroids for mycosis fungoides. Experience in 79 patients. *Arch Dermatol* 1998;134(8):949–954.
22. Kim YH. Management with topical nitrogen mustard in mycosis fungoides. *Dermatol Ther* 2003;16:288–298.
23. Zackheim HS. Topical carmustine (BCNU) in the treatment of mycosis fungoides. *Dermatol Ther* 2003;16(4):299–302.
24. Breneman D, Duvic M, Kuzel T, et al. Phase 1 and 2 trial of bexarotene gel for skin-directed treatment of patients with cutaneous T-cell lymphoma. *Arch Dermatol* 2002;138(3):325–332.
25. Gathers RC, Scherschun L, Malick F, et al. Narrowband UVB phototherapy for early-stage mycosis fungoides. *J Am Acad Dermatol* 2002;47(2):191–197.
26. Hermann JJ, Roenigk HH Jr, Hurria A, et al. Treatment of mycosis fungoides with photochemotherapy (PUVA): long-term follow-up. *J Am Acad Dermatol* 1995;33(2 Pt 1):234–242.
27. Specht L, Dabaja B, Illidge T, et al. Modern radiation therapy for primary cutaneous lymphomas: field and dose guidelines from the International Lymphoma Radiation Oncology Group. *Int J Radiat Oncol Biol Phys* 2015;92(1):32–39.
28. Wilson LD, Kacinski BM, Jones GW. Local superficial radiotherapy in the management of minimal stage IA cutaneous T-cell lymphoma (mycosis fungoides). *Int J Radiat Oncol Biol Phys* 1998;40(1):109–115.
29. Jones GW, Kacinski BM, Wilson LD, et al. Total skin electron radiation in the management of mycosis fungoides: consensus of the European Organization for Research and Treatment of Cancer (EORTC) Cutaneous Lymphoma Project Group. *J Am Acad Dermatol* 2002;47(3):364–370.
30. Cotter GW, Baglan RJ, Wasserman TH, et al. Palliative radiation treatment of cutaneous mycosis fungoides–a dose response. *Int J Radiat Oncol Biol Phys* 1983;9(10):1477–1480.
31. Neelis KJ, Schimmel EC, Vermeer MH, et al. Low dose palliative radiotherapy for cutaneous B- and T-cell lymphomas. *Int J Radiat Oncol Biol Phys* 2009;74(1):154–158.
32. Thomas TO, Agrawal P, Guitart J, et al. Outcome of patients treated with a single-fraction dose of palliative radiation for cutaneous T-cell lymphoma. *Int J Radiat Oncol Biol Phys* 2013;85(3):747–753.
33. Chen Z, Agostinelli AG, Wilson LD, et al. Matching the dosimetry characteristics of a dual-field Stanford technique to a customized single-field Stanford technique for total skin electron therapy. *Int J Radiat Oncol Biol Phys* 2004;59(3):872–885.
34. Hoppe RT, Fuks Z, Bagshaw MA. Radiation therapy in the management of cutaneous T-cell lymphomas. *Cancer Treat Rep* 1979;63:625–632.
35. Kim JH, Nisce LZ, D'Anglo GJ. Dose-time fractionation study in patients with mycosis fungoides and lymphoma cutis. *Radiology* 1976;119(2):439–442.
36. Hoppe RT, Fuks Z, Bagshaw MA. The rationale for curative radiotherapy in mycosis fungoides. *Int J Radiat Oncol Biol Phys* 1977;2:843–851.
37. Harrison C, Young J, Navi D, et al. Revisiting low dose total skin electron beam therapy in mycosis fungoides. *Int J Radiat Oncol Biol Phys* 2011;81(4):e651–e657.
38. Hoppe RT, Harrison C, Tavallaee M, et al. Low-dose total skin electron beam therapy as an effective modality to reduce disease burden in patients with mycosis fungoides: results of a pooled analysis from 3 phase-II clinical trials. *J Am Acad Dermatol* 2015;72(2):286–292.
39. Karmstrup M, Lindahl M, Gniadecki R, et al. Low-dose total skin electron beam therapy as a debulking agent for cutaneous T-cell lymphoma: an open-label prospective phase II study. *Br J Dermatol* 2012;166(2):399–404.
40. Yu JB, Khan AM, Jones AW, et al. Patient perspectives regarding the value of total skin electron beam therapy for cutaneous T-cell lymphoma/mycosis fungoides: a pilot study. *Am J Clin Oncol* 2009;32(2):142–144.
41. Price NM. Electron beam therapy. Its effect on eccrine gland function in mycosis fungoides patients. *Arch Dermatol* 1979;115:1068–1070.
42. Price NM. Radiation dermatitis following electron beam therapy. An evaluation of patients ten years after total skin irradiation for mycosis fungoides. *Arch Dermatol* 1978;114:63–66.
43. Licata AG, Wilson LD, Braverman IM, et al. Malignant melanoma and other second cutaneous malignancies in cutaneous T-cell lymphoma. The influence of additional therapy after total skin electron beam radiation. *Arch Dermatol* 1995;131:432–435.
44. Desai KR, Pezner RD, Lipsett JA, et al. Total skin electron irradiation for mycosis fungoides. Relationship between acute toxicities and measured dose at different anatomic sites. *Int J Radiat Oncol Biol Phys* 1988;15:641–645.
45. Lloyd S, Chen Z, Foss FM, et al. Acute toxicity and risk of infection during total skin electron beam therapy for mycosis fungoides. *J Am Acad Dermatol* 2013;69:537–543.
46. Jones GW, Hoppe RT, Glatstein E, et al. Electron beam treatment for cutaneous T-cell lymphoma. *Hematol Oncol Clin North Am* 1995;9:1057–1076.
47. Kim YH, Jensen RA, Watanabe GL, et al. Clinical stage IA (limited patch and plaque) mycosis fungoides. A long-term outcome analysis. *Arch Dermatol* 1996;132:1309–1313.
48. Jones G, Wilson LD, Fox-Goguen L. Total skin electron beam radiotherapy for patients who have mycosis fungoides. *Hematol Oncol Clin North Am* 2003;17:1421–1434.
49. Quiros PA, Jones GW, Kacinski BM, et al. Total skin electron beam therapy followed by adjuvant psoralen/ultraviolet-A light in the management of patients with T1 and T2 cutaneous T-cell lymphoma (mycosis fungoides). *Int J Radiat Oncol Biol Phys* 1997;38:1027–1035.
50. Chinn DM, Chow S, Kim YH, et al. Total skin electron beam therapy with or without adjuvant topical nitrogen mustard or nitrogen mustard alone as initial treatment of T2 and T3 mycosis fungoides. *Int J Radiat Oncol Biol Phys* 1999;43:951–958.
51. Wilson LD, Licata AL, Braverman IM, et al. Systemic chemotherapy and extracorporeal photochemotherapy for T3 and T4 cutaneous T-cell lymphoma patients who have achieved a complete response to total skin electron beam therapy. *Int J Radiat Oncol Biol Phys* 1995;32:987–995.
52. Jones GW, Rosenthal D, Wilson LD. Total skin electron radiation for patients with erythrodermic cutaneous T-cell lymphoma (mycosis fungoides and the Sezary syndrome). *Cancer* 1999;85:1985–1995.
53. Wilson LD, Jones GW, Kim D, et al. Experience with total skin electron beam therapy in combination with extracorporeal photopheresis in the management

Section III

of patients with erythrodermic (T4) mycosis fungoides. *J Am Acad Dermatol* 2000;43:54–60.

54. Introcaso CE, Micaily B, Richardson SK, et al. Total skin electron beam therapy may be associated with improvement of peripheral blood disease in Sezary syndrome. *J Am Acad Dermatol* 2008;58:592–595.
55. Hansen JE, Wilson LD, Carlson K, et al. Addition of TSEBT to ECP reduces circulating malignant cells in leukemic cutaneous T-cell lymphoma. *Int J Radiat Oncol Biol Phys* 2009;75(3 Suppl):S480–S481.
56. Wilson LD, Quiros PA, Kolenik SA, et al. Additional courses of total skin electron beam therapy in the treatment of patients with recurrent cutaneous T-cell lymphoma. *J Am Acad Dermatol* 1996;35:69–73.
57. Becker M, Hoppe RT, Knox SJ. Multiple courses of high-dose total skin electron beam therapy in the management of mycosis fungoides. *Int J Radiat Oncol Biol Phys* 1995;32:1445–1449.
58. Duvic M, Martin AG, Kim Y, et al. Phase 2 and 3 clinical trial of oral bexarotene (Targretin capsules) for the treatment of refractory or persistent early-stage cutaneous T-cell lymphoma. *Arch Dermatol* 2001;137(5):581–593.
59. Duvic M, Hymes K, Heald P, et al. Bexarotene is effective and safe for treatment of refractory advanced- stage cutaneous T-cell lymphoma. Multinational phase II-III trial results. *J Clin Oncol* 2001;19:2456–2471.
60. Olsen E, Duvic M, Frankel A, et al. Pivotal phase III trial of two dose levels of denileukin diftitox for the treatment of cutaneous T-cell lymphoma. *J Clin Oncol* 2001;19:376–388.
61. Olsen EA, Kim YH, Kuzel TM, et al. Phase IIb multicenter trial of vorinostat in patients with persistent, progressive, or treatment refractory cutaneous T-cell lymphoma. *J Clin Oncol* 2007;25:3109–3115.
62. Whittaker SJ, Demierre MF, Kim EJ, et al. Final results from a multicenter, international, pivotal study of romidepsin in refractory cutaneous T-cell lymphoma. *J Clin Oncol* 2010;28(29):4485–4491.
63. Kennedy GA, Seymour JF, Wolf M, et al. Treatment of patients with advanced mycosis fungoides and Sézary syndrome with alemtuzumab. *Eur J Haematol* 2003;71(4):250–256.
64. Bernengo MG, Martin AG, Kim Y, et al. Low-dose intermittent alemtuzumab in the treatment of Sézary syndrome: clinical and immunologic findings in 14 patients. *Haematologica* 2007;92(6):784–794.
65. Ross C, Tingsgaard P, Jorgensen H, et al. Interferon treatment of cutaneous T-cell lymphoma. *Eur J Haematol* 1993;51:63–72.
66. Jumbou O, N'Guyen JM, Tessier MH, et al. Long-term follow-up in 51 patients with mycosis fungoides and Sezary syndrome treated by interferon-alpha. *Br J Dermatol* 1999;140:427–431.
67. Roenigk HH Jr, Kuzel TM, Skoutelis AP, et al. Photochemotherapy alone or combined with interferon alpha-2a in the treatment of cutaneous T-cell lymphoma. *J Invest Dermatol* 1990;95:198S–205S.
68. Kuzel TM, Roenigk HH Jr, Samuelson E, et al. Effectiveness of interferon-alpha-2a combined with phototherapy for mycosis fungoides and the Sezary syndrome. *J Clin Oncol* 1995;13:257–263.
69. Chiarion-Sileni V, Bononi A, Fornasa CV, et al. Phase II trial of interferon-alpha-2a plus psolaren with ultraviolet light A in patients with cutaneous T-cell lymphoma. *Cancer* 2002;95:569–575.
70. Wollina U, Looks A, Meyer J, et al. Treatment of stage II cutaneous T-cell lymphoma with interferon alfa-2a and extracorporeal photochemotherapy: a prospective controlled trial. *J Am Acad Dermatol* 2001;44:253–260.
71. Stadler R, Otte HG, Luger T, et al. Prospective randomized multicenter clinical trial on the use of interferon -2a plus acitretin versus interferon-2a plus PUVA in patients with cutaneous T-cell lymphoma stages I and II. *Blood* 1998;92:3578–3581.
72. Lim HW, Edelson RL. Photopheresis for the treatment of cutaneous T-cell lymphoma. *Hematol Oncol Clin North Am* 1995;9:1117–1126.
73. Kim YH, Tavallaee M, Sundram U, et al. Phase II investigator-initiated study of brentuximab vedotin in mycosis fungoides and Sezary syndrome with variable CD30 expression level: a multi-institution collaborative project. *J Clin Oncol* 2015;33(32):3750–3758.
74. Koizumi K, Sawada K, Nishio M, et al. Effective high-dose chemotherapy followed by autologous peripheral blood stem cell transplantation in a patient with the aggressive form of cytophagic histiocytic panniculitis. *Bone Marrow Transplant* 1997;20:171.
75. Foss FM, Ihde DC, Breneman DL, et al. Phase II study of pentostatin and intermittent high-dose recombinant interferon alfa-2a in advanced mycosis fungoides/Sezary syndrome. *J Clin Oncol* 1992;10:1907.
76. Foss FM, Ihde DC, Linnoila IR, et al. Phase II trial of fludarabine phosphate and interferon alfa-2a in advanced mycosis fungoides/Sezary syndrome. *J Clin Oncol* 1994;12:2051.
77. Duvic M, Talpur R, Wen S, et al. Phase II evaluation of gemcitabine monotherapy for cutaneous T-cell lymphoma. *Clin Lymphoma Myeloma* 2006;7:51.
78. Duvic M, Forero-Torres A, Foss F, et al. Oral forodesine is clinically active in refractory cutaneous T-cell lymphoma: results of a phase I/II study. *Blood* 2006;108:2467.
79. Wollina U, Dummer R, Brockmeyer NH, et al. Multicenter study of pegylated liposomal doxorubicin in patients with cutaneous T-cell lymphoma. *Cancer* 2003;98(5):993–1001.
80. Foss FM. Evaluation of the pharmacokinetics, preclinical and clinical efficacy of pralatrexate for the treatment of T-cell lymphoma. *Expert Opin Drug Metab Toxicol* 2011;7(9):1141–1152.
81. Molina A, Zain J, Arber DA, et al. Durable clinical, cytogenetic, and molecular remissions after allogeneic hematopoietic cell transplantation for refractory Sezary syndrome and mycosis fungoides. *J Clin Oncol* 2005;23:6163.
82. Whittaker S, Hoppe R, Prince GM. How I treat mycosis fungoides and Sezary syndrome. *Blood* 2016;127(25):3142–3153.
83. Wu PA, Kim YH, Lavori PW, et al. A meta-analysis of patients receiving allogeneic or autologous hematopoietic stem cell transplant in mycosis fungoides and Sézary syndrome. *Biol Blood Marrow Transplant* 2009;15(8):982–990.
84. Jacobsen ED, Kim HT, Ho VT, et al. A large single-center experience with allogeneic stem cell transplantation for peripheral T-cell non-Hodgkin lymphoma and advanced mycosis fungoides/Sezary syndrome. *Ann Oncol* 2011;22(7):1608–1613.
85. Duvic M, Donato M, Dabaja B, et al. Total skin electron beam and non-myeloablative allogeneic hematopoietic stem-cell transplantation in advanced mycosis fungoides and Sezary syndrome. *J Clin Oncol* 2010;28(14):2365–2372.
86. National Comprehensive Cancer Network Guidelines Version 2.2017, Mycosis fungoides/Sezary syndrome.
87. Gerami P, Rosen S, Kuzel T, et al. Folliculotropic mycosis fungoides: an aggressive variant of cutaneous T-cell lymphoma. *Arch Dermatol* 2008;144(6): 738–746.
88. van Santen S, van Doorn R, Keelis KJ, et al. Recommendations for treatment in folliculotropic mycosis fungoides: report of the Dutch cutaneous lymphoma group. *Br J Dermatol* 2017;177(1):223–228. doi: 10.1111/bjd.15355.
89. Lee J, Viakhireva N, Cesca C, et al. Clinicopathologic features and treatment outcomes in Woringer-Kolopp disease. *J Am Acad Dermatol* 2008;59(4):706–712.
90. Kempf W, Ostheeren-Michaelis S, Paulli M, et al. Granulomatous mycosis fungoides and granulomatous slack skin: a multicenter study of the cutaneous lymphoma histopathology task force group of the European Organization For Research and Treatment of Cancer (EORTC). *Arch Dermatol* 2008;144(12):1609–1617.
91. Neuhaus IM, Ramos-Caro FA, Hassanein AM. Hypopigmented mycosis fungoides in childhood and adolescence. *Pediatr Dermatol* 2000;17(5):403–406.
92. El-Shabrawi-Caelen L, Cerroni L, Medeiros LJ, et al. Hypopigmented mycosis fungoides: frequent expression of a CD8+ T-cell phenotype. *Am J Surg Pathol* 2002;26(4):450–457.
93. Kim YH, Willemze R, Pimpinelli N, et al. TNM classification system for primary cutaneous lymphomas other than mycosis fungoides and Sezary syndrome: a proposal of the International Society for Cutaneous Lymphomas (ISCL) and the cutaneous lymphoma task force of the European Organization of Research and Treatment of Cancer (EORTC). *Blood* 2007;110(2):479–484.
94. Yu JB, Blitzblau RC, Decker RH, et al. Analysis of primary CD30+ cutaneous lymphoproliferative disease and survival from the surveillance, epidemiology, and end results database. *J Clin Oncol* 2008;26(9):1483–1488.
95. Kempf W, Pfaltz K, Vermeer MH, et al. European Organization for Research and Treatment of Cancer (EORTC), International Society of Cutaneous Lymphoma (ISCL) and United States Cutaneous Lymphoma Consortium (USCLC) consensus recommendations for the treatment of primary cutaneous CD30-positive lymphoproliferative disorders: lymphomatoid papulosis and primary cutaneous anaplastic large-cell lymphoma. *Blood* 2011;118(15):4024–4035.
96. Woo DK, Jones CR, Vanoli-Storz MN, et al. Prognostic factors in primary cutaneous anaplastic large cell lymphoma: characterization of clinical subset with worse outcome. *Arch Dermatol* 2009;145(6):667–674.
97. Yu JB, McNiff JM, Lund MW, et al. Treatment of primary cutaneous CD30+ anaplastic large-cell lymphoma with radiation therapy. *Int J Radiat Oncol Biol Phys* 2008;70(5):1542–1545.
98. Million L, Yi EJ, Wu F, et al. Radiation therapy for primary cutaneous anaplastic large cell lymphoma: an international Lymphoma Radiation Oncology Group multi-institutional experience. *Int J Radiat Oncol Biol Phys* 2016;95(5):1454–1459.
99. Liu HL, Hoppe RT, Kohler S, et al. CD30+ cutaneous lymphoproliferative disorders. The Stanford experience in lymphomatoid papulosis and primary cutaneous anaplastic large cell lymphoma. *J Am Acad Dermatol* 2003;49: 1049–1058.
100. Li YX, Wang H, Jin J, et al. Radiotherapy alone with curative intent in patients with stage I extranodal nasal-type NK/T-cell lymphoma. *Int J Radiat Oncol Biol Phys* 2012;82(5):1809–1815.
101. Jaccard A, Hermine O. Extranodal/natural killer T-cell lymphoma: advances in the management. *Curr Opin Oncol* 2011;23(5):429–435.
102. Mraz-Gernhard S, Natkunam Y, Hoppe RT, et al. Natural killer/natural killer-like T-cell lymphoma, CD56+, presenting in the skin: an increasingly recognized entity with an aggressive course. *J Clin Oncol* 2001;19:2179–2188.
103. Guitart J, Martinez-Escala ME, Subtil A, et al. Primary cutaneous aggressive epidermotropic cytotoxic T-cell lymphomas: reappraisal of a provisional entity in the 2016 WHO classification of cutaneous lymphomas. *Mod Pathol* 2017;30(5):761–772. doi: 10.1038/modpathol.2016.240.
104. Senff NJ, Hoefnagel JJ, Jansen PM, et al. Reclassification of 300 primary cutaneous B-cell lymphomas according to the new WHO-EORTC classification for cutaneous lymphomas: comparison with previous classifications and identification of prognostic markers. *J Clin Oncol* 2007;25(12):1581–1587.
105. Kutting B, Bonsmann G, Metze D, et al. Borrelia burgdorferi-associated primary cutaneous B cell lymphoma: complete clearing of skin lesions after antibiotic pulse therapy or intralesional injection of interferon alpha-2a. *J Am Acad Dermatol* 1997;36(2 Pt 2):311–314.
106. Aberer E, Fingerle V, Wutte N, et al. Within European margins. *Lancet* 2011;377(9760):178.
107. Smith BD, Smith GL, Cooper DL, et al. The cutaneous B-cell lymphoma prognostic index: a novel prognostic index derived from a population-based registry. *J Clin Oncol* 2005;23(15):3390–3395.
108. Mian M, Marcheselli L, Luminari S, et al. CLIPI: a new prognostic index for indolent cutaneous B cell lymphoma proposed by the International Extranodal Lymphoma Study Group (IELSG 11). *Ann Hematol* 2011;90(4):401–408.
109. Senff NJ, Noordijk EM, Kim YH, et al. European Organization for Research and Treatment of Cancer and International Society for Cutaneous Lymphoma consensus recommendations for the management of cutaneous B-cell lymphomas. *Blood* 2008;112(5):1600–1609.
110. National Comprehensive Cancer Network Guidelines Version 1.2017, Primary cutaneous B-cell lymphoma.
111. Morales AV, Advani R, Horwitz SM, et al. Indolent primary cutaneous B-cell lymphoma: experience using systemic rituximab. *J Am Acad Dermatol* 2008;59(6):953–957.

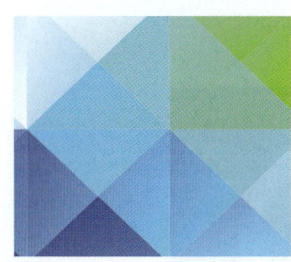

CHAPTER 84

Leukemia

Kenneth B. Roberts, Gottfried von Keudell, and Nikolai Podoltsev

INTRODUCTION

The leukemias are a group of neoplastic disorders of the hematopoietic system, characterized by aberrant or arrested differentiation. The role of radiotherapy (RT) in conventional curative treatment is largely to deliver central nervous system (CNS) treatment in combination with systemic therapy for patients with acute lymphocytic leukemia (ALL). Although the role of CNS prophylaxis has declined over the last 15 years because of toxicity concerns, it remains an important component of therapy for high-risk patients. Radiation oncologists must also be familiar with certain palliative situations unique to the leukemias as well as total body irradiation (TBI) (discussed elsewhere), as the latter is often part of a stem cell transplant program.

Childhood ALL can now be cured in 80% to 89% of cases, with initial remissions generally occurring in about 90%.[1-4] In adults, initial remission rates are generally equally high, but cure rates are only in the 30% to 45% range.[5] In contrast to the situation in pediatric ALL, pediatric acute myeloid leukemia (AML) generally fairs less well, with 60% cure rates, although this represents a marked improvement since the 1970s when cure rates were roughly 20%.[3] Adult AML cures are less frequent in the overall population, in large part a reflection that this disease principally afflicts older individuals. About 21,000 new cases are diagnosed per year in the United States with 10,000 patients dying from the disease.[2] Allogeneic stem cell transplantation has specifically targeted refractory/recurrent ALL and AML. Reduced-intensity transplants are being investigated to address the needs of high-risk or elderly patients with acute leukemia.

Chronic myelogenous leukemia (CML) and chronic lymphocytic leukemia (CLL) are primarily diseases of adults and have natural histories measured in years to decades. Both have the ability to transform to more aggressive diseases, though CML, in particular, reliably progresses to a more acute disease or blast crisis in its terminal phase. Allogeneic stem cell transplantation is associated with a high cure rate for patients with CML if conducted early in the chronic phase of the disease. However, because of the widespread use of the ABL tyrosine kinase inhibitors (TKIs), the use of allogenic transplant for CML has declined dramatically over the past decade.[6]

ANATOMIC CONSIDERATIONS

The radiation oncologist must be knowledgeable about the anatomy of the CNS, particularly the meninges (dura mater, arachnoid, and pia mater) and subarachnoid space for the proper design of CNS-directed radiation treatments. The epidural space lies between periosteum and the dura, whereas the potential space between the dura and arachnoid is called the subdural space. The pia and arachnoid are often described as a combined membrane called the leptomeninges. Between the arachnoid and pia is the subarachnoid space, which is filled with cerebrospinal fluid (CSF). The pia hugs the surface of the brain extending into sulci, fissures, and the internal cavities or ventricles, whereas the bulk of the arachnoid follows along the dura except for the fine trabeculations and into some of the major fissures of the brain. Arachnoid sheathes both nerves and blood vessels penetrating the pia and exiting the CNS, creating relatively short segments of subarachnoid space, which is of particular anatomical importance in the vertebral column. In the design of the inferior aspect of craniospinal radiation fields, the subarachnoid space extends laterally to the spinal ganglia, which are located within the intervertebral foramina.[7,8] Thus, coverage of the entire sacroiliac joints in such spinal field design is excessive. The caudad extent of the subarachnoid space is variable within the sacrum.[9] Clinically, the end of the thecal sac is now routinely determined on magnetic resonance image scanning. Pathologically, CNS leukemia originates as a perivascular infiltrate along the subpial blood vessels. As this progresses, the leukemia infiltrates preferentially into the subarachnoid space as well as into the brain parenchyma.[10]

Base of skull anatomy is also of importance to the radiation oncologist in the design of lateral cranial fields. The middle cranial fossa and temporal lobe project over the sphenoid sinuses on lateral radiographs. The cribriform plate projects along the roof of the orbit along an imaginary line that connects to the inferior aspect of the frontal sinuses. Several radiologic–anatomic studies have pointed out how the eye's lens in this "beam's eye view" is <1 cm away from the cribriform plate, having implications in field design. Insuring coverage of the entire subarachnoid space should supersede the concerns of radiation-induced cataracts as this is a readily manageable complication.[11,12] Moreover, because subarachnoid space extends as a sheath along the optic nerve, it is standard to include the posterior half of the eye globes within cranial radiation fields by using the anterolateral aspect of the bony orbit as an anatomic landmark, as it typically lies along a line that roughly bisects the eye[12] (Figs. 84.1 and 84.2).

To compensate for the blood–brain barrier, certain drugs are administered directly into the subarachnoid space either via lumbar puncture or via an intraventricular reservoir

FIGURE 84.1. Cranial irradiation field outlining treatment that encompasses the entire cranial subarachnoid space. The radiopaque markers outline the anterior aspect of the bony orbit so as to demarcate inclusion of the posterior aspect of the eye within the treatment fields.

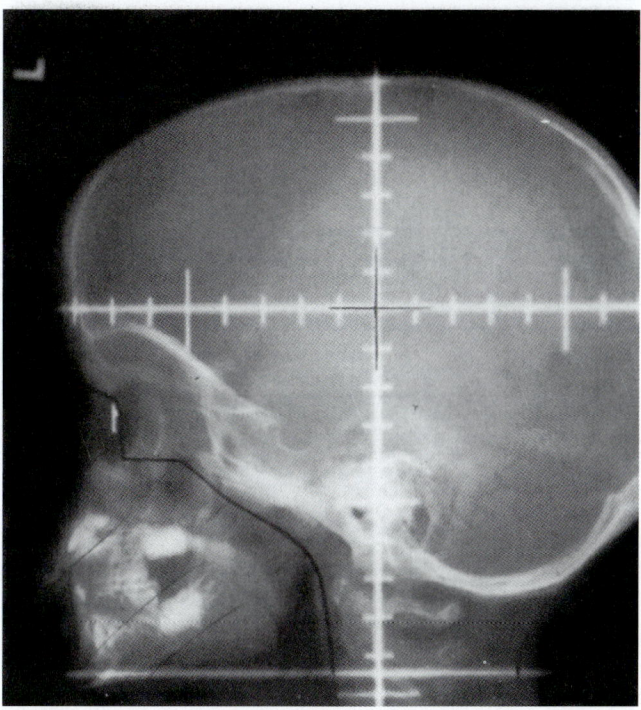

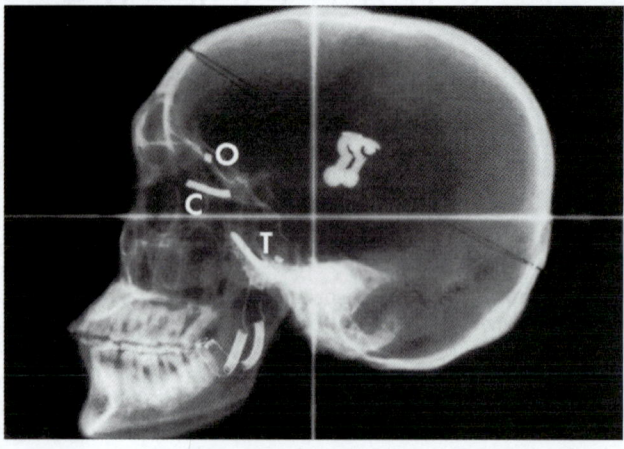

FIGURE 84.2. Skull views outlining anatomic limits of the base of skull for inclusion of the cranial subarachnoid space. **A:** Radiopaque markers have been placed at the cribriform plate (*C*), roof of the orbit (*O*), and the temporal fossa (*T*). **B:** Plain lateral radiograph shows the projection of the cribriform plate, orbital roof, and temporal fossa.

(e.g., an Ommaya reservoir). Intrathecal (IT) drugs distribute unevenly, however, throughout the subarachnoid space.[13,14] This is not surprising given the knowledge of brain anatomy and CSF circulation. CSF is mainly formed in the brain ventricles by the choroid plexuses, which are specialized capillary-rich tufted structures. This fluid then flows through the intraventricular foramina and the cerebral aqueduct of the midbrain into the fourth ventricle, from where it communicates with the rest of the subarachnoid space. CSF is resorbed principally in the dural sinuses via button-like projections called arachnoid villi. Thus, IT therapy theoretically undertreats the ventricular spaces and cerebral/cerebellar sulci as well as any gross disease extending into the brain substance. This concern has led to the concept of combining cranial RT with IT chemotherapy; the latter to cover the spinal subarachnoid space. Similarly, when craniospinal irradiation (CSI) is needed to treat a higher burden of CNS leukemia, IT therapy allows the spine to be treated to a lower dose than the brain.

ACUTE LEUKEMIAS

Classification Systems, Pathology, and Risk Stratification

Acute leukemias have traditionally been classified using the French-American-British (FAB) morphologic criteria. AML and its subtypes can most often be identified microscopically by the presence of Auer rods, staining for myeloperoxidase or monocyte-associated esterases, and other cytologic features of differentiation. Certain chromosome translocations are common to each AML subtype (Table 84.1). AML with

minimal or no myeloid differentiation (M1 and M0 subtypes) can be confused with ALL but for flow cytometric identification of early myeloid antigens. The more differentiated AML subtypes M2-M6 are usually recognizable by morphology and cytochemistry.

The FAB assignment of subtypes was replaced by the World Health Organization (WHO) classification scheme for myeloid neoplasms.[15] The WHO classification creates four key subgroups: AML with recurrent genetic abnormalities (including t(8;21), inv(16), t(15;17), t(9;11) among others), AML with myelodysplasia-related changes, therapy-related myeloid neoplasms, and AML not otherwise specified. See Table 84.2. The new subgroups are meant to highlight meaningful biologic and genetic differences between disease entities with differing prognoses and clinical behavior. In addition, in the WHO scheme, the number of blasts in the blood or bone marrow required to confirm a diagnosis of AML is 20%, instead of the 30% specified by the older FAB criteria. The WHO classification has been recently updated in 2016, reflecting advances in molecular subtyping, which is beyond the scope of this chapter.[16]

The FAB classification for ALL specified three subtypes based on morphology, which is largely of historical interest. L1 is the predominant type in 85% of childhood ALL. It is characterized by small cells with scanty cytoplasm and inconspicuous nucleoli. L2 is common in ALL of adults and is identified morphologically by blasts that show prominent nucleoli, abundant cytoplasm, and more variability in size. L3 lymphoblasts are large cells with cytoplasmic basophilia and vacuolization, similar to Burkitt lymphoma cells. The common ALL antigen (CALLA, CD10) is expressed in about 85% of ALL cases. At least with childhood ALL, this FAB system has not proved to be terribly useful with high interobserver variability and a lack of correlation with the more prognostically important immunologic and genetic features for ALL.[17] In the WHO classification, most of these entities, with the exception

TABLE 84.1 CORRELATION OF FRENCH-AMERICAN-BRITISH (FAB) CLASSIFICATION OF ACUTE MYELOGENOUS LEUKEMIA (AML) WITH COMMON CYTOGENETIC AND MOLECULAR ABNORMALITIES

FAB Type	Some Cytogenetic and Molecular Features	AML Cases (%)
M0, M1 (undifferentiated AML)	Trisomy 11, t(10;11)	31
M2 (acute myeloid leukemia)	t(8;21); RUNX1-RUNX1T1	25
M3 (acute promyelocytic leukemia)	t(15;17), t(11;17), t(5;17); PML/RARα	28
M4Eo (acute myelomonocytic leukemia with eosinophilia)	inv(16); CBFβ/MYH11	21
M5 (acute monocytic leukemia)	t(11;23), t(9;11)(p21.3;q23.3); MLLT3-KMT2A	15
M6 (acute erythroleukemia)	t(3;5)	4
M7 (acute megakaryocytic leukemia)	t(3;3), t(3;12), t(1;22) (p13.3;q13.3); RBM15-MKL1	1

TABLE 84.2 2016 WHO CLASSIFICATION OF AML

- AML with recurrent genetic abnormalities
  - t(8;21)(q22;q22); RUNX1-RUNX1T1
  - inv(16)(p13q22) or t(16;16)(p13q22); CBFβ-MYH11
  - t(15;17)Q22;Q12); PML/RARα
  - t(9;11)(p22;q23); MLLT3-KMT2A
  - AML with mutated NPM1
  - AML with mutated CEBPA
- AML with myelodysplasia-related changes
- AML, not otherwise specified

Adapted from Arber DA, Orazi A, Hasserjian R, et al. The 2016 revision to the World Health Organization classification of myeloid neoplasms and acute leukemia. *Blood* 2016;127:2391–2405.

of Burkitt's, fall under the category of precursor lymphoid neoplasms. These are subcategorized into B-cell lymphoblastic leukemia/lymphoma, not otherwise specified; B-cell leukemia/lymphoma with recurrent genetic abnormalities; and T-lymphoblastic leukemia/lymphoma.[16]

As may be apparent from the above discussion of the transition from the FAB to the WHO criteria for categorization, immunophenotyping and molecular markers have become very important in the classification of leukemia. Flow cytometry using specific monoclonal antibodies can be used to assay for a panel of antigens, often known as *cluster of differentiation (CD) molecules*, that define leukocyte maturation. For instance, CD19 and cytoplasmic CD79a define B-cell lineage, whereas cytoplasmic or surface CD3 defines T-cell lineage. Myeloid blasts are correlated with positivity for CD13, CD33, but cytoplasmic myeloperoxidase is required to definitively assign the cell to myeloid linage. With other markers defining different degrees of differentiation and maturation, ALL is now conventionally divided into T-cell and B-cell lineage. B-cell leukemia has four distinct subclasses: early pre-B, pre-B, transitional pre-B, and the more mature B cell.

Cytogenetic or chromosomal abnormalities occur in up to 90% of ALL cases. Of these, roughly two-thirds are nonrandom, falling into distinct patterns. Specific cytogenetic abnormalities have important prognostic and therapeutic implications in ALL. Chromosomal translocations occur in approximately 15% of pediatric ALL, and a bit higher in adult cases. The oldest known is the t(9;22) *BCR/ABL* translocation that forms the Philadelphia chromosome. This translocation is associated with a higher risk of CNS involvement and overall poorer prognosis. Adult and childhood forms of ALL have distinctly different patterns of genetic abnormalities as well as immunophenotyping (see Table 84.3). This may partially explain the poorer prognosis in older patients. For example, the t(9;22) *BCR/ABL* translocation occurs in 4% of childhood ALL cases compared to about 25% in adults; moreover, this genetic lesion now represents an important therapeutic target with the development of TKIs and may be associated with improved outcomes.

The *TEL/AML1* fusion gene expression (cryptic t(12;21) translocation) is a common translocation, occurring in 22% of pediatric ALL patients, in which an in utero event juxtaposes the *RUNX1* gene on chromosome 21 with the *ETV6* gene on chromosome 12. The resulting chimeric protein impairs normal hematopoietic differentiation, increasing the self-renewal capacity of early progenitor cells. On balance, it is associated with a relatively better prognosis. Conversely, the MLL rearrangement tends to be found in infants and is associated with poor prognosis; it can arise from t(4;11), t(11;10), or t(9;11) translocations. About 6% of ALL patients have the t(1;19) translocation that creates the E2A-PBX1 fusion gene. Rarer genetic abnormalities include the t(4;11) translocation

associated with African American children who have high WBC counts, the t(8;14) MYC defect in cases of mature B-cell ALL (2%), and t(11;14) associated with T-cell ALL with extramedullary involvement. One of the most recently identified genetic abnormalities is the IKAROS family zinc finger 1 (IKZF1) deletion found in 15% of precursor B-cell ALL cases. These are associated with older patients who have higher WBC count at diagnosis, and, as such, are also associated with a high-risk prognosis. IKZF1 deletions are also associated with higher chance of a BCR-ABL1 abnormality or Down syndrome.[18,19] CRLF2 overexpression and JAK mutations are also associated with IKZF1 deletion and poorer prognosis. A CRLF2 abnormality has been found to independently confer worse prognosis, even in adult ALL[19-21] BCR-ABL1–negative patients with a gene expression profile similar to BCR-ABL1–positive patients have been referred to as Ph-like ALL. This occurs in 10% to 15% of pediatric ALL patients, increasing in frequency with age, and is also associated with a poor prognosis related to IKZF1 deletion/mutations. The leukemias in this subgroup have activated kinase signaling, with 50% containing CRLF2 genomic alterations and 25% concomitant JAK mutations. Many other cases of Ph-like ALL have analogous translocations involving ABL1, JAK2, PDGFRB, or EPOR. The resulting fusion proteins may prove to be therapeutic targets using existing TKIs or those under development.

Abnormal DNA ploidy is extremely common, but two patterns seem to be clinically important. Hyperdiploidy with >51 chromosomes per cell (or DNA index >1.6) occurs in 25% of children with ALL. Although there is some association with favorable clinical factors (age >10 years and low presenting leukocyte counts), hyperdiploidy is an independent favorable factor; however, in adults with ALL, outcomes are poor even in presence of hyperdiploidy. In childhood ALL, the most common trisomies involve chromosomes 4, 10, and 17 and are associated with a good prognosis. Conversely, hypodiploidy of fewer than 45 chromosomes conveys a more unfavorable outcome.

The aforementioned laboratory assessment and clinical disease features have led to distinct risk stratification categories, at least as far as childhood ALL is concerned. Clinical prognostic features of B-cell leukemias have been commonly used to place patients into risk groups. Using the National Cancer Institute's (NCI) risk classification scheme, standard risk includes patients (two-thirds of pediatric B-cell ALL patients) whose age at diagnosis is between 1 and 10 years as well as a presenting leukocyte count of <50,000/μL, in the absence of CNS involvement, was historically associated with an 80% 4-year disease-free survival (DFS).[22] High-risk patients—defined as a high white blood cell (WBC) count, age below 1 year or above 10 years, or CNS involvement at diagnosis—had a corresponding 65% 4-year DFS. T-cell phenotype occurs in 12% to 15% of pediatric ALL cases and was once thought to convey a relatively poorer prognosis. This prejudice has been due to numerous unfavorable clinical correlations, including older age, male sex, elevated WBC count, extensive extramedullary disease including mediastinal and peripheral adenopathy or hepatosplenomegaly, and a higher tendency for relapse in the CNS and testes in males.[23] Current clinical practice is for T-cell leukemias to be treated on different protocols than B-lineage ALL. Nevertheless, when one factors out unfavorable clinical features, the prognostic difference between T- and B-cell ALL is difficult to discern. In regard to B-cell ALL, current protocols assign patients to low, standard, and high risk. Low-risk patients are operationally defined by standard-risk features along with a rapid early response to induction chemotherapy.[24] Age is also an important prognostic factor. Apart from this, the intensity of the treatment program is of importance as shown by the fact that adolescents treated on pediatric leukemia regimens have had better outcomes than those treated on adult programs.[25]

TABLE 84.3 FREQUENCY AND DISEASE CONTROL ASSOCIATED WITH IMMUNOPHENOTYPES AND CYTOGENETIC ABNORMALITIES AND SURVIVAL IN ACUTE LYMPHOBLASTIC LEUKEMIA IN CHILDREN (AGES 1–18) VS. ADULTS (AGES 18 AND OLDER)

Pattern	Frequency (%)		5-Year Disease-Free Survival (%)	
	Children	Adults	Children	Adults
Pre-B cell	80–85	75–80	80	30–40
B cell	2	3–5	45–85	45–65
T cell	15	20–25	65–75	40–60
TEL/AML1 t(12;21)	20–25	1–3	90	Rare
MLL/AF4 t(4;11)	2	5–7	20	20
BCR/ABL t(9;22)	5	25–30	20–40	<10
Hyperdiploid	25	5	80–90	10–40
Normal karyotype	9–37	30	70–87	40

Adapted with permission of American Society of Hematology from DeAngelo DJ. The treatment of adolescents and young adults with acute lymphoblastic leukemia. Hematology 2005;1: 123–130; permission conveyed through Copyright Clearance Center, Inc.

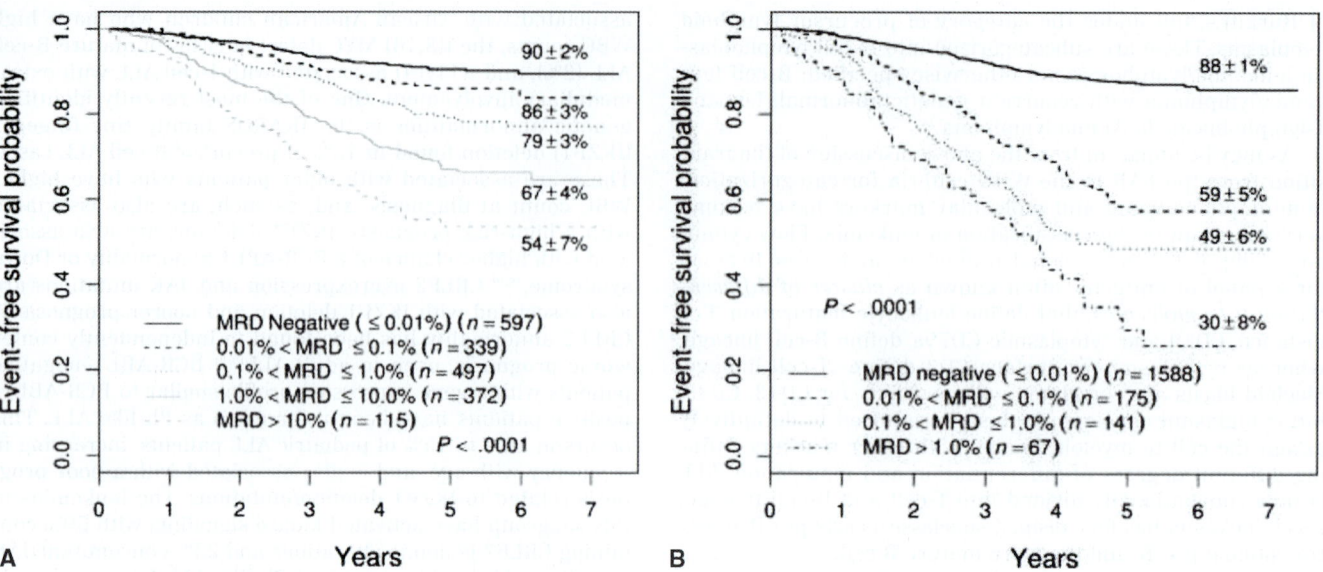

FIGURE 84.3. The prognostic importance of minimal residual disease (MRD) after induction chemotherapy for ALL. **A:** EFS of ALL patients as a function of level of day 8 PB MRD. **B:** EFS of ALL patients as a function of level of day 29 marrow MRD. (Republished with permission of American Society of Hematology from Borowitz MJ, Devidas M, Hunger SP, et al. Clinical significance of minimal residual disease in childhood acute lymphoblastic leukemia and its relationship to other prognostic factors: a Children's Oncology Group study. *Blood* 2008;111[12]:5477–5485; permission conveyed through Copyright Clearance Center, Inc.)

The response to induction chemotherapy has also been proven to be an extremely important prognostic category. In pediatric ALL, the concept of minimal residual disease (MRD) detected by flow cytometry or polymerase chain reaction (PCR) of postinduction peripheral blood or marrow aspirates has led to critical prognostic stratification. A contemporary analysis of MRD in a pediatric cooperative group trial showed that even up to 0.01% blasts from day 8 postinduction mononuclear peripheral blood cells conferred a poorer prognosis.[26] Moreover, day 29 and end of consolidation bone marrow MRD was able to further segregate unfavorable patient subgroups taking into account other prognostic factors such as *TEL/AML1*, trisomies 4 and 10, and NCI risk class. See Figure 84.3. From the assessment of MRD, the concept of risk-adapted therapy has allowed for improved outcomes with the intensification of therapy in those patients who continue to have detectable lymphoblasts after initial chemotherapy.

Assessment of CNS involvement at diagnosis in acute lymphoblastic leukemia (ALL) is critical for risk stratification, which is of course of particular importance to the radiation oncologist. Unfortunately, a traumatic lumbar puncture has been noted to be associated with a worse prognosis.[27] Regardless, CNS involvement has been unequivocally defined by a CSF leukocyte count of ≥5 WBC/μL along with either blast cells on cytospin or the presence of cranial nerve palsy. By convention, this is now classified as CNS-3. CNS-1 is defined as no blast cells on CSF cytology, whereas CNS-2 is <5 WBC/μL with blast cells present. Clinical data are conflicting as to the prognostic importance of CNS-2, reflecting the fact that CNS involvement is not simply a distinction of being present or absent but that it has also been associated with improved control with more intensive systemic and IT therapies.[28,29] Patients with CNS-3 disease who have more intensive IT chemotherapy along with cranial radiation within the first year of therapy have similar event-free survival as CNS-2 patients. For patients in remission who undergo surveillance lumbar punctures, there is even controversy regarding the prognostic importance of finding low numbers of blast or atypical cells in the CSF.[30,31]

More recent Children's Oncology Group stratification of CNS involvement has added complexity, taking into account a correction formula for traumatic lumbar punctures (so-called

Steinherz/Bleyer algorithm).[32] CNS-2 and CNS-3 are further subgrouped. Regardless, patients with CNS-3 disease are allocated to high-risk treatment protocols. See Table 84.4.

AML patient risk stratification is based on cytogenetic and molecular characteristics of the underlying driver mutations of the disease. Table 84.5 is an authoritative risk stratification scheme from the European Leukemia Network, which classifies patients into favorable, intermediate, and adverse risk categories based on the current understanding of molecular and genetic prognostic factors. Presence of complex karyotype abnormalities, FLT3-ITD and TP53 mutations among others, may justify more aggressive treatment approach. In addition, presence of MRD after induction chemotherapy is associated with significant risk of relapse and may dictate need for allo SCT rather than chemotherapy consolidation.[33] Selecting treatment

TABLE 84.4 ASSIGNMENT OF CNS STATUS AT DIAGNOSIS OF PEDIATRIC ALL

CNS-1	In cerebrospinal fluid (CSF), absence of blasts on cytospin preparation, regardless of the number of white blood cells (WBCs).
CNS-2	In CSF, presence of <5/μL WBCs and cytospin positive for blasts, or ≥5/μL WBCs but negative by Steinherz/Bleyer algorithm[b]
CNS-2a	<10/μL red blood cells (RBCs); <5/μL WBCs and cytospin positive for blasts
CNS-2b[a]	≥10/μL RBCs; <5/μL WBCs and cytospin positive for blasts
CNS-2c[a]	≥10/μL RBCs; ≥5/μL WBCs and cytospin positive for blasts but negative by Steinherz/Bleyer algorithm
CNS-3	In CSF, presence of ≥5/μL WBCs and cytospin positive for blasts and/or clinical signs of CNS leukemia:
CNS-3a	<10/μL RBCs; ≥5/μL WBCs and cytospin positive for blasts
CNS-3b[a]	≥10/μL RBCs; ≥5/μL WBCs and positive by Steinherz/Bleyer algorithm
CNS-3c	Clinical signs of CNS leukemia (such as facial nerve palsy, brain/eye involvement, or hypothalamic syndrome)

A patient with CSF WBC ≥5/μL blasts, whose CSF WBC/RBC is 2× greater than the blood WBC/RBC ratio, has CNS disease at diagnosis.
[a]CNS status that can be assigned after a TLP with blasts.
[b]The Steinherz/Bleyer algorithm provides a method of evaluating initial traumatic lumbar punctures: If the patient has leukemic cells in the peripheral blood and the lumbar puncture is traumatic and contains ≥5 WBC/μL and blasts, the following algorithm should be used to distinguish between CNS-2 and CNS-3 disease:
CSF WBC/CSF RBC >2× Blood WBC/Blood RBC.
Adapted from the Children's Oncology Group protocol AALL0331 with permission, © Children's Oncology Group.

TABLE 84.5 2017 EUROPEAN LEUKEMIA NETWORK AML RISK STRATIFICATION BY GENETICS

Risk Group	Genetic Characteristics
Favorable	t(8;21)(q22;q22.1); RUNX1-RUNX1T1
	inv(16)(p13/1;q22) or t(16;16)(p13.1;q22); CBFβ-MYH11
	Mutated NPM1 with FLT3-ITD or with FLT3-ITD^{low}
	Biallelic mutated CEBPA
Intermediate	Mutated NPM1 and FLT3-ITD^{high}
	Wild-type NPMI without FLT3-ITD or with FLT3-ITD^{low} (without adverse-risk genetic lesions)
	t(9;11)(p21.3;q23.3); MLLT3-KMT2A
	Cytogenetic abnormalities not classified as favorable or adverse
Adverse	t(6;9)(p23;q34.1); DEK-NUP214
	t(v;11q23/3); KMT2A rearranged
	t(9;22)(q34.1;q11.2); BCR-ABL1
	inv(3)(q21.3;q26.2) or t(3;3)(q21.3;q26.2); GATA2, MECOM(EVI1)
	−5 or del(5q); −7; −17/abn(17p)
	Complex karyotype, monosomal karyotype
	Wild-type NPM1 and FLT3-ITD^{high}
	Mutated RUNX1
	Mutated ASXL1
	Mutated TP53

Adapted with permission of American Society of Hematology from Döhner H, Estey E, Grimwade D, et al. Diagnosis and management of AML in adults: 2017 ELN recommendations from an international expert panel. *Blood* 2017;129(4):424–447; permission conveyed through Copyright Clearance Center, Inc.

for older AML patients should take into consideration not only disease characteristics but also patient's characteristics like age, comorbidities, and performance status with induction chemotherapy reserved for fit patients and low-intensity regimens aimed at preserving quality of life for others.[34]

Radiotherapeutic Emergencies

The radiation oncologist will be called on to assist with certain emergencies when the patient first presents with leukemia or at the time of relapse. Mediastinal adenopathy causing airway compression or spinal cord compression from epidural disease are clear indications for emergent RT. Generally, only one to three 1.5- to 2.0-Gy fractions are required while the diagnosis is being established, and systemic therapy is being initiated (Fig. 84.4). Glucocorticoids are an important adjunct to CNS RT but can produce rapid lysis of some lymphoblastic lymphomas/leukemias, which may hamper diagnostic evaluation. In the presence of cranial nerve palsies at diagnosis, some radiation oncologists recommend 10 to 15 Gy to the base of skull early in the treatment course to try and reverse the neurologic deficits.[35,36] Extreme leukocytosis with blast counts over 50,000 to 100,000/μL is a concern with myeloid leukemia, as leukostasis may occur, particularly in the vessels of the brain or lung. Lymphoid blasts are less adhesive to vessel walls, and blast counts of up to 400,000/μL or more are often well tolerated. In decades past, RT directed at the whole brain was employed using low doses on the order of 6 to 10 Gy in various fractionations. However, the role of RT in this setting has been questioned,[17,37,38] but may be considered when leukopheresis is contraindicated or unavailable. Nevertheless, one recent report suggests reconsideration of the role of cranial RT for leukostasis. Eighteen patients received WBRT in one to three fractions for a mean total dose of 5.63 Gy (range 2 to 9 Gy). Thirteen patients were treated to control neurologic symptoms rather than in a preventative manner resulting in 92% achieving prompt resolution of symptoms during RT or immediately thereafter. There was no toxicity above grade 2. Two (6%) patients developed an intracranial bleed following therapy from underlying leukostasis, whereas historically this leukostasis syndrome has been associated with a 20% acute mortality rate from stroke or heart failure.[39]

Treatment of Acute Myeloid Leukemias

A classical induction therapy for AML consists of an anthracycline on days 1 to 3 along with cytarabine (cytosine arabinoside, ara-C) for 7 days. Acute promyelocytic leukemia

FIGURE 84.4. Computed tomography scans of chest before (**A**) and after (**B**) palliative radiotherapy (RT) for mediastinal mass associated with T-cell acute lymphocytic leukemia. A 16-year-old boy presented with dyspnea and chest pain. A chest x-ray showed a mediastinal mass, whereas blood counts revealed a lymphocytosis. Diagnosis was established by flow cytometry of blood. Initial treatment with steroids, doxorubicin, vincristine, and methotrexate failed to produce immediate response. Megavoltage RT with anterior and posterior opposed beams for 6 Gy in three fractions was administered, subsequently relieving acute symptoms and allowing for general anesthesia to take place without risk for complete airway obstruction in order for central line placement and lumbar puncture to be performed.

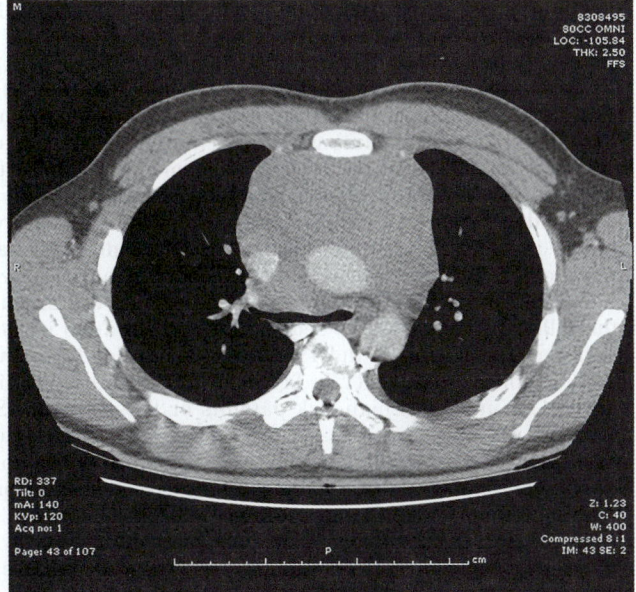
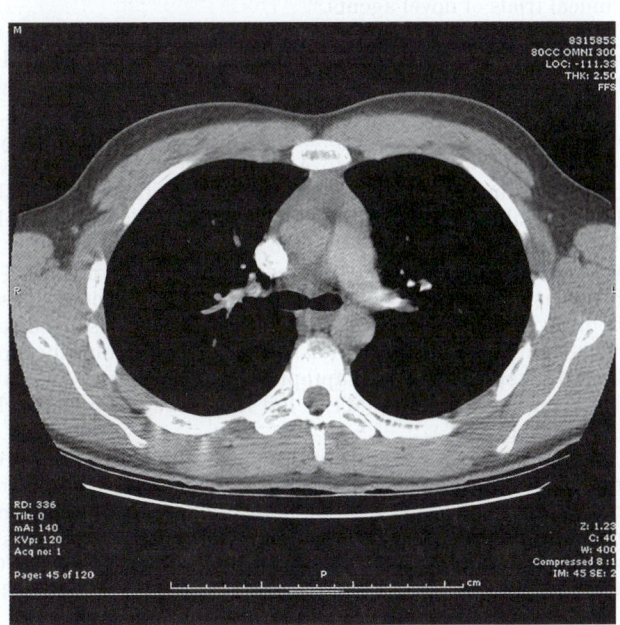

(M3 AML, APML) represents an exception to this rule. In many cases, the disseminated intravascular coagulation and associated PML-RAR fusion in APL are best managed with a combination of all-*trans* retinoic acid and arsenic trioxide, which promote differentiation and apoptosis of malignant promyelocytes.[40,41] Patients with high-risk APML defined by WBC > 10,000/μL are treated with the combination of differentiating agents and chemotherapy including anthracyclines.[42] For the remainder of the AML subtypes, daunorubicin and idarubicin are the anthracyclines most commonly used in induction chemotherapy regimens. Although a meta-analysis of multiple trials suggested that idarubicin has a higher complete response (CR) rate and survival over daunomycin,[43] more recent data from dose escalation trials using daunorubicin as part of the induction regimen suggest that when equivalently dosed, responses are similar.[44] Remission rates vary from 30% to 80% depending on patient age, karyotype, and subtype of AML.

Patients younger than age 60 have CR rates of 70% to 80%, whereas older patients tend to have lower CR rates of 30% to 50%. Patients who develop secondary AML following chemotherapy for other cancers have CR rates in the 30% to 50% range. Some induction regimens in children have added other drugs such as etoposide. Adding other chemotherapy drugs to anthracycline and cytarabine was evaluated in many studies without convincing survival benefit for AML induction in adults.[45] A double-blind, placebo-controlled trial in 717 patients with previously untreated FLT3 mutation-positive (FLT3+) AML randomized patients to either placebo or midostaurin 50 mg orally twice daily on days 8 to 21 of each cycle of induction and consolidation chemotherapy followed by continuous daily midostaurin for up to 12 cycles. The trial demonstrated a statistically significant improvement in overall survival (OS) for patients receiving midostaurin compared with those on the placebo-containing arm (HR 0.77, P = .016).[46] The FDA approved midostaurin for the treatment of adult patients with newly diagnosed AML who are FLT3+ in combination with standard cytarabine and daunorubicin induction and cytarabine consolidation.

Adults older than 60 years of age with AML and intermediate or unfavorable cytogenetics who are not candidates for hematopoietic stem cell transplantation are generally considered suitable for treatment with low-intensity palliative therapies such as low dose subcutaneous cytarabine, azacitidine, or decitabine. Alternatively, such patients may be referred for clinical trials of novel agents.[34]

Once remission is achieved, the need for additional therapy has been well documented in large randomized trials. Current data suggest that optimal postremission consolidative therapy begins with high dose ara-C for up to four cycles.[47] Alternatively, additional cycles of anthracycline for 2 days along with conventional dose cytarabine for 5 days have been used in both younger and older individuals with AML. Lumping all types of AML together as one group, the roughly 10% to 20% of patients who then remain in remission for 3 years, have a high likelihood of being cured. High dose ara-C has considerable CNS toxicity in elderly patients and has also been avoided in pediatric protocols. Other drugs used for consolidative treatment or for second-line induction therapy include etoposide, 6-mercaptopurine, amsacrine, 5-azacytidine, and methotrexate (MTX), but no one regimen is clearly advantageous.

The role of CNS prophylaxis is not well defined for AML, particularly because CNS relapse rates are relatively infrequent (at roughly 5% to 10%). Some studies show no difference in relapse rates with cranial radiation. Nevertheless, many pediatric regimens employ IT drugs such as ara-C. Patients without neurologic symptoms who have a high WBC count (>40.000/μL) at diagnosis, extramedullary involvement, high-risk APML, mixed phenotype acute leukemia, or monocytic variants of AML are believed to have a higher risk for CNS involvement, and screening CSF evaluation with prophylactic IT chemotherapy administration may be considered even after accomplishing remission. At least one study of childhood AML demonstrated a lower systemic relapse rate after cranial radiation.[48] This observation has been replicated in the Berlin-Frankfurt-Munster (BFM) group, which has studied the role of prophylactic cranial RT in childhood AML in a similar manner to their ALL studies described below. In combination with increasing intensity of induction therapy emphasizing anthracycline chemotherapy and cytarabine IT chemotherapy, cranial irradiation has helped to reduce the risk of CNS relapse. Results from study Childhood Acute Myelogenous Leukemia Study BFM-87 including nonrandomized patients showed an increased risk of CNS and/or bone marrow relapses in nonirradiated patients. Five-year DFS for patients who received cranial RT was 69% compared to 46% those not receiving RT. In later studies, there is evidence that 12 Gy resulted in the same relapse rate as 18 Gy.[49]

The radiation oncologist may be called on to treat myeloid or granulocytic sarcoma, which may predate a diagnosis of leukemia or be a harbinger of systemic relapse, and are typically associated with AML, but may also be seen with myeloproliferative disorders.[50-52] Also called a chloroma, these solid masses of leukemic infiltrates are responsive to modest doses of RT. The name chloroma derives from the fact that myeloid cells contain myeloperoxidase, which manifests a greenish color on gross inspection. These may occur in all varieties of extramedullary sites including periosteum, skin, soft tissues, gastrointestinal tract, the spine, and in epidural spaces or meninges.[53-56] Pathologic misclassifications are common, as this is a rare clinicopathologic disorder. Based on various case reports in the literature, symptomatic problems from chloromas may be readily relieved with doses of 10 to 24 Gy. The fractionation and total dose needs to take into consideration any normal tissue toxicities and the potential for future TBI should the patient be a potential candidate for an allotransplant. Recent reviews and commentary have suggested a prescription dose of 24 Gy in 12 fractions for most patients.[52,57] Although overall survival may be better than AML in many chloromas, long-term disease control requires systemic therapy used for AML.[50,58-60] Outcomes among patients with chloromas are defined by cytogenetic and molecular testing results, and selection of systemic treatment strategy should be similar to other AML patients.[61]

Treatment of Acute Lymphoblastic Leukemia

The four components of specific ALL therapy are (a) induction of remission, (b) intensification and/or consolidation, (c) maintenance therapy, and (d) CNS prophylaxis. In the 1960s, the problem of CNS recurrence was addressed with CNS radiation and IT chemotherapy. Subsequent improvements in ALL cure rates over the last 2 to 3 decades have resulted from improved risk stratification of patients with more effective, tailored multidrug regimens. As discussed in the following text, the late sequela of 24-Gy cranial irradiation was recognized in the 1980s and 1990s, leading to the elimination of cranial RT in favor of intermediate- or high dose MTX in all but high-risk patients or those with CNS-3 disease. Although not a standard worldwide, investigators at St. Jude Children's Research Hospital (SJCRH) have completely eliminated the use of upfront cranial RT in their protocols of pediatric ALL, accepting a small incidence of CNS relapse even in their high-risk patients.[62] In addition, with the improvements in systemic therapy, testicular relapse in males has become a rare event.[63] Testicular irradiation is rarely necessary except in the setting of testicular relapse or bone marrow transplantation.

Induction therapy for pediatric and young adult patients with ALL as a minimum typically includes a glucocorticoid, anthracycline, vincristine, and L-asparaginase. Other four or greater multidrug regimens have been used, all of which has resulted in initial remission rates of 95% to 99% in children and 75% to 90% in adults. Dexamethasone is now the preferred systemic steroid treatment as suggested in two clinical reports comparing it to prednisone, with dexamethasone reducing both CNS and systemic relapse in pediatric ALL.[64,65] This may be related to dexamethasone's better penetration into the CSF and longer half-life, providing enhanced protection against CNS relapse.[66]

Following induction and achieving CR, patients then receive intensification therapies that have been developed by cooperative groups in the United States and Europe.[67,68] This may consist of high doses of antimetabolites such as MTX, ara-C, or L-asparaginase. Additional anthracycline therapy is beneficial in high-risk patients.[69] It is believed that high dose MTX helps control CNS disease, which has allowed for less use of cranial radiation in some pediatric programs.

For high-risk ALL patients receiving anthracycline therapy, cardiomyopathy is a significant late side effect. American cooperative group investigators reported a randomized trial in patients with newly diagnosed T-cell acute lymphoblastic leukemia (T-ALL) who were planned to receive a threshold cumulative dose of doxorubicin of 360 mg/m^2 known to have increased cardiac risks to randomly receive dexrazoxane, as a bolus infusion immediately before every dose of doxorubicin. Of 537 patients, the 5-year event-free survival did not differ between groups: 76.7% for the dexrazoxane group versus 76.0% for the doxorubicin-only group ($P = .9$). The frequencies of severe grade 3 or 4 hematologic toxicity, infection, CNS events, and toxic deaths were similar in both groups. A nonstatistically significant trend with a low incidence of secondary malignancies were seen in the dexrazoxane group. Cardiac function as assessed by mean left ventricular fractional shortening, wall thickness, and thickness-to-dimension ratio z scores were all significantly better in those patients receiving the investigational cardioprotectant. The investigators concluded that dexrazoxane was an effective cardioprotective that did not compromise antitumor efficacy nor increase the frequencies of toxicities. As such, they stated that there should be wider use of dexrazoxane should be considered for children and adolescents who have malignancies including ALL when at risk for late cardiac disease from anthracycline treatment.[70]

In high-risk pediatric ALL cases, there continues to be much progress in developing postinduction intensification phases of therapy. For instance, in a Dutch and Australian trial of 111 children with high-risk features or high MRD, patients received three novel intensive chemotherapy agents followed by allogeneic transplantation. Thirty of these patients were at high risk by MRD and had an improved 5-year EFS of 64%.[71] Following intensification therapy, patients undergo a phase of maintenance treatment. In all but mature B-cell ALL, maintenance therapy over 2 to 3 years with agents such as weekly low dose MTX and mercaptopurine appears to be quite important, albeit for unclear reasons. In high-risk patients, cooperative group studies have demonstrated a benefit to an additional "delayed" intensification after a period of maintenance therapy.[67,72]

For ALL in adults, particularly those with the Burkitt subtype, patients have experienced improved remission rates with multiagent induction regimens that include high dose MTX, cyclophosphamide, and sometimes ara-C. These drugs

in combination with vincristine, steroids, L-asparaginase, and sometimes doxorubicin have been associated with 68% to 85% CR rates.

For relapsed ALL, a second induction generally consists of multiple drugs including vincristine, prednisone, L-asparaginase, an anthracycline with or without MTX, VP-16, or teniposide, and ara-C. If the CNS is involved, IT treatment is given along with RT.[73] If testicular relapse occurs, bilateral testicular irradiation is administered. When isolated CNS or testicular relapse develops, systemic therapy is indicated along with local RT.[74]

If a second remission develops, as occurs in 70% to 90% of cases, subsequent treatment includes either allogeneic transplantation or consolidative chemotherapy.[74,75] There are no randomized trials to indicate which is better, but comparative analysis suggests that survival is improved with allogeneic transplantation, particularly in ALL patients who had brief initial remissions.[75,76]

For high-risk ALL patients (particularly in childhood) who would benefit from an allotransplant, availability of a donor frequently limits this option. A pool of unrelated donors is now available through the National Bone Marrow Tumor Registry, markedly improves the ability to provide this curative albeit high-risk therapy. An ongoing debate, however, has revolved around the theoretically increased risk of toxicity from the use of matched unrelated donors. A comparative study was untaken among 411 children with high-risk ALL, in the prospective multinational Berlin-Frankfurt-Muenster (BFM) study group trial: ALL-SCT-BFM 2003 (Allogeneic Stem Cell Transplantation in Children and Adolescents with Acute Lymphoblastic Leukemia) who underwent conditioning with total-body irradiation and etoposide. Depending on donor availability, grafts originated from HLA-genoidentical siblings or from HLA-matched unrelated donors who were identified and matched by high-resolution allelic typing and were compatible in at least 9 of 10 HLA loci. The investigators found that the 4-year event-free survival did not differ between patients with transplantations from unrelated or sibling donors (67% vs. 71%, $P = .41$), with cumulative incidences of nonrelapse mortality 10% and 3% ($P = .02$) and relapse rates of 22% and 24% ($P = .73$), respectively. Among recipients of transplantations from unrelated donors, no significant differences in event-free survival, overall survival, or nonrelapse mortality were observed between 9/10 and 10/10 matched grafts or between peripheral blood stem cells and bone marrow. The absence of chronic graft versus host disease had no effect on event-free survival. The only observed advantage for sibling related donors was that engraftment was faster after bone marrow transplantation and associated with fewer severe infections and pulmonary complications. Thus, among high-risk pediatric patients with ALL, allogeneic hematopoietic stem cell transplantation was not affected by donor type. Standardized myeloablative conditioning using TBI and etoposide produced a low incidence of treatment-related mortality and effective control of leukemia.[77]

In a Pediatric Oncology Group (POG) study of induction therapy comprising intensive asparaginase (weekly PEG-L-asparaginase or 12 doses of non pegylated *Escherichia coli* [*E. coli*] asparaginase) with prednisone, vincristine, and doxorubicin for patients with first relapse, the second complete remission rate was 86% for those receiving PEG-L-asparaginase and 81% for those receiving *E. coli* asparaginase.[78]

CNS Prophylaxis of Acute Leukemia and the Role of Cranial Radiotherapy

Historically, as multiagent chemotherapy proved to be highly effective in producing remissions in childhood ALL, numerous investigators noted a significant increase in CNS relapses.

The CNS was recognized as a sanctuary site, protected from chemotherapy by the blood–brain barrier. In addition, CNS recurrences invariably led to systemic recurrence suggesting that CNS disease was capable of reseeding the blood and marrow.

This observation led to a long series of CNS preventative therapy trials, which initially utilized CSI. For instance, studies V and VI from 1962 to 1967 at the SJCRH established that CSI for 24 Gy in 15 to 16 fractions reduced the isolated CNS relapse rate from 67% to 4%.[79,80] CSI doses of 12 Gy did not appear to be effective with the early chemotherapy regimens from this time.[81] Concerns that full spinal RT would be associated with more acute myelosuppression, late musculoskeletal hypoplasia, as well as the technical difficulties of CSI led SJCRH investigators to compare CSI with cranial radiation plus IT MTX in study VII.[82] Here, the two CNS preventative regimens were found to be equivalent with roughly an 8% risk of CNS relapse.

In SJCRH study VIII (1972 to 1975), all patients received 24-Gy cranial radiation plus IT MTX. Patients were randomized to one of four maintenance regimens: (a) weekly intravenous (IV) MTX begun during cranial radiation, (b) oral MTX and 6-mercaptopurine, (c) oral MTX, mercaptopurine, and cyclophosphamide, and (d) same three drugs plus ara-C.[83] The incidence of CNS relapse was 5.0%, 1.5%, 20%, and 11.4%, respectively. More troublesome, however, was the development in some patients of leukoencephalopathy, a disabling syndrome of lethargy, seizures, spasticity, paresis, and ataxia. The incidence of leukoencephalopathy in the four randomization groups was 55%, 0%, 7.1%, and 1.4%, respectively. Thus, standard maintenance with oral MTX and mercaptopurine following CNS treatment with cranial radiation along with IT MTX to treat the spinal subarachnoid space was found to have the lowest CNS relapse rate and the least toxicity. The major lesson learned was that IV MTX and cranial radiation in close temporal proximity should be avoided.

In the 1970s and 1980s, additional phase III trials further defined appropriate preventative CNS therapy for childhood ALL. The Children's Cancer Study Group (CCSG) trial 101 compared the following: (a) 24-Gy CSI plus extended field RT encompassing the liver, spleen, and gonads; (b) 24-Gy CSI alone; (c) 24-Gy cranial RT plus IT MTX; and (d) IT MTX alone. Overall, the different radiation regimens were comparable in preventing CNS relapse while statistically superior to IT chemotherapy alone.[84] This finding was further confirmed in a cross-study comparison[85] as well as a Cancer and Leukemia Group B trial.[63] The CCSG further compared cranial RT plus IT MTX with CSI in high-risk patients, defined by a WBC at diagnosis of >50,000/μL; cranial irradiation and IT MTX proved to be significantly superior with respect to both CNS and systemic relapse rates.

Further cooperative group trials have refined the efficacy of CNS-directed therapies within patient groups stratified by risk. Several trials have compared cranial RT with intermediate- or high dose IV MTX along with IT chemotherapy (some with the addition of IT hydrocortisone and ara-C to MTX known as "triple" IT therapy).[63,86,87] The essential findings have been that in patients with low- or standard-risk ALL (e.g., age 3 to 6 years and WBC count <10,000/μL) who are managed without cranial radiation by substituting IT MTX throughout induction, consolidation, and maintenance therapy, CNS relapse rates have remained at a low level of 5% or less.[88–90] Additionally, with triple IT chemotherapy, there was a trend toward fewer systemic failures as well as excellent CNS control when given throughout consolidation and maintenance therapy. This may be at the expense of increased neurotoxicity, however, when given in conjunction with intermediate dose IV MTX.[90]

Moreover, a meta-analysis of 65 randomized trials of pediatric ALL worldwide initiated prior to 1993 that evaluated the role cranial RT concluded that in the vast majority of patients, cranial RT may be avoided with the use of extended IT therapy.[91] IV MTX was particularly advantageous in reducing systemic relapse. One notable exception to the conclusions of aggregated trials of this meta-analysis was the CCG-105 trial of intermediate-risk ALL. In CCG-105, 1,388 patients (with a complex matrix of adverse risk factors defined by patient age, presenting WBC count, and FAB subtype) were randomly assigned to receive either IT MTX alone or cranial radiation for CNS treatment.[92] A secondary complex randomization scheme allocated patients to standard or intensive chemotherapy. Intensive chemotherapy included either more drugs for induction or the addition of a delayed intensification chemotherapy phase after consolidative and CNS therapies. CNS recurrence rates were comparable in all groups at roughly 5% to 7% except in those patients receiving standard chemotherapy without cranial radiation, where the CNS recurrence was 20%. Thus, more intensive systemic therapy can lower CNS recurrence rates, abrogating any benefit to cranial irradiation. Finally, one interesting subanalysis of this systematic review of cranial RT for ALL looked at 809 patients across seven trials[93–97] that compared different doses of radiation (generally 18 to 21 Gy vs. 24 Gy). There were no differences in CNS or non-CNS relapse rates that could be discerned.

Regarding present-day use of prophylactic cranial RT, investigators have been focusing on patients who are at the highest risk for CNS relapse. At one extreme is the St. Jude's group that has become particularly concerned about the late effects of 24 Gy to the brain in terms of neurocognitive disabilities, hypothalamic/pituitary dysfunction, and secondary malignancies. With risk-adapted intensification of chemotherapy, Pui et al.[62] have reported favorable results with the complete elimination of cranial RT in all newly diagnosed ALL patients. In their St. Jude Total XV trial, 498 patients were treated without cranial RT yielding an 86.6% 5-year event-free survival, which was comparable to their prior studies that had included cranial RT. CNS-directed therapy used five cycles of high dose MTX including, as part of induction therapy, dexamethasone, and extended IT chemotherapy. High-risk ALL patients received up to 16 to 25 IT chemotherapy sessions, whereas low-risk patients received 13 to 18 doses of IT chemotherapy. Patients who were at increased risk of CNS relapse were those who had positive CSF cytology (CNS-2 or -3) or T-cell ALL. Moreover, a relatively high 7% of patients in first remission went on to undergo an allogeneic stem cell transplant correlating with high-risk features of MRD and adverse cytogenetic markers.

Elsewhere worldwide, the philosophy on the use of cranial RT in pediatric ALL has been to use it judiciously in high-risk patients while at the same time also reducing radiation doses to address the concerns about late effects, which includes learning disabilities and other cognitive defects, growth retardation, hypopituitarism, secondary malignancies, and the aforementioned leukoencephalopathy. The European BFM-ALL trials since 1990 have reduced the cranial radiation dose to 12 Gy with their risk-adapted intensification schemes, although those with CNS-3 disease received 24 Gy in their BFM-90 trial and 18 Gy in the more recent BFM-95 trial. Currently, the Children's Oncology Group (COG) has followed suit with a reduction in cranial radiation doses in its current ALL trials.

High-risk B-cell ALL patients for whom cranial radiation is a consideration are defined by age and high presenting WBC counts per NCI criteria, by adverse cytogenetics (e.g., bcr-abl, MLL, and hypodiploidy), by MRD after induction chemotherapy, and by CNS-3 disease. Recent COG trials of high-risk bcr-abl–positive ALL patients, however, have now eliminated the routine use of cranial RT. Most T-cell ALL patients are at increased risk for CNS relapse because of accompanying risk factors and, therefore, continue to receive cranial irradiation. An analysis of T-cell ALL patients (generally with other poor-risk features) treated within several POG protocols suggested that omitting cranial radiation had an adverse impact on CNS relapse rates.[98] Specifically, the 3-year CNS relapse rate was 18% for those who did not receive RT compared to 7% who did. On the other hand, a European report looking at a subgroup of favorable T-cell ALL patients, generally those with young age and low WBCs, suggests that it may be safe to omit cranial radiation in this subgroup.[88] However, as most T-cell ALL patients present with high WBC counts, Conter et al.[88] published a relevant comparison of the AIEOP-91 trial with the BFM-90 trial in which similar backbone chemotherapy is used. The AIEOP-91 trial omits cranial RT albeit with more IT chemotherapy, leading to a significantly higher CNS relapse along with a 3-year event-free survival of 62% compared to 88% for the BFM-90 patients who received cranial RT. Multivariate analysis showed that age younger than 10 years and WBC >100,000 in particular defined a group of T-cell ALL patients who should receive cranial RT.

To reduce the toxicity of prophylactic cranial radiation, several investigations have explored a reduction in radiation dose. The use of 18 Gy in 9 or 10 fractions along with IT MTX yields comparable disease control rates as 24 Gy.[99] Although there were some initial reports of reduced cognitive dysfunction even with such a dose reduction,[100] this issue is by no means completely settled.[101-103] The Dana Farber Cancer Institute ALL Consortium has studied the role of hyperfractionated cranial radiation (0.9 Gy twice daily) compared to standard daily fractionated treatments (1.8 Gy daily) to 18 Gy in high-risk patients.[104,105] Results from Dana Farber ALL 87-04 show excellent CNS control rates with both the standard or hyperfractionated treatments. Late neurocognitive sequela has been similar in which systemic therapy emphasizes L-asparaginase and omits high dose MTX. A follow-up Dana Farber ALL trial 95-01 compared hyperfractionated 18 Gy cranial RT to extended IT chemotherapy without cranial RT. The interesting finding here is that quantitative measurements of neurocognitive function were similar in both groups.[106] The German-Austrian-Swiss ALL-BFM ("Berlin-Frankfurt-Munich") Study Group has further reduced the radiation dose to 12 Gy, initially in a selected group of standard-risk pediatric patients.[89] With modern chemotherapy regimens as opposed to the older SJCRH experience, this further reduction in radiation dose was associated with excellent CNS control. Moreover, the ALL-BFM 90 protocol stopped using cranial RT in low- or standard-risk patients, but both the medium- and high-risk patients received 12-Gy prophylactic cranial radiation resulting in CNS recurrence rates well below 5%.[69] For the ALL-BFM 95 trial, cranial RT was deleted for the intermediate-risk B-cell ALL patients. This has resulted in a small increased risk for CNS relapse, which is considered clinically acceptable in order to avoid the late effects of such RT.[107] Specifically comparing intermediate-risk BFM 90 to BFM 95 patients, the isolated CNS relapse rate at 6 years is 0.5% versus 1.9%, $P < .01$. The 6-year "any-CNS" relapse rate was also statistically different at 2.2% versus 4.4%. Further follow-up and additional experience within the COG with this lower cranial radiation dose will be of interest in the years to come, hopefully seeing a reduction in late toxicity without compromising efficacy as cranial RT continues as used in a subset of high-risk pediatric ALL patients.

For adults with ALL, various protocols have used 24 Gy, whereas others employ 18 Gy.[101,102,108] Some programs such as Hyper-CVAD omit the use of cranial RT in the face of high dose MTX and ara-C, which effectively penetrate the blood–brain barrier.

Meningeal Leukemia at Diagnosis

At the time of diagnosis of ALL, approximately 3% to 5% of patients will present with clinically detectable CNS involvement (i.e., CNS-3 disease). Meningeal leukemia at diagnosis is typically managed as high-risk leukemia with cranial RT. The St. Jude investigators may disagree with the use of RT even here, but their results of the Total XV protocol included nine patients with CNS-3 disease whose 5-year event-free survival was only 43%.[62] These high-risk patients receive chemotherapy programs that include dose-intensive therapy with agents that penetrate the blood–brain barrier as well as IT therapy. Cranial radiation doses may vary from 18 to 25 Gy. Historically, CSI has been used, but modern practice has dispensed with the spine fields as the IT and systemic chemotherapy programs appear to be effective in assisting with CNS control. In children with ALL, meningeal involvement no longer carries a dire prognosis, as 5-year DFS rates approaching 70% are commonly seen.[109]

Within the older Children's Cancer Study Group (CCG) clinical trials for ALL, CSI has been consistently used in the management of CNS-3 disease. Until 1983, the cranial and spinal doses were 24 Gy and 12 Gy, respectively. Subsequent trials through 1989 utilized more intensive consolidation chemotherapy with a decrease in spinal radiation doses to 6 Gy. This allowed for a nonrandomized comparison of 6- and 12-Gy doses to the spine (in 2-Gy fractions). Interestingly, the patients who received a reduced spinal dose did just as well as those who received 12 Gy with less intensive chemotherapy. The 5-year event-free survival rate for patients with CNS-3 disease was 69%, compared to 67% for patients enrolled in all CCG ALL protocols in 1983 to 1989 who were without CNS-3 disease.[109]

Delay in RT up to 12 months has been found to be safe as long as intensive chemotherapy is being given first.[110,111] This avoids the marrow compromise that could potentially occur with early spine irradiation. In addition, with doses <16 Gy to the spine, myelosuppression has not been a major problem. Musculoskeletal hypoplasia would not be expected to be a significant problem for long-term survivors. The sequencing of RT *after* rather than *before* potentially neurotoxic drug therapy such as MTX may theoretically result in a lower incidence of cognitive dysfunction or encephalopathy. Some pediatric protocols will also tailor the dose to the brain based on patient age. For instance, the ALL-BFM 90 protocol, which utilizes cranial rather than CSI, avoids any RT for those younger than 1 year of age, 18 Gy for ages 1 to 2 years, and 24 Gy for older patients. In this large multicenter trial, 54 patients presented with CNS-3 disease and achieved a 48% 6-year event-free survival.[69] Arguably, this is inferior to protocols that use CSI, such as those reported by the CCG.[109] However, in the ALL-BFM 95, there were 64 patients with CNS-3 disease who had a 6-year event-free survival of 57.7% in which therapy included cranial radiation to 18 Gy without irradiation of the spine.

Some investigators in addition to those at SJCRH continue to try to avoid cranial RT in all cases including those with CNS-3 disease. The Dutch Childhood Oncology Group (DCOG) and the European Organization for Research and Treatment of Cancer (EORTC) have omitted cranial radiation by also using more high dose MTX during postinduction consolidation and by an increased frequency of IT chemotherapy. The SJCRH study also included higher cumulative doses of anthracycline than on Children's Oncology Group (COG) trials, and frequent vincristine/dexamethasone pulses and intensified dosing of L-asparaginase, whereas the EORTC trials included multiple doses of high dose cytarabine, during postinduction treatment phases for CNS-3 patients. On the DCOG-9 trial, 21 CNS-3 patients treated without cranial radiation had a 5-year EFS of 67% ± 10%. On the EORTC trial, the 8-year EFS of 49 CNS-3 patients treated without cranial radiation was 68%. The cumulative incidence of isolated CNS relapse for those patients was 9.4%. This CNS-3 subgroup is relatively uncommon, and further studies will be required to see if CNS irradiation can be safely eliminated.[112,113]

Summary of Cranial RT for Initial ALL Management

In summary, cranial RT may be used to prevent CNS relapse of leukemia. From a historical perspective that considered the brain as a sanctuary site, cranial RT has been well documented to improve outcomes for selected patients with pediatric ALL. With concerns about late sequela and improvements in systemic therapy including agents that can better penetrate the blood–brain barrier, cranial RT is used much less frequently in the upfront management of ALL. Overall, only 15% to 20% of pediatric ALL patients who have high-risk features require cranial RT currently. In current practice, cranial radiation is employed selectively in high-risk ALL patients. Although the definition of high risk has been shifting, one needs to take into account the intensity and specifics of risk-adapted chemotherapy. Nevertheless, ALL patients who benefit from cranial RT include older age (e.g., older than 10 years of age, and probably increasing benefit at ages older than 13 years); T-cell phenotype, especially in older patients with high presenting WBC over 100,000; and risk groups CNS-2 or -3 by CSF findings. Additionally, among B-cell patients, those with MRD and adverse cytogenetics should be strongly considered for cranial RT. Moreover, a recent meta-analysis supports the concept that a relatively small cohort of high-risk pediatric ALL patients require cranial RT as part of initial CNS-directed therapy.[114] All adults with ALL may be considered to be at high risk for CNS relapse, but there are no standard recommendations on cranial RT. Patients with AML, except for specific subtypes such as monocytic variants, are not generally treated with prophylactic cranial radiation at the present as the risk for CNS relapse is <5%. Unless otherwise indicated, in a specific treatment protocol, the radiation prescription for prophylactic cranial radiation to prevent ALL relapse is 18 Gy in 9 or 10 fractions. When BFM-type chemotherapy programs are used, the radiation dose has been reduced to 12 Gy with favorable outcomes. The spinal region is specifically treated by IT chemotherapy rather than RT, although an open question is whether there would be an incremental benefit to low radiation doses to the spine with meningeal leukemia at diagnosis.

The use of prophylactic cranial irradiation (PCI) in pediatric ALL is undergoing continued restriction and even abandonment because of concerns for limited efficacy and a historical body of evidence for neurocognitive, endocrine, and secondary tumor toxicities despite the recent trends in lower radiation doses for this indication. A group of international investigators performed a detailed meta-analysis of PCI use from 10 cooperative groups involving 16,623 patients age 1 to 18 years old with newly diagnosed ALL treated between 1996 and 2007. The proportion of patients eligible for PCI varied from 0% to 33% by trial, unrelated to eligibility for allogeneic stem cell transplantation in first complete remission. A meta-analysis using PCI as a dichotomous covariate compared event-free survival and cumulative incidence of isolated or any CNS relapse and isolated bone marrow relapse in high-risk subgroups of patients who either did or did not receive PCI. Results showed that only a small subgroup of patients with overt CNS disease at diagnosis had a plausible benefit from RT with a significantly lower risk of isolated CNS relapse of 4% with PCI compared to 17% who did not receive RT, $P = .02$; moreover, there was a trend toward lower risk of any CNS relapse (7% with PCI vs. 17% without, $P = .09$). These investigators, however, still questioned the role of PCI even in this or other high-risk groups of pediatric ALL receiving contemporary risk-adapted therapy as systemic relapse and death were equally high occurring in roughly one-third of patients regardless of RT usage.

The authors nicely summarized the current cooperative group use of PCI. In the current AIEOP-BFM ALL 2009 study, approximately 10% of patients receive PCI. In the current COG studies, prophylactic CRT is given only to the 2% to 3% of patients with CNS-3 status and approximately 10% of patients with T-ALL with high levels of MRD after 3 months of therapy.

Bcr-abl mutations and other high-risk molecular markers are no longer an indication for PCI by itself. In the current DFCI Consortium study, approximately 20% of patients (all patients with T-ALL and patients with B-cell precursor ALL with CNS-3, high level of MRD at the end of remission induction, MLL rearrangement, or low hypodiploidy) receive PCI. But, in the upcoming DFCI study, only CNS-3 status will be used as a criterion for PCI for patients with B-cell ALL. In the current Cooperative Acute Lymphoblastic Leukemia (COALL) 08-09 study, PCI 12 Gy is given to approximately 6% of the patients. Only patients with CNS-3 status receive PCI in the current trial of the Japanese Pediatric Leukemia/Lymphoma Study Group. Of note, several groups have completely omitted PCI including the Dutch group, the Nordic Society of Hematology and Oncology, the European Organisation for Research and Treatment of Cancer, the UK ALL group, and the St. Jude Children's Research Hospital.[115]

Therapeutic CNS Irradiation for Meningeal Relapse

With modern chemotherapy programs incorporating CNS-directed treatment, CNS relapse rates are typically <10%. As in overt CNS leukemia at diagnosis, RT has a central role. Formally, CNS relapse was thought to have a poor prognosis. Studies in the 1970s and 1980s describe disease control rates of 25% to 50%.[116-122] More recent trials, however, utilizing more intensive chemotherapy as well as RT, have reported ALL 5-year survivals of 50% to 70%.[111,123-126] Almost all trials have employed RT; the debate has been between cranial RT alone and CSI. Doses used have generally been approximately 24 Gy to the brain and 10 to 15 Gy to the spine. Most comparisons have not been randomized, but superior outcomes seem to be achieved with CSI.[69,111,123-126] One small phase III trial did show superiority for CSI compared to cranial RT.[123]

Although CNS relapse may ostensibly occur without over systemic disease, the latter is viewed as inevitable without additional systemic therapy. Therefore, intensive chemotherapy is an essential component of the treatment of meningeal relapse.[107,127]

Several prognostic factors have been found to be of importance in the setting of CNS relapse.[128-130] Patients who were originally deemed at diagnosis to be at low risk for CNS relapse by virtue of a low initial leukocyte count (<20,000/μL), who originally did not receive cranial irradiation, or whose CNS relapse occurred at a relatively long period after the original diagnosis have a better prognosis after CNS recurrence. An isolated CNS relapse has generally been more prognostically favorable compared to combined CNS and systemic relapse. After completing chemotherapy, those children with CNS relapse have better outcomes with longer disease-free intervals. For instance, experience within the POG with isolated CNS relapse of ALL in which RT used a cranial dose of 24 Gy and a spine dose of 15 Gy. The 4-year event-free survival was 71%. Those patients who presented with >18-month disease-free interval prior to CNS relapse had a 4-year event-free survival of 83% compared to 46% for those with shorter initial remission durations.[111] This has led subsequent POG and COG trials that omit RT to the spine if there is a long disease-free interval, but if the disease-free interval is <18 months, 24 Gy is given to the brain, whereas 15 Gy is delivered to the spine. Whether the omission of spinal RT in this favorable subgroup is detrimental is unclear. However, high dose ara-C has generally been added to the management of CNS relapse of ALL. With this agent, Morra et al.[131] reported a favorable 63% CR rate. These concepts have been maintained with current COG trials for CNS relapse of ALL, but with intensification of systemic therapy, spinal RT has been proposed to be dropped even for short disease-free intervals, whereas the brain is treated to 18 Gy. As for adults with CNS leukemia, most of the published experience and commentary from medical oncologists has been opposed to the use of CSI mainly for fear of excessive myelosuppression.[101] Cranial irradiation is relatively standard, however. Quite possibly, the avoidance in treating the entire CNS is detrimental, although admittedly this is not a settled issue.

Selected high-risk patients with CNS relapse may be candidates for allogeneic transplants. TBI is often a component of the preparative regimen. One function of the TBI is to specifically treat the CNS burden of disease. Because doses on the order of 12 to 15 Gy are employed here, it makes sense to boost the head prior to TBI to bring total doses to the cranium to 18 to 25 Gy. Investigators at Stanford have evaluated the neurocognitive effects of this practice of boosting the CNS in conjunction with TBI. Forty-one pediatric patients with relapsed ALL undergoing TBI-based allogeneic transplants had the brain boosted to a total mean dose of 24 Gy. In 18 patients, the spine was also boost to a total cumulative dose of 18 Gy. Five-year DFS for all patients was 67% for this high-risk group. Patients with isolated CNS disease before transplant had a trend toward superior DFS (hazard ratio 3.64, P = .11, 5-year DFS 74%) compared with those with combined CNS and bone marrow disease (5-year DFS 59%). Neurocognitive testing revealed a mean post-SCT overall intelligence quotient of 103.7 at 4.4 years. Although relative deficiencies in processing speed and/or working memory were noted in 6 of 16 tested patients (38%), the pre- and posttransplant neurocognitive testing revealed no significant change in intelligence quotient. At a mean of 12.5 years after transplant, 11 of 13 long-term survivors (85%) had completed some college level coursework.[132]

Testicular Relapse

In boys with ALL, particularly those with T-cell subtype, testicular involvement was once a common problem. Overt testicular involvement by leukemia at diagnosis occurs in approximately 2% of males with ALL and is a particularly poor prognostic situation. Microscopic burden in the testes is estimated to be higher at 5% to 15% based on biopsy data and the historic risk for testicular relapse. With modern chemotherapy, especially the use of intermediate- to high dose MTX, this is now rare. Similar to the experience with CNS relapse, there once was speculation as to whether the testes acted as a sanctuary site because of a physiologic blood–testes barrier. In 1980, a trial of prophylactic testicular irradiation significantly reduced the risk of testicular relapse but did not improve survival.[133] But modern risk-adapted chemotherapies as promulgated by St. Judes investigators no longer require testicular RT in the upfront management of patients presenting with testicular involvement as there is no reduction in relapses nor improvement in overall or event-free survival.[134]

In cases of testicular relapse, systemic and/or CNS relapse usually follows.[135] Both intensive systemic therapy and local RT are indicated. Doses <12 Gy are generally thought to be suboptimal, whereas doses of 24 to 26 Gy over 2.5 to 3.5 weeks are considered standard. Case reports of local recurrences despite adequate RT have led some to suggest higher doses. When only one testis is clinically involved, imaging or biopsy of the contralateral testes frequently reveals bilateral disease. Similarly, unilateral irradiation or orchiectomy as local management is felt to be associated with a significant risk of contralateral testicular relapse, justifying treatment directed at both testes for leukemia management, despite the expectation of infertility from RT. Data from CCG and POG studies suggest that local irradiation and intensive systemic therapy results in prolonged event-free survival in roughly 50% to 65% of patients.[74,136] Where allogeneic transplantation is indicated, TBI is often part of the conditioning regimen. One retrospective series from the Memorial Sloan-Kettering Cancer Center suggests that for TBI/cyclophosphamide preparative regimens, the risk of testicular relapse is significantly reduced with a local boost to the scrotum of 4 Gy to bring the total testicular dose to 16 to 20 Gy.[137] Regardless, there is not universal agreement about the need for a testicular boost in this setting.

Ocular Relapse

Historically, choroidal recurrence of leukemia was sometimes associated with inadequate coverage of the optic nerve and posterior globe with cranial RT. This has led to practice patterns in which the posterior eye is included in standard cranial fields. Even so, isolated relapse in the eye is rarely seen and may even occur in the anterior chamber. RT is often used as part of retrieval therapy analogous to relapse in the brain or testes. The best report of the incidence and management of this situation comes from the United Kingdom Medical Research Council leukemia clinical trial experience.[138] Investigators found a 2.2% incidence of eye relapse in their leukemia XI and ALL97 trials between 1991 and 2001. There were 17 patients who had ocular leukemia as a first relapse, either in isolation or combined with relapse at another site, and three occurred as a poor prognosis second relapse event. Among the patients with ocular relapse as a first site of recurrence, 11 patients were long-term survivors with disease control who were treated with a full chemotherapy relapse protocol along with local RT. Disease tended to not be controlled when chemotherapy was of reduced intensity; again, a lesson that isolated leukemia recurrences is a harbinger of systemic relapse. From this limited experience and from other cooperative groups, there is a sense that posterior eye relapse should direct the RT volume to include not just the eye but the CNS comprehensively. Radiation doses to the eye ranged from 10 to 24 Gy, mostly using 24 Gy as a cumulative dose that might have also entailed TBI or cranial/craniospinal RT volumes with differential dosing. An isolated relapse in the anterior chamber is felt to have less risk for occult CNS involvement and may be managed with electron beam RT rather than photons just to the eye along with intensive chemotherapy.

THE CHRONIC LEUKEMIAS

Chronic Myelogenous Leukemia

CML is a chronic myeloproliferative disorder arising from clonal expansion of the primitive hematopoietic stem cell. It involves myeloid, erythroid, megakaryocytic, and sometimes lymphoid elements. It is the first neoplastic process to be characterized by a specific cytogenetic marker, the Philadelphia chromosome (Ph+), t(9;22) described in 1960.[139] This is detectable by cytogenetics in 90% to 95% of patients and by molecular analysis in most other patients.[140] This translocation results in a BCR-ABL1 fusion protein that has tyrosine kinase activity critical for leukemic transformation.

Clinically, the disease manifests with several phases: if untreated, an initial chronic indolent phase of 3 to 4 years will progress to an accelerated phase for about 6 months and finally will transform in to blast phase with a survival of 3 to 6 months. As the disease advances, the accelerated phase is characterized by increasing difficulty in controlling the peripheral WBC count, increasing splenomegaly, increasing blasts in the peripheral blood and bone marrow, and increasing basophilia and eosinophilia. The blast crisis resembles acute leukemia with ≥20% blasts in blood or bone marrow with symptoms such as bone pain, sweats, fever, anorexia, or weight loss. Anemia, thrombocytopenia, and extramedullary disease involving bones, skin, CNS, and lymph nodes are common. In about 20% of cases, blasts are lymphoid by phenotype. Historically, prognostic factors for CML have included age, splenic size, platelet count, and percent of basophils in blood and marrow. Poor prognosis factors are age >60 years, spleen >10 cm below the costal margin, blasts >3% in blood or marrow, basophilia >7% in blood or marrow, and platelets >700,000/μL.[141]

Therapy of CML

The first effective therapy for chronic leukemias was RT to the spleen and sometimes the liver, initiated in 1902 by Pusey[142] and assessed in 1924 by Minot et al.[143] Today, RT is primarily used in a palliative setting to relieve painful splenomegaly or other extramedullary sites when indicated. In some centers, TBI plays an important role in allogeneic transplantation.

There is a long history of treating CML in chronic phase with alkylating agents, hydroxyurea, cytarabine, and interferon alpha, which is beyond the scope of this chapter. Over the past decade, such therapies, as well as hematopoietic stem cell transplant, have largely been relegated to the salvage setting through the introduction of ABL TKIs effective in inducing and maintaining long-term remissions in CML without cumulative toxicities.[144,145] Imatinib is a relatively well-tolerated oral medication that has been shown to be effective in CML in both chronic and accelerated phases.[146,147] This agent has been a paradigm for molecularly targeted therapies and is now used as upfront therapy for CML. Second generation TKIs such as dasatinib and nilotinib may be used for resistance to imatinib or patients with poor prognostic features.[148] For those who do not respond adequately to the TKIs or who lose response, allogeneic transplantation remains an important option.[149,150] About 70% of good-risk patients achieve long-term DFS.[151] Allotransplantation and TBI are further discussed in Chapter 16.

Palliative RT may be of benefit in those patients with massive splenomegaly with responses seen with doses in the 10- to 20-Gy range or lower. The radiation oncologist is well advised to understand the extreme radiosensitivity of the malignant stem cells in CML and in other hematopoietic disorders causing splenomegaly with the admonition to use very low doses per fraction (25 to 100 cGy) once or twice a week with close monitoring of blood counts (see below).

Chronic Lymphocytic Leukemia

CLL is an indolent leukemia of B-cell origin and is characterized by the accumulation of clonal, functionally incompetent B lymphocytes. It is the most common leukemia in the western world, and the course of the disease demonstrates marked variability. While some patients live a normal life span, never require therapy, others progress rapidly despite treatment. The usual course is characterized by gradual progression from incidentally found lymphocytosis to lymphadenopathy, splenomegaly, to anemia, and thrombocytopenia because of progressive bone marrow involvement and/or autoimmune phenomena. Nonlymphoid organ involvement may occur with advanced stage of disease.

Occasionally, patients with CLL develop transformation to an aggressive large B-cell lymphoma referred to as *Richter syndrome*.[152] Its incidence ranges from 3% to 5% of CLL cases.[153] It may arise in the setting of active disease or during a remission. It is characterized by an abrupt onset of asymmetric adenopathy, splenomegaly, B symptoms, and elevated LDH. Other transformations include evolution to prolymphocytic leukemia with development of progressive refractory disease and a majority of prolymphocytes in the blood. Rarely, ALL or myeloma develop in the course of CLL.[154,155]

The clinical diagnosis is based upon the blood lymphocyte count, which must be at least $5 \times 10^3/\mu L$ in an adult. The malignant B cells have a distinct immunophenotype with expression of surface markers CD5, CD19, and CD23 in addition to immunoglobulin light chain restriction and dim CD20 positivity.[156,157] Healthy individuals may harbor monoclonal B cells of this phenotype and are classified as monoclonal B-cell lymphocytosis provided there are $<5 \times 10^3/\mu L$, and no other evidence of disease is present. Patients with lymphadenopathy or other tissue morphology and similar phenotype without leukemic involvement are diagnosed with small lymphocytic lymphoma. There have been many staging systems proposed, but the most widely used are those modified by

TABLE 84.6 CHRONIC LYMPHOCYTIC LEUKEMIA STAGING SYSTEMS

Staging System	Clinical Features	Median Survival (y)
Rai staging		
Low risk		>10
0	Lymphocytosis of blood and marrow	
Intermediate risk		7
I	Lymphadenopathy	
II	Splenomegaly	
High risk		2–4
III	Anemia, Hgb < 10 g/dL (unrelated to hemolysis)	
IV	Thrombocytopenia <100,000 platelets/µL	
Binet staging		
A	<3 areas of lymphadenopathy	12
B	≥3 involved nodal areas	7
C	Anemia and/or thrombocytopenia	2

Hgb, hemoglobin.

Rai et al.[158] and Binet et al.,[159] the former used in the United States and the latter in Europe (see Table 84.6). Clinical stage is the most important predictor of survival in patients with CLL. Numerous other factors have been reported to have an impact on survival and include age, sex, lymphocyte doubling time, pattern of marrow involvement, β-2 microglobulin levels, and immunophenotype of malignant cells.[160] Cytogenetic and molecular abnormalities have more recently emerged as powerful predictors of outcome and may impact treatment decisions.[161] For example, deletion of chromosome 17p or p53 mutation confers both an inferior overall survival as well as resistance to purine analog and alkylator-based therapy.

Asymptomatic early-stage patients are typically followed without therapy ("watch and wait" approach). About 20% of such patients will continue to have an indolent course. Of the remaining patients, the decision to intervene therapeutically is often challenging. The NCI has established guidelines for the initiation of treatment, which include constitutional symptoms (B symptoms) because of CLL, symptomatic lymphadenopathy and/or hepatosplenomegaly, anemia (hemoglobin <10 g/dL), thrombocytopenia (platelets <100,000/μL), and refractory autoimmune disease.[162] The absolute lymphocyte count should not be used as an indication for treatment, as symptoms associated with marked lymphocytosis because of leukocyte aggregation do not typically occur in patients with CLL.

For many years, the standard treatment for CLL included single-agent chlorambucil with or without prednisone.[163] The newer purine analogs, 2-deoxycoformycin, fludarabine, and 2-chloro-2'-deoxy-β-D-adenosine (cladribine or 2-CDA) have been tested in CLL and, of these, fludarabine has shown a high response rate in combination with the anti-CD20 antibody, rituximab.[164] In a phase III trial comparing fludarabine to chlorambucil, the CR rate with chlorambucil was 4% and with fludarabine 20%.[165] Overall response rates were 37% with chlorambucil and 63% with fludarabine. The median survival was 66 months (fludarabine) versus 56 months. For these reasons, fludarabine is now accepted as a backbone of therapy for CLL. More recently, a combination of fludarabine, cyclophosphamide, and rituximab has resulted in a very high complete remission rate of 70% in patients with CLL, with a median time to progression of 80 months.[166] Moreover, when compared to fludarabine and cyclophosphamide, the addition of rituximab led to a survival benefit, which made this the regimen of choice in the upfront treatment of the young and fit.[167]

For patients who are older than 65 years, have comorbidities, and/or decreased renal function bendamustine plus rituximab has been used traditionally given the increased risk for adverse events including infectious complications.[168] This regimen has a relatively low toxicity mainly confined to a mild to moderate degree of reversible myelosuppression.[169]

Over the past few years, the treatment of CLL has been revolutionized with the advent of targeted therapies. Newer approaches to the treatment of CLL involve vaccines, cell cycle inhibitors, antiapoptotic agents, immunomodulatory agents, and monoclonal antibodies. Ibrutinib—a selective irreversible inhibitor of Bruton tyrosine kinase, part of the B-cell receptor signaling cascade—is the furthest developed and has been FDA approved for the upfront treatment of older patient with CLL based on the results of the RESONATE-2 trial.[170] This was an open-label, randomized phase 3 trial, which compared ibrutinib and chlorambucil, in previously untreated older patients with CLL or small lymphocytic lymphoma, and ibrutinib resulted in a higher overall response rate was 86% vs. 35%, $P < .001$, longer progression-free survival (median, not reached vs. 18.9 months), and overall survival with a relative risk of death that was 84% lower in the ibrutinib group than in the chlorambucil group (hazard ratio, 0.16; $P = .001$). Ibrutinib has also been FDA approved for patients with relapsed/refractory CLL and for the upfront treatment of patients with CLL harboring a deletion in the chromosome 17p or a deletion on p53 who have historically a poor response to traditional chemoimmunotherapy.[171,172]

Other novel agents include idelalisib, venetoclax, and ofatumumab, which are mentioned briefly, but a full discussion is beyond the scope of this review. Idelalisib is an oral inhibitor of phosphoinositide 3′-kinase (PI3K) delta, a pathway that is crucial for the maintenance and expansion of B cells.[173] In a phase III randomized, double-blind, placebo-controlled trial, patients with relapsed CLL receiving idelalisib versus those receiving placebo along with Rituxan had improved rates of overall response (81% vs. 13%; odds ratio, 29.92; $P < .001$) and overall survival at 12 months (92% vs. 80%; hazard ratio for death, 0.28; $P = .02$).[174] Largely based on these results, the FDA approved idelalisib for the treatment of patients with relapsed CLL, in combination with rituximab, for whom rituximab alone would otherwise be considered appropriate therapy because of other comorbidities.

Venetoclax, a BH3 mimetic, specifically targets BCL2 and has been proven to have efficacy in relapsed CLL including with 17p deletion, and has a low toxicity profile except for a propensity to cause tumor lysis syndrome because of its high response rate.[175] Impressively it has led to an ORR of 79% with a 20% complete remission, which is highly unusual in this heavily pretreated patient population. Based on these results, it has been FDA approved for CLL patients with 17p deletion after at least 1 prior line of therapy. Finally, a new humanized anti-CD20 monoclonal antibody, ofatumumab, was evaluated in a phase III trial of relapsed CLL in complete or partial remission after second- or third-line treatment. Patients were randomly assigned to receive maintenance ofatumumab for up to 2 years versus observation. Ofatumumab maintenance resulted in superior estimated PFS (median 29 vs. 15 months), although this did not translate into an overall survival benefit.[176]

Allogeneic transplantation has been employed with increasing frequency in the past decade with the recognition of graft versus leukemia effects and the advent of reduced-intensity conditioning. Earlier studies of allografting showed promising results in young patients with regard to disease control at the expense of significant treatment-related toxicity.[177,178] Several groups have reported favorable disease control and survival in high-risk patients with reduced-intensity conditioning regimens that are fludarabine or low dose TBI based. Of note, patients with chromosome 17p deletion appear to respond as well to allografting as those without 17p deletion.[179,180] Indications for consideration of allografting have been proposed by the European Group for Blood and Marrow Transplantation and include early relapse following chemoimmunotherapy, resistance to fludarabine, chromosome 17p deletion, and Richter transformation.[180] It is not clear whether a survival advantage will occur with stem cell transplantation because there are no controlled trials.

RT was historically a very effective initial therapy for CLL. Prior to the plethora of modern chemotherapeutics, ultra-low dose TBI was used without stem cell support decades ago for CLL given its extraordinary radiosensitivity. This historical use of TBI used roughly 3 to 12 rad or 0.03 to 0.12 Gy/fraction several times a week with doses titrated to response, but total doses in the range of 1 to 4 Gy.[181-184] But, RT is now relegated to a palliative role for CLL, for instance used in the management of painful splenomegaly or occasionally for cytopenias associated with splenomegaly when splenectomy is not an option. It is also indicated in instances of unresponsive disease to alleviate symptomatic adenopathy or nonlymphoid organ involvement. Remarkably low doses on the order of 4 Gy in 1 to 2 fractions can be effective for palliation as used with low-grade B-cell lymphomas, although fractionated doses up to 20 Gy are also reasonable for more definitive local control.[185-187]

IRRADIATION TECHNIQUES

Cranial Radiation

The volume of treatment must include the subarachnoid space within the cranial vault. The inferior margin has by convention extended to the bottom of either the first or second cervical vertebra and includes the whole vertebral body. This may facilitate matching of potential future treatment fields to the spine. Other field boundaries typically involve "flashing" over the scalp. With regard to blocking the anterior facial structures, attention must be given to the base of skull anatomy to adequately cover the cribriform plate and the middle cranial fossa. The cribriform plate is somewhat variable as a function of the age of the patient but is generally in line with the bottom of the frontal sinuses extending posteriorly for several centimeters. The middle cranial or temporal fossa projects on lateral radiographs over the sphenoid sinuses. Figure 84.2 shows plain radiographs of an adult skull with radiopaque markers at various anatomic landmarks. The posterior globe of the eye is typically included given concerns of leukemic relapse in the posterior retina near where there is subarachnoid space extending along the optic nerves. Radiopaque markers on the anterior aspect of the bony orbit are generally a good anatomic landmark that bifurcates the globe.

Figure 84.1 shows an example of lateral fields used to treat a patient with ALL. Head immobilization with Aquaplast or similar thermoplastic material facilitates a high degree of treatment position reproducibility. Accounting for setup variation and beam penumbra leads to field design that clearly must encroach on the eye. With forward gaze of the eyes, this would imply that the superior half of the lens is within the dose build-up region of the treatment fields. With the exception of very young children who cannot cooperate, voluntary rotation of the eye downward ("looking toward one's toes") would theoretically reduce the risk of cataracts. Another important caveat in treatment technique to minimize dose to the anterior portion of the eyes is the alignment of the anterior beam edge divergence. Figure 84.5 depicts this concept of angling the gantry 3 to 5 degrees to achieve a parallel anterior beam margin behind the lens, bisecting the eye producing a relatively tight radiation dose gradient. The simple trigonometric equation to determine the proper gantry rotation is as follows:

$$\tan A = D/\text{SAD}$$

where A is the desired rotation angle, D is the anteroposterior distance between the central axis (i.e., isocenter) and the projection of the anterior aspect of the bony orbit at midplane, and SAD is the source to axis (or isocenter) distance (which is generally 100 cm for most linear accelerator geometries). Because $\tan A \cong A$ (in radians) for small angles and the conversion factor for radians to degrees is approximately 57 (i.e., 180 degrees per π radians), this further simplifies to:

$$A = (D)(0.57) \text{ for a source to axis/isocenter distance of 100 cm}$$

Section III

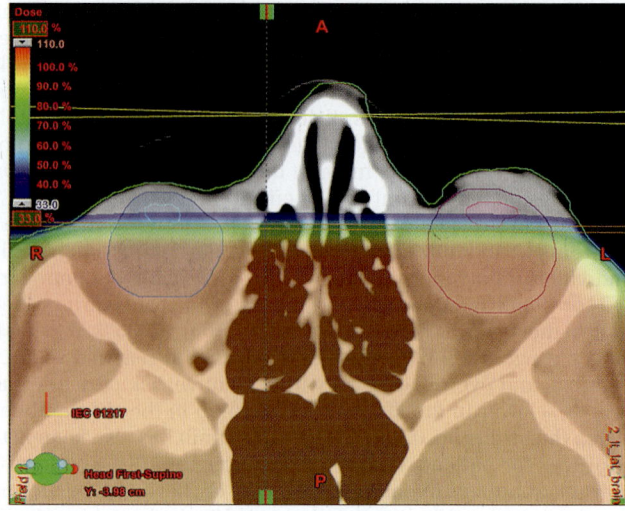

FIGURE 84.5. An 8-year-old boy with T-cell acute lymphoblastic leukemia, CNS-3 at diagnosis, requiring cranial RT to 18 Gy in 12 fractions after remission from systemic therapy. Alignment of anterior divergence of lateral cranial fields showing beam edge and color wash of radiation dose superimposed on axial CT scan at level of eyes. **A:** Parallel-opposed fields result in widened dose gradient within anterior aspect of eyes. **B:** Gantry angle of 3 to 5 degrees results in alignment of anterior margin beam divergence from lateral fields and tighter dose gradient.

Some radiation oncologists prefer to simply place the isocenter of the treatment beam just posterior to the lens so that the anterior eye is protected by a modified "half-beam block." This is a fine technique for linear accelerators equipped with independent primary collimators so that block trays are not excessively heavy. With the advent of CT simulators, alignment of beam divergence can be performed graphically without the need for trigonometric calculations. The standard radiation dose for prophylactic cranial radiation in pediatric ALL is 18 Gy in 9 to 10 fractions, but increasing use of 12 Gy in 8 fractions is based on evolving experience with selected patients being treated with BFM-type ALL programs. Although this is a reasonable dose for adults, some protocols still continue to utilize 24 Gy in 12 fractions. Photon energies >6 MV should not be used so that the dose build-up region at initial depths is superficial to the meninges.

Craniospinal Radiation and Therapeutic Cranial Radiation for CNS Leukemia

The techniques of cranial spinal radiation involve precise matching of beam divergence between a PA spine field and lateral parallel-opposed cranial fields. This topic is discussed in detail in the chapter on Central Nervous System Tumors in Children (see Chapter 88). It is recommended that there be minimal or no gap between the spine and cranial fields. The field junction may be shifted or "feathered" by 1 to 2 cm once or twice to avoid any excessive overlap of dose over the cervical spine. Some physicians prefer to place the beam isocenter at the inferior or caudad border of the initial craniocervical field so as to avoid the complexity of a couch rotation in the treatment setup. A gantry rotation to align the anterior beam divergence near the eye may still be performed. Other physicians place the isocenter near the eye to avoid divergence into the anterior globe, which can be done in conjunction with an appropriate couch rotation to match divergence with the posteroanterior spine field.

Maximum beam energy of 6 MV is recommended. Radiation doses for overt CNS leukemia are 18 to 30 Gy to the cranium in 1.5- to 1.8-Gy fractions. The authors recognize that it is increasingly rare that overt CNS leukemia for children or adults be treated with craniospinal fields, but there can be clinical circumstances where this may still be rationale. In such cases, along with the administration of IT chemotherapy, the spine may be treated to lower doses than the brain to total doses of 6 to 15 Gy depending on individual circumstances. Plans for possible TBI must be taken into account. This part of the preparative regimen for an allogeneic transplant can be conceptualized as being in part of CNS therapy.

Testicular Irradiation

For the management of leukemic infiltration of the testes, both gonads and the scrotum can be irradiated with either electrons or photons. With the patient in a "frog-leg" position and the penile shaft taped onto the abdomen, an anterior inferior oblique photon field works well. Attention to the cremaster reflex and potential ascent of the testes into the inguinal canal is important so as to avoid a geographic miss. For megavoltage photon beams, bolus may be required to avoid superficial underdosing. In young boys where the scrotum/testes thickness is under 2 cm, 250-kV orthovoltage x-rays may also be used. Alternatively, direct en face electron beams of appropriate energy work adequately. Though there are considerable dose inhomogeneities in treating such a curved surface with electrons, the relatively low doses employed in this setting translates into relatively low risks related to skin and subcutaneous soft tissue reactions. Radiation doses typically used are 24 to 26 Gy in 1.5- to 2.0-Gy fractions. When a testicular boost is given in conjunction with TBI for a hematopoietic stem cell transplant, the dose is either 4 Gy × 1 fraction or 2 Gy × 2 fractions.

Splenic Irradiation

Massive splenomegaly may be seen with CML, CLL, hairy cell leukemia, and splenic marginal zone lymphomas, where the spleen can extend into the pelvis. Significant splenomegaly may also occur with prolymphocytic leukemia, myeloproliferative disorders such as polycythemia vera or essential thrombocytosis, or myelofibrosis. One type of myelofibrosis called agnogenic myeloid metaplasia is characterized by progressive bone marrow failure, splenomegaly, and extramedullary hematopoiesis. It is therapeutically important to recognize which conditions of splenomegaly are due to extramedullary hematopoiesis rather than leukemic infiltration as whole-spleen RT with modest radiation doses can result in severe, long-lasting pancytopenia when the spleen is the primary hematopoiesis site.[188] Splenic hematopoiesis can also occur with late stages of CML, myeloproliferative disorders, and hairy cell leukemia. Extreme care is required to proceed slowly with RT in these circumstances.

Historically, splenic RT was commonly employed for palliation, but it is now uncommon, as more effective systemic treatments have been developed. Nevertheless, the radiation oncologist is called on to assist with the management of symptomatic splenomegaly from these hematologic disorders from time to time, often with excellent results.[189] Symptomatic problems include pain, early satiety, diaphragmatic irritation, and bleeding risk related to sequestration of platelets.

Leukemic infiltration of the spleen responds to relatively low doses of radiation.[190] Particularly in an elderly patient with other comorbidities, palliative splenic RT can offer significantly less risk than splenectomy.[191] Splenic irradiation has been reviewed by Weinmann et al.[192]

Anterior and posterior opposed portals for photon treatments are generally employed. In cases of leukemic infiltration, standard practice is to treat the whole spleen in 0.25- to 1.0-Gy fractions either daily or once to three times a week with doses titrated to response and hematologic tolerance.[193] As the spleen responds, one may progressively shrink the treatment fields accordingly. Generally, it is prudent to start treatment very conservatively. Blood counts may need to be monitored several times a week. Total radiation dose delivered is determined clinically by when palliation is achieved. Total doses are typically in the range of 4 to 10 Gy with usually no more than 20 Gy required. Occasionally, a large spleen that is extensively fibrotic will not response to RT. CLL and prolymphocytic leukemia are particularly radiosensitive, with occasional abscopal effects seen with splenic irradiation. One trial of CLL and splenomegaly successfully used 1.0 Gy a fraction once a week for an average of seven treatments yielding good palliation including complete normalization of blood counts in 44% of patients.[194]

In patients with extramedullary hematopoiesis, the potential for severe neutropenia or thrombocytopenia is very high with even modest radiation doses. Dose per fraction may need to be as low as 0.1 to 0.5 Gy treating several times a week to avoid severe and protracted myelosuppression. Another strategy in this situation is to treat only half of the spleen. For myelodysplastic conditions or extramedullary/intrasplenic hematopoiesis, total doses of 1 to 9 Gy are usually adequate.

With splenic irradiation, nausea is uncommon with these low dose fractions but can be readily managed with antiemetics if necessary. As there can be rapid cell lysis, allopurinol to prevent uric acid nephropathy is advised. Cumulative dose to the left kidney should be monitored, especially as retreatment in the future may be required, but it is rare for doses beyond 20 Gy to be required.

SEQUELAE OF THERAPY

Somnolence Syndrome

Approximately 1 month following cranial radiation, up to 40% to 50% of patients may develop lethargy, irritability, anorexia, and even fevers. This has been termed somnolence syndrome. It has been associated with electroencephalographic abnormalities and CSF pleocytosis.[195,196] This syndrome is self-limited and typically reverses within 1 to 3 weeks. Glucocorticoids in acute management may be helpful. Two reports suggest that the incidence of this syndrome is reduced if patients receive steroids during cranial RT.[110,197]

Pituitary Dysfunction

Hypothalamic–pituitary irradiation can impact endocrine function in a dose- and age-dependant manner. For the doses used in leukemia management, growth hormone (GH) deficiency is the most common abnormality observed. Age younger than 5 years at the time of RT is associated with particular susceptibility to the development of GH deficiency. Higher radiation doses as well as younger age correlate with an increased incidence of GH deficiency and a shorter time period for its clinical manifestations.[198] It is more common after 24 Gy than 18 Gy.[199,200] Up to 22% of adult survivors of pediatric ALL who have received cranial RT may have diminished GH responses to provocative testing.[201] Precocious puberty has been reported with radiation doses to the hypothalamic–pituitary region as low as 18 Gy, although it seems to be more prevalent in females who receive doses of 24 Gy or higher.[202] Doses <35 to 40 Gy are rarely associated with other pituitary hormone deficiencies or abnormalities. Thus, patients receiving cranial RT for

leukemia, particularly in childhood, require regular follow-up of their linear growth and sexual development. Abnormalities should then lead to appropriate endocrinologic evaluation so as to determine the need for therapy with either GH replacement or gonadotropin-releasing hormone agonists.

Cognitive Dysfunction

Intellectual and psychological impairments from the treatment of leukemia have received wide attention. Evidence that RT is to blame has been a major impetus in investigations aimed at lowering the dose delivered to the brain or eliminating it completely. Increasingly, however, there is evidence that chemotherapy may also be causing similar detriments. Objective measures of cognitive function and social functioning are inherently difficult. Nevertheless, a variety of assessment tools, intelligence quotients, or scales have been verified as useful measures of language, reasoning, and performance skills. Other descriptive measures of lowered school achievement have also been reported. Cognitive dysfunction is thought to be the result of white matter injury causing deficits in the speed of information processing.[203] These effects are most pronounced in children younger than age 5 years and probably most pronounced in those younger than 3 years of age when the brain is still undergoing growth and development especially with myelination.

Some reports have suggested a gender difference in susceptibility to radiation injury, with females more likely than males to develop intellectual impairments, although this has not been consistently reported.[204,205] The Dana Farber group has suggested that the reduction in IQ seen in girls was the result of an interaction between high dose MTX and cranial radiation.[206] Moreover, an impairment in verbal memory observed in both boys and girls was independent of cranial radiation, suggesting toxicity from systemic therapy.[206]

A reduction in radiation dose from 24 to 18 Gy has not consistently reported to result in lower cognitive difficulties.[100,101,103] Further reduction to 12 Gy is under study. Overall, for these radiation doses, the cognitive deficits have been arguably small with average full-scale IQ measures decreasing by no more than 10%, whereas other studies fail to show measurable changes. Perhaps, a more important statistic is the proportion of patients with significant reductions, say >15 points in IQ scales; the SJCRH group has reported that up to 22% to 30% of children have such deficits after 18, 24 Gy, or no cranial RT.[205] One hypothesis is that a component of cognitive difficulties is related to chemotherapy rather than RT. Regardless, a recent report from the Dana Farber group suggests that in high-risk ALL patients receiving 18-Gy cranial radiation, neurocognitive function many years after therapy is not significantly different from that of the general population.[104] Importantly, this was a group of patients who experienced a favorable 5-year DFS of 75% with a 1% CNS relapse rate. The Dana Farber group has been investigating hyperfractionated cranial radiation for CNS prophylaxis (0.9 Gy twice daily vs. 1.8 Gy daily to a total dose of 18 Gy). There are no obvious differences between standard and hyperfractionated RT in terms of late neurotoxicity reported thus far, although there are numerous methodologic problems inherent in such a comparison.[104-106] An emerging experience suggests that stimulants such as methylphenidate may be of help in managing treatment-related cognitive problems, particularly some attentional or social deficits.[207]

Leukoencephalopathy

Some early prophylactic cranial radiation studies for childhood ALL showed a significant incidence of profound encephalopathy occurring months after irradiation.[127,208] The highest incidence was seen when cranial radiation with doses as low as 24 Gy were combined with IV MTX. Leukoencephalopathy is thought to represent a demyelinating condition that may be initiated by endothelial damage and a subsequent cytokine cascade with ischemic microinfarcts.[209] Although concomitant

IV MTX seems to be a significant synergistic factor, leukoencephalopathy has been observed at low incidence rates with RT alone at doses >30 to 35 Gy, with IT MTX, or in conjunction with other chemotherapy agents. High dose chemotherapy alone is becoming increasingly recognized as causing similar dementia-like syndromes. One should also remember that after cranial RT, the blood–brain barrier is thought to be more permeable, which may contribute to chemotherapy effects on cognitive function.[210] Regardless, the risk of leukoencephalopathy is decidedly rare after doses of <20 Gy.

Secondary Malignancies

One of the larger single institution series of pediatric ALL with extended follow-up of 2,169 patients from SJCRH treated between 1962 and 1998 reported that the cumulative incidence of secondary cancers was 4.2% and 10.9% at 15 and 30 years, respectively.[211] The incidence does not appear to plateau, although second malignancies occurring after 20 years tend to be lower-grade malignancies that include meningiomas and basal cell skin cancers. The Childhood Cancer Survivor Study (CCSG) has also documented an elevated risk for nonmelanoma skin cancers in pediatric ALL survivors, with a cumulative incidence of 10% at 30 years.[212] Cranial MRI surveillance imaging may also increase the detection of asymptomatic radiation-associated meningiomas, estimated to have an incidence of 15% at 20 years and which may sometimes be multifocal.[213] Other secondary cancers attributable to RT include gliomas, parotid gland tumors, thyroid cancers, and sarcomas (bone and soft tissue).[211,214–216] The types of secondary brain tumors from RT tend to be evenly split between meningiomas and high-grade gliomas.[211] In an earlier report from the CCSG of 9,720 patients treated for ALL, 43 secondary cancers were observed after a mean follow-up of 6 years.[216] Of these, 24 were CNS tumors in patients who had previously received 24-Gy cranial RT. All but one of these patients with CNS tumors had been younger than 5 years of age at diagnosis of their acute leukemia, suggesting an age-related susceptibility. Additional data from the CCSG suggest that the risk of gliomas and meningiomas both have a linear radiation dose–response relationship.[216,217] The CCSG has now extended additional long-term follow-up of ALL patients in different treatment eras using various radiation dose prescriptions to more definitely observe that lower doses of cranial irradiation correlate with lower risk for meningiomas.[218] Age of exposure to radiation is also a significant determinant of meningioma risk as lower aged patients have higher risk. On multivariable modeling, there is an increase in hazard ratio of 1.12 per 5 Gy of cranial RT exposure. Although there is hope that a reduction in cranial radiation doses to as low as 12 Gy may reduce the incidence of secondary tumors, the German BFM group has observed in the long-term follow-up of their ALL-BFM 90 trial a 3.4% actuarial incidence of secondary brain tumors at 16 years of follow-up.[107] In comparison, for those children with ALL not receiving cranial RT, the incidence of subsequent brain tumors was 1.2% at 15 years.[214] In a review of 3,182 children treated by an allogeneic bone marrow transplant, 25 solid tumors were observed compared to an expected incidence of one case.[219] A majority of these cancers originated in the CNS or thyroid gland. Moreover, most of these patients had received TBI as part of their preparative regimen before transplant.

Testicular Effects from RT

Gonadal dysfunction is quite rare from cranial RT for leukemia management unless patients undergo retreatment that results in high cumulative doses. Direct effects from testicular irradiation, however, are very common. Doses as low as 1 Gy, even from scattered dose from adjacent external beam fields, will cause transient oligospermia or azoospermia. Higher doses, particularly those used in TBI or therapeutic testicular radiation, would be expected to cause permanent infertility. Leydig cell function, on the other hand, is more radioresistant.[220] Low

serum testosterone levels or delayed puberty are unusual with doses <29 Gy to the testes. One report of 60 male survivors of ALL showed significant germ cell dysfunction as manifested by increased FSH levels and testicular atrophy in 55% of patients treated with testicular RT and in 17% treated with craniospinal RT. The incidence of Leydig cell dysfunction was very low.[220]

REFERENCES

1. Pui CH, Evans WE. Acute lymphoblastic leukemia. *N Engl J Med* 1998;339:605–615.
2. Siegel RL, Miller KD, Jemal A. Cancer statistics, 2017. *CA Cancer J Clin* 2017;67:7–30.
3. Jemal A, Siegel R, Xu J, et al. Cancer statistics, 2010. *CA Cancer J Clin* 2010;60:277–300.
4. Hunger SP, Mullighan CG. Acute lymphoblastic leukemia in children. *N Engl J Med* 2015;373:1541–1552.
5. Laport GF, Larson RA. Treatment of adult acute lymphoblastic leukemia. *Semin Oncol* 1997;24:70–82.
6. Radich J. Stem cell transplant for chronic myeloid leukemia in the imatinib era. *Semin Hematol* 2010;47:354–361.
7. Halperin EC. Concerning the inferior portion of the spinal radiotherapy field for malignancies that disseminate via the cerebrospinal fluid. *Int J Radiat Oncol Biol Phys* 1993;26:357–362.
8. Halperin EC. Impact of radiation technique upon the outcome of treatment for medulloblastoma. *Int J Radiat Oncol Biol Phys* 1996;36:233–239.
9. Dunbar SF, Barnes PD, Tarbell NJ. Radiologic determination of the caudal border of the spinal field in cranial spinal irradiation. *Int J Radiat Oncol Biol Phys* 1993;26:669–673.
10. Price RA, Johnson WW. The central nervous system in childhood leukemia. I. The arachnoid. *Cancer* 1973;31:520–533.
11. Karlsson U, Kirby T, Orrison W, et al. Ocular globe topography in radiotherapy. *Int J Radiat Oncol Biol Phys* 1995;33:705–712.
12. Weiss E, Krebeck M, Kohler B, et al. Does the standardized helmet technique lead to adequate coverage of the cribriform plate? An analysis of current practice with respect to the ICRU 50 report. *Int J Radiat Oncol Biol Phys* 2001;49:1475–1480.
13. Rieselbach RE, Di Chiro G, Freireich EJ, et al. Subarachnoid distribution of drugs after lumbar injection. *N Engl J Med* 1962;267:1273–1278.
14. Shapiro WR, Young DF, Mehta BM. Methotrexate: distribution in cerebrospinal fluid after intravenous, ventricular and lumbar injections. *N Engl J Med* 1975;293:161–166.
15. Vardiman JW, Harris NL, Brunning RD. The World Health Organization (WHO) classification of the myeloid neoplasms. *Blood* 2002;100:2292–2302.
16. Arber DA, Orazi A, Hasserjian R, et al. The 2016 revision to the World Health Organization classification of myeloid neoplasms and acute leukemia. *Blood* 2016;127:2391–2405.
17. Pui CH. Childhood leukemias. *N Engl J Med* 1995;332:1618–1630.
18. van der Veer A, Waanders E, Pieters R, et al. Independent prognostic value of BCR-ABL1-like signature and IKZF1 deletion, but not high CRLF2 expression, in children with B-cell precursor ALL. *Blood* 2013;122:2622–2629.
19. Dorge P, Meissner B, Zimmermann M, et al. IKZF1 deletion is an independent predictor of outcome in pediatric acute lymphoblastic leukemia treated according to the ALL-BFM 2000 protocol. *Haematologica* 2013;98:428–432.
20. Feng J, Tang Y. Prognostic significance of IKZF1 alteration status in pediatric B-lineage acute lymphoblastic leukemia: a meta-analysis. *Leuk Lymphoma* 2013;54:889–891.
21. Zhang W, Kuang P, Li H, et al. Prognostic significance of IKZF1 deletion in adult B cell acute lymphoblastic leukemia: a meta-analysis. *Ann Hematol* 2017;96:215–225.
22. Smith M, Arthur D, Camitta B, et al. Uniform approach to risk classification and treatment assignment for children with acute lymphoblastic leukemia. *J Clin Oncol* 1996;14:18–24.
23. Uckun FM, Sensel MG, Sun L, et al. Biology and treatment of childhood T-lineage acute lymphoblastic leukemia. *Blood* 1998;91:735–746.
24. Gaynon PS, Desai AA, Bostrom BC, et al. Early response to therapy and outcome in childhood acute lymphoblastic leukemia: a review. *Cancer* 1997;80:1717–1726.
25. DeAngelo DJ. The treatment of adolescents and young adults with acute lymphoblastic leukemia. *Hematology* 2005;2005:123–130.
26. Borowitz MJ, Devidas M, Hunger SP, et al. Clinical significance of minimal residual disease in childhood acute lymphoblastic leukemia and its relationship to other prognostic factors: a Children's Oncology Group study. *Blood* 2008;111:5477–5485.
27. Gajjar A, Harrison PL, Sandlund JT, et al. Traumatic lumbar puncture at diagnosis adversely affects outcome in childhood acute lymphoblastic leukemia. *Blood* 2000;96:3381–3384.
28. Gilchrist GS, Tubergen DG, Sather HN, et al. Low numbers of CSF blasts at diagnosis do not predict for the development of CNS leukemia in children with intermediate-risk acute lymphoblastic leukemia: a Childrens Cancer Group report. *J Clin Oncol* 1994;12:2594–2600.
29. Mahmoud HH, Rivera GK, Hancock ML, et al. Low leukocyte counts with blast cells in cerebrospinal fluid of children with newly diagnosed acute lymphoblastic leukemia. *N Engl J Med* 1993;329:314–319.
30. Odom LF, Wilson H, Cullen J, et al. Significance of blasts in low-cell-count cerebrospinal fluid specimens from children with acute lymphoblastic leukemia. *Cancer* 1990;66:1748–1754.
31. Tubergen DG, Cullen JW, Boyett JM, et al. Blasts in CSF with a normal cell count do not justify alteration of therapy for acute lymphoblastic leukemia in remission: a Childrens Cancer Group study. *J Clin Oncol* 1994;12:273–278.

32. Shaikh F, Voicu L, Tole S, et al. The risk of traumatic lumbar punctures in children with acute lymphoblastic leukaemia. *Eur J Cancer* 2014;50:1482–1489.
33. Döhner H, Estey E, Grimwade D, et al. Diagnosis and management of AML in adults: 2017 ELN recommendations from an international expert panel. *Blood* 2017;129:424–447.
34. Podoltsev NA, Stahl M, Zeidan AM, et al. Selecting initial treatment of acute myeloid leukaemia in older adults. *Blood Rev* 2017;31:43–62.
35. Ingram LC, Fairclough DL, Furman WL, et al. Cranial nerve palsy in childhood acute lymphoblastic leukemia and non-Hodgkin's lymphoma. *Cancer* 1991;67:2262–2268.
36. Paryani SB, Donaldson SS, Amylon MD, et al. Cranial nerve involvement in children with leukemia and lymphoma. *J Clin Oncol* 1983;1:542–545.
37. Bunin NJ, Pui CH. Differing complications of hyperleukocytosis in children with acute lymphoblastic or acute nonlymphoblastic leukemia. *J Clin Oncol* 1985;3:1590–1595.
38. Nelson SC, Bruggers CS, Kurtzberg J, et al. Management of leukemic hyperleukocytosis with hydration, urinary alkalinization, and allopurinol. Are cranial irradiation and invasive cytoreduction necessary? *Am J Pediatr Hematol Oncol* 1993;15:351–355.
39. Ferro A, Jabbour SK, Taunk NK, et al. Cranial irradiation in adults diagnosed with acute myelogenous leukemia presenting with hyperleukocytosis and neurologic dysfunction. *Leuk Lymphoma* 2014;55:105–109.
40. Lo-Coco F, Avvisati G, Vignetti M, et al. Retinoic acid and arsenic trioxide for acute promyelocytic leukemia. *N Engl J Med* 2013;369:111–121.
41. Platzbecker U, Avvisati G, Cicconi L, et al. Improved outcomes with retinoic acid and arsenic trioxide compared with retinoic acid and chemotherapy in non-high-risk acute promyelocytic leukemia: final results of the randomized Italian-German APL0406 trial. *J Clin Oncol* 2017;35:605–612.
42. Iland HJ, Bradstock K, Supple SG, et al. All-trans-retinoic acid, idarubicin, and IV arsenic trioxide as initial therapy in acute promyelocytic leukemia (APML4). *Blood* 2012;120:1570–1580.
43. Wheatley K. The AML Collaborative Group: Meta-analysis of randomized trials of idarubicin (IDAR) or mitoxantrone (MITO) versus duanomycin (DNR) as induction therapy for acute myeloid leukemia (AML). *Blood* 1995;86:434a.
44. Fernandez HF, Sun Z, Yao X, et al. Anthracycline dose intensification in acute myeloid leukemia. *N Engl J Med* 2009;361:1249–1259.
45. Fernandez HF. New trends in the standard of care for initial therapy of acute myeloid leukemia. *Hematology Am Soc Hematol Educ Program* 2010;2010:56–61.
46. Stone RM, Mandrekar S, Sanford BL, et al. The multi-kinase inhibitor midostaurin (M) prolongs survival compared with placebo (P) in combination with daunorubicin (D)/cytarabine (C) induction (ind), high-dose C consolidation (consol), and as maintenance (maint) therapy in newly diagnosed acute myeloid leukemia (AML) patients (pts) age 18-60 with *FLT3* Mutations (muts): an international prospective randomized (rand) P-controlled double-blind trial (CALGB 10603/RATIFY [Alliance]). *Blood* 2015;126:6.
47. Mayer RJ, Davis RB, Schiffer CA, et al. Intensive postremission chemotherapy in adults with acute myeloid leukemia. Cancer and Leukemia Group B. *N Engl J Med* 1994;331:896–903.
48. Creutzig U, Ritter J, Zimmermann M, et al. Does cranial irradiation reduce the risk for bone marrow relapse in acute myelogenous leukemia? Unexpected results of the Childhood Acute Myelogenous Leukemia Study BFM-87. *J Clin Oncol* 1993;11:279–286.
49. Creutzig U, Zimmermann M, Dworzak MN, et al. Development of a curative treatment within the AML-BFM studies. *Klin Padiatr* 2013;225(Suppl 1):S79–S86.
50. Byrd JC, Edenfield WJ, Shields DJ, et al. Extramedullary myeloid cell tumors in acute nonlymphocytic leukemia: a clinical review. *J Clin Oncol* 1995;13:1800–1816.
51. Yamauchi K, Yasuda M. Comparison in treatments of nonleukemic granulocytic sarcoma: report of two cases and a review of 72 cases in the literature. *Cancer* 2002;94:1739–1746.
52. Bakst R, Wolden S, Yahalom J. Radiation therapy for chloroma (granulocytic sarcoma). *Int J Radiat Oncol Biol Phys* 2012;82:1816–1822.
53. Choi EK, Hyun KH, Seong HP, et al. Granulocytic sarcoma of bowel: CT findings. *Radiology* 2007;243:752–759.
54. Neiman RS, Barcos M, Berard C. Granulocytic sarcoma: a clinicopathologic study of 61 biopsied cases. *Cancer* 1981;48:1426–1437.
55. Paydas S, Zorludemir S, Ergin M. Granulocytic sarcoma: 32 cases and review of the literature. *Leuk Lymphoma* 2006;47:2527–2541.
56. Seok JH, Park J, Kim SK, et al. Granulocytic sarcoma of the spine: MRI and clinical review. *AJR Am J Roentgenol* 2010;194:485–489.
57. Yossi S, de Talhouet S, Ducastelle-Lepretre S, et al. Radiotherapy of chloroma or granulocytic sarcoma: a literature review. *Cancer Radiother* 2016;20:60–65.
58. Chevallier P, Mohty M, Lioure B, et al. Allogeneic hematopoietic stem-cell transplantation for myeloid sarcoma: a retrospective study from the SFGM-TC. *J Clin Oncol* 2008;26:4940–4943.
59. Tsimberidou AM, Kantarjian HM, Wen S, et al. Myeloid sarcoma is associated with superior event-free survival and overall survival compared with acute myeloid leukemia. *Cancer* 2008;113:1370–1378.
60. Védy D, Muehlematter D, Rausch T, et al. Acute myeloid leukemia with myeloid sarcoma and eosinophilia: prolonged remission and molecular response to imatinib. *J Clin Oncol* 2010;28:e33–e35.
61. Ganzel C, Manola J, Douer D, et al. Extramedullary disease in adult acute myeloid leukemia is common but lacks independent significance: analysis of patients in ECOG-ACRIN Cancer Research Group trials, 1980-2008. *J Clin Oncol* 2016;34:3544–3553.
62. Pui CH, Campana D, Pei D, et al. Treating childhood acute lymphoblastic leukemia without cranial irradiation. *N Engl J Med* 2009;360:2730–2741.
63. Freeman AI, Weinberg V, Brecher ML, et al. Comparison of intermediate-dose methotrexate with cranial irradiation for the post-induction treatment of acute lymphocytic leukemia in children. *N Engl J Med* 1983;308:477–484.
64. Jones B, Freeman AI, Shuster JJ, et al. Lower incidence of meningeal leukemia when prednisone is replaced by dexamethasone in the treatment of acute lymphocytic leukemia. *Med Pediatr Oncol* 1991;19:269–275.
65. Bostrom BC, Sensel MR, Sather HN, et al. Dexamethasone versus prednisone and daily oral versus weekly intravenous mercaptopurine for patients with standard-risk acute lymphoblastic leukemia: a report from the Children's Cancer Group. *Blood* 2003;101:3809–3817.
66. Balis FM, Lester CM, Chrousos GP, et al. Differences in cerebrospinal fluid penetration of corticosteroids: possible relationship to the prevention of meningeal leukemia. *J Clin Oncol* 1987;5:202–207.
67. Schorin MA, Blattner S, Gelber RD, et al. Treatment of childhood acute lymphoblastic leukemia: results of Dana-Farber Cancer Institute/Children's Hospital Acute Lymphoblastic Leukemia Consortium Protocol 85-01. *J Clin Oncol* 1994;12:740–747.
68. Reiter A, Schrappe M, Ludwig WD, et al. Chemotherapy in 998 unselected childhood acute lymphoblastic leukemia patients. Results and conclusions of the multicenter trial ALL-BFM 86. *Blood* 1994;84:3122–3133.
69. Schrappe M, Reiter A, Ludwig WD, et al. Improved outcome in childhood acute lymphoblastic leukemia despite reduced use of anthracyclines and cranial radiotherapy: results of trial ALL-BFM 90. German-Austrian-Swiss ALL-BFM Study Group. *Blood* 2000;95:3310–3322.
70. Asselin BL, Devidas M, Chen L, et al. Cardioprotection and safety of dexrazoxane in patients treated for newly diagnosed T-cell acute lymphoblastic leukemia or advanced-stage lymphoblastic non-Hodgkin lymphoma: a report of the Children's Oncology Group Randomized Trial Pediatric Oncology Group 9404. *J Clin Oncol* 2016;34:854–862.
71. Marshall GM, Dalla Pozza L, Sutton R, et al. High-risk childhood acute lymphoblastic leukemia in first remission treated with novel intensive chemotherapy and allogeneic transplantation. *Leukemia* 2013;27:1497–1503.
72. Clavell LA, Gelber RD, Cohen HJ, et al. Four-agent induction and intensive asparaginase therapy for treatment of childhood acute lymphoblastic leukemia. *N Engl J Med* 1986;315:657–663.
73. Rivera G, George SL, Bowman WP, et al. Second central nervous system prophylaxis in children with acute lymphoblastic leukemia who relapse after elective cessation of therapy. *J Clin Oncol* 1983;1:471–476.
74. Wofford MM, Smith SD, Shuster JJ, et al. Treatment of occult or late overt testicular relapse in children with acute lymphoblastic leukemia: a Pediatric Oncology Group study. *J Clin Oncol* 1992;10:624–630.
75. Torres A, Martinez F, Gomez P, et al. Allogeneic bone marrow transplantation versus chemotherapy in the treatment of childhood acute lymphoblastic leukemia in second complete remission. *Bone Marrow Transplant* 1989;4:609–612.
76. Barrett AJ, Horowitz MM, Pollock BH, et al. Bone marrow transplants from HLA-identical siblings as compared with chemotherapy for children with acute lymphoblastic leukemia in a second remission. *N Engl J Med* 1994;331:1253–1258.
77. Peters C, Schrappe M, von Stackelberg A, et al. Stem-cell transplantation in children with acute lymphoblastic leukemia: a prospective international multicenter trial comparing sibling donors with matched unrelated donors-The ALL-SCT-BFM-2003 trial. *J Clin Oncol* 2015;33:1265–1274.
78. Kelly ME, Lu X, Devidas M, et al. Treatment of relapsed precursor-B acute lymphoblastic leukemia with intensive chemotherapy: POG (Pediatric Oncology Group) study 9411 (SIMAL 9). *J Pediatr Hematol Oncol* 2013;35:509–513.
79. Aur RJ, Hustu HO, Verzosa MS, et al. Comparison of two methods of preventing central nervous system leukemia. *Blood* 1973;42:349–357.
80. Dahl GV, Simone JV, Hustu HO, et al. Preventive central nervous system irradiation in children with acute nonlymphocytic leukemia. *Cancer* 1978;42:2187–2192.
81. Hustu HO, Aur RJ. Extramedullary leukaemia. *Clin Haematol* 1978;7:313–337.
82. Simone JV. Leukaemia remission and survival. *Lancet* 1981;2:531.
83. Aur RJ, Simone JV, Hustu HO, et al. A comparative study of central nervous system irradiation and intensive chemotherapy early in remission of childhood acute lymphocytic leukemia. *Cancer* 1972;29:381–391.
84. Nesbit ME, Sather H, Robison LL, et al. Sanctuary therapy: a randomized trial of 724 children with previously untreated acute lymphoblastic leukemia: a report from Children's Cancer Study Group. *Cancer Res* 1982;42:674–680.
85. Green DM, Freeman AI, Sather HN, et al. Comparison of three methods of central-nervous-system prophylaxis in childhood acute lymphoblastic leukaemia. *Lancet* 1980;1:1398–1402.
86. Komp DM, Fernandez CH, Falletta JM, et al. CNS prophylaxis in acute lymphoblastic leukemia: comparison of two methods a Southwest Oncology Group study. *Cancer* 1982;50:1031–1036.
87. Sullivan MP, Chen T, Dyment PG, et al. Equivalence of intrathecal chemotherapy and radiotherapy as central nervous system prophylaxis in children with acute lymphatic leukemia: a Pediatric Oncology Group study. *Blood* 1982;60:948–958.
88. Conter V, Schrappe M, Arico M, et al. Role of cranial radiotherapy for childhood T-cell acute lymphoblastic leukemia with high WBC count and good response to prednisone. Associazione Italiana Ematologia Oncologia Pediatrica and the Berlin-Frankfurt-Munster groups. *J Clin Oncol* 1997;15:2786–2791.
89. Buhrer C, Henze G, Hofmann J, et al. Central nervous system relapse prevention in 1165 standard-risk children with acute lymphoblastic leukemia in five BFM trials. *Haematol Blood Transfus* 1990;33:500–503.
90. Mahoney DH Jr, Shuster J, Nitschke R, et al. Intermediate-dose intravenous methotrexate with intravenous mercaptopurine is superior to repetitive low-dose oral methotrexate with intravenous mercaptopurine for children with lower-risk B-lineage acute lymphoblastic leukemia: a Pediatric Oncology Group phase III trial. *J Clin Oncol* 1998;16:246–254.
91. Clarke M, Gaynon P, Hann I, et al. CNS-directed therapy for childhood acute lymphoblastic leukemia: childhood ALL Collaborative Group overview of 43 randomized trials. *J Clin Oncol* 2003;21:1798–1809.
92. Tubergen DG, Gilchrist GS, O'Brien RT, et al. Prevention of CNS disease in intermediate-risk acute lymphoblastic leukemia: comparison of cranial radiation and intrathecal methotrexate and the importance of systemic therapy: a Childrens Cancer Group report. *J Clin Oncol* 1993;11:520–526.
93. Schrappe M, Reiter A, Henze G, et al. Prevention of CNS recurrence in childhood ALL: results with reduced radiotherapy combined with CNS-directed chemotherapy in four consecutive ALL-BFM trials. *Klin Padiatr* 1998;210:192–199.

94. Brandalise S, Odone V, Pereira W, et al. Treatment results of three consecutive Brazilian cooperative childhood ALL protocols: GBTLI-80, GBTLI-82 and -85. ALL Brazilian Group. *Leukemia* 1993;7(Suppl 2):S142–S145.
95. Chessells JM, Durrant J, Hardy RM, et al. Medical Research Council leukaemia trial--UKALL V: an attempt to reduce the immunosuppressive effects of therapy in childhood acute lymphoblastic leukemia. Report to the Council by the Working Party on Leukaemia in Childhood. *J Clin Oncol* 1986;4:1758–1764.
96. Eden OB, Lilleyman JS, Richards S. Testicular irradiation in childhood lymphoblastic leukaemia. Medical Research Council Working Party on Leukemia in Childhoods. *Br J Haematol* 1990;75:496–498.
97. Tsukada M, Komiyama A, Nakazawa S, et al. Treatment of standard risk acute lymphoblastic leukemia in children with the Tokyo Children Cancer Study Group (TCCSG) L84-11 protocol in Japan. *Int J Hematol* 1993;57:1–7.
98. Laver JH, Barredo JC, Amylon M, et al. Effects of cranial radiation in children with high risk T cell acute lymphoblastic leukemia: a Pediatric Oncology Group report. *Leukemia* 2000;14:369–373.
99. Nesbit ME, Jr, Sather HN, Robison LL, et al. Presymptomatic central nervous system therapy in previously untreated childhood acute lymphoblastic leukaemia: comparison of 1800 rad and 2400 rad. A report for Children's Cancer Study Group. *Lancet* 1981;1:461–466.
100. Halberg FE, Kramer JH, Moore IM, et al. Prophylactic cranial irradiation dose effects on late cognitive function in children treated for acute lymphoblastic leukemia. *Int J Radiat Oncol Biol Phys* 1992;22:13–16.
101. Cortes J. Central nervous system involvement in adult acute lymphocytic leukemia. *Hematol Oncol Clin North Am* 2001;15:145–162.
102. MacLean WE, Jr., Noll RB, Stehbens JA, et al. Neuropsychological effects of cranial irradiation in young children with acute lymphoblastic leukemia 9 months after diagnosis. The Children's Cancer Group. *Arch Neurol* 1995;52:156–160.
103. Roman DD, Sperduto PW. Neuropsychological effects of cranial radiation: current knowledge and future directions. *Int J Radiat Oncol Biol Phys* 1995;31:983–998.
104. Waber DP, Shapiro BL, Carpentieri SC, et al. Excellent therapeutic efficacy and minimal late neurotoxicity in children treated with 18 grays of cranial radiation therapy for high-risk acute lymphoblastic leukemia: a 7-year follow-up study of the Dana-Farber Cancer Institute Consortium Protocol 87-01. *Cancer* 2001;92:15–22.
105. LeClerc JM, Billett AL, Gelber RD, et al. Treatment of childhood acute lymphoblastic leukemia: results of Dana-Farber ALL Consortium Protocol 87-01. *J Clin Oncol* 2002;20:237–246.
106. Waber DP, Turek J, Catania L, et al. Neuropsychological outcomes from a randomized trial of triple intrathecal chemotherapy compared with 18 Gy cranial radiation as CNS treatment in acute lymphoblastic leukemia: findings from Dana-Farber Cancer Institute ALL Consortium Protocol 95-01. *J Clin Oncol* 2007;25:4914–4921.
107. Moricke A, Reiter A, Zimmermann M, et al. Risk-adjusted therapy of acute lymphoblastic leukemia can decrease treatment burden and improve survival: treatment results of 2169 unselected pediatric and adolescent patients enrolled in the trial ALL-BFM 95. *Blood* 2008;111:4477–4489.
108. Larson RA, Dodge RK, Burns CP, et al. A five-drug remission induction regimen with intensive consolidation for adults with acute lymphoblastic leukemia: Cancer and Leukemia Group B study 8811. *Blood* 1995;85:2025–2037.
109. Cherlow JM, Sather H, Steinherz P, et al. Craniospinal irradiation for acute lymphoblastic leukemia with central nervous system disease at diagnosis: a report from the Children's Cancer Group. *Int J Radiat Oncol Biol Phys* 1996;36:19–27.
110. Mandell LR, Walker RW, Steinherz P, et al. Reduced incidence of the somnolence syndrome in leukemic children with steroid coverage during prophylactic cranial radiation therapy. Results of a pilot study. *Cancer* 1989;63:1975–1978.
111. Ritchey AK, Pollock BH, Lauer SJ, et al. Improved survival of children with isolated CNS relapse of acute lymphoblastic leukemia: a Pediatric Oncology Group study. *J Clin Oncol* 1999;17:3745–3752.
112. Sirvent N, Suciu S, Rialland X, et al. Prognostic significance of the initial cerebro-spinal fluid (CSF) involvement of children with acute lymphoblastic leukaemia (ALL) treated without cranial irradiation: results of European Organization for Research and Treatment of Cancer (EORTC) Children Leukemia Group study 58881. *Eur J Cancer* 2011;47:239–247.
113. Veerman AJ, Kamps WA, van den Berg H, et al. Dexamethasone-based therapy for childhood acute lymphoblastic leukaemia: results of the prospective Dutch Childhood Oncology Group (DCOG) protocol ALL-9 (1997-2004). *Lancet Oncol* 2009;10:957–966.
114. Richards S, Pui CH, Gayon P. Systematic review and meta-analysis of randomized trials of central nervous system directed therapy for childhood acute lymphoblastic leukemia. *Pediatr Blood Cancer* 2013;60:185–195.
115. Vora A, Andreano A, Pui CH, et al. Influence of cranial radiotherapy on outcome in children with acute lymphoblastic leukemia treated with contemporary therapy. *J Clin Oncol* 2016;34:919–926.
116. George SL, Ochs JJ, Mauer AM, et al. The importance of an isolated central nervous system relapse in children with acute lymphoblastic leukemia. *J Clin Oncol* 1985;3:776–781.
117. Kun LE, Camitta BM, Mulhern RK, et al. Treatment of meningeal relapse in childhood acute lymphoblastic leukemia. I. Results of craniospinal irradiation. *J Clin Oncol* 1984;2:359–364.
118. Ortega JA, Nesbit ME, Sather HN, et al. Long-term evaluation of a CNS prophylaxis trial--treatment comparisons and outcome after CNS relapse in childhood ALL: a report from the Childrens Cancer Study Group. *J Clin Oncol* 1987;5:1646–1654.
119. Wells RJ, Weetman RM, Baehner RL. The impact of isolated central nervous system relapse following initial complete remission in childhood acute lymphocytic leukemia. *J Pediatr* 1980;97:429–432.
120. Willoughby ML. Treatment of overt meningeal leukaemia in children: results of second MRC meningeal leukaemia trial. *Br Med J* 1976;1:864–867.
121. Pinkerton CR, Chessells JM. Failed central nervous system prophylaxis in children with acute lymphoblastic leukaemia: treatment and outcome. *Br J Haematol* 1984;57:553–561.
122. Behrendt H, van Leeuwen EF, Schuwirth C, et al. The significance of an isolated central nervous system relapse, occurring as first relapse in children with acute lymphoblastic leukemia. *Cancer* 1989;63:2066–2072.
123. Land VJ, Thomas PR, Boyett JM, et al. Comparison of maintenance treatment regimens for first central nervous system relapse in children with acute lymphocytic leukemia. A Pediatric Oncology Group study. *Cancer* 1985;56:81–87.
124. Winick NJ, Smith SD, Shuster J, et al. Treatment of CNS relapse in children with acute lymphoblastic leukemia: a Pediatric Oncology Group study. *J Clin Oncol* 1993;11:271–278.
125. Ribeiro RC, Rivera GK, Hudson M, et al. An intensive re-treatment protocol for children with an isolated CNS relapse of acute lymphoblastic leukemia. *J Clin Oncol* 1995;13:333–338.
126. Kumar P, Kun LE, Hustu HO, et al. Survival outcome following isolated central nervous system relapse treated with additional chemotherapy and craniospinal irradiation in childhood acute lymphoblastic leukemia. *Int J Radiat Oncol Biol Phys* 1995;31:477–483.
127. Evans AE. Central nervous system workshop. *Cancer Clin Trials* 1981;4(Suppl):31–35.
128. Bleyer WA. Central nervous system leukemia. *Pediatr Clin North Am* 1988;35:789–814.
129. Bleyer WA, Poplack DG. Prophylaxis and treatment of leukemia in the central nervous system and other sanctuaries. *Semin Oncol* 1985;12:131–148.
130. Bleyer WA, Sather H, Hammond GD. Prognosis and treatment after relapse of acute lymphoblastic leukemia and non-Hodgkin's lymphoma: 1985. A report from the Childrens Cancer Study Group. *Cancer* 1986;58:590–594.
131. Morra E, Lazzarino M, Alessandrino EP, et al. Central nervous system (CNS) leukemia: The role of high dose cytarabine (HDAra-C). *Bone Marrow Transplant* 1989;4:101–103.
132. Hiniker SM, Agarwal R, Modlin LA, et al. Survival and neurocognitive outcomes after cranial or craniospinal irradiation plus total-body irradiation before stem cell transplantation in pediatric leukemia patients with central nervous system involvement. *Int J Radiat Oncol Biol Phys* 2014;89:67–74.
133. Anonymous. Testicular disease in acute lymphoblastic leukaemia in childhood. Report on behalf of the Medical Research Council's Working Party on leukaemia in childhood. *Br Med J* 1978;1:334–338.
134. Hijiya N, Liu W, Sandlund JT, et al. Overt testicular disease at diagnosis of childhood acute lymphoblastic leukemia: lack of therapeutic role of local irradiation. *Leukemia* 2005;19:1399–1403.
135. Sullivan MP, Perez CA, Herson J, et al. Radiotherapy (2500 rad) for testicular leukemia: local control and subsequent clinical events: a Southwest Oncology Group study. *Cancer* 1980;46:508–515.
136. Nachman J, Palmer NF, Sather HN, et al. Open-wedge testicular biopsy in childhood acute lymphoblastic leukemia after two years of maintenance therapy: diagnostic accuracy and influence on outcome–a report from Children's Cancer Study Group. *Blood* 1990;75:1051–1055.
137. Shank B, Chu FC, Dinsmore R, et al. Hyperfractionated total body irradiation for bone marrow transplantation. Results in seventy leukemia patients with allogeneic transplants. *Int J Radiat Oncol Biol Phys* 1983;9:1607–1611.
138. Somervaille TCP, Hann IM, Harrison G, et al. Intraocular relapse of childhood acute lymphoblastic leukaemia. *Br J Haematol* 2003;121:280–288.
139. Nowell P, Hungerford D. A minute chromosome in human chronic granulocytic leukemia. *Science* 1960;132:1497.
140. Dobrovic A, Morley AA, Seshadri R, et al. Molecular diagnosis of Philadelphia negative CML using the polymerase chain reaction and DNA analysis: clinical features and course of M-bcr negative and M-bcr positive CML. *Leukemia* 1991;5:187–190.
141. Sokal JE, Cox EB, Baccarani M, et al. Prognostic discrimination in "good-risk" chronic granulocytic leukemia. *Blood* 1984;63:789–799.
142. Pusey WA. Report of cases treated with roentgen rays. *JAMA* 1902;38:911.
143. Minot GR, Buckman TE, Isaacs R. Chronic myelogenous leukemia: age incidence, duration and benefit derived from irradiation. *JAMA* 1924;82:1489.
144. O'Brien SG, Guilhot F, Larson RA, et al. Imatinib compared with interferon and low-dose cytarabine for newly diagnosed chronic-phase chronic myeloid leukemia. *N Engl J Med* 2003;348:994–1004.
145. Hochhaus A, Larson RA, Guilhot F, et al. Long-term outcomes of imatinib treatment for chronic myeloid leukemia. *N Engl J Med* 2017;376:917–927.
146. Druker BJ, Sawyers CL, Kantarjian H, et al. Activity of a specific inhibitor of the BCR-ABL tyrosine kinase in the blast crisis of chronic myeloid leukemia and acute lymphoblastic leukemia with the Philadelphia chromosome. *N Engl J Med* 2001;344:1038–1042.
147. Druker BJ, Talpaz M, Resta DJ, et al. Efficacy and safety of a specific inhibitor of the BCR-ABL tyrosine kinase in chronic myeloid leukemia. *N Engl J Med* 2001;344:1031–1037.
148. Okimoto RA, Van Etten RA. Navigating the road toward optimal initial therapy for chronic myeloid leukemia. *Curr Opin Hematol* 2011;18:89–97.
149. Thomas ED, Clift RA, Fefer A, et al. Marrow transplantation for the treatment of chronic myelogenous leukemia. *Ann Intern Med* 1986;104:155–163.
150. Gale RP, Hehlmann R, Zhang MJ, et al. Survival with bone marrow transplantation versus hydroxyurea or interferon for chronic myelogenous leukemia. The German CML Study Group. *Blood* 1998;91:1810–1819.
151. Enright H, Daniels K, Arthur DC, et al. Related donor marrow transplant for chronic myeloid leukemia: patient characteristics predictive of outcome. *Bone Marrow Transplant* 1996;17:537–542.
152. Richter MN. Generalized reticular cell sarcoma of lymph nodes associated with lymphocytic leukemia. *Am J Pathol* 1928;4:285–292.
153. Giles FJ, O'Brien SM, Keating MJ. Chronic lymphocytic leukemia in (Richter's) transformation. *Semin Oncol* 1998;25:117–125.
154. Preudhomme C, Lepelley P, Lovi V, et al. T-cell acute lymphoblastic leukemia occurring in the course of B cell chronic lymphocytic leukemia: a case report. *Leuk Lymphoma* 1995;18:361–364.
155. Brouet JC, Fermand JP, Laurent G, et al. The association of chronic lymphocytic leukaemia and multiple myeloma: a study of eleven patients. *Br J Haematol* 1985;59:55–66.

156. Swerdlow SH, Campo E, Pileri SA, et al. The 2016 revision of the World Health Organization classification of lymphoid neoplasms. *Blood* 2016;127:2375–2390.

157. Hallek M, Cheson BD, Catovsky D, et al. Guidelines for the diagnosis and treatment of chronic lymphocytic leukemia: a report from the International Workshop on Chronic Lymphocytic Leukemia updating the National Cancer Institute-Working Group 1996 guidelines. *Blood* 2008;111:5446–5456.

158. Rai KR, Sawitsky A, Cronkite EP, et al. Clinical staging of chronic lymphocytic leukemia. *Blood* 1975;46:219–234.

159. Binet JL, Auquier A, Dighiero G, et al. A new prognostic classification of chronic lymphocytic leukemia derived from a multivariate survival analysis. *Cancer* 1981;48:198–206.

160. Furman RR. Prognostic markers and stratification of chronic lymphocytic leukemia. *Hematology Am Soc Hematol Educ Program* 2010;2010:77–81.

161. Dohner H, Stilgenbauer S, Benner A, et al. Genomic aberrations and survival in chronic lymphocytic leukemia. *N Engl J Med* 2000;343:1910–1916.

162. Cheson BD, Bennett JM, Grever M, et al. National Cancer Institute-sponsored Working Group guidelines for chronic lymphocytic leukemia: revised guidelines for diagnosis and treatment. *Blood* 1996;87:4990–4997.

163. Byrd JC, Rai KR, Sausville EA, et al. Old and new therapies in chronic lymphocytic leukemia: now is the time for a reassessment of therapeutic goals. *Semin Oncol* 1998;25:65–74.

164. Byrd JC, Peterson BL, Morrison VA, et al. Randomized phase 2 study of fludarabine with concurrent versus sequential treatment with rituximab in symptomatic, untreated patients with B-cell chronic lymphocytic leukemia: results from Cancer and Leukemia Group B 9712 (CALGB 9712). *Blood* 2003;101:6–14.

165. Rai KR, Peterson BL, Applebaum FR, et al. Long-term survival analysis of the North American Intergroup Study C9011 comparing fludarabine and chlorambucil in previously untreated patients with chronic lymphocytic leukemia (CLL). *Blood* 2009;114:224.

166. Tam CS, O'Brien S, Wierda W, et al. Long-term results of the fludarabine, cyclophosphamide, and rituximab regimen as initial therapy of chronic lymphocytic leukemia. *Blood* 2008;112:975–980.

167. Hallek M, Fischer K, Fingerle-Rowson G, et al. Addition of rituximab to fludarabine and cyclophosphamide in patients with chronic lymphocytic leukaemia: a randomised, open-label, phase 3 trial. *Lancet* 2010;376:1164–1174.

168. Eichhorst B, Fink AM, Bahlo J, et al. First-line chemoimmunotherapy with bendamustine and rituximab versus fludarabine, cyclophosphamide, and rituximab in patients with advanced chronic lymphocytic leukaemia (CLL10): an international, open-label, randomised, phase 3, non-inferiority trial. *Lancet Oncol* 2016;17:928–942.

169. Fischer K, Cramer P, Busch R, et al. Bendamustine in combination with rituximab for previously untreated patients with chronic lymphocytic leukemia: a multicenter phase II trial of the German Chronic Lymphocytic Leukemia Study Group. *J Clin Oncol* 2012;30:3209–3216.

170. Burger JA, Tedeschi A, Barr PM, et al. Ibrutinib as initial therapy for patients with chronic lymphocytic leukemia. *N Engl J Med* 2015;373:2425–2437.

171. Byrd JC, Brown JR, O'Brien S, et al. Ibrutinib versus ofatumumab in previously treated chronic lymphoid leukemia. *N Engl J Med* 2014;371:213–223.

172. O'Brien S, Jones JA, Coutre SE, et al. Ibrutinib for patients with relapsed or refractory chronic lymphocytic leukaemia with 17p deletion (RESONATE-17): a phase 2, open-label, multicentre study. *Lancet Oncol* 2016;17:1409–1418.

173. Okkenhaug K, Vanhaesebroeck B. PI3K in lymphocyte development, differentiation and activation. *Nat Rev Immunol* 2003;3:317–330.

174. Furman RR, Sharman JP, Coutre SE, et al. Idelalisib and rituximab in relapsed chronic lymphocytic leukemia. *N Engl J Med* 2014;370:997–1007.

175. Roberts AW, Davids MS, Pagel JM, et al. Targeting BCL2 with venetoclax in relapsed chronic lymphocytic leukemia. *N Engl J Med* 2016;374:311–322.

176. van Oers MH, Kuliczkowski K, Smolej L, et al. Ofatumumab maintenance versus observation in relapsed chronic lymphocytic leukaemia (PROLONG): an open-label, multicentre, randomised phase 3 study. *Lancet Oncol* 2015;16:1370–1379.

177. Michallet M, Archimbaud E, Bandini G, et al. HLA-identical sibling bone marrow transplantation in younger patients with chronic lymphocytic leukemia. European Group for Blood and Marrow Transplantation and the International Bone Marrow Transplant Registry. *Ann Intern Med* 1996;124:311–315.

178. Khouri IF, Keating MJ, Vriesendorp HM, et al. Autologous and allogeneic bone marrow transplantation for chronic lymphocytic leukemia: preliminary results. *J Clin Oncol* 1994;12:748–758.

179. Sorror ML, Storer BE, Sandmaier BM, et al. Five-year follow-up of patients with advanced chronic lymphocytic leukemia treated with allogeneic hematopoietic cell transplantation after nonmyeloablative conditioning. *J Clin Oncol* 2008;26:4912–4920.

180. Dreger P, Corradini P, Kimby E, et al. Indications for allogeneic stem cell transplantation in chronic lymphocytic leukemia: the EBMT transplant consensus. *Leukemia* 2007;21:12–17.

181. Del Regato JA. Proceedings: total body irradiation in the treatment of chronic lymphogenous leukemia. *Am J Roentgenol Radium Ther Nucl Med* 1974;120:504–520.

182. Johnson RE. Total body irradiation of chronic lymphocytic leukemia: incidence and duration of remission. *Cancer* 1970;25:523–530.

183. Johnson RE. Treatment of chronic lymphocytic leukemia by total body irradiation alone and combined with chemotherapy. *Int J Radiat Oncol Biol Phys* 1979;5:159–164.

184. Johnson RE, Ruhl U. Treatment of chronic lymphocytic leukemia with emphasis on total body irradiation. *Int J Radiat Oncol Biol Phys* 1976;1:387–397.

185. Rossier C, Schick U, Miralbell R, et al. Low-dose radiotherapy in indolent lymphoma. *Int J Radiat Oncol Biol Phys* 2011;81:e1–e6.

186. Chan EK, Fung S, Gospodarowicz M, et al. Palliation by low-dose local radiation therapy for indolent non-Hodgkin lymphoma. *Int J Radiat Oncol Biol Phys* 2011;81:e781–e786.

187. Johannsson J, Specht L, Mejer J, et al. Phase II study of palliative low-dose local radiotherapy in disseminated indolent non-Hodgkin's lymphoma and chronic lymphocytic leukemia. *Int J Radiat Oncol Biol Phys* 2002;54:1466–1470.

188. Elliott MA, Tefferi A. Splenic irradiation in myelofibrosis with myeloid metaplasia: a review. *Blood Rev* 1999;13:163–170.

189. Kriz J, Micke O, Bruns F, et al. Radiotherapy of splenomegaly: a palliative treatment option for a benign phenomenon in malignant diseases. *Strahlenther Onkol* 2011;187:221–224.

190. Guiney MJ, Liew KH, Quong GG, et al. A study of splenic irradiation in chronic lymphocytic leukemia. *Int J Radiat Oncol Biol Phys* 1989;16:225–229.

191. McFarland JT, Kuzma C, Millard FE, et al. Palliative irradiation of the spleen. *Am J Clin Oncol* 2003;26:178–183.

192. Weinmann M, Becker G, Einsele H, et al. Clinical indications and biological mechanisms of splenic irradiation in chronic leukaemias and myeloproliferative disorders. *Radiother Oncol* 2001;58:235–246.

193. Wagner H, Jr, McKeough PG, Desforges J, et al. Splenic irradiation in the treatment of patients with chronic myelogenous leukemia or myelofibrosis with myeloid metaplasia. Results of daily and intermittent fractionation with and without concomitant hydroxyurea. *Cancer* 1986;58:1204–1207.

194. Chisesi T, Capnist G, Dal Fior S. Splenic irradiation in chronic lymphocytic leukemia. *Eur J Haematol* 1991;46:202–204.

195. Freeman JE, Johnston PG, Voke JM. Somnolence after prophylactic cranial irradiation in children with acute lymphoblastic leukaemia. *Br Med J* 1973;4:523–525.

196. Aronson S, Elmquist D, Garwicz S. Letter: somnolence in children with acute leukaemia. *Br Med J* 1974;3:344.

197. Uzal D, Ozyar E, Hayran M, et al. Reduced incidence of the somnolence syndrome after prophylactic cranial irradiation in children with acute lymphoblastic leukemia. *Radiother Oncol* 1998;48:29–32.

198. Birkebaek NH, Fisker S, Clausen N, et al. Growth and endocrinological disorders up to 21 years after treatment for acute lymphoblastic leukemia in childhood. *Med Pediatr Oncol* 1998;30:351–356.

199. Sklar C, Mertens A, Walter A, et al. Final height after treatment for childhood acute lymphoblastic leukemia: comparison of no cranial irradiation with 1800 and 2400 centigrays of cranial irradiation. *J Pediatr* 1993;123:59–64.

200. Stubberfield TG, Byrne GC, Jones TW. Growth and growth hormone secretion after treatment for acute lymphoblastic leukemia in childhood. 18-Gy versus 24-Gy cranial irradiation. *J Pediatr Hematol Oncol* 1995;17:167–171.

201. Steffens M, Beauloye V, Brichard B, et al. Endocrine and metabolic disorders in young adult survivors of childhood acute lymphoblastic leukaemia (ALL) or non-Hodgkin lymphoma (NHL). *Clin Endocrinol (Oxf)* 2008;69:819–827.

202. Leiper AD, Stanhope R, Kitching P, et al. Precocious and premature puberty associated with treatment of acute lymphoblastic leukaemia. *Arch Dis Child* 1987;62:1107–1112.

203. Hill JM, Kornblith AB, Jones D, et al. A comparative study of the long term psychosocial functioning of childhood acute lymphoblastic leukemia survivors treated by intrathecal methotrexate with or without cranial radiation. *Cancer* 1998;82:208–218.

204. Waber DP, Tarbell NJ, Kahn CM, et al. The relationship of sex and treatment modality to neuropsychologic outcome in childhood acute lymphoblastic leukemia. *J Clin Oncol* 1992;10:810–817.

205. Mulhern RK, Fairclough D, Ochs J. A prospective comparison of neuropsychologic performance of children surviving leukemia who received 18-Gy, 24-Gy, or no cranial irradiation. *J Clin Oncol* 1991;9:1348–1356.

206. Waber DP, Tarbell NJ, Fairclough D, et al. Cognitive sequelae of treatment in childhood acute lymphoblastic leukemia: cranial radiation requires an accomplice. *J Clin Oncol* 1995;13:2490–2496.

207. Mulhern RK, Khan RB, Kaplan S, et al. Short-term efficacy of methylphenidate: a randomized, double-blind, placebo-controlled trial among survivors of childhood cancer. *J Clin Oncol* 2004;22:4795–4803.

208. Bleyer WA. Neurologic sequelae of methotrexate and ionizing radiation: a new classification. *Cancer Treat Rep* 1981;65(Suppl 1):89–98.

209. Hong JH, Chiang CS, Campbell IL, et al. Induction of acute phase gene expression by brain irradiation. *Int J Radiat Oncol Biol Phys* 1995;33:619–626.

210. Griffin TW, Rasey JS, Bleyer WA. The effect of photon irradiation on blood-brain barrier permeability to methotrexate in mice. *Cancer* 1977;40:1109–1111.

211. Hijiya N, Hudson MM, Lensing S, et al. Cumulative incidence of secondary neoplasms as a first event after childhood acute lymphoblastic leukemia. *JAMA* 2007;297:1207–1215.

212. Friedman DL, Whitton J, Leisenring W, et al. Subsequent neoplasms in 5-year survivors of childhood cancer: the Childhood Cancer Survivor Study. *J Natl Cancer Inst* 2010;102:1083–1095.

213. Goshen Y, Stark B, Kornreich L, et al. High incidence of meningioma in cranial irradiated survivors of childhood acute lymphoblastic leukemia. *Pediatr Blood Cancer* 2007;49:294–297.

214. Loning L, Zimmermann M, Reiter A, et al. Secondary neoplasms subsequent to Berlin-Frankfurt-Munster therapy of acute lymphoblastic leukemia in childhood: significantly lower risk without cranial radiotherapy. *Blood* 2000;95:2770–2775.

215. Mody R, Li S, Dover DC, et al. Twenty-five-year follow-up among survivors of childhood acute lymphoblastic leukemia: a report from the Childhood Cancer Survivor Study. *Blood* 2008;111:5515–5523.

216. Neglia JP, Robison LL, Stovall M, et al. New primary neoplasms of the central nervous system in survivors of childhood cancer: a report from the Childhood Cancer Survivor Study. *J Natl Cancer Inst* 2006;98:1528–1537.

217. Neglia JP, Meadows AT, Robison LL, et al. Second neoplasms after acute lymphoblastic leukemia in childhood. *N Engl J Med* 1991;325:1330–1336.

218. Bowers DC, Moskowitz CS, Chou JF, et al. Morbidity and mortality associated with meningioma after cranial radiotherapy: a report from the Childhood Cancer Survivor Study. *J Clin Oncol* 2017;35:1570–1576.

219. Socié G, Curtis RE, Deeg HJ, et al. New malignant diseases after allogeneic marrow transplantation for childhood acute leukemia. *J Clin Oncol* 2000;18:348–357.

220. Sklar CA, Robison LL, Nesbit ME, et al. Effects of radiation on testicular function in long-term survivors of childhood acute lymphoblastic leukemia: a report from the Children Cancer Study Group. *J Clin Oncol* 1990;8:1981–1987.

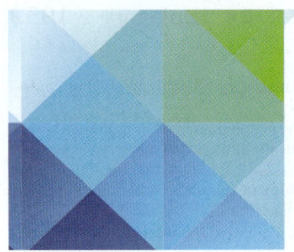

CHAPTER 85

Plasma Cell Myeloma and Plasmacytoma

David C. Hodgson, Joseph Mikhael, and Richard W. Tsang

EPIDEMIOLOGY AND ETIOLOGY

Plasma cell neoplasms account for 22% of all mature B-cell neoplasms in the Surveillance, Epidemiology, and End Results (SEER) program of the United States.[1] The majority of plasma cell neoplasms are multiple myeloma, with solitary plasmacytoma (SP) accounting for ≤6% of cases, and plasma cell leukemia occurring rarely. The incidence of multiple myeloma gradually increased in the 1970s through 2010s.[2] Data from the American Cancer Society indicate an incidence in the United States of 8 per 100,000 men per year and 5.2 per 100,000 women during the period 2009 to 2013.[3] For 2018, it is estimated that there will be 30,770 new cases and 12,770 deaths because of multiple myeloma in the United States.[3] The incidence exceeds that of Hodgkin lymphoma and is about one-third that of all malignant lymphomas. The incidence rises with advancing age, with a median age at diagnosis of 69 years,[2] and approximately 1% of cases are diagnosed in those younger than 45 years of age. Nonregistry studies usually report a lower median age ranging from 60 to 66 years.[4,5] There is a slight male predominance, and for black Americans, the incidence and mortality rates are approximately double that for whites. The 5-year relative survival rates have increased from 26% in 1975 to 30% in 1990 and almost 50% in the period 2007 to 2013.[2]

Little is known about the cause of multiple myeloma. There are studies reporting association with certain chemicals such as petroleum products.[6,7] It is now thought that all cases of myeloma are preceded by monoclonal gammopathy of unknown significance (MGUS).[8–10]

PATHOPHYSIOLOGY

Multiple myeloma arises from malignant transformation of a postgerminal center B cell. Although the full cascade of genetic abnormalities has yet to be defined, one of the earliest genetic events is the illegitimate switch recombination of partner oncogenes into the immunoglobulin heavy chain (IgH).[11] Other events may occur such as cytogenetic hyperploidy and up-regulation of cell cycle control genes. The result of these genetic abnormalities is the development and propagation of a clonal population of B cells within the bone marrow; this, however, is common and can be seen in up to 5% of the general population over the age of 70 (MGUS).[12] Most of these will not go on to develop myeloma, so there must be additional events to create the malignant phenotype of multiple myeloma. These secondary events may include mutations of kinase genes, chromosomal deletions, and up-regulation of enzymes such as c-myc.[11] Having sustained a secondary event, the malignant plasma cells begin to proliferate in the bone marrow microenvironment, producing monoclonal proteins and causing osteolytic bone disease. The slow accumulation of these malignant cells gradually results in the characteristic clinical features of myeloma: anemia, bone resorption, hypercalcemia, renal failure, and immunodeficiency. Established myeloma is sustained by a number of microenvironment features, including the bone marrow stroma itself and the cytokines interleukin-6, vascular endothelial growth factor (VEGF), and insulin-like growth factor-1.[11] The bone disease that arises in myeloma appears to be mediated in part by amplification of the RANK pathway and the inhibition of the Wnt signaling pathway.[11]

CLINICAL PRESENTATION

Multiple myeloma has a wide clinical spectrum, ranging from the preclinical condition of MGUS to the most aggressive form, plasma cell leukemia (Table 85.1). In all cases, a plasma cell clone exists, and the secretion of a monoclonal protein by these plasma cells, along with their interaction with the bone marrow environment, is the source of organ damage in patients with this illness.[11] These concepts have become particularly important, as the molecular mechanisms by which the disease progresses through these "stages" provide essential information that may help us to better understand the disease and its potential therapies.

Monoclonal Gammopathy of Unknown Significance

MGUS has traditionally been considered a benign or a premalignant condition, in which only a small proportion of patients will progress to multiple myeloma or related diseases (Table 85.1). Most are non-IgG MGUS, with 20% having light-chain immunoglobulin MGUS, and rarely IgM MGUS.[8] In

TABLE 85.1 THE SPECTRUM OF MYELOMA				
	MGUS	**Smoldering Multiple Myeloma**	**Multiple Myeloma**[a]	**Plasma Cell Leukemia**
Clinical	No organ damage	No myeloma-defining events[b] or amyloidosis	One or more myeloma-defining events[b]	Organ damage, leukocytosis, high tumor burden, and high proliferation rate
Marrow disease/M-protein features	<10% clonal plasma cells	10%–60% clonal plasma cells and/or M-protein ≥30 g/L (or urinary M = protein ≥500 mg per 24 h)	≥10% clonal plasma cells or biopsy-proven plasmacytoma[a]	Plasma cells in peripheral blood ≥2 × 10⁹/L or ≥20%. Immature plasma cells in bone marrow
Management	Monitor	Close follow-up	Chemotherapy	High-dose chemotherapy
Transformation rate	0.5%–1% per year	10% per year	–	–

[a]Multiple myeloma can be diagnosed when (a) clonal bone marrow plasma cells ≥10% or biopsy-proven bone or extramedullary plasmacytoma is present, plus (b) any one or more myeloma-defining events as outlined below.[b] Alternatively, without presence of myeloma-defining events, the presence of (a) with any one or more of the following biomarkers of malignancy also satisfies the diagnosis of multiple myeloma: clonal bone marrow plasma cell percentage ≥60%, involved:uninvolved serum light chain ratio ≥100, or >1 focal lesions on MRI (each focal lesion must be 5 mm or more in size).[13] This is also known as the SLiM (Sixty percent, Light chains, MRI) criteria.

[b]Myeloma-defining events: end-organ damage attributed to myeloma: hypercalcemia (calcium >2.75 mmol/L); renal insufficiency (creatinine >177 μmol/L or creatinine clearance <40 mL/min); anemia (hemoglobin <10 g/dL or >20 g/L below the lower limit of normal); and bone lesions (one or more osteolytic lesions on x-rays, CT, or PET scan).

MGUS, monoclonal gammopathy of unknown significance.

From Fernandez de Larrea C, Kyle RA, Durie BG, et al. Plasma cell leukemia: consensus statement on diagnostic requirements, response criteria and treatment recommendations by the International Myeloma Working Group. *Leukemia* 2013;27(4):780–791; Rajkumar SV, Dimopoulos MA, Palumbo A, et al. International Myeloma Working Group updated criteria for the diagnosis of multiple myeloma. *Lancet Oncol* 2014;15(12):e538–e548.

MGUS, the monoclonal protein is <3 g/dL, and the bone marrow clonal plasma cells are <10% with no related organ damage. This condition is likely much more common than initially thought, as it has been documented in 3% of the population and 5% in those over the age of 70 and 7.5% of those over the age of 85.[12] The risk of transformation to myeloma and related diseases (such as amyloidosis or Waldenstrom macroglobulinemia) has been estimated at 1% per year, based on a 30-year follow-up of 1,384 patients at the Mayo Clinic.[8]

Asymptomatic Multiple Myeloma (Smoldering Myeloma)

This category of myeloma represents an intermediate form of myeloma whereby patients meet serologic monoclonal protein levels ≥3 g/dL or urinary protein >500 mg per 24 hour and/or bone marrow clonal plasma cell infiltration of 10% to 60%[13] and absence of myeloma-defining events or amyloidosis (Table 85.1). These patients are not significantly anemic, do not have hypercalcemia or renal insufficiency, and do not have bony disease. Although the risk of transformation to multiple myeloma is much higher than in MGUS (20% per year), some patients' disease may remain asymptomatic without significant progression for many years. These patients generally do not require therapy but should be followed closely to monitor for progression.

Solitary Plasmacytomas

The median age at diagnosis of SP is 55 to 65 years, on average about 10 years younger than patients with multiple myeloma.[14–17] Males are affected predominately (male-to-female ratio 2:1).[14,15] A diagnosis of SP is made if all the following criteria are satisfied at presentation: a histologically confirmed single lesion with negative skeletal imaging outside the primary site, normal bone marrow biopsy (<10% monoclonal plasma cells), and no myeloma-related organ dysfunction.[13,18] A monoclonal protein is present in 30% to 75% of cases (particularly for an osseous presentation), and the level is usually minimally elevated (IgG < 3.5 g/dL, IgA < 2.0 g/dL, and urine monoclonal κ or λ < 1.0 g per 24 hours).[18–20]

The disease more commonly presents in bone (70%). Such cases are considered stage I multiple myeloma according to the original Durie Salmon staging system.[21] The most common location is the vertebra.[14,15] Patients with bone involvement often present with pain, neurologic compromise, and occasionally pathologic fracture. A lytic lesion is typical, with or without adjacent soft tissue mass. Less commonly, SP presents in an extramedullary site (20% to 30%), usually as a mass in the upper aerorespiratory passages, and produces local compressive symptoms.[14–16,22] The histologic diagnosis of extramedullary plasmacytoma (EMP) can be difficult, with the main differential diagnosis being extranodal marginal zone lymphoma (mucosa-associated lymphoid tissue type), where there can be extensive infiltration by plasmacytoid cells.[23,24]

Multiple Myeloma

By definition, myeloma involves end-organ damage as myeloma-defining events, described by the mnemonic CRAB (Calcium elevation, Renal insufficiency, Anemia, and Bone disease).[11,13] Recent modification added additional features when CRAB findings are absent, to include the SLiM criteria of 60% or more clonal plasma cells in bone marrow (S), light chains (Li) involved:uninvolved ratio >100, or MRI (M) detected number of bone lesions >1, measuring at least 5 mm in size for the diagnosis of multiple myeloma.[13] Bone pain and symptoms because of anemia, such as easy fatigability, are the most common.[5] Because of the myriad effects of the disease, other insidious symptoms can result from a combination of hypercalcemia, renal impairment, infection, neurologic

compression, and occasionally, hyperviscosity. Bone disease manifesting as generalized osteopenia and multiple lytic bone lesions can frequently lead to pathologic fractures. In the vertebral column, this often results in a diminished height. Sclerotic lesions at presentation are rare.

Laboratory evaluation generally confirms anemia, high erythrocyte sedimentation rate, and a variable degree of granulocytopenia and thrombocytopenia. An abnormal monoclonal immunoglobulin (M protein) in the blood or urine is characteristic,[5,11] most commonly IgG or IgA. Biclonal disease is also recognized, and rarely, nonsecretory disease. In up to 10% of cases, only monoclonal light chains are detected. It is important to assess for hypercalcemia, renal dysfunction, and integrity of the skeleton because these complications require appropriate management. A constellation of polyneuropathy, organomegaly, endocrinopathy, M protein, and skin changes characterizes a rare plasma cell dyscrasia known as POEMS syndrome.[25,26]

Plasma Cell Leukemia

This is a very rare variant of multiple myeloma, where the proliferation of plasma cells is not confined to the bone marrow but may be detected in the peripheral blood (plasma cell count ≥2 × 10⁹/L or ≥20%).[27] It carries a very poor prognosis, with median survival <1 year and shortest when occurring as secondary plasma cell leukemia.[27–29] There is currently no standard therapy for this condition, but patients are usually treated with high-dose, multiagent chemotherapeutic regimens or with experimental therapies, followed by autologous stem cell transplant.[27]

DIAGNOSTIC WORKUP AND STAGING

The recommended tests for the diagnosis of plasma cell neoplasms are outlined in Table 85.2. The most important components relate to the measurement and quantification of the M protein, bone marrow examination with ancillary cytogenetic studies, serum β_2 microglobulin and albumin, and diagnostic imaging.[30] The M protein should be measured with serum protein electrophoresis. Quantification of the monoclonal Ig with immunofixation techniques is also acceptable and especially useful if the M component is at a low level. If

---

TABLE 85.2 DIAGNOSTIC WORKUP FOR PLASMA CELL NEOPLASMS

General
History and physical examination
Complete blood count and blood smear, chemistry panel including calcium and creatinine

Standard Laboratory Tests
Bone marrow aspirate and trephine biopsy or biopsy of mass if solitary lesion (clonality, immunophenotype and cytogenetic studies (both conventional cytogenetics and fluorescence *in situ* hybridization), and plasma cell labeling index)
Serum β_2 microglobulin, albumin, C-reactive protein, and lactate dehydrogenase
M component measurement:
- Serum protein electrophoresis and immunofixation for quantification of immunoglobulins
- Urine protein electrophoresis
- Free light chain measurements if conventional M component is negative or equivocal (serum and urine)

Imaging Studies
Skeletal survey
Computed tomography and magnetic resonance imaging were indicated (e.g., to visualize soft tissue tumor, detailed assessment of local disease extent and bulk, assessing vertebral column osteopenia and compression fractures, and spinal cord compression)
Fluorine-18 fluorodeoxyglucose positron emission tomography or magnetic resonance imaging should be ordered to detect and quantify occult disease if present

TABLE 85.3 STAGING OF MULTIPLE MYELOMA (DURIE SALMON SYSTEM[21])

Clinical Stage	Durie and Salmon Staging System[21]
Stage I	All of the following: • Hemoglobin >10 g/dL • Serum calcium normal • Normal bone structure or solitary plasmacytoma only • Low M component (IgG < 5 g/dL, IgA < 3 g/dL, and urine light chains <4 g/24 h)[a]
Stage II	Fitting neither stage I nor stage III
Stage III	One or more of the following: • Hemoglobin <8.5 g/dL • Serum calcium >12 mg/dL • Advanced lytic bone lesions • High M component (IgG > 7 g/dL, IgA > 3 g/dL, and urine light chains >12 g/24 h)
Subclassified:	
A	Relatively normal renal function (serum creatinine <2 mg/dL)
B	Abnormal renal function (serum creatinine ≥2 mg/dL)

[a]For solitary plasmacytoma, current recommendations are IgG < 3.5 g/dL and IgA < 2 g/dL. From Durie BG, Salmon SE. A clinical staging system for multiple myeloma correlation of measured myeloma cell mass with presenting clinical features, response to treatment, and survival. *Cancer* 1975;36(3):842–854. Copyright © 1975 American Cancer Society. Reprinted by permission of John Wiley & Sons, Inc.

TABLE 85.4 STAGING OF MULTIPLE MYELOMA (THE INTERNATIONAL STAGING SYSTEM[4] AND THE REVISED INTERNATIONAL STAGING SYSTEM[36])

	International Staging System (ISS[4])	Median Survival
ISS Stage I	Serum β_2 microglobulin <3.5 mg/L and Serum albumin ≥35 g/L	62 mo
ISS Stage II	Neither I nor III i.e., β_2 microglobulin <3.5 mg/L, with albumin <35 g/L, or β_2 microglobulin 3.5–5.5 mg/L	44 mo
ISS Stage III	Serum β_2 microglobulin ≥5.5 mg/L	29 mo

	Revised International Staging System (R-ISS[36])	Median Survival
R-ISS Stage I	ISS stage I and standard risk chromosomal abnormalities[a] (by iFISH) and normal LDH	Not reached[b]
R-ISS Stage II	Neither R-ISS stage I nor III	83 mo
R-ISS Stage III	ISS stage III and either high-risk chromosomal abnormality[a] (by iFISH) or high LDH	43 mo

[a]High-risk chromosomal abnormalities are any one of Del(17p), translocation t(4;14), or translocation t(14;16).
[b]Median follow-up 46 months.
iFISH, interphase fluorescent *in situ* hybridization; LDH, lactate dehydrogenase.
Reprinted with permission from Greipp PR, San Miguel J, Durie BG, et al. International staging system for multiple myeloma. *J Clin Oncol* 2005;23(15):3412–3420. Copyright © 2005 American Society of Clinical Oncology and Palumbo A, Avet-Loiseau H, Oliva S, et al. Revised International Staging System for Multiple Myeloma: a Report From International Myeloma Working Group. *J Clin Oncol* 2015;33(26):2863–2869. Copyright © 2015 American Society of Clinical Oncology. All rights reserved.

no M protein is detectable, assays for free light chains should be performed in the serum and in the urine (Bence Jones proteinuria). The standard imaging is the skeletal survey, as radionuclide bone scan usually does not detect lytic disease and has limited value.[19] For localized areas of concern, both computed tomography (CT) and magnetic resonance imaging (MRI) can be useful. MRI is recommended to assess the extent of vertebral disease and the presence of spinal cord or nerve root compression,[31] and even if the solitary lesion is not located in the vertebra, MRI is a good screening tool to rule out additional lesions in the spine. With advances in diagnostic imaging, it is likely that "stage migration" has occurred.[32] It has been documented that some patients with presumed SP of bone will be upstaged following the detection of multiple vertebral lesions or bone marrow disease by MRI or by 18-fluorine (^{18}F) fluorodeoxyglucose positron emission tomography (FDG-PET).[33–35] PET scan is therefore a useful screening tool, as it examines the whole body in a single study and can be helpful for clarifying ambiguous CT or MRI abnormalities. The optimal role of PET in myeloma is yet to be determined but will likely evolve rapidly,[30] and it will likely be of most benefit in nonsecretory disease. The staging criteria for the historical Durie Salmon staging system are detailed in Table 85.3.[21] The newer revised International Myeloma Staging System (rISS) is simple, validated, and of importance particularly for present and future clinical trials (Table 85.4).[36] It incorporated

important cytogenetic abnormalities (e.g., del(17p), t(4;14) and t(14;16)) into the staging system. Criteria for the diagnosis of MGUS and smoldering myeloma are also well established.[13]

PROGNOSTIC FACTORS

Solitary Plasmacytoma

With respect to local control, tumor bulk appears to be an important unfavorable factor. Tumors <5 cm achieved a high level of local control with 35 Gy, whereas those ≥5 cm had a local failure rate of 58% (7 of 12 patients, total dose range 25 to 50 Gy).[17] The importance of tumor bulk is also supported by other studies.[15,37–39]

Age is a factor that affects the risk of progression to myeloma in some series[17,40–43] but not in others.[15,37–39,44,45] A bony presentation has been consistently demonstrated to have a significantly higher risk of subsequent development of myeloma with a 10-year rate of 76% compared with an extramedullary presentation where the 10-year rate was 36%[15] (Fig. 85.1). Subclinical bone disease, either detected as generalized osteopenia[46] or abnormal MRI scan of the spine,[31,47–49] predicts

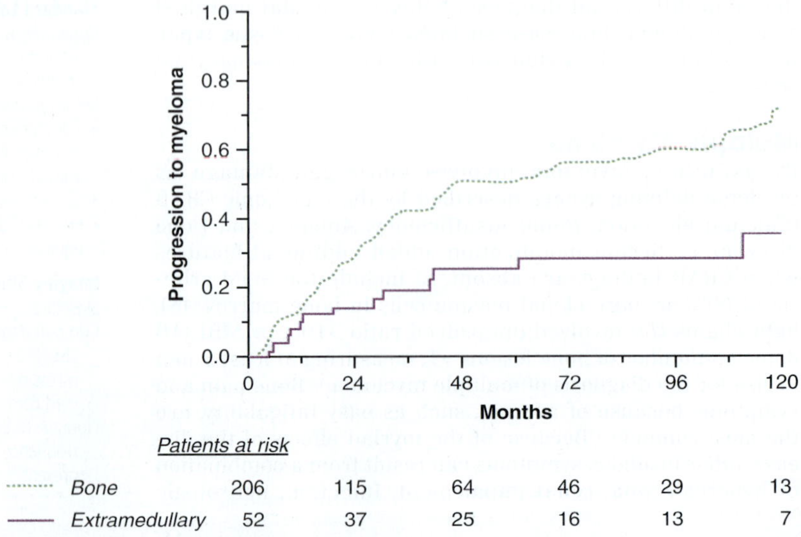

FIGURE 85.1 Probability of progression to multiple myeloma according to bone (*dotted line*) versus extramedullary (*solid line*) solitary plasmacytoma in 258 patients (*P* = .0009). (Reprinted from Ozsahin M, Tsang RW, Poortmans P, et al. Outcomes and patterns of failure in solitary plasmacytoma: a multicenter Rare Cancer Network study of 258 patients. *Int J Radiat Oncol Biol Phys* 2006;64[1]: 210–217. Copyright © 2006 Elsevier. With permission.)

Patients at risk

Bone	206	115	64	46	29	13
Extramedullary	52	37	25	16	13	7

for rapid progression to symptomatic multiple myeloma. In the updated International Myeloma Working Group (IMWG) criteria for the diagnosis of multiple myeloma, MRI detection of more than one focal lesion in bone (of 5 mm or more in size) is recognized as multiple myeloma.[13] A suppression of the normal immunoglobulin classes has been shown to correlate with a higher risk of progressing to myeloma.[46,50] Where there was an elevation of M protein pretreatment, persistence of the M protein following radiation therapy (RT) predicts for progression to myeloma.[20,51] Many of these factors reflect the presence of occult myeloma. Therefore, it is not surprising that generalized disease becomes manifest once the local disease is controlled. Pathologic factors have been examined in some studies, with the finding that anaplastic plasmacytomas (those with a higher histologic grade)[52] and those tumors expressing a high level of angiogenesis are associated with a poor outcome.[53] Anaplastic plasmacytomas share some common pathologic and clinical features with aggressive B-cell lymphomas (plasmablastic type) and can arise in the context of immunosuppression and Epstein-Barr virus infection.[54,55]

Multiple Myeloma

Analysis of over 1,000 patients evaluated at the Mayo Clinic revealed the following adverse prognostic risk factors: Eastern Cooperative Oncology Group performance status 3 or 4, serum albumin <3 g/dL, serum creatinine ≥2 mg/dL, platelet count <150,000/μL, age >70 years, β_2 microglobulin >4 mg/L, plasma cell labeling index ≥1%, serum calcium ≥11 mg/dL, hemoglobin <10 g/dL, and bone marrow plasma cell percentage ≥50%.[5] The ISS[4] and the revised ISS[36] have been validated to assist in prognostication. For the original ISS, over 10,000 patients were evaluated, and the three-stage system was developed based on two variables: serum albumin and β_2 microglobulin in the original ISS. In the revised ISS, cytogenetic abnormalities associated with a worse prognosis were also incorporated[36] (Table 85.4). These include del(17p), t(4;14), and t(14;16) detected with fluorescence *in situ* hybridization.

MANAGEMENT OF SOLITARY PLASMACYTOMA

RT is the standard treatment for SP. Surgery should be considered for structural instability of bone or rapidly progressive neurologic compromise such as spinal cord compression.[18] For patients treated with gross tumor excision, RT is still indicated because of a high likelihood of microscopic residual disease. Surgery alone without RT leads to an unacceptably high local recurrence rate.[15] A review of the literature for solitary bone plasmacytoma (Table 85.5) indicates a high local control rate with RT (79% to 95%), yet a modest overall survival rate of approximately 50% at 10 years. This is due to a high rate of progression to multiple myeloma in the bone plasmacytomas, a finding consistently reported from all series.[14,17,18,20,37,40–42,44,46,51,56,58] As shown in Table 85.5, over 60% of patients with solitary bone tumor progressed to myeloma, at a median of 2 to 3 years after treatment. When actuarial methods were not used, the progression rate is slightly lower (crude rate ranges, 53% to 54%).[37,56] Therefore, SP of bone appears to be an early form of multiple myeloma. Studies have documented about 29% to 50% of patients with apparent SP will have multiple asymptomatic lesions detected in the spine on MRI.[30,31,47,49,59] If characteristic additional lesion(s) of 5 mm or more in size are detected, the patient satisfies the diagnostic criteria for multiple myeloma and should be treated as such.[13] With more routine use of MRI and/or FDG-PET as part of the diagnostic workup to rule out multiple myeloma, going forward there is likely stage migration with truly solitary patients remaining eligible for definitive RT alone as initial treatment strategy. One of the larger series of patients with SP treated prior to 2001 showed that the progression rate to myeloma following RT is more rapid in the first 3 years (~14% per year), compared to the subsequent 7 years (~3% to 4% per year), reaching a 10-year rate of 65%.[15] This suggested that subclinical myeloma existed in up to 40% of the patients at the time of initial RT. It is likely that sensitive imaging tests initially would identify these patients and alternate

TABLE 85.5 SOLITARY PLASMACYTOMA OF BONE: REPRESENTATIVE TREATMENT RESULTS (SERIES INCLUDING MORE THAN 30 PATIENTS)

Study (Reference)	Institution	Number of Patients (median f/u)	Local Control (%)	Progression to Myeloma (10-y Rate %)	Overall Survival (10-y Rate %)
Bataille and Sany (1981)[40]	Hospital St. Eloi, France	114 (>10 y)	88	58	68[a]
Chak et al. (1987)[41]	Stanford[b]	65[b] (87 mo)	95	77	52
Frassica et al. (1989)[56]	Mayo Clinic	46 (90 mo)	89	54[a]	45
Jackson and Scarffe (1990)[50]	Christie Hospital	32 (101 mo)	97[a]	~76	~45
Holland et al. (1992)[37]	Mallinckrodt	32 (66 mo)	94	53[a]	–
Galieni et al. (1995)[46]	Siena, Italy[b]	32[b] (69 mo)	91[a]	~68	49
Tsang et al. (2001)[17]	Princess Margaret Hospital	32 (95 mo)	87	64 (8-y rate)	65 (8-y rate)
Wilder et al. (2002)[20]	MD Anderson Cancer Center	60 (94 mo)	90	62	59
Ozsahin et al. (2006)[15]	RARE Cancer Network[b]	206[b] (56 mo)	79 (10-y rate)	72	52
Kilciksiz et al. (2008)[57]	Turkish Oncology Group[b]	57[b] (29 mo)	94	37[a]	68
Reed et al. (2011)[42]	MD Anderson Cancer Center	59 (64 mo)	97	56 (5-y rate)	76 (5-y rate)
Finsinger et al. (2016)[58]	Rome, Italy	35 (107 mo)	94	57[a]	51

[a]Crude rate.
[b]Multiple institutions.

approaches such as chemotherapy with novel agents +/– RT being more appropriate.[60] The presence of low level M protein preradiation is extremely common and is not associated with a higher risk of progression to multiple myeloma. However, its persistence following radiation is highly predictive of subsequent systemic failure,[20,42,51,61] attesting to the importance of monitoring this as part of posttreatment follow-up. It has been observed that some patients recur with plasmacytoma(s) of bone or soft tissues, without bone marrow involvement.[37,40,62,63] This is infrequent, and the subsequent development of multiple myeloma is high, 75% in one series.[40]

The addition of adjuvant chemotherapy is theoretically attractive, both in enhancing local control and eradicating subclinical disease to prevent the development of myeloma. One randomized trial suggested a benefit with adjuvant melphalan and prednisone given for 3 years after RT.[64] With a median follow-up of 8.9 years, those treated with chemotherapy had a myeloma progression rate of 12%, whereas with RT alone, it was 54%. However, this was a small study, and the risk of diminishing stem cell reserve or inducing leukemia makes the prolonged use of alkylating agents an undesirable treatment option for most patients. The use of adjuvant novel agents, such as proteasome inhibitors (e.g., bortezomib) or immunomodulatory drugs (IMiDs, e.g., lenalidomide), is theoretically attractive, both in enhancing local control and eradicating subclinical disease to prevent progression to myeloma. Pilot data indicate feasibility of combining novel agents with RT,[65,66] and this approach is under active investigation in the United Kingdom in a phase III clinical trial, examining the potential role of adding lenalidomide and dexamethasone to definitive RT (https://clinicaltrials.gov/ct2/show/record/NCT02544308).

In the management of EMP, although complete surgical excision may be curative for small lesions,[67] most patients with larger lesions or with tumor location not amenable to complete excision should receive local RT. Postoperative RT is indicated for incompletely excised lesions. In contrast to bone plasmacytoma, EMPs are frequently controlled with local radiation (Table 85.6), with a lower rate of progression to myeloma, ranging from 8% to 44%,[15,16,39,52,62,67,69–72,74] indicating a significant proportion of patients are cured of their disease. Although the 10-year survival varies widely in the reported literature (range, 31% to 90%), the two larger series report survival rates of 76% at 5 years[74] and 72% at 10 years.[15] The issue of dose will be discussed later.

Initial Treatment of Symptomatic Multiple Myeloma

Patients who have symptomatic multiple myeloma require treatment of the malignant plasma cell clone. Once the decision is made to treat, however, the first step is to determine candidacy for autologous stem cell transplantation (ASCT).[11] As this modality has become the standard of care for eligible patients, it is necessary to stratify patients initially so that the ability to collect stem cells is not compromised by induction therapy.[76]

Patients Eligible for Autologous Stem Cell Transplantation

In patients who are candidates for ASCT, various regimens can be used to induce response prior to stem cell collection. Historically, most regimens were steroid based, either with high-dose dexamethasone alone or with vincristine, Adriamycin (doxorubicin), and dexamethasone (VAD).[77,78] Newer agents that have been validated in the relapse setting are now being used as initial therapy with superior results, including bortezomib and lenalidomide. Both have been routinely adopted into initial treatment[79] or for relapsed disease.

TABLE 85.6 SOLITARY EXTRAMEDULLARY PLASMACYTOMA: REPRESENTATIVE TREATMENT RESULTS (SERIES INCLUDING MORE THAN 15 PATIENTS)

Study (Reference)	Number of Patients (median f/u)	Local Control (%)	Progression to Myeloma (10-y Rate %)	Overall Survival (10-y Rate %)
Kapadia et al. (1982)[68]	17 (62 mo)	85	31[a]	31[a] (5 y)
Knowling et al. (1983)[62]	25 (71 mo)	88	28	43
Brinch et al. (1990)[69]	18	–	–	90
Soesan et al. (1992)[70]	25 (44 mo)	88	–	~50
Susnerwala et al. (1997)[52]	25 (73 mo)	79	8[a]	59 (5 y)
Liebross et al. (1999)[71]	22	95	44 (5 y)	50
Galieni et al. (2000)[72]	46[b] (118 mo)	92	15[a]	78 (15 y)
Strojan et al. (2002)[16]	26 (61 mo)	87	8	61
Chao et al. (2005)[73]	16 (66 mo)	100	31	54
Ozsahin et al. (2006)[15]	52[b] (56 mo)	74 (10 y)	36	72
Tournier-Rangeard et al. (2006)[22]	17 (80.5 mo)	73 (10 y)	36	63
Bachar et al. (2008)[74]	56 (96 mo)	88 (10 y)	28 (10 y)	56 (10 y)
Kilciksiz et al. (2008)[57]	23[b] (29 mo)	95	17[a]	89
Creach et al. (2009)[75]	18 (82 mo)	94	33[a]	55
Reed et al. (2011)[42]	25 (64 mo)	80	30 (5-y rate)	85 (5-y rate)
Sasaki et al. (2012)[63]	67 (63 mo)	87	30	56
Finsinger et al. (2016)[58]	18 (107 mo)	94	6[a]	88
Zhu et al. (2016)[39]	48 (45 mo)	86	–	60

[a]Crude rate.
[b]Multiple institutions.

Bortezomib

Bortezomib was the first proteasome inhibitor to be used in clinical trials and has demonstrated efficacy and safety in frontline therapy when used in combination. Indeed, response rates have dramatically improved when compared with VAD or dexamethasone alone. A randomized comparison of bortezomib plus dexamethasone (BD) versus VAD as induction therapy before ASCT showed that BD produced superior complete response or near-complete response: 14.8% versus 6.4%, at least very good partial response: 37.7% versus 15.1%, and overall response: 78.5% versus 62.8% than that of VAD. Median progression-free survival was 36.0 months (BD) versus 29.7 months (VAD; P = .064).[80] Even as a single agent, with dexamethasone or with doxorubicin, bortezomib has remarkable efficacy and safety in initial therapy.[81] It is often the preferred agent in patients with renal insufficiency and high-risk disease. Its greatest challenge, however, remains neuropathy, occurring in 13% to 15% of patients at ≥grade 3; this may be helped, however, with weekly use[82] or when given subcutaneously.[83]

Lenalidomide

Lenalidomide is an immunomodulatory drug derived from thalidomide that has also been shown to be effective, both as upfront therapy and in relapsed disease. It is most commonly used in combination with low-dose dexamethasone.[84]

A phase III trial of lenalidomide with low-dose dexamethasone versus lenalidomide with high-dose dexamethasone found that despite a higher rate of complete or partial response with high-dose therapy, overall 1-year survival was 87% in the high-dose group versus 96% in the low-dose group (P = .0002), largely because of the significant toxicity of the former. As a result, the trial was stopped and patients on high-dose therapy were crossed over to low-dose therapy. Three-year overall survival rates now exceed 85%. This has resulted in the extensive use of this combination in upfront myeloma.[84]

Lenalidomide has also been used in combination with conventional chemotherapy and most recently with bortezomib.[79,85] This has resulted in even higher response rates and complete response rates of >50%. The combination of lenalidomide, bortezomib, and dexamethasone (RVD) gave a complete response/very good partial response rate of 77% and is adopted as a standard of care by many centers.[79]

Thalidomide

Early reports indicate that thalidomide and dexamethasone (TD) yields a response rate of 64% (similar to VAD), without compromising the ability to collect stem cells, but with a rate of deep vein thrombosis of 12%.[86] The Medical Research Council Myeloma IX trial compared cyclophosphamide–thalidomide–dexamethasone (CTD) with cyclophosphamide–VAD as induction before ASCT. The complete response rate was 20.3% after CTD and 11.7% after cyclophosphamide–VAD,[87] lower than other regimens cited above.

In summary, preferred initial regimens include bortezomib- and/or lenalidomide-based combinations, whereas thalidomide or doxorubicin is very infrequently used in current practice.

Patients Not Eligible for Autologous Stem Cell Transplantation

In patients who will not be undergoing a transplant often because of a combination of advanced age, comorbidities, and unfit health status,[11,88] there are various options available for initial therapy. Historically, most transplant-ineligible patients received melphalan and prednisone (MP), which produced partial remissions in approximately 55% of patients, with the occasional complete response.[89] San Miguel et al.[90] reported the results of a randomized trial of 682 patients randomized to receive either nine 6-week cycles of MP or the same chemotherapy with bortezomib. The addition of bortezomib increased the proportion of patients achieving complete response (30% and 4%, P < .001) and improved median duration of response (19.9 vs. 13.1 months), time to progression (24.0 vs. 16.6 months; P < .001), and the risk of death (hazard ratio 0.61 for the bortezomib group; P = .008).

The addition of thalidomide to melphalan and prednisone (MPT) also improves outcome compared with MP alone.[91,92] However, thromboses were more common with thalidomide with an incidence of 12% (vs. 2% in the MP group). The median progression-free survival was 21.8 months for MPT and 14.5 months for MP (P = .004).[92] A meta-analysis of MP versus MPT concluded that MPT increases response rates and overall survival but with increased toxicity such as thrombosis and somnolence.[93] In the FIRST randomized trial, lenalidomide and dexamethasone (LD) when used continuously (until disease progression) gave a better median PFS (25.5 months) when compared with MPT (median PFS 21.2 months, P < .001), and 4-year overall survival was also improved (LD regimen 59%, MPT regimen 51%, P = .02).[94] These results provide several options for the initial therapy of patients who will not proceed to ASCT, with preference for a lenalidomide-based regimen approach[94,95] and elimination of alkylator (melphalan) therapy altogether.[95] Geriatric assessment with a recognized scoring system is an important part of patient evaluation for those over the age of 65 and with comorbidities or physical and/or cognitive impairment, as those who are frail tolerate treatment less well and have a poorer prognosis.[96]

Autologous Stem Cell Transplantation

ASCT has become the standard of care for eligible patients, as it has been demonstrated in multiple trials to improve the likelihood of complete response, prolong disease-free survival, and extend overall survival.[11,79,97,98] ASCT is still important even with highly effective induction therapy consisting of RVD regimen, as shown in a recently completed phase III trial of comparing RVD (eight cycles) with RVD (three cycles) followed by ASCT and then two further cycles of RVD.[79] Treatment-related mortality rates are now <2%, and often the transplant can be performed entirely as an outpatient. Melphalan 200 mg/m^2 is the most commonly used conditioning regimen, although it may be reduced in elderly patients or patients with renal insufficiency.

Tandem Transplantation

Tandem or double transplantation refers to a planned second ASCT after the patient has recovered from the first. A phase III trial in France evaluated tandem transplant versus single ASCT and demonstrated superior overall survival in the tandem group[99]; however, when further analyzed, the patients who benefited most from the second transplant were those who did not achieve a 90% reduction in their disease after the first ASCT. Therefore, it may be more prudent to consider tandem transplantation only in patients whose response to the first ASCT is suboptimal.

Allogeneic Stem Cell Transplantation

Myeloablative stem cell transplant is perhaps the only current potential cure for patients with myeloma, as the graft is not contaminated with tumor cells and may produce a profound graft versus myeloma effect.[100] However, its use is very limited because of the lack of donors, age restriction, high treatment-related mortality, and graft versus host disease. Reduced intensity nonmyeloablative allogeneic transplant following ASCT has also been investigated as a means of inducing a graft versus myeloma effect. In one study of 102 patients undergoing nonmyeloablative transplant, 5-year overall survival and progression-free survival were 64% and 36%, respectively, although the 5-year rate of nonmyeloma mortality was 18%.[101]

Maintenance Therapy

Much investigation of late has been directed at the use of maintenance therapy post-ASCT to prolong remission and survival. Two large randomized trials used maintenance lenalidomide versus placebo, with prolongation of progression-free survival by approximately 20 months.[102,103] Overall survival was similar in the European trial,[102] whereas the US trial showed a statistically improved survival with lenalidomide maintenance (3-year survival 85% vs. 77% with placebo).[103] The use of maintenance therapy post-ASCT is now considered the standard of care, with the use of lenalidomide for a duration of 1 year.[79]

Relapse after Autologous Stem Cell Transplantation

The general approach to myeloma is to provide sequential therapies to patients, knowing each will not be curative but will prolong the period of disease control. The goal is to convert the disease into a chronic illness. Whereas there used to be very limited treatment options, the armamentarium

TABLE 85.7 TREATMENT OPTIONS FOR RELAPSED MULTIPLE MYELOMA

Conventional Therapy
Repeated courses of alkylator-based therapy (melphalan)
Cyclophosphamide (IV or PO) and steroids

Transplantation
Second autologous stem cell transplant

High-Dose Chemotherapy
DTPACE
High-dose cyclophosphamide

Novel Agents
Thalidomide
Proteasome inhibitors: bortezomib, carfilzomib
IMiDs: lenalidomide, pomalidomide
Monoclonal antibodies: elotuzumab, daratumumab
Immune check point drugs: pembrolizumab and others

Combination Conventional and Novel Agent
CyBorD (cyclophosphamide, bortezomib, dexamethasone)
CRD (cyclophosphamide, lenalidomide, dexamethasone)
Vel-Doxil (bortezomib, liposomal doxorubicin)

DTPACE, dexamethasone, thalidomide, cisplatin, doxorubicin, cyclophosphamide, and etoposide; IV, intravenous; PO, by mouth.

available has grown considerably over the past few years. This has contributed to a prolongation of the median survival of patients with myeloma. Patients will relapse after a median of 2 years after the first ASCT, and several options may be pursued for treatment (Table 85.7). The most commonly used agents are again the two key drugs in myeloma: bortezomib and lenalidomide. Both have been validated extensively in relapsed disease. Even with retreatment, these agents can confer prolonged progression-free and overall survival.

The most promising agents that are being added to this list are carfilzomib,[104] pomalidomide, elotuzumab, and daratumumab. Carfilzomib is an irreversible proteasome inhibitor with significant activity in relapsed myeloma. Pomalidomide is a novel IMiD, in the family of thalidomide and lenalidomide, that has also demonstrated efficacy in relapsed myeloma, even in patients refractory to both bortezomib and lenlidomide.[105,106] Elotuzumab and daratumumab are monoclonal antibodies targeting a glycoprotein SLAMF-7[107] and CD38,[108,109] respectively, both showing activity as single agents or in combination with lenalidomide and dexamethasone.

Supportive Care

A description of therapy of myeloma would not be complete without addressing the need to treat not only the disease itself but also the complications of this disease. Erythropoietic agents assist in the management of chemotherapy-induced anemia, leading to reduction of transfusions. Bisphosphonates are critical to the optimal therapy of bone disease and may even have an effect on overall survival in certain patients.[87,110]

Local RT for bony disease remains valuable in pain control and debulking disease. Patients often present with bony disease and anemia; both of these complications are treatable, allowing an improved quality of life. Newer surgical techniques such as vertebroplasty and kyphoplasty are also being used to improve back pain and spinal symptoms.[111]

RADIATION THERAPY OF MULTIPLE MYELOMA

Total Body Irradiation

Some high-dose chemotherapy protocols for multiple myeloma incorporate total body irradiation (TBI) into the conditioning regimen. Because of toxicity concerns (mucosal and hematologic) with TBI, many programs use chemotherapy alone, most commonly melphalan. A phase III French study (IFM [Intergroupe Francophone du Mye'lome] trial 9502) examined melphalan 200 mg/m^2 alone (M200) versus melphalan 140 mg/m^2 with TBI, 8 Gy in 4 fractions (M140/TBI),[112] and found that patients in the TBI-containing arm suffered more grade 3 or 4 mucosal toxicity, heavier transfusion requirement, and longer hospitalization stay. There was a higher toxic death rate in the M140/TBI arm (3.6% vs. 0% for the M200 arm). The event-free survival was no different between the two treatments, but the 45-month overall survival favored the M200 arm (M200: 65.8%; M140/TBI: 45.5%; $P = .05$). TBI is now rarely used in conditioning regimens for ASCT, unless it is part of a research clinical trial.

Hemibody Radiation

Diffuse bone pain involving wide areas of the skeleton can be effectively palliated by half-body radiation with single doses of 5 to 8 Gy,[113–115] although this is rarely used now. The bone marrow in the unirradiated half body serves as a stem cell reserve and will slowly repopulate the irradiated marrow after treatment. The dose for upper half body should not exceed 8 Gy because of lung tolerance.[116] The main toxicity is myelosuppression. The use of hemibody radiation must be carefully considered in patients heavily pretreated with chemotherapy. Growth factor support may be helpful, whereas transfusions of blood products should be given as needed. The sequential hemibody radiation technique has been used in phase II[117,118] and phase III trials as "systemic" treatment to control myeloma, in patients with or without skeletal pain. A phase III trial by the South West Oncology Group included newly diagnosed patients treated initially with chemotherapy, with complete responders randomized to sequential hemibody radiation (7.5 Gy in 5 fractions, upper hemibody, followed 6 weeks later by lower hemibody) or further chemotherapy.[119] Survival in this trial was significantly poorer with radiation compared with chemotherapy. At present, there is no standard role for sequential hemibody radiation as systemic treatment for myeloma outside of a clinical trial.

Local External Beam for Palliation

The most common use of RT in the management of plasma cell tumors is for palliative treatment of bony disease[113,120–124] and relief of compression of the spinal cord,[125–127] cranial nerves, or peripheral nerves. It has been estimated that approximately 40% of patients with multiple myeloma will require palliative radiation therapy for bone pain at some time during the course of their disease.[128] In practice, the actual proportion is lower than estimated, varying from 24% to 34%, leading investigators in Australia to suggest that this potentially useful modality of treatment has been underutilized, even taking into account the beneficial effect of bisphosphonates, particularly for the elderly.[128] Palliative RT to the spine reduces the incidence of future vertebral fractures or the appearance of new lesions.[129] However, the role of RT in preventing impending pathologic fracture is unclear. In general, lesions at high risk for pathologic fracture should be referred for surgical stabilization, and RT can be administered after surgery for control of residual disease at the local site. Similarly, surgical intervention (decompression with or without stabilization) is indicated in patients who have structural compromise because of vertebral disease, for example, a bone fragment displaced into the spinal canal, and/or vertebral instability. Usually surgery is performed first, with radiation therapy considered in the postoperative period usually 4 to 6 weeks after surgery to allow for adequate healing.

When RT is given for pain because of disease involving a long bone, a local field suffices. It is unnecessary to treat the entire bone.[130] Doses of 10 to 20 Gy (in 5 to 10 fractions) are effective, although the pain relief is often partial.[131] Leigh et al.[121] found a symptomatic response rate of 97% (complete pain relief in 26% and partial relief in 71%) after an average dose of 25 Gy given to 306 sites in 101 patients. There was no dose–response relationship above 10 Gy. Recurrence of symptoms requiring further treatment was seen in 6% of sites after a median of 16 months. Similar results are also reported by Matuschek et al., with complete pain relief in 31% and partial relief in 54%, with median RT dose of 25 Gy.[124]

It is not clear if pain relief is better if RT is given concurrently with chemotherapy. A study by Adamietz et al.[120] reported complete pain relief in 80% of patients receiving RT with chemotherapy, compared with 40% among those receiving RT alone. In contrast, Leigh et al.[121] found no significant difference in pain relief when RT was given with or without concurrent chemotherapy. With the use of novel agent–based chemotherapy given concurrently with RT, Shin et al.[132] reported no increase in toxicity in 31 patients.

For spinal cord compression, motor improvement is expected in approximately 50% of irradiated patients. A multicenter study (not restricted to myeloma patients) suggested that a longer fractionated regimen (30 Gy in 10 fractions or higher) was associated with better neurologic recovery than 20 Gy in 5 fractions or a single 8 Gy,[133] although another recent prospective randomized trial showed that 20 Gy in 5 fractions was equivalent to 30 Gy in 10 fractions in terms of 6-month functional outcome and local control.[134] With the availability of newer drugs, the advantage of radiation-sensitizing effects with drug–radiation combinations requires continued investigation, both in terms of enhancing local control[135] and possible toxicity. Bortezomib and spinal radiation given concurrently was reported to result in severe enteritis.[136,137] The use of bisphosphonates (e.g., pamidronate) has been shown to reduce skeletal complications and pain,[138] with a reduction of the use of RT from 50% to 34% in one study.[139]

Radioimmunotherapy Approaches

Bone-seeking radiopharmaceuticals targeting the bone marrow have been studied as an alternative to TBI. Typically, a β-emitting isotope is conjugated to a phosphonate complex, such as samarium-153-ethylene diamine tetramethylene phosphonate (^{153}Sm-EDTMP or Quadramet). The isotope also emits a γ-ray, permitting scanning to locate areas of uptake. This agent has been used for palliation of bone metastasis.[140] The feasibility of this approach in a small number of myeloma patients has been reported for stem cell transplantation.[141] Another bone-seeking pharmaceutical is holmium-166-DOTMP (^{166}Ho-1,4,7,10-tetraazacyclododecane-1,4,7,10-tetramethylene-phosphonic acid), with a higher energy β emission (maximum energy 1.85 MeV) than ^{153}Sm and a shorter $T_{1/2}$ of 26.8 hours.[142] It also has a γ emission (81 KeV) suitable for imaging. With the ability to deliver much higher doses to the bone marrow than TBI, in the range of 30 to 60 Gy, yet sparing the dose-limiting normal tissues such as lung, mucosa, and kidneys, the concept of targeted radiation therapy is tantalizing. However, there remains a problem of heterogeneity of uptake in the skeleton, and the dosimetric variation may be even larger at a microscopic level because of the limited range of the β particle. Whether this approach will have a more favorable therapeutic ratio than standard conditioning regimens in the transplant setting awaits larger-scale phase II and phase III trials.

RADIATION THERAPY TECHNIQUES

Radical Radiation Therapy for Local Control of Solitary Plasmacytoma

Accurate evaluation of tumor extent is an important feature of radical RT for SP. MRI is useful to evaluate the extent of disease both within and beyond bone. This is particularly true for the paranasal sinuses, where inflammatory changes may be difficult to distinguish from tumor on CT imaging. FDG-PET is also complimentary and if available can replace MRI for screening of occult systemic disease in the spine or elsewhere.

There are few data to support specific guidelines regarding RT treatment volumes. CT and MRI imaging should be used to determine gross tumor volumes. Clinical target volumes (CTV) should encompass probable routes of microscopic spread, recognizing that barriers to the extension of local disease will vary according to anatomic location, as will the morbidity of treating adjacent normal tissues (Fig. 85.2). For the spine, the historical practice of inclusion of two vertebral bodies above and below the grossly involved vertebra(e) should be abandoned. Three-dimensional planning should always be used (except for a small skin lesion that can be treated with superficial x-rays or high-energy electrons guided by clinical examination), and the "involved field" terminology is no longer preferred, rather the "involved site" concept should be adopted similar to the published guidelines for Hodgkin[143] and non-Hodgkin lymphomas.[144,145]

For RT of a lesion involving a long bone, although coverage of the entire involved bone has been recommended by some authors, a study of palliative RT to only the symptomatic area for multiple myeloma found that recurrence in the untreated portion of the involved bone was rare.[130] Similarly, no marginal recurrences were seen among 30 patients with SP treated with RT that encompassed only the tumor with a margin.[146] Prophylactic regional nodal coverage is not necessary in SP of bone as multiple studies have found a very low risk of regional nodal failure after involved site radiation without intentional coverage of adjacent nodes (i.e., 0% to 4%).[17,51,146] For EMP, nodal involvement at presentation is observed in 10% to 20%, and occasional nodal failure in the literature led to a common practice of extending the RT coverage to the draining lymph node region.[18] Some authors specifically recommend this practice if the primary disease involves a lymphatic structure (e.g., lymph nodes or Waldeyer ring).[18,38,62] However, this is controversial as some series reported a low incidence of regional nodal failure without routine prophylactic nodal irradiation,[39,42,52,63,71] leading to variation in practices between centers.[16] After reviewing their own series of 26 patients with EMP and contrasting the results with the literature, Strojan et al.[16] concluded that prophylactic nodal radiation is probably unnecessary. With the advent of more routine use of MRI and FDG-PET, elective nodal coverage likely has little or no benefit, unless the clinical scenario is persuasive such as a very bulky primary disease in proximity to the drainage lymph node station.

In determining the CTV, using the GTV plus a margin of 1 to 3 cm is reasonable (depending on the site) respecting anatomic boundaries. A GTV to CTV expansion of 0.5 to 1 cm in the axial plane may be appropriate for covering potential microscopic extension in soft tissues, for example, in the head and neck area. However for a long bone site, for example the femur, the proximal and distant expansion should be increased to 2 to 3 cm. Planning target volumes (PTV) should account for day-to-day setup variation and will typically add 5 to 10 mm around CTV volumes depending on the immobilization technique employed (Fig. 85.2). Although parallel-opposed fields are commonly adequate to encompass disease without significant irradiation of normal tissues, CT-based planning and the

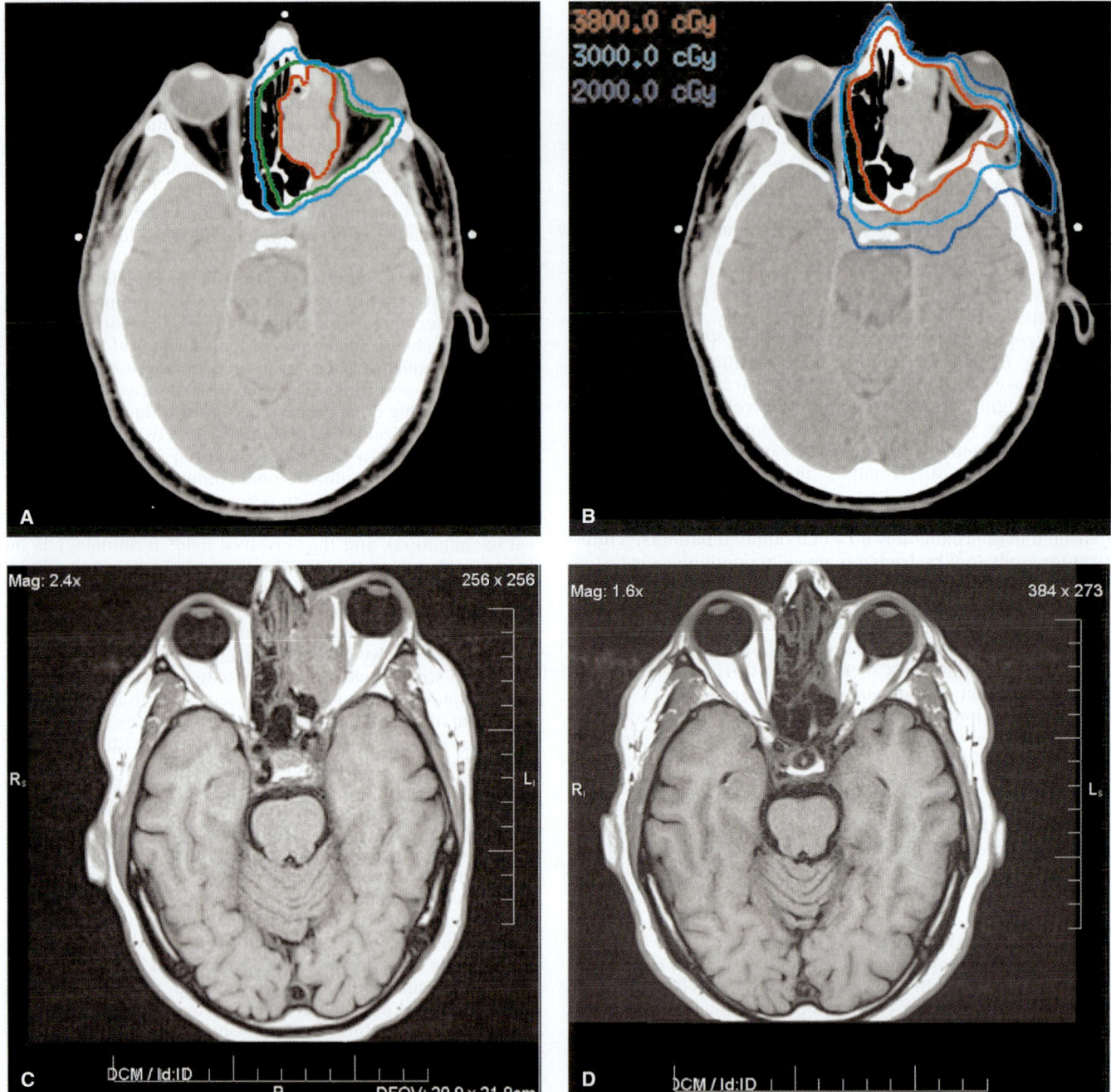

FIGURE 85.2. Radiation treatment plan for a solitary plasmacytoma of the left orbit **(A)**. The entire orbit was contoured as the clinical target volume and received 36 Gy; the gross tumor volume received a subsequent boost to a total of 40 Gy **(B)**. The initial mass on magnetic resonance imaging resolved 6 months after treatment **(C,D)**.

use of conformal techniques, including intensity-modulated radiation therapy, should be employed when needed to treat the PTV adjacent to critical structures. This can be particularly important in extramedullary disease involving the paranasal sinuses, where avoidance of the optic structures and salivary glands is desirable.

Radiation Therapy Dose

Studies evaluating RT dose–response in plasmacytoma have produced differing results. Most studies have found response rates >85% among patients treated with ≥35 Gy; some investigators have found better local control following doses ≥45 Gy,[22,56] whereas others have found no indication

of improved outcome with higher doses.[15,146] Based on a dose–response analysis of 81 patients by Mendenhall et al.[147] reported in 1980, a minimum dose of 40 Gy was recommended, including osseous and extramedullary lesions. A total dose of 40 Gy and above resulted in a local failure rate of 6% versus 31% for lower doses. Therefore, the usual practice is to administer a dose of 40 to 45 Gy or even higher for bulky tumors. However, in the largest of these studies (*n* = 258), there was no evidence of improved local control with RT doses ranging from 30 to 50 Gy, including a subset of patients with tumors >4 cm.[15] In fact, there was a worse local control rate for the group receiving total dose ≥50 Gy although not statistically significant.[15] It should be noted, however, that retrospective studies of dose–response are typically confounded by selection bias, as higher doses are prescribed to larger tumors with worse prognosis. Several studies have demonstrated durable local control in >85% of tumors <5 cm with 35 to 40 Gy, and there is little evidence that higher doses are necessary for small tumors, regardless of bone or EMP locations. In contrast, plasmacytomas >5 cm have worse local control,[15,17,39] and doses of 45 to 50 Gy are recommended in these bulkier tumors, which also tend to be EMPs. However, one should be aware that the quality of evidence supporting the use of higher RT doses is limited, and local failures are occasionally observed even after doses of 50 Gy or higher.[15,17,42]

Assessment of Response and Follow-Up

Reimaging is of greatest value in the response assessment of EMP. Repeat imaging, preferably with MRI and/or FDG-PET scan, should be done approximately 6 to 8 weeks following completion of treatment. It is rare to have symptoms suggestive of local progression that necessitate reimaging prior to this. It is common for a residual soft tissue abnormality to persist on follow-up imaging, and periodic reimaging may be required every 4 to 6 months until any residual mass disappears or remains stable on consecutive scans. It is generally not beneficial to continue to reimage a stable abnormality.

Bone destruction caused by tumor can produce persistent abnormalities on imaging following RT for painful bone metastases or isolated plasmacytoma of bone. Consequently, repeat imaging is of less value in establishing response in such cases.

With a high risk of recurrence of disease as multiple myeloma, the occurrence of new bone pain requires further investigations, including imaging as appropriate. Repeat measurement of the M protein often detects the onset of systemic disease prior to the development of symptoms and can be used as an indicator of disease burden.[20,148] Complete blood counts should be taken periodically to evaluate bone marrow function. A team of international investigators have developed recommendations for uniform response criteria for assessing the treatment of multiple myeloma.[149]

The RT doses used for myeloma are rarely associated with significant delayed side effects. Treatment of significant volumes of the parotid or submandibular glands may result in prolonged xerostomia and should be avoided. As noted previously, TBI has been associated with significant toxicity and is not widely used. Evaluation of renal function should be undertaken prior to initiating RT, which may include the kidneys, and blood counts should be evaluated prior to treating a large volume of bone marrow in the spine or pelvis. Reirradiation of vertebral metastases is possible, but careful evaluation of all prior RT records is required to ensure that the tolerance of the spinal cord is not exceeded.

REFERENCES

1. Morton LM, Wang SS, Devesa SS, et al. Lymphoma incidence patterns by WHO subtype in the United States, 1992-2001. *Blood* 2006;107(1):265–276.
2. Surveillance Epidemiology and End Results. *Cancer Facts and Figures.* Available at: https://seercancergov/statfacts/html/mulmyhtml.
3. American Cancer Society. *Cancer Facts and Figures.* 2018. https://www.cancer.org/research/cancer-facts-statistics.html.
4. Greipp PR, San Miguel J, Durie BG, et al. International staging system for multiple myeloma. *J Clin Oncol* 2005;23(15):3412–3420.
5. Kyle RA, Gertz MA, Witzig TE, et al. Review of 1027 patients with newly diagnosed multiple myeloma. *Mayo Clin Proc* 2003;78(1):21–33.
6. Bergsagel DE, Wong O, Bergsagel PL, et al. Benzene and multiple myeloma: appraisal of the scientific evidence. *Blood* 1999;94(4):1174–1182.
7. Correa A, Jackson L, Mohan A, et al. Use of hair dyes, hematopoietic neoplasms, and lymphomas: a literature review. II. Lymphomas and multiple myeloma. *Cancer Invest* 2000;18(5):467–479.
8. Kyle RA, Therneau TM, Rajkumar SV, et al. A long-term study of prognosis in monoclonal gammopathy of undetermined significance. *N Engl J Med* 2002;346(8):564–569.
9. Landgren O, Kyle RA, Pfeiffer RM, et al. Monoclonal gammopathy of undetermined significance (MGUS) consistently precedes multiple myeloma: a prospective study. *Blood* 2009;113(22):5412–5417.
10. Weiss BM, Abadie J, Verma P, et al. A monoclonal gammopathy precedes multiple myeloma in most patients. *Blood* 2009;113(22):5418–5422.
11. Palumbo A, Anderson K. Multiple myeloma. *N Engl J Med* 2011;364(11):1046–1060.
12. Kyle RA, Therneau TM, Rajkumar SV, et al. Prevalence of monoclonal gammopathy of undetermined significance. *N Engl J Med* 2006;354(13):1362–1369.
13. Rajkumar SV, Dimopoulos MA, Palumbo A, et al. International Myeloma Working Group updated criteria for the diagnosis of multiple myeloma. *Lancet Oncol* 2014;15(12):e538–e548.
14. Thumallapally N, Meshref A, Mousa M, et al. Solitary plasmacytoma: population-based analysis of survival trends and effect of various treatment modalities in the USA. *BMC Cancer* 2017;17(1):13.
15. Ozsahin M, Tsang RW, Poortmans P, et al. Outcomes and patterns of failure in solitary plasmacytoma: a multicenter Rare Cancer Network study of 258 patients. *Int J Radiat Oncol Biol Phys* 2006;64(1):210–217.
16. Strojan P, Soba E, Lamovec J, et al. Extramedullary plasmacytoma: clinical and histopathologic study. *Int J Radiat Oncol Biol Phys* 2002;53(3):692–701.
17. Tsang RW, Gospodarowicz MK, Pintilie M, et al. Solitary plasmacytoma treated with radiotherapy: impact of tumor size on outcome. *Int J Radiat Oncol Biol Phys* 2001;50(1):113–120.
18. Soutar R, Lucraft H, Jackson G, et al. Guidelines on the diagnosis and management of solitary plasmacytoma of bone and solitary extramedullary plasmacytoma. *Br J Haematol* 2004;124(6):717–726.
19. Durie BG, Kyle RA, Belch A, et al. Myeloma management guidelines: a consensus report from the Scientific Advisors of the International Myeloma Foundation. *Hematol J* 2003;4(6):379–398.
20. Wilder RB, Ha CS, Cox JD, et al. Persistence of myeloma protein for more than one year after radiotherapy is an adverse prognostic factor in solitary plasmacytoma of bone. *Cancer* 2002;94(5):1532–1537.
21. Durie BG, Salmon SE. A clinical staging system for multiple myeloma. Correlation of measured myeloma cell mass with presenting clinical features, response to treatment, and survival. *Cancer* 1975;36(3):842–854.
22. Tournier-Rangeard L, Lapeyre M, Graff-Caillaud P, et al. Radiotherapy for solitary extramedullary plasmacytoma in the head-and-neck region: a dose greater than 45 Gy to the target volume improves the local control. *Int J Radiat Oncol Biol Phys* 2006;64(4):1013–1017.
23. Alexiou C, Kau RJ, Dietzfelbinger H, et al. Extramedullary plasmacytoma: tumor occurrence and therapeutic concepts. *Cancer.* 1999;85(11):2305–2314.
24. Hussong JW, Perkins SL, Schnitzer B, et al. Extramedullary plasmacytoma. A form of marginal zone cell lymphoma? *Am J Clin Pathol* 1999;111(1):111–116.
25. Dispenzieri A. POEMS syndrome: 2017 Update on diagnosis, risk stratification, and management. *Am J Hematol* 2017;92(8):814–829.
26. Kourelis TV, Buadi FK, Kumar SK, et al. Long-term outcome of patients with POEMS syndrome: an update of the Mayo Clinic experience. *Am J Hematol* 2016;91(6):585–589.
27. Fernandez de Larrea C, Kyle RA, Durie BG, et al. Plasma cell leukemia: consensus statement on diagnostic requirements, response criteria and treatment recommendations by the International Myeloma Working Group. *Leukemia* 2013;27(4):780–791.
28. Jimenez-Zepeda VH, Reece DE, Trudel S, et al. Lenalidomide (Revlimid), bortezomib (Velcade) and dexamethasone for the treatment of secondary plasma cell leukemia. *Leuk Lymphoma* 2015;56(1):232–235.
29. Tiedemann RE, Gonzalez-Paz N, Kyle RA, et al. Genetic aberrations and survival in plasma cell leukemia. *Leukemia* 2008;22(5):1044–1052.
30. Dimopoulos M, Kyle R, Fermand JP, et al. Consensus recommendations for standard investigative workup: report of the International Myeloma Workshop Consensus Panel 3. *Blood* 2011;117(18):4701–4705.
31. Dimopoulos MA, Hillengass J, Usmani S, et al. Role of magnetic resonance imaging in the management of patients with multiple myeloma: a consensus statement. *J Clin Oncol* 2015;33(6):657–664.
32. Feinstein AR, Sosin DM, Wells CK. The Will Rogers phenomenon. Stage migration and new diagnostic techniques as a source of misleading statistics for survival in cancer. *N Engl J Med* 1985;312(25):1604–1608.
33. Even-Sapir E, Mishani E, Flusser G, et al. 18F-Fluoride positron emission tomography and positron emission tomography/computed tomography. *Semin Nucl Med* 2007;37(6):462–469.
34. Schirrmeister H, Buck AK, Bergmann L, et al. Positron emission tomography (PET) for staging of solitary plasmacytoma. *Cancer Biother Radiopharm* 2003;18(5):841–845.
35. Kim PJ, Hicks RJ, Wirth A, et al. Impact of 18F-fluorodeoxyglucose positron emission tomography before and after definitive radiation therapy in patients with apparently solitary plasmacytoma. *Int J Radiat Oncol Biol Phys* 2009;74(3):740–746.
36. Palumbo A, Avet-Loiseau H, Oliva S, et al. Revised international staging system for multiple myeloma: a report from International Myeloma Working Group. *J Clin Oncol* 2015;33(26):2863–2869.
37. Holland J, Trenkner DA, Wasserman TH, et al. Plasmacytoma. Treatment results and conversion to myeloma. *Cancer* 1992;69(6):1513–1517.
38. Mayr NA, Wen BC, Hussey DH, et al. The role of radiation therapy in the treatment of solitary plasmacytomas. *Radiother Oncol* 1990;17(4):293–303.

39. Zhu Q, Zou X, You R, et al. Establishment of an innovative staging system for extramedullary plasmacytoma. *BMC Cancer* 2016;16(1):777.

40. Bataille R, Sany J. Solitary myeloma: clinical and prognostic features of a review of 114 cases. *Cancer* 1981;48(3):845–851.

41. Chak LY, Cox RS, Bostwick DG, et al. Solitary plasmacytoma of bone: treatment, progression, and survival. *J Clin Oncol* 1987;5(11):1811–1815.

42. Reed V, Shah J, Medeiros LJ, et al. Solitary plasmacytoma: outcome and prognostic factors after definitive radiation therapy. *Cancer* 2011;117(19):4468–4474.

43. Jawad MU, Scully SP. Skeletal plasmacytoma: progression of disease and impact of local treatment; an analysis of SEER database. *J Hematol Oncol* 2009;2:41.

44. Bolek TW, Marcus RB, Mendenhall NP. Solitary plasmacytoma of bone and soft tissue. *Int J Radiat Oncol Biol Phys* 1996;36(2):329–333.

45. Shih LY, Dunn P, Leung WM, et al. Localised plasmacytomas in Taiwan: comparison between extramedullary plasmacytoma and solitary plasmacytoma of bone. *Br J Cancer* 1995;71(1):128–133.

46. Galieni P, Cavo M, Avvisati G, et al. Solitary plasmacytoma of bone and extramedullary plasmacytoma: two different entities? *Ann Oncol* 1995;6(7):687–691.

47. Mariette X, Zagdanski AM, Guermazi A, et al. Prognostic value of vertebral lesions detected by magnetic resonance imaging in patients with stage I multiple myeloma. *Br J Haematol* 1999;104(4):723–729.

48. Moulopoulos LA, Dimopoulos MA, Smith TL, et al. Prognostic significance of magnetic resonance imaging in patients with asymptomatic multiple myeloma. *J Clin Oncol* 1995;13(1):251–256.

49. Van de Berg BC, Lecouvet FE, Michaux L, et al. Stage I multiple myeloma: value of MR imaging of the bone marrow in the determination of prognosis. *Radiology* 1996;201(1):243–246.

50. Jackson A, Scarffe JH. Prognostic significance of osteopenia and immunoparesis at presentation in patients with solitary myeloma of bone. *Eur J Cancer* 1990;26(3):363–371.

51. Liebross RH, Ha CS, Cox JD, et al. Solitary bone plasmacytoma: outcome and prognostic factors following radiotherapy. *Int J Radiat Oncol Biol Phys* 1998;41(5):1063–1067.

52. Susnerwala SS, Shanks JH, Banerjee SS, et al. Extramedullary plasmacytoma of the head and neck region: clinicopathological correlation in 25 cases. *Br J Cancer* 1997;75(6):921–927.

53. Kumar S, Fonseca R, Dispenzieri A, et al. Prognostic value of angiogenesis in solitary bone plasmacytoma. *Blood* 2003;101(5):1715–1717.

54. Colomo L, Loong F, Rives S, et al. Diffuse large B-cell lymphomas with plasmablastic differentiation represent a heterogeneous group of disease entities. *Am J Surg Pathol* 2004;28(6):736–747.

55. Folk GS, Abbondanzo SL, Childers EL, et al. Plasmablastic lymphoma: a clinicopathologic correlation. *Ann Diagn Pathol* 2006;10(1):8–12.

56. Frassica DA, Frassica FJ, Schray MF, et al. Solitary plasmacytoma of bone: Mayo Clinic experience. *Int J Radiat Oncol Biol Phys* 1989;16(1):43–48.

57. Kilciksiz S, Celik OK, Pak Y, et al. Clinical and prognostic features of plasmacytomas: a multicenter study of Turkish Oncology Group-Sarcoma Working Party. *Am J Hematol* 2008;83(9):702–707.

58. Finsinger P, Grammatico S, Chisini M, et al. Clinical features and prognostic factors in solitary plasmacytoma. *Br J Haematol* 2016;172(4):554–560.

59. Moulopoulos LA, Dimopoulos MA, Weber D, et al. Magnetic resonance imaging in the staging of solitary plasmacytoma of bone. *J Clin Oncol* 1993;11(7):1311–1315.

60. Chargari C, Vennarini S, Servois V, et al. Place of modern imaging modalities for solitary plasmacytoma: toward improved primary staging and treatment monitoring. *Crit Rev Oncol Hematol* 2012;82(2):150–158.

61. Dimopoulos MA, Goldstein J, Fuller L, et al. Curability of solitary bone plasmacytoma. *J Clin Oncol* 1992;10(4):587–590.

62. Knowling MA, Harwood AR, Bergsagel DE. Comparison of extramedullary plasmacytomas with solitary and multiple plasma cell tumors of bone. *J Clin Oncol* 1983;1(4):255–262.

63. Sasaki R, Yasuda K, Abe E, et al. Multi-institutional analysis of solitary extramedullary plasmacytoma of the head and neck treated with curative radiotherapy. *Int J Radiat Oncol Biol Phys* 2012;82(2):626–634.

64. Aviles A, Huerta-Guzman J, Delgado S, et al. Improved outcome in solitary bone plasmacytomata with combined therapy. *Hematol Oncol* 1996;14(3):111–117.

65. Wiazzane N, Chargari C, Plancher C, et al. Helical tomotherapy and systemic targeted therapies in solitary plasmacytoma: Pilot study. *World J Radiol* 2013;5(6):248–252.

66. Marchand V, Decaudin D, Servois V, et al. Concurrent radiation therapy and lenalidomide in myeloma patient. *Radiother Oncol* 2008;87(1):152–153.

67. Tsang DS, Le LW, Kukreti V, et al. Treatment and outcomes for primary cutaneous extramedullary plasmacytoma: a case series. *Curr Oncol* 2016;23(6):e630–e646.

68. Kapadia SB, Desai U, Cheng VS. Extramedullary plasmacytoma of the head and neck. *Medicine* 1982;61:317–329.

69. Brinch L, Hannisdal E, Abrahamsen AF, et al. Extramedullary plasmacytomas and solitary myeloma cell tumours of bone. *Eur J Haematol* 1990;44:131–134.

70. Soesan M, Paccagnella A, Chiarion-Sileni V, et al. Extramedullary plasmacytoma: Clinical behaviour and response to treatment. *Ann Oncol* 1992;3:51–57.

71. Liebross RH, Ha CS, Cox JD, et al. Clinical course of solitary extramedullary plasmacytoma. *Radiother Oncol* 1999;52(3):245–249.

72. Galieni P, Cavo M, Pulsoni A, et al. Clinical outcome of extramedullary plasmacytoma. *Haematologica* 2000;85(1):47–51.

73. Chao MW, Gibbs P, Wirth A, et al. Radiotherapy in the management of solitary extramedullary plasmacytoma. *Intern Med J* 2005;35(4):211–215.

74. Bachar G, Goldstein D, Brown D, et al. Solitary extramedullary plasmacytoma of the head and neck—long-term outcome analysis of 68 cases. *Head Neck* 2008;30(8):1012–1019.

75. Creach KM, Foote RL, Neben-Wittich MA, et al. Radiotherapy for extramedullary plasmacytoma of the head and neck. *Int J Radiat Oncol Biol Phys* 2009;73(3):789–794.

76. Goldschmidt H, Hegenbart U, Wallmeier M, et al. Factors influencing collection of peripheral blood progenitor cells following high-dose cyclophosphamide and granulocyte colony-stimulating factor in patients with multiple myeloma. *Br J Haematol* 1997;98(3):736–744.

77. Alexanian R, Barlogie B, Tucker S. VAD-based regimens as primary treatment for multiple myeloma. *Am J Hematol* 1990;33:86–89.

78. Samson D, Gaminara E, Newland A, et al. Infusion of vincristine and doxorubicin with oral dexamethasone as first-line therapy for multiple myeloma. *Lancet* 1989;2(8668):882–885.

79. Attal M, Lauwers-Cances V, Hulin C, et al. Lenalidomide, bortezomib, and dexamethasone with transplantation for myeloma. *N Engl J Med* 2017;376(14):1311–1320.

80. Harousseau JL, Attal M, Avet-Loiseau H, et al. Bortezomib plus dexamethasone is superior to vincristine plus doxorubicin plus dexamethasone as induction treatment prior to autologous stem-cell transplantation in newly diagnosed multiple myeloma: results of the IFM 2005-01 phase III trial. *J Clin Oncol* 2010;28(30):4621–4629.

81. Richardson P, Jagannath S, Hussein M, et al. Safety and efficacy of single-agent lenalidomide in patients with relapsed and refractory multiple myeloma. *Blood* 2009;114(4):772–778.

82. Reeder CB, Reece DE, Kukreti V, et al. Once- versus twice-weekly bortezomib induction therapy with CyBorD in newly diagnosed multiple myeloma. *Blood* 2010;115(16):3416–3417.

83. Moreau P, Pylypenko H, Grosicki S, et al. Subcutaneous versus intravenous administration of bortezomib in patients with relapsed multiple myeloma: a randomised, phase 3, non-inferiority study. *Lancet Oncol* 2011;12(5):431–440.

84. Rajkumar SV, Jacobus S, Callander NS, et al. Lenalidomide plus high-dose dexamethasone versus lenalidomide plus low-dose dexamethasone as initial therapy for newly diagnosed multiple myeloma: an open-label randomised controlled trial. *Lancet Oncol* 2010;11(1):29–37.

85. Richardson PG, Weller E, Lonial S, et al. Lenalidomide, bortezomib, and dexamethasone combination therapy in patients with newly diagnosed multiple myeloma. *Blood* 2010;116(5):679–686.

86. Rajkumar SV, Hayman S, Gertz MA, et al. Combination therapy with thalidomide plus dexamethasone for newly diagnosed myeloma. *J Clin Oncol* 2002;20(21):4319–4323.

87. Morgan GJ, Davies FE, Gregory WM, et al. First-line treatment with zoledronic acid as compared with clodronic acid in multiple myeloma (MRC Myeloma IX): a randomised controlled trial. *Lancet* 2010;376(9757):1989–1999.

88. Palumbo A, Rajkumar SV, San Miguel JF, et al. International Myeloma Working Group consensus statement for the management, treatment, and supportive care of patients with myeloma not eligible for standard autologous stem-cell transplantation. *J Clin Oncol* 2014;32(6):587–600.

89. Rajkumar SV, Gertz MA, Kyle RA, et al.; Mayo Clinic Myeloma, Amyloid, and Dysproteinemia Group Current therapy for multiple myeloma. *Mayo Clin Proc* 2002;77(8):813–822.

90. San Miguel JF, Schlag R, Khuageva NK, et al. Bortezomib plus melphalan and prednisone for initial treatment of multiple myeloma. *N Engl J Med* 2008;359(9):906–917.

91. Palumbo A, Bringhen S, Caravita T, et al. Oral melphalan and prednisone chemotherapy plus thalidomide compared with melphalan and prednisone alone in elderly patients with multiple myeloma: randomised controlled trial. *Lancet* 2006;367(9513):825–831.

92. Palumbo A, Bringhen S, Liberati AM, et al. Oral melphalan, prednisone, and thalidomide in elderly patients with multiple myeloma: updated results of a randomized controlled trial. *Blood* 2008;112(8):3107–3114.

93. Fayers PM, Palumbo A, Hulin C, et al. Thalidomide for previously untreated elderly patients with multiple myeloma: meta-analysis of 1685 individual patient data from 6 randomized clinical trials. *Blood* 2011;118(5):1239–1247.

94. Benboubker L, Dimopoulos MA, Dispenzieri A, et al. Lenalidomide and dexamethasone in transplant-ineligible patients with myeloma. *N Engl J Med* 2014;371(10):906–917.

95. Weisel K, Doyen C, Dimopoulos M, et al. A systematic literature review and network meta-analysis of treatments for patients with untreated multiple myeloma not eligible for stem cell transplantation. *Leuk Lymphoma* 2017;58(1):153–161.

96. Palumbo A, Bringhen S, Mateos MV, et al. Geriatric assessment predicts survival and toxicities in elderly myeloma patients: an International Myeloma Working Group report. *Blood* 2015;125(13):2068–2074.

97. Attal M, Harousseau JL, Stoppa AM, et al. A prospective, randomized trial of autologous bone marrow transplantation and chemotherapy in multiple myeloma. *N Engl J Med* 1996;335(2):91–97.

98. Kumar A, Loughran T, Alsina M, et al. Management of multiple myeloma: a systematic review and critical appraisal of published studies. *Lancet Oncol* 2003;4(5):293–304.

99. Attal M, Harousseau JL, Facon T, et al. Single versus double autologous stem-cell transplantation for multiple myeloma. *N Engl J Med* 2003;349(26):2495–2502.

100. Mehta J, Singhal S. Graft-versus-myeloma. *Bone Marrow Transplant* 1998;22(9):835–843.

101. Rotta M, Storer BE, Sahebi F, et al. Long-term outcome of patients with multiple myeloma after autologous hematopoietic cell transplantation and nonmyeloablative allografting. *Blood* 2009;113(14):3383–3391.

102. Attal M, Lauwers-Cances V, Marit G, et al. Lenalidomide maintenance after stem-cell transplantation for multiple myeloma. *N Engl J Med* 2012;366(19):1782–1791.

103. McCarthy PL, Owzar K, Hofmeister CC, et al. Lenalidomide after stem-cell transplantation for multiple myeloma. *N Engl J Med* 2012;366(19): 1770–1781.

104. Hari P, Mateos MV, Abonour R, et al. Efficacy and safety of carfilzomib regimens in multiple myeloma patients relapsing after autologous stem cell transplant: ASPIRE and ENDEAVOR outcomes. *Leukemia* 2017;31(12): 2630–2641.

105. Lacy MQ, Hayman SR, Gertz MA, et al. Pomalidomide (CC4047) plus low-dose dexamethasone as therapy for relapsed multiple myeloma. *J Clin Oncol* 2009;27(30):5008–5014.

106. Richardson PG, Siegel DS, Vij R, et al. Pomalidomide alone or in combination with low-dose dexamethasone in relapsed and refractory multiple myeloma: a randomized phase 2 study. *Blood* 2014;123(12):1826–1832.

107. Lonial S, Dimopoulos M, Palumbo A, et al. Elotuzumab therapy for relapsed or refractory multiple myeloma. *N Engl J Med* 2015;373(7):621–631.

108. Laubach JP, Paba Prada CE, Richardson PG, et al. Daratumumab, elotuzumab, and the development of therapeutic monoclonal antibodies in multiple myeloma. *Clin Pharmacol Ther* 2017;101(1):81–88.

109. Lokhorst HM, Plesner T, Laubach JP, et al. Targeting CD38 with daratumumab monotherapy in multiple myeloma. *N Engl J Med* 2015;373(13): 1207–1219.

110. Berenson JR, Hillner BE, Kyle RA, et al. American Society of Clinical Oncology clinical practice guidelines: the role of bisphosphonates in multiple myeloma. *J Clin Oncol* 2002;20(17):3719–3736.

111. Anselmetti GC, Manca A, Montemurro F, et al. Percutaneous vertebroplasty in multiple myeloma: prospective long-term follow-up in 106 consecutive patients. *Cardiovasc Intervent Radiol* 2012;35(1):139–145.

112. Moreau P, Facon T, Attal M, et al. Comparison of 200 mg/m(2) melphalan and 8 Gy total body irradiation plus 140 mg/m(2) melphalan as conditioning regimens for peripheral blood stem cell transplantation in patients with newly diagnosed multiple myeloma: final analysis of the Intergroupe Francophone du Myelome 9502 randomized trial. *Blood* 2002;99(3):731–735.

113. Bosch A, Frias Z. Radiotherapy in the treatment of multiple myeloma. *Int J Radiat Oncol Biol Phys* 1988;15(6):1363–1369.

114. McSweeney EN, Tobias JS, Blackman G, et al. Double hemibody irradiation (DHBI) in the management of relapsed and primary chemoresistant multiple myeloma. *Clin Oncol* 1993;5(6):378–383.

115. Tobias JS, Richards JD, Blackman GM, et al. Hemibody irradiation in multiple myeloma. *Radiother Oncol* 1985;3(1):11–16.

116. van Dyk J, Keane TJ, Kan S, et al. Radiation pneumonitis following large single dose irradiation: a re-evaluation based on absolute dose to lung. *Int J Radiat Oncol Biol Phys* 1981;7:461–467.

117. Rowland CG, Garrett MJ, Crowley FA. Half body radiation in plasma cell myeloma. *Clin Radiol* 1983;34(5):507–510.

118. Singer CR, Tobias JS, Giles F, et al. Hemibody irradiation. An effective second-line therapy in drug-resistance multiple myeloma. *Cancer* 1989;63(12): 2446–2451.

119. Salmon SE, Tesh D, Crowley J, et al. Chemotherapy is superior to sequential hemibody irradiation for remission consolidation in multiple myeloma: a Southwest Oncology Group study. *J Clin Oncol* 1990;8(9):1575–1584.

120. Adamietz IA, Schober C, Schulte RW, et al. Palliative radiotherapy in plasma cell myeloma. *Radiother Oncol* 1991;20(2):111–116.

121. Leigh BR, Kurtts TA, Mack CF, et al. Radiation therapy for the palliation of multiple myeloma. *Int J Radiat Oncol Biol Phys* 1993;25(5):801–804.

122. Balducci M, Chiesa S, Manfrida S, et al. Impact of radiotherapy on pain relief and recalcification in plasma cell neoplasms: long-term experience. *Strahlenther Onkol* 2011;187(2):114–119.

123. Terpos E, Morgan G, Dimopoulos MA, et al. International Myeloma Working Group recommendations for the treatment of multiple myeloma-related bone disease. *J Clin Oncol* 2013;31(18):2347–2357.

124. Matuschek C, Ochtrop TA, Bolke E, et al. Effects of Radiotherapy in the treatment of multiple myeloma: a retrospective analysis of a Single Institution. *Radiat Oncol* 2015;10:71.

125. Rades D, Conde-Moreno AJ, Cacicedo J, et al. Excellent outcomes after radiotherapy alone for malignant spinal cord compression from myeloma. *Radiol Oncol* 2016;50(3):337–340.

126. Rades D, Douglas S, Veninga T, et al. Prognostic factors for local control and survival in patients with spinal cord compression from myeloma. *Strahlenther Onkol* 2012;188(7):628–631.

127. Wallington M, Mendis S, Premawardhana U, et al. Local control and survival in spinal cord compression from lymphoma and myeloma. *Radiother Oncol* 1997;42(1):43–47.

128. Featherstone C, Delaney G, Jacob S, et al. Estimating the optimal utilization rates of radiotherapy for hematologic malignancies from a review of the evidence: part II-leukemia and myeloma. *Cancer* 2005;103(2):393–401.

129. Lecouvet F, Richard F, Vande Berg B, et al. Long-term effects of localized spinal radiation therapy on vertebral fractures and focal lesions appearance in patients with multiple myeloma. *Br J Haematol* 1997;96(4):743–745.

130. Catell D, Kogen Z, Donahue B, et al. Multiple myeloma of an extremity: must the entire bone be treated? *Int J Radiat Oncol Biol Phys* 1998;40(1): 117–119.

131. Mill WB, Griffith R. The role of radiation therapy in the management of plasma cell tumors. *Cancer* 1980;45(4):647–652.

132. Shin SM, Chouake RJ, Sanfilippo NJ, et al. Feasibility and efficacy of local radiotherapy with concurrent novel agents in patients with multiple myeloma. *Clin Lymphoma Myeloma Leuk* 2014;14(6):480–484.

133. Rades D, Stalpers LJ, Veninga T, et al. Evaluation of five radiation schedules and prognostic factors for metastatic spinal cord compression. *J Clin Oncol* 2005;23(15):3366–3375.

134. Rades D, Segedin B, Conde-Moreno AJ, et al. Radiotherapy with 4 Gy x 5 Versus 3 Gy x 10 for metastatic epidural spinal cord compression: final results of the SCORE-2 trial (ARO 2009/01). *J Clin Oncol* 2016;34(6):597–602.

135. Goel A, Dispenzieri A, Greipp PR, et al. PS-341-mediated selective targeting of multiple myeloma cells by synergistic increase in ionizing radiation-induced apoptosis. *Exp Hematol* 2005;33(7):784–795.

136. Berges O, Decaudin D, Servois V, et al. Concurrent radiation therapy and bortezomib in myeloma patient. *Radiother Oncol* 2008;86(2):290–292.

137. Mohiuddin MM, Harmon DC, Delaney TF. Severe acute enteritis in a multiple myeloma patient receiving bortezomib and spinal radiotherapy: case report. *J Chemother* 2005;17(3):343–346.

138. Berenson JR, Lichtenstein A, Porter L, et al. Efficacy of pamidronate in reducing skeletal events in patients with advanced multiple myeloma. Myeloma Aredia Study Group. *N Engl J Med* 1996;334(8):488–493.

139. Berenson JR, Lichtenstein A, Porter L, et al. Long-term pamidronate treatment of advanced multiple myeloma patients reduces skeletal events. Myeloma Aredia Study Group. *J Clin Oncol* 1998;16(2):593–602.

140. Anderson PM, Wiseman GA, Dispenzieri A, et al. High-dose samarium-153 ethylene diamine tetramethylene phosphonate: low toxicity of skeletal irradiation in patients with osteosarcoma and bone metastases. *J Clin Oncol* 2002;20(1):189–196.

141. Dispenzieri A, Wiseman GA, Lacy MQ, et al. A Phase II study of (153)Sm-EDTMP and high-dose melphalan as a peripheral blood stem cell conditioning regimen in patients with multiple myeloma. *Am J Hematol* 2010;85(6):409–413.

142. Christoforidou AV, Saliba RM, Williams P, et al. Results of a retrospective single institution analysis of targeted skeletal radiotherapy with (166)Holmium-DOTMP as conditioning regimen for autologous stem cell transplant for patients with multiple myeloma. Impact on transplant outcomes. *Biol Blood Marrow Transplant* 2007;13(5):543–549.

143. Specht L, Yahalom J, Illidge T, et al. Modern radiation therapy for Hodgkin lymphoma: field and dose guidelines from the international lymphoma radiation oncology group (ILROG). *Int J Radiat Oncol Biol Phys* 2014;89(4): 854–862.

144. Illidge T, Specht L, Yahalom J, et al. Modern radiation therapy for nodal non-Hodgkin lymphoma-target definition and dose guidelines from the International Lymphoma Radiation Oncology Group. *Int J Radiat Oncol Biol Phys* 2014;89(1):49–58.

145. Yahalom J, Illidge T, Specht L, et al. Modern radiation therapy for extranodal lymphomas: field and dose guidelines from the International Lymphoma Radiation Oncology Group. *Int J Radiat Oncol Biol Phys* 2015;92(1): 11–31.

146. Jyothirmayi R, Gangadharan VP, Nair MK, et al. Radiotherapy in the treatment of solitary plasmacytoma. *Br J Radiol* 1997;70(833):511–516.

147. Mendenhall CM, Thar TL, Million RR. Solitary plasmacytoma of bone and soft tissue. *Int J Radiat Oncol Biol Phys* 1980;6(11):1497–1501.

148. Chang MY, Shih LY, Dunn P, et al. Solitary plasmacytoma of bone. *J Formos Med Assoc* 1994;93(5):397–402.

149. Durie BG, Harousseau JL, Miguel JS, et al. International uniform response criteria for multiple myeloma. *Leukemia* 2006;20(9):1467–1473.

CHAPTER 86

Osteosarcoma and Other Primary Tumors of Bone

Jaroslaw T. Hepel and Timothy J. Kinsella

Primary malignant tumors of bone are rare neoplasms accounting for <0.2% of all cancers. In 2010, an estimated 2,650 new cases and 1,460 related deaths were expected.[1] Osteosarcoma, chondrosarcoma, and Ewing sarcoma are the most common, comprising 35%, 30%, and 16% of cases, respectively. Other rare entities include malignant fibrous histiocytoma, fibrosarcoma, and chordoma. Ewing sarcoma is discussed in detail in Chapter 92. Osteosarcoma and the other malignant bone tumors will be discussed here.

OSTEOSARCOMA

Epidemiology

Osteosarcoma is a rare primary malignant tumor of bone, accounting for approximately 750 to 900 new cases in the United States annually. Despite its rarity, osteosarcoma is the fifth most common malignancy and the most common malignant bone tumor in children and adolescents.[2,3] It has a bimodal age distribution, with peak incidence in early adolescence and another smaller peak in adults older than 65 years of age.[4] In childhood, osteosarcoma typically occurs sporadically, whereas in adulthood, it is more commonly associated with sarcomatous degeneration of Paget disease or other benign bone lesions. There is a slight male predilection, with a ratio of 1.2:1.[2]

Pathogenesis and Risk Factors

The etiology of osteosarcoma is unknown, but there is a suggestion of a relationship with rapid bone growth. The peak incidence of osteosarcoma occurs during the adolescent growth spurt; this peak is earlier in girls corresponding to their earlier bone development. The most frequent sites of involvement correspond to the areas of greatest increase in bone length—the metaphysis of the distal femur, proximal tibia, and proximal humerus. It has been suggested that an aberration in the natural process of bone growth leads to osteosarcoma, but the specific etiology has not been elucidated. Unlike other pediatric tumors, no characteristic translocation or genetic abnormality has been defined for osteosarcoma.

Several risk factors have been associated with osteosarcoma. Development of osteosarcoma after radiation therapy exposure in childhood has been reported. The mean latency period is generally >10 years.[5–7] Similarly, chemotherapy, especially alkylating agents, has been implicated with secondary osteosarcoma.[7] Benign bone lesions, particularly Paget disease, have also been associated with osteosarcoma. Paget disease of bone is a focal skeletal disorder characterized

by accelerated bone turnover. Sarcomatous transformation is usually seen in long-standing Paget and occurs in only 0.7% to 1% of cases.[8] Other benign bone lesions have also been associated with risk of osteosarcoma, including chronic osteomyelitis, multiple hereditary exostoses, fibrous dysplasia, osteochondromas, enchondromas, sites of bone infarcts, and sites of metallic implants.[9] Several genetic conditions have been linked to an increase risk of osteosarcoma. Retinoblastoma is associated with an increased risk of secondary tumors, more than half of which are soft tissue sarcomas and osteosarcomas.[10] Li-Fraumeni syndrome is associated with a spectrum of malignancies, including breast, adrenocortical, brain, leukemia, and sarcomas, including osteosarcoma. Li-Fraumeni syndrome involves a germline inactivation of p53, a key cell cycle regulatory gene.[11] Rothmund-Thomson, Bloom, and Werner syndromes have also been associated with osteosarcoma.[12]

Clinical Presentation

Most patients present with localized pain in the affected bone. Pain is usually of several months duration and may wax and wane. There may be associated soft tissue swelling or a palpable mass. Some patients present with pathologic fracture. Osteosarcoma has a predilection for involvement of the metaphysis of long bones. The most common site of involvement is the knee (distal femur or proximal tibia), followed by the proximal humerus, mid and proximal femur, and then other bones.[13] Although most patients have micrometastatic disease at the time of presentation, only 10% to 20% of patients present with clinical evident macrometastases. The lung is the most common site of metastatic involvement, followed by bone.[14]

Diagnostic Evaluation

Plain x-ray of the affected bone classically demonstrates destruction of the normal trabecular bone with lytic and/or sclerotic lesions, osteoid formation under the periosteum (Codman triangle), and variable ossification of the associated soft tissue mass (Fig. 86.1). Magnetic resonance imaging (MRI) of the affected bone is essential to fully delineate the extent of the lesion, evaluate any soft tissue component, and evaluate for involvement of joint, nerves, and vasculature (Fig. 86.2). The entire affected bone should be imaged to evaluate for the presence of skip lesions. Skip metastases are well recognized in osteosarcoma but occur infrequently, with <5% incidence.[15,16] Systemic staging should include a computed tomography (CT) scan of the chest and radionuclide bone scan to evaluate for pulmonary and bone metastases, respectively. Positron emission tomography (PET) scan can be used as an

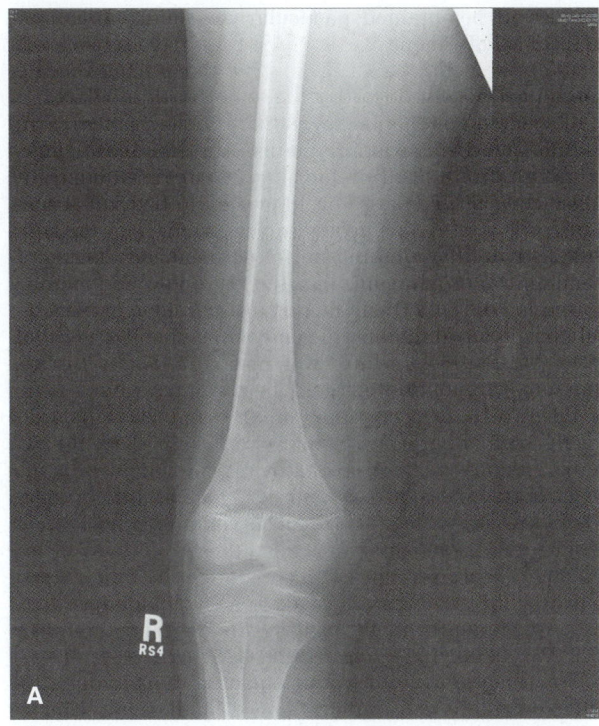
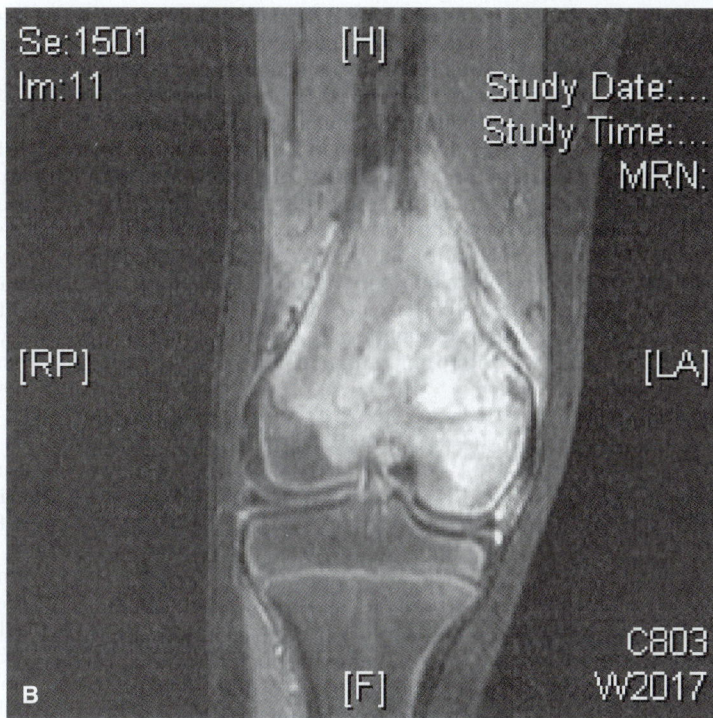

FIGURE 86.1. **A:** Plain radiograph of a distal femur osteosarcoma showing a lytic region and Codman triangle in the medial distal femur. **B:** Magnetic resonance image scan of the same lesion.

alternative for systemic staging but may have less sensitivity than CT and bone scan.[17,18] PET scan has also been used to assess response to preoperative chemotherapy.[19]

Biopsy of the tumor should be performed to confirm the diagnosis and to differentiate from other bone lesions. Similar to soft tissue sarcomas, the biopsy should be performed at a center with expertise in bone tumors and should be carried out by or in conjunction with the orthopedic surgeon who will be performing future definitive surgery in order to not jeopardize subsequent treatment, particularly a limb-preserving procedure.

Staging Systems

There are two staging systems commonly used for osteosarcoma (Table 86.1). The Musculoskeletal Tumor Society (MSTS) staging system is a surgical staging system stratifying tumors by grade and subdividing by local extent.[20] The American Joint Committee on Cancer system is less often used.[21]

FIGURE 86.2. Plain radiograph of a sclerotic pelvic osteosarcoma.

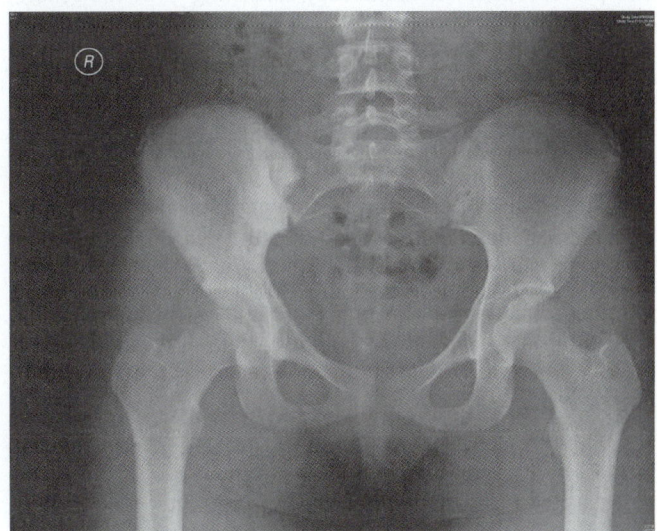

Pathology

Osteosarcoma is characterized by the presence of malignant sarcomatous stroma with associated osteoid (immature bone) production.[22] Osteosarcoma is believed to arise from mesenchymal stem cells with the capacity to have fibrous tissue, cartilage, and bone differentiation. Thus, osteosarcoma shares many features with chondrosarcomas and fibrosarcomas. However, only osteosarcoma produces woven bone matrix, a key element for diagnosis.

Osteosarcoma is classified into two main categories: conventional (intramedullary) and surface.[23] The conventional type accounts for 90% of osteosarcomas and is associated with the typical presentation in adolescence. The majority of conventional osteosarcomas are high-grade

TABLE 86.1 STAGING OF OSTEOSARCOMA

Stage	Grade	Site	Metastases
Enneking Staging System			
IA	Low	Intracompartmental	None
IB	Low	Extracompartmental	None
IIA	High	Intracompartmental	None
IIB	High	Extracompartmental	None
III	Any	Any	Present
Stage	Grade	Local extent (cm)	Metastases
AJCC Staging System[a]			
IA	Low	≤8	None
IB	Low	>8 or discontinuous	None
IIA	High	≤8	None
IIB	High	>8	None
III	High	Discontinuous	None
IVA	Any	Any	Pulmonary metastases
IVB	Any	Any	Other metastases

[a]Used with the permission of the American Joint Committee on Cancer, Chicago, Illinois. The original source for this material is *AJCC staging cancer handbook*, 7th ed. New York, NY: Springer, 2010; published by Springer Science and Business Media LLC, www.springer.com. From Edge SB, Byrd DR, Compton CC, et al., eds. *AJCC cancer staging handbook*. 7th ed. New York: Springer, 2010. Copyright © 2010 American Joint Committee on Cancer. Reproduced with permission of Springer International Publishing in the format Book via Copyright Clearance Center.

tumors. Conventional osteosarcoma is further subdivided into osteoblastic, chondroblastic, fibroblastic, and mixed subtypes. Other, less common histologic variants of conventional osteosarcoma include small cell, telangiectatic, malignant fibrous histiocytoma, and multifocal. Multifocal osteosarcoma typically carries a worse prognosis.

Surface osteosarcoma is subdivided into parosteal, periosteal, and high-grade surface.[24,25] Parosteal variant is considered to be a low-grade tumor with a low metastatic potential. Periosteal variant is intermediate in grade, with an intermediate rate of developing metastases, between parosteal and conventional osteosarcoma, about 20%. A rare variant, extraosseous osteosarcoma, arises in soft tissues and is generally associated with prior radiation exposure.[26]

Treatment

Chemotherapy plays a critical role in the management of most patients with osteosarcoma. Although only 10% to 20% of patients present with overt metastatic disease, the vast majority of patients harbor subclinical metastatic disease at the time of presentation. Before effective chemotherapy, 80% to 90% of patients subsequently developed distant metastases and died of their disease despite achieving local disease control.[27] The typical treatment sequence for intermediate- and high-grade osteosarcoma is neoadjuvant chemotherapy, followed by surgery with a limb-sparing procedure if possible and then followed by further adjuvant chemotherapy. With this approach, 60% to 70% of patients without overt metastases at diagnosis are expected to be long-term survivors.[28] Those with isolated lung metastases have an overall survival of 35% to 40%, whereas those with more extensive metastatic disease at diagnosis have <20% likelihood of long-term survival. For the less common low-grade tumors such as parosteal osteosarcoma, treatment with surgery alone is appropriate because the risk of developing metastases is low. These patients have an 80% to 90% likelihood of long-term survival.[29]

Surgery

The mainstay of surgical management is the complete *en bloc* resection of tumor. The extent and functional implications of surgery have dramatically evolved over time, with an emphasis on more conservative, limb-sparing resections with maintenance of function rather than amputation. Neoadjuvant chemotherapy has played an important role in this evolution.

For extremity lesions, limb preservation is preferred and can be accomplished in the majority of cases. Retrospective studies have shown equivalent results of limb-sparing surgery and amputation as long as adequate margins can be achieved.[30-32] Contraindications to limb-sparing surgery include nerve or vascular encasement, presence of large, biopsy-related hematoma, and pathologic fracture. Some data suggest that pathologic fracture does not increase the risk of local recurrence after limb-sparing surgery as previously believed.[33,34] Reconstructive options include use of allografts, endoprostheses, and occasionally rotationplasty.

Axial tumors, although much less common, pose a particular challenge because achieving complete surgical resection can be difficult. As a result, these lesions have a worse prognosis compared to extremity tumors. Pelvic tumors typically require a hemipelvectomy for *en bloc* resection. Some patients can undergo resection of the hemipelvis with preservation of the extremity (internal hemipelvectomy). This has a better functional outcome compared to an external hemipelvectomy, also referred to as a hindquarter amputation. Adjuvant radiation has been used to improve outcomes in patients with incomplete resections of pelvic tumors. Spinal tumors are also particularly difficult to resect with negative margins. Typically, an *en bloc* resection with vertebrectomy is performed, combined with mechanical stabilization. Postoperative radiation therapy can be used when negative margins cannot be obtained, particularly when there is microscopic dural involvement.

Chemotherapy

In the absence of chemotherapy, 80% to 90% of patients will subsequently develop distant metastases.[27] Chemotherapy thus plays an important role for all patients with intermediate- and high-grade tumors. Level I evidence for the benefit of chemotherapy was established by two randomized trials in the 1980s. Eilber et al.[35] reported on 59 patients with nonmetastatic osteosarcoma randomized to surgery followed by observation versus adjuvant chemotherapy. Disease-free survival at 2 years was 55% with chemotherapy and 20% with observation (*P* < .01). Overall survival was also superior at 2 years: 80% versus 48% with and without chemotherapy, respectively (*P* < .01). Link et al.[36] reported similar results in a group of 36 patients with nonmetastatic, high-grade osteosarcoma randomized to observation versus adjuvant chemotherapy after primary surgery. Disease-free survival at 2 years was 66% with chemotherapy and 17% with observation (*P* < .001).

The concept of neoadjuvant chemotherapy arose in conjunction with evolving surgical techniques striving for limb-preserving procedures and improved functional outcomes. This led to a randomized clinical trial by the Pediatric Oncology Group (POG).[37] POG 8651 randomized patients with nonmetastatic, high-grade osteosarcoma to neoadjuvant chemotherapy followed by surgery or surgery followed by the same chemotherapy. The 5-year relapse-free survival was not statistically different between the two groups (65% vs. 61%, respectively), nor was the rate of limb salvage (55% vs. 50%, respectively). Although this trial did not show improved outcomes with neoadjuvant chemotherapy, it did show equivalence and established a benchmark for comparison with future trials. Neoadjuvant chemotherapy is favored by most centers, with the belief that the likelihood of limb-sparing surgery and, ultimately, functional outcome can be improved with this approach. Furthermore, the response to neoadjuvant chemotherapy has been shown to be prognostic.[38] This allows for the stratification of patients for more intensive postoperative treatment.

The optimal choice of chemotherapy and administration schedule remains a subject of active research. The Memorial Sloan Kettering Cancer Center T10 regimen is frequently used for nonprotocol patients and consists of high-dose methotrexate, doxorubicin, bleomycin, cyclophosphamide, and actinomycin D.[39] EURAMOS I (AOST 0331) was an international collaborative group trial sponsored by European and American Osteosarcoma Study Group, as well as by other groups, including the Children's Oncology Group.[40] This trial sought to better define optimal chemotherapy. Patients received preoperative and postoperative chemotherapy consisting of methotrexate, doxorubicin, and cisplatin (MAP). Those with a poor response to preoperative chemotherapy, defined as ≥10% residual viable tumor, were randomized to the addition of ifosfamide and etoposide (IE), whereas those with a good response to preoperative chemotherapy were randomized to the addition of interferon. A total of 2,260 patients were enrolled. Final results were unfortunately negative with neither ifosfamide and etoposide nor interferon showing improved event-free survival. For the poor response group, at 62 months median follow-up, 3-year event-free survival was 55% for MAP and 53% MAP + IE (*P* = .69).[41] For the good response group, at 44 months median follow-up, 3-year event-free survival was 74% for MAP and 77% MAP with interferon (*P* = .214).[42]

Radiation

Historically, radiation has been used for the treatment of osteosarcoma; however, high local failure rates with the use of radiation alone; improved surgical techniques, allowing for limb preservation; and effective use of chemotherapy limit the use of radiation therapy for osteosarcoma today. With a combined approach of chemotherapy and surgery with negative margins, local control rates of 90% to 98% have been reported.[30–32,43]

Patients who have tumor resection with inadequate or positive margins or who have unresectable tumors, however, have high rates of local recurrence. The Cooperative Osteosarcoma Study (COSS) Group performed a multivariate of 1,702 analysis patients found and that poor response to neoadjuvant chemotherapy and incomplete surgical resection predicted negatively for overall survival.[38] Picci et al.[44] also reported that local recurrence was higher for limb-salvage surgery if wide, negative margins were not achieved. Furthermore, high recurrence rates have been reported in locations where complete surgery is usually not possible, including a recurrence rate of 70% in the pelvis, 68% in the spine, and 50% in the skull regions.[45–47] Radiation can potentially improve local control in these patients. Therefore, indications for integration of radiation therapy with other treatment modalities currently include incompletely resected tumors with positive margins and unresectable tumors or for palliation of symptoms.

Radiation Therapy Techniques

As with other sarcomas, proper patient position at the time of simulation and treatment is essential to achieve optimal tumor coverage and normal-tissue sparing. Customized immobilization devices may need to be constructed to achieve optimal positioning that is reproducible on a daily basis. Three-dimensional treatment planning with the aid of presurgical and postsurgical imaging is used to define gross tumor volumes and areas of subclinical disease. Typically, a 2-cm margin is used for axial tumors, which can be extended to 4 to 5 cm for extremity tumors. These margins can be restricted at natural tissue and fascial boundaries. The radiation technique used, either three-dimensional conformal or intensity-modulated radiation therapy, should be tailored to the individual patient. Dose to uninvolved organs should be minimized to prevent late organ dysfunction, as should the integral dose to minimize risk of secondary malignancy.

A prescription dose of 60 Gy in 2-Gy fractions is typically used for microscopically involved margins, whereas 66 Gy is used for macroscopic residual disease and 70 Gy is used for inoperable tumors. Chemotherapy should not be interrupted to deliver local radiation therapy. Radiation can be given concurrently but is usually delivered after chemotherapy because of increased acute toxicity with concurrent administration.

Intraoperative radiation therapy has been used to deliver dose directly to close or involved surgical margins.[48,49] Proton particle therapy has been used in an attempt to escalate radiation dose, particularly in unresectable tumors.[50,51] Radionuclide therapy with rhenium,[52] strontium,[53] and samarium[54] has been used for palliation of extensive bone metastases with good effects.

Results of Radiation Therapy

In the prechemotherapy era, Cade[55] pioneered a technique of radiotherapy with delayed amputation in patients who did not develop distant metastases. The primary tumor was controlled in some patients who refused amputation. However, the overall results were poor, with most patients dying of metastatic disease. The incorporation of chemotherapy with optimal surgery has resulted in significantly improved outcomes, obviating the need for radiation therapy for most patients. Dincbas et al.[56] evaluated the addition of preoperative radiation therapy to chemotherapy followed by limb-sparing surgery. They reported on a series of 46 patients, most of whom received 35 Gy in 10 fractions. Local control and overall survival rates at 5 years were 97.5% and 48.4%, respectively. Although the results were excellent, it is not clear whether preoperative radiation therapy improved outcomes, given that

the rate of local control with chemotherapy followed by surgery in the absence of adjuvant radiation is high, as previously summarized.

For patients who have incomplete tumor resection or unresectable tumors, the risk of local recurrence/progression is high. These patients, therefore, can potentially benefit from radiation therapy. Machak et al.[57] reported on a series of 187 patients with nonmetastatic osteosarcoma treated with induction chemotherapy. Of these, 31 patients refused surgery and were treated with radiation to a mean dose of 60 Gy. Local control was related to response to induction chemotherapy. There were no local recurrences in 11 patients who had a good response to chemotherapy. However, local progression-free survival was 31% at 3 years and 0% at 5 years for nonresponders. Schwarz et al.[58] reported on an analysis of 100 patients treated with radiation therapy in the COSS registry. Local control and overall survival for the whole group were 30% and 36%, respectively, at 5 years. Local control was significantly better when surgery was combined with radiation compared to radiation alone: 48% versus 22%, respectively ($P = .002$). Local control was also higher for primary tumors compared with recurrent tumors: 40% versus 17%, respectively. Sole et al. reported on 72 patients treated with neoadjuvant chemotherapy, resection, and postoperative radiation therapy with a median follow-up of 174 months. Local control and disease-free survival and overall survival at 10 years were 82%, 58%, and 73%, respectively. R1 resection was predictive of worse local control.[59] DeLaney et al.[31] reported on the Massachusetts General Hospital (MGH) experience. Forty-one patients with osteosarcoma underwent radiation for close or positive margins or for unresectable disease. Anatomic sites included 17 skulls, 8 extremities, 8 spines, 7 pelves, and 1 trunk. Patients received a median dose of 66 Gy (10 to 80 Gy), with about half of patients receiving a portion of their treatment with protons. The overall local control rate was 68% at 5 years. Local control was similar between patients who underwent a gross total resection or subtotal resection but was significantly better than for those who underwent biopsy only: 78% versus 78% versus 40% at 5 years, respectively ($P < .01$).

Overall, it appears that radiation is most effective when the tumor burden is small, with the best results achieved in patients who have a good response to chemotherapy or are able to undergo gross total or subtotal tumor resection. Total dose may also be an important factor. Gaitán-Yanguas[60] showed a dose–response relationship for osteosarcoma, with no lesions controlled at doses of ≤30 Gy and all lesions controlled at doses of >90 Gy. The best clinical results were reported in the MGH series.[51] A median dose of 66 Gy was used, and half of the patients received proton therapy as part of their treatment. The unique dose–depth properties of proton radiation therapy allows for dose escalation while maintaining normal-tissue sparing. This approach may explain the improved outcomes reported. However, this study did fail to show a dose–response relationship.

Whole-Lung Irradiation

Whole-lung irradiation has been shown to be beneficial in several other pediatric tumors with a propensity for lung metastases. This led to the rationale that this treatment may improve outcomes in osteosarcoma, which has a high propensity for metastases and for which the lung is the most common site of spread. Two initial small randomized trials in the prechemotherapy era showed a trend for improved disease-free and overall survival for whole-lung irradiation.[61,62] This led to the EORTC-20781/SIOP-03 phase III trial, which randomized 240 patients to three arms: chemotherapy, whole-lung irradiation, or both.[63] The whole-lung dose was 20 Gy. The 4-year disease-free survival and overall survival were 43% and 24%, respectively, with no difference between the arms. Therefore, with the recognition of the other advantages of systemic therapy, whole-lung irradiation has fallen out of favor.[64]

Surveillance and Sequelae of Treatment

Surveillance for recurrence should include imaging of the primary site with CT or MRI and chest imaging. Late complications are largely related to chemotherapy and surgical interventions. Limb functional outcomes are related to location of tumor and type of resection and reconstruction performed. Complications related to radiation therapy include joint fibrosis with decreased range of motion, bone weakening and fracture, loss of allograft, and secondary malignancy.[51] Careful consideration of radiation technique and physical rehabilitative therapy is essential to minimizing late functional impairment.

CHONDROSARCOMA

Epidemiology

Chondrosarcoma is characterized by a neoplastic process with associated cartilage matrix production that is devoid of osteoid, a characteristic of osteosarcoma. It is the second most common primary bone tumor, accounting for approximately 30% of cases.[1] Chondrosarcoma may arise at any age but typically occurs in middle-aged and older adults.[65]

Pathogenesis and Risk Factors

The etiology of chondrosarcoma is not fully understood. It is usually sporadic but can also develop from malignant transformation of benign cartilaginous lesions—osteochondromas and enchondromas. Osteochondroma is a cartilage-capped bony projection arising on the external surface of bones. It is usually located on long bones, particularly around the knee. Multiple osteochondromas are associated with hereditary multiple exostoses, an autosomal dominant syndrome. Malignant transformation occurs in 5% of patients with either solitary or multiple osteochondromas.[66,67] Enchondroma is a benign cartilaginous tumor developing in the marrow cavity of bone. Multiple enchondromas, or enchondromatosis, are usually associated with congenital disorders such as Ollier disease or Maffucci syndrome. Malignant transformation of solitary enchondromas is extremely rare, but the risk with enchondromatosis is as high as 25% to 30%.[67,68]

Clinical Presentation and Diagnostic Evaluation

Patients typically present with localized pain in the affected bone with or without associated soft tissue swelling or a palpable mass. Plain radiograph is obtained for initial evaluation, but CT and MRI are essential to characterize the lesion(s) and determine the full extent of disease.

Tissue biopsy of the tumor is necessary to confirm the diagnosis and to differentiate it from other malignant bone tumors. Biopsy should be aimed at the most aggressive portion as determined by imaging. This can help avoid biopsy of a portion of a benign precursor lesion. It also helps avoid less aggressive surgical approaches used for low-grade lesions if a high-grade component is present.[69]

The rate of metastatic disease for chondrosarcoma is very dependent on tumor grade. Low-grade lesions have a <10% risk of metastases, intermediate-grade lesions have a 10% to 50% risk, and high-grade lesion have a 50% to 70% risk.[70,71] The lungs are the main site of metastases. Staging evaluation thus should include a chest CT for intermediate- and high-grade lesions.

Staging Systems

As with osteosarcoma, both the MSTS staging system and the American Joint Committee on Cancer staging system can be used (Table 86.1). MSTS is used more often.[20,21]

Pathology

Chondrosarcoma pathologically is divided into conventional, which comprises 85% to 90% of cases, and other, uncommon variants. Conventional chondrosarcoma is further subdivided into central, peripheral, and periosteal.[72,73] Central chondrosarcoma is the most common type, accounting for 75% of all chondrosarcomas. Most are sporadic, but as many as 40% may arise for underlying enchondromas. Most commonly, the proximal femur, pelvis, and proximal humerus are involved.[74] Peripheral chondrosarcoma by definition arises from a pre-existing osteochondroma. The long bones, pelvis, and shoulder girdle are most commonly affected.[67] Periosteal chondrosarcoma arises from the surface of bone and is rare. It usually affects adults at a younger age, in their 20s and 30s, and tends to have a good prognosis.[75] Nonconventional chondrosarcoma variants include clear cell, dedifferentiated, myxoid, and mesenchymal. Clinical behavior of chondrosarcoma is highly dependent on histologic grade.[70,76,77]

Treatment

Histologic grade and tumor location are important determinates of treatment approach. Surgical excision is the primary treatment modality for chondrosarcoma. For low-grade tumors, which constitute the vast majority of chondrosarcomas, surgical resection alone is sufficient to achieve a high rate of disease control. For low-grade central tumors, intralesional excision or curettage is the preferred method of resection. This can be combined with local adjuvant chemical treatment or cryotherapy. These approaches result in good local control rates and minimize the morbidity of more extensive surgical resection.[78-81] The best outcomes are obtained with small tumors located in the extremities. Larger tumors, tumors with intra-articular or soft tissue involvement, and axial or pelvic tumors have higher local recurrence rates with these more conservative treatments and are better treated with wide excision.[82,83] For the less common intermediate- and high-grade tumors, wide *en bloc* excision is the optimal surgical approach.[77] Radiation therapy is indicated for incompletely resected high-grade or locally recurrent tumors and tumors that are unresectable. Chemotherapy is generally not very effective for chondrosarcoma, especially for the most prevalent conventional type. There is no established adjuvant chemotherapy regimen for these patients. There is some suggestion that dedifferentiated and mesenchymal chondrosarcomas may potentially benefit from chemotherapy, but phase III randomized data are lacking in these rare tumors.[84-86]

Radiation

As with osteosarcoma, no level 1 evidence exists for radiation therapy in chondrosarcoma. Based on first principles and results of published case series, radiation therapy is indicated to improve on high local failure rates after incomplete resection of high-risk tumors. These indications include intermediate- to high-grade tumors, locally recurrent tumors, and tumors in locations where surgical resection is challenging or limited. Definitive radiation can also be used for unresectable tumors. Doses of 50 Gy preoperatively and 60 to 66 Gy postoperatively for close or positive margins are typically used. Doses of ≥70 Gy are needed for definitive treatment.

Results of Radiation Therapy

Although chondrosarcoma was traditionally considered to be a "radioresistant" tumor, modern series have shown good outcomes with radiation therapy. Goda et al.[87] presented the Princess Margaret Hospital experience of combined surgery and radiation therapy for high-risk extracranial chondrosarcoma. They reported on 60 patients with a median follow-up of 75 months and showed local control rates of 100%, 94%, and 42% for R0, R1, and R2 resected patients, respectively.

Ten-year overall survival was 86%. Definitive radiation therapy has also been used for locations where complete surgical resection is difficult to achieve, that is, the spine and base of skull.[88-91] In these locations, *en bloc* resection is generally not possible, and even piecemeal resection is often not complete. Proton radiation therapy has been used in this setting. The unique depth–dose properties of protons allows for dose escalation while sparing neighboring critical structures. A large series was reported from Massachusetts General Hospital consisting of 200 patients with base-of-skull chondrosarcoma treated using a combination of photon and proton radiation therapy.[92] With median dose of 72 Cobalt Gray Equivalent (CGE), they reported a 10-year local control rate of 98%. Similar local control rates have been reported by other institutions using various conformal radiation methods to achieve a high tumor dose, including protons, fractionated stereotactic photon, and carbon ions.[91,93-95] Tables 86.2 and 86.3 summarize the results of selected studies of radiation therapy for chondrosarcoma involving the base of skull and the spine, respectively.

Surveillance and Sequelae of Treatment

Functional assessment, rehabilitation, and physical therapy are important to minimize the long-term morbidity of surgery and/or radiation therapy. Surveillance for recurrence should include history and physical exam, CT or MRI imaging of the primary area, and chest imaging on a periodic basis. Follow-up should continue for a minimum of 10 years because late recurrences are more commonly observed with chondrosarcoma than with other sarcomas.[96]

CHORDOMA

Epidemiology

Chordoma is a rare, malignant neoplasm arising from the remnant of the primitive notochord. Chordoma accounts for 1% to 4% of primary bone tumors, with an annual incidence in the United States of 0.08 cases per 100,000.[97] Median age at presentation is 60 years, but base-of-skull location typically present at a younger age, usually in the third to fourth decade of life.

Pathogenesis

In normal embryologic development, the notochord regresses as the embryo matures. Remnants can be found anywhere along the tract of the notochord from the base of skull to the sacrum. The largest foci remain at the cranial and caudal ends. This corresponds well with the anatomic distribution of chordoma, with half arising in the sacrococcygeal region and one-third at the base of skull, typically the clivus.[97] The rest occur in the vertebral bodies of the spine. Chordomas in other locations are exceedingly rare.[98]

TABLE 86.2 SELECTED STUDIES OF BASE-OF-SKULL CHORDOMA AND CHONDROSARCOMA

Institution/Study	Number of Patients	Radiation Modality	Median Dose (Range)	Median Follow-Up (Month)	Local Control	Overall Survival
MGH Terahara et al.[111]	132 chordoma	Mixed photon/ proton	68.9 CGE (66.6–79.2 CGE)	41	5 yr 59% 10 yr 44%	NR
MGH Rosenberg et al.[92]	200 chondrosarcoma	Mixed photon/ proton	72.1 CGE (64.2–79.6 CGE)	63	5 yr 99% 10 yr 98%	5 yr 99% DSS 10 yr 99% DSS
Institut Curie Noël et al.[112]	100 chordoma	Mixed photon/ proton	67 CGE	31	2 yr 86% 4 yr 54%	2 yr 94% 5 yr 81%
Institut Curie Feuvret et al.[124]	159 chondrosarcoma	Mixed photon/ proton	70.2 CGE	77	5 yr 96.4% 10 yr 93.5%	5 yr 94.9% 10 yr 87%
Paul Scherrer Institute Ares et al.[93]	64 total: 42 chordoma 22 chondrosarcoma	Mixed photon/ proton	Chordoma 73.5 CGE Chondrosarcoma 68.4 CGE	38	Chordoma 5 yr 81% Chondrosarcoma 5 yr 94%	Chordoma 5 yr 62% Chondrosarcoma 5 yr 91%
Paul Scherrer Institute Weber et al.[125]	77 chondrosarcoma	Proton	70.0 Gy RBE (64–76 Gy RBE)	69	8 yr 89.7%	8 yr 93.5%
Loma Linda University Hug et al.[91]	58 total: 33 chordoma 25 chondrosarcoma	Proton	70.7 CGE (64.8–79.2 CGE)	33	Chordoma 5 yr 76% Chondrosarcoma 5 yr 92%	Chordoma 5 yr 79% Chondrosarcoma 5 yr 100%
University of Indiana McDonald et al.[126]	39 chordoma	Proton	77.4 Gy RBE (70.2–79.2 Gy RBE)	51	5 yr 69.6%	5 yr 81.4%
University of Heidelberg Uhl et al.[95,127]	155 chordoma	Carbon ion	60 CGE	72	5 yr 72% 10 yr 54%	5 yr 85% 10 yr 75%
University of Heidelberg update Uhl et al.[92,128]	79 chondrosarcoma	Carbon ion	60 CGE	91	5 yr 88% 10 yr 88%	5 yr 96.1% 10 yr 78.9%
North American Gamma Knife Consortium Kano et al.[120]	71 chordoma	SRS-gamma knife	15 Gy (9–25 Gy)	60	5 yr 66%	5 yr 80%
North American Gamma Knife Consortium Kano et al.[129]	46 chondrosarcoma	SRS-gamma knife	15 Gy (10.5–20 Gy)	75	5 yr 85% 10 yr 70%	5 yr 86% 10 yr 76%
University of Heidelberg Debus et al.[95]	45 total: 37 chordoma 8 chondrosarcoma	F-SRT-photon	Chordoma 66.6 Gy Chondrosarcoma 64.9 Gy	27	Chordoma 2 yr 82% 5 yr 50% Chondrosarcoma 5 yr 100%	2 yr 97% 5 yr 82%
University of Toronto Sahgal et al.[130]	42 total: 24 chordoma 18 chondrosarcoma	IG-IMRT	Chordoma 76 Gy Chondrosarcoma 70 Gy	36 67	Chordoma 5 yr 65.3 Chondrosarcoma 5 yr 88.1	Chordoma 5 yr 85.6 Chondrosarcoma 5 yr 87.8

CGE, Cobalt Gray Equivalents; F-SRT; fractionated stereotactic radiation therapy; MGH, Massachusetts General Hospital; NR, not reported; RBE, relative biologic effectiveness; SRS, stereotactic radiosurgery.

TABLE 86.3 SELECTED STUDIES OF SACRAL/SPINE CHORDOMA AND CHONDROSARCOMA

Institution/Study	Number of Patients	Radiation Modality	Median Dose (Range)	Median Follow-Up (Month)	Local Control	Overall Survival
MGH DeLaney et al.[113]	29 chordoma 14 chondrosarcoma 7 other	Mixed photon/ proton	76.6 CGE (59.4–77.4 CGE)	78	5 yr 78% Chordoma 90% Chondrosarcoma 57%	5 yr 87%
Paul Scherrer Institute Rutz et al.[114]	26 chordoma	Mixed photon/ proton	72 CGE (59.4–74.4 CGE)	35	3 yr 86%	3 yr 84%
University of Florida, Jacksonville Indelicato et al.[131]	34 chordoma 17 chondrosarcoma	Proton	70.2 Gy RBE (64.2–75.6 Gy RBE)	44	4 yr 58%	3 yr 72%
University of Heidelberg Zabel-du Bois et al.[132]	34 chordoma	IMRT-photon	66 Gy (54–72 Gy)	54	2 yr 55% 5 yr 27%	2 yr 91% 5 yr 70%
Chiba RCH Imai et al.[133,134]	188 chordoma	Carbon ion	70.4 CGE (64.0–73.6 CGE)	62	5 yr 77.2%	5 yr 81.1%
Berkeley Schoenthaler et al.[135]	14 chordoma	Helium/neon ion	75.6 CGE	60	5 yr 55%	5 yr 85%

CGE, Cobalt Gray Equivalents; IMRT, intensity-modulated radiation therapy; MGH, Massachusetts General Hospital; RBE, relative biologic effectiveness; RCH, Research Center Hospital.

Clinical Presentation and Diagnostic Evaluation

Chordomas are slow-growing but locally destructive tumors. They typically present with pain at the affected area that may be of long-standing duration. Neurologic symptoms based on location are frequent. Base-of-skull tumors can present with cranial nerve deficits, particularly cranial nerve 3 or 6 palsies (Fig. 86.3). Hydrocephalus and sensorimotor deficits can also occur. In the sacral region, sacral nerve roots can be affected, resulting in bowel or bladder dysfunction. Diagnostic evaluation includes CT and MRI to characterize the extent of the primary tumor and involvement or neighboring neural structures (Fig. 86.4). Biopsy should be performed to establish the pathologic diagnosis.

Chordomas have a low metastatic potential, but metastases may occur in as many as 10% to 40% of patients.[99–103] These typically occur late in the disease course and can involve lung, bone, liver, lymph nodes, or soft tissues. Metastatic deposits tend to be slow growing, and control of local disease progression remains the major therapeutic challenge in most patients.[103]

Pathology

Chordomas are classified histologically into conventional (classic), chondroid, and dedifferentiated. The majority are conventional. Chondroid chordoma accounts for 5% to 15% and tends to have a better prognosis. Dedifferentiated chordoma account for <5% of chordomas but are more aggressive, faster growing, and more likely to metastasize.[104] Chordoma can be histologically difficult to differentiate from low-grade chondrosarcoma. The latter has a better prognosis, so the distinction is prognostically important. A careful pathologic review by a pathologist experienced in these tumors is recommended.[92]

Treatment

Although chordoma has the potential to metastasize, the dominant failure pattern is local recurrence, and this typically

FIGURE 86.3. Base-of-skull chordoma. A 50-year-old patient who presented with several months of headaches and visual field deficits. T1-weighted, postgadolinium sagittal magnetic resonance imaging of the head depicts a chordoma (*arrow*) arising from the clivus (*asterisk*) with mass effect and posterior displacement of the brainstem.

FIGURE 86.4. Sacral chordoma. A 45-year-old patient who presented with 1 year of low back pain radiating to the coccyx. T2-weighted sagittal magnetic resonance imaging of the pelvis depicts a 5-cm chordoma involving the inferior sacrum up to the level of S2.

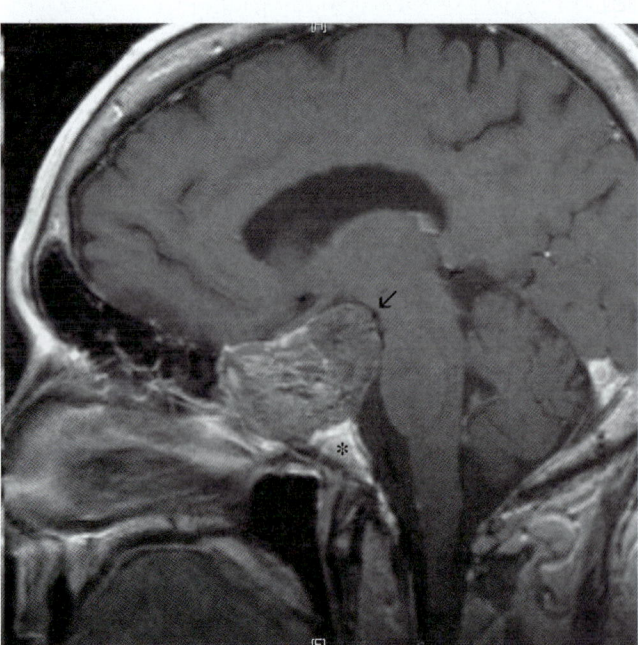

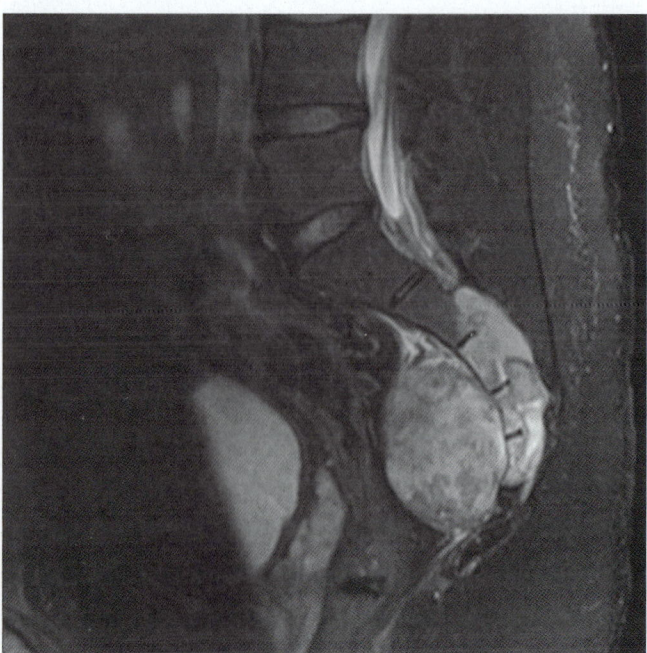

dictates morbidity and mortality for these patients. Salvage after local recurrence can achieve disease control for a period of time, but the ultimate outcomes tend to be poor. Thus, aggressive upfront treatment affords the best potential for cure. An analysis of the surveillance, epidemiology, and end results program of the National Cancer Institute consisting of 345 patients treated from 1974 to 2011 showed that 5-year overall survival of 78% to 80% was achieved with treatment using surgery +/- radiation therapy.[105]

Surgery has been the primary approach for these tumors. Complete *en bloc* resection with negative margins has been reported to achieve local control in 70% to 80% of patients.[106] However, when negative margins cannot be achieved, the failure rate is >70%.[106,107] Unfortunately, less than half of sacral tumors and even fewer base-of-skull tumors are amenable to complete resection. Aggressive surgery can also result in significant morbidity. Base-of-skull resection can result in cranial nerve deficits.[108] Resection of sacral chordomas can result in bowel and bladder dysfunction when S2 or S3 nerve roots are injured or sacrificed.[109,110]

Chordomas are considered relatively "radioresistant" tumors, and so doses of >66 Gy are required. These doses have traditionally been difficult to achieve with conventional external beam techniques, given the location of these tumors abutting sensitive neural structures. Given the advantages of the physical dose properties of the Bragg peak of charged particles, these tumors were treated early in the advent of this technology. Thus far, the best results in the treatment of chordomas have been achieved with a combination of surgery and high-dose proton radiation therapy. Local control rates of 54% to 90% have been reported.[91,93,111-114]

Chemotherapy has long been known to be inactive in chordoma, and thus, chemotherapy has not played a role in the definitive management of these patients. Recently, expression of platelet-derived growth factor and epidermal growth factor receptors on these tumors and antitumor activity of targeted therapies against these receptors have been described, renewing interest in systemic treatment.[115,116] Imatinib, cetuximab, and gefitinib have been used, but clinical experience is limited.[117,118]

Results of Radiation therapy

For base-of-skull chordomas, one of the largest experiences has been reported from Massachusetts General Hospital.[103] A crude local control of 69% was achieved in 204 patients treated using proton radiation therapy to a dose of 66.6 to 79.2 CGE. Reports of using heavier charged particle have shown similar outcomes.[119] With improvement in technology, dose escalation using conventional photons has also been achieved using intensity-modulated radiation therapy, fractionated stereotactic radiation therapy, and stereotactic radiosurgery techniques.[91,93,94,112,119,120] The outcomes with these approaches have been comparable to those reported for proton techniques. Table 86.2 summarizes the results of selected published studies for base-of-skull chordomas.

For sacral chordomas, the published literature is less robust but has shown similar results. DeLaney et al.[113] reported local control in 90% of 29 patients with sacral chordoma at a median follow-up of 4 years. Five-year actuarial local control was 100% for primary treatment versus 56% for salvage. There was no statistical difference based on extent of resection. Table 86.3 summarizes the results of published studies for spine sarcomas, including chordoma.

Sequelae of Radiation Therapy

Because of the high dose required for treatment of chordomas and the proximity of sensitive structures, late complications are not infrequent, and patients need to be followed and monitored closely. For base-of-skull chordoma, hypopituitarism, memory impairment, cranial nerve injury, sensory neural hearing loss, and central nervous system necrosis have been reported.[89,93,101] For sacral chordoma, sacral nerve root injury, erectile dysfunction, rectal bleeding, and sacral insufficiency factures have been reported.[113,121]

RARE MALIGNANT BONE TUMORS

Fibrosarcoma of bone is a very rare tumor, accounting for <5% of all primary bone tumors.[115] It is a malignant neoplasm of mesenchymal origin characterized by predominance of fibroblasts without tumor osteoid or cartilage production. It has a predilection for long bones and has a high metastatic potential. It is treated with complete surgical resection and often with adjuvant or neoadjuvant chemotherapy. Radiation therapy can be used for incompletely resected or unresectable tumors.

Malignant fibrous histiocytoma of bone also accounts for <5% of bone tumors.[122] It is characterized by a mixture of spindle-shaped fibroblastic cells in a storiform pattern and admixed with mononuclear cells with histiocytic morphology and anaplastic giant cells without tumor osteoid or cartilage production. The mainstay of treatment is complete surgical resection. Like osteosarcoma, it has a high rate of metastases. Malignant fibrous histiocytoma of bone is typically treated similarly to osteosarcoma and has been shown to benefit from chemotherapy.[123]

REFERENCES

1. Jemal A, Siegel R, Xu J, et al. Cancer statistics, 2010. *CA Cancer J Clin* 2010;60(5):277–300.
2. Gurney JG, Swensen AR, Bulterys M. *SEER pediatric monograph.* Available at: http://seer.cancer.gov/publications/childhood/bone.pdf. Accessed August 1, 2011.
3. Stiller CA, Bielack SS, Jundt G, et al. Bone tumours in European children and adolescents, 1978–1997. Report from the Automated Childhood Cancer Information System project. *Eur J Cancer* 2006;42(13):2124.
4. Dahlin DC, Unni KK. Osteosarcoma of bone and its important recognizable varieties. *Am J Surg Pathol* 1977;1(1):61–72.
5. Hawkins MM, Wilson LM, Burton HS, et al. Radiotherapy, alkylating agents, and risk of bone cancer after childhood cancer. *J Natl Cancer Inst* 1996;88(5):270.
6. Le Vu B, de Vathaire F, Shamsaldin A, et al. Radiation dose, chemotherapy and risk of osteosarcoma after solid tumours during childhood. *Int J Cancer* 1998;77(3):370.
7. Tucker MA, D'Angio GJ, Boice JD Jr, et al. Bone sarcomas linked to radiotherapy and chemotherapy in children. *N Engl J Med* 1987;317(10):588.
8. Hadjipavlou A, Lander P, Srolovitz H, et al. Malignant transformation in Paget disease of bone. *Cancer* 1992;70(12):2802.
9. Desai P, Perino G, Present D, et al. Sarcoma in association with bone infarcts. Report of five cases. *Arch Pathol Lab Med* 1996;120(5):482.
10. Draper GJ, Sanders BM, Kingston JE. Second primary neoplasms in patients with retinoblastoma. *Br J Cancer* 1986;53:661–671.
11. McIntyre JF, Smith-Sorensen B, Friend SH, et al. Germline mutations of the p53 tumor suppressor gene in children with osteosarcoma. *J Clin Oncol* 1994;12(5):925.
12. Hauben EI, Arends J, Vandenbroucke JP, et al. Multiple primary malignancies in osteosarcoma patients. Incidence and predictive value of osteosarcoma subtype for cancer syndromes related with osteosarcoma. *Eur J Hum Genet* 2003;11(8):611.
13. Meyers PA, Gorlick R. Osteosarcoma. *Pediatr Clin North Am* 1997;44(4):973.
14. Mialou V, Philip T, Kalifa C, et al. Metastatic osteosarcoma at diagnosis: prognostic factors and long-term outcome—the French pediatric experience. *Cancer* 2005;104(5):1100.
15. Kager L, Soubek A, Kastner U, et al. Skip metastases in osteosarcoma: experience of the Cooperative Osteosarcoma Study Group. *J Clin Oncol* 2006;24:1535–1541.
16. Sajadi KR, Heck RK, Neal MD. The incidence and prognosis of osteosarcoma skip metastases. *Clin Orthop Relat Res* 2004;426:92–96.
17. Franzius C, Daldrup-Link HE, Sciuk J, et al. FDG-PET for detection of pulmonary metastases from malignant primary bone tumors: comparison with spiral CT. *Ann Oncol* 2001;12(4):479.
18. Franzius C, Sciuk J, Daldrup-Link HE, et al. FDG-PET for detection of osseous metastases from malignant primary bone tumours: comparison with bone scintigraphy. *Eur J Nucl Med* 2000;27(9):1305.
19. Franzius C, Sciuk J, Brinkschmidt C, et al. Evaluation of chemotherapy response in primary bone tumors with F-18 FDG positron emission tomography compared with histologically assessed tumor necrosis. *Clin Nucl Med* 2000;25(11):874–881.

Section III

20. Enneking WF, Spanie SS, Goodman MA. A system for the surgical staging of musculoskeletal sarcoma. *Clin Orthop Relat Res* 2003;415:4–18.

21. American Joint Committee on Cancer. *Cancer staging manual.* 7th ed. New York, NY: Springer-Verlag, 2010.

22. Schajowicz F, Sissons HA, Sobin LH. The World Health Organization's histologic classification of bone tumors. A commentary on the second edition. *Cancer* 1995;75:1208–1214.

23. Inwards CY, Unni KK. Classification and grading of bone sarcomas. *Hematol Oncol Clin North Am* 1995;9(3):545.

24. Schajowicz F, McGuire MH, Santini Araujo E, et al. Osteosarcomas arising on the surfaces of long bones. *J Bone Joint Surg Am* 1988;70(4):555.

25. Raymond AK. Surface osteosarcoma. *Clin Orthop Relat Res* 1991;270:140–148.

26. Bane BL, Evans HL, Ro JY, et al. Extraskeletal osteosarcoma. A clinicopathologic review of 26 cases. *Cancer* 1990;65(12):2762.

27. Bruland OS, Høifødt H, Saeter G, et al. Hematogenous micrometastases in osteosarcoma patients. *Clin Cancer Res* 2005;11(13):4666.

28. Bacci G, Ferrari S, Donati D, et al. Neoadjuvant chemotherapy for osteosarcoma of the extremity in patients in the fourth and fifth decade of life. *Oncol Rep* 1998;5(5):1259.

29. Cesari M, Alberghini M, Vanel D, et al. Periosteal osteosarcoma: a single-institution experience. *Cancer* 2011;117(8):1731–1735.

30. Simon MA, Aschliman MA, Thomas N, et al. Limb-salvage treatment versus amputation for osteosarcoma of the distal end of the femur. *J Bone Joint Surg Am* 1986;68(9):1331.

31. Lindner NJ, Ramm O, Hillmann A, et al. Limb salvage and outcome of osteosarcoma. The University of Muenster experience. *Clin Orthop Relat Res* 1999;358:83–9.

32. Rougraff BT, Simon MA, Kneisl JS, et al. Limb salvage compared with amputation for osteosarcoma of the distal end of the femur. A long-term oncological, functional, and quality-of-life study. *J Bone Joint Surg Am* 1994;76(5):649.

33. Jaffe N, Spears R, Eftekhari F, et al. Pathologic fracture in osteosarcoma. Impact of chemotherapy on primary tumor and survival. *Cancer* 1987;59(4):701.

34. Bacci G, Ferrari S, Lari S, et al. Osteosarcoma of the limb. Amputation or limb salvage in patients treated by neoadjuvant chemotherapy. *J Bone Joint Surg Br* 2002;84(1):88.

35. Eilber F, Giuliano A, Eckardt J, et al. Adjuvant chemotherapy for osteosarcoma: a randomized prospective trial. *J Clin Oncol* 1987;5:21–26.

36. Link MP, Goorin AM, Miser AW, et al. The effect of adjuvant chemotherapy on relapse-free survival in patients with osteosarcoma of the extremity. *N Engl J Med* 1986;314(25):1600.

37. Goorin AM, Schwartzentruber DJ, Devidas M, et al. Presurgical chemotherapy compared with immediate surgery and adjuvant chemotherapy for nonmetastatic osteosarcoma: Pediatric Oncology Group POG-8651. *J Clin Oncol* 2003;21:1574–1580.

38. Bielack SS, Kempf-Bielack B, Delling G, et al. Prognostic factors in high-grade osteosarcoma of the extremities or trunk: an analysis of 1,702 patients treated on neoadjuvant cooperative osteosarcoma study group protocols. *J Clin Oncol* 2002;20(3):776–790.

39. Rosen G, Caparros B, Huvos AG, et al. Preoperative chemotherapy for osteogenic sarcoma: selection of postoperative adjuvant chemotherapy based on the response of the primary tumor to preoperative chemotherapy. *Cancer* 1982;49(6):1221.

40. European and American Osteosarcoma Study Group. Available at: http://www.ctu.mrc.ac.uk/euramos. Accessed August 8, 2011.

41. Marina NM, Smeland S, Bielack SS, et al. Comparison of MAPIE versus MAP in patients with a poor response to preoperative chemotherapy for newly diagnosed high-grade osteosarcoma (EURAMOS-1): an open-label, international, randomised controlled trial. *Lancet Oncol* 2016;17(10):1396–1408.

42. Bielack SS, Smeland S, Whelan JS, et al. Methotrexate, doxorubicin, and cisplatin (MAP) plus maintenance pegylated interferon Alfa-2b versus MAP alone in patients with resectable high-grade osteosarcoma and good histologic response to preoperative MAP: first results of the EURAMOS-1 good response randomized controlled trial. *J Clin Oncol* 2015;33(20):2279–2287.

43. Bacci G, Ferrari S, Bertoni F, et al. Long-term outcome for patients with nonmetastatic osteosarcoma of the extremity treated at the Istituto Ortopedico Rizzoli according to the Istituto Ortopedico Rizzoli/Osteosarcoma-2 Protocol: an updated report. *J Clin Oncol* 2000;18(24):4016–4027.

44. Picci P, Sangiorgi L, Bahamonde L, et al. Risk factors for local recurrences after limb-salvage surgery for high-grade osteosarcoma of the extremities. *Ann Oncol* 1997;8(9):899–903.

45. Ozaki T, Flege S, Kevric M, et al. Osteosarcoma of the pelvis: experience of the Cooperative Osteosarcoma Study Group. *J Clin Oncol* 2003;21(2):334–341.

46. Ozaki T, Flege S, Liljenqvist U, et al. Osteosarcoma of the spine: experience of the Cooperative Osteosarcoma Study Group. *Cancer* 2002;94(4):1069–1077.

47. Kassir RR, Rassekh CH, Kinsella JB, et al. Osteosarcoma of the head and neck: meta-analysis of nonrandomized studies. *Laryngoscope* 1997;107(1):56–61.

48. Oya N, Kobubo M, Mizowaki T, et al. Definitive intraoperative very high dose radiotherapy for localized osteosarcoma in the extremities. *Int J Radiat Oncol Biol Phys* 2001;51:878–893.

49. Tsuboyama T, Toguchida J, Kotoura Y, et al. Intra-operative radiation therapy for osteosarcoma in the extremities. *Int J Oncol* 2000;24:202–207.

50. Hug EB, Fitzek MM, Liebsch NJ, et al. Locally challenging osteo- and chondrogenic tumors of the axial skeleton: results of combined proton and photon radiation therapy using three dimensional treatment planning. *Int J Radiat Oncol Biol Phys* 1995;31:467–476.

51. DeLaney TF, Park L, Goldberg S, et al. Radiotherapy for local control of osteosarcoma. *Int J Radiat Oncol Biol Phys* 2005;61:492–498.

52. Sawyer EJ, Cassoni AM, Waddington W, et al. Rhenium-186 HEDP as a boost to external beam irradiation in osteosarcoma. *Br J Radiol* 1999;72:1225–1229.

53. Gompakis N, Sidi B, Salem N, et al. Strontium-89 for palliation of bone pain. *Med Pediatr Oncol* 2003;40:136.

54. Bruland OS, Skretting A, Solheim OP, et al. Targeted radiotherapy of osteosarcoma using 153Sm-EDTMP. *Acta Oncol* 1996;35:381–384.

55. Cade S. Osteogenic sarcoma. A study based on 133 patients. *Clin Orthop Relat Res* 1991;264:4–9.

56. Dincbas FO, Koca S, Mandel NM, et al. The role of preoperative radiotherapy in nonmetastatic high-grade osteosarcoma of the extremities for limb-sparing surgery. *Int J Radiat Oncol Biol Phys* 2005;62:820–828.

57. Machak GN, Tkachev SI, Solovyev YN, et al. Neoadjuvant chemotherapy and local radiotherapy for high-grade osteosarcoma of the extremities. *Mayo Clin Proc* 2003;78:147–155.

58. Schwarz R, Bruland O, Cassoni A, et al. The role of radiotherapy in osteosarcoma. *Cancer Treat Res* 2009;152:147–164.

59. Sole CV, Calvo FA, Alvarez E, et al. Adjuvant radiation therapy in resected high-grade localized skeletal osteosarcomas treated with neoadjuvant chemotherapy: long-term outcomes. *Radiother Oncol* 2016;119(1):30–34.

60. Gaitán-Yanguas M. A study of the response of osteogenic sarcoma and adjacent normal tissues to radiation. *Int J Radiat Oncol Biol Phys* 1981;7(5):593–595.

61. Breur K, Cohen P, Schweisguh O, et al. Irradiation of the lungs of an adjuvant therapy in the treatment of osteosarcoma of the limbs. An EORTC randomized study. *Eur J Cancer* 1978;14:461–471.

62. Rab GT, Ivins JC, Childs DS, et al. Elective whole lung irradiation in the treatment of osteogenic sarcoma. *Cancer* 1976;38:939–942.

63. Burgers JM, van Glabbeke M, Busson A, et al. Osteosarcoma of the limbs. Report of the EORTC-SIOP o3 trial 20781 investigating the value of adjuvant therapy with chemotherapy and/or prophylactic lung irradiation. *Cancer* 1988;61:1024–1031.

64. Whelan JS, Burcombe RJ, Janinis J, et al. A systematic review of the role of pulmonary irradiation in the management of primary bone tumors. *Ann Oncol* 2002;13:23–30.

65. Gelderblom H, Hogendoorn PC, Dijkstra SD. The clinical approach towards chondrosarcoma. *Oncologist* 2008;13(3):320–329.

66. Bovée JV. Multiple osteochondromas. *Orphanet J Rare Dis* 2008;3:3.

67. Altay M, Bayrakci K, Yildiz Y. Secondary chondrosarcoma in cartilage bone tumors: report of 32 patients. *J Orthop Sci* 2007;12(5):415.

68. Schwartz HS, Zimmerman NB, Simon MA, et al. The malignant potential of enchondromatosis. *J Bone Joint Surg Am* 1987;69(2):269.

69. Normand AN, Cannon CP, Lewis VO, et al. Curettage of biopsy-diagnosed grade 1 periacetabular chondrosarcoma. *Clin Orthop Relat Res* 2007;459:146.

70. Evans HL, Ayala AG, Romsdahl MM. Prognostic factors in chondrosarcoma of bone: a clinicopathologic analysis with emphasis on histologic grading. *Cancer* 1977;40:818.

71. Björnsson J, McLeod RA, Unni KK, et al. Primary chondrosarcoma of long bones and limb girdles. *Cancer* 1998;83(10):2105.

72. Fletcher CDM, Unni KK, Mertens F, eds. *Pathology and genetics of tumours of soft tissue and bone.* Lyon, France: IARC, 2002:233.

73. Mankin HJ, Cantley KP, Schiller AL, et al. The biology of human chondrosarcoma. II. Variation in chemical composition among types and subtypes of benign and malignant cartilage tumors. *J Bone Joint Surg Am* 1980;62(2):176–188.

74. Brien EW, Mirra JM, Kerr R. Benign and malignant cartilage tumors of bone and joint: their anatomic and theoretical basis with an emphasis on radiology, pathology and clinical biology. I. The intramedullary cartilage tumors. *Skeletal Radiol* 1997;26(6):325.

75. Murphey MD, Walker EA, Wilson AJ, et al. From the archives of the AFIP: imaging of primary chondrosarcoma: radiologic-pathologic correlation. *Radiographics* 2003;23(5):1245.

76. Giuffrida AY, Burgueno JE, Koniaris LG, et al. Chondrosarcoma in the United States (1973 to 2003): an analysis of 2890 cases from the SEER database. *J Bone Joint Surg Am* 2009;91(5):1063.

77. Fiorenza F, Abudu A, Grimer RJ, et al. Risk factors for survival and local control in chondrosarcoma of bone. *J Bone Joint Surg Br* 2002;84(1):93.

78. Veth R, Schreuder B, van Beem H, et al. Cryosurgery in aggressive, benign, and low-grade malignant bone tumours. *Lancet Oncol* 2005;6(1):25.

79. Leerapun T, Hugate RR, Inwards CY, et al. Surgical management of conventional grade I chondrosarcoma of long bones. *Clin Orthop Relat Res* 2007;463:166.

80. van der Geest IC, de Valk MH, de Rooy JW, et al. Oncological and functional results of cryosurgical therapy of enchondromas and chondrosarcomas grade 1. *J Surg Oncol* 2008;98(6):421.

81. Marcove RC. A 17-year review of cryosurgery in the treatment of bone tumors. *Clin Orthop Relat Res* 1982;(163):231–234.

82. Streitbürger A, Ahrens H, Balke M, et al. Grade I chondrosarcoma of bone: the Münster experience. *J Cancer Res Clin Oncol* 2009;135(4):543.

83. Wirbel RJ, Schulte M, Maier B, et al. Chondrosarcoma of the pelvis: oncologic and functional outcome. *Sarcoma* 2000;4(4):161.

84. Mitchell AD, Ayoub K, Mangham DC, et al. Experience in the treatment of dedifferentiated chondrosarcoma. *J Bone Joint Surg Br* 2000;82(1):55–61.

85. Cesari M, Bertoni F, Bacchini P, et al. Mesenchymal chondrosarcoma. An analysis of patients treated at a single institution. *Tumori* 2007;93(5):423–427.

86. Dantonello TM, Int-Veen C, Leuschner I, et al. Mesenchymal chondrosarcoma of soft tissues and bone in children, adolescents, and young adults: experiences of the CWS and COSS study groups. *Cancer* 2008;112(11): 2424–2431.

87. Goda JS, Ferguson PC, O'Sullivan B, et al. High-risk extracranial chondrosarcoma: long-term results of surgery and radiation therapy. *Cancer* 2011;117:2513–2519.

88. York JE, Berk RH, Fuller GN, et al. Chondrosarcoma of the spine: 1954 to 1997. *J Neurosurg* 1999;90(1 Suppl):73–78.

89. Noël G, Habrand JL, Jauffret E, et al. Radiation therapy for chordoma and chondrosarcoma of the skull base and the cervical spine. Prognostic factors and patterns of failure. *Strahlenther Onkol* 2003;179(4):241–248.

90. Austin-Seymour M, Munzenrider J, Goitein M, et al. Fractionated proton radiation therapy of chordoma and low-grade chondrosarcoma of the base of the skull. *J Neurosurg* 1989;70(1):13–17.

91. Hug EB, Loredo LN, Slater JD, et al. Proton radiation therapy for chordomas and chondrosarcomas of the skull base. *J Neurosurg* 1999;91(3): 432–439.

92. Rosenberg AE, Nielsen GP, Keel SB, et al. Chondrosarcoma of the base of the skull: a clinicopathologic study of 200 cases with emphasis on its distinction from chordoma. *Am J Surg Pathol* 1999;23(11):1370–1378.

93. Ares C, Hug EB, Lomax AJ, et al. Effectiveness and safety of spot scanning proton radiation therapy for chordomas and chondrosarcomas of the skull base: first long-term report. *Int J Radiat Oncol Biol Phys* 2009;75(4): 1111–1118.

94. Schulz-Ertner D, Nikoghosyan A, Hof H, et al. Carbon ion radiotherapy of skull base chondrosarcomas. *Int J Radiat Oncol Biol Phys* 2007;67(1): 171–177.

95. Debus J, Schulz-Ertner D, Schad L, et al. Stereotactic fractionated radiotherapy for chordomas and chondrosarcomas of the skull base. *Int J Radiat Oncol Biol Phys* 2000;47(3):591–596.

96. Lee FY, Mankin HJ, Fondren G, et al. Chondrosarcoma of bone: an assessment of outcome. *J Bone Joint Surg Am* 1999;81(3):326–338.

97. McMaster ML, Goldstein AM, Bromley CM, et al. Chordoma: incidence and survival patterns in the United States, 1973–1995. *Cancer Causes Control* 2001;12(1):1–11.

98. Tirabosco R, Mangham DC, Rosenberg AE, et al. Brachyury expression in extra-axial skeletal and soft tissue chordomas: a marker that distinguishes chordoma from mixed tumor/myoepithelioma/parachordoma in soft tissue. *Am J Surg Pathol* 2008;32(4):572–580.

99. Rich TA, Schiller A, Suit HD, et al. Clinical and pathologic review of 48 cases of chordoma. *Cancer* 1985;56(1):182–187.

100. Higinbotham NL, Phillips RF, Farr HW, et al. Chordoma: thirty-five-year study at Memorial Hospital. *Cancer* 1967;20(11):1841–1850.

101. Catton C, O'Sullivan B, Bell R, et al. Chordoma: long-term follow-up after radical photon irradiation. *Radiother Oncol* 1996;41(1):67–72.

102. Chambers PW, Schwinn CP. Chordoma. A clinicopathologic study of metastasis. *Am J Clin Pathol* 1979;72(5):765–776.

103. Fagundes MA, Hug EB, Liebsch NJ, et al. Radiation therapy for chordomas of the base of skull and cervical spine: patterns of failure and outcome after relapse. *Int J Radiat Oncol Biol Phys* 1995;33(3):579–584.

104. Chugh R, Tawbi H, Lucas DR, et al. Chordoma: the nonsarcoma primary bone tumor. *Oncologist* 2007;12(11):1344–1350.

105. Yu E, Koffer PP, DiPetrillo TA, et al. Incidence, treatment, and survival patterns for sacral chordoma in the United States, 1974–2011. *Front Oncol* 2016; 6:203.

106. Boriani S, Bandiera S, Biagini R, et al. Chordoma of the mobile spine: fifty years of experience. *Spine (Phila Pa 1976)* 2006;31(4):493–503.

107. Tzortzidis F, Elahi F, Wright D, et al. Patient outcome at long-term follow-up after aggressive microsurgical resection of cranial base chordomas. *Neurosurgery* 2006;59(2):230–237.

108. Gay E, Sekhar LN, Rubinstein E, et al. Chordomas and chondrosarcomas of the cranial base: results and follow-up of 60 patients. *Neurosurgery* 1995;36(5):887–896.

109. Devin C, Chong PY, Holt GE, et al. Level-adjusted perioperative risk of sacral amputations. *J Surg Oncol* 2006;94(3):203–211.

110. Cheng EY, Ozerdemoglu RA, Transfeldt EE, et al. Lumbosacral chordoma. Prognostic factors and treatment. *Spine (Phila Pa 1976)* 1999;24(16): 1639–1645.

111. Terahara A, Niemierko A, Goitein M, et al. Analysis of the relationship between tumor dose inhomogeneity and local control in patients with skull base chordoma. *Int J Radiat Oncol Biol Phys* 1999;45(2):351–358.

112. Noël G, Feuvret L, Calugaru V, et al. Chordomas of the base of the skull and upper cervical spine. One hundred patients irradiated by a 3D conformal technique combining photon and proton beams. *Acta Oncol* 2005;44(7): 700–708.

113. DeLaney TF, Liebsch NJ, Pedlow FX, et al. Phase II study of high-dose photon/proton radiotherapy in the management of spine sarcomas. *Int J Radiat Oncol Biol Phys* 2009;74(3):732–739.

114. Rutz HP, Weber DC, Sugahara S, et al. Extracranial chordoma: outcome in patients treated with function-preserving surgery followed by spot-scanning proton beam irradiation. *Int J Radiat Oncol Biol Phys* 2007;67(2): 512–520.

115. Tamborini E, Miselli F, Negri T, et al. Molecular and biochemical analyses of platelet-derived growth factor receptor (PDGFR) B, PDGFRA, and KIT receptors in chordomas. *Clin Cancer Res* 2006;12(23):6920–6928.

116. Weinberger PM, Yu Z, Kowalski D, et al. Differential expression of epidermal growth factor receptor, c-Met, and HER2/neu in chordoma compared with 17 other malignancies. *Arch Otolaryngol Head Neck Surg* 2005;131(8): 707–711.

117. Casali PG, Messina A, Stacchiotti S, et al. Imatinib mesylate in chordoma. *Cancer* 2004;101(9):2086–2097.

118. Hof H, Welzel T, Debus J. Effectiveness of cetuximab/gefitinib in the therapy of a sacral chondroma. *Onkologie* 2006;29(12):572–574.

119. Schulz-Ertner D, Karger CP, Feuerhake A, et al. Effectiveness of carbon ion radiotherapy in the treatment of skull-base chordomas. *Int J Radiat Oncol Biol Phys* 2007;68(2):449–457.

120. Kano H, Iqbal FO, Sheehan J, et al. Stereotactic radiosurgery for chordoma: a report from the North American Gamma Knife Consortium. *Neurosurgery* 2011;68(2):379–389.

121. Osler P, Bredella MA, Hess KA, et al. Sacral insufficiency fractures are common after high-dose radiation for sacral chordomas treated with or without surgery. *Clin Orthop Relat Res* 2016;474(3):766–772.

122. Dorfman HD, Czerniak B. Bone cancers. *Cancer* 1995;75(1 Suppl):203–210.

123. Bramwell VH, Steward WP, Nooij M, et al. Neoadjuvant chemotherapy with doxorubicin and cisplatin in malignant fibrous histiocytoma of bone: a European Osteosarcoma Intergroup study. *J Clin Oncol* 1999;17(10):3260–3269.

124. Feuvret L, Bracci S, Calugaru V, et al. Efficacy and safety of adjuvant proton therapy combined with surgery for chondrosarcoma of the skull base: a retrospective, population-based study. *Int J Radiat Oncol Biol Phys* 2016;95(1):312–321.

125. Weber DC, Badiyan S, Malyapa R, et al. Long-term outcomes and prognostic factors of skull-base chondrosarcoma patients treated with pencil-beam scanning proton therapy at the Paul Scherrer Institute. *Neuro Oncol* 2016;18(2): 236–243.

126. McDonald MW, Linton OR, Moore MG, et al. Influence of residual tumor volume and radiation dose coverage in outcomes for clival chordoma. *Int J Radiat Oncol Biol Phys* 2016;95(1):304–311.

127. Uhl M, Mattke M, Welzel T, et al. Highly effective treatment of skull base chordoma with carbon ion irradiation using a raster scan technique in 155 patients: first long-term results. *Cancer* 2014;120(21):3410–3417.

128. Uhl M, Mattke M, Welzel T, et al. High control rate in patients with chondrosarcoma of the skull base after carbon ion therapy: first report of long-term results. *Cancer* 2014;120(10):1579–1585.

129. Kano H, Sheehan J, Sneed PK, et al. Skull base chondrosarcoma radiosurgery: report of the North American Gamma Knife Consortium. *J Neurosurg* 2015;123(5):1268–1275.

130. Sahgal A, Chan MW, Atenafu EG, et al. Image-guided, intensity-modulated radiation therapy (IG-IMRT) for skull base chordoma and chondrosarcoma: preliminary outcomes. *Neuro Oncol* 2015;17(6):889–894.

131. Indelicato DJ, Rotondo RL, Begosh-Mayne D, et al. A prospective outcomes study of proton therapy for chordomas and chondrosarcomas of the spine. *Int J Radiat Oncol Biol Phys* 2016;95(1):297–303.

132. Zabel-du Bois A, Nikoghosyan A, Schwahofer A, et al. Intensity modulated radiotherapy in the management of sacral chordoma in primary versus recurrent disease. *Radiother Oncol* 2010;97(3):408–412.

133. Imai R, Kamada T, Tsuji H, et al.; Working Group for Bone and Soft Tissue Sarcomas. Effect of carbon ion radiotherapy for sacral chordoma: results of phase I-II and phase II clinical trials. *Int J Radiat Oncol Biol Phys* 2010;77(5):1470–1476.

134. Imai R, Kamada T, Araki N, et al. Carbon ion radiation therapy for unresectable sacral chordoma: an analysis of 188 cases. *Int J Radiat Oncol Biol Phys* 2016;95(1):322–327.

135. Schoenthaler R, Castro JR, Petti PL, et al. Charged particle irradiation of sacral chordomas. *Int J Radiat Oncol Biol Phys* 1993;26(2):291–298.

Section
III

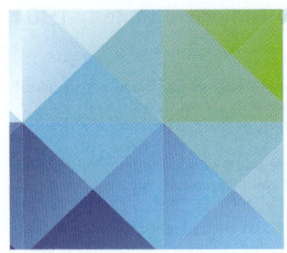

CHAPTER 87

Soft Tissue Sarcoma (Excluding Retroperitoneum)

Elizabeth H. Baldini

INCIDENCE

Soft tissue sarcomas (STS) constitute a heterogeneous group of rare malignancies that vary extensively by anatomic location, histology, and biologic behavior. They can occur at any anatomic site and may arise from many soft tissues including connective tissues, fat, muscle, vascular tissue, peripheral neural tissue, or visceral tissue. Annually, there are about 12,400 expected new cases of STS in the United States, and this accounts for approximately 0.7% of all new cancer diagnoses.[1] The median age at diagnosis for all STS is 65 years, but incidence varies by histologic subtype.[2] For example, embryonal rhabdomyosarcoma is common in children; synovial sarcoma occurs mostly in young adults; and undifferentiated pleomorphic sarcoma, liposarcoma, and leiomyosarcoma are seen mostly in older adults.

ETIOLOGY AND GENETICS

For the great majority of STS, there is no known etiology. A minority of cases can be attributed to environmental or genetic factors.[2] Associated environmental factors include radiation exposure; chemical exposures, such as vinyl chloride, dioxin, arsenical pesticides, and phenoxy herbicides; immunosuppression; lymphedema (Stewart-Treves syndrome); and viruses (human immunodeficiency virus, human herpesvirus type 8). Certain clinical syndromes are associated with a genetic predisposition for the development of sarcoma. A few examples include Li-Fraumeni syndrome and Werner syndrome, which are associated with the development of STS as well as other malignancies; neurofibromatosis type 1, which is associated with the development of malignant peripheral nerve sheath tumors; and familial adenomatous polyposis (Gardner syndrome), which is associated with the development of abdominal desmoid tumors.

HISTOLOGIC CLASSIFICATION

The World Health Organization divides soft tissue tumors into four categories: benign; intermediate, locally aggressive (e.g., desmoid fibromatosis); intermediate, rarely metastasizing (e.g., plexiform fibrohistiocytic tumor); and malignant. There are more than 50 histologic subtypes of STS. The most common subtypes include undifferentiated pleomorphic sarcoma, liposarcoma, leiomyosarcoma, myxofibrosarcoma, synovial sarcoma, and malignant peripheral nerve sheath tumor. Together, these account for about 75% of STS cases.[2] Histologic diagnosis is determined largely by tumor cell morphology. Immunohistochemical staining helps refine the diagnosis in many cases, and, increasingly, several of the histologic subtypes have characteristic chromosome translocations and gene rearrangements. Some of these characteristic translocations include Ewing sarcoma, t(11,22); synovial sarcoma, t(X,18); myxoid liposarcoma, t(12,16); and clear cell sarcoma, t(12,22).[2] There are several grading systems. The two most widely used are the US National Cancer Institute (NCI) and the French Federation Nationale des Centres de Lutte Contre le Cancer (FNCLCC) grading systems, both of which employ a three-tiered system of low, intermediate, and high grade based on mitotic activity, necrosis, and differentiation.[3] The

College of American Pathologists prefers the FNCLCC system as it is easier to use and more reproducible and may be a better predictor of prognosis.[4] Lastly, there are certain STS subtypes for which grading is not applicable.[2]

Given the rarity of STS as well as the numerous histologic subtypes, it is not surprising that diagnoses vary even among STS specialists. Several reports have examined concordance rates for histologic diagnosis or grade among pathologists. Agreement rates between nonspecialists and specialists range from 24% to 68%.[5-9] Even among sarcoma specialists, concordance rates can vary from 60% to 90%.[10,11] For this reason, it is very important to submit diagnostic slides for review by an experienced sarcoma pathologist prior to embarking on definitive treatment.

NATURAL HISTORY

STS can occur anywhere in the body. The most common site of presentation is an extremity, specifically the thigh. The approximate distribution of STS sites at presentation is extremity, 60% (lower extremity, 45%, upper extremity, 15%); trunk, 15% to 20%; retroperitoneum, 10% to 15%; and head and neck, 9%.[12] Interestingly, certain histologic subtypes have predilections for specific sites. For example, angiosarcoma commonly occurs in the head and neck, desmoid tumors frequently occur in the abdomen associated with Gardner syndrome, and epithelioid carcinoma often involves the hand or forearm.[13-15]

In the classic reports by Simon and Enneking[16] and Enneking et al.,[17] the local behavior of STS is well described. STS tends to invade longitudinally along musculoaponeurotic planes. These tumors rarely transgress fascial boundaries or invade bone. As the sarcoma grows, it compresses surrounding normal tissue to form a pseudocapsule, which contains a compression zone and a reactive zone. The latter comprises edema, inflammatory cells, and tumor cells. Furthermore, Simon and Enneking[16] have shown that microscopic tumor cells perforate through and extend beyond the pseudocapsule.

Unlike most solid tumors, STS rarely spread to lymph nodes. Three series, each with more than 1,000 consecutive patients with STS, cited only 1.8% to 3.7% of lymph node involvement at the time of initial presentation.[18-20] However, there are a few histologic subtypes for which lymph node involvement is more common. Notable lymph node involvement rates have been demonstrated for Clear cell sarcoma (10% to 18%), cutaneous Angiosarcoma (10% to 15%), Rhabdomyosarcoma (20% to 25%), and Epithelioid sarcoma (20% to 35%); these histologic subtypes can be remembered by the pneumonic "CARE."[13,19,23]

The American College of Surgeons Patterns of Care Study for adult STS showed 23% of patients had metastatic disease at presentation.[12] The single most frequent site of distant metastasis (34%) was the lung; bone, liver, and brain involvement were less common. Furthermore, as was the case for lymph node spread, certain histologic subtypes exhibit distinct patterns of recurrence. For example, myxoid liposarcoma has a predilection for spread to retroperitoneum, other extrapulmonary soft tissue sites, and bone. Among reported recurrences, about 50% occur in the retroperitoneum, 20% in other extrapulmonary soft tissue, and 15% to 17% in the bone.[24,25] For retroperitoneal STS, the most common site of recurrence is locally in the retroperitoneum.[26] These tumors also have a predilection for spread to the liver as well as the lung.[26]

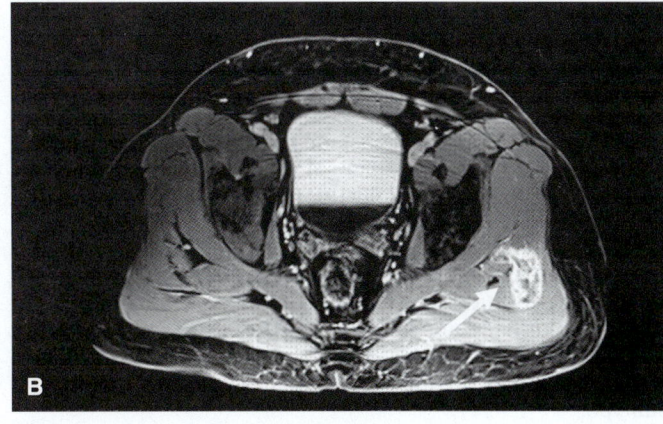

FIGURE 87.1. Comparison of computed tomography (CT) and magnetic resonance imaging (MRI) axial slices for a synovial sarcoma of the left gluteus medius muscle (denoted by *arrows*) in a 56-year-old man. **A:** The CT axial slice shows a vaguely defined soft tissue mass in the left gluteus medius muscle. **B:** The anatomic definition of the soft tissue sarcoma is seen much more clearly on the corresponding T1 postgadolinium axial slice of the MRI.

Epithelioid sarcoma can present with skip metastases involving discontiguous locations in a limb as well as lymph node involvement.[2,15,21] Lastly, myxofibrosarcoma exhibits an infiltrative growth pattern and is associated with higher rates of positive resection margins and local recurrence (LR) compared to other STS histologic subtypes; conversely, the rate of distant recurrence to lung is lower than for other STS types.[7,27–30]

INITIAL EVALUATION

Most STS cases present as a painless mass. When taking a history, one should ask how long the mass has been present, if it has changed in size and at what rate, and if there are any associated local or systemic symptoms. It is also important to ask about potential risk factors for STS, including a history of radiation exposure or a family history of malignancies including STS. On physical examination, one should assess the mass for characteristics such as size, depth, fixation to underlying structures, the presence of overlying skin changes, and potential evidence of neurovascular compromise. On the general examination, one should also note if there are any stigmata of neurofibromatosis, such as neurofibromas or café au lait spots (as there is an association between neurofibromatosis type I and malignant peripheral nerve sheath tumors).[2]

Imaging workup should include evaluation of the primary site as well as sites of potential metastatic spread. For STS of the extremity, trunk, or head and neck, evaluation of the primary tumor with a magnetic resonance imaging (MRI) scan is generally preferred to computed tomography (CT) scanning.[31,32] The T1-weighted images of the MRI scan provide excellent definition of the anatomic relation between the tumor and adjacent structures. T2-weighted images demonstrate the tumor and any associated edema. As peritumoral edema can contain malignant cells, it is important to identify this for both radiation and surgical planning.[33] Demas et al.[31] compared MRI and CT for STS lesions in the extremity and reported that for 23% of cases, the MRI scans showed tumor involvement in muscles that appeared normal on CT scan. On the other hand, a prospective study reported by Panicek et al. showed no significant difference between the two imaging modalities when performed for preoperative evaluation.[34] Nonetheless, most practitioners believe that MRI is superior to CT for evaluation of soft tissue tumors of the extremity, trunk, and head and neck. Figure 87.1 depicts a case of synovial sarcoma of the left gluteus medius muscle. The mass is difficult to discern on CT imaging (Fig. 87.1A) but very clearly delineated on MRI (Fig. 87.1B). Figure 87.2 is a second comparative example of CT and MRI and shows a leiomyosarcoma of the proximal anterior thigh. Although, the differences between the imaging modalities are not as pronounced as in Figure 87.1, the MRI again provides superior information compared to the CT scan. The MRI demonstrates probable arterial wall

FIGURE 87.2. Comparison of computed tomography (CT) and magnetic resonance imaging (MRI) axial slices for a high-grade leiomyosarcoma of the proximal anterior thigh (denoted by *arrows*) in a 53-year-old man. **A:** The CT axial slice shows a soft tissue mass in the left anterior upper thigh anterior to the superficial femoral artery and vein. **B:** The T1 postgadolinium image of the MRI at the same level provides superior resolution compared to the CT. It shows a loss of fat plane between the mass and the superficial femoral artery suggestive of arterial invasion (*long arrow*), linear fascial enhancement overlying the vastus medialis muscle (*short arrow*), and tumor spiculations into adjacent subcutaneous fat and to the skin along the biopsy tract.

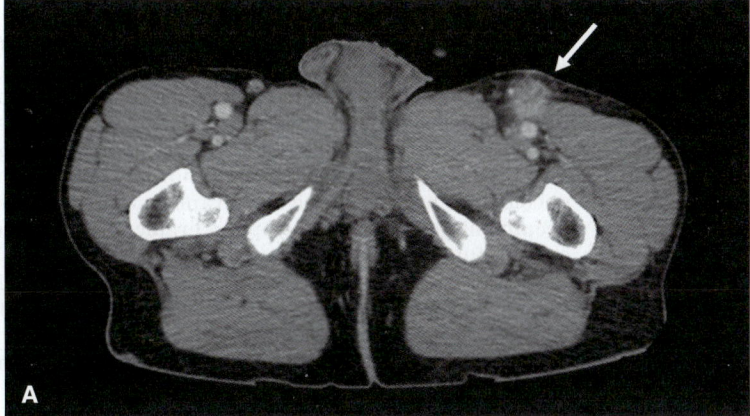
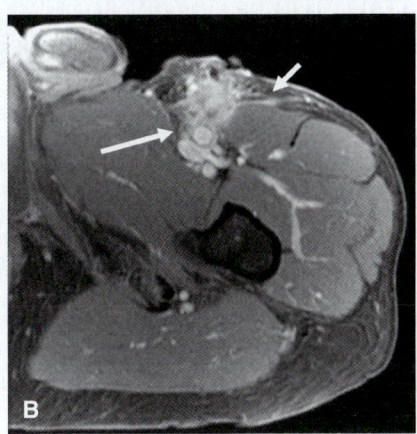

invasion, fascial enhancement of the vastus medialis muscle, and definition of tumor spiculations into the adjacent fat and along the biopsy tract. Chest CT scan is recommended to rule out pulmonary metastases for all cases except low-grade tumors or small (<5 cm) high-grade lesions, and even in these latter cases, it can be helpful to obtain a baseline chest CT at diagnosis. Currently, there is no clearly defined role for positron emission tomography (PET) as part of the diagnostic evaluation. However, PET scanning may have potential utility to help distinguish malignant peripheral nerve sheath tumors from benign neurofibromas in patients with neurofibromatosis.[35] Lastly, given that myxoid liposarcoma has a predilection for spread to bone and soft tissue, MRI of the spine and CT of the abdomen and pelvis are recommended as part of the initial evaluation for high-risk patients with this histologic subtype.[24,25,36]

CT-guided core biopsy is the desired diagnostic approach as it is accurate, safe, and expeditious.[37] Incisional biopsy is accurate and acceptable, but it is more invasive than core biopsy. If utilized, incisional biopsies should be performed carefully with the subsequent definitive resection in mind.[38] Tumor cells can potentially seed an incision, thereby necessitating removal of skin incisions at the time of surgical resection. It is important that the biopsy approach does not transgress an uninvolved compartment or joint as this would create a situation where a much more radical resection would need to be performed. Consequences of inappropriately placed incisional biopsies can be significant and include the need to perform more complex operations, with the potential for subsequent loss of function, LR, and death.[38] Fine needle aspirate (FNA) can confirm malignancy for recurrent disease, but typically does not yield enough tissue to establish an initial diagnosis.

STAGING

In 2017, the American Joint Committee on Cancer (AJCC) published the eighth edition of the TNMG (tumor, node, metastasis, grade) staging system for STS.[36] There are several changes compared to the seventh edition including new separate staging systems for STS of (a) extremity and trunk, (b) retroperitoneum, (c) head and neck, and (d) visceral sites. For the extremity and trunk sites, grade, tumor size, and lymph node and distant organ involvement all remain elements of the staging system. There are now four T size categories rather than two: ≤5 cm, >5 to 10 cm, >10 to 15 cm, and >15 cm. Depth has been removed as a staging factor. Histologic subtype is still not included as a category. Lastly, there are new stage groupings including the movement of nodal involvement (N1) from stage III to stage IV. The 8th edition AJCC extremity and trunk STS stage groupings are shown in Table 87.1.

TABLE 87.1 AMERICAN JOINT COMMITTEE ON CANCER TNMG STAGE GROUPINGS FOR EXTREMITY AND TRUNK SOFT TISSUE SARCOMA, 8TH EDITION

Stage IA	G1,X	T1	N0	M0	Low Grade, Small
Stage IB	G1,X	T2-4	N0	M0	Low grade, large
Stage II	G2,3	T1	N0	M0	Moderate/high grade, small
Stage IIIA	G2,3	T2	N0	M0	Moderate/high grade, intermediate
Stage IIIB	G2,3	T3-4	N0	M0	Moderate/high grade, large
Stage IV	Any Grade	Any T	N1	M0	Nodal involvement
	Any Grade	Any T	Any N	M1	Metastatic

G, grade; GX, grade cannot be assessed; M0, no distant metastasis; M1, distant metastasis; NX, regional lymph nodes (LN) cannot be assessed; N0, no regional LN metastasis; N1, regional LN metastasis; T1, tumor ≤5 cm; T2, tumor >5 to 10 cm; T3, tumor >10 to 15 cm; T4, tumor >15 cm. From Amin MB, Edge SB, Greene FL, et al., eds. *AJCC cancer staging manual.* 8th ed. New York: Springer, 2017. Reproduced with permission of Springer International Publishing in the format Book via Copyright Clearance Center.

PROGNOSTIC FACTORS FOR SURVIVAL AND LOCAL RECURRENCE

Many reports have evaluated patient and tumor characteristics to determine prognostic factors for disease-free survival (DFS) or overall survival (OS) and local recurrence (LR). The most powerful predictor for DFS and OS is the AJCC TNMG stage of the tumor. Survival rates are not yet available for the 8th edition, but 5-year DFS rates for AJCC seventh edition stages I, II, and III STS are 86%, 72%, and 52%, respectively.[39] The staging system incorporates most of the relevant prognostic variables. It is also valuable to consider predictive factors individually. The single most important individual prognostic factor for lower survival rates is high grade.[40-45] Five-year DFS rates range from 44% to 67% for high-grade tumors compared to 90% to 100% for low-grade tumors.[40-42] Other significant predictors for DFS include tumor size and site.[40,42-45] For a series of 1,091 patients from MD Anderson Cancer Center, 5-year OS rates were 85% for tumors ≤5 cm, 68% for tumors >5 to 15 cm, and 52% for tumors >15 cm.[44] Furthermore, patients with tumors located in the head and neck or retroperitoneum have lower survival rates than those with tumors located in the extremity or superficial trunk.[41,45,46] Histologic subtype is predictive of both OS and DFS in several reports.[40,43,44,46,47] Callegaro et al. developed two robust nomograms to predict OS and DFS for extremity STS and demonstrated adverse survivals for vascular tumors, leiomyosarcoma, synovial sarcoma and malignant peripheral nerve sheath tumor compared to all liposarcoma subtypes, myxofibrosarcoma, and undifferentiated pleomorphic sarcoma.[43] It now appears that tumor depth (superficial or deep to fascia) is not a prognostic factor, and accordingly, depth has been removed from the staging system.[43,45,48] Older age at presentation, positive resection margins, bone or neurovascular invasion, gender, and race all show mixed results regarding their predictive value for DFS.[40-46] As stated earlier, lymph node involvement for STS is rare, but if present, it is an adverse prognostic factor.[18-20]

Consistently demonstrated significant predictors for LR include positive margins of resection, presentation with locally recurrent disease, older age, and head and neck or retroperitoneal location. Rates of LR for tumors resected with positive margins range from 28% to 56% compared to 0% to 20% for those with negative margins.[30,40,41,49-54] Patients who present with locally recurrent disease are at higher risk for subsequent LR (25% to 47%) than are those who present with primary disease (11% to 21%).[40,50] Age has been analyzed with varying cutoff values including >50 years, >64 years, and as a continuous variable. Repeatedly, older age has been associated with higher LR rates.[40,41,55]

MANAGEMENT AND OUTCOME FOR SOFT TISSUE SARCOMAS OF EXTREMITY AND TRUNK

Because of the rarity of STS and the numerous forms in which it can present with respect to tumor histology, site, and size, there are many nuances related to optimal management. Furthermore, delivery of treatment requires a multimodality team that includes experienced pathologists; radiologists; surgeons from the disciplines of surgical oncology, orthopedics, and reconstructive surgery; radiation oncologists; medical oncologists; nurses; physical therapists; and social workers. Treatment goals include complete eradication of tumor with optimal function preservation and minimal treatment-related toxicities. Execution of these goals is complex, and, for this reason, STS is best treated by an experienced team at a specialized sarcoma center. Reports from Sweden, the United Kingdom, the United States, and Canada have shown superior outcomes for STS treated at specialized centers.[56-60]

Surgery

In almost all cases, appropriate surgical resection is a prerequisite for curative treatment of STS. A range of surgical procedures has been employed for the treatment of STS with varying levels of success. These procedures include marginal resection or excisional biopsy, wide resection, and radical resection or amputation. A marginal resection refers to simple removal of the tumor with its pseudocapsule. This is also often described as a "shell-out" or "whoops" procedure and is commonly performed when the diagnosis of STS is not suspected. LR rates after marginal resection range from 50% to 93%.[17,61,62] This is not surprising as it is known that microscopic tumor cells can extend beyond the pseudocapsule and up to several centimeters beyond palpable gross tumor.[16,33] Marginal resection is not an appropriate treatment.

At the other end of the spectrum is radical resection, which involves removal of all of the muscles and neurovascular structures within the compartment where the tumor resides or amputation. Reported LR rates after radical resection are much lower and range from 0% to 18%.[17,51,61,62] These LR rates are acceptable, but the cost of loss of limb (or loss of an entire compartment) is high. Amputation was a common procedure for STS of the extremities up to the 1970s.

The intermediate procedure is a wide resection. Wide resection is also described as conservative surgery (CS), limb-sparing surgery, or function-sparing surgery. It involves *en bloc* removal of tumor with a desired rim of normal tissue varying in width from about 1 cm to several centimeters depending on anatomic constraints. This procedure preserves good function (limb salvage) but as a treatment by itself is usually associated with moderately high LR rates, ranging from 25% to 60%.[17,61,62]

Wide resection/CS combined with pre- or postoperative radiation therapy (RT) is the current standard of care for most high-grade STS. Surgeons should attempt to attain negative margins at the time of definitive resection. As previously stated, the presence of positive margins is consistently associated with increased LR rates even when RT is used.[40,41,49-54,63] Because STS is so rare in comparison to benign soft tissue lesions, the initial procedure performed for an STS is often an unplanned excision (shell-out) with resulting positive margins. It is important to perform a definitive re-excision in these situations, if possible, as the likelihood of finding significant residual disease is on the order of 24% to 63%.[8,64-67] As part of the re-resection, incisions, biopsy tracts, drain sites, and any tissues contaminated by the first surgery need to be removed *en bloc* along with tumor-bed margins. Unfortunately, this often results in a greater scope of surgery and increased functional deficit than if an initial planned excision had been performed by an experienced oncologic surgeon.[38] Lastly, although the goal of resection is to attain negative margins, if this would require debilitating surgery, such as resection of a nerve, vessel, or bone, a function-sparing approach with a planned positive margin is acceptable. These decisions are best handled by experienced sarcoma surgeons. Gerrand et al.[52] compared LR rates resulting from procedures with planned positive margins (abutting critical structures) to those of procedures with unplanned (unexpected) positive margins. They found a 4% LR rate for the former compared with a 32% to 38% LR rate for the latter.

Conservative Surgery and Radiation Therapy

Three sentinel randomized trials have been performed and have established RT combined with CS as the standard management for most (high-grade) STS of the extremities and trunk (Table 87.2). The first of these trials was conducted by Rosenberg et al.[51] at the NCI. Patients with high-grade STS of the extremity were randomized to amputation or to CS and postoperative external-beam RT (60 to 70 Gy). Patients

TABLE 87.2 RANDOMIZED CONTROLLED TRIALS INCLUDING RADIATION THERAPY FOR SOFT TISSUE SARCOMAS OF THE EXTREMITIES AND TRUNK

Study	Treatment Arms	Local Recurrence	OS or DFS
Rosenberg[51] NCI 1982 N = 43 (Extremity)	Amputation vs. CS + EBRT (60–70 Gy) (both arms received doxorubicin, cyclophosphamide, methotrexate)	0% (0/16) 15% (4/27) P = .06	88% 83% P = .99 (5-year OS)
Pisters[63] MSKCC 1996 N = 164 (Extremity + trunk)	High grade (n = 119) CS vs. CS + BRT (42–45 Gy) Low grade (n = 45) CS vs. CS + BRT (42–45 Gy)	30% (19/63) 9% (5/56) P = .0025 26% (6/23) 36% (8/22) P = .49	All patients 81% 84% P = .65 (5-year DFS)
Yang[68] NCI 1998 N = 141 (Extremity)	High grade (n = 91) CS vs. CS + EBRT (63 Gy) (both arms received doxorubicin, cyclophosphamide) Low grade (n = 50) CS vs. CS + EBRT (63 Gy)	19% (9/47) 0% (0/44) P = .003 33% (8/24) 4% (1/26) P = .016	74% 75% P = .71 (10-year OS) 92% (22/24) 92% (24/26) (no. alive)
O'Sullivan[69,70] CSG 2004 N = 190 (Extremity)	Preop RT (50 Gy) + CS CS + postop RT (66 Gy)	7% 8% P = NS (5-year LR)	73% 67% P = .48 (5-year OS)

BRT, brachytherapy; CS, conservative (limb-sparing) surgery; CSG, Canadian Sarcoma Group; DFS, disease-free survival; EBRT, external-beam radiation therapy; MSKCC, Memorial Sloan-Kettering Cancer Center; NCI, National Cancer Institute; OS, overall survival; preop, preoperative; postop, postoperative.

in both treatment arms received postoperative doxorubicin, cyclophosphamide, and methotrexate; in the RT arm, chemotherapy was started 3 days prior to RT and continued concurrently with RT. LR rates were 0% (0 of 16) and 15% (4 of 27) for patients treated with amputation and with CS and RT, respectively (P = .06). There was no significant difference in survival rates. This trial was instrumental in setting a new standard for limb-sparing local management of STS. Amputations are now performed sparingly and in <15% of cases.[71,72]

The next question posed was whether adjuvant RT is necessary. Two hallmark trials randomized patients between CS alone and CS plus RT.[63,68] Both of these trials showed improved local control with the addition of RT. At the NCI, patients with high-grade STS of the extremity were randomized to treatment with CS and postoperative chemotherapy (doxorubicin and cyclophosphamide) with or without concurrent external beam RT (63 Gy). Patients with low-grade tumors were randomized to CS with or without postoperative external beam RT (63 Gy). LR rates for the high-grade tumors were 20% (9 of 44) for CS and chemotherapy compared to 0% (0 of 47) for CS, chemotherapy, and RT (P = .003). For the low-grade tumors, LR rates were 33% (8 of 24) for CS alone and 4% (1 of 26) for CS and RT (P = .016). There were no significant differences in survival rates between the two groups. An update of this trial confirmed the lack of survival difference with 20-year OS of 64% for CS alone and 71% for CS and RT (P = .22).[73] At Memorial Sloan-Kettering Cancer Center (MSKCC), patients with STS of the extremity and trunk were randomized to treatment with CS alone or CS plus adjuvant low dose rate brachytherapy (BRT).[63] BRT catheters were sewn into the tumor bed in a parallel array with 1-cm spacing between catheters and extension of catheters 1.5 to 2.0 cm beyond the tumor bed. Iridium-192 was loaded into the catheters, and a dose of 42 to 45 Gy was delivered over 4 to 6 days. LR rates for high-grade tumors were 30% (19 of 63) for CS alone compared with 9% (5 of 56) for CS plus BRT (P = .0025). No difference in LR rates by treatment was seen for low-grade tumors; rates were 26% (6 of 23) and 36% (8 of 22) for patients treated with CS alone and CS plus BRT, respectively. As in the two prior trials, there were no significant differences in survival outcomes. Given that BRT did not improve local control for low-grade tumors in this trial, BRT is typically not recommended for low-grade STS. Furthermore, for high-grade tumors treated with BRT, LR rates are higher in the setting of positive margins.[74] Therefore, BRT as monotherapy is only recommended for high-grade tumors resected with negative margins.(In the setting of positive resection margins, a combination of external beam RT and BRT or external beam RT alone is preferred.) These two randomized trials have established the role for RT combined with CS for the management of high-grade (and, in select cases, low-grade) STS. In modern series, local control following CS and RT is excellent, with most reported LR rates being <15%.[50,54,69,75–78] It is important to note that the current treatment recommendation for most low-grade STS of the extremity and trunk is wide excision alone.[79,80] As long as negative margins are obtained, LR rates are expected to be well under 20%. Relative indications for RT in the setting of low-grade tumors include situations of positive resection margins, locally recurrent disease following initial wide excision, and tumor location that would not be amenable to subsequent salvage surgery.

Radiation Therapy

Positioning the Patient

The first step of RT planning is to determine the appropriate positioning of the patient. It is important for the patient to be comfortable to ensure setup reproducibility. The multiple beam angles employed with intensity-modulated RT (IMRT)

techniques[81] enable more positioning options than would be the case for 3D-CRT techniques. In general, patients are placed in the supine position unless this places pressure on and deforms the tumor, in which case the prone position is used. Suitable positions for upper extremity lesions include supine with abduction of the arm away from the body with supination or pronation of the arm determined by the location of the tumor. Another good approach for upper extremity lesions is the "swimmer position," whereby the patient is prone with the arm extended above the head (Fig. 87.3A). For treatment of a leg, the ipsilateral leg should be straight, and the contralateral leg separated to create a gap (Fig. 87.3B). If the target is in the proximal leg, the contralateral leg can be in a frog-leg position with support under the knee. For men with proximal tumors, the genitalia should be pulled to the contralateral side (using mesh or other techniques). All men with treatment fields close to the genitalia should consider sperm banking if they wish to preserve fertility. Similarly, for cases with treatment fields close to the ovaries (e.g., tumors of proximal thigh, buttock, abdominal wall), woman interested in fertility preservation should be referred for reproductive counseling prior to starting RT. Tumors in the true anterior or posterior compartments of the leg are often the most challenging. Sometimes, the supine position with external rotation of the leg enables the use of predominantly obliquely oriented fields to achieve adequate target coverage and bone sparing. If this is not feasible, the decubitus position represents another option.

Once the position is determined, the patient must be immobilized in a reproducible fashion. A custom cast indexed to the table top is highly recommended for almost all scenarios; it

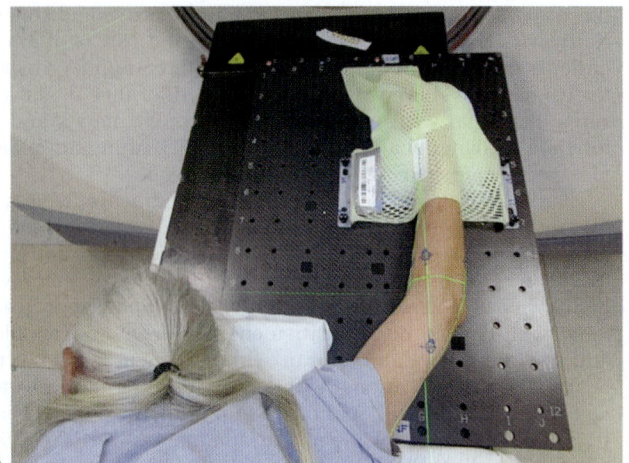

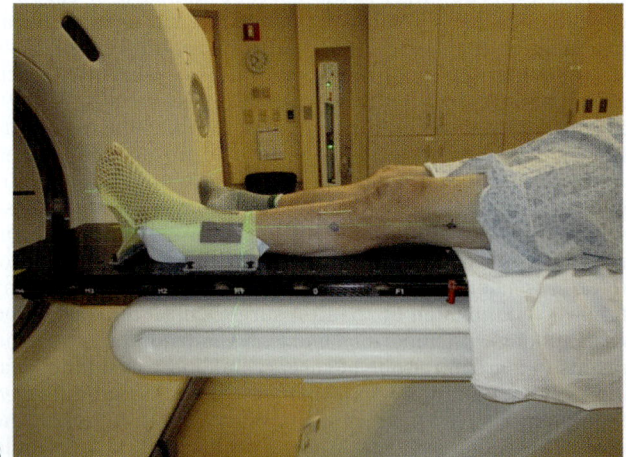

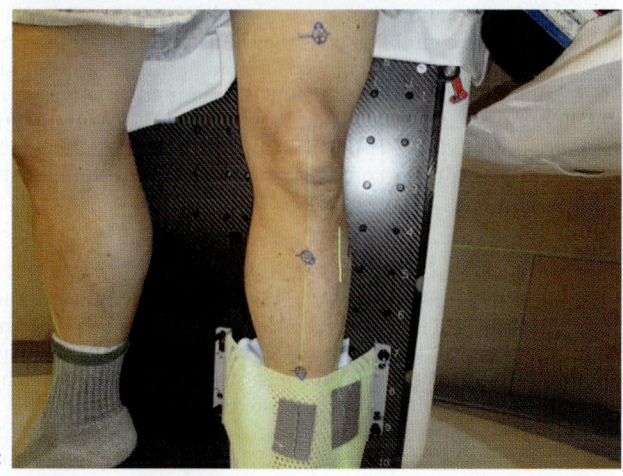

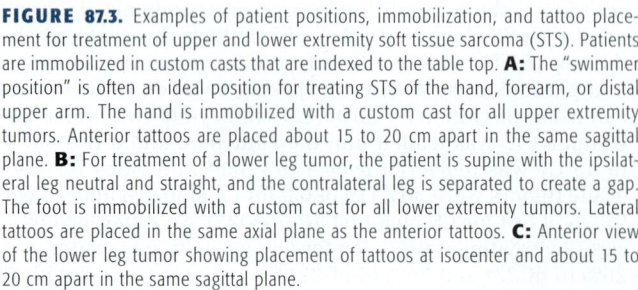

FIGURE 87.3. Examples of patient positions, immobilization, and tattoo placement for treatment of upper and lower extremity soft tissue sarcoma (STS). Patients are immobilized in custom casts that are indexed to the table top. **A:** The "swimmer position" is often an ideal position for treating STS of the hand, forearm, or distal upper arm. The hand is immobilized with a custom cast for all upper extremity tumors. Anterior tattoos are placed about 15 to 20 cm apart in the same sagittal plane. **B:** For treatment of a lower leg tumor, the patient is supine with the ipsilateral leg neutral and straight, and the contralateral leg is separated to create a gap. The foot is immobilized with a custom cast for all lower extremity tumors. Lateral tattoos are placed in the same axial plane as the anterior tattoos. **C:** Anterior view of the lower leg tumor showing placement of tattoos at isocenter and about 15 to 20 cm apart in the same sagittal plane.

is important to immobilize the foot with a custom mold for all lower extremity tumors and to immobilize the hand for all upper extremity tumors (Fig 87.3A and B). With respect to tattoo placement, a helpful protocol for extremities is to use 3 anterior tattoos and 3 lateral tattoos. The 3 anterior tattoos are placed about 15 to 20 cm apart in the same sagittal plane (Fig. 87.3A and C), and at each point, an additional lateral mark is placed in the same axial plane (Fig. 87.3B). The 6 tattoo points are all placed in a stable anatomical location for the primary purpose of reproducing the position of the entire length of the extremity, and the secondary purpose of creating a reference point for aligning the isocenter.

Target Volumes and Treatment Fields

Preoperative Radiation Therapy

Historically, treatment volumes for STS of the extremities and trunk were composed of large longitudinal margins of at least 5 cm and sometimes >10 cm with good success. Current standard of care target volumes for preoperative RT include gross tumor volume (GTV) defined as the gross tumor delineated by the T1 postgadolinium MRI. Fusion of the diagnostic MRI and planning CT for optimal target definition is strongly encouraged. Clinical target volume (CTV) is defined as the GTV plus 4-cm margins in the longitudinal directions and 1.5-cm margins radially.[82] These margins can be truncated if they extend

beyond the compartment or beyond an intact fascial barrier, bone, or skin. Editing target volumes 5 mm beneath skin surface is recommended in most scenarios to attain superficial dose avoidance. (Planned skin resection should be confirmed with the surgeon in this setting.) Peritumoral edema on T2 MRI will often be included within the CTV as defined above. If the edema is more extensive and appears suspicious, the CTV can be enlarged to include it at the discretion of the radiation oncologist. Of note, more clarity is needed to determine in which situations peritumoral edema should be included in the CTV. One report showed the presence of sarcoma cells beyond the gross tumor in 10 of 15 patients. The location of the cells varied from 1 to 4 cm beyond the tumor but did not correlate with the location or extent of peritumoral edema on MRI.[33] It is reasonable to try to include the edema in the CTV, unless so doing would require a significant increase in the treatment field. The planning target volume (PTV) is defined as the CTV plus 5 to 10 mm based on institution setup uncertainty. Figure 87.4 depicts MRI images and target volumes and for an STS of the right proximal medial thigh that was treated with preoperative IMRT.

Several series using treatment volumes similar to those described above have reported excellent local control rates on the order of 85% to 90%.[69,76–78,83] Furthermore, using these standard volumes, most LRs that occur are located within treatment fields rather than marginal to the fields.[76,77]

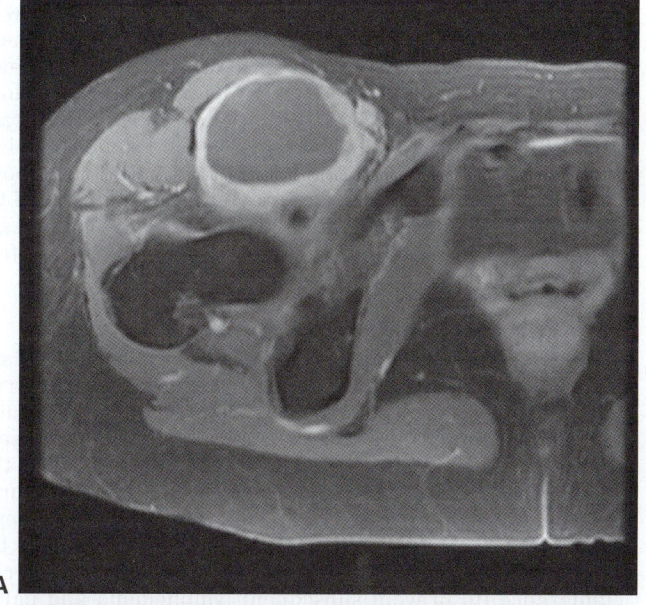

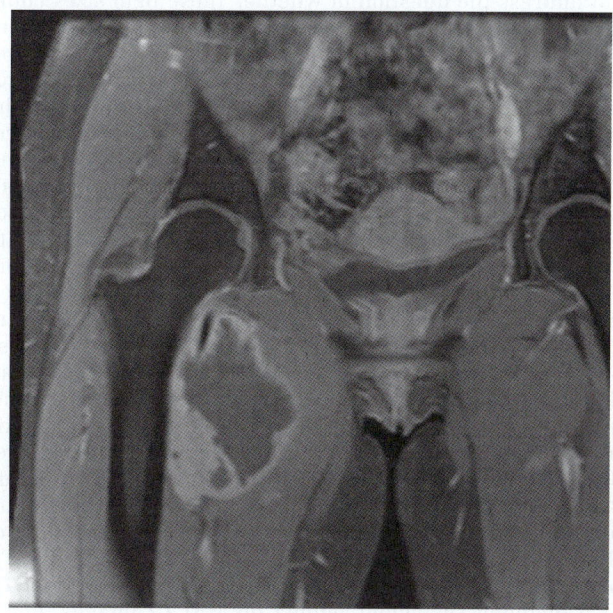

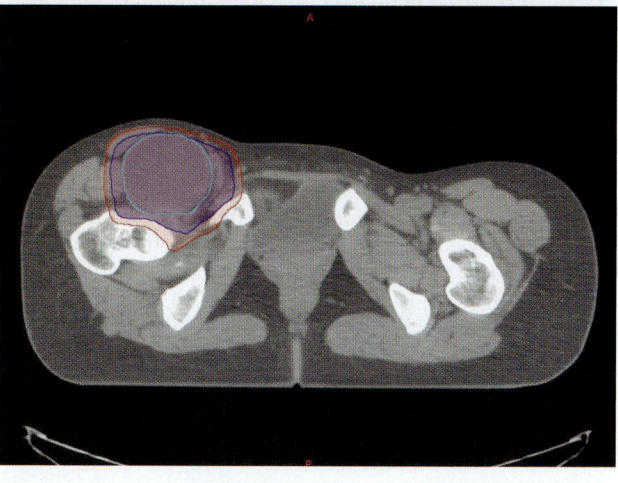

FIGURE 87.4. An unclassified pleomorphic high-grade sarcoma of the medial proximal right thigh in a 30-year-woman that was treated with preoperative IMRT (50 Gy). **A:** Axial T1 postgadolinium image of the magnetic resonance imaging (MRI) scan. **B:** Coronal T1 postgadolinium image of the MRI scan. **C:** Axial slice of the planning CT scan showing the gross tumor volume (GTV, *cyan*), clinical target volume (CTV, *purple*), and planning target volume (PTV, *red*).

Section III

Postoperative Radiation Therapy

For postoperative treatment, the nomenclature for GTV and CTV is variably described and partly a matter of semantics given that there is actually no "gross tumor." It can be helpful to draw a GTV in the location where the gross tumor was preoperatively, as sometimes this volume is used for cone-down volumes. It is also helpful to contour the operative bed. The CTV should encompass all the tissues handled during the surgery including the incision and any drain sites. (Postoperative changes seen on MRI help define the operative bed.) An additional longitudinal margin of 4 cm and a radial margin of 1.5 cm is generally added to the operative bed to form the CTV.[82] The same principles apply as listed above in terms of using the T1 postgadolinium images for GTV definition, fusing the planning CT and MRI when possible, and editing the CTV to exclude bone, an intact fascial planes, skin, or extension beyond an uncontaminated compartment. The PTV is typically CTV plus 5 to 10 mm, per institutional standard for set-up uncertainty. A second course field reduction is typically used in the postoperative setting. CTV margins for the reduced field (cone down) are generally 2 cm from the initial GTV. These postoperative treatment field definitions are associated with excellent local control rates and are the current standard of care.[69,76,83]

The excellent local control rates resulting from the use of standard preoperative and postoperative treatment fields establish that these fields are adequately large, but they do not address the question of whether these field sizes could be reduced. As such, the necessity of such large treatment fields has been called into question. Initial development of these large fields predated the CT and MRI era, when imaging modalities to define STS were suboptimal. Moreover, the BRT experience at MSKCC produced excellent local control rates using treatment volumes that extended only 1.5 to 2 cm beyond the tumor bed.[63] Lastly, several single-institution series of treatment with surgery alone have been associated with very good local control rates ranging from 0% to 20% (see the Surgery Alone section).[84–89] Specifically, Baldini et al.[85] found no recurrences in 36 patients with resection margins ≥1 cm compared to an actuarial 10-year LR rate of 13% (4 of 38) for those with margins <1 cm. Based on these observations, it is reasonable to query whether treatment field sizes can be reduced. Two studies have addressed this question. The first study is RTOG-0630, a phase II study using image-guided RT (IGRT) and reduced fields for preoperative RT for extremity STS. For tumors that were grade 2 to 3 and ≥8 cm, the CTV was defined as GTV plus 3-cm longitudinal and 1.5-cm radial margins, and for tumors that were grade 1 or <8 cm, the CTV was defined as GTV plus 2 cm longitudinal and 1 cm radial margins. The CTV also included suspicious edema on MRI T2 images. For a cohort of 79 patients, 2-year local control was 11% and all five LRs occurred within the treatment fields.[90] The authors conclude that because of the absence of marginal field recurrences, the reduced volumes were appropriate. These results are encouraging but require longer follow-up and external validation before widespread adoption of reduced volumes for preoperative RT is appropriate. The second trial is the VORTEX trial in which patients with extremity STS receiving postoperative RT were randomized to standard fields with GTV plus 5-cm longitudinal and 2-cm radial margins or to tailored fields of GTV plus 2 cm in all directions. Preliminary results presented in abstract form described a sample size of 216 patients, and 5-year local recurrence-free survival rates of 86% for standard fields and 84% for reduced fields (P = not significant).[91] Similar to the case above, these results are intriguing, but it is not appropriate to adopt reduced postoperative volumes based on early results of one study.

Brachytherapy

The CTV for BRT treatment as monotherapy should include the operative bed with a margin. The American Brachytherapy Society consensus statement describes an appropriate CTV as the surgical bed plus a 2-cm longitudinal margin and 1- to 2-cm lateral margin.[92] Similarly, the MSKCC randomized trial used margins of 1.5 to 2 cm beyond the tumor bed.[63] A more detailed description of BRT modalities, techniques, and indications is beyond the scope of this chapter. The American Brachytherapy Society consensus statement published in 2017 is a very good reference.[92]

Doses

The standard dose for preoperative external beam RT is 50 Gy delivered in 2-Gy fractions.[82] In the situation of positive margins, a postoperative external beam RT boost of 16 to 20 Gy (delivered in 1.8- to 2-Gy fractions) is sometimes delivered. The efficacy of this boost dose has not been proven and, as it may be associated with increased toxicity, its use has been called into question.[80,93,94] Other techniques to deliver an additional boost dose include BRT (both low dose rate and high dose rate) and intraoperative electron therapy. Because of variabilities in patient selection for these procedures, it is difficult to determine the relative benefit of the additional dose delivered by these modalities.[95–98] For postoperative external beam RT, treatment usually commences about 4 to 6 weeks following surgery and once the wound is fully healed. Recommended total doses are 60 to 66 Gy (delivered in 1.8- or 2-Gy fractions) for the case of negative margins and 66 to 68 Gy for positive margins.[41,99,100] The first course of treatment is typically treated to a dose of 45 to 50 Gy and the balance of the dose is given in one reduced field. The standard dose for low dose rate (LDR) BRT is 45 Gy and for high dose-rate (HDR) BRT is 30 to 50 Gy in 2- to 4-Gy bid fractions.[63,92] For treatment combining external beam RT with BRT as a boost, doses are typically 45 to 50 Gy for external beam, 15 to 25 Gy for a LDR BRT boost, and 12 to 20 Gy (in 2- to 4-Gy bid fractions) for a HDR BRT boost, for a total of approximately 65 Gy.[92,95]

Principles of Treatment Planning

As for any other malignancy, the basic principles of RT planning are to achieve good coverage of the PTV with maximal sparing of adjacent normal structures. For extremity lesions, the important normal structures are the limb itself, soft tissues, bones, and joints. For proximal thigh lesions, the perineum and genitals are also relevant. For STS of the trunk, adjacent normal structures can include small bowel, kidneys, spinal cord, stomach, liver, heart, and lung. Basic tenets for treating the extremity are to "spare a strip" of the limb circumference (to prevent subsequent lymphedema and pain), to avoid treating the whole thickness of bone to high doses (to diminish risk of fracture), and to avoid treating an entire joint to high doses (to decrease joint stiffness). It is not always possible to preserve fertility (and in any borderline situation, one should offer sperm banking or fertility consultation). Every effort should be made to place the testicles as far out of the field as possible to avoid direct treatment and to minimize the contribution from internal scatter.

Specific dosing guidelines for structures of the extremity are as follows. Spare as much as possible of the limb circumference from receiving any dose, and at a minimum, spare a 1-cm thickness to receive <20 Gy. With 3D-conformal techniques, part of the limb can usually be excluded entirely from the treatment fields. With IMRT, in order to achieve more dose conformality, the trade-off is that the volume of tissue that receives a low dose is increased; for some of these cases, the entire circumference of the limb may receive some low dose. The acceptable low dose that can be delivered to the entire limb has not been well established and will most likely vary with factors such as the total dose delivered, total volume of tissue treated, and the location in the limb. However, as a guideline, it is helpful to contour a strip of limb circumference to use as an avoidance structure in order to keep part of the treated limb dose to a minimum (<20 Gy). The whole-joint dose should be <40 to 45 Gy. Higher doses can be delivered to part of the joint if needed. Full-thickness bone irradiation should be avoided if possible, and the mean and maximum doses to the whole bone should also be kept to a minimum. Dickie et al.[101] performed a detailed analysis of dosimetric predictors for bone fracture using a matched pair analysis and found that radiation-related bone fractures were reduced if the following parameters were met: volume of bone receiving ≥40 Gy (V40) <64%, mean dose to bone <37 Gy, and maximum dose to bone <59 Gy. Normal-tissue complication probabilities for organs that may be affected by treatment of a truncal STS are listed in the Quantitative Analysis of Normal Tissue Effects in the Clinic document.[102] If RT treatment of a trunk lesion may potentially ablate ipsilateral kidney function, a renal scan should be performed to ensure adequate function of the contralateral kidney. Despite historical teaching to the contrary, tissue-equivalent bolus material is discouraged in the preoperative setting and infrequently necessary in the postoperative setting. In the preoperative setting, a paddle of skin is typically removed along with superficial tumor obviating the need for bolus; furthermore, increased surface dose appears to increase wound complication risk.[78,103] With respect to the postoperative setting, the BRT experience showed that failure to treat incision or drain sites was not associated with scar or drain site recurrences.[63]

Three-dimensional conformal RT (3D-CRT) and IMRT are both acceptable external beam treatment techniques, but IMRT has several advantages over 3D-CRT and is generally preferred. The principal dosimetric differences between these two techniques are that, compared with 3D-CRT, IMRT typically achieves comparable target coverage, improved conformality of the dose distribution around the target volume, and reduced volumes of high doses to normal tissues, but at the cost of greater volumes of low doses to normal tissues, and greater total body exposure due to increased monitor units.[104,105] Several studies show similarly excellent local control rates with IMRT compared to 3D-CRT.[69,78,83,90,103] Importantly, it also appears that IMRT is associated with a more favorable toxicity profile compared to 3D-CRT (see Chronic Radiation Therapy Toxicities). On the other hand, Hall[104] raised a caveat that IMRT may be associated with a higher rate of radiation-associated second cancers compared to 3D-CRT, resulting from the use of more monitor units with a greater total body exposure from leakage, and from a larger volume of normal tissue exposure to low doses of RT, resulting from the greater number of treatment fields. To date, there are no data suggesting higher second cancer rates dues to IMRT. Weighing all the evidence, IMRT is the preferred technique for most extremity and trunk STS.

There continue to be exciting technologic advances for treatment, which include IMRT dose painting, IGRT, adaptive RT, particle-beam radiotherapy (protons, carbon ions), and stereotactic body RT (SBRT). *Dose painting* is an application of IMRT in which differential doses are delivered to different areas of the target volume simultaneously. An interesting concept is to use dose painting to deliver higher doses to areas of the tumor believed to be more radioresistant (such as hypoxic regions), areas that may contain a higher burden of disease, or high-risk areas of the tumor that may result in positive resection margins. This appealing technique is under investigation in the setting of retroperitoneal sarcoma.[106] *Image-guided radiation therapy* refers to serial imaging of patient setup prior to treatment so that appropriate positional adjustments

can be made beforehand. Because of the increased certainty of treatment accuracy, in many cases, the added margins for "setup error" can be reduced, which allows for smaller treatment fields and potential dose escalation without undue normal tissue toxicity. For example, although spinal cord tolerance is 50 Gy, Hansen et al.[107] described the ability to treat paraspinal sarcomas to 59.4 Gy using IGRT with CT imaging to better assess patient position prior to treatment. IGRT and reduced treatment fields were also used in the phase II RTOG-0630 trial.[90] Another benefit of IGRT is that if imaging during a course of treatment demonstrates changes in patient anatomy (e.g., due to weight loss) or changes in tumor shape, a second radiation plan can be developed to adapt to these new data. This is referred to as *adaptive radiation therapy* and might be relevant for sarcomas that respond dramatically to radiation, such as myxoid liposarcoma.[108,109]

Particle beams such as protons and heavier ions (carbon ions) have more favorable physical and biologic characteristics than do photons, which make them appealing for clinical use. Specifically, because of the Bragg peak dose distribution property, treatment plans can be created with steep dose fall-off at field borders.[110] This allows for ideal sparing of adjacent critical normal structures as well as opportunities for safe dose escalation. Proton-beam treatment for malignancies has been in use at a few centers for several decades. There are published data for treatment of chordomas and chondrosarcomas of the skull base as well as for paraspinal and sacral bone tumors. There have been no randomized studies comparing photons and protons for STS, but there are several single-institution reports for protons that show very good results. Local control rates for skull-base chordomas treated with protons range from 46% to 90% and for skull-base chondrosarcomas range from 75% to 100%.[111-116] Carbon ions have been used for clinical treatment only since the 1990s. Schulz-Ertner et al.[117,118] reported a 74% 4-year local control rate for skull-base chordomas treated with carbon ions and a 90% local-control rate for skull-base chondrosarcomas. The group from Chiba, Japan, reported a 73% local-control rate for unresectable bone and STS and a 96% local-control rate for sacral chordomas.[119,120] These early results are impressive, but confirmatory long-term follow-up data are needed.

Stereotactic body radiation therapy is a technique that delivers highly focused photon radiation doses to extracranial lesions. The dose schedules are hypofractionated, with large ablative fraction sizes ranging from 6 to 30 Gy/fraction, typically for a course of 1 to 5 treatments. With respect to sarcoma, SBRT may have a role in the treatment of oligometastatic disease. Excellent local control rates, ranging from 73% to 96%, have been reported for treatment of metastases to the lung as well as other sites for a mix of tumors including sarcoma.[121-123] There are fewer data regarding the role of SBRT for definitive treatment of primary sarcomas, but there may be a role in select patients with tumors located in or adjacent to sensitive normal structures. For example, a study of SBRT for 14 patients with primary sarcoma of the spine reported local control for 5 of 7 patients treated with SBRT alone and for 5 of 7 patients treated with SBRT and surgery.[124] Figure 87.5 shows an MRI and dosimetry for a case of an unresectable leiomyosarcoma of the inferior vena cava that was treated with definitive SBRT at Brigham and Women's Hospital.

IMRT with dose painting, adaptive RT, particle beams, and SBRT all show potential dosimetric and biologic advantages compared to conventional 3D-CRT photon treatment. Promising data are available for all of these approaches, but they are limited. There will likely be appropriate places for all of these technologies in the armamentarium for sarcoma treatment, but further careful study is needed to define the optimal role of each technology and to ensure that toxicities are acceptable.

Section III

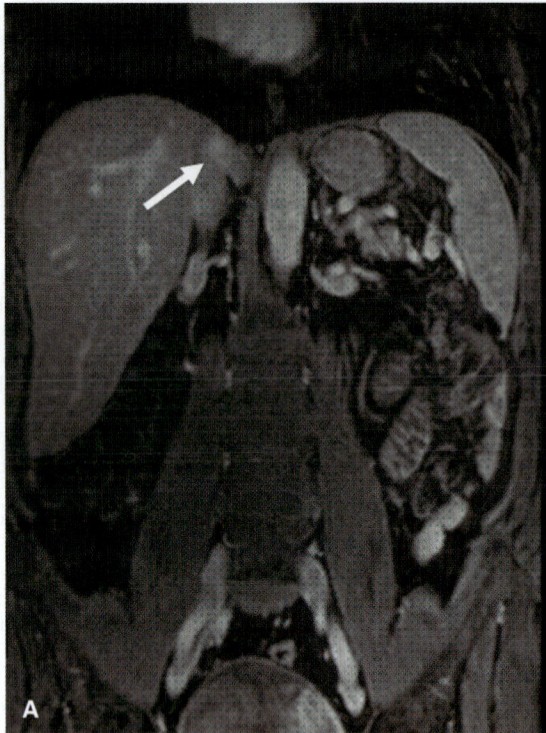
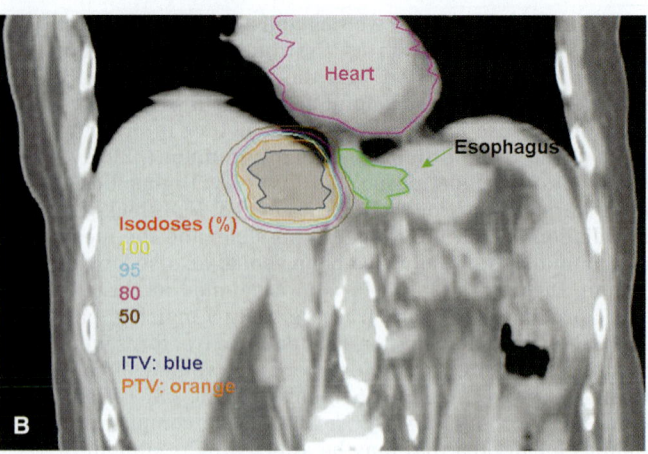

FIGURE 87.5. A 72-year-old man with a 1.8 × 1.8 cm unresectable leiomyosarcoma of the intrahepatic inferior vena cava in close proximity to the liver, esophagus, and heart that was treated with stereotactic body radiation therapy (SBRT) (60 Gy in 5 fractions). **A:** Coronal T1-weighted magnetic resonance image slice showing the tumor (denoted by the *arrow*). **B:** Coronal slice of the SBRT graphic plan showing the internal target volume (ITV, *blue*), planning target volume (PTV, *orange*), and covering isodose lines.

Radiation Therapy Toxicities

Acute Radiation Therapy Toxicities

Acute toxicities following RT treatment of the extremities include skin erythema and possible desquamation in high-dose areas, problems with wound healing, localized alopecia, and fatigue. Moist desquamation can be quite uncomfortable, but this heals typically quickly after completion of RT. Depending on tumor location, treatment of STS of the trunk can be associated with additional toxicities such as nausea, bowel irritability, or esophagitis.

The most significant of these acute sequelae is problems with wound healing. Several retrospective single-institution series have reported wound complication rates following preoperative RT of 25% to 46%.[78,125–128] Rates following postoperative RT are lower and range from 6% to 29%.[125,126] The most definitive data pertaining to wound complications are provided by the landmark randomized trial performed by the NCI Canada, in which the study endpoint was major wound complications within 120 days of surgery.[70] Major wound complications were defined as those requiring a second operation for wound repair or wound management requiring an invasive procedure, readmission, or persistent deep packing for 120 days or longer. This trial randomized 190 patients to preoperative RT (50 Gy ± 16 to 20 Gy postoperative boost) or postoperative RT (66 to 70 Gy). With a median follow-up time of 3.3 years, the study met early stopping rules and closed. Wound complication rates were 35% for patients treated with preoperative RT compared to 17% for those treated with postoperative RT (*P* = .01). Further, lower extremity site and tumor size >10 cm were independent predictors for wound complications on multivariate analysis. Others have also found large tumor size and lower extremity site to be risk factors for wound complications.[78,126] Baldini et al.[78] have reviewed the experience at Brigham and Women's Hospital

and Dana-Farber Cancer Institute for 103 patients with STS of the trunk or extremity treated with preoperative RT. On multivariate analysis, significant independent predictors for wound complications were tumor size >10 cm, tumor proximity to skin surface <3 mm, vascularized flap closure, and diabetes mellitus. In an attempt to decrease wound complications following preoperative RT, O'Sullivan et al.[103] conducted a phase II trial for 59 patients with lower extremity sarcoma. Together with the surgeon, the radiation oncologist contoured the area of the subsequent surgical flaps and designated it as an avoidance structure for IMRT planning. The resulting rate of wound complications was 30.5%, which was lower than but not statistically different from the 43% rate reported in the randomized trial. However, for patients with minimal (<1%) overlap of the flap and PTV, the wound complication rate was 14.3% compared to 39.5% for those with flap/PTV overlap (*P* = .04). The association of higher wound complications with higher flap doses is consistent with the findings in the Baldini report showing increased complications for tumors within 3 mm of the skin surface. Efforts continue to minimize postoperative wound complications.

Chronic Radiation Therapy Toxicities

The most significant chronic toxicities following RT to the extremities include edema, subcutaneous fibrosis, decreased muscle strength, decreased range of motion, pain, and, less commonly, bone fractures. Published rates of these toxicities vary, as series have different patient inclusion criteria (with respect to tumor site and treatment) and some report only moderate or severe complications, whereas others report any degree of complication. For series primarily composed of patients treated with 2-dimensional or 3D-CRT, reported rates for edema are 10% to 20%, for fibrosis they are 30% to 60%, and for bone fracture they are 0.04% to 7%.[101,129–135]

Furthermore, several of these studies correlated higher complication rates with higher doses and larger field sizes. Doses >60 or 63 Gy have been associated with higher rates of fibrosis, edema, bone fracture, pain, decreased muscle strength, and decreased range of motion.[101,129,130,132] Large RT field sizes have also been associated with more edema, fibrosis, and joint stiffness.[129,130] There have been no randomized trials comparing chronic toxicities for patients treated with 3D-CRT versus IMRT, but series composed primarily of patients treated with IMRT report lower chronic toxicities with rates for ≥ grade 2 edema of 5.3% to 11.1%, for fibrosis of 5.3% to 9.3%, and for joint stiffness of 3.5% to 5.6%.[83,90,103] Risk of bone fracture has been clearly correlated with bone doses, and IMRT enables better bone avoidance than 3D-CRT.

Radiation Timing: Preoperative Versus Postoperative

External beam RT can be delivered either prior to or following definitive resection. Reported local control rates with each approach are similar and range from 73% to 93% for preoperative RT and 72% to 92% for postoperative RT.[69,136–139] The randomized trial of preoperative versus postoperative RT conducted by the NCI Canada showed local control rates of 93% and 92% for the preoperative and postoperative groups, respectively.[69] Similarly, there is no clear difference in DFS or OS associated with either approach. The Canadian randomized trial initially showed improved survival for the preoperative RT treatment arm, but updated results showed no differences in any recurrence or survival outcomes.[69,70] One retrospective report that assessed 821 patients using the National Oncology Database showed improved DFS rates for patients treated with preoperative RT.[55] However, these results should be considered with caution given the retrospective nature of the report and associated potential selection biases.

Although the efficacy of these approaches seems to be similar, the toxicity profiles are clearly different. Preoperative RT is associated with a well-established increased risk of acute wound complications. Several retrospective reports have described wound complication rates on the order of 25% to 46%.[78,126,127] As described in detail above (see the Acute Radiation Therapy Toxicities section), the definitive data for wound complication rates come from the Canadian randomized trial in which the primary endpoint was wound complications. In that trial, wound complication rates were 35% for patients treated with preoperative RT compared to 17% for those treated with postoperative RT ($P = .01$).[70] Although wound complications adversely affected functional outcome for patients in the early postoperative period (6 weeks after surgery), this toxicity was largely reversible, as evidenced by the fact that function was equivalent between the treatment arms 1 year after resection.

On the other hand, patients treated with postoperative RT have a higher rate of chronic and generally irreversible toxicities, which include subcutaneous fibrosis, joint stiffness, edema, and bone fractures. These late toxicities have been reported in retrospective series but, again, good data come from the Canadian randomized trial.[129,130,132,140] Davis et al.[130] reported that grade 2 or higher late toxicity rates were higher for the postoperative RT group than the preoperative group. Specifically, for the postoperative and preoperative groups, respectively, rates of grade 2+ complications were as follows: subcutaneous fibrosis, 48% versus 31.5%; joint stiffness, 23% versus 18%; and edema, 23% versus 15.5%. These differences were not statistically significant, but the study was not powered to detect these differences. Statistically significant associations were seen between larger field size and rates

of fibrosis, joint stiffness, and edema. Additionally, in a retrospective series, Holt et al.[132] reported increased rates of bone fracture for patients treated postoperatively (60 to 66 Gy) compared to those treated preoperatively (50 Gy). The rates were 7% and 0.6%, respectively ($P = .007$).

It is helpful to summarize the relative advantages and disadvantages for preoperative versus postoperative RT. For preoperative RT, the advantages include the ability to treat with smaller RT fields and lower doses, both of which are associated with reduced permanent long-term toxicities. Lower RT doses are also associated with reduced treatment time, lower costs, and a hypothetical possibility of lower second-malignancy risks. Other potential advantages of preoperative RT include the ability to render unresectable or marginally resectable tumors resectable, the potential to prevent tumor seeding of the operative bed or systemic circulation, and an increased efficacy of RT from good oxygenation of tissues due to unperturbed tumor vasculature. Furthermore, in most cases, defining the tumor volume for RT planning is relatively straightforward given that it is *in situ*. The main disadvantage of preoperative RT is the higher risk of major wound complications and its concomitant increased morbidity and cost. However, most major wound complications are treatable, and therefore, this toxicity is generally considered reversible. Another disadvantage of preoperative RT is that the resected specimen is potentially less informative on pathology review because of the prior treatment.

Postoperative RT has the advantage that the complete tumor specimen is available for pathology review for determination of histology and margin status. Another important advantage is the lower risk of major wound complications. The main disadvantages of postoperative RT are the necessity for larger treatment volumes and higher doses, which are associated with higher long-term toxicities such as subcutaneous fibrosis, joint stiffness, edema, pain, and bone fractures. For the most part, these toxicities are irreversible. In theory, the interrupted vasculature related to surgery may create a hypoxic environment, rendering RT less effective (this is a potential explanation for the need for higher doses compared to the preoperative setting). Lastly, determining an RT target definition is more complex in the postoperative setting, as it requires reconstruction of where the tumor resided as well as definition of the entire operative field.

In conclusion, pre- and postoperative RT are associated with equivalent efficacies but different toxicity profiles, the most salient of which are increased (reversible) wound complications for preoperative RT and increased (irreversible) long-term toxicities of fibrosis, edema, and joint stiffness for postoperative RT. The topic is controversial, but preoperative RT is generally the preferred approach for STS of the extremities or trunk. Even when a patient is at high risk of developing a wound complication, one could argue for preoperative RT, as most wound problems are highly treatable with eventual recovery of good function.

Surgery Alone

As stated previously, CS and RT is the standard treatment for high-grade STS of the extremity and trunk. However, there are also several reports that demonstrate excellent outcomes following treatment with surgery alone. It is important to acknowledge that these are all single-institution series, all but one are retrospective, and patients were highly selected for treatment. These factors render the results less generalizable, so caution is recommended when considering this approach. Nonetheless, crude and actuarial LR rates in these select studies range from 0% to 20% and most are 10% or lower.[84–89,141] What the appropriate selection criteria for this approach are remains unclear, but potential factors can be inferred by close analysis of these reports. Excellent local control appears to be associated with wide resection performed for tumors in a subcutaneous location. Rydholm et al.[86] described only four LRs (5%) among 73 subcutaneous tumors treated with wide excision. In addition, Gibbs et al.[88] reported no LRs among 35 patients with subcutaneous STS treated with wide excision alone. Among these tumors, 47% were high grade and 32% were >5 cm. Pisters et al.[87] described a prospective series of patients with tumors <5 cm who had negative resection margins and were treated with surgery alone. The overall crude LR rate was 8%, and among the subcutaneous tumors, the rate was only 5%. Furthermore, surgical technique and margin status are important. In the series reported by Rydholm et al.,[84] a large proportion of the cases were resected without an initial biopsy and, thus, without the potential for tumor seeding of intervening tissues.

Several of the reports also describe a meticulous surgical approach to wide resection with removal of a cuff of normal tissue as well as intact fascia.[84,86,88] In the prospective trial of Pisters et al.,[87] negative resection margins were a required criterion for treatment by resection alone. The report by Baldini et al.[85] quantified surgical resection margins. In that series, 74 patients were treated with surgery alone and the overall 10-year actuarial LR rate was 7%. Interestingly, there were no recurrences seen for 36 patients with resection margins ≥1 cm compared to a 10-year actuarial LR rate of 13% (4 of 38) for those with margins <1 cm (*P* = .04).

Conversely, the authors of a retrospective study from the Institut Gustave Roussy also quantified margin status.[142] They reported a 10-year actuarial LR rate of 35% for patients treated with surgery alone who had resection margins ≥1 cm. Further, they found the addition of RT for patients with these characteristics was not associated with a significant local control benefit. As the LR rate in that series is high, it is difficult to draw meaningful conclusions except to reinforce the concept that treatment with surgery alone should be done with care.

Cahlon et al.[141] assessed 200 patients who were treated with surgery alone at MSKCC following re-resection showing no evidence of disease. Although the overall 5-year actuarial LR rate was only 9%, on multivariate analysis, age >50 and stage III disease were both predictors for higher LR rates. If both of these factors were present, the LR rate was 31%. The LR rates for low-grade tumors treated with surgery alone in these series were all very low and range from 0% to 5%.[84–88,143] In fact, the standard treatment recommendation for low-grade STS is wide resection alone. With this approach and negative margins, LR rates are typically <20%.[79] (Indications for adjuvant RT for low-grade tumors include positive resection margins, locally recurrent disease following initial treatment with surgery alone, or a tumor location that would not be amenable to subsequent salvage surgery.)

In sum, there is most certainly a subset of patients with STS of the extremity and trunk for whom wide excision alone is appropriate treatment. The selection criteria for this strategy remain undefined but will perhaps include, but not be limited to, some of the following: subcutaneous tumors; tumors resected with wide negative margins >1 cm or an intact fascia; low-grade tumors; tumors representing primary presentation of disease (e.g., not locally recurrent); tumor locations amenable to limb-sparing salvage surgery for recurrence; and patient willingness to comply with appropriate follow-up. Before surgery alone can become standard of care for select patients with STS, the eligibility criteria

need to be elucidated and tested in a prospective multi-institutional trial. Other than for low-grade tumors resected with negative margins, treatment with surgery alone should be employed cautiously.

Neoadjuvant, Concurrent, or Adjuvant Chemotherapy

Locally advanced (stage III) STS of the extremities and trunk has a significant risk of distant recurrence, and for this reason, the addition of systemic therapy to treatment algorithms is appealing. There is an established role for chemotherapy as part of the treatment for rhabdomyosarcoma and Ewing sarcoma.[144,145] For other histologies of adult STS, no clear role for chemotherapy has been defined, and this group is the subject of the discussion below. The two most standardly used drugs in the management of STS are doxorubicin and ifosfamide, with gemcitabine-based regimens increasingly used, particularly in patients with leiomyosarcoma.[146]

There are several potential benefits to a neoadjuvant chemotherapy approach. These include the potential to treat micrometastatic disease early in the treatment course; the potential to decrease the scope of the resection if sufficient response is achieved; the ability to ascertain the chemotherapy response or lack thereof for an individual patient, which could guide the use of additional (postoperative) chemotherapy; and enhanced drug delivery to the tumor with corresponding increased efficacy, given that the tumor vasculature has not been disrupted in the neoadjuvant setting. Few reports address the role of neoadjuvant chemotherapy for high-risk STS of the extremities and trunk. A prospective randomized phase II trial conducted by the European Organization for Research and Treatment of Cancer included 137 patients who were randomized to receive or not receive three cycles of doxorubicin and ifosfamide prior to resection with selective use of postoperative RT.[147] Unfortunately, the study was closed because of poor accrual and therefore lacks sufficient power for one to draw definitive conclusions. The results showed no statistically significant differences between treatment arms for DFS or OS. Specifically, the 5-year DFS rate for the chemotherapy group was 56% compared with 52% for the observation group; the corresponding 5-year OS rates were 65% and 64%, respectively. Two other retrospective reports on the use of neoadjuvant chemotherapy showed mixed results.[148,149]

Similarly, informative data are scarce regarding the use of concurrent preoperative chemotherapy and radiotherapy. Several trials have shown that treatment with RT and concurrent doxorubicin, ifosfamide, gemcitabine, or temozolomide is both feasible and safe.[150–155] There are also two reports of an interdigitated chemotherapy and RT approach. The first was a pilot trial conducted at the Massachusetts General Hospital, which enrolled 48 patients. Treatment involved an interdigitated approach of chemotherapy (mesna, doxorubicin, ifosfamide, and dacarbazine) and 44 Gy given as a split course.[156] Results were very good and associated with improved survival compared with historical controls. The RTOG subsequently enrolled 66 patients in a phase II trial with a very similar treatment approach.[157] Efficacy was somewhat comparable to that of the pilot study, but toxicities were greater, with 5% treatment-related deaths and 83% grade 4 toxicities reported.

The most data available pertain to the use of chemotherapy in the adjuvant setting. A meta-analysis reported by the Sarcoma Meta-Analysis Collaboration (SMAC) included 1,568 patients treated in 14 randomized trials using adjuvant doxorubicin-based chemotherapy. It showed that chemotherapy was associated with statistically higher rates of

LR-free survival and DFS at 10 years.[158] Ten-year LR-free survival rates were 81% and 75%, respectively, for the chemotherapy and observation groups (P = .02); the corresponding values for 10-year DFS were 55% and 45% (P = .001). For 10-year OS, there was no clear benefit, with rates of 54% for the chemotherapy group and 50% for the observation group (P = .12). However, exploratory analysis showed a significant 7% survival benefit for the subset of patients with STS of the extremities. Subsequent to this meta-analysis, several more randomized trials of adjuvant chemotherapy were performed using anthracycline or ifosfamide-based chemotherapy; many of these showed trends for survival benefits with chemotherapy, but none were statistically significant.[159–163] (One study from Italy initially reported a significant survival benefit due to chemotherapy at 4 years, but the survival benefit did not hold up with 7.5-year follow-up.)[159,160] SMAC updated their meta-analysis in 2008 with the inclusion of four additional trials (three adjuvant and one neoadjuvant).[147,159,161,162,164] The new analysis included 18 randomized trials with 1,953 patients and reported statistically significant absolute reductions of 4% for LR and 9% for distant recurrence and an absolute improvement of 6% for survival attributable to chemotherapy.[164] However, the fact that this update did not include the largest negative trial renders the results less conclusive.[163] A subsequent randomized trial of 351 patients failed to show a benefit for five cycles of adjuvant doxorubicin and ifosfamide.[165] All of the above studies included a mix of STS histologic subtypes, which is probably not appropriate as we learn more about the varied biologic behaviors of individual STS entities. There are already reports showing encouraging response rates for certain histologies and specific cytotoxic agents such as eribulin for liposarcoma,[166] trabectedin for liposarcoma and leiomyosarcoma,[167] and gemcitabine and docetaxol for uterine leiomyosarcoma.[146] Going forward, trials should include centralized pathology review and stratification by histology.

In totality, although there are hints of efficacy for certain subgroups, the available data do not support the routine use of chemotherapy for locally advanced STS. However, for select high-risk patients with high-grade and large tumors (>8 to 10 cm), it is reasonable to address the pros and cons of neoadjuvant, concurrent or interdigitated, or adjuvant chemotherapy on an individual patient basis. As toxicity can be significant, concurrent approaches are best undertaken at experienced centers.

Isolated Limb Perfusion, Isolated Limb Infusion, and Chemotherapy with Regional Hyperthermia

Isolated limb perfusion (ILP) is a complicated technique that has been used in Europe for the treatment of locally advanced STS that would otherwise require amputation. This procedure involves isolating the arterial and venous circulation of the limb by connecting it to an extracorporeal circulation, where it is oxygenated and instilled with systemic agents, most commonly, melphalan and tumor necrosis factor. A tourniquet is applied to the limb to prevent leakage into the systemic circulation and the limb is often treated with hyperthermia as well. The treatment can have significant morbidity, but reported limb salvage success rates are quite high.[168–172] *Isolated limb infusion* (ILI) employs low-flow ILP without oxygenation and has been developed as a simpler alternative to ILP. Available data suggest comparable efficacy and less toxicity for ILI compared to ILP.[173,174] Lastly, chemotherapy with regional hyperthermia (delivered via an external electromagnetic field) is another approach for locally advanced disease. A randomized trial of doxorubicin, ifosfamide, and etoposide, with or without regional hyperthermia delivered before and after local therapy, has shown superior DFS and progression-free survival rates for the regional hyperthermia group.[175] All of these techniques are complicated to deliver and associated with significant potential toxicities. However, they represent valuable potential alternatives to amputation in such settings as in transit metastases of epithelioid or clear cell sarcoma or extensive LRs after prior surgery and RT.

FUTURE DIRECTIONS

In summary, success rates for the treatment of stages I and II STS of the extremities and trunk are currently high, with local control rates of ≥85% and 5-year survival rates of 90% and 81%, respectively.[39] For these patients, we should continue to explore ways to reduce treatment-related morbidity related to surgery and RT. These strategies should include development of innovative techniques to reduce postoperative wound complications, efforts to reduce RT field sizes and to deliver more conformal therapy, and definition of patient subsets that can be effectively treated with surgery alone. For situations in which it is difficult to achieve local control, more aggressive local treatment is needed; this could include the use of RT dose escalation using IGRT, IMRT with dose painting, heavy particles, SBRT, or concurrent chemoradiation strategies. Lastly, patients with stage III disease have a high rate of distant relapse and death. For these patients, novel systemic therapies are needed. The discovery of the targeted agent imatinib mesylate for the treatment of gastrointestinal stromal tumors has been associated with great success, and similar discoveries for other histologies are anticipated.[176] As the field of STS continues to move forward, it is likely that treatment algorithms specific to various histologic subtypes will be developed.

ACKNOWLEDGMENT

I would like to acknowledge the editorial assistance of Susanna Hilfer and Mark Mackin.

REFERENCES

1. Siegel RL, Miller KD, Jemal A. Cancer Statistics, 2017. *CA Cancer J Clin* 2017;67:7–30.
2. Fletcher CDM, Bridge JA, Hogendoorn PC, et al., eds. *World Health Organization classification of tumours of soft tissue and bone.* 4th ed. Lyon, France: IARC Press, 2013.
3. Guillou L, Coindre JM, Bonichon F, et al. Comparative study of the National Cancer Institute and French Federation of Cancer Centers Sarcoma Group grading systems in a population of 410 adult patients with soft tissue sarcoma. *J Clin Oncol* 1997;15:350–362.
4. Rubin BP, Cooper K, Fletcher CD, et al. Protocol for the examination of specimens from patients with tumors of soft tissue. *Arch Pathol Lab Med* 2010;134:e31–39.
5. Raut CP, George C, Hornick JL, et al. High rates of histopathologic discordance in sarcoma with implications for clinical care. *J Clin Oncol* 2011;29:10065–10065.
6. Arbiser ZK, Folpe AL, Weiss SW. Consultative (expert) second opinions in soft tissue pathology. Analysis of problem-prone diagnostic situations. *Am J Clin Pathol* 2001;116:473–476.
7. Lehnhardt M, Daigeler A, Hauser J, et al. The value of expert second opinion in diagnosis of soft tissue sarcomas. *J Surg Oncol* 2008;97:40–43.
8. Randall RL, Bruckner JD, Papenhausen MD, et al. Errors in diagnosis and margin determination of soft-tissue sarcomas initially treated at non-tertiary centers. *Orthopedics* 2004;27:209–212.
9. Lurkin A, Ducimetiere F, Vince DR, et al. Epidemiological evaluation of concordance between initial diagnosis and central pathology review in a comprehensive and prospective series of sarcoma patients in the Rhone-Alpes region. *BMC Cancer* 2010;10:150.
10. Coindre JM, Trojani M, Contesso G, et al. Reproducibility of a histopathologic grading system for adult soft tissue sarcoma. *Cancer* 1986;58:306–309.
11. Hasegawa T, Yamamoto S, Nojima T, et al. Validity and reproducibility of histologic diagnosis and grading for adult soft-tissue sarcomas. *Hum Pathol* 2002;33:111–115.

12. Lawrence W Jr, Donegan WL, Natarajan N, et al. Adult soft tissue sarcomas. A pattern of care survey of the American College of Surgeons. *Ann Surg* 1987;205:349–359.

13. Young RJ, Brown NJ, Reed MW, et al. Angiosarcoma. *Lancet Oncol* 2010;11:983–991.

14. Galiatsatos P, Foulkes WD. Familial adenomatous polyposis. *Am J Gastroenterol* 2006;101:385–398.

15. Baratti D, Pennacchioli E, Casali PG, et al. Epithelioid sarcoma: prognostic factors and survival in a series of patients treated at a single institution. *Ann Surg Oncol* 2007;14:3542–3551.

16. Simon MA, Enneking WF. The management of soft-tissue sarcomas of the extremities. *J Bone Joint Surg Am* 1976;58:317–327.

17. Enneking WF, Spanier SS, Malawer MM. The effect of the anatomic setting on the results of surgical procedures for soft parts sarcoma of the thigh. *Cancer* 1981;47:1005–1022.

18. Fong Y, Coit DG, Woodruff JM, et al. Lymph node metastasis from soft tissue sarcoma in adults. Analysis of data from a prospective database of 1772 sarcoma patients. *Ann Surg* 1993;217:72–77.

19. Daigeler A, Kuhnen C, Moritz R, et al. Lymph node metastases in soft tissue sarcomas: a single center analysis of 1,597 patients. *Langenbecks Arch Surg* 2009;394:321–329.

20. Riad S, Griffin AM, Liberman B, et al. Lymph node metastasis in soft tissue sarcoma in an extremity. *Clin Orthop Relat Res* 2004:129–134.

21. Sakharpe A, Lahat G, Gulamhusein T, et al. Epithelioid sarcoma and unclassified sarcoma with epithelioid features: clinicopathological variables, molecular markers, and a new experimental model. *Oncologist* 2011;16:512–522.

22. La TH, Wolden SL, Rodeberg DA, et al. Regional nodal involvement and patterns of spread along in-transit pathways in children with rhabdomyosarcoma of the extremity: a report from the Children's Oncology Group. *Int J Radiat Oncol Biol Phys* 2011;80:1151–1157.

23. Guadagnolo BA, Zagars GK, Araujo D, et al. Outcomes after definitive treatment for cutaneous angiosarcoma of the face and scalp. *Head Neck* 2011;33:661–667.

24. Guadagnolo BA, Zagars GK, Ballo MT, et al. Excellent local control rates and distinctive patterns of failure in myxoid liposarcoma treated with conservation surgery and radiotherapy. *Int J Radiat Oncol Biol Phys* 2008;70:760–765.

25. Schwab JH, Boland P, Guo T, et al. Skeletal metastases in myxoid liposarcoma: an unusual pattern of distant spread. *Ann Surg Oncol* 2007;14:1507–1514.

26. Gronchi A, Miceli R, Allard MA, et al. Personalizing the approach to retroperitoneal soft tissue sarcoma: histology-specific patterns of failure and postrelapse outcome after primary extended resection. *Ann Surg Oncol* 2015;22:1447–1454.

27. Haglund KE, Raut CP, Nascimento AF, et al. Recurrence patterns and survival for patients with intermediate- and high-grade myxofibrosarcoma. *Int J Radiat Oncol Biol Phys* 2012;82:361–367.

28. Mutter RW, Singer S, Zhang Z, et al. The enigma of myxofibrosarcoma of the extremity. *Cancer* 2012;118:518–527.

29. Sanfilippo R, Miceli R, Grosso F, et al. Myxofibrosarcoma: prognostic factors and survival in a series of patients treated at a single institution. *Ann Surg Oncol* 2011;18:720–725.

30. Gundle KR, Gupta S, Kafchinski L, et al. An analysis of tumor- and surgery-related factors that contribute to inadvertent positive margins following soft tissue sarcoma resection. *Ann Surg Oncol* 2017;24:2137–2144.

31. Demas BE, Heelan RT, Lane J, et al. Soft-tissue sarcomas of the extremities: comparison of MR and CT in determining the extent of disease. *AJR Am J Roentgenol* 1988;150:615–620.

32. Aisen AM, Martel W, Braunstein EM, et al. MRI and CT evaluation of primary bone and soft-tissue tumors. *AJR Am J Roentgenol* 1986;146:749–756.

33. White LM, Wunder JS, Bell RS, et al. Histologic assessment of peritumoral edema in soft tissue sarcoma. *Int J Radiat Oncol Biol Phys* 2005;61:1439–1445.

34. Panicek DM, Gatsonis C, Rosenthal DI, et al. CT and MR imaging in the local staging of primary malignant musculoskeletal neoplasms: report of the Radiology Diagnostic Oncology Group. *Radiology* 1997;202:237–246.

35. Benz MR, Czernin J, Dry SM, et al. Quantitative F18-fluorodeoxyglucose positron emission tomography accurately characterizes peripheral nerve sheath tumors as malignant or benign. *Cancer* 2010;116:451–458.

36. Amin MB, Edge SB, Greene FL, et al., eds. *AJCC cancer staging manual*. 8th ed. Chicago, IL: Springer International Publishing, 2017.

37. Ray-Coquard I, Ranchere-Vince D, Thiesse P, et al. Evaluation of core needle biopsy as a substitute to open biopsy in the diagnosis of soft-tissue masses. *Eur J Cancer* 2003;39:2021–2025.

38. Mankin HJ, Mankin CJ, Simon MA. The hazards of the biopsy, revisited. Members of the Musculoskeletal Tumor Society. *J Bone Joint Surg Am* 1996;78:656–663.

39. Edge SB, Byrd DR, Compton CC, et al., eds. *AJCC cancer staging manual*. New York: Springer, 2010.

40. Pisters PW, Leung DH, Woodruff J, et al. Analysis of prognostic factors in 1,041 patients with localized soft tissue sarcomas of the extremities. *J Clin Oncol* 1996;14:1679–1689.

41. Zagars GK, Ballo MT, Pisters PW, et al. Prognostic factors for patients with localized soft-tissue sarcoma treated with conservation surgery and radiation therapy: an analysis of 1225 patients. *Cancer* 2003;97:2530–2543.

42. Coindre JM, Terrier P, Guillou L, et al. Predictive value of grade for metastasis development in the main histologic types of adult soft tissue sarcomas: a study of 1240 patients from the French Federation of Cancer Centers Sarcoma Group. *Cancer* 2001;91:1914–1926.

43. Callegaro D, Miceli R, Bonvalot S, et al. Development and external validation of two nomograms to predict overall survival and occurrence of distant metas-

tases in adults after surgical resection of localised soft-tissue sarcomas of the extremities: a retrospective analysis. *Lancet Oncol* 2016;17:671–680.

44. Lahat G, Tuvin D, Wei C, et al. New perspectives for staging and prognosis in soft tissue sarcoma. *Ann Surg Oncol* 2008;15:2739–2748.

45. Maki RG, Moraco N, Antonescu CR, et al. Toward better soft tissue sarcoma staging: building on American Joint Committee on Cancer Staging Systems versions 6 and 7. *Ann Surg Oncol* 2013;20:3377–3383.

46. Gutierrez JC, Perez EA, Franceschi D, et al. Outcomes for soft-tissue sarcoma in 8249 cases from a large state cancer registry. *J Surg Res* 2007;141:105–114.

47. Canter RJ, Beal S, Borys D, et al. Interaction of histologic subtype and histologic grade in predicting survival for soft-tissue sarcomas. *J Am Coll Surg* 2010;210:191.e2–198.e2.

48. Italiano A, Le Cesne A, Mendiboure J, et al. Prognostic factors and impact of adjuvant treatments on local and metastatic relapse of soft-tissue sarcoma patients in the competing risks setting. *Cancer* 2014;120:3361–3369.

49. Trovik CS, Bauer HC, Alvegard TA, et al. Surgical margins, local recurrence and metastasis in soft tissue sarcomas: 559 surgically-treated patients from the Scandinavian Sarcoma Group Register. *Eur J Cancer* 2000;36:710–716.

50. Gronchi A, Casali PG, Mariani L, et al. Status of surgical margins and prognosis in adult soft tissue sarcomas of the extremities: a series of patients treated at a single institution. *J Clin Oncol* 2005;23:96–104.

51. Rosenberg SA, Tepper J, Glatstein E, et al. The treatment of soft-tissue sarcomas of the extremities: prospective randomized evaluations of (1) limb-sparing surgery plus radiation therapy compared with amputation and (2) the role of adjuvant chemotherapy. *Ann Surg* 1982;196:305–315.

52. Gerrand CH, Wunder JS, Kandel RA, et al. Classification of positive margins after resection of soft-tissue sarcoma of the limb predicts the risk of local recurrence. *J Bone Joint Surg Br* 2001;83:1149–1155.

53. Stefanovski PD, Bidoli E, De Paoli A, et al. Prognostic factors in soft tissue sarcomas: a study of 395 patients. *Eur J Surg Oncol* 2002;28:153–164.

54. Fein DA, Lee WR, Lanciano RM, et al. Management of extremity soft tissue sarcomas with limb-sparing surgery and postoperative irradiation: do total dose, overall treatment time, and the surgery-radiotherapy interval impact on local control? *Int J Radiat Oncol Biol Phys* 1995;32:969–976.

55. Sampath S, Schultheiss TE, Hitchcock YJ, et al. Preoperative versus postoperative radiotherapy in soft-tissue sarcoma: multi-institutional analysis of 821 patients. *Int J Radiat Oncol Biol Phys* 2011;81:498–505.

56. Gustafson P, Dreinhofer KE, Rydholm A. Soft tissue sarcoma should be treated at a tumor center. A comparison of quality of surgery in 375 patients. *Acta Orthop Scand* 1994;65:47–50.

57. Clasby R, Tilling K, Smith MA, et al. Variable management of soft tissue sarcoma: regional audit with implications for specialist care. *Br J Surg* 1997;84:1692–1696.

58. Gutierrez JC, Perez EA, Moffat FL, et al. Should soft tissue sarcomas be treated at high-volume centers? An analysis of 4205 patients. *Ann Surg* 2007;245:952–958.

59. Paszat L, O'Sullivan B, Bell R, et al. Processes and outcomes of care for soft tissue sarcoma of the extremities. *Sarcoma* 2002;6:19–26.

60. Guadagnolo BA, Xu Y, Zagars GK, et al. A population-based study of the quality of care in the diagnosis of large (≥5 cm) soft tissue sarcomas. *Am J Clin Oncol* 2012;35:455–461.

61. Gerner RE, Moore GE, Pickren JW. Soft tissue sarcomas. *Ann Surg* 1975;181:803–808.

62. Leibel SA, Tranbaugh RF, Wara WM, et al. Soft tissue sarcomas of the extremities: survival and patterns of failure with conservative surgery and postoperative irradiation compared to surgery alone. *Cancer* 1982;50:1076–1083.

63. Pisters PW, Harrison LB, Leung DH, et al. Long-term results of a prospective randomized trial of adjuvant brachytherapy in soft tissue sarcoma. *J Clin Oncol* 1996;14:859–868.

64. Fiore M, Casali PG, Miceli R, et al. Prognostic effect of re-excision in adult soft tissue sarcoma of the extremity. *Ann Surg Oncol* 2006;13:110–117.

65. Zagars GK, Ballo MT, Pisters PW, et al. Surgical margins and reresection in the management of patients with soft tissue sarcoma using conservative surgery and radiation therapy. *Cancer* 2003;97:2544–2553.

66. Lewis JJ, Leung D, Espat J, et al. Effect of reresection in extremity soft tissue sarcoma. *Ann Surg* 2000;231:655–663.

67. Davis AM, Kandel RA, Wunder JS, et al. The impact of residual disease on local recurrence in patients treated by initial unplanned resection for soft tissue sarcoma of the extremity. *J Surg Oncol* 1997;66:81–87.

68. Yang JC, Chang AE, Baker AR, et al. Randomized prospective study of the benefit of adjuvant radiation therapy in the treatment of soft tissue sarcomas of the extremity. *J Clin Oncol* 1998;16:197–203.

69. O'Sullivan B, Davis A, Turcotte R, et al. Five-year results of a randomized phase III trial of pre-operative vs post-operative radiotherapy in extremity soft tissue sarcoma. ASCO Annual Meeting Proceedings 2004. *J Clin Oncol* 2004;22:Abstract 9007.

70. O'Sullivan B, Davis AM, Turcotte R, et al. Preoperative versus postoperative radiotherapy in soft-tissue sarcoma of the limbs: a randomised trial. *Lancet* 2002;359:2235–2241.

71. Williard WC, Hajdu SI, Casper ES, et al. Comparison of amputation with limb-sparing operations for adult soft tissue sarcoma of the extremity. *Ann Surg* 1992;215:269–275.

72. Enneking WF. History of orthopedic oncology in the United States: progress from the past, prospects for the future. *Cancer Treat Res* 2009;152:529–571.

73. Beane JD, Yang JC, White D, et al. Efficacy of adjuvant radiation therapy in the treatment of soft tissue sarcoma of the extremity: 20-year follow-up of a randomized prospective trial. *Ann Surg Oncol* 2014;21:2484–2489.

74. Alektiar KM, Leung D, Zelefsky MJ, et al. Adjuvant brachytherapy for primary high-grade soft tissue sarcoma of the extremity. *Ann Surg Oncol* 2002;9:48–56.

75. Lewis JJ, Leung D, Heslin M, et al. Association of local recurrence with subsequent survival in extremity soft tissue sarcoma. *J Clin Oncol* 1997;15:646–652.

76. Dickie CI, Griffin AM, Parent AL, et al. The relationship between local recurrence and radiotherapy treatment volume for soft tissue sarcomas treated with external beam radiotherapy and function preservation surgery. *Int J Radiat Oncol Biol Phys* 2012;82:1528–1534.

77. Kim B, Chen YL, Kirsch DG, et al. An effective preoperative three-dimensional radiotherapy target volume for extremity soft tissue sarcoma and the effect of margin width on local control. *Int J Radiat Oncol Biol Phys* 2010;77:843–850.

78. Baldini EH, Lapidus MR, Wang Q, et al. Predictors for major wound complications following preoperative radiotherapy and surgery for soft-tissue sarcoma of the extremities and trunk: importance of tumor proximity to skin surface. *Ann Surg Oncol* 2013;20:1494–1499.

79. Mendenhall WM, Indelicato DJ, Scarborough MT, et al. The management of adult soft tissue sarcomas. *Am J Clin Oncol* 2009;32:436–442.

80. von Mehren M, Randall RL, Benjamin RS, et al. Soft tissue sarcoma, version 2.2016, NCCN clinical practice guidelines in oncology. *J Natl Compr Canc Netw* 2016;14:758–786.

81. Alektiar KM, Brennan MF, Healey JH, et al. Impact of intensity-modulated radiation therapy on local control in primary soft-tissue sarcoma of the extremity. *J Clin Oncol* 2008;26:3440–3444.

82. Haas RL, Delaney TF, O'Sullivan B, et al. Radiotherapy for management of extremity soft tissue sarcomas: why, when, and where? *Int J Radiat Oncol Biol Phys* 2012;84:572–580.

83. Folkert MR, Singer S, Brennan MF, et al. Comparison of local recurrence with conventional and intensity-modulated radiation therapy for primary soft-tissue sarcomas of the extremity. *J Clin Oncol* 2014;32:3236–3241.

84. Rydholm A, Gustafson P, Rooser B, et al. Limb-sparing surgery without radiotherapy based on anatomic location of soft tissue sarcoma. *J Clin Oncol* 1991;9:1757–1765.

85. Baldini EH, Goldberg J, Jenner C, et al. Long-term outcomes after function-sparing surgery without radiotherapy for soft tissue sarcoma of the extremities and trunk. *J Clin Oncol* 1999;17:3252–3259.

86. Rydholm A, Gustafson P, Rooser B, et al. Subcutaneous sarcoma. A population-based study of 129 patients. *J Bone Joint Surg Br* 1991;73:662–667.

87. Pisters PW, Pollock RE, Lewis VO, et al. Long-term results of prospective trial of surgery alone with selective use of radiation for patients with T1 extremity and trunk soft tissue sarcomas. *Ann Surg* 2007;246:675–681; discussion 681–672.

88. Gibbs CP, Peabody TD, Mundt AJ, et al. Oncological outcomes of operative treatment of subcutaneous soft-tissue sarcomas of the extremities. *J Bone Joint Surg Am* 1997;79:888–897.

89. Alektiar KM, Leung D, Zelefsky MJ, et al. Adjuvant radiation for stage II-B soft tissue sarcoma of the extremity. *J Clin Oncol* 2002;20:1643–1650.

90. Wang D, Zhang Q, Eisenberg BL, et al. Significant reduction of late toxicities in patients with extremity sarcoma treated with image-guided radiation therapy to a reduced target volume: results of Radiation Therapy Oncology Group RTOG-0630 Trial. *J Clin Oncol* 2015;33:2231–2238.

91. Robinson MH, Gaunt P, Grimer R, et al. Vortex trial: a randomized controlled multicenter phase 3 trial of volume of postoperative radiation therapy given to adult patients with extremity Soft Tissue Sarcoma (STS). *Int J Radiat Oncol Biol Phys* 2016;96:S1.

92. Naghavi AO, Fernandez DC, Mesko N, et al. American Brachytherapy Society consensus statement for soft tissue sarcoma brachytherapy. *Brachytherapy* 2017;16:466–489.

93. Al Yami A, Griffin AM, Ferguson PC, et al. Positive surgical margins in soft tissue sarcoma treated with preoperative radiation: is a postoperative boost necessary? *Int J Radiat Oncol Biol Phys* 2010;77:1191–1197.

94. Pan E, Goldberg SI, Chen YL, et al. Role of post-operative radiation boost for soft tissue sarcomas with positive margins following pre-operative radiation and surgery. *J Surg Oncol* 2014;110:817–822.

95. Alektiar KM, Velasco J, Zelefsky MJ, et al. Adjuvant radiotherapy for margin-positive high-grade soft tissue sarcoma of the extremity. *Int J Radiat Oncol Biol Phys* 2000;48:1051–1058.

96. Pohar S, Haq R, Liu L, et al. Adjuvant high-dose-rate and low-dose-rate brachytherapy with external beam radiation in soft tissue sarcoma: a comparison of outcomes. *Brachytherapy* 2007;6:53–57.

97. Petera J, Soumarova R, Ruzickova J, et al. Perioperative hyperfractionated high-dose rate brachytherapy for the treatment of soft tissue sarcomas: multicentric experience. *Ann Surg Oncol* 2010;17:206–210.

98. Andrews SF, Anderson PR, Eisenberg BL, et al. Soft tissue sarcomas treated with postoperative external beam radiotherapy with and without low-dose-rate brachytherapy. *Int J Radiat Oncol Biol Phys* 2004;59:475–480.

99. Delaney TF, Kepka L, Goldberg SI, et al. Radiation therapy for control of soft-tissue sarcomas resected with positive margins. *Int J Radiat Oncol Biol Phys* 2007;67:1460–1469.

100. Ballo MT, Zagars GK, Cormier JN, et al. Interval between surgery and radiotherapy: effect on local control of soft tissue sarcoma. *Int J Radiat Oncol Biol Phys* 2004;58:1461–1467.

101. Dickie CI, Parent AL, Griffin AM, et al. Bone fractures following external beam radiotherapy and limb-preservation surgery for lower extremity soft tissue sarcoma: relationship to irradiated bone length, volume, tumor location and dose. *Int J Radiat Oncol Biol Phys* 2009;75:1119–1124.

102. Marks LB, Yorke ED, Jackson A, et al. Use of normal tissue complication probability models in the clinic. *Int J Radiat Oncol Biol Phys* 2010;76:S10–S19.

103. O'Sullivan B, Griffin AM, Dickie CI, et al. Phase 2 study of preoperative image-guided intensity-modulated radiation therapy to reduce wound and combined modality morbidities in lower extremity soft tissue sarcoma. *Cancer* 2013;119:1878–1884.

104. Hall EJ. Intensity-modulated radiation therapy, protons, and the risk of second cancers. *Int J Radiat Oncol Biol Phys* 2006;65:1–7.

105. Hong L, Alektiar KM, Hunt M, et al. Intensity-modulated radiotherapy for soft tissue sarcoma of the thigh. *Int J Radiat Oncol Biol Phys* 2004;59:752–759.

106. DeLaney TF, Chen Y-L, Baldini EH, et al. Phase 1 trial of preoperative image guided intensity modulated proton radiation therapy with simultaneously integrated boost to the high risk margin for retroperitoneal sarcomas. *Adv Radiat Oncol* 2017;2:85–93.

107. Hansen EK, Larson DA, Aubin M, et al. Image-guided radiotherapy using megavoltage cone-beam computed tomography for treatment of paraspinous tumors in the presence of orthopedic hardware. *Int J Radiat Oncol Biol Phys* 2006;66:323–326.

108. Pitson G, Robinson P, Wilke D, et al. Radiation response: an additional unique signature of myxoid liposarcoma. *Int J Radiat Oncol Biol Phys* 2004;60:522–526.

109. Engstrom K, Bergh P, Cederlund CG, et al. Irradiation of myxoid/round cell liposarcoma induces volume reduction and lipoma-like morphology. *Acta Oncol* 2007;46:838–845.

110. Kramer M, Weyrather WK, Scholz M. The increased biological effectiveness of heavy charged particles: from radiobiology to treatment planning. *Technol Cancer Res Treat* 2003;2:427–436.

111. Igaki H, Tokuuye K, Okumura T, et al. Clinical results of proton beam therapy for skull base chordoma. *Int J Radiat Oncol Biol Phys* 2004;60:1120–1126.

112. Colli B, Al-Mefty O. Chordomas of the craniocervical junction: follow-up review and prognostic factors. *J Neurosurg* 2001;95:933–943.

113. Noel G, Feuvret L, Calugaru V, et al. Chordomas of the base of the skull and upper cervical spine. One hundred patients irradiated by a 3D conformal technique combining photon and proton beams. *Acta Oncol* 2005;44:700–708.

114. Weber DC, Rutz HP, Pedroni ES, et al. Results of spot-scanning proton radiation therapy for chordoma and chondrosarcoma of the skull base: the Paul Scherrer Institut experience. *Int J Radiat Oncol Biol Phys* 2005;63:401–409.

115. Rosenberg AE, Nielsen GP, Keel SB, et al. Chondrosarcoma of the base of the skull: a clinicopathologic study of 200 cases with emphasis on its distinction from chordoma. *Am J Surg Pathol* 1999;23:1370–1378.

116. Noel G, Habrand JL, Jauffret E, et al. Radiation therapy for chordoma and chondrosarcoma of the skull base and the cervical spine. Prognostic factors and patterns of failure. *Strahlenther Onkol* 2003;179:241–248.

117. Schulz-Ertner D, Nikoghosyan A, Didinger B, et al. Carbon ion radiation therapy for chordomas and low grade chondrosarcomas—current status of the clinical trials at GSI. *Radiother Oncol* 2004;73(Suppl 2):S53–S56.

118. Schulz-Ertner D, Nikoghosyan A, Hof H, et al. Carbon ion radiotherapy of skull base chondrosarcomas. *Int J Radiat Oncol Biol Phys* 2007;67:171–177.

119. Kamada T, Tsujii H, Tsuji H, et al. Efficacy and safety of carbon ion radiotherapy in bone and soft tissue sarcomas. *J Clin Oncol* 2002;20:4466–4471.

120. Imai R, Kamada T, Tsuji H, et al. Carbon ion radiotherapy for unresectable sacral chordomas. *Clin Cancer Res* 2004;10:5741–5746.

121. Rusthoven KE, Kavanagh BD, Cardenes H, et al. Multi-institutional phase I/II trial of stereotactic body radiation therapy for liver metastases. *J Clin Oncol* 2009;27:1572–1578.

122. Milano MT, Katz AW, Schell MC, et al. Descriptive analysis of oligometastatic lesions treated with curative-intent stereotactic body radiotherapy. *Int J Radiat Oncol Biol Phys* 2008;72:1516–1522.

123. Hof H, Hoess A, Oetzel D, et al. Stereotactic single-dose radiotherapy of lung metastases. *Strahlenther Onkol* 2007;183:673–678.

124. Levine AM, Coleman C, Horasek S. Stereotactic radiosurgery for the treatment of primary sarcomas and sarcoma metastases of the spine. *Neurosurgery* 2009;64:A54–A59.

125. Pollack A, Zagars GK, Goswitz MS, et al. Preoperative versus postoperative radiotherapy in the treatment of soft tissue sarcomas: a matter of presentation. *Int J Radiat Oncol Biol Phys* 1998;42:563–572.

126. Cannon CP, Ballo MT, Zagars GK, et al. Complications of combined modality treatment of primary lower extremity soft-tissue sarcomas. *Cancer* 2006;107:2455–2461.

127. Kunisada T, Ngan SY, Powell G, et al. Wound complications following pre-operative radiotherapy for soft tissue sarcoma. *Eur J Surg Oncol* 2002;28:75–79.

128. Curtis KK, Ashman JB, Beauchamp CP, et al. Neoadjuvant chemoradiation compared to neoadjuvant radiation alone and surgery alone for Stage II and III soft tissue sarcoma of the extremities. *Radiat Oncol* 2011;6:91.

129. Stinson SF, DeLaney TF, Greenberg J, et al. Acute and long-term effects on limb function of combined modality limb sparing therapy for extremity soft tissue sarcoma. *Int J Radiat Oncol Biol Phys* 1991;21:1493–1499.

130. Davis AM, O'Sullivan B, Turcotte R, et al. Late radiation morbidity following randomization to preoperative versus postoperative radiotherapy in extremity soft tissue sarcoma. *Radiother Oncol* 2005;75:48–53.

131. Rimner A, Brennan MF, Zhang Z, et al. Influence of compartmental involvement on the patterns of morbidity in soft tissue sarcoma of the thigh. *Cancer* 2009;115:149–157.

132. Holt GE, Griffin AM, Pintilie M, et al. Fractures following radiotherapy and limb-salvage surgery for lower extremity soft-tissue sarcomas. A comparison of high-dose and low-dose radiotherapy. *J Bone Joint Surg Am* 2005;87:315–319.

Section III

133. Helmstedter CS, Goebel M, Zlotecki R, et al. Pathologic fractures after surgery and radiation for soft tissue tumors. *Clin Orthop Relat Res* 2001:165–172.

134. Alektiar KM, Zelefsky MJ, Brennan MF. Morbidity of adjuvant brachytherapy in soft tissue sarcoma of the extremity and superficial trunk. *Int J Radiat Oncol Biol Phys* 2000;47:1273–1279.

135. Bishop AJ, Zagars GK, Allen PK, et al. Treatment-related fractures after combined modality therapy for soft tissue sarcomas of the proximal lower extremity: can the risk be mitigated? *Pract Radiat Oncol* 2016;6: 194–200.

136. Cheng EY, Dusenbery KE, Winters MR, et al. Soft tissue sarcomas: preoperative versus postoperative radiotherapy. *J Surg Oncol* 1996;61:90–99.

137. Kuklo TR, Temple HT, Owens BD, et al. Preoperative versus postoperative radiation therapy for soft-tissue sarcomas. *Am J Orthop (Belle Mead NJ)* 2005;34:75–80.

138. Brant TA, Parsons JT, Marcus RB Jr, et al. Preoperative irradiation for soft tissue sarcomas of the trunk and extremities in adults. *Int J Radiat Oncol Biol Phys* 1990;19:899–906.

139. Al-Absi E, Farrokhyar F, Sharma R, et al. A systematic review and meta-analysis of oncologic outcomes of pre-versus postoperative radiation in localized resectable soft-tissue sarcoma. *Ann Surg Oncol* 2010;17:1367–1374.

140. Karasek K, Constine LS, Rosier R. Sarcoma therapy: functional outcome and relationship to treatment parameters. *Int J Radiat Oncol Biol Phys* 1992;24:651–656.

141. Cahlon O, Spierer M, Brennan MF, et al. Long-term outcomes in extremity soft tissue sarcoma after a pathologically negative re-resection and without radiotherapy. *Cancer* 2008;112:2774–2779.

142. Khanfir K, Alzieu L, Terrier P, et al. Does adjuvant radiation therapy increase loco-regional control after optimal resection of soft-tissue sarcoma of the extremities? *Eur J Cancer* 2003;39:1872–1880.

143. Fabrizio PL, Stafford SL, Pritchard DJ. Extremity soft-tissue sarcomas selectively treated with surgery alone. *Int J Radiat Oncol Biol Phys* 2000;48:227–232.

144. Crist WM, Anderson JR, Meza JL, et al. Intergroup rhabdomyosarcoma study-IV: results for patients with nonmetastatic disease. *J Clin Oncol* 2001;19:3091–3102.

145. Gaspar N, Hawkins DS, Dirksen U, et al. Ewing sarcoma: current management and future approaches through collaboration. *J Clin Oncol* 2015;33:3036–3046.

146. Hensley ML, Maki R, Venkatraman E, et al. Gemcitabine and docetaxel in patients with unresectable leiomyosarcoma: results of a phase II trial. *J Clin Oncol* 2002;20:2824–2831.

147. Gortzak E, Azzarelli A, Buesa J, et al. A randomised phase II study on neo-adjuvant chemotherapy for "high-risk" adult soft-tissue sarcoma. *Eur J Cancer* 2001;37:1096–1103.

148. Grobmyer SR, Maki RG, Demetri GD, et al. Neo-adjuvant chemotherapy for primary high-grade extremity soft tissue sarcoma. *Ann Oncol* 2004;15:1667–1672.

149. Italiano A, Penel N, Robin YM, et al. Neo/adjuvant chemotherapy does not improve outcome in resected primary synovial sarcoma: a study of the French Sarcoma Group. *Ann Oncol* 2009;20:425–430.

150. Pisters PW, Patel SR, Prieto VG, et al. Phase I trial of preoperative doxorubicin-based concurrent chemoradiation and surgical resection for localized extremity and body wall soft tissue sarcomas. *J Clin Oncol* 2004;22:3375–3380.

151. Toma S, Canavese G, Grimaldi A, et al. Concomitant chemo-radiotherapy in the treatment of locally advanced and/or metastatic soft tissue sarcomas: experience of the National Cancer Institute of Genoa. *Oncol Rep* 2003;10:641–647.

152. Cormier JN, Patel SR, Herzog CE, et al. Concurrent ifosfamide-based chemotherapy and irradiation. Analysis of treatment-related toxicity in 43 patients with sarcoma. *Cancer* 2001;92:1550–1555.

153. Jakob J, Wenz F, Dinter DJ, et al. Preoperative intensity-modulated radiotherapy combined with temozolomide for locally advanced soft-tissue sarcoma. *Int J Radiat Oncol Biol Phys* 2009;75:810–816.

154. Pisters PW, Ballo MT, Bekele N, et al. Phase I trial using toxicity severity weights for dose finding of gemcitabine combined with radiation therapy and subsequent surgery for patients with extremity and trunk soft tissue sarcomas. *J Clin Oncol* 2004;22:820s [abstract 9008].

155. Palassini E, Ferrari S, Verderio P, et al. Feasibility of preoperative chemotherapy with or without radiation therapy in localized soft tissue sarcomas of limbs and superficial trunk in the Italian Sarcoma Group/Grupo Espanol de Investigacion en Sarcomas Randomized Clinical Trial: three versus five cycles of full-dose Epirubicin Plus Ifosfamide. *J Clin Oncol* 2015;33:3628–3634.

156. DeLaney TF, Spiro IJ, Suit HD, et al. Neoadjuvant chemotherapy and radiotherapy for large extremity soft-tissue sarcomas. *Int J Radiat Oncol Biol Phys* 2003;56:1117–1127.

157. Kraybill WG, Harris J, Spiro IJ, et al. Phase II study of neoadjuvant chemotherapy and radiation therapy in the management of high-risk, high-grade, soft tissue sarcomas of the extremities and body wall: Radiation Therapy Oncology Group Trial 9514. *J Clin Oncol* 2006;24:619–625.

158. Adjuvant chemotherapy for localised resectable soft-tissue sarcoma of adults: meta-analysis of individual data. Sarcoma Meta-analysis Collaboration. *Lancet* 1997;350:1647–1654.

159. Frustaci S, Gherlinzoni F, De Paoli A, et al. Adjuvant chemotherapy for adult soft tissue sarcomas of the extremities and girdles: results of the Italian randomized cooperative trial. *J Clin Oncol* 2001;19:1238–1247.

160. Frustaci S, De Paoli A, Bidoli E, et al. Ifosfamide in the adjuvant therapy of soft tissue sarcomas. *Oncology* 2003;65(Suppl 2):80–84.

161. Brodowicz T, Schwameis E, Widder J, et al. Intensified adjuvant IFADIC chemotherapy for adult soft tissue sarcoma: a prospective randomized feasibility trial. *Sarcoma* 2000;4:151–160.

162. Petrioli R, Coratti A, Correale P, et al. Adjuvant epirubicin with or without Ifosfamide for adult soft-tissue sarcoma. *Am J Clin Oncol* 2002;25:468–473.

163. Bramwell V, Rouesse J, Steward W, et al. Adjuvant CYVADIC chemotherapy for adult soft tissue sarcoma—reduced local recurrence but no improvement in survival: a study of the European Organization for Research and Treatment of Cancer Soft Tissue and Bone Sarcoma Group. *J Clin Oncol* 1994;12:1137–1149.

164. Pervaiz N, Colterjohn N, Farrokhyar F, et al. A systematic meta-analysis of randomized controlled trials of adjuvant chemotherapy for localized resectable soft-tissue sarcoma. *Cancer* 2008;113:573–581.

165. Woll PJ, Reichardt P, Le Cesne A, et al. Adjuvant chemotherapy with doxorubicin, ifosfamide, and lenograstim for resected soft-tissue sarcoma (EORTC 62931): a multicentre randomised controlled trial. *Lancet Oncol* 2012;13:1045–1054.

166. Schoffski P, Chawla S, Maki RG, et al. Eribulin versus dacarbazine in previously treated patients with advanced liposarcoma or leiomyosarcoma: a randomised, open-label, multicentre, phase 3 trial. *Lancet* 2016;387:1629–1637.

167. Demetri GD, von Mehren M, Jones RL, et al. Efficacy and safety of trabectedin or dacarbazine for metastatic liposarcoma or leiomyosarcoma after failure of conventional chemotherapy: results of a phase III randomized multicenter clinical trial. *J Clin Oncol* 2016;34:786–793.

168. Lans TE, Grunhagen DJ, de Wilt JH, et al. Isolated limb perfusions with tumor necrosis factor and melphalan for locally recurrent soft tissue sarcoma in previously irradiated limbs. *Ann Surg Oncol* 2005;12:406–411.

169. Bonvalot S, Rimareix F, Causeret S, et al. Hyperthermic isolated limb perfusion in locally advanced soft tissue sarcoma and progressive desmoid-type fibromatosis with TNF 1 mg and melphalan (T1-M HILP) is safe and efficient. *Ann Surg Oncol* 2009;16:3350–3357.

170. Pennacchioli E, Deraco M, Mariani L, et al. Advanced extremity soft tissue sarcoma: prognostic effect of isolated limb perfusion in a series of 88 patients treated at a single institution. *Ann Surg Oncol* 2007;14:553–559.

171. van Ginkel RJ, Thijssens KM, Pras E, et al. Isolated limb perfusion with tumor necrosis factor alpha and melphalan for locally advanced soft tissue sarcoma: three time periods at risk for amputation. *Ann Surg Oncol* 2007;14:1499–1506.

172. Olofsson R, Bergh P, Berlin O, et al. Long-term outcome of isolated limb perfusion in advanced soft tissue sarcoma of the extremity. *Ann Surg Oncol* 2012;19:1800–1807.

173. Moncrieff MD, Kroon HM, Kam PC, et al. Isolated limb infusion for advanced soft tissue sarcoma of the extremity. *Ann Surg Oncol* 2008;15:2749–2756.

174. Hegazy MA, Kotb SZ, Sakr H, et al. Preoperative isolated limb infusion of Doxorubicin and external irradiation for limb-threatening soft tissue sarcomas. *Ann Surg Oncol* 2007;14:568–576.

175. Issels RD, Lindner LH, Verweij J, et al. Neo-adjuvant chemotherapy alone or with regional hyperthermia for localised high-risk soft-tissue sarcoma: a randomised phase 3 multicentre study. *Lancet Oncol* 2010;11:561–570.

176. Demetri GD, von Mehren M, Blanke CD, et al. Efficacy and safety of imatinib mesylate in advanced gastrointestinal stromal tumors. *N Engl J Med* 2002;347:472–480.

CHAPTER 88

Central Nervous System Tumors in Children

Roger E. Taylor

INTRODUCTION

Central nervous system (CNS) tumors account for 20% to 25% of all malignancies that occur in childhood. According to the North American Association of Central Cancer Registries (NAACCR), the age-standardized incidence rate was 48.47 per million in the 0- to 19-year age group for the period 2004–2007.[1] The incidence was highest among children 1 to 4 years of age and lowest among 10- to 14-year-olds.

The etiology of pediatric CNS tumors remains largely unknown. Only 2% to 5% can be ascribed to a known genetic predisposition. Included in this category are those seen in patients with neurofibromatosis types 1 (NF-1) and 2 (NF-2), tuberous sclerosis, nevoid basal cell (Gorlin's) syndrome, familial adenomatous polyposis, and Li-Fraumeni syndrome. An even smaller percentage can be attributed to ionizing radiation used for diagnostic or therapeutic purposes. For the majority of patients, no predisposing factors can be identified.

The management of children with CNS tumors has changed substantially over the past three decades. Routine use of magnetic resonance imaging (MRI), and now frequently also functional imaging, and improved neuropathologic examination and molecular diagnostics have contributed to better characterization of the different tumor types. Improved neurosurgical techniques and perioperative care permit greater degrees of surgical resection even for tumors previously considered inoperable because of their location in eloquent areas of the brain. All of these, as well as improved radiotherapy techniques, newer chemotherapy agents and regimens, and national and international clinical trials, have contributed to improved outcomes for children and adolescents with CNS tumors. According to the NAACCR, 5-year survival has increased from 62.9% for patients diagnosed in 1980 to 1989 to 75.3% for those diagnosed in 2000 to 2006.[1]

RADIOTHERAPY FOR PEDIATRIC CNS TUMORS: GENERAL ISSUES

Radiotherapy is an essential component of treatment for many children with CNS tumors. However, survivors are at significant risk for the development of long-term sequelae,[2,3] many of which, while usually multifactorial, are in large part because of radiotherapy; many of the strategies used in the management of children with CNS tumors over the past three decades have been designed to reduce the risks associated with treatment. Recent developments in radiotherapy including improved targeting and new technologies and techniques for treatment, as well as new treatment modalities such as protons, all offer important opportunities for therapeutic gain that will be discussed below and in each section of this chapter.

Long-Term Effects of Radiotherapy

The quality of survival of children with brain tumors may be compromised by long-term sequelae. Although some patients (e.g., patients with NF-1) may be at particular risk and although some sequelae (e.g., neurologic deficits) are more often due to the tumor and/or surgery, it is clear that radiotherapy is directly, alone or modulated by other factors, responsible for many late effects. A review by Kortmann et al.[4] gives an excellent account of radiation-related sequelae in children treated for low-grade glioma including effects on brain parenchyma, neurologic deficits, neurocognitive and behavioral effects, endocrine dysfunction, vasculopathy, and the development of second tumors.

The neurocognitive sequelae of radiotherapy have become much better characterized over recent years. It is now known that myelinization and functional maturation of the CNS continue until well into adolescence and even into young adulthood. Through its effect on the microvasculature as well as on the oligodendrocyte precursor cells that produce myelin, radiotherapy causes disrupted neurogenesis and cortical atrophy. Patients fail to acquire new knowledge and skills at an age-appropriate rate and show a progressive decline in IQ over time.[5] The magnitude of the deficit depends most importantly on age at treatment, but many other host (e.g., NF-1 or not), tumor (e.g., location, hydrocephalus or not), and treatment factors (e.g., radiotherapy volume and dose,[6–8] use of chemotherapy[9,10]) play a role. Moreover, the development of other deficits such as behavioral difficulties related to the location of the tumor and/or surgery or hearing impairment because of cisplatin may have a modulating effect. The end result for many patients is impaired school and social performance that deteriorates over time. There is increasing evidence that intervention using cognitive or behavioral therapy or pharmacotherapy and even exercise may be useful and that this should start soon after treatment for best results.[5,11,12]

Endocrine deficits are very common after radiotherapy.[13] Even though a substantial proportion of patients may have had deficits prior to radiotherapy because of the tumor or to surgery,[14,15] and even though there may be modulating factors such as chemotherapy that affect the frequency of deficits, radiotherapy is primarily responsible for the growth hormone deficiency that correlates with the dose of radiotherapy to the hypothalamic–pituitary axis[16–18] and the primary hypothyroidism seen after craniospinal radiotherapy. There may be direct and indirect effects on musculoskeletal development. Osteopenia is a rather common finding that may put patients, particularly those with residual neurologic deficits, at significant risk for fracture.

Radiotherapy has been implicated as well in the development of cardiovascular complications including cerebrovascular events and coronary heart disease.[15,19] Although again the etiology is likely multifactorial, it is important to be cognizant of the risks and to minimize the dose to vascular structures and the heart.

Strategies that have been used to avoid or minimize the long-term effects of treatment for pediatric brain tumors include the following:

- Avoidance of radiotherapy altogether (e.g., in patients with low-grade astrocytoma [LGA] for whom surgery alone may be a good option).
- Delay of radiotherapy for young children (i.e., those younger than age 3 to 8) by the use of chemotherapy.
- Use of daily anesthesia, improved immobilization techniques (e.g., rigid casts or a stereotactic frame), and/or daily pretreatment image verification, all of which allow the use of reduced safety margins.
- Use of image-based treatment planning using computed tomography (CT)–MRI or CT–MRI–functional imaging coregistration and better treatment planning and delivery techniques that result in greater sparing of normal brain and organs at risk.
- Use of new radiation modalities (particularly proton therapy that provides even greater sparing of the surrounding normal brain and organs at risk). Over the last 5 to 10 years, there has been a significant increase in the proportion of children with CNS tumors treated by proton therapy.
- Use of reduced radiotherapy target volumes when it is shown safe to do so (e.g., tumor bed rather than whole posterior fossa for the boost in standard-risk medulloblastoma).
- Reduction of radiotherapy dose (e.g., in young patients with standard-risk medulloblastoma for whom in the North American studies the dose for craniospinal irradiation [CSI] has been reduced progressively from 35 to 36 Gy to 23.4 Gy and, in current studies, to 18 Gy for children younger than 8).
- Use of smaller fraction sizes where appropriate (e.g., 1.5 Gy/day for patients with radiosensitive tumors such as germinoma).
- Use of hyperfractionated radiotherapy (HFRT) (e.g., as in the current European studies for standard-risk medulloblastoma).

These will be discussed later in each relevant clinical situation.

Preparation for Radiotherapy

The planning and delivery of radiotherapy for children with CNS tumors are technically challenging and labor intensive for the entire interprofessional team. The expertise of specialist personnel such as pediatric nurses and play therapists can be pivotal in encouraging a young child to lie still for the making of an immobilization device, for radiotherapy planning procedures, and for treatment itself. For children younger than age 4 or 5 years, daily anesthesia will almost always be necessary, and this will require a skilled pediatric anesthetist because anesthesia will be administered in an environment without all of the support available in an operating room.

Radiotherapy Target Volumes and Treatment Techniques

Focal, Tumor, or Tumor Bed Radiotherapy

For most tumor types, target volume definition is best accomplished using CT simulation with CT–MRI image coregistration. For patients who have undergone cerebrospinal fluid (CSF) diversion or surgical resection or in whom tumor shrinkage has occurred with chemotherapy, it will be important to take into account any anatomic shifts that may have taken place. This will be more of an issue for tumors arising in some areas than others and often adds significantly to the time required for contouring. The clinical target volume (CTV) will be tumor type specific, whereas the planning target volume (PTV) will be technique specific, ranging from 1 to 5 mm depending on the type of immobilization device used and whether daily pretreatment image verification is to be performed.

Modern radiotherapy treatment planning and delivery techniques make it easier to achieve conformity of the treated volume to the target and sparing of uninvolved normal structures than in the past. The choice of technique in an individual patient will require careful analysis of the dosimetry in the context of the available options. A review by Beltran et al.[20] provides an excellent example of the issues to be considered now when weighing alternatives.

Other options for focal treatment include brachytherapy and intracystic injection of radioactive colloids. These will be discussed in the context of the relevant clinical situation.

Whole-Ventricular Radiotherapy

Whole-ventricular irradiation is used most frequently in patients with CNS germ cell tumors. Because subependymal spread is common, the target volume logically would include the lateral, third, and fourth ventricles with a margin of 1 to 1.5 cm. If lateral opposed fields are used, the volume of brain spared will be small. Better sparing can be achieved using intensity-modulated image-guided radiotherapy[21-23] or more recently the use of proton therapy is advocated.

Craniospinal Radiotherapy

The CTV for craniospinal radiotherapy has an irregular shape that consists of the whole brain and spinal cord and their overlying meninges. In standard techniques, the lower borders of lateral whole-brain fields are matched to the cephalad border of a posterior spine field, usually with a moving junction between the brain and spine fields to minimize the risk of underdose or overdose in the cervical spinal cord. With conventional techniques, compensators may be needed to achieve dose homogeneity throughout the target volume.

Patient Positioning and Immobilization

Patients have traditionally received CSI in the prone position, but modern technology allows safe treatment in the supine position that in general is more comfortable and, if anesthesia is required, allows better control of the airway. In either case, immobilization is essential and involves the use of a head shell or full-body immobilization. Careful attention to positioning at the time of simulation is critical to minimize or even eliminate the risk of certain long-term effects. For example, using neck extension together with careful selection of the level for the junction of the brain and spine fields, it is possible to avoid including the dentition in the exit from the superior aspect of the spinal field and thus damage to developing dentition. When modern techniques are employed, it is essential to apply the relevant dose constraints in order to avoid excessive or unnecessary dose to organs at risk (OARs).

Target Volume Definition

CT simulation is necessary to ensure adequate coverage of the CTV in the subfrontal region at the cribriform plate. Traditionally, blocks have been used in the lateral fields to shield not only the facial structures but also the lenses. However, in most children, it is impossible to adequately irradiate the cribriform plate and shield the lenses (Fig. 88.1), and adequate PTV coverage should take precedence.

CT simulation is also helpful in identifying the lateral aspect of CTV for the spine field that includes the extensions

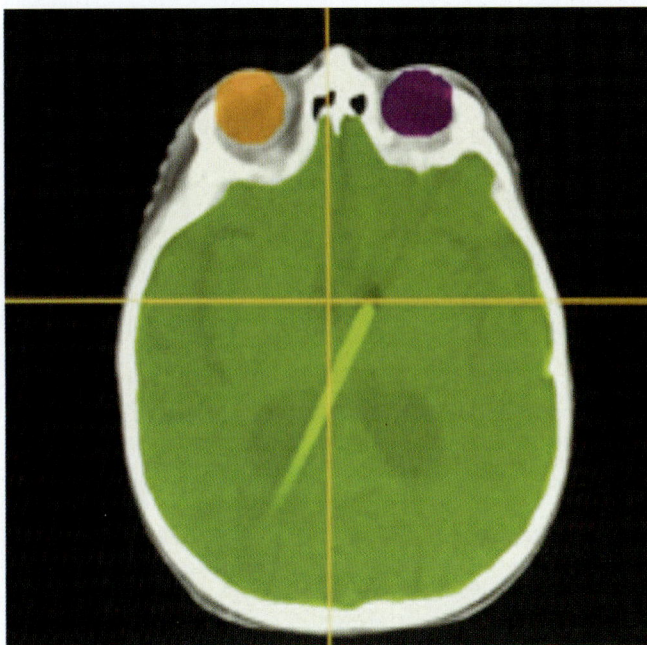

FIGURE 88.1. The use of computed tomography simulation is superior to conventional radiographs for determination of the clinical target volume for craniospinal irradiation and ensures coverage of the meninges in the subfrontal region. In most children, adequate coverage of the planning target volume precludes significant sparing of the lens.

of the meninges along the nerve roots to the lateral aspects of the spinal ganglia (Fig. 88.2). The field will be narrower in the dorsal region to avoid unnecessary irradiation of the heart and lungs and wider in the lumbar region, although here it is important to avoid an excessively wide field that will result in unnecessary irradiation of the bone marrow and gonads. The lower limit of the CTV for the spine field should be determined using MRI. The lower border of the spinal CTV should include the lower border of the thecal sac, which can be as high as L5 or as low as S3. In the interest of both CTV coverage and normal tissue sparing, it is important that the lower border be individualized according to the MRI findings.

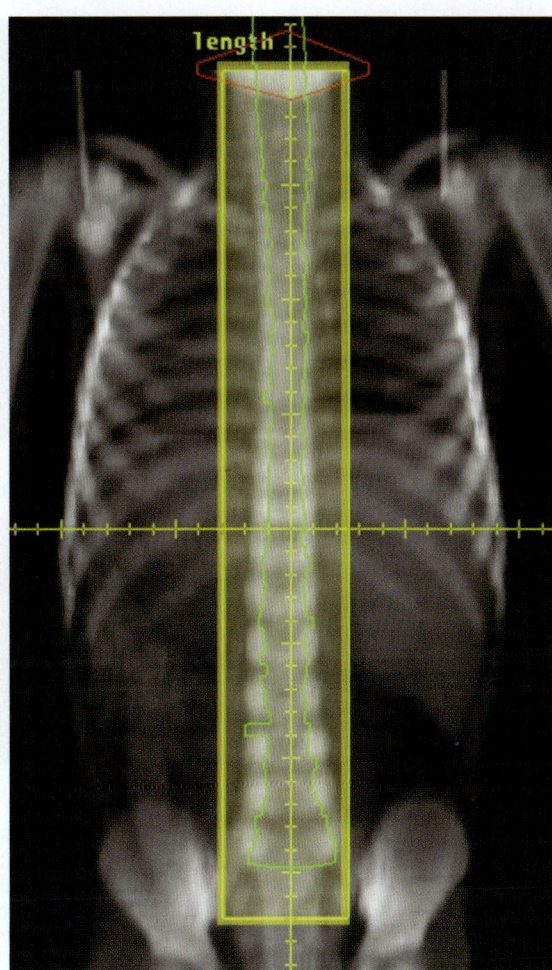

FIGURE 88.2. The use of computed tomography simulation with contouring of the cord and overlying meninges that extend laterally to the lateral aspect of the spinal ganglia results in a field width that is narrower than one based on bony anatomy. The addition of shielding further reduces the volume of normal tissues included in the treated volume.

TABLE 88.1 TECHNICAL CONSIDERATIONS FOR CRANIOSPINAL IRRADIATION	
Problem	**Possible Solutions**
Target volume definition may be difficult using conventional simulation	Use CT simulation with CT-MRI coregistration
Prone position	Supine position preferred
Uncomfortable	
Difficult to monitor airway	
Field matching over cervical spine/risk of over- or underdosage	Angle brain fields
	Use half-beam block for brain fields
	Use couch rotation or match line wedge
Choice of extended SSD or second field for treatment of spinal axis	Two fields preferred
Inhomogeneity along spinal axis	Use compensator, MLC
Irradiation of normal tissues	
Mandible/teeth	Neck extension
Thyroid	Care with level of junction
Heart	Use lower junction
GI tract	Care with width of spine field
Gonads	Use protons, IMRT, electrons
	Use protons, IMRT, electrons
	Care with lower limit and width of spine field

CT, computed tomography; GI, gastrointestinal; IMRT, intensity-modulated radiation therapy; MLC, multileaf collimator; MRI, magnetic resonance imaging; SSD, source-to-surface distance.

Treatment Planning and Delivery

There are many issues that need to be addressed in designing a CSI technique (Table 88.1). Many of the different solutions[24] add further complexity. Using modern tools for treatment planning and delivery, it is possible to greatly simplify the technique and substantially reduce planning and delivery times. One such technique is shown in Figure 88.3.[25] In general, photons in the 6- to 10-MV range provide satisfactory coverage of the PTV. A variation of dose along the spinal axis of >10% will require the use of dose compensation that can be achieved using multileaf collimation.

Electrons are used in some centers to treat the spinal axis and in fact may be of greater interest now than in the past because of improved dose calculation algorithms and even electron dose modulation techniques. However, at the same time, newer treatment planning and delivery methods such as intensity-modulated radiation therapy (IMRT) together with daily image verification allow for improved dosimetry with photons with clinically relevant dose reductions to structures anterior to the target volume such as the heart, gastrointestinal (GI) tract, and gonads.[26] The use of IMRT and smaller PTV margins raises new issues that are not as relevant as when lateral opposed fields were used, such as the need to ensure adequate coverage of all CSF extensions including those along the optic nerves and other cranial nerves (Fig. 88.4).

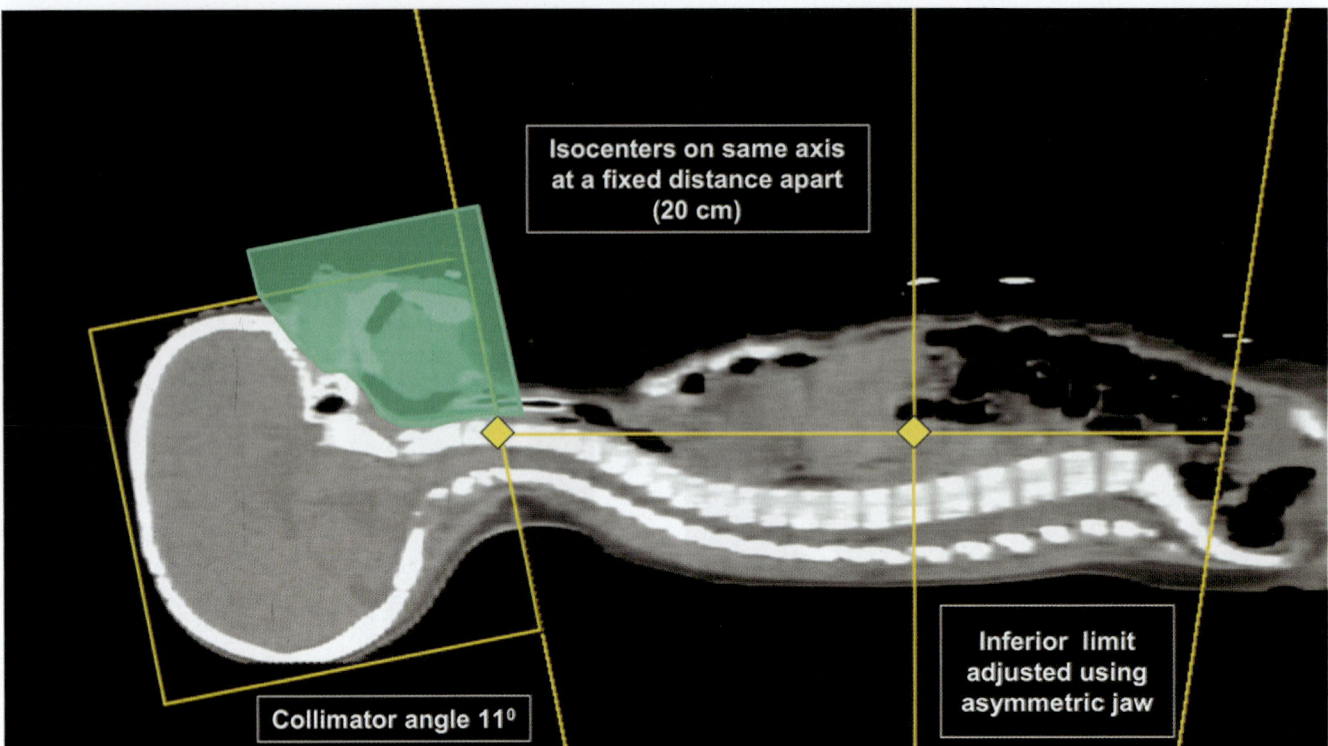

FIGURE 88.3. To cover the clinical target volume for craniospinal irradiation, lateral opposed fields are used to treat the brain and a direct posterior field is used to cover the spinal axis. Magnetic resonance imaging is used to identify the caudal extent of the thecal sac. The field junction over the cervical cord should be at a level that avoids the inclusion of the teeth in the exit of the spinal field and usually is moved weekly ("feathered") to avoid over- or underdosage. The supine position is more comfortable for the patient and safer if sedation or anesthesia is required. In the technique shown, fixed field parameters are used, which greatly facilitates treatment planning and delivery. (Reprinted from Parker WA, Freeman CR. A simple technique for craniospinal radiotherapy in the supine position. *Radiother Oncol* 2006;78[2]:217–222. Copyright © 2005 Elsevier Ireland Ltd. With permission.)

FIGURE 88.4. Postoperative axial T2-weighted magnetic resonance imaging for a patient receiving craniospinal irradiation (CSI) for medulloblastoma showing extension of cerebrospinal fluid along the optic nerves to the lamina cribrosa **(A)** and into the internal auditory canals **(B)**. Care is necessary to identify all such extensions when using intensity-modulated radiation therapy for CSI given that the margins are much tighter than when using conventional lateral opposed fields.

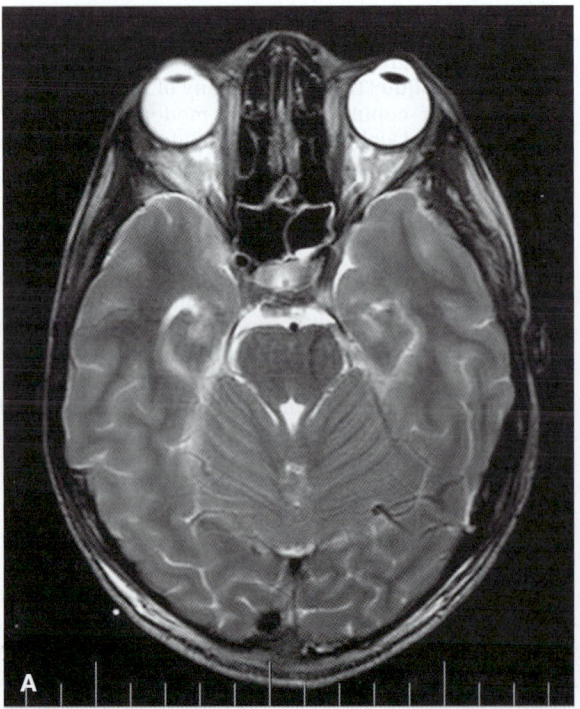
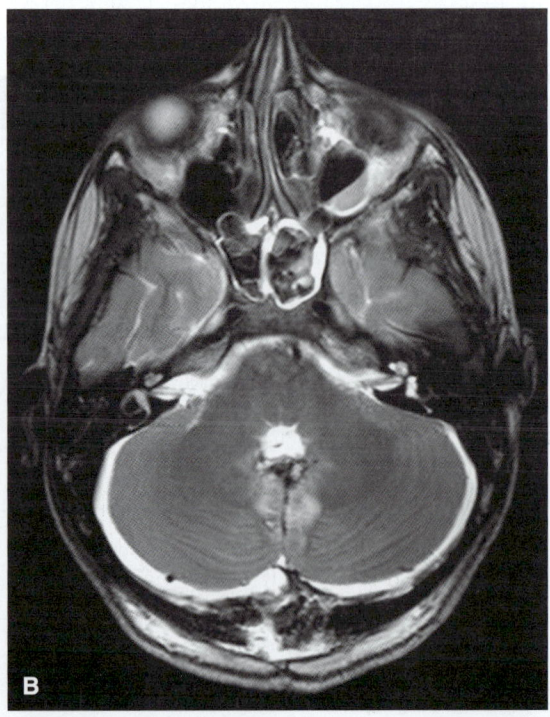

New Treatment Modalities for CSI

Protons provide a dose distribution for CSI that cannot be achieved by even the most sophisticated photon beam treatment planning, with significant reduction in low dose exposure outside the target volume.[27] There may be significant benefits from reduced irradiation of the heart and organs anterior to the spine. Currently, an increasing number of children requiring craniospinal radiotherapy are treated by proton therapy.[28]

Radiation Dose and Dose Fractionation Regimens

The conventional daily fraction size for the treatment of most pediatric CNS tumors is 1.8 Gy and the total dose typically on the order of 54 to 55.8 Gy. When treating a primary tumor of the spinal cord, it is conventional to use a lower total dose (e.g., 50.4 Gy). It is also usual to use lower doses for children younger than age 3 years to reduce the risk of neurocognitive deficits. When treating radiosensitive tumors such as intracranial germinoma, radiotherapy may be delivered using a lower dose per fraction (e.g., 1.5 Gy) and lower total doses of 30 to 45 Gy.

Many pediatric brain tumors exhibit a dose–response relationship for tumor control, and in some cases, local progression is not prevented by the use of a conventional "CNS tolerance" radiation dose. When the target contains only a small volume of normal brain tissue, dose escalation may be possible using newer treatment planning and delivery techniques. HFRT may be a useful strategy in situations where dose escalation cannot be achieved safely using conventional fractionation.

Follow-Up During and After Radiotherapy

An excellent review by Donahue[29] describes the acute reactions seen during treatment with radiotherapy and provides guidelines for their management. These days nausea and vomiting almost always can be prevented by the use of the 5HT-3 antagonists. Headache is not an expected side effect and should be investigated by physical examination for signs of raised intracranial pressure and by imaging as appropriate. Steroids, if used, usually can be tapered by the second or third week of treatment. Fatigue is a rather common symptom and is cumulative. The neurologic status of the patient, especially coordination and gait, may appear to worsen during the last weeks of treatment because of this. Children usually recover relatively quickly and often can get back to their usual routine quite soon after completion of treatment.

Predictable effects of treatment include hormonal deficits, especially primary hypothyroidism when CSI is delivered using photons and growth hormone deficit secondary to inclusion of the hypothalamic–pituitary axis. Patients should be monitored closely in follow-up and treatment instituted as appropriate. Many will also need regular follow-up in ophthalmology and audiology.

Extra pedagogic support may be necessary. Patients should have ready access to a neuropsychologist for evaluation of any special needs and in the longer term to vocational assessment and counseling.

RADIOTHERAPY FOR SPECIFIC TUMOR TYPES

The World Health Organization (WHO) classification of tumors of the nervous system that has recently been updated in 2016[30] is given in Table 88.2 and the distribution by tumor type and location in Fig. 88.5. The 2016 classification takes into account molecular characteristics of CNS tumors. There are important differences between tumors seen in childhood and those occurring in adults. In children, almost half

TABLE 88.2 WORLD HEALTH ORGANIZATION CLASSIFICATION OF TUMORS OF THE CENTRAL NERVOUS SYSTEM
Diffuse Astrocytic and Oligodendroglial Tumors
Other Astrocytic Tumors
Ependymal Tumors
Other Gliomas
Choroid Plexus Tumors
Neuronal and Mixed Neuronal–Glial Tumors
Tumors of the Pineal Region
Embryonal TumorsTumors of the Cranial and Peripheral Nerves

of all tumors arise in the infratentorial compartment. Low-grade astrocytic tumors as a group account for approximately one-third to half of all CNS tumors, but medulloblastoma is the most common distinct entity. High-grade gliomas, which account for the majority of primary brain tumors seen in adults, are much less common in children.

This chapter will follow the order of the WHO classification. Although in the past tumors arising in infants and very young children were grouped together and all managed similarly with chemotherapy in order to delay or if possible avoid radiotherapy, they are now managed according to the specific tumor type and so will be discussed here in each relevant section.

ASTROCYTIC TUMORS

- Pilocytic astrocytoma (WHO grade I)
  - Pilomyxoid astrocytoma
- Subependymal giant cell astrocytoma
- Pleomorphic xanthoastrocytoma
- Diffuse astrocytoma (WHO grade II)
  - Fibrillary astrocytoma
  - Gemistocytic astrocytoma
  - Protoplasmic astrocytoma
- Anaplastic astrocytoma (WHO grade III)
- Glioblastoma multiforme (WHO grade IV)
  - Giant cell glioblastoma
  - Gliosarcoma
- Gliomatosis cerebri

These astrocytic tumors are heterogeneous with respect to clinical presentation (age, gender, location in the CNS, imaging findings) as well as to growth potential and rate of progression. Two entities, pleomorphic xanthoastrocytoma and subependymal giant cell astrocytoma, are rare tumors. Their clinical presentation and imaging findings are quite characteristic and surgery is usually curative. They will not be discussed further here.

Low-Grade Astrocytoma (WHO Grades I and II)

So-called benign or low-grade astrocytomas (LGAs) comprise a heterogeneous group of tumors with behavior patterns that are fairly typical according to location and pathologic type. In general, in children, they follow an indolent clinical course with overall survival rates at 10 and 15 years as high as 80% to 100%. LGAs can be grouped according to their anatomic location:

- Cerebellar astrocytomas (15% to 20% of all CNS tumors)
- Hemispheric astrocytomas (10% to 15% of all CNS tumors)
- Midline supratentorial tumors, including the corpus callosum, lateral and third ventricles, and hypothalamus and thalamus (10% to 15% of all CNS tumors)
- Optic pathway tumors (approximately 5% of all CNS tumors)
- Brainstem LGAs (brainstem tumors account for 10% to 15% of all CNS tumors; 20% to 30% of these are LGAs)
- LGAs of the spinal cord (spinal cord tumors account for 3% to 6% of all CNS tumors; approximately 60% of these are LGAs)

Section III

Distribution of all childhood primary brain and CNS tumors (ages 0–19 years) by site
(n = 15,295)

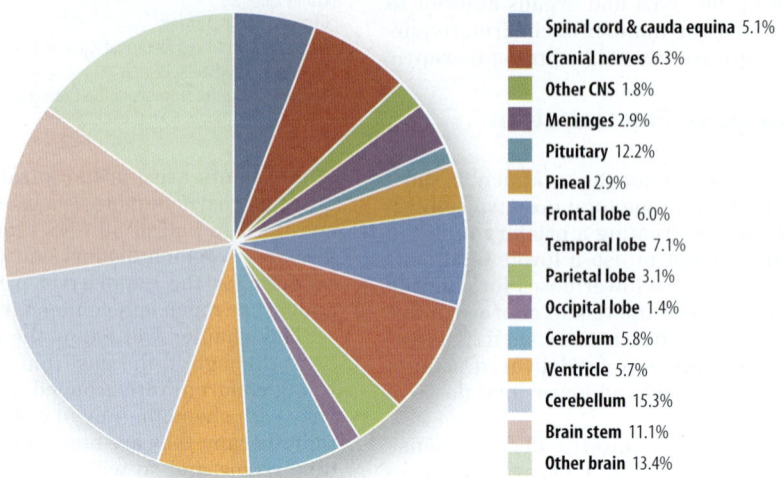

Spinal cord & cauda equina 5.1%
Cranial nerves 6.3%
Other CNS 1.8%
Meninges 2.9%
Pituitary 12.2%
Pineal 2.9%
Frontal lobe 6.0%
Temporal lobe 7.1%
Parietal lobe 3.1%
Occipital lobe 1.4%
Cerebrum 5.8%
Ventricle 5.7%
Cerebellum 15.3%
Brain stem 11.1%
Other brain 13.4%

Distribution of all childhood primary brain and CNS tumors by histology

Ages 0–14 years
(n = 11,004)

Ages 15–19 years
(n = 4,291)

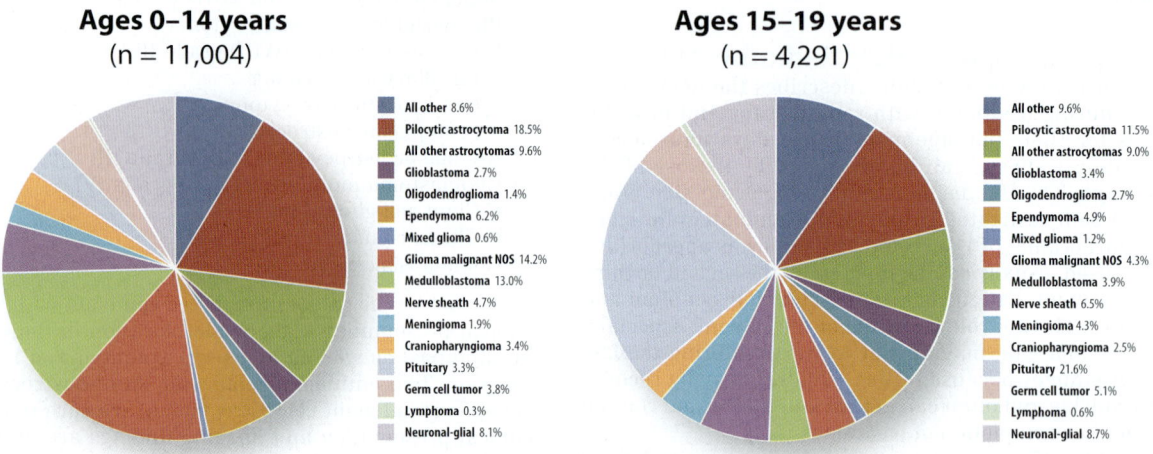

Ages 0–14 years:
All other 8.6%
Pilocytic astrocytoma 18.5%
All other astrocytomas 9.6%
Glioblastoma 2.7%
Oligodendroglioma 1.4%
Ependymoma 6.2%
Mixed glioma 0.6%
Glioma malignant NOS 14.2%
Medulloblastoma 13.0%
Nerve sheath 4.7%
Meningioma 1.9%
Craniopharyngioma 3.4%
Pituitary 3.3%
Germ cell tumor 3.8%
Lymphoma 0.3%
Neuronal-glial 8.1%

Ages 15–19 years:
All other 9.6%
Pilocytic astrocytoma 11.5%
All other astrocytomas 9.0%
Glioblastoma 3.4%
Oligodendroglioma 2.7%
Ependymoma 4.9%
Mixed glioma 1.2%
Glioma malignant NOS 4.3%
Medulloblastoma 3.9%
Nerve sheath 6.5%
Meningioma 4.3%
Craniopharyngioma 2.5%
Pituitary 21.6%
Germ cell tumor 5.1%
Lymphoma 0.6%
Neuronal-glial 8.7%

FIGURE 88.5. Distribution of central nervous system tumors by site **(A)** and histology **(B)** for the years 2004–2007. (Data from the Central Brain Tumor Registry of the United States [www.cbtrus.org].)

Pilocytic astrocytomas are the most common type in the pediatric age group, accounting for almost all of the LGAs at certain sites (e.g., the cerebellum and the anterior optic pathway). They account for a smaller proportion of LGAs arising in the deep midline structures and in the cerebral hemispheres. Macroscopically, pilocytic astrocytomas appear well circumscribed and frequently have an associated cystic component. Pilocytic astrocytomas are characterized histologically by a biphasic pattern with a varying proportion of compacted bipolar cells with Rosenthal fibers and loose-textured multipolar cells with microcysts and granular bodies. Rare mitoses, occasional hyperchromatic nuclei, microvascular proliferation, and even infiltration of the meninges are compatible with a diagnosis of pilocytic astrocytoma and not a sign of malignancy. *KIAA1549-BRAF* fusions have been identified in 75% of patients with PA using an RT-PCR assay from FFPE tissue.[31]

A variant, pilomyxoid astrocytoma, first described in infants and young children with chiasmatic/hypothalamic tumors, appears to be associated with more aggressive behavior that may include leptomeningeal seeding.[32]

Diffuse astrocytomas account for only approximately 10% to 15% of all LGAs in children but for a relatively higher proportion of those seen in infants and adolescents. Most intrinsic pontine tumors and a large proportion of astrocytomas arising in the cerebral hemispheres are diffuse astrocytomas. Diffuse astrocytomas grow by infiltration rather than destruction of anatomic structures and usually are not well circumscribed. Microscopically, they are composed of well-differentiated fibrillary or gemistocytic neoplastic astrocytes on a background of loosely structured, often microcystic, tumor matrix. Cellularity is moderately increased. The presence of nuclear atypia is a diagnostic criterion, but mitotic activity, necrosis, and microvascular proliferation are absent. The growth fraction as determined by Ki-67 and MIB-1 labeling indices is usually low. Diffuse astrocytomas may undergo malignant progression, although this is not common in the pediatric age group with the notable exception of tumors arising in the pons.

Patients with LGAs typically present with a long history of nonspecific and nonlocalizing symptoms. Symptoms and signs of raised intracranial pressure may be seen in patients with midline and cerebellar tumors. Patients with posterior fossa tumors may present with neck stiffness and a head tilt as a manifestation of raised intracranial pressure causing tonsillar herniation, altitudinal diplopia, or spinal accessory nerve irritation. Seizures are present in as many as three-quarters of patients with hemispheric lesions. Other symptoms relatively less frequent and usually of more recent onset relate to the location of the tumor. These may include, for example, focal motor deficits with hemispheric tumors, visual field deficits with tumors compressing or involving the optic pathway, neuroendocrine deficits with hypothalamic tumors, and the diencephalic syndrome (consisting of emaciation with loss of subcutaneous fat despite normal or increased appetite, alert appearance, increased vigor and euphoria, pallor without anemia, and nystagmoid movements of the eyes) in young children with chiasmatic/hypothalamic tumors.

Neuroimaging findings are usually quite characteristic. Pilocytic astrocytomas are well circumscribed, often with a cystic component that may be large relative to the size of the solid component. There is usually little edema or mass effect. The solid component enhances brightly and uniformly with contrast material. Diffuse or fibrillary astrocytomas are usually not well seen on nonenhanced CT or MRI and usually show little enhancement with contrast material. T2-weighted or fluid-attenuated inversion recovery (FLAIR) MRI sequences usually best demonstrate the extent of disease.

Management of Low-Grade Astrocytomas: General Principles

Some children with LGAs may not require any tumor-specific treatment. These include, for example, patients with NF-1, as many as 15% of whom have optic pathway tumors.[33] NF-1 patients also may have astrocytic tumors in other parts of the CNS as well as hamartomatous lesions, typically in the brainstem. These lesions may be detected on routine imaging, but even tumors that are symptomatic may remain stable over long periods so that surveillance is appropriate initial management.[34-36] A number of clinical and imaging characteristics have been correlated with a more aggressive course, but even for these patients, active intervention will usually be undertaken only at time of progressive disease that is symptomatic.

Progression-free survival without treatment may also be very good for patients with tectal plate lesions who present with hydrocephalus without localizing brainstem signs. LGA in this region may be very indolent, showing either no progression (the majority) or only very slow progression over the course of many years following CSF diversion alone. The common characteristics of these very indolent tumors are their small size (<1.5 or 2 cm) and the fact that on imaging they are hypodense/hypointense and nonenhancing. Follow-up with MRI is essential to identify patients with progressive lesions as manifested by increasing size and/or enhancement with gadolinium. Treatment (usually radiotherapy but sometimes now surgery) at time of progression is associated with a high probability of long-term tumor control.

These special situations underscore the need for careful evaluation and individualization of management of patients with LGAs depending on the specific clinical situation and tumor type. If in doubt, a period of surveillance generally will be an acceptable initial approach, reserving nonsurgical treatment for symptomatic progression.

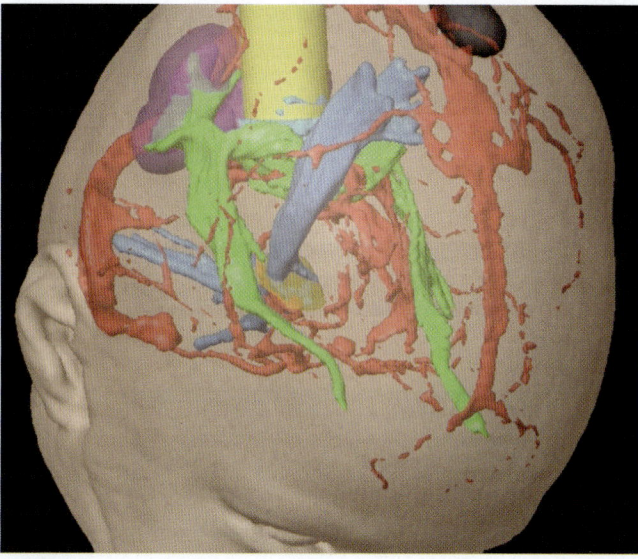

FIGURE 88.6. Surgical planning for a dysembryoplastic neuroepithelial tumor (*light blue*) in the right occipital lobe presenting with seizures. Functional magnetic resonance imaging data are used to identify the 1-degree visual cortex (*purple*). Fiber tracking identifies the optic radiations (*green*) and the corticospinal tract (*darker blue*). These data are then used to plan the trajectory (*yellow*). By identifying regions to be selectively avoided, similar information could be helpful in radiotherapy treatment planning.

Surgery is the mainstay of treatment for LGAs. Complete resection is more likely to be accomplished in patients with smaller tumors and those arising in noneloquent parts of the brain as well as in patients with the generally well-circumscribed pilocytic tumors. Modern surgical techniques that include, for example, computer-assisted resections ("neuronavigation") aided by preoperative functional MRI, MR tractography, and intraoperative mapping of eloquent areas (Fig. 88.6) together with intraoperative MRI permit greater degrees of resection in larger proportions of patients, including many who in the past would have been considered to have inoperable lesions. Complete resection is now achieved in >80% of cerebral, cerebellar, and spinal cord tumors and about 50% of diencephalic tumors.

Children with LGAs who undergo complete resection fare very well, with long-term disease-free and overall survival rates of 80% to 100%.[37-42] In most series, results are better (close to 100%) for patients with pilocytic astrocytomas than for those with diffuse or fibrillary LGAs, although some have disputed this, showing equally satisfactory results for both. In either type, postoperative adjuvant therapy is not indicated.

For children who undergo less than complete resection, the progression-free survival rate after surgery alone is less satisfactory. In a joint Children's Cancer Group (CCG)–Pediatric Oncology Group (POG) study in which such patients were observed without adjuvant treatment, any residual tumor was associated with an inferior progression-free survival rate: the 8-year progression-free survival rate was 56% for patients with <1.5 cm³ residual tumor and 45% for those with >1.5 cm³. However, the majority of patients can be salvaged with a second surgical resection and/or radiotherapy. In the CCG–POG study, overall survival at 8 years was 95% and 90%, respectively.[43]

The role of postoperative radiotherapy following less than complete resection remains unclear. In most series, the use of radiotherapy in this situation results in improved disease-free survival without any benefit in terms of overall survival. Because only approximately half of all patients will develop progressive disease, the usual recommendation for a patient who is neurologically stable will be surveillance, with MRI performed at least every 6 months for the first 3 years, the period during

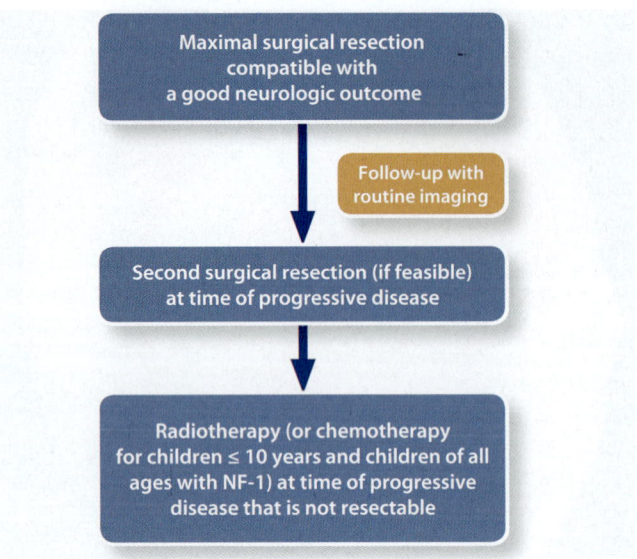

FIGURE 88.7. An algorithm for the management of patients with low-grade astrocytoma.

which risk of progression is greatest.[44] A second surgical procedure would usually be considered at time of progression, and other treatment, either radiotherapy or chemotherapy, reserved for patients with progressive, inoperable disease (Fig. 88.7).

In the past, patients with deep midline and other tumors considered surgically inaccessible were treated with radiotherapy, often even without histologic confirmation of diagnosis. However, using modern neurosurgical techniques, it is feasible to resect surgically about half of these lesions

(Fig. 88.8), and the overall strategy for these patients should now be as for patients with LGAs at other locations, albeit with the understanding that outcome is not as satisfactory. The 8-year progression-free and overall survival rates in the CCG–POG study for patients with midline chiasmatic tumors were 25% and 84%, respectively.[43]

When adjuvant therapy is indicated, the options include chemotherapy, particularly for infants and young children and for patients of all ages with NF-1 who are at greatest risk of developing neurocognitive, vasoocclusive, and neuroendocrine sequelae of treatment. The standard combination chemotherapy employed is based on a combination of carboplatin and vincristine. Complete responses to chemotherapy are not common, but overall response rates that include stable disease range from 70% to 100% and the use of chemotherapy has been shown to permit delay of radiotherapy by 2 to as many as 4+ years.[45–48] The age limit below which chemotherapy should be used is controversial. There is a trend over time for chemotherapy to be employed as initial treatment for older children. It is likely that delaying radiotherapy for 2 to 3 years will be of benefit for a child younger than age 5 to 8. However, the benefit from a similar delay for an older child is less clear, particularly when any benefit may be offset by neurologic compromise from further tumor progression as well as the need for a larger radiotherapy target volume. Moreover, recent advances in radiotherapy practice that have the potential to reduce the risks of radiotherapy have led to a reassessment of the role of radiotherapy in LGAs and better acceptance of its earlier use even in very young children.

Radiotherapy in LGAs
Due largely to improvements in surgery and to a lesser extent to successful treatment of younger children with chemotherapy, there has been a substantial decrease in the use of

FIGURE 88.8. A 12-year-old boy referred to the radiation oncology department 3 years after diagnosis of a biopsy-proven JPA of the left thalamus at another institution. He had been deemed inoperable at diagnosis and had received chemotherapy first with vincristine and carboplatin and then with weekly vinblastine. **A:** At the time of referral, he was having more frequent choreoathetotic movements of his right hand and there was evidence of progressive disease on magnetic resonance imaging (MRI). **B:** He underwent complete resection without complications and has no evidence of residual disease on his most recent MRI. This was a far better approach than radiotherapy, avoiding the neurocognitive, endocrine, and vascular complications associated with radiotherapy for tumors in this region, and with a greater probability of long-term tumor control.

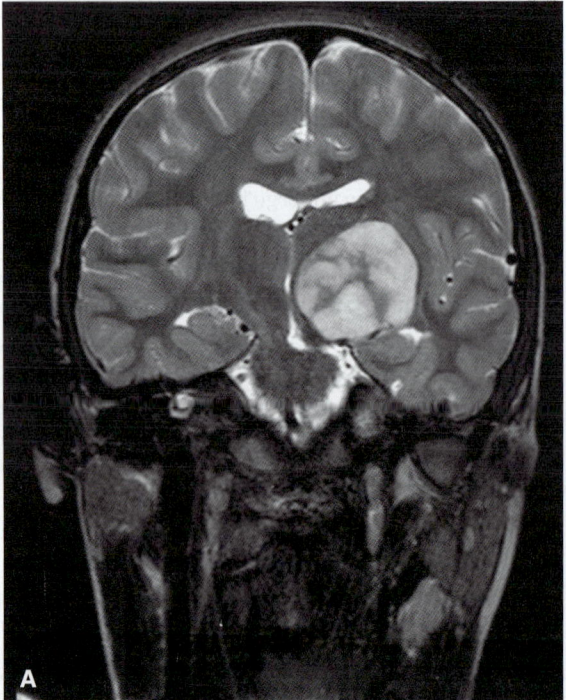
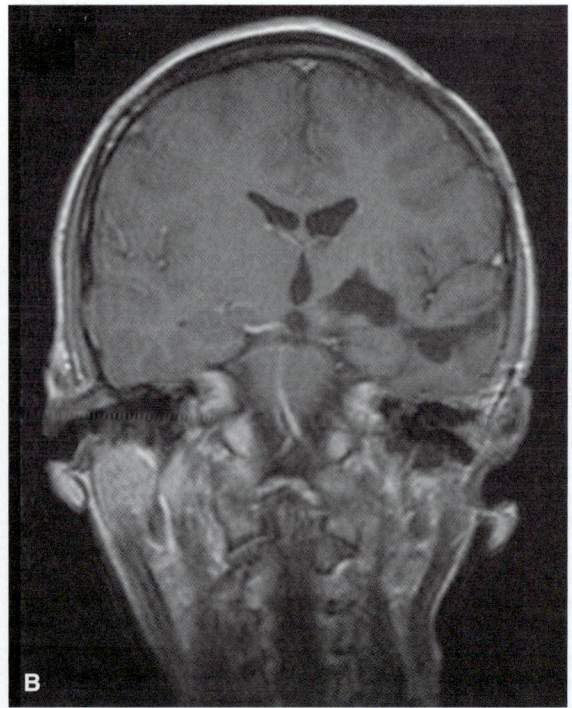

radiotherapy over recent years. Currently, only approximately 10% of all children with LGAs receive radiotherapy.

Indications for Radiotherapy

- Radiotherapy is not indicated after complete resection.
- Radiotherapy may be indicated following incomplete resection in situations when tumor progression would compromise neurologic function (e.g., "threat to vision").
- The clearest indication for radiotherapy is in patients with progressive and/or symptomatic disease that is unresectable.

Radiotherapy Target Volume

The radiotherapy target volume (the gross tumor volume or GTV) consists of all disease seen on MRI performed just prior to treatment (Fig. 88.9). The resulting treatment volume usually will be considerably smaller than one based on preoperative imaging, which until recently would have constituted standard practice. Similarly, margins that were considered standard (and still are in adult practice) are unnecessary, particularly for the well-circumscribed pilocytic tumor for which a CTV margin of 1 cm[42] or even 0 cm (i.e., CTV = GTV)[49] around the GTV as seen on T1-weighted gadolinium-enhanced images has been shown to result in excellent local control. More generous margins of 1 to 1.5 cm around the GTV as seen on T2-weighted or FLAIR images may be more appropriate for the more infiltrative diffuse fibrillary tumors. Radiotherapy planning will also take into account OARs including the hippocampus. Future protocols will specify hippocampal dose constraints.

Radiotherapy Dose

Evidence for a dose–response correlation in LGAs in children is scant. Although the European and North American studies that randomized adult patients with LGAs between low dose (45 and 50.4 Gy, respectively) and high dose (59.4 and 64.8 Gy, respectively) radiotherapy failed to demonstrate any advantage for the higher dose, it may be unwise to extrapolate that in children doses of 45 to 50 Gy are as effective as the higher doses of 54 to 55 Gy that until now have constituted standard practice. There are biologic differences between LGAs in children and in adults. As well, children who have progressed on chemotherapy may have tumors that are less sensitive. For now, the recommendation for children with LGAs would be a "standard" dose of 50 to 54 Gy depending on the age of the child and the location of the tumor and its relationship to critical normal structures such as the optic chiasm.

Radiotherapy Technique

External beam radiotherapy using a conventional dose-fractionation schedule should be considered the standard of care in LGAs and the technique to be used that which provides homogeneous irradiation of the CTV and best spares surrounding normal tissues. Increasingly proton therapy is being employed for the treatment of LGGs as a means of minimizing nontarget dose and hopefully late neurocognitive effects.

Other approaches that have been used in LGAs include radiosurgery using the gamma knife or linear accelerator–based techniques.[50] Although the use of a single fraction, typically of 10 to 20 Gy, to the periphery of the lesion or a small number of large fractions may not be optimal for diffuse or fibrillary LGAs with tumor cells embedded in rather than displacing normal brain, such treatment may be of interest for part or even all of the treatment for the less invasive pilocytic astrocytomas that are often small at time of progression.

Another option for treatment is brachytherapy, which has been used with some success particularly in European centers.[51–55] As for radiosurgery, the principal limitation with respect to the use of brachytherapy is the size of the target volume. Brachytherapy series necessarily select for smaller tumors, and there is no evidence that brachytherapy is a better treatment option than external beam radiotherapy. Radioactive solutions such as ^{32}P, ^{90}Y, ^{198}Au, and ^{186}Re may be useful in cystic LGAs, particularly for patients with recurrent disease after radiotherapy in whom symptoms not infrequently relate more to the cyst than to the solid component of tumor. Simple aspiration with or without placement of an internal shunt usually will alleviate symptoms for protracted periods, but in some cases, particularly those in which the cyst wall enhances and is felt to be biologically active, control of the cyst may be difficult, and the use of radioactive solutions could be considered. However, this is not a procedure without risks and care has to be taken to avoid leakage.

FIGURE 88.9. This patient underwent subtotal resection of a low-grade astrocytoma of the left cerebellar peduncle at age 8. **A:** Preoperative. **B:** Postoperative. **C:** Three years later, routine imaging showed evidence of progressive disease. The gross tumor volume for radiotherapy consists of the tumor as seen on magnetic resonance imaging at the time of treatment.

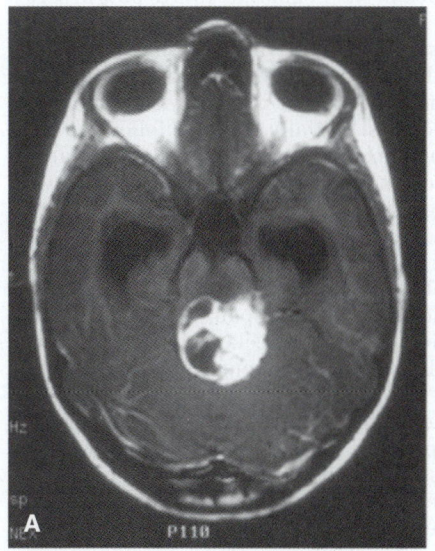
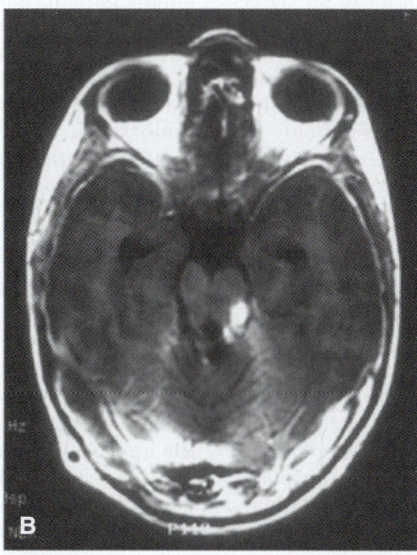
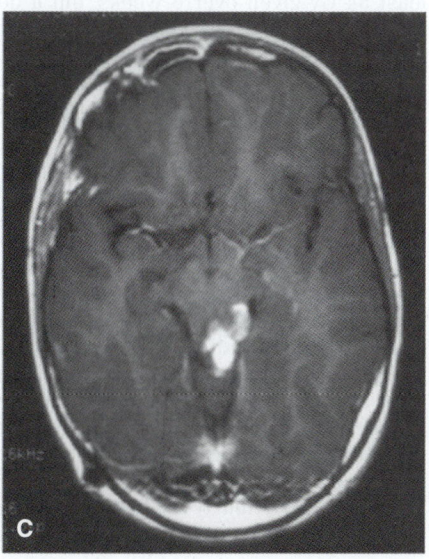

Follow-Up after Radiotherapy

Tumor regression after radiotherapy typically is slow and patients and their families need to be warned that the tumor may remain stable or sometimes even increase in size in the first months after completion of treatment. It is important not to assume that changes seen on MRI represent progressive disease. Close follow-up with early repeat imaging usually will be the best approach in this situation.

High-Grade Astrocytoma (WHO Grades III and IV)

Anaplastic astrocytoma (AA) is a diffusely infiltrating malignant astrocytoma characterized by nuclear atypia, increased cellularity, and significant proliferative activity. Glioblastoma multiforme (GBM) is the most malignant astrocytic tumor. Histopathologic features include nuclear atypia, cellular pleomorphism, mitotic activity, vascular thrombosis, microvascular proliferation, and necrosis. Both AA and GBM may develop from WHO grade II astrocytomas. However, with the exception of tumors that arise in the pons, they arise almost always in the pediatric age group *de novo* without evidence of a less malignant precursor lesion.

High-grade astrocytomas (HGAs) account for 5% of all CNS tumors in the pediatric age group. They are the most common tumor type in older adolescents. Two-thirds of HGAs are located in the cerebral hemispheres and the remainder approximately equally divided between the deep midline structures (thalamus and basal ganglia) and cerebellum. Patients with HGAs usually present with symptoms of short duration that relate to the location of the lesion.

Surgery is an important component of treatment. Because most studies show a survival advantage for patients who have undergone complete resection,[56-60] maximal surgical resection compatible with a good neurologic outcome should be the goal for all patients and a second surgical procedure should be considered if there is significant residual tumor after the first. Postoperative radiotherapy always is indicated. Although leptomeningeal seeding is seen in a substantial minority (10% to 30%) of patients, the predominant failure pattern is local and the radiotherapy target volume is local, with a GTV that consists of the tumor bed and any residual enhancing or nonenhancing residual tumor plus any abnormality seen on T2-weighted MRI with a margin for the CTV of 1.5 cm. Because these are often large tumors and doses beyond tolerance levels for structures such as the optic chiasm are required, it is usual to consider a volume reduction at 50 to 54 Gy to a CTV that consists of the tumor bed and any residual tumor plus a reduced margin of 1 cm. The dose to the CTV should be at least 54 Gy given over 6 weeks, but a dose of 59 to 60 Gy is more usual if feasible. There is no evidence that higher doses delivered using radiosurgery or stereotactic boosts, boosts with brachytherapy, or HFRT result in improved outcome, but IMRT delivering accelerated treatment to a component of the target volume (such as the GTV) may be of interest, if only to decrease the overall treatment duration.

The role of chemotherapy remains to be defined. Although responses are seen to many different agents and regimens, results have often been difficult to interpret because of small patient numbers, inconsistent inclusion criteria with respect to pathology, and confounding variables such as tumor location and extent of surgical resection. The cooperative groups in North America and Europe are investigating a number of approaches that include newer chemotherapeutic and biologic agents, some of which have radiosensitizing properties. Whenever possible, patients should be treated on such protocols. Off study, it may be difficult to make a recommendation with respect to adjuvant chemotherapy, although the poor prognosis, particularly for patients with macroscopic residual disease following surgery, usually is given as an argument for the use of the "current best" regimen, most often now temozolomide as in adults. Recent trials have explored the role of bevacizumab in addition to temozolomide, and mature outcome data are awaited.

The prognosis for children with HGAs is poor, with a median time to progression of 10 to 11 months and an overall survival at 5 years of only approximately 20%. Several factors correlate with outcome. Patients with lesions in the cerebral hemispheres fare better than those with tumors in other locations, apparently independent of extent of surgical resection. The prognosis for children with thalamic lesions appears to be particularly poor.[61] Age also may be an important factor. In contrast to most other tumor types, children younger than age 3 with HGAs fare better than older children, with overall survival at 3 to 5 years in the 33% to 50% range in the North American and United Kingdom Children's Cancer Study Group/International Paediatric Oncology Society (UKCCSG/SIOP) baby studies.[62-65] The prognosis may be even better for children younger than age 1.[66] Histologic grade (AA vs. GBM) has not been shown consistently to affect outcome, but p53 overexpression and a high MIB-1 labeling index appear to identify patients with a particularly adverse prognosis.[67]

Management of Astrocytic Tumors in Specific Locations

Optic Pathway Gliomas

Optic pathway gliomas collectively account for approximately 5% of all CNS tumors in the pediatric age group. These are tumors of young children: the peak age incidence is between 2 and 6 years and 75% of all patients are younger than 10. One-third of patients have NF-1. They may be divided into three clinicopathologic entities: tumors confined to the optic nerve(s), tumors of the optic chiasm with or without optic nerve involvement (collectively "anterior" tumors), and tumors that involve the hypothalamus or adjacent structures ("chiasmatic/hypothalamic" or "posterior" tumors). Management of patients with optic pathway gliomas is often said to be controversial but is really not when differences in behavior between the different tumor types and between patients with and without NF-1 are taken into consideration.

Optic nerve gliomas may involve one or both optic nerves. Bilateral involvement is pathognomonic of NF-1. In a substantial proportion of cases, the optic nerve tumors are incidental findings on routine imaging and patients may remain asymptomatic with nonprogressive lesions over long periods; even spontaneous regression is well documented. The frequency of progression is difficult to establish, ranging from lows of <10% among patients followed in NF-1 clinics to 40% to 50% in series reported by oncology centers. Even in patients with symptomatic tumors, the course can be quite variable: only 30% to 60% of such patients will develop progressive disease that requires treatment.[36,68] Thus, management of patients with optic nerve tumors will usually consist initially of close follow-up with regular ophthalmologic examinations and MRI, with active intervention, usually chemotherapy, reserved for patients with clear evidence of progression that is symptomatic.[68-70]

Patients with unilateral optic nerve involvement may not have NF-1. They present most frequently with proptosis that may be relatively long-standing. Findings on examination may include optic atrophy and impaired visual acuity. On MRI, optic nerve tumors are usually relatively small and well circumscribed, with bright enhancement typical for pilocytic astrocytoma. Biopsy is not necessary to make a diagnosis. Treatment usually, although not always, will be necessary and the approach will depend on whether there is useful vision. If not, then surgical resection will be the treatment of choice. If useful vision is preserved, chemotherapy would be the preferred option for infants and very young children up to age 5 and for patients of all ages with NF-1. Radiotherapy could be considered for older children. Overall, the prognosis is very good. Visual acuity remains stable or improves in the majority of cases following chemotherapy or radiotherapy. Long-term tumor control approaches 100% with either modality.[71]

Chiasmatic gliomas are tumors that involve the optic chiasm and sometimes one or both optic nerves as well. Patients typically present with loss of visual acuity and temporal field defects. On imaging, the tumors are usually relatively small and well circumscribed and enhance uniformly and brightly with contrast material, suggestive of pilocytic histology. Biopsy is usually not necessary.

A period of surveillance is appropriate initial management, particularly for patients with NF-1. For patients without NF-1, especially those who present before age 5, there is a high probability of early progression and the majority of patients will require nonsurgical treatment within a few months following diagnosis. Surgery is rarely an option for tumors in this location. As for optic nerve tumors, chemotherapy usually will be the treatment of choice for infants and young children and for patients with NF-1. Radiotherapy is reserved for salvage after chemotherapy and for definitive treatment of older children without NF-1, providing a reasonable expectation that vision will not deteriorate further and a probability of long-term progression-free survival in the 60% to 90% range.[70,72-75] Overall survival for patients with chiasmatic tumors is in the 90% to 100% range.

Posterior, or chiasmatic/hypothalamic, gliomas account for approximately 70% of all optic pathway gliomas in children. They are typically rather large lesions that probably arise in the optic chiasm and extend to involve the hypothalamus. They may extend posteriorly along the optic tracts as well. They often fill the third ventricle, eventually causing hydrocephalus. Early findings consist of nystagmus, impaired visual acuity, and visual field deficits; only later do patients present increasing head circumference and/or symptoms and signs of raised intracranial pressure.

Treatment consists of CSF diversion, if necessary, and surgical resection, particularly if tumor is growing exophytically into the basal cistern because this may provide rapid relief of symptoms. In most patients, however, resection will be incomplete. As for LGAs at other locations, a period of surveillance following surgery is reasonable, although most patients will require adjuvant therapy.[46,71] The treatment of choice for children younger than 5 and those with NF-1 usually will be chemotherapy. Progression-free survival at 3 to 5 years is rather low at 20% to at best 60%.[46-48,76] However, some patients will never need further treatment, and for those who do, the use of chemotherapy allows radiotherapy to be deferred by a median of 2 to 4+ years without jeopardizing overall survival.

The indications for radiotherapy are (a) progressive disease on chemotherapy for children younger than 10 and (b) progressive disease at diagnosis or after surgery for older patients. Radiotherapy in this situation, given to local fields to a dose of 45 to 50 Gy for younger children and of 50 to 54 Gy for those older than 5, results in local tumor control in 70% to 80% of cases.[46,71,75,77,78] Overall, however, outcomes are less satisfactory for this group of patients than for those with anterior tumors. Long-term survival is in the 50% to 80% range, and many patients will be left with significant neuroendocrine and neuropsychologic sequelae. Patients with NF-1 are particularly at risk. They may have subnormal IQ even without chemotherapy and/or radiotherapy.[79] They are also at greater risk for moyamoya syndrome, a progressive vasoocclusive process involving the circle of Willis. This may be seen without radiotherapy, but when radiotherapy is used in patients with NF-1, it is important to include MR angiography as part of the regular follow-up imaging protocol and intervene surgically if necessary to avoid a cerebrovascular accident.

Brainstem Gliomas

Tumors arising in the midbrain, pons, and medulla oblongata account for 10% to 15% of all CNS tumors in the pediatric age group. They are of several distinct types that can be broadly grouped as the more favorable low-grade focal, dorsal exophytic, and cervicomedullary tumors and the much more aggressive diffuse intrinsic pontine tumors (DIPGs).[80-82]

Focal tumors by definition are tumors of limited size (<2 cm) that on MRI are well circumscribed, without evidence of infiltration, and without edema. They may be cystic, and, as with cystic tumors at other sites, the cystic component may be large relative to the solid, biologically active, component. Focal tumors may occur at any level in the brainstem but most frequently are seen in the midbrain and medulla. They usually present with a long history of localizing findings such as an isolated cranial nerve deficit and a contralateral hemiparesis. Signs and symptoms of raised intracranial pressure are uncommon except in patients with tumors arising in the tectal region that may cause aqueduct stenosis while still small.

The management depends on the location of the tumor in the brainstem and the specific imaging characteristics of the tumor. As noted previously, patients with nonenhancing focal tumors in the tectal region who present with only hydrocephalus may do well without any treatment other than CSF diversionary procedures, usually endoscopic third ventriculostomy. Active intervention, including biopsy, is reserved for patients with clinical and radiologic evidence of progressive tumor. This is important because surgery for tumors in this location is associated with a substantial risk of morbidity even with modern techniques.

Surgery is the treatment of choice for focal tumors at other locations that are surgically accessible (meaning that they extend either toward the surface of the brainstem laterally or at the floor of the fourth ventricle) and have imaging characteristics suggestive of low-grade histology. In this regard, uniform bright enhancement with contrast material, which correlates with pilocytic histology, and the absence of peritumoral hypodensity are of particular importance. In experienced hands, the risk of morbidity for well-selected patients is low and, as with completely or subtotally resected LGAs at other sites, results may be excellent with freedom from progression in a majority of cases.[83,84] Outcomes are less satisfactory for patients with bulky tumors and for patients with tumors in the medulla with lower cranial nerve deficits who are at risk of developing postoperative feeding and/or breathing difficulties.

There are several treatment options for patients with surgically inaccessible focal lesions. By extrapolation from series reporting results of treatment using conventional radiotherapy in brainstem tumors in which outcome correlates with location (pons vs. other), imaging appearance (tumor volume, density on CT, enhancement pattern), and histology (malignant vs. benign), it is reasonable to assume that 50% to 70% of focal lesions may be permanently controlled with such treatment. Similar results have been obtained in small numbers of patients treated with HFRT and with interstitial irradiation using ^{125}I.[51,53,55] There is also some experience with the use of radiosurgery. However, standard treatment is as for LGAs at other locations, that is, external beam radiotherapy using a margin for the CTV of 0.5 cm, to a total dose on the order of 54 Gy given over 6 weeks. The risks of HFRT, radiosurgery, or stereotactic irradiation with large fraction sizes, or interstitial irradiation in inexperienced hands cannot be justified in the absence of any established superiority.

Dorsal exophytic tumors arise from the floor of the fourth ventricle. They are usually large, filling the fourth ventricle, but do not invade the brainstem to any significant extent. They present insidiously with failure to thrive in younger children and symptoms and signs of raised intracranial pressure in older patients. Cranial nerve deficits are seen in about half of the patients. On MRI, they are sharply delineated from surrounding structures. They are hypointense on T1-weighted images, are hyperintense on T2-weighted images, and enhance uniformly and brightly after gadolinium injection. Most are pilocytic astrocytomas.

Surgery is the treatment of choice for dorsal exophytic tumors. Intraoperative image guidance is essential to achieve a maximal degree of tumor resection. However, because there is usually no definite tumor–brainstem interface, even an optimal resection will leave a thin layer of tumor on the floor of the fourth ventricle. Nonetheless, the majority of children do well following surgery and routine postoperative adjuvant therapy is not indicated. Radiotherapy should be considered for the rare patient who is found to have a high-grade lesion or for patients with low-grade tumors who develop progressive disease in the early (<9 months) postoperative period. For patients whose tumors recur later, further surgery should be considered and radiotherapy reserved for those with inoperable disease. The radiotherapy volume and dose should be similar to those used for LGAs in other locations. The literature suggests that salvage is possible in the majority of cases, and overall, the prognosis for patients with dorsal exophytic tumors is excellent.[85-87]

Cervicomedullary tumors arise in the upper cervical cord and grow rostrally beyond the foramen magnum. Most are low-grade lesions whose axial growth is limited by the pyramidal decussations located ventrally at the junction of the cervical cord and medulla. At this point, the tumor grows posteriorly, causing a bulge in the dorsal aspect of the medulla, toward the fourth ventricle.[80] These tumors typically present with lower cranial nerve deficits, sleep apnea and feeding difficulties in younger children, long tract signs, and sometimes torticollis. Hydrocephalus is unusual.

Surgery is the treatment of choice. Gross total resection may be achieved in 70% to 80% of cases and subtotal removal in most of the remainder. The probability of long-term tumor control after such treatment appears to be excellent for the typical low-grade lesion. There is, therefore, no indication for routine postoperative radiotherapy for these patients.

Diffuse intrinsic pontine tumors (DIPGs) account for 70% to 80% of all brainstem tumors. They arise in the pons and cause diffuse enlargement of the brainstem. Extension to the midbrain and medulla and/or exophytic growth is seen in at least two-thirds of cases. In contrast to the other types of brainstem tumors, the majority of DIPGs are fibrillary astrocytomas with a propensity for malignant change and a very poor prognosis.

DIPGs typically present with a short duration of symptoms consisting of multiple, bilateral, cranial nerve deficits (especially VI and VII) as well as long tract signs and ataxia. About 10% of patients have hydrocephalus at diagnosis. On CT, DIPGs are isodense or hypodense, with little enhancement after contrast injection, similar to diffuse fibrillary astrocytomas at other sites. They are best seen on T2-weighted or FLAIR MRI. The presence of ring enhancement is suggestive of high-grade histology.

Surgery has no role in the management of patients with DIPGs. Outside a clinical trial, even biopsy, a relatively nonmorbid procedure now, is considered unnecessary because in the context of a typical clinical presentation, the MRI findings are characteristic and histology does not influence treatment.[88,89] Treated with conventional radiotherapy, the majority (70% or more) of patients with DIPGs will improve clinically. However, the progression-free interval is short (median <6 months) and survival is poor, with a median survival of <1 year and survival rates at 2 years <20%.

So far all attempts to improve the outcome for children with DIPGs have proved futile. HFRT was tested in a series of phase I/II studies using doses ranging from 64.8 to 78 Gy. Time to progression and overall survival were not improved

in comparison with conventional radiotherapy.[90,91] Moreover, at the higher doses of HFRT of 75.6 and 78 Gy, morbidity was considerable. This included steroid dependency, vascular events, and white matter changes outside the radiation field, as well as hearing loss, hormone deficiencies, and late-developing seizure disorders in the small number of long-term survivors.[90,92-94] Accelerated and hypofractionated radiotherapy regimens have also been tested in single-institution studies using, respectively, a total dose of 50.4 Gy given in 28 twice-daily fractions of 1.8 Gy over 3 weeks[95] and 39 Gy in 13 daily fractions and 45 Gy in 15 daily fractions.[96,97] Progression-free and overall survival rates were similar to those seen in the HFRT studies. However there are potential benefits from the reduced duration of the radiotherapy course to help facilitate rehabilitation.

Alternative approaches that use chemotherapy in combination with radiotherapy also have been disappointing. None of the many single-agent and multiagent regimens that have been tested in this patient population have been shown to provide a survival advantage compared with radiotherapy alone. New agents and novel chemotherapy–radiotherapy combinations are under investigation by the pediatric cooperative groups in North America and Europe.

Currently, standard treatment for DIPGs consists of radiotherapy given to the GTV as usually best demonstrated on T2-weighted or FLAIR MRI with a margin for the CTV of 1 to 1.5 cm to a dose of 54 Gy given in 30 daily fractions over 6 weeks that because of the initial rapid progression of neurologic deficit treatment often needs to be started on a semi-urgent basis. Because no unexpected toxicity was seen with the hypofractionated regimens, these in some cases could be considered an alternative to conventional radiotherapy that reduces the burden of treatment for the child and family.

Improvement in clinical status is usually evident as early as 2 to 3 weeks into treatment, and steroids, if used, usually can be discontinued at that point. This improvement is often impressive and well appreciated by the family, despite being of only short duration. Treatment at time of progression may include experimental chemotherapy regimens or supportive care or even retreatment with radiotherapy in selected cases.[98,99]

Astrocytoma of the Spinal Cord

Intramedullary spinal cord tumors account for 3% to 6% of all CNS tumors in the pediatric age group. About 60% are astrocytomas, the majority of which are LGAs; 30% are ependymomas; and the remainder are gangliogliomas and developmental tumors such as teratomas, lipomas, and dermoid and epidermoid cysts.

Patients typically present with pain and motor deficits, often of long duration. Rapid progression of symptoms and signs is suggestive of high-grade histology. On imaging, astrocytomas most often are seen to comprise a solid component and one or more cysts that may be intratumoral and/or extend rostrally and caudally beyond the solid component. Most enhance heterogeneously with the use of contrast material. Ependymomas, in contrast, only rarely harbor intratumoral cysts (although they may have an associated syrinx) and usually enhance homogeneously.

The management of spinal cord tumors has changed over recent years.[100] In the past, patients typically were treated with biopsy followed by radiotherapy, and there is evidence to suggest that this is effective treatment in more than half of children with LGAs.[101] However, improvements in surgery and the routine use of surgical adjuncts such as ultrasonic aspiration and support systems such as intraoperative ultrasonography and sensory and more recently motor-evoked potential monitoring improve the safety and completeness of resection so that complete or subtotal resection is now possible in approximately 80% of children with pilocytic astrocytoma (the majority), especially those with a syrinx. Resection is more difficult and less likely to be complete in patients with grade II astrocytoma because of the more infiltrative nature of these tumors and the absence of a clear interface.[100] Because outcome following complete or subtotal resection for LGAs is very good, with long-term progression-free survival in the 70% to 90% range,[102-104] routine postoperative adjuvant therapy is not indicated. For children in whom complete or subtotal resection is not possible, the options will be as for patients with LGAs in other locations, that is, early second surgery if feasible, or close follow-up with second surgery and/or radiotherapy at the time of progression. As for LGAs in other locations, chemotherapy may be an alternative to radiotherapy for young children.[105,106] The benefit of surgical resection in HGAs is less clear and the more usual approach is biopsy followed by postoperative radiotherapy.[107]

The radiotherapy target volume for LGAs consists of the solid portion of the tumor (including intratumoral cysts) with a margin for the CTV of 1 to 1.5 cm. The usual dose is 50.4 Gy given in 28 daily fractions over approximately 6 weeks. The CTV should be larger for patients with HGAs for whom a margin beyond the entire lesion of at least 1.5 cm (or one vertebral body) would be more appropriate. The dose usually will be as for LGA because of the substantial risk of morbidity at higher doses but often chemotherapy will be given as well. Although older studies[101,102] and data from the Surveillance, Epidemiology, and End Results (SEER) registry[108] and from the German cooperative group[109] all suggest that 20% to 35% of children with high-grade gliomas will survive following such treatment, a recent study from St. Jude Children's Research Hospital presents an even bleaker picture with a very high rate of both local progression and leptomeningeal spread and no long-term survivors among patients with GBM.[107]

EPENDYMAL TUMORS

The following types are seen in children:

- Myxopapillary ependymoma (WHO grade I)
- Ependymoma (WHO grade II)
- Anaplastic ependymoma (WHO grade III)

Myxopapillary Ependymoma

Myxopapillary ependymomas are slowly growing lesions almost always located in the conus filum terminale region of the spinal cord. They are the most common spinal cord tumor in this location. They usually present with back pain. On imaging, myxopapillary ependymomas are well circumscribed and usually enhance brightly after contrast injection. Despite their low-grade histology, leptomeningeal spread is not uncommon even at diagnosis and all patients should have an MRI of the whole spine and brain as part of their initial workup.

Surgical resection is the treatment of choice. If the tumor is contained within the filum, complete resection may be possible after mobilization of the filum. Whether postoperative radiotherapy is necessary after complete resection is unclear. A significant proportion of tumors recur locally and/or with leptomeningeal metastases, but salvage with further surgery and/or with radiotherapy seems to be possible in most.[110-112] If the tumor is in continuity with the conus, resection is more difficult and more likely to result in significant sequelae so that there frequently will be residual tumor. If the tumor is not resected en bloc or if there is macroscopic residual tumor, the risk of recurrence is high. Postoperative radiotherapy in this situation results in improved local control.[103,113-115] The radiotherapy target volume is local (macroscopic disease plus a margin cephalad and caudad of 1.5 cm [or one vertebral body]) for the CTV and the dose, 50.4 Gy.[115] Patients with leptomeningeal seeding at diagnosis or at relapse after surgery alone should be treated with curative intent with CSI followed by a boost to the primary site with a reasonable expectation of long-term tumor control.[103,111,114,116]

Ependymoma

Ependymoma is the third most common CNS tumor in children. About half of all cases arise in children younger than 5. Ependymoma can occur at any site in the ventricular system or in the spinal canal, but in children, approximately two-thirds arise in the ependymal lining of the fourth ventricle. Tumors in this location typically present with symptoms and signs of raised intracranial pressure. On imaging the tumor is usually large but relatively well circumscribed, with displacement rather than invasion of adjacent structures. Extension through the foramen magnum into the upper cervical region is not uncommon (Fig. 88.10). Tumors that arise in the supratentorial compartment, some of which arise outside the ventricular system, present with focal neurologic deficits. Intramedullary ependymomas, which account for approximately 30% of all spinal cord tumors arising in childhood, usually present initially with dysesthesia and sensory deficits because of their central location in the cord and only later with pain and motor deficits.

Spread of ependymoma is primarily local. However, 5% to 10% of patients have leptomeningeal seeding at diagnosis, and gadolinium-enhanced MRI of the whole CNS and CSF cytology are essential components of the workup for all patients.

Management of Ependymoma

The completeness of the surgical resection is the factor that has the greatest impact on the outcome of patients with ependymoma.[117-126] Currently, it is estimated that complete resection is achieved in 70% to 90% of supratentorial ependymomas and in a similar percentage of spinal ependymomas. Complete resection is less frequently possible in patients with infratentorial ependymomas. Most commonly, residual tumor is left behind on the floor of the fourth ventricle or laterally at the cerebellopontine angle where tumor protruding through the foramen of Luschka encircles lower cranial nerves and vessels. "Second-look" surgery may be considered, if feasible, either after the realignment of structures that takes place following resection of an initially bulky tumor in an often unstable young child or after chemotherapy.

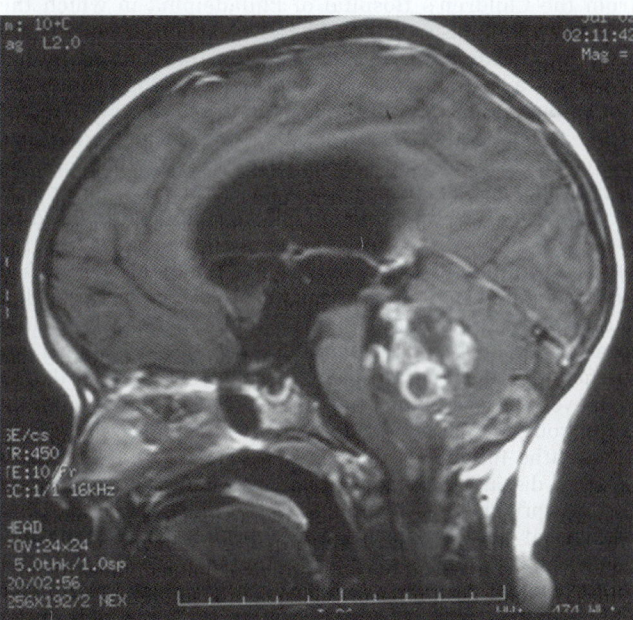

FIGURE 88.10. Typical appearance of an ependymoma that fills the fourth ventricle causing hydrocephalus and extends inferiorly below the foramen magnum over the dorsal aspect of the spinal cord to the level of C4.

Postoperative radiotherapy is the standard of care for all children with ependymoma. Some have questioned the need for such treatment for patients who have undergone complete resection.[123,127,128] However, a number of studies including studies in young children in which the goal was to delay or avoid altogether radiotherapy suggest that such a strategy results in worse disease-free and overall survival and in the long-term greater morbidity[124,129–132] and therefore can be considered acceptable only for (a) patients with ependymoma of the spinal cord who have undergone complete resection for whom disease-free survival in contemporary series approaches 100%[133–136] and (b) selected patients with supratentorial ependymoma, such as those with intraventricular tumors or with extraventricular tumors that are solid and located in noneloquent areas and can be resected with a wider margin.[128]

Radiotherapy Target Volume

Focal radiotherapy is the standard of care.[137,138] The GTV is a composite of the tumor bed, including any extension caudal to the foramen magnum and taking into account any anatomic shifts because of surgery plus any residual tumor. In the St. Jude prospective study of conformal radiotherapy that included both ependymoma and anaplastic ependymoma, the margin for the CTV was 1 cm.[126] In the subset of 107 patients in that study that received immediate postoperative radiotherapy, local control was excellent (cumulative incidence of local failure 7.8%) for patients who had undergone gross total resection, whereas patients who had undergone near-total or subtotal resection fared less well. All failures were reported to be within the 95% isodose. The current Children's Oncology Group (COG) study uses an even smaller margin for the CTV of 0.5 cm.

Radiotherapy Dose

There is evidence for a dose–response in ependymoma, with improved tumor control with doses >45 to 50 and even 54 Gy.[137] Although the lower doses may be the maximum possible for spinal ependymomas, the current standard is a dose of at least 54 Gy for children older than 18 months with infra- or supratentorial tumors. Moreover, because failure most often occurs at the site of macroscopic residual disease, even higher doses may be desirable and most would reduce the CTV at 54 Gy to respect the tolerance of the spinal cord and/or other structures and continue to a total dose of 59.4 Gy (Fig. 88.11).

HFRT has been explored in ependymoma as a strategy to more safely deliver these higher radiotherapy doses. Studies from the Children's Hospital of Philadelphia in which the majority of patients received HFRT to a mean dose of 70.7 Gy,[139] from the Italian pediatric oncology group that used a dose of 70.4 Gy,[140] and from the French pediatric oncology group that used a lower total dose of 60 Gy in 60 fractions[141] all reported HFRT to be feasible. However, in none of these studies was there any clear evidence of benefit, particularly in the context of improved surgery and modern radiotherapy.

The role of chemotherapy in ependymoma remains to be defined. There is some evidence of efficacy, but even in the more recent infant studies in which chemotherapy was used because of the desire to delay or even avoid altogether radiotherapy, more than half of the patients progressed on chemotherapy,[65,130,132,142,143] and in the COG baby study, prolonged use of chemotherapy and a delay to radiotherapy of more than 1 year were associated with a worse survival.[129] Consequently, most would now use radiotherapy for all children older than 12 months following complete resection. In patients with residual disease, chemotherapy has been justified because of the poor prognosis. As well, it may facilitate complete resection of residual disease at second-look surgery, and current North American and European trials are testing chemotherapy in this setting. Furthermore, trials are also investigating the role of adjuvant chemotherapy following complete resection.

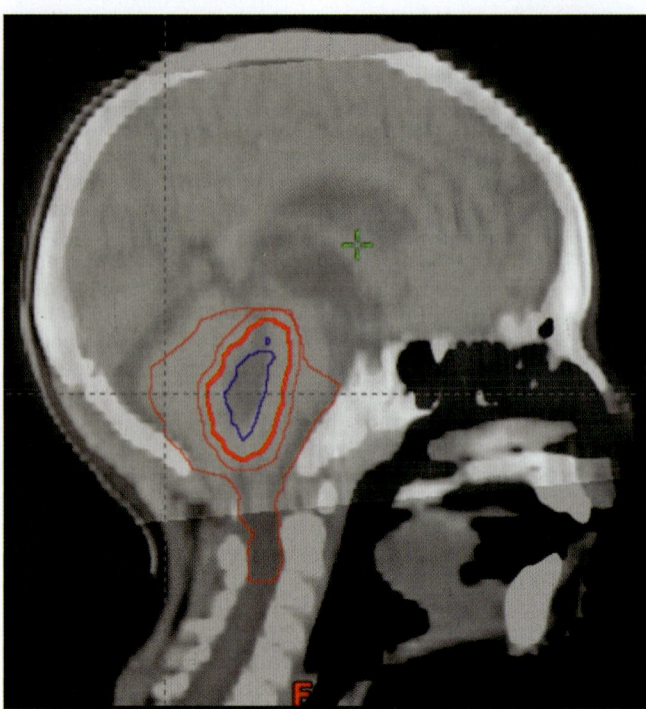

FIGURE 88.11. Care is necessary to ensure that the inferior extent of disease is included in the radiotherapy target volume. Volume reduction at 54 Gy is necessary to respect the tolerance of the spinal cord.

Reirradiation for Ependymoma

For patients who fail standard treatment with either local recurrence or, less frequently, leptomeningeal dissemination, retreatment with radiotherapy is an option that may result in durable control in a proportion of patients.[144,145]

Anaplastic Ependymoma

By definition, an anaplastic ependymoma is a malignant glioma of ependymal differentiation that is characterized by high mitotic activity, often accompanied by microvascular proliferation and pseudopalisading necrosis. There are no histopathologic features that can reliably differentiate anaplastic ependymomas from the more slowly growing and more favorable ependymomas, which probably explains the controversy in the literature with respect to the prognostic significance of tumor grade. Proliferation markers may be more useful in this regard, but several groups also are investigating genetic and expression profiles based on preliminary data that suggest that a molecular classification system can be built that will prove useful for risk stratification.

Management of anaplastic ependymoma begins with maximum surgical resection consistent with a good neurologic outcome and a workup consisting of a gadolinium-enhanced MRI of the spinal axis and CSF cytology to rule out leptomeningeal seeding, which is only slightly more frequent than in ependymoma. Postoperatively all patients receive radiotherapy. As for ependymoma, the role of chemotherapy remains to be defined but may be an option in very young children to delay the use of radiotherapy.

CSI was previously the standard of care for anaplastic ependymoma, but several institutional studies, a careful retrospective review, and prospective studies by the POG all suggest that there is no survival advantage for CSI.[118,146–150] Thus, a target volume consisting of the tumor bed and any macroscopic residual disease with a margin for the CTV of 1 cm is used for patients with localized disease and only patients with leptomeningeal seeding at diagnosis receive CSI. As for ependymoma, the dose should be at least 54 to 55 Gy and, if feasible, 59 to 60 Gy.

In contemporary series, disease-free survival for patients with anaplastic ependymoma is typically still only in the 30% to 45% range at 3 to 5 years,[140,150] although results were better in the St. Jude series, with event-free survival at 7 years of 61.3% and overall survival, 71.8%.[126] This may be in part at least because of the high rate of gross total resection in that series because, as others have shown, the prognosis is better for patients in whom complete resection has been achieved than for those with residual disease.[149,150] Patients with leptomeningeal dissemination at diagnosis fare poorly despite intensive treatment that includes CSI and chemotherapy.

CHOROID PLEXUS TUMORS

Choroid plexus tumors arise from the epithelium of the choroid plexus of the cerebral ventricles. They include:

- Choroid plexus papilloma (WHO grade I)
- Atypical choroid plexus papilloma (WHO grade II)
- Choroid plexus carcinoma (WHO grade III)

Choroid plexus tumors account for only 2% to 4% of all brain tumors that occur in children but as many as 10% to 20% of those seen in the first year of life. Choroid plexus papillomas (CPPs), which account for more than half of choroid plexus tumors in children, are composed of delicate fibrovascular connective tissue fronds covered by a single layer of uniform cuboidal columnar epithelial cells with round or oval basally situated monomorphic nuclei. Mitotic activity is low and increased mitotic activity in a CPP defines an atypical CPP. In contrast to both, choroid plexus carcinomas (CPCs) are solid tumors that tend to transgress the ventricular wall and invade the brain. Histologically, CPCs show frank evidence of malignancy including frequent mitoses (>5%/10 HPF), increased cellular density, nuclear pleomorphism, blurring of the papillary pattern with poorly structured sheets of tumor cells, and necrotic areas.

In children, most choroid plexus tumors arise in the lateral ventricles causing obstruction to CSF flow. Infants commonly present with increasing head circumference and older children with symptoms and signs of raised intracranial pressure. On neuroimaging, choroid plexus tumors are usually hyperdense, contrast-enhancing masses. Even papillomas seed into the CSF space and workup for both benign and malignant lesions should include a gadolinium-enhanced MRI of the spinal axis and CSF cytology.

Management of Choroid Plexus Tumors

Surgery is the treatment of choice for CPPs both for the primary lesion and for metastatic deposits, if feasible. Complete resection is achieved in a high percentage of cases now and outcome in this situation is excellent. Less than 10% of tumors recur and overall survival is close to 100%.[151-154] The role of radiotherapy following incomplete resection is unclear, but because not all patients will progress, follow-up without adjuvant treatment would be the usual strategy, with consideration of further surgery, if feasible, and/or radiotherapy only at the time of progression.

Results are less satisfactory for patients with CPCs. Surgery is an important component of treatment but often difficult. Blood loss may be considerable and staged procedures may be necessary to obtain maximal resection. In most series, results are better for patients who have undergone complete resection[151,155-164] and the need for adjuvant therapy in this situation is not clearly established. In one series of pooled data, survival was significantly better when radiotherapy had been given postoperatively despite a probable bias toward the use of radiotherapy in patients considered to have more unfavorable disease.[158,161] Others have reported excellent results following complete resection, in some cases with chemotherapy but

without radiotherapy.[155,156,159,160] In contrast, patients who have residual disease fare very poorly. Postoperative radiotherapy appears to be useful,[164] but the desire to avoid radiotherapy in infants and very young children may mean that chemotherapy is used instead despite less convincing evidence of efficacy. When both are used, radiotherapy is usually delivered early (following two cycles of chemotherapy) with the exception of infants and very young children in whom radiotherapy is delayed until age 3 years. Genetic and genomic analyses may in the future help guide therapy. A substantial percentage of patients with CPCs have TP53 mutations, and patients without such mutations are reported to have a more favorable prognosis and be successfully treated without radiotherapy.[165]

The radiotherapy target volume is also controversial. CSI was traditionally used in patients with CPCs, and a recent literature review showed that the use of CSI was associated with improved progression-free survival as compared with radiotherapy to the whole brain or tumor bed only.[164] Importantly, more than half of all failures occurred outside the treatment field. This is problematic given the young age of the patients, and a pragmatic approach in which local fields are used for patients with CPPs with postoperative residual (including metastatic sites) as well as for patients with atypical CPPs or CPCs without evidence of leptomeningeal seeding and only patients with atypical CPPs or CPCs with leptomeningeal seeding receive CSI would seem reasonable for now.

NEURONAL AND MIXED NEURONAL-GLIAL TUMORS

These are uncommon tumors that are characterized by the presence of both neuronal and glial elements in variable amounts. They include entities such as desmoplastic infantile astrocytoma and dysembryoplastic neuroepithelial tumor. Most will be cured by surgery, but radiotherapy may be indicated in two tumor types:

- Ganglioglioma and anaplastic ganglioglioma
- Central neurocytoma

Ganglioglioma and Anaplastic Ganglioglioma

Gangliogliomas are well-differentiated slowly growing tumors composed of mature ganglion cells in combination with neoplastic glial cells (WHO grade I or II). Tumors in which the glial component shows anaplastic features (WHO grade III) are called anaplastic gangliogliomas.

Although these tumors can arise anywhere within the CNS, most in children arise in the temporal region and typically present with seizures. Surgery is the treatment of choice. When resection is complete, the probability of long-term tumor control in patients with ganglioglioma is excellent.[166-168] The indications for radiotherapy are as for patients with LGAs, that is, for patients with progressive or recurrent disease that is not resectable, and the radiotherapy target volume and dose likewise. The significance of a high proliferation index or of the presence of anaplasia in patients with ganglioglioma is controversial. Although it seems clear that the risk of recurrence is higher in patients with these features,[166,167,169] the indications for postoperative radiotherapy remain undefined except for patients with anaplastic gangliogliomas who have undergone less than complete resection in whom the use of radiotherapy has been shown to result in improved progression-free survival.[168,170]

Central Neurocytoma

This is a neoplasm composed of uniform round cells with neuronal differentiation that arises in the lateral or third ventricles, typically the former, that is seen predominantly in adolescents and young adults. Patients usually present with symptoms and signs of raised intracranial pressure. Surgery is the treatment of choice, and when complete resection is achieved, long-term tumor control is excellent without adjuvant treatment.[171] Patients in whom complete resection cannot be achieved as well as those with tumors with atypical histology or a high mitotic rate fare less well,[171,172] and postoperative radiotherapy should be considered in these situations. Although a dose of 50 Gy appears adequate for patients with typical neurocytomas,[173] there is evidence of improved tumor control at doses of at least 54 Gy in patients with atypical neurocytoma.[174]

PINEAL PARENCHYMAL TUMORS

Pineal region tumors account for 2% to 8% of intracranial tumors in children. Approximately half are germ cell tumors, one-fourth to one-third are pineal parenchymal tumors, and most of the remainder are astrocytic tumors. Pineal parenchymal tumors are derived from pineocytoma, which are cells with photosensory and neuroendocrine functions, or their embryonal precursors. According to the WHO classification, the following entities can be distinguished:

- Pineocytoma (WHO grade I)
- Pineal parenchymal tumor of intermediate differentiation
- Pineoblastoma (WHO grade IV)

Pineocytoma

Pineocytoma is a slow-growing tumor composed of small uniform mature cells resembling pineocytes, with occasional large pineocytomatous rosettes, that accounts for approximately half of pineal parenchymal tumors and in childhood most commonly occurs in the teenage years. Patients typically present with symptoms and signs of raised intracranial pressure. Some will have symptoms of upper mesencephalic tegmental dysfunction (Parinaud syndrome), consisting of limitation of upward gaze, lid retraction, retraction nystagmus, and pupils that react more poorly to light than to accommodation. On MRI, pineocytomas are usually spherical, well-circumscribed masses, hypointense on T1- and hyperintense on T2-weighted images, with homogeneous contrast enhancement. Leptomeningeal spread has been described in pineocytoma,[175] but it is probable that the explanation for this lies in sampling error. With better imaging and more extensive surgery with more complete histologic evaluation of the tumor, it seems that leptomeningeal spread can be considered to be an uncommon event.[176]

Treatment consists of surgical resection via an occipital transtentorial or an infratentorial supracerebellar approach using modern operative adjuncts such as functional MRI and MR tractography in relation to the location of the primary visual cortex and deep MR venography. If complete or subtotal resection is accomplished, progression-free survival is in the 90% to 100% range.[177,178] Patients who undergo lesser degrees of resection or only biopsy fare less well and, although some have questioned its usefulness based on the results of a systematic review,[178] postoperative radiotherapy usually is recommended.[179] The target volume is local, consisting of macroscopic residual disease with a margin for the CTV of 1 cm, and the dose, 50 to 55 Gy over 6 weeks.

Pineal Parenchymal Tumor of Intermediate Differentiation

Pineal parenchymal tumors of intermediate differentiation are composed of diffuse sheets or large lobules of uniform cells with mild to moderate nuclear atypia and low to moderate mitotic activity. They are rare tumors, accounting for only 10% of pineal parenchymal tumors, and optimal management remains to be defined. In one series, three patients treated

with surgery alone survived free of disease.[177] At the other extreme, another group considers these to be tumors "with seeding potential" and recommends postoperative treatment with CSI as for pineoblastoma.[176]

Pineoblastoma

Pineoblastoma is a highly malignant tumor composed of patternless sheets of densely packed small cells with round to irregular nuclei and scant cytoplasm.

Pineoblastomas most frequently affect infants and very young children, who typically present with an enlarged head circumference or symptoms and signs of short duration of raised intracranial pressure. On MRI, pineoblastomas are usually multilobulated and often enhance heterogeneously, with areas of necrosis and/or hemorrhage. Infiltration of surrounding structures is common. Leptomeningeal spread is seen in as many as 50% of patients at diagnosis.

Surgery for lesions in the pineal region is difficult and complete resection is often not possible. Postoperatively, children older than 3 are treated with CSI and chemotherapy, as for high-risk medulloblastoma and supratentorial PNETs (see later). Five-year survival in this age group is in the 50% to 70% range.[176,180,181] However, infants treated with chemotherapy without radiotherapy fare extremely poorly: in prospective studies of the POG and CCG, all tumors recurred within the first 11 months (POG) and 1.2 years (CCG) and all patients died of disease.[182,183] Thus, more aggressive treatment that includes chemotherapy dose intensification is necessary. Patients with familial bilateral retinoblastoma with pineoblastoma ("trilateral retinoblastoma") also have an extremely poor prognosis, most dying within a year following diagnosis.

EMBRYONAL TUMORS

Embryonal tumors as a group are the second most common type of CNS tumor in the pediatric age group. They include medulloblastoma (MB) and atypical teratoid rhabdoid tumor (ATRT):

- Medulloblastoma
  - i. Medulloblastoma, WNT-activated
  - ii. Medulloblastoma, SHH-activated, TP53 mutant
  - iii. Medulloblastoma, SHH-activated, TP53 wild type
  - iv. Medulloblastoma, non-WNT/non-SHH, group 3
  - v. Medulloblastoma, non-WNT/non-SHH, group 4

These medulloblastoma subgroups refer to the use of conventional histopathologic features together with molecular biologic parameters in classification. Conventional histologic varieties are also recognized and are associated with particular clinical characteristics. Desmoplastic MB is associated with a better prognosis, particularly in very young children. Anaplastic and large cell MBs (A/LC MBs) appear to be adverse prognostic factors.

Medulloblastoma

Medulloblastoma accounts for 15% to 20% of all CNS tumors in children with a median age at presentation of 6 years. It is a malignant invasive embryonal tumor of the cerebellum with predominantly neuronal differentiation and an inherent tendency to metastasize via CSF pathways.

It is accepted that medulloblastomas are defined according to four subgroups based on a combination of histopathology and molecular biology.

The WNT subgroup is associated with a very good prognosis with long-term survival in excess of 90%. The majority of WNT subgroup MBs have classic histology, and a particular feature is that these tumors demonstrate beta-catenin nucleopositivity, CTNNB1 gene mutations, and monosomy-6. Rarely, the WNT subgroup may include large-cell/anaplastic cases.

WNT MB can arise at all ages but is infrequent in infants. Although overall MB is more common in males, the male to female (M:F) ratio for the WNT subgroup is approximately 1:1. Germ-line mutations of the WNT pathway inhibitor APC predispose to Turcot syndrome, which includes a predisposition to MB.

The SHH MB subgroups include *TP53* mutant and *TP53* wild-type subgroups. They are named after the sonic hedgehog signaling pathway, which is considered to drive tumor initiation in the majority of cases. The age incidence of SHH subgroups of MB is bimodal and is frequent in both infants aged <3 years and adults. The M:F ratio is approximately 1:1. The majority of nodular/desmoplastic MBs are included within the SHH subgroup. However, around 50% of SHH subgroup MB have other histologic subtypes, including classical and large-cell/anaplastic varieties. The prognosis for SHH appears to be similar to group 4 (see below) and intermediate between WNT and group 3. Individuals with germ-line mutations of the SHH receptor PTCH have Gorlin syndrome, which for several decades has been recognized as carrying a predisposition to the development of MB. Preliminary clinical trials are being designed to target the SHH pathway to improve outcome for this subgroup.

Group 3 MB represents the subgroup of MB with the poorest prognosis. The majority of MBs in group 3 are classical MB and include the majority of large cell/anaplastic tumors. They are more frequent in males than females. They arise in infants and older children, but only rarely in adults and frequently present with metastases. Group 3 MB is typically characterized by high-level amplification of the *MYC* proto-oncogene, and almost all cases exhibit aberrant *MYC* expression.

Patients with group 4 MB have an intermediate to good prognosis similar to patients with SHH tumors. They include classical and large cell/anaplastic histologies and account for approximately 30% to 40% of cases. This subgroup represents the archetypal MB, exemplified by a 7-year-old boy with a classical histology MB who has an isochromosome 17q. The M:F ratio is approximately 3:1. The molecular pathogenesis of group 4 MB is not currently clear.

Improvements in the understanding of the molecular mechanisms of MB tumorigenesis are emerging as important factors in clinical trial design leading to a tailored approach for different histologic and molecular biologic subtypes. Collaborative clinical trial groups are developing studies that will investigate prospectively the stratification of therapy according to pathologic, biologic, as well as the more traditional clinical parameters. In particular, clinical studies are beginning to involve a cautious lowering of the treatment intensity for patients with WNT MB and maintaining intensity for those in group 3. This approach requires a timely and well-coordinated approach to tumor sample collection and analysis of biologic parameters prior to treatment decisions.[184]

In most cases of MB, the tumor arises in the cerebellar vermis and projects into the fourth ventricle. Patients typically present with symptoms and signs of raised intracranial pressure (i.e., headache and morning vomiting). On MRI, medulloblastomas appear as solid masses that enhance usually fairly homogeneously with contrast material (Fig. 88.12). The frequency of leptomeningeal seeding at diagnosis is approximately 30% to 35%, and investigation at diagnosis must include a gadolinium-enhanced MRI of the spinal axis and CSF cytology. The former should be obtained whenever possible preoperatively or else at least 2 weeks postoperatively because of the artifactual changes that may be seen in the early postoperative period. CSF cytology, which should be obtained by lumbar puncture, usually cannot be obtained safely preoperatively because of the presence of raised intracranial pressure and more commonly is obtained at least 2 weeks postoperatively to avoid false positives that may be seen in the early postoperative period. Medulloblastoma is one of the few CNS tumors to spread outside the CNS (to lymph nodes, bone), but this is a very uncommon event at diagnosis, and other studies such as a bone scan or bone marrow aspiration or biopsy are not justified as a routine.

FIGURE 88.12. T1 axial **(A)** and T1 gadolinium-enhanced sagittal **(B)** magnetic resonance images of a medulloblastoma in an 11-year-old boy. Note the typical midline location of the tumor that is causing ventricular outlet obstruction with dilatation of the third and lateral ventricles.

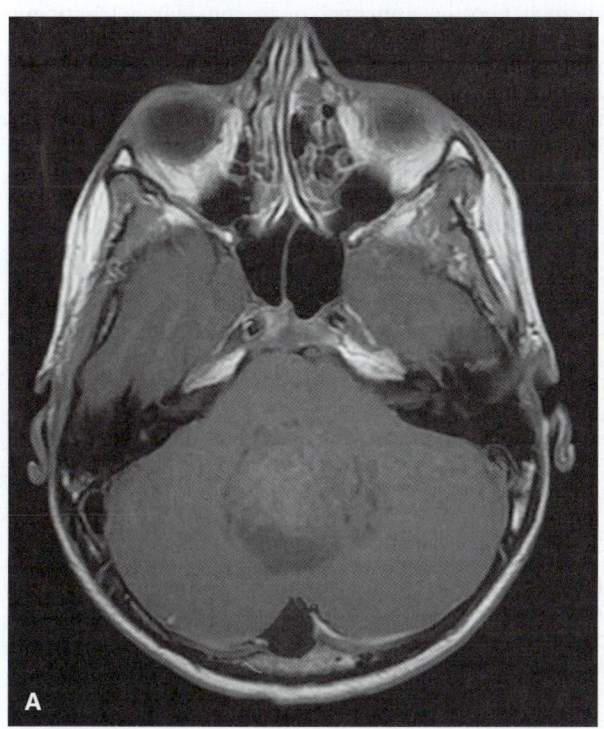

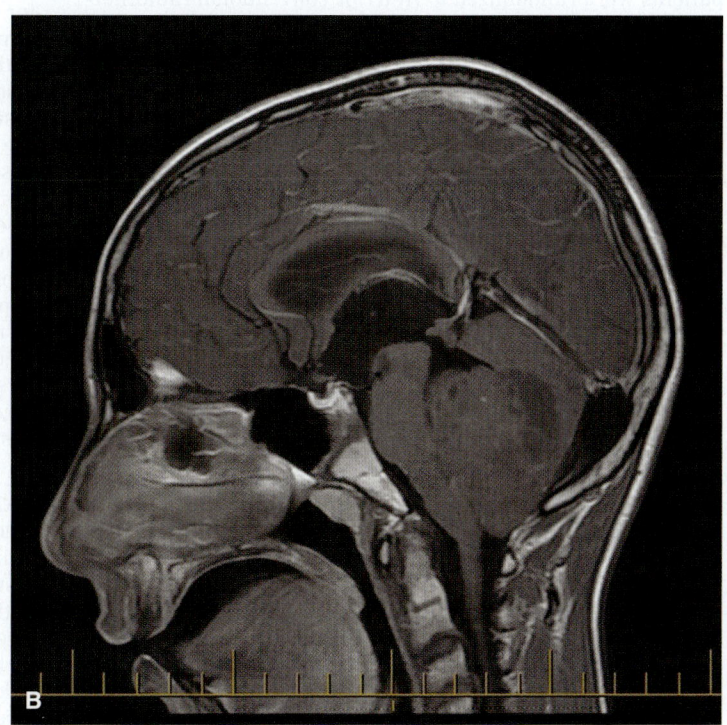

In addition to molecular biologic parameters, conventional factors that correlate with outcome include age at diagnosis, the presence or absence of leptomeningeal spread at diagnosis, and the completeness of the surgical resection. Patients are allocated to one of two overall risk categories: standard and high risk. Those who have undergone complete or subtotal resection with <1.5 cm^2 of residual tumor on postoperative MRI performed within 48 to 72 hours of surgery, and no evidence of CSF dissemination (M0) are considered to have standard-risk disease, whereas patients who have larger-volume residual tumor and those with evidence of CSF dissemination at diagnosis are characterized as high risk. With contemporary neurosurgical techniques, complete or near-total resection is accomplished in approximately 80% of cases. Overall, approximately two-thirds of patients will be standard risk and one-third will be high risk.

Management of Standard-Risk Medulloblastoma

Until the 1990s, the standard of care for patients older than 3 years with standard-risk disease consisted of postoperative radiotherapy to the craniospinal axis to a dose of 35 to 36 Gy followed by a boost to the whole posterior fossa to a total dose of 54 to 55.8 Gy. In multi-institution studies, such treatment results in long-term event-free survival in 60% to 65% of patients.[10,185,186] Sequelae of treatment include hormonal deficits, decreased bone growth, and neurocognitive deficits that correlate with the age of the child and the radiation dose.[7]

Several treatment strategies designed to reduce the morbidity associated with the use of radiotherapy have been tested. An attempt by the French Cooperative Group (SFOP) to reduce the radiotherapy target volume to avoid supratentorial radiation produced disastrous results,[187] and CSI remains the standard of care. The use of reduced-dose CSI (23.4 Gy) alone (without chemotherapy) in the North American intergroup study (CCG-923/POG#8631) resulted in a significantly increased risk of isolated neuraxis failure and an event-free survival at 5 and 8 years of only 52%.[186] HFRT may be a more promising strategy. In an SFOP pilot study that tested HFRT to a CSI dose of 36 Gy without chemotherapy, early toxicity was reduced and progression-free survival at 3 years was 81%.[188] The results of the European SIOP PNET-4 study in which patients were randomized to HFRT or conventional radiotherapy are pending.

An alternative strategy consists of reduced-dose CSI followed by a boost to the posterior fossa to a total dose of 55.8 Gy in combination with systemic chemotherapy. Progression-free survival was 79% at 5 years in a CCG pilot study that used CSI to a dose of 23.4 Gy in combination with weekly vincristine followed by adjuvant systemic chemotherapy consisting of vincristine 1.5 mg/m^2, CCNU 75 mg/m^2, and cisplatin 75 mg/m^2.[189] In the joint CCG/POG phase III randomized study (A9961) that followed, this regimen was compared to a regimen in which the CCNU was replaced by cyclophosphamide. Event-free survival at 4 years was approximately 85% in both arms,[190] and such an approach is now considered to be the standard of care for children with standard-risk medulloblastoma in North America. The recently presented COG ACNS 0331 trial evaluated the safety of an even lower dose of CSI (18 Gy) in children aged 3 to 8 years and of a reduced-volume posterior fossa boost in children of all ages.

This compared a boost to the whole posterior fossa with a tumor/surgical bed plus margin boost. Preliminary results have recently been reported.[190a] There was no significant difference in EFS for patients treated with a tumor/surgical bed plus margin boost compared with those treated with a whole posterior fossa boost. However, patients treated with 18 Gy CSRT had a reduced 5-year EFS of 71.4% compared with 82.1% for those treated with 23.4 Gy. Currently, the standard of care for children with standard-risk MB is with CSRT 23.4 Gy with a boost to the tumor bed to a total dose of 54.0 Gy, followed by eight cycles of chemotherapy with vincristine, CCNU, and cisplatin.

In the latest generation of trials in medulloblastoma such as the recently opened European PNET-trial, risk stratification is based on biologic parameters in addition to clinical and pathologic features. Patients with anaplastic large-cell histology are no longer included in the standard-risk group given their poorer outcome. Furthermore, evidence suggests that WNT medulloblastoma with β-catenin nucleopositivity is associated with a better prognosis and MYC gene amplification with a worse one, opening up the possibility of reduced-intensity radiotherapy and chemotherapy for patients with WNT medulloblastoma and the evaluation of additional treatment intensity for patients with less favorable prognosis.[191]

Management of High-Risk Medulloblastoma

Patients with residual disease >1.5 cm^2 and/or those with leptomeningeal seeding are considered to have high-risk disease. This is the group of patients in which the use of chemotherapy was shown in the prospective randomized phase III studies conducted in the 1970s to result in significant improvement in disease-free survival. Research since then has largely focused on the chemotherapy regimens, including changes in scheduling in relation to radiotherapy and in doses and routes of delivery of chemotherapy. Some have used higher-dose CSI or altered radiotherapy fractionation schedules. An overview of studies performed by the North American and European cooperative groups up until the early 2000s is given in Freeman et al.[192]

It is important to note that the definition of risk factors has evolved considerably over the past two decades, making comparison of published data quite problematic. Better postoperative imaging and more complete staging as well as identification of unfavorable pathologic features (e.g., large cell and anaplastic histology) have led to transfer of patients from the standard-risk to the high-risk category, which may partly explain the improving results for both standard-risk and high-risk disease. The category of high-risk disease is heterogeneous and includes more favorable subsets such as patients with postoperative residual disease without leptomeningeal spread, and even those with M1 (cytology-positive) disease, for whom it may be appropriate to consider a treatment approach different from that for patients with M2/3 disease with nodular seeding. For example, for patients with residual disease, M0, it would be logical to consider using a boost to residual disease in the posterior fossa to a dose higher than the standard 55.8 Gy. Management of patients with M1 disease remains controversial, but the weight of evidence suggests that they should be treated similarly to those with M2/3 disease.[193] Results for patients with M2/3 disease remain quite poor, although an impressive 81% 4-year overall survival was reported for patients treated on a COG pilot study using carboplatin daily during radiotherapy as a radiosensitizer. This forms the backbone of the current COG study for high-risk medulloblastoma, whereas the standard of care in many centers in Europe is now a hyperfractionated accelerated radiotherapy (HART) regimen given in combination with pre- and postradiotherapy chemotherapy.[194]

Management of Medulloblastoma in Infants

Medulloblastoma accounts for 20% to 40% of all CNS tumors in infants. Although up to half of infants have more favorable histologic types (desmoplastic/nodular or medulloblastoma with extensive nodularity), the prognosis overall is worse than in older children. The explanation for this is likely multifactorial. In addition to biology, the rate of complete resection is lower in this age group, and the frequency of leptomeningeal seeding at diagnosis is higher (as much as 50%), but also, many patients do not receive optimal treatment.[195] Because of the significant risks with respect to neurocognitive function associated with the use of radiotherapy in infants and very young children, chemotherapy has been used in an attempt to either delay or avoid radiotherapy altogether. Infants with M0 disease who have undergone total resection may do well with chemotherapy alone, with a 5-year overall survival of 69% in the first POG infant study[196] and of 93% in the German study,[197] although it is noteworthy that treatment in the latter included intraventricular methotrexate for which there are also concerns about the risk of neurocognitive sequelae. In other studies results were less satisfactory, in some because of the need for aggressive salvage regimens that were associated with significant long-term sequelae.[198] In fact, with the possible exception of very young children with desmoplastic/nodular medulloblastoma without residual disease, evidence suggests that radiotherapy is an important component of treatment,[64] and because recurrences are generally early (6 to 12 months) and local,[64,196,199] the recently completed North American study used early radiotherapy to a limited treatment volume consisting of the tumor bed plus an anatomically confined margin for the CTV of 1 cm for patients without leptomeningeal seeding. Infants with M2/3 disease generally are treated with intensive chemotherapy regimens. Although patients with desmoplastic/nodular histology may do quite well, with an overall survival at 5 years of 52.9% in the UKCCSG/SIOP baby study, for example,[65] the prognosis for those with other subtypes is much less satisfactory. Despite this, the goal of treatment generally will still be to avoid radiotherapy (especially CSI) and the decision to use it highly individualized based on the clinical situation and the wishes of the parents.

Radiotherapy for Medulloblastoma

CSI is the standard of care, and careful attention to coverage of the entire target volume that includes the meninges overlying the brain and spine including extensions along nerve roots is critical. In the SFOP M-7 protocol, 50% of relapses could be correlated with targeting deviations. In the subsequent studies (MSFOP-93 and MSFOP-98), the relapse rate was 17% in patients who had inadequate coverage of only one part of the CTV (a typical example being the cribriform plate), 28% for patients who had inadequate coverage at two sites, and 67% for patients who had inadequate coverage at three or more sites.[200,201] In an SFOP pilot study that tested reduced-dose CSI for standard-risk disease, overall survival at 5 years was significantly worse for patients with inadequate coverage at two or more sites as compared with no or only one major deviation (54.4% vs. 79.3%).[202]

CSI is followed by a boost to the tumor bed or posterior fossa. Previously, the entire posterior fossa had been treated to a total dose of 54 to 55.8 Gy. Using conformal treatment techniques, it is possible to reduce the dose to the cochlea, which is important in children who will also be receiving cisplatin-based chemotherapy. Better sparing of the cochlea,[203] pituitary and hypothalamus, and the temporal lobes can be achieved using a reduced target volume for the boost (Fig. 88.13). Fukunaga-Johnson et al.[204] found a low risk of isolated failure outside the tumor bed in the posterior fossa in a cohort of 114 patients, and data from several other centers as well as an SFOP pilot study that used a conformal boost limited to the tumor bed similarly support such an approach.[188,205-208] The optimal CTV for a reduced-volume posterior fossa boost remains to be defined, although an anatomically confined expansion of 1.5 cm around the GTV (any macroscopic residual tumor and the surgical bed) until recently has been regarded as reasonable and this was the margin employed in the COG ACNS 0331 trial.

Based on outcomes from this trial, the standard of care for the boost is tumor bed irradiation.

Delay to radiotherapy may be associated with poorer outcomes, and CSI should ideally start within 28 to 40 days following surgical resection. There is also evidence that it is important to deliver radiotherapy in a timely fashion, avoiding unnecessary gaps in treatment resulting from machine servicing, holidays, and the like. In the SIOP PNET-3 study event-free and overall survival were significantly worse when the duration of treatment exceeded 50 days as compared with the results for children treated as planned over 45 to 47 days.[209] When CSI has to be interrupted, for example, because of hematologic toxicity, treatment should continue to the posterior fossa boost volume while waiting for the blood counts to recover. Granulocyte colony-stimulating factor may be used to hasten recovery of the counts.

Supratentorial Primitive Neuroectodermal Tumor

Recent molecular analysis of case series has established that the group of tumors previously referred to as supratentorial primitive neuroectodermal tumor (stPNET) are now more correctly allocated to various different histologic groups, including other embryonal tumors such as ATRT (see below) or sometimes those of astrocytic lineage. This has led to confusion over how best to manage these patients.

Traditionally, the conventional usual approach for a child older than 3 with a stPNET without leptomeningeal spread consisted of maximal surgical resection followed by postoperative radiotherapy (CSI followed by a boost) and chemotherapy. Experimental regimens such as high dose chemotherapy with stem cell rescue are used in infants and young children and in patients with M+ disease. In view of current knowledge, patients who would previously have been diagnosed as having stPNET require multidisciplinary discussion including detailed expert review of pathology to determine optimum management of the individual case.

Atypical Teratoid/Rhabdoid Tumor

Atypical teratoid/rhabdoid tumor (ATRT) is a highly malignant embryonal tumor seen in very young children with a peak incidence in the birth to 2-year age group, at which age in one population-based study ATRT was as common as PNET and medulloblastoma.[210] Composed of rhabdoid cells with or without fields resembling a classical PNET, ATRT is diagnosed on the basis of the characteristic molecular findings, namely, deletion and/or mutation of the INI1 locus on chromosome 22. ATRT can arise at any location within the CNS, including the spine. Leptomeningeal seeding is seen at diagnosis in a quarter to a third of patients.

Since recognition of ATRT as a separate entity with a high frequency of early relapse and a very poor prognosis, patients have been treated with increasingly intensive chemotherapy regimens. Radiotherapy appears to be an important component of treatment.[211-217] In a series of 37 patients treated at St. Jude, early use of radiotherapy and the use of CSI were found to be associated with improved outcomes,[215] and it has been suggested that the worse survival reported for children younger than age 3 may be due in part to the less frequent use of radiotherapy and, when used, to the use of local radiotherapy rather than CSI in this age group. However, in a recent update limited to patients who received age- and risk-stratified radiotherapy, delay to radiotherapy was found to be the important factor.[218] In the current COG study, the treatment plan calls for early radiotherapy (after completion of two cycles of induction chemotherapy), although in practice, the use and timing of radiotherapy depend on the age of the child, the location (infra- or supratentorial), and the extent of disease at diagnosis (M0 or M+). Thus, children younger than 6 months at completion of chemotherapy with an infratentorial tumor and those younger than 12 months with a supratentorial

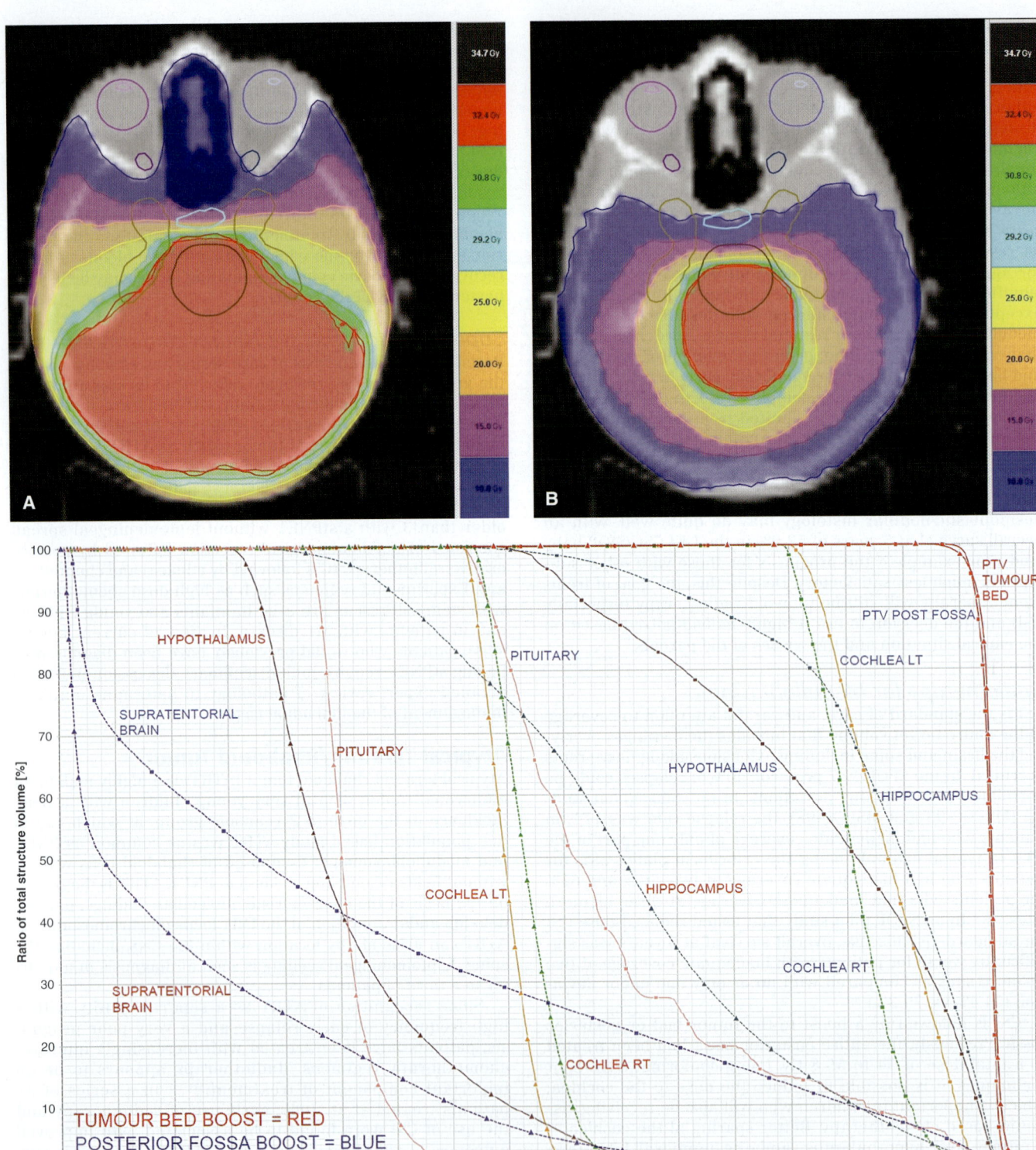

FIGURE 88.13. Axial images of an intensity-modulated radiation therapy/image-guide radiation therapy plan for a whole posterior fossa (**A**) and a reduced-volume posterior fossa boost (**B**) for a patient with medulloblastoma. **C:** Dose–volume histograms show significant sparing of organs at risk with the reduced-volume boost.

tumor receive radiotherapy later, upon completion of both induction and consolidation chemotherapy. The radiotherapy target volume is local (tumor bed and any macroscopic residual disease plus a margin for the CTV of 1 cm) for children with localized disease and CSI followed by a boost for those with leptomeningeal spread. Doses are age dependent for both local radiotherapy and CSI (50.4 vs. 54 Gy and 23.4 vs. 36 Gy for children younger and older than 3 years, respectively). In Europe, patients with nonmetastatic ATRT receive doxorubicin-based chemotherapy and local radiotherapy to a dose of 54 Gy, whereas those with metastatic disease receive CSI. An ATRT registry (EURHAB) has been established to collect multi-institutional and multinational data on patient management and outcome.

Embryonal Tumors with Multilayer Rosette

In 2000, Eberhart et al.[218a] described a variant of StPNET, the embryonal tumor with abundant neuropil and true rosettes (ETANTR) as a tumor exhibiting prominent ependymoblastic rosettes, neuronal differentiation, and a neuropil background. This tumor was predominantly recognized in young children and was associated with a very poor prognosis. More recently, in 2014, it has been recognized that there is a group of tumors that are distinct from other embryonal tumors and are referred to as embryonal tumors with multilayer rosettes (ETMRs). ETMR is now recognized as containing the three histologic variants ETANTR, ependymoblastoma, and medulloepithelioma.[219] These newly recognized tumors are yet to have a universally accepted mode of management.

GERM CELL TUMORS

Germ cell tumors of the CNS constitute a group of rare tumors that are morphologic homologs of germinal neoplasms arising in the gonads and at other extragonadal sites. They include the following entities although in many cases more than one tumor type is present:

- Germinoma
- Embryonal carcinoma
- Yolk-sac tumor (endodermal sinus tumor)
- Choriocarcinoma
- Teratoma
  - Mature
  - Immature
  - Teratoma with malignant transformation
- Mixed germ cell tumor

A teratoma is a tumor composed of an admixture of different tissue types representative of ectoderm, endoderm, and mesoderm. A mature teratoma is composed exclusively of fully differentiated tissues, sometimes arranged in such a manner as to resemble normal tissue relationships. Mitoses are absent or rare. An immature teratoma is composed of incompletely differentiated tissues resembling those of the fetus. Mitoses typically are present.

In the West, CNS germ cell tumors are relatively rare, accounting for 3% to 5% of all CNS tumors in the pediatric age group. They are more common in Asia, where they account for as many as 15% to 18% of all CNS tumors occurring in childhood. The peak age incidence is 10 to 12 years. Boys are affected more frequently than girls, with a ratio of approximately 3:1. CNS germ cell tumors arise from primordial germ cells in structures about the third ventricle, with the region of the pineal gland being the most common site of origin followed by the suprasellar region. Nongerminomatous germ cell tumors (NGGCTs) are the most common tumor type in the former area and germinomas in the latter.

The presenting symptoms and signs depend on the tumor type and the location of the tumor. Tumors in the pineal region cause obstruction to CSF flow at the aqueduct of Sylvius resulting in hydrocephalus, and most patients with tumors in this region present with a relatively short history with symptoms and signs of raised intracranial pressure. Another characteristic presentation of tumors in this region is Parinaud syndrome as a result of dorsal midbrain compression. In contrast, patients with tumors in the suprasellar region usually present with a longer history initially of neuroendocrine deficits, especially diabetes insipidus, growth failure, and precocious puberty, and only later of visual field deficits and, later still, of symptoms and signs of raised intracranial pressure. On imaging, most germ cell tumors appear as solid masses. Teratomas are more heterogeneous with cysts, areas of calcification, and sometimes fat, whereas choriocarcinomas often contain areas of hemorrhage. Bi- or multifocal disease around the third ventricle is seen in approximately 10% of patients with germinomas. Gadolinium-enhanced MRI of the spinal axis is an essential part of the workup to exclude leptomeningeal dissemination, which is found at diagnosis in approximately 10% of patients with germinomas and 10% to 15% of patients with NGGCTs. Measurement of serum and CSF tumor markers is another essential part of the initial workup. Modest elevation of β-human chorionic gonadotropin (β-hCG) (<100 IU/mL) may be seen with pure germinomas that may contain syncytiotrophoblastic cells. Higher levels of β-hCG are more suggestive of a choriocarcinoma. An elevated α-fetoprotein (α-FP) is diagnostic of a yolk-sac tumor.

In the past, many lesions arising in or about the third ventricle were treated without histologic confirmation of diagnosis. This is no longer considered acceptable practice because the differential diagnosis includes many disparate entities (such as Langerhans cell histiocytosis, astrocytoma, and ependymoma), and all patients should undergo biopsy unless CSF and/or serum markers confirm the presence of an NGGCT (elevated α-FP and/or β-hCG > 100 IU/mL) or unless a histologic diagnosis is made by other means (e.g., CSF cytology). For tumors in the pineal region with hydrocephalus, the usual surgical approach is an endoscopic third ventriculostomy, which allows access to the lesion for biopsy purposes. Intraventricular lesions have to be biopsied with care because hemorrhage, which is not infrequent, may be difficult to manage endoscopically. A stereotactic approach is also possible, but this may be quite challenging because of the proximity of deep cerebral veins and, moreover, may be suboptimal for diagnosis because of the potential for sampling error. Occasionally, complete resection will be possible; this would be a reasonable strategy for patients with NGGCTs if it can be accomplished without major morbidity because it would ensure complete characterization of the pathology and may even obviate the need for further therapy.

Germinoma

In the past, standard treatment for patients with germinoma, whether localized or disseminated, was radiotherapy alone. Results of treatment using CSI followed by a boost to the primary site are excellent, with long-term disease-free survival rates of 100% in some series.[220-224] For patients with unifocal disease without leptomeningeal spread, radiotherapy alone to limited volumes, that is, whole brain[225,226] or whole ventricle,[220,222,227] results in a high probability of local control and a low (0% to 5%) risk of failure in the spinal axis. Experience with local radiotherapy (tumor plus a margin) alone generally has been less satisfactory,[225-229] although some have reported excellent results.[230] To reduce the risk of morbidity associated with radiotherapy, chemotherapy has been considered another option, either alone or in combination with reduced-volume and/or reduced-dose radiotherapy. Several studies have shown clearly that the former, that is, the use of chemotherapy alone, is not acceptable: only 40% to 50% of patients remain disease free, and although salvage using further chemotherapy together with radiotherapy is possible in most cases and overall survival is high, this is achieved at the cost of considerable toxicity.[231-234]

In contrast, a combined approach using platinum-based chemotherapy followed by reduced-volume, reduced-dose radiotherapy is an attractive option that results in disease-free survival rates in the 90% to 96% range.[232,235-237] The optimal radiotherapy target volume using such an approach remains to be defined. Local failures were seen in 10 of 60 patients treated in the SFOP TGM-TC-90 study with chemotherapy followed by local radiotherapy[238] and with even greater frequency in some single-institution studies, which, although with a patient population with a median age in adolescence, included adult patients.[229,239] Local failure appears to be less frequent after whole ventricular radiotherapy[239] and this is becoming generally accepted as the appropriate volume in this context (Fig. 88.14), but prospective data are lacking for now.

For patients with leptomeningeal spread at diagnosis, radiotherapy alone using CSI with boosts to macroscopic disease is certainly an option, although in North America and Europe, chemotherapy followed by CSI followed by a boost to all sites of involvement would now be the more usual approach. Management of patients with bi- or multifocal midline tumors is controversial. In the past, these patients were

FIGURE 88.14. Target volume definition for whole ventricular irradiation as per the guidelines for the current Children's Oncology Group study for central nervous system germ cell tumors. Planning computed tomography and T2-weighted magnetic resonance images at the level of lateral ventricles **(A)**, hypothalamus and pineal cistern **(B)**, and fourth ventricle and prepontine cistern **(C)**. Note that this volume needs to be expanded to include the primary tumor and any other sites of involvement. Whether the suprasellar, basal, and prepontine cisterns need to be included is controversial for now. Better sparing of nontarget tissues will be achieved with the use of a four-field technique or intensity-modulated radiation therapy than with lateral opposed fields. (Courtesy of Dr. Shannon MacDonald.)

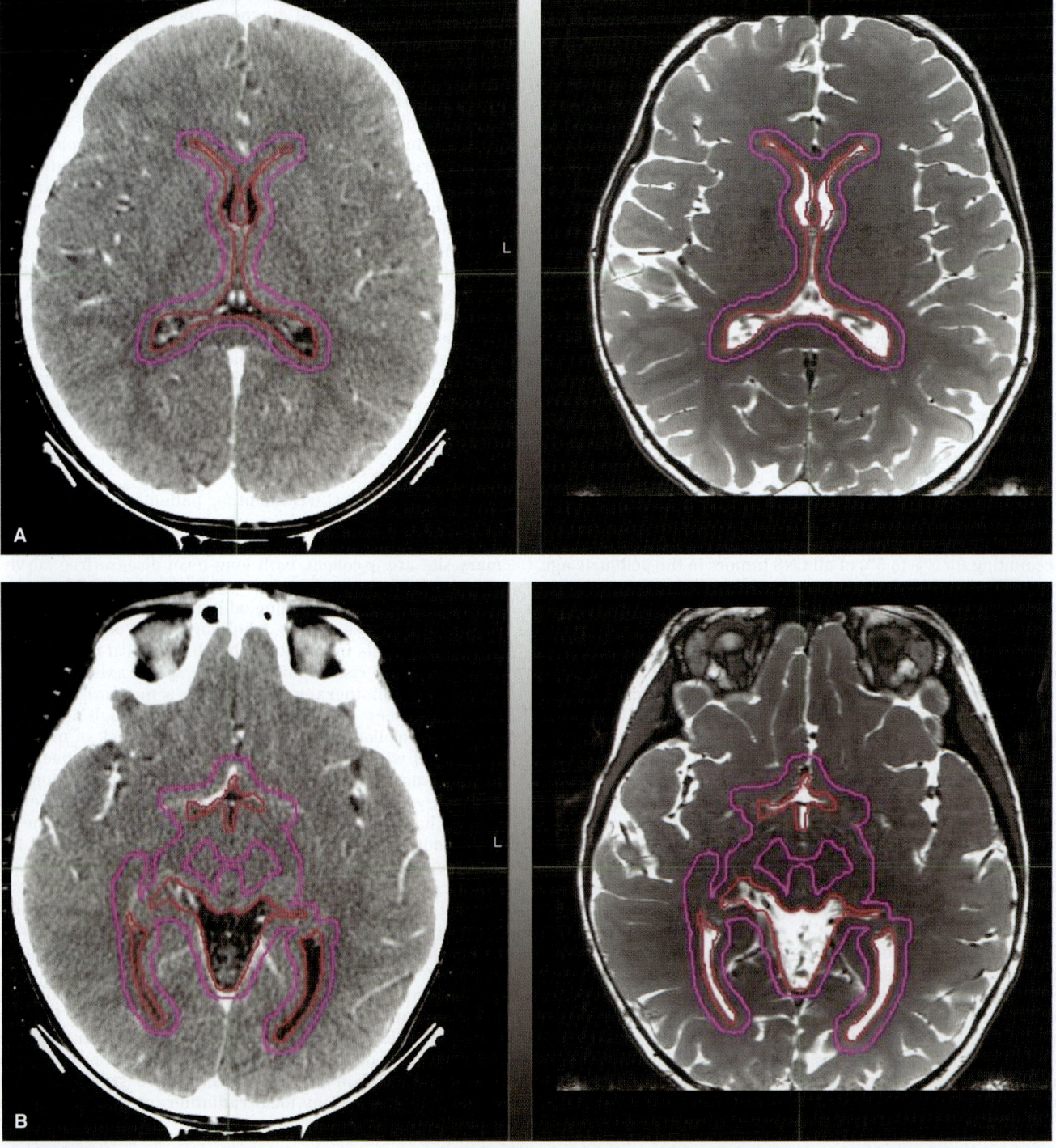

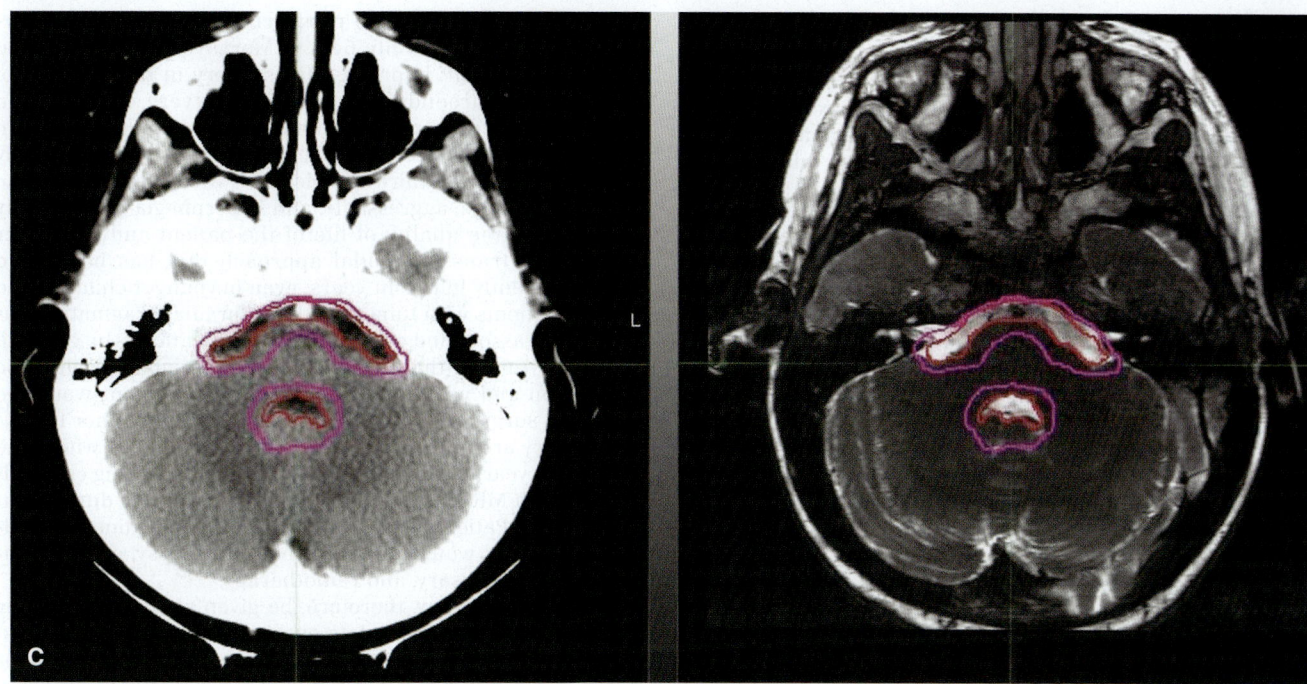

FIGURE 88.14. *(Continued)*

treated as having disseminated disease, but at least some, that is, those with bifocal disease by imaging or by inference (e.g., in a patient with a pineal region primary who has diabetes insipidus), are now more usually treated with chemotherapy and whole ventricular radiotherapy.

There is less controversy now with regard to the radiotherapy dose and dose-fractionation schedule for germinoma. Results are excellent with a CSI dose as low as 21 Gy even in patients with leptomeningeal spread. The total dose to the primary site has typically been 40 to 45 Gy but probably can be safely reduced to 30 Gy or even to 24 Gy[232,237] in patients treated with a combined chemotherapy–radiotherapy regimen who have had a complete response to chemotherapy. Finally, because germinoma is a very radiosensitive tumor, a fraction size of 1.5 Gy can be used, which, in theory, further reduces the risk of injury to normal structures.

Nongerminomatous Germ Cell Tumors

For NGGCTs, the diagnosis can be made in as many as one-third of all patients on the basis of imaging findings (location and appearance) plus tumor markers. NGGCTs are of several different histopathologic types that carry different prognoses (Table 88.3). Patients with mature teratomas without any

associated malignant elements can be managed with surgery alone, whereas those with mature teratoma with germinomatous elements will be treated as germinomas. All other patients with intermediate- and poor-prognosis tumor types[240] require more aggressive treatment. The results of treatment using radiotherapy alone are very poor, with overall survival in the 10% to 30% range. Results are better with chemotherapy alone, although 40% to 60% of patients relapse following chemotherapy and will be subjected to aggressive salvage regimens.[231,241,242] A multimodality approach that includes both chemotherapy and radiotherapy appears to be associated with the best outcome. Event-free survival was 81% in the German/Italian pilot study that led to the most recent SIOP CNS GCT study.[243] The current standard of care therefore consists of platinum-based chemotherapy followed by radiotherapy.

There is controversy with respect to the radiotherapy target volume for NGGCT. Although good results have been reported by some groups using chemotherapy followed by local radiotherapy,[179] others show a high rate of failure outside the primary site.[242,244–248] Thus, as for germinoma, a whole-ventricle volume may be a better option for more favorable patients (e.g., the intermediate-risk group, α-FP $< 1,000$ ng/mL), whereas CSI would be used for those with less favorable or disseminated disease. The usual dose to the whole ventricle volume or CSI is 30 to 36 Gy and to the primary site, 54 Gy.

Patients who have less than a complete response to chemotherapy fare poorly. Second-look surgery may be useful to both exclude the possibility that the residual imaging abnormality represents mature teratoma and/or resect residual viable tumor. This would be followed by CSI and more intensive chemotherapy such as high dose chemotherapy with stem cell rescue.

TUMORS OF THE SELLAR REGION

Tumors arising in the sellar region in children include the following:

- Craniopharyngioma
  - Adamantinomatous
  - Papillary
- Pituitary adenomas

TABLE 88.3 CLASSIFICATION OF NONGERMINOMATOUS GERM CELL TUMORS

Good Prognosis
Mature teratoma

Intermediate Prognosis
Immature teratoma
Mixed germ cell tumors consisting of germinoma with either mature or immature teratoma

Poor Prognosis
Teratoma with malignant transformation
Embryonal carcinoma
Yolk sac tumor
Choriocarcinoma
Mixed germ cell tumors including a component of embryonal carcinoma, yolk sac tumor, choriocarcinoma, or teratoma with malignant transformation

Adapted from Sawamura Y, Ikeda J, Shirato H, et al. Germ cell tumours of the central nervous system: treatment consideration based on 111 cases and their long-term clinical outcomes. *Eur J Cancer* 1998;34(1):104–110. Copyright © 1997 Elsevier. With permission.

Craniopharyngioma

By definition, craniopharyngiomas are benign partly cystic epithelial tumors that arise in the sellar region from remnants of Rathke pouch. In children, almost all are of the adamantinomatous type. They account for approximately 5% of intracranial tumors in the pediatric age group with a peak incidence between the ages of 5 and 14 years.

In the majority of patients, craniopharyngiomas have both suprasellar and intrasellar components. Children typically present with neuroendocrine deficits, especially diabetes insipidus and growth failure. Visual field deficits often go unnoticed initially. Cognitive and behavioral changes are not uncommon. Compression of or tumor growth within the third ventricle may lead to hydrocephalus and symptoms and signs of raised intracranial pressure. On neuroimaging, the findings are very typical, with solid and cystic areas in varying proportions. Calcification is seen in the majority of cases. The solid portion(s) and the cyst capsule usually enhance with the use of contrast material.

Treatment of craniopharyngiomas, although long considered a controversial issue,[249] in practice depends on the characteristics of the tumor and the availability of the surgical expertise required. The argument for surgical resection is based on single-institution (mostly specialist center) reports of long-term tumor control after complete resection as confirmed on postoperative imaging in 85% to 100% of patients.[250]

However, in a three-nation prospective study event-free survival at 3 years was only 64%.[251] Moreover, although visual deficits, if present, improve after surgery in the majority of cases, new neuroendocrine deficits are very common and hypothalamic damage is a major concern particularly in patients with tumors that have grown retro-chiasmatically into the floor of the third ventricle.[252–254] Devastating sequelae that include rage, aggressivity, and hyperphagia permanently compromise the quality of life of the patient and his or her family. The transsphenoidal approach that has been used more frequently in recent years, even in younger children and even in patients with tumors with a supradiaphragmatic component, is associated with fewer complications. In general, therefore, tumors that are smaller and/or subdiaphragmatic in location and without hypothalamic involvement would be managed surgically. Patients who have residual tumor following surgery are at high risk for progressive disease within the first 2 to 3 years following surgery,[251,255–258] mandating close follow-up with MRI performed at 3-month intervals during that time period. Patients at greater risk for complications secondary to surgery would be managed with biopsy, cyst decompression, if necessary, and radiotherapy.[259–264]

Radiotherapy may, therefore, be given as the sole therapy after biopsy, after incomplete surgery, or at time of progression/recurrence after surgery, and the heterogeneity of tumor

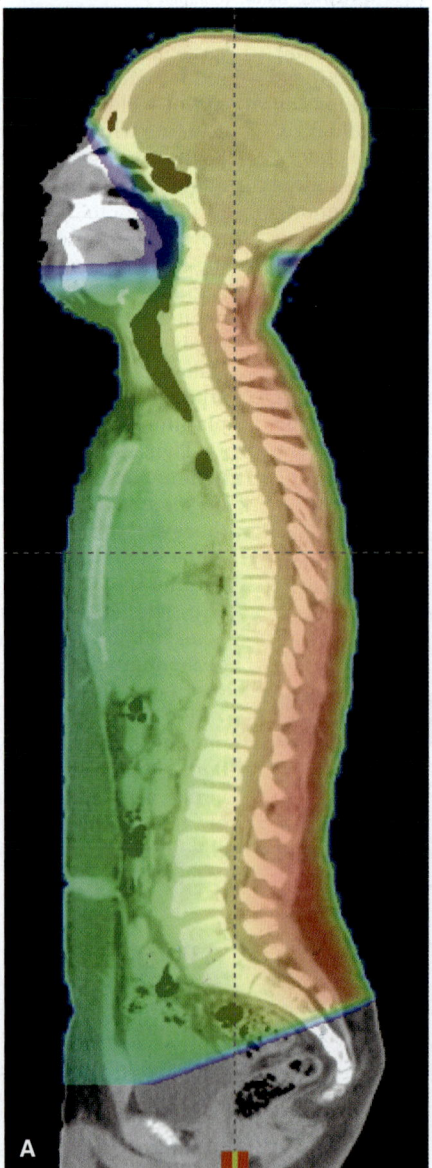
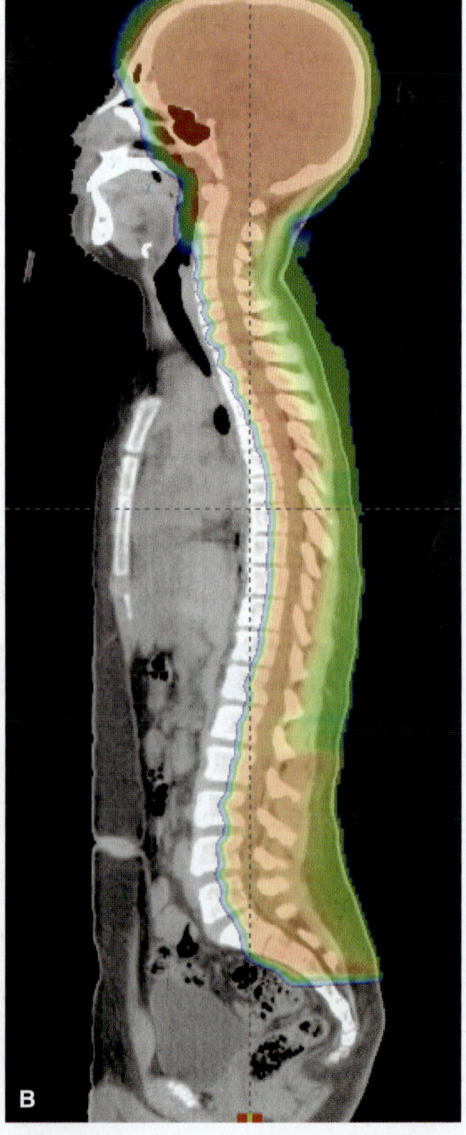

FIGURE 88.15. A: Craniospinal radiotherapy for young adult with conventional photon radiotherapy—exit from spinal field delivers low to intermediate dose to structures anterior to spine. **B:** Craniospinal radiotherapy for young adult with proton therapy—no exit dose beyond Bragg peak avoiding dose to structures anterior to spine. (Figure courtesy of Dr. D. Indelicato, University of Florida, Jacksonville.)

types and situations means that one of several approaches may be used. For example, a lesion with a small solid component and a simple cyst may be well treated with intracavitary injection of liquid radioactive material. Most contemporary experience is with β emitters such as ^{32}P and ^{90}Y delivering a high dose (i.e., 200 Gy) to the cyst wall. Intracavitary injection of radioactive material is not always easy.[265] Sometimes, the cyst fluid is very thick in consistency and there may be little or no communication between multiple cysts. It is essential to use contrast material to ensure that the catheter is well placed in the cavity and that there is no leakage of material outside the cyst before injecting radioactive material. This could be combined with radiosurgery or fractionated stereotactic irradiation to the associated solid component, although it may be reasonable to do so only later and only if there is evidence of progressive disease. Special care is needed if, as is usually the case, the tumor is in close proximity to the optic chiasm or optic nerves.[266] Tumor control rates using this approach are good for carefully selected patients.[267] However, conventionally fractionated external beam radiotherapy may be a better option for all except very small tumors, with a lower risk of morbidity.[249,268]

The target volume for external beam radiotherapy consists of the entire lesion (i.e., both the solid and cystic components) as demonstrated on MRI performed just prior to treatment. Although some have used a margin for the CTV of 1 cm,[269] a smaller margin of 0.5 cm or even 0 cm (i.e., CTV = GTV) can be justified on the basis of excellent tumor control using such margins.[270-272] A dose of 54 to 55 Gy given in 30 daily fractions over 6 weeks appears to be necessary to achieve a high probability of tumor control. Cyst enlargement during treatment or within the first 2 to 3 months after completion of radiotherapy is not uncommon. Early recognition and appropriate management consisting usually of cyst decompression is essential to avoid further neurologic compromise or even death.[273] The long-term prognosis is good, with event-free survival of 80% to 100% in most series.[251,269,272,274,275]

There is increasing interest in the use of proton therapy to reduce nontarget dose, which would be predicted to minimize late neurocognitive effects (Fig. 88.15).

Pituitary Adenomas

Pituitary adenomas are rare in childhood. Almost all cases arise in adolescence. Most are functioning adenomas that present with endocrine dysfunction, most often menstrual irregularities and galactorrhea in girls and delayed puberty in boys. They may be quite large, with extrasellar extension, and appear to be more invasive than those seen in adults.[276-278] Visual loss, when present, may be more severe and more likely to be associated with optic atrophy.[277]

Management will, in general, parallel that for adult patients. Prolactin- and growth hormone–secreting adenomas are managed medically as in adults. When surgery is necessary, a transsphenoidal approach using neuronavigation appears to be feasible and safe in children, even in those with poor pneumatization of the sphenoid sinus.[276,278] Radiotherapy is indicated if surgical resection is not possible or if hormone levels remain elevated following surgery. Highly conformal treatment with a margin for the CTV of 0.5 cm beyond macroscopic disease is appropriate in most cases, the technique used being that which optimally spares adjacent critical structures including major vessels. The usual dose, as in adults, will be 45 Gy over 5 weeks. Close follow-up by an endocrinologist is essential to ensure appropriate management of hormone deficits.

REFERENCES

1. Kohler BA, Ward E, McCarthy BJ, et al. Annual report to the nation on the status of cancer, 1975–2007, featuring tumors of the brain and other nervous system. *J Natl Cancer Inst* 2011;103(9):714–736.
2. Armstrong GT, Liu Q, Yasui Y, et al. Long-term outcomes among adult survivors of childhood central nervous system malignancies in the Childhood Cancer Survivor Study. *J Natl Cancer Inst* 2009;101(13):946–958.
3. Vinchon M, Baroncini M, Leblond P, et al. Morbidity and tumor-related mortality among adult survivors of pediatric brain tumors: a review. *Childs Nerv Syst* 2011;27(5):697–704.
4. Kortmann RD, Timmermann B, Taylor RE, et al. Current and future strategies in radiotherapy of childhood low-grade glioma of the brain. Part II: treatment-related late toxicity. *Strahlenther Onkol* 2003;179(9):585–597.
5. Mulhern RK, Merchant TE, Gajjar A, et al. Late neurocognitive sequelae in survivors of brain tumours in childhood. *Lancet Oncol* 2004;5(7):399–408.
6. Miralbell R, Lomax A, Bortfeld T, et al. Potential role of proton therapy in the treatment of pediatric medulloblastoma/primitive neuroectodermal tumors: reduction of the supratentorial target volume. *Int J Radiat Oncol Biol Phys* 1997;38(3):477–484.
7. Mulhern RK, Kepner JL, Thomas PR, et al. Neuropsychologic functioning of survivors of childhood medulloblastoma randomized to receive conventional or reduced-dose craniospinal irradiation: a Pediatric Oncology Group study. *J Clin Oncol* 1998;16(5):1723–1728.
8. Grill J, Renaux VK, Bulteau C, et al. Long-term intellectual outcome in children with posterior fossa tumors according to radiation doses and volumes. *Int J Radiat Oncol Biol Phys* 1999;45(1):137–145.
9. Ris MD, Packer R, Goldwein J, et al. Intellectual outcome after reduced-dose radiation therapy plus adjuvant chemotherapy for medulloblastoma: a Children's Cancer Group study. *J Clin Oncol* 2001;19(15):3470–3476.
10. Taylor RE, Bailey CC, Robinson K, et al. Results of a randomized study of preradiation chemotherapy versus radiotherapy alone for nonmetastatic medulloblastoma: the International Society of Paediatric Oncology/United Kingdom Children's Cancer Study Group PNET-3 Study. *J Clin Oncol* 2003;21(8):1581–1591.
11. Butler RW, Mulhern RK. Neurocognitive interventions for children and adolescents surviving cancer. *J Pediatr Psychol* 2005;30(1):65–78.
12. Mabbott DJ, Spiegler BJ, Greenberg ML, et al. Serial evaluation of academic and behavioral outcome after treatment with cranial radiation in childhood. *J Clin Oncol* 2005;23(10):2256–2263.
13. Meacham L. Endocrine late effects of childhood cancer therapy. *Curr Probl Pediatr Adolesc Health Care* 2003;33(7):217–242.
14. Merchant TE, Williams T, Smith JM, et al. Preirradiation endocrinopathies in pediatric brain tumor patients determined by dynamic tests of endocrine function. *Int J Radiat Oncol Biol Phys* 2002;54(1):45–50.
15. Gurney JG, Kadan-Lottick NS, Packer RJ, et al. Endocrine and cardiovascular late effects among adult survivors of childhood brain tumors: Childhood Cancer Survivor Study. *Cancer* 2003;97(3):663–673.
16. Sklar CA, Constine LS. Chronic neuroendocrinological sequelae of radiation therapy. *Int J Radiat Oncol Biol Phys* 1995;31(5):1113–1121.
17. Schmiegelow M, Lassen S, Weber L, et al. Dosimetry and growth hormone deficiency following cranial irradiation of childhood brain tumors. *Med Pediatr Oncol* 1999;33(6):564–571.
18. Adan L, Trivin C, Sainte-Rose C, et al. GH deficiency caused by cranial irradiation during childhood: factors and markers in young adults. *J Clin Endocrinol Metab* 2001;86(11):5245–5251.
19. Jakacki RI, Goldwein JW, Larsen RL, et al. Cardiac dysfunction following spinal irradiation during childhood. *J Clin Oncol* 1993;11(6):1033–1038.
20. Beltran C, Naik M, Merchant TE. Dosimetric effect of setup motion and target volume margin reduction in pediatric ependymoma. *Radiother Oncol* 2010;96(2):216–222.
21. Roberge D, Kun LE, Freeman CR. Intracranial germinoma: on whole-ventricular irradiation. *Pediatr Blood Cancer* 2005;44(4):358–362.
22. Raggi E, Mosleh-Shirazi MA, Saran FH. An evaluation of conformal and intensity-modulated radiotherapy in whole ventricular radiotherapy for localised primary intracranial germinomas. *Clin Oncol (R Coll Radiol)* 2008;20(3):253–260.
23. Chen MJ, Santos AS, Sakuraba RK, et al. Intensity-modulated and 3D-conformal radiotherapy for whole-ventricular irradiation as compared with conventional whole-brain irradiation in the management of localized central nervous system germ cell tumors. *Int J Radiat Oncol Biol Phys* 2010;76(2):608–614.
24. Urie M, FitzGerald TJ, Followill D, et al. Current calibration, treatment, and treatment planning techniques among institutions participating in the Children's Oncology Group. *Int J Radiat Oncol Biol Phys* 2003;55(1):245–260.
25. Parker WA, Freeman CR. A simple technique for craniospinal radiation in the supine position. *Radiother Oncol* 2006;78(2):217–222.
26. Parker W, Filion E, Roberge D, et al. Intensity-modulated radiotherapy for craniospinal irradiation: target volume considerations, dose constraints, and competing risks. *Int J Radiat Oncol Biol Phys* 2007;69(1):251–257.
27. St Clair WH, Adams JA, Bues M, et al. Advantage of protons compared to conventional X-ray or IMRT in the treatment of a pediatric patient with medulloblastoma. *Int J Radiat Oncol Biol Phys* 2004;58(3):727–734.
28. Yock TI, Yeap BY, Ebb DH, et al. Long-term toxic effects of proton radiotherapy for paediatric medulloblastoma: a phase 2 single-arm study. *Lancet Oncol* 2016;17:287–298.
29. Donahue B. Short- and long-term complications of radiation therapy for pediatric brain tumors. *Pediatr Neurosurg* 1992;18(4):207–217.
30. Louis DN, Perry A, Reifenberger G, et al. The 2016 World Health Organization Classification of Tumors of the Central Nervous System: a summary. *Acta Neuropathol* 2016;131:803–820.
31. Faulkner C, Ellis HP, Shaw A, et al. BRAF Fusion Analysis in Pilocytic Astrocytomas: KIAA1549-BRAF 15-9 Fusions are more frequent in the midline than within the cerebellum. *J Neuropathol Exp Pathol* 2015;74:867–872.
32. Komotar RJ, Burger PC, Carson BS, et al. Pilocytic and pilomyxoid hypothalamic/chiasmatic astrocytomas. *Neurosurgery* 2004;54(1):72–79.
33. Listernick R, Charrow J, Greenwald M, et al. Natural history of optic pathway tumors in children with neurofibromatosis type 1: a longitudinal study. *J Pediatr* 1994;125(1):63–66.
34. Pollack IF, Shultz B, Mulvihill JJ. The management of brainstem gliomas in patients with neurofibromatosis 1. *Neurology* 1996;46(6):1652–1660.

35. Farmer JP, Khan S, Khan A, et al. Neurofibromatosis type 1 and the pediatric neurosurgeon: a 20-year institutional review. *Pediatr Neurosurg* 2002;37(3):122–136.
36. King A, Listernick R, Charrow J, et al. Optic pathway gliomas in neurofibromatosis type 1: the effect of presenting symptoms on outcome. *Am J Med Genet A* 2003;122A(2):95–99.
37. Hirsch JF, Sainte RC, Pierre-Kahn A, et al. Benign astrocytic and oligodendrocytic tumors of the cerebral hemispheres in children. *J Neurosurg* 1989;70(4):568–572.
38. Pollack IF, Claassen D, al-Shboul Q, et al. Low-grade gliomas of the cerebral hemispheres in children: an analysis of 71 cases. *J Neurosurg* 1995;82(4):536–547.
39. Sgouros S, Fineron PW, Hockley AD. Cerebellar astrocytoma of childhood: long-term follow-up. *Childs Nerv Syst* 1995;11(2):89–96.
40. Gajjar A, Sanford RA, Heideman R, et al. Low-grade astrocytoma: a decade of experience at St. Jude Children's Research Hospital. *J Clin Oncol* 1997;15(8): 2792–2799.
41. Fernandez C, Figarella-Branger D, Girard N, et al. Pilocytic astrocytomas in children: prognostic factors—a retrospective study of 80 cases. *Neurosurgery* 2003;53(3):544–553.
42. Merchant TE, Kun LE, Wu S, et al. Phase II trial of conformal radiation therapy for pediatric low-grade glioma. *J Clin Oncol* 2009;27(22):3598–3604.
43. Wisoff JH, Sanford RA, Heier LA, et al. Primary neurosurgery for pediatric low-grade gliomas: a prospective multi-institutional study from the Children's Oncology Group. *Neurosurgery* 2011;68(6):1548–1554; discussion 54–55.
44. Saunders DE, Phipps KP, Wade AM, et al. Surveillance imaging strategies following surgery and/or radiotherapy for childhood cerebellar low-grade astrocytoma. *J Neurosurg* 2005;102(2 Suppl):172–178.
45. Reddy AT, Packer RJ. Chemotherapy for low-grade gliomas. *Childs Nerv Syst* 1999;15(10):506–513.
46. Fouladi M, Wallace D, Langston JW, et al. Survival and functional outcome of children with hypothalamic/chiasmatic tumors. *Cancer* 2003;97(4):1084–1092.
47. Laithier V, Grill J, Le Deley MC, et al. Progression-free survival in children with optic pathway tumors: dependence on age and the quality of the response to chemotherapy—results of the first French prospective study for the French Society of Pediatric Oncology. *J Clin Oncol* 2003;21(24):4572–4578.
48. Gnekow AK, Kortmann RD, Pietsch T, et al. Low grade chiasmatic-hypothalamic glioma-carboplatin and vincristine chemotherapy effectively defers radiotherapy within a comprehensive treatment strategy—report from the multicenter treatment study for children and adolescents with a low grade glioma—HIT-LGG 1996—of the Society of Pediatric Oncology and Hematology (GPOH). *Klin Padiatr* 2004;216(6):331–342.
49. Marcus KJ, Goumnerova L, Billett AL, et al. Stereotactic radiotherapy for localized low-grade gliomas in children: final results of a prospective trial. *Int J Radiat Oncol Biol Phys* 2005;61(2):374–379.
50. Kano H, Niranjan A, Kondziolka D, et al. Stereotactic radiosurgery for pilocytic astrocytomas part 2: outcomes in pediatric patients. *J Neurooncol* 2009;95(2):219–229.
51. Mundinger F, Braus DF, Krauss JK, et al. Long-term outcome of 89 low-grade brain-stem gliomas after interstitial radiation therapy. *J Neurosurg* 1991;75(5):740–746.
52. Scerrati M, Montemaggi P, Iacoangeli M, et al. Interstitial brachytherapy for low-grade cerebral gliomas: analysis of results in a series of 36 cases. *Acta Neurochir (Wien)* 1994;131(1–2):97–105.
53. Kreth FW, Faist M, Warnke PC, et al. Interstitial radiosurgery of low-grade gliomas. *J Neurosurg* 1995;82(3):418–429.
54. Korinthenberg R, Neuburger D, Trippel M, et al. Long-term results of brachytherapy with temporary iodine-125 seeds in children with low-grade gliomas. *Int J Radiat Oncol Biol Phys* 2011;79(4):1131–1138.
55. Ruge MI, Simon T, Suchorska B, et al. Stereotactic brachytherapy with iodine-125 seeds for the treatment of inoperable low-grade gliomas in children: long-term outcome. *J Clin Oncol* 2011;29(31):4151–4159.
56. Finlay JL, Boyett JM, Yates AJ, et al. Randomized phase III trial in childhood high-grade astrocytoma comparing vincristine, lomustine, and prednisone with the eight-drugs-in-1-day regimen. Childrens Cancer Group. *J Clin Oncol* 1995;13(1):112–123.
57. Campbell JW, Pollack IF, Martinez AJ, et al. High-grade astrocytomas in children: radiologically complete resection is associated with an excellent long-term prognosis. *Neurosurgery* 1996;38(2):258–264.
58. Heideman RL, Kuttesch J Jr, Gajjar AJ, et al. Supratentorial malignant gliomas in childhood: a single institution perspective. *Cancer* 1997;80(3):497–504.
59. Wisoff JH, Boyett JM, Berger MS, et al. Current neurosurgical management and the impact of the extent of resection in the treatment of malignant gliomas of childhood: a report of the Children's Cancer Group trial no. CCG-945. *J Neurosurg* 1998;89(1):52–59.
60. Qaddoumi I, Sultan I, Gajjar A. Outcome and prognostic features in pediatric gliomas: a review of 6212 cases from the Surveillance, Epidemiology, and End Results database. *Cancer* 2009;115(24):5761–5770.
61. Kramm CM, Butenhoff S, Rausche U, et al. Thalamic high-grade gliomas in children: a distinct clinical subset? *Neuro Oncol* 2011;13(6):680–689.
62. Geyer JR, Finlay JL, Boyett JM, et al. Survival of infants with malignant astrocytomas. A report from the Childrens Cancer Group. *Cancer* 1995;75(4): 1045–1050.
63. Duffner PK, Krischer JP, Burger PC, et al. Treatment of infants with malignant gliomas: the Pediatric Oncology Group experience. *J Neurooncol* 1996;28(2–3): 245–256.
64. Geyer JR, Sposto R, Jennings M, et al. Multiagent chemotherapy and deferred radiotherapy in infants with malignant brain tumors: a report from the Children's Cancer Group. *J Clin Oncol* 2005;23(30):7621–7631.
65. Grundy RG, Wilne SH, Robinson KJ, et al. Primary postoperative chemotherapy without radiotherapy for treatment of brain tumours other than ependymoma in children under 3 years: results of the first UKCCSG/SIOP CNS 9204 trial. *Eur J Cancer* 2010;46(1):120–133.
66. Sanders RP, Kocak M, Burger PC, et al. High-grade astrocytoma in very young children. *Pediatr Blood Cancer* 2007;49(7):888–893.
67. Pollack IF, Boyett JM, Yates AJ, et al. The influence of central review on outcome associations in childhood malignant gliomas: results from the CCG-945 experience. *Neuro Oncol* 2003;5(3):197–207.
68. Grill J, Laithier V, Rodriguez D, et al. When do children with optic pathway tumours need treatment? An oncological perspective in 106 patients treated in a single centre. *Eur J Pediatr* 2000;159(9):692–696.
69. Cohen BH, Kaplan AM, Packer RJ. Management of intracranial neoplasms in children with neurofibromatosis type 1 and 2. The Children's Cancer Study Group. *Pediatr Neurosurg* 1990;16(2):66–72.
70. Jenkin D, Angyalfi S, Becker L, et al. Optic glioma in children: surveillance, resection, or irradiation? *Int J Radiat Oncol Biol Phys* 1993;25(2): 215–225.
71. Khafaga Y, Hassounah M, Kandil A, et al. Optic gliomas: a retrospective analysis of 50 cases. *Int J Radiat Oncol Biol Phys* 2003;56(3):807–812.
72. Horwich A, Bloom HJ. Optic gliomas: radiation therapy and prognosis. *Int J Radiat Oncol Biol Phys* 1985;11(6):1067–1079.
73. Bataini JP, Delanian S, Ponvert D. Chiasmal gliomas: results of irradiation management in 57 patients and review of literature. *Int J Radiat Oncol Biol Phys* 1991;21(3):615–623.
74. Tao ML, Barnes PD, Billett AL, et al. Childhood optic chiasm gliomas: radiographic response following radiotherapy and long-term clinical outcome. *Int J Radiat Oncol Biol Phys* 1997;39(3):579–587.
75. Grabenbauer GG, Schuchardt U, Buchfelder M, et al. Radiation therapy of optico-hypothalamic gliomas (OHG)—radiographic response, vision and late toxicity. *Radiother Oncol* 2000;54(3):239–245.
76. Janss AJ, Grundy R, Cnaan A, et al. Optic pathway and hypothalamic/chiasmatic gliomas in children younger than age 5 years with a 6-year follow-up. *Cancer* 1995;75(4):1051–1059.
77. Combs SE, Schulz-Ertner D, Moschos D, et al. Fractionated stereotactic radiotherapy of optic pathway gliomas: tolerance and long-term outcome. *Int J Radiat Oncol Biol Phys* 2005;62(3):814–819.
78. Benesch M, Lackner H, Sovinz P, et al. Late sequela after treatment of childhood low-grade gliomas: a retrospective analysis of 69 long-term survivors treated between 1983 and 2003. *J Neurooncol* 2006;78(2):199–205.
79. Lacaze E, Kieffer V, Streri A, et al. Neuropsychological outcome in children with optic pathway tumours when first-line treatment is chemotherapy. *Br J Cancer* 2003;89(11):2038–2044.
80. Epstein FJ, Farmer JP. Brain-stem glioma growth patterns. *J Neurosurg* 1993;78(3):408–412.
81. Freeman CR, Farmer JP. Pediatric brain stem gliomas: a review. *Int J Radiat Oncol Biol Phys* 1998;40(2):265–271.
82. Fisher PG, Breiter SN, Carson BS, et al. A clinicopathologic reappraisal of brain stem tumor classification. Identification of pilocystic astrocytoma and fibrillary astrocytoma as distinct entities. *Cancer* 2000;89(7):1569–1576.
83. Lesniak MS, Klem JM, Weingart J, et al. Surgical outcome following resection of contrast-enhanced pediatric brainstem gliomas. *Pediatr Neurosurg* 2003;39(6):314–322.
84. Farmer JP, Montes JL, Freeman CR, et al. Brainstem gliomas. A 10-year institutional review. *Pediatr Neurosurg* 2001;34(4):206–214.
85. Pollack IF, Hoffman HJ, Humphreys RP, et al. The long-term outcome after surgical treatment of dorsally exophytic brain-stem gliomas. *J Neurosurg* 1993;78(6):859–863.
86. Khatib ZA, Heideman RL, Kovnar EH, et al. Predominance of pilocytic histology in dorsally exophytic brain stem tumors. *Pediatr Neurosurg* 1994;20(1): 2–10.
87. Hoffman HJ. Dorsally exophytic brain stem tumors and midbrain tumors. *Pediatr Neurosurg* 1996;24(5):256–262.
88. Albright AL, Packer RJ, Zimmerman R, et al. Magnetic resonance scans should replace biopsies for the diagnosis of diffuse brain stem gliomas: a report from the Children's Cancer Group. *Neurosurgery* 1993;33(6):1026–1029.
89. Albright AL. Diffuse brainstem tumors: when is a biopsy necessary? *Pediatr Neurosurg* 1996;24(5):252–255.
90. Freeman CR, Bourgouin PM, Sanford RA, et al. Long term survivors of childhood brain stem gliomas treated with hyperfractionated radiotherapy. Clinical characteristics and treatment related toxicities. The Pediatric Oncology Group. *Cancer* 1996;77(3):555–562.
91. Freeman CR, Kepner J, Kun LE, et al. A detrimental effect of a combined chemotherapy-radiotherapy approach in children with diffuse intrinsic brain stem gliomas? *Int J Radiat Oncol Biol Phys* 2000;47(3):561–564.
92. Freeman CR, Krischer JP, Sanford RA, et al. Final results of a study of escalating doses of hyperfractionated radiotherapy in brain stem tumors in children: a Pediatric Oncology Group study. *Int J Radiat Oncol Biol Phys* 1993;27(2): 197–206.
93. Packer RJ, Boyett JM, Zimmerman RA, et al. Outcome of children with brain stem gliomas after treatment with 7800 cGy of hyperfractionated radiotherapy. A Childrens Cancer Group Phase I/II Trial. *Cancer* 1994;74(6): 1827–1834.
94. Prados MD, Wara WM, Edwards MS, et al. The treatment of brain stem and thalamic gliomas with 78 Gy of hyperfractionated radiation therapy. *Int J Radiat Oncol Biol Phys* 1995;32(1):85–91.
95. Lewis J, Lucraft H, Gholkar A. UKCCSG study of accelerated radiotherapy for pediatric brain stem gliomas. United Kingdom Childhood Cancer Study Group. *Int J Radiat Oncol Biol Phys* 1997;38(5):925–929.
96. Janssens GO, Gidding CE, Van Lindert EJ, et al. The role of hypofractionation radiotherapy for diffuse intrinsic brainstem glioma in children: a pilot study. *Int J Radiat Oncol Biol Phys* 2009;73(3):722–726.
97. Negretti L, Bouchireb K, Levy-Piedbois C, et al. Hypofractionated radiotherapy in the treatment of diffuse intrinsic pontine glioma in children: a single institution's experience. *J Neurooncol* 2011;104(3):773–777.

98. Fontanilla HP, Pinnix CC, Ketonen LM, et al. Palliative reirradiation for progressive diffuse intrinsic pontine glioma. *Am J Clin Oncol* 2012;35(1)51–57.

99. Wolff JE, Rytting ME, Vats TS, et al. Treatment of recurrent diffuse intrinsic pontine glioma: the MD Anderson Cancer Center experience. *J Neurooncol* 2012;106(2)391–397.

100. Nadkarni TD, Rekate HL. Pediatric intramedullary spinal cord tumors. Critical review of the literature. *Childs Nerv Syst* 1999;15(1):17–28.

101. Rodrigues GB, Waldron JN, Wong CS, et al. A retrospective analysis of 52 cases of spinal cord glioma managed with radiation therapy. *Int J Radiat Oncol Biol Phys* 2000;48(3):837–842.

102. Constantini S, Miller DC, Allen JC, et al. Radical excision of intramedullary spinal cord tumors: surgical morbidity and long-term follow-up evaluation in 164 children and young adults. *J Neurosurg* 2000;93(2 Suppl):183–193.

103. Merchant TE, Kiehna EN, Thompson SJ, et al. Pediatric low-grade and ependymal spinal cord tumors. *Pediatr Neurosurg* 2000;32(1):30–36.

104. Jallo GI, Freed D, Epstein F. Intramedullary spinal cord tumors in children. *Childs Nerv Syst* 2003;19(9):641–649.

105. Lowis SP, Pizer BL, Coakham H, et al. Chemotherapy for spinal cord astrocytoma: can natural history be modified? *Childs Nerv Syst* 1998;14(7):317–321.

106. Doireau V, Grill J, Zerah M, et al. Chemotherapy for unresectable and recurrent intramedullary glial tumours in children. Brain Tumours Subcommittee of the French Society of Paediatric Oncology (SFOP). *Br J Cancer* 1999;81(5):835–840.

107. Tendulkar RD, Pai Panandiker AS, Wu S, et al. Irradiation of pediatric high-grade spinal cord tumors. *Int J Radiat Oncol Biol Phys* 2010;78(5):1451–1456.

108. Milano MT, Johnson MD, Sul J, et al. Primary spinal cord glioma: a Surveillance, Epidemiology, and End Results database study. *J Neurooncol* 2010;98(1):83–92.

109. Wolff B, Ng A, Roth D, et al. Pediatric high grade glioma of the spinal cord: results of the HIT-GBM database. *J Neurooncol* 2012;107(1):139–146.

110. Bagley CA, Wilson S, Kothbauer KF, et al. Long term outcomes following surgical resection of myxopapillary ependymomas. *Neurosurg Rev* 2009;32(3):321–334.

111. Al-Halabi H, Montes JL, Atkinson J, et al. Adjuvant radiotherapy in the treatment of pediatric myxopapillary ependymomas. *Pediatr Blood Cancer* 2010;55(4):639–643.

112. Benesch M, Weber-Mzell D, Gerber NU, et al. Ependymoma of the spinal cord in children and adolescents: a retrospective series from the HIT database. *J Neurosurg Pediatr* 2010;6(2):137–144.

113. Rezai AR, Woo HH, Lee M, et al. Disseminated ependymomas of the central nervous system. *J Neurosurg* 1996;85(4):618–624.

114. Fassett DR, Pingree J, Kestle JR. The high incidence of tumor dissemination in myxopapillary ependymoma in pediatric patients. Report of five cases and review of the literature. *J Neurosurg* 2005;102(1 Suppl):59–64.

115. Pica A, Miller R, Villa S, et al. The results of surgery, with or without radiotherapy, for primary spinal myxopapillary ependymoma: a retrospective study from the rare cancer network. *Int J Radiat Oncol Biol Phys* 2009;74(4):1114–1120.

116. Chinn DM, Donaldson SS, Dahl GV, et al. Management of children with metastatic spinal myxopapillary ependymoma using craniospinal irradiation. *Med Pediatr Oncol* 2000;35(4):443–445.

117. Healey EA, Barnes PD, Kupsky WJ, et al. The prognostic significance of postoperative residual tumor in ependymoma. *Neurosurgery* 1991;28(5):666–671.

118. Vanuytsel LJ, Bessell EM, Ashley SE, et al. Intracranial ependymoma: long-term results of a policy of surgery and radiotherapy. *Int J Radiat Oncol Biol Phys* 1992;23(2):313–319.

119. Pollack IF, Gerszten PC, Martinez AJ, et al. Intracranial ependymomas of childhood: long-term outcome and prognostic factors. *Neurosurgery* 1995;37(4):655–666.

120. Foreman NK, Love S, Thorne R. Intracranial ependymomas: analysis of prognostic factors in a population-based series. *Pediatr Neurosurg* 1996;24(3):119–125.

121. Perilongo G, Massimino M, Sotti G, et al. Analyses of prognostic factors in a retrospective review of 92 children with ependymoma: Italian Pediatric Neuro-oncology Group. *Med Pediatr Oncol* 1997;29(2):79–85.

122. Robertson PL, Zeltzer PM, Boyett JM, et al. Survival and prognostic factors following radiation therapy and chemotherapy for ependymomas in children: a report of the Children's Cancer Group. *J Neurosurg* 1998;88(4):695–703.

123. Horn B, Heideman R, Geyer R, et al. A multi-institutional retrospective study of intracranial ependymoma in children: identification of risk factors. *J Pediatr Hematol Oncol* 1999;21(3):203–211.

124. van Veelen-Vincent ML, Pierre-Kahn A, Kalifa C, et al. Ependymoma in childhood: prognostic factors, extent of surgery, and adjuvant therapy. *J Neurosurg* 2002;97(4):827–835.

125. Rogers L, Pueschel J, Spetzler R, et al. Is gross-total resection sufficient treatment for posterior fossa ependymomas? *J Neurosurg* 2005;102(4):629–636.

126. Merchant TE, Li C, Xiong X, et al. Conformal radiotherapy after surgery for paediatric ependymoma: a prospective study. *Lancet Oncol* 2009;10(3):258–266.

127. Nazar GB, Hoffman HJ, Becker LE, et al. Infratentorial ependymomas in childhood: prognostic factors and treatment. *J Neurosurg* 1990;72(3):408–417.

128. Palma L, Celli P, Mariottini A, et al. The importance of surgery in supratentorial ependymomas. Long-term survival in a series of 23 cases. *Childs Nerv Syst* 2000;16(3):170–175.

129. Duffner PK, Krischer JP, Sanford RA, et al. Prognostic factors in infants and very young children with intracranial ependymoma. *Pediatr Neurosurg* 1998;28(4):215–222.

130. Grill J, Le Deley MC, Gambarelli D, et al. Postoperative chemotherapy without irradiation for ependymoma in children under 5 years of age: a multicenter trial of the French Society of Pediatric Oncology. *J Clin Oncol* 2001;19(5):1288–1296.

131. Massimino M, Giangaspero F, Garre ML, et al. Salvage treatment for childhood ependymoma after surgery only: Pitfalls of omitting "at once" adjuvant treatment. *Int J Radiat Oncol Biol Phys* 2006;65(5):1440–1445.

132. Massimino M, Gandola L, Barra S, et al. Infant ependymoma in a 10-year AIEOP (Associazione Italiana Ematologia Oncologia Pediatrica) experience with omitted or deferred radiotherapy. *Int J Radiat Oncol Biol Phys* 2011;80(3):807–814.

133. Lonjon M, Goh KY, Epstein FJ. Intramedullary spinal cord ependymomas in children: treatment, results and follow-up. *Pediatr Neurosurg* 1998;29(4):178–183.

134. Hanbali F, Fourney DR, Marmor E, et al. Spinal cord ependymoma: radical surgical resection and outcome. *Neurosurgery* 2002;51(5):1162–1172.

135. Gomez DR, Missett BT, Wara WM, et al. High failure rate in spinal ependymomas with long-term follow-up. *Neuro Oncol* 2005;7(3):254–259.

136. Lin YH, Huang CI, Wong TT, et al. Treatment of spinal cord ependymomas by surgery with or without postoperative radiotherapy. *J Neurooncol* 2005;71(2):205–210.

137. Taylor RE. Review of radiotherapy dose and volume for intracranial ependymoma. *Pediatr Blood Cancer* 2004;42(5):457–460.

138. Merchant TE, Fouladi M. Ependymoma: new therapeutic approaches including radiation and chemotherapy. *J Neurooncol* 2005;75(3):287–299.

139. Needle MN, Goldwein JW, Grass J, et al. Adjuvant chemotherapy for the treatment of intracranial ependymoma of childhood. *Cancer* 1997;80(2):341–347.

140. Massimino M, Gandola L, Giangaspero F, et al. Hyperfractionated radiotherapy and chemotherapy for childhood ependymoma: final results of the first prospective AIEOP (Associazione Italiana di Ematologia-Oncologia Pediatrica) study. *Int J Radiat Oncol Biol Phys* 2004;58(5):1336–1345.

141. Conter C, Carrie C, Bernier V, et al. Intracranial ependymomas in children: society of pediatric oncology experience with postoperative hyperfractionated local radiotherapy. *Int J Radiat Oncol Biol Phys* 2009;74(5):1536–1542.

142. Evans AE, Anderson JR, Lefkowitz-Boudreaux IB, et al. Adjuvant chemotherapy of childhood posterior fossa ependymoma: cranio-spinal irradiation with or without adjuvant CCNU, vincristine, and prednisone: a Childrens Cancer Group study. *Med Pediatr Oncol* 1996;27(1):8–14.

143. Bouffet E, Foreman N. Chemotherapy for intracranial ependymomas. *Childs Nerv Syst* 1999;15(10):563–570.

144. Merchant TE, Boop FA, Kun LE, et al. A retrospective study of surgery and reirradiation for recurrent ependymoma. *Int J Radiat Oncol Biol Phys* 2008;71(1):87–97.

145. Zacharoulis S, Ashley S, Moreno L, et al. Treatment and outcome of children with relapsed ependymoma: a multi-institutional retrospective analysis. *Childs Nerv Syst* 2010;26(7):905–911.

146. Goldwein JW, Corn BW, Finlay JL, et al. Is craniospinal irradiation required to cure children with malignant (anaplastic) intracranial ependymomas? *Cancer* 1991;67(11):2766–2771.

147. Merchant TE, Haida T, Wang MH, et al. Anaplastic ependymoma: treatment of pediatric patients with or without craniospinal radiation therapy. *J Neurosurg* 1997;86(6):943–949.

148. Schild SE, Nisi K, Scheithauer BW, et al. The results of radiotherapy for ependymomas: the Mayo Clinic experience. *Int J Radiat Oncol Biol Phys* 1998;42(5):953–958.

149. Timmermann B, Kortmann RD, Kuhl J, et al. Combined postoperative irradiation and chemotherapy for anaplastic ependymomas in childhood: results of the German prospective trials HIT 88/89 and HIT 91. *Int J Radiat Oncol Biol Phys* 2000;46(2):287–295.

150. Timmermann B, Kortmann RD, Kuhl J, et al. Role of radiotherapy in anaplastic ependymoma in children under age of 3 years: results of the prospective German brain tumor trials HIT-SKK 87 and 92. *Radiother Oncol* 2005;77(3):278–285.

151. Pencalet P, Sainte-Rose C, Lellouch-Tubiana A, et al. Papillomas and carcinomas of the choroid plexus in children. *J Neurosurg* 1998;88(3):521–528.

152. Krishnan S, Brown PD, Scheithauer BW, et al. Choroid plexus papillomas: a single institutional experience. *J Neurooncol* 2004;68(1):49–55.

153. Jeibmann A, Wrede B, Peters O, et al. Malignant progression in choroid plexus papillomas. *J Neurosurg* 2007;107(3 Suppl):199–202.

154. Lafay-Cousin L, Keene D, Carret AS, et al. Choroid plexus tumors in children less than 36 months: the Canadian Pediatric Brain Tumor Consortium (CPBTC) experience. *Childs Nerv Syst* 2011;27(2):259–264.

155. Packer RJ, Perilongo G, Johnson D, et al. Choroid plexus carcinoma of childhood. *Cancer* 1992;69(2):580–585.

156. Pierga JY, Kalifa C, Terrier-Lacombe MJ, et al. Carcinoma of the choroid plexus: a pediatric experience. *Med Pediatr Oncol* 1993;21(7):480–487.

157. Chow E, Reardon DA, Shah AB, et al. Pediatric choroid plexus neoplasms. *Int J Radiat Oncol Biol Phys* 1999;44(2):249–254.

158. Wolff JE, Sajedi M, Coppes MJ, et al. Radiation therapy and survival in choroid plexus carcinoma. *Lancet* 1999;353(9170):2126.

159. Berger C, Thiesse P, Lellouch-Tubiana A, et al. Choroid plexus carcinomas in childhood: clinical features and prognostic factors. *Neurosurgery* 1998;42(3):470–475.

160. Fitzpatrick LK, Aronson LJ, Cohen KJ. Is there a requirement for adjuvant therapy for choroid plexus carcinoma that has been completely resected? *J Neurooncol* 2002;57(2):123–126.

161. Wolff JE, Sajedi M, Brant R, et al. Choroid plexus tumours. *Br J Cancer* 2002;87(10):1086–1091.

162. Meyers SP, Khademian ZP, Chuang SH, et al. Choroid plexus carcinomas in children: MRI features and patient outcomes. *Neuroradiology* 2004;46(9):770–780.

Section
III

163. Wrede B, Liu P, Ater J, et al. Second surgery and the prognosis of choroid plexus carcinoma—results of a meta-analysis of individual cases. *Anticancer Res* 2005;25(6C):4429–4433.

164. Mazloom A, Wolff JE, Paulino AC. The impact of radiotherapy fields in the treatment of patients with choroid plexus carcinoma. *Int J Radiat Oncol Biol Phys* 2010;78(1):79–84.

165. Tabori U, Shlien A, Baskin B, et al. TP53 alterations determine clinical subgroups and survival of patients with choroid plexus tumors. *J Clin Oncol* 2010;28(12):1995–2001.

166. Lang FF, Epstein FJ, Ransohoff J, et al. Central nervous system gangliogliomas. Part 2: clinical outcome. *J Neurosurg* 1993;79(6):867–873.

167. Luyken C, Blumcke I, Fimmers R, et al. Supratentorial gangliogliomas: histopathologic grading and tumor recurrence in 184 patients with a median follow-up of 8 years. *Cancer* 2004;101(1):146–155.

168. Rades D, Zwick L, Leppert J, et al. The role of postoperative radiotherapy for the treatment of gangliogliomas. *Cancer* 2010;116(2):432–442.

169. Rumana CS, Valadka AB, Contant CF. Prognostic factors in supratentorial ganglioglioma. *Acta Neurochir (Wien)* 1999;141(1):63–68.

170. Selch MT, Goy BW, Lee SP, et al. Gangliogliomas: experience with 34 patients and review of the literature. *Am J Clin Oncol* 1998;21(6):557–564.

171. Rades D, Schild SE. Treatment recommendations for the various subgroups of neurocytomas. *J Neurooncol* 2006;77(3):305–309.

172. Leenstra JL, Rodriguez FJ, Frechette CM, et al. Central neurocytoma: management recommendations based on a 35-year experience. *Int J Radiat Oncol Biol Phys* 2007;67(4):1145–1154.

173. Rades D, Schild SE. Is 50 Gy sufficient to achieve long-term local control after incomplete resection of typical neurocytomas? *Strahlenther Onkol* 2006;182(7):415–418.

174. Rades D, Fehlauer F, Ikezaki K, et al. Dose-effect relationship for radiotherapy after incomplete resection of atypical neurocytomas. *Radiother Oncol* 2005;74(1):67–69.

175. D'Andrea AD, Packer RJ, Rorke LB, et al. Pineocytomas of childhood. A reappraisal of natural history and response to therapy. *Cancer* 1987;59(7):1353–1357.

176. Schild SE, Scheithauer BW, Schomberg PJ, et al. Pineal parenchymal tumors. Clinical, pathologic, and therapeutic aspects. *Cancer* 1993;72(3):870–880.

177. Jouvet A, Fevre-Montange M, Besancon R, et al. Structural and ultrastructural characteristics of human pineal gland, and pineal parenchymal tumors. *Acta Neuropathol (Berl)* 1994;88(4):334–348.

178. Clark AJ, Ivan ME, Sughrue ME, et al. Tumor control after surgery and radiotherapy for pineocytoma. *J Neurosurg* 2010;113(2):319–324.

179. Schild SE, Scheithauer BW, Haddock MG, et al. Histologically confirmed pineal tumors and other germ cell tumors of the brain. *Cancer* 1996;78(12):2564–2571.

180. Jakacki RI, Zeltzer PM, Boyett JM, et al. Survival and prognostic factors following radiation and/or chemotherapy for primitive neuroectodermal tumors of the pineal region in infants and children: a report of the Childrens Cancer Group. *J Clin Oncol* 1995;13(6):1377–1383.

181. Cohen BH, Zeltzer PM, Boyett JM, et al. Prognostic factors and treatment results for supratentorial primitive neuroectodermal tumors in children using radiation and chemotherapy: a Childrens Cancer Group randomized trial. *J Clin Oncol* 1995;13(7):1687–1696.

182. Geyer JR, Zeltzer PM, Boyett JM, et al. Survival of infants with primitive neuroectodermal tumors or malignant ependymomas of the CNS treated with eight drugs in 1 day: a report from the Childrens Cancer Group. *J Clin Oncol* 1994;12(8):1607–1615.

183. Duffner PK, Cohen ME, Sanford RA, et al. Lack of efficacy of postoperative chemotherapy and delayed radiation in very young children with pineoblastoma. Pediatric Oncology Group. *Med Pediatr Oncol* 1995;25(1):38–44.

184. Pizer BL, Clifford SC. The potential impact of tumor biology on improved clinical practice for medulloblastoma: progress towards biologically driven clinical trials. *Br J Neurosurg* 2009;23:364–375.

185. Bailey CC, Gnekow A, Wellek S, et al. Prospective randomised trial of chemotherapy given before radiotherapy in childhood medulloblastoma. International Society of Paediatric Oncology (SIOP) and the (German) Society of Paediatric Oncology (GPO): SIOP II. *Med Pediatr Oncol* 1995;25(3):166–178.

186. Thomas PR, Deutsch M, Kepner JL, et al. Low-stage medulloblastoma: final analysis of trial comparing standard-dose with reduced-dose neuraxis irradiation. *J Clin Oncol* 2000;18(16):3004–3011.

187. Bouffet E, Bernard JL, Frappaz D, et al. M4 protocol for cerebellar medulloblastoma: supratentorial radiotherapy may not be avoided. *Int J Radiat Oncol Biol Phys* 1992;24(1):79–85.

188. Carrie C, Muracciole X, Gomez F, et al. Conformal radiotherapy, reduced boost volume, hyperfractionated radiotherapy, and online quality control in standard-risk medulloblastoma without chemotherapy: results of the French M-SFOP 98 protocol. *Int J Radiat Oncol Biol Phys* 2005;63(3):711–716.

189. Packer RJ, Goldwein J, Nicholson HS, et al. Treatment of children with medulloblastomas with reduced-dose craniospinal radiation therapy and adjuvant chemotherapy: a Children's Cancer Group Study. *J Clin Oncol* 1999;17(7):2127–2136.

190. Packer RJ, Gajjar A, Vezina G, et al. Phase III study of craniospinal radiation therapy followed by adjuvant chemotherapy for newly diagnosed average-risk medulloblastoma. *J Clin Oncol* 2006;24(25):4202–4208.

190a. Michalski J, Vezina G, Burger P, et al. Preliminary results of COG ACNS 0331: a phase III trial of involved field radiotherapy (IFRT) and low dose craniospinal irradiation (LD-CSI) with chemotherapy in average risk medulloblastoma: a report from the Children's Oncology Group. *Neurooncology* 2016;18(Suppl 3):iii122.

191. Ellison DW, Kocak M, Dalton J, et al. Definition of disease-risk stratification groups in childhood medulloblastoma using combined clinical, pathologic, and molecular variables. *J Clin Oncol* 2011;29(11):1400–1407.

192. Freeman CR, Taylor RE, Kortmann RD, et al. Radiotherapy for medulloblastoma in children: a perspective on current international clinical research efforts. *Med Pediatr Oncol* 2002;39(2):99–108.

193. Sanders RP, Onar A, Boyett JM, et al. M1 medulloblastoma: high risk at any age. *J Neurooncol* 2008;90(3):351–355.

194. Gandola L, Massimino M, Cefalo G, et al. Hyperfractionated accelerated radiotherapy in the Milan strategy for metastatic medulloblastoma. *J Clin Oncol* 2009;27(4):566–571.

195. Saran FH, Driever PH, Thilmann C, et al. Survival of very young children with medulloblastoma (primitive neuroectodermal tumor of the posterior fossa) treated with craniospinal irradiation. *Int J Radiat Oncol Biol Phys* 1998;42(5):959–967.

196. Duffner PK, Horowitz ME, Krischer JP, et al. The treatment of malignant brain tumors in infants and very young children: an update of the Pediatric Oncology Group experience. *Neuro Oncol* 1999;1(2):152–161.

197. Rutkowski S, Bode U, Deinlein F, et al. Treatment of early childhood medulloblastoma by postoperative chemotherapy alone. *N Engl J Med* 2005;352(10):978–986.

198. Grill J, Lellouch-Tubiana A, Elouahdani S, et al. Preoperative chemotherapy in children with high-risk medulloblastomas: a feasibility study. *J Neurosurg* 2005;103(4 Suppl):312–318.

199. Hong TS, Mehta MP, Boyett JM, et al. Patterns of treatment failure in infants with primitive neuroectodermal tumors who were treated on CCG-921: a phase III combined modality study. *Pediatr Blood Cancer* 2005;45(5):676–682.

200. Carrie C, Alapetite C, Mere P, et al. Quality control of radiotherapeutic treatment of medulloblastoma in a multicentric study: the contribution of radiotherapy technique to tumour relapse. The French Medulloblastoma Group. *Radiother Oncol* 1992;24(2):77–81.

201. Carrie C, Hoffstetter S, Gomez F, et al. Impact of targeting deviations on outcome in medulloblastoma: study of the French Society of Pediatric Oncology (SFOP). *Int J Radiat Oncol Biol Phys* 1999;45(2):435–439.

202. Oyharcabal-Bourden V, Kalifa C, Gentet JC, et al. Standard-risk medulloblastoma treated by adjuvant chemotherapy followed by reduced-dose craniospinal radiation therapy: a French Society of Pediatric Oncology Study. *J Clin Oncol* 2005;23(21):4726–4734.

203. Fukunaga-Johnson N, Sandler HM, Marsh R, et al. The use of 3D conformal radiotherapy (3D CRT) to spare the cochlea in patients with medulloblastoma. *Int J Radiat Oncol Biol Phys* 1998;41(1):77–82.

204. Fukunaga-Johnson N, Lee JH, Sandler HM, et al. Patterns of failure following treatment for medulloblastoma: is it necessary to treat the entire posterior fossa? *Int J Radiat Oncol Biol Phys* 1998;42(1):143–146.

205. Merchant TE, Happersett L, Finlay JL, et al. Preliminary results of conformal radiation therapy for medulloblastoma. *Neuro Oncol* 1999;1(3):177–187.

206. Wolden SL, Dunkel IJ, Souweidane MM, et al. Patterns of failure using a conformal radiation therapy tumor bed boost for medulloblastoma. *J Clin Oncol* 2003;21(16):3079–3083.

207. Douglas JG, Barker JL, Ellenbogen RG, et al. Concurrent chemotherapy and reduced-dose cranial spinal irradiation followed by conformal posterior fossa tumor bed boost for average-risk medulloblastoma: efficacy and patterns of failure. *Int J Radiat Oncol Biol Phys* 2004;58(4):1161–1164.

208. Merchant TE, Kun LE, Krasin MJ, et al. Multi-institution prospective trial of reduced-dose craniospinal irradiation (23.4 Gy) followed by conformal posterior fossa (36 Gy) and primary site irradiation (55.8 Gy) and dose-intensive chemotherapy for average-risk medulloblastoma. *Int J Radiat Oncol Biol Phys* 2008;70(3):782–787.

209. Taylor RE, Bailey CC, Robinson KJ, et al. Impact of radiotherapy parameters on outcome in the International Society of Paediatric Oncology/United Kingdom Children's Cancer Study Group PNET-3 study of preradiotherapy chemotherapy for M0-M1 medulloblastoma. *Int J Radiat Oncol Biol Phys* 2004;58(4):1184–1193.

210. Woehrer A, Slavc I, Waldhoer T, et al. Incidence of atypical teratoid/rhabdoid tumors in children: a population-based study by the Austrian Brain Tumor Registry, 1996–2006. *Cancer* 2010;116(24):5725–5732.

211. Weiss E, Behring B, Behnke J, et al. Treatment of primary malignant rhabdoid tumor of the brain: report of three cases and review of the literature. *Int J Radiat Oncol Biol Phys* 1998;41(5):1013–1019.

212. Hilden JM, Meerbaum S, Burger P, et al. Central nervous system atypical teratoid/rhabdoid tumor: results of therapy in children enrolled in a registry. *J Clin Oncol* 2004;22(14):2877–2884.

213. Reddy AT. Atypical teratoid/rhabdoid tumors of the central nervous system. *J Neurooncol* 2005;75(3):309–313.

214. Strother D. Atypical teratoid rhabdoid tumors of childhood: diagnosis, treatment and challenges. *Expert Rev Anticancer Ther* 2005;5(5):907–915.

215. Tekautz TM, Fuller CE, Blaney S, et al. Atypical teratoid/rhabdoid tumors (ATRT): improved survival in children 3 years of age and older with radiation therapy and high-dose alkylator-based chemotherapy. *J Clin Oncol* 2005;23(7):1491–1499.

216. Chen YW, Wong TT, Ho DM, et al. Impact of radiotherapy for pediatric CNS atypical teratoid/rhabdoid tumor (single institute experience). *Int J Radiat Oncol Biol Phys* 2006;64(4):1038–1043.

217. Athale UH, Duckworth J, Odame I, et al. Childhood atypical teratoid rhabdoid tumor of the central nervous system: a meta-analysis of observational studies. *J Pediatr Hematol Oncol* 2009;31(9):651–663.

218. Pai Panandiker AS, Merchant TE, Beltran C, et al. Sequencing of local therapy affects the pattern of treatment failure and survival in children with atypical teratoid rhabdoid tumors of the central nervous system. *Int J Radiat Oncol Biol Phys* 2012;82(5):1756–1763.

218a. Eberhart CG, Brat DJ, Cohen KJ, et al. Pediatric neuroblastic brain tumors containing abundant neuropil and true rosettes. *Pediatr Dev Pathol* 2000;3:346–352.

219. Sturm D, Orr BA, Toprak UH, et al. New brain tumor entities emerge from molecular classification of CNS-PNETs. *Cell* 2016;164(5):1060–1072.

220. Shirato H, Nishio M, Sawamura Y, et al. Analysis of long-term treatment of intracranial germinoma. *Int J Radiat Oncol Biol Phys* 1997;37(3):511–515.

221. Merchant TE, Sherwood SH, Mulhern RK, et al. CNS germinoma: disease control and long-term functional outcome for 12 children treated with craniospinal irradiation. *Int J Radiat Oncol Biol Phys* 2000;46(5):1171–1176.

222. Haas-Kogan DA, Missett BT, Wara WM, et al. Radiation therapy for intracranial germ cell tumors. *Int J Radiat Oncol Biol Phys* 2003;56(2):511–518.

223. Maity A, Shu HK, Janss A, et al. Craniospinal radiation in the treatment of biopsy-proven intracranial germinomas: twenty-five years' experience in a single center. *Int J Radiat Oncol Biol Phys* 2004;58(4):1165–1170.

224. Schoenfeld GO, Amdur RJ, Schmalfuss IM, et al. Low-dose prophylactic craniospinal radiotherapy for intracranial germinoma. *Int J Radiat Oncol Biol Phys* 2006;65(2):481–485.

225. Haddock MG, Schild SE, Scheithauer BW, et al. Radiation therapy for histologically confirmed primary central nervous system germinoma. *Int J Radiat Oncol Biol Phys* 1997;38(5):915–923.

226. Ogawa K, Shikama N, Toita T, et al. Long-term results of radiotherapy for intracranial germinoma: a multi-institutional retrospective review of 126 patients. *Int J Radiat Oncol Biol Phys* 2004;58(3):705–713.

227. Shirato H, Aoyama H, Ikeda J, et al. Impact of margin for target volume in low-dose involved field radiotherapy after induction chemotherapy for intracranial germinoma. *Int J Radiat Oncol Biol Phys* 2004;60(1):214–217.

228. Aoyama H, Shirato H, Kakuto Y, et al. Pathologically-proven intracranial germinoma treated with radiation therapy. *Radiother Oncol* 1998;47(2):201–205.

229. Jensen AW, Laack NN, Buckner JC, et al. Long-term follow-up of dose-adapted and reduced-field radiotherapy with or without chemotherapy for central nervous system germinoma. *Int J Radiat Oncol Biol Phys* 2010;77(5):1449–1456.

230. Shibamoto Y, Sasai K, Oya N, et al. Intracranial germinoma: radiation therapy with tumor volume-based dose selection. *Radiology* 2001;218(2):452–456.

231. Balmaceda C, Heller G, Rosenblum M, et al. Chemotherapy without irradiation—a novel approach for newly diagnosed CNS germ cell tumors: results of an international cooperative trial. The First International Central Nervous System Germ Cell Tumor Study. *J Clin Oncol* 1996;14(11):2908–2915.

232. Matsutani M. Combined chemotherapy and radiation therapy for CNS germ cell tumors—the Japanese experience. *J Neurooncol* 2001;54(3):311–316.

233. Kellie SJ, Boyce H, Dunkel IJ, et al. Intensive cisplatin and cyclophosphamide-based chemotherapy without radiotherapy for intracranial germinomas: failure of a primary chemotherapy approach. *Pediatr Blood Cancer* 2004;43(2):126–133.

234. da Silva NS, Cappellano AM, Diez B, et al. Primary chemotherapy for intracranial germ cell tumors: results of the third international CNS germ cell tumor study. *Pediatr Blood Cancer* 2010;54(3):377–383.

235. Sawamura Y, Shirato H, Ikeda J, et al. Induction chemotherapy followed by reduced-volume radiation therapy for newly diagnosed central nervous system germinoma. *J Neurosurg* 1998;88(1):66–72.

236. Bouffet E, Baranzelli MC, Patte C, et al. Combined treatment modality for intracranial germinomas: results of a multicentre SFOP experience. Societe Francaise d'Oncologie Pediatrique. *Br J Cancer* 1999;79(7–8):1199–1204.

237. Aoyama H, Shirato H, Ikeda J, et al. Induction chemotherapy followed by low-dose involved-field radiotherapy for intracranial germ cell tumors. *J Clin Oncol* 2002;20(3):857–865.

238. Alapetite C, Brisse H, Patte C, et al. Pattern of relapse and outcome of non-metastatic germinoma patients treated with chemotherapy and limited field radiation: the SFOP experience. *Neuro Oncol* 2010;12(12):1318–1325.

239. Nakamura H, Takeshima H, Makino K, et al. Recurrent intracranial germinoma outside the initial radiation field: a single-institution study. *Acta Oncol* 2006;45(4):476–483.

240. Sawamura Y, Ikeda J, Shirato H, et al. Germ cell tumours of the central nervous system: treatment consideration based on 111 cases and their long-term clinical outcomes. *Eur J Cancer* 1998;34(1):104–110.

241. Baranzelli MC, Patte C, Bouffet E, et al. An attempt to treat pediatric intracranial alphaFP and betaHCG secreting germ cell tumors with chemotherapy alone. SFOP experience with 18 cases. Societe Francaise d'Oncologie Pediatrique. *J Neurooncol* 1998;37(3):229–239.

242. Kellie SJ, Boyce H, Dunkel IJ, et al. Primary chemotherapy for intracranial nongerminomatous germ cell tumors: results of the second international CNS germ cell study group protocol. *J Clin Oncol* 2004;22(5):846–853.

243. Calaminus G, Andreussi L, Garre ML, et al. Secreting germ cell tumors of the central nervous system (CNS). First results of the cooperative German/Italian pilot study (CNS sGCT). *Klin Padiatr* 1997;209(4):222–227.

244. Matsutani M, Sano K, Takakura K, et al. Primary intracranial germ cell tumors: a clinical analysis of 153 histologically verified cases. *J Neurosurg* 1997;86(3):446–455.

245. Robertson PL, DaRosso RC, Allen JC. Improved prognosis of intracranial non-germinoma germ cell tumors with multimodality therapy. *J Neurooncol* 1997;32(1):71–80.

246. Aoyama H, Shirato H, Yoshida H, et al. Retrospective multi-institutional study of radiotherapy for intracranial non-germinomatous germ cell tumors. *Radiother Oncol* 1998;49(1):55–59.

247. Ogawa K, Toita T, Nakamura K, et al. Treatment and prognosis of patients with intracranial nongerminomatous malignant germ cell tumors: a multiinstitutional retrospective analysis of 41 patients. *Cancer* 2003;98(2):369–376.

248. Calaminus G, Bamberg M, Jurgens H, et al. Impact of surgery, chemotherapy and irradiation on long term outcome of intracranial malignant non-germinomatous germ cell tumors: results of the German Cooperative Trial MAKEI 89. *Klin Padiatr* 2004;216(3):141–149.

249. Brada M, Thomas DG. Craniopharyngioma revisited. *Int J Radiat Oncol Biol Phys* 1993;27(2):471–475.

250. Tomita T, McLone DG. Radical resections of childhood craniopharyngiomas. *Pediatr Neurosurg* 1993;19(1):6–14.

251. Muller HL, Gebhardt U, Schroder S, et al. Analyses of treatment variables for patients with childhood craniopharyngioma—results of the multicenter prospective trial KRANIOPHARYNGEOM 2000 after three years of follow-up. *Horm Res Paediatr* 2010;73(3):175–180.

252. Yasargil MG, Curcic M, Kis M, et al. Total removal of craniopharyngiomas. Approaches and long-term results in 144 patients. *J Neurosurg* 1990;73(1):3–11.

253. Sands SA, Milner JS, Goldberg J, et al. Quality of life and behavioral follow-up study of pediatric survivors of craniopharyngioma. *J Neurosurg* 2005;103(4 Suppl):302–311.

254. Pierre-Kahn A, Recassens C, Pinto G, et al. Social and psycho-intellectual outcome following radical removal of craniopharyngiomas in childhood. A prospective series. *Childs Nerv Syst* 2005;21(8–9):817–824.

255. Hoffman HJ, De SM, Humphreys RP, et al. Aggressive surgical management of craniopharyngiomas in children. *J Neurosurg* 1992;76(1):47–52.

256. Fisher PG, Jenab J, Gopldthwaite PT, et al. Outcomes and failure patterns in childhood craniopharyngiomas. *Childs Nerv Syst* 1998;14(10):558–563.

257. Khafaga Y, Jenkin D, Kanaan I, et al. Craniopharyngioma in children. *Int J Radiat Oncol Biol Phys* 1998;42(3):601–606.

258. Fahlbusch R, Honegger J, Paulus W, et al. Surgical treatment of craniopharyngiomas: experience with 168 patients. *J Neurosurg* 1999;90(2):237–250.

259. Backlund EO. Treatment of craniopharyngiomas: the multimodality approach. *Pediatr Neurosurg* 1994;21(Suppl 1):82–89.

260. Albright AL, Hadjipanayis CG, Lunsford LD, et al. Individualized treatment of pediatric craniopharyngiomas. *Childs Nerv Syst* 2005;21(8–9):649–654.

261. Thompson D, Phipps K, Hayward R. Craniopharyngioma in childhood: our evidence-based approach to management. *Childs Nerv Syst* 2005;21(8–9):660–668.

262. Tomita T, Bowman RM. Craniopharyngiomas in children: surgical experience at Children's Memorial Hospital. *Childs Nerv Syst* 2005;21(8–9):729–746.

263. Scott RM. Craniopharyngioma: a personal (Boston) experience. *Childs Nerv Syst* 2005;21(8–9):773–777.

264. Habrand JL, Saran F, Alapetite C, et al. Radiation therapy in the management of craniopharyngioma: current concepts and future developments. *J Pediatr Endocrinol Metab* 2006;19(Suppl 1):389–394.

265. Pollock BE, Lunsford LD, Kondziolka D, et al. Phosphorus-32 intracavitary irradiation of cystic craniopharyngiomas: current technique and long-term results. *Int J Radiat Oncol Biol Phys* 1995;33(2):437–446.

266. Lunsford LD, Pollock BE, Kondziolka DS, et al. Stereotactic options in the management of craniopharyngioma. *Pediatr Neurosurg* 1994;21(Suppl 1):90–97.

267. Hasegawa T, Kondziolka D, Hadjipanayis CG, et al. Management of cystic craniopharyngiomas with phosphorus-32 intracavitary irradiation. *Neurosurgery* 2004;54(4):813–820.

268. Tarbell NJ, Barnes P, Scott RM, et al. Advances in radiation therapy for craniopharyngiomas. *Pediatr Neurosurg* 1994;21(Suppl 1):101–107.

269. Merchant TE, Kiehna EN, Kun LE, et al. Phase II trial of conformal radiation therapy for pediatric patients with craniopharyngioma and correlation of surgical factors and radiation dosimetry with change in cognitive function. *J Neurosurg* 2006;104(2 Suppl):94–102.

270. Combs SE, Thilmann C, Huber PE, et al. Achievement of long-term local control in patients with craniopharyngiomas using high precision stereotactic radiotherapy. *Cancer* 2007;109(11):2308–2314.

271. Minniti G, Saran F, Traish D, et al. Fractionated stereotactic conformal radiotherapy following conservative surgery in the control of craniopharyngiomas. *Radiother Oncol* 2007;82(1):90–95.

272. Schulz-Ertner D, Frank C, Herfarth KK, et al. Fractionated stereotactic radiotherapy for craniopharyngiomas. *Int J Radiat Oncol Biol Phys* 2002;54(4):1114–1120.

273. Rajan B, Ashley S, Thomas DG, et al. Craniopharyngioma: improving outcome by early recognition and treatment of acute complications. *Int J Radiat Oncol Biol Phys* 1997;37(3):517–521.

274. Rajan B, Ashley S, Gorman C, et al. Craniopharyngioma—a long-term results following limited surgery and radiotherapy. *Radiother Oncol* 1993;26(1):1–10.

275. Scott RM, Hetelekidis S, Barnes PD, et al. Surgery, radiation, and combination therapy in the treatment of childhood craniopharyngioma—a 20-year experience. *Pediatr Neurosurg* 1994;21(Suppl 1):75–81.

276. Fraioli B, Ferrante L, Celli P. Pituitary adenomas with onset during puberty. Features and treatment. *J Neurosurg* 1983;59(4):590–595.

277. Lee AG, Sforza PD, Fard AK, et al. Pituitary adenoma in children. *J Neuroophthalmol* 1998;18(2):102–105.

278. Chang CZ, Wang CJ, Howng SL. Pituitary adenomas in adolescence—ten-year experience and literature review. *Kaohsiung J Med Sci* 1999;15(12):691–696.

Section
III

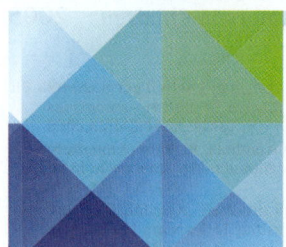

CHAPTER 89

Wilms Tumor

John A. Kalapurakal

INTRODUCTION

Wilms tumor (WT, nephroblastoma) is a highly curable childhood neoplasm. The prognosis of children with WT has improved considerably from a very high mortality rate at the beginning of the 20th century to the current cure rate of >90%.[1] The management of WT is a paradigm for successful interdisciplinary treatment of solid tumors of childhood to maximize cure rates and minimize treatment-related complications.

EPIDEMIOLOGY

WT is the most common malignant renal tumor of childhood. It occurs with an annual incidence of 7 cases per million children <15 years of age. Approximately 500 new cases are diagnosed each year in North America. The peak incidence is between 3 and 4 years of age. WT may arise as sporadic or hereditary tumors or in the setting of specific genetic disorders.[2] Most WTs are solitary lesions, multifocal within a single kidney in 12% and bilateral in 7%.[3] The clinical syndromes associated with WT include WAGR syndrome (*WT*, *A*niridia, *G*enitourinary malformations, mental *R*etardation), Denys-Drash syndrome (pseudohermaphroditism, mesangial sclerosis, renal failure, and WT), and overgrowth syndromes like Beckwith-Wiedemann syndrome (somatic gigantism, omphalocele, macroglossia, genitourinary abnormalities, ear creases, hypoglycemia, hemihypertrophy, and a predisposition to WT and other malignancies) and Simpson-Golabi-Behmel syndrome.[4,5]

BIOLOGY

Among the various genetic changes implicated in the development of WT, the most widely studied involves *WT1*, which is a tumor suppressor gene at chromosome 11p13 that was isolated from a child with WAGR syndrome.[6] *WT1* is likely to play a specific role in glomerular and gonadal development.[7] *WT1* can also act as a dominant negative oncogene resulting in abnormal cell growth such as in Denys-Drash syndrome.[8] Germ-line *WT1* mutations are observed in approximately 82% of WT patients who have genitourinary anomalies or renal failure. The frequency of *WT1* mutations in sporadic and familial WT is much lower at approximately 20% and approximately 4%, respectively.[9] Beckwith-Wiedemann syndrome maps to chromosome 11p15.5; this locus is also referred to as *WT2*.[10]

Patients with loss of heterozygosity (LOH) at 16q and 1p have higher relapse and mortality rates.[11] The National Wilms Tumor Study-5 (NWTS-5) prospectively evaluated the prognostic significance of LOH on 16q and 1p. When the effects of LOH for both 1p and 16q were considered jointly, the RR for relapse in stage I and II FH diseases was 2.9 (*P* = .001) and for stage III and IV FH diseases was 2.4 (*P* = .01). The RR for death for patients with stage I and II FH diseases with LOH for both regions was 4.3 (*P* = .01) and for stages III and IV was 2.7 (*P* = .04). Based on these results, it was proposed that in future WT trials, the therapy for children with LOH at both 1p and 16q be augmented by the addition of doxorubicin to regimen EE4A (discussed below) for early-stage (stages I

and II) tumors and cyclophosphamide/etoposide to regimen DD4A (discussed below) for advanced-stage tumors (stages III and IV).[12]

A novel WT suppressor gene on the X chromosome, *WTX*, was recently discovered. This gene is inactivated in approximately one-third of sporadic WT cases.[13] Anaplastic tumors have shown changes on 17p consistent with *TP53* deletion and specific genomic loss or underexpression on 4q and 14q and focal gain of *MYCN*.[14] Rhabdoid tumors are characterized by the genetic loss of the *SMARCB1/hSNF5/INI-1* gene located at chromosome 22q11. Global gene expression studies have shown that loss of *SMARCB1* results in repression of neural crest development and loss of cyclin-dependent kinase inhibition.[15] In children with very low-risk WT treated with just surgery alone, the presence of *WT1* mutation and 11p15 loss has been prospectively validated to be an important predictor of relapse. These biomarkers may be used to stratify patients to receive reduced chemotherapy in the future.[16] Recent gene expression studies have shown that VLRWT is composed of at least two biologically distinct clusters of tumors. Cluster 1 is composed of epithelial differentiated tubular histology tumors without nephrogenic rests and lack of LOH for 1p, 16q, and 11p. These tumors have a unique gene expression profile consistent with renal developmental arrest following mesenchymal to epithelial transition. None of these tumors relapsed. Cluster 2 is composed of mixed histology tumors with nephrogenic rests and a heterogenous gene expression pattern including down-regulation of WT1. WT1 mutation and 11p15LOH were significant predictors of relapse in VLRWTs. Prospective validation of these novel biomarkers will enable refinement of the current arbitrary definition of VLRWT based on age and tumor weight.[17,18]

Another recent COG study demonstrated that gain of 1q is a promising biomarker for patients with favorable histology WT. In a report of 1,114 patients on NWTS-5, 317 (28%) patients displayed 1q gain. The 8-year EFS with and without 1q gain was 77% and 90%, respectively (*P* < .001). The 8-year overall survival (OS) with and without 1q gain was 88% and 96%, respectively (*P* < .001). 1q gain was associated with a higher relative risk of relapse (2.4, *P* < .001).[19] Similar results were obtained by the SIOP WT2001 study after preoperative chemotherapy and nephrectomy. Among 586 patients, 28% had 1q gain. The 5-year EFS was 75% and 88% (*P* < .001), and OS was 88% and 94% (*P* = 0.01), with and without 1 q gain, respectively. Other molecular aberrations associated with poorer outcomes included *MYCN* gain and *TP53* loss.[20]

PATHOLOGIC CLASSIFICATION

Although histopathologists had attempted to relate appearance to prognosis, no generally acceptable classification was available until the report of Beckwith and Palmer[21] from the National Wilms Tumor Study-1 (NWTS-1). The NWTS classifies all tumors as having either FH or unfavorable histology (UH). The UH tumors include anaplastic tumors, clear cell sarcoma, and rhabdoid tumor of the kidney. Of 1,465 patients randomly assigned on NWTS-3, 163 (11.1%) had UH.[22] WTs are usually sharply demarcated, spherical masses with a "pushing" border and a surrounding distinct intrarenal pseudocapsule. Histologically, WT reflects the development of the normal kidney, consisting of three components, blastemal, epithelial (tubules), and stromal elements, in varying proportions.[21] The proportion of the different components has prognostic significance.[23] Nephrogenic rests consist of embryonal nephroblastic tissue and are found in 35% of kidneys with unilateral WT and in nearly 100% of kidneys with bilateral WT (BWT).[24] Nephrogenic rests may be intralobar or perilobar based on their location within the kidney.[25] Most nephrogenic rests undergo spontaneous regression and only a small proportion (1% to 5%) transform into WT.[26] The histologic feature of greatest clinical significance in WT is anaplasia.[27] Anaplasia may be focal (FA) or diffuse (DA). The definitions of FA and DA have been revised to reflect the distribution of anaplastic cells in the tumor rather than their quantitative density. These revised definitions are of prognostic significance. The 4-year survival rates for patients with stage II, III, and IV FA were 90%, 100%, and 100%, compared with 55%, 45%, and 4%, respectively, for patients with similar stage DA WT.[28]

Clear cell sarcoma of the kidney (CCSK) and malignant rhabdoid tumor of kidney (RTK) are no longer considered true WT, but they have been included in NWTS protocols.[21] CCSK has a propensity to metastasize to bone, and a skeletal survey and bone scan should be performed. RTK is the most lethal renal neoplasm in children. Primitive neuroepithelial tumors of the cerebellum or pineal region may be seen in 10% to 15% of patients with RTK.[29]

CLINICAL PRESENTATION

The classic presentation for WT is that of a healthy child in whom abdominal swelling is discovered by the child's mother or by a physician during a routine physical examination. A smooth, firm, nontender mass on one side of the abdomen is felt. Gross hematuria occurs in as many as 25% of these cases.[30] The child may be hypertensive or have nonspecific symptoms such as malaise or fever.[31] Only rarely does a patient present with symptomatic metastases.

DIAGNOSTIC WORKUP

The differential diagnosis of WT includes other malignant childhood lesions of the kidney, neuroblastoma, and benign conditions such as hydronephrosis, polycystic disease, and splenomegaly in left-sided tumors. Plain films of the abdomen may demonstrate calcifications, which occur in 60% to 70% of neuroblastomas but in only 5% to 10% of WT. Excretory urography (intravenous pyelography) was once the mainstay of imaging in WT and now has largely been replaced by ultrasonography and computed tomography (CT) scanning. Ultrasonography is very useful because it is readily available and is cost-effective.[32] A specific advantage of ultrasonography is its ability to assess vessels for flow and tumor thrombus with duplex and color Doppler.[33] Routine use of Doppler sonography after abdominal CT scans was not found to be useful in detecting cavoatrial thrombus in a Children's Oncology Group (COG) study.[34] Abdominal CT scans can demonstrate gross extrarenal spread, lymph node involvement, liver metastases, and the status of the opposite kidney (Fig. 89.1).[35] Magnetic resonance imaging (MRI) has several advantages over CT scans, especially in identifying renal origin and vascular extension of the tumor.[36] CT and MRI are useful in the detection and followup of patients with nephrogenic rests.[37] Clinical and imaging impressions do not, however, obviate the need for inspection at laparotomy.[38] Plain chest radiography and chest CT are also essential because asymptomatic pulmonary metastases are common.[39] A complete blood cell count and urinalysis should

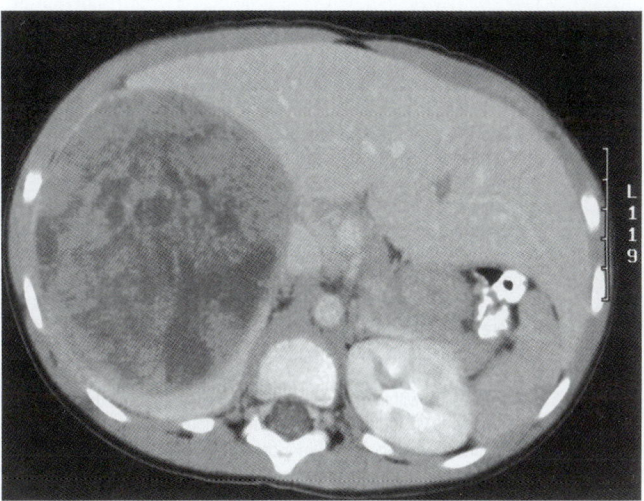

FIGURE 89.1. Computed tomography scan of a 4-year-old girl with a large right-sided Wilms tumor measuring 10.5 × 8.4 × 13.5 cm. The left kidney did not show any lesions. At laparotomy, the tumor was found to invade the diaphragm. She underwent a right radical nephrectomy. Surgical margins of resection were positive and she had metastases in the para-aortic lymph nodes. The tumor was classified as stage III favorable histology and received 10.8 Gy to the right flank and chemotherapy with vincristine, dactinomycin, and doxorubicin.

be performed. Patients with WT can be anemic from hematuria. Serum blood urea nitrogen and creatinine levels and liver function tests are routine. If neuroblastoma is not ruled out, a test for urinary catecholamines should be performed. Table 89.1 outlines the pretreatment investigations recommended by the COG.

NATURAL HISTORY

The disease is often localized at diagnosis, as evidenced by the fact that surgery and radiation therapy (RT) are curative in almost 50% of cases.[40] The first signs of local tumor spread beyond the pseudocapsule are invasion into the renal sinus or the intrarenal blood and lymphatic vessels. Spread throughout the peritoneal cavity may also occur, especially if there has been preoperative rupture or the disease has been spilled at surgery.[41,42] The most common sites of metastases of WT are in the lungs, lymph nodes, and liver. Among patients with stage IV disease, lungs were the only metastatic site in approximately 80% and 15% had liver metastases.[43] The NWTS-2 study demonstrated the prognostic importance of lymph node involvement. The 2-year relapse-free survival (RFS) with and without lymph node involvement was 54% and 82%, respectively.[41]

TABLE 89.1	PRETREATMENT WORKUP
History	Record preexisting conditions, family history of cancer, or congenital defects
Physical examination	Blood pressure, weight, height, presence of abdominal masses, congenital anomalies particularly genitourinary, hemihypertrophy, and aniridia
Laboratory	Hemoglobin, white cell, and differential counts, platelets, urinalysis, serum blood urea nitrogen, creatinine, protein, alanine, and aspartate aminotransferases, alkaline phosphatase, bilirubin
Radiology	CT or MRI scan of the abdomen and pelvis, abdominal ultrasonography, chest CT scan, chest x-ray
	Bone scan and MRI of the brain (CCSK, RTK, and renal cell carcinoma)

CT, computed tomography; CCSK, clear cell sarcoma of the kidney; MRI, magnetic resonance imaging; RTK, rhabdoid tumor of the kidney.

TABLE 89.2 CHILDREN'S ONCOLOGY GROUP STAGING OF WILMS TUMOR, RHABDOID TUMOR, AND CLEAR CELL SARCOMA OF THE KIDNEY

Stage I: Tumor limited to the kidney, completely resected. The renal capsule is intact. The tumor was not ruptured or biopsied prior to removal. The vessels of the renal sinus are not involved. There is no evidence of tumor at or beyond the margins of resection. *Note*: For a tumor to qualify for certain therapeutic protocols as stage I, regional lymph nodes must be examined microscopically

Stage II: The tumor is completely resected and there is no evidence of tumor at or beyond the margins of resection. The tumor extends beyond the kidney, as is evidenced by any one of the following criteria[a]:
- There is regional extension of the tumor (i.e., penetration of the renal capsule or extensive invasion of the soft tissue of the renal sinus)
- Blood vessels within the nephrectomy specimen outside the renal parenchyma, including those of the renal sinus, contain tumor

Stage III: Residual nonhematogenous tumor present following surgery and confined to the abdomen. Any one of the following may occur:
- Lymph nodes within the abdomen or pelvis are involved by tumor (lymph node involvement in the thorax or other extra-abdominal sites is a criterion for stage IV)
- The tumor has penetrated through the peritoneal surface
- Tumor implants are found on the peritoneal surface
- Gross or microscopic tumor remains postoperatively (e.g., tumor cells are found at the margin of surgical resection on microscopic examination)
- The tumor is not completely resectable because of local infiltration into vital structures
- Tumor spillage occurring either before or during surgery
- The tumor was biopsied (whether Tru-Cut, open, or fine needle aspiration) before removal
- Tumor is removed in more than one piece (e.g., tumor cells are found in a separately excised adrenal gland; a tumor thrombus within the renal vein is removed separately from the nephrectomy specimen)

Stage IV: Hematogenous metastases (i.e., lung, liver, bone, brain) or lymph node metastases outside the abdominal–pelvic region are present (the presence of tumor within the adrenal gland is not interpreted as metastasis and staging depend on all other staging parameters present)

Stage V: Bilateral renal involvement by tumor is present at diagnosis. An attempt should be made to stage each side according to the criteria here on the basis of the extent of disease

[a]Rupture or spillage confined to the flank, including biopsy of the tumor, is no longer included in stage II and is now included in stage III.

STAGING

Tumor staging is performed after examining the radiologic, operative, and histopathologic findings.[42,43] In NWTS-1 and NWTS-2, a tumor grouping system was used for staging and treatment stratification. After analyzing the prognostic significance of several clinical–pathologic factors in NWTS-1 and NWTS-2, a new staging system was adopted in NWTS-3. The presence of lymph node involvement was upstaged to stage III instead of group II, and local tumor spill was downstaged from group III to stage II.[42] In NWTS-5, the most significant change was the distinction between stages I and II. The criteria for stage I were revised to accommodate an important subset of WT that is being managed by nephrectomy alone. Before NWTS-5, the distinction between stages I and II in the renal sinus was established by the hilar plane, which was an imaginary plane connecting the most medial aspects of the upper and lower poles of the kidney. This criterion was difficult to apply because of tumor distortion, and thus, the hilar plane criterion has been replaced with renal sinus vascular or lymphatic invasion. This definition includes not only the involvement of vessels within the hilar soft tissue but also the vessels located in the radial extensions of the renal sinus into the renal parenchyma.[44,45] The COG staging guidelines for WT are shown in Table 89.2. The major change from NWTS-5 is that children with tumor spillage are upstaged from stage II to stage III because of the higher risk for relapse with two-drug chemotherapy alone.[46] The COG risk group classification for treatment assignment in the new generation of WT protocols is shown in Table 89.3. In addition to tumor stage, this classification will also consider the patient's age, tumor weight, presence or absence of LOH at 1p and 16q, and response to chemotherapy in children with FH tumors and lung metastases.

GENERAL MANAGEMENT

The diagnosis of WT is usually made before surgery and confirmed at surgery. A transverse transabdominal, transperitoneal incision is recommended for adequate exposure and thorough abdominal exploration.[47] The surgeon must excise all tumors without spillage, if possible. Lymph node sampling from the para-aortic, celiac, and iliac areas must be performed. The use of titanium clips to identify residual tumor and margins of resection is also recommended. Routine exploration of the contralateral kidney was mandated in the past, but it is no longer recommended because of better imaging of the contralateral kidney with CT and MRI scans.

The chemotherapy and RT regimens for WT in the COG protocols are outlined in Tables 89.4 and 89.5.

RADIATION THERAPY TECHNIQUES

RT guidelines used for primary and recurrent WT in the COG protocols are shown in Table 89.5.

TABLE 89.3 CHILDREN'S ONCOLOGY GROUP RISK GROUP CLASSIFICATION FOR FAVORABLE HISTOLOGY WILMS TUMORS

Age	Tumor Weight	Stage	LOH	Rapid Response	Risk Group	COG Study	Treatment
<2 y	<550 g	I	Any	N/A	Very low	AREN0532	Surgery only
Any	≥550 g	I	None	N/A	Low	AREN0532	EE4A
≥2 y	Any	I	None	N/A	Low	AREN0532	EE4A
Any	Any	II	None	N/A	Low	AREN0532	EE4A
≥2 y	Any	I	Yes	N/A	Standard	AREN0532	DD4A
Any	≥550 g	I	Yes	N/A	Standard	AREN0532	DD4A
Any	Any	II	Yes	N/A	Standard	AREN0532	DD4A
Any	Any	III	None	Any	Standard	AREN0532	DD4A
Any	Any	III	Yes	Any	Higher	AREN0533	M
Any	Any	IV	Yes	Any	Higher	AREN0533	M
Any	Any	IV	None	Yes	Standard	AREN0533	DD4A
Any	Any	IV	None	No	Higher	AREN0533	M

DD4A (V [vincristine] A [dactinomycin], D [doxorubicin]); EE4A (VA); LOH, loss of heterozygosity at both 1p and 16q; M (VAD/Cy [cyclophosphamide], E [etoposide]); N/A, not applicable.

TABLE 89.4 OUTLINE OF CHILDREN'S ONCOLOGY GROUP RENAL TUMOR STUDY

Tumor Risk Classification	Multimodality Treatment
Very Low-Risk FH Wilms Tumor	
<2 y, stage I, tumor weight <550 g	Nephrectomy without adjuvant therapy, if node sampling and central pathology review have been performed
Low-Risk FH Wilms Tumor	
≥2 y, stage I, tumor weight ≥550 g, stage II without LOH	Nephrectomy, no RT, regimen EE4A
Standard-Risk FH Wilms Tumor	
Stage I and II with LOH	Nephrectomy, no RT, regimen DD4A
Stage III without LOH	Nephrectomy, RT, regimen DD4A
Stage IV FH: rapid responders of lung metastases at week 6 with regimen DD4A, without LOH	Nephrectomy, RT, regimen DD4A; no WLI
Higher-Risk FH Wilms Tumor	
Stage III with LOH	Nephrectomy, RT, regimen M
Stage IV slow responders (lung) and nonpulmonary metastases, with LOH	Nephrectomy, RT, regimen M, WLI and RT to metastases
High-Risk UH Renal Tumors	
Stage I–IV focal anaplasia	Nephrectomy, RT, regimen DD4A
Stage I diffuse anaplasia	Nephrectomy, RT, regimen DD4A
Stage I–III CCSK	Nephrectomy, RT, regimen I
Stage II–IV diffuse anaplasia	Nephrectomy, RT, regimen UH1, RT to all metastatic sites
Stage IV CCSK	Nephrectomy, RT, regimen UH1, RT to all metastatic sites
Stage I–IV RTK	Nephrectomy, RT, regimen UH1, RT to all metastatic sites

CCSK, clear cell sarcoma of the kidney; FH, favorable histology; LOH, loss of heterozygosity at 1p and 16q; regimen DD4A (V [vincristine], A [dactinomycin], D [doxorubicin]); regimen EE4A (VA); regimen M (VAD/Cy [cyclophosphamide], E [etoposide]); RT, flank or abdominal irradiation; RTK, rhabdoid tumor of the kidney; regimen I (alternating VDCy/CyE); regimen UH1 (alternating VDCy/CyC [carboplatin] E); UH, unfavorable histology; WLI, whole-lung irradiation.

TABLE 89.5 CHILDREN'S ONCOLOGY GROUP RENAL TUMOR PROTOCOL RADIATION THERAPY GUIDELINES

Abdominal Tumor Stage and Histology	RT Dose/RT Field[a]
Stage I and II FH Wilms tumor	None
Stage III FH, stage I–III focal anaplasia	10.8 Gy to the flank[b]
Stage I–II DA, stage I–III CCSK[c]	10.8 Gy to the flank[b]
Stage III DA, stage I–III RTK	19.8 Gy flank[b] RT, infants ≤12 months 10.8 Gy
Recurrent abdominal Wilms tumor	12.6–18 Gy (<12 months)[b]
	21.6 Gy (older children, previous RT ≤ 10.8 Gy)
	Boost dose of 9 Gy to gross residual tumor
Lung metastases (favorable histology)	12 Gy WLI in 8 fractions[d]
Lung metastases (unfavorable histology)	12 Gy WLI in 8 fractions
Brain metastases	30.6 Gy whole brain in 17 fractions
	21.6 Gy whole brain + 10.8 Gy IMRT or stereotactic boost
Liver metastases	19.8 Gy whole liver in 11 fractions
Bone metastases	25.2 Gy to the lesion plus 3-cm margin
Unresected lymph node metastases	19.8 Gy

[a]Timing of RT (RT delay): RT should begin as close to the beginning of chemotherapy as possible, preferably by day 9 (surgery is day 0), but no later than day 14, unless medically contraindicated or when there is a delay in central pathology review.
[b]Whole-abdomen irradiation (WAI) is indicated when there is diffuse tumor spillage, preoperative or intraperitoneal tumor rupture, peritoneal tumor seeding, or hemorrhagic or cytology positive ascites. When WAI dose is >10 Gy, renal shielding is required to limit the dose to the remaining kidney to <14.4 Gy. Gross residual disease after surgery should receive a boost of 10 Gy. WAI dose is not to exceed 10 Gy in infants ≤12 months.
[c]COG protocol (AREN0321) is studying the possibility of eliminating RT in children with stage I CCSK tumors who have lymph node sampling and central pathology review.
[d]COG protocol (AREN0533) is studying the possibility of eliminating WLI in children with lung metastases who are rapid responders (complete response of lung metastasis after three-drug chemotherapy on central review of computed tomography [CT] scans at week 6). Tumor size, number of lesions, and CT or x-ray detectability are not considered indications for WLI in FH tumors. CCSK, clear cell sarcoma of the kidney; DA, diffuse anaplasia; FH, favorable histology; IMRT, intensity-modulated RT; RT, radiation therapy; RTK, rhabdoid tumor of the kidney; WLI, whole-lung irradiation.

Timing of Radiation Therapy

The NWTS has shown that although RT does not need to be given immediately after surgery,[40] a delay of ≥10 days after surgery was associated with a significantly higher abdominal relapse rate, particularly among patients with UH tumors.[48–51] Because the pathologist cannot always rule out UH quickly, all patients with WT should be scheduled to start RT no later than day 9, the day of surgery being day 0. Although most patients may not be irradiated, it is easier to cancel than to make arrangements to start RT for a small child on short notice. The influence of RT delay on abdominal tumor recurrence in patients with FH tumors treated on NWTS-3 and NWTS-4 has been reported. The mean RT delay was 10.9 days. Although univariate and multivariate analysis did not reveal RT delay of ≥10 days to adversely influence flank and abdominal recurrence, it is important to note that in 59% of children, the RT delay ranged from 8 to 12 days.[52] For the COG protocols, it is recommended that RT be given preferably by day 9 but no later than day 14 after surgery.

Radiation Therapy Dose

In NWTS-1 and NWTS-2, RT dosages to the operative bed were given according to the age of the patient; however, no significant dose–response association was detected.[49,51] In NWTS-3, there was a randomization for patients with FH tumors that resulted in elimination of RT for stage II FH and a reduction of dose to 10 Gy for stage III patients.[50] NWTS-3 and NWTS-4 data showed no RT dose response for CCSK and anaplastic tumors.[53] Therefore, it was decided to treat all abdominal disease with 10 Gy. In the COG protocols, the dose is 10 Gy for most indications except for stage III DA and stage I to III RTK, where a higher dose of 19.8 Gy is recommended (Table 89.5).[54,55]

Radiation Therapy Volume

Parallel-opposed fields using 4- or 6-MV photons are preferred. The flank RT field is determined by the CT or MRI scan performed at diagnosis before any chemotherapy is administered. The planning target volume is the tumor bed (outline of the kidney and associated tumor on the initial CT or MRI) with a 1-cm margin. The medial border must cross the midline to include the entire width of the vertebrae so as to minimize growth disturbances. An example of a flank RT portal is shown in Figure 89.2.[48] When whole-abdomen RT is administered, the femoral heads and acetabulum must be shielded (Fig. 89.3). Whole-lung irradiation (WLI) portals are shown in Figure 89.4. If the lungs and either the flank or whole abdomen have to be treated simultaneously, it is preferable to include them in one treatment portal.

Intensity-Modulated Radiation Therapy for Lung and Liver Irradiation

A multiinstitutional prospective clinical trial was conducted to determine the feasibility of cardiac-sparing lung intensity-modulated radiation therapy (IMRT). All centers were credentialed. The IMRT PTV was the 4-D minIP total lung volume plus 1cm. All target volumes, cardiac contours, and treatment plans were centrally reviewed (QARC) for preapproval prior to treatment. 20 patients were accrued. The majority had pediatric sarcomas or WTs. Lung IMRT was feasible in all patients. Median RT dose was 15 Gy (12 to 15 Gy). Pretreatment review resulted in target contour changes in 7, replanning in 3, and minor dose deviations in 2 patients. There were no major deviations. The mean cardiac (whole heart, ventricles, atria, coronary arteries, myocardium) volume doses were significantly lower after IMRT compared to AP–PA techniques. The 4-D lung volumes were significantly larger than 3-D volumes (<0.0001), and thus, standard AP–

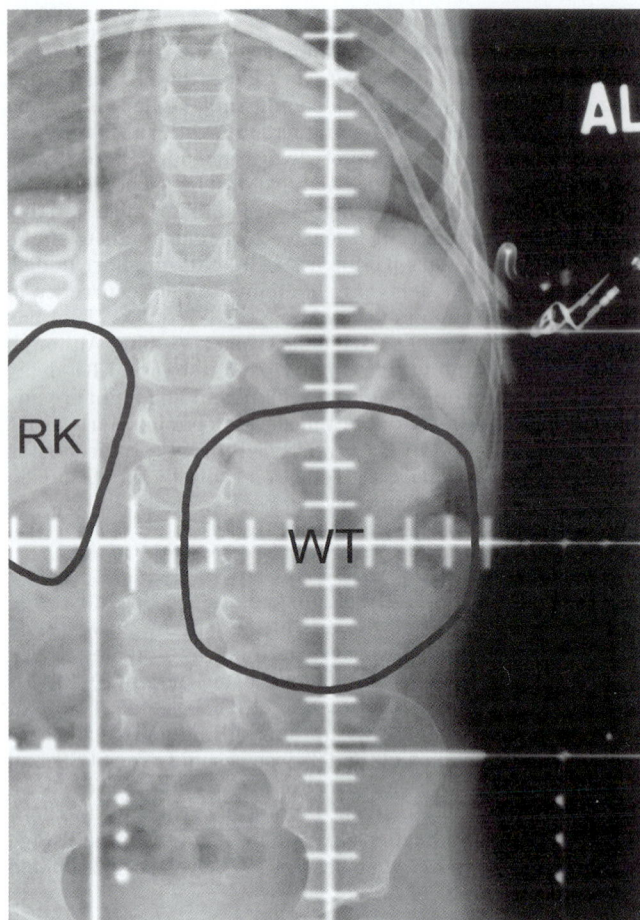

FIGURE 89.2. Anteroposterior flank irradiation portal in a 2-year-old child with a left-sided stage III favorable histology Wilms tumor (WT), showing inclusion of the entire width of the vertebral body in the irradiated volume. The outline of the right kidney (RK) and the WT from the preoperative computed tomography scan is shown.

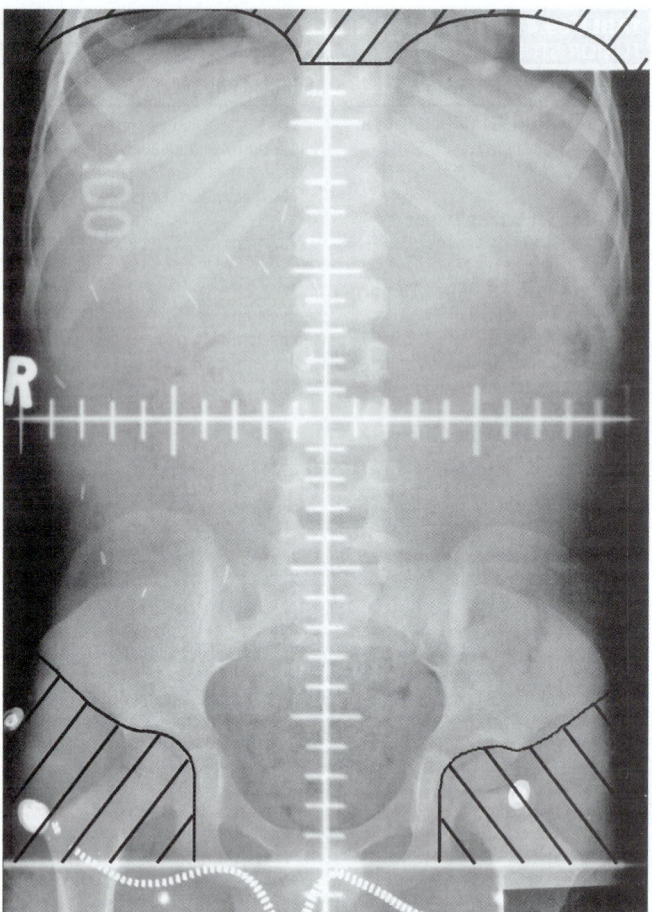

FIGURE 89.3. Anteroposterior whole-abdomen irradiation portal in a patient with stage III Wilms tumor and diffuse peritoneal tumor spillage. The upper margin of the abdominal field must include the diaphragm. The acetabulum and femoral head should be excluded from the irradiated volume to decrease the probability of slipped femoral capital epiphysis. The pants zipper can be seen low on the hips. In general, it is advisable to remove the trousers completely to ensure a reproducible setup.

FIGURE 89.4. Anteroposterior whole-lung irradiation portal in a patient with stage IV favorable histology Wilms tumor. The axial, coronal, and sagittal chest computed tomography simulation scans should be carefully reviewed to ascertain inclusion of the anterior and posterior costophrenic angles at the inferior edge of the treatment volume with a 1-cm margin.

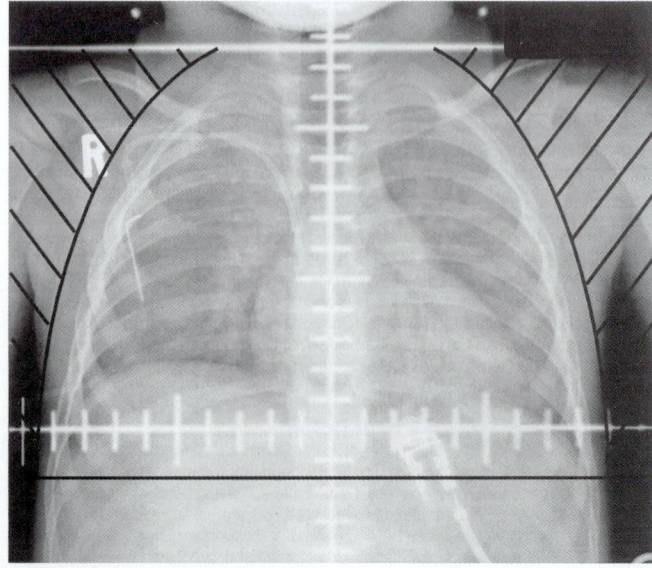

PA RT would have significantly underdosed 4-D lung volumes ($P = 0.008$). IMRT was well tolerated. No patient had radiation pneumonitis, pulmonary consolidation, or fibrosis after a minimum 2-year follow-up. The 2- and 3-year OS and lung metastasis progression-free survival were 90% and 90% and 65% and 52%, respectively. This trial demonstrated the feasibility, dosimetric advantages, safety, and efficacy of lung IMRT with chemotherapy.[56,57] The dosimetric advantages of whole-liver IMRT compared to AP–PA techniques have also been published.[58] In future WT protocols, IMRT targeting 4-D lung and liver volumes with QARC central review will be utilized for stage IV patients with lung and liver metastases.

SUMMARY OF CLINICAL TRIALS

No tumor has been studied by clinical trials as thoroughly and effectively as WT. The NWTS has been active in North America since 1969. There have also been successful studies run by the International Society of Pediatric Oncology (SIOP). The long-term results of NWTS-3 and NWTS-4 are shown in Table 89.6.

First National Wilms Tumor Study (1969–1974)

NWTS-1 showed that postoperative RT was not necessary for children younger than 2 years of age with group I tumors and that combined dactinomycin and vincristine for irradiated patients with group II and III tumors was better than therapy with either agent alone. The RFS with and without RT among patients with group I tumors younger than 2 years of age was 90% and 88%, respectively.[48]

TABLE 89.6 LONG-TERM RESULTS OF NATIONAL WILMS TUMOR STUDIES 3 AND 4[a]

Category	Number of Patients	10-Year RFS (%)	10-Year OS (%)
Stage I FH	1,582	91.4	96.6
Stage II FH	1,006	85.5	93.4
Stage III FH	1,038	84.2	89.5
Stage IV FH	592	75.2	80.7
Stage V FH	344	65.1	77.9
All FH	4,562	84.4	90.8
Clear cell sarcoma	170	67.1	77.1
Stage II–III anaplasia	128	43.0	49.2
Stage IV anaplasia	55	18.2	18.2
Rhabdoid tumor	88	27.3	28.4

[a]National Wilms Tumor Study unpublished data.
FH, favorable histology; OS, overall survival; RFS, relapse-free survival.

Second National Wilms Tumor Study (1974–1979)

NWTS-2 showed that in patients with group I tumors, there was no survival difference between 6 months and 15 months of dactinomycin plus vincristine. Patients with group II to IV tumors had a superior 2-year RFS of 77% with doxorubicin, dactinomycin, and vincristine compared with 63% with dactinomycin and vincristine alone.[41]

Third National Wilms Tumor Study (1979–1985)

The overall objective of NWTS-3 was to reduce therapy for low-risk patients (stage I to III FH) and to intensify treatment by adding a fourth drug, cyclophosphamide, for stage IV tumors with FH and all UH tumors. The results of this study demonstrated that RT and doxorubicin could be eliminated in children with stage II FH tumors. Patients with stage III FH tumors who received doxorubicin or 20 Gy had fewer abdominal relapses than those receiving 10 Gy without doxorubicin.[50] The addition of cyclophosphamide in high-risk patients did not improve outcomes.[53]

Fourth National Wilms Tumor Study (1986–1994)

By the conclusion of NWTS-3, it was clear that the treatment of WT had been refined for the majority of patients; 62% of patients with WT have stage I or II FH disease and therefore require neither flank RT nor the potentially cardiotoxic doxorubicin. NWTS-4 was designed with cost containment in mind. The results proved that the survival was similar among patients who received standard course (5 days) or single-dose, pulse-intensive (PI) dactinomycin chemotherapy. Further, PI therapy was associated with less hematologic toxicity and marked reduction of treatment costs.[59,60]

Fifth National Wilms Tumor Study (1995–2001)

One of the major goals of the NWTS-5 trial was to prospectively analyze the prognostic significance of LOH at chromosomes 1p and 16q. These results have been discussed elsewhere.[12] Patients with stage I FH and anaplastic histology and stage II FH tumors were treated with 18 weeks of dactinomycin and vincristine without RT. Stage I FH tumors in children younger than 24 months of age and with tumor weight <550 g were treated with surgery alone. Stage III and IV FH and stage II to IV focal anaplastic tumors were treated with 24 weeks of dactinomycin, vincristine, doxorubicin, and irradiation. Stage II to IV diffuse anaplastic tumors and stage I to IV CCSK were treated with cyclophosphamide, vincristine, doxorubicin, and etoposide along with irradiation. Stage I to IV RTK was treated with carboplatin, etoposide, cyclophosphamide, and irradiation. The RT guidelines in NWTS-5 were

similar to those used in NWTS-4 except for anaplastic tumors, where a dose of 10.8 Gy to the flank and abdomen was recommended compared to an age-adjusted schedule used in NWTS-1 to NWTS-4.

Children's Oncology Group Studies (2002–)

The COG renal tumor committee is the successor of the NWTS. The COG staging and risk group classification for treatment assignment in the new generation of WT protocols are shown in Tables 89.2 and 89.3. This classification will, in addition to tumor stage, also consider the patient's age, tumor weight, presence or absence of LOH at 1p and 16q, and response to chemotherapy in children with FH tumors and lung metastases. The main objectives of the first generation of COG protocols are listed below. The COG chemotherapy regimens and RT guidelines are outlined in Tables 89.4 and 89.5, respectively.

AREN0321

This was a study for children with high-risk renal tumors. This study was designed to determine whether a regimen (UH 1, 2) of cyclophosphamide/carboplatin/etoposide alternating with vincristine/doxorubicin/cyclophosphamide improves the survival of patients with DA and RTK. This study would also determine whether the excellent event-free survival in stage I CCSK can be maintained without the use of abdominal RT. Preliminary results: A higher than expected severe toxicity rate was encountered in these young children with UH tumors after treatment with these intensive multimodality treatment regimens. Despite reductions in chemotherapy dosages and large-field RT doses in young infants, severe toxicities continued to be observed and thus the study was permanently closed in 2013. In a report of AREN0321, a total of 24 patients with stage IV DA tumors were enrolled on the phase 2 window with vincristine and irinotecan. The partial response rate was 79% indicating that this regimen has high response rate in patients with diffuse anaplasia.[61] Among 66 stage II to IV DA tumors, 4-year EFS and OS were 75% and 76%, respectively. Four-year EFS for stage II, III, and IV diseases were 86%, 85%, and 54%, respectively. These results were superior to NWTS-5, where after vincristine, doxorubicin, cyclophosphamide, and etoposide, plus radiotherapy (XRT) (regimen I), the 4-year EFS for stage II to IV DA tumors was 58% (COG unpublished data).

AREN0532

This was a study for children with very low- and standard-risk FH WT. The main objectives were (a) to demonstrate that very low-risk patients treated by nephrectomy and observation alone will have a 4-year RFS of ≥85% and OS of ≥95%; (b) to document continued excellent outcome for patients with stage III WT without LOH of 1p and 16q treated with vincristine, dactinomycin, doxorubicin, and RT (regimen DD4A); and (c) to improve the current 4-year RFS for patients with stage I and II WT with LOH of 1p and 16q by adding doxorubicin but not RT to the standard dactinomycin and vincristine regimen. Preliminary results: A total of 116 children with very low-risk WTs were treated with nephrectomy alone on this study, and their 4-year event-free and OS rates were 90% and 100%, respectively. Tumor 11p15 methylation status was highly predictive of relapse.[62] Among patients with stage I/II tumors with LOH at 1p and 16q, the 4-year event-free survival after augmentation of therapy with DD4A was 84% compared to 75% with regimen EE4A.[63]

AREN0533

This was a study for higher-risk FH WT. The main objectives were (a) to demonstrate that patients with stage IV tumors with pulmonary metastases only, who have complete resolution of the pulmonary lesions after 6 weeks of regimen DD4A chemotherapy (rapid complete responders), would have a 4-year RFS of 85% with additional chemotherapy (regimen DD4A) and without WLI; (b) to demonstrate that stage IV patients who do not have resolution of pulmonary metastases by week 6 (slow incomplete responders) would have a 4-year RFS of 85% with the addition of cyclophosphamide and etoposide to a modified regimen DD4A (regimen M) and WLI; and (c) to improve the 4-year RFS to 75% for patients with stage III or IV FH WT with LOH of chromosomes 1p and 16q. Preliminary results: Among patients with stage III/IV tumors with LOH at 1p and 16q, the 4-year event-free survival after augmentation of therapy with regimen M was 92% compared to 66% with regimen DD4A.[64] Among 296 patients with lung metastasis, 105 (39%) had a complete response at week 6. Their 4-year event-free and OS rates were 78% and 95%, respectively, without WLI. Although these results were inferior to the event-free survival of 85% with WLI and DD4A, the difference was not statistically significant.[65] Among patients who had a slow incomplete response (SIR) at week 6, the augmentation of therapy with regimen M and WLI resulted in a 3-year event-free and OS of 88% and 92%, respectively. These outcomes were significantly superior to the estimated event-free survival of 75% with regimen DD4A and WLI.[66]

AREN0534

This was a study for patients with bilateral, multicentric, or bilaterally predisposed unilateral WT. The main objectives were (a) to improve 4-year RFS to 73% for patients with BWT; (b) to prevent complete removal of at least one kidney in 50% of patients with BWT by using prenephrectomy three-drug chemotherapy induction with vincristine, dactinomycin, and doxorubicin; and (c) to have 75% of children with BWT undergo definitive surgical treatment by 12 weeks after initiation of chemotherapy. Preliminary results: Two hundred and forty-nine patients were enrolled on this study, 88% were younger than 48 months, and 20% had a genetic syndrome. The 4-year RFS and OS were 81% and 94%, respectively. A total of 143 (74%) patients completed prenephrectomy chemotherapy and 60% had complete removal of at least one kidney. Among BWT patients, 84% had definitive surgical treatment by 12 weeks after initiation of chemotherapy. Surgical approaches included unilateral total nephrectomy with contralateral partial nephrectomy (48%), bilateral partial nephrectomy (35%), unilateral total nephrectomy (10.5%), unilateral partial nephrectomy (4%), and bilateral total nephrectomies (2.5%) (COG unpublished data).

Outcomes of Children with Wilms Tumor

Lung Metastases

Patients with stage IV FH with lung metastases had a 4-year survival of 80% on NWTS-3, whereas survival for those with stage IV UH was 55%.[22,43,53] In a United Kingdom Children's Cancer Study Group (UKCCSG) trial, patients with stage IV FH were spared WLI if they had complete resolution of pulmonary metastases after chemotherapy. The 6-year RFS and OS were 50% and 65%, respectively.[67] These results appear to be somewhat worse than the 4-year survival rate of 82% on NWTS-3 and 75% in the second UKCCSG Wilms tumor study because of the greater use of WLI.[22,68] In children with FH tumors enrolled in NWTS-3 and NWTS-4 who had negative chest radiographs and CT scans positive for pulmonary metastases, the 4-year RFS with and without WLI was similar at 89% and 80%, respectively.[69] In a report from NWTS-4 and NWTS-5, among children with lung metastases detected only by CT scans, the 5-year RFS after three drugs with or without WLI was significantly higher than those receiving two drugs (80% vs. 56%). There was no difference seen in 5-year OS between the three-drug and two-drug subsets (87% vs. 86%). There were no significant differences in RFS (82% vs.

72%) or OS (91% vs. 83%) based on whether these patients did or did not receive WLI. This report concluded that in patients with CT-only lung lesions, the addition of doxorubicin may improve RFS but not OS, and there was no added benefit from WLI.[70] In COG protocol AREN0533, chemotherapy response at week 6 was be used to determine whether WLI is delivered or not. Patients with FH tumors and lung metastasis who achieved a complete radiologic response to three-drug chemotherapy at week 6 did not receive WLI; all others received WLI. All patients with UH WT and lung metastases received WLI, regardless of response to chemotherapy (Tables 89.4 and 89.5).

Liver Metastases

Patients with liver metastasis undergo hepatic RT if the metastatic lesions are not completely resected at the time of initial diagnosis before any chemotherapy is delivered. Whole-liver RT is given for diffuse disease, with supplementary boosts to gross disease as indicated. When possible, however, more limited RT fields are used if the disease is more localized in the liver. In a report from NWTS-4 and NWTS-5, the RFS for patients with FH WT and liver metastases was 76%, and this was similar to the RFS in patients with lung metastases (76%), liver and lung metastases (70%), and metastases to other sites (64%).[71]

Bilateral Wilms Tumor

The goals of treatment in BWT are to maximize cure rates and to preserve functional renal parenchyma; thus, the role of radical nephrectomy and RT has been restricted. Initial surgical resections should be performed only if more than two-thirds of each kidney can be preserved.[72] The initial surgery should confirm histologic diagnosis, assess extent of disease in the kidney, and perform a lymph node biopsy. Systemic chemotherapy is then delivered, after which second-look surgery is done in order to perform tumor resection with maximal preservation of renal function. Unpublished 10-year data from the NWTS-3 and NWTS-4 showed that BWT patients, compared with those who have stage I to IV unilateral FH tumors, had lower RFS (65% and 86%) and OS (78% and 92%). In NWTS-4, the 8-year RFS and OS were 74% and 89%, respectively, for FH and 40% and 45%, respectively, for UH BWT. The incidence of end-stage renal disease was 12% among stage V patients.[73] In NWTS-5, BWT patients had a 4-year RFS and OS of only 61% and 80%, respectively. The factors that might have contributed to these poor outcomes were understaging or undertreatment, delay in definitive surgical resection, and increased incidence of anaplasia.[74,75] The current COG protocol (AREN0534) recommends earlier biopsies or resection of nonresponsive tumors so that ineffective therapies for patients with DA could be avoided. This study will intensify chemotherapy upfront (three drugs), require second-look surgery at 6 weeks and definitive surgery at 12 weeks, and recommend chemotherapy based on histologic response after definitive surgery. RT is indicated for stage III FH tumors, stage I to III UH tumors, or when chemotherapy and several surgeries do not result in complete tumor resection with negative margins. Unlike in unilateral WT, the performance of a tumor biopsy or the use of chemotherapy before definitive surgery is not an indication for flank RT in BWT.

Effect of Tumor Spillage on Outcome in Patients with Stage II and III Diseases

Operative tumor spillage was identified in 24% of patients in NWTS-3 and NWTS-4, and 22% of the spills were classified as diffuse.[46,76,77] An analysis was undertaken to determine the influence of RT and chemotherapy on abdominal tumor recurrence caused by spilled cells in abdominal stage II and III FH WT. The odds ratio for the risk of recurrence relative to no RT was 0.35 for 10 Gy (*P* = .01) and 0.08 for 20 Gy (*P* = .01). Thus, RT (10 or 20 Gy) significantly reduced abdominal tumor recurrence rates following tumor spillage. After adjusting for RT, the effect of doxorubicin on tumor recurrence was not significant. For stage II patients (NWTS-4), the 8-year RFS and OS with and without spillage were 74% and 85% (*P* = .02) and 90% and 94% (*P* = .4), respectively. The higher relapse rate among stage II children with spillage was the reason for upstaging patients with tumor spillage to stage III in the new COG staging system (Table 89.2). These patients will now receive three drugs and flank RT.[46]

Nephrectomy Only for Patients with Stage I Favorable Histology Wilms Tumor

In NWTS-5, a single-arm study was conducted to evaluate the efficacy of nephrectomy alone in children younger than 24 months of age with small (<550 g) stage I FH WT. A total of 75 children were enrolled and the 2-year RFS and OS were 87% and 100%, respectively. This study was ended because of stringent stopping rules.[78] In a recent update, the 5-year RFS and OS for these children treated with just surgery alone were 85% and 98%, respectively. These outcomes were similar after treatment with surgery and two-drug chemotherapy (regimen EE4A).[79]

Wilms Tumor with Peritoneal Implants

The outcome of 57 patients with FH WT and peritoneal implants at the time of nephrectomy in NWTS-4 and NWTS-5 was analyzed. All children received multimodality therapy with three-drug chemotherapy and RT. Forty-seven patients (82%) received whole-abdominal RT to a dose of 10.5 Gy. The overall abdominal and systemic tumor control rates were 97% and 93%, respectively. The detection of peritoneal implants was not associated with inferior survival. The 5-year RFS with and without peritoneal implants was 90% and 83%, respectively.[80]

Clear Cell Sarcoma

In the NWTS-1 through NWTS-4 experience for 351 patients with CCSK, the OS rate was 69%. Multivariate analysis revealed four independent prognostic factors for survival: treatment with doxorubicin, tumor stage, age at diagnosis, and tumor necrosis.[81] In NWTS-4, there was no significant difference among those patients initially randomized to PI or standard chemotherapy with vincristine, dactinomycin, and doxorubicin. The 8-year RFS and OS were 72% and 87% for PI and 70% and 84% for standard chemotherapy, respectively. The second randomization to short-duration and long-duration chemotherapy also did not show any significant difference in survival between the two arms. The survival in NWTS-4 was significantly superior to that of NWTS-3 (83% vs. 67%). The PI chemotherapy administration of dactinomycin and doxorubicin in NWTS-4 was presumed to be one of the reasons for the improvement in outcomes.[82]

Rhabdoid Tumor of the Kidney

A total of 142 children with RTK were enrolled in the NWTS-1 through NWTS-5 trials. The OS at 4 years was 23%. The survival rate for children with stage I or II tumors (42%) was significantly higher than for those with stage II or III tumors (16%; *P* = .014). The survival rate in infants <6 months of age was 9% compared with 41% in children >2 years of age (*P* < .001). Children who received a higher dose of RT (>25 Gy) had a significantly better outcome. However, the dose of RT was not an independent predictor of survival.[55]

Anaplastic Wilms Tumor

In NWTS-5, among 2,596 patients who were enrolled, 281 (11%) had anaplastic WT. The 4-year RFS and OS for patients with stage I anaplasia treated with vincristine and dactinomycin without RT were 70% and 83%, respectively. The 4-year RFS for anaplastic tumor patients who underwent immediate nephrectomy and regimen I chemotherapy was 83%, 65%, and 33% for stage II, III, and IV tumors, respectively. The 4-year RFS and OS for stage V tumors were 44% and 55%, respectively. Based on these results, the therapy for stage I, III, IV, and V tumors was augmented in the new COG protocols (Tables 89.4 and 89.5).[54]

Recurrent Wilms Tumor

Children with relapsed FH WT have a variable prognosis depending on the site of relapse, the time from initial diagnosis to relapse, and their previous therapy. The favorable prognostic factors include no previous treatment with doxorubicin, relapse more than 12 months after diagnosis, and intra-abdominal relapse in a patient not previously treated with abdominal RT.[83] In NWTS-5 relapse protocol, patients who relapsed after initial treatment with vincristine and dactinomycin only without RT were treated on stratum "B" with regimen "I" chemotherapy, surgery, and RT. The 4-year RFS and OS were 71% and 81% for all patients, 68% and 81% for those who relapsed in the lung only, and 78% and 83% for those who relapsed in the operative bed with or without lung metastasis.[84] Patients who relapsed after treatment with vincristine, dactinomycin, doxorubicin, and RT were treated on stratum "C" of NWTS-5 protocol, with alternating courses of drug pairs, cyclophosphamide/etoposide and carboplatin/etoposide, surgery, and RT. The 4-year RFS and OS were 42% and 48% for all patients and 49% and 53% for those who relapsed in the lung only.[85] The COG protocol (Table 89.5) recommends postoperative RT for all children with abdominal relapse because these tumors are generally large and infiltrative and surgical resection with negative margins is unlikely.

Wilms Tumor in Older Patients

WT is rarely seen in patients ≥16 years of age. Their survival is similar to that of children and they should be treated similarly.[86,87]

International Society of Pediatric Oncology Trials

The International Society of Pediatric Oncology (SIOP) studies have primarily used preoperative therapy. The goals of administering preoperative therapy are to facilitate surgical removal of the tumor without rupture, to allow for early treatment of micrometastases, and to stratify patients for postoperative therapy based on pathologic tumor response at the time of surgery. The first SIOP trial found that preoperative RT reduced the incidence of tumor spillage but did not increase survival.[88] SIOP-5, reported in 1983, showed that preoperative chemotherapy with vincristine and dactinomycin was as effective as preoperative RT plus dactinomycin in preventing tumor rupture.[89] In SIOP-6, patients with stage I disease were randomly assigned to either 17 or 38 weeks of vincristine and dactinomycin and showed no difference in survival. Among patients with stage II disease and negative lymph nodes (SIOP staging is not identical to NWTS staging) who were randomly assigned to not receive RT, there was a higher recurrence rate.[90] In SIOP-9, there was a randomization of the duration of prenephrectomy therapy with vincristine and dactinomycin (4 weeks vs. 8 weeks). No advantage was noted for 8 weeks of therapy. Among patients with stage II disease with negative lymph nodes, the rate of abdominal relapse was reduced to 7% by the addition of epirubicin.[91] SIOP 93-01 further stratified treatment according to the pathologic response to preoperative chemotherapy. The recommended dose of RT in SIOP-9 and SIOP 93-01 was 15 Gy in patients with low- and intermediate-risk stage III disease and 30 Gy in high-risk patients.[92] SIOP 93-01 showed that the amount of postoperative chemotherapy of stage I patients with either intermediate-risk histology or anaplasia could be reduced to four doses of vincristine and one course of dactinomycin with 5-year RFS and OS rates of 87% and 95%, respectively.[93] Among 1,090 patients in SIOP 93-01, 5% had tumor progression during preoperative chemotherapy. These tumors were generally smaller at diagnosis, more often stage III after surgery, and associated with higher-grade histology. They had significantly poorer event-free and OS compared to those who responded to chemotherapy.[94] A pathologic review of stage II tumors in SIOP 93-01 revealed that there was a significantly higher survival among patients who were stage II because of nonviable tumor in the renal sinus or perirenal fat compared to those with viable tumor in these sites (100% vs. 91%). It was proposed that the definition of stage II be revised.[95] In a report from SIOP WT2001 trial, after preoperative chemotherapy (VA) and surgery, patients with stage II to III intermediate-risk tumors were randomized to receive AVD (actinomycin D, vincristine, doxorubicin) versus AV without doxorubicin. Stage III patients received 14.4-Gy flank RT and 10-Gy boost to positive lymph nodes or macroscopic residual tumor. The 2-year EFS was 93% and 88%; and 5-year OS was 97% and 96%, respectively, with no statistical significant difference between these two regimens. They concluded that doxorubicin was not required for these patients.[96] In another WT2001 report for blastemal-type WTs after VA chemotherapy and surgery, stage I patients received AVD for 26 weeks, and stage II to III patients received etoposide, carboplatin, doxorubicin, and cyclophosphamide for 26 weeks. Local RT was recommended only for stage III patients. The 5-year EFS and OS were for 80% and 88%, respectively, in WT2001 compared to 67% ($P = 0.006$) and 84% ($P = 0.4$), respectively, in SIOP 93-01 trials.[97]

United Kingdom Children's Cancer Study Group

The first UKCCSG Wilms tumor study (UKW1) showed that vincristine could be used alone in patients with stage I FH disease. Among patients with lung metastases, the 6-year survival rate of 65% was significantly worse than the 4-year survival rate of 82% on NWTS-3, probably because of the inclusion of routine WLI in the NWTS.[67] In the second UKCCSG WT study (UKW2), stage I FH patients had similar survival rates as NWTS stage I patients after 10 weekly doses of vincristine. The 4-year survival rate in patients with stage IV disease was higher than in UKW1, at 75%, probably because of the greater use of WLI. The flank RT doses used for stage III FH and UH tumors are 20 and 30 Gy, respectively.[68] The UKW3 trial conducted a randomized comparison of a primary nephrectomy followed by adjuvant therapy based on surgical stage (NWTS approach) and a preoperative chemotherapy followed by nephrectomy and adjuvant therapy (SIOP approach). The 4-year RFS and OS were equivalent in the primary nephrectomy arm (80% and 85%) and in the preoperative chemotherapy arm (79% and 95%), respectively. The UKCCSG has now joined the current SIOP clinical study.[98]

LATE EFFECTS OF TREATMENT

The study of late effects is of paramount importance to prevent survivors of childhood cancer from becoming chronically sick adults.

Scoliosis

A series from Washington University showed a high incidence of scoliosis in 54% of patients who were treated with a median dose of 30 Gy. However, there was minimal functional disability.[99] In another report, the incidence of scoliosis after 10 to 12 Gy, 12.1 to 23.9 Gy, and 24 to 40 Gy was 8%, 46%, and 63%,

respectively.[100] Thus, at present, with the use of megavoltage x-rays, lower doses, and coverage of the entire width of the vertebra, the incidence of scoliosis should be low.

Congestive Heart Failure

The cumulative frequency of congestive heart failure among patients on NWTS-1 through NWTS-4 was 4.4% at 20 years among patients treated initially with doxorubicin and 17.4% among patients treated with doxorubicin for their first or subsequent relapse. The factors that were significantly associated with the incidence of heart failure were female sex, cumulative doxorubicin dose, WLI, and left abdominal RT.[101]

Pregnancy Outcome in Wilms Tumor Survivors

The NWTS Long-Term Follow-Up Study analyzed pregnancy outcomes among WT survivors. Malposition of the fetus and premature labor were significantly more frequent among previously irradiated women. The offspring of female patients who received flank RT were more likely to be of low birth weight (<2,500 g), to be premature (<36 weeks of gestation), and to have congenital malformations. A flank RT dose response was identified with higher complication rates at doses >25 Gy. A number of radiation-induced side effects involving the spine, uterus, and ovaries may all have been responsible.[102-104] The pregnancy outcomes in survivors who received abdominal RT on NWTS protocols were also analyzed. Fertility could be preserved in children with upper abdominal RT that did not include the pelvis. In rare instances, fertility could be preserved after whole-abdominal RT to 10.5 Gy. However, higher doses to the abdomen and pelvis resulted in miscarriages and fetal deaths.[105]

END-STAGE RENAL DISEASE

The 20-year cumulative incidence of end-stage renal disease among WT survivors after unilateral nephrectomy on NWTS protocols was 74% for children with Denys-Drash syndrome, 36% for children with WAGR syndrome, 7% for children with genitourinary anomalies, and 0.6% for patients with none of these conditions. The importance of long-term screening for high-risk children to facilitate early detection and treatment of impaired renal function was emphasized.[106]

Second Malignant Neoplasm

Among NWTS patients, the 15-year cumulative risk of second malignant neoplasm (SMN) was 1.6%. The risk of developing a lymphoma or leukemia was 0.4% at 8 years, after which no cases occurred. However, the risk of developing a solid tumor continued to rise sharply with time. Approximately 73% of solid tumors arose within a previous RT field. Higher doses of abdominal RT, doxorubicin use, and treatment for relapse were the significant factors correlated with the development of second tumors.[107] In another NWTS report, the standardized mortality ratio was 24.3 within 5 years of diagnosis, 12.6 for the next 5 years, and >3.0 thereafter. The main cause of mortality within the first 5 years was the original disease (91%). However, beyond 5 years, the two important causes of mortality were the original disease (40%) and late effects of treatment (39%). The three common treatment-related late effects that contributed to mortality were SMNs, congestive heart failure, and end-stage renal disease. The risk of death, particularly from treatment-related late effects, remained elevated even 20 years after diagnosis.[108] Similar results have been shown recently by the Childhood Cancer Survivor Study after a follow-up of 25 years.[109] In the British Cancer Survivor Study, the cumulative incidence of a second primary neoplasm at 30, 40, and 50 years of age was 2%, 7%, and 12%, respectively.[110] In another NWTS report, female survivors who received WLI had nearly a 15% risk of developing invasive breast cancer by age 40 years. This report highlighted the need for reevaluating current COG guidelines that recommend breast cancer screening only for those who received >20 Gy to the chest.[111]

FUTURE DIRECTIONS

The first generation of WT protocols conducted by the COG has been completed and detailed analyses are underway. Study proposals for the second generation of COG protocols are presently being considered. All of these proposals are aimed at further refining the treatment of low-risk patients to decrease treatment-related toxicity and intensify treatment of high-risk tumors to improve outcomes. The following are some of the proposals under consideration by COG and others: to include tumor molecular signatures (1q gain, LOH 1p and 16q, LOH11p15) as part of the COG risk stratification system to further refine treatment, to use cardiac-sparing IMRT in children receiving WLI to reduce cardiac toxicity,[56,57] to use IMRT to reduce renal toxicity in children receiving whole-liver irradiation,[58] to reevaluate the necessity of irradiating all children who receive chemotherapy before nephrectomy, to reevaluate the current recommendation for using whole-abdomen RT in children with localized preoperative tumor rupture limited to the flank without any ascites or peritoneal implants, to add new biologic agents to the currently used chemotherapy regimens in children with diffuse anaplastic WT and rhabdoid tumors, to intensify therapy for children with FH WT and lymph node metastases who have a higher risk of tumor relapse, to evaluate the role of proton therapy for WT; to determine the value of surgical resection or focal RT boost doses to residual lung lesions after WLI, and to explore the role of intraoperative RT in selected cases of unilateral, bilateral, and recurrent WT. The biologic sample banks of COG will continue to be a valuable source of tissue for studies aimed at identifying new biologic markers that may be of prognostic significance.

REFERENCES

1. Coppes MJ, Ritchey ML, D'Angio GJ. Preface: the path to progress in medical science: a Wilms' tumor conspectus. *Hematol Oncol Clin North Am* 1995;9:xiii–xviii.
2. Birch JM, Breslow N. Epidemiologic features of Wilms' tumor. *Hematol Oncol Clin North Am* 1995;9:1157–1178.
3. Breslow N, Beckwith JB, Ciol M, et al. Age distribution of Wilms' tumor: report from the National Wilms' Tumor Study. *Cancer Res* 1988;48:1653–1657.
4. Breslow NE, Olshan A, Beckwith JB, et al. Epidemiology of Wilms' tumor. *Med Pediatr Oncol* 1983;21:172–181.
5. Coppes MJ, Egeler RM. Genetics of Wilms' tumor. *Semin Urol Oncol* 1999;17:2–10.
6. Call KM, Glaser T, Ito CY, et al. Isolation and characterization of a zinc finger polypeptide gene at the human chromosome 11 Wilms' tumor locus. *Cell* 1990;60:509–520.
7. Pritchard-Jones K, Fleming S, Davidson D, et al. The candidate Wilms' tumor gene is involved in genitourinary development. *Nature* 1990;346:194–197.
8. Pelletier J, Bruening W, Kashtan CE, et al. Germline mutations in the Wilms' tumor suppressor gene are associated with abnormal urogenital development in Denys-Drash syndrome. *Cell* 1991;67:437–447.
9. Huff V. Wilms' tumor genetics. *Am J Hum Genet* 1998;79:260–267.
10. Koufos A, Grundy P, Morgan K, et al. Familial Wiedemann-Beckwith syndrome and a second Wilms' tumor locus both map to 11p15.5. *Am J Hum Genet* 1989;44:711–719.
11. Grundy PE, Telzerow PE, Breslow N, et al. Loss of heterozygosity for chromosomes 16q and 1p in Wilms' tumors predicts an adverse outcome. *Cancer Res* 1994;54:2331–2333.
12. Grundy PE, Breslow NE, Li S, et al. Loss of heterozygosity for chromosomes 1p and 16q is an adverse prognostic factor in favorable histology Wilms tumor: a report from the National Wilms' Tumor Study Group. *J Clin Oncol* 2005;23:7312–7321.
13. Rivera MN, Kim WJ, Wells J, et al. An X chromosome gene, WTX, is commonly inactivated in Wilms tumor. *Science* 2007;315:642–645.
14. Williams RD, Al-Saadi R, Natrajan R, et al. Molecular profiling reveals frequent gain of *MYCN* and anaplasia-specific loss of 4q and 14q in Wilms' tumor. *Genes Chromosomes Cancer* 2011;50:982–995.
15. Gadd S, Sredni ST, Huang CC, et al. Rhabdoid tumor: gene expression clues to pathogenesis and potential therapeutic targets. *Lab Invest* 2010;90:724–738.
16. Perlman EJ, Grundy PE, Anderson JR, et al. *WT1* mutation and 11p15 loss predict relapse in very low-risk Wilms' tumor treated with surgery alone: a Children's Oncology Group Study. *J Clin Oncol* 2010;26:698–703.
17. Sredni ST, Gadd S, Huang CC, et al. Subsets of very low risk Wilms tumor show distinctive gene expression, histologic and clinical features. *Clin Cancer Res* 2009;15:6800–6809.
18. Perlman EJ, Grundy PE, Anderson JR et al. WT1 mutation and 11P15 loss of heterozygosity predict relapse in very low-risk Wilms tumors treated with surgery alone: a Children's Oncology Group Study. *J Clin Oncol* 2011;29:698–703.
19. Gratias EJ, Dome JS, Jennings LJ, et al. Association of chromosome 1q gain with inferior survival in favorable histology Wilms tumor: a report from the Children's Oncology Group. *J Clin Oncol* 2016;34:3184–3189.
20. Chagtai G, Zill C, Dainese L, et al. Gain of 1q gain as a prognostic biomarker in Wilms tumors treated with preoperative chemotherapy by the International Society of Pediatric Oncology (SIOP) WT 2001 trial: a SIOP renal tumors biology consortium study. *J Clin Oncol* 2016;34:3195–3203.
21. Beckwith JB, Palmer NJ. Histopathology and prognosis of Wilms' tumor: results from the first National Wilms' Tumor Study. *Cancer* 1978;41:1937–1948.
22. D'Angio GJ, Breslow N, Beckwith JB, et al. The treatment of Wilms' tumor: results of the Third National Wilms' Tumor Study. *Cancer* 1989;64:349–360.
23. Beckwith JB, Zuppan CE, Browning NG, et al. Histological analysis of aggressiveness and responsiveness in Wilms' tumor. *Med Pediatr Oncol* 1996;27:422–428.
24. Beckwith JB. Precursor lesions of Wilms' tumor: clinical and biological implications. *Med Pediatr Oncol* 1993;21:158–168.
25. Beckwith JB. Nephrogenic rests and the pathogenesis of Wilms' tumor: developmental and clinical considerations. *Am J Med Genet* 1998;79:268–273.
26. Coppes MJ, Arnold M, Beckwith JB, et al. Factors affecting the risk of contralateral Wilms' tumor development: a report from the National Wilms' Tumor Study Group. *Cancer* 1999;85:1616–1625.
27. Bonadio JF, Storer B, Norkool P, et al. Anaplastic Wilms' tumor: clinical and pathologic studies. *J Clin Oncol* 1985;3:513–520.
28. Faria P, Beckwith JB, Mishra K, et al. Focal versus diffuse anaplasia in Wilms' tumor: new definitions with prognostic significance. A report from the National Wilms' Tumor Study Group. *Am J Surg Pathol* 1996;20:909–910.
29. Schmidt D, Beckwith JB. Histopathology of childhood renal tumors. *Hematol Oncol Clin North Am* 1995;9.1179–1200.
30. Ledlie EM, Mynors LS, Draper GJ, et al. Natural history and treatment of Wilms' tumor: an analysis of 335 cases occurring in England and Wales 1962–1966. *BMJ* 1970;4:195–200.
31. Sukarochana K, Tolentino W, Kiesewetter WB. Wilms' tumor and hypertension. *J Pediatr Surg* 1972;7:573–576.
32. Hartman DS, Sanders RC. Wilms' tumor versus neuroblastoma: usefulness of ultrasound in differentiation. *J Ultrasound Med* 1982;1:117–122.
33. Ramos IM, Taylor KJW, Kier R, et al. Tumor vascular signals in renal masses: detection with Doppler US. *Radiology* 1988;168:633.
34. Khanna G, Rosen N, Anderson JR, et al. Evaluation of diagnostic performance of CT for detection of tumor thrombus in children with Wilms tumor: a report from the Children's Oncology Group. *Pediatr Blood Cancer* 2012;58(4):551–555.
35. Reiman TAH, Siegel MJ, Shackelford GD. Wilms' tumor in children: abdominal CT and US evaluation. *Radiology* 1986;160:501–505.
36. Belt TG, Cohen MD, Smith JA, et al. MRI of Wilms' tumor: promise as the primary imaging modality. *AJR Am J Roentgenol* 1986;146:955–961.
37. Gylys-Morin V, Hoffer FA, Kozakewich H, et al. Wilms' tumor and nephroblastomatosis: imaging characteristics at gadolinium-enhanced MR imaging. *Radiology* 1993;188:517–521.
38. Ritchey ML, Green DM, Breslow NB, et al. Accuracy of current imaging modalities in the diagnosis of synchronous bilateral Wilms' tumor: a report from the National Wilms' Tumor Study Group. *Cancer* 1995;75:600–604.
39. Cohen MD. Current controversy: is computed tomography scan of the chest needed in patients with Wilms' tumor? *Am J Pediatr Hematol Oncol* 1994;16:191–193.
40. Gross RE, Neuhauser EBD. Treatment of mixed tumors of the kidney in childhood. *Pediatrics* 1950;6:843.
41. D'Angio GJ, Evans AE, Breslow NE, et al. The treatment of Wilms' tumor: results of the Second National Wilms' Tumor Study. *Cancer* 1981;47:2302–2311.
42. Farewell VT, D'Angio GJ, Breslow N, et al. Retrospective validation of a new staging system for Wilms' tumor. *Cancer Clin Trials* 1981;4:167–171.
43. Breslow N, Churchill G, Nesmith B, et al. Clinicopathologic features and prognosis for Wilms' tumor patients with metastases at diagnosis. *Cancer* 1986;58:2501–2511.
44. Beckwith JB. National Wilms' Tumor Study: an update for pathologists. *Pediatr Dev Pathol* 1998;1:79–84.
45. Weeks DA, Beckwith JB, Luckey DW. Relapse-associated variables in stage I favorable histology Wilms' tumor: a report of the National Wilms' Tumor Study. *Cancer* 1987;60:1204–1212.
46. Kalapurakal JA, Li SM, Breslow NE, et al. Intraoperative spillage of favorable histology Wilms tumor cells: influence of irradiation and chemotherapy regimens on abdominal recurrence: a report from the National Wilms Tumor Study. *Int J Radiat Oncol Biol Phys* 2010;76:201–206.
47. Leape LL, Breslow NE, Bishop HC. The surgical treatment of Wilms' tumor: results of the National Wilms' Tumor Study. *Ann Surg* 1978;187:351–356.
48. D'Angio GJ, Evans AE, Breslow NE, et al. The treatment of Wilms' tumor: results of the National Wilms' Tumor Study. *Cancer* 1976;38:633–646.
49. D'Angio GJ, Tefft M, Breslow NE, et al. Radiation therapy of Wilms' tumor: results according to dose, field, postoperative timing and histology. *Int J Radiat Oncol Biol Phys* 1978;4:769–780.
50. Thomas PRM, Tefft M, Compaan PJ, et al. Results of two radiotherapy randomizations in the third National Wilms' Tumor Study (NWTS-3). *Cancer* 1991;68:1703–1707.
51. Thomas PRM, Tefft M, Farewell VT, et al. Abdominal relapses in the Second National Wilms' Tumor Study patients. *J Clin Oncol* 1984;2:1098–1101.
52. Kalapurakal JA, Li SM, Breslow NE, et al. Influence of radiation therapy delay on abdominal tumor recurrence in patients with favorable histology Wilms tumor treated on NWTS-3 and -4: a report from the National Wilms Tumor Study Group. *Int J Radiat Oncol Biol Phys* 2003;57:495–499.
53. Green DM, Beckwith JB, Breslow NE, et al. The treatment of children with stages II–IV anaplastic Wilms' tumor: a report from the National Wilms' Tumor Study Group. *J Clin Oncol* 1994;12:2126–2131.

54. Dome JS, Cotton CA, Perlman EJ, et al. Treatment of anaplastic histology Wilms tumor: results from the Fifth National Wilms Tumor Study. *J Clin Oncol* 2006;24:2352–2358.

55. Tomlinson GE, Breslow NE, Dome J, et al. Rhabdoid tumor of the kidney in the National Wilms Tumor Study: age at diagnosis as a prognostic factor. *J Clin Oncol* 2005;23:7641–7645.

56. Kalapurakal JA, Gopalakrishnan M, Walterhouse D, et al. Final report of a prospective clinical trial of cardiac sparing whole-lung intensity modulated radiation therapy in patients with metastatic pediatric tumors. *Int J Radiat Oncol Biol Phys* 2016; 96: S118–S119.

57. Kalapurakal JA, Zhang Y, Kepka AG, et al. Advantages of cardiac-sparing whole lung IMRT in children with lung metastasis. *Int J Radiat Oncol Biol Phys* 2013;85:761–767.

58. Kalapurakal JA, Pokhrel D, Goplakrishnan M, et al. Advantages of whole-liver intensity modulated radiation therapy in children with Wilms tumor and liver metastasis. *Int J Radiat Oncol Biol Phys* 2013;85:754–760.

59. Green DM, Breslow NE, Beckwith JB, et al. Comparison between single-dose and divided-dose administration of dactinomycin and doxorubicin for patients with Wilms' tumor: a report from the National Wilms' Tumor Study Group. *J Clin Oncol* 1998;16:237–245.

60. Green DM, Breslow NE, Evans I, et al. The effect of chemotherapy dose intensity on the hematological toxicity of the treatment for Wilms' tumor: a report from the National Wilms' Tumor Study. *Am J Pediatr Hematol Oncol* 1994;16:207–212.

61. Daw NC, Anderson JR, Hoffer FA et al. A phase 2 study of vincristine and irinotecan in metastatic diffuse anaplastic Wilms tumor: results from the Children's Oncology Group AREN0321 study. *J Clin Oncol* 2014;32(suppl; abstr 10032):5s.

62. Fernandez CV, Perlman E, Mullen EA, et al. Clinical outcome and biological predictors of relapse following nephrectomy only for very low risk Wilms tumor (VLR WT): a report from Children's Oncology Group AREN0532. *J Clin Oncol* 2015;33(suppl; abstr 10023).

63. Fernandez CV, Mullen EA, Ehrlich PA, et al. Outcome and prognostic factors in stage III favorable histology Wilms tumor: a report from the Children's Oncology Group AREN0532 study. *J Clin Oncol 2015 ASCO Annual Meeting Abstracts*. Vol. 33: No. 15 suppl.

64. Dix DB, Fernandez CV, Chi YY, et al. Augmentation of therapy for favorable-histology Wilms tumor with combined loss of heterozygosity of chromosomes 1p and 16q: a report from the Children's Oncology Group AREN0533 study. *J Clin Oncol 2015 ASCO Annual Meeting Abstracts*. Vol. 33: No. 15 suppl.

65. Dix DB, Gratias EJ, Seibel N, et al. Omission of lung radiation in patients with stage IV favorable histology Wilms Tumor (FHWT) showing complete lung nodule response after chemotherapy: a report from Children's Oncology Group study AREN0533. *J Clin Oncol* 2015;33(suppl; abstr 10011).

66. Dix DB, Gratias EJ, Seibel N, et al. Treatment of stage IV favorable histology Wilms tumor with incomplete lung metastasis response after chemotherapy: a report from Children's Oncology Group study AREN0533. *J Clin Oncol* 2014;32(suppl; abstr 10001):5s.

67. Pritchard J, Imeson J, Barnes J, et al. Results of the United Kingdom Children's Cancer Study Group First Wilms' Tumor Study. *J Clin Oncol* 1995;13:124–133.

68. Mitchell C, Jones PM, Kelsey A, et al. The treatment of Wilms' tumor: results of the United Kingdom Children's Cancer Study Group (UKCCSG) second Wilms' tumor study. *Br J Cancer* 2000;83:602–608.

69. Meisel JA, Guthrie KA, Breslow NE, et al. Significance and management of computed tomography detected pulmonary nodules: a report from the National Wilms' Tumor Study Group. *Int J Radiat Oncol Biol Phys* 1999;44:579–585.

70. Grundy P, Li SM, Green DM, et al. Event free but not overall survival is improved for Wilms tumour patients with pulmonary lesions detectable only by computed tomography by the addition of doxorubicin but not from pulmonary irradiation: results of National Wilms Tumour Studies 4 and 5. *Pediatr Blood Cancer* 2012;59(4):631–635.

71. Ehrlich PF, Ferrerar F, Ritchey M, et al. Hepatic metastasis at diagnosis in favorable histology Wilms tumor is not an independent adverse prognostic factor. A report from the National Wilms Tumor Study Group. *Ann Surg* 2009;250:642–648.

72. Blute ML, Kelalis PP, Offord KP, et al. Bilateral Wilms' tumor. *J Urol* 1987;138:968–973.

73. Hamilton TE, Ritchey ML, Haase GL, et al. The management of synchronous bilateral Wilms tumor: a report from the National Wilms' Tumor Study Group. *Ann Surg* 2011;253:1004–1010.

74. Shamberger RC, Haase GC, Argani P, et al. Bilateral Wilms tumors with progressive or nonresponsive disease. *J Pediatr Surg* 2006;41:652–657.

75. Hamilton TE, Green DM, Perlman EJ, et al. Bilateral Wilms tumor with anaplasia: lessons from the National Wilms Tumor Study. *J Pediatr Surg* 2006;41:1641–1644.

76. Breslow NE, Beckwith JB, Haase GM, et al. Radiation therapy for favorable histology Wilms' tumor: prevention of flank recurrence did not improve survival on National Wilms Tumor Studies 3 and 4. *Int J Radiat Oncol Biol Phys* 2006;65:203–209.

77. Shamberger RC, Guthrie KA, Ritchey ML, et al. Surgery-related factors and local recurrence of Wilms' tumor in National Wilms' Tumor Study 4. *Ann Surg* 1999;229:292–297.

78. Green DM, Breslow NE, Beckwith JB, et al. Treatment with nephrectomy only for small, stage I/favorable histology Wilms' tumor: a report from the National Wilms' Tumor Study Group. *J Clin Oncol* 2001;19:3719–3724.

79. Shamberger RC, Anderson JR, Breslow NE, et al. Long term outcomes of infants with very low risk Wilms tumor treated with surgery alone on National Wilms Tumor Study-5. *Ann Surg* 2010;251:555–558.

80. Kalapurakal JA, Green DM, Haase G, et al. Outcomes of children with favorable histology Wilms 'tumor and peritoneal implants treated on National Wilms' Tumor Studies-4 and -5. *Int J Radiat Oncol Biol Phys* 2010;77:554–558.

81. Argani P, Perlman EJ, Breslow NE, et al. Clear cell sarcoma of the kidney: a review of 351 cases from the National Wilms' Tumor Study Group Pathology Center. *Am J Surg Pathol* 2000;24:4–18.

82. Seibel N, Li S, Breslow NE, et al. Effect of duration of treatment on treatment outcome for patients with clear-cell sarcoma of the kidney: a report from the National Wilms' Tumor Study Group. *J Clin Oncol* 2004;22:468–473.

83. Grundy P, Breslow NE, Green DM, et al. Prognostic factors of children with recurrent Wilms' tumor: results from the second and third National Wilms' Tumor Study. *J Clin Oncol* 1989;7:638–647.

84. Green DM, Cotton CA, Malogolowkin M, et al. Treatment of Wilms tumor relapsing after initial therapy with vincristine and actinomycin D. A report from the National Wilms Tumor Study Group. *Pediatr Blood Cancer* 2007;48: 493–499.

85. Malogolowkin M, Cotton CA, Green DM, et al. Treatment of Wilms tumor relapsing after initial treatment with vincristine, actinomycin D and doxorubicin. A report from the National Wilms tumor Study Group. *Pediatr Blood Cancer* 2008;50:236–241.

86. Kalapurakal JA, Nan B, Norkool P, et al. Treatment outcomes in adults with favorable histologic type Wilms tumor: an update from the National Wilms Tumor Study Group. *Int J Radiat Oncol Biol Phys* 2004;60:1379–1384.

87. Segers H, van den Heuvel-Eibrink MM, Pritchard-Jones K, et al Management of adults with Wilms' tumor: recommendations based on international consensus. *Expert Rev Anticancer Ther* 2011;11:1105–1113.

88. Lemerle J, Vote PA, Tournade MF, et al. Preoperative versus postoperative radiotherapy, single versus multiple courses of actinomycin D in the treatment of Wilms' tumor. *Cancer* 1976;38:647–654.

89. Lemerle J, Vote PA, Tournade MF, et al. Effectiveness of preoperative chemotherapy in Wilms' tumor: results of an International Society of Pediatric Oncology (SIOP) trial. *J Clin Oncol* 1983;1:604–609.

90. Jereb B, Burgers MV, Tournade M-F, et al. Radiotherapy in the SIOP (International Society of Paediatric Oncology) nephroblastoma studies: a review. *Med Pediatr Oncol* 1994;22:221–227.

91. DeKraker J, Weitzman S, Vote PA. Preoperative strategies in the management of Wilms' tumor. *Hematol Oncol Clin North Am* 1995;9:1275–1285.

92. Graf N, Tournade MF, de Kraker J. The role of preoperative chemotherapy in the management of Wilms' tumor. The SIOP studies. *Urol Clin North Am* 2000;27:443–454.

93. De Kraker J, Graf N, van Tinteren H, et al. Reduction of postoperative chemotherapy in children with stage I intermediate-risk and anaplastic Wilms tumor (SIOP-93-01): a randomized trial. *Lancet* 2004;364:1229–1235.

94. Ora I, van Tinteren H, Bergeron C, et al. Progression of localized Wilms' tumor during preoperative chemotherapy is an independent prognostic factor: a report from the SIOP 93-01 nephroblastoma trial and study. *Eur J Cancer* 2007;43:131–136.

95. Vujanic GM, Harms D, Bohoslavsky R, et al. Nonviable tumor tissue should not upstage Wilms' tumor from stage I to stage II: a report from the SIOP 93-01 nephroblastoma trial and study. *Pediatr Dev Pathol* 2009;12:111–115.

96. Pritchard-Jones K, Bergeron C, de Camargo B, et al. Omission of doxorubicin from stage II-III intermediate risk Wilms tumor (SIOP WT2001): an open labeled, non-inferiority, randomized controlled trial. *Lancet* 2015;386:1156–1164.

97. Van den Heuvel-Eibrink MM, van Tinteren H, Bergeron C, et al. Outcome of localized blastemal-type Wilms tumor patients treated according to intensified treatment in the SIOP-WT 2001 protocol, a report of the SIOP renal tumor study group (SIOP-RTSG). *Eur J Cancer* 2015;51:498–506.

98. Mitchell C, Shannon R, Vujanic GM, et al. The treatment of Wilms tumor: results of the United Kingdom Children's Cancer Study group third Wilms Tumor Study. *Med Pediatr Oncol* 2003;41:289.

99. Thomas PRM, Griffith KD, Fineberg BB, et al. Late effects of treatment for Wilms' tumor. *Int J Radiat Oncol Biol Phys* 1983;9:651–657.

100. Paulino AC, Wen BC, Brown CK, et al. Late effects in children treated with radiation therapy for Wilms' tumor. *Int J Radiat Oncol Biol Phys* 2000;46: 1239–1246.

101. Green DM, Grigoriev YA, Nan B, et al. Congestive heart failure after treatment for Wilms' tumor: a report from the National Wilms' Tumor Study Group. *J Clin Oncol* 2001;19:1926–1934.

102. Critchley HOD. Factors of importance for implantation and problems after treatment for childhood cancer. *Med Pediatr Oncol* 1999;33:9–14.

103. Green DM, Peabody EM, Nan B, et al. Pregnancy outcome after treatment for Wilms' tumor. *J Clin Oncol* 2002;20:2506–2513.

104. Green DM, Lange JM, Peabody EM, et al. Pregnancy outcome after treatment for Wilms tumor: a report from the national Wilms tumor long-term follow-up study. *J Clin Oncol* 2010;28:2824–2830.

105. Kalapurakal JA, Peterson S, Peabody EM, et al. Pregnancy outcomes after abdominal irradiation that included or excluded the pelvis in childhood Wilms tumor survivors: a report of the National Wilms Tumor Study. *Int J Radiat Oncol Biol Phys* 2004;58:1364–1368.

106. Breslow NE, Collins AJ, Ritchey ML, et al. End stage renal disease in patients with Wilms tumor: results from the National Wilms Tumor Study Group and the United States renal data system. *J Urol* 2005;174:1972–1975.

107. Breslow NE, Takashima JR, Whitton JA, et al. Second malignant neoplasms following treatment for Wilms' tumor: a report from the National Wilms' Tumor Study Group. *J Clin Oncol* 1995;13:1851–1859.

108. Cotton CA, Peterson S, Norkool PA, et al. Early and late mortality after diagnosis of Wilms tumor. *J Clin Oncol* 2009;27:1304–1309.

109. Termhuhlen AM, Tersak JM, Liu Q, et al. Twenty-five year follow up of childhood Wilms tumor. A report from the Childhood Cancer Survivor Study. *Pediatr Blood Cancer* 2011;57:1210–1216.

110. Taylor AJ, Winter DL, Pritchard-Jones K, et al. Second primary neoplasms in survivors of Wilms tumor: a population-based cohort study from the British Cancer Survivor Study. *Int J Cancer* 2008;122:2085–2093.

111. Lange JM, Takashima JR, Peterson SM et al. Breast cancer in female survivors of Wilms tumor: a report from the National Wilms Tumor Late Effects Study. *Cancer* 2014;120: 3722–3730.

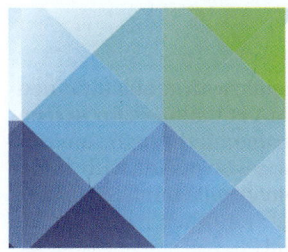

CHAPTER 90

Neuroblastoma

Arnold C. Paulino and Anita Mahajan

INTRODUCTION

Neuroblastoma is an enigmatic malignant neoplasm. In its early stages, it can be readily cured with surgery or, in some circumstances, can even spontaneously regress or mature to a benign ganglioneuroma. In the more common advanced stages, the disease can be fatal. The unique biology of neuroblastoma has attracted the interest of many researchers and is one of the first malignancies in which molecular biologic assays have influenced treatment and prognosis.

EPIDEMIOLOGY

Neuroblastoma is the most common extracranial tumor of childhood. Approximately 90% of cases occur in children <10 years old. The median age at diagnosis is 18 months. The relatively good prognosis of infants diagnosed with early-stage neuroblastoma prompted the initiation of infant-screening studies.[1]

Screening of infants for neuroblastoma has been studied systematically in large clinical trials conducted in Japan, North America, and Europe.[2-5] Excretion of catecholamine metabolites in the urine of children with neuroblastoma has served as the basis of these screening tests. Urine samples were collected and dried on filter paper and returned to screening centers to be tested qualitatively for vanillylmandelic acid (VMA) levels or quantitatively for VMA and homovanillic acid (HVA) measured by high-performance liquid chromatography and normalized to urinary creatinine levels. Children with elevated levels of these metabolites subsequently were referred for further diagnostic evaluation. The incidences of the diagnosis and death rates from neuroblastoma in the screened populations were compared to control populations in the same country or continent. The study populations generally were chosen because of access to an existing screening infrastructure that could readily be adapted to neuroblastoma. The Japanese study screened children at 6 months of age. The Quebec study screened children at 3 weeks and 6 months of age. The German study tested children at their first year's birthday.

The results and conclusions of these three large screening trials on three continents are remarkably similar. In Japan, 1,142,519 children were screened using a qualitative test, and another 550,331 were screened with the quantitative test; they all were compared to 713,025 children in a control population. The incidence rates per 100,000 were 1.12 in the control group compared to 5.69 in the qualitative group and 17.81 in the quantitative group. Despite this increased incidence in the screened group, the neuroblastoma mortality rates were unchanged by the screening.[5] In Germany, 1,475,773 children were screened between 1994 and 1999. Screening detected neuroblastoma in 149 children, 3 of whom died. Despite the screening at 12 months, another 55 children subsequently developed neuroblastoma, 14 of whom died. Compared to the control group, the incidence of stage 4 neuroblastoma was similar. The death rate from neuroblastoma was unaffected by the screening.[3] In Quebec, a total of 425,838 children were enrolled in the neuroblastoma screening trial (89% of births during a 5-year study period from 1989 to 1994). The standardized incidence ratios of neuroblastoma death in the Quebec cohort were nearly identical to those in control groups in Ontario, Minnesota, Florida, and the Greater Delaware Valley.[4] In summary, each of these trials demonstrates that screening does not affect the mortality rate of neuroblastoma. Furthermore, the overdiagnosis of clinically insignificant disease may lead to significant financial, emotional, and physical burdens on the children and their families when one considers that this tumor has high frequency of spontaneous regression in infancy. The mass screening programs have led to the diagnosis of biologically favorable and clinically insignificant tumors.[6,7]

NATURAL HISTORY

Neuroblastoma, along with ganglioneuroma and ganglioneuroblastoma, may arise from any site in the sympathetic nervous system. The most common sites of origin are the adrenal medulla (30% to 40%) and paraspinal ganglia in the abdomen or pelvis (25%). Thoracic (15%) and head and neck primary tumors (5%) are slightly more common in infants than in older children. More than 70% of patients have metastatic disease at presentation. The most frequent metastatic sites are lymph nodes, bone, bone marrow, skin (or subcutaneous tissues), and liver.[8] The lung and central nervous system are rare sites of involvement.

Neuroblastoma has the highest spontaneous remission rate of any human neoplasm, usually by maturation to ganglioneuroma.[9] Microscopic neuroblastomas have been found in the autopsy material of the adrenal glands of young infants at >40 times the expected rate. It has been suggested that most potential neuroblastomas remain clinically silent, because of spontaneous regression.[10] Despite these peculiarities, clinically obvious neuroblastoma is frequently a progressive and relentless disease.

CLINICAL PRESENTATION

Pain is the most common presenting symptom. This frequently is caused by bone, liver, or bone marrow metastases or local visceral invasion by the primary tumor. Other constitutional symptoms may include weight loss, anorexia, malaise, and fever. Respiratory distress may accompany massive hepatomegaly, especially in infants with stage IV-S disease.[8] Horner syndrome can accompany a primary tumor originating in the neck. Spinal cord compression with paralysis of the lower extremities can accompany the so-called dumbbell-shaped tumor that extends from its origin along the sympathetic ganglia through the adjacent neural foramina. Orbital metastases are not uncommon and can cause proptosis and ecchymosis. Skin metastases may have a bluish tinge, giving the classic "blueberry muffin" sign. When pressed, the release of catecholamine into the tissue causes transient blanching of the adjacent skin. An unusual presentation of localized neuroblastoma is the opsoclonus–myoclonus syndrome, manifested by truncal ataxia and cerebellar encephalopathy. This syndrome typically indicates a favorable prognosis from the tumor, but patients may have persistent neurologic sequelae after successful tumor therapy.[11,12]

DIAGNOSTIC WORKUP

As in the case of any suspected malignant neoplasm in children, the diagnosis of neuroblastoma must be established by pathologic evaluation. Tumor tissue may be obtained from the suspected primary tumor site or from involved lymph nodes by excision (if the tumor is resectable) or incisional biopsy. Bone marrow aspirate and biopsy frequently show metastatic tumor deposits that can establish the diagnosis. Pathologic evaluation of bone marrow is also a requirement for staging of neuroblastoma. Characteristically, neuroblastoma in bone marrow appears in clumps and pseudorosettes. The absence of pseudorosettes does not eliminate the possibility of neuroblastoma.

Laboratory studies should include measurement of urinary catecholamines and their metabolites. Either HVA or VMA (metabolites of dopa/norepinephrine and epinephrine, respectively) is elevated in >90% of patients with stage IV neuroblastoma. A ratio of VMA to HVA of >1.5 is associated with a favorable prognosis in patients with metastatic neuroblastoma. An assay for urinary VMA is the basis for screening studies of infants in Japan, Europe, and North America. Anemia secondary to bone marrow involvement with tumor can be evaluated with a complete blood cell count. Serum ferritin, lactate dehydrogenase (LDH), and other liver function indicators should be assayed routinely.

Appropriate use of imaging studies assists in staging and in planning an approach to therapy. X-ray studies demonstrate intrinsic speckled calcifications in 85% of neuroblastomas. Computed tomography (CT) of the abdomen with intravenous contrast is more sensitive than intravenous pyelography and provides more information about lymph node or hepatic metastases as well as tumor resectability.[13] High-quality magnetic resonance imaging (MRI) scans are being used to better evaluate blood vessel encasement, intraspinal extension (dumbbell tumors), diffuse hepatic replacement, and bone marrow involvement (Fig. 90.1). Each of these findings

FIGURE 90.1. Magnetic resonance imaging scans of a 4-month-old child with a thoracic neuroblastoma. The dumbbell shape of the paraspinal mass can be appreciated on axial **(A)**, coronal **(B)**, and sagittal **(C)** images. The intraspinal component is indicated by *arrows*. The three views of this child's tumor are helpful in radiation therapy field design.

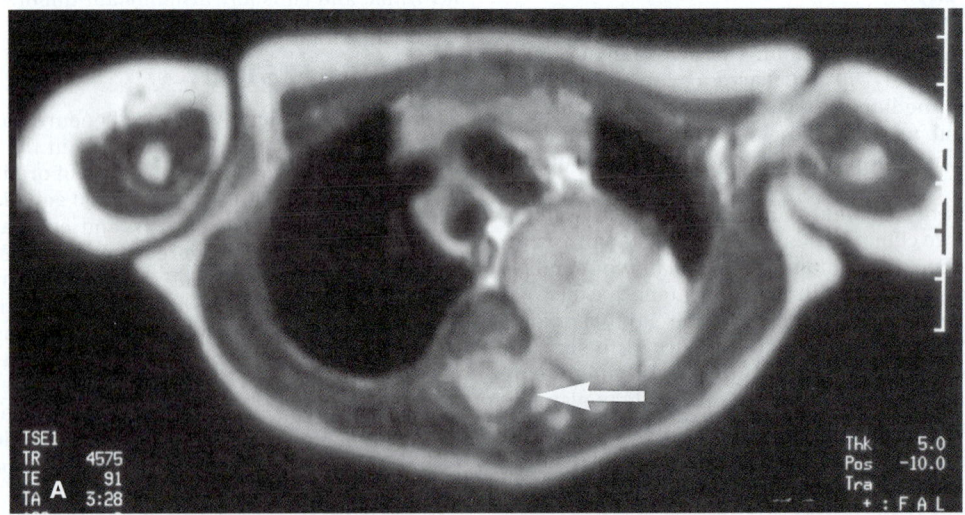

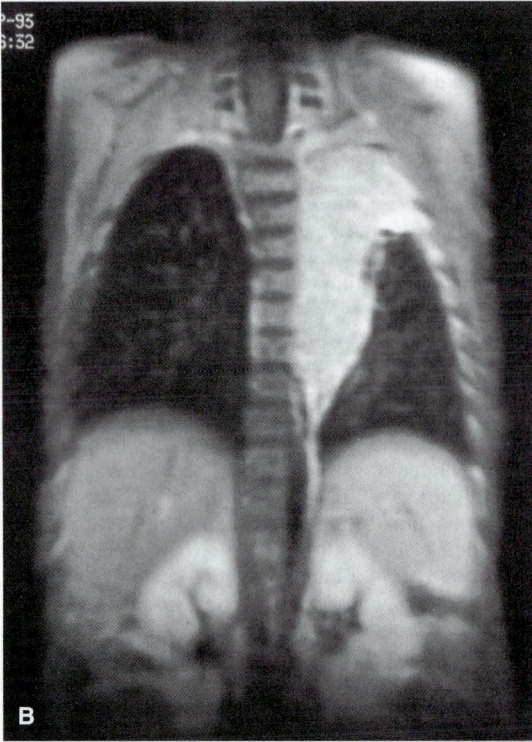

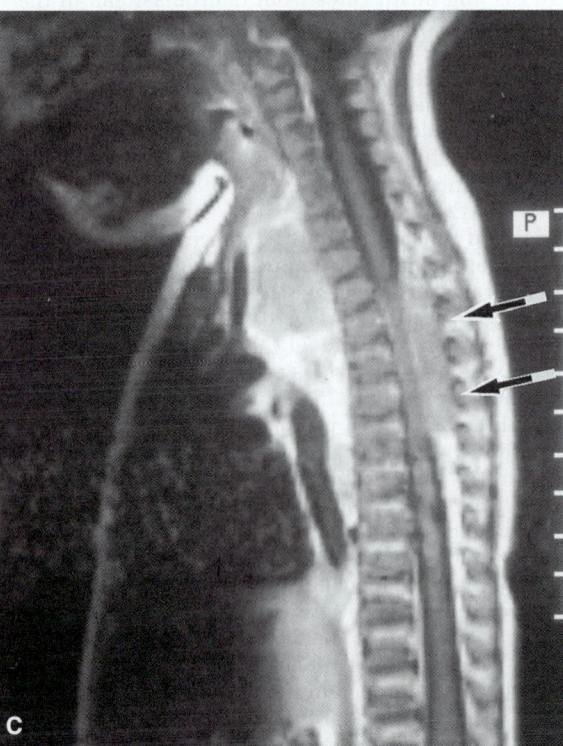

improves staging accuracy and facilitates the decision-making process regarding appropriate surgical interventions.[14–17]

Nuclear medicine scans are helpful in determining the extent of metastatic disease. Because neuroblastoma has a predilection for bony metastases, a radionuclide bone scan has been part of routine workup. A recent study from Boston questions the value of a bone scan when *meta*-iodobenzylguanidine (MIBG) scan is used.[18] In this report, 132 patients underwent both MIBG and bone scans. In the 78 cases with metastatic disease, 74% were both skeletal MIBG and bone scan positive. Only 3 had a negative skeletal MIBG and positive bone scan, but all 3 had other sites of metastatic disease. In no case did a positive bone scan alone determine a stage 4 designation. MIBG is concentrated by neurosecretory granules of both normal and neoplastic tissues of neural crest origin and can be used to image primary and metastatic sites of neuroblastoma. MIBG labeled with either ^{131}I or ^{123}I has a sensitivity of 85% to 90% and a specificity of almost 95% in the detection of metastatic neuroblastoma.[19] Poor scintigraphic response on ^{123}I-MIBG scans after induction chemotherapy has been shown to predict for a poor event-free survival in patients undergoing high-dose chemotherapy with stem cell rescue.[20] Like other neural crest–derived neoplasms, neuroblastoma can express somatostatin receptors. The long-acting somatostatin analog octreotide labeled with ^{123}I has been used to image neuroblastoma with a sensitivity comparable to that of ^{131}I-MIBG.[21] The expression of somatostatin receptors by neuroblastoma tissues is a favorable prognostic factor.[22]

The Radiology Diagnostic Oncology Group enrolled 96 children with newly diagnosed neuroblastoma in a multicenter prospective cohort study prior to surgery. CT, MRI, and bone scintigraphy were used to evaluate tumor stage. The results show that MRI is more accurate than CT for detection of stage 4 disease (sensitivities 0.83 and 0.43, respectively). When combined with bone scintigraphy, both imaging tests have high accuracy for the detection of metastases. Figures 90.2–90.4 illustrate the value of CT and MRI in staging patients with metastatic disease. The prevalence of determinants of local disease was relatively low in this study because patients who had extensive disease at the time of entry underwent delayed surgery after induction chemotherapy. Although the numbers are small, the data suggest the following: (a) In stage 1 tumor, abdominal extent was more likely to be staged correctly with CT than with MRI, which often overstaged tumor; (b) for stage 2 and 3 tumors, both CT and MRI were more likely to understage than overstage tumor; and (c) for stage 2 tumor, understaging was more likely with CT than MRI (Fig. 90.5).

STAGING

The most commonly used staging system is the International Neuroblastoma Staging System (INSS). It is based on clinical,

FIGURE 90.2. Neuroblastoma with nodal involvement in a 3-year-old boy. **A:** Computed tomography (CT) through the upper abdomen shows a large soft tissue mass (*T*) arising in the right adrenal gland and extending to the midline (aorta, *arrow*). **B:** A CT scan several centimeters lower shows several small nodes (*N*) in the right pararenal area. **C:** T2-weighted axial image shows a high–signal intensity tumor (*T*) in the right suprarenal area. **D:** T2-weighted image at a lower level shows enlarged, mildly enhancing paracaval lymph nodes (*N*). RK, right kidney. (Courtesy of Dr. Marilyn Siegel, Mallinckrodt Institute of Radiology, St. Louis, MO.)

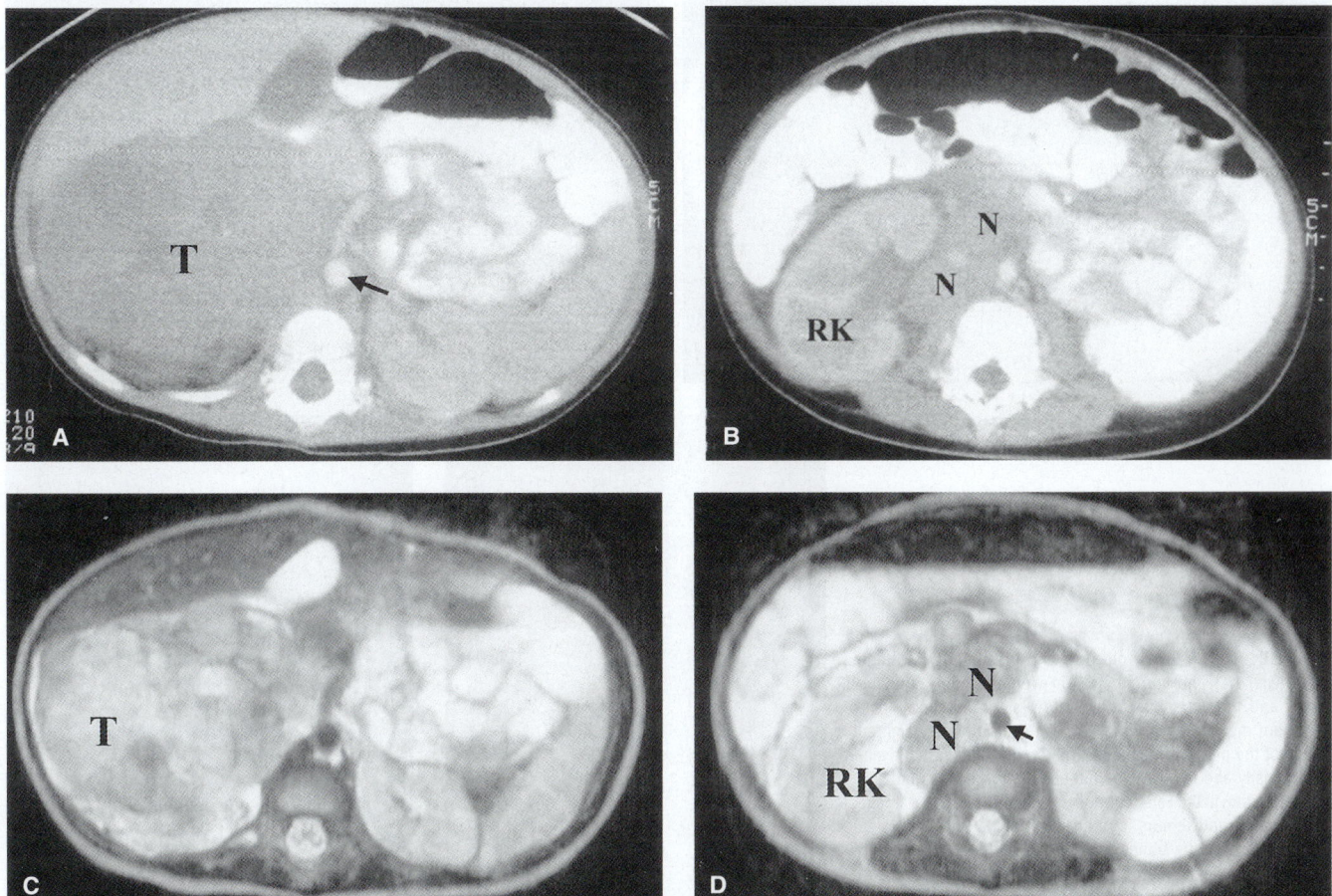

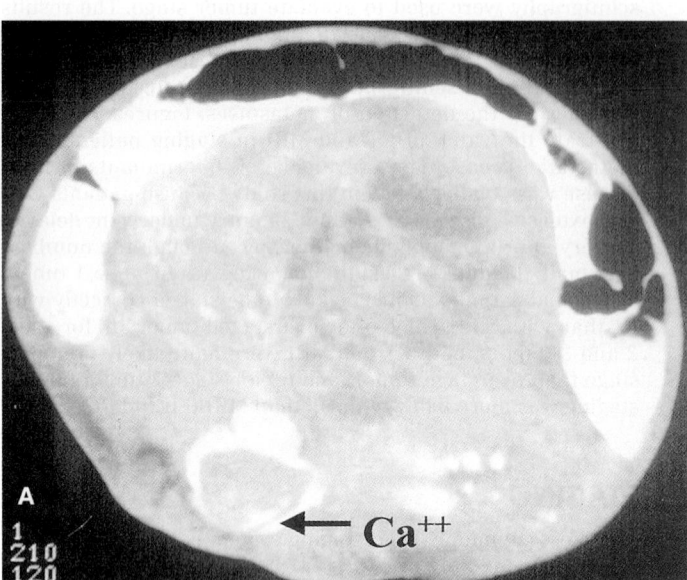

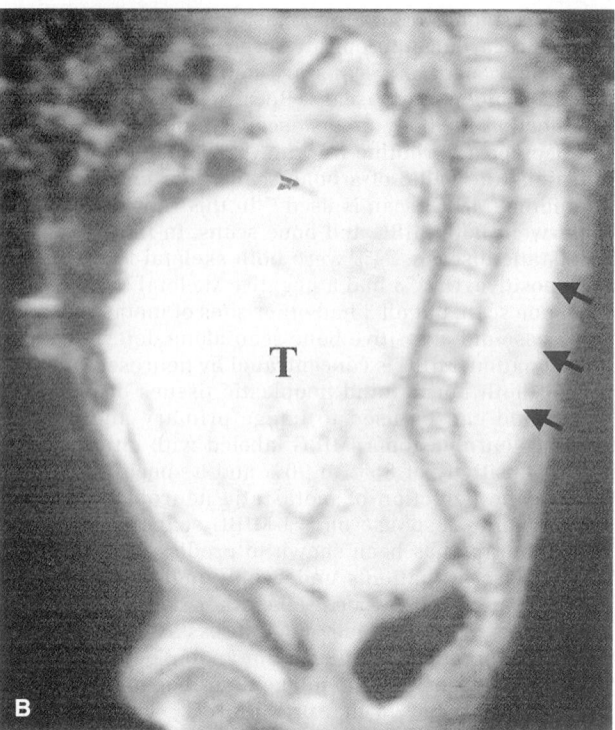

FIGURE 90.3. A 1-year-old child with constipation and a palpable mass, also noted to have lower leg weakness. **A:** Computed tomography shows a large soft tissue mass with calcifications and necrosis filling the retroperitoneum. Tumor calcification (*arrow*) is noted in the spinal cord. **B:** Sagittal, short tau inversion recovery image shows the large prevertebral mass (T) displacing bowel loops superiorly. Intraspinal tumor extends from the lower thoracic level through the lumbar level. The patient underwent emergent resection of the intraspinal tumor (*arrows*). (Courtesy of Dr. Marilyn Siegel, Mallinckrodt Institute of Radiology, St. Louis, MO.)

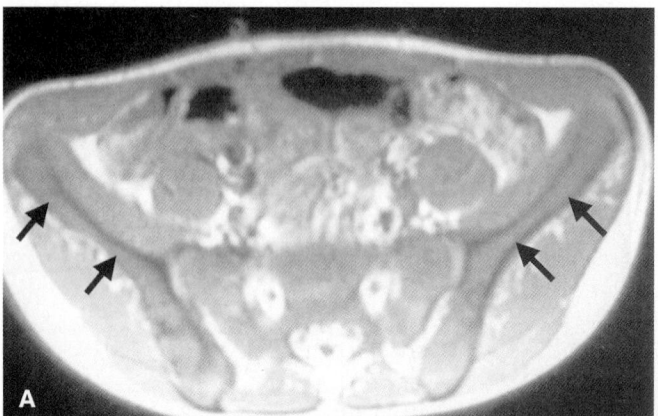

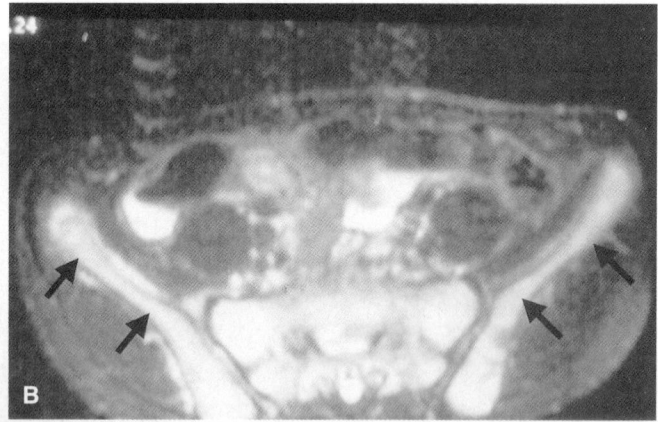

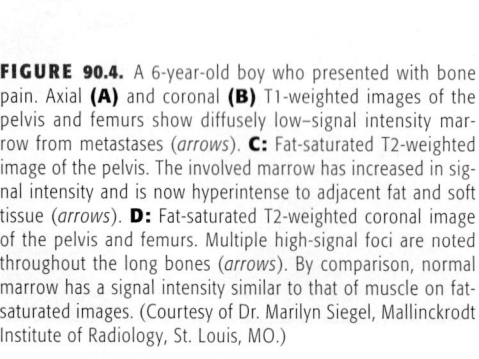

FIGURE 90.4. A 6-year-old boy who presented with bone pain. Axial **(A)** and coronal **(B)** T1-weighted images of the pelvis and femurs show diffusely low–signal intensity marrow from metastases (*arrows*). **C:** Fat-saturated T2-weighted image of the pelvis. The involved marrow has increased in signal intensity and is now hyperintense to adjacent fat and soft tissue (*arrows*). **D:** Fat-saturated T2-weighted coronal image of the pelvis and femurs. Multiple high-signal foci are noted throughout the long bones (*arrows*). By comparison, normal marrow has a signal intensity similar to that of muscle on fat-saturated images. (Courtesy of Dr. Marilyn Siegel, Mallinckrodt Institute of Radiology, St. Louis, MO.)

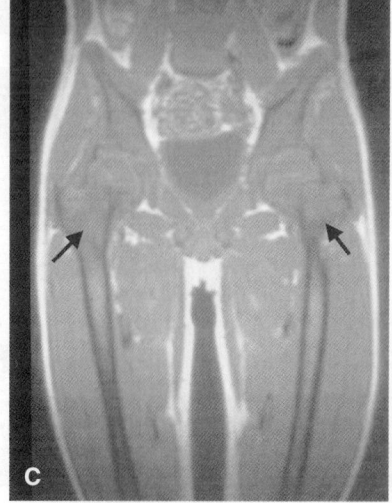

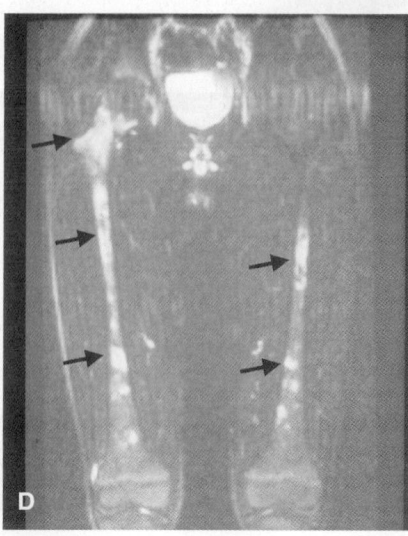

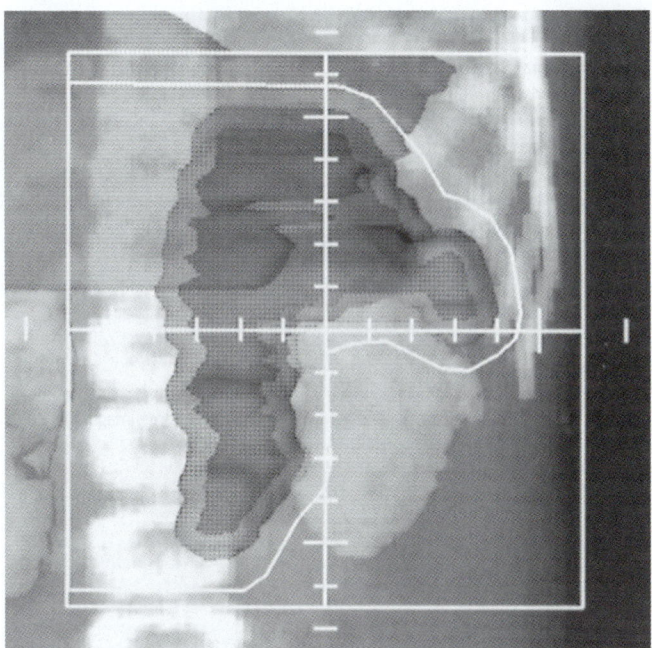

FIGURE 90.5. Radiation therapy treatment field for a child with a left adrenal primary neuroblastoma and para-aortic lymph node metastases. The beam's-eye–view display with a digital reconstructed radiograph allows for adequate coverage of the target volume and lymph node region with sparing of the ipsilateral kidney and liver while homogeneously irradiating the adjacent spine.

radiographic, and surgical findings.[23] The INSS integrates many of the concepts of previous staging systems promoted by the Children's Cancer Group (CCG) and Pediatric Oncology Group (POG)[24,25] and unifies them into a single system. Because the INSS is a postsurgical staging system, the International Neuroblastoma Risk Group (INRG) Classification System was established to stage patients before any treatment. The INRG staging system is based on clinical criteria and image-defined risk factors.[26] Each of these systems is summarized in Table 90.1.

PATHOLOGIC CLASSIFICATION

Neuroblastomas are derived from primitive neural crest cells arising from within sympathetic ganglia. Three types of tumors, representing different degrees of differentiation, are recognized. *Ganglioneuroma* consists of mature ganglion cells, Schwann cells, and nerve bundles and is benign in appearance and nature. It frequently is calcified and may represent a matured neuroblastoma.[26] Cases of maturation of proven neuroblastomas to ganglioneuromas, either spontaneously or after therapy, have been reported.[9] *Ganglioneuroblastoma* is the intermediate form between ganglioneuroma and neuroblastoma. Both mature ganglion cells and undifferentiated neuroblasts are evident.

Neuroblastoma is at the undifferentiated end of the spectrum of neural crest tumors. It is a small, round, blue cell tumor composed of dense nests of hyperchromatic cells. Homer Wright rosettes with a central fibrillary core can be present. Areas of necrosis, hemorrhage, and calcium are frequently present. Immunohistochemical stains may help distinguish neuroblastoma from other undifferentiated malignant neoplasms of childhood. Neuroblastoma characteristically stains positive for neurofilaments, neuron-specific enolase (NSE), synaptophysin, and chromogranin A and negative for muscle and leukocyte common antigens. The use of electron microscopy to demonstrate neurosecretory granules is required infrequently to establish the diagnosis.

A grading system has been proposed by Shimada et al.[27] and its significance has been confirmed by the CCG.[28,29] This clinicopathologic staging system evaluates tumor specimens for stromal development (i.e., stromal-rich and stromal-poor tumors), neuroblastic differentiation, and mitosis–karyorrhexis index of neuroblastic cells. These three histologic features and the patient's age at diagnosis divide children into favorable and unfavorable prognostic groups. The stroma-rich tumors are characterized by an extensive Schwann cell stroma. The well-differentiated stroma-rich tumors may correspond to ganglioneuroma, and the "inter-mixed" stroma-rich tumors may correspond to the ganglio-neuroblastomas. To be reliable, the Shimada classification requires pretreatment evaluation of the entire primary tumor specimen. However, primary tumors often are not completely resectable, or the presence of widespread metastases makes thorough tumor resection inappropriate before introduction of initial systemic therapy, thereby limiting the usefulness of this system.

PROGNOSTIC FACTORS

Patient age and stage at initial presentation remain the two most important factors that influence outcome (Table 90.2). In general, >75% of infants and children <2 years old survive, as do 90% to 100% of children with INSS stages 1 and 2.[30–40] The presence of tumor in regional lymph nodes is a poor prognostic factor and was recognized as such by the POG in their staging system.[41] Infants <12 months old with metastatic disease confined to the liver, bone marrow (not bone), or skin (stage IV-S) have a remarkably good prognosis; <75% of these children survive with little or no treatment.[8,42] Treatment should be directed at relief of the acute presenting event (often respiratory distress secondary to hepatomegaly), and the temptation to aggressively treat these patients in the absence of other bad prognostic factors should be avoided.

Patients with more differentiated tumors (e.g., ganglio-neuroma, ganglioneuroblastoma) fare better than do children with poorly differentiated or undifferentiated neuroblastomas. A favorable Shimada stage is associated with 90% survival, compared with 22% with unfavorable Shimada stages. Elevated serum ferritin (>142 ng/mL), NSE (>100 ng/mL), and LDH (>1,500 IU) are all associated with advanced disease and a poor prognosis.[32,43–46]

MYCN (N-*myc*) is a proto-oncogene that resides on the short arm of chromosome 2. An amplification of *MYCN* gene is associated with an extremely poor prognosis (5% survival).[46,47] *MYCN* amplification has been associated with the multidrug resistance gene, which may account for this tumor's notorious resistance to therapy.[48] A tumor with a DNA index of 1 (diploid or near-diploid) paradoxically gives a worse prognosis than tumors that are aneuploid.[49] Hyperdiploid tumors occur more often in lower stages and are associated with better chemotherapy responsiveness. Allelic loss of the short arm of chromosome 1 represents a loss of heterozygosity of a tumor suppressor gene and is also associated with a poor prognosis independent of age and stage. It reliably identifies patients with stage 1, 2, or 4S disease who have a high risk of relapse and require aggressive therapy.[50] Mutations in *ALK* (encoding anaplastic lymphoma kinase) have also been described in neuroblastoma and have been identified as the predisposition gene for familial neuroblastoma. About 14% of high-risk neuroblastoma will have somatic mutations in *ALK*.[51]

GENERAL MANAGEMENT

Because of the biologic heterogeneity of neuroblastoma, the following treatment recommendations should be considered as guidelines. The prognostic implications of a tumor's

TABLE 90.1 NEUROBLASTOMA STAGING SYSTEMS

Evans and D'Angio	Pediatric Oncology Group	International Staging System	International Neuroblastoma Risk Group
Stage I Tumor confined to the organ or structure of origin	**Stage A** Complete gross resection of primary tumor, with or without microscopic residual; intracavitary lymph nodes, not adhered to and removed with primary (nodes adhered to or within tumor resection may be positive for tumor without upstaging patient to stage C), histologically free of tumor; if primary in the abdomen or pelvis, liver histologically free of tumor	**Stage 1** Localized tumor with complete gross excision, without microscopic residual disease; representative ipsilateral lymph nodes negative for tumor microscopically (nodes attached to and removed with the primary tumor may be positive)	**L1** Localized tumor not involving vital structures as defined by the list of image-defined risk factors and confined to one body compartment
Stage II Tumor extending in continuity beyond the organ midline; regional lymph nodes on the ipsilateral side may be involved	**Stage B** Grossly unresected primary tumor; nodes and liver same as stage A	**Stage 2A** Localized tumor with incomplete gross excision; representative ipsilateral nonadherent lymph nodes negative for tumor microscopically	**L2** Locoregional tumor with presence of one or more image-defined factors
Stage III Tumor extending in continuity beyond the midline; regional lymph nodes may be involved bilaterally	**Stage C** Complete or incomplete resection of primary, intracavitary nodes not adhered to primary histologically positive for tumor; liver as in stage A	**Stage 2B** Localized tumor with or without complete gross excision, with ipsilateral nonadherent lymph nodes positive for tumor; enlarged contralateral lymph nodes must be negative microscopically	
Stage IV Remote disease involving skeleton, bone marrow, soft tissue, distant lymph node groups, etc. (see stage IV-S)	**Stage D** Any dissemination of disease beyond intracavitary nodes (i.e., extracavitary nodes, liver, skin, bone marrow, bone)	**Stage 3** Unresectable unilateral tumor infiltrating across the midline,[a] with or without regional lymph node involvement; or localized unilateral tumor with contralateral regional lymph node involvement; or midline tumor with bilateral extension by infiltration (unresectable) or by lymph node involvement	**M** Distant metastatic disease (except stage MS)
Stage IV-S Patients who would otherwise be stage I or II but who have remote disease confined to the liver, skin, or bone marrow (without radiographic evidence of bone metastases on complete skeletal survey)	**Stage DS** Infants <1 year of age with stage IV-S disease (see Evans and D'Angio)	**Stage 4** Any primary tumor with dissemination to distant lymph nodes, bone, bone marrow, liver, skin, and/or other organs (except as defined for stage 4S)	**MS** Metastatic disease in children younger than 18 months with metastasis confined to the skin, liver, and/or bone marrow
		Stage 4S Localized primary tumor as defined for stage 1, 2A, or 2B with dissemination limited to skin, liver, and/or bone marrow[b] (limited to infants <1 year of age)	

Multifocal primary tumors (e.g., bilateral adrenal primary tumors) should be staged according to the greatest extent of disease, as defined in the table, and followed by a subscript letter M (e.g., 3_M).
[a]The midline is defined as the vertebral column. Tumors originating on one side and crossing the midline must infiltrate to or beyond the opposite side of the vertebral column.
[b]Marrow involvement in stage 4S should be minimal, that is, <10% of total nucleated cells identified as malignant on bone marrow biopsy or on marrow aspirate. More extensive marrow involvement would be considered to be stage 4. The *meta*-iodobenzylguanidine scan (if performed) should be negative in the marrow.
Modified from Halperin EC, Constine LS, Tarbell NJ, et al., eds. *Pediatric radiation oncology.* 2nd ed. New York: Raven Press, 1994:171–214. With permission..

TABLE 90.2 PROGNOSTIC VARIABLES IN NEUROBLASTOMA

Prognostic Factor	Favorable	Unfavorable	Survival (%) Favorable	Survival (%) Unfavorable
Age	<2 y	>2 y	77	38
Stage	I, II, IV-S	III, IV	90–100	50, 30
Pathology (Shimada)	Favorable	Unfavorable	90	23
Ferritin	<143 ng/mL	>143 ng/mL	83	19
Neuron-specific enolase	<100	>100	79	10
Chromogranin	<190 ng/mL	>190 ng/mL	69	30
GD2 ganglioside	<103 pmol/mL	>568 pmol/mL	70	24
Urine VMA/HVA	<1	>1	84	44
gp 140TRK-A	High expression	Low expression	78	14
N-*myc*	Single copy	Amplified	70	5
DNA index	>1.1	1	100	10
1p deletion	No 1p deletion	1p deletion	90	10

HVA, homovanillic acid; VMA, vanillylmandelic acid.
Modified from Matthay KK. Neuroblastoma. A clinical challenge and biologic puzzle. *CA Cancer J Clin* 1995;45(3):179–192. Copyright © 1995 American Cancer Society. Reprinted by permission of John Wiley & Sons, Inc.

biologic indices, such as *MYCN* amplification and DNA index, may warrant more aggressive therapy in young patients with otherwise a favorable stage (Table 90.3).

Low-Risk Disease

Low-stage, resectable tumors (INSS stage 1, 2, or 3 with negative nodes) have an excellent prognosis after complete gross surgical excision. Adjuvant chemotherapy or irradiation has not improved the outcome in children with completely resected tumors with favorable biologic features.[38,52–54] Positive surgical margins or microscopic residual disease does not uniformly require more aggressive therapy. Patients with *MYCN* amplification or low DNA index may require adjuvant therapy and should be enrolled in clinical trials.[49]

Unresectable tumors that are otherwise of low stage (INSS stages 1 to 3 with negative lymph nodes) may require preoperative chemotherapy and occasionally radiation therapy to convert them into a resectable status. Second-look surgery is performed to remove a previously unresectable primary tumor and achieve a complete remission

TABLE 90.3 NEUROBLASTOMA RISK ASSESSMENT

Risk	Stage	Age	MYCN	Ploidy	Histology	Other
Low	1	Any	Any	Any	Any	
Low	2a/2b	Any	Nonamp	Any	Any	Resection ≥50%
Inter	2a/2b	Any	Nonamp	Any	Any	Resection <50%
Inter	2a/2b	Any	Nonamp	Any	Any	Biopsy only
	2a/2b	Any	Amp	Any	Any	Any degree of resection
Inter	3	<547 d	Nonamp	Any	Any	
Inter	3	≥547 d	Nonamp	Any	FH	
High	3	Any	Amp	Any	Any	
High	3	≥547 d	Nonamp	Any	UH	
High	4	<365 d	Amp	Any	Any	
Inter	4	<365d	Nonamp	Any	Any	
High	4	365 to <547 d	Amp	Any	Any	
High	4	365 to <547 d	Any	DI = 1	Any	
High	4	365 to <547 d	Any	Any	UH	
Inter	4	365 to <547 d	Nonamp	DI > 1	FH	
High	4	>547 d	Any	Any	Any	
Low	4s	<365 d	Nonamp	DI > 1	FH	Asymptomatic
Inter	4s	<365 d	Nonamp	DI = 1	Any	Asymptomatic or symptomatic
Inter	4s	<365 d	Missing	Missing	Missing	Too sick for biopsy
Inter	4s	<365 d	Nonamp	Any	Any	Symptomatic
Inter	4s	<365 d	Nonamp	Any	UH	Asymptomatic or symptomatic
High	4s	<365 d	Amp	Any	Any	Asymptomatic or symptomatic

amp, amplified; DI, DNA index; FH, favorable Shimada histology; UH, unfavorable Shimada histology.

after induction chemotherapy. Complete resection can be achieved in almost two-thirds of previously unresectable stage III to IV primary tumors.[55] The CCG reported that eventual complete resection of the primary tumor in advanced disease may have a favorable impact on outcome.[55] The benefit to complete resection in patients with advanced disease has not been uniformly established. Patients with biologically favorable tumors may be more amenable to surgery after chemotherapy, and the apparent benefit of complete resection may be a result of patient selection.[56] POG-8104 enrolled patients with INSS stage 1 (POG stage A) disease. In that trial, *MYCN* amplification and DNA index were not evaluated uniformly. Treatment was surgery only. Regardless of the presence of residual microscopic disease, the 2-year disease-free survival rate was 89%.[25] In the CCG experience (CCG trial 3881) with stage 1 disease, the 4-year event-free and overall survival rates for children treated initially with surgery alone were 93% and 99%, respectively. For patients with stage 2 disease, the event-free and overall survival rates were 81% and 98%, respectively. In that trial, only 13% of patients with stage 2 disease received any chemotherapy or radiotherapy, despite the fact that 104 patients had INSS stage 2b disease. The authors ascribe the favorable results to improved surgical management and better staging with MIBG scanning.[57]

Intermediate-Risk Disease
Locally advanced and regionally metastatic tumors (INSS stage 2b to 3 with positive lymph nodes) require more intensive therapy. Infants <1 year of age should undergo complete resection of the primary tumor and receive adjuvant chemotherapy.[56,58–60] In unresectable cases, chemotherapy may be administered at diagnosis followed by surgical resection after response to systemic treatment. In older children with lymph node metastases, adjuvant radiation therapy to the primary

and regional lymph nodes has improved the disease-free and overall survival rates. A prospective, randomized trial of postoperative chemotherapy or chemotherapy plus regional irradiation demonstrated 31% disease-free survival in children treated with chemotherapy, compared with 58% in those who also received radiation therapy.[61] However, the value of radiation therapy in intermediate-risk patients is not universally accepted. De Bernardi et al.[62] failed to demonstrate a benefit from the addition of radiotherapy in 29 children >1 year of age with postoperative residual tumor or positive regional lymph nodes. Children in that randomized study received two cycles of Peptichemio with or without radiation. Progression-free survival was 64% in the radiotherapy arm and 73% in the arm without radiotherapy.[62] Coupled with the risk of late effects from even moderate radiotherapy doses, this small trial provided an argument that systematic radiation therapy, even for POG stage C patients, may not be necessary. Current COG trials reflect this bias because the use of radiation therapy is decreasing.

Patients with intraspinal extension of neuroblastoma pose a unique problem. They frequently have severe neurologic compromise resulting from spinal cord compression. Historically, these patients were treated with laminectomy and surgical debulking with or without radiation therapy and chemotherapy.[63] Because the morbidity of this approach is significant, with a high rate of spinal growth deformity, a number of investigators have proceeded with treatment of these patients using primary chemotherapy.[55] A prospective series of 42 patients treated with primary chemotherapy demonstrated a 92% improvement in neurologic deficits, allowing children to avoid neurosurgical decompression in >60% of cases when receiving courses of carboplatin and etoposide alternating with cyclophosphamide, vincristine, and doxorubicin.

The POG experience (POG trials 8742 and 9244) with stages 2b to 3 disease demonstrates an 85% event-free survival with completely resected tumors at diagnosis, compared to 70% with incomplete resection at diagnosis (P = .259). In both of these studies, patients underwent maximum safe tumor resection followed by five courses of induction chemotherapy. In POG-8742, they received cis-platinum and etoposide alternating with cyclophosphamide and doxorubicin. In POG-9244, they received alternating cycles of vincristine, cis-platinum, etoposide, and cyclophosphamide (OPEC) and vincristine, carboplatin, etoposide, and cyclophosphamide. After second-look surgery, the same chemotherapy was given as maintenance. Radiotherapy was given to patients with viable residual tumor discovered at the time of the second-look operation. Children age 12 to 24 months at the time of radiation therapy received 24 Gy in 1.5-Gy fractions to the primary tumor site. Older children received 30 Gy in 1.5-Gy fractions. Of the 37 patients on these two protocols who survived "event free," 11 (30%) received radiotherapy. Patients with favorable Shimada histology tumors had a 92% event-free survival, compared with 58% with unfavorable tumors (P = .009). Patients with *MYCN* amplification did poorly, with outcomes comparable to those for stage D patients.[27]

Based on CCG and POG data, patients with intermediate-risk neuroblastoma have an estimated 3-year survival of between 75% and 98%. Cyclophosphamide, doxorubicin, carboplatin, and etoposide are the four most active agents.[64–66] Surgery plays a critical role in the primary management of neuroblastoma. The goals of surgery are to establish a diagnosis; provide tissue for evaluation of prognostic biologic markers; stage the disease according to INSS criteria; and attempt to totally excise the primary, if feasible. The extent of surgery has an important impact on outcome. O'Neill et al.[67] reported that 55 of 59 patients with a complete or near-complete resection were alive and free of disease 2 years after surgery, compared to only 13 of 24 cases with a subtotal resection.

Just as Haase had reported, Grosfeld and Baehner[34] found evidence for improved outcome in stage 4 patients attaining complete resection of primary tumor at delayed second-look procedures.

High-Risk Disease

The majority of patients with neuroblastoma present with metastatic disease. Many clinical trials have sought to intensify treatment of metastatic neuroblastoma through the use of high-dose myeloablative chemotherapy with stem cell rescue or bone marrow transplantation (BMT). The French Lyon-Marseille-Curie East group reported a 40% progression-free survival at 2 years and 20% at 5 years in 62 patients proceeding to autologous bone marrow transplant (ABMT).[68] The CCG reported a 43% 2-year event-free survival in 43 children undergoing consolidation melphalan, cisplatin, teniposide, doxorubicin, and total-body irradiation (TBI) to 10 Gy in 3 fractions of 3.3 Gy/day. The toxic death rate was 22%.[69] Australian investigators tested a less intense preparative regimen with a TBI regimen consisting of 12 Gy in 6 twice-daily fractions.[70] Of 28 patients registered, 19 achieved complete remission after induction chemotherapy. Seventeen of these nineteen patients underwent ABMT and fifteen (87%) remained free of disease at 5 years from ABMT. Of the 28 patients registered, 50% have survived 5 years.

Uncertain that ABMT could be studied successfully in a cooperative group, the CCG conducted two pilot studies for children with stage 4 disease. In CCG-321, patients received induction chemotherapy consisting of cisplatin, etoposide, doxorubicin, and cyclophosphamide. Of 207 patients, 159 remained disease free during induction chemotherapy. Of these patients, 67 received myeloablative chemotherapy and ABMT, whereas 74 continued conventional chemotherapy for a total of 13 cycles. The patients receiving the ABMT had a higher event-free survival than patients continuing standard chemotherapy (40% vs. 19%, $P = .019$).[71] Because they are not randomized trials, these studies potentially may have allowed a biased allocation of patients to one arm based on clinical concerns or prognostic risk factors. The POG failed to show a benefit to BMT in high-risk metastatic neuroblastoma (POG 8340).[45]

The European Neuroblastoma Study Group studied the role of consolidative ABMT with high-dose melphalan versus no further treatment following induction chemotherapy with the OPEC regimen in patients with stage 3 and 4 diseases.[72,73] With a median follow-up of 14.3 years for surviving children, they report an improvement in event-free survival (38% vs. 27%) and overall survival (47% and 30%) for the high-dose melphalan arm, but these differences did not reach statistical significance. The subset of patients with stage IV disease who were >1 year of age, however, did show statistically significant improvement in event-free survival (33% vs. 17%, $P = .01$) and overall survival (46% vs. 21%, $P = .03$).

The CCG conducted a randomized trial comparing continued chemotherapy with myeloablative therapy (including 10 Gy TBI in 3 daily fractions) and ABMT in children with high-risk neuroblastoma. All patients received radiation therapy to the primary site and select metastatic sites. A second randomization following cytotoxic therapy included 6 cycles of 13-*cis*-retinoic acid or no further therapy. Initial results demonstrated an event-free survival advantage to both BMT and 13-*cis*-retinoic acid therapy, but no overall survival advantage.[74] However, after a median follow-up of more than 7 years, a statistically significant advantage to overall survival was demonstrated for the cohort treated with both myeloablative therapy and 13-*cis*-retinoic acid therapy.[75]

Berthold et al.[76] in Germany reported results of a prospective, randomized trial in children with high-risk neuroblastoma comparing myeloablative therapy with melphalan, etoposide, and carboplatin and autologous stem cell rescue

with maintenance chemotherapy with cyclophosphamide. When analyzed as-treated, statistically significantly improved 3-year event-free survival (53% vs. 30%) and overall survival (68% vs. 53%) were seen with myeloablative therapy.

Immunotherapy with ch14.18, a monoclonal antibody against tumor-associated disialoganglioside GD2, has been shown to have activity against neuroblastoma. A randomized trial comparing 6 cycles of isotretinoin versus immunotherapy (6 cycles of isotretinoin and 5 concomitant cycles of ch14.18 in combination of alternating GM-CSF and interleukin-2) resulted in a 2-year event-free survival (47% vs. 67%) and 2-year overall survival (76% vs. 86%) with the use of immunotherapy.[77]

A recent trial compared single autologous stem cell transplant (ASCT) with carboplatin, etoposide, and melphalan (CEM) or tandem ASCT with thiotepa, cyclophosphamide ACST followed by a modified CEM regimen. For single and tandem transplant without immunotherapy, there was improvement in 3-year event-free survival (49% vs. 62%). For single and tandem transplant with immunotherapy, there was improvement in 3-year event-free survival (55% vs. 74%) and 3-year overall survival (76% vs. 86%).[78]

Local control of the primary tumor in stage 4 neuroblastoma is an important element of patient management. The role of surgical resection in metastatic disease remains controversial. Many authors have reported more favorable outcome in patients undergoing complete resection.[79] There is a strong association between chemotherapy dose intensity and surgical resectability, which reduces the significance of aggressive resection as an independent favorable factor. It can be assumed that tumors that are amenable to resection may have an inherently less aggressive biology.

In the CCG-321-P3 pilot, there was a 33% rate of local relapse in patients not undergoing a complete resection at their initial surgery, irrespective of their ultimate surgical resection status, including second-look operations.[80] This high local failure rate suggests that there is a role for local radiation therapy. In that pilot study, patients received radiotherapy only if they had gross residual disease after second-look surgery. Although the local control in patients receiving radiotherapy was the same as in unirradiated patients, one should note that only patients with gross residual disease received this local treatment, suggesting that the radiotherapy (RT) was beneficial.

In a reanalysis of CCG-3891, Hass-Kogan et al.[81] compared locoregional control rates in patients on the non-ABMT arm who received 10 to 20 Gy to gross residual disease after induction therapy to patients in the ABMT arm who received similar RT to residual disease but also received 10-Gy TBI in 3.33-Gy daily fractions in their conditioning regimen The patients in the ABMT arm had a lower locoregional recurrence rate (33% vs. 51%, $P = .004$). Although this effect may be due to the higher dose of RT delivered in this group of patients, it is not possible to separate the RT effect from that of the more intense systemic therapy also given to these patients in the ABMT arm.

Laprie et al.[82] analyzed locoregional control in MYCN-amplified INSS stage 2 and 3 patients treated with different regimens over different eras. Their approach varied from conventional chemotherapy and RT only to gross residual disease after surgery in patients >1 year of age, to high-dose chemotherapy with ABMT, to local radiation therapy to all patients. They noted an improvement in event-free survival with ABMT and RT (83% vs. 25%, $P = .001$). Again, conclusions regarding the effect of RT independent of the intensified systemic therapy are difficult to make because this was not a randomized comparison.

Multiple studies have shown that locoregional control rates with RT for high-risk neuroblastoma range from 84% to 100%, utilizing doses of 21 to 24 Gy.[83-85] For patients who have an incomplete resection, it is unclear whether a higher dose of RT is warranted. Some studies show a worse local control rate with 21 to 21.6 Gy for patients with gross disease at the primary site. A German trial showed better event-free survival and locoregional progression-free survival for patients receiving RT; in this study, a subset of patients who had subtotal resection received a median dose of 36 Gy, whereas others including those who had gross total resection did not receive RT[86]

Local therapy to the primary tumor and metastatic sites may be beneficial in the curative therapy of children with disseminated disease. Surgical resection of the primary tumor has been associated with improved survival and local control after aggressive systemic therapy.[55,80] There is a predilection for recurrence in previous sites of disease, and it is conceivable that additional local therapy with irradiation to the primary tumor site and distant metastases may enhance tumor control and cure rates.[80,84,87] Currently, patients with MIBG-avid metastatic sites after induction chemotherapy and surgery are treated with RT to 21.6 Gy. In one study, children with two or more postinduction MIBG-avid sites have a worse progression-free and overall survival despite RT to sites of persistent distant metastasis.[84]

Radiation therapy plays an extremely important role in the palliative management of patients with end-stage symptomatic neuroblastoma. Pain from bone or other visceral metastases often can be relieved with external beam radiation therapy. Mass effect from a rapidly enlarging tumor can respond dramatically to radiation therapy. In a series of 10 patients treated at Duke University Medical Center, Halperin[88] reported 7 complete responses to radiation therapy, either alone or in conjunction with chemotherapy. Radiation doses ranged from 4 to 24.4 Gy at a rate of 1 to 1.5 Gy/fraction. The seven patients with complete response survived without recurrence.

Systemic radionuclide therapy with ^{131}I-MIBG has been tested in several European and US centers with early encouraging results. This radioactive agent produced objective responses in previously treated and chemoresistant stage 4 neuroblastoma.[89,90] These early positive results prompted some investigators to test this agent in previously untreated metastatic neuroblastoma. De Kraker et al.[91] reported that a combination of ^{131}I-MIBG and second-look surgery produced response rates comparable to those of multidrug chemotherapy. Preliminary research on the combination of ^{131}I-MIBG with systemic chemotherapy and/or TBI with BMT demonstrated that this is a safe treatment and worthy of more investigation.[92-94]

The current approach by the Children's Oncology Group for patients with high-risk disease is to combine induction chemotherapy, surgical resection, autologous stem cell rescue, and radiation therapy to the primary site and select metastatic sites13-*cis*-retinoic acid and immunotherapy in an attempt to improve outcome in these patients. The current protocol utilizes a higher radiation total dose of 36 Gy for patients with gross residual disease at their primary sites.

RADIATION THERAPY TECHNIQUES: TREATMENT PLANNING AND FIELD DESIGN

Treatment of children with neuroblastoma can be challenging because of their young age and immature tissues. Most tumors will be located in the abdomen with the kidneys, liver, and spine as the usual dose-limiting organs. AP/PA fields have been previously recommended for well-lateralized lesions because of lower dose to the contralateral kidney and more homogeneous dose to the spine, whereas intensity-modulated radiation therapy (IMRT) may be more advantageous for

midline tumors.[95] Recently, proton therapy has been used and may have a dosimetric advantage to minimize dose to anterior structures beyond the retroperitoneum and posterior mediastinum.[96]

When defining the volume for the tumor bed, the postinduction chemotherapy, preoperative CT, or MRI scan is used for tumor volume delineation. Unlike other pediatric solid tumors, the initial tumor volume tumor bed is not treated with RT. The clinical target volume (CTV) is the tumor bed and residual tumor with a 1- to 1.5-cm margin, with attention to anatomic barriers of spread. A planning target volume of 0.5 cm may be used depending on the institutional experience. The CTV and PTV are typically treated to 21.6 Gy in 12 fractions. The question of whether a higher dose is needed for patients with residual tumor is currently being investigated in COG ANBL12P1 study where patients with residual disease receive a boost of 14.4 Gy in 8 fractions to the residual tumor with a 1-cm margin (CTV boost). An additional margin of 0.5 to 1 cm beyond the CTV boost is used for the PTV boost.

Persistent activity in metastatic sites after induction therapy can be treated with radiotherapy as long as the patient can tolerate the treatment. The dose is 21.6 Gy in 12 fractions over 2.4 weeks and follows the same CTV and PTV guidelines for the primary site.

Low-dose TBI has been used with variable success in the curative management of children with metastatic neuroblastoma.[97,98] In the past, TBI was part of the preparative regimen for patients undergoing BMT for high-risk metastatic disease. The patterns of failure in high-risk neuroblastoma were analyzed by Li and colleagues.[99] In this multi-institutional report, patients who had TBI were less likely to have relapse in prior sites of disease compared to those who did not have TBI. The authors conclude that radiopharmaceutical therapies may be helpful and needs to be further investigated.

Other investigators have used intraoperative radiation therapy (IORT) in patients with high-risk neuroblastoma. Haas-Kogan[100] described the results of IORT in 23 patients with high-risk disease. A single fraction of 7 to 16 Gy (median 10 Gy) to the primary tumor bed was associated with a local control rate of 100% in patients who had gross total resection, whereas IORT was unable to control any patients with gross residual disease.

Radiotherapy can also be used for palliation of painful and/or enlarging bone and soft tissue metastasis[35,101,102] with about two-thirds or more of patients having symptomatic response. Low-dose, short-fractionation schedules are appropriate if the child is not expected to live beyond 6 to 12 months. In these instances, minimizing a child's visits to the radiation therapy facility while rapidly relieving symptoms is a worthwhile goal. If the likelihood of long survival is small, 5 to 20 Gy in 1- to 5-daily fractions can allow rapid palliation.

RESULTS OF THERAPY

Low-Risk Disease

Survival rates after surgery alone of 85% to 90% or better can be expected.[25,52,53,57] Additional therapy usually is not indicated unless unfavorable biologic features are present.

Intermediate-Risk Disease

Children with large, initially unresectable tumors often respond to primary chemotherapy with combinations of drugs, including cyclophosphamide, vincristine, cisplatin, etoposide, doxorubicin, or teniposide. Children with unresponsive, unresectable gross residual disease may require external beam irradiation. Frequently, these children can undergo resection of the tumor at a second-look operation[55] and achieve a survival rate of 60% to 90%.[54]

High-Risk Disease

Children >1 year of age with metastatic neuroblastoma continue to have an unfavorable prognosis, with expected 3- or 4-year survival rates of 30%. For patients who have not progressed after induction therapy and surgery, tandem transplant with immunotherapy was associated with 3-year EFS of 74% and 3-year overall survival of 86%.[78]

Infants with metastatic disease confined to the liver, skin, and bone marrow have a uniquely favorable outcome. In stage 4S, survival rates can be as high as 75% to 90%.[60,103,104] In these patients, the goal of therapy should be limited to the relief of acute presenting symptoms. Halperin[88] reported 7 complete responses to hepatic radiation in 10 infants with symptomatic liver metastases. All 7 of these children survived. The recommended dose for symptomatic liver metastasis is 4.5 to 6 Gy in 3 to 4 fractions.

SEQUELAE OF TREATMENT

Early Complications

Acute side effects of radiation therapy depend on tumor site and fields of treatment. The short-term effects are those that can be expected for any patient receiving radiation therapy. Acute effects, especially skin reactions and mucositis, may be enhanced if concurrent chemotherapy or a hyperfractionated irradiation schedule is used.

Late Effects

Long-term effects depend on the site irradiated and the total dose of both radiation and chemotherapy agents used. Age at the time of treatment may influence the risk and severity of skeletal anomalies,[105] which may include spinal deformities such as kyphosis, scoliosis, or limb shortening. Generally, younger children are more prone to late radiation injury than older children. In one study, children irradiated at <6 months have more musculoskeletal abnormalities.[106] Both laminectomy and RT dose >17.5 Gy were risk factors for development of scoliosis in children with abdominal neuroblastoma.[105] A report from Memorial Sloan Kettering Cancer Center showed no cases of chronic renal insufficiency in 266 patients treated with techniques minimizing RT dose to bilateral kidneys.[107] A report from the Childhood Cancer Survivor Study showed the 20-year cumulative incidences of neurologic, sensory, endocrine, and musculoskeletal toxicities were 29.8%, 8.6%, 8.3%, and 7.8%. The cumulative incidence of secondary malignancies was 3.5% at 25 years after diagnosis.[108]

REFERENCES

1. Woods WG, et al. Screening for neuroblastoma in North America. 2-year results from the Quebec Project. *Am J Pediatr Hematol Oncol* 1992;14(4):312–319.
2. Schilling FH, et al. Population-based and controlled study to evaluate neuroblastoma screening at one year of age in Germany: interim results. *Med Pediatr Oncol* 2000;35(6):701–704.
3. Schilling FH, et al. Neuroblastoma screening at one year of age. *N Engl J Med* 2002;346(14):1047–1053.
4. Woods WG, et al. Screening of infants and mortality due to neuroblastoma. *N Engl J Med* 2002;346(14):1041–1046.
5. Yamamoto K. et al. Marginal decrease in mortality and marked increase in incidence as a result of neuroblastoma screening at 6 months of age: cohort study in seven prefectures in Japan. *J Clin Oncol* 2002;20(5):1209–1214.
6. Murphy SB, et al. Do children benefit from mass screening for neuroblastoma? Consensus Statement from the American Cancer Society Workshop on Neuroblastoma Screening. *Lancet* 1991;337(8737):344–346.
7. Yamamoto K, et al. Mass screening and age-specific incidence of neuroblastoma in Saitama Prefecture. *J Clin Oncol* 1995;13(8):2033–2038.
8. Evans AE, et al. A review of 17 IV-S neuroblastoma patients at the Children's Hospital of Philadelphia. *Cancer* 1980;45(5):833–839.
9. Everson T, Cole W. *Spontaneous regression of cancer.* 1st ed. Philadelphia, PA: WB Saunders, 1966.
10. Beckwith JB, Perrin EV. In situ neuroblastomas: a contribution to the natural history of neural crest tumors. *Am J Pathol* 1963;43:1089–1104.
11. Bray PF, et al. The coincidence of neuroblastoma and acute cerebellar encephalopathy. *Trans Am Neurol Assoc* 1969;94:106–109.
12. Pranzatelli MR. The neurobiology of the opsoclonus–myoclonus syndrome. *Clin Neuropharmacol* 1992;15(3):186–228.
13. Boechat MI, et al. Computed tomography in stage III neuroblastoma. *AJR Am J Roentgenol* 1985;145(6):1283–1287.
14. Couanet D, et al. Bone marrow metastases in children's neuroblastoma studied by magnetic resonance imaging. *Prog Clin Biol Res* 1988;271:547–555.
15. Fletcher BD, et al. Abdominal neuroblastoma: magnetic resonance imaging and tissue characterization. *Radiology* 1985;155(3):699–703.
16. Petrus LV, et al. The pediatric patient with suspected adrenal neoplasm: which radiological test to use? *Med Pediatr Oncol* 1992;20(1):53–57.
17. Siegel MJ, et al. MR imaging of intraspinal extension of neuroblastoma. *J Comput Assist Tomogr* 1986;10(4):593–595.
18. Gauguet JM, et al. Evaluation of the utility of (99m) Tc-MDP bone scintigraphy versus MIBG scintigraphy and cross-sectional imaging for staging patients with neuroblastoma. *Pediatr Blood Cancer* 2017;64(11).
19. Shapiro B. Imaging of catecholamine-secreting tumours: uses of MIBG in diagnosis and treatment. *Baillieres Clin Endocrinol Metab* 1993;7(2):491–507.
20. Katzenstein HM, et al. Scintigraphic response by 123I-metaiodobenzylguanidine scan correlates with event-free survival in high-risk neuroblastoma. *J Clin Oncol* 2004;22(19):3909–3915.
21. O'Dorisio MS, Hauger M, Cecalupo AJ. Somatostatin receptors in neuroblastoma: diagnostic and therapeutic implications. *Semin Oncol* 1994;21(5 Suppl 13):33–37.
22. Moertel CL, et al. Expression of somatostatin receptors in childhood neuroblastoma. *Am J Clin Pathol* 1994;102(6):752–756.
23. Brodeur GM, et al. International criteria for diagnosis, staging, and response to treatment in patients with neuroblastoma. *J Clin Oncol* 1988;6(12):1874–1881.
24. Evans AE, D'Angio GJ, Randolph J. A proposed staging for children with neuroblastoma. Children's cancer study group A. *Cancer* 1971;27(2):374–378.
25. Nitschke R, et al. Localized neuroblastoma treated by surgery: a Pediatric Oncology Group Study. *J Clin Oncol* 1988;6(8):1271–1279.
26. Monclair T, et al. The International Neuroblastoma Risk Group (INRG) staging system: an INRG Task Force report. *J Clin Oncol* 2009;27(2):298–303.
27. Shimada H, et al. Histopathologic prognostic factors in neuroblastic tumors: definition of subtypes of ganglioneuroblastoma and an age-linked classification of neuroblastomas. *J Natl Cancer Inst* 1984;73(2):405–416.
28. Chatten J, et al. Prognostic value of histopathology in advanced neuroblastoma: a report from the Childrens Cancer Study Group. *Hum Pathol* 1988;19(10):1187–1198.
29. Jacobson GM, Sause WT, O'Brien RT. Dose response analysis of pediatric neuroblastoma to megavoltage radiation. *Am J Clin Oncol* 1984;7(6):693–697.
30. Carlsen NL, et al. Prognostic factors in neuroblastomas treated in Denmark from 1943 to 1980. A statistical estimate of prognosis based on 253 cases. *Cancer* 1986;58(12):2726–2735.
31. Coldman AJ, et al. Neuroblastoma: influence of age at diagnosis, stage, tumor site, and sex on prognosis. *Cancer* 1980;46(8):1896–1901.
32. Evans AE, et al. Prognostic factor in neuroblastoma. *Cancer* 1987;59(11):1853–1859.
33. Evans AE, et al. A comparison of four staging systems for localized and regional neuroblastoma: a report from the Childrens Cancer Study Group. *J Clin Oncol* 1990;8(4):678–688.
34. Grosfeld JL, Baehner RL. Neuroblastoma: an analysis of 160 cases. *World J Surg* 1980;4(1):29–37.
35. Halperin EC, Cox EB. Radiation therapy in the management of neuroblastoma: the Duke University Medical Center experience 1967-1984. *Int J Radiat Oncol Biol Phys* 1986;12(10):1829–1837.
36. Hayes FA, Green AA. Neuroblastoma. *Pediatr Ann* 1983;12(5):366–367, 370–373.
37. Hayes FA, et al. Chemotherapy as an alternative to laminectomy and radiation in the management of epidural tumor. *J Pediatr* 1984;104(2):221–224.
38. Ninane J, Wese FX. Treatment of localized neuroblastoma. *Am J Pediatr Hematol Oncol* 1986;8(3):248–252.
39. Rosen EM, et al. Neuroblastoma: the Joint Center for Radiation Therapy/Dana-Farber Cancer Institute/Children's Hospital experience. *J Clin Oncol* 1984;2(7):719–732.
40. Simone JV. The treatment of neuroblastoma. *J Clin Oncol* 1984;2(7):717–718.
41. Hayes FA, et al. Surgicopathologic staging of neuroblastoma: prognostic significance of regional lymph node metastases. *J Pediatr* 1983;102(1):59–62.
42. Evans AE, Baum E, Chard R. Do infants with stage IV-S neuroblastoma need treatment? *Arch Dis Child* 1981;56(4):271–274.
43. Berthold F, et al. Prognostic factors in metastatic neuroblastoma. A multivariate analysis of 182 cases. *Am J Pediatr Hematol Oncol* 1992;14(3):207–215.
44. Brodeur G, Castleberry R. Neuroblastoma. In: Pizzo P, Polplack D, eds. *Principles and practice of pediatric oncology.* Philadelphia, PA: Lippincott Williams & Wilkins, 1993.
45. Shuster JJ, et al. Serum lactate dehydrogenase in childhood neuroblastoma. A Pediatric Oncology Group recursive partitioning study. *Am J Clin Oncol* 1992;15(4):295–303.
46. Seeger RC, et al. Association of multiple copies of the N-myc oncogene with rapid progression of neuroblastomas. *N Engl J Med* 1985;313(18):1111–1116.
47. Brodeur GM, et al. Amplification of N-myc in untreated human neuroblastomas correlates with advanced disease stage. *Science* 1984;224(4653):1121–1124.
48. Norris MD, et al. Expression of the gene for multidrug-resistance-associated protein and outcome in patients with neuroblastoma. *N Engl J Med* 1996;334(4):231–238.
49. Look AT, et al. Clinical relevance of tumor cell ploidy and N-myc gene amplification in childhood neuroblastoma: a Pediatric Oncology Group study. *J Clin Oncol* 1991;9(4):581–591.

50. Caron H, et al. Allelic loss of chromosome 1p as a predictor of unfavorable outcome in patients with neuroblastoma. *N Engl J Med* 1996. 334(4):225–230.

51. Bresler SC, et al. ALK mutations confer differential oncogenic activation and sensitivity to ALK inhibition therapy in neuroblastoma. *Cancer Cell* 2014;26(5):682–694.

52. Kushner BH, et al. International neuroblastoma staging system stage 1 neuroblastoma: a prospective study and literature review. *J Clin Oncol* 1996;14(7):2174–2180.

53. Matthay KK, et al. Excellent outcome of stage II neuroblastoma is independent of residual disease and radiation therapy. *J Clin Oncol* 1989;7(2):236–244.

54. Nitschke R, et al. Postoperative treatment of nonmetastatic visible residual neuroblastoma: a Pediatric Oncology Group study. *J Clin Oncol* 1991;9(7):1181–1188.

55. Haase GM, et al. Aggressive surgery combined with intensive chemotherapy improves survival in poor-risk neuroblastoma. *J Pediatr Surg* 1991;26(9):1119–1123; discussion 1123–4.

56. Shorter NA, et al. The role of surgery in the management of stage IV neuroblastoma: a single institution study. *Med Pediatr Oncol* 1995;24(5):287–291.

57. Perez CA, et al. Biologic variables in the outcome of stages I and II neuroblastoma treated with surgery as primary therapy: a children's cancer group study. *J Clin Oncol* 2000;18(1):18–26.

58. Bowman LC, et al. Impact of intensified therapy on clinical outcome in infants and children with neuroblastoma. The St Jude Children's Research Hospital experience, 1962 to 1988. *J Clin Oncol* 1991;9(9):1599–1608.

59. Castleberry RP, et al. Infants with neuroblastoma and regional lymph node metastases have a favorable outlook after limited postoperative chemotherapy: a Pediatric Oncology Group study. *J Clin Oncol* 1992;10(8):1299–1304.

60. Guglielmi M, et al. Resection of primary tumor at diagnosis in stage IV-S neuroblastoma: does it affect the clinical course? *J Clin Oncol* 1996;14(5):1537–1544.

61. Castleberry RP, et al. Radiotherapy improves the outlook for patients older than 1 year with Pediatric Oncology Group stage C neuroblastoma. *J Clin Oncol* 1991;9(5):789–795.

62. de Bernardi B, et al. Localized neuroblastoma. Surgical and pathologic staging. *Cancer* 1987;60(5):1066–1072.

63. Plantaz D, et al. The treatment of neuroblastoma with intraspinal extension with chemotherapy followed by surgical removal of residual disease. A prospective study of 42 patients—results of the NBL 90 Study of the French Society of Pediatric Oncology. *Cancer* 1996;78(2):311–319.

64. Castleberry RP, et al. Phase II investigational window using carboplatin, iproplatin, ifosfamide, and epirubicin in children with untreated disseminated neuroblastoma: a Pediatric Oncology Group study. *J Clin Oncol* 1994;12(8):1616–1620.

65. Ettinger LJ, et al. A phase II study of carboplatin in children with recurrent or progressive solid tumors. A report from the Childrens Cancer Group. *Cancer* 1994;73(4):1297–1301.

66. Philip T, et al. Phase II studies of combinations of drugs with high dose carboplatin in neuroblastoma (800 mg/m² to 1 g 250/m²): a report from the LMCE group. *Prog Clin Biol Res* 1988;271:573–582.

67. O'Neill JA, et al. The role of surgery in localized neuroblastoma. *J Pediatr Surg* 1985;20(6):708–712.

68. Philip T, et al. Improved survival at 2 and 5 years in the LMCE1 unselected group of 72 children with stage IV neuroblastoma older than 1 year of age at diagnosis: is cure possible in a small subgroup? *J Clin Oncol* 1991;9(6):1037–1044.

69. Seeger RC, et al. Intensive chemoradiotherapy and autologous bone marrow transplantation for poor prognosis neuroblastoma. *Prog Clin Biol Res* 1991;366:527–533.

70. McCowage GB, et al. Autologous bone marrow transplantation for advanced neuroblastoma using teniposide, doxorubicin, melphalan, cisplatin, and total-body irradiation. *J Clin Oncol* 1995;13(11):2789–2795.

71. Stram DO, et al. Consolidation chemoradiotherapy and autologous bone marrow transplantation versus continued chemotherapy for metastatic neuroblastoma: a report of two concurrent Children's Cancer Group studies. *J Clin Oncol* 1996;14(9):2417–2426.

72. Pinkerton CR. ENSG 1-randomised study of high-dose melphalan in neuroblastoma. *Bone Marrow Transplant* 1991;7(Suppl 3):112–113.

73. Pritchard J, et al. High dose melphalan in the treatment of advanced neuroblastoma: results of a randomised trial (ENSG-1) by the European Neuroblastoma Study Group. *Pediatr Blood Cancer* 2005;44(4):348–357.

74. Matthay KK, et al. Treatment of high-risk neuroblastoma with intensive chemotherapy, radiotherapy, autologous bone marrow transplantation, and 13-cis-retinoic acid. Children's Cancer Group. *N Engl J Med* 1999;341(16):1165–1173.

75. Matthay KK, et al. Long-term results for children with high-risk neuroblastoma treated on a randomized trial of myeloablative therapy followed by 13-cis-retinoic acid: a children's oncology group study. *J Clin Oncol* 2009;27(7):1007–1013.

76. Berthold F, et al. Myeloablative megatherapy with autologous stem-cell rescue versus oral maintenance chemotherapy as consolidation treatment in patients with high-risk neuroblastoma: a randomised controlled trial. *Lancet Oncol* 2005;6(9):649–658.

77. Yu AL, et al. Anti-GD2 antibody with GM-CSF, interleukin-2, and isotretinoin for neuroblastoma. *N Engl J Med* 2010;363(14):1324–1334.

78. Park JR, et al. A phase III randomized clinical trial (RCT) of tandem myeloablative autologous stem cell transplant (ASCT) using peripheral blood stem cell (PBSC) as consolidation therapy for high-risk neuroblastoma (HR-NB): A Children's Oncology Group (COG) study. *J Clin Oncol* 2016;34 (15 suppl):LBA3–LBA3.

79. La Quaglia MP, et al. Stage 4 neuroblastoma diagnosed at more than 1 year of age: gross total resection and clinical outcome. *J Pediatr Surg* 1994;29(8):1162–1165; discussion 1165–1166.

80. Matthay KK, et al. Patterns of relapse after autologous purged bone marrow transplantation for neuroblastoma: a Childrens Cancer Group pilot study. *J Clin Oncol* 1993;11(11):2226–2233.

81. Haas-Kogan DA, et al. Impact of radiotherapy for high-risk neuroblastoma: a Children's Cancer Group study. *Int J Radiat Oncol Biol Phys* 2003;56(1):28–39.

82. Laprie A, et al. High-dose chemotherapy followed by locoregional irradiation improves the outcome of patients with international neuroblastoma staging system Stage II and III neuroblastoma with MYCN amplification. *Cancer* 2004;101(5):1081–1089.

83. Gatcombe HG, et al. Excellent local control from radiation therapy for high-risk neuroblastoma. *Int J Radiat Oncol Biol Phys* 2009;74(5):1549–1554.

84. Mazloom A, et al. Radiation therapy to the primary and postinduction chemotherapy MIBG-avid sites in high-risk neuroblastoma. *Int J Radiat Oncol Biol Phys* 2014;90(4):858–862.

85. Casey DL, et al. Local control with 21-Gy radiation therapy for high-risk neuroblastoma. *Int J Radiat Oncol Biol Phys* 2016;96(2):393–400.

86. Simon T, et al. Role of surgery in the treatment of patients with stage 4 neuroblastoma age 18 months or older at diagnosis. *J Clin Oncol* 2013;31(6):752–758.

87. Polishchuk AL, et al. Likelihood of bone recurrence in prior sites of metastasis in patients with high-risk neuroblastoma. *Int J Radiat Oncol Biol Phys* 2014;89(4):839–845.

88. Halperin EC. Hepatic metastasis from neuroblastoma. *South Med J* 1987;80(11):1370–1373.

89. Hutchinson RJ, et al. 131-I-metaiodobenzylguanidine treatment in patients with refractory advanced neuroblastoma. *Am J Clin Oncol* 1992;15(3):226–232.

90. Lashford LS, et al. Phase I/II study of iodine 131 metaiodobenzylguanidine in chemoresistant neuroblastoma: a United Kingdom Children's Cancer Study Group investigation. *J Clin Oncol* 1992;10(12):1889–1896.

91. De Kraker J, et al. First line targeted radiotherapy, a new concept in the treatment of advanced stage neuroblastoma. *Eur J Cancer* 1995;31A(4):600–602.

92. Gaze MN, et al. Multi-modality megatherapy with [131I]meta-iodobenzylguanidine, high dose melphalan and total body irradiation with bone marrow rescue: feasibility study of a new strategy for advanced neuroblastoma. *Eur J Cancer* 1995;31A(2):252–256.

93. Mastrangelo R, et al. A new approach in the treatment of stage IV neuroblastoma using a combination of [131I]meta-iodobenzylguanidine (MIBG) and cisplatin. *Eur J Cancer* 1995;31A(4):606–611.

94. Yanik GA, et al. Pilot study of iodine-131-metaiodobenzylguanidine in combination with myeloablative chemotherapy and autologous stem-cell support for the treatment of neuroblastoma. *J Clin Oncol* 2002;20(8):2142–2149.

95. Paulino AC, et al. Comparison of conventional to intensity modulated radiation therapy for abdominal neuroblastoma. *Pediatr Blood Cancer* 2006;46(7):739–744.

96. Hattangadi JA, et al. Proton radiotherapy for high-risk pediatric neuroblastoma: early outcomes and dose comparison. *Int J Radiat Oncol Biol Phys* 2012;83(3):1015–1022.

97. GJ DA, Evans AE. Cyclic, low-dose total body irradiation for metastatic neuroblastoma. *Int J Radiat Oncol Biol Phys* 1983;9(12):1961–1965.

98. Kun LE. Fractionated total body irradiation for metastatic neuroblastoma. *Int J Radiat Oncol Biol Phys* 1981;7(11):1599–1602.

99. Li R, et al. Patterns of relapse in high-risk neuroblastoma patients treated with and without total body irradiation. *Int J Radiat Oncol Biol Phys* 2017;97(2):270–277.

100. Haas-Kogan DA, et al. Intraoperative radiation therapy for high-risk pediatric neuroblastoma. *Int J Radiat Oncol Biol Phys* 2000;47(4):985–992.

101. Caussa L, et al. Role of palliative radiotherapy in the management of metastatic pediatric neuroblastoma: a retrospective single-institution study. *Int J Radiat Oncol Biol Phys* 2011;79(1):214–219.

102. Paulino AC. Palliative radiotherapy in children with neuroblastoma. *Pediatr Hematol Oncol* 2003;20(2):111–117.

103. Nickerson HJ, et al. Comparison of stage IV and IV-S neuroblastoma in the first year of life. *Med Pediatr Oncol* 1985;13(5):261–268.

104. Strother D, et al. Results of pediatric oncology group protocol 8104 for infants with stages D and DS neuroblastoma. *J Pediatr Hematol Oncol* 1995;17(3):254–259.

105. Paulino AC, Fowler BZ. Risk factors for scoliosis in children with neuroblastoma. *Int J Radiat Oncol Biol Phys* 2005;61(3):865–869.

106. Paulino AC, et al. Locoregional control in infants with neuroblastoma: role of radiation therapy and late toxicity. *Int J Radiat Oncol Biol Phys* 2002;52(4):1025–1031.

107. Beckham TH, et al. Renal function outcomes of high-risk neuroblastoma patients undergoing radiation therapy. *Int J Radiat Oncol Biol Phys* 2017;99(2):486–493.

108. Laverdiere C, et al. Long-term outcomes in survivors of neuroblastoma: a report from the Childhood Cancer Survivor Study. *J Natl Cancer Inst* 2009;101(16):1131–1140.

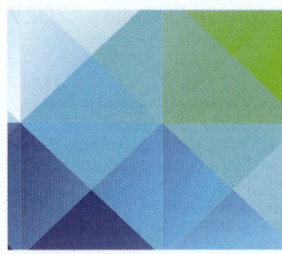

CHAPTER 91

Rhabdomyosarcoma

Dana L. Casey, John C. Breneman, Sarah S. Donaldson, and
Suzanne L. Wolden

GENERAL TREATMENT PARADIGM

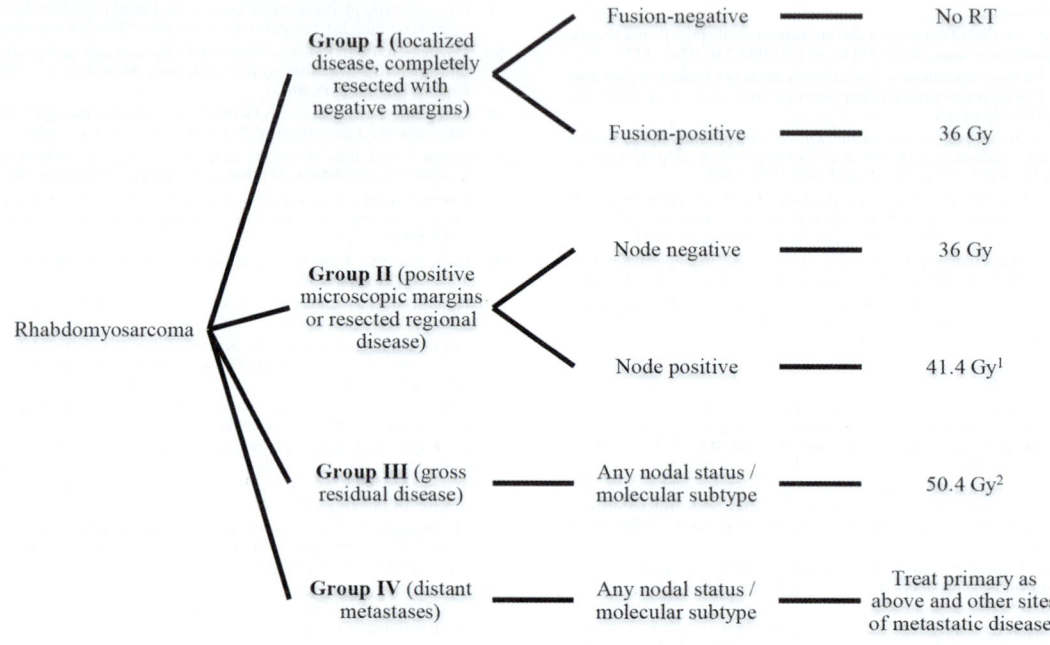

Ongoing Investigations

1. Reducing the dose to 36 Gy for patients with group II node-positive disease.
2. For patients with group III disease, treating the prechemotherapy volume to 36 Gy followed by a boost to 50.4 or 59.4 Gy if the initial size is >5 cm.
3. Treating bone metastases with stereotactic body radiation therapy.

ANATOMY

Rhabdomyosarcoma (RMS) is a highly malignant soft tissue sarcoma that arises from unsegmented, undifferentiated mesoderm or myotome-derived skeletal muscle. It may occur at any site in the body, but the most frequently involved sites are the orbit (9%); head and neck (excluding parameningeal tumors) (7%); parameningeal (25%); genitourinary (31%); extremity (13%); trunk (5%); retroperitoneum (7%); and other sites (3%).[1]

Epidemiology and Risk Factors

RMS is the most common of the childhood soft tissue sarcomas, with an annual incidence of 4.4 per 1 million whites and 1.3 per 1 million blacks. The male-to-female ratio is approximately 1.5 to 1.0, and males may have slightly better overall survival.[2]

The great majority of patients are <10 years of age at the time of diagnosis, and approximately 5% are <1 year of age. There are two peak age frequencies, at ages 2 to 6 and in adolescence. Tumors in the younger age group are likely to be of embryonal histology. About 25% of patients are ≥10 years at diagnosis and their tumors are more commonly of alveolar histology. Age has been identified as an independent predictor of prognosis, with children <1 year and >10 years having inferior survival.[3] Adults with RMS have been reported to have poor outcomes, although there is evidence that when they are treated aggressively using pediatric-type protocols, the prognosis may be similar to that of younger patients.[4–6]

The cause of RMS is unknown; however, it is associated with disorders in development, including central nervous system, genitourinary, gastrointestinal, and cardiovascular anomalies, and with congenital disorders including congenital pulmonary cysts, Gorlin basal cell nevus syndrome, and neurofibromatosis. In addition, RMS is the most frequently occurring childhood cancer in families with Li-Fraumeni syndrome, and its incidence is increased in children with neurofibromatosis type 1, Beckwith-Wiedemann syndrome, and Costello syndrome.

Recent developments in cytogenetics and molecular genetics now provide a more comprehensive understanding of the origin and biologic behavior of RMS. The classic distinction of embryonal versus alveolar histology has been largely replaced by the PAX/FOXO1 fusion status (fusion-negative vs. fusion-positive) for both prognostic and therapeutic decision-making. These details are discussed in more detail later.

NATURAL HISTORY AND PATTERNS OF SPREAD

There are unexplained associations of site of primary tumor with age at diagnosis and tumor histology. For example, tumors arising in the urinary bladder and vagina occur primarily in infants and often are of the embryonal or botryoid histologic type. Tumors arising in the trunk and extremity occur in adolescents and are often alveolar. Tumors of the head and neck area occur throughout childhood and are commonly of the embryonal type.

RMS, a locally invasive tumor often with a pseudocapsule, has the potential for local spread along fascial or muscle planes, lymphatic extension, and hematogenous dissemination. The overall risk of regional lymphatic spread is approximately 15% but varies with the site of the primary lesion. Lymph node metastases are rare in orbital tumors, but they occur in approximately 15% of tumors at other head and neck sites, most commonly the nasopharynx. Accounting for staging inaccuracies, regional lymph node extension occurs in approximately 25% of children with paratesticular, extremity, and truncal tumors and in approximately 50% of children with perineal and perianal tumors.[7,8] The risk for lymph node involvement also correlates with primary tumor invasiveness and large tumor size.

Hematogenous metastases are detected at the time of presentation in approximately 15% of patients, particularly those with truncal and extremity primary tumors. The most common sites of hematogenous dissemination are lungs, bone marrow, and bone. Malignant pleural and peritoneal effusions may also accompany tumors primary to the chest and abdomen or pelvis, respectively.[9]

CLINICAL PRESENTATION

Because RMS occurs in multiple primary sites, there are many site-specific clinical signs and symptoms. It usually presents, however, as an asymptomatic mass. When symptoms are present, they relate to mass effect on associated organs and tissues. Tumors of the orbit may cause proptosis and ophthalmoplegia. Patients with parameningeal tumors often present with nasal, aural, or sinus obstruction; cranial nerve palsy; and headache. Genitourinary tumors may cause hematuria, urinary obstruction, or constipation.

DIAGNOSTIC WORKUP

Determination of tumor extent is best done with a multidisciplinary approach by a radiation oncologist, pediatric oncologist, and appropriate subspecialty surgeon. An expeditious local and systemic workup is essential because these tumors have the potential to grow rapidly. The initial assessment by all members of the team permits accurate staging and the formation of a uniform treatment plan. Table 91.1 provides recommendation for diagnostic workup at various sites. Early experience with combined positron emission tomography (PET) and computed tomography (CT) scanning indicates this modality may be a valuable component of staging[10] and may in fact provide more accurate staging than conventional imaging.[11] PET-CT may be especially valuable in assessing response to therapy and in predicting outcomes, as conventional imaging has not shown a good correlation of tumor response to long-term clinical outcome.[12–14] Some children whose tumors exhibit characteristic fusion transcripts can be shown to have micrometastatic disease using reverse transcriptase polymerase chain reaction techniques, even when there is no evidence of metastases from routine diagnostic procedures. The clinical significance of this is, however, unknown.[15]

TABLE 91.1 RECOMMENDED WORKUP FOR TUMORS AT VARIOUS SITES

All Patients	Optional
All sites	
History	
Physical examination by several observers (including a pediatric oncologist, surgical oncologist, and radiation oncologist)	Examination under anesthesia for infants and youngsters
Laboratory studies	Plain films of bones abnormal on scans
Complete blood count	
Liver function tests	Abdomen/pelvis CT, MRI, or ultrasound
Renal function tests	
Urinalysis	
Imaging studies	
PET-CT (this study can likely replace chest/abdomen/pelvis CT and bone scan studies)	
MRI or CT of primary tumor	
Bone marrow biopsy and aspirate	
Head and neck	
MRI or CT of primary tumor (with contrast)	Plain films of area
Lumbar puncture with cytologic examination of fluid (in parameningeal primary tumors)	Dental evaluation and x-rays
	Paranasal sinus and skull films
	MRI of spine if cerebrospinal fluid is positive or patient is symptomatic
Genitourinary	
CT of MRI of abdomen/pelvis (with contrast)	Ultrasound of pelvis
Pelvic examination under anesthesia	Cystoscopy
Extremity and truncal lesions	
MRI or CT of primary lesion (with contrast)	Plain films of primary site
	Ultrasound
	Barium gastrointestinal contrast studies

CT, computed tomography; MRI, magnetic resonance imaging; PET, positron emission tomography.

STAGING SYSTEMS

The clinical grouping classification used extensively by the Intergroup Rhabdomyosarcoma Study Group (now known as the Children's Oncology Group Soft Tissue Sarcoma [COG STS] committee) investigators is somewhat of a misnomer because it actually requires surgical pathologic evaluation (Table 91.2). It is not a staging system and does not accurately reflect the biology of the disease; rather, it reflects the surgical procedure selected for an individual patient. It is, however, useful for guiding decisions for radiotherapy, based on the amount of residual tumor after the initial surgical procedure. A more valid pretreatment staging system uses a TNM

TABLE 91.2 INTERGROUP RHABDOMYOSARCOMA STUDY CLINICAL GROUPING CLASSIFICATION

Group I	Localized disease, completely resected
A	Confined to organ or muscle of origin
B	Infiltration outside organ or muscle of origin; regional nodes not involved
Group II	Compromised or regional resection
A	Grossly resected tumor with microscopic residual disease
B	Regional disease, completely resected, in which nodes may be involved or extension of tumor into adjacent organ may exist
C	Regional disease with involved nodes, grossly resected, but with evidence of microscopic residual disease
Group III	Incomplete resection or biopsy with gross residual disease
Group IV	Distant metastases at diagnosis

Adapted from Mauer HM. The Intergroup Rhabdomyosarcoma Study: objectives and clinical staging classification. *J Pediatr Surg* 1980;15:371–372. Copyright © 1980 Elsevier. With permission.

TABLE 91.3 INTERGROUP RHABDOMYOSARCOMA STUDY PRETREATMENT STAGING SYSTEM

Stage	Site[a]	Invasiveness	Size	Nodal Status	Metastases
I	Favorable	T1 or T2	a or b	N0 or N1	M0
II	Unfavorable	T1 or T2	a	N0	M0
III	Unfavorable	T1 or T2	b	N0	M0
			a or b	N1	M0
IV	Any site		T1 or T2	N0 or N1	M1

[a]Favorable sites: orbit, head and neck (nonparameningeal), genitourinary (non–bladder–prostate); unfavorable sites: genitourinary (bladder–prostate), extremity, parameningeal, other. T1, tumor confined to site or organ of origin; T2, regional extension beyond the site or organ of origin; a, ≤5 cm; b, >5 cm; N0, no evidence of regional node involvement; N1, evidence of regional node involvement (enlargement of nodes on radiographic imaging is considered evidence of involvement, although histologic confirmation is recommended when possible); M0, no distant metastasis; M1, evidence of distant metastasis.

(tumor, node, metastasis) approach, which emphasizes characteristics of the primary tumor, size and invasiveness, nodal status, and systemic spread. Noninvasiveness, small size, and an absence of metastases have been shown to influence prognosis.[16] The site of primary tumor also has a significant impact on survival.[17,18] The Intergroup Rhabdomyosarcoma Study IV (IRS-IV) prospectively demonstrated the validity of a staging system incorporating TNM classification along with primary tumor site (Table 91.3). Three-year failure-free survival was 86% for stage 1 tumors, 80% for stage 2, 68% for stage 3, and 25% for stage 4.[1,9] Of note, the clinical grouping did not correlate as well with survival. In fact, failure-free survival for clinical group II patients in the IRS-IV study was superior to that for clinical group I patients (86% vs. 83%), probably reflecting the routine use of radiotherapy for group II patients.

PATHOLOGIC CLASSIFICATION

The histogenesis of RMS can be traced from mesoderm to mesenchyme and ultimately to striated muscle tissue. The classification of RMS initially used by the IRS investigators consisted of four histologic subtypes: embryonal, botryoid subtype of embryonal, alveolar, and pleomorphic. Embryonal histologies constitute approximately two-thirds of all cases, with most of the rest having alveolar histology.[19] Other variants including a "solid" alveolar pattern, considered a subtype of alveolar RMS, a spindle cell subtype of embryonal RMS, and a diffuse anaplastic variant have also been described.[20]

To improve reproducibility of pathologic subtyping and prognostic utility, pediatric pathologists developed an updated classification system: the International Classification of Rhabdomyosarcoma. This system is based on a review of IRS-II data, and it groups pathologic subtypes into distinct prognostic groups. The International Classification of Rhabdomyosarcoma system appears to be predictive of outcome and has been reproduced by several reference pediatric pathologists.[20,21] The superior prognosis group, consisting of two subsets (botryoid and spindle cell), carries a projected 5-year survival rate of 88% to 95%.[21] The botryoid subtype, a polypoid variant of embryonal RMS, has a grape-like appearance. The stroma consists of loose cellular tissue with a myxoid appearance. Under the superficial stroma is a hypercellular zone of tumor cells called the cambium layer of Nicholson. Botryoid tumors are usually noninvasive and localized and occur in mucosal-lined organs such as the vagina, urinary bladder, middle ear, biliary tree, and nasopharynx. The spindle cell subtype of embryonal RMS has a spindled appearance, often with a storiform pattern. It is frequently found in paratesticular sites.

Patients with embryonal RMS have an intermediate prognosis, with an 83% failure-free survival at 3 years.[17] The embryonal type consists of blastemal mesenchymal cells that tend to differentiate into cross-striated muscle cells. There is often a considerable variation in degree of cytoplasmic development, ranging from primitive mesenchymal to highly differentiated muscle tumor cells. Most of the tumor cells have eosinophilic cytoplasm, which is positive by periodic acid–Schiff staining. Immunohistochemistry may demonstrate actin- or desmin-positive reactions. Ultrastructural studies exhibit evidence of myogenesis with the presence of thick and thin cytoplasmic intermediate filaments or Z-band material. Ribbon or strap-shaped cells and tadpole cells are characteristic. The presence of cross-striations confirms the diagnosis. The embryonal form may be distinguished from the other subtypes by specific structural abnormalities. A consistent loss of heterozygosity at the chromosome 11p15.5 locus suggests that this site is specific for the embryonal subtype,[22] although, unlike alveolar histology, no characteristic translocation has been identified. Immunohistochemical presence of epidermal growth factor receptor and fibrillin-2 appears to be highly specific for embryonal histology and is predictive of a favorable outcome.[23,24] Dysregulation of the RAS pathway has also been found in some patients and may be involved in the pathogenesis of this subtype.[25] The embryonal histology is found most commonly in the orbit, head and neck, and genitourinary sites.

The group with poor prognosis includes alveolar, diffuse anaplastic, and undifferentiated sarcomas. With routine use of immunohistochemistry and molecular genetic analysis, about one-third of RMSs are now classified as alveolar; it is most commonly found in adolescents with truncal, retroperitoneal, and extremity tumors. The alveolar subtype is characterized by a pseudoalveolar pattern of connective tissue trabeculae, lined by large rhabdomyoblasts and multinucleated giant cells. The "solid" variant of alveolar RMS grows as solid nests of closely aggregated tumor cells with less alveolar pattern. Alveolar histology is strongly associated with hyperdiploid content.[26] Approximately 75% of children with alveolar RMS exhibit a characteristic translocation involving chromosomes 2 and 13, t(2;13)(q35;q14), and occasionally a 1;13 translocation.[22,27] These translocations correspond to abnormal fusion genes involving *PAX3-FKHR* and *PAX7-FKHR*, respectively, and are probably the initial oncogenic events in these tumors.[28,29] Immunohistochemical presence of AP2-β and P-cadherin is also highly specific for alveolar histology.[23,24] The projected 3-year failure-free survival for children with the alveolar subtype is 66%.[1]

Undifferentiated sarcoma is largely a diagnosis of exclusion; it consists of a diffuse cell population of primitive, noncommitted mesenchymal cells. The 3-year failure-free survival rate of patients with undifferentiated sarcoma is 55%.[1] Today, sarcomas that lack characteristics of differentiation are most appropriately managed as non-RMS soft tissue sarcomas, though their outcomes have been similar to alveolar RMS.

The pleomorphic type is extremely rare; many cases formerly classified as pleomorphic RMS are currently considered to be malignant fibrous histiocytoma. Previously, tumors classified as extraosseous Ewing sarcoma were treated using guidelines for RMS. These are more appropriately considered in the Ewing family of tumors and are managed as such.

As more is learned about the molecular biology of RMS, fusion status rather than histology may be the more important driver of clinical outcomes. Recent data suggest that fusion-negative alveolar RMS is more similar to embryonal histology both clinically and molecularly.[30] On COG D9803, there was a trend toward improved event-free survival (EFS) among patients with fusion-negative alveolar RMS when compared to those with embryonal RMS (EFS 90% vs. 77%).[31] Other studies have confirmed that fusion status may be more important prognostically than histology.[30,32] As such, modern COG clinical trials account for fusion status in addition to histology for risk stratification.

PROGNOSTIC FACTORS AND THERAPEUTIC CONSIDERATIONS

Because RMS is protean in presentation, factors such as age, site, stage, extent of disease, and pathologic characteristics of the tumor influence therapeutic decisions. These prognostic factors are interrelated and are best discussed as a function of the specific site (Fig. 91.1). Although most treatment failures occur within 3 years of diagnosis, about 10% of children who are free of disease at 5 years will subsequently experience disease recurrence.[33]

Orbit

The orbit has long been recognized as a favorable prognostic site. In addition to prompt recognition of the tumor, the paucity of lymphatics in this area means that lymphatic extension is rare. Most tumors in this site have embryonal histology, and hematogenous metastasis at the time of diagnosis is uncommon. Approximately 10% are alveolar histology, however, and the prognosis for these children is more guarded.[34]

When treatment for orbital tumors is individualized, it is generally agreed that no surgical procedure should be used that may compromise vision or loss of function. In most patients, this means that biopsy only should be performed to provide the diagnosis. Primary treatment typically consists of vincristine, actinomycin-D, and cyclophosphamide (VAC) or vincristine and actinomycin-D (VA) chemotherapy with local radiotherapy beginning after the 12th week of treatment. Radiation doses of approximately 50 Gy are often used. Dose reduction to 45 Gy was tested on D9602, resulting in a local failure rate of 13% (compared to 5% seen on IRS IV).[35,36] A dose of 45 Gy was shown to result in unacceptable rates of local control for orbital RMS again on ARST0331 in those without a complete response to chemotherapy. As discussed later, orbital tumors should be treated with similar doses as other primary sites.

Chemotherapy without irradiation has resulted in local relapse and inferior EFS.[37] Although salvage radiotherapy for these patients can still be curative, functional vision in this setting is often poor.[38] Orbital exenteration should be reserved for salvage treatment and enucleation for management of posttreatment ocular complications.

With a combined-modality approach, radiotherapy can be directed to the tumor plus a margin without necessarily irradiating the entire orbit. Technique is very important for minimizing corneal and lacrimal gland dose and for preserving useful vision, ocular function, and appearance. Photon

FIGURE 91.1. Survival curves for 883 children with nonmetastatic disease entered into the fourth Intergroup Rhabdomyosarcoma Study are shown by anatomic site of the primary tumor. GU, genitourinary. (Adapted with permission from Crist WM, Anderson JR, Meza JL, et al. The Intergroup Rhabdomyosarcoma Study-IV: results for patients with non-metastatic disease. *J Clin Oncol* 2001;19[12]:3091–3102. Copyright © 2001 American Society of Clinical Oncology. All rights reserved.)

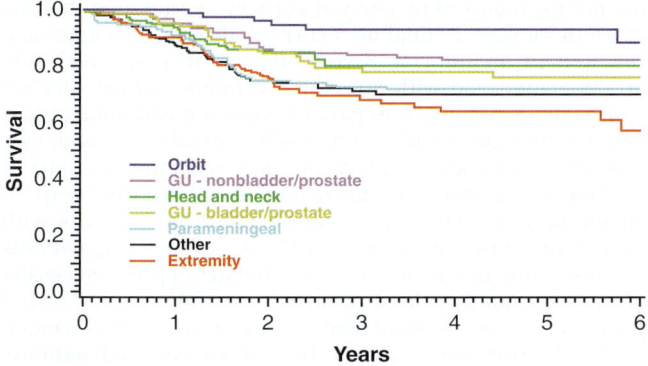

irradiation with the eyelid open can minimize the corneal dose when an anterior field is used and may be associated with improved long-term functional outcome.[39] Three-dimensional conformal or intensity-modulated radiotherapy technique is optimal for treating the target volume and sparing normal structures, and proton radiation has also been used successfully.[40]

Head and Neck: Parameningeal Sites

Nonorbital RMS of the head and neck is grouped into parameningeal sites (nasopharynx, nasal cavity, paranasal sinuses, middle ear, pterygopalatine fossa, and infratemporal fossa) and nonparameningeal sites based on differences in natural history, treatment, and prognosis. Parameningeal RMS represent the majority of nonorbital head and neck RMS, and radiotherapy is essential for maximizing the chance of cure.[17,41] These tumors have a propensity for invading the base of the skull, creating a potential for cranial nerve palsy and direct extension into the central nervous system, a pattern of spread that is seen in as many as 41% of these patients.[42] Historically, as many as 35% of children with tumor arising in a parameningeal site would later have meningeal extension, and previous irradiation regimens called for whole-brain irradiation as part of central nervous system prophylaxis.[43] However, the prognosis of these patients is markedly improved with appropriate imaging, multiagent chemotherapy, and adequate irradiation of the primary tumor and adjacent meninges, and studies demonstrate that whole-brain irradiation is not necessary, even in the presence of direct intracranial tumor extension.[44] Patients with known meningeal dissemination should receive craniospinal irradiation. A radiation dose of 50.4 Gy in 28 fractions to the primary site is commonly used. Data from the IRS studies show improved local control in patients with intracranial tumor extension when radiotherapy is started within 2 weeks of diagnosis,[42] although other reports show no disadvantage with delayed radiotherapy.[45]

Aggressive surgery is rarely indicated because complete resection usually is not possible, does not obviate the need for high-dose radiation therapy, and often results in a delay of systemic chemotherapy because of postoperative complications. Surgical approaches to these tumors have been described by proponents of multispecialty skull base surgery, but the efficacy of these approaches has not been firmly established.[46] Delayed surgical resection has been proposed as beneficial for children with residual tumor after completing chemotherapy and radiotherapy but is not considered standard of care.[47,48] The role of postradiation surgical resection is being investigated in select intermediate-risk patients enrolled onto IRS-V.

Five-year survival for patients with parameningeal RMS is approximately 75% with adequate radiotherapy.[49] For the subset of parameningeal tumors arising in the nasopharynx or nasal cavity, middle ear, and parapharyngeal locations, survival may be even higher,[44] and functional and cosmetic outcome can be good in spite of an aggressive treatment regimen (Figs. 91.2 and 91.3).

Head and Neck: Nonparameningeal Sites

Children with tumors in nonparameningeal head and neck sites tend to have a better outcome than their parameningeal counterparts (80% 5-year failure-free survival in IRS-IV) and require less-intensive chemotherapy.[1,17] These sites include the scalp, parotid, oral cavity, larynx, oropharynx, and cheek. These tumors may be more amenable to complete gross surgical excision compared with their parameningeal counterparts. Approximately 15% of these patients present with regional lymph node metastases. Radiotherapeutic management is based on the amount of residual tumor after surgery.

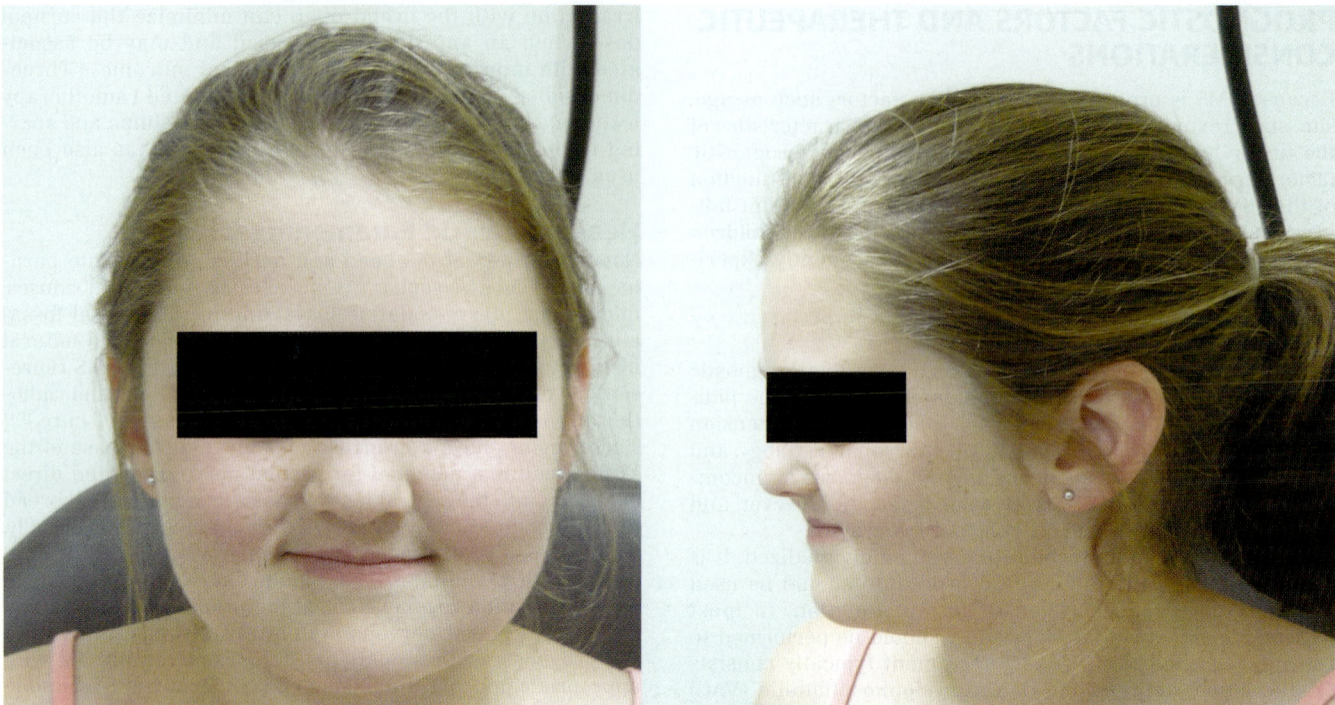

FIGURE 91.2. This 12-year-old girl was treated at age 3 years for an embryonal rhabdomyosarcoma of the nasal cavity. Her treatment consisted of excisional biopsy, followed by VAC (vincristine, actinomycin-D, and cyclophosphamide) chemotherapy and 41.4-Gy radiotherapy. Slight hypoplasia of the midface is evident, but overall cosmesis is excellent.

Draining regional lymph nodes are not routinely irradiated unless they are considered to be involved with tumor by clinical or pathologic assessment.

Pelvis

Pelvic tumors usually are divided into anatomic subgroups because the natural history, treatment, and prognosis are

FIGURE 91.3. Isodose distribution from the treatment of the child in Figure 91.2 (doses in cGy).

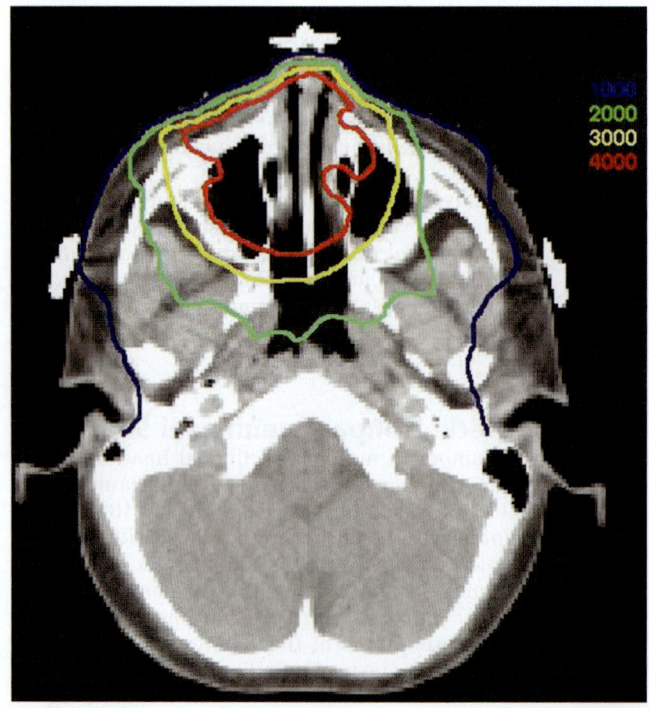

different for each site. Some children present with locally advanced pelvic tumors for which an exact site of origin cannot be determined. These large tumors are associated with an unfavorable prognosis.

Bladder and Prostate Tumors

Bladder and prostate primary tumors account for about half of all pelvic RMS[41]; 75% of patients are age <5 years at presentation, and more than 90% of these tumors are of the embryonal histologic subtype, with approximately one-third having a botryoid morphology. In boys, it is often difficult to differentiate a tumor of prostatic origin from one of bladder origin because disease usually involves both structures. However, patients with tumors arising in the prostate have significantly inferior survival compared with those with tumor confined to the bladder.[50]

Historically, anterior pelvic exenteration (or partial cystectomy for small tumors arising from the dome of the bladder) combined with chemotherapy and irradiation for microscopic or gross residual disease has been associated with a survival rate of approximately 70%.[18] More recently, emphasis has been on limited surgery to preserve bladder function. The IRS-II study treated these patients primarily with chemotherapy followed by delayed surgery or radiation therapy when there was residual or recurrent disease. This approach resulted in an inferior 3-year disease-free survival rate of 52%, compared with 80% for a primary radical surgical approach and only 22% of patients survived with intact bladders.[51] Subsequently, IRS-III intensified the therapy with systematic use of planned irradiation 6 weeks after the start of treatment and added cisplatin and doxorubicin (Adriamycin) chemotherapy.[52] The 5-year survival rate for patients with locoregional disease was 82%, with 64% of surviving patients retaining functional bladders, demonstrating the necessity of routine radiation therapy early in treatment.[53] Survival of patients with locoregional bladder or prostate tumors treated on IRS-IV was similar, with 40% of all enrolled patients reporting normal bladder function at follow-up.[54] A more recent analysis showed maintenance of continence in 69% treated with conservative surgery in a multimodality treatment program.[55]

The German Cooperative Weichteilsarkom Studiengruppe CWS-96 protocol treated children with bladder or prostate RMS using multiagent chemotherapy followed by response-adapted radiotherapy and surgery. Children with complete resection did not have radiotherapy, whereas others received 32 to 44.8 Gy using 1.6 Gy twice a day, depending on the tumor's IRS group and response to chemotherapy. Five-year EFS was 70%.[56]

A pooled analysis of patients treated prospectively on several cooperative group trials from North America and Europe showed improved local control for those who received radiotherapy as part of their initial treatment, but this did not translate into improvement in overall survival.[57]

Paratesticular Tumors

Paratesticular tumors represent approximately 7% of all RMS and may arise anywhere along the spermatic cord, from the intrascrotal area through the inguinal canal.[58] At presentation, the tumor usually is a painless scrotal or inguinal mass that does not transilluminate. Most boys with paratesticular RMS present with early-stage disease that is amenable to complete resection and is associated with cure rates approaching 90%. As with prostatic primary tumors, the lymphatic network is rich, draining directly to the retroperitoneal nodes along the external iliac and spermatic vessels, the aorta, and the vena cava. The incidence of retroperitoneal lymph node involvement varies with the age of the patient and method of staging (surgical vs. nonsurgical). In the IRS-III study, retroperitoneal lymph node sampling was done in most patients, showing a 14% incidence of node involvement for children <10 years of age and a 47% incidence for those ≥10 years. In IRS-IV, thin-cut CT without surgical sampling was used for staging, and the incidence of detected nodes dropped to 4% and 13% for the two age groups, respectively.[58]

The recommended surgical procedure for the primary tumor is inguinal orchiectomy. If there is no evidence of invasion into the scrotum and the proximal spermatic cord is free of tumor, this procedure is considered equivalent to an amputation, and no further local therapy is necessary. Surgical staging of retroperitoneal lymph nodes is controversial. European investigators do not recommend retroperitoneal lymph node sampling for these patients, preferring to treat with intensified chemotherapy in high-risk patients and salvage radiotherapy, if necessary.[59,60] In the IRS, the high risk of nodal involvement in certain subsets of these patients has led to the recommendation for ipsilateral retroperitoneal nerve-sparing node dissection for staging of all children ≥10 years of age.[58] In the absence of histologic documentation, enlargement of retroperitoneal lymph nodes on thin-section CT imaging is considered evidence of tumor involvement.

Patients with nodal disease have a 5-year survival rate of 69%, compared with 96% for those without regional nodal disease ($P < .001$). Regional lymph node irradiation to the periaortic and ipsilateral iliac nodes is recommended when there is nodal involvement.[61] Surgical violation of the scrotum or tumor extension to the structure is an indication for hemiscrotectomy or, less commonly, scrotal irradiation. If scrotal irradiation is used, orchiopexy should be considered prior to treatment to protect the remaining testes. Treatment programs must be planned to reduce morbidity, particularly among this group with high likelihood of cure.

Gynecologic Tumors

Tumors arising in the vulva, vagina, cervix, and uterus are about one-third as common as bladder and prostate primary tumors and account for 4% of all RMS.[62] Within this group, the vagina is the most common site of origin.

Patients with vaginal tumors are often much younger than those with other pelvic RMS, with most girls diagnosed before the age of 3 years. Most present with a vaginal mass or discharge; botryoid morphology is common. Initial surgery is used primarily for diagnosis, although gross tumor resection is occasionally possible without cosmetic or functional deformity. These tumors are often quite sensitive to chemotherapy, and treatment regimens have previously used a strategy of chemotherapy only, reserving surgery and radiotherapy for persistent or recurrent tumor.[62-64] However, analysis of data from the IRS-IV and IRS-V studies have revealed high rates of local failure for vaginal tumors when local control with surgery or radiotherapy is omitted.[36,65] Current guidelines from the COG STS committee call for radiotherapy in all patients with postsurgical microscopic or macroscopic tumor.

Uterine, cervical, and vulvar tumors receive chemotherapy and radiotherapy based on the amount of tumor present after initial surgery. Intracavitary and interstitial brachytherapy are useful irradiation techniques in some of these patients.[66] Data are limited, but with proper patient selection, disease control is excellent and late normal tissue effects may be significantly less with brachytherapy than is seen with external beam techniques.[67] Permanent implants with iodine-125 and temporary low dose rate and high dose rate brachytherapy have all been used, and there are no clear differences among these techniques in terms of disease control or late effects. When temporary implants are used, high dose rate brachytherapy has the practical advantage of minimizing radiation exposure to the family and medical personnel caring for the child.

Survival after treatment is excellent. Children aged 1 to 9 years have a 98% 5-year survival. Survival for infants and adolescents approaches 90%, although these patients may require more intensive systemic therapy for cure.[62]

Other Pelvic Sites

These tumors include perianal, perirectal, and perineal primary sites. The location of these primary tumors creates surgical and irradiation challenges. Combined chemotherapy and radiation therapy programs are favored over primary surgical procedures if excision requires exenteration with urinary and fecal diversion procedures or is associated with organ or sphincter dysfunction. In general, tumors in these locations are associated with poor prognostic features, high rates of regional nodal involvement, and dismal outcomes, especially in children >10 years of age.[8]

Extremity

Tumors arising in the extremity are often of the alveolar or undifferentiated subtypes, large, deeply invasive, and associated with a high probability of lymphatic and hematogenous metastasis.[68] Complete surgical resection is difficult to achieve, usually requires extensive dissection, and is associated with a high risk of residual disease. Because radiation therapy and multiagent chemotherapy have been shown to provide excellent local control, it is advisable to avoid disfiguring and mutilating surgical procedures, with their attendant functional disabilities, and to recommend limb-salvage procedures including irradiation and chemotherapy.

Regional lymph node involvement is present in approximately 24% of patients and confers a more guarded prognosis.[68] Aggressive surgical staging of draining lymph node basins is important to define extent of involvement, although if lymph node dissection is performed, it is for the purpose of staging, not for treatment. Sentinel lymph node mapping and biopsy are being investigated for their diagnostic and prognostic value.[69,70] Radiotherapy of involved regional lymphatics is mandatory, and aggressive treatment of in-transit nodal sites may improve overall local control.[71]

Radiation therapy for extremity primary tumors requires careful immobilization techniques, sparing of nonirradiated skin for lymphatic drainage, and use of shrinking fields. Routine physical therapy during and after radiation therapy is important for obtaining an optimal functional result. Overall survival at 3 years for these patients is about 70%, although failure-free survival is only 55%.[72]

Other Sites

Patients with tumors arising in sites such as a paraspinal, retroperitoneal, or intrathoracic location have a poor outcome compared with other patients.[17] Most patients with tumors in these locations are unable to undergo complete resection of the tumor. Both local and distant relapse are common. These patients should be treated aggressively with high-dose radiation therapy and multiagent chemotherapy.

Metastatic Disease

Hematogenous or distant lymph node metastasis at the time of diagnosis is an ominous finding, although not all these children do poorly. The subset of patients who are <10 years of age and have only one or two sites of metastatic disease may have long-term survival chances of >50%.[9] Intensive multiagent chemotherapy plays a major role in the treatment of these patients, although marrow ablative techniques have not improved efficacy compared with conventional chemotherapy approaches.[73,74] Local control of the primary tumor is site specific, as previously described. Metastatic sites should be treated with radiotherapy whenever feasible and control rates after radiation are similar to local control rates at the primary site.[75] The role of stereotactic body radiotherapy (SBRT) for bony sites of metastatic disease is currently being explored. Whole lung irradiation for lung metastases is currently the standard of care, although SBRT for lung metastases is also an area of active investigation.[76,77]

GENERAL MANAGEMENT

A multidisciplinary approach using surgery, irradiation, and chemotherapy is important in the management of RMS; however, the optimal sequence and specific application of each modality continue to be investigated. Although the primary goal remains long-term cure, improvement in therapeutic results necessitates considerations of quality of life, with particular attention to maximization of functional and cosmetic results.

Surgery

Before the era of multidisciplinary therapy, surgical ablation resulted in a long-term survival rate of approximately 20% of those patients able to undergo resection.[78] Certain primary sites represented exceptions to these data; for example, approximately 50% of those with localized disease of the orbit survived after orbital exenteration.[79] However, with the introduction of effective adjunctive treatment, preservation of function and appearance became major goals. The concept of reasonable surgery has evolved. It involves removal of the bulk of tumor with maximal conservation of anatomic structures, including preservation of bladder, bowel, and sexual function in patients with tumors of genitourinary origin; limb function in patients with extremity tumors; and vision, voice, deglutition, and appearance in patients with head and neck tumors.

Resection of RMS from normal surrounding tissues is often technically challenging. Only 20% of tumors are located in sites where complete excision can readily be accomplished without an undesirable loss of function or cosmesis.[17] An additional 20% of patients have compromised surgical procedures, leaving microscopic residual disease. Sixty percent of patients have tumors amenable to biopsy only or present with metastatic disease and are not candidates for primary resection. When the IRS surgical grouping system is used, patients with tumor amenable to complete excision fare better than those who have subtotal resection or biopsy alone. However, the tumors that are most accessible to surgical excision are small and noninvasive and are confined to the organ or structure of origin. Assessment using a TNM system demonstrates that prognosis is dictated by tumor size and invasiveness rather than by the initial surgical approach.[80] Furthermore, combined-modality therapy provides good local control of the primary tumor, even after subtotal excision.[81] For these reasons, the trend has been toward less-aggressive surgical resection, with more reliance on radiation therapy and chemotherapy to provide local control.[17]

In cases of suspected RMS, the initial surgical procedure should be an incisional biopsy. Surgical excision is indicated if it can be done without compromise of function or cosmesis. Normal tissue margins of at least 5 mm around the tumor are usually required to consider the resection complete (IRS group I), although this is sometimes not feasible in some anatomic sites and smaller margins may suffice. If microscopic disease remains after initial resection, a primary re-excision can be considered prior to beginning chemotherapy. Those children who can be rendered microscopically free of disease by this procedure have an improved outcome, compared with children who remain in clinical group II following initial surgery.[82,83] Amputation of an extremity, orbital exenteration, mutilating surgery of the head and neck area, therapeutic lymphadenectomy, and radical neck dissection are procedures reserved in case initial therapy fails.

Second-look operations (also termed delayed primary excisions, DPE) may be useful for converting partial responses after chemotherapy into complete responses, and there is evidence that these procedures may improve survival.[48] However, data regarding efficacy of second-look operations are mixed, with some finding no benefit with this procedure.[12] The IRS-V study evaluated whether DPE might allow a reduction in the amount of radiotherapy that is necessary to provide local tumor control; local control following DPE and reduced-dose radiation for bladder dome, extremity, and trunk tumors was similar to historic results after higher doses of definitive radiation. Some investigators have used second-look operations in an attempt to eliminate radiotherapy, although this approach has resulted in inferior local control and survival.[84] Second-look operations may be used to evaluate therapeutic response after chemotherapy or radiation therapy. In the IRS-III study, 28% of patients categorized as having clinical partial response and 43% of those scored as having no response to induction chemotherapy were reclassified as having pathologic complete response after second-look operation.[85] These children enjoyed a survival rate similar to that of children who were able to undergo complete surgical excision at the time of initial diagnosis. Therefore, a clinical or radiographic evaluation indicating residual tumor after initial therapy may be misleading and is not associated with worse outcomes.

CHEMOTHERAPY

Chemotherapy is necessary in all cases. Several drugs have demonstrated single-agent activity measured as a percentage response rate, including vincristine (59%), dactinomycin (24%), cyclophosphamide (54%), cisplatin (15% to 21%), dacarbazine (11%), mitomycin-C (36%), etoposide (15% to 21%), ifosfamide (86%), irinotecan (23%), and topotecan (46%).[86-88] Agents with known activity against central nervous system tumors, such as the nitrosoureas and methotrexate, have not shown activity against RMS.

The most extensive experience in combination chemotherapy is with VAC or VAC plus doxorubicin (VACA). Some studies have suggested that patients with embryonal histology tumors in favorable sites who have no gross residual disease or lymph node involvement after the initial surgical resection may be adequately treated with VA for 1 year, provided that irradiation is given for microscopic residual disease.[17] However, data from the recently completed IRS-V study suggest that local control may be compromised when alkylating agents are omitted.[35,36] Patients with unresectable pelvic tumors may benefit from the addition of doxorubicin and cisplatin to VAC, but tumors in other sites do not seem to benefit from the addition of these drugs compared with an intensive regimen of VAC alone.

Some subsets of patients, such as those with tumors of unfavorable histology or unfavorable site and those with extensive tumor burden, continue to fare poorly. Some of these patients with embryonal histology may benefit from intensification of the cyclophosphamide or ifosfamide component of their chemotherapy, although there are conflicting data regarding this.[89,90] Patients with metastatic RMS benefit from the addition of ifosfamide and etoposide to the standard VAC regimen.[91] High-dose chemotherapy with total-body irradiation and autologous bone marrow transplantation has not improved the outcome in these high-risk patients.[73,74]

Initial intensive chemotherapy has been used as a means of pharmacologic debulking, potentially allowing for a more conservative surgical approach or less-aggressive radiation therapy.[51,92,93] However, data fail to consistently show that response to induction chemotherapy predicts ultimate outcome.[14,94] When chemotherapy alone is used for tumors in sites such as the head and neck or pelvis, most children require radiation therapy with or without a follow-up surgical procedure because of incomplete response or local recurrence.[18,37,95,96] Omission of radiotherapy in these patients may result in inferior survival.[84,97] Even patients with only microscopic disease after initial resection (group II) require radiotherapy to achieve optimal local control.[98] In patients with group II disease who routinely receive radiotherapy, local control is 92%.[99] The approach of initial chemotherapy followed by limited irradiation or less radical surgery may be appropriate in the management of infants and very young children, in whom late effects of aggressive surgery or high-dose, large-volume irradiation are particularly severe, although this may lead to inferior local control and survival.

Radiation Therapy

Adequate irradiation implies careful attention to volume and dose. It is essential to evaluate the soft tissue extent of the primary lesion by CT scan or magnetic resonance imaging. Because RMS tends to infiltrate tissue planes widely, tumors often extend beyond a fascial compartment and beyond the obvious visible margins. Careful examination by a radiation oncologist at the time of initial diagnosis, even if the treatment plan calls for neoadjuvant chemotherapy, is essential to establish the appropriate tumor volume.

Treatment portals are designed to encompass the involved region at the time of presentation (before chemotherapy) with margins that encompass surgical sites and biopsy tracts. A biopsy should be performed of clinically suspicious lymph nodes, or they should be included in the radiation therapy portal. Prophylactic lymph node irradiation is not necessary in children with clinically negative findings who will be receiving combination chemotherapy. The gross tumor volume is defined as the tumor as seen at the time of initial diagnosis. A clinical target volume of 1 cm is added and can be modified to account for anatomic barriers to tumor spread (such as the bony orbit in primary orbital tumors) or to account for regression of "pushing" the tumor border after chemotherapy, such as may occur in large pelvic tumors that initially displace contents of the peritoneal cavity. The planning target volume adds a patient-specific margin, which is typically about 5 mm. Many current treatment protocols use a cone down boost or simultaneous integrated boost to any gross posttreatment tumor volume after a microscopic tumor dose has been delivered. Patients with tumors at parameningeal sites (middle ear, paranasal sinuses, nasopharynx, nasal cavity, infratemporal fossa, and parapharyngeal area) have developed meningeal extension of tumor when inadequate irradiation portals were used.[44] Radiation therapy portals that cover the adjacent meninges in these patients can prevent meningeal relapse.[17,42]

Three-dimensional conformal and intensity-modulated radiotherapy treatment planning techniques are valuable for ensuring adequate treatment of the tumor volume and minimizing acute and chronic toxicity from the irradiation of uninvolved, adjacent structures.[42,100-102] Proton-beam radiotherapy is being increasingly utilized as access to this form of therapy increases,[40] and dosimetric studies consistently demonstrate decreases of integral dose to normal structures compared to photon-based techniques for many children with RMS (Fig. 91.4).[103,104] Local control and survival outcomes appear similar after proton radiation compared to historical cohorts treated with photon radiation. In addition, acute and early late toxicity rates with protons appear quite promising, especially for tumors in the head and neck region.[105] Follow up is limited, though, and long-term toxicity data are necessary to follow for adverse events that may take >4 years to develop.

Immobilization techniques that ensure reproducible portals are essential. Sedation or anesthesia may be necessary to ensure adequate implementation of the treatment plan. These complex programs are best conducted in regional centers by an experienced team of physicians, including a pediatric surgeon, pediatric anesthesiologist, pediatric oncologist, and radiation oncologist.

Radiation is necessary to ensure local tumor control in patients who are unable to undergo complete surgical resection. Local control of gross disease in most anatomic sites requires doses of 50 to 55 Gy. In the IRS-IV study, investigators studied the efficacy of a higher radiation dose, 59.4 Gy, given in 1.1-Gy fractions twice daily at 6-hour intervals for children with gross residual disease.[106] This hyperfractionated regimen was compared in a prospective, randomized fashion to a standard radiotherapy regimen consisting of 50.4 Gy given as 1.8 Gy once daily. There was no difference in locoregional disease control, failure-free survival, or overall survival between the two groups. Therefore, the standard of care for group III RMS continues to be conventionally fractionated radiation with chemotherapy.

Ninety percent of patients with microscopic residual tumor achieve local control with 41.4 Gy, and the D9602 study results suggest that 36 Gy may be adequate for microscopically positive margins that are not associated with lymph node

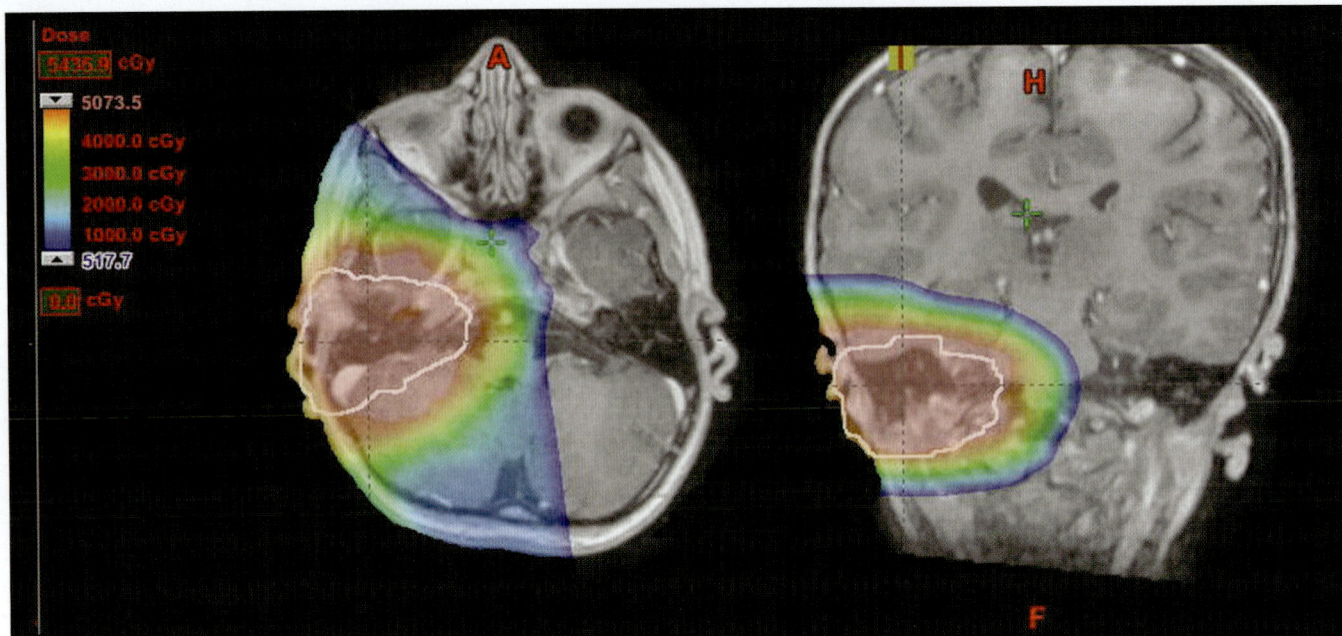

FIGURE 91.4. Isodose distribution in the axial and coronal planes for treatment of a middle ear RMS using protons. The physical properties of protons permit complete sparing of the contralateral structures and ipsilateral eye. (Courtesy of Danny Indelicato, MD.)

involvement as described in more detail below. Investigators have been unable to generate a strict dose–response curve but have observed an association with age that suggests that lower doses, often given to infants and youngsters, are associated with higher relapse rates.[107] They also suggest that local tumor control is greater for tumors <5 cm in diameter than for larger lesions, supporting the adult experience with soft tissue sarcomas.[108–110]

Results of the IRS-I study had indicated that radiotherapy was not needed for patients whose tumors were completely resected at diagnosis (group I). Subsequently, a reanalysis of data from the IRS-I to IRS-III studies suggested that the subset of group I patients with alveolar or undifferentiated histology had improved overall and failure-free survival when radiotherapy was given to the primary tumor site.[111] A more recent analysis using data from IRS-IV did not, however, show a significant advantage for radiotherapy in group I alveolar tumors. This practice is currently under review for the next generation of RMS protocols, with fusion status playing a critical role in risk stratification.[112]

Interstitial radiation therapy may play a role as primary treatment or as a boost after external beam therapy for selected sites.[46,67] The advantages of precise shaping of the dose distribution, sharp falloff of radiation dose, and shortening of overall treatment time are especially attractive in dealing with infants and young children. Some investigators report a decrease in late normal tissue effects when compared with external beam techniques.[113] There are no data regarding comparative efficacy or toxicity between high dose rate and low dose rate techniques. However, high dose rate remote brachytherapy may be particularly attractive in this patient population for logistical reasons. These children often require extensive care from family members and medical personnel during their treatment, and high dose rate techniques can eliminate radiation exposure to these caregivers.

The timing of radiation therapy must be carefully coordinated with planned surgical intervention and combination chemotherapy scheduling to optimize local control and ensure optimization of drug doses and unimpaired postoperative healing. Although radiation therapy is often delayed for several weeks to allow administration of neoadjuvant chemotherapy, some data suggest that earlier irradiation, particularly in high-risk patients, may provide better local tumor control and survival.[42,114,115] Interaction between radiation and some of the commonly used chemotherapeutic drugs can produce undesirable early and late effects. This is particularly true of dactinomycin and doxorubicin. Radiation therapy given concurrently with these agents is usually avoided. In contrast, systemic treatment with drugs such as vincristine and cyclophosphamide can usually be continued concurrently with the administration of irradiation.

Retrieval Therapy

Salvage after recurrence of RMS is difficult, which probably accounts for the inferior survival seen with treatment approaches that do not maximize therapy at the time of initial diagnosis.[97,116] Because local recurrence is the most common pattern of failure, surgery and radiotherapy play especially important roles in the treatment of these children. Aggressive treatment programs utilizing radical resection and brachytherapy have had success in selected patients with head and neck RMS.[46] There is evidence that salvage is more successful if radiotherapy was not used in the initial treatment and can be maximized for salvage therapy. Care must be taken when evaluating patients for local recurrence. Residual masses can be seen in as many as 40% of children who are shown to be pathologically free of tumor.[117]

RESULTS OF THERAPY: SUMMARY OF CLINICAL TRIALS

Because of the low incidence of RMS, much of what has been learned about its treatment has come from cooperative group trials performed in North America and Europe. Various cooperative groups have used different philosophies of treatment. In general, the North American IRS studies have emphasized the role of local control measures and European studies have focused more on chemotherapeutic approaches.

Intergroup Rhabdomyosarcoma Studies

The IRS began intergroup clinical trials for RMS in 1972 and has enrolled several thousand children with this disease since then. A primary goal has been to test the efficacy of chemotherapy and radiation therapy as a function of surgical stage. In the first IRS study (IRS-I), radiation therapy was given initially for patients with group I and II disease and was delayed until week 6 for those with group III and IV disease. All patients received multiagent chemotherapy for 2 years. This study made several important observations[118]:

1. For localized tumors amenable to complete resection (IRS group I), postoperative radiation therapy is unnecessary if the patient is given 2 years of VAC. For these patients, the relapse-free survival rate in IRS-I at 5 years was 80%, and the 5-year survival rate was 81% to 93%. Subsequent analysis has shown a benefit to postoperative radiation therapy for patients with group I tumors of alveolar or undifferentiated histology.[111]
2. VAC failed to improve results obtained with intensive VA for patients with group II disease if postoperative radiation therapy was given. For these patients, the relapse-free survival rate at 5 years was 65% to 72%, and the overall 5-year survival rate was 72%.
3. VACA provided no advantage over VAC for patients with group III disease (gross residual) or group IV disease (metastasis) if routine radiation therapy was used in addition. The complete remission rate for group III patients was 69%, and for group IV patients, it was 50%. Those who achieved complete remission had a 60% chance of staying in remission for 5 years in group III and a 30% chance in group IV. The survival rate at 5 years was 52% for group III and 20% for group IV patients.
4. The 5-year survival rate for the entire group was 55%.
5. Survival after relapse was poor—32% at 1 year and 17% at 2 years.
6. The risk of distant metastasis was much greater than the risk of local recurrence.
7. Primary tumors of the orbit and genitourinary tract carried the best prognoses, and tumors of the retroperitoneum had the worst.
8. The alveolar histologic subset had a poor prognosis, especially in extremity lesions.

A second IRS study (IRS-II) was built on the findings of IRS-I.[41] The results from this study include the following:

1. The 5-year survival rate for the IRS-II group was 62%, a 7% improvement over the IRS-I rate.
2. Patients in group I (excluding alveolar extremity patients) had better disease-free status with VAC (82%) than did those who received only VA (68%), but they had similar survival rates (82% and 88%) at 5 years. Cyclophosphamide could not be withdrawn safely from the standard VAC regimen if irradiation was omitted from patients with group I disease.
3. Intensive (cyclic-sequential) VA therapy was as effective as repetitive pulse VAC therapy for patients with group II disease, if all patients received postoperative irradiation. At 5 years, 68% to 75% remained disease free and 77% to 90% were alive, with no differences between the two therapy groups.
4. Repetitive pulse chemotherapy for 2 years increased survival in children with group III disease but not in those with group IV disease; doxorubicin and dactinomycin had comparable efficacy in the pulse regimens used. The complete remission rates were 72%.

At 5 years, 70% remained in complete remission and 64% were surviving.
5. In IRS-I, patients having tumors in parameningeal sites with high-risk factors (cranial nerve palsy, erosion of the base of the skull, or intracranial extension) had a high incidence of central nervous system relapse. In IRS-II, whole-brain radiotherapy irradiation, with or without intrathecal chemotherapy, was introduced. This prevented meningeal recurrence and increased survival in these patients with high-risk parameningeal primary tumors.
6. Primary repetitive pulse VAC for patients with special pelvic primary tumors (i.e., bladder, prostate, uterus, vagina) did not reduce the frequency of total cystectomy or produce durable bladder salvage, although survival was not compromised.
7. Survival after relapse was only 17% at 5 years.

The third IRS study (IRS-III) covered the period 1984 to 1991. This study revealed the following[17]:

1. The 5-year survival rate for the IRS-III group was 71%, an 8% improvement over the IRS-II rate. The 5-year progression-free survival rate was 65%, a 10% improvement over IRS-II.
2. Patients with group I favorable-histology tumors fared as well on a 1-year regimen of VA as did a comparable group treated with VA plus cyclophosphamide. The 5-year progression-free survival rates were 83% and 76%, respectively ($P - .18$).
3. Results for patients with group II favorable-histology tumors, excluding orbit, head, and paratesticular sites, were not improved with the addition of doxorubicin over VA chemotherapy × 1 year and radiation therapy.
4. Patients with group III tumors, excluding those in special pelvic, orbit, and other selected head sites (scalp, parotid, oral cavity, larynx, oropharynx, and cheek), fared better on the more intensive regimens of IRS-III than on pulsed VAC or VAC vincristine and doxorubicin (VADR) in IRS-II; the 5-year progression-free survival rates were 62% and 52%, respectively. The intensive regimen from IRS-III included multiple agents (VAC + doxorubicin + cisplatin + etoposide) plus radiation therapy plus second-look surgery. There were no differences in outcome among the three chemotherapy programs on IRS-III.
5. Patients with group IV tumors did not benefit from the aggressive therapy of IRS-III.
6. Patients with tumors in the bladder, vagina, and central pelvis in clinical group III had significantly improved outcome as compared with IRS-II patients, primarily because of the routine administration of early radiation therapy, which improved the bladder salvage rate from 25% in IRS-II to 60% in IRS-III.
7. Patients with unfavorable histology, in clinical groups I and II, who received VADR-VAC + cisplatin and radiation therapy had improved outcome over patients in IRS-II receiving VA or VAC and irradiation.
8. Patients with favorable-histology group II paratesticular tumors and those with favorable-histology orbit and head tumors in groups II and III do not require cyclophosphamide when VA × 1 year plus radiation therapy is used.
9. Whole-brain radiotherapy was omitted for patients with parameningeal primary tumors and cranial nerve palsy or base of skull erosion (although patients with intracranial extension of tumor still received this treatment). Risk of central nervous system relapse and survival were not compromised by this change if adequate local fields were used.

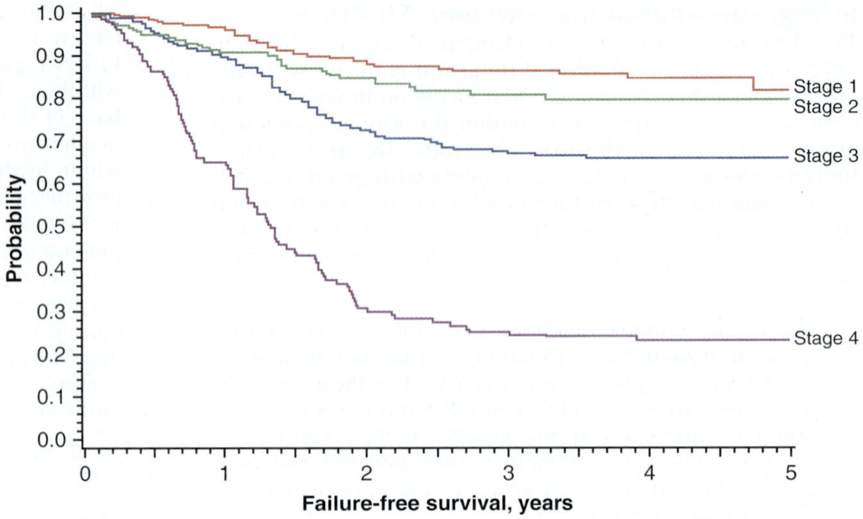

FIGURE 91.5. Survival curves of 1,010 children with rhabdomyosarcoma entered into the fourth Intergroup Rhabdomyosarcoma Study are shown by stage. (Adapted from Breneman JC, Lyden E, Pappo AS, et al. Prognostic factors and outcome in children with metastatic rhabdomyosarcoma: a report from the Intergroup Rhabdomyosarcoma Study IV. *J Clin Oncol* 2003;21: 78–84; and from Crist WM, Anderson JR, Meza JL, et al. The Intergroup Rhabdomyosarcoma Study-IV: results for patients with non-metastatic disease. *J Clin Oncol* 2001;19:3091–3102.)

The fourth IRS study (IRS-IV) was conducted from 1991 to 1997 (Fig. 91.5).[1] Results from this study are as follows:

1. For patients with group III tumors, hyperfractionated radiotherapy was no more effective than conventional radiotherapy for tumor control and survival.
2. There was no difference in survival between VAC and vincristine/actinomycin/ifosfamide and vincristine/ifosfamide/etoposide in children with nonmetastatic disease.
3. Failure-free survival at 3 years for patients with embryonal histology was superior to results seen in IRS-III (83% vs. 74%), but no difference was seen for alveolar or undifferentiated subtypes.
4. Survival for patients with group I or II orbit or eyelid tumors was excellent when treated with VA and radiotherapy for group II disease.
5. Prognostic subsets of patients based on histologic subtype, stage, and group could be identified as follows: low-risk patients had embryonal histology and were stage 1 (all groups), or stage 2 or 3 and group I or II. All other patients with locoregional disease were intermediate risk.
6. Survival for patients with metastatic disease was superior with the drug pair ifosfamide/etoposide when compared with vincristine/melphalan.[91]
7. Whole-brain radiotherapy was omitted for all patients with parameningeal primary tumors except when there was cytologic evidence of cerebrospinal fluid involvement. Survival was not compromised by this approach.

The fifth IRS studies (IRS-V) were conducted from 1997 to 2005. They studied a number of questions that included the following:

1. Can a subset of the most favorable patients be treated without alkylating agents?
2. Can radiation dose be reduced to 36 Gy for microscopic disease and 45 Gy for gross tumor in the subset of patients with orbital primaries?
3. Can radiation be omitted in patients with vaginal tumors who achieve a complete response?
4. Can radiation dose be reduced for group III patients after induction chemotherapy and second-look operation?
5. What is the activity of topotecan and irinotecan in the treatment of RMS?

Results from some of these studies are now available and show that failure-free survival for low-risk patients (treated without cyclophosphamide and given decreased radiation doses as described above) was similar to results seen in IRS-III, which also did not use cyclophosphamide, but was inferior to results from IRS-IV where cyclophosphamide or ifosfamide was given. The conclusion of this study was that reduced radiotherapy doses with 36 Gy for microscopic disease did not appear to compromise local control, but the inclusion of an alkylating chemotherapy agent in the treatment regimen may be important for maximizing outcomes in these patients.

For group III orbital tumors, dose reduction to 45 Gy resulted in an unacceptably high rate of local failure rate at 13% (compared to 5% seen on IRS IV). As such, 50.4 Gy remains the standard of care for orbital tumors with gross disease, though 45 Gy may be sufficient if there is a complete response to induction chemotherapy.[35,36] For vaginal tumors treated without radiation, local failure rates were also unacceptably high (26% on D9602 and 43% on ARST003).[65] Omission of radiation therapy for these children is not advisable, and intravaginal brachytherapy may be the preferred modality of treatment given the high dose gradient and subsequent sparing of surrounding normal tissue.

For patients who undergo second-look surgery after induction chemotherapy, radiation dose can be successfully reduced to 36 Gy for negative margins and 41.4 Gy for microscopically positive margins without compromising local control.[119] For patients with intermediate-risk disease, the addition of topotecan to the standard VAC regimen did not improve failure-free survival.[120]

Societe Internationale D'oncologie Pediatrique Studies

SIOP (the French acronym for the International Society of Pediatric Oncology) began multi-institutional trials for RMS in 1975 and has reported results from three studies to date.[95,121,122] The focus of these studies has been to minimize local therapy by using risk-adapted intensification of chemotherapy, with attempted salvage of patients who fail locally.

The first SIOP study (RMS-75) used VAC chemotherapy plus doxorubicin. Group III patients were randomized to early local therapy versus response-based delayed local therapy (surgery preferred over radiotherapy) after maximal chemotherapy response. No survival difference was seen between these arms, although overall survival was only 40%.

The second SIOP study, MMT-84 (malignant mesenchymal tumor), used a similar strategy of limited radiotherapy only when there was residual tumor after chemotherapy and surgery. Overall survival at 5 years was 68%, although EFS was only 53%, and 29% of patients had isolated local relapse.

The third SIOP study, MMT-89, concluded that alkylating agents can be omitted for patients with the most favorable prognosis. The use of radiotherapy was again limited, resulting in a local failure rate of 34%.

The SIOP and IRS studies differ significantly in their use of local therapy, with IRS studies emphasizing early introduction of radiotherapy for patients with residual tumor after surgery, and SIOP studies avoiding radiotherapy except for proven residual tumor after chemotherapy and surgery. A comparison of the results of the two studies has been performed, and although it is clear that some children can be cured without radiotherapy, the routine use of radiotherapy for residual tumor after initial surgery as used in the IRS studies results in higher survival rates for most subsets of patients.[97]

Cooperative Weichteilsarkom Studiengruppe Studies

The German-based CWS studies have taken an approach to local control that is intermediate between that of the IRS and SIOP trials. The CWS-81 trial used response-adapted radiotherapy after chemotherapy and second-look surgery with children receiving no radiotherapy, 40 or 50 Gy depending on tumor status. Results of this study showed that children who have a complete response to chemotherapy have a prognosis equal to those who have an initial complete resection of their tumor. However, those patients who do not have a complete response to chemotherapy by week 9 should have early surgery or radiotherapy. Overall disease-free survival after 5 years was 68% for children with nonmetastatic disease.[92,123] Local recurrence was the most common cause of failure.

The CWS-86 study used ifosfamide for all patients, with an abbreviated course of chemotherapy for favorable patients with early-stage disease, and altered the way radiotherapy was given.[124] Patients who had an early complete response to chemotherapy did not receive radiotherapy. Most received hyperfractionated accelerated radiotherapy of 1.6 Gy twice daily concurrent with ifosfamide and doxorubicin containing chemotherapy, using 32 Gy after a good response and 54.4 Gy after a poor response. Conclusions from this study were as follows:

1. Duration of chemotherapy can be reduced to as little as 16 weeks for the most favorable patients.
2. Ifosfamide gives improved response rates compared with cyclophosphamide.
3. Hyperfractionated accelerated radiotherapy concurrent with chemotherapy as used in the study is tolerable and provided acceptable local control.

Like CWS-81, the majority of failures in this study were local, with an especially high local recurrence rate in those group II and III patients who did not receive radiotherapy.

The CWS-91 study continued the strategy of risk-adapted therapy.[125] Patients were initially stratified for treatment according to IRS group, tumor site, and histologic subtype. After induction chemotherapy, second-look surgery was encouraged, and those with a complete resection and no high-risk features did not receive radiotherapy. Others received 32 or 48 Gy (1.6 Gy twice daily) depending on risk factors and response to initial chemotherapy. Outcomes were compared to historical controls from the CWS-86 study. Major findings were as follows:

1. Local control and EFS were improved in those patients who received radiotherapy when compared to those who did not receive radiotherapy, in spite of more unfavorable risk factors in the former group.
2. Results for patients receiving 32 or 48 Gy on CWS-91 were similar to results in similar patients treated with higher radiation doses on the CWS-86 study.

3. Patients with group I and group II tumors and favorable risk factors had equivalent outcomes with decreased intensity chemotherapy compared with similar patients treated in CWS-86.

SEQUELAE OF TREATMENT

Acute Effects

Acute side effects from surgery are primarily postoperative complications that are usually reversible and not serious. The acute toxicity from chemotherapy includes nausea, vomiting, mucositis, alopecia, and hematopoietic suppression. Drug-induced granulocytopenia significantly increases the risk of fever and infection, although the routine use of granulocyte colony–stimulating factor has lessened these risks. Newer protocols using more aggressive therapy, including topoisomerase inhibitors, ifosfamide, etoposide, and other agents, have other acute side effects, including renal and electrolyte imbalance, which demand close monitoring.

Acute radiation toxicity is related to the regions irradiated and the dose administered. It can be especially pronounced for tumors of the head and neck, abdomen, and pelvis. The synergistic effect of chemotherapeutic drugs such as dactinomycin and doxorubicin can be severe and may require modification of the treatment plan. Both dactinomycin and doxorubicin are known to accentuate a "recall" of radiation injury if given during or immediately after the course of radiation therapy.

Prompt attention to skin care is important. Moisturizers and steroid creams are effective symptomatic treatments for erythema and dry desquamation. Moist desquamation may be treated with aluminum acetate soaks or hydrocolloid dressings. Occasionally, a delay in radiation therapy is necessary to permit healing.

After orbital irradiation, an acute inflammatory reaction of the cornea and conjunctiva may be seen within weeks of completion of treatment. This can result in pain and photophobia. Topical steroids should be administered under the direction of an ophthalmologist for these symptoms.

Acute otitis externa or media with hyperemia and swelling of the membranes of the eustachian tube is common during or soon after treatment of head and neck areas. Decongestants are helpful in reducing the swelling. Erythematous mucositis, leading to a patchy, fibrinous exudate, is seen after head and neck irradiation, after drug therapy, and almost universally if the two are used simultaneously. Mouthwashes such as baking soda, 1% hydrogen peroxide, or combinations of diphenhydramine elixir, hydrocortisone, and antibiotics partially alleviate the reaction. Bacterial or fungal superinfection requires specific drug management. Pretreatment evaluation by a dentist is important to correct pre-existing problems and help guide preventive therapy such as dental hygiene and fluoride applications.

Acute gastrointestinal sequelae, such as vomiting and diarrhea, are usually managed by supportive care. Parenteral nutritional support may be necessary to prevent protein or calorie malnutrition.

Late Effects

Life-threatening late events occur in approximately 9% of survivors after treatment.[33] A higher percentage experience lesser degrees of late morbidity, with the risks dependent on factors such as primary tumor site, disease stage, and the treatment modalities employed.

Long-term sequelae related to specific chemotherapy drugs are usually site specific, and the morbidity may be accentuated by radiation therapy. Cyclophosphamide may induce hemorrhagic cystitis, and doxorubicin is implicated in late myocardiopathies.[126] Cisplatin carries a high incidence of hearing impairment. Alkylating agents and topoisomerase inhibitors are associated with the development of secondary neoplasms, particularly acute myeloid leukemia.[127,128]

Late radiation effects are related to the irradiated site, the dose of radiation, and the age of the child at the time of treatment. Effects include bone and soft tissue growth disturbances, dental abnormalities, cataract, hypopituitarism, gonadal dysfunction, induction of second malignant tumors (particularly bone sarcomas), and chronic organ dysfunction.[55,127,129-131] Long-term follow-up and treatment are important to minimize the impact of these, particularly for endocrine and dental complications.[132] Combined-modality treatment programs are significantly implicated in many of these complications.

Late surgical complications depend mainly on the choice of surgical procedure for primary treatment of the tumor. They include disfigurement and loss of function. Serious late effects of surgical treatment include the consequences of fecal and urinary diversion as well as ejaculatory impotence after retroperitoneal lymph node dissection.

FUTURE DIRECTIONS AND RESEARCH

Advances in molecular biology are providing a more comprehensive understanding of the biologic behavior of RMS and direct new research initiatives.

Chromosome aberrations are common in RMS. A consistent loss of heterozygosity at 11p15.5 is seen in embryonal RMS. Cytogenetic studies of alveolar RMS often demonstrate a translocation involving chromosomes 2 and 13, which affects the *PAX3* gene in band 2q35 and the *FKHR* gene in band 13q14.[133,134] The reciprocal translocation t(2;13) fuses *PAX3* to the *FKHR* gene, resulting in a chimeric structure that functions as an oncoprotein, resulting in dysregulation of cell growth and transformation.[135] Similarly, t(1;13) juxtaposes the *PAX7* gene on chromosome 1p36 with the *FKHR* gene on chromosome 13q14, again producing a chimeric transcript. These findings suggest that there may be a set of target genes involved in the pathogenesis of RMS, and work is currently under way to engineer vaccines against the resulting fusion proteins.[29] The identification of genes in alveolar RMS has permitted the development of molecular diagnostic assays, including reverse transcriptase polymerase chain reaction and fluorescence *in situ* hybridization, for improved detection of alveolar RMS cells.[136]

Proto-oncogene research has focused on nuclear transcription factors. Embryonal RMS does not reveal amplification of either N-*myc* or c-*myc*; however, the majority of alveolar cases do have N-*myc* amplification. Survival among N-*myc*–amplified patients is poor.[137] Recent investigations link N-*myc* regulation to the *PAX3-FKHR* fusion gene present in many patients with alveolar RMS and may suggest targets for biologic manipulations.[138] Overexpression of the histone H3 lysine 9 (H3K9) methyltransferase KMT1A has been shown to block differentiation of alveolar RMS by repressing a myogenic gene expression program and is a potential target for novel therapies.[139]

The hedgehog pathway has been found to be activated in a subset of patients with embryonal and fusion-negative alveolar RMS.[140] These children have a significantly worse outlook than those with similar phenotypes without hedgehog activation. Inhibitors of the hedgehog pathway may offer therapeutic options in this group of patients. STAT3 is also an important signaling pathway in the oncogenesis of RMS, and targeting of this cascade is also being explored.[141]

Increased expression of the insulinlike growth factor 1 receptor (IGF1R) has been demonstrated in several RMS cell lines, and IGF1R inhibitors have shown significant preclinical antitumor activity.[142] Future studies will examine the efficacy of these drugs in the clinical setting.[143] Antibodies to the death receptor DR-5, present on many RMS cells, have also shown significant preclinical activity.[144]

Alteration of tumor suppressor genes is described in RMS, although their significance is unclear. Investigators have reported that >50% of both alveolar and embryonal RMS in established cell lines contain a mutant *p53* tumor

---

What is a Fusion Gene?

Fusion genes, such as the PAX3-FOXO1 fusion gene discussed in this chapter, play a critical role in tumorigenesis. A fusion gene forms from the combination of two genes secondary to chromosomal aberrations including translocations, insertions, inversions, and interstitial deletions. As a result, fusion transcripts and proteins are created that can lead to the abnormal proliferation of cells and subsequently oncogenesis. Gene fusions are thought to be responsible for the pathogenesis of approximately 20% of cancer cases.[1]

The first fusion gene discovered was the BCR-ABL1 fusion gene characteristic of chronic myeloid leukemia (CML). This fusion results from the translocation between chromosomes 9 and 22 (the Philadelphia chromosome) and results in a constitutively active tyrosine kinase that acts as the driver mutation for CML. Since the initial characterization of the Philadelphia chromosome in the 1960s, there have been over 10,000 fusion genes identified, including the reciprocal translocation between chromosomes 2 and 13 (t2;13, or occasionally t1;13) that fuses the PAX3 (or PAX7) gene to the FOXO1 (FKHR) gene in alveolar RMS; the interstitial deletion on chromosome 21 that results in the formation of the *TMPRSS2-ERG fusion gene seen in approximately 50% of patients with prostate cancer*; the translocation between chromosome 8 and 21 (t8;21) that is characteristic of acute myeloid leukemia; the EWSR1-FLI1 fusion in Ewing sarcoma; *and the ELM4-ALK fusion seen in a small percentage of patients with lung cancer.*[2]

Fusion genes are important not only for oncogenesis but also for clinical utility. The detection of fusion genes may be used for diagnostic purposes; for example, urine *TMPRSS2-ERG can be used for screening and diagnosing prostate cancer.*[3,4] For tumors in which there is heterogeneity with respect to gene fusion status (such as RMS), fusion genes play a significant role in risk stratification. Importantly, therapeutic agents targeted at fusion proteins have changed the treatment paradigm and outcomes for many tumors (e.g., imatinib for CML and crizotinib for ALK fusion-positive lung cancer). In alveolar RMS, vaccines targeted against the PAX-FOXO1 fusion protein are currently under development.[5]

In summary, fusion genes can serve as the driver mutation for different cancer types and can play a critical role clinically for diagnosis, prognostication, and as a target for therapy. As molecular techniques continue to advance, the role of fusion genes in cancer development and therapy will continue to grow.

1. Mitelman F, Johansson B, Mertens F. The impact of translocations and gene fusions on cancer causation. *Nat Rev Cancer* 2007;7(4):233–245.
2. Mertens F, Johansson B, Fioretos T, et al. The emerging complexity of gene fusions in cancer. *Nat Rev Cancer* 2015;15(6):371–381.
3. Tomlins SA, Rhodes DR, Perner S, et al. Recurrent fusion of TMPRSS2 and ETS transcription factor genes in prostate cancer. *Science* 2005; 310(5748):644–648.
4. Sanguedolce F, Cormio A, Brunelli M, et al. Urine TMPRSS2: ERG fusion transcript as a biomarker for prostate cancer: literature review. *Clin Genitourin Cancer* 2016;14(2):117–121.
5. van den Broeke LT, Pendleton CD, Mackall C, et al. Identification and epitope enhancement of a PAX-FKHR fusion protein breakpoint epitope in alveolar rhabdomyosarcoma cells created by a tumorigenic chromosomal translocation inducing CTL capable of lysing human tumors. *Cancer Res* 2006;66(3):1818–1823.

suppressor gene.[145] However, more recent data indicate that the actual incidence of mutant *p53* in tissue derived directly from patient biopsies is much lower, and data regarding its predictive value for survival are mixed.[146,147] Studies of multiple drug–resistant genes, which encode P-glycoprotein, suggest that in RMS, high levels of P-glycoprotein lead to tumor resistance. In these tumors, there appears to be a correlation between P-glycoprotein positivity and poor outcome.[148]

The current generation of COG STS studies tests a number of clinical hypotheses. These include testing the ability to reduce the duration of chemotherapy for favorable prognosis of tumors, studying the effect of delivering radiotherapy at week 13 of treatment concurrently with temsirolimus for intermediate-risk patients, boosting tumors initially measuring >5 cm to 59.4 Gy total, and evaluating the prognostic value of early treatment response as assessed by PET imaging.

Future directions and research in RMS are being driven by many exciting molecular biologic and technologic advances. Such new findings provide hope for more refined risk-based therapy in RMS and potentially for gene therapy to be added to the therapeutic armamentarium.

REFERENCES

1. Crist WM, Anderson JR, Meza JL, et al. Intergroup rhabdomyosarcoma study-IV: results for patients with nonmetastatic disease. *J Clin Oncol* 2001;19:3091–3102.
2. Ognjanovic S, Linabery AM, Charbonneau B, et al. Trends in childhood rhabdomyosarcoma incidence and survival in the United States, 1975–2005. *Cancer* 2009;115:4218–4226.
3. Joshi D, Anderson JR, Paidas C, et al. Age is an independent prognostic factor in rhabdomyosarcoma: a report from the Soft Tissue Sarcoma Committee of the Children's Oncology Group. *Pediatr Blood Cancer* 2004;42:64–73.
4. Ferrari A, Dileo P, Casanova M, et al. Rhabdomyosarcoma in adults. A retrospective analysis of 171 patients treated at a single institution. *Cancer* 2003;98:571–580.
5. Ogilvie CM, Crawford EA, Slotcavage RL, et al. Treatment of adult rhabdomyosarcoma. *Am J Clin Oncol* 2010;33:128–131.
6. Gerber NK, Wexler LH, Singer S, et al. Adult rhabdomyosarcoma survival improved with treatment on multimodality protocols. *Int J Radiat Oncol Biol Phys* 2013;86(1):58–63.
7. La TH, Wolden SL, Rodeberg DA, et al. Regional nodal involvement and patterns of spread along in-transit pathways in children with rhabdomyosarcoma of the extremity: a report from the Children's Oncology Group. *Int J Radiat Oncol Biol Phys* 2011;80:1151–1157.
8. Casey DL, Wexler LH, LaQuaglia MP, et al. Patterns of failure for rhabdomyosarcoma of the perineal and perianal region. *Int J Radiat Oncol Biol Phys* 2014;89(1):82–87.
9. Breneman JC, Lyden E, Pappo AS, et al. Prognostic factors and clinical outcomes in children and adolescents with metastatic rhabdomyosarcoma—a report from the Intergroup Rhabdomyosarcoma Study IV. *J Clin Oncol* 2003;21:78–84.
10. McCarville MB, Christie R, Daw NC, et al. PET/CT in the evaluation of childhood sarcomas. *AJR Am J Roentgenol* 2005;184:1293–1304.
11. Tateishi U, Hosono A, Makimoto A, et al. Comparative study of FDG PET/CT and conventional imaging in the staging of rhabdomyosarcoma. *Ann Nucl Med* 2009;23:155–161.
12. Rodeberg DA, Stoner JA, Hayes-Jordan A, et al. Prognostic significance of tumor response at the end of therapy in group III rhabdomyosarcoma: a report from the Children's Oncology Group. *J Clin Oncol* 2009;27:3705–3711.
13. Burke M, Anderson JR, Kao SC, et al. Assessment of response to induction therapy and its influence on 5-year failure-free survival in group III rhabdomyosarcoma: the Intergroup Rhabdomyosarcoma Study-IV experience—a report from the Soft Tissue Sarcoma Committee of the Children's Oncology Group. *J Clin Oncol* 2007;25:4909–4913.
14. Casey DL, Wexler LH, Fox JJ, et al. Predicting outcome in patients with rhabdomyosarcoma: role of [(18)f]fluorodeoxyglucose positron emission tomography. *Int J Radiat Oncol Biol Phys* 2014;90(5):1136–1142.
15. Kelly KM, Womer RB, Barr FG. Minimal disease detection in patients with alveolar rhabdomyosarcoma using a reverse transcriptase-polymerase chain reaction method. *Cancer* 1996;78:1320–1327.
16. Lawrence W Jr, Gehan EA, Hays DM, et al. Prognostic significance of staging factors of the UICC staging system in childhood rhabdomyosarcoma: a report from the Intergroup Rhabdomyosarcoma Study (IRS-II). *J Clin Oncol* 1987;5:46–54.
17. Crist W, Gehan EA, Ragab AH, et al. The third Intergroup Rhabdomyosarcoma Study. *J Clin Oncol* 1995;13:610–630.
18. Rodary C, Gehan EA, Flamant F, et al. Prognostic factors in 951 nonmetastatic rhabdomyosarcoma in children: a report from the International Rhabdomyosarcoma Workshop. *Med Pediatr Oncol* 1991;19:89–95.
19. Perez EA, Kassira N, Cheung MC, et al. Rhabdomyosarcoma in children: a SEER population based study. *J Surg Res* 2011;170(2):e245–e251.
20. Qualman SJ, Coffin CM, Newton WA, et al. Intergroup Rhabdomyosarcoma Study: update for pathologists. *Pediatr Dev Pathol* 1998;1:550–561.
21. Asmar L, Gehan EA, Newton WA, et al. Agreement among and within groups of pathologists in the classification of rhabdomyosarcoma and related childhood sarcomas. Report of an international study of four pathology classifications. *Cancer* 1994;74:2579–2588.
22. Pappo AS, Shapiro DN, Crist WM, et al. Biology and therapy of pediatric rhabdomyosarcoma. *J Clin Oncol* 1995;13:2123–2139.
23. Wachtel M, Runge T, Leuschner I, et al. Subtype and prognostic classification of rhabdomyosarcoma by immunohistochemistry. *J Clin Oncol* 2006;24:816–822.
24. Grass B, Wachtel M, Behnke S, et al. Immunohistochemical detection of EGFR, fibrillin-2, P-cadherin and AP2beta as biomarkers for rhabdomyosarcoma diagnostics. *Histopathology* 2009;54:873–879.
25. Martinelli S, McDowell HP, Vigne SD, et al. RAS signaling dysregulation in human embryonal rhabdomyosarcoma. *Genes Chromosomes Cancer* 2009;48:975–982.
26. Shapiro DN, Parham DM, Douglass EC, et al. Relationship of tumor-cell ploidy to histologic subtype and treatment outcome in children and adolescents with unresectable rhabdomyosarcoma. *J Clin Oncol* 1991;9:159–166.
27. Shapiro DN, Valentine MB, Sublett JE, et al. Chromosomal sublocalization of the 2;13 translocation breakpoint in alveolar rhabdomyosarcoma. *Genes Chromosomes Cancer* 1992;4:241–249.
28. Scheidler S, Fredericks WJ, Rauscher FJ 3rd, et al. The hybrid PAX3-FKHR fusion protein of alveolar rhabdomyosarcoma transforms fibroblasts in culture. *Proc Natl Acad Sci U S A* 1996;93:9805–9809.
29. van den Broeke LT, Pendleton CD, Mackall C, et al. Identification and epitope enhancement of a PAX-FKHR fusion protein breakpoint epitope in alveolar rhabdomyosarcoma cells created by a tumorigenic chromosomal translocation inducing CTL capable of lysing human tumors. *Cancer Res* 2006;66:1818–1823.
30. Williamson D, Missiaglia E, de Reynies A, et al. Fusion gene-negative alveolar rhabdomyosarcoma is clinically and molecularly indistinguishable from embryonal rhabdomyosarcoma. *J Clin Oncol* 2010;28:2151–2158.
31. Skapek SX, Anderson J, Barr FG, et al. PAX-FOXO1 fusion status drives unfavorable outcome for children with rhabdomyosarcoma: a children's oncology group report. *Pediatr Blood Cancer* 2013;60(9):1411–1417.
32. Arnold MA, Anderson JR, Gastier-Foster JM, et al. Histology, fusion status, and outcome in alveolar rhabdomyosarcoma with low-risk clinical features: a report from the Children's Oncology Group. *Pediatr Blood Cancer* 2016;63(4):634–639.
33. Sung L, Anderson JR, Donaldson SS, et al. Late events occurring five years or more after successful therapy for childhood rhabdomyosarcoma: a report from the Soft Tissue Sarcoma Committee of the Children's Oncology Group. *Eur J Cancer* 2004;40:1878–1885.
34. Kodet R, Newton WA Jr, Hamoudi AB, et al. Orbital rhabdomyosarcomas and related tumors in childhood: relationship of morphology to prognosis—an Intergroup Rhabdomyosarcoma Study. *Med Pediatr Oncol* 1997;29:51–60.
35. Raney R, Walterhouse DO, Meza JL, et al. Results of the Intergroup Rhabdomyosarcoma Study Group D9602 protocol, using vincristine and dactinomycin with or without cyclophosphamide and radiation therapy, for newly diagnosed patients with low-risk embryonal rhabdomyosarcoma: a report from the Soft Tissue Sarcoma Committee of the Children's Oncology Group. *J Clin Oncol* 2011;29:1312–1318.
36. Breneman J, Meza J, Donaldson S, et al. Local control with reduced dose radiotherapy for low-risk rhabdomyosarcoma: a report from the Children's Oncology Group D9602 study. *Int J Radiat Oncol Biol Phys* 2012;83(2):720–726.
37. Rousseau P, Flamant F, Quintana E, et al. Primary chemotherapy in rhabdomyosarcomas and other malignant mesenchymal tumors of the orbit: results of the International Society of Pediatric Oncology MMT 84 Study. *J Clin Oncol* 1994;12:516–521.
38. Oberlin O, Rey A, Anderson J, et al. Treatment of orbital rhabdomyosarcoma: survival and late effects of treatment—results of an international workshop. *J Clin Oncol* 2001;19:197–204.
39. Sagerman RH. Orbital rhabdomyosarcoma: a paradigm for irradiation. *Radiology* 1993;187:605–607.
40. Yock T, Schneider R, Friedmann A, et al. Proton radiotherapy for orbital rhabdomyosarcoma: clinical outcome and a dosimetric comparison with photons. *Int J Radiat Oncol Biol Phys* 2005;63:1161–1168.
41. Maurer HM, Gehan EA, Beltangady M, et al. The Intergroup Rhabdomyosarcoma Study-II. *Cancer* 1993;71:1904–1922.
42. Michalski JM, Meza J, Breneman JC, et al. Influence of radiation therapy parameters on outcome in children treated with radiation therapy for localized parameningeal rhabdomyosarcoma in Intergroup Rhabdomyosarcoma Study Group trials II through IV. *Int J Radiat Oncol Biol Phys* 2004;59:1027–1038.
43. Tefft M, Fernandez CH, Donaldson M. Incidence of meningeal involvement by rhabdomyosarcoma of the head and neck in children: a report of the Intergroup Rhabdomyosarcoma Study (IRS). *Cancer* 1978;48(Suppl 2):253–258.
44. Raney RB, Meza J, Anderson JR, et al. Treatment of children and adolescents with localized parameningeal sarcoma: experience of the Intergroup Rhabdomyosarcoma Study Group protocols IRS-II through -IV, 1978–1997. *Med Pediatr Oncol* 2002;38:22–32.
45. Douglas JG, Arndt CA, Hawkins DS. Delayed radiotherapy following dose intensive chemotherapy for parameningeal rhabdomyosarcoma (PM-RMS) of childhood. *Eur J Cancer* 2007;43:1045–1050.
46. Blank LE, Koedooder K, Pieters BR, et al. The AMORE protocol for advanced-stage and recurrent nonorbital rhabdomyosarcoma in the head-and-neck region of children: a radiation oncology view. *Int J Radiat Oncol Biol Phys* 2009;74:1555–1562.
47. Blatt J, Snyderman C, Wollman MR, et al. Delayed resection in the management of non-orbital rhabdomyosarcoma of the head and neck in childhood. *Med Pediatr Oncol* 1997;28:294–298.
48. Bisogno G, De Rossi C, Gamboa Y, et al. Improved survival for children with parameningeal rhabdomyosarcoma: results from the AIEOP Soft Tissue Sarcoma Committee. *Pediatr Blood Cancer* 2008;50:1154–1158.

49. Benk V, Rodary C, Donaldson SS, et al. Parameningeal rhabdomyosarcoma: results of an international workshop. *Int J Radiat Oncol Biol Phys* 1996;36:533–540.

50. La Quaglia MP, Ghavimi F, Herr H, et al. Prognostic factors in bladder and bladder-prostate rhabdomyosarcoma. *J Pediatr Surg* 1990;25:1066–1072.

51. Raney RB Jr, Gehan EA, Hays DM, et al. Primary chemotherapy with or without radiation therapy and/or surgery for children with localized sarcoma of the bladder, prostate, vagina, uterus, and cervix. A comparison of the results in Intergroup Rhabdomyosarcoma Studies I and II. *Cancer* 1990;66:2072–2081.

52. Hays DM. Bladder/prostate rhabdomyosarcoma: results of the multi-institutional trials of the Intergroup Rhabdomyosarcoma Study. *Semin Surg Oncol* 1993;9:520–523.

53. Lobe TE, Wiener E, Andrassy RJ, et al. The argument for conservative, delayed surgery in the management of prostatic rhabdomyosarcoma. *J Pediatr Surg* 1996;31:1084–1087.

54. Arndt C, Rodeberg D, Breitfeld PP, et al. Does bladder preservation (as a surgical principle) lead to retaining bladder function in bladder/prostate rhabdomyosarcoma? Results from Intergroup Rhabdomyosarcoma Study IV. *J Urol* 2004;171:2396–2403.

55. Raney B, Anderson J, Jenney M, et al. Late effects in 164 patients with rhabdomyosarcoma of the bladder/prostate region: a report from the international workshop. *J Urol* 2006;176:2190–2194; discussion 4–5.

56. Seitz G, Dantonello TM, Int-Veen C, et al. Treatment efficiency, outcome and surgical treatment problems in patients suffering from localized embryonal bladder/prostate rhabdomyosarcoma: a report from the cooperative soft tissue sarcoma trial CWS-96. *Pediatr Blood Cancer* 2011;56(5):718–724.

57. Rodeberg DA, Anderson JR, Arndt CA, et al. Comparison of outcomes based on treatment algorithms for rhabdomyosarcoma of the bladder/prostate: combined results from the Children's Oncology Group, German Cooperative Soft Tissue Sarcoma Study, Italian Cooperative Group, and International Society of Pediatric Oncology Malignant Mesenchymal Tumors Committee. *Int J Cancer* 2011;128:1232–1239.

58. Wiener ES, Anderson JR, Ojimba JI, et al. Controversies in the management of paratesticular rhabdomyosarcoma: is staging retroperitoneal lymph node dissection necessary for adolescents with resected paratesticular rhabdomyosarcoma? *Semin Pediatr Surg* 2001;10:146–152.

59. Olive D, Flamant F, Zucker JM, et al. Paraaortic lymphadenectomy is not necessary in the treatment of localized paratesticular rhabdomyosarcoma. *Cancer* 1984;54:1283–1287.

60. Stewart RJ, Martelli H, Oberlin O, et al. Treatment of children with nonmetastatic paratesticular rhabdomyosarcoma: results of the Malignant Mesenchymal Tumors studies (MMT 84 and MMT 89) of the International Society of Pediatric Oncology. *J Clin Oncol* 2003;21:793–798.

61. Wiener ES, Lawrence W, Hays D, et al. Retroperitoneal node biopsy in paratesticular rhabdomyosarcoma. *J Pediatr Surg* 1994;29:171–177; discussion 8.

62. Arndt CA, Donaldson SS, Anderson JR, et al. What constitutes optimal therapy for patients with rhabdomyosarcoma of the female genital tract? *Cancer* 2001;91:2454–2468.

63. Andrassy RJ, Wiener ES, Raney RB, et al. Progress in the surgical management of vaginal rhabdomyosarcoma: a 25-year review from the Intergroup Rhabdomyosarcoma Study Group. *J Pediatr Surg* 1999;34:731–734; discussion 4–5.

64. Martelli H, Oberlin O, Rey A, et al. Conservative treatment for girls with nonmetastatic rhabdomyosarcoma of the genital tract: a report from the Study Committee of the International Society of Pediatric Oncology. *J Clin Oncol* 1999;17:2117–2122.

65. Walterhouse DO, Meza JL, Breneman JC, et al. Local control and outcome in children with localized vaginal rhabdomyosarcoma: a report from the Soft Tissue Sarcoma Committee of the Children's Oncology Group. *Pediatr Blood Cancer* 2011;57(1):76–83.

66. Magne N, Oberlin O, Martelli H, et al. Vulval and vaginal rhabdomyosarcoma in children: update and reappraisal of Institut Gustave Roussy brachytherapy experience. *Int J Radiat Oncol Biol Phys* 2008;72:878–883.

67. Nag S, Tippin D, Ruymann FB. Intraoperative high-dose-rate brachytherapy for the treatment of pediatric tumors: the Ohio State University experience. *Int J Radiat Oncol Biol Phys* 2001;51:729–735.

68. Mandell L, Ghavimi F, LaQuaglia M, et al. Prognostic significance of regional lymph node involvement in childhood extremity rhabdomyosarcoma. *Med Pediatr Oncol* 1990;18:466–471.

69. McMulkin HM, Yanchar NL, Fernandez CV, et al. Sentinel lymph node mapping and biopsy: a potentially valuable tool in the management of childhood extremity rhabdomyosarcoma. *Pediatr Surg Int* 2003;19:453–456.

70. Weiss BD, Dasgupta R, Gelfand MJ, et al. Use of sentinel node biopsy for staging parameningeal rhabdomyosarcoma. *Pediatr Blood Cancer* 2011;57:520–523.

71. La TH, Wolden SL, Rodeberg DA, et al. Regional nodal involvement and patterns of spread along in-transit pathways in children with rhabdomyosarcoma of the extremity: a report from the Children's Oncology Group. *Int J Radiat Oncol Biol Phys* 2010;80:1151–1157.

72. Neville HL, Andrassy RJ, Lobe TE, et al. Preoperative staging, prognostic factors, and outcome for extremity rhabdomyosarcoma: a preliminary report from the Intergroup Rhabdomyosarcoma Study IV (1991–1997). *J Pediatr Surg* 2000;35:317–321.

73. Horowitz ME, Kinsella TJ, Wexler LH, et al. Total-body irradiation and autologous bone marrow transplant in the treatment of high-risk Ewing's sarcoma and rhabdomyosarcoma. *J Clin Oncol* 1993;11:1911–1918.

74. McDowell HP, Foot AB, Ellershaw C, et al. Outcomes in paediatric metastatic rhabdomyosarcoma: results of The International Society of Paediatric Oncology (SIOP) study MMT-98. *Eur J Cancer* 2010;46:1588–1595.

75. Casey DL, Wexler LH, Meyers PA, et al. Radiation for bone metastases in Ewing sarcoma and rhabdomyosarcoma. *Pediatr Blood Cancer* 2015;62(3):445–449.

76. Rodeberg D, Arndt C, Breneman J, et al. Characteristics and outcomes of rhabdomyosarcoma patients with isolated lung metastases from IRS-IV. *J Pediatr Surg* 2005;40(1):256–262.

77. Yang JC, Wexler LH, Meyers PA, et al. Intensity-modulated radiation therapy with dose-painting for pediatric sarcomas with pulmonary metastases. *Pediatr Blood Cancer* 2013;60(10):1616–1620.

78. Lacey SR, Jewett TC Jr, Karp MP, et al. Advances in the treatment of rhabdomyosarcoma. *Semin Surg Oncol* 1986;2:139–146.

79. Jones IS, Reese AB, Krout J. Orbital rhabdomyosarcoma: an analysis of sixty-two cases. *Trans Am Ophthalmol Soc* 1965;63:223–255.

80. Pedrick TJ, Donaldson SS, Cox RS. Rhabdomyosarcoma: the Stanford experience using a TNM staging system. *J Clin Oncol* 1986;4:370–378.

81. Donaldson SS, Castro JR, Wilbur JR, et al. Rhabdomyosarcoma of head and neck in children. Combination treatment by surgery, irradiation, and chemotherapy. *Cancer* 1973;31:26–35.

82. Cecchetto G, Carli M, Sotti G, et al. Importance of local treatment in pediatric soft tissue sarcomas with microscopic residual after primary surgery: results of the Italian Cooperative Study RMS-88. *Med Pediatr Oncol* 2000;34:97–101.

83. Hays DM, Lawrence W Jr, Wharam M, et al. Primary reexcision for patients with "microscopic residual" tumor following initial excision of sarcomas of trunk and extremity sites. *J Pediatr Surg* 1989;24:5–10.

84. Cecchetto G, Carretto E, Bisogno G, et al. Complete second look operation and radiotherapy in locally advanced non-alveolar rhabdomyosarcoma in children: a report from the AIEOP Soft Tissue Sarcoma Committee. *Pediatr Blood Cancer* 2008;51:593–597.

85. Wiener E, Lawrence W, Hays D. Survival is improved in clinical group III children with complete response established by second look operations in the Intergroup Rhabdomyosarcoma Study (IRS) III. *Med Pediatr Oncol* 1992;19:399.

86. Pappo AS, Etcubanas E, Santana VM, et al. A phase II trial of ifosfamide in previously untreated children and adolescents with unresectable rhabdomyosarcoma. *Cancer* 1993;71:2119–2125.

87. Pappo AS, Lyden E, Breneman J, et al. Up-front window trial of topotecan in previously untreated children and adolescents with metastatic rhabdomyosarcoma: an Intergroup Rhabdomyosarcoma Study. *J Clin Oncol* 2001;19:213–219.

88. Pratt CB, Stewart C, Santana VM, et al. Phase I study of topotecan for pediatric patients with malignant solid tumors. *J Clin Oncol* 1994;12:539–543.

89. Baker KS, Anderson JR, Link MP, et al. Benefit of intensified therapy for patients with local or regional embryonal rhabdomyosarcoma: results from the Intergroup Rhabdomyosarcoma Study IV. *J Clin Oncol* 2000;18:2427–2434.

90. Spunt SL, Smith LM, Ruymann FB, et al. Cyclophosphamide dose intensification during induction therapy for intermediate-risk pediatric rhabdomyosarcoma is feasible but does not improve outcome: a report from the Soft Tissue Sarcoma Committee of the Children's Oncology Group. *Clin Cancer Res* 2004;10:6072–6079.

91. Breitfeld PP, Lyden E, Raney RB, et al. Ifosfamide and etoposide are superior to vincristine and melphalan for pediatric metastatic rhabdomyosarcoma when administered with irradiation and combination chemotherapy: a report from the Intergroup Rhabdomyosarcoma Study Group. *J Pediatr Hematol Oncol* 2001;23:225–233.

92. Koscielniak E, Jurgens H, Winkler K, et al. Treatment of soft tissue sarcoma in childhood and adolescence. A report of the German Cooperative Soft Tissue Sarcoma Study. *Cancer* 1992;70:2557–2567.

93. Regine WF, Fontanesi J, Kumar P, et al. Local tumor control in rhabdomyosarcoma following low-dose irradiation: comparison of group II and select group III patients. *Int J Radiat Oncol Biol Phys* 1995;31:485–491.

94. Breitfeld PP, Anderson J, Kao SC. Assessment of response to induction therapy and its influence on 5-year failure-free survival (FFS) in group III rhabdomyosarcoma (RMS): Intergroup Rhabdomyosarcoma Study (IRS)-IV experience. *J Clin Oncol* 2004;22(14 Suppl):8513.

95. Stevens MC, Rey A, Bouvet N, et al. Treatment of nonmetastatic rhabdomyosarcoma in childhood and adolescence: third study of the International Society of Paediatric Oncology—SIOP Malignant Mesenchymal Tumor 89. *J Clin Oncol* 2005;23:2618–2628.

96. Wharam M, Beltangady M, Hays D, et al. Localized orbital rhabdomyosarcoma. An interim report of the Intergroup Rhabdomyosarcoma Study Committee. *Ophthalmology* 1987;94:251–254.

97. Donaldson SS, Anderson JR. Rhabdomyosarcoma: many similarities, a few philosophical differences. *J Clin Oncol* 2005;23:2586–2587.

98. Schuck A, Mattke AC, Schmidt B, et al. Group II rhabdomyosarcoma and rhabdomyosarcomalike tumors: is radiotherapy necessary? *J Clin Oncol* 2004;22:143–149.

99. Smith LM, Anderson JR, Qualman SJ, et al. Which patients with microscopic disease and rhabdomyosarcoma experience relapse after therapy? A report from the Soft Tissue Sarcoma Committee of the Children's Oncology Group. *J Clin Oncol* 2001;19:4058–4064.

100. Wolden SL, Wexler LH, Kraus DH, et al. Intensity-modulated radiotherapy for head-and-neck rhabdomyosarcoma. *Int J Radiat Oncol Biol Phys* 2005;61:1432–1438.

101. Lin C, Donaldson SS, Meza JL, et al. Effect of radiotherapy techniques (IMRT vs. 3D-CRT) on outcome in patients with intermediate-risk rhabdomyosarcoma enrolled in COG D9803—a report from the Children's Oncology Group. *Int J Radiat Oncol Biol Phys* 2012;82(5):1764–1770.

102. Curtis AE, Okcu MF, Chintagumpala M, et al. Local control after intensity-modulated radiotherapy for head-and-neck rhabdomyosarcoma. *Int J Radiat Oncol Biol Phys* 2009;73:173–177.

103. Cotter SE, Herrup DA, Friedmann A, et al. Proton radiotherapy for pediatric bladder/prostate rhabdomyosarcoma: clinical outcomes and dosimetry compared to intensity-modulated radiation therapy. *Int J Radiat Oncol Biol Phys* 2011;81(5):1367–1373.

104. Ladra MM, Edgington SK, Mahajan A, et al. A dosimetric comparison of proton and intensity modulated radiation therapy in pediatric rhabdomyosarcoma patients enrolled on a prospective phase II proton study. *Radiother Oncol* 2014;113(1):77–83.

105. Ladra MM, Szymonifka JD, Mahajan A, et al. Preliminary results of a phase II trial of proton radiotherapy for pediatric rhabdomyosarcoma. *J Clin Oncol* 2014;32(33):3762–3770.

106. Donaldson SS, Meza J, Breneman JC, et al. Results from the IRS-IV randomized trial of hyperfractionated radiotherapy in children with rhabdomyosarcoma—a report from the IRSG. *Int J Radiat Oncol Biol Phys* 2001;51:718–728.

107. Malempati S, Rodeberg DA, Donaldson SS, et al. Rhabdomyosarcoma in infants younger than 1 year: a report from the Children's Oncology Group. *Cancer* 2011;117(15):3493–3501.

108. Wharam MD, Hanfelt JJ, Tefft MC, et al. Radiation therapy for rhabdomyosarcoma: local failure risk for clinical group III patients on Intergroup Rhabdomyosarcoma Study II. *Int J Radiat Oncol Biol Phys* 1997;38:797–804.

109. Wharam MD, Meza J, Anderson J, et al. Failure pattern and factors predictive of local failure in rhabdomyosarcoma: a report of group III patients on the third Intergroup Rhabdomyosarcoma Study. *J Clin Oncol* 2004;22:1902–1908.

110. Wolden SL, Lyden ER, Arndt CA, et al. Local control for intermediate-risk rhabdomyosarcoma: results from D9803 according to histology, group, site, and size: a report from the Children's Oncology Group. *Int J Radiat Oncol Biol Phys* 2015;93(5):1071–1076.

111. Wolden SL, Anderson JR, Crist WM, et al. Indications for radiotherapy and chemotherapy after complete resection in rhabdomyosarcoma: a report from the Intergroup Rhabdomyosarcoma studies I to III. *J Clin Oncol* 1999;17:3468–3475.

112. Raney RB, Anderson JR, Brown KL, et al. Treatment results for patients with localized, completely resected (group I) alveolar rhabdomyosarcoma on Intergroup Rhabdomyosarcoma Study Group (IRSG) protocols III and IV, 1984–1997: a report from the Children's Oncology Group. *Pediatr Blood Cancer* 2010;55:612–616.

113. Gerbaulet A, Panis X, Flamant F, et al. Iridium afterloading curietherapy in the treatment of pediatric malignancies. The Institut Gustave Roussy experience. *Cancer* 1985;56:1274–1279.

114. Minn AY, Lyden ER, Anderson JR, et al. Early treatment failure in intermediate-risk rhabdomyosarcoma: results from IRS-IV and D9803—a report from the Children's Oncology Group. *J Clin Oncol* 2010;28:4228–4232.

115. Puri DR, Wexler LH, Meyers PA, et al. The challenging role of radiation therapy for very young children with rhabdomyosarcoma. *Int J Radiat Oncol Biol Phys* 2006;65:1177–1184.

116. Dantonello TM, Int-Veen C, Winkler P, et al. Initial patient characteristics can predict pattern and risk of relapse in localized rhabdomyosarcoma. *J Clin Oncol* 2008;26:406–413.

117. Raney B, Stoner J, Anderson J, et al. Impact of tumor viability at second-look procedures performed before completing treatment on the Intergroup Rhabdomyosarcoma Study Group protocol IRS-IV, 1991–1997: a report from the Children's Oncology Group. *J Pediatr Surg* 2010;45:2160–2168.

118. Maurer HM, Beltangady M, Gehan EA, et al. The Intergroup Rhabdomyosarcoma Study-I. A final report. *Cancer* 1988;61:209–220.

119. Rodeberg DA, Wharam MD, Lyden ER, et al. Delayed primary excision with subsequent modification of radiotherapy dose for intermediate-risk rhabdomyosarcoma: a report from the Children's Oncology Group Soft Tissue Sarcoma Committee. *Int J Cancer* 2015;137(1):204–211.

120. Arndt CA, Stoner JA, Hawkins DS, et al. Vincristine, actinomycin, and cyclophosphamide compared with vincristine, actinomycin, and cyclophosphamide alternating with vincristine, topotecan, and cyclophosphamide for intermediate-risk rhabdomyosarcoma: Children's Oncology Group Study D9803. *J Clin Oncol* 2009;27:5182–5188.

121. Flamant F, Rodary C, Rey A, et al. Treatment of non-metastatic rhabdomyosarcomas in childhood and adolescence. Results of the second study of the International Society of Paediatric Oncology: MMT84. *Eur J Cancer* 1998;34:1050–1062.

122. Rodary C, Rey A, Olive D, et al. Prognostic factors in 281 children with non-metastatic rhabdomyosarcoma (RMS) at diagnosis. *Med Pediatr Oncol* 1988;16:71–77.

123. Treuner J, Kuhl J, Beck J, et al. New aspects in the treatment of childhood rhabdomyosarcoma: results of the German Cooperative Soft-Tissue Sarcoma Study (CWS-81). *Prog Pediatr Surg* 1989;22:162–173.

124. Koscielniak E, Harms D, Henze G, et al. Results of treatment for soft tissue sarcoma in childhood and adolescence: a final report of the German Cooperative Soft-Tissue Sarcoma Study CWS-86. *J Clin Oncol* 1999;17:3706–3719.

125. Dantonello TM, Int-Veen C, Harms D, et al. Cooperative trial CWS-91 for localized soft tissue sarcoma in children, adolescents, and young adults. *J Clin Oncol* 2009;27:1446–1455.

126. Punyko JA, Mertens AC, Gurney JG, et al. Long-term medical effects of childhood and adolescent rhabdomyosarcoma: a report from the childhood cancer survivor study. *Pediatr Blood Cancer* 2005;44:643–653.

127. Heyn R, Haeberlen V, Newton WA, et al. Second malignant neoplasms in children treated for rhabdomyosarcoma. Intergroup Rhabdomyosarcoma Study Committee. *J Clin Oncol* 1993;11:262–270.

128. Sandoval C, Pui CH, Bowman LC, et al. Secondary acute myeloid leukemia in children previously treated with alkylating agents, intercalating topoisomerase II inhibitors, and irradiation. *J Clin Oncol* 1993;11:1039–1045.

129. Abramson DH, Notis CM. Visual acuity after radiation for orbital rhabdomyosarcoma. *Am J Ophthalmol* 1994;118:808–809.

130. Paulino AC, Simon JH, Zhen W, et al. Long-term effects in children treated with radiotherapy for head and neck rhabdomyosarcoma. *Int J Radiat Oncol Biol Phys* 2000;48:1489–1495.

131. Raney B Jr, Heyn R, Hays DM, et al. Sequelae of treatment in 109 patients followed for 5 to 15 years after diagnosis of sarcoma of the bladder and prostate. A report from the Intergroup Rhabdomyosarcoma Study Committee. *Cancer* 1993;71:2387–2394.

132. Estilo CL, Huryn JM, Kraus DH, et al. Effects of therapy on dentofacial development in long-term survivors of head and neck rhabdomyosarcoma: the Memorial Sloan-Kettering Cancer Center experience. *J Pediatr Hematol Oncol* 2003;25:215–222.

133. Barr FG, Galili N, Holick J, et al. Rearrangement of the PAX3 paired box gene in the paediatric solid tumour alveolar rhabdomyosarcoma. *Nat Genet* 1993;3:113–117.

134. Shapiro DN, Sublett JE, Li B, et al. Fusion of PAX3 to a member of the forkhead family of transcription factors in human alveolar rhabdomyosarcoma. *Cancer Res* 1993;53:5108–5112.

135. Douglass EC, Shapiro DN, Valentine M, et al. Alveolar rhabdomyosarcoma with the t(2;13): cytogenetic findings and clinicopathologic correlations. *Med Pediatr Oncol* 1993;21:83–87.

136. Anderson J, Gordon T, McManus A, et al. Detection of the PAX3-FKHR fusion gene in paediatric rhabdomyosarcoma: a reproducible predictor of outcome? *Br J Cancer* 2001;85:831–835.

137. Driman D, Thorner PS, Greenberg ML, et al. MYCN gene amplification in rhabdomyosarcoma. *Cancer* 1994;73:2231–2237.

138. Mercado GE, Xia SJ, Zhang C, et al. Identification of PAX3-FKHR-regulated genes differentially expressed between alveolar and embryonal rhabdomyosarcoma: focus on MYCN as a biologically relevant target. *Genes Chromosomes Cancer* 2008;47:510–520.

139. Lee MH, Jothi M, Gudkov AV, et al. Histone methyltransferase KMT1A restrains entry of alveolar rhabdomyosarcoma cells into a myogenic differentiated state. *Cancer Res* 2011;71(11):3921–3931.

140. Zibat A, Missiaglia E, Rosenberger A, et al. Activation of the hedgehog pathway confers a poor prognosis in embryonal and fusion gene-negative alveolar rhabdomyosarcoma. *Oncogene* 2010;29:6323–6330.

141. Reed S, Li H, Li C, et al. Celecoxib inhibits STAT3 phosphorylation and suppresses cell migration and colony forming ability in rhabdomyosarcoma cells. *Biochem Biophys Res Commun* 2011;407:450–455.

142. Mayeenuddin LH, Yu Y, Kang Z, et al. Insulin-like growth factor 1 receptor antibody induces rhabdomyosarcoma cell death via a process involving AKT and Bcl-x(L). *Oncogene* 2010;29:6367–6377.

143. Kolb EA, Gorlick R, Lock R, et al. Initial testing (stage 1) of the IGF-1 receptor inhibitor BMS-754807 by the pediatric preclinical testing program. *Pediatr Blood Cancer* 2011;56:595–603.

144. Kang Z, Chen J, Yu Y, et al. Drozitumab, a human antibody to death receptor 5, has potent anti-tumor activity against rhabdomyosarcoma with the expression of caspase-8 predictive of response. *Clin Cancer Res* 2011;17(10):3181–3192.

145. Felix CA, Kappel CC, Mitsudomi T, et al. Frequency and diversity of p53 mutations in childhood rhabdomyosarcoma. *Cancer Res* 1992;52:2243–2247.

146. Ayan I, Dogan O, Kebudi R, et al. Immunohistochemical detection of p53 protein in rhabdomyosarcoma: association with clinicopathological features and outcome. *J Pediatr Hematol Oncol* 1997;19:48–53.

147. Taylor AC, Shu L, Danks MK, et al. P53 mutation and MDM2 amplification frequency in pediatric rhabdomyosarcoma tumors and cell lines. *Med Pediatr Oncol* 2000;35:96–103.

148. Chan HS, Thorner PS, Haddad G, et al. Immunohistochemical detection of P-glycoprotein: prognostic correlation in soft tissue sarcoma of childhood. *J Clin Oncol* 1990;8:689–704.

Section III

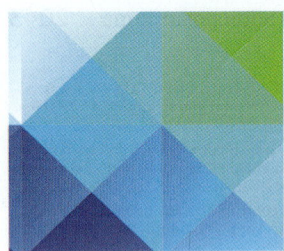

CHAPTER 92

Ewing Tumor

Line Claude, Ronan Tanguy, and Marie-Pierre Sunyach

EPIDEMIOLOGY

Ewing sarcoma family of tumor (ESFT) is the second most common primary tumor of the bone in childhood. ESFT primarily afflicts adolescents/young adults and is uncommon before 8 years and after 25 years.[1] The incidence is estimated to be 3/1,000,000 per year in White Caucasian population[2] but is rarer in Africans and Asians.[3]

Overall survival (OS) has improved mainly in localized disease since a few decades, thanks to a multidisciplinary approach. Five-year OS in localized ESFT increased from about 45% to 60%–68% after the 1990s. Five-year OS in metastatic disease has also increased but remains quite poor, about 30% to 40%,[3] especially for patients with other metastasis than isolated lung lesions.

PATHOLOGY AND CYTOGENETICS

Light microscopy shows a tumor of small, round blue cells that lack markers for lymphoma, neuroblastoma, or rhabdomyosarcoma. Cytogenetics has shown that ESFTs of the bone and soft tissue are the most undifferentiated members of a tumor family that shares a common neuroectodermal precursor cell, arrested at different stages of differentiation.[4] Cells are periodic acid–Schiff (PAS) positive, vimentin positive, and also often cytokeratin positive.[5,6] Approximately 95% of ESFTs have a translocation between the EWS gene on chromosome 22 and the FLI1 gene on chromosome 11 (t[11;22][q24;q12]) or the ERG gene on chromosome 21 (t[21;22][q22;q12]). In an analysis of 222 consecutive tumors at the Rizzoli Institute in Italy with a presumptive diagnosis of Ewing tumor, an occasional other translocation was noted.[7] The translocations are present only in tumor cells and occur in bone and soft tissue ESFT, primitive neuroectodermal tumors of the bone and soft tissue, peripheral primitive neuroectodermal tumors, Askin tumors, some esthesioneuroblastomas in children, and some central nervous system (CNS) tumors.[8]

The t(11;22) juxtaposes the EWS gene with the FLI gene (EWS/FLI gene), which seems to act as an aberrant transcription factor, resulting in tumorigenesis.[9] The t(11;22) breakpoint location has been reported as prognostic factor in some publications,[10] but both recent reports from EURO-EWING 99 (EE99) study and Children's Oncology Group (COG) study have not confirmed this impact.[11,12]

More recently, other translocations were identified involving EWS gene and non-ETS genes (NFATc2, SMARCA5, PATZ1, SP3). Moreover, CIC-DUX4 fusion transcript positive or BCOR-CCNB3 fusion with an X chromosomal inversion has been also identified in ESFT. These translocations may be associated with different mechanisms of oncogenesis and may have different clinical impacts, which are currently studied.[13,14]

CLINICAL PRESENTATION

Locoregional pain is the most common presenting symptom in patients with ESFT, reported in about 90% of cases. Pain can be intermittent and variable in intensity. Pain often does not completely disappear during the night.[15] As the majority of ESFT patients are in their second decades of life and physically active, pain is often mistaken for "bone growth" or injuries. Tumor growth eventually leads to a visible or palpable swelling of the affected site. The tumor bulk, however, may be indiscernible for a long time in patients with pelvic, chest wall, or femoral tumors. Significant limitation of movement has been described in 25% of presentations.[15]

As ESFT may arise in virtually any bone and in soft tissue, additional symptoms, depending on the affected site, may vary considerably. Patients with chest wall or pelvic primaries may experience significant complaints only at a very late stage. Neurologic symptoms or signs occur in 15% of children, either as spinal cord compression or as peripheral nerve compression.

Unlike other bone sarcomas, constitutional symptoms such as fever, weight loss, and fatigue are occasionally noted at presentation mostly on more advanced and/or metastatic stages, affecting about one-third of patients.[16] The duration of symptoms prior to the definitive diagnosis can be weeks to months, or rarely even years, with a median of 3 to 9 months.[17]

DIAGNOSTIC WORKUP: LOCAL AND SYSTEMIC

Local Workup

The initial imaging investigation when an osseous lesion is suspected is usually a simple radiograph. ESFTs are defined as a destructive lesion of the bone. Tumor-related osteolysis, detachments of the periosteum from the bone (Codman triangle), and spiculae of calcification in soft tissue tumor masses suggest the diagnosis of a malignant bone tumor. Diaphyseal location suggests an ESFT, as compared with the metaphyseal location more common in osteosarcoma.[18]

Local computed tomography (CT) and magnetic resonance imaging (MRI) are needed and complementary (Figs. 92.1

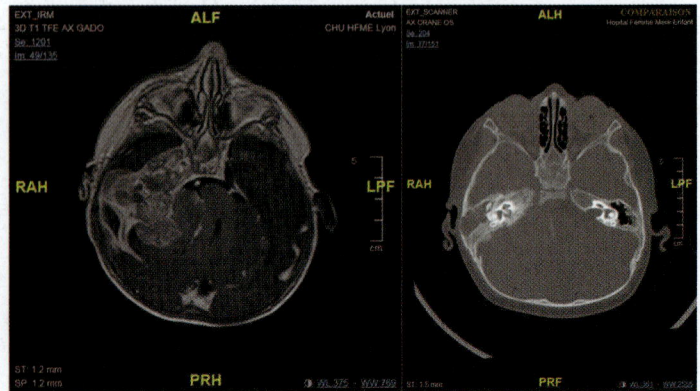

FIGURE 92.1. Ewing sarcoma of the right bone rock in a 2-year-old boy.

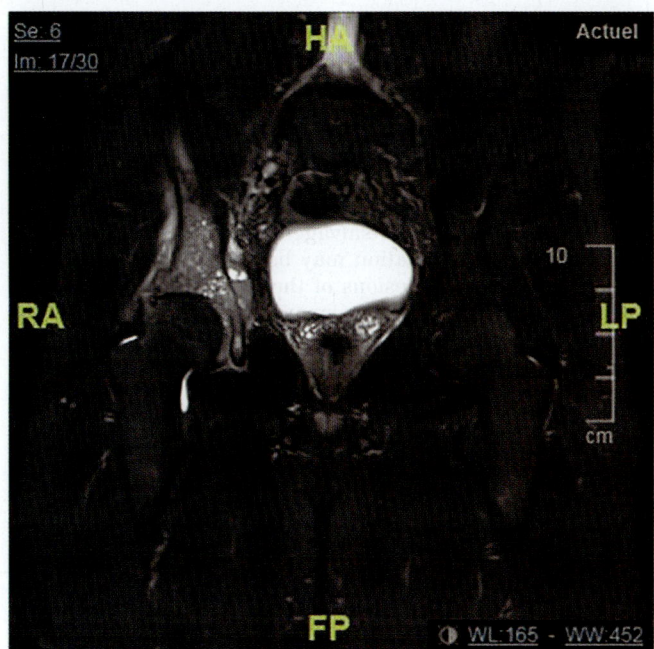

FIGURE 92.2. Localized Ewing sarcoma of the right acetabulum cup in a 16-year-old boy on magnetic resonance imaging (MRI)—Example of the planning treatment using TomoTherapy for exclusive radiotherapy (patient refused surgery)

and 92.2). CT outlines better the bone and soft tissue extent of central ESFT. The most precise definition of the local extent of disease, including the intramedullary portion and the relation of the lesion to adjacent blood vessels and nerves, is provided by MRI.[19]

Systemic Workup

Nonspecific signs of tumor or inflammation may be noted, such as an elevated erythrocyte sedimentation rate, moderate anemia, or leukocytosis. The pretreatment serum lactate dehydrogenase (LDH) rate is a prognostic factor.[20]

Whole-body MRI has also been reported to be superior to bone scan in detecting bone metastases in patients with Ewing tumors, particularly diffusion-weighted images or short-time inversion recovery (STIR) images.[19]

Currently, fluorodeoxyglucose positron emission tomography (FDG-PET-CT) is still an optional staging modality but is used more and more frequently. It has demonstrated high sensitivity and specificity in ESFT. FDG-PET-CT has been shown to detect more bone metastases than traditional bone scans do, both at diagnosis and at recurrence.[21] Because few lesions <8 mm are not detectable using FDG-PET-CT imaging, CT scans are still more accurate for the screening of lung metastases.[21]

The EWS-FLI1 transcript can sometimes be detected in the peripheral blood or bone marrow, where it may indicate residual occult disease.[22]

In conclusion, the systemic workup should include blood studies including LDH, a chest CT scan, bone marrow aspirate/biopsies, and a bone scan, or better if available a FDG-PET-CT.

Results of Workup

Approximately 53% of ESFT have a primary site in an extremity, and 47% have central primaries.[2,23] ESFT can be localized everywhere, but the most frequent sites are the pelvis (23% to 25%), femur (16% to 18%), below the knee (10% to 16%), ribs (12% to 13%), spine (8%), and humerus (5%).[24]

On the whole, the proportion of metastatic patients at diagnosis is about 20% to 25% in large prospective studies.

Metastasis is more frequent in pelvic primaries as compared with tumors of the extremities or ribs.[2,25,26]

Most frequent metastatic sites are the lungs (40%) and bones (40%), with less common disease involving the bone marrow, lymph nodes, soft tissue, and visceral sites. Rarely, the CNS is involved.[2,20]

PROGNOSTIC FEATURES

Metastatic Situation

Metastatic status at diagnosis is the strongest prognostic factor across different treatment strategies, whereas the 5-year disease-free survival (DFS) remains <30% for metastatic patients. However, patients with only lung metastasis have a better clinical outcome than those with metastases in other sites (EFS 29% to 52%).[27] In addition, other prognostic factors were identified to build a prognostic score in the EE99-R3 study.[25] After a median follow-up of 3.8 years on 281 patients, event-free survival (EFS) and OS at 3 years were still disappointing (27% and 34%, respectively). Cox regression analyses demonstrated increased risk at diagnosis for patients older than 14 years, a primary tumor volume over 200 mL, more than one bone metastatic site, bone marrow metastases, and additional lung metastases. An up-front risk score based on these factors identified three groups with EFS rates of 50% for score <3 (82 patients), 25% for score more than 3 to <5 (102 patients), and 10% for score >5 (70).

Metastases to uncommon sites (i.e., brain, liver, spleen) were associated with a worse prognosis in a retrospective study of 30 patients.[28]

Localized Disease

Most important parameters of favorable prognosis include a distal/peripheral site of primary disease, tumor volume <200 mL (or/and maximum tumor size <8 cm), normal LDH level at presentation, and a younger age at diagnosis.[2,23,29–34]

Poor histologic/radiologic response to chemotherapy has also been identified as a major adverse prognostic factor, even when chemotherapy was followed by R0 resection.[34–37]

ESFTs in the spine and sacrum are associated with significantly worse outcome and prognosis than primary ESFT in other sites,[37] but multidisciplinary approach is encouraging.[38] Similarly, the results of the Intergroup Ewing's Sarcoma Study (IESS) show that patients with primary tumors in pelvic bones have lower survival rates compared with patients with lesions in distal bones of the extremities.[39]

Ewing tumors with p53, p16/p14ARF alterations, or the presence of vascular endothelial growth factor respond poorly to chemotherapy and have a poor prognosis.[40–42] The matricellular protein CCN3, which plays an important role in bone formation, has been reported to be associated with a worse prognosis if fully expressed.[42]

Although in the past the type 1 fusion abnormality, which is the EWS-FLI1 transcript created as a result of fusion between exons 7 of *EWS* and 6 of *FLI1*, has been reported to have a favorable prognosis, more recent analyses do not confirm this. A reexamination of this association in a prospective cohort of patients with ESFT treated according to current COG protocols using more intensive chemotherapy shows no advantage.[11] In a report from the EE99 trial, no type of translocation impacted disease progression or relapse.[12]

GENERAL MANAGEMENT

Effective local *and* systemic therapy is necessary for the cure of ESFTs. Most chemotherapy regimens combine cyclophosphamide, doxorubicin, vincristine, dactinomycin, ifosfamide, and etoposide.[20,24,43–48] Induction chemotherapy is often preferred over starting the systemic therapy and local therapy concomitantly. There are several advantages to this approach:

1. Administering the chemotherapy first allows an evaluation of the effectiveness of the regimen, to adapt postoperative chemotherapy and radiotherapy.
2. Shrinkage of the soft tissue mass may help the surgeon or radiation oncologist decrease the volume of the local therapy.
3. Shrinkage of the soft tissue mass may allow the surgeon to achieve better margins.
4. Some bone healing takes place during the chemotherapy, which may diminish the risk of pathologic fracture if radiation therapy is used to treat the primary lesion.

Response rates to induction chemotherapy are high, with radiologic complete response and partial response rates of up to 90% reported.[49–51] For institutions that use surgery for the treatment of the primary lesion, excellent necrosis rates have been reported in many patients.[30,45]

The biopsy should be performed at the same institution where the treatment will be performed, and the biopsy specimen should only be taken from the soft tissue component, if present. Enough tissue should be collected for light and electron microscopy as well as cytogenetics. In experienced hands, a large-needle biopsy may be sufficient, although usually a larger sample is preferred, particularly because cytogenetics is becoming increasingly important.

Considering local treatment, the strategy has gradually moved from exclusive radiotherapy (RT) to surgery with or without RT.[2] For example, the Italian experience reports a percentage of patients treated with surgery increasing from 32% in the first protocols to 72% in the most recent studies. During the same period, RT followed an inverse evolution from 68% to 28% (P = .0001).[52,53]

There are no randomized studies to confirm the superiority of surgery compared to RT, but lots of retrospective studies demonstrate better local control (LC) and EFS after complete surgery (+/– followed by radiotherapy) as compared with RT

alone.[29,37,54–56] Patients treated with exclusive RT often come from older protocols and generally have a lower prognosis: larger tumors, more pejorative sites, and poor response to chemotherapy.[56–58]

Currently, tumor resection is performed whenever a marginal or wide resection seems possible. Intralesional resection or debulking procedures followed by RT do not offer increased LC or DFS compared with definitive RT and should be avoided.[56] Limb-salvage surgery is preferable over amputation, but amputation may be an option especially for younger patients with lesions of the fibula, tibia, and foot. In older patients, lesions of the proximal fibula, ribs, scapula, clavicle, and wing of the ilium are easier to resect than other sites. Other sites may be resectable with major reconstructive procedures and significant morbidity.[59]

However, exclusive RT is a reasonable alternative if complete surgery is difficult, especially in case of small volume. In the German series, for example, central tumors, volume <100 cm³, have a local recurrence rate after RT similar to tumors operated, with or without postoperative RT: 12.3% versus 15.9% and 11.1%.[56] In contrast, tumors larger than 100 cm³ have a local relapse rate of 26.4% after exclusive RT versus 15.4% and 6.6% after surgery with or without RT.

RADIOTHERAPY TECHNIQUES

Radiation Indication and Doses

Exclusive RT

For gross disease, standard treatment is a total dose of 55.8 to 59.40 Gy and 1.8 Gy/day. A dose of 45 to 50.4 Gy is usually recommended, although 36 Gy may be adequate for the initial field, including microscopic disease.[60–63] Local control rates of 53% to 93% have been reported with these doses (Table 92.1). Local control at doses <40 Gy is significantly worse, even for small lesions.[73] An example of exclusive RT is shown in Figure 92.3

TABLE 92.1 SURVIVAL AND LOCAL CONTROL BY METHOD OF TREATMENT TO PRIMARY LESIONS IN MAJOR COOPERATIVE GROUP TRIALS (LOCALIZED LESIONS ONLY)

Trial	Years Open	Local Control (%)			5-Year Survival (%)			
		RT	Surgery	Both	RT	Surgery	Both	Overall
IESS-I[20]	1973–1978	–	–	–	–	–	–	50[a]
IESS-II[46]	1978–1982	–	–	–	–	–	–	70[a]
IESS-II (pelvic)[46]	1978–1982	85	91	100	59	73	62	63
CESS 81[64]	1981–1985	53	91	80	44	55	67	50
CESS 86[35]	1986–1991	86	100	95	70	66	74	70
UKCCSG ET-2[65]	1987–1993	82	71	100	–	–	–	62
CESS 81, CESS 86, EICESS 92[b,56]	1981–1999	74	96	92	–	–	–	–
SE 91-CNR[c,66]	1991–1997	93	93	94	75[a]	77[a]	87[a]	–
CCG/POG Intergroup II[24]	1995–1998	–	–	–	–	–	–	79
CCG/POG Intergroup II[d,67]	1995–1998	75	75	89.5	52	41.7	47.4	49
Scandinavian and Italian group phase III[68]	1999–2006	–	–	–	–	–	–	75
INT 0054[69]	1995–1998	91,8	94,9	98	–	–	–	78
Pilot COG[70]	2008–2015	–	–	–	–	–	–	88
INT 0091 POG 8850 VACA IE	1988–1992	–	–	–	–	–	–	72
INT 0091 POG 8850 VACA[24]								61
EURO-EWING 99-R1[71]	2000–2010	–	–	–	–	–	–	3 y: 86
COG NCT00006734[72]	2001–2005	–	–	–	–	–	–	3 y: 83
VDC-IE/2 wk vs. VDC-IE/3 wk								3 y: 77

[a]Estimated from results of individual arms.
[b]Combined; data for EICESS 92 alone not available.
[c]Only 3-year survival available.
[d]Pelvic primaries only.
CCG/POG, Children's Cancer Group and Pediatric Oncology Group; CESS, Cooperative Ewing's Sarcoma Study; COG, Children's Oncology Group; EICESS, European Intergroup Cooperative Ewing Sarcoma Study; ET, Ewing tumor; IESS, Intergroup Ewing's Sarcoma Study; RT, radiotherapy; SE 91-CNR, Italian Cooperative Study of Ewing Sarcoma; UKCCSG, United Kingdom Children's Cancer Study Group; VACA-IE, vincristine, actinomycin D, cyclophosphamide, and doxorubicin and ifosfamide–etoposide; VDC-IE, vincristine, doxorubicin, cyclophosphamide, and ifosfamide–etoposide.

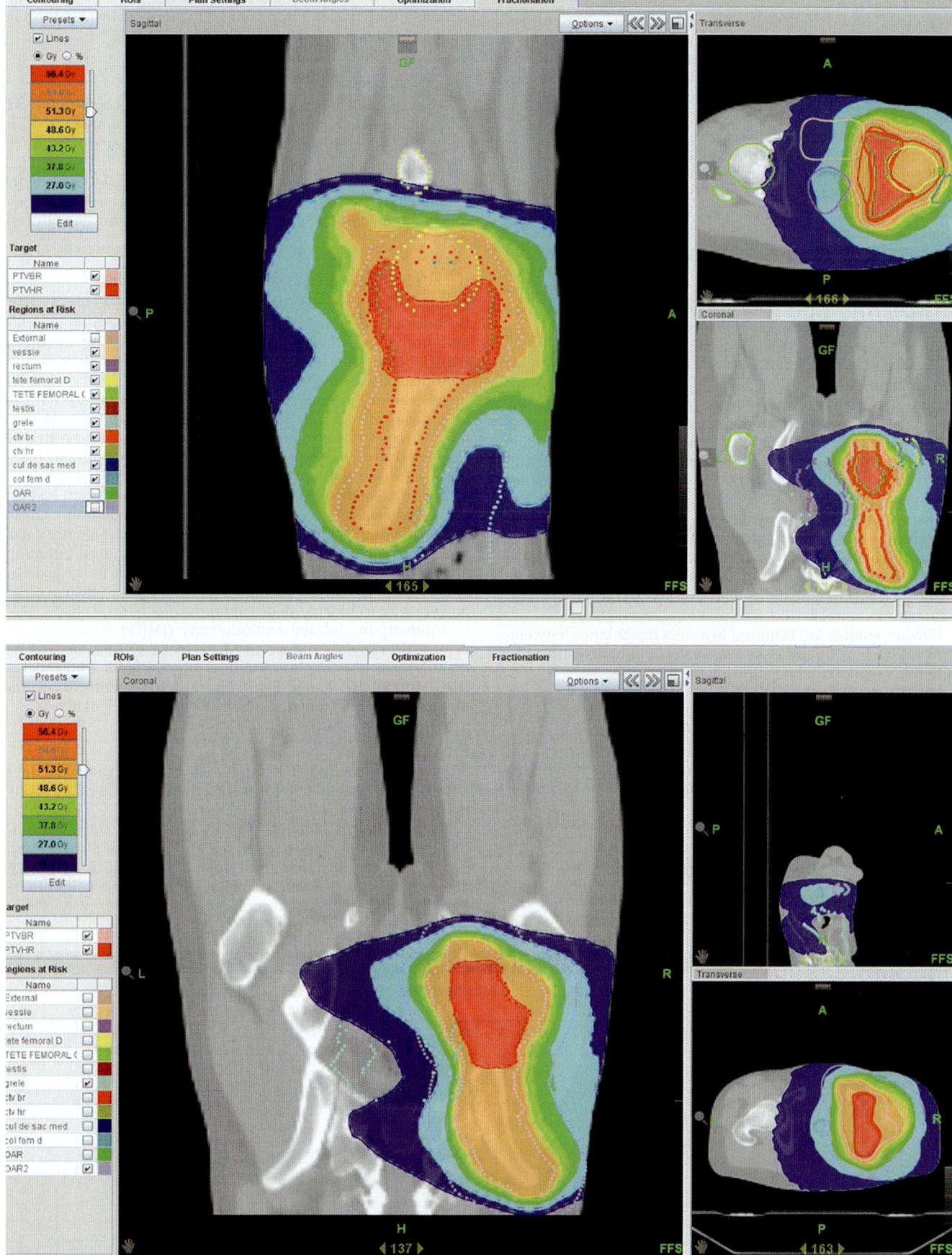

FIGURE 92.3. Example of the planning treatment using TomoTherapy for exclusive radiotherapy (patient refused surgery).

Adjuvant Radiotherapy

Jereb et al.[74] found that the local recurrence rate after conservative surgery was high without RT. Ozaki et al.[75] also reported a slight advantage for adding postoperative RT for patients with inadequate margins. Dunst and Schuck[76] reported that patients with a wide resection alone but a poor histologic response had a local failure rate of 12%, in comparison with 6% for similar patients who received postoperative RT.

As a consequence, all patients with marginal margins and all patients with a poor histologic response receive RT.

In addition, taking into account competing events, a recent analysis of the EE99 trial showed that adjuvant RT improves LC for all the patients, even after good response to induction chemotherapy.[77] With a median follow-up of 6 years, 8-year local relapse incidence was 12%. A statistically significant reduction of local relapse was shown in patients treated with surgery and RT compared to surgery alone (P = .02). The benefit of RT was particularly marked for tumors larger than 200 mL at diagnosis and 100% necrosis. A nonsignificant trend for benefit associated with postoperative RT for DFS, EFS, and OS was reported.

As a consequence, in the currently ongoing EE2012 protocol, postoperative RT is considered for all patients except for those who have had a wide local excision, defined as negative resection margins of at least 1 mm, and a good histologic response (>90% necrosis) to preoperative chemotherapy and with removal of all tissues originally involved by the prechemotherapy tumor volume.

Postoperative RT is however not recommended for those in whom the anticipated adverse side effects of RT are sufficiently high to outweigh the additional benefit of RT for local control. Reasons for deciding against RT include young age, risk of surgical complications following RT, and predisposition to cancer.

Further studies are required to assess the balance between adjuvant RT benefit and risks, especially in patients with complete R0 resection and good histologic response.

For the dose, in the COG trials, a dose of 50.4 Gy (1.8 Gy once a day) is given if postoperative RT is indicated. Doses in the range of 30 to 44.8 Gy at 1.8 Gy a day have also been reported to be effective for subclinical disease.[75,78] Intralesional resections should be treated to the same dose as in patients receiving radiotherapy alone, with doses to residue or microscopic resection up to 54 to 59.4 Gy.

Table 92.2 lists the recommended doses and fields for different clinical situations.

In a review of 153 patients treated with surgery followed by postoperative RT from Cooperative Ewing Sarcoma Study (CESS) 86 and EICESS 92, Schuck et al. showed that the interval between surgery and RT did not influence survival, although there was a slight trend for improved local control in patients receiving RT < 90 days postoperatively.[79]

Neoadjuvant RT

Good results have also been reported with preoperative RT for patients with a poor response (<50% reduction of the evaluable soft tissue mass) after two cycles of chemotherapy.[75,80] Doses of 36 to 63 Gy have been used.[75]

The total dose for preoperative RT is usually 50.4 Gy (1.80/fr) in a single phase to the PTV. If there are concerns about organ tolerance or wound healing, then this dose can be reduced to 45 Gy.

RT After High Dose Chemotherapy with Busulfan

Because of the high risk of toxicity of the association of RT and high dose chemotherapy (HDCT) including busulfan (HDCT-BuMel), both indications should be early discussed in multidisciplinary meetings.

In case of patients receiving HDCT-BuMel before RT, the total dose will often be limited (generally at 45 Gy), whereas the dose constraints to major critical organs have to be strictly respected to avoid severe toxicity. Using conventional fractions, RT doses will not exceed 30 Gy to the spinal cord[81] and 45 Gy on a small volume of the gastrointestinal tract, including the bowel, colon, rectum, stomach, and duodenum.[82] Large irradiated lung volumes should be also avoided. Hemithoracic lung or whole-lung RT is not recommended in first intention after HDCT-BuMel, because of the risk of respiratory toxicity. Spacer devices can be discussed in the pelvis to displace the bowel away from treatment volumes.

Intensity-modulated radiotherapy (IMRT) techniques or proton therapy should be used to spare critical organs as much as possible in this situation. For patients who receive HDCT-BuMel, RT should begin later. EE2012 protocol recommends to begin RT at least 10 weeks after HDCT delivery.

Fractionation

Standard fractionation delivers 1.8 to 2 Gy per fraction, 5 days a week. In very young children, fractionation using 1.6 Gy/day may be considered.

Twice-a-day RT has been used in several trials. To treat ESFTs, radiation oncologists at the University of Florida used 1.2 Gy twice a day to a total dose of 50.4, 55.2, or 60 Gy, depending on the tumor response to induction chemotherapy, and showed that late effects could be decreased while

TABLE 92.2 RECOMMENDATIONS FOR RADIATION THERAPY FIELDS AND DOSES

Clinical Situation		Total Dose (%)	Dose Per Fraction (%)	Volume
Gross target volume = GTV (after biopsy only or intralesional resection) Treatment once a day	Microscopic involvement (CTV)	36–50.4 Gy	1.8–2 Gy/fraction	Original bone and soft tissue mass
	Boost field (GTV, residue)	5.4–18 Gy[a] (total dose 54–59.4 Gy to GTV)	1.8–2 Gy/fraction	Original bone and *residual* soft tissue mass
Treatment twice a day	Initial field	36 Gy	1.2 bid	Original bone and soft tissue mass
	Boost field	14.4–19.2 Gy	1.2 bid	Original bone and *residual* soft tissue mass
Postoperative radiation (especially after marginal resection and/or poor histologic response at surgery)		45–54 Gy	1.8 qd	Original bone and soft tissue mass plus surgical scars and drains if feasible
Preoperative radiotherapy		45–50.4 Gy (Doses as low as 35 have been successful)	1.8 qd	Original bone and soft tissue mass

[a]Depending on initial dose.
bid, twice a day; CTV, clinical target volume; GTV, gross target volume; qd, once a day.

maintaining good LC, even for large primary tumors.[62,63] In CESS 86, doses of 1.6 Gy twice a day to a total of 60 Gy were given, although not in a continuous course. The Italian SE-91 trial also used 1.6 Gy twice a day to a total of 60.8 Gy, but in a continuous course. The CESS 86 trial showed no advantage for the accelerated hyperfractionated approach, but the early results of SE-91 are promising with regard to local control.[66,76] Both of the latter regimens would be theoretically expected to increase late effects.

Radiation Volumes

The Pediatric Oncology Group (POG 8346) trial showed, in a randomized fashion, that the traditional approach of irradiating the entire marrow cavity was not necessary.[54] Although "tailored" fields are the standard of care today, attention to the requisite volume is critical to obtaining maximal control rates; geographic miss has been a frequent source of failure in cooperative group studies.[54,64] Three-dimensional treatment planning is essential.

Growth tumor volume (GTV) is defined as the visible tumor on imaging at its maximal extent (using CT, FDG-PET-CT, bone and MRI scans, as available) prior to any chemotherapy or surgery.

Clinical target volume (CTV) 1 should encompass any sites of potential microscopic extension of GTV, or of contamination by GTV, including metallic prostheses, drain sites, and surgical scars (if feasible), and should be at least GTV + 1 cm.

Planning target volume (PTV) 1 is defined from CTV1, with a margin to account for day-to-day set-up variation and, if relevant, internal organ motion. This will vary according to tumor location in the body and is specific to individual institutions. PTV1 will be typically CTV1 + 0.5 to 1.0 cm.

The boost is delivered to the residual tumor volume (GTV) at the time of RT plus a 1-cm margin to CTV2. Any initial bone or bone marrow abnormalities in the primary bone should be included in GTV. CTV2 does not need to include scars and drain sites. It should take into account anatomical barriers to tumor spread such as facial boundaries and bone. PTV2 will be typically CTV2 + 0.5 to 1.0 cm. These margins are much tighter than in previous studies, and only additional follow-up will show whether they will be adequate.

The use of MRI is essential to identify the tumor extent, at the diagnosis and after the induction chemotherapy. PET-CT may be helpful for planning.

Extremity lesions require sparing at least a 1- to 2-cm strip of tissue to prevent lymphedema, which can be very difficult at times, particularly in arm lesions, although the arm is less likely to develop lymphedema than the leg. It may be necessary to consider surgery as an alternative if a strip of tissue cannot be spared. It is more important to cover the tumor adequately than to spare adjacent growth plates and joints.[83]

With the high doses of cyclophosphamide or ifosfamide given in chemotherapy regimens for Ewing tumor, it is important to minimize the dose to the bladder. Radiation cystitis can be a significant risk even at doses as low as 20 Gy. Because pelvic lesions rarely infiltrate into the tissues around the bladder, but instead tend to push aside those structures, neoadjuvant chemotherapy allows additional bladder to be spared if good shrinkage is obtained. A 1-cm medial margin on the residual disease at the time of treatment is adequate from the beginning of radiation therapy.

Radiation therapy doses are shown in Table 92.2.

RT in Special Sites

Ribs

Rib lesions should be treated conformally with a minimum of lung and heart in the high dose field. However, rib primary

tumors often present with pleural effusions. In the EICESS 92 trial, the 7-year rate of EFS was 63% with hemithorax RT versus 46% without.[84] Claren et al. recently confirmed that pleural effusion at diagnosis and incomplete resection were both independent risk factors for survival in localized tumor of the rib. Eighty-two French patients, median age 13.6 years and median follow-up 8.4 years, were treated in EE99 protocol and reviewed. Five-year DFS was 69%. Pleural effusion and incomplete surgical resection (R1 or R2) were independent prognostic factors for DFS and OS. In case of initial pleural effusion, documented or not, OS was 27% without RT versus 68% after RT ($P = .01$).[85]

Spine

The type of local treatment remains a pending question in this site. A large-scale retrospective study on patients diagnosed with ESFT of the spine in the Surveillance, Epidemiology, and End Results (SEER) registry from 1973 to 2012 was recently published. Age, surgical resection, tumor size, and extent of disease (OS $P < .001$, DSS $P < .001$) were independent factors of survival. RT trended toward improved survival but did not achieve statistical significance.[86]

A French cohort of 75 patients with localized spinal ESFT treated between 1988 and 2009 was reported. Seventy-nine percent presented initial neurologic compression and 69% had inaugural decompressive surgery. Local treatment modality was surgery and RT in 50 patients, RT alone in 19, and surgery alone in 6. After a 7-year median follow-up, the 5-year LC, EFS, and OS were 78.0%, 57.0%, and 70.0% (95% CI: 59.1–81.0), respectively. Vertebral compartment involved was the only prognostic factor.[38]

The standard dose for vertebral lesions is usually 45 Gy, but modern techniques including protons or dynamic IMRT allow nowadays to increase the dose of RT in many situations while sparing the spinal cord. The average dose used in the CESS 81, CESS 86, and EICESS 92 trials was 49.6 Gy, although sometimes spinal shielding was used.[80,87] In these trials, neurologic late effects were seen in 1 of 47 patients irradiated, occurring at a dose of 44.8 Gy at 1.6 Gy twice a day.

Sacral lesions should be treated to the full dose. The Scandinavian Sarcoma Group confirmed recently a better prognosis for sacral lesions on 29 patients. Seventy-nine percent received exclusive RT, with a 5-year DFS of 66%.[88]

Doxorubicin and dactinomycin given during the course of RT will often cause moist desquamation, particularly with beams of 6 MV or less, tangential irradiation, or skin folds. These drugs may also cause a "recall" phenomenon of the dry or moist desquamation when given after the end of radiation therapy. HDCT-BuMel should not be given before RT for spinal lesions if RT dose to the spinal cord is expected to be over 30 Gy, because of the risk of myelitis.[81]

RESULTS OF THERAPY

The majority of studies reported in the literature reflect the results of therapy only for ESFT of the bone, because before 1991 soft tissue ESFTs were treated on Intergroup Rhabdomyosarcoma Study (IRS) Group protocols. The addition of chemotherapy to local therapy increased the survival for ESFT of the bone from <10% to >40% at 5 years for patients with localized disease at diagnosis.[94] Modern protocols show better results and SEER data confirm this gradual improvement in survival rates over time. Five-year survival improved from 36% for patients treated from 1973 to 1977 to 59% for patients treated from 1993 to 1997.[3] However, late recurrences and deaths from complications continue to occur for years, yielding 10- and 15-year survival rates 10% to 15% lower than 5-year rates.[51,95]

LC and survival rates are shown in Table 92.1 for patients treated with different LC strategies in cooperative group trials that reported appropriate data. Surgery has become the treatment of choice for the primary lesion at most centers, and many series report superior local control for patients receiving surgery as a component of their local treatment, particularly if RT compliance was poor.[54,64] The influence of different LC strategies on survival is less certain. In CESS 86, with good RT compliance, survival rates were not influenced by the method of therapy to the primary tumor,[96] nor was there an advantage for surgery in pelvic primary lesions treated in Intergroup 0091.[67] Other trials show an advantage for surgery or a combination of surgery and RT. With no randomized studies addressing this question and considerable selection going into the choice of local treatment, conclusions regarding the relative influence of different local therapies on survival are based more on opinion than fact.[64]

However, systemic therapy does influence the rate of detectable local relapse. The first Intergroup Ewing's Sarcoma Study (IESS-I) reported that the addition of doxorubicin improved local control.[97] The first Children's Cancer Group/Pediatric Oncology Group (CCG/POG) intergroup study showed an improvement in survival in the intensified arm for patients with localized disease and large primary or pelvic tumors. The improvement with the more intensive regimen resulted from a decrease in the rate of local relapse; the rate of distant metastases was similar in both arms.[24] The time interval between initiation of chemotherapy and start of RT has also been reported to influence survival (local control was not evaluated), with early RT preferable to late RT.[76]

RESULTS OF CLINICAL TRIALS FOR PATIENTS WITH LOCALIZED DISEASE AT DIAGNOSIS

The first reports of drug treatment of ESFT come from the 1960s with cyclophosphamide-based protocols. In 1974, Rosen et al. published the first results of a trial of RT given with a four-drug regimen consisting of vincristine, actinomycin D, cyclophosphamide, and doxorubicin used in combination rather than sequentially, leading to long-term survival in 12 patients with EFST.[98] The VACA scheme then became a standard therapy in numerous clinical trials.

IESS-I showed that VACA chemotherapy (vincristine, dactinomycin, cyclophosphamide, and doxorubicin) produced superior results over a VAC (vincristine, dactinomycin, and cyclophosphamide) regimen alone in terms of effectiveness of local control (96% vs. 86%) and EFS (60% vs. 24%). The third arm combined bilateral whole-lung irradiation (WLI) with VAC and produced survival rates better than VAC alone, but less than VACA, indicating that bilateral WLI is an effective adjuvant, although it has not been studied in any subsequent trial except in patients with lung metastases at diagnosis.[20]

Intensifying systemic therapy in IESS-II improved the results for pelvic tumors. IESS-II also showed that induction chemotherapy was a viable option.[46] A trial at St. Jude Children's Research Hospital (Memphis, TN) confirmed this approach, and it has since been the standard of care.[49]

Based on data from previous trials, both the University of Florida and the German Cooperative Ewing Sarcoma Study (CESS) stratified ESFTs by tumor size and intensified treatment for large localized tumors. Although neither approach was randomized, both the University of Florida studies and CESS 86 found that intensifying treatment improved survival.[35,51,63]

On the basis of phase II results achieved with the combination of ifosfamide and etoposide (IE),[99] in the Pediatric

Oncology Group–Children's Cancer Group (POG-CCG) study, INT-0091 patients were randomized to receive either VACD or VACD-IE. The VACD arm achieved a 5-year EFS rate of 54% in patients with localized disease versus a 69% EFS rate in the experimental arm with the addition of IE.[24] This first CCG/POG intergroup study starting in 1988 showed that adding etoposide–ifosfamide improved the survival rates, particularly for patients with primary tumors of the pelvis.

The United Kingdom Children's Cancer Study Group trials ET-1 and ET-2 showed a better survival rate in the ET-2 trial if ifosfamide was substituted for most of the cyclophosphamide used in ET-1; however, the dose intensity in ET-2 was also higher.[65]

The first COG trial used the more standard doses but decreased the interval of chemotherapy to 2 weeks if there was blood count recovery. In this randomized trial for patients younger than 50 years with localized ESFT ($n = 568$), Womer et al. reported that VAC-IE given on an every-2-week schedule was found to be more effective than VAC-IE given on an every-3-week schedule, with no increase in toxicity; median 5-year EFS was 73% and 65%, respectively.[72]

Because of the results of the interval compression study, the five-drug standard of vincristine, cyclophosphamide, doxorubicin, ifosfamide, and etoposide with interval compression is now considered the standard ESFT regimen in North American institutions.

The EICESS 92 study investigated whether cyclophosphamide has a similar efficacy as ifosfamide in patients with standard-risk ESFT (small localized tumors) and whether the addition of etoposide to a regimen already containing ifosfamide improves survival in patients with high-risk disease (large tumors or metastatic disease at diagnosis).[100]

Patients with standard-risk disease were randomly assigned to VAIA (vincristine, dactinomycin, ifosfamide, and doxorubicin; $n = 76$) followed by either VAIA or VACA (vincristine, dactinomycin, cyclophosphamide, and doxorubicin; $n = 79$). The 3-year EFS rates were 73% and 74%, respectively, for VACA and VAIA, suggesting that cyclophosphamide has the same efficacy as ifosfamide in this group of patients. Patients with high-risk disease were randomly assigned to VAIA or VAIA plus etoposide (EVAIA). The 3-year EFS rate was not significantly different between the two treatment groups (52% and 47%, respectively, for EVAIA and VAIA). However, there was some evidence that the addition of etoposide was associated with a greater survival benefit in the subgroup of patients without metastases ($P = .18$) than in those with metastases ($P = .84$).[101] So, the EICESS 92 trial showed that for standard-risk patients (<100 mL and no metastases at diagnosis), a regimen substituting cyclophosphamide (VACA) for ifosfamide (VAIA) was equivalent.

As a follow-up to the EICESS 92 study, the EE-R1 trial evaluated cyclophosphamide as a replacement for ifosfamide as a part of consolidation therapy that also included vincristine and dactinomycin (VAC vs. VAI) after VIDE (vincristine, ifosfamide, doxorubicin, and etoposide) induction chemotherapy in 856 patients with standard-risk ESFT. VAC was statistically not inferior to VAI, but was associated with a slight increase in events (-2.8% decrease in 3-year EFS). The proportion of patients experiencing severe hematologic toxicity was slightly higher in the VAC arm, but renal tubular function impairment was more significant for patients receiving VAI.[101] The comparative evaluation of long-term renal and gonadal toxicity is ongoing and will be crucial to decisions regarding future patients.

Raney et al.[102] reported the results of treating extraosseous ESFT on the IRS until 1991. Long-term survival of these patients was probably better than for patients with bony primaries, with 10-year survival of 62%, 61%, and 77% for IRS-I, IRS-II, and IRS-III therapeutic protocols, respectively. Survival rates were better for patients with primary lesions of the head and neck, extremities, and trunk and for those with gross tumor removal. Extraosseous primary lesions are now treated on the same protocol as osseous lesions.

RESULTS OF CLINICAL TRIALS FOR PATIENTS WITH METASTATIC DISEASE AT DIAGNOSIS

Patients with metastatic disease at diagnosis have a poor prognosis. In a report from the EICESS, the 5-year EFS for patients with lung metastases only was 29%; for patients with bone and bone marrow metastases, it was 19%; and for patients with both lung and bone metastases at diagnosis, it was only 8%.[2] Although there was an improvement in survival rates in patients with localized disease treated in the first intergroup CCG/POG trial, adding ifosfamide–etoposide did not improve survival for patients with metastatic disease at diagnosis.[103]

WLI improved survival in the CESS 81, CESS 86, and EICESS 92 trials for patients with lung metastases as the only site of metastatic disease at diagnosis.[104] The CESS 81 and 86 studies also showed increasing survival rates with an increasing RT dose to the lung fields, particularly with a dose of >18 Gy (corrected for lung transmission) at either 1.5 Gy once a day or 1.25 Gy twice a day. Bölling et al. reported 99 patients from EICESS 92 with pulmonary metastasis. WLI was performed with a dose between 12 and 21 Gy. Seventy patients were treated with WLI, thirteen of them received a further boost to their primary tumor in the thorax up to a cumulative dose of 54 Gy. OS showed a trend toward better results for patients with WLI (5-year OS 61% vs. 49% without WLI, P = .36).[105] Some institutions only use WLI in patients with lung metastases who respond poorly to chemotherapy.[106]

In patients with disseminated disease, results are better with adequate treatment of the primary as well as all the metastases. EE99 showed that the 3-year EFS was better (47%) for patients receiving both surgery and radiation to the primary lesion versus either surgery alone (25%) or radiation

therapy alone (23%). Without local therapy, the EFS was 13%.[107] Obviously, selection bias cannot be excluded. At Memorial Sloan Kettering Cancer Center (New York, NY), LC was worse for patients with metastatic disease (61%) than those with localized disease (84%)[108] although in a large series from St. Jude Children's Hospital, the LC in the two groups was equal.[29]

Recent evidence shows improved survival in patients with disseminated bone metastases if all the lesions are treated. Of 120 patients enrolled on arm R3 of EURO-EWING, which suggested but did not mandate local therapy (RT, surgery, or both) to all sites of disease, 40% received local therapy (either surgery or RT) or both to all sites of metastatic disease, and 60% received no local therapy. Three-year EFS was 35% in those patients who received RT to metastatic sites compared to 16% in those who received no local therapy.[107] Paulino et al. show similar results with local therapy to all sites of metastatic disease.[28] It is acceptable to delay the RT until close to the end of chemotherapy if a significant amount of bone marrow would be treated.

HIGH DOSE THERAPY WITH STEM CELL RESCUE

Many institutions have investigated end-intensification with HDCT and stem cell rescue with and without total-body irradiation (TBI), concerning patients with high-risk localized disease, in metastatic situations, or for recurrence. TBI has been largely abandoned as part of the conditioning regimen. Many different regimens have been used, mostly a combination of melphalan with etoposide, busulfan, carboplatin, and thiotepa.[109]

Metastatic Tumors

Table 92.3 presents results of the most recent studies in metastatic situations. Patients with metastatic disease treated on EICESS studies between 1990 and 1995 had a superior 4-year EFS when HDCT was added to the end of therapy, but CCG-7951 showed no improvement with this approach over a

TABLE 92.3	SURVIVAL IN METASTATIC EWING SARCOMA: MOST RECENT PROSPECTIVE STUDIES					
Study	**Induction Chemotherapy**	**Local Treatment +/− WLI**	**HDCT or Adjuvant Chemotherapy**	**5-Year PFS (%)**	**5-Year OS (%)**
Loschi[89] N = 18 PDMES 2002–2013	VIDE × 6 HDCT Thiotepa	Surgery +/− RT or RT on primary tumor	BuMel	3 y: 11	3 y: 22
Paulussen[90] N = 171 1981–1997	VAIA × 6–10	Surgery +/− RT or RT on primary tumor WLI 15–18 Gy (N = 57)	HDCT (with or without TBI)	4 y: 27	4 y: 32
Ladenstein[25] N = 281 1999–2005	VIDE × 6 + VAI × 1	Surgery +/− RT or RT on primary tumor	HDCT-(BuMel or others)	3 y: 27	3 y: 34
Oberlin[91] N = 97 1991–1999	VA × 5 + IE × 2		HDCT-BuMel	38	37
Grier[24] N = 120 1988–1992	VACA × 17 VACA + IE × 17	Surgery +/− RT or RT on primary tumor	VIDE, VACA VACA + IE	22 22	35 34
Luksch[92] N = 102 1999–2005	VACA × 2 IE × 2	Surgery +/− RT or RT on primary tumor	VAC × 2 IE × 2 HDCT-BuMel WLI	43	52
Dirksen[93] (only lung metastasis) N = 576 2000–2014	VIDE × 6	Surgery +/− RT or RT on primary tumor	HDCT-BuMel vs. VAI × 7 + WLI	3 y: 55.7 3 y: 50.3	3 y: 55.9 3 y: 51.5

BuMel, busulfan/melphalan; HDCT, high dose chemotherapy; IE, ifosfamide–etoposide; N, number of patients; OS, overall survival; PFS, progression-free survival; TBI, total-body irradiation; VAC, vincristine, dactinomycin, and cyclophosphamide; VACA, vincristine, actinomycin D, cyclophosphamide, doxorubicin; VAI, vincristine, dactinomycin, ifosfamide; VAIA, vincristine, dactinomycin, ifosfamide, and doxorubicin; VDC-IE, vincristine, doxorubicin, cyclophosphamide, ifosfamide–etoposide; VIDE, vincristine, ifosfamide, doxorubicin, etoposide; WLI, whole-lung irradiation.

matched cohort from other Ewing tumor studies for patients with bone or bone marrow metastases.[90,110] Some institutional pilot studies without strict selection criteria show promising but not conclusive results.[48,51,91,111–113]

The survival of patients with bone metastases at diagnosis appears much better than with standard therapy in some reports. EFS rates as high as 43% have been reported in a French monocentric study. In patients with lung metastasis, EFS reached 52%.[91] The use of whole-body MRI to detect bone metastases followed by compartmental irradiation to doses up to 54 Gy and HDCT has also been reported to produce a 5-year survival rate of 45%.[113] Although it was a small series, over half the patients had lung metastases and multiple bone metastases.

The Italian Sarcoma Group and the Scandinavian Sarcoma Group designed a joint prospective study for 102 patients with metastatic ESFT (lungs, pleura, or single bone).[92] Intensive combination chemotherapy, surgery, and/or RT and consolidation treatment with HCDT-BuMel and WLI were planned. Only 71 patients on 102 received the whole therapeutic program, mostly because of disease progression. With a median follow-up of 62 months, 5-year OS and PFS for the whole group were 52% and 43%. However, for the patients with only lung metastases who completed the therapeutic program, 5-year OS and PFS were 66% and 53%, respectively.[92]

The EE99-R2 (lung) trial evaluated in a randomized way the question of the best consolidation treatment after initial chemotherapy with VIDE, comparing WLI with conventional VAI chemotherapy versus HDCT-BuMel. Two hundred and sixty-five patients were randomized: 132 received VAI-RT and 133 received HDCT. Three-year EFS was 56% after HDCT versus 50.3% for conventional arm patients (P = .21). Significantly, more patients in HDCT experienced severe acute toxicities than in the standard arm. The authors concluded that in ES with lung metastases, there is no clear benefit associated with HDCT-BuMel compared to conventional chemotherapy combined with WLI.[93]

The EURO-EWING 99-R3 study also evaluated the efficacy of induction chemotherapy (six courses of VIDE), local treatment (surgery and/or RT), and HDCT in 281 patients with ESFT with primary disseminated disease. After a median follow-up of 3.8 years, the 3-year EFS for the entire study cohort was disappointing (27%), but the EFS rates were 57% and 25% for patients with complete and partial response after HDCT, respectively. The comparison of the outcome of patients with and without HDCT was not possible because of the bias introduced in the nontransplant group: 82% of patients without HDCT died after a median time of 1 year.[25]

High-Risk Localized Tumors

A few institutions have used a single transplant to treat high-risk patients (large primary tumors or tumors of the pelvis or trunk) with localized disease. Five-year survival rates of 48% to 71% have been reported.[48,51,114] Although the results are clearly better than standard treatment for similar high-risk groups treated historically, recent intensified regimens without end-intensification appear to give similar results[24,30,51] showing that intensifying systemic therapy for patients with high-risk localized disease has improved survival rates, whether the intensification is with an ablative approach or more intensive conventional chemotherapy.

Two cooperative groups used HDCT-BuMel as consolidation treatment for high-risk localized ES, defined by poor histologic response to induction chemotherapy,[68,115] which have reported encouraging results. These studies were the basis of EE99-R2 (localized disease). Results of this trial were present in ASCO 2016.[116] Between 2000 and 2013, from 477 patients classified as high-risk patients, 216 were randomized to VAI or HDCT-BuMel. Some patients requiring RT to the primary site

were excluded to avoid excess organ toxicity from interaction between RT and busulfan. In an intention to treat analysis, the risk of an event was significantly decreased by HDCT-BuMel compared to VAI: 3-year EFS was 67% using BuMel versus 53% after VAI (P = .023). OS was also significantly better after HDCT-BuMel.

TREATMENT AFTER RELAPSE

The prognosis after relapse is poor, with a 5-year OS of only 13% for patients recurring after treatment in the CESS 81, CESS 86, and EICESS 92 studies. Patients experiencing either late (>2 years) strictly localized relapses fared slightly better.[2,117] Relapse occurring only at the local site warrants aggressive attempts at salvage.[117] To date, no standard treatment has been defined in such situation. Patients who relapse only with lung metastases can sometimes be salvaged with additional chemotherapy and WLI. Resecting the lung metastases, if there are fewer than four lesions, may also be beneficial.[118] Patients with late pulmonary relapses fare better than those with early relapses.[65] Patients who relapse with bone metastases, however, are essentially incurable with standard therapy.

Interesting response rates have been reported in retrospective studies or in phase II trials, including topotecan–cyclophosphamide,[119] temozolomide–irinotecan,[120] gemcitabine–docetaxel,[121] and high dose ifosfamide.[122] The role of HDCT for tumors, which respond to second-line therapy, is controversial, with both positive and negative results reported in retrospective and single-arm studies.[123]

SEQUELAE OF TREATMENT

ESFT has been reported to have an actuarial complication rate of 70% at 35 years.[124] Paulino et al. reported that 10 (53%) of 19 patients receiving RT alone, 4 (25%) of 16 receiving surgery alone, and 2 (40%) of 5 undergoing combined surgery and RT therapy had significant late effects.[41]

More recently, a retrospective chart review of 101 pediatric patients reported the most common complications were musculoskeletal abnormalities (50%) and cardiac toxicity (28%).[125]

Neither study included loss of function related to planed surgical resection as a complication.

The most common skeletal complication of RT is abnormal growth and development of the irradiated tissues. RT can cause premature closure of active epiphyses, producing growth deficits and limb-length discrepancies. The degree of discrepancy depends on the RT dose, patient's age, and epiphysis radiated. Because 65% of leg growth is from the distal femoral (37%) and proximal tibial (28%) epiphyses, typical RT doses to the knee in boys younger than 14 years of age and girls younger than 12 years of age will usually cause a severe enough leg-length discrepancy to require intervention.[126] Deficits of 2 to 6 cm can usually be managed by a shoe lift; larger deficits require surgical treatment.

Approximately 15% of long bone lesions develop pathologic fractures at some time in their course, 5% at diagnosis, and 10% after RT, although approximately one-third of the latter are caused by tumor recurrence or occasionally a secondary malignancy.[127] Whether the fracture is disease or treatment related, the most common site is the femur, particularly the proximal femur. RT-related fractures usually occur within 24 months after treatment, but can be much later. Doses below 40 Gy using once-a-day doses of 1.8 to 2.0 Gy appear to have a very low risk, as does a hyperfractionated approach using 1.2 Gy twice a day from 50.4 to 55.2 Gy.[60,127]

Extremity weakness, decreased range of motion secondary to fibrosis, pain in the extremity (particularly in the early morning), discoloration of the skin, and lymphedema can also occur after RT, even with careful planning and sparing of an adequate strip of tissue.

The risk of secondary neoplasia at the site of the primary lesion is related to RT dose, with an increased risk at doses >60 Gy. Sarcomas, often osteosarcoma, are the most common second tumor, and the risk for megavoltage treatment has been reported as 1% to 5% at 20 years.[20,125,128,129] The Italian Sarcoma Group Experience was reported, following 543 patients with ESFT, treated between 1983 and 2006. Fifteen patients (2.8%) experienced a secondary cancer. The cumulative 10- and 20-year incidence was 3.4% ± 0.9% and 4.7% ± 1.6%. The most common SMN in the ESFT group was RT-induced osteosarcoma ($n = 6$).[130]

In a recent paper, the British Childhood Cancer Survivor Study reported cause-specific mortality and risk of secondary neoplasms for 664 bone sarcoma survivors.[131] Beyond 25 years of follow-up, the risk of dying from all causes was comparable to the general population. In contrast, before 25 years, the risk was 12.7-fold than expected. Survivors were four times more likely to develop a secondary cancer than expected (bone and breast mainly), but the excess was restricted to 5 to 24 years post diagnosis.

The quality of life of 618 long-term survivors of ESFT was recently reported. Median observation time was 12.9 years from primary diagnosis. Survivors were less active than control subjects, but the recommended level for an active lifestyle was achieved. Pelvic tumor location was the major inferior disease-specific prognostic factor as well as older age at diagnosis and female sex.[132]

FUTURE CONSIDERATIONS

Although the 5-year survival rate of patients with ESFT appears to have improved since 1970, almost half of all patients diagnosed with Ewing tumor die of it within 10 years.[3] Outcomes for patients with metastatic disease and recurrent ESFT especially remain poor with current strategies.[125] Several randomized trials are ongoing for localized ES. The VIDE induction chemotherapy is considered the standard chemotherapy for ES in Europe, whereas the compressed VDC-IE is the standard in North America. The ongoing EE2012 trial is comparing those two regimens to define the international standard chemotherapy for ESFT. The benefit of adding zoledronic acid to maintenance conventional chemotherapy is also randomized in this trial, as well as in the Ewing 2008 study by GPOH.

The COG-AEWS1031 trial is currently evaluating the addition of cyclophosphamide/topotecan to the compressed VDC-IE. The Italian group ISG/AIEOP EW-1 trial randomizes a prolonged treatment versus a shorter dose-intense treatment.

For high-risk patients, HDCT has proven better results for patients with high-risk localized disease at diagnosis, but the limits of intensification have probably been reached with the presently available drugs. Other drugs are being tested for metastatic patients and recurrences.

The Ewing family of tumors is characterized by the t(11;22)(q24;q12) translocation that generates the EWS-FLI1 fusion transcription factor producing the malignant EWS cell. Because continued expression of EWS-FLI1 is believed to be critical for ESFT cell survival, clinically effective small molecule inhibitors have been sought.

Mithramycin has been reported to inhibit expression of EWS-FLI1 downstream targets at the messenger RNA and protein levels.[133] YK-4-279, a small molecule found by researchers at Georgetown University (Washington, DC) in a library of small molecules supplied by the National Cancer Institute, stops EWS-FLI1's fusion protein from sticking to RNA helicase A, inducing apoptosis in ESFT cells, and reduces

the growth of tumor cells.[134] The most promising targeted therapies are those acting on the microenvironment and are under research.[27]

With regard to local therapy, the focus should be on improving function and decreasing the incidence of long-term sequelae. The use of IMRT therapy and proton therapy, as well as smaller margins, should spare significantly more normal tissues than older techniques, probably decreasing late effects. However, it is unlikely that refinements in local therapy with RT or surgery will significantly improve the cure rate for patients with apparent localized disease, although treating all metastases with RT or surgery appears to be promising for high-risk patients. Stereotactic body radiation therapy (SBRT) may help treat some patients, especially in case of oligometastatic situation. Feasibility and toxicity are currently under evaluation in pediatric patients (ongoing French National protocol 2013-A01176-39).

REFERENCES

1. Karski EE, Matthay KK, Neuhaus JM, et al. Characteristics and outcomes of patients with Ewing sarcoma over 40 years of age at diagnosis. *Cancer Epidemiol* 2013;37:29–33.
2. Cotterill SJ, et al. Prognostic factors in Ewing's tumor of bone: analysis of 975 patients from the European Intergroup Cooperative Ewing's Sarcoma Study Group. *J Clin Oncol* 2000;18:3108–3114.
3. Esiashvili N, Goodman M, Marcus RB. Changes in incidence and survival of ewing sarcoma patients over the past 3 decades. *J Pediatr Hematol Oncol* 2008;30:425–430.
4. Dunst J, Paulussen M, Jürgens H. Lung irradiation for Ewing's sarcoma with pulmonary metastases at diagnosis: results of the CESS-studies. *Strahlenther Onkol* 1993;169:621–623.
5. Ambros IM, et al. MIC2 is a specific marker for Ewing's sarcoma and peripheral primitive neuroectodermal tumors. Evidence for a common histogenesis of Ewing's sarcoma and peripheral primitive neuroectodermal tumors from MIC2 expression and specific chromosome aberration. *Cancer* 1991;67:1886–1893.
6. Delattre O, et al. The Ewing family of tumors—a subgroup of small-round-cell tumors defined by specific chimeric transcripts. *N Engl J Med* 1994;331:294–299.
7. Gamberi G, et al. Molecular diagnosis in Ewing family tumors: the Rizzoli experience—222 consecutive cases in four years. *J Mol Diagn* 2011;13:313–324.
8. Hadfield MG, Quezado MM, Williams RL, et al. Ewing's family of tumors involving structures related to the central nervous system: a review. *Pediatr Dev Pathol* 2000;3:203–210
9. Denny CT. Gene rearrangements in Ewing's sarcoma. *Cancer Invest* 1996;14:83–88.
10. de Alava E, et al. EWS-FLI1 fusion transcript structure is an independent determinant of prognosis in Ewing's sarcoma. *J Clin Oncol* 1998;16:1248–1255.
11. van Doorninck JA, et al. Current treatment protocols have eliminated the prognostic advantage of type 1 fusions in Ewing sarcoma: a report from the Children's Oncology Group. *J Clin Oncol* 2010;28:1989–1994.
12. Le Deley M-C, et al. Impact of EWS-ETS fusion type on disease progression in Ewing's sarcoma/peripheral primitive neuroectodermal tumor: prospective results from the cooperative Euro-E.W.I.N.G. 99 trial. *J Clin Oncol* 2010;28:1982–1988.
13. Specht K, et al. Distinct transcriptional signature and immunoprofile of CIC-DUX4 fusion-positive round cell tumors compared to EWSR1-rearranged Ewing sarcomas: further evidence toward distinct pathologic entities. *Genes Chromosomes Cancer* 2014;53:622–633.
14. Cohen-Gogo S, et al. Ewing-like sarcomas with BCOR-CCNB3 fusion transcript: a clinical, radiological and pathological retrospective study from the Société Française des Cancers de L'Enfant. *Pediatr Blood Cancer* 2014;61:2191–2198.
15. Widhe B, Widhe T. Initial symptoms and clinical features in osteosarcoma and Ewing sarcoma. *J Bone Joint Surg Am* 2000;82:667–674.
16. Burchill SA. Ewing's sarcoma: diagnostic, prognostic, and therapeutic implications of molecular abnormalities. *J Clin Pathol* 2003;56:96–102.
17. Sneppen O, Hansen LM. Presenting symptoms and treatment delay in osteosarcoma and Ewing's sarcoma. *Acta Radiol* 1984;23:159–162.
18. Kaste SC. Imaging pediatric bone sarcomas. *Radiol Clin North Am* 2011;49:749–765.
19. Mentzel HJ, et al. Comparison of whole-body STIR-MRI and 99mTc-methylene-diphosphonate scintigraphy in children with suspected multifocal bone lesions. *Eur Radiol* 2004;14:2297–2302.
20. Nesbit ME, et al. Multimodal therapy for the management of primary, nonmetastatic Ewing's sarcoma of bone: a long-term follow-up of the First Intergroup study. *J Clin Oncol* 1990;8:1664–1674.
21. Györke T, et al. Impact of FDG PET for staging of Ewing sarcomas and primitive neuroectodermal tumours. *Nucl Med Commun* 2006;27:17–24.
22. Avigad S, et al. The predictive potential of molecular detection in the nonmetastatic Ewing family of tumors. *Cancer* 2004;100:1053–1058.

23. Glaubiger DL, Makuch R, Schwarz J, et al. Determination of prognostic factors and their influence on therapeutic results in patients with Ewing's sarcoma. *Cancer* 1980;45:2213–2219.

24. Grier HE, et al. Addition of ifosfamide and etoposide to standard chemotherapy for Ewing's sarcoma and primitive neuroectodermal tumor of bone. *N Engl J Med* 2003;348:694–701.

25. Ladenstein R, et al. Primary disseminated multifocal Ewing sarcoma: results of the Euro-EWING 99 trial. *J Clin Oncol* 2010;28:3284–3291.

26. Jenkin RD, et al. Metastatic Ewing sarcoma/PNET of bone at diagnosis: prognostic factors—a report from Saudi Arabia. *Med Pediatr Oncol* 2001;37:383–389.

27. Gaspar N, et al. Ewing sarcoma: current management and future approaches through collaboration. *J Clin Oncol* 2015;33:3036–3046.

28. Paulino AC, Mai WY, Teh BS. Radiotherapy in metastatic ewing sarcoma. *Am J Clin Oncol* 2013;36:283–286.

29. Rodríguez-Galindo C, et al. Prognostic factors for local and distant control in Ewing sarcoma family of tumors. *Ann Oncol* 2008;19:814–820.

30. Ahrens S, et al. Evaluation of prognostic factors in a tumor volume-adapted treatment strategy for localized Ewing Sarcoma of bone: the CESS 86 experience. *Med Pediatr Oncol* 1999;32:186–195.

31. Indelicato DJ, et al. Impact of local management on long-term outcomes in ewing tumors of the pelvis and sacral bones: the University of Florida Experience. *Int J Radiat Oncol Biol Phys* 2008;72:41–48.

32. Aparicio J, et al. Long-term follow-up and prognostic factors in Ewing's sarcoma. A multivariate analysis of 116 patients from a single institution. *Oncology* 1998;55:20–26.

33. Göbel V, et al. Prognostic significance of tumor volume in localized Ewing's sarcoma of bone in children and adolescents. *J Cancer Res Clin Oncol* 1987;113:187–191.

34. Oberlin O, et al. Prognostic factors in localized Ewing's tumours and peripheral neuroectodermal tumours: the third study of the French Society of Paediatric Oncology (EW88 study). *Br J Cancer* 2001;85:1646–1654.

35. Paulussen M, et al. Localized Ewing tumor of bone: final results of the Cooperative Ewing's Sarcoma Study CESS 86. *J Clin Oncol* 2001;19:1818–1829.

36. Pan HY, et al. Prognostic factors and patterns of relapse in ewing sarcoma patients treated with chemotherapy and R0 resection. *Int J Radiat Oncol Biol Phys* 2015;92:349–357.

37. Bacci G, et al. Prognostic factors in nonmetastatic Ewing's sarcoma of bone treated with adjuvant chemotherapy: analysis of 359 patients at the Istituto Ortopedico Rizzoli. *J Clin Oncol* 2000;18:4–11.

38. Vogin G, et al. Local control and sequelae in localised Ewing tumours of the spine: a French retrospective study. *Eur J Cancer* 2013;49:1314–1323.

39. Kissane JM, Askin FB, Foulkes M, et al. Ewing's sarcoma of bone: clinicopathologic aspects of 303 cases from the Intergroup Ewing's Sarcoma Study. *Hum Pathol* 1983;14:773–779.

40. Fuchs B, Inwards CY, Janknecht R. Vascular endothelial growth factor expression is up-regulated by EWS-ETS oncoproteins and Sp1 and may represent an independent predictor of survival in Ewing's sarcoma. *Clin Cancer Res* 2004;10:1344–1353.

41. Paulino AC, Nguyen TX, Mai WY. An analysis of primary site control and late effects according to local control modality in non-metastatic Ewing sarcoma. *Pediatr Blood Cancer* 2007;48:423–429.

42. Perbal B, et al. Prognostic relevance of CCN3 in Ewing sarcoma. *Hum Pathol* 2009;40:1479–1486.

43. Bacci G, et al. Predictive factors of histological response to primary chemotherapy in Ewing's sarcoma. *Acta Oncol* 1998;37:671–676.

44. Lee JA, et al. Treatment outcome of Korean patients with localized Ewing sarcoma family of tumors: a single institution experience. *Jpn J Clin Oncol* 2011;41:776–782.

45. Wunder JS, et al. The histological response to chemotherapy as a predictor of the oncological outcome of operative treatment of Ewing sarcoma. *J Bone Joint Surg Am* 1998;80:1020–1033.

46. Evans RG, et al. Multimodal therapy for the management of localized Ewing's sarcoma of pelvic and sacral bones: a report from the second intergroup study. *J Clin Oncol* 1991;9:1173–1180.

47. Burgert EO, et al. Multimodal therapy for the management of nonpelvic, localized Ewing's sarcoma of bone: intergroup study IESS-II. *J Clin Oncol* 1990;8:1514–1524.

48. Horowitz ME, et al. Total-body irradiation and autologous bone marrow transplant in the treatment of high-risk Ewing's sarcoma and rhabdomyosarcoma. *J Clin Oncol* 1993;11:1911–1918.

49. Hayes FA, et al. Therapy for localized Ewing's sarcoma of bone. *J Clin Oncol* 1989;7:208–213.

50. Oberlin O, et al. The response to initial chemotherapy as a prognostic factor in localized Ewing's sarcoma. *Eur J Cancer Clin Oncol* 1985;21:463–467.

51. Marcus Jr RB, Berrey BH, Graham-Pole J, et al. The treatment of Ewing's sarcoma of bone at the University of Florida: 1969 to 1998. *Clin Orthop Relat Res* 2002;(397):290–297.

52. Bacci G, et al. The role of surgical margins in treatment of Ewing's sarcoma family tumors: experience of a single institution with 512 patients treated with adjuvant and neoadjuvant chemotherapy. *Int J Radiat Oncol Biol Phys* 2006;65:766–772.

53. Bacci G, et al. Prognostic factors in non-metastatic Ewing's sarcoma tumor of bone: an analysis of 579 patients treated at a single institution with adjuvant or neoadjuvant chemotherapy between 1972 and 1998. *Acta Oncol* 2006;45:469–475.

54. Donaldson SS, et al. A multidisciplinary study investigating radiotherapy in Ewing's sarcoma: end results of POG #8346. Pediatric Oncology Group. *Int J Radiat Oncol Biol Phys* 1998;42:125–135.

55. Obata H, et al. Clinical outcome of patients with Ewing sarcoma family of tumors of bone in Japan: the Japanese Musculoskeletal Oncology Group cooperative study. *Cancer* 2007;109:767–775.

56. Schuck A, et al. Local therapy in localized Ewing tumors: results of 1058 patients treated in the CESS 81, CESS 86, and EICESS 92 trials. *Int J Radiat Oncol Biol Phys* 2003;55:168–177.

57. Balamuth NJ, Womer RB. Ewing's sarcoma. *Lancet Oncol* 2010;11:184–192.

58. Krasin MJ, et al. Definitive surgery and multiagent systemic therapy for patients with localized Ewing sarcoma family of tumors: local outcome and prognostic factors. *Cancer* 2005;104:367–373.

59. Scully SP, et al. Role of surgical resection in pelvic Ewing's sarcoma. *J Clin Oncol* 1995;13:2336–2341.

60. Bolek TW, Marcus RB, Mendenhall NP, et al. Local control and functional results after twice-daily radiotherapy for Ewing's sarcoma of the extremities. *Int J Radiat Oncol Biol Phys* 1996;35:687–692.

61. Donaldson SS. Ewing sarcoma: radiation dose and target volume. *Pediatr Blood Cancer* 2004;42:471–476.

62. Korah MP, et al. Incidence, risks, and sequelae of posterior fossa syndrome in pediatric medulloblastoma. *Int J Radiat Oncol Biol Phys* 2010;77:106–112.

63. Marcus RB, et al. Local control and function after twice-a-day radiotherapy for Ewing's sarcoma of bone. *Int J Radiat Oncol Biol Phys* 1991;21:1509–1515.

64. Sauer R, et al. Prognostic factors in the treatment of Ewing's sarcoma. The Ewing's Sarcoma Study Group of the German Society of Paediatric Oncology CESS 81. *Radiother Oncol* 1987;10:101–110.

65. Craft A, et al. Ifosfamide-containing chemotherapy in Ewing's sarcoma: the second United Kingdom Children's Cancer Study Group and the Medical Research Council Ewing's Tumor Study. *J Clin Oncol* 1998;16:3628–3633.

66. Rosito P, et al. Italian Cooperative Study for the treatment of children and young adults with localized Ewing sarcoma of bone: a preliminary report of 6 years of experience. *Cancer* 1999;86:421–428.

67. Yock TI, et al. Local control in pelvic Ewing sarcoma: analysis from INT-0091--a report from the Children's Oncology Group. *J Clin Oncol* 2006;24:3838–3843.

68. Ferrari S, et al. Nonmetastatic Ewing family tumors: high-dose chemotherapy with stem cell rescue in poor responder patients. Results of the Italian Sarcoma Group/Scandinavian Sarcoma Group III protocol. *Ann Oncol* 2011;22:1221–1227.

69. Granowetter L, et al. Dose-intensified compared with standard chemotherapy for nonmetastatic Ewing sarcoma family of tumors: a Children's Oncology Group Study. *J Clin Oncol* 2009;27:2536–2541.

70. Mascarenhas L, et al. Pilot study of adding vincristine, topotecan, and cyclophosphamide to interval-compressed chemotherapy in newly diagnosed patients with localized Ewing sarcoma: a report from the Children's Oncology Group. *Pediatr Blood Cancer* 2016;63:493–498.

71. Le Deley M-C, et al. Cyclophosphamide compared with ifosfamide in consolidation treatment of standard-risk Ewing sarcoma: results of the randomized noninferiority Euro-EWING99-R1 trial. *J Clin Oncol* 2014;32:2440–2448.

72. Womer RB, et al. Randomized controlled trial of interval-compressed chemotherapy for the treatment of localized Ewing sarcoma: a report from the Children's Oncology Group. *J Clin Oncol* 2012;30:4148–4154.

73. Krasin MJ, et al. Definitive irradiation in multidisciplinary management of localized Ewing sarcoma family of tumors in pediatric patients: outcome and prognostic factors. *Int J Radiat Oncol Biol Phys* 2004;60:830–838.

74. Jereb B, Ong RL, Mohan M, et al. Redefined role of radiation in combined treatment of Ewing's sarcoma. *Pediatr Hematol Oncol* 1986;3:111–118.

75. Ozaki T, et al. Significance of surgical margin on the prognosis of patients with Ewing's sarcoma. A report from the Cooperative Ewing's Sarcoma Study. *Cancer* 1996;78:892–900.

76. Dunst J, Schuck A. Role of radiotherapy in Ewing tumors. *Pediatr Blood Cancer* 2004;42:465–470.

77. Foulon S, et al. Can postoperative radiotherapy be omitted in localised standard-risk Ewing sarcoma? An observational study of the Euro-E.W.I.N.G group. *Eur J Cancer* 2016;61:128–136.

78. Merchant TE, Kushner BH, Sheldon JM, et al. Effect of low-dose radiation therapy when combined with surgical resection for Ewing sarcoma. *Med Pediatr Oncol* 1999;33:65–70.

79. Schuck A, et al. Postoperative radiotherapy in the treatment of Ewing tumors: influence of the interval between surgery and radiotherapy. *Strahlenther Onkol* 2002;178:25–31.

80. Schuck A, et al. Radiotherapy in Ewing tumors of the vertebrae: treatment results and local relapse analysis of the CESS 81/86 and EICESS 92 trials. *Int J Radiat Oncol Biol Phys* 2005;63:1562–1567.

81. Seddon BM, Cassoni AM, Galloway MJ, et al. Fatal radiation myelopathy after high-dose busulfan and melphalan chemotherapy and radiotherapy for Ewing's sarcoma: a review of the literature and implications for practice. *Clin Oncol (R Coll Radiol)* 2005;17:385–390.

82. Bölling T, et al. Radiation toxicity following busulfan/melphalan high-dose chemotherapy in the EURO-EWING-99-trial: review of GPOH data. *Strahlenther Onkol* 2009;185(Suppl 2):21–22.

83. Talleur AC, et al. Limited margin radiation therapy for children and young adults with Ewing sarcoma achieves high rates of local tumor control. *Int J Radiat Oncol Biol Phys* 2016;96:119–126.

84. Schuck A, et al. Hemithorax irradiation for Ewing tumors of the chest wall. *Int J Radiat Oncol Biol Phys* 2002;54:830–838.

85. Claren J, Doyen E, Mascard A, et al. Treatment of localized Ewing sarcomas of the rib: Euro-EWING 99 analysis of French patients. *SIOP Congr* 2017:ABSTRACT 7-0568.

86. Arshi A, et al. Prognostic determinants and treatment outcomes analysis of osteosarcoma and Ewing sarcoma of the spine. *Spine J* 2017;17:645–655.

87. Venkateswaran L, et al. Primary Ewing tumor of the vertebrae: clinical characteristics, prognostic factors, and outcome. *Med Pediatr Oncol* 2001;37:30–35.

88. Hesla AC, et al. Improved prognosis for patients with Ewing sarcoma in the sacrum compared with the innominate bones: the Scandinavian Sarcoma Group Experience. *J Bone Joint Surg Am* 2016;98:199–210.

89. Loschi S, et al. Tandem high-dose chemotherapy strategy as first-line treatment of primary disseminated multifocal Ewing sarcomas in children, adolescents and young adults. *Bone Marrow Transplant* 2015;50:1083–1088.

90. Paulussen M, et al. Primary metastatic (stage IV) Ewing tumor: survival analysis of 171 patients from the EICESS studies. European Intergroup Cooperative Ewing Sarcoma Studies. *Ann Oncol* 1998;9:275–281.

91. Oberlin O, et al. Impact of high-dose busulfan plus melphalan as consolidation in metastatic Ewing tumors: a study by the Société Française des Cancers de l'Enfant. *J Clin Oncol* 2006;24:3997–4002.

92. Luksch R, et al. Primary metastatic Ewing's family tumors: results of the Italian Sarcoma Group and Scandinavian Sarcoma Group ISG/SSG IV Study including myeloablative chemotherapy and total-lung irradiation. *Ann Oncol* 2012;23:2970–2976.

93. Uta Dirksen et al. Efficacy of busulfan-melphalan high dose chemotherapy consolidation (BuMel) compared to conventional chemotherapy combined with lung irradiation in ewing sarcoma (ES) with primary lung metastases: Results of EURO-EWING 99-R2pulm randomized trial (EE99R2pu). *ASCO Congr* 2016:Abstract no 11001.

94. Chan RC, et al. Management and results of localized Ewing's sarcoma. *Cancer* 1979;43:1001–1006.

95. Gasparini M, et al. Long-term outcome of patients with monostotic Ewing's sarcoma treated with combined modality. *Med Pediatr Oncol* 1994;23:406–412.

96. Dunst J, et al. Radiation therapy in Ewing's sarcoma: an update of the CESS 86 trial. *Int J Radiat Oncol Biol Phys* 1995;32:919–930.

97. Perez CA, et al. Radiation therapy in the multimodal management of Ewing's sarcoma of bone: report of the Intergroup Ewing's Sarcoma Study. *Natl Cancer Inst Monogr* 1981;(56):263–271.

98. Rosen G, et al. Disease-free survival in children with Ewing's sarcoma treated with radiation therapy and adjuvant four drug sequential chemotherapy. *Cancer* 1974;33:384–393.

99. Miser JS, et al. Ifosfamide with mesna uroprotection and etoposide: an effective regimen in the treatment of recurrent sarcomas and other tumors of children and young adults. *J Clin Oncol* 1987;5:1191–1198.

100. Paulussen M, et al. EICESS 92 (European Intergroup Cooperative Ewing's Sarcoma Study)—preliminary results. *Klin Padiatr* 1999;211:276–283.

101. Paulussen M, et al. Results of the EICESS-92 Study: two randomized trials of Ewing's sarcoma treatment—cyclophosphamide compared with ifosfamide in standard-risk patients and assessment of benefit of etoposide added to standard treatment in high-risk patients. *J Clin Oncol* 2008;26:4385–4393.

102. Raney RB, et al. Ewing's sarcoma of soft tissues in childhood: a report from the Intergroup Rhabdomyosarcoma Study, 1972 to 1991. *J Clin Oncol* 1997;15:574–582.

103. Miser JS, et al. Treatment of metastatic Ewing's sarcoma or primitive neuroectodermal tumor of bone: evaluation of combination ifosfamide and etoposide—a Children's Cancer Group and Pediatric Oncology Group study. *J Clin Oncol* 2004;22:2873–2876.

104. Paulussen M, et al. Ewing's tumors with primary lung metastases: survival analysis of 114 (European Intergroup) Cooperative Ewing's Sarcoma Studies patients. *J Clin Oncol* 1998;16:3044–3052.

105. Bölling T, et al. Whole lung irradiation in patients with exclusively pulmonary metastases of Ewing tumors. Toxicity analysis and treatment results of the EICESS-92 trial. *Strahlenther Onkol.* 2008;184:193–197.

106. Spunt SL, et al. Selective use of whole-lung irradiation for patients with Ewing sarcoma family tumors and pulmonary metastases at the time of diagnosis. *J Pediatr Hematol Oncol* 2001;23:93–98.

107. Haeusler J, et al. The value of local treatment in patients with primary, disseminated, multifocal Ewing sarcoma (PDMES). *Cancer* 2010;116:443–450.

108. La TH, et al. Radiation therapy for Ewing's sarcoma: results from Memorial Sloan-Kettering in the modern era. *Int J Radiat Oncol Biol Phys* 2006;64:544–550.

109. Rosenthal J, et al. High-dose therapy with hematopoietic stem cell rescue in patients with poor prognosis Ewing family tumors. *Bone Marrow Transplant* 2008;42:311–318.

110. Meyers PA, et al. High-dose melphalan, etoposide, total-body irradiation, and autologous stem-cell reconstitution as consolidation therapy for high-risk Ewing's sarcoma does not improve prognosis. *J Clin Oncol* 2001;19:2812–2820.

111. Kushner BH, Meyers PA. How effective is dose-intensive/myeloablative therapy against Ewing's sarcoma/primitive neuroectodermal tumor metastatic to bone or bone marrow? The Memorial Sloan-Kettering experience and a literature review. *J Clin Oncol* 2001;19:870–880.

112. Pinkerton CR, et al. Treatment strategies for metastatic Ewing's sarcoma. *Eur J Cancer* 2001;37:1338–1344.

113. Burdach S, et al. Total body MRI-governed involved compartment irradiation combined with high-dose chemotherapy and stem cell rescue improves long-term survival in Ewing tumor patients with multiple primary bone metastases. *Bone Marrow Transplant* 2010;45:483–489.

114. Madero L, et al. Megatherapy in children with high-risk Ewing's sarcoma in first complete remission. *Bone Marrow Transplant* 1998;21:795–799.

115. Gaspar N, et al. Risk adapted chemotherapy for localised Ewing's sarcoma of bone: the French EW93 study. *Eur J Cancer* 2012;48:1376–1385.

116. Jeremy Whelan et al. Efficacy of busulfan-melphalan high dose chemotherapy consolidation (BuMel) in localized high-risk Ewing sarcoma (ES): Results of EURO-EWING 99-R2 randomized trial (EE99R2Loc). *ASCO Congr.* 2016:Abstract no 11000.

117. Stahl M, et al. Risk of recurrence and survival after relapse in patients with Ewing sarcoma. *Pediatr Blood Cancer* 2011;57:549–553.

118. Lanza LA, Miser JS, Pass HI, et al. The role of resection in the treatment of pulmonary metastases from Ewing's sarcoma. *J Thorac Cardiovasc Surg* 1987;94:181–187.

119. Hunold A, et al. Topotecan and cyclophosphamide in patients with refractory or relapsed Ewing tumors. *Pediatr Blood Cancer* 2006;47:795–800.

120. Casey DA, et al. Irinotecan and temozolomide for Ewing sarcoma: the Memorial Sloan-Kettering experience. *Pediatr Blood Cancer* 2009;53:1029–1034.

121. Fox E, et al. Phase II study of sequential gemcitabine followed by docetaxel for recurrent ewing sarcoma, osteosarcoma, or unresectable or locally recurrent chondrosarcoma: results of sarcoma alliance for research through Collaboration Study 003. *Oncologist* 2012;17:e321–e329.

122. Ferrari S, et al. Response to high-dose ifosfamide in patients with advanced/recurrent Ewing sarcoma. *Pediatr Blood Cancer* 2009;52:581–584.

123. Gardner SL, et al. Myeloablative therapy with autologous stem cell rescue for patients with Ewing sarcoma. *Bone Marrow Transplant* 2008;41:867–872.

124. Fuchs B, Valenzuela RG, Inwards C, et al. Complications in long-term survivors of Ewing sarcoma. *Cancer* 2003;98:2687–2692.

125. Hamilton SN, Carlson R, Hasan H, et al. Long-term outcomes and complications in pediatric Ewing sarcoma. *Am J Clin Oncol* 2017;40:423–428.

126. Anderson M, Green WT, Messner MB. Growth and predictions of growth in the lower extremities. *J Bone Joint Surg Am* 1963;45–A:1–14.

127. Wagner LM, et al. Fractures in pediatric Ewing sarcoma. *J Pediatr Hematol Oncol* 2001;23:568–571.

128. Kuttesch JF, et al. Second malignancies after Ewing's sarcoma: radiation dose-dependency of secondary sarcomas. *J Clin Oncol* 1996;14:2818–2825.

129. Tucker MA, et al. Bone sarcomas linked to radiotherapy and chemotherapy in children. *N Engl J Med* 1987;317:588–593.

130. Longhi A, et al. Late effects of chemotherapy and radiotherapy in osteosarcoma and Ewing sarcoma patients: the Italian Sarcoma Group Experience (1983-2006). *Cancer* 2012;118:5050–5059.

131. Fidler MM, et al. Long-term adverse outcomes in survivors of childhood bone sarcoma: the British Childhood Cancer Survivor Study. *Br J Cancer* 2015;112:1857–1865.

132. Ranft A, et al. Quality of survivorship in a rare disease: clinicofunctional outcome and physical activity in an Observational Cohort Study of 618 long-term survivors of Ewing sarcoma. *J Clin Oncol* 2017;35:1704–1712.

133. Grohar PJ, et al. Identification of an inhibitor of the EWS-FLI1 oncogenic transcription factor by high-throughput screening. *J Natl Cancer Inst* 2011;103:962–978.

134. Erkizan HV, et al. A small molecule blocking oncogenic protein EWS-FLI1 interaction with RNA helicase A inhibits growth of Ewing's sarcoma. *Nat Med* 2009;15:750–756.

Section III

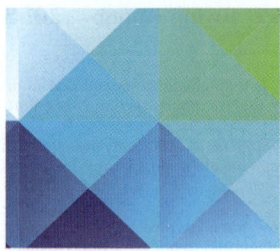

CHAPTER 93

Lymphomas in Children

Avani Dholakia Rao, Louis S. Constine, Stacy Lorine Cooper, and Stephanie A. Terezakis

INTRODUCTION

Childhood lymphomas, a broad spectrum of cancers, have become increasingly curable as treatment regimens have evolved in tandem with improvements in radiation and chemotherapy, pathology, and imaging. The challenge has been to optimally balance treatment intensity with its attendant toxicity. Treatment with adult regimens, although effective, caused unacceptable morbidities in children, such as impaired musculoskeletal development, increased risks of secondary benign and malignant neoplasms, cardiopulmonary toxicities, and other organ toxicities. Consideration given to mitigation of therapy toxicity is paramount to the design of modern pediatric trials. Although there is a focus on intensification of therapy in children with unfavorable prognosis, the field is also moving to refine and even deescalate treatment in children with a favorable prognosis. In addition, recent data have established early response to therapy as a tool to identify patients with more sensitive disease in whom therapy can be reduced or patients with more aggressive disease in whom therapy should be escalated.

Commensurate with the identification of prognostic and predictive factors, widespread use of modern imaging techniques, and the increasingly effective use of chemotherapy has been a more restrictive role for radiotherapy. Our recognition of the long-term sequelae of therapy has led to the refinement of both chemotherapy and radiation therapy (RT) strategies.

HODGKIN LYMPHOMA

Hodgkin lymphoma (HL) constitutes a class of diseases that arise in both children and adults. Although histologic similarities between adult and pediatric subtypes exist, there are a number of differences to suggest that the biology is only partially shared. For example, the clinical presentations vary in terms of the gender ratio, distribution of histologic subtypes, hypotheses of etiology, and the role of Epstein-Barr virus (EBV), as well as the potential for cure.[1] Historic therapies, though successful in adults, caused substantial morbidities in children.[2,3] As patients were often cured, children with pediatric HL have served as models for understanding the long-term toxicity of RT and chemotherapy. High dose extended field RT causing musculoskeletal hypoplasia and cytotoxic therapy with certain alkylating agents prompted the first generation of studies examining combined modality therapy using lower doses and/or smaller fields during RT with the expectation that cycles of multiagent chemotherapy could eradicate microscopic foci of disease in children staged with laparotomy.[4–9] The unacceptable rates of secondary malignancies attributed to the offending alkylating agents led to the second generation of investigations using doxorubicin-containing chemotherapy regimens to replace more toxic alkylating agents. Overall, recent 5-year survival rates of children and adolescents with HL have increased to 97% from 87% in the late 1970s.[10]

Today's treatment of children with lymphoma employs thoughtful chemotherapy regimens and nuanced radiation approaches in an effort to mitigate long-term toxicity (Table 93.1). Decisions for treatment are determined using a risk-adapted approach in which patients receive varying intensities of multiagent chemotherapy and low dose involved field RT, with the most recent studies using treatment response to guide elimination of RT in certain patients.[5,6,8,9,11–36] Future directions will aim to identify and subsequently integrate biologic factors to guide therapy in patients with very good or very poor outcomes.

Epidemiology

Pediatric HL has unique epidemiologic presentations that vary based on age, geography, gender, and socioeconomic status. The most common subtype, nodular sclerosing or classic

TABLE 93.1 RECOMMENDATIONS FOR TREATMENT APPROACH IN CLASSIC PEDIATRIC HODGKIN LYMPHOMA

Clinical Presentation	Stage	Recommended Treatment Approach
Low risk Localized disease involving <3–4 nodal regions in the absence of "B" symptoms, bulky disease, or extranodal extension.	IA, IIA	**Recommended therapy** 2–4 cycles non–cross-resistant chemotherapy (OEPA, VAMP, COPP–ABV, AV–PC). Response-based low dose ISRT (1,500–2,550 cGy). **Other considerations** If complete response after 2 cycles of OEPA, no need for ISRT.
Intermediate risk Localized disease involving ≥3–4 nodal regions in the presence of bulky lymphadenopathy (mediastinal ratio ≥33%; lymph node mass ≥6–10 cm) and extranodal extension.	IA, IIA, IIB[a] IIIA	**Recommended therapy** 3–6 cycles compacted, dose-intensive, non–cross-resistant chemotherapy (OEPA/COPP, ABVE–PC) plus low dose ISRT (1,500–2,550 cGy). **Other considerations** ABVE–PC x 4 without RT for rapid early responders after 2 cycles and complete response after cycle 4.
High risk Stage II patients with constitutional symptoms of fevers or weight loss or any patient with advanced disease.	IIB[a] IIIB IV	**Recommended therapy** 4–6 compacted, dose-intensive cycles of non–cross-resistant chemotherapy (COPP/OEPA, ABVE–PC) plus low dose ISRT (1,500–2,550 cGy). **Other considerations** 8 cycles non–cross-resistant chemotherapy alone (BEACOPP) for high-risk, poor early response.

Note: In treatment centers where prechemotherapy, postchemotherapy, and radiation simulation imaging are all obtained in the same position with the radiation simulation immobilization device, then involved-node radiation therapy (INRT) can be considered instead of ISRT.

[a]Stage IIB patients have been variably treated as intermediate or unfavorable risk. Some studies use associated factors, for example, weight loss, bulk disease, and extranodal extension, for further risk stratification.

ABV, doxorubicin, bleomycin, and vinblastine; AV–PC, doxorubicin, vincristine, prednisone, and cyclophosphamide; BEACOPP, bleomycin, etoposide, doxorubicin, cyclophosphamide, vincristine, procarbazine, prednisone; COPP, cyclophosphamide, vincristine, procarbazine, prednisone; ISRT, involved-site radiation therapy; OEPA, vincristine, etoposide, prednisone, and doxorubicin; VAMP, vinblastine, doxorubicin, methotrexate, and prednisone.

HL, is separated into childhood HL, which occurs in patients ages 14 years or younger and young adult HL, which affects patients ages 15 to 34. In the United States, childhood HL is the eighth most common cancer in children (ages 0 to 14), and young adult HL is the most common malignancy of adolescence (ages 15 to 16).[10] Although the incidence of non-Hodgkin lymphoma (NHL) is slightly more common than childhood HL in children younger than 14, comprising 6% versus 4% of all cancer diagnoses, young adult HL constitutes 15% of new cancer diagnoses compared to 8% being NHL in adolescents.

The childhood form of classic HL is rare in children < 4 years of age, usually occurring in children >10 years. Incidence is associated with male gender, increasing family size, and decreasing socioeconomic status.[37–40] In the United States, although whites have the highest overall incidence rates for both males and females, the male gender association of childhood HL is strongest in black males (M:F ratio 4:1). There is a marked variation in international incidence of HL, with an inverse relationship between the occurrence of childhood and young adult forms of the disease.[41–43] Countries with a high incidence of childhood HL demonstrate a low incidence of young adult HL and vice versa. Early and intense exposure to an infectious agent has been speculated to increase the risk for the childhood form of HL.[44,45]

In contrast to childhood HL, young adult classic HL is associated with a higher socioeconomic status, smaller family size, and later birth order.[37,38,45] There is a roughly equal incidence between older adolescent males and females.[46] Similarities between HL and paralytic poliomyelitis suggest that delayed exposure to an infectious agent may be a risk factor for the development of young adult HL, with the risk of oncogenesis increasing with later age of infectious exposure.[38] Interestingly, there also seems to be an association of early exposure to children at nursery school and day care decreasing the risk of young adult HL, most likely by facilitating childhood exposure to common infections and promoting maturation of cellular immunity.[45]

A less common subtype, nodular lymphocyte-predominant HL (NLPHL), represents approximately 5% of pediatric HL diagnoses. It is associated with a much higher incidence in males, Caucasians, and younger children (<10 years) and does not have a strong association with income or birth order. The other subtypes of HL, such as mixed cellularity (MC), lymphocyte-rich, and lymphocyte-depleted, are extremely rare in children and young adults.[47]

Pathologic Classification

As in adults, pediatric HL follows the same WHO classification into two major groups of HL: classic HL and NLPHL. Distinctions between groups are made according to their biologic and clinical features, which will be discussed later in following sections.[48,49] Classic HL is further subclassified into nodular sclerosing (NS), MC, lymphocyte-rich (LR), and lymphocyte-depleted (LD) histologies based on their unique morphology. NLPHL appears to have a better outcome, and treatment typically varies from those with classic HL.

The relative distribution of the subtypes differs in younger children compared with adolescents and adults.[40,50] Although NS is the most common subtype in all age groups, it constitutes a significantly larger proportion of cases of adolescent (77%) and adult (72%) HL than in children < age 10 (44%). Conversely, MC subtype is more common in younger children (33%) than in adolescents (11%) or adults (17%). Similarly, NLPHL is more common (13%) in children younger than 10 years than in adolescents (8%) and adults (5%). LD subtype is rare in all age groups.[40]

Biology

Similar to adult HL, both pediatric HL and NHL are neoplasms arising from the germinal center of lymph nodes.

HL is unique among the lymphomas because the malignant Hodgkin and Reed-Sternberg (HRS) cells, lymphocytic and histiocytic (L and H) cells, and their variants account for <1% of the tumor cell population. Identical immunologic gene rearrangements in HRS and L and H cells support their origin from a single transformed B cell that subsequently undergoes monoclonal expansion.[51–53] There are two distinct immunophenotypes of HL, which distinguish the differentiation of HL into World Health Organization's classifications of classic HL and NLPHL.[48] The first immunophenotype associated with classic HL is characteristic of HRS cells that consistently express CD30 and often express CD15 but lack J chain expression.[48,54] The second immunophenotype associated with NLPHL is characteristic of L and H cells that consistently express CD20 and J chain and do not express CD30 and CD15.[53,55]

Considerable evidence suggests an etiologic role of the EBV in the pathogenesis of both childhood and young adult HL.[56,57] Early serologic studies linked EBV to HL.[56,57] Delayed early adolescent exposure to EBV is frequently associated with development of infectious mononucleosis, and studies show an increased risk of HL in patients diagnosed with infectious mononucleosis.[58–63] Additionally, increased EBV antibody titers have been observed in patients with HL several years prior to HL diagnosis.[64] The incidence of EBV-associated HL varies by age, gender, ethnicity, histologic subtype, and regional economic level.[57] EBV-positive tumor genomes are more frequent in children <10 years of age and in those who live in low-income countries.[57] EBV positivity is most common in the MC and lymphocyte-depleted HL subtypes, observed in approximately 80% of children ages 0 to 14 with these subtypes of HL. Tumors of children with nodular sclerosing HL were found to be EBV-positive in nearly 40% (childhood HL) and 20% (young adult HL) of cases.[57] A detailed description of the histologic subtypes of HL is discussed below.

HL is also associated with congenital (e.g., ataxia-telangiectasia)[65] and acquired (e.g., human immunodeficiency virus [HIV]) immunodeficiencies, and EBV appears to be an important cofactor in the development of HL in these patients.[66] Concordance of HL has been observed in first-degree siblings to have a 3-fold increase risk in HL[67] with other studies suggesting as high as a 9-fold increased risk in siblings of the same gender. As high as a 99-fold increased risk in monozygotic twins of patients with HL has been reported, with no increased risk in dizygotic twins.[68] These familial cases of HL suggest a genetic predisposition to the disease or a common environmental exposure.

Clinical Presentation

Typical presenting signs and symptoms include lymphadenopathy, mediastinal mass, or systemic symptoms. Up to 90% of patients will demonstrate contiguous lymphatic spread with 80% of pediatric HL patients presenting with cervical lymphadenopathy.[69] The lymph nodes are often fixed, firm, rubbery, and painless. Mediastinal involvement is present in 76% of adolescents but only in 33% of children aged 1 to 10 years.[69] If mediastinal lymphadenopathy is present, it may be associated with a nonproductive cough, respiratory distress, or other symptoms of tracheal or bronchial obstruction. Isolated infradiaphragmatic HL is rare, occurring in <5% of patients.

As a result of cytokine production by the HRS cells, one-third of patients may have one or more of the so-called B symptoms at diagnosis. These include recurrent unexplained fevers >38.3°C during the previous month, drenching night sweats, or weight loss of more than 10% in the 6 months preceding diagnosis.[69,70] Other cytokine-mediated systemic symptoms may also include anorexia, pruritus, fibrosis, eosinophilia, thrombocytosis, plasmacytosis, and immunodeficiency.[71]

Diagnostic Workup

The diagnosis of HL is made based on morphology, immunohistochemistry, and flow cytometry reviewed by experienced lymphoma pathologists. When appropriate, molecular studies may be needed for further characterization. The diagnosis is facilitated through an excisional lymph node biopsy to provide adequate tissue for evaluation of the malignant HRS and L and H cells and the characteristic architectural changes associated with the specific histologic subtypes. Although less desirable, core needle biopsy can be considered when excisional biopsy is not possible; however, lack of adequate tissue sampled and inappropriate tissue sampling are common causes of failure of this diagnostic approach.[72] Fine needle aspiration (FNA) is neither helpful nor cost-effective and may even misguide treatment as diagnoses based on FNA often do not correlate with evaluations on subsequent excisional biopsies.[73]

A detailed history should evaluate the age, sex, and absence or presence of B symptoms, each of which may alter the management of a child with HL. Fatigue, pruritus, and alcohol-induced pain should be noted. Though these symptoms do not direct treatment, their recurrence may be an early indication of disease relapse. Physical exam involves a detailed lymph node exam, including assessment of Waldeyer ring, as well as measurement of the liver and spleen. Laboratory evaluation should include a complete blood count with white blood cell differential and platelet count, erythrocyte sedimentation rate, albumin, renal and liver function tests, and lactate dehydrogenase.

An upright posterior–anterior chest radiograph is required for assessment of mediastinal bulk defined as mediastinal adenopathy measuring 33% or more of the maximum intrathoracic cavity. Chest radiograph is highly concordant with chest computed tomography (CT),[74] although chest radiograph is still required to define bulk in the majority of protocols including those run by the Children's Oncology Group (COG). Contrast-enhanced CT is recommended for evaluation of the thorax as it can detect lymphadenopathy involving the subcarinal, hilar, and cardiophrenic angles as well as extranodal sites including the pleura, chest wall, or pericardium, which may change management.[75]

Infradiaphragmatic disease is best assessed by CT scan with oral and intravenous contrast to distinguish lymphadenopathy from other structures. CT evaluation of the abdomen and pelvis may be limited, however, with suboptimal contrast administration or in children who lack retroperitoneal fat. In such cases, magnetic resonance imaging (MRI) may provide better assessment of disease involvement in the retroperitoneal lymph nodes.

Essentially all cases of HL demonstrate (18)fluorine-fluorodeoxyglucose (^{18}F-FDG) avidity,[76] and thus ^{18}F-FDG positron emission tomography (PET) is included as standard staging for HL.[77] ^{18}F-FDG-PET scans lead to a change in stage in 10% to 30% of patients, more often upstaging.[78] ^{18}F-PET-CT is furthermore critical in monitoring treatment response, particularly in cases with persistent radiographic abnormalities[79] or "rebound" thymic growth after completion of therapy.[80] Splenic and hepatic involvement by HL is suggested by the presence of enlarged organs with areas of abnormal density on CT or MRI scans, as well as increased ^{18}F-FDG uptake on PET scan.

Traditionally, bone marrow biopsy was standard in lymphoma staging; however, given the low rate of bone marrow involvement at initial presentation, particularly in the setting of a negative ^{18}F-PET-CT for bone marrow involvement, bone marrow biopsy can be restricted to patients with B symptoms or stage III or IV disease.[77]

TABLE 93.2 REVISED ANN ARBOR STAGING SYSTEM

Stage	Involvement	Extranodal (IE) Status
Limited		
I	One node or a group of adjacent nodes	Single extranodal lesions without nodal involvement
II	Two or more nodal groups on the same side of the diaphragm	Stage I or II by nodal extent with limited contiguous extranodal involvement
II Bulky[a]	II + "bulky" disease[a]	
Advanced		
III	Nodes on both sides of the diaphragm	
	Nodes above the diaphragm + spleen involvement	
IV	Additional noncontiguous extralymphatic involvement	
Modifications	**If Present**	**If Absent**
B symptoms	B	A
Bulky disease[a]	X	–
Extranodal spread	E	–
Splenic involvement	S	–

Positron emission tomography–computed tomography used to define extent of disease in HL. Tonsils, Waldeyer ring, and spleen are considered nodal tissue.
[a]Bulky definition varies across protocols but most commonly as a mass of more than one-third of the maximum intrathoracic diameter or extramediastinal mass >6–10 cm.

Staging Systems

As for adults, children with HL are staged according to the system devised at the Ann Arbor Staging Conference in 1970 and revised at the Cotswolds meeting.[81] Patients are typically treated based on limited (stages I and II, nonbulky) or advanced (stages III or IV) disease, with stage II bulky considered limited or advanced based on other prognostic factors as shown in Table 93.2.

Prognostic Factors

A discussion of prognostic factors in pediatric HL is complicated for several reasons. First, prognostic factors such as disease stage, bulk, and biologic aggressiveness are frequently codependent.[82] Second, identification of prognostic factors is confounded by the impact of therapy, with higher-intensity therapies negating previously determined adverse risk factors.[83] Third, different institutions and different cooperative groups have various risk stratification schemes within pediatric HL protocols,[33,35,36,84–90] and within these determinations, patients with early-stage disease have different prognosticators than patients with advanced-stage disease.[82]

The following are some generalizations regarding prognostic variables derived from both adult and pediatric data:

- *Stage of disease* is the most significant prognosticator of treatment outcome. Advanced-stage disease, particularly stage IV disease with multiple organ involvement, confers an exceptionally poor prognosis when managed with conventional therapy.[91,92]
- *Bulk of disease* is reflective of both the number of disease sites and the volume of involvement at each site. Patients with several sites of involvement, typically three or more, have an inferior relapse-free (RFS) and overall survival (OS) in some, but not all, reports.[93] Bulky mediastinal adenopathy and nonmediastinal sites have historically been associated with an increased risk of disease recurrence, particularly when managed with RT alone.[93–96] Bulky mediastinal adenopathy has been defined using a variety of definitions, most commonly as a mass of more than one-third of the maximum intrathoracic diameter.[96–99] Other common definitions include

a ratio of greater than 1/3 of the mediastinal mass to the intrathoracic width at T5-6[100] or an absolute mass of >10 cm,[101] ≥5 cm,[102] or ≥6 cm[103,104] depending on the protocol. In Europe, a volume definition of bulk is used, recently defined as 200 mL estimated using an ellipsoid volume formula where $V = (xyz)/2$ where x, y, and z are the diameters of the mass in three dimensions.[105]

- *Presence of systemic symptoms* (B symptoms), which result from cytokine secretion, reflects biologic aggressiveness and correlates with an increased risk of relapse compared with the absence of such symptoms (A disease).[70,92]
- *Abnormally high levels of certain serum markers*, including ESR, hemoglobin, serum albumin, and white blood cell count, have been reported to be negative prognostic factors.[82,92] As these are confounded by increased tumor volume, it is unclear if elevated serum markers are independently prognostic for more malignant biology of disease.[82,92]
- *Histologic subtype* may correlate with prognosis. Patients with NLPHL have a unique biology and improved outcomes compared to other classic HL histologies. LD histology confers a worse outcome than do the other subtypes, but it is exceedingly rare.[96] Patients with LP histology are more commonly early stage and have an excellent outcome.[106] A recent COG study reported a survival advantage for patients with mixed cellularity HL,[107] however, most modern combined modality trials do not show any histology survival differences.[27,92]
- *Patient age* appears to be a determinant of patient outcome with children <10 years of age seemingly faring better than older patients with 5- and 10-year survival rates of 94% and 92%, respectively, compared with 93% and 86% for adolescents and 84% and 73% for adults.[40,50] This may be due to the higher prevalence of stage "A" disease in children compared to adults.[50]
- *Response to initial therapy* has recently been identified as a prognostic factor, observed in pediatric patients with advanced-stage HL treated on Pediatric Oncology Group (POG) 8725, where 93% of patients who attained a complete response after three cycles of chemotherapy remained disease free.[8] A similar finding was also observed in low-risk patients.[108] Early treatment response has since become the foundation for new trials and recommendations for response-based therapy that are discussed separately in the section "Risk-Adapted Combined Modality Therapy for Classic Hodgkin Lymphoma" to follow. As this is an emerging prognostic factor and stratification for treatment, definitions for complete response, partial response, and progressive disease based on CT or PET-CT are varied across studies.[33,35,84,109-111] Recently, a visual five-point score known as the Deauville criteria has been shown to be a reproducible approach to score response on PET-CT in adult HL and is being applied as a standard reporting criterion in clinical trials and practice in both pediatric and adult HL.[112,113]

In efforts to define a prognostic risk scoring group for pediatric HL patients treated with modern-era combined modality therapy, a retrospective analysis of the most recent COG study AHOD0031, which analyzed response-based therapy in intermediate-risk patients, was introduced. The Childhood Hodgkin International Prognostic Score (CHIPS) is a new scoring system that allocates one point each for fever, stage IV disease, albumin < 3.5, and large mediastinal adenopathy (defined as mass of more than one-third of the maximum intrathoracic diameter).[114] CHIPS was highly predictive of event-free survival (EFS), and the scoring system identified a subset (CHIPS 2 or 3) that comprised 27% of intermediate-risk patients with inferior outcomes (EFS < 80%) who may benefit from early intensification of therapy.

The use of prognostic factors is reflected in the risk grouping that various pediatric trials employ for assignment of

therapy. Such stratifications are discussed below in the "Risk-Adapted Combined Modality Therapy for Classic Hodgkin Lymphoma" section and are reflected in the summary of treatment recommendations.

General Management

Pediatric HL is a highly curable disease. Given the longevity of patients with pediatric HL, treatment is complicated by their increased risk for adverse treatment-related side effects over time.

For patients with early-stage disease, RT to extended fields to a curative dose range of 30 to 40 Gy produced the first cures in patients with HL, and similar treatment paradigms were used for adults and children. In children undergoing surgical staging with early-stage disease, 5-year disease-free survival (DFS) rates following extended-field RT ranged from 60% to 80% when treated with RT alone.[6,12,13,115] For patients with advanced-stage disease, the development of non–cross-resistant chemotherapy combinations provided the first effective therapy; however, the specific chemotherapeutic combinations have changed as their gonadotoxic and leukemogenic properties have become better understood. Although treatment approaches of the past involving large radiation fields, including total lymphoid RT, and toxic alkylating chemotherapy are archaic, the observed late morbidity and mortality as a result of second malignancies, cardiopulmonary disease, musculoskeletal growth retardation, and gonadal toxicity caused by these treatments have steered the management of pediatric HL to balance the efficacy and morbidity of treatments to children at this critical time in their development.[16,94,115-126]

A summary of chemotherapy-alone and combined modality therapy trials for the treatment of pediatric HL is summarized in Tables 93.3 and 93.4. Current management paradigms for pediatric HL involve a risk-adapted and an emerging response-adapted approach to treatment. Therapy typically involves multiagent chemotherapy followed by low dose RT for slowly responding, bulky, residual, or recurrent disease. The development of this treatment approach with the refinement of combination chemotherapy regimens and reduced-field, low dose RT is discussed in the sections to follow.

Combination Chemotherapy

The first effective systemic therapy for HL was MOPP (mechlorethamine, vincristine, procarbazine, prednisone),[144-146] although treatment was associated with ovarian failure in women, infertility in both sexes, and a high rate of secondary acute myeloid leukemia (s-AML).[147,148] The cumulative risk of secondary malignancy is 4% to 8% after MOPP-based therapy,[149] with incidence peaking 5 to 10 years after treatment and plateauing to a cumulative risk of 2% more than 10 years following treatment.[150] A regimen substituting cyclophosphamide for mechlorethamine (COPP) has been associated with a lower incidence of s-AML.[149]

Subsequently, an alternative regimen using ABVD (doxorubicin, bleomycin, vinblastine, and dacarbazine) was shown to result in superior disease control compared to MOPP chemotherapy.[151,152] Despite improvements in chemotherapeutic side effects, bleomycin and doxorubicin cause pulmonary and cardiovascular damage, respectively, each enhanced when combined with RT to the lungs and heart.[14,95,119,153] One approach to reduce the risk of cardiomyopathy caused by doxorubicin, an anthracycline agent, is to limit the cumulative dose of anthracyclines for pediatric HL patients to a maximum cumulative dose of 250 mg/m², particularly in the case of favorable risk disease. Bleomycin-induced pulmonary toxicity is manifested as a chronic pneumonitis or pulmonary fibrosis and typically occurs at doses higher than 400 U/m².[154] Most modern pediatric HL regimens use doses in the range of 60 to 100 U/m². Although such doses typically result in subclinical pulmonary

TABLE 93.3 TREATMENT RESULTS OF MODERN CHEMOTHERAPY-ALONE TRIALS IN CLASSIC PEDIATRIC HODGKIN LYMPHOMA

Reference	Group	# Patients	Stage	Chemotherapy	Percent Outcome (Year)	
					EFS, DFS, or RFS	Survival
LOW RISK						
Metzger, 2012[127]	Stanford/St. Jude/ Dana-Farber	47	IA-IIA	4 VAMP alone if CR	89 (2)	100 (2)
Keller, 2010[128]	COG AHOD 0431	175	IA, IIA	3 AV–PC alone if CR	80 (2)	100 (2)
Mauz-Korholz, 2010[32]	GPOH-HD 2002	62	IA, IB, and IIA	2 OPPA or OEPA alone if CR	93 (5)	99 (5)
Kung, 2006[108]	POG 8625	78	IA-IIIA1	4 MOPP/4 ABVD	83 (8)	94 (8)
Hakyoort-Cammel, 2004[129]	Rotterdam HD-84	23	I-IIA	6 EBVD	96 (10)	100 (10)
Dörffel, 2003, 2013[56,57]	GPOH-HD 95	66	IA/B-IIA	2 OPPA or OEPA and CR	97 (10)	99 (10)
Nachman, 2002; Wolden, 2012[36,90]	USA-CCG 5942	113	IA/B, IIA	4 COPP/ABV and CR	89 (10)	100 (3)
Sackmann-Muriel, 1997[24]	GATLA	10	IA, IIA	3 CVPP	86 (7)	
		16	IB, IIB	6 CVPP	87 (7)	
INTERMEDIATE/HIGH RISK						
Jayabose, 2016[130]	Madurai, India	9	I or II with B symptoms and/or bulk, IIIA	4 m-BEACOPP + 4 ABVD	100 (3)	100 (3)
		17	IIIB, IV	4 ABVE–PC +2 ABVD	100 (3)	100 (3)
Arya, 2006[131]	New Delhi, India	133	I-IV	4 COPP/4 ABVD	88 (50	92 (5)
Hakyoort-Cammel, 2004[129]	Rotterdam HD-84	23	IIB-IV	3–5 EBVD/MOPP	87 (10)	91 (10)
Dörffel, 2003, 2013[56,57]	GPOH-HD 95	46	IAE, IBE, IIIAE, IIB, IIIA	2 OPPA or OEPA + 2 COPP and CR	69 (10)	98 (10)
		56	IIEB, IIIEA/B, IIIB, IVA/B	2 OPPA or OEPA + 4 COPP and CR	83 (10)	100 (10)
Nachman, 2002; Wolden, 2012[36,90]	USA-CCG 5942	122	I/II w/risk factors, IIB, III	6 COPP/ABV and CR	78 (10)	100 (3)
		30	IV	COPP/ABV + CHOP +Ara-C/VP-16 and CR	80 (10)	94 (3)
Alta, 2002[132]	United Kingdom Children's Cancer Study Group	67	IV	6–8 ChlVPP	55 (5)	80 (5)
Ekert, 1999[15]	Australia/New Zealand	53	I-IV	5–6 VEEP	78 (5)	92 (5)
Hutchinson, 1998[7]	USA-CCG	57	III-IV	6 MOPP/6 ABVD	77 (4)	84 (4)
Weiner, 1997[8]	USA-POG 8725	81	IIB, IIIA2, IIIB, IV	4 MOPP/4 ABVD	79 (5)	96 (5)

ABV, doxorubicin, bleomycin, vinblastine; ABVD, doxorubicin, bleomycin, vinblastine, dacarbazine; COP, cyclophosphamide, vincristine, prednisone; CHOP, cyclophosphamide, doxorubicin, vincristine, prednisone; ChlVPP, chlorambucil, vinblastine, procarbazine, and prednisolone; COPP, cyclophosphamide, vincristine, procarbazine, prednisone; CVPP, lomustine, vinblastine, procarbazine, and prednisone; DFS, disease-free survival; EBVD, epirubicin, bleomycin, vinblastine, and dacarbazine; EFS, event-free survival; EVAP, etoposide, vinblastine, doxorubicin, and prednisone; FFP, freedom from progression; MOPP, mechlorethamine, vincristine, procarbazine, prednisone; RFS, relapse-free survival; VEEP, vincristine, etoposide, epirubicin, prednisolone.

TABLE 93.4 TREATMENT RESULTS OF MODERN COMBINED MODALITY TRIALS IN CLASSIC PEDIATRIC HODGKIN LYMPHOMA

Reference	Group	# Patients	Stage	Chemotherapy	Radiation Therapy (Gy)	Percent Outcome (Year)	
						EFS, DFS, or RFS	Survival
LOW RISK							
Keller, 2013[105]	COG AHOD 0431	275	IA, IIA	3 AV–PC	21, IF for PR; no RT if CR	PR 88/CR 80 (2)	PR/CR 100 (2)
Metzger, 2012[127]	Stanford/St. Jude/ Dana-Farber	88	IA-IIA	4 VAMP	25.5, IF, no RT for CR	PR 92/CR 89 (2)	PR/CR 100 (2)
Tebbi, 2012[133]	USA COG 9426	112	I, IIA, IIIA	RER: ABVE x 2	25.5, IF	87 (8)	97 (8)
		135	I, IIA, IIIA	SER: ABVE x 4	25.5, IF	85 (8)	96 (8)
Mauz-Korholz, 2010[134]	GPOH-HD 2002	195	IA, IB, and IIA	2 OPPA or OEPA	19.8, IF for PR, no RT for CR	PR 92/CR 93 (5)	PR/CR 99 (5)
Tebbi, 2006[135]	USA POG 9226	46	IA-IIIA1	4 ABVE	25.5, IF	91 (6)	98 (6)
Kung, 2006[108]	USA POG 8625	81	IA-IIIA1	2 MOPP/2 ABVD	25.5, IF	91 (8)	97 (8)
Hudson, 2004[136]	Stanford/St. Jude/ Dana-Farber	77	I, II	3 VAMP/3 COP (2 cycles/RT/2 cycles/ RT/2 cycles/RT)	15, IF for CR; 25.5, IF for PR	100/78 (6)	93 (6)
Dörffel, 2003, 2013[56,57]	GPOH-HD 95	328	IA/B-IIA	2 OPPA or OEPA	20–35, IF for PR; no RT if CR	PR 97/CR 93 (10)	PR 99 CR/99 (10)
Nachman, 2002; Wolden, 2012[36,90]	USA-CCG 5942	94	IA/B, IIA	4 COPP/ABV	21, IF	91 (10)	98 (3)
Donaldson, 2002, 2007[115,137]	Stanford/St. Jude/ Dana-Farber	110	CS I/II	4 VAMP	15–25.5 IF	89 (10)	96 (10)
Landman-Parker, 2000[19]	SFOP MDH-90	171	I-II	4 VBVP, good responders	20, IF	91 (5)	98 (5)
		27	I-II	4 VBVP + 1–2 OPPA poor responders	20, IF	78 (5)	
Schellong, 1999[88]	GPOH-HD 90	275	IA/IB-IIA	2 OEPA or OPPA	25, IF	94/95 (5)	99 (5)
		124	IIB-IIIA	2 OEPA or OPPA + 2 COPP	25, IF	90/96 (5)	97 (5)
Shankar, 1998[138]	United Kingdom Children's Cancer Study Group	46	I-III	8 VEEP	30–35, IF	82 (5)	93 (5)
Shankar, 1997[27]	United Kingdom Children's Cancer Study Group	125	II	6–10 ChlVPP	35, IF	85 (10)	92 (10)
Hunger, 1997[17]	Stanford	44	I-III	3 MOPP/3 ABVD	15–25.5 IF	100 (10)	100 (10)

TABLE 93.4 TREATMENT RESULTS OF MODERN COMBINED MODALITY TRIALS IN CLASSIC PEDIATRIC HODGKIN LYMPHOMA (*Continued*)

Reference	Group	# Patients	Stage	Chemotherapy	Radiation Therapy (Gy)	Percent Outcome (Year) EFS, DFS, or RFS	Survival
Schellong, 1992[139]	GPOH-HD 82	100	IA/IB-IIA	2 OPPA	35, IF	98 (9)	100 (9)
	GPOH-HD 85	53	IA/IB-IIA	2 OPA	35, IF	85 (6)	98 (6)
	GPOH-HD 87	104	IA/IB-IIA	2 OPA	30, IF	88 (5)	100 (5)
INTERMEDIATE/HIGH RISK							
Friedman, 2014[140]	USA-COG AHOOD 0031	361	IB, IAE, IIB, IIAE, IIIA, IVA with or without bulk disease, and IA or IIA with bulk disease	RER w/CR: 4 ABVE–PC	No RT	89 (4)	99 (4)
		355			21, IF	84 (4)	99 (4)
		151		SER: 4 ABVE–PC	21, IF	75 (4)	94 (4)
		153		SER: 2 ABVE–PC + DECA + 2 ABVE–PC	21, IF	79 (4)	97 (4)
Mauz-Korholz, 2010[32]	GPOH-HD 2002	139	IE, IIB, IIAE, and IIIA	2 OPPA or OEPA + 2 COPP or COPDAC	19.8, IF	88 (5)	99 (5)
		239	IIBE, IIIAE, IIIB, IVA, IVB, and IVE	2 OPPA or OEPA + 4 COPP or COPDAC		87 (5)	95 (5)
Schwartz, 2009[35]	USA-POG 9425	216	IBX-IV	RER: 3 ABVE–PC	21, IF	86 (5)	95 (5)
				SER: 5 ABVE–PC	21, IF	83 (5)	95 (5)
Hudson, 2004[136]	Stanford/St. Jude/ Dana-Farber	82	III, IV	3 VAMP/3 COP	15, IF for CR; 25.5, IF for PR	68 (6)	93 (6)
Dörffel, 2003, 2013[56,57]	GPOH-HD 95	256	IAE, IBE, IIIAE, IIB, IIIA	2 OPPA or OEPA + 2 COPP	20–35, IF for PR, no RT for CR	PR 91/CR 69 (10)	PR 98/CR 98 (10)
		341	IIEB, IIIEA/B, IIIB, IVA/B	2 OPPA or OEPA + 4 COPP		PR 89/CR 83 (10)	PR 95/CR 100 (10)
Nachman, 2002; Wolden, 2012[36,90]	USA-CCG 5942	103	I/II w/adverse features, IIB, III	6 COPP/ABV and CR	21, IF	84 (10)	95 (3)
		36	IV	COPP/ABV + CHOP +Ara-C/VP-16 and CR		89 (10)	100 (3)
Kelly, 2002, 2011[85,141]	USA-CCG 59704	99	IIBX, IIIBX, IV	4 BEACOPP then if RRR: 4 COPP/ABV (girls) or 4 ABVD (boys); Rest: 4 BEACOPP	Female RER, no RT; male RER, 21–35, IF Rest: 21, EF + boost to residual to 35	94 (5)	97 (5)
Friedmann, 2002[142]	Stanford/St. Jude/Dana-Farber Consortium	56	I/IIX, III, IV	6 VEPA	15–25.5, IF	68 (5)	82 (5)
Schellong, 1999[88]	GPOH-HD 90	124	IIB-IIIA	2 OEPA or OPPA + 2 COPP	25, IF	90/96 (5)	97 (5)
		179	IIEB, IIIEA/B, IIIB, IVA/B	2 OEPA or OPPA + 4 COPP	20–35, IF	86 (5)	94 (5)
Weiner, 1997[8]	USA-POG 8725	80	IIB, IIIA2, IIIB, IV	4 MOPP/4 ABVD	21, EF	80 (5)	87 (5)
Shankar, 1997[27]	United Kingdom Children's Cancer Study Group	80	III	6–10 ChIVPP	35, IF	73 (10)	84 (10)
		27	IV			38 (10)	71 (10)
Hunger, 1997[17]	Stanford	13	III–IV	3 MOPP/3 ABVD	15–25.5, IF	69 (10)	85 (10)
Sackmann-Muriel, 1997[24]	GATLA	43	Intermediate risk[a]	6 CVPP	30–40, IF	87 (5)	
		21		6 AOPE		67 (5)	
		24	High risk[a]	CCOPP/CAPTe		83 (5)	
Schellong, 1992[139]	GPOH-HD 82	53	IIEA, IIB, IIIA	2 OPPA + 2 COPP	30, IF	94 (9)	–
		50	IIEB, IIIEA/B, IIIB, IIIVA/B	2 OPPA + 4 COPP	25, IF	86 (9)	–
	GPOH-HD 85	21	IIEA, IIB, IIIA	2 OPA + 2 COMP	30, IF	55 (6)	95 (6)
		24	IIEB, IIIEA/B, IIIB, IIIVA/B	2 OPA + 4 COMP	25, IF	49 (6)	100 (6)
	GPOH-HD 87	34	IIEA, IIB, IIIA	2 OPA + 2 COPP	25, IF	79 (5)	–
		58	IIEB, IIIEA/B, IIIB, IIIVA/B	2 OPA + 4 COPP	20, IF	91 (5)	–
Oberlin, 1992[143]	SFOP MDH-82	31	IB-IIB	3 MOPP/3 ABVD	20–40, EF	–	–
		40	III			82 (6)	–
		21	IV			62 (6)	–
Weiner, 1991[9]	USA-POG 8426	62	IIB, IIA2, IIIB, IV	4 MOPP/4 ABVD	21, TLI	77 (3)	91 (3)
Donaldson, 1987[4]	Stanford	28	III–IV	6 MOPP	15–25.5, IF	84 (7.5)	78 (7.5)

[a]Risk groups defined by Pavlovsky S, Santarelli MT, and Maschio M, for Grupo Argentino de Tratamiento de la Leucemia Aguda (GATLA). Definition of valuable prognostic index in Hodgkin disease based on a multivariate analysis in 945 patients. *Proc of ASCO* 7:240 (Abstract #928), 198.

ABV, doxorubicin, bleomycin, vinblastine; ABVD, doxorubicin, bleomycin, vinblastine, dacarbazine; ABVE, doxorubicin, bleomycin, vinblastine, etoposide; ABVE–PC, doxorubicin, bleomycin, vincristine, etoposide, cyclophosphamide, and prednisone; AOEP, doxorubicin, vincristine, prednisone, and etoposide; AV–PC, doxorubicin, vincristine, prednisone, and cyclophosphamide; BEACOPP, bleomycin, etoposide, doxorubicin, cyclophosphamide, vincristine, procarbazine, prednisone; CAPT3, cyclophosphamide, doxorubicin, prednisone, teniposide; ChIVPP, chlorambucil, vinblastine, procarbazine, and prednisolone; CHOP, cyclophosphamide, doxorubicin, vincristine, prednisone; COP, cyclophosphamide, vincristine, prednisone; COPP, cyclophosphamide, vincristine, procarbazine, prednisone; CVPP, lomustine, vinblastine, procarbazine, and prednisone; DECA, dexamethasone, etoposide, cisplatin, and cytarabine; DFS, disease-free survival; EFS, event-free survival; FFP, freedom from progression; MOPP, mechlorethamine, vincristine, procarbazine, prednisone; OEPA, vincristine, etoposide, prednisone, doxorubicin; OPPA, vincristine, prednisone, procarbazine, doxorubicin; RER, rapid early response (criteria dependent on trial); RFS, relapse-free survival; SER, slow early response (criteria dependent on trial); VAMP, vinblastine, doxorubicin, methotrexate, and prednisone; VBVP, etoposide, bleomycin, vinblastine, and prednisone; VEEP, vincristine, etoposide, epirubicin, prednisolone; VEPA, vinblastine, etoposide, prednisone, and doxorubicin.

Section III

restriction and diffusion defects, toxicity can be exacerbated by thoracic RT. Serial pulmonary function tests during therapy are recommended, and if a compromise in function of 20% or more from baseline is observed, bleomycin can be held.[155]

To reduce the treatment-related toxicities associated with six cycles of either MOPP or ABVD, strategies alternating the two regimens, and using fewer cycles of each, have been developed. The combined ABVD and MOPP regimens used for children have produced excellent disease control with apparent diminished toxicity.[26,68,156]

Etoposide, a topoisomerase II inhibitor, has been incorporated into the treatment regimens for advanced and unfavorable HL to intensify therapy and as an alternative to alkylating agents to reduce gonadal toxicity (e.g., ABVE–PC, doxorubicin, bleomycin, vinblastine, etoposide, prednisone, cyclophosphamide).[19,24,35,88,138,142] The secondary malignancy risk with topoisomerase II inhibitors is due to a unique pathogenesis from the alkylator-related s-AML described above,[157] and the risk is compounded with the use of multiple topoisomerase II inhibitors as seen in the POG trial of dexrazoxane (topoisomerase II inhibitor) as a cardiopulmonary protectant during treatment with ABVE or ABVE–PC with unacceptably high rates of s-AML attributed to the use of multiple topoisomerase II inhibitors.[158] Risk of s-AML is low when etoposide is limited to 5.0 g/m^2 or less. Although chemotherapy intensification may be justifiable in intermediate- and unfavorable-risk patients, the risk of secondary malignancies raises questions about its appropriateness for treatment of children with favorable-risk HL.

Not only is the patient's risk level an important consideration for the balance of toxicity for disease control in the selection of chemotherapy regimens, but gender-adapted therapy has been considered given the differing susceptibility to infertility caused by procarbazine in boys compared to girls. The German Society for Paediatric Oncology and Haematology (GPOH) evaluated a gender-adapted therapy approach using an OEPA (vincristine, etoposide, prednisone, doxorubicin) regimen for boys to limit alkylator exposure, whereas girls received OPPA (vincristine, procarbazine, prednisone, doxorubicin) substituting procarbazine for etoposide.[156,159] The gender-adapted regimen is more commonly utilized in Europe.

Contemporary therapy for pediatric HL using chemotherapy alone or combined modality therapy produces long-term DFS in 85% to 100% of patients with localized disease and 70% to 90% of patients with advanced disease.[5,8,9,11,14–17,19–24,26,28–31,86,87,90,108,117,143,160–162] Multiagent chemotherapy alone is an effective treatment approach for the treatment of pediatric HL.[8,9,11,14,20,24,29,132,163] A chemotherapy alone paradigm eliminates the risk of radiation-specific toxicities such as musculoskeletal complications, thyroid and cardiopulmonary dysfunction, and solid tumor carcinogenesis; however, regimens typically require more cycles and/or higher doses of chemotherapy, and thus, patients are at an increased risk of cardiopulmonary toxicity, infertility, and s-AML. Furthermore, chemotherapy alone may be less effective than combined modality therapy for treatment of bulky and intermediate- or unfavorable-risk disease.[9,87]

In total, three trials in North America have evaluated chemotherapy alone compared to combined modality therapy in pediatric HL patients.[6,7,84,90] Two studies, the first a Children's Cancer Study Group (CCG) study evaluating 12 cycles of alternating MOPP/ABVD versus 6 cycles of ABVD plus low dose (21 Gy) RT[7] and the second POG trial of four cycles alternating MOPP and ABVD with or without low dose RT,[8] failed to show a significant advantage in EFS and OS with the addition of RT. The third study was a CCG-randomized controlled trial comparing outcomes in patients treated with contemporary risk-adapted combined modality therapy with COPP/ABV (cyclophosphamide, vincristine, prednisone, procarbazine/doxorubicin, bleomycin, vinblastine) hybrid chemotherapy

and low dose, involved field RT to those treated with COPP/ABV chemotherapy alone. The study was closed early based on a significantly higher 3-year EFS in patients randomized to also receive RT.[90] However, longer follow-up did not demonstrate a significant difference in OS among the groups because of the successful treatment of relapsed patients following intense, salvage therapy.

In the European experience, the German HL-DAL-90 protocol treated intermediate- and high-risk patients with two cycles of OPPA or OEPA (girls or boys, respectively), followed by two to four cycles of COPP. All patients received 20- to 35-Gy involved field radiation therapy (IFRT). Five-year EFS in the intermediate- and high-risk groups was 93% and 86%, respectively, which was comparable to that seen in the low-risk group. Five-year OS for all three risk groups was ≥94%.[23,26,87,164] In the subsequent HL-95 trial, which employed the same chemotherapy but omitted IFRT in complete responders, the EFS for intermediate- and high-risk patients who did not receive radiotherapy dropped to 79% compared to 91% for those who did get radiotherapy.[87]

Newer agents are emerging and are under evaluation for use in patients with high-risk classic HL, relapsed HL, or NLPHL. Rituximab is an anti-CD20 monoclonal antibody that is being evaluated for its role in NLPHL[165] and NHL.[166,167] Brentuximab vedotin is a conjugate antibody that combines an anti-CD30 antibody with a synthetic tubulin disruptor, has been evaluated for salvage HL and certain NHLs, and is currently being evaluated for its role in the up-front setting in the treatment of high-risk HL in a current COG study.[168]

Thus, although the current consensus regarding the optimal therapy for children and adolescents with HL has not been firmly established, contemporary practice of low dose IFRT (and now involved-site or involved node RT) has substantially reduced the risks of many of the undesirable radiation-associated toxicities while limiting the cycles of chemotherapy through a combined modality treatment. Still, the field is gaining success in identifying select patients who may be treated with multiagent chemotherapy alone using modern refined regimens with reduced s-AML and infertility risks.[33] The current generation of COG studies in pediatric HL evaluates risk- and response-adapted approaches to intensify or deescalate based on risk factors at presentation and response to therapy.

Techniques of Radiation Therapy

Commensurate with the increasingly effective use of chemotherapy has been a more tailored approach to radiation utilizing significant reductions in prescription dose and irradiation volume, particularly over the recent years. Still, RT remains an important component of pediatric HL treatment to complement chemotherapy for slowly responding, residual, or bulky disease and to reduce chemotherapy intensity in selected patients where the predicted late toxicity risk for RT is small.

Unlike the treatment of most adults with HL, children are typically treated at academic or tertiary care centers, often as part of or per the protocol of a clinical trial. Studies have shown that outcomes of patients with HL treated with RT alone were superior at institutions with higher volumes[99] and when patients were treated in compliance with radiation protocols.[169,170] Thus, it is the responsibility of the treating radiation oncologist to confirm the workup, to review and comply with protocol requirements, and to seek experienced guidance when necessary to achieve the best outcomes for patients.

The technique of RT has long since progressed from extended fields, which included total lymphoid, mantle field, and pelvic radiation to IFRT volumes over the last few decades because of concerns of cardiac toxicity and secondary malignancies. Additionally, over the past few years, there has been an even more dramatic shift to involved-node (INRT) or involved-site radiation therapy (ISRT) as the new standard

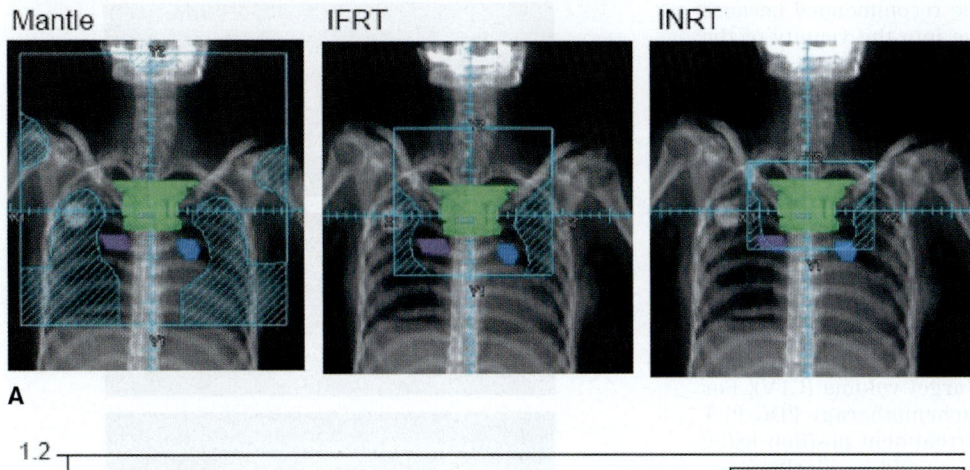

Mantle   IFRT   INRT

A

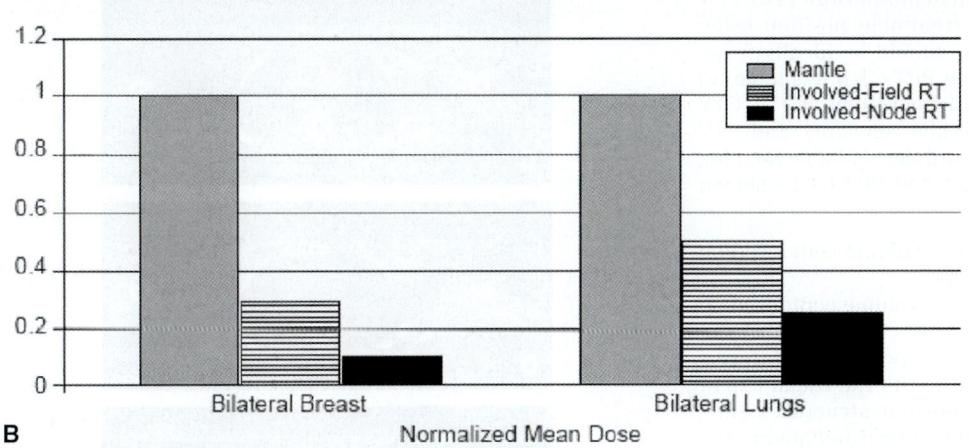

B   Normalized Mean Dose

FIGURE 93.1. **A:** Digitally reconstructed radiographs showing typical RT fields for historic mantle RT, contemporary involved field RT (IFRT), and involved-node RT (INRT) for a patient with stage I disease involving the upper mediastinum. The postchemotherapy volume of initially involved mediastinal nodes is shown in green. Hila are shown in *blue* and *violet*. **B:** Reduction in dose to breast and lung for the female patient shown in **A**. For each volume, the prescribed dose to the CTV is the same. The resulting mean dose to breast and lung tissue with mantle RT is a set value = 1. The proportional reduction in normal tissue dose occurs as a result of the reduction in treated volume with IFRT and INRT. (Reprinted with permission from Hodgson DC, Hudson MM, Constine LS. Pediatric Hodgkin lymphoma: maximizing efficacy and minimizing toxicity. *Semin Radiat Oncol* 2007;17[3]:230–242. Copyright © 2007 Elsevier. With permission.)

approach for defining the irradiation volume (Fig. 93.1). Instrumental in this progression toward smaller volumes is a balance of the increasing recognition of the late effects of early radiation fields and the high curability and salvage rates of pediatric HL.

The new field designs take into consideration modern technology, including the use of staging PET-CT scans, 3-D and 4-D treatment planning with CT scanning, conformal treatment techniques, and image guidance, replacing IFRT based on 2-D treatment planning and bony anatomy. Historically, IFRT included not just the involved lymph nodes but also the entire lymph node region containing the involved nodes and adjacent uninvolved lymph nodes.[171] These fields are no longer appropriate for modern, more focused RT aimed at reducing normal tissue exposure.

In an effort to rationally reduce the treatment fields of RT, a review of relapses in patients with HL has shown that recurrence occurs most often in initially involved nodes.[172–174] This suggests that chemotherapy is sufficient to treat microscopic disease in lymph nodes that do not appear abnormal on imaging, and RT is needed to treat sites of gross involvement. Thus, with sophisticated imaging techniques, a concerted effort to scan patients in the radiation treatment position, and more accurate RT delivery, the practice of INRT emerged as an effort by the European Organisation for Research and Treatment of Cancer and Group d'Etude des Lymphomes de l'Adulte (EORTC-GELA) investigators to customize delivery of RT to the radiographically involved regions.[175,176] Such reduction in treatment volumes is feasible largely because of FDG-PET scanning. FDG-PET has been shown to identify involved lymph nodes that were radiographically occult on CT scan in a study of patients with early-stage HL. As such, prechemotherapy FDG-PET can delineate the full extent of disease.[177] Although clinical outcomes with the use of INRT are only just emerging, a study of patients with limited-stage HL treated with INRT revealed no marginal or locoregional recurrences when margins of ≤5 cm were used.[178] Importantly, these margins are significantly larger than those prescribed in the present-day INRT practice. Currently, INRT is being practiced on both the standard and experimental arms of HL studies in Europe,[175] and INRT is being compared to IFRT in a randomized fashion in the German Hodgkin Study Group HD17 trial in unfavorable, early-stage disease in adults.

Paramount to successful INRT is the acquisition of prechemotherapy and postchemotherapy CT and FDG-PET scans with the patient in the treatment position for RT. In North America, ISRT, in contrast to INRT, has recently been introduced and readily accepted as the standard conformal therapy. Although ISRT has not been as formally evaluated as INRT, it is more conservative, designing fields and margins to account for suboptimal imaging information.

Radiation Simulation

When possible, CT simulation for the treatment of children with HL should be carried out with intravenous contrast to best delineate nodal stations and differentiate vessels. Oral contrast may be helpful for treatment of certain abdominal and pelvic tumors. Four-dimensional CT can help assess for target motion and aid in the selection of appropriate margins because of respiratory movement. If the patient is able to participate with breathhold techniques, deep inspiration breath hold at the time of simulation and treatment can allow for significant sparing of the heart and lung.[179]

Careful consideration of immobilization to be used at the time of simulation can offer significant advantages of increasing the set-up reproducibility, translating into smaller margins needed for set-up uncertainty with the planning target volume (PTV). Additionally, thoughtful patient positioning with the arms above the head to move the axillary lymph nodes away from the lungs, allowing greater lung shielding, may aid in reducing the dose to normal structures. When treating the axilla of patients who are still growing, positioning of the arms above the head may not be recommended because the axillary lymph nodes then move into the vicinity of the humeral heads, which should be blocked in growing children. Thus, the position chosen involves weighing concerns regarding tumor volume coverage and dose delivered to the lung and humeral heads.

Radiation Therapy Target Delineation

Guidelines for INRT and ISRT have been recently published to aid the radiation oncologist in defining treatment volumes.[175,180] The principles of target volume delineation for INRT and ISRT are largely the same, with differences in the quality and accuracy of prechemotherapy imaging suggesting that the margins for ISRT are larger to allow for uncertainties in contouring the clinical target volume (CTV). For both approaches, the pre- and postchemotherapy FDG-PET and CT, if possible obtained in the treatment position using the planned immobilization devices, should be ideally fused with the simulation CT (or simulation PET-CT if available) in the RT planning system. The gross tumor volume (GTV), CTV (and internal target volume [ITV] when relevant), and PTV should be delineated as follows using all the available imaging information on contrast-enhanced CT and PET-CT as shown in Figure 93.2 and described below:

- Prechemotherapy GTV: Gross tumor volume contoured on prechemotherapy CT and PET scans.
- Postchemotherapy GTV: Gross tumor volume contoured on postschemotherapy CT and PET scans.
- CTV: A volume encompassing the superior and inferior extent of the prechemotherapy GTV with the radial extent respecting overtly uninvolved, normal structures (i.e., lungs, kidneys, muscles) based on clinical judgment. The CTV should also take into account the quality and accuracy of imaging, pattern or spread of disease, changes in the volume of disease since imaging, risk of subclinical involvement, and nearby structures. Nodal volumes that are more than 5 cm apart can be treated as separate fields and do not need to be connected volumes. The CTV for ISRT will generally be larger than that for INRT because of the lack of optimal imaging information. Furthermore, if RT is being used as the sole treatment modality as in NLPHL, the CTV should be more generous as microscopic disease is likely more extensive in the absence of treatment with chemotherapy.
- ITV: Target motion should be accounted for using an ITV as defined in the ICRU Report 62 as the CTV with a margin to consider organ motion for an individual patient.[182] A 4-D CT simulation can be useful to obtain the ITV margins. If unavailable, 1.5- to 2-cm margins may be necessary in the chest or upper abdomen where respiratory movements are significant.
- PTV: This margin should account for uncertainty in setup based on patient factors or immobilization that varies across institutions.

Radiation Therapy Dose

The dose of RT prescribed is in part determined by the intensity and regimen of chemotherapy used in the combined modality approach. Typical doses in the current era of low dose RT are 15 to 25 Gy, with doses rarely exceeding 25 Gy in the pediatric setting.[17,19,31,36,90,115,136,143,155] In North America, the COG has set the standard dose as 21 Gy in 14 fractions.[33,107,183]

Radiation Therapy Planning

Although the anterior–posterior/posterior–anterior (AP/PA) beam arrangement is still commonly utilized in the delivery of RT for pediatric HL, 3-D conformal RT using nonopposed beams, intensity-modulated RT (IMRT), or proton therapy may be considered when the increase in conformality or the unique dose distribution may be favorable for the specific clinical

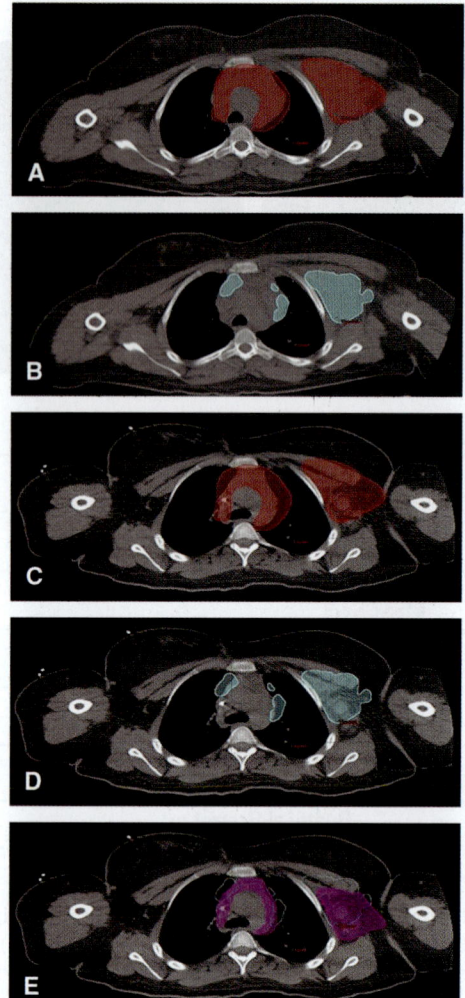

FIGURE 93.2. Illustration of the method of contouring the initially involved lymphoma gross tumor volume (GTV) on the postchemotherapy planning computed tomography (CT) scan, with information from fusion with the prechemotherapy positron emission tomography/CT scan. **A:** Prechemotherapy GTV$_{CT}$ on prechemotherapy CT scan. **B:** Prechemotherapy GTV$_{PET}$ on prechemotherapy CT scan. **C:** Prechemotherapy GTV$_{CT}$ on postchemotherapy CT scan. **D:** Prechemotherapy GTV$_{PET}$ on postchemotherapy CT scan. **E:** Clinical target volume, created by modifying GTV$_{CT}$ and GTV$_{PET}$, on the postchemotherapy CT scan. (Reprinted by permission from Springer: Hutchings M, Berthelsen AK, Barrington SF. The role of imaging in radiotherapy for Hodgkin lymphoma. In: Specht L, Yahalom J, eds. *Radiotherapy for Hodgkin lymphoma*. Heidelberg, Germany: Springer, 2011:81–89. Copyright © 2011 Springer Berlin Heidelberg.[181])

scenario. IMRT and proton therapy may be particularly useful in cases of prior RT or radiation to the thorax to spare dose to the heart, lungs, and developing breast tissue or the abdomen and pelvis to reduce dose to the reproductive organs. IMRT remains controversial in the treatment of children as a result of the concerns that increased integral dose and radiation scatter within the smaller body habitus of a child could lead to an increase in the development of secondary malignancies.[184,185] Proton therapy may offer the advantage of both reduced mean dose to normal surrounding tissue without the increase in volume of normal tissue receiving integral dose through IMRT.[186]

As always, we should strive to achieve dosimetric parameters that are as low as reasonably achievable. Data suggest that the volume getting 5 Gy or more (V5) to the breast and lung tissue may be important in the treatment of young patients with HL.[187] A mean lung dose < 15 Gy has also been shown to result in low rates of radiation pneumonitis.[188]

Gender-based use of RT has been considered, given the predisposition of females to secondary radiation-related cancers. The CCG 59704 high-risk study did include a gender-based consolidation phase with all patients receiving escalated BEACOPP up front. Slow responders received four additional cycles of BEACOPP and IFRT, but rapidly responding males were treated with ABVD with IFRT, whereas females received four cycles of COPP/ABV without radiotherapy to avoid the risks of breast cancer with mantle fields and infertility with pelvic radiation fields.[189-191]

Complications of Radiation Therapy

Acute Effects

The acute side effects of RT are related to the involved site treated. Because of the lower doses used in pediatrics, the most common toxicities include temporary loss or change in taste, xerostomia, esophagitis, low posterior scalp epilation, skin erythema, and occasionally dyspepsia, nausea, and vomiting, all depending on the location treated. Acute effects of para-aortic irradiation include early-onset nausea and vomiting, which usually abates after the second or third treatment without antiemetic therapy. Patients who receive larger fields may be subject to bone marrow suppression, the severity of which may be influenced by the systemic regimen preceding radiation.

Long-Term Effects

Musculoskeletal

Height reduction is a potential long-term consequence of irradiation, most frequently with doses > 20 Gy and most severe in prepubertal children. Growth arrest or delay is modest with the low doses currently used in modern pediatric HL treatment strategies.[192-194] Interclavicular shortening and hypoplasia of the neck muscles may occur in children irradiated before puberty, which is particularly dependent on dose delivered. Avascular necrosis of the femoral or humeral heads is rare if appropriate shielding is provided. Radiation doses of 20 to 40 Gy to the mandible may result in dental abnormalities, such as stunted tooth development, incomplete calcification, premature apical closure or eruption, and root tapering with apical constriction if in the irradiated field.[195]

Cardiovascular

Radiation-associated pericardial and myocardial diseases are related to dose (including fraction size) and volume and are complicated by the use of anthracyclines. Cardiac sequelae, including pericarditis and effusion, valvular thickening, biventricular dysfunction, and coronary artery disease, all are observed with irradiation to the heart.[26,116,119,135] Increase in mortality risk, because of premature coronary artery disease and acute myocardial infarction, has been demonstrated in patients who received mediastinal radiation in doses > 30 Gy before 20 years of age.[117]

Conversely, modern treatment approaches based on tailored low dose radiation and less cardiotoxic chemotherapy, sometimes including cardioprotectants, will optimistically reduce such effects. Radiation doses of <30 Gy and techniques that use adequate cardiac shielding and avoid anterior weighting of the treatment fields appear to reduce the risk of cardiac complications, particularly pericarditis and myocarditis.[116,119] The 45-fold excess mortality risk historically reported from acute myocardial infarction associated with higher radiation doses has diminished substantially with current approaches.[155] Also, dose to the heart can now be calculated using advanced radiation techniques, and dose can be constrained using conformal techniques in order to keep the risk of long-term development of cardiac injury to a minimum. Unfortunately, the impact of low dose RT to the heart may not become apparent until larger cohorts of survivors treated with modern combined modality regimens have longer follow-up.

Pulmonary

Use of bleomycin can increase the risk of acute pulmonary pneumonitis and late pulmonary fibrosis in patients receiving pulmonary RT. In a report from the CCG, 9% of children treated with ABVD and 21 Gy of mantle irradiation exhibited clinically significant pulmonary damage.[5] These results were confirmed recently in a study evaluating pediatric patients with any chest RT who developed radiation pneumonitis. The incidence was found to be low and most often related to therapies including bleomycin.[196]

Thyroid

Thyroid dysfunction may result from neck or upper mediastinal irradiation and most often is manifested by an elevated serum concentration of thyroid-stimulating hormone (TSH). The incidence of hypothyroidism varies, but it appears to be directly related to irradiation dose. Constine et al.[197] noted an increased serum TSH in 4 of 24 (17%) children who received mantle irradiation of ≤26 Gy and in 74 of 95 (78%) who received >26 Gy. Approximately one-fourth of these children had a concomitant low thyroxine level. In this series, 36% of children experienced spontaneous improvement in thyroid function.

In a Childhood Cancer Survivor Study, thyroid abnormalities were self-reported by 34% of patients surveyed. Hypothyroidism was the most common thyroid disturbance, with a relative risk of 17.1 (*P* < .0001) compared with sibling controls. Risk factors for hypothyroidism include increased dose of radiation, older age at diagnosis of HL, female sex, and Caucasian race.[198] The estimated actuarial risk of hypothyroidism for survivors treated with ≥45 Gy was 50% at 20 years from diagnosis. Other thyroid abnormalities identified in excess from sibling controls included hyperthyroidism (8-fold excess risk), thyroid nodules (27-fold excess risk), and thyroid cancer (18-fold excess risk).[199]

Pelvic Late Effects

Gonadal injuries, including infertility and impaired secretion of sex hormones, are potential complications of pelvic RT.[200] In women, irradiation of the pelvis can affect the ovaries, resulting in premature menopause or fertility impairment.[173] In a report of female HL survivors by the Late Effects Study Group, 42% of women treated with alkylating agent chemotherapy and subdiaphragmatic radiation had experienced menopause by age 31 years, compared with 5% of control subjects.[201] In childhood cancer survivors who continued to have spontaneous menses more than 5 years after their cancer diagnosis, the cumulative incidence of nonsurgical menopause was 8% by age 40 years, representing a 13-fold higher risk compared with a sibling control group. Risk factors for premature menopause include exposure to increasing doses of ovarian radiation, increasing exposure to alkylating agents (based on the number of agents and cumulative dose), and diagnosis of HL.[199] Normal pregnancies, without increased risk of fetal spontaneous abortion or birth defects, have been reported after pelvic irradiation.[200] In an effort to preserve ovarian function, the ovaries can be transposed via oophoropexy to a shielded area laterally or inferomedially near the uterine cervix prior to the initiation of radiation.

In boys irradiated to the pelvis, oligospermia is common, but it is reversible (usually by 18 to 24 months) in most cases if the radiation dose scattered to the shielded testes is small.[3,148,202] Permanent oligospermia may occur, however, after full-dose pelvic irradiation.[202] Several investigations have demonstrated that fertility is compromised in boys treated with gonadotoxic chemotherapy combinations like COPP, even when cycles of alkylating agent chemotherapy are limited.[156,203] Anthracycline-based regimens such as ABVD (or a similar hybrid) are associated with recovery of spermatogenesis after a temporary period of azoospermia.[204,205] In the modern treatment era, risk-adapted strategies seek to reduce or eliminate gonadotoxic treatments, resulting in excellent potential to preserve fertility in boys.[156]

Secondary Malignant Neoplasms

The 15-year actuarial risk of second malignant neoplasms ranges from 8% to 15%.[117,150,155,187,206–214] Patients are at risk for developing secondary malignancies including leukemias (e.g., acute myeloblastic leukemia) and solid tumors, most commonly breast, thyroid, bone, and soft tissues. The risk of leukemia, which exhibits a peak frequency in the first 5 to 10 years after treatment, is associated primarily with the use of alkylating agents.[206,207] In contrast to secondary hematopoietic malignancies, the risk of developing a second solid tumor increases with time after therapy, with a latency usually exceeding 10 years from diagnosis.

Several studies reveal an increased ratio of observed to expected risk of second tumors for girls compared with boys, with a median follow-up of 10 to 16 years.[189,215,216] A portion of this risk results from breast cancer, which is the most common solid second malignant neoplasm following the treatment of children. The increased risk of breast cancer is a significant concern for women treated for HL at a younger age. This increase in risk of breast cancer is related to the patient's age at the time of RT and has also been shown to decrease with a decrease in radiation dose.[217,218] In a large case-control study of 105 women who developed breast cancer from a cohort of more than 3,800 female survivors diagnosed with HL at age ≤ 30 years, the relative risk of breast cancer for a HL survivor treated at age 25 with chest radiation of at least 40 Gy without alkylating agents, the estimated cumulative risks of breast cancer by age 35, 45, and 55 years were 1.4%, 11.1%, and 29.0%.[217]

Multiple studies have now demonstrated that lower RT dose and smaller treatment fields should translate into a reduction in late effects when used judiciously.[123,125,219,220] Historical extended-field treatments included a substantial amount of breast tissue in the field design, which were then exposed to full-dose RT. Interestingly, breast tissue exposure was most significant when the axillae were irradiated in a typical mantle field as opposed to the mediastinal and hilar region. The practice of prophylactically irradiating the axillae is no longer performed, and, thus, the volume of breast tissue exposed to RT using involved-site or involved-node radiotherapy approaches is substantially less.[123] Using CT-based planning, the breast tissue can also be contoured as an avoidance structure and thereby shielded appropriately when designing RT fields in the region, a practice that was not used 30 years ago.

Current recommendations for the screening of late effects of therapy after childhood cancer can be found in the long-term follow-up guidelines developed by the COG, which are frequently updated (http://www.survivorshipguidelines.org).

Risk-Adapted Combined Modality Therapy for Classic Hodgkin Lymphoma

The sequence of therapy in the setting of combined chemotherapy and irradiation generally utilizes chemotherapy as the first modality. This allows assessment of drug response, maximization of the amount of drug treatment, and shrinkage of disease with more limited fields of irradiation. Rarely, focal irradiation prior to chemotherapy is necessary because of significant symptomatic compromise such as airway obstruction.

Current recommendations for therapy follow a risk-adapted approach based on features at presentation including B symptoms, mediastinal and peripheral lymph node bulk, extranodal extension of disease, number of involved nodal regions, Ann Arbor stage, and gender.[27,50,70,82,91–98,100,106,107] The

most recent COG risk stratification defines patients into risk groups as follows:

- Favorable risk: stages IA and IIA without bulk
- Intermediate risk: stages I to IIA with bulk, I to IIAE, I to IIB, IIIA, and IVA
- High risk: stages IIIB and IVB

In Europe, an integrated EuroNet cooperative group most recently has categorized patients into treatment groups (TGs) based on risk as follows[105]:

- TG-1: stages IA/B and IIA, without bulk ≥200 mL, and ESR < 30 mm/h
- TG-2: stages IEA/B, IIEA, IIB, or IIIA and stages IA/B and IIA with bulk ≥200 mL or ESR ≥ 30 mm/h
- TG-3: stages IIEB, IIIEA/B, IIIB, or IVA/B

The response to chemotherapy as assessed on CT and FDG-PET has been found to be a significant prognostic factor.[8,108] As a result, it has prompted the most recent series of trials to determine if response, either early during chemotherapy or after its completion, can be used to guide a reduction or intensification of therapy.[9,33,35,84,108–111,140,221,222] Although final reports for low- and high-risk groups have not yet been published, response-based therapy is now the standard approach for treatment of children with intermediate-risk HL as discussed below.[33]

Favorable Risk

Favorable-risk disease is defined differently by various clinical trial groups, but for the most part, favorable-risk disease encompasses patients with localized stage I and II disease without adverse prognostic features. Treatment typically involves two to four cycles of chemotherapy and low dose ISRT. In some regimens, the RT dose has been reduced or eliminated based on a favorable response to chemotherapy.

Response-based therapy involves either intensification of RT, chemotherapy, or both for patients with slow early response (SER) or poor response to chemotherapy while omitting RT for patients with rapid early response (RER) or good response to chemotherapy. Low-risk patients are the natural group in which to consider de-escalation of therapy because of their excellent outcomes. Early investigations of response-based therapy in the French Society of Pediatric Oncology MDH90 trial included 202 children with stage I/II HL.[19] Patients were treated with four cycles of vinblastine, bleomycin, etoposide, and prednisone (VBEP), and CT was obtained to assess response to therapy. A good response was defined as either complete remission or more than a 70% reduction in tumor size. Good responders received 20 Gy of RT to initially involved fields. The remaining patients (poor responders) were given one or two cycles of OPPA and were evaluated after each cycle. If no response was obtained after one cycle of OPPA, RT was administered to 40 Gy. If the response after the first or the second cycle exceeded 70%, the patient received 20 Gy to involved fields. Eighty-five percent of patients were good responders, and the overall 5-year OS and EFS of the entire cohort were 97.5% and 91.1%, respectively. These results were comparable to the prior French Society of Pediatric Oncology (MDH82) in which all patients received chemotherapy consisting of alkylating agents and anthracycline followed by low dose RT.[143]

The GPOH pioneered the use of risk- and gender-adapted therapy featuring the OEPA regimen for males in order to limit the amount of alkylators, whereas females received OPPA. In the GPOH-HD 95 trial, RT was successfully omitted in patients achieving complete response to chemotherapy with early-stage disease.[87] Complete response was defined as a volume reduction of ≥95% and ≤2 mL of the initial volume or unconfirmed complete response if volume reduction was

≥75% or <2 mL; fewer than 30% of patients fell into this category of good responders. There was no difference in outcome between favorable-risk patients treated with chemotherapy alone and those treated with combined modality therapy. Notably, the cohort consisted of classic HL and NLPHL. These outcomes were confirmed in the GPOH-HD 2002 study that excluded NLPHL patients in which all patients were treated with IFRT to 19.8 Gy except early-stage (IA/B and IIA without extranodal involvement) patients with complete response as defined in the prior GPOH-HD 95 study.[32] If <75% response was noted, a boost to 30 Gy was delivered, and residual disease >100 mL was boosted to 35 Gy.

Several North American investigators have demonstrated excellent treatment results using combined modality therapy for favorable-risk HL. Investigators from Stanford University Medical Center, St. Jude Children's Research Hospital, and Dana-Farber Cancer Institute reported results using a nonalkylator regimen, VAMP (vinblastine, doxorubicin, methotrexate, and prednisone), for children with clinical I/II, nonbulky HL.[137] Following four cycles of VAMP, patients were treated with 15-Gy IFRT if they achieved a complete response or 25.5 Gy for those with a partial response after two cycles of VAMP. At a median follow-up of 9.6 years, 5- and 10-year EFS rates were 92.7% and 89.4%, respectively. The POG evaluated the feasibility of combined modality therapy using four courses of DBVE (doxorubicin, bleomycin, vincristine, and etoposide) followed by IFRT to 25.5 Gy to treat stage IA, IIA, and IIIA HL.[135] At a median follow-up of 8.4 years, nearly all patients (98%) achieved complete remission after completion of therapy, and 6-year OS and EFS rates were 98% and 91%, respectively. This DBVE regimen was used by the POG and the COG to support reduction of chemotherapy via an early-response–based treatment algorithm evaluated on P9426.[133] Patients received only two courses of DBVE if they achieved an early complete response (45% of all patients) versus four courses of DBVE if they were slower responders. All patients were treated with IFRT to 25.5 Gy. Five-year OS and EFS were 98% and 88%, respectively.

To compare a chemotherapy-alone regimen to a risk-adapted combined modality treatment approach with low dose IFRT in low-risk patients achieving a complete response, the CCG trial 5942 treated patients with COPP/ABV. Those achieving a complete response to chemotherapy were randomized to receive low dose IFRT or no further therapy. Given a significantly higher number of relapses in patients who were treated with chemotherapy alone, the trial was terminated early. Although 3-year OS estimates were no different between groups, salvage therapy is a known risk for neoplastic complications and early mortality.[16] This trial was compromised by the use of less intensive chemotherapy than is used in most contemporary trials.

To better select low-risk patients who may benefit from the omission of RT, the COG AHOD0431 single-arm study incorporated interim PET-CT when possible to assess disease response and identified a group of very early responders (negative PET scan after one cycle) who may have favorable outcomes even without adjuvant RT. Two hundred and eighty-seven stage IA/IIA patients were treated with three cycles of AV–PC (doxorubicin, vincristine, prednisone, and cyclophosphamide). Those who achieved a complete response after three cycles received no further therapy, whereas partial responders received 21-Gy IFRT. Two-year OS was 100%; however, 2-year EFS for those with complete response to chemotherapy and no RT was 80% compared to 88% of those with partial response who received IFRT ($P = .11$). A subset analysis suggested the utility of interim PET-CT after one cycle (PET1) of chemotherapy in identifying patients who may be treated without RT after three cycles of AV–PC. Of the patients with complete response who did not receive RT, the 2-year EFS rate for those with a positive/equivocal PET1 versus those who had a negative PET1 was 65%

compared to 87%, respectively ($P = .005$). Similarly, 2-year EFS in partially responding patients with a positive/equivocal PET1 versus a negative PET1 was 82% versus 96%, respectively ($P = .047$).[84] These data highlight the importance of the added information gained by the interim FDG-PET scan when evaluating low-risk patients for response-adapted therapy. We await final publication of this study with long-term results.

Intermediate Risk

Patients with localized stage IA and IIA disease with unfavorable features including bulk and extranodal extension are grouped into an intermediate-risk category that also includes patients with stage IIIA disease. Treatment typically involves four cycles of chemotherapy and low dose ISRT. As in low-risk disease, RT dose generally has been reduced or eliminated based on a favorable response to chemotherapy.

In the GPOH-HD 2002 study, all patients were treated with two cycles of chemotherapy (OEPA for males and OPPA for females) with intermediate- and high-risk treatment group patients (TG-2 and TG-3) receiving two cycles of COPP for females and COPDAC for males in order to spare fertility by reducing alkylator exposure.[134] All patients were treated with IFRT to 19.8 Gy except early-stage (IA/B and IIA without extranodal involvement) patients with complete response as discussed above. If <75% CT response was noted, a boost to 30 Gy was delivered, and residual disease >100 mL was boosted to 35 Gy. The two regimens, procarbazine-free OEPA–COPDAC in boys and the standard OPPA–COPP in girls, had comparative effectiveness supporting the use of a reduced gonadotoxic regimen for boys.

The COG has completed two trials to evaluate a response-based approach. The first, POG9425, evaluated the prospect of reducing the number of chemotherapy cycles based on response to therapy.[35] The second trial, AHOD0031, evaluated a regimen to omit RT in patients with a rapid early response and complete response to chemotherapy and to intensify therapy for those with a slow response.[33]

In POG9425, intermediate- and high-risk patients received three and five cycles of ABVE–PC followed by 21-Gy regional (mantle, para-aortic, or pelvic) RT for RER and SER, respectively. There was no difference in EFS between the two groups.[35] This study provided encouraging clinical outcomes using response-based therapy.

The recently published COG AHOD0031 study[33] was the first randomized trial to compare standard and response-based treatment arms in order to risk stratify selected groups of patients for omission of RT or augmentation of systemic therapy (Fig. 93.3). Early response to therapy was determined by CT scan, and complete response status was determined by CT and gallium or FDG-PET scanning. Functional imaging was obtained after two cycles (at the time of early-response assessment), and as the availability of PET scanning increased, more patients were able to obtain interim PET-CT scans as well. All 1,712 patients received two cycles of ABVE–PC followed by response assessment. Patients with RER received two additional cycles of ABVE–PC followed by a second response assessment. Those with a CR were randomized to receive 21-Gy IFRT or no further therapy. Patients with a RER who did not have a CR were all assigned to receive IFRT. SER patients were all randomized to either two additional cycles of ABVE–PC or dexamethasone, etoposide, cisplatin, and cytarabine (DECA) followed by an additional two cycles of ABVE–PC. All SER patients received 21-Gy IFRT after chemotherapy. Four-year EFS rates were 85% overall and 86.9% for RER patients versus 77.4% for SER patients ($P < .001$). The 4-year OS for the entire cohort was 97.8% and 98.5% for RER patients versus 95.3% for the SER patients ($P < .001$). The 4-year EFS rate was 87.9% for RER/CR patients randomized to receive IFRT versus 84.3% for those randomized to no IFRT ($P = .11$).[33]

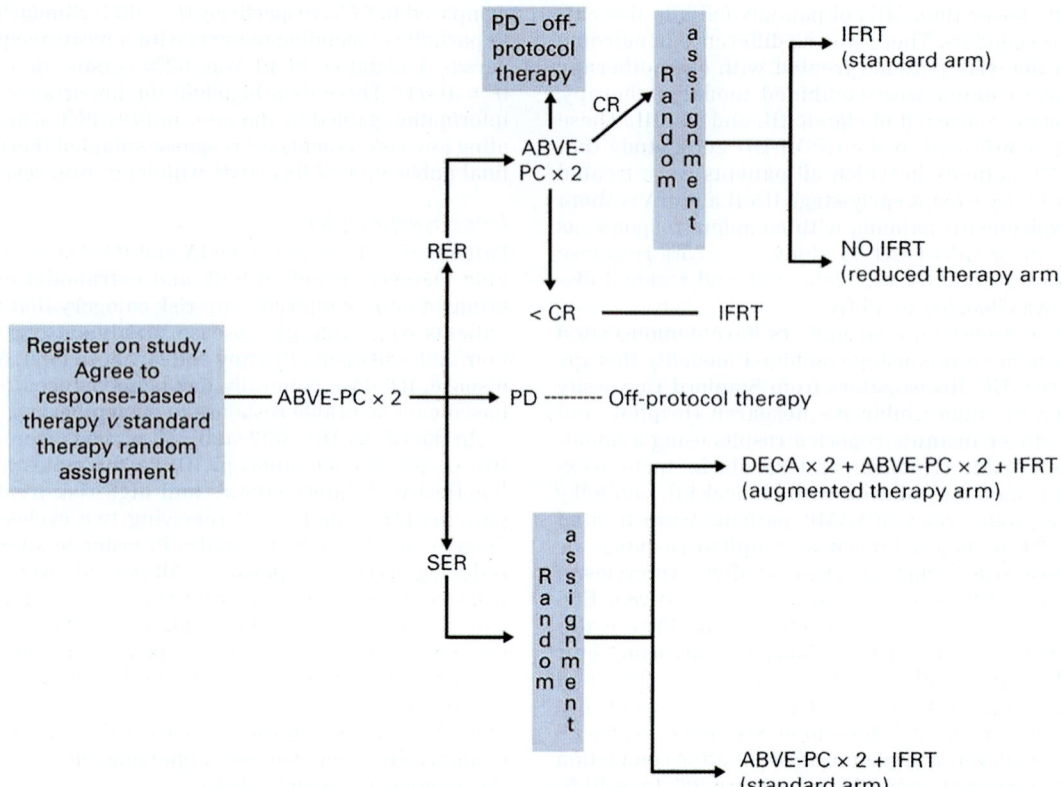

FIGURE 93.3. Study schema of COG AHOD0031, a phase III study of dose-intensive response-based chemotherapy and radiation therapy for children and adolescents with newly diagnosed intermediate-risk Hodgkin disease. RER was defined as a 60% or greater reduction in the product of perpendicular diameters (PPD) for all target lesions, or there was a return to normal size after two ABVE–PC cycles on CT scan. CR was defined as an 80% or greater reduction in the PPD or a return to normal size for all target lesions and a negative gallium or FDG-PET scan. A 50% or greater increase in the PPD of any nodal mass or organ lesions or a new lesion(s) was considered progressive disease. ABVE–PC, doxorubicin, bleomycin, vincristine, etoposide, cyclophosphamide, and prednisone; CR, complete response; DECA, dexamethasone, etoposide, cisplatin, and cytarabine; IFRT, involved field radiation therapy; PD, progressive disease; RER, rapid early responder; SER, slow early responder. (From Friedman DL, Chen L, Wolden S, et al. Dose-intensive response-based chemotherapy and radiation therapy for children and adolescents with newly diagnosed intermediate risk Hodgkin lymphoma: a report from the Children's Oncology Group Study AHOD0031. *J Clin Oncol* 2014;32[32]:3651–3658. Reprinted with permission. Copyright © 2014 American Society of Clinical Oncology. All rights reserved.)

Because of the study era, FDG-PET was not required for early-response determination, but interim PET after two cycles of ABVE–PC (PET-2) was obtained in 1,135 (66%) patients of whom 746 were eligible for the two random assignments in the study. Of the 550 patients with available PET-2 imaging that had a RER/CR, there was no difference in EFS with and without IFRT to those with a negative PET-2 (86.7% vs. 87.3%, respectively; $P = .87$). Among patients with PET-2–positive results, there was also no difference in EFS with and without IFRT (83.1% vs. 78.1%, respectively; $P = .80$). Of the 196 patients with SER with available PET-2 results, there was no difference in EFS in patients treated with or without DECA when PET-2 was negative (90.1% vs. 85.6%, respectively; $P = .54$). However, among patients with SER with PET-2–positive results, EFS with DECA was marginally superior to those treated without DECA (70.7% vs. 54.6%, respectively, $P = .05$).[33]

In a secondary analysis of the patterns of failure of AHOD0031, first relapses rarely occurred outside of the irradiated field only, and relapses commonly occurred in previously involved disease sites (94% of relapses), suggesting that INRT or ISRT may be sufficient to determine irradiation volumes without compromising local control.[221] Additionally, recurrences occurred both in bulky and nonbulky initial sites of disease, suggesting that in intermediate-risk HL, irradiation of bulky sites alone may not be a recommended treatment strategy.[221]

The results of AHOD0031 suggest that early response to chemotherapy defined by early reduction (60%) in tumor size based on CT after two cycles can be a powerful predictor of outcome and help optimize subsequent treatment. A secondary analysis of PET response after two cycles of ABVE–PC demonstrated that PET may further assist with treatment optimization. If validated, a pediatric-specific prognostic score, CHIPS, proposed using the data from AHOD0031 discussed in the "Prognostic Factors" section may also guide early therapy reduction or augmentation as the components of this score are known at diagnosis.[223] As a result of the primary outcomes of AHOD0031, response-adapted treatment is the current standard of care of patients with intermediate-risk HL.

High Risk

The criteria for high-risk clinical presentation are typically restricted to stage III or IV disease with "B" symptoms and may also include extranodal extension to contiguous structures. Combined modality therapy is the standard approach to treatment. Historically, chemotherapy was administered over the course of 6 to 8 months on a twice-monthly schedule.[7,8,35,85,90,224] An alternative strategy condenses the chemotherapy component of treatment into 3 to 5 months to enhance dose intensity and reduce the risk of developing resistant disease. RT for high-risk HL is variable and protocol dependent.

Dose-intensified treatment regimens may increase the risk of acute and late side effects. The GOPH-HD 2002 study discussed above included patients with high-risk disease and demonstrated that a procarbazine-free regimen of OEPA–COPDAC administered to boys yielded comparable outcomes as those observed in girls receiving the standard OPPA–COPP regimen.[134] The European Network for Pediatric Hodgkin Lymphoma (EuroNet-PHL)-C1 trial is testing whether equivalent results can be achieved with the procarbazine-free regimen in a non–gender-stratified approach. All patients on the trial received OEPA, and intermediate- and high-risk groups (TG-2 and TG-3) were randomly assigned to receive COPP or COPDAC. Interim results of the TG-2 and TG-3 patients randomized between the COPP and COPDAC regimen showed no difference in 4-year EFS rates between the two groups.[225] Final results will definitively inform if the less gonadotoxic regimen results in equivalent results.[105]

As in the cases of other risk groups, there is increasing interest in developing a response-adapted treatment approach for children with high-risk HL. In the GPOH-HD 95 trial outlined previously, RT was omitted in patients achieving complete response after OEPA–COPP chemotherapy.[86] Progression-free survival (PFS) for intermediate- and high-risk patients who experienced a complete response and did not receive RT was significantly lower than observed in patients without a complete response who received RT (69% and 83%, respectively, $P = .01$). This study highlighted the need for more refined criteria and modalities for response assessment than those used on GPOH-HD 95 to successfully identify intermediate- and high-risk patients for whom treatment without RT may suffice.[86]

A recent assessment of a dose-intense, response-based regimen using BEACOPP (bleomycin, etoposide, doxorubicin, cyclophosphamide, vincristine, procarbazine, and prednisone) in children with high-risk disease was reported by the COG 59704 trial. Females with a rapid response received four cycles of COPP/ABV following BEACOPP without IFRT, and males received two cycles of ABVD and IFRT. All patients with a slow response received four additional cycles of BEACOPP and IFRT. A high 5-year EFS rate of 94% was achieved, and the 5-year OS rate was 97% with significant acute hematologic toxicity and two patients developing secondary leukemia.[85]

AHOD0831 was the first COG trial for high-risk patients evaluating a risk-adapted approach to chemotherapy intensification and RT volumes based on early response to chemotherapy.[226] Patients were treated with two cycles of ABVE–PC and then assigned to one of two consolidation therapy regimens based on response to induction therapy. Patients with rapid early response received two more courses of ABVE–PC. Those with slow early response received intensification of therapy with the addition of two cycles of ifosfamide/vinorelbine followed by two courses of ABVE–PC. Patients with a continued response after completion of chemotherapy proceeded to risk-adapted RT (21 Gy in 14 fractions of IFRT) delivered only to initial sites of bulky disease in rapid responders and to PET-avid sites and sites with >2.5 cm of residual disease in slow responders. Although the study has closed, final results have not yet been reported. Preliminary analysis revealed that the approach did not meet the predefined high goal of 95% EFS.[227]

The current ongoing high-risk HL study with the COG is AHOD1331 that is evaluating the role of brentuximab in the up-front setting based on its effectiveness in the salvage setting. The trial also incorporates a response-adapted approach to RT.[226] Patients are treated with five cycles of AVE–PC with or without brentuximab with interim PET-CT after two cycles. RT of 21 Gy in 14 fractions will be given to patients with sites of disease that do not show a rapid response after two cycles of chemotherapy and to all patients with bulky mediastinal disease. The RT being administrated on this trial incorporates ISRT and allows for protons and IMRT. Although not a study question, the approach to radiation therapy varies from the established standard for pediatric RT including dose escalation from 21 to 30 Gy for patients with residual FDG-avid disease at the end of chemotherapy and delivery of RT to large

mediastinal adenopathy regardless of response to chemotherapy. The results of this trial will be enlightening not only with regard to its primary study question on the role of brentuximab in the up-front setting but also in the outcomes using a refined approach to RT for children with high-risk HL.

The ongoing EuroNet-PHL-C2 trial is also evaluating a risk-stratified and response-adapted approach in children with high-risk HL.[228] Using the Deauville score (DV) for PET response assessment,[112] patients with adequate response after two cycles of initial OEPA chemotherapy (i.e., PET-negative DV 1 to 3) will not receive RT, and those with inadequate response to chemotherapy (i.e., DV ≥ 4 or <50% volume reduction in bulky site) will receive a modified IFRT to 19.8 Gy with 10-Gy boost to sites with DV3 or higher PET avidity at the end of all chemotherapy. All intermediate- and high-risk patients will receive consolidation chemotherapy based on randomization between two and four cycles of standard COPDAC-28 (cyclophosphamide, vincristine, prednisone, dacarbazine) or intensified DECOPDAC-21 (doxorubicin, etoposide, cyclophosphamide, vincristine, prednisone, dacarbazine). This study will evaluate (a) whether intensified DECOPDAC-21 consolidation chemotherapy improves EFS as compared to standard COPDAC-28 in early responders and (b) if DECOPDAC-21 combined with radiotherapy restricted to sites that remain FDG-PET positive at the end of all chemotherapy has comparable EFS compared to COPDAC-28 plus RT as in the C1 trial.

Therapy for Lymphocyte-Predominant Hodgkin Lymphoma

NLPHL is considered indolent with a favorable prognosis with OS rates of close to 100%, typically presenting as a localized, early-stage disease. Relapses are typically late and curable with 10- and 15-year cumulative relapse rates of 4.8% and 8.3%, respectively, with similar OS rates in patients with relapsing and nonrelapsing patients.[229] Historically, patients with NLPHL have been treated on protocols for patients with classic HL; however, there are several reports in the adult and pediatric literature suggesting that they can be cured with less aggressive therapies. Adult patients are typically treated with RT alone to 30 to 40 Gy.[230,231]

Given the concern for late toxicity of RT to curative doses in children, resection has been considered as a treatment approach for localized pediatric NLPHL. A meta-analysis of French, United Kingdom, and German trial series showed that surgery alone was a feasible option for localized disease and yielded a long-term relapse-free survival of 67%.[232] The COG AHOD03P1 study prospectively evaluated 52 stage IA patients who were observed after surgery only.[222] Five-year EFS was 77% with 13 patients experiencing relapse. Twelve of the relapses were stage IA, occurring at the site or in adjacent nodes or nodal regions; one relapse was stage IIA. Nine of these patients received salvage chemotherapy with AV–PC, all achieving a complete response. Four patients relapsed after the salvage chemotherapy arm was closed and received chemotherapy per institutional choice.

The EuroNet is conducting a clinical trial to prospectively validate this "watch-and-wait" approach for children with completely resected disease and low dose chemotherapy for patients with residual disease after resection (EuroNet-PHL-LP1).[233,234]

Therapy for Refractory or Relapsed Hodgkin Lymphoma

Treatment failures in pediatric HL patients typically develop within the first 3 years, although late relapses have been reported, particularly in patients with NLPHL. The most common site of relapse following risk-adapted therapies remains the primary site of disease.[216] Generally, favorable prognostic factors include the site of relapse (nodal better than extranodal), stage at relapse (early better than advanced), histology, and response to first-line salvage chemotherapy.

Treatment options include standard-dose chemotherapy (with or without RT), RT alone, or high dose chemotherapy (with or without RT), followed by stem cell transplant, clinical trials, or palliative therapy. When pursuing transplant, RT may also be used pre- or posttransplant depending on the clinical scenario. The selection of the most appropriate salvage regimen is based on whether a complete remission was achieved, the durability of the remission, the extent of disease at relapse, and the intensity of the frontline therapy given.

Because of the excellent outcome for the majority of children and adolescents with HL, investigations regarding salvage strategy have been limited. For higher-risk relapses, a combination of ifosfamide and vinorelbine for pediatric patients in first relapse was studied by the COG (AHOD00P1). This regimen showed a very good overall response rate (CR/PR) of 78% and achieved good stem cell mobilization for future autologous stem cell transplant once remission is achieved, because studies have shown that patients undergoing autologous stem cell transplant with active disease have a worse outcome.[235] Claviez et al.[236] reported observations of 91 pediatric patients with relapsed or refractor HL treated with allogeneic hematopoietic stem cell transplantation. Relapse at 2 and 5 years is 36% and 44%, respectively. PFS rates were 40% and 30% and OS rates were 54% and 45% at 2 and 5 years, respectively.

Patients with primary refractory disease (i.e., those unresponsive to initial therapy or who relapse within 1 year of primary therapy) have a very poor prognosis. Intensive cytoreductive chemotherapy followed by myeloablation and autologous hematopoietic stem cell transplantation is reported to salvage 30% to 60% of these patients, but relapses after 5 years have been observed, and long-term treatment complications may predispose to early mortality.[237–239]

Newer targeted agents promise great efficacy with less toxicity. Brentuximab vedotin, an antibody drug conjugate that targets CD30 and is bound to an antitubulin agent monomethyl auristatin E, has shown excellent results in early clinical trial in relapsed and refractory Hodgkin lymphoma.[240,241] Given promising results, brentuximab vedotin is being incorporated in larger studies and in the up-front setting in combination with multiagent chemotherapy.[168] mTOR inhibitors, histone deacetylase inhibitors like panobinostat,[242] and nivolumab (programmed death-1 pathway inhibition)[242] are currently under investigation and may prove to be active alone or when used in combination with other agents.

Future Investigations

To build on the current era of risk- and response-adapted trials in pediatric HL, future studies should focus on refining our ability to better stratify therapies at diagnosis by validating pediatric-specific prognostic factors and identifying patients at high risk of serious toxicity from treatment.[35] Preliminary data suggest a genetic risk factor for the development of radiation-associated breast cancer in patients treated with thoracic RT for HL,[243] whereas other investigators have identified genetic variants associated with anthracycline-induced cardiotoxicity in children.[244] Such exemplary research will enable future clinicians to develop personalized treatments for patients based on risk profiles informed by both stage of disease and individual genetic presentations.

Newer drugs also promise great efficacy with less toxicity. Future studies are likely to move targeted agents, such as brentuximab vedotin, histone deacetylase inhibitors, and immunotherapy agents such as PDL-1 inhibitors into the up-front treatment of patients, starting with patients with high-risk disease. These evaluations of new agents and the applications of genetic information in future studies are

novel approaches to achieve the same decade-old goal of balancing the toxicity and efficacy of treatments for children with HL.

NON-HODGKIN LYMPHOMA

Childhood NHLs are a heterogeneous group of malignancies with variable histopathology, site of origin, and clinical manifestations. Childhood NHLs are diffuse, high grade, and poorly differentiated; extranodal involvement is common, and dissemination occurs early and often.[245] This is in striking contrast to adult NHL, in which low- and intermediate-grade nodal disease predominates.[245,246] The common low-grade lymphomas seen in adults, such as follicular and marginal zone lymphomas, are rare in children. These differences in pathology and clinical behavior observed between children and adults explain the markedly different presentations, staging practices, and treatment strategies for these age groups.

Epidemiology

In the United States, NHL is diagnosed in approximately 800 children and adolescents younger than 20 years of age, each year. According to the Surveillance, Epidemiology, and End Results Program of the National Cancer Institute, NHL accounts for about 8% of all cases of childhood cancer.[247] The incidence increases with age, being rare in the child <3 years old; incidence is higher in males than in females (ratio of 3 to 1) and higher in Caucasians than in African Americans (ratio of 1.5 to 1). In younger children, NHL is more frequent than HL, whereas the reverse is true for adolescents.

Although NHL is related to several genetic and environmental factors, its cause and pathogenesis remain unclear.[245,248] A small proportion of cases are seen in association with inherited immunodeficiencies (e.g., Wiskott-Aldrich syndrome, X-linked lymphoproliferative disease, ataxia-telangiectasia, and common variable immunodeficiency)[249,250] or acquired immunodeficiencies (e.g., HIV infection or immunosuppressive therapy in patients receiving solid organ or bone marrow transplants).[251,252]

There is geographic variation in the incidence and pathogenesis of NHL. In equatorial Africa, evidence of EBV infection has been demonstrated in the majority of endemic Burkitt tumors, but in only 10% to 15% of sporadic cases (outside of Africa). This suggests a significant role for the EBV virus in lymphomagenesis through unknown mechanisms that leads to the same oncogenic chromosomal translocations as those seen in non–EBV-associated sporadic cases of Burkitt lymphomas.[253–255] EBV infection has also been associated with the development of posttransplant lymphoproliferative disease (PTLD), a B-cell lymphoproliferative disorder seen in patients after solid organ or hematopoietic stem cell transplantation.[256,257]

Pathologic Classification

Pediatric NHL cases are divided into four major histopathologic subtypes based on morphology and immunophenotype in the order of frequency: (a) Burkitt lymphoma (BL); (b) lymphoblastic lymphoma (LL), including B-cell LL and T-cell LL; (c) large B-cell lymphoma including the subtypes diffuse large B-cell lymphoma (DLBCL) and primary mediastinal (thymic) large B-cell lymphoma (PMBL); and (d) anaplastic large-cell lymphoma (ALCL).[49,247,248,258] The distribution of histologies is shown in Table 93.5.

The classification of NHL by the WHO was updated in 2016.[48,49] It increasingly incorporates immunophenotyping and cytogenetics in important diagnostic, prognostic, and therapeutic distinctions. A few notable changes with respect to pediatric NHL exist in the updated WHO classification. Pediatric follicular lymphoma (FL) became a distinct

TABLE 93.5 CLINICAL CHARACTERISTICS OF CHILDHOOD NON-HODGKIN LYMPHOMA

Histologic Subtype	Proportion of Cases (%)	Most Common Sites of Presentation
Burkitt lymphoma	35–40	Abdomen or head and neck
T-lymphoblastic lymphoma	15–20	Mediastinum
B-lymphoblastic lymphoma	3	Cutaneous masses, isolated nodes, and bone
Diffuse large B-cell lymphoma	15–20	Nodes, abdomen, and bone
Mediastinal large B-cell lymphoma	1–2	Mediastinum
Anaplastic large-cell lymphoma	15–20	Skin, nodes, and bone

Adapted from Sandlund JT. Childhood lymphoma. In: Abeloff MD, Armitage JO, Lichter AS, et al., eds. *Clinical oncology*. 2nd ed. New York: Churchill Livingstone, 2000:2438. Copyright © 2000 Elsevier. With permission.

subtype, now known as pediatric-type FL.[48,258,260] It is characterized by large expansile highly proliferative follicles that often have prominent blastoid follicular center cells rather than classic centroblasts and a lack of MYC, BCL6, and BCL2 rearrangements; however, BCL2 protein may be expressed. Large B-cell lymphoma with IRF4 rearrangement, which commonly occurs in children and young adults, was added as a new provisional entity. Most have IG/IRF4 rearrangements, some with BCL6 rearrangements, but uniformly lack BCL2 rearrangements. These lymphomas typically occur in Waldeyer ring and/or cervical lymph nodes and are more aggressive than other pediatric-type FL. Burkitt-like lymphoma with 11q aberration was added as a provisional entity to distinguish a subset of lymphomas that have more complex karyotypes and lack MYC rearrangements with lower levels of MYC expression than Burkitt lymphomas. Instead, this subtype is notable for chromosome 11q changes with proximal gains and telomeric losses.[261,262] The clinical course seems similar to that of BL.

Overall, identification of large numbers of monoclonal antibodies directed against surface antigens has allowed subclassification of the NHLs according to immunophenotype (Table 93.6).[263] Thorough and efficient evaluation of histology and immunophenotype is key to the determination of diagnosis, prognosis, and appropriate course of treatment because pediatric NHLs are usually aggressive. Cytogenetic analysis and identification of molecular markers provide a more precise means of characterization of these tumors and will likely contribute to the understanding of pathogenesis as well as the development of novel therapeutic approaches.[264–266]

Clinical Presentation

In many cases, clinical manifestations and sites of disease correlate with NHL subtype. A mediastinal mass, which can cause wheezing, stridor, cough, or dyspnea, is present in 25% of children with NHL, commonly associated with DLBCL or T-lymphoblastic lymphoma.[267] Clinical presentation is different between endemic and sporadic BL. The abdomen is the most common site of disease in sporadic BL, which presents with abdominal pain, distension, palpable mass, nausea, vomiting, and gastrointestinal bleeding, followed by head-and-neck region involvement. Bone marrow involvement is seen in about 20% of patients with sporadic BL and LL sporadic disease.[268] However, in endemic BL, jaw involvement is the most common, and bone marrow involvement is rare.[269]

The majority (50% to 70%) of children with precursor T-cell LL present with rapidly enlarging neck and mediastinal lymphadenopathy.[248,264] Mediastinal masses can cause respiratory symptoms (e.g., cough, wheezing, shortness of breath, and orthopnea) by compressing airways or cause neck, face, and upper extremity swelling because of obstruction of the superior vena cava (SVC). Hemodynamic compromise because of pericardial effusions may also occur. However, children and

TABLE 93.6 IMMUNOPHENOTYPIC, CYTOGENIC, AND MOLECULAR MARKERS OF PEDIATRIC NHL

Marker	BL (50%–60%)	LBCL (10%–15%)		LL (20%–25%)		ALCL (10%–12%)
		DLBCL	**PMBL**	**B-LL**	**T-LL**	
Immunohistochemistry[a]						
MIB1	~100%	40%–90%	30%–90%	Not informative	Not informative	Not informative
CD10	+	+/–	–/+	+/–	+/–	–
CD19	+	+	+	+	–	–
CD20	+	+	+	+/–	–	–
CD79a	+	+	+	+	–	–
sig	+	+/–	–	–	–	–
Bcl-6	+	+/–	+/–	–	–	+/–
MUM1	–	–/+	+	–	–	–
MAL	–	–/+	+	–	–	–
TdT	–	–	–	+	+	–
cCD3	–	–	–	–	+	–/+
CD4	–	–	–	–	+/–	–/+
CD8	–	–	–	–	+/–	–/+
CD7	–	–	–	–	+	–/+
CD5	–	–/+	–	–	+/–	+/–
CD30	–	[b]	+/–	–	–	+
ALK	–	[c]	–	–	–	+
Cytogenetic	t(8;14)(q24;q32)t(2;8)(p12;q24)t(8;22)(q24;q11)	R8q24 (~30%)	Few data	Few data	Translocations involving 14q11-13; few other data	t(2;5)(p23;q35) > 90% or variants involving 2p23
Molecular biology	MYC/IGH IGK/MYC MYC/IGL		Nuclear factor-κB pathway dysregulation	IGH/TCR rearrangements	NOTCH/FBXW7, PTEN IGH/TCR rearrangements	NPM/ALK > 90% or variants

[a]+, >90% of patients; +/–, >50% of patients; –/+, <50% of patients; –, <10% of patients.
[b]Positive especially in the rare anaplastic variant.
[c]Positive in the ALK-positive LBCL.
Note: Other NHLs, such as peripheral T-cell lymphoma, extranodal natural killer/T-cell lymphoma, nasal type, and pediatric follicular lymphoma, represent <5% of pediatric NHLs and are not indicated in the table.
ALCL, anaplastic large-cell lymphoma, ALK positive; BL, Burkitt lymphoma; B-LL, B-cell lymphoblastic lymphoma; DLBCL, diffuse large B-cell lymphoma; LBCL, large B-cell lymphoma; NHL, non-Hodgkin lymphoma; PMBL, primary mediastinal (thymic) large B-cell lymphoma; T-LL, T-cell lymphoblastic lymphoma.
From Minard-Colin V, Brugières L, Reiter A. Non-Hodgkin lymphoma in children and adolescents: progress through effective collaboration, current knowledge, and challenges ahead. *J Clin Oncol* 2015;33(27):2963–2974. Reprinted with permission. Copyright © 2015 American Society of Clinical Oncology. All rights reserved.

adolescents with precursor B-cell LL tend to have limited disease in sites including the skin, bone, and peripheral lymph nodes.[270,271]

DLBCL usually presents with nodal disease, especially in the abdomen, although the bone (single or multiple sites) is also a relatively common site.[272,273] Primary mediastinal large B-cell lymphoma can be locally invasive and may present with SVC syndrome.[31]

The most frequent sites of involvement in systemic ALCL are peripheral nodes, mediastinal lymph nodes, and extranodal sites such as the skin, soft tissue, and bone.[274,275] Spontaneous regression or waxing and waning of disease has been observed.

Diagnostic Evaluation

Tissue diagnosis and investigation to determine the clinical extent of disease should be completed expeditiously. It is important that appropriate therapy be initiated promptly because of the extremely rapid growth rate of pediatric NHL.[245] Histology, immunophenotype, karyotype, and molecular studies are vital for implementation of an optimal treatment plan.[258,276] Thus, it is critical that an adequate amount of tissue be obtained at biopsy by performing either open biopsy or core needle biopsy. The use of irradiation or steroids before biopsy in the case of a symptomatic mass may result in rapid shrinkage and subsequent improvement in symptoms, but may jeopardize the ability to establish a tissue diagnosis.[277,278]

Bone marrow biopsy (BMB) has been a standard in lymphoma staging (Table 93.7).[81] Bone marrow biopsies are superior to a single aspirate or biopsy for identifying bone marrow involvement, which is often patchy in distribution in NHL.[248] In DLBCL, FDG-PET-CT has been shown to be more sensitive than BMB, but does miss low-volume diffuse involvement of 10% to 20% of the marrow.[279–281] Thus, in pediatric patients with DLBCL, FDG-PET-CT indicating bone marrow involvement is typically sufficient, and BMB is not required. If FDG-PET-CT is negative in patients with DLBCL, BMB is indicated if relevant for a clinical trial or in cases where identifying a discordant histology is important for patient management. For all other NHL histologies, a 2.5-cm unilateral BMB, along with immunohistochemistry and flow cytometry, is still standard practice because of lack of conclusive data guiding the utility of FDG-PET-CT.[77]

TABLE 93.7 INVESTIGATIONS REQUIRED FOR ACCURATE STAGING AND DIAGNOSIS OF CHILDHOOD LYMPHOMAS

History and physical examination
Complete blood count
Chemistry panel
Serum electrolytes with calcium, phosphorus, and magnesium
Liver enzymes with bilirubin
BUN, serum creatinine, LDH, and uric acid
Imaging studies
Chest radiograph
Neck, chest, abdominal, and pelvis CT scan
Fluorine-18 FDG-PET imaging
Core biopsy
Morphology (fixed)
Immunophenotypic analysis (fresh or fixed)
Cytogenetics (fresh)
Molecular analysis (fresh or fixed)
FISH for specific translocation (fresh or fixed)
Immunoglobulin gene rearrangements (fresh or fixed)
Bone marrow examination (bilateral aspirates and biopsies)
Cerebrospinal fluid examination (cell counts and cytology)

BUN, blood urea nitrogen; CT, computed tomography; FDG-PET, fluorodeoxyglucose positron emission tomography; FISH, fluorescence *in situ* hybridization; LDH, lactate dehydrogenase.
Adapted from Shad A, Magrath I. Non-Hodgkin's lymphoma. *Pediatr Clin North Am* 1997;44(4):863–890, and Gross TG, Perkins SL. Malignant non-Hodgkin lymphomas in children. In: Pizzo PA, Poplack DG, eds. *Principles and practice of pediatric oncology*. 6th ed. Philadelphia: Lippincott Williams & Wilkins, 2011:663–682. With permission.

TABLE 93.8 FDG AVIDITY ACCORDING TO WHO CLASSIFICATION

Histology	No. of Patients	FDG Avid (%)
HL	489	97–100
DLBCL	446	97–100
FL	622	91–100
Mantle cell lymphoma	83	100
Burkitt lymphoma	24	100
Marginal zone lymphoma, nodal	14	100
Lymphoblastic lymphoma	6	100
Anaplastic large T-cell lymphoma	37	94–100[a]
NK/T-cell lymphoma	80	83–100
Angioimmunoblastic T-cell lymphoma	31	78–100
Peripheral T-cell lymphoma	93	86–98
MALT marginal zone lymphoma	227	54–81
Small lymphocytic lymphoma	49	47–83
Enteropathy-type T-cell lymphoma	20	67–100
Marginal zone lymphoma, splenic	13	53–67
Marginal zone lymphoma, unspecified	12	67
Mycosis fungoides	24	83–100
Sézary syndrome	8	100[b]
Primary cutaneous anaplastic large T-cell lymphoma	14	40–60
Lymphomatoid papulosis	2	50
Subcutaneous panniculitis-like T-cell lymphoma	7	71
Cutaneous B-cell lymphoma	2	0

[a]Only 27% of cutaneous sites.
[b]Only 62% of cutaneous sites.
Note: Data adapted from Uccini S, Monardo F, Stoppacciaro A, et al. High frequency of Epstein-Barr virus genome detection in Hodgkin's disease of HIV-positive patients. *Int J Cancer* 1990;46(4):581–585, with additional updates.[18,33,34,49,67,68]
DLBCL, diffuse large B-cell lymphoma; FDG, [18F]fluorodeoxyglucose; FL, follicular lymphoma; HL, Hodgkin lymphoma; MALT, mucosa-associated lymphoid tissue; NK, natural killer.
From Barrington SF, Mikhaeel NG, Kostakoglu L. Role of imaging in the staging and response assessment of lymphoma: consensus of the International Conference on Malignant Lymphomas Imaging Working Group. *J Clin Oncol* 2014;32(27):3048–3058. Reprinted with permission. Copyright © 2014 American Society of Clinical Oncology. All rights reserved.

FDG-PET-CT should be used for staging FDG-avid NHLs.[282] Contrast-enhanced CT is indicated for all nonavid histologies. The avidity of the different NHL subtypes is reported in Table 93.8. Data in adults with HL and NHL and children with HL suggest that PET scanning to assess the rapidity of response may be prognostic.[195,283] However, further confirmation is needed to determine whether FDG-PET response has predictive value for detecting recurrence of pediatric NHL.

Laparotomy is generally no longer performed for staging as combination chemotherapy is part of the primary treatment. MRI may be helpful in detecting disease at specific sites, particularly the nervous system, but it is not routinely used.

Staging Systems

Pediatric NHL is currently staged using the Murphy/St. Jude's Children's Research Hospital system from 1980, which incorporates extent of disease and clinical patterns.[246] Since the introduction of the St. Jude staging system, the pathologic classification of NHL has changed significantly. New subtypes of pediatric NHL, some of which display unique patterns of organ involvement, including mucosal sites, skin, bone, ovary, and kidney, have been identified. The Ann Arbor staging system[81] (commonly used in adult NHL) has proved to be of limited use in pediatric NHL because of the unique clinical presentation and course of the disease in children with predominant involvement in the extranodal primary sites and a tendency to evolve into leukemia and to involve the central nervous system (CNS).

The Lugano lymphoma staging classification similarly focuses on adult lymphomas.[77] As a result, a Revised International Pediatric NHL Staging System Classification was recently developed by a multidisciplinary multinational consortium, incorporating new histologic entities, extranodal dissemination, improved diagnostic methods, and advanced imaging techniques (Table 93.9). The revised staging will enable more precise, reproducible comparisons of efficacy of treatment strategies across cooperative groups.[284]

TABLE 93.9 STAGING AND GROUPING SYSTEM FOR CHILDHOOD NON-HODGKIN LYMPHOMA

Stage/Group	Description	
	Murphy Staging System	**International Pediatric Non-Hodgkin Lymphoma Staging System**
I	Single EN tumor or single anatomic N area, excluding the mediastinum or abdomen	Single tumor excluding the mediastinum or abdomen (N; EN; B or S: EN-B, EN-S)
II	Single EN tumor with regional lymph node involvement Two or more N areas on the same side of the diaphragm Two single EN tumors + regional node involvement on the same side of the diaphragm Primary GI tract tumor (usually in ileocecal area), + involvement of associated mesenteric nodes only	Single EN tumor with regional node involvement Two or more N areas on the same side of the diaphragm Primary GI tract tumor (usually in ileocecal area), + involvement of associated mesenteric nodes, that is completely resectable (if malignant ascites or extension of tumor to adjacent organs, it should be regarded as stage III)
III	Two single EN tumors on opposite sides of the diaphragm Two or more N areas above and below the diaphragm All primary intrathoracic tumor (mediastinal, pleural, thymic) All extensive primary intra-abdominal disease including disease with spread via lymphatics to para-aortic and retroperitoneal nodes via intraperitoneal dissemination to form implants and plaques along the mesentery or peritoneum or by direct infiltration of structures adjacent to primary tumor. Ascites may be present, and complete resection of all gross tumor is not possible All paraspinal or epidural tumors, regardless of other tumor sites	Two or more EN tumors (including EN-B or EN-S) above and/or below the diaphragm Two or more N areas above and below the diaphragm Any intrathoracic tumor (mediastinal, hilar, pulmonary, pleural, or thymic) Intra-abdominal and retroperitoneal disease, including liver, spleen, kidney, and/or ovary localizations, regardless of degree of resection (except primary GI tract tumor [usually in ileocecal region] involvement of associated mesenteric nodes that is completely resectable) Any paraspinal or epidural tumor, regardless of whether other sites are involved Single B lesion with concomitant involvement of EN and/or nonregional N sites
IV	Any of the above with initial CNS or BM involvement (<25% blasts)	Any of the above findings with initial CNS involvement (stage IV CNS), BM (stage IV BM), or both (stage IV combined) based on conventional methods

Group Classification in the B-Cell Lymphomas

A	Completely resected stage I or completely resected abdominal stage II lesions
B	All cases not eligible for group A or group C (Murphy stage III and non-CNS stage IV)
C	Any CNS involvement and/or bone marrow involvement ≥25% blasts. For CNS involvement, one or more of the following applies: (1) Any L3 blasts in CSF (2) Cranial nerve palsy (if not explained by extracranial tumor) (3) Clinical spinal cord compression (4) Isolated intracerebral mass (5) Parameningeal extension: cranial and/or spinal

B, bone; BM, bone marrow; CNS, central nervous system; CSF, cerebrospinal fluid; EN, extranodal; N, nodal; S, skin.
Data from Murphy SB. Classification, staging and end results of treatment of childhood non-Hodgkin's lymphomas: dissimilarities from lymphomas in adults. *Semin Oncol* 1980;7:332–339; Patte C, et al. The Societe Francaise d'Oncologie Pediatrique LMB89 protocol: highly effective multiagent chemotherapy tailored to the tumor burden and initial response in 561 unselected children with B-cell lymphomas and L3 leukemia. *Blood* 2001;97:3370–3379; Rosolen A, Perkins SL, Pinkerton CR, et al. Revised International Pediatric Non-Hodgkin Lymphoma Staging System. *J Clin Oncol* 2015;33(18):2112–2118.

Prognostic Factors

The most important factor in determining prognosis in childhood NHL is stage, which takes into account other known prognostic variables such as tumor burden, site, and extent of involvement.[285–287]

Other clinical prognostic factors in NHL include LDH level and CNS involvement. Biologic characteristics including the presence of 13q abnormalities, MYC/8q24 rearrangement in DLBCL, and minimal disseminated disease (MDD) and minimal residual disease (MRD) in BL seem to be of prognostic relevance.[286–288] Prospective validation of these prognostic factors in patients with B-cell NHLs is planned in the ongoing Inter-B-NHL Ritux 2010 study.[166,167]

As most cases of pediatric NHL are of the diffuse, high-grade, and aggressive subtypes, only few reports support the role of histologic subtype as a prognostic factor. Response to therapy is also being investigated as a prognostic factor,[289] and attempts are being made to incorporate a standardized international pediatric NHL response criteria to facilitate communication and future investigations.[290]

Treatment of Non-Hodgkin Lymphoma

The OS of children with NHL was poor before the advent of multiagent chemotherapy in the mid-1970s.[285] Even in cases in which the disease apparently was localized, cure rates as low as 20% were reported. Failure, in most cases, was caused by early systemic dissemination of disease. In modern regimens, chemotherapy is the primary therapeutic modality for all histologies and stages of childhood NHL. The dramatic improvement in the overall rate of survival of those with childhood NHL can be attributed not only to the development of highly effective, multiagent chemotherapy regimens but also to the systematic evaluation of these diseases and their treatment by pediatric cooperative group clinical trials. Cure rates of 85% to 95% in patients with limited disease (Table 93.10) and 70% to 90% in those with extensive involvement (Table 93.11) have been reported.[291,292,295,298–321]

Burkitt Lymphoma

As a result of several consecutive prospective trials, outcomes for BL have dramatically improved.[289,291,292,295,298,309,312,322,323] Treatment consists of 2 to 6 months of multiagent, cyclophosphamide-based

TABLE 93.10 MODERN TREATMENT OUTCOMES FOR LIMITED-STAGE NON-HODGKIN LYMPHOMA BASED ON RECENT TRIALS

Histology (# Patients)	Protocol	Stage/Group	Event-Free Survival
BL (40) B-like L (15) DLBCL (43) Total = 132	FAB/LMB96[291]	A	4 yr = 98%
BL (148) DLBCL (60) NOS (21) Total = 229	NHL-BFM 95[292]	I/II, III (LDH < 500)	3 yr = 94%
ALCL (82)	HM 89 and HM 91[293]	I–IV (I/II, n = 23)	3 yr = 94% (stage I/II)
T-cell and B-cell LL (55)	AIEOP LNH 92[294]	I–IV (I/II, n = 5)	3 yr = 100% (stage I/II)
B-NHL (119, subtypes unspecified)	SFOP LMB 89[295]	I II	5 yr = 93% 5 yr = 99%

AIEOP, Italian Association of Pediatric Hematology and Oncology; ALCL, anaplastic large-cell lymphoma; BFM, Berlin-Frankfurt-Muenster Study Group; BL, Burkitt lymphoma; B-like L, Burkitt-like lymphoma; DLBCL, diffuse large B-cell lymphoma; FAB, French-American-British Study Group; HM, French protocols for pediatric ALCL; LL, lymphoblastic lymphoma; LMB, protocol for mature B-cell lymphomas; LNH, protocol for childhood lymphoblastic lymphomas; NHL, non-Hodgkin lymphomas; NOS, not otherwise specified; SFOP, Societe Francaise d'oncologie Pediatrique.

TABLE 93.11 MODERN TREATMENT OUTCOMES FOR ADVANCED-STAGE NON-HODGKIN LYMPHOMA BASED ON RECENT TRIALS

Histology (N)	Protocol	Stage/Group	Event-Free Survival
BL (25) DLBL (10) PMBCL (4) Other B-NHL (6) Total = 45	ANHL01P1 pilot[296]	III/IV	3 yr = 95%
BL (67) DLBL (15) Other B-NHL (5) Total = 87	R + B-NHL BFM 04[297]	I/II/IV/IV	3 yr =94%
BL (450) DLBL (151) PMLBL (32) Other B-NHL (4) Total = 637	FAB/LMB 96[289,291,298]	Intermediate risk (nonresected stage II/I and CNS-negative advanced stage III/IV)	4 yr = 92%
BL/BLL/B-ALL (168) DLBL/TCRLCL (13) Other B-NHL (9) Total = 190		High risk (CNS or BM positive)	Full intensity arm: 4 yr = 90% Reduced intensity arm: 4 yr = 80%
BL (108) DLBL (11) B-cell ALL (80) Other B-NHL (16) Total = 215	NHL-BFM 95[292,299]	III (LDH 500–1,000) IV (CNS−) III (LDH > 1,000) IV (CNS+)	3 yr = 85% 3 yr = 81%
LL Total = 156		III/IV[a]	5 yr = 82%
B-NHL (340, subtypes unspecified)	SFOP LMB 89 [295]	III IV	5 yr = 91% 5 yr = 87%
T-cell and B-cell LL (55)	AIEOP LNH 92[294]	III–IV (I/II, n = 50)	3 yr = 62% (stage III) 3 yr =75% (stage IV)
T-cell LL Total = 137	POG 9404[300] With HD-MTX Without HD-MTX	III/IV	5 yr with HD-MTX = 82% 5 yr without HD-MTX = 88%
ALCL Total = 217	ALCL99[301]	High risk (mediastinal, lung, liver, or spleen involvement or biopsy-proven skin lesion)	2 yr = 71%
ALCL Total = 352	EICNHL[302]	All	2 yr = 74%
ALCL (144) PTCL (28) LCL[b] (75) LCL NOS (9) Total = 175	POG 9315–APO vs. IDM/HiDAC[303]	III/IV	4 yr = 67%
ALCL (82)	HM89 and HM91[293]	I–IV (III/IV=59)	3 yr = 55% (stage III/IV)
DLBL Total = 120	POG 8615–APO vs. ACOP+[304]	III/IV	8 yr (III) = 68% 8 yr (IV) = 59%

[a]Excludes patients with central nervous system–positive disease and those who had insufficient response on day 33.
[b]Includes DLBL, follicular lymphoma and mucosal associated lymphoid tissue lymphoma.
ALCL, anaplastic large-cell lymphoma; ALL, acute lymphoblastic leukemia; BFM, Berlin-Frankfurt-Muenster Study Group; BL, Burkitt lymphoma; BM, bone marrow; B-NHL, B-cell non-Hodgkin lymphoma; CNS, central nervous system; DLBL, diffuse large B-cell lymphoma; EICNHL, European Inter-group cooperation on childhood and adolescent non-Hodgkin lymphoma; FAB, French-American-British Study Group; HM, French protocols for pediatric ALCL; HD-MTX, high-dose methotrexate; LL, lymphoblastic lymphoma; LCL, large-cell lymphoma; LDH, lactate dehydrogenase; LMB, protocol for mature B-cell lymphomas; NOS, not otherwise specified; PMBCL, primary mediastinal B-cell lymphoma; POG, Pediatric Oncology Group; PTCL, primary T-cell lymphoma; SFOP, Societe Francaise d'oncologie Pediatrique; TCRLCL, T-cell–rich large-cell lymphoma; yr, years.

chemotherapy. Relapses tend to occur within the first year. The current paradigm has been established through collaborative efforts across consortiums such as the French Society of Pediatric Oncology and French-American-British (FAB), Lymphomes Malins B (LMB), and the oligonational Berlin-Frankfurt-Munster (BFM) studies.[289,291,292,295,298,309,312,322,323] As BL frequently occurs in resource-deprived countries, treatments have been adapted in some regions to balance toxicity, efficacy, and cost. Still, over half of patients are cured with suboptimal, resource-adapted protocols.[324,325]

In health systems with available resources, the current standard frontline therapy for advanced BL is based on the FAB/LMB96 regimen.[289] Patients received cyclophosphamide, vincristine, prednisone, high dose methotrexate, doxorubicin, and cytarabine. Although 20% to 25% of patients present with advanced-stage disease involving the bone marrow and/or CNS, the current treatment approach results in EFS of approximately 90%. Of note, involvement of >25% of the marrow by Burkitt is classified as Burkitt leukemia, but

should still be treated using a high-risk lymphoma treatment paradigm, and not therapy for acute lymphoblastic leukemia. High dose methotrexate with or without high-dose cytarabine and intrathecal methotrexate with or without cytarabine can effectively serve as CNS prophylaxis or treatment of CNS-positive disease, eliminating the need for CNS irradiation.[289,291,292,295,298,309,312,322,323] Testicular involvement at diagnosis is uncommon but does occur in about 5% of children with disseminated BL and Burkitt-like NHL.[326] Testicular disease does not seem to confer a poor prognosis, and it is curable with intensive combination chemotherapy alone. Local treatment (i.e., surgery or radiation) is avoidable; therefore, gonadal function can be preserved.

Both DLBCL and BL express CD20. As such, the most recent era of studies involves incorporating the anti-CD20 monoclonal antibody (rituximab) into a conventional multiagent chemotherapy regimen. In 2004, the COG implemented ANHL01P1, a pilot study evaluating the toxicity of adding rituximab to standard therapy for patients with newly diagnosed, pediatric BL and DLBCL.[327] Survival rates were similar to the 4-year reported EFS in patients treated on FAB/LMB96, the current standard therapy.[289] In a multicenter European phase II study, 136 pediatric patients with newly diagnosed B-cell NHL received 1 dose of rituximab in an up-front window prior to starting standard chemotherapy to assess the possibility of a future phase II trial to test if rituximab could substitute for chemotherapy. An ambitious response rate of higher than 65% was set for classification of favorable activity of rituximab; however, only 41% of patients experienced disease improvement after a single dose of rituximab.[297] The current phase II/III intergroup trial, ANHL1131, will test the efficacy of frontline rituximab therapy in pediatric patients with B-cell NHL.[328] The phase II component of the study has closed and the target accrual of the phase III component is 600 patients. No data are available to date.

Large B-Cell Lymphoma

Diffuse Large B-Cell Lymphoma

The treatment of DLBCL follows the same protocols as that for BL. Follow-up for patients with DLBCL, however, should be focused on the possibility of comparatively later relapses, occurring up to 3 years following treatment.[295,309,323] The role of frontline rituximab therapy in DLBCL, as well as BL, is being investigated in the studies outlined above.

Primary Mediastinal B-Cell Lymphoma

Primary mediastinal B-cell lymphoma (PMBL) has a significantly inferior EFS approaching 70% using standard FAB/LMB96 chemotherapy.[329] It typically presents in adolescents and young adults, and therefore, pediatric-specific protocols have not been established. As the biology of disease appears similar across age groups, a reasonable alternative regimen to rituximab, cyclophosphamide, doxorubicin, and prednisone (R–CHOP) with good outcomes in adults is dose-adjusted etoposide, doxorubicin, and cyclophosphamide with vincristine, prednisone, and rituximab (DA–EPOCH–R) and may obviate the need for RT therapy in patients with PMBL.[330] This DA–EPOCH–R regimen is currently being investigated in children with PMBL.[331]

Lymphoblastic Lymphoma

Lymphoblastic lymphoma consists of both precursor T-cell (T-LL) and B-cell (B-LL) NHLs, with the majority (80% to 90%) being T-LL. T-LL typically presents at an advanced stage with a mediastinal mass and occasionally bone marrow involvement. B-LL is typically localized and presents in various locations including the bone, skin, soft tissue, and peripheral nodes.[332] Treatment approach follows an ALL-based paradigm with the addition of high-dose methotrexate and/or intrathecal injections for CNS prophylaxis,[300,333,334] rather than CNS RT.[299,335] Overall, regimens include early intensified multiagent chemotherapy consisting of vincristine, prednisone, L-asparaginase, doxorubicin, cytarabine, cyclophosphamide, and high dose methotrexate, followed by maintenance chemotherapy for 2 years.[294,299,300,315,316,333,334,336–339] Long-term EFS with current treatment protocols approaches 85%. The prognostic value of extent of disease dissemination at diagnosis and MRD identified using advanced PCR and flow cytometry technologies is being evaluated as a basis of treatment stratification in the ongoing COG study ALL0932.[340,341]

Anaplastic Large-Cell Lymphoma

Anaplastic large-cell lymphoma presents in either a systemic or primary cutaneous form. Systemic ALCL is frequently associated with "B" symptoms and extranodal disease. Advanced systemic ALCL has been treated with short-pulse chemotherapy, proven effective in B-cell lymphomas, or with modifications of high-risk ALL protocols.[302,303,321] Long-term EFS ranges from 65% to 75%[301–303,319,342,343]; however, recurrences are comparatively more responsive to salvage therapies than relapsed disease in other NHL subtypes.[258] Treatment of recurrent ALCL involves chemotherapy followed by hematopoietic stem cell transplant or weekly vincristine and yields survival rates of >90%.[301,302,344–347]

Role of Radiation Therapy

With the development of effective multiagent chemotherapy regimens, RT for local control of primary disease[305,348] (exclusive of primary bone lesions) or for CNS prophylaxis has been virtually eliminated.[298,299,349] Indications for cranial irradiation are currently limited to patients with overt symptomatic CNS lymphoma at diagnosis, particularly when unresponsive to initiation of chemotherapy or dexamethasone or when there is CNS relapse.[350]

Historically, radiation was incorporated as standard in the treatment of primary lymphomas of the bone. Localized RT to the involved bone was included as part of standard management in early chemotherapy trials.[305] In a prospective randomized trial evaluating the need for local RT in early-stage NHL, all patients with primary lymphoma of the bone received 37.5 Gy and were not included in the randomization to "no radiation."[305] Given the rarity of these entities, the patterns of failure of all early-stage primary lymphomas of the bone treated on three consecutive POG studies were examined to determine the impact on outcome of radiotherapy as an adjuvant treatment in children receiving chemotherapy. Across the three studies, a total of 31 patients with primary lymphoma were analyzed. Seven patients had both chemotherapy and radiation, whereas the remaining 24 were treated with chemotherapy only. There were no local relapses identified in this subset analysis.[348] With these data, it is reasonable to treat patients with primary lymphoma of the bone with chemotherapy alone without adjuvant RT.

Radiation is used for some cases of relapsed or refractory disease, either as palliation or consolidation, for emergency treatment of mediastinal disease or symptomatic neurologic compromise such as spinal cord compression, palliation of pain, and treatment of overt symptomatic CNS lymphoma at diagnosis or relapse.

For persistent disease after chemotherapy or relapse disease, children are often treated with high dose chemotherapy with stem cell rescue.[351] RT to the site of residual or relapsed disease can be considered pre- or posttransplant, typically to at least 20 to 30 Gy. One must take into account potential preparatory regimens for transplant particularly if total-body irradiation (TBI) will be incorporated. Persistent disease after chemotherapy is overall rare in NHL; however, it is more common in PMBL. Consolidative ISRT in the case of residual disease following induction chemotherapy for PMBL is debated, but should be strongly considered.[330,352,353]

Emergent palliative radiation for superior vena cava syndrome, airway compromise, or spinal cord compression can produce dramatic and rapid responses, typically within 48 hours of treatment. Treatments can be daily with 1.5 to 2 Gy per fraction or hyperfractionated with twice-daily treatments of 1.2 to 1.5 Gy per day. For palliation, total doses as low as 4 Gy in 2-Gy fractions can result in rapid relief from symptoms associated with such conditions as SVC syndrome, acute respiratory distress, spinal cord compression, and orbital proptosis.[354] Local radiotherapy delivered at a dose range of 20 to 30 Gy may be more appropriate for palliation of cranial nerve deficits.[355] Steroids, ideally after confirmation of a histologic diagnosis, can also cause dramatic shrinkage of the tumor. Every attempt at biopsy should be made before steroids are administered given the potential to reduce yield in diagnosis. If steroids must be started emergently, then biopsy should be obtained within 48 hours to have the greatest chance at yielding a diagnosis in this setting.

Future Investigations

Given the high overall success rates of the current multiagent chemotherapy regimens, future trials will aim to develop more targeted therapeutic regimens that include new types of active chemical agents, monoclonal antibodies, and molecularly targeting agents. The obstacle that exists for improving NHL therapy for children is the small number of relapsed or refractory pediatric patients available to participate in early-phase trials. Given the diversity of histologies in pediatric NHL, the population is further limited given the relative rarity of the entities. Still, over the last decade, there has been progress in identifying potential targets and utilizing novel therapies for pediatric NHL. For example, ALCL tumor cells strongly express CD30 on their surface, making them a target for antibody therapy. Brentuximab vedotin, a conjugate antibody that combines an anti-CD30 antibody with a synthetic tubulin disruptor, has been evaluated in a phase II study of adults and pediatric patients with relapsed or refractory ALCL with good response rates.[356] Targeted therapy using crizotinib may also be an area of future interest in patients with ALCL as the majority demonstrate rearrangements involving the *ALK* gene. Early studies show tolerability of crizotinib in a small cohort of pediatric ALCL patients, paving the path for future efficacy studies.[357]

CD20 is expressed on the surface of cells with DLBCL and BL. Currently, most clinical experience with monoclonal antibodies in adult and pediatric B-cell NHLs exists with rituximab (anti-CD20). Several second- and third-generation anti-CD20 monoclonal antibodies are in development and undergoing trials in adult patients with NHL but with no pediatric experience. Future studies with these newer anti-CD20 antibodies should be evaluated in pediatric patients if adult trials are promising.[358]

Immunotherapeutic approaches also show promise in some subtypes of NHL. Specifically, blockage of the PD-1 (programmed death) pathway in PMBCL recently demonstrated good tolerability and efficacy in the relapsed/refractory setting.

Such new targeted treatments hold promise for improving outcomes in children with refractory and relapsed lymphoma. If successful, it may be possible to move therapies to the frontline and possibly reduce treatment intensity and chemotherapy-related toxicities.

REFERENCES

1. Punnett A, Tsang RW, Hodgson DC. Hodgkin lymphoma across the age spectrum: epidemiology, therapy, and late effects. *Semin Radiat Oncol* 2010;20(1):30–44.
2. Donaldson SS, Hancock SL, Hoppe RT. The Janeway lecture. Hodgkin's disease—finding the balance between cure and late effects. *Cancer* 1999;5(6):325.
3. Hays DM. An evaluation of long-term survival and treatment complications in children with Hodgkin's disease. *J Pediatr Surg* 1983;18(5):652.
4. Donaldson SS, Link MP. Combined modality treatment with low-dose radiation and MOPP chemotherapy for children with Hodgkin's disease. *J Clin Oncol* 1987;5(5):742–749.
5. Fryer CJ, Hutchinson RJ, Krailo M, et al. Efficacy and toxicity of 12 courses of ABVD chemotherapy followed by low-dose regional radiation in advanced Hodgkin's disease in children: a report from the Children's Cancer Study Group. *J Clin Oncol* 1990;8(12):1971–1980.
6. Gehan EA, Sullivan MP, Fuller LM, et al. The intergroup Hodgkin's disease in children. A study of stages I and II. *Cancer* 1990;65(6):1429–1437.
7. Hutchinson RJ, Fryer CJ, Davis PC, et al. MOPP or radiation in addition to ABVD in the treatment of pathologically staged advanced Hodgkin's disease in children: results of the Children's Cancer Group Phase III Trial. *J Clin Oncol* 1998;16(3):897–906.
8. Weiner MA, Leventhal B, Brecher ML, et al. Randomized study of intensive MOPP-ABVD with or without low-dose total-nodal radiation therapy in the treatment of stages IIB, IIIA2, IIIB, and IV Hodgkin's disease in pediatric patients: a Pediatric Oncology Group study. *J Clin Oncol* 1997;15(8):2769–2779.
9. Weiner MA, Leventhal BG, Marcus R, et al. Intensive chemotherapy and low-dose radiotherapy for the treatment of advanced-stage Hodgkin's disease in pediatric patients: a Pediatric Oncology Group study. *J Clin Oncol* 1991;9(9):1591–1598.
10. Ward E, DeSantis C, Robbins A, et al. Childhood and adolescent cancer statistics, 2014. *CA Cancer J Clin* 2014;64(2):83–103.
11. Baez F, Ocampo E, Conter V, et al. Treatment of childhood Hodgkin's disease with COPP or COPP-ABV (hybrid) without radiotherapy in Nicaragua. *Ann Oncol* 1997;8(3):247–250.
12. Barrett A, Crennan E, Barnes J, et al. Treatment of clinical stage I Hodgkin's disease by local radiation therapy alone. A United Kingdom Children's Cancer Study Group study. *Cancer* 1990;66(4):670–674.
13. Bayle-Weisgerber C, Lemercier N, Teillet F, et al. Hodgkin's disease in children. Results of therapy in a mixed group of 178 clinical and pathologically staged patients over 13 years. *Cancer* 1984;54(2):215–222.
14. Behrendt H, Brinkhuis M, Van Leeuwen EF. Treatment of childhood Hodgkin's disease with ABVD without radiotherapy. *Med Pediatr Oncol* 1996;26(4):244–248.
15. Ekert H, Toogood I, Downie P, et al. High incidence of treatment failure with vincristine, etoposide, epirubicin, and prednisolone chemotherapy with successful salvage in childhood Hodgkin disease. *Med Pediatr Oncol* 1999;32(4):255–258.
16. Hudson MM, Poquette CA, Lee J, et al. Increased mortality after successful treatment for Hodgkin's disease. *J Clin Oncol* 1998;16(11):3592–3600.
17. Hunger SP, Link MP, Donaldson SS. ABVD/MOPP and low-dose involved-field radiotherapy in pediatric Hodgkin's disease: the Stanford experience. *J Clin Oncol* 1994;12(10):2160–2166.
18. Jenkin D, Doyle J, Berry M, et al. Hodgkin's disease in children: Treatment with MOPP and low-dose, extended field irradiation without laparotomy. Late results and toxicity. *Med Pediatr Oncol* 1990;18(4):265–272.
19. Landman-Parker J, Pacquement H, Leblanc T, et al. Localized childhood Hodgkin's disease: response-adapted chemotherapy with etoposide, bleomycin, vinblastine, and prednisone before low-dose radiation therapy-results of the French Society of Pediatric Oncology Study MDH90. *J Clin Oncol* 2000;18(7):1500.
20. Lobo-Sanahuja F, García I, Barrantes JC, et al. Pediatric Hodgkin's disease in Costa Rica: twelve years' experience of primary treatment by chemotherapy alone, without staging laparotomy. *Med Pediatr Oncol* 1994;22(6):398–403.
21. Oberlin O, Sarrazin D, Lemerle J, et al. Clinical staging, primary chemotherapy and involved field radiotherapy in childhood Hodgkin's disease. *Eur Paediatr Haematol Oncol* 1985;2(1):65–70.
22. Olweny CL, Katongole-Mbidde E, Kiire C, et al. Childhood Hodgkin's disease in Uganda: a ten year experience. *Cancer* 1978;42(2):787–792.
23. Rühl U, Albrecht M, Dieckmann K, et al. Response-adapted radiotherapy in the treatment of pediatric Hodgkin's disease: an interim report at 5 years of the German GPOH-HD 95 trial. *Int J Radiat Oncol Biol Phys* 2001;51(5):1209–1218.
24. Sackmann-Muriel F, Zubizarreta P, Gallo G, et al. Hodgkin disease in children: results of a prospective randomized trial in a single institution in Argentina. *Med Pediatr Oncol* 1997;29(6):544–552.
25. Schellong G. The balance between cure and late effects in childhood Hodgkin's lymphoma: the experience of the German-Austrian Study-Group since 1978. *Ann Oncol* 1996;7(Suppl 4):S72.
26. Schellong G, Dorffel W, Claviez A, et al. Salvage therapy of progressive and recurrent Hodgkin's disease: results from a multicenter study of the pediatric DAL/GPOH-HD study group. *J Clin Oncol* 2005;23(25):6181–6189.
27. Shankar AG, Ashley S, Radford M, et al. Does histology influence outcome in childhood Hodgkin's disease? Results from the United Kingdom Children's Cancer Study Group. *J Clin Oncol* 1997;15(7):2622–2630.
28. Sripada PVSS, Tenali SG, Vasudevan M, et al. Hybrid (COPP/ABV) therapy in childhood Hodgkin's disease: a study of 53 cases during 1989–1993 at the Cancer Institute, Madras. *Pediatr Hematol Oncol* 1995;12(4):333–341.
29. Berg vdH, Stuve W, Behrendt H. Treatment of Hodgkin's disease in children with alternating mechlorethamine, vincristine, procarbazine, and prednisone (MOPP) and adriamycin, bleomycin, vinblastine, and dacarbazine (ABVD) courses without radiotherapy. *Med Pediatr Oncol* 1997;29(1):23–27.
30. Berg Hvd, Zsiros J, Behrendt H. Treatment of childhood Hodgkin's disease without radiotherapy. *Ann Oncol* 1997;8(Suppl 1):15–17.
31. Vecchi V, Pileri S, Burnelli R, et al. Treatment of pediatric Hodgkin disease tailored to stage, mediastinal mass, and age. An Italian (AIEOP) multicenter study on 215 patients. *Cancer* 1993;72(6):2049–2057.
32. Christine M-K, Dirk H, Wolfgang D, et al. Procarbazine-free OEPA-COPDAC chemotherapy in boys and standard OPPA-COPP in girls have comparable effectiveness in pediatric Hodgkin's lymphoma: the GPOH-HD-2002 study. *J Clin Oncol* 2010;28(23):3680–3686.
33. Friedman DL, Chen L, Wolden S, et al. Dose-intensive response-based chemotherapy and radiation therapy for children and adolescents with newly diagnosed intermediate-risk Hodgkin lymphoma: a report from the Children's Oncology Group Study AHOD0031. *J Clin Oncol* 2014;32(32):3651–3658.
34. Charpentier A-M, Friedman DL, Wolden S, et al. Predictive factor analysis of response-adapted radiation therapy for chemotherapy-sensitive pediatric Hodgkin lymphoma: analysis of the Children's Oncology Group AHOD 0031 Trial. *Int J Radiat Oncol Biol Phys* 2016;96(5):943–950.
35. Schwartz CL, Constine LS, Villaluna D, et al. A risk-adapted, response-based approach using ABVE-PC for children and adolescents with intermediate- and high-risk Hodgkin lymphoma: the results of P9425. *Blood* 2009;114(10):2051–2059.
36. Wolden SL, Chen L, Kelly KM, et al. Long-term results of CCG 5942: a randomized comparison of chemotherapy with and without radiotherapy for children with Hodgkin's lymphoma—a report from the Children's Oncology Group. *J Clin Oncol* 2012;30(26):3174–3180.
37. Gutensohn N, Cole P. Epidemiology of Hodgkin's disease in the young. *Int J Cancer* 1977;19(5):595–604.
38. Gutensohn N, Cole P. Childhood social environment and Hodgkin's disease. *N Engl J Med* 1981;304(3):135.
39. Westergaard T, Melbye M, Pedersen JB, et al. Birth order, sibship size and risk of Hodgkin's disease in children and young adults: a population-based study of 31 million person-years. *Int J Cancer* 1997;72(6):977–981.
40. Cleary SF, Link MP, Donaldson SS. Hodgkin's disease in the very young. *Int J Radiat Oncol Biol Phys* 1994;28(1):77–83.
41. Correa P, O'Conor GT. Epidemiologic patterns of Hodgkin's disease. *Int J Cancer* 1971;8(2):192–201.
42. Doll R, Parkin DM. *Cancer incidence in five continents*. Vol. 164. Lyon, France: International Agency for Research on Cancer, 2014.
43. Grufferman S, Delzell E. Epidemiology of Hodgkin's disease. *Epidemiol Rev* 1984;6:76–106.
44. Glaser SL, Jarrett RF. The epidemiology of Hodgkin's disease. *Baillieres Clin Haematol* 1996;9(3):401.
45. Ellen TC, Scott MM, Lorenzo R, et al. Number of siblings and risk of Hodgkin's lymphoma. *Cancer Epidemiol Biomarkers Prev* 2004;13(7):1236–1243.
46. Spitz MR, Sider JG, Johnson CC, et al. Ethnic patterns of Hodgkin's disease incidence among children and adolescents in the United States, 1973-82. *J Natl Cancer Inst* 1986;76(2):235.
47. Hall G, Katzilakis N, Pinkerton C, et al. Outcome of children with nodular lymphocyte predominant Hodgkin lymphoma—a Children's Cancer and Leukaemia Group report. *Br J Haematol* 2007;138(6):761–768.
48. Swerdlow SH. *WHO classification of tumours of haematopoietic and lymphoid tissues.* Lyon, France: World Health Organization, 2008.

49. Swerdlow SH, Campo E, Pileri SA, et al. The 2016 revision of the World Health Organization classification of lymphoid neoplasms. *Blood* 2016;127(20):2375–2390.
50. Bazzeh F, Rihani R, Howard S, et al. Comparing adult and pediatric Hodgkin lymphoma in the Surveillance, Epidemiology and End Results Program, 1988–2005: an analysis of 21 734 cases. *Leuk Lymphoma* 2010;51(12):2198–2207.
51. Haluska FG, Brufsky AM, Canellos GP. The cellular biology of the Reed-Sternberg cell. *Blood* 1994;84(4):1005.
52. Küppers R, Rajewsky K. The origin of Hodgkin and Reed/Sternberg cells in Hodgkin's disease. *Annu Rev Immunol* 1998;16(1):471–493.
53. Pileri SA, Ascani S, Leoncini L, et al. Hodgkin's lymphoma: the pathologist's viewpoint. *J Clin Pathol* 2002;55(3):162–176.
54. Stein H. Hodgkin lymphomas: introduction. In: *World Health Organization classification of tumours pathology & genetics: tumours of haematopoietic and lymphoid tissues*, 2001.
55. Mason DY, Banks PM, Chan J, et al. Nodular lymphocyte predominance Hodgkin's disease. A distinct clinicopathological entity. *Am J Surg Pathol* 1994;18(5):526–530.
56. Ambinder RF, Browning PJ, Lorenzana I, et al. Epstein-Barr virus and childhood Hodgkin's disease in Honduras and the United States. *Blood* 1993;81(2):462.
57. Glaser SL, Lin RJ, Stewart SL, et al. Epstein-Barr virus-associated Hodgkin's disease: epidemiologic characteristics in international data. *Int J Cancer* 1997;70(4):375–382.
58. Connelly RR, Christine BW. A cohort study of cancer following infectious mononucleosis. *Cancer Res* 1974;34(5):1172–1178.
59. Carter CD, Brown JTM, Herbert JT, et al. Cancer incidence following infectious mononucleosis. *Am J Epidemiol* 1977;105(1):30–36.
60. Kvåle G, Høiby EA, Pedersen E. Hodgkin's disease in patients with previous infectious mononucleosis. *Int J Cancer* 1979;23(5):593–597.
61. Miller RW, Beebe GW. Infectious mononucleosis and the empirical risk of cancer. *J Natl Cancer Inst* 1973;50(2):315.
62. Muñoz N, Davidson RJL, Witthoff B, et al. Infectious mononucleosis and Hodgkin's disease. *Int J Cancer* 1978;22(1):10–13.
63. Nils R, Larsen SO, Clemmesen J. Hodgkin's disease in patients with previous infectious mononucleosis: 30 years' experience. *Br Med J* 1974;2(5913):253–256.
64. Mueller N, Evans A, Harris NL, et al. Hodgkin's disease and Epstein-Barr virus. Altered antibody pattern before diagnosis. *N Engl J Med* 1989;320(11):689–695.
65. Filipovich AH, Mathur A, Kamat D, et al. Primary immunodeficiencies: genetic risk factors for lymphoma. *Cancer Res* 1992;52(19 Suppl):5465s–5467s.
66. Uccini S, Monardo F, Stoppacciaro A, et al. High frequency of Epstein-Barr virus genome detection in Hodgkin's disease of HIV-positive patients. *Int J Cancer* 1990;46(4):581–585.
67. Goldin LR, Pfeiffer RM, Gridley G, et al. Familial aggregation of Hodgkin lymphoma and related tumors. *Cancer* 2004;100(9):1902–1908.
68. Mack TM, Cozen W, Shibata DK, et al. Concordance for Hodgkin's disease in identical twins suggesting genetic susceptibility to the young-adult form of the disease. *N Engl J Med* 1995;332(7):413–419.
69. Kaplan HS. Hodgkin's disease: unfolding concepts concerning its nature, management and prognosis. *Cancer* 1980;45(10):2439–2474.
70. Crnkovich MJ, Leopold K, Hoppe RT, et al. Stage I to IIB Hodgkin's disease: the combined experience at Stanford University and the Joint Center for Radiation Therapy. *J Clin Oncol* 1987;5(7):1041–1049.
71. Kadin ME, Liebowitz DN. Cytokines and cytokine receptors in Hodgkin's disease. In: *Hodgkin's disease*. Philadelphia, PA: Lippincott Williams & Wilkins, 1999:139.
72. Pappa VI, Hussain HK, Reznek RH, et al. Role of image-guided core-needle biopsy in the management of patients with lymphoma. *J Clin Oncol* 1996;14(9):2427–2430.
73. Sean TH, Thomas MG, Thomas PM. Utility of fine-needle aspiration as a diagnostic technique in lymphoma. *J Clin Oncol* 2004;22(15):3046–3052.
74. Bradley AJ, Carrington BM, Lawrance JAL, et al. Assessment and significance of mediastinal bulk in Hodgkin's disease: comparison between computed tomography and chest radiography. *J Clin Oncol* 1999;17(8):2493.
75. Rostock RA, Siegelman SS, Lenhard RE, et al. Thoracic CT scanning for mediastinal Hodgkin's disease: results and therapeutic implications. *Int J Radiat Oncol Biol Phys* 1983;9(10):1451–1457.
76. Michal W-S, Olga B, Ron E, et al. ^{18}F-FDG avidity in lymphoma readdressed: a study of 766 patients. *J Nucl Med* 2010;51(1):25.
77. Cheson BD, Fisher RI, Barrington SF, et al. Recommendations for initial evaluation, staging, and response assessment of Hodgkin and non-Hodgkin lymphoma: the Lugano classification. *J Clin Oncol* 2014;32(27):3059–3067.
78. Bruce DC. Role of functional imaging in the management of lymphoma. *J Clin Oncol* 2011;29(14):1844–1854.
79. Quarles van Ufford H, Hoekstra O, de Haas M, et al. On the added value of baseline FDG-PET in malignant lymphoma. *Mol Imaging Biol* 2010;12(2):225–232.
80. Rhodes MM, Delbeke D, Whitlock JA, et al. Utility of FDG-PET/CT in follow-up of children treated for Hodgkin and non-Hodgkin lymphoma. *J Pediatr Hematol Oncol* 2006;28(5):300–306.
81. Lister TA, Crowther D, Sutcliffe SB, et al. Report of a committee convened to discuss the evaluation and staging of patients with Hodgkin's disease: Cotswolds meeting. *J Clin Oncol* 1989;7(11):1630–1636.
82. Specht L. Prognostic factors in Hodgkin's disease. *Semin Radiat Oncol* 1996;6(3):146–161.
83. Dieckmann K, Pötter R, Hofmann J, et al. Does bulky disease at diagnosis influence outcome in childhood Hodgkin's disease and require higher radiation doses? Results from the German-Austrian Pediatric Multicenter Trial DAL-HD-90. *Int J Radiat Oncol Biol Phys* 2003;56(3):644–652.
84. Keller FG, Nachman J, Constine L, et al. A phase III study for the treatment of children and adolescents with newly diagnosed low risk Hodgkin lymphoma (HL). *Blood* 2010;116(21):767.
85. Kelly KM, Sposto R, Hutchinson R, et al. BEACOPP chemotherapy is a highly effective regimen in children and adolescents with high-risk Hodgkin lymphoma: a report from the Children's Oncology Group. *Blood* 2011;117(9):2596–2603.
86. Dörffel W, Rühl U, Lüders H, et al. Treatment of children and adolescents with Hodgkin lymphoma without radiotherapy for patients in complete remission after chemotherapy: final results of the multinational trial GPOH-HD95. *J Clin Oncol* 2013;31(12):1562–1568.
87. Dörffel W, Lüders H, Rühl U, et al. Preliminary results of the multicenter trial GPOH-HD 95 for the treatment of Hodgkin's disease in children and adolescents: analysis and outlook. *Klin Padiatr* 2003;215(3):139–145.
88. Schellong G, Pötter R, Brämswig J, et al. High cure rates and reduced long-term toxicity in pediatric Hodgkin's disease: the German-Austrian multicenter trial DAL-HD-90. The German-Austrian Pediatric Hodgkin's Disease Study Group. *J Clin Oncol* 1999;17(12):3736–3744.
89. Kelly KM. Management of children with high-risk Hodgkin lymphoma. *Br J Haematol* 2012;157(1):3–13.
90. Nachman JB, Sposto R, Herzog P, et al. Randomized comparison of low-dose involved-field radiotherapy and no radiotherapy for children with Hodgkin's disease who achieve a complete response to chemotherapy. *J Clin Oncol* 2002;20(18):3765–3771.
91. Bader SB, Weinstein H, Mauch P, et al. Pediatric stage IV Hodgkin disease. Long-term survival. *Cancer* 1993;72(1):249–255.
92. Smith RS, Chen Q, Hudson MM, et al. Prognostic factors for children with Hodgkin's disease treated with combined-modality therapy. *J Clin Oncol* 2003;21(10):2026.
93. Mauch PM. Controversies in the management of early stage Hodgkin's disease. *Blood* 1994;83(2):318.
94. Behar RA, Hoppe RT. Radiation therapy in the management of bulky mediastinal Hodgkin's disease. *Cancer* 1990;66(1):75–79.
95. Maity A, Goldwein JW, Lange B, et al. Mediastinal masses in children with Hodgkin's disease. An analysis of the Children's Hospital of Philadelphia and the Hospital of the University of Pennsylvania experience. *Cancer* 1992;69(11):2755–2760.
96. Specht L, Nordentoft AM, Cold S, et al. Tumor burden as the most important prognostic factor in early stage Hodgkin's disease. Relations to other prognostic factors and implications for choice of treatment. *Cancer* 1988;61(8):1719–1727.
97. Hopper K, Diehl L, Lynch J, et al. Mediastinal bulk in Hodgkin disease method of measurement versus prognosis. *Invest Radiol* 1991;26(12):1101–1109.
98. Gospodarowicz MK, Sutcliffe SB, Clark RM, et al. Analysis of supradiaphragmatic clinical stage I and II Hodgkin's disease treated with radiation alone. *Int J Radiat Oncol Biol Phys* 1992;22(5):859–865.
99. Hoppe RT, Hanlon AL, Hanks GE, et al. Progress in the treatment of Hodgkin's disease in the United States, 1973 versus 1983. The patterns of care study. *Cancer* 1994;74(12):3198–3203.
100. Bonfante V, Santoro A, Viviani S, et al. Early stage Hodgkin's disease: ten-year results of a non-randomised study with radiotherapy alone or combined with MOPP. *Eur J Cancer* 1993;29(1):24–29.
101. Hagemeister FB, Purugganan R, Fuller L, et al. Treatment of early stages of Hodgkin's disease with novantrone, vincristine, vinblastine, prednisone, and radiotherapy. *Semin Hematol* 1994;31(2 Suppl 3):36–43.
102. Bartlett NL, Rosenberg SA, Hoppe RT, et al. Brief chemotherapy, Stanford V, and adjuvant radiotherapy for bulky or advanced-stage Hodgkin's disease: a preliminary report. *J Clin Oncol* 1995;13(5):1080–1088.
103. Fabian CJ, Mansfield CM, Dahlberg S, et al. Low-dose involved field radiation after chemotherapy in advanced Hodgkin disease. A Southwest Oncology Group randomized study. *Ann Intern Med* 1994;120(11):903–912.
104. Thar TL, Million RR, Hausner RJ, et al. Hodgkin's disease, stages I and II: relationship of recurrence to size of disease, radiation dose, and number of sites involved. *Cancer* 1979;43(3):1101.
105. Körholz D, Wallace W, Landman-Parker J. Euro-Net-Paediatric Hodgkin's Lymphoma Group (Euro-Net-PHL-C1): first international inter-group study for classic Hodgkin's lymphoma in children and adolescents, 2012. Retrieved from http://clinicaltrials.gov/ct/show/NCT00433459:2012.
106. Bodis S, Kraus MD, Pinkus G, et al. Clinical presentation and outcome in lymphocyte-predominant Hodgkin's disease. *J Clin Oncol* 1997;15(9):3060–3066.
107. Castellino S, Keller F, Voss S, et al. Outcomes and Patterns of Failure in Children/Adolescents with Low Risk Hodgkin Lymphoma (HL) who are FDG-PET (PET3) Positive after AVPC Therapy. *Klin Padiatr* 2014;226(2).
108. Kung FH, Schwartz CL, Ferree CR, et al. POG 8625: a randomized trial comparing chemotherapy with chemoradiotherapy for children and adolescents with stages I, IIA, IIIA1 Hodgkin disease. *J Pediatr Hematol Oncol* 2006;28(6):362–368.
109. Keller F, Nachman J, Castellino S. Very early response as measured by (18F)-fluorodeoxyglucose-positron emission tomography (FDG-PET) after one cycle of chemotherapy in newly diagnosed pediatric/adolescent low risk Hodgkin lymphoma (HL). *Hematologica* 2013;98:37.
110. Raemaekers JM, André MP, Federico M, et al. Omitting radiotherapy in early positron emission tomography–negative stage I/II Hodgkin lymphoma is associated with an increased risk of early relapse: clinical results of the preplanned interim analysis of the randomized EORTC/LYSA/FIL H10 trial. *J Clin Oncol* 2014;32(12):1188–1194.
111. Radford J, Illidge T, Counsell N, et al. Results of a trial of PET-directed therapy for early-stage Hodgkin's lymphoma. *N Engl J Med* 2015;372(17):1598–1607.
112. Meignan M, Gallamini A, Itti E, et al. Report on the Third International Workshop on Interim Positron Emission Tomography in Lymphoma held in Menton, France, 26–27 September 2011 and Menton 2011 consensus. *Leuk Lymphoma* 2012;53(10):1876–1881.
113. Biggi A, Gallamini A, Chauvie S, et al. International validation study for interim PET in ABVD-treated, advanced-stage Hodgkin lymphoma: interpretation criteria and concordance rate among reviewers. *J Nucl Med* 2013;54(5):683–690.
114. Schwartz CL, Chen L, McCarten K, et al. Childhood Hodgkin International Prognostic Score (CHIPS) predicts event-free survival in Hodgkin lymphoma: a report from the Children's Oncology Group. *Pediatr Blood Cancer* 2017;64(4).
115. Sarah SD, Melissa MH, Kathleen RL, et al. VAMP and low-dose, involved-field radiation for children and adolescents with favorable, early-stage Hodgkin's disease: results of a prospective clinical trial. *J Clin Oncol* 2002;20(14):3081–3087.
116. Adams MJ, Hardenbergh PH, Constine LS, et al. Radiation-associated cardiovascular disease. *Crit Rev Oncol Hematol* 2003;45(1):55–75.

117. Daniel MG, Andrew H, Catherine SC, et al. Cancer and cardiac mortality among 15-year survivors of cancer diagnosed during childhood or adolescence. *J Clin Oncol* 1999;17(10):3207–3215.

118. Hancock SL, Tucker MA, Hoppe RT. Factors affecting late mortality from heart disease after treatment of Hodgkin's disease. *JAMA* 1993;270(16):1949–1955.

119. Hancock SL, Donaldson SS, Hoppe RT. Cardiac disease following treatment of Hodgkin's disease in children and adolescents. *J Clin Oncol* 1993;11(7):1208–1215.

120. Aleman B, Belt-Dusebout A, Bruin M, et al. Late cardiotoxicity after treatment for Hodgkin lymphoma. *Blood* 2007;109(5):1878–1886.

121. Avilés A, Neri N, Nambo MJ, et al. Late cardiac toxicity secondary to treatment in Hodgkin's disease. A study comparing doxorubicin, epirubicin and mitoxantrone in combined therapy. *Leuk Lymphoma* 2005;46(7):1023–1028.

122. Girinsky T, Cosset JM. Pulmonary and cardiac late effects of ionizing radiations alone or combined with chemotherapy. *Cancer Radiother* 1997;1(6):735–743.

123. Hodgson DC, Hudson MM, Constine LS. Pediatric Hodgkin lymphoma: maximizing efficacy and minimizing toxicity. *Semin Radiat Oncol* 2007;17(3):230–242.

124. Andrea KN, Bernardo MVP, Edie W, et al. Second malignancy after Hodgkin disease treated with radiation therapy with or without chemotherapy: long-term risks and risk factors. *Blood* 2002;100(6):1989–1996.

125. Ng AK, Travis LB. Radiation therapy and breast cancer risk. *J Natl Compr Canc Netw* 2009;7(10):1121.

126. Anthony JS, Ama ZSR, David CL, et al. Myocardial infarction mortality risk after treatment for Hodgkin disease: a collaborative British cohort study. *J Natl Cancer Inst* 2007;99(3):206–214.

127. Metzger ML, Weinstein HJ, Hudson MM, et al. Association between radiotherapy vs no radiotherapy based on early response to VAMP chemotherapy and survival among children with favorable-risk Hodgkin lymphoma. *JAMA* 2012;307(24):2609–2616.

128. Keller FG, Nachman J, Constine L, et al. A phase III study for the treatment of children and adolescents with newly diagnosed low risk Hodgkin lymphoma (HL). *Blood* 2010;116:A767.

129. Hakvoort-Cammel FG, Buitendijk S, van den Heuvel-Eibrink M, et al. Treatment of pediatric Hodgkin disease avoiding radiotherapy: excellent outcome with the Rotterdam-HD-84-protocol. *Pediatr Blood Cancer* 2004;43(1):8–16.

130. Jayabose S, Viswanathan K, Kumar V, et al. ABVE-PC and modified BEACOPP regimen in Indian children with Hodgkin lymphoma: feasibility and efficacy. *Indian J Med Paediatr Oncol* 2016;37(2):106.

131. Arya LS, Dinand V, Thavaraj V, et al. Hodgkin's disease in Indian children: outcome with chemotherapy alone. *Pediatr Blood Cancer* 2006;46(1):26–34.

132. Atra A, Higgs E, Capra M, et al. ChlVPP chemotherapy in children with stage IV Hodgkin's disease: results of the UKCCSG HD 8201 and HD 9201 studies. *Br J Haematol* 2002;119(3):647–651.

133. Tebbi CK, Mendenhall NP, London WB, et al. Response-dependent and reduced treatment in lower risk Hodgkin lymphoma in children and adolescents, results of P9426: a report from the Children's Oncology Group. *Pediatr Blood Cancer* 2012;59(7):1259–1265.

134. Mauz-Körholz C, Hasenclever D, Dörffel W, et al. Procarbazine-free OEPA-COPDAC chemotherapy in boys and standard OPPA-COPP in girls have comparable effectiveness in pediatric Hodgkin's lymphoma: the GPOH-HD-2002 study. *J Clin Oncol* 2010;28(23):3680–3686.

135. Tebbi CK, Mendenhall N, London WB, et al. Treatment of stage I, IIA, IIIA1 pediatric Hodgkin disease with doxorubicin, bleomycin, vincristine and etoposide (DBVE) and radiation: a Pediatric Oncology Group (POG) study. *Pediatr Blood Cancer* 2006;46(2):198–202.

136. Melissa MH, Matthew K, Michael PL, et al. Risk-adapted, combined-modality therapy with VAMP/COP and response-based, involved-field radiation for unfavorable pediatric Hodgkin's disease. *J Clin Oncol* 2004;22(22):4541–4550.

137. Sarah SD, Michael PL, Howard JW, et al. Final results of a prospective clinical trial with VAMP and low-dose involved-field radiation for children with low-risk Hodgkin's disease. *J Clin Oncol* 2007;25(3):332–337.

138. Shankar AG, Ashley S, Atra A, et al. A limited role for VEEP (vincristine, etoposide, epirubicin, prednisolone) chemotherapy in childhood Hodgkin's disease. *Eur J Cancer* 1998;34(13):2058–2063.

139. Schellong G, Brämswig J, Hörnig-Franz I. Treatment of children with Hodgkin's disease—results of the German Pediatric Oncology Group. *Ann Oncol* 1992;3(Suppl 4):S73–S76.

140. Friedman D, Wolden S, Constine L, et al. AHOD0031: a phase III study of dose-intensive therapy for intermediate risk Hodgkin lymphoma: a report from the Children's Oncology Group. *Blood* 2010;116.

141. Kelly K, Hutchinson R, Sposto R, et al. Feasibility of upfront dose-intensive chemotherapy in children with advanced-stage Hodgkin's lymphoma: preliminary results from the Children's Cancer Group Study CCG-59704. *Ann Oncol* 2002;13(Suppl 1):107–111.

142. Alison MF, Melissa MH, Howard JW, et al. Treatment of unfavorable childhood Hodgkin's disease with VEPA and low-dose, involved-field radiation. *J Clin Oncol* 2002;20(14):3088–3094.

143. Oberlin O, Leverger G, Pacquement H, et al. Low-dose radiation therapy and reduced chemotherapy in childhood Hodgkin's disease: the experience of the French Society of Pediatric Oncology. *J Clin Oncol.* 1992;10(10):1602–1608.

144. Vincent T. Devita JR, Arthur A S, et al. Combination Chemotherapy in the Treatment of Advanced Hodgkin's Disease. *Ann Intern Med.* 1970;73(6):881–895.

145. Longo DL, Young RC, Wesley M, et al. Twenty years of MOPP therapy for Hodgkin's disease. *J Clin Oncol.* 1986;4(9):1295–1306.

146. DeVita VT, Canellos GP, Moxley JH. A decade of combination chemotherapy of advanced Hodgkin's disease. *Cancer* 1972;30(6):1495–1504.

147. Pedersen-Bjergaard J, Specht L, Larsen SO, et al. Risk of therapy-related leukaemia and preleukaemia after Hodgkin's disease. Relation to age, cumulative dose of alkylating agents, and time from chemotherapy. *Lancet* 1987;2(8550):83–88.

148. Sy Ortin TT, Shostak CA, Donaldson SS. Gonadal status and reproductive function following treatment for Hodgkin's disease in childhood: the Stanford experience. *Int J Radiat Oncol Biol Phys* 1990;19(4):873–880.

149. Schellong G, Riepenhausen M, Creutzig U, et al. Low risk of secondary leukemias after chemotherapy without mechlorethamine in childhood Hodgkin's disease. German-Austrian Pediatric Hodgkin's Disease Group. *J Clin Oncol* 1997;15(6):2247–2253.

150. Bhatia S, Robison LL, Oberlin O, et al. Breast Cancer and Other Second Neoplasms after Childhood Hodgkin's Disease. *N Engl J Med.* 1996;334(12):745–751.

151. Santoro A, Bonadonna G, Valagussa P, et al. Long-term results of combined chemotherapy-radiotherapy approach in Hodgkin's disease: superiority of ABVD plus radiotherapy versus MOPP plus radiotherapy. *J Clin Oncol* 1987;5(1):27–37.

152. Canellos GP, Anderson JR, Propert KJ, et al. Chemotherapy of advanced Hodgkin's disease with MOPP, ABVD, or MOPP alternating with ABVD. *N Engl J Med* 1992;327(21):1478–1484.

153. Hutchison RE, Berard CW, Shuster JJ, et al. B-cell lineage confers a favorable outcome among children and adolescents with large-cell lymphoma: a Pediatric Oncology Group study. *J Clin Oncol* 1995;13(8):2023–2032.

154. Kreisman H, Wolkove N. Pulmonary toxicity of antineoplastic therapy. *Semin Oncol* 1992;19(5):508–520.

155. Hudson MM, Greenwald C, Thompson E, et al. Efficacy and toxicity of multiagent chemotherapy and low-dose involved-field radiotherapy in children and adolescents with Hodgkin's disease. *J Clin Oncol* 1993;11(1):100–108.

156. Brämswig JH, Heimes U, Heiermann E, et al. The effects of different cumulative doses of chemotherapy on testicular function. Results in 75 patients treated for Hodgkin's disease during childhood or adolescence. *Cancer* 1990;65(6):1298–1302.

157. Malcolm AS, Lawrence R, James RA, et al. Secondary leukemia or myelodysplastic syndrome after treatment with epipodophyllotoxins. *J Clin Oncol* 1999;17(2):569–577.

158. Cameron KT, Wendy BL, Debra F, et al. dexrazoxane-associated risk for acute myeloid leukemia/myelodysplastic syndrome and other secondary malignancies in pediatric Hodgkin's disease. *J Clin Oncol* 2007;25(5):493–500.

159. Hassel JU, Brämswig JH, Schlegel W, et al. Testicular function after OPA/COMP chemotherapy without procarbazine in boys with Hodgkin's disease. Results in 25 patients of the DAL-HD-85 study. *Klin Padiatr* 1991;203(4):268–272.

160. Maity A, Goldwein JW, Lange B, and D'Angio G. Comparison of high-dose and low-dose radiation with and without chemotherapy for children with Hodgkin's disease: an analysis of the experience at the Children's Hospital of Philadelphia and the Hospital of the University of Pennsylvania. *J Clin Oncol* 1992;10(6):929–935.

161. Ekert H, Fok T, Dalla-Pozza L, et al. A pilot study of EVAP/ABV chemotherapy in 25 newly diagnosed children with Hodgkin's disease. *Br J Cancer* 1993;67(1):159.

162. Schwartz CL. The management of Hodgkin disease in the young child. *Curr Opin Pediatr* 2003;15(1):10–16.

163. Ekert H, Waters KD, Smith PJ, et al. Treatment with MOPP or ChlVPP chemotherapy only for all stages of childhood Hodgkin's disease. *J Clin Oncol* 1988;6(12):1845–1850.

164. Ruhl U, Albrecht MR, Lueders H, et al. The German multinational GPOH-HD 95 trial: treatment results and analysis of failures in pediatric Hodgkins disease using combination chemotherapy with and without radiation. *Int J Radiat Oncol Biol Phys* 2004;60(1):S131.

165. Advani RH, Horning SJ, Hoppe RT, et al. Mature results of a phase II study of rituximab therapy for nodular lymphocyte-predominant Hodgkin lymphoma. *J Clin Oncol* 2014;32(9):912–918.

166. Intergroup Randomized Trial for Children or Adolescents With B-Cell Non Hodgkin Lymphoma or B-Acute Leukemia: Rituximab Evaluation in High Risk Patients, 2012. Retrieved from https://clinicaltrials.gov/ct2 (Identification No. NCT01516580).

167. Hvizdala EV, Berard C, Callihan T, et al. Nonlymphoblastic lymphoma in children—histology and stage-related response to therapy: a Pediatric Oncology Group study. *J Clin Oncol* 1991;9(7):1189–1195.

168. Brentuximab Vedotin and Combination Chemotherapy in Treating Children and Young Adults With Stage IIB or Stage IIIB-IVB Hodgkin Lymphoma, 2014. Retrieved from http://clinicaltrials.gov/ct2 (Identification No. NCT02166463).

169. Dieckmann K, Pötter R, Wagner W, et al. Up-front centralized data review and individualized treatment proposals in a multicenter pediatric Hodgkin's disease trial with 71 participating hospitals: the experience of the German–Austrian pediatric multicenter trial DAL-HD-90. *Radiother Oncol* 2002;62(2):191–200.

170. FitzGerald TJ, Bishop-Jodoin M, Cicchetti MG, et al. quality of radiotherapy reporting in randomized controlled trials of Hodgkin's lymphoma and non-Hodgkin's lymphoma: in regard to Bekelman and Yahalom (Int J Radiat Oncol Biol Phys 2009;73:492–498). *Int J Radiat Oncol Biol Phys* 2010;77(1):315–316.

171. Yahalom J, Mauch P. The involved field is back: issues in delineating the radiation field in Hodgkin's disease. *Ann Oncol* 2002;13(Suppl 1):79–83.

172. Campbell B, Voss N, Pickles T, et al. 6002 ORAL involved-field radiotherapy (IFRT) and involved-nodal radiotherapy (INRT) as a component of combination therapy for limited stage Hodgkin lymphoma: a question of field size. *EJC Suppl* 2007;5(4):345–346.

173. Dhakal S, Bates JE, Casulo C, et al. Patterns and Timing of Failure for Diffuse Large B-Cell Lymphoma After Initial Therapy in a Cohort Who Underwent Autologous Bone Marrow Transplantation for Relapse. *Int J Radiat Oncol Biol Phys* 2016;96(2):372–378.

174. Shahidi M, Kamangari N, Ashley S, et al. Site of relapse after chemotherapy alone for stage I and II Hodgkin's disease. *Radiother Oncol* 2006;78(1):1–5.

175. Girinsky T, van der Maazen R, Specht L, et al. Involved-node radiotherapy (INRT) in patients with early Hodgkin lymphoma: concepts and guidelines. *Radiother Oncol* 2006;79(3):270–277.

176. Girinsky T, Specht L, Ghalibafian M, et al. The conundrum of hodgkin lymphoma nodes: to be or not to be included in the involved node radiation fields. The EORTC-GELA lymphoma group guidelines. *Radiother Oncol* 2008;88(2):202–210.

177. Girinsky T, Ghalibafian M. Radiotherapy of Hodgkin lymphoma: indications, new fields, and techniques. *Semin Radiat Oncol* 2007;17(3):206–222.

178. Belinda AC, Nick V, Tom P, et al. Involved-nodal radiation therapy as a component of combination therapy for limited-stage Hodgkin's lymphoma: a question of field size. *J Clin Oncol* 2008;26(32):5170–5174.

179. Paumier A, Ghalibafian M, Gilmore J, et al. Dosimetric benefits of intensity-modulated radiotherapy combined with the deep-inspiration breath-hold

technique in patients with mediastinal Hodgkin's lymphoma. *Int J Radiat Oncol Biol Phys* 2012;82(4):1522–1527.

180. Specht L, Yahalom J, Illidge T, et al. Modern radiation therapy for Hodgkin lymphoma: field and dose guidelines from the international lymphoma radiation oncology group (ILROG). *Int J Radiat Oncol Biol Phys* 2014;89(4):854–862.

181. Hutchings M, Berthelsen AK, Barrington SF. The role of imaging in radiotherapy for Hodgkin lymphoma. In: Specht L, Yahalom J, eds. *Radiotherapy for Hodgkin lymphoma.* Heidelberg, Germany: Springer, 2011:81–89.

182. International Commission on Radiation Units and Measurements. *Prescribing, recording, and reporting photon beam therapy.* Bethesda, MD: International Commission on Radiation Units and Measurements, 1993.

183. Appel BE, Chen L, Buxton A, et al. Impact of low-dose involved-field radiation therapy on pediatric patients with lymphocyte-predominant Hodgkin lymphoma treated with chemotherapy: a report from the Children's Oncology Group. *Pediatr Blood Cancer* 2012;59(7):1284–1289.

184. Plowman PN, Cooke K, Walsh N. Indications for tomotherapy/intensity-modulated radiation therapy in paediatric radiotherapy: extracranial disease. *Br J Radiol* 2008;81(971):872–880.

185. Hall EJ. Intensity-modulated radiation therapy, protons, and the risk of second cancers. *Int J Radiat Oncol Biol Phys* 2006;65(1):1–7.

186. Hoppe BS, Flampouri S, Su Z, et al. Effective dose reduction to cardiac structures using protons compared with 3DCRT and IMRT in mediastinal Hodgkin lymphoma. *Int J Radiat Oncol Biol Phys* 2012;84(2):449–455.

187. Travis LB, Hill DA, Dores GM, et al. Breast cancer following radiotherapy and chemotherapy among young women with Hodgkin disease. *JAMA* 2003;290(4):465–475.

188. Koh E-S, Sun A, Tran TH, et al. Clinical dose-volume histogram analysis in predicting radiation pneumonitis in Hodgkin's lymphoma. *Int J Radiat Oncol Biol Phys* 2006;66(1):223–228.

189. Constine LS, Tarbell N, Hudson MM, et al. Subsequent malignancies in children treated for Hodgkin's disease: associations with gender and radiation dose. *Int J Radiat Oncol Biol Phys* 2008;72(1):24–33.

190. Omer B, Kadan-Lottick NS, Roberts KB, et al. Patterns of subsequent malignancies after Hodgkin lymphoma in children and adults. *Br J Haematol* 2012;158(5):615–625.

191. O'Brien MM, Donaldson SS, Balise RR, et al. Second malignant neoplasms in survivors of pediatric Hodgkin's lymphoma treated with low-dose radiation and chemotherapy. *J Clin Oncol* 2010;28(7):1232–1239.

192. Jhanwar YS, Straus DJ. The role of PET in lymphoma. *J Nucl Med* 2006;47(8):1326.

193. Eichenauer DA, Bredenfeld H, Haverkamp H, et al. Hodgkin's lymphoma in adolescents treated with adult protocols: a report from the German Hodgkin study group. *J Clin Oncol* 2009;27(36):6079–6085.

194. Reinhardt MJ, Herkel C, Altehoefer C, et al. Computed tomography and 18F-FDG positron emission tomography for therapy control of Hodgkin's and non-Hodgkin's lymphoma patients: when do we really need FDG-PET? *Ann Oncol* 2005;16(9):1524–1529.

195. Cheson BD, Pfistner B, Juweid M, et al. Revised response criteria for malignant lymphoma. *J Clin Oncol* 2007;25(5):579–586.

196. Hua C, Hoth KA, Wu S, et al. Incidence and correlates of radiation pneumonitis in pediatric patients with partial lung irradiation. *Int J Radiat Oncol Biol Phys* 2010;78(1):143–149.

197. Constine LS, Donaldson SS, McDougall IR, et al. Thyroid dysfunction after radiotherapy in children with Hodgkin's disease. *Cancer* 1984;53(4):878–883.

198. Metzger ML, Hudson MM, Somes GW, et al. White race as a risk factor for hypothyroidism after treatment for pediatric Hodgkin's lymphoma. *J Clin Oncol* 2006;24(10):1516–1521.

199. Sklar CA, Mertens AC, Mitby P, et al. Premature menopause in survivors of childhood cancer: a report from the childhood cancer survivor study. *J Natl Cancer Inst* 2006;98(13):890–896.

200. Floch OL, Donaldson SS, Kaplan HS. Pregnancy following oophoropexy and total nodal irradiation in women with Hodgkin's disease. *Cancer* 1976;38(6):2263–2268.

201. Byrne J, Fears TR, Gail MH, et al. Early menopause in long-term survivors of cancer during adolescence. *Am J Obstet Gynecol* 1992;166(3):788–793.

202. Pedrick TJ, Hoppe RT. Recovery of spermatogenesis following pelvic irradiation for Hodgkin's disease. *Int J Radiat Oncol Biol Phys* 1986;12(1):117–121.

203. Hobbie WL, Ginsberg JP, Ogle SK, et al. Fertility in males treated for Hodgkins disease with COPP/ABV hybrid. *Pediatr Blood Cancer* 2005;44(2):193–196.

204. Viviani S, Santoro A, Ragni G, et al. Gonadal toxicity after combination chemotherapy for Hodgkin's disease. comparative results of MOPP vs ABVD. *Eur J Cancer Clin Oncol* 1985;21(5):601–605.

205. Anselmo AP, Cartoni C, Bellantuono P, et al. Risk of infertility in patients with Hodgkin's disease treated with ABVD vs MOPP vs ABVD/MOPP. *Haematologica* 1990;75(2):155–158.

206. Beaty O, Hudson MM, Greenwald C, et al. Subsequent malignancies in children and adolescents after treatment for Hodgkin's disease. *J Clin Oncol* 1995;13(3):603–609.

207. Bhatia S, Yasui Y, Robison LL, et al. High risk of subsequent neoplasms continues with extended follow-up of childhood Hodgkin's disease: report from the Late Effects Study Group. *J Clin Oncol* 2003;21(23):4386.

208. Mertens AC, Yasui Y, Liu Y, et al. Pulmonary complications in survivors of childhood and adolescent cancer. *Cancer* 2002;95(11):2431–2441.

209. Rooney CM, Ng C, Loftin S, et al. Use of gene-modified virus-specific T lymphocytes to control Epstein-Barr-virus-related lymphoproliferation. *Lancet* 1995;345(8941):9–13.

210. Sankila R, Garwicz S, Olsen J, et al. Risk of subsequent malignant neoplasms among 1,641 Hodgkin's disease patients diagnosed in childhood and adolescence: a population-based cohort study in the five Nordic countries. Association of the Nordic Cancer Registries and the Nordic Society of Pediatric Hematology and Oncology. *J Clin Oncol* 1996;14(5):1442–1446.

211. van Leeuwen FE, Klokman W, Hagenbeek A, et al. Second cancer risk following Hodgkin's disease: a 20-year follow-up study. *J Clin Oncol* 1994;12(2):312–325.

212. van Leeuwen FE, Klokman WJ, Veer MBvt, et al. Long-term risk of second malignancy in survivors of Hodgkin's disease treated during adolescence or young adulthood. *J Clin Oncol* 2000;18(3):487–487.

213. Van Leeuwen FE, Klokman WJ, Stovall M, et al. Roles of radiation dose, chemotherapy, and hormonal factors in breast cancer following Hodgkin's disease. *J Natl Cancer Inst* 2003;95(13):971–980.

214. Wolden SL, Lamborn KR, Cleary SF, et al. Second cancers following pediatric Hodgkin's disease. *J Clin Oncol* 1998;16(2):536–544.

215. Armstrong GT, Sklar CA, Hudson MM, et al. Long-term health status among survivors of childhood cancer: does sex matter? *J Clin Oncol* 2007;25(28):4477–4489.

216. Tarbell NJ, Mauch P, Gelber RD, et al. Sex differences in risk of second malignant tumours after Hodgkin's disease in childhood. *Lancet* 1993;341(8858):1428–1432.

217. Travis LB, Hill DA, Dores GM, et al. Cumulative absolute breast cancer risk for young women treated for Hodgkin lymphoma. *J Natl Cancer Inst* 2005;97(19):1428–1437.

218. Elkin EB, Klem ML, Gonzales AM, et al. Characteristics and outcomes of breast cancer in women with and without a history of radiation for Hodgkin's lymphoma: a multi-institutional, matched cohort study. *J Clin Oncol* 2011;29(18):2466–2473.

219. Travis LB, Rabkin CS, Brown LM, et al. Cancer survivorship—genetic susceptibility and second primary cancers: research strategies and recommendations. *J Natl Cancer Inst* 2006;98(1):15–25.

220. De Bruin ML, Sparidans J, van't Veer MB, et al. Breast cancer risk in female survivors of Hodgkin's lymphoma: lower risk after smaller radiation volumes. *J Clin Oncol* 2009;27(26):4239–4246.

221. Dharmarajan KV, Friedman DL, Schwartz CL, et al. Patterns of relapse from a phase 3 study of response-based therapy for intermediate-risk Hodgkin lymphoma (AHOD0031): a report from the Children's Oncology Group. *Int J Radiat Oncol Biol Phys* 2015;92(1):60–66.

222. Appel BE, Chen L, Buxton AB, et al. Minimal Treatment of Low-Risk, Pediatric Lymphocyte-Predominant Hodgkin Lymphoma: A Report From the Children's Oncology Group. *J Clin Oncol* 2016;34(20):2372–2379.

223. Schwartz CL, Chen L, McCarten K, et al. Childhood Hodgkin International Prognostic Score (CHIPS) predicts event-free survival in Hodgkin lymphoma: a report from the Children's Oncology Group. *Pediatr Blood Cancer* 2017;64(4):e26278.

224. Mauz-Krholz C, Metzger ML, Kelly KM, et al. Pediatric hodgkin lymphoma. *J Clin Oncol* 2015;33(27):2975–2985.

225. Landman-Parker J, Wallace H, Hasenclever D, et al. First international intergroup study for classic Hodgkin lymphoma in children and adolescents: EuroNet PHL C1 report of the latest interim analysis *International symposium on Hodgkin lymphoma,* 2016, Cologne, Germany, October 22–25, 2016.

226. Combination Chemotherapy and Radiation Therapy in Treating Young Patients With Newly Diagnosed Hodgkin Lymphoma, 2009. Retrieved from http://clinicaltrials.gov/ct2 (Identification No. NCT01026220).

227. Kelly KM, Cole PD, Chen L, et al. *Phase III study of response adapted therapy for the treatment of children with newly diagnosed very high risk Hodgkin lymphoma (Stages IIIB/IVB) (AHOD0831): a report from the Children's Oncology Group. Blood* 2015;126(23):3927.

228. Second International Inter-Group Study for Classic Hodgkin Lymphoma in Children and Adolescents, 2015. Retrieved from http://clinicaltrials.gov/ct2 (Identification No. NCT02684708).

229. Bodis S, Henry-Amar M, Bosq J, et al. Late relapse in early-stage Hodgkin's disease patients enrolled on European Organization for Research and Treatment of Cancer protocols. *J Clin Oncol* 1993;11(2):225–232.

230. Wirth A, Yuen K, Barton M, et al. Long-term outcome after radiotherapy alone for lymphocyte-predominant Hodgkin lymphoma—a retrospective multicenter study of the Australasian Radiation Oncology Lymphoma Group. *Cancer* 2004;101(4):1221–1229.

231. Nogova L, Reineke T, Eich HT, et al. Extended field radiotherapy, combined modality treatment or involved field radiotherapy for patients with stage IA lymphocyte-predominant Hodgkin's lymphoma: a retrospective analysis from the German Hodgkin Study Group (GHSG). *Ann Oncol* 2005;16(10):1683–1687.

232. Mauz-Körholz C, Gorde-Grosjean S, Hasenclever D, et al. Resection alone in 58 children with limited stage, lymphocyte-predominant Hodgkin lymphoma—experience from the European network group on pediatric Hodgkin lymphoma. *Cancer* 2007;110(1):179–185.

233. Terezakis SA, Metzger ML, Hodgson DC, et al. ACR appropriateness Criteria® pediatric Hodgkin lymphoma. *Pediatr Blood Cancer* 2014;61(7):1305–1312.

234. *Surgery Alone, Surgery With Cyclophosphamide, Vinblastine, and Prednisolone (CVP), or CVP Alone in Treating Young Patients With Stage IA or Stage IIA Nodular Lymphocyte-Predominant Hodgkin Lymphoma,* 2010. Retrieved from http://clinicaltrials.gov/ct2 (Identification No. NCT01088750).

235. Trippett TM, Chen A. Treatment of relapsed/refractory Hodgkin lymphoma. In: *Pediatric lymphomas.* Springer; 2007:67–84.

236. Claviez A, Canals C, Dierickx D, et al. Allogeneic hematopoietic stem cell transplantation in children and adolescents with recurrent and refractory Hodgkin lymphoma: an analysis of the European Group for Blood and Marrow Transplantation. *Blood* 2009;114(10):2060–2067.

237. Williams CD, Goldstone AH, Pearce R, et al. Autologous bone marrow transplantation for pediatric Hodgkin's disease: a case-matched comparison with adult patients by the European Bone Marrow Transplant Group Lymphoma Registry. *J Clin Oncol* 1993;11(11):2243–2249.

238. Schmitz N, Pfistner B, Sextro M, et al. Aggressive conventional chemotherapy compared with high-dose chemotherapy with autologous haemopoietic stem-cell transplantation for relapsed chemosensitive Hodgkin's disease: a randomised trial. *Lancet* 2002;359(9323):2065–2071.

239. Claviez A, Sureda A, Schmitz N. Haematopoietic SCT for children and adolescents with relapsed and refractory Hodgkin's lymphoma. *Bone Marrow Transplant* 2008;42(S2):S24.

240. Locatelli F, Neville K, Rosolen A, et al. Phase 1/2 Study of Brentuximab Vedotin in Pediatric Pts with Relapsed/Refractory (R/R) Hodgkin Lymphoma (HL) or Systemic Anaplastic Large-Cell Lymphoma (sALCL): Preliminary Phase 2 HL Data. *Klin Padiatr* 2014;226(2).

241. Anas Y, Ajay KG, Scott ES, et al. Results of a pivotal phase II study of brentuximab vedotin for patients with relapsed or refractory Hodgkin's lymphoma. *J Clin Oncol* 2012;30(18):2183–2189.

242. Stephen MA, Alexander ML, Ivan B, et al. PD-1 blockade with nivolumab in relapsed or refractory Hodgkin's lymphoma. *N Engl J Med* 2015;372(4):311–319.

243. Ma YP, van Leeuwen FE, Cooke R, et al. FGFR2 genotype and risk of radiation-associated breast cancer in Hodgkin lymphoma. *Blood* 2012;119(4):1029–1031.

244. Henk V, Colin JDR, Rassekh SR, et al. Pharmacogenomic prediction of anthracycline-induced cardiotoxicity in children. *J Clin Oncol* 2012;30(13):1422–1428.

245. Gross T, Perkins S. Malignant non-Hodgkin lymphomas in children. In: Pizzo PA, Poplack DG, eds. *Principles and practice of paediatric oncology*. 6th ed. Philadelphia, PA: Lippincott Williams & Wilkins, 2011:663–682.

246. Murphy SB. Classification, staging and end results of treatment of childhood non-Hodgkin's lymphomas: dissimilarities from lymphomas in adults. *Semin Oncol* 1980;7(3):332–339.

247. Percy CL, Smith MA, Linet M, et al. Lymphomas and reticuloendothelial neoplasms *(ICCC II): Cancer incidence and survival among children and adolescents: United States SEER Program 1975–1995*, Bethesda, MD: NIH publication 99–4649, 1999:35–50.

248. Sandlund JT, Downing JR, Crist WM. Non-Hodgkin's lymphoma in childhood. *N Engl J Med* 1996;334(19):1238–1248.

249. Gatti RA, Good RA. Occurrence of malignancy in immunodeficiency diseases. A literature review. *Cancer* 1971;28(1):89–98.

250. Kersey JH, Spector BD, Good RA. Cancer in children with primary immunodeficiency diseases. *J Pediatr* 1974;84(2):263–264.

251. Grulich AE, van Leeuwen MT, Falster MO, et al. Incidence of cancers in people with HIV/AIDS compared with immunosuppressed transplant recipients: a meta-analysis. *Lancet* 2007;370(9581):59–67.

252. Pollock BH, Jenson HB, Leach CT, et al. Risk factors for pediatric human immunodeficiency virus–related malignancy. *JAMA* 2003;289(18):2393–2399.

253. Epstein MA, Achong BG, Barr YM. Virus particles in cultured lymphoblasts from Burkitt's lymphoma. *Lancet* 1964;283(7335):702–703.

254. Cohen JI. Epstein-Barr virus infection. *N Engl J Med* 2000;343(7):481–492.

255. Denis B. Determining the climatic limitations of a children's cancer common in Africa. *Br Med J* 1962;2(5311):1019–1023.

256. Gross TG, Savoldo B, Punnett A. Posttransplant lymphoproliferative diseases. *Pediatr Clin N Am* 2010;57(2):481–503.

257. Webber SA, Naftel DC, Fricker FJ, et al. Lymphoproliferative disorders after paediatric heart transplantation: a multi-institutional study. *Lancet* 2006;367(9506):233–239.

258. Minard-Colin V, Brugières L, Reiter A, et al. Non-Hodgkin Lymphoma in Children and Adolescents: Progress Through Effective Collaboration, Current Knowledge, and Challenges Ahead. *J Clin Oncol* 2015;33(27):2963–2974.

259. Sandlund J. *Childhood lymphoma*. Vol. 2. New York, NY: Churchill Livingstone, 2000.

260. Liu Q, Salaverria I, Pittaluga S, et al. Follicular lymphomas in children and young adults: a comparison of the pediatric variant with usual follicular lymphoma. *Am J Surg Pathol* 2013;37(3):333.

261. Ferreiro JF, Morscio J, Dierickx D, et al. Post-transplant molecularly defined Burkitt lymphomas are frequently MYC-negative and characterized by the 11q-gain/loss pattern. *Haematologica* 2015;100(7):e279.

262. Salaverria I, Martin-Guerrero I, Wagener R, et al. A recurrent 11q aberration pattern characterizes a subset of MYC-negative high-grade B-cell lymphomas resembling Burkitt lymphoma. *Blood* 2014;123(8):1187.

263. Jaffe ES. The role of immunophenotypic markers in the classification of non-Hodgkin's lymphomas. *Semin Oncol* 1990;17(1):11–19.

264. Burkhardt B. Paediatric lymphoblastic T-cell leukaemia and lymphoma: one or two diseases? *Br J Haematol* 2010;149(5):653–668.

265. Margit H, Ralf H, Dieter B. Severe Chlamydia pneumoniae infection in a patient with mild neutropenia during treatment of Hodgkin's disease. *Ann Hematol* 2004;83(7):441–443.

266. Grever MR, Tran T, Botstein D, et al. Distinct types of diffuse large B-cell lymphoma identified by gene expression profiling. *Nature* 2000;403(6769):503–511.

267. Weinstein HJ, Vance ZB, Jaffe N, et al. Improved prognosis for patients with mediastinal lymphoblastic lymphoma. *Blood* 1979;53(4):687–694.

268. Murphy SB, Bowman WP, Abromowitch M, et al. Results of treatment of advanced-stage Burkitt's lymphoma and B cell (SIg+) acute lymphoblastic leukemia with high-dose fractionated cyclophosphamide and coordinated high-dose methotrexate and cytarabine. *J Clin Oncol* 1986;4(12):1732–1739.

269. Magrath IT. African Burkitt's lymphoma. History, biology, clinical features, and treatment. *Am J Pediatr Hematol Oncol* 1991;13(2):222.

270. Neth O, Seidemann K, Jansen P, et al. Precursor B-cell lymphoblastic lymphoma in childhood and adolescence: clinical features, treatment, and results in trials NHL-BFM 86 and 90. *Med Pediatr Oncol* 2000;35(1):20–27.

271. Link MP, Roper M, Dorfman RF, et al. Cutaneous lymphoblastic lymphoma with pre-B markers. *Blood* 1983;61(5):838.

272. Sandlund JT, Santana V, Abromowitch M, et al. Large cell non-Hodgkin lymphoma of childhood: clinical characteristics and outcome. *Leukemia* 1994;8(1):30–34.

273. Cairo MS, Sposto R, Hoover-Regan M, et al. Childhood and adolescent large-cell lymphoma (LCL): a review of the Children's Cancer Group experience. *Am J Hematol* 2003;72(1):53–63.

274. Sandlund JT, Pui CH, Santana VM, et al. Clinical features and treatment outcome for children with CD30+ large-cell non-Hodgkin's lymphoma. *J Clin Oncol* 1994;12(5):895–898.

275. Kadin ME, Sako D, Berliner N, et al. Childhood Ki-1 lymphoma presenting with skin lesions and peripheral lymphadenopathy. *Blood* 1986;68(5):1042.

276. van Vuren A, Meyer-Wentrup F. New targets for antibody therapy of pediatric B cell lymphomas. *Pediatr Blood Cancer* 2014;61(12):2158–2163.

277. Loeffler JS, Leopold KA, Recht A, et al. Emergency prebiopsy radiation for mediastinal masses: impact on subsequent pathologic diagnosis and outcome. *J Clin Oncol* 1986;4(5):716–721.

278. Borenstein SH, Gerstle T, Malkin D, et al. The effects of prebiopsy corticosteroid treatment on the diagnosis of mediastinal lymphoma. *J Pediatr Surg* 2000;35(6):973–976.

279. Carr R, Barrington SF, Madan B, et al. Detection of lymphoma in bone marrow by whole-body positron emission tomography. *Blood* 1998;91(9):3340.

280. Pelosi E, Penna D, Douroukas A, et al. Bone marrow disease detection with FDG-PET/CT and bone marrow biopsy during the staging of malignant lymphoma: results from a large multicentre study. *Q J Nucl Med Mol Imaging* 2011;55(4):469.

281. Khan AB, Barrington SF, Mikhaeel NG, et al. PET-CT staging of DLBCL accurately identifies and provides new insight into the clinical significance of bone marrow involvement. *Blood* 2013;122(1):61.

282. Barrington SF, Mikhaeel NG, Kostakoglu L, et al. Role of imaging in the staging and response assessment of lymphoma: consensus of the International Conference on Malignant Lymphomas Imaging Working Group. *J Clin Oncol* 2014;32(27):3048–3058.

283. Furth C, Steffen IG, Amthauer H, et al. Early and late therapy response assessment with [18F]fluorodeoxyglucose positron emission tomography in pediatric Hodgkin's lymphoma: analysis of a prospective multicenter trial. *J Clin Oncol* 2009;27(26):4385–4391.

284. Rosolen A, Perkins SL, Pinkerton CR, et al. Revised international pediatric non-Hodgkin lymphoma staging system. *J Clin Oncol* 2015;33(18):2112–2118.

285. Murphy SB, Fairclough DL, Hutchison RE, et al. Non-Hodgkin's lymphomas of childhood: an analysis of the histology, staging, and response to treatment of 338 cases at a single institution. *J Clin Oncol* 1989;7(2):186–193.

286. Poirel HA, Cairo MS, Heerema NA, et al. Specific cytogenetic abnormalities are associated with a significantly inferior outcome in children and adolescents with mature B-cell non-Hodgkin's lymphoma: results of the FAB LMB 96 international study. *Leukemia* 2009;23(2):323–331.

287. Lara M, Marta P, Valentino C, et al. Prognostic role of minimal residual disease in mature B-cell acute lymphoblastic leukemia of childhood. *J Clin Oncol* 2007;25(33):5254–5261.

288. Lara M, Marta P, Emanuele SGdA, et al. Minimal disseminated disease in high-risk Burkitt's lymphoma identifies patients with different prognosis. *J Clin Oncol* 2011;29(13):1779–1784.

289. Patte C, Auperin A, Gerrard M, et al. Results of the randomized international FAB/LMB96 trial for intermediate risk B-cell non-Hodgkin lymphoma in children and adolescents: it is possible to reduce treatment for the early responding patients. *Blood* 2007;109(7):2773–2780.

290. Sandlund JT, Guillerman RP, Perkins SL, et al. International pediatric non-Hodgkin lymphoma response criteria. *J Clin Oncol* 2015;33(18):2106–2111.

291. Gerrard M, Cairo MS, Weston C, et al. Excellent survival following two courses of COPAD chemotherapy in children and adolescents with resected localized B-cell non-Hodgkin's lymphoma: results of the FAB/LMB 96 international study. *Br J Haematol* 2008;141(6):840–847.

292. Woessmann W, Seidemann K, Mann G, et al. The impact of the methotrexate administration schedule and dose in the treatment of children and adolescents with B-cell neoplasms: a report of the BFM Group Study NHL-BFM95. *Blood* 2005;105(3):948–958.

293. Brugieres L, Deley MC, Pacquement H, et al. CD30(+) anaplastic large-cell lymphoma in children: analysis of 82 patients enrolled in two consecutive studies of the French Society of Pediatric Oncology. *Blood* 1998;92(10):3591–3598.

294. Pillon M, Piglione M, Garaventa A, et al. Long-term results of AIEOP LNH-92 protocol for the treatment of pediatric lymphoblastic lymphoma: a report of the Italian Association of pediatric hematology and oncology. *Pediatr Blood Cancer* 2009;53(6):953–959.

295. Patte C, Auperin A, Michon J, et al. The Societe Francaise d'Oncologie Pediatrique LMB89 protocol: highly effective multiagent chemotherapy tailored to the tumor burden and initial response in 561 unselected children with B-cell lymphomas and L3 leukemia. *Blood* 2001;97(11):3370–3379.

296. Goldman S, Smith L, Anderson JR, et al. Rituximab and FAB/LMB 96 chemotherapy in children with stage III/IV B-cell non-Hodgkin lymphoma: a Children's Oncology Group report. *Leukemia* 2013;27(5):1174–1177.

297. Meinhardt A, Burkhardt B, Zimmermann M, et al. Phase II window study on rituximab in newly diagnosed pediatric mature B-cell non-Hodgkin's lymphoma and Burkitt leukemia. *J Clin Oncol* 2010;28(19):3115–3121.

298. Cairo MS, Gerrard M, Sposto R, et al. Results of a randomized international study of high-risk central nervous system B non-Hodgkin lymphoma and B acute lymphoblastic leukemia in children and adolescents. *Blood* 2007;109(7):2736–2743.

299. Burkhardt B, Woessmann W, Zimmermann M, et al. Impact of cranial radiotherapy on central nervous system prophylaxis in children and adolescents with central nervous system–negative stage III or IV lymphoblastic lymphoma. *J Clin Oncol* 2006;24(3):491–499.

300. Asselin BL, Devidas M, Wang C, et al. Effectiveness of high-dose methotrexate in T-cell lymphoblastic leukemia and advanced-stage lymphoblastic lymphoma: a randomized study by the Children's Oncology Group (POG 9404). *Blood* 2011;118(4):874–883.

301. Le Deley M-C, Rosolen A, Williams DM, et al. Vinblastine in children and adolescents with high-risk anaplastic large-cell lymphoma: results of the randomized ALCL99-vinblastine trial. *J Clin Oncol* 2010;28(25):3987–3993.

302. Brugières L, Le Deley M-C, Rosolen A, et al. Impact of the methotrexate administration dose on the need for intrathecal treatment in children and adolescents with anaplastic large-cell lymphoma: results of a randomized trial of the EICNHL Group. *J Clin Oncol* 2009;27(6):897–903.

303. Laver JH, Kraveka JM, Hutchison RE, et al. Advanced-stage large-cell lymphoma in children and adolescents: results of a randomized trial incorporating intermediate-dose methotrexate and high-dose cytarabine in the maintenance phase of the APO regimen: a Pediatric Oncology Group phase III trial. *J Clin Oncol* 2005;23(3):541–547.

304. Laver JH, Mahmoud H, Pick TE, et al. Results of a randomized phase III trial in children and adolescents with advanced stage diffuse large cell non Hodgkin's lymphoma: a Pediatric Oncology Group study. *Leuk Lymphoma* 2001;42(3):399–405.

305. Link MP, Shuster JJ, Donaldson SS, et al. Treatment of children and young adults with early-stage non-Hodgkin's lymphoma. *N Engl J Med* 1997;337(18):1259–1266.

306. Meadows AT, Sposto R, Jenkin RD, et al. Similar efficacy of 6 and 18 months of therapy with four drugs (COMP) for localized non-Hodgkin's lymphoma of children: a report from the Children's Cancer Study Group. *J Clin Oncol* 1989;7(1):92–99.

307. Anderson JR, Jenkin RD, Wilson JF, et al. Long-term follow-up of patients treated with COMP or LSA2L2 therapy for childhood non-Hodgkin's lymphoma: a report of CCG-551 from the Childrens Cancer Group. *J Clin Oncol* 1993;11(6):1024–1032.
308. Brecher ML, Schwenn MR, Coppes MJ, et al. Fractionated cyclophosphamide and back to back high dose methotrexate and cytosine arabinoside improves outcome in patients with stage III high grade small non-cleaved cell lymphomas (SNCCL): a randomized trial of the Pediatric Oncology Group. *Med Pediatr Oncol* 1997;29(6):526–533.
309. Reiter A, Schrappe M, Tiemann M, et al. Improved treatment results in childhood B-cell neoplasms with tailored intensification of therapy: a report of the Berlin-Frankfurt-Münster Group Trial NHL-BFM 90. *Blood* 1999;94(10):3294–3306.
310. Cairo MS, Sposto R, Perkins SL, et al. Burkitts and Burkitt-like lymphoma in children and adolescents: a review of the Childrens Cancer Group Experience. *Br J Haematol* 2003;120(4):660–670.
311. Jaume M, Daniel AF, Jing Q, et al. Lymphoblastic lymphoma of childhood and the LSA2-L2 protocol: the 30-year experience at Memorial-Sloan-Kettering Cancer Center. *Cancer* 2003;98(6):1283–1291.
312. Reiter A, Schrappe M, Parwaresch R, et al. Non-Hodgkin's lymphomas of childhood and adolescence: results of a treatment stratified for biologic subtypes and stage—a report of the Berlin-Frankfurt-Münster Group. *J Clin Oncol* 1995;13(2):359–372.
313. Reiter A, Schrappe M, Ludwig WD, et al. Intensive ALL-type therapy without local radiotherapy provides a 90% event-free survival for children with T-cell lymphoblastic lymphoma: a BFM group report. *Blood* 2000;95(2):416.
314. Goldberg JM, Silverman LB, Levy DE, et al. Childhood T-cell acute lymphoblastic leukemia: the Dana-Farber Cancer Institute acute lymphoblastic leukemia consortium experience. *J Clin Oncol* 2003;21(19):3616–3622.
315. Amylon MD, Shuster J, Pullen J, et al. Intensive high-dose asparaginase consolidation improves survival for pediatric patients with T cell acute lymphoblastic leukemia and advanced stage lymphoblastic lymphoma: a Pediatric Oncology Group study. *Leukemia* 1999;13(3):335–342.
316. Abromowitch M, Sposto R, Perkins S, et al. Shortened intensified multi-agent chemotherapy and non-cross resistant maintenance therapy for advanced lymphoblastic lymphoma in children and adolescents: report from the Childrens Oncology Group. *Br J Haematol* 2008;143(2):261–267.
317. Reiter A, Schrappe M, Tiemann M, et al. Successful treatment strategy for Ki-1 anaplastic large-cell lymphoma of childhood: a prospective analysis of 62 patients enrolled in three consecutive Berlin-Frankfurt-Munster group studies. *J Clin Oncol* 1994;12(5):899–908.
318. Sposto R, Meadows AT, Chilcote RR, et al. Comparison of long-term outcome of children and adolescents with disseminated non-lymphoblastic non-Hodgkin lymphoma treated with COMP or daunomycin-COMP: a report from the Children's Cancer Group. *Med Pediatr Oncol* 2001;37(5):432–441.
319. Brugières L, Deley MC, Pacquement H, et al. CD30(+) anaplastic large-cell lymphoma in children: analysis of 82 patients enrolled in two consecutive studies of the French Society of Pediatric Oncology. *Blood* 1998;92(10):3591–3598.
320. Cairo MS, Krailo MD, Morse M, et al. Long-term follow-up of short intensive multiagent chemotherapy without high-dose methotrexate ('Orange') in children with advanced non-lymphoblastic non-Hodgkin's lymphoma: a Children's Cancer Group Report. *Leukemia* 2002;16(4):594.
321. Seidemann K, Tiemann M, Schrappe M, et al. Short-pulse B-non-Hodgkin lymphoma-type chemotherapy is efficacious treatment for pediatric anaplastic large cell lymphoma: a report of the Berlin-Frankfurt-Münster Group Trial NHL-BFM 90. *Blood* 2001;97(12):3699–3706.
322. Patte C, Philip T, Rodary C, et al. High survival rate in advanced-stage B-cell lymphomas and leukemias without CNS involvement with a short intensive polychemotherapy: results from the French Pediatric Oncology Society of a randomized trial of 216 children. *J Clin Oncol* 1991;9(1):123–132.
323. Tsurusawa M, Mori T, Kikuchi A, et al. Improved treatment results of children with B-cell non-Hodgkin lymphoma: a report from the Japanese Pediatric Leukemia/Lymphoma Study Group B-NHL03 study. *Pediatr Blood Cancer* 2014;61(7):1215–1221.
324. Traoré F, Coze C, Atteby JJ, et al. Cyclophosphamide monotherapy in children with Burkitt lymphoma: a study from the French–African Pediatric Oncology Group (GFAOP). *Pediatr Blood Cancer* 2011;56(1):70–76.
325. Harif M, Barsaoui S, Benchekroun S, et al. Treatment of B-cell lymphoma with LMB modified protocols in Africa—report of the French-African Pediatric Oncology Group (GFAOP). *Pediatr Blood Cancer* 2008;50(6):1138–1142.
326. Dalle JH, Mechinaud F, Michon J, et al. Testicular disease in childhood B-cell non-Hodgkin's lymphoma: the French Society of Pediatric Oncology experience. *J Clin Oncol* 2001;19(9):2397.
327. Barth MJ, Goldman S, Smith L, et al. Rituximab pharmacokinetics in children and adolescents with de novo intermediate and advanced mature B-cell lymphoma/leukaemia: a Children's Oncology Group report. *Br J Haematol* 2013;162(5):678–683.
328. Combination Chemotherapy With or Without Rituximab in Treating Younger Patients With Stage III-IV Non-Hodgkin Lymphoma or B-Cell Acute Leukemia. (2012). Retrieved from http://clinicaltrials.gov/ct2(Identification No. HYPERLINK "http://asheducationbook.hematologylibrary.org/external-ref?link_type=CLINTRIALGOV&access_num=NCT01595048" NCT01595048)
329. Gerrard M, Waxman IM, Sposto R, et al. Outcome and pathologic classification of children and adolescents with mediastinal large B-cell lymphoma treated with FAB/LMB96 mature B-NHL therapy. *Blood* 2013;121(2):278–285.
330. Dunleavy K, Pittaluga S, Maeda LS, et al. Dose-adjusted EPOCH-rituximab therapy in primary mediastinal B-cell lymphoma. *N Engl J Med* 2013;368(15):1408.
331. Intergroup Trial for Children or Adolescents With Primary Mediastinal Large B-Cell Lymphoma: DA-EPOCH-Rituximab Evaluation. (2012). Retrieved from http://clinicaltrials.gov/ct2(Identification No. NCT01516567)
332. Ducassou S, Ferlay C, Bergeron C, et al. Clinical presentation, evolution, and prognosis of precursor B-cell lymphoblastic lymphoma in trials LMT96, EORTC 58881, and EORTC 58951. *Br J Haematol* 2011;152(4):441–451.
333. Termuhlen AM, Smith LM, Perkins SL, et al. Disseminated lymphoblastic lymphoma in children and adolescents: results of the COG A5971 trial: a report from the Children's Oncology Group. *Br J Haematol* 2013;162(6):792–801.
334. Patte C, Kalifa C, Flamant F, et al. Results of the LMT81 protocol, a modified LSA2L2 protocol with high dose methotrexate, on 84 children with non-B-cell (lymphoblastic) lymphoma. *Med Pediatr Oncol* 1992;20(2):105–113.
335. Uyttebroeck A, Suciu S, Laureys G, et al. Treatment of childhood T-cell lymphoblastic lymphoma according to the strategy for acute lymphoblastic leukaemia, without radiotherapy: long term results of the EORTC CLG 58881 trial. *Eur J Cancer* 2008;44(6):840–846.
336. Tubergen DG, Krailo MD, Meadows AT, et al. Comparison of treatment regimens for pediatric lymphoblastic non-Hodgkin's lymphoma: a Childrens Cancer Group study. *J Clin Oncol* 1995;13(6):1368–1376.
337. Bergeron C, Cline S, Pacquement H, et al. Childhood T cell lymphoblastic lymphoma (TLL) results of the SFOP LMT96 strategy. *Pediatr Blood Cancer* 2006;46(7):867.
338. Reiter A, Burkhardt B, Zimmermann M, et al. Results of the European intergroup trial EURO-LB02 on lymphoblastic lymphoma (LBL) in children/adolescents. *Br J Haematol* 2012;159:38.
339. Michel D, Stefan S, Alina F, et al. Comparison of Escherichia coli-asparaginase with Erwinia-asparaginase in the treatment of childhood lymphoid malignancies: results of a randomized European Organisation for Research and Treatment of Cancer-Children's Leukemia Group phase 3 trial. *Blood* 2002;99(8):2734–2739.
340. Elaine C-S, John TS, Sherrie LP, et al. Minimal disseminated disease in childhood T-cell lymphoblastic lymphoma: a report from the children's oncology group. *J Clin Oncol* 2009;27(21):3533–3539.
341. Risk-Adapted Chemotherapy in Treating Younger Patients With Newly Diagnosed Standard-Risk Acute Lymphoblastic Leukemia or Localized B-Lineage Lymphoblastic Lymphoma(2010). Retrieved from http://clinicaltrials.gov/ct2(Identification No. HYPERLINK "https://clinicaltrials.gov/show/NCT01190930"NCT01190930)
342. Williams DM, Hobson R, Imeson J, et al. Anaplastic large cell lymphoma in childhood: analysis of 72 patients treated on The United Kingdom Children's Cancer Study Group chemotherapy regimens. *Br J Haematol* 2002;117(4):812–820.
343. Rosolen A, Pillon M, Garaventa A, et al. Anaplastic large cell lymphoma treated with a leukemia-like therapy—report of the Italian Association of Pediatric Hematology and Oncology (AIEOP) LNH-92 protocol. *Cancer* 2005;104(10):2133–2140.
344. Brugières L, Quartier P, Le Deley M, et al. Relapses of childhood anaplastic large-cell lymphoma: treatment results in a series of 41 children—a report from the French Society of Pediatric Oncology. *Ann Oncol* 2000;11(1):53–58.
345. Laurence B, Helene P, Marie-Cecile Le D, et al. Single-drug vinblastine as salvage treatment for refractory or relapsed anaplastic large-cell lymphoma: a report from the French Society of Pediatric Oncology. *J Clin Oncol* 2009;27(30):5056–5061.
346. Woessmann W, Zimmermann M, Lenhard M, et al. Relapsed or refractory anaplastic large-cell lymphoma in children and adolescents after Berlin-Frankfurt-Muenster (BFM)–type first-line therapy: a BFM-group study. *J Clin Oncol* 2011;29(22):3065–3071.
347. Woessmann W, Brugires L, Rosolen A, et al. Risk-adapted therapy for patients with relapsed or refractory ALCL-interim-results of the prospective EICNHL-Trial ALCL-relapse. *Br J Haematol* 2012;159:41.
348. Kaveri S, Jonathan JS, Sarah SD, et al. Treatment of localized primary non-Hodgkin's lymphoma of bone in children: a pediatric oncology group study. *J Clin Oncol* 1999;17(2):456.
349. Sandlund JT, Pui CH, Zhou Y, et al. Effective treatment of advanced-stage childhood lymphoblastic lymphoma without prophylactic cranial irradiation: results of St Jude NHL13 study. *Leukemia* 2009;23(6):1127–1130.
350. Julio CB, Meenakshi D, Stephen JL, et al. Isolated CNS relapse of acute lymphoblastic leukemia treated with intensive systemic chemotherapy and delayed CNS radiation: a pediatric oncology group study. *J Clin Oncol* 2006;24(19):3142–3149.
351. Griffin TC, Weitzman S, Weinstein H, et al. A study of rituximab and ifosfamide, carboplatin, and etoposide chemotherapy in children with recurrent/refractory B-cell (CD20+) non-Hodgkin lymphoma and mature B-cell acute lymphoblastic leukemia: a report from the Children's Oncology Group. *Pediatr Blood Cancer* 2009;52(2):177–181.
352. Vassilakopoulos TP, Pangalis GA, Katsigiannis A, et al. Rituximab, cyclophosphamide, doxorubicin, vincristine, and prednisone with or without radiotherapy in primary mediastinal large B-cell lymphoma: the emerging standard of care. *Oncologist* 2012;17(2):239–249.
353. Giri S, Bhatt VR, Pathak R, et al. Role of radiation therapy in primary mediastinal large B-cell lymphoma in rituximab era: a US population-based analysis. *Am J Hematol* 2015;90(11):1052–1054.
354. Haas RLM, Poortmans P, de Jong D, et al. Effective palliation by low dose local radiotherapy for recurrent and/or chemotherapy refractory non-follicular lymphoma patients. *Eur J Cancer* 2005;41(12):1724–1730.
355. Ingram LC, Fairclough DL, Furman WL, et al. Cranial nerve palsy in childhood acute lymphoblastic leukemia and non-Hodgkin's lymphoma. *Cancer* 1991;67(9):2262–2268.
356. Pro B, Advani R, Brice P, et al. Brentuximab vedotin (SGN-35) in patients with relapsed or refractory systemic anaplastic large-cell lymphoma: results of a phase II study. *J Clin Oncol* 2012;30(18):2190–2196.
357. Mosse YP, Lim MS, Voss SD, et al. Safety and activity of crizotinib for paediatric patients with refractory solid tumours or anaplastic large-cell lymphoma: a Children's Oncology Group phase 1 consortium study. *Lancet Oncol* 2013;14(6):472–480.
358. Zinzani PL, Ribrag V, Moskowitz CH, et al. Safety and tolerability of pembrolizumab in patients with relapsed/refractory primary mediastinal large B-cell lymphoma. *Blood* 2017;130(3):267–270.

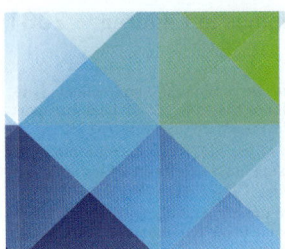

CHAPTER 94

Unusual Tumors in Children

Zachary Buchwald and Natia Esiashvili

INTRODUCTION

Many rare childhood tumors are comparable to those that occur in the adult population and require the similar therapeutic strategy, with particular attention given to late sequelae. There are groups of rare tumors, however, diagnosed predominantly in children and require specific treatment strategies including radiotherapy.

NASOPHARYNGEAL CARCINOMA IN CHILDHOOD

Nasopharyngeal carcinoma (NPC) is a rare malignant tumor in childhood and adolescence (<1% of pediatric malignancies). The frequency differs greatly by geographic area: 1 case per 100,000 in Europe, the United States, and Australia; 10 per 100,000 in North Africa; and 80 per 100,000 in South China, Malaysia, and Greenland. Interestingly, although the absolute numbers are lower in nonendemic countries (United States, Turkey, Israel), childhood NPC is 6% to 18% of all cases compared to <1% to 2% in endemic countries/regions (southern China, Southeast Asia, Mediterranean basin).[1] A study from 2016 found that NPC in children has different demographic distribution relative to adults and is associated with low socioeconomic status, rural location, and more advanced disease at presentation.[2] The World Health Organization formerly divided NPC into three distinct classification groups: type I, keratinizing squamous cell carcinoma; type II, nonkeratinizing carcinoma; and type III, undifferentiated carcinoma. A recent change in terminology instead divides them into two broad categories: keratinizing and nonkeratinizing with the latter subdivided into differentiated and undifferentiated. Most pediatric NPC cases are type III (undifferentiated).[3] As in older patients, Epstein-Barr virus is associated with this type of NPC in addition to certain human leukocyte antigen (HLA) haplotypes/alleles (A2 Bsin2, Aw19, Bw46, and B17). The virus is found in the tumor cells and not in the surrounding lymphocytes. Antibody and antigen titers are useful for both diagnosis and follow-up (Table 94.1).[4] The association between dietary factors and NPC has been suspected in China and seems to be confirmed in a case–control study published by Jia et al.[5]

Clinical Presentation

The mean age at presentation is 13 years, and it has a male (1.8:1) and black predominance.[6] Typically, the initial presentation is a painless mass in the upper neck. There can be associated nasal obstruction, epistaxis, otitis, and neck and facial pain. The tumor usually originates in the fossa of Rosenmüller, followed early on by locoregional extension, including extensive pharyngeal involvement and often bone, lung, and cervical lymph node metastases.

On clinical examination, bilateral lymphadenopathy and cranial nerve palsies are found; a nasopharyngeal mass can be seen by direct or indirect nasopharyngoscopy, and sometimes, a protruding mass can be seen in the oral cavity.

The diagnostic workup must include a cranial and neck computed tomography (CT) scan with contrast, magnetic resonance imaging (MRI), and a positron emission tomography-computed tomography (PET-CT). Pathologic confirmation is obtained by biopsy. Commonly used staging systems are the tumor-node-metastasis (TNM)/American Joint Committee on Cancer (AJCC), Kyoto, and Ho classifications. The Ho and Kyoto systems are based on topographic extension; the more commonly used TNM/AJCC classification is based on tumor volume and CT information.[7]

Treatment

In adult NPC, concomitant radiotherapy (RT) and chemotherapy (cisplatin and 5-fluorouracil) are the standard of care.[8,9] Because of the scarcity of pediatric NPC cases, it is difficult to perform randomized studies in this age group. Based on adult trials, multimodality treatment is generally accepted as the standard of care for children for stage II or greater with potentially RT alone for stage I.[10] Usually, two courses of 5-fluorouracil/cis-diamminedichloroplatinum II (cisplatin) are given on weeks 1 and 5 of RT, whereas others prefer the standard adult regimen of three cycle.[11,12] Others have used neoadjuvant cisplatin-based chemotherapy, followed by radiation or chemoradiotherapy.[13] A recent phase II study comparing two cisplatin-based induction regimens (docetaxel plus cisplatin and 5-fluorouracil vs. cisplatin and 5-fluorouracil) did not demonstrate a difference in toxicity or efficacy.[14]

Radiation Therapy

A dose–response relationship for local control with a threshold at 60 Gy has been reported in a number of series.[11,15,16] However, Habrand et al.[17] reported interesting results with lower doses of radiation therapy (50 Gy) in patients with a good response to chemotherapy. These results are in accordance with the reports of Polychronopoulou et al.[18] and Orbach et al.[19] In this series, 70% of children achieved local control with doses of <60 Gy (50% received only 52 Gy). A study from St. Jude also reported a better outcome for patients receiving cisplatin and doses of radiation >50 Gy.[20] Techniques include three-dimensional (3D) dosimetry, customized blocking, and, if possible, MRI/CT scan image fusion for intensity-modulated radiotherapy (IMRT). Proton beam therapy is appropriate where available.

The target volume encompasses the tumor site and the neck (even in N0 disease) because of the severity of late

	IgG VCA	Ig EA	IgM VCA	IgA VCA	IgA EA	EBNA
TABLE 94.1 ANTIGEN AND ANTIBODY EPSTEIN-BARR VIRUS TITERS						
Naive patient	0	0	0	0	0	0
Immune patient	Mild	0	0	0	0	Mild
Burkitt lymphoma	Raised	Raised	0	0	0	Raised
AIDS	Very raised	Raised	0	0	0	0
NC	Very raised	Very raised	Mild	Raised	Raised	Very raised

AIDS, acquired immunodeficiency syndrome; EA, early antigen (active disease); EBNA, EBV-associated nuclear antigen (cellular immunity); Ig, immunoglobulin; NC, nasopharynx carcinoma; VCA, vision capsid antigen (immune status).

sequelae after standard techniques. The standard of care for radiotherapy is IMRT, if available.[20] A 2017 retrospective analysis comparing 2D-CRT to IMRT demonstrated that IMRT has improved overall survival with reduced grade 2 to 4 xerostomia and hearing loss.[21] High dose rate, pulsed low dose rate, or conventional low dose rate intraluminal brachytherapy is used for the boost at some institutions. For some physicians, hyperfractionated radiotherapy is believed to be standard of care. One publication examining hyperfractionated radiotherapy showed an increased rate of neurologic complication.[22] The overall survival for T1-T2 disease is 70% to 90% at 5-years. The survival for T3-T4 disease using combined modality is 50% to 60%. For advanced stage, innovative targeted therapies are being evaluated. These include induction of the lytic viral cycle with ganciclovir, gene therapy, antitumor vaccination against the viral protein LMP2, and more recently other immunomodulatory approaches including the adoptive transfer of EBV-specific T cells.[23-25]

Late Effects

Xerostomia is the main side effect of treatment, followed by dental caries, trismus, muscular atrophy, nerve palsies, and endocrine dysfunction resulting from pituitary irradiation. Significant auditory late toxicity and sporadic cases of visual morbidity, secondary to radiotherapy with or without cisplatin-based chemotherapy, have been reported.[26] The St. Jude retrospective analysis reported a rate of 8.5% of subsequent malignancies 8.6 to 27 years after treatment.[20]

New techniques such as IMRT have been shown to decrease the late sequelae including xerostomia.[21]

OTHER HEAD AND NECK TUMORS

Carcinoma of the Oropharynx and Salivary Glands

Schwaab et al.[27] reported the largest pediatric series, with only 2% squamous cell carcinoma among 380 head and neck tumors. The more frequent sites of disease are the tongue, lip, tonsil, palate, and salivary glands. Cigarette smoking or use of smokeless tobacco has been shown to be an etiologic factors for adolescent tongue carcinoma.[28] For other sites, passive smoking, poor oral hygiene, or genetic predispositions (xeroderma pigmentosum or retinoblastoma) have been suggested.

Special attention must be paid to larynx carcinoma because some of the cases may develop from juvenile papillomatosis, a benign condition of the aerodigestive tract that may undergo malignant degeneration. Guidelines for surgery and radiation therapy are the same as those for adults. Combined chemotherapy and radiation can be attempted for organ conservation.[29] The node area to treat does not differ from adults and must follow the Gregoire definition.[30] Psychological support and rehabilitation programs are an essential part of the comprehensive treatment for children who undergo major surgical resection.

HPV-positive oropharyngeal cancer is not a significant problem in this age group as HPV exposure is associated with sexual activity. However, in one series, the HPV prevalence in the oral cavity/oropharynx of children was 1.9%.[31] This should help guide vaccine recommendations that may help reduce the incidence of HPV-positive disease in the future.

Esthesioneuroblastoma

Esthesioneuroblastoma is a malignant tumor arising from the olfactory nerve in the upper nasal cavity. Intracranial extension is common at the time of diagnosis. Esthesioneuroblastoma is mostly seen in patients in their 20s or 60s. Positive S100 and neuron-specific enolase stains combined with negative epithelial markers strongly suggest a neurogenic origin.[32] The clinical presentation includes nasal obstruction, loss of smell, epistaxis, and, sometimes, enlarged cervical lymph nodes.

Bony structures are often involved, as well as the ethmoid and maxillary sinuses. The most commonly used staging/grouping system is by Kadish et al.[32] and is based on degree of local tumor extension. Tumors are also graded according to the Hyams system.[33]

There is no universally agreed-upon standard of care. For localized disease, tumors are resected, if possible. Because of a high risk of recurrence, postoperative radiotherapy is usually offered and has been shown to reduce recurrence risk. Earlier studies have shown local control can be obtained in >75% of cases.[34] Eich et al.[35] and Broich et al.[36] recommend combined surgery and radiotherapy in all stages. Demiroz et al.[37] reviewed 26 patients treated between 1995 and 2007. The relapse rate for patients treated with surgery alone was 29% versus 0% for those treated by surgery and postoperative radiotherapy. The recommended dose is 50 to 60 Gy.

More recently, for previously untreated disease, Hollen et al. showed local control rates at 5 years of 79%. The age range for these 26 patients was 3 to 82 years.[38] One large retrospective study from China examined long-term outcomes for 113 patients from 1979 to 2014. The majority of patients were Kadish stage C, and they were treated with multimodality therapy and different sequencing including 51 who received preoperative radiotherapy. The local control for preoperative radiotherapy followed by surgery was 91% at 5-years.[39]

Elective neck irradiation or dissection is not typically advocated because <10% of early-stage cases exhibit nodal involvement. However, node metastases are frequent if the tumor extends beyond the paranasal sinuses, and Hollen et al.[38] show that elective nodal irradiation reduces the risk of regional relapse for stage B and C disease. Therefore, lymph node dissection or prophylactic irradiation may be considered under certain clinical circumstances. Chemotherapy has yet to be accepted as part of routine first-line treatment for early-stage disease, although responses to chemotherapy have been reported.[40] It can reduce tumor volume prior to surgery or radiotherapy and can be used for palliative purposes in advanced cases. Promising results with cyclophosphamide, doxorubicin, vincristine, cis-platinum, and etoposide, combined with radiotherapy and stem cell support, have been reported by Mishima et al.[41] They obtained 8 complete responses in 12 Kadish stage C and D patients. Neoadjuvant concurrent chemoradiotherapy as preoperative treatment for locally advanced esthesioneuroblastoma has been reported by Sohrabi et al.[42] with very promising results.

Recently, data evaluating the role of proton therapy have begun to accumulate. Lucas et al. retrospectively evaluated eight patients (4 to 21 years old), the majority of whom were treated with different surgery, chemotherapy, and radiotherapy sequencing; however, all received proton treatment (59.4 to 70 GyE). The results are encouraging with a 5-year overall survival of 87.5% and local control of 100% with acceptable toxicities.[43]

Juvenile Nasopharyngeal Angiofibroma

Juvenile nasopharyngeal angiofibroma (JNA) is a malignant vascular tumor most often arising from the posterior lateral wall of the nasopharynx in adolescent males. The lesion tends to extend into the nasal cavities, maxillary and sphenoid sinuses, orbit, and infratemporal fossa. Several classifications have been proposed, but the classification of Radkowski et al.[44] appears to be the most appropriate, at least for surgical purposes (Table 94.2). Common symptoms are epistaxis, cheek swelling, a visible orbital tumor, and cranial nerve palsies. JNA is more frequent in familial adenomatous polyposis patients. A mutation in the cluster region of the APC gene was reported in several studies, suggesting that JNA is perhaps a familial adenomatous polyposis tumor.[45,46]

Treatment consists of surgery for small lesions, often with preoperative embolization or hormone therapy. Surgery carries a risk of significant operative blood loss. For localized

TABLE 94.2 STAGING CLASSIFICATION FOR JUVENILE NASOPHARYNGEAL ANGIOFIBROMA

Stage	Description
Ia	Limited to the nose and/or nasopharynx
Ib	Same as Ia, but with extension into one or more paranasal sinuses
IIa	Minimal extension through the sphenopalatine foramen, into and including a minimal part of the medialmost part of pterygomaxillary fossa
IIb	Full occupation of the pterygomaxillary fossa, displacing the posterior wall of the maxillary antrum forward; lateral and/or anterior displacement of branches of the maxillary artery; superior extension may occur, eroding orbital bones
IIc	Extension through the pterygomaxillary fossa into the cheek and temporal fossa or posterior to the pterygoid plates
IIIa	Erosion of the skull base with minimal intracranial extension
IIIb	Erosion of the skull base with extensive intracranial extension with or without cavernous sinus invasion

Based on the classification of Radkowski D, McGill T, Healy GB, et al. Angiofibroma. Changes in staging and treatment. *Arch Otolaryngol Head Neck Surg* 1996;122:122–129.

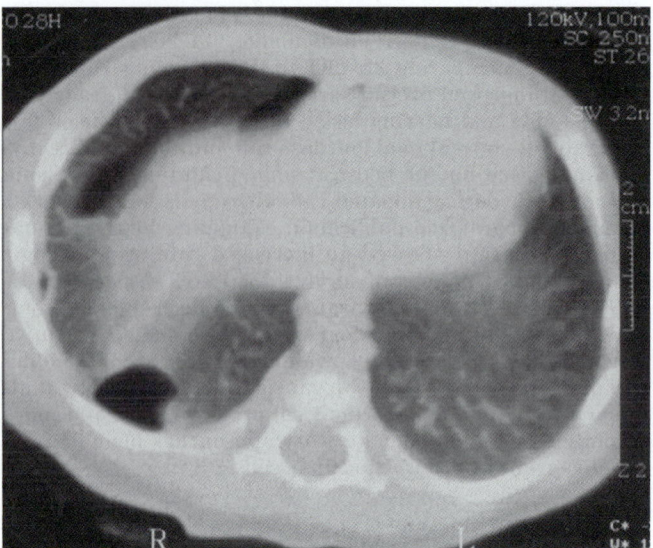

FIGURE 94.1. Pleuropneumoblastoma in a 1-year-old girl.

JNA, the cure rate obtained by surgery alone can be as high as 90%. Resection with negative margins is required because inadequate margins will result in a high local failure rate.[47] Minimally invasive endoscopic resection has been proposed for early-stage JNA. Lesions limited to the nasal cavity and/or nasopharynx or lesions with minimal extension through the sphenopalatine foramen are suitable for this procedure. A craniofacial approach is recommended for lesions extending into the pterygoid plates.[48,49] For tumors with intracranial extension, there are recent data demonstrating near-total tumor resections with good outcomes.[50] Radiation therapy is used either as adjuvant treatment or as sole treatment in locally advanced lesions extending into unresectable areas. IMRT have been successfully applied in unresectable and recurrent tumors.[51] A wide range of doses have been used, but there is no evidence that doses of >36 Gy are advantageous. Chakraborty et al.[52] treated eight patients with IMRT with a median dose of 39 Gy. The local control rate was 87% with a mean follow-up of 2 years. Mallick et al.[53] looked at long-term outcomes for patients treated with radiotherapy for refractory residual or unresectable disease from 1990 to 2012 with a median dose of 30 Gy and showed a 10-year progression-free survival of 70.7%. There is no role for cytotoxic chemotherapy in JNA. The role of antiangiogenic agents is speculative, although a recent complete molecular profile suggests other potential targets.[54]

LUNG CANCER

Bronchogenic Carcinoma

Pediatric bronchogenic carcinoma is extremely rare, and its management does not differ from that of adults. Most of the tumors occur during adolescence. Histology is more frequently undifferentiated adenocarcinoma or carcinoid tumors rather than squamous cell carcinoma.[55]

Of 230 cases of primary pulmonary neoplasms of childhood reviewed by Hartman and Shochat,[56] <25% were bronchogenic carcinoma. The survival rate was very similar to that of adults, stage for stage. Treatment strategies of these patients should be similar to adults.

Pleuropulmonary Blastoma

According to the International Pleuropulmonary Blastoma (PPB) Registry (IPBBR), there have been 425 confirmed cases of PPB. This tumor can occur from the neonatal period up to 12 years of age and is the most common primary malignancy of the lung in childhood.[57] PPB was often mixed with pulmonary blastoma until it was accepted that PPB is purely a pediatric tumor. The main histologic difference between pulmonary blastoma and PPB is the absence of epithelial carcinomatous components in PPB; PPB consists of mesenchymal stroma only. The tumor usually begins in pulmonary tissue, but it can also originate in the pleura or mediastinum.[58] According to the Dehner et al.[59] classification, three pathologic features can occur: cystic (type I), mixed (type II), and solid (type III). According to the IPPBR, the 5-year overall survival rates are 91%, 71%, and 53% for types I, II, and III, respectively, with the PPB type shown to be strongest predictor of outcome.[60,61] A germ-line mutation in DICER1 is the known cause of the majority of PPB cases,[62] and Messinger et al. concluded that surveillance of DICER1 carriers may be reasonable to detect PPB before it progresses. Some reports described PPB association with a preexisting pulmonary cyst.[63] It is unclear whether PPB arises in preexisting malformation or whether PPB induces cystic lesion formation. The report from the IPPBR showed that great vessel or cardiac extension is present at diagnosis in 3% of cases.[64]

Clinically, PPB exhibits no specific symptoms. The usual presentation is cough, thoracic pain, and fever. Respiratory impairment is unusual. Radiologic findings depend on the extent of the cystic component (Fig. 94.1). The standard treatment is surgery alone with chemotherapy included and radiotherapy used in a minority of cases.

Priest et al.[57] reported an only 8% survival rate at 5 years among 50 patients[65]; however, large cohorts described earlier showed superior outcomes. Multimodal therapy with surgery followed by chemotherapy and radiotherapy (10.5 Gy) has been reported[66]; however, the IPPBR study examining the largest patient cohort demonstrated no benefit from adjuvant radiotherapy.[61] The value of chemotherapy is somewhat controversial for type I PPB. Because of higher metastatic potential, multiagent combinations such as actinomycin D, cyclophosphamide, cisplatin, etoposide, doxorubicin, and vincristine have been used in type II and III PPB.[58,67–70] Long-term survival can be achieved for patients treated with surgery and chemotherapy; however, the optimal combination of chemotherapy drugs or their direct impact on outcomes is less clear.

BREAST TUMORS

Malignant breast tumors account for <1% of all childhood cancers and <0.1% of all breast cancers.[71–74]

A review of adolescents seen at the MD Anderson Cancer Center during a 40-year period identified breast cancer in 16 patients <20 years of age. Ten patients had primary adenocarcinoma of the breast, four had cystosarcoma phyllodes, and two had breast metastases from other primary tumors. Four of the 16 patients had a family history of breast disease.[75] Roisman et al.[76] reported seven female patients, ages 14 to 17 years, who were treated in various hospitals in Israel for malignancy of the breast between 1967 and 1989. There were two cases of undifferentiated carcinoma with positive axillary lymph nodes, two cases of cystosarcoma phyllodes, one case of rhabdomyosarcoma, and two cases of malignant lymphoma, one of them Burkitt type. Umanah et al.[77] reported 1 case (1.2%) of an invasive ductal carcinoma among 84 breast tumor materials from patients aged 10 to 19 years in a Nigerian city.

Ultrasonography is the most appropriate initial investigation in any adolescent patient with a breast mass because dense breast tissue adversely affects the quality of mammography.[78] MRI is recommended for diagnosing breast cancer when conventional imaging is complex and indeterminate, especially in young patients with dense mammographies.

Juvenile secretory carcinoma of the breast is rare and was first described by McDivitt and Stewart[79] in 1966 in seven girls ages 3 to 15 years, all of whom had a benign clinical course. The tumor cells are characterized by abundant mucin- and mucopolysaccharide-containing materials.[80] Hormonal receptors are generally negative.[81] Local tumor excision alone may be adequate therapy, although simple and radical mastectomies have also been used.[81–83]

The histology and patterns of spread of adenocarcinoma of the breast in children and adolescents are similar to those in adults. Because most publications refer to isolated cases, neither a consensus of opinion nor specific guidelines exist with regard to treatment. In general, principles of clinical management established for adults should be adopted. Because recurrences were found in 25% of patients treated with excisional biopsy alone, this seems inadequate, and a simple mastectomy with axillary lymph node dissection should probably be performed.[84] Sentinel lymph node biopsy offers an approach to stage the axillary lymphatic drainage with a lower complication rate than formal dissection.[85] On the other hand, McDivitt and Stewart[79] believed that the disease tends to run a relatively favorable course and that radical therapy is therefore unnecessary. Hartman and Magrish[86] considered it important to avoid radiotherapy in young children, and instead, they recommended radical mastectomy.

Inflammatory carcinoma of the breast is extremely rare in children.[87,88]

There have been case reports of primary lymphoma, rhabdomyosarcoma, adenoid cystic carcinoma, radiation-induced sarcoma, and cystosarcoma phyllodes of the breast in children.[89–94]

Cystosarcoma phyllodes appears as a large breast mass; in 25% of cases, it is bilateral. Norris and Taylor[93] were the first to separate benign from malignant lesions in this disorder. The distinction is based on tumor size, stromal invasion, cellular atypia, degree of mitotic activity, focal calcification, and/or patterns of infiltration. Metastases occur in the lungs and bones. Lymph node metastases are extremely rare. Simple or wide local excision or simple mastectomy, with rare local recurrences, may adequately treat histologically benign lesions. In malignant cystosarcoma phyllodes, some authors recommend radical mastectomy with or without axillary lymph node dissection, and others are in favor of simple mastectomy.[95–99] The use of radiotherapy and postoperative chemotherapy in cystosarcoma phyllodes is controversial. These modalities should be reserved for locally advanced, palliative, and disseminated cases.

Rhabdomyosarcoma of the breast, either primary or metastatic, is rare. Billroth[100] reported the first case of primary rhabdomyosarcoma in a 16-year-old girl in 1860. In a series of 108 patients <20 years of age with this malignancy, Howarth et al.[101] reported 7 patients who had metastatic tumors to the breast with primary rhabdomyosarcoma located on an extremity or buttock. Six of the seven patients had alveolar histology. Rhabdomyosarcoma of the breast and other sarcomas of the breast are treated primarily by surgery followed, in most cases, by adjuvant radiation and chemotherapy.

Breast metastases in the pediatric age group include hepatocarcinoma, non-Hodgkin lymphoma, rhabdomyosarcoma Hodgkin disease, neuroblastoma, and adenocarcinoma.[102]

GASTROINTESTINAL TUMORS OF CHILDHOOD

Gastrointestinal tract malignant tumors are relatively rare in children. Carcinoid and hepatobiliary tumors are the most common.[103] Others are adenocarcinoma, lymphoma, and leiomyosarcoma. More common are benign tumors such as hamartoma, leiomyoma, neurofibroma, and hemangioma.

Esophagus

In most cases, an esophageal tumor is of epithelial origin, either squamous cell carcinoma or adenocarcinoma. Rarely, sarcomas may develop in the esophagus (leiomyosarcoma, carcinosarcoma, malignant schwannoma). Malignization of a chemical injury to the esophagus has been described.[104] Carcinoma of the esophagus may develop in association with Barrett esophagus and Cornelia de Lange syndrome.[105,106] McGill et al.[107] reported on a 16-year-old 3-year survivor of gastroesophageal junction cancer following resection and chemotherapy. The most common benign tumor of the esophagus in the pediatric age group is leiomyoma; desmoid and teratoma may also occur.[108–110] The management of esophageal cancer in the pediatric age group follows the same guidelines of treatment as in adults.[111]

Stomach

Adenocarcinoma is extremely rare representing <0.05% of pediatric gastrointestinal malignancies; it may arise in association with Peutz-Jeghers syndrome.[112] *Helicobacter pylori* infection also appears to be a risk factor.[113] In children, the prognosis is exceedingly poor with a median survival of 5 months.[114] A report from 2015 describes an *H. pylori*–positive antral tumor in a 16-year-old boy.[115]

Non-Hodgkin lymphoma is the most frequent gastric malignancy in the pediatric age group, followed by leiomyosarcoma and leiomyoblastoma.[116] The management of non-Hodgkin lymphoma follows the treatment guidelines of non-Hodgkin lymphoma in adults. There is also some evidence that primary gastric Burkitt lymphoma may also be associated with *H. pylori*.[117]

Leiomyosarcoma of the stomach is treated primarily with surgery. Postoperative irradiation is given to patients with a high risk of local recurrence (such as positive surgical margins or extension into the retroperitoneum).

As in the adult age group, subtotal gastrectomy with resection of associated lymph nodes is the treatment of choice for children with gastric carcinoma. No data are available on adjuvant radiation–chemotherapy in the pediatric age group. In adults, there are multiple randomized studies that show a benefit to adjuvant chemoradiotherapy compared to chemotherapy alone if the patient has a D2 dissection with positive lymph nodes.[118] A sandwich regimen of chemo, surgery, and chemotherapy has also demonstrated a progression-free and overall survival benefit.[119]

Radiotherapy guidelines are similar to those for the adult age group. At the time of radiotherapy planning, attention should be given to vital structures such as spinal cord, kidneys, small bowel, and liver. During treatment, acute side effects may occur, such as nausea, weight loss, and fatigue.

Several combination chemotherapy regimens have been used in the adjuvant setting and for locally advanced or metastatic gastric carcinoma. More than 20% of gastric cancers and up to 33% of gastroesophageal junction tumors show HER2 overexpression.[120] A phase II trial examining the role of trastuzumab demonstrated encouraging efficacy.[121]

Small Bowel

According to the Surveillance, Epidemiology, and End Results (SEER) data, the incidence of malignant small intestine tumors is low in patients <30 years of age.[122] The most common malignancy of the small intestine in children is non-Hodgkin lymphoma.[123] Sarcomas of the small bowel and carcinoids may also develop in children. Small intestine adenocarcinoma may develop spontaneously or in association with Peutz-Jeghers syndrome.[124]

Treatment guidelines are similar to those of the adult age group. Adjuvant radiation can be given after surgery for duodenal sarcomas or adenocarcinomas arising in the segment fixed to the retroperitoneum or for palliative purposes such as for pain or bleeding.

Colorectal Cancer

Carcinoma of the rectum and the large bowel is rare in children and adolescents. Recent SEER data for 2014 record a rate of around 0.4 per 100,000 for patients <20 years of age.[125] Young patients with long-standing ulcerative colitis have an increased risk of developing colorectal cancer.[126,127] Several genetic conditions may also be associated with colorectal carcinoma in childhood and adolescence. These include familial polyposis, Turcot syndrome, Oldfield syndrome, and Gardner syndrome.[120,122-126,128-134] The genetic events associated with the development of colorectal carcinoma in familial adenomatous polyposis syndrome, from epithelial proliferation, through formation of adenomas, to the sequential development of colorectal malignancy, have been described by Vogelstein et al.,[135] and more recently, the associated mutations have been well characterized.[136]

Similar to the adult age group, signs and symptoms of colorectal cancer are related to the segment of the large bowel where the tumor is located. Because of its rarity in the pediatric and adolescent age groups, diagnosis of colorectal carcinoma is often delayed, and patients usually present with acute symptoms that necessitate urgent laparotomy. Colorectal cancer in the young is usually diagnosed at an advanced stage with metastases involving the omentum, peritoneum, mesenteric lymph nodes, liver, ovaries, and sometimes lungs, brain, and bones, and therefore, it carries a poor prognosis.[137]

Colorectal carcinoma is diagnosed by direct fiberoptic colonoscopy. Radiographic studies include barium enema with air contrast, CT scan, and radioisotope studies (fluorodeoxyglucose–positron emission tomography [FDG-PET]) to determine metastatic spread. Preoperative carcinoembryonic antigen (CEA) level is important both as a prognosticator and for follow-up purposes. CA19-9 has been less valuable, although some tumors produce CA19-9 without CEA production.

Adenocarcinoma of the colorectum may be well, moderately, or poorly differentiated. The mucinous variety and signet cell types are associated with an extremely poor prognosis. Mucinous adenocarcinoma is the most common histotype in the pediatric age group.[138] Unlike adult patients, in whom 60% of colonic cancers are located within 25 cm of the anus and in whom the rectum and sigmoid are also common sites for mucinous adenocarcinoma, tumors in children are probably more evenly distributed in all parts of the colon.[109,139,140] In a series reported by Andersson and Bergdahl,[141] the most common area was the transverse colon (39%). In a series of 20 patients reported by Karnak et al.[142] from Turkey, the rectosigmoid area was the most frequent site of location of the primary tumor (65%, the same as in adults). Another series from St. Jude's evaluated 24 adolescents with colorectal,

21 of whom had poorly differentiated mucin-producing adenocarcinoma. The disease-free survival reported was extremely poor.[143]

Surgery alone is the primary and most effective treatment for early-stage colorectal carcinoma. Because of late diagnosis, the rate of complete resection has been less than optimal in children. In the series of Karnak et al.,[142] complete resection was possible in only 6 of 20 patients. The surgical guidelines are similar to those of adult patients. Similarly, the use of chemotherapy and radiotherapy follows the guidelines of the adult age group with the Sauer et al.[144] demonstrating superiority for preoperative chemoradiotherapy for T3, T4, or node-positive rectal cancer. Special attention should be given to radiochemotherapy sequelae on the reproductive system, as both the ovaries and testes are exquisitely radiosensitive.

Appendix

The most frequent malignant tumors of the appendix in the pediatric age group are carcinoids. These tumors are usually diagnosed incidentally during surgery for acute appendicitis or during other abdominal surgery. Complete surgical removal is the treatment of choice.[145,146]

Pancreas

Pancreatic tumors are rare in children. The most important types are the functional tumors, pancreatoblastomas, and solid papillary epithelial neoplasms.[147,148] The adult form of pancreatic adenocarcinoma rarely occurs in children.

Functional islet cell tumors are characterized by their hormonal activity. The diagnostic procedures and management follow the same guidelines set for adults.

Pancreatoblastoma, a rare tumor, accounting for 25% of pancreatic cancer in children <10 years old, has an annual incidence of 0.004 per 100,000 persons.[149] The mean age of diagnosis is 5.[150] The European Cooperative Study Group for pediatric rare tumors analyzed 20 patients diagnosed between 2000 and 2009.[151] The tumor is characterized by adenocarcinomatous tissue with ductal cells, acinar cells, squamoid corpuscles, and sometimes islet cell differentiation. These tumors stain positively by periodic acid–Schiff, α-trypsin, and α-keratin and in many cases can be associated with increased levels of α-fetoprotein (AFP).[152-154] Familial adenomatous polyposis and Beckwith-Wiedemann syndrome are associated with neonatal cases.[150] The SEER database from 1973 to 2004 reports 10 cases, and the United Kingdom National Registry of Childhood Tumors reports 11 cases.[155]

In most cases, the tumor is located in the head of the pancreas. In patients with a solitary noninfiltrative tumor, complete local resection without radical pancreatoduodenectomy is recommended. Unlike patients with local disease, in whom local resection can be curative, in many other cases, the tumor is clearly malignant, with porta hepatis or vascular invasion, local recurrences, and nodal and disseminated metastases. The prognosis for these patients is very poor.[156,157] For unresectable disease, neoadjuvant chemotherapy may be recommended with adjuvant chemotherapy to follow resection.

Radiation therapy is used in the postoperative setting, in locoregional recurrences, and in the neoadjuvant setting. A dose of 40 to 50 Gy is recommended.[154,158] Technical guidelines of radiotherapy planning are similar to those of the adults. Intraoperative radiotherapy for recurrent disease has also been used.

Chemotherapy has been used for unresectable tumors, to treat metastatic disease, or in the adjuvant setting. 5-fluorouracil, cyclophosphamide, actinomycin D, vincristine, vinblastine, mitomycin C, bleomycin, ifosfamide, etoposide, cisplatin, doxorubicin, and gemcitabine, alone or in combination, have been used with very modest results.[150,159,160] Because the disease is so rare, it is impossible to set firm guidelines and treatment policies for chemotherapy in pediatric pancreatoblastoma; however, there are case reports of long-term survival and tolerance of aggressive surgical and chemotherapy regimens for locally advanced disease.[161] There is also evidence that a combination of vinorelbine and oral cyclophosphamide may be effective for relapsed disease.[162]

Papillary cystic tumors of the pancreas, also known as Frantz tumors or solid pseudopapillary tumors, are usually encapsulated lesions that can develop throughout the pancreas. They are characterized by cystic or pseudocystic spaces surrounded by residual solid tissue. Only 15% of these tumors are malignant, and they usually occur in female patients at a mean age of 24 years at diagnosis.[163]

These tumors usually present as an upper abdominal mass. Unlike other malignant pancreatic tumors, their prognosis is excellent after complete surgical excision.[164] In a retrospective analysis, Hwang et al. showed that CT scan findings of an increased solid component indicated the disease was more likely to be malignant and a more radical resection should be recommended.[165]

The adult type of pancreatic adenocarcinoma is extremely rare in the pediatric and adolescent age groups. Signs and symptoms are similar to those of adult carcinoma of the pancreas.[158] These tumors are managed according to guidelines of treatment set for adult patients with surgery for resectable disease.

Hepatobiliary Tumors

Hepatobiliary tumors are the most common neoplasms of the gastrointestinal tract to occur in children. They constitute 0.5% to 2% of pediatric cancer in Europe and in the United States. Hepatocellular carcinoma (HCC) occurs more frequently in Saharan Africa and the Asia.[77,166,167] This geographic clustering may be explained by the high rates of hepatitis B infection and hepatitis B serum antigen positivity.[168] This is supported by the dramatic decrease in the rate of HCC in Taiwan from 10% to 1% 10 years after a nationwide hepatitis B vaccination program was launched.[169]

Benign hepatic tumors are more frequent than malignant tumors in young children. In older children, malignant tumors become more common. Benign tumors are classified according to the cell of origin: mesenchymal (hemangioma, hemangioendothelioma, hamartoma, peliosis hepatis) or epithelial (cysts, focal nodal hyperplasia, adenoma).[170] On rare occasions, radiation therapy may be used for the treatment of hemangiomas.

Malignant tumors of the liver are classified according to the tissue of origin, with hepatocellular tumors (hepatoblastoma [HBL] and HCC) most common, constituting 75% to 90% of primary hepatic malignant tumors of childhood. Other tumors include malignant mesenchymoma, undifferentiated embryonal sarcoma, primary hepatic malignant tumors with rhabdoid features, leiomyosarcoma, angiosarcoma, hepatic sinusoid tumors, carcinoid, and non-Hodgkin lymphoma.

Bile duct adenocarcinoma (cholangiocarcinoma) is extremely rare before the age of 30. This tumor has been associated with certain rare congenital biliary anomalies, ulcerated colitis, cystic fibrosis, and sclerosing cholangitis.[170,171] The liver is also a common site for metastatic disease.

Of the malignant tumors of the liver in childhood, HBL is the most common. HBL occurs almost exclusively in small infants, although isolated instances in older children and in young adolescents have been reported. These tumors occur more frequently among males.

HBL is associated with Beckwith-Wiedemann syndrome, familial adenomatous polyposis, and congenital anomalies like hemihypertrophy and cleft palate, Wilms tumor, and glycogen storage diseases.[172-174] Although the association between HBL and Beckwith-Wiedemann syndrome indicates abnormalities on chromosome 11 and loss of heterozygosity of 11p, increased incidence of HBL in families with familial adenomatous polyposis indicates abnormalities of chromosome 5q.[174,175]

More recently, it has been shown that familial adenomatous polyposis cases with HBL are associated with germ-line mutations of APC, located on 5q. However, the sporadic cases of HBL instead demonstrate mutations in the Wnt–β-catenin pathway.[176] Others have shown that activation of the telomerase gene, TERT, and MYC expression are associated with the more aggressive HBL phenotypes.[177]

The presenting signs and symptoms are distension of the abdomen, anorexia, vomiting, anemia, fever, and jaundice. Isosexual precocity secondary to human chorionic gonadotropin (HCG) secretion or testosterone production by the tumor can be seen in some cases.[178]

Serum AFP produced by the embryonal endoderm is increased in 84% to 90% of patients with HBL.[179] HCG and cystathionase may also serve as tumor markers.[180] Histologically, HBLs (Fig. 94.2) are classified into five subtypes (Table 94.3). These subtypes can occur together in varying proportions, but present definitions do not take this into account, which makes it difficult to relate a specific histologic subtype with prognosis. Pure fetal histology has a better outcome, but the histologic definition of "pure fetal" is not clear.[182] The prognosis of the rare (3%) small cell undifferentiated subtype is poor. In long-term survivors of HBL, the most common histologic variant is the conventional type with predominantly fetal cell patterns. A German study (HB 89–94)[183] identified several poor prognostic factors in HBL: metastatic disease, AFP > 1,000,000 ng/mL, extrahepatic and intrahepatic vascular invasion, multifocal disease, involvement of both liver lobes, stage (TNM), and poorly differentiated epithelial histology. More informative molecular data have begun to accumulate.[176] Sumazin et al. performed whole-exome sequencing, mRNA and miRNA expression arrays, and high-resolution copy number arrays. They found three distinct molecular clusters with prognostic biomarkers including NOTCH1 and NFE2L2.[184] They demonstrate, from clustering of mRNA profiles, the high-risk group has a difference in cumulative survival relative to the low- and intermediate-risk groups.

HCC is the second most common primary malignant liver tumor in the pediatric age group and accounts for about one-fourth to one-third of hepatic malignancies. Although reported in children as young as 21 months, most reports indicate that HCC usually develops in early adolescence.[185,186] This is in contrast to HBL, which occurs primarily in infancy and is seldom seen in children older than 3 years. Similar to HBL, HCC occurs mainly in males.[187,188] The fibrolamellar carcinoma variant of HCC occurs mainly in young adults around the age of 20 years but has also been reported in childhood.[189,190]

Approximately 25% of HCC cases in childhood are associated with cirrhosis secondary to biliary atresia, Fanconi anemia, glucose-6-phosphatase deficiency, and hereditary tyrosinemia.[191] The most important known etiologic factor for HCC is the high incidence of maternal transmission of the hepatitis B surface antigen in Africa and Asia.[192,193] Other etiologic factors include exposure to aflatoxins, hepatic fibrosis, anabolic steroids, inherited disorders of metabolism, membranous obstruction of the inferior vena cava, and possibly ethanol abuse.[167,188,194] However, these etiologic factors apply mostly to HCC in the adult age group. In adult black South African patients, deletions of alleles on chromosome 17p and P53 (codon 249) have been identified[195,196]; the exact molecular mechanisms responsible for the development of HCC are not known.

Similar to HBL, two-thirds of children with HCC have an elevated AFP.[197] AFP levels are high in the healthy newborn and drop rapidly by the age of 1 month and should not be detectable by age 2 years.[198] Initial AFP level is a significant prognostic factor: In a study performed by the Radiation Therapy Oncology Group,[199] the mortality in HCC was 1.8 times higher in patients with strongly positive AFP. AFP is an indicator of tumor growth and can serve as a valuable marker

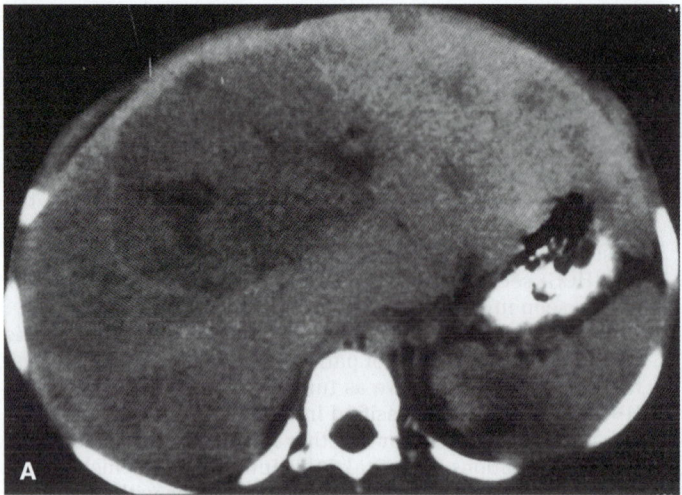
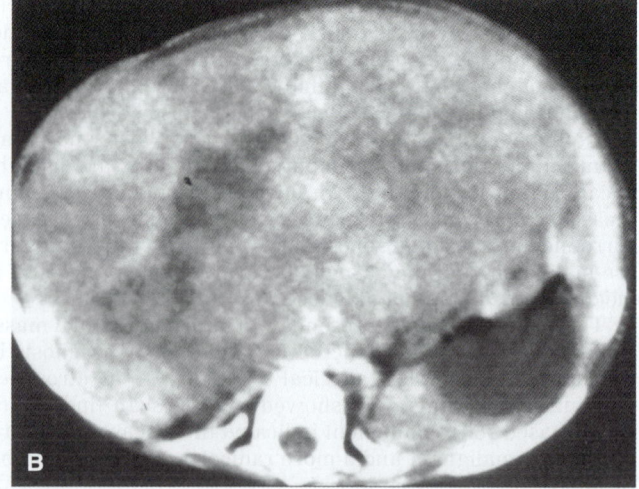
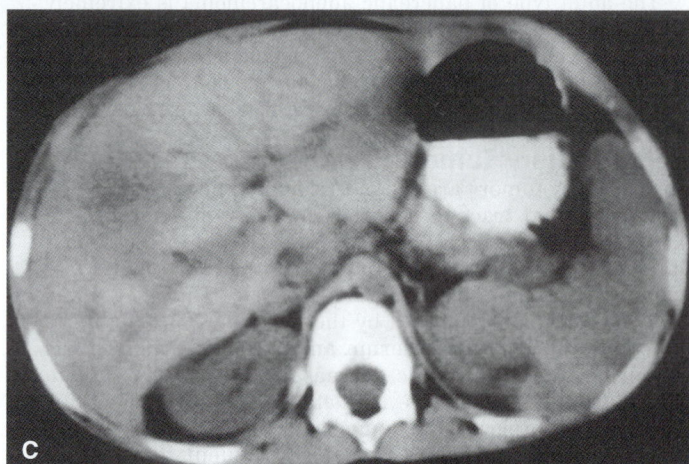

FIGURE 94.2. A 7-year-old girl with hepatoblastoma at diagnosis **(A)**, after one cycle of chemotherapy **(B)**, and after four cycles of chemotherapy before right hepatic lobectomy **(C)**.

of response to therapy. After complete tumor resection, AFP level should return to normal within 2 months.[200] Increasing levels of AFP during the follow-up period after surgery indicate local recurrence or metastatic disease.[197]

The Children's Cancer Study Group (CCSG) intergroup and Pediatric Oncology Group (POG) staging systems for primary malignant liver tumors are based on resectability and on the histologic subtype (Table 94.4[201] and Table 94.5[203]).

Successful therapy of localized HBL or HCC depends mainly on the feasibility of complete surgical excision.[183] Up to two-thirds of HBL patients have resectable tumors at presentation because these tumors are usually unifocal and encapsulated. Cure can be achieved in one-third of the successfully operated patients, typically those with fetal HBL.[172,182,204]

In contrast, only 30% of the cases of HCC are suitable for complete resection at the time of diagnosis because of the multifocal involvement or size. From 50% to 75% of the fibrolamellar variant of HCC is amenable to complete resection at the time of presentation.[205,206] In principle, tumor resectability is determined by the tumor size, the existence of

bilobar involvement necessitating the resection of more than three liver segments, vascular invasion, or metastatic spread. Patients with advanced disease who are not suitable for primary surgery may be considered for neoadjuvant preoperative cytoreductive chemotherapy. In these cases, the diagnosis can be based on clinical presentation; on imaging findings, including FDG-PET scan[207] and tumor markers; or on tissue diagnosis obtained via open biopsy or CT/ultrasound-guided needle biopsy, although there are some concerns that a needle

TABLE 94.3 HISTOLOGIC CLASSIFICATION OF HEPATOBLASTOMA

Epithelial type (56%)	Mixed epithelial and mesenchymal type (44%)
Fetal pattern (31%)	Without teratoid features (34%)
Embryonal and fetal pattern (19%)	With teratoid features (10%)
Macrotrabecular pattern (3%)	
Small cell undifferentiated pattern (3%)	

Modified from Stocker JT. Hepatoblastoma. *Semin Diagn Pathol* 1994;11(2):136–143. Copyright © 1994 Elsevier. With permission..

TABLE 94.4 CHILDREN'S CANCER STUDY GROUP STAGING SYSTEM FOR PRIMARY MALIGNANT LIVER TUMORS

Stage	Description
I	Complete excision
A	Favorable histology (fetal HBL)
B	Unfavorable histology (embryonal HBL, HCC)
II	Microscopic residual disease
A	In liver
B	Extrahepatic
III	Gross residual disease ± node involvement ± spilled tumor
A	Tumor completely removed; tumor spilled, residual gross disease in nodes, or both
B	Gross tumor not completely removed ± positive nodes ± spill
IV	Metastatic disease
A	Primary tumor completely excised
B	Primary tumor not completely excised

HBL, hepatoblastoma; HCC, hepatocellular carcinoma.
Data derived from Cohen MD, Bugaieski EM, Haliloglu M, et al. Visual presentation of the staging of pediatric solid tumors. *Radiographics* 1996;16:523–545.; Perilongo G., S.D., Meadown A.T., et al. *Liver tumors.* New York: Wiley-Liss, 1992. References 201 and 202.

TABLE 94.5 PEDIATRIC ONCOLOGY GROUP STAGING SYSTEM FOR PRIMARY MALIGNANT LIVER TUMORS

Stage	Description
I	Complete resection achieved
II	Microscopic residual tumor remaining
III	Gross residual tumor remaining
IV	Metastatic disease present at diagnosis

Modified from Bowman LC, Riely CA. Management of pediatric liver tumors. *Surg Oncol Clin N Am* 1996;5(2):451–459. Copyright © 1996 Elsevier. With permission.

biopsy may cause a significant hemorrhage. Preoperative cytoreductive chemotherapy can reduce the size of the tumor in the majority of HBL patients and in a significant percentage of HCC patients, rendering them resectable. A variety of chemo regimens exist including cisplatin, vincristine, and 5-fluorouracil,[208] the camptothecin analogues topotecan and irinotecan; oxaliplatin; and liposomal doxorubicin (Doxil).[183] Sorafenib, a tyrosine kinase inhibitor, is available for unresectable HCC. In animal models of pediatric HCC, sorafenib has shown promising efficacy.[209] A phase II trial also demonstrated a good toxicity profile for sorafenib in children.[210] Bevacizumab has shown a survival benefit in a phase II trial.[211,212] In one center's experience, bevacizumab plus conventional platinum-based chemotherapy was effective and safe.[213] If resectability cannot be achieved using chemotherapy, there is still a chance to render unresectable tumors resectable by radiotherapy.[205] The perioperative mortality of hepatic lobectomy is on the order of 5% to 10% in specialized centers applying improved surgical techniques, modern methods of anesthesia, and state-of-the-art postoperative intensive care.[214]

Surgical resection of pulmonary metastases can be attempted if they persist after chemotherapy and if the primary tumor can be completely resected. Patients who are successfully operated on for stage I disease and later develop a solitary lung metastasis are also suitable for metastasectomy.

Total hepatectomy and liver transplantation can be attempted in unresectable HBL (about 10% after chemotherapy) and HCC (>50% are unresectable at diagnosis) with tumor confined to the liver without penetration of the capsule and in the absence of lymph node and distant metastases. The overall survival is between 50% and 83%, with a minimum follow-up of 2 years. The best outcome was achieved in patients with a good response to chemotherapy who had a "first-line transplant" (i.e., not after an unsuccessful attempt at resection).[183,215–217]

Although it has been used preoperatively and postoperatively in children with HBL and HCC, radiation therapy has a limited role in curative management.

Preoperative radiation was given to children who remained unresectable after initial chemotherapy.[205,218,219] In the postoperative setting, it has been shown that patients with residual disease after surgery may benefit from postoperative irradiation. In a combined POG-CCSG protocol,[182] patients with microscopic residual disease after surgery received postoperative chemotherapy and limited field irradiation, 45 Gy to the tumor bed. Their 3-year progression-free survival was 60%. Patients who were unable to undergo complete resection after preoperative chemotherapy received whole-liver irradiation, 30 Gy. Their 3-year progression-free survival was 22%.

According to the Institut Gustave Roussy protocol,[205] children were treated with preoperative chemotherapy followed by surgery. If there was evidence for microscopic or gross persistent tumor at surgery, more chemotherapy was given and limited field irradiation was administered to the site of residual tumor, 25 to 45 Gy. Fifteen patients were reported by Habrand et al.,[205] 11 with HBL, 2 with HCC, and 2 without tissue diagnosis. Nine patients who underwent surgical resection of the primary tumor received either preoperative or postoperative chemotherapy consisting of vincristine, doxorubicin, and cyclophosphamide, alternating with vincristine, cyclophosphamide, and *cis*-platinum. Radiotherapy with a median dose of 40 Gy was given to eight incompletely resected patients. Six of eight patients were alive at a median of 45 months from the time of diagnosis. One inoperable patient was rendered operable by whole-liver irradiation (24 Gy) and concurrent 5-fluorouracil and *cis*-platinum. This patient was alive at 68 months after radiation therapy. Of four unresectable primaries, one was controlled by radiotherapy. Two children received whole-lung irradiation, 18 to 20 Gy, for pulmonary metastases; neither of them was controlled. One of these two patients underwent pulmonary metastasectomy and was alive without evidence of disease 41 months after surgery.

When radiotherapy is given to children with HBL or HCC, careful assessment of the tumor volume is essential to reduce the amount of normal liver tissue irradiated. Parallel-opposed high-energy beams or multiple-field techniques, using 3D treatment planning systems or IMRT, should be employed. When limited irradiation volume is administered, a dose of 35 to 45 Gy is appropriate for bulky disease and 25 to 45 Gy for microscopic residual disease. For children treated with a palliative intent, whole-liver irradiation, 20 to 25 Gy in 2 to 2.5 weeks, is adequate.

The results of whole-lung irradiation for macroscopic pulmonary metastases are discouraging. A total dose of 12- to 13-Gy whole-lung irradiation might be considered in patients with microscopic residual pulmonary metastatic disease after chemotherapy or surgery and chemotherapy.

A number of multicenter trials have been performed by cooperative study groups to test the value of preoperative and postoperative combination chemotherapy in HBL and HCC. In some of the studies, radiotherapy was included as part of the treatment protocol. It has been demonstrated that a significant number of initially unresected tumors could be surgically removed after chemotherapy and that complete resection followed by adjuvant chemotherapy was superior to surgery alone.

In CCG trial 831,[220] patients with residual disease in one lobe after surgery received actinomycin D, vincristine, and cyclophosphamide combination chemotherapy and involved-field irradiation. Patients with disseminated tumors received chemotherapy alone. Of 40 children entered into the study, there were only 7 long-term survivors: those with either stage I disease or minor residual tumor who received irradiation.

In CCG trial 881,[220] doxorubicin and 5-fluorouracil were added to the actinomycin D, vincristine, and cyclophosphamide combination used in CCG 831. A response rate of 44% was observed in patients with measurable disease, and 83% of patients receiving the drug combination as an adjuvant treatment were disease-free at 30 months.

In CCG trial 823F,[220] patients with HBL (33 children) or HCC (14 children) confined to the liver received doxorubicin and cisplatin prior to definitive surgery. Although only 2 of 14 HCC patients survived, 78% of 25 HBL patients who completed chemotherapy and were eligible for surgery were alive without evidence of disease. In 16 patients, complete resection was performed, and no viable tumor was found in 9 of them at the time of surgery. Fifteen of these patients were alive and disease free. It was found that, for children with unresectable or metastatic HBL entered into this study, early changes in AFP levels were a reliable predictor of outcome and could identify poor responders to therapy. The authors suggested that if the AFP level failed to decrease by two logs prior to surgery, a surgical approach should probably not be attempted.[221]

In a trial performed by the Pediatric Hepatoma Study Intergroup (CCG 8881/POG 8945),[222] patients were allocated to receive either cisplatin, vincristine, and 5-fluorouracil or cisplatin and doxorubicin. Both chemotherapy regimens were

Section III

equally effective in terms of overall and disease-free survival; however, the cisplatin plus doxorubicin combination was significantly more toxic.

POG study 8,679[223] enrolled children with stage I to IV HBL. Children with stage I favorable histology received surgery alone. Children with stage I unfavorable histology or stage II disease received surgery and adjuvant cisplatin, vincristine, and 5-fluorouracil. Children with stage III or IV disease received five cycles of chemotherapy, after which they were evaluated for surgery. Unresectable patients received limited field irradiation, 33 to 39 Gy, and additional chemotherapy. The 3-year disease-free survival for stage I unfavorable histology and stage II patients was 91; for stage III, it was 67; and for stage IV patients, it was 13. Three of five irradiated patients underwent complete resection and were free of disease.

The International Society of Pediatric Oncology (SIOP) designed a series of clinical trials based on a risk-adapted treatment approach philosophy. In the SIOPEL-1 trial, patients underwent a preoperative cisplatin–doxorubicin (PLADO) regimen.[224] The investigators concluded that the extent of pretreatment hepatic disease and the presence of pulmonary metastases were significant prognosticators of 5-year event-free survival. Survival for HCC patients was significantly inferior to that of children with HBL, and complete tumor excision remained the only realistic chance of cure. A novel staging system was developed called PRETEXT (pretreatment extent of disease), and two risk clusters for treatment failure were identified: a "standard-risk" group, comprising patients with disease confined to the liver and involving up to three hepatic sectors, and a "high-risk" group, with disease extending to all four hepatic sectors or with extrahepatic spread. It was suggested that PLADO chemotherapy followed by delayed surgery and a short course of postoperative chemotherapy used in the SIOPEL-1 trial should be regarded as best treatment for children with HBL and that future treatment programs should be measured against this standard.[225,226]

In the SIOPEL-2 trial, patients were stratified according to standard- and high-risk groups. For high-risk HBL patients, treatment was intensified by adding carboplatin to the cisplatin/doxorubicin regimen used in the SIOPEL-1 trial, in a rapidly alternating sequence of administration. For standard-risk HBL patients, 3-year overall and progression-free survivals were 91% and 89%, and for the high-risk HBL group, they were 53% and 48%, respectively. Despite chemotherapy intensification, only half of the high-risk HBL patients were long-term survivors.[227]

SIOPEL-3 standard-risk HBL trial compared doxorubicin plus cisplatin versus cisplatin alone with cisplatin monotherapy achieving similar rates of complete resection and survival[228]. For the high-risk patients, they were treated with alternating cycles of cisplatin and carboplatin plus doxorubicin and delayed tumor resection with results showing an improved survival compared to previous results.

Finally, SIOPEL-4, a prospective single-arm trial for high-risk HBL, evaluated a dose-dense cisplatin regimen with results showing feasibility and efficacy for this cohort. Complete resection of all tumor lesions was achieved in 74% with 3-year event-free survival of 76%.[229]

SIOPEL-5 was focused exclusively on HCC and was closed because of poor accrual, and SIOPEL-6 is a randomized trial evaluating the efficacy of STS in reducing ototoxicity for standard-risk HBL patients receiving cisplatin. Final results are pending although there were no adverse outcomes related to STS reported.[230]

An ongoing phase III COG trial, AHEP-0731, has the primary objective of evaluating survival for HBL based on the stage treated with surgical resection followed by two cycles of cisplatin, 5-FU, and vincristine. The guidelines of the study recommend surgical resection only for PRETEXT I and II

tumors and specific imaging findings with the intention of more effectively systematizing surgical decisions rather than relying on individual practitioners.[231]

Investigators from the United States analyzed the effectiveness of intrahepatic chemotherapy[232] and intrahepatic chemoembolization.[233] They concluded that these treatment modalities can halt the progression and possibly downstage advanced hepatic malignancies.

Japanese investigators used transarterial chemoembolization with Lipiodol and cisplatin/etoposide, concluding that this treatment modality was particularly useful in potentiating the cytoreductive effect of antitumor drugs and also useful in reducing toxicities.[234]

Other Japanese investigators analyzed the survival outcome for patients with HBL treated by preoperative and/or postoperative chemotherapy using a combination of cisplatin and tetrahydropyranyl–Adriamycin.[235] They concluded that preoperative chemotherapy resulted in an improved resectability of the tumor, whereas postoperative chemotherapy played an important role in the increased cure rate of patients with an incomplete tumor resection or metastasis.

In the prospective, multicenter, single-arm German Liver Tumor Study HB94, children undergoing primary surgery received ifosfamide, cisplatin, and Adriamycin (IPA) chemotherapy and/or etoposide and carboplatin. Treatment was risk stratified according to stage: stage I patients receive IPA ×2; stage II patients receive IPA ×2 to 3; and stage III or IV patients receive carboplatin/etoposide plus IPA. Growth pattern of the liver tumor, vascular tumor invasion, occurrence of distant metastases, initial AFP level, and surgical radicality were found to be pretreatment prognostic factors.[236]

In an interim analysis of the German Liver Tumor Study HB 99, it was shown that adding high-dose carboplatin and etoposide to the regimen for high-risk HBL patients was highly efficient and induced a remission in the majority of patients with advanced and metastasized high-risk HBL.[237]

LANGERHANS CELL HISTIOCYTOSIS

Langerhans cell histiocytosis (LCH), a dendritic disorder, is believed to affect fewer than 1 in 200,000 children; however, any age group can be affected.[238]

Other terms for LCH include histiocytosis X, eosinophilic granuloma, Letterer-Siwe disease, and Hand-Schüller-Christian disease; however, the preferred term is LCH.

The pathogenesis is not completely understood, but excessive production of interleukin-1, interleukin-17a prostaglandin, and metalloproteases MMP9 and MMP12,[239] as well as of prostaglandin E_2, has been demonstrated in affected bone. These factors can play a major role in osteoclast activation. Controversy exists regarding whether the clonal proliferation of LCH cells results from a malignant transformation or is the result of an immunologic stimulus. Regardless of the mechanism responsible for the clonal proliferation, the primary treatment, if necessary, involves chemotherapeutic agents. Select chemotherapeutic drugs also have immunomodulatory activity. The diagnosis of LCH is based on a histologic and immunophenotypical examination of tissue. The main feature is the morphologic identification of the characteristic Langerhans cells. In addition, positive staining of the lesional cells with CD1a, langerin (CD207), or both are required for a definitive diagnosis. The expression of langerin confirms the presence of Birbeck granules, the cytoplasmic organelles typically found in Langerhans cells.[240]

In children older than 2 years, the disease is less aggressive, with widespread bone granulomas causing pain, otitis, diabetes insipidus (42%), and exophthalmos. Eosinophilic granuloma is characterized by bone involvement only and with symptoms related to the location of the granuloma. Central nervous system (CNS) involvement is possible; most frequently, meningeal and pituitary lesions occur, but intraparenchymal lesions, especially hypothalamic and cerebellar, can also be encountered.

Staging procedures include a skeletal survey (rather than isotopic bone scan). Many prognostic scores have been proposed, all based on the extent of disease, age at diagnosis, and demonstrable organ dysfunction.[241] Patients are classified into the following groups:

Single system	Unifocal or multifocal organ system involvement
	Unifocal or multifocal bone involvement
	Skin
	Lymph node
	Hypothalamic/pituitary/CNS
	Other (e.g., thyroid)
Multisystem	Involvement of ≥2 organs or systems[242]

Treatment decisions are based on whether the high- or low-risk organs are involved and whether the disease is single system or multisystem. Many cases of LCH are indolent or resolve spontaneously. Aggressive treatment therefore should not be given if there is no organ dysfunction. International efforts during the last 20 years have shown that combination therapy with vinblastine/prednisone is an effective therapy for multisystem LCH. Trials conducted by the Histiocyte Society confirmed this regimen as standard therapy for multisystem LCH with and without risk organ involvement.[243,244]

Risk organs and their involvement were defined according to modified Lahey criteria as follows:

- Hematopoietic: Anemia and/or leukopenia and/or thrombocytopenia
- Liver: Enlargement >3 cm below the costal margin, dysfunction, or both
- Spleen: Enlargement >2 cm below the costal margin
- Lung: Typical changes via high-resolution CT, histopathologic diagnosis, or both[245]

Local Therapy

The POG 8047 study demonstrated that a similar control rate can be achieved (70% to 90%) with biopsy, curettage, or tumor excision.[246] Wide excision is recommended for expendable bones (clavicle, ribs) and biopsy for other sites. Curettage is not indicated if there is a risk of instability (cervical vertebra, femoral neck) or if a poor cosmetic or orthopedic outcome is likely.

Radiation therapy was widely used in the 1960s but is no longer indicated in the large majority of cases. Radiation therapy could be discussed in a case of resistant cerebral location. Tumors are very radiosensitive; however, wide range of dose has been reported for treatment of LCH (3 to 50 Gy).[247–251]

It appears that 9 Gy for bone lesions and 15 Gy for soft tissues will result in very high response and local control rates; however, they may be still consequential for children and should be only considered in selected cases.

Systemic Treatment

In Situ Injection of Steroids

The procedure is performed under general anesthesia and fluoroscopic guidance. Methylprednisolone is injected directly into the granuloma.[252] It has not been proven whether the steroid or the local trauma is responsible for the effects.

Chemotherapy

The exact point in the course of the disease at which chemotherapy should be considered is controversial. There is little agreement on the factors that should be considered as bad prognostic signs. Only organ dysfunction and/or multiorgan disease have been generally accepted as indications for chemotherapy. Initially, high-dose steroids are used and followed, when necessary, by

vinblastine. The international study LCH2 compared vinblastine and etoposide, with no benefit seen for the latter. Thus, because of the risk of etoposide-induced leukemia, the drug should not be used as first-line therapy.[253] The LCH3 protocol failed also to find any advantage for methotrexate.[244] There is no proof that a multidrug regimen is more effective than single-agent chemotherapy as first-line therapy. Furthermore, it is unknown whether early treatment prevents the development of diabetes insipidus at a later stage.[254,255] Recently, promising results were reported using thalidomide for treatment of disseminated LCH.[256]

For resistant disease (especially in infants), a more aggressive approach, including cyclosporine, liver transplantation, bone marrow transplantation, and/or monoclonal antibody therapy, is under investigation.[257,258] Pamidronate has been shown to be effective in reducing bone pain secondary to skeletal involvement by LCH.[259]

The reported overall incidence of the long-term consequences of LCH ranges from 20% to 70%. The reason for this wide variation is due to sample size, therapy used, duration of follow-up, and method of data collection. Children at low risk for organ involvement have approximately a 20% likelihood of developing long-term sequelae.[260] The most commonly reported permanent consequences are diabetes insipidus, orthopedic abnormalities, hearing loss, and neurologic issues.

Rosai-Dorfman disease (RDD), also known as sinus histiocytosis with massive lymphadenopathy, is nonmalignant histiocytic disorder. Histology and immunohistochemistry help differentiate RDD from malignant disorders such as lymphoma and LCH.

Patients typically present with fever, leukocytosis, and nonpainful cervical lymphadenopathy. Although the disease has a predilection for the lymph nodes in the head and neck, RDD can also present in any extranodal site, with common sites including the skin and soft tissue, the CNS, and, less commonly, the gastrointestinal tract.

RDD is usually self-limiting and eventually recedes, making systemic therapy rarely required. In patients with RDD requiring systemic treatment, steroids are a first-line therapeutic option.

In patients with RDD, radiation can be used for symptomatic steroid-resistant disease. Although no standard radiation guidelines have been established for patients with RDD, lymphoma-like approaches with total doses ranging between 30 and 50 Gy have been employed.[261]

ENDOCRINE TUMORS

Adrenocortical Carcinoma

Adrenocortical carcinoma (ACC) accounts for 0.2% of childhood cancer and in 75% of the cases occurs in children younger than 5 years, more commonly in females.[262–267] ACC is sometimes associated with Beckwith-Wiedemann syndrome and hemihypertrophy.[268]

Children with ACC may present with abdominal pain and a palpable mass. More than 75% of the tumors are functional, secreting one or more hormones: androgens, cortisol, aldosterone, or estrogens. The most common presenting sign is virilization, with deepening of the voice, hirsutism, premature pubic hair, clitoromegaly, phallumegaly, excessive muscular development, and advanced bone age. Pure Cushing syndrome (moon face, plethora, hypertension, striae, weight gain, acne, and "buffalo hump") is rare in children. Feminization or aldosterone-secreting tumors are also rare.[266]

Urinary 17-ketocorticosteroids and 17-hydroxycorticosteroids are usually elevated, with steroid production not influenced by adrenocorticotropic hormone suppression.

Diagnostic imaging studies include CT and/or MRI. It is sometimes difficult to separate ACC from adenoma. However, at presentation, most carcinomas are >6 cm and calcified, whereas benign adenomas are small and nonfunctional. A characteristic echogenic star pattern can be seen on ultrasonography, and CT scan shows an inhomogeneous tumor with irregular contrast material. Recently, the use of 18-FDG-PET has been shown to be effective in discriminating between benign and malignant adrenal lesions.[269,270] Because both benign adenomas and ACC may exhibit abnormal mitoses and cellular and nuclear pleomorphism, malignancy is determined by the finding of capsular penetration, invasion of the inferior vena cava up to the right atrium, lymph node, and distant metastases.[262]

Generally, the prognosis of ACC is poor.[271–273] Small, well-encapsulated, and easily excised tumors can be cured by surgery alone. In locally advanced cases, there is a significant risk of locoregional and metastatic relapse.[266,267] Repeat complete resection of local recurrences and discrete metastatic lesions can improve survival.[274]

The literature on adjuvant radiation therapy after resection of ACC is scarce and relatively old and consists of small series or case reports. Postoperative whole-abdominal irradiation (15 to 30 Gy) was administered by Stewart et al.[275] Three of four irradiated patients were long-term survivors. Percarpio and Knowlton[276] used preoperative irradiation, 45 to 50 Gy, to treat two patients and postoperative irradiation to treat four patients with unresectable tumors or spillage at the time of surgery. One patient who was treated preoperatively was rendered operable; three of four postoperatively treated patients relapsed in the field of radiation and one outside the field.

Magee et al.[277] reported a series of 15 patients with ACC, 9 of whom received postoperative irradiation. Three of the irradiated patients were girls under the age of 2 years, who received 30 Gy in 4 weeks. Two of these girls died as the result of a second malignancy arising in the irradiated volume.

Based on these results and the results of similar small retrospective series,[263,278–280] it is difficult to make any firm recommendations on the role of radiotherapy in ACC. Investigators from the United Kingdom reported a relatively high frequency of second, fatal, primary tumors, especially if radiotherapy was part of the treatment protocol.[281]

Mitotane (o,p-DDD) is the most frequently used chemotherapeutic agent for recurrent or metastatic ACC, with a response rate of approximately 20%. Other agents include suramin, doxorubicin, 5-fluorouracil, streptozotocin, cisplatin, and etoposide, alone or in combination, with response rates of 20% to 30%.[282] The administration of adjuvant chemotherapy is controversial. Some investigators advocate the use of adjuvant mitotane after surgery[278]; however, the administration of this drug is associated with significant gastrointestinal, neuromuscular, and skin toxicity, as well as with abnormal platelet aggregation and prolongation of bleeding time. There is also a significant decrease in urinary 17-hydroxysteroids and 17-ketosteroids. The response rates to mitotane are highly dependent on obtaining adequate serum levels (>10 to 14 mcg/mL), and the therapeutic window between toxicity and efficacy is quite narrow. Hence, most authorities agree that in the absence of solid data based on randomized, well-controlled clinical trials, it is difficult to justify the administration of radiation or chemotherapy in the adjuvant setting.[187,281,283]

PHEOCHROMOCYTOMA AND PARAGANGLIOMA

Pheochromocytoma and paraganglioma are rare tumors of childhood and adolescence.[284–288] Pediatric pheochromocytoma occurs usually between 8 and 14 years of age, more frequently in males. More than 90% of all pheochromocytomas in adults, and 70% of pheochromocytomas in children, originate in the adrenal gland, but the tumor can occur at any site in the sympathetic chain, most commonly below the diaphragm. The most common sites of occurrence of extra-adrenal pheochromocytoma are the superior paraaortic region, between the diaphragm and the lower renal poles, in the paraganglia, the organs of Zuckerkandl, and the bladder. Extra-abdominal tumors may develop in the brain, thorax, and the bladder.[284,287,289,290] Approximately 10% of all patients with pheochromocytoma are children, but several characteristics distinguish them from their adult counterparts. Unlike pheochromocytomas of the adult age group, children with pheochromocytoma have a higher incidence of bilaterality, a higher association with the multiple endocrine neoplasia (MEN) syndromes, and a lower incidence of malignant neoplasms.[284,289,291,292]

Familial pheochromocytoma is associated with other endocrine tumors in the MEN IIA and IIB syndromes.[289,293–295]

In addition to the familial syndrome of isolated pheochromocytomas, pheochromocytomas in the pediatric age group can be associated with other inherited diseases, such as von Hippel-Lindau disease (retinocerebral angiomatosis), tuberous sclerosis, and von Recklinghausen neurofibromatosis.

Malignant pheochromocytomas occur in 10% of the pediatric cases of pheochromocytoma. The definition of malignancy is based on biologic and clinical behavior and not on histologic features alone.

Pheochromocytoma is responsible for 1% of cases of childhood hypertension, which, unlike the situation in adults, is sustained and not paroxysmal. Other signs and symptoms include diaphoresis, flushing, fatigue, headache, and convulsions.[296]

Adrenal pheochromocytomas produce epinephrine and norepinephrine, but most extra-adrenal pheochromocytomas produce only norepinephrine.

Urinary epinephrine, norepinephrine, metanephrine, and vanillylmandelic acid values remain the gold standard for biochemical screening of pheochromocytoma. On some occasions, urinary catecholamine levels may be normal, whereas serum levels are elevated. Imaging studies include ultrasonography, CT scan, and/or MRI. Iodine-131 metaiodobenzylguanidine (MIBG) scan provides the most accurate and direct method of diagnosing adrenal, extra-adrenal, or metastatic pheochromocytoma because MIBG, which has a molecular structure similar to that of norepinephrine, is actively concentrated and stored in catecholamine storage vesicles of pheochromocytoma cells.[284,289,297–299]

Surgery is the definitive therapy. The most significant reduction in preoperative and postoperative mortality has come from the control of perioperative hypertension using alpha- and beta-blockers.[34,300]

External beam irradiation is used for palliation of lymph node, bone, brain, and spinal cord metastases. High-dose iodine-131 MIBG has been used with modest results in metastatic disease. Streptozotocin or cyclophosphamide, vincristine, and dacarbazine may produce modest decreases in catecholamine secretion in patients with malignant pheochromocytoma.[282] Patients with malignant pheochromocytoma require chronic medical control of their elevated blood pressure by alpha and beta blockade or inhibition of catecholamine synthesis with α-methyl-para-tyrosine.[301–303]

THYROID CARCINOMA

Thyroid carcinoma accounts for 1% to 1.5% of all cases of cancer in the pediatric and adolescent age groups, with between 0.4 and 1.5 cases per million, two to three times as frequent in girls as in boys.[304] After the April 26, 1986, Chernobyl nuclear reactor accident, a remarkable incidence increase was observed in children exposed to radioactive iodine (RAI) fallout.[305,306] The incidence of thyroid cancer in Belarus and Ukraine began to rise sharply in 1989 to 1990: in adults, the number of new cases increased twofold to threefold; and in

TABLE 94.6 HISTOLOGIC TYPES OF CHILDHOOD THYROID CANCER

Type	Frequency (%)	Characteristics
1. Differentiated carcinoma		
A. Papillary carcinoma	70–80	Infiltrative and multicentric; lymph node metastases in 70%–90% of cases; hematogenous spread (mainly lung) in 5%–10% of cases
B. Follicular carcinoma	16–20	Vascular invasion
2. Medullary carcinoma	Rare	Occurs in isolation, but more frequently associated with one of the MEN syndromes; usually aggressive and can be fatal
3. Undifferentiated carcinoma	Rare	Aggressive, usually fatal within 6 months of diagnosis
4. Insular carcinoma	Very rare	A variant of the poorly differentiated carcinoma; aggressive, poor prognosis

children <20 years of age, and particularly during the first 5 years of life, the number of new cases increased 20- to 30-fold.[305] Almost all new pediatric cases were papillary tumors (94% to 98%), with a relatively high incidence of lymph node (65%) and lung (5%) metastases at presentation (Table 94.6). Lubin et al.[307] reported pooled data from nine cohort studies of childhood external radiation exposure and thyroid cancer with individualized dose estimates, ≥1,000 irradiated subjects or ≥10 thyroid cancer cases, with data limited to individuals receiving doses <0.2 gray.

Estimates of threshold dose ranged from 0.0 to 0.03 gray, with an upper 95% confidence bound of 0.04 gray. The increasing dose–response trend persisted >45 years after exposure, was greater at younger age at exposure and younger attained age, and was similar by sex and number of treatments.

Follicular carcinoma accounts for 16% to 20% of cases and usually has favorable behavior and outcome. The papillary thyroid carcinoma (PTC) is a tumor named for its papillary growth pattern, although the defining diagnostic criteria are actually the nuclear features of neoplastic cells. In addition to enhanced screening, the important factor contributing to increased incidence of PTC is the increase in diagnosis of a variant of PTC known as the follicular variant of PTC (FVPTC). Among two main subtypes, infiltrative (or nonencapsulated) and encapsulated, encapsulated FVPTC (EFVPTC) has increased in incidence by an estimated two- to threefold over the past two to three decades and makes up 10% to 20% of all thyroid cancers currently diagnosed in Europe and North America.[308,309] In a recent international, multidisciplinary, retrospective study of patients with thyroid nodules diagnosed as EFVPTC, including 109 patients with noninvasive EFVPTC observed for 10 to 26 years and 101 patients with invasive EFVPTC observed for 1 to 18 years found that thyroid tumors currently diagnosed as noninvasive EFVPTC have a very low risk of adverse outcome and should be termed as noninvasive follicular thyroid neoplasm with papillary-like nuclear features (NIFTP).[310] This reclassification will affect a large population of patients worldwide and result in a significant reduction in psychological and clinical consequences associated with the diagnosis of cancer.[311]

Medullary carcinomas are rare and tend to be more aggressive than the differentiated carcinomas and can be fatal. They are associated with the immunoreactive thyrocalcitonin marker. Because of the aggressive clinical course, experts advocate genetic testing to identify affected individuals with specific mutations in the ret oncogene that predict for MEN syndromes. Those individuals could be candidates for prophylactic thyroidectomy at an earlier age than if the increase in serum calcitonin was used to identify C-cell

hyperplasia or early carcinoma. At present, genetic testing should be performed at birth in children suspected of having the MEN IIA syndrome and no later than 1 year of age for those with possible MEN IIB.[312–314]

Children with thyroid cancer are commonly euthyroid and usually present with a thyroid nodule or palpable cervical lymph node. Conventional radiographs may show calcifications in the region of the thyroid gland (psammoma bodies). Iodine radionuclide scan may show a cold nodule.

Paradoxically, despite the fact that 70% to 80% of patients present with regional lymph node involvement and approximately 20% have distant metastases at diagnosis, the prognosis of differentiated thyroid cancer in children and adolescents is excellent.[3,314–316]

Thyroid carcinoma is treated primarily by surgery. The extent of surgery for the primary tumor (subtotal lobectomy, lobectomy, total thyroidectomy) and involved lymph nodes (node picking, modified or radical neck dissection) is controversial.[317]

The arguments in favor of total thyroidectomy include the multifocality of the tumor, decrease in neck recurrences, the ability to use serum thyroglobulin as a tumor marker after radical surgery, and the ability to detect pulmonary metastases by RAI scan earlier. The arguments for more limited surgery are mainly the increased complication rate of radical surgery, with apparently no clear survival advantage.[3,313–315,318–323]

The use of RAI for routine ablation of remaining thyroid tissue after surgery in patients without any known metastatic disease is another area of controversy. However, many support the administration of RAI in this setting because of the high incidence of nodal and systemic metastases of thyroid cancer in the young.[324]

RAI is indicated in patients with cervical lymph node involvement or distant metastases. The radiopharmaceutical is taken up by 50% to 80% of well-differentiated tumors and is able to deliver high focal doses of irradiation to any remaining thyroid tissue.

Side effects of RAI include nausea, xerostomia, taste alterations, increases in caries, stomatitis, candidiasis, glossalgia, hypogeusia, thyroiditis, and gastrointestinal discomfort.[325,326] Potential and rare long-term complications include myelosuppression, leukemia, bladder cancer, salivary cancer, gastric cancer, breast cancer, and infertility. These complications occur rarely with today's treatment doses and protocols.[324]

Exogenous thyroid hormone is given to suppress thyroidstimulating hormone production and to decrease the probability of tumor recurrence. Exogenous thyroid hormone is also given as replacement therapy to keep the patients euthyroid despite thyroidectomy.[318,327,328]

External beam irradiation in children with differentiated thyroid cancer is indicated for unresectable primary tumor or cervical or mediastinal lymph nodes that do not take up RAI. It also has a role in advanced locoregional disease, with extensive extrathyroid extension, or where there is gross residual tumor after attempted surgical excision, or when definitive resection has not been possible. Although external beam irradiation is useful for palliative therapy of advanced or metastatic disease, the lack of randomized controlled studies makes its role as part of initial adjuvant treatment controversial, and it is rarely indicated for microscopic residual disease. Radiotherapy, with or without chemotherapy, can be administered in children with anaplastic thyroid carcinoma.[316]

The volume of irradiation is designed according to operative and pathologic findings and can range from whole-neck and upper mediastinal irradiation to just treating the thyroid gland or thyroid bed. CT-based planning, 3D treatment planning, or IMRT is advocated to allow the administration of curative doses (in the range of 55 to 65 Gy) to the target volume without compromising spinal cord tolerance. This can be achieved by a variety of techniques.[329]

In the Mayo Clinic series, survival rates for children did not differ significantly from those of matched controls at 20 to 30 years.[330] In the Royal Marsden series,[318] the median overall survival was 53 years, and the median survival for patients who developed recurrence was 30 years. The only presenting feature predictive of poorer survival was the presence of metastases at diagnosis. According to a study reported by the Surgical Discipline Committee of the Children's Cancer Group, the overall survival for children presenting with distant metastases was 100% at 10 years. The progression-free survival rate was 76% at 5 years and 66% at 10 years. In a series of 14 children with papillary thyroid cancer and pulmonary metastases treated at the Mayo Clinic[328] by various surgical procedures, RAI, external beam irradiation (one patient), and suppressive hormone therapy, at a mean follow-up time of 19.3 years, 50% were alive completely free of disease and 50% were alive and asymptomatic with residual pulmonary disease.

GERM CELL TUMORS

Gonadal or extragonadal germ cell tumors (GCTs) represent <2% of pediatric cancer. The tumor is the result of neoplastic transformation of primitive germ cells or totipotent embryonal cells (Fig. 94.3).[331] The GCTs can arise from the brain to the sacrococcygeal region with the most common site presentation in the testis, ovary, sacrococcygeal region, retroperitoneum, and mediastinum. Aberrant migration can explain unusual tumor sites.[332] The Children's Oncology Group evaluated the link between a family history of cancer and pediatric GCT in a case–control study of 274 cases. The risk of GCT decreased among female cases with a family history with onset before 40 years but increased for boys, especially for those with a family history of melanoma.[333] The most frequent cytogenetic abnormality is the isochromosome 12p for both gonadal and extragonadal GCT, except for children <3 years of age at diagnosis. Klinefelter syndrome can be associated with GCT in boys.[305] Intracranial germ cell tumors are discussed in Chapter 84.

TABLE 94.7 GERM CELL TUMOR AND CLINICAL MARKERS

Tumor Type	β-HCG	AFP	LDH	CEA	PLAP
Embryonal carcinoma	+	+		+	
Mature teratoma					
Immature teratoma	+	+	+	+	
Yolk sac tumor		+++	+	+	
Choriocarcinoma	+++		+		
Germinoma	+		+	+	+++

AFP, α-fetoprotein; β-HCG, beta-human chorionic gonadotropin; CEA, carcinoembryonic antigen; LDH, lactate dehydrogenase; PLAP, placental alkaline phosphatase.

Clinical Presentation

Abdominal pain, abdominal distension, and sacrococcygeal or buttock swelling are the frequent presenting signs.[334] Staging includes imaging both of the primary tumor and most frequent sites of metastatic dissemination (lungs, liver, brain, and bone). Serum AFP, β-HCG, lactate dehydrogenase, CEA, and placental alkaline phosphatase levels are mandatory prior to the initiation of any treatment. Serum AFP level must be interpreted according to patient age (level >1,000 mg/mL is normal until the age of 1 month). Clinical markers are strongly correlated with some histologic features (Table 94.7); however, high AFP levels can be detected in infectious diseases of the liver, and increased β-HCG level can be associated with malignancies other than choriocarcinoma. The half-life time of AFP is 5 to 7 days and that of β-HCG is 24 to 36 hours. Both are very useful tools for predicting and monitoring treatment response, progression of disease, and relapse.[335]

Treatment

Their cure rate is high and strongly correlated with adherence to strict treatment guidelines.

Surgery is the standard treatment for mature teratomas and sacrococcygeal tumors (with complete removal of the tumor and the coccyx), but it may be combined with chemotherapy to limit the extent of irradiation. Surgery is often the first treatment for malignant gonadal GCT: orchiectomy with

FIGURE 94.3. Classification of germ cell tumors.

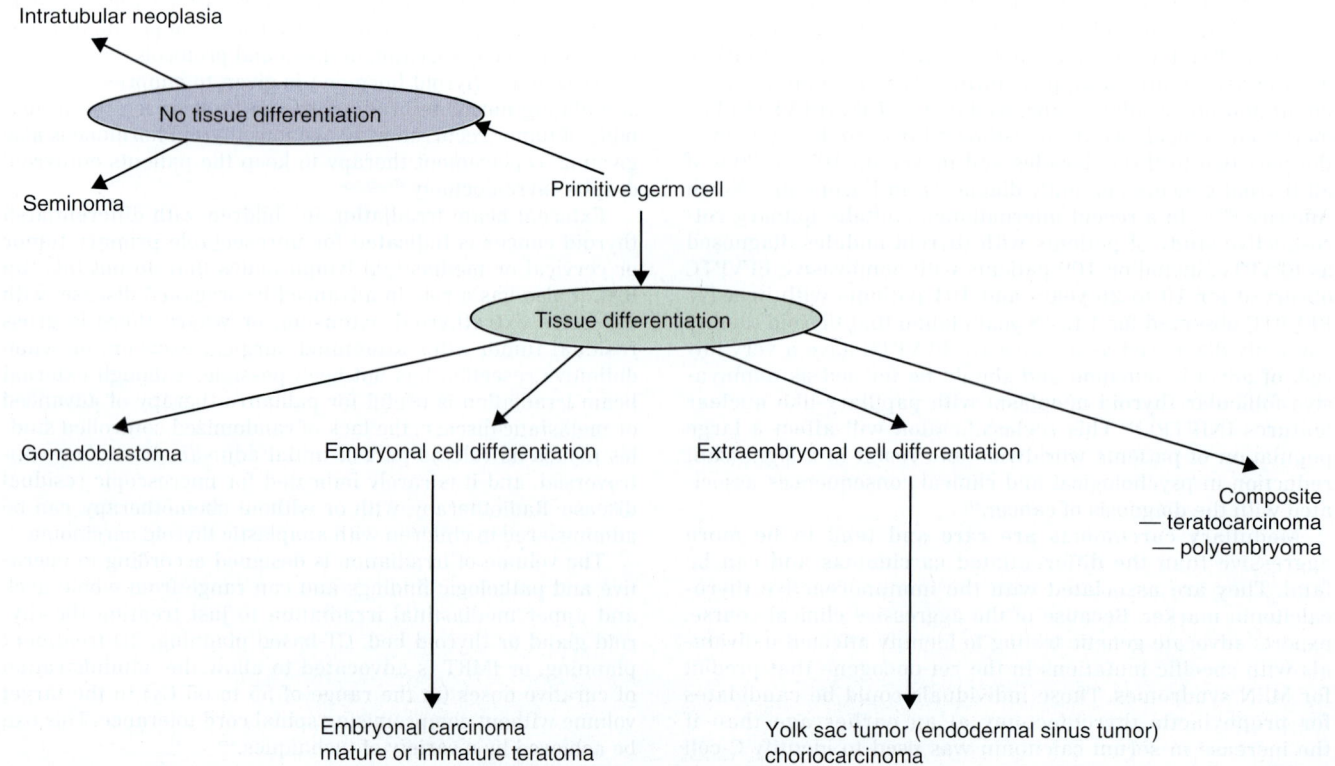

high inguinal ligation or ovariectomy with careful peritoneal cavity exploration. Lymph node dissection is not recommended in early-stage GCT, especially in germinomas. Second-look surgery can be indicated in cases of residual disease (clinical or biochemical) after chemotherapy.

Since the introduction of cisplatin-based chemotherapy, the survival rate of GCT has risen from 60% to 90%,[336] and regimens used are similar to those used in the adult age group. There is now a trend to use carboplatin in order to reduce late toxicities.[337] The rate of decline of serum tumor markers has demonstrated prognostic significance and must be used in the management of poor-risk patients.[225] Radiotherapy is rarely indicated except for some cases of early-stage ovarian germinoma in adolescents (dose, 20 to 25 Gy). The use of radiotherapy for ovarian germinoma in the young, however, must be compared with salvage chemotherapy after surgery alone. In advanced cases of ovarian dysgerminoma, careful surgical staging followed by conservative resection and chemotherapy without radiotherapy results in an overall survival rate as high as 85% without compromising the possibility of future pregnancy.[65] There is no indication for radiotherapy after complete response in extragonadal GCT. For stage IA ovarian dysgerminoma, conservative surgery is the gold standard, even in a case of incomplete staging, and chemotherapy is given only in the event of relapse, according to the last Italian group report.[338]

BENIGN VASCULAR TUMORS

Hemangiomas

Infantile hemangiomas, congenital hemangiomas, and kaposiform hemangioendotheliomas constitute vasculoproliferative tumors. They are subdivided on the basis of presence or absence of endothelial cell glucose transporter 1 (GLUT1) isoform protein. Infantile hemangioma is the most common benign vascular tumor in children and affects approximately

40% of all infants. The skin, subcutaneous, and soft tissue of the head and neck are the site of origin in 60% of patients, followed by the trunk, extremities, and viscera (e.g., liver, lung, gastrointestinal tract).

In some cases, their development can be associated with adverse cosmetic effects, unacceptable symptoms, and organ compression that in certain cases could be life threatening. Such cases require therapy. There are two distinct types of hemangiomas[339]: dynamic lesions, which include cellular hemangiomas, capillary hemangiomas, and cavernous hemangiomas; and adynamic lesions, which include port-wine stains, telangiectasias, and venous lakes. Vascular malformations are subdivided into two major groups, low or slow flow and high or fast flow.[340]

Radiation therapy is very rarely used in the treatment of hemangiomas. Treatment of infantile hemangiomas depends on the location and number of lesions as well as associated symptoms. Laser therapy is available for skin ulceration, the most frequent complication. For hemangiomas with symptoms, including thrombocytopenia or hypothyroidism, as well as heart failure caused by numerous hepatic hemangiomas, treatment is typically started with antiangiogenic drugs (propranolol, steroids, and less often vincristine) followed by gradually more aggressive treatments, such as embolization and rarely surgery. External beam radiotherapy was used in the past for patients not responding to steroids or interferon. Total doses of 300 to 750 cGy, and rarely exceeding 1,000 cGy, at 10 to 20 cGy per fraction could achieve good local control.[341]

Recently, radiotherapy fell out of favor because of concerns for potential late effects, like scarring, bone growth abnormalities, dental and periodontal problems, and secondary neoplasms.[342-345 346,347]

Higher doses (30 to 40 Gy) are used in older patients for large and progressive lesions for achieving lasting local control.[348]

Special attention must be given to the Kasabach-Merritt syndrome (KMS) (Fig. 94.4), which is defined as combination

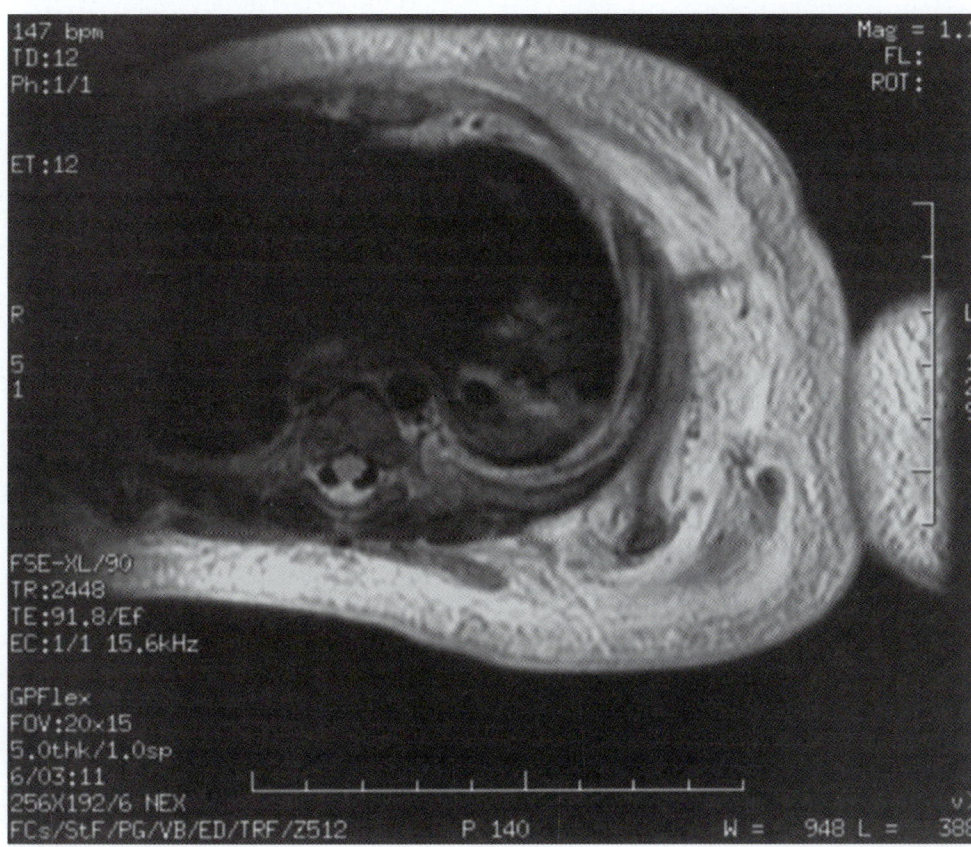

FIGURE 94.4. Kasabach-Merritt syndrome. Massive left hemithorax infiltration and involvement of the left arm.

Section III

of cutaneous vascular abnormalities with or without visceral involvement and thrombopenia because of intravascular coagulopathy. KMS is associated only with Kaposi-like hemangioendothelioma or tufted angioma. Kaposi-like hemangioendothelioma must be distinguished from infantile hemangioma, which disappears spontaneously.[349,350] These are alarming hemangiomas with life-threatening lesions (mediastinum, lower extremities, abdomen) either because of compression or secondary to a thrombocytic coagulopathy or high-output cardiac failure. Cavernous hemangiomas can be located in the epidural space and cause spinal cord compression. Surgical resection is the standard treatment.[351]

Radiotherapy is used in a rare setting for unresectable cases and should be considered very cautiously because of its late effects. A dose of 10 Gy in 10 fractions can be given; it is not mandatory to encompass the whole hemangioma in the target volume.[352,353]

Lymphangiomas

Histologically, lymphangiomas are a benign proliferation of lymph vessels. Four types are recognized: (a) capillary lymphangiomas, (b) cavernous lymphangiomas, (c) cystic hygromas, and (d) lymphangeal hemangiomas. Surgery is the treatment of choice.

Special attention must be given to the Gorham syndrome, also known as the bone-vanishing syndrome or massive osteolysis of bone.[354] Gorham syndrome is a bone hamartoma with various percentages of lymphangioma and hemangioma, characterized by well-margined osteolytic scattered lesions that progressively affect the cortex, with no respect for joint boundaries (Fig. 94.5). All bones can be affected (vertebrae, ribs, scapula). Progression is unpredictable, from spontaneous remission to bone absorption and sometimes even death. The prognosis is very poor when pleural or visceral involvement develops. Some encouraging results have been reported using antiresorptive therapy such as calcitonin or biphosphonates.[355] Although radiotherapy is the last resort

for the patient, encouraging results have been reported for patients with chylothorax and in patients with rib, thorax, and vertebral body involvement. The usual dose is approximately 18 Gy to the hemithorax. Affected bones have been treated to approximately 40 Gy with good response.[356]

DESMOPLASTIC SMALL ROUND CELL TUMOR

Desmoplastic small round cell tumor (DSRCT) was first described in 1989.[357] It is a rare aggressive neoplasm with typical clinical, histologic, karyotypic, and biologic characteristics. DSRCT mainly affects male adolescents and young adults, but it sometimes occurs in young females. Clinically, patients present with a bulky abdominal or pelvic mass, but intracranial, testicular, renal soft tissue, and bone DSRCTs have also been described.[358-361]

The tumor is characterized by a desmoplastic stroma with circumscribed tumor cells and encased nests of primitive undifferentiated cells. The tumoral cells express epithelial (keratin, EMA), conjunctival (vimentin), muscular (desmin), and neuroendocrinal markers.

Reciprocal translocation (11:22) (p13:q12) has been described, which results from a fusion between the terminal part of the Ewing sarcoma gene (EWS) and the carboxy terminus part of the Wilms tumor gene (WT1).[362]

The DSRCTs are highly chemosensitive, but the prognosis is still poor. Kretschmar et al.[363] reviewed 101 cases of DSRCT: after 2 years, only 2 patients were still alive, and the median survival was 17 months.

More recently, investigators from the Memorial Sloan Kettering Cancer Center reported a series of 66 patients treated with high dose alkylating agent–based chemotherapy with autologous bone marrow transplantation, surgical debulking, and whole-abdominopelvic radiotherapy. The dose to the whole abdomen was 30 Gy (1.5 Gy twice daily), and patients with gross residual disease received a boost of 6 to 15 Gy. The

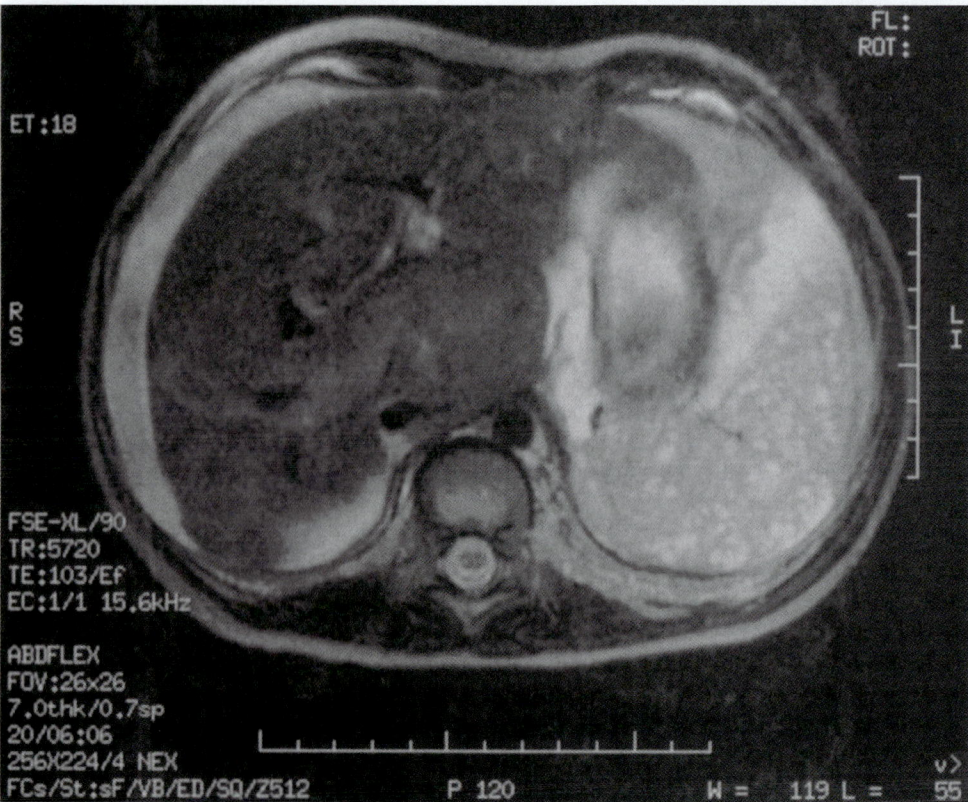

FIGURE 94.5. Gorham disease in a 3-year-old girl. Diffuse lymphangiomatosis affecting pelvic bones, ribs, spleen, and liver.

3-year overall survival was 48%, but the progression-free survival was only 35% in the first report.[363] In a more recent publication, a slightly better survival rate at 3 years (55%) was reported.[364] Survival at 3 years was only 27% when the three modalities were not used, with only 10 patients surviving without evidence of disease at a median follow-up of 2.4 years.

The MD Anderson Cancer Center published an outpatient and home chemotherapy program, including neoadjuvant chemotherapy, continuous hyperthermic peritoneal perfusion with cisplatin, and abdominal radiation (30 Gy) with simultaneous temozolomide with an overall survival at 3 years of 71% among eight patients.[365,366]

NONMELANOMA SKIN CANCER

Basal and squamous cell carcinomas are rare in children and adolescents. When they occur in the pediatric and adolescent age groups, there is usually an underlying predisposing genetic disorder, such as basal cell nevus syndrome (BCNS) or Gorlin-Goltz syndrome and xeroderma pigmentosum. Basal and squamous carcinomas have also been reported to arise in nevus sebaceous[367] and after radiation for benign or malignant conditions.[368,369]

BCNS or Gorlin-Goltz syndrome[370–372] is an autosomal dominant disorder with variable penetrance characterized by a "coarse face" with hypertelorism and frontal bossing, multiple basal cell carcinomas presenting at a young age, pits on the palms and soles, skeletal abnormalities (e.g., bifid ribs, hemivertebrae, fusion of vertebral bodies), jaw cysts, epidermic cysts and hamartomas, oculoneurologic abnormalities, and ectopic calcification of the falx cerebri and other structures. Skin lesions located in the head and neck tend to invade the deep structures. Several patients with BCNS were reported to have developed medulloblastoma at early childhood and ovarian fibromas.[164,370,373–377]

Mutation of the human homologue of *Drosophila*-patched (PTC) gene is considered the molecular defect in BCNS.[377,378] The Gorlin-Goltz syndrome is a unique example of the genetic–environmental interaction for the production of malignancies: children treated for medulloblastoma by craniospinal irradiation developed multiple skin cancers in the irradiated area, an unusual and special illustration of multihit mutagenesis, suggesting that radiotherapy should probably be omitted or limited in children with BCNS.[377]

Xeroderma pigmentosum (XP) is an extremely rare, autosomal recessive inherited disease characterized by abnormal pigmentation and >1,000-fold increase in nonmelanoma skin cancer (basal cell carcinoma and squamous cell carcinoma) on sun-exposed skin. XP patients are also at a significant risk to develop melanoma.[379,380] Neurologic abnormalities such as areflexia and mental retardation are sometimes associated with XP. The genetic abnormality underlying XP leads to defects in nucleotide excision repair of ultraviolet-induced DNA damage.[379,381,382]

Skin cancer in affected children is treated by standard techniques (such as surgery, cryosurgery, chemosurgery). There should not be any contraindication to using radiotherapy to treat skin cancer or any other malignancy in XP patients because ionizing radiation damage is normally repaired in these patients.[383]

MALIGNANT MELANOMA

Childhood melanoma can sometimes be associated with large congenital nevocytic nevi, dysplastic nevus syndrome, immunosuppression, transplacental malignant melanoma, and xeroderma pigmentosum.[384–389] Pediatric malignant melanoma should be distinguished from the juvenile melanoma or Spitz nevus characterized by a relatively benign course and long-term survival.[390–392]

The management of childhood melanoma follows the guidelines set for adult patients.[393] The prognosis is related to the Breslow or Clark thickness of the primary lesion and nodal status. Chemotherapy regimens usually have a poor activity against melanoma in adults. However, St. Jude Children's Research Hospital (SJCRH) has reported a complete or partial response in 8 of 18 (44%) pediatric patients receiving cyclophosphamide, vincristine, and dacarbazine.[394] Immunotherapy has been explored with promising results. Given the favorable results with the use of interferon α-2b in adults, 15 patients <18 years of age with stage III melanoma, defined as having a primary tumor thickness >4 mm or having lymph node or in-transit metastases, were included in a SJCRH feasibility study.[395] Another group from Toronto used the high dose interferon in children with metastatic disease.[396] Most of the patients in both studies did complete their therapy with some alterations in dosage because of toxicity. Intergroup Study of Cancer and Leukemia Group B, Children's Oncology Group, Eastern Cooperative Oncology Group, and Southwest Oncology Group (S0008) studied the role of biochemotherapy, which provided statistically significant improvement in RFS but no difference in OS patients with high-risk melanoma.[397] Targeted therapies, such as BRAF and MEK inhibitors that are approved for the treatment of patients with advanced melanoma who harbor *BRAF* V600E mutation–positive tumors, result in a significant survival advantage compared to chemotherapy.[398]

Recently, drugs blocking immune checkpoints, such as cytotoxic T-lymphocyte–associated antigen 4 (CTLA-4) and the programmed cell death protein 1 (PD-1) have been used to enhance antitumor immunity and have drawn huge interest.[399,400] Overall, the pediatric age group represented a very small proportion of patients studied for systemic therapy. Therefore, treatment plans for children are mainly extrapolated from adult studies.

Radiotherapy has a role mainly for palliation of metastatic disease or in locally advanced lesions. Again, data here should extrapolate from the adult literature; however, high dose per fraction regimens will need to be evaluated with caution because of toxicity concerns.

REFERENCES

1. Ayan I, Kaytan E, Ayan N. Childhood nasopharyngeal carcinoma: from biology to treatment. *Lancet Oncol* 2003;4:13–21.
2. Richards MK, et al. Factors associated with mortality in pediatric vs adult nasopharyngeal carcinoma. *JAMA Otolaryngol Head Neck Surg* (2016);142:217–222.
3. Shanmugartnam K, Sobin LH. *Histological typing of hyper-respiratory tract tumors.* Geneva, Switzerland: World Health Organization, 1978:32.
4. Neel HB III, Pearson GR, Taylor WF. Antibodies to Epstein-Barr virus in patients with nasopharyngeal carcinoma and in comparison groups. *Ann Otol Rhinol Laryngol* 1984;93:477–482.
5. Jia WH, et al. Traditional Cantonese diet and nasopharyngeal carcinoma risk: a large-scale case-control study in Guangdong, China. *BMC Cancer* 2010;10:446.
6. Ayan I, Altun M. Nasopharyngeal carcinoma in children: retrospective review of 50 patients. *Int J Radiat Oncol Biol Phys* 1996;35:485–492.
7. American Joint Committee for Cancer Staging and End Results Reporting. *Manual for staging of cancer.* 8th ed. Philadelphia, PA: JB Lippincott, 2017.
8. Al-Sarraf M, et al. Chemoradiotherapy versus radiotherapy in patients with advanced nasopharyngeal cancer: phase III randomized intergroup study 0099. *J Clin Oncol* 1998;16:1310–1317.
9. Cheng SH, et al. Long-term survival of nasopharyngeal carcinoma following concomitant radiotherapy and chemotherapy. *Int J Radiat Oncol Biol Phys* 2000;48:1323–1330.
10. Saba NF, Salama JK, Beitler JJ, et al. ACR Appropriateness criteria for nasopharyngeal carcinoma. *Head Neck* 2016;38:979–986.
11. Wolden SL, et al. Improved long-term survival with combined modality therapy for pediatric nasopharynx cancer. *Int J Radiat Oncol Biol Phys* 2000;46:859–864.
12. Zaghloul MS, et al. Does primary tumor volume predict the outcome of pediatric nasopharyngeal carcinoma?: A prospective single-arm study using neoadjuvant chemotherapy and concomitant chemotherapy with intensity modulated radiotherapy. *Asia Pac J Clin Oncol* 2016;12:143–150.
13. Arush MW, Stein ME, Rosenblatt E, et al. Advanced nasopharyngeal carcinoma in the young: the Northern Israel Oncology Center experience, 1973–1991. *Pediatr Hematol Oncol* 1995;12:271–276.
14. Casanova M, et al. International randomized phase 2 study on the addition of docetaxel to the combination of cisplatin and 5-fluorouracil in the induction treatment for nasopharyngeal carcinoma in children and adolescents. *Cancer Chemother Pharmacol* 2016;77:289–298.

Section III

15. Serin M, Erkal HS, Elhan AH, et al. Nasopharyngeal carcinoma in childhood and adolescence. *Med Pediatr Oncol* 1998;31:498–505.

16. Uzel O, Yoruk SO, Sahinler I, et al Nasopharyngeal carcinoma in childhood: long-term results of 32 patients. *Radiother Oncol* 2001;58:137–141.

17. Habrand J, Valls DG, Petras S, et al Carcinoma of the nasopharynx in children and adolescents treated with initial chemotherapy (CT) followed by adapted doses of radiotherapy (RT). *Int J Radiat Oncol Phys* 2004;69:191–s247.

18. Polychronopoulou S, et al. Nasopharyngeal carcinoma in childhood and adolescence: a single institution's experience with treatment modalities during the last 15 years. *Pediatr Hematol Oncol* 2004;21:393–402.

19. Orbach D, et al. Radiation and chemotherapy combination for nasopharyngeal carcinoma in children: radiotherapy dose adaptation after chemotherapy response to minimize late effects. *Pediatr Blood Cancer* 2008;50:849–853.

20. Cheuk DK, et al. Prognostic factors and long-term outcomes of childhood nasopharyngeal carcinoma. *Cancer* 2011;117:197–206.

21. Qiu WZ, et al. A retrospective study comparing the outcomes and toxicities of intensity-modulated radiotherapy versus two-dimensional conventional radiotherapy for the treatment of children and adolescent nasopharyngeal carcinoma. *J Cancer Res Clin Oncol* 2017;143:1563–1572.

22. Teo PM, et al. Final report of a randomized trial on altered-fractionated radiotherapy in nasopharyngeal carcinoma prematurely terminated by significant increase in neurologic complications. *Int J Radiat Oncol Biol Phys* 2000;48:1311–1322.

23. Feng WH, Israel B, Raab-Traub N, et al Chemotherapy induces lytic EBV replication and confers ganciclovir susceptibility to EBV-positive epithelial cell tumors. *Cancer Res* 2002;62:1920–1926.

24. Li JH, et al. Efficacy of targeted FasL in nasopharyngeal carcinoma. *Mol Ther* 2003;8:964–973.

25. Smith C, et al. Effective treatment of metastatic forms of Epstein-Barr virus-associated nasopharyngeal carcinoma with a novel adenovirus-based adoptive immunotherapy. *Cancer Res* 2012;72:1116–1125.

26. Rosenblatt E, et al. Late visual and auditory toxicity of radiotherapy for nasopharyngeal carcinoma. *Tumori* 2003;89:68–74.

27. Schwaab G, Bouzouita K, Janot F, et al. [ORL cancer in the child. Histologic and topographic distribution. Therapeutic indications (apropos of 380 IGR cases 1975–1987)]. *Bull Cancer* 1989;76:757–762.

28. Johnson GK, Squier CA. Smokeless tobacco use by youth: a health concern. *Pediatr Dent* 1993;15:169–174.

29. Torossian JM, Beziat JL, Philip T, et al Squamous cell carcinoma of the tongue in a 13-year-old boy. *J Oral Maxillofac Surg* 2000;58:1407–1410.

30. Gregoire V, et al. CT-based delineation of lymph node levels and related CTVs in the node-negative neck: DAHANCA, EORTC, GORTEC, NCIC, RTOG consensus guidelines *Radiother Oncol* 2003;69:227–236.

31. Smith EM, et al. Prevalence of human papillomavirus in the oral cavity/oropharynx in a large population of children and adolescents. *Pediatr Infect Dis J* 2007;26:836–840.

32. Kadish S, Goodman M, Wang CC. Olfactory neuroblastoma. A clinical analysis of 17 cases. *Cancer* 1976;37:1571–1576.

33. Hyams VJ, Batsakis JG, Michaels L. *Tumors of the upper respiratory tract and ear*. Washington, DC: Armed Forces Institute of Pathology, 1988.

34. Foote RL, et al. Esthesioneuroblastoma: the role of adjuvant radiation therapy. *Int J Radiat Oncol Biol Phys* 1993;27:835–842.

35. Eich HT, et al. Radiotherapy of esthesioneuroblastoma. *Int J Radiat Oncol Biol Phys* 2001;49:155–160.

36. Broich G, Pagliari A, Ottaviani F. Esthesioneuroblastoma: a general review of the cases published since the discovery of the tumour in 1924. *Anticancer Res* 1997;17:2683–2706.

37. Demiroz C, et al. Esthesioneuroblastoma: is there a need for elective neck treatment? *Int J Radiat Oncol Biol Phys* 2011;81:e255–e261.

38. Hollen TR, et al. Esthesioneuroblastoma of the nasal cavity. *Am J Clin Oncol* 2015;38:311–314.

39. Yin ZZ, et al. Long-term outcomes of patients with esthesioneuroblastomas: a cohort from a single institution. *Oral Oncol* 2016;53:48–53.

40. Sheehan JM, Sheehan JP, Jane JA Sr, et al Chemotherapy for esthesioneuroblastomas. *Neurosurg Clin N Am* 2000;11:693–701.

41. Mishima Y, et al. Combination chemotherapy (cyclophosphamide, doxorubicin, and vincristine with continuous-infusion cisplatin and etoposide) and radiotherapy with stem cell support can be beneficial for adolescents and adults with estheisoneuroblastoma. *Cancer* 2004;101:1437–1444.

42. Sohrabi S, et al. Neoadjuvant concurrent chemoradiation for advanced esthesioneuroblastoma: a case series and review of the literature. *J Clin Oncol* 2011;29:e358–e361.

43. Lucas JT Jr, et al. Proton therapy for pediatric and adolescent esthesioneuroblastoma. *Pediatr Blood Cancer* 2015;62:1523–1528.

44. Radkowski D, McGill T, Healy GB, et al. Angiofibroma. Changes in staging and treatment. *Arch Otolaryngol Head Neck Surg* 1996;122:122–129.

45. Abraham SC, Montgomery EA, Giardiello FM, et al. Frequent beta-catenin mutations in juvenile nasopharyngeal angiofibromas. *Am J Pathol* 2001;158:1073–1078.

46. Valanzano R, et al. Genetic evidence that juvenile nasopharyngeal angiofibroma is an integral FAP tumour. *Gut* 2005;54:1046–1047.

47. Cummings BJ, et al. Primary radiation therapy for juvenile nasopharyngeal angiofibroma. *Laryngoscope* 1984;94:1599–1605.

48. Enepekides DJ. Recent advances in the treatment of juvenile angiofibroma. *Curr Opin Otolaryngol Head Neck Surg* 2004;12:495–499.

49. Wormald PJ, Van Hasselt A. Endoscopic removal of juvenile angiofibromas. *Otolaryngol Head Neck Surg* 2003;129:684–691.

50. Kumar AR, Nayak JV, Janisiewicz AM, et al The combined subtemporal-transfacial approach for the resection of juvenile nasopharyngeal angiofibromas with intracranial extension. *Otol Neurotol* 2015;36:151–155.

51. Kuppersmith RB, Teh BS, Donovan DT, et al. The use of intensity modulated radiotherapy for the treatment of extensive and recurrent juvenile angiofibroma. *Int J Pediatr Otorhinolaryngol* 2000;52:261–268.

52. Chakraborty S, Ghoshal S, Patil VM, et al. Conformal radiotherapy in the treatment of advanced juvenile nasopharyngeal angiofibroma with intracranial extension: an institutional experience. *Int J Radiat Oncol Biol Phys* 2011;80:1398–1404.

53. Mallick S, Benson R, Bhasker S, et al. Long-term treatment outcomes of juvenile nasopharyngeal angiofibroma treated with radiotherapy. *Acta Otorhinolaryngol Ital* 2015;35:75–79.

54. Pandey P, et al. Current molecular profile of juvenile nasopharyngeal angiofibroma: first comprehensive study from India. *Laryngoscope* 2017;127:E100–E106.

55. La Salle AJ, Andrassy RJ, Stanford W. Bronchogenic squamous cell carcinoma in childhood; a case report. *J Pediatr Surg* 1977;12:519–521.

56. Hartman GE, Shochat SJ Primary pulmonary neoplasms of childhood: a review. *Ann Thorac Surg* 1983;36:108–119.

57. Priest JR, et al. Pleuropulmonary blastoma: a clinicopathologic study of 50 cases. *Cancer* 1997;80:147–161.

58. Romeo C, Impellizzeri P, Grosso M, et al Pleuropulmonary blastoma: long-term survival and literature review. *Med Pediatr Oncol* 1999;33:372–376.

59. Dehner LP, Watterson J, Priest J. Pleuropulmonary blastoma. A unique intrathoracic pulmonary neoplasm of childhood. *Perspect Pediatr Pathol* 1995;1995:214–216.

60. Schultz KA, Williams GM, Stewart D, et al. Association of recurrent or progressive p of form types II and III pleuropulmonary blastoma (PPB) with poor outcome: a report from the international PPB registry. *J Clin Oncol* 2015;33:Abstract 10014.

61. Messinger YH, et al. Pleuropulmonary blastoma: a report on 350 central pathology-confirmed pleuropulmonary blastoma cases by the International Pleuropulmonary Blastoma Registry. *Cancer* 2015;121:276–285.

62. Hill DA, et al. DICER1 mutations in familial pleuropulmonary blastoma. *Science* 2009;325:965.

63. Dosios T, et al. Pleuropulmonary blastoma in childhood. A malignant degeneration of pulmonary cysts. *Pediatr Surg Int* 2004;20:863–865.

64. Priest JR, et al. Great vessel/cardiac extension and tumor embolism in pleuropulmonary blastoma: a report from the International Pleuropulmonary Blastoma Registry. *Pediatr Blood Cancer* 2011;56:604–609.

65. Ayhan A, Bildirici I, Gunalp S, et al. Pure dysgerminoma of the ovary: a review of 45 well staged cases. *Eur J Gynaecol Oncol* 2000;21:98–101.

66. Pinarli FG, Oguz A, Ceyda K, et al. Type II pleuropulmonary blastoma responsive to multimodal therapy. *Pediatr Hematol Oncol* 2005;22:71–76.

67. Indolfi P, et al. Pleuropulmonary blastoma: management and prognosis of 11 cases. *Cancer* 2000;89:1396–1401.

68. Kotiloglu E, Kaya H, Guney I, et al The Mckusick-Kaufman syndrome: report of a case with some associations. *Turk J Pediatr* 2002;44:176–179.

69. Ozkaynak MF, Ortega JA, Laug W, et al. Role of chemotherapy in pediatric pulmonary blastoma. *Med Pediatr Oncol* 1990;18:53–56.

70. Parsons SK, et al. Aggressive multimodal treatment of pleuropulmonary blastoma. *Ann Thorac Surg* 2001;72:939–942.

71. Altman AJ, Schwartz A. *Malignant diseases of infancy, childhood and adolescence*. 2nd ed. Philadelphia, PA: WB Saunders, 1983:505.

72. De Cholnoky T. Mammary cancer in youth. *Surg Gynecol Obstet* 1943;77:55–60.

73. Farrow JH, Hiroyuki A. Breast lesions in young girls. *Surg Clin North Am* 1969;49:261–269.

74. Haagensen CD. *The relation of age to the frequency of breast carcinoma in diseases of the breast*. 3rd ed. Philadelphia, PA: WB Saunders, 1986.

75. Corpron CA, Black CT, Singletary SE, et al. Breast cancer in adolescent females. *J Pediatr Surg* 1995;30:322–324.

76. Roisman I, Barak V, Robinson E, et al Breast malignancies in adolescents in Israel (1967–1989). *Breast Dis* 1992;5:149–168.

77. Umanah IN, Akhiwu W, Ojo OS. Breast tumours of adolescents in an African population. *Afr J Paediatr Surg* 2010;7:78–80.

78. Templeman C, Hertweck SP. Breast disorders in the pediatric and adolescent patient. *Obstet Gynecol Clin North Am* 2000;27:19–34.

79. McDivitt RW, Stewart FW. Breast carcinoma in children. *JAMA* 1966;195:388–390.

80. Dugue G, Bock G, Molho L, et al Breast cancer in the young. *J Natl Med Assoc* 1989;81:1184, 1187–1188.

81. Eskelinen M, et al. Carcinoma of the breast in children. *Z Kinderchir* 1990;45:52–55.

82. Bower R, Bell MJ, Ternberg JL. Management of breast lesions in children and adolescents. *J Pediatr Surg* 1976;11:337–346.

83. Sears JB, Schlesinger MJ. Carcinoma of the breast in a ten-year-old girl: report of a case. *N Engl J Med* 1940;223:760–761.

84. Karl SR, Ballantine TV, Zaino R. Juvenile secretory carcinoma of the breast. *J Pediatr Surg* 1985;20:368–371.

85. Bond SJ, Buchino JJ, Nagaraj HS, et al. Sentinel lymph node biopsy in juvenile secretory carcinoma. *J Pediatr Surg* 2004;39:120–121.

86. Hartman AW, Magrish P. Carcinoma of breast in children; case report: six-year-old boy with adenocarcinoma. *Ann Surg* 1955;141:792–798.

87. Chamadol W, Pesie M, Puapairoj A. Inflammatory carcinoma of the breast in a 12-year-old Thai girl. *J Med Assoc Thai* 1987;70:543–548.

88. Nichini FM, et al. Inflammatory carcinoma of the breast in a 12-year-old girl. *Arch Surg* 1972;105:505–508.

89. Blichert-Toft M, Hansen JP, Hansen OH, et al. Clinical course of cystosarcoma phyllodes related to histologic appearance. *Surg Gynecol Obstet* 1975;140:929–932.

90. McDivitt RW, Urban JA, Farrow JH. Cystosarcoma phyllodes. *Johns Hopkins Med J* 1967;120:33–45.

91. Miliauskas JR, Leong AS. Adenoid cystic carcinoma in a juvenile male breast. *Pathology* 1991;23:298–301.

92. Mollitt DL, Golladay ES, Gloster ES, et al Cystosarcoma phyllodes in the adolescent female. *J Pediatr Surg* 1987;22:907–910.

93. Norris HJ, Taylor HB. Relationship of histologic features to behavior of cystosarcoma phyllodes. Analysis of ninety-four cases. *Cancer* 1967;20:2090–2099.

94. Squire R, Bianchi A, Jakate SM. Radiation-induced sarcoma of the breast in a female adolescent. Case report with histologic and therapeutic considerations. *Cancer* 1988;61:2444–2447.

95. Halverson JD, Hori-Rubaina JM. Cystosarcoma phyllodes of the breast. *Am Surg* 1974;40:295–301.

96. Long RT, Hesker AE, Johnson RE. Surgical management of cystosarcoma phyllodes with a report of 8 cases. *Mo Med* 1962;59:1179–1181.

97. Schmidt B, Lantsberg L, Goldstein J, et al Cystosarcoma phyllodes. *Isr J Med Sci* 1981;17:895–898.

98. Treves N, Sunderland DA. Cystosarcoma phyllodes of the breast. A malignant and a benign tumor. A clinicopathological study of seventy-seven cases. *Cancer* 1951;4:1386–1332.

99. West TL, Weiland LH, Clagett OT. Cystosarcoma phyllodes. *Ann Surg* 1971;173:520–528.

100. Billroth T. Untersuchungen uber den feineren Bau und die Entwicklung der Brustdrusengeschwulste. *Virchows Arch Pathol Anat Physiol* 1860;18:51–81.

101. Howarth CB, Caces JN, Pratt CB. Breast metastases in children with rhabdomyosarcoma. *Cancer* 1980;46:2520–2524.

102. Rogers DA, et al. Breast malignancy in children. *J Pediatr Surg* 1994;29:48–51.

103. Garcia Marcilla JA, Sanchez Bueno F, Aguilar J, et al Primary small bowel malignant tumors. *Eur J Surg Oncol* 1994;20:630–634.

104. Schettini ST, Ganc A, Saba L Esophageal carcinoma secondary to a chemical injury in a child. *Pediatr Surg Int* 1998;13:519–520.

105. DuVall GA, Walden DT. Adenocarcinoma of the esophagus complicating Cornelia de Lange syndrome. *J Clin Gastroenterol* 1996;22:131–133.

106. Hassall E. Barrett's esophagus: new definitions and approaches in children. *J Pediatr Gastroenterol Nutr* 1993;16:345–364.

107. McGill TW, Downey EC, Westbrook J, et al. Gastric carcinoma in children. *J Pediatr Surg* 1993;28:1620–1621.

108. Bourque MD, et al. Esophageal leiomyoma in children: two case reports and review of the literature. *J Pediatr Surg* 1989;24:1103–1107.

109. Pratt CB, et al. Colorectal carcinoma in adolescents implications regarding etiology. *Cancer* 1977;40:2464–2472.

110. Vade A, Nolan J. Posterior mediastinal teratoma involving the esophagus. *Gastrointest Radiol* 1989;14:106–108.

111. Brenner B, Ilson DH, Minsky BD. Treatment of localized esophageal cancer. *Semin Oncol* 2004;31:554–565.

112. Harting MT, et al. Treatment issues in pediatric gastric adenocarcinoma. *J Pediatr Surg* 2004;39:e8–e10.

113. Subbiah V, Varadhachary G, Herzog CE, et al Gastric adenocarcinoma in children and adolescents. *Pediatr Blood Cancer* 2011;57:524–527.

114. Sasaki H, et al. Adenocarcinoma at the esophageal gastric junction arising in an 11-year-old girl. *Pathol Int* 1999;49:1109–1113.

115. Lin CH, et al. Pediatric gastric cancer presenting with massive ascites. *World J Gastroenterol* 2015;21:3409–3413.

116. Jaeger HJ, Schmitz-Stolbrink A, Albrecht M, et al. Gastric leiomyosarcoma in a child. *Eur J Radiol* 1996;23:111–114.

117. Moschovi M, Menegas D, Stefanaki K, et al. Primary gastric Burkitt lymphoma in childhood: associated with *Helicobacter pylori?* *Med Pediatr Oncol* 2003;41:444–447.

118. Lee J, et al. Phase III trial comparing capecitabine plus cisplatin versus capecitabine plus cisplatin with concurrent capecitabine radiotherapy in completely resected gastric cancer with D2 lymph node dissection: the ARTIST trial. *J Clin Oncol* 2012;30:268–273.

119. Cunningham D, et al. Perioperative chemotherapy versus surgery alone for resectable gastroesophageal cancer. *N Engl J Med* 2006;355:11–20.

120. Albarello L, Pecciarini L, Doglioni C. HER2 testing in gastric cancer. *Adv Anat Pathol* 2011;18:53–59.

121. Takashima T, et al. Phase II study of S-1 in combination with trastuzumab for HER2-positive metastatic breast cancer. *Anticancer Res* 2014;34:3583–3588.

122. Weiss NS, Yang CP. Incidence of histologic types of cancer of the small intestine. *J Natl Cancer Inst* 1987;78:653–656.

123. Azab MB, et al. Prognostic factors in primary gastrointestinal non-Hodgkin's lymphoma. A multivariate analysis, report of 106 cases, and review of the literature. *Cancer* 1989;64:1208–1217.

124. Tovar JA, Eizaguirre I, Albert A, et al. Peutz-Jeghers syndrome in children: report of two cases and review of the literature. *J Pediatr Surg* 1983;18:1–6.

125. National Cancer Institute. *Surveillance, epidemiology, and end results.* Bethesda, MD: National Institutes of Health, 2014.

126. Hinton JM. Risk of malignant change in ulcerative colitis. *Gut* 1966;7:427–432.

127. Rogler G. Chronic ulcerative colitis and colorectal cancer. *Cancer Lett* 2014;345:235–241.

128. MacDonald V, Hilton BA. Postoperative pain management in frail older adults. *Orthop Nurs* 2001;20:63–76.

129. Sulkes A. Chemotherapy in gastric cancer: a brief chronicle with emphasis on recent developments. *Isr Med Assoc J* 2004;6:415–419.

130. Jiang Y, Ajani JA. Multidisciplinary management of gastric cancer. *Curr Opin Gastroenterol* 2010;26:640–646.

131. Church JM, McGannon E, Burke C, et al Teenagers with familial adenomatous polyposis: what is their risk for colorectal cancer? *Dis Colon Rectum* 2002;45:887–889.

132. Gardner EJ. Follow-up study of a family group exhibiting dominant inheritance for a syndrome including intestinal polyps, osteomas, fibromas and epidermal cysts. *Am J Hum Genet* 1962;14:376–390.

133. Hamilton SR, et al. The molecular basis of Turcot's syndrome. *N Engl J Med* 1995;332:839–847.

134. Oldfield MC. The association of familial polyposis of the colon with multiple sebaceous cysts. *Br J Surg* 1954;41:534–541.

135. Vogelstein B, et al. Genetic alterations during colorectal-tumor development. *N Engl J Med* 1988;319:525–532.

136. Morin PJ, Kinzler KW, Sparks AB. Beta-Catenin Mutations: Insights into the APC Pathway and the Power of Genetics. *Cancer Res* 2016;76:5587–5589.

137. Hill DA, et al. Colorectal carcinoma in childhood and adolescence: a clinicopathologic review. *J Clin Oncol* 2007;25:5808–5814.

138. Kravarusic D, et al. Colorectal carcinoma in childhood: a retrospective multi-center study. *J Pediatr Gastroenterol Nutr* 2007;44:209–211.

139. Chen LK, Hwang SJ, Li AF, et al Colorectal cancer in patients 20 years old or less in Taiwan. *South Med J* 2001;94:1202–1205.

140. Symonds DA, Vickery AL. Mucinous carcinoma of the colon and rectum. *Cancer* 1976;37:1891–1900.

141. Andersson A, Bergdahl L. Carcinoma of the colon in children: a report of six new cases and a review of the literature. *J Pediatr Surg* 1976;11:967–971.

142. Karnak I, Ciftci AO, Senocak ME, et al Colorectal carcinoma in children. *J Pediatr Surg* 1999;34:1499–1504.

143. Odone V, Chang L, Caces J, et al. The natural history of colorectal carcinoma in adolescents. *Cancer* 1982;49:1716–1720.

144. Sauer R, et al. Preoperative versus postoperative chemoradiotherapy for rectal cancer. *N Engl J Med* 2004;351:1731–1740.

145. Field JL, Adamson LF, Stoeckle HE. Review of carcinoids in children. Functioning carcinoid in a 15-year-old male. *Pediatrics* 1962;29:953–960.

146. Moertel CG, Weiland LH, Nagorney DM, et al. Carcinoid tumor of the appendix: treatment and prognosis. *N Engl J Med* 1987;317:1699–1701.

147. Nadler EP, et al. The use of endoscopic ultrasound in the diagnosis of solid pseudopapillary tumors of the pancreas in children. *J Pediatr Surg* 2002;37:1370–1373.

148. Shorter NA, Glick RD, Klimstra DS, et al. Malignant pancreatic tumors in childhood and adolescence: the Memorial Sloan-Kettering experience, 1967 to present. *J Pediatr Surg* 2002;37:887–892.

149. Vilaverde F, Reis A, Rodrigues P, et al. Adult pancreatoblastoma—case report and review of literature. *J Radiol Case Rep* 2016;10:28–38.

150. Glick RD, Pashankar FD, Pappo A, et al. Management of pancreatoblastoma in children and young adults. *J Pediatr Hematol Oncol* 2012;34(Suppl 2):S47–S50.

151. Bien E, et al. Pancreatoblastoma: a report from the European cooperative study group for paediatric rare tumours (EXPeRT). *Eur J Cancer* 2011;47:2347–2352.

152. Chun Y, Kim W, Park K, et al. Pancreatoblastoma. *J Pediatr Surg* 1997;32:1612–1615.

153. Klimstra DS, Wenig BM, Adair CF, et al. Pancreatoblastoma. A clinicopathologic study and review of the literature. *Am J Surg Pathol* 1995;19:1371–1389.

154. Willnow U, Willberg B, Schwamborn D, et al Pancreatoblastoma in children. Case report and review of the literature. *Eur J Pediatr Surg* 1996;6:369–372.

155. Perez EA, et al. Malignant pancreatic tumors: incidence and outcome in 58 pediatric patients. *J Pediatr Surg* 2009;44:197–203.

156. Mah PT, Loo DC, Tock EP. Pancreatic acinar cell carcinoma in childhood. *Am J Dis Child* 1974;128:101–104.

157. Mielcarek PA. Primary Adenocarcinoma of the Pancreas in a Fifteen Year Old Boy. *Am J Pathol* 1935;11:527–533.

158. Murakami T, et al. Pancreatoblastoma: case report and review of treatment in the literature. *Med Pediatr Oncol* 1996;27:193–197.

159. Defachelles AS, et al. Pancreatoblastoma in childhood: clinical course and therapeutic management of seven patients. *Med Pediatr Oncol* 2001;37:47–52.

160. Sheng L, Weixia Z, Longhai Y, et al. Clinical and biologic analysis of pancreatoblastoma. *Pancreas* 2005;30:87–90.

161. Yonekura T, et al. Aggressive surgical and chemotherapeutic treatment of advanced pancreatoblastoma associated with tumor thrombus in portal vein. *J Pediatr Surg* 2006;41:596–598.

162. Dhamne C, Herzog CE. Response of Relapsed Pancreatoblastoma to a Combination of Vinorelbine and Oral Cyclophosphamide. *J Pediatr Hematol Oncol* 2015;37:e378–e380.

163. Mao C, et al. Papillary cystic and solid tumors of the pancreas: a pancreatic embryonic tumor? Studies of three cases and cumulative review of the world's literature *Surgery* 1995;118:821–828.

164. Kimonis VE, et al. Clinical manifestations in 105 persons with nevoid basal cell carcinoma syndrome. *Am J Med Genet* 1997;69:299–308.

165. Hwang J, Kim DY, Kim SC, et al. Solid-pseudopapillary neoplasm of the pancreas in children: can we predict malignancy? *J Pediatr Surg* 2014;49:1730–1733.

166. Gelfand M, Castle WM, Buchanan WM. Primary carcinoma of the liver (hepatoma) in Rhodesia: a clinical study. *S Afr Med J* 1972;46:527–532.

167. Weinberg AG, Finegold MJ. Primary hepatic tumors of childhood. *Hum Pathol* 1983;14:512–537.

168. Leuschner I, Harms D, Schmidt D. The association of hepatocellular carcinoma in childhood with hepatitis B virus infection. *Cancer* 1988;62:2363–2369.

169. Chang MH, et al. Universal hepatitis B vaccination in Taiwan and the incidence of hepatocellular carcinoma in children. Taiwan Childhood Hepatoma Study Group. *N Engl J Med* 336, 1855–1859 (1997).

170. Takano H, Smith WL. Gastrointestinal tumors of childhood. *Radiol Clin North Am* 1997;35:1367–1389.

171. Halperin EC, Constine LS, Tarbell NJ, et al. *Pediatric radiation oncology.* Philadelphia, PA: Lippincott Williams & Wilkins, 2012.

172. Bhattacharya S, Lobo FD, Pai PK, et al. Hepatic neoplasms in childhood—a clinicopathologic study. *Pediatr Surg Int* 1998;14:51–54.

173. Ito E, et al. Type 1a glycogen storage disease with hepatoblastoma in siblings. *Cancer* 1987;59:1776–1780.

174. Kingston JE, Herbert A, Draper GJ, et al Association between hepatoblastoma and polyposis coli. *Arch Dis Child* 1983;58:959–962.

Section III

175. Koufos A, et al. Loss of heterozygosity in three embryonal tumours suggests a common pathogenetic mechanism. *Nature* 1985;316:330–334.
176. Cairo S, et al. Hepatic stem-like phenotype and interplay of Wnt/beta-catenin and Myc signaling in aggressive childhood liver cancer. *Cancer Cell* 2008;14:471–484.
177. Ueda Y, et al. Wnt signaling and telomerase activation of hepatoblastoma: correlation with chemosensitivity and surgical resectability. *J Pediatr Surg* 2011;46:2221–2227.
178. Galifer RB, Sultan C, Margueritte G, et al Testosterone-producing hepatoblastoma in a 3-year-old boy with precocious puberty. *J Pediatr Surg* 1985;20:713–714.
179. Weinberg AG, Finegold MJ Primary hepatic tumors in childhood. In: Finegold MJ, Bennington JL, eds. *Pathology of neoplasia in children and adolescents*. Philadelphia, PA: WB Saunders, 1986:333–372.
180. Voute PA, Penkerton R. Liver tumors. In: Peckham M, Pinedo H, Umberto V, eds. *Oxford textbook of oncology*. New York: Oxford Press, 1995:2036–2039.
181. Stocker JT. Hepatoblastoma. *Semin Diagn Pathol* 1994;11:136–143.
182. Haas JE, et al. Histopathology and prognosis in childhood hepatoblastoma and hepatocarcinoma. *Cancer* 1989;64:1082–1095.
183. Plaschkes J. Proceedings of an international research workshop on pediatric liver tumours, 18–20 March 1999, Berne, Switzerland. Into the year 2000. *Med Pediatr Oncol* 2001;36:380–382.
184. Sumazin P, et al. Genomic analysis of hepatoblastoma identifies distinct molecular and prognostic subgroups. *Hepatology* 2017;65:104–121.
185. Exelby PR, Filler RM, Grosfeld JL. Liver tumors in children in the particular reference to hepatoblastoma and hepatocellular carcinoma: American Academy of Pediatrics Surgical Section Survey—1974. *J Pediatr Surg* 1975;10:329–337.
186. Newman KD. Malignant liver tumors of children. *Semin Pediatr Surg* 1992;1:145–151.
187. Dickstein G, Shechner C, Arad E, et al. Is there a role for low doses of mitotane (o,p'-DDD) as adjuvant therapy in adrenocortical carcinoma? *J Clin Endocrinol Metab* 1998;83:3100–3103.
188. Kew MC. Hepatocellular carcinoma with and without cirrhosis. A comparison in southern African blacks. *Gastroenterology* 1989;97:136–139.
189. Craig JR, Peters RL, Edmondson HA, et al. Fibrolamellar carcinoma of the liver: a tumor of adolescents and young adults with distinctive clinico-pathologic features. *Cancer* 1980;46:372–379.
190. Lack EE, Neave C, Vawter GF. Hepatocellular carcinoma. Review of 32 cases in childhood and adolescence. *Cancer* 1983;52:1510–1515.
191. Lack EE, Neave C, Vawter GF. Hepatoblastoma. A clinical and pathologic study of 54 cases. *Am J Surg Pathol* 1982;6:693–705.
192. Bellani FF, Massimino M. Liver tumors in childhood: epidemiology and clinics. *J Surg Oncol Suppl* 1993;3:119–121.
193. Harvey VJ, Woodfield DG, Probert JC. Maternal transmission of hepatocellular carcinoma. *Cancer* 1984;54:1360–1363.
194. Ames BN, Durston WE, Yamasaki E, et al Carcinogens are mutagens: a simple test system combining liver homogenates for activation and bacteria for detection. *Proc Natl Acad Sci U S A* 1973;70:2281–2285.
195. Bressac B, Kew M, Wands J, et al Selective G to T mutations of p53 gene in hepatocellular carcinoma from southern Africa. *Nature* 1991;350:429–431.
196. Hsu IC, et al. Mutational hotspot in the p53 gene in human hepatocellular carcinomas. *Nature* 1991;350:427–428.
197. Giacomantonio M, Ein SH, Mancer K, et al. Thirty years of experience with pediatric primary malignant liver tumors. *J Pediatr Surg* 1984;19:523–526.
198. Smith WL, Franken EA, Mitros FA. Liver tumors in children. *Semin Roentgenol* 1983;18:136–148.
199. Stillwagon GB, et al. Prognostic factors in unresectable hepatocellular cancer: Radiation Therapy Oncology Group Study 83-01. *Int J Radiat Oncol Biol Phys* 1991;20:65–71.
200. Gauthier F, Valayer J, Thai BL, et al. Hepatoblastoma and hepatocarcinoma in children: analysis of a series of 29 cases. *J Pediatr Surg* 1986;21:424–429.
201. Cohen MD, Bugaieski EM, Haliloglu M, et al. Visual presentation of the staging of pediatric solid tumors. *Radiographics* 1996;16:523–545.
202. Perilongo G., S.D., Meadown A.T., et al. *Liver tumors*. New York: Wiley-Liss, 1992).
203. Bowman LC, Riely CA. Management of pediatric liver tumors. *Surg Oncol Clin N Am* 1996;5:451–459.
204. Nagasue N, et al. Active uptake of testosterone by androgen receptors of hepatocellular carcinoma in humans. *Cancer* 1986;572162–2167.
205. Habrand JL, et al. Is there a place for radiation therapy in the management of hepatoblastomas and hepatocellular carcinomas in children? *Int J Radiat Oncol Biol Phys* 1992;23:525–531.
206. Schmidt D, Harms D, Lang W. Primary malignant hepatic tumours in childhood. *Virchows Arch A Pathol Anat Histopathol* 1985;407:387–405.
207. Mody RJ, Pohlen JA, Malde S, et al. FDG PET for the study of primary hepatic malignancies in children. *Pediatr Blood Cancer* 2006;47:51–55.
208. Reynolds M, Douglass EC, Finegold M, et al Chemotherapy can convert unresectable hepatoblastoma. *J Pediatr Surg* 1992;27:1080–1083; discussion 1083–1084.
209. Nagel C, Armeanu-Ebinger S, Dewerth A, et al. Anti-tumor activity of sorafenib in a model of a pediatric hepatocellular carcinoma. *Exp Cell Res* 2015;331:97–104.
210. Kim A, et al. Phase 2 trial of sorafenib in children and young adults with refractory solid tumors: a report from the Children's Oncology Group. *Pediatr Blood Cancer* 2015;62:1562–1566.
211. Cheng AL, et al. Efficacy and safety of sorafenib in patients in the Asia-Pacific region with advanced hepatocellular carcinoma: a phase III randomised, double-blind, placebo-controlled trial. *Lancet Oncol* 2009;10:25–34.
212. Sun W, et al. Phase 2 trial of bevacizumab, capecitabine, and oxaliplatin in treatment of advanced hepatocellular carcinoma. *Cancer* 2011;117:3187–3192.
213. DE Pasquale MD, de Ville de Goyet J, Monti L, et al. Bevacizumab Combined with Chemotherapy in Children Affected by Hepatocellular Carcinoma: a Single-center Experience. *Anticancer Res* 2017;37:1489–1493.
214. Guglielmi M, et al. Rationale and results of the International Society of Pediatric Oncology (SIOP) Italian pilot study on childhood hepatoma: surgical resection d'emblee or after primary chemotherapy? *J Surg Oncol Suppl* 1993;3:122–126.
215. Hertl M, Cosimi AB. Liver transplantation for malignancy. *Oncologist* 2005;10:269–281.
216. Superina R, Bilik R. Results of liver transplantation in children with unresectable liver tumors. *J Pediatr Surg* 31, 835–839 (1996).
217. Tagge EP, et al. Resection, including transplantation, for hepatoblastoma and hepatocellular carcinoma: impact on survival. *J Pediatr Surg* 1992;27: 292–296; discussion 297.
218. Berry CL, Keeling JW. Hepatoblastoma. In: *Pediatric pathology*. Berlin, Germany: Springer-Verlag, 1981:660–662.
219. Clatworthy HW Jr, Schiller M, Grosfeld JL. Primary liver tumors in infancy and childhood. 41 cases variously treated. *Arch Surg* 1974;109:143–147.
220. Pazdur R, Bready B, Cangir A. Pediatric hepatic tumors: clinical trials conducted in the United States. *J Surg Oncol Suppl* 1993;3:127–130.
221. Van Tornout JM, et al. Timing and magnitude of decline in alpha-fetoprotein levels in treated children with unresectable or metastatic hepatoblastoma are predictors of outcome: a report from the Children's Cancer Group. *J Clin Oncol* 1997;15:1190–1197.
222. Ortega JA, Douglass EC, Feusner JH, et al Randomized comparison of cisplatin/vincristine/fluorouracil and cisplatin/continuous infusion doxorubicin for treatment of pediatric hepatoblastoma: a report from the Children's Cancer Group and the Pediatric Oncology Group. *J Clin Oncol* 2000;18:2665–2675.
223. Douglass EC, Reynolds M, Finegold M, et al Cisplatin, vincristine, and fluorouracil therapy for hepatoblastoma: a Pediatric Oncology Group study. *J Clin Oncol* 1993;11:96–99.
224. Czauderna P, et al. Hepatocellular carcinoma in children: results of the first prospective study of the International Society of Pediatric Oncology group. *J Clin Oncol* 2002;20:2798–2804.
225. Mazumdar M, et al. Predicting outcome to chemotherapy in patients with germ cell tumors: the value of the rate of decline of human chorionic gonadotrophin and alpha-fetoprotein during therapy. *J Clin Oncol* 2001;19:2534–2541.
226. Pritchard J, et al. Cisplatin, doxorubicin, and delayed surgery for childhood hepatoblastoma: a successful approach—results of the first prospective study of the International Society of Pediatric Oncology. *J Clin Oncol* 2000;18:3819–3828.
227. Perilongo G, et al. Risk-adapted treatment for childhood hepatoblastoma. Final report of the second study of the International Society of Paediatric Oncology—SIOPEL 2. *Eur J Cancer* 2004;40:411–421.
228. Perilongo G, et al. Cisplatin versus cisplatin plus doxorubicin for standard-risk hepatoblastoma. *N Engl J Med* 2009;361:1662–1670.
229. Zsiros J, et al. Dose-dense cisplatin-based chemotherapy and surgery for children with high-risk hepatoblastoma (SIOPEL-4): a prospective, single-arm, feasibility study. *Lancet Oncol* 2013;14:834–842.
230. Brock Penelope Rachel, Maibach Rudolf, Childs Margaret, et al. Anti-tumor efficacy in SIOPEL 6: A multi-centre open label randomised phase III trial of the efficacy of sodium thiosulphate (STS) in reducing ototoxicity in patients receiving cisplatin (Cis) monotherapy for standard risk hepatoblastoma (SR-HB). *J Clin Oncol* 2015;33(Suppl 15):10039.
231. Meyers RL, Czauderna P, Otte JB. Surgical treatment of hepatoblastoma. *Pediatr Blood Cancer* 2012;59:800–808.
232. Gerber DA, et al. Use of intrahepatic chemotherapy to treat advanced pediatric hepatic malignancies. *J Pediatr Gastroenterol Nutr* 2000;30:137–144.
233. Arcement CM, et al. Intrahepatic chemoembolization in unresectable pediatric liver malignancies. *Pediatr Radiol* 2000;30:779–785.
234. Ogita S, Tokiwa K, Taniguchi H, et al. Intraarterial injection of anti-tumor drugs dispersed in lipid contrast medium: a choice for initially unresectable hepatoblastoma in infants. *J Pediatr Surg* 22, 412–414 (1987).
235. Suita S, et al. Improved survival outcome for hepatoblastoma based on an optimal chemotherapeutic regimen—a report from the study group for pediatric solid malignant tumors in the Kyushu area. *J Pediatr Surg* 2004;39:195–198; discussion 195–198.
236. Fuchs J, et al. Pretreatment prognostic factors and treatment results in children with hepatoblastoma: a report from the German Cooperative Pediatric Liver Tumor Study HB 94. *Cancer* 2002;95:172–182.
237. Haberle B, Bode U, von Schweinitz D. [Differentiated treatment protocols for high- and standard-risk hepatoblastoma—an interim report of the German Liver Tumor Study HB99]. *Klin Padiatr* 2003;215:159–165.
238. Arceci RJ. The histiocytoses: the fall of the Tower of Babel. *Eur J Cancer* 1999;35:747–767; discussion 767–749.
239. Coury F, et al. Langerhans cell histiocytosis reveals a new IL-17A-dependent pathway of dendritic cell fusion. *Nat Med* 2008;14:81–87.
240. Lau SK, Chu PG, Weiss LM. Immunohistochemical expression of Langerin in Langerhans cell histiocytosis and non-Langerhans cell histiocytic disorders. *Am J Surg Pathol* 2008;32:615–619.
241. Halperin EC, C.L.S., Tarbell N.J., Kun L.E. Langerhans' cell histiocytosis. In: *Pediatric radiative oncology*. 446–472 (Raven Press, New York, 1994).
242. Broadbent V, Gadner H. Current therapy for Langerhans cell histiocytosis. *Hematol Oncol Clin North Am* 1998;12:327–338.
243. McClain KL. Drug therapy for the treatment of Langerhans cell histiocytosis. *Expert Opin Pharmacother* 2005;6:2435–2441.
244. Gadner H, et al. Improved outcome in multisystem Langerhans cell histiocytosis is associated with therapy intensification. *Blood* 2008;111:2556–2562.
245. Lahey, M.E. Prognostic factors in histiocytosis X. *Am J Pediatr Hematol Oncol* 1981;3:57–60.
246. Berry DH, Gresik M, Maybee D, et al. Histiocytosis X in bone only. *Med Pediatr Oncol* 1990;18:292–294.
247. Kriz J, et al. Radiotherapy in langerhans cell histiocytosis—a rare indication in a rare disease. *Radiat Oncol* 2013;8:233.
248. Selch MT, Parker RG. Radiation therapy in the management of Langerhans cell histiocytosis. *Med Pediatr Oncol* 1990;18:97–102.

249. Olschewski T, Seegenschmiedt MH. Radiotherapy of Langerhans' Cell Histiocytosis: Results and Implications of a National Patterns-of-Care Study. *Strahlenther Onkol* 2006;182:629–634.

250. Olschewski T, Seegenschmiedt MH. Radiotherapy for bony manifestations of Langerhans cell histiocytosis. Review and proposal for an international registry. *Strahlenther Onkol* 2006;182:72–79.

251. Micke O, Seegenschmiedt MH, German Cooperative Group on Radiotherapy for Benign Diseases. Radiotherapy in painful heel spurs (plantar fasciitis)—results of a national patterns of care study. *Int J Radiat Oncol Biol Phys* 2004;58:828–843.

252. Cohen M, Zornoza J, Cangir A, et al. Direct injection of methylprednisolone sodium succinate in the treatment of solitary eosinophilic granuloma of bone: a report of 9 cases. *Radiology* 1980;136:289–293.

253. Gadner H, et al. A randomized trial of treatment for multisystem Langerhans' cell histiocytosis. *J Pediatr* 2001;138:728–734.

254. Dunger DB, et al. The frequency and natural history of diabetes insipidus in children with Langerhans-cell histiocytosis. *N Engl J Med* 1989;321:1157–1162.

255. Gadner H, Heitger A, Grois N, et al. Treatment strategy for disseminated Langerhans cell histiocytosis. DAL HX-83 Study Group. *Med Pediatr Oncol* 1994;23:72–80.

256. Mauro E, et al. A case of disseminated Langerhans' cell histiocytosis treated with thalidomide. *Eur J Haematol* 2005;74:172–174.

257. Akkari V, et al. Hematopoietic stem cell transplantation in patients with severe Langerhans cell histiocytosis and hematological dysfunction: experience of the French Langerhans Cell Study Group. *Bone Marrow Transplant* 2003;31:1097–1103.

258. Frost JD, Wiersma SR. Progressive Langerhans cell histiocytosis in an infant with Klinefelter syndrome successfully treated with allogeneic bone marrow transplantation. *J Pediatr Hematol Oncol* 1996;18:396–400.

259. Farran RP, Zaretski E, Egeler RM. Treatment of Langerhans cell histiocytosis with pamidronate. *J Pediatr Hematol Oncol* 2001;23:54–56.

260. Haupt R, et al. Permanent consequences in Langerhans cell histiocytosis patients: a pilot study from the Histiocyte Society-Late Effects Study Group. *Pediatr Blood Cancer* 2004;42:438–444.

261. Toguri D, et al. Radiotherapy for steroid-resistant laryngeal Rosai-Dorfman disease. *Curr Oncol* 2011;18:e158–e162.

262. Abramson SJ Adrenal neoplasms in children. *Radiol Clin North Am* 1997;35:1415–1453.

263. Bradley EL III. Primary and adjunctive therapy in carcinoma of the adrenal cortex. *Surg Gynecol Obstet* 1975;141:507–516.

264. Honour JW, Price DA, Grant DB. Virilizing adrenocortical tumors in childhood. *Pediatrics* 1986;78:547.

265. Jones GS, Shah KJ, Mann JR. Adreno-cortical carcinoma in infancy and childhood: a radiological report of ten cases. *Clin Radiol* 1985;36:257–262.

266. Michalkiewicz EL, et al. Clinical characteristics of small functioning adrenocortical tumors in children. *Med Pediatr Oncol* 1997;28:175–178.

267. Sabbaga CC, Avilla SG, Schulz C, et al. Adrenocortical carcinoma in children: clinical aspects and prognosis. *J Pediatr Surg* 1993;28:841–843.

268. Lee PD, Winter RJ, Green OC. Virilizing adrenocortical tumors in childhood: eight cases and a review of the literature. *Pediatrics* 1985;76:437–444.

269. Tenenbaum F, et al. 18F-fluorodeoxyglucose positron emission tomography as a diagnostic tool for malignancy of adrenocortical tumours? Preliminary results in 13 consecutive patients. *Eur J Endocrinol* 2004;150:789–792.

270. Zettinig G, et al. Positron emission tomography imaging of adrenal masses: (18) F-fluorodeoxyglucose and the 11beta-hydroxylase tracer (11)C-metomidate. *Eur J Nucl Med Mol Imaging* 2004;31:1224–1230.

271. Bellantone R, et al. Role of reoperation in recurrence of adrenal cortical carcinoma: results from 188 cases collected in the Italian National Registry for Adrenal Cortical Carcinoma. *Surgery* 1997;122:1212–1218.

272. Crucitti F, Bellantone R, Ferrante A, et al The Italian Registry for Adrenal Cortical Carcinoma: analysis of a multiinstitutional series of 129 patients. The ACC Italian Registry Study Group. *Surgery* 1996;119:161–170.

273. Godine LB, Berdon WE, Brasch RC, et al Adrenocortical carcinoma with extension into inferior vena cava and right atrium: report of 3 cases in children. *Pediatr Radiol* 1990;20:166–168; discussion 169.

274. Schulick RD, Brennan MF. Long-term survival after complete resection and repeat resection in patients with adrenocortical carcinoma. *Ann Surg Oncol* 6, 719–726 (1999).

275. Stewart DR, Jones PH, Jolleys A. Carcinoma of the adrenal gland in children. *J Pediatr Surg* 1974;9:59–67.

276. Percarpio B, Knowlton AH. Radiation therapy of adrenal cortical carcinoma. *Acta Radiol Ther Phys Biol* 1976;15:288–292.

277. Magee BJ, Gattamaneni HR, Pearson D. Adrenal cortical carcinoma: survival after radiotherapy. *Clin Radiol* 1987;38:587–588.

278. Kasperlik-Zaluska AA, Migdalska BM, Zgliczynski S, et al. Adrenocortical carcinoma. A clinical study and treatment results of 52 patients. *Cancer* 1995;75:2587–2591.

279. Markoe AM, Serber W, Micaily B, et al. Radiation therapy for adjunctive treatment of adrenal cortical carcinoma. *Am J Clin Oncol* 1991;14:170–174.

280. Zografos GC, Driscoll DL, Karakousis CP, et al Adrenal adenocarcinoma: a review of 53 cases. *J Surg Oncol* 1994;55:160–164.

281. Driver CP, Birch J, Gough DC, et al. Adrenal cortical tumors in childhood. *Pediatr Hematol Oncol* 1998;15:527–532.

282. Norton JA. Adrenal tumors. In: DeVita VT Jr, Hellman S, Rosenberg SA. *Cancer: principles and practice of oncology.* Philadelphia, PA: Lippincott Williams & Wilkins, 2005:1528–1539.

283. Luton JP, et al. Clinical features of adrenocortical carcinoma, prognostic factors, and the effect of mitotane therapy. *N Engl J Med* 1990;322:1195–1201.

284. Caty MG, Coran AG, Geagen M, et al. Current diagnosis and treatment of pheochromocytoma in children. Experience with 22 consecutive tumors in 14 patients. *Arch Surg* 1990;125:978–981.

285. Kaufman BH, et al. Pheochromocytoma in the pediatric age group: current status. *J Pediatr Surg* 1983;18:879–884.

286. Khafagi FA, et al. Phaeochromocytoma and functioning paraganglioma in childhood and adolescence: role of iodine 131 metaiodobenzylguanidine. *Eur J Nucl Med* 18, 191–198 (1991).

287. Perel Y, et al. Pheochromocytoma and paraganglioma in children: a report of 24 cases of the French Society of Pediatric Oncology. *Pediatr Hematol Oncol* 1997;14:413–422.

288. Stackpole RH, Melicow MM, Uson AC. Pheochromocytoma in children. Report of 9 case and review of the first 100 published cases with follow-up studies. *J Pediatr* 1963;63:314–330.

289. Fonkalsrud EW. Pheochromocytoma in childhood. *Prog Pediatr Surg* 1991;26:103–111.

290. Whalen RK, Althausen AF, Daniels GH Extra-adrenal pheochromocytoma. *J Urol* 1992;147:1–10.

291. Schwartz DL, Gann DS, Haller JA Jr. Endocrine surgery in children. *Surg Clin North Am* 1974;54:363–385.

292. Telander RL, Zimmerman D, Kaufman BH, et al. Pediatric endocrine surgery. *Surg Clin North Am* 1985;65:1551–1587.

293. Fassbender WJ, et al. Multiple endocrine neoplasia (MEN)—an overview and case report—patient with sporadic bilateral pheochromocytoma, hyperparathyroidism and marfanoid habitus. *Anticancer Res* 2000;20:4877–4887.

294. Gagel RF, et al. The clinical outcome of prospective screening for multiple endocrine neoplasia type 2a. An 18-year experience. *N Engl J Med* 1988;318:478–484.

295. Gifford RW Jr, Manger WM, Bravo EL. Pheochromocytoma. *Endocrinol Metab Clin North Am* 23, 387–404 (1994).

296. Mayo CH. Paroxysmal hypertension with tumor of retroperitoneal nerve: report of a case. *JAMA* 1927;1927:1047–1050.

297. Leung A, et al. Specificity of radioiodinated MIBG for neural crest tumors in childhood. *J Nucl Med* 1997;38:1352–1357.

298. Welbourn RB. Early surgical history of phaeochromocytoma. *Br J Surg* 1987;74:594–596.

299. McEwan AJ, Shapiro B, Sisson JC, et al Radio-iodobenzylguanidine for the scintigraphic location and therapy of adrenergic tumors. *Semin Nucl Med* 1985;15:132–153.

300. Raum WJ. Pheochromocytoma. *Curr Thor Endocrinol Metab* 1994;5;172–178.

301. Coutant R, et al. Prognosis of children with malignant pheochromocytoma. Report of 2 cases and review of the literature. *Horm Res* 1999;52:145–149.

302. Laporte R, et al. [Severe arterial hypertension and pheochromocytoma in childhood. Case report and review of the literature]. *Arch Mal Coeur Vaiss* 2000;93:627–630.

303. Ram CV. Pheochromocytoma. *Cardiol Clin* 1988;6:517–535.

304. Storm HH, Plesko I. Survival of children with thyroid cancer in Europe 1978–1989. *Eur J Cancer* 2001;37:775–779.

305. Antonelli A, et al. Epidemiologic and clinical evaluation of thyroid cancer in children from the Gomel region (Belarus). *World J Surg* 1996;20:867–871.

306. Leenhouts HP, Brugmans MJ, Chadwick KH. Analysis of thyroid cancer data from the Ukraine after 'Chernobyl' using a two-mutation carcinogenesis model. *Radiat Environ Biophys* 2000;39:89–98.

307. Lubin JH, et al. Thyroid Cancer Following Childhood Low Dose Radiation Exposure: A Pooled Analysis of Nine Cohorts. *J Clin Endocrinol Metab* 2017;102:2575–2583.

308. Jung CK, et al. The increase in thyroid cancer incidence during the last four decades is accompanied by a high frequency of BRAF mutations and a sharp increase in RAS mutations. *J Clin Endocrinol Metab* 2014;99:E276–E285.

309. Lupi C, et al. Association of BRAF V600E mutation with poor clinicopathological outcomes in 500 consecutive cases of papillary thyroid carcinoma. *J Clin Endocrinol Metab* 2007;92:4085–4090.

310. Nikiforov YE, et al. Nomenclature Revision for Encapsulated Follicular Variant of Papillary Thyroid Carcinoma: A Paradigm Shift to Reduce Overtreatment of Indolent Tumors. *JAMA Oncol* 2016;2:1023–1029.

311. Haugen BR, et al. 2015 American Thyroid Association Management Guidelines for Adult Patients with Thyroid Nodules and Differentiated Thyroid Cancer: The American Thyroid Association Guidelines Task Force on Thyroid Nodules and Differentiated Thyroid Cancer. *Thyroid* 2016;26:1–133.

312. Alsanea O, Clark OH. Familial thyroid cancer. *Curr Opin Oncol* 2001;13:44–51.

313. Geiger JD, Thompson NW. Thyroid tumors in children. *Otolaryngol Clin North Am* 1996;29:711–719.

314. La Quaglia MP, Corbally MT, Heller G, et al. Recurrence and morbidity in differentiated thyroid carcinoma in children. *Surgery* 1988;104:1149–1156.

315. Vassilopoulou-Sellin R, Goepfert H, Raney B, et al Differentiated thyroid cancer in children and adolescents: clinical outcome and mortality after long-term follow-up. *Head Neck* 1998;20:549–555.

316. Ben Arush MW, Stein ME, Perez Nahum M, et al Pediatric thyroid carcinoma: 22 years of experience at the Northern Israel Oncology Center (1973–1995). *Pediatr Hematol Oncol* 2000;17:85–92.

317. Segal K, Shvero J, Stern Y, et al Surgery of thyroid cancer in children and adolescents. *Head Neck* 1998;20:293–297.

318. Landau D, Vini L, A'Hern R, et al Thyroid cancer in children: the Royal Marsden Hospital experience. *Eur J Cancer* 2000;36:214–220.

319. Klopp CT, Rosvoll RV, Winship T. Is destructive surgery ever necessary for treatment of thyroid cancer in children? *Ann Surg* 1967;165:745–751.

320. La Quaglia MP, Telander RL. Differentiated and medullary thyroid cancer in childhood and adolescence. *Semin Pediatr Surg* 1997;6:42–49.

321. Gerfo PL, Chabot J, Gazetas P. The intraoperative incidence of detectable bilateral and multicentric disease in papillary cancer of the thyroid. *Surgery* 1990;108:958–962; discussion 962–953.

322. Ontai S, Straehley CJ. The surgical treatment of well-differentiated carcinoma of the thyroid. *Am Surg* 1985;51:653–657.

323. Webb AJ, Brewster S, Newington D. Problems in diagnosis and management of goitre in childhood and adolescence. *Br J Surg* 1996;83:1586–1590.

Section III

324. Yeh SD, La Quaglia MP. 131I therapy for pediatric thyroid cancer. *Semin Pediatr Surg* 1997;6:128–133.

325. Caglar M, Tuncel M, Alpar R. Scintigraphic evaluation of salivary gland dysfunction in patients with thyroid cancer after radioiodine treatment. *Clin Nucl Med* 2002;27:767–771.

326. Mandel SJ, Mandel L. Radioactive iodine and the salivary glands. *Thyroid* 2003;13:265–271.

327. Desjardins JG, et al. A twenty-year experience with thyroid carcinoma in children. *J Pediatr Surg* 1988;23:709–713.

328. Brink JS, et al. Papillary thyroid cancer with pulmonary metastases in children: long-term prognosis. *Surgery* 2000;128:881–886; discussion 886–887.

329. Baker DL, B.N.J. *Germ cell tumors.* New York: Wiley-Liss, 1992).

330. Zimmerman D, et al. Papillary thyroid carcinoma in children and adults: long-term follow-up of 1039 patients conservatively treated at one institution during three decades. *Surgery* 1988;104:1157–1166.

331. Oliver RT, Leahy M, Ong J. Combined seminoma/non-seminoma should be considered as intermediate grade germ cell cancer (GCC). *Eur J Cancer* 1995;31A:1392–1394.

332. Berney DM, et al. The frequency of intratubular embryonal carcinoma: implications for the pathogenesis of germ cell tumours. *Histopathology* 2004;45:155–161.

333. Poynter JN, et al. Family history of cancer and malignant germ cell tumors in children: a report from the Children's Oncology Group. *Cancer Causes Control* 2010;21:181–189.

334. Powles TB, Bhardwa J, Shamash J, et al. The changing presentation of germ cell tumours of the testis between 1983 and 2002. *BJU Int* 2005;95:1197–1200.

335. Yolk sac carcinoma. Tumor Board of the Children's Hospital of Philadelphia. *Med Pediatr Oncol* 1987;15:96–101

336. Einhorn LH, et al. Evaluation of optimal duration of chemotherapy in favorable-prognosis disseminated germ cell tumors: a Southeastern Cancer Study Group protocol. *J Clin Oncol* 1989;7:387–391.

337. Pinkerton CR, et al. 'JEB'—a carboplatin based regimen for malignant germ cell tumours in children. *Br J Cancer* 1990;62:257–262.

338. Mangili G, et al. Is surgical restaging indicated in apparent stage IA pure ovarian dysgerminoma? The MITO group retrospective experience. *Gynecol Oncol* 2011;121:280–284.

339. Pasyk KA, Argenta LC, Austad ED. Histopathology of human expanded tissue. *Clin Plast Surg* 1987;14:435–445.

340. Garzon M. Hemangiomas: update on classification, clinical presentation, and associated anomalies. *Cutis* 2000;66:325–328.

341. Ogino I, et al. Radiation therapy for life- or function-threatening infant hemangioma. *Radiology* 2001;218:834–839.

342. Furst CJ, Lundell M, Holm LE, et al Cancer incidence after radiotherapy for skin hemangioma: a retrospective cohort study in Sweden. *J Natl Cancer Inst* 1988;80:1387–1392.

343. Furst CJ, Silversward C, Holm LE. Mortality in a cohort of radiation treated childhood skin hemangiomas. *Acta Oncol* 1989;28:789–794.

344. Lundell M, Hakulinen T, Holm LE. Thyroid cancer after radiotherapy for skin hemangioma in infancy. *Radiat Res* 1994;140:334–339.

345. Lundell M. Holm LE. Risk of solid tumors after irradiation in infancy. *Acta Oncol* 1995;34:727–734.

346. Lundell M, Mattsson A, Hakulinen T, et al. Breast cancer after radiotherapy for skin hemangioma in infancy. *Radiat Res* 1996;145:225–230.

347. Haddy N, et al. Thyroid adenomas and carcinomas following radiotherapy for a hemangioma during infancy. *Radiother Oncol* 2009;93:377–382.

348. Portnow LH, et al. Fractionated radiotherapy in the management of benign vascular tumors. *Am J Clin Oncol* 2012;35:557–561.

349. Browning J, Frieden I, Baselga E, et al. Congenital, self-regressing tufted angioma. *Arch Dermatol* 2006;142:749–751.

350. Jones EW, Orkin M. Tufted angioma (angioblastoma). A benign progressive angioma, not to be confused with Kaposi's sarcoma or low-grade angiosarcoma. *J Am Acad Dermatol* 1989;20:214–225.

351. Minh NH. Cervicothoracic spinal epidural cavernous hemangioma: case report and review of the literature. *Surg Neurol* 2005;64:83–85; discussion 85.

352. Bistolfi F, et al. [Role of low-dose radiotherapy in the multimodal treatment of Kasabach-Merritt syndrome]. *Radiol Med* 1995;90:162–166.

353. Enjolras O, Riche MC, Merland JJ, et al. Management of alarming hemangiomas in infancy: a review of 25 cases. *Pediatrics* 1990;85:491–498.

354. Moller G, et al. The Gorham-Stout syndrome (Gorham's massive osteolysis). A report of six cases with histopathological findings. *J Bone Joint Surg Br* 1999;81:501–506.

355. Moller G, et al. [Gorham-Stout idiopathic osteolysis—a local osteoclastic hyperactivity?]. *Pathologe* 1999;20:177–182.

356. Mawk JR, et al. Successful conservative management of Gorham disease of the skull base and cervical spine. *Childs Nerv Syst* 1997;13:622–625.

357. Gerald WL, Rosai J. Case 2. Desmoplastic small cell tumor with divergent differentiation. *Pediatr Pathol* 1989;9:177–183.

358. Adsay V, Cheng J, Athanasian E, et al. Primary desmoplastic small cell tumor of soft tissues and bone of the hand. *Am J Surg Pathol* 1999;23:1408–1413.

359. Cummings OW, et al. Desmoplastic small round cell tumors of the paratesticular region. A report of six cases. *Am J Surg Pathol* 1997;21:219–225.

360. Goodman KA, Wolden SL, La Quaglia MP, et al. Whole abdominopelvic radiotherapy for desmoplastic small round-cell tumor. *Int J Radiat Oncol Biol Phys* 2002;54:170–176.

361. Su MC, Jeng YM, Chu YC. Desmoplastic small round cell tumor of the kidney. *Am J Surg Pathol* 2004;28:1379–1383.

362. Gerald WL, et al. Clinical, pathologic, and molecular spectrum of tumors associated with t(11;22)(p13;q12): desmoplastic small round-cell tumor and its variants. *J Clin Oncol* 1998;16:3028–3036.

363. Kretschmar CS, Colbach C, Bhan I, et al. Desmoplastic small cell tumor: a report of three cases and a review of the literature. *J Pediatr Hematol Oncol* 1996;18:293–298.

364. Lal DR, et al. Results of multimodal treatment for desmoplastic small round cell tumors. *J Pediatr Surg* 2005;40:251–255.

365. Aguilera D, et al. Outpatient and home chemotherapy with novel local control strategies in desmoplastic small round cell tumor. *Sarcoma* 2008;2008:261589.

366. Hayes-Jordan A, Anderson PM. The diagnosis and management of desmoplastic small round cell tumor: a review. *Curr Opin Oncol* 2011;23:385–389.

367. Hughes JR, O'Donnell PJ, Pembroke AC. Basal cell carcinoma arising in a naevus sebaceous in a 5-year-old girl. *Clin Exp Dermatol* 1995;20:177.

368. Scerri L, Navaratnam AE. Basal cell carcinoma presenting as a delayed complication of thorium X used for treating a congenital hemangioma. *J Am Acad Dermatol* 1994;31:796–797.

369. Yoshihara T, Ikuta H, Hibi S, et al. Second cutaneous neoplasms after acute lymphoblastic leukemia in childhood. *Int J Hematol* 1993;59:67–71.

370. Boutimzine N, et al. [Gorlin-Goltz phacomatosis: ophthalmological aspects in one case]. *J Fr Ophtalmol* 2000;23:180–186.

371. Binkley GW, Johnson HH Jr. Epithelioma adenoides cysticum; basal cell nevi, agenesis of the corpus callosum and dental cysts; a clinical and autopsy study. *AMA Arch Derm Syphilol* 1951;63:73–84.

372. Gorlin RJ, Goltz RW. Multiple nevoid basal-cell epithelioma, jaw cysts and bifid rib. A syndrome. *N Engl J Med* 1960;262:908–912.

373. Dowling PA, Fleming P, Saunders ID, et al. Odontogenic keratocysts in a 5-year-old: initial manifestations of nevoid basal cell carcinoma syndrome. *Pediatr Dent* 2000;22:53–55.

374. Jose Tincani A, Santos Martins A, Gomes Andrade R, et al. Nevoid basal-cell syndrome: literature review and case report in a family. *Sao Paulo Med J* 1995;113:917–921.

375. Lasso JM, Garcia-Tutor E, Bazan A. Aggressive basal cell carcinoma of the temporal region in a patient with Gorlin-Goltz syndrome. *Ann Plast Surg* 2000;44:429–434.

376. Stavrou T, Dubovsky EC, Reaman GH, et al. Intracranial calcifications in childhood medulloblastoma: relation to nevoid basal cell carcinoma syndrome. *AJNR Am J Neuroradiol* 2000;21:790–794.

377. Walter AW, Pivnick EK, Bale AE, et al. Complications of the nevoid basal cell carcinoma syndrome: a case report. *J Pediatr Hematol Oncol* 1997;19:258–262.

378. Zedan W, Robinson PA, High AS. A novel polymorphism in the PTC gene allows easy identification of allelic loss in basal cell nevus syndrome lesions. *Diagn Mol Pathol* 2001;10:41–45.

379. Copeland NE, Hanke CW, Michalak JA. The molecular basis of xeroderma pigmentosum. *Dermatol Surg* 1997;23:447–455.

380. Kocabalkan O, Ozgur F, Erk Y, et al. Malignant melanoma in xeroderma pigmentosum patients: report of five cases. *Eur J Surg Oncol* 1997;23:43–47.

381. Berneburg M, Lehmann AR. Xeroderma pigmentosum and related disorders: defects in DNA repair and transcription. *Adv Genet* 2001;43:71–102.

382. Slor H, et al. Clinical, cellular, and molecular features of an Israeli xeroderma pigmentosum family with a frameshift mutation in the XPC gene: sun protection prolongs life. *J Invest Dermatol* 2000;115:974–980.

383. Sakata K, et al. Radiation therapy for patients with xeroderma pigmentosum. *Radiat Med* 1996;14:87–90.

384. Gari LM, Rivers JK, Kopf AW. Melanomas arising in large congenital nevocytic nevi: a prospective study. *Pediatr Dermatol* 1988;5:151–158.

385. Handfield-Jones SE, Smith NP. Malignant melanoma in childhood. *Br J Dermatol* 1996;134:607–616.

386. McWhirter WR, Dobson C, Ring I. Childhood cancer incidence in Australia, 1982–1991. *Int J Cancer* 1996;65:34–38.

387. Naasan A, al-Nafussi A, Quaba A. Cutaneous malignant melanoma in children and adolescents in Scotland, 1979–1991. *Plast Reconstr Surg* 1996;98:442–446.

388. Pratt CB, Palmer MK, Thatcher N, et al. Malignant melanoma in children and adolescents. *Cancer* 1981;47:392–397.

389. Reintgen DS, Vollmer R, Seigler HF. Juvenile malignant melanoma. *Surg Gynecol Obstet* 1989;168:249–253.

390. Barnhill RL, Flotte TJ, Fleischli M, et al. Cutaneous melanoma and atypical Spitz tumors in childhood. *Cancer* 1995;76:1833–1845.

391. Helm KF, Schwartz RA, Janniger CK. Juvenile melanoma (Spitz nevus). *Cutis* 1996;58:35–39.

392. Spitz S. Melanomas of childhood. 1948. *CA Cancer J Clin* 1991;41:40–51.

393. Rao BN, et al. Malignant melanoma in children: its management and prognosis. *J Pediatr Surg* 1990;25:198–203.

394. Hayes FA, Green AA. Malignant melanoma in childhood: clinical course and response to chemotherapy. *J Clin Oncol* 1984;2:1229–1234.

395. Navid F, et al. The feasibility of adjuvant interferon alpha-2b in children with high-risk melanoma. *Cancer* 2005;103:780–787.

396. Shah NC, Gerstle JT, Stuart M, et al. Use of sentinel lymph node biopsy and high-dose interferon in pediatric patients with high-risk melanoma: the Hospital for Sick Children experience. *J Pediatr Hematol Oncol* 2006;28:496–500.

397. Flaherty LE, et al. Southwest Oncology Group S0008: a phase III trial of high-dose interferon Alfa-2b versus cisplatin, vinblastine, and dacarbazine, plus interleukin-2 and interferon in patients with high-risk melanoma—an intergroup study of cancer and leukemia Group B, Children's Oncology Group, Eastern Cooperative Oncology Group, and Southwest Oncology Group. *J Clin Oncol* 2014;32:3771–3778.

398. Larkin J, et al. Combined vemurafenib and cobimetinib in BRAF-mutated melanoma. *N Engl J Med* 2014;371:1867–1876.

399. Hodi FS, et al. Improved survival with ipilimumab in patients with metastatic melanoma. *N Engl J Med* 2010;363:711–723.

400. Postow MA, et al. Nivolumab and ipilimumab versus ipilimumab in untreated melanoma. *N Engl J Med* 2015;372:2006–2017.

PART N
Benign Diseases

CHAPTER 95
Nonmalignant Diseases

Simon A. Brown, Jerry J. Jaboin, Tony Y. Eng, Jose G. Bazan, and Charles R. Thomas Jr.

Benign diseases generally include a class of localized tumors or growths that have a low potential for progression and do not invade surrounding tissue or metastasize to distant sites. Pathologically, they are composed of well-differentiated cells that are considered nonmalignant and usually do not require any treatment. However, clinically, not all benign diseases have benign consequences. Some untreated benign diseases can produce bothersome mass or secretory effects. Others can be locally aggressive and cause secondary debilitating symptoms. For example, Graves ophthalmopathy can lead to local pain and visual impairment without therapeutic intervention[1]; a hormonally active pituitary adenoma may cause growth abnormality in addition to blindness[2]; desmoid tumors can be locally persistent even after surgical resection and grow uncontrollably similar to their malignant counterparts.[3]

Documented empirical use of radiation in imaging and the treatment of benign diseases or conditions occurred soon after the discovery of x-rays by Wilhelm Röntgen in 1895.[4] Between 1920 and 1960, over a million Americans, mostly young adults and children, received x-ray treatments to the head and neck region for benign conditions.[5] The efficacy of painless x-ray treatment led to the treatment of many benign conditions with radiation: acne, body hair, scalp ringworm, enlarged tonsils, enlarged thymus, enlarged neck lymph nodes, whooping cough, and others. Radiation therapy was used in some instances because of a lack of effective alternative therapies.

Over the past decades, advances in medical and surgical therapies have provided new treatment options for many diseases. With improved awareness of late radiation sequelae on normal tissue, particularly radiation carcinogenesis, use of radiation therapy for treatment of benign conditions has gradually declined. However, with modern radiation therapy techniques and better understanding of radiobiology, judicial use of radiation provides good local control with minimal toxicity and relief of associated symptoms.

RADIOBIOLOGIC EFFECTS ON BENIGN DISEASES

The precise radiobiologic mechanisms of radiation effects on benign diseases are not well defined. Radiation is believed to work through a complex of multicellular interactions that affect different cell types in our body system.[6,7] Specific cellular and functional mechanisms depend on the specific disease and site. Although most benign lesions have no known stimuli or causes, some benign lesions may be triggered by trauma as seen in keloid formation after body piercing or heterotopic bone formation after surgery. In conditions that arise following trauma, local inflammation and repair occur, which is often characterized by stimulation of growth factors and accelerated cellular proliferation. For example, in the development of keloids, fibroblast proliferation is responsible for most of the hyperproliferative process. Even with the lower doses commonly used in benign diseases, radiotherapy is clinically effective in inhibiting cell proliferation and suppressing cell differentiation without inducing cell death as is typically seen with tumoricidal doses of radiation. Yet, radiation can induce apoptosis in selected target cells by influencing the expression of cytokines in macrophages, leukocytes, endothelial, and other cells and thereby modulating the inflammatory cascade.

Among the major sites of radiation effects are the blood vessels; vascular endothelial cells respond rapidly to radiation damage by up-regulating the cytokine-mediated cellular reactions responsible for inflammatory tissue response. Low-dose irradiation (total dose <12 Gy using 1.0 Gy or less per fraction) exerts anti-inflammatory effects on the endothelial cells of capillaries and mononuclear cells of the immune system.[8]

Cell adhesion molecules, selectins, are mobilized to the cell membrane and change the capillary permeability allowing the inflammatory cells (lymphocytes, macrophages, monocytes) to migrate into interstitial space. The anti-inflammatory effect is attributed to the modulation of cytokine and adhesion molecule expression on the activated endothelial cells and leukocytes. These cells are known to be radiosensitive. They express proinflammatory cytokines (e.g., interleukin-1, interleukin-6) or necrosis factors (e.g., tumor necrosis factor-α), which influence the complement cascade and enzymes of inflammatory reaction. Interleukin-1 stimulates the production and release of proinflammatory prostaglandins leading to a change in synthesis of inducible nitric oxide synthetase.

The radiation-induced modulation of nitric oxide production and oxidative burst in activated macrophages and native granulocytes lead to modification of the immune response and inflammatory process as well as clinical analgesic effects. Although endothelial cells possess a high proliferative potential and are sensitive to radiation damage at high doses, they are not prone to rapid mitotic radiation death at low doses.

Chronic inflammatory processes are triggered by antigen–antibody reactions and mediated by mononuclear peripheral blood cells in the immune system. Ionizing radiation helps suppress some of these cell populations, such as T lymphocytes, in the inflammation process or modulate their effects. Although low doses of radiation can exert an anti-inflammatory response, high doses of radiation as used in malignant tumors can elicit proinflammatory effects and fibrotic change in normal tissue.[9] At higher single or total doses, endothelial cell damage can lead to sclerosis and obliteration of blood vessels. In vascular disorders such as hemangiomas or arteriovenous malformations, high radiation doses may induce occlusion of pathologic vessels. In addition to inhibition of cell proliferation, cell killing may play a part in the management of benign meningiomas, pituitary adenomas, or neuromas where higher, tumoricidal doses of radiation may be required.

RISK OF SECOND MALIGNANCIES

The induction of cancer or genetic defects by radiation exposure is attributed to stochastic effects where there is no threshold level of radiation exposure below which cancer induction or genetic effects will not occur. Increasing the radiation dose or the volume of exposure will increase the probability that a cancer or genetic effect will occur. Sometimes, the radiation effects are difficult to separate from inherent genetic effects. For example, in patients with retinoblastoma, the *Rb1* gene plays an important role in the development of radiation-induced sarcomas.[10,11] In a study of 384 retinoblastoma patients treated with radiation, the actuarial risk for developing a sarcoma in the treatment field 18 years after treatment was 6.6%.[10] In another study of 693 patients, the cumulative risk for any sarcoma 50 years after radiotherapy was 13.1%.[11] Although most sarcomas were within the irradiated fields, 18 out of 69 sarcomas developed outside of the treatment fields. *Rb1* mutations appear to confer a genetic predisposition to developing sarcomas especially after radiation exposure.

The risk of the induction of secondary tumors was overestimated in the past.[12] Trott and Kamprad used the epidemiologic data from long-term follow-up studies on patients treated with radiotherapy for benign diseases to estimate the risk of cancer induction.[13] Taking all known modifying and organ-specific factors into account, including doses of radiation and volume irradiated, the estimated absolute lifetime risk for sarcoma induction was <0.0001% for 1 Gy and a 100-cm² field. Table 95.1 lists the absolute lifetime risk for other malignancies.

Jansen et al.[14] applied the effective dose concept and estimated the carcinogenic risk in patients after radiotherapy of benign diseases (heterotopic ossification [HO], omarthrosis, gonarthrosis, heel spurs, and hidradenitis suppurativa). Special risk-modifying factors, including age at exposure and gender, were taken into account. For an average-aged population, the estimated number of radiation-induced fatal tumors was between 0.5 and 40 persons per 1,000 patients treated. The range of effective doses was also found to be large (5 to 400 mSv). In addition to age and gender, the individual risk also depends on individual inherent sensitivity, anatomic site, type of disease, and treatment techniques, such as dose and fractionation. The International Commission on Radiological Protection estimates the incidence of cancer from ionizing radiation increases linearly and is about 5.5%/Sv.[15] Thus, for a patient exposed to 20 mSv—the typical limit for radiation workers per year—irradiation increases the lifetime cancer risk by about $0.020 \times 5.5/\text{Sv} = 0.1\%$.[7]

TABLE 95.1 THE ESTIMATED ABSOLUTE LIFETIME RISK FOR MALIGNANCIES AFTER RADIATION THERAPY FOR BENIGN DISEASES

Types	Absolute Lifetime Risk
Skin (basal cell carcinoma)	0.1% for 100-cm² field
Osteosarcoma	<0.0001% for 1 Gy and a 100-cm² field
Leukemia	1% for 1-Gy TBI
Brain tumor	0.2% after 20 Gy for endocrine orbitopathy
Thyroid carcinoma	1% per Gy for children <10 yr
Breast carcinoma	5% for one breast, 1 Gy, age <35 (<3% for age 35–45)
Lung carcinoma	1% within 25 y after a mean lung dose of 1 Gy

INDICATION FOR RADIOTHERAPY

The majority of benign diseases can be classified as inflammatory, degenerative, hyperproliferative, or functional. Therefore, therapeutic approaches vary widely and are regionally customized, in part because of geographic traditions and differences in clinical training. Radiation treatment of benign diseases is less commonly used in the United States than in some other parts of the world where variations in indications and treatment schedules are institutionally based.[16] Within Germany, a pattern of care study revealed significant geographic and institutional differences.[17] Although most radiation treatments for benign disease are delivered in the low-dose range (<10 to 15 Gy), the prescribed dose varied widely and inconsistently within geographic regions and between institutions.

Degenerative processes in tendons, ligaments, and joints can cause pain by chronic inflammation and trigger secondary functional impairment of the involved musculoskeletal system. Although radiation does not halt the degenerative process, it may reduce the inflammation and provide partial or complete pain relief. This clinical effect is well established in reports of osteoarthritis, synovitis, and bursitis, where low-dose radiation therapy has improved the function of affected joints.[17,18]

Benign diseases may have a significant effect on self-image and self-esteem because of cosmetic appearance (e.g., facial keloids, juvenile angiofibroma) or lasting impact on quality of life because of chronic pain or other secondary symptoms (e.g., heterotopic bone, macular degeneration). When benign diseases become locally invasive with aggressive growth, therapeutic intervention can prevent or limit functional loss of organs. In rare cases of large hemangioma with associated thrombocytopenia and consumption coagulopathy (Kasabach-Merritt syndrome [KMS]), potentially fatal complications can occur, and timely therapeutic intervention can be life-saving.[19]

Despite lack of an international consensus, the German Working Group on Radiotherapy of Benign Diseases published their consensus guidelines for radiation therapy of nonmalignant diseases. The guidelines were to serve as a starting point for quality assessment, prospective clinical trials, and outcomes research.[7,18,20-22] In brief, treatment is indicated when benign diseases are symptomatic or potentially symptomatic. When other methods are unavailable or have failed, radiation therapy should be considered. As medical professionals, we remain mindful of therapeutic gain and potential treatment side effects and complications. A thorough risk–benefit analysis is always pertinent. Organ-specific acute and chronic toxicities including potential effects on fertility and induction of secondary tumors in the future must be explained to and discussed with patients, especially those who are young and have a long life expectancy. Informed consent that is required for all medical interventions is certainly required for treatment of benign diseases and should be obtained prior to the delivery of radiation therapy.

The current chapter covers some of the more common benign conditions that we still encounter in the practice of radiation oncology. Details on the therapeutic approaches and data on radiation dose regimens for different benign diseases are summarized in the individual corresponding sections.

BENIGN NEOPLASMS OF THE BRAIN, HEAD, AND NECK

Nonmalignant tumors of the central nervous system (CNS) and neck can lead to severe, life-threatening symptoms because of pressure and mass effect on critical structures from tumor growth. However, depending on growth rate and location, the surrounding tissue may adapt leading to a delay in the clinical diagnosis.

Meningioma

Background and Clinical Aspects

Meningiomas are the most common tumors of the CNS. The incidence peaks in the seventh decade of life with a 2 to 3:1 female-to-male predominance. The lowest incidence is among those of American Indian/Alaskan Native backgrounds, approximately 35% greater for Whites and Asian and Pacifica Islanders and nearly double for Blacks.[23] The majority (>90%, Central Brain Tumor Registry of the United States (CBTRUS) 2008–2012) of meningiomas are benign and classified by the World Health Organization (WHO) as grade I tumors.[24] They can be heritable in some genetic syndromes (e.g., neurofi-bromatosis type 2; SMARCE1-related meningioma, multiple endocrine neoplasia type 1), which present in childhood but make up a minimal percentage of these tumors.[25] These WHO grade II meningiomas (4.6% by CBTRUS) have a higher tendency for local recurrence, and WHO grade III/malignant meningiomas (anaplastic, rhabdoid, papillary) are exceedingly rare.

The most common presenting symptom is headache, but patients may present with other localizing symptoms depending on the tumor location. The radiographic diagnosis of meningioma is often made on computed tomography (CT) or magnetic resonance imaging (MRI) based upon the appearance of a homogeneously and intensely enhancing extra-axial mass with or without the presence of a dural tail.

Surgical Management

Surgical resection is the treatment of choice for most patients with dual benefits of symptomatic relief and pathologic diagnosis. The primary goal of surgery is to remove as much tumor burden as possible while minimizing the risk of neurologic deficits (maximal safe resection). Gross total resection (GTR) is generally attempted for patients with tumors in locations such as the convexity and olfactory groove.[26,27] After GTR, the relapse rate is as low as 10%, but depends upon the Simpson classification, which grades tumors according to extent of resection and degree of dural involvement (Table 95.2).[28] Local recurrence rates are as high as 40% for patients with incomplete resection,[28] though these rates can be substantially reduced with the use of adjuvant radiotherapy. Notably, endoscopic endonasal approaches have allowed for access to anterior cranial base tumors with reasonable morbidity rates.[29]

Meningiomas tend to be highly vascularized tumors. In select patients, preoperative embolization is used to decrease blood loss and improve the extent of resection.[30,31]

TABLE 95.2 SIMPSON GRADING SYSTEM FOR POSTOPERATIVE MENINGIOMAS WITH ASSOCIATED RATES OF RECURRENCE

Simpson Grade	Description	Recurrence Rate
I	Complete macroscopic tumor removal with adherent dura as well as the possibly affected part of the cranial calotte	8.9% (8/90 patients)
II	Complete macroscopic tumor removal with adherent dura via diathermia	15.8% (18/114 patients)
III	Complete macroscopic tumor removal without adherent dura or possibly additional extradural parts	29.2% (7/24 patients)
IV	Partial macroscopic tumor removal while leaving intradural tumor parts	39.2% (20/51 patients)
V	Simple decompressive and bioptic removal of tumor	88.9% (8/9 patients)

Adapted from Simpson D. The recurrence of intracranial meningiomas after surgical treatment. *J Neurol Neurosurg Psychiatry* 1957;20(1):22–39, with permission from BMJ Publishing Group Ltd.

Active Surveillance

Asymptomatic patients with small meningiomas may be observed clinically. At the time of tumor growth or the development of symptoms, patients can be treated with surgery or radiation therapy. The safety and reasoning for this approach were established in a large retrospective series from Japan that demonstrated that the majority of patients do not require intervention in the short-term.[32]

Systemic Therapy

Interest in the use of medical therapy to treat meningiomas stems from the observation that up to 67% of meningiomas express the progesterone receptor or androgen receptor and approximately 10% express the estrogen receptor.[33] However, response rates to antihormonal agents are low. Overall, studies that have investigated the role of chemotherapy, such as hydroxyurea, in the management of recurrent disease have demonstrated little efficacy.[33]

Radiotherapy

Primary radiotherapy (RT) is indicated for tumors in locations in which complete resection is not feasible (i.e., optic nerve, cavernous sinus, major venous sinus) or for patients who are poor surgical candidates. Adjuvant RT is indicated for patients with STR, recurrent disease, or WHO grade II/III tumors. RT techniques include conventionally fractionated three-dimensional conformal radiotherapy (3DRT), conventionally fractionated intensity-modulated radiation therapy (IMRT), frame-based or linear accelerator–based fractionated stereotactic radiotherapy (FSRT), stereotactic radiosurgery (SRS), or protons and heavy ions.

The MRI sequences that best delineate the gross tumor volume (GTV) should be coregistered with the treatment planning CT scan for optimal treatment planning and delivery. Particularly for patients receiving FSRT or SRS, it is important that a neuroradiologist and neurosurgeon be involved in assisting with GTV delineation, as enhancement from residual tumor versus postoperative change is often difficult to ascertain.

For 3DRT or IMRT treatments, the clinical target volume (CTV) is constructed by adding a symmetric margin (0 to 1 cm for WHO grade I; 1 to 2 cm for WHO grade II/III) around the GTV, respecting normal tissue boundaries and accounting for the imaging characteristics of the tumor. An additional 3 to 5 mm is added for the final planning target volume (PTV). These margins may be modified based on institutional policy and other considerations, such as the availability of daily image guidance (i.e., kV imaging or cone-beam CT).

For benign meningiomas, the typical dose prescription to the PTV is 50 to 54 Gy given in 1.8- to 2-Gy daily fractions. Retrospective data suggest that local control is inferior for patients treated with doses of <52 Gy.[34] For patients with more aggressive histology (WHO grade II/III tumors), a higher dose prescription in the range of 59.4 to 63 Gy is used. Several modern series of radiotherapy show 5-year local control rates ranging approximately 89% to 98%, with three-dimensional conformal therapy demonstrating local control rates >95% (Table 95.3).[34–38] Although there is still no consensus on the benefits of adjuvant radiotherapy for WHO grade II meningioma, a National Cancer Database (NCDB) analysis demonstrated a survival benefit for adjuvant radiotherapy in patients with subtotal resection.[39]

SRS and FSRT are increasingly being used in the treatment of meningiomas. The decision to fractionate depends largely upon tumor size and proximity to critical structures, such as the optic apparatus or brainstem. Typical dose prescriptions for frame-based SRS range from 12 to 16 Gy prescribed to the 50% isodose line (IDL) and 14 to 18 Gy prescribed to the 80% IDL for a frameless robotic radiosurgery platform. In patients with

Section III

TABLE 95.3 CLINICAL OUTCOMES OF STEREOTACTIC RADIOSURGERY OR EXTERNAL BEAM RADIOTHERAPY (WITH OR WITHOUT SURGERY) FOR MENINGIOMAS IN MODERN SERIES

Study (Year)	No. of Patients	Radiation	S + R/R	Dose (Median or Mean)	Local Control (%)
Ganz et al. (2009)[44]	97	SRS	NA	12 Gy	100 (2 y)
Takanashi et al. (2009)[50]	101	SRS	24%/76%	13.2 Gy	97 (1 y)
Han et al. (2008)[45]	98	SRS	36%/64%	12.7 Gy	90 (5 y)
Iwai et al. (2008)[47]	108	SRS	NA	12 Gy	93 (5 y)
					83 (10 y)
Kondziolka et al. (2008)[49]	972	SRS	49%/51%	14 Gy	87 (10 y)
Davidson et al. (2007)[42]	36	SRS	100%/0%	16 Gy	100 (5 y)
					95 (10 y)
Feigl et al. (2007)[43]	214	SRS	43%/57%	13.6 Gy	86.3 (4 y)
Hasegawa et al. (2007)[46]	115	SRS	57%/43%	13 Gy	87 (5 y)
					73 (10 y)
Kollova et al. (2007)[48]	368	SRS	30%/70%	12.5 Gy	98 (5 y)
Zachenhofe et al. (2006)[51]	36	SRS	70%/30%	17 Gy	94 (9 y)
Goldsmith et al. (1994)[34]	117	EBRT	100%/0%	54 Gy	89 (5 y)
					77 (10 y)
Mendenhall et al. (2003)[35]	101	EBRT	35%/65%	54 Gy	95 (5 y)
					92 (10 y)
Nutting et al. (1999)[37]	82	EBRT	100%/0%	55–60 Gy	92 (5 y)
					83 (10 y)
Vendrely et al. (1999)[38]	156	EBRT	51%/49%	50 Gy	79 (5 y)

EBRT, external beam radiotherapy; R, radiation; S, surgery; SRS, stereotactic radiosurgery.
Adapted from Minniti G, Amichetti M, Enrici RM. Radiotherapy and radiosurgery for benign skull base meningiomas. *Radiat Oncol* 2009;4:42.

tumors that require fractionated treatment, dose prescriptions vary and are dependent upon the individual case. Additionally, a select group of perioptic tumors, including meningiomas, can be treated with a prescription of 24 to 30 Gy in 3 to 5 fractions (to the 80% IDL) resulted in high rates of tumor control and visual preservation (Fig. 95.1).[40] There is nonrandomized, prospective evidence indicating that FSRT should be the treatment of choice for optic nerve sheath meningiomas because of the high rate of preservation of visual acuity.[41]

Reported results with SRS are excellent, with 5-year local control rates as high as 98% to 100% (Table 95.3).[42–51] DiBiase et al.[52] demonstrated that male gender, conformality index <1.4, and size >10 mL predict for worse outcome after SRS. Improved disease-free survival in patients was also noted for coverage of the dural tail as part of the target volume, though benefits should be weighed against toxicity.[52] In Ferraro et al.,[53] additional poor prognosticators included high mitotic rate, nuclear atypia, spontaneous necrosis, and WHO grade III pathology.

Because of their physical properties, protons and heavy ions (i.e., carbon) are attractive choices for the treatment of meningiomas, particularly for those located near critical structures. Several studies have shown excellent local control rates with the combination of protons and photons or protons alone.[54–56]

Pituitary Adenoma
Background and Clinical Aspects
Pituitary adenomas are the second most common intracranial tumors with a US incidence of 11,700.[23] Approximately 65% to 70% of these tumors are functional (secretory), thereby producing increased amounts of hormones. Prolactinomas and growth hormone (GH)–secreting adenomas are the most frequently encountered. Functional adenomas are more common in women, whereas nonfunctioning and GH-secreting adenomas are more common in men.

Adenomas are often classified by size with a picoadenoma <0.3 cm, microadenoma <1 cm, and macroadenoma >1cm. Clinical presentation can vary, but nonfunctional adenomas (mostly consisting of gonadotrophs) are most commonly with visual symptoms (often bitemporal hemianopsia from compression of the optic chiasm). Less commonly, patients complain of headaches (~20%), and with larger tumor extent,

there can be cranial nerve involvement or hypopituitarism (second to hypothalamic extension).

Patients with functional adenomas present with signs and symptoms that correspond to the excess hormone: galactorrhea, amenorrhea, diminished libido, and infertility in patients with prolactinomas, acromegaly or gigantism in patients with GH-secreting adenomas, Cushing disease in adrenocorticotropic hormone (ACTH)-secreting adenomas, and hyperthyroidism in patients with thyroid-stimulating hormone (TSH)-secreting adenomas. In patients who have had bilateral adrenalectomy, up to 40% will develop Nelson syndrome, which is characterized by an ACTH-secreting adenoma and increased skin pigmentation secondary to increased release of alpha-melanocyte–stimulating hormone.

In addition to history and detailed physical examination (H&P), workup of a pituitary tumor includes laboratory analysis of pituitary hormone levels, contrast-enhanced MRI with thin slices through the pituitary (Fig. 95.2A and B), and tissue diagnosis to rule out other causes of pituitary masses including craniopharyngioma, meningioma, suprasellar germ cell tumor, metastatic disease, or a benign lesion (i.e., cyst).

Surgical Management
Transsphenoidal surgery is generally the treatment of choice for pituitary adenomas, providing immediate relief of compressive symptoms and potentially decreasing hormone secretion. In some cases, a more aggressive surgery (i.e., extended transsphenoidal approach, frontal craniotomy) may be indicated for patients with extensive intracranial and skull-based involvement. Overall, local control rates range from 50% to 80% after surgery alone for both functioning and nonfunctioning adenomas.[57] In patients that continue to have abnormally elevated hormones after surgical resection, adjuvant treatment with pharmacotherapy and/or radiation therapy is pursued.

Pharmacotherapy
For unsuccessful or contraindicated surgeries, pharmacotherapy, such as bromocriptine and cabergoline for prolactinomas, octreotide for GH adenomas and TSH adenomas, and ketoconazole for ACTH adenomas, has been used as an adjunct for patients with functioning adenomas. The SEISMIC study, a 24-week multicenter open-label trial after failed

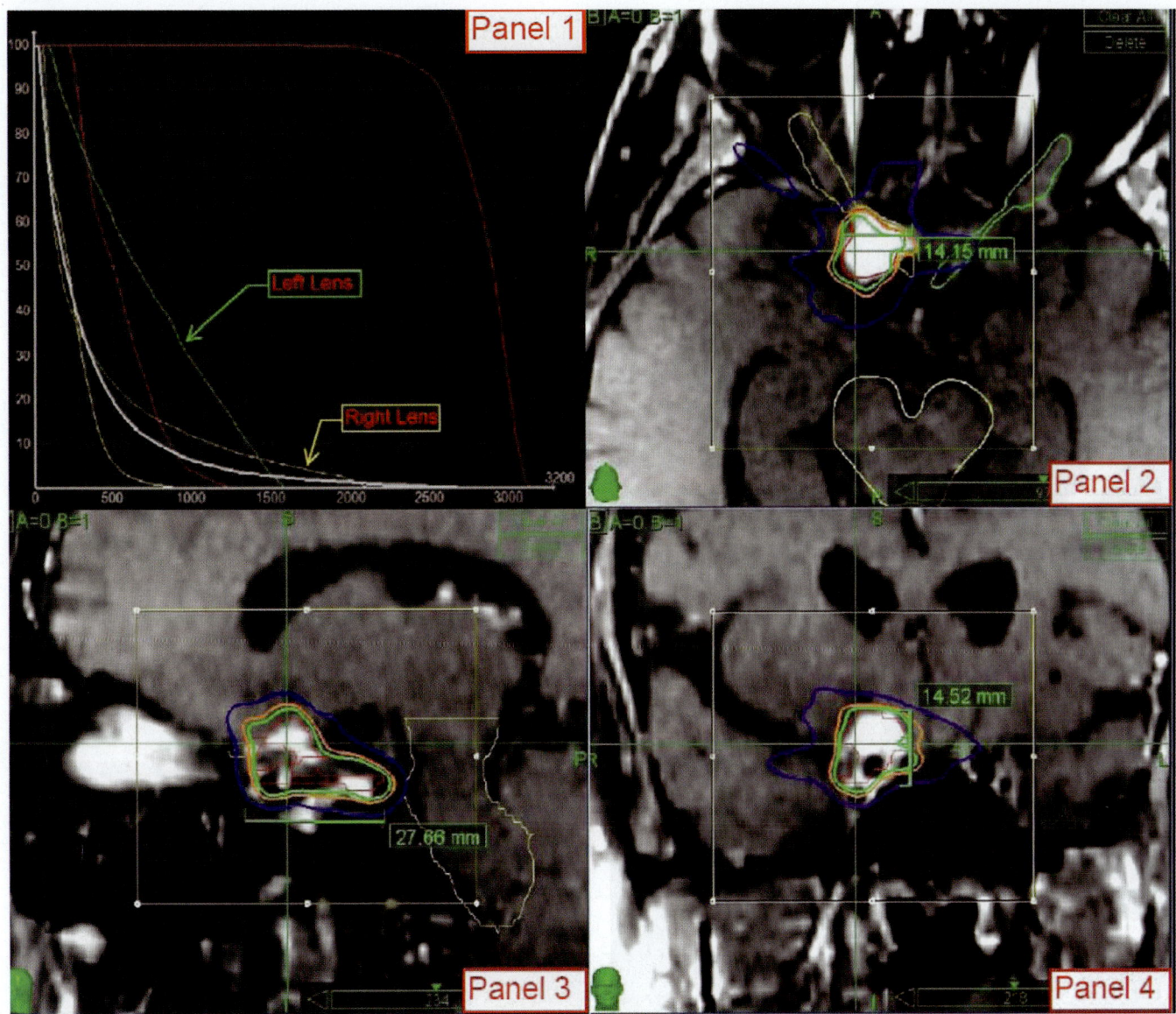

FIGURE 95.1. Radiosurgery treatment plan of a patient with a right optic nerve sheath meningioma treated to a dose of 24 Gy in 3 fractions. The lesion is intensely enhancing on the postcontrast stereotactic MRI sequences. *Panel 1* demonstrates the dose–volume histogram for the patient. The maximum dose to the ipsilateral optic nerve was 22.3 Gy. *Panels 2 to 4* demonstrate the isodose curves for the treatment in the axial, sagittal, and coronal planes. The 100% (24 Gy) isodose line is *green*, the 88% (21 Gy) isodose line is in *orange*, and the 50% (12 Gy) isodose line is *blue*.

multimodality therapy, demonstrated that mifepristone could produce significant clinical and metabolic improvement in patients with Cushing syndrome with an acceptable risk profile.[58] However, with the exception of prolactinomas, the use of these drugs as monotherapy is generally not curative. Prolactinomas can often be managed with pharmacotherapy alone, but a high proportion of patients are unable to tolerate bromocriptine for long periods of time because of nausea, headache, and fatigue.

Radiotherapy

Except for medically inoperable patients in which RT is used in the primary setting, the role of RT is generally in the adjuvant setting with the following indications: recurrent tumor after surgery, persistence of hormone elevation after surgery, and residual disease after STR/debulking procedure. Tumor growth control is excellent, particularly for patients with nonfunctioning adenomas.[59–61] Endocrine control after treatment of functioning adenomas, as demonstrated by normalization of pituitary hormone levels, takes years to develop. At a median

of 2 years after RT, growth hormone levels stabilize quickest; normalization is slowest for TSH-secreting adenomas.[62] Pharmacologic therapy should be discontinued 1 to 2 months prior to the initiation of RT based on evidence demonstrating lower RT sensitivity with concurrent medical treatment.[63]

RT techniques include 3DRT, IMRT, single-fraction SRS, SBRT (or HSRT), and FSRT. Delineation of the GTV (or preoperative GTV in the case of GTR) should be performed by coregistration of the postoperative MRI to the treatment planning CT scan. CTV is the gross disease and subclinical extent of the tumor; an additional 3 to 5 mm is added to the CTV to create the PTV. These margins may be modified based on institutional policy and other considerations, such as the availability of daily image guidance. Nonfunctional adenomas are typically prescribed a dose of 45 to 50.4 Gy given in 1.8- to 2.0-Gy daily fractions (Fig. 95.2C–E). Higher doses in the range of 50.4 to 54 Gy are recommended for secretory adenomas, as these are felt to be more locally aggressive and less radioresponsive. Prolactinomas, in particular, rarely achieve biochemical normalization with radiation monotherapy.

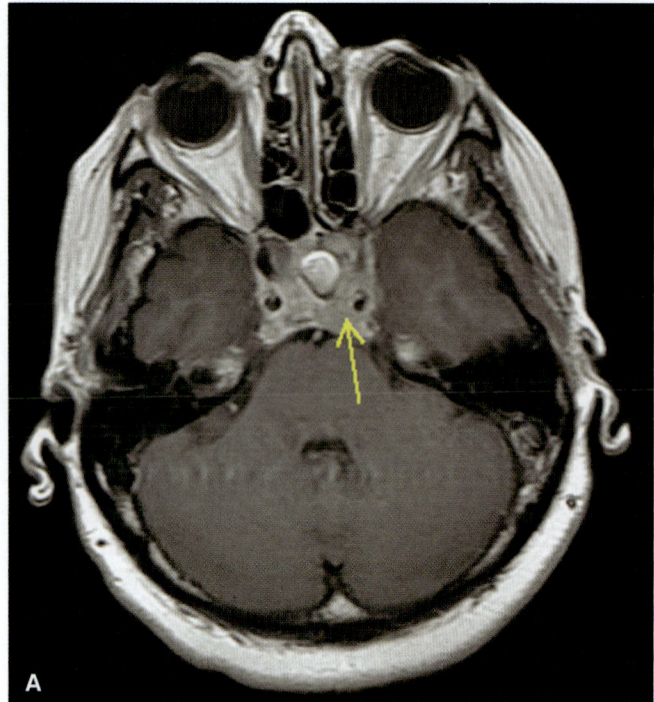

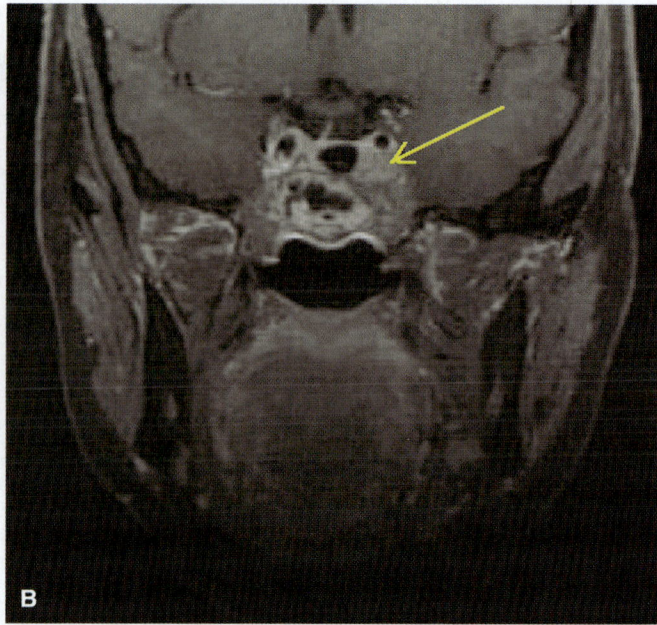

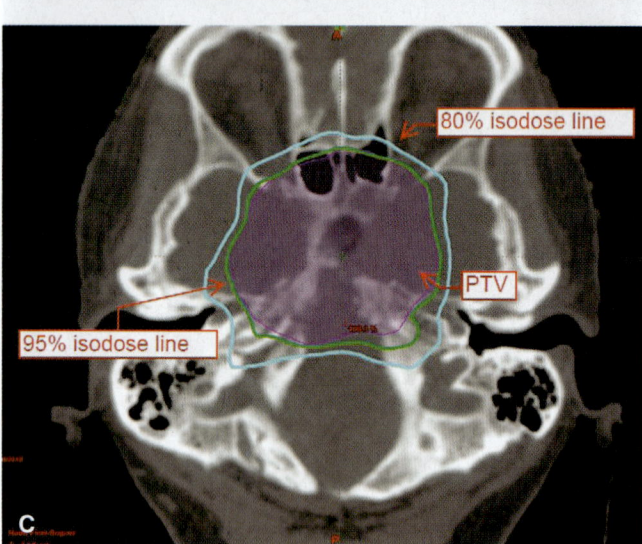

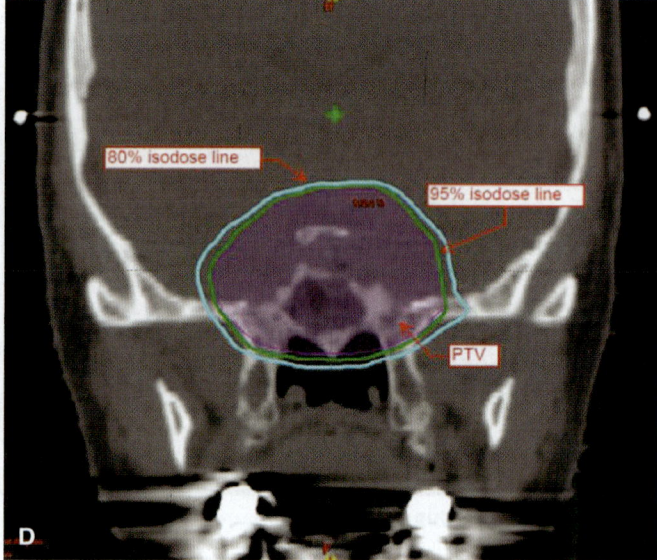

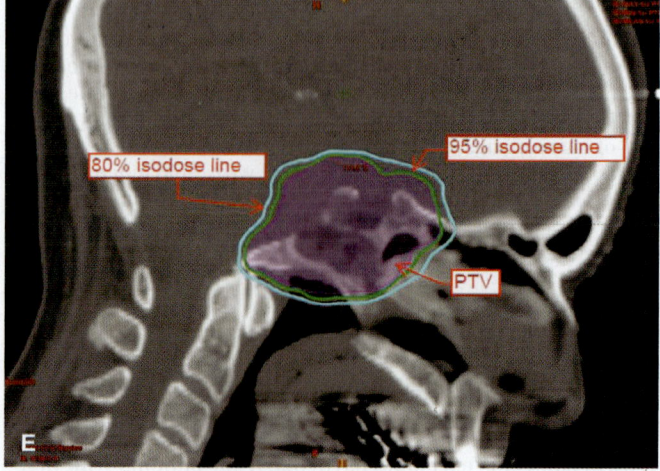

FIGURE 95.2. **A** and **B:** A recurrent nonfunctioning pituitary adenoma 7 years after surgical resection in the axial **(A)** and coronal **(B)** planes. The *yellow arrows* denote invasion into the left cavernous sinus. **C–E:** Rapid arc intensity-modulated radiotherapy treatment plan for the same patient in the axial **(C)**, coronal **(D)**, and sagittal **(E)** planes. The PTV (*purple-shaded area*) was prescribed 50.4 Gy in 28 fractions.

SRS has become the more attractive option for the treatment of pituitary adenomas. General principles apply in that FSRT is used over SRS for large lesions (i.e., >3 cm) or lesions near critical structures (i.e., <1 to 2 mm from the chiasm). Similar to 3DRT/IMRT, higher doses are needed for functional adenomas compared to nonfunctional adenomas. Numerous retrospective studies have demonstrated excellent local control rates of 92% to 100% for nonfunctional adenomas using doses of 14 to 25 Gy (at the edge of the tumor) in a single fraction.[64] Commonly used prescriptions are 16 to 20 Gy in a single fraction for nonfunctional adenomas and 20 to 25 Gy in a single fraction for functional adenomas using a frameless robotic radiosurgery platform. Hypofractionated regimens can also be applied. In a 25-year experience of 1,837 patients undergoing SRS for benign tumors, there were neither radiation-induced tumors nor malignant transformation noted in the 188 pituitary adenomas identified.[65]

Craniopharyngioma

Background and Clinical Aspects

Craniopharyngiomas make up 6% to 10% of pediatric CNS tumors, or approximately 350 to 400 cases per year in the United States.[23] The median age of diagnosis is 5 to 10 years with a second peak in patients >40 years old and an equal male:female ratio.

These benign tumors are epithelial, arising from remnants of Rathke pouch (hypophyseal–pharyngeal duct), and are most commonly located in the suprasellar region, though they may be found in the sella proper. Craniopharyngiomas generally abut the hypothalamus and third ventricle. Histologically, they are divided into the adamantinomatous and squamous subtypes. The adamantinomatous subtype is characterized by a solid and cystic pattern with the well-known description of "machine oil–like" cystic fluid.

Presenting signs and symptoms include headache, nausea and vomiting, bitemporal hemianopsia, and endocrine dysfunction (diabetes insipidus [DI], dwarfism, fat tissue disturbance, adrenal cortical insufficiency). The most common hormone deficiency is lack of GH. The workup is similar to that of pituitary adenoma and includes H&P, pituitary hormone levels, and brain MRI with thin slices through the sella (Fig. 95.3).

Surgery

The primary goal of surgery is complete resection. However, GTR may be associated with high rates of neurologic sequelae including visual impairment and panhypopituitarism. In order

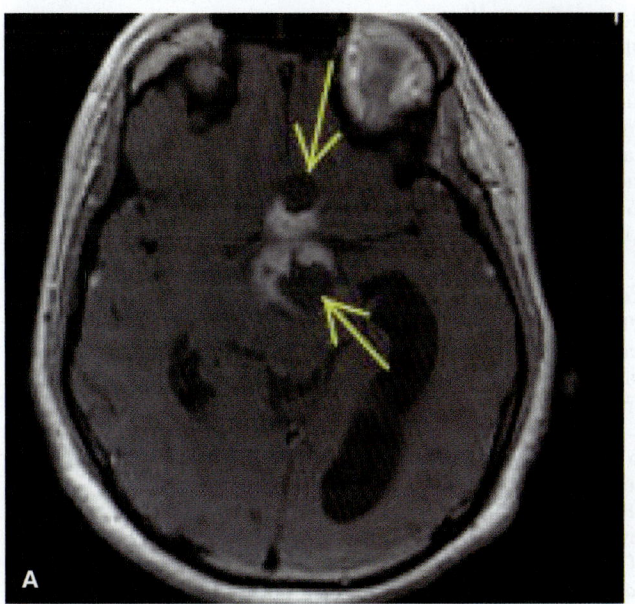
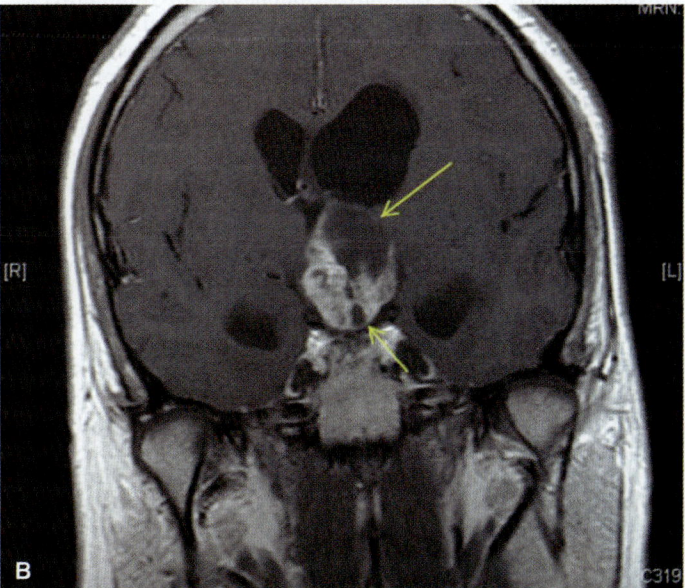
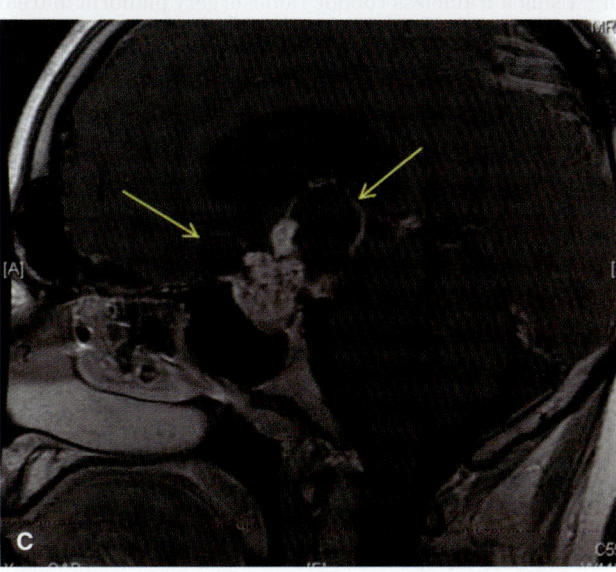

FIGURE 95.3. Axial **(A)**, coronal **(B)**, and sagittal **(C)** MRI images of a patient with multicystic (*yellow arrows*) craniopharyngioma prior to treatment.

to minimize morbidity, most patients are treated with maximal safe resection followed by adjuvant RT.

Intracavitary Therapies

Intralesional bleomycin may be directly injected into the cyst to decrease the rate of cyst recurrence.[66] Cystic craniopharyngiomas may also be managed by the use of intralesional radioactive isotope injection using a beta emitter (yttrium 90, phosphorus 32). Typical prescriptions range from 200 to 250 Gy prescribed to the cyst wall. Optimal results are seen in patients whose tumors have one cyst and lack a large solid component.[67,68]

External Beam Radiotherapy

External beam radiation therapy is often used in the adjuvant setting. In select patients (i.e., <3 years old), observation following STR may be an option as local control rates are similar with RT at the time of relapse ("salvage" RT) compared with adjuvant RT with no compromise in overall survival.[69]

RT techniques include 3DRT, IMRT, FSRT, proton therapy, and intralesional RT with beta-emitting isotopes. The GTV is the postoperative residual tumor volume, including the cyst wall, if present. The postoperative MRI should be fused with the treatment planning CT scan for optimal target delineation. The CTV includes the gross tumor and subclinical disease with a GTV for set-up margins. Dose prescriptions for 3DRT and IMRT are typically at least 54 Gy given in 1.8-Gy daily fractions.

Fractionated proton radiotherapy has demonstrated excellent results. The Loma Linda series treated 15 patients to a total dose of 50.4 to 59.4 gray equivalents (GyE) given in 1.8 GyE daily fractions.[70] Local control was achieved in 14 out of 15 patients with few long-term complications. In a series from the Massachusetts General Hospital (MGH), no failures were seen in 24 patients that received fractionated proton radiotherapy to a total dose of 52.2 to 54 GyE in 1.8 GyE per fraction.[71] Overall survival and recurrence outcomes have been mixed when comparing proton to conformal photon radiotherapy.[72]

It has been well established that cysts may regrow during the several weeks of fractionated treatment. The MGH proton study recommends that reimaging (CT or MRI if cyst is not well visualized on CT) be performed within 2 weeks of the treatment planning scan and every 2 weeks thereafter; for large cysts or those that demonstrate growth during RT, weekly reimaging is recommended.[71] Image-guided radiotherapy techniques now allow for the convenient monitoring of cyst regrowth with cone beam CT scans while patients are on the treatment table.

SRS and FSRT have been used with success in the treatment of craniopharyngioma. In one series from Stanford using a frameless robotic platform,[73] 16 patients were treated postoperatively with doses of 18 to 38 Gy given over 3 to 10 fractions prescribed to mean IDL of 75%. Local control was 91% in this cohort of patients with no visual or neuroendocrine complications. Similar results have been demonstrated with use of a frame-based platform.[74–77]

Vestibular Schwannoma (Acoustic Neuroma)

Background and Clinical Aspects

Acoustic neuromas (AN) are derived from the neurilemmal of the vestibulocochlear nerve (CN VIII) and represent 5% to 8% of primary CNS brain tumors. The vast majority of cases (90%) are unilateral and sporadic, and when bilateral (10% of cases), they are associated with neurofibromatosis type II (NF-2).

Clinical presentation can include symptoms of sensorineural hearing loss, tinnitus, and vertigo. Hearing loss is correlated with tumor location (intracanalicular) rather than tumor size. In a minority of patients (5%), facial nerve symptoms may be present. As the AN grows, it may affect the trigeminal nerve (CN V) and brainstem.

During the initial workup, physical examination should include the Rinne test (air conduction > bone conduction on the affected side) and Weber test (vibratory sound louder on the unaffected side) to test for sensorineural hearing loss, as well as detailed examination of CN V and CN VII. All patients should undergo audiometry when the diagnosis of AN is suspected; this will often reveal asymmetric hearing loss more prominent at high frequencies as well as impairments in speech discrimination score. Imaging should include a contrast-enhanced MRI with thin slices through the internal auditory canal. The entire neuraxis should be imaged in patients with NF-2.

Surgery

Surgery is the mainstay of management of vestibular schwannomas, particularly for patients with large, symptomatic lesions. The standard approaches are retromastoid suboccipital, translabyrinthine, and middle fossa with each providing unique advantages and risks. Most patients can undergo a complete resection and have low recurrence risk. Though cases of subtotal resection are associated with an approximately 15% risk of recurrence, surgical mortality is approximately 0.5% based on a NCDB analysis of 10,136 patients.[78] Hearing preservation is approximately 50% to 60% after surgery, and facial nerve preservation ranges from 80% to 90%.[79,80]

Active Surveillance

Observation is appropriate management for some individuals; indications include age >60, multiple comorbidities, small tumor size, and risk of hearing loss. Serial MRI and audiometry (every 6 to 12 months) should be performed in this patient cohort for surveillance. Treatment is initiated when the lesion demonstrates rapid and significant growth or when the patient becomes symptomatic. Overall, a growth rate of <1 mm/year is expected for most patients.[81]

Radiotherapy

RT in the form of SRS or FSRT is an option for the primary treatment of AN, often with higher rates of hearing preservation and facial nerve presentation compared with surgery. Proton therapy has also been used to treat AN.

SRS doses using frame-based platforms are generally 12 to 13 Gy prescribed to the 50% IDL. Although earlier studies demonstrated lower hearing preservation rates with higher SRS doses,[82] current results are significantly improved at these lower margin doses. Flickinger demonstrated local control rate of 98.6%, hearing preservation rate of 70.3%, 4.4% rate of trigeminal neuropathy, and no incidence of facial nerve dysfunction.[83] Using a frameless robotic radiosurgery platform to treat 383 ANs to a dose of 18 to 21 Gy given in 3 fractions, Stanford demonstrated 98% local control, 76% hearing preservation, 2% incidence of trigeminal nerve dysfunction (transient in 4 of the 8 affected patients), and no facial nerve dysfunction.[84]

Common dose prescriptions employing FSRT include 25 Gy in 5 fractions, 30 Gy in 10 fractions, and 50 to 55 Gy in 25 to 30 fractions. A nonrandomized, prospective trial compared SRS (10 to 12.5 Gy) to FSRT (20 to 25 Gy in 5 fractions). This study demonstrated comparable rates of local control, hearing preservation, and CN V and CN VII preservation between the two groups.[85]

Proton beam SRS has also been used to treat AN, though with low rates of hearing preservation compared to other RT techniques. In a series from MGH, 88 patients were treated to a median dose of 12 GyE given in a single fraction prescribed to a median IDL of 70%. Tumor control rates at 2 and 5 years were 95.3% and 93.6%, respectively. Facial and trigeminal nerve preservation rates were 90%. Only 33% of patients retained serviceable hearing.[86] In a study of FSRT using proton beam, local control was excellent, but the hearing preservation rate was also poor at 42%.[87]

Chordoma

Background and Clinical Aspects

Chordomas are rare, representing <1% of intracranial lesions. They are slowly growing and locally aggressive midline tumors originating from the embryonal notochord remnants. Hence, they occur along the axial skeleton in the skull base (35%), vertebral column (15%), or sacral regions (50%).[88] The most common sites of skull-based tumors include the clivus, dorsum sella, and nasopharynx.

Patients typically present with signs and symptoms attributable to the primary site of the tumor. Workup includes MRI with contrast enhancement. CT may complement MRI to assess local bony destruction. A biopsy is necessary primarily to distinguish chordoma from chondrosarcoma, which has a better prognosis, and other malignancies. In children, biopsy is essential to distinguish chordoma from rhabdomyosarcoma, which can frequently present in the same location.

Surgery

Complete surgical resection is the mainstay of treatment. However, because of their location, GTR is often not possible. Relapse rates are as high as 50% even after surgical resection with negative margins.[89] Poor prognostic factors include large tumors, recurrent tumors, older age, clinical visual deficits, and presence of necrosis on biopsy.[90–92]

Systemic Therapy

Approximately 25% of chordomas metastasize to the lungs, liver, or bone. In these patients, or in patients with recurrent disease after surgical resection and radiation therapy, molecularly targeted agents may be considered. Several small studies have demonstrated some benefit to the use of sorafenib and imatinib or the combination of imatinib and sirolimus in this situation.[93–96]

Radiotherapy

Adjuvant radiation therapy is indicated to reduce recurrence rates for skull-based chordomas regardless of resection status. Retrospective data suggest that salvage RT is inferior to adjuvant RT with 5- and 10-year overall survival rates of 50% and 0%, respectively, for those treated with salvage RT compared to 80% and 65%, respectively, for patients treated with adjuvant RT.[97] RT techniques for treatment of skull-based chordomas include conventionally fractionated EBRT and IMRT, fractionated charged particle therapy (protons, carbon ions), and FSRT.

Determination of the GTV should be made by coregistration of the preoperative and/or postoperative MRI to the treatment planning CT scan. Particularly for pediatric cases in which IMRT will be used with tight margins, a neuroradiologist should be available at the time of treatment planning to assist in creating the GTV. Margins for CTV should be 1 to 2 cm with an additional 3 to 5 mm for the PTV. Dose prescriptions to the PTV for patients receiving photon-based treatment should be at least 60 Gy given in 1.8 to 2.0-Gy daily fractions.

Proton-based therapy can achieve higher doses with good results. In a series of 195 chordomas treated at the MGH, 5-year PFS was 70% with doses of 63 to 79.2 GyE given in 1.8 to 2.0 GyE daily fractions.[98] Among the 28 patients with primary spinal chordomas who underwent preoperative RT and en bloc resection, no local recurrences were seen.[99] Loma Linda examined 33 cases of chordomas treated with a median of 70 GyE and found 76% 5-year local control and 79% 5-year overall survival.[91]

In a report of 96 chordomas treated using carbon ion therapy at the University of Heidelberg with median total dose of 60 GyE (range, 60 to 70 GyE) delivered in 20 fractions within 3 weeks, good local control rates of 81% at 3 years and 70% at 5 years were observed.[100] In a recent report of 188 patients who received >60 GyE, the 5-year local control, overall survival,

and disease-free survival rates were 77.2%, 81.1%, and 50.3%, respectively.[101]

FSRT and SRS are less well established than charged particle therapy. The North American Gamma Knife Consortium published the experience of 71 patients that underwent gamma knife SRS as primary, adjuvant, or salvage therapy for skull base chordomas.[102] The median dose to the tumor margin was 15 Gy (range, 9 to 25 Gy). Five-year local control was 66% for the entire cohort (69% for the no prior RT group and 62% for the prior RT group). Debus et al.[103] reported on 37 patients with chordomas treated with FSRT to a median dose of 66.6 Gy given in 1.8-Gy daily fractions; the target volume was encompassed by 90% of the dose. Local control was 82% at 2 years and 50% at 5 years.

Glomus Tumor/Chemodectoma/ Paraganglioma

Background and Clinical Aspects

Glomus tumors are rare, benign tumors that originate from chromaffin-negative chemoreceptor cells derived from the embryonic neural crest. They occur particularly along the carotid artery near the bifurcation (carotid body tumor), the jugular bulb (glomus jugulare), or the middle ear (glomus tympanicum). The peak age is in the fifth decade of life. Bilateral or multiple tumors occur in 10% to 20% of affected patients.

Symptoms include headache, cranial nerve dysfunction, dysphagia, pulsatile tinnitus, vertigo, and large, pulsating masses in the neck. In rare cases, patients present with episodic hypertension, which may be related to the secretion of vasoactive substances by the tumor. In this situation, urine and serum metanephrines should be measured. The clinical presentation coupled with imaging (high-resolution CT, MRI, and/or angiography) often establishes the diagnosis. In patients in which multiple tumors are suspected, imaging with metaiodobenzylguanidine (MIBG) may be useful.

Surgery

In the carotid region, primary tumor resection after previous embolization is the therapy of choice. At the skull base or tympanum, neurosurgical intervention is often deferred because of the high rates of complications, including stroke and cranial nerve injury.[104]

Radiotherapy

RT is indicated for patients with tumors in unsuitable locations (i.e., skull base), as adjuvant therapy after STR, or as salvage therapy at the time of relapse after surgery. A retrospective comparative analysis of 41 patients with jugular paraganglioma treated by conventional radiotherapy and 47 patients by surgery showed similar outcomes, 96% and 86%, local control rates, respectively, but the radiotherapy patients achieved tumor control with less morbidity.[105] RT techniques include conventionally fractionated 3DRT/IMRT, SRS, and FSRT.

The diagnostic MRI should be coregistered with the treatment planning CT scan. The GTV is delineated, and 1 to 1.5 cm is added for clinical and set-up margin. With conventional techniques, doses are often 45 to 55 Gy given in 1.8- to 2-Gy daily fractions with local control rates near or >90% in several series.[106–108]

Results with SRS have been comparable to that of conventionally fractionated RT. Using a frame-based platform, reported tumor margin doses range from 12.5 to 20 Gy prescribed to the 50% IDL [109–111] and 15 to 25 Gy for LINAC-based SRS.[104] Local control rates in these series range from 90% to 100%. A recent meta-analysis of SRS published by the Johns Hopkins Hospital reviewed 335 patients treated with SRS across 19 different studies.[112] In the eight studies with median follow-up of >3 years, clinical control was 95% and tumor control was 96%. The control rates were equal among patients treated with LINAC-based platforms and frame-based platforms. Complications were rare and often transient in each of the studies examined. On the basis of these findings, the authors advocate for the use of SRS as primary treatment of glomus jugulare tumors.[112]

Juvenile Nasopharyngeal Angiofibroma

Background and Clinical Aspects

Juvenile nasopharyngeal angiofibroma (JNA) is a rare, benign, vascularized tumor in the head and neck, affecting mostly male adolescents. It originates from the first branchial arch artery. JNAs typically occur in the sphenoethmoidal suture and spread from the nasal cavity to the sphenopalatine foramen and pterygopalatine fossa. Other routes of local spread include the paranasal sinuses, infratemporal fossa, orbital space, and middle cranial fossa.

Symptoms initially include recurrent epistaxis and impaired nose breathing. As local extension occurs, patients may develop facial swelling, orbital symptoms (blindness), cranial nerve deficits, and headaches from intracranial extension.

Diagnosis is often made with the clinical presentation and CT- or MRI-based imaging. Biopsy may cause massive bleeding. Several staging systems are used to categorize the tumors based on extent of local extension (Table 95.4).[113–115]

Surgery

Surgery combined with embolization is the preferred treatment. Through surgery, most JNAs without intracranial extension have local control rates of near 100%. In patients with intracranial extension, complete resection is often not possible.

Radiotherapy

Tumors with intracranial extension or tumors in patients that are medically inoperable are generally treated with RT as the primary modality. Indications for postoperative RT include relapse after surgery. Fractionated IMRT is currently the RT technique of choice to limit collateral radiation to critical structures near the target volume.

The PTV is generally treated to 30 to 50 Gy given in fraction sizes of 2 to 3 Gy/day. In modern series, local control rates range from 85% to 100% (Table 95.5).[116–119] After RT, JNA remission is slow, and late recurrences may occur.

Langerhans Cell Histiocytosis (Histiocytosis X)

Background and Clinical Aspects

Langerhans cell histiocytosis (LCH) is a rare disorder that affects approximately 300 individuals with a higher incidence in children (3 to 5 per million) than adults (1 to 2 per million). Age is an important prognostic factor with children having better outcomes than adults. In the past, it was felt that children younger than 2 years old had a poor prognosis, but recent data from the LCH-II study now refute that point.[120]

The disease is due to an accumulation and/or proliferation of cells that phenotypically resemble the Langerhans skin cell and can cause tissue damage by production of cytokines and infiltration. The actual Langerhans cell is a myeloid dendritic cell that expresses the same antigens (CD1a and CD207) as the Langerhans skin cell.[121] On electron microscopy, Birbeck granules are the classic finding.

LCH can affect a variety of organ systems. Patients are typically stratified into groups based on the extent of disease: single-system disease at a single site, single-system disease involving multiple sites, or multisystem disease. The clinical presentation is dependent upon the sites of disease. Involvement of the skeletal system is the most common site for children and may manifest as pain, palpable mass, or motion deficit or chronic otitis in the case of mastoid or middle ear involvement. Bony lesions from LCH are predominantly lytic in appearance, and the skull is the most frequently involved bony structure.

Cutaneous involvement affects primarily the skin of the scalp and groin and resembles a seborrheic dermatitis. Patients with cranial involvement (posterior pituitary or hypothalamus) may present with DI. The disease may also involve the cervical lymph nodes. Pulmonary involvement is more typically seen in adults. Hepatomegaly, splenomegaly, bone marrow infiltration, and involvement of the gastrointestinal tract are further potential sites of disease.

Evaluation of the patient with suspected LCH should include complete history and physical examination. Routine laboratory work should include CBC with differential. Patients that have symptoms of DI should also undergo a water restriction test. A skeletal survey with or without bone scan should be performed to assess for potential lytic lesions. Further imaging with CT of the head should be performed in patients with skull, orbital, or mastoid involvement. MRI of the head is indicated for patients with DI and those suspected of having brain parenchymal disease involvement. CT of the chest is performed to evaluate patients with pulmonary involvement. An MRI abdomen should be performed for patients with palpable hepatomegaly or splenomegaly.

Surgery

Treatment of LCH depends upon the site and extent of disease. Asymptomatic lesions may be observed. For patients with involvement of only the skeletal system, treatment options include curettage, excision, or intralesional steroid injection. Response rates with curettage or excision alone range from 70% to 90%.[122] Single-system multifocal bone disease may be effectively treated with corticosteroids or chemotherapy, such as vinblastine. For skin-only disease, topical nitrogen mustard and methotrexate are considered effective treatments.

Systemic Therapy

In patients with multisystem disease with symptoms (fever, pain, failure to thrive)

TABLE 95.5 CLINICAL RESULTS OF RADIOTHERAPY IN JUVENILE NASOPHARYNGEAL ANGIOFIBROMA

Study	No. Patients	Study Period	Dose (Gy)	Local Control	Side Effects
Chakraborty et al. (2011)[116]	9	2006–2009	30–46	87.5% (2 y)	No late toxicity
Mcafee et al. (2006)[118]	22	1975–2003	30–36	90% (10 y)	Cataracts (6), transient CNS syndrome (2), "in-field" BCC (2)
Lee et al. (2002)[117]	27	1960–2000	30–55	85% (5 y)	15% late toxicity (growth retardation, panhypopituitarism, TLN, cataracts)
Reddy et al. (2001)[119]	15	1980–1991	30–35	85% (5 y)	Cataracts (3), CNS syndrome (1), BCC (1)

BCC, basal cell carcinoma; CNS, central nervous system; TLN, temporal lobe necrosis.

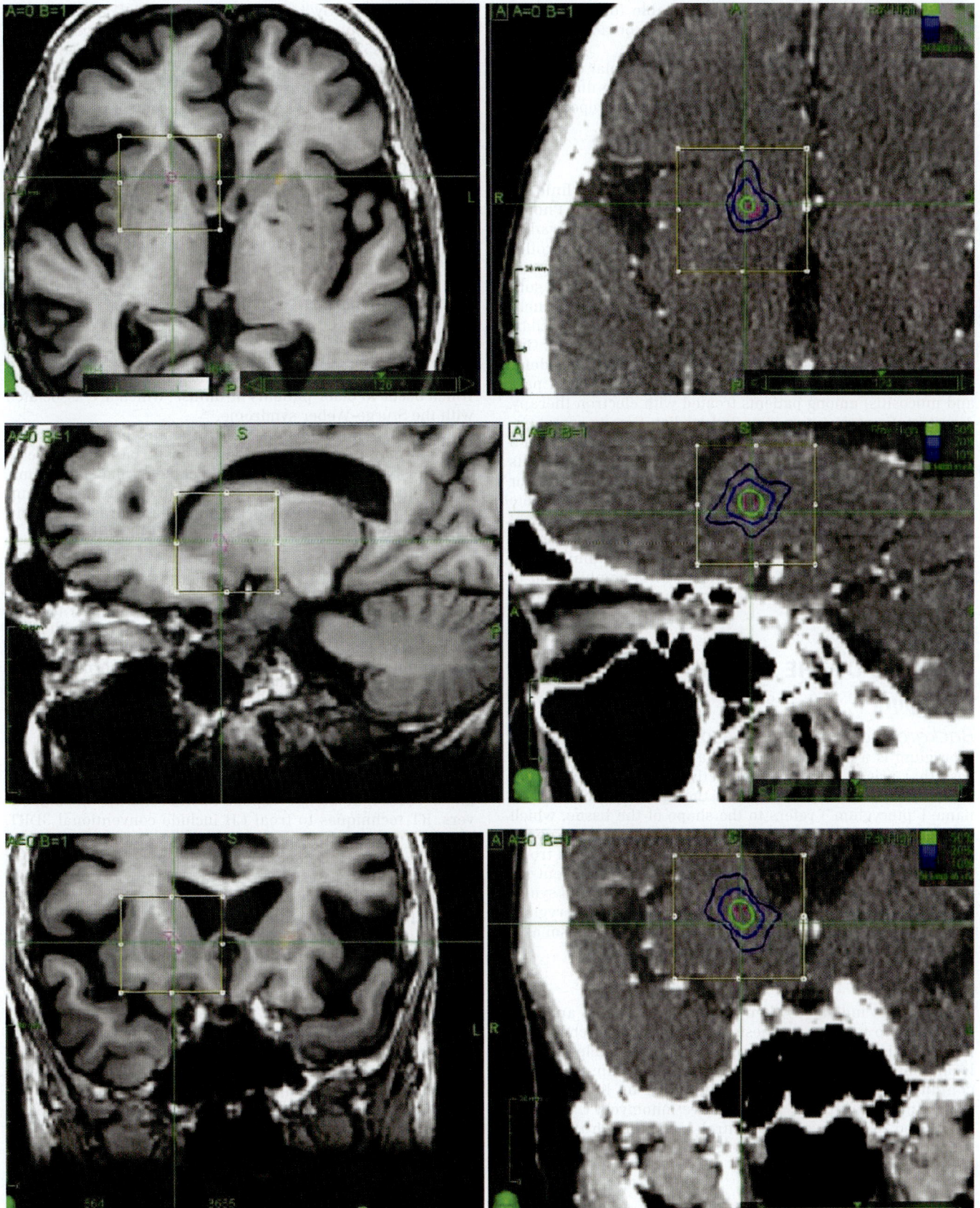

FIGURE 95.5. Stereotactic MRI sequences (**Left**) demonstrating the contoured anterior limbs of the internal capsule bilaterally and the corresponding treatment plan for the right internal capsule (**Right**) for a patient with refractory OCD. The right internal capsule was prescribed 70 Gy to the 50% IDL (140-Gy maximum dose) in a single fraction.

has been shown to have a more favorable toxicity profile regarding central side effects and can also be administered subcutaneously.[176-179]

Botulism can be injected into the submandibular or parotid glands under ultrasound guidance. Because the duration of effect can range from 3 to 7 months, the need for repeat injections is often necessary.[178,180]

Radiotherapy

Electron-based and photon therapy are both techniques deployed in delivering radiotherapy for sialorrhea. Photon therapy is typically delivered with parallel opposed radiation targeting the inferior two-thirds of the bilateral parotids and the entire bilateral submandibular glands. Most common electron field arrangement targeted the entire bilateral submandibular and parotid glands. The durability of treatment effect is variable, but the side effects of treatment are characteristic of patients receiving head and neck radiation. Guy et al.[181] compared the two treatment techniques and demonstrated longer durability and less acute toxicity (oral pain and mucositis) among patients treated with electron therapy. A systematic review demonstrated median time to symptomatic improvement was 2 months with efficacy ranging from 3 months to over 5 years.[179] Assouline et al.[182] treated 50 patients with 6MeV photons to a regimen of 20 Gy in 4 fractions or 10 Gy in 2 fractions with 92% of patients achieving a complete response with no difference in toxicity.[168] In this cohort eight of nine patients receiving a second RT course were treated initially with the lower-dose (10Gy) regimen. Optimal treatment is likely a 3-D conformal plan with a combination of mixed photon–electron beams using an oral cavity avoidance to minimize toxicity.

DISEASES OF THE EYE AND ORBIT

Pterygium

Background and Clinical Aspects

Pterygium is a chronic fibrovascular and degenerative process that arises from the conjunctival–corneal border that extends from the nasal corner of the eye to the cornea. Its name ("pterygium") refers to the shape of the tissue, which is winglike. The exact prevalence of this problem is unknown, but it is well established that the frequency is higher in tropical regions. Most patients are asymptomatic and present for medical attention on the basis of cosmetic concerns, but symptoms may include redness and irritation of the eye. Pterygium may impair vision by producing an irregular astigmatism as it grows onto the cornea.

Surgery

Treatment is indicated when vision is threatened and less commonly to improve cosmesis. The treatment of choice for pterygium is surgical excision with an adjunct to help improve local control rates (i.e., sliding conjunctival flap; rotational conjunctival autograft; free conjunctival or limbal autograft). Intraoperative or postoperative mitomycin C has also been used to improve local control rates, though this leads to increased risk of scleral ulceration, secondary glaucoma, iritis, and cataracts.

Radiotherapy

Local radiation therapy with strontium 90 plays an important role as an adjunct to surgery to prevent relapse. Fractionation schemes of 3 Gy × 10 to 6 Gy × 10 once per week have been commonly used with rates of local recurrence after surgery ranging from 5% to 12%.[183,184] In the most recent randomized study, Nakamatsu et al.[185] evaluated 73 pterygia in 71 patients

and compared 30 Gy/3 fractions versus 40 Gy/4 fractions. The 2-year local control rate was nonsignificantly higher in the 30-Gy arm (85% vs. 75%). In a prospective randomized trial of single-dose postoperative radiotherapy (25 Gy × 1) delivered within 24 hours of surgery compared to sham RT, patients that received radiotherapy had a local control rate of 93.2% compared to 33.3% in the placebo.[186] In another randomized study, Viani et al.[187] compared low fractionation dose (2 Gy in 10 fractions) to high fractionation dose (5 Gy in 7 fractions) beta radiotherapy in the postoperative settings. Control rates were similar between the two groups (93.8% vs. 92.3%) with a significantly lower incidence of poorer cosmesis, photophobia, eye irritation, and scleromalacia in the low fractionation dose arm.

Choroidal Hemangioma

Background and Clinical Aspects

Choroidal hemangiomas (CH) are rare vascular tumors that arise from the choroid. CH can be classified as circumscribed, which occur in older patients or diffuse, which are associated with the Sturge-Weber syndrome.[188]

Clinically, these lesions are often asymptomatic, but patients may present with a visual disturbance by several mechanisms, including retinal detachment, macular edema, and retinal pigment changes.[189] Lesions are detected on fundoscopic exam. Further workup includes ultrasonography, angiography with fluorescent dyes, and CT or MRI.

Surgery

Among the surgical treatment options available, CH that are not near the central visual structures (macula and papilla) are often treated with photodynamic therapy (PDT) with a low rate of complications.[188] Other treatment modalities include laser photocoagulation and transpupillary thermotherapy. In general, radiation therapy is preferred over PDT for the treatment of diffuse CH, though several small studies have reported encouraging results with the use of PDT.[188]

Radiation Therapy

RT is indicated to treat lesions near the macula and papilla and in cases that did not respond to other therapeutic maneuvers. RT techniques to treat CH include conventional 3DRT, proton beam therapy, and brachytherapy. Data for the use of radiosurgery for this condition are scarce[190].

Typical dose prescriptions for 3DCRT are 18 to 20 Gy for circumscribed CH and 30 Gy for diffuse CH given in 1.8- to 2-Gy daily fractions. Schilling irradiated 36 circumscribed CH with 20 Gy in 10 fractions.[191] Retinal reattachment occurred in 64% of the cases with improved vision in 50% and stable vision in 50%.

Fractionated proton radiotherapy doses range from 16.4 to 30 Gy in four fractions.[192-194] In the study by Zografos et al.,[194] all 54 cases experienced retinal reattachment and visual acuity was improved in 70%. Levy-Gabriel et al.[195] demonstrated a 100% rate of retinal reattachment and substantial improvement in visual acuity using proton beam therapy.

Plaque brachytherapy using cobalt 60, iodine 125, or ruthenium 106 has been used to treat circumscribed lesions.[189,194,196,197] Typical doses prescribed to the apex of the lesion range from 25 to 50 Gy. Each isotope has advantages and disadvantages depending on the physical properties (i.e., energy, half-life), and there is no evidence to support the use of one over the other.

Age-Related Macular Degeneration

Age-related macular degeneration (AMD) is the leading cause of blindness in the developed world.[198] The development of AMD is dependent on age, with a prevalence of up to 35%

in the eighth decade of life. External beam radiotherapy with photons or protons and brachytherapy have been used in the past to treat macular degeneration. Overall, results of radiotherapy in the management of this disease have been mixed. A Cochrane meta-analysis in 2010 analyzed 14 randomized trials utilizing RT as a treatment for AMD and concluded that the review "does not provide convincing evidence that radiotherapy is an effective treatment for neovascular AMD."[199]

However, there is renewed interest in radiation therapy for AMD based on results of the IRay in Conjunction with Anti-VEGF Treatment for Patients with Wet AMD (INTREPID) trial.[200] In this study, 230 participants that had received at least 3 injections with anti-VEGF therapy were randomized to 16 Gy, 24 Gy, or sham SRT. The primary endpoint was mean number of pro re nata (PRN) intravitreal ranibizumab injections over 52 weeks. With 2 years of follow-up, patients that received 16 or 24 Gy had fewer PRN treatments compared to the sham SRT group. SRT was found to induce microvascular change, but this affected vision in only 1% of patients.[200] This trial supports SRT as a potential method to stop or slow down the visual loss associated with continued intravitreal injections of anti-VEGF therapy.

Graves Ophthalmopathy

Background and Clinical Aspects

Graves ophthalmopathy (GO), also referred to as Graves orbitopathy or thyroid eye disease, is an autoimmune disorder affecting the musculature of the orbits. The presence of activated T lymphocytes leads to an inflammatory reaction secondary to the release of cytokines. It is estimated that up to 50% of patients with Graves disease will develop orbitopathy, but 10% of patients are euthyroid and some are hypothyroid at presentation.[1] Smoking is the greatest risk factor for the development of GO and also predicts for a poorer response to therapy.[1]

A multidisciplinary team including an ophthalmologist, endocrinologist, and radiation oncologist should be involved in the evaluation of the patient with GO. Clinical features of patients with GO include proptosis (measured by the Hertel exophthalmometer on physical exam), photophobia, upper eyelid retraction, periorbital edema (because of the accumulation of collagen and hyaluronan, which attract water), conjunctival erythema, and tearing and visual impairment (Fig. 95.6A and B). Patients may complain of a "gritty" sensation in their eyes. Several classification systems are available to document the extent of disease, though the one favored at our institution is the SPECS Ophthalmic Index (Table 95.7), which assigns a score of 1 to 3 on the basis of six categories: *S*oft tissue involvement, *P*roptosis, *E*xtraocular movements, *C*orneal involvement, and *S*ight (visual acuity).

Imaging studies, such as CT or MRI, will demonstrate abnormalities, including enlargement of the extraocular muscles and fatty infiltration, in 70% to 80% of cases.[1] The most commonly involved muscles include the inferior and medial rectus muscles.[201]

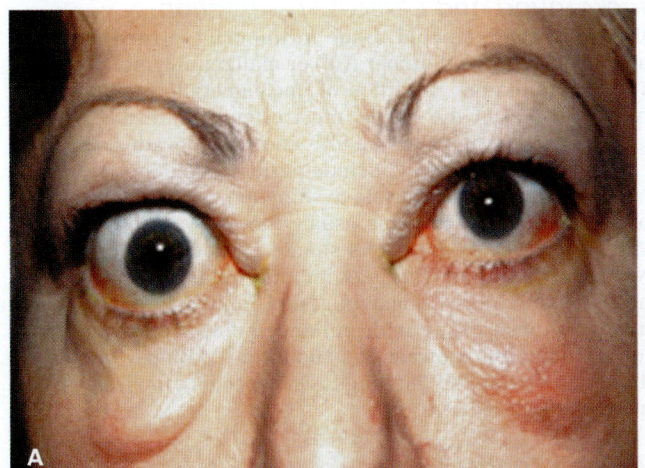

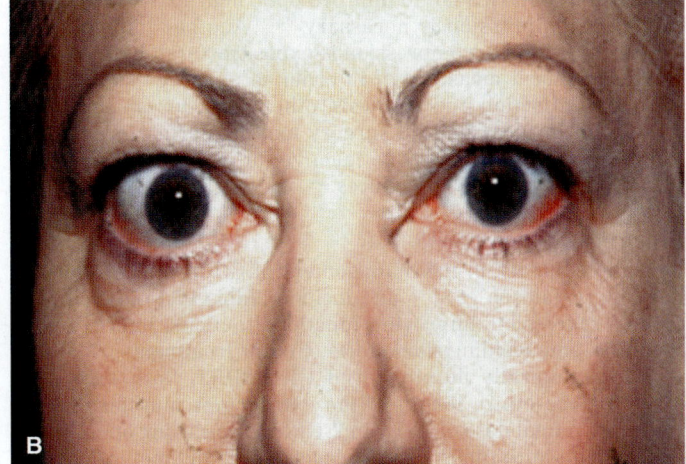

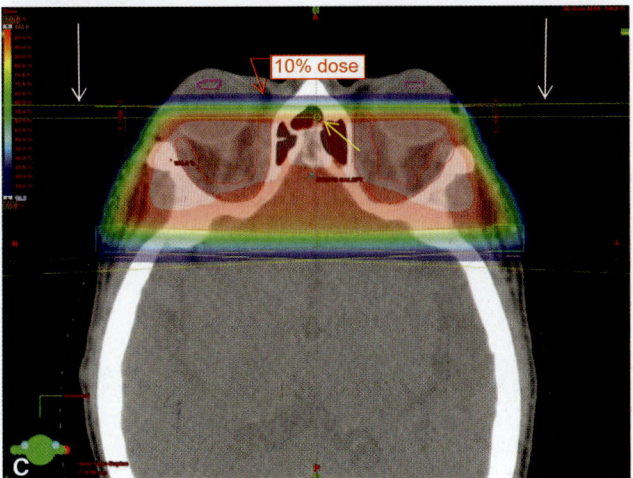

FIGURE 95.6. **A** and **B:** A 50-year-old woman with Graves ophthalmopathy before **(A)** and after **(B)** treatment with corticosteroids and radiotherapy for prominent eyelid edema and strabismus. **C:** 3-D conformal radiotherapy treatment plan for a patient with Graves ophthalmopathy. The isocenter (*yellow arrow*) is placed a few mm posterior to the lenses (*magenta*), and the opposing fields are beam split anteriorly (*white arrows*). The extraocular muscles are contoured in *red*. The color wash display demonstrates that <10% of the dose reaches the lens.

TABLE 95.7 SPECS CLASSIFICATION SYSTEM FOR GRAVES OPHTHALMOPATHY

Clinical Feature	Grade 1 (1 Point)	Grade 2 (2 Points)	Grade 3 (3 Points)
S (soft tissue involvement)	Minimal objective symptoms: redness, chemosis, slight periorbital edema	Moderate objective symptoms: redness, chemosis, moderate periorbital edema	Severe objective symptoms: conjunctival exposition, prominent periorbital edema
P (proptosis)	>20–23 mm	24–27 mm	>27 mm
E (eye muscle dysfunction)	Rare diplopia; none in primary position	Frequent diplopia; moderate mobility impairment	Severe constant muscular dysfunction
C (corneal involvement)	Slight corneal changes and no symptoms	Prominent corneal changes and moderate symptoms	Keratitis or other severe eye symptoms
S (sight loss)	20/25–20/40	20/45–20/100	>20/100

Management Overview

Treatment options for GO include glucocorticoids, orbital radiotherapy, and surgery (orbital decompression, eye muscle surgery, eyelid surgery). Smokers should be encouraged to quit. Prior to the initiation of treatment, the patient's thyroid function should be normalized. Radioiodine therapy, but not antithyroid drugs, may cause worsening of GO.[202] Once thyroid function is stabilized, the treatment of GO depends upon the severity of the disease.

Medical Management (Glucocorticoids)

Glucocorticoids (GCs) are a mainstay of treatment for GO. Immediate treatment with high-dose steroids (IV or oral) is required for patients whose vision is threatened by optic neuropathy.[203] GCs may also be used to treat patients with moderate to severe active ophthalmopathy.[203]

Surgery

In the event that GCs fail to improve optic neuropathy, urgent orbital decompression is necessary.[204,205] Another indication for urgent orbital decompression is exposure keratopathy not relieved by local measures.[204] In order to improve extraocular muscle function and cosmesis, other procedures such as strabismus surgery and lid surgery may be performed. It is recommended that the GO be inactive for at least 6 months before pursuing these procedures.[204]

Radiotherapy

Indications for RT in the management of GO have been outlined by Donaldson et al.[206] and include (Table 95.8) inducing clinical regression, improving functional deficits, improving cosmesis, and avoiding side effects of other treatments.

RT is generally administered with 3DRT. Both orbits, including the entire length of the extraocular muscles, are treated to a total dose of 20 Gy in 2-Gy fractions using opposed lateral fields with the isocenter placed a few millimeters posterior to the lenses using a beam-split technique (Fig. 95.6C).

For patients with progressive GO, retrospective data suggest that orbital RT is an effective treatment modality. Marquez et al.[207] reviewed the records of 197 patients treated at Stanford, all of whom received 20 to 30 Gy to the bilateral retrobulbar

region. Outcomes assessed included SPECS score and patient satisfaction. There was a 96% overall response rate and 98% patient satisfaction rate with the largest improvements in soft tissue findings (89%), extraocular muscle dysfunction (85%), and corneal abnormalities (96%). In a more recent study, Matthiesen et al.[208] reported on 211 patients that received orbital RT between 2000 and 2010 for GO. Overall, 97% of patients had stabilization of disease and 84% reported symptomatic improvement. Steroids were discontinued in 98% of patients who received them as initial therapy. A subset of 14 patients received orbital reirradiation for persistent symptoms, with 5 achieved a complete response and 9 had disease stabilization. These 14 patients did not experience increased toxicity compared to the rest of the cohort.[208]

Reactive Lymphoid Hyperplasia/Orbital Pseudotumor

Background and Clinical Presentation

Disease of the lymphoid tissue in the orbit is rare and may include orbital pseudotumor (OP) or malignant lymphomas. OP is an inflammatory condition of unclear etiology that affects the soft tissue of the orbits, most often unilaterally.[201] Most patients present between the fifth and sixth decades of life.[209]

Clinical features of OP include periorbital edema, retrobulbar pain, extraocular muscle dysfunction, palpable mass, and exophthalmos.[201] Symptoms usually develop acutely. Imaging with CT or MRI of the orbits should be obtained for further evaluation. Imaging findings include enlarged extraocular muscles, optic nerve thickening, and infiltrates in the retrobulbar adipose tissue with enhancement after administration of iodinated contrast or gadolinium.[201] Biopsy should be obtained to establish the diagnosis, especially for lesions that are easily accessible.

Medical Therapy

Corticosteroids are the treatment of choice for the majority of patients. Response rates for optic neuropathy are as high as 92% with an overall response rate of 78%.[201] However, only 33% of patients experience long-term control with a single course of steroids.[210]

TABLE 95.8 CLINICAL GUIDELINES FOR USE OF RADIOTHERAPY IN GRAVES OPHTHALMOPATHY (GO)

Radiotherapy Goal	Precondition/Indications	Contraindications
Induce clinical regression	*Pretherapeutic diagnostics*: evidence of autoimmune thyroid disease; CT/MRI	Stable GO without clinical progression
Reduce/eliminate functional deficits	*Ophthalmologic diagnostics*: documented progressive disease	Lack of euthyrosis
Improve cosmetics/esthetics	*Subjective/objective findings*: evidence of functional deficits and disorders	"Cosmetic" indication alone without functional impairment
Avoid/decrease undesired effects of other measures	*Exclusion of risk factors*: no other eye disease (i.e., diabetic retinopathy)	No consent to planned therapy

Smitt MC, Donaldson SS. Radiation therapy for benign diseases of the orbit. *Semin Radiat Oncol* 1999;19(2):259–264.

Surgery

Surgical excision may be used for easily accessible lesions. Relapses are common after surgery.

Radiation Therapy

Indications for RT include recurrent lesions after surgery, steroid-refractory lesions, and lesions not amenable to other treatments. The RT technique of choice is 3DRT.

A planning CT should be obtained and coregistered with the diagnostic MR or diagnostic CT to delineate the target volume, when visible. Unilateral treatment is typically performed with a single lateral field or with an anterior and lateral field, weighted more heavily laterally. Bilateral orbital involvement is treated in a manner similar to GO. Occasionally, superficial lesions may be treated with electrons. Typically, the prescription dose is 20 Gy given in 10 fractions.[201]

Two modern series demonstrate the efficacy of orbit RT on OP. In a study by Matthiesen et al.,[211] 20 orbits in 16 patients were treated with RT for OP. With a mean dose of 20 Gy in 10 fractions, 87.5% of the patients experienced a response (clinical improvement and/or tapering of corticosteroid dose). Corticosteroid use was stopped or reduced in 81% of the patients. No significant late effects were reported. Similarly, Prabhu et al.[212] reported on 26 orbits affected with OP in 20 patients treated with radiation therapy (25.2 to 30.6 Gy) between 2002 and 2011. The majority (85%) demonstrated a response to RT, and 70% of the patients initially on steroids were completely off steroids by the last follow-up visit. Long-term complications occurred in seven patients, the majority of which were cataracts.[212]

BENIGN DISEASES OF SOFT TISSUE AND BONES

General Overview of Inflammatory Conditions of Joints and Tendons

The role of radiation therapy in the treatment of benign inflammatory conditions involving the joints and/or tendons is controversial. Osteoarthritis (OA), tendonitis, bursitis, rotator cuff syndrome, and tennis elbow are examples of inflammatory conditions for which radiation therapy has been used in the past. These soft tissue syndromes may result from repetitive activities that cause overuse or injury to the joint areas, incorrect posture, stress on the soft tissues because of an abnormal or poor positioned joint or bone, or other diseases, such as autoimmune diseases or infection.

Although the cause of each disorder may be different, the clinical presentation and general treatment plan are frequently similar. Symptoms include pain, swelling, or inflammation in the tissues and structures around a joint, such as the tendons, ligaments, bursae, and muscles. Treatment generally involves a combination of exercise, lifestyle modification, and analgesics. If pain becomes debilitating, joint replacement surgery may be used to improve the quality of life. In rare instances, low-dose radiation therapy (<10 to 15Gy) can be employed. The low dose required to improve symptoms suggests the possible mechanism of action for radiation therapy (Table 95.9).

Osteoarthritis

Osteoarthritis (OA), the most common joint disorder, is a chronically debilitating musculoskeletal disorder, which predominately affects older people. It presents with pain associated with cartilage destruction, bone modification, and structural changes of capsule and synovia. Symptoms are caused by reactive inflammation of joint surface and joint capsule lining (synovia). Risk factors include age, genetic predisposition, bone fracture or joint injury whether by an

TABLE 95.9 RADIATION THERAPY MECHANISM OF ACTION DOSE CONCEPTS

Mechanisms of Action	Single Dose (Gy)	Total Dose (Gy)
Cellular gene and protein expression (e.g., eczemas)	<2.0	<2
Inhibition of inflammation in lymphocytes (e.g., in pseudotumor orbitae)	0.3–1.0	2–6
Inhibition of fibroblast proliferation (e.g., in keloids)	1.5–3.0	8–12
Inhibition of proliferation in benign tumors (e.g., in desmoids)	1.8–3.0	45–60

accident of overuse from work or sports, and increased BMI.[213] The incidence of OA is expected to rise worldwide because of an aging population and the increasing prevalence of obesity compared to previous decades.

Nonradiotherapeutic Treatment

Hunter et al.[214] provide a general overview of the diagnosis, investigation, and treatment of OA. The treatment of early OA is intended to reduce the primary symptoms of joint pain and stiffness with the goal of maintaining and improving the functional capacity of the affected joint(s).[215] Exercise, weight reduction, and joint braces, among other measures, have shown some success at unloading damaged joints and improving symptoms.[216] For osteoarthritis of the hip and knee, exercises that strengthen muscles and improve aerobic condition are most effective.[217]

Oral analgesics are the mainstay of treatment for OA. Although acetaminophen is frequently offered due to its relative safety and effectiveness, a nonsteroidal anti-inflammatory drug (NSAID) may be added or substituted.[218] NSAIDs can be used in patients with symptomatic OA of the hand, hip, or knee. The goal is to administer the lowest effective dose for the shortest duration. The use of stronger analgesics, such as weak opioids and narcotic, may be considered when other methods have been ineffective or if certain drugs are contraindicated.[216] Glucosamine and chondroitin sulfate are over-the-counter remedies that are frequently used to reduce pain, but their efficacy has not been proven.[219] Corticosteroids and other analgesics may be injected directly into the joint; injections may temporarily reduce swelling and pain. Acupuncture and other complementary and alternative treatment modalities have been used, but their efficacy has yet to be proven.[220]

Surgery is reserved for patients with severe OA and those who have not responded to noninvasive therapies. Total or partial joint replacement is most commonly used for OA involving the knee, hip, and shoulder and is considered when structural damage is visible on x-rays. However, there are modern surgical procedures that can obviate or delay the need for joint replacement, including osteotomies, and joint resurfacing.[221] Joint fusion or arthrodesis may be used to treat arthritis of the spine, ankles, hands, and feet. Arthroscopy, or arthroscopic surgery, is a minimally invasive surgical procedure that can be used to examine and treat the interior surface of a damaged joint. Arthroscopic procedures can help relieve pain for a short time and allow the joints to move better. Although arthroscopy may delay the need for joint replacement surgery, it does not improve the arthritis itself.[222]

Radiotherapeutic Options

In nonsurgical candidates, low-dose RT may be considered if pharmacotherapy has failed. RT can lead to primary freedom from pain and secondary to improved joint function.[223] Several single-institution studies have been published that report long-term pain relief and functional gain in 50% to 75% of patients. In Germany, a pattern of care study investigated the use of RT for the treatment of OA of the knee (gonarthrosis) from the years 2006 to 2008.[224] Almost 80% of institutions in Germany have used RT to treat OA in the 2-year period analyzed. Treatment of 4,544 patients was performed annually at 188 institutions. The median total dose was 6 Gy (range 3 to 12 Gy), with a median single dose of 1 Gy (0.25 to 3 Gy). Long-term clinical outcomes were available in 5,069 cases. The majority of patients experienced pain reduction for at least 3 months, but pain management for up to 12 months was reported. In 30% of patients, a second course of RT was used for inadequate pain response or early pain recurrence.[224] Micke et al.[225] published a prospective study on elderly patients with gonarthrosis using a similar RT regimen demonstrating a good analgesic effect of low-dose RT with minimal side effects.

As with arthroscopy, radiation may reduce pain and pain-related dysfunction, but it does not improve the arthritis itself. Because of its efficacy and relative safety, RT may provide an alternative to conventional conservative treatment for patients who are not surgical candidates.

Gorham-Stout Syndrome

Gorham-Stout syndrome, also known as disappearing bone disease or massive osteolysis, is a rare bone disorder of unknown etiology. It is characterized by progressive proliferation of small blood or lymph vessels resulting in destruction and resorption of the bone matrix. The symptoms are non-specific, but include muscular weakness, limb tenderness, and pathologic fracture occurring minimal trauma. Involvement of the cervical spine or skull base could be fatal. Case reports indicate limited efficacy of systemic therapies such as zoledronic acid and interferon-α.[226,227] Radiation therapy has also been used.[228] Heyd et al.[229] completed a national patterns-of-care study and literature review that summarizes the scant data available for this rare disorder. The 38 articles listed therein provide evidence from treatment of 44 patients that conventionally fractionated external beam RT (total dose of 36 to 45 Gy) may prevent disease progression in 75% to 80% of cases.

Pigmented Villonodular Synovitis

Pigmented villonodular synovitis or tenosynovial giant cell tumor is a rare proliferative disorder of synovial tissue. Symptoms include sudden onset, unexplained joint swelling and pain that frequently involves a single joint. The knee and foot are most commonly affected, but there are reports of shoulder, hand, and hip involvement.[230] Decreased motion, joint stiffness, and increased pain occur as the disorder progresses. Surgical resection with either synovectomy or joint replacement is the treatment of choice.[231]

Radiation therapy is indicated in cases of diffuse disease, bulky disease resulting in bone destruction, or in the rare instance of multiple recurrences after resection. Although intrasynovial injection of radioactive isotopes postoperatively has been used in the past for high-risk patients,[232] most institutions use external beam radiation therapy. RT to a dose of 36 to 50 Gy has been effective.[21,233,234] MRI is essential for delineating disease pre- and postoperatively. Final dose of RT should be tailored to the amount of residual disease.[235]

Vertebral Hemangiomas

Hemangiomas are benign proliferations of blood vessels that can affect any tissue and are typically asymptomatic. About 50% of hemangiomas involving the vertebral body are associated with pain and therefore may require treatment. Treatment options include surgical resection or more conservative interventions such as transarterial embolization, vertebroplasty, or intralesional injections.[236] Radiation therapy either alone or postoperatively has been successful in reducing pain caused by vertebral hemangiomas.[237] In a German multicenter trial, a total of 84 patients with 96 symptomatic lesions were irradiated for a symptomatic vertebral hemangioma. At a median 68-month follow-up, 90% of patients had either complete or partial pain relief. Radiation doses ≥34 Gy resulted in significantly improved pain relief. A total radiation dose of 36 to 40 Gy delivered in 2 Gy per fraction has been recommended.[238]

DISEASES OF CONNECTIVE TISSUE AND SKIN

Desmoid Tumors

Background and Clinical Aspects

Desmoid tumors (also called aggressive fibromatosis or deep musculoaponeurotic fibromatosis) are benign tumors of connective tissue tumors that arise from muscle fascias, aponeuroses, tendons, and scar tissue. They are slightly more predominant in females and tend to occur during the third and fourth decades of life, although children and the elderly can be affected. In the general population, desmoids are rare; the estimated incidence is 2 to 4 per million per year. Genetic factors, trauma, and/or surgery predisposes the development of desmoids. Most desmoids arise sporadically, with 85% of cases associated with CTNNB1 gene mutation in the Wnt/β-catenin signaling pathway. Mutations in the APC genes result in desmoid tumors affecting 10% to 20% of patients with familial adenomatous polyposis (FAP) and are a manifestation of Gardner syndrome.[239,240]

Tumors can develop anywhere in the body, but most commonly involve in the trunk/extremity, abdominal wall, and intra-abdominal sites, including the bowel and mesentery. Approximately 30% of patients with desmoid tumors have a history of prior desmoid tumors.[241,242] Sporadic cases commonly involve the extremities, the shoulder girdle, and the buttock.[242] In patients with FAP, intra-abdominal desmoids predominate and tend to be associated with surgical sites and anastomoses following colectomy.[243] Desmoid tumors in women can occur during or after pregnancy and therefore may be associated with high estrogen states. Women who have been pregnant are more likely to have abdominal desmoid tumors that develop within 10 years of the last pregnancy.[244]

Although desmoids have no known potential for metastasis or dedifferentiation, they are locally aggressive and commonly have a high rate of recurrence even after complete resection. Diagnostics workup with MRI helps to estimate size and infiltration into other organs and should be obtained prior to incisional biopsy that is obtained to confirm diagnosis.

Nonradiotherapeutic Treatment

Observation is a viable option for stable, asymptomatic desmoids. Treatment is indicated for symptomatic patients, if there is risk to adjacent structures, or to improve cosmesis. Complete surgical resection of the tumor with negative microscopic margins is the treatment of choice for most desmoid tumors. Because of the size and infiltrative nature of extra-abdominal desmoids, resection may result in significant morbidity requiring skin grafting or flap reconstruction. Desmoid tumors have a high rate of recurrence following even complete surgical removal. Recent meta-analysis of 1,295 patients demonstrated that risk of recurrence in patients with positive surgical margins was almost twofold higher.[245] Although resection does not alter survival in most patients, given the histologically benign nature of desmoids, the overall surgical strategy should still be an attempt at complete removal using function-preserving surgical approaches to minimize major morbidity (functional and/or cosmetic).[246]

Although extra-abdominal desmoid tumors can generally be treated effectively with local therapy, surgical intervention tends to be counterproductive in intra-abdominal variants, especially the ones associated with FAP. In some instances, systemic therapy may achieve significant and durable cytoreduction, obviating the need for resection. Patients with desmoid tumors have been treated with NSAIDs. The most widely used NSAID for treatment of desmoid tumors is sulindac. Hormonal agents such as tamoxifen, raloxifene, and progesterone have been used, often in combination with NSAIDs. Tamoxifen has been used most widely and is typically prescribed at doses similar to those used for breast cancer (10 mg daily). Much higher doses (120 mg daily) have been recommended,[247] but high-dose tamoxifen is difficult to tolerate, and there is no evidence to suggest that higher doses of tamoxifen are better than lower doses.

A variety of palliative chemotherapeutic regimens have been used.[248-251] With the waxing and waning natural history of desmoids, it is difficult to say whether systemic therapy provides much benefit over observation. In one series, 142 patients presented with either a primary ($n = 74$) or recurrent ($n = 68$) desmoid tumor. Eighty-three patients were treated with observation along, and fifty-nine received either hormone therapy or chemotherapy. There was no statistically significant difference in progression-free rates between the two groups.

Desmoid tumors also respond to the tyrosine kinase inhibitor imatinib.[252,253] The response is thought to be due to expression of one of Gleevec's molecular targets, PDGF receptor, on desmoid tumors.[254] Phase II clinical trials have demonstrated efficacy of imatinib in the treatment of progressive and recurrent aggressive fibromatosis. Although response rates are low, the 2-year progression-free rate in responders is about 50% with a favorable toxicity profile.[253,255] Kasper et al.[255] prospectively administered imatinib (800 mg/daily) to patients with desmoid tumors not amenable to R0 resection without significant function loss and demonstrated a 2-year progression arrest rate of 45%.

Intralesional injections[256] and radiofrequency ablation[257] have also been used. Although the techniques led to some tumor shrinkage, the experience to date is limited and the long-term results are not yet known.

Radiotherapeutic Options

Radiation therapy is a viable option for inoperable patients and may also be used in combination with surgery or chemotherapy. Spear et al.[258] retrospectively compared the efficacy of surgery-alone, radiation-alone, and combined modality therapy (radiation and surgery) in the treatment of desmoid tumors. Five-year local control rates among surgery, radiation therapy, and combined modality groups were 69%, 93%, and 72%, respectively. More recently, Janssen et al.[245] performed a meta-analysis on the influence of surgical margin and adjuvant RT on local recurrence and found that RT reduces the risk of recurrence in patients with microscopically positive resection margins. The association of adjuvant RT benefit was even stronger for resection of recurrent tumors with positive margins. Of note, adjuvant radiotherapy for patients with negative margins did not affect recurrence rates.

The general recommended radiation dose for inoperable or recurrent desmoids is 60 to 65 Gy.[21] However, long-term results at another institution show increased posttreatment toxicity in patients who receive RT doses >56 Gy.[246,259]

Young age (≤30 years) was also associated with increased late toxicity. In a retrospective study of 30 patients under the age of 30, younger age (<18) is associated with inferior locoregional control following RT. Although actuarial control rates were better with RT doses of ≥55Gy, almost 50% of patients experienced grade III and IV complications, including pathologic fractures, impaired range of motion, pain, and in-field skin cancers.[260] Because long-term results suggest that unresectable tumors respond to 56 Gy with a 75% expectation of local control, the lower dose may be more appropriate in this population.

When an R0 resection is not possible, doses of 50 to 60 Gy postoperatively should be given to improve local control. RT is often not considered for intra-abdominal tumors because of the dose and increased field size required increase risk of bowel injury. Because of the complexities involved in managing the disease, a multidisciplinary approach must be taken.[261]

Peyronie Disease

Background and Clinical Aspects

Peyronie disease (also known as "induratio penis plastica") is a chronic inflammatory connective tissue disorder involving the penile tunica albuginea that results in tissue proliferation and the development of hard plaques, most commonly on the dorsal surface of the penis, which may cause a curvature and changes in the length or circumference of the penis while erect. Symptoms may lead to difficult intercourse, penile pain, and erectile dysfunction.

Peyronie disease (PYD) affects up to 10% of men, although a recent population-based study suggests the condition may be underreported in the United States.[262] Although PYD can affect teenagers, men between the ages 40 to 70 are mostly affected, with a peak incidence at 50 years of age. The cause is unknown, but is often associated with prior penile trauma. Diabetes mellitus and arterial and venous vascular disease are risk factors, along with an assumed genetic predisposition. PYD results in pain, abnormal curvature, erectile dysfunction, indentation, loss of girth, and shortening. Slow progression over several months is typical, with spontaneous remission occurring in <15% of men.[263]

Nonradiotherapeutic Treatment

Results of nonsurgical treatment of PYD are mixed and controversial.[264,265] Some success has been reported with vitamin E supplementation, but results have not been confirmed in larger studies.[266] A combination of vitamin E and colchicine may delay disease progression.[267] Other agents that specifically target inflammatory pathways have also shown mixed benefit, including TGFβ1 inhibitors,[268] coenzyme Q10,[269] and sildenafil, among others.[270] Topical therapies have largely been ineffective, but penile injection with verapamil or collagenase, intended to break up scar tissue formed by the inflammation, has shown some efficacy.[271] Physical therapy and extracorporeal shock treatments have also had limited benefit.

Surgical options for PYD are complex procedures that should only be performed by experienced urologists and are reserved for patients not responding to other therapies.[272] Although the nonsurgical treatments discussed may not reliably treat the disease, they can be used to stabilize the scarring process and may result in some reduction of deformity. A combination of nonsurgical techniques may have even more efficacy.[273]

Radiotherapeutic Options

The largest experience with the use of RT in the treatment of PYD has been in Europe. Retrospective studies report varied symptom improvement with the use of RT in terms of pain, curvature reduction, plaque volume, and sexual functioning.[274] These data also suggest that any benefit of RT is best in the treatment of early stages of disease, when radioresponsive inflammatory cells and fibroblasts are still active in the disease. RT in later stages of PYD once the plaques have fully formed is thought to yield worse outcomes.

The current recommendation for RT in PYD is a total dose of 10 to 20 Gy in daily single fractions of 2 to 3 Gy using a direct ventral field with the penis laying on the scrotum and a lead or polyethylene layer between the scrotum and testes. Orthovoltage, low-energy photons and/or electrons may be used. One retrospective study from the Netherlands indicated that low-dose RT, either 13.5 Gy (9 × 1.5 Gy, 3 fractions per week) or 12 Gy (6 × 2 Gy, daily fractions), resulted in pain relief in the majority of the 179 patients evaluated.[275] Sexual dysfunction was a reported side effect, although this is confounded by the underlying disease.

As experimental models improve our understanding of the pathogenesis of PYD, the use of RT for plaque development in this highly complex vascular organ may further decline given concerns regarding radiation-induced vascular fibrosis, and more effective therapies emerge.[276,277]

Dupuytren Contracture

Background and Clinical Aspects

Dupuytren contracture, also known as Morbus Dupuytren (MD) and Morbus Ledderhose (ML) depending on involvement of the hands or feet, respectively, is a connective tissue disorders that affects the palmar or plantar fascia. Some authors estimate a global prevalence of Dupuytren disease to be between 3% and 6%. Incidence increases after the age of 40 and the condition affects men more often than women. A genetic predisposition along with a number of environmental factors (smoking, alcohol use) can lead to local ischemia and free radical release, which, in turn, stimulates fibroblast proliferation and cytokine production, particularly IL-1.

In the early stage, subcutaneous nodules appear, which may be fixed to the overlying skin. As the disease progresses, cords develop and become visibly predominant. With further progression, the cords reach the periosteum of the bones and lead to the characteristic appearance of palmar or plantar contraction. The fourth/fifth phalanges of the hand (MD) or the first/second toes of the foot (ML) are most commonly affected digits (Fig. 95.7). With increased thickening of the fascia and progressive contracture, the fingers and toes begin to curl, resulting in significant functional deficits, for example, difficulty grabbing (MD) or walking (ML).

Nonradiotherapeutic Treatment

Excision of diseased cords and fascia via limited or selective fasciectomy is widely considered the gold standard treatment for Dupuytren contracture.[278,279] A 20-year review of open surgery for Dupuytren contracture showed that major complications occurred in 15.7% of cases and wound complications were seen in 22% of cases.[280] Even with excellent surgical resection, relapse is common, with 30% to 50% recurrence rate at 3 years.

Modern minimally invasive techniques have substantially reduced the complication rates. Percutaneous needle fasciotomy is a technique where cords are weakened through the insertion and manipulation of a small 25-gauge needle mounted on a 10-mL syringe.[281] The procedure is performed under local anesthesia and patients may return to full usage of the affected limb within 24 hours. Because the cords and nodules are not fully excised, minimally invasive surgery has an even higher recurrence rate than surgical excision. A randomized study comparing percutaneous needle fasciotomy with limited fasciectomy showed an 85% recurrence rate after 5 years with the minimally invasive procedure.[282]

During the early stage of Dupuytren's, medication (steroids, allopurinol, nonsteroidals, vitamin E) may provide benefit, but the effects are temporary. Collagenase *Clostridium histolyticum* (CCH) injections are an FDA-approved nonsurgical treatment option for adult Dupuytren contracture patients with a palpable cord. Injections of this collagenase enzyme weaken the cords through breakdown of the peptide bonds in collagen, which subsequently allows for finger manipulation and release of contractures.[283–285] Although CCH has proven to be a useful minimally invasive technique for patients with later-stage DC, recurrence rates of 35% at 3 years of follow-up have been reported.[285,286]

Radiotherapeutic Options

Radiotherapy is currently used in the treatment of Dupuytren's exclusively for early-stage patients (who have a <10-degree deformity) and is considered standard of care for prevention of Dupuytren progression. Low-dose radiotherapy hinders fibroblast proliferation and the cascade of inflammatory markers that induce collagen formation and fibroblast differentiation into fibronectin. Many studies have demonstrated patient-reported effectiveness of radiation preventing further Dupuytren progression with minimal toxicity.[287–290] Adamietz et al. reviewed 176 hands treated with low-dose radiotherapy. Of those patients with <5-degree deformity, 82% had a patient-hand–reported disease progression-free survival at 10-year follow-up. Betz et al. retrospectively reviewed 208

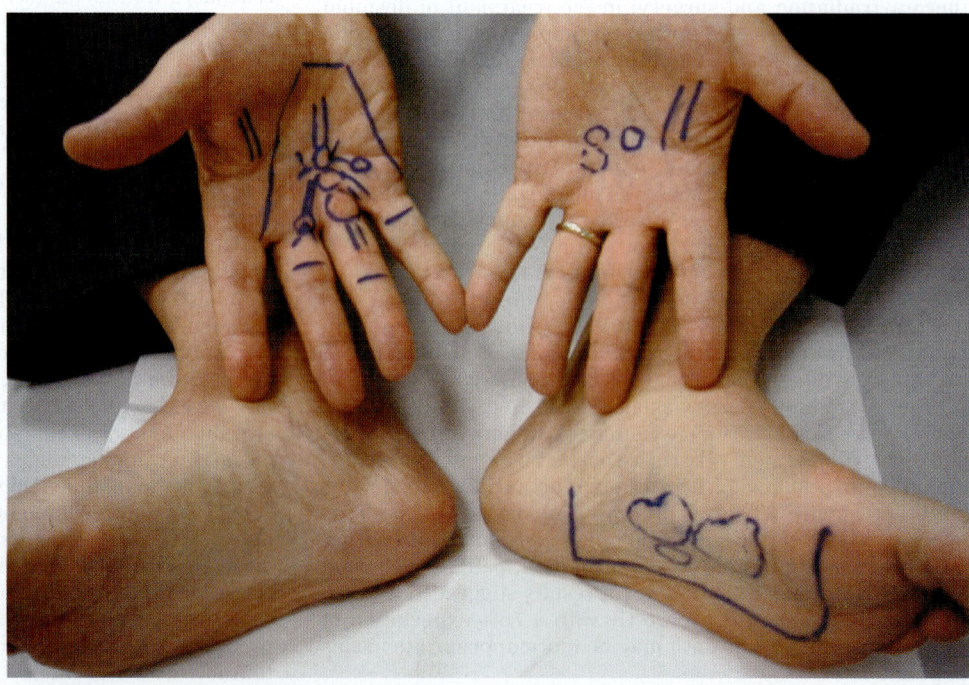

FIGURE 95.7. Dupuytren contracture of both hands and the left foot.

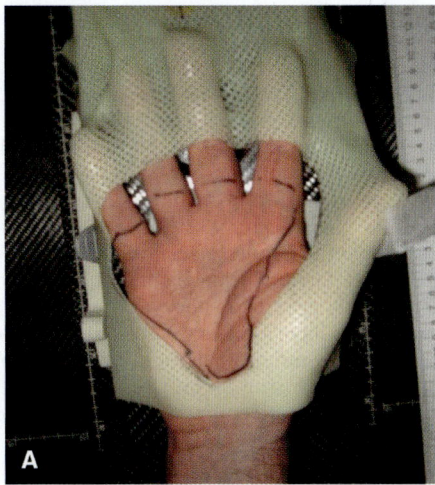
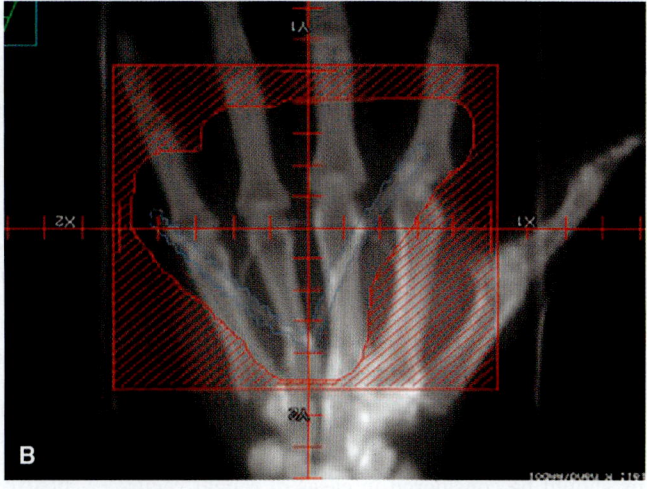

FIGURE 95.8. A: Immobilization for treatment of Dupuytren contracture with electrons. **B:** Block formation with clinical margin. (Courtesy of Barbara Agrimson CMD, RT (R) (T) Oregon Health & Science University.)

hands treated with low-dose radiation and found that patients with <5-degree deformity had an 87% patient-hand–reported disease progression-free survival at 13-year follow-up. Most recently in 2015, a prospective study by Schuster et al. published the largest US patient-reported outcomes after low-dose radiation for early-stage Dupuytren's. In this study, 45 patients had received low-dose radiation via electrons directed en face. After 31 months, 94% of surveyed patients reported the RT was successful with minimal toxicity.

Seegenschmiedt et al.[290] performed a randomized clinical trial comparing the safety and efficacy of two different dose regimens with an untreated control group.[21] Group A received 10 × 3 Gy (30 Gy) via a split course (5 × 3 Gy) repeated at intervals of 12 weeks; in Group B, patients were treated with 7 × 3 Gy (21 Gy) delivered over 2 weeks. Regardless of the dose regimen, approximately 90% of treated patients had stable or improved disease. After a mean follow-up of 8 years, the extension deficit increased in 35% of the control group, in 7% of the 21-Gy group, and in only 4% of the 30-Gy group. Acute toxicity was more pronounced in group B, but long-term toxicity was comparable and included dryness, desquamation, skin atrophy, and altered sensation. The results of this study indicate that the prophylactic RT is well tolerated by patients and effective at preventing disease progression, and the 30-Gy

regimen may be superior.[21] Irrespective of dose regimen, the target volume should include palpable or detectable nodules and cords surrounded by a 3- to 5-mm margin; and appropriate immobilization and shielding of unaffected joints are required (Fig. 95.8).

Keloids and Hypertrophic Scars

Background and Clinical Aspects

Keloids are an excessive tissue proliferation after scars after skin injury from surgery, heat, chemical burns, inflammation (e.g., acne), or even spontaneous proliferation. They differ from hypertrophic scars by their typical infiltrative growth pattern, causing local pain and inflammatory reactions, and sometimes long-term progression; hypertrophic scars show thickening without surrounding reaction and can flatten spontaneously. Keloids appear mostly in the upper body and in regions with high skin tension (e.g., sternum, ear lobes). The cause is still unknown, although there is a genetic and race-specific predisposition that is already noted during adolescence. Keloids at the ear lobe after piercing are typical. In some patients, the resulting lesions are severely disfiguring and painful (Fig. 95.9). Recurrence is common after treatment.

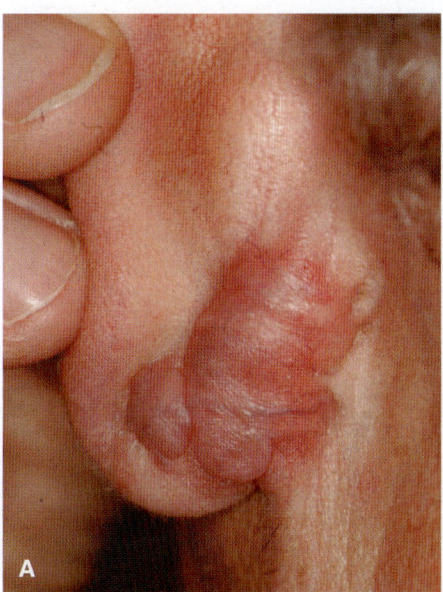
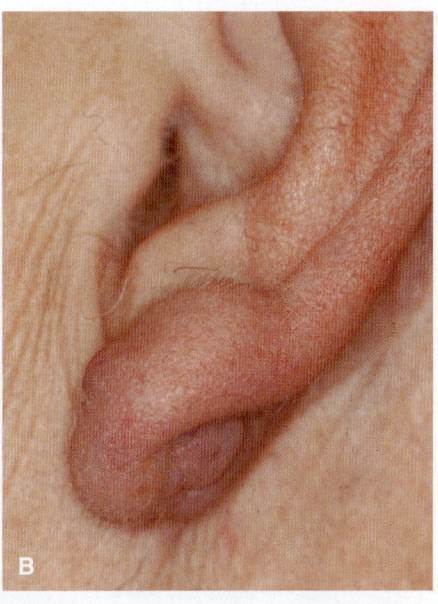

FIGURE 95.9. A: Keloid behind left ear lobe. **B:** Status of keloid following resection plus 4 × 4-Gy radiotherapy.

Nonradiotherapeutic Treatment

Silicone bandages, pressure dressings, and cryosurgery have all been used to treat for keloids with varying efficacy.[291,292] Intralesional injections remain the first-line therapy for most keloids. Corticosteroids, 5-FU, and verapamil have all been directly injected into keloid lesions with symptom improvement. Up to 70% of patients respond to intralesional corticosteroid injection with flattening of keloids, although the recurrence rate is high in some studies (up to 50% at 5 years).[293]

Surgical excision may be indicated if injection therapy alone does not result in improvement. In patients treated with excision alone, recurrence rates range from 45% to 100%[294]; therefore, excision is typically combined with perioperative and postoperative injections of either triamcinolone or interferon.[293]

Radiotherapeutic Options

Radiotherapy should be considered in cases of repeat recurrences postoperatively or where there is a high-risk of recurrence (e.g., marginal resection, large lesion, unfavorable location). Primary RT can be considered in instances where resection would result in functional impairment and in actively proliferating disorders within about 6 months after the triggering trauma. Because proliferating fibroblasts and mesenchymal and inflammatory cells are the target cells for RT, fully matured keloids have minimal response to RT alone. Prophylactic RT immediately following excision (within the first 24 hours) is most effective and reduces the risk of recurrence to 15% to 25% in most series.

Among different modalities for postexcisional radiotherapy, brachytherapy was found to have a lower recurrence rate when compared to electron and x-ray therapy by meta-analysis.[295] The target volume is limited to the scar plus a 1-cm margin; lead shielding can be constructed to protect normal tissue. An analysis of multicenter data on the use of postoperative RT for earlobe keloids shows that higher dose per fraction and use of deeper-penetrating electrons are preferable to standard 2-Gy fractionation schemes.[296] Achieving a BED of 15 to 22.5 Gy (at α/β of 10) with 10, 12, or 20 Gy delivered within 1 week over 2, 3, or 4 fractions, respectively, is sufficient for efficacy evaluated by relapse rate and good cosmesis. Common side effects include erythema and changes in skin pigmentation.

Heterotopic Ossification

Background and Clinical Aspects

Heterotopic ossification (HO) is a common complication of total hip arthroplasty, hip trauma, or acetabular fracture. HO occurs when the soft tissues around the hip become ossified. Following trauma, primitive mesenchymal cells in the surrounding soft tissues are transformed into osteoblastic tissue that then forms mature bone. The hip is the most common joint affected; HO typically occurs around the femoral neck and adjacent to the greater trochanter. The risk factors for development of HO are unknown, but the incidence is greater in men and occurs in more than 80% of patients who have a history of ipsilateral or contralateral HO. It is also more common in patients with a known history of osteoarthritis, ankylosing spondylitis, and Paget disease.[297] Hip stiffness is the primary symptom and the diagnosis is made radiographically. Pain is typically not associated with HO.

Nonradiotherapeutic Treatment

The treatment for HO is surgical excision followed by some form of HO prophylaxis. Prophylaxis is only applied to patients at high risk for developing HO. A meta-analysis showed that NSAIDs are effective in reducing the risk of postoperative HO.[298] Indomethacin is the most commonly used nonselective NSAID for HO prophylaxis. Indomethacin is a prostaglandin synthase inhibitor that also suppresses mesenchymal cells. The limited data available have not shown a clear benefit to the use of selective cyclooxygenase-2 (COX-2) inhibitors in HO prophylaxis.[299,300] Kan et al. performed a meta-analysis comparing selective NSAIDs (COX-2 inhibitors) and nonselective NSAIDs versus placebo in HO prevention. Efficacy was the same among the two classes with similar rates of discontinuation from gastrointestinal side effects.[301] Bisphosphonates have been used for prophylaxis because they delay mineralization of osteoid and appear to have some efficacy in preventing HO if used at the appropriate time. In one study, the cost of bisphosphonate use was prohibitive for routine use when compared to indomethacin.[302]

Radiotherapeutic Options

External beam radiation is an effective method for prevention of HO after total hip arthroplasty. Prophylactic radiation therapy for the prevention of HO has been used since the 1970s. A single fraction of 700 or 800 cGy to the at-risk region (Fig. 95.10) is recommended and should be delivered in the

FIGURE 95.10. Typical treatment field for HO. **A:** Field set up for elbow after radial head replacement. **B:** Field setup of acetabulum with active HO and after hip arthroplasty.

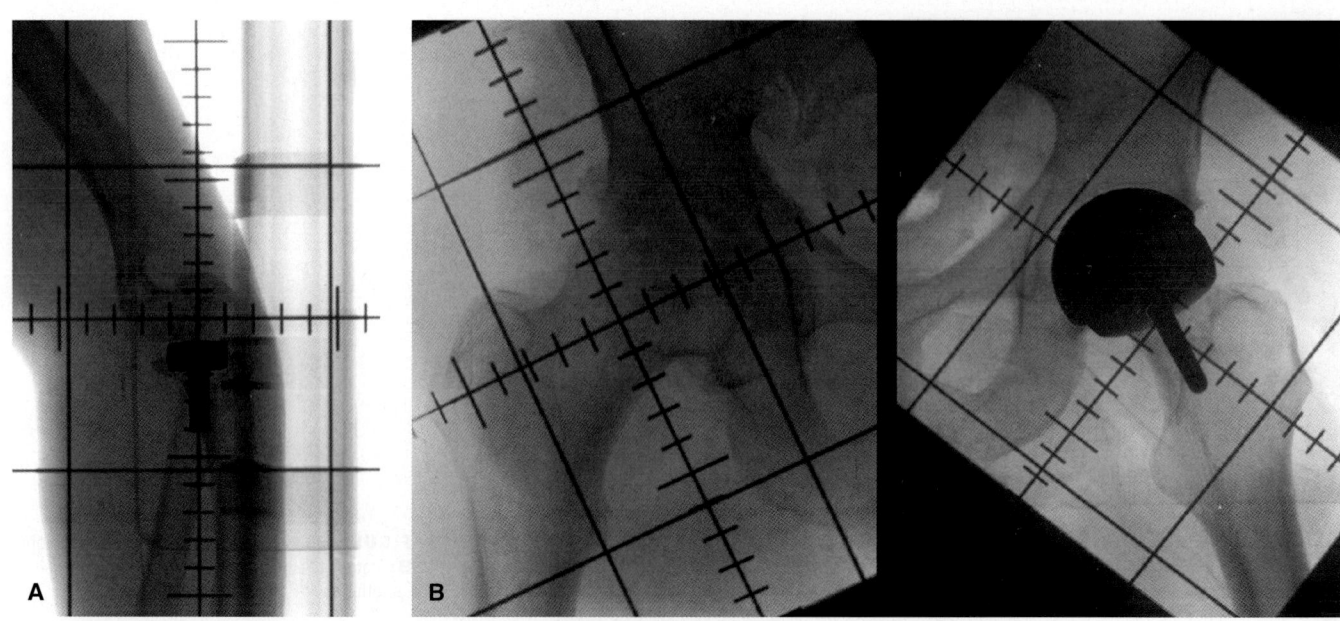

A   B

perioperative period, either preoperatively (within 4 hours) or postoperatively (within 72 hours).[22] Typically, an AP-PA field size measures 14 × 14 cm with the cranial field border approximately 3 cm above the acetabulum and the caudal field border encompassing two-thirds of the proximal implant. The dose is prescribed to the body midplane.[22]

When comparing radiation therapy and NSAIDs, there is no clear benefit for use of one modality over another. A prospective, randomized study demonstrated that radiation therapy and indomethacin are both effective in the prevention of postoperative HO.[303] Although one meta-analysis of seven randomized studies concluded that radiotherapy is more effective than NSAIDs for HO prophylaxis,[304] a more recent analysis of 9 studies involving 1,295 patients found no statistically significant difference between the two.[305] An economic analysis using the same nine studies and the meta-analysis suggest that radiation therapy is not cost-effective when compared to use of NSAIDs.[306] This analysis has yet to be validated.

REFERENCES

1. Bahn RS. Graves' ophthalmopathy. *N Engl J Med* 2010;362(8):726–738.
2. Platta CS, Mackay C, Welsh JS. Pituitary adenoma: a radiotherapeutic perspective. *Am J Clin Oncol* 2010;33(4):408–419.
3. Shields CJ, Winter DC, Kirwan WO, et al. Desmoid tumours. *Eur J Surg Oncol* 2001;27(8):701–706.
4. Hessenbruch A. A brief history of x-rays. *Endeavour* 2002;26(4):137–141.
5. Inskip PD. Thyroid cancer after radiotherapy for childhood cancer. *Med Pediatr Oncol* 2001;36(5):568–573.
6. Trott KR, Kamprad F. Radiobiological mechanisms of anti-inflammatory radiotherapy. *Radiother Oncol* 1999;51(3):197–203.
7. Reichl B, Block A, Schafer U, et al. DEGRO practical guidelines for radiotherapy of non-malignant disorders: part I: physical principles, radiobiological mechanisms, and radiogenic risk. *Strahlenther Onkol* 2015;191(9):701–709.
8. Rodel F, Keilholz L, Herrmann M, et al. Radiobiological mechanisms in inflammatory diseases of low-dose radiation therapy. *Int J Radiat Biol* 2007;83(6):357–366.
9. Hill RP, Rodemann HP, Hendry JH, et al. Normal tissue radiobiology: from the laboratory to the clinic. *Int J Radiat Oncol Biol Phys* 2001;49(2):353–365.
10. Draper GJ, Sanders BM, Kingston JE. Second primary neoplasms in patients with retinoblastoma. *Br J Cancer* 1986;53(5):661–671.
11. Kleinerman RA, Tucker MA, Abramson DH, et al. Risk of soft tissue sarcomas by individual subtype in survivors of hereditary retinoblastoma. *J Natl Cancer Inst* 2007;99(1):24–31.
12. Leer JW, van Houtte P, Seegenschmiedt H. Radiotherapy of non-malignant disorders: where do we stand? *Radiother Oncol* 2007;83(2):175–177.
13. Trott KR, Kamprad F. Estimation of cancer risks from radiotherapy of benign diseases. *Strahlenther Onkol* 2006;182(8):431–436.
14. Jansen JT, Broerse JJ, Zoetelief J, et al. Estimation of the carcinogenic risk of radiotherapy of benign diseases from shoulder to heel. *Radiother Oncol* 2005;76(3):270–277.
15. The 2007 Recommendations of the International Commission on Radiological Protection. ICRP publication 103. *Ann ICRP* 2007;37(2–4):1–332.
16. Leer JW, van Houtte P, Davelaar J. Indications and treatment schedules for irradiation of benign diseases: a survey. *Radiother Oncol* 1998;48(3):249–257.
17. Seegenschmiedt MH, Katalinic A, Makoski H, et al. Radiation therapy for benign diseases: patterns of care study in Germany. *Int J Radiat Oncol Biol Phys* 2000;47(1):195–202.
18. Micke O, Seegenschmiedt MH. Consensus guidelines for radiation therapy of benign diseases: a multicenter approach in Germany. *Int J Radiat Oncol Biol Phys* 2002;52(2):496–513.
19. Mitsuhashi N, Furuta M, Sakurai H, et al. Outcome of radiation therapy for patients with Kasabach-Merritt syndrome. *Int J Radiat Oncol Biol Phys* 1997;39(2):467–473.
20. Ott OJ, Niewald M, Weitmann HD, et al. DEGRO guidelines for the radiotherapy of non-malignant disorders. Part II: painful degenerative skeletal disorders. *Strahlenther Onkol* 2015;191(1):1–6.
21. Seegenschmiedt MH, Micke O, Niewald M, et al. DEGRO guidelines for the radiotherapy of non-malignant disorders: part III: hyperproliferative disorders. *Strahlenther Onkol* 2015;191(7):541–548.
22. Reinartz G, Eich HT, Pohl F; German Cooperative Group on Radiotherapy for Benign Diseases. DEGRO practical guidelines for the radiotherapy of non-malignant disorders—part IV: symptomatic functional disorders. *Strahlenther Onkol* 2015;191(4):295–302.
23. Ostrom QT, Gittleman H, Fulop J, et al. CBTRUS Statistical Report: Primary Brain and Central Nervous System Tumors Diagnosed in the United States in 2008–2012. *Neuro Oncol* 2015;17(Suppl 4):iv1–iv62.
24. Louis DN, Ohgaki H, Wiestler OD, et al. *WHO classification of the tumours of the central nervous system.* Revised 4th ed. Lyon, France: IARC Press, 2016.
25. Gerkes EH, Fock JM, den Dunnen WF, et al. A heritable form of SMARCE1-related meningiomas with important implications for follow-up and family screening. *Neurogenetics* 2016;17(2):83–89.
26. Morokoff AP, Zauberman J, Black PM. Surgery for convexity meningiomas. *Neurosurgery* 2008;63(3):427–433; discussion 433–424.
27. Nakamura M, Struck M, Roser F, et al. Olfactory groove meningiomas: clinical outcome and recurrence rates after tumor removal through the fronto-lateral and bifrontal approach. *Neurosurgery* 2007;60(5):844–852; discussion 844–852.
28. Simpson D. The recurrence of intracranial meningiomas after surgical treatment. *J Neurol Neurosurg Psychiatry* 1957;20(1):22–39.
29. Zhang Q, Wang Z, Guo H, et al. Resection of anterior cranial base meningiomas with intra- and extracranial involvement via a purely endoscopic endonasal approach. *ORL J Otorhinolaryngol Relat Spec* 2012;74(4):199–207.
30. Dowd CF, Halbach VV, Higashida RT. Meningioma: the role of preoperative angiography and embolization. *Neurosurg Focus* 2003;15(1):E10.
31. Oka H, Kurata A, Kawano N, et al. Preoperative superselective embolization of skull-base meningiomas: indications and limitations. *J Neurooncol* 1998;40(1):67–71.
32. Yano S, Kuratsu J. Indications for surgery in patients with asymptomatic meningiomas based on an extensive experience. *J Neurosurg* 2006;105(4):538–543.
33. Wen PY, Quant E, Drappatz J, et al. Medical therapies for meningiomas. *J Neurooncol* 2010;99(3):365–378.
34. Goldsmith BJ, Wara WM, Wilson CB, et al. Postoperative irradiation for subtotally resected meningiomas. A retrospective analysis of 140 patients treated from 1967 to 1990. *J Neurosurg* 1994;80(2):195–201.
35. Mendenhall WM, Morris CG, Amdur RJ, et al. Radiotherapy alone or after subtotal resection for benign skull base meningioma. *Cancer* 2003;98(7):1473–1482.
36. Minniti G, Amichetti M, Enrici RM. Radiotherapy and radiosurgery for benign skull base meningiomas. *Radiat Oncol* 2009;4:42.
37. Nutting C, Brada M, Brazil L, et al. Radiotherapy in the treatment of benign meningioma of the skull base. *J Neurosurg* 1999;90(5):823–827.
38. Vendrely V, Maire JP, Darrouzet V, et al. [Fractionated radiotherapy of intracranial meningiomas: 15 years' experience at the Bordeaux University Hospital Center]. *Cancer Radiother* 1999;3(4):311–317.
39. Wang C, Kaprealian TB, Suh JH, et al. Overall survival benefit associated with adjuvant radiotherapy in WHO grade II meningioma. *Neuro Oncol* 2017;19(9):1263–1270.
40. Adler JR Jr, Gibbs IC, Puataweepong P, et al. Visual field preservation after multisession cyberknife radiosurgery for perioptic lesions. *Neurosurgery* 2008;62(Suppl 2):733–743.
41. Paulsen F, Doerr S, Wilhelm H, et al. Fractionated stereotactic radiotherapy in patients with optic nerve sheath meningioma. *Int J Radiat Oncol Biol Phys* 2012;82(2):773–778.
42. Davidson L, Fishback D, Russin JJ, et al. Postoperative Gamma Knife surgery for benign meningiomas of the cranial base. *Neurosurg Focus* 2007;23(4):E6.
43. Feigl GC, Samii M, Horstmann GA. Volumetric follow-up of meningiomas: a quantitative method to evaluate treatment outcome of gamma knife radiosurgery. *Neurosurgery* 2007;61(2):281–286; discussion 286–287.
44. Ganz JC, Reda WA, Abdelkarim K. Gamma Knife surgery of large meningiomas: early response to treatment. *Acta Neurochir (Wien)* 2009;151(1):1–8.
45. Han JH, Kim DG, Chung HT, et al. Gamma knife radiosurgery for skull base meningiomas: long-term radiologic and clinical outcome. *Int J Radiat Oncol Biol Phys* 2008;72(5):1324–1332.
46. Hasegawa T, Kida Y, Yoshimoto M, et al. Long-term outcomes of Gamma Knife surgery for cavernous sinus meningioma. *J Neurosurg* 2007;107(4):745–751.
47. Iwai Y, Yamanaka K, Ikeda H. Gamma Knife radiosurgery for skull base meningioma: long-term results of low-dose treatment. *J Neurosurg* 2008;109(5):804–810.
48. Kollova A, Liscak R, Novotny J Jr, et al. Gamma Knife surgery for benign meningioma. *J Neurosurg* 2007;107(2):325–336.
49. Kondziolka D, Mathieu D, Lunsford LD, et al. Radiosurgery as definitive management of intracranial meningiomas. *Neurosurgery* 2008;62(1):53–58; discussion 58–60.
50. Takanashi M, Fukuoka S, Hojyo A, et al. Gamma Knife radiosurgery for skull-base meningiomas. *Prog Neurol Surg* 2009;22:96–111.
51. Zachenhofer I, Wolfsberger S, Aichholzer M, et al. Gamma-Knife radiosurgery for cranial base meningiomas: experience of tumor control, clinical course, and morbidity in a follow-up of more than 8 years. *Neurosurgery* 2006;58(1):28–36; discussion 28–36.
52. DiBiase SJ, Kwok Y, Yovino S, et al. Factors predicting local tumor control after Gamma knife stereotactic radiosurgery for benign intracranial meningiomas. *Int J Radiat Oncol Biol Phys* 2004;60(5):1515–1519.
53. Ferraro DJ, Funk RK, Blackett JW, et al. A retrospective analysis of survival and prognostic factors after stereotactic radiosurgery for aggressive meningiomas. *Radiat Oncol* 2014;9:38.
54. Combs SE, Hartmann C, Nikoghosyan A, et al. Carbon ion radiation therapy for high-risk meningiomas. *Radiother Oncol* 2010;95(1):54–59.
55. Halasz LM, Bussiere MR, Dennis ER, et al. Proton stereotactic radiosurgery for the treatment of benign meningiomas. *Int J Radiat Oncol Biol Phys* 2011;81(5):1428–1435.
56. Noel G, Bollet MA, Calugaru V, et al. Functional outcome of patients with benign meningioma treated by 3D conformal irradiation with a combination of photons and protons. *Int J Radiat Oncol Biol Phys* 2005;62(5):1412–1422.
57. Laws ER, Sheehan JP, Sheehan JM, et al. Stereotactic radiosurgery for pituitary adenomas: a review of the literature. *J Neurooncol* 2004;69(1–3):257–272.
58. Fleseriu M, Biller BM, Findling JW, et al. Mifepristone, a glucocorticoid receptor antagonist, produces clinical and metabolic benefits in patients with Cushing's syndrome. *J Clin Endocrinol Metab* 2012;97(6):2039–2049.
59. Breen P, Flickinger JC, Kondziolka D, et al. Radiotherapy for nonfunctional pituitary adenoma: analysis of long-term tumor control. *J Neurosurg* 1998;89(6):933–938.

Section III

60. Estrada J, Boronat M, Mielgo M, et al. The long-term outcome of pituitary irradiation after unsuccessful transsphenoidal surgery in Cushing's disease. *N Engl J Med* 1997;336(3):172–177.

61. Gittoes NJ, Bates AS, Tse W, et al. Radiotherapy for non-function pituitary tumours. *Clin Endocrinol (Oxf)* 1998;48(3):331–337.

62. Littley MD, Shalet SM, Beardwell CG, et al. Hypopituitarism following external radiotherapy for pituitary tumours in adults. *Q J Med* 1989;70(262):145–160.

63. Landolt AM, Haller D, Lomax N, et al. Octreotide may act as a radioprotective agent in acromegaly. *J Clin Endocrinol Metab* 2000;85(3):1287–1289.

64. Sheehan JP, Kondziolka D, Flickinger J, et al. Radiosurgery for residual or recurrent nonfunctioning pituitary adenoma. *J Neurosurg* 2002;97(5 Suppl):408–414.

65. Pollock BE, Link MJ, Stafford SL, et al. The risk of radiation-induced tumors or malignant transformation after single-fraction intracranial radiosurgery: results based on a 25-year experience. *Int J Radiat Oncol Biol Phys* 2017;97(5):919–923.

66. Hukin J, Steinbok P, Lafay-Cousin L, et al. Intracystic bleomycin therapy for craniopharyngioma in children: the Canadian experience. *Cancer* 2007;109(10):2124–2131.

67. Hasegawa T, Kondziolka D, Hadjipanayis CG, et al. Management of cystic craniopharyngiomas with phosphorus-32 intracavitary irradiation. *Neurosurgery* 2004;54(4):813–820; discussion 820–812.

68. Voges J, Sturm V, Lehrke R, et al. Cystic craniopharyngioma: long-term results after intracavitary irradiation with stereotactically applied colloidal beta-emitting radioactive sources. *Neurosurgery* 1997;40(2):263–269; discussion 269–270.

69. Stripp DC, Maity A, Janss AJ, et al. Surgery with or without radiation therapy in the management of craniopharyngiomas in children and young adults. *Int J Radiat Oncol Biol Phys* 2004;58(3):714–720.

70. Luu QT, Loredo LN, Archambeau JO, et al. Fractionated proton radiation treatment for pediatric craniopharyngioma: preliminary report. *Cancer J* 2006;12(2):155–159.

71. Winkfield KM, Linsenmeier C, Yock TI, et al. Surveillance of craniopharyngioma cyst growth in children treated with proton radiotherapy. *Int J Radiat Oncol Biol Phys* 2009;73(3):716–721.

72. Bishop AJ, Greenfield B, Mahajan A, et al. Proton beam therapy versus conformal photon radiation therapy for childhood craniopharyngioma: multi-institutional analysis of outcomes, cyst dynamics, and toxicity. *Int J Radiat Oncol Biol Phys* 2014;90(2):354–361.

73. Lee M, Kalani MY, Cheshier S, et al. Radiation therapy and CyberKnife radiosurgery in the management of craniopharyngiomas. *Neurosurg Focus* 2008;24(5):E4.

74. Chiou SM, Lunsford LD, Niranjan A, et al. Stereotactic radiosurgery of residual or recurrent craniopharyngioma, after surgery, with or without radiation therapy. *Neuro Oncol* 2001;3(3):159–166.

75. Kobayashi T, Kida Y, Mori Y, et al. Long-term results of gamma knife surgery for the treatment of craniopharyngioma in 98 consecutive cases. *J Neurosurg* 2005;103(6 Suppl):482–488.

76. Selch MT, DeSalles AA, Wade M, et al. Initial clinical results of stereotactic radiotherapy for the treatment of craniopharyngiomas. *Technol Cancer Res Treat* 2002;1(1):51–59.

77. Ulfarsson E, Lindquist C, Roberts M, et al. Gamma knife radiosurgery for craniopharyngiomas: long-term results in the first Swedish patients. *J Neurosurg* 2002;97(5 Suppl):613–622.

78. McClelland S III, Kim E, Murphy JD, et al. Operative Mortality Rates of Acoustic Neuroma Surgery: A National Cancer Database Analysis. *Otol Neurotol* 2017;38(5):751–753.

79. Gormley WB, Sekhar LN, Wright DC, et al. Acoustic neuromas: results of current surgical management. *Neurosurgery* 1997;41(1):50–58; discussion 58–60.

80. Samii M, Matthies C. Management of 1000 vestibular schwannomas (acoustic neuromas): the facial nerve—preservation and restitution of function. *Neurosurgery* 1997;40(4):684–694; discussion 694–685.

81. Bakkouri WE, Kania RE, Guichard JP, et al. Conservative management of 386 cases of unilateral vestibular schwannoma: tumor growth and consequences for treatment. *J Neurosurg* 2009;110(4):662–669.

82. Kondziolka D, Lunsford LD, McLaughlin MR, et al. Long-term outcomes after radiosurgery for acoustic neuromas. *N Engl J Med* 1998;339(20):1426–1433.

83. Flickinger JC, Kondziolka D, Niranjan A, et al. Acoustic neuroma radiosurgery with marginal tumor doses of 12 to 13 Gy. *Int J Radiat Oncol Biol Phys* 2004;60(1):225–230.

84. Hansasuta A, Choi CY, Gibbs IC, et al. Multi-session stereotactic radiosurgery for vestibular Schwannomas: single institution experience with 383 cases. *Neurosurgery* 2011;69(6):1200–1209.

85. Meijer OW, Vandertop WP, Baayen JC, et al. Single-fraction vs. fractionated linac-based stereotactic radiosurgery for vestibular schwannoma: a single-institution study. *Int J Radiat Oncol Biol Phys* 2003;56(5):1390–1396.

86. Weber DC, Chan AW, Bussiere MR, et al. Proton beam radiosurgery for vestibular schwannoma: tumor control and cranial nerve toxicity. *Neurosurgery* 2003;53(3):577–586; discussion 586–578.

87. Vernimmen FJ, Mohamed Z, Slabbert JP, et al. Long-term results of stereotactic proton beam radiotherapy for acoustic neuromas. *Radiother Oncol* 2009;90(2):208–212.

88. Smoll NR, Gautschi OP, Radovanovic I, et al. Incidence and relative survival of chordomas: the standardized mortality ratio and the impact of chordomas on a population. *Cancer* 2013;119(11):2029–2037.

89. Tzortzidis F, Elahi F, Wright D, et al. Patient outcome at long-term follow-up after aggressive microsurgical resection of cranial base chordomas. *Neurosurgery* 2006;59(2):230–237; discussion 230–237.

90. Fagundes MA, Hug EB, Liebsch NJ, et al. Radiation therapy for chordomas of the base of skull and cervical spine: patterns of failure and outcome after relapse. *Int J Radiat Oncol Biol Phys* 1995;33(3):579–584.

91. Hug EB, Loredo LN, Slater JD, et al. Proton radiation therapy for chordomas and chondrosarcomas of the skull base. *J Neurosurg* 1999;91(3):432–439.

92. Choy W, Terterov S, Kaprealian TB, et al. Predictors of recurrence following resection of intracranial chordomas. *J Clin Neurosci* 2015;22(11):1792–1796.

93. Casali PG, Messina A, Stacchiotti S, et al. Imatinib mesylate in chordoma. *Cancer* 2004;101(9):2086–2097.

94. Ferraresi V, Nuzzo C, Zoccali C, et al. Chordoma: clinical characteristics, management and prognosis of a case series of 25 patients. *BMC Cancer* 2010;10:22.

95. Stacchiotti S, Marrari A, Tamborini E, et al. Response to imatinib plus sirolimus in advanced chordoma. *Ann Oncol* 2009;20(11):1886–1894.

96. Bompas E, Le Cesne A, Tresch-Bruneel E, et al. Sorafenib in patients with locally advanced and metastatic chordomas: a phase II trial of the French Sarcoma Group (GSF/GETO). *Ann Oncol* 2015;26(10):2168–2173.

97. Carpentier A, Polivka M, Blanquet A, et al. Suboccipital and cervical chordomas: the value of aggressive treatment at first presentation of the disease. *J Neurosurg* 2002;97(5):1070–1077.

98. Debus J, Hug EB, Liebsch NJ, et al. Brainstem tolerance to conformal radiotherapy of skull base tumors. *Int J Radiat Oncol Biol Phys* 1997;39(5):967–975.

99. Rotondo RL, Folkert W, Liebsch NJ, et al. High-dose proton-based radiation therapy in the management of spine chordomas: outcomes and clinicopathological prognostic factors. *J Neurosurg Spine* 2015;23(6):788–797.

100. Schulz-Ertner D, Karger CP, Feuerhake A, et al. Effectiveness of carbon ion radiotherapy in the treatment of skull-base chordomas. *Int J Radiat Oncol Biol Phys* 2007;68(2):449–457.

101. Imai R, Kamada T, Araki N; Working Group for Bone and Soft Tissue Sarcomas. Carbon Ion Radiation Therapy for Unresectable Sacral Chordoma: An Analysis of 188 Cases. *Int J Radiat Oncol Biol Phys* 2016;95(1):322–327.

102. Kano H, Iqbal FO, Sheehan J, et al. Stereotactic radiosurgery for chordoma: a report from the North American Gamma Knife Consortium. *Neurosurgery* 2011;68(2):379–389.

103. Debus J, Schulz-Ertner D, Schad L, et al. Stereotactic fractionated radiotherapy for chordomas and chondrosarcomas of the skull base. *Int J Radiat Oncol Biol Phys* 2000;47(3):591–596.

104. Li G, Chang S, Adler JR, Jr., et al. Irradiation of glomus jugulare tumors: a historical perspective. *Neurosurg Focus* 2007;23(6):E13.

105. Huy PT, Kania R, Duet M, et al. Evolving Concepts in the Management of Jugular Paraganglioma: A Comparison of Radiotherapy and Surgery in 88 Cases. *Skull Base* 2009;19(1):83–91.

106. de Jong AL, Coker NJ, Jenkins HA, et al. Radiation therapy in the management of paragangliomas of the temporal bone. *Am J Otol* 1995;16(3):283–289.

107. Hinerman RW, Amdur RJ, Morris CG, et al. Definitive radiotherapy in the management of paragangliomas arising in the head and neck: a 35-year experience. *Head Neck* 2008;30(11):1431–1438.

108. Mendenhall WM, Parsons JT, Stringer SP, et al. Radiotherapy in the management of temporal bone chemodectoma. *Skull Base Surg* 1995;5(2):83–91.

109. Foote RL, Pollock BE, Gorman DA, et al. Glomus jugulare tumor: tumor control and complications after stereotactic radiosurgery. *Head Neck* 2002;24(4):332–338; discussion 338–339.

110. Gerosa M, Visca A, Rizzo P, et al. Glomus jugulare tumors: the option of gamma knife radiosurgery. *Neurosurgery* 2006;59(3):561–569; discussion 561–569.

111. Poznanovic SA, Cass SP, Kavanagh BD. Short-term tumor control and acute toxicity after stereotactic radiosurgery for glomus jugulare tumors. *Otolaryngol Head Neck Surg* 2006;134(3):437–442.

112. Guss ZD, Batra S, Limb CJ, et al. Radiosurgery of glomus jugulare tumors: a meta-analysis. *Int J Radiat Oncol Biol Phys* 2011;81(4):e497–e502.

113. Chandler JR, Goulding R, Moskowitz L, et al. Nasopharyngeal angiofibromas: staging and management. *Ann Otol Rhinol Laryngol* 1984;93(4 Pt 1):322–329.

114. Fisch U. The infratemporal fossa approach for nasopharyngeal tumors. *Laryngoscope* 1983;93(1):36–44.

115. Radkowski D, McGill T, Healy GB, et al. Angiofibroma. Changes in staging and treatment. *Arch Otolaryngol Head Neck Surg* 1996;122(2):122–129.

116. Chakraborty S, Ghoshal S, Patil VM, et al. Conformal radiotherapy in the treatment of advanced juvenile nasopharyngeal angiofibroma with intracranial extension: an institutional experience. *Int J Radiat Oncol Biol Phys* 2011;80(5):1398–1404.

117. Lee JT, Chen P, Safa A, et al. The role of radiation in the treatment of advanced juvenile angiofibroma. *Laryngoscope* 2002;112(7 Pt 1):1213–1220.

118. McAfee WJ, Morris CG, Amdur RJ, et al. Definitive radiotherapy for juvenile nasopharyngeal angiofibroma. *Am J Clin Oncol* 2006;29(2):168–170.

119. Reddy KA, Mendenhall WM, Amdur RJ, et al. Long-term results of radiation therapy for juvenile nasopharyngeal angiofibroma. *Am J Otolaryngol* 2001;22(3):172–175.

120. Gadner H, Grois N, Arico M, et al. A randomized trial of treatment for multisystem Langerhans' cell histiocytosis. *J Pediatr* 2001;138(5):728–734.

121. Allen CE, Li L, Peters TL, et al. Cell-specific gene expression in Langerhans cell histiocytosis lesions reveals a distinct profile compared with epidermal Langerhans cells. *J Immunol* 2010;184(8):4557–4567.

122. Berry DH, Gresik M, Maybee D, et al. Histiocytosis X in bone only. *Med Pediatr Oncol* 1990;18(4):292–294.

123. Gadner H, Grois N, Potschger U, et al. Improved outcome in multisystem Langerhans cell histiocytosis is associated with therapy intensification. *Blood* 2008;111(5):2556–2562.

124. Rosenzweig KE, Arceci RJ, Tarbell NJ. Diabetes insipidus secondary to Langerhans' cell histiocytosis: is radiation therapy indicated? *Med Pediatr Oncol* 1997;29(1):36–40.

125. Kriz J, Eich HT, Bruns F, et al. Radiotherapy in langerhans cell histiocytosis—a rare indication in a rare disease. *Radiat Oncol* 2013;8:233.

126. Selch MT, Parker RG. Radiation therapy in the management of Langerhans cell histiocytosis. *Med Pediatr Oncol* 1990;18(2):97–102.

127. Minehan KJ, Chen MG, Zimmerman D, et al. Radiation therapy for diabetes insipidus caused by Langerhans cell histiocytosis. *Int J Radiat Oncol Biol Phys* 1992;23(3):519–524.

128. Maruyama K, Kawahara N, Shin M, et al. The risk of hemorrhage after radiosurgery for cerebral arteriovenous malformations. *N Engl J Med* 2005;352(2):146–153.

129. Pollock BE, Meyer FB. Radiosurgery for arteriovenous malformations. *J Neurosurg* 2004;101(3):390–392; discussion 392.

130. Flickinger JC, Pollock BE, Kondziolka D, et al. A dose-response analysis of arteriovenous malformation obliteration after radiosurgery. *Int J Radiat Oncol Biol Phys* 1996;36(4):873–879.

131. Sinclair J, Chang SD, Gibbs IC, et al Multisession CyberKnife radiosurgery for intramedullary spinal cord arteriovenous malformations. *Neurosurgery* 2006;58(6):1081–1089; discussion 1081–1089.

132. Drolet BA, Esterly NB, Frieden IJ. Hemangiomas in children. *N Engl J Med* 1999;341(3):173–181.

133. Enjolras O, Wassef M, Mazoyer E, et al. Infants with Kasabach-Merritt syndrome do not have "true" hemangiomas. *J Pediatr* 1997;130(4):631–640.

134. Leaute-Labreze C, Dumas de la Roque E, Hubiche T, et al. Propranolol for severe hemangiomas of infancy. *N Engl J Med* 2008;358(24):2649–2651.

135. Sans V, de la Roque ED, Berge J, et al. Propranolol for severe infantile hemangiomas: follow-up report. *Pediatrics* 2009;124(3):e423–e431.

136. Pope E, Chakkittakandiyil A. Topical timolol gel for infantile hemangiomas: a pilot study. *Arch Dermatol* 2010;146(5):564–565.

137. Leong E, Bydder S. Use of radiotherapy to treat life-threatening Kasabach-Merritt syndrome. *J Med Imaging Radiat Oncol* 2009;53(1):87–91.

138. Ogino I, Torikai K, Kobayasi S, et al. Radiation therapy for life- or function-threatening infant hemangioma. *Radiology* 2001;218(3):834–839.

139. Burchiel KJ. A new classification for facial pain. *Neurosurgery* 2003;53(5):1164–1166; discussion 1166–1167.

140. Eller JL, Raslan AM, Burchiel KJ. Trigeminal neuralgia: definition and classification. *Neurosurg Focus* 2005;18(5):E3.

141. Miller JP, Acar F, Burchiel KJ. Classification of trigeminal neuralgia: clinical, therapeutic, and prognostic implications in a series of 144 patients undergoing microvascular decompression. *J Neurosurg* 2009;111(6):1231–1234.

142. Singh R, Davis J, Sharma S. Stereotactic Radiosurgery for Trigeminal Neuralgia: A Retrospective Multi-Institutional Examination of Treatment Outcomes. *Cureus* 2016;8(4):e554.

143. Brisman R, Mooij R. Gamma knife radiosurgery for trigeminal neuralgia: dose-volume histograms of the brainstem and trigeminal nerve. *J Neurosurg* 2000;93(Suppl 3):155–158.

144. Cheuk AV, Chin LS, Petit JH, et al. Gamma knife surgery for trigeminal neuralgia: outcome, imaging, and brainstem correlates. *Int J Radiat Oncol Biol Phys* 2004;60(2):537–541.

145. Kondziolka D, Lunsford LD, Flickinger JC, et al. Stereotactic radiosurgery for trigeminal neuralgia: a multiinstitutional study using the gamma unit. *J Neurosurg* 1996;84(6):940–945.

146. Maesawa S, Salame C, Flickinger JC, et al. Clinical outcomes after stereotactic radiosurgery for idiopathic trigeminal neuralgia. *J Neurosurg* 2001;94(1):14–20.

147. Nicol B, Regine WF, Courtney C, et al. Gamma knife radiosurgery using 90 Gy for trigeminal neuralgia. *J Neurosurg* 2000;93(Suppl 3):152–154.

148. Pollock BE, Phuong LK, Foote RL, et al. High-dose trigeminal neuralgia radiosurgery associated with increased risk of trigeminal nerve dysfunction. *Neurosurgery* 2001;49(1):58–62; discussion 62–54.

149. Smith ZA, De Salles AA, Frighetto L, et al. Dedicated linear accelerator radiosurgery for the treatment of trigeminal neuralgia. *J Neurosurg* 2003;99(3):511–516.

150. Regis J, Tuleasca C, Resseguier N, et al. Long-term safety and efficacy of Gamma Knife surgery in classical trigeminal neuralgia: a 497-patient historical cohort study. *J Neurosurg* 2016;124(4):1079–1087.

151. Tuleasca C, Carron R, Resseguier N, et al. Repeat Gamma Knife surgery for recurrent trigeminal neuralgia: long-term outcomes and systematic review. *J Neurosurg* 2014;121 Suppl:210–221.

152. Lee JY, Sandhu S, Miller D, et al. Higher dose rate Gamma Knife radiosurgery may provide earlier and longer-lasting pain relief for patients with trigeminal neuralgia. *J Neurosurg* 2015;123(4):961–968.

153. Marshall K, Chan MD, McCoy TP, et al. Predictive variables for the successful treatment of trigeminal neuralgia with gamma knife radiosurgery. *Neurosurgery* 2012;70(3):566–572; discussion 572–563.

154. Flickinger JC, Pollock BE, Kondziolka D, et al. Does increased nerve length within the treatment volume improve trigeminal neuralgia radiosurgery? A prospective double-blind, randomized study. *Int J Radiat Oncol Biol Phys* 2001;51(2):449–454.

155. Adler JR Jr, Bower R, Gupta G, et al. Nonisocentric radiosurgical rhizotomy for trigeminal neuralgia. *Neurosurgery* 2009;64(2 Suppl):A84–A90.

156. Wiebe S, Blume WT, Girvin JP, et al. A randomized, controlled trial of surgery for temporal-lobe epilepsy. *N Engl J Med* 2001;345(5):311–318.

157. Regis J, Rey M, Bartolomei F, et al. Gamma knife surgery in mesial temporal lobe epilepsy: a prospective multicenter study. *Epilepsia* 2004;45(5):504–515.

158. Barbaro NM, Quigg M, Broshek DK, et al. A multicenter, prospective pilot study of gamma knife radiosurgery for mesial temporal lobe epilepsy: seizure response, adverse events, and verbal memory. *Ann Neurol* 2009;65(2):167–175.

159. Young RF, Jacques S, Mark R, et al. Gamma knife thalamotomy for treatment of tremor: long-term results. *J Neurosurg* 2000;93(Suppl 3):128–135.

160. Young RF, Li F, Vermeulen S, et al. Gamma Knife thalamotomy for treatment of essential tremor: long-term results. *J Neurosurg* 2010;112(6):1311–1317.

161. Elaimy AL, Arthurs BJ, Lamoreaux WT, et al. Gamma knife radiosurgery for movement disorders: a concise review of the literature. *World J Surg Oncol* 2010;8:61.

162. Rand RW, Jacques DB, Melbye RW, et al. Gamma Knife thalamotomy and pallidotomy in patients with movement disorders: preliminary results. *Stereotact Funct Neurosurg* 1993;61(Suppl 1):65–92.

163. Friedman JH, Epstein M, Sanes JN, et al. Gamma knife pallidotomy in advanced Parkinson's disease. *Ann Neurol* 1996;39(4):535–538.

164. Young RF, Vermeulen S, Posewitz A, et al. Pallidotomy with the gamma knife: a positive experience. *Stereotact Funct Neurosurg* 1998;70(Suppl 1):218–228.

165. Friehs GM, Park MC, Goldman MA, et al. Stereotactic radiosurgery for functional disorders. *Neurosurg Focus* 2007;23(6):E3.

166. Kondziolka D, Flickinger JC, Hudak R. Results following gamma knife radiosurgical anterior capsulotomies for obsessive compulsive disorder. *Neurosurgery* 2011;68(1):28–32; discussion 23–23.

167. Lopes AC, Greenberg BD, Noren G, et al. Treatment of resistant obsessive-compulsive disorder with ventral capsular/ventral striatal gamma capsulotomy: a pilot prospective study. *J Neuropsychiatry Clin Neurosci* 2009;21(4):381–392.

168. Xia P, Kotecha R, Sharma N, et al. A Treatment Planning Study of Stereotactic Body Radiotherapy for Atrial Fibrillation. *Cureus* 2016;8(7):e678.

169. Bhatt N, Fogarty T, Maguire P. Cardiac Radiosurgery for the Treatment of Atrial Fibrillation. *World J Cardiovasc Dis* 2016;6:143–155.

170. Bode F, Blanck O, Gebhard M, et al. Pulmonary vein isolation by radiosurgery: implications for non-invasive treatment of atrial fibrillation. *Europace* 2015;17(12):1868–1874.

171. Blanck O, Ipsen S, Chan MK, et al. Treatment Planning Considerations for Robotic Guided Cardiac Radiosurgery for Atrial Fibrillation. *Cureus* 2016;8(7):e705.

172. Ipsen S, Blanck O, Lowther NJ, et al. Towards real-time MRI-guided 3D localization of deforming targets for non-invasive cardiac radiosurgery. *Phys Med Biol* 2016;61(22):7848–7863.

173. Ipsen S, Blanck O, Oborn B, et al. Radiotherapy beyond cancer: target localization in real-time MRI and treatment planning for cardiac radiosurgery. *Med Phys* 2014;41(12):120702.

174. Sharma A, Wong D, Weidlich G, et al. Noninvasive stereotactic radiosurgery (CyberHeart) for creation of ablation lesions in the atrium. *Heart Rhythm* 2010;7(6):802–810.

175. Wang L, Fahimian B, Soltys SG, et al. Stereotactic Arrhythmia Radioablation (STAR) of Ventricular Tachycardia: A Treatment Planning Study. *Cureus* 2016;8(7):e694.

176. Loo BW Jr, Soltys SG, Wang L, et al. Stereotactic ablative radiotherapy for the treatment of refractory cardiac ventricular arrhythmia. *Circ Arrhythm Electrophysiol* 2015;8(3):748–750.

177. Cvek J, Neuwirth R, Knybel L, et al. Cardiac radiosurgery for malignant ventricular tachycardia. *Cureus* 2014;6(7):e190. doi:10.7759/cureus.190.

178. Banfi P, Ticozzi N, Lax A, et al. A review of options for treating sialorrhea in amyotrophic lateral sclerosis. *Respir Care* 2015;60(3):446–454.

179. Hawkey NM, Zaorsky NG, Galloway TJ. The role of radiation therapy in the management of sialorrhea: A systematic review. *Laryngoscope* 2016;126(1):80–85.

180. Stokholm MG, Bisgard C, Vilholm OJ. Safety and administration of treatment with botulinum neurotoxin for sialorrhoea in ALS patients: review of the literature and a proposal for tailored treatment. *Amyotroph Lateral Scler Frontotemporal Degener* 2013;14(7–8):516–520.

181. Guy N, Bourry N, Dallel R, et al. Comparison of radiotherapy types in the treatment of sialorrhea in amyotrophic lateral sclerosis. *J Palliat Med* 2011;14(4):391–395.

182. Assouline A, Levy A, Abdelnour-Mallet M, et al. Radiation therapy for hypersalivation: a prospective study in 50 amyotrophic lateral sclerosis patients. *Int J Radiat Oncol Biol Phys* 2014;88(3):589–595.

183. Monteiro-Grillo I, Gaspar L, Monteiro-Grillo M, et al, Postoperative irradiation of primary or recurrent pterygium: results and sequelae. *Int J Radiat Oncol Biol Phys* 2000;48(3):865–869.

184. Nishimura Y, Nakai A, Yoshimasu T, et al. Long-term results of fractionated strontium-90 radiation therapy for pterygia. *Int J Radiat Oncol Biol Phys* 2000;46(1):137–141.

185. Nakamatsu K, Nishimura Y, Kanamori S, et al. Randomized clinical trial of postoperative strontium-90 radiation therapy for pterygia: treatment using 30 Gy/3 fractions vs. 40 Gy/4 fractions. *Strahlenther Onkol* 2011;187(7):401–405.

186. Jurgenliemk-Schulz IM, Hartman LJ, Roesink JM, et al. Prevention of pterygium recurrence by postoperative single-dose beta-irradiation: a prospective randomized clinical double-blind trial. *Int J Radiat Oncol Biol Phys* 2004;59(4):1138–1147.

187. Viani GA, De Fendi LI, Fonseca EC, et al. Low or High Fractionation Dose beta-Radiotherapy for Pterygium? A Randomized Clinical Trial. *Int J Radiat Oncol Biol Phys* 2011.

188. Singh AD, Kaiser PK, Sears JE. Choroidal hemangioma. *Ophthalmol Clin North Am* 2005;18(1):151–161, ix.

189. Lopez-Caballero C, Saornil MA, De Frutos J, et al. High-dose iodine-125 episcleral brachytherapy for circumscribed choroidal haemangioma. *Br J Ophthalmol* 2010;94(4):470–473.

190. Kim YT, Kang SW, Lee JI. Gamma knife radiosurgery for choroidal hemangioma. *Int J Radiat Oncol Biol Phys* 2011;81(5):1399–1404.

191. Schilling H, Sauerwein W, Lommatzsch A, et al. Long-term results after low dose ocular irradiation for choroidal haemangiomas. *Br J Ophthalmol* 1997;81(4):267–273.

Section
III

192. Hannouche D, Frau E, Desjardins L, et al. Efficacy of proton therapy in circumscribed choroidal hemangiomas associated with serious retinal detachment. *Ophthalmology* 1997;104(11):1780–1784.

193. Lee V, Hungerford JL. Proton beam therapy for posterior pole circumscribed choroidal haemangioma. *Eye (Lond)* 1998;12 (Pt 6):925–928.

194. Zografos L, Egger E, Bercher L, et al. Proton beam irradiation of choroidal hemangiomas. *Am J Ophthalmol* 1998;126(2):261–268.

195. Levy-Gabriel C, Rouic LL, Plancher C, et al. Long-term results of low-dose proton beam therapy for circumscribed choroidal hemangiomas. *Retina* 2009;29(2):170–175.

196. Madreperla SA, Hungerford JL, Plowman PN, et al. Choroidal hemangiomas: visual and anatomic results of treatment by photocoagulation or radiation therapy. *Ophthalmology* 1997;104(11):1773–1778; discussion 1779.

197. Shields CL, Honavar SG, Shields JA, et al. Circumscribed choroidal hemangioma: clinical manifestations and factors predictive of visual outcome in 200 consecutive cases. *Ophthalmology* 2001;108(12):2237–2248.

198. Bressler NM. Age-related macular degeneration is the leading cause of blindness. *JAMA* 2004;291(15):1900–1901.

199. Evans JR, Sivagnanavel V, Chong V. Radiotherapy for neovascular age-related macular degeneration. *Cochrane Database Syst Rev* 2010(5):CD004004.

200. Jackson TL, Chakravarthy U, Slakter JS, et al. Stereotactic radiotherapy for neovascular age-related macular degeneration: year 2 results of the INTREPID study. *Ophthalmology* 2015;122(1):138–145.

201. Smitt MC, Donaldson SS. Radiation therapy for benign disease of the orbit. *Semin Radiat Oncol* 1999;9(2):179–189.

202. Bartalena L, Marcocci C, Bogazzi F, et al. Relation between therapy for hyperthyroidism and the course of Graves' ophthalmopathy. *N Engl J Med* 1998;338(2):73–78.

203. Bartalena L, Tanda ML. Clinical practice. Graves' ophthalmopathy. *N Engl J Med* 2009;360(10):994–1001.

204. Bartalena L, Baldeschi L, Dickinson AJ, et al. Consensus statement of the European group on Graves' orbitopathy (EUGOGO) on management of Graves' orbitopathy. *Thyroid* 2008;18(3):333–346.

205. Wakelkamp IM, Baldeschi L, Saeed P, et al. Surgical or medical decompression as a first-line treatment of optic neuropathy in Graves' ophthalmopathy? A randomized controlled trial. *Clin Endocrinol (Oxf)* 2005;63(3):323–328.

206. Donaldson SS, McDougall IR. *Radiotherapy of intraocular and orbital tumors.* Berlin, Germany: Springer, 2002.

207. Marquez SD, Lum BL, McDougall IR, et al. Long-term results of irradiation for patients with progressive Graves' ophthalmopathy. *Int J Radiat Oncol Biol Phys* 2001;51(3):766–774.

208. Matthiesen C, Thompson JS, Thompson D, et al. The efficacy of radiation therapy in the treatment of Graves' orbitopathy. *Int J Radiat Oncol Biol Phys* 2012;82(1):117–123.

209. Yan J, Wu Z, Li Y. A clinical analysis of idiopathic orbital inflammatory pseudotumor. *Yan Ke Xue Bao* 2000;16(3):208–213.

210. Mombaerts I, Schlingemann RO, Goldschmeding R, et al. Are systemic corticosteroids useful in the management of orbital pseudotumors? *Ophthalmology* 1996;103(3):521–528.

211. Matthiesen C, Bogardus C Jr, Thompson JS, et al. The efficacy of radiotherapy in the treatment of orbital pseudotumor. *Int J Radiat Oncol Biol Phys* 2011;79(5):1496–1502.

212. Prabhu RS, Kandula S, Liebman L, et al. Association of clinical response and long-term outcome among patients with biopsied orbital pseudotumor receiving modern radiation therapy. *Int J Radiat Oncol Biol Phys* 2013;85(3):643–649.

213. Minten MJ, Mahler E, den Broeder AA, et al. The efficacy and safety of low-dose radiotherapy on pain and functioning in patients with osteoarthritis: a systematic review. *Rheumatol Int* 2016;36(1):133–142.

214. Hunter DJ, Lo GH. The management of osteoarthritis: an overview and call to appropriate conservative treatment. *Med Clin North Am* 2009;93(1):127–143, xi.

215. Wesseling J, Dekker J, van den Berg WB, et al. CHECK (Cohort Hip and Cohort Knee): similarities and differences with the Osteoarthritis Initiative. *Ann Rheum Dis* 2009;68(9):1413–1419.

216. Zhang W, Nuki G, Moskowitz RW, et al. OARSI recommendations for the management of hip and knee osteoarthritis: part III: Changes in evidence following systematic cumulative update of research published through January 2009. *Osteoarthritis Cartilage* 2010;18(4):476–499.

217. Roddy E, Zhang W, Doherty M. Aerobic walking or strengthening exercise for osteoarthritis of the knee? A systematic review. *Ann Rheum Dis* 2005;64(4):544–548.

218. Zhang W, Doherty M, Leeb BF, et al. EULAR evidence based recommendations for the management of hand osteoarthritis: report of a Task Force of the EULAR Standing Committee for International Clinical Studies Including Therapeutics (ESCISIT). *Ann Rheum Dis* 2007;66(3):377–388.

219. Black C, Clar C, Henderson R, et al. The clinical effectiveness of glucosamine and chondroitin supplements in slowing or arresting progression of osteoarthritis of the knee: a systematic review and economic evaluation. *Health Technol Assess* 2009;13(52):1–148.

220. Lapane KL, Sands MR, Yang S, et al. Use of complementary and alternative medicine among patients with radiographic-confirmed knee osteoarthritis. *Osteoarthritis Cartilage* 2012;20(1):22–28.

221. Ronn K, Reischl N, Gautier E, et al. Current surgical treatment of knee osteoarthritis. *Arthritis* 2011;2011:454873.

222. Laupattarakasem W, Laopaiboon M, Laupattarakasem P, et al. Arthroscopic debridement for knee osteoarthritis. *Cochrane Database Syst Rev* 2008(1):CD005118.

223. Niewald M, Fleckenstein J, Naumann S, et al. Long-term results of radiotherapy for periarthritis of the shoulder: a retrospective evaluation. *Radiat Oncol* 2007;2:34.

224. Mucke R, Seegenschmiedt MH, Heyd R, et al. [Radiotherapy in painful gonarthrosis. Results of a national patterns-of-care study]. *Strahlenther Onkol* 2010;186(1):7–17.

225. Micke O, Seegenschmiedt MH, Adamietz IA, et al. Low-Dose Radiation Therapy for Benign Painful Skeletal Disorders: The Typical Treatment for the Elderly Patient? *Int J Radiat Oncol Biol Phys* 2017;98(4):958–963.

226. Hagberg H, Lamberg K, Astrom G. Alpha-2b interferon and oral clodronate for Gorham's disease. *Lancet* 1997;350(9094):1822–1823.

227. Kuriyama DK, McElligott SC, Glaser DW, et al. Treatment of Gorham-Stout disease with zoledronic acid and interferon-alpha: a case report and literature review. *J Pediatr Hematol Oncol* 2010;32(8):579–584.

228. Mawk JR, Obukhov SK, Nichols WD, et al. Successful conservative management of Gorham disease of the skull base and cervical spine. *Childs Nerv Syst* 1997;13(11–12):622–625.

229. Heyd R, Micke O, Surholt C, et al. Radiation therapy for Gorham-Stout syndrome: results of a national patterns-of-care study and literature review. *Int J Radiat Oncol Biol Phys* 2011;81(3):e179–e185.

230. Mankin H, Trahan C, Hornicek F. Pigmented villonodular synovitis of joints. *J Surg Oncol* 2011;103(5):386–389.

231. Hamlin BR, Duffy GP, Trousdale RT, et al. Total knee arthroplasty in patients who have pigmented villonodular synovitis. *J Bone Joint Surg Am* 1998;80(1):76–82.

232. Chin KR, Barr SJ, Winalski C, et al. Treatment of advanced primary and recurrent diffuse pigmented villonodular synovitis of the knee. *J Bone Joint Surg Am* 2002;84-A(12):2192–2202.

233. Horoschak M, Tran PT, Bachireddy P, et al. External beam radiation therapy enhances local control in pigmented villonodular synovitis. *Int J Radiat Oncol Biol Phys* 2009;75(1):183–187.

234. Blanco CE, Leon HO, Guthrie TB. Combined partial arthroscopic synovectomy and radiation therapy for diffuse pigmented villonodular synovitis of the knee. *Arthroscopy* 2001;17(5):527–531.

235. Berger B, Ganswindt U, Bamberg M, et al. External beam radiotherapy as postoperative treatment of diffuse pigmented villonodular synovitis. *Int J Radiat Oncol Biol Phys* 2007;67(4):1130–1134.

236. Acosta FL Jr, Dowd CF, Chin C, et al. Current treatment strategies and outcomes in the management of symptomatic vertebral hemangiomas. *Neurosurgery* 2006;58(2):287–295; discussion 287–295.

237. Heyd R, Seegenschmiedt MH, Rades D, et al. Radiotherapy for symptomatic vertebral hemangiomas: results of a multicenter study and literature review. *Int J Radiat Oncol Biol Phys* 2010;77(1):217–225.

238. Rades D, Bajrovic A, Alberti W, et al. Is there a dose-effect relationship for the treatment of symptomatic vertebral hemangioma? *Int J Radiat Oncol Biol Phys* 2003;55(1):178–181.

239. Crago AM, Chmielecki J, Rosenberg M, et al. Near universal detection of alterations in CTNNB1 and Wnt pathway regulators in desmoid-type fibromatosis by whole-exome sequencing and genomic analysis. *Genes Chromosomes Cancer* 2015;54(10):606–615.

240. Kasper B, Baumgarten C, Bonvalot S, et al. Management of sporadic desmoid-type fibromatosis: a European consensus approach based on patients' and professionals' expertise—a sarcoma patients EuroNet and European Organisation for Research and Treatment of Cancer/Soft Tissue and Bone Sarcoma Group initiative. *Eur J Cancer* 2015;51(2):127–136.

241. Lopez R, Kemalyan N, Moseley HS, et al. Problems in diagnosis and management of desmoid tumors. *Am J Surg* 1990;159(5):450–453.

242. Schlemmer M. Desmoid tumors and deep fibromatoses. *Hematol Oncol Clin North Am* 2005;19(3):565–571, vii–viii.

243. Lefevre JH, Parc Y, Kerneis S, et al. Risk factors for development of desmoid tumours in familial adenomatous polyposis. *Br J Surg* 2008;95(9):1136–1139.

244. Gansar GF, Markowitz IP, Cerise EJ. Thirty years of experience with desmoid tumors at Charity Hospital. *Am Surg* 1987;53(6):318–319.

245. Janssen ML, van Broekhoven DL, Cates JM, et al. Meta-analysis of the influence of surgical margin and adjuvant radiotherapy on local recurrence after resection of sporadic desmoid-type fibromatosis. *Br J Surg* 2017;104(4):347–357.

246. Ballo MT, Zagars GK, Pollack A, et al. Desmoid tumor: prognostic factors and outcome after surgery, radiation therapy, or combined surgery and radiation therapy. *J Clin Oncol* 1999;17(1):158–167.

247. Hansmann A, Adolph C, Vogel T, et al. High-dose tamoxifen and sulindac as first-line treatment for desmoid tumors. *Cancer* 2004;100(3):612–620.

248. Gega M, Yanagi H, Yoshikawa R, et al. Successful chemotherapeutic modality of doxorubicin plus dacarbazine for the treatment of desmoid tumors in association with familial adenomatous polyposis. *J Clin Oncol* 2006;24(1):102–105.

249. Garbay D, Le Cesne A, Penel N, et al. Chemotherapy in patients with desmoid tumors: a study from the French Sarcoma Group (FSG). *Ann Oncol* 2012;23(1):182–186.

250. Constantinidou A, Jones RL, Scurr M, et al. Advanced aggressive fibromatosis: effective palliation with chemotherapy. *Acta Oncol* 2011;50(3):455–461.

251. Azzarelli A, Gronchi A, Bertulli R, et al. Low-dose chemotherapy with methotrexate and vinblastine for patients with advanced aggressive fibromatosis. *Cancer* 2001;92(5):1259–1264.

252. Chugh R, Wathen JK, Patel SR, et al. Efficacy of imatinib in aggressive fibromatosis: results of a phase II multicenter Sarcoma Alliance for Research through Collaboration (SARC) trial. *Clin Cancer Res* 2010;16(19):4884–4891.

253. Penel N, Le Cesne A, Bui BN, et al. Imatinib for progressive and recurrent aggressive fibromatosis (desmoid tumors): an FNCLCC/French Sarcoma Group phase II trial with a long-term follow-up. *Ann Oncol* 2011;22(2):452–457.

254. Wcislo G, Szarlej-Wcislo K, Szczylik C. Control of aggressive fibromatosis by treatment with imatinib mesylate. A case report and review of the literature. *J Cancer Res Clin Oncol* 2007;133(8):533–538.

255. Kasper B, Gruenwald V, Reichardt P, et al. Imatinib induces sustained progression arrest in RECIST progressive desmoid tumours: final results of a phase II study of the German Interdisciplinary Sarcoma Group (GISG). *Eur J Cancer* 2017;76:60–67.

256. Clark TW. Percutaneous chemical ablation of desmoid tumors. *J Vasc Interv Radiol* 2003;14(5):629–634.

257. Ilaslan H, Schils J, Joyce M, et al. Radiofrequency ablation: another treatment option for local control of desmoid tumors. *Skeletal Radiol* 2010;39(2):169–173.

258. Spear MA, Jennings LC, Mankin HJ, et al. Individualizing management of aggressive fibromatoses. *Int J Radiat Oncol Biol Phys* 1998;40(3):637–645.

259. Guadagnolo BA, Zagars GK, Ballo MT. Long-term outcomes for desmoid tumors treated with radiation therapy. *Int J Radiat Oncol Biol Phys* 2008;71(2):441–447.

260. Rutenberg MS, Indelicato DJ, Knapik JA, et al. External-beam radiotherapy for pediatric and young adult desmoid tumors. *Pediatr Blood Cancer* 2011;57(3):435–442.

261. Lev D, Kotilingam D, Wei C, et al. Optimizing treatment of desmoid tumors. *J Clin Oncol* 2007;25(13):1785–1791.

262. Dibenedetti DB, Nguyen D, Zografos L, et al. A Population-Based Study of Peyronie's Disease: Prevalence and Treatment Patterns in the United States. *Adv Urol* 2011;2011:282503.

263. Tan RB, Sangkum P, Mitchell GC, et al. Update on medical management of Peyronie's disease. *Curr Urol Rep* 2014;15(6):415.

264. Levine LA. Review of current nonsurgical management of Peyronie's disease. *Int J Impot Res* 2003;15(Suppl 5):S113–S120.

265. Hauck EW, Diemer T, Schmelz HU, et al. A critical analysis of nonsurgical treatment of Peyronie's disease. *Eur Urol* 2006;49(6):987–997.

266. Mynderse LA, Monga M. Oral therapy for Peyronie's disease. *Int J Impot Res* 2002;14(5):340–344.

267. Prieto Castro RM, Leva Vallejo ME, Regueiro Lopez JC, et al. Combined treatment with vitamin E and colchicine in the early stages of Peyronie's disease. *BJU Int* 2003;91(6):522–524.

268. Safarinejad MR, Asgari MA, Hosseini SY, et al. A double-blind placebo-controlled study of the efficacy and safety of pentoxifylline in early chronic Peyronie's disease. *BJU Int* 2010;106(2):240–248.

269. Safarinejad MR. Efficacy and safety of omega-3 for treatment of early-stage Peyronie's disease: a prospective, randomized, double-blind placebo-controlled study. *J Sex Med* 2009;6(6):1743–1754.

270. Trost LW, Gur S, Hellstrom WJ. Pharmacological Management of Peyronie's Disease. *Drugs* 2007;67(4):527–545.

271. Kuehhas FE, Weibl P, Georgi T, et al. Peyronie's Disease: Nonsurgical Therapy Options. *Rev Urol* 2011;13(3):139–146.

272. Kendirci M, Hellstrom WJ. Critical analysis of surgery for Peyronie's disease. *Curr Opin Urol* 2004;14(6):381–388.

273. Abern MR, Larsen S, Levine LA. Combination of penile traction, intralesional verapamil, and oral therapies for Peyronie's disease. *J Sex Med.* 2012;9(1):288–295.

274. Mulhall JP, Hall M, Broderick GA, et al. Radiation therapy in Peyronie's disease. *J Sex Med* 2012;9(5):1435–1441.

275. Incrocci L, Wijnmaalen A, Slob AK, et al. Low-dose radiotherapy in 179 patients with Peyronie's disease: treatment outcome and current sexual functioning. *Int J Radiat Oncol Biol Phys* 2000;47(5):1353–1356.

276. Gonzalez-Cavid NF, Rajfer J. Experimental models of Peyronie's disease. implications for new therapies. *J Sex Med* 2009;6(2):303–313.

277. Mulhall JP, Branch J, Lubrano T, et al. Radiation increases fibrogenic cytokine expression by Peyronie's disease fibroblasts. *J Urol* 2003;170(1):281–284.

278. Khashan M, Smitham PJ, Khan WS, et al. Dupuytren's Disease: Review of the Current Literature. *Open Orthop J* 2011;5(Suppl 2):283–288.

279. Skoff HD. The surgical treatment of Dupuytren's contracture: a synthesis of techniques. *Plast Reconstr Surg* 2004;113(2):540–544.

280. Denkler K. Surgical complications associated with fasciectomy for Dupuytren's disease: a 20-year review of the English literature. *Eplasty* 2010;10:e15.

281. van Rijssen AL, Werker PM. Percutaneous needle fasciotomy in Dupuytren's disease. *J Hand Surg Br* 2006;31(5):498–501.

282. van Rijssen AL, Ter Linden H, Werker PM. Five-year results of randomized clinical trial on treatment in Dupuytren's disease: percutaneous needle fasciotomy versus limited fasciectomy. *Plast Reconstr Surg* 2012;129(2):469–477.

283. Gilpin D, Coleman S, Hall S, et al. Injectable collagenase *Clostridium histolyticum*: a new nonsurgical treatment for Dupuytren's disease. *J Hand Surg* 2010;35(12):2027–2038 e2021.

284. Hurst LC, Badalamente MA, Hentz VR, et al. Injectable collagenase *Clostridium histolyticum* for Dupuytren's contracture. *N Engl J Med* 2009;361(10):968–979.

285. Schulze SM, Tursi JP. Postapproval clinical experience in the treatment of Dupuytren's contracture with collagenase *Clostridium histolyticum* (CCH): the first 1,000 days. *Hand* 2014;9(4):447–458.

286. Peimer CA, Blazar P, Coleman S, et al. Dupuytren contracture recurrence following treatment with collagenase *Clostridium histolyticum* (CORDLESS study): 3-year data. *J Hand Surg* 2013;38(1):12–22.

287. Adamietz B, Keilholz L, Grunert J, et al. [Radiotherapy of early stage Dupuytren disease. Long-term results after a median follow-up period of 10 years]. *Strahlenther Onkol* 2001;177(11):604–610.

288. Keilholz L, Seegenschmiedt MH, Sauer R. Radiotherapy for prevention of disease progression in early-stage Dupuytren's contracture: initial and long-term results. *Int J Radiat Oncol Biol Phys* 1996;36(4):891–897.

289. Betz N, Ott OJ, Adamietz B, et al. Radiotherapy in early-stage Dupuytren's contracture. Long-term results after 13 years. *Strahlenther Onkol* 2010;186(2):82–90.

290. Seegenschmiedt MH, Olschewski T, Guntrum F. Radiotherapy optimization in early-stage Dupuytren's contracture: first results of a randomized clinical study. *Int J Radiat Oncol Biol Phys* 2001;49(3):785–798.

291. O'Brien L, Pandit A. Silicon gel sheeting for preventing and treating hypertrophic and keloid scars. *Cochrane Database Syst Rev* 2006;(1):CD003826.

292. Russell R, Horlock N, Gault D. Zimmer splintage: a simple effective treatment for keloids following ear-piercing. *Br J Plast Surg* 2001;54(6):509–510.

293. Shaffer JJ, Taylor SC, Cook-Bolden F. Keloidal scars: a review with a critical look at therapeutic options. *J Am Acad Dermatol.* 2002;46(2 Suppl Understanding):S63–S97.

294. Berman B, Bieley HC. Adjunct therapies to surgical management of keloids. *Dermatol Surg* 1996;22(2):126–130.

295. Mankowski P, Kanevsky J, Tomlinson J, et al. Optimizing Radiotherapy for Keloids: A Meta-Analysis Systematic Review Comparing Recurrence Rates Between Different Radiation Modalities. *Ann Plast Surg* 2017;78(4):403–411.

296. Flickinger JC. A radiobiological analysis of multicenter data for postoperative keloid radiotherapy. *Int J Radiat Oncol Biol Phys* 2011;79(4):1164–1170.

297. Iorio R, Healy WL. Heterotopic ossification after hip and knee arthroplasty. risk factors, prevention, and treatment. *J Am Acad Orthop Surg* 2002;10(6):409–416.

298. Fransen M. Preventing chronic ectopic bone-related pain and disability after hip replacement surgery with perioperative ibuprofen. A multicenter, randomized, double-blind, placebo-controlled trial (HIPAID). *Control Clin Trials* 2004;25(2):223–233.

299. Saudan M, Saudan P, Perneger T, et al. Celecoxib versus ibuprofen in the prevention of heterotopic ossification following total hip replacement: a prospective randomised trial. *J Bone Joint Surg Br* 2007;89(2):155–159.

300. Barthel T, Baumann B, Noth U, et al. Prophylaxis of heterotopic ossification after total hip arthroplasty: a prospective randomized study comparing indomethacin and meloxicam. *Acta Orthop Scand* 2002;73(6):611–614.

301. Kan SL, Yang B, Ning GZ, et al. Nonsteroidal Anti-inflammatory Drugs as Prophylaxis for Heterotopic Ossification after Total Hip Arthroplasty: A Systematic Review and Meta-Analysis. *Medicine (Baltimore)* 2015;94(18):e828.

302. Vasileiadis GI, Sakellariou VI, Kelekis A, et al. Prevention of heterotopic ossification in cases of hypertrophic osteoarthritis submitted to total hip arthroplasty. Etidronate or Indomethacin? *J Musculoskelet Neuronal Interact* 2010;10(2):159–165.

303. Kienapfel H, Koller M, Wust A, et al. Prevention of heterotopic bone formation after total hip arthroplasty: a prospective randomised study comparing postoperative radiation therapy with indomethacin medication. *Arch Orthop Trauma Surg* 1999;119(5–6):296–302.

304. Pakos EE, Ioannidis JP. Radiotherapy vs. nonsteroidal anti-inflammatory drugs for the prevention of heterotopic ossification after major hip procedures: a meta-analysis of randomized trials. *Int J Radiat Oncol Biol Phys* 2004;60(3):888–895.

305. Vavken P, Castellani L, Sculco TP. Prophylaxis of heterotopic ossification of the hip: systematic review and meta-analysis. *Clin Orthop Relat Res* 2009;467(12):3283–3289.

306. Vavken P, Dorotka R. Economic evaluation of NSAID and radiation to prevent heterotopic ossification after hip surgery. *Arch Orthop Trauma Surg* 2011;131(9):1309–1315.

Section III

Palliative and Supportive Care

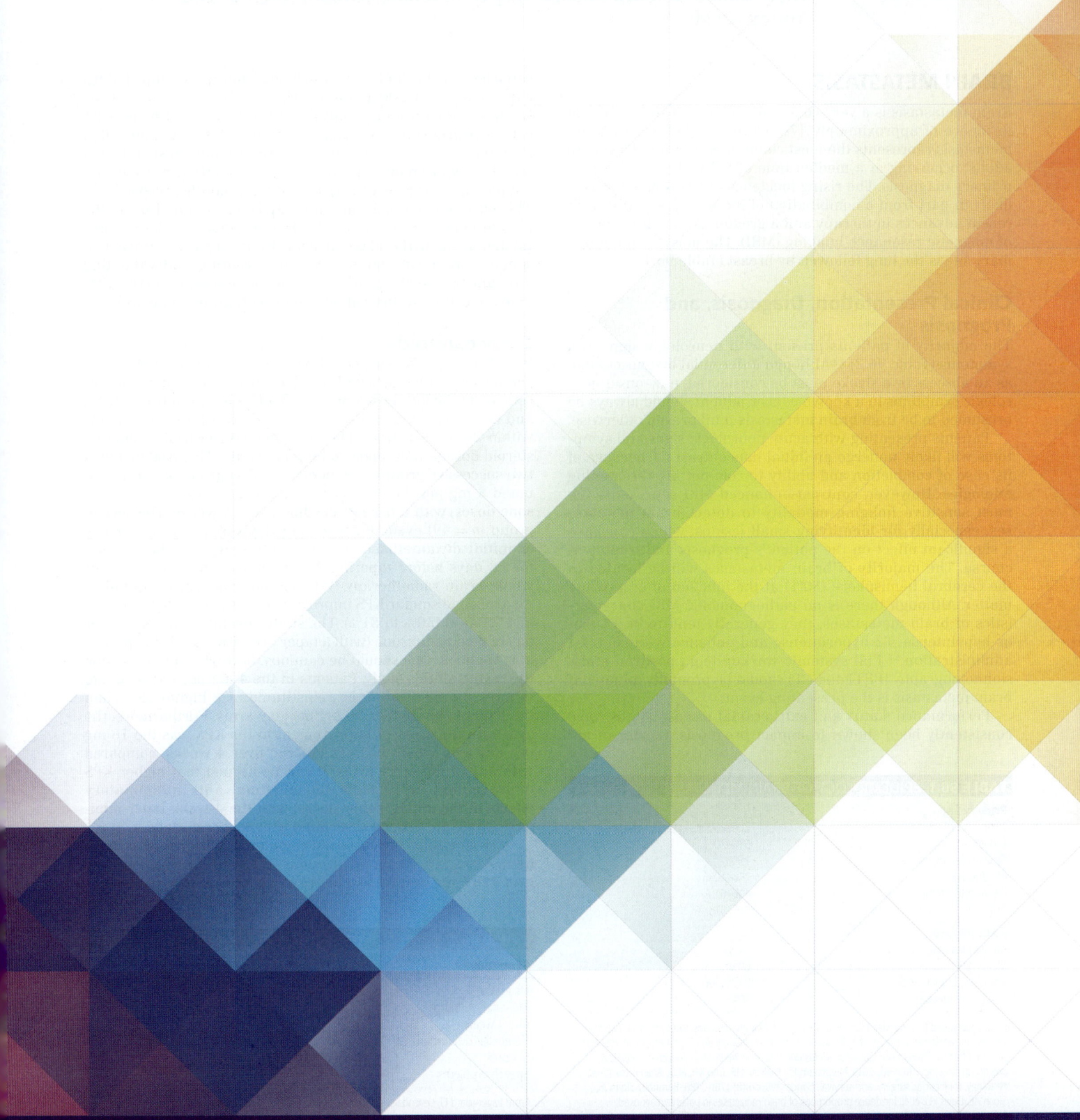

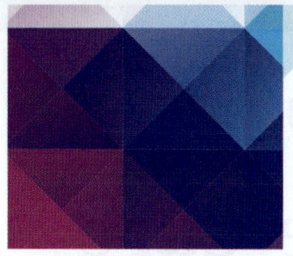

CHAPTER 96

Palliation of Brain and Spinal Cord Metastases

Arpit Chhabra, Mark Mishra, Roy A. Patchell, William Regine, and Young Kwok

BRAIN METASTASIS

Brain metastasis is a very common diagnosis, with an annual incidence of approximately 170,000 to 300,000 cases. Brain metastasis represents the most common intracranial lesion in adults, occurring at a median time of 8.5 to 12 months from primary diagnosis. The rising incidence of brain metastasis is likely in part from a combination of increasing survival from recent advances in therapy and a greater availability and use of magnetic resonance imaging (MRI). The most common primary site is the lung followed by breast (Table 96.1).[1-4]

Clinical Presentation, Diagnosis, and Prognosis

The majority of patients present with neurologic signs and symptoms (Table 96.2).[1,5] Although differential diagnoses such as an abscess or a stroke must be considered, new-onset neurologic symptoms in a known cancer patient should always be presumed to be from brain metastasis until proven otherwise.

Patients presenting with acute neurologic signs and symptoms will likely undergo an initial noncontrast CT because of its ease of completion and ability to rule out life-threatening etiologies. However, contrast-enhanced MRI represents the most sensitive imaging modality to detect brain metastases, especially for identifying small lesions, which can have a significant effect on the patient's prognosis and treatment course. The majority of brain metastases will be located in the cerebral hemisphere (80%) at the junction of gray-white matter. Although there is no pathognomonic MRI characteristics of brain metastases, they generally tend to be T1 iso- or hypointense, T2 hyperintense and enhance with contrast administration.[6,7] Full systemic workup (e.g., positron emission tomography [PET] and CT) should be promptly initiated if brain metastasis is the presenting event.

Performance status and extracranial disease status have consistently been shown to impact prognosis. Gaspar et al.[8]

reported on the Radiation Oncology Therapy Group (RTOG) experience of 1,200 patients. This analysis revealed three recursive partitioning analysis (RPA) classes, with the RPA class I (Karnofsky performance score [KPS] ≥ 70, controlled primary, age < 65 years, no extracranial metastases), II (not meeting requirements of classes I or III), and III (KPS < 70) having median survivals of 7.1, 4.2, and 2.3 months, respectively. This class scheme has subsequently been validated using the patient cohort from RTOG 91-04.[9] Contemporary series have further refined the class division by incorporating disease-specific prognostic factors, thereby creating and validating a diagnosis-specific graded prognostic assessment (DS-GPA) index to estimate survival outcomes with brain metastases.[10]

Corticosteroids

Initial therapy for suspected or confirmed brain metastases should promptly start with corticosteroids (e.g., dexamethasone or methylprednisolone), which effectively improve edema and neurologic deficits in approximately two-thirds of patients within 24 to 48 hours.[11] The only randomized trial evaluating steroid dosage was reported by Vecht et al.[12] This trial included two successive groups of patients. The first group (n = 47) evaluated 8 mg per day versus 16 mg per day initial dexamethasone doses, with tapering schedules over 4 weeks. The second group (n = 49) evaluated 4 mg per day versus 16 mg per day of initial dexamethasone, with continuation of these doses for 28 days before tapering. The patients were scheduled for whole-brain radiotherapy (WBRT) and concurrent ranitidine. All arms had similar KPS improvements at 7 days (54% to 70%) and 28 days (50% to 81%). The study concludes that 4 mg per day of dexamethasone (with a taper over 4 weeks) is the preferable regimen. One should be cautious, however, in interpreting the results of this study. Patients in the 4 mg per day arm had to have the medication be reinstituted at a higher rate than the patients in the 8 or 16 mg per day arms. Furthermore, the arm with the greatest improvement in the KPS was the 16 mg per day arm when this was tapered over 4 weeks, compared with any of the other arms. It can be argued that higher KPS improvement arose from the maximal anti-inflammatory effects of the initial higher doses, with the 4-week taper minimizing the late toxicity associated with corticosteroids.

A reasonable corticosteroid regimen in patients with brain metastases is a 10 mg intravenous (IV) or oral bolus, followed by a 4 to 6 mg every 6 to 8 hours of dexamethasone equivalent

TABLE 96.1 EPIDEMIOLOGY OF BRAIN METASTASIS

Primary Site	
Lung	20%–50%
Breast	5%–20%
Small cell lung cancer	15%
Melanoma	7%–10%
Renal cell carcinoma	4%–6%
Colon	2%–5%
Relevant Facts	
Median survival	<1 yr
Mean age	60 yr
Annual U.S. incidence	>170,000
Clinical incidence	30%

From Lagerwaard FJ, Levendag PC, Nowak PJ, et al. Identification of prognostic factors in patients with brain metastases: a review of 1292 patients. *Int J Radiat Oncol Biol Phys* 1999;43(4):795–803; Suh JH, Chao ST, Peereboom DM, et al. *Metastatic cancer to the brain in cancer–principles & practice of oncology.* 10th ed., 2015; Nussbaum ES, Djalilian HR, Cho KH, et al. Brain metastases. Histology, multiplicity, surgery, and survival. *Cancer* 1996;78(8):1781–1788; Barnholtz-Sloan JS, Sloan AE, Davis FG, et al. Incidence proportions of brain metastases in patients diagnosed (1973 to 2001) in the Metropolitan Detroit Cancer Surveillance System. *J Clin Oncol* 2004;22(14):2865–2872.

TABLE 96.2 CLINICAL PRESENTATION OF BRAIN METASTASIS

Symptom	Percentage of Patients
Headache	24–53
Mental disturbance	14–32
Motor weakness	20–40
Cerebellar dysfunction	7–26
Seizures	12–22
Speech problems	14

From Lagerwaard FJ, Levendag PC, Nowak PJ, et al. Identification of prognostic factors in patients with brain metastases: a review of 1292 patients. *Int J Radiat Oncol Biol Phys* 1999;43(4):795–803 and Posner JB. Brain metastases: 1995. A brief review. *J Neurooncol* 1996;27(3):287–293.

TABLE 96.3 SELECTED RANDOMIZED TRIALS EXAMINING VARIOUS FRACTIONATION SCHEDULES FOR BRAIN METASTASIS

Author/Study Group (Reference)	Dose/ Fractions	N	Median Survival	P
Borgelt et al./RTOG[18]				
First study (1971–1973)	30 Gy/10	233	21 wk	NS
	30 Gy/15	217	18 wk	
	40 Gy/15	233	18 wk	
	40 Gy/20	227	16 wk	
Second study (1973–1976)	20 Gy/5	447	15 wk	NS
	30 Gy/10	228	15 wk	
	40 Gy/15	227	18 wk	
Haie-Meder et al./French	25 Gy/10	110	4.2 mo	NS
(1986–1989)[19]	36 Gy/6[a]	106	5.3 mo	
Priestman et al./Royal College of	30 Gy/10	263	84 day	.04
Radiology (1990–1993)[20]	12 Gy/2	270	77 day	
Murray et al./RTOG-91-04	30 Gy/10	213	4.5 mo	NS
(1991–1995)[21]	54.4 Gy/34[b]	216	4.5 mo	
Graham et al./Australia	40 Gy/20[c]	57	6.1 mo	NS
(1996–2006)[22]	20 Gy/4	56	6.6 mo	

[a]18 Gy/3 split course with another 18 Gy/3 within 1 month.
[b]32 Gy in 1.6 Gy twice a day hyperfractionation to the whole brain followed by boost of 22.4 Gy in 1.6 twice a day hyperfractionation to visible lesions with a 2-cm margin.
[c]40 Gy in 1.0 Gy twice a day hyperfractionation for the entire course of therapy.
NS, not significant; RTOG, Radiation Therapy Oncology Group.

dose (with a concurrent proton-pump inhibitor [PPI]), before this is tapered in a clinically cautious manner. The trial by Vecht et al., however, did demonstrate that 4 mg per day (e.g., 2 mg BID) of dexamethasone is probably acceptable in select, symptomatic patient's minimal mass effect. In asymptomatic patients with little peritumoral edema or mass effect, initial corticosteroids may be reserved until the first sign of neurologic symptoms.

Anticonvulsants

Patients may present to the radiation oncologist already started on prophylactic anticonvulsants. This represents one of the most preventable causes of neurocognitive decline in brain tumor patients given the known negative impact on quality of life and neurocognition with anticonvulsants. In a study of 156 patients with low-grade glioma (85% experiencing a seizure), Klein et al.[13,14] analyzed the impact of antiepileptic treatment on quality of life and neurocognitive function. This study convincingly demonstrates the significant correlation between the use of anticonvulsants (even with lack of seizures) and a decrease in quality of life and neurocognitive function.

Based on four negative randomized trials, the American Academy of Neurology in 2000 recommended that prophylactic anticonvulsants not be initiated in newly diagnosed brain tumor patients who have not experienced a seizure.[15] This recommendation continues to be relevant as there has now been a fifth randomized trial that has shown no benefit in newly diagnosed brain tumors.[16]

Whole-Brain Radiotherapy

WBRT continues to be a standard of care in select patients with diffuse brain metastasis (≥5 brain metastases). WBRT is well known to provide improvement in neurologic symptoms with overall response rates of 70% to 93%.[17] Unfortunately, there exists no agreement on the optimal dose and fractionation schedule for WBRT, despite numerous studies are designed to determine the optimal delivery. Table 96.3 summarizes selected randomized fractionation studies.[18–22] A total of 30 Gy in 10 fractions or 37.5 Gy in 15 fractions continue to remain the standards for a vast majority of patients receiving WBRT.[2] As reported by Nieder et al., the radiographic overall response rate with this fractionation scheme is 59% (24% CR and 35% PR).[23]

For patients with poor performance status, and/or uncontrolled extracranial disease burden, a shorter fractionation scheme (e.g., 20 Gy in 5 fractions) can be considered. For this patient cohort, a supportive care–alone strategy may also be considered. Most recently, a phase III randomized, noninferiority study, the QUARTZ (Quality of Life after Treatment of Brain Metastases) trial, compared the Quality Adjusted Life Years (QALY) between optimal supportive care (OSC) alone and OSC + WBRT (20 Gy in 5 daily fractions) for NSCLC patients with brain metastases unsuitable for resection or stereotactic radiotherapy. OSC consisted of dexamethasone titrated based on patient's symptoms as well as patient access to palliative care clinicians and nurses. Results revealed a difference in mean QALY of 4.7 days (46.4 QALY days for OSC + WBRT vs. 41.7 QALY days for OSC), which was within the prespecified noninferiority margin of 7 days. Overall survival was not significantly different between randomization arms (OSC + WBRT: 9.2 weeks vs. OSC alone: 8.5 weeks). Subgroup analysis suggested a survival benefit in favor of OSC + WBRT for patients younger than 60, KPS ≥ 70, and controlled extracranial primary.[24] However, serious concerns about patient selection, methodology, and trial design have been pointed out.[25,26] Therefore, although WBRT may be omitted in select patients with very poor prognosis, it still remains an important therapeutic strategy.

Historically, WBRT has been frequently cited as the major cause of neurocognitive decline in cancer patients. One of the most misinterpreted studies on this subject is the Memorial Sloan-Kettering Cancer Center experience reported by DeAngelis et al.[27] who reported an 11% risk of radiation-induced dementia in patients undergoing WBRT for brain metastasis. The 11% figure is very misleading. Of the 47 patients who survived 1 year after WBRT, 5 patients (11%) developed severe dementia. When these 5 patients were examined, all were treated in a fashion that would significantly increase the risk of late radiation toxicity (i.e., large daily fractions and concurrent radiosensitizer). Three patients received 5 and 6 Gy daily fractions, whereas a fourth patient received 6 Gy fractions with concurrent Adriamycin. Only 1 patient received what is considered a standard radiation fractionation scheme (i.e., 30 Gy in 10 fractions), but this patient received a concurrent radiosensitizer (lonidamine). No patient who received the standard 30 Gy in 10 fractions WBRT alone experienced dementia.

Additionally, this trial did not address the potential neurocognitive changes in WBRT patients resulting from any underlying disease progression. Li et al. have attempted to further elucidate the true incidence of WBRT-related neurocognitive changes while controlling for brain metastasis response. All patients received WBRT in 30 Gy in 10 fractions and were subjected to a battery of neurocognitive tests monthly for 6 months and then every 3 months thereafter until death. The neurocognitive tests covered domains of memory, verbal fluency, and executive function. Additionally, patients underwent serial MRI with the summed volume of up to six brain metastases used for assessment of good or poor response. Good or poor response was defined as reduction of the summed volume at 2 months being >45% or <45%, respectively. Results revealed that volume regression was associated with preservation of neurocognitive function, primarily in the domains of executive function and fine motor coordination. Tumor volume changes, however, had weaker association with preservation of memory function (recall and delayed recall), which were domains most susceptible to changes from WBRT use.[28]

The RTOG subsequently completed RTOG 0933 and 0614, evaluating the role of hippocampal avoidance WBRT (HA-WBRT) and use of WBRT + memantine, respectively, in an effort to preserve memory-related dysfunction as was identified by Li et al.[28] RTOG 0933 was a phase II trial comparing the 4-month decline in HVLT-delayed recall scores with HA-WBRT (30 Gy in 10 fractions) relative to a historical control group receiving standard WBRT (30 Gy in 10 fractions). HA-WBRT resulted in a mean decline of 7% in HVLT-DR scores from baseline to 4 months, which was significantly lower than the mean decline of 30%

Section IV

for historical controls.[29] RTOG 0614 was a phase III placebo-controlled trial randomizing patients to WBRT (37.5 Gy in 15 fractions) with or without 24 weeks of memantine administration. The primary end point was the effect of memantine use on delayed recall at 24 weeks, which trended in favor of memantine use, though was not statistically significant ($P = .059$). Use of memantine, nonetheless, resulted in superior results in various other domains including delayed recognition, executive function, and processing speed.[30] These results have prompted the ongoing trial (NRG-CC001) evaluating the role of WBRT with or without hippocampal avoidance in patients all of whom receive memantine. Until there are mature data from this trial, it is hard to justify the routine use of memantine or HA-WBRT.

Targeted Agents as an Alternative to WBRT in NSCLC

Historically, the use of systemic chemotherapy for control of NSCLC brain metastasis has been limited by the poor penetration of these agents through the blood brain barrier (BBB). However, with a greater understanding of the BBB and the many oncogenic drivers present in NSCLC, contemporary targeted therapies have begun to pay a larger role in the management of brain metastases. Epidermal growth factor receptor (EGFR) mutations as well as anaplastic lymphoma kinase (ALK) rearrangements, which occur in 15% to 20% of advanced NSCLC cases,[31] represent two commonly targeted mutations. Zimmerman et al. identified a brain metastasis response rate of 74% to 89% with the use of EGFR tyrosine kinase inhibitors

(TKIs).[32] Similarly, Rusthoven et al. note response rates of 36% to 67% with next-generation TKI's, such as alectinib, in ALK-positive NSCLC brain metastases.[33] Magnuson et al. have reported the largest pooled multi-institutional analysis to date evaluating the optimal sequencing of EGFR-TKI's and radiation therapy in patients with EGFR-mutant NSCLC brain metastases. TKI naive patients who had developed brain metastases underwent one of three treatment regimens: SRS followed by EGFR-TKI, WBRT followed by EGFR-TKI, or EGFR-TKI followed by SRS or WBRT at a time of intracranial progression. At baseline, patients receiving upfront EGFR-TKI had smaller (<1 cm) and less symptomatic intracranial disease. Median OS for the upfront SRS, WBRT, and EGFR-TKI arms was 46, 30, and 25 months, respectively ($P < .001$). Both upfront SRS and WBRT use were independently associated with improved OS relative to upfront EGFR-TKI. Use of upfront SRS or WBRT was also associated with a trend toward lower risk of intracranial progression, highlighting the potential for inferior outcomes with deferral of early radiotherapy.[34] On the contrary, Gerber et al. found equivalent survival outcomes with use of upfront EGFR-TKI or WBRT in patients with EGFR mutant brain metastases.[35] As such, prospective trials remain critically warranted at this time to address the role of targeted agents.

Surgical Resection

Surgical resection can aid in obtaining a pathologic diagnosis of intracranial lesions, provide immediate relief of tumor mass effect (Fig. 96.1), and may cure a small percentage of

Preoperative T1 axial MRI

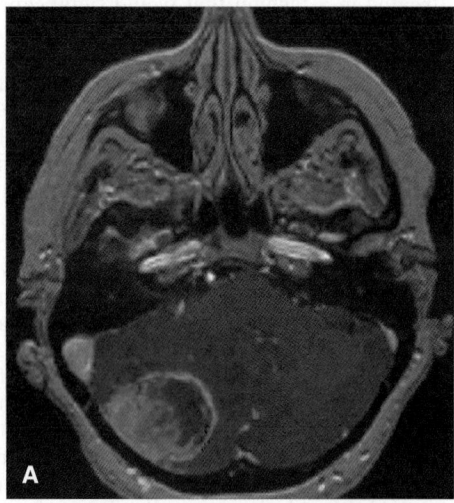

Preoperative T2 axial MRI

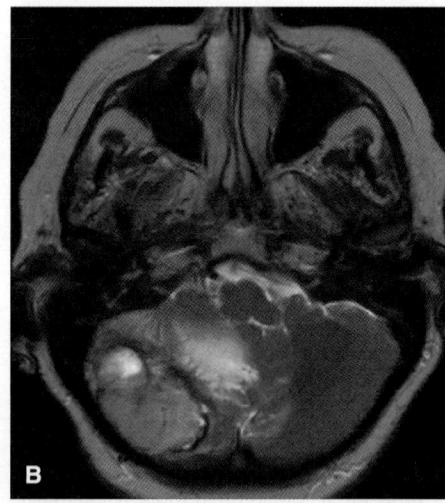

Postoperative T1 axial MRI

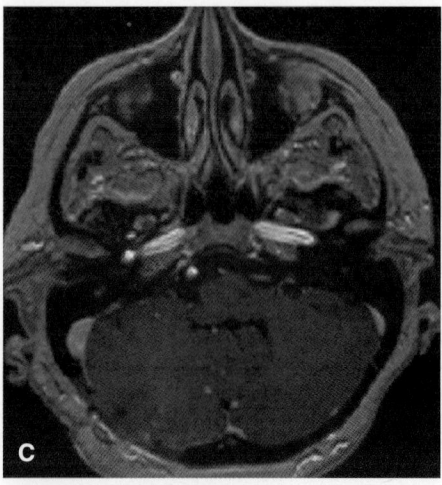

FIGURE 96.1. **A:** Six months after definitive therapy for stage IIIB non–small-cell lung carcinoma (NSCLC), a patient presented with progressively worsening headache, nausea, vomiting, and coordination difficulties. T1-gadolinium-enhanced axial magnetic resonance imaging (MRI) demonstrates a large, necrotic right cerebellar mass. **B:** T2-axial MRI reveals large area of vasogenic edema, with resultant mass effect causing fourth ventricular compression and hydrocephalus (not shown). **C:** Patient was taken immediately for a craniotomy, and a gross total resection was achieved. Pathology revealed metastatic NSCLC. Postoperative T1-gadolinium-enhanced axial MRI reveals no residual tumor, decompression of the mass effect, and reexpansion of the fourth ventricle.

patient with single or solitary lesions. On the other hand, radiation typically takes several days to work. Radiobiologically, 30 Gy in 10 fractions to a solid tumor (excluding radiosensitive tumors) is not adequate to achieve long-term tumor control.

Given that up to 50% of brain metastases can present as a single lesion, there has been historical interest in evaluating the role of surgery in the management of brain metastases.[36] There have now been three phase III trials testing the hypothesis that surgical resection to single brain metastasis is potentially beneficial. All three trials included patients with either a single lesion, defined as the presence of only one intracranial lesion regardless of the extracranial disease status, or a solitary lesion, defined as the intracranial lesion being the only site of metastatic disease. Table 96.4 summarizes the three trials.[37–39] The studies by Patchell et al.[37] (KPS ≥ 70) and Noordijk et al.[38] (World Health Organization grade ≤ 2) included better performance status patients compared with the Mintz et al.[39] study (KPS ≥ 50), which may have contributed to the differences in the outcomes between these studies. Additionally, 45% of patients in the study by Mintz et al. had extracranial metastases, as compared to 37.5% and 31.7% in the studies by Patchell et al. and Noordijk et al., respectively. Similarly, as highlighted by Noordijk et al., the survival benefit to the addition of surgery to WBRT was most pronounced in the patient with inactive or stable extracranial disease, with no survival benefit present for patients with active or progressive extracranial disease. The results of these studies suggest that surgical resection should be reserved for lesions causing life-threatening complications, requiring pathologic confirmation or in patients with good performance status (i.e., KPS ≥ 70) with controlled extracranial disease burden.

TABLE 96.4 RANDOMIZED TRIALS OF SURGICAL RESECTION OF SINGLE BRAIN METASTASIS

Author/Study Group (Reference)			P
Patchell et al./University of Kentucky (n = 48)[37]			
Primary end point	Surgery + RT (36 Gy/12 fx)	RT Alone (36 Gy/12 fx)	
Overall survival	40 wk	15 wk	<.01
Secondary end points			
Local control			
Local failure	20%	52%	<.02
Time to local failure	>59 wk	21 wk	<.0001
Time to neurologic death	62 wk	26 wk	<.0009
KPS ≥ 70 maintenance	38 wk	8 wk	<.005
Noordijk et al./Dutch (n = 63)[38]	Surgery + RT (40 Gy/20 fx)[a]	RT Alone (40 Gy/20 fx)[a]	
Primary end points			
Overall survival	10 mo	6 mo	.04
FIS[1b]	7.5 mo	3.5 mo	.06
Mintz et al./Canadian (n = 84)[39]	Surgery + RT (30 Gy/10 fx)	RT Alone (30 Gy/10 fx)	
Primary end point			
Overall survival	5.6 mo	6.3 mo	NS
Secondary end points			
FIS (proportion of days, mean)[2b]	32%	32%	NS
Quality of life (Spitzer score)			
1–3 months (mean)	6.38	5.36	NS
4–6 months (mean)	6.32	6.15	NS

[a]40 Gy total in 2 Gy twice a day hyperfractionation for the entire course of therapy.
[b]Functionally independent survival as defined by:
  [1]WHO performance status ≤ 1 and neurologic condition ≤ 1.
  [2]KPS ≥ 70.
fx, fraction number; KPS, Karnofsky performance score; RT, whole-brain radiotherapy; WHO, World Health Organization.

Radiosurgery Boost Trials

Radiosurgery provides a suitable alternative to conventional surgery. The three aforementioned randomized trials of surgical resection were all performed before the widespread availability of stereotactic radiosurgery (SRS). Although no randomized trials have been performed comparing surgery with SRS, SRS boost appears to provide at least comparable, if not improved, local control rates (80% to 90% when combined with WBRT). Therefore, in the setting of limited intracranial disease burden, unless emergent surgery is warranted, SRS alone or as a boost can serve as a noninvasive alternative. Additionally, although two of the three aforementioned surgery trials have shown a survival benefit in single brain metastasis, there have been no randomized trials addressing the role of surgery for multiple lesions. In contrast, three randomized trials have assessed the efficacy of SRS boost in the treatment of multiple metastases (Table 96.5).

The first randomized trial was reported by Kondziolka et al.[41] from the University of Pittsburgh. This small study was stopped early at a planned interim analysis of 60% patient accrual because the authors reported having found a large difference in the primary end point of 1-year local control in favor of SRS (92% vs. 0%; P = .0016). Unfortunately, the study used nonstandard end points to measure recurrence, defining it as any increase in the lesion size on MRI. Furthermore, no attempt was made to control for steroid use, radiation changes, or other factors that might produce small fluctuations in the lesion size on MRI. Median overall survival was not significantly different between arms (WBRT alone: 7.5 months vs. WBRT + SRS: 11 months, P = .22). Therefore, this study is difficult to interpret.

Chougule et al.[42] from Brown University reported the second trial, although this has to date only been published in abstract form. This trial had three treatment arms and randomized patients to treatment with SRS alone, SRS plus WBRT, or WBRT alone. This trial suffers from several methodologic problems. Although the authors conclude that the survival times among the treatment arms were similar and that patients treated with SRS experienced superior local control, no probability values are given. Furthermore, 51 of the patients had surgical resection for at least one symptomatic brain metastasis prior to entry into the study, and no attempt was made to stratify for previous surgery. The inclusion of the surgically resected patients effectively made this a six-arm trial and, therefore, the size of this trial was not large enough to support a meaningful analysis. Finally, the radiation doses used in the SRS arms cannot be considered conventional because the peripheral dose was not individualized based on the tumor size or volume.

In the third study, RTOG-95-08, inclusion was limited to 1 to 3 metastases, with maximum diameter of 4 cm for the largest lesion with additional lesions not exceeding 3 cm. WBRT dose was 37.5 Gy in 15 fractions, whereas SRS boost dose was lesion size based in accordance with the results of RTOG 90-05. The primary end point was overall survival, which was not statistically different between the WBRT plus SRS and WBRT-alone arms (6.5 and 5.7 months, respectively; P = .1356), although the SRS boost improved the survival in the subgroup (planned analysis) of patients with single metastasis.[40] For secondary end points, the local control and performance measures were higher in the SRS boost arm, but this did not translate into a lower death rate from neurologic progression. Multiple unplanned subgroup analyses were completed, and an overall survival benefit with SRS boost was found in several subgroups that included patients with RPA class 1, tumor size ≥2 cm, and non–small cell lung cancer or metastatic squamous histology from any site. Unfortunately, these subset analyses were not planned or prespecified, and the probability values needed for significance should have

TABLE 96.5 RANDOMIZED TRIALS OF STEREOTACTIC RADIOSURGERY BOOST IN BRAIN METASTASES

Author/Study Group (Reference)				P
Andrews/RTOG 95-08 (n = 333; 1–3 lesions)[40]	**RT** (37.5 Gy/10 fx)	**RT Alone** (37.5 Gy/10 fx)		
Primary end point (overall survival)				
1–3 lesions	5.7 mo	6.5 mo		NS
Single brain metastasis	6.5 mo	4.9 mo		.04
(planned subgroup analysis)				
Secondary end points				
Local control (1 yr)	82%	71%		.01
Neurologic death rate	28%	31%		NS
Performance outcome				
KPS stable/improve				
At 3 mo	50%	33%		.02
At 6 mo	43%	27%		.03
Mental status				NS
Unplanned subgroup analysis				
(overall survival)				
Largest tumor > 2 cm	6.5 mo	5.3 mo		.04
RPA class I	11.6 mo	9.6 mo		.05
Squamous/NSCLC	5.9 mo	3.9 mo		.05
Other outcomes				
Response rate (3 mo)				
Tumor	73%	62%		.04
Edema	70%	47%		.002
Kondziolka et al./University of Pittsburgh (n = 27; 2–4 lesions)[41]	**RT** (30 Gy/12 fx)	**RT Alone** (30 Gy/12 fx)		
Primary end point				
Local control (1 yr)	92%	0%		.0016
Time to local failure	36 mo	6 mo		.005
Time to any brain failure	34 mo	5 mo		.002
Secondary end points				
Overall survival	11 mo	7.5 mo		NS
Treatment morbidity	0	0		
Progression-free survival	Not reported			
Need for retreatment	Not reported			
Chougule et al./Brown University (n = 109; 1–3 lesions)[42]	**RT + SRS** (30 Gy/10 fx + 20 Gy SRS)	**RT Alone** (30 Gy/10 fx)	SRS Alone (30 Gy SRS)	
End points (abstract only)				
Overall survival	5 mo	9 mo	7 mo	Not reported
Local control	91%	62%	87%	Not reported
New brain lesions	19%	23%	43%	Not reported

fx, fraction number; KPS, Karnofsky performance score; NS, not significant; NSCLC, non–small-cell lung cancer; RPA, recursive partitioning analysis; RT, whole-brain radiotherapy; SRS, stereotactic radiosurgery.

been adjusted for inflation of the type I error. When this was done, none of these subgroup analyses showed a positive benefit for SRS. On the other hand, this trial did demonstrate that SRS boost is associated with lower edema and corticosteroid use, countering a commonly held notion that SRS actually increases the edema risk. However, regarding the major end points for multiple metastases, this study should be considered a negative trial.

More recently, Sperduto et al. completed a secondary analysis of RTOG 95-08 to determine the efficacy of SRS boost with patients restratified by DS-GPA scores. Their secondary analysis predominantly included lung cancer primaries (84%). Results revealed an overall survival benefit to SRS boost in patients with DS-GPA score of 3.5 to 4, irrespective of number of metastases (WBRT alone: 10.3 months vs. WBRT + SRS: 21 months, $P = .05$). No survival benefit for SRS boost was observed with DS-GPA scores <3.5. These results should be interpreted with caution, however, given the small sample size and potential nonrandom selection of patients in the secondary analysis.[43]

In conclusion, although SRS boost is indicated (from RTOG-95-08 and from the extrapolation of surgical resection data) in patients with a single metastasis, it is difficult to justify its routine use in patients with multiple metastases in light of the equivocal phase III SRS boost trials.

Postoperative or Postradiosurgery Radiotherapy

An ongoing controversy in the treatment of brain metastasis is the role of WBRT postoperatively or post-SRS. In a multiinstitutional retrospective SRS study, Sneed et al.[44] argue for the omission of upfront WBRT because this does not compromise overall survival. Unfortunately, only an overall survival analysis was performed, and no local control or detailed retreatment data were given. In an earlier study by Sneed et al.[45] on the University of California–San Francisco SRS experience, patients who were initially treated with SRS alone without WBRT experienced worse freedom from new brain metastasis and overall brain freedom from progression despite the imbalance of the prognostic factors that favored the SRS-alone group, although the overall survival was not different. Because of the equivalency of overall survival, many have advocated withholding upfront WBRT with salvage therapies including repeat SRS or delayed WBRT for failures. One caveat to this approach is that recurrent brain failure can lead to unacceptable consequences and symptoms. For example, Regine et al.[46] reported on 36 patients with planned observation after initial SRS alone. Even with close follow-up with examinations and high-resolution MRIs, 47% of patients experienced brain failure, with 71% and 59% experiencing symptomatic relapse and neurologic deficits, respectively.

The omission of upfront WBRT may have even more serious consequences for patients with more radioresistant tumors such as renal-cell carcinoma (RCC). The SRS dose given is typically limited by tumor size and volume, not by whether the patient received additional dose with WBRT. Therefore, a patient treated with WBRT plus SRS receives much higher tumor dose than SRS alone. It is then not surprising that the Eastern Cooperative Oncology Group protocol E6397 demonstrated very disappointing results.[47] In this phase II trial that evaluated SRS alone in radioresistant tumors (RCC, melanoma, sarcoma), Manon et al.[47] reported a 6-month total brain failure rate of 48.3% with 6-month local failure within the SRS volume of 32.2%, which is elevated relative to other histologies. The authors correctly conclude that routine avoidance of WBRT should be approached judiciously.

Fortunately, there have been seven phase III trials that have assessed the use of postoperative or postradiosurgery radiation (Table 96.6). Patchell et al.[48] evaluated upfront WBRT (50.4 Gy in 28 fractions) versus observation in resected metastatic lesions with a primary end point comparing local and distant intracranial

TABLE 96.6 RANDOMIZED TRIALS OF POSTOPERATIVE/POSTRADIOSURGERY WHOLE-BRAIN RADIOTHERAPY

Study (Reference)			*P*
Patchell et al./University of Kentucky (*n* = 95; single lesion)[48]	**Surgery + RT** (50.4 Gy/28 fx)	**Surgery Only**	
Primary end point			
Brain tumor recurrence			
Total brain recurrence	18%	70%	<.001
Original site only	4%	33%	
Distant site only	8%	24%	
Original and distant	6%	13%	
Distant site total	14%	37%	<.01
Original site total	10%	46%	<.001
Secondary end points			
Cause of death			
Neurologic	14%	44%	.003
Systemic	84%	46%	<.001
Functional independence[a]	37 wk	35 wk	NS
Overall survival	48 wk	43 wk	NS
Aoyama et al./Japanese JROSG-99-1 (*n* = 132; 1–4 lesions)[49]	**SRS + WBRT** (30 Gy/10 fx)	**SRS Alone**	
Primary end point			
Overall survival			
1 year[b]	39%	28%	NS
Median	7.5 mo	8.0 mo	NS
Secondary end points			
Brain recurrence (total)[b]	47%	76%	<.001
Functional preservation[a,b]	34%	27%	NS
Neurologic death	23%	19%	NS
Need for salvage therapy	10 patients	29 patients	<.001
Radiation morbidity			
Acute	4 patients	8 patients	NS
Late	7 patients	3 patients	NS
Muacevic et al./German (*n* = 70; 1 lesion)[c, 50]	**Microsurgery + WBRT** (40 Gy/20 fx)	**SRS Alone**	
Primary end point			
Overall survival	9.5 ms	10.3 ms	NS
Secondary end point			
Brain recurrence			
Local (1 yr)	18%	3.2%	.06
Distant (1 yr)	3%	25.8%	.04
Kocher et al./EORTC-22952-26001 (*n* = 359; 1–3 lesions)[51]	**SRS or S + WBRT** (30 Gy/10 fx)	**SRS or Surgery (S) Alone**	
Primary end point			
Functional independence	9.5 mo	10 mo	NS
Secondary end points			
Brain tumor recurrence			
Original site: SRS	19%	31%	.040
Distant site: SRS	33%	48%	.023
Original site: S	27%	59%	<.001
Distant site: S	23%	42%	.008
Progression-free survival	4.6 mo	3.4 mo	NS
Overall survival	10.7 mo	10.9 mo	NS
Chang et al./MDACC (*n* = 58; 1–3 lesions)[52]	**SRS + WBRT** (30 Gy/12 fx)	**SRS Alone**	
Primary end point			
Neurocognitive function (HVLT-R drop at 4 months)	52%	24%	Significant
Secondary end points			
Local control (1 yr)	100%	67%	.012
Distant brain control (1 yr)	73%	45%	.02
Overall survival	5.7 mo	15.2 mo	.003

[a]As defined by KPS ≥ 70 maintenance.
[b]One-year actuarial rates.
[c]SRS alone versus microsurgery plus WBRT.
fx, fraction number; HVLT-R, Hopkins Verbal Learning Test-Revised; JROSG, Japanese Radiation Oncology Study Group; KPS, Karnofsky performance score; NS, not significant; RT, whole brain radiotherapy; S, surgery; SRS, stereotactic radiosurgery.

control rates. Results demonstrated that surgical resection without WBRT led to a failure rate at the original site and distant brain/leptomeningeal recurrence of 46% and 37%, respectively. In comparison, surgical resection with upfront WBRT led to a significantly lower failure rate at the original site and

distant brain/leptomeningeal recurrence of 10% and 14%, respectively. More importantly, 44% of the patients in the surgery-alone arm died as a result of neurologic sequelae from brain failure as compared to 14% of patients receiving upfront WBRT (*P* = .003). Overall survival was not significantly different between arms (surgery alone: 43 weeks vs. surgery + WBRT: 48 weeks, *P* = .39). The results of this study have been frequently misinterpreted in the literature. Some have justified the withholding of upfront WBRT based on the fact that this study demonstrated equivalent survivals. In fact, this study was designed with brain tumor recurrence rate as the primary end point and not overall survival. To show an overall survival difference, this trial needed to enroll over 2,000 patients. This study met its primary end point and confirmed the importance of postoperative WBRT in preventing brain failure and death from neurologic causes.

Given the long-term cognitive impact attributed to WBRT, however, contemporary series have evaluated the efficacy of postoperative SRS as an alternative to upfront WBRT. No phase III trials have been published to date, though two prospective trials have recently completed and reported in presentation form. Mahajan et al. prospectively evaluated local tumor control rates of resected metastases receiving postoperative cavity SRS vs. observation in 1 to 3 brain metastases. All lesions not resected received definitive SRS. Secondary objectives included distant brain control and overall survival. Results revealed 1-year local control rates for observation and postoperative SRS of 45% and 72%, respectively (*P* = .01). One-year freedom from distant brain failure with observation and postoperative SRS was 33% and 43%, respectively (*P* = .29). Similarly, overall survival did not differ with use of postoperative cavity SRS (observation: 17 months vs. postoperative SRS: 17 months, *P* = .37).[53]

Additionally, Brown et al. recently reported the results of NCCTG N107C/RTOG 1270, which randomized patients to postoperative SRS vs. postoperative WBRT in a prospective

Section IV

trial. This trial included 1 to 4 brain metastases with surgical resection of one lesion, and subsequent randomization to postoperative cavity SRS vs. postoperative WBRT with all unresected metastases receiving SRS in both arms. Preliminary results reveal that 77% of enrolled patients had single brain metastasis with 59% being of lung primary. Primary end points were cognitive deterioration-free survival and overall survival. Use of postoperative WBRT resulted in a shorter cognitive deterioration-free survival vs. SRS (median 2.8 vs. 3.2 months, respectively, $P < .0001$) with 6-month cognitive deterioration rates of 85.7% and 53.8% for WBRT and SRS, respectively. However, long-term follow-up in the WBRT group will be critical to assess the percentage of patients in whom these early neurocognitive changes are transient and resolve over time. Additionally, limitations to these results include that the WBRT sample size (numbers at risk) in whom cognitive impact was evaluated was significantly smaller with time than the sample size randomized to WBRT and that factors known to result in cognitive decline, such as antiepileptic and corticosteroid use, were not reported as stratification variables. Use of WBRT did, however, provide improved 1-year intracranial control rates of 78.6% and 54.7% for WBRT and SRS, respectively ($P < .0001$). Although median surgical bed relapse-free rates were similar (WBRT: 7.7 months vs. SRS: 7.5 months, $P = .04$), use of WBRT trended for improved long-term surgical bed control. Median overall survival rates did not differ between arms (WBRT: 11.5 months vs. SRS 11.8 months, $P = .65$).[54] Complete analyses of these trials remain pending and will further elucidate the role of postoperative SRS an alternative to WBRT, though postoperative WBRT continues to remain the standard of care. Furthermore, it remains difficult to justify the current routine use of surgery with postoperative cavity SRS for lesions not causing significant mass effect, as these patients should be strongly considered for SRS treatment alone.

There have now been four phase III trials that have evaluated the role of SRS alone versus the addition of WBRT. In the Japanese Radiation Oncology Study Group JROSG-99-1 phase III trial of one to four lesions, the SRS-only arm experienced increased 1-year total brain recurrence rate ($P < .001$), increased 1-year rate of distant brain relapse ($P = .003$), and increased 1-year local tumor failure ($P = .002$). This resulted in more frequent use of salvage therapy ($P < .001$) in the SRS-alone arm.[49] Furthermore, the average time until Mini-Mental State Examination (MMSE) deterioration was significantly longer for the WBRT plus SRS arm (16.5 months vs. 7.6 months; $P = .05$), in large part due to increased recurrence in the SRS group.[55] Median overall survival did not differ between groups (WBRT + SRS: 7.5 months vs. SRS alone: 8 months, $P = .42$). Despite, no overall survival benefit for the entire group, this study demonstrates the importance of WBRT in decreasing brain failure, corroborating the findings of the Patchell et al.[48] study.

Subsequently, this group has performed a secondary analysis evaluating the outcomes of post-SRS WBRT in non–small-cell lung primaries restratified by DS-GPA. Significantly increased median overall survival was observed with DS-GPA score of 2.5 to 4 (WBRT + SRS: 16.7 months vs. SRS alone: 10.6 months, $P = .04$), whereas no survival differential was observed with DS-GPA scores <2.5. No significant difference in neurocognitive function, as assessed by the MMSE, was observed at baseline or during follow-up for WBRT + SRS or SRS-alone arms for either DS-GPA scores <2.5 or >2.5.[56] The results of the secondary analyses of the RTOG 95-08 and JROSG-99-1 trials therefore indicate that patients with brain metastases from NSCLC primary with favorable DS-GPA scores may benefit more from combined treatment (WBRT + SRS) than either treatment alone. Future prospective examination of this conclusion is warranted.

Muacevic et al.[50] randomized single brain metastasis patients (KPS ≥ 70, size ≤ 3 cm, stable systemic disease) to SRS alone versus resection plus WBRT. Although this trial is not exactly an SRS ± WBRT trial, it addresses the benefit of WBRT

to local therapies. Those randomized to SRS alone experienced worse distant ($P = .04$) recurrences, but there were no differences in neurologic death rates or overall survival.

The results of EORTC-22952-26001 have been reported with the primary end point of evaluating duration of functional independence.[51] In this study, patients with one to three brain metastases underwent local therapy with either surgery or SRS and were then randomized to the addition of WBRT versus observation. WBRT did not improve duration of functional independence or overall survival but was associated with a significant decrease in 2-year local and distant brain relapse rate versus observation with either surgery or SRS. This resulted in a 16% decrease in the risk of neurologic death. Although there was no difference in duration of functional independence between the two arms, the authors conclude that this is likely because of a variety of factors, including the subjective definition of functional independence, the routine use of MRI imaging rendering the majority of recurrences as asymptomatic, and the potential impact of systemic progression on performance status.

Chang et al.[52] reported on a series of 58 patients with one to three brain metastases randomized to SRS with or without WBRT. The primary end point of the study was neurocognitive function, which was assessed using the Hopkins Verbal Learning Test-Revised at 4 months after therapy. They found that patients receiving combined therapy were more likely to have a decline in learning and memory function at 4 months compared with patients who did not receive WBRT. The median survival was 15.2 months for the SRS-alone group and 5.7 months for the WBRT/SRS group ($P = .003$). However, the local (100% vs. 67%; $P = .012$) and distant (73% vs. 45%; $P = .02$) brain control rates were worse in the SRS-alone group compared with the WBRT/SRS group. There are multiple criticisms of this study worth noting.[57] First, because the primary end point was neurocognitive function, the authors did not stratify by baseline neurocognitive function or other factors known to impact neurocognition. Second, the authors chose a single test at a single time point. Ideally, a whole battery of tests should be performed at multiple time points to adequately assess the trend of something as complex as neurocognition. Most importantly, the combined arm inexplicably had a shorter survival, contrary to the four previously mentioned trials that demonstrated equivalent survivals. The median survival of 5.7 months was within 2 months of the primary end point mark, which classically falls within the time point of progressively worsening cognition seen in terminally ill patients.[58,59] The superior survival in spite of inferior local and distant brain control is unprecedented and can possibly be explained by an improper randomization, which is possible in a small study.

In summary, four of the five phase III local with or without WBRT trials unequivocally show a meaningful benefit of WBRT in terms of preventing neurologic deaths or brain failure. It is difficult to ignore the level I evidence provided by these phase III trials. Adjuvant WBRT, therefore, should be strongly considered after local therapy with surgical resection or SRS. However, this has become very controversial. Therefore, it is critical for radiation oncologists to help patients navigate through the risks and benefits of additional WBRT.

Repeat Whole-Brain Radiotherapy

Occasionally, patients will fail in the brain after initial WBRT. Salvage surgery, SRS, or repeat WBRT should strongly be considered. Wong et al.[60] reported on a series of 86 patients who underwent repeat WBRT. The median dose for the first course was 30 Gy in 10 fractions, whereas the median dose for the second course was 20 Gy. A total of 70% experienced neurologic improvement, with 27% experiencing complete neurologic resolution whereas 43% had partial improvement after repeat WBRT. Median survival was 4 months after second course of WBRT, with a retreatment dose of >20 Gy associated with a significantly longer survival. Clinically significant radiation-related complications were rare.

Son et al.[61] similarly reported on a series of 17 patients who underwent whole brain reirradiation. The median RT dose for the first course of treatment was 35 Gy in 14 fractions and for the second course 21.6 Gy in 1.8 Gy per fraction. The median survival time for all patients after retreatment WBRT was 5.2 months. In patients with stable extracranial disease, the median survival time after retreatment was 19.8 months compared with 2.5 months in patients with progressive extracranial disease. Eighty percent of patients experienced improved symptoms, with acute mild to moderate adverse reactions seen in 70.5% of patients.

Therefore, repeat WBRT is relatively safe and highly effective for recurrent or progressive brain metastases after initial WBRT. A minimum of 20 Gy in 1.8 to 2 Gy fractions should be given.

Concurrent Radiosensitizers

Although a majority of patients with brain metastases ultimately succumb to systemic progression, a significant percentage will die from neurologic progression. Multiple randomized trials of concomitant radiosensitizers have been performed in an attempt to optimize brain control (Table 96.7).[62–70] No trial has demonstrated a survival advantage, although a few have demonstrated an increased response rate. The trials with temozolomide show promise. Temozolomide is an oral alkylating agent with excellent CNS penetration. However, the findings of these relatively small trials need to be confirmed in a larger trial. Otherwise, a patient should be treated with a concomitant radiosensitizer only on a prospective trial.

Causes of Neurocognitive Decline in Brain Tumor Patients

Historically, brain radiation has been frequently cited as a major cause of neurocognitive decline in cancer patients. As

previously discussed, the experience reported by DeAngelis et al.[27] initially reported an 11% risk of radiation-induced dementia in patients undergoing WBRT for brain metastasis. The accuracy of this dementia rate is questioned by the nature of the statistical interpretation utilized. Although the study included 232 patients in the initial analysis, it only examined the 47 patients who survived at least 1 year. The principles of conditional probability dictate that the 11% risk is accurate only if a patient survives 1 year, which is significantly longer than most reported series. Therefore, a radiation-induced dementia risk of 2% (5 of 232) would reflect the true probability *ab initio* for patients presenting with brain metastasis. Indeed, in a separate study of a larger cohort, DeAngelis et al.[71] estimated the risk of radiation-induced dementia to be 1.9% to 5.2% for all patients presenting with brain metastasis.

Additionally, the increased local control achieved with use of adjuvant WBRT may actually improve neurocognition in a significant number of patients, as brain recurrence or progression is associated with a decrease in neurocognitive function.[72] In a neurocognitive analysis of RTOG-91-04, Regine et al.[73] demonstrated that approximately one-third of patients treated with WBRT experienced improvement in their MMSE; most importantly, those who had uncontrolled brain metastases had an average decrement of 6 points on the MMSE, which was a significantly greater drop than those with controlled brain metastases ($P = .02$).

Although it is certainly possible that subtle neurocognitive decline may result from WBRT, evaluating these changes will require more sophisticated battery of testing than has historically been employed. Additionally, appreciating the baseline cognitive dysfunction in patients with brain metastases will provide the most accurate assessment of the decline resulting from additional WBRT. In the large phase III motexafin gadolinium study, the neurocognitive battery examined memory recall, memory recognition, memory delayed recall, verbal fluency, pegboard hand coordinate, and executive function.[74] This study demonstrated that 21.0% to 65.1% of patients had impaired functioning *at baseline* before treatment with WBRT. Furthermore, patients who progressed in the brain after treatment experienced significantly worse scores in all of these individual tests.

There are now strong data that other confounding factors, such as anticonvulsants, benzodiazepines, opioids, chemotherapy, surgery, and tumor progression, contribute significantly to the neurocognitive decline of patients with brain tumor. It will be vital to control for these factors when interpreting ongoing studies evaluating alternative WBRT strategies (e.g., HA-WBRT, concurrent memantine).

SPINAL CORD COMPRESSION

In the United States, more than 20,000 cases of metastatic spinal cord compression (MSCC) are diagnosed annually, and it is estimated to develop in approximately 5% to 10% of all cancer patients.[75,76] MSCC is a devastating complication of cancer. It is considered a true medical emergency, and immediate intervention is required. Even with aggressive therapy, results can often be unsatisfactory. Although most patients with MSCC have limited survival, up to one-third will survive beyond 1 year.[77] Therefore, aggressive therapy should always be considered to preserve or improve the quality of life.

Pathophysiology

MSCC develops primarily in one of four ways: (a) continued growth and expansion of vertebral bone metastasis into the epidural space; (b) neural foramina extension by a paraspinal mass; (c) destruction of vertebral cortical bone, causing vertebral body collapse with displacement of bony fragments into the epidural space; or (d) rarely primary hematogenous seeding to the epidural space. Although complex, the most significant

TABLE 96.7 SELECTED RANDOMIZED TRIALS OF RADIOSENSITIZERS IN BRAIN METASTASIS

Author/Study Group (Reference)	Arms	Response Rate (%)	P	Median Survival	P
Komarnicky et al./ RTOG 79-16[62] (n = 859)	RT (30 Gy/10 fx)	45[a]	NS	4.5 mo	NS
	RT + misonidazole	42[a]	NS	3.9 mo	NS
	RT (30 Gy/6 fx)	42[a]		4.1 mo	
	RT + misonidazole	45[a]		3.1 mo	
Ushio et al./ Japan[69,b] (n = 88)	RT (40 Gy/20 fx)	36	<.05	27 wk	NS
	RT + nitrosourea	69		29 wk	
	RT + nitrosourea + tegafur	74		30.5 wk	
Phillips et al./ RTOG-89-05[63] (n = 72)	RT (37.5 Gy/15 fx)	50[d]	NS	6.1 mo	NS
	RT + BrdUrd	63[d]		4.3 mo	
Guerrieri et al./ Australia[70,b] (n = 42)	RT (20 Gy/5 fx)	10	NS	4.4 mo	NS
	RT + carboplatin	29		3.7 mo	
Antonadou et al./ Greece[64] (n = 52)	RT (40 Gy/20 fx)	67	.017	7.0 mo	NS
	RT + temozolomide	96		8.6 mo	
Verger et al./Spain[65] (n = 82)	RT (30 Gy/10 fx)	54[c]	.03	3.1 mo	NS
	RT + temozolomide	72[c]		4.5 mo	
Mehta et al./ SMART Trial[66] (n = 401)	RT (30 Gy/10 fx)	51	NS	4.9 mo	NS
	RT + MGd	46		5.2 mo	
Suh et al./REACH Trial[67] (n = 515)	RT (30 Gy/10 fx)	38	NS	4.4 mo	NS
	RT + efaproxiral	46		5.4 mo	
Knisely et al./ RTOG-01-18[68] (n = 175)	RT (37.5 Gy/15 fx)			3.9 mo	NS
	RT + thalidomide			3.9 mo	

[a]Percentage of survival time in KPS 90–100 range.
[b]Only lung cancer patients.
[c]Ninety-day freedom from brain metastasis.
[d]Overall complete and partial response rate.
BrdUrd, bromodeoxyuridine; fx, fractions; KPS, Karnofsky performance score; MGd, motexafin gadolinium; NS, not significant; RT, wholebrain radiotherapy; RTOG, Radiation Therapy and Oncology Group; SWOG, South West Oncology Group.

damage caused by MSCC appears to be vascular in nature as opposed to mechanical. Epidural tumor extension causes epidural venous plexus compression, which leads to intramedullary edema. This increase in vascular permeability and edema cause increased pressure on the small arterioles. Capillary blood flow diminishes as the disease progresses, leading to white matter ischemia. Prolonged ischemia eventually results in white matter infarction and permanent cord damage.[78]

Clinical Presentation, Diagnosis, and Prognosis

The vast majority of patients with MSCC have a cancer diagnosis history. As highlighted by Prasad et al.,[79] the most common tumor types are breast cancer, lung cancer, and prostate cancer, accounting for 15% to 20% of all cases. This reflects the high natural incidence of these tumors and their propensity for osseous metastasis. New-onset back pain in cancer patients needs to be taken seriously and worked up. Even without a prior cancer diagnosis, MSCC should be suspected in anyone who presents with progressively worsening back pain, incontinence, or paraplegia, especially in the high-risk population such as long-time smokers. The most common level of the MSCC involvement is in the thoracic spine (60% to 80%), followed by lumbar (15% to 30%) and cervical spine (<10%), whereas multiple levels can be involved in up to half of the patients.[79] Back pain is the most common presenting symptom (70% to 94%), followed by weakness (61% to 91%), sensory deficits (46% to 90%), and autonomic dysfunction (40% to 57%).[79]

MRI is the standard modality for spine imaging. It has a very high sensitivity, specificity, and accuracy in diagnosing MSCC.[80,81] Because patients can have synchronous, multifocal MSCC, an MRI of the entire spine with and without contrast should be promptly performed in anyone suspected of having MSCC. High-resolution CT scan or CT myelogram of the spine should be performed for those with contraindications to MRI.

One of the most important prognostic factors predicting ambulatory outcome is the rapidity of symptom onset. Other important prognostic factors include radiosensitive histology (e.g., multiple myeloma, germ cell tumors, small cell carcinoma) and pretherapy ambulatory function. In a prospective study of 98 patients with MSCC reported by Rades et al.,[82] the single strongest predictor for ambulatory status after therapy on multivariate analysis was time to development of motor deficits before radiation (P < .001) from the start of any symptoms. This cohort was separated into three groups according to the time to motor deficits before radiation therapy: 1 to 7 days (group A), 8 to 14 days (group B), and >14 days (group C). The ambulatory rates after therapy for groups A, B, and C were 35%, 55%, and 86% (P < .001), respectively. The symptom improvement rates for groups A, B, and C were 10%, 29%, and 86% (P = .026), respectively. The other factor significant on the multivariate analysis for post-therapy ambulatory status was favorable histology (P = .005), and there was a trend regarding pre-therapy ambulatory status (P = .076). Acute, rapid deterioration is predictive of irreversible spinal cord infarction. Only 10% of the patients in group A had symptom improvement; therefore, prompt diagnosis and treatment of MSCC are essential.

Corticosteroids

Corticosteroids must be started as soon as possible in anyone suspected of having MSCC, even before radiographic diagnosis, because this can be rapidly discontinued if a negative diagnosis is obtained. Corticosteroids effectively decrease cord edema and serve as an effective bridge to definitive treatment. Although multiple retrospective studies have demonstrated their clinical efficacy, Sorensen et al.[83] reported the only randomized controlled study (n = 57) on the utility of high-dose corticosteroids before definitive radiotherapy in MSCC from solid tumors. The treatment arm consisted of 96 mg of IV bolus of dexamethasone followed by 96 mg oral per day for 3 days and a 10-day taper versus no corticosteroid therapy. This study demonstrated 3-month and 6-month ambulatory rates of 81% versus 63% and 59% versus 33% (P < .05), respectively, in favor of high-dose dexamethasone.

The optimal maintenance dose of corticosteroids is unknown. Vecht et al.[84] reported the only randomized study (n = 37) comparing corticosteroid doses in patients with MSCC, but this study only evaluated the IV loading dose. It compared IV loading doses of 10 mg versus 100 mg, followed in both arms by the same oral regimen of 16 mg per day. Both arms demonstrated significant reductions in pain from baseline (P < .001); however, there was no difference between the two arms with respect to pain reduction, ambulation, or bladder function.

Very high doses of corticosteroids are associated with significant side effects. The Sorensen et al.[83] phase III study reported an 11% incidence of serious side effects for patients in the treatment arm, whereas Heimdal et al.[85] reported a 14.3% incidence of serious gastrointestinal (GI) side effects in 28 consecutive patients treated with 96 mg of IV dexamethasone per day. The toxicities in the Heimdal et al. report included one fatal ulcer hemorrhage, one rectal bleeding, and two bowel perforations. Subsequently, the dexamethasone dose was decreased to 16 mg per day for the next 38 consecutive patients, and there were no incidences of serious side effects (P < .05). Most importantly, the ambulatory rates were not different between the two dexamethasone doses.

Based on these data, a loading dose of 10 mg of IV dexamethasone followed by a maintenance dose of 4 to 6 mg every 6 to 8 hours should be sufficient before being tapered. Patients can be safely switched to an oral regimen after 24 to 48 hours because there is good oral bioavailability of corticosteroids. Furthermore, patients should be started on a PPI for GI prophylaxis. Although here has been no randomized trial utilizing PPIs in patients receiving corticosteroids, there have been multiple studies demonstrating the protective effects of PPIs against peptic ulcers in patients receiving chronic nonsteroidal anti-inflammatory drugs (NSAIDs).[86] NSAIDs and corticosteroids both cause GI mucosal injury by decreasing mucosal-protective prostaglandin levels. Therefore, it is not an unreasonable extrapolation to assume that PPIs provide a similar mucosal protective effect with corticosteroids, especially considering that the morbidity of GI toxicity can be life-threatening. Additionally, multiple comparative series reveal the superiority of PPI's to histamine H2 receptor antagonists for ulcer prophylaxis.[87] Use of oral antacids is not recommended as they have not been shown to protect against injury.[86]

Surgery

Radiation for nonradiosensitive tumors typically takes several days to have an effect and does not stabilize the spine, whereas surgery allows for immediate cord decompression and provides an opportunity to stabilize the spine intraoperatively. At some institutions, surgery was used infrequently because several retrospective studies and one small randomized study showed no benefit to surgery plus radiation over radiation alone. Young et al.[88] randomized 29 patients with MSCC to decompressive laminectomy followed by radiation versus radiation alone. Although this trial showed no benefit to surgery in terms of pain relief, ambulation, or sphincter function, it is difficult to draw any conclusion because of the small sample size. All of these studies used posterior laminectomy in conjunction with radiotherapy; however, most of the lesions in MSCC involve the anterior portion of the vertebral body. Therefore, a laminectomy may not effectively relieve the compression simply by opening the spinal canal and may actually worsen the stability of the spine.

Therefore, authors have advocated the use of direct surgical decompression, tumor debulking, and spinal stabilization via instrumentation to improve on the results from radiation alone. Patchell et al.[89] reported the first phase III randomized trial testing the efficacy of direct decompressive surgery in patients with MSCC (Table 96.8). The study compared radiation alone (standard 30 Gy in 10 fractions) versus circumferential

TABLE 96.8 KEY FINDINGS OF A PHASE III STUDY OF PATIENTS WITH METASTATIC SPINAL CORD COMPRESSION

	Surgery + Radiation (*n* = 50)	Radiation Alone (*n* = 51)	*P*
Primary end point			
Ability to walk post treatment			
Rate	84% (42/50)	57% (29/51)	.001
Time[c]	122 days	13 days	.003
Secondary end points[c]			
Maintenance of continence	156 days	17 days	.016
Maintenance of ASIA score[a]	566 days	72 days	.001
Maintenance of Frankel score[a]	566 days	72 days	.0006
Overall survival	126 days	100 days	.033
Other end points			
Mean daily morphine[b]	0.4 mg	4.8 mg	.002
Mean daily dexamethasone[b]	1.6 mg	4.2 mg	.0093
In patients ambulatory at study entry			
Ability to walk (maintaining)			
Rate	94% (32/34)	74% (26/34)	.024
Time[c]	153 days	54 days	.024
In patients nonambulatory at study entry			
Ability to walk (regaining)			
Rate	62% (10/16)	19% (3/16)	.012
Time[c]	59 days	0 days	.04

[a]Measures of spinal function after injury.
[b]Converted into equivalent doses.
[c]Reported time (days) are median values.
ASIA, American Spinal Injury Association.

decompressive and stabilization surgery within 24 hours of diagnosis followed by the same radiotherapy (within 2 weeks of surgery). The trial was terminated early when early-stopping rules were met regarding the primary end point of ambulation after treatment. This trial definitively demonstrated an advantage to surgery for every end point at statistically significant levels. For nonambulatory patients, the combined treatment patients had a significantly higher chance of regaining the ability to walk after therapy. Maintenance of continence, maintenance of American Spinal Cord Injury (ASIA) and Frankel scores (measures of spinal function after injury), median overall survival, and median mean daily dexamethasone and morphine equivalent doses all favored the surgery arm.

If operable, patients should undergo surgical decompression and stabilization followed by radiotherapy. Even for radiosensitive tumors, surgery can often stabilize the spine. Therefore, all patients with MSCC should be evaluated by a surgeon. Effective multidisciplinary teamwork is critical to the rapid evaluation and management of patients with MSCC.

Radiotherapy

Palliative radiotherapy has been the standard of care in the treatment of patients with MSCC. Although a total of 30 Gy in 10 fractions is the most frequently employed fractionation schedule, multiple fractionation schemes have been reported, which undoubtedly reflects the heterogeneity in the patient population and tumor histology. In one of the largest studies to date, Rades et al.[90] reported a retrospective series of 1,304 patients with MSCC. The patients were separated into five schedules: 8 Gy × 1 in 1 day (*n* = 261, group 1), 4 Gy × 5 in 1 week (*n* = 279, group 2), 3 Gy × 10 in 2 weeks (*n* = 274, group 3), 2.5 Gy × 15 in 3 weeks (*n* = 233, group 4), and 2 Gy × 20 in 4 weeks (*n* = 257, group 5). All of the groups had similar posttreatment ambulatory rates (63% to 74%) and motor function improvements (26% to 31%). However, in-field recurrence rates were much lower for the protracted schedules. The 2-year in-field recurrence rates for groups 1, 2, 3, 4, and 5 were 24%, 26%, 14%, 9%, and 7% (*P* < .001), respectively. They recommend that a single fraction of 8 Gy should be used in MSCC patients with limited survival expectations and that 30 Gy in 10 fractions should be used for all other patients.

Maranzano et al. have reported on two randomized trials evaluating short, radiation schedules. However, it is very difficult to interpret these results because neither trial included a fractionation that would be considered a standard of care.[77,91] A more relevant randomized trial was reported by Rades et al.[92] comparing a short course regimen (4 Gy × 5) to 30 Gy × 10 in patients with poor to intermediate survival prognosis, defined as having an estimated 6-month survival of 14% to 56% based on a validated scoring system. Primary end point was motor function response rate showing improvement or no progression of motor deficits at 1 month. Seventy-five percent of patients survived > 1 month. One-month response rates were similar for both radiation regimens (87.2% to 89.6%, *P* = .73). Both regimens also had similar RT effects on motor function at 3 and 6 months post treatment. Ambulatory status at 1, 3, and 6 months was not significantly different between regimens. Local progression-free survival and overall survival (median: 3.2 months) were also similar for both arms. Based on this trial results, 4 Gy × 5 was deemed noninferior to 30 Gy × 10 and should be strongly considered for patients in whom poor prognosis in whom limiting treatment time and discomfort should be a high priority.

For patients receiving radiotherapy for MSCC from solid tumors, 30 Gy in 10 fractions is considered the standard of care. Shorter fractionation schedules, such as 8 Gy × 1 or 4 Gy × 5, should only be reserved for those with clear evidence of progressive disease refractory to systemic therapy in whom survival expectations are poor. These short schedules should be clearly avoided in newly diagnosed, chemotherapy naïve patients because the clinical course can be quite variable and prolonged. Chemotherapy may be considered in select, newly diagnosed patients with excellent neurologic functional status and very chemosensitive tumors (e.g., lymphoma, multiple myeloma, germ cell tumors), but this is still considered outside the accepted standard as these tumors also respond very effectively to radiotherapy. If the patient is found to have a good performance status, oligometastatic disease, and controlled primary disease, then consideration should be made to escalate the total dose beyond 30 Gy because in an effort to achieve greater long-term gross tumor control while respecting dose constraints. Special techniques such as intensity-modulated radiation therapy (IMRT) or fractionated stereotactic body radiation therapy (SBRT) should be considered to safely escalate the total dose (Fig. 96.2).

Caution against Short, Hypofractionated Radiotherapy

A common mistake made by those who advocate a short hypofractionated regimen (e.g., 8 Gy × 1 to 2 or 4 Gy × 5) for MSCC is equating the safety and equivalency of these abbreviated schedules in bone and lung metastases trials as a justification for the safety of such regimens in MSCC. The consequence of progression of a bone metastasis despite prior radiotherapy (i.e., 8 Gy × 1) is an increase in pain, which leads to an increased need for pain medications and usually reirradiation. By contrast, the consequences of MSCC progression despite prior radiotherapy are an increase in pain, paralysis, and incontinence, which usually contribute significantly to the direct demise of the patient. Because some studies, but not all, suggest that single fraction radiotherapy for bone metastasis is associated with a higher retreatment rate than fractionated therapy, a note of caution is appropriate for single fraction radiotherapy for MSCC.[93]

Therefore, these abbreviated schedules should be routinely avoided unless the patient is refractory to multiple lines of systemic therapy and has convincing evidence of progressive systemic disease with limited expected survival.

Pediatric Spinal Cord Compression

MSCC in the pediatric population differs from adult MSCC. Histologic subtypes commonly encountered in children (e.g., neuroblastoma, Wilms tumor, and Ewing sarcoma) rarely occur in adults. In adults, most cases of MSCC are caused by

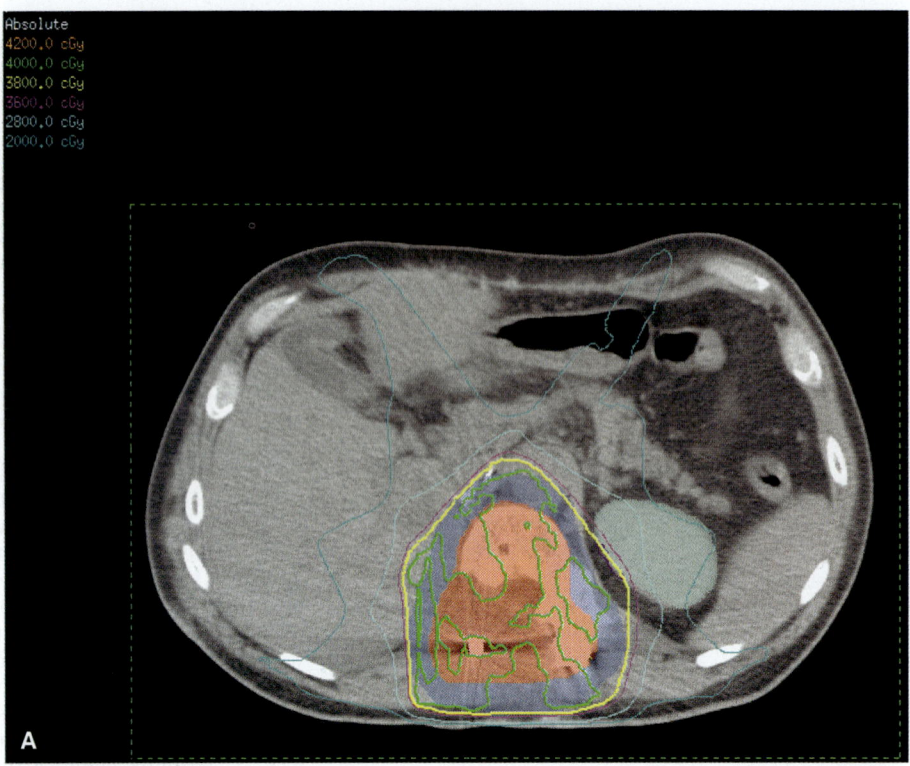

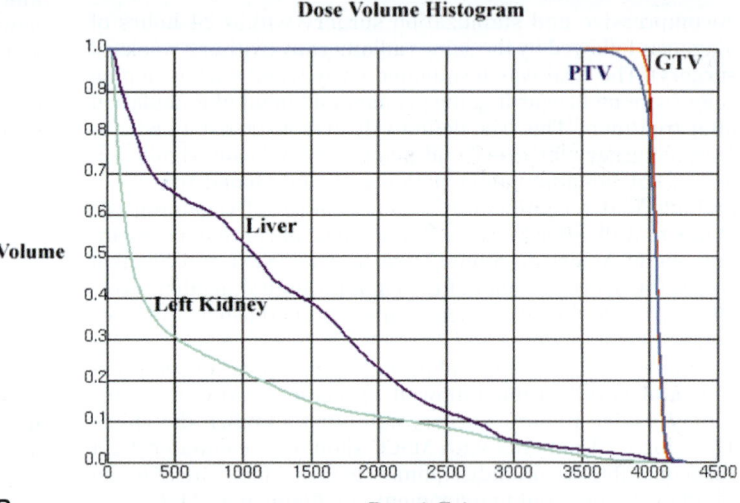

Dose Volume Histogram

FIGURE 96.2. A: Five years after undergoing a right nephrectomy for a stage I renal call carcinoma (RCC), patient presented with progressively worsening midback pain. Magnetic resonance image of the spine revealed a T11–12 right-sided paraspinal mass invading the right lateral T12 vertebral body and neural foramina causing T12 spinal cord compression. Patient underwent a gross total resection and instrumentation to stabilize the spine. A full metastatic workup revealed the vertebral disease as the solitary site of recurrent RCC. Chemistries revealed a mild chronic renal insufficiency, with a creatinine level of 2.1 mg/dL. Intensity-modulated radiation therapy (IMRT) was used to minimize the dose to the left kidney. The figure shows an axial computed tomography image of the IMRT plan generated, with the *red* and *blue* color washes representing gross tumor volume (GTV) and planning target volume (PTV), respectively. **B:** The dose–volume histogram of the IMRT plan is shown. A total of 40 Gy in 20 fractions was delivered to the PTV (GTV + 1 cm). The PTV was modified so the margin was decreased to 8 mm along the left lateral edge of the vertebral body next to the left kidney.

direct invasion into the epidural space by metastatic vertebral body tumors, although, in children, most are caused by direct neural foraminal invasion, causing the characteristic "dumbbell" tumor. Chemotherapy plays a central role in the treatment of pediatric MSCC.[94]

Neuroblastoma is the most common histology of pediatric MSCC. Hayes et al.[95] (nine cases of neuroblastoma and five cases of Ewing sarcoma) and Sanderson et al.[96] (four cases of neuroblastoma) demonstrated that chemotherapy alone allowed complete recovery of spinal cord function in all cases. The French Society of Pediatric Oncology protocol NBL-90 included 42 nonmetastatic neuroblastoma patients with intraspinal extension and consequent MSCC.[97] All were treated with initial chemotherapy, and this resulted in intraspinal tumor shrinkage, avoidance of surgery, and neurologic deficit improvement in 58%, 60%, and 92% of the patients, respectively. Severe neurologic sequelae occurred in only six patients (15%).

Emergent surgery should be offered to any pediatric patient with rapid neurologic progression at initial presentation or while on chemotherapy. In most circumstances, this should be followed by definitive chemotherapy. In stable or mildly symptomatic patients, chemotherapy can obviate the need for surgery, which is often associated with long-term skeletal deformities. Radiation should be reserved only for those who require palliation for progressive disease after failure of multiple systemic regimens, those who progress neurologically despite the initial treatment with chemotherapy or surgery, and those who present with primary vertebral tumors (e.g., primary vertebral Ewing sarcoma) in which definitive surgery is rarely feasible.

Intramedullary Spinal Cord Metastasis

Intramedullary spinal cord metastasis (ISCM) is rare, representing only 1% of all intramedullary tumors but being more greatly recognized as an entity given enhanced radiographic techniques. According to a review by Kalayci et al.,[98] ISCM is most commonly secondary to a lung primary (54%), followed by breast cancer (11%). Although back pain is common in >90% of MSCC patients, back or neck pain was seen in only 38% with ISCM. However, high sensory deficits (79%), sphincter dysfunction (60%), and weakness (91%) are more common in ISCM. The most striking difference between ISCM and MSCC is the high incidence of synchronous brain metastasis (41%) in patients presenting with ISCM. This is not surprising when one considers the route of spread and the high incidence of lung primaries in patients with ISCM. An MRI of the brain should be obtained.

The treatment of ISCM should be approached very similarly to MSCC, except for the role of surgery. Most surgeons are reluctant to operate in ISCM because surgery carries a high morbidity rate. Corticosteroids as well as radiation therapy should be promptly initiated. Unfortunately, a diagnosis of ISCM portends a poor prognosis with median survival of 1 to 5.5 months.[99]

Leptomeningeal Carcinomatosis

Leptomeningeal carcinomatosis (LCM) is a rare complication of multiple cancers, occurring in approximately 5% of metastatic cancer. A diagnosis of LCM portends a poor prognosis with medial survival of 2.3 to 4.7 months in modern series.[100] The most frequent cancers associated with LCM are lung and breast. In breast cancer, it is often seen in patients who have *HER2-neu* overexpression or infiltrating lobular histology.[101] In lung cancer, it is most commonly involved by NSCLC with adenocarcinoma histology accounting for 50% to 78% of cases.[102]

The majority of patients present with signs and symptoms. According to the review by Gleissner and Chamberlain,[103] spinal symptoms (>60%) are the most common, followed by cerebral (50%) and cranial nerve symptoms (40%). Contrast-enhanced MRI is the radiographic modality of choice. The entire neuroaxis must be imaged if LCM is clinically suspected in a patient with a known malignancy as multifocal involvement is common. In most patients, the MRI will reveal leptomeningeal enhancement that is frequently associated with cranial nerve enhancement and gross tumor deposits. MRI can provide a diagnosis of LCM with a sensitivity and specificity of 76% and 77%, respectively.[104] A radiographic diagnosis of LCM may be limited, however, in the setting of hematopoietic tumors as the rate of positive neuroimaging is approximately 50%, thereby requiring CSF cytology for confirmation.[100]

CSF cytology is also warranted in a setting when suspicion for LCM is high but MRI is equivocal. Multiple samples may need to be obtained because the initial yield of a lumbar tap may be only 50%.[103] Neurosurgery must be consulted to evaluate the need for (a) shunting if hydrocephalus is suspected and (b) placement of Rickham or Ommaya reservoir for possible intrathecal (IT) chemotherapy. Gleissner and Chamberlain[103] argue that CSF flow studies should be performed with indium-111 or technetium-99, because up to 40% of patients have abnormal

CSF flow from gross tumor deposits that may disrupt adequate IT chemotherapy delivery. However, flow studies are not performed by many centers because gross tumor nodules, most likely to cause flow disruption and not effectively treated by IT chemotherapy, are treated with radiation anyway. Thus, CSF flow studies typically do not change the overall management of patients with LCM who require treatment decisions to be made in an expedient manner.

There is no consensus on the optimal management of patients with LCM. This is mainly because of the lack of large published experiences, limited number of randomized trials, nonuniform treatment regimens in single institution experiences, and inclusion of various primary tumor histologies in the clinical trials. However, most would agree that an aggressive treatment with radiation (either WBRT or focal spinal radiation to symptomatic sites) and IT chemotherapy are indicated in patients with good performance status. The optimal dose and fractionation schedule of radiation therapy delivered in the setting of LCM remains unknown; however, similar to WBRT and MSCC, 30 Gy in 10 fractions is the most typical scheduled used. In patients with poor performance status, larger fractions may be more advantageous because these patients will rarely live long enough to experience late radiation toxicity and larger fractions may result in a faster symptomatic response. In a large published experience on LCM from small cell lung cancer ($n = 36$), the dismal median survival of 1.3 months is a direct result of only 14 patients being offered some kind of therapy ($n = 9$ for radiation, $n = 5$ for chemotherapy).[105] In contrast, Chamberlain and Kormanik,[106] in a series of patients with LCM from non–small-cell lung cancer ($n = 32$), treated patients prospectively with radiotherapy followed by IT chemotherapy. The median survival for the entire cohort was 5 months, while patients with normal CSF flow had a significantly longer median survival compared with patients with interrupted CSF flow (6 months vs. 4 months; $P < .05$). This suggests that an aggressive multimodality approach can produce survival times that are comparable to patients with multiple brain parenchymal metastases.

All of the randomized clinical trials on patients with LCM from solid tumors have included IT methotrexate (MTX)-based regimens (Table 96.9).[107-111] The only trial that compared IT versus non-IT (i.e., systemic) chemotherapy was reported by Boogerd et al.[111] However, this negative trial only included patients with breast primaries. Glantz et al.[109] reported that IT DepoCyt (cytarabine liposome injection) led to a greater median time to neurologic progression (8 weeks vs. 4 weeks; $P = .007$), although the overall survival was not statistically different. The only positive trial reported to date has been by Kim et al.[110] from Seoul National University. Patients randomized to IT MTX, Ara-C (arabinofuranosyl cytidine), and hydrocortisone had a significantly longer survival than those randomized to IT MTX alone (18.2 weeks vs. 10.4 weeks; $P = .029$). Patients with adenocarcinoma of the lung in the multiagent arm had a significant, longer survival (23.9 weeks vs. 10.4 weeks; $P = .038$). Multiple other agents have been studied, but none have demonstrated significant responses.

There is ample evidence that focal radiation, such as WBRT or spinal radiation, provides added

TABLE 96.9 RANDOMIZED TRIALS OF SOLID TUMOR PATIENTS WITH LEPTOMENINGEAL CARCINOMATOSIS

Study (Ref.)	N	Histology	Arms[a]	RR[b] (%)	Median Survival	Survival (P-value)
Hitchins et al. (1987)[107]	44	Solid tumors	IT MTX 15 mg	61	12 wk	.08
			IT MTX + Ara-C 50 mg/m²	45	7 wk	
			Concurrent RT (not randomized)	75		
			No concurrent RT	35		<.05
Grossman et al. (1993)[108]	52	Nonleukemic[c]	IT MTX 10 mg	0	16 wk	NS
			IT thiotepa 10 mg	0	14 wk	
Glantz et al. (1999)[109]	61	Solid tumors	IT MTX 10 mg	20	2.6 wk	.15
			IT DepoCyt 50 mg	26	3.5 wk	
Kim et al. (2003)[110]	55	Solid tumors	IT MTX 15 mg	14	10 wk	.03
			IT MTX + Ara-C 30 mg/m² + hydrocortisone 15 mg/m²	39	19 wk	
			Concurrent RT (not randomized)	82	19 wk	
			No concurrent RT	50	11 wk	.47
Boogerd et al. (2004)[111]	35	Breast	IT chemotherapy[d]	41	18 wk	.32
			Non-IT chemotherapy	39	30 wk	

[a]All studies allowed palliative radiation when necessary.
[b]RR determination by neurologic and CSF improvements as predefined by each study.
[c]Fourteen patients (19%) had lymphoma and the rest had solid tumors.
[d]All patients started with MTX and switched to Ara-C if no response.
Ara-C, cytarabine; DepoCyt, sustained-release cytarabine; IT, intrathecal; MTX, methotrexate; NS, not significant; RR, response rate.

benefit to IT chemotherapy. This is particularly true in patients with bulky meningeal disease because IT chemotherapy only penetrates 2 to 3 mm. In the randomized IT chemotherapy trial reported by Hitchins et al.,[107] patients who received concurrent CNS radiation had a higher response rate compared with those who did not (73% vs. 35%; $P < .05$). Likewise, in the randomized trial reported by Kim et al.,[110] those who received concurrent CNS radiation had a significant higher neurologic response rate (81.5% vs. 50.0%; $P = .014$). There is a concern that concurrent radiation and IT chemotherapy could potentially increase toxicity. However, the vast majority of patients do not survive long enough to see the late neurologic toxicity manifest.

CONCLUSION

A significant percentage of cancer patients will require palliative radiation therapy at some point during their natural history. On the basis of randomized data, patients with a limited number of brain metastases should be treated with local therapy such as surgery or SRS with or without whole-brain irradiation whereas those with numerous brain metastases should be treated with whole-brain irradiation alone. In patients with spinal cord compression, surgical decompression should be strongly considered in patients with single-level disease and good performance status followed by radiation therapy. Radiation therapy alone can also be considered for all patients with spinal cord compression with the most common fractionation scheme being 30 Gy in 10 fractions. Leptomeningeal carcinomatosis continues to have an unfavorable prognosis, and the use of radiation therapy should be based on the palliation of individual signs and symptoms.

REFERENCES

1. Lagerwaard FJ, Levendag PC, Nowak PJ, et al. Identification of prognostic factors in patients with brain metastases: a review of 1292 patients. *Int J Radiat Oncol Biol Phys* 1999;43(4):795–803.
2. Suh JH, Chao ST, Peereboom DM, et al. Metastatic cancer to the brain. In: DeVita VT, Lawrence TS, Rosenberg SA, eds. *DeVita, Hellman, and Rosenberg's Cancer: Principles & Practice of Oncology*. 10th ed. Philadelphia: Wolters Kluwer; 2015.
3. Nussbaum ES, Djalilian HR, Cho KH, et al. Brain metastases. Histology, multiplicity, surgery, and survival. *Cancer* 1996;78(8):1781–1788.
4. Barnholtz-Sloan JS, Sloan AE, Davis FG, et al. Incidence proportions of brain metastases in patients diagnosed (1973 to 2001) in the Metropolitan Detroit Cancer Surveillance System. *J Clin Oncol* 2004;22(14):2865–2872.
5. Posner JB. Brain metastases: 1995. A brief review. *J Neurooncol* 1996;27(3):287–293.
6. Fink KR, Fink JR. Imaging of brain metastases. *Surg Neurol Int* 2013;4(Suppl 4):S209–S219.
7. Soffietti R, Cornu P, Delattre JY, et al. EFNS Guidelines on diagnosis and treatment of brain metastases: report of an EFNS Task Force. *Eur J Neurol* 2006;13(7):674–681.
8. Gaspar L, Scott C, Rotman M, et al. Recursive partitioning analysis (RPA) of prognostic factors in three Radiation Therapy Oncology Group (RTOG) brain metastases trials. *Int J Radiat Oncol Biol Phys* 1997;37(4):745–751.
9. Gaspar LE, Scott C, Murray K, et al. Validation of the RTOG recursive partitioning analysis (RPA) classification for brain metastases. *Int J Radiat Oncol Biol Phys* 2000;47(4):1001–1006.
10. Sperduto PW, Kased N, Roberge D, et al. Summary report on the graded prognostic assessment: an accurate and facile diagnosis-specific tool to estimate survival for patients with brain metastases. *J Clin Oncol* 2012;30(4):419–425.
11. Ruderman NB, Hall TC. Use of glucocorticoids in the palliative treatment of metastatic brain tumors. *Cancer* 1965;18:298–306.
12. Vecht CJ, Hovestadt A, Verbiest HB, et al. Dose-effect relationship of dexamethasone on Karnofsky performance in metastatic brain tumors: a randomized study of doses of 4, 8, and 16 mg per day. *Neurology* 1994;44(4):675–680.
13. Klein M, Engelberts NH, van der Ploeg HM, et al. Epilepsy in low-grade gliomas: the impact on cognitive function and quality of life. *Ann Neurol* 2003;54(4):514–520.
14. Klein M, Heimans JJ, Aaronson NK, et al. Effect of radiotherapy and other treatment-related factors on mid-term to long-term cognitive sequelae in low-grade gliomas: a comparative study. *Lancet* 2002;360(9343):1361–1368.
15. Glantz MJ, Cole BF, Forsyth PA, et al. Practice parameter: anticonvulsant prophylaxis in patients with newly diagnosed brain tumors. Report of the Quality Standards Subcommittee of the American Academy of Neurology. *Neurology* 2000;54(10):1886–1893.
16. Wu AS, Trinh VT, Suki D, et al. A prospective randomized trial of perioperative seizure prophylaxis in patients with intraparenchymal brain tumors. *J Neurosurg* 2013;118(4):873–883.
17. Coia LR. The role of radiation therapy in the treatment of brain metastases. *Int J Radiat Oncol Biol Phys* 1992;23(1):229–238.
18. Borgelt B, Gelber R, Kramer S, et al. The palliation of brain metastases: final results of the first two studies by the Radiation Therapy Oncology Group. *Int J Radiat Oncol Biol Phys* 1980;6(1):1–9.
19. Haie-Meder C, Pellae-Cosset B, Laplanche A, et al. Results of a randomized clinical trial comparing two radiation schedules in the palliative treatment of brain metastases. *Radiother Oncol* 1993;26(2):111–116.
20. Priestman TJ, Dunn J, Brada M, et al. Final results of the Royal College of Radiologists' trial comparing two different radiotherapy schedules in the treatment of cerebral metastases. *Clin Oncol (R Coll Radiol)* 1996;8(5):308–315.
21. Murray KJ, Scott C, Greenberg HM, et al. A randomized phase III study of accelerated hyperfractionation versus standard in patients with unresected brain metastases: a report of the Radiation Therapy Oncology Group (RTOG) 9104. *Int J Radiat Oncol Biol Phys* 1997;39(3):571–574.
22. Graham PH, Bucci J, Browne L. Randomized comparison of whole brain radiotherapy, 20 Gy in four daily fractions versus 40 Gy in 20 twice-daily fractions, for brain metastases. *Int J Radiat Oncol Biol Phys* 2010;77(3):648–654.
23. Nieder C, Berberich W, Schnabel K. Tumor-related prognostic factors for remission of brain metastases after radiotherapy. *Int J Radiat Oncol Biol Phys* 1997;39(1):25–30.
24. Mulvenna P, Nankivell M, Barton R, et al. Dexamethasone and supportive care with or without whole brain radiotherapy in treating patients with non-small cell lung cancer with brain metastases unsuitable for resection or stereotactic radiotherapy (QUARTZ): results from a phase 3, non-inferiority, randomised trial. *Lancet* 2016;388(10055):2004–2014.
25. Cagney DN, Alexander BM, Aizer AA. Whole brain radiotherapy for non-small cell lung cancer. *Lancet* 2017;389(10077):1394–1395.
26. Zhu J, Kang M, Fan X. Whole brain radiotherapy for non-small cell lung cancer. *Lancet* 2017;389(10077):1395.
27. DeAngelis LM, Mandell LR, Thaler HT, et al. The role of postoperative radiotherapy after resection of single brain metastases. *Neurosurgery* 1989;24(6):798–805.
28. Li J, Bentzen SM, Renschler M, et al. Regression after whole-brain radiation therapy for brain metastases correlates with survival and improved neurocognitive function. *J Clin Oncol* 2007;25(10):1260–1266.
29. Gondi V, Pugh SL, Tome WA, et al. Preservation of memory with conformal avoidance of the hippocampal neural stem-cell compartment during whole-brain radiotherapy for brain metastases (RTOG 0933): a phase II multi-institutional trial. *J Clin Oncol* 2014;32(34):3810–3816.
30. Brown PD, Pugh S, Laack NN, et al. Memantine for the prevention of cognitive dysfunction in patients receiving whole-brain radiotherapy: a randomized, double-blind, placebo-controlled trial. *Neuro Oncol* 2013;15(10):1429–1437.
31. Barlesi F, Mazieres J, Merlio JP, et al. Routine molecular profiling of patients with advanced non-small-cell lung cancer: results of a 1-year nationwide programme of the French Cooperative Thoracic Intergroup (IFCT). *Lancet* 2016;387(10026):1415–1426.
32. Zimmermann S, Dziadziuszko R, Peters S. Indications and limitations of chemotherapy and targeted agents in non-small cell lung cancer brain metastases. *Cancer Treat Rev* 2014;40(6):716–722.
33. Rusthoven CG, Doebele RC. Management of brain metastases in ALK-positive non-small-cell lung cancer. *J Clin Oncol* 2016;34(24):2814–2819.
34. Magnuson WJ, Lester-Coll NH, Wu AJ, et al. Management of brain metastases in tyrosine kinase inhibitor-naive epidermal growth factor receptor-mutant non-small-cell lung cancer: a retrospective multi-institutional analysis. *J Clin Oncol* 2017;35(10):1070–1077.
35. Gerber NK, Yamada Y, Rimner A, et al. Erlotinib versus radiation therapy for brain metastases in patients with EGFR-mutant lung adenocarcinoma. *Int J Radiat Oncol Biol Phys* 2014;89(2):322–329.
36. Delattre JY, Krol G, Thaler HT, et al. Distribution of brain metastases. *Arch Neurol* 1988;45(7):741–744.
37. Patchell RA, Tibbs PA, Walsh JW, et al. A randomized trial of surgery in the treatment of single metastases to the brain. *N Engl J Med* 1990;322(8):494–500.
38. Noordijk EM, Vecht CJ, Haaxma-Reiche H, et al. The choice of treatment of single brain metastasis should be based on extracranial tumor activity and age. *Int J Radiat Oncol Biol Phys* 1994;29(4):711–717.
39. Mintz AH, Kestle J, Rathbone MP, et al. A randomized trial to assess the efficacy of surgery in addition to radiotherapy in patients with a single cerebral metastasis. *Cancer* 1996;78(7):1470–1476.
40. Andrews DW, Scott CB, Sperduto PW, et al. Whole brain radiation therapy with or without stereotactic radiosurgery boost for patients with one to three brain metastases: phase III results of the RTOG 9508 randomised trial. *Lancet* 2004;363(9422):1665–1672.
41. Kondziolka D, Patel A, Lunsford LD, et al. Stereotactic radiosurgery plus whole brain radiotherapy versus radiotherapy alone for patients with multiple brain metastases. *Int J Radiat Oncol Biol Phys* 1999;45(2):427–434.
42. Chougule P, Burton-Williams M, Saris S, et al. Randomized treatment of brain metastasis with gamma knife radiosurgery, whole brain radiotherapy or both. *Int J Radiat Oncol Biol Phys* 2000;3(48):114.
43. Sperduto PW, Shanley R, Luo X, et al. Secondary analysis of RTOG 9508, a phase 3 randomized trial of whole-brain radiation therapy versus WBRT plus stereotactic radiosurgery in patients with 1–3 brain metastases; poststratified by the graded prognostic assessment (GPA). *Int J Radiat Oncol Biol Phys* 2014;90(2):526–531.
44. Sneed PK, Suh JH, Goetsch SJ, et al. A multi-institutional review of radiosurgery alone vs. radiosurgery with whole brain radiotherapy as the initial management of brain metastases. *Int J Radiat Oncol Biol Phys* 2002;53(3):519–526.
45. Sneed PK, Lamborn KR, Forstner JM, et al. Radiosurgery for brain metastases: is whole brain radiotherapy necessary? *Int J Radiat Oncol Biol Phys* 1999;43(3):549–558.
46. Regine WF, Huhn JL, Patchell RA, et al. Risk of symptomatic brain tumor recurrence and neurologic deficit after radiosurgery alone in patients with newly diagnosed brain metastases: results and implications. *Int J Radiat Oncol Biol Phys* 2002;52(2):333–338.
47. Manon R, O'Neill A, Knisely J, et al. Phase II trial of radiosurgery for one to three newly diagnosed brain metastases from renal cell carcinoma, melanoma, and sarcoma: an Eastern Cooperative Oncology Group study (E 6397). *J Clin Oncol* 2005;23(34):8870–8876.
48. Patchell RA, Tibbs PA, Regine WF, et al. Postoperative radiotherapy in the treatment of single metastases to the brain: a randomized trial. *JAMA* 1998;280(17):1485–1489.

49. Aoyama H, Shirato H, Tago M, et al. Stereotactic radiosurgery plus whole-brain radiation therapy vs stereotactic radiosurgery alone for treatment of brain metastases: a randomized controlled trial. *JAMA* 2006;295(21):2483–2491.
50. Muacevic A, Wowra B, Siefert A, et al. Microsurgery plus whole brain irradiation versus Gamma Knife surgery alone for treatment of single metastases to the brain: a randomized controlled multicentre phase III trial. *J Neurooncol* 2008;87(3):299–307.
51. Kocher M, Soffietti R, Abacioglu U, et al. Adjuvant whole-brain radiotherapy versus observation after radiosurgery or surgical resection of one to three cerebral metastases: results of the EORTC 22952-26001 study. *J Clin Oncol* 2011;29(2):134–141.
52. Chang EL, Wefel JS, Hess KR, et al. Neurocognition in patients with brain metastases treated with radiosurgery or radiosurgery plus whole-brain irradiation: a randomised controlled trial. *Lancet Oncol* 2009;10(11):1037–1044.
53. Mahajan A, Ahmed S, Li J, et al. Postoperative stereotactic radiosurgery versus observation for completely resected brain metastases: results of a prospective randomized study. *Int J Radiat Oncol Biol Phys* 2016;96(2S):S2.
54. Brown P, Ballman K, Cerhan J, et al. N107C/CEC. 3: a phase III trial of postoperative stereotactic radiosurgery (SRS) compared with whole brain radiotherapy (WBRT) for resected metastatic brain disease. *Int J Radiat Oncol Biol Phys* 2016;96(5):937–940.
55. Aoyama H, Tago M, Kato N, et al. Neurocognitive function of patients with brain metastasis who received either whole brain radiotherapy plus stereotactic radiosurgery or radiosurgery alone. *Int J Radiat Oncol Biol Phys* 2007;68(5):1388–1395.
56. Aoyama H, Tago M, Shirato H; Japanese Radiation Oncology Study Group I. Stereotactic radiosurgery with or without whole-brain radiotherapy for brain metastases: secondary analysis of the JROSG 99-1 Randomized Clinical Trial. *JAMA Oncol* 2015;1(4):457–464.
57. Mahmood U, Kwok Y, Regine WF, et al. Whole-brain irradiation for patients with brain metastases: still the standard of care. *Lancet Oncol* 2010;11(3):221–222; author reply 223.
58. Lawlor PG, Gagnon B, Mancini IL, et al. Occurrence, causes, and outcome of delirium in patients with advanced cancer: a prospective study. *Arch Intern Med* 2000;160(6):786–794.
59. Pereira J, Hanson J, Bruera E. The frequency and clinical course of cognitive impairment in patients with terminal cancer. *Cancer* 1997;79(4):835–842.
60. Wong WW, Schild SE, Sawyer TE, et al. Analysis of outcome in patients reirradiated for brain metastases. *Int J Radiat Oncol Biol Phys* 1996;34(3):585–590.
61. Son CH, Jimenez R, Niemierko A, et al. Outcomes after whole brain reirradiation in patients with brain metastases. *Int J Radiat Oncol Biol Phys* 2012;82(2):e167–e172.
62. Komarnicky LT, Phillips TL, Martz K, et al. A randomized phase III protocol for the evaluation of misonidazole combined with radiation in the treatment of patients with brain metastases (RTOG-7916). *Int J Radiat Oncol Biol Phys* 1991;20(1):53–58.
63. Phillips TL, Scott CB, Leibel SA, et al. Results of a randomized comparison of radiotherapy and bromodeoxyuridine with radiotherapy alone for brain metastases: report of RTOG trial 89-05. *Int J Radiat Oncol Biol Phys* 1995;33(2):339–348.
64. Antonadou D, Paraskevaidis M, Sarris G, et al. Phase II randomized trial of temozolomide and concurrent radiotherapy in patients with brain metastases. *J Clin Oncol* 2002;20(17):3644–3650.
65. Verger E, Gil M, Yaya R, et al. Temozolomide and concomitant whole brain radiotherapy in patients with brain metastases: a phase II randomized trial. *Int J Radiat Oncol Biol Phys* 2005;61(1):185–191.
66. Mehta MP, Rodrigus P, Terhaard CH, et al. Survival and neurologic outcomes in a randomized trial of motexafin gadolinium and whole-brain radiation therapy in brain metastases. *J Clin Oncol* 2003;21(13):2529–2536.
67. Suh JH, Stea B, Nabid A, et al. Phase III study of efaproxiral as an adjunct to whole-brain radiation therapy for brain metastases. *J Clin Oncol* 2006;24(1):106–114.
68. Knisely JP, Berkey B, Chakravarti A, et al. A phase III study of conventional radiation therapy plus thalidomide versus conventional radiation therapy for multiple brain metastases (RTOG 0118). *Int J Radiat Oncol Biol Phys* 2008;71(1):79–86.
69. Ushio Y, Arita N, Hayakawa T, et al. Chemotherapy of brain metastases from lung carcinoma: a controlled randomized study. *Neurosurgery* 1991;28(2):201–205.
70. Guerrieri M, Wong K, Ryan G, et al. A randomised phase III study of palliative radiation with concomitant carboplatin for brain metastases from non-small cell carcinoma of the lung. *Lung Cancer* 2004;46(1):107–111.
71. DeAngelis LM, Delattre JY, Posner JB. Radiation-induced dementia in patients cured of brain metastases. *Neurology* 1989;39(6):789–796.
72. Taylor BV, Buckner JC, Cascino TL, et al. Effects of radiation and chemotherapy on cognitive function in patients with high-grade glioma. *J Clin Oncol* 1998;16(6):2195–2201.
73. Regine WF, Scott C, Murray K, et al. Neurocognitive outcome in brain metastases patients treated with accelerated-fractionation vs. accelerated-hyperfractionated radiotherapy: an analysis from Radiation Therapy Oncology Group Study 91-04. *Int J Radiat Oncol Biol Phys* 2001;51(3):711–717.
74. Meyers CA, Smith JA, Bezjak A, et al. Neurocognitive function and progression in patients with brain metastases treated with whole-brain radiation and motexafin gadolinium: results of a randomized phase III trial. *J Clin Oncol* 2004;22(1):157–165.
75. Byrne TN. Spinal cord compression from epidural metastases. *N Engl J Med* 1992;327(9):614–619.
76. Quinn JA, DeAngelis LM. Neurologic emergencies in the cancer patient. *Semin Oncol* 2000;27(3):311–321.
77. Maranzano E, Bellavita R, Rossi R, et al. Short-course versus split-course radiotherapy in metastatic spinal cord compression: results of a phase III, randomized, multicenter trial. *J Clin Oncol* 2005;23(15):3358–3365.
78. Kato A, Ushio Y, Hayakawa T, et al. Circulatory disturbance of the spinal cord with epidural neoplasm in rats. *J Neurosurg* 1985;63(2):260–265.
79. Prasad D, Schiff D. Malignant spinal-cord compression. *Lancet Oncol* 2005;6(1):15–24.
80. Loughrey GJ, Collins CD, Todd SM, et al. Magnetic resonance imaging in the management of suspected spinal canal disease in patients with known malignancy. *Clin Radiol* 2000;55(11):849–855.
81. Loblaw DA, Laperriere NJ. Emergency treatment of malignant extradural spinal cord compression: an evidence-based guideline. *J Clin Oncol* 1998;16(4):1613–1624.
82. Rades D, Heidenreich F, Karstens JH. Final results of a prospective study of the prognostic value of the time to develop motor deficits before irradiation in metastatic spinal cord compression. *Int J Radiat Oncol Biol Phys* 2002;53(4):975–979.
83. Sorensen S, Helweg-Larsen S, Mouridsen H, et al. Effect of high-dose dexamethasone in carcinomatous metastatic spinal cord compression treated with radiotherapy: a randomised trial. *Eur J Cancer* 1994;30A(1):22–27.
84. Vecht CJ, Haaxma-Reiche H, van Putten WL, et al. Initial bolus of conventional versus high-dose dexamethasone in metastatic spinal cord compression. *Neurology* 1989;39(9):1255–1257.
85. Heimdal K, Hirschberg H, Slettebo H, et al. High incidence of serious side effects of high-dose dexamethasone treatment in patients with epidural spinal cord compression. *J Neurooncol* 1992;12(2):141–144.
86. Lanza FL, Chan FK, Quigley EM; Practice Parameters Committee of the American College of Gastroenterology. Guidelines for prevention of NSAID-related ulcer complications. *Am J Gastroenterol* 2009;104(3):728–738.
87. Mo C, Sun G, Wang YZ, et al. PPI versus histamine H2 receptor antagonists for prevention of upper gastrointestinal injury associated with low-dose aspirin: systematic review and meta-analysis. *PLoS One* 2015;10(7):e0131558.
88. Young RF, Post EM, King GA. Treatment of spinal epidural metastases. Randomized prospective comparison of laminectomy and radiotherapy. *J Neurosurg* 1980;53(6):741–748.
89. Patchell RA, Tibbs PA, Regine WF, et al. Direct decompressive surgical resection in the treatment of spinal cord compression caused by metastatic cancer: a randomised trial. *Lancet* 2005;366(9486):643–648.
90. Rades D, Stalpers LJ, Veninga T, et al. Evaluation of five radiation schedules and prognostic factors for metastatic spinal cord compression. *J Clin Oncol* 2005;23(15):3366–3375.
91. Maranzano E, Trippa F, Casale M, et al. 8 Gy single-dose radiotherapy is effective in metastatic spinal cord compression: results of a phase III randomized multicentre Italian trial. *Radiother Oncol* 2009;93(2):174–179.
92. Rades D, Segedin B, Conde-Moreno AJ, et al. Radiotherapy with 4 Gy × 5 versus 3 Gy x 10 for metastatic epidural spinal cord compression: final results of the SCORE-2 trial (ARO 2009/01). *J Clin Oncol* 2016;34(6):597–602.
93. Wu JS, Wong R, Johnston M, et al.; Cancer Care Ontario Practice Guidelines Initiative Supportive Care Group. Meta-analysis of dose-fractionation radiotherapy trials for the palliation of painful bone metastases. *Int J Radiat Oncol Biol Phys* 2003;55(3):594–605.
94. Klein SL, Sanford RA, Muhlbauer MS. Pediatric spinal epidural metastases. *J Neurosurg* 1991;74(1):70–75.
95. Hayes FA, Thompson EI, Hvizdala E, et al. Chemotherapy as an alternative to laminectomy and radiation in the management of epidural tumor. *J Pediatr* 1984;104(2):221–224.
96. Sanderson IR, Pritchard J, Marsh HT. Chemotherapy as the initial treatment of spinal cord compression due to disseminated neuroblastoma. *J Neurosurg* 1989;70(5):688–690.
97. Plantaz D, Rubie H, Michon J, et al. The treatment of neuroblastoma with intraspinal extension with chemotherapy followed by surgical removal of residual disease. A prospective study of 42 patients—results of the NBL 90 Study of the French Society of Pediatric Oncology. *Cancer* 1996;78(2):311–319.
98. Kalayci M, Cagavi F, Gul S, et al. Intramedullary spinal cord metastases: diagnosis and treatment—an illustrated review. *Acta Neurochir (Wien)* 2004;146(12):1347–1354; discussion 1354.
99. Lee SS, Kim MK, Sym SJ, et al. Intramedullary spinal cord metastases: a single-institution experience. *J Neurooncol* 2007;84(1):85–89.
100. Clarke JL, Perez HR, Jacks LM, et al. Leptomeningeal metastases in the MRI era. *Neurology* 2010;74(18):1449–1454.
101. Lamovec J, Zidar A. Association of leptomeningeal carcinomatosis in carcinoma of the breast with infiltrating lobular carcinoma. An autopsy study. *Arch Pathol Lab Med* 1991;115(5):507–510.
102. Morris PG, Reiner AS, Szenberg OR, et al. Leptomeningeal metastasis from non-small cell lung cancer: survival and the impact of whole brain radiotherapy. *J Thorac Oncol* 2012;7(2):382–385.
103. Gleissner B, Chamberlain MC. Neoplastic meningitis. *Lancet Neurol* 2006;5(5):443–452.
104. Straathof CS, de Bruin HG, Dippel DW, et al. The diagnostic accuracy of magnetic resonance imaging and cerebrospinal fluid cytology in leptomeningeal metastasis. *J Neurol* 1999;246(9):810–814.
105. Seute T, Leffers P, ten Velde GP, et al. Leptomeningeal metastases from small cell lung carcinoma. *Cancer* 2005;104(8):1700–1705.
106. Chamberlain MC, Kormanik P. Carcinoma meningitis secondary to non-small cell lung cancer: combined modality therapy. *Arch Neurol* 1998;55(4):506–512.
107. Hitchins RN, Bell DR, Woods RL, et al. A prospective randomized trial of single-agent versus combination chemotherapy in meningeal carcinomatosis. *J Clin Oncol* 1987;5(10):1655–1662.
108. Grossman SA, Finkelstein DM, Ruckdeschel JC, et al. Randomized prospective comparison of intraventricular methotrexate and thiotepa in patients with previously untreated neoplastic meningitis. Eastern Cooperative Oncology Group. *J Clin Oncol* 1993;11(3):561–569.
109. Glantz MJ, Jaeckle KA, Chamberlain MC, et al. A randomized controlled trial comparing intrathecal sustained-release cytarabine (DepoCyt) to intrathecal methotrexate in patients with neoplastic meningitis from solid tumors. *Clin Cancer Res* 1999;5(11):3394–3402.
110. Kim DY, Lee KW, Yun T, et al. Comparison of intrathecal chemotherapy for leptomeningeal carcinomatosis of a solid tumor: methotrexate alone versus methotrexate in combination with cytosine arabinoside and hydrocortisone. *Jpn J Clin Oncol* 2003;33(12):608–612.
111. Boogerd W, van den Bent MJ, Koehler PJ, et al. The relevance of intraventricular chemotherapy for leptomeningeal metastasis in breast cancer: a randomised study. *Eur J Cancer* 2004;40(18):2726–2733.

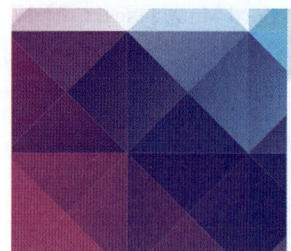

CHAPTER 97

Palliation of Bone Metastases

Alexander A. Harris and William F. Hartsell

BACKGROUND AND INCIDENCE

Metastatic disease to the bone is a common cause of pain and other significant symptoms that are detrimental to quality of life. The exact incidence of bone metastases is difficult to determine, but estimates are that >100,000 people in the United States will develop osseous metastatic disease annually.[1,2] The incidence of bone metastases varies significantly, depending on the primary site, with breast and prostate cancer accounting for up to 70% of patients with metastatic disease.[3] Bone metastases may be found in up to 85% of patients dying from breast, prostate, or lung cancer. Other primary sites with a propensity for bone metastases include thyroid, melanoma, and kidney. On the other hand, gastrointestinal sites of primary malignancy give rise to bone metastasis in only 3% to 15% of patients with metastatic disease.[4] Some hematologic malignancies, including myeloma and lymphoma, can also cause significant pain and bone destruction.

The ultimate prognosis for patients with bone metastases is poor, with median survival typically measured in months rather than years. Overall survival depends on the primary site and the presence or absence of visceral metastases. Patients with bone metastases from lung cancer have short median survival durations of 6 months. However, patients with bone metastases from breast or prostate primary sites may have significantly longer survival times. In patients with bone-only metastatic prostate or breast cancer, median survivals of 2 to 4 years have been reported.[3,5,6] Whether the survival time is only a few months or extends to multiple years, these patients will often require active treatment because of pain, difficulty with ambulation and immobility, hypercalcemia, pathologic fractures, neurologic deficits, anxiety, depression, spinal cord or nerve root compression, fatigue, insomnia or sleep disturbances, and general deterioration of quality of life.[4,7,8]

The axial skeleton is the most common site of bone metastasis, with metastasis most frequently occurring in the spine, pelvis, and ribs. The lumbar spine is the most frequent site of bone metastasis.[9-12] In the appendicular skeleton, the proximal femurs are the most common site of metastatic disease, and humeral lesions also occur frequently. The acral sites (feet and hands) are rarely involved. Certain skeletal sites are associated with specific types of metastatic cancer. For example, scapular metastases are seen more frequently from renal primaries.[13] Involvement of the skull is more common with breast primaries. The distal appendicular skeleton (tibia, fibula) and acral sites (especially the hands) are more common with lung primaries, and involvement of the toes is seen more commonly with genitourinary primaries.

The most common symptom of bone metastases is slowly progressive, insidious pain that is fairly well localized. The pain may be worse at night. Pain from the femur or acetabulum may worsen with weight bearing or ambulation. In contrast, pain from the inferior ischium or sacrum may be worse with sitting but less bothersome with ambulation. Although the pain is frequently localized, pain may radiate to other areas. This is most frequently seen with pain in the lower back, pelvis, or hips that may radiate down the legs. Pain that radiates does not necessarily indicate nerve impingement because radicular pain can also be caused by spasm of muscles that originate or insert near the area of disease (e.g., pain in the hip radiating to the knee).

The concept of "oligometastases" was proposed by Hellman and Weichselbaum in 1995.[14] This has been used as a justification for aggressive treatment of a small number of visceral metastases, and there is some evidence of benefit in certain patients with a few lung, liver, or brain metastases. This principle has also been applied to bone metastases, primarily in the setting of stereotactic body radiotherapy. Although some patients have achieved long-term disease-free survival, there is a question as to whether this simply is a factor of patient selection rather than a separate and distinct subgroup of patients.[15] The treatment for bone metastases remains in the realm of palliative and supportive care, but as more studies are performed with long-term follow-up, it is possible that the goals of treatment may change to curative in a subset of patients.

PATHOPHYSIOLOGY

There are primarily three types of cells within mature bone: osteocytes, osteoblasts, and osteoclasts. Osteoblasts originate from osteogenic cells, found in the periosteum or endosteum. The osteogenic cells differentiate into osteoblasts when there is a mechanical or chemical stimulus for remodeling or repair. The osteoblasts build bone by depositing collagen type I into the extracellular space. An inorganic complex of calcium and phosphate (hydroxyapatite) is laid down within this organic matrix to provide the strength and density of the bone. The osteoblasts then mature into osteocytes, which maintain the bone structure. Osteoclasts are multinucleated giant cells that originate from pluripotent hematopoietic bone marrow cells and adhere to the bone surface.[16] These cells create an acidophilic environment that causes dissolution of the hydroxyapatite crystals and proteolysis of the bone matrix.

The differentiation and activation of osteoclasts occur because of the effects of a group of proteins that are related to tumor necrosis factor; including osteoprotegerin, receptor activator of nuclear factor-κB (RANK), and the RANK ligand (RANKL). Osteoblasts, stromal cells, and activated T cells express and release RANKL. The RANKL binds to the RANK receptor on osteoclast precursors, which then induces the formation of mature osteoclasts. This may occur through up-regulation of RANKL expression in osteoblasts via a hedgehog signaling pathway.[17] Osteoprotegerin is a decoy receptor for RANKL and inhibits the differentiation and activation of osteoclasts.[16] The destruction of bone by osteolytic metastases is mediated by the osteoclasts, not by the tumor cells. However, the factors that activate the osteoclasts are likely produced by the tumor cells, including RANKL, interleukin-1, interleukin-6, parathyroid hormone-related peptide (PTHrP), transforming growth factor β (TGF-β), and macrophage inflammatory protein 1α.[18-20]

Normal bone is constantly being remodeled in a cycle lasting about 120 to 200 days (3 to 6 months). For the first 20 to 40 days of the cycle, the bone is resorbed by osteoclasts. The bone is then rebuilt by osteoblasts during the next 100 to 150 days.[21]

The structure of the bone changes during growth and development. At the time of birth, all bones are immature, woven bone. Woven bone is more cellular, with no organized orientation to the collagen fibers of the bone. As bones age, the woven bone is absorbed and is replaced by lamellar bone. The lamellar bone is organized circumferentially around neurovascular canals. This cylindrical structure provides much more strength than the haphazard orientation of woven bone. Most adult bone is lamellar.

Adult bone has three distinct layers; cortical, cancellous, and bone marrow. The cortical bone is the dense, compact exterior portion of the bone. This portion of the bone comprises most of the mass and strength of the skeleton. Internal to the cortical bone is the porous, haphazard network of bone tissue known as cancellous bone, which is also known as trabecular or spongy bone. Inside the porous cancellous bone is the bone marrow. There are two different types of bone marrow, red marrow and yellow marrow. Red marrow produces red blood cells, white blood cells, and platelets. Red marrow is highly vascular. Yellow marrow produces fat, cartilage, and bone. Yellow marrow is scantly vascular. At birth, all marrow is red marrow, but as bone ages, red marrow is slowly replaced by yellow marrow.

In the adult body, there are five different types of bone: long, short, flat, sesamoid, and irregular bone. Long bones consist of the epiphyses, metaphyses, and a diaphysis. The diaphysis is the long shaft of the bone, consisting of a hard cortical exterior encapsulating a central cavity consisting of cancellous bone and bone marrow, known as the medullary cavity. The epiphyses are at the ends of the bone. These are composed of hyaline cartilage initially, which becomes ossified during puberty. The metaphysis is the area between the epiphysis and diaphysis. Most of the bones of the limbs are made of long bones. Short bones are cuboid in shape and make up the bones of the wrist and ankle. Flat bones are thin and curved bones. They make up the skull and sternum. Sesamoid bones are found suspended in tendons, such as the patella. Irregular bones are oddly shaped bones that contain a thin layer of cortical tissue surrounding an interior of active cancellous and bone marrow. The majority of the axial skeleton, including the spine and pelvis, is made up of irregular bones.

Metastases to the bone most often occur in the red marrow, which is found in highest concentration in the skull, irregular bones of the axial skeleton, and the medullary portion of the appendicular skeleton. This most often occurs by hematogenous spread but may occur by direct extension as well. Involvement of adjacent bone by direct extension (e.g., mandibular involvement from an oral cavity cancer) does not necessarily imply that there is a higher likelihood of distant bone metastases, and its management is very different from that of bone metastases from hematogenous spread.

The relatively high proportion of hematogenous metastasis to bone compared with other sites in the body cannot simply be explained by blood flow, which is >30 times greater in the lung than in red bone marrow.[22] The predilection of certain tumor sites to metastasize to bone may be related to local growth factors in the bone such as TGF-β, insulin-like growth factors I and II, fibroblastic growth factors, platelet-derived growth factors, preferential adherence to endothelial surfaces in certain bones by cell adhesion molecules, or chemotactic attraction from bone cells by osteocalcin or type I collagen.[4,16,23]

Bone metastases are often described as either osteolytic or osteoblastic. However, these are different representations of abnormalities in the normal bone-remodeling process. Breast and lung cancers more commonly cause osteolytic-appearing lesions. Prostate and thyroid cancers more often have osteoblastic-appearing lesions. Only myeloma is associated with purely osteolytic lesions.[16] Most other tumors have a combination of osteolytic and osteoblastic components.

The mechanism of pain from bone metastases is not clearly understood. Possible mechanisms include mechanical instability, irritation of periosteal stretch receptors, tumor-directed osteoclast-mediated osteolysis, tumor cells themselves, tumor-induced nerve injury, production of nerve growth factor, or stimulation of other cytokine receptors.[2,3,24,25] Because the mechanisms of pain may be multifactorial, a combination of therapies may be superior to any one therapy alone.[24]

EVALUATION

The most common symptom associated with bone metastasis is pain. Therefore, the physical examination is an important step in evaluating a patient with bone metastases. The physical examination may help make decisions regarding appropriate subsequent imaging studies. Firm palpation will often elicit the specific area of pain, with "point tenderness" often pointing directly to the affected area in the bone. It is important to carefully evaluate the entire skeletal system with examination because intense pain at one site often masks subjective reports of pain at other sites. A careful physical examination may reveal hidden pain in other locations. A thorough neurologic examination is also important, especially in patients with spinal metastases, to carefully evaluate for the possibility of spinal cord, cauda equina, or nerve root compression.

Technetium-99m bone scintigraphy (nuclear medicine bone scan) is the best method for screening patients at risk for bone metastasis who may not present with bone pain. It is also useful to evaluate the extent of metastatic disease in the bone (Fig. 97.1). Bone scintigraphy is an indicator of osteoblastic activity. Because multiple myeloma is frequently purely osteolytic, bone scans are less useful for evaluating extent of disease in myeloma. Bone scintigraphy is not specific for metastatic disease, and positive findings must often be confirmed using other imaging studies. A confirmatory study is especially important in a weight-bearing bone such as the proximal femur. False-positive readings may be seen in areas of arthritis, trauma, prior fractures, or Paget's disease. In addition, the osteoblastic activity in healing bone after treatment may give the appearance of progressive disease. False-negative readings may occur in fast-growing, highly aggressive tumors, especially if these are mainly osteolytic.

For symptomatic patients with point tenderness or for patients with an abnormal bone scan, plain radiographs are typically the most appropriate first or next imaging study.[26]

FIGURE 97.1. Nuclear medicine bone scan from a woman with metastatic breast cancer. The bone scan shows the abnormality in multiple osseous sites, as well as in the right breast and axilla.

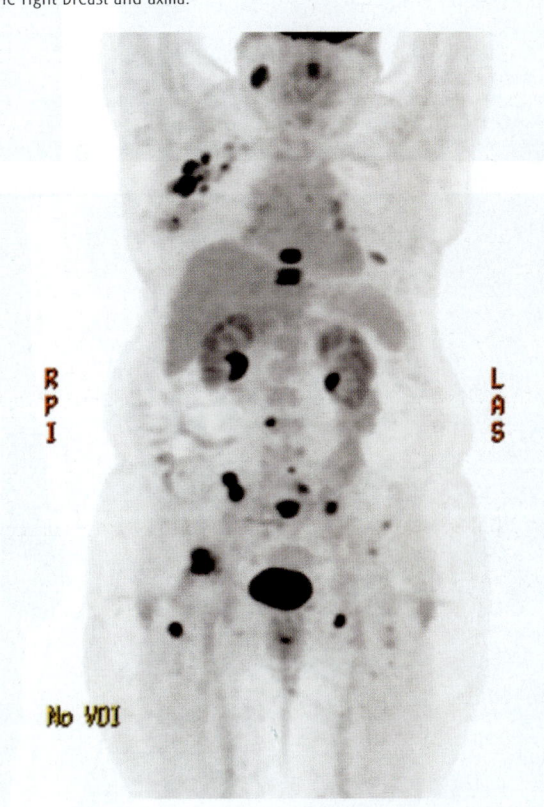

Radiographs are easy to obtain and inexpensive. The appearance of bone metastases on x-rays varies depending on the primary site and histology, with some appearing osteolytic and some osteoblastic. However, nearly all bone metastases have components of both osteolytic and osteoblastic processes. The primary disadvantage of plain radiographs is that small lesions are rarely seen. Approximately 30% to 50% of the bone mineral content must be lost before the lesion will be apparent on x-rays.

Computed tomography (CT) scans are more sensitive than plain radiographs and may be better able to localize the lesion within the bone. However, CT scans are more expensive and more time-consuming and may not be useful as a screening tool for skeletal metastasis. The CT may be useful in defining the extent of cortical destruction and helping to assess the risk of a pathologic fracture.[27] In addition, the CT scan may be used to guide needle biopsies to obtain a tissue diagnosis (Fig. 97.2A and B). CT scans have limited usefulness in detecting marrow involvement but are much better than plain radiographs at evaluating soft tissue extension of disease.

Magnetic resonance imaging (MRI) is better than plain radiography or nuclear medicine bone scintigraphy at assessing

FIGURE 97.2. Images from a patient with metastatic prostate cancer. Nuclear medicine bone scan **(A)** shows uptake in the right pedicle of L4, seen as an osteoblastic lesion on axial CT **(B)**. This was biopsy confirmed as metastatic prostate cancer. The bone scan does not demonstrate the lesion in the L2 vertebral body, which is demonstrated on the sagittal **(C)** and axial **(D)** magnetic resonance images.

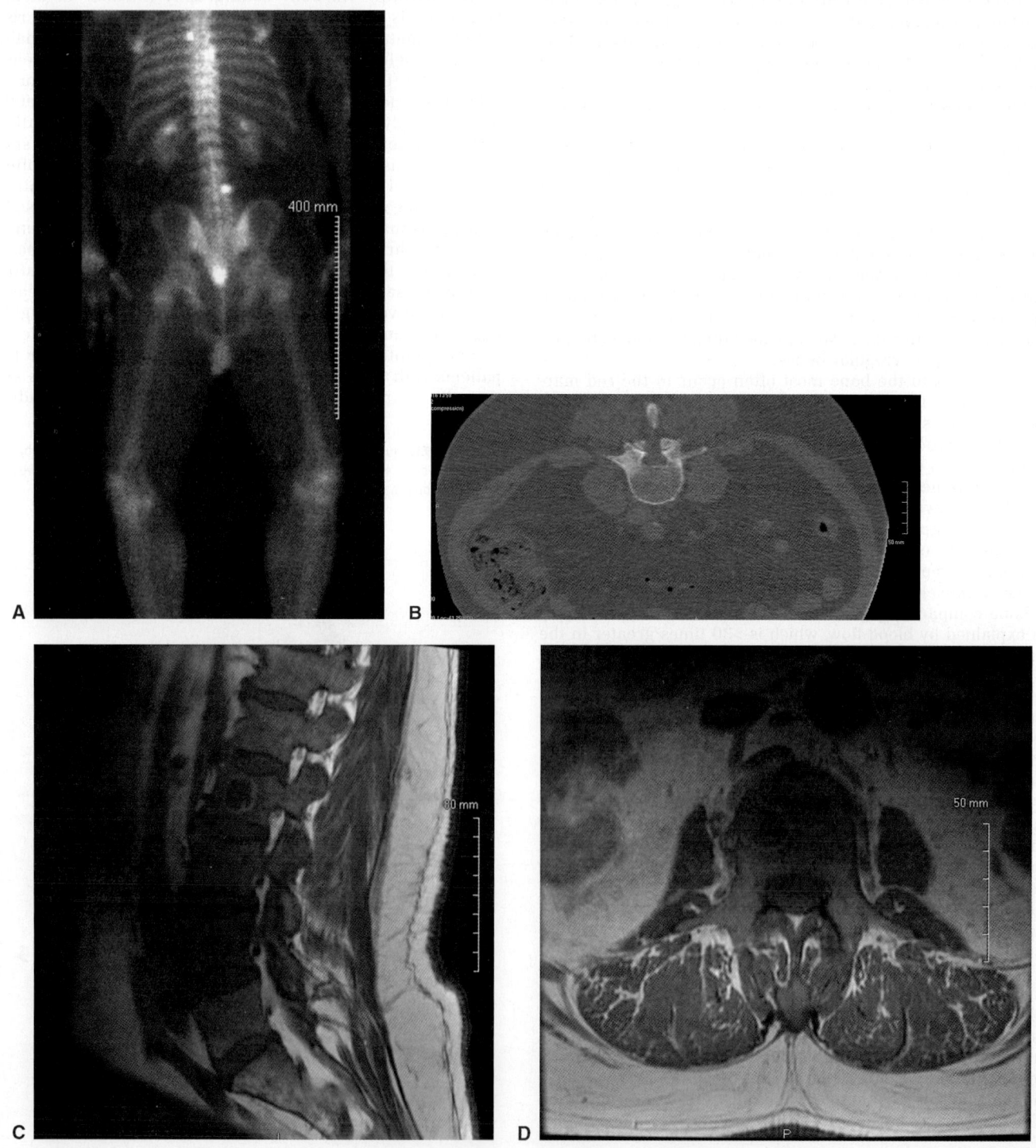

the involvement of trabecular bone and bone marrow, especially in the vertebral bodies (Fig. 97.2C and D). The findings are typically best seen on T1 contrast-enhanced images and short-tau inversion recovery (STIR) images. Metastatic prostate cancer is visible as high-intensity lesions on the STIR images and is visible prior to its appearance on bone scintigraphy.[28] In addition, MRI scans are useful in determining the involvement of neurovascular structures. MRI scans are not useful as a screening tool for bone metastases because of the high cost and lengthy time of the exam. However, MRI scans may be more sensitive than bone scintigraphy in the vertebral body region. The sensitivity of MRI scanning has been reported as 91% to 100%, compared with 62% to 85% for bone scintigraphy.[28,29] In addition, MRI images can help distinguish whether a vertebral body compression fracture is from malignancy or from osteoporosis.

Positron emission tomography (PET) scanning evaluates areas of increased metabolic activity, most commonly using the 18-fluorodeoxyglucose (FDG) isotope. These scans are useful in detecting highly metabolic osteolytic bone metastases but are less sensitive for the less metabolically active osteoblastic metastases. In addition, precise determination of the location of lesions is difficult with PET scans, but the use of simultaneous CT scans allows for much better localization of the abnormal FDG uptake.[30] PET scans may be useful as a whole-body screening tool.[30,31] Comparative studies have shown PET scans to be more sensitive than Tc-99m scintigraphy or whole-body MRI scans in detecting bone metastases.[32,33] There may be limitations in the sensitivity of PET scanning in certain areas such as the skull, where the intense physiologic metabolic uptake from the adjacent brain parenchyma may obscure small skull metastases. 18-FDG-PET scans have been used for many epithelial tumor types, but less frequently for prostate cancers. There are multiple new PET scan isotopes, which may be more sensitive and more specific for metastatic prostate cancer, including ^{18}F-NaF, ^{11}C-choline, ^{11}C-acetate, and ^{18}F-fluciclovine.[34]

PAIN MANAGEMENT

The majority of patients with bone metastases will experience pain during their disease course, and pain control can significantly improve their quality of life. Pain management may be achieved either by debulking disease using cytotoxic therapy or by symptomatic control with pharmacologic interventions.

Despite increasing understanding about the effective treatment of pain, patients with pain from bone metastases frequently have inadequate pain management. Barriers to pain treatment include physician underestimation of the patient's pain and reluctance by the patient to report pain.[35] In addition, concerns about opioid abuse and dependence may lead to undertreatment of cancer pain. There is a significant discrepancy between the physician estimate of pain and the pain level reported by the patient.[36] The use of a validated pain scale, such as the Brief Pain Inventory, gives the patient an opportunity to describe both the severity of pain and the interference it has with daily functioning in a manner that can be understood both by the patient and the physician.[35] This also allows for distinguishable comparisons of pain levels over time, to better assess the effectiveness of treatments.

Pain control can be achieved in the majority of patients using the World Health Organization analgesic ladder. Step I uses nonopioid analgesics such as acetaminophen or nonsteroidal anti-inflammatory drugs; step II uses weak opioids such as codeine; step III uses strong opioids such as morphine or oxycodone. These medications are increased as necessary until the patient is free of pain. Typically, the medications are given on a routine schedule ("by the clock") rather than waiting until a certain level of pain is reached ("on demand").

Using this schedule, 70% to 76% of patients will have good pain relief.[37,38] Adjuvant medications such as gabapentin, pregabalin, or amitriptyline may be added for neuropathic pain. Antianxiety or antidepressant medications may also be of benefit in selected patients.

The opioid-based pain medications frequently cause constipation and may cause nausea. Patients using opioid medications should routinely be administered a fiber medication with or without a stool softener to minimize constipation. Other side effects of the opioid analgesics may include sedation, mental status changes, and mood changes.

SURGICAL MANAGEMENT

Surgical management of bone metastases is performed primarily to prevent or treat pathologic fractures. The goals of surgical intervention are to prevent or relieve pain, improve motor function, and improve overall quality of life. Treatment techniques are simpler and more effective when the procedure is performed prophylactically for an impending fracture rather than after the occurrence of a pathologic fracture. The risk of pathologic fracture depends on multiple factors, including location and extent of the lesion; whether the lesion is osteolytic, osteoblastic, or mixed; and the primary cancer site.

Fractures of the weight-bearing bones are the most likely to cause significant functional deficits. The proximal femur may have a higher propensity for fracture than other sites, but some authors have suggested that the fracture risk in upper limbs is similar to the risk in the femur. Whether or not there is a difference in the risk of fracture, the peritrochanteric femur is the site most likely to cause serious morbidity, and therefore, the threshold for prophylactic intervention should be relatively low. The femur accounts for 65% of pathologic fractures requiring surgical intervention.[39] The humerus and vertebral bodies are also sites that require special attention because of the potential functional deficits from pathologic fractures.

The size of the bone metastasis is an important predictor of risk of fracture, especially with regard to the extent of cortical destruction. Various models have been used to predict the risk of pathologic fracture based on the size of the lesion. In series using plain radiographs, lesions ≥2.5 cm in the cortex of the femur were significantly more likely to fracture.[40] The proportion of cortical destruction is important as well. The risk of pathologic fracture of the femur begins to significantly increase when there is destruction of >50% of the cortex; the risk of fracture is 80% when >75% of the cortex is destroyed.[41] Femoral lesions with axial cortical destruction >30 mm had a 23% risk of pathologic fracture, compared with 3% risk of fracture for cortical destruction ≤30 mm.[42] The location within the bone is important as well. An experimental model has shown that the greatest reduction in strength of the femur occurs with lesions in the inferior and medial aspect of the femoral neck, and posterior lesions have the least impact (Fig. 97.3).[43]

A scoring system proposed by Mirels[44] has a 12-point scale based on the location of the lesion, pain, extent of cortical destruction, and radiographic appearance (Table 97.1). The risk of fracture is 15% for a score of 8 and 33% for a score of 9. He proposed that prophylactic fixation is indicated for a score of ≥9.

The decision to proceed with surgery should be based on a number of factors, which include but are not limited to the estimated risk of pathologic fracture and overall life expectancy. For patients with a very limited life expectancy, surgery may not be indicated even if the risk of pathologic fracture is relatively high.[39] Clinical prediction of survival may be more accurate than relying on specific parameters such as

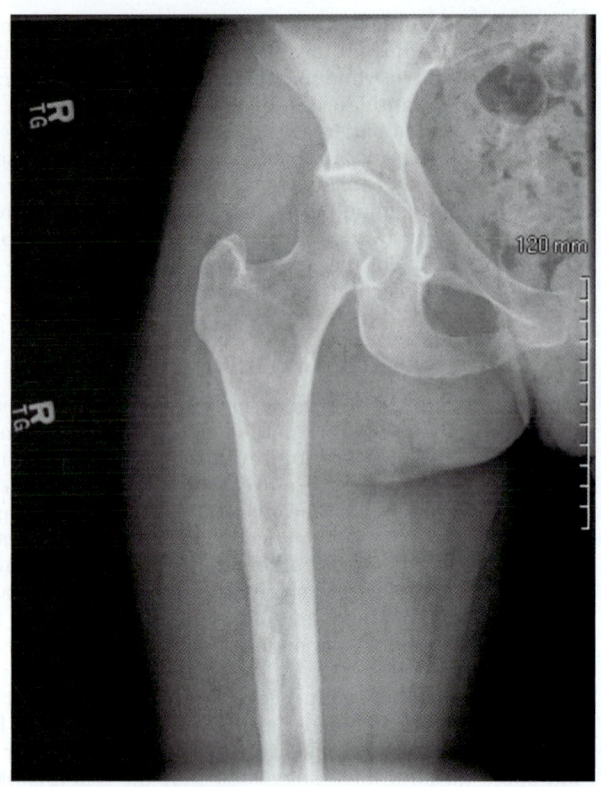
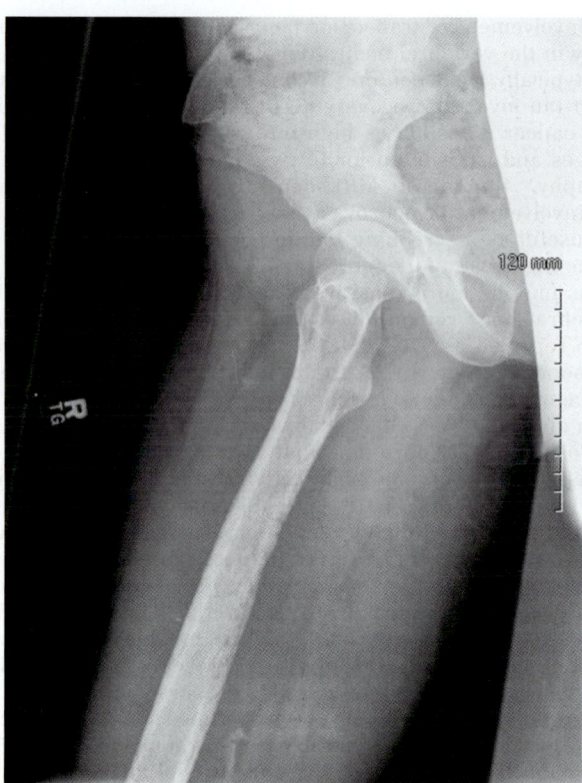

FIGURE 97.3. Anterior–posterior **(A)** and oblique **(B)** radiographs of the right femur in a patient with metastatic breast cancer. Note the significant destruction of the posterior cortex from the proximal to mid diaphysis of the femur, in a "moth-eaten" appearance.

diagnosis (primary site), performance status, number of bone metastases, presence of visceral metastases, and hemoglobin level.[45]

Femoral fractures are the most common site of surgical correction. Fractures of the femoral neck can be managed either by total hip arthroplasty (which replaces both the femoral head and acetabulum) or a proximal femoral endoprosthesis alone.[39] Fractures of the intertrochanteric area may be managed by open reduction and internal fixation without the use of a prosthesis. This may allow for better long-term gait because of preservation of the hip flexor and adductor strength.[39] Lytic disease that extends below the intertrochanteric area is treated with a long intramedullary rod that provides stability throughout the length of the femur. If there is significant destruction of the greater trochanter and femoral neck or head in addition to subtrochanteric involvement, a prosthetic replacement would be more appropriate than a reconstruction nail.[46] Fractures of the distal femur may be managed either with a plate and compression screw or with an intracondylar nail and screws augmented by intramedullary methyl methacrylate cement. The latter method may reduce the risk of late failure of the repair, especially in patients receiving postoperative radiation therapy.[39]

Repair of pathologic fractures of the humerus may be more problematic because of the small intramedullary canal and because of the proximity of the radial nerve, which may require extensive dissection.[39] Pathologic fractures of the proximal humerus will frequently require prosthetic replacement.[39] Fractures in the diaphysis may be repaired with a compression plate and screws. An alternative is to use a segmental diaphyseal replacement prosthetic device, which involves a prosthetic device than can be cemented into an allograft.[46] Supracondylar fractures are difficult to manage because the shape of the bone is not conducive to a plate and screws; these lesions may require intramedullary rods inserted in a retrograde manner through both the medial and lateral condyles, supplemented by intramedullary cement.[39]

Most pathologic fractures of the pelvis do not require surgical intervention, except for those involving the acetabulum.[39] Repair of acetabular fractures may involve the use of a total hip acetabular prosthesis, but more extensive lesions may require reconstruction that transfers the load-bearing stresses into more structurally intact bone in the iliac bone or sacroiliac joint.[39]

INTERVENTIONAL TECHNIQUES

Vertebroplasty is an effective method of palliating pain from vertebral body metastases, even in patients who have received prior radiotherapy.[47] Most patients experience pain relief within 48 hours. The procedure involves percutaneous injection of methyl methacrylate under CT or fluoroscopic guidance. Retropulsion of bone, epidural tumor, or collapse of the bone to less than one-third of its original height are relative contraindications to percutaneous vertebroplasty because of the risk of extrusion of the cement into the spinal canal, potentially causing neurologic complications. In some patients with epidural tumor, percutaneous vertebroplasty can be performed safely and effectively with a relatively low

TABLE 97.1 MIRELS' SCORING SYSTEM OF PREDICTION OF PATHOLOGIC FRACTURE RISK				
Score	Pain	Location	Cortical Destruction	Radiographic Appearance
1	Mild	Upper limb	<1/3	Blastic
2	Moderate	Lower limb	1/3–2/3	Mixed
3	Severe	Peritrochanteric	>2/3	Lytic

A score is assigned for each of the four categories, and the sum of those scores is used to estimate the risk of pathologic fracture.
Reprinted from Mirels H. Metastatic disease in long bones: a proposed scoring system for diagnosing impending pathologic fractures. *Clin Relat Orthop Res* 1989;249:256–264. With permission.

risk of serious complications.[48,49] However, the procedure should be considered with some caution; in a systematic review of 987 patients, there were 5 deaths and 19 other serious complications.[50]

Kyphoplasty involves percutaneous placement of a balloon-like device into a symptomatic spinal metastasis (most commonly into a fractured or compressed vertebral body).[51] The balloon is then inflated to restore the height of the vertebral body, and methyl methacrylate is subsequently injected into this cavity. This procedure may provide significant relief of pain and improve overall functioning, especially in patients with mechanical instability of the vertebral body.[52,53] Kyphoplasty may be a better option than vertebroplasty in patients with vertebral wall deficiency.[52]

An ablative procedure is frequently coupled with vertebroplasty or kyphoplasty.[54] Radiofrequency ablation (RFA) may be used to ablate the tumor but is most effective for tumors that are osteolytic or mixed osteolytic and blastic. The RFA may not be as effective in tumors that are primarily sclerotic. Cryoablation may be used for larger lesions or those that are sclerotic. For both of these procedures, special attention to cord and nerve temperatures is required to minimize the risk of complications.

SYSTEMIC TREATMENT

The rationale for using systemic therapy in the management of bone metastasis is compelling. The pathophysiology of bone metastasis involves hematogenous dissemination, and most patients with bone metastasis suffer from multiple synchronous sites of disease. In theory, administering systemic cytotoxic therapy should deliver palliative benefit by simultaneously addressing all sites of bone metastasis. A localized therapy such as external-beam radiation may be most appropriate for palliation if symptoms are localized. On the other hand, systemic chemotherapy may offer palliative benefit if symptoms are diffuse or constitutional and disease is widespread. The chemotherapy drugs are frequently given with bisphosphonates and corticosteroids, which may affect the response rates.

Measurement of response to systemic therapy has generally been with the same criteria used for solid metastatic tumors: a measurable radiographic change. This works well for lung and liver metastasis but not as well for bone metastasis. For bone metastases, the definition of a complete response is complete disappearance of all lesions on radiographs for at least 4 weeks. This is unlikely to occur even if all tumor cells are eradicated. A partial response requires some recalcification of lytic lesions, which may not be evident for 6 months or more.[55] PET scans may be more accurate at assessing response in a timely manner but are too expensive to be used as a routine follow-up evaluation for bone metastases. Markers of bone resorption may be a good way to detect response to therapy but are not clinically available at this time. Response to therapy for other modalities (i.e., radiotherapy, bisphosphonates) is measured in terms of pain relief and quality-of-life measures. Unfortunately, there is not much literature on accurate and reliable response criteria to palliative systemic therapy for bone metastasis. Most of the studies of chemotherapy for metastatic disease involve patients with visceral as well as osseous metastases. The responses in terms of pain are typically reported for all patients, not just those with bone metastases, so pure bone metastatic pain is difficult to ascertain. There is more information regarding response to chemotherapy for patients with metastatic prostate cancer because this more frequently involves bone-only metastatic disease.

Tannock et al.[56] recommended using more relevant end points of palliation. They performed a randomized trial of mitoxantrone plus prednisone versus prednisone alone for patients with hormone-refractory prostate cancer and pain. Improvement in pain was seen in 29% of patients receiving the chemotherapy, compared with 12% of those who received prednisone alone. In a subsequent study, they compared mitoxantrone and prednisone plus or minus clodronate for a similar group of patients. Most had mild pain at study entry (160 of 209; 77%), and the remainder had moderate pain scores. The patients with moderate pain who received chemotherapy and clodronate had a 58% response rate ($\geq$2-point improvement in pain score) compared with 26% for those who received chemotherapy alone. The median duration of pain response was 6 months. The TAX327 phase III trial was conducted in 1,006 men with hormone-resistant metastatic prostate cancer and randomized patients to receive prednisone combined with either docetaxel or mitoxantrone. The docetaxel arm showed an improvement in overall survival, lower cancer-induced bone pain, and better objective tumor response.[57]

In patients with bone metastasis, there is seldom reason to combine chemotherapy with concurrent radiation therapy because of the potential for increased toxicity when both modalities are delivered concurrently.

A number of hormonal therapies are available in the management of metastatic prostate and breast cancer. In properly selected patients, hormonal therapy has the potential for providing excellent palliation of metastatic disease with limited morbidity. In 1984, the Medical Research Council started a prospective, randomized trial in which 938 patients who either had asymptomatic metastatic prostate cancer or were not medical candidates for definitive therapy were randomized to immediate versus delayed hormone ablation therapy. Hormone ablation was achieved using either a luteinizing hormone–releasing hormone agonist or by orchiectomy. This study showed that immediate versus delayed initiation of hormone ablation therapy in the subset of patients with metastatic prostate cancer helped to prevent serious complications from metastatic disease. Serious complications including pathologic fracture, spinal cord compression, development of extraskeletal metastases, and ureteral obstruction were twofold more frequent in patients whose hormonal therapy was deferred compared with patients who received immediate hormone ablation therapy.[58]

Osteoclast inhibitors are also often used in conjunction with other systemic treatments. The bisphosphonates are pyrophosphate analogs that bind to calcium phosphate with high affinity and are potent agents affecting bone resorption through osteoclast inhibition.[59] The nitrogen-containing bisphosphonates inhibit the key enzyme farnesyl diphosphate synthase in the mevalonate pathway.[60] This prevents the action of several additional enzymes required for bone resorption. The bisphosphonates include pamidronate, alendronate, ibandronate, risedronate, and zoledronic acid. Zoledronic Acid is much more potent than the other bisphosphonates, in part because it also inhibits tumor cell adhesion to the extracellular matrix. There is evidence that the bisphosphonates also induce apoptosis in cancer cells.[61]

The initial studies of bisphosphonate usage were primarily in women with metastatic breast cancer. Pamidronate was evaluated in multiple randomized, prospective studies of women with osteolytic bone metastases from breast cancer. The Aredia Breast Cancer Study Group Protocols 18 and 19 enrolled women receiving either chemotherapy (P19) or hormonal therapy (P18). In the P18 study, 372 women randomized to receive either placebo or pamidronate 90 mg as a 2-hour infusion every 4 weeks for 24 cycles.[62] The primary end point was the prevention of "skeletal-related complications" (pathologic fractures, spinal cord compression, hypercalcemia, or the requirement for surgery or radiation therapy on bone). There were fewer skeletal-related complications in the pamidronate arm (475 events vs. 648 in the placebo group), but the benefit in reducing pathologic fractures and hypercalcemia was not significant until 18 to 24 months of treatment. The primary difference was that twice as many placebo patients required radiation therapy for palliation of pain, most often in the first 6 to 12 months. There was no difference in survival, although pain levels and serum markers of bone resorption were significantly lower in the group receiving pamidronate. In the P19 study, women with stage IV breast cancer who were receiving chemotherapy and had lytic bone metastasis were given placebo or pamidronate for 12 monthly cycles.[63] Patients in the pamidronate arm suffered fewer overall skeletal complications and had a greater median time to first skeletal complication when compared with patients in the placebo arm of the study. Women treated with pamidronate maintained better performance status and had less bone pain secondary to metastasis.

Rosen et al.[64] evaluated 773 patients with bone metastases from solid tumors, including lung cancer, renal cell carcinoma, head and neck cancers, thyroid, and other primary sites (exclusive of breast and prostate cancer). They compared placebo with zoledronic acid in doses of either 4 or 8 mg given every 3 weeks for 9 months. The primary end point was proportion of patients developing a skeletal-related event (SRE), including pathologic fracture, spinal cord compression, or the need for surgery or radiation therapy. The proportion of patients developing an SRE was 44% in the placebo group compared with 38% in the 4-mg zoledronic acid group ($P = .127$) and 35% in the 8-mg group ($P = .023$). The time to development of an SRE was significantly longer with zoledronic acid compared with placebo (230 vs. 163 days; $P = .017$). The dose of the 8-mg group was reduced to 4 mg during the latter part of the study because of safety concerns, and thus 25% of patients in the 8-mg treatment arm actually received only 4 mg per dose. In addition, only 25% of patients received the full 9-month course of treatment because of death (27%), adverse events (21%), patient decision to discontinue (15%), or "insufficient efficacy" (7%). There was no improvement in two specific events—surgery to bone and spinal cord compression—in the patients receiving zoledronic acid compared with placebo. In addition, the need for analgesics gradually increased and functional capacity decreased from baseline to month 9 in all groups, with no differences between zoledronic acid and placebo.

The Medical Research Council PRO4 and PRO5 were two prospective, randomized trials conducted to evaluate sodium clodronate in men with prostate cancer. Long-term data showed that sodium clodronate improved overall survival in men with metastatic prostate cancer who were starting hormone therapy, but there was no improvement in overall survival for men with nonmetastatic disease.[65]

Complications of supportive therapy with bisphosphonates include osteoradionecrosis (particularly of the jaw) and renal insufficiency.[66] The mechanism of bisphosphonate-induced osteoradionecrosis is not known. Risk factors include the intravenous use of pamidronate and zoledronic acid, duration of treatment of 36 months or longer, older age in patients with multiple myeloma, and need for periodontal procedures.[67] Bisphosphonates are not metabolized by the body and are excreted by the kidneys. Bisphosphonate therapy can lead to renal toxicity. The incidence of renal toxicity is 9% to 15% in trials when 4 mg of zoledronic acid is delivered intravenously during 15 minutes.[66] Moreover, the rate of renal toxicity depends on underlying renal disease, dose of bisphosphonate used, and duration of the infusion.

Another form of systemic therapy is the use of agents that target the RANK pathway. Denosumab is a human monoclonal antibody specific for the RANKL. The antibody binds to RANKL and thus inhibits the formation, activation, maturation, and survival of osteoclasts.[68] In randomized, prospective comparisons of denosumab with zoledronic acid in patients with metastatic breast or prostate cancer, denosumab was superior to zoledronic acid in delaying or preventing the time to skeletal-related events.[69,70]

RADIATION THERAPY

Radiation therapy has been reported to be effective in palliating painful bone metastases, with partial pain relief seen in 60% to 90% of patients and complete pain relief in 30% to 50% of patients. These data are primarily from meta-analyses of studies using physician evaluation of pain. When patient evaluation of pain is used, pain improvement is seen in 60% to 80% of patients and complete pain relief is seen in 15% to 40% of patients.[71] The response to treatment depends on a large number of factors, including sex, primary site and histology, performance status, type of lesion (osteolytic vs. osteoblastic), location of the metastases, weight-bearing versus non–weight-bearing site, extent of disease, number of painful sites, marital status, and level of pain prior to treatment. The effectiveness of the treatment also depends on the goal: palliation of pain, prevention of pathologic fracture, avoidance of future treatments, or local control of the disease. The doses required and volumes treated may be quite different for each of these goals. In addition to pain relief, other symptoms may also be relieved by radiotherapy. Patients who have improvement in pain after radiotherapy may also have improvement in emotional functioning, decreased insomnia, decreased constipation, and overall improvement in quality-of-life scores.[72] Radiation therapy should be an integral part of palliative treatment for bone metastases to treat pain and prevent other symptoms.[73]

Local-field external-beam radiation therapy is typically used for palliation of a few discrete areas of painful metastases (Fig. 97.4). The first large randomized study evaluating different dose and fractionation schemes was the Radiation Therapy Oncology Group (RTOG) 74-02 trial.[74] Patients with solitary bone metastases were randomized to 40.5 Gy in 15 fractions versus 20 Gy in 5 fractions. Patients with multiple painful metastases were allocated to one of four treatment schedules: 30 Gy in 10 fractions, 15 Gy in 5 fractions, 20 Gy in 5 fractions, or 25 Gy in 5 fractions. The initial analysis by Tong et al.[74] in 1982 showed no statistically significant difference in response rates between any of the treatment arms, with complete responses in 49% to 61% of patients. These results were questioned by Blitzer,[75] who reanalyzed the data using different criteria for complete response, which excluded patients who received repeat treatment, and defined complete response as no pain and no analgesic usage. With this adjustment in response definition, there was a significant difference in response favoring the longer treatment courses: 40.5 Gy in 15 fractions for the solitary metastases and 30 Gy in 10 fractions for multiple metastases. This was offered as evidence that higher doses were necessary for optimal palliation, even though one of the highest biologic doses for multiple fractions (25 Gy in 5 fractions) had one of the lower response rates. This reanalysis highlighted the importance of retreatment in this group of patients, especially in those given lower total doses during the initial course of radiation therapy.

There have been multiple randomized, prospective trials evaluating different dose and fractionation schemes.[74,76-88] Most of the earlier studies evaluated different multifraction treatment regimens (Table 97.2). No significant difference was seen between longer-course treatments and the shorter-duration, lower-total-dose treatment courses. Two randomized studies evaluated single doses of radiation therapy for palliation of bone metastases. Hoskin et al.[89] randomized patients to 4 versus 8 Gy, and Jeremic et al.[90] randomized patients to one of three dose levels, 4 versus 6 versus 8 Gy. In both of these studies, the 8-Gy arm was superior to 4 Gy,

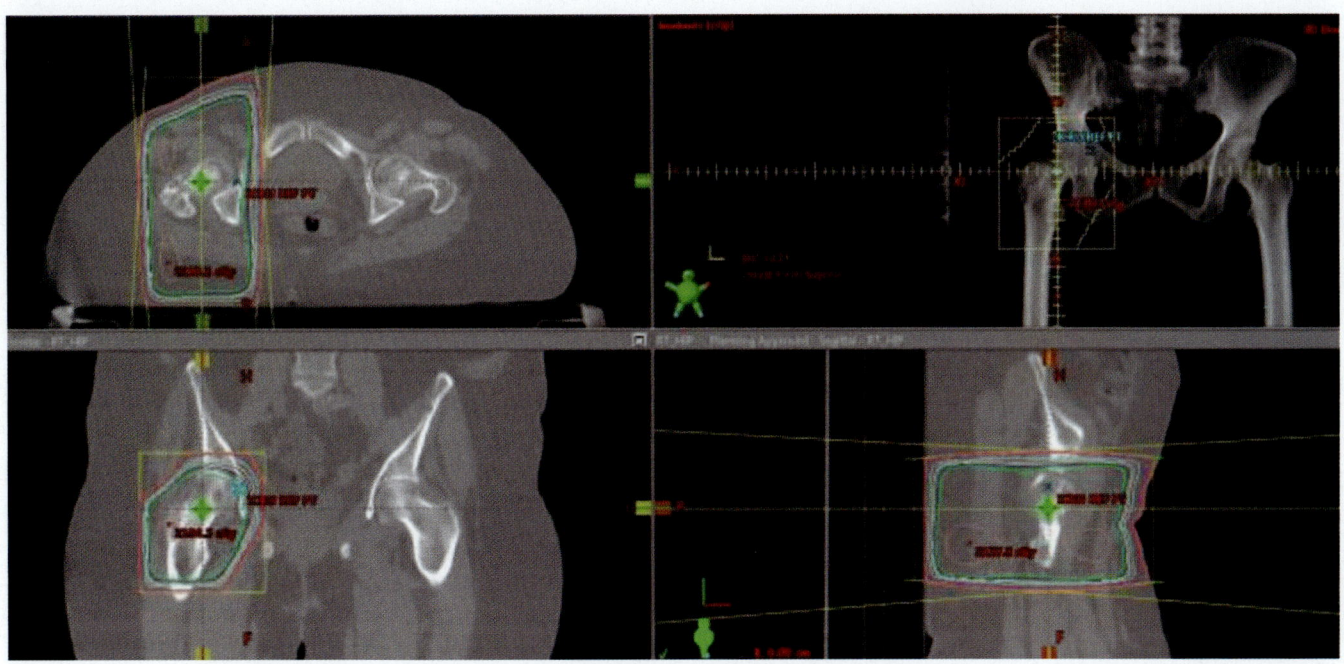

FIGURE 97.4. Isodose plan for a patient receiving radiation therapy to the right hip, showing axial and coronal projections of the doses as well as a digitally reconstructed radiograph of the treatment fields.

indicating that there is a threshold dose necessary to achieve adequate palliation. Most of the randomized trials during the last 15 years used a multiple-fraction treatment scheme as the control arm and a single dose of 8 to 10 Gy as the study arm (Tables 97.3 and 97.4).

Two large studies compared single-dose treatment to longer courses of radiation therapy. The Dutch trial evaluated patients with bone metastases from solid tumors, primarily breast (39%), prostate (23%), and lung (25%); patients with metastatic melanoma and renal cell carcinomas were excluded.[88] The primary end point was patient-assessed pain relief, evaluated on an 11-point scale (0 = no pain, 10 = worst imaginable pain). A total of 1,171 patients were randomized to either 8 Gy in a single fraction or 24 Gy in six fractions. The painful areas had to be included in a single-treatment volume. The spine (36%) and pelvis (30%) were the two most common sites of treatment. The median pain score was 6.3, with a minimum score of 2. About half of the patient were receiving narcotic pain medications prior to randomization, and slightly more than half (53%) were receiving systemic therapy. The median survival after treatment was 30 weeks, with no difference between the two treatment groups.

There was no difference in overall or complete response rates between the single-dose versus longer-course treatment arms. Overall, 71% of patients achieved a response to therapy during follow-up, with 35% achieving a complete response. Most of the responses occurred within the first 4 to 6 weeks after treatment. Complete response rates were higher for patients with breast and prostate primaries than with lung or other primary sites (44% and 41% vs. 21% and 16%, respectively).

There were two significant differences between the two treatment groups: retreatment rates and pathologic fracture rates. The rate of pathologic fracture in the treated area was 4% for the 8-Gy single-treatment arm compared with 2% for the 24 Gy/six fraction group. The median time to fracture was similar for the two groups at 21 and 17 weeks. Although there was a significant difference in pathologic fracture between the two groups, these rates are still relatively low. There was also a significant difference in retreatment rates between the two arms of the study, with a much higher likelihood of a second course of treatment in the single-treatment group. The group of patients receiving 24 Gy in six fractions initially was given a second course of treatment 7% of the time, whereas 25% of the 8-Gy single-fraction group was given retreatment. Retreatment occurred more commonly with lung/other tumors than with breast/prostate primaries. In addition, the retreatment was given at a lower pain score (median 6.8 for 8-Gy single-fraction compared with 7.5 for the multiple-fraction group) and at an earlier time (14 weeks after initial treatment compared with 23 weeks). This may indicate a greater willingness to reirradiate after a single dose of 8 Gy or more reluctance to give retreatment after a higher initial dose of radiation therapy.

TABLE 97.2 RANDOMIZED TRIALS WITH ≥100 EVALUABLE PATIENTS COMPARING MULTIPLE-FRACTION TREATMENTS FOR PALLIATION OF BONE METASTASES

Study	Number of Patients (Number Evaluable)	Dose (Gy)/Number of Fractions	Complete Response[a] (%)	Overall Response[a] (%)	Pathologic Fractures (%)
Tong et al.,[74] 1982, U.S. (solitary treatment site)	266 (146)	20/5	53	82	4
		40/15	61	85	18
Tong et al.,[74] 1982, U.S. (multiple sites)	750 (613)	15/5	49	87	5
		20/5	56	85	7
		25/5	49	83	9
		30/10	57	78	8
Hirokawa et al.,[80] 1988, Japan	128 (128)	25/5	NA	75	NA
		30/10		75	
Rasmusson et al.,[87] 1995, Denmark	217 (127)	15/3	NA	69	NA
		30/10		66	
Niewald et al.,[86] 1996, Germany	100 (100)	20/5	33	77	8
		30/15	31	86	13

[a]Response rates listed are for pain relief.
Number of patients entered on study and number of patients evaluable for response; dosage schedule; complete and overall responses; and proportion of patients with pathologic fractures after treatment. NA, not available from published report.

TABLE 97.3 RANDOMIZED TRIALS OF SINGLE VERSUS MULTIPLE FRACTIONS WITH ≥100 EVALUABLE PATIENTS: DEMOGRAPHICS AND STUDY DESIGN

Study	Number of Patients (Number Evaluable)	Primary End Point	Secondary End Point(s)	Primary Site	Treatment Site	Response Evaluation Time[a]	Percentage Severe Pain Pretreatment[b]
Foro Arnalot et al.,[77] 2008, Spain	160	Pain and relief analgesics	—	Breast, 27% Lung, 26% Prostate, 25%	Pelvis, 39% Spine, 36% Long bones, 14%	—	50 (median pain score of 7)
Kaasa et al.,[81] 2006, Norway/Sweden	376	Pain relief	Fatigue, quality of life	Prostate, 38% Breast, 30% Lung, 11%	Spine, 38% Pelvis, 35% Extremities, 20%	—	35–41
Hartsell et al.,[79] 2005, U.S./Canada	949 (898)	Pain relief	Analgesic use, toxicity, path, fracture rate, retreatment rate	Breast, 50% Prostate, 50%	C spine, 5% T spine, 19% L spine, 27%	3 mo	72–73
Kirkbride et al.,[82] 2000, Canada	398 (287)	Pain relief and analgesics	—	Breast, 40% Lung, 26% Prostate, 23%	Spine, 30% Pelvis, 29%	3 mo	—
Steenland et al.,[88] 1999, Netherlands	1,171 (1,073)	Pain relief	Quality of life	Breast, 39% Lung, 25% Prostate, 23%	TL spine, 30% Pelvis, 36% Femur, 10% Ribs, 8% Humerus, 6%	During first year	Mean pain score: 6.3 (moderate)
Bone Pain Working Group,[76] 1999, U.K./New Zealand	765	Pain relief	Nausea and vomiting	Breast, 36% Prostate, 34% Lung, 12%	Pelvis/hip, 28% L spine, 20% Ribs, 11% T spine, 9% Femur, 6%	—	22–23
Koswig and Budach,[83] 1999, Germany	107	Pain relief	Recalcification	Breast, 58% Lung, 24% Prostate, 10% Kidney, 7%	Spine, 81% Extremities, 13%	6 wk	—
Nielsen et al.,[85] 1998, Denmark	241 (239)	Pain relief	Quality of life, analgesic use	Breast, 39% Prostate, 34% Lung, 13%	TL spine, 42% Pelvis, 21% Hips/femur, 18% Other, 19%	12 wk	—
Gaze et al.,[78] 1997, U.K.	265 (240)	Pain relief	Side effects, quality of life	Any epithelial tumor	—	—	—

[a]Time from study entry to assessment of response.
[b]Proportion of patients with severe pain scores at the time of study entry.
C, cervical; L, lumbar; NA, not available from published report; T, thoracic.

The second large study of single-dose versus longer-course treatment for palliation of bone metastases was RTOG study 9714, which was conducted in the United States and Canada.[79] This was limited to patients with painful bone metastases from breast or prostate primaries, with up to three painful sites allowed. Pain was evaluated using the Brief Pain Inventory, an 11-point scale. At the time of randomization, the patient was required to have a minimum pain score of 5 or a high narcotic pain medication requirement of the equivalent of >60 mg of morphine per day. More than 70% of the patients had severe

TABLE 97.4 RANDOMIZED TRIALS OF SINGLE VERSUS MULTIPLE FRACTIONS: RESULTS

Study	Number of (Number Patients Evaluable)	Dose (Gy)/ Fractions	Median Survival (mo)	Complete Response[a]	Overall Response[a]	Retreatment Rate (%)	Pathologic Fractures[b] (%)	Toxicity
Foro Arnalot et al.,[77] 2008, Spain	160	8/1 vs. 30/10	6.5 7.6	15 13	75 86	2 28	NA	12% 18%
Kaasa et al.,[81] 2006, Norway/Sweden	376	8/1 vs. 30/10	9.6 7.9	NA	No difference	16 4	4 11	NA
Hartsell et al.,[79] 2005, U.S./Canada	949 (898)	8/1 vs. 30/10	9.1 9.3	15 18	65 66	18 9	5 4	10% grade 2–4 17% P = .002
Kirkbride et al.,[82] 2000, Canada	398 (287)	8/1 vs. 20/5	NA	22 29	51 48	NA	NA	NA
Steenland et al.,[88] 1999, Netherlands	1171 (1073)	8/1 vs. 20/5	7	37 33	72 69	25 7	4 2	No difference
Bone Pain Working Party,[76] 1999, U.K./New Zealand	761 (681)	8/1 vs. 20/5[c]	NA	57 58	78 78	23 10	2 <1	No difference
Koswig and Budach,[83] 1999, Germany	107 (107)	8/1 vs. 30/10	NA	33 31	81 78	NA	NA	NA
Nielsen et al.,[85] 1998, Denmark	241 (239)	8/1 vs. 20/5	NA	15 15	73 76	21 12	NA	No difference
Gaze et al.,[78] 1997, U.K.	265 (240)	10/1 vs. 22.5/5	NA	37 47	81 76	NA	NA	21% P = NS 26% emesis

[a]Proportion of patients with pathologic fractures after treatment.
[b]Response rates listed are for pain relief.
[c]A regimen of 30 Gy/10 was also allowed; 98% of patients received 20 Gy/5.
NA, not available from published report; NS, not statistically significant.

pain at study entry (pain scores of 7 to 10). Patients were randomized to 8 Gy in a single fraction versus 30 Gy in 10 treatments. The median survival was 9.3 months. Overall toxicity rates were low, with fewer patients in the 8-Gy treatment group experiencing acute toxicity. There were no significant differences in complete (17%) and partial pain response rates (49%) between the two treatment groups. Complete pain and narcotic response (0 pain score and no narcotic pain medication use) was seen in 11%; these responses were all determined at the 3-month posttreatment evaluation. As in the Dutch trial, the rate of retreatment was higher in the 8-Gy treatment group, with 18% in that group receiving retreatment compared with 9% in the 30-Gy group. This disparity in the rate of retreatment occurred despite nearly identical rates of stable (26% vs. 24%) or progressive pain scores (9% vs. 10%) and similar rates of narcotic use between the two groups.

In contrast to the Dutch trial, there was no difference in the rate of pathologic fractures between the two groups (5% for 8 Gy vs. 4% for 30 Gy). Further analysis of this study has shown that certain subgroups may benefit from the longer course of palliative radiation therapy. Konski et al.[91] showed that although married men and both single and married women were more likely to receive retreatment after receiving 8 versus 30 Gy of palliative radiation therapy, there was no difference in retreatment rates among single men. The authors suggest that social support factors may significantly affect the ability of some patients to access repeat therapies for painful bone metastasis, especially as their health declines. Such subgroups of patients may benefit from the longer 10-fraction course of therapy.

These two large prospective, randomized trials comparing single-fraction to multiple-fraction palliative radiation therapy have similar results and help to clarify the role of palliative radiotherapy for bone metastases. The assessment of pain was performed by the patients rather than by physicians or other health care providers. The studies with the highest response rates generally used physician assessment of pain response (e.g., the RTOG 7402 study). Even with patient assessment of response, the single-fraction treatment yields similar response rates to the longer-course treatment. The patients in the Dutch trial were treated when their pain was in the moderate range, with only half on narcotic pain medications, compared with severe pain and high dose narcotic pain medication for most of the patients entered on the RTOG trial. This may account for the higher rates of complete response on the Dutch trial. In the RTOG trial, the group of patients with a single area of pain or with moderate pain scores at the time of study entry had higher complete response rates. Thus, it appears that the outcome is much better if patients are treated with palliative radiotherapy earlier in the course of their bone metastases rather than waiting until pain is severe or narcotic pain medication requirements are significant. There was no difference in pain response whether the treated bone metastases were in the spine or in extremity sites. The rates of pathologic fracture after treatment are relatively low, but it is not clear whether higher doses provide greater protection from fractures. The rates of retreatment are significantly higher with the single-dose schedules, but there may be some physician bias partially accounting for this difference because the retreatment tends to be offered at an earlier time and at lower levels of pain following the single-dose treatment.

There have been multiple randomized, prospective trials in the last 40 years comparing shorter-course, lower–total-dose treatment to the more "standard" longer-course, higher-dose treatment. Several conclusions are clear from these studies:

1. Single-dose treatments of 8 Gy provide similar pain relief to longer treatment regimens (30 Gy in 10 fractions or 20 to 24 Gy in five to eight treatments).
2. The retreatment rates are higher after short-course treatment by a factor of two to three.
3. Response rates are lower when scored by the patient instead of by the treating physician.
4. Response rates are better when the initial pain scores are lower, that is, when the patients are treated for moderate pain rather than severe pain.
5. There is no consistent dose–response relationship for palliation of bone metastases.

The lack of a dose–response relationship suggests that the mechanism of initial pain relief is not a reduction in tumor burden but more likely a change in the local environment that has caused activation of bone resorption by osteoclasts.[2] This helps to explain the seeming paradox of similar pain improvement with single-dose treatment compared with higher–total-dose, longer-course treatment. The treatment paradigm for bone metastases may be more analogous to treatments for certain benign conditions such as prevention of heterotopic ossification or keloid formation. In those conditions, a single or few treatments are given to diminish the activation of osteoblasts or fibroblasts.

This mechanism of pain relief may also help to explain the higher rates of retreatment after single-dose 8-Gy treatment because there will be less cell kill with this dose compared with 30 Gy in 10 fractions. Thus, for patients with a longer life span, there is a greater opportunity for regrowth of the tumor, which may again affect the local milieu, causing osteoclast activation.

For patients with a poor performance status, difficulty making multiple trips for treatment, extensive nonosseous metastases, and/or a short life expectancy, the most appropriate treatment is a single fraction of 8 Gy. Even with a limited expectancy (<3 months), the majority of patients experience pain relief, and palliative radiotherapy should still be considered for those patients.[92,93] For patients with a longer life expectancy, bone-only metastases, and good performance status, a longer course of treatment (30 Gy in 10 fractions) may be more appropriate to minimize the risk of retreatment. For selected patients with a solitary bone metastasis ("oligometastasis"), an even higher dose of treatment may be indicated, although this must be tempered by potential weakening of surrounding normal bone.

The single large-fraction treatment may be more likely to cause a "flare" reaction, with a temporary increase in pain at the site of the metastases.[94] The risk of this side effect may be diminished by the use of anti-inflammatory medications, either corticosteroids or nonsteroidal anti-inflammatory medications. Although the risk of significant acute toxicity has been low in the randomized trials, another potential concern is the risk of nausea or emesis if a significant portion of the stomach is within the treatment field (e.g., with a field covering the lower thoracic spine). It may be beneficial to give prophylactic antiemetics 1 to 2 hours before the treatment to minimize the possibility of this side effect.

For select patients that do not respond to the initial treatment course or for those with pain recurrence after an initial successful treatment, reirradiation to the painful metastatic sites can be administered.[95] Approximately 60% of retreated patients experienced an improvement of their pain, with 16% to 28% of patients experiencing a complete resolution of pain.[96] Patients also experienced an improved overall quality of life, and decrease in pain associated functional limitations after retreatment of a painful bone metastasis.[97] A randomized, controlled, noninferiority study compared single-dose treatment to longer courses of radiation therapy for the retreatment of previously irradiated painful metastatic bone cancer. 425 patients were randomized to receive either 20 Gy over multiple fractions or 8 Gy over one fraction. The single-fraction course was found to be noninferior to the multiple-fraction course, and resulted in a lower frequency of acute toxicity. There was no difference in pathologic fracture or spinal cord compression between these two groups.[95]

An economic analysis comparing shorter course treatment plans (8 Gy x1) to longer-course treatment plans (30 Gy x 10) was done in order to assess whether the longer treatment course is cost-effective in treating patients with bone metastasis by preventing further retreatment. The mean cost of the single-fraction treatment group was $998 with a quality-adjusted survival of 7.26 months, as compared to mean cost of $2316 and a quality-adjusted survival of 9.53 months for the longer treatment group. The incremental cost-effectiveness ratio was found to be $6972.95 per quality-adjusted life year. This study showed that the short, single-fraction treatment course with potential subsequent retreatments is both the less expensive, and more cost-effective treatment course for treating painful bone metastasis.[98]

Stereotactic radiosurgery has also been evaluated for the treatment of bone metastasis, particularly in the spinal region. A prospective, nonrandomized cohort study conducted at the University of Pittsburgh in 500 cases of spinal metastasis treated with single-fraction radiosurgery to a maximum intratumor dose of 12.5 to 25 Gy demonstrated long-term pain level improvement in 86% of cases. Long-term tumor control was demonstrated in 90% of cases when radiosurgery was used as the primary treatment modality.[99]

The Radiation Therapy Oncology Group (RTOG) 0631 is a phase II/III study evaluating the role of stereotactic radiosurgery for patients with spine metastasis. Patients on this trial are randomized to either single-fraction external-beam radiation to 8 Gy or to single-fraction image-guided stereotactic radiosurgery to 16 Gy. The primary end point of this study is assessment of pain control at the treated site(s). The phase II portion of this study demonstrated the feasibility and accurate use of stereotactic radiosurgery to treat spinal metastases.[100] The primary end point of the phase III portion of the study will compare the pain relief at the treated site(s) and improvement in quality of life between the two groups. The results of the phase III portion of the study are pending.

The use of bisphosphonates with external-beam radiotherapy may further improve the outcome in terms of both pain and bone healing. A prospective trial by Vassiliou et al.[101] evaluated 45 patients who received both external-beam irradiation and monthly ibandronate for painful bone metastases from solid tumors. All of the patients had improvement in pain, with 57% complete responses and 43% partial responses when using the same response criteria as RTOG 9714. The average pain score decreased from 6.3 to 0.8, and opioid pain medication use decreased from 84% of the patients before treatment to 24% after treatment. Bone density in the area of the metastases increased by 73% by 10 months after treatment. A similar study using pamidronate and 30 Gy of external-beam radiotherapy in women with painful bone metastases from breast cancer found that 88% of patients had complete radiographic response by International Union Against Cancer criteria.[102]

The majority of patients with osseous metastases have multiple lesions. Although radiation therapy is effective at palliating pain in a few sites, it cannot be used to treat widespread disease. Two techniques that have been used to treat more-diffuse metastases are hemibody irradiation (HBI) and intravenous radiopharmaceuticals.

Hemibody Radiation Therapy

HBI, or wide-field radiation therapy, refers to the technique of treating a large portion of the body with external-beam irradiation. Although the term *hemibody irradiation* is used, typically the field does not cover half of the body, but more accurately treats about one-third of the body. The treatment has been used for palliation of symptoms and as an adjuvant to prevent the development of new bone metastases. The treatment for palliation of pain is most useful in patients who have diffuse, widespread bone metastases.

The treatment volumes have been divided into upper, middle, and lower HBI. The fields for upper HBI cover the thorax and abdomen from the neck to the top of the iliac crests. For midbody HBI, the fields include the abdomen and pelvis from the diaphragm to the ischial tuberosities. For lower HBI treatment, the field borders are from the top of the pelvis to the inferior portion of the femurs. The toxicities from each of the fields depend on the critical structures included. The most problematic of these is the risk of radiation pneumonitis with upper HBI. This is the dose-limiting toxicity for upper HBI, and dose-inhomogeneity corrections for the lung are necessary to minimize the risk of fatal pneumonitis. A lower total dose can be given to the upper hemibody fields compared with the middle or lower hemibody areas.

RTOG 78-10 was a dose-searching prospective protocol evaluating the maximum tolerated dose (MTD) for single-dose HBI.[103] The MTD for middle and lower hemibody treatment was 8 Gy. The MTD for the upper HBI was 6 Gy if the lung dose was uncorrected and 7 Gy if lung corrections were used. Improvement in pain was noted in 80% of patients with breast cancer and 90% of patients with prostate cancer. Overall, the response rate in terms of pain relief was 73%, with complete relief of symptoms seen in 19%. Pain relief was seen relatively rapidly, with 50% of responses occurring within 2 days and 95% of responses within 2 weeks. The subsequent study RTOG 82-06 evaluated the use of HBI in addition to local radiotherapy to determine whether the HBI would prevent the development of new sites of disease.[104] All of the patients received involved-field irradiation to one or more painful sites, and half of the patients were randomly assigned to receive single-dose HBI as well. The median time to progression was 6.3 months in the local-treatment-only group compared with 12.6 months for those receiving HBI. Fewer patients receiving HBI required additional treatment. The incidence of severe hematologic toxicity was low and transitory but was seen only in the group receiving HBI.

Both the RTOG and the International Atomic Energy Agency performed trials evaluating multifraction courses of HBI.[105,106] The doses per fraction ranged from 2.5 to 4 Gy to a total of 8 to 20 Gy. The maximum tolerated dose on the RTOG 88-08 study was 17.5 Gy in seven fractions. On the International Atomic Energy Agency study, 3 Gy twice daily for 2 days (12 Gy total) or 3 Gy daily for 5 days (15 Gy total) was more effective than 4 Gy daily for 2 days. The primary toxicities were hematologic and gastrointestinal. The rationale for these doses was to decrease the acute toxicity. However, each of these regimens requires multiple treatments during several days, and the acute toxicities are not appreciably different than the single-dose treatment. With the use of appropriate antiemetic premedications and with cytokines to aid in hematologic recovery, there does not appear to be any appreciable benefit to the fractionated HBI compared with the single dose.

Premedication with antiemetics and anti-inflammatory medications significantly reduce the acute side effects of treatment. Before the development of the 5-HT3 receptor antagonists, nausea was a significant side effect of treatment, even with pretreatment and posttreatment use of steroids, prochlorperazine, and intravenous hydration. With the use of ondansetron, granisetron, or other 5-HT3 receptor antagonists, the incidence of acute nausea and emesis has been minimized and HBI is well tolerated.[107] A typical premedication regimen consists of dexamethasone, 8 to 16 mg, and ondansetron, 8 to 16 mg, 1 hour before treatment with HBI.[108]

Radiopharmaceuticals

The concept of radiopharmaceutical treatment is compelling.[109] Calcium (and to a lesser extent phosphorous) analogs will preferentially accumulate in bone, especially in areas of active bone turnover. A radioactive isotope that is a β-emitter or low-energy γ-source will allow localized treatment in the areas in which the radiopharmaceutical accumulates, thus minimizing side effects and giving an excellent therapeutic ratio. The radiopharmaceuticals are given in a single injection that is easily administered. The treatment can be combined with other modalities, including chemotherapy or external-beam radiation therapy.

The first radiopharmaceutical used for treatment of bone metastases was phosphorous-32 (P-32). Treatment with P-32 for diffuse bone metastases was successful in giving subjective pain relief but with unacceptable bone marrow toxicity. Other radioisotopes have been used for the palliation of diffuse osseous metastases with a better therapeutic ratio than P-32. Strontium-89 (Sr-89) is chemically similar to calcium and is deposited in the bone matrix, preferentially in sites of active osteogenesis. Sr-89 is a pure β-emitter with an energy of 1.4 MeV and a half-life of 50.6 days.[110] Samarium-153 (Sm-153) is primarily a β-emitter but also has a component of gamma emission, which is useful for imaging purposes. The Sm-153 ethylenediamine tetra-methylenephosphonic acid (EDTMP) is concentrated in areas of high bone turnover, accumulating in areas of hydroxyapatite. The physical half-life of Sr-153 is 46.3 hours, but the biologic half-life is much shorter because about half of the compound is excreted in the urine within 8 hours of injection.[111] These two isotopes have been evaluated in multiple prospective trials. There are other, newer isotopes that are being evaluated, including rhenium-186, rhenium-188, and tin-117m. All of these isotopes accumulate in areas of osteoblastic activity, especially in areas of increased uptake on bone scintigraphy; for this reason, most of the patients entered on prospective trials have metastatic prostate cancer.

Strontium-89

The first study of Sr-89 with substantial numbers of patients was a randomized, prospective trial of Sr-89 versus placebo in 126 men with metastatic prostate cancer, reported by Porter and McEwan[112] in 1993. The patients were randomized after involved-field radiation therapy in a double-blind fashion to 400 MBq of Sr-89 versus placebo. Although there was no statistically significant difference in the primary end point of pain relief, there were several secondary end points that were improved with the Sr-89. More patients were able to discontinue pain medications (17% vs. 2%), and there were fewer sites of new pain requiring additional radiotherapy in the patients who received Sr-89. Smeland et al.[113] reported on a similar study of Sr-89 versus placebo after involved-field radiation therapy, which showed no difference in outcome between the two groups. In this study, the dose of Sr-89 was only 150 MBq.

There have been two randomized trials of Sr-89 versus external-beam radiation therapy. A study by Quilty et al.[114] from the United Kingdom evaluated Sr-89 given in a dose of 200 MBq compared with external-beam radiotherapy. For patients with a few bone metastases, the randomization was Sr-89 versus local-field radiation therapy. Patients with more widespread metastases were randomized to Sr-89 versus HBI of 8 Gy to the lower hemibody or 6 Gy to the upper hemibody.

There was no difference in pain relief, toxicity, or median survival between the groups. In the patients with diffuse disease, there were fewer new pain sites after Sr-89 than HBI. The trial by Oosterhof et al.[115] evaluated 203 patients with hormone-refractory metastatic prostate cancer, randomly assigning patients to receive local-field radiation therapy or 150 MBq of intravenous Sr-89. There was no difference in pain relief or toxicity between the two treatment arms.

Sr-89 can be given concomitantly with chemotherapy. Two randomized, prospective trials evaluated concomitant chemotherapy with Sr-89 for patients with hormone-refractory metastatic prostate cancer. In the trial by Sciuto et al.,[116] 70 patients received 148 MBq of Sr-89 on day 0. They were randomly assigned to receive cisplatin, 18 mg/m² intravenously on day 0 and 16 mg/m² on days 10 and 11, or placebo on the same days. The group that received cisplatin and Sr-89 had significantly more patients with pain relief (91% vs. 63%), longer duration of pain palliation (120 vs. 60 days), longer median survival (9 vs. 6 months), and a significantly greater proportion of patients with improvement in performance status (66% vs. 26%), with no significant difference in toxicity. Tu et al.[117] performed a phase II randomized study of doxorubicin, 20 mg/m² per week given intravenously, with randomization between 2.035 MBq/kg of intravenous Sr-89 versus placebo. Neutropenia and anemia were common in the combined Sr-89 plus doxorubicin group compared with doxorubicin alone, but the median survival was also significantly better (28 vs. 17 months).

An economic evaluation of the Trans-Canada randomized study found Sr-89 treatment to be cost-effective.[118] The patients who received the Sr-89 had significantly lower subsequent costs for palliative medications, hormonal therapy, and subsequent radiation therapy. However, Oosterhof et al.[115] found that Sr-89 was associated with higher costs than external-beam radiotherapy.

Samarium-153

Samarium-153 is chelated with ethylenediamine tetra-methylenephosphonic acid to form Sm-153 EDTMP, a compound that is preferentially taken up in newly formed bone. The unbound remainder of the drug is rapidly cleared via urinary excretion. Phase I/II studies showed that doses of >2.5 mCi/kg are associated with neutropenia. In a dose-escalation study, Collins et al.[119] evaluated doses from 0.5 to 3.0 mCi/kg. There was no significant difference in clinical response between 1.0 and 2.5 mCi. There have been at least five randomized, prospective evaluations of Sm-153 for metastatic cancers (primarily for prostate cancers).[111,120-123] Two of these studies used a placebo arm in comparison to 1.0 mCi/kg[122] or 0.5 and 1.0 mCi/kg.[111] In both of these studies, the 1.0-mCi/kg dose gave significant improvement in pain relief compared to placebo. The average opioid dose decreased for the patients receiving Sm-153, compared to an increase in the patients receiving placebo. Transient marrow suppression was seen, with a nadir at 4 to 6 weeks and recovery by 8 weeks; this primarily manifested as grade ≥3 neutropenia (14% compared with 0% for placebo).

The other phase III study evaluated three dose levels of Sm-153 (0.5, 1.0, and 1.5 mCi/kg). Olea et al.[120] reported no difference in response rates among the different dose levels, with an overall pain relief response rate of 73%. Two randomized phase II studies compared doses of 0.5 with 1.0 mCi/kg, with no placebo arm.[121,123] In these two studies, there was no significant difference between the two dose levels for response or toxicity. There was no difference in response by primary site, although the numbers of patients were small for each primary site. The study by Tian et al.[123] is the only one in which metastatic prostate cancer patients did not comprise the majority of patients included.

Radium-223

Radium-223 dichloride is a pharmaceutical that emits alpha particles and selectivity targets bone metastases. The ALSYMPCA trial was a phase III, prospective randomized study of men with castrate-resistant prostate cancer with bone metastases. Patients were randomized to receive 6 injections every 4 weeks of either radium-223 or placebo. The randomization was 2:1, with 614 patients receiving Ra-223 and 307 patients receiving placebo. The primary end point of the study was survival, which was significantly greater in the patients treated with Ra-223 (14.9 months) compared to placebo (11.3 months).[124] Multiple secondary end points were improved with the Ra-223 compared to placebo: (1) time to first symptomatic skeletal event (15.6 vs. 9.8 months), (2) decreased risk of spinal cord compression, (3) lower use of external radiation therapy for bone pain, and (4) decrease in certain biomarkers (total alkaline phosphatase and lactic dehydrogenase, although there was not a statistically significant difference in prostate specific antigen).[124,125] There was no difference between the groups in pathologic bone fractures or the need for orthopedic intervention. The rates of significant adverse events were low, as was the risk of myelosuppression, in the patients receiving Ra-223.[125] Radium-223 has been used concomitantly with abiraterone, enzalutamide, and denosumab in an open-label prospective but nonrandomized study, with relatively low significant toxicity rates (grade $\geq$ 3 hematologic toxicity was <10%).[126] Radium-223 is the only bone-directed radionuclide, which has shown improvement not only in pain and quality of life but also in overall survival.

Patient Selection

Radiopharmaceuticals, specifically Ra-223, Sr-89, and Sm-153, are effective in providing pain relief for patients with diffuse osseous metastases. This is primarily true for metastases that have an osteoblastic component. In general, if a Tc-99m nuclear medicine bone scan shows localized areas of increased uptake, then radiopharmaceutical treatment is likely to be of benefit. An advantage of radioisotope treatment is that it can be combined with other modalities, such as external-beam radiation therapy or chemotherapy. Because the targets of treatment are similar, treatment with bisphosphonates should not be given simultaneously with radioisotopes because this may reduce the efficacy of both medications. However, there is evidence that the Radium-223 can be given concomitantly with denosumab. Relative contraindications to therapy would be impaired renal or hepatic function or inadequate hematologic reserve.

Radiopharmaceuticals: Summary

The primary advantages of Sm-153 compared with Sr-89 are reduced radiation safety issues (because of the much shorter half-life) and the ability to image the distribution of the Sm-153. Although there has not been a randomized comparison of Sr-89 and Sm-153, there does not appear to be a significant difference in the incidence, severity, onset, or duration of hematologic toxicity, despite the short half-life of the Sm-153. Both radiopharmaceuticals appear equally effective at palliating pain from bone metastasis. Radium-223 offers not only palliation of pain but also the possibility of improved overall survival, at least in patients with castrate-resistant metastatic prostate cancer. These radiopharmaceuticals add to the growing armamentarium of therapies designed to palliate pain and improve the quality of life of patients with bone metastasis from cancer.

CONCLUSION

Palliative radiation therapy is of significant benefit to patients with painful bone metastasis, with most patients experiencing relief in the magnitude of pain following treatment. Response rates to palliative radiation therapy for localized sites of pain are consistently higher than response rates from palliative systemic therapy, and palliative external-beam radiation therapy remains the mainstay of treatment for clinically localized painful bone metastasis. Providing shorter, single-fraction palliative treatment schedules (i.e., 800 cGy × one fraction) for properly selected patients with bone metastasis can help better integrate palliative radiation therapy into the multidisciplinary management of patients with metastatic cancer and offer equivalent palliation compared with longer courses of palliative radiation therapy. Systemic targeted therapies including Ra-223, Sm-153, and Sr-89 offer yet another means to target painful sites of bone metastasis without limiting the ability to use localized external-beam radiation therapy and systemic chemotherapy.

REFERENCES

1. Ratanatharathorn V, Powers WE, Moss WT, et al. Bone metastasis: review and critical analysis of random allocation trials of local field treatment. *Int J Radiat Oncol Biol Phys* 1999;44:1–18.
2. Smith HS. Painful osseous metastases. *Pain Physician* 2011;14:E373–E405.
3. Coleman RE. Skeletal complications of malignancy. *Cancer* 1997;80(Suppl 8):1588–1594.
4. Nielsen OS, Munro AJ, Tannock IF. Bone metastases: pathophysiology and management policy. *J Clin Oncol* 1991;9:509–524.
5. Coleman RE, Rubens RD. The clinical course of bone metastases from breast cancer. *Br J Cancer* 1987;55:61–66.
6. Singh D, Yi WS, Brasacchio RA, et al. Is there a favorable subset of patients with prostate cancer who develop oligometastases? *Int J Radiat Oncol Biol Phys* 2004;58:3–10.
7. Khan L, Uy C, Nguyen L, et al. Self-reported rates of sleep disturbance in patients with symptomatic bone metastases attending an outpatient radiotherapy clinic. *J Palliat Med* 2011;14:708–714.
8. Nguyen J, Cramarossa G, Bruner D, et al. A literature review of symptom clusters in patients with breast cancer. *Expert Rev Pharmacoecon Outcomes Res* 2011;11:533–539.
9. Asdourian PL, Weidenbaum M, DeWald RL, et al. The pattern of vertebral involvement in metastatic vertebral breast cancer. *Clin Orthop Relat Res* 1990;250:164–170.
10. Hitchins RN, Philip PA, Wignall B, et al. Bone disease in testicular and extragonadal germ cell tumours. *Br J Cancer* 1988;58:793–796.
11. Matsuyama T, Tsukamoto N, Imachi M, et al. Bone metastasis from cervix cancer. *Gynecol Oncol* 1989;32:72–75.
12. Steinmetz MP, Mekhail A, Benzel EC. Management of metastatic tumors of the spine: strategies and operative indications. *Neurosurg Focus* 2001;11:e2.
13. Gurney H, Larcos G, McKay M, et al. Bone metastases in hypernephroma. Frequency of scapular involvement. *Cancer* 1989;64:1429–1431.
14. Hellman S, Weichselbaum R. Oligometastases. *J Clin Oncol* 1995;13:8–10.
15. Palma DA, Salama JK, Lo SS, et al. The oligometastatic state—separating truth from wishful thinking. *Nat Rev Clin Oncol* 2014;11:549–557
16. Roodman GD. Mechanisms of bone metastases. *N Engl J Med* 2004;350:1655–1664.
17. Cannonier SA, Sterling JA. The role of hedgehog signaling in tumor induced bone disease. *Cancers (Basel)* 2015;7:1658–1683.
18. Roodman GD. Biology of osteoclast activation in cancer. *J Clin Oncol* 2001;19:3562–3571.
19. Park SI, Lee C, Sadler WD, et al. Parathyroid hormone-related protein drives a CD11b+Gr1+ cell-mediated positive feedback loop to support prostate cancer growth. *Cancer Res* 2013;73:6574–6583.
20. Ding X, Park SI, McCauley LK, et al. Signaling between transforming growth factor β (TGF-β) and transcription factor SNAI2 represses expression of microRNA miR-203 to promote epithelial-mesenchymal transition and tumor metastasis. *J Biol Chem* 2013;288:10241–10253.
21. Eriksen EF. Cellular mechanisms of bone remodeling. *Rev Endocr Metab Disord* 2010;11:219–227.
22. Zetter BR. The cellular basis of site-specific tumor metastasis. *N Engl J Med* 1990;322:605–612.
23. Ratanatharathorn V, Powers WE, Temple HT. In: Perez CA, Brady LW, Halperin EC, et al., eds. *Principles and practice of radiation oncology*, 4th ed. Philadelphia, PA: JB Lippincott, 2003:2385–2404.
24. Goblirsch MJ, Zwolak PP, Clohisy DR. Biology of bone cancer pain. *Clin Cancer Res* 2006;12:6231s–6235s.

25. Hoskin PJ, Stratford MRL, Folkes LK, et al. Effect of local radiotherapy for bone pain on urinary markers of osteoclast activity. *Lancet* 2000;355:1428–1429.

26. Costelloe CM Rohren EM, Madewell JE, et al. Imaging bone metastases in breast cancer: techniques and recommendations for diagnosis. *Lancet Oncol* 2009;10:606–614.

27. Schmidt GP, Schoenberg SO, Reiser MF, et al. Whole-body MR imaging of bone marrow. *Eur J Radiol* 2005;55:33–40.

28. Flickinger FW, Sanal SM. Bone marrow MRI: techniques and accuracy for detecting breast cancer metastases. *Magn Reson Imaging* 1994;12: 829–835.

29. Hamaoka T, Madewell JE, Podoloff DA, et al. Bone imaging in metastatic breast cancer. *J Clin Oncol* 2004;22:2942–2953.

30. Evan-Sapr E, Mester U, Mishani E, et al. The detection of bone metastases in patients with high-risk prostate cancer: 99mTc-MDP Planar bone scintigraphy, single- and multi-field-of-view SPECT, 18F-fluoride PET, and 18F-fluoride PET/CT. *J Nucl Med* 2006;47:287–297.

31. Fujimoto R, Higashi T, Nakamoto Y, et al. Diagnostic accuracy of bone metastases detection in cancer patients: comparison between bone scintigraphy and whole-body FDG-PET. *Ann Nucl Med* 2006;20:399–408.

32. Daldrup-Link HE, Franzius C, Link TM. Whole-body MR imaging for detection of bone metastases in children and young adults: comparison with skeletal scintigraphy and FDG PET. *Am J Roentgenol* 2001;177:229–236.

33. Ohta M, Tokuda Y, Suzuki Y, et al. Whole body PET for the evaluation of bony metastases in patients with breast cancer: comparison with 99Tcm-MDP bone scintigraphy. *Nucl Med Commun* 2001;22:875–879.

34. Schuster DM, Nanni C, Fanti S. PET tracers beyond FDG in prostate cancer. *Semin Nucl Med* 2016;46:507–521.

35. Cleeland CS. The measurement of pain from metastatic bone disease: capturing the patient's experience. *Clin Cancer Res* 2006;12:6236s–6242s.

36. Cleeland CS, Gonin R, Hatfield AK, et al. Pain and its treatment in outpatients with metastatic cancer. *N Engl J Med* 1994;330:592–596.

37. Meuser T, Pietruck C, Radbruch L, et al. Symptoms during cancer pain treatment following WHO-guidelines: a longitudinal follow-up study of symptom prevalence, severity and etiology. *Pain* 2001;93:247–257.

38. Zech DF, Grond S, Lynch J, et al. Validation of World Health Organization guidelines for cancer pain relief: a 10-year prospective study. *Pain* 1995;63: 65–76.

39. Harrington KD. Orthopaedic management of extremity and pelvic lesions. *Clin Orthop Relat Res* 1995;312:136–147.

40. Beals RK, Lawton GD, Snell WE. Prophylactic internal fixation of the femur in metastatic breast cancer. *Cancer* 1971;28:1350–1354.

41. Fidler M. Incidence of fracture through metastases in long bones. *Acta Orthop Scand* 1981;52:623–627.

42. Van der Linden Y, Dijkstra PD, Kroon HM, et al. Comparative analysis of risk factors for pathological fracture with femoral metastases. *J Bone Joint Surg Br* 2004;86:566–573.

43. Cheal EJ, Hipp JA, Hayes WC. Evaluation of finite element analysis for prediction of the strength reduction due to metastatic lesions in the femoral neck. *J Biomech* 1993;26:251–264.

44. Mirels H. Metastatic disease in long bones: a proposed scoring system for diagnosing impending pathologic fractures. *Clin Orthop Relat Res* 1989;249:256–264.

45. Nathan SS, Healey JH, Mellano D, et al. Survival in patients operated on for pathologic fractures: implication for end-of-life orthopedic care. *J Clin Oncol* 2005;23:6072–6082.

46. Sim FH, Frassica FJ, Chao EYS. Orthopaedic management using new devices and prostheses. *Clin Orthop Relat Res* 1995;312:160–172.

47. Chow E, Holden L, Danjoux C, et al. Successful salvage using percutaneous vertebroplasty in cancer patients with painful spinal metastases or osteoporotic compression fractures. *Radiother Oncol* 2004;70:265–267.

48. Hentschel SJ, Burton AW, Fourney DR, et al. Percutaneous vertebroplasty and kyphoplasty performed at a cancer center: refuting proposed contraindications. *J Neurosurg Spine* 2005;2:436–440.

49. Shimony JS, Gilula LA, Zeller AJ, et al. Percutaneous vertebroplasty for malignant compression fractures with epidural involvement. *Radiology* 2004;232:846–853.

50. Chew C, Craig L, Edwards R, et al. Safety and efficacy of percutaneous vertebroplasty in malignancy: a systematic review. *Clin Radiol* 2011;66: 63–72.

51. Kassamali RH, Ganeshan A, Hoey ET, et al. Pain management in spinal metastases: the role of percutaneous vertebral augmentation. *Ann Oncol* 2011;22:782–786.

52. Qian Z, Sun Z, Gu Y, et al. Kyphoplasty for the treatment of malignant vertebral compression fractures caused by metastasis. *J Clin Neurosci* 2011;18: 763–767.

53. Tancioni F, Lorenzetti MA, Navarria P, et al. Percutaneous vertebral augmentation in metastatic disease: state of the art. *J Support Oncol* 2011;9: 4–10.

54. Callstrom MR, Charboneau JW. Image guided palliation of painful metastases using percutaneous ablation. *Tech Vasc Interv Radiol* 2007;10: 120–131.

55. Houston SJ, Rubens RD. The systemic treatment of bone metastases. *Clin Orthop Relat Res* 1995;312:95–104.

56. Tannock IF, Osoba D, Stockler MR, et al. Chemotherapy with mitoxantrone plus prednisone or prednisone alone for symptomatic hormone-resistant prostate cancer: a Canadian randomized trial with palliative end points. *J Clin Oncol* 1996;14:1756–1764.

57. Berthold, DR, Pond, GR, Soban, F, et al. Docetaxel plus prednisone or mitoxantrone and prednisone for advanced refractory prostate cancer: updated survival in the TAX327 study. *J Clin Oncol* 2008;26:242–245.

58. Medical Research Council Prostate Cancer Working Party Investigators Group. Immediate versus deferred treatment for advanced prostatic cancer: initial results of the MRC trial. *Br J Urol* 1997;79:235–246.

59. Michaelson MD, Smith MR. Bisphosphonates for treatment and prevention of bone metastases. *J Clin Oncol* 2005;23:8219–8224.

60. Russell RG, Rogers MJ, Frith JC, et al. The pharmacology of bisphosphonates and new insights into their mechanisms of action. *J Bone Miner Res* 1999;14(Suppl 2):53–65.

61. Senaratne SG, Pirianov G, Mansi JL, et al. Bisphosphonates induce apoptosis in human breast cancer cell lines. *Br J Cancer* 2000;82:1459–1468.

62. Theriault RL, Lipton A, Hortobagyi GN, et al. Pamidronate reduces skeletal morbidity in women with advanced breast cancer and lytic bone lesions: a randomized, placebo-controlled trial. Protocol 18 Aredia Breast Cancer Study Group. *J Clin Oncol* 1999;17:846–854.

63. Hortobagyi GN, Theriault RL, Porter L. Efficacy of pamidronate in reducing skeletal complications in patients with breast cancer and lytic bone metastases. Protocol 19 Aredia Breast Cancer Study Group. *N Engl J Med* 1996;335:1785–1791.

64. Rosen LS, Gordon L, Tchekmedyian NS, et al. Long-term efficacy and safety of zoledronic acid in the treatment of skeletal metastases in patients with nonsmall cell lung carcinoma and other solid tumors: a randomized, phase III, double-blind, placebo-controlled trial. *Cancer* 2004;100: 2613–2621.

65. Dearnaley DP, Mason, MD, Parmar, MK, et al. Adjuvant therapy with oral sodium clodronate in locally advanced and metastatic prostate cancer: long-term overall survival results from the MRC PRO4 and PRO5 randomized controlled trials. *Lancet Oncol* 2009;10:872–876.

66. Mehrotra B, Ruggiero S. Bisphosphonate complications including osteonecrosis of the jaw. *Hematology* 2006;1:356–360.

67. Migliorati CA, Siegel MA, Elting LS. Bisphosphonate-associated osteonecrosis: a long-term complication of bisphosphonate treatment. *Lancet Oncol* 2006;7:508–514.

68. Lipton A, Goessl C. Clinical development of anti-RANKL therapies for treatment and prevention of bone metastases. *Bone* 2011;48:96–99.

69. Fizazi K, Carducci M, Smith M, et al. Denosumab compared with zoledronic acid for treatment of bone metastases in men with castration-resistant prostate cancer: a randomized, double-blind study. *Lancet* 2011;377: 813–822.

70. Stopeck AT, Lipton A, Body JJ, et al. Denosumab compared with zoledronic acid for the treatment of bone metastases in patients with advanced breast cancer: a randomized, double-blind study. *J Clin Oncol* 2010;28: 5132–5139.

71. Chow E, Harris K, Fan G, et al. Palliative radiotherapy trials for bone metastases: a systematic review. *J Clin Oncol* 2007;25:1423–1436.

72. Caissie A, Zeng L, Nguyen J, et al. Assessment of health-related quality of life with European Organization for Research and Treatment of Cancer QLQ-C15-PAL after palliative radiotherapy of bone metastases. *Clin Oncol (R Coll Radiol)* 2012;24:125–133.

73. Lutz S, Berk L, Chang E, et al. Palliative radiotherapy for bone metastases: an ASTRO evidence-based guideline. *Int J Radiat Oncol Biol Phys* 2011;79:965–976.

74. Tong D, Gillick L, Hendrickson FR. The palliation of symptomatic osseous metastases: final results of the study by the Radiation Therapy Oncology Group. *Cancer* 1982;50:893–899.

75. Blitzer P. Reanalysis of the RTOG study of the palliation of symptomatic osseous metastasis. *Cancer* 1985;55:1468–1472.

76. Bone Pain Trial Working Party. 8 Gy single fraction radiotherapy for the treatment of metastatic skeletal pain: randomised comparison with a multifraction schedule over 12 months of patient follow-up. *Radiother Oncol* 1999;52:111–121.

77. Foro Arnalot P, Fontanals AV, Galcerán JC. Randomized clinical trial with two palliative radiotherapy regimens in painful bone metastases: 30 Gy in 10 fractions compared to 8 Gy in single fraction. *Radiother Oncol* 2008;89: 150–155.

78. Gaze MN, Kelly CG, Kerr GR, et al. Pain relief and quality of life following radiotherapy for bone metastases: a randomized trial of two fractionation schedules. *Radiother Oncol* 1997;45:109–116.

79. Hartsell WF, Scott CB, Bruner DW, et al. Randomized trial of short- versus long-course radiotherapy for palliation of painful bone metastases. *J Natl Cancer Inst* 2005;97:798–804.

80. Hirokawa Y, Wadasaki K, Kashiwado K, et al. A multiinstitutional prospective randomized study of radiation therapy of bone metastases [in Japanese]. *Nippon Igaku Hoshasen Gakkai Zasshi* 1988;48:1425–1431.

81. Kaasa S, Brenne E, Lund JA, et al. Prospective randomized multicenter trial on single fraction radiotherapy (8 Gy × 1) versus multiple fractions (3 Gy × 10) in the treatment of painful bone metastases. *Radiother Oncol* 2006;79: 278–284.

82. Kirkbride P, Warde RR, Panzarella T, et al. A randomized trial comparing the efficacy of a single radiation fraction with fractionated radiation therapy in the palliation of skeletal metastases. *Int J Radiat Oncol Biol Phys* 2000;48 (Suppl 1):185.

83. Koswig S, Budach V. Remineralization and pain relief in bone metastases after different radiotherapy fractions (10 time 3 Gy vs 1 time 8 Gy). A prospective study. *Strahlenther Onkol* 1999;175:500–508.

84. Madsen EL. Painful bone metastasis: efficacy of radiotherapy assessed by the patients—a randomized trial comparing 4 Gy × 6 versus 10 Gy × 2. *Int J Radiat Oncol Biol Phys* 1983;9:1775–1779.

85. Nielsen OS, Bentzen SM, Sandberg E, et al. Randomized trial of single dose versus fractionated palliative radiotherapy of bone metastases. *Radiother Oncol* 1998;47:233–240.

86. Niewald M, Tkocz HJ, Abel U, et al. Rapid course radiation therapy vs. more standard treatment: a randomized trial for bone metastases. *Int J Radiat Oncol Biol Phys* 1996;36:1085–1089.

87. Rasmusson B, Vejborg I, Jensen AB, et al. Irradiation of bone metastases in breast cancer patients: a randomized study with 1 year follow-up. *Radiother Oncol* 1995;34:179–184.

88. Steenland E, Leer JW, van Houwelingen H, et al. The effect of a single fraction compared to multiple fractions on painful bone metastases: a global analysis of the Dutch Bone Metastases Study. *Radiother Oncol* 1999;52: 101–109.

89. Hoskin PJ, Price P, Easton D, et al. A prospective randomized trial of 4 Gy or 8 Gy single doses in the treatment of metastatic bone pain. *Radiother Oncol* 1992;23:74–78.

90. Jeremic B, Shibamoto Y, Acimovic L, et al. A randomized trial of three single-dose radiation therapy regimens in the treatment of metastatic bone pain. *Int J Radiat Oncol Biol Phys* 1998;42:161–167.

91. Konski A, DeSilvio M, Hartsell W, et al. Continuing evidence for poorer treatment outcomes for single male patients: retreatment data from RTOG 97 14. *Int J Radiat Oncol Biol Phys* 2006;66:229–233.

92. Dennis K, Wong K, Zhang L, et al. Palliative radiotherapy for bone metastases in the last 3 months of life: worthwhile or futile? *Clin Oncol (R Coll Radiol)* 2011;23:709–715.

93. Meeuse JJ, van der Linden YM, van Tienhoven G, et al. Efficacy of radiotherapy for painful bone metastases during the last 12 weeks of life: results from the Dutch Bone Metastasis Study. *Cancer* 2010;116:2716–2725.

94. Loblaw DA, Wu JS, Kirkbride P, et al. Pain flare in patients with bone metastases after palliative radiotherapy—a nested randomized control trial. *Support Care Cancer* 2007;15:451–455.

95. Chow E, van der Linden YM, Roos D, et al. Single versus multiple fractions of repeat radiation for painful bone metastases: a randomised, controlled, non-inferiority trial. *Lancet Oncol* 2014;15:164–171.

96. Huisman M, van den Bosch MA, Wijlemans JW, et al. Effectiveness of reirradiation for painful bone metastases: a systematic review and meta-analysis. *Int J Radiat Oncol Biol Phys* 2012;84:8–14.

97. Chow E, Meyer RM, Bingshu E, et al. Impact of reirradiation of painful osseous metastases on quality of life and function: a secondary analysis of NCIC CTG SC.20 randomized trial. *J Clin Oncol* 2014;32:3867–3873.

98. Konski A, James J, Hartsell W, et al. Economic analysis of Radiation Therapy Oncology Group (RTOG) 97-14: multiple versus single fraction radiation treatment of patients with bone metastases. *Am J Clin Oncol* 2009;32: 423–428.

99. Gerszten PC, Burton SA, Ozhasoglu C, et al. Radiosurgery for spinal metastases: clinical experience of 500 cases from a single institution. *Spine* 2007;15:193–199.

100. Ryu S, Pugh SL, Gerszten PC, et al. ROGT 0631 phase II/III study of image-guided stereotactic radiosurgery for localized (1-3) spine metastases: phase II results. *Pract Radiat Oncol* 2014;4:76–81.

101. Vassiliou V, Kalogeropoulou G, Christopoulos C, et al. Combination ibandronate and radiotherapy for the treatment of bone metastases: clinical evaluation and radiographic assessment. *Int J Radiat Oncol Biol Phys* 2007;67: 264–272.

102. Kouloulias V, Matsopoulos G, Kouvaris J, et al. Radiotherapy in conjunction with intravenous infusion of 180 mg of disodium pamidronate in management of osteolytic metastases from breast cancer: clinical evaluation, biochemical markers, quality of life, and monitoring of recalcification using assessments of gray-level histogram in plain radiographs. *Int J Radiat Oncol Biol Phys* 2003;57:143–157.

103. Salazar OM, Rubin P, Hendrickson F, et al. Single dose half-body irradiation for palliation of multiple bone metastases from solid tumors: final Radiation Therapy Oncology Group Report. *Cancer* 1986;58:29–36.

104. Poulter C, Cosmatos D, Rubin P, et al. A report of RTOG 82-06: a phase III study of whether the addition of single dose hemibody irradiation is more effective than local field irradiation alone in the treatment of symptomatic osseous metastases. *Int J Radiat Oncol Biol Phys* 1992;23: 207–214.

105. Salazar OM, Sandhu T, da Motta NW, et al. Fractionated half-body irradiation (HBI) for the rapid palliation of widespread, symptomatic, metastatic bone disease: a randomized phase III trial of the International Atomic Energy Agency (IAEA). *Int J Radiat Oncol Biol Phys* 2001;50:765–775.

106. Scarantino CW, Caplan R, Rotman M, et al. A phase I/II study to evaluate the effect of fractionated hemibody irradiation in the treatment of osseous metastases—RTOG 88-22. *Int J Radiat Oncol Biol Phys* 1996;36:37–48.

107. Scarantino C, Omitz, RD, Hoffman LG, et al. On the mechanism of radiation induced emesis: the role of serotonin. *Int J Radiat Oncol Biol Phys* 1994;30:825–830.

108. Sarin R, Budrukkar A. Efficacy, toxicity and cost-effectiveness of single-dose versus fractionated hemibody irradiation (HBI) [Letter]. *Int J Radiat Oncol Biol Phys* 2002;52:1146.

109. Bauman G, Charette M, Reid R, et al. Radiopharmaceuticals for the palliation of painful bone metastasis—a systemic review. *Radiother Oncol* 2005;75: 258–270.

110. Siegel HJ, Luck JV Jr, Siegel ME. Advances in radionuclide therapeutics in orthopaedics. *J Am Acad Orthop Surg* 2004;12:55–64.

111. Serafini AN, Houston SJ, Resche I, et al. Palliation of pain associated with metastatic bone cancer using samarium-153 lexidronam: a double-blind placebo controlled clinical trial. *J Clin Oncol* 1998;16:1574–1581.

112. Porter AT, McEwan AJ. Strontium-89 as an adjuvant to external beam radiation improves pain relief and delays disease progression in advanced prostate cancer: results of a randomized controlled trial. *Semin Oncol* 1993;20: 38–43.

113. Smeland S, Erikstein B, Aas M, et al. Role of strontium-89 as adjuvant to palliative external beam radiotherapy is questionable: results of a double-blind randomized study. *Int J Radiat Oncol Biol Phys* 2003;56:1397–1404.

114. Quilty PM, Kirk D, Bolger JJ, et al. A comparison of the palliative effects of strontium-89 and external beam radiotherapy in metastatic prostate cancer. *Radiother Oncol* 1994;31:33–40.

115. Oosterhof GON, Roberts JT, De Reijke T, et al. Strontium89 chloride versus palliative local field radiotherapy in patients with hormonal escaped prostate cancer: a phase III study of the European organisation for research and treatment of cancer genitourinary group. *Eur Urol* 2003;44:519–526.

116. Sciuto R, Festa A, Rea S, et al. Effects of low-dose cisplatin on 89Sr therapy for painful bone metastases from prostate cancer: a randomized clinical trial. *J Nucl Med* 2002;43:79–86.

117. Tu S-M, Delpassand ES, Jones D, et al. Strontium-89 combined with doxorubicin in the treatment of patients with androgen independent prostate cancer. *Urol Oncol* 1996;2:191–197.

118. McEwan AJ, Amyotte GA, McGowan DG, et al. A retrospective analysis of the cost effectiveness of treatment with Metastron (89Sr-chloride) in patients with prostate cancer metastatic to bone. *Nucl Med Commun* 1994;15:499–504.

119. Collins C, Eary JF, Donaldson G, et al. Samarium-153-EDTMP in bone metastases of hormone refractory prostate carcinoma: a phase I/II trial. *J Nucl Med* 1993;34:1839–1844.

120. Olea E, Riccabona G, Tian J, et al. Efficacy and toxicity of 153Sm EDTMP in the palliative treatment of painful skeleton metastases: results of an IAEA international multicenter study [Abstract]. *J Nucl Med* 2000;51:146P.

121. Resche I, Chatal JF, Pecking A, et al. A dose-controlled study of 153Sm-ethylenediaminetetramethylenephosphonate (EDTMP) in the of treatment patients with painful bone metastases. *Eur J Cancer* 1997;33: 1583–1591.

122. Sartor O, Quick D, Reid R, et al. A double blind placebo controlled study of 153samarium-EDTMP for palliation of bone pain in patients with hormone-refractory prostate cancer [Abstract]. *J Urol* 1997;157:321.

123. Tian JH, Zhang JM, Hou QT, et al. Multicentre trial on the efficacy and toxicity of single-dose samarium-153-ethylene diamine tetramethylene phosphonate as a palliative treatment for painful skeletal metastases in China. *Eur J Nucl Med* 1999;26:2–7.

124. Parker C, Nilsson S, Heinrich D, et al. Alpha emitter radium-223 and survival in metastatic prostate cancer. *N Engl J Med* 2013;369:213–223.

125. Sartor O, Coleman R, Nilsson S, et al. Effect of radium-223 dichloride on symptomatic skeletal events in patients with castration-resistant prostate cancer and bone metastases: results from a phase 3, double-blind, randomised trial. *Lancet Oncol* 2014;15:738–746.

126. Saad F, Carles J, Gillessen S, et al. Radium-223 and concomitant therapy in patients with metastatic castration-resistant prostate cancer: an international, early-access, open-label, single arm phase 3b trial. *Lancet Oncol* 2016;17:1306–1316.

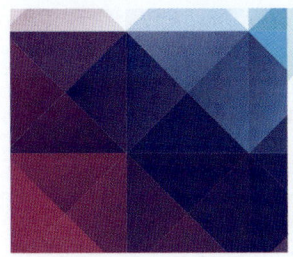

CHAPTER 98

Palliation of Visceral Recurrences and Metastases and Treatment of Oligometastatic Disease

Alexander A. Harris and William F. Hartsell

INTRODUCTION

The 5-year survival and overall cure rates for many cancers have significantly improved over the past 40 years. Unfortunately, there is still a substantial minority of patients who develop recurrent or metastatic disease. The most common sites of metastatic disease are bones, brain, lungs, and liver. In addition, there are other visceral sites of recurrence or metastatic disease that may cause significant symptoms. Palliative radiation therapy for treatment of bone and brain metastases is well established, with multiple randomized prospective trials evaluating best treatment practices. However, there is less information on treatment of visceral metastases, although radiation oncologists recognize that radiation therapy is frequently effective at palliating symptoms from visceral metastases.

The specific goals of treatment will depend on the symptoms, treatment site, functional status of the patient, and other patient-specific factors. The indications for treatment may include pain, visceral obstruction, bleeding, or other symptoms that negatively impact the quality of life. In general, this treatment is given with the goal of improving the quality of life, not the quantity of life. For some disease sites, this can be done with a very short course, low-dose treatment. For other sites, this will require higher doses given to control the local disease.

Some visceral metastases will cause pain. For example, liver or adrenal metastases may cause significant pain. Splenic metastases from hematologic metastases may cause abdominal pain, early satiety, and abdominal distention. In contrast, pulmonary metastases rarely cause pain. Instead, these lesions may cause airway obstruction or hemoptysis. Metastatic lesions in the gastrointestinal system may cause bleeding or obstructive symptoms (esophageal obstruction, gastric outlet obstruction, gastric bleeding, biliary obstruction, rectal obstruction). In addition to rectal obstruction, pelvic masses may cause ureteral obstruction, bleeding (vaginal, bladder, or rectal), or pain from involvement of the sacrum or sacral nerves.

There has been a revolution in the understanding of the metastatic process in the past decade. Traditionally in solid tumor biology, cancer cells are thought to undergo some genetic change that potentiates them to grow into tumors and cause daughter cells to spread through the lymphatic or circulatory system to lymph nodes and distant sites. However, recent understanding of the epithelial–mesenchymal transition demonstrates that cancer cells develop embryonic stem cell–like properties that allow them to disseminate to distant sites. The microenvironment surrounding the primary tumor and metastatic sites can regulate the metastatic process. In addition, metastasis occurs much earlier than clinical detection of lymphadenopathy and radiographic or symptomatic evidence of the development of distant visceral disease.[1] Treatment of visceral metastases in the oligometastatic setting may allow for improved palliation and may also improve the overall survival in carefully selected patients.

MALIGNANT LOWER AIRWAY OBSTRUCTION

The lower airway is generally defined as being below the first tracheal ring. Upper airway obstructions can be emergently treated with a tracheostomy. The lower airway can become compromised from either primary or metastatic malignancy. Patients may have intrinsic compression caused by an endobronchial tumor or extrinsic airway compression by a tumor mass in the lung parenchyma or bulky lymphadenopathy during the course of their illness. Clinical symptoms, bronchoscopy, and radiographic imaging are used to determine the extent of luminal obstruction. It is important to determine whether the airway obstruction is endobronchial or from external compression of the airway in order to select the most appropriate treatment. For intrinsic compression of a tumor mass growing inside the bronchial lumen, interventional bronchoscopy techniques offer immediate benefit in many patients. These interventional techniques can result in relief of dyspnea, decreased risk of postobstructive pneumonia, and improved functional status.[2-4] Either laser resection of tumor or endobronchial stent placement, along with radiation therapy, is effective in maintaining the patency of the lower airway.[5,6] The additional treatment of the airway can be given with either external-beam radiation therapy, endobronchial brachytherapy, or photodynamic therapy. Brachytherapy is typically the best option in patients who have recurred after prior external-beam radiation therapy. For endobronchial therapy, the recommended doses are 7.5 Gy × 3 or 10 Gy × 2.[7] In a prospective observational study, de Aquino Gorayeb et al. utilized high-dose-rate endobronchial brachytherapy for palliation of malignant airway obstruction. The study protocol consisted of three fractions of 7.5 Gy weekly or biweekly, with over half of the patients having been previously treated with external beam radiation. Of the 78 patients treated, 70% reported an improvement in performance status and 87% noted improvement of one or more of their presenting complaints (dyspnea, cough, infection, and/or hemoptysis). Of the patients who presented with one or more of the above symptoms, 57% noted improvement in their dyspnea, 34% noted improvement in their cough, 80% noted improvement in their infection symptoms, and 100% noted improvement in their hemoptysis.[8]

External-beam radiation therapy is typically used for treatment of airway compromise caused by extrinsic compression of a bronchus. Endobronchial brachytherapy typically does not improve symptoms when there is external compression of the airways.[9,10] The highest doses from brachytherapy will be given to the (relatively) normal mucosa of the airway, with a much lower dose to the extrinsic tumor that is causing the compression.

There is no standard fractionation scheme or total dose for palliative external-beam treatment for lung cancer. A review by Fairchild et al.[11] found the best results, in terms of palliation of symptoms, are achieved with relatively high doses of radiation therapy: 3 Gy per fraction to a total of 30 to 45 Gy, or 2 Gy per fraction to 50 to 60 Gy. The trade-off is that there is a higher rate of acute esophagitis with these higher doses. The American Society for Radiation Oncology clinical practice guideline consensus statement recommends doses equivalent to 30 Gy in 10 fractions or greater.[12] For patients with a poor performance status or who have difficulty traveling for multiple treatments, shorter fractionation schemes such as 20 Gy in 5 fractions can be used. Very short regimens (17 Gy in 2 fractions or 10 Gy in 1 fraction) may be useful in certain situations; however, there are reports of radiation myelopathy with these regimens (17 Gy in 2 fractions).[12]

In most patients who receive radiation therapy for palliation of pulmonary symptoms, there is no benefit to the addition of chemotherapy. Combined chemotherapy and radiation therapy may improve response rates slightly, but with significantly greater acute toxicity.[12]

LIVER METASTASES

The liver is a common metastatic site. It is the most frequent site of distant metastatic disease from gastrointestinal tumors, especially colorectal, but also including esophageal, stomach, and pancreatic cancers. The liver is also a frequent site of metastases from lung cancer, breast cancer, and melanoma. A patient with liver metastases may have symptoms of anorexia or early satiety, weight loss, nausea, right upper quadrant or epigastric pain, jaundice, and fever.

For patients with few metastatic lesions in the liver and no evidence of extrahepatic metastases, 12% to 36% may be cured with surgical resection.[13] The risk factors associated with the best outcome are clear resection margins, low levels of carcinoembryonic antigen, a single metastatic deposit, metachronous presentation of the liver metastasis, and node-negative disease (with the original primary).[13] There are multiple other treatments that can be used for patients with one or a few hepatic metastases, including radiofrequency ablation, microwave coagulation therapy, transarterial chemoembolization, and stereotactic body radiotherapy (SBRT).[14]

Most patients with liver metastases are found to have multiple lesions, extrahepatic disease, or other risk factors that make them unsuitable for these surgical or interventional procedures. It is common for these patients to undergo multiple courses of systemic therapy prior to being seen and evaluated by a radiation oncologist. For many years, the only viable chemotherapy option for metastatic gastrointestinal tumors was 5-fluorouracil, often given in combination with leucovorin. More recently, multiple drug regimens including oxaliplatin or irinotecan have significantly improved the response rates and increased the median duration of survival. Targeted agents such as cetuximab or bevacizumab may improve the response rates even further. These new combinations have changed the goal of treatment from palliation to prolonging survival; with this new paradigm, the multiple drug regimens are given as neoadjuvant therapy with the goal of downsizing tumor bulk in order to facilitate a resection.[15] Hepatic arterial infusion of chemotherapy gives higher local concentrations of the chemotherapy agents and also gives higher response rates. A meta-analysis of hepatic arterial infusion chemotherapy for liver metastases demonstrated a significantly higher response rate but showed no improvement in survival duration.[16]

The group of patients who are referred to a radiation oncologist for palliation of liver metastases tend to be the patients who have more medical comorbidities, a greater tumor burden, and who have been previously treated with multiple other therapies. Despite these poor prognostic factors, radiation therapy can be effective in palliating symptoms (Fig. 98.1).[17]

FIGURE 98.1. Axial **(A)** and coronal **(B)** isodose plots in a patient with diffuse metastases in an enarged liver, causing significant pain.

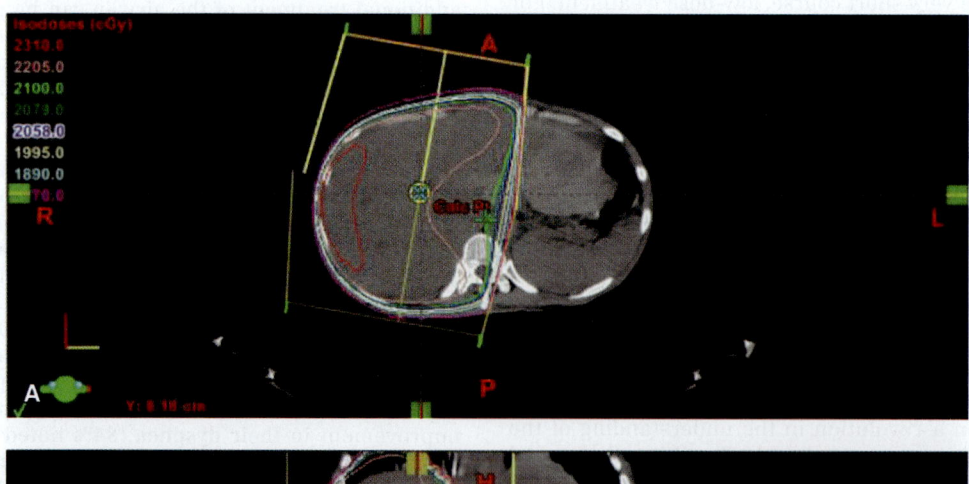

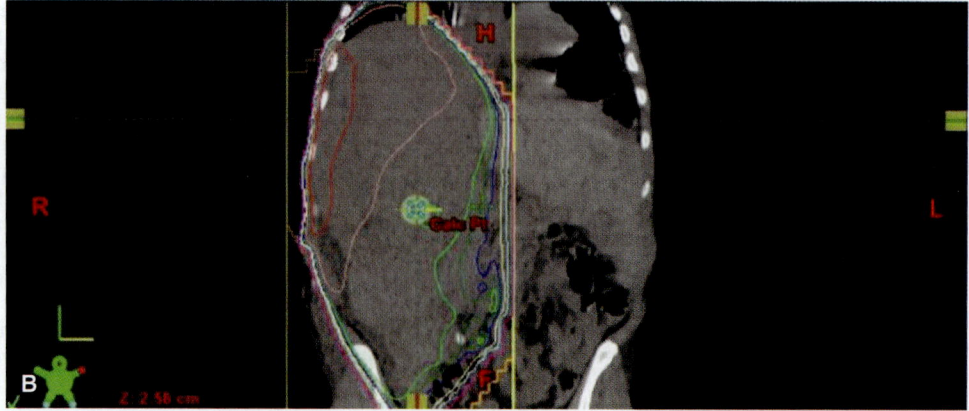

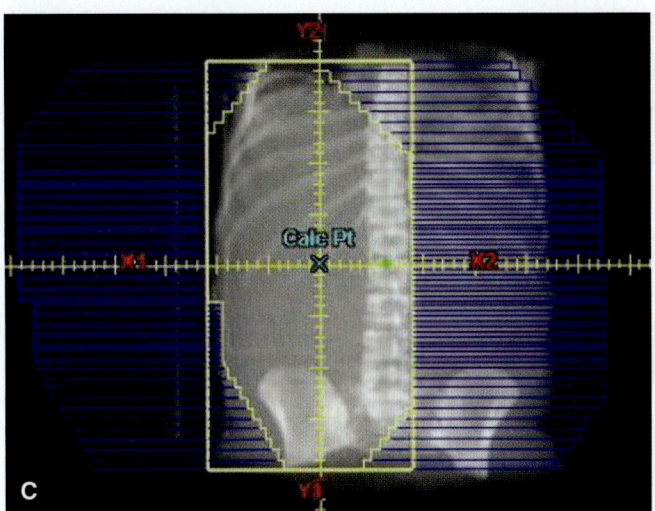

FIGURE 98.1. (*Continued*) Treatment field is shown in **(C)**. This patient was given 21 Gy in 7 fractions, and had significant improvement in pain within 4 weeks.

Palliative treatment of the liver is limited by radiation-induced liver toxicity (RILD). This toxicity becomes apparent 1 week to 3 months after treatment and may result in liver failure and death.[18] Both dose and volume of liver irradiated are important in avoiding RILD. For treatment of the whole liver, the threshold for RILD is approximately 30 Gy in 2 Gy fractions or 33 Gy in 1.5 Gy twice daily fractions.[19,20] The Radiation Therapy Oncology Group's trial RTOG-7605 evaluated multiple regimens in patients with multiple liver metastases: 30 Gy in 15 fractions, 25.6 Gy in 16 fractions, 20 Gy in 10 fractions, and 21 Gy in 7 fractions.[21] Improvement in symptoms was seen in 55% of the patients, with no difference among the four treatment regimens. A subsequent RTOG trial evaluated whole-liver radiation therapy with a dose of 21 Gy in 7 fractions; patients were randomized to receive the radiation alone or with the addition of misonidazole to the radiation.[22] There was minimal toxicity and a rapid symptomatic response in the majority of patients. Complete pain relief was reported in 54% of the patients, and 80% of the patients noted an improvement in pain following treatment. Overall, there was no significant benefit with the addition of misonidazole. The best response rates were seen in patients with colorectal primaries. Bydder et al.[23] reported on a series of 28 patients treated with a hypofractionated regimen of 10 Gy in 2 fractions to the whole liver. The overall response rate was 54%, with 2 patients experiencing grade 3 toxicity (emesis and diarrhea).

If a smaller portion of the liver is irradiated, higher doses can be given with low risk for RILD. A 5% risk of RILD is associated with 90, 47, and 31 Gy with uniform irradiation of one-third, two-thirds, and the whole liver, respectively. If the effective liver volume irradiated is <25%, doses >100 Gy can be given with little risk of RILD.[24,25]

Selective internal radiation therapy (SIRT) is another option for patients with diffuse liver metastases. This technique involves the use of yttrium-90 (^{90}Y) glass or resin microspheres that are given through intra-arterial infusions into the liver. A phase III trial of patients with liver metastases from colorectal cancer evaluated intra-arterial floxuridine alone compared to intra-arterial floxuridine plus SIRT with ^{90}Y resin microspheres.[26] The patients who received SIRT had a significantly better overall response rate, time-to-tumor progression, and overall survival. The addition of SIRT did not increase grade 3 or 4 toxicity.

In summary, patients with multiple symptomatic liver metastases may be palliated by whole-liver radiation therapy. Relatively low doses of 21 Gy in 7 fractions or 30 Gy in 15 fractions are generally well tolerated and provide symptomatic relief for the majority of patients.[17–22] Treatment to high doses can be done if a smaller percentage of the liver is radiated.

BILIARY OBSTRUCTION

Malignant biliary obstruction may be caused either by a tumor mass causing extrinsic compression onto the bile duct or intrinsic compression from tumor progression within the bile duct lumen. This obstruction can lead to hyperbilirubinemia and jaundice, which can cause pruritus, anorexia, and weight loss. The biliary obstruction may be a life-threatening emergency. Emergent drainage of the bile duct is achieved initially by external stent. These stents are later converted to internal endoprostheses; however, these catheters typically only remain patent for 4 to 8 months.[27] The patency of these stents can be extended with the use of intraluminal brachytherapy, photodynamic therapy, or external-beam radiation therapy. Intraluminal brachytherapy extends stent patency and lengthens survival duration in patients with inoperable cholangiocarcinoma.[28,29] Although there are few data specifically for the use of external-beam radiation therapy for palliative treatment of metastatic biliary obstruction, it may be of benefit especially for treatment of extrinsic bile duct compression by a tumor mass.[30]

PAINFUL ADRENAL METASTASES

The adrenal glands are a common site of metastatic disease from many types of cancer, primarily due to the rich blood supply of the adrenal gland. Lung cancer is the most common source of adrenal metastases. These metastases are frequently asymptomatic, but occasionally may cause pain. For patients with a good performance status and few sites of metastatic disease, surgical management may be appropriate. Radiation therapy is also appropriate for palliative treatment.

Palliative radiotherapy typically has been given with conventional external-beam techniques. Soffen et al.[31] reported the results in 16 patients with painful adrenal metastases treated with palliative radiation therapy. The majority of the patients received 30 Gy in 10 to 12 treatments. A response was seen in 12 of 16 patients (75%), with 6 of those patients having complete response for the duration of their survival. Nearly half of the patients (44%) experienced nausea, which may have been related to the technique of treatment with anterior and posterior fields. No late toxicity was seen, but the median survival was only 3 months. A multicenter retrospective study assessed results from 134 patients treated with 3D conformal (88%), intensity-modulated radiation therapy (IMRT) (6%), or SBRT (6%) for adrenal metastasis from hepatocellular carcinoma. Treatment regimens ranged from 20 to 60 Gy (median of 45 Gy) with dose per fraction of 1.8 to 15 Gy (median 2.5 Gy). A complete response was seen in 6 patients, a partial response seen in 48 patients, for an objective response rate of 39%. Seventy-eight patients (55%) were noted to have stable disease.[32]

There are multiple recent reports evaluating the use of intensity-modulated radiation therapy techniques or stereotactic body radiation therapy techniques for treatment of adrenal metastases. Most of these patients were treated for asymptomatic adrenal metastases, rather than for palliation of symptoms. These treatments appear to provide a high rate of local control. SBRT studies have shown local control rates ranging from 73% to 100% after 1 year, with minimal toxicity.[33–35] These newer radiotherapy treatments may be appropriate for patients with limited volume disease (oligometastases) (Fig. 98.2). In the palliative setting, there is a benefit with a dose of 30 Gy in 10 to 12 treatments using conventional techniques.

Section
IV

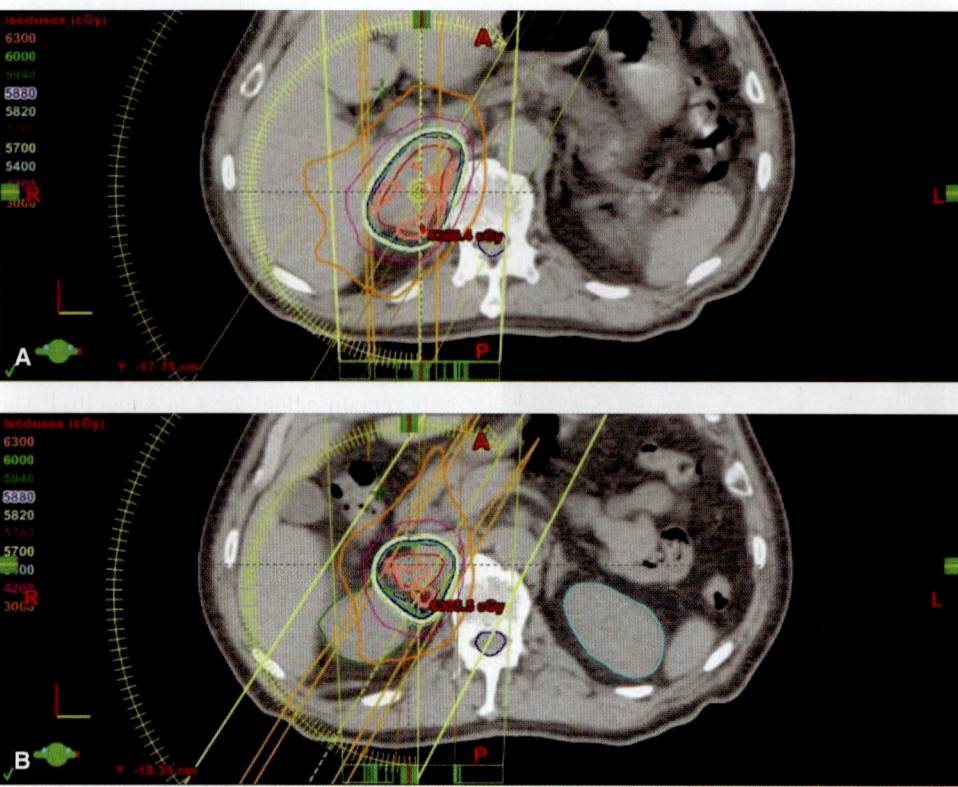

FIGURE 98.2. Axial isodose plots from superior **(A)** and inferior **(B)** aspect of SBRT fields for an adrenal metastasis. This patient was given 50 Gy in 5 fractions.

SPLENIC METASTASES

It is relatively uncommon for solid tumors to metastasize to the spleen. Splenomegaly is more often associated with hematologic malignancies and disorders such as leukemia or myeloproliferative diseases. The spleen can become massively enlarged, causing pain, early satiety, nausea, or emesis. These symptoms may also occur when the spleen is enlarged because of extramedullary hematopoiesis due to marrow failure.[36]

Treatment with radiation therapy can be very effective at reducing the size of the spleen and palliating the other symptoms associated with splenomegaly. The doses required for palliation of symptoms are much lower than the doses typically used for palliation of other visceral metastases. The response may be quite rapid as well, which necessitates evaluation of the field sizes on a frequent basis. The regimens frequently used include doses of 0.25 to 1 Gy given two to three times per week. It is important to evaluate blood counts on a frequent basis, since anemia and thrombocytopenia may occur rapidly with precipitous drops in the counts over a very short period. A typical regimen is the one reported by McFarland et al.[37] Their patients were treated twice-weekly beginning at 0.5 Gy per fraction the first week, increasing to 0.75 Gy per fraction in the 2nd week and 1 Gy per fraction on the 3rd week. A complete blood count was obtained prior to each treatment. The total dose was typically <5 Gy. Even with these low doses, 14 of 16 patients had subjective improvement in their symptoms, and 12 of 16 patients had objective decrease in the splenomegaly.

A recent systemic review of palliative splenic radiation for the treatment of splenomegaly in the setting of hematologic malignancy showed that the treatment was effective at reducing splenic size, splenic pain, and improving cytopenias. Over the 27 articles reviewed, the average partial response rate was 85%, with 72% of the treatment courses resulting in splenic size reduction, 59% resulting in pain relief, and 78% resulting in improvement in cytopenia. Of the total of 766 treatment courses assessed, 33% resulted in acute toxicities, with the most common being a grade 3 to 4 leukopenia/neutropenia or thrombocytopenia. No long-term toxicities were noted.[38] Treatment of the spleen may cause an abscopal effect as well, with decrease in size of involved lymph nodes distant to the treated spleen.[37]

VAGINAL BLEEDING OR DISCHARGE

Vaginal bleeding is a common symptom at diagnosis in several gynecologic tumors, especially cervical, uterine, and vaginal tumors.[39] The initial treatment should be with vaginal packing.[40] Radiation therapy is also effective at controlling this type of vaginal bleeding. A hypofractionated treatment course is typically used, usually with 2.5 to 4 Gy per fraction. A typical course of treatment would be 30 Gy in 10 fractions.[39] Often, the bleeding will slow or stop after 3 to 5 treatments. The treatment can be continued to definitive doses at that point, using more standard fractionation of 1.8 to 2.0 Gy per fraction (Fig. 98.3). An alternative method of palliating bleeding and vaginal discharge is to use a single large fraction of 10 Gy.[41–43] This will result in a high likelihood of reducing or stopping the bleeding, often within 24 to 48 hours of the first dose. This dose of 10 Gy can be repeated at 1-month intervals. The risk of complications increases when this dose is repeated a third or fourth time, so this should be limited to one to two fractions.[44]

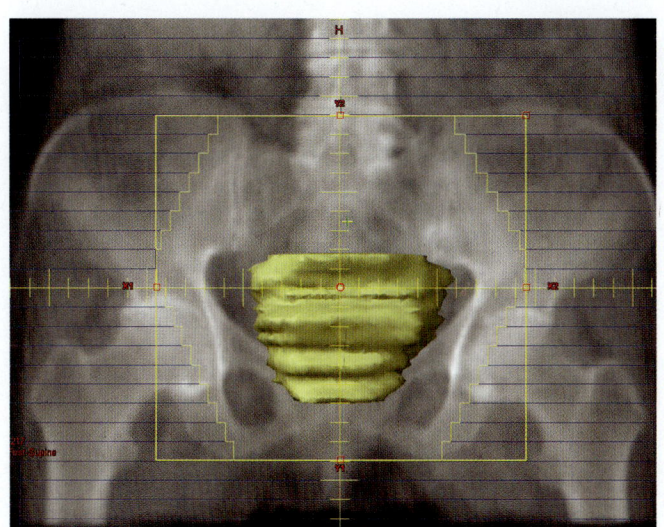

FIGURE 98.3. Digitally reconstructed anterior-posterior radiograph of a palliative pelvic field. This palliative field arrangement would be appropriate to treat a patient with hemorrhage from a cervical or bladder cancer.

PELVIC RECURRENCE

Recurrent pelvic malignancies may cause significant symptoms, including pain, bleeding, or obstruction. The choice of the appropriate palliative treatment depends on multiple factors, including the type and amount of prior treatment. In contrast to palliative treatment of other sites of recurrent disease, aggressive combined modality treatment may provide the best chance of palliation of symptoms for recurrent pelvic malignancies.

Recurrent colorectal cancer may cause life-threatening problems from bowel obstruction. For most patients in this circumstance, surgical intervention is the most appropriate treatment. This may involve complete surgical removal of the disease, if possible, or a diverting colostomy to alleviate the symptoms of obstruction.[45] There is a high risk of perioperative complications in this group of patients, primarily because it is frequently difficult to perform an adequate bowel preparation prior to surgery.

Hydronephrosis and severe pain may be signs of a more advanced tumor and are relative contraindications to surgical resection.[46] The majority of patients with recurrent rectal cancers have posterior or posterolateral involvement of the pelvis, which makes surgery more difficult.[47] The presence of severe pain may indicate invasion of the sacrum or sacral nerve roots. Tumors that invade these structures are more difficult to resect completely. Melton et al.[48] and Wells et al.[49] reported that patients who underwent an aggressive surgical resection of locally recurrent rectal cancers had a high risk of significant complications. Patients who had sacral resection as part of the surgical treatment had a 42% risk of significant complications.[49]

Patients with bulky pelvic recurrences who have not previously received radiation therapy are appropriate candidates for combined chemotherapy and radiation therapy. A prospective randomized Danish trial evaluated radiation therapy alone (50 Gy in 25 fractions, with a boost of 10 to 20 Gy in 5 to 10 fractions) compared with the same radiation therapy with concomitant weekly bolus dose of 5-fluorouracil.[50] This treatment was given to patients with locally recurrent or inoperable rectal cancers. There was no improvement in survival with the addition of chemotherapy, but there was a higher rate of acute complications (33% with chemotherapy vs. 13% with radiation alone). In several retrospective studies, the addition of chemotherapy was beneficial. Ito et al.[51] reported on 30 patients with symptomatic intrapelvic recurrent rectal

cancers. They noted a higher pain relief rate in the patients receiving chemotherapy (100% vs. 77% for radiation alone) and a near doubling of the median survival time (7.8 vs. 4 months). For these patients with locally recurrent rectal cancers, combined modality therapy is usually recommended to improve the likelihood of local control.

Relatively high doses of radiation therapy are required for palliation of symptoms. A review by Wong et al.[52] showed that total dose was important in achieving a response, with the highest responses seen in patients receiving ≥ 50 Gy. In their series, the patients with the best prognostic factors received higher doses, but the dose–response relationship was still predictive of local control and survival in a multivariate analysis. Bae et al.[53] also found improvement in the rate and duration of symptom control in patients who received higher doses. They recommended a biologic effective dose >40 Gy$_{10}$ when possible.

Patients who have received prior irradiation and subsequently develop locally recurrent rectal cancer are frequently treated with surgery, chemotherapy, or a combination of the two. However, there are circumstances in which additional radiation therapy may be beneficial. The radiation therapy may be given as hyperfractionated external-beam radiation, intraoperative radiation therapy (IORT), or brachytherapy. Lingareddy et al.[54] utilized hyperfractionation with 1.2 Gy twice a day to a median dose of 30.6 Gy for reirradiation of patients with locally recurrent rectal cancer; these patients had received full-dose pelvic radiation therapy as part of their initial treatment. They used limited fields for the reirradiation, excluding the bladder and small bowels. Most of the patients (90%) received concurrent 5-fluorouracil chemotherapy. There was improvement in pain in 65% of these patients and cessation of bleeding in 100%. The late toxicity of treatment was significantly lower in patients who received hyperfractionated treatment compared to single daily treatments (18% vs. 47%). The most frequent late toxicities were small bowel obstruction (17%) and fistula formation (8%). An Italian prospective study evaluated patients with recurrent rectal cancer who had previously received radiation therapy.[55] Patients with biopsy-proven recurrent disease were given preoperative combined modality treatment, with hyperfractionated radiation therapy (30.6 Gy using 1.2 Gy twice a day, followed by a 10.8 Gy boost also with 1.2 Gy twice a day) and continuous infusion 5-fluorouracil. The patients were then evaluated for resection, and surgery was performed at 4 to 6 weeks following the chemoradiotherapy, when feasible. Fifty-one (86%) of the patients completed the preoperative treatment as planned, and 30 (50.8%) underwent resection. The overall median survival was 42 months, and the 5-year survival was 39%. Seven patients had late grade 3 toxicity, and there were no grade 4 toxicities.

SBRT has shown promising results for treating previously irradiated pelvic cancers; however the majority of the literature is limited to small, single institution studies.[56,57] Dewas et al.[57] reviewed 16 patients with lateral pelvic recurrences of anal, rectal, endometrial or bladder cancer. The patients received reirradiation of 36 Gy over 6 treatments to the lateral pelvic recurrence. The 1-year local control rate was approximately 50%, with a median disease free survival of 8 months, with toxicities limited to $\leq$grade 2. Defoe et al.[58] reported on 14 patients with presacral tumors from rectal cancer who received SBRT treatment after prior radiotherapy. The patients were retreated to a dose of 36 Gy over 3 fractions. Local control rates were 91% at 1 year, and 68% at 2 years, with overall survival of 90% and 79%, respectively. Toxicities were limited to $\leq$grade 2. Jerezek-Fossa et al. treated 34 patients with recurrent prostate cancer, localized to pelvic lymph nodes. The patients were retreated on average to 30 Gy over 4.5 fractions. About half of the treated patients received androgen deprivation therapy.[59] Biochemical response was noted in 84% of cases. In patients that received SBRT without androgen deprivation therapy, the biochemical response rate was 81%, with a complete prostate-specific antigen (PSA) response rate of 56%. Most toxicity was acute, with 18% of treated patients experiencing acute urinary toxicity, and 3% experiencing acute rectal toxicity. Late urinary toxicity occurred in 20% of patients, and late rectal toxicity in 6%.

Intraoperative radiation therapy may be useful in some patients with locally recurrent rectal cancer. The patients who may benefit from this treatment are those with locally advanced recurrent rectal cancer who have no evidence of metastatic disease. Haddock et al.[60] reported on a series of 51 previously irradiated patients with recurrent rectal cancer who underwent maximal resection followed by intraoperative radiation therapy using electrons. The dose given was 10 to 30 Gy, with a median of 20 Gy. Thirty-seven patients received additional external-beam radiation therapy (median 25.2 Gy) following the surgery and IORT. The 2-year survival rate was 48%, but the 5-year survival rate was only 12%. The local control rate was 60% at 2 years, with a trend toward better local control in patients who received ≥30 Gy external-beam treatment in addition to the IORT (81% local control vs. 54% for those who received no external-beam treatment or doses <30 Gy). The toxicity included peripheral neuropathy in 32% of patients and ureteral narrowing or obstruction in 14%.

Brachytherapy is another alternative method to deliver radiation dose to a relatively limited volume. Alektiar et al.[61] reported on 74 patients with locally recurrent colorectal cancers. The patients underwent surgical resection of the recurrence, followed by high-dose-rate intraoperative brachytherapy, with doses of 10 to 18 Gy. The 5-year overall survival rate was 23% with a 5-year local control rate of 39%. The primary toxicity was peripheral neuropathy, which occurred in 16% of the patients. Patients with negative margins of resection had a higher likelihood of local control compared to those who had positive margins (43% vs. 28%). Kolotas et al.[62] evaluated palliative interstitial high-dose-rate brachytherapy in a group of 38 patients. Only four of the patients had the catheters implanted intraoperatively; most were placed using computed tomography guidance, with the catheters implanted through the perineum or sacrum. This group of patients had bulky disease at the time of implant. The median survival was 15 months following brachytherapy, with most deaths caused by distant metastases. There was stable disease in 28 of 38 patients, with pain relief in 89.5% of patients.

In summary, palliative radiation therapy is effective in reducing pain or bleeding from recurrent pelvic malignancies. Because of the location and nature of pelvic recurrences, combined modality treatment with chemotherapy, radiation therapy, and surgery may be needed. Relatively high doses of radiation may also be needed to provide the palliative benefits of treatment.

RADIATION THERAPY IN THE SETTING OF OLIGOMETASTATIC DISEASE

As reviewed in the preceding sections, the radiotherapeutic management of metastatic disease has historically been limited to palliation, typically utilizing relatively low overall doses and abbreviated treatment schedules. The goal of this approach has been to provide short- to moderate-term palliation, while limiting treatment-related toxicity and minimizing duration of therapy. Until recently, this paradigm has been generalized to nearly all patients staged as metastatic, with an essentially uniform treatment strategy applied to a widely heterogeneous group of patients, presentations, and disease biology. The paradigm shift of "curative" local therapy, including radiation therapy for select presentations of "oligometastatic" disease, was first proposed by Weichselbaum and Hellman in a 1995 editorial.[63] According to this concept, select patients with controlled locoregional disease and a limited number of metastatic sites may theoretically be cured with definitive local therapy, especially in the setting of effective systemic therapy. During the era of Weichselbaum and Hellman's writing, limitations in radiotherapy technique precluded effective ablation of most sites of oligometastatic disease without significant toxicity. Furthermore, available systemic therapy was largely ineffective in eliminating microscopic systemic disease. However, interval advances in highly conformal image-guided radiotherapy and the increased efficacy of systemic and molecular therapies have allowed for the translation of this theoretical concept into clinical investigation and practice.

Early investigations of definitive radiation therapy for metastatic disease included isolated metastatic liver disease.[64] Investigators at the University of Michigan first pioneered the paradigm of high-dose three-dimensional conformal radiation therapy in a cohort of patients that included both primary hepatocellular carcinoma and hepatic metastasis, achieving acceptable local control and toxicity (Fig. 98.4). With the advent of image-guided SBRT, the definitive treatment of isolated hepatic metastasis has been the focus of intense clinical investigation and practice.[65] A multi-institutional phase I and II trial of 47 patients with one to three liver lesions (each <6 cm in size) tested dose-escalated SBRT of 36 to 60 Gy in 3 fractions, reporting a 2-year local control of 92% for all lesions. Local control rates of 100% for lesions ≤3 cm and 77% for lesions >3 cm were also achieved in the 60-Gy cohort. With a median follow-up of 16 months, an overall survival of 20.5 months was reported, with no documented radiation-induced liver disease and grade ≥3 toxicity of 2%.[66] A pooled analysis of 65 patients from three institutions has also demonstrated an excellent efficacy and toxicity profile for SBRT in the definitive treatment of colorectal liver metastasis, recommending a prescription dose of at least 48 Gy for a 3-fraction regimen for optimal

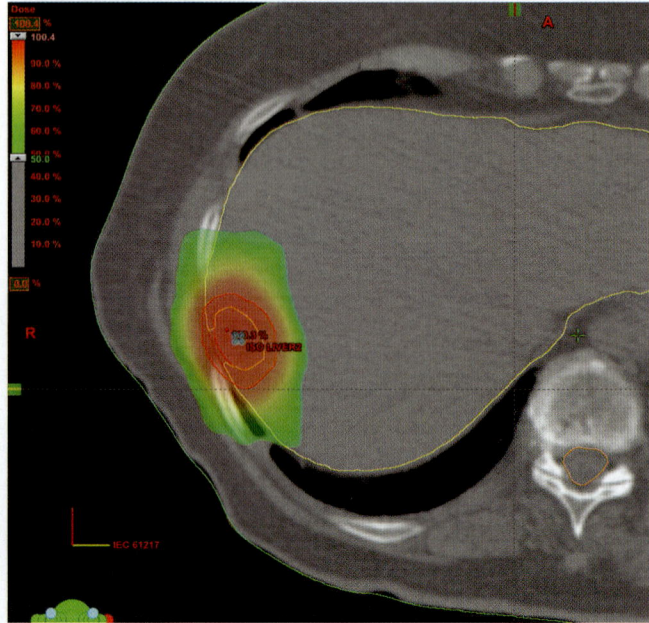

FIGURE 98.4. Axial computed tomography images showing the dose distribution from stereotactic body radiotherapy treatment of a liver metastasis.

local control.[67] More recently, Goodman et al. evaluated the long term safety and efficacy of SBRT treatment for oligometastatic liver disease. Eighty-one patients, with 1 to 3 liver metastases were treated with a median dose of 54 Gy in 3 to 5 fractions. They found that local control was 94% after 33 months, and a partial or complete response was observed in 69% of lesions treated. Grade 3 liver toxicity occurred in 5% of the cases.[33]

With rapid advances in SBRT technique and experience in the definitive treatment of primary lung malignancies, the definitive SBRT treatment of oligometastatic disease involving the lung has also been the subject of numerous clinical reports.[68,69] A multi-institutional phase I and II trial of SBRT for lung metastasis dose-escalated 38 patients with one to three lesions and cumulative maximal tumor diameters of <7 cm from 48 to 60 Gy in 3 fractions. A median survival of 19 months and local control rate of 96% at 2 years were achieved, while symptomatic radiation pneumonitis was uncommon (2.6%) and grade ≥3 toxicity was reported as 8%.[70] A German multi-institutional pooled database of 700 patients with oliogmetastic lung cancer treated with SBRT showed a 2-year local control rate of 81.2% and overall survival rate of 54.4%. Radiation-induced pneumonitis grade 2 or higher was observed in 6.5% of patients.[71]

The curative treatment of oligometastatic sites in addition to lung and liver has also shown promise in published clinical reports. In most series, the oligometastatic state has been defined as one to five sites of metastatic disease, with inconsistent application of primary disease status, overall disease volume, or maximal lesion size as constraints for oligometastatic disease (Fig. 98.5). Investigators from the University of Chicago have reported a dose-escalation trial of 29 patients with one to five sites of metastatic disease, concluding that there was minimal toxicity and potential clinical benefit from this approach.[72] Another prospective study of 121 curative-intent SBRT with five or fewer oligometastatic lesions yielded 4-year survival rates of 28%, progression-free survival of 20%, and local control of 60%.[73] Twenty-nine patients were alive and with no evidence of disease at last follow-up, leading the authors to conclude that "oligometastatic disease is a potentially curable state of distant cancer spread."

FIGURE 98.5. PET scan showing a solitary lung metastasis from a patient with a renal cell carcinoma **(A)**, with axial **(B)** and coronal **(C)** iosdose images.

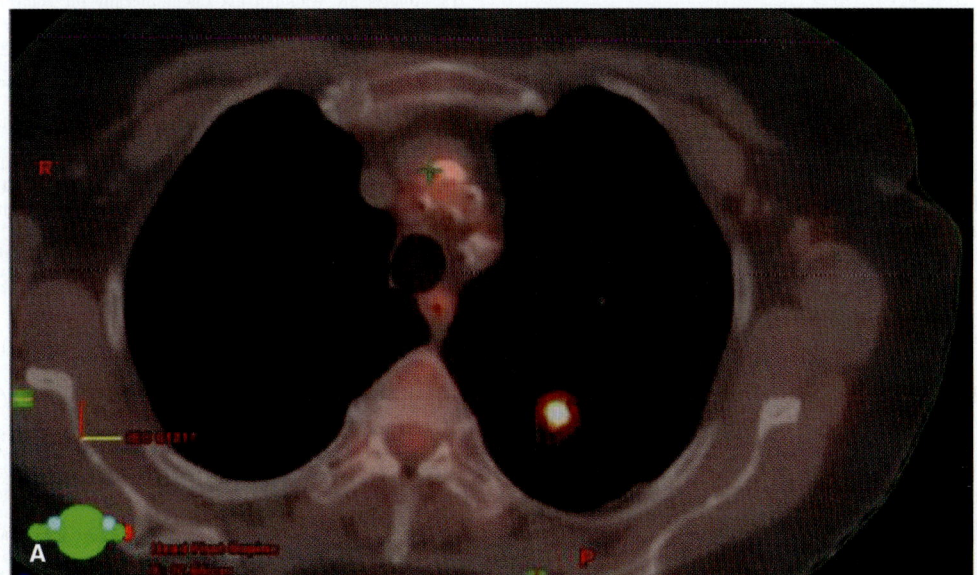

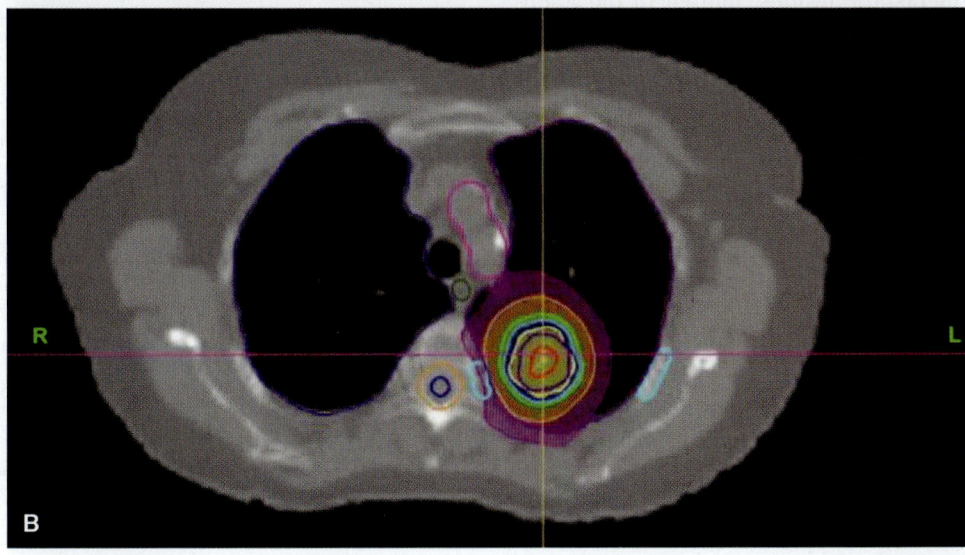

(Continued)

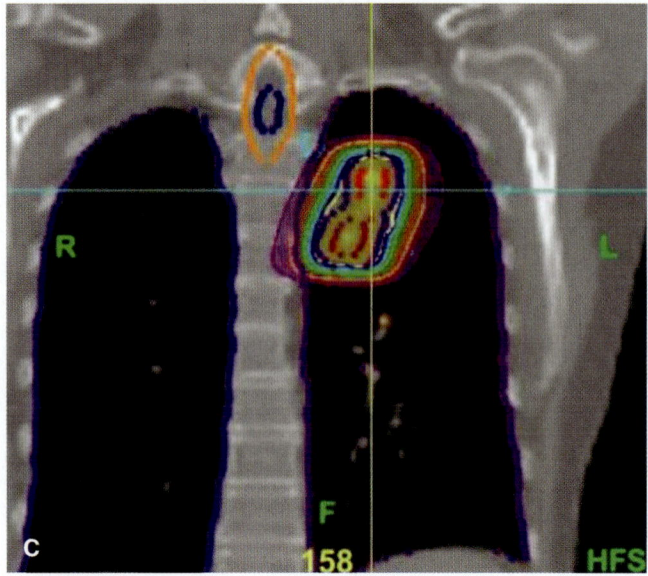

FIGURE 98.5. (Continued)

Other investigators have also examined the curative role of oligometastatic disease for specific primary sites of disease. Milano et al.[74] examined the role of curative SBRT for 51 metastatic breast cancer patients, concluding prolonged survival and possible cure for select patients with limited metastatic disease, as well as the utility of palliative-intent SBRT for symptomatic or potentially symptomatic sites. International guideline statements have also addressed the management of select oligometastatic breast cancer patients in consensus recommendations, stating "a small but very important subset of metastatic breast cancer patients, for example those with a solitary metastatic lesion, can achieve complete remission and a long survival."[75] Similarly, the role of curative SBRT for the treatment of limited metastatic prostate cancer shows promise. Prospective studies have shown good rates of local and PSA control in limited boney and nodal metastatic disease.[76,77]

While these studies show promising results, toxicity from SBRT remains a significant concern. To address this, an NRG trial (NRG-BR001) is currently underway to investigate recommended treatment doses for oligometastatic non-small cell lung cancer, breast cancer, and prostate cancer. The study is accruing patients with less than or equal to four metastatic lesions, limited to the abdomen and pelvis, central and peripheral lung, mediastinal and cervical lymph nodes, liver, bone, or spine. Results are pending.[78]

Early reports have also documented the potential utility of curative SBRT for oligometastatic disease from gynecological and non–small cell lung primary sites, as well as involved oligometastatic sites such abdominal nodal metastases and adrenal gland metastasis.[79–84]

In summary, SBRT may be beneficial in selected patients with a small number of metastatic sites; these patients should be treated on prospective trials in order to obtain a better understanding of the appropriate use of this technology.

REFERENCES

1. Hendrix MJC. Charting a course to a distant site. *Nat Rev Cancer* 2009;9:237.
2. Ferrell B, Koczywas M, Grannis F, et al. Palliative care in lung cancer. *Surg Clin North Am* 2011;91:403–417
3. Jung B, Murgu S, Colt H. Rigid bronchoscopy for malignant central airway obstruction from small cell lung cancer complicated by SVC syndrome. *Ann Thorac Cardiovasc Surg* 2011;17:53–57.
4. Ranu H, Madden BP. Endobronchial stenting in the management of large airway pathology. *Postgrad Med J* 2009;85:682–687
5. Canak V, Zarić B, Milivancev A, et al. Combination of interventional pulmonology techniques (Nd:YAG laser resection and brachytherapy) with external beam radiotherapy in the treatment of lung cancer patients with Karnofsky index ≤50. *J BUON* 2006;11:447–456.
6. Zarić B, Canak V, Milivancev A, et al. The effect of Nd:YAG laser resection on symptom control, time to progression and survival in lung cancer patients. *J BUON* 2007;12:361–368.
7. Nag S, Kelly JF, Horton JL, et al. Brachytherapy for carcinoma of the lung. *Oncology* 2001;15:371–381.
8. de Aquino Gorayeb MM, Gregório MG, de Oliveira EQ, et al. High-dose-rate brachytherapy in symptom palliation due to malignant endobronchial obstruction: a quantitative assessment. *Brachytherapy* 2013;12(5):471–478.
9. Suh J, Dass KK, Pagliaccio L, et al. Endobronchial radiation therapy with or without neodymium yttrium aluminum garnet laser resection for managing malignant airway obstruction. *Cancer* 1994;73:2583–2588.
10. Allen MD, Baldwin JC, Fish VJ, et al. Combined laser therapy and endobronchial radiotherapy for unresectable lung carcinoma with bronchial obstruction. *Am J Surg* 1985;150:71–77.
11. Fairchild A, Harris K, Barnes E, et al. Palliative thoracic radiotherapy for lung cancer: a systematic review. *J Clin Oncol* 2008;26:4001–4011.
12. Rodrigues G, Videtic GMM, Sur R, et al. Palliative thoracic radiotherapy in lung cancer: an American Society for Radiation Oncology evidence-based clinical practice guideline. *Pract Radiat Oncol* 2011;1:60–71.
13. Abbas S, Lam V, Hollands M. Ten-year survival after liver resection for colorectal metastases: systematic review and meta-analysis. *ISRN Oncol* 2011;2011:763245.
14. Qian J. Interventional therapies of unresectable liver metastases. *J Cancer Res Clin Oncol* 2011;137:1763–1772.
15. Alberts SR, Wagman LD. Chemotherapy for colorectal liver metastases. *Oncologist* 2008;13:1063–1073.
16. Mocellin S, Pilati P, Lise M, et al. Hepatic arterial infusion (HAI) compared to systemic chemotherapy for the treatment of unresectable liver metastases from colorectal carcinoma: a systematic review and meta-analysis of randomized controlled trials. *J Clin Oncol* 2007;25:5649–5654.
17. Malik U, Mohiuddin M. External-beam radiotherapy in the management of liver metastases. *Semin Oncol* 2002;29:196–201.
18. Lawrence TS, Robertson JM, Anscher MS, et al. Hepatic toxicity from cancer treatment. *Int J Radiat Oncol Biol Phys* 1995;31:1237–1248.
19. Ingold JA, Reed GB, Kaplan HS, et al. Radiation hepatitis. *Am J Roentgenol Radium Ther Nucl Med* 1965;93:200–208.
20. Russell AH, Clyde C, Wasserman TH, et al. Accelerated hyperfractionated hepatic irradiation in the management of patients with liver metastases: results of the RTOG dose escalating protocol. *Int J Radiat Oncol Biol Phys* 1993;27:117–123.
21. Borgelt BB, Gelber R, Brady LW, et al. The palliation of hepatic metastases: results of the Radiation Therapy Oncology Group pilot study. *Int J Radiat Oncol Biol Phys* 1981;7:587–591.
22. Leibel SA, Pajak TF, Massullo V, et al. A comparison of misonidazole sensitized radiation therapy to radiation therapy alone for the palliation of hepatic metastases: results of a Radiation Therapy Oncology Group randomized prospective protocol. *Int J Radiat Oncol Biol Phys* 1987;13:1057–1064.
23. Bydder S, Spry NA, Christie DR, et al. A prospective trial of short-fractionation for the palliation of liver metastases. *Australas Radiol* 2003;47:284–288.
24. Dawson LA, Ten Haken RK, Lawrence TS. Partial irradiation of the liver. *Semin Radiat Oncol* 2001;11:240–246.
25. Dawson LA, Ten Haken RK. Partial volume tolerance of the liver to radiation. *Semin Radiat Oncol* 2005;15:279–283.
26. Gray B, Van Hazel G, Hope M, et al. Randomised trial of SIR-spheres plus chemotherapy vs. chemotherapy alone for treating patients with liver metastases from primary large bowel cancer. *Ann Oncol* 2001;12:1711–1720.
27. Shapiro MJ. Management of malignant biliary obstruction: nonoperative and palliative techniques. *Oncology* 1995;9:493–496.
28. Shinohara ET, Mitra N, Guo M, et al. Radiotherapy is associated with improved survival in adjuvant and palliative treatment of extrahepatic cholangiocarcinomas. *Int J Radiat Oncol Biol Phys* 2009;74:1191–1198.
29. Eschelman DJ, Shapiro MJ, Bonn J, et al. Malignant biliary duct obstruction: long-term experience with Gianturco stents and combined-modality radiation therapy. *Radiology* 1996;200:717–724.
30. Johnson DW, Safai C, Goffinet DR. Malignant obstructive jaundice: treatment with external-beam and intracavitary radiotherapy. *Int J Radiat Oncol Biol Phys* 1985;11:411–416.
31. Soffen EM, Solin LJ, Rubenstein JH, et al. Palliative radiotherapy for symptomatic adrenal metastases. *Cancer* 1990;65:1318–1320.
32. Jung J, Yoon SM, Park HC, et al. Radiotherapy for Adrenal Metastasis from Hepatocellular Carcinoma: A Multi-Institutional Retrospective Study (KROG 13-05). *PLoS One* 2016;11(3):e0152642.
33. Goodman BD, Mannina EM, Althouse SK, et al. Long-term safety and efficacy of stereotactic body radiation therapy for hepatic oligometastases. *Pract Radiat Oncol* 2016;6:86–95.
34. Holy R, Piroth M, Pinkawa M, et al. Stereotactic body radiation therapy (SBRT) for treatment of adrenal gland metastases from non-small cell lung cancer. *Strahlenther Onkol* 2011;187:245–251.

35. Ahmed KA, Barney BM, Macdonald OK, et al. Stereotactic body radiotherapy in the treatment of adrenal metastases. *Am J Clin Oncol* 2013;36:509–513.

36. Barosi G, Rosti V, Vannucchi AM. Therapeutic approaches in myelofibrosis. *Expert Opin Pharmacother* 2011;12:1597–1611.

37. McFarland JT, Kuzma C, Millard FE, et al. Palliative irradiation of the spleen. *Am J Clin Oncol* 2003;26:178–183.

38. Zaorsky NG, Williams GR, Barta SK, et al. Splenic irradiation for splenomegaly: a systematic review. *Cancer Treat Rev* 2016;53:47–52.

39. Mishra SK, Laskar S, Muckaden MA, et al. Monthly palliative pelvic radiotherapy in advanced carcinoma of uterine cervix. *J Cancer Res Ther* 2005;1:208–212.

40. Smith SC, Koh WJ. Palliative radiation therapy for gynaecological malignancies. *Best Pract Res Clin Obstet Gynaecol* 2001;15:265–278.

41. Adelson MD, Wharton JT, Delclos L, et al. Palliative radiotherapy for ovarian cancer. *Int J Radiat Oncol Biol Phys* 1987;13:17–21.

42. Onsrud M, Hagen B, Strickert T. 10-Gy single-fraction pelvic irradiation for palliation and life prolongation in patients with cancer of the cervix and corpus uteri. *Gynecol Oncol* 2001;82:167–171.

43. Tinger A, Waldron T, Peluso N, et al. Effective palliative radiation therapy in advanced and recurrent ovarian carcinoma. *Int J Radiat Oncol Biol Phys* 2001;51:1256–1263.

44. Konski A, Feigenberg S, Chow E. Palliative radiation therapy. *Semin Oncol* 2005;32:156–164.

45. Hahnloser D, Nelson H, Gunderson LL, et al. Curative potential of multimodality therapy for locally recurrent rectal cancer. *Ann Surg* 2003;237:502–508.

46. deWilt JHW, Vermaas M, Ferenschild FTJ, et al. Management of locally advanced primary and recurrent rectal cancer. *Clin Colon Rectal Surg* 2007;20:255–263.

47. Moriya Y. Treatment strategy for locally recurrent rectal cancer. *Jpn J Clin Oncol* 2006;36:127–131.

48. Melton GB, Paty PB, Boland PJ, et al. Sacral resection for recurrent rectal cancer: analysis of morbidity and treatment results. *Dis Colon Rectum* 2006;49:1099–1107.

49. Wells BJ, Stotland P, Ko MA, et al. Results of an aggressive approach to resection of locally recurrent rectal cancer. *Ann Surg Oncol* 2007;14:390–395.

50. Overgaard M, Bertelsen K, Dalmark M, et al. A randomized feasibility study evaluating the effect of radiotherapy alone or combined with 5-fluorouracil in the treatment of locally recurrent or inoperable colorectal carcinoma. *Acta Oncol* 1993;32:547–553.

51. Ito Y, Ohtsu A, Ishikura S, et al. Efficacy of chemoradiotherapy on pain relief in patients with intrapelvic recurrence of rectal cancer. *Jpn J Clin Oncol* 2003;33:180–185.

52. Wong R, Thomas G, Cummings B, et al. In search of a dose-response relationship with radiotherapy in the management of recurrent rectal carcinoma in the pelvis: a systematic review. *Int J Radiat Oncol Biol Phys* 1998;40:437–446.

53. Bae SH, Park W, Choi DH, et al. Palliative radiotherapy in patients with a symptomatic pelvic mass of metastatic colorectal cancer. *Radiat Oncol* 2011;6:52.

54. Lingareddy V, Ahmad NR, Mohiuddin M. Palliative reirradiation for recurrent rectal cancer. *Int J Radiat Oncol Biol Phys* 1997;38:785–790.

55. Valentini V, Morganti AG, Gambacorta MA, et al. Preoperative hyperfractionated chemoradiation for locally recurrent rectal cancer in patients previously irradiated to the pelvis: a multicentric phase II study. *Int J Radiat Oncol Biol Phys* 2006;64:1129–1139.

56. Mantel F, Flentje M, Guckenberger M. Stereotactic body radiation therapy in the re-irradiation situation—a review. *Radiat Oncol* 2013;8:7.

57. Dewas S, Bibault JE, Mirabel X, et al. Robotic image-guided reirradiation of lateral pelvic recurrences: preliminary results. *Radiat Oncol* 2011;6:77.

58. Defoe SG, Bernard ME, Rwigema JC, et al. Stereotactic body radiotherapy for the treatment of presacral recurrences from rectal cancers. *J Cancer Res Ther* 2011;7:408–411.

59. Jereczek-Fossa BA, Beltramo G, Fariselli L, et al. Robotic image-guided stereotactic radiotherapy, for isolated recurrent primary, lymph node or metastatic prostate cancer. *Int J Radiat Oncol Biol Phys* 2012;82:889–897.

60. Haddock MG, Gunderson LL, Nelson H, et al. Intraoperative irradiation for locally recurrent colorectal cancer in previously irradiated patients. *Int J Radiat Oncol Biol Phys* 2001;49:1267–1274.

61. Alektiar KM, Zelefsky MJ, Paty PB, et al. High-dose-rate intraoperative brachytherapy for recurrent colorectal cancer. *Int J Radiat Oncol Biol Phys* 2000;48:219–226.

62. Kolotas C, Röddiger S, Strassmann G, et al. Palliative interstitial HDR brachytherapy for recurrent rectal cancer. Implantation techniques and results. *Strahlenther Onkol* 2003;179:458–463

63. Hellman S, Weichselbaum RR. Oligometastases. *J Clin Oncol* 1995;13:8–10.

64. Dawson LA, McGinn CJ, Normolle D, et al. Escalated focal liver radiation and concurrent hepatic artery fluorodeoxyuridine for unresectable intrahepatic malignancies. *J Clin Oncol* 2000;18:2210–2218.

65. Sawrie SM, Fiveash JB, Caudell JJ. Stereotactic body radiation therapy for liver metastases and primary hepatocellular carcinoma: normal tissue tolerances and toxicity. *Cancer Control* 2010;17:111–119.

66. Rusthoven KE, Kavanagh BD, Cardenes H, et al. Multi-institutional phase I/II trial of stereotactic body radiation therapy for liver metastases. *J Clin Oncol* 2009;27:1572–1578.

67. Chang DT, Swaminath A, Kozak M, et al. Stereotactic body radiotherapy for colorectal liver metastases: a pooled analysis. *Cancer* 2011;117:4060–4069.

68. Norihisa Y, Nagata Y, Takayama K, et al. Stereotactic body radiotherapy for oligometastatic lung tumors. *Int J Radiat Oncol Biol Phys* 2008;72:398–403.

69. Siva S, MacManus M, Ball D. Stereotactic radiotherapy for pulmonary oligometastases: a systematic review. *J Thorac Oncol* 2010;5:1091–1099.

70. Rusthoven KE, Kavanagh BD, Burri SH, et al. Multi-institutional phase I/II trial of stereotactic body radiation therapy for lung metastases. *J Clin Oncol* 2009;27:1579–1584.

71. Rieber J, Streblow J, Uhlmann L, et al. Stereotactic body radiotherapy (SBRT) for medically inoperable lung metastases—a pooled analysis of the German working group "stereotactic radiotherapy." *Lung Cancer* 2016;97:51–58.

72. Salama JK, Chmura SJ, Mehta N, et al. An initial report of a radiation dose-escalation trial in patients with one to five sites of metastatic disease. *Clin Cancer Res* 2008;14:5255–5259.

73. Milano MT, Katz AW, Muhs AG, et al. A prospective pilot study of curative-intent stereotactic body radiation therapy in patients with 5 or fewer oligometastatic lesions. *Cancer* 2008;112:650–658.

74. Milano MT, Zhang H, Metcalfe SK, et al. Oligometastatic breast cancer treated with curative-intent stereotactic body radiation therapy. *Breast Cancer Res Treat* 2009;115:601–608.

75. Cardoso F, Winer EP, Fallowfield LJ. Metastatic breast cancer. Recommendations proposal from the European School of Oncology (ESO)-MBC Task Force. *Breast* 2007;16:9–10.

76. Muacevic A, Kufeld M, Rist C, et al. Safety and feasibility of image-guided robotic radiosurgery for patients with limited bone metastases of prostate cancer. *Urol Oncol* 2013;31:455-460.

77. Casamassima F, Masi L, Menichelli C, et al. Efficacy of eradicative radiotherapy for limited nodal metastases detected with choline PET scan in prostate cancer patients. *Tumori* 2011;97:49–55.

78. https://www.rtog.org/ClinicalTrials/ProtocolTable/StudyDetails.aspx?study=1311

79. Higginson DS, Morris DE, Jones EL, et al. Stereotactic body radiotherapy (SBRT): technological innovation and application in gynecologic oncology. *Gynecol Oncol* 2011;120:404–412.

80. Yano T, Haro A, Yoshida T, et al. Prognostic impact of local treatment against postoperative oligometastases in non-small cell lung cancer. *J Surg Oncol* 2010;102:852–855.

81. Khan AJ, Mehta PS, Zusag TW, et al. Long term disease-free survival resulting from combined modality management of patients presenting with oligometastatic, non-small cell lung carcinoma (NSCLC). *Radiother Oncol* 2006;81:163–167.

82. Bignardi M, Navarria P, Mancosu P, et al. Clinical outcome of hypofractionated stereotactic radiotherapy for abdominal lymph node metastases. *Int J Radiat Oncol Biol Phys* 2010;81:831–838.

83. Casamassima F, Livi L, Masciullo S, et al. Stereotactic radiotherapy for adrenal gland metastases: University of Florence experience. *Int J Radiat Oncol Biol Phys* 2012;82:919–923.

84. Scorsetti M, Bignardi M, Alongi F, et al. Stereotactic body radiation therapy for abdominal targets using volumetric intensity modulated arc therapy with RapidArc: feasibility and clinical preliminary results. *Acta Oncol* 2011;50:528–538.

Section IV

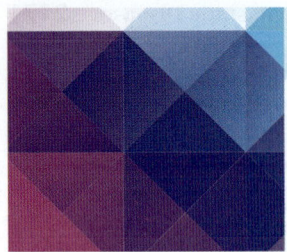

C H A P T E R 9 9

Cancer Pain: Assessment and Management

Esther Yu, Paul Koffer, and Tracy A. Balboni

INTRODUCTION

The most common cancer-related symptom that radiation oncologists are called upon to assess and manage is cancer-related pain. More than half of patients undergoing radiotherapy (RT) experience pain.[1] Notably, majorities of patients and physicians feel that patients' pain is suboptimally controlled[2] highlighting the need for oncologists to have a comprehensive understanding of and facility with cancer pain assessment and management.

PAIN AS A MULTIDIMENSIONAL CONSTRUCT

Pain is a complex symptom that is dynamically related to physical, emotional, social, and spiritual aspects of illness and quality of life. For example, the young parent with metastatic cancer who is struggling emotionally with concerns of how this will impact his/her young children may experience bone pain heralding progressive disease with much greater intensity than a patient who has experienced acceptance of his/her illness. Dame Cicely Saunders, founder of the modern hospice movement, termed this comprehensive concept, "total pain" (Fig. 99.1).[3] Such an approach is critical

to holistic pain assessment and management, addressing the multidimensionality of pain and drawing upon multidimensional resources for its mitigation. In the patient examples above, physical strategies to address pain, such as pharmacologic agents and palliative radiation therapy, should be considered together with psychosocial/spiritual assessment and care as part of a comprehensive approach to pain management, an approach discussed further in Chapter 100. Such an approach is fostered by multidisciplinary management of patients with cancer pain, including palliative and psychosocial specialists, social work, and chaplaincy.

PHYSICAL ETIOLOGIES OF CANCER-RELATED PAIN

Though cancer can be asymptomatic within the normal tissues, symptoms arise once sufficient disruption of normal tissues has occurred, with pain being the most common manifestation. Cancer pain has been hypothesized to be multifactorial in its etiology (Fig. 99.2).[4] It is hypothesized to arise from induction of local inflammatory cytokines within the microenvironment with recruitment of inflammatory cells. These in turn promote sensitization and activation of primary afferent neurons. Additionally, cancer pain can arise from

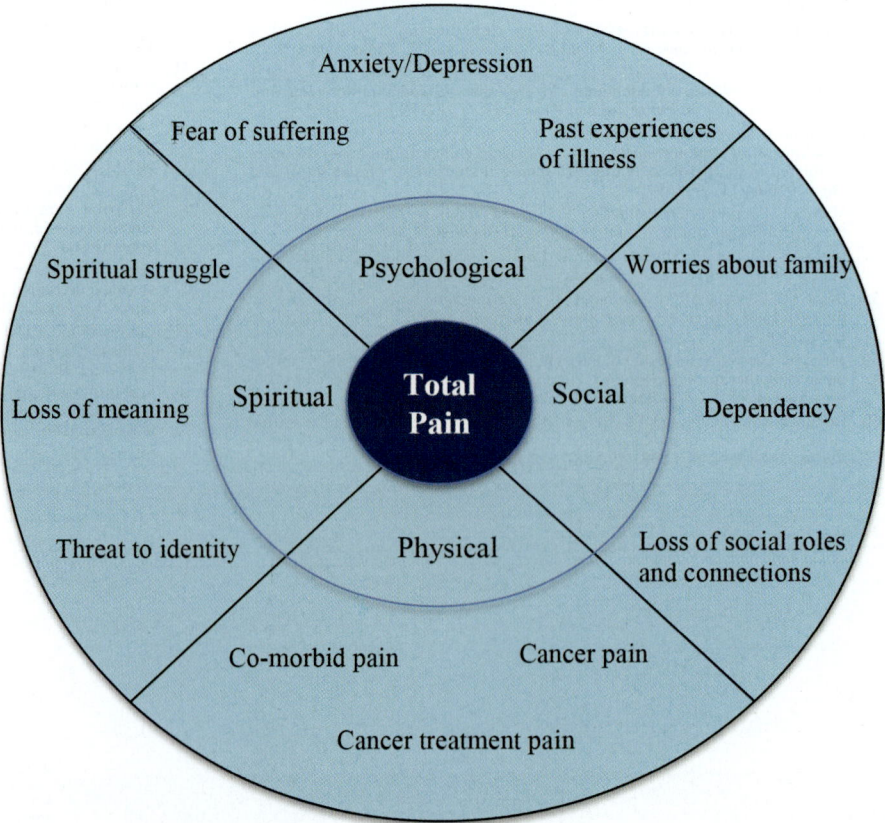

FIGURE 99.1. Dame Cicely Saunders[3] conceptual model of total pain, with examples of factors contributing to the physical, psychological, social, and spiritual pain domains. (Reprinted by permission from Saunders C. The treatment of intractable pain in terminal cancer. *Proc R Soc Med* 1963;56:195–197. Copyright © 1963 SAGE Publications.)

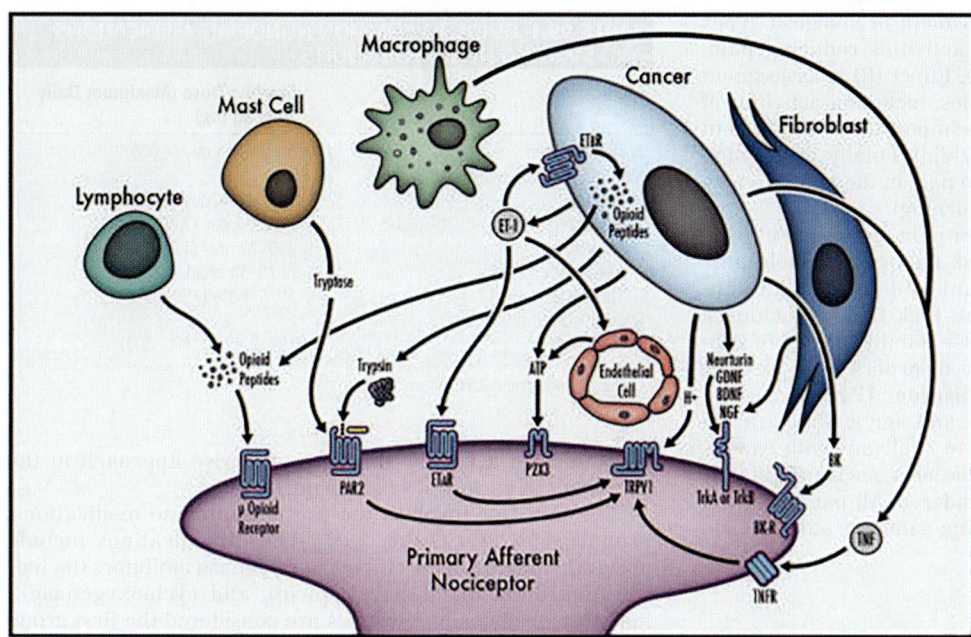

FIGURE 99.2. Schmidt[4] model of the mechanisms of cancer pain. Cancer cells are hypothesized to secrete mediators that sensitize and/or activate primary afferent neurons within the local microenvironment. Cancer cells are posited to secrete chemoattractants that recruit lymphocytes, mast cells, macrophages, and fibroblasts that secrete mediators modulating cancer pain. BDNF, brain-derived neurotrophic factor; BK, bradykinin; BK-R, bradykinin receptor; ET-1, endothelin-1; ET_AR, endothelin A receptor; ET_BR, endothelin B receptor; GDNF, glial-derived neurotrophic factor; NGF, nerve growth factor; PAR2, protease-activated receptor 2; TrkA, tyrosine kinase receptor A; TrkB, tyrosine kinase receptor B; TRPV1, transient receptor potential vanilloid 1. (Reprinted by permission from Schmidt BL. The neurobiology of cancer pain. *Neuroscientist* 2014;20[5]:546–562. Copyright © 2014 SAGE Publications.)

Section IV

mechanical disruption and/or mass effect on normal tissues. This includes normal tissue destruction resulting in pain, such as lytic disease causing bone instability as well as local tissue compression or expansion resulting in pain, such as back pain from malignant spinal cord compression or capsular stretch pain from extensive liver metastases.

Cancer-related pain can also result from the delivery of RT and subsequent complications to normal tissues. Acutely, irradiation of normal tissues with a rapid growth rate causes cell death and triggers a cascade of cytokines and thrombotic and growth factors, propagating local painful reactions.[5,6] Examples include RT-related mucositis and dermatitis. RT can also cause pain because of late or chronic tissue damage such as fibrosis and damage to local microvasculature. Pain management in the setting of acute RT toxicities typically requires a strategy conducive to dynamic pain management needs, including rapid uptitration with gradual downtitration of pain interventions, as symptoms resolve. In the setting of pain related to the long-term effects of RT, pain management strategies should reflect the frequent long-term nature of these pain syndromes given that they often are caused by permanent damage to normal tissues.

This chapter provides an overview of cancer pain assessment, management, and guidelines critical to the practice of radiation oncology. RT is often a valuable component of a treatment plan for cancer-related pain given its efficacy in palliating symptomatic cancers involving bone, nerves, and other soft tissues.[7] The application of RT for the palliation of cancer-related pain and other symptoms is covered in their respective chapters elsewhere in this book.

Types of Cancer-Related Pain

Pain is generally classified as nociceptive or neuropathic or can present as a combination of these pain types. For example, lumbar vertebral body involvement at L1 with tumor compressing the L1 exiting nerve root can cause both local somatic pain (e.g., mid to lower back pain) because of bone involvement by tumor as well as referred neuropathic pain down the L1 dermatomal distribution to the lateral hip. Nociceptive pain refers to the nervous system response that is proportional to the tissue damage initiating the response. Nociceptive pain is subcategorized into somatic pain and visceral pain depending on the location and symptoms of the painful stimulus. Somatic pain generally is a local response to

damage to normal tissues such as skin, muscle, or connective tissue. It often presents as a dull or achy pain that is localizable to its source. Conversely, visceral pain is typically due to irritation of viscera (e.g., colic from gallstones) and may be difficult to localize, though it can also have a somatic component. Visceral pain often is characterized as a dull, sharp, and/or cramping pain.

Neuropathic pain results from irritation and activation of peripheral or central nerves. Patients may complain of burning, shooting, tingling, or numbness, which generally occurs along a nerve distribution.[8] Neuropathic pain can result in pain out of proportion to the pain stimulus where there is abnormal pain processing by the peripheral or central nervous system.

Cancer Pain Assessment

All patients should be screened for pain at each point of clinical contact. Typically, screening is performed with the 0 to 10 pain intensity scale. A comprehensive pain assessment should be performed at initial consultation and at each subsequent evaluation of their ongoing pain management.[9] A comprehensive pain assessment is critical for determining the etiology of pain and for informing strategies for symptom management, both pharmacologically and with local interventions such as radiation therapy. Each type of pain syndrome is amenable to treatment with different modalities. For example, localized, somatic pain may be better treated with nonsteroidal anti-inflammatory drugs (NSAIDs) and/or with opioid medications, whereas neuropathic pain may be more effectively managed with anticonvulsants or antidepressants with or without opiates.

Comprehensive pain assessment should include assessment of the following factors, captured in the acronym "PAINED" to aid in application to clinical practice. Place (P) is assessment of the location of pain, including any pain radiation. Activators (A) are determining factors that make the pain worse, such as positions (e.g., lying down), actions (e.g., walking), or time of day. Intensity and interval (I) are assessment of the intensity of the pain, typically assessed with the 0 to 10 pain scale from 0 (none) to 10 (worst possible pain) together with the interval of time the pain has been present; this includes assessment of changes in pain intensity over time. Asking about the range of pain intensity and intensity changes with aggravating factors can also be informative. Nullifier (N) is assessment of those factors that reduce pain, including analgesics (with full assessment of analgesic types used and quantity), positions and activities reducing pain, or other practices (e.g., meditation). Effect (E) is assessment of the effect of pain on daily activities, including activities of daily living and additional activities important to the patient (e.g., being able to pick up a grandchild). Finally, description (D) is assessment of the quality of the pain in the patient's own words (e.g., dull, stabbing, aching, burning).

Assessment of the patient goals for pain management (e.g., activity goals) and evaluation of risk factors for opioid misuse and diversion are also important to determine an optimal strategy for pain management. Risk factors include a prior history of drug or alcohol abuse, family history of substance abuse, history of psychiatric disorders (e.g., anxiety, depression, posttraumatic stress disorder [PTSD]), history of legal problems or incarceration, and age < 45 years.[9] In patients with risk factors, referrals to clinicians with experience in managing pain in high-risk patients, such as palliative medicine specialists, should be considered. All patients given opiates should be educated regarding safe use, storage, and disposal of opiates.

Cancer Pain Management

A comprehensive pain assessment guides the application of workup and treatment strategies. For example, a patient with metastatic cancer and low back pain radiating to the lower extremities should have a magnetic resonance imaging (MRI) of the spine to assess for possible etiology of cord/cauda compression, with the treatment strategy based on the etiology. Wherever possible, the etiology of the pain should be addressed (e.g., radiation therapy for bone metastasis–related pain) in addition to pharmacologic intervention. The roles of radiation therapy in alleviating cancer-related pain are addressed elsewhere. Herein, guidelines to approach pharmacologic and other non–cancer-directed therapies to alleviate pain are outlined.

GUIDELINES FOR PAIN MANAGEMENT

Many national and international organizations have developed guidelines for pain management. Despite variations in the details, the principles and approaches are consistent across guidelines. The World Health Organization (WHO), American Pain Society (APS), and National Comprehensive Cancer Network (NCCN) guidelines are discussed here.

WHO Pain Ladder. The WHO guidelines for analgesic management of cancer pain, first described in the early 1980s,[10,11] consist of a three-step approach that has been validated in clinical trials.[12] Despite some debate on its effectiveness,[13]

TABLE 99.1 GUIDE TO COMMON NONOPIATE MEDICATIONS AND STARTING DOSES FOR ADULTS

Medication	Starting Dose (Maximum Daily Dose in mg)
Acetaminophen	500, 3–4 × day (4,000)
Nonsteroidal anti-inflammatory drugs	
Aspirin	325, 3–4 × day (4,000)
Ibuprofen	200, 3 × day (2,400)
Naproxen	250, 2 × day (1,250)
Ketorolac	IV 15–30 up to 4 doses
Diclofenac	50, 3 × day (150 mg)
Specific COX-2 inhibitors	
Celecoxib	100, 2 × day (400–800)

COX-2, cyclooxygenase-2; IV, intravenous.

it establishes a widely practiced, stepwise approach in the treatment of various levels of pain severity.

The first tier involves the use of nonopiate medications, primarily NSAIDs (Table 99.1). These medications include acetaminophen, nonspecific cyclooxygenase inhibitors (including ibuprofen, diclofenac, aspirin), and cyclooxygenase-2 inhibitors (celecoxib).[14] NSAIDs are considered the first group of medications to administer. If the patient's pain persists or worsens, the second tier adds a weak opioid in addition to the nonopiate. Finally, continued treatment for worsening pain includes the addition of a strong opioid to replace the weak opiate, the third tier (Table 99.2).

Five simple principles are recommended to make the pharmacologic treatments effective: (a) Oral administration of analgesics should be used whenever possible; (b) analgesics should be given at regular intervals; (c) analgesics should be prescribed according to pain intensity as evaluated with a pain scale; (d) dosing of analgesics should be adapted to the individual; and (e) analgesics should be prescribed with a constant concern for detail.[17]

Over time, adaptations of the WHO ladder have been proposed. In refractory pain or crises of chronic pain, a fourth step may be considered. This fourth step includes invasive techniques such as nerve blocks, neurolysis, or surgical or other interventions.[10,18] Adjuvant medications including steroids, anxiolytics, antidepressants, hypnotics, anticonvulsants, antiepileptic-like gabapentinoids (gabapentin and pregabalin), membrane stabilizers, sodium channel blockers, N-methyl-D-aspartate receptor antagonists, and cannabinoids may be used in the treatment of neuropathic pain.[19,20]

APS and NCCN Guidelines. Although the WHO guidelines are a good initial step in pain management, other organizations have expanded these strategies to improve treatment for cancer pain. These guides provide initial medication dosages, the addition of adjuvant medications, and information on appropriate dose increases, allowing the radiation oncologist to further develop pain management skills.

The 2005 APS *Guideline for the Management of Cancer Pain in Adults and Children* contains detailed discussions of cancer pain management algorithms, pharmacologic strategies, coanalgesics, psychological strategies, supportive therapy, integration of nonpharmacologic and

TABLE 99.2 GUIDE TO COMMON WEAK AND STRONG OPIOID MEDICATIONS AND POTENTIAL STARTING DOSES[a]

Opioid	PO Starting Dose (mg)	PO Conversion (mg)	IV Conversion (mg)
Weak			
Tramadol	50, 2–3 × day	–	–
Codeine	30, 4–6 × day	–	–
Hydrocodone	5, 4–6 × day	–	–
Strong			
Morphine	15, 4–6 × day	30	10
Hydromorphone	2–4, 4–6 × day	8	2
Methadone	2.5–5, 2–3 × day	2	1
Fentanyl	Transdermal 25 µg/d	NA	0.2
Oxycodone	5–15, 4–6 × day	20	NA

[a]Opiate medication must be titrated for adequate pain relief and minimal side effects. For the strong opiates, equivalent doses for conversion are given, with methadone IV as the base dose of 1 mg.[9,15,16] The conversion factors can be used to change PO or IV doses among the different opiates (i.e., 2 mg of PO methadone is roughly equivalent to 30 mg of PO morphine). Similarly, 2 mg of PO methadone is equivalent to 1 mg of IV methadone. When changing from one opiate to another, a reduction factor is sometimes applied (usually 25% to 50% of the original medication's dose) because of less tolerance to the new medication. For example, if a patient is using 60 mg of PO morphine every 4 hours, an equivalent oxycodone dose may be 40 mg × a 50% reduction, leading to 20 mg every 4 hours.
IV, intravenous; NA, not applicable; PO, by mouth.

pharmacologic treatments, physical strategies, nerve blocks, surgical strategies, radiation therapy, chemotherapy, and pain management in special populations. It also discusses patient education and the importance of patients' adherence to the pain management plan as well as how to improve quality of care in pain management.[21]

The latest (2017) NCCN guidelines[9] for adult cancer pain outline the following management principles: (a) Patients should be screened for pain at each point of contact; (b) pain intensity must be quantified and quality described by the patient whenever possible; (c) a formal comprehensive pain assessment must be performed for new or worsening pain; (d) reassessment of pain intensity must be performed at specified intervals to ensure that the therapy selected is having the desired effect; (e) education must be provided to the patient to ensure safe use and disposal of opiates and other analgesics; and (f) all patients should be screened for potential opiate misuse, abuse, or diversion. The guidelines provide specific suggestions for dosing of NSAIDs, opioids, and coanalgesics, as well as titrating and rotating of opioids, escalating of opioid dosage, managing opioid adverse effects, and deciding when and how to proceed to other techniques/interventions for the management of cancer pain.

Role of Oncologists and Pain Specialists in Managing Cancer-Related Pain

Radiation oncologists, together with other oncology clinical practitioners, are responsible for assessing and managing pain for their patients by utilizing the guidelines as noted above. However, this raises the question of when to call upon palliative medicine or acute pain specialists in pain management. Randomized trials have shown a quality of life benefit of early involvement of palliative medicine clinicians in the care of cancer patients, and hence, American Society of Clinical Oncology recommendations call for the early integration of palliative care into standard oncology care.[22] Oncologists should have a low threshold to call upon palliative care providers to guide pain management strategies, particularly in the setting of refractory pain, complex pain syndromes, and/or difficult-to-manage side effects. Integration of palliative medicine into oncology care, and when to refer patients to palliative medicine specialists, is discussed in more detail in Chapter 100.

Routes of Administration

Chemotherapy, surgery, and RT often produce significant side effects that can limit oral administration of pain medications. Furthermore, cancer-related pain can be so severe that acute pain management requires hospital admission and intravenous (IV) pain medication administration. Both opiate and nonopiate pain medications come in formulations that can be delivered via nonoral routes such as transdermal, IV, or rectal. When changing from oral to another delivery mode, care must be taken to give equipotent analgesic doses. Conversion charts for opioids are readily available in the literature.[23] When switching opiate agents, a 25% to 50% dose reduction should be applied to account for incomplete cross tolerance between distinct opioid agents. Such complicated pain management scenarios may require an inpatient stay and/or the assistance of pain management specialists.

Opiate Side Effects

Treating a patient's pain is a balance of maximizing analgesic effects and minimizing side effects.[24] Common opioid side effects include gastrointestinal (constipation, nausea, and emesis), respiratory (decreased respiratory rate), dermatologic (pruritus and dry mouth), and peripheral/central nervous system (myoclonus, sedation, hallucinations, and seizures) effects.

General management strategies include the pharmacologic treatment of the side effects. These include the standard inclusion of strategies to mitigate constipation such as high water intake, dietary fiber, and a daily regimen of stool softeners and laxatives. Consideration of peripherally acting opioid antagonist methylnaltrexone is made in the case of constipation refractory to these measures. Nausea can be mitigated through the use of antiemetics, though care must be taken in the use of antiemetics that can cause constipation such as ondansetron. Another important opiate side effect mitigation strategy is to reduce the dose of opiates required to achieve analgesia through the use of adjunctive medications for pain management, including agents such as glucocorticoids, anticonvulsants, and antidepressants. These medications are discussed further in the next section. A third strategy is opioid rotation as some opiate side effects such as pruritis and myoclonus can be mitigated by rotating to another opioid agent. Opioid rotation should follow the principles of an approximate 25% to 50% dose reduction based on an equianalgesic table given incomplete cross-tolerance of different opiate agents.[9]

Adjuvant Therapies and Interventions for Pain Management

Using the WHO ladder, pain related to cancer can be managed with oral medications in 70% to 85% of patients.[12,25] At any point on the WHO analgesic ladder, adjuvant therapy can be initiated to supplement NSAIDs and opioid treatment. Benefits of adjuvant therapy include use of medications tailored to specific causes of nociceptive responses (i.e., neuropathic pain) and reduction of opiate side effects.

Adjuvant Therapies in Neuropathic Pain

Because neuropathic pain often is not responsive to opioid medications unless high doses are applied, other classes of medications often are prescribed.[26] Glucocorticoids (e.g., dexamethasone) are effective for the short-term management of tumor-related neuropathic pain and often are the initial agent of choice when managing neuropathic pain while awaiting an anticipated response to palliative RT. If glucocorticoids are insufficient to control neuropathic pain, and/or palliative RT does not sufficiently resolve neuropathic pain symptoms, typically anticonvulsants or antidepressants are considered.

Anticonvulsants such as gabapentin, carbamazepine, and pregabalin are effective in managing neuropathic symptoms.[8] Both gabapentin and pregabalin are renally excreted and have minimal drug–drug interactions, which renders these medications effective first-line treatments for neuropathic pain.[8] Like anticonvulsants, antidepressants are a broad category of medications that stabilize neurons involved in neuropathic pain. Tricyclic antidepressants in low doses, such as amitriptyline, have been well-studied and can be effective for pain relief.[27] Serotonin reuptake inhibitors and newer classes of antidepressants, including selective serotonin and norepinephrine reuptake inhibitors (milnacipran, duloxetine, and venlafaxine), are less well-studied but are often prescribed for neuropathic pain. Because many patients with neuropathic pain experience depression or anxiety, antidepressants may play a dual treatment role and improve efficacy of pain control.[27]

Topical agents can also be effective in management of neuropathic pain and often have minimal side effects. These include capsaicin cream and transdermal lidocaine, both found to be effective in the management of neuropathic pain.[28-30]

Muscle relaxants are another class of agents that can be used both in neuropathic pain and other pain syndromes. Because painful muscle spasm can add to the pain etiology

TABLE 99.3 COMMON ADJUVANT MEDICATIONS WITH STARTING DOSAGES AND COMMON SIDE EFFECTS

Medication	Starting Dose (PO unless Otherwise Specified; mg)	Significant Side Effects
Antidepressants		
Amitriptyline	10–25 at night	Cardiac, CNS
Nortriptyline	10–25 at night	Cardiac, CNS
Venlafaxine	37.5 every day	CNS
Duloxetine	60 every day	Nausea, somnolence
Anticonvulsants		
Gabapentin	100, 3 × day	CNS, sedation
Carbamazepine	100, 2 × day	Bone marrow, liver, CNS
Pregabalin	75, 2 × day	CNS, sedation
Topicals		
Lidocaine 5%	1–3 patches for 12 h	CNS, cardiac
Capsaicin	0.025% cream	Burning
Muscle relaxants		
Baclofen	5, 3 × day	CNS
Cyclobenzaprine	5, 3 × day	Drowsiness, dry mouth
Tizanidine	2 every night (4 mg tid)	Weakness, dry mouth
N-Methyl-D-aspartate antagonist		
Ketamine	Intravenous infusion	Hallucinations, CNS

PO, by mouth; tid, three times a day.

in both neuropathic and other pain syndromes (e.g., somatic pain from vertebral body fracture), muscle relaxants can have a role in mitigating pain in this setting. Agents typically used include baclofen and cyclobenzaprine.

Finally, agents that antagonize the NMDA (N-methyl-D-aspartate) receptor are also considered in the management of neuropathic pain; however, prescription of these medications is typically limited to pain specialists. The NMDA receptor has a role in modulating pain signals throughout the nervous system. Methadone is a long-acting opioid receptor antagonist, which is hypothesized to also act as an NMDA receptor antagonist, preventing morphine tolerance and NMDA hyperalgesia effects.[31] Ketamine, a specific NMDA receptor antagonist, is also employed by pain management specialists to relieve cancer and neuropathic pain, especially refractory pain.[32]

Other adjuvant analgesic drug classes used in cancer therapy include local anesthetics, steroids, muscle relaxants, benzodiazepines, α-adrenergic agonists, and bisphosphonates.[32] In recent years, there has been a resurgence in clinical trials of cannabis extracts and analogs in the treatment of refractory cancer pain.[33] Many of these medications are used in specific pain syndromes, which may be useful for the radiation oncologist (Table 99.3).

INTERVENTIONAL PAIN MANAGEMENT STRATEGIES

Although most cancer pain can be managed medically, some patients require interventional procedures to achieve pain relief. Such interventions include neuroablative techniques and implantable neuroaxial drug delivery devices. These strategies should be considered in patients with refractory pain despite pharmacologic management via traditional administration routes (e.g., oral) escalated according to WHO guidelines or among patients with severe side effects despite optimization of pharmacologic agents.

Neuroablative Techniques

Neuroablative techniques can be excellent options for patients who have pain along discrete nerve distributions when chronic and/or insufficiently controlled by conventional systemic pharmacologic management. Interventional pain management specialists offer a myriad of neurolytic procedures that can be highly efficacious and can reduce or even obviate the need for systemic pharmacologic pain medications.

Common nerves targeted include intercostal nerves for thoracic chest wall or abdominal wall pain, maxillary and mandibular nerves for facial pain, and median branch nerves for facet arthropathy.[34] Cryoanalgesia techniques apply subzero temperatures to induce wallerian degeneration of neurons while allowing normal regrowth of axons. Radiofrequency techniques use heat to induce nerve damage. Chemical neurolysis can be achieved with phenol or alcohol preparations.

Pain signals initiating from the perineal, pelvic, and abdominal regions may be transmitted via visceral afferents following the sympathetic nervous system. Along with these fibers, the sympathetic nerves coalesce at specific ganglia (impar, superior and inferior hypogastric, and celiac plexus). At these sites, image-guided neurolytic procedures can be performed.[35] When pain fibers are destroyed in this process, the associated region is also sympathetically denervated.

Implantable Neuroaxial Drug Delivery Devices

Implantable neuroaxial drug delivery devices are indicated when oral opioid doses are escalated without sufficient pain relief and/or when side effects are intolerable.[36] Either semipermanent epidural systems or permanent intrathecal delivery systems can be used to deliver local anesthetic and opiate medications in low concentrations to appropriate spinal cord root levels.[37] The benefits of these methods include decreased side effects than systemic pain pharmacologic agents and often superior pain control.[38]

Electrostimulation techniques also may be applied to disrupt the flow of pain signals in the spinal cord. Transcutaneous electrical nerve stimulation, spinal cord stimulation at thoracic and lumbar regions, and deep brain stimulation at the thalamus or motor cortex can interfere with the conduction of pain signals.[39] The stimulation of large motor fibers inhibits the conduction of pain signals by small nerve fibers and has shown efficacy for various pain syndromes.[40]

Neurosurgical techniques are generally reserved for refractory pain and specific indications. Plexus root avulsions may be responsive to dorsal root entry zone lesioning, but the indications and success rates are limited.[41] More specific lesions at the spinal cord and central nervous system (e.g., thalamotomy and deep brain stimulation) have also been used with variable success and significant side effects.[42] Finally, various chemoneurolytic medications can be delivered intrathecally for destruction of specific nerve roots or parts of the spinal cord for the treatment of refractory cancer pain.[43]

COMPLEMENTARY THERAPIES

Conventional medical regimens may not satisfactorily treat cancer-related pain syndromes. Several complementary modalities such as hypnosis, biofeedback, massage, music therapy, mind–body exercises, and dietary supplementation have been shown to reduce anxiety and chronic pain,[44] yet more multi-institutional, randomized, controlled trials are needed to confirm their efficacy in this setting.[45]

Acupuncture is perhaps the most extensively studied alternative method for pain control.[46] Acupuncture can relieve both acute pain (e.g., postoperative dental pain) and chronic pain (e.g., headache, osteoarthritis).[47–49] Acupuncture also appears effective against cancer-related pain. A randomized, placebo-controlled trial tested auricular acupuncture for patients with cancer pain despite medication. Pain intensity decreased by 36% at 2 months from baseline in the treatment group, a statistically significant difference compared with the two control groups for whom little pain reduction was seen.[50] Most patients in this study had neuropathic pain, which is often refractory to conventional treatment. Neurophysiologic studies show that acupuncture-induced analgesia appears to be mediated by endogenous opioids and other neurotransmitters.[51]

Functional brain imaging studies suggest that acupuncture also modulates the affective–cognitive aspect of pain perception.[52] Correlations between functional magnetic resonance imaging signal intensities and analgesic effects induced by acupuncture have been reported.[53]

SPECIFIC SCENARIOS FOR THE RADIATION ONCOLOGIST

The following section identifies some common pain scenarios and syndromes specific to the setting of radiation oncology and proposes strategies for their management. As previously noted, radiation oncologists are generalist palliative care providers who should readily reach out for the expertise of pain specialists (e.g., palliative medicine and anesthesia pain services) to ensure optimal pain control and quality of life for their patients.

Pain during Radiotherapy Planning and Treatment

Radiation oncologists regularly encounter patients who cannot tolerate RT positioning secondary to pain. The first goal should be to optimize treatment positioning and to decrease time on the treatment table to minimize pain. Often, simple modifications in treatment setup (e.g., cushion under the knees and/or neck), where feasible without compromising radiation delivery, can greatly mitigate incident pain. Next, overall pain management using the aforementioned guidelines should be optimized. Premedication with additional dosing of the breakthrough pain agent such as short-acting opiates approximately 1 hour prior to the simulation or treatment should be performed to anticipate incident pain. Not infrequently, patients will require IV pharmacologic management as an inpatient and hence IV premedication can be given. For such inpatients with severe pain, pain specialists should be involved to optimize pain management using specialized strategies. Among patients with pain that is severe only with the positioning and who may become overmedicated with traditional short-acting opiates, fast-acting opiates can also be considered. For example, transmucosal preparations of fentanyl are optimal because of their pharmacologic properties of fast onset and resolution of effect.

Mucositis and Proctitis

Pain associated with mucositis (up to 75% of patients treated with radiation) can be debilitating and, if not sufficiently controlled, may result in treatment delays and/or dose limitations of RT.[54] Pain control strategies for patients with mucositis follow the aforementioned pain management guidelines, but with some adaptations given the particular needs of this patient population. Topical analgesics, such as viscous lidocaine preparations (e.g., 1:1:1 solution of magnesium and aluminum hydroxide, diphenhydramine, and lidocaine), can provide relief from incident pain when swallowing.[55] When systemic pain management is required, often liquid short-acting opiate preparations and transdermal long-acting agents (e.g., fentanyl patch) are required given difficulty swallowing pills. Mucositis prevention and management will be discussed in greater detail in Chapter 100.

Similar to oral mucosa, the rectum is susceptible to acute and chronic proctitis, with patients typically presenting with tenesmus and rectal pain. In addition to systemic pain control, topical-directed therapies are often used in this setting, including hydrocortisone topical preparations and the use of sucralfate.[56] Management of constipation and diarrhea is also critical in these patients as either can worsen local irritation. Acute proctitis in the setting of RT most often heals within several weeks of RT completion without clinical sequelae, but particularly among patients receiving high-dose RT to the rectum, chronic proctitis can occur. These patients have chronic mucosal irritation that can be painful with rectal mucosal thinning and aberrant blood vessel formation that can result in rectal bleeding. Novel therapies, including hyperbaric oxygen and laser therapy, have been used successfully to heal rectal mucosa and reduce associated symptoms.[57–59]

Plexopathy

Nerve plexopathies are a frequent problem encountered by radiation oncologists, often because of tumor involving the nerve plexus. This scenario is typically managed with radiation therapy directed at the culprit tumor site for palliation together with the aforementioned pharmacologic processes for managing neuropathic pain. Though less common, radiation therapy can also cause plexopathies. Similar to muscle fibers, nerve bundles exposed to dose equivalents of more than approximately 60 Gy in 2 Gy fractions undergo significant decreases in large nerve fiber density.[60] Significant pain may ensue months to years after RT, especially in the brachial plexus distribution.[61] Rates of radiation-induced plexopathy range from 1% to 5% in selected patient populations. Among these patients, 10% will have complicated pain syndromes.[62] Treatments involve physical and occupational therapy, together with pain management strategies, generally overseen by a pain specialist. Typical strategies include multimodality pain regimens (opioid and neuropathic pain medications as previously discussed), with consideration of interventional pain procedures and other novel interventions.[63]

Radiation-Related Muscle Spasm

Muscle fibers, once thought to be radioresistant, may undergo significant change, especially months to years after radiation exposure.[64] One-time muscle exposures to 10 to 20 Gy or fractionated doses >55 Gy are associated with myokymia, pain, and decreased muscle strength and range of motion.[64] Specific cancer locations susceptible to muscle complications include head and neck cancers and soft tissue cancers (e.g., Ewing sarcoma).[64] Treatment regimen includes early physical therapy and orthopedic exercises and pharmacologic therapy such as muscle relaxants such as baclofen or cyclobenzaprine. Novel treatments involve the use of botulinum toxin injected in small doses (15 to 25 units) into the muscle to relieve contracture or spasm.[65,66]

Summary

Pain is a common problem in patients with advanced cancer. RT is frequently utilized to treat pain caused by the underlying cancer. A multimodal management approach should be applied, starting with oral analgesics administered according to clinical practice guidelines, with simultaneous attention to the psychosocial and spiritual aspects of pain and illness. For patients who experience refractory pain despite medical management according to pain management guidelines, pain specialists (e.g., palliative medicine and/or anesthesia pain services) should be involved and specialty pain interventions (e.g., interventional procedures) considered, where applicable. Complementary therapies may be helpful in some patients, although their efficacy has not been definitively established.

REFERENCES

1. Pignon T, Fernandez L, Ayasso S, et al. Impact of radiation oncology practice on pain: a cross-sectional survey. *Int J Radiat Oncol Biol Phys* 2004;60(4):1204–1210.
2. Cleeland CS, Janjan NA, Scott CB, et al. Cancer pain management by radiotherapists: a survey of radiation therapy oncology group physicians. *Int J Radiat Oncol Biol Phys* 2000;47(1):203–208.
3. Saunders C. The treatment of intractable pain in terminal cancer. *Proc R Soc Med* 1963;56:195–197.
4. Schmidt BL. The neurobiology of cancer pain. *Neuroscientist* 2014;20(5):546–562.
5. Maria OM, Eliopoulos N, Muanza T. Radiation-Induced Oral Mucositis. *Front Oncol* 2017;7:89.

6. Lalla RV, Bowen J, Barasch A, et al. MASCC/ISOO clinical practice guidelines for the management of mucositis secondary to cancer therapy. *Cancer* 2014;120(10):1453–1461.

7. Friedland J. Local and systemic radiation for palliation of metastatic disease. *Urol Clin North Am* 1999;26(2):391–402, x.

8. Irving GA. Contemporary assessment and management of neuropathic pain. *Neurology* 2005;64(12 Suppl 3):S21–S27.

9. NCCN Clinical Practice Guidelines in Oncology: Adult Cancer Pain (ver 2.2017). *NCCN Guidelines 2017*, 2017; https://www.nccn.org/professionals/physician_gls/pdf/pain.pdf. Accessed July 28, 2017.

10. Jadad AR, Browman GP. The WHO analgesic ladder for cancer pain management. Stepping up the quality of its evaluation. *JAMA* 1995;274(23):1870–1873.

11. Ventafridda V, Saita L, Ripamonti C, et al. WHO guidelines for the use of analgesics in cancer pain. *Int J Tissue React* 1985;7(1):93–96.

12. Zech DF, Grond S, Lynch J, et al. Validation of World Health Organization Guidelines for cancer pain relief: a 10-year prospective study. *Pain* 1995;63(1):65–76.

13. Azevedo Sao Leao Ferreira K, Kimura M, Jacobsen Teixeira M. The WHO analgesic ladder for cancer pain control, twenty years of use. How much pain relief does one get from using it? *Support Care Cancer* 2006;14(11):1086–1093.

14. Bruera E. Mechanism of action of nonsteroidal anti-inflammatory drugs. *Cancer Invest* 1998;16(7):538–539.

15. Malhotra V, Moryl N, Sudbury MA. *Palliative cancer care*. Sudbury, MA: Jones and Bartlett Publishers, 2006.

16. American Pain. *Principles of analgesic use in the treatment of acute pain and cancer pain*. 6th ed. Glenview, Illinois: American Pain Society, 2008.

17. Organization TWH. *WHO guidelines cancer pain relief*. 2nd ed. Geneva, Switzerland: World Health Organization, 1996.

18. Cahana A, Mavrocordatos P, Geurts JWM, et al. Do minimally invasive procedures have a place in the treatment of chronic low back pain? *Expert Rev Neurother* 2004;4(3):479–490.

19. Moulin DE, Clark AJ, Gilron I, et al. Pharmacological management of chronic neuropathic pain—consensus statement and guidelines from the Canadian Pain Society. *Pain Res Manag* 2007;12(1):13–21.

20. Dworkin RH, O'Connor AB, Backonja M, et al. Pharmacologic management of neuropathic pain: evidence-based recommendations. *Pain* 2007;132(3):237–251.

21. Gordon DB, Dahl JL, Miaskowski C, et al. American pain society recommendations for improving the quality of acute and cancer pain management: American Pain Society Quality of Care Task Force. *Arch Intern Med* 2005;165(14):1574–1580.

22. Ferrell BR, Temel JS, Temin S, et al. Integration of Palliative Care Into Standard Oncology Care: American Society of Clinical Oncology Clinical Practice Guideline Update. *J Clin Oncol* 2017;35(1):96–112.

23. Cherny NI, Portenoy RK. Cancer pain management. Current strategy. *Cancer* 1993;72(11 Suppl):3393–3415.

24. Cherny NI. The management of cancer pain. *CA Cancer J Clin* 2000;50(2): 70–116; quiz 117–120.

25. Ventafridda V. A validation study of the WHO method for cancer pain relief. *Cancer* 1987;59(4):850–856.

26. Milch RA. Neuropathic pain: implications for the surgeon. *Surg Clin North Am* 2005;85(2):225–236.

27. Hainline B. Chronic pain: physiological, diagnostic, and management considerations. *Psychiatr Clin North Am* 2005;28(3):713–735.

28. Priano L, Gasco MR, Mauro A. Transdermal treatment options for neurological disorders: impact on the elderly. *Drugs Aging* 2006;23(5):357–375.

29. Sawynok J. Topical analgesics in neuropathic pain. *Curr Pharm Des* 2005;11(23):2995–3004.

30. Jones VM, Moore KA, Peterson DM. Capsaicin 8% topical patch (Qutenza)—a review of the evidence. *Palliat Care Pharmacother* 2011;25(1):32–41.

31. Inturrisi CE. Pharmacology of methadone and its isomers. *Minerva Anestesiol* 2005;71(7–8):435–437.

32. Lussier D, Huskey AG, Portenoy RK. Adjuvant analgesics in cancer pain management. *Oncologist* 2004;9(5):571–591.

33. Farquhar-Smith WP. Do cannabinoids have a role in cancer pain management? *Curr Opin Support Palliat Care* 2009;3(1):7–13.

34. Trescot AM. Cryoanalgesia in interventional pain management. *Pain Physician* 2003;6(3):345–360.

35. de Leon-Casasola OA. Critical evaluation of chemical neurolysis of the sympathetic axis for cancer pain. *Cancer Control* 2000;7(2):142–148.

36. Mercadante S. Neuraxial techniques for cancer pain: an opinion about unresolved therapeutic dilemmas. *Reg Anesth Pain Med* 1999;24(1):74–83.

37. Lordon SP. Interventional approach to cancer pain. *Curr Pain Headache Rep* 2002;6(3):202–206.

38. Smith TJ, Coyne PJ, Staats PS, et al. An implantable drug delivery system (IDDS) for refractory cancer pain provides sustained pain control, less drug-related toxicity, and possibly better survival compared with comprehensive medical management (CMM). *Ann Oncol* 2005;16(5):825–833.

39. McNicol E, Horowicz-Mehler N, Fisk RA, et al. Management of opioid side effects in cancer-related and chronic noncancer pain: a systematic review. *J Pain* 2003;4(5):231–256.

40. Rushton DN. Electrical stimulation in the treatment of pain. *Disabil Rehabil* 2002;24(8):407–415.

41. Sindou M, Mertens P. Neurosurgical management of neuropathic pain. *Stereotact Funct Neurosurg* 2000;75(2–3):76–80.

42. Slavik E, Ivanovic S. Cancer pain (neurosurgical management). *Acta Chir Iugosl* 2004;51(4):15–23.

43. Candido K, Stevens RA. Intrathecal neurolytic blocks for the relief of cancer pain. *Best Pract Res Clin Anaesthesiol* 2003;17(3):407–428.

44. Deng G, Cassileth BR. Integrative oncology: complementary therapies for pain, anxiety, and mood disturbance. *CA Cancer J Clin* 2005;55(2):109–116.

45. Bardia A, et al. Efficacy of complementary and alternative medicine therapies in relieving cancer pain: a systematic review. *J Clin Oncol* 2006;24(34):5457–5464.

46. Park J, et al. The status and future of acupuncture clinical research. *J Altern Complement Med* 2008;14(7):871–881.

47. Berman BM. Effectiveness of acupuncture as adjunctive therapy in osteoarthritis of the knee: a randomized, controlled trial. *Ann Intern Med* 2004;141(12):901–910.

48. NIH Consensus Conference. Acupuncture. *JAMA* 1998;280(17):1518–1524.

49. Melchart D. Acupuncture for recurrent headaches: a systematic review of randomized controlled trials. *Cephalalgia* 1999;19(9):779–786; discussion 765.

50. Alimi D, Rubino C, Pichard-Leandri E, et al. Analgesic effect of auricular acupuncture for cancer pain: a randomized, blinded, controlled trial. *J Clin Oncol* 2003;21(22):4120–4126.

51. Han JS. Acupuncture and endorphins. *Neurosci Lett* 2004;361(1–3):258–261.

52. Wu MT. Central nervous pathway for acupuncture stimulation: localization of processing with functional MR imaging of the brain—preliminary experience. *Radiology* 1999;212(1):133–141.

53. Zhang WT, et al. Relations between brain network activation and analgesic effect induced by low vs. high frequency electrical acupoint stimulation in different subjects a functional magnetic resonance imaging study. *Brain Res* 2003;982(2):168–178.

54. Scully C, Epstein J, Sonis S. Oral mucositis: a challenging complication of radiotherapy, chemotherapy, and radiochemotherapy: part 1, pathogenesis and prophylaxis of mucositis. *Head Neck* 2003;25(12):1057–1070.

55. Scully C, Epstein J, Sonis S. Oral mucositis: a challenging complication of radiotherapy, chemotherapy, and radiochemotherapy. Part 2. Diagnosis and management of mucositis. *Head Neck* 2004;26(1):77–84.

56. Denton AS, et al. Systematic review for non-surgical interventions for the management of late radiation proctitis. *Br J Cancer* 2002;87(2):134–143.

57. Colwell JC, Goldberg M. A review of radiation proctitis in the treatment of prostate cancer. *J Wound Ostomy Continence Nurs* 2000;27(3):179–187.

58. Jones K. Treatment of radiation proctitis with hyperbaric oxygen. *Radiother Oncol* 2006;78(1):91–94.

59. Clarke RE, et al. Hyperbaric oxygen treatment of chronic refractory radiation proctitis: a randomized and controlled double-blind crossover trial with long-term follow-up. *Int J Radiol Oncol Biol Phys* 2008;72(1):134–143.

60. Vujaskovic Z, et al. Ultrastructural morphometric analysis of peripheral nerves after intraoperative irradiation. *Int J Radiat Biol* 1995;68(1):71–76.

61. Galecki J. Radiation-induced brachial plexopathy and hypofractionated regimens in adjuvant irradiation of patients with breast cancer-a review. *Acta Oncol* 2006;45(3):280–284.

62. Jaeckle KA. Neurological manifestations of neoplastic and radiation-induced plexopathies. *Semin Neurol* 2004;24(4):385–393.

63. Schierle C, Winograd JM. Radiation-induced brachial plexopathy: review. Complication without a cure. *J Reconstr Microsurg* 2004;20(2):149–152.

64. Gillette EL, et al. Late radiation injury to muscle and peripheral nerves. *Int J Radiat Oncol Biol Phys* 1995;31(5):1309–1318.

65. Lou JS, Pleninger P, Kurlan R. Botulinum toxin A is effective in treating trismus associated with postradiation myokymia and muscle spasm. *Mov Disord* 1995;10(5):680–681.

66. Van Daele DJ, et al. Head and neck muscle spasm after radiotherapy: management with botulinum toxin A injection. *Arch Otolaryngol Head Neck Surg* 2002;128(8):956–959.

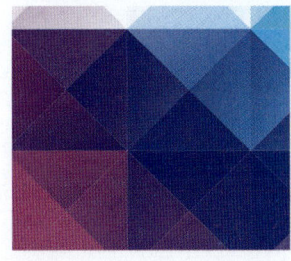

CHAPTER 100

Palliative and Supportive Care

Paul Koffer, Esther Yu, and Tracy A. Balboni

INTRODUCTION: PALLIATIVE AND SUPPORTIVE CARE IN ONCOLOGY

Definitions

The National Consensus Project defines palliative care as "patient and family-centered care that optimizes quality of life by anticipating, preventing, and treating suffering. Palliative care throughout the continuum of illness involves addressing physical, intellectual, emotional, social, and spiritual needs and to facilitate patient autonomy, access to information, and choice."[1] Palliative care may be delivered in a variety of settings including inpatient and outpatient care as well as throughout the patient's disease course, from initial diagnosis to the end of life. The National Consensus Project has defined eight domains of palliative care (Table 100.1) critical to quality palliative care provision.

Palliative care delivered in definitive cancer care settings is at times separately referred to as "supportive care." Furthermore, in some cancer care settings, regardless of the treatment intent, the term "supportive care" is used. To ensure clarity and comprehensiveness, this chapter defines "palliative and supportive care" as care that addresses the biopsychosocial and spiritual dimensions of patient quality of life throughout the cancer care continuum.

EVIDENCE AND CLINICAL GUIDELINES: PALLIATIVE CARE IN ONCOLOGY

In the oncology setting, there is a strong body of evidence supporting the integration of specialty palliative care into oncology care. The American Society of Clinical Oncology (ASCO) set forth the 2012 ASCO Provisional Clinical Opinion based on the randomized controlled trial by Temel et al.[2] This study of 151 advanced lung cancer patients randomized to receive either concurrent palliative care at the time of diagnosis or usual care showed that integration of palliative care into oncology care resulted in better quality of life and fewer depressive symptoms. Additionally, despite receiving less aggressive medical interventions, patients randomized to early palliative care had longer median survival.[2] A survival benefit was also seen in the ENABLE III trial, which randomized patients to early or delayed palliative care. Survival at 1 year was 63% for patients who enrolled early versus 48% for those who enrolled 3 months later.[3] Caregivers may also experience lower levels of depression and stress burden with early enrollment.[4] In the realm of everyday life, early consultation can improve symptom severity and ongoing quality of life for patients.[5] These studies clearly demonstrate that early initiation of palliative care has wide-ranging benefits for patients and caregivers.

Based on these findings and others, ASCO set forth the 2017 ASCO Clinical Practice Guideline Update.[6] These guidelines call for the early integration of palliative care in the treatment of advanced cancer patients and incorporation of palliative care for patients across the cancer care trajectory with attention to triggers based on regular screening for palliative and supportive care needs.

The ASCO Clinical Practice Guidelines call for oncologists

NCP Domain	Domain Description
Domain 1: Structure and Processes of Care	This domain addresses interdisciplinary team engagement and collaboration with patients and families, with an emphasis on coordinated assessment and continuity of care across healthcare settings. Clarity and specificity of interdisciplinary composition, team member qualifications, necessary education, training, and support are described. This section includes quality assessment process and improvement according to the mandates under the Patient Protection and Affordable Care Act.
Domain 2: Physical Aspects of Care	This domain addresses the assessment of physical symptoms with appropriate, validated tools and the multidimensional management of symptoms with pharmacological, interventional, behavioral, and complementary interventions. Explicit policies for the treatment of pain and symptom management and safe prescribing of controlled medications are recommended.
Domain 3: Psychological and Psychiatric Aspects of Care	This domain addresses the collaborative assessment process for psychological concerns and psychiatric diagnoses. Essential elements are described and include patient–family communication on assessment, diagnosis, and treatment options for common conditions in context of respect for goals of care of the patient and family. The domain also includes description and required elements of a bereavement program.
Domain 4: Social Aspects of Care	This domain addresses interdisciplinary engagement and collaboration with patients and families to identify, support, and capitalize on patient and family strengths. The essential elements of a palliative care social assessment are defined. The role of the professional social worker (e.g., with a bachelor's or master's degree) is described.
Domain 5: Spiritual, Religious, and Existential Aspects of Care	This domain defines spirituality and describes assessment, access, and staff collaboration in attending to spiritual concerns throughout the illness trajectory. Requirements for staff training and education are set forth, and responsibility of the interdisciplinary team—including a chaplain—to explore, assess, and attend to spiritual issues of patients and families are discussed. Spiritual and religious rituals and practices to promote comfort are promoted.
Domain 6: Cultural Aspects of Care	This domain defines culture and cultural competence for the interdisciplinary team, with culture understood as a source of resilience and strength for patients and families. This domain accentuates cultural and linguistic competence using plain language, literacy, and linguistically appropriate care delivery.
Domain 7: Care of the Patient at the End of Life	This domain highlights communication and documentation of signs and symptoms of the dying process for the patient, the family, and involved health providers. Meticulous assessment and management of patient pain and other symptoms and attention to family guidance as to what to expect in the dying process and post death period are emphasized. Bereavement support, beginning with anticipatory grief, is emphasized, together with social, spiritual, and cultural aspects of care throughout the dying process.
Domain 8: Ethical and Legal Aspects of Care	This domain is subdivided into advance care planning, ethics, and legal aspects of care. Under advance care planning, the responsibilities of palliative care teams to promote ongoing discussion regarding goals of care together with completion and documentation of advance care planning. In ethical issues, the frequency and complexity of ethics issues are acknowledged and team competencies in identifying and resolving commonly encountered ethical issues are described. The importance of seeking guidance from ethical committees is also emphasized. Finally, under legal issues, the complex legal and regulatory issues in palliative care are acknowledged, together with an emphasis on team members understanding scope of practice within the provision of palliative care. There is also an emphasis on the necessity of and access to expert legal counsel that are essential to navigating the intricate and sensitive legal and regulatory issues in palliative care.

TABLE 100.1 DOMAINS FROM THE NATIONAL CONSENSUS PROJECT GUIDELINES[a]

[a]National Consensus Project for Quality Palliative Care. *Clinical practice guidelines for quality palliative care.* 3rd ed. Pittsburgh: National Consensus Project for Quality Palliative Care, 2013. Available from https://www.nationalcoalitionhpc.org/ncp-guidelines-2013/; Note that the *NCP Clinical Practice Guidelines for Quality Palliative Care.* 4th ed. will be published in Fall of 2018. More information can be found at www.nationalcoalitionhpc.org/ncp

to act as generalist providers of palliative and supportive care.[6] Specific to radiation oncology, radiation oncologists provide specialty expertise in the use of radiation therapy for the management of cancers, both definitively and palliatively. Together with this specialist role, radiation oncologists must have a basic competency in addressing the aforementioned domains of palliative and supportive care that can arise at all phases of cancer treatment. Palliative medicine teams may then be viewed as corresponding specialist providers working in tandem with the oncology team. Notably, some cancer care centers do not have ready access to palliative care teams. In this setting, the oncology care team is called upon to gain more in-depth facility in providing palliative and supportive care. Though advocacy for establishment of palliative medicine resources is needed, care teams in those settings are encouraged to seek out continuing medical education experiences that deepen palliative and supportive care knowledge. Organizations such as the American Society for Radiation Oncology, the American Society of Clinical Oncology, and the American Academy of Hospice and Palliative Medicine sponsor educational opportunities for oncology clinicians using a variety of formats such as online or conferences.

As generalist providers of palliative care, oncologists have a role in the initial screening, assessment, and management of several palliative care domains including physical, psychological, social, and spiritual aspects of quality of life. To this end, patient-reported outcome measures (PROMs) are surveys that allow patients to comprehensively and systematically report and rate their symptoms and psychosocial/spiritual distress. PROMs aid in informing when clinicians are needed to provide additional supportive care and interventions to improve symptom control and overall patient well-being.[7] A recent trial of electronic integration of PROMs in patients with metastatic cancer demonstrated improved measures of quality of life[8] and a significant survival benefit with the addition of PROMs, with results guiding supportive care intervention.[8] These findings point to the need for the standard integration of PROMs in oncology settings as a means of screening patients for palliative and supportive care needs.

In the ensuing sections, we will review common palliative and supportive care issues that arise in the radiation oncology setting and strategies for their management. These include fatigue (both cancer and radiation related), weight loss and cachexia, radiation-induced salivary gland injury, radiation-related mucosal injury, radiation-induced nausea and vomiting, radiation-related diarrhea and other intestinal injury, radiation-induced skin injury, and radiation-related genitourinary injury, including male and female sexual function. Given its frequency and complexity, cancer pain management is addressed with a dedicated chapter (Chapter 99). Radiation oncology clinicians can be expected to provide more in-depth expertise and management for common palliative supportive care issues that arise among their patients. Palliative and supportive care issues with which radiation oncologists have less familiarity (e.g., psychosocial and spiritual issues) should be addressed with established screening tools such as PROMs that provide thresholds to prompt referrals to specialty providers for intervention.

Cancer-Related Fatigue

Cancer-related fatigue (CRF) affects a majority of patients with a cancer diagnosis including those receiving active treatment as well as cancer survivors.[9] The National Comprehensive Cancer Network (NCCN) defines CRF as "a distressing, persistent, subjective sense of physical, emotional, and/or cognitive tiredness or exhaustion related to cancer or cancer treatment that is not proportional to recent activity and that interferes with usual function." CRF is often multifactorial and can be related to the cancer treatments themselves (including radiotherapy and chemotherapy), tumor burden, and up-regulation proinflammatory cytokines including Il-1, Il-6, and TNF-α.[10,11]

The most recent NCCN guideline at the time of this publication (Version 2.2017) recommends screening for CRF in all patients undergoing treatment for cancer at regular intervals with the simple question, "How would you rate your fatigue on a scale of 0 to 10 over the past 7 days?" For those with fatigue scores of 4 or greater, a more focused history should be obtained with an emphasis on possible contributing or related factors including pain, medication side effects, emotional distress, sleep disturbances, hypothyroidism, anemia, and nutritional deficits.[12] Primary management of CRF should be focused on correcting any of these contributing factors. Nutrition deficits and imbalance often occur and may be overlooked in these patients. Weight, caloric intake, fluid intake, electrolyte abnormalities, and micronutrient deficiency from an imbalanced diet should be identified and nutritional counseling provided. One of the most common causes of fatigue is inadequate and/or poor-quality sleep. Control of stimulus, optimizing sleep environment, and promotion of sleep hygiene are all important. Massage therapy to reduce tension and stress is often helpful. Patient should be counseled on self-monitoring of fatigue levels, energy conservation techniques, and the use of distraction. Simple behavioral changes in daily life, such as setting priorities, pacing daily activities, delegating as much as possible, scheduling activities at times of peak energy, and structuring a daily routine to promote quality of sleep, can go a long way to reduce fatigue.

Many nonpharmacologic interventions have proven successful in managing CRF. A meta-analysis of 113 studies examined the effect of exercise, psychological interventions, and pharmacologic interventions for CRF.[13] This analysis showed significant reduction in fatigue scores in cancer patients with both exercise and psychological interventions but not with pharmacologic interventions. Specifically, there is randomized evidence in support of the use of yoga in reduction of CRF in patients being treated for breast and colorectal cancer.[14,15] Cognitive behavioral therapy (CBT) has also been found to be effective in the treatment of CRF in a randomized trial of cancer survivors.[16]

Pharmacologic interventions can also be implemented in carefully selected patients for whom nonpharmacologic interventions are not effective.[17] Short-term uses of glucocorticoids such as dexamethasone and methylprednisolone have been evaluated in several randomized trials. Dexamethasone 4 mg/twice daily for 14 days was compared to placebo in 84 patients with advanced cancer showing short-term improvement in fatigue scores, quality of life, and physical well-being.[18] A separate randomized trial of methylprednisolone 32 mg/daily for 14 days was also compared to placebo again showing short-term improvement in fatigue.[19] However, long-term use of glucocorticoids is limited by their significant side effect profile including hyperglycemia, psychological symptoms including anxiety and agitation, insomnia, GI bleeding, and adrenal insufficiency upon withdrawal.[20,21]

Psychostimulants such as methylphenidate and modafinil have also been evaluated in CRF with conflicting results. A meta-analysis of 5 randomized controlled trials (298 patients) in the treatment of CRF showed improvement fatigue scores with methylphenidate over placebo but not in cognition or quality of life and with increased rates of vertigo, anxiety, nausea, and anorexia.[22] Modafinil was compared to placebo in 208 patients with advanced lung cancer showing no difference in fatigue, depression, sleepiness, or quality of life.[23] In general, these medications should only be considered in patients refractory to more established treatment modalities, and a referral to palliative care should be strongly considered in these cases.

Radiotherapy-Associated Fatigue

Radiotherapy can also be directly responsible for worsening fatigue in cancer patients. Radiation-related fatigue is often difficult to distinguish from generalized CRF resulting from multiple aforementioned etiologies. Radiotherapy fatigue has been demonstrated in patients treated to multiple different body sites including treatment for prostate, breast, and head and neck cancer. Radiation-associated fatigue typically is short lived and less severe than chemotherapy-generated fatigue. Compared with women who received adjuvant radiation, women receiving adjuvant chemotherapy were more than twice as likely to develop fatigue during the course of therapy.[24] In a prospective study of 28 men receiving radical external beam radiation for prostate cancer, the prevalence of moderate to severe fatigue increased from 7% at baseline to 32% at completion of radiation. Fatigue significantly interfered with walking ability, normal work, daily chores, and enjoyment of life, but only at the end of radiation. Improvement occurred after completion of treatment, but remained higher than baseline at 6.5 weeks of follow-up.[25] Similar results are seen in studies of breast cancer patients. In 38 women alive with no evidence of disease 2.5 years after adjuvant radiation for localized breast cancer, there was no significant difference between chronic fatigue levels after radiation and pretreatment values.[26] In another cohort of breast cancer patients, during and for 3 months after adjuvant radiation for breast cancer, fatigue increased from 33% to 93% and gradually improved during the following 3 months.[27] In patients with advanced cancer, fatigue levels initially worsened with radiation, stabilized at week 8, and returned to baseline by week 27.[28]

The size of the radiotherapy field also relates to the likelihood of developing fatigue. For example, patients treated with whole-breast radiotherapy are more likely to experience fatigue compared to those treated with partial breast radiotherapy.[26] In addition, in a survey of patients with brain metastases treated with whole brain radiation or radiosurgery, 69% of patients receiving whole-brain radiation experienced severe fatigue and problems with cognition. Only 5% of radiosurgery patients reported fatigue.[29]

Cancer-Related Weight Loss and Cachexia

Weight loss and anorexia are a commonly encountered problem among cancer patients and has been associated with poor overall survival.[30] Cancer-related cachexia is a distinct category within weight loss and anorexia categorized by a metabolic syndrome associated with a proinflammatory state resulting in loss of muscle with or without associated loss of fat. This syndrome can occur even in the absence of decreased caloric intake or malabsorption.[31] Increases in Il-1, Il-6, and TNF-α have all been associated with increased protein catabolism resulting in skeletal muscle breakdown and a worsening cachexia syndrome.[32] The exact definition and diagnostic criteria for cancer-related cachexia have been previously ill-defined. An international panel of experts published a definition and classification of cancer-related cachexia in 2011 defining cachexia as "patients who have more than 5% loss of stable body weight over the past 6 months, or a body mass index (BMI) less than 20 kg/m^2 and ongoing weight loss of more than 2%, or sarcopenia and ongoing weight loss of more than 2%."[33]

The data regarding the optimum treatment of cancer-related cachexia are limited. Patients with cachexia should be managed by a multimodality approach with emphasis on identifying potentially reversible factors. Although there is mixed evidence on intensive nutritional intervention, all patients with cancer-related cachexia should be evaluated by a nutritionist for advice on diet modification and liquid meal supplementation.[33,34] Dietary counseling has been shown to improve outcomes in selected populations.[35] Patients should be encouraged to take in multiple smaller, calorie-dense meals throughout the day.[34] Liquid meal supplements seem to have the greatest impact if they are taken in between, rather than with meals, with reduction in early satiety and improved overall caloric intake.[36]

Cancer patients tend to have a higher protein turnover. Adequate protein intake is critical in patients undergoing cancer treatment. Daily intake of 1.5 to 2.0 g of protein per kilogram of ideal body weight generally maintains a positive nitrogen balance. Caloric intake helps maintain the weight. Between 30% and 90% of total calories can come from carbohydrates. Fat provides energy, serves as a vehicle for other nutrients, and performs other important biologic functions. It usually makes up around 30% of the content in enteral formulas. Vitamins, minerals, and other micronutrients should be included. Sufficient water intake is required to offset the 2.5-L daily fluid loss. Body weight and serum markers (albumin, transferrin, and prealbumin) can be monitored to assess whether the nutritional support is adequate.[37-39]

In patients with moderate to severe radiation-induced oral mucositis or esophagitis, oral nutritional support can be challenging. Tube feeding bypasses the injured tissues and provides direct access to the absorption surface. Nasogastric or nasojejunal tubes enable short-term access. For longer-term access (>30 days), gastrostomy, gastrojejunostomy, and jejunostomy tubes can be placed endoscopically, radiologically, or surgically. Percutaneous endoscopic gastrostomy is increasingly the method of choice, often placed prophylactically when severe upper GI toxicity is anticipated.[40-43] Gastrostomy tube placement is not without risk. Some series suggest a 17% morbidity rate. In 3% of patients, serious complications such as peritonitis, sepsis, perforation, and dislodgement were reported.[44,45] For patients with reflux esophagitis, gastroparesis, aspiration pneumonia, or limited stomach volume, a jejunostomy tube may be placed instead. The feeding tube should be cared for properly to prevent displacement or malfunctioning such as clogging.

When adequate nutrition intake can be achieved, enteral intake is preferred over parenteral support because it uses and helps maintain the existing alimentary functions. It is less expensive, safer, and associated with fewer side effects. However, in patients without a functioning GI tract because of obstruction, poor GI motility, intractable vomiting, severe diarrhea, short bowel syndrome, or severe pancreatitis, total parenteral nutrition may be appropriate. Implementation of total parenteral nutrition requires special expertise and is done in a concerted manner between the cancer-treating team and the nutrition support team.[46,47]

Pharmacologic interventions have also been studied to improve appetite, weight gain, and quality of life in patients with cancer-related cachexia, particularly those who have failed intensive nutritional support. Short-term uses of glucocorticoids (such as prednisone and dexamethasone) have shown modest benefits in improving appetite and weight gain, but do not seem to improve quality of life and can result in significant side effects such as hyperglycemia, psychological side effects such as anxiety and agitation, insomnia, adrenal insufficiency, and gastrointestinal bleeding.[20,21] Megestrol acetate, a progestin with antiandrogen activity, has also been shown to modestly improve appetite compared to placebo in randomized trials at a dose of 800 mg/daily.[48] A head-to-head comparison of megestrol acetate and dexamethasone showed them to be equivalent in the induction of weight gain.[21] Dronabinol, a cannabinoid, which has been examined for treatment of nausea and anorexia, has not been shown to be superior to placebo in inducing weight gain in cancer patients and has been shown to be inferior to megestrol acetate.[49] In general, short-term use of glucocorticoids and more sustained use of megestrol acetate can be considered for management of cachexia in patients who have failed conservative nutritional management.

SALIVARY GLAND INJURY: XEROSTOMIA

Xerostomia, the subjective experience of dry mouth, is among the most common complaints experienced by cancer patients treated with radiotherapy to the head and neck area. It is caused by salivary gland dysfunction as a result of damage in the field of radiation. Histologically, irradiated salivary glands demonstrate acinar atrophy and chronic inflammation. Inflammatory changes and fibrosis are observed in periductal and intralobular areas, whereas the ductal system remains relatively intact.[50,51]

Salivary dysfunction develops immediately and predictably. A 50% to 60% decrease in salivary flow occurs during the first week. As radiotherapy continues and the total radiation dose increases, salivary function decreases accordingly in a dose-dependent fashion. After initial deterioration, a recovery phase may be seen, with patients reporting reduced xerostomia even though salivary flow remains depressed. This may result from adaptation to the sensation of xerostomia and compensatory response from surviving functional glandular tissues. However, salivary function usually continues to decline for 6 to 8 months after therapy, and many patients show no recovery even at 12 months.[52,53] In some patients, xerostomia may be permanent.

In addition to oral discomfort, radiation-induced salivary gland injury contributes to systemic problems, including loss of appetite, chronic esophagitis, gastroesophageal reflux, and sleep disruption because of the need for frequent mouth moistening and subsequent polyuria.[54] The lubricating, buffering, and antimicrobial effects of saliva maintain the integrity of oral tissue (dental and mucosal). Saliva also assists in speech, taste perception, mastication, bolus formation, and swallowing.[55] Decreased salivation can lead to dental caries, periodontal diseases, a shift of oral flora, poor tolerability to dental prosthesis and inflammation, and atrophy and ulceration of mucosa. As a result, radiation-induced xerostomia has a debilitating impact on health and overall quality of life in head and neck cancer patients and survivors.[56]

Xerostomia Prevention

The extent of radiation-induced salivary dysfunction is influenced by radiation field, radiation dose, and initial volume and function of the salivary gland. Several approaches have been developed to prevent or minimize injury to salivary glands. They include salivary gland transplantation, intensity-modulated radiation therapy, and amifostine therapy.[57] In several earlier studies, surgical transfer of submandibular glands into the submental space prior to radiation therapy resulted in prevention of xerostomia.[58-61] A 2-year follow-up showed that 83% to 92% of patients reported no or minimal xerostomia.[61,62] Advances in three-dimensional conformal radiation therapy and intensity-modulated radiation therapy make it possible to conduct gland-sparing radiotherapy. Several studies showed that both subjective and objective measures of salivatory function are preserved. Limiting the mean dose of the parotid glands to ≤26 Gy decreases the risk of long-term xerostomia. Local treatment failure rates do not appear to be compromised by the use of salivary gland-sparing intensity-modulated RT.[63-68]

Intravenous (IV) amifostine, a thiol-containing radioprotectant, administered at 200 mg/m[2] daily 15 to 30 minutes before irradiation, reduced acute and chronic xerostomia in an open-label phase III study.[69] Antitumor treatment efficacy was preserved; however, oral mucositis was not reduced. Nausea, vomiting, hypotension, and allergic reactions were the most common side effects.[70] Subcutaneous administration of amifostine has been explored for reduced side effects.[71-73] A multicentered phase III randomized trial failed to show that subcutaneous amifostine is superior to IV amifostine in terms of patient compliance or efficacy.[74] Other agents are less promising. Pilocarpine during radiation therapy was compared to salivary gland transfer in the prevention of xerostomia and found to be inferior.[75,76] Cevimeline, a muscarinic agonist, was evaluated in randomized controlled trial with conflicting results.[77,78]

Management of Radiation-Induced Xerostomia

Current treatment of radiation-induced xerostomia includes dietary and oral hygiene, saliva substitution, or stimulation of salivation by moistening agents or medications.[57,79,80] Cold, tepid, soft food and beverages are preferred. Hard, spicy foods should be avoided. In patients without residual salivary function, saliva substitutes are used to relieve xerostomia. Water is commonly used and preferred by patients. Other types of mouthwash such as saline, bicarbonate, glycerol, or commercial formulations are available. Artificial saliva has been designed to mimic natural saliva. It may contain carboxymethylcellulose, porcine and bovine mucin, or xanthan gum. In patients with residual salivary function, increased flow of natural saliva can be achieved by stimulation with chewing gum, sucking ointment, sugarless candies, menthol, acid, vitamin C, or lozenges developed to provide antimicrobial enzymes.

Several sialogogues, defined as systemic salivary gland stimulants, have been tested with mixed results. They are typically muscarinic agonists such as pilocarpine, bethanechol, carbachol, or cevimeline. Other classes of agents include neostigmine, physostigmine, nicotinic acid, potassium iodide, bromhexine (a mucolytic), and anethole trithione.[51] Current data support the use of pilocarpine. Further studies are needed to determine the long-term efficacy and safety of cevimeline and bethanechol.[57]

The most extensively studied pharmacologic treatment for xerostomia is pilocarpine. Oral administration at 5 to 10 mg, three times daily, is the standard regimen. Several randomized, double-blind, placebo-controlled trials have shown clinical efficacy and safety of pilocarpine in treating radiation-induced xerostomia.[81,82] In a multicenter study, 54% of the 207 study subjects reported reduction in the overall severity of xerostomia. Only 25% of those receiving placebo reported improvement. Speaking ability improved in 33% of patients receiving pilocarpine versus 18% of those receiving placebo. Saliva production also improved, but this did not correlate with subjective symptom relief.[81] In another multicenter trial that involved 162 patients, both subjective symptom and objective measurement of saliva flow improved significantly in those receiving pilocarpine versus placebo. Best results were obtained with continuous treatment for 8 to 12 weeks.[83]

Some patients require pilocarpine treatment for 2 months or longer to achieve maximum effect. Sweating, the most common side effect, is experienced by 37% to 65% of patients. In one study, 6% and 29% of patients in the 5- and 10-mg groups, respectively, dropped out because of the adverse effects.[81] Because of the cholinergic activity of pilocarpine, it is not recommended for patients with cardiovascular disease, and it is contraindicated in patients with narrow-angle glaucoma and uncontrolled asthma.[84]

Acupuncture has been shown to stimulate saliva production.[85-87] It even shows some benefit in pilocarpine-resistant xerostomia.[88] Patients with more severe symptoms appear to benefit more from acupuncture treatment.[89] Acupuncture given concurrently with radiotherapy was shown to significantly reduce xerostomia and improve quality of life.[90] Yet, an acupuncture-like transcutaneous electrical nerve stimulation given concomitantly with radiation failed to do the same.[91] Acupuncture appears to modulate the function of the autonomic nervous system, which may stimulate salivary gland function and induce salivary flow.[92-95] Functional magnetic resonance imaging changes in the brain were associated with acupuncture treatment.[96] In summary, acupuncture appears to be a low-risk intervention that offers a potential future treatment for radiation-induced xerostomia.[57,97]

MUCOSAL INJURY: ORAL MUCOSITIS, NAUSEA AND VOMITING, DIARRHEA, AND OTHER GASTROINTESTINAL TOXICITY

Radiation therapy causes mucosal injury. When such injury occurs in the oral cavity, as commonly seen in patients irradiated at the head and neck area, it is called *stomatitis* or *oral mucositis*. When the injury occurs in nonoral alimentary tract mucosa, it presents as esophagitis, gastritis, enteritis, colitis, or proctitis. These injuries manifest as pain, dysphagia, odynophagia, nausea, vomiting, and diarrhea, typically described as GI toxicity. Mucosal injuries by radiation appear to share the same underlying molecular pathogenesis, regardless of anatomic location.[98–100] Some favor the terminology of *alimentary mucositis* to describe the hierarchy and constellation of toxicity to the oral and GI mucosa.[101] Depending on the site of irradiation, dosage, and fractionation, patients' risks of mucositis vary. More than 50% of patients receiving radiation to the head and neck, abdomen, or the pelvis will experience moderate to severe mucositis. Stem cell transplant recipients who received total-body irradiation have more severe and prolonged symptoms.[102]

Recent research indicates that the pathogenesis of mucositis is not simply the result of nonspecific epithelial cell death. Rather, it may involve a more complex pan–tissue process.[103–105] The complexity of the pathogenesis of mucositis reflects the dynamic interactions of all of the cell and tissue types that comprise the epithelium and submucosa. Genetic predisposition, circadian variables, epithelial type and characteristics, and local microbial environment all play a role in determining the risk of mucosal injury.[106–108] Novel therapies are being developed based on these new findings.[107,109]

A practice guideline developed in 2004 by the Multinational Association of Supportive Care in Cancer and International Society of Oral Oncology was updated in 2014.[104,110] These guidelines provide an excellent and evidence-based reference in the prevention and management of chemotherapy and radiotherapy-related mucositis.

Oral Mucositis Prevention

Topical benzydamine, a drug with anti-inflammatory, analgesic, and antimicrobial effects, has been shown to reduce the frequency and severity of oral ulcers and pain in a randomized controlled trial.[111] It inhibits the production of proinflammatory cytokines, including tumor necrosis factor-α.[111,112] Chlorhexidine failed to prevent radiation-induced oral mucositis (Fig. 100.1).[113–115]

Basic oral care is the foundation of care for oral mucositis. There is a lack of evidence supporting one protocol over another. Therefore, feasibility, adherence, performance, and outcomes are more important than the use of specific agents. Three randomized and three nonrandomized trials showed that implementation of a systematic protocol improved outcome.[116–121] Protocols consisting of brushing, flossing, bland rinses, and moisturizers should be implemented for all patients. An interdisciplinary approach to oral care (nurse, physician, dentist, dental hygienist, dietician, pharmacist, and others as relevant) is preferred. Dental examinations and treatment are important prior to the start of cancer therapy, especially for those with head and neck cancer, and should continue throughout active treatment and follow-up.[122]

Studies testing amifostine for oral mucositis have been disappointing. Although it appeared useful in the prevention of xerostomia, inconsistent results have been reported for its use for oral symptoms.[123] New classes of agents are being investigated. Recombinant human keratinocyte growth factor-1 (rhuKGF-1, palifermin) was shown to reduce mucositis in patients with hematologic malignancies receiving high-dose chemotherapy and total-body irradiation with autologous stem cell transplantation.[124] Palifermin reduces incidence of severe oral mucositis in head and neck cancer patients receiving definitive chemoradiotherapy and delays the onset of severe symptoms when compared to placebo. Yet, the differences are not significant after multivariate analysis.[125] Its use in non–stem cell transplantation settings is not recommended based on current data.

On the other hand, a local granulocyte–macrophage colony–stimulating factor mouthwash should *not* be used in efforts to prevent oral mucositis in the transplant setting. Other growth factors and cytokines are in early stage of development, including epidermal growth factor, transforming growth factor-β, glucagonlike peptide-2, lactoferrin, anti-inflammatory amino acid decapeptide, recombinant human interleukin 11, and insulin-like growth factor 1.[126] Natural product and dietary supplements such as glutamine, PV701 (milk-derived protein extract), several vitamins (A, B_{12}, E), folate, aloe vera (a plant extract), probiotics, and curcumin, an extract from turmeric, were shown to hold promise in reducing radiation-induced mucositis. Most of the studies are not of sufficient quality to support a recommendation.

Oral Mucositis Treatment

Pain management is an important component of the management of oral mucositis. Most studies were done in the setting of chemotherapy-induced mucositis, instead of radiation-induced oral mucositis. Systemic and topical analgesics are used, as are coating agents. The use of opioids, nonopioids, and adjuvant medications is covered in more detail in Chapter 99. These agents can be given via oral, transmucosal, transdermal, or IV routes. Use of topical agents is widespread in practice, with practices and institutions using their own favorite formulation. Typically, these are compounded mixtures with nicknames such as "magic mouthwash." Common ingredients include viscous lidocaine, diphenhydramine, and Maalox. Despite their popularity, there is little evidence supporting their effectiveness.[115,127–132] Doxepin rinses have also been evaluated for the treatment of oral mucositis. In a randomized, placebo-controlled trial of 155 patients being receiving head and neck radiotherapy, doxepin was found to modestly improve painful mucositis.[133] The MASCC/ISOO 2014 guideline currently suggests doxepin 0.5% solution or 2% morphine mouthwash for the treatment of radiotherapy-associated oral mucositis but provide no guidance on the use of lidocaine-based mixtures.[110]

FIGURE 100.1. A, B: Radiotherapy-induced oral mucositis.

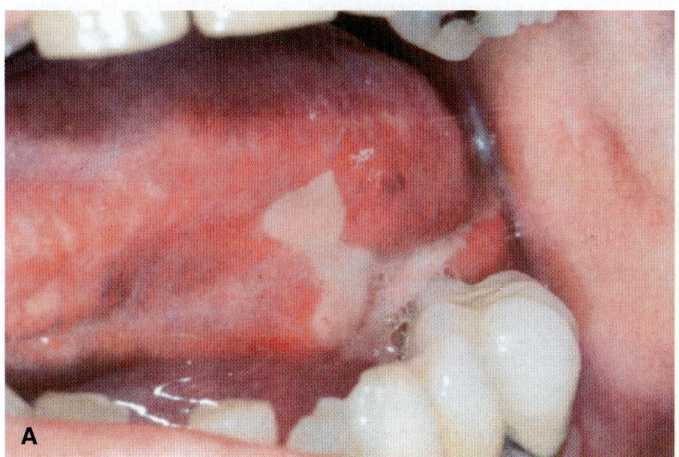

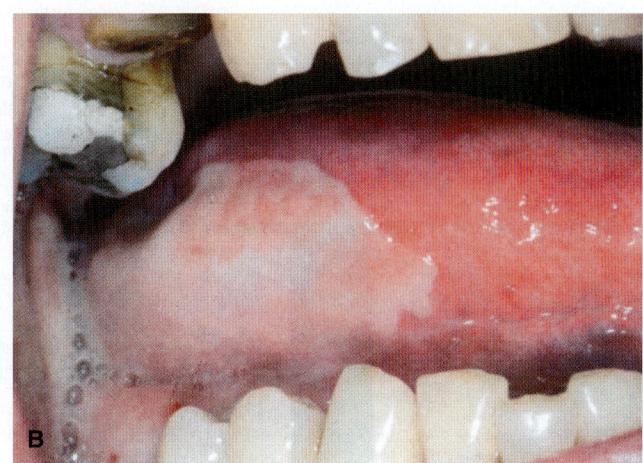

Gastrointestinal Mucositis Prevention

Several medications have been shown to significantly reduce the frequency and severity of radiation-induced GI mucositis, which usually presents as diarrhea and pain. Depending on the location, the GI mucositis may be termed *esophagitis*, *enteritis*, *colitis*, *proctosigmoiditis*, or *proctitis*. External beam irradiation to the pelvis as part of treatment for prostate, rectal, or cervical cancer produces lower GI injury in the majority of patients.

In a randomized, controlled trial of pelvic irradiation, sulfasalazine 1 g orally twice daily reduces GI toxicity from 93% to 80% and diarrhea from 86% to 55% when compared with placebo. Grade 4 diarrhea was reduced from 16% of the patients to none.[134] Amifostine is an antioxidant that appears to protect normal cells from radiation injury preferentially to cancer cells.[135] Amifostine was shown in several studies to prevent proctitis in patients receiving standard-dose radiation for rectal cancer.[123] The frequency, onset, and duration of acute rectal toxicity were reduced.[136–138] When used in patients receiving combined chemoradiation for non–small cell lung cancer, amifostine significantly reduced the need for morphine to control pain from severe esophagitis,[139] but its efficacy was mixed in other settings.[136,140,141] IV amifostine is not without side effects. Other routes of administration that might reduce side effects are under study.

Other agents that did not show significant benefit include glutamine,[140] oral sucralfate,[142,143] rectal administration of sucralfate,[144] and other anti-inflammatories commonly used in ulcerative colitis, such as 5-aminosalicylates,[145] mesalazine,[146] and olsalazine.[147] They should not be used to prevent radiation GI toxicity.

Gastrointestinal Mucositis Treatment

Nausea and Vomiting

In addition to measures discussed here that aim to treat the underlying pathology of radiation-induced mucosal injury, symptomatic treatment should also be provided. Radiation-induced nausea and emesis tend to be undertreated. Factors that influence radiation-induced emesis include single and total dose rate, fractionation, field-size and irradiated volume, site of irradiation and organs included in the radiation field, patient positioning, radiation technique, energy and beam quality, previous or simultaneous influencing therapy, and general health status

of the patient.[148] Evidence-based practice guidelines developed by national organizations differ in specific recommendations and in, when recommendations apply, reflecting the limited amount of high-level evidence available to date. The updated guidelines from the Multinational Association of Supportive Care in Cancer[149] American Society of Clinical Oncology,[150] and NCCN[151] are summarized in Table 100.2.

Diarrhea

Symptomatic management of radiation-induced diarrhea is similar to that of chemotherapy-induced diarrhea.[152,153] Diarrhea usually occurs during the third week of fractionated abdomen or pelvic radiotherapy. Guidelines were developed by an expert panel and updated in 2004.[154]

For mild to moderate diarrhea, the initial management should include dietary modifications.[155] Patients should eat small, frequent, protein-rich meals. Adequate fluid intake (35 mL/kg/day) is necessary. Liquids should be taken primarily between meals. Soluble fibers such as oats, pectin, guar, and psyllium help retain stool consistency. Spices, alcohol, caffeine, high-osmolar beverages, and high-lactose food should be avoided.[155]

Loperamide remains the mainstay of pharmacologic treatment. It should be started at 4 mg followed by 2 mg every 4 hours or after every unformed stool (maximum 16 mg per day). Unlike in chemotherapy, where loperamide may be discontinued after initial response, standard doses of loperamide should be continued for the duration of radiation. This is because the long duration of fractionated radiation may cause repeated injury to the intestinal mucosa. The dose is increased to 2 mg every 2 hours if the diarrhea persists for more than 24 hours.

If diarrhea has not resolved after another 24 hours on the higher dose of loperamide, the drug should be continued and a second-line agent, such as tincture of opium (paregoric), an antimotility agent, can be added. Diphenoxylate and atropine can also be used, although they do not have as favorable a side effect profile as loperamide. Patients with diarrhea may require outpatient evaluation and IV fluid. Antibiotics and complete stool and blood workup are usually not necessary in the absence of signs of dehydration or infection. Octreotide and glutamine have been studied and found of no benefit.[156,157] Probiotic supplementation showed beneficial effect in the prevention and treatment of radiation-induced diarrhea in

TABLE 100.2 GUIDELINES FOR PREVENTION AND TREATMENT OF RADIATION-INDUCED NAUSEA AND VOMITING

	Risk			
	High	**Moderate**	**Low**	**Minimal**
MASCC/ESMO risk category	Total body	Upper abdomen, craniospinal	Cranium, craniospinal, H&N, thorax, pelvis	Breast, extremities
MASCC/ESMO recommendation	Prophylaxis with 5-HT₃ receptor antagonists + dexamethasone	Prophylaxis with 5-HT₃ receptor antagonists + optional dexamethasone	Prophylaxis or rescue with 5-HT₃ receptor antagonists, dopamine receptor antagonist, or dexamethasone	Rescue with dexamethasone, dopamine receptor antagonists, or 5-HT₃ receptor antagonists
ASCO risk category	Total body	Upper abdomen, craniospinal	Brain, H&N, thorax, pelvis	Breast, extremities
ASCO recommendation	Prophylactic 5-HT₃ receptor antagonist before each fraction and the day after RT; Prophylactic dexamethasone prior to fraction 1–5	Prophylactic 5-HT₃ receptor antagonist before each fraction; Prophylactic dexamethasone prior to fraction 1–5	A 5-HT₃ receptor antagonist, dopamine receptor antagonist or dexamethasone as rescue therapy	Dopamine, dexamethasone or 5-HT₃ receptor antagonists as rescue
NCCN risk category	Total body	Upper abdomen/localized sites	–	–
NCCN recommendation	Prophylactic ondansetron, 8 mg oral twice or 3 times a day or granisetron, 2 mg oral daily ± dexamethasone, 4 mg oral every day	Same as in total-body radiation	–	–
NCCN recommendation for breakthrough treatment	The same in chemo-induced nausea vomiting	The same in chemo-induced nausea vomiting	–	The same in chemo-induced nausea vomiting

5-HT₃, 5-hydroxytryptamine 3; ASCO, American Society of Clinical Oncology; H&N, head and neck; MASCC, Multinational Association of Supportive Care in Cancer; NCCN, National Comprehensive Cancer Network; RT, radiotherapy.

animal studies, but high-quality clinical studies are lacking. If diarrhea is severe, persistent, or complicated, hospitalization may be considered.[154]

SKIN INJURY: ACUTE DERMATITIS AND CHRONIC SKIN CHANGES

Radiation-induced skin injury can lead to acute dermatitis or chronic skin changes.[158,159] These changes can occur at both the entrance and exit sites of the irradiation beam. Severity is determined by the dose, fractionation, beam, volume, and surface area. Patient-specific factors such as poor nutrition status, preexisting vascular condition or connective tissue disease, excessive skin folds, and genetics also play a role.[160] The pathophysiology is a combination of direct radiation injury and a subsequent inflammatory response. Free radicals from ionizing radiation cause alteration of DNA, proteins, lipids, and carbohydrates. Epithelial basal cells, vascular endothelial cells, and Langerhans cells are damaged. A cascade of proinflammatory cytokines, thrombotic factors, growth factors, and other molecules is activated.[161]

Acute skin changes may become visible after 10 to 14 hours. Grade 1 changes include mild generalized erythema and dry desquamation, pruritus, scaling, dyspigmentation, and hair loss. After 4 or 5 weeks of radiotherapy and radiation doses to the skin of 40 Gy or greater, grade 2 dermatitis may develop, with tender or edematous erythema, moist desquamation in skin folds, and considerable pain. They tend to peak 1 to 2 weeks after the last treatment and start healing 3 to 5 weeks after radiation. Complete healing may take 1 to 3 months. Occasionally, dermatitis may progress to grade 3, characterized by confluent moist desquamation, or even grade 4, with ulcers, hemorrhage, and necrosis.[158,162] Chronic changes may develop months or years after the initial exposure. Postinflammatory hypo- or hyperpigmentation, textural changes (xerosis and hyperkeratosis), loss of hair follicles and sebaceous glands, atrophy, telangiectasia, or subcutaneous fibrosis are among the manifestations. Fibrosis can result in tissue retraction, pain, and limitation of movement. The scalp appears more tolerant to radiation injury than the skin of the face, neck, trunk, and extremities. The affected skin can be predisposed to ulcers and skin breakdown.[163,164] In some patients, radiation recall dermatitis may occur. This happens when a patient who has completed radiation encounters a drug and develops skin reaction similar to an acute radiation dermatitis. The offending drugs are usually cytotoxic agents. Radiation recall dermatitis is probably due to local cutaneous immunologic responses to the challenging agent.[165]

Mild acute dermatitis is treated symptomatically. Washing with water, gentle cleansing with a mild agent, wearing loose, nonbinding clothing, and avoidance of irritants, antiperspirants, and ultraviolet exposure all help. When erythema and dry desquamation occur, creams or ointments (petrolatum-based, castor oil, balsam of Peru, trypsin, trolamine) can be used. Topical sucralfate or hyaluronic acid was shown to be efficacious in some controlled studies.[166,167] In a phase III study in breast cancer patients receiving postoperative radiotherapy, an extract from the calendula plant significantly reduced the occurrence of moderate to severe acute dermatitis from 63% to 41% when compared with trolamine, a nonsteroidal agent.[168] Other topical agents containing aloe vera, D-panthenol, almond, or chamomile can also be tried. The use of these agents is supported only by uncontrolled studies or anecdotal evidence.[169,170]

The value of topical antioxidants has not been established, and topical steroids are controversial, with research producing conflicting results. There are concerns of infection and skin atrophy, known side effects of topical steroids. At best, steroids may ameliorate the symptoms, but they do not prevent the dermatitis.[171] Topical ascorbic acid lotion (vitamin C)

did not show discernible benefit for the prevention of radiation dermatitis.[172]

When acute dermatitis becomes severe, usual wound care should be applied to the erosions and ulcerations. Key measures are keeping the site clean and moist, pain management, protection from contamination, debridement, and infection control.[164,173] During radiation treatment, hydrogel dressings, hydrocolloid dressing, burn pads, or foam dressings can be applied. If the wound is infected, ionic silver powder, topical antibiotics, cadexomer iodine, or maltodextrin powder can be added. Referral to wound care specialists should be made in these cases.[169] In recent years, more specific agents have been investigated, such as topical granulocyte–macrophage colony–stimulating factor, tacrolimus, pimecrolimus, and platelet-derived growth factor, though these are not included in the standard of care.[158]

Chronic skin changes from radiation injury are harder to treat. Chronic fibrosis is associated with high incidence of skin breakdown and infection. A team approach should be adopted that includes wound care, physical therapy, deep massage, and pain management to address cosmetic and quality of life issues. Pentoxifylline appears to have an antifibrotic effect. Oral pentoxifylline (800 mg/day) and vitamin E (1,000 IU/day) for 6 months significantly reduce radiation-induced fibrosis.[174] Prophylactic use of pentoxifylline significantly reduces late skin changes, fibrosis, and soft tissue necrosis in a randomized controlled study, possibly through its protective effect against vascular pathology.[175] Intramuscular liposomal copper or zinc superoxide dismutase, subcutaneous interferon-γ, or hyperbaric oxygen therapy has also been used.

GENITOURINARY TRACT INJURY

Urinary Symptoms

Irradiation to the pelvic region as part of treatment for cancer of the prostate, uterus, ovary, cervix, rectum, or urinary bladder can cause urinary problems because of injury to mucosa, vasculature, and smooth muscles.[176,177] Acute reactions occur within 3 to 6 months of treatment. Chronic changes occur later. Acute reactions present as dysuria, frequency, and urgency. They are usually not as severe as some of the cystitis caused by chemotherapy. Strictures or fistula can develop during the years following radiotherapy.[178,179]

Once infection is ruled out, symptomatic relief with phenazopyridine is usually the first-line treatment for acute symptoms. It is given at 200 mg orally, three times a day. Phenazopyridine accumulates in the urine essentially unchanged and acts as a topical analgesic within the bladder. Patients should be warned that phenazopyridine turns the urine into a bright orange color and can stain clothing. If the symptoms are not adequately relieved, antispasmodics can be added. Oxybutynin or flavoxate help relax the smooth muscles and reduce urinary urgency and frequency.[180] Tolterodine is a cholinergic antagonist that is also effective for overactive bladder. It causes less dry mouth, but its response rate is lower.[181] Trospium was documented to improve symptoms in radiation-induced cystitis and is significantly better tolerated than immediate-release oxybutynin.[182]

Intravesical infusion of hyaluronic acid or chondroitin sulfate, injection of botulinum toxin A into bladder wall, and hyperbaric oxygen therapy have shown benefit.[183–186] Intravenous WF10 (tetrachlorodecaoxide), an immunomodulator, was reported to be beneficial.[187,188] In patients with severe pain, aggressive pain control with opioids may be needed.

Symptomatic management of chronic changes is similar to that of acute reactions. Dilatation or placement of a permanent catheter may be required for significant obstruction. Patients not responding to less aggressive treatment may be candidates for reconstructive surgery to repair the stricture, sphincter failure, or fistula.

Section IV

Female Sexuality

High-dose radiation to the pelvis causes varying degrees of sexual dysfunction related to injury to the ovaries and vagina.[189,190] Ovarian failure as a result of pelvis irradiation leads to postmenopausal changes. Acute injury occurs during the course of radiation therapy and the following few months. It usually presents as vaginal and vulvar mucositis, pain, and ulceration. Chronic changes are less frequent than acute changes, which can develop more than 3 months after the completion of treatment. Chronic changes include fibrosis, loss of elasticity and sensation, susceptibility to trauma and infection, postcoital bleeding, and dyspareunia.[191-193]

Maintenance of local hygiene, aggressive treatment of infection, and regular dilatation of the vaginal canal help reduce the acute reaction. Hormone replacement therapy and application of lubricants for mucosal dryness can be used to treat acute injury. To prevent chronic changes, uses of vaginal dilators, lubricants, and supplemental estrogen were shown to be helpful. When fibrosis is established, treatment may require more drastic measures, such as hyperbaric oxygen therapy or surgical reconstruction. Although these are common options in clinical practice, the level of evidence supporting their use varies.[189]

Most studies of use of topical estrogen showed benefit.[194,195] Radiation causes damage to the epithelium, which may persist for another 3 to 6 months after therapy. Topical estrogen promotes epithelial regeneration. Benzydamine is an antiinflammatory that also has analgesic, local anesthetic, and antimicrobial effects. It can be applied topically to achieve a higher local tissue concentration. It reduced both subjective symptoms and objective observation of vaginal mucositis.[196,197] There have been several uncontrolled studies of hyperbaric oxygen therapy in the treatment of established necrotic wound resulting from perineal and vaginal radiation; the strength of evidence is modest.[198,199] In women with severe radiation damage, such as perineal defect or obliteration of the vagina, reconstructive surgery may be considered. All reported studies are retrospective.[189]

Male Sexuality

When planning radiation for prostate cancer, its effect on male sexual function must be considered and discussed with the patient. Although the rate of erectile dysfunction (ED) is lower in patients receiving radiotherapy versus radical prostatectomy, sexual dysfunctions remain one of the most important posttreatment quality of life issues.[200,201] A survey showed that 68% of men aged 45 to 70 years were willing to trade off a 10% or greater advantage in 5-year survival to maintain sexual potency.[202] Onset of ED is gradual, usually beginning about 6 months posttreatment and continuing to deteriorate for 4 years.[203]

Radiation does not appear to reduce testosterone production or cause pelvic nerve injury.[204] In addition to psychological reasons, vascular changes after radiation appear to be the predominant cause of postradiation male sexual dysfunction. As such, smoking and hypertension are risk factors.[205,206] With external beam radiation, the rates of ED vary from 7% to 72%, a wide range attributed to the differing study populations. Brachytherapy is associated with 2% to 89% of ED.[207] Diminished sexual desire, decreased orgasmic pleasure, and a reduced ejaculation volume are other problems reported by patients.[208]

The rising use of androgen deprivation therapy (ADT) for the treatment of intermediate-risk, high-risk, and metastatic prostate cancer has also had a dramatic impact on male sexuality. Rapid drops in testosterone brought on by the initiation of ADT can cause decrease or result in the complete loss of libido and sexual desire in up to 90% of men being treated for prostate cancer as well physical and emotional changes such as weight gain, gynecomastia, genital shrinkage, depression, and emotional lability.[209] Sexual side effects related to ADT can begin almost immediately and can last for several years after completion of therapy. A quality of life analysis of a prospective, definitive prostate cancer trial demonstrated that at 2 years after completion of the therapy, 75.4% patients receiving 4 to 8 months of ADT in conjunction with definitive radiotherapy stated that their ability to function sexually was poor or very poor versus only 44.0% treated with radiotherapy alone.[210] Patients and their partners are often unprepared for the profound side effects related to ADT. In a survey of 79 patients and their partners recently prescribed ADT, 30% to 50% were unaware that low of libido, erectile dysfunction, and genital shrinkage were possible side effects of ADT. Care should be taken by physicians to communicate all of these side effects to both patients and their partners and to facilitate consultation with couple counseling, sex therapy, and men's health clinics when appropriate.

Treatment of postradiotherapy sexual dysfunction should take a multidisciplinary approach, including psychosocial evaluation and counseling, pharmacologic intervention, and exploration of the use of mechanical devices.[207,211] The mainstay of pharmacologic treatment is phosphodiesterase inhibitors in patients with arteriogenic ED. A randomized double-blinded, placebo-controlled crossover trail suggests a positive response to sildenafil. Yet, the overall response rate is low. Only 21% of patients improved during sildenafil treatment but not during placebo treatment.[212] Tadalafil is found beneficial in these patient populations too.[213,214]

Intracavernosal injection of prostaglandins or phentolamine papaverine is also effective. For patients who are refractory to pharmacologic intervention, implantation of a penile prosthesis can be considered. Minimal intraoperative and postoperative complications and an excellent patient satisfaction rate were reported.[215] Vacuum devices are another option.

REFERENCES

1. *Clinical Practice Guidelines for Quality Palliative Care.* 3rd ed. National Consensus Project for Quality Palliative Care, 2013.
2. Temel JS, Greer JA, Muzikansky A, et al. Early palliative care for patients with metastatic non-small-cell lung cancer. *N Engl J Med* 2010;363(8):733–742.
3. Bakitas MA, Tosteson TD, Li Z, et al. Early versus delayed initiation of concurrent palliative oncology care: patient outcomes in the ENABLE III randomized controlled trial. *J Clin Oncol* 2015;33(13):1438–1445.
4. Dionne-Odom JN, Azuero A, Lyons KD, et al. Benefits of early versus delayed palliative care to informal family caregivers of patients with advanced cancer: outcomes from the ENABLE III randomized controlled trial. *J Clin Oncol* 2015;33(13):1446–1452.
5. Zimmermann C, Swami N, Krzyzanowska M, et al. Early palliative care for patients with advanced cancer: a cluster-randomised controlled trial. *Lancet* 2014;383(9930):1721–1730.
6. Ferrell BR, Temel JS, Temin S, et al. Integration of palliative care into standard oncology care: American Society of Clinical Oncology Clinical Practice Guideline Update. *J Clin Oncol* 2017;35(1):96–112.
7. Kotronoulas G, Kearney N, Maguire R, et al. What is the value of the routine use of patient-reported outcome measures toward improvement of patient outcomes, processes of care, and health service outcomes in cancer care? A systematic review of controlled trials. *J Clin Oncol* 2014;32(14):1480–1501.
8. Basch E, Deal AM, Dueck AC, et al. Overall Survival Results of a Trial Assessing Patient-Reported Outcomes for Symptom Monitoring During Routine Cancer Treatment. *JAMA* 2017;318(2):197–198.
9. Stone P, Richards M, Hardy J. Fatigue in patients with cancer. *Eur J Cancer* 1998;34(11):1670–1676.
10. Kurzrock R. The role of cytokines in cancer-related fatigue. *Cancer* 2001;92(6 Suppl):1684–1688.
11. Jager A, Sleijfer S, van der Rijt CC. The pathogenesis of cancer related fatigue: could increased activity of pro-inflammatory cytokines be the common denominator? *Eur J Cancer* 2008;44(2):175–181.
12. Ahlberg K, Ekman T, Gaston-Johansson F, et al. Assessment and management of cancer-related fatigue in adults. *Lancet* 2003;362(9384):640–650.
13. Mustian KM, Alfano CM, Heckler C, et al. Comparison of pharmaceutical, psychological, and exercise treatments for cancer-related fatigue: a meta-analysis. *JAMA Oncol* 2017;3(7):961–968.
14. Cramer H, Pokhrel B, Fester C, et al. A randomized controlled bicenter trial of yoga for patients with colorectal cancer. *Psychooncology* 2016;25(4):412–420.
15. Chandwani KD, Perkins G, Nagendra HR, et al. Randomized, controlled trial of yoga in women with breast cancer undergoing radiotherapy. *J Clin Oncol* 2014;32(10):1058–1065.
16. Gielissen MF, Verhagen S, Witjes F, et al. Effects of cognitive behavior therapy in severely fatigued disease-free cancer patients compared with patients waiting for cognitive behavior therapy: a randomized controlled trial. *J Clin Oncol* 2006;24(30):4882–4887.

17. Yennurajalingam S, Bruera E. Review of clinical trials of pharmacologic interventions for cancer-related fatigue: focus on psychostimulants and steroids. *Cancer J* 2014;20(5):319–324.
18. Yennurajalingam S, Frisbee-Hume S, Palmer JL, et al. Reduction of cancer-related fatigue with dexamethasone: a double-blind, randomized, placebo-controlled trial in patients with advanced cancer. *J Clin Oncol* 2013;31(25):3076–3082.
19. Bruera E, Roca E, Cedaro L, et al. Action of oral methylprednisolone in terminal cancer patients: a prospective randomized double-blind study. *Cancer Treat Rep* 1985;69(7–8):751–754.
20. Miller S, McNutt L, McCann MA, et al. Use of corticosteroids for anorexia in palliative medicine: a systematic review. *J Palliat Med* 2014;17(4):482–485.
21. Loprinzi CL, Kugler JW, Sloan JA, et al. Randomized comparison of megestrol acetate versus dexamethasone versus fluoxymesterone for the treatment of cancer anorexia/cachexia. *J Clin Oncol* 1999;17(10):3299–3306.
22. Gong S, Sheng P, Jin H, et al. Effect of methylphenidate in patients with cancer-related fatigue: a systematic review and meta-analysis. *PLoS One* 2014;9(1):e84391.
23. Spathis A, Fife K, Blackhall F, et al. Modafinil for the treatment of fatigue in lung cancer: results of a placebo-controlled, double-blind, randomized trial. *J Clin Oncol* 2014;32(18):1882–1888.
24. Andrykowski MA, Schmidt JE, Salsman JM, et al. Use of a case definition approach to identify cancer-related fatigue in women undergoing adjuvant therapy for breast cancer. *J Clin Oncol* 2005;23(27):6613–6622.
25. Truong PT, Berthelet E, Lee JC, et al. Prospective evaluation of the prevalence and severity of fatigue in patients with prostate cancer undergoing radical external beam radiotherapy and neoadjuvant hormone therapy. *Can J Urol* 2006;13(3):3139–3146.
26. Geinitz H, Zimmermann FB, Thamm R, et al. Fatigue in patients with adjuvant radiation therapy for breast cancer: long-term follow-up. *J Cancer Res Clin Oncol* 2004;130(6):327–333.
27. Knobf MT, Sun Y. A longitudinal study of symptoms and self-care activities in women treated with primary radiotherapy for breast cancer. *Cancer Nurs* 2005;28(3):210–218.
28. Brown P, Clark MM, Atherton P, et al. Will improvement in quality of life (QOL) impact fatigue in patients receiving radiation therapy for advanced cancer? *Am J Clin Oncol* 2006;29(1):52–58.
29. Kondziolka D, Niranjan A, Flickinger JC, et al. Radiosurgery with or without whole-brain radiotherapy for brain metastases: the patients' perspective regarding complications. *Am J Clin Oncol* 2005;28(2):173–179.
30. Dewys WD, Begg C, Lavin PT, et al. Prognostic effect of weight loss prior to chemotherapy in cancer patients. Eastern Cooperative Oncology Group. *Am J Med* 1980;69(4):491–497.
31. Evans WJ, Morley JE, Argiles J, et al. Cachexia: a new definition. *Clin Nutr* 2008;27(6):793–799.
32. Argiles JM, Busquets S, Stemmler B, et al. Cancer cachexia: understanding the molecular basis. *Nat Rev Cancer* 2014;14(11):754–762.
33. Fearon K, Strasser F, Anker SD, et al. Definition and classification of cancer cachexia: an international consensus. *Lancet Oncol* 2011;12(5):489–495.
34. Dev R, Wong A, Hui D, et al. The evolving approach to management of cancer cachexia. *Oncology (Williston Park)* 2017;31(1):23–32.
35. Ravasco P, Monteiro-Grillo I, Vidal PM, et al. Dietary counseling improves patient outcomes: a prospective, randomized, controlled trial in colorectal cancer patients undergoing radiotherapy. *J Clin Oncol* 2005;23:1431–1438.
36. Wilson MM, Purushothaman R, Morley JE. Effect of liquid dietary supplements on energy intake in the elderly. *Am J Clin Nutr* 2002;75(5):944–947.
37. Buzby K. In: Bloch A, ed. *Overview: screening, assessing, and monitoring*. Vol. 1990. Rockville, MD: SRC—GoogleScholar, 1990.
38. Colasanto JM, et al. Nutritional support of patients undergoing radiation therapy for head and neck cancer. *Oncology (Williston Park)* 2005;19:371–379.
39. Trujillo E, Matarese L, Gottschlich M, et al. Enteral nutrition: a comprehensive overview. In: Matarese LE, Gottschlich MM, eds. *Contemporary nutrition support practice a clinical guide*. Philadelphia, PA: W.B. Saunders Co., 1998.
40. Byrne KR, Fang JC. Endoscopic placement of enteral feeding catheters. *Curr Opin Gastroenterol* 2006;22(5):546–550.
41. Gopalan S, Khanna S. Enteral nutrition delivery technique. *Curr Opin Clin Nutr Metab Care* 2003;6(3):313–317.
42. Marcy PY. Systematic percutaneous fluoroscopic gastrostomy for concomitant radiochemotherapy of advanced head and neck cancer: optimization of therapy. *Support Care Cancer* 2000;8:410–413.
43. Senft M. The influence of supportive nutritional therapy via percutaneous endoscopically guided gastrostomy on the quality of life of cancer patients. *Support Care Cancer* 1993;1(5):272–275.
44. Grant MD, Rudberg MA, Brody JA. Gastrostomy placement and mortality among hospitalized Medicare beneficiaries. *JAMA* 1998;279(24):1973–1976.
45. Safadi BY, Marks JM, Ponsky JL. Percutaneous endoscopic gastrostomy. *Gastrointest Endosc Clin N Am* 1998;8:551–568.
46. Mahaffey SM, Copeland EM III. Total parenteral nutrition in the cancer patient. *Adv Surg* 1987;20:47–67.
47. Shike M. Nutrition therapy for the cancer patient. *Hematol Oncol Clin North Am* 1996;10(1):221–234.
48. Loprinzi CL, Ellison NM, Schaid DJ, et al. Controlled trial of megestrol acetate for the treatment of cancer anorexia and cachexia. *J Natl Cancer Inst* 1990;82(13):1127–1132.
49. Jatoi A, Windschitl HE, Loprinzi CL, et al. Dronabinol versus megestrol acetate versus combination therapy for cancer-associated anorexia: a North Central Cancer Treatment Group study. *J Clin Oncol* 2002;20(2):567–573.
50. Berk LB, Shivnani AT, Small W, Jr. Pathophysiology and management of radiation-induced xerostomia. *J Support Oncol* 2005;3(3):191–200.
51. Guchelaar HJ, Vermes A, Meerwaldt JH. Radiation-induced xerostomia: pathophysiology, clinical course and supportive treatment. *Support Care Cancer* 1997;5(4):281–288.
52. Eisbruch A, Kim HM, Terrell JE, et al. Xerostomia and its predictors following parotid-sparing irradiation of head-and-neck cancer. *Int J Radiat Oncol Biol Phys* 2001;50(3):695–704.
53. Valdez IH. Radiation-induced salivary dysfunction: clinical course and significance. *Spec Care Dentist* 1991;11(6):252–255.
54. Vissink A PA, Gravenmade EJ, et al. The causes and consequences of hyposalivation. *Ear Nose Throat J* 1988;67(3):166–168, 173–176.
55. Pedersen AM, Bardow A, Jensen SB, et al. Saliva and gastrointestinal functions of taste, mastication, swallowing and digestion. *Oral Dis* 2002;8(3): 117–129.
56. Ship JA, Hu K. Radiotherapy-induced salivary dysfunction. *Semin Oncol* 2004;31(6 Suppl 18):29–36.
57. Jensen SB, Pedersen AM, Vissink A, et al. A systematic review of salivary gland hypofunction and xerostomia induced by cancer therapies: management strategies and economic impact. *Support Care Cancer* 2010;18(8):1061–1079.
58. Al-Qahtani K, Hier MP, Sultanum K, et al. The role of submandibular salivary gland transfer in preventing xerostomia in the chemoradiotherapy patient. *Oral Surg Oral Med Oral Pathol Oral Radiol Endod* 2006;101(6):753–756.
59. Jha N, Seikaly H, Harris J, et al. Prevention of radiation induced xerostomia by surgical transfer of submandibular salivary gland into the submental space. *Radiother Oncol* 2003;66(3):283–289.
60. Rieger J, Seikaly H, Jha N, et al. Submandibular gland transfer for prevention of xerostomia after radiation therapy: swallowing outcomes. *Arch Otolaryngol Head Neck Surg* 2005;131(2):140–145.
61. Zhang Y, Guo CB, Zhang L, et al. Prevention of radiation-induced xerostomia by submandibular gland transfer. *Head Neck* 2012;34(7):937–942.
62. Seikaly H, Jha N, Harris JR, et al. Long-term outcomes of submandibular gland transfer for prevention of postradiation xerostomia. *Arch Otolaryngol Head Neck Surg* 2004;130(8):956-961.
63. Amosson CM, Teh BS, Van TJ, et al. Dosimetric predictors of xerostomia for head-and-neck cancer patients treated with the smart (simultaneous modulated accelerated radiation therapy) boost technique. *Int J Radiat Oncol Biol Phys* 2003;56(1):136–144.
64. Eisbruch A, Dawson LA, Kim HM, et al. Conformal and intensity modulated irradiation of head and neck cancer: the potential for improved target irradiation, salivary gland function, and quality of life. *Acta Otorhinolaryngol Belg* 1999;53(3):271–275.
65. Lee N, Xia P, Fischbein NJ, et al. Intensity-modulated radiation therapy for head-and-neck cancer: the UCSF experience focusing on target volume delineation. *Int J Radiat Oncol Biol Phys* 2003;57(1):49–60.
66. Münter MW, Karger CP, Hoffner SG, et al. Evaluation of salivary gland function after treatment of head-and-neck tumors with intensity-modulated radiotherapy by quantitative pertechnetate scintigraphy. *Int J Radiat Oncol Biol Phys* 2004;58(1):175–184.
67. Parliament MB, Scrimger RA, Anderson SG, et al. Preservation of oral health-related quality of life and salivary flow rates after inverse-planned intensity-modulated radiotherapy (IMRT) for head-and-neck cancer. *Int J Radiat Oncol Biol Phys* 2004;58(3):663–673.
68. Little M, Schipper M, Feng FY, et al. Reducing xerostomia after chemo-IMRT for head and neck cancer: beyond sparing the parotid glands. *Int J Radiat Oncol Biol Phys* 2012;83(3):1007–1014.
69. Brizel DM, Wasserman TH, Henke M, et al. Phase III randomized trial of amifostine as a radioprotector in head and neck cancer. *J Clin Oncol* 2000;18(19):3339–3345.
70. Mosteller F, Jennifer F-T. *Institute of Medicine: quality of life and technology assessment*. Washington, DC: National Academy Press, 1989.
71. Anne PR, Machtay M, Rosenthal DI, et al. A phase II trial of subcutaneous amifostine and radiation therapy in patients with head-and-neck cancer. *Int J Radiat Oncol Biol Phys* 2007;67(2):445–452.
72. Bardet E, Martin L, Calais G, et al. Preliminary data of the GORTEC 2000-02 phase III trial comparing intravenous and subcutaneous administration of amifostine for head and neck tumors treated by external radiotherapy. *Semin Oncol* 2002;29(6 Suppl 19):57–60.
73. Koukourakis MI, Kyrias G, Kakolyris S, et al. Subcutaneous administration of amifostine during fractionated radiotherapy: a randomized phase II study. *J Clin Oncol* 2000;18(11):2226–2233.
74. Bardet E, Martin L, Calais G, et al. Subcutaneous compared with intravenous administration of amifostine in patients with head and neck cancer receiving radiotherapy: final results of the GORTEC2000-02 phase III randomized trial. *J Clin Oncol* 2011;29(2):127–133.
75. Jha N, Seikaly H, Harris J, et al. Phase III randomized study: oral pilocarpine versus submandibular salivary gland transfer protocol for the management of radiation-induced xerostomia. *Head Neck* 2009;31(2):234–243.
76. Rieger JM, Jha N, Lam Tang JA, et al. Functional outcomes related to the prevention of radiation-induced xerostomia: oral pilocarpine versus submandibular salivary gland transfer. *Head Neck* 2012;34(2):168–174.
77. New approaches to preventing xerostomia. *J Support Oncol* 2006;4(2):87–88.
78. Chambers MS, Jones CU, Biel MA, et al. Open-label, long-term safety study of cevimeline in the treatment of postirradiation xerostomia. *Int J Radiat Oncol Biol Phys* 2007;69(5):1369–1376.
79. Nieuw Amerongen AV, Veerman EC. Current therapies for xerostomia and salivary gland hypofunction associated with cancer therapies. *Support Care Cancer* 2003;11(4):226–231.
80. Kahn ST, Johnstone PA. Management of xerostomia related to radiotherap for head and neck cancer. *Oncology (Williston Park)* 2005;19(14):1827–1 discussion 1832–1834, 1837–1839.
81. Johnson JT, Ferretti GA, Nethery WJ, et al. Oral pilocarpine for diation xerostomia in patients with head and neck cancer. *N* 1993;329(6):390-395.
82. Rieke JW, Hafermann MD, Johnson JT, et al. Oral pilocarp induced xerostomia: integrated efficacy and safety results from randomized clinical trials. *Int J Radiat Oncol Biol Phys* 1995;31(

Section IV

83. LeVeque FG, Montgomery M, Potter D, et al. A multicenter, randomized, double-blind, placebo-controlled, dose-titration study of oral pilocarpine for treatment of radiation-induced xerostomia in head and neck cancer patients. *J Clin Oncol* 1993;11(6):1124–1131.

84. Wiseman LR, Faulds D. Oral pilocarpine: a review of its pharmacological properties and clinical potential in xerostomia. *Drugs* 1995;49(1):143–155.

85. Blom M, Dawidson I, Fernberg JO, et al. Acupuncture treatment of patients with radiation-induced xerostomia. *Eur J Cancer B Oral Oncol* 1996;32B(3):182–190.

86. Blom M, Lundeberg T. Long-term follow-up of patients treated with acupuncture for xerostomia and the influence of additional treatment. *Oral Dis* 2000;6(1):15–24.

87. Johnstone PA, Niemtzow RC, Riffenburgh RH. Acupuncture for xerostomia: clinical update. *Cancer* 2002;94(4):1151–1156.

88. Johnstone PA, Peng YP, May BC, et al. Acupuncture for pilocarpine-resistant xerostomia following radiotherapy for head and neck malignancies. *Int J Radiat Oncol Biol Phys* 2001;50(2):353–357.

89. Pfister DG, Cassileth BR, Deng GE, et al. Acupuncture for pain and dysfunction after neck dissection: results of a randomized controlled trial. *J Clin Oncol* 2010;28(15):2565–2570.

90. Meng Z, Garcia MK, Hu C, et al. Randomized controlled trial of acupuncture for prevention of radiation-induced xerostomia among patients with nasopharyngeal carcinoma. *Cancer* 2012;118(13):3337–3344.

91. Wong RK, Sagar SM, Chen BJ, et al. Phase II Randomized Trial of Acupuncture-Like Transcutaneous Electrical Nerve Stimulation to Prevent Radiation-Induced Xerostomia in Head and Neck Cancer Patients. *J Soc Integr Oncol* 2010;8(2):35–42.

92. Haker E, Egekvist H, Bjerring P. Effect of sensory stimulation (acupuncture) on sympathetic and parasympathetic activities in healthy subjects. *J Auton Nerv Syst* 2000;79(1):52–59.

93. Kimura A, Sato A. Somatic regulation of autonomic functions in anesthetized animals--neural mechanisms of physical therapy including acupuncture. *Jpn J Vet Res* 1997;45(3):137–145.

94. Loaiza LA, Yamaguchi S, Ito M, et al. Electro-acupuncture stimulation to muscle afferents in anesthetized rats modulates the blood flow to the knee joint through autonomic reflexes and nitric oxide. *Auton Neurosci* 2002;97(2):103–109.

95. Middlekauff HR, Shah JB, Yu JL, et al. Acupuncture effects on autonomic responses to cold pressor and handgrip exercise in healthy humans. *Clin Auton Res* 2004;14(2):113–118.

96. Deng G, Hou BL, Holodny AI, et al. Functional magnetic resonance imaging (fMRI) changes and saliva production associated with acupuncture at LI-2 acupuncture point: a randomized controlled study. *BMC Complement Altern Med* 2008;8:37.

97. O'Sullivan EM, Higginson IJ. Clinical effectiveness and safety of acupuncture in the treatment of irradiation-induced xerostomia in patients with head and neck cancer: a systematic review. *Acupunct Med* 2010;28(4):191–199.

98. Eilers J, Epstein JB. Assessment and measurement of oral mucositis. *Semin Oncol Nurs* 2004;20(1):22–29.

99. Keefe DM. Gastrointestinal mucositis: a new biological model. *Support Care Cancer* 2004;12(1):6–9.

100. Sonis ST, Peterson DE, McGuire DB, et al. Prevention of mucositis in cancer patients. *J Natl Cancer Inst Monogr* 2001(29):1–2.

101. Peterson DE, Keefe DM, Hutchins RD, et al. Alimentary tract mucositis in cancer patients: impact of terminology and assessment on research and clinical practice. *Support Care Cancer* 2006;14(6):499–504.

102. Trotti A, Byhardt R, Stetz J, et al. Common toxicity criteria: version 2.0. an improved reference for grading the acute effects of cancer treatment: impact on radiotherapy. *Int J Radiat Oncol Biol Phys* 2000;47(1):13–47.

103. Blijlevens NM, Donnelly JP, De Pauw BE. Mucosal barrier injury: biology, pathology, clinical counterparts and consequences of intensive treatment for haematological malignancy: an overview. *Bone Marrow Transplant* 2000;25(12):1269–1278.

104. Sonis ST, Elting LS, Keefe D, et al. Perspectives on cancer therapy-induced mucosal injury: pathogenesis, measurement, epidemiology, and consequences for patients. *Cancer* 2004;100(9 Suppl):1995–2025.

105. Yeoh AS, Bowen JM, Gibson RJ, et al. Nuclear factor kappaB (NFkappaB) and cyclooxygenase-2 (Cox-2) expression in the irradiated colorectum is associated with subsequent histopathological changes. *Int J Radiat Oncol Biol Phys* 2005;63(5):1295–1303.

106. Anthony L, Bowen J, Garden A, et al. New thoughts on the pathobiology of regimen-related mucosal injury. *Support Care Cancer* 2006;14(6):516–518.

107. Sonis ST. The pathobiology of mucositis. *Nat Rev Cancer* 2004;4(4):277–284.

108. Peterson DE, Lalla RV. Oral mucositis: the new paradigms. *Curr Opin Oncol* 2010;22(4):318–322.

109. Spielberger R, Stiff P, Bensinger W, et al. Palifermin for oral mucositis after intensive therapy for hematologic cancers. *N Engl J Med* 2004;351(25):2590–2598.

110. Lalla RV, Bowen J, Barasch A, et al. MASCC/ISOO clinical practice guidelines for the management of mucositis secondary to cancer therapy. *Cancer* 2014;120(10):1453–1461.

111. Epstein JB, Silverman S Jr, Paggiarino DA, et al. Benzydamine HCl for prophylaxis of radiation-induced oral mucositis: results from a multicenter, randomized, double-blind, placebo-controlled clinical trial. *Cancer* 2001;92(4):875–885.

112. Kim JH, Chu FC, Lakshmi V, et al. Benzydamine HCl, a new agent for the treatment of radiation mucositis of the oropharynx. *Am J Clin Oncol* 1986;9(2):132–134.

113. Foote RL, Loprinzi CL, Frank AR, et al. Randomized trial of a chlorhexidine mouthwash for alleviation of radiation-induced mucositis. *J Clin Oncol* 1994;12(12):2630–2633.

114. Samaranayake LP, Robertson AG, MacFarlane TW, et al. The effect of chlorhexidine and benzydamine mouthwashes on mucositis induced by therapeutic irradiation. *Clin Radiol* 1988;39(3):291–294.

115. Spijkervet FK, van Saene HK, Panders AK, et al. Effect of chlorhexidine rinsing on the oropharyngeal ecology in patients with head and neck cancer who have irradiation mucositis. *Oral Surg Oral Med Oral Pathol* 1989;67(2):154–161.

116. Beck S. Impact of a systematic oral care protocol on stomatitis after chemotherapy. *Cancer Nurs* 1979;2(3):185–199.

117. Borowski B, Benhamou E, Pico JL, et al. Prevention of oral mucositis in patients treated with high-dose chemotherapy and bone marrow transplantation: a randomised controlled trial comparing two protocols of dental care. *Eur J Cancer B Oral Oncol* 1994;30B(2):93–97.

118. Cheng KK, Molassiotis A, Chang AM, et al. Evaluation of an oral care protocol intervention in the prevention of chemotherapy-induced oral mucositis in paediatric cancer patients. *Eur J Cancer* 2001;37(16):2056–2063.

119. Dudjak LA. Mouth care for mucositis due to radiation therapy. *Cancer Nurs* 1987;10(3):131–140.

120. Kenny SA. Effect of two oral care protocols on the incidence of stomatitis in hematology patients. *Cancer Nurs* 1990;13(6):345–353.

121. Levy-Polack MP, Sebelli P, Polack NL. Incidence of oral complications and application of a preventive protocol in children with acute leukemia. *Spec Care Dentist* 1998;18(5):189–193.

122. Keefe DM, Schubert MM, Elting LS, et al. Updated clinical practice guidelines for the prevention and treatment of mucositis. *Cancer* 2007;109(5):820–831.

123. Bensadoun RJ, Schubert MM, Lalla RV, et al. Amifostine in the management of radiation-induced and chemo-induced mucositis. *Support Care Cancer* 2006;14(6):566–572.

124. Hensley ML, Hagerty KL, Kewalramani T, et al. American Society of Clinical Oncology 2008 clinical practice guideline update: use of chemotherapy and radiation therapy protectants. *J Clin Oncol* 2009;27(1):127–145.

125. Le QT, Kim HE, Schneider CJ, et al. Palifermin reduces severe mucositis in definitive chemoradiotherapy of locally advanced head and neck cancer: a randomized, placebo-controlled study. *J Clin Oncol* 2011;29(20):2808–2814.

126. Bültzingslöwen Iv, Brennan MT, Spijkervet FKL, et al. Growth factors and cytokines in the prevention and treatment of oral and gastrointestinal mucositis. *Support Care Cancer* 2006;14(6):519–527.

127. Carnel SB, Blakeslee DB, Oswald SG, et al. Treatment of radiation- and chemotherapy-induced stomatitis. *Otolaryngol Head Neck Surg* 1990;102(4):326–330.

128. Coetzee MJ, Boshoff B, Goedhals L, et al. Formula C—popular, cheap and readily available relief for radiation and cancer chemotherapy mucositis. *S Afr Med J* 1997;87(1):80–81.

129. Dodd MJ, Dibble SL, Miaskowski C, et al. Randomized clinical trial of the effectiveness of 3 commonly used mouthwashes to treat chemotherapy-induced mucositis. *Oral Surg Oral Med Oral Pathol Oral Radiol Endod* 2000;90(1):39–47.

130. Dodd MJ, Larson PJ, Dibble SL, et al. Randomized clinical trial of chlorhexidine versus placebo for prevention of oral mucositis in patients receiving chemotherapy. *Oncol Nurs Forum* 1996;23(6):921–927.

131. Rothwell BR, Spektor WS. Palliation of radiation-related mucositis. *Spec Care Dentist* 1990;10(1):21–25.

132. Turhal NS, Erdal S, Karacay S. Efficacy of treatment to relieve mucositis-induced discomfort. *Support Care Cancer* 2000;8(1):55–58.

133. Leenstra JL, Miller RC, Qin R, et al. Doxepin rinse versus placebo in the treatment of acute oral mucositis pain in patients receiving head and neck radiotherapy with or without chemotherapy: a phase III, randomized, double-blind trial (NCCTG-N09C6 [Alliance]). *J Clin Oncol* 2014;32(15):1571–1577.

134. Kilic D, Egehan I, Ozenirler S, et al. Double-blinded, randomized, placebo-controlled study to evaluate the effectiveness of sulphasalazine in preventing acute gastrointestinal complications due to radiotherapy. *Radiother Oncol* 2000;57(2):125–129.

135. Koukourakis MI. Amifostine: is there evidence of tumor protection? *Semin Oncol* 2003;30(6 Suppl 18):18–30.

136. Athanassiou H, Antonadou D, Coliarakis N, et al. Protective effect of amifostine during fractionated radiotherapy in patients with pelvic carcinomas: results of a randomized trial. *Int J Radiat Oncol Biol Phys* 2003;56(4):1154–1160.

137. Kouvaris J, Kouloulias V, Malas E, et al. Amifostine as radioprotective agent for the rectal mucosa during irradiation of pelvic tumors. A phase II randomized study using various toxicity scales and rectosigmoidoscopy. *Strahlenther Onkol* 2003;179(3):167–174.

138. Myerson R, Zobeiri I, Birnbaum E, et al. Early results from a phase I/II radiation dose-escalation study with concurrent amifostine and infusional 5-fluorouracil chemotherapy for preoperative treatment of unresectable or locally recurrent rectal carcinoma. *Semin Oncol* 2002;29(6 Suppl 19):29–33.

139. Komaki R, Lee JS, Kaplan B, et al. Randomized phase III study of chemoradiation with or without amifostine for patients with favorable performance status inoperable stage II-III non-small cell lung cancer: preliminary results. *Semin Radiat Oncol* 2002;12(1 Suppl 1):46–49.

140. Leong SS, Tan EH, Fong KW, et al. Randomized double-blind trial of combined modality treatment with or without amifostine in unresectable stage III non-small-cell lung cancer. *J Clin Oncol* 2003;21(9):1767–1774.

141. Movsas B, Scott C, Langer C, et al. Randomized trial of amifostine in locally advanced non–small-cell lung cancer patients receiving chemotherapy and hyperfractionated radiation: radiation therapy oncology group trial 98-01. *J Clin Oncol* 2005;23(10):2145–2154.

142. Kneebone A, Mameghan H, Bolin T, et al. The effect of oral sucralfate on the acute proctitis associated with prostate radiotherapy: a double-blind, randomized trial. *Int J Radiat Oncol Biol Phys* 2001;51(3):628–635.

143. Martenson JA, Bollinger JW, Sloan JA, et al. Sucralfate in the prevention of treatment-induced diarrhea in patients receiving pelvic radiation therapy: a North Central Cancer Treatment Group phase III double-blind placebo-controlled trial. *J Clin Oncol* 2000;18(6):1239–1245.

144. O'Brien PC, Franklin CI, Dear KB, et al. A phase III double-blind randomised study of rectal sucralfate suspension in the prevention of acute radiation proctitis. *Radiother Oncol* 1997;45(2):117–123.

145. Baughan CA, Canney PA, Buchanan RB, et al. A randomized trial to assess the efficacy of 5-aminosalicylic acid for the prevention of radiation enteritis. *Clin Oncol (R Coll Radiol)* 1993;5(1):19–24.

146. Resbeut M, Marteau P, Cowen D, et al. A randomized double blind placebo controlled multicenter study of mesalazine for the prevention of acute radiation enteritis. *Radiother Oncol* 1997;44(1):59–63.

147. Martenson JA, Jr., Hyland G, Moertel CG, et al. Olsalazine is contraindicated during pelvic radiation therapy: results of a double-blind, randomized clinical trial. *Int J Radiat Oncol Biol Phys* 1996;35(2):299–303.

148. Feyer PC, Stewart AL, Titlbach OJ. Aetiology and prevention of emesis induced by radiotherapy. *Support Care Cancer* 1998;6(3):253–260.

149. Roila F, Molassiotis A, Herrstedt J, et al. 2016 MASCC and ESMO guideline update for the prevention of chemotherapy- and radiotherapy-induced nausea and vomiting and of nausea and vomiting in advanced cancer patients. *Ann Oncol* 2016;27(Suppl 5):v119–v133.

150. Hesketh PJ, Kris MG, Basch E, et al. Antiemetics: American Society of Clinical Oncology Clinical Practice Guideline Update. *J Clin Oncol* 2017;35(28):3240–3261.

151. Urba S. Radiation-induced nausea and vomiting. *J Natl Compr Canc Netw* 2007;5(1):60–65.

152. Gwede CK. Overview of radiation- and chemoradiation-induced diarrhea. *Semin Oncol Nurs* 2003;19(4 Suppl 3):6–10.

153. O'Brien BE, Kaklamani VG, Benson AB III. The assessment and management of cancer treatment-related diarrhea. *Clin Colorectal Cancer* 2005;4(6):375–381; discussion 382–383.

154. Benson AB III, Ajani JA, Catalano RB, et al. Recommended guidelines for the treatment of cancer treatment-induced diarrhea. *J Clin Oncol* 2004;22(14):2918–2926.

155. Stern J, Ippoliti C. Management of acute cancer treatment-induced diarrhea. *Semin Oncol Nurs* 2003;19(4 Suppl 3):11–16.

156. Martenson JA, Halyard MY, Sloan JA, et al. Phase III, double-blind study of depot octreotide versus placebo in the prevention of acute diarrhea in patients receiving pelvic radiation therapy: results of North Central Cancer Treatment Group N00CA. *J Clin Oncol* 2008;26(32):5248–5253.

157. Kozelsky TF, Meyers GE, Sloan JA, et al. Phase III double-blind study of glutamine versus placebo for the prevention of acute diarrhea in patients receiving pelvic radiation therapy. *J Clin Oncol* 2003;21(9):1669–1674.

158. Hymes SR, Strom EA, Fife C. Radiation dermatitis: clinical presentation, pathophysiology, and treatment 2006. *J Am Acad Dermatol* 2006;54(1):28–46.

159. Wickline MM. Prevention and treatment of acute radiation dermatitis: a literature review. *Oncol Nurs Forum* 2004;31(2):237–247.

160. Harper JL, Franklin LE, Jenrette JM, et al. Skin toxicity during breast irradiation: pathophysiology and management. *South Med J* 2004;97(10):989–993.

161. Denham JW, Hauer-Jensen M. The radiotherapeutic injury—a complex 'wound'. *Radiother Oncol* 2002;63(2):129–145.

162. Malkinson FD, Keane JT. Radiobiology of the skin: review of some effects on epidermis and hair. *J Invest Dermatol* 1981;77(1):133–138.

163. Dutreix J. Human skin: early and late reactions in relation to dose and its time distribution. *Br J Radiol Suppl* 1986;19:22–28.

164. Mendelsohn FA, Divino CM, Reis ED, et al. Wound care after radiation therapy. *Adv Skin Wound Care* 2002;15(5):216–224.

165. Camidge R, Price A. Characterizing the phenomenon of radiation recall dermatitis. *Radiother Oncol* 2001;59(3):237–245.

166. Liguori V, Guillemin C, Pesce GF, et al. Double-blind, randomized clinical study comparing hyaluronic acid cream to placebo in patients treated with radiotherapy. *Radiother Oncol* 1997;42(2):155–161.

167. Maiche A, Isokangas OP, Grohn P. Skin protection by sucralfate cream during electron beam therapy. *Acta Oncol* 1994;33(2):201–203.

168. Pommier P, Gomez F, Sunyach MP, et al. Phase III randomized trial of Calendula officinalis compared with trolamine for the prevention of acute dermatitis during irradiation for breast cancer. *J Clin Oncol* 2004;22(8):1447–1453.

169. Hom DB, Adams G, Koreis M, et al. Choosing the optimal wound dressing for irradiated soft tissue wounds. *Otolaryngol Head Neck Surg* 1999;121(5):591–598.

170. Maiche AG, Grohn P, Maki-Hokkonen H. Effect of chamomile cream and almond ointment on acute radiation skin reaction. *Acta Oncol* 1991;30(3):395–396.

171. Schmuth M, Wimmer MA, Hofer S, et al. Topical corticosteroid therapy for acute radiation dermatitis: a prospective, randomized, double-blind study. *Br J Dermatol* 2002;146(6):983–991.

172. Halperin EC, Gaspar L, George S, et al. A double-blind, randomized, prospective trial to evaluate topical vitamin C solution for the prevention of radiation dermatitis. CNS Cancer Consortium. *Int J Radiat Oncol Biol Phys* 1993;26(3):413–416.

173. Dormand EL, Banwell PE, Goodacre TE. Radiotherapy and wound healing. *Int Wound J* 2005;2(2):112–127.

174. Delanian S, Balla-Mekias S, Lefaix J-L. Striking regression of chronic radiotherapy damage in a clinical trial of combined pentoxifylline and tocopherol. *J Clin Oncol* 1999;17(10):3283–3290.

175. Aygenc E, Celikkanat S, Kaymakci M, et al. Prophylactic effect of pentoxifylline on radiotherapy complications: a clinical study. *Otolaryngol Head Neck Surg* 2004;130(3):351–356.

176. Kagan AR. Bladder, testicle, and prostate irradiation injury. *Front Radiat Ther Oncol* 1989;23:323–337; discussion 338–340.

177. Marks LB, et al. The response of the urinary bladder, urethra, and ureter to radiation and chemotherapy. *Int J Radiat Oncol Biol Phys* 1995;31:1257–1280.

178. Greskovich FJ, et al. Complications following external beam radiation therapy for prostate cancer: an analysis of patients treated with and without staging pelvic lymphadenectomy. *J Urol* 1991;146:798–802.

179. Perez CA. Radiation therapy alone in the treatment of carcinoma of the uterine cervix: a 20-year experience. *Gynecol Oncol* 1986;23:127–140.

180. Milani R, et al. Flavoxate hydrochloride for urinary urgency after pelvic radiotherapy: comparison of 600 mg versus 1200 mg daily dosages. *J Int Med Res* 1988;16:71–74.

181. Diokno AC. Prospective, randomized, double-blind study of the efficacy and tolerability of the extended-release formulations of oxybutynin and tolterodine for overactive bladder: results of the OPERA trial. *Mayo Clin Proc* 2003;78(6):687–695.

182. Rovner ES. Trospium chloride in the management of overactive bladder. *Drugs* 2004;64(21):2433–2446.

183. Shao Y, Lu GL, Shen ZJ. Comparison of intravesical hyaluronic acid instillation and hyperbaric oxygen in the treatment of radiation-induced hemorrhagic cystitis. *BJU Int* 2012;109:691–694.

184. Hazewinkel MH, et al. Prophylactic vesical instillations with 0.2 chondroitin sulfate may reduce symptoms of acute radiation cystitis in patients undergoing radiotherapy for gynecological malignancies. *Int Urogynecol J* 2011;22:725–730.

185. Smit SG, Heyns CF. Management of radiation cystitis. *Nat Rev Urol* 2010;7:206–214.

186. Chuang YC, et al. Bladder botulinum toxin A injection can benefit patients with radiation and chemical cystitis. *BJU Int* 2008;102:704–706.

187. Veerasarn V, Boonnuch W, Kakanaporn C. A phase II study to evaluate WF10 in patients with late hemorrhagic radiation cystitis and proctitis. *Gynecol Oncol* 2006;100:179–184.

188. Veerasarn V. Reduced recurrence of late hemorrhagic radiation cystitis by WF10 therapy in cervical cancer patients: a multicenter, randomized, two-arm, open-label trial. *Radiother Oncol* 2004;73(2):179–185.

189. Denton AS, Maher EJ. Interventions for the physical aspects of sexual dysfunction in women following pelvic radiotherapy. *Cochrane Database Syst Rev* 2003;(1):CD003750.

190. Stead ML. Sexual function after treatment for gynecological malignancy. *Curr Opin Oncol* 2004;16(5):492–495.

191. Cartwright-Alcarese F. Addressing sexual dysfunction following radiation therapy for a gynecologic malignancy. *Oncol Nurs Forum* 1995;22:1227–1232.

192. Shell JA. Evidence-based practice for symptom management in adults with cancer: sexual dysfunction. *Oncol Nurs Forum* 2002;29(1):53–69.

193. Wilmoth MC, Spinelli A. Sexual implications of gynecologic cancer treatments. *J Obstet Gynecol Neonatal Nurs* 2000;29:413–421.

194. Hintz BL. Systemic absorption of conjugated estrogenic cream by the irradiated vagina. *Gynecol Oncol* 1981;12(1):75–82.

195. Pitkin RM, VanVoorhis LW. Postirradiation vaginitis. An evaluation of prophylaxis with topical estrogen. *Radiology* 1971;99:417–421.

196. Bentivoglio G, Diani F. Use of topical benzydamine in gynecology. *Clin Exp Obstet Gynecol* 1981;8(3):103–110.

197. Volterrani F, Tana S, Trenti N. Topical benzydamine in the treatment of vaginal radiomucositis. *Int J Tissue React* 1987;9:169–171.

198. Bui QC, et al. The efficacy of hyperbaric oxygen therapy in the treatment of radiation-induced late side effects. *Int J Radiat Oncol Biol Phys* 2004;60:871–878.

199. Williams JA Jr, Clarke D, Dennis WA, et al. The treatment of pelvic soft tissue radiation necrosis with hyperbaric oxygen. *Am J Obstet Gynecol* 1992;167(2):412–415; discussion 415–416.

200. Robinson JW, Dufour MS, Fung TS. Erectile functioning of men treated for prostate carcinoma. *Cancer* 1997;79(3):538–544.

201. Donovan JL, Hamdy FC, Lane JA, et al. Patient-Reported Outcomes after Monitoring, Surgery, or Radiotherapy for Prostate Cancer. *N Engl J Med* 2016;375(15):1425–1437.

202. Singer PA, et al. Sex or survival: trade-offs between quality and quantity of life. *J Clin Oncol* 1991;9:328–334.

203. Fransson P, Widmark A. Self-assessed sexual function after pelvic irradiation for prostate carcinoma. Comparison with an age-matched control group. *Cancer* 1996;78:1066–1078.

204. Tomic R. Some effects of orchiectomy, oestrogen treatment and radiation therapy in patients with prostatic carcinoma. *Scand J Urol Nephrol Suppl* 1983;77:1–37.

205. Goldstein I. Radiation-associated impotence. A clinical study of its mechanism. *JAMA* 1984;251:903–910.

206. Zelefsky MJ, Eid JF. Elucidating the etiology of erectile dysfunction after definitive therapy for prostatic cancer. *Int J Radiat Oncol Biol Phys* 1998;40:129–133.

207. Incrocci L, Slob AK, Levendag PC. Sexual (dys)function after radiotherapy for prostate cancer: a review. *Int J Radiat Oncol Biol Phys* 2002;52:681–693.

208. Helgason AR, et al. Decreased sexual capacity after external radiation therapy for prostate cancer impairs quality of life. *Int J Radiat Oncol Biol Phys* 1995;32:33–39.

209. Higano CS. Sexuality and intimacy after definitive treatment and subsequent androgen deprivation therapy for prostate cancer. *J Clin Oncol* 2012;30(30):3720–3725.

210. Gay HA, Sanda MG, Liu J, et al. External beam radiation therapy or brachytherapy with or without short-course neoadjuvant androgen deprivation therapy: results of a multicenter, prospective study of quality of life. *Int J Radiat Oncol Biol Phys* 2017;98(2):304–317.

211. Merrick GS, Wallner KE, Butler WM. Management of sexual dysfunction after prostate brachytherapy. *Oncology (Williston Park)* 2003;17:52–62; discussion 62, 67–70, 73.

212. Watkins Bruner D, et al. Randomized, double-blinded, placebo-controlled crossover trial of treating erectile dysfunction with sildenafil after radiotherapy and short-term androgen deprivation therapy: results of RTOG 0215. *J Sex Med* 2011;8:1228–1238.

213. Ricardi U, et al. Efficacy and safety of tadalafil 20 mg on demand vs. tadalafil 5 mg once a day in the treatment of postradiotherapy erectile dysfunction in prostate cancer men a randomized phase II trial. *J Sex Med* 2010;7:2851–2859.

214. Incrocci L, et al. A randomized, double-blind, placebo-controlled, cross-over study to assess the efficacy of tadalafil (Cialis) in the treatment of erectile dysfunction following three-dimensional conformal external-beam radiotherapy for prostatic carcinoma. *Int J Radiat Oncol Biol Phys* 2006;66:439–444.

215. Dubocq FM, et al. Outcome analysis of penile implant surgery after external beam radiation for prostate cancer. *J Urol* 1997;158:1787–1790.

Section IV

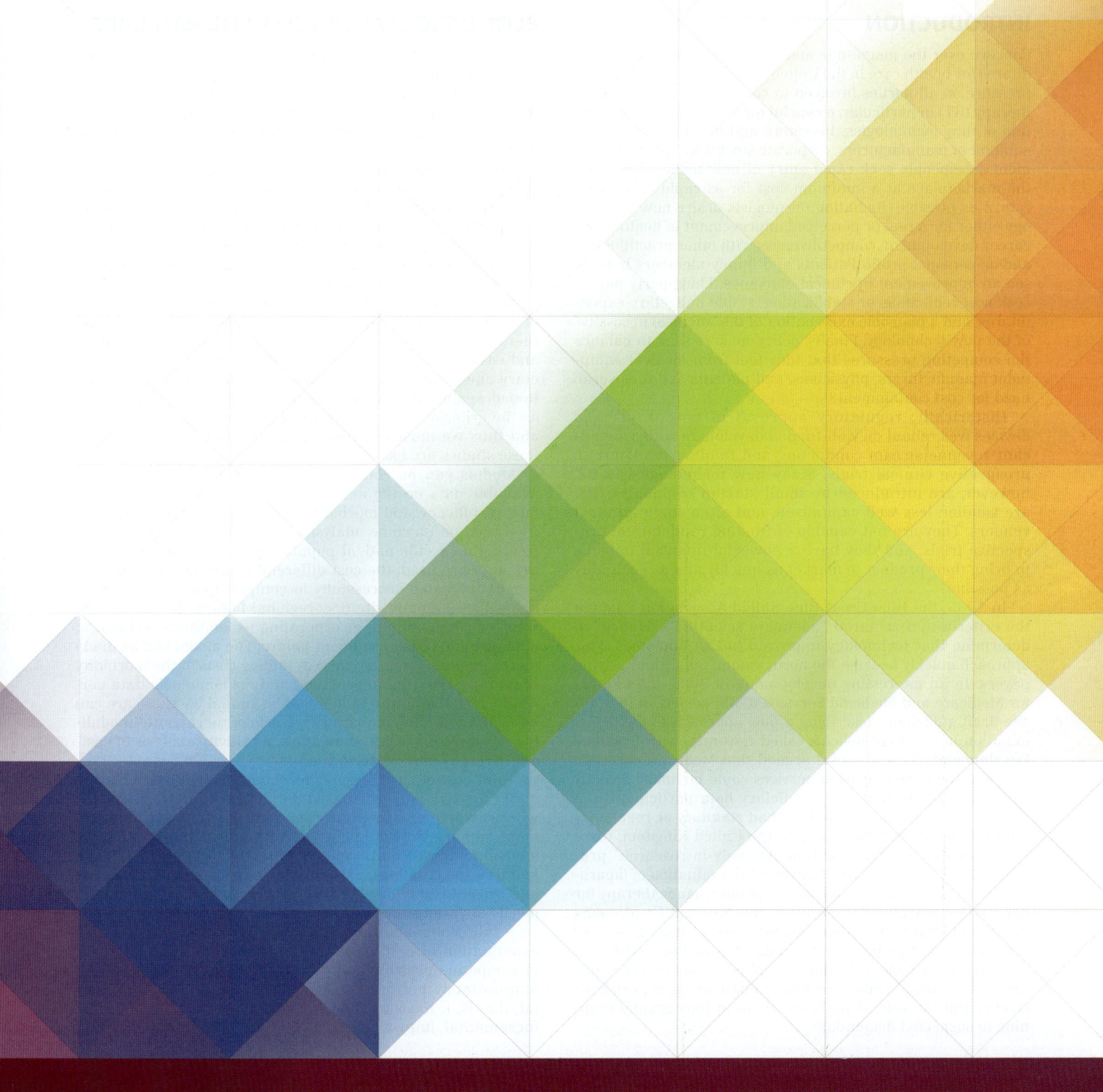

SECTION V
Economics, Education, Ethics, and Technology Assessment

CHAPTER 101

Technology Assessment, Outcome Analysis Research, Comparative Effectiveness, and Evidence-Based Radiation Oncology

Peter A. S. Johnstone, Carlos A. Perez, Edward C. Halperin, Yolande Lievens, and Andre A. Konski

INTRODUCTION

Concern over the magnitude and continued growth of expenditures for health care in the United States has led to economic pressure on all parties involved to contain costs. In radiation therapy (RT) in particular, powerful forces affect the introduction of new technologies. Inventors and developers, medical equipment manufacturers, corporate stockholders, and equipment salespeople seek rapid entry of new technologies into the marketplace at a minimum cost for as rapid a financial return as possible. Radiation oncologists desire new technology either for a real or perceived improvement in health care, career development, competitiveness with other practitioners, and/or personal profit. Patients and family members hope to see an improvement in clinical outcomes. Third-party payers seek cost reductions or stabilization, stable budgetary expenditures, and a plausible explanation of the "medical necessity" of the new technology. Finally, policy makers seek to balance the competing pressures that they feel from medical equipment manufacturers, physicians, and patients and the overall need for cost containment.[1]

Historically, regulatory approval of new drugs and devices was reliant on well-funded developers with a significant revenue stream conducting and funding randomized, prospective clinical trials. Many new technologies in RT, however, are introduced by small startup companies that are smaller, less well capitalized, and often single-product vendors. They are not capable of funding randomized, prospective trials, and they have a powerful financial impetus to bring their product to market as quickly and as profitably as possible.

In 1985, the Blue Cross Blue Shield Association adopted the criteria that required "adequate scientific evidence" to determine that technology improved health outcomes. This approach quickly became the norm among public and private payers. In an interesting development, in 2005, the Centers for Medicare and Medicaid Services (CMS) posted on its website draft guidelines describing a new approach to the determination of coverage policies called Coverage with Evidence Development.[1] This proposal argued that Medicare coverage of promising technologies or services could be linked directly to a requirement that the beneficiary be a participant in a trial or registry and that the CMS had statutory or regulatory authority for that requirement. In the United Kingdom, there was a similar proposal for funding "only-in-research" programs. Such programs were used for the evaluation of laparoscopic surgery for colorectal cancer, photodynamic therapy for age-related macular degeneration, the National Emphysema Treatment Trial to determine whether lung reduction surgery was superior to pulmonary rehabilitation without surgery, a comparison of balloon angioplasty plus carotid artery stenting versus carotid endarterectomy in patients at high risk for stroke, and the role of positron-emission tomography scanning in suspected dementia.[2]

ECONOMIC EVALUATION IN HEALTH CARE

Economic evaluation is routinely becoming an important criterion for evaluation of therapeutic strategies. Unfortunately, consistent criteria are not followed for evaluation of the economics of treatment, which reduces the usefulness and credibility of comparative cost and other financial data/statistics across studies or over time.[3]

The potential contribution of more complex and expensive procedures to the outcome of cancer therapy thus must be carefully evaluated.[4] Obviously, a significant portion of the increase in health care costs is linked to new technology. Although much of this technology is welcome, cost–benefit should be demonstrated. Some technologic advances improve health care and can be justified economically if we document a positive impact on tumor control, patient survival, morbidity of treatment, and quality of life. The efficacy of diagnostic and therapeutic procedures can be related to outcome studies, and costs should be carefully evaluated based on both monetary and health-related considerations. Doubilet et al.[11] cautioned against the indiscriminate use of "cost-effectiveness" as the criterion on which medical decisions should be made, and thus we must carefully define the end points on which these studies are based.

Models can be constructed using a Markov model and available data on the natural history of a tumor, prognostic factors, efficacy, and morbidity of a given therapeutic modality (based on outcome analysis) and reimbursement data for treating a specific patient population. When patterns-of-failure data are used, the cost differential can be calculated for a patient treated successfully in contrast to one who fails in a specific anatomic site (locoregional failure, distant metastasis, or combination), incorporating expenditures related to management of the treatment failure. The model can be made more complete (and complex) by adding costs of the morbidity of therapy. With the information and epidemiologic data currently available in the United States, annual costs of care can be computed and compared for various therapeutic modalities. Using Monte Carlo simulation, sensitivity analysis of cost-effectiveness may be performed.

Total cost-of-care projections should be carried out using a Markov-type analysis based on clinical experience, which will provide more accurate cost data for different management options. Providing cost–benefit information to patients (consumers) will be necessary when evaluating diagnostic and treatment options, particularly in carcinoma of the breast and prostate, in which great controversy exists regarding the merits of various modalities.

A full economic evaluation typically involves quantitative examination of both costs and outcomes, or consequences, of competing possible options, including no intervention. An appropriately performed economic evaluation is incremental, that is, it measures the extra cost incurred to obtain the incremental improvement in outcome. Drummond et al.[6]

TABLE 101.1 LEVELS OF EVIDENCE AND GRADING OF EVIDENCE FOR RECOMMENDATIONS

	Type of Evidence
Level	
I	Evidence obtained from meta-analysis of multiple, well-designed, controlled studies or from high-power randomized, controlled clinical trials
II	Evidence obtained from at least one well-designed experimental study or low-power randomized, controlled clinical trial
III	Evidence obtained from well-designed, quasi-experimental studies such as nonrandomized, controlled, single-group, pre/post, cohort, time, or matched case–control series
IV	Evidence from well-designed, nonexperimental studies, such as comparative and correlational descriptive and case studies
V	Evidence from case reports and clinical examples
Grade	
A	There is evidence of type I or consistent findings from multiple studies of type II, III, or IV
B	There is evidence of type II, III, or IV and findings are generally consistent
C	There is evidence of type II, III, or IV but findings are inconsistent
D	There is little or no systematic empirical evidence

Adapted from Drummond M, Sculpher MJ, Torrance GW, et al. *Methods for the economic evaluation of health care programmes.* 3rd ed. Oxford, UK: Oxford University Press, 2005:105. Reproduced by permission of Oxford University Press.

identified different types of full economic evaluation based on the denominator chosen (Table 101.1).

In evaluating medical care, the term *efficacy* is not interchangeable with *effectiveness*. The maximum possible reduction in a disease because of the use of medical intervention is properly termed efficacy, which is generally measured with randomized, controlled trials, which will achieve the maximum possible benefit when patients are carefully selected and stratified, randomization arms are properly designed, compliance is high, and trial participants are often free of other diseases or conditions that might interfere with the intervention being evaluated. The benefits established in a randomized, controlled trial are only partially applicable to day-to-day practice in a general population. The value of a medical intervention in the general population is termed effectiveness. The difference between efficacy and effectiveness can be very large, and obtaining a realistic measurement of effectiveness is often difficult.[7]

There are four approaches to health economic evaluation for comparing two therapies: (a) incremental cost-effectiveness; (b) cost minimization, in which one assumes or observes no difference in effectiveness; (c) cost–utility analysis (CUA); and (d) incremental cost–benefit analysis. The last can be expressed in units of either effectiveness or costs. When analyzing data from a clinical trial, expressing incremental net benefit in units of cost allows the investigator to examine all the approaches in a single graph, complete with the corresponding statistical inferences.

The most widely used approach, *cost-effectiveness analysis* (CEA), compares the incremental costs of a new technology or intervention to the incremental gain or loss of clinical outcome of the new intervention, ideally measured in life years gained (LYG). Other potential denominators in a CEA are disease-free survival or number of cancers prevented or detected, but the use of such intermediary outcome measures hampers comparison among different CEAs and should therefore be discouraged. The evaluation will result in a ratio of the cost/outcome, for example, cost/life year gained ($/LYG, €/LYG), called the incremental cost-effectiveness ratio. Assuming a well-defined comparison of two RT approaches and a sufficiently long follow-up, LYG may be measured, but it can be questioned whether this metric has most relevance to patients.

When the outcome of the evaluated interventions is expected to be the same, the economic evaluation will be limited to a cost comparison called cost-minimization analysis (CMA). Provided that there is sufficient evidence that the outcome of interest for the experimental treatment or intervention does not differ from the standard treatment, a CMA is undertaken. This simply requires a cost comparison, with the intervention resulting in the lower cost being favored from a health economics perspective.

The third type of full economic evaluation, *cost–utility analysis* (CUA), acknowledges quality of life after an intervention by weighting the LYG with a "utility factor" typically ranging from 0 (death) to 1 (perfect health). For example, if a patient had a utility or preference for a health state of 0.5 and he survived in that state for 1 year, then he would have had a quality-adjusted survival of 6 months. A CUA employs quality-adjusted life years (QALYs) in the denominator, with the result expressed as cost/QALY. Utilities or patient preferences for a certain health outcome can be measured with instruments such as the Health Utilities Index III[8] and EuroQol[9] or tests such as Time Trade-Off or Standard Gamble.[10] CUAs are helpful in trying to compare nonsimilar health interventions, such as a prostate cancer–screening program with a child immunization program. CUA calculates the value of an intervention as the ratio of its incremental cost divided by its incremental survival benefit, with survival weighted by utilities to produce QALYs. Many studies are at variance with current standards; only 20% of studies took a societal perspective, more than one-third failed to discount both the costs and QALYs, and utilities were often simply estimates from the investigators or other physicians. There remains much room for improvement in the methodologic rigor with which utilities are measured. Considering quality of life effects by incorporating utilities into economic studies is particularly important in oncology, when many therapies obtain modest improvements in response or survival at the expense of nontrivial toxicity.

The last type of full economic evaluation is *cost–benefit analysis*, in which both cost and outcome are valued in terms of currency. Where the benefit in monetary units is greater than the cost, the medical intervention is considered worthwhile. Putting a dollar value on the quantity and quality of a life is, however, a highly specialized and controversial area. Full economic evaluation in RT, requiring detailed input on short- and long-term costs and outcomes, can be difficult to perform. One such approach addresses costs and outcomes separately and leads to cost and outcome descriptions, respectively.[6] However, there are dangers with separating costs and outcomes, and one must be cautious that the information generated will not be misused.

Stinnett and Mullahy[11] introduced the concept of net health benefit as an alternative to cost-effectiveness ratios for the statistical analysis of patient-level data on the costs and health effects of competing interventions. Net health benefit addresses a number of problems associated with cost-effectiveness ratios by assuming a value for the willingness to pay for a unit of effectiveness. Willan[12] extended the concept of net health benefit to demonstrate that standard statistical procedures can be used for the analysis power and sample size determines cost-effectiveness data. He showed that by varying the value of the willingness to pay, the point estimate and confidence interval for the increment cost-effectiveness ratio can be determined.

The most useful descriptions of outcome of a new treatment strategy, particularly from the patient's perspective, result from the conduct of clinical trials. Randomized and controlled phase III trials have been categorized as efficacy or effectiveness evaluations.[6] It can be argued, however, that such comparisons may indirectly lead to the increased cost of health care as funders come under pressure to broadly adopt new interventions with only marginal clinical benefit and no consideration of the opportunity cost. A pure cost comparison, in contrast, entails the opposite risk. If the tendency to reduce

Section V

health care spending is strong, this might result in the simple choice of the cheapest approach, which may, in turn, lead to reduced quality, hence inferior outcome.

There are many reasons why data and conclusions from cost-based studies may be suspect. For example, in a computerized literature search of >14,000 articles published since 1994 having *cost* as a keyword, critiques focused on three areas:

1. Costs are not measured correctly[13-15] because most studies use charge or reimbursement dollars as a proxy for cost. This is an incorrect measure because neither value is representative of the resources consumed or foregone in the process of providing a good service. Neither is a cost: the former is a construct, and the latter is the result of a negotiation between a payer and a provider.

2. Costs are not compiled using a proper perspective and scope.[14,16] Most studies only tabulate the cost to the health care provider and not that to the patient, the family, or society.

3. There is a lack of consistency in reporting results,[13,17,18] which prevents interstudy and interinstitutional comparison.[19]

Clearly, a better costing method is required. Russell[20] emphasized that to serve its purpose, a model must produce accurate predictions and low probability for substantial variation in the factors that influence costs and effects. He identified three aspects of modeling: validating effectiveness estimates, modeling costs, and the implications of common statistical forms. Validation procedures similar to those for effectiveness estimates are proposed for costs. Modelers need to ensure that the events described by a model represent costs and effects. Modelers can also help improve the epidemiologic and clinical research on which cost-effectiveness analyses depend by showing the implications for resource allocation of the statistical forms conventionally used in these fields.

Comparative effectiveness research (CER) aims to improve the quality, effectiveness, and efficiency of health care and to help patients, health care professionals, and purchasers make informed decisions regarding various treatment options, particularly for chronic illnesses or cancer. CER is moving forward, with recently defined priorities and a newly funded Patient-Centered Outcomes Research Institute (PCORI). Economic analyses are most valuable to health policy analysts and health care managers who must allocate resources and establish benefit packages. An economic health care analysis tries to directly relate the incremental cost of an intervention to its potential benefit. The intervention is always evaluated relative to an alternative form of treatment.[3]

CER must be focused on patient outcomes. One cannot assume that a higher dose of radiation to a target field or a more conformal dose distribution will result in better survival or improved tolerance. Outcomes of significance to the patient such as survival, disease-free survival, quality of life, or specific side effects must be the focal points of research.[21] It is particularly important for radiation oncologists to remember that an improved dose distribution achieved through intensity-modulated radiotherapy (IMRT), conformal techniques, or particle therapy is not the same as an improved outcome. The presence of an improved outcome as the result of a difference in dose distribution must be proven, not assumed.

TYPES OF COST IN HEALTH CARE

The numerator in economic analysis is cost. A number of studies on the costs of treating cancer patients with RT[22-25] used either relevant costs defined in a number of ways or different proxies for actual costs (billed charges, revenue received, Medicare allowable). Recent reviews illustrate the wide variety of cost information and cost methods used in the literature and call for a consistent method for estimating site- and intent-specific treatment costs.[3,15,16,19,26] In estimating costs of health care interventions, several decision tools, including cost analysis, cost-effectiveness, and cost–utility and cost–benefit analysis, seek to define a unit of health outcome per unit input of cost. Before employing any of these decision tools, proper definition and calculation of cost are essential. Cost of medical care can be calculated in many different ways as highlighted below.

Costs during Treatment

Direct medical costs include the value of all the goods and services consumed in the provision of an intervention or dealing with the side effects of treatment. These costs include the consumption of all capital and human resources such as professional time, diagnostics, treatment, and medications.

Direct non–health care costs include all costs as a consequence of undergoing a treatment but not related to the treatment itself. Examples are the cost of transportation while patients are receiving treatment. Other costs sometimes included are *changes in the use of informal caregiver time* (including the cost of family or other providers to provide health care in the home or continuous nursing care for disabled individuals) and *patient time costs* (referring to the time patients spend receiving care, including the value of the time consumed in receiving the treatment as well as travel and waiting time).

Indirect medical costs include all costs in the time after the treatment has been terminated and include costs of late toxicity or related diseases. In RT, these costs can differ quite substantially between different approaches if the side effects are very different or if one of the interventions has a higher curative potential. Typically, however, these costs occur many years after termination of the treatment.

Indirect nonmedical costs refer to costs that are important for society, in that they measure loss of productivity because of long-term disability or premature death. Costs to the family or society can be substantial. These include the patient's travel costs, the patient's or care provider's time off from work, and the considerable strain on caregivers. There may also be "downstream" effects. If a caregiver is devoting time to an ill spouse, he or she is taking time away from work or child care responsibilities, for example.

Global cost estimates of the cost of RT are the aggregate costs of the human and capital resources consumed in the delivery of an RT service. They do not contain the fine detail required when comparing, say, one RT protocol with another. However, they can have value as a background to allocating national health care budgets between different classes of medical intervention.

Data reveal that even in countries with optimal infrastructure, the budget assigned to RT is roughly 5% of the total amount spent on cancer care.[27] In the early 1990s, the European Union estimated the average cost per course of RT at about 3,000€, compared to roughly 7,000€ and 17,000€ for surgical and chemotherapy treatments, respectively. However, in spite of the perception of high capital costs, it is the personnel cost that dominates the cost of the provision of the service (about 70%), with capital investment typically representing <30% of the total RT budget.[10,28,29]

Reimbursement-Based Costs

Although economic evaluation theoretically advocates the use of cost figures that reflect actual resource consumption, this is frequently not achievable, and charges for service are used as a proxy. It should, however, be realized that large discrepancies may exist between the reimbursement of treatments and the costs of resources consumed while delivering a treatment.

Because of the fact that reimbursement often lags behind the introduction of novel technologies, in many countries, there is a tendency for high-tech treatments to be underreimbursed. The inverse seems to hold for the United States, where the reimbursement is likely to be higher for new technologies, although it decreases with time.

Besides numerical differences between costs and charges, other, more practical and theoretical problems may arise when utilizing reimbursement figures for economic evaluation. This was observed by the Radiation Therapy Oncology Group when performing an economic evaluation based on combining clinical trial data with cost data obtained from Medicare for each patient.[30] The first problem was that Medicare-managed care products do not have individual claims because managed care companies receive capitated payments and therefore may not record and/or report individual claims to Medicare. A more accurate estimation of costs would result from using administrative claims data to calculate costs, provided that they contain all claims of care a patient received. Another potential problem is that an underestimation of costs could occur if codes with only a cancer diagnosis were used, thus neglecting costs related to treatment toxicity or indirect medical costs occurring in the further follow-up of the patient. It may also be difficult to generalize the results of an analysis based on Medicare patients older than 65 years to the general population. Finally, it is apparent that obtaining administrative claims data from Medicare can be a costly procedure in itself.[31]

ACTIVITY-BASED COST ANALYSIS

Activity-based costing (ABC) is a system widely used in manufacturing but rarely in health care. ABC dissects the process of providing patient care into a series of microlevel tasks and assigns costs to these tasks. As a result, ABC directly identifies resources consumed by cost objects (treatments, patients, or health care providers).[8] Tabulating these tasks and resources consumed allows for comparison of cost values across institutions and time in a consistent and credible way. From this, the economic impact of differences in operating policies can be quantified, and the comparison of cost to health outcome will be improved.

The traditional cost models that hospitals have used are outdated and ill equipped to provide accurate information on costs of a specific medical procedure or global cost of medical care for a patient from initial diagnosis to death. Cost models break organizations into departments for financial oversight and budgetary control. The focus of these cost models is departmental budgets, and they are not specific for a patient or a procedure, although patients and procedures (not the department) trigger costs. For example, the accounting system of a hospital may be able to provide a fair assessment of the total budget (cost) of its radiation oncology department. However, the same system is of little help in assessing the actual cost of treating a patient with prostate cancer using RT. This lack of applicability of cost information at the patient or the procedure level often leads to faulty decision-making because analysis of the whole department does not necessarily translate into data about an individual patient.

ABC is concerned with measuring resource consumption by an individual patient. There are two general advantages of using ABC: increased accuracy of cost measurements and transparency of cost-incurring sections. The latter advantage—increased accounting transparency—means that there is a more lucid and readily apparent correlation between costs and actions. This allows managers to evaluate each step of the process, perceive inefficiencies in the system, and quantify economic benefits of process improvements.

The cost data of any technology should reflect the facilities and equipment costs (including depreciation and replacement), space (including housekeeping and utilities), and recorded time and effort of all professional staff on hospital payroll treating patients. Specific technical approaches should be identified, for example, in patients undergoing definitive RT, standard two-dimensional (2-D) or three-dimensional (3-D) conformal RT (CRT) or IMRT or image-guided RT (IGRT). Time and effort observations for multiple tasks must be recorded by the respective staff members as they take place. The numbers of observations provide a representative sample of treatment procedures.

Technical cost is defined as the actual expenditures recorded in hospital accounting records. The total technical cost of a course of therapy includes staff time and effort, compensation including fringe benefits, space, utilities, maintenance, equipment depreciation, supplies, support services, liability cost, and administrative overhead. The ABC method[32–35] was used to derive technical (hospital) resource utilization costs for treatment procedures in treating localized prostate cancer.[3,24] The costing method consists of four major steps:

1. Creating a process flow map that identifies and defines all of the activities and steps associated with the treatment of patients with standard irradiation or with 3DCRT (Fig. 101.1).
2. Collecting and recording the staff time expended on each activity
3. Identifying and accumulating all hospital costs from the general accounting ledger system related to the patients treated at a radiation oncology center in a given period
4. Allocating actual cost to each activity to derive total specific costs of technical resource utilization for a course of 2D- or 3DCRT, IMRT, or IGRT

An example of an ABC cost calculation model is the one developed in by Lievens et al.[29] Because it was felt that current RT protocols, with a shift toward more complex treatment planning and delivery techniques and more thorough quality assurance procedures, were no longer accurately captured within the original model, a novel version has recently been developed.[36] Because evolving technology over the last decade was more complex, it was found that the introduction of IMRT compared to 3DCRT translated into an almost doubling of procedure costs. ABC analysis allowed the authors to identify exactly where these extra costs were incurred. It was shown that the cost increase was the consequence not of the IMRT technique as such but of the combined effect of IMRT using more fields and delivering dose escalation and the introduction of more frequent online imaging guidance for position verification.

If, however, techniques such as IMRT or gated radiotherapy delivery make it possible to reduce the number of fractions using simultaneous integrated boosts or accelerated hypofractionation, the resulting costs may decrease while yielding potentially improved treatment outcomes.[31] This phenomenon has been discussed in some detail by Konski and colleagues.[37]

Time and Effort Analysis

An integral phase of ABC is identifying process flow, listing each individual involved in the process, and recording the actual amount of time spent to perform an activity by each person involved using electronic or paper daily activity logs. Determining the participant's task time should follow the monopolizing rule: Timing begins when a specific patient requires the participant's attention and stops when he or she is no longer doing so. Whether or not the patient is still present in the activity area is immaterial. For example, for an office visit, the nurse's time to prepare the patient's paperwork

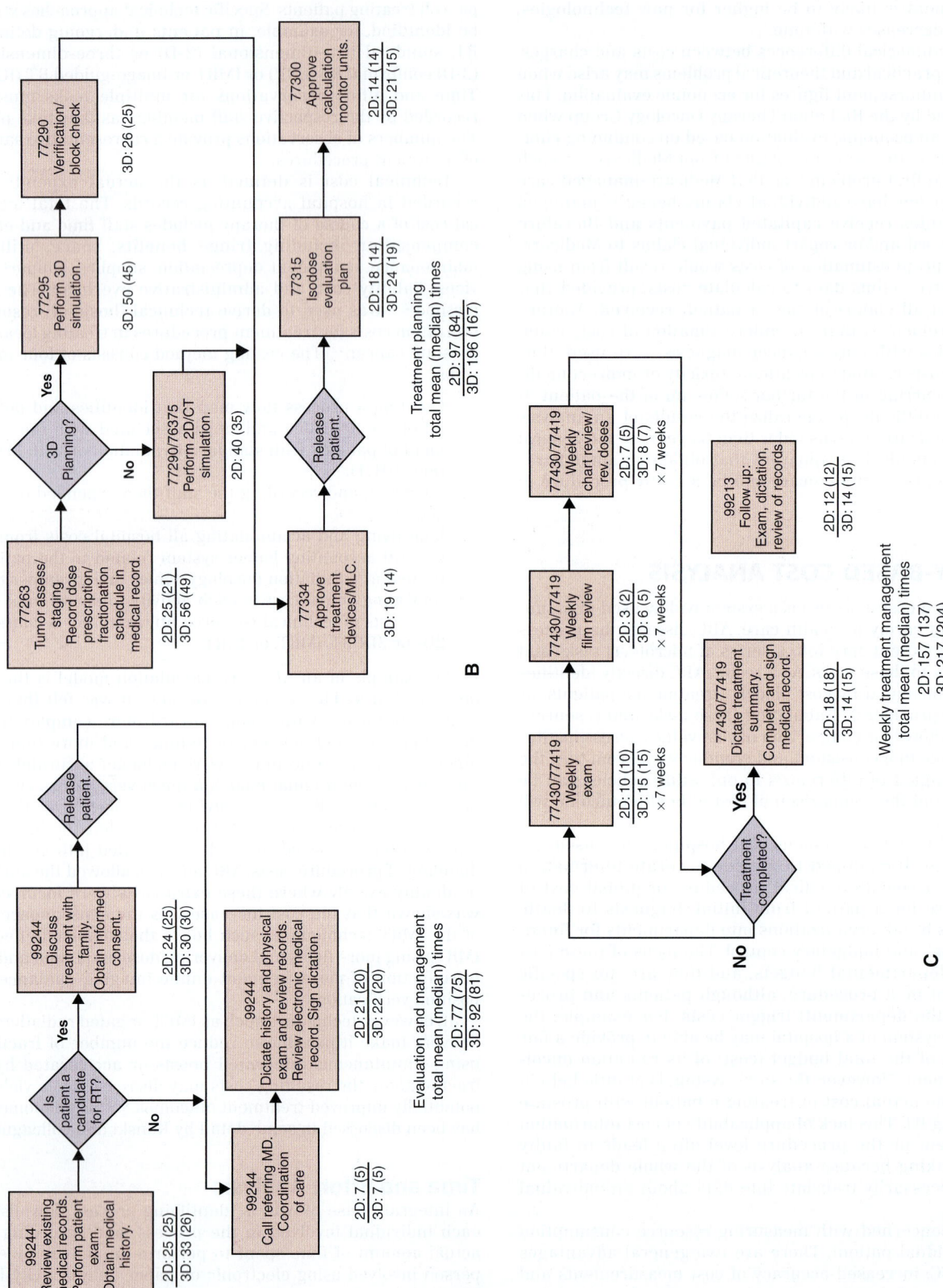

FIGURE 101.1. Process flow chart. Activity map and corresponding mean (median) times for definitive irradiation of cancer of the prostate. **A:** Evaluation and management. **B:** Treatment planning. **C:** Weekly management. MLC, multileaf collimator.

should be attributed to the patient, even before the patient arrives or after he or she has left the office. The actual activity time may be adjusted upward to recognize some normal unproductive time of activity participants, such as time spent in work breaks. Tables are generated to show the time and effort involved in each of the functions necessary to register and evaluate the patient, perform treatment planning, deliver external beam irradiation, and supervise the management, as well as in preparation of the appropriate records to document all information, including quality assurance requirements.

Times are collected for each activity in the treatment process beginning with the initial consultation through the first follow-up visit after full treatment. These data points are analyzed and used to generate average times for patients treated with a specific technique along with the standard deviation of times.

RESOURCE UTILIZATION COSTS

Four types of resources should be catalogued and measured for each task:

1. Activity participants (e.g., radiation oncologists, physicists, therapists, dosimetrists, nurses, receptionists)
2. Physical resources (e.g., space, equipment, machines)
3. Supplies (e.g., x-ray films, office supplies)
4. Support services (e.g., administration, centralized information system)

Patient-related expenses include salaries and fringe benefits of the staff, Social Security contributions, retirement annuities, health, life disability and long-term care, dental insurance, tuition and child care benefits, and disability insurance. Average hourly salary and related costs for each staff member are computed.

There are many supplies, such as office paper and latex gloves, for which the cost is trivial, and it is not economically worthwhile to track their specific use for individual patients. An average cost rate can be computed for such supplies by dividing their total cost by the total number of patients, which is applied to each patient. However, supplies used only by patients with specific diseases or procedures (e.g., contrast material, immobilization devices) need to be recorded for individual patients.

For hospital-based departments, indirect operating costs are classified into general hospital operating expenses and administrative overhead, which includes hospital liability insurance and administrative costs such as shared activities (administrative personnel for purchasing and payroll functions, human resources, public relations, and financial operations). The allocation of indirect operating costs among different departments of the hospital is complex. Models include allocating them as a proportion of personnel costs and many others.

The allocation of cost among various units in a hospital can also be the source of discord between different units. In many hospitals, allocation of costs is a mechanism of cross-subsidization among different departments (e.g., the surgery department subsidizing primary care). Administrative cost can be determined by computing prorated allocation, dividing the total hospital indirect expenses by the proportion of the radiation oncology center technical budget to the total hospital annual budget.

Technical equipment expenses for treatment of patients are included using American Hospital Association standard depreciation schedules. The cost of depreciation of all equipment involved in the management of these patients, including treatment planning and delivery, should be accounted for on a prorated basis.

Because an increasing proportion of the health insurance market is being controlled by managed care, with its cost-cutting pressures, there may be a tendency to de-emphasize the importance of quality of care. Under such conditions, it is critical to document any decreased morbidity of treatment with advanced technology in comparison with conventional external beam RT (see Chapters 69 and 70 for prostate cancer). This potential benefit is of great financial significance because treatment of major therapy complications may be costly.

Owen et al.[38] conducted economic studies for two phase III Radiation Therapy Oncology Group (RTOG) studies comparing different irradiation fractionation schedules: 1-04 and 90-03 (brain metastasis and head and neck cancer, respectively). Expected numbers of current procedural terminology codes and relative value units (RVUs) were modeled. Institutions retrospectively provided procedure codes, quantities, and components, which were converted to RVUs used for Medicare payments. The median and mean RVUs were within the range predicted by the model for all arms of one study and above the predicted range for the other study. The model predicted resource use well for patients who completed treatment per protocol. Some institutions experienced difficulty collecting retrospective data; prospective collection of data is necessary to validate such studies.

This information also will be very helpful in contract negotiations with health care organizations and third-party payers and in setting policies for establishing therapy guidelines and justification of health care expenditures.

OUTCOMES IN ECONOMIC ANALYSIS

Outcomes, such as survival or year of life gained, are the denominator in economic analyses. Ways to identify outcomes are highlighted below.

OUTCOME RESEARCH

Outcome research focuses on identifying variations in medical procedures and associated health outcomes. Figure 101.2 illustrates the interplay of outcome research and clinical trials with clinical and policy decision-making.

The term *outcome* is frequently used to describe a variety of end points or products of health care. Areas of specific focus of outcome analysis include the following:

1. Structure of care (such as features of health care facilities, staffing, equipment)
2. Process of care (such as type of studies performed, services provided)
3. Patient characteristics (gender, age, race, ethnic group)
4. Disease focus (such as location and type of tumor, histology, pathologic features)
5. Treatment-related factors (type of treatment, tumor response, disease-free survival, overall survival, morbidity of therapy)
6. Socioeconomics (such as cost–benefit, quality of life, financial impact of the disease, recovery, and rehabilitation)

Meta-analysis is another mechanism to systematically research and collect published/unpublished randomized clinical trial data and quantitatively summarize results to obtain objective assessment of efficacy. The process should be (a) hypothesis driven, (b) protocol based, and (c) reproducible and comprehensive. However, meta-analysis has some potential shortcomings, such as uncontrolled testing conditions, sample heterogeneity, unrecorded interventions, ambiguous end points, lack of independence of determinant factors, synergistic interactions, and sometimes contradictory experimental results.

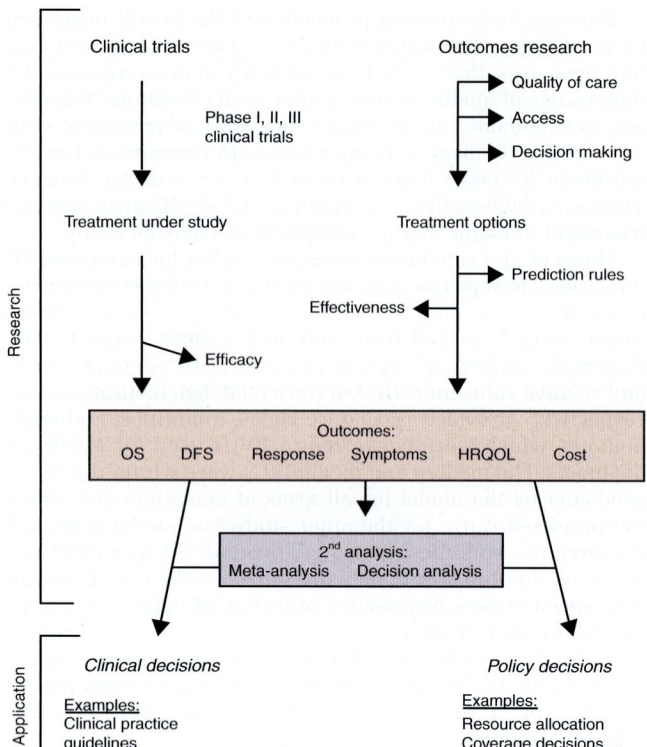

FIGURE 101.2. Conceptual framework of outcome research. Interaction is shown between research topics, end points, analytic techniques, and applications in defining outcomes research. Depicted in the upper left corner are the classic clinical trials and analytic techniques that are not outcomes research. In the upper right corner are shown the study topics, end points, and analytic techniques that are considered to be outcomes research. Outcomes depicted in the center box may or may not constitute outcomes research, depending on the context. For example, overall survival as measured in a phase III trial is not an outcomes study (efficacy), whereas it is if observed in a large community cohort (effectiveness). Symptoms have both efficacy and outcomes influences. Applications are indicated in italics and may emanate from either clinical trials or outcomes research. See text for further details. (From Lee SJ, Earle CC, Weeks JC. Outcomes research in oncology: history, conceptual framework, and trends in the literature. *J Natl Cancer Inst* 2000;92[3]:195–204. Reproduced by permission of Oxford University Press.)

Efforts have intensified during the last 20 years to promote outcome research in oncology, and there is a critical need to continue to support randomized, controlled studies. Patient and physician acceptance of participation in outcome research studies must be improved because only 10% to 20% of patients with newly diagnosed cancer participate in these important studies.[39] There is considerable variation in participation of patients in research studies as a function of patient age and disease site. In general, compliance with participation in studies is much higher among pediatric patients than adults.

Among the most commonly used data are those of the Surveillance, Epidemiology, and End Result (SEER) program. SEER is a continuing project of the biometry branch of the U.S. National Cancer Institute. The program draws data from several population-based cancer reporting systems covering approximately 14% of the total population of the United States. When linked to Medicare and other insurance administrative files, it has been extremely valuable in assessing the quality of care of the elderly and other insured populations. Although an excellent data source, SEER has been criticized as being inadequate to represent the diversity of systems of care throughout the country and in general does not have data that may more accurately define patient- or tumor-specific prognostic characteristics or treatment details.

The National Cancer Database, a joint project of the American College of Surgeons' Commission on Cancer and the American Cancer Society, holds information on more than half of all newly diagnosed cases of cancer in the United States and includes many of the demographic, clinical, and health systems data elements necessary to assess quality of care. A serious limitation of the National Cancer Database is the absence of complete information on outpatient care; its data have not been widely used to assess quality of care, but it has great potential for doing so.

An effective national system to collect this type of information should be established in the United States to collect data about the following:

1. Demographics of individuals with cancer (e.g., age, ethnic group, socioeconomic status, and insurance or health plan coverage)
2. Type of cancer (stage, histologic type, grade, comorbid conditions)
3. Treatment, including outcome of procedures, such as adjuvant chemotherapy and RT
4. Specialty training of care providers
5. Site of care delivery (such as community hospital or specialized cancer center)
6. Type of care delivery system (such as managed care, fee for service, government agency)
7. Outcomes (tumor control, survival, complications of treatment, quality of life, satisfaction with services provided)

WAYS TO MEASURE OUTCOMES INDICATIVE OF SURVIVAL AND TUMOR RESPONSE

Survival can be measured as overall survival, disease-free survival, progression-free survival, or event-free survival. It is clearly the most important outcome in cancer treatment. It is also clear, however, that survival alone is insufficient as a measure of outcome. The quality of survival and the cost of maintaining and improving survival must also be assessed.[40]

Making a choice between alternative treatment approaches often involves a tradeoff between length of survival and quality of life. A survival measurement alone might not answer the question of whether gains in survival justify toxicity. Quality-adjusted survival attempts to adjust the absolute length of life to reflect the patient's quality of life. Quality-adjusted survival provides a framework within which tradeoffs that influence treatment choices can be defined as in decision and cost-effective analysis to assess the effectiveness of alternative therapies.[41,42]

Quality of Life Outcome Measures

Quality of life considers the impact of cancer and its treatment on the physical, psychological, and social components of patient's lives. Cancer-related quality of life is a family of outcomes including the global quality of life as well as physical, psychological, and social dimensions, each one of which is a potentially separate outcome. Because of its subjective nature, the assessment of quality of life generally should include an evaluation by the patient. Quality of life measures should be characterized by reliability and validity.[42–44]

Toxicity Measures of Outcome

Toxicities are subjective, objective, or both. An example of a subjective toxicity would be a symptom such as nausea that is often not associated with overt signs or laboratory abnormalities. Evaluation of toxicities of this sort rests with the patient's report. Objective toxicities are measured by physical examination or laboratory tests. The common toxicity criteria use a system for categorizing toxicity from cancer treatment according to its severity. Such systems are widely used in cooperative group trials.

Measures of Cancer Response Outcomes

Measures of tumor response include complete response, response to radiation, and time to progression. Response may also be measured by biomarkers and changes in cancer-induced abnormalities and common blood tests. Some studies demonstrated the positive relationship between response rate and quality of life, but others did not. It is clear that freedom from progression may not be a convincing indication of the benefits of treatment if it does not predict significantly improved survival or cure. Freedom from progression is therefore not an adequate measure of quality of life.[39]

Cost-Effectiveness as a Cancer Outcome

Cost is not an outcome. It is, instead, what we spend to produce an outcome. Cost-effectiveness, in contrast, is often an important outcome. Cost-effectiveness may be reported in terms of cost per year of life saved or cost per quality-adjusted year of life saved. Clinical practice guidelines are generally informed by cost-effectiveness considerations.[41,42] If all that matters is minimizing expense, then the lowest-cost treatment—or no treatment in some cases—would be preferred. However, cost–benefit, which incorporates the incremental impact of a new technology on outcome, and cost–utility, which also relates additional costs to impact on survival as well as on the patient's quality of life and productivity, are important parameters in the assessment of new technology.[3] The projected cost of treating a patient who initially has control of the local tumor and no distant metastases is about one-third of that for a patient who develops a treatment failure.[45]

Health technology assessment (HTA) plays an essential role in modern health care by supporting evidence-based decision-making in policy and practice. HTA involves addressing five questions[46]:

1. Can a health care intervention achieve its expected goal when used in optimal circumstances? (Efficacy)
2. Does the intervention do more good than harm when used in routine practice? (Effectiveness)
3. What is the balance between the health outcome obtained and the resources required to deliver the intervention? (Efficiency or Cost-Effectiveness)
4. Is the supply of services matched to locations where they are accessible to persons that need them? (Availability)
5. Who gains and who loses by choosing to allocate resources to one health care program instead of another? (Distribution)

Technology assessment, cost–benefit outcome analysis, clinical trials supported by evidence-based medicine (EBM), and comparative effectiveness together can enhance the rationale and quality of medical care provided to patients at a competitive cost.

TECHNOLOGY ASSESSMENT

Technologic change is the key driver of health care expenditure growth because it is generally associated with increased rather than reduced cost. As the economist Henry Aaron is quoted as saying, "Rapid scientific advance always raises expenditures even as it lowers prices. Those who think otherwise need only to turn their historical eyes to automobiles, airplanes, television, and computers. In each case, massive technologic advance drove down the price of services, the total outlay soared."[47] A good example in medicine of this phenomenon is laparoscopic cholecystectomy. Although the price of a laparoscopic procedure is less than the price of an open cholecystectomy, after the introduction of the new technology, the rates of both types of surgery increased, and the growth in the quantity of services overwhelmed the impact of per unit reduction in price. Similar examples can be found

in the widespread use of magnetic resonance imaging, computed tomography, coronary artery bypass grafting, angioplasty, cardiac intensive care units, neonatal intensive care units, and positron-emission tomography and the growth of radiation oncology facilities. Technology may also increase costs by either premature adoption of the technology without adequate evidence that it improves outcome or overuse of technology, regardless of value, to provide a competitive market advantage or to generate revenues.[48]

Technology assessment is undertaken to determine (a) the appropriateness of adopting a new procedure consistent with the health care organization's mission and strategic plan; (b) the safety, efficacy, and cost-effectiveness of the new technology; (c) distinctions between appropriate and inappropriate use of the new technology; and (d) quality improvement methods to optimize the use of the new technology.[49] Technology assessment is a complex process that involves financial considerations; a given therapeutic outcome; treatment-induced morbidity; quality of life; impact on caregivers, family, and coworkers; and lost opportunity costs.

When new technology emerges and priorities for allocation of increasingly scarce resources are considered, it is imperative to carry out economic analyses and also to assess the positive effects to the population who will benefit from the new technology compared with standard treatment techniques. The U.S. Centers for Medicare Management concluded that cost-effectiveness should be considered in approving reimbursement by Medicare for new technology procedures.

Halperin[50] pointed out the importance of technology assessment in determining the merits of new devices or modalities and the impact they may have on the cost of health care. In a provocative editorial, Lee[51] pointed out that although technology is ubiquitous in radiation oncology, it is our professional responsibility to critically evaluate the merits of new technologic developments. Yet, technology assessment can be a thorny and complex subject. Many of the technologic advances in radiation oncology have not undergone a strict test of worthiness in formal clinical trials. Simulation, positioning techniques, computed tomography scanning for treatment planning, online imaging, intensity-modulated RT, adaptive planning, and daily image guidance have had multiple dosimetric validations, but no randomized trial has documented their impact on outcome of large numbers of patients. However, lack of this evidence would not lead us to discontinue any of these procedures, which have been shown to improve in some way (i.e., less toxicity) the quality of care provided to patients.

Many nations have agencies to conduct HTA, and there is an international network of agencies for HTA that can share such data. The United States, however, has no national coordinating body on HTA. Assessments are conducted through organizations such as the Veterans Administration, the Blue Cross Blue Shield Association, and professional organizations like the American College of Radiology, the Medicare Coverage Advisory Committee, and HMOs.

Health care organizations use a variety of models to assess and acquire technology, some of which include outcome. Reliable data for such benchmarking are frequently scarce. Some compare new and emerging technology against existing technology, although reliable outcome data are rare. Most institutions or individuals buy what physicians, advocacy groups, philanthropists, or governing boards want and use manufacturers and physicians as the primary sources of technology information. Cowan and Berkowitz[48] pointed out several key mistakes that occur during the diffusion of technology:

1. Technologies are adopted simply because they are new, without assessing their impact on outcomes.
2. Equipment is replaced solely because of its age. To avoid overuse of technology, health care organizations must

carefully match the capacity of existing technology with projected utilization in a world of limited resources.

3. Applications of technology expand without adequate justification based on outcome or cost considerations.

4. Numerous vendors are used, and numerous models of products with duplicative specifications are purchased. Reducing the number of brands and models of devices used may provide an opportunity to reduce purchasing and inventory costs, as well as maintenance and repair costs. On the other hand, competitive pressures in the marketplace may provide downward pressure on equipment prices and favor multiple vendors.

5. Economies of scale in regionalizing technology decisions are missed because of lack of consolidation of services. This is sometimes related to inadequate systems for patient transport to treatment centers.

Duplication of services may add cost without significant increase in work volume.

The benefit of 3DCRT, IMRT, or IGRT is hypothetically linked to (a) improved local tumor control because of better coverage of the target volume with a specific dose of irradiation, (b) less acute and late morbidity, and (c) the possibility of carrying out dose escalation studies if morbidity is held to an acceptable level, resulting in improved survival.[45] Several institutions, the RTOG, and 10 institutions under cooperative agreement with the National Cancer Institute conducted phase I/II dose escalation studies in carcinoma of the prostate and are carrying out a study on carcinoma of the lung. Depending on the results, the cost–benefit of 3DCRT, IMRT, or IGRT must be further evaluated in dose escalation and in larger multi-institutional phase III studies, comparing it with standard techniques to justify its somewhat higher initial cost. Cases most likely to benefit from 3DCRT, IMRT, or IGRT include patients with (a) tumors in sites with complex anatomy, (b) irregular-shaped tumors, (c) tumors adjacent to radiation-sensitive normal structures, (d) tumors that undergo significant changes in volume during treatment, and (e) small-volume or high-dose treatment.

A recent workshop convened by the National Cancer Policy Forum in July 2015[52] specifically concerned itself with "value" as the relationship between clinical effectiveness and cost. The panel described the rapid market saturation of IMRT with only small, recent randomized trials assessing moist desquamation in breast cancer[53] and xerostomia in head and neck cancer.[54] This was due in large part to consensus among radiation oncologists of the dosimetric advantages provided by the technique. Nevertheless, Medicare expenses for IMRT were estimated to increase fourfold between 2002 and 2010, from about \$200B to about \$800B.[55]

Another example is the recent adoption of particle therapy—most commonly proton therapy in the United States. The literature on the cost-effectiveness of particle therapy for cancer is scarce, studies are often not comparable, and many studies are not performed according to standard health assessment criteria. Evidence on the cost-effectiveness of particle therapy is, therefore, limited.

Consensus also exists for some proposed uses for proton therapy such as pediatrics, again absent randomized data. In this case, initial centers were built not only by university-based cancer programs but by regional or venture capital–based entities. Because early centers were quite expensive, protons became a convenient example of rampant health care costs,[56] and in some cases, the accusations were valid. Clearly, despite the value of protons in complex and pediatric cases, most centers required a large number of "simple" treatments for which no clinical benefit could be proven simply in order to service debt.[57] The ultimate result of proton facility locations being driven by available venture capital, geographic ego, and academic marketeers is that the expansion

became unsustainable,[58] evidenced by closing of the Indiana University Health Proton Therapy Center in 2014. Although smaller proton facilities and vendor competition have greatly reduced entrance costs, more upheaval is expected within the proton space in the United States before settling.[59] Given limited success with existing grant systems in the United States, it is unclear that adequate reimbursement will be found to support such innovative and costly treatments to learn whether it is truly more efficacious.

The introduction of protons and heavy ions (hadrons) into the RT armamentarium has brought additional controversy in technology assessment because of the higher cost of facilities, equipment, and operation, with much dispute as to the cost-effectiveness of these innovative modalities. A 2008 review of the literature showed that only 17 publications (out of 777 on particle therapy) dealt with economic aspects, and only 5 of them were on cost-effectiveness.[60] Many articles have been published on the physical advantages of protons or heavy ions in comparison with photons, resulting in better dose distribution in the target volume with less radiation administered to normal tissues, which may decrease morbidity and eventually the risk of second malignancies.[61,62] However, there is a lack of randomized trials documenting superior clinical outcomes with these particles.

Opinions on the need for or ethical considerations to subjecting patients to prospective trials have been expressed.[63,64] Perrier et al.[65] used an ABC approach similar to the examples discussed previously to evaluate the cost of carbon ion therapy. It allowed an in-depth definition of the cost of treatment preparation and the actual irradiation, depending on various parameters such as actual treatment time and patient setup time. The approach of Peeters et al.,[66] conversely, was more aggregate, using a spreadsheet model that assumes that treatment costs scale linearly with the number of fractions. This, obviously, is a somewhat simple approximation of reality, which results in less accurate estimates.[29]

The American Society for Radiation Oncology maintains the position that new technologies and modifications of existing technologies representing significant paradigmatic shifts in treatment approach should be implemented into clinical practice in such a manner as to ensure safety, efficacy, and, ideally, cost-effectiveness.[67]

EVIDENCE-BASED MEDICINE AND EVIDENCE-BASED ONCOLOGY

There have been significant scientific advances in biologic sciences and health care. At the same time, there has been increased accountability and in some instances attempts to ration services; as a mechanism to accomplish this, arbitrary clinical practice guidelines have been promulgated. A more rational effort to define optimal heath care should be based on identification of innovative approaches, outcome analysis in properly designed clinical trials, and careful assessment of current practice; more importantly, we have a dire need for solid and credible clinical research and evidence-based decision-making in medicine.

The growth in basic and translational research data to guide medical practice has made it critical for clinicians to appraise and use published data for medical decisions. EBM is the compelling idea that any recommendation of a specific medical procedure should be supported by empirical evidence for its superior efficacy/toxicity ratio compared with alternative treatment options in a patient with a given presentation.[68–70]

EBM helps correct an imbalance in contemporary medicine in which clinicians are being trained to maintain high standards of critical consciousness in methodologic domains but not in the broader historic and sociocultural domains that surround them.[71]

Evidence-based health care is the conscious use of current best evidence in making decisions about the care of individuals or the delivery of health services. Current best evidence is up-to-date information from relevant valid research about the effects of different forms of health care, the potential for harm from exposure to particular agents, the accuracy of diagnostic tests, and the predictive power of prognostic factors.

Evidence-based clinical practice is an approach to decision-making in which the clinician uses the best evidence available, in the context of consultation with the patient, to decide on which option suits the patient best. EBM is a conscientious, explicit, and judicious use of current best evidence in making decisions about the care of individual patients.

Such evidence-based practice aims to apply the best available evidence gained from the scientific method to clinical decision-making. It seeks to assess the strength of evidence of the risks and benefits of treatment or lack of treatment and diagnostic tests. Evidence quality will range from more rigorous—meta-analysis and systematic reviews of double-blind, placebo clinical trials—to less (conventional wisdom).

The systematic review of published research is the major method used for evaluating particular treatments. The Cochrane Collaborations are among the best known and respected examples of systematic reviews. Like other collections of systematic reviews, it requires authors to provide a detailed and repeatable plan of literature search and evaluation of the evidence. Once all the evidence is assessed, treatment is categorized as "likely to be beneficial," "likely to be harmful," or "evidence did not support either benefit or harm."

EBM categorizes different types of clinical evidence and rates or grades them according to the strengths of their freedom from the various biases that have beset medical research. The strongest evidence for therapeutic intervention is provided by systematic review of randomized, triple-blind, placebo-controlled trials with allocation concealment and complete follow-up involving a homogeneous patient population and medical condition. In contrast, patient testimonials, case reports, or even expert opinion has little value as proof because of the placebo effect, the biases inherent in observation in reporting cases, and difficulty in ascertaining who is an expert.

Randomized, controlled trials are highly desirable to answer questions about technology assessment, but there are alternatives. Carefully controlled observational studies are good predictors of the outcome of randomized trials as long as enough essential information is collected to ensure that the patients are standardized. It is equally important in an observational series to understand which patients have been excluded.[21]

The American College of Radiology (ACR) has created a product named Appropriateness Criteria. These are exceptional medical practice guidelines that have been used by the Agency for Healthcare Research and Quality as designated by the Institute of Medicine. The ACR adopted the AQA's[72] definition of appropriateness: "The concept of appropriateness, as applied to health care, balances risk and benefit of treatment, test, or procedure in the context of available resources for an individual patient with specific characteristics. Appropriateness criteria provides guidance to supplement the clinician's judgment as to whether a patient is a reasonable candidate for the given treatment, test, or procedure." Specifically for radiation oncology treatments and procedures, there are published ACR appropriateness guidelines that one can consult to garner an opinion about the "consensus view."[72]

The Delphi methodology is a technique used to arrive at appropriateness ratings. A series of surveys is conducted to elicit members of the expert panel's interpretation of the evidence concerning the appropriateness of a therapeutic procedure for specific clinical scenario. The panelist receives a survey with an evidence table and narrative. Each panelist is asked to interpret the available evidence and rank each procedure. The survey is completed by each panelist without consulting fellow panel members. Ratings are done on a scale of 1 through 9, which is further divided into three categories: 1 to 3 is defined as usually not appropriate; 4 to 6 is defined as maybe appropriate; and 7 to 9 is defined as usually appropriate. Each panel member assigns one rating for each RT procedure or intervention per survey round. Surveys are collected and the results are tabulated, deidentified, and redistributed after each round. A maximum of three rounds is conducted. This modified Delphi technique enables each panelist to express individual interpretations of the evidence and his or her expert opinion without receiving bias from fellow panelists in a simple, standardized, and economical process. A consensus is defined as 80% agreement within a rating category.

Practicing EBM requires recognition that, in most encounters with patients, questions arise that should be answered to provide the patient with the best available medical care. Appropriate and relevant clinical questions contain four elements: (a) a patient or problem, (b) an intervention, (c) a comparison intervention (if necessary), and (d) an outcome. Important practical steps in practicing EBM include the following:

1. Formulation of the patient's clinical problem
2. Search of literature for relevant and reliable data
3. Evaluation of validity and usefulness of data
4. Integration of critical evaluation of evidence with clinical judgment
5. Implementation of useful information
6. Assessment of outcome to improve medical practice

Once the right questions have been formulated, the best source for finding most types of best evidence is by searching Medline (National Library of Medicine), PubMed (National Library of Medicine), OVID, the Cochrane Database, or a similar database by computer.

The quality (strength) of evidence is based on a hierarchy, proceeding from the most reliable results of systematic reviews of well-designed prospective clinical trials to results of one or more well-designed meta-analysis studies, results of large retrospective case series, expert opinion, and personal experience.[73] Once the best data have been found, the EBM approach involves critically appraising the quality of the evidence, determining its magnitude and precision, and applying it to a specific patient.[74,75]

The Cochrane Collaboration was established in 1993 as an international network to help health care providers, policy makers, patients, their advocates, and their caregivers make well-informed decisions about health care by preparing, updating, and promoting the success of Cochrane reviews. More than 4,500 such reviews have been published so far online in the Cochrane Library.[76]

The Cochrane Collaboration traces its origins to a 1972 publication by the British epidemiologist A. Cochrane entitled *Effectiveness and Efficiency: Random Reflections on Health Services*.[77] This book called attention to the collective ignorance concerning the effects of health care. In 1979, Cochrane published an essay in which he suggested that "it is surely a great criticism of our profession that we have not organized a critical summary, by specialty or subspecialty, adapted periodically, of all relevant randomized controlled trials."[78] Responding to Cochrane's charge, the Cochrane Collaboration undertook such a crucial but enormous undertaking.

There are >28,000 people working within the Cochrane Collaboration in >100 countries. Its central functions are funded by royalties of its publisher, which comes from sales from subscription to the Cochrane Library. The individual entities of the Cochrane Collaboration are funded by a large variety of governmental, institutional, and private funding sources and are bound by organization policy limiting uses of funds from corporate sponsors.

Section V

EBM promotes rule-based behavior on the part of physicians in an effort, among other things, to eliminate variations in medical practice. However, professionals do not follow rules per se; they intuit what is right in a situation, including, sometimes, that it is right to defer to a rule.[79]

The practice of EBM (careful clinical judgment in evaluating the "best available data") should be differentiated from the special collection of data regarded as "suitable evidence." The new collection of best available information has major constraints for the care of individual patients; derived almost exclusively from randomized trials and meta-analyses, the data do not include many types of treatments or patients seen in clinical practice, and the results show comparative efficacy of treatment for an "average" randomized patient, not for pertinent subgroups formed by such cogent clinical features as severity of symptoms, illness, comorbidity, and other clinical nuances. The intention-to-treat analyses in clinical trial reporting do not reflect important postrandomization events leading to altered treatment, and the results seldom provide suitable background data when therapy is given prophylactically rather than remedially. The authoritative aura given to the "collection of data" may lead to abuses that produce inappropriate guidelines or poorly supported doctrinaire dogmas for clinical practice.[80]

There are a variety of mechanisms to apply EBM to clinical practice, including formulation of treatment pathways, practice guidelines, appropriateness criteria, consensus conferences, patterns of care, and institutional peer review. A fundamental part of EBM is the filtering of evidence through the clinical skill of the clinician. It is not easy to determine which level of evidence is required, and it is estimated that only 20% of medical procedures currently in practice can be justified by evidence-based medical standards. When does a new cancer therapy cease being experimental and become a component of the standard of care? This distinction is subject to powerful influences for for-profit pharmaceutical companies and medical equipment manufacturers wanting to increase their sales and financial return to shareholders, advocacy groups, politicians, and a public anxiously awaiting the next "cancer breakthrough." A dispassionate set of systems for technology assessment of cancer therapies is essential to evidence-based oncology practice.

In 1993 in the United States, the American Society of Clinical Oncology (ASCO) formed a Health Services Research Committee (HSRC) to perform technology assessments and to develop guidelines for cancer treatment. The committee is composed of clinical researchers and clinicians from academic centers and private practice and performs technology assessment after hearing from expert advisors. The committee does not develop guidelines; it assembles expert panels to develop guidelines.[41]

Among the most important initial tasks of the HSRC was to create an outcome working group to define the outcomes of cancer treatment that should be considered for technology assessment in forming cancer treatment guidelines. Not surprisingly, patients, physicians, researchers, payers, and policy makers all have different ideas about which outcomes of cancer treatment are important. The main purpose of ASCO's technology assessments and guidelines is to define what constitutes the best cancer treatment, not to inform policy development and payment decisions. The working group on outcomes, therefore, considered outcomes primarily from the perspective of the clinical investigators who produced evidence for the guidelines, individual doctors and patients who have to make decisions about treatment, and health service researchers who evaluate the quality and cost of care produced by the guidelines. Because it is clear that there are health policy implications of ASCO's technology assessments and guidelines, the working group also considered outcomes that would convince health policy makers that ASCO's tech-

nology assessment was sound and that its guidelines represented worthwhile treatment.[41,49] For technology assessment, the ASCO working group is composed of members of the Health Services Research Committee and selected members. They conduct a literature review and analyze the outcome-based evidence. Testimony is collected from invited experts and interested parties. After evaluating the information, the working group defines specific questions and provides a report outlining conditions under which the proposed procedures are warranted to assist both physicians and patients in making informed decisions regarding the technologist or procedures.

The working group identifies specific questions to be addressed by the technology assessment, develops a strategy for completing the assessment, and reviews the available literature and evidence. The process may include face-to-face meetings of available working groups and members, circulation of draft forms of the technology assessment, and opportunities for comment. Working groups do not attempt to codify established practice. They review the available evidence and add their best clinical judgment to make final recommendations.

Making a treatment selection involves defining the patient's condition, identifying management options and outcome, collecting and summarizing evidence, and applying value judgments or preferences to arrive at an optimal course of action.[81] The randomized, controlled clinical trial has become the "gold standard" for evaluating the efficacy of health care intervention. In the 30-year period starting in 1966, >80,000 journal articles from randomized, controlled trial results were registered in the Medline database. The first 5 years of that period contributed <1% of the total number of articles, whereas the last half decade contributed more than the previous 25 years combined. (For more detailed review of the principles of design in clinical trials, the reader is referred to Bentzen.)[92] A proposal for structured reporting of randomized clinical trials was described in the consolidation of standards for reporting trial guidelines[42] that have been accepted by many medical journals. For instance, the journal *Radiotherapy and Oncology* adopted a set of guidelines for reporting clinical research (Table 101.2).[82] Linking management options to known outcomes in clinical trials or obtained through systematic reviews is becoming a common procedure (Fig. 101.2).

Clinical decisions are complex and based on many sources of information (Fig. 101.3).[42] Patient management decisions are always a function of both scientific evidence and individual preferences (physicians, health care providers, patients). A development to improve the basis for clinical decision-making is an international movement to improve the reporting of clinical research results, particularly in randomized, controlled trials and method analyses. New data on current molecular biology and genetics investigations have broadened the scope of evidence-based oncology.

Hunt et al.[83] reported on an analysis of 68 controlled medical trials, 40 of which were published since 1992, to assess the effects of computer-based clinical decision support systems on physician performance and patient outcome. They observed that, in 43 of 65 studies (66%) on physician performance, a benefit was found, including drug dosing systems, use of diagnostic aids, preventive care assistance, and other medical care procedures. Only 6 of 14 studies assessing patient outcome found a benefit, indicating that the impact of clinical decision support systems on patient outcome has been insufficiently studied. Furthermore, very few reports dealt with cancer-related treatment issues; most reports centered on prevention, activities, and cancer screening.[84,85]

Although oncologists, patients, and national organizations recognize that communication is very important in cancer care, evidence-based data on the subject are scarce.

TABLE 101.2 GUIDELINES FOR REPORTING CLINICAL OUTCOME STUDIES IN THE JOURNAL *RADIOTHERAPY AND ONCOLOGY*

Heading	Subheading	Item	Was It Reported? Yes/No/NA[a]	If Yes, on What Page Number?
Title		1. Identify the study as a randomized trial	_____	_____
Introduction		2. State the prospectively defined hypothesis, clinical objectives, and planned subgroup or covariate analyses	_____	_____
Methods	Study design	3. Define the patient population, inclusion and exclusion criteria	_____	_____
		4. Planned treatments and their timing	_____	_____
	Radiotherapy	5. Radiotherapy dose prescription method, dose planning procedure	_____	_____
		6. Target volume definition, critical organs considered, simulation and verification procedures	_____	_____
		7. Dose fractionation details	_____	_____
		8. Planned radiotherapy quality assurance procedures	_____	_____
	End points and analysis	9. Primary and secondary end points, specific follow-up procedures, the minimum clinically relevant difference, the target sample size and how it was decided	_____	_____
		10. Statistical analyses, their purpose and methods used, and whether the intention-to-treat principle was used	_____	_____
		11. Trial monitoring, early-stopping rules	_____	_____
	Randomization	12. Method used for randomization	_____	_____
		13. Method of concealment and time of randomization	_____	_____
		14. Method to separate the generator of random treatment assignments from the treating physician	_____	_____
Results	Masking patient flow and follow-up analysis	15. Describe any blinding procedures (if relevant)	_____	_____
		16. Provide an overview of number of patients randomized, compliance with treatment, radiotherapy quality assurance results	_____	_____
		17. State the effect of treatment on primary and secondary tumor outcome measures, including effect estimates with confidence intervals	_____	_____
		18. Describe the incidence and grade of treatment-induced early and late toxicity by treatment group	_____	_____
		19. State frequencies as absolute numbers when feasible (e.g., 10/20 and not just 50%)	_____	_____
		20. Present summary data with appropriate statistics to permit alternative analyses or interpretations and comparisons with other trials on the same problem	_____	_____
		21. Describe prognostic variables by treatment group, check if they were balanced, and if not describe attempts to adjust for them	_____	_____
		22. Describe protocol deviations from the study as planned, together with reasons	_____	_____
Discussion		23. State the interpretation of the study findings, including sources of bias and imprecision, and discuss how this trial compares with other similar studies	_____	_____
Conclusion		24. State the general interpretation of the trial in view of all available evidence in the literature	_____	_____

These guidelines meet the minimum criteria defined in the CONSORT statement for reporting of randomized clinical trials.
[a]NA, not applicable; certain items apply to randomized studies only.
Reprinted from Bentzen SM. Towards evidence based radiation oncology: improving the design, analysis, and reporting of clinical outcome studies in radiotherapy. *Radiother Oncol* 1998;46(1):5–18. Copyright © 1998 Elsevier Science Ireland Ltd. With permission.

Section V

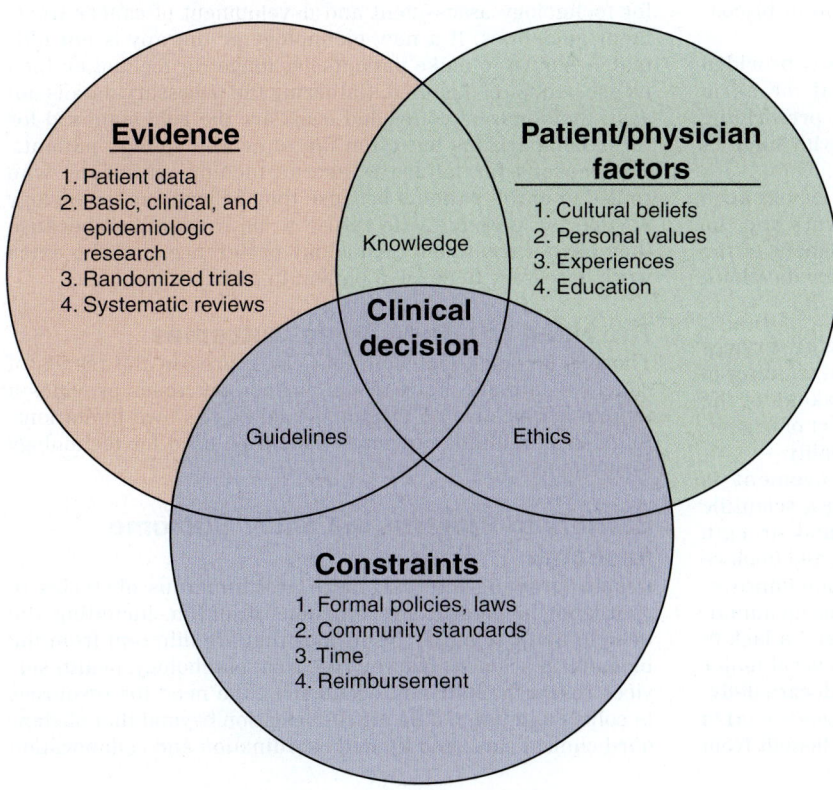

Evidence
1. Patient data
2. Basic, clinical, and epidemiologic research
3. Randomized trials
4. Systematic reviews

Patient/physician factors
1. Cultural beliefs
2. Personal values
3. Experiences
4. Education

Knowledge

Clinical decision

Guidelines

Ethics

Constraints
1. Formal policies, laws
2. Community standards
3. Time
4. Reimbursement

FIGURE 101.3. Factors that enter into clinical decisions. (From Mulrow CD, Cook DJ, Davidoff F. Systematic reviews: critical links in the great chain of evidence. In: Mulrow CD, Cook DJ, eds. *Systematic reviews: synthesis of best evidence for health care decisions*. Philadelphia, PA: American College of Physicians, 1998:1–4. Copyright © 1998 American College of Physicians. Reprinted by permission.)

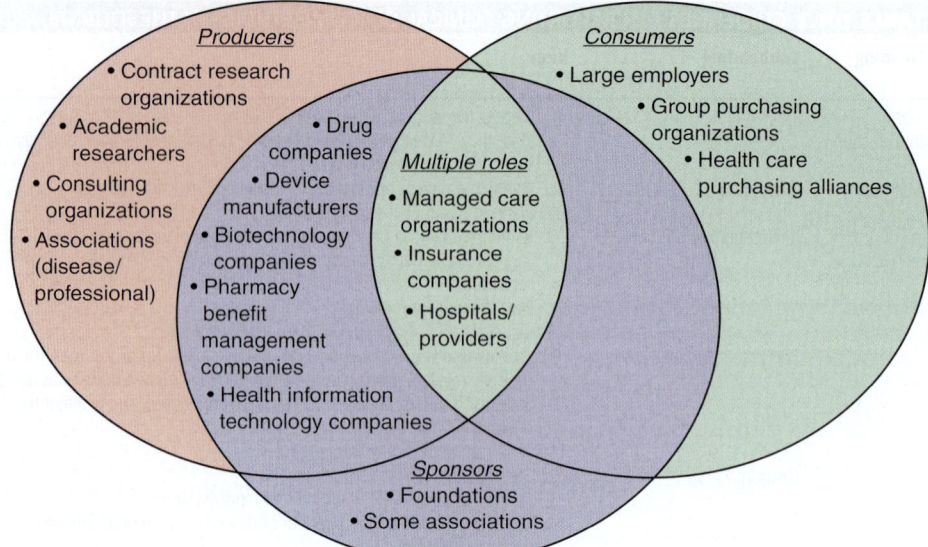

FIGURE 101.4. Stakeholders in outcomes and effectiveness research. (Adapted from Lewin Group. *Outcomes and effectiveness research in the private sector: final report.* Fairfax, VA: Lewin Group, 1997; and Mulrow CD, Cook DJ, Davidoff F. Systematic reviews; critical links in the great chain of evidence. In: *Systematic reviews: synthesis of best evidence for health care decisions.* Philadelphia, PA: American College of Physicians, 1998:1–4.)

Oncologists should use a patient-centered interview approach, ask patients what level of involvement they want in medical decision-making, develop a caring attitude, and consider that patient–physician encounters should provide both cognitive data of patient understanding and feelings.[86]

QUALITY OF MEDICAL CARE AND EVIDENCE-BASED MEDICINE

Continuous quality improvement emerged from the industrial sector as an effective means of reducing production errors. The quality of health care can be precisely defined and measured with a degree of scientific accuracy comparable to that of most measures in clinical medicine.[87] Health care quality problems can be classified into three categories:

1. *Underuse* is the failure to provide a health care service when it would have produced a favorable outcome for a patient, such as not administering irradiation in breast-conserving therapy.
2. *Overuse* occurs when a health care service is provided under circumstances in which its potential for harm exceeds the possible benefit—for example, prescribing postoperative pelvic irradiation to a patient with stage IA G1 endometrial carcinoma.
3. *Misuse* takes place when an appropriate service has been selected but a preventable complication occurs and the patient does not receive the full potential benefit of the service; avoidable complications of surgery, medications, or irradiation are important misuse problems.[88]

Other issues influencing the inadequate use of services include geographic variation in the rate of use, training of general practice or specialist physicians, the makeup of the nonphysician health care workforce, and the effect of organization of medical services as a determinant of quality.

In health care, continuous quality improvement is most effective when used as an integral part of a scientific approach to improving clinical practice. A potential strength is the ability to motivate good performers to excel and to place emphasis on generating new methods for achieving improvement. Among its limitations are a too-narrow focus on administrative (as opposed to clinical) aspects of care and a lack of attention to problems of overuse or underuse. Several major strategies have been advocated to move the health care delivery system toward improving quality. The challenges are (a) to always provide effective care of those who could benefit from

it, (b) to always refrain from providing inappropriate services, and (c) to eliminate all preventable complications.[89] Skeptics point out that no health care market currently competes on the basis of improving quality, and there is little theoretical basis in economics to predict that this success will occur.[88] Mendelson et al.[43] noted that there are many parties involved in outcome and effectiveness research (Fig. 101.4) and that payers and providers of health care may in the future use outcome research as a basis for coverage of services, including procedures, devices, or drugs.

HOW ONE MIGHT USE OUTCOMES FOR TECHNOLOGY ASSESSMENT AND GUIDELINE DEVELOPMENT

Priority of Outcomes

Patient outcomes are more important than cancer outcomes for technology assessment and development of cancer treatment guidelines. If a new technology or therapy is not ultimately shown to make patients live longer or feel better, then its use cannot be justified. Gathering the necessary data is not easy. Randomized, controlled trials are the gold standard for these comparisons but often fail to accrue enough patients. The reasons for failure to accrue include physicians who refuse to enroll patients because they believe one technology is superior, patients who refuse to be randomized because they have a treatment/technology preference, and the extra work necessary to enroll a patient in a trial.[21]

The Need to Use Multiple Outcomes

There is no single outcome that can represent the results of cancer treatment. Each of the various outcomes provides a unique perspective on treatment and has its own limitations. In general, multiple outcomes should be used for technology assessment.

Barriers to Progress in Cancer Outcome Research

Despite growing interest, there are numerous obstacles to overcome in health care outcome research, including the need to apply scientific disciplines that are different from the biomedical sciences (survey research, psychology, health services research, statistics, economics), the need for resources to collect additional data and information beyond that of standard clinical care, and limited coordination and collaboration among researchers working in the field. Other barriers are intrinsic to a specific cancer, including heterogeneity of patients, type of tumor, phases of the disease, and ethnic and socioeconomic characteristics. Furthermore, many institutions do not give a high priority to or adequately fund outcome research because this activity is considered a cost, not a revenue center, and there is a lack of conviction that this effort will reduce health care spending.[88,90]

Data sharing and increased collaboration in data collection and analysis should be promoted among health care providers and the various groups conducting outcome research. Creative approaches to educating providers and patients about outcome studies are needed, as well as mechanisms to ensure that patients and health professionals have ready access to the results of outcome research.

Making a treatment selection involves defining the patient's condition, identifying management options and outcome, collecting and summarizing evidence, and applying value judgments or preferences to arrive at an optimal course of action.[4] The randomized, controlled clinical trial, the first of which was published in 1952, has become the "gold standard" for evaluating the efficacy of health care intervention.

Clinical decisions are complex and based on many sources of information (Fig. 101.3).[29] Patient management decisions are always a function of both scientific evidence and individual preferences (physicians, health care providers, patients).

Although oncologists, patients, and national organizations recognize that communication is very important in cancer care, evidence-based data on the subject are scarce. Oncologists should use a patient-centered interview approach, ask patients what level of involvement they want in medical decision-making, develop a caring attitude, and consider that patient–physician encounters should provide both cognitive data of patient understanding and feelings.[41]

The Complexity of Randomized, Prospective Clinical Trials

Randomized, prospective, controlled trials are held forth as the gold standard for determining the appropriateness of introducing technology into clinical practice. One must be cognizant, however, of adverse influences upon the generalizability of randomized, controlled trials. If the age, gender, severity of the disease, risk factors, comorbidity, ethnicity, or socioeconomic status of the patients in the randomized, prospective trial is not representative of the general population, it may be inappropriate to generalize the results of the clinical trial to that population. Similarly, if the dose, timing of administration, duration of therapy, quality of care, or comedications of the patients in the trial are not similar to those of the general population, the results may not be applicable.[20]

There is a long-standing joke that one does not need a randomized, prospective trial to ascertain the efficacy of a parachute. In medicine, there are long lists of new technologies that were introduced into general practice based on historical controls without randomized, prospective trials. These include, for example, the use of thyroxin for myxedema, insulin for diabetes, vitamin B12 for pernicious anemia, sulfonamides for puerperal sepsis, penicillin for lobar pneumonia, streptomycin for tuberculosis, defibrillation for ventricular fibrillation, and cisplatin, vinblastine, and bleomycin for disseminated testicular cancer. The analysis of a randomized clinical trial has traditionally been based on a hypothesis that presumes that there is no difference between treatments. The hypothesis is tested by estimating the probability of obtaining a result as extreme as or more extreme than the one observed if the hypothesis is true. The hypothesis may be irrelevant if there had been previous studies demonstrating that the treatment had some benefits. Those who criticize randomized, prospective trials will quickly argue that "no one ever did a randomized trial to prove that a linear accelerator was better than a cobalt machine, that port films were necessary, or that simulation was preferable to a clinical setup." These arguments are, to some extent, true. One must remember, however, that there is a considerable financial difference between using and not using a port film compared to using a linear accelerator versus a $200 million proton apparatus.[85]

Nonetheless, prospective, randomized clinical trials have come to occupy a prominent role in clinical research in radiation oncology. The most commonly used clinical end points are summarized in Table 101.3. Unfortunately, many published reports have unclear definitions or lack some of the fundamental end points.

Clinical trials are time consuming and costly. Randomization is the only method that may guarantee that comparisons of treatment outcome are, on average, unbiased. Not all

TABLE 101.3 MOST COMMONLY USED CLINICAL END POINTS IN RADIATION THERAPY TRIALS

End Point	Definition of Event	Comments
Local control	No evidence of disease at the primary site (T position)	Statistically, this is the absence of an event (i.e., local recurrence); estimated at a given time as the local recurrence–free rate
Local failure rate	Recurrence in T position	Estimated as 1 minus the local recurrence–free rate
Locoregional control	No evidence of disease in T and N positions	See above, but for T or N recurrence, whichever comes first; sometimes defined as in-field control (i.e., control within the treated volume)
Survival or overall survival	Death irrespective of cause	–
Cancer-specific survival or cause-specific survival	Death of cancer	Often defined as death of cancer or with active disease
Disease-free survival	Any recurrence or death from any cause, whichever comes first	A composite end point combining survival and disease control
Local recurrence–free survival	Local recurrence or death from any cause, whichever comes first	As above, but with local recurrence as the relevant event
Disease-free rate	Any recurrence	Death without recurrence is a cause of censoring
Local relapse-free rate	Local recurrence	As above
Early reactions	Signs or symptoms of a specific early reaction; defined by measuring scale	Typically defined inside a time window; actuarial methods normally not used
Late reactions	Signs or symptoms of a specific late reaction; defined by measuring scale	Actuarial methods should be used
Palliation	Typically defined by measuring scale	May require special statistical considerations
Quality of life	Typically defined by measuring scale	May require special statistical considerations

All definitions involving local recurrence are defined for nodal recurrence (N position) or distant recurrence (M) by analogy.
Reprinted from Bentzen SM. Towards evidence based radiation oncology: improving the design, analysis, and reporting of clinical outcome studies in radiotherapy. *Radiother Oncol* 1998;46(1):5–18.
Copyright © 1998 Elsevier Science Ireland Ltd. With permission.

clinical trials yield positive results, and not all new therapies are improvements compared with the standard therapy.[69,74] As an example, a recent analysis of outcome data from 57 randomized, controlled trials, including a total of 12,734 patients, conducted between 1968 and 2002 by the RTOG[73] showed that overall, experimental and standard radiotherapies were equally successful (odds ratio for survival, 1.01; $P = .5$); however, treatment-related mortality was significantly greater in the experimental arm of the trials (odds ratio, 1.76; $P = .008$). A drawback of randomized trials for the evaluation of a new technology in radiation oncology is that to detect small improvements in morbidity from, for example, an alleged improved dose distribution, an enormous number of patients will need to be accrued and followed for a considerable length of time. Radiation oncologists must, therefore, give serious consideration to the development of novel paradigms for HTAs without meeting, in some cases, the ideal requirement of randomization.[73]

Practice Guidelines

Guidelines for health services resulting from valid and appropriate outcome studies have the potential to promote consistency and quality of care. In the United States, clinical practice guidelines have been promulgated by the American Cancer Society, the American College of Radiology, the American Society of Clinical Oncology, the National Cancer Centers Network, and other professional organizations (Table 101.4).[21,44] Sisk[90] observed that for such guidelines to be successful, it is very important to involve local physicians in the process, to get their views and ultimately their support. The values of practice guidelines in medicine include minimizing inappropriate practice variations, providing reference points for education/practice, improving patient care and outcomes, providing criteria for self-evaluation, setting indicators for external quality review, assisting with service coverage and reimbursement, and decreasing overall cost of medical care. Perceived drawbacks to such guidelines include overregulation and loss of autonomy for both physicians and patients. The conflicting needs and motivations of physicians, patients, third-party carriers, and society bring into play a variety of ethical perspectives. Although contrasting ethical foundations likely will lead to significantly different solutions to the health care resource problem, it is only through educated and reasoned discussion that this problem can be tackled.[91]

Courts in the United States have ruled that guideline developers can be held liable for faulty guidelines and that doctors cannot pass off their liability by claiming that adherence to guidelines corrupted clinical judgment. Protocols and guidelines provide the courts with examples of clinical standards across a wide range of medical practice. However, adherence to guidelines has not automatically been equated with reasonable practice, and the courts seem unlikely to follow the standards enunciated in clinical guidelines without critically evaluating their authority, flexibility, and scope of application.[92]

TABLE 101.4 AMERICAN COLLEGE OF RADIOLOGY APPROPRIATENESS GUIDELINES LITERATURE EVIDENCE TABLE KEY

Strength of recommendation (quality of the study design)
- *Good* evidence to support recommendation that procedure be performed
- *Fair* evidence to support recommendation be performed
- *Poor* evidence to support recommendation but may be made on other grounds
- *Fair* evidence to support recommendation not be performed
- *Good* evidence to support recommendation not be performed

Reprinted from Leibel SA. ACR appropriateness criteria. Expert Panel on Radiation Oncology. American College of Radiology. *Int J Radiat Oncol Biol Phys* 1999;43(1):125–168. Copyright © 1999 American College of Radiology. With permission.

CONCLUSIONS

Technology assessment, outcome analysis, cost–benefit, comparative effectiveness, and clinical trials supported by EBM should be strengthened and fostered to enhance the rationale and quality of medical care provided to patients at a competitive cost. Basic and translational laboratory research and properly designed, relevant, and timely prospective clinical trials should be strongly promoted, and patient participation must be increased to acquire more accurate information to develop innovative therapeutic strategies in oncology. Methods for accurate cost accounting of medical care and comparative effectiveness studies need further development. Technology assessment will substantially contribute to better utilization of scarce health care resources and will be invaluable in determining the potential value of innovative therapeutic approaches.

REFERENCES

1. Centers for Medicare and Medicaid Services. Coverage with evidence development. Available at: http://www.cms.gov/Medicare/Coverage/Coverage-with-Evidence-Development/index.html
2. Wallner PE, Konski A. A changing paradigm in the study and adoption of emerging health care technologies: coverage with evidence development. *J Am Coll Radiol* 2008;5:1125–1129.
3. Hayman J, Weeks J, Mauch P. Economic analyses in health care: an introduction to the methodology with an emphasis on radiation therapy. *Int J Radiat Oncol Biol Phys* 1996;35:827–841.
4. Brook RH, Kamberg CJ, McGlynn EA. Health system reform and quality. *JAMA* 1996;276:476–480.
5. Fuchs VR, Garber AM. The new technology assessment. *N Engl J Med* 1990;323:673–677.
6. Drummond M, Sculpher MJ, Torrance GW, et al. *Methods for the economic evaluation of health care programmes.* Oxford, UK: Oxford University Press, 2005.
7. Feeny D, Furlong W, Boyle M, et al. Multi-attribute health status classification systems. Health Utility Index. *Pharmacoeconomics* 1995;7:490–502.
8. Harngren CT, Foster G, Datar SM. *Cost accounting. a managerial emphasis,* 9th ed. Upper Saddle River, NJ: Prentice-Hall, 1996.
9. EQ-5D. Available at: www.euroqol.org.
10. Perez CA. Methodology of research and practice for the third millennium: evidence-based medicine. *Rays* 2000;25:285–308.
11. Doubilet P, Weinstein MC, McNeil BJ. Use and misuse of the term "cost effective" in medicine. *N Engl J Med* 1986;314:253–256.
12. Stinnett AA, Mullahy J. Net health benefits: a new framework for the analysis of uncertainty in cost-effectiveness analysis. *Med Decis Making* 1998;18:S68–S80.
13. Meltzer MI. Introduction to health economics for physicians. *Lancet* 2001;358:993–998.
14. Clancy CM, Kamerow DB. Evidence-based medicine meets cost-effectiveness analysis. *JAMA* 1996;276:329–330.
15. Neilson AR, Davies HT. Interpreting reported health-care costs. *Hosp Med* 1998;59:803–806.
16. Siegel JE, Weinstein MC, Russell LB, et al. Recommendations for reporting cost-effectiveness analyses. Panel on Cost-Effectiveness in Health and Medicine. *JAMA* 1996;276:1339–1341.
17. Russell LB, Gold MR, Siegel JE, et al. The role of cost-effectiveness analysis in health and medicine. Panel on Cost-Effectiveness in Health and Medicine. *JAMA* 1996;276:1172–1177.
18. Rigby K, Silagy C, Crockett A. Health economic reviews. Are they compiled systematically? *Int J Technol Assess Health Care* 1996;12:450–459.
19. Smith JM. Effectively costing out options. *JAMA* 1996;276:1180.
20. Weinstein MC, Siegel JE, Gold MR, et al. Recommendations of the panel on cost-effectiveness in Health and Medicine. *JAMA* 1996;276:1253–1258.
21. Berkwits M. From practice to research: the case for criticism in an age of evidence. *Soc Sci Med* 1998;47:1539–1545.
22. Lee WR. Technology assessment: vigilance required. *Int J Radiat Oncol Biol Phys* 2008;70:652–653.
23. Cotter GW. Surgery or radiation therapy: a comparative cost analysis for early carcinoma of the prostate and breast. *Appl Radiol* 1990;19:25–28.
24. Penn CR. Megavoltage irradiation in a district general hospital remote from a main oncology centre: the Torbay experience reviewed. *Clin Oncol (R Coll Radiol)* 1992;4:108–113.
25. Perez CA, Kobeissi B, Smith BD, et al. Cost accounting in radiation oncology: a computer-based model for reimbursement. *Int J Radiat Oncol Biol Phys* 1993;25(5):895–906.
26. Ringborg U, Bergqvist D, Brorsson B, et al. The Swedish Council on Technology Assessment in Health Care (SBU) systematic overview of radiotherapy for cancer including a prospective survey of radiotherapy practice in Sweden 2001—summary and conclusions. *Acta Oncol* 2003;42:357–365.
27. Smith TJ, Hillner BE, Desch CE. Efficacy and cost-effectiveness of cancer treatment: rational allocation of resources based on decision analysis. *J Natl Cancer Inst* 1993;85:1460–1474.

28. Organisation for Economic Co-operation and Development. OECD health data 2011. Available at: http://www.oecd.org/document/16/o,3343,en_2649_34631_2085200_1_1_1_1,00.html

29. Norlund A. Cost of radiotherapy. *Acta Oncol* 2003;42:411–415.

30. Lievens Y, Van Den Bogaert W, Kesteloot K. Activity-based costing: a practical model for cost calculation in radiotherapy. *Int J Radiat Oncol Biol Phys* 2003;57:522–535.

31. Konski A, Bhargavan M, Owen J, et al. Feasibility of economic analysis of Radiation Therapy Oncology Group (RTOG) 91-11 using Medicare data. *Int J Radiat Oncol Biol Phys* 2010;79:436–442.

32. Lievens Y, Dunscombe P, Konski A. Promises and pitfalls of health technology assessment. In: Levit SH, Purdy JA, Perez CA, et al., eds. *Technical basis of radiation therapy*. 5th ed. New York: Springer, 2012:549–564.

33. Antos J, Brimson JA. *Activity-based management for service industries, government entities and nonprofit organizations*. New York: Wiley, 1994.

34. Cooper R. *Elements of activity-based costing, emerging practices in cost management*. New York: Warren, Gorham & Lamont, 1990.

35. Cooper R, Kaplan RS. *The design of cost management systems*. Upper Saddle River, NJ: Prentice-Hall, 1991.

36. Foster G, Gupta M. Activity accounting: an electronics industry implementation. In: Kaplan RS, ed. *Measures for manufacturing excellence*. Boston, MA: Harvard Business School Press, 1990:225–268.

37. Konski A, Yu JB, Freedman G, et al. ReCAP: radiation oncology practice: adjusting to a new reimbursement model. *J Oncol Pract* 2016;12(5):e576–e583.

38. Sackett DL, Straus S, Richardson S, et al. *Evidence-based medicine: how to practice and teach EBM*. 2nd ed. London: Churchill Livingston, 2000.

39. Mendelson DN, Goodman CS, Ahn R, et al. Outcomes and effectiveness research in the private sector. *Health Aff (Millwood)* 1998;17:75–90.

40. Newman L, ed. *Medical outcomes and guidelines sourcebook*. New York: Faulkner & Gray, 1999.

41. Feinstein AR, Horwitz RI. Problems in the "evidence" of "evidence-based medicine". *Am J Med* 1997;103:529–535.

42. Bentzen SM. Towards evidence based radiation oncology: improving the design, analysis, and reporting of clinical outcome studies in radiotherapy. *Radiother Oncol* 1998;46:5–18.

43. Chassin MR, Galvin RW. The urgent need to improve health care quality. Institute of Medicine National Roundtable on Health Care Quality. *JAMA* 1998;280:1000–1005.

44. Panek WC. Ethical considerations related to outcome studies-based clinical practice guidelines. *J Glaucoma* 1999;8:267–272.

45. Van der Werf E, Verstraete J, Lievens Y. The cost of radiotherapy in a decade of technology evolution. *Radiother Oncol* 2012;102(1):148–153.

46. Detsky AS, Naglie IG. A clinician's guide to cost-effective analysis. *Ann Intern Med* 1990;113:147–154.

47. Bodenheimer T. High and rising health care costs. Part 2: Technologic innovation. *Ann Intern Med* 2005;142:932–937.

48. Russell LB. Modelling for cost-effectiveness analysis. *Stat Med* 1999;18:3235–3244.

49. Cowan J, Berkowitz D. Technology assessment at work: part I—principles and a case study. *Physician Exec* 1996;22:5–6, 8–9.

50. Chlebowski RT, Collyar DE, Somerfield MR, et al. American Society of Clinical Oncology technology assessment on breast cancer risk reduction strategies: tamoxifen and raloxifene. *J Clin Oncol* 1999;17:1939–1955.

51. Halperin EC. Overpriced technology in radiation oncology. *Int J Radiat Oncol Biol Phys* 2000;48:917–918.

52. Smith GL, Ganz PA, Bekelman JE, et al. "Promoting appropriate use of advanced radiation technologies in oncology: summary of a National Cancer Policy Forum Workshop." *Int J Radiat Oncol Biol Phys* 2017;97:450–461.

53. Pignol JP, Olivotto I, Rakovitch E et al. A multicenter randomized trial of breast intensity-modulated radiation therapy to reduce acute radiation dermatitis. *J Clin Oncol* 2008;26:2085–2092.

54. Nutting CM, Morden JP, Harrington KJ, et al. Parotid-sparing versus intensity modulated versus conventional radiotherapy in head and neck cancer (PARSPORT): A phase 3 randomized controlled trial. *Lancet Oncol* 2011;12:127–136.

55. Shen X, Showalter TN, Mishra MV et al. Radiation oncology services in the modern era: Evolving patterns of usage and payments in the office setting for Medicare patients from 2000 to 2010. *J Oncol Pract* 2014;10:e201–e207.

56. Emanuel EJ. The problem with single payer plans. *Hastings Cent Rep* 2008;38:38–41.

57. Johnstone PAS, Kerstiens J, Helsper R. Proton facility economics: The importance of "simple" treatments. *J Am Coll Radiol* 2012;9:560–563.

58. Kerstiens J, Johnstone PAS. Proton therapy expansion under current United States reimbursement models. *Int J Radiat Oncol Biol Phys* 2014;89:235–240.

59. Johnstone PAS, Kerstiens J. Reconciling reimbursement for proton therapy. *Int J Radiat Oncol Biol Phys* 2016;95:9–10.

60. Willan AR. Analysis, sample size, and power for estimating incremental net health benefit from clinical trial data. *Control Clin Trials* 2001;22:228–237.

61. Pijls-Johannesma M, Pommier P, Lievens Y. Cost-effectiveness of particle therapy: current evidence and future needs. *Radiother Oncol* 2008;89:127–134.

62. Goitien M, Cox JD. Should randomized clinical trials be required for proton radiotherapy? *J Clin Oncol* 2008;26:175–176.

63. Lodge M, Pijls-Johannesma M, Stirk L, et al. A systematic literature review of the clinical and cost-effectiveness of hadron therapy in cancer. *Radiother Oncol* 2007;83:110–122.

64. Glatstein E, Glick J, Kaiser L, et al. Should randomized clinical trials be required for proton radiotherapy? An alternative view. *J Clin Oncol* 2008;26:2438–2439.

65. Suit H, DeLaney T, Goldberg S, et al. Proton vs carbon ion beams in the definitive radiation treatment of patients with cancer. *Radiother Oncol* 2010;95:3–22.

66. Perrier L, Combs SE, Aurberger T, et al. A decision-making tool for a costly innovative technology. The case for carbon ion radiotherapy. *J Econ Med* 2007;25:367–380.

67. Peeters A, Grutters JP, Pijls-Johannesma M, et al. How costly is particle therapy? Cost analysis of external beam radiotherapy with carbon-ions, protons and photons. *Radiother Oncol* 2010; 95:45–53.

68. Perez CA, Kobeissi BJ, Chao KSC, et al. *3-D conformal and intensity modulated radiation therapy: physics and clinical applications*. Madison, WI: Advanced Medical Publishing, 2001.

69. Buyyounouski MK, Price RA, Harris EER, et al. Stereotactic body radiotherapy for primary management of early stage low to intermediate risk prostate cancer: report of ASTRO Emerging Technology Committee. *Int J Radiat Oncol Biol Phys* 2010;76:1297–1304.

70. Bentzen SM, Wasserman TH. Balancing on a knife's edge: evidence-based medicine and the marketing of new technology. *Int J Radiat Oncol Biol Phys* 2008;72:12–13.

71. Bigby M. Evidence-based medicine in a nutshell. A guide to finding and using the best evidence in caring for patients. *Arch Dermatol* 1998;134:1609–1618.

72. Newcomer LN. Finding the answers we need: comparative effectiveness. *Practical Radiat Oncol* 2011;1:83–84.

73. Leibel SA. ACR appropriateness criteria. Expert Panel on Radiation Oncology. American College of Radiology. *Int J Radiat Oncol Biol Phys* 1999;43:125–168.

74. Guyatt GH, Sinclair J, Cook DJ, et al. Users' guides to the medical literature: XVI. How to use a treatment recommendation. Evidence-Based Medicine Working Group and the Cochrane Applicability Methods Working Group. *JAMA* 1999;281:1836–1843.

75. Bentzen SM Randomized controlled trials in health technology assessment: overkill or overdue? *Radiother Oncol* 2008;86:142–147.

76. Eifel PJ, Moughan J, Erickson B, et al. Patterns of radiotherapy practice for patients with carcinoma of the uterine cervix: a pattern of care study. *Int J Radiat Oncol Biol Phys* 2004;60:1144–1153.

77. Cochrane collaboration. *Preparing, maintaining, and promoting the accessibility of systemic reviews of the effects of healthcare interventions*. Oxford: Cochrane Collaboration, 1999.

78. Cochrane A. *Effectiveness and efficiency: random reflection on health services*. London: Royal Society of Medicine Press Limited; 2004.

79. Cochrane AL. 1931–1971: A critical review, with particular reference to the medical profession. In: *Medicine for the year 2000*. London: Office of Health Economics; 1979:1–11.

80. Tanenbaum SJ. Evidence and expertise: the challenge of the outcomes movement to medical professionalism. *Acad Med* 1999;74:757–763.

81. Owen JB, Grigsby PW, Caldwell TM, et al. Can costs be measured and predicted by modeling within a cooperative clinical trials group? Economic methodologic pilot studies of the radiation therapy oncology group (RTOG) studies 90-03 and 91-04. *Int J Radiat Oncol Biol Phys* 2001;49:633–639.

82. American Society of Clinical Oncology. Outcomes of cancer treatment for technology assessment and cancer treatment guidelines. *J Clin Oncol* 1996;14:671–670.

83. Mulrow CD, Cook DJ, Davidoff F. Systematic reviews; critical links in the great chain of evidence. In: *Systematic reviews: synthesis of best evidence for health care decisions*. Philadelphia, PA: American College of Physicians, 1998:1–4.

84. Hunt DL, Haynes RB, Hanna SE, et al. Effects of computer-based clinical decision support systems on physician performance and patient outcomes: a systematic review. *JAMA* 1998;280:1339–1346.

85. McAlister FA, Straus SE, Guyatt GH, et al. Users' guides to the medical literature: XX. Integrating research evidence with the care of the individual patient. Evidence-Based Medicine Working Group. *JAMA* 2000;283:2829–2836.

86. Rawlins M. De testimonio: on the evidence for decisions about the use of therapeutic interventions. *Clin Med* 2008;8:579–588.

87. Back A. Patient-physician communication in oncology: what does the evidence show? *Oncology* 2006;20:67–74.

88. Pommier P, Lievens Y, Feschet F et al. Simulating demand for innovative radiotherapies: an illustrative model based on carbon ion and proton radiotherapy. *Radiother Oncol* 2010;96:243–249.

89. Sisk JE. Increased competition and the quality of health care. *Milbank Q* 1998;76:687–707, 512.

90. American Society of Clinical Oncology. Recommended breast cancer surveillance guidelines. *J Clin Oncol* 1997;15:2149–2156.

91. Sisk JE. How are health care organizations using clinical guidelines? *Health Aff (Millwood)* 1998;17:91–109.

92. Bentzen S. Radiation oncology health technology assessment—the best is the enemy of the good. *Nat Clin Pract Oncol* 2008;5:563.

Section V

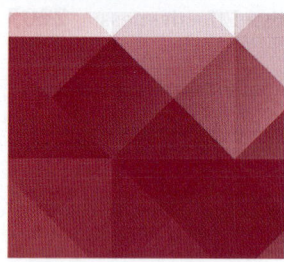

CHAPTER 102

Error Avoidance*

Bhishamjit S. Chera, Lukasz Mazur, Prithima Mosaly, and Lawrence B. Marks

INTRODUCTION

Improving the quality of health care is garnering enthusiastic support in the current social and political environment. The Institute of Medicine (IOM) published two seminal reports highlighting that (a) there is a large gap between what we know to be good quality care and what actually exists in practice and (b) patient safety is an urgent quality problem.[1,2] The IOM defines quality as the degree to which health services for individuals and populations increase the likelihood of desired health outcomes and are consistent with current professional knowledge and that health care should be (a) safe, (b) effective, (c) patient centered, (d) timely, (e) efficient, and (f) equitable.

The concept of safety in health care is not new. The ethical standard of *first, do no harm*, given to us by Hippocrates in the 5th century BC[3] and mandated as a key principle in the practice of medicine by Florence Nightingale[4] in the late 19th century has been taught in medical education for years.[5] However, patients suffer iatrogenic harm from medical treatment every day. In 1999, the IOM reported that 44,000 to 98,000 people die each year in the United States as a result of preventable medical errors, which roughly equates to 3 jumbo-jet crashes every 2 days.[1,5]

Public awareness of radiation delivery errors has increased in a number of developed countries such as the United States, because of articles in *The New York Times*, a World Health Organization report,[6–10] and an accident in Épinal, France.[11] Society (e.g., patients, politicians, attorneys) is demanding *safe* health care. Highly publicized medical errors are driving our profession to prioritize quality

---

*Portions of this chapter were adopted from Marks L, et al. *Engineering patient safety in radiation oncology: University of North Carolina's pursuit for high reliability and value creation*. Boca Raton, FL: Taylor & Francis, 2015.

and safety. Our professional societies responded by publishing numerous quality and safety publications, such as the ASTRO-sponsored *Safety is no Accident*, and holding several safety-focused meetings.[12] Serious accidents have also been reported in the 1990s in the United Kingdom, triggering a strong response by their National Health Service. One result was the publication of the report "An Organisation with a Memory."[13] Similarly, the European Radiation Oncology Safety Information System (ROSIS) project started in the early 2000s to promote safety through systematic incident reporting and analysis.[14]

Furthermore, it is also known that the quality of radiation delivery affects patient outcomes. Post hoc analyses of noncompliance with clinical protocol radiotherapy guidelines show associations between deviations, disease control, and overall survival in patients treated on clinical trials.[15–17] Ohri et al.[15] analyzed 8 clinical trials and observed that deviations in the radiation plans were associated with decreases in overall survival (HR = 1.74, 95% CI = 1.28 to 2.35, P < .001). In addition, spreading treatment protocols from the research environment to the broader, routine clinical setting is affected by a systematic loss of efficacy, chiefly because of a relaxation of the tight constraints in schedule, treated volumes, doses, etc. that prevail in the research setup (i.e., efficacy in clinical trial vs. effectiveness in clinical practice).[18] Thus, quality assurance (QA) of radiotherapy plans is important to ensure the delivery of effective care.

Radiation oncology is a modest-sized field with approximately 4,000 practicing radiation oncologists in the United States. Nevertheless, the clinical impact of radiation therapy (RT) is large. Approximately 50% of patients with cancer receive RT, with ≈ 600,000 patients treated annually in the United States alone. A reasonable estimate is that there is an incident during the course of treatment in ≈1% to 3% of patients, but the vast majority of these are not clinically relevant (Table 102.1). However, ≈1 in 1,000 to 10,000 treated

---

TABLE 102.1 EVENT RATES IN RADIOTHERAPY

	Event Rates (%)			
	Per Treatment	**Per Course**	**Per Fraction**	**Per Field**
Multiple Center Series				
United Kingdom, 2006		0.04 (0.003)		
Pennsylvania State, 2009	0.0025 (0.0006)[a]			
NY State[b], 2009	0.06 (0.01)[a]			
Single-Institution Series				
Fraass, 1998	0.44	1.20		
Macklis, 1998		3.06		0.18 (0)
Barthelemt-Brichant, 1999				3.22
Patton, 2003	0.17	3.3		
Huang, 2005		1.97	0.29	
Yeung, 2005		4.66	0.25	
French, 2006			0.32 (0.05)[a]	0.037 (0.005)[a]
Marks, 2007	0.10			

[a]Estimated "serious" incident rate.
[b]NY state regions outside of the Metropolitan NY City area.

patients is affected by a reportable event with potentially serious consequences. This rate may compare unfavorably with highly reliable industries such as commercial aviation (≈ 1 death in 4.7 million passenger flights) or other areas of medicine such as anesthesiology (≈ 1 death in 200,000 procedures).

RT is a highly technical field and the inappropriate application of radiation can have severe consequences. There is a broad understanding of the need for strict technical standards (e.g., defining the accuracy of the planning and delivery systems). The American Association of Physicists in Medicine (AAPM) and other professional groups provide many guidelines (e.g., Task Group reports) to help guide the technical aspects of our work. However, technical accuracy alone is not enough to ensure quality and safety. The practice of radiation oncology is a human endeavor that requires the coordinated efforts of many people with diverse, yet synergistic, skills. For example, numerous handoffs are routine in our work; thus, there is great need for clarity in our communications. Other industries facing similar challenges have learned that quality and safety require addressing both the technical and human aspects of their processes. As the technical aspects are largely understood and accepted, our focus here will be on the human-based aspects (see Fig. 102.1). This emphasis is not intended to minimize the importance of these technical aspects nor the leadership role of physicists and other "technically focused" team members. We acknowledge the critical importance of these technical components but believe the human-based aspects deserve special highlighting at this time.

In this chapter, we discuss the practical application of error-avoidance strategies from nonmedical high-reliability organizations (HROs). As a primer, Table 102.2 defines several keywords and terms formally utilized among safety experts. In the vernacular, this specificity is often lost, and the overall meaning and understanding of these keywords may broadly overlap.

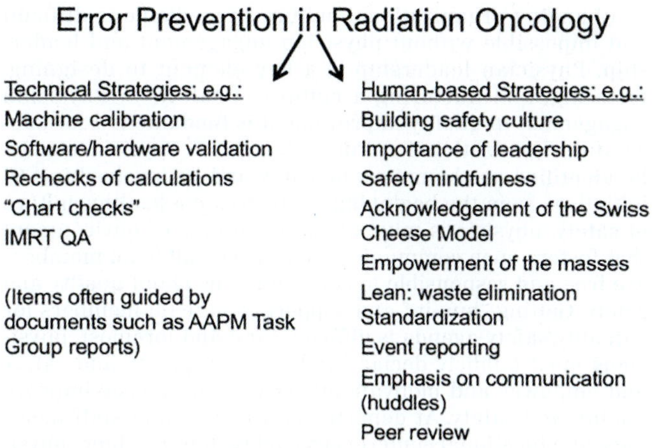

Error Prevention in Radiation Oncology

Technical Strategies; e.g.:
Machine calibration
Software/hardware validation
Rechecks of calculations
"Chart checks"
IMRT QA

(Items often guided by documents such as AAPM Task Group reports)

Human-based Strategies; e.g.:
Building safety culture
Importance of leadership
Safety mindfulness
Acknowledgement of the Swiss Cheese Model
Empowerment of the masses
Lean: waste elimination Standardization
Event reporting
Emphasis on communication (huddles)
Peer review

FIGURE 102.1. There are many technical-based strategies to prevent errors in radiation oncology (e.g., AAPM Task Group reports). In this chapter, we focus on human-based strategies.

PHYSICIAN LEADERSHIP

Transformational physician leadership is absolutely necessary for error avoidance strategies to be successful.

Traditionally, the quality of radiation delivery has been the responsibility of the "technical personnel," for example, physicists, dosimetrists, and radiation therapists. QA has historically been largely focused on the mechanical performance of the radiation therapy devices, the accuracy of the treatment planning system, and the physical and mental tasks of the radiation therapists. This is clearly insufficient as the experience from HROs demonstrates that quality can only be achieved by a multipronged effort to define robust and consistent procedures, the monitoring of quality indicators to assess reliability of these procedures, and a culture to support these ongoing activities.

Radiation oncologists' participation in continuous quality improvement (CQI) has generally been limited. Though the majority of radiation oncology clinic and department leaders are radiation oncologists, CQI has not been a priority in their work. This current arrangement will not support the culture needed to build robust and sustainable improvements. Radiation oncologists have unique clinical perspectives that are needed during CQI initiatives, and as leaders, they must be actively involved to motivate others and build an optimal culture to support this work.[19] Furthermore, the expanding complexity of the broader health system and the rapid adoption of increasingly complicated radiotherapy technologies compel radiation oncologists to be involved in the CQI effort.[19]

TABLE 102.2 COMMON TERMS, KEYWORDS, AND VERNACULAR OF ERROR AVOIDANCE/PREVENTION

Keyword/Term	Definition/Explanation
Quality	The IOM defines quality as "the degree to which health services for individuals and populations increase the likelihood of desired health outcomes and are consistent with current professional knowledge"
Safety	Safety (or patient safety) is the prevention of errors and adverse effects to patients associated with health care
Error	An error is a preventable adverse effect of care, whether or not it is evident or harmful to the patient. Slips, lapses, and mistakes are all considered forms of error, mainly human error
Near-error	An event or situation that could have resulted in an accident, injury, or illness but did not either by chance or through timely intervention
Quality control	All planned operational techniques necessary to retrospectively verify if a provided product or service met the requirements of quality
Quality assurance	All planned proactive (i.e., prospective) processes, techniques, and actions necessary to ensure adequate confidence that a product or service meets the requirement for quality
Incident reporting system	A program/system by which any individual of an organization can report incidents (safety events, error, near-errors, etc.) that occur in their daily work for analysis and shared learning in a secure and nonpunitive environment with the goal of improving quality and safety
Hierarchy of effectiveness	Human factors engineering concept for error reduction strategies
Lean	A systematic approach to identify and eliminate waste (non–value-added activities) through continuous improvement
Human factors engineering	An engineering knowledge domain that covers three main areas: (1) physical ergonomics concerned with physical activity, (2) cognitive (or information processing) ergonomics concerned with mental process, and (3) organizational (or macroergonomics) ergonomics concerned with sociotechnical system design
Normal accident theory	Theory that hypothesized that systems in which elements are tightly coupled and interactively complex would be subjected to accidents in the normal course of operations
Swiss cheese model	A conceptual error causation model based on four failure domains: organizational influences, supervision, preconditions, and specific acts

Changing organizational culture in medicine is difficult and impossible without physician engagement and leadership. Physician leadership is a key element to designing, fostering, and nurturing a culture of safety.[19-22] Physician engagement in quality improvement is fundamental for successful organizational cultural change.[21,22] Physicians must be identified as champions of safety and be involved in CQI initiatives from the beginning.[21,22] To create a healthy culture of safety, physicians must adopt a "no-blame" environment that fosters open communication in which all team members are free and responsible to raise concerns about quality and safety. Getting "buy-in" and support from team members for a quality/safety agenda is difficult. First and foremost, physicians must publicly declare and support quality and safety and empower and motivate others to continuously improve quality and safety. At departmental faculty and staff meetings, at educational conferences, and within the clinic, physicians should dialogue about the importance of quality and safety and celebrate those who are actively engaging in initiatives and improvements. Physicians should not be on the "sidelines" as observers but should visibly and actively serve as leaders of quality and safety.

According to change management experts, successful CQI efforts require that physician leaders demonstrate a blend of *transactional* and *transformational* leadership behaviors.[23,24] Transactional leadership is a task-oriented, command-and-control approach emphasizing what needs to be done and how to do it. This approach seems to be most useful when organizations are operating within well-defined constraints and seek to further efficiencies within existing structures. Transformational leadership focuses on the relationship between the leader and follower and is largely concerned with motivating and inspiring followers to do more than expected. It is contingent on followers' strong levels of trust, admiration, loyalty, and respect for the leader. This approach is most useful when organizations are attempting to adapt, innovate, and change in order to address new opportunities and challenges. Transformational leadership appears to result in greater job satisfaction and a more collaborative/helpful environment among workers as well as higher trust in the leader.[25]

In summary, physician leaders must actively work with others to promote quality and safety with high levels of urgency for change, charisma, vision, et cetera. The behaviors, actions, and words of physician leaders can carry great weight as others may emulate them. A physician leader who does not consistently and overtly espouse these principles may inadvertently discourage others from embracing these concepts. Physician leaders need to continuously inspire people to go beyond their regular duties and identify ways to improve quality and safety.

SYSTEMS THINKING

The effective and safe application of radiotherapy requires many team members, technologies, and processes to function reliably. The ever-present risk of errors including unforeseen errors and interactions in our systems is complex, for example, failure patterns are not always predictable. Sustainable advances in quality and safety require that we adopt a *systems-based approach* for error avoidance and prevention.[26-29]

The Problem with Systems Thinking in Medicine

Medical training and education have developed a culture with a powerful tenant that quality and safety are the personal responsibility of the physician. Physicians are taught that if we work and study hard enough, we won't make a mistake. Thus, many physicians believe that quality and safety improvements are a personal endeavor to be conducted in their autonomous microsystem. This credence does not allow for a system-based perspective and naturally leads to a "blame culture." Physicians are socialized in medical school and residency to strive for error-free practice, are taught that mistakes are unacceptable, and thus condition themselves to be infallible. Physicians are motivated to not commit errors, in part, for fear of punishment via social/peer disapproval. Errors are seen as character flaws and as someone's fault, and blame is used to encourage proper performance. This desire to be infallible may result in physicians not reporting errors, because of embarrassment/shame by colleagues, fear of patient reaction, and fear of litigation. Also, as errors are not discussed, potential lessons learned are not shared with team members and processes and systems are not improved.

Unfortunately, the culture of medicine is based on individuals not making errors rather than (appropriately) acknowledging that they will, that is, that physicians are humans performing in imperfect systems. Dr. Lucian Leape has stated that "The single greatest impediment to error prevention is...that we *punish* people for making mistakes."[5]

Errors Will Occur and Are Due to System Flaws, Not Character Flaws

Professors Popper and McIntyre published an enlightening paper in 1983 entitled "The critical attitudes in Medicine: The need for a new ethics," including the following principle assertions: (a) "Errors by doctors are common," (b) "We (physicians) are all fallible, and it is impossible for anybody to avoid all mistakes, even avoidable ones. The old idea that we must avoid them, has to be revised. It is mistaken and it has led to hypocrisy," and, (c) "But whereas doctors may acknowledge this responsibility in principle, there is little evidence that they spend much time analyzing their error, either in clinical practice or even during their training."[30]

Radiation oncologists must understand that errors will occur (as part of the human condition) and that we must design systems to minimize errors, identify them efficiently, and prevent them from reaching the patient. Error-free performance is unachievable and the mentality of infallibility will inevitably result in system failure. From the cognitive psychology viewpoint, making mistakes is, in fact, a "normal" behavior, a condition for learning which gains experience on how to interact with the world. Remember the saying "good judgment comes from experience, experience comes from bad judgment."

In addition, the belief that an error-free practice is a realistic objective is a source of great stress and ultimately results in professional burnout. Expecting errors to occur and realizing that they are a manageable part of everyday practice allow us to practice in a no-blame culture focusing on the underlying root causes of system failures. Although the proximal error is often a human error, the root causes of the error are often due to poor system and organizational design. Workers are not so much the actors of their own errors; rather, they are victims of a poorly designed environment. Errors are indicative of system flaws rather than character flaws. The medical approach to error avoidance has been with superficial investigations of the often downstream causes of errors resulting in solutions to prevent specific individuals from repeating the error. This approach often results in work-arounds that may only temporarily prevent errors. Understanding the underlying root causes and creating system solutions will lead to sustainable improvements. For example, though a radiation delivery error may be immediately attributed to a performance issue with a radiation therapy technologist, the underlying root cause may be due to inadequate supervision or training, workload (too much or not enough), nonstandardized/ambiguous communications, or poorly designed human–machine/computer interfaces. Management decisions can have unintended consequences creating workplace situations that predispose team members to errors, that is, "accidents waiting to happen." Systems should be designed to incorporate a series of safety barriers that make it difficult for an individual to err. In other words, our systems and environment should make it easy to do the right thing. This concept does not imply that character flaws are nonexistent. Repeated mistakes by the same individual should raise concerns regarding his or her ability to carry such a function but only after the root cause problems have been honestly and properly addressed. Furthermore, team members should be held accountable for participating in quality improvement work (e.g., reporting errors, participating in improvement discussions) and in fostering a safety culture (e.g., not ostracizing others for reporting or making errors).

Focusing on Making Better Systems ("It's the Process, Not the Person")

Human error has been extensively studied by psychologists and engineers in HRO (e.g., aviation, nuclear power, automobile manufacturing). Two theories that are particularly instructive to medicine are the Swiss cheese model (SCM) and normal accident theory (NAT).

Swiss Cheese Model

Although errors are often attributed to human error, their root causes are often poor system and organizational design (James Reason, Swiss cheese model [SCM][31]) (Fig. 102.2). The successful practice of radiation oncology relies on people and their ability to repeatedly perform diverse tasks in a reliable and accurate manner. However, people do not perform tasks in a vacuum. From the SCM perspective, peoples' actions (Fig. 102.2) are influenced by "upstream" latent failure pathways (contributory factors that may lie dormant for long periods of time) at the organizational, workplace, and people levels (e.g., policies, programs, schedules, workflows, training, perceptions). The worker's action that is linked to the incident (e.g., forgetting to do something) is

FIGURE 102.2. Adaptation of James Reason's Swiss cheese model. (From Marks L, Mazur L. *Engineering patient safety in radiation oncology: University of North Carolina's pursuit for high reliability and value creation.* Boca Raton, FL: Taylor & Francis, 2015:256. Copyright ©2015 Taylor and Francis Group, LLC. Reproduced by permission of Taylor and Francis Group, LLC, a division of Informa plc.)

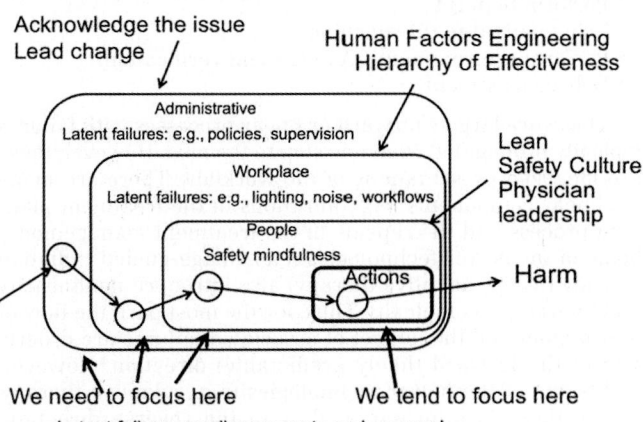

often referred to as the "active failure." Often, during root cause analyses, too much emphasis is placed on the person's active failure and not enough attention to the "upstream" layers of the SCM.

Human Factors Analysis and Classification System

From a system thinking perspective, it is critical to analyze both the active and latent failure pathways to fully understand root causes of patient harm. The human factors analysis and classification system (HFACS) model is perhaps the most widely used method, having been applied in civil and military aviation,[32,33] helicopter maintenance,[34] coal mining,[35] rail transportation,[36] maritime,[37] construction,[38] health care,[39] and road transportation.[40] HFACS was developed by Shappell and Wiegmann,[32] based on Reason's SCM (Fig. 102.3). HFACS investigates events using 4 main levels of failure and 12 additional sublevels (Fig. 102.3).[31] To classify an event into the various categories of the HFACS model, a user starts at the first level (unsafe act, mandatory to select) and then proceeds to the corresponding sublevels (e.g., unintended vs. intended violation), followed by the nanocodes (unintended violation, skill based vs. decision-based vs. perceptual; intended violation, routine violation vs. exceptional violation). Although these categorizations are somewhat arbitrary and inexact, they can help drive improvement work by providing a framework to better analyze and understand system behaviors.

We will apply this approach to an incident that occurred in our clinic. The patient was scheduled to receive a bilateral lung treatment: first to the left lung and then the right lung. When the radiation therapist downloaded the patient's right lung treatment plan, the digital reconstructed radiograph for the right lung plan was the same as the digital reconstructed radiograph from the left lung plan. Using HFACS at the action level, the failure investigation team identified an *unintended action* where the planner demonstrated an attention failure as one of the causes (forgot to change the right lung digital reconstructed radiographs). At the precondition for unsafe act level, the team found the planner was under an increased workload. At the unsafe supervision level, the team identified both the physician and planner failed to check digital reconstructed radiographs before approving the plan. Finally, at the organization influence level, the team identified the lack of a formal policy for digital reconstructed radiograph checks. In summary, application of the HFACS model may help identify and foster discussion on latent failures and their pathways, reduce the temptation for finger pointing, and develop a culture of safety.

Normal Accident Theory

Substantial work in non–health care settings has been performed to better understand the causes of accidents and investigate potential mitigation strategies. One of the nation's leading theorists in the area of safety, Dr. Charles Perrow, coined the term normal accident theory (NAT, Fig. 102.4).[41] He argues that failures in systems occur often and are indeed expected and part of the normal operations (hence the name *normal*). He categorizes systems based on how these failures interact within the larger system and lead to major accidents. Systems in which failures propagate and interact predictably are considered *linear* and those where failures behave unpredictably are *interactively complex*.

He further categorizes systems in their ability to detect and respond to failures. Systems that are relatively slow with more opportunity to detect and respond to failures are termed *loosely coupled*, whereas those that are fast with less opportunity to detect and respond to failures are termed *tightly coupled*.

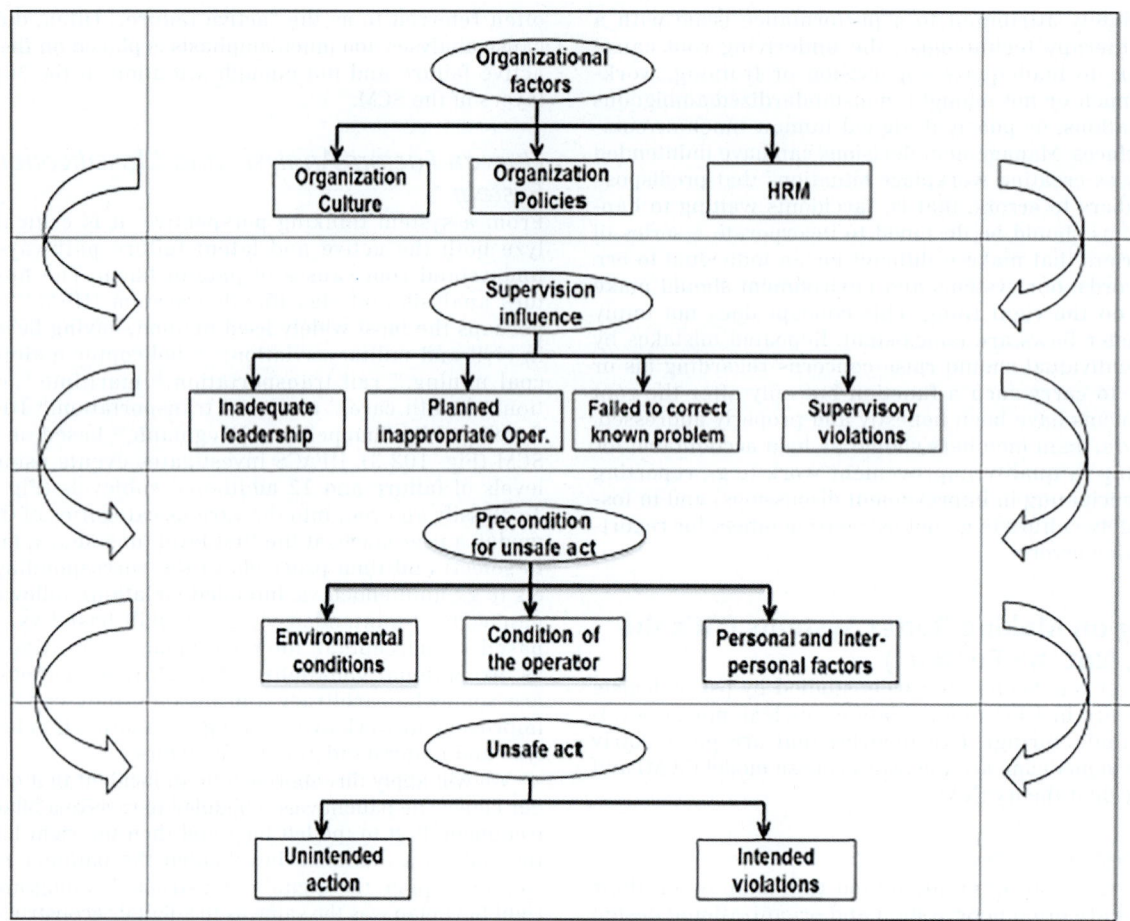

FIGURE 102.3. HFACS model with categories, subcategories, and hierarchy. (Reprinted from Mosaly P, Mazur LM, Burkhardt K, et al. Application of Human Factors and Classification System [HFACS] Model to Event Analysis in Radiation Oncology. *Pract Radiat Oncol* 2015;5[2]:113–119. Copyright © 2015 Elsevier. With permission.)

For example, the post office is linear (failures have predictable consequences) and is loosely coupled (failures are largely corrected and most of the mail ultimately gets delivered). Dams are also linear, but are tightly coupled. A dam breach will likely lead to a flood because the time scale required to fix the breach is too long to mitigate the (literally) downstream effects. Universities are interactively complex because events in their varied components (e.g., multiple departments, schools, social events, athletics, etc.) interact in unforeseen ways (Fig. 102.4).

Perrow argues that systems that are both interactively complex and tightly coupled have a particular propensity for catastrophic failure. Failures in these subsystems are assuredly going to occur, and because these will propagate in unforeseen ways that cannot be mitigated, major global system failures are probable. In other words, complex systems cannot be fully understood and their behavior will always have some element of chaos. He argues that only a change in their structure such as reducing coupling, or reducing interactive complexity, can help reduce the probability of a catastrophic event.

Applying NAT Constructs to Radiation Oncology

Is radiation oncology linear or nonlinear (Fig. 102.4)? From the provider's perspective, workflow in the clinic might be broadly simplified as:

- Evaluate the patient and medical records.
- Make treatment recommendations.
- Perform radiation treatment planning.

- Review treatment plans (often iterate).
- Initiate therapy.
- Conduct treatment management (i.e., monitor/continue therapy, repeat).

Similarly, on the technical side (e.g., physicist/dosimetrist/therapist), workflow for a radiosurgery case might be broadly simplified as:

- Gather planning images.
- Fuse planning images with diagnostic images.
- Generate image segmentations.
- Review desired dose/volume parameters with the provider.
- Perform treatment planning.
- Perform plan QA.
- Bring patient to the machine.
- Perform pretreatment QA/alignment verification.
- Deliver treatment.

These are largely forward or linear processes with failures typically propagated from one step to the next. However, these are idealized presentations of the workflow. There are many nonlinear components (e.g., iterations in the treatment planning process and the repeats in the treatment management). Some of the newer technologies (e.g., image-guided radiation therapy [IGRT], adaptive therapy) also introduce nonlinearity and interactive complexity. Thus, for the most part, the flow of information and the impact of associated failures are orderly and in the forward (likely predictable) direction. However, with some of the newer technologies (e.g., adaptive therapy, IGRT), there is information flow in the reverse direction, essentially causing some procedures to be repeated. Further,

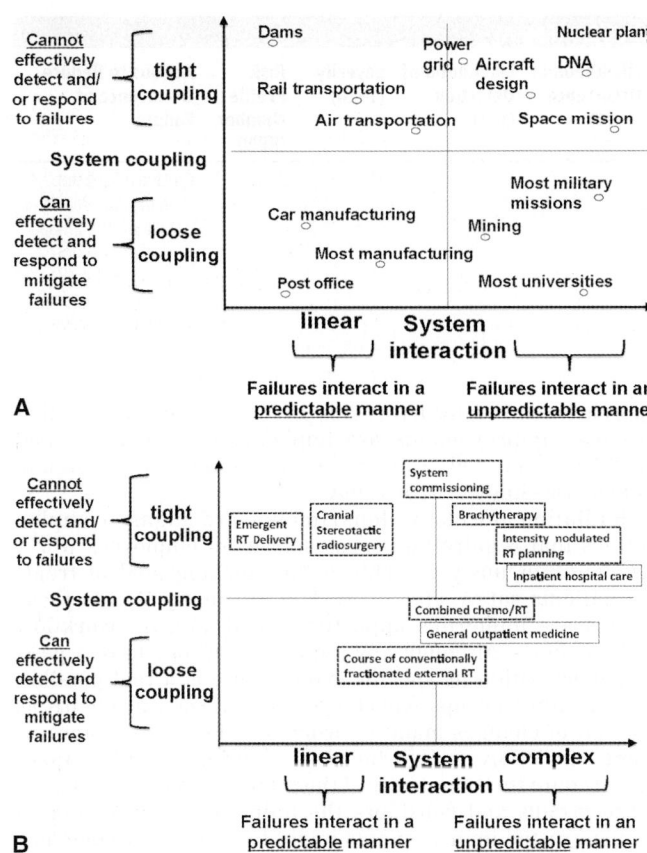

relatively slow pace tends to soften the impact of failure (i.e., reduce their clinical impact).

Are there parts of our practice that are tightly coupled (Fig. 102.4)? Yes, consider intraoperative radiotherapy, brachytherapy, and radiosurgery settings where the entire procedure is often compressed into a few hours. In these instances, some steps have near-immediate impacts on other steps. Furthermore, portions of our routine processes are very fast. Consider the setup and delivery steps for each individual fraction of radiation: patient identification, setup, image verification, and treatment delivery. This sequence of steps occurs very rapidly, which leaves the potential for many human errors. Also, failures in some processes can be difficult to detect and may affect many treatments or patients downstream (e.g., system commissioning) and thus may be considered tightly coupled. As we introduce more components to the processes such as combined chemoradiotherapy and adaptive therapy, the number of steps and people involved increases. Interactions become more complex (unusual interactions between failures become more likely) and coupling becomes tighter. It may become more difficult to detect and address these failures.

So, what is the relevance of this discussion? Can we use these constructs to guide QA strategies? Safety experts suggest there are global optimal QA strategies applicable to all types of systems (e.g., leadership-driven safety mindfulness, the application of automation and forcing functions wherever able, etc.). However, there are particular QA considerations for different systems depending where they lie on this paradigm of linear versus interactively complex and loosely coupled versus tightly coupled.

For example, a course of conventionally fractionated external RT (mostly linear, modestly coupled, and generally slow) might be amenable to employee-based CQI strategies. For interactively complex systems that are loosely coupled, their behavior is less predictable than the linear systems. Failures and their interactive effects can be detected, but corrective actions often have further unforeseen effects. Thus, to assure quality, a strategy of continuous comprehensive monitoring (perhaps with forcing functions) is best. Any changes or interventions need to be carefully considered as they may result in unexpected consequences. CQI-based improvement cycles may be useful in some areas but may be more challenging because there are more stakeholders and interactive effects can be difficult to predict. Thus, these systems may appear to be sometimes chaotic, as leadership responds to continual iterations. Because their pace is somewhat slow, observers have the luxury to analyze system behavior retrospectively and to second-guess previous actions (because interactions may seem obvious in hindsight). Processes that are both interactively complex and tightly coupled can be unpredictable. Failures and their interactive effects are often not detected until they manifest as a catastrophic event given that their character may be unknown (e.g., it is hard to monitor and thus detect an unforeseen type of failure). Even if failure effects are detected, human-based corrections are unreliable as system behavior is interactively complex. Thus, quality is best assured by rather strict adherence to process standardization in all areas. System performance needs to be comprehensively monitored because the nature or type of a failure cannot be reliably predicted. Ideally, this monitoring process should be automated to assure compliance; human intervention is too slow and often misguided. Vigilant testing and verification are needed before any changes in the system or its processes are made. The adoption of automation and forcing functions (where possible), end-to-end testing, strict QA, and redundant checks for IMRT planning, brachytherapy, and system commissioning reflects our field's recognition that these systems are interactively complex and tightly coupled.

FIGURE 102.4. Normal accident theory concepts of loose versus tight coupling (*y*-axis) and linear versus interactively complex **(A)**. Several nonmedical systems from Perrow's original description are plotted according to normal accident theory concepts. (Adapted from Perrow C. *Normal accidents: living with high-risk technologies.* Princeton paperbacks. Princeton, NJ: Princeton University Press, 1999.) Car manufacturing processes (assembly lines) are considered as linear and loosely coupled systems. Things tend to happen in an orderly fashion (linear), and failures can often be detected and corrected in a timely fashion. Water dams are thought of as linear and tightly coupled systems. A failure at one dam (e.g., a breech) typically has predictable downstream (quite literally) consequences (linear). The system is tightly coupled because this is almost certainly going to manifest (e.g., cause a flood). Even though the breech is readily apparent, it is usually not humanly possible to prevent the flood (the time scale for corrective action is much slower than the flow of the water). Universities are seen as complex and loosely coupled systems. Decisions in broad areas of the university often affect each other (interactively complex). The unforeseen impacts of these complex interactions are often detected and can be addressed and averted in a timely fashion (loosely coupled). Nuclear power plants are examples of interactively complex and tightly coupled systems. The interactions between the various components are hard to predict; things can happen very fast, much faster than the response time of a human monitoring the system (tightly coupled). In **B**, we map several radiation oncology processes to approximate locations on the normal accident theory grid. (Adapted from Marks L, et al. *Engineering patient safety in radiation oncology: University of North Carolina's pursuit for high reliability and value creation.* Boca Raton, FL: Taylor & Francis, 2015.)

some of the processes are long, with many steps (e.g., intensity-modulated radiation therapy [IMRT] planning and delivery), thus increasing the possibility of unexpected interactions of different failures.

Is radiation oncology coupled or uncoupled (Fig. 102.4)? Broadly speaking, most radiation oncology processes are modestly coupled. The pace of the work is generally slow enough for unexpected interactions between failures to be evident. For example, suboptimal decisions about patient positioning and immobilization are typically evident early in the course of therapy and can be addressed. In many areas of radiation oncology, as well as other areas of medicine, the

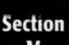

TABLE 102.3 SIMPLISTIC EXAMPLE OF FAILURE MODES AND EFFECTS ANALYSIS (FMEA)

Steps in the Process	Failure Mode	Failure Causes	Failure Effect	Likelihood of Occurrence (1–10)	Likelihood of Detection (1–10)	Severity (1–10)	Risk Profile Number (RPN)	Actions to Reduce Occurrence of Failure
3Ps (pacemaker, pregnancy, prior radiation)	Increase in patients treated without accounting for 3Ps	Information entered in an electronic medical record by the nurse cannot be transferred automatically into the planning system	Damage to the pacemaker thus leading to cardiac complications, miscarriage, or excess radiation toxicity	6	5	10	300	Created a hard stop in the data transfer system. The physician must choose yes or no for 3Ps before proceeding with the process

These processes are made safe for clinical use through QA initiatives. Further, our field embraces automated technologies aimed to enhance accuracy and patient safety (e.g., automatic tracking, gating). If this is copied verbatim, that is fine; we just need to be sure that we say so in the acknowledgments and be sure that we get permission from the publisher of our book.

Failure Modes and Effects Analysis

Failure Modes and Effects Analysis (FMEA) is a prospective way to conduct failure analysis and is based on trying to predict where failures will occur (vs. HFACS, a retrospective approach). The FMEA technique is a well-established and widely used tool for safety and improvement in many industries[42] including health care[43–45] and, specifically, radiation therapy.[46,47] The FMEA technique consists of three steps. First, it requires generating or selecting process steps for analysis. Second, it lists all possible failure modes per each process step. Third, a numeric value is assigned for each failure mode based on (a) likelihood of occurrence, (b) likelihood of detection, and (c) potential severity. The numeric values usually range from 1 and 10, with 1 meaning "very unlikely to occur/detect" and 10 meaning "very likely to occur/detect." Finally, a risk priority number (RPN) for each failure mode is calculated by multiplying the three scores. The lowest possible score could be 1 and the highest 1,000. Identifying the failure modes with highest RPNs should help teams prioritize improvement opportunities (e.g., see Table 102.3).

Ford et al.[47] applied this FMEA approach to processes within their radiation oncology clinic. Only approximately 50% of the actual incidents occurring in their clinic were predicted by the formal FMEA analysis. This observation highlights the complex nature of our systems, that is, failure modes cannot always be predicted as there are often unforeseen failures and failure interactions. The utility of FMEA for error avoidance and prevention in radiation oncology requires further study.

CONTINUOUS QUALITY IMPROVEMENT

Processes in many HROs and in most areas of medicine are continually evolving. Even if systems were "perfect" at one instance in time, they will assuredly drift toward imperfection as workflows change. Further, given the complexities of these systems, changes in processes may have unforeseen consequences. For these reasons, it is generally understood that continuous incremental improvements are needed to adapt to evolving systems and to carefully evaluate the consequences of any changes as well as minimize the risk of unforeseen problems. A cornerstone of quality improvement work is improvement *cycles* with ongoing monitoring informing additional cycles in a never-ending iterative manner. This

approach continually drives change forward and ensures that proposed improvements are implemented, sustained, and modified (as needed) over time. Often, this cycle is referred to as Plan–Do–Study–Act, or PDSA.

Radiation oncology departments are highly complex entities that require numerous subsets of employees working simultaneously to achieve the common goal of treating patients safely, effectively, and efficiently. Within these groups are numerous opportunities to improve workflow and outcomes. Although any improvement may have a positive effect within its specific group, there is a real possibility that other groups will develop unforeseen problems as a result of changes made in order to achieve that improvement. The PDSA cycle, when correctly implemented, takes into account the complexity of the interrelationships between these groups and considers the unintended consequences that suggested improvements might have on the system as a whole instead of just one part. The major steps in the PDSA cycle are:

- *Plan*: This is the start of the cycle. In the planning stage, a problem within the system is identified and described in detail so that a set of goals and expected outcomes can be determined.
- *Do*: This is the initial implementation stage. Corrections that result from the planning step are implemented, and data are collected that relate to the efficacy of these corrections.
- *Study*: This is the step of the cycle that takes the data collected in the previous step and analyzes how well everything is working. Here, the outcomes of the changes are compared to expectations, that is, if the changes made were actually the ones intended. Analyses completed here are carried forward to the next step.
- *Act*: This is sometimes considered the "adjust" phase of the cycle. The focus is to assess the analyses from the study phase and determine what adjustments can or should be made in order to better address the identified problem.

Transforming Individuals into Effective Problem Solvers

The challenge is *how* radiation oncology professionals will respond to latent and active failures when they occur, not *whether* they will respond. Radiation oncology professionals are dedicated employees who take pride in the safety of their patients. Human nature and working conditions often predispose radiation oncologists to develop quick fixes and work-arounds when faced with latent and active failures. Prospective PDSA problem-solving behavior is difficult to cultivate in individual workers, but this type of problem-solving is the most effective and most likely to result in long-term quality improvement. Furthermore, empowerment of frontline staff (i.e., nonphysician staff) is crucial to the

CQI process. Given that there are more nonphysician staff than physician staff in a radiation oncology department, there are a greater number of ideas that can be generated for problem-solving and PDSA cycles if they are given the support to participate in and/or lead quality improvement efforts. In addition to supportive and engaged leadership and a strong culture of safety, additional driving forces acting on individuals transforming their behaviors include the following[32]:

- *Standard operating procedures*: Support employees with detection of failures. When standard operating procedures continuously "fail," this should conflict with the desire to conform to existing ways of operating. This, in turn, should spur individual motivation for change.
- *Positive feedback*: Employees need to know their improvement efforts are valued even under circumstances of suboptimal final results. If feedback is positive, employees are more likely to invest in future improvement efforts.
- *Role models*: Employees need to see that problem-solving behaviors are rewarded. The exact nature of the reward, that is, monetary, title, or other nonmonetary recognition, is not as important as the reward's meaning to the recipient and the value placed by the members of the organization. This creates tangible examples for others to emulate.
- *Job-related autonomy*: Without a sense of autonomy, employees tend to follow the rules, especially if the rules are perceived to be good enough and do not openly cause harm. Without autonomy, conformance is viewed as a safe choice.
- *Support from direct supervisor*: This is needed to create an appealing work environment for problem-solving behaviors. Employees must be empowered by supervisors to take action.
- *Individualized attributes of the employee*: Employees with a strong sense of care and concern for patients, coworkers, and the organization are more likely to break free from the status quo and take improvement actions based on problem-solving behaviors.
- *Critical thinking skills*: Employees must be trained to skillfully conceptualize and assess situations, question assumptions, determine options for responding to the situation, apply improvement tools, and make intelligent decisions.
- *Organizational accountability*: This accountability refers to becoming a continuous improvement organization. In the presence of failures, it is leadership's role to set improvement expectations at a high but attainable level. In the absence of failures, leadership must develop a sense of urgency to improve and communicate its importance.

Although understanding, developing, and promoting the driving forces for positive change is of high importance, careful consideration must also be given to restraining forces, which can act as barriers to the transition to problem-solving behaviors.

- *Low staffing levels and high work efficiency requirements*: If employees are to become initiators or enhancers, they must have time in their workdays to take necessary actions for improvements. If staffing levels are low and the demands for efficiency and productivity are high, the perception is there is not sufficient time to institute real improvements. Thus, making quick fixes, expediting, or conforming is more likely to happen.
- *Burdensome defect reporting systems*: When reporting systems are too administratively burdensome, employees are less inclined to report a defect, which, in turn, decreases an organizations ability to learn.
- *Concerns related to psychological safety*: Employees' ability to think and act freely without fear of negative consequences to self-image, status, or career is repeatedly identified as a significant restraining force. Prior research has demonstrated that higher psychological safety increases the willingness of individuals to engage in failure reporting and improvement behaviors even though such efforts are inherently risky and can have negative personal and career consequences.[48,49]
- *Gratification and burnout*: Naturally, initial reactions to quickly fixed problems or procedural shortcuts under time pressure can bring some satisfaction. This feeling of instant gratification can be a powerful motivator for continuing to use work-arounds to get rapid resolution of problems. Such "firefighting behavior" becomes the norm and the desire for true improvement is dampened. However, in the long run, when employees find themselves solving the same problems, a more insidious restraining force arises due to personal burnout.
- *Culture of conforming to work procedures*: When organizational pressure to conform to work procedures is strong, employees will not be motivated to engage in process improvement efforts. Note that this force does not imply abandoning efforts to develop standard operating procedures. Rather, it implies that the desire to comply with work procedures may motivate employees to keep doing their jobs in the same way.
- *Suboptimal training on improvement philosophy*: If employees have not been exposed to an improvement philosophy at work, they are less likely to know the mechanics of how to continuously improve. The specialized methods, tools, and mind-set required to succeed at initiating and enhancing behaviors must be disseminated to frontline workers. This requires dedicated training and a sustained commitment by the leadership team.
- *Lack of dedicated improvement time*: Without time to invest in problem-solving behavior, employees may find it difficult to sustain this behavior over time.
- *Lack of knowledge of improvement methods/tools*: Those who are effective at initiating and enhancing need to be trained in these areas and gain experience over time in applying tools and methods.
- *Lack of operational visibility*: Certain systems in radiation oncology centers are tightly coupled where the actions of one professional group tend to affect or be affected by actions of other professional groups. The lack of visibility of how their local work areas are connected to the larger operating system can limit employees' ability to be effective at problem-solving behaviors. Without sufficient visibility and understanding, it is difficult for employees to identify sources of defects and make system-wide improvements.
- *Lack of employee's social network for improvement*: Outside of senior leadership, direct supervision, and explicit continuous improvement role models, potential initiators and enhancers need a support system of colleagues. Employees who strive to enhance will experience inevitable setbacks and challenges. The support and encouragement of colleagues can be invaluable to continuous improvement initiatives.

"Lean" Approach to CQI

Lean is a management philosophy derived from the Toyota Production System.[50,51] The heart of Lean is preserving value with less work by the identification and elimination of "waste" and developing highly reliable processes. This is performed in a context of connectedness, respect, and growth of all employees who are trained to identify waste and errors and suggest possibilities for improvements that will be tested using scientific methods. Categories of waste include defects, overproduction, waiting, overprocessing, excessive inventory and motion, and (most damaging) failure to use employees to their highest potential. Waste reduction results in quality improvement and reduction in time and cost. The Institute for Healthcare Improvement believes that Lean principles can and are being successfully applied to the delivery of health care. Hence, it makes sense to take a closer look at Toyota to learn how they have developed their processes.[52] A few of the more common process engineering practices are:

- *Just-in-time*: Producing only what is needed, when it is needed, and in only the necessary quantities; reducing work-in-process inventory.
- *Kanban*: A card that signals production of a set quantity of goods once that number of goods has been used by a customer process.
- *Production leveling (or heijunka)*: Spreading production evenly over time; reducing batch sizes to one.
- *Set-up time reduction*: Reducing the time to changeover between producing different products; required to make production more even.
- *Standardized work*: Documented and detailed work procedures strictly followed by everyone doing the job such that the work is performed the same way every time.
- *Multiskilled workers*: Workers trained in multiple job tasks so work can be assigned flexibly to balance the line dynamically.
- *Kaizen*: An activity with a purpose to remove the waste ("muda") and to humanize the workplace by eliminating overly hard work ("muri").

At the operational level, Lean is equipped with two basic tools: *value-stream mapping*[53] and the *A3 problem-solving tool*.[54,55] Value-stream maps graphically represent key people, material, and information required to deliver a product or service. They are designed to distinguish value-adding from non–value-adding steps. A3s are a problem-solving tool where the user documents the problem area, current state, root cause analysis of the problem, target condition, countermeasures, implementation plan (who, what, when, outcome, metrics), and follow-up plan (30-, 60-, 90-day assessment) on a sheet of paper (the name "A3" is derived from the paper size). These basic tools are often used during Kaizen events, which are usually 1- to 4-day activities where employees engage in small cycles of improvement that promote Lean thinking and behavior. Kaizen events are a critical component in implementing lean because they directly eliminate unnecessary waste and bring the organization closer to desired performance outputs.

Six-Sigma Approach to CQI

Six Sigma is a business management philosophy for quality improvement that originated in the US manufacturing industry. It seeks to improve efficiency and reliability of processes by identifying and removing the causes of failures and minimizing process variability. The approach is heavily dependent on quantitative data; thus, the process can take many months to quantitatively assess the multiple components of the current state, design an improvement plan, and assess its impact. The term Six Sigma reflects the desire for critical errors to occur at a rate approximating six standard deviations away from the desired performance. Six-Sigma approaches require experts in data generation, analysis, and associated statistical knowledge. It uses the DMAIC process (define, measure, analyze, improve, and control) to conduct improvement projects:

- **Define:** To clearly articulate the problem under investigation while focusing on the voice of the customer (VOC) and critical to quality (CTQs) drivers. In addition, to establish project goal, potential resources, project scope, and project timeline and milestones.
- **Measure:** To objectively establish baselines as the basis for improvement. This data collection step establishes process performance baselines.
- **Analyze:** To identify, validate, and select root causes for elimination.
- **Improve:** To identify, test, and implement a solution to the problem, in part or in whole. Lean and Six Sigma are often combined at this step, especially when the goal is to reduce operational waste.
- **Control:** To sustain gains and monitor improvements to ensure continued and sustainable success. Control charts are often used during this stage to assess the stability of the improvements over time.

Compared to Lean, there is relatively little empirical research on the utility of Six Sigma to effectively improve quality and safety, other than "best practice" studies by consultants or practitioners. Further, Six Sigma is a more time-consuming and complicated process compared to Lean-based approaches and, when applied to complex systems within health care, can be particularly challenging because quantitative data may be needed from *many* interactive areas, thus complicating analysis. In practice, the length and difficulty of this approach can make physicians and other stakeholders disillusioned with and resistant to CQI work. Nevertheless, this "ultra–data-driven" approach can be very helpful in settings where the simpler Lean-based approaches cannot be applied. This may include settings where iterative trial-and-error approaches are not safe (e.g., where any failure can be catastrophic such as with nuclear power plants or NASA) and where such detailed multifaceted data are needed to even understand the current state.

PATIENT SAFETY CULTURE

The concept of safety culture originated in HROs such as nuclear power, aviation, and manufacturing. High-reliability organizations maintain a commitment to safety at all levels from frontline workers to managers. The safety culture of an organization is defined "…as the product of individual and group values, attitudes, perceptions, competencies, and patterns of behavior that determine the commitment to, and the style and proficiency of, an organization's health and safety management".[56] Creating a patient safety culture is a critical component of any type of safety improvement program. Outside of health care, a strong safety culture is noted as a critical underpinning in other high-reliability organizations.[56–58]

The key features of a culture of safety are (a) acknowledging the high-risk nature of processes, (b) having a blame-free environment where workers can report errors/near-errors without fear of punishment, (c) encouraging collaboration across ranks and disciplines to improve safety, and (d) organizational/leadership commitment of resources to address safety concerns. In non–health care high-reliability organizations, the safety of workers themselves is the focus of the safety culture. In health care, a culture of safety for health care professionals is pertinent as is prioritizing the safe delivery of health care to the patient, hence the concept of *patient* safety culture. Assessing the safety culture in an organization can be challenging. The Agency for Healthcare Research and Quality (AHRQ) administers a patient safety culture survey that is generally regarded as a reasonable measure.[59] Interestingly, there are some data, albeit limited, to support the notion that centers with better safety culture scores, as assessed by their own staff, have lower rates of severe adverse events.[60]

The following are some of the key components of the safety culture within commercial aviation[61–65]:

- *Training*: Most commercial airline carriers encourage, reward, and pay staff to attend required quality/safety training. If an employee misses or fails training/proficiency checks, they usually face restrictions until their underperformance has been rectified. Training focuses on the inevitability of errors and the importance of culture, teamwork, and communication in avoiding errors as well as containing their spread and mitigating their effects before they lead to serious or catastrophic harm.

- *Policies and procedures that enforce safe operations*: There must always be two physiologically and psychologically sound pilots to fly a plane. This minimum safety requirement *always* applies. No exceptions are granted. This is often audited by random drug and alcohol tests. Further, during the safety-critical phases of a flight such as flying below an altitude of 10,000 feet, the pilots and cabin crew must adhere to strict standard operating procedures and refrain from all nonessential activities (e.g., reading newspapers or chatting idly). This safety requirement is known as the sterile cockpit rule. Crew members are taught how to call, without awkwardness, for implementation of the sterile cockpit rule at additional times when particular concentration becomes necessary. The entire crew is informed about the enforced rule through warnings or alert systems. Adoption of comparable policies in radiation oncology centers would be controversial, but they might better ensure patient safety.

- *Flight recorders*: These recorders, also known as black boxes, monitor key flight parameters throughout each flight. This data is analyzed by computers *after every flight*. Readings outside of predetermined acceptable ranges trigger warning signals that can initiate an investigation. The full exploration of flight recording is only conducted in catastrophic circumstances, but pilots and staff know that all of their actions are being monitored and that everything they do and say is being recorded.

How do we build an infrastructure to support a culture of safety in radiation oncology centers? Where do we start? Perhaps, not with flight recorders right away. However, one could consider posttreatment assessments of the quality of patient setups by a computer-based analysis of pretreatment images (e.g., cone beam CT or surface mappings) as analogous to flight recorders. More importantly, we believe that our field (and frankly all of medicine) needs to develop and maintain a high level of urgency toward change and innovation to improve quality and safety. We need to acknowledge our challenges and build a robust set of tools to drive improvement work as well as nurture the culture to support and apply these tools. Several examples of our initiatives include:

- *Incident learning*: Many HROs have incident learning systems in which any individual can report errors/incidents that occur in the processes they work with, and these incidents are studied and analyzed to identify targets for process improvement. Learning from these errors/incidents plays a key role in improving quality and safety. The *Good Catch Program* is our departmental incident reporting system. In effect since 2012, it is custom-built, enabling users to easily report any types of system failures (e.g., waste, work-arounds, incidents reaching the

patients). Reporting can be done anonymously, if desired, if people are reluctant/anxious about reporting. Over time, with a "just culture," very few of our reported issues are anonymous. Reporting is encouraged and celebrated; the person(s) reporting the "best" good catches each month are publicly celebrated with their names and pictures posted in several places throughout the department. They are given a modest gift certificate for our hospital's eatery, and they are asked to sign the department basketball that is on display in our trophy case. The event reporting system is purposefully named "Good Catch" to provide a positive connotation to participation.[66,67] The American Society of Radiation Oncology launched the Radiation Oncology Incident Learning System (RO-ILS) in 2014 to provide a standardized system for analyzing incidents/errors and providing shared learning across the radiation oncology profession.

- *Safety rounds*: Departmental leaders speak with front-line employees about their work, for example, what is good, what can be better, how we can improve things for them, and do they have the tools they need to work safety, efficiently, and reliability? These discussions occur *at their workstations*, not in a conference room or office, as a sign of respect for the workers, and so leadership can better appreciate the issues being discussed. The goal is to improve performance of the overall system, empower workers to think about how they can make improvements, and help build a culture of respect and improvement. Safety rounds, with visits to several locations in our department, occur every 3 months with the goal of reaching all areas at least annually.[48,68]

- *Huddles*: Suboptimal communication is one of the most common factors implicated in root cause analyses of critical events. Huddles, brief meetings among various members of work teams, held at regularly scheduled times, is an approach attempting to improve communication. For example, we ask our clinical teams (e.g., nurses, residents, and faculty) to briefly huddle at the start of a clinic day to review the schedule and identify any anticipated challenges (e.g., conflicts, double-bookings) that may be mitigated or accommodated. We also have a daily department-wide huddle where that day's planned clinical work is reviewed, again to identify and plan for anticipated challenges. The daily list of patients due for treatment planning and CT simulation is reviewed. Staff have the opportunity to seek clarifications regarding ambiguities in any of the directives, and the names of the doctor, resident, physicist, and dosimetrist "of the day" are reviewed. It is a time for announcements, introductions of visitors, and brief discussions of any items of broad interest or concern. These daily departmental huddles serve a social function, can help improve interpersonal and organizational communication, and break down unnecessary hierarchies.[56,69,70]

- *Time-outs*: These are formal standardized methods to help review the most crucial aspects of the radiation planning and delivery process (similar to a presurgery checklist in an operating room). Our dosimetrists and faculty perform a time-out at the time of signing the treatment plan and prescription to review the dose per fraction, number of fractions, treatment site, and the presence or absence of receipt of prior radiation, which aids in identifying possible overlap issues. Our radiation therapists perform a similar time-out on the first day of a patient setup on the treatment machine.[71–73]

- *Peer review*: Peer review can be loosely defined as the process whereby providers evaluate the quality of their colleague's work to ensure that prevailing care standards are met. Typically, peer review is most valuable for the

Goal: High Reliability and Value Creation

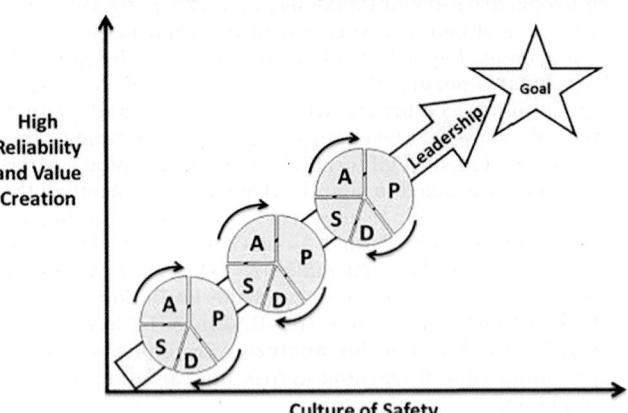

Improvement Cycle: P - Plan **D** - Do **S** - Study **A** - Act

FIGURE 102.5. This conceptual figure illustrates the symbiotic relationship between the culture of safety (*x*-axis), high reliability and value creation (*y*-axis), and continuous improvement cycles (PDSA). Each of these components is mutually dependent and reinforces the other. As such, the relative positions of the three components are somewhat arbitrary. At the organization level, leaders must be the driving force behind improvement cycles, which promote the culture of safety (e.g., safety mindfulness among the staff and robust systems). Similarly, there must be some degree of a culture of safety in order to successfully perform the PDSA cycles. Building a culture of safety and systematically improving processes through the PDSA approach will increase reliability and value creation. The sizes of the pie charts on the leadership arrow pointing toward the goal (shown using a star symbol in the top right corner) are deliberate, with Plan (P) being the largest, indicating the need for thoughtful planning and readiness of all stakeholders before relatively rapid improvements, Doing (D), Studying (S), and Acting (A), as no major improvement can be typically achieved in one leap. (The figure is conceptually adopted from teaching of Mark Chassin, President and Chief Executive Officer at Joint Commission, 2012 Institute for Healthcare Improvement (IHI) Annual Conference.)

somewhat subjective aspects of work that are not readily amenable to objective assessment. In medicine, this is often done retrospectively through chart review *after* patients complete their treatment. This retrospective approach can be helpful to detect shortcomings that can be addressed or to reinforce positive actions to improve care for future patients. However (obviously), for an individual patient's case, peer review done *prior* to therapy or early during the course of therapy is better than peer review done later or after therapy is completed.

Peer review in radiation oncology appears to be a useful tool to improve patient care[74–76] and has been strongly endorsed by several national and international organizations.[72] As in medicine in general, peer review done prior to, or early in the course of radiation treatment, is likely to be most useful. Indeed, radiation treatment plans that deviate from standard protocols are associated with inferior patient outcomes (i.e., cancer control and survival), and prospective peer review holds promise to improve patient outcomes.[15,16]

Despite the promise of peer review, our field has not broadly embraced its full potential. For example, a recent survey of North American academic radiation oncology centers noted marked variation in the use of peer review.[77] Further, based on discussions with colleagues nationally, it is our impression that most peer review is done after treatment has been initiated, rather than prior to treatment. Because there is much effort required to make adjustments after therapy has been initiated, many suggested adjustments may not be made (or perhaps some suggestions are not even offered because the potential associated rework is so high). To address this issue in our clinic, we perform pretreatment peer review of essentially all cases. For patients undergoing

conventional 3-D or IMRT planning the broad treatment plan and goals are discussed. All image segmentations are reviewed prior to planning, for the IMRT cases. This work is performed daily, immediately prior to our department huddle, and both meetings are often blended together (e.g., if the treatment planning computers are slow in bringing up the next patient for peer review, we will perform parts of the huddle during that hiatus).

CONCLUSIONS

Our field is highly technical and errors can result from technical failures. However, the practice of radiation oncology is largely a human endeavor, and most errors are strongly linked to "human-based aspects" (e.g., workflows, communication, human–machine interactions). Our systems currently behave somewhat unpredictably (because of many interactive variables), and the resulting complexity requires an ongoing robust embrace of CQI; there are no easy fixes. Our field can only achieve very high levels of reliability if we acknowledge these complexities and our challenges as human beings working in a complex system. We need to embrace a culture of safety, where leaders and workers together openly identify existing waste or shortcomings and generate improved systems that are more reliable and efficient (Fig. 102.5). For example, we can, and should, more systematically standardize our processes as a means to reduce complexity. A greater understanding is needed of the multifaceted causes of errors as well as systematically and openly discussing and addressing our latent failures. They occur all around us and are currently tolerated given they largely do not lead to major problems (except when they do). The many strategies outlined in this chapter, proven successful in many industries, can be more broadly applied in our field to reduce the risks of errors. We owe this to our patients and to ourselves.

REFERENCES

1. Kohn LT, Corrigan J, Donaldson MS. *To err is human: building a safer health system.* Washington, DC: National Academy Press, 2000:xxi, 287 p.
2. Institute of Medicine (U.S.). Committee on Quality of Health Care in America. *Crossing the quality chasm: a new health system for the 21st century.* Washington, DC: National Academy Press, 2001:xx, 337 p.
3. Edelstein L. *The Hippocratic Oath: text, translation and interpretation by Ludwig Edelstein.* Baltimore, MD: The Johns Hopkins Press (1943), 1994:1.
4. Nightingale F. *Notes on hospitals.* 3rd ed. London, UK: Longman, Green, Longman, Roberts, and Green, 1863:ix p., 1 l., 187 p.
5. Leape LL. Error in medicine. *JAMA* 1994;272(23):1851–1857.
6. World Health Organization. *Radiotherapy risk profile. Technical manual.* Geneva: WHO Publishing, 2007.
7. Bogadanich W. Safety features planned for radiation machines. *New York Times,* 2010.
8. Bogadanich W. VA is fined over errors in radiation at hospital. *New York Times,* 2010.
9. Bogadanich W. Radiation errors reported in Missouri. *New York Times,* 2010.
10. Bogadanich W. Radiation offers new cures and ways to do harm. *New York Times,* 2010.
11. Peiffert D, Simon JM, Eschwege F. Epinal radiotherapy accident: passed, present, future. *Cancer Radiother* 2007;11(6–7):309–312.
12. ASTRO. *Safety is no accident: a framework for quality radiation oncology and care,* 2012. https://www.astro.org/uploadedFiles/Main_Site/Clinical_Practice/Patient_Safety/Blue_Book/SafetyisnoAccident.pdf
13. NHS Department of Health Expert Group (Chairman, CMO). An organization with a memory. *Report of an expert group on learning from adverse events in the NHS,* 2000:92. http://webarchive.nationalarchives.gov.uk/20130105144251/http://www.dh.gov.uk/prod_consum_dh/groups/dh_digitalassets/@dh/@en/documents/digitalasset/dh_4065086.pdf
14. Cunningham J, et al. Radiation Oncology Safety Information System (ROSIS)—profiles of participants and the first 1074 incident reports. *Radiother Oncol* 2010;97(3):601–607.
15. Ohri N, et al. Radiotherapy protocol deviations and clinical outcomes: a meta-analysis of cooperative group clinical trials. *J Natl Cancer Inst* 2013; 105(6):387–393.

16. Peters LJ, et al. Critical impact of radiotherapy protocol compliance and quality in the treatment of advanced head and neck cancer: results from TROG 02.02. *J Clin Oncol* 2010;28(18):2996–3001.

17. Weber DC, et al. QA makes a clinical trial stronger: evidence-based medicine in radiation therapy. *Radiother Oncol* 2012;105(1):4–8.

18. Scalliet PG. Effect of clinical routine on patients' outcome. *Lancet* 2004;363(9414):1079.

19. Marks LB, et al. The need for physician leadership in creating a culture of safety. *Int J Radiat Oncol Biol Phys* 2011;79(5):1287–1289.

20. Potters L, Bloom B. Our pledge to achieve safety. *Int J Radiat Oncol Biol Phys* 2012;82(4):1310–1311.

21. Chera BS, et al. Improving quality of patient care by improving daily practice in radiation oncology. *Semin Radiat Oncol* 2012;22(1):77–85.

22. Reinertsen JL, Gosfield AG, Rupp W, et al. *Engaging physicians in a shared quality agenda. IHI Innovation Series white paper.* Cambridge, MA: Institute for Healthcare Improvement, 2007.

23. Bass BM. *Leadership and performance beyond expectations.* New York/London: Free Press/Collier Macmillan, 1985: xvi, 256 p.

24. Burns JM. *Leadership.* 1st ed. New York, NY: Harper & Row, 1978:ix, 530 p.

25. Podsakoff PM, MacKenzie SB, Bommer WH. Transformational leader behaviors and substitutes for leadership as determinants of employee satisfaction, commitment, trust, and organizational citizenship. *J Air Waste Manage Assoc* 1996;22(2):259–298.

26. Aiken LH, et al. An international perspective on hospital nurses' work environments: the case for reform. *Policy Politics Nurs Pract* 2001;2(4):255–263.

27. Bogdanich W. Medical group urges new rules on radiation. *New York Times*, 2010.

28. Bogdanich W. As technology surges, radiation safeguards lag. *New York Times*, 2010:A1.

29. Bono JE, Anderson MH. The advice and influence networks of transformational leaders. *J Appl Psychol* 2005;90(6):1306.

30. McIntyre N, Popper K. The critical attitude in medicine: the need for a new ethics. *Br Med J (Clin Res Ed)* 1983;287(6409):1919–1923.

31. Reason J. *Human error.* Cambridge, UK: Cambridge University Press, 1990.

32. Shappel SA, Wiegmann DA. *The human factors analysis and classification system—HFACS.* Washington, DC. U.S. Federal Aviation Administration, Office of Aviation Medicine, 2000.

33. Portaluri M, et al. Incidents analysis in radiation therapy: application of the human factors analysis and classification system. *Ann Ist Super Sanita* 2008;45(2):128–133.

34. Rashid H, Place C, Braithwaite G. Helicopter maintenance error analysis: beyond the third order of the HFACS-ME. *Int J Ind Ergon* 2010;40(6):636–647.

35. Patterson JM, Shappell SA. Operator error and system deficiencies: analysis of 508 mining incidents and accidents from Queensland, Australia using HFACS. *Accid Anal Prev* 2010;42(4):1379–1385.

36. Baysari MT, McIntosh AS, Wilson JR. Understanding the human factors contribution to railway accidents and incidents in Australia. *Accid Anal Prev* 2008;40(5):1750–1757.

37. Celik M, Cebi S. Analytical HFACS for investigating human errors in shipping accidents. *Accid Anal Prev* 2009;41(1):66–75.

38. Walker D. Applying the human factors analysis and classification system (HFACS) to incidents in the UK construction industry, 2007. *Master's Thesis*, Cranfield University, Bedford, UK.

39. ElBardissi AW, et al. Application of the human factors analysis and classification system methodology to the cardiovascular surgery operating room. *Ann Thorac Surg* 2007;83(4):1412–1419.

40. Iden R, Shappell SA. A human error analysis of US fatal highway crashes 1990–2004. *Proceedings of the Human Factors and Ergonomics Society Annual Meeting.* Sage Publications, 2006.

41. Perrow C. *Normal accidents: living with high-risk technologies.* Princeton paperbacks. Princeton, NJ: Princeton University Press, 1999:x, 451 p.

42. Stamatis DH. *Failure mode and effect analysis: FMEA from theory to execution.* Milwaukee, WI: ASQ Quality Press, 2003.

43. Sheridan-Leos N, Schulmeister L, Hartranft S. Failure mode and effect analysis (TM): a technique to prevent chemotherapy errors. *Clin J Oncol Nurs* 2006;10(3):393.

44. Duwe B, Fuchs BD, Hansen-Flaschen J. Failure mode and effects analysis application to critical care medicine. *Crit Care Clin* 2005;21(1):21–30.

45. Wetterneck TB, et al. Using failure mode and effects analysis to plan implementation of smart iv pump technology. *Am J Health Syst Pharm* 2006;63(16):1528–1538.

46. Huq MS, et al. A method for evaluating quality assurance needs in radiation therapy. *Int J Radiat Oncol Biol Phys* 2008;71(1):S170–S173.

47. Ford EC, et al. Evaluation of safety in a radiation oncology setting using failure mode and effects analysis. *Int J Radiat Oncol Biol Phys* 2009;74(3):852–858.

48. Edmondson A, Moingeon B. From organizational learning to the learning organization. *Manage Learn* 1998;29(1):5–20.

49. Edmondson A. Psychological safety and learning behavior in work teams. *Adm Sci Q* 1999;44(2):350–383.

50. Ohno T. *Toyota production system: beyond large-scale production.* Boca Raton, FL: CRC Press, 1988.

51. Shah R, Ward PT. Defining and developing measures of lean production. *J Oper Manage* 2007;25(4):785–805.

52. Miller D. *Going lean in health care.* IHI Innovation Series White Paper. Cambridge, MA: Institute for Healthcare Improvement, 2005:2013.

53. Mazur LM, Chen S-JG. Understanding and reducing the medication delivery waste via systems mapping and analysis. *Health Care Manage Sci* 2008;11(1):55–65.

54. Mazur LM. Evaluation of industrial engineering students' competencies for process improvement in hospitals. *J Ind Eng Manage* 2010;3(3):603.

55. Mazur LM, Chen S-JG, Prescott B. Pragmatic evaluation of the Toyota Production System (TPS) analysis procedure for problem solving with entry-level nurses. *J Ind Eng Manage* 2008;1(2):240–268.

56. Roberts KH. Some characteristics of high reliability organizations. *Org Sci* 1990;1:160–177.

57. Roberts KH, Bea R. Must accidents happen? Lessons from high-reliability organizations. *Acad Manage Exec* 2001;15:70–79.

58. Leape L, et al. Transforming healthcare: a safety imperative. *Qual Saf Health Care* 2009;18(6):424–428.

59. Agency for Healthcare Research and Quality. Surveys on patient safety culture, 2015. [cited 2015]; Available: http://www.ahrq.gov/professionals/quality-patient-safety/patientsafetyculture/index.html

60. Mardon RE, et al. Exploring relationships between hospital patient safety culture and adverse events. *J Patient Saf* 2010;6(4):226–232.

61. Chassin MR, Loeb JM. The ongoing quality improvement journey: next stop, high reliability. *Health Aff* 2011;30(4):559–568.

62. La Porte TR. High reliability organizations: unlikely, demanding and at risk. *J Conting Crisis Manage* 1996;4(2):60–71.

63. Perrow C. *Normal accidents: living with high-risk technologies.* New York, NY: Basic Books, 1984

64. Roberts KH, Bea R, Bartles DL. Must accidents happen? Lessons from high-reliability organizations. *Acad Manage Exec* 2001;15(3):70–78.

65. Roberts KH. Some characteristics of one type of high reliability organization. *Org Sci* 1990;1(2):160–176.

66. Das P, et al. Rate of radiation therapy events in a large academic institution. *J Am Coll Radiol* 2013;10(6):452–455.

67. Herzer KR, et al. Patient safety reporting systems: sustained quality improvement using a multidisciplinary team and "good catch" awards. *Jt Comm J Qual Patient Saf* 2012;38(8):339–347.

68. Lukasz M, Mazur JKM, Chen S-J. Quality improvement in hospitals: identifying and understanding behaviors. *J Healthcare Eng* 2012;3(4):621–648.

69. Fine BA, et al. Leading lean: a Canadian healthcare leader's guide. *Healthcare Q* 2009;12(3):32–41.

70. Montgomery VL. Impact of staff-led safety walk rounds. In: Henriksen K, Battles JB, Keyes MA, et al., eds. *Advances in patient safety: new directions and alternative approaches (Vol. 3: Performance and tools).* Agency for Healthcare Research and Quality, 2008.

71. Gawande A. *The checklist manifesto: how to get things right.* 1st ed. New York, NY: Metropolitan Books, 2010:x, 209 p.

72. Marks LB, et al. Enhancing the role of case-oriented peer review to improve quality and safety in radiation oncology: executive summary. *Pract Radiat Oncol* 2013;3(3):149–156.

73. Marks L, et al. Improving safety for patients receiving radiotherapy: the successful application of quality assurance initiatives. *Int J Radiat Oncol Biol Phys* 2008;72(1):S143.

74. Brundage MD, et al. A real-time audit of radiation therapy in a regional cancer center. *Int J Radiat Oncol Biol Phys* 1999;43(1):115–124.

75. Shakespeare TP, et al. Evaluation of an audit with feedback continuing medical education program for radiation oncologists. *J Cancer Educ* 2005;20(4):216–221.

76. Boxer M, et al. Impact of a real-time peer review audit on patient management in a radiation oncology department. *J Med Imaging Radiat Oncol* 2009;53(4):405–411.

77. Lawrence YR, et al. Quality assurance peer review chart rounds in 2011: a survey of academic institutions in the United States. *Int J Radiat Oncol Biol Phys* 2012;84(3):590–595.

78. Marks L, et al. *Engineering patient safety in radiation oncology: University of North Carolina's pursuit for high reliability and value creation.* Boca Raton, FL: Taylor & Francis, 2015.

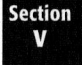

Section
V

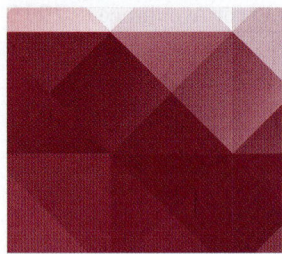

CHAPTER 103

Radiation Oncology Education

Daniel W. Golden and Paris-Ann Ingledew

INTRODUCTION

Radiation oncology is a unique specialty that requires a broad knowledge base, as it is one of the few specialties that deliver care to patients from all age groups and all genders and interfaces with a multitude of medical specialties. The radiation oncologist must have the requisite clinical skills necessary to evaluate a new patient at the time of consultation, appropriately stage a tumor,[1] assess treatment planning scans for extent of tumor to delineate target volumes and organs at risk accurately,[2] and evaluate patients during and after treatment for radiation toxicities and signs of tumor recurrence.[3] In order to do this, radiation oncologists must not only have a solid foundational knowledge of oncology, tumor biology, physics, and radiation delivery but also be versed in a variety of additional areas including communication, collaboration, patient advocacy, and health system management.[4,5] Other professions that work as part of the radiation oncology care team, including medical physics,[6,7] dosimetry,[8] radiation therapy,[9] nursing,[10,11] social work,[12] and physical therapy,[13] also have specific skill sets that are acquired during training and continue to develop while working in the radiation oncology clinic. Although the focus of this chapter is education for radiation oncologists, to provide optimal patient-centered care, the educational process for all of these professions ideally is coordinated in a complementary fashion, with each member of the interprofessional and interdisciplinary radiation oncology team optimally trained to deliver high-quality, effective, and compassionate patient care (Fig. 103.1).

Descriptions of radiation oncology educational training programs can be found in the literature dating from the 1950s,[14] and currently, radiation oncology training programs exist worldwide.[15–23] Despite the abundance of established training programs, there is little literature discussing the core aspects of medical education and its application to radiation oncology. The goals of this chapter therefore are to describe fundamental educational theory and processes necessary to develop an effective radiation oncology educational curriculum, to review current educational practices in radiation oncology, and to identify potential areas for radiation oncology educational scholarship. Physician training at the undergraduate (medical school), graduate (residency and fellowship), and continuing medical education (CME) (attending physician) levels primarily will be used to frame this discussion, but the concepts, theory, and methods described can be applied to education of other health professions involved in radiation oncology clinical care.

BACKGROUND

The day-to-day practice of medical education in radiation oncology needs to be considered within the broader context of learning theories. It is essential to look beyond the oncology

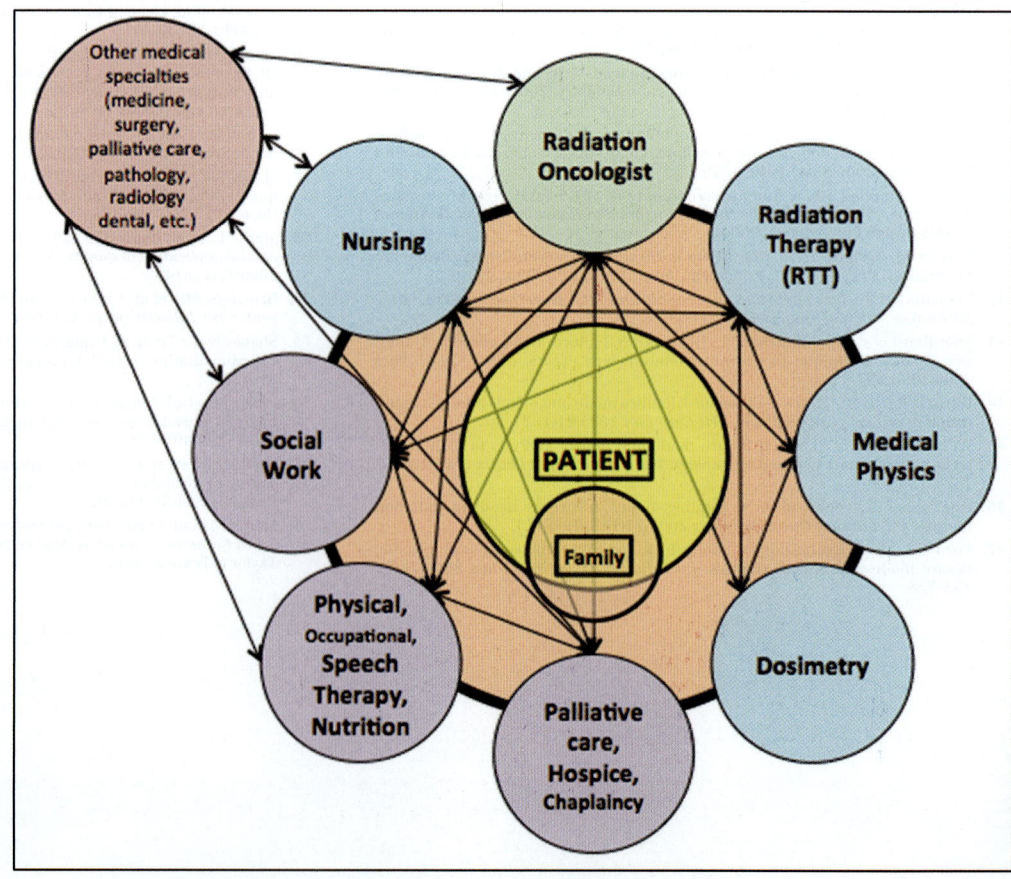

FIGURE 103.1. Interprofessional care of the radiation oncology patient.

literature, and even outside of the medical literature, to understand the best practices for medical education and curriculum development.

Learning Theory

Much of the literature surrounding learning has differentiated between "andragogy," or adult learning defined as "the method and practice of teaching adult learners," viewed as unique from "pedagogy," which is defined as "the method and practice of teaching" but which literally means "leading children." There is considerable debate surrounding this differentiation. Rather than present a detailed discussion of the history and controversies in learning theory, concepts of learning theories will be discussed in relation to the range of adult learners in radiation oncology from medical student to practicing radiation oncologists. The basic concepts of most learning theories are based on behavioral change and transformative experiences. The goal of any educational intervention is to effect a behavioral change in the learner through some form of experience. Examples within radiation oncology include improving physician–patient interactions (behavior) through an objective simulated clinical exam (experience),[24] improving brachytherapy technique (behavior) through simulation-based education (experience),[25] and improving contour accuracy (behavior) through a simulated contouring workshop (experience).[2]

To help understand the process by which educational interventions can result in changes in behaviors, learning models can be informative. Kolb's experiential learning model (Fig. 103.2) describes a four-step cycle of learning that includes a concrete experience, reflective observation, abstract conceptualization, and active experimentation.[26] Similarly, Merriam et al.[27] describe three keys to transformational learning including (a) experience, (b) critical reflection, and (c) development. Collins[28] frames adult learning in the context of studying theory and applying it to practice. Others propose that the two fundamental components of adult learning are critical thinking and self-directed learning.[29,30]

Taken together, educational opportunities that allow for concrete experiences, application, and the opportunity for reflection are best aligned with these principles.

Learning theory can be enhanced by an understanding of the six assumptions regarding characteristics of the adult learner as defined by Knowles et al.[31] (Fig. 103.3). These six assumptions can be applied to learning in radiation oncology. For example, in the case of a radiation oncology residency training program, the residents must understand why, what, and how they are going to learn their chosen profession. They need to have some autonomy and control over their learning within the structure of the residency training program. Therefore, when the radiation oncology educator is developing an adult learning experience, consideration should be given to Knowles' six assumptions, what behavior the curriculum or educational intervention intends to change, and how the learning experiences will stimulate critical thinking, self-directed learning, and transformation.

Lastly, to optimize learning, it is important for medical educators to consider the learning environment when designing an educational program. The Hebbian version of the Yerkes-Dodson law suggests that learners have an optimal level of arousal, or stress, that will promote optimal learning (Fig. 103.4).[32,33] At very low levels of stress and arousal, the learner is not stimulated enough to learn. An example is an early morning resident lecture with no postlecture knowledge assessment. The stakes for the resident learner are low, and the resident may not engage with the presentation to learn. As arousal increases, an optimal point is encountered on the learning curve where stress optimally enhances learning without negatively impacting it. As stress continues to increase, learning begins to decline because of stress impeding higher-level cognitive process such as attention, working memory, and problem-solving. Thus, the radiation oncology educator must consider stressors on the trainees (both positive and negative) and determine if the amount of stress within a given learning environment will facilitate optimal learning. Examples of

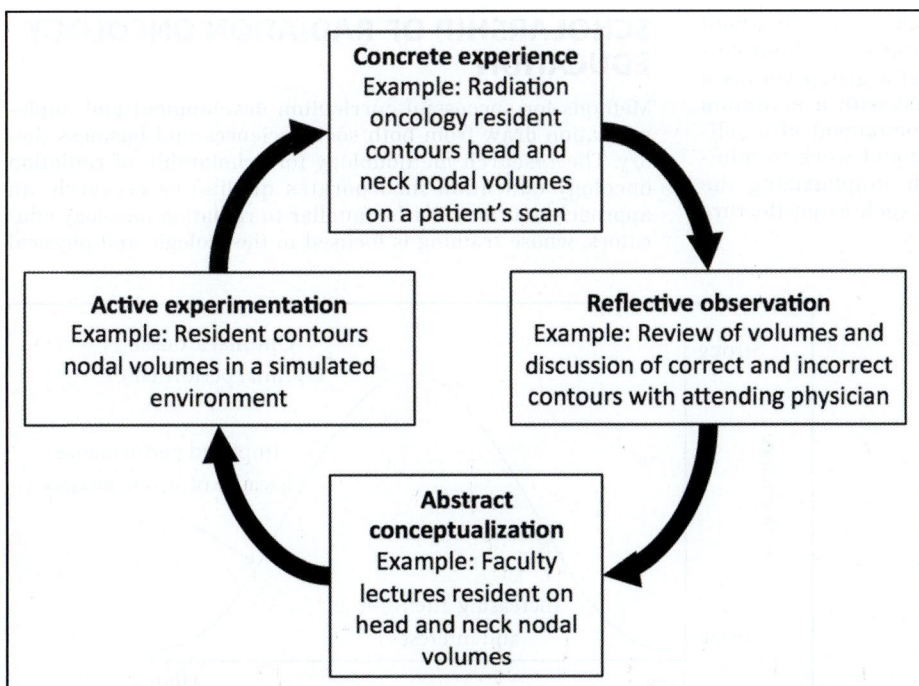

FIGURE 103.2. Kolb's experiential learning model in relation to radiation oncology educational activities. (Adapted from Kolb DA. *Experiential learning: Experience as the source of learning and development.* 2nd ed. Upper Saddle River, NJ: Pearson Education, 2015:51. Copyright © 2015. Reprinted by permission of Pearson Education, Inc., New York.)

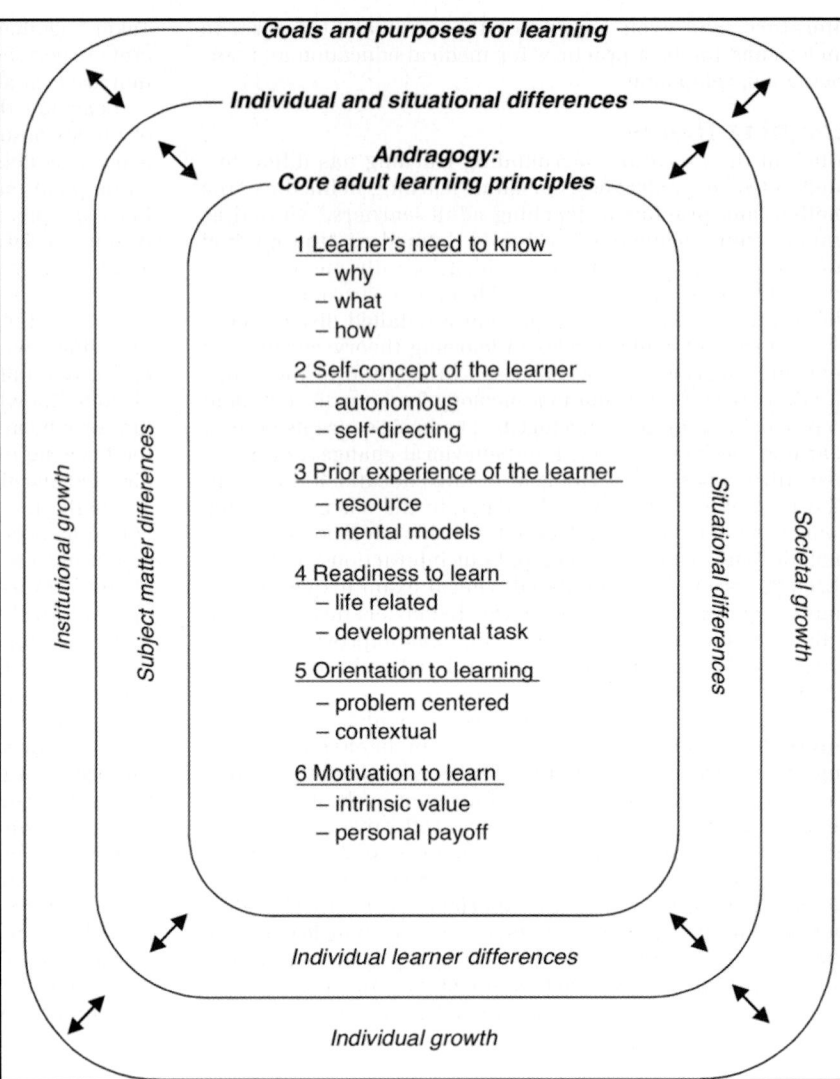

FIGURE 103.3. Knowles and Swanson's six assumptions of adult learning. (From Knowles MS, Holton EF III, Swanson RA. *The adult learner: the definitive classic in adult education and human resource development.* 8th ed. New York: Routledge, 2014:6. Copyright © 2015 Knowles MS, Holton EF III, Swanson RA. Reproduced by permission of Taylor and Francis Group, LLC, a division of Informa plc.)

pertinent stressors include medical student anxiety about securing a residency position, resident anxiety about certification boards, presenting in front of a group versus a single listener, or a multiple-choice test with a minimum score required to obtain credit as a component of a self-assessment CME module. Educators should work to minimize undue (negative) stressors while emphasizing the rationale for planned positive stressors such as postlecture knowledge assessments.

SCHOLARSHIP OF RADIATION ONCOLOGY EDUCATION

Methods for successful curriculum development and implementation draw from both social sciences and business theory. The research methodology for scholarship of radiation oncology education incorporates qualitative research, an approach that may not be familiar to radiation oncology educators, whose training is focused in the biologic and physical

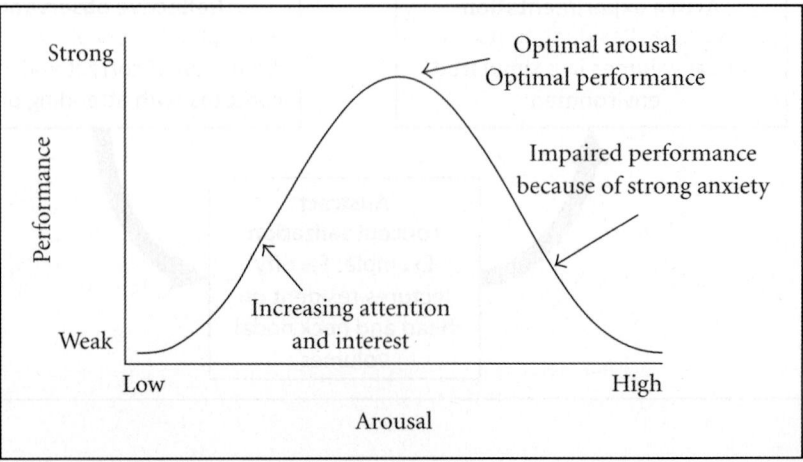

FIGURE 103.4. Hebbian version of the Yerkes-Dodson law correlating arousal with performance.

sciences. This section reviews the concepts of scholarship as relevant to radiation oncology education and provides an introduction to qualitative methods and conceptual frameworks useful to radiation oncology educational scholarship.

Scholarship in Medical Education

When undertaking any medical education intervention, careful attention should be given at the outset for opportunities for scholarship.[34] Boyer[35] defines four types of scholarship including the scholarship of discovery, the scholarship of application, the scholarship of integration, and the scholarship of teaching. The scholarship of discovery refers to scholarly activities for the purpose of finding new knowledge and best encompasses our traditional view of research.[35,36] The scholarship of integration refers to scholarship that draws on other research and draws across disciplines or extends research to new areas and beyond boundaries helping to illuminate relationships.[35,36] The scholarship of application takes knowledge and applies it in new and practical ways.[35,37] Finally, the scholarship of teaching refers to teaching practices approached with a scholarly lens. This expanded definition of scholarship allows for many activities in medical education to be viewed as grounds for scholarship outside of research projects.

Scholarship is defined as a tangible product of knowledge or its presentation that is peer-reviewed and disseminated publicly.[38] Hutchings and Shulman[39] define the following three essential criteria for scholarship:

1. The work must be made public.
2. The work must be available for peer review and critique according to accepted standards.
3. The work must be able to be reproduced and built on by other scholars.

Criteria for excellence in scholarship can be applied to educational scholarship and help to assess the quality of scholarship. Glassick[40] defines six criteria to assess scholarship:

1. Clear goals
2. Adequate preparation
3. Appropriate methods
4. Significant results
5. Effective presentation
6. Reflective critique

Application of these criteria assists the radiation oncology educator to evaluate the potential to turn a medical education project into a work of scholarship. For example, a novel resident training curriculum implemented at a single institution and not disseminated in peer-reviewed literature does not qualify as scholarship based on the above definition. However, if the residency program director publishes learner assessment and program evaluation data in a peer-reviewed journal or disseminates the curriculum materials using MedEdPORTAL, the implementation and evaluation of the curriculum qualify as scholarship.

The difference between scholarly teaching and the scholarship of teaching must also be defined. Fincher and Work[41] define three levels of teaching (Fig. 103.5). The first level is basic teaching. In radiation oncology, basic teaching examples include giving a lecture, facilitating a case conference, demonstrating proper history-taking technique or brachytherapy technique to trainees, or educating patients regarding the radiation treatment process and potential toxicities.

The next level is scholarly teaching. This implies that the instructor is using evidence-based practices when teaching trainees. Examples in radiation oncology could include using best practices when delivering a PowerPoint presentation,[42] providing patient educational materials at or below the sixth grade reading level,[43] or using the 1-minute preceptor model to teach a clinical pearl to a resident after an initial consultation.[44]

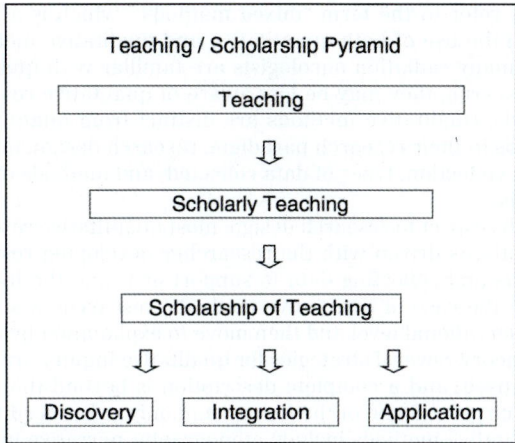

FIGURE 103.5. Fincher and Work's pyramid of teaching and scholarship. (From E Fincher R-M, Work JA. Perspectives on the scholarship of teaching. *Med Educ* 2006;40[4]:293–295. Copyright © 2006 Blackwell Publishing Ltd. Reprinted by permission of John Wiley & Sons, Inc.)

The third tier is scholarship of teaching, which includes developing and disseminating new knowledge through discovery, integration, or application. Drawing from Boyer,[35,40] discovery refers to obtaining new knowledge in a discipline. Scholarship examples in this context include the evaluation of new innovations or interventions. Examples in radiation oncology include demonstrating that students who participate in a radiation oncology clerkship with a didactic curriculum report increased confidence to function as a resident,[45] utilizing a novel Internet-based contouring tool that can improve target delineation accuracy,[46] and demonstrating that inclusion of a radiation oncology lecture in the medical school curriculum is feasible and increases objective knowledge of the specialty.[47]

Scholarship of integration refers to making connections across scholarship and synthesizing data across studies.[40] Examples include a literature review of radiation oncology teaching in the undergraduate setting[48] or a Best Evidence in Medical Education systematic review on faculty development initiatives aimed to improve teaching effectiveness.[49] The scholarship of application bridges theory with practice often drawing together fields and disciplines.[35,50] In the context of radiation oncology, this could include assessing the value of simulation in brachytherapy training,[25] bringing simulation which is well utilized in other specialties to radiation oncology, and evaluating the impact on learner performance.

Without scholarship in radiation oncology education, educational programs will advance slowly. Individual training programs will be unaware of the best practices implemented at other training programs and may develop redundant educational material, which introduces inefficiency in a process that is already limited in resources. Just as clinical oncology and basic science research is disseminated as manuscripts in peer-reviewed journals, novel radiation oncology educational initiatives must be rigorously developed and evaluated in preparation for dissemination to the international radiation oncology community.[34] However, because of limitations of journal publication alone in effecting change,[51] programs such as the Radiation Oncology Education Collaborative Study Group[52] have been established to improve dissemination and implementation of educational research and programs. These processes allow other institutions to adopt or adapt novel educational initiatives and subsequently build on them for further dissemination.

Qualitative Versus Quantitative Research

For health profession educators, scholarly research comes from both quantitative and qualitative sources, and many studies benefit from the use of both simultaneously.[53] Some studies refer to the term "mixed methods," which is a reference to the use of both quantitative and qualitative methods. While many radiation oncologists are familiar with quantitative research, they may be less aware of qualitative research methods. Qualitative methods are distinct from quantitative methods in their research paradigm, research design, method of data collection, types of data collected, and methods of data analysis.

With respect to research design, most quantitative research is hypothesis driven with the researcher developing research methods and collecting data to support or refute the hypothesis. In the case of qualitative methods, researchers start at the observational level and then move to explanation by building a theory. Several strategies for qualitative inquiry are commonly used, and a complete description is beyond the scope of this chapter. Some of the more commonly referenced terms in qualitative methods include ethnography, narrative inquiry, and grounded theory approach. Ethnographic research encompasses a variety of research techniques aimed at characterizing the authentic everyday experiences of subjects through observation and interviews.[54,55] An example of ethnographic research is a study utilizing detailed interviews with teaching faculty and observations of their teaching patterns on the ward to identify the characteristics of effective clinical teachers.[56] Narrative research is the study of participants through the analysis of documents.[55] Usually the participant describes one or more pivotal life events and the researcher looks to describe these events. Finally, grounded theory is a term used in qualitative methods to describe the process in which a "theory" is generated from data of the experiences of the participants.[55] Unlike quantitative research that starts with a theory, the grounded approach uses data to generate theory by looking for emerging themes through a process of constant comparative analysis.[54] Data are collected through interviews, document analysis, and focus groups. In a grounded theory approach, as data are collected, a theory is generated, then more data are collected, and the theory is revised as needed, continuing the process until it appears that the theory is relatively robust. An example of grounded theory methodology in radiation oncology is the use of focus groups and in-depth interviews to develop a four-step learning process for implementation of high-precision radiation technology: (a) Anxiety as new skills are acquired, (b) learning to interpret new imaging and findings while continuing to experience uncertainty, (c) questioning assumptions and critical reflection resulting in new understanding, and (d) constructing new knowledge through research, development, and dialogue.[57]

The processes and methods used in qualitative studies include distinguishable methods that help to build observations to support explanations.[58] Methods of data collection include focus groups, one-on-one interviews, surveys with open-ended questions, observations of behaviors, and document analysis (e.g., themes in portfolios). Unlike quantitative data that are numeric, the data collected in a qualitative study are usually text or words. For example, data may be collected in the form of words, or even pictures, rather than numbers. The analysis of qualitative data is an iterative process to conceptualize and reduce data, analyze it to develop themes, elaborate on categories, and find relationships.[54] Common to qualitative methods, steps are taken to ensure reliability of the themes developed through stages of analysis. This may include having coraters of themes, peer review from others not involved in the study, checking the themes with study participants, and triangulation with established literature. Ultimately the goal of qualitative research is to develop hypotheses, building theory through descriptions of observations, and to describe and explain complex phenomena by analyzing data for themes and relationships. Table 103.1 summarizes key differences between quantitative and qualitative methods.

TABLE 103.1 SUMMARY OF DIFFERENCES BETWEEN QUALITATIVE AND QUANTITATIVE RESEARCH

	Quantitative Research	Qualitative Research
Research paradigm	– Deductive Research – Collect data to test hypothesis	– Inductive Research – Observations to explain and then develop theory
Research method examples	– Closed-ended surveys (i.e., demographics of current radiation training programs) – Observations of time taken to complete a task (i.e., contouring)	– Open-ended surveys (i.e., resident descriptions of current challenges in training programs) – Observational study (i.e., observations of differences of learner's contouring abilities at different stages of training) – Document analysis (i.e., analysis of learner's portfolio reflections on dealing with difficult cancer patients)
Data	– Numeric data	– Words as data

Qualitative research is important to medical education. There are certain educational research questions that are best approached using qualitative research methods[59] such as:

1. "How does charting influence the quality and quantity of communication between different health care professionals?
2. How do health care professionals learn to teach on the job?
3. What constitutes "professional competence" and how is that different from "professional identity"?
4. What influences patients' adherence with their doctor's suggestions?"

Qualitative methods can be used specifically for radiation oncology scholarship in multiple settings (Table 103.2). For example, qualitative methods can be used to develop and evaluate a program to teach radiation oncology residents communication skills with elderly cancer patients. One-on-one interviews, focus groups, and surveys with open-ended questions could be used to conduct a targeted needs assessment of learners (see curriculum development below) prior to developing a new educational program. The results would inform the development of the program. Later, reflections on the new training program, collected through repeated one-on-one interviews, surveys, and analysis of reflective writing exercises, could be used to systematically evaluate the program once implemented. Years later, the clinical behaviors of oncologists in practice could be observed to reflect on the

TABLE 103.2 EXAMPLES OF USE OF QUALITATIVE METHODS IN RADIATION ONCOLOGY EDUCATION

Educational Issue	Qualitative Approach
Analyzing "memorable" in-training experiences of medical students on radiation oncology rotations[248]	Thematic analysis of written narratives to describe the training experiences of learners in a clinical education program
Needs assessment for development of a radiation oncology curriculum for medical students[174]	Analysis of written responses to open-ended surveys to analyze for gaps and strengths in current training Thematic analysis of one-on-one interviews with stakeholders
Establishing needs and priorities in a global radiation oncology training programs[249]	Facilitated group discussion with analysis of themes to develop consensus on possible goals and objectives for a training program
Evaluation of a contouring boot camp[18]	Thematic analysis of open-ended survey questions to provide evaluation data
Evaluation of a didactic curriculum for a radiation oncology medical student clerkship[181]	Thematic analysis of open-ended survey questions to provide evaluation data

retention of skills in learners and the impact of the program on their communication skills. Utilizing both qualitative and quantitative methods for program development facilitates development and improvement of a training program in a scholarly manner.

Conceptual Frameworks

When approaching radiation oncology medical education endeavors through a scholarly lens, it is critical to define one or more conceptual frameworks used to guide the educational process. While medical education scholars often employ conceptual frameworks in curriculum development and program evaluation, it is helpful to be able to identify them. A systematic review found that a lack of a conceptual framework is one of the most common reasons education scholarship is rejected for publication.[60]

Conceptual frameworks are "ways of thinking about a problem or a study, or ways of representing how complex things work the way they do. Different frameworks will emphasize different variables and outcomes, and their inter-relatedness."[61] Conceptual frameworks are not mutually exclusive, and there is the potential to apply multiple conceptual frameworks to a single curriculum development endeavor. For example, a radiation oncology educator developing a simulation-based education curriculum to train residents how to perform interstitial breast brachytherapy may use the six-step approach to curriculum development[62] to guide the overarching curriculum development process, the theory of deliberate practice from Ericsson et al.[63] when developing the specific educational method to develop adequate breast brachytherapy psychomotor skills, and Kirkpatrick's four-step framework[64] when developing a plan for program evaluation. Bordage defines 11 key points pertaining to conceptual frameworks (Table 103.3) that clarify the critical nature of conceptual frameworks to educational scholarship, both to guide curriculum development and move the field of radiation oncology education forward in a logical and coherent manner.[61]

There are numerous conceptual frameworks in the medical education and general education literature that can be applied to radiation oncology educational scholarship. If an applicable conceptual framework is not available for a particular curriculum development program, existing conceptual frameworks can be modified and adapted to fit, or a new conceptual framework can be developed and reported in the peer-reviewed literature. To help guide the development of new literature in radiation oncology education, Table 103.4

TABLE 103.3 KEY POINTS REGARDING CONCEPTUAL FRAMEWORKS

1. Conceptual frameworks help understand (illuminate) problems.
2. Different conceptual frameworks emphasize (magnify) different aspects of the problem or elements of the solutions.
3. More than one conceptual framework may be relevant to a given situation.
4. Any given conceptual framework, or combination of frameworks, can lead to a variety of alternative solutions.
5. Conceptual frameworks can come from theories, models, or evidence-based best practices.
6. Scholars need to apply the principles outlined in the conceptual framework(s) selected.
7. Conceptual frameworks help identify important variables and their potential relationships; this also means that some variables are disregarded.
8. Conceptual frameworks are dynamic entities and benefit from being challenged and altered as needed.
9. Conceptual frameworks allow scholars to build upon one another's work and allow individuals to develop programs of research.
10. Programmatic, conceptually based research helps accumulate deeper understanding over time and thus moves the field forward.
11. Relevant conceptual frameworks can be found outside one's specialty or field.

Adapted from Bordage G. Conceptual frameworks to illuminate and magnify. *Med Educ* 2009;43(4):312–319. Copyright © 2009 Blackwell Publishing Ltd. Reprinted by permission of John Wiley & Sons, Inc.

TABLE 103.4 EXAMPLES OF CONCEPTUAL FRAMEWORKS APPLICABLE TO DOMAINS OF RADIATION ONCOLOGY EDUCATION

Education Domain	Conceptual Framework Examples
Curriculum development	*Six-step approach to curriculum development*[62] 1. Problem identification 2. Needs assessment of the learners 3. Goals and objectives 4. Educational strategies 5. Implementation 6. Evaluation and feedback
Goals and objectives	*Bloom's revised taxonomy of learning objectives*[109,110] 1. Knowledge → Remember 2. Comprehension → Understand 3. Application → Apply 4. Analysis → Analyze 5. Synthesis → Evaluate 6. Evaluation → Create
Educational methods/ learning theory	*Miller's pyramid of clinical competence*[116,117] – Knows – Knows how – Shows – Does *Kolb's experiential model*[26] – Concrete experience – Reflective observation – Analysis and integration – Application to new situations *Ericsson's theory of deliberate (mixed) practice with feedback*[63] – Motivate through improvement in real-life performance – Take into account the learner's pre-existing knowledge (difficulty of the task tailored to the individual) – Allow repetition of the skills multiple times – Accompanied by feedback that is constructive and timely *Merrill's first principles*[250] Learning is facilitated when: 1. Problem—Learners are engaged in solving real-world problems 2. Activation—Existing knowledge is activated as a foundation for new knowledge 3. Demonstration—New knowledge is demonstrated to the learner 4. Application—New knowledge is applied by the learner 5. Integration—New knowledge is integrated into the learner's world
Skills acquisition/ simulation-based education	*Mastery learning*[251] – Baseline testing – Clear objectives – Engagement in educational activities – Clear minimum passing standards – Formative testing – Advancement dependent on achievement – Individualized time frame *Features of effective simulation education*[252] – Feedback to the learner – Repetition – Simulation integrated into the overall curriculum – Learners practice with increasing difficulty and complexity – Simulations adapted to multiple learning strategies – Clinical variation built into the sessions – Control of the environment – Individualized learning options – Defined outcomes, benchmarks – Simulation closely represents practice *Kneebone's evaluation criteria for simulation programs*[253] Simulations should: – Allow for sustained, deliberate practice within a safe environment, ensuring that recently acquired skills are consolidated within a defined curriculum, which assures regular reinforcement – Provide access to expert tutors when appropriate, ensuring that such support fades when no longer needed – Map onto real-life clinical experience, ensuring that learning supports the experience gained within communities of actual practice – Provide a supportive, motivational, and learner-centered milieu, which is conducive to learning

(Continued)

TABLE 103.4 EXAMPLES OF CONCEPTUAL FRAMEWORKS APPLICABLE TO DOMAINS OF RADIATION ONCOLOGY EDUCATION (Continued)

Education Domain	Conceptual Framework Examples
Assessment	*National Council on Measurement in Education (NCME) standards: 5 sources of validity evidence*[130,254] 1. Content 2. Response process 3. Internal structure 4. Relationship to other variables 5. Consequences *Criteria for good assessment*[255] 1. Validity or coherence 2. Reproducibility or consistency 3. Equivalence 4. Feasibility 5. Educational effect 6. Catalytic effect 7. Acceptability
Evaluation	*Kirkpatrick's four levels of program evaluation*[64] 1. Reaction 2. Learning 3. Behavior 4. Results *Grant's ACTION model for evaluating new technologies for learning*[256] – Access – Cost – Types of learning – Integration – Organization – Novelty
Continuing medical education	*Davis' characteristics of effective (best practice) CME programs*[239] 1. Needs assessment that can be either subjective (e.g., questionnaires) or objective (e.g., literature review) 2. Focused initiative to meet the needs of the physician 3. Interactive educational programs 4. Multiple educational strategies 5. Multiple sessions 6. Time for feedback and practice 7. Outcome evaluation *Harden's Crisis Criteria for effective CME*[238] 1. Convenience 2. Relevance 3. Individualization 4. Self-assessment 5. Independent learning 6. Systematic
Interprofessional education	*Ivey's categorization of interprofessional practices*[257] – Parallel practice – Coordination – Consultation – Collaboration – Multidisciplinary teams – Interdisciplinary teams *Parsell and Bligh's elements of interprofessional education*[258] – Relationships – Collaboration and teamwork – Roles and responsibilities – Benefits *MUSC spiral theory*[259,260] Teamwork–Prepare–think–practice Transforming ways of knowing–Absolute–transitional–independent–contextual Ever-increasing acquisition, application, demonstration
Professionalism	*Assessment of professionalism*[261] – Evaluations by faculty supervisors – Nurses and patients – Peer evaluation – Self-evaluation – Standardized patients – Longitudinal observations

provides examples of conceptual frameworks that may be applied when approaching common radiation oncology education issues. In summary, the radiation oncology educator should be able to identify the conceptual framework that applies to their educational intervention.

CURRICULUM DEVELOPMENT

Using the background medical education theory and key principles to medical education scholarship, the radiation oncology educator can begin curriculum development. The objective of this section is to discuss the educational theory relevant to curriculum development, review curriculum development models, and then explore approaches to curriculum development with application to radiation oncology.

A curriculum can be defined as any planned educational experience.[62] In this context, radiation oncology curriculum examples include a 1-hour lecture on the history of radiation oncology for medical students, a residency training program's annual clinical rotation and didactic lecture schedule, a patient seminar on late effects of radiation oncology, or a national meeting on hands-on brachytherapy simulation workshop. The common thread through all of these examples is that the educator has a goal for the curriculum—that is, some type of knowledge transfer.

Curriculum theory proposes three types of curricula in any educational setting (Table 103.5). The first type of curriculum is the "set" or explicit curriculum. The set curriculum is what the educator defines a priori as the instructional plan. A radiation oncology clerkship will have goals and objectives defined for participating medical students to orient them to the experience. The overarching goal of the clerkship is likely "to learn the fundamentals of clinical radiation oncology." A syllabus may be prepared, and the educational strategies employed are chosen to reach the explicit curricular goal.

The second curriculum in any educational setting is the "hidden" or implicit curriculum. The hidden curriculum is what the learner comes to "know" based on interactions that occur outside of formal learning environments.[65] Examples in radiation oncology could include a medical student in a resident workroom overhearing a resident disparaging a referring service or a department choosing not to allocate resident education time to quality and safety or communication skills. The hidden curriculum often is referred to with a negative connotation, but there are positive effects of the hidden curriculum. For example, a resident may observe their attending

TABLE 103.5 EDUCATIONAL THEORY'S THREE COEXISTING CURRICULUM TYPES

Type of Curriculum	Radiation Oncology Examples
Set, formal, or explicit curriculum	– Medical student clerkship lecture series – Residency lecture series and rotation schedule – Goals and objectives for society meeting educational session
Hidden or implicit curriculum	– Radiation oncology resident disparages a referring specialty in front of a medical student – Radiation oncology attending models superb compassion when counseling a patient regarding terminal diagnosis – Radiation oncology attending belittles a dosimetrist in front of a resident and medical student
Null curriculum	– Medical school does not include any radiation oncology in their formal curriculum – Residency program director decides to forgo a formal treatment planning rotation because of training time constraints – Society does not include a session on palliative radiation because of space constraints at conference center

physician during a particularly compassionate patient encounter and take away a positive lesson on how to interact with a similar patient in the future. Radiation oncology educators must consider their departmental and institutional hidden curriculum when developing a novel set of curriculum. Individual educators may be encouraged to view their behaviors as modeling and note the potential impacts on the hidden curriculum. Areas to consider relating to the hidden curriculum include policy development, evaluation, resource allocation, and institutional slang.[65] These four areas within a radiation oncology department can teach trainees both positive and negative lessons without the trainee ever being exposed to a formal learning environment.

The third type of curriculum is the "null" curriculum, which is defined as what is not taught.[66] The classic example in childhood education is removing art class from a grammar school curriculum, which results in a negative impact on the children by sending a message that art is not important and can therefore be ignored. Medical educators within radiation oncology are faced with limited time for education. Thus, during the curriculum planning process, radiation oncology educators must strive for a balance of including material that is important to their learners while not overburdening the learner or institutional resources. Topics that are important to functioning as a radiation oncologist but are often not taught formally during training because of resource constraints include (but are not limited to) treatment planning and plan evaluation, diagnostic radiology interpretation skills, communications, collaboration, and leadership skills. The Accreditation Council for Graduate Medical Education (ACGME) permits residency programs to count resident attendance at multidisciplinary tumor boards as adequate training in medical oncology, radiology, and pathology in place of formal clinical rotations.[4] Because of training time constraints, this capitulation is necessary, but it may send a message to US radiation oncology residents that knowledge pertaining to these specialties is less important. This may lead to the long-term detriment of patient care.[67] Radiation oncology itself suffers from the consequences of the null curriculum. Radiation oncology's status as a subspecialty means the formal medical school curriculum frequently does not include radiation oncology material leading to reduced knowledge of the specialty[68,69] and residency training programs outside of radiation oncology frequently do not provide formal lectures or training pertaining to radiation oncology.[70,71] Radiation oncology educators must carefully consider the institutional and departmental educational milieu when deciding on which educational initiatives to pursue or cut.

Curriculum Development Models

Curriculum development should be a logic and rational process. Often in medical education, curriculum development is a haphazard process or occurs in a reactive, rather than proactive, manner. Multiple curriculum development models are proposed. These include empirical/analytical/systematic curriculum inquiry, deliberative curriculum inquiry, and reconceptualist curriculum inquiry.[72]

Systematic curriculum inquiry is perhaps the most commonly utilized curriculum development model. Systematic curriculum development has been in the literature for over 60 years with multiple educators, medical and nonmedical, contributing to the current iteration.[62,73,74] The six-step approach to medical education curriculum development[62] provides a systematic approach to curriculum development and, if followed, helps medical educators ensure critical components necessary for effective curriculum planning are not missed. One criticism of the systematic approach is that it can be a top–down process with curriculum deans, residency program directors, or clerkship directors dictating curriculum content and structure.

Deliberative curriculum inquiry focuses on the process of curriculum planning, implementation, and evaluation.[75] To be effective, deliberative curriculum inquiry requires a structure for "deliberation."[76] Curriculum stakeholders are given an opportunity to evaluate the curriculum goals and objectives, propose modification to educational methods, and suggest methods for assessment and evaluation. For example, a radiation oncology residency program choosing to employ deliberative curriculum inquiry would create an opportunity for stakeholders within the program (residency, chairperson, program director, department faculty, institution, and patients) to provide feedback on the program. The ACGME now requires US radiation oncology residency programs to have a program evaluation committee conduct an annual evaluation of the program.[4] Members of the program evaluation committee must include department faculty and residents. To improve the deliberative nature of this process, inclusion of other stakeholders can be considered (e.g., patients, institution, etc.).

The final curriculum development model is reconceptualist curriculum inquiry.[77] This model of curriculum inquiry aims to explore how the curriculum relates to society. How does the curriculum interact with economic, cultural, and political institutions? An example of reconceptualist curriculum inquiry in radiation oncology is a program director's decision whether to include formal education (e.g., a lecture) on health economics in a radiation oncology residency program. By choosing to educate the program's trainees about the economic implications of different radiation treatment modalities, the residency program can have a future societal impact on economic and political institutions.

The systematic, deliberative, and reconceptualist models of curriculum development are not mutually exclusive. Rather, these models can be used simultaneously to achieve the most effective radiation oncology curriculum possible that is properly structured, includes consideration of stakeholder viewpoints, and has potential for societal impact. Further discussion of curriculum development will focus on the systematic model,[62] but implications of the deliberative and reconceptualist models should be considered as well.

Systematic Curriculum Development

Systematic curriculum development for medical education is most clearly defined by the "six-step approach" from Thomas et al.[62] The six steps are (a) problem identification and general needs assessment, (b) needs assessment of targeted learners, (c) goals and specific objectives, (d) educational strategies, (e) implementation, and (f) evaluation and feedback (Fig. 103.6). Although these six steps are presented in a sequential order, in practice they often are occurring simultaneously. Each step can have effects on or be affected by the other steps. The following discussion will focus on each of the six steps with relevant examples from radiation oncology cited where applicable.

Problem Identification and General Needs Assessment

When beginning to develop an educational intervention, an initial problem identification and general needs assessment is done. With respect to radiation oncology, sample problems could include variability in the delineation of radiation target volumes between radiation oncologists[78–81] or lack of exposure to oncology training in medical school curriculum.[82] In either case, once the problem is identified, a general needs assessment is done. This includes determining the current approach to the problem and defining the ideal approach. Often, an educator may identify a problem in their local educational and clinical environment but on review of the literature discovers that another institution or organization is addressing the problem adequately. Rather than develop a new curriculum

Section
V

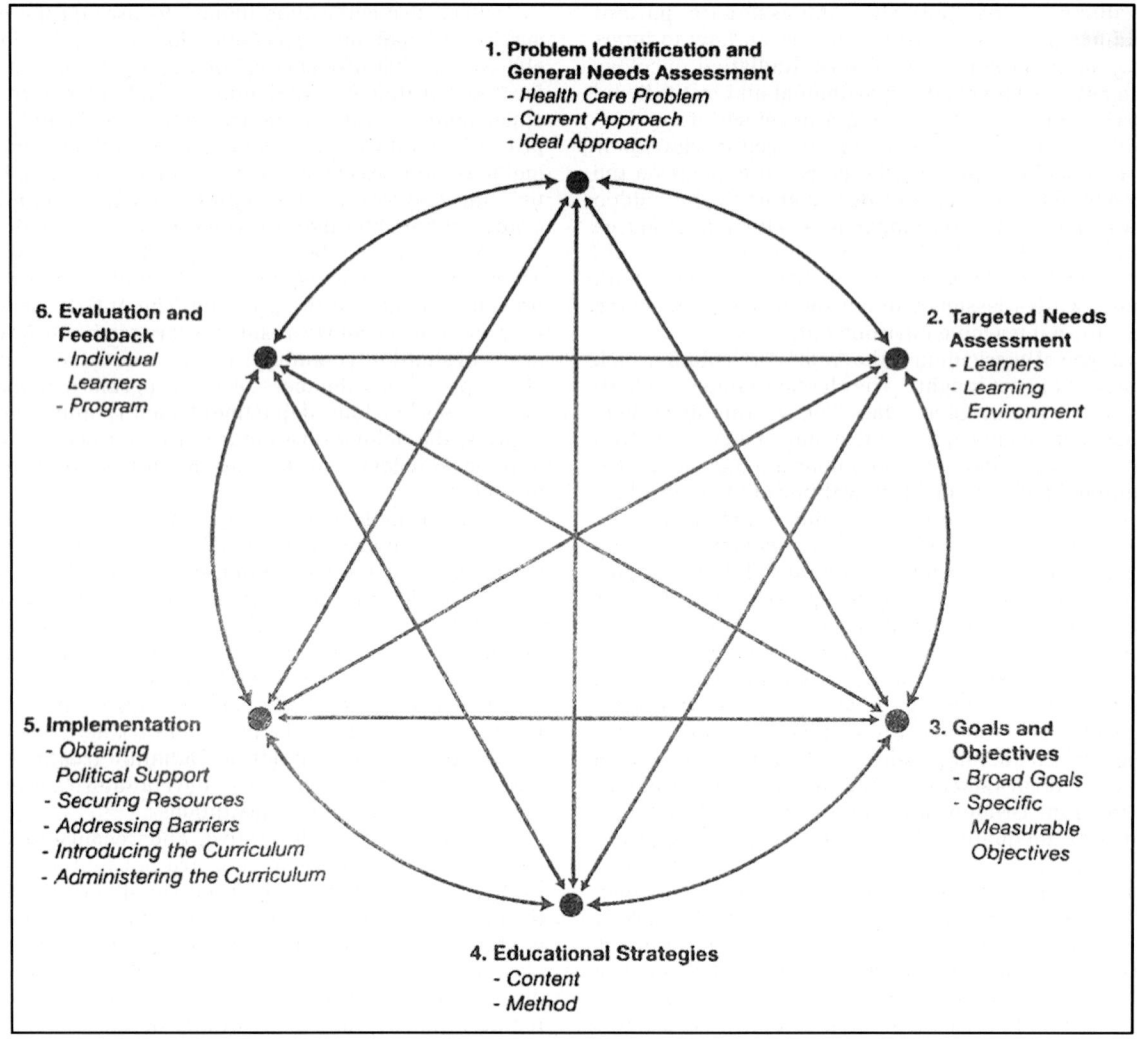

FIGURE 103.6. The six-step approach to systematic curriculum development. (From Thomas PA, Kern DE, Hughes MT, et al. *Curriculum development for medical education: a six-step approach.* 3rd ed. Baltimore: Johns Hopkins University Press, 2016: Figure 1, p. 7. © 1998, 2009, 2016 Johns Hopkins University Press. Reprinted with permission of Johns Hopkins University Press.)

for the identified problem, the educator can adopt or adapt the existing curriculum to their local needs.

A systematic literature review is an excellent method to identify the current approach to a problem. A systematic literature review may not identify any published approach in which case there is no curriculum precedent for the educator to follow. Conversely, the systematic review may identify other approaches to the identified problem and thereby provide the educator with a starting point for their curriculum development process. When conducting a medical education systematic review, it is necessary to review resources beyond the usual peer-reviewed literature databases (e.g., MedEdPORTAL[83]) to ensure approaches to the identified problem are not previously published. Methodology for systematic reviews is defined in the Preferred Reporting Items for Systematic Reviews and Meta-Analyses (PRISMA) statement[84] and the Institute of Medicine's "Finding What Works in Health Care: Standards for Systematic Reviews"[85] and is beyond the scope of this text. A systematic review of the medical education literature for curriculum development should follow the same rigorous approach used for a systematic review of clinical research.

Subsequent to identifying the current approach to the problem, the ideal approach should be defined. This is an opportunity to incorporate aspects of deliberative and reconceptualist curriculum inquiry. Stakeholders representing the targeted learners (e.g., medical students or residents),

patients, health care professionals, medical educators, and society can be included in this step of curriculum development to ensure all relevant parties agree with the proposed ideal approach. In the previous examples (i.e., variability in contouring and lack of oncology undergraduate education), there would be different stakeholders. The contouring variability example could include residents, faculty, and dosimetrists. For the undergraduate oncology education, stakeholders could include medical students, university faculty, teaching faculty, and accreditation bodies. Educators in radiation oncology must also consider accreditation bodies (e.g., Liaison Committee on Medical Education [LCME], ACGME, Accreditation Council for Continuing Medical Education [ACCME]) and certifying organizations (e.g., American Board of Radiology (ABR), the Royal College of Physicians and Surgeons of Canada (RCPSC), Canadian Medical Education Directions for Specialists (CanMEDS), the Royal Australian and New Zealand College of Radiologists (RANZCR), and the Royal College of Radiologists in the United Kingdom, etc.) when considering the ideal approach to a problem. Training program requirements from these accrediting and certification bodies may direct the ideal approach to an educational problem. New information can be obtained from stakeholders through in-person interviews, focus groups, and questionnaires or surveys. Qualitative and quantitative methods can be used to collect date to define the problem and define goals for the ideal approach to achieve.

By obtaining input from all stakeholders, the educator minimizes the chance of overlooking a key component of the ideal approach to the problem and can begin to generate momentum with the stakeholders for eventual implementation of their new curriculum. The identified differences between the current and ideal approach to a specific health care problem should be the target of any subsequent curriculum development.

Lastly, based on the problem identification and general needs assessment, the educator can decide the amount of time and effort to dedicate to curriculum development. If the potential for a positive impact on targeted learners, patients, and society is high, then more time and effort may be devoted to curriculum development. Conversely, if there is a low likelihood of significant impact on learners, patients, or society, less time and effort may be necessary to obtain an acceptable curriculum.

Problem identification and general needs assessments in the radiation oncology literature include surveys identifying a deficiency in medical student knowledge of radiation oncology,[68,69] an analysis of average volume of brachytherapy cases performed by resident volume,[86] studies showing failure of practicing physicians to implement best practices based on high-level evidence,[87,88] or evaluation of critical safety events.[89] These studies identify a problem and indicate a general need for curricular development to solve the problem. However, they do not provide detailed information regarding how best to design the curriculum to solve the problem.

Targeted Needs Assessment

Once the educational problem is identified and the differences between the current and ideal approach are realized, the educator should conduct a targeted needs assessment of the learning environment and learners. In radiation oncology, the targeted learner could be a medical student, resident, attending physician, patient, nurse, dosimetrist, physicist, etc. The learning environment may be a clerkship, residency program, society meeting, or any other myriad learning environments. The goal of this step in systematic curriculum development is to determine the specific needs of the radiation oncology educators, learners, and environment that differ from the ideal approach identified in the prior step. For example, the physics curriculum proposed by the American Society for Radiation Oncology (ASTRO) for radiation oncology residents[90] may not be feasible in a specific training program's learning environment. Alternatively, the literature reviewed in the general needs assessment may not be current, and educational methods will require updating and modification to be relevant to current learners. For example, a radiation oncology residency program developed in 2002 in Singapore[91] may not cover all aspects of radiation oncology training necessary in 2017. Additionally, the program was designed to satisfy accreditation requirements of RANZCR and may need to be modified if implemented by a program in the United States or Canada because of different accreditation requirements set forth by the ACGME or RCPSC, respectively. However, the design and implementation of the Singapore residency program can provide a starting point for a new residency program followed by a targeted needs assessment within the new program's educational milieu.

Detailed information about the targeted learners and the targeted environment is necessary to develop an effective curriculum. Table 103.6 summarizes characteristics about the targeted learner and environment that are necessary to understand before proceeding further with curriculum development. For example, if the targeted learner is a junior radiation oncology resident, understanding that they have limited or no prior education about contouring a prostate fossa will lead to a different curriculum design compared to if the targeted learner is an attending physician attending

TABLE 103.6 CONTENT RELEVANT TO A TARGETED NEEDS ASSESSMENT

Content About Targeted Learners
Expectations regarding the scope of knowledge and skills needed
Previous training and experiences relevant to the curriculum
Already planned training and experiences relevant to the curriculum
Existing characteristics/proficiencies/practices
  Cognitive: knowledge, problem-solving abilities
  Affective: attitudes, values, beliefs, role expectations
  Psychomotor: skills/capabilities (e.g., history, physical examinations, procedures, counseling, current behaviors/performance/practices)
Perceived and measured deficiencies and learning needs
Attitudes and motivations of learners to improve performance
Preferences and experiences regarding different learning strategies
  Synchronous (educator sets time, such as noon lecture)
  Asynchronous (learner decides on learning time, such as with e-learning)
  Duration (amount of time the learner think is needed to learn or that he/she can devote to learning)
  Methods (e.g., readings, lectures, online learning resources, large and small group discussions, problem-based learning, team-based learning, peer teaching, demonstrations, role-plays/simulations, supervised experience)

Content About Targeted Learning Environment
Related existing curricula
Needs of stakeholders other than the learners (course directors, clerkship directors, program directors, faculty, accrediting bodies, others)
Barriers, enablers, and reinforcing factors that affect learning by the targeted learners
  Barriers (e.g., time, unavailability, or competition for resources)
  Enablers (e.g., learning portfolios, electronic medical record reminders)
  Reinforcing factors (e.g., incentives such as grades, awards, recognition)
Resources (e.g., patients and clinical experiences, faculty, role models and mentors, information resources, access to hardware and software technology, audiovisual equipment, simulation center)
Informal and collateral curriculum

Thomas PA, Kern DE, Hughes MT, et al. *Curriculum development for medical education: a six-step approach.* 3rd ed. Baltimore: Johns Hopkins University Press, 2016: Table 3.1, p. 32. © 1998, 2009, 2016 Johns Hopkins University Press. Reprinted with permission of Johns Hopkins University Press.

a refresher course. Similarly, the resources available within a targeted learning environment dictate how a curriculum is structured. A residency program with a proton center and busy pediatric service will design their resident rotation schedule differently than a training program that does not have a proton center and refers all pediatric cases to an out-of-area proton facility.

Given the critical nature of the targeted needs assessment to developing an effective curriculum, methods to obtain the necessary information must be carefully considered. Results of the National Resident Match Program (NRMP), Association of Residents in Radiation Oncology (ARRO) chief resident survey, and the ASTRO workforce survey can provide a starting point for curriculum development. These surveys can provide information on past experiences of targeted learners, work environment, and intrinsic and extrinsic motivation. In addition, these surveys frequently include information on the learning environment in residency programs for graduate medical education (GME) curriculum development or practice settings for CME curriculum development. An educator must consider how broadly they want their curriculum to be applicable. If the curriculum is developed specifically for a problem identified within their own institution, it may not be applicable to other institutions or educational programs. Thus, reviewing national survey data of training programs[22] and practice environments[92] will inform the radiation oncology educator how they can develop their curriculum in a manner such that it satisfies the needs at their local institution and will be beneficial to other educators in need of a similar curriculum. Table 103.7 summarizes methods commonly employed when conducting a needs assessment of targeted learners.

Surveys represent the most common method for a radiation oncology targeted needs assessment published in the

TABLE 103.7 METHODS FOR NEEDS ASSESSMENT OF TARGETED LEARNERS

Needs Assessment Method	Radiation Oncology Example
Informal discussion or interviews with individual learners, supervisors, or other stakeholders (in person, over the phone, or by e-mail)	Development of an integrated interdisciplinary oncology elective[174]
Focus group discussions	Focus group discussions with oncologists on patient- and family-centered care[262]
Formal interviews	Interviews of radiation oncology professions regarding uptake of high-precision radiotherapy[57]
Formal questionnaires	Targeted needs assessment for radiation oncology medical student clerkship curriculum[45,98]
Direct observation of targeted learners	Mini-CEX[263]
Pretests of knowledge, attitudes, or skills	Pretest of prostate fossa contouring ability[2]
Audits of current performance	Analysis of brachytherapy procedure volume at US residency programs[86]
Strategic planning sessions for the curriculum	Development of medical school oncology educational goals and objectives[176]

Thomas PA, Kern DE, Hughes MT, et al. *Curriculum development for medical education: a six-step approach.* 3rd ed. Baltimore: Johns Hopkins University Press, 2016: Table 3.2, pp. 37–38. © 1998, 2009, 2016 Johns Hopkins University Press. Reprinted with permission of Johns Hopkins University Press.

literature. Numerous resources are available to guide a radiation oncology educator designing a survey or questionnaire for a targeted needs assessment including resources from the Association for Medical Education in Europe (AMEE)[93,94] and textbooks.[62,95,96] Surveys include interviews, focus groups, and questionnaires. Radiation oncology educators should decide which method best suits the needs of their curriculum development process. Advantages and disadvantages and basic techniques of each method are summarized elsewhere.[62] General considerations when designing a survey include paying careful attention to the goal of the survey (questions should have clear justification for inclusion) and avoiding subjective questions, sensitive questions, or lengthy surveys as the response rate will decrease with increasing survey length or sensitivity of questions asked. The survey population should be informed of the purpose of the survey and whether responses are confidential. Surveys represent research, and therefore local Institutional Review Board (IRB) approval or exemption should be obtained prior to survey dissemination. A survey should be pilot-tested to ensure clarity and understandability.[62] In addition, the pilot data should be analyzed to determine if the data collection format would allow the educator to obtain the desired needs assessment results.

Survey response rate is critical to obtaining representative data. Survey responses can suffer when either the targeted learner does not receive the survey (e.g., requesting that a residency program coordinator forward survey invitations on to residents) or when the targeted learner elects not to complete the survey because of length, sensitivity of question topics, unclear questions, or other factors that inadvertently discourage responses. Methods by which to improve survey responses (unit response rate) and question responses (item response rate) are summarized elsewhere.[94]

Targeted needs assessments at the undergraduate medical education (UGME), GME, and CME levels are frequently reported in the literature, although many do not identify themselves as such. At the UGME level, targeted needs assessments provide perspective and guidance on radiation oncology education in the general medical school curriculum[68,97] and for radiation oncology clerkships.[45,98] At the GME level, examples of needs assessments include those investigating general residency experiences,[22,99] resident education in IMRT,[100] resident knowledge of caring for elderly patients with cancer,[101]

palliative care training,[102,103] brachytherapy experience,[86,104] radiation physics education,[105] and radiobiology education.[106] Numerous other GME needs assessments for specific educational goals are reported in the literature. Finally, at the CME level, surveys of practicing physicians can inform educators regarding deficiencies in clinical knowledge that should be addressed. An example of a CME targeted needs assessment is assessing expert consensus on involved-site radiation for lymphoma and determining that there is a lack of consensus.[79] Although these studies provide some guidance, it is critical to incorporate alternative methods for the needs assessment including focused interviews, discussion with multiple stakeholders, and evaluation of available resources.

Goals and Objectives

Once the radiation oncology educator has defined the health care problem, performed a general needs assessment, and conducted a targeted needs assessment, they can begin to formulate goals and objectives for the curriculum. Alternatively, the educator may begin the entire curriculum development process with a general goal or specific objective for their targeted learners. Goals and objectives are key to curriculum development because they help guide the choice of curricular content, educational strategies, learner assessment methods, and curriculum evaluation methods and communicate to others what the curriculum addresses and aims to achieve.[62] Curriculum goals are broad and general.

In contrast, curriculum objectives are Specific, Measurable, Attainable, and Relevant and have a Time frame (SMART).[107] Specific and measurable objectives help to refine the curriculum content and guide learner assessment and curriculum evaluation methods. Objectives should contain five basic elements: "(a) *Who* (b) *will do* (c) *how much (how well)* (d) *of what* (e) *by when?*"[108] By defining specific measurable objectives, the radiation oncology educator can determine the ideal educational, assessment, and evaluation methods that will demonstrate efficacy of the curriculum.

Learner objectives can be in one of three learning domains: cognitive, affective, or psychomotor. Within the three learning domains, cognitive refers to "knowledge," affective to "attitudinal," and psychomotor to "skill" or "behavioral" objectives.[62] Bloom's taxonomy for the cognitive domain defined six levels of the cognitive domain: knowledge, comprehension, application, analysis, synthesis, and evaluation (Fig. 103.7A).[109] The cognitive domain taxonomy was subsequently modified to remembering, understanding, applying, analyzing, evaluating, and creating.[110] One of the modifications included changing the domains to verbs rather than nouns to emphasize the active nature of the learning process. The cognitive taxonomy was further refined to four levels: retrieval of knowledge, comprehension, analysis, and use of knowledge.[111] Taxonomies for the affective domain[112] (Fig. 103.7B) and psychomotor domain[113–115] (Fig. 103.7C) are also defined in the literature. Another conceptual framework used to define progressive levels of learning objectives is Miller's pyramid of clinical competence, which progresses through four phases: Knows, Knows how, Shows, and Does (Fig. 103.8).[116,117]

When writing objectives, verbs that are open to fewer interpretations should be used. For example, "to list" or "to demonstrate" is better than "to know" or "be able to." Examples of action verbs that can be used to define objectives for the cognitive, affective, and psychomotor domains can be found in medical education texts.[117a] The action verb used in the objective can guide what type of assessment method is used to determine if the learner meets the objective. The radiation oncology educator should not overlook the critical nature of writing specific and measurable objectives. These represent the linchpin of any curriculum. Unfocused, unattainable, or unclear objectives will lead to confusion regarding educational, assessment, and evaluation methods.

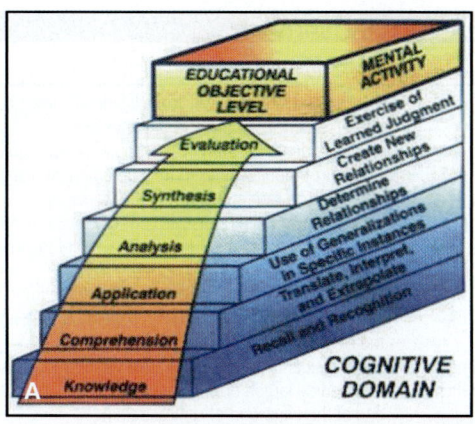

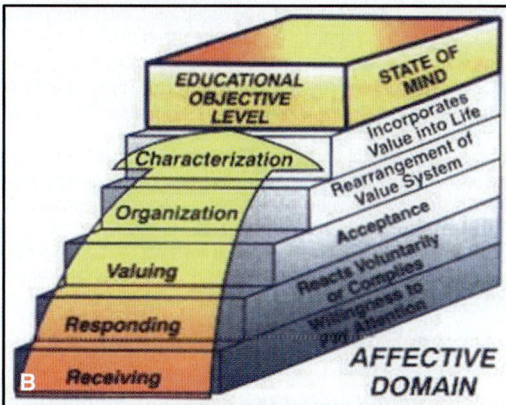

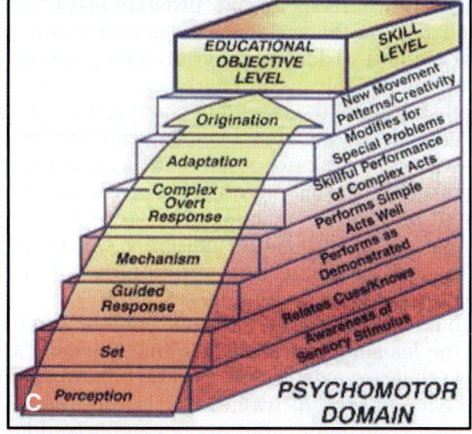

FIGURE 103.7. A–C: Taxonomy for cognitive, affective, and psychomotor learning domains.

Learner objectives are generally written to the highest order expected of the learner. However, the radiation oncology educator needs to consider any enabling objectives at lower levels on the pyramid that are required to achieve the higher-order target objective.[62] In addition to learner objectives, the curriculum designer may also define process objectives in relation to curriculum implementation. Table 103.8 provides examples of learner and related process objectives relevant to radiation oncology. Finally, outcome objectives can be specified that relate to patient or societal outcomes.[62] Demonstrating a positive effect of an educational curriculum on patient or societal health outcomes is the ultimate goal for any medical educator. However, measuring the direct effect of an educational intervention for medical trainees on outcome objectives can be challenging because of the numerous variables that determine health outcomes.

Within the context of educational goals and objectives, competency-based education is gaining popularity. Competency-based education is defined as:

> *… an approach to preparing physicians for practice that is fundamentally oriented to graduate outcome abilities … It deemphasizes time-based training and promises greater accountability, flexibility, and learner-centeredness and focuses on the competencies required of learners driven by needs of the health care system.*[118]

With respect to radiation oncology competency-based education, national accrediting bodies have developed structured guidelines to assist with defining goals and objectives for program graduates. In the United States, as a component of the Next Accreditation System,[119] the ACGME worked with a number of stakeholder groups, including the ABR, to develop the Radiation Oncology Milestones. The Milestones define competency levels for residents within the six competency domains of Patient Care, Medical Knowledge, Systems-Based Practice, Practice-Based Learning and Improvement, Professionalism, and Interpersonal and Communication Skills.[120] Competency objectives for levels of training are defined within the six domains. Level one is the knowledge or skill level expected of an incoming resident, level four is that of a graduating resident, and level five is above that of a graduating resident. The ACGME currently mandates that a program's clinical competency committee assess residents using the Milestone framework semiannually. The learner objective is to achieve or outperform the ACGME Milestone commensurate with their training level, and the process objective is to have all residents at or above their training level.

Similarly, the RCPSC has developed the Canadian Medical Education Directions for Specialists (CanMEDS) framework.[5,121] The CanMEDS competencies include Medical Expert,

FIGURE 103.8. Miller's pyramid of clinical competence as interpreted by Mehay and Burns. (From Miller GE. The assessment of clinical skills/competence/performance. *Acad Med J Assoc Am Med Coll* 1990;65:S63–S67; From Mehay R. *The essential handbook for GP training and education*. CRC Press, 2012. Copyright © 2012 The UK Association of Programme Directors. Reproduced by permission of Taylor and Francis Group, LLC, a division of Informa plc.)

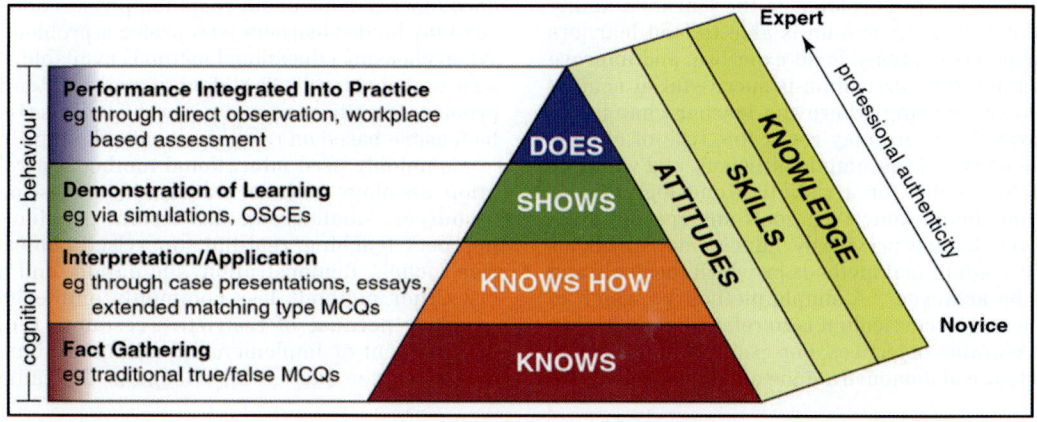

TABLE 103.8 SAMPLE LEARNER AND PROCESS OBJECTIVES FOR RADIATION ONCOLOGY EDUCATION

Domain	Level on Domain Taxonomy	Learner Objective	Process Objective
Cognitive	Remembering	The medical student will correctly identify three radiation emergencies at the end of the lecture	80% of medical students will correctly identify three radiation emergencies at the end of the lecture
	Applying	The resident will correctly compute the appropriate number of monitor units to treat an emergency spinal cord compression at the end of the workshop	100% of residents will correctly compute the appropriate number of monitor units to treat an emergency spinal cord compression at the end of the workshop
	Evaluating	The radiation oncologist will correctly revise incorrect head and neck target volumes at the end of the interactive contouring workshop	80% of radiation oncologists will correctly revise incorrect head and neck target volumes at the end of the interactive contouring workshop
Affective	Receiving	The medical student will acknowledge the importance of using nonmedical jargon with patients at the end of the clerkship	100% of medical students will acknowledge the importance of using nonmedical jargon with patients at the end of the clerkship
	Valuing	The resident will demonstrate a willingness to use nonmedical jargon during patient consultations at the end of their first year of clinical training	100% of residents will demonstrate a willingness to use nonmedical jargon during patient consultations at the end of their first year of clinical training
	Characterization	The radiation oncologist will modify their discussions with patients to minimize use of medical jargon after completing the communication workshop	100% of radiation oncologists will modify their discussions with patients to minimize use of medical jargon after completing the communication workshop
Psychomotor	Perception	The medical student will correctly identify the bevel side of a brachytherapy needle after observing a permanent prostate implant	100% of medical students will correctly identify the bevel side of a brachytherapy needle after observing a permanent prostate implant
	Guided response	The resident will correctly reproduce the attending physician's needle placement technique after a lecture on technique and observing a complete permanent prostate implant	80% of residents will correctly reproduce the attending physician's needle placement technique after a lecture on technique and observing a complete permanent prostate implant
	Origination	The brachytherapy fellow will correctly and independently construct a new HDR catheter implant pattern after encountering pubic arch interference by halfway through their 1-year fellowship	100% of brachytherapy fellows will correctly and independently construct new HDR catheter implant patterns after encountering pubic arch interference by halfway through their 1-year fellowship

Communicator, Collaborator, Scholar, Health Advocate, Leader, and Professional. Currently the RCPSC is defining the CanMEDS competencies within the constructs of Entrustable Professional Activities and Milestones in the Competency by Design Project.[122] Similar to the ACGME Milestone project, there will be specific Entrustable Professional Activities (EPAs) and milestones for four levels of residency training including transition to discipline, foundations of discipline, core of discipline, and transition to practice.

Instruction/Educational Strategies

As discussed in the learning theory section of this chapter, effective learning can be facilitated by addressing preconceptions, building expertise, and developing a metacognitive approach to learning.[123] Learners have prior experiences that shape their attitude and motivation toward learning new knowledge or a new skill. These experiences lead to preconceptions that may need to be addressed prior to engaging the learner. Building expertise requires repeatedly exposing learners to specific conceptual frameworks so they can develop fluency of retrieval known as "automatism."[62] As the learners gain experience, they improve their ability to utilize the specific knowledge or skill until they have achieved expertise. Metacognition refers to the learners' ability to recognize what they know or need to know in a specific problem-solving situation. This concept is related to the learner's ability for self-reflection.[62] If a curriculum is able to lead learners to identify their preconceptions, build expertise, and improve their metacognition, the curriculum is successful in achieving transformative learning where the learner changes in a meaningful way. Learners may resist this type of change because it challenges their assumptions, beliefs, and values.[62]

Educational strategies for a radiation oncology educational curriculum should match the goals and specific measurable objectives defined previously. Educational strategies refer to both the content and methods by which the goals and objectives will be achieved.[62] A simple method by which to choose the content of a curriculum is to refer to the nouns in the specific measurable objectives. For example, if the objective is "the resident will demonstrate the ability to contour the prostate fossa by the end of the workshop," then the content of the curriculum will focus on the "prostate fossa." Although this seems obvious on the surface, a large curriculum such as that of a clerkship or residency program may have numerous subgoals and specific objectives. There is a risk of bias toward easily implementable and assessable content. If each specific objective is not considered when choosing content and educational strategies, the educator risks omitting content critical to one or more of the specific objectives. To prevent omission of content in a larger educational program with multiple goals and objectives, curriculum mapping can be pursued. A detailed discussion of curriculum mapping is beyond the scope of this text and can be found elsewhere.[62]

Educational methods to relay specific content must also be matched to the learning styles of individual learners. Multiple learning style theories exist in the literature.[124] An example of a learning style conceptual framework is Dunn and Dunn's visual, auditory, kinesthetic, and tactile categorization.[125] It is not usually feasible to create a specific curriculum for each individual learner's preferred learning style. In addition, most learners will learn from multiple different educational strategies. Thus, radiation oncology educators should include multiple educational methods that will allow learners with different learning styles to achieve the learning objective. For example, utilizing only slide-based didactic lectures to teach radiation oncology residents about radiation physics and radiation biology may hinder learners who prefer a problem-based format. When choosing educational methods available, resources must also be considered. The ideal approach identified after the problem identification and general needs assessment may not be feasible based on resources available (time, money, etc.).

Commonly used educational methods in relation to radiation oncology include readings, lectures, online learning resources, small group discussion, problem-based learning, peer teaching, real-life supervised clinical experiences, role models, demonstration, simulation, and artificial models. Other methods less commonly employed in radiation oncology because of restrictive resource requirements for development or implementation, limited numbers of faculty or learners, or lack of knowledge in the radiation oncology educator community of the educational method include large group discussion, team-based learning, reflection on experience, role-play, standardized patients, audio/video review of the learner, and behavioral/environmental interventions.[62]

Educational methods can be divided based on the domain objectives they aim to achieve. Cognitive objectives may be best achieved through readings, lectures, or discussion; affective objectives through standardized patients, reflection on experience, and role-play; and psychomotor objectives may be best achieved through real-life and supervised clinical experiences, simulation and artificial models, or demonstration.

Radiation oncology educators face unique challenges when choosing appropriate educational methods. At the UGME and GME training levels, the number of learners is often small. Medical school clerkships may have one to three students rotating at any given time. Residency training programs also have limited numbers of trainees, often at different training levels. The limited number of trainees translates into limited resources (faculty time, money, space, clinical volume) that can be dedicated to educational methods. Thus, radiation oncology educators must utilize educational methods that efficiently utilize limited resources while achieving the goal and specific objectives of their curriculum.

To overcome the challenge of limited resources, individuals, collaborative groups, societies, and certifying organizations have developed curriculum proposals and specific educational methods to assist individual radiation oncology educators in achieving their local educational goals and objectives. Table 103.9 summarizes selected curricula and educational methods. In addition, educational methods utilized by other medical specialties to teach knowledge and skills that are not specific to radiation oncology (e.g., breaking bad news, diagnostic radiology knowledge, etc.) should be adopted or adapted by radiation oncology educator so as not to reinvent the wheel.

Implementation

Once a curriculum is developed with content and educational methods are selected to accomplish the specified goals and objectives, implementation must occur. All too often, well-designed educational interventions are unsuccessful because of barriers encountered during the implementation phase. Consideration of barriers to successful implementation should start at the outset of the curriculum planning process. The general and targeted needs assessment phase of curriculum development is a useful opportunity to begin establishing rapport with stakeholders who will need to provide support for successful implementation. For example, during the development of a new 1-month international clinical experience for radiation oncology residents, a program director must consider stakeholders (e.g., the chairman, teaching faculty, GME office, and residents) for a needs assessment but also use the opportunity to develop relations that will be important for successful implementation. For example, if early in the development of the 1-month international clinical experience the residency program director fails to discuss the required funds with the chairman and/or international rotation requirements with the GME office, the resulting decrease in available residents for service coverage or the requirements for an international rotation with the GME office may present insurmountable barriers at the time of implementation. Additionally, if the residents themselves were not made aware of the proposed experience prior to an attempt at implementation, they may choose not to participate, thus negating the effort put into the curriculum development.

Resources for successful implementation must be identified and obtained. These include personnel, time, facilities, and funding.[62] Successful implementation requires appropriate resources, and as Figure 103.6 demonstrates, barriers to implementation must be considered during the earlier phases of curriculum development. Table 103.10 provides a checklist

TABLE 103.9 SELECTED RADIATION ONCOLOGY CURRICULA AND EDUCATIONAL METHODS

Topic	Citation
Medical student oncology curriculum	Tam et al.[176] Hirsch et al.[47]
Medical student radiation oncology clerkship curriculum	Radiation Oncology Education Collaborative Study Group (ROECSG)[82]
Radiation oncology residency clinical curriculum	1. Accreditation Council for Graduate Medical Education (ACGME)[4] 2. European Society for Radiotherapy and Oncology (ESTRO)[265] 3. Royal Australian and New Zealand College of Radiologists (RANZCR)[266] 4. Royal College of Radiologists (RCR)[185]
Radiation oncology residency program physics curriculum	Burmeister et al.[90]
Contouring education	Alfieri et al.[205] Gunther et al.[2] Gillespie et al.[46]
Communications	Ju et al.[24]
Treatment planning	Golden et al.[179]
Proton therapy physics	Winey et al.[212]
Safety	Abdel-Wahab et al.[267]
Brachytherapy	Thaker et al.[25]
Pediatric radiation oncology	Ahern et al.[268]
Anatomy	Cabrera et al.[188,269]
Palliative care curriculum for radiation oncology residency	Garcia et al.[270]

TABLE 103.10 CHECKLIST FOR IMPLEMENTATION

- Identify resources
  - Personnel: faculty, audiovisual, computing, information technology, secretarial and other support staff, patients
  - Time: curriculum director, faculty, support staff, learners
  - Facilities: space, clinical sites, clinical equipment, educational equipment, virtual space (servers, content management software)
  - Funding/costs: direct financial costs, hidden or opportunity costs, faculty compensation, costs of scholarship
- Obtain support
  - Internal
    From: those with administrative authority (dean's office, hospital administration, department chair, program director, division director, etc.), faculty, learners, other stakeholders
    For: curricular time, personnel, resources, political support
  - External
    From: government, professional societies, philanthropic organizations or foundations, accreditation bodies, other entities (e.g., managed care organizations), individual donors
    For: funding, political support, external requirements, curricular or faculty development resources
- Develop administrative mechanisms to support the curriculum
  - Administrative structure: to delineate responsibilities and decision-making
  - Communication
    Content: rationale; goals and objectives; information about the curriculum, learners, faculty, facilities and equipment, scheduling; changes in the curriculum; evaluation results; etc.
    Mechanisms: websites, social media, memos, meetings, syllabus materials, site visits, reports, etc.
  - Operations: preparation and distribution of schedules and curricular materials; collection, collation, and distribution of evaluation data; curricular revisions and changes, etc.
  - Scholarship: plans for presenting and publishing about curriculum; human subject protection considerations; IRB approval, if necessary
- Anticipate and address barriers
  - Financial and other resources
  - Competing demands
  - People: attitudes, job/role security, power and authority, etc.
- Pilot
  - Phase-in
  - Full implementation
- Plan for curriculum enhancement and maintenance

Thomas PA, Kern DE, Hughes MT, et al. *Curriculum development for medical education: a six-step approach.* 3rd ed. Baltimore: Johns Hopkins University Press, 2016: Table 6.1, p. 103. © 1998, 2009, 2016 Johns Hopkins University Press. Reprinted with permission of Johns Hopkins University Press.

TABLE 103.11 KANTER'S SIX STEPS TO LEADING POSITIVE CHANGE

1. Show up
2. Speak up
3. Look up
4. Team up
5. Never give up
6. Lift others up

Source: TEDxtalk given by Rosabeth Moss Kanter in 2013 (https://youtu.be/owU5aTNPJbs). Copyright © Rosabeth Moss Kanter. Professor Kanter is a Harvard Professor.

that can be used early in the curriculum development process to streamline the implementation phase.

Any new or modified educational curriculum represents a change in the status quo, and therefore radiation oncology educators must become familiar with methods to effect successful change. Kanter's six steps to leading positive change[126] (Table 103.11) and Kotter's eight steps to leading change[127] (Fig. 103.9) are two examples of conceptual frameworks that can be employed to garner support from necessary stakeholders and successfully develop and implement a new curriculum or changes to an existing curriculum. One unifying theme in both conceptual frameworks is that to effect change, others must be involved in the process of change. Further discussion of leadership theory[128] and organizational culture[129] is beyond the scope of this text.

Evaluation

Per the six-step framework,[62] evaluation is a final step in curriculum development. Evaluation takes place both at the learner and the program level. In education parlance, "assessment" refers to a test or survey to provide feedback to the learner, whereas "evaluation" refers to methods used to evaluate the educational program. These can include stakeholder surveys, review of aggregate assessment data to determine if the specific and measurable objectives were achieved, etc. In

this section, assessment of the individual learner is referred to as distinct from the evaluation of an educational program, although both are intimately linked.

Learner Assessment. Key to the delivery of any educational intervention is a clear plan for learner assessment. Assessment is defined as "any systematic method of obtaining information from tests and other sources, used to draw inferences about characteristics of people, objects of programs."[130] The purposes of learner assessment are multifold.[131] Many of the educational attributes or traits that educators assess are hypothetical concepts. Assessments allow educators to assign a measure or degree of quantification to such attributes. Assessments aim to document achievement of what was learned or taught, which is helpful to assess the competency of learners and generate learner feedback for areas of improvement. Assessments can also be useful to measure aptitude to gauge learner performance, assign grades or provide ranking, and predict future performances or suitability for certain educational programs (i.e., MCAT for admission to medical school). Ultimately, in many settings, assessments are a requirement for accreditation and can inform decisions about the effectiveness of medical education programs and be integral to a programmatic evaluation (see below). To be meaningful, learner assessment must be clearly linked to objectives, define standards for performance, and include measurements that are reliable.

Assessments may be formative or summative. Formative assessments provide the learner with feedback with the intent to allow the learner to identify what they have learned and areas for improvement.[131,132] Formative assessments should occur at multiple defined points throughout a training program or course. In radiation oncology residency programs, formative assessments could include in-house written exams for physics or radiation biology, objective structured clinical examinations (OSCEs) to assess communication skills and end-of-life discussions administered midway through a clerkship rotation in medical school, or annual in-service training

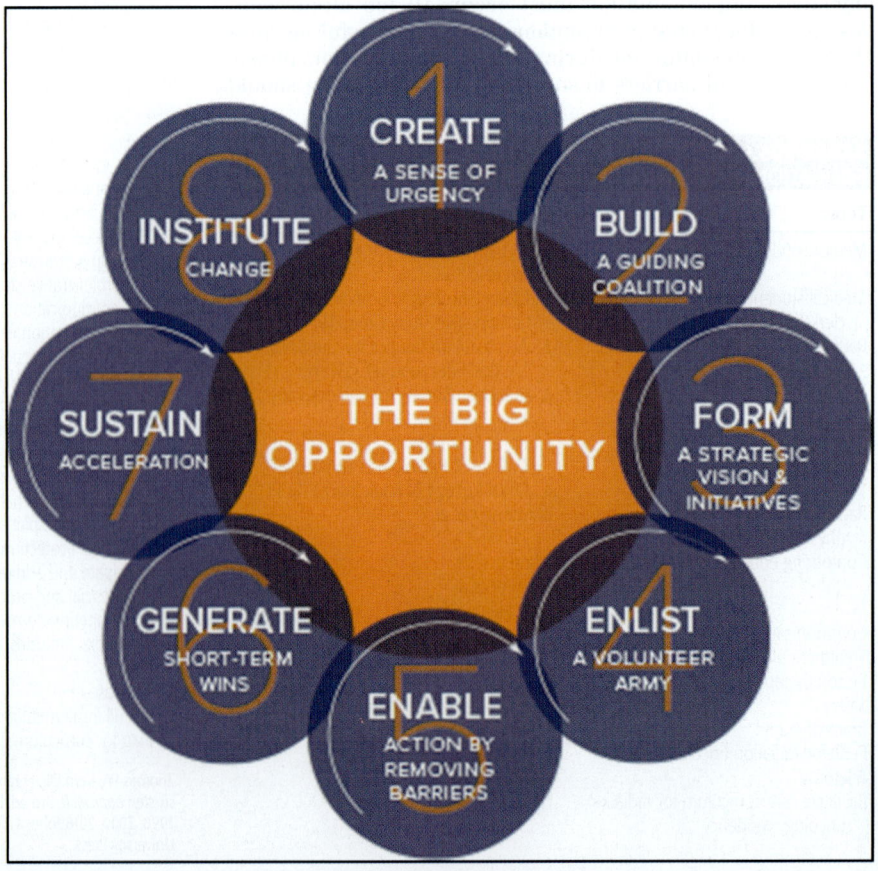

FIGURE 103.9. Kotter's eight steps to leading change. (From Kotter JP. *Leading change, with a new preface by the author*. Boston, MA: Harvard Business Review Press, 2012. Reprinted by permission of Kotter International.)

exams to assess clinical knowledge. Summative assessments are intended to provide an overall summary of a learner's achievement. They are generally done at the end of a defined curricular period. With respect to radiation oncology, this may include licensing exams at the end of residency such as those administered by the ABR or RCPSC. Assessments can be "low stakes" and "high stakes." These are often linked, but not always, to formative and summative evaluations, respectively. The consequences of the exam define the stakes of the exam. High-stakes exams have "a serious impact on the examinee," whereas low stakes have significantly lower potential for impact on the trainee.[132,133] Assessments can also be norm-referenced (e.g., percentile determines performance) or criterion-referenced, which are interpreted in the context of specific objectives or learning standards (e.g., "Pass/Fail" or "Meets Standard, Standard in Progress, Does not Meet Standard"). The annual in-service training exam is an example of a norm-referenced test, whereas competency-based assessment is usually criterion-referenced. Methods to set the pass threshold including the Angoff Method (used for the ABR certifying exams) are discussed elsewhere.[132]

Assessment Methods.
There is a wide range of assessment methods reported in the medical education literature.[62,133,134] Although not an exhaustive list, the following provides a sample of assessment methods. Downing and Yudkowsky[132] propose that there are four major types of assessment methods. Table 103.12 summarizes these methods with examples relevant to radiation oncology. The four groups include written tests, performance tests, clinical observations, and miscellaneous or other forms not classified. Written tests are among the most commonly used forms of assessment. Written tests may include open-ended (a.k.a. constructed responses, short or long answer, essay) responses or closed-ended (a.k.a. selected responses, matching, true or false, multiple choice). Closed-ended multiple-choice questions offer the advantage of being easy to administer and grade but may lack the ability to assess diagnostic reasoning. Well-constructed written tests may overcome this problem and allow for more detailed assessments of knowledge and reasoning.[133,135,136]

Performance tests are those assessments that allow for direct observation of the learner. They allow the learner to demonstrate "what they can do."[132] The most common examples are the OSCEs or simulations. An OSCE consists of a series of stations with a distinct focus on a clinical task.[133] Many OSCEs use standardized patients trained to portray a patient and relevant medical scenario.[134] For the purposes of assessment at an OSCE station, an observer will assess the performance of the learner based on a checklist or global rating tool. Although this type of assessment can be constructed to be realistic and reliable, they can be expensive and highly dependent on checklist quality and observer consistency. The term simulation refers to a realistic representation of a real-world task.[132] High-fidelity simulations can be used to assess

procedural skills or teamwork scenarios. They provide a relatively low-risk environment to assess high-risk and low-frequency scenarios.[137] Simulations can be realistic and provide reliable assessments. However, they can be expensive and do not provide a "real-time/real-world" assessment.

Clinical observations are assessments made based on performance in the clinical setting.[132] The clinical performance evaluation or global assessment rating is one of the most common methods utilized during training. The ACGME toolbox distinguishes the global rating from other assessment methods in that "A rater judges the general categories of ability instead of specific skills or behavior and the ratings are completed retrospectively based on general impressions collected over a period of time derived from multiple sources or information."[138] These are easy to carry out for the rater and usually done in real time. There has been considerable literature, however, on the subjectivity of the raters and the variability in the assessments coupled with issues with rating tools.[139]

The final category of assessment includes tools not well positioned in any of the categories above. These include assessment tools such as portfolios, formal oral exams, and bedside oral exams. A portfolio is a purposeful sampling of work to support attestation of meeting a required level of training or competency. Portfolios are combined with self-reflection and allow the learner to demonstrate areas of strengths and potential areas for improvement.[133,140] Portfolios can include a broad sampling of a learner's experiences including dictations, procedure logs, sample contouring logs, quality improvement projects, and even videos of procedural techniques or consults. Mentoring is integral to the interpretation of the portfolio. Portfolios can provide a broad sampling to support assessment but can be labor intensive and dependent on faculty development.

Selection of Assessment Methods.
Numerous resources provide guidance on the selection of specific assessment methods. From a conceptual perspective, the ACGME defined five characteristics integral to an assessment instrument or approach including that the approach should provide valid and reliable data, be feasible, apply to the assessment circumstances, and finally provide valuable information.[141] Van Der Vleuten and Schuwirth[142] developed a conceptual model that mirrors these criteria. Their model describes five criteria to help select an appropriate assessment tool. The criteria included are validity (if the assessment measures what it is intended to measure), reliability (does the tool reproducibly measure what it is intended to measure), educational impact (what are the effects of using the tool on learners and the educators), acceptability to learners and faculty, and costs. This model proposes that each of the criteria are weighted depending on the intended purpose of the assessment data and that all factors are multiplied together. For example, if the assessment would be for a certifying exam (e.g., ABR licensing exam), then more weight may be given to reliability and

TABLE 103.12 COMMON ASSESSMENT METHODS AND RELEVANT RADIATION ONCOLOGY EXAMPLES		
Assessment Method	**Example**	**Radiation Oncology Example with Relevant Literature if Applicable**
Written exam	Multiple-choice exam Essay exam Short-answer exam	– American College of Radiology (ACR) Radiation Oncology In-Training (TXIT) Exam[196] – Pre- and Posttest Written Exams after e-learning module[271] – American Board of Radiology Qualifying Exam – Royal College of Physicians and Surgeons of Canada Radiation Oncology Written Exam
Performance Test	OSCE Simulation	– Cancer Pain Management OSCE for Medical Students[272] – Standardized Patients to Assess Communication Skills in Radiation Oncology Residents[24] – Prostate Fossa Contouring Simulation[2] – Prostate or Gynecologic Brachytherapy Insertion Simulation on Phantom
Clinical observation	Structured clinical observation	– Mini-CEX – Direct Observation of Medical Student and Resident in Radiation Oncology Clinic rotations
Miscellaneous	Portfolio review Chart simulation	– Portfolio review to include clinical encounter notes, collection of clinical evaluations, sample of contouring tasks, quality improvement projects[273]

validity as opposed to an in-house physics exam intended to provide the learner with formative feedback where more weight may be given to costs and educational impact. This model is useful to conceptualize that each assessment method has inherent advantages and disadvantages and many factors should be both considered and relatively weighted in choosing a method appropriate to the educational context.

In the context of selecting an assessment method that measures what it is intended to, Miller's pyramid of clinical competence can help to provide a framework.[116,132] As discussed previously, Miller's pyramid (Fig. 103.8) progresses through four levels of clinical competence: knows, knows how, shows, and does. It can be useful to map assessment methods to each of these levels. At the base level of "know," a learner may be asked to simply demonstrate factual knowledge of a concept. At this level, assessment methods examine the ability of the learner to recite knowledge. Examples of assessment methods include traditional written tests such as true or false. "Knows how" implies that learner can use factual knowledge for the purposes of interpretation or application. This level may be assessed by more detailed written tests including short or long written answers or oral exams where the learner is required to show not only their knowledge but its application. The "shows" level implies an ability to demonstrate learned skills. Assessment methods include simulations or OSCEs. Finally, the "does" level moves the learner's performance into clinical practice. Assessments in this setting take place in the "real world" and include direct observations in a clinical setting and multisource feedback. Figure 103.10 depicts the selection of assessment methods in radiation oncology based on Miller's pyramid.

Although a multitude of assessment methods exist, the role of the medical educator is to select methods that provide a broad sampling of performance and are reliable, reproducible, and free of bias. No single assessment can give a perfect measure

TABLE 103.13	PRACTICAL QUESTIONS TO ASK WHEN DEVELOPING AN ASSESSMENT FRAMEWORK
Question	**Subset of Questions**
What is the goal of assessment?	What is the intended purpose of the assessment data? Is the data meant to be formative or summative?
What are you trying to assess?	Where does the entity being assessed exist on the Miller's pyramid[116]? How best can the learner demonstrate what you are trying to measure (i.e., written test or clinical observation)? How many measurements and methods would provide an adequate sampling of the entity to be measured?
When will you assess?	How often should assessments take place? If the assessments are formative, what frequency is needed for the learner to improve their performance? Are assessments too frequent and thus not feasible or sustainable?
Who will conduct the assessments?	How will you ensure the assessments are similar and reproducible? Will you need faculty development? How many assessments do different observers need?
Who will manage the assessment data?	Where will the assessment data be kept? Who will collate, distribute, and review the assessment data? How will the security of the assessment data be maintained? How will feedback be given in a timely fashion?

of performance or knowledge, and the application of several methods will provide the most reliable data. Assessment should be mapped to the objectives and instructional methods within a curriculum map (see objectives section).[143,144] A purposeful discussion of assessment methods should happen at the time of curriculum development with the intent of clearly defining what needs to be measured, how this will be measured, who will measure (and how will their skills be developed to support this), and how will the data be used.[133,137] Table 103.13 summarizes some of the practical questions a radiation oncology educator could ask themselves when developing an assessment plan.

FIGURE 103.10. Miller's pyramid[116] applied to assessment methods in radiation oncology.

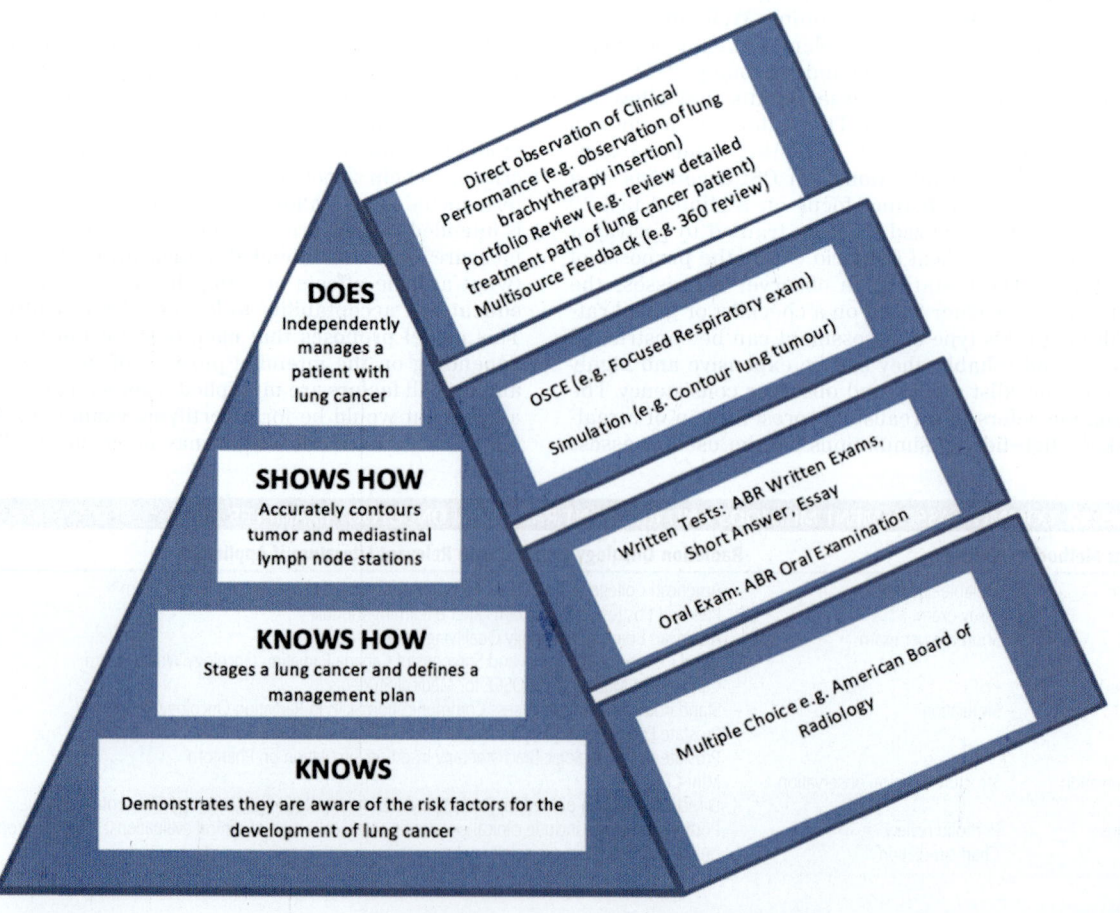

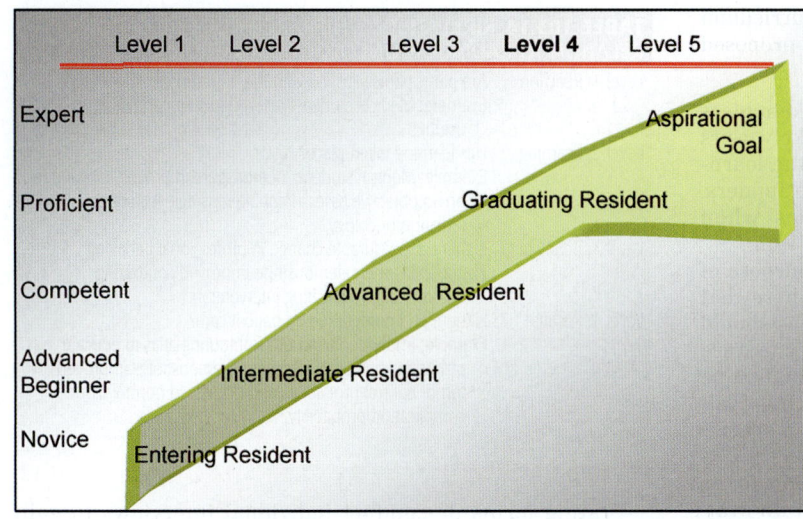

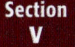

Section V

FIGURE 103.11. ACGME milestone levels of expectation. (From Ling L, Derstine P, Cohen N. *Implementing milestones and clinical competency committees.* 2013. Reprinted with permission of Accreditation Council for Graduate Medical Education.)

Competency and Assessment. As discussed previously in the Goals and Objectives section, medical training is shifting to competency-based frameworks.[118] Within radiation oncology GME, relevant frameworks include the RCPSC CanMEDS framework[5] and ACGME/ABR Radiation Oncology Milestone.[120] In Canada, the RCPSC is developing specialty-specific competency frameworks for all specialties including radiation oncology through the Competence by Design project.[122,145] Both the ACGME Milestone Project (Fig. 103.11) and the Radiation Oncology Competence by Design (Fig. 103.12) define competencies related to the various roles (i.e., Communicator, Collaborator, etc.) and specific to level of training. By the end of a specific level of training, a learner is expected to demonstrate competency through the accomplishment of a number or training level–specific EPAs.[146] An EPA is a clinical task that is demonstrable and typically includes multiple milestones.

Each of the competency-based frameworks in the United States (ACGME) and Canada (CanMEDS) has toolboxes that may help the educator to select assessment methods by competency.[138,147] With the evolving competency-based curriculum, there will be changes to these toolboxes, but the foundations will likely remain similar. Although these toolboxes divide assessment methods by competency, it is well established that many of the competencies overlap and their assessment on an individual level is artificial at best. Competencies are not stable through training and develop

with experience.[148] The most robust assessment of competencies will rely on features mentioned previously and will include broad, purposeful, and frequent sampling with reliable and reproducible methods. In the context of competency-based assessments, the assessment data can be used both "for learning" and allow self-reflection and to "assess learning" to ensure accountability to training programs and society.[149] Lastly, both the RCPSC and the ACGME mandate the involvement of a clinical competence committee to review competency assessments on a regular basis and help to provide feedback to the learner and the program. With a shift to competency-based training and assessment, a considerable amount of faculty development will need to occur to ensure that the assessments are performed in a consistent and reliable manner and accomplish the intended outcomes.

Program Evaluation. Program evaluation is a key step in curriculum development. The purposes of evaluation are multifold. Program evaluation can be performed[150,151]:

...to determine the effectiveness of the curriculum for learners
...to document that curricular objectives have been met
...to enable faculty to make changes to improve the program
...to provide data to track program management, evaluate efficiency, to support accountability and dissemination

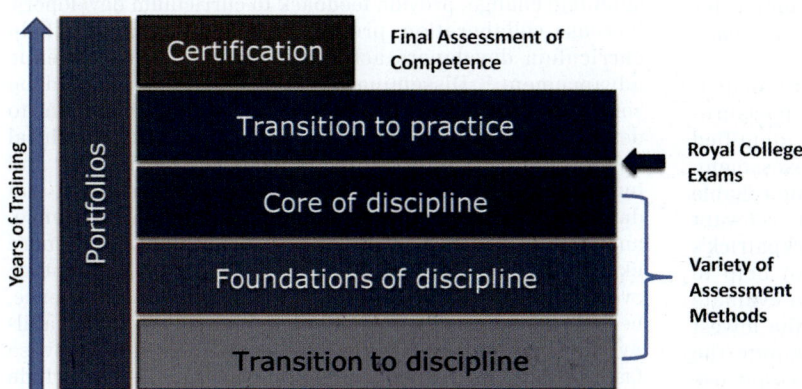

FIGURE 103.12. College of Physicians and Surgeons of Canada Competence by Design Conceptual Framework for Residency Training. (Adapted from Royal from The Royal College of Physicians and Surgeons of Canada. Accessed May 16, 2018.)

Eight practical steps adapted from the six-step curriculum approach,[62] Fitzpatrick,[152] and AMEE guides[151,153] are proposed to guide program evaluation:

1. Identification of users: As a first step, the stakeholders should be identified. Stakeholders refer to the likely users of the evaluation data. This will often include the learners, the faculty, the curriculum developers, the funders, the university, and the accreditation bodies when appropriate.

2. Determine the purpose of the evaluation: The purpose of the evaluation should be clearly defined. It is here that the approaches to evaluation and the dimensions should be reviewed as discussed above. Key questions to ask are what approach is this evaluation? Will this evaluation be summative or formative? How will the results of this evaluation impact the program and how will the data specifically be used?

3. Identify resources and select and an evaluation team: Resources will need to be allocated to conduct an evaluation. Such resources can include personnel, time, equipment (e.g., computers, access to secure databases), and funding. Many medical schools and residency programs may have existing evaluation units, and it can be useful to identify this at the outset. With respect to choosing an evaluation team, it is useful to consider if an evaluation team is best composed of internal or external reviewers. Additionally depending on the approach to evaluation, it may be useful to include participants, faculty, learners, and health care consumers, among others.

4. Determine the evaluation questions: The evaluation questions depend on the approach to the evaluation. With respect to an objective-oriented approach, evaluation should be linked to the process and outcome objectives of a curriculum (see Goals and Objectives). As such, the evaluation will examine the *who will do how much of what and when*. It is best when writing program objectives that a lens is given to the evaluation questions to ensure they are in fact measurable and clear. If a participant-oriented approach is taken, evaluation questions could be directed to participants, and the questions asked are related to the perceived effectiveness of the program and the relative strengths and weaknesses.

5. Select an evaluation design: A variety of evaluation approaches can be taken. For the most part, these are dependent on the approach to evaluation and are well summarized elsewhere.[151] Some of the most common evaluation designs relate to an objective approach to document that learning objectives have been met. These can include a posttest design, a pre-posttest design, or a controlled pre- and posttest design (i.e., where an experimental group is exposed to a curricular intervention). As the degree of control increases, the complexity to administer also increases. There are well-known limitations to each design approach.[62]

6. Select a measurement method and relevant instruments to collect data: It is essential that the measurement method be aligned with the questions identified in the evaluation. Similar to the section on assessment, evaluation methods should be chosen to provide reliable and reproducible data that evaluate questions relevant to making appropriate judgments. In part, Kirkpatrick's hierarchy of evaluation[64] (Table 103.14) can help to frame the possible methods one might use to evaluate a program examining learner outcomes. At the lowest level of the hierarchy, one could simply evaluate the participation and reaction of learners. One could use

TABLE 103.14	KIRKPATRICK'S HIERARCHY OF EVALUATION[64] IN RELATION TO RADIATION ONCOLOGY EDUCATION
Level 1: Reaction	Are participants satisfied with the educational experience?
	Example: Medical students rate a clerkship curriculum as useful.[82]
Level 2: Learning	Has learning taken place?
	Example: Medical students demonstrate improved knowledge on an objective assessment after a single lecture on radiation oncology.[165]
Level 3: Behavior	Is there a measurable change in professional behavior?
	Example: Learners demonstrate improved contouring accuracy after a teaching intervention.[46]
Level 4: Results	Is there an improvement in patient care?
	Example: Implementation of a contouring atlas to educate physicians on contour accuracy demonstrates improved tumor control probability and decreased normal tissue complication probability.[274]

rating forms or conduct individual interviews to gain information on the satisfaction of learners (or stakeholders). To demonstrate that learning had taken place, one could examine the results of written or oral exams. With respect to documenting a change in behavior, this would likely be best done in the context of direct observation. Finally, improved patient care could be done through direct observation and performance audits. The most robust evaluation data would be both quantitative and qualitative.

7. Collect and analyze the data: The data must be both collected and analyzed. As part of curriculum design, it is essential to define the frequency with which evaluations will be done and how the data will be stored and analyzed. Data may require analysis with both descriptive statistics and qualitative analysis. When established standards are in existence, the data may be compared to these or the literature can be reviewed to relate the experience to other programs or institutions.

8. Dissemination and feedback: The last stage of program evaluation is the act of collating the results and dissemination. Evaluations should be timely and distributed to the relevant stakeholders. It is useful to review the purposes of the evaluation in order to assess who should receive the results and in what format.

Overall, program evaluation is a key component of curriculum development. Table 103.15 provides specific examples of radiation oncology program evaluation.

Dissemination

To qualify as scholarship, any curriculum development project must be disseminated to the public.[39] Dissemination of a novel curriculum can help address a health care problem, stimulate change, provide feedback to curriculum developers, increase collaboration, prevent redundant work, and help curriculum developers achieve recognition and academic advancement.[62] Dissemination of a curriculum should be considered during all phases of curriculum development to develop a coherent strategy for dissemination, address ethical and legal issues related to protection of the participants and intellectual property, identify what curriculum material and data will be disseminated, identify the target audience, and identify venues for dissemination.[62] Innovations are more likely to be adopted if there is a perceived relative advantage over existing practice; compatibility with previous experience, beliefs, and values; simplicity of the innovation; trial ability allowing the innovation to be implemented in a stepwise fashion; and observability.[154] Ethical and legal issues include

TABLE 103.15 EXAMPLES OF EDUCATIONAL EVALUATION STUDIES IN RADIATION ONCOLOGY

Study Summary	Evaluation Approaches	Evaluation Methods
Evaluation of a Radiation Safety Initiative for Nurses[275]	Objectives oriented	Pre- and postwritten tests to assess for changes in knowledge and attitudinal objectives
Evaluation of Theoretical Radiation Oncology Training Programs[23]	Participant oriented	Written user satisfaction surveys
Evaluation of a Contouring Bootcamp[18]	Objectives oriented Participant oriented	Pre- and post written tests Written learner satisfaction surveys
Longitudinal Study to Assess Adherence to Clinical Pathways[276]	Objectives oriented	Pre- and post written tests using Clinical Performance and Value Vignettes
10-Year review of student accomplishments in rapid response radiotherapy program[277]	Objectives oriented/ management oriented Participant oriented	Number of first authored papers produced by students in the program Written learner satisfaction surveys

consideration of whether local IRB exemption or approval is required prior to disseminating the curriculum. In the United States, many educational projects qualify as "exempt" from IRB review based on Health and Human Services Office for Human Research Protections guidelines for exemption.[155] Projects that are exempted include:

Category 1: Research conducted in established or commonly accepted educational settings, involving normal educational practices, such as (i) research on regular and special education instructional strategies or (ii) research on the effectiveness of or the comparison among instructional techniques, curricula, or classroom management methods.

Category 2: Research involving the use of educational tests (cognitive, diagnostic, aptitude, achievement), survey procedures, interview procedures, or observation of public behavior, unless (i) information obtained is recorded in such a manner that human subjects can be identified, directly or through identifiers linked to the subjects, and (ii) any disclosure of the human subjects' responses outside the research could reasonably place the subjects at risk of criminal or civil liability or be damaging to the subjects' financial standing, employability, or reputation.

Radiation oncology educators are encouraged to speak with their institutional IRB representatives to obtain advice on whether IRB exemption or full review is required for an educational project. Professional ramifications for not obtaining proper IRB approval of a scholarship project can be significant.

Consideration of intellectual property issues is also important. Images, figures, and tables used in lectures may be subject to copyright protection. Publishers can be contacted for permissions, or more simply, when developing an educational product, care can be taken to avoid copyrighted materials. In addition, institutions may have copyright protections for patient images or photographs, and the curriculum developer is advised to discuss possible copyright issues with the appropriate institutional representative.

Multiple components of the curriculum development process can be disseminated including a systematic review performed as a general needs assessment, a survey focus group done as the targeted needs assessment, the curriculum materials themselves including goals and objectives with

educational methods (e.g., lecture, workshop, small group), and then the assessment and evaluation data. Methods for dissemination include presentations at national meetings, publication in peer-reviewed journals, and dissemination via the Internet (e.g., MedEdPORTAL[83]). A more detailed discussion of curriculum dissemination strategies is available elsewhere.[62]

Curriculum Maintenance, Renewal, and Reform

Radiation oncology educational programs must adapt and evolve to accommodate changes in accrediting body requirements, learner preferences, turnover of faculty and staff, and changes in clinical practice. Additionally, novel systemic therapies and radiation oncology techniques are continually being developed and implemented. As such, training programs must continually address these changes. A seminal paper by Abrahamson describes nine "diseases" of the curriculum. Examples include "carcinoma of the curriculum" characterized by uncontrollable growth of one segment or component of the curriculum, "iatrogenic curriculitis" where the curriculum suffers from excessive tampering or meddling, "curriculum hypertrophy" with an increasingly crowded curriculum due to more and more content crammed into limited educational time, bad teaching leading to "idiopathic curriculitis," and "curriculum ossification" where the curriculum is "cast in concrete" and is characterized by comments such as "What do you want to change anything for?" or "Well, we've always done it this way."[156] These "diseases," although humorous on the surface, affect many radiation oncology educational programs including medical school clerkships, residency training programs, educational sessions at society meetings, and CME programs. To prevent or treat Abrahamson's diseases of the curriculum, radiation oncology educators should routinely re-evaluate their curriculum for deficiencies and areas in need of improvement. A curriculum is never "done" and can be re-evaluated utilizing the six-step model[62] or by applying Harden's ten questions.[74] Without regular re-evaluation, radiation oncology educators are at risk for curricular ossification or any of Abrahamson's other diseases of the curriculum.

To achieve success when revising or reforming an existing curriculum, methods discussed previously for implementation should be employed. In particular, utilizing a deliberative curriculum development model that includes as many stakeholders as possible will help to garner political support for curriculum reform.[157]

CURRENT PRACTICES IN RADIATION ONCOLOGY TRAINING

Having a basic understanding of the principles of medical education can help to facilitate the careful development, implementation, and evaluation of a new curriculum and educational scholarship. The following section focuses on the real-world application of medical education principles to UGME, GME, and CME in radiation oncology. This review will focus on the current educational landscape in each setting and identify areas for potential future educational development and scholarship.

Undergraduate Medical Education in Radiation Oncology

Radiation oncology education as a specific discipline begins during the undergraduate phase of medical training. Students enter medical school with varied experiences and preconceptions about which specialty they plan to pursue. As a small specialty, radiation oncology may be relatively unknown to

Section V

medical students relative to larger core clerkship specialties (internal medicine, pediatrics, surgery, obstetrics and gynecology, psychiatry, family medicine) or specialties that are commonly portrayed in popular culture (surgery, emergency medicine, etc.). Therefore, radiation oncology educators must work to ensure that the specialty is represented in their institution's core curriculum. In one US needs assessment for radiation oncology education, only 30% of respondents reported receiving a lecture in their medical school on radiation oncology, and 1% reported a mandatory radiation oncology educational experience.[45] A survey of students, primary care providers, and radiation oncology attendings at seven US medical schools demonstrated persistent misconceptions regarding radiation oncology.[97] For example, 23% of fourth year medical students and 19% of primary care providers responded that radiation oncologists "push a button to deliver RT every day," indicating a lack of knowledge regarding the daily clinical duties of a radiation oncologist. Similarly, in a survey at two US medical schools, medical students reported increasing comfort regarding their knowledge of medical oncology, surgical oncology, and hospice/palliative care, but not radiation oncology or survivorship care.[69] A survey of Canadian medical schools demonstrates similar deficiencies in radiation oncology education with 17% of students reporting no radiation oncology training, a majority reporting ≤2 hours of radiation oncology teaching, and 19% reporting they were deterred from considering radiation oncology as a career choice because of lack of knowledge about the specialty.[158] Combined, these data indicate that medical students are not being adequately exposed to clinical aspects of radiation oncology during their core medical school curriculum and are uncomfortable with their radiation oncology knowledge. This deficiency may lead to potential negative consequences. First, students who may otherwise choose radiation oncology as their specialty are not being exposed early and in enough depth in medical school to consider pursuing the specialty. Second, for the majority of students who pursue specialties other than radiation oncology, lack of a basic understanding of the specialty may negatively impact future patient care, including recognizing the need for a radiation oncology consultation or toxicities commonly caused by radiation.

Radiation Oncology Education for All Medical Students

Multiple efforts to develop radiation oncology educational experiences for the general UGME curriculum are reported.[158-171] General exposure to radiation oncology can be achieved through development of a preclinical oncology interest group[172] or through tumor board shadowing experience.[171]

Hirsch et al.[47,163,165] at Boston University developed a 1.5-hour didactic lecture on radiation oncology during the radiology clerkship. All students at their institution received the lecture. A pre- and postclerkship multiple-choice exam was administered to assess objective knowledge improvement. The average exam score increased, most significantly on the radiation oncology scores (56.5% to 71.8% correct, $P < .001$), demonstrating that a single lecture can have a significant impact on knowledge of radiation oncology. The same group has developed the Oncology Education Initiative for preclinical students that includes a radiation oncologist-led oncology education block for second year medical students.[173] Students rate the oncology block favorably and specifically report that the oncology block "was effective in contributing to [their] overall medical education."

The group at Thomas Jefferson University has taken a different approach offering an optional 3-week radiation oncology elective during the third year surgery clerkship.[166,168] Overall objective test scores improved after the rotation (64% to 82%) and within the subdomains of clinical (63% to 79%), biology (70% to 77%), and physics (62% to 88%) knowledge (all values $P < .001$).[166] On a follow-up survey, an average of 1.5 years after completion of the elective, improvements in knowledge persisted, with some decay seen for clinical and physics knowledge. Students felt that the elective helped them to understand when to consult a radiation oncologist, identify emergent situations where radiation is needed, and how to take care of patients with cancer, among other benefits.[168]

At the University of British Columbia, other approaches have been used to increase medical student exposure to radiation oncology. During the third year surgery clerkship rotation, only 10% to 15% of medical students partake in radiation oncology electives. As a result, upwards of 85% to 90% of graduating medical students receive no clinical exposure to radiation oncology. A targeted needs assessment of learners identified that, relative to other areas of clinical training, medical students felt unprepared to take care of cancer patients and that supplemental online resources were needed.[174] Based on the six-step method for curriculum development,[62] Ingledew and colleagues developed and implemented a series of online modules, supported by virtual patient vignettes and educational whiteboard videos to provide basic oncology instruction to medical students. User satisfaction surveys demonstrated that medical students completing the modules feel more prepared to deal with oncology in clinical scenarios.[175] The online modules are now being examined for impact on knowledge. The online materials are being utilized throughout Canada and in selected universities in the United States and elsewhere. New modules are being added to meet the objectives of the Canadian Oncology Education Goal and Objectives for medical students.[176]

The aforementioned programs represent methods by which a radiation oncology educator can include a radiation oncology educational experience in their school's core curriculum. Other institutions worldwide report strategies to include radiation oncology in the medical school curriculum.[167,169,177] Radiation oncology primers are available to supplement a course or lecture.[3] Oncology curricula for medical schools have also been proposed that include radiotherapy.[164,176] The primary challenge to implementing radiation oncology education within the core curriculum of a medical school is resource scarcity, in particular student time. Thus, it is critical that the radiation oncology educator utilize the methods discussed above to ensure successful implementation.

Education for Students Pursuing a Career in Radiation Oncology

Medical students interested in pursuing a career in radiation oncology represent a different group of learners than the general medical student population. Prior to their first formal rotation in a radiation oncology department, the majority of US medical students spend time in a radiation oncology department shadowing physicians (69%), work in a radiation oncology department conducting research (clinical, translational, or basic science) (60%), or had a lecture on radiation oncology during the first or second year of medical school (30%). Only 26% report no prior radiation oncology clinical or research experience.[45] However, 23% of fourth year medical students who have not completed a rotation in radiation oncology still believe that radiation oncologists push a button every day to deliver radiation.[97] Thus, the radiation oncology clerkship is a critical educational experience for students considering radiation oncology as a specialty choice to ensure they understand what their clinical activities and professional responsibilities will entail once they complete residency training. Additionally, the clerkship likely represents the student's first significant formal radiation oncology educational experience and is thus the beginning of their radiation oncology training.

The traditional radiation oncology clerkship in the United States and Canada employs the apprenticeship model. Students spend time working with attending and resident physicians in the clinic observing daily clinical activities including consultations, simulations, treatment planning, contouring, plan review and approval, management of on-treatment patients, and follow-up visits to manage acute and late toxicities. Students report opportunities to participate in clinical care including performing an oncologic history and physical independently without resident or faculty supervision (90%), write or dictate a consult (73%), contour at a planning station for a clinical case (78%), participate in a brachytherapy case (60%), participate in a stereotactic radiosurgery case (57%), participate in a stereotactic body radiation therapy (SBRT) case (49%), and review port films (52%).[45] However, merely participating in these clinical experiences does not mean the medical student is learning the basic background knowledge associated with the experience. For example, participating in a plan review of a base of tongue squamous cell carcinoma being treated with intensity-modulated radiation therapy (IMRT) does not mean the student learns the clinical, radiobiologic, and physics aspects of external beam radiation treatment. Students are encouraged to read primary and secondary literature outside of clinic, but as discussed previously, students will have different learning styles,[124] and thus educational strategies other than clinical observation and outside reading should be incorporated into the clerkship experience.

Students may attend resident-level didactics (clinical, physics, radiation biology) and shadow physicians at tumor boards, but the majority of clerkships did not include formal didactics at the medical student training level.[45,98] This apprenticeship model is not unique to radiation oncology and is frequently used in other subspecialty clerkships where there are limited students at any one time.

These clerkships are also sometimes referred to as "audition rotations" where one of the student's goals for the clerkship is to secure a competitive residency position. There are multiple critiques of the practice of audition rotations. First, audition rotations potentially waste valuable educational time during the final year of medical school when the student could be broadening their medical education before focusing on radiation oncology. Second, audition rotations outside of the geographic location where the medical student resides require the student to have sufficient funds to travel and pay for room and board during the elective clerkship. Therefore,

wealthier students may be more likely to take audition rotations. Because in the US economic status correlates with race, selecting students for residency positions based on performance during an audition rotation may discriminate against minority groups. Lastly, audition rotations may be difficult to arrange for students with significant home and family responsibilities, thus discriminated against married students or students with children. Residency training programs must be cognizant of the pitfalls of using audition rotations to select future residents and, rather, should holistically evaluate each applicant's medical school performance, letters of recommendation, and personal statement for potential fit with the training program.[178]

In a national radiation oncology clerkship needs assessment in the United States, students reported giving a departmental talk on a topic of their choice at 87% of clerkship experiences, whereas 72% of clerkships had no medical student lectures, and 52% of clerkships had no formal lecture, case discussion, or hands-on didactic session at the medical student training level.[98] This disparity suggests that clerkships may place an emphasis on the audition aspect of the experience rather than the educational experience.

Based on these data demonstrating a lack of structured didactics for the medical student clerkship, the Radiation Oncology Education Collaborative Study Group (ROECSG) developed a structured, didactic curriculum for the radiation oncology medical student clerkship. Using the six-step model for curriculum development,[62] a series of targeted needs assessments were conducted to determine the target learners' (medical students) needs and preferred learning methods (Fig. 103.13).[45,98] Based on these data, a structured, didactic curriculum was developed incorporating three lectures (Introduction to Radiation Oncology, Radiation Biology and Physics, and Simulations/Radiation Emergencies) and a hands-on treatment planning workshop.[179] The needs assessment demonstrated that students want the opportunity to give a lecture to the department (perhaps for the purposes of auditioning for residency) and to give formal case presentations. These activities were not removed from the clerkship but rather supplemented by the addition of the formalized lectures and a treatment planning workshop. The curriculum was piloted at 2 institutions in 2012[180] and subsequently expanded to 11 academic medical centers in 2013.[82,181] 88 students completed the curriculum in 2013 and subjective evaluation of the curriculum was positive. All lectures and the treatment planning workshop were rated as "quite" to

FIGURE 103.13. Survey respondent perspectives on the utility of specific curricular components of an ideal radiation oncology clerkship: median Likert scale (interquartile range). EBM, evidence-based medicine; MS4, fourth year medical student. (Reprinted from Jagadeesan VS, Raleigh DR, Koshy M, et al. A national radiation oncology medical student clerkship survey: didactic curricular components increase confidence in clinical competency. *Int J Radiat Oncol Biol Phys* 2014;88[1]:51–56. Copyright © 2014 Elsevier. With permission.)

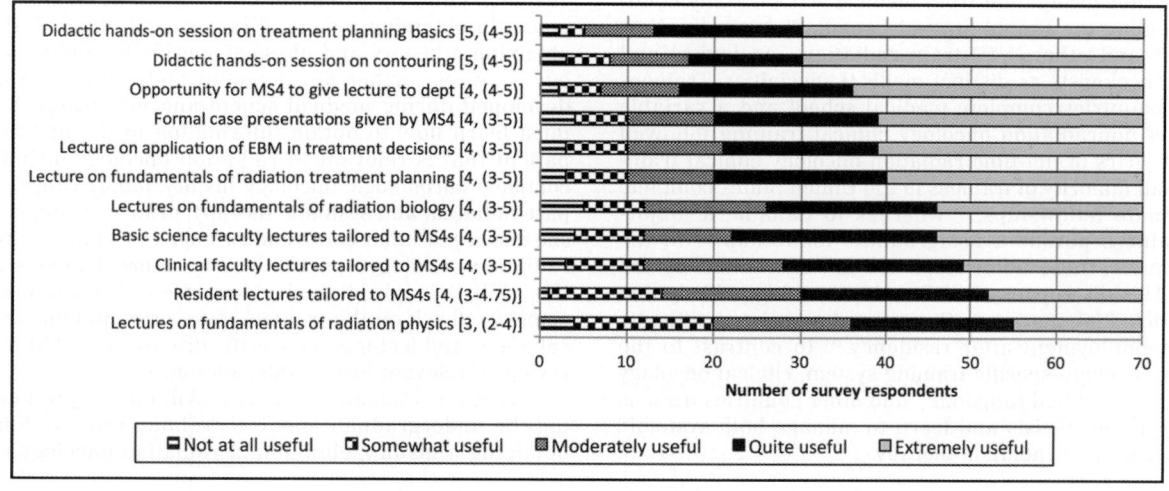

"extremely" useful. Students rated the curriculum as helping them to better understand radiation oncology as a specialty, increase their comfort with their specialty decision, and help the transition to radiation oncology residency.[82] The curriculum subsequently expanded to 22 academic medical centers with 146 students completing it in 2017. Mean objective multiple-choice question test scores pre- and postcurriculum were 63% and 80%, respectively ($P < .01$). Postscores for students rotating de novo at ROECSG institutions ($n = 30$) were higher compared with prescores for students with 1 or more prior rotations at non-ROECSG institutions ($n = 55$) (77% vs. 69%, $P = .01$).[181a] This exploratory analysis showing students completing a clerkship at ROECSG institutions perform objectively better when compared with students who completed clerkships at non-ROECSG institutions supports a structured didactic curriculum as a standard component of a radiation oncology clerkship.

Based on the needs assessment indicating students desired hands-on training for contouring,[45] an additional module was developed that teaches fundamental concepts of atlas-based contouring of the prostate fossa.[182] Using a treatment planning station, students first contoured the prostate fossa on a standardized CT scan with no prior instruction. Utilizing Kolb's experiential learning model[26] (Fig. 103.3), this represents the concrete experience. The student then receives a lecture on the CT anatomy of the prostate fossa and how to follow atlas-based instructions for contouring the target volume (reflective observation and abstract conceptualization). The student then repeats the contouring exercise using the atlas and their new knowledge from the lecture (active experimentation and concrete experience). Finally, the student turns on a "gold standard" contour as determined by experts in genitourinary radiation oncology (reflective observation). Students reported subjective improvements in comfort contouring a prostate fossa, ability to find references for contouring, knowledge of CT prostate/pelvis anatomy, and ability to use contouring software tools. In addition, objective analysis of contour accuracy when compared to the gold standard showed significant improvements after the educational intervention.[2]

Formal UGME curriculum development remains nascent in radiation oncology. Implementation of a formal didactic curriculum and hands-on planning and contouring workshops represent methods by which the UGME radiation oncology educator can ensure medical students are making the best career choice while enhancing the students' clinical knowledge to ease the transition to residency training.

Graduate Medical Education in Radiation Oncology

Clinical training in radiation oncology primarily occurs during GME after graduation from medical school. Many countries including the United States,[4] Canada,[121] Australia, New Zealand,[16] and others[15,19-21] train radiation oncologists and medical oncologists as distinct medical specialties. Trainees in these countries complete medical school and a variable amount of nonradiation oncology clinical training followed by 3 to 4 years of full-time radiation oncology clinical training. A small minority of trainees in the United States complete postgraduate fellowships,[183] whereas in Canada, a majority of trainees pursue a postgraduate fellowship.[184] In the United States, these fellowships are not accredited by the ACGME. This discrepancy in fellowship training is likely due to a restricted job market in Canada and associated difficulty securing employment after residency.[184] In contrast to the radiation oncology–specific training system, clinical oncology trainees in the United Kingdom[185] and other countries train as nonsurgical oncologists and learn to manage both systemic chemotherapy and radiation therapy.

Although certain disease sites such as pediatric malignancies and treatment techniques such as interstitial brachytherapy have relatively few numbers of cases and are nonuniformly geographically distributed, trainees in the United States continue to be certified to treat all disease sites. This raises a dilemma of whether these trainees are adequately prepared to treat rare diseases or use specialized treatment modalities. US residency program directors address this problem by allowing residents to train at other centers that see higher volumes of rare cases or use specialized treatment procedures. Although in an ideal training environment all trainees would see high volumes of rare cases or specialized procedures, analysis of radiation oncology training programs suggests that subspecialty certification is unlikely in radiation oncology.[186] Thus, programs must continue to develop novel training methods including simulation-based education and case-based education to provide sufficient training for rare cases and techniques. By ensuring trainees are competent in the clinical and technical fundamentals of radiation oncology as applied to any disease site or therapeutic technique, training programs will ensure that their graduates are competent to treat rare tumors (e.g., pediatric malignancies) or use specialized techniques (e.g., interstitial brachytherapy) when required.

Regardless of whether trainees focus solely on radiation oncology or learn radiation and medical oncology as in the UK system, during residency, trainees must become competent in all aspects of clinical radiation oncology including obtaining a focused radiation oncology history and physical, the treatment decision process, simulation, contouring, treatment planning, plan review, and treatment and toxicity management. Residents must learn fundamental scientific knowledge of radiation biology and physics, research methods, and biostatistics. Residents in the United States are assessed semiannually by their department's clinical competency committee using the ACGME Radiation Oncology Milestones,[120] which, as described previously, are divided into the ACGME core competencies including Patient Care, Medical Knowledge, Systems-Based Practice, Practice-Based Learning and Improvement, Professionalism, and Interpersonal and Communication Skills. In Canada, an almost analogous set of core competencies is represented by the CanMEDS framework and include Medical Expert, Communicator, Collaborator, Scholar, Leader, and Health Advocate.[5] Finally, residents must be responsible to themselves, their chosen profession, society, and the patient. Based on these complementary learning goals, a conceptual framework of GME radiation oncology education is presented (Fig. 103.14). Educational scholarship related to the clinical care path outlined in this conceptual framework is discussed henceforth.

History and Physical

Trainees entering radiation oncology GME should be competent in obtaining a focused history and physical. However, obtaining a history and physical specific for radiation oncology requires further development and refinement of skills developed during medical school and internship. A trainee must learn how to obtain information in the history of the patient that is relevant to radiation oncology including the complete chronologic oncology history, family cancer history, past radiation and systemic therapy, history of connective tissue disease or other contraindications for radiation, and other radiation oncology–specific history items. Trainees acquire this skill through clinical observation of attending physicians, feedback on the trainee's case presentations and clinical notes, and lectures on specific disease sites that include a review of relevant history information.

Physical examination is also a skill that is developed during the undergraduate medical training process. Similar to obtaining a history, obtaining a radiation oncology physical

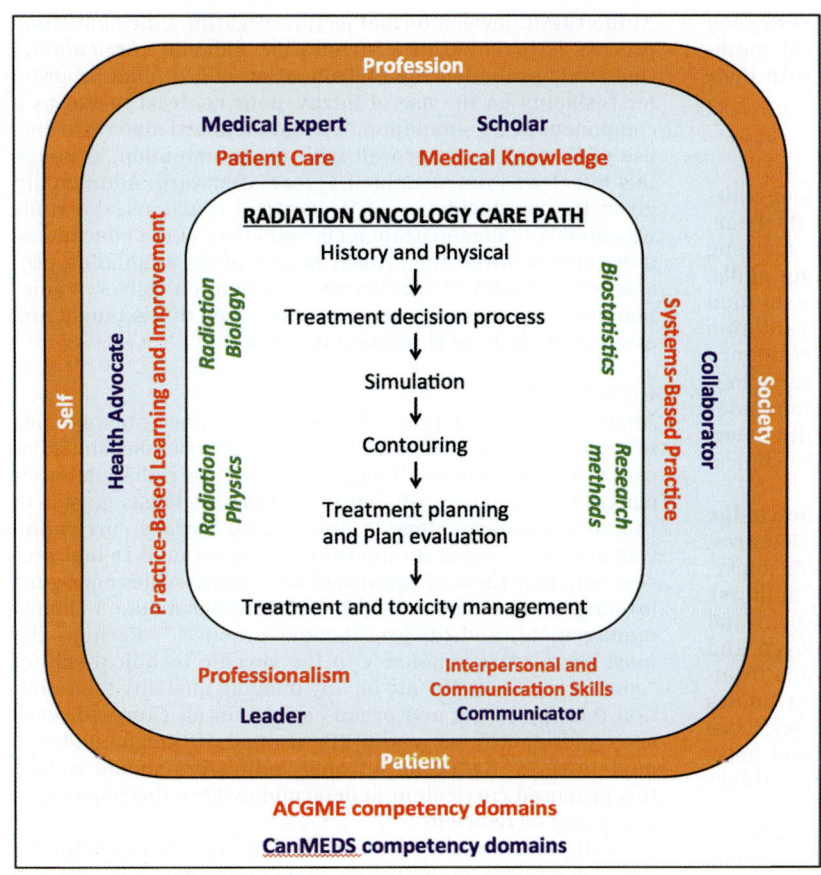

FIGURE 103.14. Conceptual framework for radiation oncology clinical education structured on learner obligations, Accreditation Council for Graduate Medical Education (ACGME) and Canadian Medical Education Directives for Specialists (CanMEDS) core competencies, fundamental knowledge of physics/radiation biology and research methodology knowledge, and the patient's clinical care path.

exam requires additional skill refinement. For example, trainees must learn to carefully examine the supraclavicular fossa in a patient with cervical cancer and periaortic lymphadenopathy on imaging, whereas patients with anal cancer must be assessed for inguinal lymphadenopathy, and patients with nasopharyngeal squamous cell carcinoma should have a thorough cranial nerve exam. Similar to the patient history, these skills are most commonly taught through faculty clinical observation and lecture format.

To perform an appropriate physical exam, anatomic knowledge relevant to oncology is critical.[187] Time spent learning about anatomy is heavily frontloaded in the UGME curriculum with minimal time allotted during residency training, whereas the need for applied anatomy knowledge increases drastically at the start of residency training (Fig. 103.15). To address this need for applied anatomy knowledge, Duke University developed an oncoanatomy course for resident trainees that included a 1-hour didactic session followed by a 1-hour session in the gross anatomy lab with cadaveric prosections. Implementation of this course demonstrated a significant improvement in objective anatomic knowledge, and residents rated the course as highly effective.[188]

Communication skills are also necessary during the history and physical process. The University of Pennsylvania developed a novel OSCE with the goal of improving resident skills with regard to breaking bad news.[24] Residents were presented with two case scenarios and given the opportunity to work through the cases with standardized patients. Residents worked through an initial case and then underwent an evaluation by and feedback from the standardized patient, faculty, and residents themselves using the Kalamazoo Essential Elements Communication Checklist—Adapted.[189,190] The residents then completed a second case scenario. Although there was no difference demonstrated in resident performance between scenarios 1 and 2, barriers to developing strong

interpersonal relationships were revealed including perceived lack of empathy, absence of shared decision-making, and use of excessive medical jargon. Resident feedback included the suggestion to allow the resident to review the video recording of the encounter and then repeat the same encounter to try

FIGURE 103.15. Schematic of time spent in anatomic instruction and the need to apply knowledge of anatomy for the radiation oncologist in training. There is a large temporal separation between instruction and application. IORT, intraoperative radiation therapy; PGY, postgraduate year; Rad Onc, radiation oncology; SBRT, stereotactic body radiation therapy; SRS, stereotactic radiosurgery. (Reprinted from Chino J, Doyle S, Marks LB. The anatomy of radiation oncology residency training. *Int J Radiat Oncol Biol Phys* 2014;88[1]:3–4. Copyright © 2014 Elsevier. With permission.)

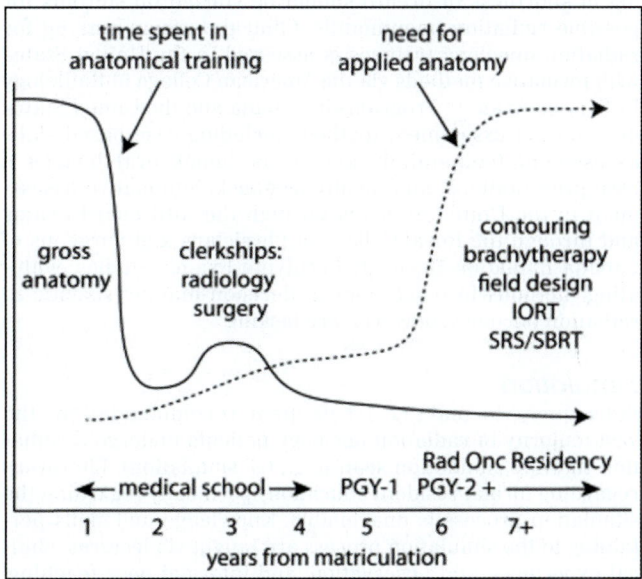

new wording.[24] An OSCE encounter represents a novel method by which radiation oncology trainees can be taught methods to develop strong interpersonal relationships with their patients at the first clinical encounter.

Clinical Decision-Making

Once the trainee obtains a focused radiation oncology history and physical, they must make a treatment decision. Determining a treatment recommendation requires a strong fund of medical knowledge and clinical reasoning skills. Ensuring that graduating trainees obtain the requisite fund of medical knowledge required of a competent radiation oncologist is perhaps the most important role of residency training program. Without knowledge of treatment guidelines and the primary literature supporting those recommendations, a radiation oncology trainee will have difficulty determining the optimal treatment approach for a specific clinical scenario.

Trainees most commonly learn medical knowledge through a variety of methods including readings, lectures, online learning resources, peer teaching, and real-life supervised clinical experiences (personal observations of authors). Other teaching methods such as small group discussions and problem-based learning are less commonly employed and represent novel educational methods that may provide trainees with varying learning styles and additional opportunities to assimilate the material. Outside of radiation oncology, there is a substantive body of literature on clinical decision-making[191–194] with recommendations to clearly define critical thinking objectives in a course or curriculum.[195]

Trainee knowledge and clinical decision-making skills for radiation oncology are unique compared to internal medicine, surgery, or other core specialties. However, the same principles for teaching clinical decision-making in these specialties apply to radiation oncology. The most important clinical decision made by the radiation oncologist is whether or not a patient should receive radiation therapy. The radiation oncologist must evaluate clinical data to determine if radiation therapy is indicated and how best to integrate it with other forms of therapy. However, radiation oncologists also utilize clinical decision-making skills on a daily basis when determining the threshold to order a magnetic resonance imaging (MRI) of the brain in a patient with locally advanced node-positive breast cancer complaining of headaches midway through adjuvant breast radiation, whether a complaint of dysuria during prostate radiation should prompt a urinalysis or if a patient who completed radiation for lung cancer and is complaining of shortness of breath should be started on steroids for possible radiation pneumonitis. Clinical decision-making for radiation oncology trainees is assessed in the United States with formative methods via the American College of Radiology In-Service Exam.[196] Programs in Canada and the United States use internal assessment methods including case-based skills assessment (colloquially known as "mock oral boards"), case presentations, and faculty feedback. Summative assessment in the United States is through the ABR board exams and through the Royal College of Physicians and Surgeons of Canada Radiation Oncology Certifying Exams. Studies evaluating methods to teach clinical decision-making specific to radiation oncology, however, are lacking.

Simulation

Subsequent to making a treatment recommendation, the vast majority of radiation oncology patients undergo a radiation therapy simulation scan (e.g., CT simulation). Literature regarding formal resident education specifically regarding the simulation process is unavailable. Knowledge and skills pertaining to the simulation process are taught via lectures, clinical experience and observation, and informal peer teaching.

At the UGME level, a formal lecture regarding the simulation process is included in a structured, didactic curriculum.[82] One study evaluated the efficacy of an educational program for residents on the use of intravenous contrast media as a component of CT simulation.[197] Resident knowledge regarding use of IV contrast improved with the intervention, although this effect was not sustained 1 year afterward. Additionally, given the low incidence of IV contrast reactions, the study was unable to demonstrate a clinical effect of the educational intervention. Given the critical nature of the simulation process to the quality of effectiveness of radiation delivery, radiation oncology educators must consider how this is taught and assessed in their local training program.

Contouring

After a patient undergoes simulation, a trainee must be able to accurately and efficiently contour target volumes and adjacent critical structures. "Imaging literacy" for radiation oncologists likely requires collaboration from specialists outside of radiation oncology alone.[198] An imaging literacy curriculum was developed using an international two-round Delphi process with four thematic groups of key competencies emerging: (a) imaging fundamentals, (b) clinical application, (c) clinical management, and (d) professional practice.[199] Perhaps the most pertinent competency to the specific technical skill of "contouring" is "Delineate on any imaging modality the radiation therapy target and organs at risk in all cancer disease sites and identify targets in 2D, 3D, and 4D image guidance modalities."[199] Radiation oncology educators should review this proposed curriculum to determine where their local program may be deficient.

Multiple educational methods are reported to improve radiologic interpretation skills and contouring skills. Trainee daily clinical activities should include contouring to allow residents to gain a hands-on "concrete" experience per the Kolb experiential learning model.[26] If a program requires trainees to spend significant amounts of time seeing patients in clinic while attending physicians or dosimetrists complete contouring duties, the trainees may graduate deficient in this skill.

To address this curriculum gap, based on a pilot study at a single institution,[200] a two-and-a-half-day National Anatomy and Radiology Contouring Boot Camp was implemented in Canada with significant improvements in knowledge assessment scores and Dice similarity coefficients comparing contour accuracy.[18] In the United States, Memorial Sloan Kettering Cancer Center developed a contouring training module for head and neck cancer demonstrating improvements in contouring accuracy, although there were still significant deviations in contours indicating a need for repeated exposure and possibly refinement of the curriculum.[201] This is similar to the prostate fossa contouring module developed for medical students.[2] Other contouring educational interventions are also published.[202–205]

Web-based educational methods are also under development. EduCase[206] (access with subscription at EduCase.com) was demonstrated to have a high usability as assessed by resident trainees for head and neck nodal station educational modules.[207] In a randomized study, the use of eContour[208] (access free with registration at eContour.org) compared with any other available contouring materials improved objective assessment of target delineation of the high-risk volume and contralateral parotid gland.[46] Of note, the high-risk volume showed consistently high variability in the Memorial Sloan Kettering study[201] suggesting that the eContour educational format might further enhance the learning experience. Residents using eContour demonstrated greater knowledge of contour delineation and radiographic anatomy on an objective knowledge assessment, and the mean usability score was high.[46]

Treatment Planning and Treatment Plan Evaluation

Subsequent to accurately delineating contours, a radiation oncology trainee must become proficient in treatment planning and treatment plan evaluation. Working collaboratively with dosimetrists and physicists, the trainee must learn to create a treatment plan, and evaluate treatment plan quality, specifically, to determine when it is not meeting appropriate dosimetric constraints or adequately covering the target volume. Although the treatment plan will nearly always be created by the dosimetrist or physicist in clinical practice, an understanding of how the plan is created, along with the limitations and uncertainties involved, will be exceptionally valuable to the resident when he/she enters clinical practice. In the United States, the current ACGME program requirements state that the educational program must include "regularly scheduled didactic sessions" with "instruction in medical physics that includes practical demonstrations of ... the use of state-of-the-art treatment planning systems."[4] In the ACGME Radiation Oncology Milestones, each "patient care" milestone includes a competency stating that the resident "critically evaluates treatment plan options."[120] Similarly, the Royal College of Radiologists in the United Kingdom calls for "comprehensive teaching of radiotherapy planning ... including simulation, virtual simulation, three-dimensional conformal planning, image fusion and IMRT, Volumetric Modulated Arc Therapy (VMAT) and image-guided radiation therapy (IGRT),"[185] and similar content is found in the Royal College of Physicians and Surgeons of Canada Radiation Oncology Objectives of training documents.[121]

Currently, treatment planning and treatment plan evaluation concepts are taught in the course of regular clinical duties, didactic lectures,[90] and peer-to-peer teaching. The ASTRO physics curriculum developed by the ASTRO Physics Core Curriculum Subcommittee recommends 7 hours dedicated to "Photon beam characteristics and dosimetry," 2 hours dedicated to "Electron beam characteristics and dosimetry," 3 hours dedicated to "Intensity modulated radiation therapy," and 1 hour dedicated to "Prescribing, reporting, and evaluating radiation therapy treatment plans."[90] Training programs may include a treatment planning rotation for their residents, but given the competing demands for resident time, most programs do not offer a formal dosimetry rotation.[105] In the recent ARRO chief resident survey, only two-thirds of graduating residents reported receiving adequate experience in treatment planning.[22]

Given the critical nature of radiation treatment plan evaluation for all modalities (three-dimensional conformal radiation, intensity-modulated radiation treatment, SBRT, radiosurgery, etc.), there are limited reports of formal educational methods to teach treatment plan evaluation. A series of self-directed modules teaching fundamentals of dosimetry and plan evaluation including AP/PA spine, three-field breast, and intensity-modulated radiation were developed at the University of Chicago.[179] These modules provide an opportunity for "active experimentation" within Kolb's experiential learning model.[26] Completion of the modules by the resident physicians was associated with improved resident comfort with AP/PA treatment planning, three-field breast treatment planning, and IMRT planning. Resident understanding of dosimetry concepts including dose grid, beam energy selection, calculation point, iterations, segments, optimization, and ring structure was also significantly improved.[209] Additional structured educational methods to teach and assess competence with treatment planning and dosimetry are needed to ensure that trainees are graduating with the skills necessary to adequately evaluate and constructively critique treatment plans in independent practice. The ASTRO physics curriculum provides an outline for additional dosimetry module development.[90]

Treatment and Toxicity Management

Once a patient begins radiation treatment, the trainee must be proficient in evaluating portal images as well as volumetric image data and images from other modalities for image-guided radiation, adjusting treatment plans as needed, managing acute toxicity of treatment, and coordinating care with other specialties including medical oncology and surgical specialties. Similar to how other steps in the clinical care path are taught, treatment and toxicity management is primarily taught through a combination of clinical experience, lectures, and reading. Investigations of novel educational methods to teach skills necessary for treatment and toxicity management are limited. A review of methods by which to assess residents' clinical skills proposes the use of OSCEs, standardized patients, and patient management problems in addition to the standard assessment methods of "ward" evaluation, multiple-choice question tests, and oral examinations.[210] An OSCE to teach residents communication skills was developed at the University of Pennsylvania.[24] Two cases representing treatment or toxicity management were developed including telling a patient 2 months out from radiation treatment that there is a tumor recurrence and telling the family of an 8-year-old patient that the proton machine is out of commission and the remainder of treatment will be IMRT. Residents received formative feedback from standardized patients and faculty observers. Educational strategies such as OSCEs and standardized patients represent novel and effective methods by which to teach radiation oncology trainees about management of patients receiving radiation and management of acute and late toxicity, which is essential as toxicities from modern treatments become less common. Further development of teaching material for this component of the care path is needed.

Medical Physics

Medical physics is a key component of training in radiation oncology with the ACGME,[4] RCPSC,[121] and Royal College of Radiologists (RCR)[185] including medical physics as a required training. According to a recent survey of residency program directors in the United States, 100% of residency programs provide a didactic course in radiation physics,[211] and >85% of US residents report adequate formal courses in radiation biology and physics.[22] Didactic lectures represent one of many educational strategies to teach the concepts and knowledge required of a practicing radiation oncologist. Medical physics training for radiation oncology residents in the United States is heterogeneous with a median of 42 lectures but a range from 10 to 90 per year and only approximately one-third of programs reporting physics rotations.[105] Additional educational strategies should be considered to allow optimal adult learning to occur. Providing an opportunity for hands-on experiences allows for learning in the context of Kolb's experiential learning cycle.[26] Didactic lectures alone cannot accomplish this.

The ASTRO Physics Core Curriculum Subcommittee developed a comprehensive recommended curriculum for medical physics education consisting of 56 hours of didactic sessions.[90] The curriculum also provides recommended references, a set of suggested practical clinical radiation oncology physics modules, and a set of suggested practical modules for radiation therapy treatment planning. The group recommends that training programs ensure residents complete the course at least twice during their training. A detailed physics curriculum for proton therapy is also proposed.[212]

A novel medical physics educational strategy is used at one training program in the UK where radiation oncology registrars (the equivalent of residents in the United States) spend 6 months completing a medical physics rotation.[213] These trainees continue to spend 1 day per week in clinic to maintain their clinical skills. The goal of the program is that by the end of the 6-month block, the trainee is competent in planning any case with the exception of total-body irradiation. This novel educational strategy utilizing a combination of continued clinical training and hands-on medical physics training could be adapted at other training programs. Importantly, the emphasis on advanced dosimetry over basic physical interactions has become more relevant to clinical practice in the setting of robust modern treatment planning systems.

Radiation Biology

Similar to radiation physics, radiation biology is a key component of training in radiation oncology with the ACGME,[4] RCPSC,[121] and RCR[185] requiring a fundamental understanding of radiobiologic concepts. All US radiation oncology training programs report formal radiation biology courses[211] with residents reporting sufficient training in radiation biology.[22] A survey of US and Canadian radiation biology educators indicates that many are not completely familiar with relevant radiation biology materials, some do not receive adequate departmental support, and more than 50% are not routinely provided with resident radiation biology performance on the in-training exam.[106] Many residents use the ASTRO radiation biology study guide as a learning resource.[214] In addition, the American College of Radiology in-training exam can be used as a teaching and assessment tool.[215] In recent years, incorporation of mechanisms of systemic therapies, some of which are delivered concurrent with radiation therapy, represents information that is more applicable to daily practice.

Continuing Medical Education in Radiation Oncology

For the practicing radiation oncologist, lifelong learning to ensure clinical knowledge and skills are up to date is critical. Perhaps even more so than some other areas of medicine, radiation oncology is constantly evolving due to the development of new technologies and treatment techniques and new treatment paradigms for cancer. The continued maintenance and acquisition of skills in radiation oncology is a complex process, and the implementation of new techniques and maintenance of competency can be challenging.[57] Evidence supporting the efficacy of CME for the maintenance of competency is mixed. Early studies suggested CME has a positive impact on physician performance and patient outcomes.[216] More recent studies failed to demonstrate a significant improvement in patient outcomes for physicians engaging in ongoing maintenance of competency activities.[217,218] A series of Cochrane literature reviews suggest that the impacts of CME may be linked with the type of CME activity, with isolated didactic lectures less effective as compared to interactive sessions, well-planned educational meetings, and quality improvement activities.[219-221] Within radiation oncology, the role for maintenance of certification programs administered by certification organizations remains controversial.[222] However, maintaining an up-to-date fund of clinical knowledge and ensuring clinical skills remain current are characteristics of any good physician. In addition, effective education of practicing physicians to drive a change in practice patterns to high-quality and high-value care is needed.[87,88] Thus, programs that educate practicing radiation oncologists are valuable, regardless of whether they are mandated by certifying organizations.

To encourage practicing radiation oncologists to engage in lifelong learning, certifying organizations such as the ABR and RCPSC has established maintenance of certification standards. In the United States, the ABR maintenance of certification process includes four parts: (a) Professional Standing, (b) Lifelong Learning and Self-Assessment, (c) Cognitive Expertise, and (d) Practice Quality Improvement.[223] Professional Standing requires a valid, unrestricted licensure in all states of practice. CME applies most directly to Lifelong

Learning and Self-Assessment and Cognitive Expertise components of the ABR's maintenance of certification process. Lifelong Learning and Self-Assessment requirements include completing 75 American Medical Association Category 1 CME credits every 3 years. Twenty-five of these credits must be "Self-Assessment" CME (SA-CME) credits. The general CME credits can be obtained by attending local tumor boards, CME-accredited resident lectures, or any other AMA Category 1 accredited activity. The SA-CME credits can be completed at approved lectures or through journal CME offerings. A by-product of the SA-CME requirement is that residency training programs are now certifying resident didactics for SA-CME to encourage faculty to attend the resident lectures.[224] Cognitive expertise was traditionally assessed by the ABR with a multiple-choice question recertification exam every 10 years. Because radiation oncology does not have any ACGME accredited subspecialty fellowships, the exam covered all disease sites. In 2015, the ABR began to allow practicing physicians to select specific disease sites for the recertification exam to satisfy cognitive expertise, but this ended in 2017.[225] The ABR is currently transitioning to an ongoing longitudinal assessment that will replace the 10-year recertification exam. This will include weekly multiple-choice questions that aim to test "walking around knowledge" in response to the efficacy demonstrated by the Maintenance of Certification in Anesthesiology (MOCA) Program referred to as the MOCA Minute.[226] Finally, to satisfy the requirement for practice and quality improvement (PQI), a practice quality improvement project or other participatory quality improvement activity must be completed every 3 years.

CME requirements in the RCPSC construct are similar to the ABR lifelong learning and self-assessment. CME in Canada represents the culmination of the Competence by Design competence continuum.[227] In contrast to the United States (until recently), in Canada, there is no recertification exam. The RCPSC maintenance of certification program requires radiation oncologists to obtain 400 credits and a minimum of 25 credits in each maintenance of competency program section per 5-year cycle. RCPSC maintenance of competency credits fall into one of three categories/program sections including (a) group learning, (b) self-learning, and (c) assessment.[228] With a transition to Competence by Design (Fig. 103.12), the RCPSC maintenance of competency system will likely undergo significant changes. As such, the maintenance of competency will need to allow for continuous ongoing demonstration of competency with ongoing feedback to facilitate learning in practice.[229]

CME activities cover a broad range of educational strategies including didactic learning, interactive sessions, and practice audit and feedback. These activities often mirror those discussed previously for UGME and GME education. Some of the most commonly recognized CME activities include didactic learning activities at educational meetings (e.g., American Society for Radiation Oncology [ASTRO], European Society for Radiotherapy and Oncology [ESTRO], and Canadian Association of Radiation Oncology [CARO] annual society meetings). A variety of interactive activities including large contouring workshops,[230] provided through national societies, are also used in CME. Many national society meetings include seminars and workshops and allow for the discussion of or dissemination of new techniques. In Europe, the ESTRO School has developed the Fellowship in Anatomic Delineation and Contouring (FALCON), which incorporates web-based contouring into their educational programs.[230] CME can also be delivered in a small group learning environment such as weekly tumor boards, simulation-based education, or local grand rounds and lectures.[231,232] Despite the frequency with which such activities are offered, there is a relative paucity of scholarship. Very few publications have robust program evaluation from these CME activities, and the majority evaluate user satisfaction[232] as opposed to change in knowledge or behavior.

Although historically CME was designed to deliver educational content to individual physicians, a primary goal of CME is now systems-based or quality improvement.[233] Quality improvement and "audit with feedback" CME programs are becoming more common.[220] Shakespeare et al.[234] examined the effects of audit with feedback for practicing radiation oncologist's changes in behavior. Their audit included an assessment of patient charting and radiation plans. Radiation oncologists were provided individualized feedback. The audit with feedback resulted in improvements in some aspects of patient charting and documentation and radiation planning. These effects were retained through time and demonstrated that audit with feedback may be a useful CME exercise. As peer-review and quality assurance programs are developed at radiation oncology centers,[235,236] careful attention should be paid to not only improve consistency and quality in radiation plans[237] but also design programs that allow for continuous practice improvement. By educating individual physicians, CME can drive organizational change and overall improvements in health care delivery. Additionally, when deficiencies are noted through the process of peer-review, individual or group educational programs may be required, and review of medical education principles previously discussed may be helpful.

In order to develop CME activities, similar to other areas of radiation oncology education, guiding principles and frameworks can help to provide valuable perspective. CME activities include a broad range of educational interventions. These can include, among others, didactic programs (e.g., lectures and journal clubs with question and answer session), interactive instruction (e.g., interactive case discussion, group role-play), audit and feedback, and academic detailing (i.e., individual education delivered by a trained professional to education on evidence-based techniques). Harden describes six criteria for effective CME: (a) convenience, (b) relevance, (c) individualization, (d) self-assessment, (e) independent learning, and (f) systematic.[238] The development of effective curriculum for CME programs can be based on the six-step model[62] and enhanced by Davis et al.'s[239] description of the seven characteristics of effective CME programs including (a) needs assessment, (b) focused initiative, (c) interactive educational programs, (d) multiple educational strategies, (e) multiple sessions, (f) time for feedback and practice, and (g) outcome evaluation. The application of established frameworks to any CME activity or program should allow for robust development, implementation, and evaluation.

Although there is a significant body of literature examining the best practices in development, implementation, and outcomes of CME activities in a variety of other areas in medicine, radiation oncology remains ripe for educational scholarship. Work can be done to improve existing CME curricula and to develop novel CME educational strategies. Potential areas for scholarship include the application of established educational frameworks to CME development and evaluation outcomes linked to changes in knowledge, behavior, and clinical outcomes.

Areas for Further Scholarship in Radiation Oncology Education

Radiation oncology education at the UGME, GME, and CME levels continues to evolve. There remain a myriad of scholarship opportunities to rationally and methodically improve radiation oncology education. Examples include further developing and validating competency frameworks such as the ACGME Milestones[120] and CanMEDS Competence by Design.[5,122] Development of EPAs also represents an opportunity to move radiation oncology forward.[240] Looking beyond the medical profession, there is ample opportunity to develop interprofessional educational activities at all training levels.[241,242]

Simulation-based medical education is no longer a new concept[243] and is being rapidly adopted by other specialties. Within radiation oncology, there is ample evidence that increasing experience can improve outcomes for brachytherapy[244] and head and neck treatment, particularly in the IMRT era.[80] Reports of decreasing case volume for brachytherapy,[86] reports of limited pediatric cases,[186] and reports from graduating residents of inadequate training in intraoperative radiation, brachytherapy, and proton therapy[22] suggest that development of simulation-based education specific to radiation oncology may provide a solution to the dilemma of how to safely train residents and assess competency for case scenarios or procedures that are less common or require high technical skill. Many educational reports within radiation oncology represent simulation-based medical education, even though they are not identified as such. For example, there are multiple reports of contouring training on a standardized case.[2,46,201,202,207,230] This represents simulation-based education because the trainee is working in a simulated environment with no real-world consequences when making an error, though reports in radiation oncology less often self-identify as simulation-based medical education, with the few examples including brachytherapy training,[25] interprofessional team simulation,[245] and preparation for on-call emergencies.[246]

CONCLUSION

Radiation oncology is a unique field within medicine. Although much of the essential cognitive, affective, and psychomotor knowledge acquired during medical school is useful to a radiation oncology trainee, the knowledge and skills required of a competent and compassionate radiation oncologist are unique and iterative. Curricula to teach this radiation oncology knowledge and skill set must be developed in a logical and rational manner to ensure desired goals and objectives of the learning process are achieved. Furthermore, curricula must be continually updated to meet changes in modern radiation oncology. For example, training in radiographic anatomy and treatment plan evaluation is critical in the modern era but often is relegated to the null curriculum in UGME, GME, and CME. Meanwhile, the approach to educational programs must reflect changes in information technology, with the potential to increase simulation-based training over traditional didactic lectures and for longitudinal assessments to replace exams performed once every decade. Dissemination of curricular innovations is essential to ensure the radiation oncology educational community is aware of the progress and can further build and improve radiation oncology education while ensuring the educator receives appropriate academic recognition. The radiation oncology profession must place value on medical education scholarship to encourage the advancement of the entire discipline.

Radiation oncology educators must critically evaluate the local, national, and international training milieu and consider disruptive innovation to ensure vigorous and active curriculum revision and renewal. Disruptive innovation is defined in the business sense as follows:

> *"Dominant players in most markets focus on sustaining innovations... That makes a market ripe for upstart companies seeking to introduce disruptive innovations... more convenient products or services."*[247]

The concept of disruptive innovation can be applied to radiation oncology education. Current radiation oncology curricula across the globe evolved to satisfy the requirements set forth by accrediting bodies but are not necessarily the most effective and efficient methods for teaching a particular radiation oncology topic or concept. Educational innovations that are demonstrated as effective through rigorous curriculum inquiry, learner assessment, and program evaluation and are disseminated have the potential to disrupt the status quo radiation oncology curriculum on a large scale with the ultimate goal of improving the quality of patient care.

ACKNOWLEDGMENTS

The authors thank Joanne Alfieri MD, Georges Bordage MD MSc PhD, Steve Braunstein MD PhD, Jay Burmeister PhD, Graeme Duncan MB ChB FRCPC, Erin Gillespie MD, Jillian Gunther MD PhD, Ariel Hirsch MD, W. Robert Lee MD MEd, Malcolm Mattes MD, Meredith Giuliani MBBS Med FRCPC, Dan Pratt PhD, Joseph Rencic MD, Charles Thomas Jr. MD, Theresa Trotter MD, Paul Wallner DO, Susan Wu MD, and Jason Chao Ye MD for the critical input and feedback during the writing of this chapter.

REFERENCES

1. Rosenthal DI, et al. Importance of patient examination to clinical quality assurance in head and neck radiation oncology. *Head Neck* 2006;28:967–973.
2. Gunther JR, et al. A Prostate Fossa Contouring Instructional Module: Implementation and Evaluation. *J Am Coll Radiol* 2016;13:835–841.e1.
3. Berman AT, Plastaras JP, Vapiwala N. Radiation oncology: a primer for medical students. *J Cancer Educ* 2013;28:547–553.
4. *ACGME program requirements for graduate medical education in radiation oncology*, 2016. https://www.acgme.org/Portals/0/PFAssets/ProgramRequirements/430_radiation_oncology_2016_TCC.pdf
5. Frank JR, Snell L, Sherbino J. *CanMEDS 2015 physician competency framework*. Canada: Royal College of Physicians and Surgeons of Canada, 2015. http://www.royalcollege.ca/rcsite/documents/canmeds/canmeds-full-framework-e.pdf
6. Caruana CJ, Christofides S, Hartmann GH. European Federation of Organisations for Medical Physics (EFOMP) policy statement 12.1: recommendations on medical physics education and training in Europe 2014. *Phys Med* 2014;30:598–603.
7. Prisciandaro JI, et al. Essentials and guidelines for clinical medical physics residency training programs: executive summary of AAPM Report Number 249. *J Appl Clin Med Phys* 2014;15:4763.
8. Medical dosimetry training curriculum. American Association of Medical Dosimetrists. *Med Dosim* 1998;23:311–332.
9. Coffey M, Leech M, Poortmans P; ESTRO RTT Committee. Benchmarking Radiation TherapisT (RTT) education for safe practice: the time is now. *Radiother Oncol* 2016;119:12–13.
10. Carper E, Haas M. Advanced practice nursing in radiation oncology. *Semin Oncol Nurs* 2006;22:203–211.
11. Gosselin-Acomb TK. Role of the radiation oncology nurse. *Semin Oncol Nurs* 2006;22:198–202.
12. Miller JJ, et al. Role of a medical social worker in improving quality of life for patients with advanced cancer with a structured multidisciplinary intervention. *J Psychosoc Oncol* 2007;25:105–119.
13. Holtgrefe KM. Twice-weekly complete decongestive physical therapy in the management of secondary lymphedema of the lower extremities. *Phys Ther* 2006;86:1128–1136.
14. Introduction of radiation medicine into the undergraduate medical curriculum; fifth report of the Expert Committee on Professional and Technical Education of Medical and Auxiliary Personnel. *World Health Organ Tech Rep Ser* 1958;108:1–24.
15. Corn BW, Symon Z, Gamzu R. The state of radiation therapy in the state of Israel. *Int J Radiat Oncol Biol Phys* 2014;90:975–978.
16. Duchesne GM, Turner SL, Cronje S. Around the globe—radiation oncology in Australia. *Int J Radiat Oncol Biol Phys* 2014;90:1–6.
17. Mineikyte R, Janulionis E, Liutkeviciute-Navickiene J, et al. Cancer education in Lithuania. *Ecancermedicalscience* 2014;8:487.
18. Jaswal J, et al. Evaluating the impact of a Canadian national anatomy and radiology contouring boot camp for radiation oncology residents. *Int J Radiat Oncol Biol Phys* 2015;91:701–707.
19. Amendola B, Amendola M. Status of Radiation Therapy in Uruguay: Past, Present, and Future. *Int J Radiat Oncol Biol Phys* 2016;94:428–434.
20. Kabolizadeh P, Aghili M, Balakhanlou B. A Time for Optimism? The State of Radiation Oncology in Iran. *Int J Radiat Oncol Biol Phys* 2016;94:221–227.
21. Kannan V, Bajpai R. Conforming Modern Radiation Oncology Facilities to the Irregular Contours of the Vast and Varied Nation of India. *Int J Radiat Oncol Biol Phys* 2016;94:645–651.
22. Nabavizadeh N, et al. Results of the 2013–2015 Association of Residents in Radiation Oncology Survey of Chief Residents in the United States. *Int J Radiat Oncol Biol Phys* 2016;94:228–234.
23. Faivre J-C, et al. Evaluation of the Theoretical Teaching of Postgraduate Radiation Oncology Medical Residents in France: A Cross-Sectional Study. *J Cancer Educ* 2017;1–8. doi: 10.1007/s13187-017-1170-2.
24. Ju M, et al. Assessing interpersonal and communication skills in radiation oncology residents: a pilot standardized patient program. *Int J Radiat Oncol Biol Phys* 2014;88:1129–1135.
25. Thaker NG, et al. Establishing high-quality prostate brachytherapy using a phantom simulator training program. *Int J Radiat Oncol Biol Phys* 2014;90:579–586.
26. Kolb DA. *Experiential learning: experience as the source of learning and development*. Englewood Cliffs, NJ: Prentice Hall, 1983.
27. Merriam SB, Caffarella RS, Baumgartner LM. *Learning in adulthood: a comprehensive guide*. San Francisco, CA: Jossey-Bass, 2007. https://books.google.com/books?id=ffaKVcPVC84C&lpg=PR3&ots=JWlWxaqCWH&dq=Learning%20in%20adulthood%3A%20a%20comprehensive%20guide&lr&pg=PR3#v=onepage&q=Learning%20in%20adulthood:%20a%20comprehensive%20guide&f=false
28. Collins M. *Adult education as vocation: a critical role for the adult educator.* Routledge, UK: Chapman and Hall, Inc., 1991.
29. Garrison DR. Critical Thinking and Self-Directed Learning in Adult Education: An Analysis of Responsibility and Control Issues. *Adult Educ Q* 1992;42:136–148.
30. Owen TR. *Self-directed learning in adulthood: a literature review*, 2002. https://eric.ed.gov/?id=ED461050
31. Knowles MS III, Holton EF, Swanson RA. *The adult learner: the definitive classic in adult education and human resource development*. Abingdon, UK: Routledge, 2014.
32. Yerkes RM, Dodson JD. The relation of strength of stimulus to rapidity of habit-formation. *J Comp Neurol Psychol* 1908;18:459–482.
33. Hebb DO. Drives and the C. N. S. (conceptual nervous system). *Psychol Rev* 1955;62:243–254.
34. Golden DW, Langer M. Education: the third, but not last, pillar of academic radiation oncology. *Int J Radiat Oncol Biol Phys* 2012;83:1353–1354.
35. Boyer E. *Scholarship reconsidered: priorities of the professoriate*. Stanford, CA: The Carnegie Foundation for the Advancement of Teaching, 1990. http://www.hadinur.com/paper/BoyerScholarshipReconsidered.pdf
36. Beckman TJ, Cook DA. Developing scholarly projects in education: a primer for medical teachers. *Med Teach* 2007;29:210–218.
37. Grady EC, et al. Defining scholarly activity in graduate medical education. *J Grad Med Educ* 2012;4:558–561.
38. Diamond RM. *The disciplines speak: rewarding the scholarly, professional, and creative work of faculty*. Forum on faculty roles & rewards, 1995. https://eric.ed.gov/?id=ED406957
39. Hutchings P, Shulman LS. The Scholarship of Teaching: *New Elaborations, New Developments*. *Change Mag High Learn* 1999;31:10–15.
40. Glassick CE. Boyer's expanded definitions of scholarship, the standards for assessing scholarship, and the elusiveness of the scholarship of teaching. *Acad Med* 2000;75:877–880.
41. E Fincher R-M, Work JA. Perspectives on the scholarship of teaching. *Med Educ* 2006;40:293–295.
42. Holzl J. Twelve tips for effective PowerPoint presentations for the technologically challenged. *Med Teach* 1997;19:175–179.
43. Byun J, Golden DW. Readability of patient education materials from professional societies in radiation oncology: are we meeting the national standard? *Int J Radiat Oncol Biol Phys* 2015;91:1108–1109.
44. Aagaard E, Teherani A, Irby DM. Effectiveness of the one-minute preceptor model for diagnosing the patient and the learner: proof of concept. *Acad Med* 2004;79:42–49.
45. Jagadeesan VS, et al. A national radiation oncology medical student clerkship survey: didactic curricular components increase confidence in clinical competency. *Int J Radiat Oncol Biol Phys* 2014;88:51–56.
46. Gillespie EF, et al. Multi-institutional Randomized Trial Testing the Utility of an Interactive Three-dimensional Contouring Atlas among Radiation Oncology Residents. *Int J Radiat Oncol Biol Phys* 2017;98(3):547–554. doi:10.1016/j.ijrobp.2016.11.050
47. Hirsch AE, et al. Quantitatively and qualitatively augmenting medical student knowledge of oncology and radiation oncology: an update on the impact of the oncology education initiative. *J Am Coll Radiol* 2012;9:115–120.
48. Dennis KEB, Duncan G. Radiation oncology in undergraduate medical education: a literature review. *Int J Radiat Oncol Biol Phys* 2010;76:649–655.
49. Steinert Y, et al. A systematic review of faculty development initiatives designed to enhance teaching effectiveness: a 10-year update: BEME Guide No. 40. *Med Teach* 2016;38:769–786.
50. Hofmeyer A, Newton M, Scott C. Valuing the scholarship of integration and the scholarship of application in the academy for health sciences scholars: recommended methods. *Health Res Policy Syst* 2007;5:5.
51. Grimshaw JM, Russell IT. Effect of clinical guidelines on medical practice: a systematic review of rigorous evaluations. *Lancet* 1993;342:1317–1322.
52. Radiation Oncology Education Collaborative Study Group. Available at: https://roecsg.uchicago.edu/. Accessed April 13, 2017.
53. Bordage G. Moving the field forward: going beyond quantitative–qualitative. *Acad Med* 2007;82:S162–S168.
54. Corbin J, Strauss A. *Basics of qualitative research*. Thousand Oaks, CA: SAGE Publications, Inc., 2015.
55. Fraenkel J, Wallen N, Hyun H. *How to design and evaluate research in education*. 8th ed. New York, NY: McGraw Hill, 2014.
56. Irby DM. What clinical teachers in medicine need to know. *Acad Med* 1994;69:333–342.
57. Kane GM. Step-by-step: a model for practice-based learning. *J Contin Educ Health Prof* 2007;27:220–226.
58. Harris IB. Qualitative methods. In: Norman GR, et al., eds. *International handbook of research in medical education*. the Netherlands: Springer, 2002:45–95. doi: 10.1007/978-94-010-0462-6_3.
59. Pratt DD. *Sample qualitative research questions*. Extract from handout for Harvard Macy Institute for Health Professionals, 2015.
60. Bordage G. Reasons reviewers reject and accept manuscripts: the strengths and weaknesses in medical education reports. *Acad Med* 2001;76:889–896.
61. Bordage G. Conceptual frameworks to illuminate and magnify. *Med Educ* 2009;43:312–319.
62. Thomas PA, Kern DE, Hughes MT, et al. eds. *Curriculum development for medical education: a six-step approach*. Johns Hopkins University Press, 2016. https://www.amazon.com/Curriculum-Development-Medical-Education-Six-Step/dp/1421418525/
63. Ericsson KA. Deliberate practice and the acquisition and maintenance of expert performance in medicine and related domains. *Acad Med* 2004;79:S70–S81.
64. Kirkpatrick JD, Kirkpatrick WK. *Kirkpatrick's four levels of training evaluation*. Alexandria, VA: Association for Talent Development, 2016

65. Hafferty FW. Beyond curriculum reform: confronting medicine's hidden curriculum. *Acad Med* 1998;73:403–407.
66. Flinders DJ, Noddings N, Thornton SJ. The null curriculum: its theoretical basis and practical implications. *Curric Inq* 1986;16:33–42.
67. Mattes MD. Multidisciplinary oncology education: going beyond tumor board. *J Am Coll Radiol* 2016;13:1239–1241.
68. Mattes MD, Patel KR, Burt LM, et al. A Nationwide Medical Student Assessment of Oncology Education. *J Cancer Educ* 2016;31:679–686.
69. Oskvarek J, et al. Medical Student Knowledge of Oncology and Related Disciplines: A Targeted Needs Assessment. *J Cancer Educ* 2016;31(3):529–532. doi: 10.1007/s13187-015-0876-2.
70. Shaverdian N, et al. Gaps in radiation therapy awareness: results from an educational multi-institutional survey of United States internal medicine residents. *Int J Radiat Oncol Biol Phys* 2017;98(5):1153–1161.
71. Akthar AS, et al. Interdisciplinary Oncology Education: A National Survey of Trainees and Program Directors in the United States. *J Cancer Educ* 2016. doi: 10.1007/s13187-016-1139-6.
72. Harris IB. Contributions to professional education from the field of curriculum studies: research and practice with new traditions of investigation. *Prof Educ Res Q* 1991;13:3–13.
73. Tyler RW. *Basic principles of curriculum and instruction*. Chicago, IL: The University of Chicago Press, 1949.
74. Harden RM. Ten questions to ask when planning a course or curriculum. *Med Educ* 1986;20:356–365.
75. Harris IB. Deliberative inquiry: the arts of planning. In: Short EC, ed. *Forms of curriculum inquiry*. New York, NY: SUNY Press, 1991:285–307.
76. Short EC. *Forms of curriculum inquiry*. New York, NY: SUNY Press, 1991.
77. Schubert WH. *Curriculum: perspective, paradigm, and possibility*. New York, NY: Macmillan Publishing Company, 1986.
78. Wu DH, et al. Interobserver variation in cervical cancer tumor delineation for image-based radiotherapy planning among and within different specialties. *J Appl Clin Med Phys* 2005;6:106–110.
79. Hoppe BS, Hoppe RT. Expert radiation oncologist interpretations of involved-site radiation therapy guidelines in the management of Hodgkin lymphoma. *Int J Radiat Oncol Biol Phys* 2015;92:40–45.
80. Boero IJ, et al. Importance of Radiation Oncologist Experience Among Patients With Head-and-Neck Cancer Treated With Intensity-Modulated Radiation Therapy. *J Clin Oncol* 2016;34:684–690.
81. Joo JH, et al. Variability in target delineation of cervical carcinoma: a Korean radiation oncology group study (KROG 15-06). *PLoS One* 2017;12:e0173476.
82. Radiation Oncology Education Collaborative Study Group; Radiation Oncology Education Collaborative Study Group Writing Committee; et al. Multi-Institutional Implementation and Evaluation of a Curriculum for the Medical Student Clerkship in Radiation Oncology. *J Am Coll Radiol* 2016;13:203–209.
83. MedEdPORTAL. Available at: https://www.mededportal.org/. Accessed April 14, 2017.
84. Liberati A, et al. The PRISMA statement for reporting systematic reviews and meta-analyses of studies that evaluate health care interventions: explanation and elaboration. *Ann Intern Med* 2009;151:W65–W94.
85. Institute of Medicine (US) Committee on Standards for Systematic Reviews of Comparative Effectiveness Research. *Finding what works in health care: standards for systematic reviews*. Washington, DC: National Academies Press (US), 2011.
86. Compton JJ, et al. Resident-reported brachytherapy experience in ACGME-accredited radiation oncology training programs. *Brachytherapy* 2013;12: 622–627.
87. Bekelman JE, et al. Uptake and costs of hypofractionated vs conventional whole breast irradiation after breast conserving surgery in the United States, 2008–2013. *JAMA* 2014;312:2542–2550.
88. Bekelman JE, Epstein AJ, Emanuel EJ. Single- vs multiple-fraction radiotherapy for bone metastases from prostate cancer. *JAMA* 2013;310:1501–1502.
89. Bissonnette J-P, Medlam G. Trend analysis of radiation therapy incidents over seven years. *Radiother Oncol* 2010;96:139–144.
90. Burmeister J, et al. The American Society for Radiation Oncology's 2015 Core Physics Curriculum for Radiation Oncology Residents. *Int J Radiat Oncol Biol Phys* 2016;95:1298–1303.
91. Shakespeare TP, Back MF, Lu JJ, et al. Design of an internationally accredited radiation oncology resident training program incorporating novel educational models. *Int J Radiat Oncol Biol Phys* 2004;59:1157–1162.
92. Pohar S, et al. American Society for Radiation Oncology (ASTRO) 2012 Workforce Study: the radiation oncologists' and residents' perspectives. *Int J Radiat Oncol Biol Phys* 2013;87:1135–1140.
93. Artino AR, La Rochelle JS, Dezee KJ, et al. Developing questionnaires for educational research: AMEE Guide No. 87. *Med Teach* 2014;36:463–474.
94. Phillips AW, Reddy S, Durning SJ. Improving response rates and evaluating nonresponse bias in surveys: AMEE Guide No. 102. *Med Teach* 2016;38:217–228.
95. Fowler FJ. *Survey research methods*. Thousand Oaks, CA: SAGE Publications, Inc., 2013.
96. Fink AG. *How to conduct surveys: a step-by-step guide*. Thousand Oaks, CA: SAGE Publications, Inc., 2016.
97. Zaorsky NG, et al. What Are Medical Students in the United States Learning About Radiation Oncology? Results of a Multi-Institutional Survey. *Int J Radiat Oncol Biol Phys* 2016;94:235–242.
98. Golden DW, Raleigh DR, Chmura SJ, et al. Radiation oncology fourth-year medical student clerkships: a targeted needs assessment. *Int J Radiat Oncol Biol Phys* 2013;85:296–297.
99. Gondi V, et al. Results of the 2005 to 2008 Association of Residents in Radiation Oncology surveys of chief residents in the United States: didactics and research experience. *Am J Clin Oncol* 2012;35:32–39.
100. Malik R, Oh JL, Roeske JC, et al. Survey of resident education in intensity-modulated radiation therapy. *Technol Cancer Res Treat* 2005;4:303–309.
101. Morris L, Thiruthaneeswaran N, Lehman M, et al. Are Future Radiation Oncologists Equipped With the Knowledge to Manage Elderly Patients With Cancer? *Int J Radiat Oncol Biol Phys* 2017;98(4):743–747. doi: 10.1016/j.ijrobp.2017.01.001.
102. Wei RL, et al. Palliative care and palliative radiation therapy education in radiation oncology: a survey of US radiation oncology program directors. *Pract Radiat Oncol* 2017;7(4):234–240. doi: 10.1016/j.prro.2016.11.009.
103. Krishnan M, et al. Radiation oncology resident palliative education. *Pract Radiat Oncol* 2017;7(6):e439–e448.
104. Gaudet M, Jaswal J, Keyes M. Current state of brachytherapy teaching in Canada: a national survey of radiation oncologists, residents, and fellows. *Brachytherapy* 2015;14:197–201.
105. Das IJ, Moskvin V. Variability of physics education in radiation oncology medical residency programs. *J Am Coll Radiol* 2012;9:835–838.
106. Rosenstein BS, Held KD, Rockwell S, et al. American Society for Radiation Oncology (ASTRO) survey of radiation biology educators in U.S. and Canadian radiation oncology residency programs. *Int J Radiat Oncol Biol Phys* 2009;75:896–905.
107. Latham GP. Goal Setting: A Five-Step Approach to Behavior Change. *Org Dynam* 2003;32:309–318.
108. Green LW. *Health education planning: a diagnostic approach*. California City, CA: Mayfield Publishing Company, 1979.
109. Bloom BS. *Taxonomy of educational objectives: the classification of educational goals*. New York, NY: D. McKay, 1956.
110. Krathwohl DR. A Revision of Bloom's Taxonomy: An Overview. *Theory Pract* 2002;41:212–218.
111. *The new taxonomy of educational objectives*. Corwin, 2006.
112. Kraftwohl DR, Bloom BS, Masia BB. *Taxonomy of educational objectives, the classification of educational goals : handbook II: affective domain*. New York, NY: David McKay Company, 1967.
113. Simpson EJ. *The classification of educational objectives, psychomotor domain*, Urbana, IL: University of Illinois, 1966.
114. Dave RH. Psychomotor levels. In: Robert J. Armstrong ed. *Developing and writing behavioral objectives*. Tucson, AZ: Educational Innovators Press, 1970:20–21.
115. Harrow AJ. *A taxonomy of the psychomotor domain: a guide for developing behavioral objectives*. New York, NY: David McKay Co., 1972.
116. Miller GE. The assessment of clinical skills/competence/performance. *Acad Med* 1990;65:S63–S67.
117. Mehay R. *The essential handbook for GP training and education*. Boca Raton, FL: CRC Press, 2012.
117a. Ledlow GR, Coppola MN. *Leadership for health professionals*. Burlington, MA: Jones & Bartlett Publishers, 2010.
118. Frank JR, et al. Toward a definition of competency-based education in medicine: a systematic review of published definitions. *Med Teach* 2010;32:631–637.
119. Nasca TJ, Philibert I, Brigham T, et al. The next GME accreditation system—rationale and benefits. *N Engl J Med* 2012;366:1051–6.
120. The Radiation Oncology Milestone Project, 2014. http://www.acgme.org/Portals/0/PDFs/Milestones/RadiationOncologyMilestones.pdf
121. Objectives of Training in the Specialty of Radiation Oncology, 2014. http://www.royalcollege.ca/cs/idcplg?IdcService=GET_FILE&dID=227814&dDocName=TZTEST3RCPSCED000945
122. *Competence by design: reshaping Canadian medical education*. Ottawa, Canada: Royal College of Physicians and Surgeons of Canada, 2014. http://www.royalcollege.ca/rcsite/documents/cbd/competency-by-design-ebook-e.pdf
123. National Research Council Committee on Developments in the Science of Learning with additional material from the Committee on Learning Research and Educational Practice. *How people learn: brain, mind, experience, and school: expanded edition*. Washington, DC: National Academies Press, 2000.
124. Coffield F, Moseley D, Hall E, et al. *Learning styles and pedagogy in post-16 learning: a systematic and critical review*. Great Britain: Learning and Skills Research Centre (LSRC), 2004.
125. Dunn RS, Dunn KJ. *Teaching students through their individual learning styles: a practical approach*. Reston, VA: Prentice Hall College Div, 1978.
126. Kanter RM. *Six keys to leading positive change*, 2013. TEDx Talks. https://www.youtube.com/watch?v=owU5aTNPJbs
127. Kotter JP. *Leading change, with a new preface by the author*. Harvard, MA: Harvard Business Review Press, 2012.
128. Northouse PG. *Leadership: theory and practice*. 7th ed. Thousand Oaks, CA: SAGE Publications, Inc., 2015.
129. Bolman LG, Deal TE. *Reframing organizations: artistry, choice, and leadership*. San Francisco, CA: Jossey-Bass, 2013.
130. American Educational Research Association (AERA); American Psychological Association (APA); National Council on Measurement in Education (NCME). *Standards for educational and psychological testing*. Washington, DC: American Educational Research Association, 2014.
131. Alliance for Clinical Education. *Handbook on medical student evaluation and assessment*. Syracuse, NY: Gegensatz Press, 2015.
132. Downing SM, Yudkowsky R. *Assessment in health professions education*. New York and Abingdon: Routledge, 2009.
133. Epstein RM. Assessment in medical education. *N Engl J Med* 2007;356:387–396. http://dx.doi.org/10.1056/NEJMra054784
134. Norcini JJ, McKinley DW. Assessment methods in medical education. *Teach Teach Educ* 2007;23:239–250.
135. Farmer EA, Page G. A practical guide to assessing clinical decision-making skills using the key features approach. *Med Educ* 2005;39:1188–1194.
136. Charlin B, Roy L, Brailovsky C, et al. The Script Concordance test: a tool to assess the reflective clinician. *Teach Learn Med* 2000;12:189–195.
137. Swing SR. Assessing the ACGME general competencies: general considerations and assessment methods. *Acad Emerg Med* 2002;9:1278–1288.
138. Accreditation Council for Graduate Medical Education [ACGME]. Outcome project. *Toolbox of assessment methods*, 2000. Available at: http://njms.rutgers.edu/culweb/medical/documents/ToolboxofAssessmentMethods.pdf. Accessed April 18, 2017.

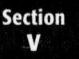

139. Williams RG, Klamen DA, McGaghie WC. Cognitive, social and environmental sources of bias in clinical performance ratings. *Teach Learn Med* 2003;15:270–292.

140. Carraccio C, Englander R. Evaluating competence using a portfolio: a literature review and web-based application to the ACGME competencies. *Teach Learn Med* 2004;16:381–387.

141. Lynch DC, Swing SR. Accreditation Council for Graduate Medical Education & American Board of Medical Specialties. Key Considerations for Selecting Assessment Instruments and Implementing Assessment Systems. Available at: http://www.acgme.org/outcome/assess/keyConsider.as. Accessed September 24 2007.

142. Van Der Vleuten CPM, Schuwirth LWT. Assessing professional competence: from methods to programmes. *Med Educ* 2005;39:309–317.

143. Zelenitsky S, et al. Using curriculum mapping to engage faculty members in the analysis of a pharmacy program. *Am J Pharm Educ* 2014;78:139.

144. Harden RM. AMEE Guide No. 21: curriculum mapping: a tool for transparent and authentic teaching and learning. *Med Teach* 2001;23:123–137.

145. Royal College of Physicians and Surgeons competency by design, 2017. Available at: http://www.royalcollege.ca/rcsite/cbd/competence-by-design-cbd-e

146. Ling L, Derstine P, *Cohen N.* Implementing milestones and clinical competency committees, 2013. https://www.acgme.org/Portals/0/PDFs/ACGMEMilestones-CCC-AssesmentWebinar.pdf

147. CanMEDS 2015 tools, 2015. Available at: http://canmeds.royalcollege.ca/en/tools. Accessed April 18, 2017.

148. Ginsburg S, McIlroy J, Oulanova O, et al. Toward authentic clinical evaluation: pitfalls in the pursuit of competency. *Acad Med* 2010;85:780–786.

149. van der Vleuten CPM, et al. A model for programmatic assessment fit for purpose. *Med Teach* 2012;34:205–214.

150. Muraskin LD. *Understanding evaluation: the way to better prevention programs.* Washington, DC: Department of Education, 1993:1–103.

151. Goldie J. AMEE Education Guide no. 29: evaluating educational programmes. *Med Teach* 2006;28:210–224.

152. Fitzpatrick JL, Sanders JR, Worthen BR. *Program evaluation: alternative approaches and practical guidelines.* Upper Saddle River, NJ: Pearson, 2010.

153. Frye AW, Hemmer PA. Program evaluation models and related theories: AMEE Guide No. 67. *Med Teach* 2012;34:e288–e299.

154. Rogers EM. *Diffusion of innovations.* 4th ed. New York, NY: Free Press, 1995.

155. 45 CFR 46. *HHS.gov,* 2016. Available at: https://www.hhs.gov/ohrp/regulations-and-policy/regulations/45-cfr-46/index.html. Accessed April 14, 2017.

156. Abrahamson S. Diseases of the curriculum. *J Med Educ* 1978;53:951–957.

157. Bordage G, Harris I. Making a difference in curriculum reform and decision-making processes. *Med Educ* 2011;45:87–94.

158. Clayton R, Trotter T. The impact of undergraduate education in radiation oncology. *J Cancer Educ* 2013;28:192–196.

159. Hansen JT, Rubin P. Clinical anatomy in the oncology patient: a preclinical elective that reinforces cross-sectional anatomy using examples of cancer spread patterns. *Clin Anat* 1998;11:95–99.

160. Fukuchi SG, Offutt LA, Sacks J, et al. Teaching a multidisciplinary approach to cancer treatment during surgical clerkship via an interactive board game. *Am J Surg* 2000;179:337–340.

161. Barrett WL, Aron BS, Breneman JC, et al. Clinical oncology clerkship for third-year medical students. *J Cancer Educ* 2001;16:182–184.

162. Abacioglu U, Sarikaya O, Iskit S, et al. Integration of a problem-based multidisciplinary clinical cancer management course into undergraduate education. *J Cancer Educ* 2004;19:144–148.

163. Hirsch AE, Singh D, Ozonoff A, et al. Educating medical students about radiation oncology: initial results of the oncology education initiative. *J Am Coll Radiol* 2007;4:711–715.

164. Ideal oncology curriculum for medical schools, 2007. Available at: http://www.cancer.org.au/Healthprofessionals/OncologyEducation/IdealOncology.htm. Accessed November 30, 2011.

165. Hirsch AE, Mulleady Bishop P, Dad L, et al. An increase in medical student knowledge of radiation oncology: a pre-post examination analysis of the oncology education initiative. *Int J Radiat Oncol Biol Phys* 2009;73:1003–1008; quiz 1008.e1–1008.e2.

166. Zaorsky NG, et al. Assessing the value of an optional radiation oncology clinical rotation during the core clerkships in medical school. *Int J Radiat Oncol Biol Phys* 2012;83:e465–e469.

167. Tamaki Y, et al. Long-term results of radiation oncology seminar for medical students and residents held between 1995 and 2011: career paths of the participants. *Jpn J Radiol* 2013;31:755–759.

168. Zaorsky NG, et al. Impact of a radiation oncology elective on the careers of young physicians: update on a prospective cohort study. *Int J Radiat Oncol Biol Phys* 2013;86:214–215.

169. Matkowski R, Szelachowska J, Szewczyk K, et al. Improvements in undergraduate oncology education introduced at Polish medical universities between 2004 and 2010 under Poland's 'National Program for Combating Neoplastic Diseases'. *J Cancer Educ* 2014;29:428–433.

170. Agarwal A, DeNunzio NJ, Ahuja D, et al. Beyond the standard curriculum: a review of available opportunities for medical students to prepare for a career in radiation oncology. *Int J Radiat Oncol Biol Phys* 2014;88:39–44.

171. Mattes MD, Gerbo R, Dattola RM. Tumor Board Shadowing for Medical Students as a Means of Early Exposure to Multidisciplinary Oncology Education. *J Am Coll Radiol* 2017;14:253–255.

172. Agarwal A, Shah A, Byler S, et al. Cultivating Interest in Oncology Through a Medical Student Oncology Society. *J Cancer Educ* 2017;32:31–34.

173. Agarwal A, Koottappillil B, Shah B, et al. Medical Student—Reported Outcomes of a Radiation Oncologist—Led Preclinical Course in Oncology: A Five-Year Analysis. *Int J Radiat Oncol Biol Phys* 2015;92:735–739.

174. Lai L, Ingledew P. Development of an integrated interdisciplinary oncology elective. *J Investig Med* 2011;59:183.

175. Ingledew P, et al. Helping to bridge the gap: the development of online learning resources to supplement oncology education.. *Radiother Oncol* 2015;116(s1):80.

176. Tam VC, Ingledew P-A, Berry S, et al. Developing Canadian oncology education goals and objectives for medical students: a national modified Delphi study. *CMAJ Open* 2016;4:E359–E364.

177. Arenas M, Sabater S, Biete A, et al. Radiation Oncology Teaching Programmes as Part of the Undergraduate Degree in Medicine in Spanish Universities: the Need for an Update of the Contents and Structure. *J Cancer Educ* 2018;33(2):352–358. doi: 10.1007/s13187-016-1106-2.

178. Halperin EC. The audition elective. *Int J Radiat Oncol Biol Phys* 1988;15:791–792.

179. Golden DW, Stepaniak CJ, Chmura SJ. Radiation Oncology Self-Directed Dosimetry Workshops: AP/PA Spine, 3-Field Breast, and IMRT. *MedEdPORTAL,* 2012. Available at: www.mededportal.org/publication/9297

180. Golden DW, et al. Radiation oncology medical student clerkship: implementation and evaluation of a bi-institutional pilot curriculum. *Int J Radiat Oncol Biol Phys* 2014;88:45–50.

181. Ye JC, et al. Medical Student Perspectives on a Multi-institutional Clerkship Curriculum: A Report From the Radiation Oncology Education Collaborative Study Group. *Int J Radiat Oncol Biol Phys* 2015;92:217–219.

182. Gunther J, et al. Post-Operative Prostate and Seminal Vesicle Fossae Contouring Module: Evaluation of Medical Student Target Delineation Before and After a Teaching Intervention. *MedEdPORTAL Publ,* 2015;11:10199. doi: 10.15766/mep_2374-8265.10199.

183. Bland RE, Hodges JC, Folkert MR, et al. Employment After Radiation Oncology Residency: A Survey of the Class of 2014. *Int J Radiat Oncol Biol Phys* 2015;92:969–970.

184. Loewen SK, et al. Delayed Workforce Entry and High Emigration Rates for Recent Canadian Radiation Oncology Graduates. *Int J Radiat Oncol Biol Phys* 2015;93:251–256.

185. Specialty Training Curriculum for Clinical Oncology, 2016. https://www.rcr.ac.uk/sites/default/files/2016_curriculum_-_clinical_oncology_15_november_2016.pdf

186. Donaldson SS, Halperin EC. Subspecialty training and certification for radiation oncology. *J Am Coll Radiol* 2004;1:488–492.

187. Chino J, Doyle S, Marks LB. The anatomy of radiation oncology residency training. *Int J Radiat Oncol Biol Phys* 2014;88:3–4.

188. Cabrera AR, et al. Incorporating gross anatomy education into radiation oncology residency: a 2-year curriculum with evaluation of resident satisfaction. *J Am Coll Radiol* 2011;8:335–340.

189. Makoul G. Essential elements of communication in medical encounters: the Kalamazoo consensus statement. *Acad Med* 2001;76:390–393.

190. Joyce BL, Steenbergh T, Scher E. Use of the kalamazoo essential elements communication checklist (adapted) in an institutional interpersonal and communication skills curriculum. *J Grad Med Educ* 2010;2:165–169.

191. Croskerry P. From mindless to mindful practice—cognitive bias and clinical decision making. *N Engl J Med* 2013;368:2445–2448.

192. Schmidt HG, Mamede S. How to improve the teaching of clinical reasoning: a narrative review and a proposal. *Med Educ* 2015;49:961–973.

193. Rencic J. Twelve tips for teaching expertise in clinical reasoning. *Med Teach* 2011;33:887–892.

194. *Teaching clinical reasoning.* USA: American College of Physicians, 2015. https://www.amazon.com/Teaching-Clinical-Reasoning-Acp-Medicine/dp/1938921054/

195. Abrami PC, et al. Instructional Interventions Affecting Critical Thinking Skills and Dispositions: A Stage 1 Meta-Analysis. *Rev Educ Res* 2008;78:1102–1134.

196. Hatch SS, et al. Radiation Oncology Resident In-Training Examination. *Int J Radiat Oncol Biol Phys* 2015;92:532–535.

197. Barker CA, et al. Contrast media use in radiation oncology: a prospective, controlled educational intervention study with retrospective analysis of patient outcomes. *J Am Coll Radiol* 2010;7:967–974.

198. Gillan C, Uchino M, Giuliani M, et al. Defining imaging literacy in radiation oncology interprofessionally: toward a competency profile for Canadian residency programs. *J Med Imaging Radiat Sci* 2013;44:150–156.

199. Giuliani ME, et al. Determining an imaging literacy curriculum for radiation oncologists: an international Delphi study. *Int J Radiat Oncol Biol Phys* 2014;88:961–966.

200. Labranche L, Johnson M, Palma D, et al. Integrating anatomy training into radiation oncology residency: considerations for developing a multidisciplinary, interactive learning module for adult learners. *Anat Sci Educ* 2015;8:158–165.

201. Bekelman JE, Wolden S, Lee N. Head-and-neck target delineation among radiation oncology residents after a teaching intervention: a prospective, blinded pilot study. *Int J Radiat Oncol Biol Phys* 2009;73:416–423.

202. Dewas S, et al. Delineation in thoracic oncology: a prospective study of the effect of training on contour variability and dosimetric consequences. *Radiat Oncol* 2011;6:118.

203. Awan M, et al. Prospective assessment of an atlas-based intervention combined with real-time software feedback in contouring lymph node levels and organs-at-risk in the head and neck: quantitative assessment of conformance to expert delineation. *Pract Radiat Oncol* 2013;3:186–193.

204. D'Souza L, et al. Evaluating the impact of an integrated multidisciplinary head & neck competency-based anatomy & radiology teaching approach in radiation oncology: a prospective cohort study. *BMC Med Educ* 2014;14:124.

205. Alfieri J, et al. Development and impact evaluation of an e-learning radiation oncology module. *Int J Radiat Oncol Biol Phys* 2012;82:e573–e580.

206. EduCase. Available at: https://www.educase.com/. Accessed April 16, 2017.

207. Deraniyagala R, Amdur RJ, Boyer AL, et al. Usability study of the EduMod eLearning Program for contouring nodal stations of the head and neck. *Pract Radiat Oncol* 2015;5:169–175.

208. eContour. Available at: https://econtour.org/. Accessed April 16, 2017.

209. Melotek JM, Stepaniak CJ, Chmura SJ, et al. Implementation and Evaluation of a Self-directed Dosimetry Curriculum for Radiation Oncology Residents. *Int J Radiat Oncol Biol Phys* 2015;93:E379–E380.

210. Reddy S, Vijayakumar S. Evaluating clinical skills of radiation oncology residents: parts I and II. *Int J Cancer* 2000;90:1–12.
211. Jani AB, Marshall D, Vapiwala N, et al. Results of the 2014 Survey of the Association of Directors of Radiation Oncology Programs (ADROP). *Pract Radiat Oncol* 2015;5(6):e673–e678. doi: 10.1016/j.prro.2015.06.007.
212. Winey B, et al. Core physics competencies for proton therapy training of radiation oncology and medical physics residents and fellows. *Int J Radiat Oncol Biol Phys* 2014;88:971–972.
213. Nikapota A, Rogers S, Sevitt T, et al. Six months in physics—a useful training opportunity? *Br J Radiol* 2007;80:766.
214. ARRO Certification Resources Physics and Radiation Biology Curriculum. Available at: https://www.astro.org/Affiliate/ARRO/Resident-Resources/Certification-Resources/Physics-and-Radiation-Biology-Curriculum/. Accessed April 21, 2017.
215. Dynlacht JR, Zeman EM. Recent initiatives for radiation oncology resident education in radiation and cancer biology. *Radiat Res* 2007;168:262–265.
216. Davis DA, Thomson MA, Oxman AD, et al. Evidence for the effectiveness of CME. A review of 50 randomized controlled trials. *JAMA* 1992;268:1111–1117.
217. Hayes J, et al. Association between physician time-unlimited vs time-limited internal medicine board certification and ambulatory patient care quality. *JAMA* 2014;312:2358–2363.
218. Gray BM, et al. Association between imposition of a Maintenance of Certification requirement and ambulatory care-sensitive hospitalizations and health care costs. *JAMA* 2014;312:2348–2357.
219. Thomson O'Brien MA, et al. Continuing education meetings and workshops: effects on professional practice and health care outcomes. *Cochrane Database Syst Rev* 2001;(2):CD003030. doi: 10.1002/14651858.CD003030.
220. Jamtvedt G, Young JM, Kristoffersen DT, et al. Audit and feedback: effects on professional practice and health care outcomes. *Cochrane Database Syst Rev* 2006;(2):CD000259. doi: 10.1002/14651858.CD000259.pub2.
221. Forsetlund L, et al. Continuing education meetings and workshops: effects on professional practice and health care outcomes. *Cochrane Database Syst Rev* 2009;(2):CD003030. doi: 10.1002/14651858.CD003030.pub2.
222. Sandhu A. Maintenance of Certification: From Realism to Skepticism. *Int J Radiat Oncol Biol Phys* 2015;93:209–210.
223. Maintenance of Certification—The American Board of Radiology. Available at: https://www.theabr.org/moc-gen-landing. Accessed April 21, 2017.
224. Kim H, et al. Increasing faculty participation in resident education and providing cost-effective self-assessment module credit to faculty through resident-generated didactics. *Pract Radiat Oncol* 2017;7(4):241–245. doi: 10.1016/j.prro.2016.12.003.
225. Wallner PE, Gerdeman A, Willis JM, et al. The American Board of Radiology radiation oncology Maintenance of Certification Part 3 Modular Examination: evaluation of the first administration. *Pract Radiat Oncol* 2016;6:436–438.
226. Sun H, et al. Association between Participation in an Intensive Longitudinal Assessment Program and Performance on a Cognitive Examination in the Maintenance of Certification in Anesthesiology Program®. *Anesthesiology* 2016;125:1046–1055.
227. The Royal College of Physicians and Surgeons of Canada: Competence by Design. Available at: http://www.royalcollege.ca/rcsite/cbd/competence-by-design-cbd-e. Accessed April 22, 2017.
228. The Royal College of Physicians and Surgeons of Canada: Framework of Continuing Professional Development Activities. Available at: http://www.royalcollege.ca/rcsite/cpd/moc-program/moc-framework-e. Accessed April 22, 2017.
229. Campbell CM, Parboosingh J. The Royal College experience and plans for the maintenance of certification program. *J Contin Educ Health Prof* 2013;33(Suppl 1):S36–S47.
230. Eriksen JG, et al. Four years with FALCON—an ESTRO educational project: achievements and perspectives. *Radiother Oncol* 2014;112:145–149.
231. Khoo ELH, et al. Prostate contouring variation: can it be fixed? *Int J Radiat Oncol Biol Phys* 2012;82:1923–1929.
232. Szumacher E, et al. Multidisciplinary radiation oncology palliative care rounds as a continuing educational activity implementing the rapid response radiotherapy program at the Toronto Sunnybrook Regional Cancer Centre. *J Cancer Educ* 2003;18:86–90.
233. Price D. Continuing medical education, quality improvement, and organizational change: implications of recent theories for twenty-first-century CME. *Med Teach* 2005;27:259–268.
234. Shakespeare TP, Mukherjee RK, Lu JJ, et al. Evaluation of an audit with feedback continuing medical education program for radiation oncologists. *J Cancer Educ* 2005;20:216–221.
235. Marks LB, et al. Enhancing the role of case-oriented peer review to improve quality and safety in radiation oncology: executive summary. *Pract Radiat Oncol* 2013;3:149–156.
236. Canadian Partnership for Quality Radiotherapy Quality Assurance Guidelines for Canadian Radiation Treatment Programs, 2015. Available at: http://www.cpqr.ca/wp-content/uploads/2013/09/QRT2015-12-03.pdf. Accessed May 10, 2017.
237. Rouette J, et al. Directly Improving the Quality of Radiation Treatment Through Peer Review: A Cross-sectional Analysis of Cancer Centers Across a Provincial Cancer Program. *Int J Radiat Oncol Biol Phys* 2017;98(3):521–529. doi: 10.1016/j.ijrobp.2016.10.017.
238. Harden RM. A new vision for distance learning and continuing medical education. *J Contin Educ Health Prof* 2005;25:43–51.
239. Davis N, Davis D, Bloch R. Continuing medical education: AMEE Education Guide No. 35. *Med Teach* 2008;30:652–666.
240. Ten Cate O. Nuts and bolts of entrustable professional activities. *J Grad Med Educ* 2013;5:157–158.
241. Thistlethwaite J. Interprofessional education: a review of context, learning and the research agenda. *Med Educ* 2012;46:58–70.
242. Core competencies for interprofessional collaborative practice: report of an expert panel, 2011. https://nexusipe-resource-exchange.s3-us-west-2.amazonaws.com/IPEC_CoreCompetencies_2011.pdf
243. Gaba DM. The future vision of simulation in healthcare. *Simul Healthc* 2007;2:126–135.
244. Merrick GS, et al. The effect of pro-qura case volume on post-implant prostate dosimetry. *Int J Radiat Oncol Biol Phys* 2011;81:e727–e734.
245. Giuliani M, et al. Evaluation of high-fidelity simulation training in radiation oncology using an outcomes logic model. *Radiat Oncol* 2014;9:189.
246. Brown LC, Laack TA, Ma DJ, et al. Multidisciplinary medical simulation: a novel educational approach to preparing radiation oncology residents for oncologic emergent on-call treatments. *Int J Radiat Oncol Biol Phys* 2014;90:705–706.
247. Christensen CM, Bohmer RMJ, Kenagy J. Will Disruptive Innovations Cure Health Care? *Harvard Business Review*, 2000. Available at: https://hbr.org/2000/09/will-disruptive-innovations-cure-health-care. Accessed April 10, 2017.
248. Ingledew P. Experiencing Cancer: Exploring Themes in Oncology Clerkship Narratives. *Med Educ* 2010;S2:52.
249. Turner S, et al. Establishing a Global Radiation Oncology Collaboration in Education (GRaCE): objectives and priorities. *Radiother Oncol* 2015;117:188–192.
250. Merrill MD. First principles of instruction. *Educ Technol Res Dev* 2002;50:43–59.
251. McGaghie WC, Siddall VJ, Mazmanian PE, et al.; American College of Chest Physicians Health and Science Policy Committee. Lessons for continuing medical education from simulation research in undergraduate and graduate medical education: effectiveness of continuing medical education: American College of Chest Physicians Evidence-Based Educational Guidelines. *Chest* 2009;135:62S–68S.
252. Issenberg SB, McGaghie WC, Petrusa ER, et al. Features and uses of high-fidelity medical simulations that lead to effective learning: a BEME systematic review. *Med Teach* 2005;27:10–28.
253. Kneebone R. Evaluating clinical simulations for learning procedural skills: a theory-based approach. *Acad Med* 2005;80:549–553.
254. Downing SM. Validity: on meaningful interpretation of assessment data. *Med Educ* 2003;37:830–837.
255. Norcini J, et al. Criteria for good assessment: consensus statement and recommendations from the Ottawa 2010 Conference. *Med Teach* 2011;33:206–214.
256. Stanton F, Grant J. Approaches to experiential learning, course delivery and validation in medicine. A background document. *Med Educ* 1999;33:282–297.
257. Ivey SL, Brown KS, Teske Y, et al. A model for teaching about interdisciplinary practice in health care settings. *J Allied Health* 1988;17:189–195.
258. Parsell G, Bligh J. Interprofessional learning. *Postgrad Med J* 1998;74:89–95.
259. Medical University of South Carolina: Creating Collaborative Care (C3) A Quality Enhancement Plan (QEP), 2007. Available at: http://academicdepartments.musc.edu/c3/publications/qep_final.pdf. Accessed November 2, 2014.
260. Blue AV, Mitcham M, Smith T, et al. Changing the future of health professions: embedding interprofessional education within an academic health center. *Acad Med* 2010;85:1290–1295.
261. Ginsburg S, et al. Context, conflict, and resolution: a new conceptual framework for evaluating professionalism. *Acad Med* 2000;75:S6–S11.
262. Nguyen TK, Bauman GS, Watling CJ, et al. Patient- and family-centered care: a qualitative exploration of oncologist perspectives. *Support Care Cancer* 2017;25:213–219.
263. Alfieri J, Sultanem K. Implementation of mini-CEX assessments in an outpatient clinic-oriented specialty. *16th Ott. Conf. 12th Can. Conf. Med. Educ.—Transform. Healthc. Excell. Assess. Eval.—Abstr. Book*, 2014:169.
264. Anderson LW, et al. *A taxonomy for learning, teaching, and assessing: a revision of Bloom's taxonomy of educational objectives. Complete edition*. New York, NY: Pearson, 2000.
265. Eriksen JG, et al. The updated ESTRO core curricula 2011 for clinicians, medical physicists and RTTs in radiotherapy/radiation oncology. *Radiother Oncol* 2012;103:103–108.
266. Turner S, Seel M, Berry M. Radiation Oncology Training Program Curriculum developments in Australia and New Zealand: design, implementation and evaluation—what next? *J Med Imaging Radiat Oncol* 2015;59:728–735.
267. Abdel-Wahab M, Rosenblatt E, Holmberg O, et al. Safety in radiation oncology: the role of international initiatives by the International Atomic Energy Agency. *J Am Coll Radiol* 2011;8:789–794.
268. Ahern V, Klein L, Bentvelzen A, et al. An evaluation of a paediatric radiation oncology teaching programme incorporating a SCORPIO teaching model. *J Med Imaging Radiat Oncol* 2011;55:213–219.
269. Chino JP, et al. Teaching the anatomy of oncology: evaluating the impact of a dedicated oncoanatomy course. *Int J Radiat Oncol Biol Phys* 2011;79:853–859.
270. Garcia MA, Braunstein SE, Anderson WG. A Palliative Care Didactic Course for Radiation Oncology Residents. *Int J Radiat Oncol Biol Phys* 2017;97(5):884–885.
271. Pham D, et al. A Multidisciplinary Evaluation of a Web-based eLearning Training Programme for SAFRON II (TROG 13.01): a Multicentre Randomised Study of Stereotactic Radiotherapy for Lung Metastases. *Clin Oncol* 2016;28:e101–e108.
272. Sloan PA, et al. Cancer pain management skills among medical students: the development of a Cancer Pain Objective Structured Clinical Examination. *J Pain Symptom Manage* 2001;21:298–306.
273. International Atomic Energy Agency. Clinical Training of Medical Physicists Specializing in Radiation Oncology. Available at: http://www-pub.iaea.org/MTCD/publications/PDF/TCS-37_web.pdf. Accessed April 18, 2017.
274. Mavroidis P, et al. Consequences of anorectal cancer atlas implementation in the cooperative group setting: radiobiologic analysis of a prospective randomized in silico target delineation study. *Radiother Oncol* 2014;112:418–424.
275. Dauer LT, Kelvin JF, Horan CL, et al. Evaluating the effectiveness of a radiation safety training intervention for oncology nurses: a pretest-intervention-posttest study. *BMC Med Educ* 2006;6:32.
276. Kubal T, et al. Longitudinal cohort study to determine effectiveness of a novel simulated case and feedback system to improve clinical pathway adherence in breast, lung and GI cancers. *BMJ Open* 2016;6:e012312.
277. McDonald R, et al. Student Accomplishments in the Rapid Response Radiotherapy Program: A 10-Year Review. *J Cancer Educ* 2015;30:693–698.

CHAPTER 104

Ethics, Professional Values, and Legal Considerations in Radiation Oncology

Brian D. Kavanagh, Laurel J. Lyckholm, and Jeremy Sugarman

INTRODUCTION

Although progress in medical science has improved the quality and duration of life for some patients with cancer and other serious illnesses, technical expertise alone does not fully account for the upsurge in the societal standing of medical doctors during the past 100 years.[1]

High regard for physicians is contingent on the trust that doctors act unselfishly in a patient's best interests, a role sometimes called moral fiduciary.[2] Essential to this role are medical knowledge and a firm grasp of ethics. Derived from the Greek ηθος (ethos), meaning character, ethics refers to the process of applying values and principles in professional interactions and particularly in medical decision-making on behalf of patients. Although not a routine requirement for admission, many medical schools encourage undergraduate applicants to take an introductory course in ethics, and the curriculum of most medical schools now includes coursework in ethics.

To foster an appreciation for the intellectual underpinnings of modern medical ethics, this chapter begins with an overview of scholarly approaches to ethics. Next is a discussion of selected proclamations and codes of ethics published by professional societies, federal commissions, and other authorities as guidelines for medical practice and research. Finally, common practical ethical issues in radiation oncology are addressed, including relevant medicolegal considerations.

CONCEPTUAL APPROACHES USED IN BIOMEDICAL ETHICS

The term bioethics, coined in the early 1970s, refers to the academic inquiry and public policy movement addressing the application of science and medicine from a humanistic perspective.[3] Medical ethics may be most accurately viewed as a branch of bioethics, but the terms are commonly used interchangeably. Among the more influential theoretical approaches that are used in bioethics are *utilitarianism, deontology, casuistry, virtue theory, principlism, and feminism.*

Utilitarianism is based on the premise that, in any situation, the best course of action is the one that produces the maximum net positive value (or least negative value). Utilitarianism can be applied to an individual patient's case or to matters of health policy, in which decisions might be made to achieve the greatest overall benefit for the largest number of people.

Unlike utilitarianism, deontology is an ethical theory based on the morality of actions themselves rather than their net result. Deontology, sometimes called Kantianism in recognition of the influence of Immanuel Kant,[4] calls for consistent standards of behavior at all times, regardless of the consequences. One simple example of the difference between utilitarianism and deontology is the issue of educating patients about their diagnosis, especially if the prognosis is very poor. Whereas a deontologist would always feel obliged to tell the truth even at the risk of causing distress, a utilitarian considers whether telling a patient the complete truth about the disease does or does not really benefit the patient. In daily practice, finding the right balance between purely utilitarian and purely deontologic perspectives in a situation like this one requires consideration of case-specific factors. Respect for the patient's autonomy, for example, is one of the *prima facie* ethical principles discussed in the next section. Truth-telling is an integral component, and overriding this principle requires justification.

Casuistry is an approach to ethics that emphasizes inductive reasoning based on established precedents, and it is a common practice in both law and medicine. The proper course of action in any individual case is decided by recalling decisions made in prior similar cases. The major weakness of casuistry is the lack of a reference benchmark or settled opinion on novel technologies.

Virtue theory focuses on the character of moral agents, in this case physicians and other health care providers, focusing less on actions or outcomes. As such, virtue theory captures the way in which correct moral actions occur. For example, it is not only important to tell patients the truth about their diagnoses, but it is also critical to do so in a compassionate manner. In this case, the virtue is compassion. Accordingly, although virtue is a critical part of assessing moral action, virtues themselves have little guiding force.

Principlism is a system of applied ethics through which core principles ideally govern behavior in the absence of compelling reasons to override them. Principlism can be integrated with the other philosophical approaches already mentioned and serves as a unifying influence.

Feminism concentrates on the concerns of those who are vulnerable and marginalized, as well as categorized unjustly according to particular hierarchies. Frameworks such as structural violence aid in analyzing various practices and policies that perpetuate oppression and injustice. Narrative practice provides a voice to those who may be marginalized on the basis of sex, race, gender, age, disability, susceptibility or presence of stigmatized diseases, imprisonment, health status, and other social categorizations. As such, feminism does not focus solely on women's issues, but on those who are traditionally subject to discrimination.

ETHICAL PRINCIPLES IN BIOMEDICAL ETHICS

A *prima facie* obligation may be defined as one that is "binding unless overridden or outweighed by competing moral obligations."[4] Four *prima facie* principles of bioethics are highlighted here: *respect for autonomy, beneficence, nonmaleficence,* and *justice.*

Respect for a patient's autonomy is based on respect for the right to individual liberty. A patient's voluntary decision to seek medical care or comply with referral to a specialist is the starting point of most patient–physician relationships, and competent patients should remain free to forgo therapy or change physicians at any time. The responsibility to respect patients' autonomy is established not only in ethics but also in law. An example is the requirement to obtain a patient's informed consent for proposed medical therapy. In a landmark case involving postmastectomy chest wall radiation therapy, a patient who sustained soft tissue necrosis won a lawsuit against her radiation oncologist for negligence and for lack of proper disclosure regarding possible treatment-related toxicity. The Kansas Supreme Court ruled that doctors should explain "in language as simple as necessary" the side effects associated with any recommended therapy.[5]

The principle of *beneficence* is intertwined with that of *nonmaleficence*. Some authors have offered nuanced distinctions between the two principles,[4] but the key point is that physicians should act for the benefit of patients and should not harm their patients. Beneficence and nonmaleficence are typically concordant objectives, but sometimes an intervention that is helpful also entails a high risk of adverse treatment-induced sequelae. For example, administering high dose morphine to a patient severely dyspneic from an incurable lung malignancy can relieve symptoms but at the same time risks fatally suppressing respiratory drive. Here the quality of remaining life might be improved by a measure that also hastens death. Such an action can sometimes be justified by the principle of double effect, the earliest expression of which is generally attributed to St. Thomas Aquinas.[6]

In recent years, a number of states in the United States have enacted so-called Death with Dignity legislation that permits physicians to prescribe life-ending medications to certain patients with terminal illness when pain or other distress from the illness becomes intolerable to the patient. Generally, there is a stipulation that the patient must be able to self-administer the medication, and there is also a requirement that the patient is competent to make the decision to end his or her life. Individual hospitals and health systems retain local administrative authority regarding whether these statutes are implemented within the institution and, if so, what specific local regulatory requirements apply.

The principle of justice refers to fairness, typically the equitable distribution of health care resources. Justice-related questions often arise concerning matters of public policy. One specific example is the challenge of determining the means to allocate scarce organs for transplantation. A more global problem faced by all governments is the calculus of distributive justice implies that persons ought to be afforded medical care according to their medical needs and the ability of the system to provide.

FORMAL OATHS AND CODES OF ETHICS

There are many published declarations of medical ethics authored by physicians. Not surprisingly, the tone and language of each reflect the social mores and sometimes historical events of the era in which it was composed.

The Hippocratic Oath

I will prescribe regimen for the good of my patients according to my ability and my judgment and never do harm to anyone

The *Corpus Hippocraticum* is a collection of medical treatises dating from around the fifth century BCE, believed to be the work of philosopher–physicians from the Greek island of Cos (Fig. 104.1). Contained within the *Corpus* is the well-known oath of Hippocrates, an ancient physician's pledge of professionalism. Curiously, the oath is inconsistent with some other sections of the *Corpus,* perhaps because it was added later. Comments about abortion and surgery, for example, are at variance with teachings elsewhere in the collected works.[7] Nevertheless, timeless themes are included, and the oath has survived in various modernized versions. The oath is often recited by medical students at the time of graduation—even if its contents are not always well remembered.[8,9]

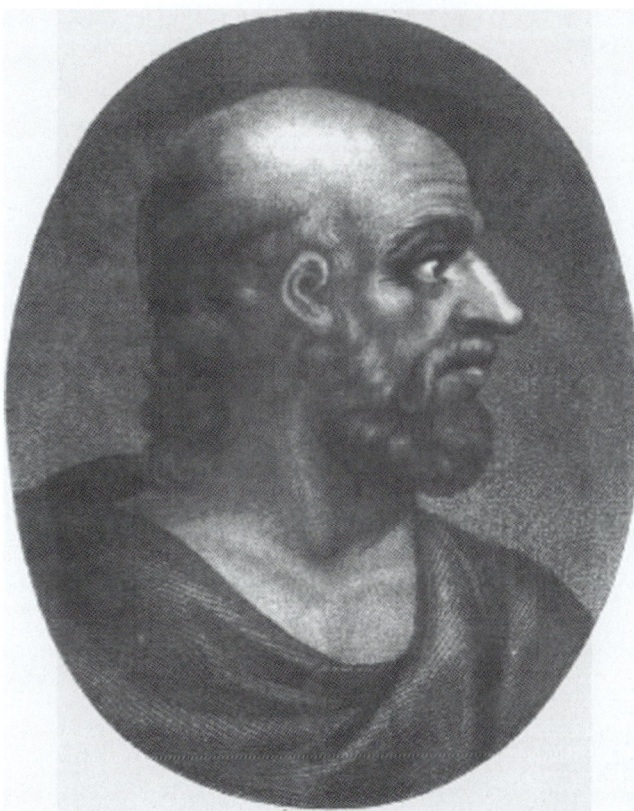

FIGURE 104.1. Early19th-century engraving depicting a likeness of Hippocrates, closely resembling images of ancient coins found on the island of Cos bearing his likeness. (Image Courtesy of the U.S. National Library of Medicine.)

Percival's Medical Ethics

Hospital physicians and surgeons should minister to the sick, with due impressions of the importance of their office, reflecting that the ease, the health, and the lives of those committed to their charge depend on their skill, attention, and fidelity.

Thomas Percival (1740–1804) (Fig. 104.2) published *Medical Ethics* at a time when there were considerable tension among clinicians in his community.[10] In the 1760s, Manchester, England, was a prosperous urban society that comfortably supported public health initiatives, including an infirmary serving as a charity hospital and teaching institution. But as the city grew and became crowded by the 1790s, tensions arose between rival groups in the medical community. Percival was prompted to draft a code of ethics after a contentious dispute about enlarging the infirmary's staff, a threat to the controlling physician faction.[11]

When he began writing *Medical Ethics,* Percival was already a well-known writer and moralist whose *A Father's Instructions to His Children*, published in 1775, included essays promoting personal virtues and social awareness to young readers. While completing *Medical Ethics,* Percival suffered devastating personal tragedies, bereaving the untimely deaths of two of his own sons. The finished work was dedicated to a third son studying medicine at the time.

Ultimately, *Medical Ethics* provided a template for the codes of ethics adopted by the American Medical Association (AMA) and other societies in the 19th century. Early 20th-century pundits criticized Percival's work as merely a book of medical *etiquette* rather than medical *ethics.* However, revisionist historians have subsequently argued that although Percival focused on interprofessional relationships, he also taught that a physician's duty toward the patient outweighs obligations of civility toward other health care professionals.

Section
V

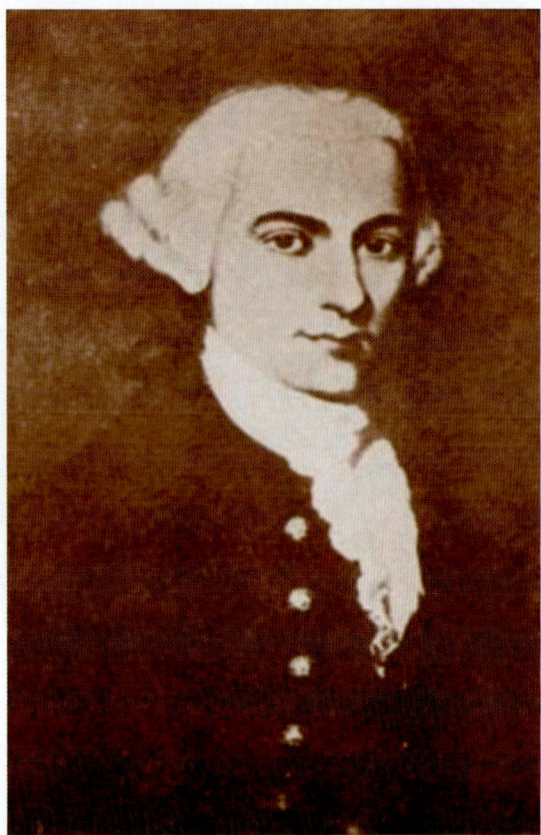

FIGURE 104.2. Thomas Percival (1740–1804). (From Brockbank EM. *Sketches of the lives and work of the honorary medical staff of the Manchester Infirmary, from its foundation in 1752 to 1830 when it became the Royal Infirmary.* Manchester: Manchester University Press, 1904.)

Furthermore, Percival advanced the enlightened view that indigent patients should receive the same quality of care as affluent patients.[12]

The American Medical Association Code of Ethics

The AMA first adopted a code of ethics at its inaugural meeting in 1847. The initial code was modeled on the work of Percival, but subsequent updates have reflected societal changes and technologic progress. The 2016 update begins with an articulation of basic principles[13]:

I. *A physician shall be dedicated to providing competent medical care, with compassion and respect for human dignity and rights.*

II. *A physician shall uphold the standards of professionalism, be honest in all professional interactions, and strive to report physicians deficient in character or competence, or engaging in fraud or deception, to appropriate entities.*

III. *A physician shall respect the law and also recognize a responsibility to seek changes in those requirements, which are contrary to the best interests of the patient.*

IV. *A physician shall respect the rights of patients, colleagues, and other health professionals and shall safeguard patient confidences and privacy within the constraints of the law.*

V. *A physician shall continue to study, apply, and advance scientific knowledge; maintain a commitment to medical education; make relevant information available to patients, colleagues, and the public, obtain consultation; and use the talents of other health professionals when indicated.*

VI. *A physician shall, in the provision of appropriate patient care, except in emergencies, be free to choose whom to serve, with whom to associate, and the environment in which to provide medical care.*

VII. *A physician shall recognize a responsibility to participate in activities contributing to the improvement of the community and the betterment of public health.*

VIII. *A physician shall, while caring for a patient, regard responsibility to the patient as paramount.*

IX. *A physician shall support access to medical care for all people.*

Among the numerous topics discussed in more detail in the eleven chapters of the code are conflicts of interest in patient care. The AMA code states that "Under no circumstances may physicians place their own financial interests above the welfare of their patients...Treatment or hospitalization that is willfully excessive or inadequate constitutes unethical practice."

The Nuremberg Code and the Declaration of Geneva

During World War II, odious crimes were committed by Nazi physicians who conducted horrific experiments on concentration camp prisoners who were coerced to submit. The Nuremberg Code was a formal response to these World War II–era human rights atrocities disguised as medical experiments.[14] Issued from the military tribunal that tried some of the Nazi doctors who conducted these experiments, the Nuremberg Code acknowledges that medical investigations are important. However, for a medical experiment to be morally permissible, it must meet 10 criteria, paraphrased as follows:

- Voluntary consent of the human subject
- Necessity to yield results helpful to society
- Appropriate design based on knowledge of the disease under study
- Avoidance of unnecessary physical and mental suffering and injury
- Absence of reason to believe that death or disabling injury will occur
- Overall degree of risk in proportion to the nature of the problem to be solved
- Adequate precautions against the possibility of the subject's injury, disability, or death
- Qualified persons conducting the study
- Unrestricted freedom of the subject to end the experiment if he or she reaches the physical or mental state where continuation of the experiment seems impossible
- Willingness of the investigator to discontinue the study at any time if there is reason to believe that continuing the experiment is likely to result in injury or death to the subject.

In the aftermath of the war, the international medical community was especially sensitized to the need for universal adherence to high standards of ethical behavior. The Declaration of Geneva was adopted in 1948 by the World Medical Association and has been updated since then. The text includes the physician's vow to ignore "considerations of age, disease or disability, creed, ethnic origin, gender, nationality, political affiliation, race, sexual orientation, or social standing" in the treatment of a patient and to uphold "even under threat ... the utmost respect for human life."

Case Study

Despite publicity about the Nuremberg Code and the Geneva declaration, controversial large-scale, government-sponsored medical studies took place in the years following World War

II. Experimentation on the effects of radiation exposure on humans was conducted in the United States during the Cold War, when fears of nuclear warfare prompted inquiry into the carcinogenic and other adverse health effects of environmental exposure to ionizing radiation. In response to public concern about thousands of federally funded studies conducted from the 1940s through 1970s without consent of the subjects, in 1994, President Bill Clinton established the Advisory Committee on Human Radiation Experiments (ACHRE). ACHRE was comprised of ethicists, radiation oncologists, and others with relevant expertise. It was charged with evaluating the experiments' ethical and scientific standards and recommending actions to ensure that any mistakes of the past would not be repeated. ACHRE reviewed all available documentation and also conducted an oral history project in which scientists described prevailing sentiments regarding human research ethics during the era of interest.

ACHRE found that government officials and investigators were in some cases culpable "for not having had policies and practices in place to protect the rights and interests of human subjects who ... could not possibly derive direct medical benefit."[15] One example was the observational study of uranium mine workers exposed to radon levels known to be hazardous, without warning and without efforts to reduce the radon levels by ventilating the mines. As a result, lung cancer developed in hundreds of workers, and appropriate compensation was recommended for the individuals affected.

The Belmont Report

In 1972, Jean Heller exposed the injustices of the U.S. Public Health Services (USPHS) Study of Untreated Syphilis in the Negro Male that was conducted in Tuskegee, Alabama.[16] During a 40-year period beginning in the 1930s, 399 indigent African American sharecroppers with syphilis and 200 without syphilis were subjects in a natural history study of the disease. The men mistakenly believed that diagnostic blood tests and lumbar punctures composed treatment for their "bad blood" when in reality, these were done solely to monitor the course of the infection. Moreover, years later when penicillin was discovered and found to be effective in the treatment of syphilis, it was withheld intentionally from the men. Subsequently, public awareness of the USPHS study likely contributed to enduring reluctance among some members of minority groups to participate in clinical trials,[17,18] and the political backlash provoked action by the federal government.

The 1974 National Research Act established the National Commission for the Protection of Human Subjects of Biomedical and Behavioral Research. The commission met at the Belmont Conference Center in Maryland to develop ethical guidelines for the conduct of biomedical and behavioral research. In 1979, the commission published *Ethical Principles and Guidelines for the Protection of Human Subjects of Research*, commonly known as the Belmont Report.[19]

In the Belmont Report, a clear distinction is made between medical research and clinical practice. The term *practice* describes interventions intended "to enhance the well-being of an individual patient ... that have a reasonable expectation of success," whereas *research* is "designed to test an hypothesis, permit conclusions to be drawn, and ... contribute to generalizable knowledge." Sometimes, a clinician uses good judgment and departs from standard methods for the benefit of an individual patient in special circumstances. However, if major innovations are proposed as replacement for standard techniques, then a formal investigation should be conducted to assess safety and efficacy. The National Commission embraced a principlist perspective in drafting the report, emphasizing in particular respect for persons, beneficence, and justice. The Belmont Report's definition of respect for persons incorporates respect for autonomy and special concern for individuals with diminished capacity to exercise their autonomy. Involving prisoners in research activity is cited as an example. Although it is inappropriate to deny prisoners the possible benefit of experimental interventions, any direct or indirect pressure on prisoners to participate in clinical studies must be avoided. For instance, a promise of clemency in return for study enrollment is unacceptable. The report also addresses the nature of justice in medical research, emphasizing that the process of selecting subjects for a research study must be carefully examined. Investigators should minimize the chance that socioeconomically disadvantaged groups are represented disproportionately as a result of a vulnerability to manipulation in the health care environment.

National Electrical Manufacturers Association Code of Ethics

The makers of equipment and software used in the practice of radiation oncology are not required to demonstrate clinical efficacy of a new device or software through the same sort of clinical testing that is required by the U.S. Food and Drug Administration (FDA) for approval of a new drug or implantable medical device. Rather, most treatment devices are approved after demonstration of safety and substantial equivalence to an approved device that is already commercially available. A company that wishes to sell a new device submits a premarket notification to the FDA at least 90 days before commercial distribution is to begin, in accordance with Section 510(k) of the FDA Modernization Act of 1997. Because devices may be introduced into the market without proof of superiority in any given clinical situation, manufacturers may promote their products to physicians by emphasizing intuitively attractive features that might or might not provide meaningful clinical advantage to patients.

On January 1, 2005, members of the National Electrical Manufacturers Association (NEMA) adopted a code of ethics regarding interactions between makers of medical imaging and treatment equipment and physicians (www.nema.org). Individual sections of the NEMA code address member-sponsored product training and education, support for third-party educational conferences, sales and promotional meetings, arrangements with consultants, gifts, provision of reimbursement and other economic information, charitable donations, and research grants. The guidelines are essentially consistent with the AMA policy on gifts and applicable federal regulations. NEMA members are allowed to support educational conferences and advertise their wares in these venues, and also they may provide educational support for individual customers in the safe use of their products. However, hospitality provided by NEMA member at conferences and meeting should be "modest in value and ... subordinate in time and focus to the purpose of the meeting." When it is necessary to demonstrate nonportable equipment, members may pay for reasonable travel costs of attendees with a *bona fide* professional interest but not for their guests.[20]

COMMON ETHICAL ISSUES IN RADIATION ONCOLOGY

Doctors wear a lot of hats these days; besides the usual physician role, we are expected to be a researcher, financial counselor, administrator, gatekeeper, patient advocate in the medicolegal system, ethicist, and Lord knows what else.

—*Thomas J. Smith*[21]

Financial Relationships with Hospitals and Referring Physicians

Reimbursement for radiation oncology services or other procedure-intensive subspecialties can be a major revenue source for hospitals. At the same time, subspecialists depend on other physicians to refer patients for evaluation and management. These situations can tempt hospital administrators to reward subspecialists for practicing in their facility and might tempt the subspecialists to induce referrals with financial incentives. In either case, a conflict of interests emerges: Treatment recommendations can be influenced not only appropriately by patient-centered beneficence but also inappropriately by the physician's interest in personal gain. In the United States, the Anti-Kickback Statute and the Stark Law make it illegal to engage in such unscrupulous medical business practices.

The Anti-Kickback Statute (42 U.S.C. §1320a-7b) includes criminal penalties for acts involving Medicare or state health care programs. Section (b) makes it a felony punishable by a fine up to $25,000 and up to 5 years in prison to solicit or receive "any remuneration (including any kickback, bribe, or rebate) directly or indirectly ... in return for referring an individual to a person for ... any item or service" reimbursed in whole or in part through Medicare or a state health care program. The Anti-Kickback Statute also bans other fraudulent transactions supported through the same funding sources.

Named for its leading congressional author, Rep. Pete Stark of California, the Stark Law (42 U.S.C. §1395nn; "Limitation on certain physician referrals") bans other misconduct involving Medicare and Medicaid patients. The Stark Law prohibits a physician from referring a patient for a "designated health service" to a clinic or other facility with which the physician or an immediate family member of the physician has a financial relationship. Radiation therapy is considered a designated health service, but it is clarified that a request by a radiation oncologist for radiation therapy is considered integral to the consultation request from the (nonradiation oncologist) referring physician and does not constitute a self-referral *per se* in most situations. Sanctions for violations of the numerous Stark Law regulations may include civil prosecution.

Self-Referral for Radiation Oncology Services

In addition to being considered a designated health service per Stark Law language, radiation therapy is also considered in the category of in-office ancillary service exemptions for Medicare coverage. The implication is that radiation therapy is grouped with a number of less complex services such as simple blood tests or antibiotic injections that a physician might reasonably do in his or her office for the convenience of rendering a quick diagnosis or managing a simple medical problem on an outpatient basis. Because of this classification for radiation therapy, nonradiation oncologists may own linear accelerators and derive profit from the utilization of this technology on patients referred for treatment. One of the most contentious issues to emerge in recent years is the debate over the legitimacy and ethics of business arrangements in which nonradiation oncologists own radiotherapy delivery technology and derive profit from self-referring patients for treatment.

In 2013, Jean Mitchell reported a study in *The New England Journal of Medicine* in which patterns of IMRT utilization for prostate cancer were analyzed. Urologists were grouped according to whether they purchased radiotherapy equipment. For those who purchased equipment (the self-referring group), the use of IMRT in the periods before and during ownership were compared. To account for the changing baseline trends in prostate cancer management, the use of IMRT among patients seen by non–self-referring urologists who did not own radiotherapy equipment was also analyzed,

and a "difference-in-differences" methodology was employed. It was observed that men treated by self-referring urologists, as compared with men treated by non–self-referring urologists, were significantly more likely to be treated with IMRT rather than less expensive options.[22] Other similarly constructed studies have yielded concordant results.[23,24]

Terry Wall offers a perspective on both the legal and ethical aspects of this issue.[25] He points out that advocacy efforts by the American Society for Radiation Oncology (ASTRO) over the last decade to remove radiation therapy from the list of in-office ancillary service exemptions have been unsuccessful, and there is unlikely to be a legislative resolution. Dr. Wall poses the question of whether an individual radiation oncologist who is the potential recipient of a self-referral is "eating fruit from a poisonous tree." He offers guidance for the individual practitioner to ensure that self-referral arrangements put the patient's interest first, including a mandate to disclose the financial interests to the patient and inform patients of their alternative to receive care elsewhere.

Electronic Record-Keeping and Billing Practices

The principles of respect for autonomy and nonmaleficence oblige confidentiality in physician–patient communications. Publicizing private details of a patient's condition can create social and economic harms for the patient. With the advent of electronic medical records and Internet communication, there is a greater need for vigilance in this respect.

In the United States, the Health Insurance Portability and Accountability Act of 1996 (HIPAA) empowered the Department of Health and Human Services to codify standards for storage and transmission of an individual patient's health information. Penalties for violations vary in proportion to their severity. In the worst case of wrongful disclosure of information with intent to sell it, a fine of up to $250,000 and a prison term of up to 10 years can be imposed.

Submitting fraudulent claims to the government for reimbursement of health care services is illegal. The False Claims Act (31 U.S.C. §3729) provides that any person who knowingly presents fraudulent claims to the US government may be fined $5,000 to $10,000 and may be liable for three times the amount of any damages sustained by the government.

Applications of New Technology

Innovative treatment delivery methods such as stereotactic body proton therapy (SBRT), proton therapy, adaptive therapy, and other new treatment techniques can be intuitively appealing but cannot be assumed to provide meaningful clinical benefit unless tested properly against existing standard treatment methods. A recent example underscoring this need is the lack of benefit of proton therapy over photon therapy for non–small cell lung cancer in the first randomized trial comparing these modalities.[26] Ideally, it is best that such innovations are tested in formal research protocols in which a clinical problem is identified and the new technology is proposed as a solution so that toxicity and efficacy can be monitored closely. A prospective clinical trial approved and monitored by an institutional review board affords the opportunity to advance knowledge in the field with ethical oversight.[27]

Clinical Trial Conduct

Instances of flagrantly improper clinical research taint the annals of medical history. The USPHS study of syphilis mentioned earlier and the human radiation experiments conducted during the Cold War without the consent of the participants are dark reminders of the need for ethical oversight of research.

Obtaining a participant's informed consent is of paramount importance in conducting most clinical research. Despite the recognized importance of informed consent, precisely how much information should be conveyed to a potential clinical trial participant is debatable. The Belmont Report offers this criterion: "the extent and nature of information should be such that persons, knowing that the procedure is neither necessary for their care nor perhaps fully understood, can decide whether they wish to participate" in the study. In certain situations, the nature of a study requires that there is incomplete disclosure of information to the participant to sustain the integrity of the study. The Belmont Report condones such research only when "i) incomplete disclosure is truly necessary to accomplish the goals of the research, ii) there are no undisclosed risks to subjects that are more than minimal, and iii) there is an adequate plan for debriefing subjects, when appropriate, and for dissemination of research results to them." The federal rules governing research (45 CFR 46) reflect these arguments.

Advances in the biosciences, such as stem cell research, cloning, and manipulations of the human genome, have been associated with contentious public debate. Federal government and professional policies on such matters have sometimes been constructed as a compromise between scientific opportunity and political ideology.[28] Extra safeguards have been imposed in some settings; for example, the federal government requires an extra level of review for gene-transfer experiments.[29]

Genetics

The management of some cancer patients can involve assessment of genetic markers that might predict treatment response and reveal a predisposition to the development of certain cancers among the patient's family members. The National Society of Genetic Counselors has published a guideline concerning genetic cancer risk assessment, counseling, and testing.[30] It is recommended that the process of obtaining informed consent for genetic testing should include, among other considerations, an explanation to the patient of possible implications on the ability to obtain health or disability insurance in the future.

Relationships with Industry Sponsors

Incentives from industry representatives to prescribe pharmaceuticals or purchase equipment threaten the fiduciary obligations physicians have to their patients. The AMA code of ethics states that physicians should decline cash gifts in any amounts from any entity with a financial interest in the physicians' treatment recommendations.[13] The AMA code allows for accepting an in-kind gift that will directly benefit patients and is of minimal value and allows for support for educational programs with certain restrictions.

Advertising items such as patient education pamphlets and anatomic models bearing a sponsor's name are commonly found in radiation oncology clinics.[31] Physicians should be aware of any real or perceived influence on the patient–physician relationships resulting from their tacit compliance with such marketing activities.

Pharmaceutical companies may be prosecuted for kickback schemes or other illegal enticements to physicians, and the civil and criminal penalties paid by the corporations held responsible have ranged up to hundreds of millions of dollars.[32] Brennan et al.[33] contend that voluntary self-regulation by physicians, industry, and government is an insufficient safeguard against the conflict of interests nurtured by close relationships between practicing doctors and sellers of pharmaceuticals and medical products. These authors argue that academic medical centers should set an example for the rest of the medical community by establishing policies that forbid

gifts to physicians, funds for travel, unjustified consulting fees, participation in speakers' bureaus, and the practice of "ghostwriting" medical articles, among other things. Substantial attention has focused on implementing policies related to these issues.[34,35]

Prasad and Rajkumar recommend a forward-looking strategy of transparency and full disclosure to as a means of minimizing the impact of conflict of interest in academic publications and presentations.[36] Their suggestions include excluding authors of reviews, editorials, and practice guidelines from having any financial interest that exceed a reasonable threshold[37]; stopping the practice of having professional medical writers funded by industry serve to prepare manuscripts; and open disclosure of the amount of support given to professional organizations by individual industry sponsors.

CASE-SPECIFIC DILEMMAS: THE ROLE OF AN ETHICS CONSULTANT OR COMMITTEE

The radiation oncology–related ethical issues discussed thus far relate primarily to general practice and research guidelines. However, individual cases can also pose uncertainties regarding the proper choice of action for a specific patient.

Case Study

A 37-year-old woman undergoes modified radical mastectomy for a pathologic T3N2M0 breast cancer; postoperative chemotherapy and locoregional radiation therapy are recommended. The patient wishes to receive the therapy only if she can periodically interrupt it to alternate with what she calls a "natural herbal" therapy.

In this case, respect for a patient's autonomy conflicts with what is believed to be in the patient's best interests, but a physician cannot ethically abrogate the fiduciary responsibility to a patient simply for reasons of unfamiliarity with alternative medicine or prejudice against its worth.[38] Similar situations may arise when patients do not adhere to standard treatment recommendations because of a particular religious faith or cultural heritage. Although physicians must respect patients' choices, there is no strict obligation for a physician to accept a particular individual as a patient, especially if there are foreseeable personal conflicts that might adversely affect the patient–physician relationship, unless the treatment is needed urgently and/or there are no other physicians with the same skills or knowledge to treat the patient.

Pediatric oncology also requires special considerations. Parents are the chief decision makers, but sometimes their wishes can seem discordant with the best interests of the child. In a different context, what should be done if the adult children of a patient with a heritable trait for malignancy inquire of the patient's diagnosis, but the patient has instructed the physician not to reveal any information to them? The obligation to patient–physician confidentiality conflicts with a potentially overriding obligation toward the family members who might benefit from guidance toward screening.

In cases such as these in which it is difficult to choose between two defensible courses of action, individuals and committees with experience in clinical medical ethics can provide the expertise needed to sort through the ethical, legal, and social issues involved.[39]

PALLIATIVE MEDICINE

Palliative medicine has become a well-established component of clinical practice, and numerous academic medical centers offer accredited fellowship programs in this field.

Palliative medicine places emphasis on symptom management and on the goals of care, not only at the end of life but also in the treatment of serious illnesses. An exclusively palliative approach is ethically justified when fully aggressive therapy might be intolerable or futile, but the use of early concurrent palliative care can also be beneficial for patients with metastatic cancer or cancer with high symptom burden who are still receiving aggressive anti-cancer therapy.

Case Study

A 92-year-old woman presented with stage IVa maxillary sinus cancer. She complained of sinus fullness and a painful 4-cm neck node. Radical radiation therapy to the primary and neck was recommended, and the patient underwent placement of a percutaneous gastric feeding tube and full dental extraction. Midway through the course of treatment, the patient required a lengthy hospitalization for failure to thrive and severe mucositis.

In retrospect a less aggressive course of radiation therapy intended to reduce the sinus and neck symptoms would have likely been a better choice for this patient, who was frail and unable to withstand intense treatment. Palliative medicine pays careful attention to a patient's individual needs, quality of life, and a discussion of goals of care. A recent randomized study demonstrated improved quality of life and overall survival when palliative care was given early alongside standard cancer treatment for metastatic lung cancer.[40] In many cases, aggressive symptom management and good communication among patient, family, and provider may result in better quality and, perhaps, quantity of life than would antineoplastic therapy that has little expectation of efficacy but significant risk of morbidity.[41]

ETHICS AND MEDICAL ERRORS

Soon after the discovery of x-rays by Wilhelm Röntgen more than 100 years ago, the first cases of malpractice involving the clinical use of radiation therapy were tried in the US court system.[42] During the early 20th century, severe dermatitis was a frequent plaintiff's complaint—not surprising in view of the physical limitations of the low-energy machines available at the time.

In 1999, the Institute of Medicine published a report on medical errors, elevating the level of public awareness and stimulating inquiry into this topic.[43] One recent study has suggested that medical errors might be the third leading cause of death in the United States.[44]

Physicians are often reluctant to discuss errors. It has been suggested that doctors and patients "harbor deep within themselves the expectation that the physician will be perfect."[45] Other reasons for reticence include uncertainty about whether an event really is an error, concern for the patient's well-being, and fear of litigation.[46]

If a patient has an undesirable treatment outcome, careful review of the case can help distinguish error from untoward but unsurprising occurrence. For example, severe pneumonitis after breast radiation therapy is uncommon but not necessarily proof of negligence. Concern that disclosing an error causes a patient undue anxiety is contradicted by studies revealing that patients prefer physicians to acknowledge errors[47] and that they might even sue for lack of apology.[48] In cases of alleged or suspected error leading to injury, the institutional risk management service should usually be contacted for advice. However, fear of litigation should be mitigated by the fact that a low overall percentage of patients who suffer negligent injuries actually file malpractice claims.[46]

Nondisclosure of error can weaken the trust at the core of the patient–physician relationship. The argument for disclosure is especially strong when there is a specific preventive intervention that might lessen the severity of possible future injury. Nevertheless, the question still remains: Are physicians ethically obliged to disclose an error, even if there is no immediate harm to the patient?

Case Study

A patient with T3N1M0 squamous cell carcinoma of the left retromolar trigone received concurrent cisplatin plus intensity-modulated radiation therapy to the gross disease, with elective coverage of adjacent nodal echelons. The intent was to give 54 Gy to adjacent uninvolved lymph nodes at a rate of 1.8 Gy/day and 66 Gy to the gross disease at a rate of 2.2 Gy/day using a synchronous integrated boost technique, with all treatment completed in 30 fractions. After the spinal cord was contoured as an organ at risk, the structure was inadvertently deleted on all planning computed tomography slices below the level of the gross disease. As a result, when the intensity-modulated radiation therapy inverse planning software optimized the dose distribution according to the constraint of limiting the maximum dose to the spinal cord to 50 Gy, the entire cross-section of a 6-cm length of cervical spinal cord received the full prescription dose. The error was not detected until 1 week after the patient completed treatment, during a routine quality assurance check.

In this example, no injury has yet occurred, but the patient is at increased risk for radiation myelitis. Although there is currently no available proven preventive measure, if the escalated risk of myelitis is unknown to the patient, he or she might later undergo misguided management by another physician if symptoms develop. For instance, if the patient develops arm and leg weakness, a magnetic resonance imaging scan showing nonspecific enhancement and edema in the cervical spinal cord might be interpreted as evidence of metastatic intramedullary or epidural tumor rather than radiation change. Unaware of the prior treatment error, the patient would be unable to inform the other physician involved about the high risk for radiation injury. As a result, the patient might be given only minimal supportive care on the assumption of incurable recurrent disease rather than appropriate efforts toward rehabilitation.

Evans and Decker[49] have offered practical suggestions on how to address the issue of a medical error in radiation oncology once the event has been recognized. They advise disclosure for any errors that result in a perceptible clinical effect, change in diagnosis or treatment course, or a chance of future harm. Their two-phase response recommendation involves initial attention to the patient's immediate needs and an apology that avoids giving an impression of defensiveness. Later, after a more thorough analysis of the situation has been completed with the involvement of the hospital's risk management team, a carefully prepared discussion with the patient and other interested parties can occur.

Toward the goal of fostering a culture of safety across the field of radiation oncology and facilitating the identification of preventable systematic errors with different treatment delivery platforms, ASTRO and the American Association of Physicists in Medicine (AAPM) have created a national Radiation Oncology Incident Learning System.[50] This program allows for anonymous, privacy-protected self-reporting of incidents and near misses. The information can be used locally to inform root cause analysis projects that identify ways of improving patient safety. Industrial engineering-based principles for minimizing errors in a busy radiation oncology clinic are now becoming widely implemented, and entire texts devoted to this topic are available.[51,52]

CONCLUSION

Society's view concerning medical ethics has shifted over time to adapt to the forces of advancing knowledge. Ethical guidelines have sometimes been constructed as formal documents or mandated as law, but no single system comprehensively predicts and resolves all situational dilemmas. The core principles of medical ethics remain essential foundations for the practice of medicine.

REFERENCES

1. Starr P. *The social transformation of American medicine*. New York: Basic Books, 1982.
2. Chervenak FA, McCullough LB. The moral foundation of medical leadership: the professional virtues of the physician as fiduciary of the patient. *Am J Obstet Gynecol* 2001;184:875–879.
3. Reich WT. The word "bioethics": its birth and the legacies of those who shaped it. *Kennedy Inst Ethics J* 1994;4:319–335.
4. Beauchamp TL, Childress JF. *Principles of biomedical ethics*. 4th ed. New York: Oxford University Press, 1994.
5. *Natanson v Kline*, 350 P. 2d 1093 (Kan 1960).
6. Aquinas T. *Summa Theologica* II-II, Q64, art. 7, "Of Killing." In: Baumgarth WP, Regan RJ, eds. *On law, morality, and politics*. Indianapolis, IN: Hackett, 1988:226–227.
7. Lyons AS. Hippocrates. In: Lyons AS, Petrucelli RJ, eds. *Medicine: an illustrated history*. Hong Kong: Abrams, 1987:207–217.
8. Halperin EC. Physician awareness of the contents of the Hippocratic Oath. *J Med Humanit* 1989;2:107–114.
9. Moffic HS, Coverdale J, Bayer T. The Hippocratic Oath and clinical ethics. *J Clin Ethics* 1992;1:287–289.
10. Leake CD, ed. *Percival's medical ethics*. Huntington, NY: Krieger, 1975.
11. Pickstone JV. Thomas Percival and the production of medical ethics. In: Baker R, Porter D, Porter R, eds. *The codification of medical morality: historical and philosophical studies of the formalization of Western medical morality in the eighteenth and nineteenth centuries, vol 1. Medical ethics and etiquette in the eighteenth century (Philosophy and Medicine, vol 45)*. Boston, MA: Kluwer Academic, 1993:164–176.
12. Baker R. Deciphering Percival's code. In: Baker R, Porter D, Porter R, eds. *The codification of medical morality: historical and philosophical studies of the formalization of Western medical morality in the eighteenth and nineteenth centuries, vol 1. Medical ethics and etiquette in the eighteenth century (Philosophy and Medicine, vol 45)*. Boston, MA: Kluwer Academic, 1993:188–214.
13. AMA Code of Medical Ethics. www.ama-assn.org/delivering-care/ama-code-medical-ethics. Accessed July 5, 2017.
14. Trials of War Criminals before the Nuremberg Military Tribunals under Control Council Law No. 10. Nuremberg, October 1946–April 1949. *Washington*, DC: U.S. Government Printing Office, 1949–1953.
15. Advisory Committee on Human Radiation Experiments. *Final Report of the Advisory Committee on Human Radiation Experiments (stock number 061-000-00-848-9)*. Washington, DC: Government Printing Office, 1995.
16. Heller J. Syphilis victims in the U.S. study went untreated for 40 years. *The New York Times*. July 26, 1972:1, 8. [The story was also reported in part in *The Evening Star and Washington Daily News*. July 25, 1972:A1.]
17. Corbie-Smith G, Thomas S, Williams M, et al. Attitudes and beliefs of African Americans toward participation in medical research. *J Gen Intern Med* 1999;14:537–546.
18. Corbie-Smith G. The continuing legacy of the Tuskegee Syphilis Study: implications for clinical research. *Am J Med Sci* 1999;317:5–8.
19. National Commission for the Protection of Human Subjects of Biomedical and Behavioral Research. Belmont Report: Ethical Principles and Guidelines for the Protection of Human Subjects of Research. Available at: www.hhs.gov/ohrp/humansubjects/guidance/belmont.html. Accessed January 17, 2013.
20. National Electronic Manufacturers Association. NEMA Code of Ethics on Interactions with Health Care Providers. Adopted November 30, 2004. Available at: www.nema.org/news/Documents/nema+codeofethics-faq-adopted.pdf. Accessed January 17, 2013.
21. Smith TJ. A piece of my mind: which hat do I wear? *JAMA* 1993;270:1657–1659.
22. Mitchell JM. Urologists' use of intensity-modulated radiation therapy for prostate cancer. *N Engl J Med* 2013;369(17):1629–1637.
23. Bekelman JE, Suneja G, Guzzo T, et al. Effect of practice integration between urologists and radiation oncologists on prostate cancer treatment patterns. *J Urol* 2013;190(1):97–101.
24. Williams SB, Huo J, Chapin BF, et al. Impact of urologists' ownership of radiation equipment in the treatment of prostate cancer. *Prostate Cancer Prostatic Dis* 2017;20(3):300–304.
25. Wall TJ. Ethics in the legal and business practices of radiation oncology. *Int J Radiat Oncol Biol Phys*. 2017;99(2):265–268. doi: 10.1016/j.ijrobp.2017.06.2462.
26. Liao ZX, Lee JJ, Komaki R, et al. Bayesian randomized trial comparing intensity modulated radiation therapy versus passively scattered proton therapy for locally advanced non-small cell lung cancer. *J Clin Oncol* 2016;34(15 suppl):8500. doi: 10.1200/JCO.2016.34.15_suppl.8500
27. Dunn CM, Chadwick G. *Protecting study volunteers in research: a manual for investigative sites*. Boston, MA: CenterWatch, 1999.
28. Marwick C. President Bush sidesteps critics in stem cell debate. *BMJ* 2001;323:357.
29. *National Institutes of Health (NIH) Guidelines for Research Involving Recombinant DNA Molecules, Appendix M*. Washington, DC: Department of Health and Human Services, 2002.
30. Riley BD, Culver JO, Skrzynia C, et al. Essential elements of genetic cancer risk assessment, counseling, and testing: updated recommendations of the National Society of Genetic Counselors. *J Genet Couns* 2012;21(2):151–161.
31. Hutchinson P, Halperin EC. The hidden persuaders: subtle advertising in radiation oncology. *Int J Radiat Oncol Biol Phys* 2002;54:989–991.
32. Studdert DM, Mello MM, Brennan TA. Financial conflict of interest in physician relationships with the pharmaceutical industry: self-regulation in the shadow of federal prosecution. *N Engl J Med* 2004;351:1891–1900.
33. Brennan TA, Rothman DJ, Blank L, et al. Health industry practices that create conflicts of interest: a policy proposal for academic medical centers. *JAMA* 2006;295:429–433.
34. Wasserstein AG, Brennan PJ, Rubenstein AH. Institutional leadership and faculty response: fostering professionalism at the University of Pennsylvania School of Medicine. *Acad Med* 2007;82(11):1049–1056.
35. Coleman DL. Establishing policies for the relationship between industry and clinicians: lessons learned from two academic health centers. *Acad Med* 2008;83(9):882–887.
36. Prasad V, Rajkumar SV. Conflict of interest in academic oncology: moving beyond the blame game and forging a path forward. *Blood Cancer J* 2016;6:e489. doi: 10.1038/bcj.2016.101
37. Drazen JM, Curfman GD. Financial associations of authors. *N Engl J Med* 2002;346:1901–1902.
38. Sugarman J, Burk L. Physicians' ethical obligations regarding alternative medicine. *JAMA* 1998;280:1623–1625.
39. Lo B. *Resolving ethical dilemmas: a guide for clinicians*. 2nd ed. Philadelphia: Lippincott Williams & Wilkins, 2000.
40. Temel JS, Greer JA, Muzikansky A, et al. Early palliative care for patients with metastatic non-small-cell lung cancer. *N Engl J Med* 2010;363:733–742.
41. Ferris FD, Bruera E, Cherny N, et al. Palliative cancer care a decade later: accomplishments, the need, next steps—from the American Society of Clinical Oncology. *J Clin Oncol* 2009;27(18):3052–3058.
42. Halperin EC. X-rays at the bar, 1896–1910. *Invest Radiol* 1988;23:639–646.
43. Kohn LT, Corrigan JM, Donaldson MS, eds. *To err is human: building a safer health system*. Washington, DC: Institute of Medicine, 1999.
44. Makary MA, Daniel M. Medical error—the third leading cause of death in the US. *BMJ* 2016;353:i2139.
45. Hilfiker D. Facing our mistakes. *N Engl J Med* 1984;310:118–122.
46. Baylis F. Errors in medicine: nurturing truthfulness. *J Clin Ethics* 1997;8:336–340.
47. Whitman AB, Park DM, Hardin SB. How do patients want physicians to handle mistakes? A survey of internal medicine patients in an academic setting. *Arch Intern Med* 1996;156:2565–2569.
48. Vincent C, Young M, Phillips A. Why do people sue doctors? A study of patients and relatives taking legal action. *Lancet* 1994;343:1609–1613.
49. Evans SB, Decker R. Disclosing medical errors: a practical guide and discussion of radiation oncology-specific controversies. *Int J Radiat Oncol Biol Phys* 2011;80(5):1285–1288.
50. Hoopes DJ, Dicker AP, Eads NL, et al. RO-ILS: Radiation Oncology Incident Learning System: A report from the first year of experience. *Pract Radiat Oncol* 2015;5(5):312–318.
51. Marks L, Mazur L, Chera B, Adams R. *Engineering patient safety in radiation oncology: University of North Carolina's Pursuit for High Reliability and Value Creation*. Boca Raton, FL: CRC Press, 2015.
52. Dicker AP, Ford EC, Williams TR, eds. *Quality and safety in radiation oncology: implementing tools and best practices for patients, providers, and payers*. New York: Demos Medical, 2016.

Section
V

CHAPTER 105

Health Economics and Health Policy

Ann C. Raldow, Eric M. Chang, and Michael L. Steinberg

INTRODUCTION

The 21st century has been marked by a continued increase in health expenditure in the United States, estimated at 16.9% of the country's gross domestic product (GDP) in 2015—the highest ranked in data collected from the Organization for Economic Cooperation and Development (OECD) member countries and nearly twice the OECD average[1] (Fig. 105.1). Furthermore, national health spending is only expected to continue its rise in the coming years, with the Centers for Medicare and Medicaid Services (CMS) National Health Expenditures projecting health spending to grow 1.2% points faster than GDP per year over the 2016 to 2025 period, amounting to 19.9% share of GDP by 2025.[2] The cost of cancer care is escalating precipitously, estimated at $24.7 billion in 1987 (in 2007 US dollars) versus $48.1 billion in the 2001 to 2005 period.[3] Although the double-digit growth rates in US cancer expenditures observed prior to the Great Recession began to decline substantially in 2007, associated costs of cancer care are still projected to rise from $124.57 billion to $157.77 billion from 2010 to 2020 (in 2010 US dollars) assuming constant incidence, survival, and cost.[4,5]

There are many factors contributing to this rise in costs, including aging of the population, with anticipated increases in both the number and the percentage of elderly patients and commensurate increases in new diagnoses, magnified by persistence of risk-increasing behaviors and earlier diagnoses via improved cancer screening.[6,7] These demographic factors warrant discussion regarding the allocation and prioritization of resources. Yet, the increasing cost to the individual patient merits further consideration as well. Driven partly by innovation—new advances in systemic therapies, radiotherapy techniques, surgical devices, and diagnostic tools—these investments pose a particular dilemma, as efforts to cut costs would potentially slow the development of lifesaving medications and technologies. However, in the setting of limited resources, these rising costs are not benign. In 2011, roughly 40% of expenditures in cancer care were publicly funded (34.1% by Medicare and 5.3% by Medicaid), and by 2030, more than 70% of cancer diagnoses will be made in persons eligible for Medicare.[6,8] Thus, from a societal perspective, we must consider whether our expenditure in cancer care is reasonable when balanced with other priorities in medical care and other areas. Furthermore, substantial out-of-pocket costs directly impact patients' ability to access medical care and to afford other nonmedical life necessities, with having insurance often not enough to protect patients from the impact of the high costs of treatment.[9] Estimates by the Congressional Budget Office (CBO) indicate that aging explains less than half of the estimated increase in spending for major health care programs as a share of GDP from 2016 to 2046, with the majority resulting from rising health care costs per person—indicating that these challenging questions and the need for the transformation of health care delivery will not go away.[10]

In this setting of mounting health care costs, interest in health policy and health economics has flourished in the past decades. Broadly, health policy as a discipline encompasses questions of access, cost, and quality of health care.[11] As a function of health policy, health economics addresses difficult questions regarding the appropriate and efficient allocation of resources in the health care setting as well as the behavior of stakeholders in the face of competing choices for financial

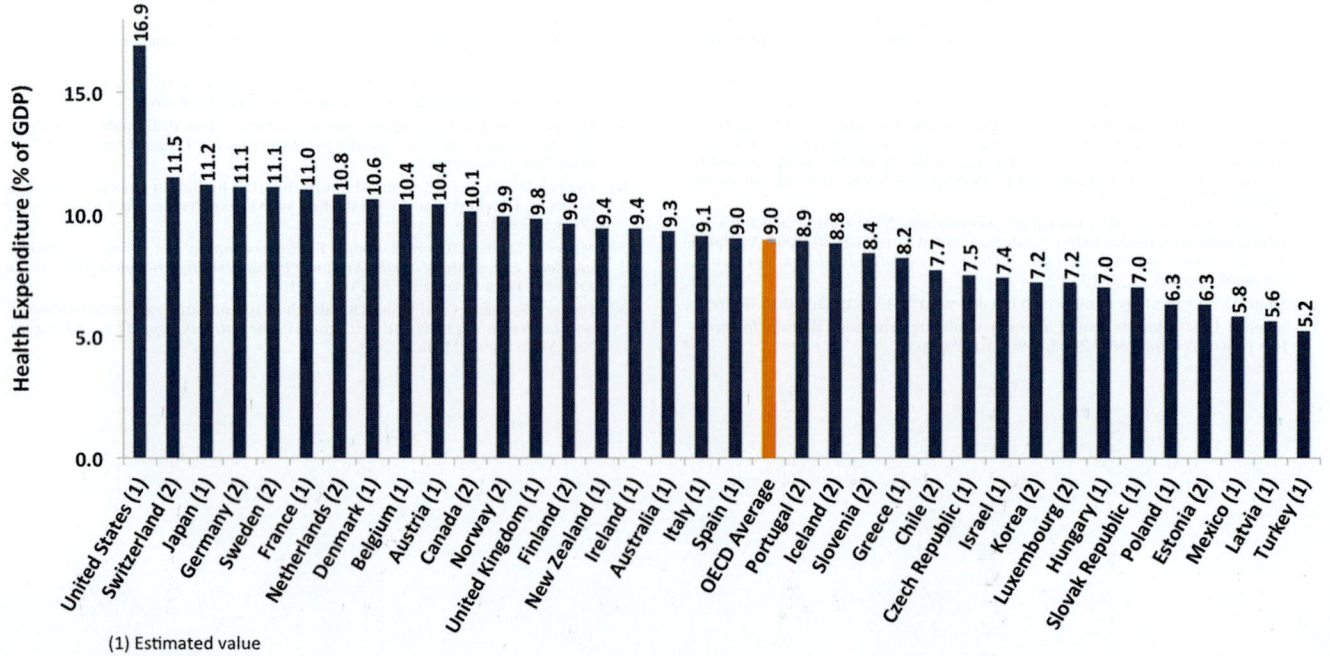

FIGURE 105.1. Health expenditure expressed as a percentage of gross domestic product (GDP) among the Organization for Economic Cooperation and Development (OECD) member countries. (Source: OECD Health Statistics 2016.)

(1) Estimated value
(2) Provisional value

resources. In his seminal article, "Uncertainty and the Welfare Economics of Medical Care," Kenneth Arrow, often credited with the birth of health care economics, distinguishes between health and other goods, noting that health care, in contrast with other goods and the free market ideal, is marked by uncertainty on behalf of the patient in evaluating the quality of care provided by their physician, leading to asymmetric information.[12] Physicians, serving as agents for their patients, are expected to act in their patients' best interests, though this system, based on trust, permits for misaligned incentives. Moreover, health care is awash in externalities or costs and benefits externally imposed by the purchaser on others not party to the transaction. Given these notable exceptions, it is imperative that health policy ensures symmetric access to quality health care. As defined by Steinberg, ideal health policy should ensure (1) that all patients get all necessary care, (2) that equivocal and nonindicated treatment be excluded, (3) that cost of care be socially responsible, (4) that variation in the quality of care be so small from a technical perspective that does not matter from which facility or provider a patient receives treatment, and (5) that when competition occurs, it should be over the quality of the art of care, such as how patient centered it is and how well staff and physicians communicate with patients.[11]

Radiation oncology, in particular, has been labeled as an outlier in its contribution to health care spending and as such has often been targeted in policy discussions. Though Medicare's sustainable growth rate (SGR) formula for physician payment was permanently repealed in April 2015, radiation oncology was notable for exceeding its SGR target over the 2003 to 2009 period by nearly 300% expressed as a percentage of 2002 expenditure.[13,14] Between 2000 and 2009, the total Medicare expenditures for external beam radiation therapy (RT) increased from $256 million to $1.08 billion, mainly owing to reimbursement for intensity-modulated radiation therapy (IMRT).[15] Additionally, the code for IMRT demonstrated the fourth highest percent increase of all Medicare codes between 2010 and 2011.[16] Although there are likely multiple underlying causes for the field's disparate contributions to health care spending, including the employment of advanced technologies and the complex teams required for their safe and effective use, they were at least in part secondary to our primarily resource-based payment system, in which hospitals and clinics are reimbursed for discrete elements of care.[17] In this system, there is incentive to maximize billable units, such as by using advanced treatment modalities when not clinically indicated and by dividing dose over an increased number of fractions— all facilitated by the technologic and complex nature of radiation oncology. This engenders further inefficiency as payers invest in the creation of guidelines to restrict payments and providers in turn require significant resources to guarantee appropriate billing. Although radiation oncology's role as a beneficiary of this system could be interpreted as cause for blame, it may also be seen as a charge for leadership by the field in health care reform discussions and in the development and use of modern methods for assessing quality of care and the comparative effectiveness of various treatment modalities.

RT plays a fundamental role in the curative and palliative treatment of cancer. Its continued value in cancer care will depend on the advancement of not only clinical evidence but also health services research. Toward this end, this chapter will provide an overview of the value proposition in health care as it relates to radiation oncology, with a focus on modern methods for assessing comparative and cost-effectiveness, including decision analysis and cost-effectiveness analysis. These techniques provide an alternative method for approaching clinical questions not readily answered with standard data analyses and aim to maximize the value of each health care dollar spent. Thus, understanding their employ will be of importance in the establishment of the value of RT in health policy discussions moving forward.

VALUE IN RADIATION ONCOLOGY

Remarkable advances in RT have been made in the past decades, allowing for extraordinary precision in treatment delivery and the attainment of dose escalation paired with decreased morbidity to surrounding normal tissues. In particular, IMRT achieves highly conformal dose distributions using computer-based treatment planning and delivery. The advent of stereotactic body radiation therapy (SBRT) has further provided the ability to deliver large doses of radiation with extreme precision using complex methods of patient immobilization and tumor localization, at times supplanting or offering an alternative definitive treatment to surgery in multiple disease sites. Coupled with RT, concomitant advances in oncologic surgery, medical oncology, and diagnostic testing have ushered in an era of personalized medicine, with the promise of more effective, tailored therapy with reduced toxicity. However, historically in cancer care, as in most fields of medicine, doing more for patients has not always equated to improved outcomes. Rising health care spending has not necessarily met with a proportional improvement in outcomes, with the US ranking 13th out of 32 OECD countries in mortality from cancer per 100,000 persons in 2013, leading to calls for an increased focus on "high-value care" by policy makers, providers, professional societies, payers, and patient groups in the context of health care reform.[18-20] The value proposition in health care is not merely an exercise in cost containment, but it also strives toward a delivery system that incentivizes high-quality, evidence-based, and cost-effective treatments.[21] In this section, we will discuss the value proposition as it applies to the specialty of radiation oncology, describing current challenges and future directions in the advancement toward value-based care. Given the many stakeholders involved, it is important to note that the patient's voice is a highly valued component of value-based health care delivery. We therefore address these issues with a focus on the patient perspective of high-value care.

DEFINING VALUE IN RADIATION ONCOLOGY

In order to discuss value and the metrics used to measure it, we must first establish a mutual understanding of what is meant by the term *value*.[21] Outside of the world of health care, a "good value" can be described as a desirable product or service that can be purchased for a fair price.[22] Definitions of *value* from the Merriam-Webster dictionary center on the fair return in goods, services, or money for something exchanged, with clear parallels in the definition of value as it applies to medicine in terms of relative worth, cost, and quality of care.[23] These issues are reflected in the definitions of value as put forth by multiple governing bodies in health care from around the world, including the European Observatory on Health Systems and Policies, which describes value to include "patient preferences, quality, equity, efficiency, and product acceptability among a wide range of stakeholders," and the United Kingdom's National Institute for Health and Clinical Excellence (NICE), which defines value as "based on scientific value judgments, including clinical evaluation and an economic evaluation, and social value judgments, including considerations of efficiency and effectiveness."[24,25]

THE VALUE EQUATION

In order to unify the often-conflicting goals of the numerous stakeholders in health care delivery, Michael Porter and Elizabeth Olmsted Teisberg established a working definition of value in health care as health outcomes achieved per dollar spent (value = outcomes/cost)[26,27] (Fig. 105.2). Outcomes in

$$Value = \frac{Outcomes}{Cost}$$

FIGURE 105.2. The value equation as defined by Porter. (From Porter ME. What is value in health care? *N Engl J Med* 2010;363[26]:2477–2481. Copyright © 2010 Massachusetts Medical Society. Reprinted with permission from Massachusetts Medical Society.)

this equation are specified to include both near-term and longer-term health in order to cover the ultimate results of care and are noted to be condition-specific and multitiered, with adequate measurement of risk factors and baseline condition to enable for risk adjustment. Costs are defined to include the total costs of the complete cycle of care as opposed to individual services; as Porter notes, narrowly targeted cost containment efforts may not maximize value for the patient, with at times the best approach to increasing value being spending more on some services to reduce the need for others.[27] As both outcomes and costs are dependent on results as opposed to inputs, the challenge in value-based care is to shift focus away from the volume of services as is typical in traditional fee-for-service systems.

As described by Porter, "Value should always be defined around the customer, and… the creation of value for patients should determine the rewards for all other actors in the system."[27] Recognizing the importance of the patient in the value proposition, Teckie and colleagues, in setting forth a framework for value in the field of radiation oncology, further expanded the numerator toward a more comprehensive definition of quality to include structure and process along with outcomes, in line with the classic Donabedian model[22,28] (Fig. 105.3). The Donabedian model is a conceptual framework for evaluating the quality of medical care, in which assessments are drawn from three dimensions of care: structure, process, and outcomes. Structure encompasses the context in which care is delivered, including the physical facility, human resources, organizational characteristics, and, of particular importance in radiation oncology, the equipment and technology. Process includes all acts of health care delivery, including interactions between the patient and physician and the technical delivery of care. In the Donabedian model, outcomes include not just objective measures, such as survival and functional status, but also subjective measures, such as quality of life and patient satisfaction. By this expanded framework (value = quality/cost), efforts to improve structure, process, and outcomes can all be seen as strides toward improving value.

STRUCTURE

Donabedian defines structure as "concerned with such things as the adequacy of facilities and equipment; the qualifications of medical staff and their organization; the administrative structure and operations of programs and institutions providing care; fiscal organization and the like."[28] Radiation oncology, as a field, has become increasingly complex in recent years, with advances in treatment modalities involving multifaceted structural elements requiring multidisciplinary teams and state-of-the-art technology for adequate delivery. This complexity has allowed for wide variation in structural practices. Although at times this variation is indicated based on an individual patient's needs, critics have noted that deviations may not be associated with increased quality of care, with an opportunity for enhancement of value via standardization.[8] In 2010, the American Society for Radiation Oncology (ASTRO) convened a total of 12 multidisciplinary societies to develop a guidance document describing the elements necessary for the safe delivery of RT. This document, entitled "Safety is No Accident," was published in 2012 and sets forth specific requirements for a radiation oncology facility in terms of structure, personnel, and technical process.[29] In 2014, in an effort to expand adoption of these principles and further unify variations in care delivery, ASTRO launched the ASTRO Accreditation Program for Excellence (APEx), which provides impartial third-party review of practices' personnel, equipment, treatment planning, medical records, patient safety policies, and quality control/quality assessment activities against an established set of performance standards with focus on structure and process elements.[30] Radiation oncology practices (including freestanding single facilities, multisite organizations, and practices that are part of a hospital facility) that apply undergo a process of self-assessment and third-party review against a set of 16 established standards with accreditation granted for a 4-year cycle. The Commission on Cancer (COC) and the National Accreditation Program for Breast Centers (NAPBC) both accept APEx accreditation as fulfilling the RT component of their accreditation programs. Accreditation ideally demonstrates achievement of a threshold level of quality and safety to referring physicians, peers, prospective patients, regulatory agencies, and payers. However, it remains to be seen whether these various stakeholders value accreditation or understand what the evaluation process involves. Moreover, without appropriate economic incentives

FIGURE 105.3. Components of value as defined by Teckie and colleagues, adapted from the Porter equation including elements from the Donabedian model. (Adapted with permission from Teckie S, McCloskey SA, Steinberg ML. Value: a framework for radiation oncology. *J Clin Oncol* 2014;32[26]:2864–2870. Copyright © 2014 American Society of Clinical Oncology. All rights reserved.)

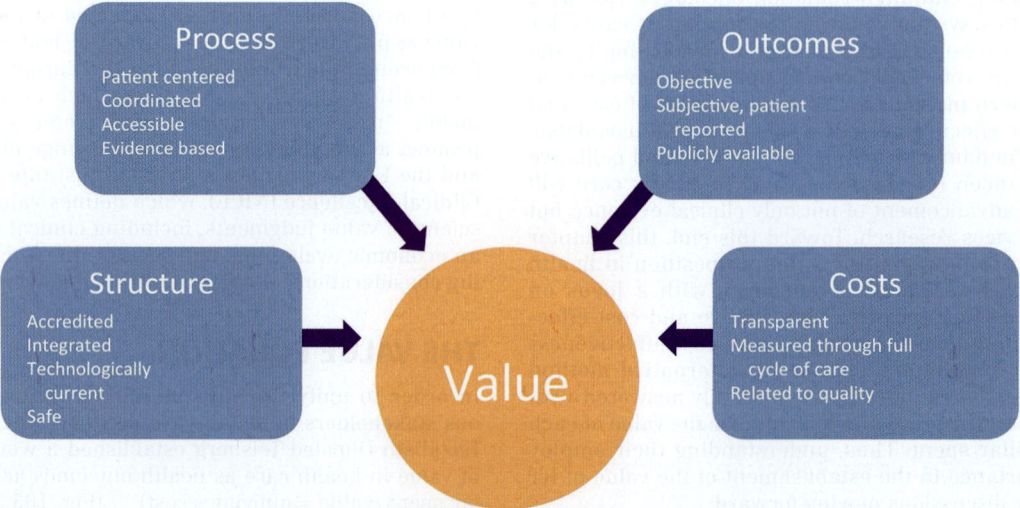

to pursue and maintain accreditation, it is unclear how many radiation oncology practices will elect to participate. At the time of writing (April 1, 2017), 36 facilities have obtained APEx practice accreditation, though more are undergoing the painstaking application and accreditation process.[31]

Integration of Care

In traditional organizational structure of medical care, delivery of care is siloed according to separate medical specialties or departments. However, in the past decades, there has been a shift toward medical practices centered around the patients' perspective of their medical condition integrated across the continuum of care; additionally falling under the realm of structure, this strategy has received attention for promoting high-value care.[32] In the integrated practice unit (IPU) model, clinical and nonclinical personnel deliver care according to evidence-based care pathways and treatment directives with responsibility for the full cycle of care, including inpatient, outpatient, rehabilitative care, and supporting services, such as nutrition and social work. Importantly, the team measures outcomes, costs, and processes for each patient with feedback mechanisms for refinement of care delivery, economic efficiency, and patient convenience, all relevant to the value proposition. This integration promotes value not only by limiting overuse of tests and procedures but also by increasing use of patient-centered shared decision-making. Specific to oncology, the multidisciplinary clinic model centers a team of multiple specialties, including medical oncologists, radiation oncologists, radiologists, surgical oncologists, and pharmacists, around a specific tumor site.[33] While requiring significant reorganization and reassessment of traditional interactions between subspecialists and ancillary staff, adaptation of these models has been successful at many high-volume centers, with suggestion of both improved outcomes and reduced costs compared to similar community groups.[34,35] For instance, comparison of a consecutive sample of 104 melanoma patients with localized disease treated in the Michigan community with 104 blindly selected patients treated at the University of Michigan Multidisciplinary Melanoma Clinic during an identical time period matched for Breslow depth and melanoma body site indicated cost savings of $1,600 per patient for patients treated in the multidisciplinary clinic.[34] Via coordination between multiple specialties in complex decision-making, the multidisciplinary model may allow for higher attainment of benchmark measures for quality care in accordance with national practice guidelines. For example, a study of 609 patients with nonmetastatic breast cancer treated in the University of California, Los Angeles multidisciplinary breast clinic indicated increased appropriate referral rates for genetic testing for family history–based (62% vs. 92%) and overall (80% vs. 96%) indications after the inclusion of a genetic counselor in the multidisciplinary clinic.[36] Although limited primarily to observational studies because of difficulty in recruiting patients from practices in which the multidisciplinary model is not standard of care and confounded by parallel improvements in therapies, multiple studies have demonstrated potentially increased survival in patients treated in the multidisciplinary care setting.[37,38] Variations of care for complex patients and for those from underserved backgrounds or rural areas would ideally be minimized in the multidisciplinary setting.[39]

Alternative Payment Models

Newer coverage models, under the umbrella of the Donabedian definition of structure, offer an opportunity to incentivize value by linking reimbursement to quality metrics as well as encouraging patients to select high-value centers or providers. Traditional fee-for-service reimbursement, in linking payment to the volume of services provided, has been criticized for incentivizing overutilization of care, often without proportionate benefit. The technologic focus of radiation oncology, in particular, allows for a surplus of discrete billable units per treatment episode.[17] Pure prospective payment, proposed as an alternative to the traditional fee-for-service payment, reimburses providers a fixed amount independent of the volume of services provided, with aim of promoting efficiency via incentivizing providers away from costly treatments.[40] However, by shifting the marginal cost of care—and associated financial risk—to providers, pure prospective payment may incentivize providers to select patients with lower risk of complications ("cherry picking"), or to provide less care than would best treat the patient ("stinting on care"), and to avoid treating patients whose optimal treatment involves costly interventions.[40] Thus, the ideal reimbursement system would fall in between these two extremes, with payment linked to value while still allowing for evenly distributed access to high-quality care.[41]

Unfortunately, even with an established definition of value, deriving applicable metrics for quantifying value in oncology remains elusive. Although there are widely accepted measurements of outcomes (e.g., prostate-specific antigen progression-free survival in prostate cancer) and toxicities associated with treatment (e.g., the Common Terminology Criteria for Adverse Events [CTCAE]), adequately assessing these metrics may require multiple years of follow-up, impractical for adaptation to a reasonable payment cycle. Likewise, it is often difficult to assess whether adverse effects are the result of surgery, chemotherapy, radiation, or something unrelated to treatment.[17] As noted before, linking payment to outcomes metrics without accurate risk adjustment algorithms could also discourage providers from treating sicker patients. In the field of medical oncology, the American Society of Clinical Oncology (ASCO), the European Society for Medical Oncology (ESMO), and the National Comprehensive Cancer Network (NCCN) have each put forth frameworks for the evaluation of value, with notable overlap in their attempts to quantify the gradients of benefit associated with drug regimens, toxicity, and quality of life, though formal cost-effectiveness analyses are deemphasized.[42] Radiation oncology has been late in the development of its own value metrics, with many measures of quality advanced through more broadly focused organizations. In parallel with the efforts of the American Medical Association's Physicians Consortium for Performance Improvement and other similar organizations to develop, implement, and validate quality metrics, the National Quality Forum (NQF) was funded by Congress with aim of evaluating quality measures for transmission to the CMS for inclusion in eventual value-based penalties and bonuses. ASTRO has endeavored to establish a series of best practice guidelines, based on evidence and expert review, as well as determining a list of five interventions to only be used in specific situations because of proven lack of value as part of the American Board of Internal Medicine Foundation's *Choosing Wisely* initiative[43] (Fig. 105.4). Although admirable steps toward the value proposition, early quality indicators have been criticized for representing little more than enforcers of current standard of care, with persistence of many low-bar measures such as documentation of stage of disease or presence of normal tissue dose constraints. These measures are further debilitated by minimal correlation with reimbursement, without tracking by payers or accrediting bodies, thus effectively having limited impact on patients or society with call to focus metrics on true gaps in care.[44] Furthermore, care must be taken to ensure adherence to guidelines does not limit patients whose unique clinical situations call for individualized care or slow clinically meaningful advancement if innovation outpaces updates to guidelines.[17]

1	Don't initiate whole breast radiotherapy as a part of breast conservation therapy in women age ≥50 with early stage invasive breast cancer without considering shorter treatment schedules.
2	Don't initiate management of low-risk prostate cancer without discussing active surveillance.
3	Don't routinely use extended fractionation schemes (>10 fractions) for palliation of bone metastases.
4	Don't routinely recommend proton beam therapy for prostate cancer outside of a prospective clinical trial or registry.
5	Don't routinely use intensity modulated radiotherapy (IMRT) to deliver whole breast radiotherapy as part of breast conservation therapy.

FIGURE 105.4. The American Society for Radiation Oncology's list of five radiation oncology–specific treatments that are commonly ordered but may not always be appropriate as part of the national American Board of Internal Medicine Foundation's Choosing Wisely campaign. (Reprinted from Hahn C, Kavanagh B, Bhatnagar A, et al. Choosing wisely: the American Society for Radiation Oncology's top 5 list. *Pract Radiat Oncol* 2014;4[6]:349–355. Copyright © 2014 American Society for Radiation Oncology. With permission.)

With clear quality metrics still under development, payment reform thus far has mostly occurred in the form of narrow or tiered networks offered by health plans, often based on price or provider relationships with the larger market-dominant entity.[22] However, several alternative payment schemes, such as population-based shared savings arrangements, clinical pathways, and bundles of care and episodes of care payments, have been examined in oncology, accelerated by their inclusion in accountable care organizations (ACOs).[17] In population-based shared savings arrangements, providers are reimbursed via similar fee schedules though are rewarded when their fee-for-service payments are below a predefined target, often via the provider receiving a percentage of the savings. These risk-sharing arrangements have been implemented as elements of oncology-focused ACOs with report of decreased spending growth and high scores on quality metrics. In the clinical pathway approach, best practices are established for each clinical scenario with providers rewarded for adherence with higher fee-for-service payments, bonuses, or other incentives. Providers are expected to adhere to pathways for 60% to 80% scenarios to allow for individualization of care. This has demonstrated success in reducing treatment variation, drug trend, and hospitalizations in medical oncology; however, its application has been criticized as ill-suited to radiation oncology given the field's anatomic and technologic focus, which allows for potentially larger number of branch points in the decision-making process with a greater role for patient preference in the selection of treatment modality. Lastly, bundled or episodic payment has been described as a middle ground between fee-for-service and pure prospective payment, in which providers are reimbursed upfront based on the expected costs for a clinically defined episode of care thereby incentivizing efficient use of resources. CMS has devoted significant focus to experiments in episodic payment systems, though with focus in oncology primarily on comprehensive bundles that include medical, surgical, and radiation services as well as the complications of care. Multiple companies have experimented with specialty-specific episodic bundles in radiation oncology with reported improvements in administrative efficiencies, though in this model attention to quality measurement will be necessary to ensure implementation actually yields higher-value care without incentivizing providers away from high-risk populations. Likewise, to properly incentivize high-value care, bundled payment schemes will likely require context-specific models for different clinical scenarios as well as cost calculations based on updated RT codes that more accurately reflect current clinical practice.[45]

In July 2015, Turning the Tide Against Cancer, an initiative convened by the American Association for Cancer Research, the Personalized Medicine Coalition, and Feinstein Kean

Healthcare to identify policy solutions that will sustain medical innovation while addressing the issue of rising health care costs, held a roundtable consisting of a multidisciplinary group of stakeholders to review key considerations for oncology-focused alternative payment models.[46,47] Noting reliance on annually calculated spending benchmarks and only intermittently updated episode-of-care definitions, the panel highlighted the importance of having alternative payment models keep pace with emerging science via incentivizing adoption of innovative medicine and technologies that have the potential to improve patient outcomes and make health care more efficient. Toward this end, it stressed the avoidance of unintended barriers to patient access to novel therapies, particularly those that may be expensive in the short term but that may result in savings in the long term. Given the trend toward more personalized medicine, the roundtable acknowledged that a critical step in this is the coverage of diagnostics that will enable identification of patients that respond best to targeted therapies and thus avoiding the cost of treating patients who will not benefit or will be harmed by adverse effects or delays in initiating more effective treatments. Likewise, the participants suggested that alternative payment models incentivize the physician's ability to appropriately tailor treatment to an individual patient's needs and preferences, furthermore noting that there is no one-size-fits-all model, with the impact of a payment system at times dependent on geographic region, practice characteristics, setting, and other factors. Finally, the panel indicated that alternative payment models should include mechanisms to encourage participation in clinical trials and ongoing postmarket clinical research. Given the potential for models to incentivize patients toward rigorous care protocols or clinical pathways, the panel indicated that care should be taken to make it financially feasible for practices to enroll patients and participate in clinical trials to support continued development of cancer treatment.

PROCESS

Process includes all components of health care delivery, including both the technical processes in how health care is delivered as well as the interpersonal processes that describe the manner in which care is delivered, with focus on patient-centered, accessible, and coordinated care.[28] As defined by Donabedian, process can be measured via review of medical records, interviews with patients and providers, and direct observation of health care visits with measurement intrinsically tied to metrics of quality. In a technologically focused specialty such as radiation oncology, the measurement of process goes beyond those components immediately noticeable by patients, such as the quality of the patient–physician interaction and the timeliness of care, to include less tangible components, such as physician expertise and medical physics quality assurance oversight for treatment planning and delivery.[22] Thus, structural efforts to establish patient-centered and safety-focused process standards, such as the previously mentioned APEx accreditation program, are directly linked with process improvement. The Radiation Therapy Oncology Group (RTOG) cooperative group clinical trials, which specify treatment planning specifics such as contouring guidelines, dose constraints, and planning techniques as enforced by centralized review processes, are another example of process standardization, with evidence suggesting protocol deviations are associated with poorer outcomes.[22] In this light, ASTRO's previously mentioned best practice initiative, which establishes clinical practice guidelines based on the RAND/University of California Los Angeles appropriateness criteria, looks beyond defining guidelines to support the indication of radiation to include evidence-based and expert panel–devised assessment of the technical processes underlying the delivery of therapy.[48]

Physician Expertise

Regarding physician expertise, similar to surgical procedures, multiple studies have described the presence of a learning curve in the application of advanced radiation oncology techniques, including IMRT volume delineation, technical IMRT delivery, and brachytherapy procedures. For instance, in a single-institution study from the Department of Radiation Oncology at CancerCare Manitoba, the number of prostate cancer patients treated with I 125 interstitial implant with D90 < 140 Gy, a metric for the dosimetric quality of the brachytherapy implant, which correlates with decreased biochemical relapse-free survival, declined with increasing experience at the program, with brachytherapy team experience found to be a more important predictive factor of implant quality than size of the prostate.[49] Furthermore, with regard to IMRT, a population-based analysis by Boero and colleagues identified radiation providers from Medicare claims of 6,212 Medicare beneficiaries with head and neck cancer treated between 2000 and 2009 and found that among patients undergoing IMRT, those treated by higher-volume providers had increased survival compared with those treated by lower-volume providers. Specifically, for every five additional patients treated per provider per year, the risk of all-cause mortality decreased by 21%.[50] Patients treated by higher-volume physicians additionally had decreased head and neck cancer–specific mortality and decreased risk of aspiration pneumonia. Of note, no significant relationship between provider volume and patient survival or toxicity was observed among patients treated with conventional RT. Such results highlight the importance of improved training or novel educational resources for practicing physicians, with focus on skills-based education, in the establishment of value in radiation oncology, particularly as technology continues to advance at a rapid rate. Other advancements, such as in semiautomated target delineation, knowledge-based planning, and telemedicine, may also assist toward this end without necessitating physician or patient travel.

OUTCOMES

Outcomes span all of the effects of health care on patients or populations. These include objective outcomes providers and payers have traditionally assessed, such as survival, disease control, functional status, disease recurrence, and complications of treatment. Subjective outcomes, such as patient-reported outcomes, psychosocial ramifications of disease or treatment, ability to maintain employment status, and patient's understanding of disease, although considered

by some as more difficult to assess via traditional scientific methods, are also included and hold equal import in the value discussion. Of the components in the value equation, the medical community is best at assessing objective outcomes, with wide support for furthering our understanding of the objective impact of particular interventions via high-level clinical research. However, given the expense of such research, there is a need for additional methods to assess objective outcomes at the population level in real-world settings, with multiple specialty-based and multidisciplinary real-time observation registries under development to meet this need.[51] The advancement of accurate methods for risk stratification is of particular importance if these outcomes are to be reported on an individual provider level to enhance patient selection of providers or if they are to be connected with reimbursement. This consideration is also relevant for comparisons between treatment modalities, with wider use of multiple research methods for comparative effectiveness in oncology; some of these methods will be detailed in this chapter's section on research methods.

The Outcome Measures Hierarchy

As described by Porter, the outcomes for any medical condition can be arranged in a three-tiered hierarchy[27] (Fig. 105.5). Each tier includes two levels, each described by one or more distinct outcomes dimensions, with success for each dimension measured through specific metrics. In this hierarchy, Tier 1 represents the health status achieved or retained, and it includes levels of survival and degree of health or recovery. Specific to cancer care, common metrics in Tier 1 include 5-year overall survival and functional status. Tier 2 relates to the recovery process and includes levels of time required to achieve recovery and disutility of care. Common metrics specific to cancer care include time to remission and rates of adverse effects related to the treatment process. Lastly, Tier 3 describes the sustainability of health and includes the levels of recurrence of the original disease and associated complications as well as new health issues caused by treatment. Common metrics in cancer include cancer recurrence and incidence of second primary cancers. In this hierarchy schema, Tier 1 is generally considered the most important with lower-tier outcomes dependent on success at higher tiers. However, trade-offs between tiers may exist—such as sacrificing survival benefit in favor of a less morbid treatment modality—and mapping these trade-offs is an important part in furthering innovation in care.

Patient-Reported Outcomes

The study of subjective outcomes, by comparison, is less mature in its development than traditional clinical research in radiation oncology. While initially falling under the purview of dedicated health services research, patient-reported outcomes are increasingly included in clinical research in oncology, in part spearheaded by the RTOG, which has developed a model for the inclusion of patient-reported outcomes as endpoints in clinical trials.[52] The U.S. Food and Drug Administration (FDA) provides a broad definition of patient-reported outcomes as "any report of the status of a patient's health condition that comes directly from the patient, without interpretation of the patient's response by a clinician or anyone else."[53] With respect to their inclusion in clinical trials, however, patient-reported outcomes typically include health-related quality of life (HRQOL) instruments, with hundreds of validated generic and disease-specific instruments available and radiation oncology-specific instruments currently in development.[54,55] For instance, the National Cancer Institute (NCI) developed a patient-reported outcome measurement system for use in cancer clinical trials, named the Patient-Reported Outcomes version of the Common Terminology

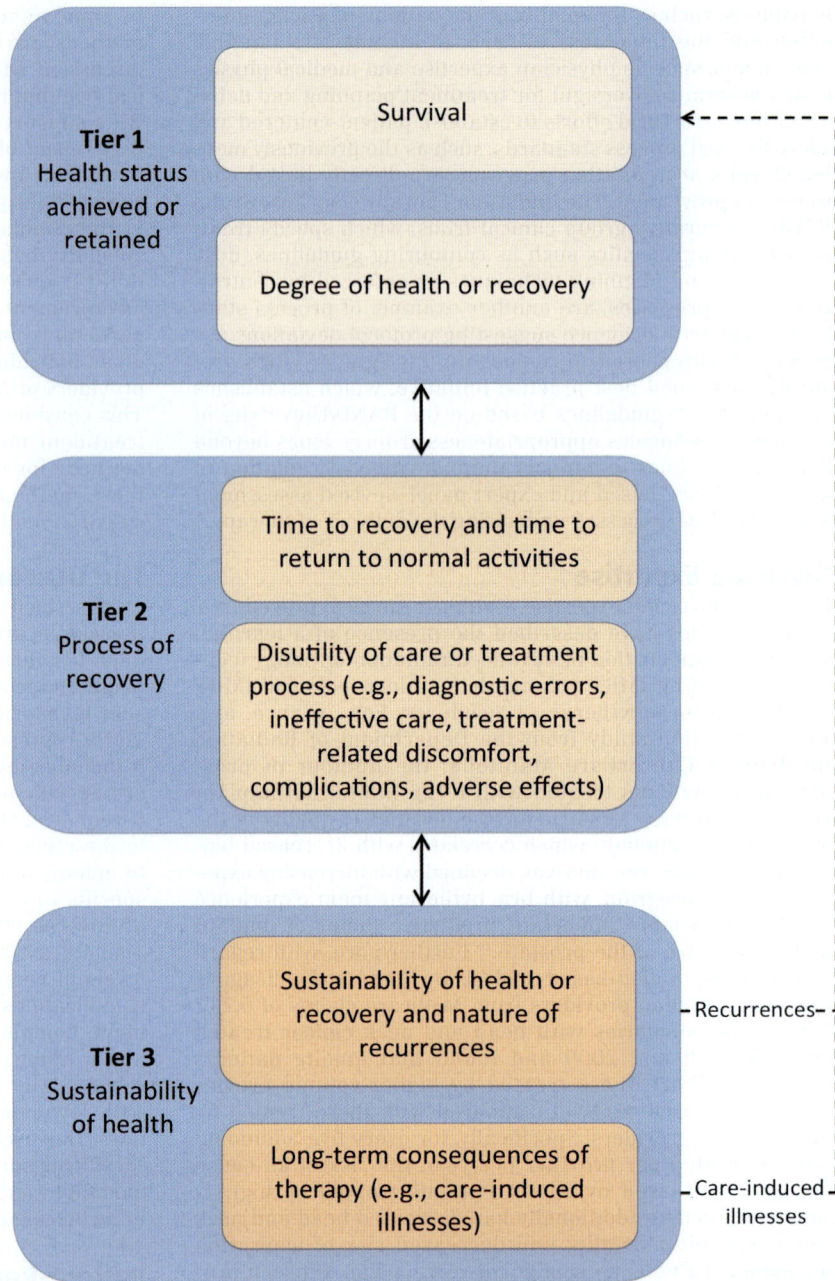

FIGURE 105.5. The outcome measures hierarchy as defined by Porter. (From Porter ME. What is value in health care? *N Engl J Med* 2010;363[26]:2477–2481. Copyright © 2010 Massachusetts Medical Society. Adapted with permission from Massachusetts Medical Society.)

Criteria for Adverse Events (PRO-CTCAE). Designed to be used as a companion to the CTCAE, the PRO-CTCAE includes an item library of 124 items representing 78 symptomatic toxicities drawn from the CTCAE and has been tested in a consortium of academic- and community-based cancer treatment sites in the NCI-sponsored clinical trial network.[56] Many challenges exist regarding the optimal application of such instruments, including refining the validation process, establishing the clinical meaningfulness of their results, and deciding how to handle missing data; further research to understand their utility in drawing conclusions in the trial setting, such as with regard to dose-limiting toxicity and overall/comparable tolerability, is necessary as well. Nevertheless, these tools offer an opportunity to inform translational and comparative effectiveness research, health care technology assessment, and quality assurance, as well as to quantify value from the patient perspective. Another patient-reported outcome commonly measured is patient satisfaction, which refers to the patient's perception of the quality of care received.[57] Although limited by patients' relative inability to assess the technical

quality of their care and inevitable dependence on patients' initial expectations, patient satisfaction remains an important part of the patient experience, and its inclusion in the value proposition reflects the greater shift in mindset in health care toward patient-centered care.

VALUE: A PATIENT-CENTERED APPROACH

Paralleling the rise of value-based care, patient-centered cancer care has received increasing focus in recent decades, as advocated by the Institute of Medicine (IOM), patient groups, and professional societies.[58] Patient-centered care, as defined by the Picker Institute, describes care that address multiple dimensions of patient care including patient preference, emotional support, physical comfort, information and communication needs, continuity and transition, care coordination, involvement of family and friends, and access to care.[59] Patient-centered care, while inherently aligned with value-based care via a shared focus on high-quality care,

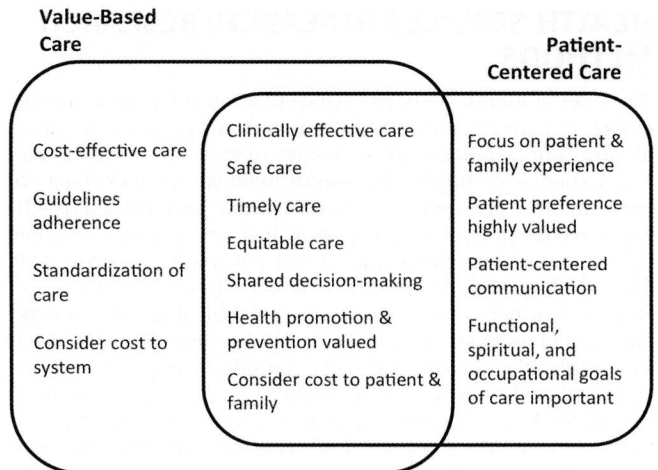

Value-Based Care / **Patient-Centered Care**

Cost-effective care	Clinically effective care	Focus on patient & family experience
Guidelines adherence	Safe care	
	Timely care	Patient preference highly valued
Standardization of care	Equitable care	
	Shared decision-making	Patient-centered communication
Consider cost to system	Health promotion & prevention valued	Functional, spiritual, and occupational goals of care important
	Consider cost to patient & family	

FIGURE 105.6. Attributes of value-based care and patient-centered care. (Adapted by permission from Springer: Tseng EK, Hicks LK. Value based care and patient-centered care: divergent or complementary? *Curr Hematol Malig Rep* 2016;11[4]:303–310. Copyright © 2016 Springer Science+Business Media New York.)

has distinct attributes not typically included in discussions of value, such as patient experience and preference measures as well as conceptions of cost that are payer–as opposed to patient-focused[20] (Fig. 105.6). Patients themselves appear to intuit these contradictions: in a series of focus groups, interviews, and online surveys of health care consumers undertaken by the American Institutes for Research, respondents in general were unfamiliar with concepts related to evidence-based care, believing medical guidelines to reflect an "inflexible, bargain-basement approach" to treating unique individual patients.[60] Thus, for the transition to value-based care to be accepted and effective on a population level, patients—as recipients, codecision-makers, and cofinanciers of this care—will need to be included in the discussion, with patient-centered outcomes, perspectives, and preferences explicitly incorporated into the definitions and metrics of quality and cost.[61]

Aligning Patient-Centered and Value-Based Care

Challenging the alignment of patient-centered and value-based care is the relative inability to assess cost in health care. Under the traditional fee-for-service–based system, although providers and administrators may have knowledge of individual billing charges and the direct costs of running a radiation oncology clinic, it is more difficult to calculate the total cost of care administered at a patient level. Furthermore, in our free market system, the charge for the same procedure can vary widely between providers, with no consistent correlation with the quality or outcome of care.[22] In comparison with how their purchasing decisions are made outside of health care, patients are left to make important health care decisions with a relative deficiency of information, unable to assess the real costs or quality of care offered by different providers; this is exacerbated in a system where the majority of patients are insured by a third party and bear only a small fraction of the total cost of care. Patients thus cannot function as "utility maximizers," choosing products that provide the highest utility for the lowest dollar. This discrepancy in effect removes the market pressure toward high-value care, in part contributing to increased cost, over- and underutilization, and decreased quality in health care. In effort to recreate this market pressure on patients, health plans have responded by increasing cost sharing via higher deductibles and copays. This practice, however, can counteract the achievement

of value by preventing patients from pursuing necessary, high-cost sharing treatments, ultimately worsening patients' health and increasing the overall cost of care.

The Financial Burden of Cancer Care

Oncology care, in particular, has been presumed to be relatively shielded from the downward pressure of cost on demand, though evidence suggests that even cancer patients consider treatment cost in their decision-making, suggesting that the cost of care should receive greater emphasis in assessments of value from a patient perspective.[62] Multiple studies have reinforced the detrimental effect that out-of-pocket costs have on patients' access to medical care as well as ability to pay for other nonmedical life necessities, with a report from the NCI indicating between 33% and 80% of cancer patients depleting their savings to finance medical expenses.[22,63] In a population-based study from Western Washington State, a cancer diagnosis was associated with a 2.65-times greater likelihood of declaring personal bankruptcy. Upon further analysis, cancer patients declaring personal bankruptcy additionally demonstrated a 79% greater mortality risk than those who did not.[64] This relationship between extreme financial distress and greater mortality risk is likely multifactorial, partly explained by overall poorer well-being, impaired health-related quality of life, or subpar quality of care.[65] Likely, further exacerbating the patient's sense of well-being, the burden of financial hardship for cancer care is not borne by the patient alone, with between 2% and 34% of patients borrowing money from friends or family to pay for care.[63] Unfortunately, as multiple forms of cancer are currently incurable with many patients eventually succumbing to disease, at least a portion of these expenses are likely exhausted on futile care at the end of life. Although the administration of chemotherapy in patients in their last weeks of life has been well documented—indeed, chemotherapy administered the last 2 weeks of life is an emerging quality indicator employed by the ASCO Quality Oncology Practice Initiative—evidence indicates that the field of radiation oncology is not immune to potential contributions to futile care, with a population-based study of Surveillance, Epidemiology, and End Results (SEER) Medicare and Texas Cancer Registry Medicare databases indicating an increase in use of advanced RT techniques in patients in the last 30 days of life from 2000 to 2009, with the proportion of patients treated with IMRT increasing from 0% to 6.2% and with stereotactic radiosurgery from 0% to 5.0%.[66–68] Although further research is necessary to determine whether these shifts in practice patterns improve palliative outcomes and to better identify patients that may benefit from advanced techniques in the palliative setting, consideration should be given toward the potential impact of the cost of these therapies on patients and their families.

Financial Toxicity

Building evidence describing the deleterious effect of the cost of cancer care on patient well-being has led to a push for the inclusion of "financial toxicity," described as the harmful personal financial burden faced by patients receiving cancer treatment, in physicians' discussions with patients of the side effects associated with a particular treatment, with both the IOM and ASCO categorizing cost of care discussions as an essential component of high-quality care.[26,69–71] Clearly, numerous potential obstacles currently preclude effective cost of care discussions between patients and physicians, including uncertainty about the appropriateness of the topic and inability to accurately assess the cost of care.[72] Comprehensive intervention will likely require further research on the measurement of the material, psychological, and behavioral effects of financial toxicity and the identification of potential modifiable risk factors as well as further inclusion of these metrics at a policy level.[73] Composite scores using summary measures of multiple

Section V

components of financial hardship, such as the Comprehensive Score for Financial Toxicity (COST) and Personal Financial Wellness Scale (PFW Scale), have been employed in clinical studies as a patient-reported outcome though results can be difficult to interpret with unclear application to the general population.[63]

Decisional Regret

As previously discussed, the effective measurement of more subjective outcomes in radiation oncology remains an area in need further research, and their greater inclusion in assessments of value is a critical challenge in the alignment of value-based and patient-centered care.[20] Validated metrics of patient-reported outcomes, in which patients report directly on perceptions of their own health, have been developed and are now more broadly included in clinical trials, providing essential patient-centered data on the impact of interventions; likewise, development of validated instruments to assess patient-reported experience measures, or their perception of their experience with health care delivery, is underway. An intriguing example of a validated and well-studied patient-reported outcome with applications to radiation oncology is decisional regret, defined as the negative emotion experienced when we suspect that an alternative course of action would have resulted in a better outcome.[74] Cancer-related decision-making is complex, requiring an understanding of both the medical and psychosocial impacts of treatment in the context of one's personal values and beliefs; given the complexity and multifactorial nature of these choices, decisional regret offers a broad measure of a patient's treatment experience and quality of life and has been shown to be a more sensitive outcome than patient satisfaction in certain settings. In prostate cancer, multiple factors have been associated with treatment regret, including poor health-related and global posttreatment quality of life. Interestingly, specific treatment modalities have also been associated with increased posttreatment regret. For example, at the University of California, Los Angeles, survey of patients with localized prostate cancer treated with IMRT, SBRT, or high dose rate (HDR) brachytherapy suggested that patients treated with SBRT experienced significantly less treatment regret compared with patients treated with IMRT or HDR.[75] Thus, when comparing modalities—particularly with equivalent long-term survival and comparable toxicity profiles—further understanding of the patient experience is informative in assessing the value of specific medical interventions.

VALUE IN RADIATION ONCOLOGY: CONCLUSIONS

Regardless of the volume of ongoing debate surrounding health care reform, in many ways, the transition to some form of value-based care is inevitable. Enacted in April 2015, the Medicare Access and CHIP Reauthorization Act (MACRA) repealed the SGR to establish the Quality Payment Program to encourage physician participation in alternative payment models that utilize value-based payment; in response to unsustainable rising health care costs, multiple private payers have begun experimenting with alternative payment models already.[17,76] This transition offers an opportunity to serve patients, providers, society, and shareholders alike through better alignment of incentives among stakeholders and reduced administrative costs. Whatever method of payment reform ultimately takes ahold will arise from iterative experimentation; radiation oncologists and the patients they treat will be best served by taking an active role in this collaborative process, both via participation in health care advocacy and contribution to novel health services research.

HEALTH SERVICES RESEARCH: RESEARCH METHODS

The field of health services research, often referred to as outcomes research, refers to the study of access to care, costs of care, and quality of care. Access to care concerns factors that expedite or hinder the use of medical services. Costs of care include payments by insurers and patients for medical services as well as the cost of lost productivity because of time away from work and decreased wages. As previously discussed, quality of medical care incorporates elements of structure, process, and outcomes. Although there are several methods of analysis relevant to health services research, decision analysis and cost-effectiveness analysis, in particular, are standard techniques used to evaluate and compare medical therapies. As the costs of oncologic care rise, it is vital to evaluate the cost-effectiveness of RT. Cost-effectiveness analyses assess the costs relative to health outcomes for a particular medical intervention. This chapter section will explain the theoretical aspects of decision and cost-effectiveness analyses.

DECISION ANALYSIS

Although randomized clinical trials are the "gold standard" for gathering evidence, they have several limitations.[77] For instance, randomized trials often necessitate lengthy follow-up before showing differences between various treatments, and their results may not be available until the therapy itself is out of date. In addition, randomized trials report the best treatment for the "average person"; patient preferences are not considered.[78]

Decision analysis uses a set of mathematical tools designed to determine the most favorable outcome with regard to a particular endpoint (such as overall survival or time without recurrence) for individuals with a given starting situation under many different sets of circumstances, using existing data or assumptions regarding the effectiveness and toxicities of treatments. Decision models can help outline the trade-offs for different treatments in clinical situations when no good evidence is available.

METHODOLOGY OF DECISION ANALYSIS

To make a model, a decision tree is created to symbolize the results of clinical choices. The model requires making simplifying assumptions while still being sufficiently complex to correctly illustrate the important aspects of the decision. Figure 105.7 depicts a scenario in which a patient is faced with the treatment dilemma of whether or not to undergo RT for illness X.[78] Decision nodes are signified by squares in the decision tree, chance nodes by circles, and terminal nodes by triangles.

Subsequent to choosing a treatment, there is a chance node after which all potential events are shown as branches. The probability of a particular outcome following a chance node is determined from data from the literature or expert opinion. The probabilities of events at each chance node must add to 1. In Figure 105.7, if the patient with illness X chooses RT, he has a 90% chance of surviving the treatment and a 10% chance of dying from the treatment. If the patient survives the treatment, he then has an 80% chance of remaining alive and a 20% chance of dying. If the patient forgoes treatment, he has a 70% chance of living and a 30% chance of dying.

The terminal nodes depict the final outcomes states of each pathway. Next to each of the terminal nodes is a value associated with that state. In our example, the only two outcome states are living and dying. Being alive and dead are associated with values of 1 and 0, respectively. When calculating the expected survival rate for RT, we see that if a patient survives

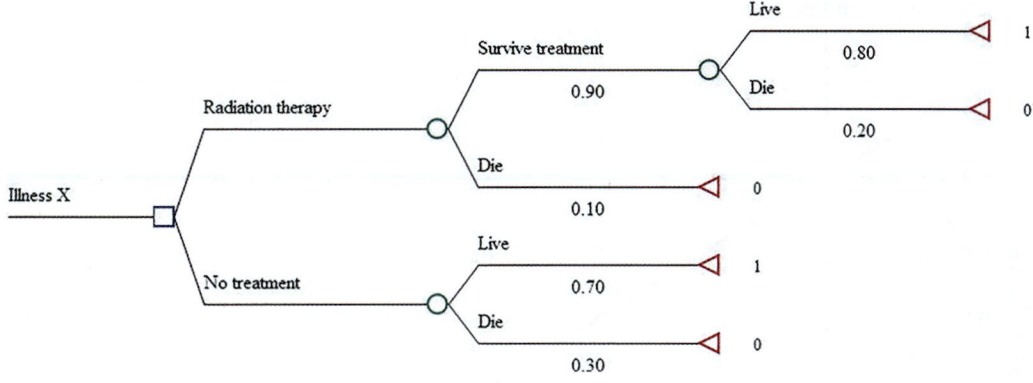

FIGURE 105.7. Decision tree of a patient with illness X. (Adapted from Sher DJ, Punglia RS. Decision analysis and cost-effectiveness analysis for comparative effectiveness research: a primer. *Semin Radiat Oncol* 2014;24[1]:14–24. Copyright © 2014 Elsevier. With permission.)

treatment, he has an 80% chance of living (outcome of 1) and a 20% chance of dying (outcome of 0). The value at this chance node is calculated by multiplying the probability of the outcome with the associated value, resulting in a value of 0.80. We then substitute the value of 0.80 as the value associated with surviving treatment and multiply this value by its probability of 0.90. The resulting value (0.72) is then combined with that of dying from treatment (outcome of 0 with probability of 0.10), for an expected value of 0.72. The expected survival rate for no treatment is calculated by multiplying the likelihood of living (0.70) with its outcome of 1 and combining that to the product of the likelihood of dying (0.30) and its outcome of 0, to obtain a value of 0.70.

OUTCOME VALUES

In our simple example, the outcome value was the likelihood of survival with or without treatment for illness X. However, decision analyses can also model values associated with different health states. A utility is an econometric construct that describes how an individual values a given health state versus death (0) and perfect health (1).[79] The worse the health state, the worse the utility. For instance, experiencing a rectal toxicity may be associated with a utility of 0.7, and living with distant metastasis may be associated with a utility of 0.6. This ability to describe utilities for different outcomes states allows modelers to incorporate side effects of treatments into their model, an important consideration given that many cancer treatments affect a patient's quality of life. The benefit associated with various cancer treatments depends on the trade-offs between the fear and consequences of recurrence versus the inconvenience and potential toxicity of treatment.

Utilities are different from more familiar, descriptive quality of life measures as they reflect how a respondent values a state under conditions of *uncertainty*. Although there are several techniques for assessing utilities, the most firmly grounded in expected utility theory is the standard gamble. The standard gamble assesses the utility for a health state by asking how high a risk of death a participant would accept to improve it (Fig. 105.8). The respondent is asked to choose between a certain life in an intermediate health state and a gamble between optimal health and immediate death. The probabilities in the gamble are varied systematically until the respondent feels that the two choices (life in an intermediate health state and the gamble) are equally desirable. At the "point of indifference," the respondent's utility for the health state is given by the probability of optimal health in the gamble. The utility of the health state is given by the probability of perfect health in the gamble such that the respondent is indifferent between the gamble and the certain intermediate outcome.

Utilities can also be used to calculate quality-adjusted life-years (QALYs), an index of survival that is adjusted to account for the patient's quality of life during a specific period. The quality-adjusted life-year (QALY) is the standard effectiveness measure.[80] A QALY is determined by multiplying the time spent in a certain health state with the utility associated with that state. For example, 2 years of time spent in a state whose utility is 0.5 would be the equivalent of 1 QALY.

SENSITIVITY ANALYSIS

The published literature and expert opinion provide the basis for probabilities at the nodes of a decision tree. However, these estimates are often quite uncertain. Sensitivity analyses are therefore usually a critical part of decision models. Sensitivity analyses vary a certain parameter (e.g., the probability of recurrence of prostate cancer) over the entire plausible range of its values and then study the effect of varying the parameter on the outcome. Sensitivity analyses provide a measure of the robustness of a conclusion in a similar way to confidence intervals and *P* values in biostatistics. They may

FIGURE 105.8. The standard gamble assesses the utility for a health state by asking how high a risk of death a participant would accept to improve it.

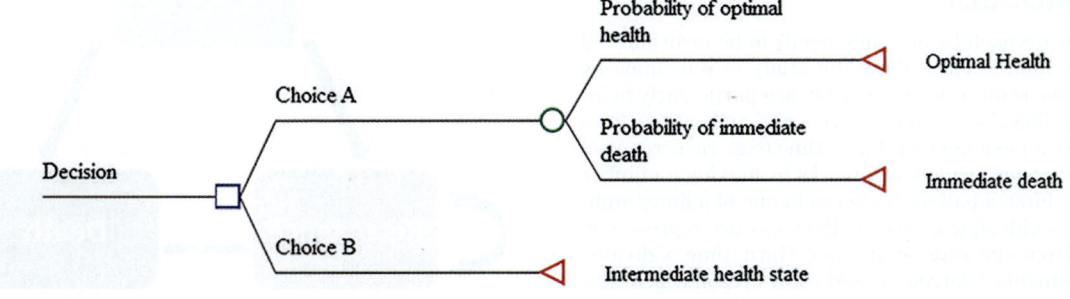

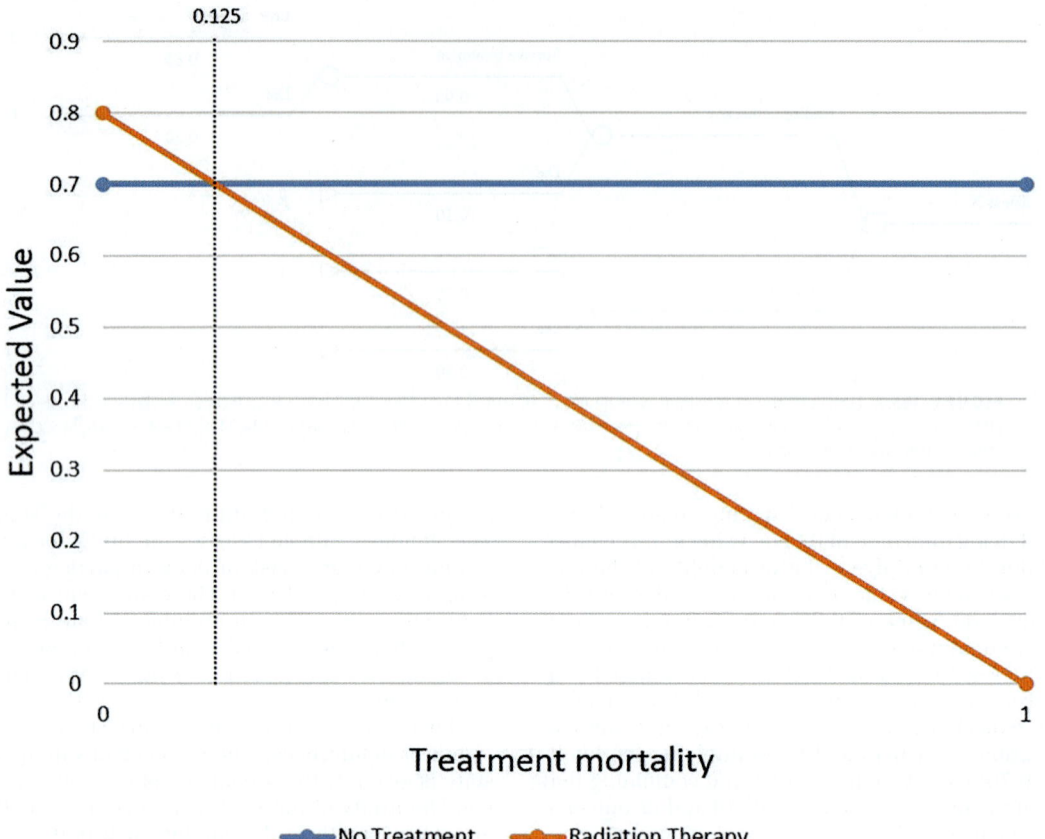

FIGURE 105.9. Sensitivity analysis of mortality from treatment for illness X. (Adapted from Sher DJ, Punglia RS. Decision analysis and cost-effectiveness analysis for comparative effectiveness research: a primer. *Semin Radiat Oncol* 2014;24[1]: 14–24. Copyright © 2014 Elsevier. With permission.)

also increase the level of confidence by confirming the lack of significant dependence of an outcome on a certain transition parameter. In addition, sensitivity analyses may also identify areas where further research may be valuable by revealing dependence of an outcome measure on the variable studied.[18] One-way sensitivity analyses provide threshold values. Two-way and three-way sensitivity analyses systematically vary two to three parameters simultaneously; the outcomes for each combination of variables can then be assessed.

In the example shown in Figure 105.7, we may not know the likelihood of treatment mortality for illness X. It may also vary by physician or with patient characteristics. In order to determine the optimal treatment strategy for a given treatment mortality, we can conduct a one-way sensitivity analysis. As shown in Figure 105.9, the expected value of RT decreases as the treatment mortality increases. The threshold mortality at which RT and no treatment yield equivalent expected outcomes is 0.125. Below this mortality threshold, RT is associated with the best expected value, but no treatment becomes the optimal strategy above this value.

MARKOV MODELS

Markov models are useful when time needs to be incorporated into a decision model. They allow the study of outcomes by describing events as discrete states. They are particularly helpful in modeling clinical situations where a patient is at risk for a given event over an extended period of time (e.g., recurrence of prostate cancer). Markov modeling works by making a number of assumptions. First, a patient is always in one of a finite number of discrete health states. Second, all events are represented as transitions from one state to another. Third, time is divided into equal increments referred to as Markov cycles, which may

be days, months, or years depending on the clinical situation. Fourth, transitions between health states occur only once per cycle. Finally, all patients in a given health state face the same transition probabilities, no matter when they entered that particular health state.[18] Patients start the model in a single health state. As the model cycles, the patients travel through time and may remain in their previous health state or transition to a different health state with a certain transition probability.

Figure 105.10 shows a simplified prostate cancer model.[78] Patients who have completed initial therapy start in the "no-disease" health state. At each cycle, the patients may

FIGURE 105.10. Markov model with three health states. (Adapted from Sher DJ, Punglia RS. Decision analysis and cost-effectiveness analysis for comparative effectiveness research: a primer. *Semin Radiat Oncol* 2014;24[1]:14–24. Copyright © 2014 Elsevier. With permission.)

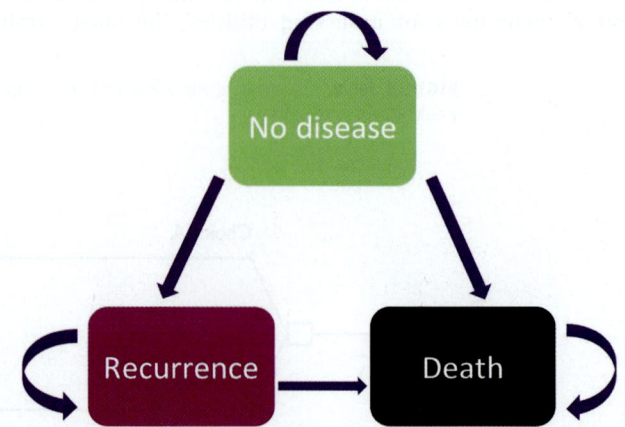

either remain in the "no-disease" health state, have a finite probability of having a recurrence and transition to the "recurrence" health state, or have a finite probability of dying of causes unrelated to their cancer and transition to the "death" health state. Once in the "recurrence" health state, patients may remain there or with a certain probability die from their recurrent disease and enter the "death" health state. Once the patients enter the "death" health state, they may not exit. (This is an example of an "absorbing" health state.) A type of a Markov model called an absorbing model runs until all patients are in the "death" health state and can be used to calculate residence times in transient states allowing for life expectancy and time spent without recurrence.

One common method to evaluate a Markov model is the Monte Carlo simulation, where simulated patients enter the model one by one. The computer program then randomly selects a value for a variable in the decision analysis using a probability distribution and tracks the outcome. The process is repeated thousands of times (simulating thousands of patients), and the mean and standard deviation for a result (e.g., mean overall survival) are obtained.

COST-EFFECTIVENESS ANALYSIS

Cost-effectiveness analysis is a set of mathematical tools designed to compare the relative costs and benefits of treatment alternatives. The most common type of cost-effectiveness analysis uses a model-based study, which is nearly identical to a classic decision analysis. A Markov model is created, and QALYs are accumulated over the time scope of the study. Costs are also accumulated during each stage, such that by the end of the analysis, there is a cost and QALY associated with each strategy. One then orders the strategies by effectiveness.

The end result of any cost-effectiveness analysis is reported as an incremental cost-effectiveness ratio (ICER), which is the ratio of the change in costs to incremental benefits of a therapeutic intervention or treatment.[81] The ICER is usually reported as a cost per QALY (e.g., $55,000 per QALY). Treatments are considered "cost-effective" or not based on whether or not the ICER passes a particular threshold, the societal "willingness to pay" (WTP). $50,000 per QALY is a commonly accepted value above which treatments are not considered cost-effective in the United States.[82] A new treatment is said to "dominate" the standard treatment if is more effective and less costly.[81]

COSTS

Costs included in a cost-effectiveness analysis depend on the perspective of the analysis. In the societal perspective, every cost needs to be measured, including capital expenses and the lost economic productivity of both the patient and caregivers.[81] In the payer perspective, only costs paid by the payer are pertinent. Analyses from the payer perspective primarily take health care reimbursements into account. Costs associated with RT can be divided into fixed costs and variable costs. Fixed costs consist of costs of the facility, physics and engineering maintenance of the machine, and salaried labor.[83] The capital cost of purchasing a linear accelerator or building a proton therapy center makes up a substantial fraction of the fixed costs. The estimated cost of a linear accelerator is approximately $4 million. The market price of a proton unit is estimated to be on the order of $120 million.[84]

The variable costs of RT vary substantially by radiation treatment modality. They can be broken down into three basic categories: treatment simulation, treatment planning,

and treatment delivery.[83] IMRT and three-dimensional conformal radiation therapy (3D-CRT) simulations involve a CT simulation, which necessitates more effort on the part of physicians, physicists, and therapists than a two-dimensional (2D) simulation, which is done using a simple fluoroscopic simulator. Whereas the planning process for a 2D plan involves calculations that can be performed using a calculator, a three-dimensional (3D) plan requires more work by the dosimetrist. An IMRT plan is even more complex and, for that reason, more costly. Moreover, quality assurance programs for IMRT plans often entail "dry runs" to guarantee that the planned dose approximates the delivered dose, adding to costs.[85] Because each Lucite compensator is custommade for each proton patient, compensators used in proton beam therapy (PBT) are more expensive than the wedges used in conventional RT. By the same token, delivering a simple 2D plan is considerably less expensive than a 3D-CRT or IMRT treatment, and PBT is even more expensive (producing protons in a cyclotron is more resource-intensive than producing photon from a linear accelerator). In addition, the daily image guidance associated with IMRT incurs additional costs.

WHAT TYPES OF COST-EFFECTIVENESS QUESTIONS ARE THERE WITHIN RADIATION ONCOLOGY?

There are three types of questions that can be answered within the field of radiation oncology with cost-effectiveness models.[78] First, what is the cost-effectiveness of using RT, compared to other types of treatments, such as surgery? Second, what is the cost-effectiveness of using RT, as compared to observation? Finally, what is the cost-effectiveness of using different RT modalities or fractionation regimens?

Examples of Cost-Effectiveness Studies within Prostate Radiation Oncology

These questions (particularly the last category) have inspired research within the field of prostate cancer, as the explosion of new and expensive technologies such as IMRT, SBRT, and PBT calls for careful analyses of their cost-effectiveness. For example, Konski and colleagues developed a Markov model comparing PBT with IMRT for a 70-year-old man with intermediate-risk prostate cancer from the payer perspective.[86] Their model included four health states: alive without disease, alive on hormonal therapy, alive on chemotherapy, and death. The model assumed that the conformality of proton therapy would permit dose escalation with the same risk of toxicity as IMRT, resulting in 5-year freedom from biochemical relapse for patients treated with IMRT and PBT of 83% and 93%, respectively. Utilities for a patient treated with IMRT were obtained from patients with intermediate-risk prostate cancer undergoing IMRT (without hormone therapy) randomly assigned to treatment in a phase III clinical trial at Fox Chase Cancer Center (Philadelphia, PA). Utility values for patients receiving hormone therapy and chemotherapy were obtained from the literature. Costs for the technical component of the treatment were obtained from ambulatory payment classification rates for 2005. Physician-expected reimbursement was calculated from the corresponding resource value units multiplied by the 2005 conversion factor. The cost of hormones was obtained from the Drug Red Book, and the cost of chemotherapy in the last year of life was estimated based on the literature. Even with the unproven assumption of improved biochemical response with a 10-Gy dose escalation, proton therapy was not cost-effective. For a 70-year-old man, the ICER was US$63,000 with a 15-year time window. The probabilistic sensitivity analysis revealed that there was only a 49% likelihood that PBT was cost-effective at a societal WTP of US$50,000/QALY and there was only an approximately 60% chance of cost-effectiveness at a WTP of US$100,000/QALY. If the cancer outcomes were assumed to be identical between IMRT and PBT, there was only 24% likelihood that PBT was cost-effective. One limitation of this study is that the assumption that dose escalation using PBT results in a 10% reduction in 5-year freedom from biochemical relapse and equal toxicity as compared to IMRT is unproven. In addition, the study was performed from the payer's perspective, and costs of building the facilities were not included in the calculation.

In another study, Sher and colleagues developed a Markov model comparing the cost-effectiveness of robotic (R-) and nonrobotic (NR-) SBRT to IMRT for a 65-year-old man with low-risk prostate cancer from the payer perspective.[87] Their model included the six health states of alive with no evidence of disease, alive with asymptomatic local recurrence, alive with symptomatic local recurrence, alive with distant metastases, death from unrelated causes, and death from prostate cancer. Over time, the patient could also experience toxicity. Patients were allowed to have any combination of sexual, rectal, and urinary toxicities, with the assumption that the development of any toxicity was independent of the others. All toxicities from treatment were assumed to occur within 5 years of therapy; after 5 years, they assumed no new onset of toxicity. Given the lack of robust follow-up, it was assumed that the recurrence risk after SBRT was the same as the recurrence risk after IMRT. Each health state was associated with a cost and a utility derived from the published literature. Patients were followed until death. The baseline costs of each radiotherapy treatment were defined by the 2012 Medicare payment schedule for hospital-based practice. The total costs of IMRT, NR-SBRT, and R-SBRT were $27,564.21, $10,108.93, and $19,275.41, respectively. Costs after local or distant recurrence were taken from Bayoumi and colleagues, and costs for the management of proctopathy, bladder toxicity, and impotence were extracted from the Institute for Clinical and Economic Review. Quality-adjusted life expectancy after IMRT was slightly higher than after SBRT, because worse toxicity was assumed after SBRT. The ICERs for IMRT over R-SBRT and NR-SBRT were $285,000 and $591,100/QALY, respectively. On sensitivity analysis, SBRT was almost always the cost-effective therapy, in which the ICER for IMRT was generally over $100,000/QALY. Treatment efficacy, rectal toxicity, and impotence and the potential for unforeseen SBRT late effects were the most critical parameters in the model. When including these uncertain parameters in a probabilistic sensitivity analysis, SBRT was still most likely to be cost-effective at a WTP of $100,000/QALY. The authors concluded that SBRT clearly contained more value than IMRT for external beam treatment. One limitation of this study is that although outcomes are well established after IMRT, they are less mature after SBRT, with prospective trials reporting recurrence and toxicity data at relatively short follow-up.

In a third cost-effectiveness study, Hayes and colleagues developed a Markov model comparing observation versus initial treatment for men aged 65 and 75 years with newly diagnosed low-risk prostate cancer using the societal perspective.[88] Brachytherapy (BT), IMRT, radical prostatectomy (RP), active surveillance (AS), and watchful waiting (WW) were modeled. Men were aged 65 or 75 years on model entry, and they exited at death. The AS strategy comprised PSA tests every 3 months, digital rectal examinations every 6 months, and biopsies at 1 year and every 3 years thereafter. Men who progressed to more aggressive disease or selected treatment received IMRT. Ten percent of men who developed a Gleason score of 7 had "unfavorable risk" disease and received 6 months of androgen deprivation therapy with IMRT. The WW strategy reproduced the Prostate Cancer Intervention Versus Observation Trial (PIVOT) experience.[89] Men were followed with visits and PSA tests every 6 months and bone scans every 5 years, and 20.4% of men were treated over 10 years (49% with RP, 39% with IMRT, and 12% with BT). Model inputs were generated from a systematic review and from PIVOT; probabilities were estimated using a random effects model from a meta-analysis.[89,90] All men treated initially were assumed to have the hazard ratio (HR) point estimate of 1.48 reported in PIVOT for prostate cancer–specific death, compared with WW.[89] The publication assumed that AS would provide 25% additional benefit compared with WW in preventing prostate cancer–specific death and used an HR for prostate cancer–specific death for treatment compared with AS of 1.85. The annual probability of Gleason progression on AS was 2.3%, and the annual probability of developing other signs of disease progression was 5.2%.[90] Adverse effects of treatment were classified as short term (occurring and resolving within 90 days) and long term (occurring or persisting at least 90 days after treatment and persisting for life). Utilities for health states were elicited using a time–trade-off method from men without prostate cancer.[90] Costs were derived from Medicare reimbursements and average wages for age-matched men. Observation was more effective and less costly than initial treatment. Compared with AS, WW provided 2 additional months of quality-adjusted life expectancy (9.02 vs. 8.85 years) at a savings of $15,374 ($24,520 vs. $39,894) in men aged 65 years and 2 additional months (6.14 vs. 5.98 years) at a savings of $11,746 ($18,302 vs. $30,048) in men aged 75 years. BT was the most effective and least expensive initial treatment. Treatment became more effective than observation when it led to more dramatic reductions in prostate cancer death (HR 0.47 vs. WW and 0.64 vs. AS). Active surveillance became as effective as WW in men aged 65 years when the probability of progressing to treatment on AS decreased below 63% or when the quality of life with AS versus WW was 4% higher in men aged 65 years or 1% higher in men aged 75 years. WW remained least expensive in all analyses. The authors concluded that, for men aged 65 and 75 years with newly diagnosed low-risk prostate cancer, observation is more effective and costs less than initial treatment and WW is most cost-effective. One important limitation of the study is that the base-case results depend on a HR for prostate cancer–specific mortality of 1.48 for treatment versus WW, which was obtained from a subgroup analysis of the low-risk patients in PIVOT. However, the 95% confidence interval on this HR was large (0.42 to 5.24) because only 10 deaths from prostate cancer occurred in this subgroup.

HEALTH SERVICES RESEARCH: CONCLUSIONS

Although randomized clinical trials are the gold standard for obtaining level I evidence, the dearth of long-term data directing therapeutic choices is one reason to perform decision analysis, which allows assumptions to be made and then varied over a wide range to determine their effects on results. To date, only a handful of properly constructed cost-effectiveness analyses studying radiation have been reported in the literature. There is a pressing need for additional cost-effectiveness studies within the field of radiation oncology. As our treatments become more technical and expensive, it is our responsibility to prove that these treatments lead to benefits (either better survival or improved quality of life) that warrant the increased cost.

Kenneth J. Arrow, MA, PhD
(August 23, 1921–February 21, 2017)

Kenneth J. Arrow, MA, PhD, was an American scholar, world-renowned for his work in economic theory and often credited with inventing the field of health economics. Although he had not previously written about health care, in 1963 Arrow was invited by the Ford Foundation to apply his theories to medical markets as part of a larger effort to address policy areas with significant public–private overlap, such as health, education, and welfare. The resultant paper, entitled "Uncertainty and the Welfare Economics of Medical Care," was published in *The American Economic Review* and first described the ways in which health care delivery fundamentally differs from the classical free market. The article has since become one of the most cited articles in the field of health economics, and its principles—such as asymmetric information, in which consumers and sellers do not share mutual information—have been broadly applied to fields outside of health and have served as an influence in widely impacting legislation. Outside of health care, Arrow's 1951 book *Social Choice and Individual Values* was credited with serving as the basis of social choice theory, which addresses matters of collective decision-making. For his contributions to general equilibrium analysis and welfare theory, Arrow was awarded the Nobel Memorial Prize in Economic Sciences in 1972—at age 51, the youngest Laureate in Economic Sciences to date.

Arrow earned a bachelor's degree from the City College of New York and master's degree and doctorate from Columbia University. He served on the economics faculties at the University of Chicago, Stanford University, and Harvard University, prior to retiring from Stanford in 1991. He served as the president of the American Economic Association in 1973 and was the recipient of numerous honorary degrees and awards, including the National Medal of Science in 2004.

REFERENCES

1. Organisation for Economic Co-operation and Development. OECD Health Statistics 2016. Available at: http://www.oecd.org/els/health-systems/health-data.htm

2. Centers for Medicare and Medicaid Services. CMS National Health Expenditures 2015. Available at: https://www.cms.gov/research-statistics-data-and-systems/statistics-trends-and-reports/nationalhealthexpenddata/nationalhealthaccountshistorical.html

3. Tangka FK, Trogdon JG, Richardson LC, et al. Cancer treatment cost in the United States: has the burden shifted over time? *Cancer* 2010;116(14):3477–3484.

4. Lee JA, Roehrig CS, Butto ED. Cancer care cost trends in the United States: 1998 to 2012: US Cancer Care Cost Trends: 1998–2012. *Cancer* 2016;122(7):1078–1084.

5. Mariotto AB, Yabroff KR, Shao Y, et al. Projections of the cost of cancer care in the United States: 2010–2020. *J Natl Cancer Inst* 2011;103(2):117–128.

6. Raghavan D, Legnini MW. Value in oncology: balance between quality and cost. In: Dizon DS, ed. *American Society of Clinical Oncology 2016 Educational Book*. Alexandria, VA: American Society of Clinical Oncology, Inc., 2016:9–13.

7. Sullivan R, Peppercorn J, Sikora K, et al. Delivering affordable cancer care in high-income countries. *Lancet Oncol* 2011;12(10):933–980.

8. Fratt L. The new economics of radiation oncology. *Health Imaging*. Available at: http://www.healthimaging.com/topics/healthcare-economics/new-economics-radiation-oncology. Published May 6, 2013. Accessed April 1, 2017.

9. Meropol NJ, Schrag D, Smith TJ, et al. American Society of Clinical Oncology guidance statement: the cost of cancer care. *J Clin Oncol* 2009;27(23):3868–3874.

10. Niu X, Topoleski J. Spending for social security and major health care programs in the long-term budget outlook. Congressional Budget Office Blog. Available at: https://www.cbo.gov/publication/51840. Published August 1, 2016. Accessed April 1, 2017.

11. Steinberg ML. Introduction: health policy and health care economics observed. *Semin Radiat Oncol* 2008;18(3):149–151.

12. Arrow KJ. Uncertainty and the welfare economics of medical care. *Am Econ Rev* 1963;53(5):941–973.

13. Steinbrook R. The repeal of Medicare's sustainable growth rate for physician payment. *JAMA* 2015;313(20):2025.

14. Alhassani A, Chandra A, Chernew ME. The sources of the SGR "hole." *N Engl J Med* 2012;366(4):289–291.

15. Shen X, Showalter TN, Mishra MV, et al. Radiation oncology services in the modern era: evolving patterns of usage and payments in the office setting for Medicare patients from 2000 to 2010. *J Oncol Pract* 2014;10(4):e201–e207.

16. Mohideen N. Medicare scrutinizes radiation oncology reimbursement. *ASTRO News* 2013;16:28.

17. Falit BP, Chernew ME, Mantz CA. Design and implementation of bundled payment systems for cancer care and radiation therapy. *Int J Radiat Oncol Biol Phys* 2014;89(5):950–953.

18. Organisation for Economic Co-operation and Development. *Health at a glance 2015: OECD indicators*. Paris, France: OECD Publishing, 2015.

19. Brooks GA, Li L, Sharma DB, et al. Regional variation in spending and survival for older adults with advanced cancer. *J Natl Cancer Inst* 2013;105(9):634–642.

20. Tseng EK, Hicks LK. Value based care and patient-centered care: divergent or complementary? *Curr Hematol Malig Rep* 2016;11(4):303–310.

21. Institute of Medicine. *Assessing and improving value in cancer care: workshop summary*. Washington, DC: National Academies Press, 2009.

22. Teckie S, McCloskey SA, Steinberg ML. Value: a framework for radiation oncology. *J Clin Oncol* 2014;32(26):2864–2870.

23. Merriam-Webster. Value. Merriam-Webster Online Dictionary. Available at: https://www.merriam-webster.com/dictionary/value. Published 2016. Accessed November 12, 2016.

24. Sorenson C, Drummond M, Kanavos P. *Ensuring value for money in health care: the role of health technology assessment in the European union*. Copenhagen, Denmark: The European Observatory on Health Systems and Policies, 2008.

25. Rawlins MD. National Institute for Clinical Excellence and its value judgments. *BMJ* 2004;329(7459):224–227.

26. Porter ME, Teisberg EO. *Redefining health care: creating value-based competition on results*. Boston, MA: Harvard Business School Press, 2006.

27. Porter ME. What is value in health care? *N Engl J Med* 2010;363(26):2477–2481.

28. Donabedian A. Evaluating the quality of medical care. *Milbank Q* 2005;83(4):691–729.

29. American Society for Radiation Oncology. Safety is No Accident: A Framework for Quality Radiation Oncology and Care. American Society for Radiation Oncology. Available at: https://www.astro.org/uploadedFiles/Main_Site/Clinical_Practice/Patient_Safety/Blue_Book/SafetyisnoAccident.pdf. Published 2012. Accessed April 1, 2017.

30. American Society for Radiation Oncology. APEx Program Guidance. American Society for Radiation Oncology. Available at: https://www.astro.org/uploaded-Files/Main_Site/Practice_Management/Practice_Accrediation/GuidanceBook.pdf. Published January 2015. Accessed April 1, 2017.

31. American Society for Radiation Oncology. APEX Accredited Facilities. American Society for Radiation Oncology. Available at: https://www.astro.org/Daily-Practice/Accreditation/APEx-Accredited-Faclities. Published April 1, 2017. Accessed April 1, 2017.

32. Porter ME, *Lee TH*. The strategy that will fix healthcare. *Harvard Business Review*, 2013.

33. Horvath LE, Yordan E, Malhotra D, et al. Multidisciplinary care in the oncology setting: historical perspective and data from lung and gynecology multidisciplinary clinics. *J Oncol Pract* 2010;6(6):e21–e26.

34. Fader DJ, Wise CG, Normolle DP, et al. The multidisciplinary melanoma clinic: a cost outcomes analysis of specialty care. *J Am Acad Dermatol* 1998;38(5 Pt 1):742–751.

35. Pollock RE. Value-based health care: the MD Anderson experience. *Ann Surg* 2008;248(4):510–516.

36. Kishan AU, Gomez CL, Dawson NA, et al. Increasing appropriate BRCA1/2 mutation testing: the role of family history documentation and genetic counseling in a multidisciplinary clinic. *Ann Surg Oncol* 2016;23(S5):634–641.

37. Birchall MA, Bailey D, Lennon A. Performance and standards for the process of head and neck cancer care: South and West audit of head and neck cancer 1996–1997 (SWAHN I). *Br J Cancer* 2000;83(4):421–425.

38. Junor EJ, Hole DJ, Gillis CR. Management of ovarian cancer: referral to a multidisciplinary team matters. *Br J Cancer* 1994;70(2):363–370.

39. Conron M, Denton E. Improving outcomes in lung cancer: the value of the multidisciplinary health care team. *J Multidiscip Healthc* 2016;9:137–144.

40. Bekelman JE, Epstein AJ, Emanuel EJ. Getting the next version of payment policy "right" on the road toward accountable cancer care. *Int J Radiat Oncol Biol Phys* 2014;89(5):954–957.

41. Raghavan D. Costs of cancer care: rhetoric, value, and steps forward. *Semin Oncol* 2013;40(6):659–661.

42. Schnipper LE, Bastian A. New frameworks to assess value of cancer care: strengths and limitations. *Oncologist* 2016;21(6):654–658.

43. Hahn C, Kavanagh B, Bhatnagar A, et al. Choosing wisely: the American Society for Radiation Oncology's top 5 list. *Pract Radiat Oncol* 2014;4(6):349–355.

44. Wallner PE, Steinberg ML. "Feeding the beast" is not the road to value. *Int J Radiat Oncol Biol Phys* 2015;93(1):13–15.

Section V

45. Mohideen N, Kavanagh BD, Beyer D, et al. Radiation oncology: a perspective on health reform and value-based initiatives. *J Oncol Pract* 2014;10(4): e212–e214.

46. Turning the Tide Against Cancer. The Initiative. Turning the Tide Against Cancer. http://www.turningthetideagainstcancer.org/initiative. Published 2013. Accessed April 1, 2017.

47. Miller AM, Omenn GS, Kean MA. The impact of alternative payment models on oncology innovation and patient care. *Clin Cancer Res* 2016;22(10): 2335–2341.

48. American Society for Radiation Oncology. Clinical Practice Statements. American Society for Radiation Oncology. Available at: https://www.astro.org/Clinical-Practice-Statements.aspx. Accessed April 1, 2017.

49. Liu HW, Malkoske K, Sasaki D, et al. The dosimetric quality of brachytherapy implants in patients with small prostate volume depends on the experience of the brachytherapy team. *Brachytherapy* 2010;9(3):202–207.

50. Boero IJ, Paravati AJ, Xu B, et al. Importance of radiation oncologist experience among patients with head-and-neck cancer treated with intensity-modulated radiation therapy. *J Clin Oncol* 2016;34(7):684–690.

51. Jagsi R, Bekelman JE, Chen A, et al. Considerations for observational research using large data sets in radiation oncology. *Int J Radiat Oncol Biol Phys* 2014;90(1):11–24.

52. Scott CB, Stetz J, Bruner DW, et al. Radiation Therapy Oncology Group quality of life assessment: design, analysis, and data management issues. *Qual Life Res* 1994;3(3):199–206.

53. U.S. Department of Health and Human Services FDA Center for Drug Evaluation and Research; U.S. Department of Health and Human Services FDA Center for Biologics Evaluation and Research; U.S. Department of Health and Human Services FDA Center for Devices and Radiological Health. Guidance for industry: patient-reported outcome measures: use in medical product development to support labeling claims: draft guidance. *Health Qual Life Outcomes* 2006;4:79.

54. Siddiqui F, Liu AK, Watkins-Bruner D, et al. Patient-reported outcomes and survivorship in radiation oncology: overcoming the cons. *J Clin Oncol* 2014;32(26):2920–2927.

55. Dueck AC, Mendoza TR, Mitchell SA, et al. Validity and reliability of the US National Cancer Institute's Patient-Reported Outcomes Version of the Common Terminology Criteria for Adverse Events (PRO-CTCAE). *JAMA Oncol* 2015;1(8):1051–1059.

56. National Cancer Institute. Patient-Reported Outcomes version of the Common Terminology Criteria for Adverse Events (PRO-CTCAE™). National Cancer Institute. Available at: https://healthcaredelivery.cancer.gov/pro-ctcae. Accessed April 1, 2017.

57. Litwin MS. Health services research. *Semin Radiat Oncol* 2008;18(3): 152–160.

58. Abrahams E, Foti M, Kean MA. Accelerating the delivery of patient-centered, high-quality cancer care. *Clin Cancer Res* 2015;21(10):2263–2267.

59. Picker Institute. Principles of patient-centered care. Picker Institute. http://pickerinstitute.org/about/picker-principles. Accessed April 1, 2017.

60. Carman KL, Maurer M, Yegian JM, et al. Evidence that consumers are skeptical about evidence-based health care. *Health Aff (Millwood)* 2010;29(7): 1400–1406.

61. Abraham I, McBride A, MacDonald K. Arguing (about) the value of cancer care. *J Natl Compr Canc Netw* 2016;14(11):1487–1489.

62. Wong YN, Egleston BL, Sachdeva K, et al. Cancer patients' trade-offs among efficacy, toxicity, and out-of-pocket cost in the curative and noncurative setting. *Med Care* 2013;51(9):838–845.

63. PDQ Adult Treatment Editorial Board. Financial toxicity and cancer treatment (PDQ®): health professional version. In: *PDQ cancer information summaries*. Bethesda, MD: National Cancer Institute (US), 2016. http://www.ncbi.nlm.nih.gov/books/NBK384502. Accessed April 1, 2017.

64. Ramsey SD, Bansal A, Fedorenko CR, et al. Financial insolvency as a risk factor for early mortality among patients with cancer. *J Clin Oncol* 2016;34(9):980–986.

65. Zafar SY. Financial toxicity of cancer care: it's time to intervene. *J Natl Cancer Inst* 2016;108(5):djv370.

66. Earle CC, Neville BA, Landrum MB, et al. Trends in the aggressiveness of cancer care near the end of life. *J Clin Oncol* 2004;22(2):315–321.

67. Campion FX, Larson LR, Kadlubek PJ, et al. Advancing performance measurement in oncology: Quality Oncology Practice Initiative participation and quality outcomes. *J Oncol Pract* 2011;7(3S):31s–35s.

68. Guadagnolo BA, Liao KP, Giordano SH, et al. Increasing use of advanced radiation therapy technologies in the last 30 days of life among patients dying as a result of cancer in the United States. *J Oncol Pract* 2014;10(4): e269–e276.

69. Zafar SY, Peppercorn JM, Schrag D, et al. The financial toxicity of cancer treatment: a pilot study assessing out-of-pocket expenses and the insured cancer patient's experience. *Oncologist* 2013;18(4):381–390.

70. Ubel PA, Abernethy AP, Zafar SY. Full disclosure: out-of-pocket costs as side effects. *N Engl J Med* 2013;369(16):1484–1486.

71. Ganz PA, Levit LA. Charting a new course for the delivery of high-quality cancer care. *J Clin Oncol* 2013;31(36):4485–4487.

72. O'Connor JM, Kircher SM, de Souza JA. Financial toxicity in cancer care. *J Community Support Oncol* 2016;14(3):101–106.

73. Tucker-Seeley RD, Yabroff KR. Minimizing the "financial toxicity" associated with cancer care: advancing the research agenda. *J Natl Cancer Inst* 2016;108(5):djv410.

74. Feldman-Stewart D, Siemens DR. What if?: regret and cancer-related decisions. *Can Urol Assoc J* 2015;9(9–10):295–355.

75. Shaverdian N, Verruttipong D, Wang P-C, et al. Exploring value from the patient's perspective between modern radiation therapy modalities for localized prostate cancer. *Int J Radiat Oncol Biol Phys* 2017;97(3):516–525.

76. American Society for Radiation Oncology. MIPS/APM Proposed Rule Summary. American Society for Radiation Oncology. Available at: https://www.astro.org/uploadedFiles/_MAIN_SITE/News_and_Publications/What_Is_Happening_In_Washington/2016/MIPSAPMSummary.pdf. Published May 11, 2016. Accessed April 1, 2017.

77. Meyer AM, Carpenter WR, Abernethy AP, et al. Data for cancer comparative effectiveness research: past, present, and future potential. *Cancer* 2012;118(21):5186–5197.

78. Sher DJ, Punglia RS. Decision analysis and cost-effectiveness analysis for comparative effectiveness research: a primer. *Semin Radiat Oncol* 2014;24(1):14–24.

79. Stiggelbout AM, de Haes JC. Patient preference for cancer therapy: an overview of measurement approaches. *J Clin Oncol* 2001;19(1):220–230.

80. Gold MR, Siegel JE, Russell LB, et al., eds. *Cost-effectiveness in health and medicine*. Oxford, USA: Oxford University Press, 1996.

81. Hunink MGM, Glasziou PP, Siegel JE. *Decision making in health and medicine: integrating evidence and values*. Cambridge, UK: Cambridge University Press, 2001.

82. Winkelmayer WC, Weinstein MC, Mittleman MA, et al. Health economic evaluations: the special case of end-stage renal disease treatment. *Med Decis Making* 2002;22(5):417–430.

83. Sher DJ. Cost-effectiveness studies in radiation therapy. *Expert Rev Pharmacoecon Outcomes Res* 2010;10(5):567–82.

84. ProCure. *Developing proton therapy centers*. USA: ProCure O, 2009.

85. Van de Werf E, Lievens Y, Verstraete J, et al. Time and motion study of radiotherapy delivery: economic burden of increased quality assurance and IMRT. *Radiother Oncol* 2009;93(1):137–140.

86. Konski A, Speier W, Hanlon A, et al. Is proton beam therapy cost effective in the treatment of adenocarcinoma of the prostate? *J Clin Oncol* 2007;25(24):3603–3608.

87. Sher DJ, Parikh RB, Mayo Jackson S, et al. Cost effectiveness analysis of SBRT versus IMRT for low-risk prostate cancer. *Am J Clin Oncol* 2014;37(3): 215–21.

88. Hayes JH, Ollendorf DA, Pearson SD, et al. Observation versus initial treatment for men with localized, low-risk prostate cancer: a cost-effectiveness analysis. *Ann Intern Med* 2013;158(12):853–860.

89. Wilt TJ, Brawer MK, Jones KM, et al. Radical prostatectomy versus observation for localized prostate cancer. *N Engl J Med* 2012;367(3):203–213.

90. Hayes JH, Ollendorf DA, Pearson SD, et al. Active surveillance compared with initial treatment for men with low-risk prostate cancer: a decision analysis. *JAMA* 2010;304(21):2373–2380.

Index

(Note: Page numbers followed by "f" indicate figure, page numbers followed by "t" indicate table, and page numbers followed by "b" indicate box.)